D0879468

AHFS® DRUG INFORMATION® 2020

Published by Authority of the Board of the
AMERICAN SOCIETY OF HEALTH-SYSTEM PHARMACISTS®
American Hospital Formulary Service®

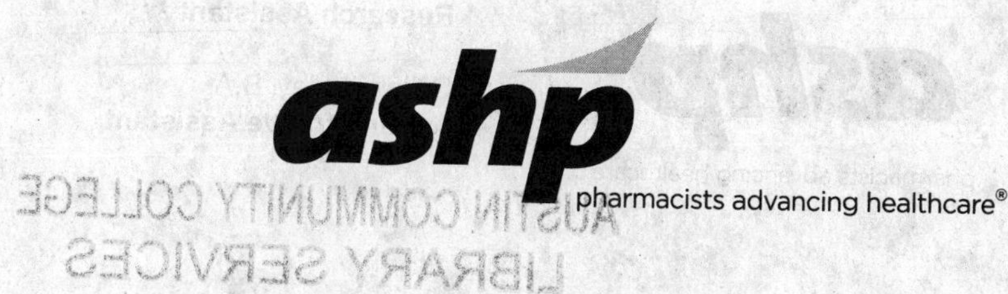

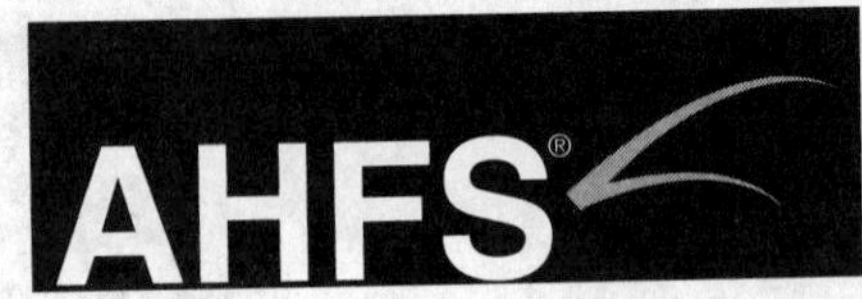

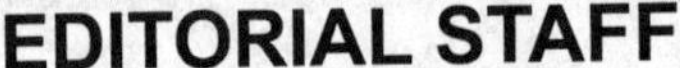

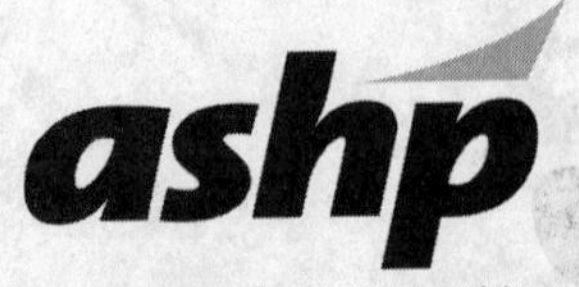

pharmacists advancing healthcare®

LIBRARY OF CONGRESS CATALOG CARD NUMBER: 59-7620

INTERNATIONAL STANDARD BOOK NUMBER (ISBN): 978-1-58528-611-9

INTERNATIONAL STANDARD SERIAL NUMBER (ISSN): 8756-6028

Printed in Canada

For Ordering Information

Write

American Society of Health-System Pharmacists
Customer Service Department
4500 East-West Highway, Suite 900
Bethesda, MD 20814 USA

Phone

Toll Free: 1-866-279-0681
International: 001-301-664-8700

Email

custserv@ashp.org

Fax

800-665-ASHP

Web

http://www.ahfsdruginformation.com

Payments to ASHP are not deductible as charitable contributions for federal income tax purposes. However, they may be deductible under other provisions of the Internal Revenue Code.

Notices

Notice of Warning Concerning Patent and Trade-Mark Rights and Listing of Manufacturer, Labeler, and/or Distributor—The inclusion in the text of the *AHFS Drug Information 2020®* of any drugs in respect to which patent or trademark rights may exist shall not be deemed, and is not intended as a grant of, or authority to exercise, any right or privilege protected by such patent or trademark. All such rights and privileges are vested in the patent or trademark owner, and no other person may exercise the same without express permission, authority, or license secured from such patent or trademark owner. Listing of proprietary titles for the drugs covered in the monographs in *AHFS Drug Information®* is for the purpose of information only. It is not to be interpreted as constituting or implying the right or privilege to dispense any product, other than the one prescribed or ordered under the trademark specified in a prescription order without the consent of the prescriber or as dictated by appropriate laws, regulations, and practices governing such practice. FDA regulations establish specific criteria under which a firm may present itself as the manufacturer, labeler, and/or distributor of a specific drug product. The listing of firms in the text of *AHFS Drug Information®* is for informational purposes only and may not necessarily be consistent with FDA regulations. Readers should refer to FDA regulations and the agency for specific information on this subject.

The use of portions of the text, including some of the graphic formulas, of the *United States Pharmacopeia*, Twenty-fourth Revision, and the *National Formulary*, Nineteenth Edition, official January 1, 1994®, and of previous revisions official at the time the *AHFS Drug Information 2020®* monographs were published, and of current and previous editions of the *USP Dictionary of USAN and International Drug Names* is by permission received from the United States Pharmacopeial Convention, Inc. The Convention is not responsible for any inaccuracy of quotation or for any false or misleading implication that may arise due to the text or formulas as used or due to the quotation of revisions no longer official.

The nature of drug information is that it is constantly evolving because of ongoing research and clinical experience and is often subject to interpretation and the uniqueness of each clinical situation and patient. While care has been taken to ensure the accuracy of the information presented, the reader is advised that the authors, editors, reviewers, contributors, and publishers cannot be responsible for the continued currency of the information or for any errors or omissions in this book or for any consequences arising therefrom. Because of the dynamic nature of drug information, readers are advised that decisions regarding drug therapy must be based on the independent judgment of the clinician, changing information about a drug (e.g., as reflected in the literature), and changing medical practices.

PREFACE

An Evidence-based Foundation for Safe and Effective Drug Therapy

With this edition, *AHFS Drug Information®* (*AHFS® DI™*) marks 62 years of continuous publication as the premier evidence-based drug compendium. The mission of *AHFS® DI™* is to provide an evidence-based foundation for safe and effective drug therapy. Widely trusted for its established record in refuting unfounded efficacy claims, its rigorous science-based editorial process, and its independence from the influence of pharmaceutical manufacturers, *AHFS® DI™* has remained true to its mission since the first edition was published in 1959. This notable achievement of more than six decades of evidence-based medical publishing has gained *AHFS® DI™* the unique distinction of being the longest published federally designated drug compendium issued by a scientific and professional society.

As such, *AHFS® DI™* maintains a unique role in establishing medically accepted uses of drugs, both labeled and off-label, and advancing evidence-based clinical practice. In addition, unlike most compendia, recognition of the authority of *AHFS® DI™* in establishing medically accepted uses of drugs extends far beyond just cancer uses to include the full spectrum of drug therapy.

With the 2020 edition, the *American Hospital Formulary Service®* (*AHFS®*) marks its 62nd year of continuous publication by the American Society of Health-System Pharmacists® (ASHP®). First published in 1959, the *Formulary Service®* has evolved to address increasingly complex issues related to drug therapy and formulary management.

AHFS® DI™ is a collection of drug monographs kept current by ongoing electronic updates (e.g., AHFS®*first*Releases™ on new molecular entities, MedWatch notices, http://www.ahfsdruginformation.com) and by a revised master print volume issued each year. The *AHFS® DI™* database is maintained continuously throughout the year for the purpose of disseminating comprehensive, evaluative drug information to the entire medical and paramedical community, and updates are issued frequently on an ongoing basis in electronic formats. (See AHFS® Clinical Drug Information™ [AHFS® CDI™].)

AHFS® was first published in 1959 as an adaptation from the *Hospital Formulary of Selected Drugs* by Don E. Francke. *AHFS®* had its roots in the hospital formulary system, which was intended to establish a sound therapeutic and economic basis for drug policy. In fact, the evidence-based assessments of medically accepted uses of drugs by *AHFS®* predated the US Food and Drug Administration's (FDA's) own authority to evaluate drug effectiveness claims, and established *AHFS®* as one of the first authoritative sources of critical evaluations of drug therapy. Today, it is the sole independent, non-commercial source of such evaluations in the US.

Originally, the *Formulary Service™* was conducted through the Committee of Pharmacy and Pharmaceuticals of the American Society of Hospital (now Health-System) Pharmacists to assist the pharmacy and therapeutics committee of each hospital in preparing its hospital formulary. Since then, *AHFS® DI™* has developed beyond its original purpose to become the most comprehensive, authoritative source of evaluative, evidence-based drug information available. Paramount to providing such information is the critical, evidence-based evaluation of pertinent clinical data concerning drugs, with a focus on assessing thoroughly the advantages and disadvantages of various therapies, including interpretation of various claims of drug efficacy.

As a result of its foundation in a professional and scientific society, the values, editorial standards, and professional priorities of *AHFS® DI™* differ importantly from those of commercial drug information publishers. The critical evidence-based assessment and provision of drug information is a core professional activity of ASHP and competency of its members. Despite increased emphasis on provision of evidence-based drug information in all pharmacy practice settings, ASHP and its members remain at the forefront of disseminating such information.

As a professional society, ASHP takes a leadership position in influencing health policy, practice, and education toward the goal of assuring that patient care is grounded in accurate, timely, unbiased, and evidence-based drug information. ASHP has been at the forefront of efforts to improve medication use and enhance patient safety for more than 75 years, a notable milestone. ASHP's mission is to help people achieve optimal health outcomes and its vision is that medication use will be optimal, safe, and effective for all people all of the time. Publication of *AHFS® DI™* has been a key component in support of ASHP's mission and vision.

■ AHFS® Patient Medication Information™ (PMI™)

ASHP has a long history of providing patients with meaningful information about medications. *AHFS®* Patient Medication Information™ (*PMI™*) had its origins in 1976 as a collaboration among ASHP, the American Hospital Association (AHA), the US Department of Health, Education, and Welfare (DHEW; now DHHS), and the US Center for Disease Control (CDC; now the Centers for Disease Control and Prevention) and is the only trusted and objective compendium-based database of PMI published by a professional and scientific society in the US. *AHFS® PMI™* previously was referred to as *AHFS® Consumer Medical Information™* (*CMI™*).

Credibility of sources has been ranked by physicians and other clinicians as the most important characteristic of the Internet related to health information. Consumers also are emphasizing credibility of the health information they obtain on the Internet, trusting safe and effective treatment information from professional societies like ASHP the most and that from pharmaceutical companies the least. AHFS® has a clear reputation for credible, valid information based on its history, references, and evidence basis. *AHFS® PMI™* hosted by the National Institutes of Health (NIH), is one of only a few such sites of trusted, accurate medication information, with an outreach to over 100 million consumers annually. *AHFS® PMI™* is ASHP's most expansive public outreach.

The trust placed in *AHFS® PMI™* has resulted in strategic alliances with groups such as the National Library of Medicine (MedlinePlus® and MedlinePlus® Connect) and Consumers Union (Consumer Reports Health and Best Buy Drugs), groups that also place a high priority on the credibility that *AHFS® PMI™* provides. In collaboration with Consumer Reports Best Buy Drugs, ASHP has developed a series of off-label drug use reports through a grant from the state Attorney General Consumer and Prescriber Education Grant Program, which was funded by a multistate settlement of consumer fraud claims regarding the marketing of the prescription drug Neurontin® (gabapentin). When accessing any of these sites, consumers can be assured that they are receiving the most trusted and credible medication information available. *AHFS® PMI™* also is accessible through ASHP's own website—http://www.safemedication.com.

AHFS® PMI™ also includes links within the context of each of its drug monographs in support of CDC's PROTECT initiative on safe medication use. Through PROTECT, CDC, the Consumer Healthcare Products Association Educational Foundation, and other organizations support the Up and Away and Out of Sight campaign aimed at educating families and other caregivers about the importance of storing medications in a safe place to prevent inadvertent overdoses by children.

AHFS® PMI™ also has been adopted as the trusted source of patient medication information by a leading provider of bedside patient engagement and education resources in hospitals—Sonifi® Healthcare (formerly LodgeNet® Healthcare). This service focuses on improving patient satisfaction, outcomes, and quality as measured by the Hospital Consumer Assessment of Healthcare Providers and Systems (HCAHPS) survey, care measures, and other indicators.

■ Off-Label Drug Reviews for Oncology

In 2008, *AHFS® DI™* introduced a process for publishing structured, codified, evidence-based determinations for off-label cancer uses. The decision to create a separate method resulted from the unique characteristics of evidence-based decisions that are applied to serious and life-threatening conditions such as cancer. This process supplements the long-standing evidence-based process used by AHFS® to evaluate off-label uses of drugs and biologics and incorporates the desirable characteristics for cancer-specific compendia outlined by the Medicare Evidence Development and Coverage Advisory Committee (MedCAC). The cancer-specific codified method developed by AHFS® is consistent with distinctions applied to evidence-based assessments of cancer treatments by other authoritative sources such as the National Cancer Institute (NCI) and FDA.

The principles of the *AHFS® DI™* evidence-based editorial development process have not changed with this oncology process. However, the codified determinations supplement and enhance the traditional *AHFS® DI™* evaluation of off-label uses with structured determinations that summarize ongoing assessments of new and changing evidence. ASHP appointed an Oncology Expert Committee, comprised of oncologists, oncology pharmacists, and oncology nurses, to assist with the independent review and final recommendations for off-label cancer determinations. Final decisions are made solely by the Oncology Expert Committee for determinations emanating from this supplementary process for oncology uses and by AHFS® staff for other information, taking into account the advice of other expert reviewers. All processes related to the review and publication of determinations are transparent and designed to mitigate any potential conflict of interest in order to preserve the integrity of *AHFS® DI™* and to minimize bias.

Federal regulations for transparency and conflict of interest disclosure and management became effective January 1, 2010 for off-label oncology determinations. AHFS® employs a process for evaluating therapies that is publicly transparent as defined by CFR Section 414.930(a) and that includes criteria used to evaluate the use, a listing of evidentiary materials reviewed by the compendium, and a listing of all individuals who participated substantively in the development, review, or disposition of the request. In the case of balloted determinations made by the AHFS® Oncology Expert Committee as of this date, conflict of interest disclosure policies follow the definition of a publicly transparent process for identifying potential conflicts of interest as established in this section of the CFR.

Documents describing this process for off-label oncology uses, including levels of evidence, transparency, and conflict of interest disclosure and management, may be viewed under the Off-label Uses section of the *AHFS® DI™* website at http://www.ahfsdruginformation.com. Subscribers may access details about specific determinations of medical acceptance for these uses at this website location.

■ Editorial Independence

Information included in *AHFS® DI™* shapes treatment decisions made by clinicians and influences public and private health-care policies and decisions. As a result, it is important that the information be authoritative, objective, and free of undue influence from pharmaceutical companies and other third parties who may seek to use the compendium to promote their own vested interests. Editorial decisions are evidence-based and made independent of such third parties.

AHFS® DI™ is the only remaining official drug compendium published by a non-commercial, nonprofit professional and scientific society. ASHP is an IRS 501(c)(6) tax-exempt entity. ASHP is the national professional organization that represents pharmacists who serve as patient care providers on health-care teams in acute and ambulatory settings spanning the full spectrum of medication use. ASHP has a long history of fostering evidence-based medication use as well as patient medication safety. *AHFS® DI™* and *PMI™* are published in part to support the mission of pharmacists in helping people achieve optimal health outcomes.

AHFS® DI™ is published by ASHP under the authority of its elected Board of Directors. As such, the Board exercises oversight through its ongoing Society considerations. This oversight by the Board also involves review and approval of relevant recommendations originating from its appointed Council on Therapeutics and the advisory and best practices developments of its other Councils, House of Delegates, and other policy-recommending bodies.

In addition, a wide array of experts, principally physicians but also other clinicians, medical scientists, pharmacists, pharmacologists, and other professionally qualified individuals, participate in an ongoing extramural review process for *AHFS® DI™*. Participation is solicited but voluntary, and no honorarium nor other benefit other than limited access to the *AHFS® DI™* database is provided. These experts must provide full disclosure of interest, including any affiliation with or financial involvement with the manufacturer of the drug(s) under consideration and directly competitive products.

ASHP considers it essential that interactions between AHFS® staff and pharmaceutical companies be limited to the legitimate exchange of the scientific and medical information needed to fulfill the mission of *AHFS® DI™*. To maintain independence from the undue influence of the promotional interests of pharmaceutical companies, communications are directed to the scientific and medical information areas within the companies; contact with marketing areas is avoided.

ASHP holds in high regard the responsibilities attendant to the public and private trust placed in the evidence-based editorial deliberations of *AHFS® DI™*. As such, ASHP also considers it essential to protect the integrity and independence of the editorial decisions of AHFS® staff by separating the Society's business activities with pharmaceutical companies (e.g., exhibits at educational meetings, journal advertising) from the editorial activities of its drug compendium. An editorial independence statement, approved by ASHP's Board of Directors and available at http://www.ahfsdruginformation.com, outlines the principles that AHFS® staff apply in ensuring such independence.

■ Comparative, Unbiased, Evaluative Drug Information

AHFS® DI™ is a tested and proven source of comparative, unbiased, and evidence-based drug information containing a monograph on virtually every molecular drug entity available in the US. Drug monographs are prepared by a professional editorial and analytical staff, who critically evaluate published evidence on the drug. The monographs incorporate the advice of leading medical experts in the specific field of therapy under consideration, including experts from major research and clinical institutions as well as public bodies such as the National Institutes of Health (NIH) and US Centers for Disease Control and Prevention (CDC) and professional associations with therapeutic authority. It is this process for establishing medically accepted uses of drugs that makes *AHFS® DI™* monographs unbiased and authoritative.

Using an independent, evidence-based, evaluative process, *AHFS® DI™* monographs incorporate information from pertinent references in the literature and expert therapeutic guidelines. The monographs also address the labeling approved by FDA, in some cases challenging outdated and clinically irrelevant information that may persist in the approved labeling. *AHFS® DI™* monographs continue to include information on uses, dosages, and routes and/or methods of administration that may not be included in the FDA-approved labeling for the drug ("off-label/unlabeled uses"). (See Uses in the Users Guide, p. xiii.) Monographs often incorporate information from several hundred published references, and some general statements and individual monographs incorporate information from several thousand references.

The current *AHFS® DI™* database includes more than 94,000 uniquely cited references linked to more than 700,000 statements and provides direct links to more than 61,000 supporting evidence sources. Tens-of-thousands of additional references from the *AHFS®* archives provide support for monographs on drugs introduced into the US market prior to 1984. It is this point-by-point analysis and evaluation of the literature that make *AHFS® DI™* monographs comprehensive, evaluative, and considerably beyond the FDA-approved labeling in their scope.

■ Widely Vetted Editorial Process in Support of Compendial Recognition

The *American Hospital Formulary Service®* grew out of the concept of the formulary system in institutions. The ASHP Minimum Standard for Pharmacies in Hospitals, which described principles of the formulary system, was approved in 1951 by ASHP and the American Pharmaceutical Association, American Hospital Association, American Medical Association, and American College of Surgeons and served as the cornerstone for Joint Commission standards on formularies.

The broad-based vetting and recognition of ASHP's editorial standards over several decades are unparalleled. (See also the section "Highly Recognized Authority" below.)

In the mid-1960s through the mid-1970s, recommendations from the US Department of Health, Education, and Welfare (DHEW), including DHEW's Task Force on Prescription Drugs and FDA's Bureau of Drugs, proposed the creation of a Federal drug compendium. Key people involved in promoting the concept of a national formulary included FDA Commissioner James Goddard and DHEW Secretary Caspar Weinberger. Congressional Committees involved included the Senate Monopoly Committee (Senator Gaylord Nelson, Chair) and the Senate Subcommittee on Health. Various physician proponents of the quality and scope of *AHFS®* and others corresponded and met with most of the Federal principals involved in these deliberations and proposed *AHFS®* as meeting the goals for such a compendium. ASHP also provided comments at the Drug Information Association's symposium on a Federal Drug Compendium held in Washington, DC June 11–12, 1970. At the time, *AHFS®* was "the only constantly updated compendium of edited, organized, unbiased, and evaluated information on virtually all drugs used in the United States."

The National Academy of Sciences–National Research Council (NAS–NRC) was contracted by FDA in 1966 to evaluate efficacy claims being made by manufacturers for drugs cleared for marketing from 1938–1962 (prior to Kefauver-Harris amendments). Analysis of existing conclusions in *AHFS®* found remarkable similarities with the NAS–NRC findings and spoke well for *AHFS®* as an evaluative, unbiased drug compendium. (*Am J Hosp Pharm.* 1968; 25:483-4.)

Based on ASHP's demonstrated expertise as a scientifically based group that reviewed drug data in an ongoing program and that could provide a continuum of experience and evaluation of drug information, FDA contracted with ASHP in 1975 to develop a class prescription labeling system. ASHP exhaustively applied this system to 20 major therapeutic classes and subclasses of drugs (e.g., antipsychotics, antidepressants, various anti-infective and endocrine classes, analgesics, antihypertensives), developing standard, objective professional class labeling for safe and effective use that FDA applied to numerous individual drug products included in these classes. At the time, pharmaceutical company labeling for drug products within the same class and even for the same generic drug included inconsistent information, including that about efficacy of the drugs.

The Medicare Catastrophic Health Coverage Act of 1988 (Public Law 100-360) required that the Secretary of the Department of Health and Human Services (DHHS) establish outpatient standards for prescribing drugs that were based on accepted medical practice. In establishing such, the Secretary was directed to incorporate standards from current authoritative compendia for the prescribing, dispensing, and utilization of covered outpatient drugs. The editorial policies and procedures, scope, and evidence-based analyses applied to *AHFS® DI™* content were exhaustively scrutinized by Congressional staff as part of this process. To assist the Secretary in making a determination of official compendial designation, *AHFS® DI™* was required to establish that it met the criteria identified by the Conference Committee as an appropriate source of information for establishing the prescribing standards based on accepted medical practice. The activities surrounding this legislation, including intense analysis by Congressional staff and that of the Health Care Financing Administration (HCFA; now the Centers for Medicare & Medicaid Services [CMS]), ultimately resulted in the designation of *AHFS® DI™* as a source for establishing these drug prescribing standards. This set the precedent for recognition by Federal, State, and private sector entities of *AHFS® DI™* as an authoritative source for establishing drug use standards in subsequent legislation (e.g., Omnibus Budget Reconciliation Act [OBRA] of 1990 and 1993) and guidelines. Federal compendial recognition continues under part 456 of CMS regulations governing utilization control for Medicaid and under section 1927 of the Social Security Act.

In January 1989, HCFA began developing regulations to implement section 202 of the Medicare Catastrophic Coverage Act of 1988 aimed at establishing standards for prescribing outpatient drugs based on accepted medical practice. In establishing these standards, HCFA required ASHP to describe the extent to which *AHFS® DI*™ met each of the criteria outlined in the Congressional Conference Report. HCFA was required by Congress to designate as official only those compendia that based such medical practice standards on review of published scientific and medical information and that provided adequate assurances that the expert reviewers who assisted in establishing the standards were free of financial (or other) conflicts of interest. ASHP participated in a public hearing conducted by HCFA's Bureau of Eligibility, Reimbursement, and Coverage on the use of authoritative compendia to determine prescribing standards for the new Medicare outpatient drug coverage. In September 1989, HCFA published its determination that *AHFS® DI*™ met the selection criteria as an official compendium. HCFA's determination was subject to broad-based public scrutiny and comment via the *Federal Register* (1989; 172:37190-246). HCFA also established the expectation that such designation of any compendium in the future would require evaluation by the Agency as to whether the compendium met the established standards as well as publication for public comment in the *Federal Register* of their selection decision in the form of a proposed rule.

In 1989, the Health Insurance Association of America (HIAA; now America's Health Insurance Plans [AHIP]) recommended that insurers use *AHFS® DI*™ as well as certain other resources (e.g., peer-reviewed literature, medical specialty organizations, consultants) for making determinations about off-label uses. In 1994, ASHP met with the HIAA Health Care Technology Committee regarding the use of *AHFS® DI*™ as a standard for making determinations on reimbursement of off-label uses.

In 1989, ASHP also was invited to the National Blue Cross and Blue Shield Association's Technology Management Conference for the purpose of addressing the individual member Plan Medical Directors and senior Plan management regarding the use of the compendia for evaluating the efficacy of off-label uses. As a result, the National Blue Cross and Blue Shield Association changed its previous position that off-label uses be considered investigational and therefore ineligible for reimbursement. The revised position stated that off-label uses should be eligible for reimbursement based on evaluation of efficacy and that *AHFS® DI*™ was a valuable resource for use in the evaluation process.

In September 1991, ASHP was invited to participate in Medicaid's National Medical Directors' Conference to provide information on the use of *AHFS® DI*™ for making decisions regarding which drugs to pay for and under what clinical circumstances. This conference was a forum for the medical directors to discuss HCFA's national drug coverage determinations.

Section 4401 of OBRA 90 (Public Law 101-508) specified requirements for a Drug Use Review program as part of Medicaid. As a result of OBRA 90, section 1927(g) of Title XIX of the Social Security Act required State Medicaid programs to assess data on drug use against standards established by ASHP, the American Medical Association (AMA), and the United States Pharmacopeia (USP) (the latter 2 no longer publish a drug compendium). Once again, the *Federal Register* (1992; 57:49397-412) provided an opportunity for public comment; the rule was finalized in September 1994.

Section 9401 of HCFA's State Medicaid Manual required that State Medicaid programs use *AHFS® DI*™ as a predetermined standard against which to assess drug use. In June 1992, this revision to the Manual was submitted to the State Medicaid Directors for comment prior to being finalized. The authority of *AHFS® DI*™ as an official compendium was further recognized under OBRA 93 for use by State Medicaid programs for information on medically accepted off-label uses of drugs and under the Medicare provisions of this Act for medically accepted indications of antineoplastic drugs.

Section 1861(t) of the Social Security Act established *AHFS® DI*™ as an official compendium for use in determining medically accepted indications of drugs and biologics used in anti-cancer chemotherapeutic regimens under Medicare Part B and section 1927(k) established such compendial recognition for all Medicare Part D drugs.

Because of its long-standing record in evidence-based evaluation of information on drug use, ASHP was requested by FDA in 1993 to assist the Agency in attempting to identify important off-label uses. ASHP was the only professional pharmacy organization requested to assist FDA in this effort.

In 2003, *AHFS® DI*™ was specified by the National Association of Insurance Commissioners as a standard reference compendia in their model Health Carrier Prescription Drug Benefit Management Act that provides standards for the establishment, maintenance, and management of prescription drug formularies and other pharmaceutical benefit management procedures used by health plans that provide prescription drug benefits.

In 2013 and 2014, ASHP's AHFS® staff, as part of a team of highly specialized Life Sciences Subject Matter Experts, led by Reed Technology, performed a key role in the Prescription Drug Labeling Improvement and Enhancement Initiative (PDLI-EI) under a contract (Contract # HHSF223201310225C) with FDA. The purpose of this contract was to provide FDA's Center for Drug Evaluation (CDER) with the necessary services to complete a number of projects aimed at improving and enhancing prescription drug labeling.

■ Widely Used in Print and Electronic Formats

AHFS® DI™ and its point-of-care derivative database *AHFS® DI*™ *Essentials*™ are used widely as sources of authoritative drug information by physicians, pharmacists, dentists, nurses, and other health care professionals and by schools of pharmacy, nursing, and medicine and are available in a variety of formats. Electronic formats include eBroselow's SafeDose®, Lexicomp® Online; First DataBank's AHFS Drug Information® monographs available from multiple vendors; *AHFS Drug Information®* from STAT!Ref®, Pepid's Pharmacist Pro with *AHFS® DI*™, and Medicines-Complete®; *Drug Information Fulltext®* (*DIF®*); and *AHFS® DI*™ Powered by Skyscape Medpresso. *AHFS® DI*™ *Essentials*™ is available electronically in online and mobile applications.

In hospitals, clinics, extended-care facilities, nursing homes, health maintenance organizations, and other organized health-care settings, *AHFS® DI*™ as print and/or electronic databases is accessible in patient-care areas for ready use by physicians, nurses, pharmacists, and other healthcare professionals. *AHFS® DI*™ also is used in community pharmacies, chain drugstores, and other ambulatory care and professional practice settings and is available in most medical libraries.

■ AHFS® Clinical Drug Information™ (AHFS® CDI™)

In 2016, ASHP released a comprehensive, electronic suite of its leading drug information databases, including *AHFS® DI*™. The new product, AHFS® Clinical Drug Information™ (AHFS® CDI™), expands the availability of these trusted ASHP resources, providing clinicians with real-time drug and safety updates and direct links to more than 61,000 supporting evidence sources, as well as easy access to the detailed drug information and in-depth coverage of off-label uses found in *AHFS® DI*™. In addition to the monographs of *AHFS® DI*™, subscribers to AHFS® CDI™ have access to *AHFS® DI*™ *Essentials*™, which offers quick, point-of-care answers. Additional ASHP drug information resources are included in the new product, including ASHP's drug shortages resources (which are prepared in conjunction with the University of Utah Drug Information Service). ASHP's *Handbook on Injectable Drugs®* also can be integrated into the suite. AHFS® CDI™ features links to 20 additional specialty databases of drug-specific information, including prescribing information, drug images and imprints, FDA's latest boxed warnings, safety labeling changes, REMS, pharmacogenomic data, a specialty breast-feeding database, and other clinical resources.

AHFS® Clinical Drug Information™ is available for individual and institutional subscribers via web browser and is mobile-optimized for use on iOS and Android devices. AHFS® CDI™ also is available as an iOS app. In addition, the user interface will integrate into clinical workflow solutions in hospitals and ambulatory care settings. An application programming interface (API) is available.

■ Highly Recognized Authority

AHFS® DI™ is supported solely through subscriptions. *AHFS® DI*™ has been officially adopted by the US Public Health Service and the Department of Veterans Affairs; recommended by the National Association of Boards of Pharmacy as part of the standard reference library; recommended by the American College of Physicians as part of a library for internists; included in the Standards for Medicare; approved by the American Pharmaceutical (now Pharmacists) Association, American Health Care Association, American Hospital Association, and Catholic Health Care Association of the United States; recognized by the US Congress, CMS, AHIP, National Blue Cross and Blue Shield Association, National Association of Insurance Commissioners, and various third-party healthcare insurance providers for coverage decisions on off-label (unlabeled) uses; and included as a required or recommended standard reference for pharmacies in many states.

The authority of *AHFS® DI*™ also includes Federal recognition through legislation and regulation as an "official" compendium for information on medically accepted uses of drugs. The Federal compendial recognition for *AHFS® DI*™ originated in the Medicare Catastrophic Coverage Act. HCFA (now CMS) determined that *AHFS® DI*™ met the compendial selection criteria established by Congress and adopted the compendium for carrying out certain aspects of the Act and in meeting the need of the US Secretary of HHS to establish standards based on accepted medical practice for the prescribing, dispensing, and utilization of covered drugs. This established the Federal precedent for use of *AHFS® DI*™ as a compendial standard in subsequent legislative and regulatory initiatives, including for drug coverage under Medicaid and Medicare Parts B and D.

For additional information on official recognition, see the section on Widely Vetted Editorial Process in Support of Compendial Recognition above.

Continuously Updated and Revised

The *AHFS® DI™* database and annual print edition are updated extensively, incorporating revised information on uses, therapeutic perspectives, cautions, drug interactions, new products, and other new developments. In addition, the database is expanded by dozens of new drug monographs over the course of the year.

■ Recognition and Increased Granularity of the AHFS® Pharmacologic-Therapeutic Classification©

The *AHFS®* Pharmacologic-Therapeutic Classification© is the most widely used formulary-structure drug classification in the US and Canada. The AHFS® classification is maintained continuously by ASHP and allows the grouping of drugs with similar pharmacologic, therapeutic, and/or chemical characteristics in a 4-tier hierarchy.

Additional subdivision of the *AHFS®* Pharmacologic-Therapeutic Classification© to provide more specific subgroupings of certain drugs along therapeutic and pharmacologic lines is implemented with the 2020 edition. New this year are subclasses: 8:12.06.28 Siderophore Cephalosporins; 8:12.28.26 Pleuromutilins; 28:32.12 Calcitonin Gene-related Peptide (CGRP) Antagonists; and 92:22 Bone Anabolic Agents. **For additional details on the new subclasses and affected drug monographs, see the link to the AHFS® Classification Drug Assignments and Reassignments on the homepage at http://www.ahfsdruginformation.com.**

In the printed version of the classification in *AHFS® DI™*, a drug monograph generally is only printed under one classification; however, multiple classifications may apply based on a drug's pharmacology or therapeutic uses. Multiple classifications for a drug in print are represented by cross-references in the table of contents for each chapter/class. If cross-referenced, the drug name is given followed by the classification number that it is printed under. Electronically, all applicable classes for a drug are listed.

CMS' "Guidelines for Reviewing Prescription Drug Plan Formularies and Procedures" and "Medicare Prescription Drug Benefit Manual: Part D Drugs and Formulary Requirements" describe use of the *AHFS®* Pharmacologic-Therapeutic Classification© as the only named alternative to USP's Model Guidelines for use by prescription drug plans (PDPs) in implementing the formulary portion of the outpatient prescription drug benefit in the Medicare Modernization Act (MMA) of 2003. These Guidelines are part of the MMA Final Guidelines for Formularies that address the "CMS Strategy for Affordable Access to Comprehensive Drug Coverage."

The AHFS® Classification is a registered external code system in the HL7 Vocabulary Repository. (OID: 2.16.840.1.113883.6.234.)

The AHFS® Classification also is an approved value code of the External Code List for use in the Formulary & Benefit, Telecommunication, Post-Adjudication, & SCRIPT e-Prescribing standards of the National Council for Prescription Drug Programs (NCPDP).

■ Evolving Therapeutic Guidance and Perspective

The *AHFS® DI™* database is expanded, revised, and updated extensively throughout the year to add new monographs and address evolving therapeutic guidance and perspective through review of newly published studies and authoritative guidelines from government and professional organizations. This information is reflected in the revised print edition published each January.

■ Major Cautionary Information

The *AHFS® DI™* database is revised and updated extensively throughout the year to address evolving information on medication safety. Manufacturer labeling, FDA safety communications such as MedWatch notices and Risk Evaluation and Mitigation Strategy (REMS) information, published studies and reports, and other safety information are addressed throughout the course of the year. Through semi-automated processes, much of this information is updated on an ongoing basis in electronic versions of the database to reflect more contemporaneously changes made by FDA.

■ Retirement of Dr. Gerald K McEvoy

On March 31, 2019, Dr. Gerald K McEvoy retired after almost 38 years as the leader of AHFS DI and related drug information resources. During this time, Gerry led the AHFS group through various transitions, moving AHFS DI from its original loose-leaf print edition to an annual bound edition and on into various digital formats. He also led efforts to provide patients with meaningful information about medications. Gerry has a passion for ensuring that healthcare professionals have an unbiased, evidence-based foundation to provide safe and effective drug therapy for their patients. His passion and vision have been inspirations to the staff of AHFS, ASHP, and many others throughout the healthcare and public policy communities. We thank him for his many contributions.

■ The Editorial staff wishes to express appreciation to the many consultants and reviewers for their excellent guidance and cooperation and to our subscribers for their support and comments.

■ www.ahfsdruginformation.com

Some monographs have been omitted from the print version of *AHFS® DI™* because of space limitations. Copies of these monographs are available on the "For Subscribers" page of the AHFS Drug Information® website, www.ahfsdruginformation.com, in the "Electronic Only Monographs" section. A username and password are required to access the subscriber-only portions of the website. For the 2020 edition, the username and password for accessing electronic-only content are as follows:

- **username: ahfs2020**
- **password: ASHP94498**

Associated index entries for monographs that appear on the website are followed by the symbol "§" rather than by a page number. This symbol refers the user to a footnote in the index that also provides the above username and password for the 2020 edition.

AHFS® Pharmacologic-Therapeutic Classification©

0:01 Front Matter

4:00 Antihistamine Drugs

- 4:04 First Generation Antihistamines
  - 4:04.04 Ethanolamine Derivatives*
  - 4:04.08 Ethylenediamine Derivatives*
  - 4:04.12 Phenothiazine Derivatives*
  - 4:04.16 Piperazine Derivatives*
  - 4:04.20 Propylamine Derivatives*
  - 4:04.92 Miscellaneous Derivatives*
- 4:08 Second Generation Antihistamines
- 4:92 Other Antihistamines*

8:00 Anti-infective Agents

- 8:08 Anthelmintics
- 8:12 Antibacterials
  - 8:12.02 Aminoglycosides
  - 8:12.06 Cephalosporins
    - 8:12.06.04 First Generation Cephalosporins
    - 8:12.06.08 Second Generation Cephalosporins
    - 8:12.06.12 Third Generation Cephalosporins
    - 8:12.06.16 Fourth Generation Cephalosporins
    - 8:12.06.20 Fifth Generation Cephalosporins
    - 8:12.06.28 Siderophore Cephalosporins*
  - 8:12.07 Miscellaneous β-Lactams
    - 8:12.07.04 Carbacephems*
    - 8:12.07.08 Carbapenems
    - 8:12.07.12 Cephamycins
    - 8:12.07.16 Monobactams
  - 8:12.08 Chloramphenicol
  - 8:12.12 Macrolides
    - 8:12.12.04 Erythromycins
    - 8:12.12.12 Ketolides*
    - 8:12.12.92 Other Macrolides
  - 8:12.16 Penicillins
    - 8:12.16.04 Natural Penicillins
    - 8:12.16.08 Aminopenicillins
    - 8:12.16.12 Penicillinase-resistant Penicillins
    - 8:12.16.16 Extended-spectrum Penicillins
  - 8:12.18 Quinolones
  - 8:12.20 Sulfonamides
  - 8:12.24 Tetracyclines
    - 8:12.24.04 Aminomethylcyclines
    - 8:12.24.08 Fluorocyclines
    - 8:12.24.12 Glycylcyclines
  - 8:12.28 Antibacterials, Miscellaneous
    - 8:12.28.04 Aminocyclitols*
    - 8:12.28.08 Bacitracins
    - 8:12.28.12 Cyclic Lipopeptides
    - 8:12.28.16 Glycopeptides
    - 8:12.28.20 Lincomycins
    - 8:12.28.24 Oxazolidinones
    - 8:12.28.26 Pleuromutilins
    - 8:12.28.28 Polymyxins
    - 8:12.28.30 Rifamycins
    - 8:12.28.32 Streptogramins
    - 8:12.28.92 Other Miscellaneous Antibacterials*
- 8:14 Antifungals
  - 8:14.04 Allylamines
  - 8:14.08 Azoles
  - 8:14.16 Echinocandins
  - 8:14.28 Polyenes
  - 8:14.32 Pyrimidines
  - 8:14.92 Antifungals, Miscellaneous
- 8:16 Antimycobacterials
  - 8:16.04 Antituberculosis Agents
  - 8:16.92 Antimycobacterials, Miscellaneous
- 8:18 Antivirals
  - 8:18.04 Adamantanes
  - 8:18.08 Antiretrovirals
    - 8:18.08.04 HIV Entry and Fusion Inhibitors
    - 8:18.08.08 HIV Protease Inhibitors
    - 8:18.08.12 HIV Integrase Inhibitors
    - 8:18.08.16 HIV Nonnucleoside Reverse Transcriptase Inhibitors
    - 8:18.08.20 HIV Nucleoside and Nucleotide Reverse Transcriptase Inhibitors
    - 8:18.08.92 Antiretrovirals, Miscellaneous*
  - 8:18.20 Interferons
  - 8:18.24 Monoclonal Antibodies
  - 8:18.28 Neuraminidase Inhibitors
  - 8:18.32 Nucleosides and Nucleotides
  - 8:18.40 HCV Antivirals
    - 8:18.40.04 HCV Cyclophilin Inhibitors*
    - 8:18.40.08 HCV Entry Inhibitors*
    - 8:18.40.16 HCV Polymerase Inhibitors
    - 8:18.40.20 HCV Protease Inhibitors
    - 8:18.40.24 HCV Replication Complex Inhibitors
    - 8:18.40.92 HCV Antivirals, Miscellaneous*
  - 8:18.92 Antivirals, Miscellaneous
- 8:30 Antiprotozoals
  - 8:30.04 Amebicides
  - 8:30.08 Antimalarials
  - 8:30.92 Antiprotozoals, Miscellaneous
- 8:36 Urinary Anti-infectives
- 8:92 Anti-infectives, Miscellaneous*

10:00 Antineoplastic Agents

12:00 Autonomic Drugs

- 12:04 Parasympathomimetic (Cholinergic) Agents
- 12:08 Anticholinergic Agents
  - 12:08.04 Antiparkinsonian Agents*
  - 12:08.08 Antimuscarinics/Antispasmodics
- 12:12 Sympathomimetic (Adrenergic) Agents
  - 12:12.04 α-Adrenergic Agonists
  - 12:12.08 β-Adrenergic Agonists
    - 12:12.08.04 Nonselective β-Adrenergic Agonists
    - 12:12.08.08 Selective β_1-Adrenergic Agonists
    - 12:12.08.12 Selective β_2-Adrenergic Agonists
  - 12:12.12 α- and β-Adrenergic Agonists
- 12:16 Sympatholytic (Adrenergic Blocking) Agents
  - 12:16.04 α-Adrenergic Blocking Agents
    - 12:16.04.04 Nonselective α-Adrenergic Blocking Agents
    - 12:16.04.08 Nonselective α_1-Adrenergic Blocking Agents*
    - 12:16.04.12 Selective α_1-Adrenergic Blocking Agents
  - 12:16.08 β-Adrenergic Blocking Agents*
    - 12:16.08.04 Nonselective β-Adrenergic Blocking Agents*
    - 12:16.08.08 Selective β-Adrenergic Blocking Agents*
- 12:20 Skeletal Muscle Relaxants
  - 12:20.04 Centrally Acting Skeletal Muscle Relaxants
  - 12:20.08 Direct-acting Skeletal Muscle Relaxants
  - 12:20.12 GABA-derivative Skeletal Muscle Relaxants
  - 12:20.20 Neuromuscular Blocking Agents
  - 12:20.92 Skeletal Muscle Relaxants, Miscellaneous
- 12:92 Autonomic Drugs, Miscellaneous

16:00 Blood Derivatives

20:00 Blood Formation, Coagulation, and Thrombosis

- 20:04 Antianemia Drugs
  - 20:04.04 Iron Preparations
  - 20:04.08 Liver and Stomach Preparations*
- 20:12 Antithrombotic Agents
  - 20:12.04 Anticoagulants
    - 20:12.04.08 Coumarin Derivatives
    - 20:12.04.12 Direct Thrombin Inhibitors
    - 20:12.04.14 Direct Factor Xa Inhibitors
    - 20:12.04.16 Heparins
    - 20:12.04.92 Anticoagulants, Miscellaneous
  - 20:12.14 Platelet-reducing Agents
  - 20:12.18 Platelet-aggregation Inhibitors
  - 20:12.20 Thrombolytic Agents
  - 20:12.92 Antithrombotic Agents, Miscellaneous
- 20:16 Hematopoietic Agents
- 20:24 Hemorrheologic Agents
- 20:28 Antihemorrhagic Agents
  - 20:28.08 Antiheparin Agents
  - 20:28.16 Hemostatics
  - 20:28.92 Antihemorrhagic Agents, Miscellaneous
- 20:92 Blood Formation, Coagulation, and Thrombosis Agents, Miscellaneous

24:00 Cardiovascular Drugs

- 24:04 Cardiac Drugs
  - 24:04.04 Antiarrhythmic Agents
    - 24:04.04.04 Class Ia Antiarrhythmics
    - 24:04.04.08 Class Ib Antiarrhythmics
    - 24:04.04.12 Class Ic Antiarrhythmics
    - 24:04.04.16 Class II Antiarrhythmics*
    - 24:04.04.20 Class III Antiarrhythmics
    - 24:04.04.24 Class IV Antiarrhythmics
    - 24:04.04.92 Antiarrhythmics, Miscellaneous
  - 24:04.08 Cardiotonic Agents
  - 24:04.92 Cardiac Drugs, Miscellaneous
- 24:06 Antilipemic Agents
  - 24:06.04 Bile Acid Sequestrants
  - 24:06.05 Cholesterol Absorption Inhibitors
  - 24:06.06 Fibric Acid Derivatives
  - 24:06.08 HMG-CoA Reductase Inhibitors
  - 24:06.24 Proprotein Convertase Subtilisin Kexin Type 9 (PCSK9) Inhibitors
  - 24:06.92 Antilipemic Agents, Miscellaneous
- 24:08 Hypotensive Agents
  - 24:08.04 α-Adrenergic Blocking Agents*
  - 24:08.08 β-Adrenergic Blocking Agents*
  - 24:08.12 Calcium-Channel Blocking Agents*
    - 24:08.12.08 Dihydropyridines*
    - 24:08.12.92 Calcium-Channel Blocking Agents, Miscellaneous*
  - 24:08.16 Central α-Agonists
  - 24:08.20 Direct Vasodilators
  - 24:08.24 Diuretics*
    - 24:08.24.04 Carbonic Anhydrase Inhibitors*
    - 24:08.24.08 Loop Diuretics*
    - 24:08.24.12 Osmotic Diuretics*
    - 24:08.24.16 Potassium-sparing Diuretics*
    - 24:08.24.20 Thiazide Diuretics*
    - 24:08.24.24 Thiazide-like Diuretics*
    - 24:08.24.92 Diuretics, Miscellaneous*
  - 24:08.32 Peripheral Adrenergic Inhibitors

24:08.44 Renin-Angiotensin-Aldosterone System Inhibitors*
24:08.44.04 Angiotensin-Converting Enzyme Inhibitors*
24:08.44.08 Angiotensin II Receptor Antagonists*
24:08.44.20 Mineralocorticoid (Aldosterone) Receptor Antagonists*
24:08.92 Hypotensive Agents, Miscellaneous*
24:12 Vasodilating Agents
24:12.08 Nitrates and Nitrites
24:12.12 Phosphodiesterase Type 5 Inhibitors
24:12.92 Vasodilating Agents, Miscellaneous
24:16 Sclerosing Agents
24:20 α-Adrenergic Blocking Agents
24:24 β-Adrenergic Blocking Agents
24:28 Calcium-Channel Blocking Agents
24:28.08 Dihydropyridines
24:28.92 Calcium-Channel Blocking Agents, Miscellaneous
24:32 Renin-Angiotensin-Aldosterone System Inhibitors
24:32.04 Angiotensin-Converting Enzyme Inhibitors
24:32.08 Angiotensin II Receptor Antagonists
24:32.20 Mineralocorticoid (Aldosterone) Receptor Antagonists
24:32.40 Renin Inhibitors
24:32.92 Renin-Angiotensin-Aldosterone System Inhibitors, Miscellaneous

26:00 Cellular Therapy*

28:00 Central Nervous System Agents

28:04 General Anesthetics
28:04.04 Barbiturates
28:04.16 Inhalation Anesthetics*
28:04.92 General Anesthetics, Miscellaneous
28:08 Analgesics and Antipyretics
28:08.04 Nonsteroidal Anti-inflammatory Agents
28:08.04.08 Cyclooxygenase-2 (COX-2) Inhibitors
28:08.04.24 Salicylates
28:08.04.92 Other Nonsteroidal Anti-inflammatory Agents
28:08.08 Opiate Agonists
28:08.12 Opiate Partial Agonists
28:08.92 Analgesics and Antipyretics, Miscellaneous
28:10 Opiate Antagonists
28:12 Anticonvulsants
28:12.04 Barbiturates
28:12.08 Benzodiazepines
28:12.12 Hydantoins
28:12.16 Oxazolidinediones*
28:12.20 Succinimides
28:12.92 Anticonvulsants, Miscellaneous
28:16 Psychotherapeutic Agents
28:16.04 Antidepressants
28:16.04.12 Monoamine Oxidase Inhibitors
28:16.04.16 Selective Serotonin- and Norepinephrine-reuptake Inhibitors
28:16.04.20 Selective-serotonin Reuptake Inhibitors
28:16.04.24 Serotonin Modulators
28:16.04.28 Tricyclics and Other Norepinephrine-reuptake Inhibitors
28:16.04.92 Antidepressants, Miscellaneous
28:16.08 Antipsychotics
28:16.08.04 Atypical Antipsychotics
28:16.08.08 Butyrophenones
28:16.08.24 Phenothiazines
28:16.08.32 Thioxanthenes
28:16.08.92 Antipsychotics, Miscellaneous
28:16.92 Psychotherapeutic Agents, Miscellaneous*
28:20 Anorexigenic Agents and Respiratory and CNS Stimulants
28:20.04 Amphetamines
28:20.08 Anorexigenic Agents
28:20.08.04 Amphetamine Derivatives
28:20.08.32 Selective Serotonin Receptor Agonists
28:20.08.92 Anorexigenic Agents, Miscellaneous
28:20.32 Respiratory and CNS Stimulants
28:20.80 Wakefulness-promoting Agents
28:20.92 Anorexigenic Agents and Stimulants, Miscellaneous*
28:24 Anxiolytics, Sedatives, and Hypnotics
28:24.04 Barbiturates
28:24.08 Benzodiazepines
28:24.92 Anxiolytics, Sedatives, and Hypnotics, Miscellaneous
28:28 Antimanic Agents
28:32 Antimigraine Agents
28:32.12 Calcitonin Gene-related Peptide (CGRP) Antagonists
28:32.28 Selective Serotonin Agonists
28:32.92 Antimigraine Agents, Miscellaneous*
28:36 Antiparkinsonian Agents
28:36.04 Adamantanes
28:36.08 Anticholinergic Agents
28:36.12 Catechol-*O*-Methyltransferase (COMT) Inhibitors
28:36.16 Dopamine Precursors
28:36.20 Dopamine Receptor Agonists
28:36.20.04 Ergot-derivative Dopamine Receptor Agonists
28:36.20.08 Nonergot-derivative Dopamine Receptor Agonists
28:36.32 Monoamine Oxidase B Inhibitors
28:40 Fibromyalgia Agents
28:56 Vesicular Monoamine Transporter 2 (VMAT2) Inhibitors
28:92 Central Nervous System Agents, Miscellaneous

32:00 Contraceptives (foams, devices)*

34:00 Dental Agents*

36:00 Diagnostic Agents

36:04 Adrenocortical Insufficiency
36:06 Allergenic Extracts*
36:08 Amyloidosis*
36:10 Appendicitis*
36:12 Blood Volume*
36:16 Brucellosis*
36:18 Cardiac Function
36:24 Circulation Time*
36:26 Diabetes Mellitus*
36:28 Diphtheria*
36:30 Drug Hypersensitivity*
36:32 Fungi
36:34 Gallbladder Function
36:36 Gastric Function*
36:38 Intestinal Absorption*
36:40 Kidney Function
36:44 Liver Function
36:46 Lymphatic System*
36:48 Lymphogranuloma Venereum*
36:52 Mumps
36:56 Myasthenia Gravis
36:58 Ocular Disorders*
36:60 Thyroid Function*
36:61 Pancreatic Function
36:62 Phenylketonuria*
36:64 Pheochromocytoma*
36:66 Pituitary Function
36:68 Roentgenography*
36:70 Respiratory Function*
36:72 Scarlet Fever*
36:76 Sweating*
36:80 Trichinosis*
36:84 Tuberculosis
36:88 Urine and Feces Contents*
36:88.12 Ketones*
36:88.20 Occult Blood*
36:88.24 pH*
36:88.28 Protein*
36:88.40 Sugar*

38:00 Disinfectants (for agents used on objects other than skin)*

40:00 Electrolytic, Caloric, and Water Balance

40:04 Acidifying Agents
40:08 Alkalinizing Agents
40:10 Ammonia Detoxicants
40:12 Replacement Preparations
40:18 Ion-removing Agents
40:18.16 Sodium-removing Agents*
40:18.17 Calcium-removing Agents
40:18.18 Potassium-removing Agents
40:18.19 Phosphate-removing Agents
40:18.92 Other Ion-removing Agents
40:20 Caloric Agents
40:24 Salt and Sugar Substitutes*
40:28 Diuretics
40:28.04 Carbonic Anhydrase Inhibitors*
40:28.08 Loop Diuretics
40:28.12 Osmotic Diuretics
40:28.16 Potassium-sparing Diuretics
40:28.20 Thiazide Diuretics
40:28.24 Thiazide-like Diuretics
40:28.28 Vasopressin Antagonists
40:28.92 Diuretics, Miscellaneous*
40:36 Irrigating Solutions
40:40 Uricosuric Agents
40:92 Electrolytic, Caloric, and Water Balance Agents, Miscellaneous

44:00 Enzymes

48:00 Respiratory Tract Agents

48:02 Antifibrotic Agents
48:04 Antihistamines*
48:04.04 First Generation Antihistamines*
48:04.08 Second Generation Antihistamines*
48:08 Antitussives
48:10 Anti-inflammatory Agents
48:10.08 Corticosteroids*
48:10.08.04 Nasal Preparations*
48:10.08.08 Orally Inhaled Preparations*
48:10.20 Interleukin Antagonists
48:10.24 Leukotriene Modifiers
48:10.32 Mast-cell Stabilizers
48:12 Bronchodilators*
48:12.04 Adrenergic Agents*
48:12.04.08 Nonselective β-Adrenergic Agonists*
48:12.04.12 Selective β_2-Adrenergic Agonists*
48:12.04.16 α- and β-Adrenergic Agonists*
48:12.08 Anticholinergic Agents*
48:12.12 Xanthine Derivatives*
48:14 Cystic Fibrosis Transmembrane Conductance Regulator Modulators
48:14.04 Cystic Fibrosis Transmembrane Conductance Regulator Correctors

52:00 Eye, Ear, Nose, and Throat (EENT) Preparations

56:00 Gastrointestinal Drugs

60:00 Gold Compounds

64:00 Heavy Metal Antagonists

68:00 Hormones and Synthetic Substitutes

72:00 Local Anesthetics

76:00 Oxytocics

78:00 Radioactive Agents*

80:00 Antitoxins, Immune Globulins, Toxoids, and Vaccines

84:00 Skin and Mucous Membrane Agents

86:00 Smooth Muscle Relaxants

88:00 Vitamins

92:00 Miscellaneous Therapeutic Agents

94:00 Devices*

96:00 Pharmaceutical Aids*

* Category is currently not in use in the printed version of *AHFS Drug Information*®.

AHFS Reviewers

Susan M. Abdel-Rahman, Pharm.D.
Andre Abitbol, M.D.
Stephen E. Abram, M.D.
David G. Addiss, M.D.
Traci D. Adkins, Pharm.D.
Naurang M. Agrawal, M.D.
Joseph Aisner, M.D.
Jaffer A. Ajani, M.D.
David S. Alberts, M.D.
Paolo Alboni, M.D.
M. Al-Sarraf, M.D.
Mary G. Amato, Pharm.D.
Guy W. Amsden, Pharm.D.
J. V. Anandan, Pharm.D.
Allan M. Arbeter, M.D.
George L. Arnold, Pharm.D.
Tamra Arnold, M.D.
David A. Ashford, D.V.M.
Frédéric Assal, M.D.
Michael B. Atkins, M.D.
Robert C. Bahler, M.D.
John G. Bartlett, M.D.
Bryan N. Becker, M.D.
Elinor Ben-Menachem
Ellin Berman, M.D.
David I. Bernstein, M.D.
Elana J. Bernstein, M.D., MSc
Tulio Bertorini, MD.
Robert F. Betts, M.D.
Karl R. Beutner, M.D., Ph.D.
Stephen J. Bickston, MD
William J. Binder, M.D.
Richard J. Bing, M.D.
Nina H. Bjarnason, M.D.
Henry R. Black, M.D.
Eugene R. Bleecker, M.D.
Andrew Blitzer, M.D.
Charles D. Bluestone, M.D.
Joanne L. Blum, M.D., Ph.D.
Elizabeth Bolyard, R.N., M.P.H.
Rachel Bongiorono, Pharm.D.
Philip Bonomi, M.D.
Mark V. Boswell, M.D.
Athos Bousvaros, M.D.
Allison Brashear, M.D.
Mark E. Brecher, M.D.
Rubin Bressler, M.D.
Michael A. Brodsky, M.D.
Stuart Brown, M.D.
Rebecca H. Buckley, M.D.
Daniel R. Budman, M.D.
Paul A. Bunn, Jr., M.D.
Mark R. Burge, M.D.
Craig G. Burkhart, M.D.
Craig N. Burkhart, M.D.
Gilbert Burnham, M.D.
Harold J. Burstein, M.D.
Aman U. Buzdar, M.D.
Karim Anton Calis, Pharm.D., M.P.H.
Carl B. Camras, M.D.
Denise M. Cardo, M.D.
Charles C. J. Carpenter, M.D.
Craig Cheetham, Pharm.D.
Adam Cheifitz, M.D.
Melvin D. Cheitlin, M.D.
Judy Cheng, Pharm.D.
Joanne Chia, Pharm.D.
Linda A. Chiarello, R.N.
James Chin, M.D.
Aram V. Chobanian, M.D.
Hak Choy, M.D.
Chelsea O. Church, Pharm.D.
Allison Chung, M.D.
Sebastian Ciancio, D.D.S.
Leslie Citrome, M.D.
Nathan G. Clark, M.D.
Dennis A. Clements, M.D., Ph.D.
Jerome D. Cohen, M.D.
Lawrence J. Cohen, Pharm.D, BCPP, FASHP, FCCP
Michael R. Cohen, M.S.
Monte S. Cohon, Pharm.D.
Gregory B. Collins, M.D.
Marcela Contreras, M.D.
Joseph P. Costantino, Dr.P.H.
Michael Coyne, M.S.
Burke A. Cunha, M.D.
Samir Damani, M.D., Pharm.D.
Richard Dart, M.D., Ph.D.
Ezra Davidson, M.D.
Barry R. Davis, M.D.
John M. Davis, M.D.
Mellar P. Davis, M.D.
David Dennis, M.D., M.P.H.
John P. DiMarco, M.D., Ph.D.
Magdalene Dohil, M.D.
Dan Douer, M.D.
Robert Dreicer, M.D.
Andreas duBois, M.D.
Janice P. Dutcher, M.D.
Keith R. Edwards, M.D.
Libby Edwards, M.D.
Megan Ehret, Pharm.D., BCPP
Lawrence F. Eichenfield, M.D.
Elizabeth A. Eisenhauer, M.D.
Mervyn L. Elgart, M.D.
Vicki Ellingrod, Pharm.D.
Janet A Englund, M.D.
Jay Epstein, M.D.
Erika J. Ernst, Pharm.D.
Brian L. Erstad, Pharm.D.
Francisco J. Esteva, M.D.
Martin Evans, M.D.
Michael D. Ezekowitz, M.B., Ch.B., D.Phil., FRCP
Gerald Faich, M.D., M.P.H.
Matthew Falagas, M.D.
Lameh Fananapazir, M.D.
Margaret Fang, MD, MPH
Jessica Farrell, PharmD
Ralph D. Feigin, M.D.
Ronald M. Ferdman, M.D.
Robert A. Figlin, M.D.
S. Edwin Fineberg, M.D.
Sydney M. Finegold, M.D.
Jordan N. Fink, M.D.
John Finlayson, Ph.D.
Marc Fischer, M.D.
Douglas Fish, Pharm.D.
Lawrence E. Flaherty, M.D.
Charles Flexner, M.D.
David A. Fox, M.D.
Erin Fox, Pharm.D.
Barbara Frankowski, M.D.
Thomas J. Franz, M.D.
Robert J. Frazen, M.D.
Maisha Kelly Freeman, Pharm.D., BCPS
Mitchell H. Friedlaender, M.D.
Edward S. Friedman, M.D.
Matthew A. Fuller, Pharm.D.
Susan E. Fugate, Pharm.D.
Curt D. Furberg, M.D., Ph.D.
Daniel E. Furst, M.D.
Brian F. Gage, MD, MSc
Ann Gaines, Ph.D.
Joel E. Gallant, M.D., M.P.H.
Barry J. Gales, Pharm.D.
Bernard J. Gersh, M.B., Ch.B., D.Phil.
Anne Gershon, M.D.
Tracy Glauser, M.D.
Robert L. Goldenberg, M.D.
Joseph A. Golish, M.D.
Mildred D. Gottwald, Pharm.D.
Elena Govorkova, M.D.
William J. Gradishar, M.D.
J. Andrew Grant, M.D.
Cristina D. Gray, Pharm.D.
John R. Graybill, M.D.
Gordon R. Greenberg, M.D.
Sara R. Grimsley, Pharm.D.
Moses Grossman, M.D.
Michael P. Gulseth, Pharm.D., BCPS, FASHP
Sally K. Guthrie, Pharm.D.
Thomas Guttuso, M.D.
David W. Haas, M.D.
John D. Hainsworth, M.D.
Stephen B. Hanauer, M.D.
Scott D. Hanes, Pharm.D.
Jacklyn A. Harris
Christopher J. Harrison, M.D
Edward A. Hartshorn, Ph.D.
Patrick Haslett, M.D.
Jimmi Hatton, Pharm.D.
Ernest Hawk, M.D.
C. J. Hawkey
Frederick G. Hayden, M.D.
Ned Hayes, M.D.
Robert P. Heaney, M.D
Amy M. Heck, Pharm.D.
David H. Henry, M.D.
Keith Henry, M.D.
D. Gray Heppner, M.D.
Harry W. Herr, M.D.
Mary Hess, Pharm.D.
Charles B. Hicks, M.D.
Gerald M. Higa, Pharm.D.
Eve Higginbotham, M.D.
Steven Hirsch, M.D
Monto Ho, M.D.
P. Michael Ho, M.D., Ph.D., FACC
Christopher Holtzer, Pharm.D.
Jay H. Hoofnagle, M.D.
Ed Horton, M.D
Patricia Howard, Pham.D.
Elaine Hylek, M.D.
Thomas Iannucci, M.D.
Robert J. Ignoffo, Pharm.D.
David Ilson, M.D.
Timothy J. Ives, Pharm.D., M.P.H.
Bruce Ivins, Ph.D.
Lisa Jackson, M.D.
Judith Jacobi, Pharm.D.
Robert R. Jacobson, M.D.
Joseph Jankovic, M.D.
Sean M. Jeffery, Pharm.D.
Joohi Jimenez-Shahed, M.D.
Bankole A. Johnson, DSc., M.D., Ph.D., FRCPsych
Candace Johnson, M.D., Ph.D.
David H. Johnson, M.D
Todd Johnson, Pharm.D.
David R. Jones, M.D.
Jeffrey Jones, M.D.
S. Christopher Jones, Pharm.D.
Rose Jung, Pharm.D.
Sophia N. Kalantaridou, M.D, Ph.D.
Pramodini B. Kale-Pradhan, Pharm.D.
James Kalus, Pharm.D., BCPS, FASHP
William B. Kannel, M.D.
Norman M. Kaplan, M.D.
Herbert E. Kaufman, M.D.
Paul L. Kaufman, M.D.
Carol A. Kauffman, M.D.
Sanjay Kaul, M.D.
J. J. Kavanaugh, M.D.
H. William Kelly, Pharm.D.
George A. Kenna, Ph.D., BSPharm
Karl Kieburtz, M.D.
Evan D. Kharasch, M.D., Ph.D.
Paul E. Kilgore, M.D.
Michael B. Kimmey, M.D.
W. James King, M.D.
Gerald L. Klein, M.D
Jerome O. Klein, M.D
Lloyd W. Klein, M.D.
Alan S. Kliger, M.D.
Dennis M. Klinman, M.D., Ph.D.
Robert A. Kloner, M.D., Ph.D.
Denise R. Kockler, Pharm.D.
Mary Anne Koda-Kimble, Pharm.D.
L. Andrew Koman, M.D.
Burton I. Korelitz, M.D.
Mori J. Krantz, M.D.
Sanford B. Krantz, M.D.
Sanjeev Krishna, MBChB
Susan E. Krown, M.D.
Theodore Krupin, M.D.
Peter J. Kudenchuk, M.D.
Lewis H. Kuller, M.D, Ph.D.
Matthias C. Kurth, M.D., Ph.D.
Cynthia LaCivita, Pharm.D.
Frank Lanza, M.D.
Marc Lapointe, B.S., Pharm.D.
Elaine Larson, R.N., Ph.D.
Sewa Legha, M.D.
Jerrold B. Leikin, M.D.
Martha L. Lepow, M.D.
Jack L. Lesher, Jr., M.D.
Gary M. Levin, Pharm.D., BCPP, FCCP
Bernard Levin, M.D.
Jay F. Levine, D.V.M., M.P.H.
A. Michael Lincoff, M.D.
Richard B. Lipton, M.D.
David Litvak, M.D.
Elizabeth Loder, M.D.
K. Y. Look, M.D.
Sherry Luedtke, Pharm.D.
Edward G. Lufkin, M.D.
Noni E. MacDonald, M.D.
Iftekhar Mahmood, Ph.D
Gerard A. Malanga, M.D.
Mark E. Mallatt, D.D.S., M.S.D.
George A. Mansoor, M.D.
Cosme Manzarbeitia, M.D.
Lisa Maragakis, M.D.
Thomas H. Maren, M.D.
Kim A. Margolin, M.D.
Maurie Markman, M.D.
Michael F. Marmor, M.D.
Alan Matarasso, M.D.
Karl Matuszewski, M.S., Pharm.D.
S. James Matthews, Pharm.D.
Gary R. Matzke, Pharm.D.
Jeannine S. McCune, Pharm.D.
Donald P. McDonnell, Ph.D.
Thomas J. McGinnis
Roger S. McIntyre, M.D., FRCPC
William P. McGuire III, M.D.
Anthony E. Mega, M.D.
Terri Meinking, M.D.
Aaron E. Miller, M.D.
John Miller, M.D.
Lisa J. Miller, Pharm.D., BCPP, CGP
Robert W. Miller, M.D.
Larry E. Millikan, M.D.
Robert Mocharnuk, M.D.
Maryam R. Mohassel, Pharm.D.
David J. Moliterno, M.D.
Gilles R. G. Monif, M.D.
Malcolm J. Moore, M.D.
Brigitta Mueller, M.D.
Meryl Nass, M.D.
Harold S. Nelson, M.D.
Herbert Newton, M.D., FAAN
Faizan Niazi, Pharm.D.
Allen R. Nissenson, M.D.
Nicholas B. Norgard, Pharm.D., BCPS
Gary D. Novack, Ph.D.
John Nowakowski, M.D.
Unyime O. Nseyo, M.D.

Thomas B. Nutman, M.D.
Martin Offringa, M.D., Ph.D.
Arinze Nkemdirim Okere, Pharm.D., M.S., BCPS
Brian Olshansky, M.D.
Joyce A. O'Shaughnessy, M.D.
James C. Overall, M.D.
Lance J. Oyen, Pharm.D.
Richard L. Page, M.D.
Kishan J. Pandya, M.D.
Adelisa Panlilio, M.D.
Timothy R. Pasquale, Pharm.D
Robin Patel, M.D.
Michele L. Pearson, M.D.
Jeffrey F. Peipert, M.D., M.P.H.
Mark Peppercorn, M.D.
John R. Perfect, M.D.
Mark Pescovitz, M.D.
William A. Peters III, M.D.
Ronald F. Pfeiffer, M.D.
Jonathan P. Piccini, M.D.
Michael F. Pichichero, M.D.
L. Ross Pierce, M.D.
Philip J. Podrid, M.D.
William G. Powderly, M.D.
Bayard L. Powell, M.D.
Sheldon H. Preskorn, M.D.
Frederick J. Raal, M.D., Ph.D.
James Rahal, Pharm.D.
Judith L. Rapoport, M.D.
Murray A. Raskind, M.D.
Michael D. Reed, Pharm.D.
Darrel A. Regier, M.D.
Marc S. Rendell, M.D.
Michael X. Repka, M.D.
Kenneth E. Resztak, Pharm.D.
Lois Reynolds, B.S.
D. D. Richman, M.D.
Jim Riser
Ian Roberts, M.D.
David Robertson, M.D.
Rose Marie Robertson, M.D.
Matthew Roe, M.D.
Peter G. Rose, M.D.
Bruce J. Roth, M.D.
Ronald J. Ruggiero, Pharm.D.
Dennis Russell, Pharm.D.
Rosalie Sagraves, Pharm.D.
Mary C. Sano, Ph.D.
Paul F. Schellhammer, M.D.
Arthur A. Schuna, M.S.
Paula K. Schweitzer, Ph.D.
Alan B. Scott, M.D.
Andrew Seidman, M.D.
Edmund C. Settle, Jr., M.D.
Stephen D. Shafran, M.D.
Edward J. Shannon, M.D.
Fadia T. Shaya, Ph.D.
Walter B. Shelley, M.D.
Sheldon G. Sheps, M.D.
William U. Shipley, M.D.
Leonard H. Sigal, M.D.
Paul Singh, MD, PMH
Joyce G. Small, M.D.
Peter Small, M.D.
Ralph E. Small, Pharm.D.
Edgar B. Smith, M.D.
Lewis J. Smith, M.D.
Michael B.H. Smith, M.D.
Miriam Smith, M.D.
Philip Smith, D.D.S.
Marcus Snow, M.D.
David R. Snydman, M.D.
Jack D. Sobel, M.D.
Magdalena Socieszczyk, M.D.
Richard S. Sohn, M.D.
Anil K. Sood, M.D.
Joseph A. Sparano, M.D.
Monica Spaulding, M.D.
Sheldon L. Spector, M.D.
Sarah A. Spinler, Pharm.D., FASHP, BCPS
Jerry L. Spivak, M.D.
Julie Stading, Pharm.D.
Walter M. Stadler, M.D.
Rod Starke, M.D.
Stuart E. Starr, M.D.
Russell W. Steele, M.D.
Virginia Steen, M.D.
Allen C. Steere, M.D.
Evan A. Stein, M.D., Ph.D.
Katherine M. Stone, M.D.
Pamela Stratton, M.D.
Beth H. Stover, R.N.
K. N. Siva Subramanian, M.D.
Samy Suissa, Ph.D.
Neil M. Sussman, M.D.
Morton N. Swartz, M.D.
Martin Tallman, M.D.
Karen T. Tashima, M.D.
Hugh R. Taylor, M.D.
Nana Tchabo, M.D.
William Tester, M.D.
Tate Thigpen, M.D.
Dennis Thompson, Pharm.D.
Gary D. Tollefson, M.D., Ph.D.
Eric J. Topol, M.D.
William J. Tremaine, M.D.
Edward L. Trimble, M.D.
Richard G Trohman, M.D.
Melvin D. Trousdale, M.D.
James Trussell, Ph.D.
Joseph K.C. Tsui, M.D.
Frederick Varricchio, M.D., Ph.D.
David L. Veenestra, Pharm.D.
Jean Venable-Goode, Pharm.D.
C. F. Verschraegen, M.D.
Donald G. Vidt, M.D.
Peter H. Vlasses, Pharm.D.
Victor G. Vogel, M.D., M.H.S.
Nicholas J. Vogelzang, M.D.
Ralph Vogler, M.D.
Paul Volberding, M.D.
Nicholas A. Votolato, M.D.
Richard J. Wallace, Jr., M.D.
Cheryl H. Waters, M.D.
Barbara Watson, M.D.
Martin B. Wax, M.D.
Guy F. Webster, M.D.
John M. Weiler, M.D.
Robert N. Weinreb, M.D.
Arthur Weinstein, M.D.
Susan Welkos, M.D.
Anthony H. Wheeler, M.D.
John S. Wheeler, M.D.
C. Michael White, Pharm.D.
Nicholas J. White, M.D.
William B. White, M.D.
Peter H. Wiernik, M.D.
Sabrina L. Wilbur, M.D.
Andrew Wiznia, M.D.
Michael H. Woo, Pharm.D.
Kimberly A. Workowski, M.D.
Gary P. Wormser, M.D.
Julie Wright, Pharm.D.
James P. Wymer
Robert Yarchoan, M.D.
Gary C. Yee, Pharm.D.
Jerry Yee, M.D.
Hui-Ling Yen, M.D.
Ram Yogev, M.D.
Florence H. Yong, M.S.
William B. Young, M.D.
Joseph M. Zeterberg, M.D.
Peter Zimetbaum, M.D.
Kai Zwingenberger, M.D.

AHFS Oncology Expert Committee

Current Members

Massimo Cristofanilli, M.D., FACP
Marc Earl, Pharm.D., BCOP
Beth Faiman, Ph.D., R.N., ANP-BC, AOCN
Mandy Gatesman, Pharm.D., BCOP
Christine Gegeckas, R.Ph., BCOP
Raymond Hohl, M.D., Ph.D
LeAnne Kennedy, Pharm.D., BCOP
Sandra E. Kurtin, R.N., M.S., AOCN, ANP-C
Jeffrey Liticker, B.S., BCOP
Robert Mancini, Pharm.D., BCOP
LeAnn B. Norris, Pharm.D., BCPS, BCOP
Peter Rosen, M.D.
Rowena Schwartz, Pharm.D., BCOP
Ronald Walters, M.D., MBA, MHA

Past Members

David Frame, Pharm.D., BCOP
Mark Huberman, M.D.
Thomas Hughes, Pharm.D., BCOP
Patrick Medina, Pharm.D., BCOP
Thien Oo, M.D.
Danielle Roman, Pharm.D., BCOP
Eric Seifter, M.D.
J. Andrew Skirvin, Pharm.D., BCOP
Gamini Soori, M.D., MBA
James Anthony Trovato, Pharm.D., MBA, BCOP, FASHP

For additional details about the work of this Committee, see information on Off-label Uses, including Supporting Documents and Oncology Final Determinations, on the AHFS website at http://www.ahfsdruginformation.com.

Former Editors

Charles B. Cleveland
Donald E. Francke
William M. Heller
Judith A. Kepler
George P. Provost
Mary Jo Reilly
Gerald K. McEvoy

AHFS Drug Information® Users Guide

Organization of Content

AHFS Drug Information® (*AHFS® DI™*) is a collection of drug monographs on virtually every single-drug entity available in the United States. *AHFS Drug Information®* is a tested and proven source of comparative, unbiased, and evaluative drug information.

AHFS® DI™ monographs are written principally on single-drug entities; information on various trademarked preparations and brands of a drug is contained in a single monograph. Drug *combinations* are described in the monographs on the principal ingredients or, rarely, appear as separate monographs (e.g., Co-trimoxazole 8:12.20) when the combinations are considered important because of therapeutic rationale and/or frequency of use. There also are general statements on groups of drugs (e.g., Salicylates 28:08.04.24) whose activities and uses permit their discussion as a class. Information on older and prototype drugs is another feature of *AHFS® DI™*.

■ Organization of the Book

In the annual print edition of *AHFS® DI™*, drug monographs are arranged by the widely recognized and used *AHFS®* Pharmacologic-Therapeutic Classification©. (See p. viii.) This arrangement permits easy review of information on a group of drugs with similar activities and uses and allows the reader to determine quickly the similarities and differences among drugs within a group.

A *table of contents* precedes each major class of drugs (e.g., 8:00 Anti-infective Agents) in the book. The table of contents lists each drug monograph included in that major class according to the specific subclass (e.g., Cephalosporins 8:12.06). Within each subclass, monographs are arranged alphabetically by nonproprietary (generic) name and are preceded by the general statement, when present, for that subclass. The names of the drugs are the United States Adopted Names (USAN) and other names for drugs as described in the *USP Dictionary of USAN and International Drug Names.*

In the print edition of *AHFS® DI™*, a monograph must be printed within a single class section. However, multiple classifications may apply to a drug (based on its pharmacology or therapeutic uses); these are represented by cross-references provided in the table of contents for each class to the location of the monograph in the book. Although the print version of *AHFS® DI™* does not include reference notations, all statements appearing in the publication are documented. (See the discussion on References.)

Because of the unique arrangement of the book, information on a particular drug can be located by several methods. Information can be located via the Index by using any of the following index terms:

- proprietary (trade) name
- nonproprietary (generic) name
- synonym (e.g., British Approved Name [BAN])
- abbreviation (e.g., INH for isoniazid)
- pharmacy equivalent name (PEN) (e.g., co-triamterzide for the fixed combination of hydrochlorothiazide and triamterene)
- former name (e.g., glyceryl guaiacolate for guaifenesin)

The Index also includes entries for all *AHFS®* Pharmacologic-Therapeutic Classification© terms; therefore, a specific class of drugs (e.g., cephalosporins) can be located by referring to the Index. Once the table of contents for a specific major class of drugs has been located, the page number for the beginning of each drug monograph is listed alongside the monograph title in the table; thus, the list of drug monographs in a given subclass can be quickly scanned to locate a specific drug or drugs of interest. Synonyms for drug classes and other cross-references for classes of drugs (e.g., ACE inhibitors) also may be included in the Index.

Some monographs have been omitted from the print version of *AHFS® DI™* because of space limitations. Associated index entries and listings in the table of contents for each major class of drugs in the printed book refer users to the website www.ahfsdruginformation.com to see these monographs. A username and password are required to access these electronic-only monographs. (See the Preface and the Index for information on subscriber access to this website.)

Each year after publication of the print edition of *AHFS® DI™*, new monographs are created, and revisions to existing monographs continue. At the end of the subscription year, any new or revised monographs that were published electronically usually will become incorporated into the upcoming annual edition of *AHFS® DI™* within the appropriate AHFS® Pharmacologic-Therapeutic class©. Revised monographs carry the statement "Selected Revisions January 2020" or some other appropriate revision date in the Copyright notice at the end of the monograph. Because information about a drug frequently changes, the manufacturer's labeling should be reviewed periodically.

■ Organization of Full-length Monographs—Information within each full-length drug monograph is divided into the sections and subsections described below; the types of information that may be included in each major section and subsection within a monograph also are described. Not all sections or subsections are included in each monograph; such subdivisions are used when applicable and necessary. Some information may appear in one or more sections, depending on the type of discussion (e.g., pharmacogenomics information may appear under Dosage, Cautions, and/or Pharmacokinetics depending on the specific information presented). Individual monographs may not contain all of the information described below, or other subsections may be used as needed to organize the text; the absence of specific information within an individual monograph does not imply that such information is unavailable.

The presence or absence of a particular drug or use should *not* be interpreted as indicating any judgment by *AHFS® DI™* on its merits.

Monograph Title and Synonyms

Lists the USAN name or other name for the drug(s) described; salts generally are included even when omitted from the USAN name. If multiple forms (e.g., salts, esters) of the same drug are available, all forms are described within the monograph; the title may include all forms (if only a few) or just the base (active moiety). Occasionally, when several drug entities are described in a single monograph, an alternative title descriptive of the group (e.g., Antacids 56:04) is used. Common synonyms for the drug are listed alongside the USAN or other names.

When recommended by the US Food and Drug Administration (FDA) or the Institute for Safe Medication Practices (ISMP), "tall man" (mixed case) lettering is used for drug names in titles or synonyms (e.g., "diazePAM").

When a graphic formula of the drug or prototype (if multiple drugs) is present, it is in the style adopted by the USAN Council and United States Pharmacopeial Convention.

Occasionally, certain synonyms (e.g., pharmacy equivalent names [PENs]) that apply to specific preparations or combinations rather than to the drug itself are noted parenthetically alongside various preparation headings. (See the discussion on Preparations.)

Introductory Description

Provides a brief chemical, structural, and/or pharmacologic/therapeutic description for the purpose of orientation and introduction.

REMS

Provides a brief description of a Risk Evaluation and Mitigation Strategy (REMS) approved by FDA, including a list of the components. Because REMS frequently are modified or rescinded, a cross reference to FDA's list of "Approved Risk Evaluation and Mitigation Strategies (REMS)" is provided to refer users to the most current information. REMS for drug *combinations* are described in the monographs on the principal ingredient that requires the REMS.

Uses

Provides information on uses that are included in the labeling approved by FDA and those that are not (i.e., "off-label" [unlabeled] uses). Off-label uses are identified with daggers† within the text of the monograph; a footnote that describes the use as unlabeled appears at the end of the monograph. The authority of *AHFS® DI™* to establish medically accepted uses of drugs is recognized through designation as an official federal compendium. (See the Preface for additional information.) Comparisons with other forms of therapy and limitations on use are included when appropriate. This section usually is subdivided by major indication.

Under the Federal Food, Drug, and Cosmetic (FD&C) Act, the labeling approved by FDA for a drug is limited to those uses for which the sponsor has submitted information regarding the safety and efficacy of that product and which has been reviewed by FDA; other uses for which the sponsor has chosen not to submit data to FDA may be demonstrated in the clinical literature before and after the product is approved by FDA. The FD&C Act does not, however, limit the manner in which a clinician may use an approved drug. Once a drug has been approved for marketing, the clinician may prescribe it for uses or in treatment regimens or patient populations (e.g., children) that are not included in approved labeling. Such off-label uses may be appropriate and rational, and may reflect approaches to drug therapy that have been reported extensively in the medical literature.

Valid new uses for drugs often are first discovered via serendipitous observations and therapeutic innovations, and then subsequently may be confirmed by well-designed and controlled studies. Inclusion of such new uses in the FDA-approved labeling for a drug may take considerable time and, without the initiative of the sponsor whose product is involved, may never occur. Therefore, accepted medical practice (state-of-the-art) often includes drug use that is not included in FDA-approved labeling.

Accordingly, *AHFS® DI™* monographs attempt to describe most uses for a drug, whether or not they are included in FDA-approved labeling; however, the presence or absence of a particular use should *not* be interpreted as indicating any judgment by *AHFS® DI™* on its merits. Coverage of off-label uses in *AHFS Drug Information®*, an official Federal drug compendium, has been recognized by the US Congress (e.g., in OBRA 90 and OBRA 93), the Centers for Medicare & Medicaid Services (CMS; Section 1861 and 1927 of the Social Security Act), third-party health-care providers, and others. (See Off-label Uses at http://www.ahfsdruginformation.com for additional information.)

AHFS® DI™ is the longest published official drug compendium and the only remaining one published by a non-commercial, nonprofit scientific and professional society. ASHP is an IRS 501(c)(6) tax-exempt entity.

Drugs designated as orphan drugs by FDA and those otherwise considered as orphans are described. An orphan drug is one that is used for the treatment of a rare disease or condition that either occurs in fewer than 200,000 individuals in the US or is more prevalent but for which there is no reasonable expectation that the cost of developing and marketing the drug in the US for such disease or condition would be recovered from US sales. An orphan drug also may be a vaccine, diagnostic drug, or preventive drug if the individuals to whom it will be administered in the US are fewer than 200,000 per year.

AHFS Grades of Recommendation. During 2008, *AHFS® DI™* introduced a new process for publishing structured, codified, evidence-based determinations for off-label cancer uses. In some monographs that subsequently were revised based on Final Off-label Determinations for cancer uses, text describing such uses based on *AHFS®* Grades of Recommendation may be noted. Following are the categories of *AHFS®* Grades of Recommendation and the definitions of each:

A: Recommended (Accepted) (e.g., should be used, is recommended/indicated, is useful/effective/beneficial in most cases)

B: Reasonable Choice (Accepted, with Possible Conditions) (e.g., treatment option) (e.g., is reasonable to use under certain conditions [e.g., in certain patient groups], can be useful/effective/beneficial, is probably recommended/indicated)

C: Not Fully Established (Unclear risk/benefit, equivocal evidence, inadequate data and/or experience) (e.g., usefulness/effectiveness unknown/unclear/uncertain or not well established relative to standard of care)

D: Not Recommended (Unaccepted) (e.g., considered inappropriate, obsolete, or unproven; is not recommended/indicated/useful/effective/beneficial; or may be harmful)

Dosage and Administration

Includes information on reconstitution and administration of specific dosage forms and on dosage. In addition, restricted distribution programs for certain drugs may be described when special requirements for prescribing and dispensing a drug exist or where distribution is otherwise limited (e.g., orphan drugs).

The Administration subsection describes the routes of administration and, when necessary for clarity, the appropriate dosage form for each route. Instructions for administering the drug (e.g., after meals, with food) and specialized methods of administration are given. Occasionally, instructions for extemporaneous preparation of a dosage form that is not commercially available (e.g., preparation of a pediatric oral suspension from the contents of capsules) are included. For injectable drugs or other dosage forms requiring reconstitution, the Administration subsection is replaced by the Reconstitution and Administration subsection. In addition to information described for the Administration subsection, instructions for reconstitution and, when applicable, further dilution of the dosage form are presented. The rate of injection or infusion of the drug is described, as well as any precautions associated with administration. Generally, compatibility and stability information is described under Chemistry and Stability.

The Dosage subsection describes recommended and alternative dosage schedules for each dosage form and route of administration and condition being treated. Information in this subsection often is divided by use. When applicable, dosage equivalencies are described. The initial, maintenance, and maximum dosages are given. When available and applicable, specific dosages for children, geriatric or debilitated patients, or patients with renal and/or hepatic impairment are described. Occasionally, when use of a fixed-dosage combination preparation or concomitant use of the drug with another drug is considered rational, specific regimens may be described. Because information about a drug frequently changes, the manufacturer's labeling should be reviewed periodically.

Cautions

Includes information about adverse effects, precautions and contraindications, pediatric and geriatric precautions, mutagenicity and carcinogenicity, and pregnancy, fertility, and lactation precautions.

Adverse reactions of a drug are undesirable effects, reasonably associated with use of the drug, that may occur as part of its pharmacologic action or may be unpredictable in occurrence. The general Adverse Effects subsection usually is replaced by multiple subsections that are specifically divided by body system affected (e.g., GI, CNS, Hematologic) or by type of effect (e.g., Sensitivity Reactions).

The Precautions and Contraindications subsection includes any special care to be taken by practitioners and/or patients for safe and effective use of the drug and describes serious adverse effects and potential safety hazards, limitations on use imposed by them, and actions that should be taken if they occur. Those situations or conditions for which the drug should not be used because the risk clearly outweighs any possible benefit also are described. Additional precautions and contraindications are included in other appropriate sections of the drug monograph (e.g., Pediatric Precautions; Pregnancy, Fertility, and Lactation; Drug Interactions). Because precautionary information about a drug frequently changes, the manufacturer's labeling should be reviewed periodically.

The Pediatric Precautions subsection describes those pediatric age groups for which safety and/or efficacy of the drug have not been established from adequate and well-controlled studies. Risks associated with use of the drug in pediatric age groups also are described.

The Geriatric Precautions subsection includes precautions, warnings, and contraindications associated with use of the drug in geriatric individuals and provides some perspective regarding study and experience in this population, including factors that may affect response and tolerance.

Pediatric and geriatric information also may be described within the appropriate major sections of the monograph. For example, information on age-dependent pharmacokinetics of the drug would be described within the Pharmacokinetics section and that on age-specific dosage recommendations would be described in the Dosage and Administration section of the monograph. When relevant information on use of the drug in pediatric or geriatric patients is readily available in the medical literature and/or the drug is labeled specifically for use in this age group, details about efficacy generally are described in the Uses section.

The Mutagenicity and Carcinogenicity subsection describes data derived from long-term animal studies evaluating carcinogenic potential of the drug as well as data derived from in vitro tests of mutagenic potential. Pertinent evidence from human data regarding the mutagenic and/or carcinogenic potential of the drug also is included.

The Pregnancy, Fertility, and Lactation subsection describes the safety of the drug in pregnant and/or lactating women and any potential effects on male and female reproduction capacity. Precautionary information regarding use of the drug during pregnancy, which is based on FDA's previously designated pregnancy categories A, B, C, D, and X, is included when available. (See Overviews: Pregnancy Precautions for a description of the previously used FDA categories.) In 2014, FDA amended the requirements for pregnancy and lactation labeling, eliminating these long-recognized lettered categories and replacing the letters with a narrative structure for pregnancy labeling. Therefore, *AHFS® DI™* monographs may have varying styles depending on the available information. Additional pertinent information regarding use of the drug during pregnancy or effects on labor and delivery also is presented.

A description of whether the drug is distributed into milk is included when available, and any associated precautions regarding use of the drug in nursing women are described. Effects of the drug on lactation and/or the nursing infant also are described.

Evidence from animal studies regarding effects of the drug on fertility is given, and relevant advice regarding the importance of these animal findings is included when available. Pertinent evidence from humans regarding effects of the drug on fertility also is described.

Acute Toxicity

Describes toxic effects of the drug associated with intentional or accidental ingestion or administration of a large dose. Information on the amount of drug in a single dose that usually is associated with symptoms of overdosage and the amount of drug in a single dose that is likely to be life-threatening is included when available. Manifestations, laboratory findings, and potential complications of acute overdosage are described. Plasma concentrations associated with toxicity are included when well described.

Recommendations for management of acute toxicity, including those for supportive and symptomatic treatment, are described.

Chronic Toxicity

Includes well-described toxic effects of the drug associated with prolonged use. When information on chronic toxicity is limited, it often is described in the appropriate subsection under Cautions. The pathogenesis, manifestations, and treatment of chronic toxic effects are discussed. Also included is a description of tolerance to and/or physical or psychologic dependence on the drug. Adverse effects associated with abrupt withdrawal of the drug are described, and appropriate measures for management are included.

Drug Interactions

Describes clinically important drug/drug and drug/food interactions, including adverse and therapeutically useful interactions. The mechanism of the interaction, associated clinical importance, precautions to be observed, and management of the interaction are described. Generally, potential interactions supported only by animal or in vitro data are not described. Occasionally, theoretical interactions are presented because of the likelihood of their occurrence (e.g., based on evidence from similar drugs) or the potential severity of the effect should it occur.

Laboratory Test Interferences

Includes information on common, well-established drug/laboratory test interferences. The mechanism of the interaction, effects on test results, and effects on interpretation of these results are included. Alternative laboratory tests are described when appropriate. Alterations in laboratory test results that reflect a pathologic effect of the drug (e.g., aminoglycoside-induced increase in serum creatinine concentration) are described in the appropriate subsections under Cautions. Because of the nature of information on laboratory tests, appropriate specialized references on laboratory methods should be consulted when detailed information is required.

Pharmacology

Includes a brief statement of pharmacologic activity and/or mechanism of action, often compared with other similar drugs, for the purpose of orientation and introduction. Expanded descriptions of pharmacologic activities and effects are included. When relevant to human pharmacology and therapeutics, animal or in vitro data are presented. Data from human studies are not specified as such unless needed for clarification. Quantitative and qualitative comparative (with other drugs) information is provided when appropriate. Pharmacology usually is subdivided by pharmacologic effect (e.g., Anti-inflammatory, Analgesic) and/or body system affected (e.g., CNS, GI, Hematologic).

For anti-infectives, pharmacology is described under Mechanism of Action, Spectrum, and Resistance.

Mechanism of Action

Describes the mechanism of anti-infective activity for anti-infective agents.

Spectrum

Describes the in vitro spectra of activity of anti-infectives. The subsection on Susceptibility Testing describes factors (e.g., pH, test media, inoculum size) affecting susceptibility tests and defines susceptible and resistant organisms in terms of in vitro susceptibility test results (e.g., zone diameters for the Kirby-Bauer method, MICs for the tube dilution method). MIC values for clinically important organisms are included in the spectra subsections. Spectra often are divided according to class of organism (e.g., Gram-negative Bacteria, Anaerobic Bacteria).

In general, nomenclature for microorganisms follows that presented in *Bergey's Manual of Systematic Bacteriology* and the *Approved Lists of Bacterial Names* and validation lists and notification lists published in the *International Journal of Systematic and Evolutionary Bacteriology*. Other standard sources of current approved bacterial names (e.g., Prokaryotic Nomenclature Up-to-date at http://www.dsmz.de/bacterial-diversity/prokaryotic-nomenclature-up-to-date.html, List of Prokaryotic Names with Standing in Nomenclature at http://www.bacterio.net/), as described by the American Society for Microbiology in Instructions to Authors for *Antimicrobial Agents and Chemotherapy*, also are used. When available, in vitro susceptibility information generally is described according to the Clinical and Laboratory Standards Institute (CLSI) and/or the manufacturer's labeling.

Resistance

Describes the mechanism of resistance of microorganisms to anti-infective agents. Microbiologic tolerance to these agents also is described. Information on cross-resistance with other anti-infective agents is included. Definition of resistance in terms of in vitro susceptibility test results is described in the Spectrum section. Descriptions of resistant organisms are included in the Resistance section and/or in the spectra subsections of Spectrum.

Resistance of cells to antineoplastic agents generally is described in the Pharmacology section. Resistance or tolerance to the pharmacologic and/or therapeutic effects (e.g., tachyphylaxis) of other drugs generally is described in Pharmacology and/or Uses. Tolerance to the pharmacologic effects of some drugs (e.g., opiate agonists) also may be described in the Chronic Toxicity section.

Pharmacokinetics

Describes absorption, distribution, and elimination (biotransformation and excretion) characteristics of a drug.

The Absorption subsection includes information on extent (bioavailability) and rate of absorption by usual routes of administration and factors (e.g., product formulation) that might influence them. Applicable comparative information on doses, dosage forms, and routes of administration is included. Information on serum concentrations achieved and on the period of time for onset, peak, and duration of pharmacologic and/or therapeutic effect also is included, even when an absorption phase per se does not occur (e.g., following IV administration). Ranges for therapeutic and/or toxic concentrations (e.g., plasma, serum) of the drug are described when established.

The Distribution subsection describes the usual distribution of the drug into body tissue and fluids. Information describing the drug's propensity to cross the blood-brain barrier and placenta and to distribute into milk is included. Protein binding characteristics are presented.

The Elimination subsection describes the biotransformation and excretory characteristics of the drug. Information on elimination half-life and factors influencing it, clearance, site and extent of biotransformation, metabolic products and their activities, and routes of elimination from the body (e.g., urine, feces via bile) and factors affecting them is included. The effect of peritoneal dialysis and hemodialysis on elimination of the drug also is discussed.

Chemistry and Stability

Includes a brief chemical, structural, and/or pharmacologic description, often compared with other similar drugs, for the purpose of orientation and introduction. Structure-activity relationships are described when applicable. A physical description of drug entities includes physical appearance, taste, odor, and solubility. Solubilities are described according to USP descriptive terms (see the current edition of the *United States Pharmacopeia–National Formulary* [*USP–NF*]) or as appropriate specific solubilities (i.e., amount of solute per volume of solvent).

If the drug is ionizable, the pK_a is given. Other chemical and/or physical constants such as pH and osmolarity/osmolality of commercially available preparations are included. Preservatives and other important excipients in a commercial preparation also are described. Dosage equivalencies (e.g., units per mg of drug, mg of base per mg of salt) are given when the dosage of a drug differs from the commercially available form (e.g., salt, ester). Amounts of important ions (e.g., mg/mEq of potassium, sodium) in commercial preparations also are included.

Applicable stability information such as the effect of pH, autoclaving, heat, light, moisture, air, freezing, and microwave thawing is described. Storage requirements (i.e., recommended environmental storage conditions) also are described. Stability information about reconstituted and/or diluted preparations is provided. Physical and/or chemical compatibility information may be included. Additional detailed compatibility information on injectable drugs is available in the *Handbook on Injectable Drugs*® (available from the American Society of Health-System Pharmacists; go to www.ashp.org for details).

Preparations

Lists commercially available preparations of the drug. Preparations are described under the appropriate heading by USAN or other nonproprietary (generic) name. Combination preparations are described under a separate heading (e.g., Aspirin Combinations) following the appropriate single-entity subsection (e.g., Aspirin); official USP combination names (e.g., Metoprolol Tartrate and Hydrochlorothiazide) are used whenever possible.

Although USP has changed its naming conventions to eliminate salt forms in many official monograph titles (active moiety nomenclature concept), the American Society of Health-System Pharmacists continues to oppose this nomenclature change because of resulting confusion and loss of important chemical identity cues, and therefore *AHFS® DI*™ will continue to include salts in the Preparations headings for clarity. When recommended by FDA or the Institute for Safe Medication Practices (ISMP), "tall man" (mixed case) lettering is used for generic or brand (trade) names (e.g., "diazePAM").

When established by USP, pharmacy equivalent names (PENs) (e.g., co-careldopa for levodopa and carbidopa) are listed parenthetically alongside the corresponding combination heading. PENs are short and simple names that can be used for convenience by practitioners when it would be impractical to use the complete nonproprietary combination name. PENs are informational rather than official (*USP–NF*) in the US, but are offered by USP as standardized terms intended to discourage the proliferation of trivial names and undefined abbreviations for combinations. This abbreviated nomenclature was pioneered by the *British Pharmacopoeia* (*BP*) and subsequently adopted by USP.

Preparations are listed hierarchically by route of administration (alphabetically), dosage form (alphabetically), and strength (in order of increasing strength). When potency is described in terms other than those listed in the drug heading (e.g., potency of cefotaxime sodium is expressed in terms of cefotaxime), the labeled moiety is described parenthetically after the strength [e.g., 1 g (of cefotaxime)].

Route of administration and dosage form listings may be modified (e.g., Injection, for IM use only; Tablets, chewable; Capsules, extended-release). Following each preparation description, the proprietary (trade) names are listed alphabetically and include the corresponding manufacturers. Generally, preparations that are available by nonproprietary (generic) name do not include the names of the manufacturers/labelers; these preparations are listed under the generic name and described as being "available by nonproprietary name."

Generally, dosage forms used in the Preparations sections are the pharmaceutical dosage forms described in USP. (See the current edition of the *United States Pharmacopeia–National Formulary*.) Several dosage forms (i.e., elixir, extract, fluidextract, spirit, tincture) are used only when the preparation is official (USP or NF). Solution generally is used to describe all liquid preparations of dissolved drug, regardless of solvent; although syrups occasionally are official (USP or NF), these are listed as solutions and syrup is included only as part of the proprietary name.

Applicable legal descriptions (e.g., drugs subject to control under the Federal Controlled Substances Act of 1970, drugs subject to restricted distribution programs) are included.

References

Includes the bibliography for cited references. Information included in *AHFS® DI*™ is thoroughly referenced. Access to referenced statements and the References section of individual drug monographs for *AHFS® DI*™ and its point-of-care derivative database *AHFS® DI™Essentials*™ can be gained through electronic versions (e.g., AHFS® Clinical Drug Information™ [AHFS® CDI™], eBroselow's SafeDose®, Lexicomp® Online®; First DataBank's AHFS Drug Information® monographs available from multiple vendors; *AHFS Drug Information*® from STAT!Ref®, Pepid's Pharmacist Pro with AHFS DI®, and MedicinesComplete®; *Drug Information Fulltext*® [*DIF*®]; *AHFS® DI*™ Powered by Skyscape Medpresso).

Reference citations currently are electronically accessible for all monographs published after March 1984. For monographs originally published prior to that time, bibliographic citations are accessible only for selected revisions occurring since 1984. To determine whether a monograph was published or revised after March 1984, see the copyright notice at the end of the monograph in question. In electronic versions of *AHFS® DI*™, approximately 90% of the monographs currently are completely or partially referenced.

For additional information on searching the electronic versions of *AHFS® DI*™, contact the eHealth Solutions Division in the ASHP Publishing Office by phone at 301-657-3000 or by FAX at 301-664-8857 or by email at *pdiso@ashp.org*.

■ **AHFS®*first*Releases™**—Certain monographs in *AHFS® DI*™ are designated as AHFS®*first*Releases™. This designation appears in a boldface footnote preceding the Preparations section of the monograph. The AHFS®*first*Releases™ disseminate timely information on new molecular entities (NMEs) in an expedited format as soon as possible after FDA approval; the principal limitation is availability of final labeling from the manufacturer.

Scope

AHFS®*first*Releases™ are descriptions about new molecular entities that include information drawn from the manufacturer's labeling (package insert); however, the descriptions are not intended to be comprehensive. When additional information on such drugs is needed before publication of a more detailed monograph, the manufacturer's labeling should be consulted. AHFS®*first*Releases™ are intended to provide information that can answer typical basic questions about newly approved drugs. As such, the descriptions are limited to highlights of boxed warnings in labeling; a brief description of a REMS (if one is approved by FDA for the drug); the brand name; an introductory sentence providing a brief pharmacologic/therapeutic description; highlights of labeled dosage and administration information; highlights of labeled contraindications; labeled warnings and precautions, including those for specific populations; highlights of common adverse effects; highlights of interactions; highlights of the actions and spectrum of the drug; manufacturer-recommended advice to patients; and a product description. As a result, the AHFS®*first*Releases™ do not provide full disclosure about the respective drugs, and therefore it is essential that the manufacturer's labeling be consulted for more detailed information on usual uses, dosage and administration, cautions, precautions, contraindications, potential drug interactions, laboratory test interferences, and acute toxicity. Sections for Preparations and References are similar to those previously described for full-length monographs.

■ **Overviews**—Certain monographs in *AHFS® DI*™ are designated as Overviews. This designation appears in a boldface footnote preceding the Preparations section of the monograph.

Scope

The Overview drug monographs are summary descriptions that include information drawn principally from the manufacturer's labeling (package insert) and the principal clinical studies that supported approval of the drug. Pertinent information from other sources such as authoritative therapeutic guidelines, secondary references (e.g., review articles), and a limited number of primary references also are included; however, the overviews are not intended to be comprehensive.

The Overviews are intended to provide subscribers to *AHFS® DI*™ with summaries on new molecular entities (NMEs) that can answer most common questions about these drugs. As such, the Overviews are limited to basic information on the drugs, including brief descriptions (chemical and pharmacologic) of the type of drug, its labeled uses and associated dosages, administration instructions, product availability, cautionary information (e.g., contraindications; warnings and precautions; sensitivity reactions; cautions applicable to specific populations, common adverse effects), drug interactions, and important advice for patients. Some Overviews have been expanded to include important "unlabeled/off-label" uses. While selected information appears in these monographs, the scope of the Overview format limits the extent of discussion. As a result, the Overviews do not provide full disclosure about the respective drugs, and therefore it is essential that the manufacturer's labeling be consulted for more detailed information on pharmacodynamics, pharmacokinetics, adverse reactions, laboratory test interferences, and acute and chronic toxicity. Sections for Preparations and References are similar to those previously described for full-length monographs.

Pregnancy Precautions

The pregnancy precautions in the Overviews historically have followed FDA's lettered categories (A, B, C, D, or X), as stated in the manufacturer's labeling. Because of the summary format of the Overviews, only the letter designation previously appeared. However, as noted previously FDA amended the requirements for pregnancy and lactation labeling in 2014, eliminating these lettered categories and replacing the letters with a narrative structure for pregnancy labeling. Therefore, some *AHFS® DI*™ Overviews now contain text descriptions of information about use of a drug during pregnancy when the lettered category has not been provided in the labeling.

Following are definitions of the categories FDA previously had designated:

Category A. Adequate and well-controlled studies in pregnant women have failed to demonstrate a risk to the fetus in the first trimester and there is no evidence of risk in later trimesters. If the drug were used during pregnancy, the possibility of fetal harm appears remote.

Category B. Either animal reproduction studies have failed to demonstrate a risk to the fetus and there are no adequate and well-controlled studies in pregnant women or animal reproduction studies have shown an adverse effect (other than on fertility) but adequate and well-controlled studies in pregnant women have failed to demonstrate a risk to the fetus in the first trimester and there is no evidence of risk in later trimesters. In either case, the drug should be used during pregnancy only when clearly needed.

Category C. Either animal reproduction studies have revealed evidence of an adverse fetal effect and there are no adequate and well-controlled studies in pregnant women or animal reproduction studies have not been performed and it is not known whether the drug can cause fetal harm when administered to pregnant women. In the first case, the drug should be used during pregnancy only when the potential benefits justify the possible risks to the fetus. In the latter case, the drug should be used during pregnancy only when clearly needed.

Category D. There is positive evidence of human fetal risk based on adverse reaction data from investigational or postmarketing experience or studies in humans, but the potential benefits from use of the drug in pregnant women may be acceptable in certain conditions despite the possible risks to the fetus. The drug should be used during pregnancy only in life-threatening situations or severe disease for which safer drugs cannot be used or are ineffective. When the drug is administered during pregnancy or if the patient becomes pregnant while receiving the drug, the patient should be informed of the potential hazard to the fetus.

Category X. The drug may (can) cause fetal toxicity when administered to pregnant women based on animal or human studies demonstrating fetal abnormalities or positive evidence of human fetal risk from adverse reaction data from investigational or postmarketing experience, or both, and the risk of use of the drug during pregnancy clearly outweighs any benefit (e.g., safer drugs or alternative therapies are available). Since the risks clearly outweigh any possible benefits in women who are or may become pregnant, the drug is contraindicated in such women. If the drug is inadvertently administered during pregnancy or if the patient becomes pregnant while receiving the drug, the patient should be informed of the potential hazard to the fetus.

■ **SumMons®** Certain monographs in *AHFS® DI*™ are designated as SumMons® (summary monographs). This designation appears in a boldface footnote preceding the Preparations section of the monograph. SumMons® are summary descriptions about a drug, which include information that is drawn principally from the manufacturer's labeling (package insert) and/or other pertinent information (such as secondary references [e.g., review articles] and a limited number of primary references [e.g., the principal clinical studies]); however, no attempt is made to be complete, and the information may *not* be evaluative. When additional information on such drugs is needed pending development and publication of a more detailed *AHFS® DI*™ monograph, the manufacturer's labeling should be consulted.

The summaries are intended to provide only basic information on the drugs, and therefore are limited to brief descriptions (chemical and pharmacologic) of the type of drug, its labeled uses and associated dosages, and product availability. While selected precautionary information occasionally may appear in these summaries, no attempt is made to be complete, and therefore it is *essential* that the labeling be consulted for detailed information on the usual cautions, precautions, and contraindications. Some SumMons® have been expanded to include a detailed Cautions section, but it remains *essential* that the labeling be consulted for information on potential drug interactions, laboratory test interferences, and acute toxicity for such expanded descriptions. Some SumMons® also have been expanded to include important "unlabeled/off-label" uses. Sections for Preparations and References are similar to those previously described for full-length monographs.

■ **Notices**

Copyright

Other Notices

For other notices of warning, see Notices on p. iii of the master volume issued in January of each year.

4:00 Antihistamine Drugs

§ Omitted from the print version of *AHFS Drug Information*® because of space limitations. This monograph is available on the *AHFS Drug Information*® website, http://ahfsdruginformation.com. Username: ahfs2020; Password: ASHP94498.

* Please see the full AHFS Pharmacologic-Therapeutic Classification© on p. viii. Not all classes are used in the printed edition.

Antihistamine Drugs 4:00

Antihistamines General Statement

■ Antihistamines, which inhibit the effects of histamine at H_1 receptors, have been classified as first generation (i.e., relatively sedating) or second generation (i.e., relatively nonsedating).

Uses

Antihistamines are most often used to provide symptomatic relief of allergic symptoms caused by histamine release. The drugs are not curative and merely provide palliative therapy. Antihistamines are used only as adjunctive therapy to epinephrine and other standard measures in the treatment of anaphylactic reactions and laryngeal edema after the acute manifestations have been controlled. Individual patients vary in their response to antihistamines. A specific antihistamine that provides dramatic relief without adverse effects to one patient may produce intolerable adverse effects in another patient. Trial of various antihistamines may be necessary to determine which drug will provide relief while causing minimal adverse effects.

■ **Nasal Allergies and the Common Cold** Antihistamines are most beneficial in the management of nasal allergies. Seasonal allergic rhinitis (e.g., hay fever) and perennial (nonseasonal) allergic rhinitis are benefited more than perennial nonallergic (vasomotor) rhinitis. Orally administered antihistamines generally provide symptomatic relief of rhinorrhea, sneezing, oronasopharyngeal irritation or itching, lacrimation, and red, irritated, or itching eyes associated with the early response to histamine. The drugs generally are not effective in relieving symptoms of nasal obstruction, which are characteristic of the late allergic reaction, although limited data indicate that cetirizine and levocetirizine may relieve some symptoms of late allergic reactions. Antihistamines (e.g., azelastine) also may be administered intranasally for the symptomatic relief of seasonal allergic rhinitis. (See Uses in Azelastine 52:02.) In comparative studies, intranasal azelastine was more effective than placebo and at least as effective as oral antihistamines (e.g., cetirizine, terfenadine [no longer commercially available in the US]) or intranasal corticosteroids in relieving allergic rhinitis. However, unlike intranasal corticosteroids, azelastine does not appear to exhibit local histologic anti-inflammatory activity; therefore, beneficial effects on nasal obstruction appear to result principally from antihistaminic and/or other activity.

Chronic nasal congestion and headache caused by edema of the paranasal sinus mucosa are often refractory to antihistamine therapy. In the treatment of hay fever, antihistamines are more likely to be beneficial when therapy is initiated at the beginning of the hay fever season when pollen counts are low (e.g., before pollination begins) and if used regularly during the pollen season. Antihistamines are less likely to be effective when pollen counts are high, when pollen exposure is prolonged, and when nasal congestion is prominent.

Although antihistamines frequently are used for symptomatic relief in the common cold, evidence of effectiveness remains to be clearly established. Antihistamines cannot prevent, cure, or shorten the course of the common cold, but may provide some symptomatic relief. Conventional (prototypical, first generation) antihistamines (e.g., those with anticholinergic activity) are considered effective in relieving rhinorrhea and sneezing associated with the common cold, but evidence of efficacy in relieving oronasopharyngeal itching, lacrimation, or itching eyes associated with this condition currently is lacking. Nonsedating (second generation) antihistamines do not appear to be effective in relieving rhinorrhea, suggesting that histamine is not a principal mediator of this manifestation. The extent to which histamine contributes to other manifestations of the common cold currently is unclear, but pathogenesis of the full constellation of symptoms that constitute the common cold appears to be complex, involving a number of mediators and neurologic mechanisms.

Routine, prolonged administration of fixed combinations containing antihistamines, nasal decongestants, anticholinergics, analgesic-antipyretics, caffeine, antitussives, and/or expectorants has been questioned. Single-ingredient products generally are safer than combination products, while also facilitating dosage adjustment. There is no evidence that combinations containing 2 or more antihistamines are more effective than one antihistamine or that combinations of subtherapeutic doses of 2 or more antihistamines are more effective than therapeutic doses of one antihistamine. Oral antihistamine combinations containing an analgesic-antipyretic and/or nasal decongestant; an antitussive and nasal decongestant; an analgesic-antipyretic, antitussive, and nasal decongestant; or an antitussive may be rational if each ingredient has demonstrated clinical effectiveness and is present in therapeutic dosage. Selective use of such combinations can provide a convenient and rational approach for relief of concurrent symptoms (e.g., rhinorrhea, nasal congestion, cough), which often are present in allergic rhinitis and other conditions (e.g., common cold), by allowing the patient to use a single combination rather than multiple single-entity preparations. Combination preparations generally should be used only when symptoms amenable to each ingredient are present concurrently. Combinations containing an antihistamine and an expectorant, anticholinergic agent, or bronchodilator are *not* considered rational.

Although cough and cold preparations that contain antihistamines, nasal decongestants, cough suppressants, and/or expectorants commonly were used in pediatric patients younger than 2 years of age, systematic reviews of controlled trials have concluded that nonprescription (over-the-counter, OTC) cough and cold preparations are *no* more effective than placebo in reducing acute cough and other symptoms of upper respiratory tract infection in these patients. Furthermore, adverse events, including deaths, have been (and continue to be) reported in pediatric patients younger than 2 years of age receiving these preparations. (See Cautions: Pediatric Precautions.)

■ **Other Allergic Conditions** Antihistamines are often effective in the treatment of allergic dermatoses and other dermatoses associated with histamine release, but effectiveness varies with the causative agent and symptoms may return when the drug is stopped. Antihistamines have been used in the symptomatic treatment of chronic idiopathic urticaria; occasionally, patients who do not experience adequate relief with an antihistamine (H_1-receptor antagonist) alone may benefit from the addition of an H_2-receptor antagonist.

However, in one study, the addition of an H_2-receptor antagonist did not provide a substantial increase in response (as determined by reduction in whealing). Some antihistamines also may symptomatically relieve pruritus accompanying atopic dermatitis, contact dermatitis, pruritus ani or vulvae, and insect bites. Some evidence suggests that first generation antihistamines such as hydroxyzine and diphenhydramine may be more effective than second generation antihistamines (e.g., terfenadine [no longer commercially available in the US], loratadine) for the relief of pruritus associated with certain allergic dermatoses (e.g., atopic dermatitis), but additional study is needed to elucidate further the relative efficacy of these drugs as antipruritics. Antihistamines also may be used in the treatment of dermatographism. Patients with dermatographism or other urticarial conditions who do not experience adequate relief with an antihistamine (H_1-receptor antagonist) alone may benefit from the addition of an H_2-receptor antagonist to enhance relief of pruritus and wheal formation.

Antihistamines are useful in the management of allergic conjunctivitis caused by foods or inhaled allergens. Allergic or hypersensitivity reactions to penicillin, streptomycin, sulfonamides, and other drugs may be amenable to antihistamine therapy. Pruritus and urticaria accompanying these conditions usually are temporarily relieved; edema is more resistant and serum sickness is not benefited.

Symptoms of mild transfusion reactions not caused by ABO incompatibility or pyrogens may be alleviated by antihistamines. The drugs should *not* be added to blood being transfused. Antihistamines may be administered prophylactically to patients with a history of transfusion reactions, but the drugs should not be given routinely to patients receiving blood. Antihistamines also may be useful to prevent sequelae following desensitization procedures and allergic reactions to radiographic contrast media. It must be kept in mind that prophylactic use of antihistamines may mask incipient signs of allergic reactions, and the patient's hypersensitivity may not be recognized until a serious reaction occurs.

Although epinephrine is the initial drug of choice for patients with anaphylactic or anaphylactoid reactions, antihistamines are useful in the ancillary treatment of pruritus, urticaria, angioedema, and bronchospasm associated with these reactions. Concurrent use of H_1- and H_2-receptor antagonists appears to reduce the adverse effects of histamine on the peripheral vasculature and myocardium during anaphylaxis.

■ **Asthma** Antihistamines may provide some benefit in certain asthmatic patients, but the drugs usually are not effective in treating bronchial asthma per se and should *not* be used in the treatment of severe acute asthma attacks. In addition, antihistamines are not included in the usual recommended regimens for the management of asthma, including long-term control of the disease. Antihistamine and decongestant combinations may provide symptomatic relief (e.g., of rhinitis) in patients with chronic rhinitis and persistent asthma, but the drugs have not been shown to have a protective effect on lower airways; other agents (e.g., inhaled corticosteroids) are for protective effects on lower airways. In general, patients with predictable seasonal asthma should receive long-term anti-inflammatory therapy (e.g., inhaled corticosteroids, mast-cell stabilizers), initiated prior to the anticipated onset of exposure to allergens and continued throughout the season. The drugs may be used with caution to treat hay fever or other airway disorder with a histamine-mediated component in patients with such disorders and asthma. Although some clinicians believe that the anticholinergic effects (e.g., reduction of nasal secretions) of some of these drugs may cause thickening of bronchial secretions resulting in further airway obstruction in asthmatics, especially those with status asthmaticus, most experts consider complete avoidance of currently available antihistamines in asthmatics unjustified. (See Cautions: Precautions and Contraindications.)

■ **Motion Sickness and Vertigo** Some antihistamines (e.g., dimenhydrinate, diphenhydramine, meclizine, promethazine) are useful for the prevention and treatment of nausea, vomiting, and/or vertigo associated with motion sickness and they are considered the drugs of choice for the management of this condition. For additional information on the use of antihistamines for the management of motion sickness, see Dimenhydrinate and see Meclizine Hydrochloride in 56:22.08. Dimenhydrinate and meclizine have also been used in the symptomatic treatment of vertigo associated with diseases affecting the vestibular system (e.g., labyrinthitis, Ménière's disease). Nonphenothiazine antihistamines are less effective than the phenothiazines in controlling nausea and vomiting not related to vestibular stimulation.

■ **Nausea and Vomiting of Pregnancy** Doxylamine succinate is used in fixed combination with pyridoxine hydrochloride for the management of nausea and vomiting of pregnancy in women who have not responded to conservative management. (See Uses in Doxylamine 4:04.)

■ **Chemotherapy-induced Nausea and Vomiting** Some antihistamines (e.g., diphenhydramine) may be useful as adjunctive antiemetic agents to prevent chemotherapy-induced nausea and vomiting†; however, the American Society of Clinical Oncology currently does not recommend that antihistamines be used alone as antiemetic agents in patients receiving chemotherapy.

■ **Insomnia** Some antihistamines, especially the ethanolamines such as diphenhydramine and doxylamine, are used for their sedative effects as nighttime sleep aids. The US Food and Drug Administration (FDA) states that diphenhydramine currently is the only antihistamine commercially available in the US that has been shown to be both safe and effective for *self-medication* as a nighttime sleep aid. In individuals who experience occasional sleeplessness or those who have difficulty falling asleep, diphenhydramine (administered as either the citrate or hydrochloride salt) is more effective than placebo in reducing sleep onset (i.e., time to fall asleep) and increasing the depth and quality of sleep. Although the safety and efficacy of doxylamine as a nighttime sleep aid have not been fully established, the FDA states that, pending further accumulation of data, doxylamine-containing nighttime sleep aids that have been approved for this use may continue to be marketed in the US. Some proprietary sleep aids also may continue to contain pyrilamine despite a lack of substantial evidence of safety and efficacy for use of this antihistamine as a nighttime sleep aid; however, many such preparations have been or are likely to be reformulated with other antihistamines (e.g., diphenhydramine).

■ **Other Systemic Uses** Some antihistamines such as diphenhydramine have been used effectively as antitussives. Diphenhydramine also may be useful in the management of tremor early in the course of parkinsonian syndrome and in the management of drug-induced extrapyramidal reactions.

■ **Topical and Other Local Uses** Diphenhydramine and tripelennamine (no longer commercially available in the US; extemporaneous formulation would be necessary) are used topically for temporary relief of pruritus and pain associated with various skin conditions including minor burns, sunburn, minor cuts or scrapes, insect bites, or minor skin irritations. The drugs may provide effective localized antipruritic activity when applied topically if pruritus and discomfort are histamine mediated; the weak local anesthetic action of the drugs also may contribute to the overall effect. However, many clinicians suggest that topical diphenhydramine not be used on large areas of the body or more often than directed, since increased percutaneous absorption of the drug may occur that can result in systemic adverse effects and toxicity. (See Acute Toxicity: Manifestations.) Topical diphenhydramine also should not be used for *self-medication* in the management of varicella (chickenpox) or measles without first consulting a clinician.

Some antihistamines also have been used for their topical or local anesthetic effects in ophthalmic, urologic, proctologic, gastroscopic, otolaryngologic, and dental procedures. However, topical use of antihistamines generally is discouraged because sensitivity reactions (e.g., sensitization, hypersensitivity) may result. (See Cautions: Sensitivity Reactions.) In addition, use of certain antihistamines (e.g., diphenhydramine) for local anesthesia via local infiltration also is discouraged because of the risk of local tissue necrosis. If the drugs are used topically as antipruritics, therapy generally should be short-term (i.e., for no longer than 7 days) because of the increasing risk of sensitivity reactions from prolonged or repeated use. Antihistamines are more effective, especially if pruritus is generalized, and are less likely to cause sensitivity reactions when the drugs are administered systemically rather than applied topically.

Dosage and Administration

■ **Administration** Antihistamines usually are administered orally. Although some of these drugs may be given IV, IM, or subcutaneously, most antihistamines are not administered parenterally because they frequently cause local irritation. Some antihistamines also may be administered topically or intranasally. Topical use of antihistamines generally is discouraged since sensitivity reactions (e.g., sensitization, hypersensitivity) may result. In addition, topical preparations containing diphenhydramine should not be used more often than directed for any condition, applied on large areas of the body, or used concomitantly with other preparations containing diphenhydramine, including those used orally, since increased serum concentrations of diphenhydramine may occur that can result in CNS toxicity. (See Acute Toxicity: Manifestations.) Topical diphenhydramine also should not be used for *self-medication* in the management of varicella (chickenpox) or measles without first consulting a clinician.

■ **Dosage** Dosage of antihistamines should be individualized according to the patient's response and tolerance.

Cautions

Adverse effects, which vary in incidence and severity with the individual drug, are caused by all antihistamines, although serious toxicity rarely occurs. Individual patients vary in their susceptibility to the adverse effects of these drugs, and such effects may disappear despite continued therapy. Geriatric patients may be particularly susceptible to dizziness, sedation, and hypotension. Most mild reactions may be relieved by a reduction in dosage or changing to another antihistamine.

Severe cardiovascular effects, including prolongation of the QT interval, arrhythmias, cardiac effects, hypotension, palpitations, syncope, dizziness and/or death have been reported in patients receiving astemizole (no longer commercially available in the US) or terfenadine (no longer commercially available in the US). These cardiotoxic effects usually were associated with higher than recommended dosages and/or increased plasma concentrations of the drugs and their active metabolites.

■ **CNS Effects** CNS depression is common with usual dosage of antihistamines, especially with the ethanolamine derivatives. Sedation, ranging from mild drowsiness to deep sleep, occurs most frequently; however, in the treatment of allergies, this effect may be therapeutically useful. Dizziness, lassitude, disturbed coordination, and muscular weakness may also occur. In some patients, the sedative effects disappear spontaneously after the antihistamine has been administered for 2–3 days. Individuals who perform potentially hazardous tasks requiring mental alertness or physical coordination (e.g., operating machinery, driving a motor vehicle) should be warned about possible drowsiness, dizziness, or weakness. Patients also should be warned to avoid consuming alcoholic beverages while taking antihistamines, since alcohol may potentiate these CNS effects. In addition, patients already receiving other CNS depressants (e.g., sedatives, tranquilizers) should be warned not to undertake *self-medication* with an antihistamine without first consulting their clinician. Patients using diphenhydramine or doxylamine for *self-medication* should be warned that the drugs may cause *marked* drowsiness. Acrivastine, desloratadine, fexofenadine, loratadine, and, possibly, cetirizine and levocetirizine appear to cause fewer adverse CNS effects, including effects on psychomotor performance and reactivity, than other currently available (first generation) antihistamines and therefore commonly have been referred to as relatively "nonsedating" or second generation antihistamines. However, while most second generation antihistamines do not appear to potentiate the effects of CNS depressants, including alcohol, acrivastine, cetirizine, and levocetirizine may potentiate such effects, although less prominently than first generation antihistamines.

Some patients, especially children, receiving antihistamines may experience paradoxical excitement characterized by restlessness, insomnia, tremors, euphoria, nervousness, delirium, palpitation, and even seizures. There have been several reports of toxic psychosis in children who received concomitant oral and topical diphenhydramine for relief of pruritus associated with varicella (chickenpox), poison ivy, or sunburn. (See Acute Toxicity: Manifestations.) In addition, central anticholinergic syndrome characterized by hallucinations, agitation, and confusion occurred in several children receiving usual or excessive dosages of cyproheptadine. Patients should be warned that phenindamine may be particularly likely to occasionally cause insomnia and nervousness in some individuals. Antihistamines also may precipitate epileptiform seizures in patients with focal lesions of the cerebral cortex, and the drugs should be administered with caution in patients with seizure disorders.

An acute dystonic reaction, which consisted of trismus, difficulty in swallowing, dysarthria, rigidity, and motor incoordination, and was accompanied by mental confusion and tremors, was reported in at least 1 patient receiving IV diphenhydramine.

■ **GI and Hepatic Effects** Adverse GI effects of antihistamines include epigastric distress, anorexia, nausea, vomiting, diarrhea, or constipation. GI symptoms may be decreased by administering the drug with meals or with milk. Cholestasis, hepatitis, hepatic failure, hepatic function abnormality, and jaundice have been reported rarely in patients receiving antihistamines (e.g., cyproheptadine, terfenadine).

■ **Sensitivity Reactions** Antihistamines can cause sensitivity reactions (e.g., sensitization, hypersensitivity) following topical application or systemic administration, but such reactions are more likely following topical use of the drugs, especially ethylenediamine derivatives. Antihistamines can act as haptens and cause IgE-mediated (type I) hypersensitivity reactions or T cell-mediated (type IV) sensitization reactions. Type I reactions appear to occur rarely, but type IV reactions occur more frequently, particularly following topical application of the drugs. Sensitization following topical use of antihistamines results in allergic contact dermatitis, which may be manifested as eczema, pruritus, and inflammation, at the site of application. Once local sensitization to an antihistamine occurs, the dermatitis can recur following subsequent topical or systemic exposure to the drug or a chemically related drug (including local anesthetics). Photosensitivity (principally photoallergic dermatitis) reactions, which may be manifested as eczema, pruritus, papular rash, and erythema on exposed skin, also have occurred following topical or systemic administration of antihistamines, and cross-sensitivity with chemically related drugs can occur.

■ **Cardiovascular Effects** Although antihistamines exhibit anticholinergic and local anesthetic effects, including quinidine-like effects on cardiac conduction, and certain drugs have been investigated for potential antiarrhythmic activity, adverse cardiovascular effects are uncommon and usually limited to overdosage situations. When adverse cardiac effects have occurred, they generally were characteristic anticholinergic and/or local anesthetic (quinidine-like) effects such as tachycardia, palpitation, ECG changes (e.g., widened QRS), and arrhythmias (e.g., extrasystole, heart block). Other cardiovascular effects reported with antihistamines include hypotension and hypertension; in some cases, hypotension may result in part from α-adrenergic blocking activity of the antihistamine.

Serious cardiac effects, including prolongation of the QT interval corrected for rate (QT_c), ST-U abnormalities, arrhythmias (e.g., ventricular tachycardia, atypical ventricular tachycardia [torsades de pointes], ventricular fibrillation, heart block), arrest, hypotension, palpitations, syncope, dizziness, and/or death (secondary to ventricular tachyarrhythmia), have been reported rarely in patients receiving terfenadine or astemizole. Astemizole and terfenadine are no longer commercially available in the US. These cardiotoxic effects usually were associated with higher than recommended dosages and/or increased plasma concentrations of the drugs and their active metabolites, although serious cardiac effects also have been reported occasionally at usual astemizole or terfenadine dosages. While patients with impaired liver function and, possibly, geriatric patients may have been at particular risk of accumulation of these antihistamines and associated cardiotoxic effects, these effects have been reported rarely in apparently healthy individuals with no associated risk factors.

Patients who were receiving concomitant therapy with an azole (including imidazole derivative [e.g., ketoconazole] and triazole derivative [e.g., itraconazole]) antifungal, a macrolide (e.g., clarithromycin, erythromycin, troleandomycin) anti-infective, mibefradil (no longer commercially available in the US), quinine, or grapefruit juice also appeared to be at substantial risk of such toxicity, probably secondary to interference with metabolism of the antihistamine. In addition, concomitant use of terfenadine or astemizole with most human immunodeficiency virus (HIV) protease inhibitors, quinupristin and dalfopristin, zileuton, or serotonin-reuptake inhibitors has not been recommended since HIV protease inhibitors, quinupristin and dalfopristin, zileuton, and serotonin-reuptake inhibitors have been associated with increased plasma concentrations of these antihistamines and potentially serious and/or life-threatening adverse effects could have occurred as a result of these drugs' effects on the metabolism of astemizole or terfenadine.

The potential for similar drug interactions and cardiac effects with loratadine remains to be elucidated more fully. However, acrivastine and loratadine have not been shown to prolong the QT interval when administered alone. Prolongation of the QT_c interval has been reported in a limited number of healthy adults receiving desloratadine dosages of 45 mg daily (9 times the recommended daily dosage) for 10 days; however, the manufacturer states that no clinically relevant adverse events were reported.

The manufacturer of cetirizine states that no clinically important prolongation of the QT_c interval has been reported in healthy adult men receiving cetirizine during controlled clinical studies. The manufacturer of levocetirizine (the *R* enantiomer of cetirizine) states that no clinically important prolongation of the QT_c interval has been reported following administration of a single dose of levocetirizine. The effects of multiple-dose administration are not known, but levocetirizine is not expected to have clinically important effects on the QT_c interval based on results of QT_c studies with cetirizine and the lack of reports of QT_c interval prolongation during postmarketing surveillance of that drug. The manufacturer of cetirizine also states that concomitant administration of the antihistamine with drugs known to inhibit cytochrome P-450 microsomal enzymes (e.g., azithromycin, erythromycin, ketoconazole) has not been associated with clinically important changes in ECG parameters (e.g., QT_c intervals) and that no clinically important interactions have been reported in patients receiving cetirizine concomitantly with azithromycin, erythromycin, or ketoconazole.

The manufacturer of fexofenadine states that no statistically significant mean increases in the QT_c interval have been reported in healthy adults or patients with seasonal allergic rhinitis receiving fexofenadine hydrochloride dosages up to 400 mg twice daily (for 6 days) or 60–240 mg twice daily (for 2 weeks), respectively, during controlled clinical studies.

The mechanism of the cardiotoxic effects of astemizole and terfenadine has not been fully understood, and it appeared to be contrary to what would have been expected from studies on cardiac histamine H_1-receptors; the possibility that H_3-receptors (mediating a regulatory feedback mechanism) may have been involved had been suggested. Limited evidence from animal models using terfenadine has suggested that the cardiotoxic effects of the drug may have resulted at least in part from blockade of the potassium channel involved in repolarization of cardiac cells (i.e., blockade of the delayed rectifier potassium current I_K). Unlike other antihistamines, anticholinergic and/or local anesthetic effects appeared to be unlikely causes of the cardiac effects of these 2 second generation (relatively "nonsedating") antihistamines.

It has been recommended that usual dosages of terfenadine (i.e., 60 mg twice daily) and astemizole (i.e., 10 mg daily) *not* be exceeded because of the risk of potentially life-threatening cardiotoxic effects. Because of this risk, patients were advised *not* to temporarily increase (e.g., double) the prescribed dosage in an attempt to accelerate or improve symptomatic relief provided by these drugs.

Patients with hepatic impairment, geriatric patients, those receiving drugs or who had underlying conditions that might have prolonged the QT interval, and those who were receiving drugs that could have produced electrolyte abnormalities such as hypokalemia or hypomagnesemia may have been at increased risk of cardiac arrhythmias during terfenadine or astemizole therapy. Therefore, administration of these antihistamines was *not* recommended in such patients. Terfenadine or astemizole also should *not* have been used in patients receiving a macrolide (e.g., clarithromycin, erythromycin, troleandomycin) anti-infective, an azole antifungal (including imidazole [e.g., itraconazole] and triazole [e.g., itraconazole] derivatives), or mibefradil; in addition, use of these antihistamines in patients receiving any other drug (e.g., quinine, most HIV protease inhibitors, serotonin-reuptake inhibitors, zileuton) that potentially could inhibit their metabolism was *not* recommended. It also has been recommended that astemizole or terfenadine not be taken with grapefruit juice. Concomitant administration of astemizole with therapeutic doses of quinine was contraindicated.

■ **Other Adverse Effects** Adverse anticholinergic effects of antihistamines include dryness of mouth, nose, and throat; dysuria; urinary retention; impotence; vertigo; visual disturbances; blurred vision; diplopia; tinnitus; acute labyrinthitis; insomnia; tremors; nervousness; irritability; and facial dyskinesia. Tightness of the chest, thickening of bronchial secretions, wheezing, nasal stuffiness, sweating, chills, early menses, toxic psychosis, headache, faintness, and paresthesia have occurred.

Rarely, agranulocytosis, hemolytic anemia, leukopenia, thrombocytopenia, and pancytopenia have been reported in patients receiving some antihistamines. Increased appetite and/or weight gain also occurred in patients receiving antihistamines (cyproheptadine).

■ **Precautions and Contraindications** Antihistamines having substantial anticholinergic activity (usually conventional [prototypical, first generation] including ethanolamines) should be administered with caution, if at all, in patients with angle-closure glaucoma, prostatic hypertrophy (which may result in difficulty in urination), stenosing peptic ulcer, pyloroduodenal obstruction, or bladder neck obstruction. Because it was suggested that the anticholinergic effect of antihistamines might reduce the volume and cause thickening of bronchial secretions and thus result in obstruction of respiratory passages, it had been recommended that the drugs be used with caution and only under the direction of a clinician in patients with asthma or chronic obstructive pulmonary disease if clearance of bronchial secretions was a problem. While some clinicians and manufacturers continue to warn against use of the drugs in patients with asthma because of potential effects of anticholinergic activity on the volume and fluidity of bronchial secretions, most experts and clinicians believe that there currently is little, if any, direct evidence of antihistamine-induced exacerbation of asthma secondary to bronchial drying nor substantiation for avoiding use of currently available antihistamines in asthmatic patients. Antihistamines usually should not be used, unless under the direction of a clinician, in patients who have a breathing problem (e.g., emphysema, chronic bronchitis), and these drugs generally should not be used in asthmatics who previously experienced a serious antihistamine-induced adverse bronchopulmonary effect. In addition, antihistamines should be used with caution in patients with increased intraocular pressure, hyperthyroidism, cardiovascular disease, or hypertension. The drugs are contraindicated in patients with asthmatic attacks. For *self-medication*, cough preparations containing an antihistamine (e.g., diphenhydramine) should not be used for persistent or chronic cough or breathing problems such as those occurring with smoking, asthma, chronic bronchitis, or emphysema, or for cough accompanied by excessive phlegm, unless directed by a clinician. A persistent cough may be indicative of a serious condition. If cough persists for more than one week, is recurrent, or is accompanied by fever, rash, or persistent headache, a clinician should be consulted.

Patients should be advised that CNS depression (e.g., drowsiness) is common with first generation antihistamines, even at usual dosages and particularly with ethanolamine derivatives. (See Cautions: CNS Effects.) In addition, patients should be warned that additive CNS depression may occur when first generation antihistamines or possibly, cetirizine or levocetirizine is administered concomitantly with other CNS depressants, including alcohol. (See Drug Interactions: CNS Depressants.) Patients receiving acrivastine, a second generation antihistamine, also should be warned of the possibility of such effects.

Diphenhydramine toxicity (e.g., dilated pupils, facial flushing, hallucinations, ataxic gait, urinary retention) has been reported in pediatric patients following topical application of diphenhydramine to large areas of the body (often areas with broken skin) or following concomitant use of topical and oral preparations containing diphenhydramine. (See Acute Toxicity: Manifestations.) Therefore, the US Food and Drug Administration (FDA) and many clinicians warn that oral diphenhydramine should *not* be used concomitantly with any other preparations containing the drug, including those used topically. (See Cautions, in Diphenhydramine 4:04.) In addition, topical preparations containing diphenhydramine should not be used more often than directed for any condition, applied on large areas of the body, or used concomitantly with other preparations containing diphenhydramine, including those used orally, since increased serum concentrations of diphenhydramine may occur that can result in CNS toxicity. (See Acute Toxicity: Manifestations.) Patients should be advised to consult a clinician prior to use of topical diphenhydramine for the management of varicella (chickenpox) or measles.

Although diphenhydramine appears to have low abuse potential, several children, adolescents, and at least one adult with chronic hematologic and antineoplastic diseases have exhibited drug-seeking behavior and anticholinergic effects after chronic intermittent rapid IV administration of the drug.

While astemizole and terfenadine were commercially available in the US, individuals receiving these second generation antihistamines were warned that patients with hepatic impairment (e.g., cirrhosis, hepatitis); geriatric patients; those who were concomitantly receiving an azole-derivative anti-infective (e.g., fluconazole, itraconazole, ketoconazole, metronidazole, miconazole), a macrolide antibiotic (e.g., clarithromycin, erythromycin, troleandomycin), mibefradil (no longer commercially available in the US), or other potent inhibitors of the cytochrome P-450 isoenzyme (CYP3A) (including most HIV protease inhibitors, quinupristin and dalfopristin, zileuton, or serotonin-reuptake inhibitors) responsible for the metabolism of astemizole or terfenadine (see Drug Interactions); those who were having underlying conditions that might prolong the QT interval corrected for rate (QT_c) (e.g., hypokalemia, hypomagnesemia, bradycardia, congenital QT syndrome); those who were receiving drugs that might prolong the QT_c interval (e.g., certain antiarrhythmic agents, bepridil hydrochloride, certain psychotropic agents, probucol [no longer commercially available in the US], cisapride, sparfloxacin, pentamidine); or those who were receiving drugs (e.g., diuretics) that could produce electrolyte abnormalities, such as hypokalemia or hypomagnesemia, may have experienced prolongation of the QT_c interval and may have been at increased risk of cardiac arrhythmias (e.g., ventricular tachycardia, atypical ventricular tachycardia [torsades de pointes], ventricular fibrillation) when they were receiving recommended dosages of astemizole or terfenadine. Therefore, administration of astemizole or terfenadine was not recommended in such patients.

In addition, astemizole or terfenadine was contraindicated in patients with disease states (e.g., severe hepatic impairment) or receiving concomitant therapy (e.g., itraconazole, ketoconazole, clarithromycin, erythromycin, troleandomycin, mibefradil) known to impair metabolism of the antihistamine. Astemizole also was contraindicated in patients receiving concomitant therapy with quinine.

For additional cautions, contraindications, and drug interactions with the phenothiazine derivatives, see the Phenothiazines General Statement 28:16.08.24.

■ Pediatric Precautions Antihistamines should not be administered to premature or full-term neonates. Young children may be more susceptible than adults to the toxic effects of antihistamines. (See Acute Toxicity.) Adults responsible for the supervision of a child receiving an antihistamine should be warned that children may be at increased risk for experiencing CNS stimulant effects with antihistamines. (See Cautions: CNS Effects.) Although the relationship and possible mechanism(s) have not been elucidated, respiratory depression, sleep apnea, and sudden infant death syndrome (SIDS) have occurred in a number of infants and young children who were receiving usual dosages of phenothiazine-derivative antihistamines (i.e., promethazine, trimeprazine [no longer commercially available in the US]). (See Cautions: Pediatric Precautions, in Promethazine 4:04.) In addition, death has been reported in children younger than 2 years of age receiving carbinoxamine-containing preparations or cough and cold preparations containing an antihistamine with or without other agents (e.g., cough suppressants, expectorants, nasal decongestants). (See Uses: Regulations Governing Carbinoxamine-containing Preparations, in Carbinoxamine Maleate 4:04 and also see Cautions: Pediatric Precautions, in Pseudoephedrine Hydrochloride 12:12.12.)

In a report published by the US Centers for Disease Control and Prevention (CDC), cough and cold preparations containing carbinoxamine, pseudoephedrine, acetaminophen, and/or dextromethorphan were determined by medical examiners or coroners to be the underlying cause of death in 3 infants 6 months of age or younger during 2005. The actual cause of death might have been overdosage of one drug, interaction of different drugs, an underlying medical condition, or a combination of drugs and underlying medical conditions. In addition, an estimated 1519 children younger than 2 years of age were treated in emergency departments in the US during 2004–2005 for adverse events, including overdoses, associated with cold and cough preparations.

The dosages at which cold and cough preparations can cause illness or death in pediatric patients younger than 2 years of age are not known, and there are no specific dosage recommendations (i.e., approved by the US Food and Drug Administration [FDA]) for the symptomatic treatment of cold and cough for patients in this age group. Because of the absence of dosage recommendations, limited published evidence of effectiveness, and risks for toxicity (including fatal overdosage). FDA stated that nonprescription cough and cold preparations should not be used in children younger than 2 years of age; the agency continues to assess safety and efficacy of these preparations in older children. Meanwhile, because children 2–3 years of age also are at increased risk of overdosage and toxicity, some manufacturers of oral nonprescription cough and cold preparations agreed to voluntarily revise the product labeling to state that such preparations should not be used in children younger than 4 years of age. FDA recommends that parents and caregivers adhere to the dosage instructions and warnings on the product labeling that accompanies the preparation if administering to children and consult with their clinician about any concerns. Clinicians should ask caregivers about use of nonprescription cough and cold preparations to avoid overdosage.

Because antihistamines may cause drowsiness that can be potentiated by other CNS depressants (e.g., sedatives, tranquilizers), an antihistamine should be used in children receiving one of these drugs only under the direction of a clinician. Antihistamines should not be used in children who have a breathing problem (e.g., chronic bronchitis) or glaucoma unless otherwise directed by a clinician. It also has been recommended that antihistamines not be used in children with asthma, liver disease, or seizure disorder unless under the direction of a clinician. Overdosage of doxylamine has been reported in children. Manifestations of doxylamine overdosage in children have included coma, generalized tonic-clonic (grand mal) seizures, cardiorespiratory arrest, and death. Children appear to be at high risk for cardiorespiratory arrest secondary to doxylamine overdosage. For additional information, see the individual monographs in 4:00.

Acute toxicity has been reported in pediatric patients following topical application of diphenhydramine to large areas of the body (often areas with broken skin) or following concomitant use of topical and oral preparations containing diphenhydramine. (See Cautions: Precautions and Contraindications, and also see Acute Toxicity.)

While it is desirable to avoid the use of alcohol-containing antihistamine preparations in children because of potential toxicity, inclusion of alcohol in some preparations may be a pharmaceutical necessity (e.g., as a solvent) and therefore complete avoidance of such preparations may not be possible. According to a final rule issued in 1995 by FDA, over-the-counter (OTC) oral preparations intended for use in children younger than 6 years of age, children 6–11 years of age, or children 12 years of age and older may contain up to 0.5, 5, or 10% alcohol, respectively.

■ Pregnancy and Lactation Antihistamines should not be used in women who are or may become pregnant unless the potential benefits justify the possible risks to the fetus. Some manufacturers caution that antihistamines should not be used during the third trimester because of the risk of severe reactions (e.g., seizures) to the drugs in neonates and premature infants. For additional information, see the individual monographs in 4:00.

Doxylamine succinate in fixed combination with pyridoxine hydrochloride is intended for use in the management of nausea and vomiting of pregnancy. Historically, there was considerable controversy regarding the teratogenic potential, if any, of doxylamine succinate; however, after evaluating extensive data and information concerning the possible teratogenicity of the drug, FDA concluded that it is unlikely that doxylamine succinate is teratogenic. In addition, FDA states that the removal of products containing doxylamine succinate that previously were commercially available for the management of nausea and vomiting of pregnancy was not for reasons of safety or effectiveness. Numerous epidemiologic studies (including cohort studies, case-control studies, and meta-analyses) have been performed to investigate possible teratogenic effects of doxylamine succinate in fixed combination with pyridoxine hydrochloride in pregnant women and have found no evidence of an increased risk of fetal malformations.

Most manufacturers state that antihistamines should not be administered to nursing women, since the drugs may inhibit lactation and small amounts appear to be distributed into milk. Adverse effects (e.g., excitement, irritability, and sedation) have been reported in infants presumably exposed to antihistamines (e.g., doxylamine) through human milk. Infants with apnea or other respiratory syndromes may be particularly vulnerable to the sedative effects of antihistamines (e.g., doxylamine).

Because of the potential for serious adverse reactions (e.g., CNS effects) to antihistamines in nursing infants, a decision should be made whether to discontinue nursing or antihistamines, taking into account the importance of the drugs to the woman. The manufacturer of doxylamine in fixed combination with pyridoxine states that this preparation should *not* be used in nursing women.

Drug Interactions

■ **CNS Depressants** Additive CNS depression may occur when antihistamines are administered concomitantly with other CNS depressants including barbiturates, tranquilizers, and alcohol. If antihistamines are used concomitantly with other depressant drugs, caution should be used to avoid overdosage. Patients should be advised to avoid alcoholic beverages during antihistamine therapy. Patients already receiving another CNS depressant (e.g., sedatives, tranquilizers) should not undertake *self-medication* with an antihistamine without first consulting a physician. Unlike first generation antihistamines, most second generation antihistamines (e.g., astemizole [no longer commercially available in the US], loratadine, terfenadine [no longer commercially available in the US]) do not appear to potentiate the sedative effects of CNS depressants; however, acrivastine, cetirizine, and levocetirizine, which also have been classified as second generation antihistamines, may potentiate such effects, although less prominently than first generation antihistamines.

It also should be considered that monoamine oxidase (MAO) inhibitors may prolong and intensify some anticholinergic effects (e.g., dryness) of antihistamines. The manufacturer of doxylamine in fixed combination with pyridoxine hydrochloride states that the drug is contraindicated in patients receiving MAO inhibitors.

■ **Epinephrine** Phenothiazine-type antihistamines (e.g., methdilazine [no longer commercially available in the US], promethazine, trimeprazine [no longer commercially available in the US]) may block and reverse the vasopressor effect of epinephrine. If patients receiving phenothiazines require a vasopressor agent, norepinephrine or phenylephrine should be used; *epinephrine should not be used.*

■ **Drugs and Foods Affecting Hepatic Microsomal Enzymes** Concomitant administration of astemizole or terfenadine with drugs that can inhibit the metabolism of these antihistamines has resulted in accumulation of potentially cardiotoxic concentrations of astemizole or terfenadine and/or their active metabolites. (See Cautions: Cardiovascular Effects.) Both human and animal data have indicated that associated cardiotoxic effects resulted principally from accumulation of unchanged astemizole (and its main metabolite desmethylastemizole) or unchanged terfenadine.

Serious, potentially life-threatening cardiac effects have occurred when astemizole or terfenadine was used concomitantly with certain azole antifungal (including imidazole derivative [e.g., ketoconazole] and triazole derivative [e.g., itraconazole]) or macrolide (e.g., clarithromycin, erythromycin, troleandomycin) anti-infectives, mibefradil (no longer commercially available in the US), or quinine sulfate (a single dose of 430 mg), probably secondary to inhibition of metabolism of the antihistamine by these drugs. Therefore, while astemizole or terfenadine was commercially available in the US, concomitant therapy with these or other known inhibitors of astemizole or terfenadine metabolism was contraindicated. No clinically adverse effects or changes in the QT_c intervals were reported after concomitant administration of erythromycin or ketoconazole with fexofenadine, the active metabolite of terfenadine. The increased safety profile of fexofenadine compared with the parent drug, terfenadine, may result from the lack of fexofenadine-induced cardiotoxicity in addition to only minimal metabolism of fexofenadine in the liver by the cytochrome P-450 microsomal enzyme system.

Concomitant use of terfenadine or astemizole with other chemically related azole-derivative anti-infective (e.g., fluconazole, miconazole, metronidazole), most human immunodeficiency virus (HIV) protease inhibitors, quinupristin and dalfopristin, zileuton, or serotonin-reuptake inhibitors has not been recommended since these drugs may have increased plasma concentrations of terfenadine and/or astemizole and potentially serious and/or life-threatening adverse effects could have occurred.

Grapefruit juice also may have inhibited metabolism of terfenadine. Increased oral bioavailability of unchanged terfenadine observed with concomitant administration of the drug and grapefruit juice has been associated with prolongation of the QT interval averaging 3.3% (range: −1.6 to 9.5%); mean QT interval corrected for rate (QT_c) increased by 4–14 msec compared with administration of terfenadine with water. Therefore, it has been recommended that astemizole or terfenadine not be taken concomitantly with grapefruit juice.

Ketoconazole and Other Azole Antifungal Agents Prolongation of the QT interval and QT interval corrected for rate (QT_c) and, rarely, serious cardiovascular effects, including arrhythmias (e.g., ventricular tachycardia, atypical ventricular tachycardia [torsades de pointes, ventricular fibrillation]), cardiac arrest, palpitations, hypotension, dizziness, syncope, and death, have been reported in patients receiving recommended dosages of astemizole or terfenadine concomitantly with ketoconazole. Ketoconazole has markedly inhibited the metabolism of astemizole or terfenadine, probably via inhibition of the cytochrome P-450 microsomal enzyme system, which resulted in increased plasma concentrations of unchanged astemizole (and its principal metabolite desmethylastemizole) or unchanged terfenadine; clearance of the active carboxylic acid metabolite of terfenadine also may have been reduced. Increased plasma concentrations of unchanged astemizole (and its principal metabolite desmethylastemizole) or unchanged terfenadine has been associated with prolongation of the QT and QT_c intervals. Similar alterations in astemizole or terfenadine pharmacokinetics and adverse cardiac effects (prolongation of the QT_c interval, cardiac arrest, and ventricular arrhythmias [e.g., torsades de pointes]) have been reported in patients receiving the antihistamine concomitantly with itraconazole. Therefore, while commercially available in the US, astemizole and terfenadine were contraindicated in patients receiving ketoconazole or itraconazole. In addition, it has been recommended that astemizole and terfenadine also not be used in patients receiving drugs that are structurally related to these antifungals (e.g., triazoles such as fluconazole, imidazoles such as miconazole, nitroimidazoles such as metronidazole).

Increased plasma concentrations of loratadine and its active metabolite desloratadine (descarboethoxyloratadine) also have been reported in controlled clinical studies in healthy men receiving 10 mg of loratadine once daily concomitantly with ketoconazole dosages of 200 mg every 12 hours. In these studies, area under the plasma concentration-time curve (AUC) of loratadine increased by 307% following concomitant administration with ketoconazole while AUC of desloratadine increased by 73% following concomitant administration with ketoconazole. However, no clinically important changes, as measured by ECG and laboratory evaluations, vital signs, and adverse effects, were reported after concomitant administration of ketoconazole with loratadine. In addition, no changes in QT_c intervals, sedation, or syncope were reported in these individuals. Plasma concentrations of ketoconazole appeared to be unchanged in individuals receiving loratadine concomitantly. In addition, increased plasma concentrations of loratadine (AUC increased by 180%) and desloratadine (AUC increased by 56%) have been reported in a limited number of individuals receiving a single 20-mg dose of loratadine concomitantly with a ketoconazole dosage of 200 mg twice daily. However, no changes in QT_c intervals were reported 2, 6, and 24 hours after concomitant administration of the drugs. Adverse effects were similar in individuals receiving loratadine alone compared with those receiving loratadine concomitantly with ketoconazole.

Increased plasma concentrations of desloratadine and 3-hydroxydesloratadine have been reported in a controlled clinical study in healthy individuals receiving 7.5 mg of desloratadine once daily concomitantly with ketoconazole dosages of 200 mg every 12 hours for 10 days. In this study, AUC of desloratadine or 3-hydroxydesloratadine increased by 39 or 72%, respectively, while peak plasma concentrations increased by 45 or 43%, respectively, following concomitant administration with ketoconazole. However, no clinically important changes, as measured by ECG and laboratory evaluations, vital signs, and adverse effects, were reported after concomitant administration of ketoconazole with desloratadine.

The manufacturer of cetirizine states that no clinically important drug interactions have been reported in patients receiving cetirizine concomitantly with ketoconazole.

Increased plasma concentrations of fexofenadine have been reported in 2 studies in healthy individuals receiving 120 mg of fexofenadine twice daily concomitantly with ketoconazole 400 mg once daily. In these studies, AUC of fexofenadine increased by 164% following concomitant administration with ketoconazole while peak plasma concentrations of fexofenadine increased by 135%. However, no clinically important adverse effects or changes in the QT_c intervals were reported after concomitant administration of ketoconazole with fexofenadine.

Macrolides Erythromycin and clarithromycin have altered the metabolism of astemizole or terfenadine. In some individuals, concomitant administration of erythromycin with astemizole or terfenadine has resulted in increased plasma concentrations of unchanged astemizole (and its principal metabolite desmethylastemizole) or unchanged terfenadine (and its active carboxylic metabolite fexofenadine). Prolongation of the QT_c, ST-U abnormalities, and ventricular tachycardia, including torsades de pointes, have been reported in some patients receiving astemizole or terfenadine concomitantly with erythromycin or the structurally related macrolides clarithromycin, troleandomycin, or josamycin. Cardiac arrest and death have occurred in patients receiving erythromycin concomitantly with astemizole or terfenadine. Therefore, while commercially available in the US, astemizole or terfenadine was contraindicated in patients receiving clarithromycin, erythromycin, or troleandomycin.

Limited data have suggested that azithromycin and dirithromycin did not appear to alter the metabolism of terfenadine.

Increased plasma concentrations of loratadine and its active metabolite desloratadine have been reported in controlled clinical studies in healthy men receiving 10 mg of loratadine once daily concomitantly with erythromycin dosages of 500 mg every 8 hours for 10 days. In these studies, AUC of loratadine increased by 40% following concomitant administration with erythromycin, while AUC of desloratadine increased by 46%. However, no clinically important changes, as measured by ECG and laboratory evaluations, vital signs, and adverse effects, were reported after concomitant administration of erythromycin with loratadine. In addition, no changes in QT_c intervals, sedation, or syncope were reported in these individuals. Although the clinical importance has not been established, decreased plasma concentrations of erythromycin (AUC decreased by 15–18%) have been reported in these patients receiving loratadine concomitantly.

Increased plasma concentrations of loratadine and desloratadine also have been reported in a controlled drug interaction study in healthy men receiving 10 mg of loratadine every 24 hours concomitantly with clarithromycin dosages of 500 mg every 12 hours for 10 days. In this study, peak steady-state plasma concentrations and AUC of loratadine increased by 36 and 76%, respectively, following concomitant administration with clarithromycin for 10 days while peak steady-state plasma concentrations and AUC of desloratadine increased by 69 and 49%, respectively, compared with administration of loratadine alone. Although mean maximum QT_c interval was modestly increased (by less than 3% and not exceeding 439 msec) when loratadine was administered concomitantly with clarithromycin, such increase was similar to that observed when loratadine was administered alone and probably was not clinically important. The pharmacokinetics of clarithromycin were not affected by concomitant loratadine.

Increased plasma concentrations of desloratadine and 3-hydroxydesloratadine have been reported in a controlled clinical study in healthy individuals receiving 7.5 mg of desloratadine once daily concomitantly with erythromycin dosages of 500 mg every 8 hours for 10 days. In this study, AUC of desloratadine or 3-hydroxydesloratadine increased by 14 or 40%, respectively, while peak plasma concentrations increased by 24 or 43%, respectively, following concomitant administration with erythromycin. In another study in healthy individuals receiving 5 mg of desloratadine once daily concomitantly with azithromycin (500 mg followed by 250 mg once daily for 4 days), AUC of desloratadine or 3-hydroxydesloratadine increased by 5 or 4%, respectively, while peak plasma concentrations increased by 15%. However, no clinically important changes, as measured by ECG and laboratory evaluations, vital signs, and adverse effects, were reported after concomitant administration of erythromycin or azithromycin with desloratadine.

The manufacturer of cetirizine states that no clinically important drug interactions have been reported in patients receiving cetirizine concomitantly with azithromycin or erythromycin.

Increased plasma concentrations of fexofenadine have been reported in 2 studies in healthy individuals receiving 120 mg of fexofenadine twice daily concomitantly with erythromycin dosages of 500 mg every 8 hours. In these studies, AUC of fexofenadine increased by 109% following concomitant administration with erythromycin, while peak plasma concentrations of fexofenadine increased by 82%. However, no clinically important adverse effects or changes in the QT_c intervals were reported after concomitant administration of erythromycin with fexofenadine.

HIV Protease Inhibitors In vitro, ritonavir has been shown to inhibit the metabolism of terfenadine, but the clinical importance of this in vitro finding is not known. Several manufacturers of HIV protease inhibitors and some clinicians state that specific in vivo pharmacokinetic drug interaction studies between these antihistamines and HIV protease inhibitors currently are not available. Concomitant use of astemizole or terfenadine with HIV protease inhibitors (e.g., indinavir, nelfinavir, ritonavir, saquinavir) has not been recommended, because of the theoretical risk that the HIV protease inhibitor could produce substantially increased plasma concentrations of unchanged astemizole or terfenadine resulting in potentially serious and/or life-threatening adverse effects. The manufacturers of indinavir and ritonavir state that concomitant use of either drug with astemizole or terfenadine is contraindicated because such use may precipitate potentially life-threatening adverse effects.

Serotonin-reuptake Inhibitors In vitro, fluvoxamine, nefazodone, or sertraline and/or their metabolites have been shown to inhibit metabolism of terfenadine probably secondary to inhibition of the cytochrome P-450 (CYP34A) enzyme system, but the clinical importance of these in vitro findings is not known. Concomitant administration of astemizole or terfenadine and any of the serotonin-reuptake inhibitors (i.e., fluoxetine, fluvoxamine, nefazodone, paroxetine, sertraline) has not been recommended since substantially increased plasma concentrations of unchanged astemizole or terfenadine could occur resulting in an increased risk of serious adverse cardiac effects. The manufacturer of fluvoxamine and some clinicians state that concomitant use of the antidepressant with terfenadine or astemizole is contraindicated. However, at least one manufacturer (i.e., of sertraline) states that in vivo drug interaction studies with sertraline and terfenadine have failed to confirm any important alteration in plasma terfenadine concentrations by the antidepressant and that a clinically important interaction is unlikely.

Increased plasma concentrations of desloratadine and 3-hydroxydesloratadine have been reported in a controlled clinical study in healthy individuals who were pretreated with fluoxetine for 23 days prior to receiving 5 mg of desloratadine once daily concomitantly with fluoxetine 20 mg once daily for 7 days. In this study, peak plasma concentrations of desloratadine or 3-hydroxydesloratadine increased by 15 or 17%, respectively, while AUC of 3-hydroxydesloratadine increased by 13%, following concomitant administration with fluoxetine. However, no clinically important changes, as measured by ECG and laboratory evaluations, vital signs, and adverse effects, were reported after concomitant administration of fluoxetine with desloratadine.

Zileuton Increased plasma concentrations of terfenadine have been reported in one study in healthy individuals receiving 60 mg of terfenadine every 12 hours concomitantly with zileuton dosages of 600 mg every 6 hours for 7 days. In this study, AUC and peak plasma concentrations of terfenadine increased by about 35%, resulting from a 22% decrease in the clearance of unchanged terfenadine. Although no adverse cardiac effects (e.g., substantial changes in QT_c intervals) were reported in these individuals, concomitant administration of astemizole or terfenadine with zileuton is not recommended since pharmacokinetics of the antihistamines may be impaired resulting in an increased risk of serious adverse cardiac effects.

Quinine and Chemically Related Drugs There has been some evidence indicating that quinine may alter the pharmacokinetics of astemizole. Quinine is extensively metabolized in the liver; however, only limited information exists about the specific cytochrome P-450 microsomal isoenzymes responsible for the drug's metabolism. Increased plasma concentrations of astemizole and desmethylastemizole were reported in a study in healthy men receiving 10 mg of astemizole orally once daily for 24 days and 20 mg of quinine sulfate every 4 hours for 4 consecutive doses on the 22nd day and then a single 430-mg dose on the 24th day of the study. In this study, slight increases in the maximum plasma concentration and AUC of astemizole were associated with concomitant administration of the 20-mg doses of quinine sulfate; however, no clinically or statistically significant changes in QT interval were observed. Maximum plasma concentrations and AUCs of astemizole and desmethylastemizole increased threefold following concomitant administration of the antihistamine and the 430-mg dose of quinine sulfate; these increases were associated with increases in the QT interval. Therefore, the manufacturer of astemizole has stated that concomitant administration of astemizole and therapeutic doses (i.e., more than 80 mg daily) of quinine sulfate were contraindicated.

Although increases in plasma concentrations of astemizole and its desmethyl metabolite also may occur in patients receiving the antihistamine concomitantly with food products containing quinine (e.g., tonic water), such increases are small and not associated with clinically or statistically significant prolongation of the QT interval when consumption is limited to approximately 1 L (32 oz) of tonic water a day (about 80 mg of quinine sulfate). Since consumption of larger daily amounts of quinine in tonic water may be associated with risk in patients receiving astemizole, patients who consume large amounts of tonic water daily may wish to consult their clinician.

Histamine H_2-Receptor Antagonists and Xanthine Derivatives The manufacturer of terfenadine has stated that detectable plasma concentrations of unchanged terfenadine were not present and mean pharmacokinetic parameters (e.g., AUC, elimination half-life, peak plasma concentration) for the carboxylic acid metabolite fexofenadine did not appear to be affected in a study in which a single dose of terfenadine was given to individuals receiving multiple doses of cimetidine. Other data also suggest that an interaction between the drugs seems unlikely. While the potential for such a drug interaction has not been established, cardiotoxic effects also occurred following a terfenadine overdosage in at least one patient who was receiving cimetidine. In addition, torsades de pointes and prolongation of QT interval were reported in a patient receiving terfenadine 60 mg twice daily concomitantly with cimetidine 400 mg twice daily, and some clinicians state that concomitant use of terfenadine and cimetidine is not recommended.

Increased plasma concentrations of loratadine and its active metabolite desloratadine have been reported in controlled clinical studies in healthy men receiving 10 mg of loratadine once daily concomitantly with cimetidine dosages of 300 mg 4 times daily (every 6 hours) for 10 days. In these studies, AUC of loratadine increased by 103% following concomitant administration with cimetidine, while AUC of descarboethoxyloratadine increased by 6% following concomitant administration with cimetidine. However, no clinically important changes, as measured by ECG and laboratory evaluations, vital signs, and adverse effects, were reported after concomitant administration of cimetidine with loratadine. In addition, no changes in QT_c intervals, sedation, or syncope were reported in these individuals. Plasma concentrations of cimetidine appeared to be unchanged in individuals receiving loratadine concomitantly.

Increased plasma concentrations of desloratadine have been reported in a controlled clinical study in healthy individuals receiving 5 mg of the drug once daily concomitantly with cimetidine (600 mg every 12 hours for 14 days under steady-state conditions). In this study, peak plasma concentrations and AUC of desloratadine increased by 12 and 19%, respectively, following concomitant administration with cimetidine. However, no clinically important changes, as measured by ECG and laboratory evaluations, vital signs, and adverse effects, were reported after concomitant administration of cimetidine with desloratadine.

Other Drugs To date, the number of patients receiving loratadine concomitantly with ranitidine or theophylline has been too small to rule out a possible drug interaction between loratadine and such drugs and therefore, the manufacturers have recommended that loratadine be used with caution in patients receiving them.

Grapefruit Juice Concomitant oral administration of grapefruit juice with terfenadine has been reported to increase bioavailability of terfenadine. This increased bioavailability of terfenadine was associated with prolongation of the QT interval averaging 3.3% (range: −1.6 to 9.5%); mean QT_c intervals increased by 4–14 msec compared with administration of terfenadine with water. The interaction between grapefruit juice and terfenadine bioavailability appears to result from inhibition, probably prehepatic, of the cytochrome P-450 enzyme system by some constituent(s) in the juice. Patients have been discouraged to ingest grapefruit juice concomitantly with terfenadine; in addition, concomitant administration of astemizole with grapefruit juice has not been recommended since substantially increased plasma concentrations of unchanged astemizole also could occur resulting in an increased risk of serious adverse cardiac effects.

Concomitant oral administration of grapefruit juice with desloratadine does not appear to alter bioavailability of the drug.

Laboratory Test Interferences

Antihistamines may suppress inhalation-challenge testing with histamine or antigen as well as the wheal and flare reactions to antigen skin testing. Considerable interindividual variation in the extent and duration of suppression has been reported, depending on the antigen and test technique, antihistamine and dosage regimen, time since the last dose, and individual response to testing. In one study, usual oral dosages of chlorpheniramine or diphenhydramine suppressed the wheal response for about 2 days after the last dose, promethazine or tripelennamine suppressed whealing for about 3 days, and hydroxyzine suppressed whealing for about 4 days. Combined use of an H_1- and H_2-antagonist appears to have a synergistic suppressive effect on immediate and late cutaneous reactions to skin test antigens. Whenever possible, antihistamines should be discontinued about 4 days prior to skin testing procedures since they may prevent otherwise positive reactions to dermal reactivity indicators. Some evidence suggests that loratadine or terfenadine should be discontinued at least 7 days prior to such testing and that the results of such tests should be interpreted with caution even if testing were performed 4–6 weeks after astemizole discontinuance.

In one study, topical application of an antihistamine (i.e., 2% pyrilamine maleate cream) to the skin test site 10 minutes after antigen testing decreased pruritus but did not suppress wheal or flare 10 minutes after application.

Acute Toxicity

■ **Manifestations** Although antihistamines have relatively high therapeutic indexes, overdosage may result in death, especially in infants and children. There have been several reports of toxicity, often occurring within 24–48 hours of repeated topical application of diphenhydramine, in children with pruritus associated with varicella (chickenpox), poison ivy, or sunburn. Such toxicity included toxic psychosis (sometimes mimicking varicella encephalitis) and occurred in children who received oral and topical diphenhydramine concomitantly. The toxicity usually was associated with increased (60–1900 ng/mL) serum concentration of diphenhydramine. Topical diphenhydramine usually was applied to large areas of the body and usually was contained in Caladryl®, a commercially available lotion containing 1% diphenhydramine and 8% calamine; such combination is no longer commercially available in the US since Caladryl® has been reformulated by the manufacturer to contain pramoxine hydrochloride with calamine or zinc acetate. In general, overdosage of diphenhydramine may cause CNS stimulation and/or depression; in young children, CNS stimulation is dominant. Symptoms of antihistamine toxicity in children may resemble atropine overdosage and include fixed dilated pupils, abnormal eye movements, flushed face, dry mouth, urinary retention, fever, excitation, hallucinations, disorientation, delusions, agitation, bizarre behavior, confusion, jitteriness, restlessness, irritability, hyperactivity, delirium, twitching, tiredness, abnormal tongue movement, unsteady gait, trembling extremities, slurred speech, ataxia, incoordination, athetosis, tonic-clonic seizures, and postictal depression. Children recovered gradually from these adverse CNS effects, usually within 24–48 hours following removal of the topical preparation and discontinuance of all diphenhydramine-containing preparations.

Overdosage in adults usually causes CNS depression with drowsiness or coma which may be followed by excitement, seizures, and finally postictal depression. In children and adults, cerebral edema and upper nephron nephrosis, a deepening coma, tachycardia, QRS widening, heart block, cardiorespiratory collapse/arrest, cardiogenic shock, and death may occur. The risk of cardiotoxicity has been particularly likely with astemizole and terfenadine; however, these 2 antihistamines are no longer commercially available in the US. (See Cautions: Cardiovascular Effects.) Symptoms of overdosage occur within 30 minutes to 2 hours after ingestion; death may occur within 18 hours. Toxic effects may persist for prolonged (e.g., several days) periods after acute overdosage of antihistamines (e.g., astemizole) with long elimination half-lives. Rhabdomyolysis (evidenced by myoglobinuria) has been associated with overdosage of doxylamine. Acute toxicity has been reported following topical overdosage of diphenhydramine or tripelennamine (no longer commercially available in the US) in children.

■ **Treatment** Treatment of acute antihistamine overdosage consists of symptomatic and supportive therapy including artificial respiration, if necessary. If the patient is conscious, has not lost the gag reflex, and is not having seizures, emesis should be induced; however, the manufacturer of trimeprazine (no longer commercially available in the US) stated that emesis should not be induced because dystonic reaction of the head and neck may cause aspiration of gastric contents. The manufacturer of carbinoxamine maleate also states that emesis should not be induced; activated charcoal should be administered and gastric lavage should be considered following ingestion of a potentially life-threatening amount of carbinoxamine maleate.

While phenothiazine-type antihistamines may exhibit an antiemetic effect, ipecac syrup still may be effective in oral poisonings with these agents if given early (usually within 1 hour) before toxic or antiemetic effects appear. If emesis cannot be induced, gastric lavage and administration of activated charcoal are indicated; an endotracheal tube with cuff inflated should be in place to prevent aspiration of gastric contents. Saline cathartics (e.g., magnesium sulfate) may be administered.

Vasopressor agents, such as norepinephrine or phenylephrine, may be administered if necessary. Epinephrine should *not* be used, especially with phenothiazine overdosage, because epinephrine may lower the blood pressure further. Analeptic agents should *not* be used since they may cause seizures. Physostigmine may be useful to counteract the CNS anticholinergic effects of antihistamine intoxication. Diazepam can be given IV in the management of seizures that do not respond to physostigmine. Hyperthermia may be treated with cold packs or sponging with tepid water; sponging with alcohol should not be used.

If hypotension and/or cardiac arrhythmias occur (reported mainly with overdosage of astemizole or terfenadine), appropriate therapy should be instituted. Antiarrhythmic agents that can prolong the QT interval (e.g., class 1A agents) should be *avoided* in treating overdosage-associated arrhythmias in which prolongation of the QT_c interval is a manifestation. While arrhythmias may resolve spontaneously following discontinuance of the antihistamine, when necessary, therapy for ventricular tachyarrhythmias with associated QT prolongation (e.g., torsades de pointes) can include temporary atrial or ventricular pacing, IV magnesium sulfate, IV isoproterenol, and/or DC cardioversion (for initial management of sustained, symptomatic runs).

Pharmacology

Histamine is a physiologically active, endogenous substance (autacoid) that binds to and activates histamine H_1- and H_2-receptors at various sites in the body. H_3-receptors, which may be involved in feedback control of histamine synthesis and release, also have been described. The principal pharmacologic effects of histamine involve the cardiovascular system, extravascular smooth muscle (e.g., bronchial tree), and exocrine glands (e.g., stimulation of salivary, gastric, lacrimal, and bronchial secretions). Histamine also can stimulate some nerve endings and thus causes pruritus. Characteristic cardiovascular effects of histamine include direct and indirect microvascular dilation, hypotension, tachycardia, and flushing (involving H_1- and H_2-receptors) and increased vascular permeability (thought to principally involve H_1-receptors). Intracutaneous injection of histamine produces a "triple response" of local reddening, a bright halo or flare, and wheal formation. In allergic conditions, histamine and other substances (e.g., leukotrienes, prostaglandins, kinins, serotonin, platelet-activating factor) are secreted from mast cells, basophils, and other cells in response to antigenic stimulation. Histamine binds to and activates specific receptors in the nose, eyes, respiratory tract, and skin, causing characteristic allergic signs and symptoms.

The term antihistamine has historically been used to describe drugs that act as H_1-receptor antagonists. Although drugs that antagonize H_2-receptors also are commercially available (e.g., cimetidine, famotidine, nizatidine, ranitidine), these drugs generally are not referred to as antihistamines but rather as H_2-receptor antagonists. Antihistamines competitively antagonize most of the smooth muscle stimulating actions of histamine on the H_1-receptors of the GI tract, uterus, large blood vessels, and bronchial muscle. Contraction of the sphincter of Oddi and bile duct may be mediated in part by H_1-receptors, and opiate-induced contraction of biliary smooth muscle has been antagonized by antihistamines. The drugs only are feebly antagonistic to bronchospasm induced by antigen-antibody reactions. Antihistamines also effectively antagonize the action of histamine that results in increased capillary permeability and the formation of edema. H_1-receptor antagonists also suppress flare and pruritus that accompany the endogenous release of histamine. Antihistamines appear to act by blocking H_1-receptor sites, thereby preventing the action of histamine on the cell; they do not chemically inactivate or physiologically antagonize histamine nor do they prevent the release of histamine. Antihistamines do not block the stimulating effect of histamine on gastric acid secretion, which is mediated by H_2-receptors of the parietal cells. **For information on the effects of H_2-receptor antagonists, see Cimetidine 56:28.12, Famotidine 56:28.12, Nizatidine 56:28.12, and Ranitidine 56:28.12.**

The basic ethylamine group common to antihistamines also is common to anticholinergics, ganglionic and adrenergic blocking agents, local anesthetics, and antispasmodics; antihistamines therefore may be expected to exhibit some of the activities of these other classes of drugs. Some antihistamines also demonstrate a quinidine-like effect on myocardial conduction, and they may enhance the pressor action of norepinephrine. The antiemetic and antimotion-sickness actions of some antihistamines appear to result, at least in part, from their central anticholinergic and CNS depressant properties. The effects of diphenhydramine on parkinsonian syndrome and drug-induced extrapyramidal reactions are also apparently related to its central anticholinergic effects.

Although the antipruritic effect of systemically administered or locally applied antihistamines in conditions associated with histamine-induced pruritus appears to result from a peripheral antihistaminic effect and possibly a local anesthetic effect, the sedative effect of systemically administered antihistamines also appears to contribute to their antipruritic activity. The drugs are more effective antipruritics when administered systemically than when applied topically, especially when pruritus is generalized. Because pruritus can involve mediators other than histamine, the antipruritic efficacy of antihistamines is not routine.

Pharmacokinetics

Limited information is available on the pharmacokinetics of most antihistamines.

■ Absorption Antihistamines generally are well absorbed following oral or parenteral administration, but various salts may differ in activity and toxicity because of differences in solubility or absorption. The least soluble antihistamines are often the least toxic and may have a slow onset but prolonged duration of action. Following oral administration of antihistamines, symptomatic relief of allergic reactions usually begins within 15–30 minutes and usually is maximal within 1 hour. The duration of action is variable but symptoms usually are relieved for 3–6 hours after oral administration of most antihistamines. There may be some decrease in effectiveness with prolonged use of these drugs, although a substantial degree of tolerance to the antihistaminic effects generally does not occur. However, tolerance to the sedative effects may occur.

Some antihistamines (e.g., astemizole [no longer commercially available in the US], cetirizine, desloratadine, loratadine) exhibit a slower onset of action and/or prolonged duration of effect. Following single- and multiple-dose administration, the long-acting antihistamine loratadine exhibits antihistaminic effects beginning within 1–3 hours, reaching a maximum at 8–10 hours, and lasting in excess of 24 hours. Following single- and multiple-dose administration of a 5-mg dose of desloratadine, the antihistaminic effect of the drug is apparent within 1 hour and lasts for 24 hours. Following oral administration of a single 10-mg dose of cetirizine hydrochloride in healthy individuals, the antihistaminic effect of the drug is apparent within 20–60 minutes and lasts for at least 24 hours. Following oral administration of a 5-mg dose of levocetirizine dihydrochloride in patients with allergic rhinitis, the antihistaminic effect of the drug is apparent within 1 hour and lasts for at least 24 hours.

Topically applied antihistamines generally do not readily penetrate intact skin, especially when salts of the drugs are used. However, percutaneous absorption can occur, especially when the stratum corneum is disrupted, and rarely may result in systemic effects and toxicity.

■ Distribution The distribution of most antihistamines has not been fully characterized. Those compounds that have been studied show highest concentrations in the lungs and lower concentrations in spleen, kidneys, brain, muscle, and skin. Protein binding of these agents ranges from 50–99%.

Unlike other currently available antihistamines, second generation (also referred to as relatively "nonsedating") antihistamines such as acrivastine, astemizole, cetirizine, desloratadine, fexofenadine, levocetirizine, loratadine, and terfenadine (no longer commercially available in the US) appear to distribute poorly or not appreciably into the CNS at usual dosages. It is thought that this lack of CNS distribution results principally from the inability of these agents to cross the tightly fused outer membranes of endothelial cells lining the brain capillaries. Cetirizine, because of its substantial polarity, also does not readily cross the blood-brain barrier; however, some data indicate that the drug may cause more somnolence than other second generation antihistamines. Levocetirizine also is considered mildly sedating.

Small amounts of the drugs appear to be distributed into milk.

■ Elimination The metabolic fate of most antihistamines is not clearly established. The drugs usually appear to be extensively metabolized, mainly in the liver. Some second generation antihistamines (e.g., astemizole, loratadine, terfenadine) are metabolized principally by the cytochrome P-450 microsomal enzyme system, mainly by the isoenzyme 3A4 (CYP3A4), although other isoenzymes, including CYP1A2 and CYP2D6, also may be involved. Desloratadine also is extensively metabolized; however, the enzyme(s) responsible for metabolism of the drug has not been identified. Other second generation antihistamines (e.g., cetirizine, fexofenadine, levocetirizine) appear to be only minimally metabolized in the liver.

Metabolism of some antihistamines that are extensively metabolized in the liver (e.g., astemizole, terfenadine) may be substantially reduced in patients with hepatic impairment and possibly in geriatric patients. In addition, metabolism also may be substantially reduced in patients concomitantly receiving foods (e.g., grapefruit juice) or drugs (e.g., certain azole-derivative anti-infective agents, including fluconazole, itraconazole, ketoconazole, metronidazole, and miconazole; certain macrolide antibiotics, including clarithromycin, erythromycin, and troleandomycin; mibefradil [no longer commercially available in the US]; possibly certain human immunodeficiency virus [HIV] protease inhibitors, including indinavir, nelfinavir, ritonavir, and saquinavir; possibly some serotonin-reuptake inhibitors, including fluoxetine, fluvoxamine, nefazodone, paroxetine, and sertraline; zileuton; quinine) that affect the hepatic microsomal enzyme system. Decreased metabolism may result in accumulation of potentially toxic concentrations of the unchanged antihistamines that may be associated with serious adverse cardiac effects. (See Cautions: Cardiovascular Effects and see Drug Interactions.)

Many antihistamines are excreted in urine as inactive metabolites within 24 hours; however, some antihistamines (e.g., terfenadine, desloratadine, loratadine, astemizole, acrivastine) have active H_1-antagonist metabolites. Negligible amounts of most antihistamines are excreted unchanged in urine; however, cetirizine and levocetirizine are excreted in urine mainly as unchanged drug.

Chemistry

Antihistamines (histamine H_1-receptor antagonists) competitively inhibit most of the pharmacologic actions of histamine.

Antihistamines have been classified chemically and also have been classified according to their propensity to cause sedation, with relatively sedating antihistamines (i.e., conventional, prototypical antihistamines) being classified as first generation and relatively "nonsedating" antihistamines (e.g., acrivastine, astemizole [no longer commercially available in the US], desloratadine, fexofenadine, loratadine, terfenadine [no longer commercially available in the US]) being classified as second generation. Cetirizine also is considered a second generation antihistamine; however, some data indicate that it causes more sedation than other second generation antihistamines. Levocetirizine, the active *R* enantiomer of cetirizine, is considered a mildly sedating antihistamine and has been found to be slightly more sedating than desloratadine.

FIRST GENERATION ANTIHISTAMINES	
azatadine[a]	diphenhydramine
brompheniramine	doxylamine
carbinoxamine	hydroxyzine
chlorpheniramine	meclizine
clemastine	promethazine
cyproheptadine	triprolidine
dimenhydrinate	

SECOND GENERATION ANTIHISTAMINES	
acrivastine	fexofenadine
astemizole[a]	levocetirizine
cetirizine	loratadine
desloratadine	terfenadine[a]

[a] *no longer commercially available in the US*

Most antihistamines are substituted ethylamines. In general, these molecules consist of 3 portions: R^1 = nucleus, X = a linkage such as nitrogen, oxygen, or carbon, and the ethylamine group. Antihistamines can be depicted by a general formula:

$$R^1{-}X{-}\overset{|}{\underset{|}{C}}{-}\overset{|}{\underset{|}{C}}{-}N\begin{matrix}R^2\\ \\ R^3\end{matrix}$$

R^1 is composed of aromatic and/or heterocyclic groups, which may be separated from X by a methylene group. Hydrogenation of the rings in the R^1 portion of the molecule decreases antihistamine activity. Usually, activity of an antihistamine is increased by substitution of a halogen atom in the *para* position of the phenyl or benzyl group of R^1. For maximum activity, the terminal nitrogen of the ethylamine group should be a tertiary amine with methyl groups or a small cyclic moiety in R^2 and R^3. In optically active compounds, the *dextro* isomer (e.g., dexchlorpheniramine, dexbrompheniramine) usually is more active than the *levo* isomer.

Antihistamines can be classified on the basis of X substitution as follows:

ETHYLENEDIAMINE DERIVATIVES	
antazoline	pyrilamine
methapyrilene	tripelennamine

This group of antihistamines has nitrogen in the X position. Ethylenediamine derivatives have relatively weak CNS effects; however, drowsiness may occur in some patients. Adverse GI effects are common with this group of antihistamines.

ETHANOLAMINE DERIVATIVES (AMINOALKYL ETHERS)	
bromodiphenhydramine[a]	diphenhydramine
carbinoxamine	diphenylpyraline
clemastine	doxylamine
dimenhydrinate	phenyltoloxamine

This group of antihistamines, which has oxygen in the X position, has substantial atropine-like activity. Drugs in this group commonly cause CNS depression; with usual doses, drowsiness occurs in about 50% of patients who receive ethanolamine derivative antihistamines. The incidence of adverse GI effects with these antihistamines is relatively low. Dimenhydrinate (see 56:22.08) and diphenhydramine also are used as antiemetics.

ALKYLAMINES (PROPYLAMINE DERIVATIVES)

acrivastine
brompheniramine
chlorpheniramine
dexbrompheniramine
dexchlorpheniramine
dimethindene
pheniramine
pyrrobutamine
triprolidine

These antihistamines contain a carbon atom in the X position. Alkylamines cause less drowsiness and more CNS stimulation than the other antihistamines and thus are suitable for daytime use.

PHENOTHIAZINE DERIVATIVES

promethazine

In this group of antihistamines, nitrogen, as part of a phenothiazine nucleus, is in the X position. Most phenothiazines are used principally as antipsychotics (see 28:16.08); however, some are useful as antihistamines, antipruritics, and antiemetics.

PIPERAZINE DERIVATIVES

cetirizine
hydroxyzine
levocetirizine
meclizine

In this group, nitrogen, as part of a piperazine nucleus, is in the X position. Meclizine is used in the treatment of motion sickness. (See 56:22.08.) Hydroxyzine is used as a tranquilizer, sedative, antipruritic, and antiemetic. (See 28:24.92.)

OTHERS

astemizole[a]
azatadine[a]
cyproheptadine
desloratadine
fexofenadine
loratadine
phenindamine
terfenadine[a]

[a] *no longer commercially available in the US*

For further information on chemistry and stability, pharmacokinetics, uses, and dosage and administration of antihistamines available as single entities, see the individual monographs in 4:00.

FIRST GENERATION ANTIHISTAMINES 4:04

diphenhydrAMINE Hydrochloride

■ Diphenhydramine is an ethanolamine-derivative, first generation antihistamine.

Uses

Diphenhydramine shares the actions and uses of other antihistamines.

Diphenhydramine also is used as an antitussive for temporary relief of cough caused by minor throat and bronchial irritation such as may occur with common colds or inhaled irritants.

Diphenhydramine is effective for the prevention and treatment of nausea, vomiting, and/or vertigo associated with motion sickness.

Diphenhydramine may be useful as an adjunctive antiemetic agent to prevent chemotherapy-induced nausea and vomiting†; however, the American Society of Clinical Oncology (ASCO) currently does not recommend that antihistamines be used alone as antiemetic agents in patients receiving chemotherapy.

Diphenhydramine also is used as a nighttime sleep aid for the short-term management of insomnia. In individuals who experience occasional sleeplessness or those who have difficulty falling asleep, the drug is more effective than placebo in reducing sleep onset (i.e., time to fall asleep) and increasing the depth and quality of sleep.

Diphenhydramine, alone or in conjunction with other antiparkinsonian agents, may be useful as alternative therapy in the management of tremor early in the course of parkinsonian syndrome. The drug also may be useful in the management of drug-induced extrapyramidal reactions.

Diphenhydramine may be used topically for temporary relief of pruritus and pain associated with various skin conditions including minor burns, sunburn, minor cuts or scrapes, insect bites, minor skin irritations, or rashes associated with poison oak, poison ivy, or poison sumac. However, because systemic diphenhydramine toxicity (e.g., psychosis) has been reported in pediatric patients following topical application of the drug to large areas of the body (often areas with broken skin), many clinicians suggest that topical diphenhydramine be used only on limited areas of skin and not used more often than directed to avoid excessive percutaneous absorption of the drug. (See Acute Toxicity: Manifestations, in the Antihistamines General Statement 4:00.) Topical diphenhydramine also should not be used for *self-medication* in the management of varicella (chickenpox) or measles without first consulting a clinician.

Dosage and Administration

■ **Administration** Diphenhydramine hydrochloride usually is administered orally.

Diphenhydramine citrate usually is administered orally.

When oral therapy is not feasible, diphenhydramine hydrochloride may be given by deep IM or, preferably, IV injection. The drug should not be given subcutaneously, intradermally, or perivascularly because of its irritating effects; local necrosis has been reported following subcutaneous or intradermal administration of parenteral diphenhydramine. IV use of the drug in a home-care setting should be employed under careful supervision. Use of diphenhydramine for local anesthesia via local infiltration is discouraged because of the risk of local tissue necrosis. Diphenhydramine hydrochloride should not be given to premature or full-term neonates. (See Cautions: Pediatric Precautions.)

For the temporary relief of pruritus associated with various skin conditions and disorders, diphenhydramine hydrochloride-containing preparations are applied topically in the form of a cream, lotion, or topical solution. The possibility of clinically important percutaneous absorption of the drug following topical application should be considered. (See Cautions.)

■ **Dosage** Dosage should be individualized according to the patient's response and tolerance.

Adult Dosage **Usual Dosage.** The usual adult oral dosage of diphenhydramine hydrochloride is 25–50 mg 3 or 4 times daily at 4- to 6-hour intervals, not to exceed 300 mg in 24 hours.

The usual adult IM or IV dose of diphenhydramine hydrochloride is 10–50 mg; in a few patients, up to 100 mg may be required. Some experts recommend a dose of 25–50 mg. The rate of IV administration should not exceed 25 mg/minute.

The maximum adult IM or IV dosage of diphenhydramine hydrochloride is 400 mg daily.

Allergic Rhinitis, the Common Cold, and Cough. For temporary symptomatic relief of allergic rhinitis or for temporary relief of rhinorrhea and sneezing associated with the common cold, the usual oral dosage of diphenhydramine hydrochloride for *self-medication* in adults is 25–50 mg every 4–6 hours, not to exceed 300 mg in 24 hours.

For the temporary relief of cough caused by minor throat and bronchial irritation, the usual oral dosage of diphenhydramine hydrochloride for *self-medication* in adults is 25 mg (equivalent to 38 mg of diphenhydramine citrate) every 4 hours, not to exceed 150 mg (equivalent to 228 mg of diphenhydramine citrate) in 24 hours.

When used both for temporary symptomatic relief of allergic rhinitis or rhinorrhea and sneezing associated with the common cold and also for relief of cough caused by minor throat and bronchial irritation, the usual oral dosage of diphenhydramine hydrochloride for *self-medication* in adults is 25 mg (equivalent to 38 mg of diphenhydramine citrate) every 4–6 hours, not to exceed 150 mg (equivalent to 228 mg of diphenhydramine citrate) in 24 hours.

Motion Sickness. For the prevention and treatment of nausea, vomiting, and/or vertigo associated with motion sickness, the usual oral dosage of diphenhydramine hydrochloride for *self-medication* in adults is 25–50 mg every 4–6 hours, not to exceed 300 mg in 24 hours. For the prevention of motion sickness, a dose should be given 30 minutes before exposure to motion; subsequent doses may be given before meals and at bedtime for the duration of the exposure.

Insomnia. As a nighttime sleep aid, the usual oral dosage of diphenhydramine hydrochloride for *self-medication* in adults is 50 mg (equivalent to 76 mg of diphenhydramine citrate) at bedtime as needed, or as directed by a clinician. Higher dosages also occasionally have been used for sedative effects as directed by a clinician, but some evidence suggests that the efficacy of a 100-mg dose is not substantially greater than that of a 50-mg dose, although adverse (e.g., anticholinergic) effects may be increased.

Because insomnia may be indicative of a serious underlying physical, emotional, or psychological condition requiring professional medical attention, patients should be advised to avoid using diphenhydramine for *self-medication* for longer than 7–10 nights and to consult a clinician if insomnia persists continuously for longer than 2 weeks.

Parkinsonian Syndrome. For the symptomatic treatment of parkinsonian syndrome, some clinicians have suggested an initial oral dosage of 25 mg of diphenhydramine hydrochloride 3 times daily; if necessary, dosage is then gradually increased to 50 mg 4 times daily.

Pediatric Dosage **Usual Dosage.** When diphenhydramine was available only by prescription, the prescribing information for the drug indicated a usual oral diphenhydramine hydrochloride dosage for children weighing more than 9.1 kg of 12.5–25 mg 3 or 4 times daily at 4- to 6-hour intervals and for children weighing 9.1 kg or less an oral diphenhydramine hydrochloride dosage of 6.25–12.5 mg 3 or 4 times daily at 4- to 6-hour intervals. However, these dosage recommendations are *not* included in the current labeling of *nonprescription* oral diphenhydramine preparations, and clinicians should use caution when considering use of nonprescription oral diphenhydramine in children younger than 4 years of age. (See Cautions: Pediatric Precautions.)

Alternatively, for oral, deep IM, or IV therapy, children (other than premature or full-term neonates) may be given 5 mg/kg daily or 150 mg/m^2 daily divided in 4 doses; some experts recommend a dosage of 1–2 mg/kg daily. The rate of IV administration should not exceed 25 mg/minute.

The maximum oral, IM, or IV dosage of diphenhydramine hydrochloride in children older than 1 month of age is 300 mg daily.

Allergic Rhinitis, the Common Cold, and Cough. For *self-medication* to provide temporary symptomatic relief of allergic rhinitis or temporary relief of rhinorrhea or sneezing associated with the common cold, children 12 years of age and older may receive the dosage used in adults; children 6 to younger than 12 years of age may receive 12.5–25 mg orally every 4–6 hours, not to exceed 150 mg in 24 hours. Diphenhydramine hydrochloride should not be used for *self-medication* of these conditions in children younger than 6 years of age; when directed by a clinician, the usual oral dosage in children 2 to younger than 6 years of age is 6.25 mg every 4–6 hours, not to exceed 37.5 mg in 24 hours.

For *self-medication* of cough caused by minor throat and bronchial irritation, children 12 years of age and older may receive the dosage used in adults; children 6 to younger than 12 years of age may receive 12.5 mg (equivalent to 19 mg of diphenhydramine citrate) orally every 4 hours, not to exceed 75 mg (equivalent to 114 mg of diphenhydramine citrate) in 24 hours. Diphenhydramine hydrochloride should not be used for *self-medication* of cough in children younger than 6 years of age; when directed by a clinician, the usual oral dosage in children 2 to younger than 6 years of age is 6.25 mg (equivalent to 9.5 mg of diphenhydramine citrate) every 4 hours, not to exceed 37.5 mg (equivalent to 57 mg of diphenhydramine citrate) in 24 hours.

Motion Sickness. For *self-medication* to prevent and treat nausea, vomiting, and/or vertigo associated with motion sickness, children 12 years of age and older may receive the dosage used in adults; children 6 to younger than 12 years of age may receive 12.5–25 mg of diphenhydramine hydrochloride 30–60 minutes before travel and every 4–6 hours, not to exceed 150 mg in 24 hours. Children 2–5 years of age† may receive a dosage of 6.25 mg of diphenhydramine hydrochloride 30–60 minutes before travel and every 4–6 hours during travel, not to exceed 37.5 mg in 24 hours. (See Cautions: Pediatric Precautions.)

Insomnia. For *self-medication* as a nighttime sleep aid, children 12 years of age and older may receive the dosage used in adults. In children 2 to younger than 12 years of age with sleep disorders†, oral diphenhydramine hydrochloride doses of 1 mg/kg (up to a maximum dose of 50 mg) have been given 30 minutes before retiring. (See Cautions: Pediatric Precautions.) Diphenhydramine should not be used for *self-medication* for longer than 7–10 nights.

Topical Dosage For temporary relief of pruritus and pain associated with various skin conditions in adults and children 2 years of age or older, creams, lotions, or solutions containing 1–2% diphenhydramine hydrochloride are applied to the affected areas 3 or 4 times daily or as directed by a clinician; topical diphenhydramine should not be used more often than directed.

If the condition worsens, or if symptoms persist for longer than 7 days or resolve and then recur within a few days, topical therapy with diphenhydramine hydrochloride should be discontinued and a clinician consulted; the possibility of sensitization by, or hypersensitivity to, the drug should be considered.

Topical preparations containing diphenhydramine hydrochloride should not be used on large areas of the body or concomitantly with other preparations containing the antihistamine, including those used orally, since increased serum concentrations of diphenhydramine may occur that can result in systemic toxicity. (See Acute Toxicity: Manifestations, in the Antihistamines General Statement 4:00.) The drug also should not be used for topical *self-medication* in the management of varicella (chickenpox) or measles without first consulting a clinician.

Cautions

Diphenhydramine shares the toxic potentials of other antihistamines, and the usual precautions of antihistamine therapy should be observed. (See Cautions in the Antihistamines General Statement 4:00.)

When diphenhydramine is used in fixed combination with other agents (e.g., analgesic-antipyretics, nasal decongestants), the usual cautions, precautions, and contraindications associated with these agents must be considered in addition to those associated with diphenhydramine.

Local necrosis has occurred with subcutaneous or intradermal administration of parenteral diphenhydramine.

Diphenhydramine toxicity (e.g., dilated pupils, flushed face, hallucinations, ataxic gait, urinary retention) has been reported in pediatric patients following topical application of diphenhydramine to large areas of the body (often areas with broken skin) or following concomitant use of topical and oral preparations containing the drug. (See Acute Toxicity: Manifestations, in the Antihistamines General Statement 4:00.) Therefore, the US Food and Drug Administration (FDA) and many clinicians warn that oral diphenhydramine should *not* be used concomitantly with any other preparations containing the drug, including those used topically. In December 2002, the FDA issued a final rule requiring that a warning statement regarding such concomitant use be added to all OTC oral antiemetic, antihistamine, antitussive, and nighttime sleep aid preparations containing diphenhydramine.

Diphenhydramine hydrochloride topical solution contains a flammable vehicle, and the solution should not be exposed to an open flame or ignited materials (e.g., a lighted cigarette). Because of the potential for increased systemic exposure and subsequent toxicity, many clinicians state that topical preparations containing diphenhydramine should not be used more often than directed for any condition, applied on large areas of the body, or used concomitantly with other preparations containing the drug, including those used orally, since increased serum concentrations of diphenhydramine may occur that can result in systemic toxicity. (See Acute Toxicity: Manifestations, in the Antihistamines General Statement 4:00.) Patients should be advised to consult a clinician prior to use of topical diphenhydramine for the management of varicella (chickenpox) or measles.

Commercially available formulations of diphenhydramine may contain sodium bisulfite, a sulfite that may cause allergic-type reactions, including anaphylaxis and life-threatening or less severe asthmatic episodes, in certain susceptible individuals. The overall prevalence of sulfite sensitivity in the general population is unknown but probably low; such sensitivity appears to occur more frequently in asthmatic than in nonasthmatic individuals.

Although diphenhydramine appears to have low abuse potential and a favorable adverse effect profile, several children, adolescents, and young adults with chronic hematologic and neoplastic diseases have exhibited drug-seeking behavior or anticholinergic effects after repeated parenteral (e.g., bolus IV injection) administration of diphenhydramine over a prolonged period of time. It has been suggested that such route of administration may be associated with the development of adverse effects and the abuse potential of the drug and therefore, some clinicians recommend oral administration of diphenhydramine whenever possible. Alternatively, if the IV route is indicated, the drug should be infused over 20 minutes or longer and the lowest effective dosage of diphenhydramine should be employed. In addition, some clinicians suggest that IV diphenhydramine should not be used empirically for premedication, but should be reserved for patients with a history of reactions requiring treatment with an antihistamine. It is recommended that IV diphenhydramine be administered under careful supervision in a home-care setting.

■ **Pediatric Precautions** Diphenhydramine toxicity (e.g., dilated pupils, facial flushing, hallucinations, ataxic gait, urinary retention) has been reported in pediatric patients (19 months to 9 years of age) following topical application of diphenhydramine to large areas of the body (often areas with broken skin) or following concomitant use of topical and oral preparations containing the drug for *self-medication* in the symptomatic management of pain and pruritus associated with varicella (chickenpox), poison ivy, or sunburn. Manifestations typically resolved within 48 hours following discontinuance of the drug, and no deaths have been reported following topical use of diphenhydramine alone. For a complete discussion of acute diphenhydramine toxicity, see Acute Toxicity: Manifestations, in the Antihistamines General Statement 4:00.

Like other antihistamines, diphenhydramine should be used with caution in infants and young children and should not be used in premature or full-term neonates. (See Cautions: CNS Effects and see Pediatric Precautions, in the Antihistamines General Statement 4:00.) Children younger than 6 years of age should receive diphenhydramine only under the direction of a physician. Safety and efficacy of diphenhydramine as a nighttime sleep aid in children younger than 12 years of age have not been established. In addition, children may be more prone than adults to paradoxically experience CNS stimulation rather than sedation when antihistamines are used as nighttime sleep aids. Because diphenhydramine may cause marked drowsiness that may be potentiated by other CNS depressants (e.g., sedatives, tranquilizers), the antihistamine should be used in children receiving one of these drugs only under the direction of a physician.

Depending on the manufacturer and the particular formulation of the drug, topical preparations containing diphenhydramine should be used in children younger than 2, 6, or 12 years of age only under the direction of a clinician.

The possibility of drug-seeking behavior and anticholinergic effects in pediatric patients receiving repeated parenteral diphenhydramine over prolonged periods should be considered.

Overdosage and toxicity (including death) have been reported in children younger than 2 years of age receiving nonprescription (over-the-counter, OTC) preparations containing antihistamines, cough suppressants, expectorants, and nasal decongestants alone or in combination for relief of symptoms of upper respiratory tract infection. There is limited evidence of efficacy for these preparations in this age group, and appropriate dosages (i.e., approved by the US Food and Drug Administration [FDA]) for the symptomatic treatment of cold and cough have not been established. Therefore, FDA stated that nonprescription cough and cold preparations should not be used in children younger than 2 years of age; the agency continues to assess safety and efficacy of these preparations in older children. Meanwhile, because children 2–3 years of age also are at increased risk of overdosage and toxicity, some manufacturers of oral nonprescription cough and cold preparations agreed to voluntarily revise the product labeling to state that such preparations should not be used in children younger than 4 years of age. FDA recommends that parents and caregivers adhere to the dosage instructions and warnings on the product labeling that accompanies the preparation if administering to children and consult with their clinician about any concerns. Clinicians should ask caregivers about use of nonprescription cough and cold preparations to avoid overdosage. For additional information on precautions associated with the use of cough and cold preparations in pediatric patients, see Cautions: Pediatric Precautions in the Antihistamines General Statement 4:00.

■ **Mutagenicity and Carcinogenicity** Long-term animal studies to determine the carcinogenic and mutagenic potential of diphenhydramine have not been performed to date.

■ **Pregnancy, Fertility, and Lactation** Reproduction studies in rats and rabbits receiving diphenhydramine hydrochloride dosages up to 5 times the recommended human dosage have not revealed evidence of harm to the fetus. However, diphenhydramine has been shown to cross the placenta. In one epidemiologic study, use of bromodiphenhydramine (no longer commercially available) but not diphenhydramine was associated with an increased risk of teratogenic effects. In another epidemiologic study, there also was no evidence of increased risk of teratogenicity associated with diphenhydramine use during the first trimester, although a modest association could not be ruled out. Use of diphenhydramine during the first trimester of pregnancy has been associated with an increased risk of cleft palate alone or combined with other fetal abnormalities, and the drug has been reported to potentiate the teratogenic effect of morphine in mice. The manufacturers state that there are no adequate and controlled studies to date using diphenhydramine in pregnant women, and the drugs should be used during pregnancy only when clearly needed.

Reproduction studies in rats and rabbits receiving diphenhydramine hydrochloride dosages up to 5 times the recommended human dosage have not revealed evidence of impaired fertility.

Diphenhydramine has been detected in milk. Because of the potential for serious adverse reactions to antihistamines in nursing infants, a decision should be made whether to discontinue nursing or diphenhydramine, taking into account the importance of the drug to the woman.

Pharmacokinetics

■ **Absorption** Diphenhydramine hydrochloride is well absorbed following oral administration, but apparently undergoes first-pass metabolism in the liver and only about 40–60% of an oral dose reaches systemic circulation as unchanged diphenhydramine. Diphenhydramine can be absorbed percutaneously following topical administration and rarely may result in systemic effects and toxicity, especially following concomitant oral and topical administration of the drug or when extensive disruption of the epidermal barrier (e.g., blistered or oozing skin) is present. (See Acute Toxicity: Manifestations, in the Antihistamines General Statement 4:00.)

Following oral administration of a single dose of diphenhydramine, the drug appears in plasma within 15 minutes and peak plasma concentrations are attained within 1–4 hours. Following single oral doses of 50 and 100 mg in healthy adults, peak plasma drug concentrations of 37–83 and 81–159 ng/mL, respectively, have been reported. Following oral administration of diphenhydramine hydrochloride dosages of 25 mg every 4 hours or 50 mg every 6 hours, peak steady-state plasma concentrations of the drug were 55 or 85 ng/mL, respectively, and minimum steady-state plasma concentrations were 27.5 or 30 ng/mL, respectively. Following IV injection of a single 50-mg dose over a 1-minute period in healthy adults in one study, plasma diphenhydramine concentration 1 hour after the injection ranged from 99–196 ng/mL. The antihistamine effect, as determined by suppression of the wheal response induced by intradermal injection of histamine, appears to be maximal within 1–3 hours and may persist for up to 7 hours after administration of a single dose of the drug, and appears to be positively correlated with plasma concentration of the drug. The sedative effect also appears to be maximal within 1–3 hours after administration of a single dose of diphenhydramine and appears to be positively correlated with plasma drug concentration, with marked drowsiness and/or sleep occurring at plasma concentrations of 70 ng/mL or greater.

■ **Distribution** Distribution of diphenhydramine into human body tissues and fluids has not been fully characterized. Following IV administration in rats, highest concentrations of the drug are attained in the lungs, spleen, and brain, with lower concentrations in the heart, muscle, and liver. Following IV administration in healthy adults, diphenhydramine reportedly has an apparent volume of distribution of 188–336 L. Volume of distribution of the drug reportedly is larger in Asian (about 480 L) than white adults. The drug crosses the placenta and has been detected in milk, although the extent of distribution into milk has not been quantitated.

Diphenhydramine is approximately 80–85% bound to plasma proteins in vitro. Less extensive protein binding of the drug has been reported in healthy Asian adults and in adults with liver cirrhosis.

■ **Elimination** Plasma concentrations of diphenhydramine appear to decline in a monophasic manner, although some pharmacokinetic data suggest a polyphasic elimination. The terminal elimination half-life of diphenhydramine has not been fully elucidated, but appears to range from 2.4–9.3 hours in healthy adults. The terminal elimination half-life reportedly is prolonged in adults with liver cirrhosis.

Diphenhydramine is rapidly and apparently almost completely metabolized. Following oral administration, the drug apparently undergoes substantial first-pass metabolism in the liver. Diphenhydramine appears to be metabolized principally to diphenylmethoxyacetic acid, which may further undergo conjugation. The drug also undergoes dealkylation to form the *N*-demethyl and *N, N*-didemethyl derivatives. Diphenhydramine and its metabolites are excreted principally in urine. Following oral administration of a single 100-mg dose in healthy adults, about 50–75% of the dose is excreted in urine within 4 days, almost completely as metabolites and with most urinary excretion occurring within the first 24–48 hours; only about 1% of a single oral dose is excreted unchanged in urine.

Chemistry and Stability

■ **Chemistry** Diphenhydramine and bromodiphenhydramine (no longer commercially available) are ethanolamine-derivative antihistamines. Bromodiphenhydramine differs structurally from diphenhydramine in the *para*-substitution of a bromine atom for a hydrogen atom on one phenyl group. Diphenhydramine is commercially available as the hydrochloride or citrate salt; the citrate salt is only available in fixed-combination preparations. Diphenhydramine hydrochloride occurs as a white, odorless, crystalline powder which slowly darkens on exposure to light. Diphenhydramine hydrochloride has solubilities of approximately 1 g/mL in water and 0.5 g/mL in alcohol at 25°C. The pK_a of diphenhydramine is approximately 9. Commercially available diphenhydramine hydrochloride injection has a pH of 5–6, which may have been adjusted with either sodium hydroxide or hydrochloric acid.

■ **Stability** Diphenhydramine hydrochloride preparations generally should be stored at 15–30°C and protected from moisture; freezing of the elixir, injection, oral solution, or topical lotion should be avoided. The injection and elixir should be stored in light-resistant containers. Diphenhydramine hydrochloride capsules and elixir should be stored in tight containers and the elixir, oral solution, and tablets in well-closed containers.

Diphenhydramine hydrochloride injection is reportedly compatible with most IV infusion solutions. The injection has been reported to be physically incompatible with some drugs, but the compatibility depends on several factors (e.g., concentration of the drugs, specific diluents used, resulting pH, temperature). Specialized references should be consulted for specific compatibility information.

For further information on chemistry, pharmacology, pharmacokinetics, uses, cautions, acute toxicity, drug interactions, laboratory test interferences, and dosage and administration of diphenhydramine, see the Antihistamines General Statement 4:00.

Preparations

Excipients in commercially available drug preparations may have clinically important effects in some individuals; consult specific product labeling for details.

diphenhydrAMINE Hydrochloride

Oral		
Capsules	25 mg*	**Diphenhist®**, Rugby
		Diphenhydramine Hydrochloride Capsules
	50 mg*	**Diphenhydramine Hydrochloride Capsules**
		Sleepinal® Night-time Sleep Aid Capsules, Blairex
Capsules, liquid-filled	25 mg	**Benadryl® Allergy Dye-Free Liqui-Gels®**, McNeil Consumer
	50 mg	**Unisom® SleepGels®**, Chattem
Elixir	12.5 mg/5 mL*	**Diphenhydramine Hydrochloride Elixir**
		Hydramine® Elixir, Goldline
Solution	12.5 mg/5 mL*	**AllerMax®**, Pfeiffer
		Diphenhist®, Rugby
		Diphenhydramine Solution
Tablets	25 mg*	**Diphenhist® Captabs®**, Rugby
		diphenhydrAMINE Hydrochloride Tablets
		Nytol® QuickCaps® Caplets®, GlaxoSmithKline
		Sominex® Nighttime Sleep Aid, GlaxoSmithKline
	50 mg	**Compoz® Nighttime Sleep Aid,** Medtech
		Nighttime Sleep Aid®, Rugby
		Sominex® Nighttime Sleep Aid, GlaxoSmithKline
		Twilite® Caplets®, Pfeiffer
Tablets, film-coated	25 mg	**Benadryl® Allergy Ultratab®**, McNeil Consumer
	50 mg	**AllerMax® Caplets®**, Pfeiffer
		Sominex® Caplets® Maximum Strength, GlaxoSmithKline
Parenteral		
Injection	50 mg/mL*	**Benadryl®**, Pfizer
		diphenhydrAMINE Hydrochloride Injection

*available from one or more manufacturer, distributor, and/or repackager by generic (nonproprietary) name

diphenhydrAMINE Citrate and Acetaminophen

Oral		
For solution	38 mg/packet with 500 mg/packet Acetaminophen	**Goody's® PM Powder,** GlaxoSmithKline
Tablets, film-coated	38 mg with Acetaminophen 500 mg	**Excedrin P.M.® Caplets®**, Novartis
		Excedrin P.M.® Gelcaps®, Novartis

Other diphenhydrAMINE Citrate Combinations

Oral		
Tablets, film-coated	38 mg with Aspirin 500 mg	**Bayer® PM Extra Strength Caplets®**, Bayer

diphenhydrAMINE Hydrochloride Combinations

Oral		
Solution	12.5 mg/5 mL with Acetaminophen 160 mg/5 mL, and Phenylephrine Hydrochloride 2.5 mg/5 mL	**Children's Tylenol® Plus Cold and Allergy**, McNeil
Tablets	25 mg with Acetaminophen 500 mg	**Tylenol® PM Caplets®**, McNeil
		Tylenol® PM Geltabs®, McNeil
		Tylenol® PM Rapid Release Gels®, McNeil
Tablets, film-coated	12.5 mg with Acetaminophen 325 mg and Phenylephrine Hydrochloride 5 mg	**Sudafed® PE Severe Cold Caplets®**, Pfizer
	12.5 mg with Acetaminophen 500 mg	**Percogesic® Aspirin-Free Caplets® Extra Strength**, Medtech
		Tylenol® Severe Allergy Caplets®, McNeil
	25 mg with Acetaminophen 325 mg and Phenylephrine Hydrochloride 5 mg	**Tylenol® Allergy Multi-Symptom Nighttime Cool Burst® Caplets®**, McNeil
	25 mg with Acetaminophen 500 mg	**Tylenol® PM Caplets®**, McNeil

†Use is not currently included in the labeling approved by the US Food and Drug Administration

Promethazine Hydrochloride

■ Promethazine is a phenothiazine derivative with potent first generation antihistaminic properties.

Uses

Promethazine shares the uses of the antihistaminic drugs. (See Uses in the Antihistamines General Statement 4:00.) Promethazine's pronounced sedative effect limits the usefulness of the drug as an antihistamine in many ambulatory patients. In contrast to most other phenothiazines, promethazine is effective in the management of motion sickness.

For the use of promethazine as a sedative and antiemetic, see Promethazine Hydrochloride 28:24.92 and also see the Phenothiazines General Statement 28:16.08.24.

Dosage and Administration

■ **Administration** Promethazine hydrochloride may be administered orally, rectally, or by deep IM injection. Promethazine hydrochloride also is administered by IV injection. However, because IV administration of the drug has been associated with severe tissue injury, including gangrene requiring amputation, the US Food and Drug Administration (FDA) states that deep IM injection is the preferred method for administration of promethazine hydrochloride injections. (See Cautions: Precautions and Contraindications.) If IV administration of promethazine hydrochloride is required, FDA states that the drug should be administered through the tubing of an IV infusion set that is known to be correctly functioning; FDA also states that the *maximum* rate of IV administration is 25 mg/minute, and the *maximum* concentration of the injection is 25 mg/mL. If the patient complains of pain at the injection site during presumed IV injection of the drug, the injection should immediately be stopped, and the possibility of intra-arterial placement of the needle or perivascular extravasation should be evaluated. Promethazine hydrochloride injection is commercially available in 2 strengths: 25 mg/mL and 50 mg/mL. FDA states that the preparation containing 50 mg/mL is for IM injection *only*; the preparation containing 25 mg/mL may be administered by IM or IV injection.

Because of the risk of severe tissue injury and amputations if promethazine hydrochloride is inadvertently administered intra-arterially or if extravasation were to occur, some medication safety experts (e.g., the Institute for Safe Medication Practices [ISMP]) recommend that parenteral administration of the drug be avoided and replaced by safer alternative therapies.

Subcutaneous or intra-arterial injection of promethazine hydrochloride is contraindicated.

Promethazine hydrochloride injection should be inspected visually for particulate matter and discoloration prior to administration whenever solution and container permit. The injection should be discarded if the solution is discolored or contains a precipitate.

■ **Dosage** Dosages of promethazine hydrochloride by the various routes of administration are identical.

Because of the risk of potentially fatal respiratory depression, promethazine hydrochloride should *not* be used in children younger than 2 years of age. The drug should be used cautiously and at the lowest effective dosage in older children (See Cautions: Pediatric Precautions.)

Allergic Conditions As an antihistamine, promethazine hydrochloride usually is given at bedtime because of its pronounced sedative effects. The usual adult oral dose of promethazine hydrochloride is 25 mg before retiring; if necessary, however, 12.5 mg may be administered before meals and on retiring. Children 2 years of age and older may receive a single bedtime dose of up to 25 mg or up to 12.5 mg 3 times daily depending on the age and weight of the child. Alternatively, children 2 years of age and older may be given 0.5 mg/kg at bedtime or 0.125 mg/kg as needed. Dosage should be adjusted to the smallest amount adequate to relieve symptoms.

When the oral route is not feasible, 25 mg of promethazine hydrochloride may be given rectally or IM; if required, the drug may be administered by IV injection (see Dosage and Administration: Administration and see Cautions: Precautions and Contraindications). This dose may be repeated within 2 hours if necessary, but oral therapy should be instituted as soon as possible if further medication is necessary.

To prevent or control minor allergic transfusion reactions in adults, 25 mg of promethazine hydrochloride may be administered prior to or during a blood transfusion.

Motion Sickness For the management of motion sickness, adults may be given 25 mg of promethazine hydrochloride and children may receive 12.5–25 mg or 0.5 mg/kg. The first dose should be given at least 30–60 minutes prior to departure. A second dose may be given 8–12 hours later if necessary. Additional doses may be given on arising in the morning and before the evening meal for the duration of the journey.

Common Cold For the temporary relief of rhinorrhea or sneezing associated with the common cold in adults and children 12 years of age and older, an oral promethazine hydrochloride dosage of 6.25 mg every 4–6 hours, not to exceed 37.5 mg in 24 hours, has been suggested. In children 6 to younger than 12 years of age, an oral dosage of 3.125 mg every 4–6 hours, not to exceed 18.75 mg in 24 hours, has been suggested. When directed by a clinician, an oral dosage of 1.56 mg every 4–6 hours, not to exceed 9.36 mg in 24 hours, has been suggested for children 2 to younger than 6 years of age. (See Cautions: Pediatric Precautions.) Because the toxic potential of long-term therapy with promethazine for the symptomatic relief of the common cold has not been fully elucidated, the drug currently is recommended only for short-term use.

Cautions

■ **Adverse Effects** Promethazine has adverse effects similar to those of other antihistamines and shares the toxic potentials of the phenothiazines; the usual precautions of antihistamine and phenothiazine therapy should be observed. (See Cautions in the Antihistamines General Statement 4:00 and in the Phenothiazines General Statement 28:16.08.24.) Although the risk of adverse reactions (e.g., blood dyscrasias, hepatotoxicity, reactivation of psychotic processes, tachycardia, cardiac arrest, endocrine disturbances, dermatologic disorders, ocular changes, hypersensitivity reactions) that have occurred during long-term administration of antipsychotic phenothiazines appears to be minimal, the possibility that they could occur with prolonged administration of promethazine should be considered.

The most common adverse reactions of promethazine are pronounced sedative effects and confusion or disorientation. Adverse anticholinergic effects of the drug include dryness of mouth, blurring of vision, and, rarely, dizziness. Extrapyramidal reactions may occur with high doses and usually subside with dosage reduction. Lassitude, fatigue, incoordination, tinnitus, diplopia, oculogyric crises, insomnia, excitation, nervousness, euphoria, hysteria, tremors, abnormal movements, nightmares, delirium, agitation, seizures, hallucinations, torticollis, tongue protrusion, oversedation, dystonic reactions, and catatonic-like states have been reported. Restlessness, akathisia, and, occasionally, marked irregular respiration have occurred. Neuroleptic malignant syndrome (NMS) also may occur. Patients with pain who have received inadequate or no analgesia have developed athetoid-like movements of the upper extremities following parenteral administration of promethazine. These symptoms usually disappeared when the pain was controlled.

Leukopenia, thrombocytopenia, thrombocytopenic purpura, and agranulocytosis have been reported in patients receiving promethazine.

Tachycardia, bradycardia, increased or decreased blood pressure, and faintness have occurred in patients receiving promethazine. Although rapid IV administration of promethazine may produce a transient fall in blood pressure, blood pressure usually is maintained or slightly elevated when the drug is given slowly. Venous thrombosis at the injection site also has been reported.

Promethazine has been associated with obstructive jaundice, which was usually reversible following discontinuance of the drug. Cholestatic jaundice, nausea, and vomiting have been reported in patients receiving promethazine. Photosensitivity has been reported and may be a contraindication to further promethazine therapy. Urticaria, dermatitis, angioedema, dermatologic reactions, and asthma also have been reported. Nasal stuffiness, respiratory depression (may be fatal), cardiac arrest, and apnea (may be fatal) also may occur.

Local Reactions Associated with Promethazine Hydrochloride Injection Severe chemical irritation and damage to tissues (e.g., burning, pain, erythema, swelling, severe spasm of distal vessels, thrombophlebitis, venous thrombosis, phlebitis, abscesses, tissue necrosis, gangrene) may occur with administration of promethazine injection, regardless of the route of administration. Such irritation and damage also may result from perivascular extravasation, unintentional intra-arterial injection, and intraneuronal or perineuronal infiltration. Parenteral administration of promethazine may produce nerve damage (ranging from temporary sensory loss to palsies and paralysis) while injection near or into a nerve may result in permanent tissue damage. In some cases, surgical intervention (e.g., fasciotomy, skin graft, amputation) may be needed. (See Dosage and Administration: Administration and see also Cautions: Precautions and Contraindications.)

■ Precautions and Contraindications Promethazine has adverse effects similar to those of other antihistamines and shares the toxic potentials of the phenothiazines; the usual precautions of antihistamine and phenothiazine therapy should be observed. (See Cautions: Precautions and Contraindications in the Antihistamines General Statement 4:00 and in the Phenothiazines General Statement 28:16.08.24.)

Some commercially available formulations of promethazine hydrochloride contain sulfites that may cause allergic-type reactions, including anaphylaxis and life-threatening or less severe asthmatic episodes, in certain susceptible individuals. The overall prevalence of sulfite sensitivity in the general population is unknown but probably low; such sensitivity appears to occur more frequently in asthmatic than in nonasthmatic individuals.

Ambulatory patients should be warned that promethazine may impair their ability to perform hazardous tasks requiring mental alertness or physical coordination such as operating machinery or driving a motor vehicle. It should be kept in mind that the antiemetic effect of promethazine may obscure signs of overdosage of other drugs or of symptoms of conditions such as intestinal obstruction or brain tumor, and thereby interfere with diagnosis.

Promethazine should be used with caution in patients with cardiovascular disease or impaired liver function or who are having an asthmatic attack. Some manufacturers state that the drug should be used cautiously in individuals with peptic ulcer. Some manufacturers also state that the drug should be used with caution in patients with acute or chronic respiratory impairment, particularly children, because the cough reflex may be suppressed. Promethazine should be used with caution, if at all, in patients with a history of sleep apnea. (See Cautions: Pediatric Precautions.)

Because IV administration of the drug has been associated with severe tissue injury, including gangrene requiring amputation, the US Food and Drug Administration (FDA) states that deep IM injection is the preferred method for administration of promethazine hydrochloride injections. If IV administration of promethazine hydrochloride is required, extreme care should be exercised to avoid extravasation or inadvertent intra-arterial injection. (See Dosage and Administration: Administration and see Local Reactions Associated with Promethazine Hydrochloride Injection under Cautions: Adverse Effects.) If the patient complains of pain at the injection site during presumed IV injection of the drug, the injection should immediately be stopped, and the possibility of intra-arterial placement of the needle or perivascular extravasation should be evaluated. Clinicians should be alert for signs and symptoms of potential tissue injury, including burning or pain at the site of injection, phlebitis, swelling, and blistering, and patients should be informed that adverse effects may occur immediately (i.e., while receiving the injection) or may develop hours to days after an injection of promethazine. Although there are no proven successful treatment regimens for the management of extravasation or inadvertent intra-arterial injection of promethazine, sympathetic block and administration of heparin are commonly employed during the acute management.

Because of the risk of severe tissue injury and amputations if promethazine hydrochloride is inadvertently administered intra-arterially or if extravasation were to occur, some medication safety experts (e.g., the Institute for Safe Medication Practices [ISMP]) recommend that parenteral administration of the drug be avoided and replaced by safer alternative therapies.

FDA states that subcutaneous or intra-arterial administration of promethazine hydrochloride is contraindicated. Promethazine hydrochloride should *not* be administered intra-arterially, because chemical irritation may be severe and cause severe arteriospasm, possibly resulting in impairment of circulation and gangrene requiring amputation. Since promethazine discolors blood on contact, aspiration of dark blood at the site of injection does *not* rule out the possibility of intra-arterial placement of the needle.

Promethazine is contraindicated in patients who have exhibited hypersensitivity or idiosyncrasy to promethazine or other phenothiazines. Promethazine also is contraindicated in pediatric patients younger than 2 years of age, because of the risk of developing potentially fatal respiratory depression. (See Cautions: Pediatric Precautions.) In addition, the drug is contraindicated in patients who have received large doses of other CNS depressants and/or who are comatose. The manufacturers state that the drug is contraindicated for use in the treatment of lower respiratory tract symptoms (e.g., asthma). There is some evidence that epileptic patients may experience increased severity of seizures if treated with promethazine, and the drug may be contraindicated in these patients. Since increases in blood pressure may occur, promethazine should be administered with extreme caution, if at all, to patients in hypertensive crisis. Some manufacturers state that promethazine also is contraindicated in patients with bone marrow depression, angle-closure glaucoma, prostatic hypertrophy, stenosing peptic ulcer, pyloroduodenal obstruction, or bladder neck obstruction, while others state that the drug may be used with caution in such patients. Some experts do *not* recommend administering promethazine to pediatric patients who are vomiting, unless the vomiting is prolonged and there is a known cause.

■ Pediatric Precautions Promethazine (like other antihistamines) should not be used in premature or full-term neonates. (See Cautions: CNS Effects and see Pediatric Precautions, in the Antihistamines General Statement 4:00.)

Because respiratory depression (sometimes fatal) has been reported in pediatric patients younger than 2 years of age receiving a wide range of weight-adjusted doses of promethazine hydrochloride during postmarketing surveillance, the drug is *contraindicated* in this pediatric age group.

Promethazine should be administered with caution in children 2 years of age and older, because of possible respiratory depression and/or apnea that may be fatal. The lowest effective dose of the drug should be used. Concomitant use of promethazine with other respiratory depressants should be avoided.

Children receiving promethazine should be closely supervised while performing hazardous activities such as bike riding. Adults responsible for the supervision of a child receiving promethazine should be warned that children may be at increased risk for experiencing CNS-stimulant effects with antihistamines. The drug should not be used in acutely ill or dehydrated children or in those with acute infections, since these patients have an increased susceptibility to dystonias. Use of promethazine also should be avoided in children with signs and symptoms that suggest Reye's syndrome, since the potential extrapyramidal effects produced by the drug may obscure the diagnosis of or be confused with the CNS signs and symptoms of this condition, and in children with signs and symptoms of other hepatic disease. Because promethazine may cause marked drowsiness that may be potentiated by other CNS depressants (e.g., sedatives, tranquilizers), the antihistamine should be used in children receiving one of these drugs only under the direction of a clinician. Promethazine should not be used in children with asthma, liver disease, a seizure disorder, or glaucoma unless otherwise directed by a clinician.

Excessively high dosages of promethazine hydrochloride have caused sudden death in pediatric patients, although sleep apnea, and sudden infant death syndrome (SIDS) have been reported in a number of infants and young children who were receiving usual dosages of promethazine hydrochloride or trimeprazine (no longer commercially available in the US). The relationship to the drugs and possible mechanism(s) of such effects have not been elucidated. In one study, the number but not the duration of central apneas during sleep was increased and obstructive apnea during sleep (accompanied by decreased heart rate and arterial oxygen pressure) developed in 4 healthy infants who were receiving 1 mg/kg of promethazine hydrochloride daily for 3 days. Promethazine should be used with caution in children with a history of sleep apnea, those with a family history of SIDS, and those who are less prone than usual to spontaneous arousal from sleep.

Overdosage and toxicity (including death) have been reported in children younger than 2 years of age receiving nonprescription (over-the-counter, OTC) preparations containing antihistamines, cough suppressants, expectorants, and nasal decongestants alone or in combination for relief of symptoms of upper respiratory tract infection. Clinicians should ask caregivers about use of nonprescription cough and cold preparations to avoid overdosage. For additional information on precautions associated with the use of cough and cold preparations in pediatric patients, see Cautions: Pediatric Precautions, in the Antihistamines General Statement 4:00.

■ Geriatric Precautions Clinical studies of promethazine did not include sufficient numbers of patients 65 years of age and older to determine whether geriatric patients respond differently than younger patients. While clinical experience generally has not revealed age-related differences in response to the drug, care should be taken in dosage selection of promethazine. Because of increased risk of sedative effects and confusion (associated with promethazine) and the greater frequency of decreased hepatic, renal, and/or cardiac function and of concomitant disease and drug therapy in geriatric patients, the manufacturers suggest that patients in this age group receive initial dosages of the drug in the lower end of the usual range.

■ Mutagenicity and Carcinogenicity Long-term animal studies to determine the carcinogenic potential of promethazine have not been performed to date. There was no evidence of promethazine-induced mutagenesis in the Ames microbial mutagen test. There are no human or other animal data concerning the carcinogenic or mutagenic potentials of the drug. For information on the carcinogenic potential of phenothiazines, see Cautions: Carcinogenicity, in the Phenothiazines General Statement 28:16.08.24.

■ Pregnancy, Fertility, and Lactation Safe use of promethazine during pregnancy (except during labor) with respect to possible adverse effects on fetal development has not been established. Although there are no adequate and controlled studies to date in humans, promethazine has not been shown to be teratogenic in rats receiving oral dosages of 6.25–12.5 mg/kg daily (about 2.1–4.2 times the maximum recommended human dosage, depending on the use of the drug). The drug has been shown to produce fetal mortality in rats receiving intraperitoneal dosages of 25 mg/kg daily. Antihistamines, including promethazine, have been fetocidal in rodents, but the pharmacologic effects of histamine in rodents differ from those in humans. Promethazine has been reported to possibly ameliorate the effects of hemolytic disease of the newborn† (erythroblastosis fetalis) when administered during pregnancy in Rh-sensitized women, but the safety and efficacy of the drug for this use have not been clearly established; other methods of management are preferred. Promethazine should be used during pregnancy only when the potential benefits justify the possible risks to the fetus.

There are no animal or human data concerning the effect of promethazine on fertility.

It is not known whether promethazine is distributed into milk. Because many drugs are distributed in human milk and because of the potential for serious adverse reactions to promethazine in nursing infants if it were distributed, a decision should be made whether to discontinue nursing or the drug, taking into account the importance of the drug to the woman.

Drug Interactions

■ **CNS Depressants** Promethazine hydrochloride is additive with or may potentiate the sedative and respiratory depressant actions of opiates or other analgesics and other CNS depressants such as barbiturates or other sedatives, antihistamines, tranquilizers, or alcohol. When promethazine is used concomitantly with other depressant drugs, caution should be used to avoid overdosage. When promethazine is used concomitantly with barbiturates or opiates, dosage of these drugs should be reduced by at least 50 or 25–50%, respectively.

■ **Epinephrine** Although reversal of the vasopressor effect of epinephrine has not been reported with promethazine, such possibility should be considered. If patients receiving promethazine require a vasopressor agent, norepinephrine or phenylephrine should be used; *epinephrine should not be used* since it may further decrease blood pressure in patients with partial adrenergic blockade.

■ **Anticholinergic Agents** Caution should be used during concomitant use of promethazine with drugs having anticholinergic properties.

■ **Monoamine Oxidase (MAO) Inhibitors** An increased incidence of extrapyramidal effects has been reported in patients receiving phenothiazines concomitantly with MAO inhibitors.

Laboratory Test Interferences

Promethazine may interfere with several immunologic urinary pregnancy tests. The drug may elicit a false-positive Gravindex® test and false-negative Prepurex® and Dap® test. Promethazine may interfere with blood grouping in the ABO system. The drug significantly alters the flare response in intradermal allergen tests.

Acute Toxicity

■ **Manifestations** In adults, overdosage of promethazine may range from mild depression of the CNS and cardiovascular system to profound hypotension, respiratory depression, seizures, deep sleep, unconsciousness, and sudden death. Hyperreflexia, hypertonia, ataxia, athetosis, and extensor-plantar reflexes (Babinski reflex) also may occur. In children, a paradoxical reaction characterized by hyperexcitability, abnormal movements, nightmares, and respiratory depression may occur. A 12-year-old patient who had taken 200 mg of the drug exhibited numbness and pain in the left leg, tactile hallucinations, extreme hyperesthesia and hyperalgesia, and sinus tachycardia.

■ **Treatment** Treatment of promethazine overdosage is similar to that of other phenothiazines. Treatment of phenothiazine overdosage generally involves symptomatic and supportive care. General physiologic measures such as maintenance of adequate ventilation should be instituted if necessary. There is no specific antidote for phenothiazine intoxication; however, anticholinergic antiparkinsonian drugs may be useful in controlling extrapyramidal reactions associated with phenothiazine overdosage.

Following acute ingestion of the drugs, the stomach should be emptied by gastric lavage and consideration also should be given to repeated doses of activated charcoal. If the patient is comatose, having seizures or a dystonic reaction, or lacks the gag reflex, gastric lavage may be performed if an endotracheal tube with cuff inflated is in place to prevent aspiration of gastric contents. Gastric lavage may be useful even several hours after the drug has been ingested, since GI motility may be greatly reduced following overdosage of phenothiazines. Induction of emesis generally should not be attempted, since a phenothiazine-induced dystonic reaction of the head or neck may result in aspiration of vomitus during emesis; centrally acting emetics are of little value in the management of promethazine overdosage. Administration of a saline cathartic may be beneficial in enhancing evacuation of the drug from the GI tract.

Cardiovascular monitoring should begin immediately and should include continuous ECG monitoring to detect possible arrhythmias. Treatment may include correction of electrolyte abnormalities and acid-base balance, lidocaine, phenytoin, isoproterenol, ventricular pacing, and defibrillation. Antiarrhythmic agents that can prolong the QT interval (e.g., class IA [disopyramide, procainamide, quinidine] or III agents) should be avoided in treating overdosage-associated arrhythmias in which prolongation of QT_c is a manifestation.

Appropriate therapy (IV fluids and a vasopressor [norepinephrine, phenylephrine]) should be instituted if hypotension occurs; epinephrine, bretylium, or dopamine should not be used. See Cautions: Cardiovascular Effects in the Phenothiazines General Statement 28:16.08.24. For the management of refractory hypotension, vasopressors such as phenylephrine, levarterenol, or metaraminol may be used. Acidosis and electrolyte imbalances should be corrected.

Appropriate therapy should be instituted if excessive sedation occurs; CNS stimulants that may cause seizures should be avoided. If seizures occur, treatment should not include barbiturates because these drugs may potentiate phenothiazine-induced respiratory depression. However; pentobarbital and secobarbital have been used in acute overdosage of promethazine. Hypothermia is common and sometimes difficult to control. Naloxone does not appear to reverse the depressant effects of promethazine overdosage.

In some patients with acute toxicity, exchange transfusions may be useful, but hemodialysis, forced diuresis, hemoperfusion, or manipulation of urine pH is of little value in enhancing elimination of phenothiazines.

Pharmacology

Promethazine is a phenothiazine derivative with potent antihistaminic properties and shares the actions of the antihistamines.

Although the drug can produce either CNS stimulation or CNS depression, CNS depression manifested by sedation is more common with therapeutic doses of promethazine. The precise mechanism of the CNS effects of the drug is not known. Promethazine also has antiemetic, anticholinergic, and local anesthetic effects. In contrast to most other phenothiazines, promethazine also has an anti-motion sickness action, possibly as a result of a central anticholinergic effect on the vestibular apparatus and the integrative vomiting center and medullary chemoreceptive trigger zone of the midbrain. Although it has been reported that the drug has slight antitussive activity, this may result from its anticholinergic and CNS-depressant effects. In therapeutic doses, promethazine appears to have no significant effect on the cardiovascular system. Although rapid IV administration of promethazine may produce a transient fall in blood pressure, blood pressure usually is maintained or slightly elevated when the drug is given slowly.

Promethazine has been reported to inhibit collagen-induced neonatal platelet aggregation in vitro and collagen-induced platelet aggregation in neonates whose mothers had received the drug during labor; however, the clinical importance of this effect is not known. Promethazine also has been reported to possibly ameliorate the effects of hemolytic disease of the newborn (erythroblastosis fetalis) when administered during pregnancy in Rh-sensitized women. The exact mechanism(s) has not been elucidated, but several mechanisms may be involved. In vitro studies indicate that promethazine inhibits the ability of fetal macrophages to bind Rh-positive erythrocytes; inhibits phagocytosis and hexose monophosphate shunt activity in polymorphonuclear leukocytes; inhibits lysis of fetal Rh-positive erythrocytes mediated by lymphocytes and polymorphonuclear leukocytes; and stabilizes the erythrocyte membrane against hemolysis. Promethazine also has been shown to have immunosuppressive activity in animals. Although some data suggested that the drug may reduce the number and function of fetal T-cells when administered chronically during pregnancy, other data indicate that the drug does not affect the number of fetal T- or B-cells; further studies on the potential effects of promethazine on fetal immunocompetence are needed.

Pharmacokinetics

■ **Absorption** Promethazine is well absorbed from the GI tract and from parenteral sites. Plasma concentrations of promethazine required for antihistaminic effects are unknown. The onset of antihistaminic effects occurs within 20 minutes following oral, rectal, or IM administration, and within 3–5 minutes following IV administration. The duration of antihistaminic effects usually is about 4–6 hours (depending on the dose and route of administration), but such effects may persist for 12 hours or more.

■ **Distribution** Promethazine is widely distributed in body tissues. Compared with other organs, lower concentrations of the drug are found in the brain, but this concentration is higher than the plasma concentration. Promethazine has been reported to be 93% protein bound when determined by gas chromatography and 76–80% bound when determined by high-performance liquid chromatography.

Promethazine readily crosses the placenta. It is not known whether the drug is distributed into milk.

■ **Elimination** Promethazine is metabolized in the liver. The drug is excreted slowly in the urine (mainly) and feces principally as inactive promethazine sulfoxide and glucuronides.

Chemistry and Stability

■ **Chemistry** Promethazine hydrochloride is an ethylamino derivative of phenothiazine and occurs as a racemic mixture. The drug occurs as a white to faint yellow, practically odorless, crystalline powder that slowly oxidizes and turns blue on prolonged exposure to air. The drug is very soluble in water and in hot dehydrated alcohol. Promethazine hydrochloride injection has a pH of 4–5.5. The pK_a of the drug is 9.1.

■ **Stability** Promethazine hydrochloride preparations should be protected from light. Promethazine hydrochloride oral solution and tablets should be stored in tight, light-resistant containers at 15–30 and 20–25°C, respectively, while the rectal suppositories should be stored in well-closed containers at 2–8°C. Freezing of the oral solution should be avoided. Following the date of manufacture, commercially available promethazine preparations have expiration dates of 2–5 years depending on the dosage form and manufacturer.

Promethazine hydrochloride injection should be stored in tight, light-resistant containers at 20–25°C with excursions of 15–30°C permitted. The injection should be discarded if the solution is discolored or contains a precipitate. Promethazine hydrochloride injection has been reported to be chemically incompatible with several drugs, especially those with an alkaline pH. However, the compatibility depends on several factors (e.g., concentration of the drugs, specific diluents used, resulting pH, temperature). Specialized references should be consulted for specific compatibility information.

Preparations

Excipients in commercially available drug preparations may have clinically important effects in some individuals; consult specific product labeling for details.

Promethazine Hydrochloride

Oral		
Solution	6.25 mg/5 mL*	**Promethazine Hydrochloride Syrup**
Tablets	12.5 mg*	**Phenergan**® (scored), Wyeth
		Promethazine Hydrochloride Tablets
	25 mg*	**Phenergan**® (scored), Wyeth
		Promethazine Hydrochloride Tablets
	50 mg*	**Phenergan**®, Wyeth
		Promethazine Hydrochloride Tablets
Parenteral		
Injection	25 mg/mL*	**Promethazine Hydrochloride Injection**
Injection, for IM use only	50 mg/mL*	**Promethazine Hydrochloride Injection**
Rectal		
Suppositories	12.5 mg*	**Phenadoz**®, Paddock
		Phenergan®, Wyeth
		Promethazine Hydrochloride Suppositories
	25 mg*	**Phenadoz**®, Paddock
		Phenergan®, Wyeth
		Promethazine Hydrochloride Suppositories
	50 mg*	**Phenergan**®, Wyeth
		Promethazine Hydrochloride Suppositories
		Promethegan®, G&W

*available from one or more manufacturer, distributor, and/or repackager by generic (nonproprietary) name

Promethazine Hydrochloride Combinations

Oral		
Solution	6.25 mg/5 mL with Phenylephrine Hydrochloride 5 mg/5 mL*	**Prometh**® **VC Syrup**, Actavis

*available from one or more manufacturer, distributor, and/or repackager by generic (nonproprietary) name

†Use is not currently included in the labeling approved by the US Food and Drug Administration

SECOND GENERATION ANTIHISTAMINES 4:08

Loratadine

■ Loratadine, a derivative of azatadine, is a second generation antihistamine.

Uses

Loratadine shares the uses of other antihistamines, including the management of allergic rhinitis and chronic idiopathic urticaria. For additional information on these and other uses of antihistamines, see Uses in the Antihistamines General Statement 4:00.

■ **Allergic Rhinitis** Loratadine alone or in fixed combination with pseudoephedrine sulfate is used for *self-medication* to provide symptomatic relief of seasonal allergic rhinitis (e.g., hay fever). Antihistamines are not curative and merely provide palliative therapy; since seasonal allergic rhinitis may be a chronic, recurrent condition, successful therapy often may require long-term, intermittent use of these drugs. In the treatment of seasonal allergic rhinitis, antihistamines are more likely to be beneficial when therapy is initiated at the beginning of the hay fever season when pollen counts are low. Antihistamines are less likely to be effective when pollen counts are high, when pollen exposure is prolonged, and when nasal congestion is prominent. Chronic nasal congestion and headache caused by edema of the paranasal sinus mucosa often are refractory to antihistamine therapy. Antihistamines generally are not effective in relieving symptoms of nasal obstruction.

In patients with seasonal allergic rhinitis, loratadine alone or in fixed combination with pseudoephedrine hydrochloride generally provides symptomatic relief of rhinorrhea, sneezing, oronasopharyngeal irritation or itching, lacrimation, and red, irritated, or itching eyes. Tablets containing loratadine in fixed combination with pseudoephedrine hydrochloride also provide symptomatic relief of nasal congestion; loratadine alone may provide some relief, but is generally less effective in relieving nasal congestion than other symptoms of seasonal allergic rhinitis. Tablets containing loratadine in fixed combination with pseudoephedrine hydrochloride generally should only be used when both the antihistaminic and nasal decongestant activity of the combination preparation are needed concurrently.

Relief of symptoms associated with rhinitis usually begins within about 1 hour following initiation of loratadine therapy. Loratadine is more effective than placebo in providing symptomatic relief and appears to be as effective as other currently available antihistamines, including astemizole (no longer commercially available in the US), azatadine, chlorpheniramine, clemastine, or terfenadine (no longer commercially available in the US). However, loratadine reportedly is associated with a lower incidence of adverse effects, especially CNS effects, than azatadine, cetirizine, chlorpheniramine, or clemastine, and the incidence of CNS adverse effects appears to be similar to that associated with astemizole, terfenadine, or placebo. Although the incidence of adverse CNS effects is low when loratadine is administered at the recommended dosage of 10 mg daily, there is evidence that drowsiness may occur at higher dosages (e.g., 20–40 mg). The incidence of adverse anticholinergic effects (e.g., dry mouth) also is low and comparable to that reported for placebo. In one controlled study comparing 4 weeks of oral loratadine therapy (10 mg daily) to that with intranasal administration of fluticasone (200 mcg daily) in patients 12–17 years of age with moderate to severe seasonal allergic rhinitis, fluticasone was more effective than loratadine in providing relief from rhinitis nasal symptoms (e.g., nasal itching, nasal obstruction, sneezing, rhinorrhea) as reflected in both mean symptom severity scores and the median percentage of symptom-free days; however, there was no substantial difference between the loratadine and fluticasone treatment groups in the relief of ocular irritation manifestations.

Loratadine also is used for *self-medication* to provide symptomatic relief of seasonal allergic rhinitis in children 2–12 years of age. Efficacy of loratadine for symptomatic management of seasonal allergic rhinitis in children 2–12 years of age is based on extrapolation of the demonstrated efficacy of loratadine in adults and the likelihood that the disease course, pathophysiology, and drug activity are substantially similar between the 2 populations. Safety of loratadine in children 2–5 and 6–12 years of age is based on clinical trials in which the drug was administered orally once daily at dosages of 5 and 10 mg, respectively, for 2 weeks. Recommended pediatric doses were based on cross-study comparisons of the pharmacokinetics of loratadine in adults and children and on safety profiles of the drug from studies in adults and children at recommended or higher doses.

Loratadine also has been used for the symptomatic treatment of perennial allergic rhinitis†. In several short-term (3–4 week) studies, loratadine (10 mg once daily) was as effective as clemastine (1 mg twice daily), or terfenadine (60 mg twice daily) and more effective than placebo in providing symptomatic relief of perennial allergic rhinitis. In a long-term (6 month) study comparing the efficacy of loratadine (10 mg daily) and clemastine (1 mg twice daily) in patients with perennial allergic rhinitis, loratadine was as effective as clemastine in providing symptomatic relief of perennial allergic rhinitis, and was more effective in relieving nasal obstruction than clemastine after 1 week of treatment. Limited data indicate that loratadine (2.5–5 mg daily) was as effective as dexchlorpheniramine (0.5–1 mg every 8 hours) in relieving the symptoms of perennial allergic rhinitis in children. Further study is needed to determine the exact role of loratadine in the treatment of perennial allergic rhinitis. Although the efficacy of loratadine has not been determined, antihistamines generally are less effective in the treatment of perennial nonallergic (vasomotor) rhinitis† than in allergic rhinitis.

■ **Chronic Idiopathic Urticaria** Loratadine is used for *self-medication* to provide symptomatic relief of pruritus, erythema, and urticaria associated with chronic idiopathic urticaria (e.g., hives). Safety and efficacy of loratadine were established in controlled studies of patients 12 years of age and older with chronic idiopathic urticaria receiving the drug at a dosage of 10 mg daily or placebo. In these studies, loratadine was superior to placebo in relieving associated pruritus, erythema, and urticaria. The manufacturer states that loratadine does not *prevent* chronic idiopathic urticaria or allergic skin reactions.

Loratadine also is used for *self-medication* to provide symptomatic relief of pruritus, erythema, and urticaria associated with chronic idiopathic urticaria in children 6–12 years of age. Loratadine is not recommended for *self-medication* in children younger than 6 years of age. The drug formerly was commercially available in the US only as a prescription drug. At that time, loratadine was approved for the management of chronic idiopathic urticaria in children 2 years of age and older, and the drug can continue to be used in this age group under the direction of a clinician. Efficacy of loratadine for symptomatic relief of chronic idiopathic urticaria in children 2–12 years of age is based on extrapolation of the demonstrated efficacy of loratadine in adults and the likelihood that the disease course, pathophysiology, and drug activity are substantially similar between the 2 populations. Recommended pediatric doses are based on cross-study comparisons of the pharmacokinetics of loratadine in adults and children and on safety profiles of the drug from studies in adults and children at recommended or higher doses.

Dosage and Administration

■ **Administration** Loratadine is administered orally. Loratadine conventional tablets, orally disintegrating tablets, and the commercially available tablets containing the drug in fixed combination with pseudoephedrine sulfate can be administered without regard to meals.

Although the oral bioavailability of loratadine is increased when the drug is administered as the orally disintegrating tablet *without* water, the bioavailability of the active metabolite desloratadine (descarboethoxyloratadine) is unaffected, and the manufacturers state that the orally disintegrating tablets can be administered with or without water. The orally disintegrating tablets are administered by placing a tablet on the tongue, where it disintegrates within a few seconds, and then subsequently swallowing with or without water. Tablets containing loratadine in fixed combination with pseudoephedrine sulfate should be swallowed intact and patients should be instructed not to break, chew, or dissolve such tablets. Patients also should be instructed to take Claritin-D® 24 Hour extended-release tablets with a full glass of water.

■ **Dosage** ***Allergic Rhinitis and Chronic Idiopathic Urticaria*** For symptomatic relief of seasonal allergic rhinitis, the usual dosage of loratadine for *self-medication* in adults and children 6 years of age and older is 10 mg once daily. The usual dosage for *self-medication* in children 2 to under 6 years of age is 5 mg once daily as the syrup. When loratadine is used in fixed combination with pseudoephedrine sulfate in a twice-daily (12-hour) formulation for symptomatic relief of allergic rhinitis in adults and children 12 years of age and older, the usual dosage for *self-medication* is 5 mg of loratadine twice daily (every 12 hours). Alternatively, when the fixed combination containing loratadine with pseudoephedrine sulfate (Claritin-D® 24-Hour) in a once-daily (24-hour) formulation is used for symptomatic relief of allergic rhinitis in adults and children 12 years of age and older, the usual dosage for *self-medication* is 10 mg of loratadine once daily.

For the management of chronic idiopathic urticaria, the usual dosage of loratadine for *self-medication* in adults and children 6 years of age and older is 10 mg once daily. Although loratadine currently is not labeled for *self-medication* in children younger than 6 years of age, the drug can be used under the direction of a clinician at a prescribed dosage of 5 mg once daily for the management of chronic idiopathic urticaria in children 2–5 years of age.

While the risk of adverse CNS effects (e.g., drowsiness) appears to be low with the usual dosage of loratadine, the risk is dose related, increasing with dosages 2–4 times the usual dosage. The risk of such effects may be particularly likely in geriatric patients and in those with hepatic or renal impairment, even at usual dosages. The adverse effect profile in pediatric patients 6–12 years of age receiving 10 mg of the drug daily was similar to that of adults.

■ **Dosage in Renal and Hepatic Impairment** In patients with chronic renal impairment (creatinine clearance of 30 mL/minute or less), both oral bioavailability and peak plasma concentrations of loratadine and desloratadine may be increased compared with individuals with normal renal function. However, elimination half-lives of the drug and its active metabolite appear to be similar to those of individuals with normal renal function. Patients with renal impairment receiving loratadine for *self-medication* should be advised to consult a clinician before initiating therapy, since a different dosage may be recommended. Therapy with loratadine conventional or orally disintegrating tablets or oral solution should be initiated at a dosage of 10 mg *every other day* in adults and children 6 years of age and older with a glomerular filtration rate less than 30 mL/minute and at a dosage of 5 mg *every other day* in children 2–5 years of age with renal insufficiency. In addition, therapy with the commercially available tablets containing loratadine in fixed combination with pseudoephedrine sulfate should be initiated in adults and children 12 years of age and older with a glomerular filtration rate less than 30 mL/minute at a dosage of 5 mg *once daily* when the 12-hour formulation is used or at a dosage of 10 mg *every other day* when the 24-hour formulation is used, since clearance of both loratadine and pseudoephedrine are decreased in such patients. Hemodialysis does not appear to affect the pharmacokinetics of loratadine or desloratadine.

The pharmacokinetics of loratadine and its active metabolite also may be altered in patients with hepatic impairment and dosage adjustment may be necessary. Therefore, patients with hepatic impairment receiving loratadine for *self-medication* should be advised to consult a clinician before initiating therapy, since a different dosage may be recommended. Therapy with loratadine conventional or orally disintegrating tablets or oral solution should be initiated at a dosage of 10 mg *every other day* in adults and children 6 years of age and older with hepatic failure and at a dosage of 5 mg *every other day* in children 2–5 years of age with hepatic failure. Since fixed-ratio combination preparations do not permit individual titration of dosages, and clearance of loratadine is decreased more substantially than that of pseudoephedrine sulfate in patients with hepatic impairment, the manufacturer recommends that tablets containing loratadine in fixed combination with pseudoephedrine sulfate generally *not* be used in such patients.

Cautions

Adverse reactions to loratadine occur relatively infrequently, are dose related, and usually are transient and mild in severity. During controlled clinical trials in adolescent and adult patients 12 years of age and older receiving conventional tablets, solution, or orally disintegrating tablets orally, the incidence of loratadine-induced adverse effects was similar to that reported with placebo. The incidence of adverse reactions (except for the increased incidence of insomnia and dry mouth) reported with 12-hour extended-release tablets containing loratadine 5 mg in fixed combination with pseudoephedrine sulfate 120 mg also was similar to that reported with placebo, and the incidence of adverse reactions reported with 24-hour extended-release tablets containing loratadine 10 mg in fixed combination with pseudoephedrine sulfate 240 mg was similar to that reported in patients receiving twice-daily 120-mg extended-release pseudoephedrine alone. About 2% of patients 12 years of age or older receiving either loratadine or placebo and less than 1% of patients 6–12 years of age receiving loratadine discontinued therapy before completion of their respective studies. Adverse effects in pediatric patients 6–12 years of age were similar in type and frequency to those observed in adult patients receiving loratadine. Adverse effects in children 2–5 years of age receiving loratadine 5 mg orally once daily for 2 weeks in a double-blind, placebo-controlled clinical trial were consistent with the known safety profile of the drug and likely adverse effects in the population studied.

Although loratadine metabolism, like that of terfenadine (no longer commercially available in the US), is inhibited by certain drugs (e.g., azole antifungal agents) that affect hepatic microsomal enzymes, unchanged loratadine does *not* appear to share the cardiotoxic potential of unchanged terfenadine. (See Cautions: Cardiovascular Effects.)

■ **CNS Effects** The most frequent adverse effects reported with loratadine are nervous system effects. Headache occurred in about 12% of patients receiving loratadine in clinical trials. In clinical trials in patients receiving the 12-hour extended-release dosage form of loratadine in fixed combination with pseudoephedrine sulfate, headache occurred in 19% of patients receiving loratadine 5 mg and pseudoephedrine sulfate 120 mg, 18% of those receiving loratadine alone, and 17% of those receiving pseudoephedrine sulfate alone. Although headache occurred in more than 2% of patients receiving 24-hour extended-release tablets containing loratadine 10 mg in fixed combination with pseudoephedrine sulfate 240 mg in clinical trials, this effect was reported more frequently in those receiving placebo. Sedation (e.g., drowsiness, fatigue) occurred in about 12% (e.g., 8 and 4%, respectively) of patients receiving loratadine in clinical trials. The incidence of drowsiness appears to be dose related; although the incidence of drowsiness in patients receiving 10 mg of loratadine is no greater than that in patients receiving placebo, dose-related drowsiness becomes more prominent with doses of 20–40 mg. In studies of patients receiving extended-release dosage forms of loratadine in fixed combination with pseudoephedrine sulfate, drowsiness occurred in 6–7% of patients receiving the combination, 4–8% of those receiving loratadine alone, and 5% of those receiving pseudoephedrine sulfate alone.

Insomnia occurs in 5–16% of patients receiving extended-release dosage forms of loratadine in fixed combination with pseudoephedrine sulfate, in 1–4% of those receiving loratadine alone, and 9–19% of those receiving pseudoephedrine sulfate alone. Nervousness occurred in 3–5% of patients receiving extended-release dosage forms of the drug in fixed combination, in 1–3% of those receiving loratadine alone, and 4–7% of those receiving pseudoephedrine sulfate alone. In children 6–12 years of age receiving loratadine 10 mg daily or placebo, nervousness occurred in 4 or 2%, fatigue in 3 or 2%, hyperkinesia in 3 or 1%, dysphonia in 2 or less than 1% of patients, respectively. Malaise occurred in 2% of patients 6–12 years of age receiving loratadine, but did not occur in those receiving placebo, and occurred in at least one adult or pediatric patient in other clinical studies. Fatigue occurred in 2–3% of children 2–5 years of age receiving loratadine in controlled clinical trials and more frequently in patients receiving loratadine than in those receiving placebo.

Adverse nervous system effects occurring in at least one pediatric or adult patient receiving loratadine in clinical trials include hypoesthesia, asthenia, dizziness, dysphonia, hypertonia, migraine, paresthesia, tremor, vertigo, agitation, amnesia, anxiety, confusion, decreased libido, depression, impaired concentration,irritability, and morbid dreaming. Seizures were reported rarely during postmarketing surveillance of the drug.

■ **Pulmonary Effects** In patients 6–12 years of age receiving loratadine in clinical trials, wheezing occurred in 4 or 2% of patients receiving loratadine or placebo, respectively, and upper respiratory tract infection occurred in 2 or less than 1%, respectively, in this age group. Bronchitis, bronchospasm, coughing, dyspnea, hemoptysis, and hiccup occurred in at least one pediatric or adult patient in clinical trials of loratadine.

■ **Oronasopharyngeal Effects** The most frequent adverse oronasopharyngeal effect reported with loratadine was dry mouth, which occurred in about 3% of patients; dry mouth occurred in 8–14% of patients receiving 12- or 24-hour extended-release tablets containing loratadine and pseudoephedrine, but in only 2–4, 7–9, or 2–3%, respectively, of patients receiving loratadine, pseudoephedrine, or placebo in control groups. Epistaxis and pharyngitis occurred in 2–3% of children 2–5 years of age receiving loratadine in controlled clinical trials and more frequently in patients receiving loratadine than in those receiving placebo. Adverse orónasopharyngeal effects occurring in at least one patient in clinical trials of pediatric and adult patients receiving loratadine included altered salivation, altered taste, laryngitis, nasal dryness, sinusitis, and sneezing. Repeated application of loratadine orally disintegrating tablets to the buccal mucosa of animals did not result in local irritation, and there was no increased frequency of mouth or tongue irritation when loratadine was administered as orally disintegrating tablets in clinical trials.

■ **GI Effects** Abdominal pain occurred in about 2% of patients 6–12 years of age receiving loratadine, but not in those receiving placebo. Diarrhea, stomatitis, and tooth disorder occurred in 2–3% of children 2–5 years of age receiving loratadine in controlled clinical trials and more frequently in patients receiving loratadine than in those receiving placebo. Adverse GI effects occurring in at least one patient in clinical trials of pediatric and adult patients receiving loratadine included anorexia, constipation, dyspepsia, flatulence, gastritis, increased appetite, loose stools,nausea, and vomiting.

Mechanical upper GI obstruction after ingestion of a Claritin-D® 24 Hour tablet, including obstruction requiring endoscopic removal of the tablet, was reported rarely during postmarketing surveillance. Many of the individuals in whom upper GI obstruction occurred after ingesting the Claritin-D® 24 Hour preparation had a history of difficulty in swallowing tablets, a known upper GI narrowing, or abnormal esophageal peristalsis.It is not known whether use of the currently available reformulated Claritin-D® 24 hour tablet is associated with an increased risk of GI obstruction.

■ **Ocular and Otic Effects** Conjunctivitis occurred in 2% of patients 6–12 years of age receiving loratadine in controlled trials, and in less than 1% of patients receiving placebo. Earache occurred in 2–3% of children 2–5 years of age receiving loratadine in controlled clinical trials and more frequently in patients receiving loratadine than in those receiving placebo. Blepharospasm, altered lacrimation, blurred vision, ocular pain, earache, and tinnitus occurred in at least one pediatric or adult patient receiving loratadine.

■ **Sensitivity Reactions** Rash occurred in 2–3% of children 2–5 years of age receiving loratadine in controlled clinical trials and more frequently in those receiving loratadine than in patients receiving placebo. In clinical trials of pediatric and adult patients receiving loratadine, angioedema, photosensitivity reaction, pruritus, purpura, and urticaria occurred in at least one patient. Anaphylaxis and erythema multiforme occurred rarely in postmarketing surveillance of loratadine.

■ **Cardiovascular Effects** In clinical trials of adults and children 6 years of age and older receiving loratadine, hypertension, hypotension, palpitations, supraventricular tachyarrhythmias, syncope, and tachycardia occurred in at least one patient. Peripheral edema occurred rarely in postmarketing surveillance of loratadine.

Syncope associated with prolonged QT interval corrected for rate (QT_c) and ventricular arrhythmias were reported within 24 hours after adding loratadine to an existing drug regimen in a geriatric patient. However, the patient had a history of similar arrhythmias and was receiving quinidine, and return to normal sinus rhythm occurred within hours after discontinuance of both quinidine and loratadine. The time course of resolution is consistent with rapidly declining plasma quinidine concentrations and inconsistent with the long half-life of loratadine and its active metabolite desloratadine (descarboethoxyloratadine). In addition, loratadine did not appear to increase the patient's plasma quinidine concentration, since a specimen obtained at the time of the event produced results similar to those obtained 5 weeks prior to the event, and dosage of quinidine was unchanged. Although blockade of the delayed rectifier potassium channel I_k has been demonstrated for quinidine, astemizole (no longer commercially available in the US), and terfenadine (no longer commercially available in the US), and is considered by some clinicians to be the mechanism responsible for torsades de pointes, loratadine does not block this potassium channel at plasma concentrations up to 875 times greater than those obtained with recommended dosage of the drug. Therefore, loratadine does not appear to have cardiotoxic effects, even at dosages substantially greater than the recommended dosage, and does not appear to be responsible for the reported adverse cardiac effect in this patient.

Although serious cardiac effects, including ventricular fibrillation and death associated with prolonged QT interval and atypical ventricular arrhythmia (torsades de pointes) have been reported in patients receiving other "second generation" antihistamines (e.g., astemizole, terfenadine), loratadine administered alone to adults at 4 times the recommended daily dosage for 90 days has not been associated with prolongation of the QT_c interval. In a clinical study, administration of loratadine in single doses up to 160 mg (16 times the maximum daily dosage) was not associated with prolongation of the QT_c interval. Concomitant administration of the drug with other drugs known to inhibit cytochrome P-450 (CYP) microsomal enzymes (e.g., ketoconazole, erythromycin, clarithromycin, cimetidine) is associated with substantially increased loratadine and/or desloratadine plasma concentrations in healthy individuals, but there are no clinically relevant changes in ECG parameters (e.g., QT_c intervals) associated with such administration. For more information, see Drug Interactions: Drugs Affecting Hepatic Microsomal Enzymes and also see Cautions: Cardiovascular Effects in the Antihistamines General Statement.

■ **Hepatic Effects** Abnormal hepatic function, including jaundice, hepatitis, and hepatic necrosis were reported rarely during postmarketing surveillance of loratadine.

■ **Other Adverse Effects** Influenza-like symptoms and viral infections occurred in 2–3% of children 2–5 years of age receiving loratadine in controlled clinical trials and more frequently in patients receiving loratadine than in those receiving placebo. Flushing, increased sweating, dermatitis, dry hair, dry skin, thirst, fever, weight gain, back pain, chest pain, leg cramps, rigors, arthralgia, myalgia, breast pain, dysmenorrhea, menorrhagia, vaginitis, impotence, altered micturition, urinary discoloration, urinary incontinence, and urinary retention occurred in at least one patient in clinical trials of loratadine. Alopecia, thrombocytopenia, and breast enlargement occurred rarely in postmarketing surveillance of loratadine.

■ **Precautions and Contraindications** The incidence of adverse effects associated with loratadine use generally appears to be less than that associated with the use of first generation (prototypical, sedating) antihistamines, but similar effects have been reported, and the potential for typical adverse effects induced by these agents should be considered during loratadine therapy. Pharmacologic studies indicate that loratadine does not have appreciable anticholinergic effects at doses exceeding those required for antihistaminic activity, and anticholinergic-like effects (e.g., dryness of the nose) either did not occur, or occurred with a frequency similar to placebo, in clinical studies. If a fixed-combination preparation containing loratadine and pseudoephedrine hydrochloride is used, the precautions and contraindications associated with pseudoephedrine must be considered.

Patients with hepatic impairment or renal insufficiency (e.g., glomerular filtration rate less than 30 mL/minute), including geriatric patients, have decreased clearance of the drug, and should be given a lower initial dose of loratadine. Because patients with hepatic impairment experience greater decreases in clearance of loratadine than pseudoephedrine, and the doses of loratadine and pseudoephedrine in the fixed-combination preparations cannot be individually adjusted, these preparations generally should not be used in patients with hepatic insufficiency. Patients with renal insufficiency should receive a lower initial dosage of the fixed-combination preparations. (See Dosage and Administration: Dosage.)

Patients receiving loratadine in fixed combination with pseudoephedrine sulfate for *self-medication* should be advised to consult a clinician before initiating therapy if they have heart disease, hypertension, thyroid disease, diabetes mellitus, or difficulty in urination resulting from enlargement of the prostate.

Patients receiving loratadine should be instructed to take the drug only as needed and not to exceed the recommended dosage, because taking more than the recommended dosage may cause drowsiness. Patients also should be questioned about other drugs (both prescription and those for self-medication) that they are receiving and should be advised against concurrent use of the fixed-combination preparations of loratadine with over-the-counter (OTC) antihistamines and decongestants. Patients should be instructed to store the drug in a tightly closed container in a cool, dry place, away from heat or direct sunlight, and away from children.

Patients receiving loratadine in fixed combination with pseudoephedrine sulfate for *self-medication* should be instructed to discontinue therapy and contact their clinician if symptoms do not improve within 7 days or are accompanied by fever or if nervousness, dizziness, or sleeplessness occurs.

Patients receiving loratadine as *self-medication* for management of chronic idiopathic urticaria (e.g., hives) should be informed that the drug does not *prevent* hives resulting from any known cause (e.g., food, drug, insect sting, latex or rubber gloves), and that avoidance of the cause is the only way to prevent occurrence of this dermatologic reaction. Prior to initiating loratadine therapy, patients should consult a clinician if they have hives that are unusual in color, that look bruised or blistered, or that do not itch. Patients should be warned that hives may present with other severe allergic reactions, including anaphylactic shock (e.g., trouble swallowing, swelling of the tongue, trouble speaking, wheezing or trouble breathing, dizziness or loss of consciousness, swelling in or around the mouth, drooling). These manifestations may occur when hives first appear or up to several hours later and can be life-threatening if not treated immediately. If anaphylactic shock occurs in conjunction with hives, patients should be advised to seek emergency help *immediately*. Patients should be instructed to discontinue loratadine therapy and contact their clinician if manifestations of chronic idiopathic urticaria do not improve within 3 days or if the hives have persisted for more than 6 weeks. In addition, patients who have been prescribed an epinephrine auto-injector for management of anaphylaxis or severe allergic reactions associated with chronic idiopathic urticaria should be advised to carry the epinephrine auto-injector at all times; loratadine should *not* be used as a substitute for this device.

Patients should be advised to discontinue loratadine therapy immediately and to contact their clinician if any signs of an allergic reaction occur. (See Cautions: Sensitivity Reactions.)

Individuals who must restrict their intake of phenylalanine should be warned that Alavert® rapidly disintegrating tablets contain aspartame, which is metabolized in the GI tract following oral administration, to provide 8.4 mg of phenylalanine per tablet.

Loratadine is contraindicated in patients who are hypersensitive to the drug or any ingredient in its formulation. Because of rare postmarketing reports of mechanical upper GI obstruction (including that requiring endoscopic removal) caused by ingestion of Claritin-D® 24 Hour tablets, individuals with a history of difficulty in swallowing tablets, a known upper GI narrowing, or abnormal esophageal peristalsis should *not* use the Claritin-D® 24 Hour tablet preparation.

■ **Pediatric Precautions** Safety of loratadine in children 2–5 and 6–12 years of age is based on clinical trials in which the drug was administered orally at dosages of 5 and 10 mg daily, respectively, for 2 weeks. (See Uses.)

Safety and efficacy of loratadine in children younger than 2 years of age have not been established.

Safety and efficacy of loratadine in fixed combination with pseudoephedrine sulfate in children younger than 12 years of age also have not been established.

Overdosage and toxicity (including death) have been reported in children younger than 2 years of age receiving preparations containing antihistamines, cough suppressants, expectorants, and nasal decongestants alone or in combination for relief of symptoms of upper respiratory tract infection. There is limited evidence of efficacy for these preparations in this age group, and appropriate dosages (i.e., approved by the US Food and Drug Administration [FDA]) for symptomatic treatment of cold and cough have not been established. Therefore, FDA stated that nonprescription cough and cold preparations should not be used in children younger than 2 years of age; the agency continues to assess safety and efficacy of these preparations in older children. FDA recommends that parents and caregivers adhere to the dosage instructions and warnings on the product labeling that accompanies the preparation if administering to children and consult with their clinician about any concerns. Clinicians should ask caregivers about use of nonprescription cough and cold preparations to avoid overdosage. For additional information on precautions associated with the use of cough and cold preparations in pediatric patients, see Cautions: Pediatric Precautions in the Antihistamines General Statement 4:00.

■ **Geriatric Precautions** Although limited data from a study of patients 66–78 years of age indicate that the peak plasma concentration and AUC of loratadine and desloratadine are increased in geriatric patients, safety and efficacy of the drug in geriatric patients have not been studied specifically to date. Because geriatric patients frequently have decreased renal function (e.g., glomerular filtration), particular attention should be paid to evaluating renal function prior to initiation of loratadine and subsequently thereafter in this age group. If evidence of renal impairment exists or develops, appropriate adjustments in dosage should be made. (See Dosage and Administration: Dosage in Renal Impairment.)

Safety and efficacy of loratadine in fixed combination with pseudoephedrine in geriatric patients 60 years of age and older have not been studied to date. However, geriatric patients may be especially sensitive to, and are more likely to have adverse effects from, administration of sympathomimetic amines than younger patients. Extended-release preparations containing pseudoephedrine therefore should not be administered to these patients until safety has been established by administration of a short-acting preparation. For further information about the effects of pseudoephedrine in geriatric patients, see Precautions and Contraindications in Pseudoephedrine 12:12.12.

■ **Mutagenicity and Carcinogenicity** No evidence of loratadine-induced mutagenesis was seen in the reverse (Ames) or forward point mutation (CHO-HGPRT) assays, the rat primary hepatocyte unscheduled DNA assay for DNA damage, or in 2 assays for chromosomal damage (human peripheral blood lymphocyte clastogenesis assay, mouse bone marrow erythrocyte micronucleus assay). A positive finding occurred in the nonactivated but not in the activated phase of the mouse lymphoma assay.

In animal carcinogenicity studies, mice received daily oral loratadine dosages of up to 40 mg/kg for 18 months, and rats received up to 25 mg/kg daily for 2 years, and plasma AUCs of loratadine and its active metabolite desloratadine were obtained to determine the exposure of the animals to the drug. The achieved plasma AUCs of loratadine and desloratadine were 3.6 and 18 times higher in mice given 40 mg/kg, 28 and 67 times higher in rats given 25 mg/kg, and 10 and 15 times higher in rats given 10 mg/kg, respectively, than in adults given the maximum recommended oral daily dosage. Also, the achieved plasma AUCs of loratadine and desloratadine were 5 and 20 times higher in mice given 40 mg/kg, 40 and 80 times higher in rats given 25 mg/kg, and 15 and 20 times higher in rats given 10 mg/kg, respectively, than in children given the maximum recommended oral daily dosage. Although hepatocellular tumors (combined adenomas and carcinomas) occurred more frequently in male mice administered 40 mg/kg, in male rats administered 10 mg/kg, or male and female rats administered 25 mg/kg of loratadine daily than in control animals in these studies, the clinical importance of these findings in long-term use of the drug in humans is unknown.

■ **Pregnancy, Fertility, and Lactation** An increased incidence of hypospadias in male infants born to women who received loratadine during pregnancy was reported in one study. However, analysis of data from the National Birth Defects Prevention Study (NBDPS) indicated that use of loratadine during early pregnancy was not associated with an increased risk of second- or third-degree hypospadias. In addition, in 2 small prospective cohort studies that surveyed pregnant women who contacted a teratology information service, use of loratadine during the first trimester of pregnancy was not associated with major congenital anomalies and did not affect the rate of live birth, gestational age at birth, and birth weight. Despite these findings, it should be noted that interpretation of these results is limited by the statistical limitations of the studies (i.e., small sample size, inadequate power, reliance on patient recall of drug use, exclusion criteria). The 2 prospective cohort studies were powered to detect statistical significance only if a substantial (i.e., approximately threefold) increase in the overall rate of major congenital anomalies was observed; the study that relied on NBDPS data excluded first-degree hypospadias because of the difficulty of detecting this mildest form in routine surveillance, making it difficult to determine the relationship between loratadine and this form of hypospadias. Thus, while these data may be useful, further study is needed to completely rule out the teratogenic risk of loratadine. Because there are no adequate and controlled studies to date using loratadine in pregnant women, loratadine alone or in fixed combination with pseudoephedrine hydrochloride should be used during pregnancy only when the potential benefits justify the possible risks to the fetus. Reproduction studies in rats and rabbits using loratadine dosages up to 75 and 150 times, respectively, the maximum daily human dosage on a mg/m² basis have not revealed evidence of harm to the fetus.

Decreased fertility (i.e., lower female conception rates), which was reversible by discontinuing the drug, occurred in male rats at an oral loratadine dosage of 64 mg/kg (about 50 times the maximum recommended human daily oral dosage on a mg/m² basis). Studies in female and male rats using loratadine dosages of about 24 mg/kg (20 times the maximum recommended human daily oral dosage on a mg/m² basis) have not revealed evidence of impaired fertility or reproduction.

Loratadine and desloratadine distribute readily into breast milk, achieving concentrations that are equivalent to those in plasma (i.e., a milk to plasma AUC ratio of 1.17 and 0.85, respectively). The manufacturer states that about 0.03% of a single 40-mg dose of loratadine was distributed into breast milk as loratadine and desloratadine over 48 hours. Pseudoephedrine also distributes readily into breast milk. Caution should be exercised when loratadine is administered alone or in fixed combination with pseudoephedrine to a nursing woman, and a decision should be made whether to discontinue nursing or the drug, taking into account the importance of the drug to the woman.

Drug Interactions

■ **Drugs Affecting Hepatic Microsomal Enzymes** Although increased plasma concentrations (AUC_{0-24h}) of loratadine and its active metabolite desloratadine (descarboethoxyloratadine) have been reported when the drug was concomitantly administered with therapeutic dosages of ketoconazole, erythromycin, clarithromycin, or cimetidine in controlled clinical pharmacology studies in healthy individuals, no clinically important changes in ECG or laboratory evaluations, vital signs, or adverse effects were reported. Unlike unchanged terfenadine (no longer commercially available in the US), unchanged loratadine does not appear to be cardiotoxic. (See Cautions: Cardiovascular Effects.) For further information about these and other drug interactions with loratadine, see Drug Interactions in the Antihistamines General Statement 4:00.

■ **Monoamine Oxidase Inhibitors** No specific drug interaction studies have been conducted with fixed-combination extended-release tablets containing loratadine and pseudoephedrine sulfate. Because monoamine oxidase (MAO) inhibitors potentiate the pressor effects of sympathomimetic drugs (e.g., pseudoephedrine), fixed-combination extended-release tablets containing loratadine and pseudoephedrine are contraindicated in patients receiving an MAO inhibitor, or for 2 weeks after discontinuance of an MAO inhibitor. For further information about drug interactions with pseudoephedrine, see Pseudoephedrine Hydrochloride 12:12.12.

■ **Other Drugs** Loratadine does not affect plasma protein binding of warfarin or digoxin. No apparent increase in adverse effects occurred in individuals receiving oral contraceptives concomitantly with loratadine.

Laboratory Test Interferences

In vitro addition of pseudoephedrine to sera containing the cardiac isoenzyme MB of serum creatinine phosphokinase progressively inhibits the activity of the enzyme, resulting in complete inhibition over 6 hours.

Acute Toxicity

■ **Pathogenesis** The acute lethal dose of loratadine in humans is not known. The oral LD_{50} of loratadine exceeds 5 g/kg in mature rats and in mice. No deaths occurred when loratadine was administered to mature rats or mice at doses up to 5 g/kg (approximately 2400 and 2900 times or approximately 1200 and 1400 times, respectively, the maximum recommended adult and pediatric oral daily dosages on a mg/m² basis). Similarly, when the drug was administered to monkeys at doses up to 1280 mg/kg (approximately 2100 and 1500 times, respectively, the maximum recommended adult and pediatric oral daily dosages on a mg/m² basis), no deaths occurred. However, lethality occurred when loratadine was administered to juvenile rats at a dose of 125 mg/kg (approximately 100 and 70 times, respectively, the maximum recommended adult and pediatric oral daily dosages on a mg/m² basis).

■ **Manifestations** In adults, drowsiness, tachycardia, and headache have been reported after overdoses (e.g., 40–180 mg) of loratadine tablets. In children, extrapyramidal manifestations and palpitations have been reported with overdoses (exceeding 10 mg) of loratadine syrup.

■ **Treatment** Treatment of loratadine overdosage generally involves symptomatic and supportive care, initiated promptly and maintained as long as necessary. In acute loratadine overdosage, the stomach should be emptied immediately by inducing emesis with ipecac syrup. Administration of activated charcoal after emesis may be useful in preventing absorption of loratadine. If induction of vomiting is unsuccessful or contraindicated (e.g., the patient is comatose, having seizures, or lacks the gag reflex), gastric lavage with a 0.9% sodium chloride solution may be performed if an endotracheal tube with cuff inflated is in place to prevent aspiration of gastric contents. Saline cathartics may be of value to rapidly dilute bowel contents. Loratadine is not removed by hemodialysis. It is not known if loratadine is removed by peritoneal dialysis.

Pharmacology

Loratadine is a long-acting antihistamine. The drug has been characterized as a specific, selective peripheral H_1-receptor antagonist and has been referred to as a relatively "nonsedating" or second generation antihistamine. The pharmacology of loratadine resembles that of other currently available antihistamines; however, the overall pharmacologic profile of loratadine differs from that of these other drugs. Experimental evidence indicates that the drug exhibits competitive, specific, and selective antagonism of histamine H_1-receptors. Although the exact nature of loratadine's interaction at the H_1-receptor is unknown, disposition of the drug suggests that the prolonged nature of loratadine's antagonism of histamine may result from the drug's slow dissociation from the H_1-receptors or the formation of the active metabolite, desloratadine (descarboethoxyloratadine).

In vitro, loratadine exhibits a threefold greater affinity for peripheral histamine H_1-receptors than it does for those from brain tissues, whereas terfenadine (no longer commercially available in the US) exhibits a similar affinity for H_1-receptors from peripheral and brain tissues. In vivo, unlike sedating or first generation antihistamines, loratadine does not readily cross the blood-brain barrier and therefore does not appear to interact appreciably with H_1-receptors within the CNS. The presence of a carboxyethyl ester moiety in loratadine may limit distribution of the drug into the CNS, with a resultant decreased potential for adverse CNS effects (e.g., sedation) and anticholinergic effects compared with many other antihistamines. The incidence of CNS effects (e.g., sedation, impaired psychomotor performance) associated with loratadine in clinical studies is similar to that with placebo or terfenadine (no longer commercially in the US) and less than that with currently available sedating or first generation antihistamines (e.g., azatadine, chlorpheniramine, clemastine). Although the incidence of drowsiness in patients receiving the recommended 10 mg dose of loratadine is similar to that in patients receiving placebo, dose-related drowsiness may occur in patients receiving 20–40 mg of the drug. Administration of a single 10 mg dose of loratadine does not appear to impair visual-motor coordination or cause subjective CNS impairment, and administration of a single 10 or 20 mg dose or of repeated 10-mg daily doses of loratadine does not appear to impair driving performance. However, administration of higher than recommended doses (e.g., 20 mg daily over 4 days) can result in substantial impairment of driving performance in some individuals. (See Cautions: CNS Effects.)

Unlike many other currently available antihistamines, loratadine has low affinity for cholinergic receptors in vitro, and does not possess appreciable anticholinergic effects at doses exceeding those required for antihistaminic activity in pharmacologic studies. In clinical studies of individuals receiving loratadine, anticholinergic-like effects (e.g., dryness of the nose, mouth, throat, and/or lips) either did not occur or occurred with a frequency similar to that for individuals receiving placebo. Loratadine was a more potent inhibitor of serotonin-induced bronchospasm than terfenadine in pharmacologic studies. Loratadine does not exhibit any appreciable α-adrenergic blocking activity in vitro.

Administration of a 10-mg dose of loratadine with alcohol or diazepam does not increase substantially the level of impairment observed with either drug alone. In animals, concomitant administration of large oral doses of either loratadine or terfenadine with diazepam, ethanol, hexobarbital, or phenobarbital resulted in an almost identical profile of interactions. At doses 50 times greater than their antihistamine ED_{50}, both loratadine and terfenadine potentiated the anticonvulsant effects of diazepam. At doses 80 times greater than their antihistamine ED_{50}, both antihistamines potentiated the ability of large doses of ethanol or barbiturates to induce loss of righting reflex but there was no potentiation with lower doses of ethanol or phenobarbital.

Loratadine appears to have some additional activity against inflammation mediators, but the clinical importance of this activity is unknown. Loratadine suppresses the release of histamine and leukotrienes from animal mast cells in vitro, and inhibits the release of leukotrienes (but not histamine) from human lung cell fragments. Loratadine administered orally to animals inhibits allergen- and histamine-induced bronchospasm, and suppresses changes in lung resistance and dynamic lung compliance in animals with anaphylaxis-provoked bronchospasm. Limited evidence suggests that loratadine has greater activity than terfenadine or astemizole (no longer commercially available in the US) in suppressing allergic or inflammatory responses in studies of individuals receiving allergenic skin prick tests or nasal challenges, but it is unclear to what extent these findings resulted from the antihistaminic activity of the drug, and additional clinical studies are required to elucidate the effects, if any, of loratadine in suppressing inflammatory mediator release in humans.

Although decreased efficacy (subsensitivity, tolerance), including decreased inhibition of skin reactivity to allergen or histamine, may occur within days or weeks of initiation of therapy with first generation antihistamines, tolerance to the effects of loratadine has not occurred during clinical studies of patients receiving loratadine for 2–24 weeks.

For further information on pharmacology of antihistamines, see the Antihistamines General Statement 4:00.

Pharmacokinetics

■ Absorption Loratadine is rapidly absorbed from the GI tract following oral administration. The drug appears to be well absorbed following oral administration; however, the oral bioavailability of loratadine in humans currently is not known, although at least 85% of an orally administered dose was absorbed in animals. Loratadine administered to healthy adults as the syrup, conventional tablets, or orally disintegrating tablets reportedly results in plasma concentrations of the drug and its major metabolite desloratadine (descarboethoxyloratadine) that are similar for the 3 dosage forms. Administration of loratadine 10 mg for 10 days as orally disintegrating tablets in healthy adults results in peak plasma concentrations and areas under the plasma concentration-time curve (AUCs) that average about 6 and 11% greater than those achieved with conventional loratadine tablets. The manufacturer states that tablets and orally disintegrating tablets are bioequivalent with respect to the desloratadine metabolite. Administration of loratadine and pseudoephedrine sulfate as extended-release tablets reportedly does not affect the bioavailability of either drug substantially.

Dose-independent (linear) bioavailability and pharmacokinetics of loratadine occur with increasing doses of the drug. When loratadine is administered in single doses of 10, 20, or 40 mg, the peak plasma concentration and AUC of the drug and its active metabolite desloratadine are proportional to the dose administered. The pharmacokinetics of loratadine and desloratadine also do not appear to be altered substantially by duration of administration; during a study of healthy individuals receiving 40 mg of loratadine daily for 10 days, steady-state plasma concentrations and AUCs of the drug and its metabolite were achieved by the fifth day of administration and there was little accumulation of unchanged drug. After either single or multiple dosing of loratadine, peak plasma concentrations of the drug usually exceed those of its active metabolite desloratadine, but AUCs of this metabolite usually exceed those of the parent drug.

Pharmacokinetics of loratadine in children 2–12 years old are similar to those in adults; children 8–12 years of age receiving a single loratadine dose of 10 mg as the syrup achieve peak plasma concentrations and AUCs similar to those achieved in adults receiving this dose as oral tablets or syrup, and children 2–5 years of age receiving 5 mg of loratadine as the syrup achieve peak plasma concentrations and AUCs similar to those achieved in adults and children 8 years of age and older receiving 10 mg of the drug as oral tablets or as the syrup. In patients with hepatic impairment, increased plasma concentrations and AUCs of unchanged loratadine secondary to impaired metabolism of the drug can occur. Plasma concentrations and AUCs of loratadine and desloratadine are increased in adults with impaired renal function and in geriatric adults. In clinical studies, peak plasma concentrations and AUCs of loratadine were increased by about 73% and those of desloratadine were increased by about 120% in adults with impaired renal function (e.g., creatinine clearance of 30 mL/minute or less) compared with those in adults with normal renal function, and peak plasma concentrations and AUCs of loratadine and this metabolite were increased by 50% in geriatric adults (66–78 years of age) compared with younger adults.

Food increases the extent of loratadine absorption, may increase peak plasma concentrations and AUCs of the drug, and delays time-to-peak plasma concentration of the drug and its metabolite by about 1 hour. Although the manufacturer states that food did not affect peak plasma concentrations of the drug or its metabolite in one single-dose study, food increased peak plasma loratadine concentrations by 80% in another study of individuals receiving a single dose of 24-hour extended-release tablets in fixed combination with pseudoephedrine sulfate, but did not increase substantially the peak plasma concentration of desloratadine. In another study, administration of a single dose of loratadine with food increased loratadine and desloratadine AUCs by about 40 and 15%, respectively. However, in a single-dose study of adults receiving the 24-hour extended-release tablets of loratadine in fixed combination with pseudoephedrine sulfate, administration of the drug with food increased the AUC of loratadine by 120% but did not substantially affect the AUC of desloratadine. Food increases the AUC of loratadine administered as orally disintegrating tablets by about 48% but does not affect the AUC of desloratadine and does not affect the peak plasma concentrations of the drug or its metabolite. Time-to-peak plasma concentrations of loratadine and its metabolite is delayed by about 2.4 and 3.7 hours, respectively, when the orally disintegrating tablets of the drug are administered following a meal. Administration of loratadine orally disintegrating tablets without water increases the AUC of the drug by 26% but does not affect peak plasma loratadine concentrations; oral bioavailability of desloratadine is similar when orally disintegrating tablets are administered with or without water.

Following oral administration of a single 10-mg dose of loratadine (as a capsule) in healthy adults, mean peak plasma concentrations of 4.7 and 4 ng/mL of the drug and its active metabolite were attained in about 1.5 and 3.7 hours, respectively. When loratadine was administered in a single 20-mg oral dose as a capsule to healthy adults, peak plasma concentrations of 10.8 and 9.9 ng/mL of loratadine or desloratadine were attained at 1 and 1.5 hours, respectively. Following oral administration of a single 40-mg dose of loratadine as a capsule in healthy adults, mean peak plasma concentrations of 26.1 and 16 ng/mL of the drug and its active metabolite were attained in about 1.2 and 2 hours, respectively, and when loratadine was administered in the same oral dose as a solution in healthy adults, peak plasma loratadine concentrations of 21 ng/mL were attained at 1 hour. Steady-state plasma concentrations of the drug and its active metabolite are achieved by the fifth day of administration, and there is little accumulation of unchanged drug. The AUC of loratadine is less than that of desloratadine at steady state; in one study, the AUC of the drug was about 23% of that of its metabolite at steady-state concentrations occurring from the fifth to the tenth day of administration. Following oral administration of loratadine conventional tablets at a dosage of 10 mg daily for 10 days in healthy adults, peak plasma loratadine and desloratadine concentrations occur at 1.3 and 2.5 hours, respectively. When loratadine is administered at this dosage as orally disintegrating tablets in healthy adults, peak plasma concentrations of the drug and its metabolite are attained at 1.3 and 2.3 hours, respectively. Following oral administration of loratadine capsules at a dosage of 40 mg daily for 10 days to healthy adults, peak plasma concentrations of 21.3 and 17.4 ng/mL, respectively, of loratadine and desloratadine were attained at about 1.6 and 2.9 hours on the first day; on the tenth day, peak plasma concentrations of 27.1 and 28.6 ng/mL of the drug and its active metabolite were attained at 1.4 and 3 hours, respectively.

The magnitude and duration of the antihistaminic effect (as measured by suppression of the wheal response induced by intradermal injection of histamine) of loratadine appear to increase with increasing dosage of the drug. Following oral administration of loratadine, the antihistaminic effect of the drug is apparent within 1–4 hours, and the onset of antihistaminic action appears to correlate with the rapid absorption of loratadine and formation of desloratadine. The manufacturer states that when 10 mg of the drug is administered as single or multiple doses, the antihistaminic effect is maximal within 8–12 hours; however, in a study of patients receiving loratadine dosages of 10, 20, or 40 mg twice daily, wheal suppression was maximal at 4–6 hours after administration of the first dose. The manufacturer states that when 10 mg of the drug is administered in single or multiple doses, the antihistaminic effect persists for 24 hours or longer; however, duration of response appears to depend on the dose and duration of administration. In a study in healthy individuals receiving oral loratadine 10, 20, or 40 mg twice daily for 28 days, histamine-induced wheal suppression persisted for at least 12 hours after administration of the first dose of the drug and for at least 32, 36, or 48 hours after administration of the last dose of 10, 20, or 40 mg, respectively. In another study in healthy adults receiving single doses of loratadine, suppression of histamine-induced wheal response persisted for 12 hours following oral administration of a 10 mg dose and for 48 hours after a 40 or 80 mg dose.

Although a therapeutic range for plasma loratadine concentrations has not been established, the manufacturer states that following oral administration of a therapeutic dose of loratadine, the expected plasma concentration of unchanged drug is 2.5–100 ng/mL, and that of desloratadine is 0.5–100 ng/mL.

■ **Distribution** Distribution of loratadine and its metabolites into human body tissues and fluids has not been determined. Large clearance values following oral administration of loratadine suggest extensive presystemic metabolism and/or tissue distribution of the drug in humans. Neither loratadine nor its metabolites appear to cross the blood-brain barrier appreciably in animals.

At expected plasma concentrations of the drug and its metabolite following administration of a therapeutic dose in healthy adults, loratadine and desloratadine are about 97–99 and 73–77% bound, respectively, to plasma proteins.

Loratadine and its active metabolite desloratadine are distributed into breast milk in concentrations that are equivalent to plasma concentrations. The AUCs of the drug and this metabolite in breast milk are about 117 and 85%, respectively, of maternal plasma AUCs; however, the total amount of loratadine and its active metabolite excreted into breast milk is minimal. In one study, about 0.03% (11.7 mcg) of a single 40-mg oral dose of loratadine was excreted into breast milk as loratadine and desloratadine over 48 hours.

■ **Elimination** Plasma concentrations of loratadine and desloratadine appear to decline in a biphasic manner. In healthy adults receiving either single 10-, 20-, or 40-mg doses or a daily dosage of 40 mg of the drug, the mean distribution half-life of unchanged loratadine was about 1–2 hours, and the mean elimination half-life was 8–15 hours; the mean distribution half-life of desloratadine was 2–4 hours, and the mean elimination half-life was about 17–28 hours. Plasma clearance of loratadine is high after oral administration, probably secondary to extensive first-pass metabolism and tissue distribution. Like the elimination half-life, oral clearance of loratadine does not vary greatly with dose; apparent clearance after oral administration of a single 20- or 40-mg dose of the drug in healthy adults was 202 or 142 mL/minute per kg (12.1 or 8.5 L/hour per kg), respectively.

Loratadine undergoes extensive first-pass metabolism, and is metabolized in the liver by the cytochrome P-450 (CYP) microsomal enzyme system, principally by hydrolysis of the carbamate moiety to the active metabolite desloratadine. Results of in vitro studies using human liver microsomes indicate that metabolism of loratadine is mediated principally by the isoenzyme 3A4 (CYP3A4) and to a lesser extent by CYP2D6. In the presence of a CYP3A4 inhibitor (e.g., ketoconazole), loratadine is principally metabolized to desloratadine by the CYP2D6 isoenzyme. Concomitant administration of the drug with either a CYP3A4 inhibitor (e.g., ketoconazole, erythromycin) or a CYP3A4 and CYP2D6 inhibitor (e.g., cimetidine) is associated with substantially increased plasma concentrations of unchanged drug in healthy individuals. (See Drug Interactions: Drugs Affecting Hepatic Microsomal Enzymes.)

In patients with hepatic impairment, the half-life of loratadine and desloratadine may be prolonged. In patients with chronic alcoholic liver disease, the elimination half-life of loratadine and desloratadine generally increases with increasing severity of liver disease, but usually appears to be within the range (e.g., 3–20 and 9–92 hours, respectively) reported for healthy individuals. In patients with impaired renal function, the half-lives of the drug and its active metabolite do not appear to be prolonged compared with individuals with normal renal function.

Desloratadine is pharmacologically active, and also is extensively metabolized by hydroxylation and undergoes conjugation. Limited evidence from animal studies indicates that desloratadine may have about 4 times the antihistaminic activity of the parent drug on a mg-for-mg basis, but the conjugated metabolites of desloratadine are assumed to have minimal activity.

After 10 days of daily administration of loratadine, about 80% of the drug is excreted as metabolic products equally distributed in urine and feces. After administration of a single 40-mg dose of ^{14}C-loratadine as an oral solution in healthy individuals, approximately 40% of the radiolabeled dose was recovered in the urine over 7 days. High-performance liquid chromatography (HPLC) analysis of urine radioactivity identified only small fractions of loratadine- and desloratadine-associated radioactivity, and a larger fraction that was tentatively identified as hydroxydesloratadine. Most plasma radioactivity was attributed to conjugates of desloratadine metabolites, and plasma radioactivity cleared with a half-life of 46 hours, a rate similar to the excretion of radioactivity in urine.

Plasma drug clearance may be decreased and the half-life prolonged in geriatric individuals, but differences in pharmacokinetics between geriatric and younger adults do not appear to be substantial, and some clinicians state such differences are unlikely to be clinically important. In healthy geriatric individuals, the mean elimination half-life of loratadine is increased to 18.2 hours (range: 6.7–37 hours), but that of desloratadine is decreased to 17.5 hours (range: 11–38 hours).

In patients with impaired renal function (e.g., creatinine clearance of 30 mL/minute or less) the mean elimination half-lives of loratadine and its active metabolite desloratadine appear to be similar to those in individuals with normal renal function. Neither loratadine nor desloratadine is substantially removed by hemodialysis.

Chemistry and Stability

■ **Chemistry** Loratadine is a tricyclic antihistamine. The drug is a derivative of azatadine, and is related structurally to cyproheptadine. Loratadine differs from azatadine by the presence of a carboxyethyl ester moiety on the piperidine ring and an 8-chloro group on the benzocycloheptapyridine tricyclic ring structure. Conversion of the basic tertiary amino function of azatadine to a neutral carbamate results in compounds, including loratadine, that are less basic and more polar than the parent drug, decreasing their distribution into the CNS. Although the ethyl carbamate derivative has about 1/80th the potency of azatadine, the addition of an 8-chloro group to the tricyclic ring of this compound to form loratadine increases its potency fourfold, and substantially increases its duration of action. Loratadine occurs as a white to off-white powder and is insoluble in water but very soluble in alcohol, acetone, and chloroform.

The orally disintegrating loratadine tablets differ from the conventional tablet formulation; both dosage forms contain 10 mg of the drug in each tablet, and are administered orally, but the orally disintegrating tablets are flavored and disintegrate within seconds after placement on the tongue, allowing the tablet contents to be swallowed with or without water. The fixed-combination tablets formulated for 12-hour dosing contain 5 mg of loratadine and 60 mg of pseudoephedrine sulfate in an immediate-release outer shell and 60 mg of pseudoephedrine sulfate in an extended-release matrix core that slowly releases the drug whereas the fixed-combination tablets formulated for 24-hour dosing contain 10 mg of loratadine in an immediate-release outer shell and 240 mg of pseudoephedrine sulfate in an extended-release matrix core that slowly releases the drug.

■ **Stability** Loratadine syrup, tablets, orally disintegrating tablets, and fixed-combination loratadine and pseudoephedrine sulfate extended-release tablets should be stored in tight, light-resistant containers. Loratadine tablets should be stored at 2–30°C, and the syrup and orally disintegrating tablets, should be stored at 2–25°C. The fixed-combination extended-release tablets formulated for 12- or 24-hour dosing should be stored at 15–25°C.

Loratadine preparations commercially available in blister packages for individual and institutional use should be stored in a dry place and protected from excessive moisture; the fixed-combination extended-release tablets formulated for 24-hour dosing and commercially available in unit dose blister packages for institutional use also should be protected from light. Loratadine orally disintegrating tablets commercially available in blister packages should be used within 6 months of opening the laminated foil pouch enclosing each blister card, and each tablet should be used immediately after opening an individual blister; individual orally disintegrating tablets that are not used immediately after opening the blister should be discarded.

Preparations

Excipients in commercially available drug preparations may have clinically important effects in some individuals; consult specific product labeling for details.

Loratadine

Oral		
Solution	5 mg/5 mL	**Children's Claritin® Fruit Flavored Syrup 24 Hour,** Schering-Plough
		Children's Claritin® Allergy, Grape Flavor, Schering-Plough
Tablets	10 mg*	**Alavert® Non-Drowsy Allergy Relief 24 Hour,** Wyeth
		Claritin® Hives Relief, Schering-Plough
		Claritin® 24 Hour, Schering-Plough
		Loratadine Tablets
Tablets, orally disintegrating	10 mg	**Alavert® Non-Drowsy Allergy Relief 24 Hour,** Wyeth
		Claritin® Reditabs® 24 Hour, Schering-Plough

*available from one or more manufacturer, distributor, and/or repackager by generic (nonproprietary) name

Loratadine Combinations

Oral		
Tablets, extended-release core (containing pseudoephedrine 60 mg)	5 mg with Pseudoephedrine Sulfate 120 mg	**Alavert® Allergy & Sinus D-12 Hour,** Wyeth
		Claritin-D® 12 Hour, Schering-Plough
Tablets, extended-release core (pseudoephedrine sulfate only), film-coated	10 mg with Pseudoephedrine Sulfate 240 mg	**Claritin-D® 24 Hour,** Schering-Plough

†Use is not currently included in the labeling approved by the US Food and Drug Administration

8:00 Anti-Infective Agents*

§ Omitted from the print version of *AHFS Drug Information* because of space limitations. This monograph is available on the *AHFS Drug Information* web site, http://www.ahfsdruginformation.com. See the Preface for details on accessing this site.
Username: ahfs2020; Password: ASHP94498
* Please see the full AHFS Pharmacologic-Therapeutic Classification© on p. viii. Not all classes are used in the printed edition.

ANTI-INFECTIVE AGENTS 8:00

Anti-infectives Available from CDC

Anti-infectives Available from CDC

The US Centers for Disease Control and Prevention (CDC) distributes the anti-infective agents listed below to clinicians in the US through the Drug Service, Division of Scientific Resources, and the Division of Global Migration and Quarantine. These drugs are not commercially available in the US and FDA has granted permission to CDC to distribute them to qualifying US clinicians for patients in the US. Some of these drugs are licensed by FDA and some are made available under investigational new drug (IND) status. These drugs can only be dispensed to licensed US physicians who register as clinical sub-investigators by completing form FDA-1572.

For information on how to obtain these drugs, clinicians should contact the CDC Drug Service at 404-639-3670 (during working hours) or 770-488-7100 (emergency operations center at any time). Additional information is available at the CDC Drug Service website (http://www.cdc.gov/laboratory/drugservice) or by email (drugservice@cdc.gov).

Anti-infective Agent	Uses
Artesunate	Treatment of severe malaria requiring parenteral treatment
Diethylcarbamazine citrate (DEC)	Treatment of certain filarial diseases, including lymphatic filariasis (*Wuchereria bancrofti, Brugia malayi*, B. timori), tropical pulmonary eosinophilia, loiasis; prophylaxis in individuals at increased risk for *Loa Loa* infection
Eflornithine hydrochloride (DFMO; Ornidyl®)	Treatment of second-stage African trypanosomiasis (sleeping sickness) caused by *Trypanosoma brucei gambiense* with CNS involvement
Melarsoprol (Arsobal®)	Treatment of second-stage African trypanosomiasis (sleeping sickness) with CNS involvement
Nifurtimox (Lampit®)	Treatment of American trypanosomiasis (Chagas disease) caused by *T. cruzi*
Sodium stibogluconate (Pentostam®)	Treatment of leishmaniasis
Suramin (Germanin®)	Treatment of first-stage African trypanosomiasis (sleeping sickness) caused by *T. brucei rhodesiense* without CNS involvement

ANTIBACTERIALS 8:12

AMINOGLYCOSIDES 8:12.02

Aminoglycosides General Statement

■ Aminoglycosides are antibiotics that generally are active against many aerobic gram-negative bacteria and some aerobic gram-positive bacteria and principally are used for serious infections.

Uses

■ **Parenteral** Amikacin, gentamicin, or tobramycin is used IM or IV in the short-term treatment of serious infections, including bone and joint infections, intra-abdominal infections (including peritonitis), respiratory tract infections, septicemia, or skin and soft tissue infections (including those resulting from burns), caused by susceptible gram-negative bacteria. The drugs also are effective in serious, complicated, recurrent urinary tract infections caused by susceptible gram-negative bacteria; however, they are not indicated for the initial treatment of uncomplicated urinary tract infections unless the causative organisms are resistant to other less toxic anti-infectives.

Although IM streptomycin also has been used in the treatment of urinary tract infections, respiratory tract infections, and bacteremia caused by susceptible gram-negative bacteria and IM or IV kanamycin has been used for the short-term treatment of serious infections caused by susceptible gram-negative bacteria, these drugs are not considered drugs of choice for these infections and should be used only when in vitro susceptibility has been demonstrated and other parenteral aminoglycosides or other appropriate anti-infectives are ineffective or contraindicated. When a parenteral aminoglycoside is indicated in the treatment of serious infections caused by Enterobacteriaceae or *Pseudomonas*, amikacin, gentamicin, or tobramycin usually is preferred.

Because of reported in vitro synergism (see Drug Interactions: Anti-infective Agents), aminoglycosides (amikacin, gentamicin, tobramycin) are used concomitantly with an extended-spectrum penicillin with antipseudomonal activity (e.g., carbenicillin, piperacillin and tazobactam, ticarcillin and clavulanate) in the treatment of serious *Pseudomonas* infections, especially in immunosuppressed patients. However, in vitro inactivation of aminoglycosides by β-lactam antibiotics indicates that the drugs should be administered separately and in vitro mixing of the drugs should be avoided. (See β-Lactams under Drug Interactions: Anti-infective Agents.)

In the treatment of mixed aerobic-anaerobic bacterial infections, an IM or IV aminoglycoside is used in conjunction with another appropriate anti-infective (e.g., clindamycin, metronidazole, piperacillin and tazobactam, ampicillin and sulbactam). (See Other Anti-infectives under Drug Interactions: Anti-infective Agents.) The US Centers for Disease Control and Prevention (CDC) and many clinicians suggest a regimen of IM or IV gentamicin and IV clindamycin as one of several possible parenteral regimens for the treatment of acute pelvic inflammatory disease (PID). (See Uses: Pelvic Inflammatory Disease, in Clindamycin 8:12.28.20.)

Although aminoglycosides are not usually recommended for the treatment of staphylococcal infections, the drugs have been used IM or IV in the treatment of serious infections caused by susceptible gram-positive bacteria when other less toxic anti-infectives are ineffective or contraindicated. The manufacturers state that amikacin, gentamicin, kanamycin, or tobramycin may be considered for the treatment of known or suspected staphylococcal infections in certain situations. This includes treatment of infections caused by susceptible staphylococci when other more appropriate anti-infectives are contraindicated (e.g., because of hypersensitivity) or would be ineffective because of resistance and for initial treatment of mixed infections that may involve both gram-negative bacteria and staphylococci. A regimen of vancomycin with or without gentamicin and with or without rifampin has been recommended for the treatment of oxacillin-resistant (methicillin-resistant) staphylococcal infections.

Prior to and during parenteral aminoglycoside therapy, the causative organism should be cultured and in vitro susceptibility tests conducted. In patients in whom serious gram-negative bacterial infections are suspected, aminoglycoside therapy may be started pending results of susceptibility tests. In certain serious infections when the causative organism is unknown, concomitant therapy with another anti-infective (e.g., penicillin, cephalosporin) may be indicated pending results of susceptibility tests because of the possibility of infections due to aminoglycoside-resistant gram-positive organisms. In general, the choice of a specific parenteral aminoglycoside should be based on the usual spectrum and pattern of aminoglycoside resistance in the hospital or community until results of in vitro tests are available. If the causative organism is found to be resistant to the aminoglycoside selected, another aminoglycoside or other anti-infective to which the organism is susceptible should be substituted.

Endocarditis **Enterococcal Endocarditis.** Gentamicin† or streptomycin is used in conjunction with other appropriate anti-infectives (ampicillin, penicillin G sodium, vancomycin) for the treatment of endocarditis caused by *Enterococcus* (e.g., *E. faecalis*, *E. faecium*). Enterococci usually are resistant to aminoglycosides alone and also are relatively resistant to ampicillin, penicillin G, or vancomycin. However, because antibacterial activity of the drugs may be additive or synergistic, regimens of gentamicin or streptomycin used concomitantly with ampicillin, penicillin G sodium, or vancomycin may be effective for the treatment of enterococcal endocarditis. Because enterococci generally exhibit high-level resistance to other aminoglycosides (amikacin, kanamycin, tobramycin), these aminoglycosides are not used in the treatment of enterococcal endocarditis.

Enterococcal isolates should routinely be tested for in vitro susceptibility to penicillin and vancomycin and for high-level resistance to gentamicin and streptomycin. (See Spectrum: In Vitro Susceptibility Testing.) The most appropriate regimen for the treatment of enterococcal endocarditis is selected based on results of in vitro susceptibility testing; treatment duration depends on whether native or prosthetic valves are involved and how long symptoms have been present prior to initiation of treatment. Gentamicin usually is the preferred aminoglycoside for the treatment of enterococcal endocarditis, in part because IV gentamicin may be better tolerated than IM streptomycin and because laboratory monitoring of serum gentamicin concentrations may be more readily available than laboratory monitoring of streptomycin concentrations. Streptomycin may be effective for the treatment of enterococcal endocarditis caused by gentamicin-resistant strains since some, but not all, enterococci with high-level resistance to gentamicin are susceptible to streptomycin. Vancomycin should be used only in patients unable to tolerate ampicillin or penicillin G sodium since regimens that include vancomycin and an aminoglycoside may be associated with an increased risk of ototoxicity and nephrotoxicity and may be less effective compared with regimens that include one of the β-lactams and an aminoglycoside. (See Drug Interactions: Neurotoxic, Ototoxic, or Nephrotoxic Drugs.)

Studies evaluating efficacy of once-daily aminoglycoside regimens in animal models of enterococcal endocarditis have given conflicting results. Therefore, pending further accumulation of data regarding efficacy of once-daily gentamicin or streptomycin regimens in patients with enterococcal endocarditis, the American Heart Association (AHA) and Infectious Diseases Society of America (IDSA) state that once-daily gentamicin or streptomycin regimens should *not* be used for the treatment of enterococcal endocarditis.

For the treatment of native or prosthetic valve endocarditis caused by enterococci *susceptible* to penicillin, vancomycin, and aminoglycosides, the AHA and IDSA recommend a regimen of IV ampicillin or IV penicillin G sodium given in conjunction with either IV or IM gentamicin or IM or IV streptomycin. An alternative regimen of IV vancomycin given in conjunction with IV or IM gentamicin should be used only in patients unable to tolerate penicillins. Streptomycin should be used instead of gentamicin if in vitro testing indicates the strain is gentamicin-resistant. In patients with native valve endocarditis, treatment with ampicillin or penicillin G sodium and gentamicin (or streptomycin) should be continued for 4–6 weeks; although a 4-week regimen may be used in those who have had symptoms of infection for 3 months or less prior to initiation of treatment, a 6-week regimen is recommended for those who have had symptoms for longer than 3 months. In patients with prosthetic valve or other prosthetic cardiac material, treatment should be continued for a minimum of 6 weeks. In addition, whenever a regimen of vancomycin and gentamicin (or streptomycin) is used, treatment should be continued for 6 weeks.

For the treatment of native or prosthetic valve endocarditis caused by β-lactamase-producing enterococci *resistant* to penicillin and *susceptible* to aminoglycosides and vancomycin, the AHA and IDSA recommend a regimen of IV ampicillin sodium and sulbactam sodium and IV or IM gentamicin or, alternatively, a regimen of IV vancomycin and IV or IM gentamicin. Treatment should be continued for 6 weeks; however, if the strain is resistant to gentamicin, ampicillin-sulbactam should be continued for longer than 6 weeks. A 6-week regimen of IV vancomycin and IV or IM gentamicin is recommended when enterococci are intrinsically penicillin-resistant. Consultation with an infectious disease specialist is recommended when enterococci resistant to penicillin, aminoglycosides, or vancomycin are involved.

Endocarditis Caused by Viridans Streptococci or S. bovis. Gentamicin is used in conjunction with other appropriate anti-infectives for the treatment of endocarditis caused by viridans streptococci (e.g., *S. sanguis, S. oralis, S. salivarius, S. mutans, Gamella morbillorum*) or *S. bovis* (nonenterococcal group D streptococci). The AHA and IDSA state that once-daily gentamicin regimens can be used in conjunction with other appropriate anti-infectives for the treatment of endocarditis caused by viridans streptococci or *S. bovis*.

For the treatment of native valve endocarditis caused by viridans streptococci or *S. bovis* highly susceptible to penicillin (i.e., penicillin MIC 0.12 mcg/mL or less), the AHA and IDSA recommend monotherapy with IV penicillin G sodium or IV or IM ceftriaxone given for 4 weeks. These monotherapy regimens avoid the use of gentamicin and are preferred in most patients older than 65 years of age and in those with impaired renal or eighth cranial nerve function. If necessary because of supply problems, monotherapy with ampicillin can be substituted for penicillin G sodium; if necessary in patients unable to tolerate penicillin or ceftriaxone, a 4-week regimen of IV vancomycin can be used. In *selected* patients only, the AHA and IDSA state that a 2-week regimen that consists of IV penicillin G sodium or IV or IM ceftriaxone in conjunction with once-daily IV or IM gentamicin can be used. The 2-week regimen should be used only in patients with uncomplicated native valve endocarditis caused by highly penicillin-susceptible viridans streptococci or *S. bovis* who are at low risk for gentamicin adverse effects; the 2-week regimen should *not* be used in those with known cardiac or extracardiac abscess, creatinine clearance less than 20 mL/minute, impaired eighth cranial nerve function, or infections caused by *Abiotrophia, Granulicatella,* or *Gemella.*

For the treatment of native valve endocarditis caused by viridans streptococci or *S. bovis* relatively resistant to penicillin (i.e., penicillin MIC greater than 0.12 mcg/mL and less than or equal to 0.5 mcg/mL), the AHA and IDSA recommend a 4-week regimen of IV penicillin G sodium or IV or IM ceftriaxone in conjunction with IV or IM gentamicin given during the initial 2 weeks of treatment. Alternatively, in patients unable to tolerate penicillin G sodium or ceftriaxone, IV vancomycin can be used.

In patients with prosthetic valves or other prosthetic material who have endocarditis caused by viridans streptococci or *S. bovis* highly susceptible to penicillin (i.e., penicillin MIC 0.12 mcg/mL or less), the AHA and IDSA recommend a 6-week regimen of IV penicillin G sodium or IV or IM ceftriaxone given with or without IV or IM gentamicin given during the initial 2 weeks of treatment. When highly penicillin-susceptible strains are involved, it is unclear whether the combination regimen that includes an aminoglycoside during the first 2 weeks is more effective than use of the β-lactam alone. If the strains involved are relatively or fully penicillin-resistant (i.e., penicillin MIC greater than 0.12 mcg/mL), the AHA and IDSA recommend a 6-week regimen of IV penicillin G sodium or IV or IM ceftriaxone given with a 6-week regimen of IV or IM gentamicin. Alternatively, in patients unable to tolerate penicillin G sodium or ceftriaxone, a 6-week regimen of IV vancomycin can be used.

Endocarditis caused by viridans streptococci or *S. bovis* highly resistant to penicillin (i.e., penicillin MIC greater than 0.5 mcg/mL) or caused by *Abiotrophia defectiva, Granulicatella,* or *Gamella* should be treated with a regimen recommended for enterococcal endocarditis. (See Enterococcal Endocarditis under Parenteral: Endocarditis, in Uses.)

Staphylococcal Endocarditis. Gentamicin is used in conjunction with other appropriate anti-infectives for the treatment of staphylococcal endocarditis†, including infections caused by coagulase-positive strains (*S. aureus*) or coagulase-negative strains (e.g., *S. epidermidis, S. lugdunensis*). Pending further accumulation of data, the AHA and IDSA state that once-daily gentamicin regimens should *not* be used for the treatment of staphylococcal endocarditis.

For the treatment of native valve endocarditis caused by oxacillin-susceptible staphylococci, the AHA and IDSA recommend a regimen of IV nafcillin or oxacillin with or without IV or IM gentamicin. For penicillin-allergic patients (nonanaphylactoid type only), a regimen of IV cefazolin with or without IV or IM gentamicin is recommended. In patients with complicated right-sided staphylococcal endocarditis or with left-sided staphylococcal endocarditis, a 6-week regimen of the β-lactam should be used and gentamicin given concomitantly during the first 3–5 days of treatment. In those with uncomplicated right-sided staphylococcal endocarditis (i.e., patients with no evidence of renal failure, extrapulmonary metastatic infections, aortic or mitral valve involvement, meningitis, or oxacillin-resistant strains), a 2-week regimen that includes both the β-lactam and gentamicin can be considered.

Staphylococcal endocarditis in patients with prosthetic valves or other prosthetic material usually is caused by oxacillin-resistant staphylococci, especially when endocarditis develops within 1 year after surgery, and is associated with high morbidity and mortality rates. Unless susceptibility to oxacillin has been demonstrated using in vitro susceptibility testing, it should be assumed that patients with staphylococcal prosthetic valve endocarditis have oxacillin-resistant strains. If prosthetic valve endocarditis is known to be caused by oxacillin-susceptible staphylococci, the AHA and IDSA recommend at least 6 weeks of IV nafcillin or oxacillin in conjunction with IV or oral rifampin and concomitant use of IV or IM gentamicin during the initial 2 weeks of treatment. If the strain is known to be penicillin susceptible (i.e., penicillin MIC 0.1 mcg/mL or less) and does not produce β-lactamase, IV penicillin G sodium can be substituted for nafcillin or oxacillin in this regimen; for penicillin-allergic patients (nonanaphylactoid type only), IV cefazolin can be substituted for nafcillin or oxacillin. If the strain is known or presumed to be oxacillin-resistant, the AHA and IDSA recommend at least 6 weeks of IV vancomycin in conjunction with IV or oral rifampin and concomitant use of IV or IM gentamicin during the initial 2 weeks of treatment.

Prevention of Endocarditis. Gentamicin is used in conjunction with ampicillin or with vancomycin (in penicillin-allergic patients) for prevention of bacterial endocarditis† in patients undergoing certain genitourinary and GI tract (except esophageal) surgery or instrumentation who have cardiac conditions that put them at high risk. (See Prophylaxis of Bacterial Endocarditis under Uses: Prophylaxis in the Aminopenicillins General Statement 8:12.16.08)

The current recommendations published by the AHA should be consulted for specific information on which cardiac conditions are associated with high or moderate risk of endocarditis and which procedures require prophylaxis.

Meningitis and Other CNS Infections Amikacin, gentamicin, or tobramycin is used in the treatment of meningitis caused by susceptible bacteria. However, these drugs usually are used in conjunction with other appropriate anti-infectives (e.g., β-lactams, carbapenems, vancomycin) and should not be used alone for the treatment of meningitis since CSF concentrations attained following IM or IV administration are unpredictable and generally low. Amikacin, gentamicin, or tobramycin has been used intrathecally† or intraventricularly† to supplement IM or IV administration in the treatment of CNS infections (including meningitis and ventriculitis) caused by susceptible bacteria. Although concomitant parenteral and intrathecal or intraventricular therapy may result in higher anti-infective CSF concentrations, such therapy also may be associated with increased mortality in neonates.

Mycobacterial Infections Streptomycin, kanamycin†, or amikacin† is used in conjunction with other antituberculosis agents in the treatment of clinical tuberculosis.

Streptomycin or amikacin have been used in conjunction with other antimycobacterial anti-infectives in the treatment of infections caused by some other mycobacteria, including *Mycobacterium avium* complex† (MAC), *M. abscessus*†, *M. chelonae*†, *M. fortuitum*†, and *M. kansasii*†.

Although streptomycin and kanamycin have bactericidal activity against *M. leprae* in mice and streptomycin has been used in the past for the treatment of leprosy†, aminoglycosides are not currently recommended for the treatment of leprosy.

For information on general principles in the treatment of tuberculosis and other mycobacterial diseases, see the Antituberculosis Agents General Statement 8:16.04.

Respiratory Tract Infections Amikacin, gentamicin, or tobramycin is used in the treatment of respiratory tract infections, including community-acquired pneumonia (CAP) and nosocomial pneumonia, caused by susceptible bacteria. The drugs are used in conjunction with other appropriate anti-infectives and may be included in initial empiric combination regimens in severely ill patients and/or when multidrug-resistant gram-negative bacteria may be involved.

Nosocomial Infections. The ATS, IDSA, and other clinicians recommend use of an antipseudomonal cephalosporin (cefepime, ceftazidime), antipseudomonal penicillin (piperacillin and tazobactam, ticarcillin and clavulanate), or an antipseudomonal carbapenem (imipenem or meropenem) for initial therapy of hospital-acquired pneumonia, ventilator-associated pneumonia, or health-care associated pneumonia because these drugs have a broad spectrum of activity against gram-positive, gram-negative, and anaerobic bacteria. In severely ill patients or in those with late-onset disease or risk factors for multidrug-resistant bacteria, the initial regimen should also include an aminoglycoside (amikacin, gentamicin, tobramycin) or antipseudomonal fluoroquinolone (ciprofloxacin or levofloxacin) to improve coverage against *Pseudomonas*. In hospitals where oxacillin-resistant (methicillin-resistant) *Staphylococcus* are common or if there are risk factors for these strains, the initial regimen also should include vancomycin or linezolid.

Other Infections Streptomycin or gentamicin† is used in the treatment of Brucellosis (*Brucella melitensis*), plague (*Yersinia pestis*), or tularemia (*Francisella tularensis*). Gentamicin, or to a lesser extent, streptomycin, also has been used in the treatment of *Bartonella* infections†.

Amikacin is used in the treatment of *Nocardia*† infections and infections caused by *Rhodococcus equi*†.

Streptomycin is used in the treatment of *Burkholderia*† infections (i.e., glanders) and for the treatment of rat-bite fever† caused by *Streptobacillus moniliformis* or *Spirillum minus*.

Gentamicin† is used as an adjunct in the treatment of granuloma inguinale (Donovanosis) caused by *Klebsiella granulomatis* (formerly *Calymmatobacterium granulomatis*). Streptomycin also has been used in the treatment of granuloma inguinale and in the treatment of chancroid caused by *Haemophilus ducreyi*, but is not usually recommended for these infections.

Empiric Therapy in Febrile Neutropenic Patients Aminoglycosides (amikacin, gentamicin, tobramycin) are used in conjunction with an appropriate β-lactam (e.g., ceftazidime, ceftriaxone, cefepime), carbapenem (e.g., imipenem or meropenem), or extended-spectrum penicillin (e.g., piperacillin and tazobactam, ticarcillin and clavulanate) for empiric anti-infective therapy of presumed bacterial infections in febrile neutropenic patients†. An aminoglycoside should not be used alone for empiric therapy in febrile neutropenic patients. (For a more complete discussion of this therapy, see Uses: Empiric Therapy in Febrile Neutropenic Patients, in the Cephalosporins General Statement 8:12.06)

Perioperative Prophylaxis Gentamicin is used in conjunction with clindamycin for perioperative prophylaxis† in patients undergoing head and neck surgery (incisions through oral or pharyngeal mucosa). A regimen of vancomycin with or without gentamicin has been recommended as an alternative for perioperative prophylaxis in patients undergoing vascular surgery and a regimen of clindamycin or metronidazole with gentamicin has been recommended as an alternative for perioperative prophylaxis in patients undergoing gynecologic and obstetric surgery who cannot receive β-lactams. Gentamicin also is used as an adjunct to cefoxitin in patients undergoing contaminated or dirty surgery†, such as that involving a perforated abdominal viscus. The fact that concurrent use of aminoglycosides and general anesthetics or neuromuscular blocking agents may potentiate neuromuscular blockade and cause respiratory paralysis should be considered. (See Drugs Interactions: General Anesthetics and Neuromuscular Blocking Agents.)

■ **Oral** Oral neomycin or, less frequently, oral paromomycin, is used to inhibit ammonia-forming bacteria in the GI tract as an adjunct to protein restriction and supportive therapy in adults and children with hepatic encephalopathy. The subsequent decrease in blood ammonia may result in neurologic improvement. (See Uses: Hepatic Encephalopathy in Neomycin 8:12.02.)

Neomycin is used orally as an adjunct to mechanical cleansing of the large intestines for preoperative prophylaxis in patients undergoing colorectal surgery. For patients undergoing colorectal surgery, clinicians generally recommend a regimen of oral neomycin and oral erythromycin, oral neomycin and oral metronidazole, IV cefoxitin or IV cefotetan (no longer commercially available in the US), or IV cefazolin used in conjunction with IV metronidazole. It has been suggested that an oral regimen is as effective as a parenteral regimen in patients undergoing elective colorectal surgery. Although many clinicians use both an oral and a parenteral regimen in patients undergoing colorectal surgery, there is controversy over the benefits and risks of this strategy. (See Uses: Perioperative Prophylaxis in Neomycin 8:12.02.)

Although neomycin has been used orally as an adjunct to fluid and electrolyte replacement in the treatment of bacterial GI infections†, including diarrhea caused by enteropathogenic *E. coli* (EPEC), oral neomycin is no longer recommended for the treatment of any GI infection.

Oral paromomycin is used in the treatment of various parasitic infections, including intestinal amebiasis caused by *Entamoeba histolytica*, infections caused by *Dientamoeba fragilis*†, and giardiasis†). (See Paromomycin 8:30.04.)

Oral neomycin has been used in the treatment of hypercholesterolemia†. (See Uses: Hypercholesterolemia in Neomycin 8:12.02.)

■ **Oral Inhalation** Aminoglycosides have been administered by oral inhalation for the management of bronchopulmonary *Ps. aeruginosa* infections in cystic fibrosis patients. Tobramycin is commercially available as a preservative-free solution specifically formulated for oral inhalation via a nebulizer. Gentamicin, kanamycin, and tobramycin also have been administered by oral inhalation as aerosols prepared extemporaneously from parenteral preparations of the drugs. Orally inhaled aminoglycosides generally are used for long-term suppressive therapy for prophylaxis of exacerbations of bronchopulmonary *Ps. aeruginosa* infections in cystic fibrosis patients, but are not routinely recommended for the treatment of acute exacerbations of these infections. (See Cystic Fibrosis Patients under Uses: Respiratory Tract Infections in Tobramycin 8:12.02.)

For topical uses of gentamicin, neomycin, and tobramycin, see 52:04.04 and 84:04.04.

Dosage and Administration

■ **Administration** Amikacin, gentamicin, kanamycin, and tobramycin are administered by IM injection or IV infusion. IV administration generally is recommended in patients with life-threatening infections, septicemia, shock, severe hypotension, congestive heart failure, hematologic disorders, severe burns, or reduced muscle mass. Streptomycin is administered by IM injection, but also has been given by IV infusion†.

Neomycin and paromomycin are administered orally. Although kanamycin also has been administered orally, an oral dosage form is no longer commercially available in the US.

Tobramycin solution for oral inhalation is administered via a nebulizer. Tobramycin†, kanamycin, and gentamicin† also have been administered by oral inhalation as aerosols prepared extemporaneously from parenteral preparations of the drugs.

Amikacin, gentamicin, and tobramycin have been administered intrathecally† or intraventricularly† for the treatment of CNS infections. Intraventricular administration of aminoglycosides usually is preferred to intrathecal administration, especially in cases of ventriculitis, to ensure adequate drug concentrations throughout the CSF.

Although some aminoglycosides (e.g., kanamycin, neomycin) have been administered by intraperitoneal instillation or local irrigation (abscess cavities, pleural space, peritoneal and ventricular cavities), there is an increased risk of toxicity with these routes. (See Other Precautions under Cautions: Precautions and Contraindications.)

Aminoglycosides should not be admixed with other drugs or infused simultaneously through the same tubing with other drugs.

■ **Dosage** Aminoglycoside dosage should be individualized taking into consideration the patient's pretreatment body weight, renal status, serum concentrations of the drug, severity of the infection, and susceptibility of the causative organism. Because of the potential toxicity of aminoglycosides, fixed-dosage recommendations that are not based on patient weight or serum drug concentrations are not advised.

Duration of Treatment The usual duration of IM or IV aminoglycoside therapy for the treatment of many infections is 7–10 days. Although a longer duration may be necessary in complicated infections, toxicity is more likely to occur when aminoglycoside treatment is continued for longer than 10 days. Prolonged aminoglycoside therapy should be avoided and treatment duration should be limited to short term whenever feasible. Some aminoglycoside manufacturers (e.g., amikacin) state that safety of treatment for longer than 14 days has not been established. If use of an aminoglycoside for longer than 10 days is considered, serum concentrations and renal, auditory, and vestibular functions should be monitored. (See Cautions.)

Uncomplicated infections caused by susceptible organisms generally respond to usual dosages in 24–48 hours. If definitive clinical response has not occurred within 3–5 days, the susceptibility of the causative organism should be reevaluated. Failure of the infection to respond to the aminoglycoside administered may be due to inadequate serum concentrations of the drug, resistance of the organism, or the presence of septic foci which require surgical drainage.

Once-Daily Dosing Parenteral aminoglycosides historically have been administered in dosage regimens that include multiple daily doses (usually 2–4 doses daily), and these are the only dosage regimens included in current prescribing information for parenteral amikacin, gentamicin, kanamycin, and tobramycin. However, parenteral aminoglycosides are now administered in once-daily† (single-daily) dosing regimens in selected patients based on evidence that once-daily regimens can be at least as effective as, may provide superior pharmacokinetic-pharmacodynamic parameters (peak plasma concentration/MIC ratio), and may be less toxic than conventional dosage regimens employing multiple daily doses of the drugs. Once-daily (extended interval) dosage regimens may provide rapidly effective serum aminoglycoside concentrations that maximize bactericidal activity without increasing the risk of adverse effects. Such regimens also reduce time and expense associated with aminoglycoside monitoring and therapy (e.g., decreased number of IV infusions and associated administration costs). However, once-daily parenteral aminoglycoside regimens should *not* be used in all patients. It has been suggested that once-daily regimens have not been adequately studied to date in patients with creatinine clearance less than 25 mL/minute, pediatric patients, geriatric patients, pregnant women, obese patients, or patients with burns, ascites, or certain severe infections (e.g., meningitis, osteomyelitis, skin and skin structure infections, enterococcal endocarditis). In addition, the most appropriate methods for optimizing dosage selection for once-daily regimens and monitoring serum aminoglycoside concentrations in patients receiving such regimens have not been clearly established. (See Laboratory Monitoring of Therapy under Dosage and Administration: Dosage.)

Results of several analyses of pooled data from randomized, controlled studies in adults found that once-daily administration of aminoglycosides was associated with similar or greater efficacy (e.g., bacteriologic and/or clinical cure), less nephrotoxicity, and no greater risk of ototoxicity compared with administration of multiple daily doses of these drugs. However, various definitions of nephrotoxicity were used in these studies. In addition, only a few studies to date have included infants or children, pregnant women, or patients with renal dysfunction, or life-threatening infections (e.g., endocarditis, bacteremia). Results of at least one analysis of pooled data from randomized, controlled studies in pediatric patients indicate that once-daily administration of aminoglycosides is at least as safe and as effective as regimens that involve multiple daily doses. However, additional well-controlled studies in these and other appropriate patient groups, including comparisons with individualized pharmacokinetic dosing regimens (e.g., high-dose, extended-interval regimens), are needed to fully define the optimal use of once-daily aminoglycoside dosing regimens.

Once-daily aminoglycoside regimens appear to offer several possible microbiologic advantages over multiple-daily dosing. Current pharmacodynamic data suggest that the use of larger, less frequent doses of aminoglycosides may enhance the antimicrobial efficacy of aminoglycosides. Unlike some other antibiotics (e.g., β-lactams), aminoglycosides have concentration-dependent bactericidal effects against many pathogens; higher serum concentrations are associated with increased bactericidal effects. The drugs also exhibit a prolonged, concentration-dependent postantibiotic effect (PAE) against a variety of gram-negative and gram-positive pathogens. In addition, less frequent (e.g., once-daily) dosing may minimize or prevent the occurrence of aminoglycoside-induced adaptive resistance (i.e., reversible refractoriness to the antimicrobial effects of subsequent aminoglycoside doses because of decreased uptake of the drug following the initial dose) and selection of aminoglycoside-resistant subpopulations in gram-negative bacteria by allowing a recovery period during the dosing interval in which serum aminoglycoside concentrations are negligible.

Once-daily aminoglycoside regimens also appear to offer advantages in terms of the risk of toxicity reported with the drugs. Aminoglycoside-related toxicity appears to be reduced, or at least not increased, with once-daily dosing regimens because infrequent administration of large doses results in less drug accumulation in tissue than does multiple daily dosing or continuous IV infusion.

Once-daily dosing of aminoglycosides may minimize the risk of nephrotoxicity because renal cortical uptake for most aminoglycosides appears to be saturable, reaching a plateau despite increasing serum concentrations. Although results have not been entirely consistent, evidence in animals indicates that administration of larger, less frequent doses of aminoglycosides results in lower renal cortical aminoglycoside concentrations than those found with multiple daily dosing or continuous IV infusion, while the efficacy of these dosing regimens has been reported to be similar. Limited data in humans also suggest that the renal cortical concentrations and nephrotoxicity of aminoglycosides may be reduced with once-daily dosing while efficacy comparable to that observed with multiple daily dosing is maintained. In a study in patients undergoing nephrectomy who received identical single doses of gentamicin given by IV infusion over 30 minutes or 24 hours, gentamicin concentrations in renal cortical tissue were 50% higher with the 24-hour infusion. In addition, nephrotoxicity (defined as an increase in serum creatinine concentration of approximately 0.5 mg/dL) was observed less frequently in patients with serious infections who received gentamicin as a single daily dose than in those who received the same daily dose in 3 divided doses.

Although less is known about the relationship between ototoxicity and aminoglycoside dosing regimen or maintenance of aminoglycoside serum concentrations above or below a certain level, available data suggest that once-daily dosing of aminoglycosides at least does not appear to result in increased ototoxicity compared with multiple daily dosing.

Once-daily aminoglycoside regimens have not been adequately studied to date in patients with renal impairment (e.g., creatinine clearance less than 25 mL/minute). It has been suggested that once-daily dosing regimens may be inappropriate in patients with renal dysfunction in whom aminoglycoside half-life is prolonged since such patients would be unlikely to have an aminoglycoside-free period with dosing every 24 hours and more prolonged dosing intervals or reduced dosage of the aminoglycoside should be used in such patients.

Some clinicians also suggest that once-daily aminoglycoside regimens may not be advisable in patients with serious infections and impaired host defenses (e.g., *Pseudomonas aeruginosa* infections in patients with neutropenia) and/or clinical conditions associated with rapid clearance or unpredictable pharmacokinetics of aminoglycosides (e.g., extensive burns, cystic fibrosis, ascites, severe sepsis, dialysis treatment) since such regimens could allow prolonged intervals of undetectable aminoglycoside concentrations that could outlast the PAE. Aminoglycosides usually are administered as adjunctive therapy with other anti-infective agents (e.g., β-lactam antibiotics) in patients with serious gram-negative infections to provide synergistic antimicrobial effects, and limited data from studies employing such combined therapy in neutropenic patients suggest no substantial detrimental effects on clinical outcomes.

Pending further accumulation of data, use of once-daily aminoglycoside dosing is *not* recommended in patients with enterococcal endocarditis.

There now is some evidence from a few studies that once-daily tobramycin regimens may be as effective as multiple-daily doses in some cystic fibrosis patients.

The optimum dosages for once-daily aminoglycoside regimens when the drugs are used alone or in conjunction with other anti-infectives have not been established. In most early studies, the once-daily dosage was simply the total daily dose that was given in 2 or more divided doses in the conventional regimen. In addition, other anti-infectives (e.g., β-lactam antibiotics) were administered concomitantly with the aminoglycosides in most studies of once-daily aminoglycoside therapy, confounding accurate determination of the efficacy of once-daily aminoglycoside therapy.

Although early studies of once-daily aminoglycoside dosing generally consisted of administration of the usual total daily dosage as a single daily dose, various approaches have now been used in an attempt to optimize dosage for once-daily regimens. These approaches involve individualized pharmacokinetic parameters or microbiologic end points (e.g., peak plasma concentration/MIC ratio) and a variety of dosage nomograms and computer-assisted programs designed to achieve certain serum concentrations. Specialized references should be consulted for specific information.

Laboratory Monitoring of Therapy When aminoglycosides are administered in conventional dosage regimens that involve multiple daily doses, therapeutic drug monitoring of peak and trough concentrations is recommended to ensure potentially effective serum concentrations and avoid toxicity. For gentamicin or tobramycin administered in conventional dosage regimens (i.e., multiple daily doses), peak serum concentrations of 4–10 mcg/mL and trough concentrations that do not exceed 1–2 mcg/mL usually are recommended. For amikacin and kanamycin administered in conventional dosage regimens, peak serum concentrations of 15–30 and trough concentrations less than 5–10 mcg/mL have been suggested. Suggested desirable peak and trough serum concentrations of streptomycin are 5–35 mcg/mL and less than 5–10 mcg/mL, respectively.

The ratio of the peak serum aminoglycoside concentration to the MIC of the pathogen also has been evaluated as an indicator of aminoglycoside bactericidal efficacy by which to adjust aminoglycoside dosage and serum concentrations. Limited data in patients receiving multiple daily doses of aminoglycosides have suggested an association between clinical response and a peak (i.e., one-hour postinfusion) serum concentration/MIC ratio up to 12. When MIC data are unavailable for patients receiving once-daily aminoglycoside dosing regimens, some clinicians have used a high target peak serum concentration (e.g., 20 mcg/mL for gentamicin or tobramycin) to ensure optimal peak/MIC ratios. (See Dosage: Once-Daily Dosing.) However, a causal relationship between maintenance of certain peak or trough serum concentrations or other pharmacodynamic endpoints and clinical response or toxicity has not been established to date for aminoglycoside dosing regimens.

Currently recommended therapeutic ranges for aminoglycosides generally are based on data in patients receiving aminoglycosides in multiple daily doses and often were derived by retrospective evaluation of data on efficacy and toxicity. In addition, definitions of nephrotoxicity and ototoxicity have varied among clinical studies, and toxicity often was attributed to aminoglycoside therapy without considering the potential contributory effects of concomitant anti-infective therapy. Nevertheless, pending the availability of more definitive methods for ensuring efficacy and minimizing toxicity of aminoglycoside therapy, most clinicians recommend monitoring of aminoglycoside serum concentrations and/or peak serum concentration/MIC ratio, particularly in patients with life-threatening infections, suspected toxicity or nonresponse to treatment, decreased or varying renal function, and/or when increased aminoglycoside clearance (e.g., patients with cystic fibrosis, burns) or prolonged therapy is likely.

In patients receiving conventional aminoglycoside dosage regimens that involve multiple daily doses, blood specimens for peak serum aminoglycoside concentrations usually are obtained approximately 30–60 minutes following an IM and 15–30 minutes after completion of an IV infusion; specimens for trough drug concentrations are obtained immediately prior to the next IM or IV dose.

Additional study is needed to determine the most appropriate use of therapeutic drug monitoring in patients receiving once-daily† regimens. It has been suggested that routine therapeutic drug monitoring may be unnecessary or that it may be adequate to measure only trough aminoglycoside concentrations in patients receiving once-daily aminoglycoside regimens. However, although a more favorable peak/MIC ratio may be possible with once-daily regimens and efficacy is presumed, there still is a need to monitor serum concentrations to ensure that accumulation does not occur in patients receiving once-daily regimens. The possibility that peak serum concentrations may be higher and trough concentrations lower with once-daily regimens than with conventional regimens should be considered. The ideal therapeutic ranges for once-daily dosing have not been established and the optimal time to obtain blood samples to monitor aminoglycoside concentrations in patients receiving once-daily aminoglycoside regimens is unclear, especially for critically ill patients and those with renal impairment. Specialized references should be consulted for specific information.

■ **Dosage in Renal Impairment** In patients with impaired renal function, doses and/or frequency of administration of aminoglycosides must be modified in response to serum concentrations of the drugs and the degree of renal impairment. Various formulae, tables, nomograms, and computer-assisted programs based on serum creatinine or creatinine clearance have been used to aid in dosage adjustment in patients with renal impairment. One frequently used method that has been recommended for determining dosage of amikacin, gentamicin, kanamycin, or tobramycin in patients with renal impairment is the method of Sarubbi and Hull, which is based on corrected creatinine clearance. (See Table.) However, even when one of these methods is used, peak and trough serum aminoglycoside concentrations should be monitored, especially in patients with changing renal function. These dosage calculation methods should not be used in patients undergoing hemodialysis or peritoneal dialysis; supplemental doses of aminoglycosides may be required after dialysis.

■ Aminoglycoside Dosing for Adults with Renal Impairment

(Do not use in hemodialysis or peritoneal dialysis patients or in children.)

Table 1. Select Loading Dose in mg/kg (based on estimated ideal body weight) to provide peak serum concentrations in range listed below for desired aminoglycoside

AMINOGLYCOSIDE	USUAL LOADING DOSES	EXPECTED PEAK SERUM CONCENTRATIONS
Tobramycin Gentamicin	1 to 2 mg/kg	4 to 10 mcg/mL
Amikacin Kanamycin	5.0 to 7.5 mg/kg	15 to 30 mcg/mL

$$C(c)cr\ male = \frac{(140 - age)}{serum\ creatinine}$$

$$C(c)cr\ female = 0.85 \times C(c)cr\ male$$

Table 2. Select Maintenance Dose (as percentage of chosen loading dose) to continue peak serum concentrations indicated above according to desired dosing interval and the patient's corrected (for a 70-kg ideal body weight) creatinine clearance [C(c)cr].

C(c)cr (mL/min)	Half-life [a]	8 hrs	12 hrs	24 hrs
90	3.1	84%	—	—
80	3.4	80	91%	—
70	3.9	76	88	—
60	4.5	71	84	—
50	5.3	65	79	—
40	6.5	57	72	92%
30	8.4	48	63	86
25	9.9	43	57	81
20	11.9	37	50	75
17	13.6	33	46	70
15	15.1	31	42	67
12	17.9	27	37	61
10 [b]	20.4	24	34	56
7	25.9	19	28	47
5	31.5	16	23	41
2	46.8	11	16	30
0	69.3	8	11	21

[a] Alternatively, one-half of the chosen loading dose may be given at an interval approximately equal to the estimated half-life.

[b] Dosing for patients with C(c)cr ≤ 10 mL/min should be assisted by measured serum concentrations.

Modified from Sarubbi FA Jr, Hull JH. Amikacin serum concentrations: prediction of levels and dosage guidelines. Ann Intern Med. *1978; 89:612-8.*

Alternatively, many clinicians recommend that dosage of these aminoglycosides be determined using appropriate pharmacokinetic methods for calculating dosage requirements and patient-specific pharmacokinetic parameters (e.g., elimination rate constant, volume of distribution) derived from serum concentration-time data; in determining dosage, the susceptibility of the causative organism, presence of a postantibiotic effect (PAE), severity of infection, and the patient's immune and clinical status also must be considered.

Additional study is needed to determine whether the daily dose should be decreased or the dosage interval increased in patients with elevated trough concentrations.

Cautions

Ototoxicity and nephrotoxicity are the most serious adverse effects of aminoglycoside therapy and are most likely to occur in patients with past or present histories of renal impairment (especially if dialysis is required) and in patients who are severely dehydrated, receiving high aminoglycoside dosage or prolonged aminoglycoside therapy, or also are receiving or have received other ototoxic and/or nephrotoxic drugs. (See Drug Interactions: Neurotoxic, Ototoxic, or Nephrotoxic Drugs.)

■ **Ototoxicity** Neurotoxicity manifested as auditory or vestibular ototoxicity has been reported with aminoglycosides administered by any route. Eighth cranial nerve damage may be manifested by vestibular manifestations such as dizziness, nystagmus, vertigo, and ataxia, and/or by auditory symptoms such as tinnitus, roaring in the ears, and varying degrees of hearing impairment. High-frequency deafness (detectable only by audiometric testing) usually occurs first. Patients developing cochlear damage may not have manifestations during aminoglycoside therapy to warn them of developing eighth-nerve toxicity, and total or partial irreversible bilateral deafness may occur after the drug has been discontinued. Ototoxicity usually is bilateral, may be partial or total, and usually is irreversible. The risk of aminoglycoside-associated hearing loss increases with the degree of exposure to either high peak or high trough serum concentrations.

Although the distinctions are not absolute and either or both forms of ototoxicity may occur with any of the aminoglycosides, vestibular manifestations are more frequently associated with gentamicin, tobramycin, or streptomycin and auditory manifestations are more frequently associated with amikacin, kanamycin, neomycin, or paromomycin. The manufacturer of streptomycin states that vestibular dysfunction is cumulatively related to the total daily streptomycin dose and symptoms are likely to develop within 4 weeks in a large percentage of patients receiving a streptomycin dosage of 1.8–2 g daily, especially those who are elderly or have renal impairment. The ototoxic potential of gentamicin and tobramycin appears to be similar.

Tinnitus and/or hearing loss has been reported in some patients receiving tobramycin by oral inhalation. In some reported cases, tobramycin administered by oral inhalation was used in patients who had previously received or were concurrently receiving a systemic aminoglycoside.

Ototoxicity has been reported in patients receiving oral neomycin. Although relatively small amounts of neomycin usually are absorbed following oral administration, toxicity can occur even when recommended dosage is used. The risk of ototoxicity with oral neomycin is increased in patients with renal impairment and in those receiving high dosage and/or prolonged treatment.

■ **Renal and Electrolyte Effects** Aminoglycoside-induced nephrotoxicity may be evidenced by tubular necrosis; increased serum concentrations of BUN, nonprotein nitrogen (NPN), and creatinine; decreased urine specific gravity and creatinine clearance; proteinuria or albuminuria; or cells or casts in the urine. Azotemia, oliguria, toxic nephropathy, and acute renal failure have been reported. A Fanconi-like syndrome (proximal renal tubular dysfunction) characterized by aminoaciduria and metabolic acidosis also has occurred in patients receiving aminoglycosides (e.g., gentamicin).

Hypocalcemia, hypomagnesemia, and hypokalemia have been reported with aminoglycosides. Rarely, renal electrolyte wasting manifested as hypocalcemia, hypomagnesemia, and hypokalemia that may be associated with paresthesia, tetany, confusion, and positive Chvostek and Trousseau signs has occurred. When this electrolyte wasting occurs in infants, tetany and muscle weakness appear to be the predominant manifestations. If renal effects and electrolyte abnormalities develop in patients receiving an aminoglycoside, appropriate therapy should be instituted to correct any electrolyte imbalance(s) associated with the syndrome.

Rarely, nephrotoxicity may not become apparent until the first few days after cessation of aminoglycoside therapy. Aminoglycoside-induced renal toxicity usually is reversible following discontinuance of the drug; however, death secondary to uremia has occurred rarely.

At usual dosages, streptomycin appears to be less nephrotoxic than the other aminoglycosides. The relative nephrotoxicities of the other aminoglycosides in humans have not been definitely established. In some animal and clinical studies, tobramycin appeared to be less nephrotoxic than gentamicin; in other clinical studies, there was no difference in the incidence of nephrotoxicity reported with tobramycin or gentamicin. Amikacin and gentamicin appear to be approximately equal in nephrotoxic potential.

Transient increases in serum creatinine concentrations have been reported in clinical studies in patients receiving tobramycin by oral inhalation, but the incidence was similar to that reported in those receiving placebo.

Although nephrotoxicity occurs most frequently in patients with a history of renal impairment who are treated for longer periods or with higher doses than recommended, adverse renal effects can occur in patients with initially normal renal function.

■ **Nervous System Effects** Neuromuscular blockade, apnea, respiratory depression, and respiratory paralysis have been reported when aminoglycosides were administered parenterally, orally, or by topical irrigation or instillation. Aminoglycosides produce varying degrees of neuromuscular blockade; neomycin probably is the most potent neuromuscular blocking agent of the currently available aminoglycosides followed by streptomycin, kanamycin, amikacin, gentamicin, and tobramycin. Although the blockade induced by an aminoglycoside is generally dose related and self-limiting, it rarely may result in respiratory paralysis. Neuromuscular effects are most likely to occur when an aminoglycoside is applied to serosal surfaces (as in intrapleural injection or peritoneal instillation) or is administered to patients with neuromuscular disease (e.g., myasthenia gravis or parkinsonism) or hypocalcemia or to patients who are receiving general anesthetics, neuromuscular blocking agents, or massive transfusions of citrated blood. Aminoglycoside-induced neuromuscular blockade may be partially or completely reversed by administration of calcium salts, but mechanically assisted respiration may be necessary.

Peripheral neuropathy or encephalopathy, including numbness, skin tingling, muscle twitching, seizures, and a myasthenia gravis-like syndrome, has been reported during aminoglycoside therapy. Other nervous system effects that have been reported in patients receiving an aminoglycoside include headache, tremor, lethargy, confusion or disorientation, paresthesia, peripheral neuritis, arachnoiditis, encephalopathy, pseudotumor cerebri, and acute organic brain syndrome.

CNS depression characterized by stupor and flaccidity, and in some cases, coma and respiratory depression, has been reported in very young infants receiving streptomycin dosage higher than recommended.

Visual disturbances, optic neuritis with blurred vision, scotomas, and enlargement of the blind spot have been reported with aminoglycoside therapy.

■ **Dermatologic and Sensitivity Reactions** Serious sensitivity reactions, such as anaphylaxis and dermatologic reactions including exfoliative dermatitis, toxic epidermal necrolysis, erythema multiforme, angioedema, and Stevens-Johnson syndrome, have been reported rarely in patients receiving aminoglycosides; fatalities have occurred rarely. Cross-sensitivity occurs among the aminoglycosides.

Other hypersensitivity reactions that have been reported with aminoglycosides include rash, pruritus, urticaria, stomatitis, generalized burning, fever, eosinophilia, and laryngeal edema.

Some commercially available aminoglycoside preparations for IM or IV administration (e.g., amikacin, gentamicin, kanamycin, tobramycin) contain sodium metabisulfite, which may cause allergic-type reactions (including anaphylaxis and life-threatening or less severe asthmatic episodes) in certain susceptible individuals. The overall prevalence of sulfite sensitivity in the general population is unknown but probably low; such sensitivity appears to occur more frequently in asthmatic than in nonasthmatic individuals.

The manufacturer of streptomycin cautions that contact with streptomycin solutions during handling or preparation may cause sensitization to the drug.

■ **GI Effects** Adverse GI effects, including nausea, vomiting, diarrhea, increased salivation, stomatitis, weight loss, decreased appetite, or anorexia have been reported with parenteral aminoglycosides.

The most frequent adverse reactions of orally administered aminoglycosides (neomycin, paromomycin) are nausea, vomiting, abdominal cramps, and diarrhea.

A malabsorption syndrome that affects absorption of fat, nitrogen, cholesterol, carotene, glucose, disaccharides, xylose, lactose, sodium, calcium, cyanocobalamin (vitamin B_{12}), and iron has been reported with oral neomycin or paromomycin. The malabsorption syndrome usually is dose-related and reversible and occurs most frequently when oral neomycin therapy is prolonged or when high neomycin dosage (12 g daily) is used. A sprue-like syndrome with diarrhea, steatorrhea, and azotorrhea may occur with oral neomycin dosages of 4–6 g daily.

Enterocolitis, possibly caused by neomycin-resistant staphylococci or *Clostridium difficile*, has been reported rarely with oral neomycin.

■ **Local Effects** Adverse local reactions, including pain at the injection site, local irritation, sterile abscess, subcutaneous atrophy, and fat necrosis have occurred with IM or IV administration of aminoglycosides. Infection at the site of injection, venous thrombosis or phlebitis extending from the site of injection, extravasation, and hypervolemia also have been reported. If an adverse local reaction occurs, discontinue the infusion, evaluate the patient, institute appropriate therapeutic countermeasures, and save the remainder of the infusion solution for examination if deemed necessary.

Intrathecal† or intraventricular† administration of aminoglycosides has caused local inflammation and other complications such as nerve root pain, burning at the injection site, paraplegia, radiculitis, transverse myelitis, arachnoiditis, and other complications. Changes in renal and eighth cranial nerve function, leg cramps, rash, fever, seizures, and an increase in CSF protein have been reported in patients receiving intrathecal gentamicin in conjunction with IM or IV administration of the drug.

Intravitreous† and/or subconjunctival† administration of aminoglycosides (e.g., amikacin, tobramycin) has resulted in macular infarction or necrosis, sometimes leading to permanent loss of vision.

■ **Hematologic Effects** Adverse hematologic effects reported with aminoglycosides include anemia, leukopenia, granulocytopenia, transient agranulocytosis, thrombocytopenia, eosinophilia, and increased or decreased reticulocyte counts. Pancytopenia and hemolytic anemia have been reported with streptomycin.

■ **Other Adverse Effects** Other adverse effects that have been reported with aminoglycosides include tachycardia, arthralgia or joint pain, transient hepatomegaly or splenomegaly, hepatic necrosis, myocarditis, hypotension, hypertension, mental depression, alopecia, purpura, and pulmonary fibrosis. Transient increases in serum concentrations of AST (SGOT), ALT (SGPT), LDH, alkaline phosphatase, and bilirubin have been reported.

■ **Precautions and Contraindications** ***Sensitivity Reactions*** Aminoglycosides are contraindicated in patients with a history of hypersensitivity or serious toxic reactions to any aminoglycoside. Cross-sensitivity occurs among the aminoglycosides.

Some commercially available IM or IV preparations of aminoglycosides contain sulfites which may cause allergic-type reactions (including anaphylaxis and life-threatening or less severe asthmatic episodes) in certain susceptible individuals. (See Cautions: Dermatologic and Sensitivity Reactions.)

The manufacturer states that individuals who handle or prepare streptomycin solutions should use care to avoid contact and resultant sensitization to the drug.

If an allergic reaction to an aminoglycoside occurs, the drug should be discontinued and appropriate therapy instituted as indicated.

Underlying GI Conditions Oral neomycin and oral paromomycin are contraindicated in patients with intestinal obstruction. Oral neomycin is contraindicated in patients with inflammatory or ulcerative GI disease because of the potential for enhanced GI absorption of the drug. The manufacturer states that oral paromomycin should be used with caution in patients with ulcerative bowel lesions since inadvertent absorption could cause renal toxicity.

Ototoxicity and Nephrotoxicity Patients receiving an aminoglycoside (by any route of administration) should be under close medical supervision because of the risk of ototoxicity and nephrotoxicity. Patients should be well hydrated to minimize chemical irritation of the renal tubules.

The risk of ototoxicity and nephrotoxicity is greatest in patients with past or present histories of renal impairment, dehydration, or previous exposure to ototoxic drugs and in those who receive high dosage or prolonged treatment. In addition, patients with preexisting tinnitus, vertigo, or subclinical high-frequency hearing loss are especially susceptible to ototoxicity and should be carefully observed for signs of eighth cranial nerve damage during aminoglycoside therapy.

Renal function should be assessed prior to initiation of aminoglycoside therapy. Renal and eighth-cranial nerve function should be monitored closely during aminoglycoside therapy, especially in patients with known or suspected renal impairment at the start of treatment and in those whose renal function deteriorates during treatment. When feasible, serial audiograms should be performed in patients old enough to be tested, particularly high-risk patients. Urine should be evaluated for decreased specific gravity, increased excretion of protein, and presence of cells or casts and serum BUN, serum creatinine, and creatinine clearance should be monitored. Serum calcium, magnesium, and sodium also should be monitored. (See Cautions: Renal and Electrolyte Effects and see Cautions: Ototoxicity.)

The difference between therapeutic and toxic serum concentrations of the aminoglycosides may be narrow. Although a causal relationship has not been established, ototoxicity and nephrotoxicity may be related to high peak serum aminoglycoside concentrations and/or high trough drug concentrations between doses. Prolonged peak serum concentrations of amikacin or kanamycin above 30–35 mcg/mL, gentamicin or tobramycin above 10–12 mcg/mL, or streptomycin above 40–50 mcg/mL may be associated with an increased risk of toxicity. Whenever possible, especially in patients with renal impairment, peak and trough serum concentrations of aminoglycosides should be determined periodically and dosage adjusted to maintain desired serum concentrations. (See Dosage and Administration: Dosage.)

If evidence of ototoxicity (e.g., dizziness, vertigo, tinnitus, roaring in the ears, hearing loss) occurs during aminoglycoside therapy, the drug should be discontinued or dosage reduced. The manufacturer of streptomycin states that baseline and periodic caloric stimulation tests and audiometric tests are advisable with extended streptomycin therapy and that tinnitus, roaring noises, or a sense of fullness in the ears indicates the need for audiometric examination and/or termination of streptomycin therapy. Tinnitus may be a sentinel symptom of ototoxicity and the onset of this symptom warrants caution.

If signs of renal irritation (e.g., presence of white or red blood cells, casts, or albumin in urine) occur during aminoglycoside therapy, hydration should be increased. If other evidence of nephrotoxicity (e.g., decreased creatinine clearance or urine specific gravity, increased BUN and/or serum creatinine concentrations) occurs, the aminoglycoside should be discontinued or dosage reduced. If azotemia increases or if a progressive decrease in urinary output occurs, the drug should be discontinued.

Because of an increased risk, aminoglycosides should not be used concomitantly and/or sequentially with other systemic, oral, or topical drugs that have neurotoxic, ototoxic, or nephrotoxic effects. (See Drug Interactions: Neurotoxic, Ototoxic, or Nephrotoxic Drugs.)

Neuromuscular Blockade The possibility of neuromuscular blockade and respiratory paralysis should be considered when aminoglycosides are administered by any route, especially in patients receiving anesthetics or neuromuscular blocking agents (e.g., tubocurarine, rocuronium, succinylcholine) or in those receiving massive transfusions of citrate-anticoagulated blood. (See Drug Interactions: Neurotoxic, Ototoxic, and Nephrotoxic Drugs.) Neuromuscular blockade and respiratory paralysis have been reported when the drugs were administered parenterally, orally, or by topical irrigation or instillation.

Aminoglycosides should be used with caution in patients with muscular disorders such as myasthenia gravis or parkinsonism, since the drugs may aggravate muscle weakness as a result of their potential to produce neuromuscular blockade. Calcium salts may reverse neuromuscular blockade, but mechanical respiratory assistance may be necessary. (See Cautions: Nervous System Effects.)

Selection and Use of Anti-infectives To reduce development of drug-resistant bacteria and maintain effectiveness of aminoglycosides and other antibacterials, the drugs should be used only for the treatment or prevention of infections proven or strongly suspected to be caused by susceptible bacteria. When selecting or modifying anti-infective therapy, use results of culture and in vitro susceptibility testing. In the absence of such data, consider local epidemiology and susceptibility patterns when selecting anti-infectives for empiric therapy.

Patients should be advised that antibacterials (including aminoglycosides) should only be used to treat bacterial infections and not used to treat viral infections (e.g., the common cold). Patients also should be advised about the importance of completing the full course of therapy, even if feeling better after a few days, and that skipping doses or not completing therapy may decrease effectiveness and increase the likelihood that bacteria will develop resistance and will not be treatable with aminoglycosides or other antibacterials in the future.

The use of aminoglycosides by any route may result in the overgrowth of nonsusceptible organisms, including fungi. If superinfection occurs, appropriate therapy should be instituted.

Systemic Risks Associated with Local Administration Administration of aminoglycosides by intraperitoneal instillation or local irrigation (abscess cavities, pleural space, peritoneal and ventricular cavities) is associated with an increased risk of systemic toxicity since the drugs are absorbed quickly and in substantial amounts when applied topically. (See Pharmacokinetics: Absorption.) Serious adverse systemic effects, including delayed-onset irreversible deafness, renal failure, and death resulting from neuromuscular blockade, have been reported following irrigation of small and large surgical sites with an aminoglycoside preparation.

Other Precautions Parenteral aminoglycoside solutions containing sodium should be used with caution, if at all, in patients with congestive heart failure, severe renal insufficiency, or any clinical condition that involves edema with sodium retention. In patients with decreased renal function, administration of solutions containing sodium may result in sodium retention.

The fact that oral neomycin may adversely affect GI absorption of some vitamins and drugs should be considered. (See Drug Interactions: Neomycin.)

In the event of aminoglycoside overdosage or toxic reactions, hemodialysis may aid in removal of aminoglycosides, especially if renal function is (or becomes) compromised. Peritoneal dialysis may be less effective than hemodialysis. In neonates, exchange transfusions may also be considered.

■ **Pediatric Precautions** Aminoglycosides should be used with caution and in reduced dosage in premature and full-term neonates because renal immaturity in these patients may result in prolonged serum half-lives of the drugs.

A manufacturer of gentamicin states that the risk of toxic reactions is low in neonates, infants, and children with normal renal function provided they do not receive gentamicin dosages that are higher or continued longer than recommended.

Safety and efficacy of oral neomycin have not been established in pediatric patients younger than 18 years of age. The manufacturers state that if use of oral neomycin is considered necessary in this age group, the drug should be used with caution and the duration of therapy should not exceed 3 weeks.

Safety and efficacy of tobramycin solution for oral inhalation have not been established in pediatric patients younger than 6 years of age, in patients with forced expiratory volume in 1 second (FEV_1) less than 25% or exceeding 75% of the predicted value, or in patients colonized with *Burkholderia cepacia* (formerly *Ps. cepacia*).

■ **Geriatric Precautions** Geriatric patients may be at higher risk of aminoglycoside-associated nephrotoxicity and ototoxicity than younger adults.

Aminoglycosides are substantially eliminated in urine and the risk of toxicity may be increased in patients with impaired renal function. Because of age-related decreases in renal function, dosage should be selected with caution and renal function closely monitored whenever aminoglycosides are used in geriatric patients. Measuring creatinine clearance may be more useful than determining BUN or serum creatinine concentrations in this patient population since reduced renal function may not always be evident using the routine screening tests.

■ **Pregnancy, Fertility, and Lactation** Aminoglycosides can cause fetal harm when administered to pregnant women. Aminoglycosides cross the placenta and there have been several reports of total irreversible bilateral congenital deafness in children whose mothers received streptomycin during pregnancy. Although serious adverse effects have not been reported in fetuses or neonates whose mothers received other aminoglycosides during pregnancy, the potential for fetal toxicity exists with these antibiotics.

If an aminoglycoside is administered during pregnancy or if the patient becomes pregnant while receiving the drug, the patient should be informed of the potential hazard to the fetus.

Reproduction studies in animals using subcutaneous amikacin or tobramycin have not revealed evidence of impaired fertility.

Small amounts of aminoglycosides are distributed into milk following IM or IV administration. Although it is not known whether neomycin is distributed into human milk following oral administration, it is distributed into cow milk following IM injection. It is not know whether tobramycin is distributed into milk following oral inhalation. Because of the potential for serious adverse reactions to aminoglycosides in nursing infants, a decision should be made whether to discontinue nursing or the drug, taking into account the importance of the drug to the woman.

Drug Interactions

■ **Neurotoxic, Ototoxic, or Nephrotoxic Drugs** Concomitant and/or sequential use of an aminoglycoside and other systemic, oral, or topical drugs that have neurotoxic, ototoxic, or nephrotoxic effects (e.g., other aminoglycosides, acyclovir, amphotericin B, bacitracin, capreomycin, certain cephalosporins, colistin, cisplatin, methoxyflurane, polymyxin B, vancomycin) may result in additive toxicity and should be avoided, if possible.

Because of the possibility of an increased risk of ototoxicity due to additive effects or altered serum and tissue aminoglycoside concentrations, aminoglycosides should not be given concomitantly with potent diuretics such as ethacrynic acid, furosemide, urea, or mannitol. It has been suggested that concomitant use of certain anti-emetics that suppress nausea and vomiting of vestibular origin and vertigo (e.g., dimenhydrinate, meclizine) may mask symptoms of aminoglycoside-associated vestibular ototoxicity.

■ **General Anesthetics and Neuromuscular Blocking Agents** Concurrent use of an aminoglycoside with general anesthetics or neuromuscular blocking agents (e.g., succinylcholine, rocuronium, tubocurarine) may potentiate neuromuscular blockade and cause respiratory paralysis. A single amikacin dose has potentiated the neuromuscular blocking effects of a single intubating dose of rocuronium.

Aminoglycosides should be used with caution in patients receiving anesthetics or neuromuscular blocking agents, and patients should be closely observed for signs of respiratory depression.

■ **Neomycin** Oral neomycin may potentiate the effects of oral anticoagulants, possibly by interfering with GI absorption or synthesis of vitamin K. Prothrombin times should be monitored in patients receiving concomitant oral aminoglycoside and oral anticoagulant therapy, and dosage of the anticoagulant should be adjusted as required.

Although the clinical importance is unclear, oral neomycin has been reported to decrease GI absorption of digoxin, but apparently does not affect the terminal plasma half-life of digoxin. Serum digoxin concentrations should be monitored in patients receiving oral neomycin.

Although the clinical importance is unclear, oral neomycin has been reported to decrease GI absorption of fluorouracil, methotrexate, cyanocobalamin (vitamin B_{12}), and penicillin V.

Oral neomycin may decrease the rate but not the extent of absorption of oral spironolactone.

■ **Anti-infective Agents** ***β-Lactams*** In vitro studies indicate that the antibacterial activity of aminoglycosides and β-lactam antibiotics may be additive or synergistic against some organisms including Enterobacteriaceae, *Pseudomonas aeruginosa*, enterococci, and viridans streptococci. The synergistic effect of aminoglycosides and β-lactams is used to therapeutic advantage, especially in the treatment of infections caused by enterococci or *Ps. aeruginosa*. Although the exact mechanism of this synergistic effect has not been determined, it appears that by inhibiting bacterial cell-wall synthesis the penicillin allows more effective ingress of the aminoglycoside to the ribosomal binding site. Synergism between aminoglycosides and extended-spectrum penicillins generally is unpredictable and antagonism has been reported rarely in vitro when these penicillins were used in conjunction with amikacin, gentamicin, or tobramycin. Therefore, some clinicians suggest that when concomitant therapy is indicated it may be advisable to use appropriate in vitro studies to demonstrate synergism against the isolated organism. Concomitant administration of an extended-spectrum penicillin and an aminoglycoside has resulted in decreased serum aminoglycoside concentrations and elimination $t_{1/2}$, especially in patients with renal impairment. Therefore, serum aminoglycoside concentrations should be monitored in patients receiving concomitant therapy, especially when very high doses of an extended-spectrum penicillin are used or when the patient has impaired renal function.

Concomitant use of aminoglycosides and cephalosporins may result in increased nephrotoxicity since cephalosporins may spuriously elevate creatinine concentrations. (See Drug Interactions: Neurotoxic, Ototoxic, or Nephrotoxic Drugs.)

Penicillins are physically and/or chemically incompatible with aminoglycosides and can inactivate aminoglycosides in vitro. In vitro inactivation of aminoglycosides by penicillins can occur if the drugs are administered in the same syringe or IV infusion container. If concomitant therapy is indicted, the drugs should be administered separately and should not be admixed. Penicillins can inactivate aminoglycosides in vitro in serum samples obtained from patients receiving concomitant therapy with the drug and this may result in falsely decreased aminoglycoside concentrations. Amikacin appears to be the least susceptible and tobramycin the most susceptible to inactivation by β-lactam antibiotics, and most studies indicate that carbenicillin inactivates aminoglycosides at a faster rate than do other currently available extended-spectrum penicillins. To ensure accurate serum aminoglycoside assays in patients receiving concomitant therapy, penicillinase should be added to blood collection tubes whenever samples cannot be assayed immediately for aminoglycoside concentrations.

Carbapenems The antibacterial activity of imipenem and aminoglycosides is additive or synergistic in vitro against some gram-positive bacteria including *Enterococcus faecalis*, *Staphylococcus aureus*, and *Listeria monocytogenes*. Depending on the method used to determine in vitro synergism, the combination of imipenem and an aminoglycoside is synergistic against 35–98% of *E. faecalis* tested.

Other Anti-infectives The antibacterial activity of streptomycin and vancomycin may be additive or synergistic against enterococci (e.g., *E. faecalis*). However, vancomycin and aminoglycosides have similar neurotoxic, ototoxic, and nephrotoxic effects and concomitant and/or sequential use of the drugs may result in additive toxicity and should be avoided, if possible. (See Drug Interactions: Neurotoxic, Ototoxic, or Nephrotoxic Drugs.)

Chloramphenicol, clindamycin, and tetracycline have been reported to antagonize the bactericidal activity of aminoglycosides in vitro, and some clinicians recommend that these drugs not be used concomitantly. However, in vivo antagonism has not been demonstrated, and aminoglycosides have been administered successfully in conjunction with chloramphenicol or clindamycin with no apparent decrease in activity.

■ **Nonsteroidal Anti-inflammatory Agents** Indomethacin has been reported to increase trough and peak serum aminoglycoside (e.g., amikacin, gentamicin) concentrations in premature neonates who were receiving the drugs concomitantly. Increases in serum aminoglycoside concentrations appeared to be related to indomethacin-induced decreases in urine output. It also has been postulated that inhibitors of prostaglandin synthesis (e.g., aspirin) may increase nephrotoxicity of aminoglycosides. Serum aminoglycoside concentrations and renal function should be closely monitored and aminoglycoside dosage adjusted accordingly when aminoglycosides are used concomitantly with indomethacin in premature neonates.

Laboratory Test Interferences

■ **Tests for Urinary Glucose** Streptomycin reportedly causes false-positive results in urine glucose determinations using cupric sulfate solution (Benedict's reagent, Clinitest®).

Mechanism of Action

Aminoglycosides are usually bactericidal in action. Although the exact mechanism of action has not been fully elucidated, the drugs appear to inhibit protein synthesis in susceptible bacteria by irreversibly binding to 30S ribosomal subunits.

Spectrum

In general, aminoglycosides are active against many aerobic gram-negative bacteria and some aerobic gram-positive bacteria; however, there are differences in spectra of activity of the individual drugs. Aminoglycosides are inactive against fungi, viruses, and most anaerobic bacteria.

■ **In Vitro Susceptibility Testing** When in vitro susceptibility testing is performed according to the standards of the Clinical and Laboratory Standards Institute (CLSI; formerly National Committee for Clinical Laboratory Standards [NCCLS]), clinical isolates identified as *susceptible* to an aminoglycoside are inhibited by drug concentrations usually achievable when the recommended dosage is used for the site of infection. Clinical isolates classified as *intermediate* have minimum inhibitory concentrations (MICs) that approach usually attainable blood and tissue concentrations and response rates may be lower than for strains identified as susceptible. Therefore, the intermediate category implies clinical applicability in body sites where the drug is physiologically concentrated or when a higher than usual dosage can be used. This intermediate category also includes a buffer zone which should prevent small, uncontrolled technical factors from causing major discrepancies in interpretation, especially for drugs with narrow pharmacotoxicity margins. If results of in vitro susceptibility testing indicate that a clinical isolate is *resistant* to an aminoglycoside, the strain is not inhibited by drug concentrations generally achievable with usual dosage schedules and/or MICs fall in the range where specific microbial resistance mechanisms are likely and clinical efficacy of the drug against the isolate has not been reliably demonstrated in clinical studies.

Because there are differences in the spectra of activity of amikacin, gentamicin, kanamycin, tobramycin, and streptomycin, CLSI recommends that these drugs be tested individually to determine in vitro susceptibility.

Disk Susceptibility Tests When the disk-diffusion procedure is used to test in vitro susceptibility of Enterobacteriaceae, *Pseudomonas aeruginosa*, *Acinetobacter*, or *Staphylococcus*, individual disks containing 30 mcg of amikacin, 10 mcg of gentamicin, 30 mcg of kanamycin, 10 mcg of tobramycin, or 10 mcg of streptomycin should be used. There is no class susceptibility disk that can be used to test susceptibility to all aminoglycosides.

Susceptibility of enterococci to aminoglycosides cannot be predicted using standard disk-diffusion procedures. Although enterococci may appear susceptible to aminoglycosides in vitro, the drugs are not effective clinically when used alone in these infections. Therefore, CLSI recommends that enterococci be screened for high-level resistance to gentamicin and streptomycin and these results used to predict synergy between these aminoglycosides and ampicillin, penicillin G, or vancomycin for the treatment of enterococcal infections. In vitro susceptibility of enterococci to other aminoglycosides does not need to be evaluated since other aminoglycosides are inferior to gentamicin and streptomycin for the treatment of enterococcal infections. When the disk-diffusion screening test is used to test enterococci for high-level aminoglycoside resistance, a disk containing 120 mcg of gentamicin and a disk containing 300 mcg of streptomycin should be used. When the test is performed according to CLSI standardized procedures, a growth inhibition zone of 6 mm indicates the enterococcal strain is resistant and the aminoglycoside will not be synergistic with ampicillin, penicillin G, or vancomycin. If the growth inhibition zone is 7–9 mm, results are inconclusive and the agar or broth dilution screening test for high-level aminoglycoside resistance should be performed. If the growth inhibition zone is 10 mm or larger, the enterococcal strain is susceptible to the aminoglycoside and a synergistic effect will occur with ampicillin, penicillin G, or vancomycin provided the strain also is susceptible to that drug.

Table 3. Interpretation of Disk Diffusion Zone Diameters (nearest whole mm) for Disk Susceptibility Tests Performed According to CLSI Standardized Procedures

	Resistant	Intermediate	Susceptible
Enterobacteriaceae (Note: Although *Salmonella* and *Shigella* may appear susceptible in vitro, aminoglycosides are not active clinically in these infections and results should not be reported as susceptible)			
Amikacin	≤14	15–16	≥17
Gentamicin	≤12	13–14	≥15
Kanamycin	≤13	14–17	≥18
Tobramycin	≤12	13–14	≥15
Streptomycin	≤11	12–14	≥15
Pseudomonas aeruginosa			
Amikacin	≤14	15–16	≥17
Gentamicin	≤12	13–14	≥15
Tobramycin	≤12	13–14	≥15
Acinetobacter			
Amikacin	≤14	15–16	≥17
Gentamicin	≤12	13–14	≥15
Tobramycin	≤12	13–14	≥15
Staphylococcus			
Amikacin	≤14	15–16	≥17
Gentamicin	≤12	13–14	≥15
Kanamycin	≤13	14–17	≥18
Tobramycin	≤12	13–14	≥15
Enterococcus Note: The disk-diffusion screening test for high-level aminoglycoside resistance should be performed instead of the standard disk-diffusion procedure. See text.			

Dilution Susceptibility Tests When broth or agar dilution susceptibility tests are used to test in vitro susceptibility to aminoglycosides, each drug must be tested individually.

Susceptibility of enterococci to aminoglycosides cannot be predicted using standard broth or agar dilution procedures. Although enterococci may appear susceptible to aminoglycosides in vitro, the drugs are not effective clinically when used alone in these infections. Therefore, CLSI recommends that enterococci be screened for high-level resistance to gentamicin and streptomycin and these results used to predict synergy between these aminoglycosides and ampicillin, penicillin G, or vancomycin for the treatment of enterococcal infections. In vitro susceptibility of enterococci to other aminoglycosides does not need to be evaluated since other aminoglycosides are inferior to gentamicin and streptomycin for the treatment of enterococcal infections. When the agar or broth screening test is used to test enterococci for high-level aminoglycoside resistance and is performed according to CLSI standardized procedures, the presence of more than one colony on the agar or any growth in the broth indicates the enterococcal strain is resistant and the aminoglycoside will not be synergistic with ampicillin, penicillin G, or vancomycin. The absence of growth indicates the enterococcal strain is susceptible to the aminoglycoside and a synergistic effect will occur with ampicillin, penicillin G, or vancomycin provided the strain also is susceptible to that drug.

Table 4. Interpretation of MICs (mcg/mL) For Diffusion Susceptibility Tests Performed According to CLSI Standardized Procedures

	Susceptible	Intermediate	Resistant
Enterobacteriaceae (Note: Although *Salmonella* and *Shigella* may appear susceptible in vitro, aminoglycosides are not active clinically in these infections and results should not be reported as susceptible)			
Amikacin	≤16	32	≥64
Gentamicin	≤4	8	≥16
Kanamycin	≤16	32	≥64
Tobramycin	≤4	8	≥16
Pseudomonas aeruginosa and Other Non-Enterobacteriaceae (except Acinetobacter, Burkholderia, Stenotrophomonas)			
Amikacin	≤16	32	≥64
Gentamicin	≤4	8	≥16
Tobramycin	≤4	8	≥16
Acinetobacter			
Amikacin	≤16	32	≥64
Gentamicin	≤4	8	≥16
Tobramycin	≤4	8	≥16
Staphylococcus			
Amikacin	≤16	32	≥64
Gentamicin	≤4	8	≥16
Kanamycin	≤16	32	≥64
Tobramycin	≤4	8	≥16
Enterococcus Note: The broth or agar diffusion screening test for high-level aminoglycoside resistance should be performed instead of the standard procedure. See text.			
Brucella			
Gentamicin	≤4	–	–
Streptomycin	≤8	–	–
Yersinia pestis			
Gentamicin	≤4	8	≥16
Streptomycin	≤4	8	≥16
Francisella tularensis			
Gentamicin	≤4	–	–
Streptomycin	≤8	–	–

■ **Gram-Negative Aerobic Bacteria** Aminoglycosides generally are active against *Acinetobacter*, *Citrobacter*, *Enterobacter*, *Escherichia coli*, *Klebsiella*, indole-positive and indole-negative *Proteus*, *Providencia*, *Pseudomonas*, *Salmonella*, *Serratia*, and *Shigella*. A large percentage of these organisms are susceptible to amikacin, gentamicin, and tobramycin; resistance is more common with kanamycin, and a large percentage of these organisms are resistant to streptomycin, neomycin, and paromomycin. Amikacin, gentamicin, and tobramycin are active against most strains of *Ps. aeruginosa*; however, these organisms are generally resistant to kanamycin, neomycin, paromomycin, and streptomycin. Amikacin is active against some strains of bacteria, especially *Proteus*, *Pseudomonas*, and *Serratia*, which are not susceptible to the other aminoglycosides. However, there also are strains of bacteria resistant to amikacin which may be susceptible to gentamicin and/or tobramycin.

Streptomycin and gentamicin are active against *Brucella* and *Yersinia pestis*. Although most strains of *Y. pestis* are susceptible to streptomycin, streptomycin-resistant strains have been reported rarely. Streptomycin, gentamicin, and tobramycin are active in vitro against *Francisella tularensis*.

Streptomycin is active against *Calymmatobacterium granulomatis*, *Haemophilus influenzae*, *H. ducreyi*, and *Pasteurella multocida*.

■ **Gram-Positive Bacteria** Aminoglycosides are active against some strains of *Staphylococcus aureus* and *S. epidermidis*. The drugs are only minimally active against streptococci; most strains of enterococci are resistant to the aminoglycosides alone. Streptomycin is active against *Nocardia*, *Enterococcus faecalis*, and *Erysipelothrix*.

Mycobacteria Streptomycin is active in vitro against many strains of *Mycobacterium tuberculosis* and *M. bovis* and some strains of *M. avium* complex (MAC), *M. kansasii*, *M. malmoense*, *M. marinum*, *M. szulgai*, and *M. ulcerans*.

Amikacin and kanamycin are active against many strains of *M. tuberculosis* and may be active against multidrug-resistant strains. In vitro, amikacin is active against some strains of *M. avium* complex, *M. abscessus*, *M. chelonae*, *M. fortuitum*, *M. kansasii*, *M. marinum*, and *M. ulcerans*. Kanamycin is active in vitro against some strains of *M. abscessus*.

Gentamicin and tobramycin usually are inactive against *M. tuberculosis* at clinically attainable concentrations.

Streptomycin and kanamycin have activity against *M. leprae* in experimental leprosy in mice.

Parasites Paromomycin is active against protozoa, especially *Entamoeba histolytica*, and has some anthelmintic activity against *Taenia saginata*, *Hymenolepis nana*, *Diphyllobothrium latum*, and *Taenia solium*. Limited in vitro studies indicate that neomycin and paromomycin have some activity against *Acanthamoeba*, and that neomycin concentrations of 12.5 mcg/mL or paromomycin concentrations of 5 mcg/mL may be amebistatic against these organisms. Paromomycin also appears to have some activity against *Cryptosporidium*, but no anti-infective has been found to reliably eliminate *Cryptosporidium*.

Resistance

Natural and acquired resistance to one or more of the aminoglycosides has been reported in both gram-negative and gram-positive bacteria. Resistance to a specific aminoglycoside may be due to decreased permeability of the bacterial cell wall, alterations in the ribosomal binding site, or the presence of a plasmid-mediated resistance factor which is acquired by conjugation. Plasmid-mediated resistance enables the resistant bacteria to enzymatically modify the drug by acetylation, phosphorylation, or adenylylation and can be transferred between organisms of the same or different species. Resistance to other aminoglycosides and several other anti-infectives (e.g., chloramphenicol, sulfonamides, tetracycline) may be transferred on the same plasmid.

Streptomycin-resistant *Y. pestis* have been reported rarely; resistance is plasmid-mediated and transferable. Although a streptomycin-resistant *Y. pestis* strain isolated from a human case of bubonic plague in Madagascar was susceptible to spectinomycin, tetracyclines, sulfonamides, and chloramphenicol in vitro, a multidrug-resistant strain with high-level resistance to streptomycin, kanamycin, spectinomycin, tetracyclines, sulfonamides, chloramphenicol, and ampicillin also has been isolated in Madagascar.

M. avium complex (MAC) with intermediate or high-level in vitro resistance to streptomycin has been reported. The importance of this in vitro resistance to streptomycin in terms of clinical response to treatment with multiple-drug regimens that include streptomycin and other drugs (e.g., clarithromycin, rifampin, ethambutol) is unclear.

There is partial cross-resistance among the aminoglycosides. *Mycobacterium tuberculosis* generally demonstrate complete cross-resistance between amikacin and kanamycin and partial cross-resistance between kanamycin and capreomycin. Streptomycin-resistant *M. tuberculosis* may be susceptible to amikacin, kanamycin, and capreomycin. Resistant strains of initially susceptible *M. tuberculosis* develop rapidly if an aminoglycoside is used alone in the treatment of clinical tuberculosis. When one of these drugs is combined with other antituberculosis agents in the treatment of the disease, emergence of resistant strains may be delayed or prevented.

Pharmacokinetics

Absorption Aminoglycosides are poorly absorbed from the GI tract. The drugs are well absorbed following parenteral administration; however, there may be considerable interpatient variation in serum concentrations achieved with a specific IM dose because of differences in rates of absorption from IM injection sites. Following IM administration in adults with normal renal function, peak concentrations of the drugs are usually attained within 0.5–2 hours and measurable concentrations may persist 8–12 hours.

Aminoglycosides are rapidly and almost completely absorbed following topical administration (except to the urinary bladder) during surgical procedures (e.g., from the peritoneum). Serious adverse systemic effects, including irreversible deafness, renal failure, and death resulting from neuromuscular blockade, have been reported following irrigation of small and large surgical sites with an aminoglycoside preparation. Aminoglycosides are also rapidly absorbed from the bronchial tree, wounds, or denuded skin after local instillation, or when used to irrigate joints; use of large doses at these sites may also result in substantial plasma concentrations of the drugs.

Distribution Following absorption, aminoglycosides are widely distributed into body fluids including ascitic, pericardial, peritoneal, pleural, synovial, and abscess fluids. Aminoglycosides are distributed primarily in the extracellular fluid volume. At a concentration of 15 mcg/mL, approximately 35% of streptomycin is bound to plasma proteins; other aminoglycosides are only minimally protein bound.

Aminoglycosides diffuse poorly into the CSF following IM or IV administration; even in patients with inflamed meninges, aminoglycoside concentrations in CSF are unpredictable and generally low (0–50% of concurrent serum concentrations). Following intralumbar administration, there may be limited upward diffusion of the drugs, presumably because of the direction of the CSF flow. Intraventricular administration usually produces high drug concentrations throughout the CNS. The drugs do not readily penetrate ocular tissue. Streptomycin does not penetrate thick-walled abscesses, but does penetrate tuberculosis cavities and caseous tissues. A small portion of each aminoglycoside dose accumulates in body tissues and is tightly bound intracellularly. Most body compartments and tissues including the inner ear and kidneys become progressively saturated with an aminoglycoside over the course of therapy, and the drug is slowly released from these areas. It has been postulated that this accumulation may account for the ototoxicity and nephrotoxicity associated with aminoglycosides. The individual aminoglycosides differ in their affinity for renal tissue; streptomycin has less affinity for renal tissue than the other aminoglycosides.

In general, aminoglycosides readily cross the placenta, and fetal serum concentrations of the drugs are reported to be 16–50% of maternal serum concentrations. Small amounts of the drugs are also distributed into bile, saliva, sweat, tears, sputum, and milk.

Elimination The plasma elimination half-lives ($t_{1/2}$s) of aminoglycosides are usually 2–4 hours in adults with normal renal function. Plasma concentrations are higher and plasma elimination $t_{1/2}$s are more prolonged in patients with impaired renal function. Plasma concentrations and plasma elimination $t_{1/2}$s of the drugs are not usually affected by hepatic impairment; however, the plasma elimination $t_{1/2}$ of streptomycin has been reported to be more prolonged in patients with both renal and hepatic impairment than in patients with renal impairment alone. In infants, aminoglycoside plasma elimination $t_{1/2}$s are inversely proportional to birthweight and gestational age and probably reflect renal maturity. Studies using gentamicin indicate that febrile patients may have slightly lower plasma concentrations of the drug than afebrile patients given the same dose; however, the clinical importance of this effect is unclear. Plasma concentrations of gentamicin (and presumably other aminoglycosides) may also be lower and the plasma elimination $t_{1/2}$ prolonged in patients with marked edema or pathologic fluid collections because of altered distribution of the drug.

Aminoglycosides are not metabolized and are excreted unchanged in the urine primarily by glomerular filtration. In patients with normal renal function, 40–97% of a single IM or IV dose of an aminoglycoside is excreted in the urine within 24 hours. Because a small portion of each aminoglycoside dose accumulates in body tissues, complete recovery of a single dose in urine requires approximately 10–20 days in patients with normal renal function. Terminal elimination $t_{1/2}$s of greater than 100 hours have been reported for amikacin, gentamicin, and tobramycin in adults with normal renal function following repeated IM or IV administration of the drugs. Following oral administration, unabsorbed neomycin is excreted unchanged in the feces.

Aminoglycosides are readily removed by hemodialysis and to a lesser extent by peritoneal dialysis; the amount of drug removed depends on several factors (e.g., type of coil used, flow-rate).

Chemistry and Stability

Chemistry Aminoglycosides are antibiotics and semisynthetic antibiotic derivatives obtained from cultures of *Streptomyces* or *Micromonospora*. The drugs contain 1 or 2 amino sugars glycosidically linked to an aminocyclitol nucleus and are more accurately termed aminoglycosidic aminocyclitols. Streptidine is the aminocyclitol nucleus of streptomycin, and 2-deoxystreptamine is the aminocyclitol nucleus of amikacin, gentamicin, kanamycin, neomycin, paromomycin, and tobramycin.

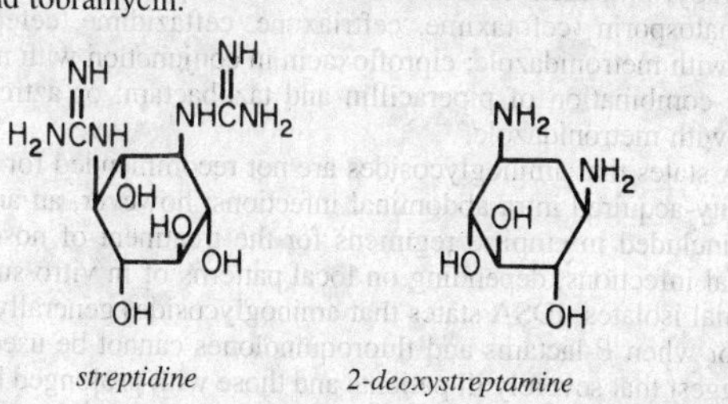

NH NH H2NCNH NHCNH2 OH HO OH OH NH2 NH2 OH HO OH

streptidine *2-deoxystreptamine*

Neomycin B and paromomycin contain 3 amino sugars attached to the central 2-deoxystreptamine nucleus. The kanamycin family (kanamycins A and B, amikacin, tobramycin) contains 2 amino sugars attached to the central 2-deoxystreptamine nucleus. The gentamicin family (C_1, C_2, and C_{1A}) contains a different 3-amino sugar (garosamine). Amikacin is a semisynthetic derivative prepared from kanamycin A with a wider spectrum of activity than the parent drug.

Amikacin, gentamicin, kanamycin, streptomycin, and tobramycin are commercially available for parenteral administration as sulfate salts; neomycin and paromomycin are commercially available for oral administration as sulfate salts; and tobramycin is commercially available as the base for oral inhalation via nebulization. Aminoglycosides are highly polar molecules and are relatively lipid insoluble.

Stability In general, aminoglycosides are stable at pH 2–11 and are most active at alkaline pH. The 2-deoxystreptamine derivatives are heat stable; however, streptomycin deteriorates if heated and should not be autoclaved. Aqueous solutions of the aminoglycosides may be discolored by light and are subject to darkening by air oxidation; discoloration does not appear to affect potency.

Aminoglycosides are potentially physically and/or chemically incompatible with many drugs including β-lactam antibiotics (e.g., penicillins, cephalosporins), but the compatibility depends on the specific drug and several other factors (e.g., concentration of the drugs, specific diluents used, resulting pH, temperature). Specialized references should be consulted for specific compatibility information. (See also Drug Interactions: Anti-infective Agents.)

For specific dosages and additional information on chemistry and stability, pharmacokinetics, and uses of the aminoglycosides, see the individual monographs in 8:12.02 and see Paromomycin 8:30.04.

†Use is not currently included in the labeling approved by the US Food and Drug Administration

Amikacin Sulfate

■ Amikacin is a semisynthetic aminoglycoside antibiotic derived from kanamycin A.

Uses

■ **Serious Bacterial Infections** Amikacin is used for the short-term treatment of serious infections caused by susceptible gram-negative bacteria, including *Acinetobacter*, *Escherichia coli*, *Enterobacter*, *Klebsiella*, *Proteus*, *Providencia*, *Pseudomonas*, or *Serratia marcescens*. Amikacin may be the preferred aminoglycoside for initial treatment of serious nosocomial gram-negative infections, especially in areas where resistance to gentamicin and tobramycin has been reported.

Although amikacin and other aminoglycosides are not usually recommended for the treatment of staphylococcal infections, the manufacturers state that amikacin may be considered for the treatment of known or suspected staphylococcal infections in certain situations. This includes initial treatment of severe infections when the causative organisms may be either gram-negative bacteria or staphylococci, treatment of infections caused by susceptible staphylococci in patients hypersensitive to other more appropriate anti-infectives, and treatment of mixed infections that may involve both gram-negative bacteria and staphylococci.

■ **Intra-abdominal Infections** Amikacin is used for the treatment of serious intra-abdominal infections (including peritonitis) caused by susceptible gram-negative bacteria, including *Acinetobacter*, *Enterobacter*, *E. coli*, *Klebsiella*, *Proteus*, *Providencia*, *Serratia*, or *Pseudomonas*. Amikacin usually is used as an adjunct to other appropriate anti-infectives (e.g., clindamycin, metronidazole, piperacillin and tazobactam, ampicillin and sulbactam).

The Infectious Diseases Society of America (IDSA) states that patients with community-acquired intra-abdominal infections of mild to moderate severity may receive initial treatment with an empiric regimen of the fixed combination of ampicillin and sulbactam, cefazolin or cefuroxime in conjunction with metronidazole, the fixed combination of ticarcillin and clavulanate, ertapenem monotherapy, or a fluoroquinolone (ciprofloxacin, levofloxacin, moxifloxacin) in conjunction with metronidazole. Patients who are immunosuppressed or have more severe community-acquired intra-abdominal infections should receive a regimen that has a broader spectrum of activity such as meropenem monotherapy; imipenem and cilastatin monotherapy; a third or fourth generation cephalosporin (cefotaxime, ceftriaxone, ceftazidime, cefepime) in conjunction with metronidazole; ciprofloxacin in conjunction with metronidazole; the fixed combination of piperacillin and tazobactam; or aztreonam in conjunction with metronidazole.

IDSA states that aminoglycosides are not recommended for *routine* use in community-acquired intra-abdominal infections; however, an aminoglycoside may be included in empiric regimens for the treatment of nosocomial intra-abdominal infections, depending on local patterns of in vitro susceptibility of nosocomial isolates. IDSA states that aminoglycosides generally should be reserved for when β-lactams and fluoroquinolones cannot be used. Other clinicians suggest that severely ill patients and those with prolonged hospitalization should receive an initial regimen that includes an antipseudomonal agent such as an antipseudomonal penicillin (ticarcillin and clavulanate, piperacillin and tazobactam), a carbapenem (imipenem or meropenem), ceftazidime, or cefepime used in conjunction with metronidazole. These clinicians state that an aminoglycoside also could be included in the empiric regimen.

■ **Meningitis and Other CNS Infections** Amikacin is used for the treatment of meningitis caused by susceptible gram-negative bacteria. Like other aminoglycosides, amikacin should not be used alone for the treatment of meningitis, but may be used in conjunction with other anti-infectives.

Amikacin has been used in conjunction with ampicillin for initial empiric treatment of meningitis caused by *Streptococcus agalactiae* (group B streptococci) in neonates or for *Listeria monocytogenes* meningitis in children. Concomitant use of amikacin and a third-generation cephalosporin also has been used for the treatment of neonatal gram-negative bacterial meningitis, including infections caused by *E. coli*. In adults, amikacin has been used concomitantly with imipenem for the treatment of meningitis caused by *E. coli*, concomitantly with meropenem for the treatment of meningitis caused by *Pseudomonas*, or concomitantly with imipenem or colistin (commercially available as colistimethate sodium) for the treatment of meningitis caused by *Acinetobacter*. To provide higher amikacin CSF concentrations for the treatment of meningitis, amikacin has been given intrathecally† or intraventricularly† concomitantly with IM or IV administration. Although concomitant parenteral and intrathecal or intraventricular therapy may result in higher anti-infective CSF concentrations, such therapy also may be associated with increased mortality in neonates.

■ **Mycobacterial Infections** ***Active Tuberculosis*** Amikacin is used in conjunction with antituberculosis agents for the treatment of active tuberculosis†.

The American Thoracic Society (ATS), US Centers for Disease Control and Prevention (CDC), and Infectious Diseases Society of America (IDSA) recommend several possible multiple-drug regimens for the treatment of culture-positive pulmonary tuberculosis. These regimens have a minimum duration of 6 months (26 weeks), and consist of an initial intensive phase (2 months) and a continuation phase (usually either 4 or 7 months).

Amikacin is considered a second-line agent for use in multiple-drug regimens in patients with relapse, treatment failure, or *Mycobacterium tuberculosis* resistant to isoniazid and/or rifampin or when first-line drugs cannot be tolerated. If amikacin is added as a new drug to a regimen in patients experiencing treatment failure who have proven or suspected drug-resistant tuberculosis, at least 2 (preferably 3) new drugs known or expected to be active against the resistant strain should be added at the same time. After results of in vitro susceptibility testing are available, the regimen can be adjusted accordingly. Streptomycin-resistant *M. tuberculosis* may be susceptible to both amikacin and kanamycin; complete cross-resistance usually occurs between amikacin and kanamycin. Patients with treatment failure or drug-resistant *M. tuberculosis* should be managed in consultation with an expert in the treatment of tuberculosis.

For information on general principles of antituberculosis therapy and recommendations regarding specific multiple-drug regimens and duration of therapy, see the Antituberculosis Agents General Statement 8:16.04.

Other Mycobacterial Infections Amikacin has been used as an alternative agent in multiple-drug regimens used for the treatment of *M. avium* complex† (MAC) infections. A regimen of amikacin, ethambutol, rifampin, and ciprofloxacin and a regimen of amikacin, ethambutol, ciprofloxacin, and clarithromycin or azithromycin has been used with some success in HIV-infected patients. However, there was no evidence that addition of amikacin to a regimen of rifampin, ethambutol, clofazimine, and ciprofloxacin provided any additional benefit in HIV-infected patients.

Amikacin is used in conjunction with other antimycobacterial anti-infectives for the treatment of nonpulmonary infections caused by *M. abscessus*†, *M. chelonae*†, and *M. fortuitum*†.

■ **Nocardia Infections** Amikacin is used in the treatment of infections caused by *Nocardia*†. Sulfonamides (usually co-trimoxazole) are the treatment of choice for most *Nocardia* infections; concomitant use of amikacin, imipenem, and/or ceftriaxone is recommended for initial treatment of severe or disseminated infections. When sulfonamides cannot be used, some clinicians recommend regimens containing amikacin, a carbapenem (imipenem or meropenem), a third-generation cephalosporin (ceftriaxone), a tetracycline (doxycycline, minocycline), fixed combination of amoxicillin and clavulanate, clarithromycin, cycloserine, or linezolid. In vitro susceptibility testing, if available, is recommended for *Nocardia* isolates from patients with invasive disease and those unable to tolerate a sulfonamide. Prolonged treatment is necessary.

■ **Rhodococcus Infections** Amikacin is used for the treatment of infections caused by *Rhodococcus equi*†. Optimum regimens for these infections have not been identified, but combination regimens have been recommended. Some clinicians suggest that the regimen of choice is vancomycin with or without a fluoroquinolone, rifampin, carbapenem (imipenem or meropenem), or amikacin.

■ **Empiric Therapy in Febrile Neutropenic Patients** Amikacin is used for empiric anti-infective therapy of presumed bacterial infections in febrile neutropenic patients†. Amikacin is used in conjunction with an appropriate antipseudomonal cephalosporin (e.g., ceftazidime, ceftriaxone, cefepime), extended-spectrum penicillin (e.g., piperacillin and tazobactam, ticarcillin and clavulanate), or carbapenem (e.g., imipenem, meropenem).

Published protocols for the treatment of infections in febrile neutropenic patients should be consulted for specific recommendations regarding selection of the initial empiric regimen, when to change the initial regimen, possible subsequent regimens, and duration of therapy in these patients. Consultation with an infectious disease expert knowledgeable about infections in immunocompromised patients also is advised.

Dosage and Administration

■ **Administration** Amikacin sulfate is administered by IM injection or IV infusion.

Amikacin sulfate has been given intrathecally† or intraventricularly† as an adjunct to IM or IV administration of the drug for the treatment of meningitis and other CNS infections.

Although amikacin has been given intraperitoneally†, the risk of toxicity associated with this route should be considered. (See Cautions in the Aminoglycosides General Statement 8:12.02.)

Patients should be well hydrated prior to and during amikacin therapy to minimize chemical irritation of renal tubules which may occur as the result of high urine amikacin concentrations.

Renal function should be assessed prior to and daily during amikacin therapy. Patients should be under close clinical observation because of the risk of ototoxicity and nephrotoxicity. (See Cautions in the Aminoglycosides General Statement 8:12.02.)

Prior to administration, amikacin solutions should be inspected visually for particulate matter or discoloration.

IM Injection For IM injection, the appropriate dose of commercially available injection containing amikacin in a concentration of 50 or 250 mg/mL should be given undiluted. IM injections of amikacin have been given into the upper outer quadrant of the buttocks.

IV Infusion IV infusions for adults are prepared by adding 500 mg of amikacin to 100–200 mL of compatible IV infusion fluid (e.g., 0.9% sodium chloride, 5% dextrose). (See Chemistry and Stability: Stability.) For pediatric patients, the volume of diluent depends on the dosage of amikacin prescribed and is chosen to provide the appropriate infusion rate.

Amikacin should not be admixed with other drugs or infused simultaneously through the same tubing with other drugs. If a β-lactam anti-infective (e.g., cephalosporin, penicillin) is administered concomitantly with amikacin, the drugs should not be admixed and should be administered separately.

Rate of Administration. In adults, IV infusions of amikacin should be given over 30–60 minutes.

In pediatric patients, the volume of infusion fluid should be sufficient to provide an infusion period of 1–2 hours in infants or 30–60 minutes in older children.

■ Dosage

Dosage of amikacin sulfate is expressed in terms of amikacin. IM and IV dosage is identical.

Like other aminoglycosides, dosage of amikacin should be individualized taking into consideration the patient's pretreatment body weight, renal status, severity of the infection, and susceptibility of the causative organism. Many clinicians recommend that amikacin dosage be determined using appropriate pharmacokinetic methods for calculating dosage requirements and patient-specific pharmacokinetic parameters (e.g., elimination rate constant, volume of distribution) derived from serum concentration-time data.

Whenever possible, especially in patients with life-threatening infections, suspected toxicity or nonresponse to treatment, decreased or varying renal function, and/or when increased aminoglycoside clearance (e.g., patients with cystic fibrosis, burns) or prolonged therapy is likely, peak and trough serum concentrations of amikacin should be determined periodically and dosage should be adjusted to maintain desired serum concentrations. (See Dosage and Administration: Dosage, in the Aminoglycosides General Statement 8:12.02.) A causal relationship between maintenance of certain peak or trough serum concentrations or other pharmacodynamic endpoints and clinical response or toxicity has not been established to date for amikacin dosing regimens. However, for amikacin administered in conventional dosage regimens (i.e., multiple daily doses), peak serum concentrations of 15–30 and trough concentrations less than 5–10 mcg/mL have been suggested. Amikacin serum concentrations greater than 30–35 mcg/mL may be associated with toxicity. The manufacturers recommend that peak serum concentrations (30–90 minutes after injection) greater than 35 mcg/mL and trough serum concentrations (just prior to the next dose) greater than 10 mcg/mL should be avoided.

Parenteral aminoglycosides historically have been administered in dosage regimens that include multiple daily doses, and current prescribing information for IM or IV amikacin only includes dosage regimens that involve multiple daily doses (usually 2 or 3 doses daily). However, there is evidence that once-daily† (single-daily) aminoglycoside dosage regimens are at least as effective as, may provide superior pharmacokinetics, and may be less toxic than conventional dosage regimens employing multiple daily doses. Once-daily parenteral aminoglycoside regimens should *not* be used in all patients. Additional controlled studies in children, patients with renal dysfunction, and other appropriate patient groups are needed to fully define the optimal use of once-daily aminoglycoside dosing regimens. In addition, the most appropriate methods for optimizing dosage selection for once-daily regimens and monitoring serum aminoglycoside concentrations in patients receiving such regimens have not been clearly established. (See Dosage and Administration: Dosage, in the Aminoglycosides General Statement 8:12.02.)

The usual duration of amikacin treatment is 7–10 days. The manufacturers state that safety of amikacin treatment for longer than 14 days has *not* been established. If a clinical response does not occur within 3–5 days, amikacin should be discontinued and in vitro susceptibility to the drug should be reassessed. In difficult and complicated infections, use of amikacin should be reevaluated if treatment longer than 10 days is being considered. If the drug is continued, serum amikacin concentrations and renal, auditory, and vestibular functions should be monitored closely.

The maximum dosage of amikacin recommended by the manufacturers is 15 mg/kg (up to 1.5 g) daily.

Adult Dosage **General Adult Dosage.** If IM or IV amikacin is used for the treatment of serious infections caused by susceptible bacteria in adults with normal renal function, the usual adult dosage recommended by the manufacturers is 15 mg/kg daily given in 2 or 3 equally divided doses (i.e., 5 mg/kg every 8 hours or 7.5 mg/kg every 12 hours).

Adults have received amikacin in a once-daily† regimen of 15 mg/kg once daily.

Active Tuberculosis. The American Thoracic Society (ATS), US Centers for Disease Control and Prevention (CDC), and Infectious Diseases Society of America (IDSA) state that the usual dosage of IM or IV amikacin for use in conjunction with other antituberculosis agents for the treatment of active tuberculosis† in adults is 15 mg/kg daily (up to 1 g) given as a single daily dose (usually 750–1000 mg daily) 5–7 times weekly for the first 2–4 months or until culture conversion; dosage can then be reduced to 15 mg/kg daily (up to 1 g) given 2 or 3 times weekly, depending on efficacy of the other drugs in the regimen.

The ATS, CDC, and IDSA recommend that adults older than 59 years of age receive a dosage of 10 mg/kg (up to 750 mg) daily.

Other Mycobacterial Infections. Amikacin has been given IM or IV in a dosage of 7.5–15 mg/kg daily in conjunction with other antimycobacterial anti-infectives for the treatment of infections caused by *Mycobacterium avium* complex† (MAC).

For the treatment of infections caused by *M. abscessus*† or *M. fortuitum*†, IV amikacin has been given in a dosage of 10–15 mg/kg daily in 2 divided doses in conjunction with other antimycobacterial anti-infectives.

Meningitis. If amikacin is used for the treatment of meningitis, some clinicians recommend that adults receive 15 mg/kg daily given in 3 divided doses.

In adults with meningitis caused by susceptible gram-negative bacteria, 4–20 mg of amikacin has been administered intrathecally† or intraventricularly† as a single daily dose in conjunction with IM or IV amikacin given in a dosage of 7.5 mg/kg every 12 hours.

Nocardiosis. For the treatment of nocardiosis†, IM or IV amikacin has been given in a dosage of 5–7.5 mg/kg every 12 hours.

Urinary Tract Infections. If amikacin is used for the treatment of uncomplicated urinary tract infections caused by susceptible bacteria when other less toxic anti-infectives cannot be used, the usual adult dosage is 250 mg twice daily.

Empiric Therapy in Febrile Neutropenic Patients. For empiric anti-infective therapy of presumed bacterial infections in febrile neutropenic patients†, adults have received IV amikacin in a dosage of 7.5 mg/kg twice daily in conjunction with IV ceftazidime or IV cefepime.

Pediatric Dosage **General Dosage for Neonates.** The manufacturers state that amikacin should be used with caution in premature and full-term neonates because renal immaturity in these patients may result in a prolonged serum half-life of the drug.

When IM or IV amikacin is used in neonates, the manufacturers recommend an initial loading dose of 10 mg/kg followed by 7.5 mg/kg every 12 hours.

The American Academy of Pediatrics (AAP) recommends that neonates younger than 1 week of age receive IM or IV amikacin in a dosage of 7.5 mg/kg every 18–24 hours if they weigh less than 1.2 kg, 7.5 mg/kg every 12 hours if they weigh 1.2–2 kg, or 7.5–10 mg/kg every 12 hours if they weigh more than 2 kg. For neonates 1–4 weeks of age, the AAP recommends a dosage of 7.5 mg/kg every 18–24 hours for those weighing less than 1.2 kg, 7.5–10 mg/kg every 8 or 12 hours for those weighing 1.2–2 kg, and 10 mg/kg every 8 hours for those weighing more than 2 kg. The AAP states that the drug is inappropriate for the treatment of mild to moderate infections.

Full-term neonates have received amikacin in a once-daily† regimen of 15 mg/kg once daily.

General Dosage for Infants and Children. The usual dosage of IM or IV amikacin recommended by the manufacturers for children and older infants with normal renal function is 15 mg/kg daily given in 2 or 3 equally divided doses (i.e., 7.5 mg/kg every 12 hours or 5 mg/kg every 8 hours).

The AAP recommends that pediatric patients beyond the neonatal period receive IM or IV amikacin in a dosage of 15–22.5 mg/kg daily given in 3 equally divided doses for the treatment of severe infections. Some clinicians suggest a dosage of 30 mg/kg daily given in 3 equally divided doses in this age group. The AAP states that the drug is inappropriate for the treatment of mild to moderate infections.

Children have received amikacin in a once-daily† regimen of 15–20 mg/kg once daily.

Active Tuberculosis. For the treatment of active tuberculosis† in children younger than 15 years of age or weighing 40 kg or less, the ATS, CDC, and IDSA state that the usual dosage of IM or IV amikacin for use in conjunction with other antituberculosis agents is 15–30 mg/kg daily (up to 1 g) given once daily or twice weekly.

For the treatment of active tuberculosis in children 15 years of age or older or weighing more than 40 kg, the ATS, CDC, and IDSA state that the usual dosage of IM or IV amikacin for use in conjunction with other antimycobacterial agents is 15 mg/kg daily (up to 1 g) given as a single daily dose (usually 750–1000 mg daily) 5–7 times weekly for the first 2–4 months or until culture conversion; dosage can then be reduced to 15 mg/kg daily (up to 1 g) given 2 or 3 times weekly, depending on efficacy of the other drugs in the regimen.

When IM or IV amikacin is used for the treatment of drug-resistant tuberculosis, the AAP recommends that infants, children, or adolescents receive a dosage of 15–30 mg/kg daily (up to 1 g).

Meningitis. If parenteral amikacin is used for the treatment of meningitis, some clinicians recommend that neonates 7 days of age or younger receive 15–20 mg/kg daily given in 2 divided doses and that older neonates and children receive 20–30 mg/kg daily given in 3 divided doses. Smaller doses and longer intervals between doses may be indicated in neonates weighing less than 2 kg.

Empiric Therapy in Febrile Neutropenic Patients. For empiric anti-infective therapy of presumed bacterial infections in febrile neutropenic patients†, children 1–17 years of age have received IV amikacin in a dosage of 20 mg/kg once daily or 6.5 mg/kg 3 times daily has been used in conjunction with IV ceftazidime.

■ **Dosage in Renal Impairment** In patients with impaired renal function, doses and/or frequency of administration of amikacin must be modified in response to serum concentrations of the drug and the degree of renal impairment. There are various methods to determine dosage and a wide variation in dosage recommendations for these patients. However, even when one of these methods is used, peak and trough serum concentrations of the drug should be monitored, especially in patients with changing renal function.

The manufacturers recommend an initial amikacin loading dose of 7.5 mg/kg. For subsequent therapy, the manufacturers state that 7.5-mg/kg doses can be given at intervals (in hours) calculated by multiplying the patient's steady-state serum creatinine (in mg/dL) by 9. Alternatively, many clinicians recommend the dosing method of Sarubbi and Hull, which is based on corrected creatinine clearance. (See Dosage and Administration: Dosage in Renal Impairment, in the Aminoglycosides General Statement 8:12.02.)

In adults with renal failure undergoing hemodialysis, some clinicians recommend supplemental doses of 50–75% of the initial loading dose at the end of each dialysis period. Others suggest that supplemental amikacin doses may not be necessary in patients undergoing short-term hemodialysis. Serum amikacin concentrations should be monitored in dialysis patients and dosage adjusted as needed to maintain desired serum concentrations.

For the treatment of active tuberculosis† in adults with renal impairment, the ATS, CDC, and IDSA recommend that usual doses be given at less frequent intervals since use of lower doses may reduce efficacy of the drug. These experts recommend that adults with renal impairment receive amikacin in a dosage of 12–15 mg/kg daily given 2 or 3 times weekly. In addition, if the patient is receiving hemodialysis, the dose should be given after the procedure is finished and serum concentrations of the drug monitored to avoid toxicity.

Pharmacokinetics

The pharmacokinetics of amikacin are similar to those of the other aminoglycosides. In all studies described in the Pharmacokinetics section, amikacin was administered as the sulfate salt; dosages and concentrations of the drug are expressed in terms of amikacin.

■ **Absorption** Amikacin is poorly absorbed from the GI tract.

Amikacin is rapidly absorbed following IM administration. Following IM administration of a single 7.5-mg/kg dose of amikacin in adults with normal renal function, peak plasma amikacin concentrations are attained within about 0.5–2 hours and average 17–25 mcg/mL; plasma concentrations 10 hours after the dose average 2.1 mcg/mL.

When a 7.5-mg/kg dose of amikacin is administered by IV infusion over 30 minutes, peak plasma concentrations of the drug average 38 mcg/mL immediately following the infusion, 18 mcg/mL at 1 hour, and 0.75 mcg/mL at 10 hours. In adults receiving 15 mg/kg once daily by IV infusion over 30 minutes, peak serum concentrations (measured 30 minutes after completion of an infusion) were 40.9 mcg/mL and trough concentrations (measured immediately before start of an infusion) were 1.8 mcg/mL.

In a study in neonates, peak serum amikacin concentrations of 17–20 mcg/mL were attained 30 minutes after a single 7.5-mg/kg IM dose of the drug. In a study in infants (mean age 3.5 months) with serious infections, serum amikacin concentrations after a single 7.5-mg/kg dose ranged from 11.8–23 mcg/mL at 30–60 minutes after the dose, averaged 4.2 mcg/mL 4 hours after the dose, and were undetectable (less than 0.8 mcg/mL) 12 hours after the dose. When this same dose was given to children up to 6 years of age (mean age 3.1 years), peak serum amikacin concentrations were attained 30–60 minutes after the dose and ranged from 9–29 mcg/mL; serum concentrations 4 hours after the dose averaged 3.7 mcg/ml and the drug was undetectable (less than 0.8 mcg/mL) 12 hours after the dose.

Plasma concentrations of amikacin may be lower in pregnant women than in nonpregnant patients, probably because of an increased volume of distribution and increased glomerular filtration rate.

Accumulation of amikacin does not appear to occur in adult or pediatric patients with normal renal function receiving usual dosages of the drug twice daily for 4–10 days.

■ **Distribution** Following administration of usual dosages of amikacin, therapeutic concentrations of the drug are achieved in bone, heart, gallbladder, and lung tissue. Amikacin also is well distributed into urine, bile, sputum, bronchial secretions, and interstitial, pleural, and synovial fluids.

In a study in adults with bronchopneumonia who received IV amikacin in a dosage of 15 mg/kg once daily or 7.5 mg/kg twice daily, mean concentrations of amikacin in bronchial secretions (3 hours after initiation of the IV infusion on day 1) were 13.6 or 4.8 mcg/mL, respectively. In the group that received the once-daily regimen, mean concentrations in bronchial secretions remained above 8 mcg/mL for 12 hours after a dose while mean concentrations in bronchial secretions remained at 3–4 mcg/mL for a 24-hour period in those receiving the twice-daily regimen.

Amikacin is distributed into CSF in low concentrations following IM or IV administration. In infants, CSF concentrations may be 10–20% of concurrent serum concentrations, but may be 50% of concurrent serum concentrations in those with inflamed meninges. In a study in children 4 months to 8 years of age with bacterial meningitis who received 7.5 mg/kg of amikacin twice daily by IV infusion over 30 minutes in conjunction with IV ceftriaxone (amikacin infusions were started 1 hour after ceftriaxone infusions were completed), CSF concentrations 3 hours after the third amikacin dose averaged 1.65 mcg/mL.

In one adult with meningitis, intrathecal administration of 4 mg of amikacin daily in conjunction with IM administration of 15 mg/kg daily for 2 weeks resulted in CSF concentrations of the drug ranging from 7–40 mcg/mL 12 hours after an intrathecal dose and 1–19 mcg/mL 24 hours after an intrathecal dose.

The apparent volume of distribution of amikacin in healthy adults averages about 24 L (28% of body weight). The apparent volume of distribution of the drug in neonates indicates that amikacin is distributed principally into the extracellular fluid volume in this age group.

Amikacin crosses the placenta and is distributed into amniotic fluid. Peak fetal serum concentrations are about 16% of peak maternal serum concentrations.

Amikacin is distributed into milk in low concentrations.

■ **Elimination** The plasma elimination half-life of amikacin usually is 2–3 hours in adults with normal renal function and is reported to range from 28–86 hours in adults with severe renal impairment.

The plasma elimination half-life of amikacin is reported to be 4–5 hours in full-term infants 7 days of age or older and 7–8 hours in low birth-weight infants 1–3 days of age. In preterm neonates, half-life is inversely related to postconceptional age and has ranged from 4.5–15.6 hours. In one study in infants and children 20 days to 6 years of age, mean plasma half-life after a single 7.5-mg/kg IM dose was about 2 hours.

In adults with normal renal function, 94–98% of a single IM or IV dose of amikacin is excreted unchanged by glomerular filtration within 24 hours. Urine concentrations of amikacin average 563 mcg/mL for 6 hours following a single 250-mg IM dose and 832 mcg/mL following a single 500-mg IM dose in adults with normal renal function.

Amikacin is removed by hemodialysis. The drug also is removed by peritoneal dialysis, including continuous ambulatory peritoneal dialysis.

Chemistry and Stability

■ **Chemistry** Amikacin is a semisynthetic aminoglycoside antibiotic derived from kanamycin A. The drug is commercially available as the sulfate salt. Amikacin sulfate occurs as a white, crystalline powder and is freely soluble in water. Commercially available amikacin sulfate injection is a colorless to light straw-colored solution; sulfuric acid is added during the manufacturing process to adjust the pH to 3.5–5.5.

■ **Stability** Amikacin sulfate injection should be stored at 15–30°C. Although amikacin sulfate solutions may become light straw-colored during storage, this does not indicate loss of potency.

Amikacin sulfate is stable for 24 hours at room temperature at concentrations of 0.25 and 5 mg/mL in most IV infusion fluids, including 0.9% sodium chloride, 5% dextrose injection, 5% dextrose in 0.2 or 0.45% sodium chloride injection, lactated Ringer's injection, Normosol-M® or Normosol-R® in 5% dextrose injection, Plasma-Lyte 56 or 148 in 5% dextrose injection. The above solutions also are stable for 24 hours at room temperature after being refrigerated at 4°C for 60 days or after being frozen for 30 days at −15°C. Amikacin sulfate injection should not be mixed with other drugs.

For further information on chemistry and stability, mechanism of action, spectrum, resistance, pharmacokinetics, uses, cautions, drug interactions, and dosage and administration of amikacin, see the Aminoglycosides General Statement 8:12.02.

Preparations

Excipients in commercially available drug preparations may have clinically important effects in some individuals; consult specific product labeling for details.

Amikacin Sulfate

Parenteral		
Injection	50 mg (of amikacin) per mL*	**Amikacin Sulfate Injection**
	250 mg (of amikacin) per mL*	**Amikacin Sulfate Injection**

*available from one or more manufacturer, distributor, and/or repackager by generic (nonproprietary) name

†Use is not currently included in the labeling approved by the US Food and Drug Administration

Gentamicin Sulfate

■ Gentamicin is an aminoglycoside antibiotic.

Uses

■ **Serious Bacterial Infections** Gentamicin is used for the treatment of serious bone and joint infections, respiratory tract infections, septicemia, skin and skin structure infections, and urinary tract infections caused by susceptible gram-negative bacteria, including *Citrobacter*, *Enterobacter*, *Escherichia coli*, *Klebsiella*, *Proteus*, *Serratia*, or *Pseudomonas aeruginosa*. The drug usually is used as an adjunct to an appropriate β-lactam (e.g., ceftriaxone, cefotaxime, cefepime, piperacillin and tazobactam, ticarcillin and clavulanate) or carbapenem (e.g., imipenem, meropenem) for empiric treatment of these infections. Gentamicin is not usually indicated for initial treatment of uncomplicated infections (e.g., uncomplicated urinary tract infections) unless the causative organism is susceptible and other less toxic anti-infectives cannot be used.

Gentamicin has been used for the treatment of serious infections, including bone and joint infections, septicemia, skin and skin structure infections, and urinary tract infections caused by susceptible *Staphylococcus aureus*. Although gentamicin and other aminoglycosides are not usually recommended for the treatment of staphylococcal infections, the manufacturers state that gentamicin may be considered for the treatment of known or suspected staphylococcal infections in certain situations. This includes treatment of infections caused by susceptible staphylococci when other more appropriate anti-infectives are contraindicated (e.g., because of hypersensitivity) or would be ineffective because of resistance and for initial treatment of mixed infections when the causative organisms may be either gram-negative bacteria or staphylococci. A regimen of vancomycin with or without gentamicin and with or without rifampin has been recommended for the treatment of oxacillin-resistant (methicillin-resistant) staphylococcal infections.

■ Intra-abdominal Infections

Gentamicin is used for the treatment of serious intra-abdominal infections (including peritonitis) caused by susceptible *Citrobacter*, *Enterobacter*, *E. coli*, *Klebsiella*, *Proteus*, *Serratia*, *Pseudomonas aeruginosa*, or *S. aureus*. Gentamicin usually is used as an adjunct to other appropriate anti-infectives (e.g., clindamycin, metronidazole, piperacillin and tazobactam, ampicillin and sulbactam).

The Infectious Diseases Society of America (IDSA) states that patients with community-acquired intra-abdominal infections of mild to moderate severity may receive initial treatment with an empiric regimen of the fixed combination of ampicillin and sulbactam, cefazolin or cefuroxime in conjunction with metronidazole, the fixed combination of ticarcillin and clavulanate, ertapenem monotherapy, or a fluoroquinolone (ciprofloxacin, levofloxacin, moxifloxacin) in conjunction with metronidazole. Patients who are immunosuppressed or have more severe community-acquired intra-abdominal infections should receive a regimen that has a broader spectrum of activity such as meropenem monotherapy; imipenem and cilastatin monotherapy; a third or fourth generation cephalosporin (cefotaxime, ceftriaxone, ceftazidime, cefepime) in conjunction with metronidazole; ciprofloxacin in conjunction with metronidazole; the fixed combination of piperacillin and tazobactam; or aztreonam in conjunction with metronidazole.

The IDSA states that aminoglycosides are not recommended for *routine* use in community-acquired intra-abdominal infections; however, an aminoglycoside may be included in empiric regimens for the treatment of nosocomial intra-abdominal infections, depending on local patterns of in vitro susceptibility of nosocomial isolates. IDSA states that aminoglycosides generally should be reserved for when β-lactams and fluoroquinolones cannot be used. Other clinicians suggest that severely ill patients and those with prolonged hospitalization should receive an initial regimen that includes an antipseudomonal agent such as an antipseudomonal penicillin (ticarcillin and clavulanate, piperacillin and tazobactam), a carbapenem (imipenem or meropenem), ceftazidime, or cefepime used in conjunction with metronidazole. These clinicians state that an aminoglycoside also could be included in the empiric regimen.

■ Endocarditis

Gentamicin is used for the treatment of bacterial endocarditis† and for prevention of bacterial endocarditis†.

Treatment **Enterococcal Endocarditis.** Gentamicin is used in conjunction with an appropriate anti-infective (ampicillin, penicillin G sodium, vancomycin) for the treatment of native or prosthetic valve endocarditis† caused by *Enterococcus* (e.g., *E. faecalis*, *E. faecium*). Enterococci usually are resistant to aminoglycosides alone and also are relatively resistant to ampicillin, penicillin G and vancomycin. However, because antibacterial activity of the drugs may be additive or synergistic, regimens of gentamicin or streptomycin used concomitantly with ampicillin, penicillin G sodium, or vancomycin may be effective in the treatment of enterococcal endocarditis.

For the treatment of native or prosthetic valve enterococcal endocarditis caused by strains *susceptible* to penicillin, vancomycin, and aminoglycosides, the American Heart Association (AHA) and IDSA recommend a regimen of IV ampicillin sodium or IV penicillin G sodium given in conjunction with either IV or IM gentamicin or IV or IM streptomycin. Streptomycin usually is used only if the strains are gentamicin-resistant. For patients unable to tolerate penicillins, an alternative regimen is IV vancomycin given in conjunction with IV or IM gentamicin or IV or IM streptomycin.

Enterococcal isolates should routinely be tested for in vitro susceptibility to penicillin and vancomycin and for high-level resistance to gentamicin and streptomycin. (See Spectrum: In Vitro Susceptibility Testing in the Aminoglycosides General Statement 8:12.02.) The most appropriate regimen for the treatment of enterococcal endocarditis is selected based on results of in vitro susceptibility testing; treatment duration depends on whether native or prosthetic valves are involved and how long symptoms have been present prior to initiation of treatment. Gentamicin usually is the preferred aminoglycoside for the treatment of enterococcal endocarditis, in part because IV gentamicin may be better tolerated than IM streptomycin and because laboratory monitoring of serum gentamicin concentrations may be more readily available than laboratory monitoring of streptomycin concentrations. However, streptomycin may be effective for the treatment of enterococcal endocarditis caused by gentamicin-resistant strains since some, but not all, enterococci with high-level resistance to gentamicin are susceptible to streptomycin. Vancomycin should be used only in patients unable to tolerate ampicillin or penicillin G since regimens that include vancomycin and an aminoglycoside may be associated with an increased risk of ototoxicity and nephrotoxicity and may be less effective compared with regimens that include one of the β-lactams and an aminoglycoside. (See Drug Interactions: Neurotoxic, Ototoxic, or Nephrotoxic Drugs, in the Aminoglycosides General Statement 8:12.02.)

Endocarditis Caused by Viridans Streptococci or S. bovis. Gentamicin is used in conjunction with other appropriate anti-infectives for the treatment of endocarditis caused by viridans streptococci† (e.g., *S. sanguis*, *S. oralis*, *S. salivarius*, *S. mutans*, *Gamella morbillorum*) or *S. bovis*† (nonenterococcal group D streptococci).

For the treatment of native valve endocarditis caused by viridans streptococci or *S. bovis* highly susceptible to penicillin (i.e., penicillin MIC of 0.12 mcg/mL or less), the AHA and IDSA recommend monotherapy with IV penicillin G sodium or IV or IM ceftriaxone given for 4 weeks. These monotherapy regimens avoid the use of gentamicin and are preferred in most patients older than 65 years of age and in those with impaired renal or eighth cranial nerve function. In *selected* patients only, the AHA and IDSA state that a 2-week regimen that consists of IV penicillin G sodium or IV or IM ceftriaxone in conjunction with IV or IM gentamicin can be used. The 2-week regimen should be used only in patients with uncomplicated native valve endocarditis caused by highly penicillin-susceptible viridans streptococci or *S. bovis* who are at low risk for gentamicin adverse effects; the 2-week regimen should *not* be used in those with known cardiac or extracardiac abscess, creatinine clearance less than 20 mL/minute, impaired eighth cranial nerve function, or infections caused by *Abiotrophia*, *Granulicatella*, or *Gemella*.

For the treatment of native valve endocarditis caused by viridans streptococci or *S. bovis* relatively resistant to penicillin (i.e., penicillin MIC greater than 0.12 mcg/mL and less than or equal to 0.5 mcg/mL), the AHA and IDSA recommend a 4-week regimen of IV penicillin G sodium or IV or IM ceftriaxone in conjunction with IV or IM gentamicin given during the initial 2 weeks of treatment. Alternatively, in patients unable to tolerate penicillin G sodium or ceftriaxone, IV vancomycin can be used.

In patients with prosthetic valves or other prosthetic material who have endocarditis caused by viridans streptococci or *S. bovis* highly susceptible to penicillin (i.e., penicillin MIC of 0.12 mcg/mL or less), the AHA and IDSA recommend a 6-week regimen of IV penicillin G sodium or IV or IM ceftriaxone with or without IV or IM gentamicin given during the initial 2 weeks of treatment. When highly penicillin-susceptible strains are involved, it is unclear whether the combination regimen that includes an aminoglycoside during the first 2 weeks is more effective than use of the β-lactam alone. If the strains involved are relatively or fully penicillin-resistant (i.e., penicillin MIC greater than 0.12 mcg/mL), the AHA and IDSA recommend a 6-week regimen of IV penicillin G sodium or IV or IM ceftriaxone given with a 6-week regimen of IV or IM gentamicin. Alternatively, in patients unable to tolerate penicillin G sodium or ceftriaxone, a 6-week regimen of IV vancomycin can be used.

Endocarditis caused by viridans streptococci or *S. bovis* highly resistant to penicillin (i.e., penicillin MIC greater than 0.5 mcg/mL) or caused by *Abiotrophia defectiva*, *Granulicatella*, or *Gamella* should be treated with a regimen recommended for enterococcal endocarditis. (See Enterococcal Endocarditis under Uses: Endocarditis.)

Staphylococcal Endocarditis. Gentamicin is used in conjunction with other appropriate anti-infectives for the treatment of staphylococcal endocarditis†, including infections caused by coagulase-positive strains (*S. aureus*) or coagulase-negative strains (e.g., *S. epidermidis*, *S. lugdunensis*).

For the treatment of native valve endocarditis caused by oxacillin-susceptible staphylococci, the AHA and IDSA recommend a regimen of IV nafcillin or oxacillin with or without IV or IM gentamicin. For penicillin-allergic patients (nonanaphylactoid type only), a regimen of IV cefazolin with or without IV or IM gentamicin is recommended. In patients with complicated right-sided staphylococcal endocarditis or with left-sided staphylococcal endocarditis, a 6-week regimen of the β-lactam should be used and gentamicin given concomitantly during the first 3–5 days of treatment. In those with uncomplicated right-sided staphylococcal endocarditis (i.e., patients with no evidence of renal failure, extrapulmonary metastatic infections, aortic or mitral valve involvement, meningitis, or oxacillin-resistant strains), a 2-week regimen that includes both the β-lactam and gentamicin can be considered.

Staphylococcal endocarditis in patients with prosthetic valves or other prosthetic material usually is caused by oxacillin-resistant staphylococci, especially when endocarditis develops within 1 year after surgery, and is associated with high morbidity and mortality rates. Unless susceptibility to oxacillin has been demonstrated using in vitro susceptibility testing, it should be assumed that patients with staphylococcal prosthetic valve endocarditis have oxacillin-resistant strains. If prosthetic valve endocarditis is known to be caused by oxacillin-susceptible staphylococci, the AHA and IDSA recommend at least 6 weeks of IV nafcillin or oxacillin in conjunction with IV or oral rifampin and concomitant use of IV or IM gentamicin during the initial 2 weeks of treatment. If the strain is known to be penicillin susceptible (i.e., penicillin MIC of 0.1 mcg/mL or less) and does not produce β-lactamase, IV penicillin G sodium can be substituted for nafcillin or oxacillin in this regimen; for penicillin-allergic patients (nonanaphylactoid type only), IV cefazolin can be substituted for nafcillin or oxacillin. If the strain is known or presumed to be oxacillin-resistant, the

AHA and IDSA recommend at least 6 weeks of IV vancomycin in conjunction with IV or oral rifampin and concomitant use of IV or IM gentamicin during the initial 2 weeks of treatment.

Prevention Gentamicin is used in conjunction with ampicillin or with vancomycin (in penicillin-allergic patients) for prevention of bacterial endocarditis† in patients undergoing certain genitourinary and GI tract (except esophageal) surgery or instrumentation who have cardiac conditions that put them at high risk. (See Prophylaxis of Bacterial Endocarditis under Uses: Prophylaxis in the Aminopenicillins General Statement 8:12.16.08)

The current recommendations published by the AHA should be consulted for specific information on which cardiac conditions are associated with high or moderate risk of endocarditis and which procedures require prophylaxis.

■ **Meningitis and Other CNS Infections** Gentamicin is used in conjunction with other anti-infectives for the treatment of CNS infections (meningitis) caused by susceptible *S. aureus*, *Citrobacter*, *Enterobacter*, *E. coli*, *Klebsiella*, *Proteus*, *Serratia*, or *Ps. aeruginosa*. Like other aminoglycosides, gentamicin should not be used alone for the treatment of meningitis, but may be used as an adjunct to other appropriate anti-infectives.

For initial empiric treatment of neonatal meningitis, especially when *Streptococcus agalactiae* (group B streptococci), *E. coli*, or *Listeria monocytogenes* might be involved, a regimen of ampicillin and cefotaxime with or without gentamicin has been recommended. For the treatment of nosocomial meningitis when *Pseudomonas* are involved, a regimen of vancomycin, an antipseudomonal cephalosporin (e.g., ceftazidime), and an aminoglycoside (amikacin, gentamicin, tobramycin) has been recommended. For the treatment of enterococcal meningitis†, a regimen of ampicillin and gentamicin has been recommended; if ampicillin-resistant enterococci are involved, a regimen of vancomycin and gentamicin has been recommended.

To provide higher gentamicin CSF concentrations for the treatment of meningitis, gentamicin has been given intrathecally† or intraventricularly† concomitantly with IM or IV administration. Although concomitant parenteral and intrathecal or intraventricular therapy may result in higher anti-infective CSF concentrations, such therapy also may be associated with increased mortality in neonates. Some clinicians state that intraventricular gentamicin should not be used routinely for the treatment of meningitis and should be reserved for patients who do not respond or are not likely to respond to parenteral anti-infectives alone.

■ **Bartonella Infections** Gentamicin has been used in the treatment of *Bartonella* infections†, including infections caused by *B. henselae* (e.g., cat scratch disease, bacillary angiomatosis, bacillary peliosis hepatitis, endocarditis), *B. quintana* (e.g., bacteremia, endocarditis, trench fever, bacillary angiomatosis), or *B. bacilliformis* (Carrion's disease).

Optimum anti-infective regimens for the treatment of *Bartonella* infections have not been identified, and various drugs have been used to treat these infections, including aminoglycosides (gentamicin), tetracyclines (doxycycline), macrolides (erythromycin, azithromycin), cephalosporins (ceftriaxone), quinolones (ciprofloxacin), chloramphenicol, vancomycin, co-trimoxazole, or rifampin. There is some evidence that effective treatment of *Bartonella* endocarditis should include an aminoglycoside (gentamicin) during at least the first 2 weeks of therapy.

Although cat scratch disease caused by *B. henselae* generally is a self-limited illness in immunocompetent individuals and localized infections may resolve spontaneously in 2–4 months, anti-infective therapy should be considered for acutely or severely ill patients with systemic manifestations, especially those with hepatic or splenic involvement, endocarditis, extensive lymphadenopathy, painful adenitis, or compromised immune function. Anti-infectives are indicated in patients with *B. quintana* infections and those who develop bacillary angiomatosis, bacillary peliosis, or trench fever. *B. quintana* infections have been reported most frequently in immunocompromised patients (e.g., individuals with HIV infection), homeless individuals in urban areas, and chronic alcohol abusers. Bartonella infections tend to persist or recur and prolonged therapy (several months or longer) usually is necessary, especially in immunocompromised patients.

■ **Brucellosis** ***Treatment*** Gentamicin is used in the treatment of brucellosis†. Tetracyclines generally are considered the drugs of choice for the treatment of brucellosis; however, concomitant use of another anti-infective (e.g., streptomycin or gentamicin and/or rifampin) is recommended to reduce the likelihood of relapse, especially for severe infections and when there are complications such as meningitis, endocarditis, or osteomyelitis. Monotherapy is no longer recommended for the treatment of brucellosis since such therapy is associated with high relapse rates.

A regimen of oral doxycycline and oral rifampin may be effective for the treatment of less severe brucellosis. For the treatment of acute, complicated brucellosis (e.g., skeletal disease, endocarditis), a regimen of oral doxycycline (or oral co-trimoxazole in children younger than 8 years of age) and oral rifampin, with IM streptomycin given during the first 2–3 weeks usually is recommended. Gentamicin can be used if streptomycin is unavailable. Although data are limited, alternative regimens that have been suggested for the treatment of brucellosis include co-trimoxazole with or without gentamicin (or streptomycin) or rifampin; ciprofloxacin (or ofloxacin) and rifampin; and chloramphenicol with or without streptomycin. For the treatment of neurobrucellosis, a regimen that includes a tetracycline, rifampin, and streptomycin is recommended.

Prophylaxis Postexposure prophylaxis with anti-infectives is not generally recommended after possible exposure to endemic brucellosis; however, use of an anti-infective regimen recommended for the treatment of brucellosis (e.g., doxycycline and rifampin) should be considered following a high-risk exposure to *Brucella*. These high-risk exposures include needlestick injuries involving the brucella vaccine available for veterinary use (a brucella vaccine for use in humans is not available), inadvertent laboratory exposure to the organism, or confirmed exposure in the context of biologic warfare or bioterrorism.

■ **Granuloma Inguinale (Donovanosis)** Gentamicin is used as an adjunct in the treatment of granuloma inguinale† (donovanosis), a sexually transmitted disease caused by *Klebsiella granulomatis* (formerly *Calymmatobacterium granulomatis*) involving genital ulcerative lesions. The CDC recommends that donovanosis be treated with a regimen of oral doxycycline or, alternatively, a regimen of oral azithromycin, oral ciprofloxacin, oral erythromycin, or oral co-trimoxazole. If lesions do not respond within the first few days of therapy, the CDC recommends that an aminoglycoside (e.g., gentamicin) be added to the treatment regimen. The CDC also states that consideration should be given to adding an aminoglycoside (e.g., gentamicin) to the treatment regimen in pregnant and lactating women and in HIV-infected individuals.

■ **Pelvic Inflammatory Disease** The CDC and many clinicians currently suggest IV clindamycin in conjunction with IV or IM gentamicin as one of several possible parenteral regimens for the treatment of acute pelvic inflammatory disease† (PID) in adults and adolescents.

For additional information on treatment of PID, see Uses: PID in Ceftriaxone Sodium 8:12.06.12.

■ **Plague** ***Treatment*** Gentamicin is used for the treatment of plague† caused by *Yersinia pestis*. Streptomycin generally has been considered the drug of choice for the treatment of bubonic, septicemia, and pneumonic plague; however, gentamicin also is considered a drug of choice since it may be as effective and is more readily available than streptomycin. Alternatives recommended when aminoglycosides are not used include doxycycline (or tetracycline), chloramphenicol, co-trimoxazole (may be less effective than other alternatives), or fluoroquinolones (ciprofloxacin, ofloxacin). Chloramphenicol generally is considered the drug of choice for the treatment of plague meningitis. Penicillins and other β-lactams are not recommended for the treatment of plague.

Anti-infective regimens recommended for the treatment of naturally occurring or endemic bubonic, septicemic, or pneumonic plague also are recommended for the treatment of plague that occurs following exposure to *Y. pestis* in the context of biologic warfare or bioterrorism. These exposures would most likely result in primary pneumonic plague. Prompt initiation of anti-infective therapy (within 18–24 hours of onset of symptoms) is essential in the treatment of pneumonic plague. Some experts (e.g., the US Working Group on Civilian Biodefense, US Army Medical Research Institute of Infectious Diseases [USAMRIID], European Commission Task Force on Biological and Chemical Agent Threats [BICHAT]) recommend that treatment of plague in the context of biologic warfare or bioterrorism should be initiated with a parenteral anti-infective such as streptomycin (or gentamicin) or, alternatively, doxycycline, ciprofloxacin, or chloramphenicol; an oral regimen (doxycycline, ciprofloxacin) may be substituted when the patient's condition improves or if parenteral therapy is unavailable.

Prompt initiation of anti-infective therapy (within 18–24 hours of onset of symptoms) is essential in the treatment of pneumonic plague. When plague is suspected, appropriate anti-infectives should be initiated immediately and not delayed for laboratory confirmation.

Prophylaxis Postexposure prophylaxis with anti-infectives is recommended after high-risk exposures to plague, including close exposure to individuals with naturally occurring plague or laboratory exposure to viable *Y. pestis*. In the context of biologic warfare or bioterrorism, some experts (e.g., the US Working Group on Civilian Biodefense, USAMRIID) recommend that asymptomatic individuals with exposure to plague aerosol or asymptomatic individuals with household, hospital, or other close contact (within about 2 m) with an individual who has pneumonic plague should receive postexposure anti-infective prophylaxis; however, any exposed individual who develops a temperature of 38.5°C or higher or new cough should promptly receive a parenteral anti-infective for treatment of the disease. An oral regimen of doxycycline or ciprofloxacin usually is recommended for such prophylaxis; although efficacy has not been established, co-trimoxazole has been recommended for prophylaxis in children younger than 8 years of age.

■ **Tularemia** ***Treatment*** Gentamicin is used in the treatment of tularemia† caused by *Francisella tularensis*. Although streptomycin generally is considered the drug of choice for this infection, gentamicin is more readily available and may be used as an alternative drug of choice when streptomycin is unavailable. Other alternatives for the treatment of tularemia include tetracyclines (doxycycline), chloramphenicol, or ciprofloxacin.

Anti-infective regimens recommended for the treatment of naturally occurring or endemic tularemia also are recommended for the treatment of tularemia that occurs following exposure to *F. tularensis* in the context of biologic warfare or bioterrorism. However, the fact that a fully virulent streptomycin-resistant strain of *F. tularensis* was developed in the past for use in biologic warfare should be considered. Exposures to *F. tularensis* in the context of biologic warfare or bioterrorism would most likely result in inhalational tularemia with pleuropneumonitis, although the organism also can infect humans through the skin, mucous membranes, and GI tract.

Prophylaxis Postexposure prophylaxis with anti-infectives usually is not recommended after possible exposure to natural or endemic tularemia (e.g., tick bite, rabbit or other animal exposure) and is unnecessary in close contacts of tularemia patients since human-to-human transmission of the disease is not known to occur. However, postexposure prophylaxis is recommended following a high-risk laboratory exposure to *F. tularensis* (e.g., spill, centrifuge accident, needlestick injury). In the context of biologic warfare or bioterrorism, some experts (e.g., the US Working Group on Civilian Biodefense, USAMRIID, BICHAT) recommend that asymptomatic individuals with exposure to *F. tularensis* receive postexposure anti-infective prophylaxis; however, any individual who develops an otherwise unexplained fever or flu-like illness within 14 days of presumed exposure should promptly receive a parenteral anti-infective for treatment of the disease. Oral doxycycline (or oral tetracycline) or oral ciprofloxacin usually is recommended for postexposure prophylaxis following such exposures; streptomycin or gentamicin also have been recommended for postexposure prophylaxis of tularemia†.

■ Empiric Therapy in Febrile Neutropenic Patients Gentamicin is used for empiric anti-infective therapy of presumed bacterial infections in febrile neutropenic patients†. Gentamicin is used in conjunction with an appropriate antipseudomonal cephalosporin (e.g., ceftazidime, ceftriaxone, cefepime), extended-spectrum penicillin (e.g., piperacillin and tazobactam, ticarcillin and clavulanate), or carbapenem (e.g., imipenem, meropenem). Gentamicin should not be used alone for empiric therapy in febrile neutropenic patients.

Published protocols for the treatment of infections in febrile neutropenic patients should be consulted for specific recommendations regarding selection of the initial empiric regimen, when to change the initial regimen, possible subsequent regimens, and duration of therapy in these patients. Consultation with an infectious disease expert knowledgeable about infections in immunocompromised patients also is advised.

■ Perioperative Prophylaxis Gentamicin is used in conjunction with clindamycin for perioperative prophylaxis† in patients undergoing head and neck surgery (incisions through oral or pharyngeal mucosa). In addition, in patients who cannot receive β-lactams, a regimen of vancomycin with or without gentamicin has been recommended as an alternative for perioperative prophylaxis in those undergoing vascular surgery and a regimen of clindamycin or metronidazole with gentamicin has been recommended as an alternative for perioperative prophylaxis in those undergoing gynecologic and obstetric surgery.

Gentamicin also is used as an adjunct to cefoxitin or cefotetan (no longer commercially available in the US) in patients undergoing contaminated or dirty surgery†, such as that involving a perforated abdominal viscus. When used in patients undergoing these procedures, anti-infective therapy often is considered treatment rather than prophylaxis and is continued postoperatively for about 5–7 days. There is some evidence that a shorter course of anti-infectives (12–24 hours) may be as effective as a 5-day regimen in patients with penetrating abdominal and intestinal injuries.

If gentamicin is used perioperatively, the fact that concurrent use of aminoglycosides and general anesthetics or neuromuscular blocking agents may potentiate neuromuscular blockade and cause respiratory paralysis should be considered. (See Drug Interactions: General Anesthetics and Neuromuscular Blocking Agents in the Aminoglycosides General Statement 8:12.02.)

Dosage and Administration

■ Administration Gentamicin sulfate is administered by IM injection or IV infusion. IV administration may be preferred in patients with septicemia, shock, congestive heart failure, hematologic disorders, severe burns, or reduced muscle mass.

Gentamicin sulfate has been administered intrathecally† or intraventricularly† as an adjunct to IM or IV administration of the drug for the treatment of meningitis and other CNS infections.

Patients should be well hydrated prior to and during gentamicin therapy since dehydration increases the risk of toxicity.

Renal function should be assessed prior to and monitored during gentamicin therapy. Patients should be under close clinical observation because of the risk of ototoxicity and nephrotoxicity. (See Cautions in the Aminoglycosides General Statement 8:12.02.)

Prior to administration, gentamicin solutions should be inspected visually for particulate matter or discoloration.

IM Injection For IM injection, the appropriate dose of commercially available injection containing gentamicin in a concentration of 10 or 40 mg/mL should be withdrawn from the vial and given undiluted.

The commercially available gentamicin injection in 0.9% sodium chloride should *not* be used for IM administration of the drug.

IV Infusion IV infusions for adults are prepared from commercially available injections containing gentamicin in a concentration of 10 or 40 mg/mL by diluting the appropriate dose of gentamicin with 50–200 mL of 0.9% sodium chloride or 5% dextrose injection. For pediatric patients, the volume of infusion fluid depends on the patient's needs, but should be sufficient to allow a gentamicin infusion period of 30 minutes to 2 hours.

Alternatively, the appropriate dose of premixed gentamicin solution in 0.9% sodium chloride injection can be used; however, these premixed solutions may not be appropriate for the dosage requirements of neonates, infants, or children. The commercially available premixed solutions should not be diluted or buffered prior to administration and should be given only by IV infusion. Premixed gentamicin solution in 0.9% sodium chloride injection is provided in single-dose flexible containers; additives should not be introduced into the injection container and the containers should not be used in series. However, if the dose needed is greater or less than that in the container, the manufacturer states that the appropriate amount of gentamicin sulfate solution can be introduced into or removed from the container. The manufacturer's instructions should be consulted for proper use of commercially available premixed gentamicin sulfate in 0.9% sodium chloride injection.

Gentamicin should not be admixed with other drugs or infused simultaneously through the same tubing with other drugs. If a β-lactam anti-infective (e.g., cephalosporin, penicillin) is administered concomitantly with gentamicin, the drugs should not be admixed and should be administered separately.

Rate of Administration. IV infusions of gentamicin should be given over 30 minutes to 2 hours.

Intrathecal or Intraventricular Administration If gentamicin is administered intrathecally† or intraventricularly†, a preservative-free preparation of the drug should be used.

■ Dosage Dosage of gentamicin sulfate is expressed in terms of gentamicin. IM and IV dosage is identical.

Like other aminoglycosides, dosage of gentamicin should be individualized taking into consideration the patient's pretreatment body weight, renal status, severity of the infection, and susceptibility of the causative organism. The manufacturers state that dosage in obese patients should be based on the patient's estimated lean body weight. Many clinicians recommend that gentamicin dosage be determined using appropriate pharmacokinetic methods for calculating dosage requirements and patient-specific pharmacokinetic parameters (e.g., elimination rate constant, volume of distribution) derived from serum concentration-time data.

Whenever possible, especially in patients with life-threatening infections, suspected toxicity or nonresponse to treatment, decreased or varying renal function, and/or when increased aminoglycoside clearance (e.g., patients with cystic fibrosis, burns) or prolonged therapy is likely, peak and trough serum concentrations of gentamicin should be determined periodically and dosage should be adjusted to maintain desired serum concentrations. (See Dosage and Administration: Dosage, in the Aminoglycosides General Statement 8:12.02.) A causal relationship between maintenance of certain peak or trough serum concentrations or other pharmacodynamic endpoints and clinical response or toxicity has not been established to date for gentamicin dosing regimens. However, for gentamicin administered in conventional dosage regimens (i.e., multiple daily doses), peak serum concentrations of 4–10 mcg/mL and trough concentrations that do not exceed 1–2 mcg/mL have been suggested. An increased risk of toxicity may be associated with peak serum gentamicin concentrations greater than 10–12 mcg/mL and/or trough concentrations greater than 2 mcg/mL. The manufacturers state that prolonged peak serum concentrations greater than 12 mcg/mL and trough concentrations greater than 2 mcg/mL should be avoided.

Parenteral aminoglycosides historically have been administered in dosage regimens that include multiple daily doses, and current prescribing information for IM or IV gentamicin only includes dosage regimens that involve multiple daily doses (usually 3 or 4 doses daily). However, there is evidence that once-daily† (single-daily) aminoglycoside dosage regimens are at least as effective as, may provide superior pharmacokinetics, and may be less toxic than conventional dosage regimens employing multiple daily doses of the drugs. Although once-daily gentamicin regimens are recommended for some indications, once-daily gentamicin regimens should *not* be used in all patients and should *not* be used for the treatment of enterococcal or staphylococcal endocarditis†. Additional controlled studies in children, patients with renal dysfunction, and other appropriate patient groups are needed to fully define the optimal use of once-daily aminoglycoside dosing regimens. In addition, the most appropriate methods for optimizing dosage selection for once-daily regimens and monitoring serum aminoglycoside concentrations in patients receiving such regimens have not been clearly established. (See Dosage and Administration: Dosage, in the Aminoglycosides General Statement 8:12.02.)

The usual duration of gentamicin treatment is 7–10 days. In difficult and complicated infections, a longer course of treatment may be necessary. However, toxicity is more likely to occur if treatment is continued for longer than 10 days and renal, auditory, and vestibular functions should be monitored closely.

Adult Dosage **General Adult Dosage.** If IM or IV gentamicin is used for the treatment of serious infections caused by susceptible bacteria in adults with normal renal function, the usual adult dosage recommended by the manufacturers is 3 mg/kg daily given in 3 equally divided doses every 8 hours. For life-threatening infections in adults with normal renal function, the manufacturers state that an IM or IV gentamicin dosage up to 5 mg/kg daily given in 3 or 4 equally divided doses may be used, but dosage should be reduced to 3 mg/kg daily as soon as clinically indicated.

If a once-daily† gentamicin regimen is used in adults with normal renal function, some clinicians recommend a dosage of 4–5 mg/kg once daily. A once-daily regimen of 5–7 mg/kg once daily also has been recommended. It has been suggested that, if gentamicin is used alone for the treatment of serious infections (e.g., without concomitant use of a β-lactam), a dosage of 7 mg/kg once daily usually is required.

Endocarditis Treatment. For the treatment of native or prosthetic valve enterococcal endocarditis†, the American Heart Association (AHA) and Infectious Diseases Society of America (IDSA) recommend that adults receive IM or IV gentamicin in a dosage of 3 mg/kg daily given in 3 equally divided doses in conjunction with IV ampicillin sodium (12 g daily in 6 equally divided doses) or IV penicillin G sodium (18–30 million units daily). In patients with native valve enterococcal endocarditis caused by strains susceptible to penicillin and gentamicin, treatment should be continued for 4–6 weeks; although a 4-week regimen may be used in those who have had symptoms of infection for 3 months or less prior to initiation of treatment, a 6-week regimen is recommended for those who have had symptoms for longer than 3 months. In patients with prosthetic valve or other prosthetic cardiac material, treatment should be continued for a minimum of 6 weeks. In those with enterococci susceptible to penicillins, gentamicin, and vancomycin who are unable to tolerate penicillins, a 6-week regimen of IM or IV gentamicin (3 mg/kg daily given in 3 equally divided doses) should be used in conjunction with a 6-week regimen of IV vancomycin (30 mg/kg daily given in 2 equally divided doses). If penicillin-resistant enterococci are involved, the AHA and IDSA recommend that adults receive a 6-week regimen of IM or IV gentamicin (3 mg/kg daily given in 3 equally divided doses) in conjunction with a 6-week regimen of IV ampicillin sodium and sulbactam sodium (12 g of ampicillin daily given in 4 equally divided doses) or IV vancomycin (30 mg/kg daily given in 2 equally divided doses). Pending further accumulation of data, the AHA and IDSA state that once-daily gentamicin regimens should *not* be used for the treatment of enterococcal endocarditis.

If a 2-week regimen is appropriate for the treatment of native valve endocarditis caused by viridans streptococci or *S. bovis*† highly susceptible to penicillin (i.e., penicillin MIC of 0.12 mcg/mL or less) (see Endocarditis Caused by Viridans Streptococci or S. bovis in Uses: Endocarditis), the AHA and IDSA recommend that adults receive IM or IV gentamicin in a dosage of 3 mg/kg given once daily or in 3 equally divided doses for 2 weeks in conjunction with a 2-week regimen of IV penicillin G sodium (12–18 million units daily) or IV or IM ceftriaxone (2 g once daily). For the treatment of native valve endocarditis caused by viridans streptococci or *S. bovis* relatively resistant to penicillins (i.e., penicillin MIC greater than 0.12 mcg/mL and less than or equal to 0.5 mcg/mL), AHA and IDSA recommend that adults receive a 2-week regimen of IM or IV gentamicin in a dosage of 3 mg/kg given once daily or in 3 equally divided doses in conjunction with a 4-week regimen of IV penicillin G sodium (24 million units daily) or IV or IM ceftriaxone (2 g once daily). If prosthetic valves or other prosthetic materials are involved and viridans streptococci or *S. bovis* is penicillin susceptible (i.e., penicillin MIC of 0.12 mcg/mL or less), the AHA and IDSA recommend a 2-week regimen of IM or IV gentamicin in a dosage of 3 mg/kg once daily or in 3 equally divided doses in conjunction with a 6-week regimen of IV penicillin G sodium (24 million units daily) or IV or IgivenM ceftriaxone (2 g once daily). However, if the organisms are relatively or fully resistant to penicillins (i.e., penicillin MIC greater than 0.12 mcg/mL), then IM or IV gentamicin in a dosage of 3 mg/kg given once daily or in 3 equally divided doses should be continued for 6 weeks in conjunction with a 6-week regimen of IV penicillin G sodium (24 million units daily) or IV or IM ceftriaxone (2 g once daily).

If gentamicin is used as an adjunct to a β-lactam for the treatment of native valve staphylococcal endocarditis†, the AHA and IDSA recommend an IM or IV gentamicin dosage of 3 mg/kg daily given in 2 or 3 equally divided doses during the first 3–5 days of a 6-week regimen of IV nafcillin or oxacillin (12 g daily given in 4–6 equally divided doses) or IV cefazolin (6 g daily given in 3 equally divided doses). For the treatment of prosthetic valve staphylococcal endocarditis, the AHA and IDSA recommend that adults receive a 2-week regimen of IM or IV gentamicin in a dosage of 3 mg/kg daily given in 2 or 3 equally divided doses in conjunction with at least 6 weeks of IV nafcillin or oxacillin (12 g daily given in 6 equally divided doses) or, for oxacillin-resistant (methicillin-resistant) strains, IV vancomycin (30 mg/kg daily given in 3 equally divided doses); either regimen should also include IV or oral rifampin (900 mg daily given in 3 equally divided doses for at least 6 weeks). Pending further accumulation of data, the AHA and IDSA state that once-daily gentamicin regimens should *not* be used for the treatment of staphylococcal endocarditis.

Endocarditis Prevention. For prevention of endocarditis† in patients at high risk undergoing certain genitourinary tract and nonesophageal GI procedures (see Prophylaxis of Bacterial Endocarditis under Uses: Prophylaxis in the Aminopenicillins General Statement 8:12.16.08), the AHA and others recommend that adults receive an IM or IV dose of gentamicin (1.5 mg/kg up to 120 mg) and a dose of ampicillin (2 g IM or IV) administered at separate sites within 30 minutes of starting the procedure; 6 hours later, adults should receive a dose of ampicillin (1 g IM or IV) or amoxicillin (1 g orally) given without gentamicin.

For prevention of endocarditis† in penicillin-allergic patients at high risk undergoing certain genitourinary tract or nonesophageal GI procedures, the AHA and others recommend that adults receive an IM or IV dose of gentamicin (1.5 mg/kg up to 120 mg) and a dose of vancomycin (1 g IV) administered at separate sites within 30 minutes of starting the procedure; follow-up doses are not necessary in these patients.

Meningitis. If gentamicin is used for the treatment of meningitis, some clinicians recommend that adults receive 5 mg/kg daily given in 3 divided doses.

An intrathecal† or intraventricular† gentamicin dosage of 4–8 mg once daily has been recommended for the treatment of meningitis in adults.

Urinary Tract Infections. If gentamicin is used for the treatment of uncomplicated urinary tract infections caused by susceptible bacteria when other less toxic anti-infectives cannot be used, a dosage of 160 mg of gentamicin IM once daily has been recommended. A single 5-mg/kg IM dose of gentamicin has been used for the treatment of uncomplicated urinary tract infections.

Pelvic Inflammatory Disease. For the treatment of acute pelvic inflammatory disease† (PID) when a parenteral regimen is indicated, adolescents and adults with normal renal function may receive an initial IM or IV gentamicin dose of 2 mg/kg followed by 1.5 mg/kg every 8 hours given in conjunction with clindamycin (900 mg IV every 8 hours). Although once-daily gentamicin regimens (e.g., 3 mg/kg once daily) have not been evaluated in the treatment of PID, such regimens have been efficacious in analogous situations. The parenteral gentamicin and clindamycin regimen can be discontinued 24 hours after clinical improvement occurs and treatment switched to an oral regimen (i.e., oral doxycycline or oral clindamycin) to complete a total of 14 days of therapy.

Bartonella Infections. For the treatment of serious *Bartonella* infections† (e.g., endocarditis known or suspected of being caused by *B. henselae*, bacteremia or pericardial infusion caused by *B. quintana*), IV gentamicin has been given in a dosage of 3 mg/kg daily in conjunction with other anti-infectives (e.g., doxycycline, ceftriaxone, amoxicillin, penicillin G benzathine, oxacillin, vancomycin). Gentamicin has been given for at least the first 14 days and the other anti-infectives continued for up to about 6 weeks.

Granuloma Inguinale (Donovanosis). When gentamicin is used as an adjunct to a recommended oral anti-infective (doxycycline, azithromycin, ciprofloxacin, erythromycin, co-trimoxazole) for the treatment of granuloma inguinale (donovanosis)† caused by *Klebsiella granulomatis* (formerly *Calymmatobacterium granulomatis*), the CDC recommends that gentamicin be given in a dosage of 1 mg/kg IV every 8 hours.

Donovanosis usually is treated with an oral anti-infective regimen given for at least 3 weeks and until all lesions have healed. If improvement is not evident within the first few days of the oral regimen, IV gentamicin should be added. Adjunctive use of IV gentamicin also should be considered for the treatment of Donovanosis in pregnant or lactating women and HIV-infected individuals. Relapse can occur 6–18 months after apparently effective therapy.

Plague. For the treatment of plague†, including pneumonic plague that occurs as the result of exposure to *Yersinia pestis* in the context of biologic warfare or bioterrorism, the recommended dosage of gentamicin in adults with normal renal function is 5 mg/kg IM or IV once daily or, alternatively, adults may receive a 2-mg/kg loading dose following by 1.75 mg/kg IM or IV every 8 hours. A dosage of 2.5 mg/kg IM twice daily has been effective in some patients.

The usual duration of therapy for the treatment of plague is 10 days; some experts recommend a duration of at least 10–14 days.

Tularemia. For the treatment of tularemia† that occurs as the result of exposure to *Francisella tularensis* in the context of biologic warfare or bioterrorism, the US Working Group on Civilian Biodefense recommends that adults with normal renal function receive a gentamicin dosage of 5 mg/kg IM or IV once daily for 10 days. The US Army Medical Research Institute of Infectious Diseases (USAMRIID) recommends that adults receive 5 mg/kg IM or IV once daily or, alternatively, a 2-mg/kg loading dose following by 1.7 mg/kg IM or IV every 8 hours for at least 10–14 days.

Perioperative Prophylaxis. For perioperative prophylaxis in patients undergoing head and neck surgery†, some clinicians recommend that a gentamicin dose of 1.5 mg/kg be given IV in conjunction with IV clindamycin (600–900 mg) immediately prior to surgery; this may be repeated if surgery is prolonged or major blood loss occurs. Postoperative doses of prophylactic drugs generally are unnecessary. Other clinicians recommend a gentamicin dose of 1.7 mg/kg given IV and a dose of clindamycin (600 mg IV) given at the time of induction of anesthesia and repeated twice at 8-hour intervals for a total of 3 doses.

For prophylaxis following contaminated or dirty surgery, such as surgery involving a perforated abdominal viscus†, gentamicin is given IV in a dosage of 1.5 mg/kg every 8 hours in conjunction with cefoxitin (1–2 g IV every 6 hours). When used in this situation, the regimen may be continued postoperatively for about 5 days and is considered treatment rather than prophylaxis.

Pediatric Dosage

General Dosage for Neonates. When IM or IV gentamicin is used in premature or full-term neonates 1 week of age or younger, the manufacturers recommend 2.5 mg/kg every 12 hours. For neonates older than 1 week of age, the manufacturers recommend a dosage of 2.5 mg/kg every 8 hours.

The American Academy of Pediatrics (AAP) recommends that neonates younger than 1 week of age receive IM or IV gentamicin in a dosage of 2.5 mg/kg every 18–24 hours if they weigh less than 1.2 kg or 2.5 mg/kg every 12 hours if they weigh 1.2 kg or more. For neonates 1–4 weeks of age, the AAP recommends a dosage of 2.5 mg/kg every 18–24 hours for those weighing less than 1.2 kg, 2.5 mg/kg every 8 or 12 hours for those weighing 1.2–2 kg, and 2.5 mg/kg every 8 hours for those weighing more than 2 kg. The AAP states that the drug is inappropriate for the treatment of mild to moderate infections.

Once-daily† gentamicin regimens have been used in neonates. Neonates have received 4–5 mg/kg of gentamicin once daily by IV infusion over 30–60 minutes.

General Dosage for Infants and Children. The usual dosage of IM or IV gentamicin recommended by the manufacturers for older infants with normal renal function is 2.5 mg/kg every 8 hours. The manufacturers recommend that children receive gentamicin in a dosage of 2–2.5 mg/kg every 8 hours.

The AAP recommends that pediatric patients beyond the neonatal period receive gentamicin in a dosage of 3–7.5 mg/kg daily given in 3 equally divided doses for the treatment of severe infections. The AAP states that the drug is inappropriate for the treatment of mild to moderate infections.

Once-daily† gentamicin regimens have been used in infants and children. The AAP states that a gentamicin regimen of 5–6 mg/kg once every 24 hours is investigational in children. In clinical studies, children have received gentamicin in a dosage of 4.5–7.5 mg/kg once daily.

Endocarditis Treatment. For the treatment of native or prosthetic valve enterococcal endocarditis†, the AHA and IDSA recommend that children receive IM or IV gentamicin in a dosage of 3 mg/kg daily given in 3 equally divided doses in conjunction with IV ampicillin sodium (300 mg/kg daily given in 4–6 equally divided doses) or IV penicillin G sodium (300,000 units/kg daily given in 4–6 equally divided doses). In patients with native valve enterococcal endocarditis caused by strains susceptible to penicillin, gentamicin, and vancomycin, treatment should be continued for 4–6 weeks; although a 4-week regimen may be used in those who have had symptoms of infection for 3 months or less prior to initiation of treatment, a 6-week regimen is recommended for those who have had symptoms for longer than 3 months. In patients with prosthetic valve or other prosthetic cardiac material, treatment should be continued for a minimum of 6 weeks. In children with enterococci susceptible to penicillin, gentamicin, and vancomycin who are unable to tolerate penicillins, a 6-week regimen of IM or IV gentamicin (3 mg/kg daily given in 3 equally divided doses) should be used in conjunction with a 6-week regimen of IV vancomycin (40 mg/kg daily given in 2 or 3 equally divided doses). If penicillin-resistant enterococci are involved, the AHA and IDSA recommend that children receive a 6-week regimen of IM or IV gentamicin (3 mg/kg daily given in 3 equally divided doses) in conjunction with a 6-week regimen of IV ampicillin sodium and sulbactam sodium (300 mg/kg daily of ampicillin given in 4 equally divided doses) or IV vancomycin (40 mg/kg daily given in 2 or 3 equally divided doses). Pending further accumulation of data, the AHA and IDSA state that once-daily gentamicin regimens should *not* be used for the treatment of enterococcal endocarditis.

If a 2-week regimen is appropriate for the treatment of native valve endocarditis caused by viridans streptococci or *S. bovis*† highly susceptible to penicillin (i.e., penicillin MIC of 0.12 mcg/mL or less) (see Endocarditis Caused by Viridans Streptococci or S. bovis in Uses: Endocarditis), the AHA and IDSA recommend that children receive IM or IV gentamicin in a dosage of 3 mg/kg daily in 1 or 3 equally divided doses for 2 weeks in conjunction with a 2-week regimen of IV penicillin G sodium (200,000 units/kg daily in 4–6 equally divided doses) or IV or IM ceftriaxone (100 mg/kg once daily). For the treatment of native valve endocarditis caused by viridans streptococci or *S. bovis* relatively resistant to penicillins (i.e., penicillin MIC greater than 0.12 mcg/mL and less than or equal to 0.5 mcg/mL), AHA and IDSA recommend that children receive IM or IV gentamicin in a dosage of 3 mg/kg daily in 1 or 3 equally divided doses for 2 weeks in conjunction with a 4-week regimen of IV penicillin G sodium (200,000 units/kg daily in 4–6 equally divided doses) or IV or IM ceftriaxone (100 mg/kg once daily). If prosthetic valves or other prosthetic materials are involved and viridans streptococci or *S. bovis* is penicillin susceptible, the AHA and IDSA recommend that children receive a 2-week regimen of IM or IV gentamicin in a dosage of 3 mg/kg daily in 1 or 3 equally divided doses in conjunction with a 6-week regimen of IV penicillin G sodium (300,000 units/kg daily given in 4–6 equally divided doses) or IM or IV ceftriaxone (100 mg/kg once daily). However, if the organisms are relatively or fully resistant to penicillins, then gentamicin (3 mg/kg daily in 1 or 3 equally divided doses) should be continued for 6 weeks in conjunction with the 6-week regimen of IV penicillin G sodium (200,000 units/kg daily in 4–6 equally divided doses) or IV or IM ceftriaxone (100 mg/kg once daily).

If gentamicin is used as an adjunct to a β-lactam for the treatment of native valve staphylococcal endocarditis†, the AHA and IDSA recommend that children receive IM or IV gentamicin in a dosage of 3 mg/kg daily given in 3 equally divided doses for the first 3–5 days of a 6-week regimen of IV nafcillin or oxacillin (200 mg/kg daily given in 4–6 equally divided doses) or IV cefazolin (100 mg/kg daily given in 3 equally divided doses). For the treatment of prosthetic valve staphylococcal endocarditis, the AHA and IDSA recommend that children receive a 2-week regimen of IM or IV gentamicin in a dosage of 3 mg/kg daily given in 3 equally divided doses in conjunction with at least 6 weeks of IV nafcillin or oxacillin (200 mg/kg daily given in 4–6 equally divided doses) or, for oxacillin-resistant strains, IV vancomycin 40 mg/kg daily given in 2 or 3 equally divided doses); either regimen should also include IV or oral rifampin (20 mg/kg daily given in 3 equally divided doses for at least 6 weeks). Pending further accumulation of data, the AHA and IDSA state that once-daily gentamicin regimens should *not* be used for the treatment of staphylococcal endocarditis.

Endocarditis Prevention. For prevention of endocarditis† in patients at high risk undergoing certain genitourinary or nonesophageal GI tract procedures (see Prophylaxis of Bacterial Endocarditis under Uses: Prophylaxis in the Aminopenicillins General Statement 8:12.16.08), the AHA, AAP, and others recommend that children receive an IM or IV dose of gentamicin (1.5 mg/kg up to 120 mg) and an IM or IV dose of ampicillin (50 mg/kg up to 2 g) administered at separate sites within 30 minutes of starting the procedure; 6 hours later, a dose of ampicillin (25 mg/kg IM or IV) or amoxicillin (25 mg/kg orally) should be given without gentamicin.

For prevention of endocarditis† in penicillin-allergic patients at high risk undergoing certain genitourinary or nonesophageal GI tract procedures, the AHA, AAP, and others recommend that children receive a dose of IM or IV gentamicin (1.5 mg/kg up to 120 mg) and a dose of vancomycin (20 mg/kg given IV over 1–2 hours) at separate sites and completed within 30 minutes of starting the procedure; follow-up doses are not necessary in these patients.

Meningitis. For the treatment of meningitis, some clinicians recommend that neonates 7 days of age or younger receive a parenteral gentamicin dosage of 5 mg/kg daily given in 2 divided doses and that older neonates and children receive a parenteral dosage of 7.5 mg/kg daily given in 3 divided doses. Smaller doses and longer intervals between doses may be indicated in neonates weighing less than 2 kg.

An intrathecal† or intraventricular† gentamicin dosage of 1–2 mg once daily has been recommended for children older than 3 months of age.

Plague. For the treatment of plague†, including pneumonic plague that occurs as the result of exposure to *Yersinia pestis* in the context of biologic warfare or bioterrorism, the US Working Group on Civilian Biodefense and USAMRIID recommend that children with normal renal function receive gentamicin in a dosage of 2.5 mg/kg IM or IV 3 times daily; neonates up to 1 week of age and premature neonates should receive a dosage of 2.5 mg/kg IV twice daily. A dosage of 2.5 mg/kg IM twice daily has been effective in some patients.

The usual duration of therapy for the treatment of plague is 10 days; some experts recommend a duration of at least 10–14 days.

Tularemia. For the treatment of tularemia† that occurs as the result of exposure to *Francisella tularensis* in the context of biologic warfare or bioterrorism, the US Working Group on Civilian Biodefense and USAMRIID recommend that children with normal renal function receive gentamicin in a dosage of 2.5 mg/kg IM or IV every 8 hours.

For the treatment of naturally occurring or endemic tularemia†, children have received gentamicin in a dosage of 5–7.5 mg/kg daily given in 3 divided doses.

The usual duration of therapy for the treatment of tularemia is 10 days; some experts recommend a duration of at least 10–14 days.

Urinary Tract Infections. For the treatment of uncomplicated urinary tract infections in children, a single 5-mg/kg IM dose† of gentamicin (up to 300 mg) has been used. The drug should not be used for uncomplicated infections unless other less toxic anti-infectives cannot be used.

■ **Dosage in Renal Impairment** In patients with impaired renal function, doses and/or frequency of administration must be modified in response to serum concentrations of the drug and the degree of renal impairment. There are various methods to determine dosage and a wide variation in dosage recommendations for these patients. However, even when one of these methods is used, peak and trough serum concentrations of the drug should be monitored, especially in patients with changing renal function.

The manufacturers recommend that adults with renal impairment receive an initial dose of 1–1.7 mg/kg. For subsequent therapy, the manufacturers state that 1 mg/kg doses can be given at intervals (in hours) calculated by multiplying the patient's steady-state serum creatinine (in mg/dL) by 8. Alternatively, many clinicians recommend the dosing method of Sarubbi and Hull, which is based on corrected creatinine clearance. (See Dosage and Administration: Dosage in Renal Impairment, in the Aminoglycosides General Statement 8:12.02.) These dosage calculation methods should not be used in patients undergoing hemodialysis or peritoneal dialysis.

In adults with renal failure undergoing hemodialysis, the manufacturers recommend supplemental doses of 1–1.7 mg/kg at the end of each dialysis period in adults and supplemental doses of 2–2.5 mg/kg at the end of each dialysis period in children. Some clinicians suggest supplemental doses of 50–75% of the initial loading dose at the end of each dialysis period. Serum gentamicin concentrations should be monitored in dialysis patients and dosage adjusted as needed to maintain desired serum concentrations.

Pharmacokinetics

The pharmacokinetics of gentamicin are similar to those of the other aminoglycosides. In all studies described in the Pharmacokinetics section, gentamicin was administered as the sulfate salt; dosages and concentrations of the drug are expressed in terms of gentamicin.

■ **Absorption** Gentamicin is poorly absorbed from the GI tract and must be administered parenterally.

Gentamicin is rapidly absorbed following IM administration. Following IM administration of a single 1-mg/kg dose of gentamicin in adults with normal renal function, peak serum gentamicin concentrations of 4–7.6 mcg/mL are attained within 30–90 minutes.

Serum concentrations attained following IV infusion over 20 minutes to 2 hours usually are similar to those attained when the same dose is given by IM injection. When gentamicin is administered by IV infusion over 2 hours, peak serum concentrations usually occur at 30–60 minutes and are measurable for 6–8 hours.

In neutropenic adults who received gentamicin in a once-daily regimen of 4.5 mg/kg once every 24 hours by IV infusion over 30 minutes, peak serum gentamicin concentrations averaged 10.9, 7.1, 4.2, 1.8, and 0.16 mcg/mL at 1, 2, 4, 8, and 24 hours after the infusion.

In infants, peak serum gentamicin concentrations of 3–5 mcg/mL are attained 30–60 minutes following a single 2.5-mg/kg IM dose. A single 1-mg/kg IV dose in children 6 months to 5 years of age, 5–10 years of age, or older than 10 years of age resulted in mean peak serum concentrations of 1.58, 2.03, and 2.81 mcg/mL, respectively.

Serum concentrations may be lower in febrile patients and in seriously ill patients, including those with anemia, severe burns, or malignancy.

Accumulation of gentamicin does not appear to occur in patients with normal renal function receiving 1-mg/kg doses every 8 hours for 7–10 days. However, accumulation may occur with higher doses and/or when the drug is given for prolonged periods, especially in patients with renal impairment.

■ **Distribution** Following parenteral administration of usual dosages of gentamicin, the drug can be detected in lymph, subcutaneous tissue, lung, sputum, and bronchial, pleural, pericardial, synovial, ascitic, and peritoneal fluids. Concentrations in bile may be low, suggesting minimal biliary excretion. In patients with ventilator-associated pneumonia receiving IV gentamicin (240 mg once daily), drug concentrations in alveolar lining fluid were 32% of serum concentrations and averaged 4.24 mcg/mL 2 hours after a dose.

Only minimal concentrations of gentamicin are attained in ocular tissue following IM or IV administration.

Gentamicin is distributed into CSF in low concentrations following IM or IV administration. CSF concentrations of gentamicin following intrathecal administration depend on the dose administered, the site of injection, the volume in which the dose is diluted, and the presence or absence of obstruction to CSF flow. There may be considerable interpatient variation in concentrations achieved. In one study, intrathecal administration of 4 mg of gentamicin resulted in CSF concentrations of the drug of 19–46 mcg/mL for 8 hours and less than 3 mcg/mL at 20 hours.

Gentamicin crosses the placenta.

Gentamicin is distributed into milk following IM administration.

■ **Elimination** The plasma elimination half-life of gentamicin is usually 2–4 hours in adults with normal renal function and is reported to range from 24–60 hours in adults with severe renal impairment.

The serum half-life of gentamicin averages 3–3.5 hours in infants 1 week to 6 months of age and 5.5 hours in full-term infants and large premature infants less than 1 week of age. In small premature infants, the plasma half-life is approximately 5 hours in those weighing over 2 kg, 8 hours in those weighing 1.5–2 kg, and 11.5 hours in those weighing less than 1.5 kg.

Gentamicin clearance may be decreased in geriatric patients compared with other adults.

In adults with normal renal function, 50–93% of a single IM dose of gentamicin is excreted unchanged by glomerular filtration within 24 hours. Peak urine concentrations of gentamicin may range from 113–423 mcg/mL 1 hour after a single IM dose of 1 mg/kg in adults with normal renal function. Complete recovery of the dose in urine requires approximately 10–20 days in patients with normal renal function, and terminal elimination half-lives of greater than 100 hours have been reported in adults with normal renal function following repeated IM or IV administration of the drug.

Gentamicin is removed by hemodialysis and peritoneal dialysis.

Chemistry and Stability

■ **Chemistry** Gentamicin is an aminoglycoside antibiotic obtained from cultures of *Micromonospora purpurea*. The commercially available drug is a mixture of the sulfate salts of gentamicin C_1, C_2, and C_{1A}. Gentamicin sulfate occurs as a white to buff powder and is freely soluble in water and insoluble in alcohol.

Commercially available gentamicin sulfate injection for IM or IV administration is a clear, colorless to slightly yellow solution; sodium hydroxide and/or sulfuric acid may be added during manufacture to adjust the pH to 3–5.5. Each mL of injection containing 40 mg of gentamicin per mL also contains 1.8 mg of methylparaben and 0.2 mg of propylparaben as preservatives, 3.2 mg of sodium metabisulfite, and 0.1 mg of edetate disodium. Each mL of injection containing 10 mg of gentamicin per mL in multiple-dose vials contains 1.3 mg of methylparaben, 0.2 mg of propylparaben, 3.2 mg of sodium metabisulfite, and 0.1 mg of edetate disodium. Injections containing 10 mg of gentamicin per mL in single-dose vials do not contain preservatives.

Commercially available premixed gentamicin sulfate in 0.9% sodium chloride injection for IV use is an isotonic solution with a pH of approximately 4 (3–5.5); sodium hydroxide and/or sulfuric acid may be added during manufacture to adjust the pH. These injections are isotonic with a calculated osmolarity of 290 mOsm/L.

■ **Stability** Commercially available gentamicin sulfate injections for IM or IV administration containing 40 mg of gentamicin per mL should be stored at 15–30°C and those containing 10 mg/mL should be stored at 20–25°C. Commercially available premixed gentamicin sulfate in 0.9% sodium chloride injection for IV use in Viaflex® Plus or PAB® plastic containers should be stored at controlled room temperature of 25°C, but may be exposed briefly to temperatures up to 40°C. These injections should not be frozen.

Gentamicin sulfate is stable for 24 hours at room temperature in most IV infusion fluids including 0.9% sodium chloride or 5% dextrose injection. Gentamicin sulfate injections should not be mixed with other drugs.

The commercially available premixed gentamicin sulfate in 0.9% sodium chloride injection for IV use is provided in plastic containers fabricated from specially formulated polyvinyl chloride (Viaflex® Plus) or from a rubberized copolymer of ethylene and propylene (PAB®). Safety of these plastics has been confirmed in tests in animals according to USP biological tests for plastic containers as well as by tissue culture toxicity studies.

For further information on chemistry and stability, mechanism of action, spectrum, resistance, pharmacokinetics, uses, cautions, drug interactions, and dosage and administration of gentamicin, see the Aminoglycosides General Statement 8:12.02. For topical uses of gentamicin, see 52:04.04 and 84:04.04.

Preparations

Excipients in commercially available drug preparations may have clinically important effects in some individuals; consult specific product labeling for details.

Gentamicin Sulfate

Parenteral		
Injection, for IM or IV use	10 mg (of gentamicin) per mL*	Gentamicin Sulfate Pediatric Injection
	40 mg (of gentamicin) per mL*	Gentamicin Sulfate Injection

*available from one or more manufacturer, distributor, and/or repackager by generic (nonproprietary) name

Gentamicin Sulfate in Sodium Chloride

Parenteral		
Injection, for IV infusion	0.4 mg (of gentamicin) per mL (40 mg) in 0.9% Sodium Chloride*	Gentamicin Sulfate Injection Isotonic (Viaflex® Plus), Baxter
	0.6 mg (of gentamicin) per mL (60 mg) in 0.9% Sodium Chloride*	Gentamicin Sulfate Injection Isotonic (Viaflex® Plus), Baxter
		Gentamicin Sulfate in 0.9% Sodium Chloride Injection (PAB®), Braun
	0.8 mg (of gentamicin) per mL (40 or 80 mg) in 0.9% Sodium Chloride*	Gentamicin Sulfate Injection Isotonic (Viaflex® Plus), Baxter
		Gentamicin Sulfate in 0.9% Sodium Chloride Injection (PAB®), Braun
	1 mg (of gentamicin) per mL (100 mg) in 0.9% Sodium Chloride*	Gentamicin Sulfate Injection Isotonic (Viaflex® Plus), Baxter
		Gentamicin Sulfate in 0.9% Sodium Chloride Injection (PAB®), Braun
	1.2 mg (of gentamicin) per mL (60 or 120 mg) in 0.9% Sodium Chloride*	Gentamicin Sulfate Injection Isotonic (Viaflex® Plus), Baxter
		Gentamicin Sulfate in 0.9% Sodium Chloride Injection (PAB®), Braun
	1.6 mg (of gentamicin) per mL (80 mg) in 0.9% Sodium Chloride*	Gentamicin Sulfate Injection Isotonic (Viaflex® Plus), Baxter
		Gentamicin Sulfate in 0.9% Sodium Chloride Injection (PAB®), Braun
	2 mg (of gentamicin) per mL (100 mg) in 0.9% Sodium Chloride*	Gentamicin Sulfate Injection Isotonic (Viaflex® Plus), Baxter
	2.4 mg (of gentamicin) per mL (120 mg) in 0.9% Sodium Chloride*	Gentamicin Sulfate Injection Isotonic (Viaflex® Plus), Baxter

*available from one or more manufacturer, distributor, and/or repackager by generic (nonproprietary) name

†Use is not currently included in the labeling approved by the US Food and Drug Administration

Tobramycin Sulfate

■ Tobramycin is an aminoglycoside antibiotic.

Uses

■ **Bone and Joint Infections** Tobramycin is used parenterally for the treatment of serious bone and joint infections caused by susceptible *Enterobacter*, *Escherichia coli*, *Klebsiella*, *Proteus*, *Pseudomonas aeruginosa*, or *Staphylococcus aureus*. Tobramycin usually is used as an adjunct to other appropriate anti-infectives.

■ **Intra-abdominal Infections** Tobramycin is used parenterally for the treatment of serious intra-abdominal infections (including peritonitis) caused by susceptible *Enterobacter*, *E. coli*, or *Klebsiella*. Tobramycin usually is used as an adjunct to other appropriate anti-infectives (e.g., clindamycin, metronidazole, piperacillin and tazobactam, ampicillin and sulbactam)

The Infectious Diseases Society of America (IDSA) states that patients with community-acquired intra-abdominal infections of mild to moderate severity may receive initial treatment with an empiric regimen of the fixed combination of ampicillin and sulbactam, cefazolin or cefuroxime in conjunction with metronidazole, the fixed combination of ticarcillin and clavulanate, ertapenem monotherapy, or a fluoroquinolone (ciprofloxacin, levofloxacin, moxifloxacin) in conjunction with metronidazole. Patients who are immunosuppressed or have more severe community-acquired intra-abdominal infections should receive a regimen that has a broader spectrum of activity such as meropenem monotherapy; imipenem and cilastatin monotherapy; a third or fourth generation cephalosporin (cefotaxime, ceftriaxone, ceftazidime, cefepime) in conjunction with metronidazole; ciprofloxacin in conjunction with metronidazole; the fixed combination of piperacillin and tazobactam; or aztreonam in conjunction with metronidazole.

The IDSA states that aminoglycosides are not recommended for *routine* use in community-acquired intra-abdominal infections; however, an aminoglycoside may be included in empiric regimens for the treatment of nosocomial intra-abdominal infections, depending on local patterns of in vitro susceptibility of nosocomial isolates. IDSA states that aminoglycosides generally should be reserved for when β-lactams and fluoroquinolones cannot be used. Other clinicians suggest that severely ill patients and those with prolonged hospitalization should receive an initial regimen that includes an antipseudomonal agent such as an antipseudomonal penicillin (ticarcillin and clavulanate, piperacillin and tazobactam), a carbapenem (imipenem or meropenem), ceftazidime, or cefepime used in conjunction with metronidazole. These clinicians state that an aminoglycoside also could be included in the empiric regimen.

■ **Meningitis and Other CNS Infections** Tobramycin is used parenterally for the treatment of CNS infections (meningitis) caused by susceptible bacteria. Like other aminoglycosides, tobramycin should not be used alone for the treatment of meningitis. To provide higher tobramycin CSF concentrations for the treatment of meningitis, tobramycin has been given intrathecally† or intraventricularly† concomitantly with IM or IV administration. Although concomitant parenteral and intrathecal or intraventricular therapy may result in higher anti-infective CSF concentrations, such therapy also may be associated with increased mortality in neonates.

■ **Respiratory Tract Infections** Tobramycin is used parenterally for the treatment of serious respiratory tract infections caused by susceptible *S. aureus, Enterobacter, E. coli, Klebsiella, Serratia,* or *Ps. aeruginosa.*

Parenteral tobramycin is used in conjunction with other appropriate anti-infectives for the treatment of community-acquired pneumonia (CAP) or nosocomial pneumonia and may be included in initial empiric combination regimens in severely ill patients and/or when multidrug-resistant gram-negative bacteria may be involved. For empiric treatment of nosocomial pneumonia, tobramycin is used as an adjunct to an appropriate β-lactam (e.g., ceftriaxone, cefotaxime, cefepime, piperacillin and tazobactam, ticarcillin and clavulanate) or carbapenem (e.g., imipenem, meropenem); if oxacillin-resistant (methicillin-resistant) staphylococci may be involved, the initial empiric regimen also should include linezolid or vancomycin.

Cystic Fibrosis Patients Tobramycin is used parenterally for management of acute exacerbations of pulmonary *Ps. aeruginosa* infections in adults and children with cystic fibrosis. Parenteral tobramycin usually is used in conjunction with an antipseudomonal β-lactam (e.g., ceftazidime) or carbapenem (e.g., imipenem, meropenem) in these patients. There is evidence from clinical studies that a once-daily tobramycin regimen is at least as effective as a 3-times daily tobramycin regimen for management of exacerbations of pulmonary *Ps. aeruginosa* infections in cystic fibrosis patients.

Oral Inhalation. Commercially available tobramycin solution for oral inhalation is administered via nebulization for the management of bronchopulmonary *Ps. aeruginosa* infections in cystic fibrosis patients 6 years of age or older. There is evidence that a regimen of tobramycin oral inhalation is more effective than placebo for early treatment of *Ps. aeruginosa* infections in cystic fibrosis patients and may improve lung function and reduce the frequency of exacerbations. Use of tobramycin oral inhalation solution can be considered for suppressive therapy in cystic fibrosis patients colonized with *Ps. aeruginosa* if they are 6 years of age or older and have a forced expiratory volume in 1 second (FEV_1) that is 25–75% of the predicted value. Safety and efficacy of the solution for oral inhalation have not been established in pediatric patients younger than 6 years of age, in patients with FEV_1 less than 25% or exceeding 75% of the predicted value, or in patients colonized with *Burkholderia cepacia* (formerly *Ps. cepacia*).

Results of randomized, double-blind, placebo-controlled studies in cystic fibrosis patients 6 years of age or older with *Ps. aeruginosa* indicate that tobramycin solution for oral inhalation given in conjunction with standard therapy for cystic fibrosis can improve lung function, decrease the density of *P. aeruginosa* in expectorated sputum, and reduce the need for hospitalization and parenteral therapy with antipseudomonal anti-infectives. At baseline, the FEV_1 in all study patients was 25–75% of the predicted value. Patients were randomized to receive 3 cycles of tobramycin solution for oral inhalation (300 mg twice daily given using a hand-held reusable nebulizer [PARI LC PLUS®] connected to a Pulmo-Aide® compressor) or placebo (sodium chloride solution flavored with 1.25 mg of quinine sulfate to mimic the taste of the active treatment); each cycle consisted of 28 days of administration of drug or placebo followed by 28 days without administration of drug or placebo. Besides tobramycin solution for oral inhalation or placebo, patients received standard therapy recommended for patients with cystic fibrosis, such as oral and parenteral anti-infectives active against *Pseudomonas*, β_2-adrenergic agonists, cromolyn sodium, orally inhaled corticosteroids, and techniques for clearance of the airway; about 77% of patients also received concurrent therapy with dornase alfa.

Tobramycin solution for inhalation was superior to placebo based on the primary end point of lung function at 20 weeks (at the end of the third cycle), measured as FEV_1 and expressed as the percentage of the predicted value. At 20 weeks, the change in lung function in patients who received the drug was an average 10% increase in FEV_1 over baseline compared with an average 2% decrease in FEV_1 in those who received placebo.

Tobramycin solution for oral inhalation also was superior to placebo based on the primary end point of the density of *P. aeruginosa* in sputum at 20 weeks, calculated as the $\log_{10}$ value for the sum of colony forming units (CFUs) per g of sputum. At 20 weeks, there was an average decrease of 0.8 $\log_{10}$ CFU per g of sputum from baseline in patients who received the drug compared with an average increase of 0.3 $\log_{10}$ CFU per g of sputum in those who received placebo. The greatest reductions in the density of *P. aeruginosa* in sputum in patients who received the drug were observed during the first 2 cycles of administration. At 4 weeks (after the initial 28-day treatment regimen), there was an average reduction of 1.9 $\log_{10}$ CFU per g of sputum in patients treated with the drug; at 12 weeks (after the second 28-day treatment regimen), there was an average reduction of 1.8 $\log_{10}$ CFU per g of sputum in those treated with the drug. During the periods when patients were alternated off of administration of tobramycin solution for oral inhalation, the density of *P. aeruginosa* in sputum in patients treated with the drug approached values calculated at the start of the first cycle of administration of the drug.

The average duration of hospitalization was 5.1 days in patients who received tobramycin solution for oral inhalation and 8.1 days in those who received placebo. Parenteral anti-infectives active against *Pseudomonas* were administered for an average of 9.6 days in patients who received tobramycin solution for oral inhalation and 14.1 days in patients who received placebo. One or more courses of parenteral anti-infectives active against *Pseudomonas* were administered to 39% of patients who received tobramycin solution for oral inhalation and 52% of patients who received placebo.

In vitro susceptibility testing of *Ps. aeruginosa* isolates obtained from patients in these clinical studies indicates that susceptibility of most isolates was not adversely affected by 3 treatment cycles of tobramycin oral inhalation therapy. However, *Ps. aeruginosa* isolates with increased tobramycin MICs were reported in some patients who received the drug. The relationship between clinical outcome and in vitro susceptibility of *Ps. aeruginosa* to tobramycin is unclear. There was no evidence of improvement in FEV_1 or reduction in the bacterial density in sputum in a limited number of patients who had clinical isolates of *P. aeruginosa* that were resistant to tobramycin (MICs of 128 mcg/mL or greater) at study entry.

■ **Septicemia** Tobramycin is used parenterally for the treatment of septicemia caused by susceptible *E. coli, Klebsiella,* or *Ps. aeruginosa.*

Tobramycin is used as an adjunct to an appropriate β-lactam (e.g., ceftriaxone, cefotaxime, cefepime, piperacillin and tazobactam, ticarcillin and clavulanate) or carbapenem (e.g., imipenem, meropenem) for empiric treatment of life-threatening septicemia.

■ **Skin and Skin Structure Infections** Tobramycin is used parenterally for the treatment of serious skin and skin structure infections caused by susceptible *S. aureus, Enterobacter, E. coli, Klebsiella, Proteus,* or *Ps. aeruginosa.* Tobramycin is used as an adjunct to other appropriate anti-infectives.

■ **Urinary Tract Infections** Tobramycin is used parenterally for the treatment of serious complicated and recurrent UTIs caused by susceptible *S. aureus, Citrobacter, Enterobacter, E. coli, Klebsiella, Proteus, Providencia, Serratia,* or *Ps. aeruginosa.* Tobramycin is used as an adjunct to other appropriate anti-infectives.

Tobramycin is not indicated for uncomplicated initial episodes of urinary tract infections unless the causative organism is resistant to other less-toxic alternatives.

■ **Empiric Therapy in Febrile Neutropenic Patients** Tobramycin is used parenterally for empiric anti-infective therapy of presumed bacterial infections in febrile neutropenic patients†. Tobramycin is used in conjunction with an appropriate antipseudomonal cephalosporin (e.g., ceftazidime, ceftriaxone, cefepime), extended-spectrum penicillin (e.g., piperacillin and tazobactam, ticarcillin and clavulanate), or carbapenem (e.g., imipenem, meropenem).

Published protocols for the treatment of infections in febrile neutropenic patients should be consulted for specific recommendations regarding selection of the initial empiric regimen, when to change the initial regimen, possible subsequent regimens, and duration of therapy in these patients. Consultation with an infectious disease expert knowledgeable about infections in immunocompromised patients also is advised.

Dosage and Administration

■ **Reconstitution and Administration** Tobramycin sulfate is administered by IM injection or IV infusion.

Commercially available tobramycin solution for oral inhalation is administered via nebulization. The oral inhalation solution should *not* be administered IV, IM, subcutaneously, or intrathecally.

Tobramycin sulfate has been administered intrathecally† or intraventricularly† in conjunction with IM or IV administration of the drug.

Patients should be well hydrated prior to and during tobramycin therapy since dehydration increases the risk of toxicity.

Renal function should be assessed prior to and periodically during amikacin therapy. Patients should be under close clinical observation because of the risk of ototoxicity and nephrotoxicity. (See Cautions in the Aminoglycosides General Statement 8:12.02.)

Parenteral Administration The commercially available pharmacy bulk packages of tobramycin sulfate powder or solution should be used for preparing solutions for IV infusion and should not be used to prepare solutions for IM injection. Commercially available premixed tobramycin sulfate solutions in 0.9% sodium chloride injection are for IV infusion only.

Tobramycin sulfate solutions should be inspected visually for particulate matter and discoloration before use.

IM Injection. For IM injection, the appropriate dose of tobramycin sulfate should be withdrawn from multiple-dose vials containing 10 or 40 mg of tobramycin per mL.

Solutions prepared from or commercially available in pharmacy bulk packages or ADD-Vantage® vials and the commercially available premixed solutions of tobramycin sulfate in 0.9% sodium chloride injection should *not* be administered IM.

IV Infusion. IV infusions of tobramycin sulfate should be given over 20–60 minutes. Infusion periods of less than 20 minutes should not be used because this infusion rate may result in peak serum tobramycin concentrations exceeding 12 mcg/mL.

For adults, IV infusions of tobramycin sulfate can be prepared from multiple-dose vials of tobramycin sulfate solution containing 10 or 40 mg of tobramycin per mL by diluting the calculated tobramycin dose in 50–100 mL of 0.9% sodium chloride injection or 5% dextrose injection. For pediatric patients, the volume of diluent should be proportionately less than for adults.

Alternatively, IV infusions can be prepared using the single-dose ADD-Vantage® vials of tobramycin sulfate. The contents of these vials should be diluted according to the manufacturer's directions using only 50 or 100 mL ADD-Vantage flexible diluent containers and should be used within 24 hours after dilution. The ADD-Vantage vials are not intended for multiple-dose or IM use and should be used only when 80-mg doses of the drug are required.

IV infusions also can be prepared using the commercially available pharmacy bulk package of tobramycin sulfate powder or the commercially available pharmacy bulk package of tobramycin sulfate solution. The sterile powder is reconstituted by adding 30 mL of sterile water for injection to a vial labeled as containing 1.2 g of tobramycin (pharmacy bulk package) to provide a solution containing 40 mg of tobramycin per mL. This solution should be refrigerated and used within 96 hours; if stored at room temperature, the solution must be used within 24 hours. If the pharmacy bulk package of tobramycin sulfate solution containing 40 mg of tobramycin per mL is used, IV infusion solutions should be prepared according to the manufacturer's directions.

Alternatively, commercially available premixed tobramycin sulfate in 0.9% sodium chloride injection containing 0.8 or 1.2 mg of tobramycin per mL can be used. These premixed solutions should not be diluted or buffered prior to administration and should be given only by IV infusion. These solutions are provided in single-dose flexible containers; additives should not be introduced into the injection container and the containers should not be used in series. However, if the dose needed is greater or less than that in the container, the manufacturer states that the appropriate amount of tobramycin sulfate solution can be introduced into or removed from the container. The manufacturer's instructions should be consulted for proper use of commercially available premixed tobramycin sulfate in 0.9% sodium chloride injection.

Tobramycin sulfate should not be admixed with other drugs or infused simultaneously through the same tubing with other drugs. If a β-lactam anti-infective (e.g., cephalosporin, penicillin) is administered concomitantly with tobramycin, the drugs should not be admixed and should be administered separately.

Oral Inhalation Commercially available tobramycin solution for oral inhalation is administered via nebulization.

Tobramycin solution for oral inhalation should be administered using a PARI LC PLUS® nebulizer (a hand-held, reusable nebulizer) connected to a DeVilbiss Pulmo-Aide® compressor.

Prior to administration of tobramycin solution for oral inhalation, the manufacturers' information should be reviewed to ensure thorough familiarity with the use and maintenance of the nebulizer and compressor. Tobramycin solution for oral inhalation should be administered while the patient is sitting or standing upright and breathing normally through the mouthpiece of the nebulizer. Patients may find that breathing through the mouth may be aided by using nose clips. A nebulizer treatment period of about 15 minutes usually is required to completely administer the usual dose of tobramycin solution for oral inhalation.

Tobramycin solution for oral inhalation should not be diluted prior to administration and should not be admixed with other drugs (e.g., dornase alfa) in the nebulizer. Patients usually receive tobramycin solution for oral inhalation in conjunction with various other standard therapies recommended for patients with cystic fibrosis. The manufacturer and some clinicians recommend that patients should receive other therapies prior to doses of tobramycin solution for oral inhalation. Based on protocols used in clinical studies evaluating tobramycin solution for oral inhalation, it has been recommended that patients receive doses of inhaled bronchodilators first, then dornase alfa administered by oral inhalation, then chest physiotherapy, then tobramycin solution administered by oral inhalation. If orally inhaled corticosteroids, cromolyn sodium, or nedocromil sodium also are indicted in the patient, these drugs should be administered following the dose of tobramycin solution for oral inhalation.

■ Dosage

Parenteral Dosage Dosage of tobramycin sulfate and tobramycin are expressed in terms of tobramycin. IM and IV dosage is identical.

Like other aminoglycosides, dosage of tobramycin should be individualized taking into consideration the patient's pretreatment body weight, renal status, severity of the infection, and susceptibility of the causative organism. The manufacturers state that dosage in obese patients may be calculated using the patient's estimated lean body weight plus 40% of the excess weight. Many clinicians recommend that tobramycin dosage be determined using appropriate pharmacokinetic methods for calculating dosage requirements and patient-specific pharmacokinetic parameters (e.g., elimination rate constant, volume of distribution) derived from serum concentration-time data.

Whenever possible, especially in patients with life-threatening infections, suspected toxicity or nonresponse to treatment, decreased or varying renal function, and/or when increased aminoglycoside clearance (e.g., patients with cystic fibrosis, burns) or prolonged therapy is likely, peak and trough serum concentrations of tobramycin should be determined periodically and dosage should be adjusted to maintain desired serum concentrations. (See Dosage and Administration: Dosage, in the Aminoglycosides General Statement 8:12.02.) A causal relationship between maintenance of certain peak or trough serum concentrations or other pharmacodynamic endpoints and clinical response or toxicity has not been established to date for tobramycin dosing regimens. However, for tobramycin administered in conventional dosage regimens (i.e., multiple daily doses), peak serum concentrations of 4–10 mcg/mL and trough concentrations that do not exceed 1–2 mcg/mL have been suggested. Tobramycin serum concentrations greater than 10–12 mcg/mL may be associated with toxicity.

Parenteral aminoglycosides historically have been administered in dosage regimens that include multiple daily doses, and current prescribing information for IM or IV tobramycin only includes dosage regimens that involve multiple daily doses (usually 3 or 4 doses daily). However, there is evidence that once-daily† (single-daily) aminoglycoside dosage regimens are at least as effective as, may provide superior pharmacokinetics, and may be less toxic than conventional dosage regimens employing multiple daily doses of the drugs. Once-daily parenteral aminoglycoside regimens should *not* be used in all patients. Additional controlled trials in children, patients with renal dysfunction, cystic fibrosis patients, and other appropriate patient groups are needed to fully define optimal use of once-daily aminoglycoside dosing regimens. In addition, the most appropriate methods for optimizing dosage selection for once-daily regimens and monitoring serum aminoglycoside concentrations in patients receiving such regimens have not been clearly established. (See Dosage and Administration: Dosage, in the Aminoglycosides General Statement 8:12.02.)

The usual duration of parenteral tobramycin therapy is 7–10 days. Although a longer course of treatment may be necessary in difficult and complicated infections, renal, auditory, and vestibular function should be closely monitored because neurotoxicity is more likely to occur when treatment is extended longer than 10 days.

General Adult Dosage. The usual IM or IV dosage of tobramycin recommended by the manufacturers for adults with normal renal function is 3 mg/kg daily given in 3 equally divided doses at 8-hour intervals. The manufacturers state that adults with life-threatening infections may receive up to 5 mg/kg daily given IM or IV in 3 or 4 equally divided doses, but dosage should be reduced to 3 mg/kg daily as soon as clinically indicated.

The manufacturers state that, to prevent increased toxicity and excessive tobramycin concentrations, dosage should not exceed 5 mg/kg daily unless serum concentrations of the drug are monitored.

Adults have received parenteral tobramycin in a once-daily† regimen of 4–5 mg/kg once daily. A parenteral dosage of 7 mg/kg once daily also has been used.

Meningitis. If parenteral tobramycin is used for the treatment of meningitis, some clinicians recommend that adults receive 5 mg/kg daily given in 3 divided doses.

Tobramycin doses of 5–20 mg have been administered intrathecally† or intraventricularly† once daily in adults.

Cystic Fibrosis Patients. When parenteral tobramycin sulfate is used in patients with cystic fibrosis, altered pharmacokinetics may result in increased clearance and reduced serum aminoglycoside concentrations. Therefore, monitoring tobramycin serum concentrations during treatment is especially important as a basis for determining appropriate dosage.

If parenteral tobramycin is used in patients with cystic fibrosis, an initial regimen of 10–15 mg/kg daily given in 3 or 4 equally divided doses usually is used and subsequent dosage adjusted based on serum tobramycin concentrations. Alternatively, a once-daily† parenteral tobramycin regimen of 7–15 mg/kg given once daily by IV infusion has been used in adults with cystic fibrosis. In some patients, this dosage was used initially and subsequent dosage adjusted based on serum tobramycin concentrations. Tobramycin usually is continued for 14 days in these patients.

For oral inhalation dosage in patients with cystic fibrosis, see Dosage: Oral Inhalation Dosage.

General Pediatric Dosage. The manufacturers recommend that pediatric patients older than 1 week of age receive IM or IV tobramycin in a dosage of 6–7.5 mg/kg daily given in 3 or 4 equally divided doses (2–2.5 mg/kg every 8 hours or 1.5–1.89 mg/kg every 6 hours). The manufacturers state that dosage in neonates 1 week of age or younger should not exceed 4 mg/kg daily given in equally divided doses at 12-hour intervals.

The American Academy of Pediatrics (AAP) recommends that neonates younger than 1 week of age receive IM or IV tobramycin in a dosage of 2.5 mg/kg every 18–24 hours if they weigh less than 1.2 kg or 2.5 mg/kg every 12 hours if they weigh 1.2 kg or more. For neonates 1–4 weeks of age, the AAP recommends a dosage of 2.5 mg/kg every 18–24 hours for those weighing less than 1.2 kg, 2.5 mg/kg every 8 or 12 hours for those weighing 1.2–2 kg, or 2.5 mg/kg every 8 hours for those weighing more than 2 kg.

The AAP recommends that pediatric patients beyond the newborn period receive IM or IV tobramycin in a dosage of 3–7.5 mg/kg daily given in 3 equally divided doses for the treatment of severe infections. The AAP states that tobramycin is inappropriate for the treatment of mild to moderate infections.

The AAP states that a once-daily† IM or IV regimen (5–6 mg/kg once every 24 hours) is investigational in children. A once-daily regimen of 7–15 mg/kg given by IV infusion once daily has been used in children with cystic fibrosis. In some patients, this dosage was used initially and subsequent dosage adjusted based on serum tobramycin concentrations.

If parenteral tobramycin is used for the treatment of meningitis, some clinicians recommend that neonates 7 days of age or younger receive 4 or 5 mg/kg daily given in 2 divided doses and that older neonates and children receive 6 or 7.5 mg/kg daily given in 3 divided doses. Smaller doses and longer intervals between doses may be indicated in neonates weighing less than 2 kg.

Oral Inhalation Dosage **Cystic Fibrosis Patients.** Dosage of commercially available tobramycin solution for oral inhalation is the same for all patients regardless of age or body weight. The drug is given in an intermittent dosage regimen that involves alternating 28-day periods when the drug is given with 28-day periods when the drug is not given.

The dosage of tobramycin solution for oral inhalation recommended for the management of acute exacerbations of pulmonary *Ps. aeruginosa* infections in adults and children 6 years of age or older with cystic fibrosis is 300 mg twice daily for 28 days. Doses should be administered using the recommended nebulizer system every 12 hours (or at intervals as close to every 12 hours as possible); doses should not be administered at intervals less than 6 hours. Each 28-day regimen of tobramycin solution for oral inhalation should be followed by a 28-day period when the drug is not administered.

■ **Dosage in Renal Impairment** In patients with impaired renal function, doses and/or frequency of administration of tobramycin must be modified in response to serum concentrations of the drug and the degree of renal impairment. There are various methods to determine dosage and a wide variation in dosage recommendations for these patients. However, even when one of these methods is used, peak and trough serum concentrations of the drug should be monitored, especially in patients with changing renal function.

The manufacturers recommend an initial loading dose of 1 mg/kg with subsequent dosage adjusted either by using reduced doses at 8-hour intervals or using usual doses at prolonged intervals. If serum concentrations of tobramycin are unavailable, dosage adjustments in patients with renal impairment may be guided by creatinine clearance or serum creatinine concentrations because these values correlate with the half-life of tobramycin. The manufacturers' information should be consulted for a nomogram based on creatinine clearance or serum creatinine concentrations that can be used to determine the amount of reduced dose that can be given at the usual dosing intervals. Alternatively, if creatinine clearance is not available and the patient's condition is stable, the manufacturers state that the usual dosage of the drug can be given at a reduced dosage frequency that is calculated by multiplying the patient's steady-state serum creatinine (in mg/dL) by 6. Many clinicians recommend the dosing method of Sarubbi and Hull, which is based on corrected creatinine clearance. (See Dosage and Administration: Dosage in Renal Impairment, in the Aminoglycosides General Statement 8:12.02.)

In adults with renal failure undergoing hemodialysis, some clinicians recommend supplemental doses of 50–75% of the initial loading dose at the end of each dialysis period. Serum tobramycin concentrations should be monitored in dialysis patients and dosage adjusted as needed to maintain desired serum concentrations.

Pharmacokinetics

The pharmacokinetics of tobramycin are similar to those of the other aminoglycosides. In all studies described in the Pharmacokinetics section, tobramycin was administered parenterally as the sulfate salt; dosages and concentrations of the drug are expressed in terms of tobramycin.

■ **Absorption** Tobramycin is poorly absorbed from the GI tract.

Tobramycin is rapidly absorbed following IM administration. Following IM administration of a single dose of tobramycin of 1 mg/kg in adults with normal renal function, peak serum tobramycin concentrations average 4–6 mcg/mL and are attained within 30–90 minutes; at 6–8 hours after the dose, serum concentrations are 1 mcg/mL or less. When the same dose is administered by IV infusion over 30–60 minutes, similar plasma concentrations of the drug are attained.

In one study in neonates receiving IM tobramycin in a dosage of 2 mg/kg every 12 hours, peak serum concentrations of the drug were attained 0.5–1 hour after a dose and ranged from 4.9–5.2 mcg/mL after the first dose and 4.5–5.1 mcg/mL after 10–16 doses. In neonates 2–7 days of age receiving tobramycin in a dosage of 2.5 mg/kg by IV infusion every 12 hours, steady-state peak serum concentrations ranged from 3.5–9.9 mcg/mL and trough serum concentrations ranged from 1.1–3.6 mcg/mL in those weighing less than 2 kg. In those weighing 2 kg or more, peak serum concentrations ranged from 5–10.2 mcg/mL and trough serum concentrations ranged from 0.7–2 mcg/mL.

Bioavailability of tobramycin administered by oral inhalation via a nebulizer may be variable because of individual differences in nebulizer performance and airway pathology. Following oral inhalation via nebulization, tobramycin remains concentrated principally in the airways; the drug does not readily cross epithelial membranes. Tobramycin sputum concentrations are highly variable following oral inhalation, but the drug does not appear to accumulate in sputum following multiple doses. Following an initial 300-mg dose of commercially available tobramycin solution for oral inhalation given via a nebulizer, sputum concentrations of the drug at 10 minutes averaged 1237 mcg/g (range: 35–7414 mcg/g). After 20 weeks of intermittent therapy (300-mg twice daily for 28 days followed by 28 days without the drug), sputum concentrations 10 minutes after administration averaged 1154 mcg/g (range: 39–8085 mcg/g) and sputum concentrations 2 hours after administration were approximately 14% of those obtained 10 minutes after administration. Following a single 300-mg dose of the commercially available tobramycin solution for oral inhalation given via nebulization in patients with cystic fibrosis, serum tobramycin concentrations averaged 0.95 mcg/mL at 1 hour after administration; after 20 weeks of intermittent therapy (300 mg twice daily for 28 days followed by 28 days without the drug), serum tobramycin concentrations averaged 1.05 mcg/mL at 1 hour after administration.

■ **Distribution** The volume of distribution of tobramycin in neonates 2–7 days of age has ranged from 0.5–1.24 L/kg.

Tobramycin is rapidly distributed into most body tissues and fluids following IM or IV administration, including bronchial secretions, sputum, and peritoneal, synovial, and abscess fluids. Low concentrations occur in bile.

Only very low concentrations of tobramycin are distributed into CSF following IM or IV administration, even in patients with meningitis. In one adult with meningitis, intrathecal administration of 3–8 mg of tobramycin every 48 hours in conjunction with IM administration of 3 mg/kg daily resulted in CSF concentrations of the drug averaging 15–46 mcg/mL during the first 24 hours and 3–9 mcg/mL at 48 hours.

Tobramycin crosses the placenta and is distributed into amniotic fluid.

Tobramycin is distributed into milk. Following IM or IV administration, tobramycin concentrations in milk are very low or undetectable.

■ **Elimination** The plasma elimination half-life of tobramycin following parenteral administration usually is 2–3 hours in adults with normal renal function and has ranged from 50–70 hours in adults with impaired renal function.

The serum elimination half-life of tobramycin is reported to average 4.6 hours in full-term infants weighing more than 2.5 kg and 8.7 hours in infants weighing less than 1.5 kg. In one study in neonates 2–7 days of age, elimination half-life ranged from 5.68–13.6 hours in those weighing less than 2 kg and 3.54–6.73 hours in those weighing 2 kg or more.

In adults with normal renal function, up to 84% of a single 1-mg/kg IM dose of tobramycin is excreted unchanged by glomerular filtration within 8 hours and up to 93% is excreted unchanged within 24 hours. Peak urine concentrations of tobramycin may range from 75–100 mcg/mL following a single IM dose of 1 mg/kg in adults with normal renal function. Complete recovery of the dose in urine requires approximately 10–20 days in patients with normal renal function, and terminal elimination half-lives of greater than 100 hours have been reported in adults with normal renal function following repeated IM or IV administration of the drug.

When tobramycin is administered by oral inhalation using a nebulizer, any drug that is not absorbed systemically probably is eliminated principally in expectorated sputum.

Total body clearance of tobramycin is approximately 20% higher in patients with cystic fibrosis than in patients without the disease; however, renal clearance is similar.

Tobramycin is removed by hemodialysis and peritoneal dialysis.

Chemistry and Stability

■ **Chemistry** Tobramycin is an aminoglycoside antibiotic obtained from cultures of *Streptomyces tenebrarius*. Tobramycin occurs as a white to off-white, hygroscopic powder and is freely soluble in water and very slightly soluble in alcohol. The drug is commercially available as the sulfate salt for parenteral administration and as the base for administration by oral inhalation via a nebulizer.

Parenteral Commercially available tobramycin sulfate solutions containing 10 or 40 mg of tobramycin per mL are clear, colorless, aqueous solutions; sulfuric acid and/or sodium hydroxide is added during manufacture to adjust the pH to 3–6.5. The solutions in multiple-dose vials or single-dose ADD-Vantage® vials contain sodium metabisulfite; some multiple-dose vials contain phenol as a preservative. Solutions in pharmacy bulk packages contain sodium metabisulfite, but do not contain other preservatives.

The commercially available powder for injection for IV infusion (pharmacy bulk package) is formulated without sodium bisulfite or preservatives; sulfuric acid and/or sodium hydroxide may be added during manufacture to adjust the pH.

The commercially available premixed solutions containing 0.8 or 1.2 mg of tobramycin per mL in 0.9% sodium chloride injection are clear, colorless solutions that do not contain a preservative; these solutions have an osmolarity of approximately 313 or 316 mOsm/L, respectively. Sulfuric acid and/or sodium hydroxide is added during manufacture to adjust the pH to 3–6.5.

Oral Inhalation Commercially available tobramycin solution for oral inhalation occurs as a clear, slightly yellow, aqueous solution. Each 5-mL single-use ampul containing 300 mg of tobramycin contains 11.25 mg of sodium chloride in sterile water for injection; sulfuric acid and sodium hydroxide are added during the manufacture of the solution to adjust the pH to 6. The solution for oral inhalation does not contain preservatives.

■ **Stability** ***Parenteral*** Tobramycin sulfate solution in multiple-dose vials should be stored at 20–25°C or 15–30°C, depending on the manufacturer. Tobramycin sulfate is stable for 24 hours at room temperature in many IV infusion solutions; however, the drug is incompatible with IV solutions containing alcohol.

Tobramycin sulfate solution in single-dose ADD-Vantage® vials should be stored at 20–25°C. After the vials have been connected to an appropriate ADD-Vantage® diluent container and activated for dilution, resultant solutions should be used within 24 hours.

Tobramycin sulfate powder for injection for IV infusion (pharmacy bulk package) should be stored at 15–30°C. Following reconstitution, solutions containing 40 mg of tobramycin per mL prepared from the pharmacy bulk package should be refrigerated and used within 96 hours; if stored at room temperature, the reconstituted solution must be used within 24 hours.

Tobramycin sulfate solution containing 40 mg of tobramycin per mL (pharmacy bulk package) should be stored at 20–25°C. After the container has been entered to prepare IV solutions, any unused portion remaining in the vial should be discarded within 4 hours.

Commercially available premixed tobramycin sulfate in 0.9% sodium chloride injection provided in single-dose flexible plastic containers should be stored at 25°C; freezing should be avoided. Although brief exposure to temperatures up to 40°C does not adversely affect these solutions, exposure to excessive heat should be avoided.

Tobramycin sulfate solutions should not be admixed with other drugs.

Oral Inhalation Commercially available tobramycin solution for oral inhalation should be stored at 2–8°C. If refrigeration is not available, intact or opened foil pouches containing ampuls of the solution for oral inhalation may be stored at room temperature up to 25°C for up to 28 days. The ampuls should not be exposed to intense light. Tobramycin solution for oral inhalation may darken if stored at room temperature, but this does not indicate a change in the quality of the preparation. Any tobramycin solution for oral inhalation that is cloudy or has visible particles should be discarded. In addition, any tobramycin solution for oral inhalation that has been stored at 2–8°C beyond the expiration date stamped on the ampul or stored for longer than 28 days at room temperature should be discarded.

For further information on chemistry and stability, mechanism of action, spectrum, resistance, pharmacokinetics, uses, cautions, drug interactions, and dosage and administration of tobramycin, see the Aminoglycosides General Statement 8:12.02.

Preparations

Excipients in commercially available drug preparations may have clinically important effects in some individuals; consult specific product labeling for details.

Tobramycin

Oral Inhalation		
Solution, for nebulization only	300 mg per 5 mL	**Tobi®**, Chiron

Tobramycin Sulfate

Parenteral		
For injection, for IV infusion only	1.2 g (of tobramycin) pharmacy bulk package*	**Tobramycin Sulfate for Injection**
For injection, concentrate for IV infusion	10 mg (of tobramycin) per mL (80 mg)*	**Tobramycin Sulfate ADD-Vantage®**, Hospira
Injection	10 mg (of tobramycin) per mL (20 mg)*	**Tobramycin Sulfate Pediatric Injection**
	40 mg (of tobramycin) per mL (80 mg or 1.2 g)*	**Tobramycin Sulfate Injection**
	40 mg (of tobramycin) per mL (2 g) pharmacy bulk package*	**Tobramycin Sulfate Injection**

*available from one or more manufacturer, distributor, and/or repackager by generic (nonproprietary) name

Tobramycin Sulfate in Sodium Chloride

Parenteral		
Injection, for IV infusion only	0.8 mg (of tobramycin) per mL (80 mg) in 0.9% Sodium Chloride*	**Tobramycin Sulfate in 0.9% Sodium Chloride Injection**
	1.2 mg (of tobramycin) per mL (60 mg) in 0.9% Sodium Chloride*	**Tobramycin Sulfate in 0.9% Sodium Chloride Injection**

*available from one or more manufacturer, distributor, and/or repackager by generic (nonproprietary) name

†Use is not currently included in the labeling approved by the US Food and Drug Administration

Selected Revisions January 2009,

CEPHALOSPORINS 8:12.06

Cephalosporins General Statement

■ Cephalosporins are semisynthetic β-lactam antibiotics that are structurally and pharmacologically related to penicillins and cephamycins (e.g., cefotetan, cefoxitin). Cephalosporins generally are divided into 5 groups ("generations") based on their spectra of activity.

Uses

Cephalosporins are used parenterally for the treatment of lower respiratory tract, skin and skin structure, urinary tract, and bone and joint infections caused by susceptible gram-positive or gram-negative bacteria and also are used parenterally for the treatment of meningitis and septicemia/bacteremia caused by susceptible gram-positive or gram-negative bacteria. Cephalosporins also are used parenterally for the treatment of intra-abdominal, biliary tract, and gynecologic infections (including pelvic inflammatory disease) caused by susceptible bacteria. Cefotaxime, cefoxitin, ceftriaxone, and cefuroxime are used parenterally for the treatment of uncomplicated gonorrhea or other gonococcal infections; cefepime, ceftazidime, and ceftriaxone are used for empiric anti-infective therapy in febrile neutropenic patients; and cefazolin, cefotaxime, ceftriaxone, and cefuroxime are used parenterally for perioperative prophylaxis.

Cephalosporins are used orally for the treatment of mild to moderate respiratory tract infections, including acute maxillary sinusitis, acute bacterial exacerbations of chronic bronchitis, secondary infections of acute bronchitis, and community-acquired pneumonia, caused by susceptible bacteria (e.g., *Streptococcus pneumoniae, Haemophilus influenzae, H. parainfluenzae, Moraxella catarrhalis*); acute bacterial otitis media caused by susceptible bacteria (e.g., *S. pneumoniae, H. influenzae, M. catarrhalis*); and pharyngitis and tonsillitis caused by *Streptococcus pyogenes* (group A β-hemolytic streptococci). Cefaclor, cefadroxil, cefdinir, cefditoren pivoxil, cefpodoxime proxetil, cefprozil, ceftibuten, cefuroxime axetil, and cephalexin also are used orally for the treatment of mild to moderate skin and skin structure infections caused by susceptible staphylococci or streptococci. In addition, cefaclor, cefadroxil, cefixime, cefpodoxime proxetil, cefuroxime axetil, and cephalexin are used orally for the treatment of mild to moderate urinary tract infections caused by susceptible gram-negative bacteria (e.g., *Escherichia coli, Klebsiella, Proteus mirabilis*). Some clinicians suggest that certain oral third generation cephalosporins (cefdinir, cefpodoxime proxetil, ceftibuten) are one of several alternatives that can be used for the outpatient treatment of recurrent urinary tract infections or urinary tract infections acquired in hospitals or nursing homes since these infections are likely to be caused by multidrug-resistant gram-negative bacilli. Certain oral cephalosporins (e.g., cefixime, cefpodoxime proxetil, cefuroxime axetil) have been used for the treatment of uncomplicated gonorrhea. (See Uses: Gonorrhea and Associated Infections.)

Prior to and during cephalosporin therapy, the causative organism should be cultured and in vitro susceptibility tests performed. In serious infections, therapy may be initiated pending results of in vitro tests. In certain serious infections when the causative organism is unknown, concomitant therapy with another anti-infective agent (e.g., an aminoglycoside) may be indicated pending results of susceptibility tests. Use of a cephalosporin does not replace surgical procedures such as incision and drainage when indicated.

■ **Gram-positive Bacterial Infections** First and second generation cephalosporins are used in the treatment of infections caused by susceptible staphylococci or streptococci. Third generation cephalosporins generally are less active than first and second generation cephalosporins against gram-positive aerobic bacteria, especially staphylococci, and usually are not used in the treatment of infections caused by gram-positive bacteria when a penicillin or a first or second generation cephalosporin could be used. Some third generation cephalosporins (e.g., cefotaxime, ceftriaxone) are considered drugs of choice for serious bacterial infections, including endocarditis or meningitis, caused by susceptible *S. pneumoniae* or viridans streptococci. Unlike other cephalosporins, fifth generation cephalosporins (e.g., ceftaroline) have activity against methicillin-resistant *S. aureus* (MRSA, also known as oxacillin-resistant *S. aureus* [ORSA]) and are used in the treatment of some MRSA infections.

■ **Gram-negative Bacterial Infections** Use of first generation cephalosporins (cefazolin) in the treatment of gram-negative bacterial infections generally is limited to infections caused by susceptible *E. coli*, *H. influenzae*, *Klebsiella*, or *P. mirabilis*. Second and third generation cephalosporins are used in the treatment of infections caused by these organisms as well as infections caused by susceptible *Enterobacter*, *Morganella morganii* (formerly *Proteus morganii*), *Neisseria*, *Providencia rettgeri* (formerly *P. rettgeri*), or *P. vulgaris*; cefotaxime, ceftazidime, and ceftriaxone also are used in the treatment of infections caused by susceptible *Serratia*. Certain parenteral third generation cephalosporins (i.e., cefepime, cefotaxime, ceftazidime, ceftriaxone) may be drugs of choice for the treatment of infections caused by susceptible Enterobacteriaceae, including susceptible *E. coli*, *Klebsiella pneumoniae*, *P. rettgeri*, *M. morganii*, *P. vulgaris*, or *P. stuartii* and are alternatives for the treatment of infections caused by susceptible *Serratia*; an aminoglycoside usually is used concomitantly in severe infections. Ceftazidime and cefepime are considered alternatives for the treatment of infections caused by susceptible *Pseudomonas aeruginosa*; an aminoglycoside may be used concomitantly. Ceftazidime is more active in vitro on a weight basis against *Ps. aeruginosa* than most other currently available cephalosporins and is active against some strains resistant to many other cephalosporins, aminoglycosides, and extended-spectrum penicillins. Ceftaroline, a fifth generation cephalosporin, generally has activity against gram-negative aerobes that is similar to that reported with third generation cephalosporins.

■ **Endocarditis** ***Treatment*** Ceftriaxone is used for the treatment of native valve or prosthetic valve endocarditis caused by viridans streptococci (e.g., *S. oralis*, *S. milleri* group, *S. mitis*, *S. mutans*, *S. salivarius*, *S. sanguis*, *Gamella morbillorum*) or *S. bovis* (nonenterococcal group D streptococcus)†. The drug also is used for the treatment of native valve or prosthetic valve endocarditis caused by slow-growing fastidious gram-negative bacilli termed the HACEK group† (i.e., *Haemophilus parainfluenzae*, *H. aphrophilus*, *H. paraphrophilus*, *H. influenzae*, *Actinobacillus actinomycetemcomitans*, *Cardiobacterium hominis*, *Eikenella corrodens*, *Kingella kingae*, *K. denitrificans*). In addition, ceftriaxone has been used for the treatment of native or prosthetic valve endocarditis caused by *E. faecalis* resistant to penicillin, aminoglycosides, and vancomycin. (See Uses: Endocarditis in Ceftriaxone Sodium 8:12.06.12.)

IV cefazolin is used as an alternative to nafcillin or oxacillin for the treatment of staphylococcal endocarditis, including infections caused by coagulase-positive strains (*S. aureus*) or coagulase-negative strains (e.g., *S. epidermidis*†, *S. lugdunensis*†) in penicillin-allergic patients (nonanaphylactoid type only). Cefazolin also is used as an alternative to penicillin G sodium for the *treatment* of endocarditis caused by susceptible *Streptococcus pyogenes* (group A β-hemolytic streptococci) or *S. pneumoniae*†. (See Uses: Endocarditis in Cefazolin Sodium 8:12.06.04.)

For empiric treatment of culture-negative endocarditis† in prosthetic valve recipients with early onset endocarditis (within 1 year after prosthetic valve placement), a multiple-drug regimen that includes vancomycin, gentamicin, cefepime, and rifampin is recommended. (See Uses: Endocarditis in Cefepime Hydrochloride 8:12.06.16.)

Prevention Certain cephalosporins (cefazolin, ceftriaxone, cephalexin, cefadroxil) are used as alternatives to amoxicillin or ampicillin for *prevention* of α-hemolytic (viridans group) streptococcal endocarditis† in penicillin-allergic adults and children undergoing certain dental or upper respiratory tract procedures who have underlying cardiac conditions that put them at the highest risk of adverse outcome from endocarditis. These cephalosporins should not be used for such prophylaxis in patients with a history of immediate-type penicillin hypersensitivity (e.g., urticaria, angioedema, anaphylaxis).

The cardiac conditions identified by the American Heart Association (AHA) as those associated with the highest risk and for which endocarditis prophylaxis is recommended are prosthetic cardiac valves, previous infective endocarditis, congenital heart disease (i.e., unrepaired cyanotic congenital heart disease including palliative shunts and conduits; a completely repaired congenital heart defect where a prosthetic material or device was placed by surgery or catheter intervention within the last 6 months; repaired congenital heart disease with residual defects at the site or adjacent to the site of a prosthetic patch or prosthetic device which inhibits endothelialization), and cardiac valvulopathy after cardiac transplantation. AHA states that endocarditis prophylaxis is recommended for such patients when they undergo dental procedures that involve manipulation of gingival tissue or the periapical region of teeth or perforation of the oral mucosa or undergo invasive procedures of the respiratory tract that involve incision or biopsy of the respiratory mucosa (e.g., tonsillectomy, adenoidectomy). Although endocarditis prophylaxis also may be indicated for such patients when they undergo surgical procedures that involve infected skin, skin structure, or musculoskeletal tissue, prophylaxis solely to prevent infective endocarditis is not recommended for GI or genitourinary tract procedures.

When selecting anti-infectives for prophylaxis of bacterial endocarditis, the current recommendations published by AHA should be consulted.

■ **GI Infections** Some parenteral third generation cephalosporins are used in the treatment of GI infections caused by *Salmonella* or *Shigella* or the treatment of other uncommon infectious diarrheal illnesses, including infections caused by *Vibrio* and *Yersinia*.

Salmonella Gastroenteritis Anti-infective therapy generally is not indicated in otherwise healthy individuals with uncomplicated (noninvasive) gastroenteritis caused by non-typhi *Salmonella* (e.g., *S. enteritidis*, *S. typhimurium*) since these infections generally subside spontaneously and there is some evidence that such therapy may prolong the duration of fecal excretion of the organisms; however, the US Centers for Disease Control and Prevention (CDC), American Academy of Pediatrics (AAP), Infectious Diseases Society of America (IDSA), and others recommend anti-infective therapy in individuals with severe *Salmonella* gastroenteritis and in those who are at increased risk of invasive disease. These individuals at increased risk include infants younger than 3–6 months of age; individuals older than 50 years of age; individuals with hemoglobinopathies, severe atherosclerosis or valvular heart disease, prostheses, uremia, chronic GI disease, or severe colitis; and individuals who are immunocompromised because of malignancy, immunosuppressive therapy, HIV infection, or other immunosuppressive illness.

When an anti-infective is considered necessary in an individual with *Salmonella* gastroenteritis, CDC, AAP, IDSA, and others recommend ceftriaxone, cefotaxime, a fluoroquinolone (should be used in children only if the benefits outweigh the risks and no other alternative exists), ampicillin, amoxicillin, co-trimoxazole, or chloramphenicol, depending on the susceptibility of the causative organism. (See Uses: Typhoid Fever and Other Salmonella Infections in Ceftriaxone 8:12.06.12.)

Shigella Infections Ceftriaxone is used for the treatment of shigellosis† caused by susceptible *Shigella sonnei* or *S. flexneri* and is an alternative to fluoroquinolones for treatment of these infections in pediatric patients or when susceptibility is unknown or strains resistant to ampicillin and co-trimoxazole are isolated. (See Shigella Infections under Uses: GI Infections, in Ceftriaxone 8:12.06.12.)

Vibrio Infections Cefotaxime is one of several alternatives recommended for the treatment of severe cases of *Vibrio parahaemolyticus*† infection when anti-infective therapy is indicated in addition to supportive care. *V. parahaemolyticus* infections can occur as the result of ingestion of contaminated undercooked or raw fish or shellfish, and some clinicians recommend use of tetracycline, doxycycline, gentamicin, or cefotaxime when treatment is considered necessary. (See Uses Vibrio Infections, in Cefotaxime 8:12.06.12.)

Cefotaxime and ceftazidime are considered drugs of choice for the treatment of infections caused by *V. vulnificus*†; these infections can occur as the result of ingesting raw or undercooked seafood (especially raw oysters) or through contamination of a wound with seawater or seafood drippings. While optimum anti-infective therapy for the treatment of *V. vulnificus* infections has not been identified, use of cefotaxime, ceftazidime, tetracycline, or doxycycline is recommended.

Yersinia Infections Cefotaxime is suggested as a possible choice for the treatment of GI infections caused by *Yersinia enterocolitica* or *Y. pseudotuberculosis*. These *Yersinia* infections usually are self-limited and anti-infective therapy unnecessary; however, AAP, IDSA, and others recommend use of anti-infectives in immunocompromised individuals or for the treatment of severe infections or when septicemia or other invasive disease occurs. GI infections caused by *Y. enterocolitica* or *Y. pseudotuberculosis* can occur as the result of ingesting undercooked pork, unpasteurized milk, or contaminated water; infection has occurred in infants whose caregivers handled contaminated chitterlings (raw pork intestines) or tofu. Use of co-trimoxazole, an aminoglycoside (amikacin, gentamicin, tobramycin), a fluoroquinolone (e.g., ciprofloxacin), doxycycline, or cefotaxime has been recommended when treatment is considered necessary; combination therapy may be necessary. Some clinicians suggest that the role of oral anti-infectives in the management of enterocolitis, pseudoappendicitis syndrome, or mesenteric adenitis caused by *Yersinia* needs further evaluation.

■ **Intra-abdominal Infections** Cefazolin, cefepime, cefotaxime, cefoxitin, ceftazidime, ceftriaxone, and cefuroxime are used for the treatment of intra-abdominal infections. The fixed combination of ceftazidime and avibactam and the fixed combination of ceftolozane and tazobactam are used for the treatment of complicated intra-abdominal tract infections. Certain cephalosporins (e.g., cefotaxime, ceftriaxone, cefotetan, cefoxitin) also are used for the treatment of various obstetric and gynecologic infections, including pelvic inflammatory disease. (See Uses: Pelvic Inflammatory Disease.) Because the prevalence of *B. fragilis* resistant to cefotetan has been increasing, some experts state that cefotetan is not recommended for empiric treatment of intra-abdominal infections.

Although monotherapy with cefazolin, ceftriaxone, or cefuroxime is an option for initial empiric treatment of mild to moderate community-acquired biliary tract infections (cholecystitis or cholangitis) and monotherapy with cefoxitin is an option for initial empiric treatment of mild to moderate community-acquired extrabiliary intra-abdominal infections, cephalosporins usually should be used in conjunction with metronidazole for initial empiric treatment of community-acquired or healthcare-associated intra-abdominal infections.

For initial empiric treatment of mild to moderately severe community-acquired extrabiliary intra-abdominal infections in adults, IDSA recommends either monotherapy with cefoxitin, ertapenem, moxifloxacin, tigecycline, or the fixed combination of ticarcillin and clavulanate sodium, or a combination regimen that includes a cephalosporin (cefazolin, cefotaxime, ceftriaxone, cefuroxime) or fluoroquinolone (ciprofloxacin, levofloxacin) in conjunction with metronidazole. For initial empiric treatment of high-risk or severe community-acquired extrabiliary intra-abdominal infections in adults (e.g., those with advanced age, immunocompromise, severe physiologic disturbance), IDSA recommends either monotherapy with a carbapenem (doripenem, imipenem, meropenem) or the fixed combination of piperacillin and tazobactam, or a combination regimen that includes either a cephalosporin (cefepime, ceftazidime) or fluoroquinolone (ciprofloxacin, levofloxacin) in conjunction with metronidazole. IDSA also recommends ceftazidime or cefepime in conjunction with metronidazole as one of several regimens that can be used for initial empiric treatment of healthcare-associated complicated intra-abdominal infections in adults and recommends a combination regimen that includes a cephalosporin (cefotaxime, ceftriaxone, ceftazidime, cefepime) in conjunction with metronidazole as one of several options that can be used for empiric treatment of community-acquired complicated intra-abdominal infections in pediatric patients.

For additional information regarding management of intra-abdominal infections, the current IDSA clinical practice guidelines available at http://www.idsociety.org should be consulted.

■ Meningitis and Other CNS Infections IV cefotaxime, ceftazidime, ceftriaxone, and cefuroxime are used in adult or pediatric patients for the treatment of meningitis caused by susceptible *H. influenzae*, *Neisseria meningitidis*, or *S. pneumoniae*; however, cefotaxime or ceftriaxone generally are preferred when a cephalosporin is indicated for the treatment of meningitis caused by these organism. IV cefotaxime and ceftriaxone are used alone or in conjunction with an aminoglycoside for the treatment of meningitis or other CNS infections caused by susceptible Enterobacteriaceae (e.g., *E. coli*, *Klebsiella*) and IV ceftazidime is used in conjunction with an aminoglycoside for the treatment of meningitis caused by susceptible *Ps. aeruginosa*.

Empiric Treatment of Meningitis Pending results of CSF culture and in vitro susceptibility testing, the most appropriate anti-infective regimen for empiric treatment of suspected bacterial meningitis should be selected based on results of CSF Gram stain and antigen tests, age of the patient, the most likely pathogen(s) and source of infection, and current patterns of bacterial resistance within the hospital and local community. When results of culture and susceptibility tests become available and the pathogen is identified, the empiric anti-infective regimen should be modified (if necessary) to ensure that the most effective regimen is being administered. There is some evidence that short-term adjunctive therapy with IV dexamethasone may decrease the incidence of audiologic and/or neurologic sequelae in infants and children with *H. influenzae* meningitis and possibly may provide some benefit in patients with *S. pneumoniae* meningitis. AAP and other clinicians suggest that use of adjunctive dexamethasone therapy should be considered during the initial 2–4 days of anti-infective therapy in infants and children 6–8 weeks of age or older with known or suspected bacterial meningitis and is recommended in those with suspected or proven *H. influenzae* infection. If used, dexamethasone should be initiated before or concurrently with the first dose of anti-infective. (See Uses: Bacterial Meningitis in the Corticosteroids General Statement 68:04 and see Dexamethasone 68:04.)

Bacterial meningitis in neonates usually is caused by *S. agalactiae* (group B streptococci), *Listeria monocytogenes*, or aerobic gram-negative bacilli (e.g., *E. coli*, *K. pneumoniae*). AAP recommends that neonates with suspected bacterial meningitis receive an empiric regimen of IV ampicillin and an aminoglycoside pending results of CSF culture and susceptibility testing. An empiric regimen of IV ampicillin and IV cefotaxime or IV ceftazidime with or without gentamicin also is recommended. Because frequent use of cephalosporins in neonatal units may result in rapid emergence of resistant strains of some gram-negative bacilli (e.g., *Enterobacter cloacae*, *Klebsiella*, *Serratia*), AAP cautions that cephalosporins should be used for empiric treatment of meningitis in neonates only if gram-negative bacterial meningitis is strongly suspected. Consideration should be given to including IV vancomycin in the empiric regimen if *S. pneumoniae*, enterococci, or *Staphylococci* is suspected. Because ceftriaxone should be used with caution in neonates who are hyperbilirubinemic (especially those born prematurely), cefotaxime may be the preferred cephalosporin for empiric treatment of meningitis is neonates. However, because premature, low-birthweight neonates are at increased risk for nosocomial infection caused by staphylococci or gram-negative bacilli, some clinicians suggest that these neonates receive an empiric regimen of IV ceftazidime and IV vancomycin.

In infants beyond the neonatal stage who are younger than 3 months of age, bacterial meningitis usually is caused by *S. agalactiae*, *L. monocytogenes*, *H. influenzae*, *S. pneumoniae*, *N. meningitidis*, or aerobic gram-negative bacilli (e.g., *E. coli*, *K. pneumoniae*). The empiric regimen recommended for infants in this age group is IV ampicillin and either IV ceftriaxone or IV cefotaxime. Consideration should be given to including IV vancomycin in the empiric regimen if *S. pneumoniae* is suspected.

In adults and children 3 months through 17 years of age, bacterial meningitis usually is caused by *N. meningitidis or S. pneumoniae* is *N. meningitidis* or *S. pneumoniae*. An empiric regimen of IV ceftriaxone or IV cefotaxime usually is used for empiric therapy of suspected bacterial meningitis in children 3 months through 17 years of age and in adults 18–50 years of age. Although an empiric regimen of IV ampicillin and IV chloramphenicol can be used as an alternative regimen in children 3 months through 17 years of age, most clinicians prefer a cephalosporin regimen unless the drugs are contraindicated. Because of the increasing prevalence of penicillin-resistant *S. pneumoniae* that also are resistant to or have reduced susceptibility to cephalosporins, AAP and others recommend that the initial empiric cephalosporin regimen include IV vancomycin (with or without rifampin) pending results of in vitro susceptibility tests; vancomycin and rifampin should be discontinued if the causative organism is found to be susceptible to the cephalosporin. CDC and some clinicians have recommended that vancomycin be added to the empiric regimen in areas where there have been reports of highly penicillin-resistant strains of *S. pneumoniae*, but other clinicians suggest that use of ceftriaxone or cefotaxime in conjunction with vancomycin provides the optimal initial empiric regimen. While *L. monocytogenes* meningitis is relatively rare in this age group, the empiric regimen should include ampicillin if *L. monocytogenes* is suspected.

In adults older than 50 years of age, bacterial meningitis usually is caused by *S. pneumoniae*, *L. monocytogenes*, *N. meningitidis*, or aerobic gram-negative bacilli, and the empiric regimen recommended for this age group is IV ampicillin given in conjunction with IV cefotaxime or IV ceftriaxone. Because of the increasing prevalence of penicillin-resistant *S. pneumoniae*, some clinicians suggest that the empiric regimen also should include IV vancomycin (with or without rifampin).

Meningitis Caused by Streptococcus pneumoniae IV ceftriaxone and IV cefotaxime are considered drugs of choice for the treatment of meningitis caused by susceptible *S. pneumoniae*. Treatment failures have been reported when these cephalosporins were used alone for the treatment of meningitis caused by *S. pneumoniae* with intermediate or high-level penicillin resistance (i.e., penicillin MIC 0.1 mcg/mL or greater). In addition, strains of *S. pneumoniae* with reduced susceptibility to cephalosporins have been reported with increasing frequency, and use of cefotaxime or ceftriaxone alone may be ineffective for the treatment of meningitis caused by these strains. For meningitis caused by *S. pneumoniae* with high-level resistance to penicillin (i.e., penicillin MIC 8 mcg/mL or greater), IV cefotaxime or IV ceftriaxone is used in conjunction with vancomycin with or without rifampin. The prevalence of *S. pneumoniae* with reduced susceptibility to penicillin and/or cephalosporins varies geographically, and clinicians should be aware of the prevalence and pattern of *S. pneumoniae* drug resistance in the local community to optimize empiric regimens and initial therapy for serious pneumococcal infections.

Because susceptibility can no longer be assumed, *S. pneumoniae* isolates should be routinely tested for in vitro susceptibility. If anti-infective therapy in a patient with meningitis is initiated with an empiric regimen of IV ceftriaxone or IV cefotaxime and IV vancomycin (with or without rifampin) and results of culture and in vitro susceptibility testing indicate that pathogen involved is a strain of *S. pneumoniae* susceptible to the cephalosporin and susceptible or resistant to penicillin, vancomycin and rifampin can be discontinued and therapy completed using ceftriaxone or cefotaxime alone. If the isolate is found to have reduced susceptibility to ceftriaxone and cefotaxime *and* penicillin, the IV cephalosporin and IV vancomycin usually are both continued. If the patient's condition does not improve or worsens or results of a second repeat lumbar puncture (performed 24–48 hours after initiation of anti-infective therapy) indicate that the anti-infective regimen has not eradicated or substantially reduced the number of pneumococci in CSF, rifampin probably should be added to the regimen or vancomycin discontinued and replaced with rifampin. If meningitis is caused by *S. pneumoniae* highly resistant to ceftriaxone (i.e., MIC 4 mcg/mL or greater), consultation with an infectious disease expert is recommended.

Meningitis Caused by Haemophilus influenzae IV ceftriaxone and IV cefotaxime are considered drugs of choice for the initial treatment of meningitis caused by susceptible *H. influenzae* (including penicillinase-producing strains). AAP suggests that children with meningitis possibly caused by *H. influenzae* can receive an initial treatment regimen of ceftriaxone, cefotaxime, or a regimen of ampicillin given in conjunction with chloramphenicol; some clinicians prefer ceftriaxone or cefotaxime for the initial treatment of meningitis caused by *H. influenzae* since these cephalosporins are active against both penicillinase-producing and nonpenicillinase-producing strains. Because of the prevalence of ampicillin-resistant *H. influenzae*, ampicillin should not be used alone for empiric treatment of meningitis when *H. influenzae* may be involved. The incidence of *H. influenzae* meningitis in the US has decreased considerably since *H. influenzae* type b conjugate vaccines became available for immunization of infants.

Meningitis Caused by Neisseria meningitidis While both IV ampicillin and IV penicillin G may be used for the treatment of meningitis caused by *N. meningitidis*, AAP and other clinicians suggest that IV penicillin G is the drug of choice for the treatment of these infections and IV ceftriaxone and IV cefotaxime are acceptable alternatives. Chloramphenicol is recommended for the treatment of *N. meningitidis* meningitis in patients with a history of anaphylactoid-type hypersensitivity reactions to penicillin.

Meningitis Caused by Enterobacteriaceae Some clinicians recommend that meningitis caused by Enterobacteriaceae (e.g., *E. coli*, *K. pneumoniae*) be treated with a third generation cephalosporins (i.e., cefotaxime, ceftazidime, ceftriaxone) with or without an aminoglycoside. Because ceftazidime (but not cefotaxime or ceftriaxone) is effective for the treatment of meningitis caused by *Ps. aeruginosa*, some clinicians suggest that a regimen of ceftazidime and an aminoglycoside may be preferred for the treatment of meningitis caused by gram-negative bacilli pending results of culture and susceptibility testing.

Meningitis Caused by Pseudomonas aeruginosa In patients with meningitis caused by *Ps. aeruginosa*, most clinicians recommend that therapy be initiated with a regimen of ceftazidime and a parenteral aminoglycoside. If the patient fails to respond to this regimen, concomitant use of intrathecal or intraventricular aminoglycoside therapy or use of an alternative parenteral anti-infective (e.g., aztreonam, meropenem, a quinolone) should be considered based on results of in vitro susceptibility tests. When treating pediatric patients with meningitis caused by *Ps. aeruginosa* or Enterobacteriaceae, consultation with an infectious disease expert may be beneficial.

Meningitis Caused by Streptococcus agalactiae For the initial treatment of meningitis or other severe infection caused by *S. agalactiae* (group B streptococci), a regimen of IV ampicillin or IV penicillin G given in conjunction with an aminoglycoside is recommended. Some clinicians suggest that IV ampicillin is the drug of choice for the treatment of group B streptococcal meningitis and that an aminoglycoside (IV gentamicin) should be used concomitantly during the first 72 hours until in vitro susceptibility testing is completed and a clinical response if observed; thereafter, ampicillin can be given alone.

Meningitis Caused by Listeria monocytogenes The optimal regimen for the treatment of meningitis caused by *L. monocytogenes* has not been established. Cephalosporins are not active against *Listeria monocytogenes*, an organism that most frequently causes meningitis in neonates or immunocompromised individuals, and the drugs should not be used alone for empiric treatment of meningitis when this organisms may be involved. AAP and other clinicians generally recommend that meningitis or other severe infection caused by *L. monocytogenes* be treated with a regimen of IV ampicillin with or without an aminoglycoside (usually gentamicin); alternatively, a regimen of penicillin G used in conjunction with gentamicin can be used. In patients hypersensitive to penicillin, the alternative regimen for treatment of meningitis caused by *L. monocytogenes* is co-trimoxazole.

Brain Abscess and Other CNS Infections Bacterial brain abscesses and other CNS infections (e.g., subdural empyema, intracranial epidural abscesses) often are polymicrobial and can be caused by gram-positive aerobic cocci, Enterobacteriaceae (e.g., *E. coli*, *Klebsiella*), and/or anaerobic bacteria (e.g., *Bacteroides*, *Fusobacterium*). The choice of anti-infectives for empiric therapy of these infections should be based on the predisposing condition and site of primary infection. Some clinicians suggest that the empiric anti-infective regimen in patients who develop the CNS infections after respiratory tract infection (e.g., otitis media, mastoiditis, paranasal sinusitis, pyogenic lung disease) should consist of an appropriate third generation IV cephalosporin (e.g., ceftriaxone, cefotaxime, ceftazidime) given in conjunction with metronidazole; employing one of these cephalosporins rather than a penicillin provides coverage against *Haemophilus* and facultative anaerobic gram-negative bacteria. If presence of staphylococci is suspected, a penicillinase-resistant penicillin (e.g., nafcillin, oxacillin) or vancomycin should be added to the empiric regimen. In patients who develop brain abscess, subdural empyema, or intracranial epidural abscess after trauma or neurosurgery, the empiric regimen should consist of an appropriate third generation IV cephalosporin (e.g., ceftriaxone, cefotaxime, ceftazidime) given in conjunction with a penicillinase-resistant penicillin or vancomycin. Prolonged anti-infective therapy (e.g., 3–6 weeks or longer) usually is required for the treatment of brain abscess, subdural empyema, or intracranial epidural abscess.

■ **Otitis Media** ***Acute Otitis Media*** Various oral cephalosporins (e.g., cefaclor, cefdinir, cefixime, cefpodoxime proxetil, cefprozil, ceftibuten, cefuroxime axetil, cephalexin) are used for the treatment of acute otitis media (AOM) caused by *S. pneumoniae*, *H. influenzae* (including β-lactamase-producing strains), or *M. catarrhalis* (including β-lactamase-producing strains). Parenteral ceftriaxone also is used for the treatment of AOM caused by *S. pneumoniae*, *H. influenzae* (including β-lactamase-producing strains), or *M. catarrhalis* (including β-lactamase-producing strains).

AOM is one of the most frequently diagnosed bacterial infection in children, and 65–95% of children will have at least one episode of AOM by 3 years of age. *S. pneumoniae*, *H. influenzae*, and *M. catarrhalis* are the bacteria most frequently recovered from middle ear fluid of patients with AOM; *S. pyogenes* and *S. aureus* also are recovered rarely. In addition, there is evidence that respiratory viruses (e.g., respiratory syncytial virus, rhinoviruses, influenza virus, parainfluenza virus, enteroviruses) may be present either alone or in combination with bacterial pathogens and may play a role in the etiology and pathogenesis of AOM in some patients.

Diagnosis and Management Strategies for AOM. AAP and American Academy of Family Physicians (AAFP) first issued evidence-based clinical practice guidelines for the diagnosis and management of AOM in 2004. In 2013, AAP revised and updated those guidelines after comprehensive reviews of more recent published evidence. The 2013 AAP evidence-based clinical practice guidelines provide recommendations for the diagnosis and management of uncomplicated AOM, including recurrent AOM, in children 6 months through 12 years of age and apply only to otherwise healthy children who do not have underlying conditions that may alter the natural course of AOM (e.g., tympanostomy tubes, cleft palate, genetic conditions with craniofacial abnormalities such as Down syndrome, immunodeficiencies, cochlear implants). These AAP guidelines should be consulted for additional information on diagnosis and management of AOM.

Accurate diagnosis of AOM is critical for clinical decision-making since it avoids unnecessary treatment. AOM involves the presence of fluid in the middle ear accompanied by a wide spectrum of signs or symptoms of acute local or systemic illness (e.g., otalgia, otorrhea, hearing loss, swelling around the ear, vertigo, nystagmus, tinnitus, fever, irritability, headache, diarrhea, lethargy, anorexia, vomiting) that evolve as the disease progresses. Older children with AOM usually have a history of rapid onset of ear pain, but preverbal infants and young children may have mild or nonspecific symptoms that overlap with those of an upper respiratory tract illness.

Current AAP evidence-based clinical practice guidelines for the diagnosis and management of uncomplicated AOM in children 6 months through 12 years of age state that clinicians should diagnose AOM in children who present with moderate to severe bulging of the tympanic membrane *or* new onset of otorrhea not due to acute otitis externa. A diagnosis of AOM also should be made in children who present with mild bulging of the tympanic membrane *and* recent (less than 48 hours) onset of ear pain (holding, tugging, rubbing of the ear in a nonverbal child) or intense erythema of the tympanic membrane. These guidelines state that a diagnosis of AOM should *not* be made in children who do not have middle ear effusion (MEE) based on pneumatic otoscopy and/or tympanometry.

Current AAP evidence-based clinical practice guidelines for the diagnosis and management of uncomplicated AOM in children 6 months through 12 years of age state that management of AOM should include an assessment of pain and, if ear pain is present, the clinician should recommend treatment to reduce the pain. AOM-associated pain can be substantial during the first few days of illness and often persists longer in young children. AAP states that pain management, especially during the first 24 hours of an AOM episode, should be addressed regardless of the use of anti-infectives. Treatment for otalgia should be selected based on a consideration of the benefits and risks and, whenever possible, incorporate parent and/or caregiver and patient preference. Acetaminophen or ibuprofen are effective for mild to moderate pain, readily available, and usually the mainstay of pain management for AOM.

Up to 60–80% of cases of AOM resolve spontaneously within 7–14 days, and *routine* administration of anti-infectives is not considered necessary for the treatment of all cases of AOM. Some clinicians have recommended that all cases of AOM be treated with an appropriate anti-infective regimen to facilitate resolution of the primary infection and associated symptoms and prevent suppurative complications or other sequelae, and state that judicious use of anti-infectives in the management of otitis media involves accurately diagnosing AOM and distinguishing AOM (which should be treated with anti-infectives) from otitis media with effusion (which usually is not treated with anti-infectives). However, for the majority of patients with uncomplicated AOM, anti-infective therapy appears to provide only minimal benefits in terms of resolution of the acute symptoms of infection (e.g., pain) and the proposed benefits of such therapy in terms of time to bacteriologic or clinical resolution of AOM or in terms of long-term consequences of otitis media (e.g., persistence of middle ear effusion, recurrence of AOM, hearing loss, need for adenoidectomy or insertion of tympanostomy tubes, mastoiditis) have never been substantiated in well-designed, placebo-controlled studies. In addition, there is evidence that overuse of anti-infectives, including overuse in the treatment of AOM, contributes to emergence of resistant bacteria (e.g., multidrug-resistant *S. pneumoniae*). Based on these considerations, many clinicians now recommend a management strategy for AOM that involves use of symptomatic care with analgesics and close observation via telephone contact or office visits for the majority of patients with uncomplicated AOM and use of anti-infectives only in those who do not have symptomatic improvement within 24–72 hours after diagnosis and in those who appear least likely to have spontaneous resolution and most likely to have poor outcomes (e.g., more acutely ill, those with 3 or more episodes of AOM in the past 18 months, history of serous otitis or tympanostomy tubes).

Current AAP evidence-based clinical practice guidelines for the diagnosis and management of uncomplicated AOM in children 6 months through 12 years of age include an initial management option of *observation with close follow-up without initial use of anti-infectives* in certain selected children with uncomplicated AOM based on age, illness severity, and assurance of follow-up. The recommendation for initial observation with close follow-up in select children provides an opportunity for the patient to improve without anti-infectives and is based on results of randomized, controlled studies with limitations and consideration of the benefits and risks of such a strategy.

Current AAP guidelines state that anti-infective treatment should be initiated in children 6 months of age or older who have AOM (bilateral or unilateral) with severe signs or symptoms (i.e., moderate or severe otalgia, otalgia for at least 48 hours, or temperature 39°C or higher) and in children 6 through 23 months of age who have nonsevere bilateral AOM without signs or symptoms (i.e., mild otalgia for less than 48 hours and temperature less than 39°C). However, these guidelines state that a management strategy of *either* initiation of anti-infective treatment *or* observation with close follow-up can be used in children 6 through 23 months of age who have nonsevere unilateral AOM without severe signs or symptoms (i.e., mild otalgia for less than 48 hours, temperature less than 39°C) and in children 24 months of age or older with nonsevere AOM (bilateral or unilateral) without severe signs or symptoms (i.e., mild otalgia for less than 48 hours, temperature less than 39°C). The strategy of observation with close follow-up should be based on joint decision-making between the clinician and the parent and/or caregiver and must include a mechanism that ensures follow-up and initiation of anti-infective therapy if AOM worsens or fails to improve within 48–72 hours after symptom onset.

If the initial management strategy was observation with close follow-up, anti-infective therapy should be initiated if symptoms worsen or there is no improvement within 48–72 hours after onset of symptoms. If the initial management strategy was anti-infective treatment, consideration should be given to changing the anti-infective regimen if symptoms worsen or fail to respond within 48–72 hours after initiation of treatment. (See Anti-infectives for AOM after Initial Treatment Failure under Uses: Otitis Media.)

After the patient has shown clinical improvement, follow-up is based on the usual clinical course of AOM. Persistent MEE is common after resolution of acute symptoms of AOM and should not be viewed as requiring anti-infective treatment. (See Otitis Media with Effusion under Uses: Otitis Media.)

Anti-infectives for Initial Treatment of AOM. When anti-infectives are indicated for treatment of AOM, the initial anti-infective agent usually is selected empirically based on efficacy against the most probable bacterial pathogens. Other considerations in the choice of an anti-infective for initial empiric treatment of AOM include pharmacokinetic data related to distribution of the drug into middle ear fluid, compliance issues related to patient acceptance of dosage formulation and dosage schedule, adverse effects profiles, and cost considerations; drug susceptibility patterns in the local community can be considered, but local surveillance data are not necessarily representative of AOM isolates found in otherwise healthy patients.

Amoxicillin usually is considered the drug of first choice for initial empiric treatment of AOM, unless the infection is suspected of being caused by β-lactamase-producing bacteria resistant to the drug, in which case amoxicillin and clavulanate potassium is recommended. The fact that multidrug-resistant *S. pneumoniae* are being reported with increasing frequency should be considered when selecting an anti-infective agent for empiric treatment of AOM. However, AAP, AAFP, CDC, and others state that, despite the increasing prevalence of multidrug-resistant *S. pneumoniae* and presence of β-lactamase-producing *H. influenzae* or *M. catarrhalis* in many communities, amoxicillin remains the anti-infective of first choice for treatment of uncomplicated AOM since amoxicillin is highly effective, has a narrow spectrum of activity, is well distributed into middle ear fluid, is well tolerated, has an acceptable taste, and is inexpensive. Amoxicillin (when given in dosages of 80–90 mg/kg daily) usually is effective in the treatment of AOM caused by *S. pneumoniae*, including infections involving strains with intermediate resistance to penicillins, and also usually is effective in the treatment of AOM caused by most strains of *H. influenzae*. Because *S. pneumoniae* is the most frequent cause of AOM (25–50% of cases) and because AOM caused by *S. pneumoniae* is more likely to be severe and less likely to resolve spontaneously than AOM caused by *H. influenzae* or *M. catarrhalis*, it has been suggested that it may be more important to choose an empiric anti-infective based on its activity against *S. pneumoniae* rather than its activity against other possible pathogens.

Various other anti-infectives, including oral cephalosporins (cefaclor, cefdinir, cefixime, cefpodoxime proxetil, cefprozil, ceftibuten, cefuroxime axetil, cephalexin), parenteral ceftriaxone, oral macrolides (azithromycin, clarithromycin, fixed combination of erythromycin and sulfisoxazole), oral co-trimoxazole, and oral loracarbef, have been used in the treatment of AOM. These anti-infectives vary in their efficacy against AOM pathogens.

Current AAP evidence-based guidelines for the diagnosis and management of uncomplicated AOM in children 6 months through 12 years of age state that high-dose amoxicillin (80–90 mg/kg daily in 2 divided doses) should be used for initial treatment when a decision has been made to use anti-infective therapy *and* the child has not received amoxicillin within the past 30 days *or* does not have concurrent purulent conjunctivitis *or* is not allergic to penicillin. These guidelines state that high-dose amoxicillin and clavulanate (90 mg/kg of amoxicillin and 6.4 mg/kg of clavulanate daily in 2 divided doses) should be used if the child received amoxicillin within the past 30 days *or* has concurrent purulent conjunctivitis *or* has a history of recurrent AOM unresponsive to amoxicillin. These AAP guidelines state that the preferred alternatives for initial treatment of AOM in penicillin-allergic patients are oral cephalosporins (cefdinir, cefpodoxime proxetil, cefuroxime axetil) or parenteral ceftriaxone.

Results of controlled clinical studies indicate that 10-day regimens of most oral anti-infectives used in the empiric treatment of AOM are equally effective, and there is no evidence that the overall response rate to anti-infectives with a broader spectrum of activity (e.g., second and third generation cephalosporins) is any better than that reported with amoxicillin or amoxicillin and clavulanate potassium. Of the currently available oral cephalosporins, cefaclor, cefdinir, cefixime, cefpodoxime proxetil, cefprozil, ceftibuten, and cefuroxime axetil have been used effectively for the treatment of AOM in pediatric patients. However, there is evidence that some cephalosporins (e.g., cefaclor, cefprozil) may be less effective than some other available agents for the treatment of AOM when β-lactamase-producing bacteria are present and some (e.g., cefixime, ceftibuten) may be less effective than some other available agents for the treatment of AOM when *S. pneumoniae* with reduced susceptibility to penicillin are present.

Duration of Initial Treatment of AOM. The optimal duration of therapy for AOM is uncertain. Anti-infectives traditionally have been administered for 7–10 days for the treatment of AOM, but shorter durations of treatment also have been used. The 10-day regimen was derived from the duration of treatment for *S. pyogenes* pharyngitis and tonsillitis. Although there is some evidence from controlled clinical studies in pediatric patients with AOM that the clinical response rate to 5-day regimens of certain oral cephalosporins (e.g., cefaclor†, cefdinir, cefpodoxime proxetil, cefprozil†, cefuroxime axetil†) is similar to that of 10-day regimens of oral cephalosporins, amoxicillin, or amoxicillin and clavulanate potassium, such regimens appear to be less effective than 10-day regimens in children younger than 2 years of age.

Current AAP evidence-based guidelines for the diagnosis and management of uncomplicated AOM in children 6 months through 12 years of age state that a 10-day regimen of an appropriate oral anti-infective is recommended for the treatment of AOM in children younger than 2 years of age and in those with severe symptoms. These guidelines state that a 7-day regimen of an appropriate oral anti-infective may be as effective as a 10-day regimen in children 2–5 years of age with mild to moderate AOM, and a 5- to 7-day regimen of an appropriate oral anti-infective may be adequate in children 6 years of age or older with mild to moderate AOM.

Other clinicians suggest that while 5-day regimens can be considered for adults and children 2 years of age and older with mild, uncomplicated AOM, further study is needed to more fully evaluate efficacy of short-term regimens in infants and young children since studies to date have included only a limited number of children younger than 2 years of age. These clinicians state that short-term anti-infective regimens (i.e., 5 days or less) may not be appropriate for the treatment of AOM in children younger than 2 years of age or for patients with underlying disease, craniofacial abnormalities, recurrent or persistent AOM, or perforated tympanic membranes and spontaneous purulent drainage.

Parenteral Ceftriaxone for Treatment of AOM. Parenteral ceftriaxone has been shown to be effective for initial or repeat treatment of AOM, and is a good choice when the patient has persistent vomiting or cannot otherwise tolerate an oral regimen. The manufacturer recommends a single dose of IM ceftriaxone for initial treatment of AOM, but cautions that the potential advantages of this single-dose parenteral regimen should be balanced against its potentially lower clinical cure rate compared with a 10-day oral anti-infective regimen. AAP states that either a 1- or 3-day regimen† of parenteral ceftriaxone can be used for initial treatment of AOM, but cautions that there is some evidence that more than a single dose of the drug may be required to prevent recurrence of middle ear infections within 5–7 days after the initial dose. A 3-day regimen† of parenteral ceftriaxone is recommended for retreatment in patients who fail to respond to initial treatment with other anti-infectives.

The single-dose IM ceftriaxone regimen offers some practical advantages over 5- to 10-day oral anti-infective regimens since it provides a more convenient dosing schedule, ensures compliance, and can be administered to patients who have nausea and vomiting; however, ceftriaxone may be more costly than oral regimens and the drug has a spectrum of activity that is broader than necessary for the treatment of AOM. Some clinicians suggest that further study of the single-dose ceftriaxone regimen is needed to more fully assess the bacteriologic eradication rate, long-term efficacy, and rate of relapse, and to determine whether the single-dose regimen contributes to emergence of resistant organisms.

Anti-infectives for AOM after Initial Treatment Failure. Consideration can be given to changing the anti-infective regimen in children who do not have clinical improvement within 48–72 hours after the initial anti-infective regimen is started. Current AAP evidence-based clinical practice guidelines for the diagnosis and management of uncomplicated AOM in children 6 months through 12 years of age state that patients who fail to respond to an initial regimen of high-dose amoxicillin (80–90 mg/kg daily in 2 divided doses) should be retreated with high-dose amoxicillin and clavulanate (90 mg/kg of amoxicillin and 6.4 mg/kg of clavulanate daily in 2 divided doses). Those who fail to respond to an initial regimen of high-dose amoxicillin and clavulanate potassium or an initial regimen of an appropriate oral cephalosporin (cefdinir, cefpodoxime proxetil, cefuroxime axetil) should be treated with parenteral ceftriaxone (50 mg/kg daily for 3 days).

There is evidence that a 3-day regimen of IM ceftriaxone (50 mg/kg once daily) can be effective for the treatment of persistent or recurrent AOM† in pediatric patients 3 months of age or older with infections that failed to respond to treatment with other anti-infectives (e.g., amoxicillin, amoxicillin and clavulanate potassium, cefaclor, cefuroxime axetil). A 3-day regimen of ceftriaxone has been shown to be more effective than a 1-day regimen for retreatment in patients who fail to respond to initial treatment with another anti-infective. The 3-day ceftriaxone regimen has been effective for the treatment of persistent or relapsing otitis media caused by *H. influenzae*, *M. catarrhalis*, *S. pyogenes*, or penicillin-susceptible *S. pneumoniae*; however, treatment failures have been reported when the causative agent was *S. pneumoniae* with reduced susceptibility to penicillin.

Clindamycin (30–40 mg/kg daily in 3 divided doses) can be used (with or without a third generation cephalosporin) as an alternative for the treatment of AOM in patients who fail to respond to an initial anti-infective regimen. Although clindamycin may be effective for penicillin-resistant *S. pneumoniae*, it may not be effective against multidrug-resistant *S. pneumoniae* and lacks efficacy against *H influenzae*. If clindamycin is used for retreatment, concomitant use of an anti-infective active against *H. influenzae* and *M. catarrhalis* (e.g., cefdinir, cefixime, cefuroxime) should be considered.

Because of reported resistance in *S. pneumoniae*, AAP states that co-trimoxazole and the fixed combination of erythromycin and sulfisoxazole should *not* be used as alternatives for the treatment of AOM in patients who fail to improve while receiving amoxicillin.

Primary treatment failure of AOM occurs most frequently in children younger than 2 years of age. While primary treatment failure and persistent AOM may be the result of infection with bacteria resistant to the anti-infective administered (e.g., penicillin-resistant *S. pneumoniae*, β-lactamase-producing *H. influenzae*), many cases appear to be related to other factors since results of tympanocentesis indicate that the causative organism(s) often are susceptible in vitro to the primary treatment regimen or, in some cases, no bacteria are isolated. Patients with AOM who fail to respond to an initial anti-infective regimen often also fail to respond to a subsequent regimen, regardless of the anti-infective used.

If AOM persists after a series of anti-infective regimens, tympanocentesis should be considered and culture of middle ear fluid performed to make a bacteriologic diagnosis and obtain in vitro susceptibility test results. If tympanocentesis is not available, a regimen of oral clindamycin with or without an anti-infective to provide coverage against *H. influenzae* and *M. catarrhalis* (e.g., cefdinir, cefixime, cefuroxime) may be considered. Consultation with a pediatric medical subspecialist (e.g., otolaryngologist) for possible tympanocentesis, drainage, and culture and consultation with an infectious disease expert before use of unconventional anti-infectives should be considered.

Recurrent AOM. Current AAP evidence-based clinical practice guidelines for the diagnosis and management of uncomplicated AOM in children 6 months through 12 years of age state that anti-infective prophylaxis should *not* be prescribed to reduce the frequency of episodes of AOM in children with recurrent AOM. Recurrent AOM is defined as 3 or more episodes of AOM within a 6-month period or 4 or more episodes of AOM within a 12-month period that includes at least 1 episode in the preceding 6 months. About 50% of children younger than 2 years of age who are treated for AOM will have a recurrence within 6 months. Winter season, male gender, and passive exposure to tobacco smoke have been associated with an increased likelihood of AOM recurrence. Other risk factors for recurrence include AOM symptoms lasting more than 10 days, a family history of the infection, group day-care outside the home during the first 2 years of life, and use of bottles or pacifiers. There is some evidence that breastfeeding for at least 4–6 months reduces episodes of AOM and recurrent AOM.

Anti-infectives (e.g., amoxicillin, sulfisoxazole) have been administered as long-term prophylaxis or suppressive therapy in children with recurrent AOM in an attempt to prevent recurrence or have been administered intermittently as prophylaxis at the first sign of an upper respiratory tract infection in children with a history of recurrent AOM. Although there is some evidence that anti-infective prophylaxis may decrease the incidence of new symptomatic episodes of AOM in some children with a history of recurrent AOM, such prophylaxis is not routinely recommended. Results of a meta-analysis indicate that use of anti-infective prophylaxis results in an average decrease of only 0.11 episodes of AOM per patient per month (slightly more than 1 episode per year). In addition, anti-infective prophylaxis does not provide any long-lasting benefit since any decrease in AOM episodes occurs only while prophylaxis is being given. AAP states that anti-infective prophylaxis is not appropriate for children with long-term MEE or for children with infrequent episodes of AOM. The small reduction in frequency of AOM must be weighed against the cost and potential adverse effects of anti-infective prophylaxis (e.g., allergic reactions, GI effects such as diarrhea) and concerns that prophylaxis may promote emergence of resistant bacteria, including multidrug-resistant *S. pneumoniae*, or alter nasopharyngeal flora and foster colonization with resistant bacteria.

Otitis Media with Effusion Anti-infectives are not usually recommended for management of otitis media with effusion (OME). OME involves liquid in the middle ear (MEE) without signs and symptoms of acute ear infection. OME may occur as an inflammatory response after an episode of AOM or may occur spontaneously as a consequence of eustachian tube dysfunction. About 60–70% of children have MEE present 2 weeks after successful treatment of AOM and 10–25% still have MEE at 3 months. It is important to differentiate OME from AOM. Management of OME usually involves observation and close monitoring until resolution. Anti-infective treatment is *not* usually indicated because OME does not represent an acute infectious process. The AAFP, American Academy of Otolaryngology-Head and Neck Surgery, and AAP Subcommittee on Otitis Media with Effusion have issued evidence-based clinical practice guidelines regarding diagnosis and management of OME in children 2 months to 12 years of age (with or without developmental disabilities or underlying conditions that predispose to OME and its sequelae). These guidelines should be consulted for information on diagnosis and management of OME.

Chronic Suppurative Otitis Media without Cholesteatoma Ceftazidime has been used with some success in the treatment of chronic suppurative otitis media (CSOM) without cholesteatoma. CSOM is defined as chronic infection of the middle ear and mastoid associated with tympanic membrane perforation and otorrhea lasting more than 6 weeks, and may occur as the result of unresolved AOM and/or eustachian tube dysfunction. The most common bacteria reported in patients with CSOM are *Ps. aeruginosa*, *Klebsiella*, *S. aureus*, *S. epidermidis*, and anaerobic bacteria, including *Bacteroides*, *Prevotella*, *Peptostreptococcus*, and *Peptococcus*. While ceftazidime has been effective in the treatment of CSOM when gram-negative bacteria were involved, it has been ineffective when gram-positive bacteria (e.g., *S. aureus*) were involved. Because CSOM often is a mixed aerobic-anaerobic infection, anti-infectives usually used in the treatment of AOM or OME would be ineffective. Topical anti-infectives (e.g., ciprofloxacin otic suspension, ofloxacin otic solution, gentamicin) used in conjunction with daily aural toilet can be effective for the treatment of uncomplicated CSOM; more severe or persistent infections require treatment with a parenteral anti-infective (e.g., ceftazidime, clindamycin, ciprofloxacin, gentamicin, ticarcillin, ticarcillin disodium and clavulanate potassium).

■ **Otitis Externa** Ceftazidime has been effective when used in the treatment of malignant otitis externa† caused by *Ps. aeruginosa*. Bacterial otitis externa usually is caused by *Ps. aeruginosa* or *S. aureus*. Although acute bacterial otitis externa localized in the external auditory canal may be effectively treated using topical anti-infectives (e.g., ciprofloxacin otic suspension, ofloxacin otic solution), malignant otitis externa is an invasive, potentially life-threatening infection, especially in immunocompromised patients such as those with diabetes mellitus or human immunodeficiency virus (HIV) infection, and requires prompt diagnosis and long-term treatment with parenteral anti-infectives (e.g., ceftazidime and/or ciprofloxacin).

■ **Pharyngitis and Tonsillitis** Oral cephalosporins (e.g., cefaclor, cefadroxil, cefdinir, cefditoren pivoxil, cefixime, cefpodoxime proxetil, cefprozil, ceftibuten, cefuroxime axetil, cephalexin) are used for the treatment of pharyngitis and tonsillitis caused by *S. pyogenes* (group A β-hemolytic streptococci). Although cephalosporins usually are effective in eradicating *S. pyogenes* from the nasopharynx, efficacy of the drugs in the subsequent prevention of rheumatic fever remains to be established.

Selection of an anti-infective for the treatment of *S. pyogenes* pharyngitis and tonsillitis should be based on the drug's spectrum of activity, bacteriologic and clinical efficacy, potential adverse effects, ease of administration, patient compliance, and cost. No regimen has been found to date that effectively eradicates group A β-hemolytic streptococci in 100% of patients.

Because the drugs have a narrow spectrum of activity, are inexpensive, and generally are effective with a low frequency of adverse effects, AAP, IDSA, American Heart Association (AHA), and other experts recommend a penicillin regimen (i.e., 10 days of oral penicillin V or oral amoxicillin or a single dose of IM penicillin G benzathine) as the treatment of choice for *S. pyogenes* pharyngitis and tonsillitis and prevention of initial attacks (primary prevention) of rheumatic fever. Other anti-infectives (e.g., oral cephalosporins, oral macrolides, oral clindamycin) are recommended as alternatives in penicillin-allergic patients.

A 10-day regimen of an appropriate oral cephalosporin is recommended for the treatment of *S. pyogenes* pharyngitis and tonsillitis in most penicillin-allergic patients; however, cephalosporins should be avoided in those with a history of immediate (anaphylactic-type) penicillin hypersensitivity. If an oral cephalosporin is used, a 10-day regimen of a first generation cephalosporin (cefadroxil, cephalexin) is preferred instead of other cephalosporins with broader spectrums of activity (e.g., cefaclor, cefdinir, cefixime, cefpodoxime proxetil, cefuroxime). The broader spectrum cephalosporins offer no advantages over penicillins or first generation cephalosporins since they generally are more expensive and more likely to result in resistant flora.

Although there is some evidence that bacteriologic and clinical cure rates reported with 10-day regimens of certain oral cephalosporins (e.g., cefaclor, cefadroxil, cefdinir, cefixime, cefpodoxime proxetil, cefprozil, cefuroxime axetil, ceftibuten, cephalexin) may be slightly higher than those reported with the 10-day oral penicillin V regimen, analysis of data from the 10-day cephalosporin studies suggests that the difference in eradication rates may have been due to a higher rate of eradication of carriers inadvertently included in the study population. In addition, although there is some evidence that a shorter duration of therapy with certain oral cephalosporins (e.g., a 5-day regimen of cefadroxil, cefdinir, cefixime, or cefpodoxime proxetil or a 4- or 5-day regimen of cefuroxime axetil) achieves bacteriologic and clinical cure rates equal to or greater than those achieved with the traditional 10-day oral penicillin V regimen, AHA and IDSA state that use of cephalosporin regimens administered for 5 days or less for the treatment of *S. pyogenes* pharyngitis and tonsillitis cannot be recommended at this time.

■ **Respiratory Tract Infections** ***Community-acquired Pneumonia*** Some oral cephalosporins (cefdinir, cefpodoxime proxetil, cefprozil, cefuroxime axetil) and some parenteral cephalosporins (cefepime, cefotaxime, ceftaroline fosamil, ceftriaxone) are used in the treatment of community-acquired pneumonia (CAP) caused by susceptible bacteria.

Initial treatment of CAP generally involves use of an empiric anti-infective regimen selected based on the most likely pathogens and local susceptibility patterns; therapy may then be changed (if possible) to provide a more specific regimen (pathogen-directed therapy) based on results of in vitro culture and susceptibility testing. The most appropriate empiric regimen varies depending on the severity of illness at the time of presentation and whether outpatient treatment or hospitalization in or out of an intensive care unit (ICU) is indicated and the presence or absence of cardiopulmonary disease and other modifying factors that increase the risk of certain pathogens (e.g., penicillin- or multidrug-resistant *S. pneumoniae*, enteric gram-negative bacilli, *Ps. aeruginosa*).

For both outpatients and inpatients, most experts recommend that an empiric regimen for treatment of CAP include an anti-infective active against *S. pneumoniae* since this organism is the most commonly identified cause of bacterial pneumonia and causes more severe disease than many other common CAP pathogens. Although monotherapy may be appropriate for empiric treatment of CAP in many outpatients and some inpatients, a combination regimen is always indicated for empiric treatment of CAP in patients requiring treatment in an ICU. Such patients require an empiric regimen that covers *S. pneumoniae*, *Legionella*, *H. influenzae*, *Mycoplasma pneumoniae*, *Chlamydophila pneumoniae* (formerly *Chlamydia pneumoniae*), and relevant gram-negative bacilli.

Outpatient Regimens for CAP. Pathogens most frequently involved in CAP infections in *outpatients* include *S. pneumoniae*, *M. pneumoniae*, *C. pneumoniae*, respiratory viruses, and *H. influenzae* (especially in cigarette smokers).

For empiric outpatient treatment of CAP in previously healthy individuals without risk factors for drug-resistant *S. pneumoniae*, IDSA and the American Thoracic Society (ATS) recommend monotherapy with a macrolide (azithromycin, clarithromycin, erythromycin) or, alternatively, doxycycline.

For empiric outpatient treatment of CAP in patients with risk factors for drug-resistant *S. pneumoniae* (e.g., comorbidities such as chronic heart, lung, liver, or renal disease, diabetes mellitus, alcoholism, malignancies, asplenia, immunosuppression, history of anti-infective treatment within the last 3 months), ATS and IDSA recommend monotherapy with a fluoroquinolone with enhanced activity against *S. pneumoniae* (gemifloxacin, levofloxacin, moxifloxacin) or, alternatively, a combination regimen that includes a β-lactam active against *S. pneumoniae* (high-dose amoxicillin or fixed combination of amoxicillin and clavulanic acid or, alternatively, ceftriaxone, cefpodoxime proxetil, or cefuroxime) given in conjunction with a macrolide (azithromycin, clarithromycin, erythromycin) or, alternatively, given in conjunction with doxycycline.

Inpatient Regimens for CAP. Pathogens most frequently involved in CAP infections in non-ICU *inpatients* include *S. pneumoniae, M. pneumoniae, C. pneumoniae, H. influenzae, Legionella,* and respiratory viruses. Patients with severe CAP admitted into the ICU usually have infections caused by *S. pneumoniae, S. aureus, Legionella,* gram-negative bacilli, or *H. influenzae*. Factors that increase the risk of Enterobacteriaceae or *Ps. aeruginosa* infection in CAP patients include severe CAP requiring treatment in an ICU, structural lung disease (bronchiectasis), severe chronic obstructive pulmonary disease (COPD), smoking, alcoholism, chronic corticosteroid therapy, and frequent anti-infective therapy. Coverage against anaerobic bacteria usually is indicated only in classic aspiration pleuropulmonary syndrome in patients who had loss of consciousness as a result of alcohol or drug overdosage or after seizures in patients with concomitant gingival disease or esophageal motility disorders.

For empiric inpatient treatment of CAP in non-ICU patients, IDSA and ATS recommend monotherapy with a fluoroquinolone with enhanced activity against *S. pneumoniae* (gemifloxacin, levofloxacin, moxifloxacin) or, alternatively, a combination regimen that includes a β-lactam (usually cefotaxime, ceftriaxone, or ampicillin) given in conjunction with a macrolide (azithromycin, clarithromycin, erythromycin) or doxycycline.

For empiric treatment of CAP in ICU patients when *Pseudomonas* and methicillin-resistant *S. aureus* (MRSA; also known as oxacillin-resistant *S. aureus* or ORSA) are *not* suspected, IDSA and ATS recommend a combination regimen that includes a β-lactam (cefotaxime, ceftriaxone, fixed combination of ampicillin and sulbactam) given in conjunction with either azithromycin or a fluoroquinolone (moxifloxacin, gemifloxacin, levofloxacin). If *Pseudomonas* is suspected, IDSA and ATS recommend an empiric combination regimen that includes an antipneumococcal, antipseudomonal β-lactam (cefepime, imipenem, meropenem, fixed combination of piperacillin and tazobactam) given in conjunction with a fluoroquinolone (ciprofloxacin, levofloxacin); a combination regimen that includes one of these antipseudomonal β-lactams, an aminoglycoside, and azithromycin; or a combination regimen that includes one of these antipseudomonal β-lactams, an aminoglycoside, and an antipneumococcal fluoroquinolone. If *Ps. aeruginosa* has been identified by appropriate microbiologic testing, the preferred treatment regimen is an antipseudomonal β-lactam (cefepime, ceftazidime, aztreonam, imipenem, meropenem, piperacillin, ticarcillin) given in conjunction with ciprofloxacin, levofloxacin, or an aminoglycoside and the preferred alternative regimen is an aminoglycoside given in conjunction with ciprofloxacin or levofloxacin. If community-acquired MRSA may be involved, vancomycin or linezolid should be included in the initial empiric regimen.

Inpatient treatment of CAP is initiated with a parenteral regimen, although therapy may be changed to an oral regimen if the patient is improving clinically, is hemodynamically stable, able to ingest drugs, and has a normally functioning GI tract. CAP patients usually have a clinical response within 3–7 days after initiation of therapy and a switch to oral therapy generally can be made during this period.

Acute Sinusitis Oral cefdinir, cefixime†, cefpodoxime proxetil, cefprozil, and cefuroxime axetil are used for the treatment of acute maxillary sinusitis caused by susceptible bacteria (e.g., *S. pneumoniae, H. influenzae, M. catarrhalis*). Parenteral ceftriaxone† and cefotaxime† are recommended as alternatives for initial treatment of severe bacterial sinusitis.

When anti-infective therapy is indicated for the treatment of acute bacterial sinusitis, IDSA recommends amoxicillin and clavulanate potassium and AAP recommends either amoxicillin or amoxicillin and clavulanate potassium as the drug of choice for initial empiric treatment. Because of variable activity against *S. pneumoniae* and *H. influenzae*, IDSA no longer recommends second or third generation oral cephalosporins for empiric monotherapy of sinusitis in adults or children. If an oral cephalosporin is used as an alternative for empiric treatment of acute bacterial sinusitis in children (e.g., in penicillin-allergic individuals), IDSA and AAP recommend a combination regimen that includes a third generation cephalosporin (cefixime or cefpodoxime) and clindamycin (or linezolid). In children who are vomiting, unable to tolerate oral therapy, or unlikely to adhere to the initial doses, treatment of acute sinusitis can be initiated with a single dose of parenteral ceftriaxone and then switched to an oral regimen if clinical improvement is observed at 24 hours. For patients with severe bacterial sinusitis requiring hospitalization, parenteral ceftriaxone and cefotaxime are preferred alternatives for initial treatment in penicillin-allergic patients who cannot receive amoxicillin and clavulanate potassium.

■ Septicemia Cefotaxime, ceftazidime, ceftriaxone, cefazolin, and cefepime† are used parenterally for the treatment of bacteremia/septicemia caused by susceptible bacteria (e.g., *S. aureus, S. pneumoniae, H. influenzae, E. coli, K. pneumoniae, Serratia*).

The choice of anti-infective for the treatment of sepsis syndrome should be based on the probable source of infection, causative organism, immune status of the patient, and local patterns of bacterial resistance. Some experts state that, although certain parenteral cephalosporins (cefepime, cefotaxime, ceftriaxone, ceftazidime) can be used for the treatment of gram-negative sepsis, ceftazidime is less active than the other cephalosporins against gram-positive cocci and most cephalosporins (except cefepime and ceftazidime) have limited activity against *Ps. aeruginosa*.

For initial treatment of life-threatening sepsis in adults, some clinicians recommend that a third or fourth generation cephalosporin (cefepime, cefotaxime, ceftazidime, ceftriaxone), the fixed combination of piperacillin and tazobactam, or a carbapenem (doripenem, imipenem, meropenem) be used in conjunction with vancomycin; some experts also suggest including an aminoglycoside or fluoroquinolone during the initial few days of treatment.

■ Urinary Tract Infections Some oral cephalosporins (cefaclor, cefadroxil, cefixime, cefpodoxime proxetil, cefuroxime axetil, cephalexin) and some parenteral cephalosporins (cefazolin, cefepime, ceftazidime, ceftriaxone, cefuroxime) are used for the treatment of uncomplicated and/or complicated urinary tract infections caused by susceptible bacteria. The fixed combination of ceftazidime and avibactam and the fixed combination of ceftolozane and tazobactam are used for the treatment of complicated urinary tract infections.

■ Chancroid Ceftriaxone is used for the treatment of genital ulcers caused by *H. ducreyi* (chancroid)†, and is considered a drug of choice for the treatment of this infection. (See Uses: Chancroid, in Ceftriaxone Sodium 8:12.06.12.)

■ Gonorrhea and Associated Infections Cefoxitin, cefotaxime, ceftriaxone, and cefuroxime are used parenterally and cefixime, cefpodoxime proxetil, and cefuroxime axetil have been used orally for the treatment of uncomplicated gonorrhea caused by susceptible *Neisseria gonorrhoeae*. Cefoxitin, cefotaxime†, ceftriaxone†, and cefuroxime also have been used parenterally for the treatment of disseminated gonorrhea and other gonococcal infections.

Ceftriaxone is considered the drug of choice for the treatment of most *N. gonorrhoeae* infections, including uncomplicated gonococcal infections of the cervix, urethra, rectum, and pharynx; disseminated gonococcal infections; gonococcal conjunctivitis; gonococcal meningitis and endocarditis; gonococcal epididymitis or proctitis in adults and adolescents; gonococcal ophthalmia neonatorum; and uncomplicated gonorrhea or disseminated gonococcal infections in neonates and children. Ceftriaxone also is used in conjunction with other agents for empiric anti-infective prophylaxis in sexual assault victims†. CDC states that ceftriaxone is the most effective cephalosporin for the treatment of gonorrhea and, unlike most other drugs, is effective for the treatment of gonorrhea at all sites, including cervical, urethral, rectal, and pharyngeal gonococcal infections. Other parenteral or oral cephalosporins do not offer any advantages over ceftriaxone.

N. gonorrhoeae with reduced susceptibility to ceftriaxone and/or cefixime or other cephalosporins have been reported with increasing frequency during the last decade in the US and elsewhere (e.g., Asia, Europe, Canada); some treatment failures have been reported. There have been rare reports of *N. gonorrhoeae* with high-level ceftriaxone resistance in some countries (Japan, France, Spain). Although the overall prevalence of isolates with reduced susceptibility to cephalosporins remains low in the US, potential emergence of high-level cephalosporin resistance in *N. gonorrhoeae* is a major concern since available treatment options are limited if cephalosporins cannot be used.

Susceptibility of *N. gonorrhoeae* in the US is being monitored by the CDC Gonococcal Isolate Surveillance Project (GISP). GISP data from 2000–2010 indicate that the percentage of US *N. gonorrhoeae* isolates with elevated ceftriaxone MICs (MICs 0.125 mcg/mL or greater) increased from 0.1 to 0.3% and the percentage with elevated cefixime MICs (MICs 0.25 mcg/mL or greater) increased from 0.2 to 1.4%. All 2009–2010 isolates with decreased susceptibility to cefixime were resistant to ciprofloxacin and tetracycline, but were susceptible to azithromycin. GISP data regarding *N. gonorrhoeae* isolates from men who have sex with men indicate that the percentage of isolates with elevated ceftriaxone MICs increased from 0% in 2006 to 1% in 2011 and the percentage of isolates with elevated cefixime MICs increased from 0.2% in 2006 to 3.8% in 2011. More recent GISP data indicate that the proportion of isolates in the US with decreased susceptibility to ceftriaxone or cefixime has remained low. During 2013, no isolates with decreased susceptibility to ceftriaxone or cefixime (i.e., MICs 0.5 mcg/mL or greater) were identified.

Because of concerns related to reports of *N. gonorrhoeae* with reduced susceptibility to cephalosporins, CDC now recommends that IM ceftriaxone be used in conjunction with oral azithromycin for the treatment of uncomplicated gonorrhea (dual treatment). The theoretical basis of this recommendation is that combination therapy using 2 anti-infectives with different mechanisms of action may improve treatment efficacy and potentially delay emergence and spread of cephalosporin resistance. In addition, CDC no longer recommends use of cefixime or any other oral cephalosporin as first-line treatment for gonococcal infections. Cefixime should *only* be used as an alternative for the treatment of urogenital or rectal gonococcal infections when ceftriaxone is unavailable or cannot be used.

CDC recommends that healthcare providers treating gonorrhea remain vigilant for treatment failures (evidenced by persistent symptoms or a positive follow-up test despite treatment) and report any occurrence of treatment failure to local or state health departments. If there is evidence of treatment failure, relevant clinical specimens should be cultured and in vitro susceptibility testing performed. In addition, an infectious disease specialist, an STD/HIV Prevention

Training Center (http://www.nnptc.org), or the CDC (404-639-8659) should be consulted for treatment advice and the case should be reported to CDC through local or state health departments within 24 hours of diagnosis.

Although a test-of-cure is not necessary for individuals with uncomplicated urogenital or rectal gonorrhea who are treated with a recommended or alternative regimen, those with pharyngeal gonorrhea who are treated with an alternative regimen should return 14 days after treatment for a test-of-cure. To minimize transmission, individuals treated for gonorrhea should be instructed to abstain from sexual activity for 7 days after treatment and until all sexual partners have been adequately treated. The patient's recent sexual partners (i.e., individuals having sexual contact with the infected patient within the 60 days preceding onset of symptoms or gonorrhea diagnosis) should be referred for evaluation, testing, and presumptive dual treatment.

Uncomplicated Gonorrhea For the treatment of uncomplicated cervical, urethral, or rectal gonorrhea in adults and adolescents, CDC states that a combination regimen that includes a single 250-mg dose of IM ceftriaxone *and* oral azithromycin (single 1-g dose) is the treatment of choice. Both drugs should be administered together on the same day, preferably simultaneously and under direct supervision.

If necessary because ceftriaxone is not available or cannot be used and the patient has urogenital or rectal gonorrhea, CDC recommends an alternative combination regimen that includes a single 400-mg dose of oral cefixime *and* oral azithromycin (single 1-g dose).

Disseminated Gonococcal Infections CDC recommends that patients with disseminated gonococcal infections be hospitalized for initial treatment, especially when compliance may be a problem, when the diagnosis is uncertain, or when the patient has purulent synovial effusions or other complications. All patients with disseminated infections should be evaluated for clinical evidence of endocarditis and meningitis. Consultation with an infectious disease expert is advised.

For treatment of disseminated gonococcal infections classified as arthritis and arthritis-dermatitis syndrome†, CDC recommends that adults and adolescents receive a combination regimen of IM or IV ceftriaxone (1 g every 24 hours) *and* oral azithromycin (single 1-g dose); the recommended alternative is IV cefotaxime (1 g IV every 8 hours) *and* oral azithromycin (single 1-g dose). At 24–48 hours after substantial improvement, therapy can be switched to an oral anti-infective selected based on in vitro susceptibility testing. Total treatment duration for gonococcal arthritis and arthritis-dermatitis syndrome is at least 7 days.

For treatment of disseminated gonococcal infections that involve meningitis and endocarditis†, CDC recommends that adults and adolescents receive a combination regimen of IV ceftriaxone (1–2 g every 12–24 hours) *and* oral azithromycin (single 1-g dose). The parenteral regimen should be continued for 10–14 days for the treatment of gonococcal meningitis or for at least 4 weeks for the treatment of gonococcal endocarditis.

For additional information on treatment of gonorrhea and associated infections, including treatment of gonococcal infections in neonates, infants, and children, see Uses: Gonorrhea and Associated Infections in Ceftriaxone 8:12.06.12.

■ Leptospirosis Ceftriaxone and cefotaxime have been used in the treatment of severe leptospirosis† caused by *Leptospira*. Leptospirosis is a spirochete infection that may range in severity from a self-limited systemic illness to a severe, life-threatening illness that includes jaundice, renal failure, hemorrhage, cardiac arrhythmias, pneumonitis, and hemodynamic collapse (Weil syndrome).

Penicillin G generally has been considered the drug of choice for the treatment of moderate to severe leptospirosis. Other anti-infectives recommended for the treatment of severe leptospirosis include cephalosporins (ceftriaxone, cefotaxime), aminopenicillins (ampicillin, amoxicillin), tetracyclines (doxycycline, tetracycline), or macrolides (azithromycin).

■ Lyme Disease Oral cefuroxime axetil, IV ceftriaxone, and IV cefotaxime are used for the treatment of Lyme disease†. First generation cephalosporins (e.g., cephalexin) are ineffective and should *not* be used for the treatment of Lyme disease. Although other second or third generation cephalosporins may be effective, the only cephalosporins currently recommended by IDSA, AAP, and other clinicians for the treatment of Lyme disease are cefuroxime axetil, ceftriaxone, and cefotaxime.

Lyme disease (Lyme borreliosis) is a tick-born spirochetal disease. In the US, Lyme disease is caused by the spirochete *Borrelia burgdorferi*, which is transmitted by the bite of *Ixodes scapularis* or *I. pacificus* ticks. In addition to *B. burgdorferi*, *I. scapularis* may be simultaneously infected with and transmit *Anaplasma phagocytophilum* (causative agent of human granulocytotropic anaplasmosis [HGA, formerly known as human granulocytic ehrlichiosis]) and/or *Babesia microti* (causative agent of babesiosis). Because coinfection with *A. phagocytophilum* and/or *B. microti* can occur in patients with Lyme disease in geographic areas where these other pathogens are endemic, these diseases should be considered in the differential diagnosis of patients being evaluated for Lyme disease. Since cephalosporins are ineffective for the treatment of HGA and/or babesiosis, diagnosing such coinfections is critical to ensure that appropriate anti-infectives are used for treatment. (See Lyme Disease in Uses: Spirochetal Infections and see Uses: Ehrlichiosis and Anaplasmosis, in the Tetracyclines General Statement 8:12.24.)

Early Lyme Disease **Erythema migrans.** IDSA, AAP, and other clinicians recommend oral doxycycline, oral amoxicillin, or oral cefuroxime axetil as first-line therapy for the treatment of the early localized or early disseminated Lyme disease† associated with erythema migrans, in the absence of specific neurologic manifestations or advanced atrioventricular (AV) heart block. IDSA states that a 14-day regimen (range 14–21 days) of any of these oral anti-infectives (doxycycline, amoxicillin, cefuroxime axetil) may be used for initial treatment of early Lyme disease since all 3 drugs have been shown to be effective for the treatment of erythema migrans and associated symptoms in prospective clinical studies. Doxycycline offers the advantage of also being effective for the treatment of HGA coinfection (but not babesiosis coinfection).

Although IV ceftriaxone is effective for early Lyme disease manifested as erythema migrans, it is not superior to the recommended oral anti-infectives and is more likely to cause serious adverse effects; therefore, IV ceftriaxone is not usually recommended for the treatment of early Lyme disease in the absence of neurologic involvement or advanced AV heart block.

Transplacental transmission of *B. burgdorferi* appears to occur rarely, if at all, and epidemiologic studies in pregnant women have not documented an association between exposure to Lyme disease prior to conception or during pregnancy and subsequent fetal death, congenital malformations, or prematurity. IDSA, AAP, and other clinicians state that pregnant or nursing women need not be treated differently than other patients with Lyme disease, except that they should not receive doxycycline.

Early Neurologic Lyme Disease. Although oral anti-infectives (e.g., doxycycline, amoxicillin, cefuroxime axetil) generally are effective for the treatment of the early Lyme disease associated with erythema migrans in the absence of specific neurologic manifestations, parenteral anti-infectives are recommended for the treatment of early Lyme disease when there are acute neurologic manifestations such as meningitis or radiculopathy. Radiculopathy, cranial neuropathy, and mononeuropathy multiplex may be manifestations of acute peripheral nervous system involvement. In the US, cranial neuropathy is the most common manifestation of early neurologic Lyme disease; seventh cranial nerve palsy is the most common of the cranial neuropathies and bilateral involvement may occur. Cranial nerve palsies in patients with Lyme disease frequently are associated with lymphocytic CSF pleocytosis, with or without symptoms of meningitis. Although anti-infectives may not hasten resolution of seventh cranial nerve palsy associated with *B. burgdorferi* infection, anti-infectives should be given to prevent further sequelae.

IDSA and other clinicians recommend a 14-day regimen (range: 10–28 days) of IV ceftriaxone as first-line therapy for the treatment of acute neurologic Lyme disease manifested by meningitis or radiculopathy; IV cefotaxime and IV penicillin G sodium are the preferred alternatives. It has been suggested that IV ceftriaxone may be preferable to IV penicillin G for serious manifestations of early disseminated or late Lyme disease (i.e., those involving major organs) based on ceftriaxone's greater in vitro and in vivo activity against *B. burgdorferi*, excellent CSF penetration, and prolonged serum concentrations achievable with once-daily administration of the drug. Although IV cefotaxime appears to be as effective as IV ceftriaxone or IV penicillin G sodium for the treatment of acute neurologic Lyme disease and does not cause the biliary complications reported with ceftriaxone, ceftriaxone has the advantage of once-daily dosing. In patients with acute neurologic manifestations who are intolerant of cephalosporins and penicillin, there is some evidence that oral doxycycline may be an adequate alternative that can be considered for use in adults and children 8 years of age or older; because doxycycline is well absorbed orally, IV doxycycline should only be needed rarely.

Some clinicians suggest that a 14-day regimen (range: 14–21 days) of oral anti-infectives (amoxicillin, doxycycline, cefuroxime axetil) may be used in patients with cranial nerve palsy without clinical evidence of meningitis (i.e., those with normal CSF examinations or those for whom CSF examination is deemed unnecessary because there are no clinical signs of meningitis); however, a 14-day parenteral regimen (range: 10–28 days) is indicated when there is both clinical and laboratory evidence of CNS involvement and meningitis. Although there is some experience using oral anti-infectives in patients with seventh cranial nerve palsy, it is unclear whether an oral regimen would be as effective for patients with other cranial neuropathies.

Lyme Carditis. IDSA states that patients with AV heart block and/or myopericarditis associated with early Lyme disease may be treated with a 14-day regimen (range: 14–21 days) of oral or parenteral anti-infectives. Although there is no evidence to date to suggest that a parenteral regimen is more effective than an oral regimen for the treatment of Lyme carditis, a parenteral regimen usually is recommended for initial treatment of hospitalized patients; an oral regimen can be used to complete therapy and for the treatment of outpatients. When a parenteral regimen is used, IV ceftriaxone or, alternatively, IV cefotaxime or IV penicillin G sodium is recommended. When an oral regimen is used, oral amoxicillin, oral doxycycline, or oral cefuroxime axetil is recommended.

Because of the potential for life-threatening complications, hospitalization and continuous monitoring is advisable for patients who are symptomatic (syncope, dyspnea, chest pain) and also is recommended for those with second- or third-degree AV block or first-degree heart block when the PR interval is prolonged to 0.3 seconds or longer. Patients with advanced heart block may require a temporary pacemaker and consultation with a cardiologist is recommended.

Borrelial Lymphocytoma. Although experience is limited, IDSA states that available data indicate that borrelial lymphocytoma† may be treated with a 14-day regimen (range: 14–21 days) of oral doxycycline, oral amoxicillin, or oral cefuroxime axetil in the dosages used for the treatment of erythema migrans.

Late Lyme Disease **Lyme Arthritis.** Patients with uncomplicated Lyme arthritis† without clinical evidence of neurologic disease generally can be treated with a 28-day regimen of oral doxycycline, oral amoxicillin, or oral cefuroxime axetil. However, patients with Lyme arthritis and concomitant neurologic disease should receive a 14-day parenteral regimen (range: 14–28 days) of IV ceftriaxone or, alternatively, IV cefotaxime or IV penicillin G sodium. While oral regimens are easier to administer, associated with fewer serious adverse effects, and less expensive than IV regimens, some patients with Lyme arthritis treated with oral anti-infectives have subsequently developed overt neuroborreliosis, which may require IV therapy for successful resolution. Therefore, additional study is needed to fully evaluate the comparative safety and efficacy of oral versus IV anti-infectives for the treatment of Lyme arthritis.

In patients who have persistent or recurrent joint swelling after a recommended oral regimen, IDSA and other clinicians recommend retreatment with the oral regimen or a switch to a parenteral regimen. Some clinicians prefer retreatment with an oral regimen for patients whose arthritis substantively improved but did not completely resolve; these clinicians reserve parenteral regimens for those patients whose arthritis failed to improve or worsened. It has been suggested that clinicians should consider allowing several months for joint inflammation to resolve after initial treatment before an additional course of anti-infectives is given.

Late Neurologic Lyme Disease. IDSA and other clinicians recommend that patients with late neurologic Lyme disease† affecting the CNS or peripheral nervous system (e.g., encephalopathy, neuropathy) receive a 14-day regimen (range: 14–28 days) of IV ceftriaxone or, alternatively, IV cefotaxime or IV penicillin G sodium. Response to anti-infective treatment usually is slow and may be incomplete in patients with late neurologic Lyme disease. IDSA states that retreatment is not recommended unless relapse is shown by reliable objective measures.

Acrodermatitis Chronica Atrophicans. IDSA states that available data indicate that acrodermatitis chronica atrophicans† may be treated with a 21-day regimen (range: 14–28 days) of oral doxycycline, oral amoxicillin, or oral cefuroxime axetil in the dosages used for the treatment of erythema migrans. It is unclear whether a parenteral regimen would be more effective than an oral regimen.

■ Nocardiosis

Cephalosporins (ceftriaxone, cefotaxime, cefoxitin, cefuroxime) have been used for the treatment of nocardiosis† caused by *Nocardia*.

Co-trimoxazole (fixed combination of sulfamethoxazole and trimethoprim) usually is considered the drug of choice for the treatment of nocardiosis. Other drugs that have been used alone or in combination regimens for the treatment of nocardiosis include a sulfonamide alone (sulfadiazine, sulfamethoxazole [not commercially available as a single-entity preparation in the US]), amikacin, tetracyclines, cephalosporins (ceftriaxone, cefotaxime, cefuroxime), cefoxitin, carbapenems (imipenem or meropenem), fixed combination of amoxicillin and clavulanate, clarithromycin, cycloserine, or linezolid.

Anti-infective agents for the treatment of invasive nocardiosis or for the treatment of nocardiosis in patients unable to tolerate sulfonamides should be selected based on results of in vitro susceptibility testing. If nocardiosis involves the CNS or if the infection is disseminated or overwhelming, some clinicians suggest that amikacin and ceftriaxone should be included in the treatment regimen during the first 4–12 weeks of therapy or until there is clinical improvement. A regimen of amikacin and ceftriaxone has been effective for the treatment of disseminated *N. asteroides* infection complicated by cerebral abscess.

■ Pelvic Inflammatory Disease

Several parenteral cephalosporins (cefotaxime, ceftriaxone) and closely related cephamycins (cefotetan, cefoxitin) have been used in the treatment of acute pelvic inflammatory disease (PID); these drugs are inactive against *C. trachomatis* and should not be used alone in the treatment of PID.

PID is an acute or chronic inflammatory disorder in the upper female genital tract and can include any combination of endometritis, salpingitis, tubo-ovarian abscess, and pelvic peritonitis. PID generally is a polymicrobial infection frequently caused by sexually transmitted organisms, especially *N. gonorrhoeae* and/or *Chlamydia trachomatis*; however, organisms that can be part of the normal vaginal flora (e.g., anaerobic bacteria, *Gardnerella vaginalis*, *H. influenzae*, enteric gram-negative bacilli, *S. agalactiae*) also have been associated with PID. In addition, cytomegalovirus or mycoplasma (e.g., *Mycoplasma hominis*, *M. genitalium*, *Ureaplasma urealyticum*) may be involved in some cases. PID is treated with an empiric regimen that provides broad-spectrum coverage. The regimen should be effective against *N. gonorrhoeae* and *C. trachomatis* and also probably should be effective against anaerobes, gram-negative facultative bacteria, and streptococci. The optimum empiric regimen for the treatment of PID has not been identified. A wide variety of parenteral and oral regimens have been shown to achieve clinical and microbiologic cure in randomized studies with short-term follow-up; however, only limited data are available to date regarding elimination of infection in the endometrium and fallopian tubes or intermediate or long-term outcomes, including the impact of these regimens on the incidence of long-term sequelae of PID (e.g., tubal infertility, ectopic pregnancy, pain).

Parenteral Regimens for PID When a parenteral regimen is indicated for the treatment of PID, CDC generally recommends a 2-drug regimen of cefoxitin (2 g IV every 6 hours) or cefotetan (2 g IV every 12 hours) given in conjunction with doxycycline (100 mg IV or orally every 12 hours) or a 2-drug regimen of clindamycin (900 mg IV every 8 hours) and gentamicin (usually a 2-mg/kg IV or IM loading dose followed by 1.5 mg/kg every 8 hours). While certain parenteral cephalosporins (e.g., cefotaxime, ceftriaxone) also have been used for the treatment of PID, CDC states that only limited data are available regarding use of these cephalosporins in patients with PID and they are less active than cefotetan or cefoxitin against anaerobic bacteria. CDC states that only limited data are available to support the use of other parenteral regimens for the treatment of acute PID, although a regimen of IV ampicillin and sulbactam given with oral or IV doxycycline provides broad-spectrum coverage and is effective against *C. trachomatis*, *N. gonorrhoeae*, and anaerobes in women with tubo-ovarian abscess.

Oral Regimens for PID Data are not available regarding use of oral cephalosporins for the treatment of PID. When acute PID that is mild to moderately severe is treated with an oral regimen, CDC recommends a regimen that consists of a single dose of IM ceftriaxone, IM cefoxitin (with oral probenecid), or IM cefotaxime given in conjunction with a 14-day regimen of oral doxycycline (with or without oral metronidazole). The optimal parenteral cephalosporin for this regimen is unclear; although cefoxitin has better anaerobic coverage, ceftriaxone has better coverage against *N. gonorrhoeae*.

For additional information regarding treatment of PID, the current CDC sexually transmitted diseases treatment guidelines available at http://www.cdc.gov/std should be consulted.

■ Syphilis

Ceftriaxone has some activity against *Treponema pallidum* and there is some limited evidence that the drug may be effective for the treatment of syphilis†. Penicillin G is the drug of choice for the treatment of all stages of syphilis and data to support the use of penicillin alternatives are limited.

CDC states that, based on limited clinical studies, biologic plausibility, and pharmacologic properties, ceftriaxone may be an effective alternative for the treatment of primary or secondary syphilis† or neurosyphilis† in penicillin-allergic patients. However, optimal dosage and duration of ceftriaxone therapy for these infections have not been defined and the possibility of cross-allergenicity with penicillin should be considered. Although ceftriaxone might be effective for the treatment of latent syphilis† in penicillin-allergic patients, CDC states that the only acceptable alternatives to penicillin for the treatment of these infections are doxycycline or tetracycline. Decisions regarding the treatment of syphilis in penicillin-allergic patients should be made in consultation with a specialist.

For the treatment of infants with clinical evidence of congenital syphilis†, CDC states that use of ceftriaxone can be considered if there is a penicillin shortage and penicillin G sodium and penicillin G procaine are unavailable. However, because studies that strongly support ceftriaxone for the treatment of congenital syphilis have not been conducted, the drug should be used with careful clinical and serologic follow-up and in consultation with a specialist in the treatment of infants with congenital syphilis.

For additional information regarding treatment of syphilis, the current CDC sexually transmitted diseases treatment guidelines available at http://www.cdc.gov/std should be consulted.

■ Empiric Therapy in Febrile Neutropenic Patients

Cefepime has been used alone or in conjunction with other anti-infectives for empiric anti-infective therapy of presumed bacterial infections in febrile neutropenic adults or pediatric patients. Ceftazidime† and ceftriaxone† also have been used for empiric anti-infective therapy in febrile neutropenic patients, but are not generally recommended. Ceftazidime is no longer considered a reliable drug for empiric monotherapy in febrile neutropenic patients because of poor activity against gram-positive bacteria and decreasing potency against gram-negative bacteria; ceftriaxone monotherapy may not provide adequate coverage against some potential pathogens (e.g., *Ps. aeruginosa*).

Successful treatment of infections in granulocytopenic patients requires prompt initiation of empiric anti-infective therapy (even when fever is the only sign or symptom of infection) and appropriate modification of the initial regimen if the duration of fever and neutropenia is protracted, if a specific site of infection is identified, or if organisms resistant to the initial regimen are present. The initial empiric regimen should be chosen based on the underlying disease and other host factors that may affect the degree of risk, on local epidemiologic data regarding usual pathogens in these patients and in vitro susceptibility of bacterial isolates recovered from other patients in the same health-care facility, and the individual patient's pattern of colonization and resistance. The fact that gram-positive bacteria have become a predominant pathogen in febrile neutropenic patients should be considered when selecting an empiric anti-infective regimen. However, although gram-positive bacteria reportedly account for about 60% and gram-negative bacteria account for about 35% of microbiologically documented infections, gram-negative infections are associated with greater mortality.

No empiric regimen has been identified that would be appropriate for initial treatment of all febrile neutropenic patients. IDSA recommends use of a parenteral empiric regimen in most febrile neutropenic patients; use of an oral regimen (e.g., oral ciprofloxacin and oral amoxicillin and clavulanate potassium) should be considered *only* for selected adults at low risk for complications who have adequate and stable renal and hepatic function, an expected duration of neutropenia less than 7 days, and no active medical comorbidities. All other patients are considered high risk and should receive an initial IV empiric regimen consisting of an antipseudomonal β-lactam (e.g., cefepime, imipenem, meropenem, fixed-combination of piperacillin and tazobactam). Other anti-infectives (e.g., aminoglycosides, fluoroquinolones, and/or vancomycin) may be added to the regimen for the management of complications (e.g., pneumonia) or when antimicrobial resistance is suspected or proven. Vancomycin and other anti-infectives active against aerobic gram-positive cocci are not usually included in the initial empiric regimen except in certain clinical scenarios, including suspected catheter-related infections, skin and soft tissue infections, pneumonia, or hemodynamic instability.

Regardless of the initial regimen selected, patients should be reassessed daily and the anti-infective regimen altered (if indicated) based on the presence or absence of fever, identification of the causative organism, and the clinical condition of the patient; anti-infectives active against gram-positive organisms may be discontinued after 2 days if there is no evidence of such infections.

Published protocols for the treatment of infections in febrile neutropenic patients should be consulted for specific recommendations regarding selection of the initial empiric anti-infective regimen, when to change the initial regimen, possible subsequent regimens, and duration of anti-infective therapy in these patients. In addition, consultation with an infectious disease expert knowledgeable about infections in immunocompromised patients is advised.

■ Perioperative Prophylaxis

Cefazolin, cefotaxime, ceftriaxone, and cefuroxime have been used perioperatively to reduce the incidence of infections in patients undergoing certain contaminated or potentially contaminated surgical procedures or undergoing certain clean surgical procedures where the development of infection at the surgical site would have severe consequences. Perioperative prophylaxis with an appropriate anti-infective agent can decrease the incidence of infection, particularly surgical site infections, after some procedures.

Because cefazolin has a narrow spectrum of activity that covers the most likely surgical site pathogens, has a moderately long serum half-life, and has been shown to be effective, it is considered by many clinicians to be the drug of choice for perioperative prophylaxis for a wide variety of procedures. Cefazolin is considered a drug of choice for perioperative prophylaxis in patients undergoing certain cardiac surgery (e.g., coronary artery bypass, placement of pacemaker or other cardiac device), noncardiac thoracic surgery (e.g., lobectomy), vascular surgery (arterial surgery involving the abdominal aorta, a prosthesis, or a groin incision or lower extremity amputation for ischemia), head and neck surgery involving incisions through oral or pharyngeal mucosa, neurosurgery (e.g., craniotomy, spinal surgery), orthopedic surgery (e.g., total joint replacement, surgical repair of closed fractures, internal fixation of compound or open fractures), GI surgery (gastroduodenal, esophageal, biliary tract, colorectal, appendectomy, bariatric), genitourinary surgery (e.g., open or laparoscopic surgery including percutaneous renal surgery, procedures with entry into the urinary tract or implantation of a prosthesis), and gynecologic and obstetric surgery (cesarean section or vaginal, abdominal, or laparoscopic hysterectomy). Cefazolin also is recommended as a drug of choice for perioperative prophylaxis in patients undergoing heart, lung, heart-lung, pancreas, and pancreas-kidney transplantation.

Cefuroxime is considered a drug of choice for cardiac procedures (e.g., coronary artery bypass, placement of pacemaker or other cardiac device). Cefuroxime also is considered a drug of choice for perioperative prophylaxis in patients undergoing clean head and neck surgery involving placement of prosthesis (excluding tympanostomy) and is a drug of choice when used in conjunction with metronidazole for perioperative prophylaxis in patients undergoing clean-contaminated cancer surgery of the head and neck or other clean-contaminated head and neck procedures (excluding tonsillectomy and functional endoscopic sinus procedures).

Cefotaxime used in conjunction with ampicillin is considered a regimen of choice for perioperative prophylaxis in patients undergoing liver transplantation†.

Ceftriaxone is recommended as one of several options for perioperative prophylaxis in patients undergoing biliary tract procedures, but should not be used in patients undergoing cholecystectomy for noninfected biliary conditions.

A first or second generation cephalosporin (cefazolin, cefuroxime) generally is preferred when a cephalosporin is used for perioperative prophylaxis. Third generation cephalosporins (cefotaxime, ceftriaxone, ceftazidime) and fourth generation cephalosporins (cefepime) are not usually recommended for perioperative prophylaxis because they are expensive, some are less active than first or second generation cephalosporins against staphylococci, they have spectrums of activity wider than necessary for organisms encountered in elective surgery, and their use for prophylaxis may promote emergence of resistant organisms.

If cefazolin is used for perioperative prophylaxis in patients undergoing certain GI procedures (e.g., colorectal surgery, appendectomy) that might involve exposure to *B. fragilis* or other anaerobic bowel bacteria or in patients undergoing head and neck surgery involving incisions through oral or pharyngeal mucosa, it should be used in conjunction with metronidazole to provide anaerobic coverage.

Published guidelines and protocols for perioperative prophylaxis should be consulted for additional information regarding specific procedures.

Cardiac Surgery

Perioperative prophylaxis can decrease the incidence of infection after cardiac surgery. For cardiac procedures lasting longer than 400 minutes, the risk of postoperative infection is decreased if intraoperative anti-infective doses are given in addition to a preoperative dose. Regarding the use of postoperative doses in patients undergoing cardiac surgery, there are data to support use of a single preoperative dose or prophylaxis continued for 24 hours postoperatively; however, there is no evidence of benefit beyond 48 hours and no evidence to support continuing prophylaxis after wound closure or until all indwelling drains and intravascular catheters are removed.

Results of a pooled analysis of 7 placebo-controlled studies indicate that perioperative prophylaxis reduces the incidence of infection after permanent pacemaker implantation. In patients receiving implantation of permanent pacemakers and cardioverter-defibrillators, studies indicate that perioperative prophylaxis reduces the incidence of wound infection, inflammation, and skin erosion.

For perioperative prophylaxis in patients undergoing cardiac surgery, many clinicians recommend IV cefazolin or IV cefuroxime. Although routine use of vancomycin for perioperative prophylaxis is not recommended, IV vancomycin is considered an alternative for perioperative prophylaxis in cardiac surgery patients at institutions where methicillin-resistant *S. aureus* (MRSA; also known as oxacillin-resistant *S. aureus* or ORSA) and methicillin-resistant *S. epidermidis* frequently cause postoperative wound infection or in patients who were previously colonized with MRSA or are allergic to penicillins or cephalosporins.

Noncardiac Thoracic Surgery

Although studies evaluating use of perioperative prophylaxis in patients undergoing pulmonary surgery are sparse, such prophylaxis is routinely used. In one randomized, double-blind, placebo-controlled study in patients undergoing noncardiac thoracic surgery, a single preoperative dose of cefazolin decreased the incidence of postoperative surgical site infection, but did not affect the incidence of postoperative empyema or nosocomial pneumonia. Although there is evidence from a placebo-controlled study that multiple doses of a cephalosporin (cefazolin) can prevent infection after closed-tube thoracostomy for chest trauma, some clinicians suggest that insertion of chest tubes for other indications, such as spontaneous pneumothorax, does not require prophylaxis.

For perioperative prophylaxis in patients undergoing noncardiac thoracic surgery, many clinicians recommend IV cefazolin or IV ampicillin and sulbactam. Although routine use of vancomycin for perioperative prophylaxis is not recommended, IV vancomycin may be considered an alternative for perioperative prophylaxis in patients undergoing noncardiac thoracic surgery at institutions where MRSA and methicillin-resistant *S. epidermidis* frequently cause postoperative wound infection or in patients who were previously colonized with MRSA or are allergic to penicillins or cephalosporins. In patients allergic to penicillins and cephalosporins, a reasonable alternative is clindamycin or vancomycin used in conjunction with gentamicin, ciprofloxacin, levofloxacin, or aztreonam.

GI Surgery

Esophageal and Gastroduodenal Surgery. Perioperative prophylaxis is not usually indicated for patients undergoing routine gastroesophageal endoscopy, but is recommended for high-risk patients undergoing esophageal or gastroduodenal procedures.

Although there are no controlled studies evaluating efficacy, perioperative prophylaxis is used routinely in patients undergoing bariatric surgery, including adjustable gastric banding, vertical banded gastroplasty, Roux-en-y bypass, and biliopancreatic diversion.

For perioperative prophylaxis in high-risk patients undergoing esophageal or gastroduodenal surgery (e.g., those who are morbidly obese or have GI obstruction, decreased gastric acidity, decreased GI motility, gastric bleeding, malignancy or perforation, or immunosuppression), many clinicians recommend IV cefazolin as the drug of choice. Dosage may need to be increased in morbidly obese patients. In patients allergic to penicillins and cephalosporins, a reasonable alternative is clindamycin or vancomycin used in conjunction with gentamicin, ciprofloxacin, levofloxacin, or aztreonam.

Biliary Tract Surgery. Perioperative prophylaxis is recommended for patients undergoing biliary tract surgery who are at high risk of infection (e.g., those older than 70 years of age or those with acute cholecystitis, a nonfunctioning gallbladder, obstructive jaundice, or common duct stones). In high-risk patients undergoing endoscopic retrograde cholangiopancreatography (ERCP), perioperative prophylaxis is recommended only if complete biliary drainage is unlikely to be achieved. Perioperative prophylaxis is not considered necessary for low-risk patients undergoing elective laparoscopic cholecystectomy since there is no evidence that such prophylaxis provides any benefit in these patients.

For perioperative prophylaxis in high-risk patients undergoing biliary tract surgery (e.g., those older than 70 years of age or those with acute cholecystitis, nonfunctioning gallbladder, obstructive jaundice, or common duct stones), many clinicians recommend IV cefazolin as the drug of choice. Alternatives include other cephalosporins (cefotetan, cefoxitin, ceftriaxone) or ampicillin and sulbactam. In patients allergic to penicillins and cephalosporins, a reasonable alternative is clindamycin or vancomycin used in conjunction with gentamicin, ciprofloxacin, levofloxacin, or aztreonam.

Colorectal Surgery. There is evidence that perioperative prophylaxis can decrease the incidence of infection after colorectal surgery, and such prophylaxis usually is recommended.

For perioperative prophylaxis in patients undergoing colorectal surgery, many clinicians recommend a parenteral regimen of IV cefoxitin or IV cefotetan, IV cefazolin (or IV ceftriaxone) used in conjunction with IV metronidazole, or IV ampicillin and sulbactam. In patients allergic to penicillins and cephalosporins, a reasonable alternative is clindamycin used in conjunction with gentamicin, ciprofloxacin, levofloxacin, or aztreonam.

Alternatively, an oral prophylaxis regimen of oral neomycin with either oral erythromycin or oral metronidazole can be used. Many clinicians use both an oral regimen and a parenteral regimen for perioperative prophylaxis in patients undergoing colorectal surgery, and there is some evidence that use of an oral regimen (with mechanical bowel preparation) in conjunction with a parenteral regimen is more effective than use of a parenteral regimen alone.

In a randomized, prospective study in patients undergoing elective colorectal surgery, the overall incidence of intra-abdominal septic complications in those who received mechanical bowel preparation and an oral regimen (erythromycin and neomycin) alone was similar to that in those who received both the oral regimen and a parenteral regimen (cefoxitin); however, the incidence of abdominal wound infection was higher in those who received the oral regimen alone (14.6%) than in those who received the combined oral and parenteral regimen (5%).

Appendectomy. There is evidence that perioperative prophylaxis can reduce the incidence of infection after surgery for acute appendicitis.

For perioperative prophylaxis in patients undergoing nonperforated appendectomy, many clinicians recommend IV cefoxitin or IV cefotetan or IV cefazolin used in conjunction with IV metronidazole. In patients allergic to penicillins and cephalosporins, a reasonable alternative is clindamycin or vancomycin used in conjunction with gentamicin, ciprofloxacin, levofloxacin, or aztreonam.

If perforation has occurred, anti-infectives are continued postoperatively for about 5 days.

Genitourinary Surgery **Cystoscopy.** Perioperative prophylaxis generally is not recommended in patients with sterile urine undergoing cystoscopy without manipulation (dilation, biopsy, fulguration, resection or ureteral instrumentation). When cystoscopy with manipulation is planned, urine cultures are positive or unavailable, or an indwelling urinary catheter is present, many clinicians recommend that patients receive treatment with an appropriate anti-infective before surgery to sterilize the urine or receive a single preoperative dose of an anti-infective selected based on the most likely infecting organisms.

If perioperative prophylaxis is indicated in individuals undergoing cystoscopy who are at high risk (urine culture positive or unavailable, preoperative urinary catheter, transrectal prostatic biopsy, placement of prosthetic material) or in individuals undergoing cystoscopy with manipulation or upper urinary tract instrumentation (shockwave lithotripsy, ureteroscopy), many clinicians recommend oral or IV ciprofloxacin, oral co-trimoxazole, or IV cefazolin.

Open or Laparoscopic Surgery. There is evidence that perioperative prophylaxis decreases the incidence of postoperative bacteriuria and septicemia in patients with sterile urine undergoing transurethral prostatectomy and transrectal prostatic biopsies. Prophylaxis also is used for patients undergoing ureteroscopy, shock wave lithotripsy, percutaneous renal surgery, or open laparoscopic procedures or undergoing placement of a urologic prosthesis (penile implant, artificial sphincter, synthetic pubovaginal sling, bone anchors for pelvic floor reconstruction).

For perioperative prophylaxis in individuals undergoing open or laparoscopic surgery (including percutaneous renal surgery, procedures with entry into the urinary tract, or procedures involving implantation of a prosthesis), many clinicians recommend IV cefazolin. In patients allergic to penicillins and cephalosporins, a reasonable alternative is clindamycin used in conjunction with gentamicin, ciprofloxacin, levofloxacin, or aztreonam.

Gynecologic and Obstetric Surgery Perioperative prophylaxis decreases the incidence of infection after vaginal and abdominal hysterectomy. In addition, there is evidence that perioperative prophylaxis can prevent infection after elective and nonelective cesarean section, including emergency cesarean section in high-risk situations (e.g., active labor, premature rupture of membranes), and after elective abortions, including second trimester abortions or first trimester abortion in high-risk women. A pooled analysis of results of randomized, placebo-controlled studies in women who underwent therapeutic abortion before 16 weeks' gestation indicates that perioperative prophylaxis reduces the overall risk of postabortal infection by 42% compared with placebo.

Many clinicians suggest that the preferred agents for perioperative prophylaxis in women undergoing vaginal, abdominal, or laparoscopic hysterectomy are IV cefoxitin, IV cefotetan, IV cefazolin, or IV ampicillin and sulbactam. IV cefazolin generally is the preferred agent for prophylaxis in women undergoing cesarean section; oral doxycycline is recommended for prophylaxis in those undergoing abortion.

Head and Neck Surgery There is evidence that perioperative prophylaxis decreases the incidence of surgical site infection after oncologic head and neck operations involving incisions through the oral or pharyngeal mucosa. Perioperative prophylaxis has not been shown to be beneficial in patients undergoing tonsillectomy, nasal septoplasty, or functional endoscopic sinus procedures. Perioperative prophylaxis is not indicated for clean head and neck surgery.

For perioperative prophylaxis in patients undergoing head or neck surgery involving incisions through oral or pharyngeal mucosa, many clinicians recommend IV clindamycin, IV cefazolin used in conjunction with IV metronidazole, or IV ampicillin and sulbactam. Other clinicians recommend cefazolin or cefuroxime for perioperative prophylaxis in patients undergoing clean head and neck surgery involving placement of prosthesis (excluding tympanostomy). For patients undergoing clean-contaminated cancer surgery of the head and neck or other clean-contaminated head and neck procedures (excluding tonsillectomy and functional endoscopic sinus procedures), these experts recommend cefazolin used in conjunction with metronidazole, cefuroxime used in conjunction with metronidazole, or ampicillin and sulbactam.

Neurosurgery There is evidence that perioperative use of an anti-infective agent active against staphylococci can decrease the incidence of infection after craniotomy. Although some studies in patients undergoing implantation of permanent CSF shunts showed lower infection rates in those receiving perioperative prophylaxis, the benefit of such prophylaxis in patients undergoing ventriculostomy placement remains uncertain.

Although the rate of postoperative infections is low in patients undergoing spinal surgery involving conventional lumbar discectomy, many clinicians use perioperative prophylaxis in such patients because of the serious consequences of a surgical site infection. The risk of infection is higher after prolonged spinal surgery or spinal procedures involving fusion or insertion of foreign material, and perioperative prophylaxis generally is used in these patients.

For perioperative prophylaxis in patients undergoing neurosurgery, many clinicians recommend IV cefazolin. Although routine use of vancomycin for perioperative prophylaxis is not recommended, IV vancomycin may be considered an alternative for perioperative prophylaxis in patients undergoing neurosurgery at institutions where MRSA and methicillin-resistant *S. epidermidis* frequently cause postoperative wound infection or in patients who were previously colonized with MRSA or are allergic to penicillins or cephalosporins.

Ophthalmic Surgery Data are limited regarding the effectiveness of anti-infective prophylaxis in patients undergoing ophthalmic surgery; however, many clinicians use a topical or subconjunctival anti-infective for prophylaxis in patients undergoing such surgery. Some clinicians state that there is no evidence that perioperative prophylaxis is needed for procedures that do not invade the globe. While there is no consensus regarding the most effective drug, route, or duration of perioperative prophylaxis in patients undergoing ophthalmic surgery, many clinicians recommend use of a topical aminoglycoside (gentamicin, tobramycin), topical fluoroquinolone (ciprofloxacin, gatifloxacin, levofloxacin, moxifloxacin, ofloxacin), or a topical preparation containing neomycin, polymyxin b sulfate, and gramicidin; some clinicians also recommend subconjunctival injection of cefazolin or intracameral cefazolin or cefuroxime.

Orthopedic Surgery There is evidence that perioperative prophylaxis with an anti-infective agent active against staphylococci can decrease the incidence of both early and delayed infection in patients undergoing joint replacement or surgical repair of closed fractures. Perioperative prophylaxis can decrease the rate of infection in patients with hip and other closed fractures undergoing procedures that involve internal fixation with nails, plates, screws, or wires and in patients with compound or open fractures. However, additional study is needed to determine whether single-dose regimens or regimens continued for 24 hours are most effective. A retrospective review concluded that anti-infective prophylaxis is not indicated for patients undergoing arthroscopic surgery procedures.

For perioperative prophylaxis in patients undergoing orthopedic surgery, many clinicians recommend IV cefazolin. Although routine use of vancomycin for perioperative prophylaxis is not recommended, IV vancomycin may be considered an alternative for perioperative prophylaxis in patients undergoing orthopedic surgery at institutions where MRSA and methicillin-resistant *S. epidermidis* frequently cause postoperative wound infection or in patients who were previously colonized with MRSA or are allergic to penicillins or cephalosporins.

Vascular Surgery There is evidence that perioperative prophylaxis with a cephalosporin can decrease the incidence of postoperative surgical site infection after arterial reconstructive surgery on the abdominal aorta, vascular operations on the leg that include a groin incision, or amputation of a lower extremity for ischemia. Many clinicians also recommend perioperative prophylaxis in patients undergoing implantation of any vascular prosthetic material (e.g., grafts for vascular access in hemodialysis); however, such prophylaxis generally is not indicated for carotid endarterectomy or brachial artery repair without prosthetic material. Although perioperative prophylaxis is not routinely recommended for endovascular stenting, prophylaxis may be justified in patients with certain risk factors (e.g., repeat intervention within 7 days, prolonged indwelling arterial sheath, procedure duration longer than 2 hours, presence of other infected implants, immunosuppression).

For perioperative prophylaxis in patients undergoing vascular surgery (e.g., arterial surgery involving a prosthesis, the abdominal aorta, or a groin incision; lower extremity amputation for ischemia), many clinicians recommend IV cefazolin. Although routine use of vancomycin for perioperative prophylaxis is not recommended, IV vancomycin may be considered an alternative for perioperative prophylaxis in patients undergoing vascular surgery at institutions where MRSA and methicillin-resistant *S. epidermidis* frequently cause postoperative wound infection or in patients who were previously colonized with MRSA or are allergic to penicillins or cephalosporins.

Timing and Number of Doses When perioperative prophylaxis is indicated in patients undergoing surgery, administration of an appropriate anti-infective should be timed to ensure that bactericidal concentrations of the drug are established in serum and tissues by the time the initial surgical incision is made; therapeutic concentrations of the drug should then be maintained in serum and tissues for the duration of the procedure.

An IV dose of the appropriate anti-infective should be given within 60 minutes before the initial incision. However, if vancomycin or a fluoroquinolone is used, the anti-infective infusion should be started within 1–2 hours before the initial incision to minimize the risk of an adverse effect occurring around the time of anesthesia induction and to ensure adequate tissue levels of the drug at the time of the initial incision.

Single-dose perioperative prophylaxis may be sufficient. However, if surgery is prolonged (more than 3–4 hours), major blood loss occurs, or other factors are present that shorten the half-life of the drug (e.g., extensive burns), additional doses should be administered during the procedure to ensure adequate serum and tissue concentrations of the anti-infective throughout the procedure. Intraoperative doses may not be warranted if there are factors that prolong the half-life of the drug (e.g., renal impairment). For prolonged procedures in patients with normal renal function, some clinicians suggest that intraoperative doses be administered during the procedure at intervals that correspond to 1–2 times the half-life of the drug. If intraoperative doses are necessary, the redosing interval should be measured from the time of administration of the preoperative dose, not from the beginning of the procedure.

For most procedures, the duration of prophylaxis should be less than 24 hours. There is no evidence to support continuing prophylaxis after wound closure or until all indwelling drains and intravascular catheters are removed.

■ Prevention of Perinatal Group B Streptococcal Disease In certain penicillin-allergic women, cefazolin is used as an alternative to penicillin G or ampicillin for prevention of perinatal group B streptococcal (GBS) disease†.

Pregnant women who are colonized with GBS in the genital or rectal areas can transmit GBS infection to their infants during labor and delivery resulting in invasive neonatal infection that can be associated with substantial morbidity and mortality. Intrapartum anti-infective prophylaxis for prevention of early-onset neonatal GBS disease is administered *selectively* to women at high risk for transmitting GBS infection to their neonates. CDC, AAP, and other experts recommend *routine* universal prenatal culture-based screening for GBS colonization (vaginal and rectal cultures) in *all* pregnant women at 35–37 weeks of gestation, unless GBS bacteriuria is known to be present during the current pregnancy or the woman had a previous infant with invasive GBS disease. These experts state that anti-infective prophylaxis to prevent perinatal GBS disease is indicated in pregnant women identified as GBS carriers during the routine prenatal GBS screening performed at 35–37 weeks during the current pregnancy, in women with GBS bacteriuria identified at any time during the current pregnancy, and in women who had a previous infant diagnosed with invasive GBS disease. Anti-infective prophylaxis to prevent perinatal GBS disease also is indicated in women with unknown GBS status at the time of onset of labor (i.e., culture not done, incomplete, or results unknown) if delivery is at less than 37 weeks of gestation, the duration of amniotic membrane rupture is 18 hours or longer, intrapartum temperature is 38°C or higher, or an intrapartum NAAT was positive for GBS.

When intrapartum prophylaxis is indicated in the mother to prevent GBS disease in the neonate, it should be given at onset of labor or rupture of membranes. CDC, AAP, and other experts recommend penicillin G (5 million units IV initially followed by 2.5–3 million units IV every 4 hours until delivery) as the regimen of choice and ampicillin (2 g IV initially followed by 1 g IV every 4 hours until delivery) as the preferred alternative. If intrapartum GBS prophylaxis is indicated in a penicillin-allergic woman who is *not* at high risk for anaphylaxis (i.e., does not have a history of anaphylaxis, angioedema, respiratory distress, or urticaria after receiving a penicillin or cephalosporin), CDC, AAP, and others recommend IV cefazolin (2 g IV initially followed by 1 g IV every 8 hours until delivery). If intrapartum prophylaxis is indicated in a penicillin-allergic woman who is at high risk for anaphylaxis (e.g., history of anaphylaxis, angioedema, respiratory distress, or urticaria after receiving a penicillin or cephalosporin), IV clindamycin (900 mg IV every 8 hours until delivery) is recommended if the GBS isolate is susceptible to the drug; alternatively, IV vancomycin (1 g IV every 12 hours until delivery) can be used if the isolate is resistant to clindamycin.

For additional information regarding prevention of perinatal group B streptococcal disease, the current CDC guidelines available at http://www.cdc.gov should be consulted.

Dosage and Administration

■ Administration Cephalosporins, in appropriate forms, may be administered orally, IV, by deep IM injection, or intraperitoneally. In general, orally administered cephalosporins should not be relied on for the treatment of the initial phase of severe infections or in patients with nausea and vomiting. Cephalosporins should be given IV in patients with meningitis, septicemia, endocarditis, or other severe or life-threatening infections. Cephalosporins have been administered by regional perfusion†, subconjunctivally†, intraventricularly†, or intrathecally†, but the risk of CNS toxicity must be considered with the latter route. (See Cautions: Other Adverse Effects.)

■ Dosage The duration of cephalosporin therapy depends on the type of infection. Generally, therapy should be continued for a minimum of 48–72 hours after the patient becomes asymptomatic or evidence of eradication of the infection has been obtained. In infections caused by β-hemolytic streptococci, therapy should be continued for at least 10 days. At least 4–6 weeks of therapy may be required in serious infections such as septicemia, endocarditis, or osteomyelitis.

■ Dosage in Renal Impairment In patients with impaired renal function, decreases in doses and/or frequency of administration of cephalosporins may be required and should be based on the degree of renal impairment, severity of the infection, susceptibility of the causative organism, and serum concentrations of the cephalosporins.

Cautions

Cephalosporins generally are well tolerated and with only a few exceptions, adverse effects reported with the various cephalosporin derivatives are similar. The most frequent adverse effects reported with oral cephalosporins include GI effects (diarrhea, nausea, vomiting), headache, and rash and the most frequent adverse effects reported with parenteral cephalosporins include local reactions at the injection site, adverse GI effects, and adverse hematologic effects. Although not reported with other cephalosporins, some previously available cephalosporins (e.g., cefamandole, cefoperazone) and structurally related cephamycins (e.g., cefotetan) that contain an *N*-methylthiotetrazole (NMTT) side chain have been associated with an increased risk of hypoprothrombinemia and disulfiram-like reactions. In addition, while the clinical importance is unclear, derivatives that contain an NMTT side chain have caused adverse testicular effects in animal studies.

■ Dermatologic and Sensitivity Reactions Hypersensitivity reactions have been reported in approximately 5% or less of patients receiving a cephalosporin. These reactions include urticaria, pruritus, rash (maculopapular, erythematous, or morbilliform), fever and chills, eosinophilia, joint pain or inflammation, edema, facial edema, erythema, genital and anal pruritus, angioedema, shock, hypotension, vasodilatation, Stevens-Johnson syndrome, erythema multiforme, toxic epidermal necrolysis, and exfoliative dermatitis. Anaphylaxis, including a few fatalities, has occurred rarely with cephalosporins.

Serum sickness-like reactions consisting of erythema multiforme or maculopapular pruritic rash or urticaria accompanied by arthritis, arthralgia, and fever have been reported rarely in patients receiving cefaclor. These reactions usually have occurred in pediatric patients younger than 6 years of age, most often with second or subsequent courses of the drug. While serum sickness-like reactions have been reported rarely in patients receiving other cephalosporins (i.e., cefprozil, cephalexin) or other β-lactam antibiotics (i.e., amoxicillin, loracarbef), these reactions been reported more frequently with cefaclor than with any other anti-infective agent. (See Cautions: Adverse Effects in Cefaclor 8:12.06.08.)

■ Hematologic Effects Positive direct and indirect antiglobulin (Coombs') test results have been reported in 3% or more of patients receiving a cephalosporin. (See Laboratory Test Interferences: Immunohematology Tests.) The mechanism of this reaction is usually nonimmunologic in nature; a cephalosporin-globulin complex coats the erythrocytes and reacts nonspecifically with Coombs' serum. Nonimmunologic positive Coombs' test results are most likely to occur in patients who have received large doses of a cephalosporin or who have impaired renal function or hypoalbuminemia.

Other adverse hematologic effects of cephalosporins include rare, mild and transient neutropenia, thrombocythemia or thrombocytopenia, leukocytosis, granulocytosis, monocytosis, lymphocytopenia, basophilia, and reversible leukopenia. Transient lymphocytosis has been reported occasionally in infants and children receiving cefaclor. Rarely, decreased hemoglobin and/or hematocrit, anemia, and agranulocytosis have been reported with some cephalosporins. Aplastic anemia, pancytopenia, hemolytic anemia, and epistaxis or hemorrhage also have been reported with cephalosporin therapy. Immune-mediated hemolytic anemia with extravascular hemolysis, including some fatalities, have been reported in patients receiving cefotaxime, ceftriaxone, or cefotetan.

Prolonged prothrombin time (PT), prolonged activated partial thromboplastin time (APTT), and/or hypoprothrombinemia (with or without bleeding) have been reported rarely with cefaclor, cefixime, cefoperazone (no longer available in the US), cefotaxime, cefotetan, cefoxitin, ceftizoxime (no longer commercially available in the US), ceftriaxone, and cefuroxime. Although the true incidence of hypoprothrombinemia and bleeding complications during therapy with these drugs has not been established, these effects have been reported most frequently with drugs that contain an NMTT side chain (e.g., cefamandole, cefoperazone [drugs no longer commercially available in the US]) and have usually occurred in geriatric, debilitated, or other patients with vitamin K deficiency or in patients with severe renal failure or following radical GI surgery. The mechanism(s) of the hypoprothrombinemic effect of these drugs has not been clearly established. While hypoprothrombinemia with some of the drugs may result in part from a reduction in vitamin K-producing bacteria in the GI tract, there is evidence that a direct effect on hepatic synthesis of prothrombin or prothrombin precursors is involved. The NMTT side chain apparently interferes with vitamin K metabolism and regeneration and inhibits γ-carboxylation of glutamic acid, the vitamin K-dependent step in the hepatic synthesis of prothrombin. Hypoprothrombinemia has usually been reversed by administration of vitamin K. Vitamin K should be administered when indicated to treat hypoprothrombinemia associated with use of other cephalosporins.

■ Renal and Genitourinary Effects Renal effects that have occurred occasionally with administration of a cephalosporin include transient increases in BUN and serum creatinine concentrations, renal dysfunction, and toxic nephropathy. Nephrotoxicity has been reported rarely with cephalexin and cefazolin and acute renal failure has been reported with cefazolin and cefixime. Reversible interstitial nephritis has occurred rarely during cefaclor therapy, and purpuric nephritis has been reported with oral cefpodoxime proxetil therapy in postmarketing experience outside the US. Renal toxicity is most likely to occur in patients older than 50 years of age, patients with prior renal impairment, or patients who are receiving other nephrotoxic drugs. (See Drug Interactions: Nephrotoxic Drugs.) All cephalosporins should be administered with caution and in reduced dosage in the presence of markedly impaired renal function. In patients with suspected renal impairment, careful clinical observation and renal function tests should be performed prior to and during cephalosporin therapy.

Genitourinary effects reported with cephalosporin therapy include vaginitis, vaginal candidiasis, genital pruritus, and menstrual irregularities.

■ Hepatic Effects Transient increases in serum AST (SGOT), ALT (SGPT), γ-glutamyl transferase (γ-glutamyl transpeptidase, GGT, GGTP), and alkaline phosphatase concentrations have occurred occasionally with cephalosporin therapy. Increased serum concentrations of bilirubin and/or LDH have been reported with many cephalosporins; decreased serum albumin and/or total protein also have been reported. Hepatic dysfunction, including cholestasis, also has been reported with cephalosporin therapy. Hepatitis and/or jaundice have been reported with cefazolin, cefixime, and ceftazidime. These hepatic effects are generally mild and disappear when cephalosporin therapy is discontinued.

Acute liver injury has been reported with oral cefpodoxime proxetil therapy in postmarketing experience outside the US.

■ GI Effects The most frequent adverse reactions to orally administered cephalosporins are nausea, vomiting, and diarrhea. These effects are usually mild and transient, but rarely may be severe enough to require discontinuance of the drug. Other adverse GI effects that have occurred with some of the oral cephalosporins include abdominal pain, tenesmus, epigastric pain/dyspepsia, decreased appetite/anorexia, glossitis, flatulence, candidiasis (e.g., oral thrush), taste alteration, decreased salivation, and heartburn. Adverse GI effects also can occur with IM or IV cephalosporins.

Treatment with anti-infectives alters the normal flora of the colon leading to overgrowth of *Clostridium difficile*. *C. difficile* infection (CDI) and *C. difficile*-associated diarrhea and colitis (CDAD; also known as antibiotic-associated diarrhea and colitis or pseudomembranous colitis) have been reported with nearly all systemic anti-infectives, including cephalosporins, and may range in severity from mild diarrhea to fatal colitis. *C. difficile* produces toxins A and B which contribute to the development of CDAD; hypertoxin-producing strains of *C. difficile* are associated with increased morbidity and mortality since they may be refractory to anti-infectives and colectomy may be required.

CDAD should be considered in the differential diagnosis in patients who develop diarrhea during or after anti-infective therapy. Careful medical history is necessary since CDAD has been reported to occur as late as 2 months or longer after anti-infective therapy is discontinued. If CDAD is suspected or confirmed, anti-infective therapy not directed against *C. difficile* should be discontinued whenever possible. Patients should be managed with appropriate supportive therapy (e.g., fluid and electrolyte management, protein supplementation), anti-infective therapy directed against *C. difficile* (e.g., metronidazole, vancomycin), and surgical evaluation as clinically indicated. Antiperistaltic agents (e.g., opiates, diphenoxylate with atropine) should be avoided since they may obscure symptoms and precipitate toxic megacolon.

■ Local Effects Local reactions are quite common following IM or IV administration of some parenteral cephalosporins; phlebitis and thrombophlebitis occasionally occur with IV administration of the drugs. Although reports are conflicting and results of many studies inconclusive, there appears to be little difference in the overall incidence of *mild* phlebitis and thrombophlebitis among the currently available IV cephalosporins.

■ Nervous System Effects Nervous system effects that have occurred following oral, IM, or IV administration of cephalosporins include dizziness, headache, malaise, fatigue, nightmares, and vertigo. Hyperactivity, nervousness or anxiety, agitation, hallucinations, insomnia, somnolence, weakness, hot flushes, alteration in color perception, confusion, and hypertonia also have been reported during therapy with some cephalosporins, although a causal relationship has not necessarily been established. Mild to moderate hearing loss has been reported in a few pediatric patients receiving cefuroxime sodium for the treatment of meningitis.

In patients with renal insufficiency, elevated concentrations of ceftazidime reportedly may lead to seizures, encephalopathy, asterixis, and neuromuscular excitability. Seizures also have been reported with cefixime and cefuroxime. Rarely, toxic paranoid reactions have occurred in patients with renal impairment receiving oral cephalexin. Life-threatening or fatal encephalopathy (disturbance of consciousness including confusion, hallucinations, stupor, and coma), myoclonus, seizures, and nonconvulsive status epilepticus have been reported in patients receiving cefepime. Most cases of cefepime-associated neurotoxicity have occurred in patients with renal impairment who received a cefepime dosage that exceeded the recommended dosage for such patients; however, some cases occurred in patients who received a dosage appropriately adjusted for renal impairment.

Intrathecal administration of cephalosporins, particularly in large doses, has resulted in CNS toxicity evidenced by hallucinations, nystagmus, and seizures. (See Cautions: Precautions and Contraindications.)

■ Other Adverse Effects Other adverse effects reported with cephalosporin therapy include chest pain, pleural effusion, pulmonary infiltrate, dyspnea or respiratory distress, cough, and rhinitis. Increased or decreased serum glucose concentration also has been reported. Fungal skin infection, exacerbation of acne, and ocular itching have been reported rarely in patients receiving oral cefpodoxime proxetil therapy.

An anamnestic photosensitivity (photo recall)-like dermatitis, characterized by a pruritic, erythematous, maculopapular eruption distributed in the area of a recent sunburn on the upper abdomen and chest, has been reported in at least one patient receiving concomitant IV therapy with cefazolin and gentamicin sulfate. Whether this phenomenon was caused by one or both drugs has not been determined; however, the reaction resolved within 48 hours following discontinuance of both drugs.

■ Precautions and Contraindications Prior to initiation of cephalosporin therapy, careful inquiry should be made concerning previous hypersensitivity reactions to cephalosporins, penicillins, and other drugs. Cephalosporins are contraindicated in patients with a history of allergic reactions to cephalosporin antibiotics. There is clinical and laboratory evidence of partial cross-sensitivity among bicyclic β-lactam antibiotics including penicillins, cephalosporins, cephamycins, and carbapenems. There appears to be little cross-sensitivity between bicyclic β-lactam antibiotics and monobactams (e.g., aztreonam). Although the true incidence of cross-sensitivity among the β-lactam antibiotics has not been definitely established, it has been clearly documented and may occur in up to 10–15% of patients with a history of penicillin hypersensitivity. Some patients have had severe reactions, including anaphylaxis, to both penicillins and cephalosporins. Cephalosporins should be used with caution in individuals hypersensitive to penicillins. Some clinicians suggest that cephalosporins should be avoided in patients who have had an immediate-type (anaphylactic) hypersensitivity reaction to penicillins and should be administered with caution to patients who have had a delayed-type (e.g., rash, fever, eosinophilia) reaction to penicillins or other drugs. If an allergic reaction occurs during cephalosporin therapy, the drug should be discontinued and the patient treated with appropriate therapy (e.g., epinephrine, corticosteroids, and maintenance of an adequate airway and oxygen) as indicated.

To reduce development of drug-resistant bacteria and maintain effectiveness of cephalosporins and other antibacterials, the drugs should be used only for the treatment or prevention of infections proven or strongly suspected to be caused by susceptible bacteria. When selecting or modifying anti-infective therapy, results of culture and in vitro susceptibility testing should be used. In the absence of such data, local epidemiology and susceptibility patterns should be considered when selecting anti-infectives for empiric therapy.

Patients should be advised that antibacterials (including cephalosporins) should only be used to treat bacterial infections and not used to treat viral infections (e.g., the common cold). Patients also should be advised about the importance of completing the full course of therapy, even if feeling better after a few days, and that skipping doses or not completing therapy may decrease effectiveness and increase the likelihood that bacteria will develop resistance and will not be treatable with cephalosporins or other antibacterials in the future.

Prolonged use of a cephalosporin may result in the overgrowth of nonsusceptible organisms, especially *Enterobacter*, *Pseudomonas*, enterococci, or *Candida*. If superinfection occurs, appropriate therapy should be instituted.

Cephalosporins should be used with caution in patients with a history of GI disease, particularly colitis. Because *C. difficile*-associated diarrhea and colitis has been reported with the use of cephalosporins, it should be considered in the differential diagnosis of patients who develop diarrhea during or following therapy with the drugs. (See Cautions; GI Effects.) Patients should be advised that diarrhea is a common problem caused by anti-infectives and usually ends when the drug is discontinued; however, they should contact a clinician if watery and bloody stools (with or without stomach cramps and fever) occur during or as late as 2 months or longer after the last dose.

Seizures have been reported with several cephalosporins (e.g., ceftazidime, cefuroxime, cefepime), particularly in patients with renal impairment in whom dosage of the drug was not reduced. (See Cautions: Nervous System Effects.) If seizures occur during cephalosporin therapy, the drug should be discontinued and anticonvulsant therapy initiated as clinically indicated. If neurotoxicity associated with cefepime therapy occurs, consideration should be given to discontinuing the drug or making appropriate dosage adjustments based on the patient's renal function.

Because some cephalosporins have been associated with a decrease in prothrombin activity, some manufacturers state that prothrombin time (PT) should be monitored when these drugs are used in patients with renal or hepatic impairment, in patients with poor nutritional status, in patients receiving a protracted course of anti-infective therapy, or in those previously stabilized on anticoagulant therapy. Vitamin K should be administered if indicated.

■ Geriatric Precautions No overall differences in safety and efficacy have been reported with use of cephalosporins in those 60 years of age and older compared with younger adults, Although clinical experience has revealed no evidence of age-related differences, the possibility of increased sensitivity in some geriatric individuals cannot be ruled out.

Cephalosporins are substantially eliminated in urine and the risk of toxicity may be increased in patients with impaired renal function. Because geriatric patients are more likely to have decreased renal function, use caution when selecting dosage for such patients and consider monitoring renal function.

■ Pregnancy, Fertility, and Lactation Although there have been no reports of adverse effects to the fetus to date, safe use of cephalosporins during pregnancy has not been definitely established. The drugs should be used during pregnancy only when clearly needed.

Adverse testicular effects (e.g., reduced testicular weight, seminiferous tubule degeneration, delayed maturity of germinal epithelium, reduced germinal cell population, vacuolation of Sertoli cell cytoplasm) have been reported in prepubertal rats receiving certain previously available cephalosporins (e.g., cefamandole, cefoperazone) and structurally related cephamycins (e.g., cefotetan) that contain an NMTT side chain; impaired fertility also has been reported, particularly with high dosages. The relevance of these findings to humans is not known.

Because cephalosporins are distributed into milk, the drugs should be used with caution in nursing women.

Drug Interactions

■ **Nephrotoxic Drugs** Concomitant use of nephrotoxic agents such as aminoglycosides, colistin, polymyxin B, or vancomycin may increase the risk of nephrotoxicity with some cephalosporins and probably should be avoided, if possible.

■ **Alcohol** Disulfiram-like reactions have occurred when alcohol was ingested within 48–72 hours after administration of some previously available cephalosporins (e.g., cefamandole, cefoperazone) and structurally related cephamycins (e.g., cefotetan) that contain an *N*-methylthiotetrazole (NMTT) side chain. The reactions appear to result from accumulation of acetaldehyde and do not occur if alcohol is ingested prior to the first dose of the antibiotic.

■ **Estrogens or Progestins** Some cephalosporins (e.g., ceftazidime) may affect gut flora, leading to lower estrogen reabsorption and reduced efficacy of oral contraceptives containing estrogen and progesterone.

■ **Probenecid** Concomitant administration of oral probenecid competitively inhibits tubular secretion resulting in higher and more prolonged serum concentrations of most cephalosporins.

■ **Other Anti-infective Agents** In vitro studies indicate that the antibacterial activity of cephalosporins may be additive or synergistic with aminoglycosides or penicillins against some organisms. Although some in vitro studies showed additive or synergistic antibacterial activity between chloramphenicol and a cephalosporin, there is more recent in vitro evidence of antagonism between cephalosporins (e.g., cefotaxime, ceftazidime, ceftriaxone) and chloramphenicol against a variety of gram-negative and -positive bacteria, particularly when chloramphenicol was added to the medium before the β-lactam. In addition, at least one case of in vivo antagonism has been reported in an infant with *Salmonella enteritidis* meningitis. Therefore, it is recommended that combined therapy with chloramphenicol and a cephalosporin be avoided, particularly when bactericidal activity is considered important.

Laboratory Test Interferences

■ **Immunohematology Tests** Positive direct and indirect antiglobulin (Coombs') test results have been reported in 3% or more of patients receiving a cephalosporin. (See Cautions: Hematologic Effects.) This reaction may interfere with hematologic studies or transfusion cross-matching procedures. In addition, positive Coombs' test results may occur in neonates whose mother received a cephalosporin prior to delivery.

■ **Tests for Urinary Glucose** Cephalosporins can cause false-positive results in urine glucose determinations using cupric sulfate solution (Benedict's reagent, Clinitest®); glucose oxidase tests (Clinistix®) are unaffected by the drugs.

■ **Tests for Creatinine** Some cephalosporins, in high concentrations, may cause falsely elevated serum or urine creatinine values when the Jaffé reaction is used. In one in vitro study, high concentrations of ceftriaxone (50 mcg/mL or greater) caused falsely elevated serum creatinine values when a manual method was used; however, other studies indicate that the drug does not interfere with automated methods for determining serum or urinary creatinine concentrations.

Mechanism of Action

Cephalosporins are usually bactericidal in action. The antibacterial activity of the cephalosporins, like penicillins and cephamycins, results from inhibition of mucopeptide synthesis in the bacterial cell wall. Although the exact mechanisms of action of cephalosporins have not been fully elucidated, β-lactam antibiotics bind to several enzymes in the bacterial cytoplasmic membrane (e.g., carboxypeptidases, endopeptidases, transpeptidases) that are involved in cell-wall synthesis and cell division. It has been hypothesized that β-lactam antibiotics act as substrate analogs of acyl-D-alanyl-D-alanine, the usual substrate for these enzymes. This interferes with cell-wall synthesis and results in the formation of defective cell walls and osmotically unstable spheroplasts. Cell death following exposure to β-lactam antibiotics usually results from lysis, which appears to be mediated by bacterial autolysins such as peptidoglycan hydrolases.

The target enzymes of β-lactam antibiotics have been classified as penicillin-binding proteins (PBPs) and appear to vary substantially among bacterial species. The affinities of various β-lactam antibiotics for different PBPs appear to explain the differences in morphology that occur in susceptible organisms following exposure to different β-lactam antibiotics and may also explain differences in the spectrum of activity of β-lactam antibiotics that are not caused by the presence or absence of β-lactamases.

Spectrum

In general, cephalosporins are active in vitro against many gram-positive aerobic bacteria, some gram-negative aerobic bacteria, and some anaerobic bacteria; however, there are substantial differences among the cephalosporins in spectra of activity as well as levels of activity against susceptible bacteria. Cephalosporins are inactive against fungi and viruses.

■ **Classification of Cephalosporins and Closely Related β-Lactam Antibiotics Based on Spectra of Activity** Currently available cephalosporins are generally divided into 5 groups based on their spectra of activity: first, second, third, fourth, and fifth generation cephalosporins. Closely related β-lactam antibiotics (e.g., cephamycins) also may be classified in these groups because of their similar spectra of activity.

First Generation Cephalosporins

cefadroxil
cefazolin
cephalexin

First generation cephalosporins usually are active in vitro against gram-positive cocci including penicillinase-producing and nonpenicillinase-producing *Staphylococcus aureus* and *S. epidermidis*; *Streptococcus pyogenes* (group A β-hemolytic streptococci); *S. agalactiae* (group B streptococci); and *S. pneumoniae*. First generation cephalosporins have limited activity against gram-negative bacteria, although some strains of *Escherichia coli*, *Klebsiella pneumoniae*, *Proteus mirabilis*, and *Shigella* may be inhibited in vitro by the drugs. First generation cephalosporins are inactive against enterococci, including *Enterococcus faecalis* (formerly *S. faecalis*), methicillin-resistant *S. aureus* (MRSA; also known as oxacillin-resistant *S. aureus*, ORSA), *Bacteroides fragilis*, *Citrobacter*, *Enterobacter*, *Listeria monocytogenes*, *Proteus* other than *P. mirabilis*, *Providencia*, *Pseudomonas*, and *Serratia*.

Susceptible strains of *S. aureus*, *S. pneumoniae*, *S. pyogenes*, or *S. agalactiae* usually are inhibited in vitro by cefazolin concentrations of 0.1–1 mcg/mL or cephalexin concentrations of 0.1–12 mcg/mL. *S. epidermidis* may be inhibited in vitro by cefazolin concentrations of 0.1–12.5 mcg/mL, although some strains require concentrations greater than 32 mcg/mL for in vitro inhibition. Susceptible strains of *E. coli*, *K. pneumoniae*, or *P. mirabilis* generally are inhibited in vitro by cefazolin concentrations of 0.8–12.5 mcg/mL.

Second Generation Cephalosporins

cefaclor
cefoxitin (a cephamycin)
cefprozil
cefuroxime

Second generation cephalosporins usually are active in vitro against bacteria susceptible to first generation cephalosporins. In addition, the second generation drugs are active in vitro against most strains of *Haemophilus influenzae* (including ampicillin-resistant strains). Although the specific spectra of activity differ, second generation cephalosporins generally are more active in vitro against gram-negative bacteria than first generation cephalosporins. However, cefaclor is less active than other second generation cephalosporins against gram-negative bacteria. The second generation drugs may be active in vitro against some strains of *Acinetobacter*, *Citrobacter*, *Enterobacter*, *E. coli*, *Klebsiella*, *Neisseria*, *Proteus*, *Providencia*, and *Serratia* that are resistant to the first generation drugs. Cefoxitin also has some activity in vitro against *B. fragilis*. Second generation cephalosporins are inactive against enterococci (e.g., *E. faecalis*), MRSA, and *Pseudomonas*.

For more complete information on the spectra of activity of cefoxitin and cefuroxime, see the individual monographs in 8:12.06.08 or 8:12.07.12.

Third Generation Cephalosporins

cefdinir
cefditoren
cefixime
cefotaxime
cefotetan (a cephamycin)
cefpodoxime
ceftazidime
ceftibuten
ceftolozane
ceftriaxone

Third generation cephalosporins usually are less active in vitro against susceptible staphylococci than first generation cephalosporins; however, the third generation drugs have an expanded spectrum of activity against gram-negative bacteria compared with the first and second generation drugs. Third generation cephalosporins generally are active in vitro against gram-negative bacteria susceptible to the first and second generation drugs, and most also are active in vitro against some strains of *Citrobacter*, *Enterobacter*, *E. coli*, *Klebsiella*, *Neisseria*, *Proteus*, *Morganella*, *Providencia*, and *Serratia* that may be resistant to first and second generation cephalosporins. Cefdinir, cefixime, and cefpodoxime are inactive against most strains of *Enterobacter* and *Pseudomonas* and have limited in vitro activity against anaerobic bacteria; cefixime also is inactive against most staphylococci. Cefditoren has increased activity, similar to first generation cephalosporins, against gram-positive bacteria, unlike other third generation cephalosporins. Third generation cephalosporins are inactive against MRSA and generally are inactive against enterococci (e.g., *E. faecalis*) and *L. monocytogenes*. Some parenteral third generation cephalosporins (ceftazidime, ceftolozane) have activity in vitro against *Ps. aeruginosa*.

Ceftazidime is available as a single-entity preparation or in fixed combination with avibactam (a non-β-lactam β-lactamase inhibitor). Ceftolozane is commercially available in the US only in fixed combination with tazobactam (a β-lactamase inhibitor). These fixed combinations containing a third generation cephalosporin and a β-lactamase inhibitor have expanded spectra of activity against gram-negative bacteria that produce extended-spectrum β-lactamases (ESBLs) and are active against some gram-negative bacteria resistant to the third generation cephalosporin alone.

For more complete information on the spectra of activity of the third generation cephalosporins, see the individual monographs in 8:12.06.12.

Fourth Generation Cephalosporins

cefepime

Fourth generation cephalosporins, like third generation cephalosporins, have an expanded spectrum of activity against gram-negative bacteria compared with the first and second generation drugs. However, fourth generation cephalosporins are active in vitro against some gram-negative bacteria, including *Pseudomonas aeruginosa* and certain Enterobacteriaceae, that generally are resistant to third generation cephalosporins. In addition, fourth generation cephalosporins may be more active against gram-positive bacteria than some third generation drugs (e.g., ceftazidime). Cefepime has a spectrum of activity against aerobic gram-positive and gram-negative bacteria that is similar to that of cefotaxime and ceftriaxone and has activity against *Ps. aeruginosa* that appears to approach that of ceftazidime. However, cefepime is more active than third generation cephalosporins against Enterobacteriaceae that produce inducible β-lactamases. The extended spectrum of activity of cefepime is related to the fact that the drug penetrates the outer membrane of gram-negative bacteria more rapidly than most other cephalosporins and the fact that the drug is more resistant to inactivation by chromosomally and plasmid-mediated β-lactamases than most other cephalosporins. In addition, inducible β-lactamases have a low affinity for cefepime and the drug is hydrolyzed by these enzymes at a slower rate than third generation cephalosporins such as ceftazidime. Cefepime is inactive against MRSA, enterococci, and *L. monocytogenes*.

Fifth Generation Cephalosporins

ceftaroline fosamil

Like third and fourth generation cephalosporins, fifth generation cephalosporins have an expanded spectrum of activity that includes both gram-positive and gram-negative bacteria. However, unlike first, second, third, and fourth generation cephalosporins, fifth generation cephalosporins have activity against methicillin-resistant *Staphylococcus aureus* (MRSA; also known as oxacillin-resistant *S. aureus*, ORSA). Ceftaroline is the only fifth generation cephalosporin commercially available in the US. Ceftobiprole medocaril (not commercially available in the US) may be available in other countries.

Ceftaroline is active against many gram-positive bacteria, including *S. aureus* (e.g., MRSA, vancomycin-resistant *S. aureus* [VRSA], daptomycin-nonsusceptible *S. aureus*), coagulase-negative staphylococci (e.g., *S. epidermidis* including methicillin-resistant [oxacillin-resistant] strains), and *Streptococcus* (e.g., *S. pneumoniae* including penicillin-resistant *S. pneumoniae* and multi-drug-resistant *S. pneumoniae* [MDRSP], *S. pyogenes*, *S. agalactiae*, viridans streptococci). Ceftaroline also is active against many Enterobacteriaceae, but is inactive against *Ps. aeruginosa*. The drug has only limited activity against *Enterococcus*. In addition, ceftaroline is inactive against gram-negative bacteria that produce extended-spectrum β-lactamases (ESBLs) from the TEM, SHV, or CTX-M families, AmpC cephalosporinases, class B metallo-β-lactamases, or serine carbapenemases (such as KPC).

■ **In Vitro Susceptibility Testing** When in vitro susceptibility testing is performed according to the standards of the Clinical and Laboratory Standards Institute (CLSI; formerly National Committee for Clinical Laboratory Standards [NCCLS]), clinical isolates identified as *susceptible* to a cephalosporin are inhibited by drug concentrations usually achievable when the recommended dosage is used for the site of infection. Clinical isolates classified as *intermediate* have minimum inhibitory concentrations (MICs) that approach usually attainable blood and tissue concentrations and response rates may be lower than for strains identified as susceptible. Therefore, the intermediate category implies clinical applicability in body sites where the drug is physiologically concentrated or when a higher than usual dosage can be used. This intermediate category also includes a buffer zone which should prevent small, uncontrolled technical factors from causing major discrepancies in interpretation, especially for drugs with narrow pharmacotoxicity margins. If results of in vitro susceptibility testing indicate that a clinical isolate is *resistant* to a cephalosporin, the strain is not inhibited by drug concentrations generally achievable with usual dosage schedules and/or MICs fall in the range where specific microbial resistance mechanisms are likely and clinical efficacy of the drug against the isolate has not been reliably demonstrated in clinical studies.

Because of differences in spectra of activity, the first generation cephalosporins (cefazolin), second generation cephalosporins (cefaclor, cefprozil, cefuroxime), third generation cephalosporins (cefdinir, cefditoren, cefixime, cefotaxime, cefpodoxime, ceftazidime, ceftibuten, ceftriaxone), fourth generation cephalosporins (cefepime), and fifth generation cephalosporins (ceftaroline) should be tested individually to determine in vitro susceptibility.

CLSI states that in vitro susceptibility test results for cephalothin (no longer commercially available in the US) should only be used to predict susceptibility of Enterobacteriaceae to certain oral cephalosporins (i.e., cefadroxil, cephalexin, cefpodoxime). Although older data suggest that cephalothin results could predict susceptibility to some other cephalosporins, recent data are not available to confirm this.

Disk Susceptibility Tests When the disk-diffusion procedure is used to test in vitro susceptibility, individual disks containing cefaclor (30 mcg), cefazolin (30 mcg), cefdinir (5 mcg), cefditoren (5 mcg), cefepime (30 mcg), cefixime (5 mcg), cefotaxime (30 mcg), cefotetan (30 mcg), cefoxitin (30 mcg), cefpodoxime (10 mcg), cefprozil (30 mcg), ceftaroline (30 mcg), ceftazidime (30 mcg), ceftibuten (30 mcg), ceftriaxone (30 mcg), or cefuroxime (30 mcg) should be used. There is no class susceptibility disk that can be used to test susceptibility to all cephalosporins.

The disk-diffusion procedure should not be used to test in vitro susceptibility of *Streptococcus pneumoniae* to cephalosporins; in vitro susceptibility should be evaluated using broth or agar dilutions tests.

See Table 1 for information on interpretation of disk diffusion zone diameters when disk-diffusion susceptibility tests are used to test in vitro susceptibility to cephalosporins.

For information on disk-diffusion procedures used to test in vitro susceptibility to the fixed combination of ceftazidime and avibactam or fixed combination of ceftolozane and tazobactam and information on interpretation of disk diffusion zone diameters for these fixed combinations, see Spectrum: In Vitro Susceptibility Testing in Ceftazidime and Avibactam Sodium 8:12.06.12 or in Ceftolozane Sulfate and Tazobactam Sodium 8:12.06.12.

Table 1. Interpretation of Disk Diffusion Zone Diameters (nearest whole mm) for Disk Susceptibility Tests Performed According to CLSI Standardized Procedures

	Resistant	Intermediate	Susceptible
Enterobacteriaceae			
(Note: Although *Salmonella* and *Shigella* may appear susceptible in vitro to first and second generation cephalosporins and cephamycins, the drugs are not active clinically in these infections and results should not be reported as susceptible)			
Cefazolin (based on dosage of 2 g every 8 hr)	≤19	20–22	≥23
Cefuroxime (based on parenteral dosage of 1.5 g every 8 hr)	≤14	15–17	≥18
Cefepime (based on dosage of 1 g every 8 hr or 2 g every 12 hr)	≤14	15–17	≥18
Cefotetan	≤12	13–15	≥16
Cefoxitin	≤14	15–17	≥18
Cefotaxime (based on dosage of 1 g every 8 hr)	≤22	23–25	≥26
Ceftaroline (community-acquired pneumonia or skin isolates)	≤19	20–22	≥23
Ceftriaxone (based on dosage of 1 g every 24 hr)	≤19	20–22	≥23
Ceftazidime	≤17	18–20	≥21
Cefuroxime axetil (oral)	≤14	15–22	≥23
Cefaclor	≤14	15–17	≥18
Cefdinir (not applicable for Citrobacter, Providencia, Enterobacter)	≤16	17–19	≥20
Cefixime (not applicable for Morganella)	≤15	16–18	≥19
Cefpodoxime (not applicable for Morganella)	≤17	18–20	≥21
Cefprozil (not applicable for Providencia)	≤14	15–17	≥18
Ceftibuten (for urine isolates only)	≤17	18–20	≥21
Pseudomonas aeruginosa			
Ceftazidime (based on dosage of 1 g every 6 hr or 2 g every 8 hr)	≤14	15–17	≥18
Cefepime (based on dosage of 1 g every 8 hr or 2 g every 12 hr)	≤14	15–17	≥18
Acinetobacter			
Ceftazidime	≤14	15–17	≥18
Cefepime	≤14	15–17	≥18
Cefotaxime	≤14	15–22	≥23
Ceftriaxone	≤13	14–20	≥21
Burkholderia cepacia			
Ceftazidime	≤17	18–20	≥21
Staphylococcus			
Cefazolin	≤14	15–17	≥18
Cefepime	≤14	15–17	≥18
Cefotaxime	≤14	15–22	≥23
Cefotetan	≤12	13–15	≥16
Ceftaroline	–	–	≥24
Ceftazidime	≤14	15–17	≥18

Ceftriaxone	≤13	14–20	≥21
Cefuroxime sodium (parenteral)	≤14	15–17	≥18
Cefaclor	≤14	15–17	≥18
Cefdinir	≤16	17–19	≥20
Cefpodoxime	≤17	18–20	≥21
Cefprozil	≤14	15–17	≥18
Cefuroxime axetil (oral)	≤14	15–22	≥23
Streptococcus (other than S. pneumoniae)			
Cefepime (β-hemolytic group)			≥24
Cefepime (viridans group)	≤21	22–23	≥24
Cefotaxime (β-hemolytic group)	–	–	≥24
Cefotaxime (viridans group)	≤25	26–27	≥28
Ceftriaxone (β-hemolytic group)	–	–	≥24
Ceftriaxone (viridans group)	≤24	25–26	≥27
Haemophilus influenzae and H. parainfluenzae			
Cefotaxime	–	–	≥26
Ceftazidime	–	–	≥26
Ceftriaxone	–	–	≥26
Cefuroxime sodium (parenteral)	≤16	17–19	≥20
Cefepime	–	–	≥26
Cefaclor	≤16	17–19	≥20
Cefprozil	≤14	15–17	≥18
Cefdinir	–	–	≥20
Cefixime	–	–	≥21
Cefpodoxime	–	–	≥21
Cefuroxime axetil (oral)	≤16	17–19	≥20
Ceftibuten	–	–	≥28
Neisseria gonorrhoeae			
Cefotaxime	–	–	≥31
Ceftriaxone	–	–	≥35
Cefotetan	≤19	20–25	≥26
Cefoxitin	≤23	24–27	≥28
Cefuroxime axetil (oral)	≤25	26–30	≥31
Cefepime	–	–	≥31
Ceftazidime	–	–	≥31
Cefixime	–	–	≥31
Cefpodoxime	–	–	≥29
Neisseria meningitidis			
Cefotaxime	–	–	≥34
Ceftriaxone	–	–	≥34

Dilution Susceptibility Tests When broth or agar dilution susceptibility tests are used to test in vitro susceptibility to cephalosporins, each drug must be tested individually.

See Table 2 for interpretation of MICs when dilution susceptibility tests are used to test in vitro susceptibility to cephalosporins.

For information on dilution susceptibility tests used to test in vitro susceptibility to the fixed combination of ceftazidime and avibactam or fixed combination of ceftolozane and tazobactam and information on interpretation of MICs for these fixed combinations, see Spectrum: In Vitro Susceptibility Testing in Ceftazidime and Avibactam Sodium 8:12.06.12 or in Ceftolozane Sulfate and Tazobactam Sodium 8:12.06.12.

Table 2. Interpretation of MICs (mcg/mL) For Diffusion Susceptibility Tests Performed According to CLSI Standardized Procedures

Enterobacteriaceae	Susceptible	Intermediate	Resistant
(Note: Although *Salmonella* and *Shigella* may appear susceptible in vitro to first and second generation cephalosporins and cephamycins, the drugs are not active clinically in these infections and results should not be reported as susceptible)			
Cefazolin (based on dosage of 2 g every 8 hr)	≤2	4	≥8
Cefuroxime sodium (based on parenteral dosage of 1.5 g every 8 hr)	≤8	16	≥32
Cefepime (based on dosage of 1 g every 8 hr or 2 g every 12 hr)	≤8	16	≥32
Cefotetan	≤16	32	≥64
Cefoxitin	≤8	16	≥32
Cefotaxime (based on dosage of 1 g every 8 hr)	≤1	2	≥4
Ceftaroline (community-acquired pneumonia or skin isolates)	<0.5	1	≥2
Ceftriaxone (based on dosage of 1 g every 24 hr)	≤1	2	≥4
Ceftazidime	≤4	8	≥16
Cefuroxime axetil (oral)	≤4	8–16	≥32
Cefaclor	≤8	16	≥32
Cefdinir	≤1	2	≥4
Cefixime	≤1	2	≥4
Cefpodoxime	≤2	4	≥8
Cefprozil	≤8	16	≥32
Ceftibuten (for urine isolates only)	≤8	16	≥32
Pseudomonas aeruginosa			
Ceftazidime (based on dosage of 1 g every 6 hr or 2 g every 8 hr)	≤8	16	≥32
Cefepime (based on dosage of 1 g every 8 hr or 2 g every 12 hr)	≤8	16	≥32
Acinetobacter			
Ceftazidime	≤8	16	≥32
Cefepime	≤8	16	≥32
Cefotaxime	≤8	16–32	≥64
Ceftriaxone	≤8	16–32	≥64
Burkholderia cepacia and Stenotrophomonas maltophilia			
Ceftazidime	≤8	16	≥32
Other Non-Enterobacteriaceae			
Ceftazidime	≤8	16	≥32
Cefepime	≤8	16	≥32
Cefotaxime	≤8	16–32	≥64
Ceftriaxone	≤8	16–32	≥64
Staphylococcus			
Cefazolin	≤8	16	≥32
Cefepime	≤8	16	≥32
Cefotaxime	≤8	16–32	≥64
Cefotetan	≤16	32	≥64
Ceftaroline	≤1		–
Ceftazidime	≤8	16	≥32
Ceftriaxone	≤8	16–32	≥64
Cefuroxime sodium (parenteral)	≤8	16	≥32
Cefaclor	≤8	16	≥32
Cefdinir	≤1	2	≥4
Cefpodoxime	≤2	4	≥8
Cefprozil	≤8	16	≥32
Cefuroxime axetil (oral)	≤4	8–16	≥32
Streptococcus pneumoniae			
Cefepime (except CSF isolates)	≤1	2	≥4
Cefepime (CSF isolates)	≤0.5	1	≥2
Cefotaxime (except CSF isolates)	≤1	2	≥4
Cefotaxime (CSF isolates)	≤0.5	1	≥2

Ceftaroline (community-acquired pneumonia isolates)	≤0.25	–	–
Ceftriaxone (except CSF isolates)	≤1	2	≥4
Ceftriaxone (CSF isolates)	≤0.5	1	≥2
Cefuroxime sodium (parenteral)	≤0.5	1	≥2
Cefaclor	≤1	2	≥4
Cefdinir	≤0.5	1	≥2
Cefpodoxime	≤0.5	1	≥2
Cefprozil	≤2	4	≥8
Cefuroxime axetil (oral)	≤1	2	≥4
Streptococcus (other than S. pneumoniae)			
Cefepime (β-hemolytic group)	≤0.5	–	–
Cefepime (viridans group)	≤1	2	≥4
Cefotaxime (β-hemolytic group)	≤0.5	–	–
Cefotaxime (viridans group)	≤1	2	≥4
Ceftriaxone (β-hemolytic group)	≤0.5	–	–
Ceftriaxone (viridans group)	≤1	2	≥4
Haemophilus influenzae and H. parainfluenzae			
Cefotaxime	≤2	–	–
Ceftazidime	≤2	–	–
Ceftriaxone	≤2	–	–
Cefuroxime sodium (parenteral)	≤4	8	≥16
Cefepime	≤2	–	–
Cefaclor	≤8	16	≥32
Cefprozil	≤8	16	≥32
Cefdinir	≤1	–	–
Cefixime	≤1	–	–
Cefpodoxime	≤2	–	–
Cefuroxime axetil (oral)	≤4	8	≥16
Ceftibuten	≤2	–	–
Neisseria gonorrhoeae			
Cefotaxime	≤0.5	–	–
Ceftriaxone	≤0.25	–	–
Cefotetan	≤2	4	≥8
Cefoxitin	≤2	4	≥8
Cefuroxime sodium (parenteral)	≤1	2	≥4
Cefepime	≤0.5	–	–
Ceftazidime	≤0.5	–	–
Cefixime	≤0.25	–	–
Cefpodoxime	≤0.5	–	–
Neisseria meningitidis			
Cefotaxime	≤0.12	–	–
Ceftriaxone	≤0.12	–	–
Anaerobes			
Cefotaxime	≤16	32	≥64
Cefotetan	≤16	32	≥64
Cefoxitin	≤16	32	≥64
Ceftriaxone	≤16	32	≥64

Resistance

Bacterial resistance to cephalosporins may be natural or acquired and may result from one or a combination of factors. Some bacteria are not affected by concentrations of a cephalosporin that are lethal to other bacteria because their cell surfaces are not permeable to the drug or because their metabolic pathways are not inhibited by the drug. A major mechanism of bacterial resistance to cephalosporins is the production of β-lactamases which inactivate the drugs by hydrolyzing the β-lactam ring. However, absence or presence of a β-lactamase does not entirely dictate susceptibility or resistance to a cephalosporin. Bacterial resistance usually results both from the production of a β-lactamase and the presence of permeability barriers to the drug. The β-lactamases produced by different bacterial species differ in physical, chemical, and functional properties. Staphylococcal β-lactamases are usually inducible, extracellular penicillinases. A variety of β-lactamases are produced by gram-negative bacteria; some are chromosome-mediated inducible cephalosporinases and a few are determined by plasmid-mediated resistance factors.

Pharmacokinetics

■ **Absorption** Cefazolin sodium, cefepime hydrochloride, cefotaxime sodium, ceftaroline fosamil, ceftazidime, ceftriaxone sodium, and cefuroxime sodium are not appreciably absorbed from the GI tract and must be given parenterally.

Cefaclor, cefadroxil, cefprozil, ceftibuten dihydrate, cephalexin, and cephalexin hydrochloride are well absorbed from the GI tract. Following oral administration, bioavailability of cefdinir averages 16–25%. Approximately 30–50% of an oral dose of cefixime and 50% of an oral dose of cefpodoxime proxetil is absorbed from the GI tract. Cefditoren pivoxil, cefpodoxime proxetil, and cefuroxime axetil are prodrugs and are inactive until hydrolyzed in vivo to cefditoren, cefpodoxime, and cefuroxime, respectively, by nonspecific esterases in the intestinal lumen and blood. Ceftaroline fosamil also is a prodrug that is inactive until it is converted in vivo to ceftaroline by a plasma phosphatase following IV administration.

Administration with food does not affect the rate of absorption or peak serum concentrations of cefadroxil. While the rate of absorption of cefixime or cefprozil may be decreased by the presence of food in the GI tract, the extent of absorption and peak plasma concentrations of the drug generally are not affected. Compared with administration in the fasting state, administration of cefdinir with a high-fat meal decreases the rate and extent of absorption of the drug. Administration of cefditoren pivoxil with a moderate- or high-fat meal increases the rate and extent of absorption, compared with administration in the fasting state. The effect of food on oral bioavailability of cefaclor, cefpodoxime proxetil, ceftibuten, and cefuroxime axetil varies depending on the formulation of the drugs administered.

■ **Distribution and Elimination** Following absorption, most cephalosporins are widely distributed to tissues and fluids, including pleural fluid, synovial fluid, and bone. Following oral administration, cefdinir, cefixime, cefpodoxime, ceftibuten, cefprozil, and cefuroxime are distributed into middle ear fluid, tonsils, sinus tissue, and bronchial mucosa. Following oral administration, cefditoren has been shown to distribute into tonsils and skin blister fluid. Although the total quantity of some cephalosporins distributed into bile is low, therapeutic concentrations of some of the drugs (e.g., cefazolin, cefepime, cefixime) generally are obtained if biliary obstruction is not present. Only low concentrations of first or second generation cephalosporins diffuse into CSF following oral, IM, or IV administration even when meninges are inflamed; however, therapeutic concentrations of cefotaxime, ceftazidime, ceftriaxone, or cefuroxime generally are attained in CSF following IM or IV administration, especially if meninges are inflamed. Cefepime also is distributed into CSF following parenteral administration.

Cephalosporins readily cross the placenta, and fetal serum concentrations may be 10% or more of maternal serum concentrations. Cephalosporins are distributed in low concentrations into milk.

Table 3. Serum Half-lives of Cephalosporins in Adults with Normal Renal Function and Approximate Degrees of Protein Binding

Drug	Serum Half-life (in hours)	% Bound to Serum Proteins
FIRST GENERATION		
Cefadroxil	1.1–2	20
Cefazolin	1.2–2.2	74–86
Cephalexin	0.5–1.2	6–15
SECOND GENERATION		
Cefaclor	0.5–1	25
Cefprozil	1–1.4	35–45
Cefuroxime	1–2	33–50
THIRD GENERATION		
Cefdinir	1.7–1.8	60–70
Cefditoren	1.4–1.6	88
Cefixime	2.4–4	65–70
Cefotaxime	0.9–1.7	13–38
Cefpodoxime	2.1–2.9	22–33
Ceftazidime	1.4–2	5–24
Ceftibuten	2–2.6	65
Ceftolozane	2.8–3.1	16–21
Ceftriaxone	5.4–10.9	58–96
FOURTH GENERATION		
Cefepime	2–2.3	20
FIFTH GENERATION		
Ceftaroline	2.7	20

Serum cephalosporin concentrations may be higher and the serum half-lives prolonged in patients with impaired renal function.

Cefaclor, cefadroxil, cefazolin, cefdinir, cefditoren, cefixime, cefpodoxime, cefprozil, ceftazidime, ceftolozane, cefuroxime, and cephalexin are not appreciably metabolized. Cefuroxime axetil, cefditoren pivoxil, and cefpodoxime proxetil are rapidly hydrolyzed to their respective microbiologically active forms, cefuroxime, cefditoren, and cefpodoxime, by nonspecific esterases in the intestinal mucosa and/or blood following oral administration. The axetil moiety of cefuroxime is metabolized to acetaldehyde and acetic acid; hydrolysis of cefditoren pivoxil results in the formation of pivalate, which is absorbed and excreted as pivaloylcarnitine in urine. Cefepime is partially metabolized in vivo. Cefotaxime is partially metabolized (presumably in the liver, kidneys, and other tissues) to desacetyl metabolites which also have antibacterial activity, although less than that of the parent compounds. Ceftriaxone is metabolized to a small extent to microbiologically inactive metabolites in the intestines after biliary excretion.

Cephalosporins and their metabolites are rapidly excreted by the kidneys. Cefaclor, cefadroxil, cefazolin, cefditoren, cefixime, cefotaxime, cefpodoxime, cefprozil, cefuroxime, and cephalexin are excreted by both glomerular filtration and tubular secretion; cefepime, ceftazidime, ceftolozane, and ceftriaxone are excreted principally by glomerular filtration. The same system of anion transport is responsible for the tubular secretion of cephalosporins as for other β-lactam antibiotics and probenecid. Oral probenecid administered shortly before or with most cephalosporins usually slows the rate of excretion of the antibiotic and produces higher and more prolonged serum concentrations, especially with those cephalosporins excreted principally by tubular secretion. Most cephalosporins are removed by hemodialysis or peritoneal dialysis.

Chemistry and Stability

■ **Chemistry**

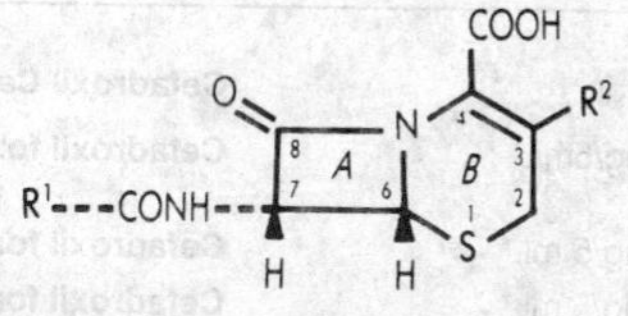

cephalosporin nucleus (A β-lactam ring) (B dihydrothiazine ring)

Cephalosporins are semisynthetic antibiotic derivatives of cephalosporin C, a substance produced by the fungus *Cephalosporium acremonium*. The drugs are β-lactam antibiotics structurally and pharmacologically related to penicillins and cephamycins (e.g., cefoxitin). All commercially available cephalosporins contain the 7-aminocephalosporanic acid (7-ACA) nucleus, which is composed of a β-lactam ring fused with a 6-membered dihydrothiazine ring instead of the 5-membered thiazolidine ring of penicillins. Cleavage at any point in the β-lactam ring system of cephalosporins results in complete loss of antibacterial activity.

Addition of various groups at R^1 (position 7) and R^2 (position 3) of the cephalosporin nucleus results in derivatives with differences in spectra of activity, stability against hydrolysis by β-lactamases, protein binding, GI absorption, or susceptibility to desacetylation. Many commercially available oral cephalosporins (e.g., cefdinir, cefditoren pivoxil, cefixime, cefpodoxime proxetil, ceftibuten) and parenteral cephalosporins (e.g., cefepime, cefotaxime, ceftazidime, ceftriaxone) contain an aminothiazolyl side chain at position 7 of the cephalosporin nucleus. The aminothiazolyl side chain enhances antibacterial activity, particularly against Enterobacteriaceae, and generally results in enhanced stability against β-lactamases. Unlike other commercially available cephalosporins, ceftaroline contains a 1,3-thiazole ring, linked to the 3-position of the cephem ring by a sulfur, which appears to contribute to activity against methicillin-resistant *Staphylococcus aureus* (MRSA; also known as oxacillin-resistant *S. aureus* or ORSA). Some previously available cephalosporins (e.g., cefamandole, cefoperazone) and structurally related cephamycins (e.g., cefotetan) contain an *N*-methylthiotetrazole (NMTT) side chain at position 6 of the cephalosporin nucleus. The NMTT side chain enhances antibacterial activity, helps to prevent metabolism of the drugs, and also may be associated with certain adverse effects (e.g., hypoprothrombinemia, disulfiram-like reactions).

■ **Stability** In solution, most cephalosporins are stable for only short periods of time unless frozen.

Cephalosporins are potentially physically and/or chemically incompatible with some drugs including aminoglycosides, but the compatibility depends on the specific drug and several other factors (e.g., concentration of the drugs, specific diluents used, resulting pH, temperature). Specialized references should be consulted for specific compatibility information.

For specific dosages and additional information on chemistry and stability, spectrum, resistance, pharmacokinetics, uses, cautions, drug interactions, and laboratory test interferences of the cephalosporins, see the individual monographs in 8:12.06.

†Use is not currently included in the labeling approved by the US Food and Drug Administration

FIRST GENERATION CEPHALOSPORINS 8:12.06.04

Cefadroxil

■ Cefadroxil is a semisynthetic, first generation cephalosporin antibiotic.

Uses

■ **Pharyngitis and Tonsillitis** Oral cefadroxil is used for the treatment of pharyngitis and tonsillitis caused by *Streptococcus pyogenes* (group A β-hemolytic streptococci). Although cefadroxil generally is effective in eradicating *S. pyogenes* from the nasopharynx, efficacy of the drug in prevention of subsequent rheumatic fever has not been established to date.

Selection of an anti-infective for the treatment of *S. pyogenes* pharyngitis and tonsillitis should be based on the drug's spectrum of activity, bacteriologic and clinical efficacy, potential adverse effects, ease of administration, patient compliance, and cost. No regimen has been found to date that effectively eradicates group A β-hemolytic streptococci in 100% of patients.

Because the drugs have a narrow spectrum of activity, are inexpensive, and generally are effective with a low frequency of adverse effects, the American Academy of Pediatrics (AAP), Infectious Diseases Society of America (IDSA), American Heart Association (AHA), and others recommend a penicillin regimen (i.e., 10 days of oral penicillin V or oral amoxicillin or single dose of IM penicillin G benzathine) as the treatment of choice for *S. pyogenes* pharyngitis and tonsillitis and prevention of initial attacks (primary prevention) of rheumatic fever. Other anti-infectives (e.g., oral cephalosporins, oral macrolides, oral clindamycin) are recommended as alternatives in penicillin-allergic individuals.

If an oral cephalosporin is used for the treatment of *S. pyogenes* pharyngitis and tonsillitis, a 10-day regimen of a first generation cephalosporin (cefadroxil, cephalexin) is preferred instead of other cephalosporins with broader spectrums of activity (e.g., cefaclor, cefdinir, cefixime, cefpodoxime, cefuroxime).

■ **Skin and Skin Structure Infections** Oral cefadroxil is used for the treatment of mild to moderate skin and skin structure infections caused by susceptible staphylococci or streptococci.

■ **Urinary Tract Infections** Oral cefadroxil is used for the treatment of mild to moderate urinary tract infections, including acute prostatitis, caused by susceptible *Escherichia coli*, *Klebsiella*, or *Proteus mirabilis*.

■ **Prevention of Bacterial Endocarditis** Oral cefadroxil is used as an alternative for prevention of α-hemolytic (viridans group) streptococcal endocarditis† in penicillin-allergic individuals undergoing certain dental or upper respiratory tract procedures who have underlying cardiac conditions that put them at highest risk of adverse outcomes from endocarditis. Cefadroxil should not be used for such prophylaxis in those with a history of immediate-type hypersensitivity to penicillins (e.g., urticaria, angioedema, anaphylaxis).

For information on which cardiac conditions are associated with highest risk of endocarditis and which procedures require prophylaxis, see Prevention under Uses: Endocarditis, in the Cephalosporins General Statement 8:12.06. When selecting anti-infectives for prophylaxis of bacterial endocarditis, the current recommendations published by the AHA should be consulted.

Dosage and Administration

■ **Reconstitution and Administration** Cefadroxil is administered orally.

Cefadroxil may be administered without regard to meals. Administration with food may minimize adverse GI effects.

Reconstitution Cefadroxil powder for oral suspension should be reconstituted at the time of dispensing by adding the amount of water specified on the container to provide a suspension containing 125, 250, or 500 mg of cefadroxil per 5 mL. The water should be added in 2 equal portions and the bottle shaken after each addition.

The oral suspension should be shaken well prior to administration of each dose.

■ **Dosage** ***Adult Dosage*** **Pharyngitis and Tonsillitis.** For the treatment of pharyngitis and tonsillitis caused by *Streptococcus pyogenes* (group A β-hemolytic streptococci), the usual adult dosage of cefadroxil is 1 g daily given as a single dose or in 2 equally divided doses for 10 days.

Skin and Skin Structure Infections. For the treatment of skin and skin structure infections, the usual adult dosage of cefadroxil is 1 g daily given as a single dose or in 2 equally divided doses.

Urinary Tract Infections. For the treatment of uncomplicated urinary tract infections (i.e., cystitis), the usual adult dosage of cefadroxil is 1 or 2 g daily given as a single dose or in 2 equally divided doses. The usual adult dosage for the treatment of other urinary tract infections is 2 g daily given in 2 equally divided doses.

Pediatric Dosage **General Pediatric Dosage.** The American Academy of Pediatrics (AAP) recommends that pediatric patients beyond the neonatal period receive cefadroxil in a dosage of 30 mg/kg daily in 2 equally divided doses for the treatment of mild or moderate infections. The AAP states that the drug is inappropriate for the treatment of severe infections.

Pharyngitis and Tonsillitis. For the treatment of group A β-hemolytic streptococcal pharyngitis and tonsillitis, the usual pediatric dosage of cefadroxil is 30 mg/kg daily given as a single dose or in 2 equally divided doses for 10 days.

Skin and Skin Structure Infections. For the treatment of impetigo, pediatric patients should receive cefadroxil in a dosage of 30 mg/kg daily given as a single dose or in 2 equally divided doses. For the treatment of other skin and skin structure infections, children should receive 30 mg/kg daily given in divided doses every 12 hours.

Urinary Tract Infections. For the treatment of urinary tract infections, the usual pediatric dosage of cefadroxil is 30 mg/kg daily given in divided doses every 12 hours.

■ **Dosage in Renal Impairment** In patients with creatinine clearances of 50 mL/minute per 1.73 m² or lower, doses and/or frequency of administration of cefadroxil must be modified in response to the degree of renal impairment. The manufacturers recommend that adults receive an initial dose of 1 g followed by 500-mg maintenance doses at the following dosage intervals based on the patient's creatinine clearance: (See Table 1.)

Table 1. Adult Dosage of Cefadroxil in Renal Impairment

Cl_{cr} (mL/min per 1.73 m²)	Initial Dose	Maintenance Dosage
25–50	1 g	500 mg every 12 hours
10–25	1 g	500 mg every 24 hours
0–10	1 g	500 mg every 36 hours

Cautions

Cefadroxil shares the toxic potentials of other cephalosporins, and the usual cautions, precautions, and contraindications associated with cephalosporin therapy should be observed. (See Cautions in the Cephalosporins General Statement 8:12.06.)

Spectrum

Based on its spectrum of activity, cefadroxil is classified as a first generation cephalosporin. For information on the classification of cephalosporins and closely related β-lactam antibiotics based on spectra of activity, see Spectrum in the Cephalosporins General Statement 8:12.06. Like other first generation cephalosporins (e.g., cefazolin, cephalexin), cefadroxil is active in vitro against many gram-positive aerobic cocci but has limited activity against gram-negative bacteria.

■ **In Vitro Susceptibility Testing** Strains of staphylococci resistant to penicillinase-resistant penicillins (methicillin-resistant [oxacillin-resistant] staphylococci) should be considered resistant to cephalexin, although results of in vitro susceptibility tests may indicate that the organisms are susceptible to the drug.

For information on interpreting results of in vitro susceptibility testing (disk susceptibility tests, dilution susceptibility tests) when cefadroxil susceptibility testing is performed according to the standards of the Clinical and Laboratory Standards Institute (CLSI; formerly National Committee for Clinical Laboratory Standards [NCCLS]), see Spectrum: In Vitro Susceptibility Testing, in the Cephalosporins General Statement 8:12.06.

Pharmacokinetics

■ **Absorption** Cefadroxil is acid-stable and is rapidly and almost completely absorbed from the GI tract. The rate of absorption and peak serum concentrations of cefadroxil are not affected when the drug is administered with food.

Following oral administration in healthy adults with normal renal function, peak serum cefadroxil concentrations are attained within 1–2 hours and average about 10–18 mcg/mL following a single 500-mg dose and 24–35 mcg/mL following a single 1-g dose.

In a group of children 13 months to 12 years of age with normal renal function, peak serum concentrations of cefadroxil averaged 13.7 mcg/mL and were attained within 1 hour after a single oral dose of 15 mg/kg; serum concentrations of the drug were 0.6–1.8 mcg/mL at 6 hours.

■ **Elimination** The serum half-life of cefadroxil is 1.1–2 hours in adults with normal renal function.

Cefadroxil is excreted unchanged in urine. In adults with normal renal function, from 70 to more than 90% of a single 500-mg or 1-g oral dose of the drug is excreted unchanged in urine within 24 hours, principally within the first 6–9 hours after administration. In adults with normal renal function, peak urine concentrations of cefadroxil of 1.8 mg/mL may be attained following a single 500-mg oral dose.

The serum half-life of cefadroxil is prolonged in patients with impaired renal function. The half-life of cefadroxil is 2.5–8.5 hours in patients with creatinine clearances of 20–50 mL/minute per 1.73 m² and 13.3–25.5 hours in patients with creatinine clearances less than 20 mL/minute per 1.73 m². Renal elimination of cefadroxil is substantially reduced in patients with creatinine clearances less than 20 mL/minute per 1.73 m², with about 10–30% of a single oral dose excreted unchanged in urine within 24 hours.

Cefadroxil is removed by hemodialysis.

Chemistry and Stability

■ **Chemistry** Cefadroxil is a semisynthetic cephalosporin antibiotic. Cefadroxil is commercially available as the monohydrate which occurs as a white to yellowish-white, crystalline powder and is soluble in water and slightly soluble in alcohol.

■ **Stability** Cefadroxil capsules and tablets should be stored in tight containers at 20–25°C.

Cefadroxil powder for oral suspension should be stored at 20–25°C. After reconstitution, cefadroxil oral suspension should be refrigerated in a tight container; any unused suspension should be discarded if not used within 14 days.

For further information on chemistry, mechanism of action, spectrum, resistance, pharmacokinetics, uses, cautions, drug interactions, laboratory test interferences, and dosage and administration of cefadroxil, see the Cephalosporins General Statement 8:12.06.

Preparations

Excipients in commercially available drug preparations may have clinically important effects in some individuals; consult specific product labeling for details.

Cefadroxil

Oral		
Capsules	500 mg*	**Cefadroxil Capsules**
For suspension	125 mg/5mL*	**Cefadroxil for Suspension**
	250 mg/5 mL*	**Cefadroxil for Suspension**
	500 mg/5 mL*	**Cefadroxil for Suspension**
Tablets	1 g*	**Cefadroxil Tablets**

*available from one or more manufacturer, distributor, and/or repackager by generic (nonproprietary) name

†Use is not currently included in the labeling approved by the US Food and Drug Administration

ceFAZolin Sodium

■ Cefazolin sodium is a semisynthetic, first generation cephalosporin antibiotic.

Uses

■ **Biliary Tract Infections** Cefazolin is used for the treatment of biliary tract infections caused by susceptible *Escherichia coli*, *Klebsiella*, *Proteus mirabilis*, *Staphylococcus aureus*, or various streptococci.

■ **Bone and Joint Infections** Cefazolin is used for the treatment of bone and joint infections caused by susceptible *S. aureus*.

■ **Endocarditis** *Treatment* **Staphylococcal Endocarditis.** Cefazolin is used as an alternative to nafcillin or oxacillin for the treatment of staphylococcal endocarditis, including infections caused by coagulase-positive strains (*S. aureus*) or coagulase-negative strains (e.g., *S. epidermidis*, *S. lugdunensis*) in penicillin-allergic patients (nonanaphylactoid type only). Cefazolin should *not* be used in patients with a history of immediate-type penicillin hypersensitivity (urticaria, angioedema, anaphylaxis).

For the treatment of native valve endocarditis caused by oxacillin-susceptible (methicillin-susceptible) staphylococci, the American Heart Association (AHA) and Infectious Diseases Society of America (IDSA) recommend a regimen of IV nafcillin or oxacillin with or without IV or IM gentamicin. For penicillin-allergic patients (nonanaphylactoid type only), a regimen of IV cefazolin with or without IV or IM gentamicin is recommended. In patients with complicated right-sided staphylococcal endocarditis or with left-sided staphylococcal endocarditis, a 6-week regimen of the β-lactam should be used and gentamicin given concomitantly during the first 3–5 days of treatment. In those with uncomplicated right-sided staphylococcal endocarditis (i.e., patients with no evidence of renal failure, extrapulmonary metastatic infections, aortic or mitral valve involvement, meningitis, or oxacillin-resistant strains), a 2-week regimen that includes both the β-lactam and gentamicin can be considered.

Staphylococcal endocarditis in patients with prosthetic valves or other prosthetic material usually is caused by oxacillin-resistant staphylococci, especially when endocarditis develops within 1 year after surgery, and is associated with high morbidity and mortality rates. Unless susceptibility to oxacillin has been demonstrated using in vitro susceptibility testing, it should be assumed that patients with staphylococcal prosthetic valve endocarditis have oxacillin-resistant strains. If prosthetic valve endocarditis is known to be caused by oxacillin-susceptible staphylococci, the AHA and IDSA recommend at least 6 weeks of IV nafcillin or oxacillin in conjunction with IV or oral rifampin and concomitant use of IV or IM gentamicin during the initial 2 weeks of treatment. If the strain is known to be penicillin susceptible (i.e., penicillin MIC 0.1 mcg/mL or less) and does not produce β-lactamase, IV penicillin G sodium can be substituted for nafcillin or oxacillin in this regimen; for penicillin-allergic patients (nonanaphylactoid type only), IV cefazolin can be substituted for nafcillin or oxacillin.

Cefazolin and other cephalosporins should *not* be used for the treatment of endocarditis caused by oxacillin-resistant staphylococci, despite the fact that in vitro testing may indicate the strains are susceptible. If the strain is known or presumed to be oxacillin-resistant, the AHA and IDSA recommend at least 6 weeks of IV vancomycin in conjunction with IV or oral rifampin and concomitant use of IV or IM gentamicin during the initial 2 weeks of treatment.

Streptococcal Endocarditis. Cefazolin is used as an alternative to penicillin G sodium for the treatment of endocarditis caused by susceptible *Streptococcus pyogenes* (group A β-hemolytic streptococci), or *S. pneumoniae*†.

For the treatment of endocarditis caused by highly penicillin-susceptible *S. pneumoniae*†, the AHA and IDSA recommend a 4-week regimen of penicillin G sodium, cefazolin, or ceftriaxone. Vancomycin should only be used in patients who cannot receive a β-lactam. It has been suggested that high-dose treatment with penicillin G sodium or a third-generation cephalosporin can be used in patients with endocarditis caused by penicillin-resistant *S. pneumoniae* provided meningitis is not present. However, penicillin-resistant *S. pneumoniae* often are cross-resistant to cephalosporins, and consultation with an infectious disease specialist is recommended whenever decisions are being made regarding treatment of pneumococcal endocarditis.

For the treatment of endocarditis caused by *S. pyogenes*, the AHA and IDSA recommend a 4-week regimen of IV penicillin G sodium. In penicillin-allergic patients (nonanaphylactoid type only), cefazolin or ceftriaxone are acceptable alternatives. Vancomycin should only be used in patients who cannot receive a β-lactam.

For the treatment of endocarditis caused by groups B, C, or G streptococci, the AHA and IDSA recommend 4–6 weeks of IV penicillin G sodium or, alternatively, a cephalosporin; some clinicians recommend that gentamicin be added to the regimen for at least the first 2 weeks. Consultation with an infections disease specialist is recommended.

Prevention Cefazolin is used for the prevention of α-hemolytic (viridans group) streptococcal endocarditis† in penicillin-allergic individuals undergoing certain dental or upper respiratory tract procedures who have cardiac conditions that put them at highest risk. Oral amoxicillin is the usual drug of choice for such prophylaxis. Cefazolin is an alternative in penicillin-allergic individuals or when an oral anti-infective cannot be used. Cefazolin should not be used in those with immediate-type penicillin hypersensitivity (e.g., urticaria, angioedema, anaphylaxis).

For information on which cardiac conditions are associated with the highest risk of endocarditis and which procedures require prophylaxis, see Prevention under Uses: Endocarditis, in the Cephalosporins General Statement 8:12.06. When selecting anti-infectives for prophylaxis of bacterial endocarditis, the current recommendations published by the AHA should be consulted.

■ **Respiratory Tract Infections** Cefazolin is used for the treatment of respiratory tract infections caused by susceptible *S. pneumoniae*, *S. pyogenes* (group A β-hemolytic streptococci), *S. aureus* (including penicillin-resistant strains), *Klebsiella*, or *Haemophilus influenzae*.

■ **Septicemia** Cefazolin is used for the treatment of septicemia caused by susceptible *S. pneumoniae*, *S. aureus* (including penicillinase-producing strains), *E. coli*, *Klebsiella*, or *P. mirabilis*.

■ **Skin and Skin Structure Infections** Cefazolin is used for the treatment of skin or skin structure infections caused by susceptible *S. aureus* (including penicillinase-producing strains), *S. pyogenes*, or other streptococci.

■ **Urinary Tract and Urogenital Infections** Cefazolin is used for the treatment of urinary tract infections caused by susceptible *E. coli*, *P. mirabilis*, *Klebsiella*, some strains of *Enterobacter*, or some strains of enterococci.

Cefazolin is used for the treatment of prostatitis or epididymitis caused by susceptible *E. coli*, *Klebsiella*, *P. mirabilis*, or some strains of enterococci.

■ **Prevention of Perinatal Group B Streptococcal Disease** In certain penicillin-allergic women, cefazolin is used as an alternative to penicillin G or ampicillin for prevention of perinatal group B streptococcal (GBS) disease†.

Pregnant women who are colonized with GBS in the genital or rectal areas can transmit GBS infection to their infants during labor and delivery resulting in invasive neonatal infection that can be associated with substantial morbidity and mortality. Intrapartum anti-infective prophylaxis for prevention of early-onset neonatal GBS disease is administered *selectively* to women at high risk for transmitting GBS infection to their neonates. The US Centers for Disease Control and Prevention (CDC), American Academy of Pediatrics (AAP), and other experts recommend *routine* universal prenatal culture-based screening for GBS colonization (vaginal and rectal cultures) in *all* pregnant women at 35–37 weeks of gestation, unless GBS bacteriuria is known to be present during the current pregnancy or the woman had a previous infant with invasive GBS disease. These experts state that anti-infective prophylaxis to prevent perinatal GBS disease is indicated in pregnant women identified as GBS carriers during the routine prenatal GBS screening performed at 35–37 weeks during the current pregnancy, in women with GBS bacteriuria identified at any time during the current pregnancy, and in women who had a previous infant diagnosed with invasive GBS disease. Anti-infective prophylaxis to prevent perinatal GBS disease also is indicated in women with unknown GBS status at the time of onset of labor (i.e., culture not done, incomplete, or results unknown) if delivery is at less than 37 weeks of gestation, the duration of amniotic membrane rupture is 18 hours or longer, intrapartum temperature is 38°C or higher, or an intrapartum nucleic acid amplification test (NAAT) was positive for GBS.

When intrapartum prophylaxis is indicated in the mother to prevent GBS disease in the neonate, it should be given at onset of labor or rupture of membranes. The CDC, AAP, and other experts recommend penicillin G as the drug of choice and ampicillin as the preferred alternative for such prophylaxis. If intrapartum prophylaxis is indicated in a penicillin-allergic woman who is *not* at high risk for anaphylaxis (i.e., does not have a history of anaphylaxis, angioedema, respiratory distress, or urticaria after receiving a penicillin or cephalosporin), IV cefazolin is recommended. If intrapartum prophylaxis is indicated in a penicillin-allergic woman who is at high risk for anaphylaxis (e.g., history of anaphylaxis, angioedema, respiratory distress, or urticaria after receiving a penicillin or cephalosporin), IV clindamycin is recommended if the GBS isolate is susceptible to the drug; alternatively, IV vancomycin can be used if the isolate is resistant to clindamycin.

For additional information regarding prevention of perinatal group B streptococcal disease, the current CDC guidelines available at http://www.cdc.gov should be consulted.

■ **Perioperative Prophylaxis** Cefazolin is used perioperatively to reduce the incidence of infection in patients undergoing certain cardiac surgery (e.g., coronary artery bypass, placement of cardiac devices), noncardiac thoracic surgery (e.g., lobectomy), vascular surgery (arterial surgery involving the abdominal aorta, a prosthesis, or a groin incision or lower extremity amputation for ischemia), head and neck surgery involving incisions through oral or pharyngeal mucosa, neurosurgery (e.g., craniotomy, spinal surgery), orthopedic surgery (e.g., total joint replacement, surgical repair of closed fractures, internal fixation of compound or open fractures), GI surgery (gastroduodenal, esophageal, biliary tract, colorectal, appendectomy, bariatric), genitourinary surgery (e.g., open or laparoscopic surgery including percutaneous renal surgery, procedures with entry into the urinary tract or implantation of a prosthesis), and gynecologic and obstetric surgery (cesarean section or vaginal, abdominal, or laparoscopic hysterectomy). Published guidelines and protocols for perioperative prophylaxis should be consulted for recommendations regarding specific procedures.

Because cefazolin has a narrow spectrum of activity that covers the most likely surgical site pathogens, has a moderately long serum half-life, and has been shown to be effective, it is considered by many clinicians to be the drug of choice for perioperative prophylaxis for a wide variety of contaminated or potentially contaminated procedures. Cefazolin also is recommended as a drug of choice for perioperative prophylaxis in patients undergoing heart, lung, heart-lung, pancreas, and pancreas-kidney transplantation.

If cefazolin is used for perioperative prophylaxis in patients undergoing certain GI procedures (e.g., colorectal surgery, appendectomy) that might involve exposure to *Bacteroides fragilis* or other anaerobic bowel bacteria or in patients undergoing head and neck surgery involving incisions through oral or pharyngeal mucosa, it should be used in conjunction with metronidazole to provide anaerobic coverage. (See Uses: Perioperative Prophylaxis, in the Cephalosporins General Statement 8:12.06.)

Dosage and Administration

■ **Reconstitution and Administration** Cefazolin sodium is administered by IV injection or infusion or by deep IM injection. The drug also has been administered intraperitoneally in dialysis solutions†.

Prior to administration, cefazolin solutions should be inspected visually for particulate matter; if particulate matter is evident, the solution should be discarded.

Intermittent IV Injection For direct IV injection, vials labeled as containing 500 mg or 1 g of cefazolin should be reconstituted with 2 or 2.5 mL, respectively, of sterile water for injection to provide solutions containing approximately 225 or 330 mg/mL, respectively. These solutions should be further diluted in approximately 5 mL of sterile water for injection, or according to the manufacturers' directions.

The appropriate dose should then be injected over a period of 3–5 minutes directly into a vein or the tubing of a freely flowing compatible IV solution.

Intermittent or Continuous IV Infusion For intermittent IV infusion, vials labeled as containing 500 mg or 1 g of cefazolin should be reconstituted with 2 or 2.5 mL, respectively, of sterile water for injection to provide solutions containing approximately 225 or 330 mg/mL, respectively. The reconstituted solutions should be further diluted in 50–100 mL of a compatible IV solution.

Alternatively, the commercially available Duplex® drug delivery system containing 1 or 2 g of cefazolin and 50 mL of dextrose 4 or 3% injection, respectively, in separate chambers should be reconstituted (activated) according to the manufacturer's directions and administered by IV infusion.

Cefazolin pharmacy bulk vials should be reconstituted according to the manufacturer's directions and then further diluted in a compatible IV solution prior to IV infusion. The reconstituted solutions should be used promptly; the pharmacy bulk vial should be discarded within 4 hours after initial entry.

Thawed solutions of the commercially available frozen premixed cefazolin sodium injection in dextrose should be given only by intermittent or continuous IV infusion. The frozen injection should be thawed at room temperature (25°C) or under refrigeration (5°C); the injection should not be thawed by warming in a water bath or by exposure to microwave radiation. Precipitates that may have formed in the frozen injection usually will dissolve with little or no agitation when the injection reaches room temperature; potency is not affected. After thawing to room temperature, the injection should be agitated and the container checked for minute leaks by firmly squeezing the bag. The injection should be discarded if container seals or outlet ports are not intact or leaks are found or if the solution is cloudy or contains an insoluble precipitate. Additives should not be introduced into the injection container. The injection should not be used in series connections with other plastic containers, since such use could result in air embolism from residual air being drawn from the primary container before administration of fluid from the secondary container is complete.

IM Injection IM injections of cefazolin sodium are prepared by reconstituting vials labeled as containing 500 mg or 1 g of cefazolin with 2 or 2.5 mL, respectively, of sterile water for injection to provide solutions containing approximately 225 or 330 mg/mL, respectively.

IM injections of cefazolin should be made deeply into a large muscle mass.

■ Dosage

Dosage of cefazolin sodium is expressed in terms of cefazolin and is identical for IM or IV administration.

To avoid unintentional overdosage, the commercially available Duplex® drug delivery system containing cefazolin and dextrose injection and the commercially available frozen premixed cefazolin injection in dextrose should *not* be used in patients who require less than the entire 1- or 2-g dose in the container.

Adult Dosage **General Adult Dosage.** The usual adult dosage of cefazolin for the treatment of mild infections caused by susceptible gram-positive cocci is 250–500 mg every 8 hours.

The usual adult dosage of cefazolin for the treatment of moderate to severe infections is 0.5–1 g every 6–8 hours.

The usual adult dosage of cefazolin for the treatment of severe, life-threatening infections (e.g., endocarditis, septicemia) is 1–1.5 g every 6 hours. In rare instances, up to 12 g daily has been used.

Endocarditis Treatment. For the treatment of endocarditis caused by staphylococci or *Streptococcus pneumoniae*, the manufacturers recommend that adults receive 1–1.5 g of cefazolin every 6 hours. Dosage up to 12 g daily has been used.

If IV cefazolin is used for the treatment of native valve staphylococcal endocarditis in penicillin-allergic patients (nonanaphylactoid type only) with oxacillin-susceptible (methicillin-susceptible) strains, the American Heart Association (AHA) and Infectious Diseases Society of America (IDSA) recommend that adults receive 6 g daily given in 3 equally divided doses; cefazolin should be given for 6 weeks and may be used with or without IM or IV gentamicin (3 mg/kg daily in 3 equally divided doses given during the first 3–5 days of the cefazolin regimen).

If IV cefazolin is used for the treatment of prosthetic valve staphylococcal endocarditis in penicillin-allergic patients (nonanaphylactoid type only) with oxacillin-susceptible strains, the AHA and IDSA recommend that adults receive 6 g daily given in 3 equally divided doses; cefazolin should be given for 6 weeks or longer and used in conjunction with IV or IM gentamicin (3 mg/kg daily given in 2 or 3 equally divided doses during the first 2 weeks of treatment) and IV or oral rifampin (900 mg daily given in 3 equally divided doses for 6 weeks or longer).

If cefazolin is used for the treatment of endocarditis caused by susceptible *S. pyogenes* or *S. pneumoniae*†, the AHA recommends a treatment duration of 4 weeks.

If cefazolin is used for the treatment of endocarditis caused by groups B, C, or G streptococci†, a treatment duration of 4–6 weeks is recommended and some clinicians also include gentamicin during at least the first 2 weeks. Consultation with an infectious disease specialist is recommended.

Endocarditis Prevention. If cefazolin is used as an alternative for *prevention* of α-hemolytic (viridans group) streptococcal endocarditis† in individuals considered to be at highest risk for bacterial endocarditis following certain dental or upper respiratory tract procedures, adults should receive a single 1-g IM or IV dose administered 0.5–1 hour prior to the procedure. Cefazolin should *not* be used for such prophylaxis in individuals with a history of immediate-type hypersensitivity reactions to penicillin.

Respiratory Tract Infections. The usual adult dosage of cefazolin for the treatment of pneumonia caused by *S. pneumoniae* is 500 mg every 12 hours.

Septicemia. The usual adult dosage of cefazolin for the treatment of septicemia is 1–1.5 g every 6 hours. Dosage up to 12 g daily has been used.

Urinary Tract Infections. The usual adult dosage of cefazolin for the treatment of acute, uncomplicated urinary tract infections is 1 g every 12 hours.

Prevention of Perinatal Group B Streptococcal Disease. If cefazolin is used for intrapartum anti-infective prophylaxis for prevention of perinatal group B streptococcal (GBS) disease in women with penicillin hypersensitivity who are not at risk for anaphylaxis, the US Centers for Disease Control and Prevention (CDC) recommends that an initial 2-g IV dose of cefazolin be given at the time of onset of labor or rupture of membranes followed by 1 g IV every 8 hours until delivery. (See Uses: Prevention of Perinatal Group B Streptococcal Disease.)

Perioperative Prophylaxis. For perioperative prophylaxis in contaminated or potentially contaminated surgery, the manufacturers recommend that adults receive 1 or 2 g of cefazolin IM or IV 30–60 minutes prior to surgery and state that additional doses of 0.5–1 g may be given IM or IV during the procedure. Although the manufacturers state that 0.5–1 g may be given IM or IV every 6–8 hours for 24 hours postoperatively and, when the occurrence of infection may be particularly devastating (e.g., open-heart surgery, prosthetic arthroplasty), prophylaxis may be continued for 3–5 days postoperatively, most clinicians state that the duration of prophylaxis should be less than 24 hours for most procedures.

For perioperative prophylaxis in adults undergoing certain cardiac surgery, noncardiac thoracic surgery, vascular surgery, head and neck surgery, neurosurgery, orthopedic surgery, GI surgery, genitourinary surgery, or gynecologic and obstetric surgery (see Uses: Perioperative Prophylaxis), cefazolin should be given within 60 minutes before surgical incision to ensure adequate serum and tissue concentrations. Some experts recommend a cefazolin dose of 1 g in adults weighing less than 80 kg and 2 g in those weighing 80 kg or more and suggest that morbidly obese patients may need higher dosage. Other experts recommend a cefazolin dose of 2 g for most adults and 3 g in those weighing 120 kg or more.

During prolonged procedures (longer than 4 hours) or if major blood loss occurs, additional intraoperative doses of cefazolin should be given every 4 hours. The duration of prophylaxis should be less than 24 hours for most procedures; there is no evidence to support continuing prophylaxis after wound closure or until all indwelling drains and intravascular catheters are removed.

If cefazolin is used for perioperative prophylaxis in patients undergoing certain GI procedures (e.g., colorectal surgery, appendectomy) that might involve exposure to *Bacteroides fragilis* or other anaerobic bowel bacteria or in patients undergoing head and neck surgery involving incisions through oral or pharyngeal mucosa, the usual cefazolin dose should be given in conjunction with IV metronidazole (0.5 g) within 60 minutes before surgical incision.

Pediatric Dosage **General Dosage for Neonates.** The manufacturers state that safety and efficacy of cefazolin have not been established in premature infants or neonates 1 month of age or younger.

The American Academy of Pediatrics (AAP) recommends that neonates 7 days of age or younger† receive IV or IM cefazolin in a dosage of 25 mg/kg every 12 hours, regardless of weight. For neonates 8–28 days of age†, the AAP recommends a dosage of 25 mg/kg every 12 hours for those weighing 2 kg or less and 25 mg/kg every 8 hours for those weighing more than 2 kg.

General Dosage for Infants and Children. The usual dosage of cefazolin recommended by the manufacturers for the treatment of mild to moderately severe infections in pediatric patients older than 1 month of age is 25–50 mg/kg daily given in 3 or 4 equally divided doses. The manufacturers state that dosage may be increased to 100 mg/kg daily in divided doses for the treatment of severe infections.

The AAP recommends that pediatric patients beyond the neonatal period receive IV or IM cefazolin in a dosage of 25–50 mg/kg daily given in 3 equally divided doses for the treatment of mild to moderate infections or 100–150 mg/kg daily given in 3 equally divided doses for the treatment of severe infections.

Endocarditis Treatment. If IV cefazolin is used for the treatment of native valve staphylococcal endocarditis in penicillin-allergic patients (nonanaphylactoid type only) with oxacillin-susceptible strains, the AHA and IDSA recommend that pediatric patients receive 100 mg/kg daily (up to 6 g daily) given in 3 or 4 equally divided doses; cefazolin should be given for 6 weeks and may be used with or without IM or IV gentamicin (3 mg/kg daily in 3 equally divided doses given during the first 3–5 days of the cefazolin regimen).

If IV cefazolin is used for the treatment of prosthetic valve staphylococcal endocarditis in penicillin-allergic patients (nonanaphylactoid type only) with oxacillin-susceptible strains, the AHA and IDSA recommend that pediatric patients receive 100 mg/kg daily (up to 6 g daily) given in 3 or 4 equally divided doses; cefazolin should be given for 6 weeks or longer and used in conjunction with IV or IM gentamicin (3 mg/kg daily given in 2 or 3 equally divided doses during the first 2 weeks of treatment) and IV or oral rifampin (20 mg/kg daily in 3 equally divided doses given for 6 weeks or longer).

If cefazolin is used for the treatment of endocarditis caused by susceptible *S. pyogenes* or *S. pneumoniae*†, the AHA recommends a treatment duration of 4 weeks.

Endocarditis Prevention. If cefazolin is used as an alternative for *prevention* of α-hemolytic (viridans group) streptococcal endocarditis† in individuals considered to be at highest risk for bacterial endocarditis following certain dental or upper respiratory tract procedures, pediatric patients should receive a single dose of 50 mg/kg given IM or IV 0.5–1 hour prior to the procedure. Cefazolin should *not* be used for such prophylaxis in individuals with a history of immediate-type hypersensitivity reactions to penicillin.

Perioperative Prophylaxis. For perioperative prophylaxis in pediatric patients undergoing certain cardiac surgery, noncardiac thoracic surgery, vascular surgery, head and neck surgery, neurosurgery, orthopedic surgery, GI surgery, or genitourinary surgery (see Uses: Perioperative Prophylaxis), some experts recommend that cefazolin should be given in a dose of 30 mg/kg within 60 minutes before surgical incision to ensure adequate serum and tissue concentrations.

During prolonged procedures (longer than 4 hours) or if major blood loss occurs, additional intraoperative doses of cefazolin should be given every 4 hours. The duration of prophylaxis should be less than 24 hours for most procedures; there is no evidence to support continuing prophylaxis after wound closure or until all indwelling drains and intravascular catheters are removed.

If cefazolin is used for perioperative prophylaxis in patients undergoing certain GI procedures (e.g., colorectal surgery, appendectomy) that might involve exposure to *B. fragilis* or other anaerobic bowel bacteria or in patients undergoing head and neck surgery involving incisions through oral or pharyngeal mucosa, pediatric patients should receive the usual cefazolin dose in conjunction with IV metronidazole (15 mg/kg) within 60 minutes before surgical incision.

■ Dosage in Renal Impairment

In patients with impaired renal function, doses and/or frequency of administration of cefazolin must be modified in response to the degree of impairment, severity of the infection, susceptibility of the causative organism, and serum concentrations of the drug.

The manufacturers recommend an initial loading dose appropriate for the severity of the infection followed by dosage based on the degree of renal impairment. (See Table 1 and Table 2.)

Table 1. Dosage for Adults with Renal Impairment

Creatinine Clearance (mL/minute)	Dosage After Initial Loading Dose
35–54	Full doses at intervals ≥8 hours
11–34	50% of usual dose every 12 hours
≤10	50% of usual dose every 18–24 hours

Table 2. Dosage for Children Older than 1 Month of Age with Renal Impairment

Creatinine Clearance (mL/minute)	Dosage After Initial Loading Dose
40–70	60% of usual daily dosage in divided doses every 12 hours
20–40	25% of usual daily dosage in divided doses every 12 hours
5–20	10% of usual daily dosage once every 24 hours

Cautions

Cefazolin shares the toxic potentials of other cephalosporins, and the usual cautions, precautions, and contraindications associated with cephalosporin therapy should be observed. (See Cautions in the Cephalosporins General Statement 8:12.06.)

Spectrum

Based on its spectrum of activity, cefazolin is classified as a first generation cephalosporin. For information on the classification of cephalosporins and closely related β-lactam antibiotics based on spectra of activity, see Spectrum in the Cephalosporins General Statement 8:12.06. Like other first generation cephalosporins (e.g., cefadroxil, cephalexin), cefazolin is active in vitro against many gram-positive aerobic cocci but has limited activity against gram-negative bacteria.

■ **In Vitro Susceptibility Testing** Strains of staphylococci resistant to penicillinase-resistant penicillins (oxacillin-resistant [methicillin-resistant] staphylococci) should be considered resistant to cefazolin, although results of in vitro susceptibility tests may indicate that the organisms are susceptible to the drug.

For information on interpreting results of in vitro susceptibility testing (disk susceptibility tests, dilution susceptibility tests) when cefazolin susceptibility testing is performed according to the standards of the Clinical and Laboratory Standards Institute (CLSI; formerly National Committee for Clinical Laboratory Standards [NCCLS]), see Spectrum: In Vitro Susceptibility Testing, in the Cephalosporins General Statement 8:12.06.

Pharmacokinetics

■ **Absorption** Cefazolin sodium is not appreciably absorbed from the GI tract and must be administered parenterally. Following IM administration of cefazolin sodium in healthy adults with normal renal function, peak serum cefazolin concentrations are attained within 1–2 hours and average 17 mcg/mL following a single 250-mg dose, 30–44 mcg/mL following a single 500-mg dose, and 64–76 mcg/mL following a single 1-g dose. Following a single 1-g IV dose in adults with normal renal function, serum concentrations of cefazolin average 188 mcg/mL at 5 minutes, 74 mcg/mL at 1 hour, and 46 mcg/mL at 2 hours. In one study in adults with normal renal function, steady-state serum concentrations of cefazolin were reached 3 hours after IV infusion of 3.5 mg/kg over 1 hour followed by 1.5 mg/kg over 2 hours.

In one study in children, peak serum concentrations of cefazolin occurred at 30 minutes and averaged 28 mcg/mL after a single cefazolin IM dose of 5–6.25 mg/kg and 42 mcg/mL after a single IM dose of 10–12.5 mg/kg.

■ **Elimination** The serum half-life of cefazolin is 1.2–2.2 hours in adults with normal renal function. In one study, half-life was 6.8 hours in 1 adult with a creatinine clearance of 26 mL/minute, 12 hours in 3 adults with creatinine clearances of 12–17 mL/minute, and 57 hours in 3 adults with creatinine clearances less than 5 mL/minute.

Cefazolin is excreted unchanged in urine. Approximately 60% of a single IM or IV dose of cefazolin is excreted within 6 hours and 80–100% of the dose is excreted within 24 hours in adults with normal renal function. In adults with normal renal function, peak urinary cefazolin concentrations of about 2 or 4 mg/mL may be attained following a single 500-mg or 1-g IM dose, respectively, of the drug.

Chemistry and Stability

■ **Chemistry** Cefazolin sodium is a semisynthetic cephalosporin antibiotic. Cefazolin sodium occurs as a white to off-white, crystalline powder which may have a faint odor or as a white to off-white lyophilized solid. The drug is freely soluble in water and very slightly soluble in alcohol. Each gram of cefazolin as the sodium salt contains 48 mg of sodium.

When the commercially available cefazolin sodium powder for injection is reconstituted as directed, solutions containing 225 or 330 mg/mL are light yellow to yellow and have a pH of 4.5–6.

When the commercially available Duplex® delivery system containing 1 or 2 g of cefazolin and 50 mL of dextrose 4 or 3% injection, respectively, in separate chambers is reconstituted (activated) according to the manufacturer's directions, the resultant solution is iso-osmotic and has an osmolality of approximately 290 mOsm/kg.

Commercially available frozen premixed cefazolin sodium injection in dextrose containing 1 g of cefazolin is a sterile, nonpyrogenic, iso-osmotic solution of the drug provided in a plastic container fabricated from specially formulated multilayered plastic (PL 2040). The 1-g frozen injection of cefazolin contains approximately 2 g of dextrose to adjust osmolality and contains sodium bicarbonate to adjust pH.

■ **Stability** Cefazolin sodium powder for injection should be stored at 20–25°C and protected from light. Following reconstitution of the commercially available powder for injection with sterile water for injection, solutions containing approximately 225 or 330 mg of cefazolin per mL are pale yellow to yellow in color and are stable for 24 hours at room temperature or 10 days at 5°C. Reconstituted solutions have a pH of approximately 4.5–6; rapid hydrolysis of the drug occurs when pH exceeds 8.5, and precipitation of the insoluble free acid may occur when pH is below 4.5.

Reconstituted solutions containing approximately 225 or 330 mg of cefazolin per mL may be frozen in their original containers immediately after reconstitution with sterile water for injection and are stable for 12 weeks when stored at −20°C. If the solutions are warmed to facilitate thawing, care should be taken to avoid heating after thawing has been completed. Once thawed, solutions should not be refrozen.

The commercially available Duplex® delivery system containing 1 or 2 g of cefazolin and 50 mL of dextrose injection in separate chambers should be stored at 20–25°C, but may be exposed to temperatures ranging from 15–30°C. Following reconstitution (activation), these IV solutions must be used within 24 hours if stored at room temperature or within 7 days if stored in a refrigerator and should not be frozen.

The commercially available frozen premixed cefazolin sodium injection in dextrose should be stored at −20°C or lower. The frozen injection should be thawed at room temperature (25°C) or under refrigeration (5°C) and, once thawed, should not be refrozen. Thawed solutions of the commercially available frozen injection are stable for 48 hours at room temperature (25°C) or 30 days under refrigeration (5°C). The commercially available frozen injection of the drug is provided in plastic containers fabricated from specially formulated multilayered plastic PL 2040 (Galaxy® containers). Solutions in contact with PL 2040 can leach out some of its chemical components in very small amounts within the expiration period of the injection; however, safety of the plastic has been confirmed in tests in animals according to USP biological tests for plastic containers as well as by tissue culture toxicity studies.

Cefazolin sodium powder and solutions of the drug tend to darken, depending on storage conditions; however, such discoloration does not indicate loss of potency.

For further information on chemistry, mechanism of action, spectrum, resistance, pharmacokinetics, uses, cautions, drug interactions, laboratory test interferences, and dosage and administration of cefazolin, see the Cephalosporins General Statement 8:12.06.

Preparations

Excipients in commercially available drug preparations may have clinically important effects in some individuals; consult specific product labeling for details.

ceFAZolin Sodium

Parenteral

For injection	500 mg (of cefazolin)*	**Cefazolin Sodium for Injection**
	1 g (of cefazolin)*	**Cefazolin Sodium for Injection**
	10 g (of cefazolin) pharmacy bulk package*	**Cefazolin Sodium for Injection**
	20 g (of cefazolin) pharmacy bulk package*	**Cefazolin Sodium for Injection**
For injection, for IV infusion	1 g (of cefazolin)*	**Cefazolin for Injection** (available in dual-chambered Duplex® drug delivery system with 4% dextrose injection), B Braun
	2 g (of cefazolin)	**Cefazolin for Injection** (available in dual-chambered Duplex® drug delivery system with 3% dextrose injection), B Braun

*available from one or more manufacturer, distributor, and/or repackager by generic (nonproprietary) name

ceFAZolin Sodium in Dextrose

Parenteral

Injection (frozen), for IV infusion	20 mg (of cefazolin) per mL (1 g) in 4% Dextrose*	**Cefazolin Sodium Iso-osmotic in Dextrose Injection** (Galaxy® [Baxter])

*available from one or more manufacturer, distributor, and/or repackager by generic (nonproprietary) name

†Use is not currently included in the labeling approved by the US Food and Drug Administration

Cephalexin

■ Cephalexin is a semisynthetic, first generation cephalosporin antibiotic.

Uses

■ **Acute Otitis Media** Oral cephalexin is used for the treatment of acute otitis media (AOM) caused by susceptible *Streptococcus pneumoniae*, *Haemophilus influenzae*, *Moraxella catarrhalis*, staphylococci, or streptococci.

When anti-infective therapy is indicated for the treatment of AOM, the American Academy of Pediatrics (AAP) recommends high-dose amoxicillin or amoxicillin and clavulanate potassium as the drugs of first choice for initial treatment. These experts recommend certain cephalosporins (cefdinir, cefpodoxime, cefuroxime, ceftriaxone) as alternatives for initial treatment in penicillin-allergic patients who do not have a history of severe and/or recent penicillin-allergic reactions.

For additional information regarding treatment of AOM, including information on diagnosis and management strategies, anti-infectives for initial treatment, duration of initial treatment, and anti-infectives after initial treatment failure, see Acute Otitis Media under Uses: Otitis Media, in the Cephalosporins General Statement 8:12.06.

■ **Pharyngitis and Tonsillitis** Oral cephalexin is used for the treatment of pharyngitis and tonsillitis caused by *S. pyogenes* (group A β-hemolytic streptococci). Although cephalexin generally is effective in eradicating *S. pyogenes* from the nasopharynx, efficacy of the drug in prevention of subsequent rheumatic fever has not been established to date.

Selection of an anti-infective for the treatment of *S. pyogenes* pharyngitis and tonsillitis should be based on the drug's spectrum of activity, bacteriologic and clinical efficacy, potential adverse effects, ease of administration, patient compliance, and cost. No regimen has been found to date that effectively eradicates group A β-hemolytic streptococci in 100% of patients.

Because the drugs have a narrow spectrum of activity, are inexpensive, and generally are effective with a low frequency of adverse effects, the AAP, Infectious Diseases Society of America (IDSA), American Heart Association (AHA), and others recommend a penicillin regimen (i.e., 10 days of oral penicillin V or oral amoxicillin or single dose of IM penicillin G benzathine) as the treatment of choice for *S. pyogenes* pharyngitis and tonsillitis and prevention of initial attacks (primary prevention) of rheumatic fever. Other anti-infectives (e.g., oral cephalosporins, oral macrolides, oral clindamycin) are recommended as alternatives in penicillin-allergic individuals.

If an oral cephalosporin is used for the treatment of *S. pyogenes* pharyngitis and tonsillitis, a 10-day regimen of a first generation cephalosporin (cefadroxil, cephalexin) is preferred instead of other cephalosporins with broader spectrums of activity (e.g., cefaclor, cefdinir, cefixime, cefpodoxime, cefuroxime).

■ **Bone and Joint Infections** Oral cephalexin is used for the treatment of bone and joint infections caused by susceptible staphylococci or *Proteus mirabilis*.

■ **Respiratory Tract Infections** Oral cephalexin is used for the treatment of mild to moderate respiratory tract infections caused by susceptible *S. pneumoniae*.

■ **Skin and Skin Structure Infections** Oral cephalexin is used for the treatment of mild to moderate skin and skin structure infections caused by susceptible staphylococci or streptococci.

■ **Urinary Tract Infections** Oral cephalexin is used for the treatment of mild to moderate urinary tract infections, including acute prostatitis, caused by susceptible *Escherichia coli*, *Klebsiella pneumoniae*, or *P. mirabilis*.

■ **Prevention of Bacterial Endocarditis** Oral cephalexin is used as an alternative for prevention of α-hemolytic (viridans group) streptococcal endocarditis† in penicillin-allergic individuals undergoing certain dental or upper respiratory tract procedures who have underlying cardiac conditions that put them at highest risk of adverse outcomes from endocarditis. Cephalexin should not be used for such prophylaxis in those with a history of immediate-type hypersensitivity to penicillins (e.g., urticaria, angioedema, anaphylaxis).

For information on which cardiac conditions are associated with highest risk of endocarditis and which procedures require prophylaxis, see Prevention under Uses: Endocarditis, in the Cephalosporins General Statement 8:12.06. When selecting anti-infectives for prophylaxis of bacterial endocarditis, the current recommendations published by AHA should be consulted.

Dosage and Administration

■ **Reconstitution and Administration** Cephalexin is administered orally.

Although food may decrease the rate of absorption of cephalexin (see Pharmacokinetics: Absorption), the manufacturers state that the drug may be administered without regard to meals.

Reconstitution Cephalexin powder for oral suspension should be reconstituted at the time of dispensing by adding the amount of water specified on the container to provide a suspension containing 125 or 250 mg of cephalexin per 5 mL. The water should be added in 2 equal portions and the bottle shaken after each addition.

The oral suspension should be shaken well prior to administration of each dose.

■ **Dosage** Cephalexin is commercially available as the monohydrate; dosage is expressed in terms of cephalexin.

Adult Dosage **General Adult Dosage.** The usual adult dosage of cephalexin ranges from 1–4 g daily given in divided doses. Dosage usually is 250 mg every 6 hours or 500 mg every 12 hours. For severe infections or those caused by less susceptible organisms, higher dosage may be needed (up to 4 g daily in adults).

If dosage greater than 4 g daily is required, initial therapy with a parenteral cephalosporin should be considered.

Pharyngitis and Tonsillitis. For the treatment of group A β-hemolytic streptococcal pharyngitis and tonsillitis in patients older than 15 years of age, the usual dosage is 500 mg of cephalexin every 12 hours given for at least 10 days.

Bone and Joint Infections. For the treatment of bone and joint infections in patients older than 15 years of age, the manufacturer recommends 250 mg every 6 hours. Higher dosages may be needed for severe infections or those caused by less susceptible bacteria.

Respiratory Tract Infections. For the treatment of respiratory tract infections in patients older than 15 years of age, the manufacturer recommends 250 mg every 6 hours for mild to moderate infections. Higher dosages may be needed for more severe infections or those caused by less susceptible bacteria.

Skin and Skin Structure Infections. For the treatment of skin and skin structure infections in patients older than 15 years of age, the usual dosage is 500 mg of cephalexin every 12 hours.

Urinary Tract Infections. For the treatment of uncomplicated cystitis in patients older than 15 years of age, the usual dosage is 500 mg of cephalexin every 12 hours given for 7–14 days.

Prevention of Bacterial Endocarditis. If cephalexin is used as an alternative to amoxicillin or ampicillin for prevention of α-hemolytic (viridans group) streptococcal endocarditis† in penicillin-allergic individuals considered to be at highest risk for bacterial endocarditis following certain dental or upper respiratory tract procedures, adults should receive a single 2-g dose administered 0.5–1 hour prior to the procedure.

Pediatric Dosage **General Pediatric Dosage.** The manufacturers state that the usual dosage of cephalexin for children is 25–50 mg/kg daily in divided doses; however, these dosages may be doubled for severe infections.

The American Academy of Pediatrics (AAP) recommends that pediatric patients beyond the neonatal period receive cephalexin in a dosage of 25–50 mg/kg daily in 2 or 4 equally divided doses for the treatment of mild or moderate infections and 75–100 mg/kg daily in 3 or 4 equally divided doses for the treatment of severe infections.

Acute Otitis Media. For the treatment of otitis media, the manufacturers recommend a pediatric dosage of 75–100 mg/kg daily in 4 equally divided doses.

Pharyngitis and Tonsillitis. The usual dosage of cephalexin for the treatment of group A β-hemolytic streptococcal pharyngitis in children older than 1 year of age is 25–50 mg/kg daily in equally divided doses every 12 hours given for at least 10 days.

Skin and Skin Structure Infections. For the treatment of skin and skin structure infections in pediatric patients, the usual dosage of cephalexin is 25–50 mg/kg daily in equally divided doses every 12 hours.

Prevention of Bacterial Endocarditis. If cephalexin is used as an alternative to amoxicillin or ampicillin for prevention of α-hemolytic (viridans group) streptococcal endocarditis† in penicillin-allergic individuals considered to be at highest risk for bacterial endocarditis following certain dental or upper respiratory tract procedures, pediatric patients should receive a single 50-mg/kg dose (no more than 2 g) administered 0.5–1 hour prior to the procedure.

■ **Dosage in Renal Impairment** The manufacturers state that cephalexin should be used with caution in patients with markedly impaired renal function, and close clinical observation and laboratory studies are recommended in such patients because safe dosage may be lower than usual dosages.

Some clinicians state that modification of the usual dosage does not appear to be necessary in patients with creatinine clearances greater than 40 mL/minute. These clinicians suggest that the usual adult dosage be used for the initial dose. Then, for subsequent doses, adults with creatinine clearances of 11–40 mL/minute should receive 500 mg every 8–12 hours, those with creatinine clearances of 5–10 mL/minute should receive 250 mg every 12 hours, and those with creatinine clearances less than 5 mL/minute should receive 250 mg every 12-24 hours.

Cautions

Cephalexin shares the toxic potentials of other cephalosporins, and the usual cautions, precautions, and contraindications associated with cephalosporin therapy should be observed. (See Cautions in the Cephalosporins General Statement 8:12.06.)

■ **Pediatric Precautions** Cephalexin is labeled for use in pediatric patients; safety and efficacy were established based on clinical trials using recommended dosages of the drug administered as capsules or oral suspension.

Cephalexin capsules should only be used in children and adolescents who are able to ingest capsules.

Spectrum

Based on its spectrum of activity, cephalexin is classified as a first generation cephalosporin. For information on the classification of cephalosporins and closely related β-lactam antibiotics based on spectra of activity, see Spectrum in the Cephalosporins General Statement 8:12.06. Like other first generation cephalosporins (e.g., cefadroxil, cefazolin), cephalexin is active in vitro against many gram-positive aerobic cocci but has limited activity against gram-negative bacteria.

■ **In Vitro Susceptibility Testing** Strains of staphylococci resistant to penicillinase-resistant penicillins (methicillin-resistant [oxacillin-resistant] staphylococci) should be considered resistant to cephalexin, although results of in vitro susceptibility tests may indicate that the organisms are susceptible to the drug.

For information on interpreting results of in vitro susceptibility testing (disk susceptibility tests, dilution susceptibility tests) when cephalexin susceptibility testing is performed according to the standards of the Clinical and Laboratory Standards Institute (CLSI; formerly National Committee for Clinical Laboratory Standards [NCCLS]), see Spectrum: In Vitro Susceptibility Testing, in the Cephalosporins General Statement 8:12.06.

Pharmacokinetics

■ **Absorption** Cephalexin (as the monohydrate) is acid-stable and is rapidly and completely absorbed from the GI tract. Following oral administration in healthy, fasting adults with normal renal function of a single 250-mg, 500-mg, or 1-g dose of cephalexin, peak serum cephalexin concentrations are attained within 1 hour and average 9, 18, or 32 mcg/mL, respectively. Serum concentrations of cephalexin were still detectable 6 hours after the dose.

Peak serum concentrations are slightly lower and are attained later when cephalexin is administered with food, although the total amount of drug absorbed is unchanged. Following oral administration of cephalexin in healthy, fasting adults, serum concentrations 15 and 30 minutes after a single 500-mg dose averaged about 0.2 and 12 mcg/mL, respectively.

Absorption of cephalexin is delayed in young children and may be decreased up to 50% in neonates. Peak serum concentrations of the drug have been reported to occur within 3 hours in infants younger than 6 months of age, within 2 hours in children 9–12 months of age, and within 1 hour in older children.

■ **Elimination** The serum half-life of cephalexin is 0.5–1.2 hours in adults with normal renal function. The serum half-life of the drug is reported to be about 5 hours in neonates and 2.5 hours in children 3–12 months of age. In one study, the serum half-life was 7.7 hours in adults with creatinine clearances of 13.5 mL/minute, 10.8 hours in adults with creatinine clearances of 9.2 mL/minute, and 13.9 hours in adults with creatinine clearances of 4 mL/minute.

Cephalexin is excreted in urine as unchanged drug via both glomerular filtration and tubular secretion. Approximately 70–90% of a single 250- or 500-mg oral dose is excreted within 8–12 hours in adults with normal renal function. Cephalexin concentrations of 0.2 (range: 0.054–0.67) or 0.11–4 mg/mL have been reported in urine collected over a 6-hour period following a single 250- or 500-mg dose, respectively, in adults with normal renal function. Peak urine concentrations of the drug averaging about 2 mg/mL occur 2 hours after a single 500-mg oral dose of cephalexin.

Chemistry and Stability

■ **Chemistry** Cephalexin is a semisynthetic cephalosporin antibiotic. Cephalexin is commercially available as the monohydrate. Cephalexin (as the monohydrate) occurs as a white to off-white, crystalline powder and is slightly soluble in water and practically insoluble in alcohol.

■ **Stability** Cephalexin capsules should be stored in tight, light-resistant containers at 20–25°C, but may be exposed to temperatures ranging from 15–30°C.

Cephalexin powder for oral suspension should be stored at 20–25°C. After reconstitution, cephalexin oral suspension should be refrigerated in a tight container; any unused suspension should be discarded if not used within 14 days.

For further information on chemistry, mechanism of action, spectrum, resistance, pharmacokinetics, uses, cautions, drug interactions, laboratory test interferences, and dosage and administration of cephalexin, see the Cephalosporins General Statement 8:12.06.

Preparations

Excipients in commercially available drug preparations may have clinically important effects in some individuals; consult specific product labeling for details.

Cephalexin

Oral		
Capsules	250 mg*	Cephalexin Capsules Keflex®, Shionogi
	333 mg*	Cephalexin Capsules
	500 mg*	Cephalexin Capsules Keflex®, Shionogi
	750 mg*	Cephalexin Capsules Keflex®, Shionogi
For suspension	125 mg/5 mL*	Cephalexin for Suspension
	250 mg/5 mL*	Cephalexin for Suspension
Tablets, film-coated	250 mg*	Cephalexin Film-coated Tablets
	500 mg*	Cephalexin Film-coated Tablets

*available from one or more manufacturer, distributor, and/or repackager by generic (nonproprietary) name

†Use is not currently included in the labeling approved by the US Food and Drug Administration

SECOND GENERATION CEPHALOSPORINS 8:12.06.08

Cefaclor

■ Cefaclor is a semisynthetic, second generation cephalosporin antibiotic.

Uses

Cefaclor is used orally for the treatment of acute otitis media caused by susceptible bacteria; pharyngitis and tonsillitis caused by *Streptococcus pyogenes* (group A β-hemolytic streptococci); mild to moderate upper and lower respiratory tract infections (including pneumonia) caused by susceptible bacteria; uncomplicated skin and skin structure infections caused by susceptible bacteria; and urinary tract infections (including pyelonephritis and cystitis) caused by susceptible bacteria. While commercially available cefaclor capsules and oral suspension can be used for any of these infections, safety and efficacy of cefaclor extended-release tablets have been established only for the treatment of mild to moderate respiratory tract infections (i.e., acute exacerbations of chronic bronchitis, secondary infections of acute bronchitis) caused by susceptible bacteria; pharyngitis and tonsillitis caused by *S. pyogenes*; and mild to moderate uncomplicated skin and skin structure infections caused by susceptible *Staphylococcus aureus* (methicillin-susceptible [oxacillin-susceptible] strains only).

■ **Acute Otitis Media** Cefaclor capsules and oral suspension are used for the treatment of acute otitis media (AOM) caused by *Streptococcus pneumoniae, Haemophilus influenzae*, staphylococci, or *S. pyogenes* (group A β-hemolytic streptococci). When selecting an anti-infective for treatment of AOM that may involve *H. influenzae*, clinicians should consider the fact that β-lactamase-negative, ampicillin-resistant (BLNAR) strains of *H. influenzae* should be considered resistant to cefaclor despite apparent in vitro susceptibility of some strains.

When anti-infective therapy is indicated for the treatment of AOM, the American Academy of Pediatrics (AAP) recommends high-dose amoxicillin or amoxicillin and clavulanate potassium as the drugs of first choice for initial treatment. These experts recommend certain cephalosporins (cefdinir, cefpodoxime, cefuroxime, ceftriaxone) as alternatives for initial treatment in penicillin-allergic patients who do not have a history of severe and/or recent penicillin-allergic reactions.

Results of controlled clinical studies in pediatric patients with AOM indicate that a 10-day regimen of oral cefaclor generally is as effective as a 10-day regimen of oral amoxicillin, oral cefixime (no longer commercially available in the US), oral cefprozil, or oral ceftibuten.

Cefaclor has been effective for the treatment of AOM in some pediatric patients when administered in a 5-day regimen†; however, the shortened regimen appears to be less effective in patients with spontaneous perforation of the tympanic membrane and purulent drainage than in those with intact tympanic membranes. In a controlled study in children with AOM who were randomized to received 5 or 10 days of oral cefaclor (20 mg/kg twice daily), the treatment failure rate in those with intact tympanic membranes at the time of diagnosis was 10% in those who received the 5-day regimen and 6% in those who received the 10-day regimen; in those with spontaneous perforation of the tympanic membrane at the time of diagnosis, the failure rate was 53 and 8%, respectively. Further study is needed to evaluate use of a 5-day regimen of oral cefaclor for the treatment of AOM. The AAP states that oral anti-infective regimens of less than 10 days' duration are not recommended for the treatment of AOM in children younger than 2 years of age or in patients with severe symptoms.

For additional information regarding treatment of AOM, including information on diagnosis and management strategies, anti-infectives for initial treatment, duration of initial treatment, and anti-infectives after initial treatment failure, see Acute Otitis Media under Uses: Otitis Media, in the Cephalosporins General Statement 8:12.06.

■ **Pharyngitis and Tonsillitis** Cefaclor capsules, oral suspension, and extended-release tablets are used for the treatment of pharyngitis and tonsillitis caused by susceptible *S. pyogenes* (group A β-hemolytic streptococci). Although cefaclor usually is effective in eradicating *S. pyogenes* from the nasopharynx, efficacy in the prevention of subsequent rheumatic fever has not been established to date.

Selection of an anti-infective for the treatment of *S. pyogenes* pharyngitis and tonsillitis should be based on the drug's spectrum of activity, bacteriologic and clinical efficacy, potential adverse effects, ease of administration, patient compliance, and cost. No regimen has been found to date that effectively eradicates group A β-hemolytic streptococci in 100% of patients.

Because the drugs have a narrow spectrum of activity, are inexpensive, and generally are effective with a low frequency of adverse effects, the AAP, Infectious Diseases Society of America (IDSA), American Heart Association (AHA), and others recommend a penicillin regimen (i.e., 10 days of oral penicillin V or oral amoxicillin or a single dose of IM penicillin G benzathine) as the treatment of choice for *S. pyogenes* pharyngitis and tonsillitis and prevention of initial attacks (primary prevention) of rheumatic fever. Other anti-infectives (e.g., oral cephalosporins, oral macrolides, oral clindamycin) are recommended as alternatives in penicillin-allergic individuals.

If an oral cephalosporin is used for the treatment of *S. pyogenes* pharyngitis and tonsillitis, a 10-day regimen of a first generation cephalosporin (cefadroxil, cephalexin) is preferred instead of other cephalosporins with broader spectrums of activity (e.g., cefaclor, cefdinir, cefixime, cefpodoxime, cefuroxime).

Although there is some evidence that a shorter duration of therapy with certain oral cephalosporins (e.g., a 5-day regimen of cefadroxil, cefdinir, cefixime, or cefpodoxime proxetil or a 4- or 5-day regimen of cefuroxime axetil) achieves bacteriologic and clinical cure rates equal to or greater than those achieved with the traditional 10-day oral penicillin V regimen, the IDSA and AHA state that use of cephalosporin regimens administered for 5 days or less for the treatment of *S. pyogenes* pharyngitis and tonsillitis cannot be recommended at this time.

A 10-day regimen of oral cefaclor is at least as effective as a 10-day regimen of oral penicillin V or a 10-day regimen of oral amoxicillin and clavulanate potassium for the treatment of *S. pyogenes* pharyngitis and tonsillitis. In an open, randomized study in adults and adolescents 12 years of age or older with acute pharyngitis caused by *S. pyogenes*, a 10-day regimen of oral cefaclor (250 mg 3 times daily) was at least as effective as a 10-day regimen of oral cefprozil (500 mg once daily); the clinical response rate was 85% for both drugs and the bacteriologic eradication rate was 95% in those who received cefaclor and 91% in those who received cefprozil. In double-blind, randomized multicenter studies designed to compare efficacy of a 10-day regimen of cefaclor capsules (250 mg 3 times daily) and a 10-day regimen of cefaclor extended-release tablets (375 mg twice daily), the clinical response rates were 98.1 and 96.7%, respectively, and the bacteriologic eradication rates were 94.1 and 93.6%, respectively.

■ **Respiratory Tract Infections** Cefaclor capsules and oral suspension are used for the treatment of lower respiratory tract infections (including pneumonia) caused by susceptible *S. pneumoniae*, *H. influenzae*, or *S. pyogenes*. Cefaclor extended-release tablets are used for the treatment of mild to moderate acute exacerbations of chronic bronchitis or secondary infections of acute bronchitis caused by susceptible *H. influenzae* (non-β-lactamase-producing strains only), *Moraxella catarrhalis* (including β-lactamase-producing strains), or *S. pneumoniae*. When selecting an anti-infective for treatment of lower respiratory tract infections that may involve *H. influenzae*, consider the fact that strains of *H. influenzae* should be considered resistant to cefaclor despite apparent in vitro susceptibility of some strains. The manufacturer cautions that data are insufficient to establish efficacy of cefaclor extended-release tablets in the treatment of acute or chronic bronchitis that is known, suspected, or potentially caused by β-lactamase-producing strains of *H. influenzae*.

The overall clinical response rate (cure or improvement) reported in adults with acute bacterial bronchitis or acute bacterial exacerbations of chronic bronchitis treated with cefaclor capsules (250 mg 3 times daily) is 92% and the overall bacteriologic elimination rate is 80–92%. When results are stratified according to causative agent, the bacteriologic elimination rate is 85% for infections caused by *H. influenzae* and 100% for those caused by *H. parainfluenzae*† or *Klebsiella pneumoniae*†; 81% for infections caused by *S. pneumoniae*; and 75% for infections caused by *M. catarrhalis*.

■ **Skin and Skin Structure Infections** Cefaclor capsules, oral suspension, and extended-release tablets are used for the treatment of uncomplicated skin and skin structure infections caused by *Staphylococcus aureus* (methicillin-susceptible [oxacillin-susceptible] strains only). Cefaclor capsules and oral suspension also can be used for the treatment of uncomplicated skin and skin structure infections caused by *S. pyogenes*; however, the manufacturer states that efficacy of cefaclor extended-release tablets for the treatment of uncomplicated skin or skin structure infections known or suspected of being caused by these bacteria has not been established.

In a multicenter, randomized study in adults and children 2 years of age or older with mild to moderate bacterial skin and skin structure infections (e.g., carbuncle, cellulitis, folliculitis, furuncle, impetigo, infected dermatitis, paronychia, pyoderma, superficial abscess, wound infection), patients were randomized to receive 5–10 days of therapy with oral cefaclor (250 mg 3 times daily in adults or 20 mg/kg daily in 3 doses) or oral cefprozil (500 mg once daily in adults or 20 mg/kg once daily in children). Results of this study indicate that cefaclor and cefprozil are equally effective for these infections and similarly tolerated; a satisfactory clinical response was attained in 92 and 93% of patients, respectively, and the bacteriologic eradication rate was 89 and 91%, respectively.

■ **Urinary Tract Infections** Cefaclor capsules and oral suspension are used for the treatment of urinary tract infections (including pyelonephritis and cystitis) caused by susceptible *Escherichia coli*, *Klebsiella*, *Proteus mirabilis*, or coagulase-negative staphylococci.

Dosage and Administration

■ **Reconstitution and Administration** Cefaclor is administered orally.

Food does not affect the extent of absorption of cefaclor administered as conventional capsules or oral solution, and these preparations may be administered without regard to meals. However, food increases the extent of absorption of cefaclor administered as extended-release tablets. (See Pharmacokinetics: Absorption.) The manufacturer recommends that cefaclor extended-release tablets be administered with meals or within 1 hour of eating to enhance GI absorption.

Cefaclor extended-release tablets should not be cut, crushed, or chewed.

Reconstitution Cefaclor powder for oral suspension should be reconstituted at the time of dispensing by adding the amount of water specified on the container to provide a suspension containing 125, 187, 250, or 375 mg of cefaclor per 5 mL. The water should be added in 2 portions and the bottle shaken well after each addition.

The oral suspension should be shaken well prior to administration of each dose.

■ **Dosage** Cefaclor is commercially available as the monohydrate; dosage is expressed in terms of anhydrous cefaclor.

Adult Dosage **Acute Otitis Media.** The usual adult dosage of cefaclor administered as capsules or oral suspension for the treatment of acute otitis media is 250 mg every 8 hours; for more severe infections or those caused by less susceptible organisms, 500 mg may be given every 8 hours. Although the daily dosage of cefaclor capsules or oral suspension usually is administered in 3 equally divided doses, the manufacturer states that daily dosage may be given in 2 equally divided doses at 12-hour intervals for the treatment acute otitis media.

Pharyngitis and Tonsillitis. The usual adult dosage of cefaclor administered as capsules or oral suspension for the treatment of pharyngitis and tonsillitis caused by *Streptococcus pyogenes* (group A β-hemolytic streptococci) is 250 mg every 8 hours for at least 10 days; for more severe infections or those caused by less susceptible organisms, 500 mg may be given every 8 hours. Although the daily dosage of cefaclor capsules or oral suspension usually is administered in 3 equally divided doses, the manufacturer states that daily dosage may be given in 2 equally divided doses at 12-hour intervals for the treatment of pharyngitis.

If cefaclor extended-release tablets are used for the treatment of pharyngitis and/or tonsillitis caused by *S. pyogenes*, the usual adult dosage is 375 mg every 12 hours for 10 days.

Respiratory Tract Infections. For the treatment of lower respiratory tract infections caused by susceptible bacteria, the usual adult dosage of cefaclor administered as capsules or oral suspension is 250 mg every 8 hours; for more severe infections (e.g., pneumonia) or those caused by less susceptible organisms, 500 mg may be given every 8 hours.

If cefaclor extended-release tablets are used for the treatment of acute bacterial exacerbation of chronic bronchitis or secondary bacterial infections of acute bronchitis caused by susceptible *Haemophilus influenzae* (non-β-lactamase-producing strains only), *Moraxella catarrhalis* (including β-lactamase-producing strains), or *S. pneumoniae*, the usual adult dosage is 500 mg every 12 hours for 7 days.

Skin and Skin Structure Infections. For the treatment of skin and skin structure infections caused by susceptible *Staphylococcus aureus* or *S. pyogenes*, the usual adult dosage of cefaclor administered as capsules or oral suspension is 250 mg every 8 hours; for more severe infections or those caused by less susceptible organisms, 500 mg may be given every 8 hours.

If cefaclor extended-release tablets are used for the treatment of uncomplicated skin and skin structure infections caused by susceptible *S. aureus*, the usual adult dosage is 375 mg every 12 hours for 7–10 days.

Urinary Tract Infections. For the treatment of urinary tract infections (including pyelonephritis and cystitis) caused by susceptible bacteria, the usual adult dosage of cefaclor administered as capsules or oral suspension is 250 mg every 8 hours; for more severe infections or those caused by less susceptible organisms, 500 mg may be given every 8 hours.

Pediatric Dosage **General Pediatric Dosage.** The American Academy of Pediatrics (AAP) recommends that pediatric patients beyond the neonatal period receive cefaclor in a dosage of 20–40 mg/kg daily in 2 or 3 equally divided doses for the treatment of mild or moderate infections. The AAP states that the drug is inappropriate for the treatment of severe infections.

A maximum cefaclor dosage of 1 g daily is recommended in pediatric patients.

Acute Otitis Media. The usual dosage of cefaclor capsules or oral suspension for the treatment of otitis media in children 1 month of age or older is 40 mg/kg daily in divided doses every 8 or 12 hours.

Pharyngitis and Tonsillitis. The usual dosage of cefaclor capsules or oral suspension for the treatment of pharyngitis or tonsillitis in children 1 month of age or older is 20 mg/kg daily in divided doses every 8 or 12 hours for at least 10 days. For more severe infections or those caused by less susceptible organisms, 40 mg/kg daily in divided doses every 8 hours can be used.

Respiratory Tract Infections. The usual dosage of cefaclor capsules or oral suspension for the treatment of lower respiratory tract infections in children 1 month of age or older is 20 mg/kg daily in divided doses every 8 hours for 10 days. For more severe infections or those caused by less susceptible organisms, 40 mg/kg daily in divided doses every 8 hours can be used.

Skin and Skin Structure Infections. The usual dosage of cefaclor capsules or oral suspension for the treatment of skin and skin structure infections in children 1 month of age or older is 20 mg/kg daily in divided doses every 8 hours for 10 days. For more severe infections or those caused by less susceptible organisms, 40 mg/kg daily in divided doses every 8 hours can be used.

Urinary Tract Infections. The usual dosage of cefaclor capsules or oral suspension for the treatment of urinary tract infections in children 1 month of age or older is 20 mg/kg daily in divided doses every 8 hours for 10 days. For more severe infections or those caused by less susceptible organisms, 40 mg/kg daily in divided doses every 8 hours can be used.

■ Dosage in Renal Impairment Modification of usual cefaclor dosage is not necessary in patients with renal impairment; however, close clinical observation and appropriate laboratory tests are recommended in patients with moderate or severe renal impairment since experience in such patients is limited.

Cautions

■ Adverse Effects Most adverse effects reported with cefaclor are similar to those reported with other oral cephalosporins. (See Cautions in the Cephalosporins General Statement 8:12.06.) The most frequent adverse effects reported with cefaclor include GI effects (diarrhea, nausea, vomiting), headache, and rash.

Serum sickness-like reactions consisting of erythema multiforme or maculopapular pruritic rash or urticaria accompanied by arthritis, arthralgia, irritability, and fever have been reported rarely in patients receiving cefaclor. These reactions differ from serum sickness type III hypersensitivity reactions since they generally are not associated with lymphadenopathy and proteinuria, circulating immune complexes have not been identified, and sequelae have not been reported. Serum sickness-like reactions have been reported most frequently in pediatric patients younger than 6 years of age receiving cefaclor oral suspension for the treatment of acute otitis media, pharyngitis and tonsillitis, or other upper respiratory tract infection and occur most often with second or subsequent courses of the drug. Signs and symptoms of the reaction usually are apparent 2–11 days after initiation of cefaclor therapy and begin to subside within a few days after the drug is discontinued. Oral antihistamines and corticosteroids provide symptomatic relief and may enhance resolution of the reaction; short-term (i.e., 2–3 days) hospitalization has been necessary in some patients because of symptoms (e.g., arthralgia) that ranged from mild to severe. The true incidence of serum sickness-like reactions in patients receiving cefaclor is unclear but has been estimated to be 0.5% or lower. While similar serum sickness-like reactions have been reported rarely in patients receiving other cephalosporins (i.e., cefprozil, cephalexin) or other β-lactam antibiotics (i.e., amoxicillin, loracarbef), these reactions have been reported more frequently with cefaclor than with any other anti-infective agent. Some clinicians recommend that cefaclor *not* be used in patients who have had a serum sickness-like reaction to the drug; however, others suggest that a history of a serum sickness-like reaction from cefaclor does not necessarily contraindicate use of other cephalosporins or other β-lactam antibiotics.

Severe hypersensitivity reactions, including Stevens-Johnson syndrome, toxic epidermal necrolysis, and anaphylaxis, have been reported rarely with cefaclor. Anaphylactic reactions may be manifested by solitary symptoms, including angioedema, asthenia, edema (including face and limbs), dyspnea, paresthesia, syncope, hypotension, or vasodilation. There has been at least one report of hypersensitivity myocarditis that appeared to be a sensitivity reaction to cefaclor. Hypersensitivity reactions rarely may persist for several months.

■ Precautions and Contraindications Cefaclor shares the toxic potentials of other cephalosporins, and the usual cautions, precautions, and contraindications associated with cephalosporin therapy should be observed. (See Cautions in the Cephalosporins General Statement 8:12.06.)

Prior to initiation of cefaclor therapy, careful inquiry should be made concerning previous hypersensitivity reactions to cephalosporins, penicillins, or other drugs. There is clinical and laboratory evidence of partial cross-allergenicity among cephalosporins and other β-lactam antibiotics, including penicillins and cephamycins. Cefaclor is contraindicated in patients who are hypersensitive to the drug or other cephalosporins and should be used with caution in patients with a history of hypersensitivity to penicillins. Use of cephalosporins should be avoided in patients who have had an immediate-type (anaphylactic) hypersensitivity reaction to penicillins. If a hypersensitivity reaction occurs during cefaclor therapy, the drug should be discontinued and the patient treated with appropriate therapy (e.g., epinephrine, corticosteroids, and maintenance of an adequate airway and oxygen) as indicated.

To reduce development of drug-resistant bacteria and maintain effectiveness of cefaclor and other antibacterials, the drug should be used only for the treatment or prevention of infections proven or strongly suspected to be caused by susceptible bacteria. When selecting or modifying anti-infective therapy, results of culture and in vitro susceptibility testing should be used. In the absence of such data, local epidemiology and susceptibility patterns should be considered when selecting anti-infectives for empiric therapy should be considered.

Patients should be advised that antibacterials (including cefaclor) should only be used to treat bacterial infections and not used to treat viral infections (e.g., the common cold). Patients also should be advised about the importance of completing the full course of therapy, even if feeling better after a few days, and that skipping doses or not completing therapy may decrease effectiveness and increase the likelihood that bacteria will develop resistance and will not be treatable with cefaclor or other antibacterials in the future.

Because *Clostridium difficile* infection (CDI) and *C. difficile*-associated diarrhea and colitis (CDAD; also known as antibiotic-associated diarrhea and colitis or pseudomembranous colitis) have been reported with the nearly all anti-infectives, including cephalosporins, it should be considered in the differential diagnosis of patients who develop diarrhea during or following cefaclor therapy. Patients should be advised that diarrhea is a common problem caused by anti-infectives and usually ends when the drug is discontinued; however, they should contact a clinician if watery and bloody stools (with or without stomach cramps and fever) occur during or as late as 2 months or longer after the last dose.

■ Pediatric Precautions Safety and efficacy of cefaclor capsules and oral suspension have not been established in children younger than 1 month of age.

Safety and efficacy of cefaclor extended-release tablets have not been established in children younger than 16 years of age.

■ Geriatric Precautions Safety and efficacy of cefaclor in geriatric adults (i.e., those older than 65 years of age) are similar to that observed in younger adults.

Cefaclor is substantially eliminated by the kidneys. Although no age-related dosage adjustments are required in geriatric patients, dosage should be selected with caution and renal function monitoring should be considered because of age-related decreases in renal function.

■ Mutagenicity and Carcinogenicity Animal studies have not been performed to date to evaluate the mutagenic and carcinogenic potential of cefaclor.

■ Pregnancy, Fertility, and Lactation Reproduction studies in mice, rats, and ferrets using doses up to 3–5 times the maximum human dosage (1500 mg daily) based on mg/m^2 have not revealed evidence of harm to the fetus. There are no adequate and controlled studies using cefaclor in pregnant women or during labor and delivery, and the drug should be used during pregnancy only when clearly needed.

Reproduction studies in animals using cefaclor have not revealed evidence of impaired fertility.

Because low concentrations of cefaclor (0.16–0.21 mcg/mL) have been detected in milk following a single 500-mg oral dose of the drug, cefaclor should be used with caution in nursing women.

Acute Toxicity

Overdosage of cefaclor may cause nausea, vomiting, epigastric distress, and diarrhea; the severity of the epigastric distress and diarrhea are dose related. If other symptoms are present, they probably are secondary to an underlying disease state, an allergic reaction, or the effects of other intoxication. The manufacturer of cefaclor capsules and oral suspension states that, in the event of cefaclor overdosage, GI decontamination is not necessary unless 5 times the normal dose of cefaclor has been ingested. The benefits of forced diuresis, peritoneal dialysis, hemodialysis, or charcoal hemoperfusion in treating cefaclor overdosage have not been established.

Spectrum

Based on its spectrum of activity, cefaclor is classified as a second generation cephalosporin. While cefaclor is less active in vitro against gram-negative bacteria than other currently available second generation cephalosporins, cefaclor is active against some gram-negative bacteria that are generally resistant to the first generation drugs (e.g., *Haemophilus influenzae*). For information on the classification of cephalosporins and closely related β-lactam antibiotics based on spectra of activity, see Spectrum in the Cephalosporins General Statement 8:12.06.

■ In Vitro Susceptibility Testing Strains of staphylococci resistant to penicillinase-resistant penicillins (methicillin-resistant [oxacillin-resistant] staphylococci) should be considered resistant to cefaclor, although results of in vitro susceptibility tests may indicate that the organisms are susceptible to the drug. In addition, β-lactamase-negative, ampicillin-resistant (BLNAR) strains of *H. influenzae* should be considered resistant to cefaclor despite the fact that results of in vitro susceptibility tests may indicate that the organisms are susceptible to the drug.

For information on interpreting results of in vitro susceptibility testing (disk susceptibility tests, dilution susceptibility tests) when cefaclor susceptibility testing is performed according to the standards of the Clinical and Laboratory Standards Institute (CLSI; formerly National Committee for Clinical Laboratory Standards [NCCLS]), see Spectrum: In Vitro Susceptibility Testing, in the Cephalosporins General Statement 8:12.06.

Pharmacokinetics

■ Absorption Cefaclor is acid-stable and is well absorbed from the GI tract. Following oral administration of cefaclor capsules in healthy, fasting adults with normal renal function, peak serum concentrations of cefaclor are attained within 30–60 minutes and average 5–7 mcg/mL following a single

250-mg dose, 13–15 mcg/mL following a single 500-mg dose, and 23–25 mcg/mL following a single 1-g dose. When 500 mg of cefaclor is administered as capsules, peak plasma concentrations are attained 0.9 hours after the dose and average 16.8 mcg/mL in fasting individuals; however, in nonfasting individuals, peak plasma concentrations are attained 1.5 hours after the dose and average 9.3 mcg/mL.

In nonfasting individuals who receive 375 mg of cefaclor as an extended-release tablet, peak plasma concentrations of the drug average 3.7 mcg/mL and are attained 2.7 hours after the dose. Following oral administration 500 mg of cefaclor as an extended-release tablet in fasting individuals, peak plasma concentrations of the drug are attained 1.5 hours after the dose and average 5.4 mcg/mL; when the same dose is given to nonfasting individuals, peak plasma concentrations are attained 2.5 hours after the dose and average 8.2 mcg/mL.

Peak serum concentrations are lower and attained later when cefaclor capsules are administered with food, although the total amount of drug absorbed is unchanged. Administration of cefaclor extended-release tablets with food increases the extent of absorption and peak plasma concentrations of the drug.

In one study in infants younger than 18 months of age, peak serum concentrations of cefaclor ranged from 2–14 mcg/mL 1 hour after a single oral dose of 10 mg/kg and 1.2–23 mcg/mL 1 hour after a single oral dose of 15 mg/kg.

■ **Elimination** The serum half-life of cefaclor is 0.6–1 hour in adults with normal renal function and 2.3–2.8 hours in anuric patients. In one study, the serum half-life of cefaclor was 1.3 hours in an adult with a creatinine clearance of 55 mL/minute, 2.5 hours in an adult with a creatinine clearance of 10.5 mL/minute, and 5.6 hours in an adult with a creatinine clearance of 8 mL/minute. In another study in functionally anephric patients who were given multiple doses of the drug, the serum half-life averaged 2.9 hours.

Cefaclor is excreted unchanged in urine. Approximately 50–85% of a single oral dose is excreted within 8 hours in adults with normal renal function; the major portion of the dose is excreted within the first 2 hours. In adults with normal renal function, peak concentrations of cefaclor average 600 mcg/mL, 900 mcg/mL, and 1.9 mg/mL in urine collected over an 8-hour period following a single 250-mg, 500-mg, or 1-g dose, respectively.

Chemistry and Stability

■ **Chemistry** Cefaclor is a semisynthetic cephalosporin antibiotic.

Cefaclor is commercially available for oral administration as capsules, powder for oral suspension, and extended-release tablets containing cefaclor monohydrate; potency is expressed on the anhydrous basis. Cefaclor occurs as a crystalline powder and is sparingly soluble in water.

■ **Stability** Cefaclor capsules should be stored at 20–25°C and protected from moisture.

Cefaclor powder for oral suspension should be stored at 20–25°C. After reconstitution, the suspension should be stored in a tight container in the refrigerator; any unused suspension should be discarded after 14 days.

Cefaclor extended-release tablets should be stored in tight, light-resistant containers at 20–25°C.

For further information on chemistry, mechanism of action, spectrum, resistance, pharmacokinetics, uses, cautions, drug interactions, laboratory test interferences, and dosage and administration of cefaclor, see the Cephalosporins General Statement 8:12.06.

Preparations

Excipients in commercially available drug preparations may have clinically important effects in some individuals; consult specific product labeling for details.

Cefaclor

Oral		
Capsules	equivalent to anhydrous cefaclor 250 mg*	Cefaclor Capsules
	equivalent to anhydrous cefaclor 500 mg*	Cefaclor Capsules
For suspension	equivalent to anhydrous cefaclor 125 mg/5 mL*	Cefaclor for Suspension
	equivalent to anhydrous cefaclor 187 mg/5 mL*	Cefaclor for Suspension
	equivalent to anhydrous cefaclor 250 mg/5 mL*	Cefaclor for Suspension
	equivalent to anhydrous cefaclor 375 mg/5 mL*	Cefaclor for Suspension
Tablets, extended-release	equivalent to anhydrous cefaclor 500 mg*	Cefaclor Extended-Release Tablets

*available from one or more manufacturer, distributor, and/or repackager by generic (nonproprietary) name

†Use is not currently included in the labeling approved by the US Food and Drug Administration

Cefprozil

■ Cefprozil is a semisynthetic, second generation cephalosporin antibiotic.

Uses

Cefprozil is used orally for the treatment of mild to moderate respiratory tract infections (i.e., acute sinusitis, secondary bacterial infections of acute bronchitis, acute exacerbations of chronic bronchitis, community-acquired pneumonia†) caused by susceptible bacteria. The drug also is used orally for the treatment of acute otitis media caused by susceptible bacteria, pharyngitis and tonsillitis caused by *Streptococcus pyogenes* (group A β-hemolytic streptococci), and mild to moderate uncomplicated skin and skin structure infections caused by susceptible bacteria.

■ **Acute Otitis Media** Oral cefprozil is used in children 6 months through 12 years of age for the treatment of acute otitis media (AOM) caused by *Streptococcus pneumoniae*, *Haemophilus influenzae* (including β-lactamase-producing strains), or *Moraxella catarrhalis* (including β-lactamase-producing strains).

When anti-infective therapy is indicated for the treatment of AOM, the American Academy of Pediatrics (AAP) recommends high-dose amoxicillin or amoxicillin and clavulanate potassium as the drugs of first choice for initial treatment. These experts recommend certain cephalosporins (cefdinir, cefpodoxime, cefuroxime, ceftriaxone) as alternatives for initial treatment in penicillin-allergic patients who do not have a history of severe and/or recent penicillin-allergic reactions.

Results of controlled clinical studies in children 6 months to 17 years of age with clinically and/or microbiologically confirmed AOM indicate that a 10-day regimen of oral cefprozil generally is as effective as a 10-day regimen of oral cefaclor, oral cefixime, oral amoxicillin and clavulanate potassium, or oral ceftibuten. In published studies, the overall clinical response rate to a 10-day regimen of oral cefprozil in pediatric patients with AOM has been 83–97% and the bacteriologic eradication rate has been 84–95%. Although the clinical and bacteriologic response rates to oral cefprozil in pediatric patients with AOM generally have been similar to those reported with oral amoxicillin and clavulanate potassium, the manufacturer cautions that, in patients with otitis media caused by β-lactamase-producing bacteria, cefprozil therapy may be associated with a slightly lower bacteriologic eradication rate than therapy with an anti-infective agent that contains a specific β-lactamase inhibitor (i.e., amoxicillin and clavulanate potassium) and that the possibility of reduced overall efficacy should be weighed carefully against *local* susceptibility patterns for common pathogens encountered in this infection when considering use of cefprozil for the treatment of otitis media.

In one study in children 6 months to 12 years of age with AOM with middle ear effusion, including patients with recurrent otitis media (i.e., 4 or more prior episodes of AOM within the last 12 months or 3 or more prior episodes within the last 6 months) or persistent AOM (i.e., symptoms of otalgia and signs of middle ear inflammation despite the fact that anti-infective agent therapy was given within the last 7 days), the overall clinical response rate to 10 days of oral cefprozil therapy (30 mg/kg daily) was 78%. When results of children with AOM caused by a single identified pathogen were stratified according to the causative organism, the clinical response rate to cefprozil was 91% in those with otitis media caused by *M. catarrhalis*, 77–81% in those with otitis media caused by *S. pneumoniae* or *H. influenzae*, and 71% in those with otitis media caused by *S. pyogenes*.

Cefprozil has been effective for the treatment of AOM in pediatric patients when administered in a 5-day regimen†, and there is some evidence that the 5-day regimen may be as effective as the usually recommended 10-day regimen for the treatment of AOM in certain pediatric patients without a history of recurrent infections. In one controlled study in children 3 months to 14 years of age with AOM who were randomized to receive 5 or 10 days of oral cefprozil (30 mg/kg daily given in 2 divided doses), a satisfactory clinical response (cure or improvement) was attained in 94.4% of those who received the 5-day regimen and 96.4% of those who received the 10-day regimen. However, in the subgroup of patients with a history of 3 or more prior episodes of AOM, the clinical response rate was 100% in those who received the 10-day regimen versus 70% in those who received the 5-day regimen. Further study is needed to evaluate use of a 5-day regimen of oral cefprozil for the treatment of AOM. The AAP states that oral anti-infective regimens of less than 10 days' duration are not recommended for the treatment of AOM in children younger than 2 years of age or in patients with severe symptoms.

For additional information regarding treatment of AOM, including information on diagnosis and management strategies, anti-infectives for initial treatment, duration of initial treatment, and anti-infectives after initial treatment failure, see Acute Otitis Media under Uses: Otitis Media, in the Cephalosporins General Statement 8:12.06.

■ **Pharyngitis and Tonsillitis** Oral cefprozil is used in adults and children 2 years of age or older for the treatment of pharyngitis and tonsillitis caused by susceptible *S. pyogenes* (group A β-hemolytic streptococci). Although cefprozil usually is effective in eradicating *S. pyogenes* from the nasopharynx, substantial data to establish efficacy of the drug for prophylaxis of subsequent rheumatic fever are not available to date.

Selection of an anti-infective for the treatment of *S. pyogenes* pharyngitis and tonsillitis should be based on the drug's spectrum of activity, bacteriologic and clinical efficacy, potential adverse effects, ease of administration, patient compliance, and cost. No regimen has been found to date that effectively eradicates group A β-hemolytic streptococci in 100% of patients.

Because the drugs have a narrow spectrum of activity, are inexpensive, and generally are effective with a low frequency of adverse effects, AAP, Infectious Diseases Society of America (IDSA), American Heart Association (AHA), and others recommend a penicillin regimen (i.e., 10 days of oral penicillin V or oral amoxicillin or a single dose of IM penicillin G benzathine) as the treatment of choice for *S. pyogenes* pharyngitis and tonsillitis and prevention of initial attacks (primary prevention) of rheumatic fever. Other anti-infectives (e.g., oral cephalosporins, oral macrolides, oral clindamycin) are recommended as alternatives in penicillin-allergic individuals.

If an oral cephalosporin is used for the treatment of *S. pyogenes* pharyngitis and tonsillitis, a 10-day regimen of a first generation cephalosporin (cefadroxil, cephalexin) is preferred instead of other cephalosporins with broader spectrums of activity (e.g., cefaclor, cefdinir, cefixime, cefpodoxime, cefuroxime).

Although there is some evidence that a shorter duration of therapy with certain oral cephalosporins (e.g., a 5-day regimen of cefadroxil, cefdinir, cefixime, or cefpodoxime proxetil or a 4- or 5-day regimen of cefuroxime axetil) achieves bacteriologic and clinical cure rates equal to or greater than those achieved with the traditional 10-day oral penicillin V regimen, the IDSA and AHA state that use of cephalosporin regimens administered for 5 days or less for the treatment of *S. pyogenes* pharyngitis and tonsillitis cannot be recommended at this time.

Results of randomized, multicenter studies in pediatric patients with streptococcal pharyngitis or tonsillitis indicate that a 10-day regimen of oral cefprozil is more effective than a 10-day regimen of oral penicillin V. In one study in children 3–18 years of age with streptococcal pharyngitis or tonsillitis randomized to receive 10 days of oral cefprozil (7.5 mg/kg twice daily) or 10 days of oral penicillin V (16.25 mg/kg 3 times daily), the clinical response rate (cure or improvement) was 95.3% in those who received cefprozil versus 88.1% in those who received penicillin V; the bacteriologic eradication rates were 89 or 84.2%, respectively. A 10-day regimen of oral cefprozil has been used effectively to eradicate *S. pyogenes* in pediatric patients who failed to respond to a 10-day regimen of oral penicillin V.

In an open, randomized study in adults and adolescents 12 years of age or older with acute streptococcal pharyngitis, a 10-day regimen of oral cefprozil (500 mg once daily) was at least as effective as a 10-day regimen of oral cefaclor (250 mg 3 times daily); the clinical response rate was 85% for both drugs and the bacteriologic eradication rate was 91% in those who received cefprozil and 95% in those who received cefaclor. In another study in adults and children 2 years of age or older randomized to receive oral cefprozil or oral cefaclor, the overall clinical response rate was 80% in those who received cefprozil and 72% in those who received cefaclor; the bacteriologic eradication rates were 83 and 76%, respectively.

■ **Respiratory Tract Infections** ***Acute Sinusitis*** Oral cefprozil is used in adults and children 6 months of age or older for the treatment of acute sinusitis caused by *S. pneumoniae*, *H. influenzae* (including β-lactamase-producing strains), or *M. catarrhalis* (including β-lactamase-producing strains). In an open-label, multicenter study in adults and children 13 years of age or older with acute maxillary sinusitis, the overall clinical response rate was 80–83% in those who received cefprozil and 78% in those who received amoxicillin and clavulanate potassium.

When anti-infective therapy is indicated for the treatment of acute bacterial sinusitis, the IDSA recommends amoxicillin and clavulanate potassium and the AAP recommends either amoxicillin or amoxicillin and clavulanate potassium as the drug of choice for initial empiric treatment. Because of variable activity against *S. pneumoniae* and *H. influenzae*, the IDSA no longer recommends second or third generation oral cephalosporins for empiric monotherapy of sinusitis in adults or children. If an oral cephalosporin is used as an alternative for empiric treatment of acute bacterial sinusitis in children (e.g., in penicillin-allergic individuals), the IDSA and AAP recommend a combination regimen that includes a third generation cephalosporin (cefixime or cefpodoxime) and clindamycin (or linezolid).

Acute and Chronic Bronchitis Oral cefprozil is used in adults and children 13 years of age or older for the treatment of secondary bacterial infections of acute bronchitis and acute bacterial exacerbations of chronic bronchitis caused by susceptible *S. pneumoniae*, *H. influenzae* (including β-lactamase-producing strains), or *M. catarrhalis* (including β-lactamase-producing strains). Safety and efficacy of the drug for the treatment of these infections in children 12 years of age or younger have not been established to date.

Results of a multicenter, open-label randomized study in adults with bronchitis indicate that oral cefprozil (500 mg every 12 hours) may be slightly more effective than oral cefuroxime axetil (500 mg every 12 hours) for these infections. The overall clinical response rate was 96% in those who received cefprozil and 82.5% in those who received cefuroxime; the bacteriologic eradication rate was 100% and 91.7%, respectively.

Community-Acquired Pneumonia Cefprozil is used in the treatment of mild to moderate community-acquired pneumonia† (CAP).

If an oral cephalosporin is used as an alternative to penicillin G or amoxicillin for treatment of CAP caused by penicillin-susceptible *S. pneumoniae*, the American Thoracic Society (ATS) and IDSA recommend cefpodoxime, cefprozil, cefuroxime, cefdinir, or cefditoren.

For additional information on treatment of CAP, see Community-acquired Pneumonia under Uses: Respiratory Tract Infections, in the Cephalosporins General Statement 8:12.06.

■ **Skin and Skin Structure Infections** Oral cefprozil is used in adults and children 2 years of age or older for the treatment of uncomplicated skin and skin structure infections caused by *Staphylococcus aureus* (including penicillinase-producing strains) and *S. pyogenes*. The drug also has been effective when used in a limited number of patients for the treatment of uncomplicated skin and skin structure infections caused by *S. epidermidis*†, *S. saprophyticus*†, group B or G streptococci†, *Escherichia coli*†, or *Klebsiella pneumoniae*†. Abscesses should be surgically drained if indicated.

Results of multicenter, randomized studies in adults and children 2 years of age or older with mild to moderate bacterial skin and skin structure infections (e.g., carbuncle, cellulitis, folliculitis, furuncle, impetigo, infected dermatitis, paronychia, pyoderma, superficial abscess, wound infection) indicate that 5–10 days of therapy with oral cefprozil (250 mg twice daily or 500 mg once daily in adults; 20 mg/kg once daily in children) is at least as effective as 5–10 days of therapy with oral cefaclor (250 mg 3 times daily in adults or 20 mg/kg daily in 3 doses). A satisfactory clinical response was attained in 93–95% of patients who received cefprozil and in 78–92% of patients who received cefaclor; the bacteriologic eradication rates were 86–91% and 74–89%, respectively.

Dosage and Administration

■ **Reconstitution and Administration** Cefprozil is administered orally.

Administration of cefprozil tablets or oral suspension with food does not affect the extent of absorption or peak plasma concentrations of the drug, but may increase the time to peak concentrations. (See Pharmacokinetics: Absorption.)

Reconstitution Cefprozil powder for oral suspension should be reconstituted at the time of dispensing by adding the amount of water specified on the container to provide a suspension containing 125 or 250 mg of cefprozil per 5 mL. The water should be added in 2 equal portions and the bottle shaken after each addition.

The oral suspension should be shaken well prior to administration of each dose.

■ **Dosage** Cefprozil is commercially available as the monohydrate; dosage is expressed in terms of anhydrous cefprozil.

Adult Dosage **Pharyngitis and Tonsillitis.** The usual dosage of cefprozil for the treatment of pharyngitis and tonsillitis caused by *Streptococcus pyogenes* (group A β-hemolytic streptococci) in adults and adolescents 13 years of age or older is 500 mg once daily for at least 10 days.

Respiratory Tract Infections. For the treatment of acute sinusitis in adults and adolescents 13 years of age or older, the usual dosage of cefprozil is 250 or 500 mg every 12 hours for 10 days; the higher dosage should be used to treat moderate to severe sinusitis.

For the treatment of secondary bacterial infections of acute bronchitis and acute bacterial exacerbations of chronic bronchitis, the usual dosage of cefprozil for adults and adolescents 13 years of age or older is 500 mg every 12 hours for 10 days.

Skin and Skin Structure Infections. For the treatment of uncomplicated skin and skin structure infections in adults and adolescents 13 years of age or older, the usual dosage of cefprozil is 250 or 500 mg every 12 hours or 500 mg once daily for 10 days.

Pediatric Dosage Children 13 years of age or older may receive the usual adult dosage of cefprozil.

General Pediatric Dosage. The American Academy of Pediatrics (AAP) recommends that pediatric patients beyond the neonatal period receive cefprozil in a dosage of 15–30 mg/kg daily in 2 equally divided doses for the treatment of mild or moderate infections. The AAP states that the drug is inappropriate for the treatment of severe infections.

Acute Otitis Media. For the treatment of acute otitis media in children 6 months through 12 years of age, the usual dosage of cefprozil is 15 mg/kg every 12 hours for 10 days.

Pharyngitis and Tonsillitis. The usual dosage of cefprozil for the treatment of pharyngitis and tonsillitis caused by *S. pyogenes* (group A β-hemolytic streptococci) in children 2–12 years of age is 7.5 mg/kg every 12 hours for at least 10 days.

Respiratory Tract Infections. For the treatment of acute sinusitis in children 6 months through 12 years of age, the usual dosage of cefprozil is 7.5 or 15 mg/kg every 12 hours for 10 days; the higher dosage should be used to treat moderate to severe infections.

Skin and Skin Structure Infections. For the treatment of uncomplicated skin and skin structure infections in children 2–12 years of age, the usual dosage of cefprozil is 20 mg/kg once daily for 10 days.

■ **Dosage in Renal and Hepatic Impairment** In patients with creatinine clearances less than 30 mL/minute, dose but not frequency of administration of cefprozil should be modified; such patients should receive 50% of the usual cefprozil dose using the usual dosing period. Because the drug is partially removed by hemodialysis, cefprozil should be administered to patients undergoing hemodialysis after the end of the dialysis period.

Modification of usual dosage of cefprozil is not necessary in patients with hepatic impairment.

Cautions

Adverse effects reported with cefprozil are similar to those reported with other cephalosporins. (See Cautions in the Cephalosporins General Statement 8:12.06.) Cefprozil generally is well tolerated; most adverse effects are transient and mild to moderate in severity. Adverse effects have been severe enough to require discontinuance in about 2% of patients. The most frequent adverse effects of cefprozil involve the GI tract. In young children, diarrhea, vomiting, and rash (principally in the diaper area) appear to be most common, while in adults, diarrhea and nausea appear to be most common.

■ **GI Effects** Nausea is one of the most common adverse effects of cefprozil, occurring in 3.5% of patients receiving the drug. Diarrhea or loose stools have occurred in 2.9% of patients receiving cefprozil. The incidence of diarrhea with cefprozil appears to be comparable to that with cefaclor but less than that with amoxicillin and clavulanate potassium, and possibly some other oral cephalosporins. Vomiting and abdominal pain or discomfort each have occurred in 1% of patients. Dyspepsia, flatulence, glossitis, and mouth pain have been reported rarely in patients receiving cefprozil; a causal relationship to the drug has not been established. Adverse GI effects may be severe enough to result in discontinuance of cefprozil.

Clostridium difficile-associated Diarrhea and Colitis Treatment with anti-infectives alters normal colon flora and may permit overgrowth of *Clostridium difficile*.

C. difficile infection (CDI) and *C. difficile*-associated diarrhea and colitis (CDAD; also known as antibiotic-associated diarrhea and colitis or pseudomembranous colitis) have been reported with nearly all anti-infectives, including cefprozil, and may range in severity from mild diarrhea to fatal colitis. *C. difficile* produces toxins A and B which contribute to development of CDAD; hypertoxin-producing strains of *C. difficile* are associated with increased morbidity and mortality since they may be refractory to anti-infectives and colectomy may be required.

CDAD should be considered in the differential diagnosis in patients who develop diarrhea during or after anti-infective therapy. Careful medical history is necessary since CDAD has been reported to occur as late as 2 months or longer after anti-infective therapy is discontinued.

If CDAD is suspected or confirmed, anti-infective therapy not directed against *C. difficile* should be discontinued whenever possible. Patients should be managed with appropriate supportive therapy (e.g., fluid and electrolyte management, protein supplementation), anti-infective therapy directed against *C. difficile* (e.g., metronidazole, vancomycin), and surgical evaluation as clinically indicated. (See Superinfection/Clostridium difficile-associated Diarrhea and Colitis under Cautions: Precautions and Contraindications.)

■ **Dermatologic and Sensitivity Reactions** Rash occurred in 0.9% of patients receiving cefprozil in clinical studies. In young children, rash associated with cefprozil therapy most commonly is a diaper rash rather than a sensitivity reaction. Urticaria and pruritus have been reported rarely. Anaphylaxis, serum-sickness-like reactions, erythema, exanthema, erythema multiforme, erythema nodosum, and Stevens-Johnson syndrome also have been reported rarely; however, a causal relationship with cefprozil has not been established. Sensitivity reactions (e.g., rash, urticaria) have been reported more frequently in children than in adults. Such reactions usually occur within a few days after initiation of therapy and subside within a few days after discontinuance of the drug. Toxic epidermal necrolysis has been reported with cephalosporins. If a severe hypersensitivity reaction occurs during cefprozil therapy, the drug should be discontinued and the patient given appropriate treatment (e.g., epinephrine, corticosteroids, maintenance of an adequate airway, oxygen) as indicated.

■ **Nervous System Effects** Dizziness has been reported in 1% of patients receiving cefprozil. Hyperactivity, headache, nervousness, insomnia, confusion, and somnolence each have been reported in less than 1% of patients receiving the drug. Lightheadedness has been reported rarely.

Although seizures have not been reported in patients receiving cefprozil, several cephalosporins have been implicated in precipitating seizures, particularly in patients with renal impairment in whom the dosage was not reduced. If seizures associated with cefprozil therapy occur, the drug should be discontinued and anticonvulsant therapy administered if clinically indicated.

■ **Hepatic Effects** Increases in serum AST (SGOT) and ALT (SGPT) concentrations have been reported in 2% of patients receiving cefprozil. Elevations in serum alkaline phosphatase and bilirubin concentrations also have been reported in 0.2% and less than 0.1%, respectively, of patients receiving the drug. Cholestatic jaundice has been reported rarely in patients receiving cefprozil. Increases in serum LDH concentrations have been reported in patients receiving cephalosporins.

■ **Hematologic Effects** Eosinophilia has been reported in 2.3% of patients receiving cefprozil. Decreased leukocyte count has been reported in 0.2% of patients receiving the drug. Although a causal relationship has not been established, neutropenia, thrombocytopenia, prolonged partial thromboplastin time, thrombocytosis,prolonged prothrombin time, prolonged prothrombin ratio, and decreased hematocrit have been reported rarely in patients receiving cefprozil.

Other adverse hematologic effects reported in patients receiving cephalosporins include positive antiglobulin (Coombs') test results, agranulocytosis, aplastic anemia, pancytopenia, hemolytic anemia, and hemorrhage.

■ **Renal Effects** Elevated BUN and serum creatinine concentrations each have been reported in 0.1% of patients receiving cefprozil. Adverse renal effects reported in patients receiving cephalosporins include renal dysfunction and toxic nephropathy.

■ **Other Adverse Effects** Vaginitis and genital pruritus have been reported in 1.6% of patients receiving cefprozil. Leukorrhea and vaginal candidiasis have been reported infrequently. Diaper rash and superinfection have been reported in 1.5% of patients receiving the drug. Although a causal relationship to cefprozil has not been established, fever, chills, sweating, tinnitus, visual field defects, generalized pain, back pain, leg pain, angioedema, and crying have been reported rarely.

■ **Precautions and Contraindications** Cefprozil shares the toxic potentials of the cephalosporins, and the usual precautions of cephalosporin therapy should be observed.

Sensitivity Reactions Prior to initiation of cefprozil therapy, careful inquiry should be made concerning previous hypersensitivity reactions to cefprozil, other cephalosporins, penicillins, or other drugs. There is clinical and laboratory evidence of partial cross-allergenicity among β-lactam antibiotics including penicillins, cephalosporins, and cephamycins.

Cefprozil is contraindicated in patients with known hypersensitivity to cephalosporins and should be used with caution in patients with a history of hypersensitivity to penicillins. Use of cephalosporins should be avoided in patients who have had an immediate-type (anaphylactic) hypersensitivity reaction to penicillins.

If a hypersensitivity reaction occurs during cefprozil therapy, the drug should be discontinued and the patient treated with appropriate therapy (e.g., epinephrine, corticosteroids, and maintenance of an adequate airway and oxygen as indicated.

Selection and Use of Anti-infectives To reduce development of drug-resistant bacteria and maintain effectiveness of cefprozil and other antibacterials, the drug should be used only for the treatment or prevention of infections proven or strongly suspected to be caused by susceptible bacteria. When selecting or modifying anti-infective therapy, results of culture and in vitro susceptibility testing should be used. In the absence of such data, local epidemiology and susceptibility patterns should be considered when selecting anti-infectives for empiric therapy.

Patients should be advised that antibacterials (including cefprozil) should only be used to treat bacterial infections and not used to treat viral infections (e.g., the common cold). Patients also should be advised about the importance of completing the full course of therapy, even if feeling better after a few days, and that skipping doses or not completing therapy may decrease effectiveness and increase the likelihood that bacteria will develop resistance and will not be treatable with cefprozil or other antibacterials in the future.

Superinfection/Clostridium difficile-associated Diarrhea and Colitis As with other anti-infective agents, prolonged use of cefprozil may result in overgrowth of nonsusceptible organisms. Careful observation of the patient during cefprozil therapy is essential. If superinfection occurs, appropriate therapy should be initiated.

Because CDI and *C. difficile*-associated diarrhea and colitis have been reported with the use of cefprozil or other cephalosporins, it should be considered in the differential diagnosis of patients who develop diarrhea during or following cefprozil therapy.

Patients should be advised that diarrhea is a common problem caused by anti-infectives and usually resolves when the drug is discontinued; however, they should contact a clinician if severe watery or bloody stools (with or without stomach cramps and fever) occur during or as late as 2 months or longer after the last dose.

Cefprozil should be used with caution in patients with a history of GI disease, especially colitis.

Other Precautions and Contraindications In patients with known or suspected renal impairment, careful observation and appropriate laboratory studies should be performed prior to and during cefprozil therapy. Because plasma concentrations of cefprozil may be higher and more prolonged in these patients, doses and/or frequency of administration should be decreased. (See Dosage and Administration: Dosage in Renal and Hepatic Impairment.) The manufacturer states that cephalosporins, including cefprozil, should be used with caution in patients receiving potent diuretics (e.g., furosemide), since concomitant use of these drugs may adversely affect renal function.

Individuals with phenylketonuria (i.e., homozygous genetic deficiency of phenylalanine hydroxylase) and other individuals who must restrict their intake of phenylalanine should be warned that oral suspensions of cefprozil contains aspartame (NutraSweet®) which is metabolized to phenylalanine in the GI tract following oral administration.

Positive direct antiglobulin (Coombs') test results have been reported in patients receiving a cephalosporin. (See Cautions: Hematologic Effects, in the Cephalosporins General Statement 8:12.06.) Patients receiving a cephalosporin, including cefprozil, may show a false-positive result in urine glucose determinations using cupric sulfate (e.g., Benedict's solution, Fehling's solution, Clinitest®).

Urinary glucose determinations using glucose oxidase methods (e.g., Clinistix®, Tes-Tape®) are unaffected by the drugs. A false-negative result may occur in the ferricyanide test for blood glucose. Cefprozil does not interfere with the alkaline picrate method used to determine plasma or urinary creatinine concentrations.

■ **Pediatric Precautions** Safety and efficacy of cefprozil for the treatment of acute otitis media or acute sinusitis in children younger than 6 months of age or the treatment of pharyngitis and tonsillitis or uncomplicated skin and skin structure infections in children younger than 2 years of age have not been established. The manufacturers caution that drug accumulation secondary to prolonged elimination has been reported in neonates receiving other cephalosporins.

Sensitivity reactions (e.g., rash, urticaria) have been reported more frequently in children than in adults. The most common adverse effects occurring in children receiving cefprozil are similar to those seen in adults and include diarrhea, nausea, vomiting, and rash.

■ **Geriatric Precautions** Of the more than 4500 adults who received cefprozil in clinical studies, 14% were 65 years of age or older, while 5% were 75 years of age and older. Although no overall differences in efficacy or safety were observed between geriatric and younger patients, and other clinical experience revealed no evidence of age-related differences, the possibility that some older patients may exhibit increased sensitivity to the drug cannot be ruled out. Cefprozil is known to be substantially excreted by the kidney, and the risk of cefprozil-induced toxicity may be greater in patients with renal impairment. Because geriatric patients may have decreased renal function, initial dosage should be selected carefully and it may be useful to monitor renal function.

■ **Mutagenicity and Carcinogenicity** Mutagenesis studies performed in appropriate prokaryotic and eukaryotic cells in vitro or in vivo have not shown cefprozil to be mutagenic. Long-term in vivo studies have not been performed to date to evaluate the carcinogenic potential of the drug.

■ **Pregnancy, Fertility, and Lactation** Reproduction studies in mice, rats, or rabbits using oral cefprozil in dosages 0.8, 8.5, or 18.5 times, respectively, the maximum daily human dose (1 g) based upon mg/m^2 have not revealed evidence of harm to the fetus. There are no adequate and well-controlled studies to date using cefprozil in pregnant women or during labor and delivery, and the drug should be used during pregnancy or labor and delivery only when clearly needed.

Reproduction studies in male or female rats receiving oral cefprozil in dosages up to 18.5 times the maximum recommended human dosage have not revealed evidence of impaired fertility.

Because trace concentrations of cefprozil (less than 0.3% of a dose) are distributed into milk, the drug should be used with caution in nursing women.

Spectrum

Based on its spectrum of activity, cefprozil is classified as a second generation cephalosporin. For information on the classification of cephalosporins and closely related β-lactam antibiotics based on spectra of activity, see Spectrum in the Cephalosporins General Statement 8:12.06.

Like other currently available second generation cephalosporins (e.g., cefaclor, cefamandole, cefuroxime), cefprozil is active in vitro against both gram-positive and gram-negative bacteria. The drug generally is more active in vitro against gram-negative bacteria than first generation cephalosporins, but has a narrower spectrum of activity against gram-negative bacteria than third generation cephalosporins. The spectrum of activity of cefprozil is similar to that of cefaclor; however, in vitro on a weight basis, cefprozil may be more active against susceptible organisms than cefaclor.

■ **In Vitro Susceptibility Testing** Strains of staphylococci resistant to penicillinase-resistant penicillins (methicillin-resistant [oxacillin-resistant] staphylococci) should be considered resistant to cefprozil, although results of in vitro susceptibility tests may indicate that the organisms are susceptible to the drug. In addition, β-lactamase-negative, ampicillin-resistant (BLNAR) strains of *H. influenzae* should be considered resistant to cefprozil despite the fact that results of in vitro susceptibility tests may indicate that the organisms are susceptible to the drug.

For information on interpreting results of in vitro susceptibility testing (disk susceptibility tests, dilution susceptibility tests) when cefprozil susceptibility testing is performed according to the standards of the Clinical and Laboratory Standards Institute (CLSI; formerly National Committee for Clinical Laboratory Standards [NCCLS]), see Spectrum: In Vitro Susceptibility Testing, in the Cephalosporins General Statement 8:12.06.

Pharmacokinetics

Some of the pharmacokinetic data described in the Pharmacokinetics section were derived from studies that involved cefprozil capsules (not commercially available in the US); however, these capsules, cefprozil oral solution (not commercially available in the US), commercially available cefprozil film-coated tablets, and commercially available cefprozil oral suspension have been shown to be bioequivalent when administered under fasting conditions. Results of high-pressure liquid chromatographic (HPLC) assays that distinguish between the *cis-* and *trans-*isomers of cefprozil indicate that the pharmacokinetics of the isomers are identical and the proportions of *cis-* and *trans-*cefprozil in plasma and urine are similar to those contained in commercially available preparations of the drug (i.e., approximately a 9:1 ratio).

In adults with normal renal function, peak plasma concentrations and area under the plasma concentration-time curve (AUC) of cefprozil increase in proportion to the dose over the dosage range of 250 mg to 1 g, and there is no evidence that the drug accumulates in plasma following multiple oral doses (up to 1 g every 8 hours for 8–10 days). Results of pharmacokinetic studies indicate that the AUC of cefprozil reported in healthy geriatric adults (i.e., adults 65 years of age or older) is 35–60% higher than that reported in younger healthy adults (20–40 years of age) and that the average AUC in adult females is 15–20% higher than that reported in adult males. Studies in adults with impaired renal function indicate that the pharmacokinetics of cefprozil are affected by the degree of renal impairment and that plasma half-life of the drug increases with decreasing renal impairment. The plasma half-life of cefprozil is increased slightly in patients with hepatic impairment, but this does not necessitate a change in dosage of the drug.

■ **Absorption** Following oral administration of cefprozil in fasting adults, bioavailability of the drug is approximately 90–95%. Studies using commercially available cefprozil tablets or oral suspension indicate that presence of food in the GI tract does not affect the extent of absorption or peak plasma concentrations of the drug; however, compared with administration in the fasting state, the time to peak plasma concentrations may be prolonged by 15–45 minutes when the drug is administered with food. Results of a crossover study using cefprozil capsules (not commercially available in the US) indicate that bioavailability of the drug is not affected by concomitant administration of an antacid containing magnesium hydroxide and aluminum hydroxide.

In healthy, fasting adults who receive a single 250-mg, 500-mg, or 1-g oral dose of cefprozil as capsules, peak plasma concentrations are attained within 1.5 hours and average 6.1, 10.5, or 18.3 mcg/mL, respectively; plasma concentrations 8 hours after the dose average 0.2, 0.4, or 1 mcg/mL, respectively.

In pediatric patients 8 months to 8 years of age who received a single 15- or 30-mg/kg oral dose of cefprozil as the oral suspension, peak plasma concentrations were attained within 1.2–1.4 hours and averaged 11.2 or 15.9 mcg/mL, respectively. In pediatric patients 6 months to 12 years of age who received a single 7.5-, 15-, or 30-mg/kg oral dose of the drug as the oral suspension, peak plasma concentrations were attained within 1–2 hours; plasma concentrations averaged 3.99, 8.47, or 17.61 mcg/mL, respectively, 2 hours after the dose and 0.91, 2.75, or 8.66 mcg/mL, respectively, 4 hours after the dose.

■ **Distribution** The steady-state volume of distribution of cefprozil is estimated to be 0.23 L/kg in healthy adults with normal renal function.

Following oral administration, cefprozil is distributed into various body tissues and fluids including blister fluid, middle ear fluid, and tonsillar and adenoidal tissue.

In pediatric patients with chronic otitis media with effusion who received a single 15- or 20-mg/kg oral dose of cefprozil as the oral suspension, concentrations of the drug in middle ear fluid collected within 6 hours of the dose ranged from 0.06–4.4 or 0.17–8.67 mcg/mL, respectively; concurrent plasma concentrations ranged from 0.38–15.97 or 1.28–21.47 mcg/mL, respectively.

In children 2–14 years of age undergoing elective tonsillectomy and/or adenoidectomy who received a single 7.5- or 20-mg/kg dose of cefprozil as the oral suspension, concentrations of the drug in tonsillar or adenoidal tissue ranged from 37–47 or 46–82% of concurrent plasma concentrations, respectively.

Information on distribution of cefprozil into CSF is not available.

Cefprozil is distributed into milk in low concentrations following oral administration (i.e., in concentrations less than 0.3% of the dose). In a study in women who received a single 1-g dose of oral cefprozil, concentrations of the drug in breast milk over the next 24 hours ranged from 0.25–3.36 mcg/mL.

Cefprozil is 35–45% bound to plasma proteins; binding is independent of drug concentration over the range of 2–20 mcg/mL.

■ **Elimination** In adults with normal renal function, the plasma half-life of cefprozil averages 1–1.4 hours and renal clearance of the drug averages 1.78–2.53 mL/minute per kg. The plasma half-life of the drug in pediatric patients 6 months to 12 years of age averages 0.94–2.1 hours.

Cefprozil is eliminated principally in urine by glomerular filtration and tubular secretion. Approximately 54–70% of a single oral dose of the drug is eliminated unchanged in urine within 24 hours. In adults with normal renal function who receive a single 250-mg, 500-mg, or 1-g oral dose of cefprozil, concentrations of the drug in urine over the first 4 hours following the dose average 700, 1000, and 2900 mcg/mL, respectively. Renal clearance of the drug following a single 1-g dose of cefprozil reportedly is 40% lower in healthy adults 65 years of age and older than in healthy adults 20–40 years of age.

The plasma half-life of cefprozil is prolonged in patients with renal impairment and, depending on the degree of impairment, may average 5.2–5.9 hours. In a study in patients with hepatic impairment who received a single 1-g oral dose of cefprozil, the plasma half-life of the drug averaged 2.2 hours.

Cefprozil is removed by hemodialysis.

Chemistry and Stability

■ **Chemistry** Cefprozil is a semisynthetic cephalosporin antibiotic. The drug is an oral cephalosporin structurally similar to cefaclor; however, cefprozil contains a *p*-hydroxyphenyl group at position 7 of the cephalosporin nucleus and contains a 1-propenyl group at position 3 instead of the chloride contained in cefaclor. Cefprozil is an isomeric mixture of the *cis*- and *trans*-isomers of the drug in approximately a 9:1 ratio. Both isomers have similar antibacterial activity against gram-positive bacteria; however, the *cis*-isomer is 8–9 times more active against gram-negative bacteria than the*trans*-isomer.

Cefprozil is commercially available as the monohydrate; potency is calculated on the anhydrous basis. Cefprozil occurs as a white to yellowish powder. The drug is slightly soluble in water and practically insoluble in alcohol. Cefprozil has a pK_as of about 2.7, 7.4, and 9.7. Following reconstitution, cefprozil oral suspension containing 125 or 250 mg of cefprozil per 5 mL occurs as a pink, bubble-gum-flavored suspension.

■ **Stability** Cefprozil tablets should be stored at 20–25°C.

Cefprozil powder for oral suspension should be stored at 20–25°C. Following reconstitution, cefprozil oral suspension should be stored in a tight container in a refrigerator; any unused suspension should be discarded after 14 days.

For further information on chemistry, mechanism of action, spectrum, resistance, uses, cautions, acute toxicity, drug interactions, or laboratory test interferences of cefprozil, see the Cephalosporins General Statement 8:12.06.

Preparations

Excipients in commercially available drug preparations may have clinically important effects in some individuals; consult specific product labeling for details.

Cefprozil

Oral		
For suspension	125 mg (of anhydrous cefprozil) per 5 mL*	**Cefprozil for Suspension**
	250 mg (of anhydrous cefprozil) per 5 mL*	**Cefprozil for Suspension**
Tablets, film-coated	250 mg (of anhydrous cefprozil)*	**Cefprozil Film-coated Tablets**
	500 mg (of anhydrous cefprozil)*	**Cefprozil Film-coated Tablets**

*available from one or more manufacturer, distributor, and/or repackager by generic (nonproprietary) name

†Use is not currently included in the labeling approved by the US Food and Drug Administration

Cefuroxime Axetil
Cefuroxime Sodium

■ Cefuroxime is a semisynthetic, second generation cephalosporin antibiotic.

Uses

Cefuroxime axetil is used orally for the treatment of mild to moderate respiratory tract infections (i.e., acute maxillary sinusitis, acute exacerbations of chronic bronchitis, secondary infections of acute bronchitis, community-acquired pneumonia†) caused by susceptible bacteria; acute bacterial otitis media; pharyngitis and tonsillitis caused by *Streptococcus pyogenes* (group A β-hemolytic streptococci); mild to moderate uncomplicated skin and skin structure infections caused by *Staphylococcus aureus* (including β-lactamase-producing strains) or *S. pyogenes*; and uncomplicated urinary tract infections caused by *Escherichia coli* or *Klebsiella pneumoniae*. Cefuroxime axetil also is used orally for the treatment of Lyme disease and has been used for the treatment of uncomplicated gonorrhea. The manufacturers of cefuroxime axetil oral suspension state that safety and efficacy of the suspension have been established only for the treatment of pharyngitis and tonsillitis, acute otitis media, and impetigo caused by susceptible bacteria. and for the treatment of Lyme disease.

Cefuroxime sodium is used parenterally in the treatment of lower respiratory tract infections (including pneumonia), serious skin and skin structure infections, genitourinary tract infections, bone and joint infections, septicemia, and meningitis caused by susceptible organisms. Cefuroxime sodium also has been used parenterally for perioperative prophylaxis.

Because cefuroxime, like other second generation cephalosporins, generally is less active against susceptible gram-positive cocci than are first generation cephalosporins, most clinicians state that cefuroxime probably should not be used in the treatment of infections caused by gram-positive bacteria when a penicillin or a first generation cephalosporin could be used. In addition, because cefuroxime generally is less active in vitro against Enterobacteriaceae than third generation cephalosporins, some clinicians state that a third generation drug such as cefotaxime or ceftriaxone generally is preferred if a parenteral cephalosporin is indicated in the treatment of infections known or suspected to be caused by these gram-negative bacteria.

Prior to initiation of cefuroxime therapy, appropriate specimens should be obtained for identification of the causative organism and in vitro susceptibility tests. If cefuroxime is started pending results of susceptibility tests, it should be discontinued if the causative organism is found to be resistant to the drug. In the treatment of known or suspected sepsis or the treatment of other serious infections when the causative organism is unknown, concomitant therapy with an aminoglycoside may be indicated pending results of in vitro susceptibility tests.

■ **Acute Otitis Media** Cefuroxime axetil is used orally for the treatment of acute otitis media (AOM) caused by *S. pneumoniae*, *H. influenzae* (including β-lactamase-producing strains), *M. catarrhalis* (including β-lactamase-producing strains), or *S. pyogenes*.

When anti-infective therapy is indicated for the treatment of AOM, the American Academy of Pediatrics (AAP) recommends high-dose amoxicillin and amoxicillin and clavulanate potassium as the drugs of first choice for initial treatment. These experts recommend certain cephalosporins (cefdinir, cefpodoxime, cefuroxime, ceftriaxone) as alternatives for initial treatment in penicillin-allergic patients who do not have a history of severe and/or recent penicillin-allergic reactions.

Results of controlled clinical studies in children 3 months to 12 years of age with AOM indicate that a 10-day regimen of oral cefuroxime axetil is as effective or more effective than a 10-day regimen of oral cefaclor, oral amoxicillin, or oral amoxicillin and clavulanate potassium. In published studies, the overall clinical response rate to a 10-day regimen of oral cefuroxime axetil in pediatric patients with AOM has ranged from 62–94%.

Cefuroxime axetil also has been effective for the treatment of AOM in pediatric patients when administered in a 5-day regimen†. In a randomized study in children 3 months to 12 years of age with AOM, a satisfactory bacteriologic response (cure or presumed cure) was obtained in 92% of those who received a 5-day regimen of cefuroxime axetil (30 mg/kg daily given in 2 divided doses), 84% of those who received a 10-day regimen or cefuroxime axetil (30 mg/kg daily given in 2 divided doses), or 95% of those who received a 10-day regimen of amoxicillin and clavulanate potassium (40 mg/kg daily given in 3 divided doses). There is evidence from a randomized study in children 6–36 months of age with AOM that a 5-day regimen of oral cefuroxime axetil is as effective as and may be better tolerated than an 8- or 10-day regimen of oral amoxicillin and clavulanate potassium. The AAP states that oral anti-infective regimens of less than 10 days' duration are not recommended for the treatment of AOM in children younger than 2 years of age or in patients with severe symptoms.

For additional information regarding treatment of AOM, including information on diagnosis and management strategies, anti-infectives for initial treatment, duration of initial treatment, and anti-infectives after initial treatment failure, see Acute Otitis Media under Uses: Otitis Media, in the Cephalosporins General Statement 8:12.06.

■ **Pharyngitis and Tonsillitis** Cefuroxime axetil is used orally for the treatment of pharyngitis and tonsillitis caused by *S. pyogenes* (group A β-hemolytic streptococci). Although cefuroxime usually is effective in eradicating *S. pyogenes* from the nasopharynx, efficacy of the drug in the subsequent prevention of rheumatic fever remains to be established.

Selection of an anti-infective for the treatment of *S. pyogenes* pharyngitis and tonsillitis should be based on the drug's spectrum of activity, bacteriologic and clinical efficacy, potential adverse effects, ease of administration, patient compliance, and cost. No regimen has been found to date that effectively eradicates group A β-hemolytic streptococci in 100% of patients.

Because the drugs have a narrow spectrum of activity, are inexpensive, and generally are effective with a low frequency of adverse effects, the AAP, Infectious Diseases Society of America (IDSA), American Heart Association (AHA), and others recommend a penicillin regimen (i.e., 10 days of oral penicillin V or oral amoxicillin or a single dose of IM penicillin G benzathine) as the treatment of choice for *S. pyogenes* pharyngitis and tonsillitis and prevention of initial attacks (primary prevention) of rheumatic fever. Other anti-infectives (e.g., oral cephalosporins, oral macrolides, oral clindamycin) are recommended as alternatives in penicillin-allergic individuals.

If an oral cephalosporin is used for the treatment of *S. pyogenes* pharyngitis and tonsillitis, a 10-day regimen of a first generation cephalosporin (cefadroxil, cephalexin) is preferred instead of other cephalosporins with broader spectrums of activity (e.g., cefaclor, cefdinir, cefixime, cefpodoxime, cefuroxime).

Although there is some evidence that a shorter duration of therapy with certain oral cephalosporins (e.g., a 5-day regimen of cefadroxil, cefdinir, cefixime, or cefpodoxime proxetil or a 4- or 5-day regimen of cefuroxime axetil) achieves bacteriologic and clinical cure rates equal to or greater than those achieved with the traditional 10-day oral penicillin V regimen, the IDSA and AHA state that use of cephalosporin regimens administered for 5 days or less for the treatment of *S. pyogenes* pharyngitis and tonsillitis cannot be recommended at this time.

A 10-day regimen of oral cefuroxime axetil is at least as effective as a 10-day regimen of oral penicillin V for the treatment of *S. pyogenes* pharyngitis and tonsillitis. In addition, results of a prospective, randomized study in children 2–15 years of age indicate that a 4-day regimen of oral cefuroxime axetil (20 mg/kg of cefuroxime in 2 divided doses daily) is as effective as a 10-day regimen of oral penicillin V (45 mg/kg daily in 3 divided doses). The clinical response rate was 94.8% in those who received the 4-day cefuroxime regimen and 96.1% in those who received the 10-day penicillin regimen; 30 days after treatment, the bacteriologic relapse rate was 2.8 and 2.3%, respectively.

■ **Respiratory Tract Infections** Cefuroxime axetil is used orally for the treatment of mild to moderate respiratory tract infections, including acute maxillary sinusitis caused by susceptible *Streptococcus pneumoniae* or *Haemophilus influenzae* (non-β-lactamase-producing strains only) and acute exacerbations of chronic bronchitis and secondary infections of acute bronchitis caused by susceptible *S. pneumoniae*, *H. influenzae* (non-β-lactamase-producing strains only), or *H. parainfluenzae* (non-β-lactamase-producing strains only).

Cefuroxime sodium is used parenterally for the treatment of lower respiratory tract infections, including pneumonia, caused by susceptible *S. pneumoniae*, *Staphylococcus aureus* (penicillinase- and nonpenicillinase-producing strains), *S. pyogenes* (group A β-hemolytic streptococci), *H. influenzae* (including ampicillin-resistant strains), *Escherichia coli*, and *Klebsiella*.

Acute Sinusitis Cefuroxime axetil is used orally for the treatment of acute maxillary sinusitis caused by susceptible *S. pneumoniae* or *H. influenzae* (non-β-lactamase-producing strains only). The manufacturers state that insufficient data exist to establish efficacy of cefuroxime axetil in the treatment of acute bacterial maxillary sinusitis that is known or suspected to be caused by β-lactamase-producing strains of *H. influenzae* or *M. catarrhalis*.

When anti-infective therapy is indicated for the treatment of acute bacterial sinusitis, the IDSA recommends amoxicillin and clavulanate potassium and the AAP recommends either amoxicillin or amoxicillin and clavulanate potassium as the drug of choice for initial empiric treatment. Because of variable activity against *S. pneumoniae* and *H. influenzae*, the IDSA no longer recommends second or third generation oral cephalosporins for empiric monotherapy of sinusitis in adults or children. If an oral cephalosporin is used as an alternative for empiric treatment of acute bacterial sinusitis in children (e.g., in penicillin-allergic individuals), the IDSA and AAP recommend a combination regimen that includes a third generation cephalosporin (cefixime or cefpodoxime) and clindamycin (or linezolid).

Community-Acquired Pneumonia Oral cefuroxime axetil is used for the treatment of mild to moderate community-acquired pneumonia† (CAP). The American Thoracic Society (ATS) and Infectious Diseases Society of America (IDSA) recommended cefuroxime as an alternative for treatment of CAP caused by penicillin-susceptible *S. pneumoniae* and as an alternative in certain combination regimens used for empiric treatment of CAP.

Initial treatment of CAP generally involves use of an empiric anti-infective regimen based on the most likely pathogens and local susceptibility patterns; therapy may then be changed (if possible) to provide a more specific regimen (pathogen-directed therapy) based on results of in vitro culture and susceptibility testing. The most appropriate empiric regimen varies depending on the severity of illness at the time of presentation and whether outpatient treatment or hospitalization in or out of an intensive care unit (ICU) is indicated and the presence or absence of cardiopulmonary disease and other modifying factors that increase the risk of certain pathogens (e.g., penicillin- or multidrug-resistant *Streptococcus pneumoniae*, enteric gram-negative bacilli, *Pseudomonas aeruginosa*). Most experts recommend that an empiric regimen for the treatment of CAP include an anti-infective active against *S. pneumoniae* since this organism is the most commonly identified cause of bacterial pneumonia and causes more severe disease than many other common CAP pathogens.

For empiric *outpatient* treatment of CAP when risk factors for drug-resistant *S. pneumoniae* are present (e.g., comorbidities such as chronic heart, lung, liver, or renal disease, diabetes, alcoholism, malignancies, asplenia, immunosuppression; use of anti-infectives within the last 3 months), ATS and IDSA recommend monotherapy with a fluoroquinolone active against *S. pneumoniae* (moxifloxacin, gemifloxacin, levofloxacin) or, alternatively, a combination regimen that includes a β-lactam active against *S. pneumoniae* (high-dose amoxicillin or fixed combination of amoxicillin and clavulanic acid or, alternatively, ceftriaxone, cefpodoxime, or cefuroxime) given in conjunction with a macrolide (azithromycin, clarithromycin, erythromycin) or doxycycline. Cefuroxime and cefpodoxime may be less active against *S. pneumoniae* than amoxicillin or ceftriaxone.

A sequential regimen of parenteral cefuroxime sodium (given for 48–72 hours) followed by oral cefuroxime axetil (given for 7 days) has been used effectively for the treatment of CAP in adults. If a parenteral cephalosporin is used as an alternative to penicillin G or amoxicillin for treatment of CAP caused by penicillin-susceptible *S. pneumoniae*, ATS and IDSA recommend ceftriaxone, cefotaxime or cefuroxime; if an oral cephalosporin is used for treatment of these infections, ATS and IDSA recommend cefpodoxime, cefprozil, cefuroxime, cefdinir, or cefditoren.

For additional information on treatment of CAP, see Community-Acquired Pneumonia under Uses: Respiratory Tract Infections, in the Cephalosporins General Statement 8:12.06.

■ **Gonorrhea and Associated Infections** IM cefuroxime sodium has been used in conjunction with oral probenecid for the treatment of uncomplicated gonorrhea and disseminated gonococcal infections caused by *Neisseria gonorrhoeae*, including penicillinase-producing strains (PPNG). Cefuroxime axetil has been used orally for the treatment of uncomplicated urethral and endocervical gonorrhea caused by *N. gonorrhoeae* and for the treatment of uncomplicated rectal gonorrhea in females caused by nonpenicillinase-producing strains of the organism. However, parenteral cefuroxime sodium and oral cefuroxime axetil are not included in current US Centers for Disease Control and Prevention (CDC) recommendations for the treatment of gonococcal infections.

Because of concerns related to recent reports of *N. gonorrhoeae* with reduced susceptibility to cephalosporins, the CDC states that oral cephalosporins are no longer recommended as first-line treatment for uncomplicated gonorrhea. For the treatment of uncomplicated urogenital, anorectal, or pharyngeal gonorrhea, the CDC recommends a combination regimen that includes a single dose of IM ceftriaxone *and* either a single dose of oral azithromycin or a 7-day regimen of oral doxycycline.

The CDC states that cefuroxime axetil at the dosage recommended by the manufacturers (single 1-g oral dose of cefuroxime) meets the minimum efficacy criteria for treatment of urogenital and rectal gonococcal infections, but the pharmacodynamics of this oral drug are less favorable than those of IM ceftriaxone, oral cefixime, or oral cefpodoxime. In addition, cefuroxime axetil has unsatisfactory efficacy in pharyngeal infections.

For additional information on current recommendations for the treatment of gonorrhea and associated infections, see Uses: Gonorrhea and Associated Infections in Ceftriaxone 8:12.06.12.

■ **Lyme Disease** Oral cefuroxime axetil is used in adults and children for the treatment of early Lyme disease manifested as erythema migrans. When an oral regimen is indicated, oral cefuroxime axetil also is used in the treatment of early neurologic Lyme disease† in patients with cranial nerve palsy alone without evidence of meningitis, Lyme carditis†, borrelial lymphocytoma†, and uncomplicated Lyme arthritis† without clinical evidence of neurologic disease.

Lyme disease is a tick-borne spirochetal disease. In the US, Lyme disease is caused by the spirochete *Borrelia burgdorferi*, which is transmitted by the bite of *Ixodes scapularis* or *I. pacificus* ticks. For additional information on Lyme disease, see Lyme Disease in Uses: Spirochetal Infections, in the Tetracyclines General Statement 8:12.24.

Early Lyme Disease **Erythema Migrans.** Oral cefuroxime axetil is used for the treatment of early Lyme disease manifested as erythema migrans.

The IDSA, AAP, and other clinicians recommend oral doxycycline, oral amoxicillin, or oral cefuroxime axetil as first-line therapy for the treatment of early localized or early disseminated Lyme disease associated with erythema migrans, in the absence of specific neurologic involvement or advanced atrioventricular (AV) heart block. The IDSA states that a 14-day regimen (range 14–21 days) of any of these oral anti-infectives (doxycycline, amoxicillin, cefuroxime axetil) may be used for initial treatment of early Lyme disease since all 3 drugs have been shown to be effective for the treatment of erythema migrans and associated symptoms in prospective clinical studies. Doxycycline offers the advantage of also being effective for the treatment of human granulocytic anaplasmosis (HGA, formerly known as human granulocytic ehrlichiosis), which may occur simultaneously with early Lyme disease.

Efficacy of cefuroxime axetil for the treatment of early Lyme disease has been evaluated in studies that included adults and pediatric patients 12 years of age or older with physician-documented erythema migrans (with or without systemic manifestations of infection), and results of these studies indicate that the drug is as effective as oral doxycycline in producing resolution of erythema migrans and preventing the development of manifestations of late Lyme disease. The clinical diagnosis of early Lyme disease in study patients was validated objectively by a blinded expert who examined available photographs of skin lesions taken before therapy and/or by serologic evidence of antibodies specific to *B. burgdorferi* identified using enzyme-linked immunosorbent assay (ELISA) and Western immunoblot. Patients were randomized to receive oral cefuroxime axetil (500 mg of cefuroxime twice daily) or oral doxycycline (100 mg 3 times daily) for 20 days and evaluated during treatment (days 8–12) and posttreatment (days 1–5, 1 month, and then at 3-month intervals for up to 1 year). In patients who were evaluated at 1 month posttreatment, a satisfactory clinical response consisting of either clinical success (defined as resolution of erythema migrans and other manifestations of infection within 5 days posttreatment and maintained through follow-up at 1 month posttreatment) or clinical improvement (defined as resolution of erythema migrans within 5 days posttreatment with incomplete resolution of other manifestations of infection at that time but further improvement or complete resolution of manifestations by follow-up at 1 month posttreatment) was attained in 91 or 93% of patients who received cefuroxime axetil or doxycycline, respectively. Clinical success was attained in 72 or 73% of patients receiving cefuroxime axetil or doxycycline, respectively; clinical improvement was attained in 19% of patients receiving either drug. In patients evaluated at 1 year, a satisfactory clinical outcome consisting of success (defined as the absence of signs or symptoms of late Lyme disease throughout the 1-year follow-up) or clinical improvement (defined as the presence of some signs or symptoms consistent with late Lyme disease but no objective evidence of active disease throughout the 1-year follow-up) was attained in 84 or 87% of patients who received cefuroxime axetil or doxycycline, respectively. Success at 1 year was attained in 73% of patients receiving either drug; clinical improvement was attained in 10% of patients receiving cefuroxime axetil and 13% of patients receiving doxycycline.

Early Neurologic Lyme Disease. Oral cefuroxime axetil is used in the treatment of early neurologic Lyme disease† in patients with cranial nerve palsy alone without evidence of meningitis. Parenteral anti-infectives (IV ceftriaxone, IV penicillin G sodium, IV cefotaxime) are recommended for the treatment of early Lyme disease when there are acute neurologic manifestations such as meningitis or radiculopathy. However, some clinicians suggest that a 14-day regimen (range: 14–21 days) of oral anti-infectives (amoxicillin, doxycycline, cefuroxime axetil) may be used in patients with cranial nerve palsy without clinical evidence of meningitis (i.e., those with normal CSF examinations or those for whom CSF examination is deemed unnecessary because there are no clinical signs of meningitis). Although there is some experience using oral anti-infectives in patients with seventh cranial nerve palsy, it is unclear whether an oral regimen would be as effective for patients with other cranial neuropathies. Although anti-infectives may not hasten resolution of seventh cranial nerve palsy associated with *B. burgdorferi* infection, anti-infectives should be given to prevent further sequelae.

Lyme Carditis. Oral cefuroxime axetil is used in the treatment of Lyme carditis†. The IDSA states that patients with AV heart block and/or myopericarditis associated with early Lyme disease may be treated with a 14-day regimen (range: 14–21 days) of oral or parenteral anti-infectives. Although there is no evidence to date to suggest that a parenteral regimen is more effective than an oral regimen for the treatment of Lyme carditis, a parenteral regimen usually is recommended for initial treatment of hospitalized patients; an oral regimen can be used to complete therapy and for the treatment of outpatients. When a parenteral regimen is used, IV ceftriaxone or, alternatively, IV cefotaxime or IV penicillin G sodium is recommended. When an oral regimen is used, oral doxycycline, oral amoxicillin, or oral cefuroxime axetil is recommended.

Borrelial Lymphocytoma. Although experience is limited, the IDSA states that available data indicate that borrelial lymphocytoma† may be treated with a 14-day regimen (range 14–21 days) of oral doxycycline, oral amoxicillin, or oral cefuroxime axetil in the dosages used for the treatment of erythema migrans.

Late Lyme Disease **Lyme Arthritis.** Patients with uncomplicated Lyme arthritis† without clinical evidence of neurologic disease generally can be treated with a 28-day regimen of oral doxycycline, oral amoxicillin, or oral cefuroxime axetil. Patients with Lyme arthritis and concomitant neurologic disease should receive a parenteral regimen of IV ceftriaxone or, alternatively, IV cefotaxime or IV penicillin G sodium. While oral regimens are easier to administer, associated with fewer serious adverse effects, and less expensive than IV regimens, some patients with Lyme arthritis treated with oral anti-infectives have subsequently developed overt neuroborreliosis, which may require IV therapy for successful resolution. Therefore, additional study is needed to fully evaluate the comparative safety and efficacy of oral versus IV anti-infectives for the treatment of Lyme arthritis.

In patients who have persistent or recurrent joint swelling after a recommended oral regimen, the IDSA and other clinicians recommend retreatment with the oral regimen or a switch to a parenteral regimen. Some clinicians prefer retreatment with an oral regimen for patients whose arthritis substantively improved but did not completely resolve; these clinicians reserve parenteral regimens for those patients whose arthritis failed to improve or worsened. It has been suggested that clinicians should consider allowing several months for joint inflammation to resolve after initial treatment before an additional course of anti-infectives is given.

■ **Meningitis** Parenteral cefuroxime has been used in neonates†, children, and adults for the treatment of meningitis caused by susceptible *S. pneumoniae, H. influenzae* (including ampicillin-resistant strains), *N. meningitidis*, or *S. aureus* (penicillinase- and nonpenicillinase-producing strains); however, cefuroxime is not considered a drug of choice for these infections. Treatment failures have been reported when cefuroxime was used in the treatment of meningitis, especially in meningitis caused by *H. influenzae*. In addition, while results of some studies in pediatric patients with meningitis indicate that the clinical cure rate with IV cefuroxime is similar to that reported for IV ceftriaxone, the bacteriologic response to cefuroxime appears to be slower, which may increase the risk for hearing loss and neurologic sequelae. In a study in children 44 days to 16 years of age with acute bacterial meningitis who were randomized to receive empiric therapy with IV ceftriaxone (100 mg/kg once daily) or IV cefuroxime (240 mg/kg daily in 4 doses), all patients in both groups were considered clinically cured; however, the rate of sterilization of CSF after the first 18–36 hours of therapy was higher in those who received ceftriaxone (98%) than in those who received cefuroxime (88%). When a cephalosporin is indicated for the treatment of bacterial meningitis, a parenteral third generation cephalosporin (usually ceftriaxone or cefotaxime) generally is recommended.

■ **Perioperative Prophylaxis** IV cefuroxime sodium is used for perioperative prophylaxis in patients undergoing cardiac surgery and is considered a drug of choice for cardiac procedures (e.g., coronary artery bypass, pacemaker or other cardiac device insertion, ventricular assist devices). IV cefuroxime also is considered a drug of choice when used alone for perioperative prophylaxis in patients undergoing clean head and neck surgery involving placement of prosthesis (excluding tympanostomy) and when used in conjunction with metronidazole for perioperative prophylaxis in patients undergoing clean-contaminated cancer surgery of the head and neck or other clean-contaminated head and neck procedures (excluding tonsillectomy and functional endoscopic sinus procedures).

IV cefuroxime also has been used for perioperative prophylaxis in patients undergoing noncardiac thoracic surgery, GI or biliary tract surgery, gynecologic or obstetric surgery (e.g., vaginal hysterectomy), orthopedic procedures, or heart transplantation. However, other anti-infectives (e.g., cefazolin) usually are recommended for perioperative prophylaxis in patients undergoing these procedures. (See Uses: Perioperative Prophylaxis, in the Cephalosporins General Statement 8:12.06.)

Dosage and Administration

■ **Reconstitution and Administration** Cefuroxime axetil is administered orally. Cefuroxime sodium is administered by IV injection or infusion or by deep IM injection. The drug should be given IV rather than IM in patients with septicemia or other severe or life-threatening infections or in patients with lowered resistance, particularly if shock is present.

Oral Administration Cefuroxime axetil oral suspension must be administered with food. Although cefuroxime axetil film-coated tablets may be given orally without regard to meals, administration with food maximizes bioavailability of the drug. (See Pharmacokinetics: Absorption.)

In children aged 3 months to 12 years who are unable to swallow tablets, cefuroxime may be administered as the commercially available oral suspension. Although commercially available cefuroxime axetil tablets have been crushed and mixed with food (e.g., applesauce, ice cream), the crushed tablets have a strong, persistent taste and the manufacturers state that the drug should not be administered in this manner. (See Cautions: Pediatric Precautions.) Cefuroxime axetil tablets also have been allowed to disintegrate in a small amount (60–90 mL) of beverage (e.g., apple juice or milk) and the beverage stirred and ingested immediately followed by additional amounts of beverage; disintegration of the tablets is optimal when the beverage is at room temperature.

Limited data from a study conducted by the manufacturer suggest that cefuroxime axetil is stable for 2 hours at room temperature when added as single 125- or 250-mg tablets to 40 mL of Tropicana® orange juice, Welch's® grape juice, or Nestle's® chocolate milk. However, extemporaneous preparation of an oral suspension of the drug intended for *multiple* dosing currently is not recommended since stability information for more prolonged periods currently is not available and because the drug is commercially available as an oral suspension.

The child's tolerance of the taste of cefuroxime axetil should be ascertained by the clinician and parent, preferably when prescription of the drug is being considered (e.g., while the child is still in the physician's office).

Reconstitution. Cefuroxime axetil powder for oral suspension should be reconstituted at the time of dispensing by adding the amount of water specified on the bottle to provide a suspension containing 125 or 250 mg of cefuroxime (as cefuroxime axetil) per 5 mL of suspension. After tapping the bottle to thoroughly loosen the powder for oral suspension, the water should be added in one portion and the suspension agitated well.

The suspension should be agitated well just prior to each use and the cap replaced securely after each opening.

Intermittent IV Injection For direct intermittent IV injection, vials labeled as containing 750 mg or 1.5 g of cefuroxime should be reconstituted with 8 or 16 mL, respectively, of sterile water for injection to provide solutions containing approximately 90 mg/mL; the entire contents of the vial should be withdrawn for each dose.

The appropriate dose should then be injected directly into a vein over a 3- to 5-minute period or injected slowly into the tubing of a freely flowing compatible IV solution.

Intermittent or Continuous IV Infusion ADD-Vantage® (TwistVial®) vials labeled as containing 750 mg or 1.5 g of cefuroxime should be reconstituted with 50 or 100 mL of 5% dextrose injection, 0.9% sodium chloride injection, or 0.45% sodium chloride injection in a compatible flexible container according to the manufacturer's directions.

Alternatively, the commercially available Duplex® drug delivery system containing 750 mg or 1.5 g of cefuroxime and 50 mL of dextrose 4.1 or 2.9% injection, respectively, in separate chambers should be reconstituted (activated) according to the manufacturer's directions and administered by IV infusion.

The 7.5-g pharmacy bulk vial should be reconstituted according to the manufacturer's directions. The pharmacy bulk vial is *not* intended for direct IV infusion.

Thawed solutions of the commercially available frozen premixed cefuroxime sodium injection should be administered only by intermittent or continuous IV infusion. The frozen injection should be thawed at room temperature (25°C) or under refrigeration (5°C); the injection should not be thawed by warming in a water bath or by exposure to microwave radiation. Precipitates that may have formed in the frozen injection usually will dissolve with little or no agitation when the injection reaches room temperature; potency is not affected. After thawing to room temperature, the injection should be agitated and the container checked for minute leaks by firmly squeezing the bag; the container may be fragile and should be handled with care. The injection should be discarded if container seals or outlet ports are not intact or leaks are found or if the solution is cloudy or contains an insoluble precipitate. Additives should not be introduced into the injection container. The injection should not be used in series connections with other plastic containers, since such use could result in air embolism from residual air being drawn from the primary container before administration of fluid from the secondary container is complete.

Other IV solutions flowing through a common administration tubing or site should be discontinued while cefuroxime is being infused unless the solutions are known to be compatible and the flow rate is adequately controlled. If an aminoglycoside is administered concomitantly with cefuroxime, the drugs should be administered at separate sites.

Rate of Administration. Intermittent IV infusions of cefuroxime generally are infused over 15–60 minutes.

IM Injection IM injections of Zinacef® are prepared by adding 3 mL of sterile water for injection to a vial labeled as containing 750 mg of cefuroxime to provide a suspension containing approximately 220 mg/mL. The suspension should be shaken gently prior to administration, and the entire contents of the vial should be withdrawn for each dose.

IM injections should be made deeply into a large muscle mass such as the gluteus or lateral aspect of the thigh. The plunger of the syringe should be drawn back before IM injection to ensure that the needle is not in a blood vessel.

■ Dosage

Dosage of cefuroxime axetil is expressed in terms of cefuroxime. Cefuroxime axetil tablets and oral suspension are *not* bioequivalent and are *not* substitutable on a mg/mg basis. (See Pharmacokinetics: Absorption.)

Dosage of cefuroxime sodium also is expressed in terms of cefuroxime and is identical for IM or IV administration.

Adult Dosage

General Oral Adult Dosage. For the treatment of uncomplicated skin and skin-structure infections in adults and adolescents 13 years of age or older, the usual oral dosage of cefuroxime given as cefuroxime axetil tablets is 250 or 500 mg twice daily for 10 days. For the treatment of uncomplicated urinary tract infections (UTIs), the usual oral dosage of cefuroxime given as cefuroxime axetil tablets is 125 or 250 mg twice daily for 7–10 days.

The usual parenteral adult dosage of cefuroxime given as cefuroxime sodium is 750 mg to 1.5 g every 8 hours. Uncomplicated UTIs, skin and skin structure infections, and uncomplicated pneumonia in adults generally respond to a parenteral dosage of 750 mg every 8 hours. Severe or complicated infections or bone and joint infections in adults generally require 1.5 g every 8 hours and life-threatening infections or infections caused by less susceptible organisms may require 1.5 g every 6 hours. Dosage of parenteral cefuroxime for the treatment of bacterial meningitis in adults should not exceed 3 g every 8 hours.

Pharyngitis and Tonsillitis. For the treatment of pharyngitis and tonsillitis caused by *Streptococcus pyogenes* (group A β-hemolytic streptococci) in adults and adolescents 13 years of age or older, the usual oral dosage of cefuroxime given as cefuroxime axetil tablets is 250 mg twice daily for 10 days.

Respiratory Tract Infections. For the treatment of acute bacterial maxillary sinusitis in adults and adolescents 13 years of age or older, the usual oral dosage of cefuroxime given as cefuroxime axetil tablets is 250 mg twice daily for 10 days. For the treatment of acute bacterial exacerbations of chronic bronchitis and secondary bacterial infections of acute bronchitis in adults and adolescents 13 years of age or older, the usual oral dosage of cefuroxime given as cefuroxime axetil tablets is 250 or 500 mg twice daily. The manufacturers recommend that therapy be continued for 10 days for the treatment of acute bacterial exacerbations of chronic bronchitis or for 5–10 days for the treatment of secondary bacterial infections of acute bronchitis. While there is evidence that a 5-day regimen of cefuroxime axetil is as effective as a 10-day regimen of the drug for the treatment of secondary bacterial infections of acute bronchitis, efficacy of the shorter regimen for the treatment of acute exacerbations of chronic bronchitis has not been established.

If cefuroxime axetil is used for the outpatient treatment of community-acquired pneumonia† (CAP) in adults, the American Thoracic Society (ATS) and Infectious Diseases Society of America (IDSA) recommend an oral dosage of 500 mg of cefuroxime twice daily. For empiric treatment of CAP, cefuroxime must be used in conjunction with other anti-infectives. (See Community-acquired Pneumonia under Uses: Respiratory Tract Infections.)

For the treatment of uncomplicated pneumonia in adults, the manufacturers recommend a parenteral cefuroxime dosage of 750 mg every 8 hours. In severe or complicated infections, a dosage of 1.5 g every 8 hours is recommended.

Gonorrhea and Associated Infections. For the parenteral treatment of uncomplicated gonorrhea caused by *Neisseria gonorrhoeae*, including penicillinase-producing strains (PPNG), the manufacturer of Zinacef® recommends that adults receive a single 1.5-g IM dose of cefuroxime and 1 g of oral probenecid; the cefuroxime dose should be divided and given at 2 different sites. For the parenteral treatment of disseminated gonococcal infections, the manufacturers recommend that adults receive 750 mg of cefuroxime IM or IV every 8 hours.

For the oral treatment of uncomplicated urethral or endocervical gonorrhea caused by *N. gonorrhoeae* or for the oral treatment of uncomplicated rectal gonorrhea in females caused by nonpenicillinase-producing strains of the organism, adults and adolescents 13 years of age or older have received a single 1-g dose of cefuroxime.

The US Centers for Disease Control and Prevention (CDC) does not recommend oral or parenteral cefuroxime for the treatment of gonococcal infections. (See Uses: Gonorrhea and Associated Infections.)

Lyme Disease. For the treatment of early Lyme disease manifested as erythema migrans, the manufacturers recommend that adults and adolescents 13 years of age or older receive 500 mg of oral cefuroxime twice daily for 20 days.

IDSA and other clinicians recommend that adults receive 500 mg of oral cefuroxime twice daily for 14 days (range: 14–21 days) for the treatment of early localized or early disseminated Lyme disease manifested as erythema migrans, in the absence of specific neurologic involvement or advanced atrioventricular (AV) heart block.

If an oral regimen is used for the treatment of early neurologic Lyme disease† in patients with cranial nerve palsy alone without clinical evidence of meningitis (see Early Neurologic Lyme Disease under Uses: Lyme Disease), Lyme carditis†, or borrelial lymphocytoma†, the IDSA recommends that adults receive 500 mg of oral cefuroxime twice daily for 14 days (range: 14–21 days).

If an oral regimen is used for the treatment of uncomplicated Lyme arthritis† in patients without clinical evidence of neurologic disease (see Late Lyme Disease under Uses: Lyme Disease), the IDSA recommends that adults receive 500 mg of oral cefuroxime twice daily for 28 days.

Perioperative Prophylaxis. For perioperative prophylaxis in adults undergoing open-heart surgery, the manufacturers recommend that a single 1.5-g dose of cefuroxime be given IV at the time of induction of anesthesia and every 12 hours thereafter for a total dosage of 6 g (i.e., up to 48 hours). Some experts recommend that 1.5 g of cefuroxime be given within 1 hour prior to surgical incision and that additional 1.5-g doses be given every 4 hours during prolonged procedures (longer than 4 hours) or if major blood loss occurs. Various data support a duration of perioperative prophylaxis ranging from a single preoperative dose to continuation of prophylaxis for 24 hours postoperatively; there is no evidence of benefit beyond 48 hours and no evidence to support continuing prophylaxis until all drains and indwelling catheters are removed.

If cefuroxime is used for perioperative prophylaxis in other clean-contaminated or potentially contaminated surgery (e.g., vaginal hysterectomy), the manufacturers recommend that adults receive 1.5 g of cefuroxime IV just prior to surgery (approximately 30–60 minutes before the initial incision) and, in lengthy operations, 750 mg of the drug IV or IM every 8 hours. For most procedures, postoperative doses are usually unnecessary and may increase the risk of bacterial resistance. If the procedure is prolonged (longer than 4 hours) or if major blood loss occurs, 1.5-g doses of cefuroxime may be given IV every 4 hours.

Pediatric Dosage

Cefuroxime axetil film-coated tablets and oral suspension are not bioequivalent and are not substitutable on a mg/mg basis. (See Pharmacokinetics: Absorption.)

General Pediatric Dosage. For the treatment of most susceptible infections (except bone and joint infections or meningitis) in children 3 months of age or older, the manufacturers recommend a cefuroxime dosage of 50–100 mg/kg daily given IM or IV in equally divided doses every 6–8 hours; the manufacturer states that 100 mg/kg should be given IM or IV for more severe infections. The IM or IV dosage of cefuroxime recommended by the manufacturers for the treatment of bone and joint infections in children 3 months of age or older is 150 mg/kg daily in 3 divided doses every 8 hours.

The American Academy of Pediatrics (AAP) recommends that neonates 7 days of age or younger receive IM or IV cefuroxime in a dosage of 50 mg/kg every 12 hours, regardless of weight. Neonates 8–28 days of age should receive a dosage of 50 mg/kg every 8–12 hours if they weigh 2 kg or less or 50 mg/kg every 8 hours if they weigh more than 2 kg.

For pediatric patients beyond the neonatal period, the AAP recommends an IM or IV cefuroxime dosage of 75–100 mg/kg daily given in 3 equally divided doses for the treatment of mild to moderate infections or 100–200 mg/kg daily in 3 or 4 equally divided doses for the treatment of severe infections. These clinicians recommend that children beyond the neonatal period receive oral cefuroxime in a dosage of 20–30 mg/kg daily in 2 equally divided doses for the treatment of mild to moderate infections. The AAP states that oral cefuroxime is inappropriate for the treatment of severe infections.

Acute Otitis Media. For the treatment of acute otitis media in children 3 months to 12 years of age who can swallow tablets whole, the usual oral dosage of cefuroxime as cefuroxime axetil film-coated tablets is 250 mg twice daily for 10 days. Alternatively, children 3 months to 12 years of age with acute otitis media can receive cefuroxime as cefuroxime axetil oral suspension in a dosage of 30 mg/kg daily (maximum 1 g daily) given in 2 divided doses for 10 days.

Cefuroxime axetil has been administered in a 5-day regimen† for the treatment of acute otitis media in children 3 months to 12 years of age. The AAP states that oral anti-infective regimens of less than 10 days' duration are not recommended for the treatment of AOM in children younger than 2 years of age or in patients with severe symptoms.

Pharyngitis and Tonsillitis. For the treatment of pharyngitis and tonsillitis caused by *S. pyogenes* (group A β-hemolytic streptococci) in children 3 months to 12 years of age who can swallow tablets whole, the usual oral dosage of cefuroxime as cefuroxime axetil film-coated tablets is 125 mg every 12 hours for 10 days. Alternatively, children 3 months to 12 years of age may receive cefuroxime as cefuroxime axetil oral suspension in a dosage of 20 mg/kg daily (maximum 500 mg daily) in 2 divided doses for 10 days.

Acute Sinusitis. For the treatment of acute bacterial maxillary sinusitis in children 3 months to 12 years of age who can swallow tablets whole, the usual oral dosage of cefuroxime as cefuroxime axetil film-coated tablets is 250 mg twice daily for 10 days. Alternatively, children 3 months to 12 years of age may receive cefuroxime as cefuroxime axetil oral suspension in a dosage of 30 mg/kg daily (maximum 1 g daily) given in 2 divided doses for 10 days.

Lyme Disease. For the treatment of early localized or early disseminated Lyme disease manifested as erythema migrans, in the absence of specific neurologic involvement or advanced AV heart block, the manufacturer, IDSA, AAP, and other clinicians recommend that children receive oral cefuroxime in a dosage of 30 mg/kg daily (up to 1 g daily) administered in 2 divided doses for 14 days (range 14–21 days).

If an oral regimen is used for the treatment of early neurologic Lyme disease† in patients with cranial nerve palsy alone without clinical evidence of meningitis (see Early Neurologic Lyme Disease under Uses: Lyme Disease), Lyme carditis†, or borrelial lymphocytoma†, the IDSA recommends that children receive oral cefuroxime in a dosage of 30 mg/kg daily in 2 equally divided doses (up to 500 mg per dose) for 14 days (range 14–21 days).

If an oral regimen is used for the treatment of uncomplicated Lyme arthritis† in patients without clinical evidence of neurologic disease (see Late Lyme Disease under Uses: Lyme Disease), the IDSA and AAP recommend that children receive oral cefuroxime in a dosage of 30 mg/kg daily in 2 equally divided doses (up to 500 mg per dose) for 28 days.

Meningitis. For the treatment of bacterial meningitis in children 3 months of age or older, the usual dosage of IV cefuroxime is 200–240 mg/kg daily given in divided doses every 6–8 hours.

Skin and Skin Structure Infections. For the treatment of impetigo in children 3 months to 12 years of age, the usual oral dosage of cefuroxime as cefuroxime axetil oral suspension is 30 mg/kg daily (maximum 1 g daily) in 2 divided doses for 10 days.

Perioperative Prophylaxis. If cefuroxime is used for perioperative prophylaxis in children, some clinicians recommend that 50 mg/kg of cefuroxime be given within 1 hour prior to surgical incision. If the procedure is prolonged (longer than 4 hours) or if major blood loss occurs, additional 50-mg/kg doses may be given IV. Various data support a duration of perioperative prophylaxis ranging from a single preoperative dose to continuation of prophylaxis for 24 hours postoperatively; there is no evidence of benefit beyond 48 hours and no evidence to support continuing prophylaxis until all drains and indwelling catheters are removed.

Duration of Therapy The duration of cefuroxime therapy depends on the type of infection but should generally be continued for at least 48–72 hours after the patient becomes afebrile or evidence of eradication of the infection is obtained.

For the treatment of uncomplicated UTIs, the manufacturers recommend that therapy with cefuroxime axetil tablets be continued for 7–10 days. For the treatment of uncomplicated skin and skin-structure infections, or acute otitis media caused by susceptible organisms, the manufacturers recommend that therapy with cefuroxime axetil tablets be continued for 10 days.

Chronic urinary tract infections may require several weeks of cefuroxime therapy, and bacteriologic and clinical assessments should be made frequently during therapy and for several months after the drug is discontinued. When cefuroxime is used in the treatment of staphylococcal and other infections involving a collection of pus, surgical drainage should be performed when indicated.

■ Dosage in Renal Impairment

Modification of usual dosage of parenteral cefuroxime is unnecessary in patients with creatinine clearances greater than 20 mL/minute. However, in patients with creatinine clearances of 20 mL/minute or less, doses and/or frequency of administration of parenteral cefuroxime must be modified in response to the degree of renal impairment, severity of the infection, and susceptibility of the causative organism. The manufacturers and some clinicians recommend that adults with creatinine clearances of 10–20 mL/minute receive 750 mg IM or IV every 12 hours and that adults with creatinine clearances less than 10 mL/minute receive 750 mg IM or IV every 24 hours. In children with impaired renal function, the manufacturers recommend that the frequency of administration of parenteral cefuroxime be modified based on the recommendations for adults with impaired renal function.

In patients undergoing hemodialysis, a supplemental dose of parenteral cefuroxime should be given after each dialysis period.

Safety and efficacy of oral cefuroxime axetil in patients with renal impairment have not been established.

Cautions

Adverse effects reported with cefuroxime axetil and cefuroxime sodium are similar to those reported with other cephalosporins.

■ Dermatologic and Sensitivity Reactions

Hypersensitivity reactions have been reported in less than 1% of patients receiving cefuroxime axetil or cefuroxime sodium. These reactions include rash (e.g., morbilliform), fever, pruritus, erythema, urticaria, Stevens-Johnson syndrome, erythema multiforme, toxic epidermal necrolysis, serum sickness-like reactions, angioedema, and anaphylaxis. At least one case of severe bronchospasm has been reported in a patient who received cefuroxime axetil. Positive direct antiglobulin (Coombs') test results have also been reported in a few patients receiving oral or parenteral cefuroxime; however, it is not clear whether the mechanism of this reaction is immunologic in nature. If a severe hypersensitivity reaction occurs during cefuroxime therapy, the drug should be discontinued and the patient given appropriate therapy (e.g., epinephrine, corticosteroids, maintenance of an adequate airway, oxygen) as indicated.

There is clinical and laboratory evidence of partial cross-allergenicity among cephalosporins and other β-lactam antibiotics including penicillins and cephamycins; however, the true incidence of cross-allergenicity among these anti-infectives has not been established. When cefuroxime axetil was used in patients with a history of delayed hypersensitivity reactions to penicillins and no history of hypersensitivity to cephalosporins, a delayed hypersensitivity reaction occurred in about 3% of these patients. The manufacturer states that when cefuroxime sodium was used in patients with a history of hypersensitivity to penicillin, rash reportedly occurred in 4.4–6.7% of these patients.

■ Local Effects

The most frequent adverse reactions to IM or IV cefuroxime sodium are local reactions at the injection site. Mild to moderate pain, which persists for less than 5 minutes, has been reported in up to 95% of patients following IM administration of cefuroxime. Severe pain has been reported occasionally. IM injections of cefuroxime reportedly are less painful when the drug is administered as a suspension rather than a solution and are also less painful when the injection is given into the buttock rather than the thigh.

Thrombophlebitis reportedly occurs in approximately 2% of patients receiving cefuroxime IV.

■ GI Effects

Nausea and vomiting have been reported in 2.6–6.7% and diarrhea or loose stools have been reported in 3.7–10.6% of patients receiving oral cefuroxime axetil. A strong, persistent, bitter taste has been reported when cefuroxime axetil was administered as crushed tablets (see Pediatric Precautions). In addition, up to 5% of children receiving the commercially available oral suspension of cefuroxime axetil disliked the taste of the suspension; during clinical trials, discontinuance of therapy because of the taste of the suspension or other problems with administration occurred in 1.4% of patients.

Gagging, epigastric burning, GI bleeding, abdominal pain, flatulence, GI infection, ptyalism, indigestion, mouth ulcers, swollen tongue, anorexia, thirst, dyspepsia, and stomach cramps also have been reported in patients receiving the drug orally.

The frequency of adverse GI effects (particularly diarrhea) may be greater with oral cefuroxime axetil than with oral cefaclor, and nausea appears to be more common when oral cefuroxime axetil is used concomitantly with oral probenecid than when the antibiotic is used alone. In addition, adverse GI effects were reported more frequently with previously available oral formulations of cefuroxime axetil, and, in part, prompted several reformulations of the product. Adverse GI effects including nausea and diarrhea have been reported in less than 1% of patients receiving IM or IV cefuroxime sodium.

Clostridium difficile-associated Diarrhea and Colitis Treatment with anti-infectives alters normal colon flora and may permit overgrowth of *Clostridium difficile.*

C. difficile infection (CDI) and *C. difficile*-associated diarrhea and colitis (CDAD; also known as antibiotic-associated diarrhea and colitis or pseudomembranous colitis) have been reported with nearly all anti-infectives, including cefuroxime, and may range in severity from mild diarrhea to fatal colitis. *C. difficile* produces toxins A and B which contribute to the development of CDAD; hypertoxin-producing strains of *C. difficile* are associated with increased morbidity and mortality since they may be refractory to anti-infectives and colectomy may be required.

CDAD should be considered in the differential diagnosis in patients who develop diarrhea during or after anti-infective therapy and managed accordingly. Careful medical history is necessary since CDAD has been reported to occur as late as 2 months or longer after anti-infective therapy is discontinued.

If CDAD is suspected or confirmed, anti-infectives not directed against *C. difficile* should be discontinued whenever possible. Patients should be managed with appropriate supportive therapy (e.g., fluid and electrolyte management, protein supplementation), anti-infective therapy directed against *C. difficile* (e.g., metronidazole, vancomycin), and surgical evaluation as clinically indicated.

■ Hematologic Effects

Decreased hemoglobin concentration and decreased hematocrit have been reported in about 10% of patients receiving cefuroxime. Transient eosinophilia occurs less frequently, and transient neutropenia, pancytopenia, thrombocytopenia, and leukopenia occur rarely. Thrombocytosis, lymphocytosis, hemolytic anemia, and increased prothrombin time also have been reported.

■ CNS Effects

Headache, dizziness, somnolence or sleepiness, hyperactivity, irritable behavior, seizures, myoclonic jerks, and generalized hyperexcitability have been reported rarely in patients receiving cefuroxime.

A psychotic reaction, consisting of disorientation, fluctuating consciousness, and episodes of restlessness, agitation, and anxiety, occurred in a geriatric patient who received IV cefuroxime sodium; symptoms resolved within 24 hours after the drug was discontinued. Some patients who experienced adverse CNS effects while receiving cefuroxime had preexisting renal impairment.

■ Hepatic Effects

Transient increases in serum AST (SGOT), ALT (SGPT), alkaline phosphatase, LDH, and bilirubin concentrations have been reported in less than 5% of patients receiving oral or parenteral cefuroxime. Jaundice has been reported rarely.

■ Renal and Genitourinary Effects

Acute renal failure and interstitial nephritis have been reported rarely in patients receiving cefuroxime. Although a causal relationship has not been established, transient increases in BUN and/or serum creatinine concentrations and decreased creatinine clearance have been reported in a few patients receiving cefuroxime. Bilateral renal cortical necrosis that appeared to be a hypersensitivity reaction has been reported in at least one patient who received cefuroxime axetil.

Urinary tract infection, kidney pain, urethral pain or bleeding, dysuria, vaginitis, vaginal candidiasis, vulvovaginal pruritus, and vaginal discharge or irritation have been reported in less than 1% of patients receiving oral cefuroxime axetil therapy.

■ Other Adverse Effects

Jarisch-Herxheimer reaction has occurred in 5.6% of patients receiving cefuroxime axetil for the treatment of Lyme disease. In a clinical study in patients with early Lyme disease, the Jarisch-Herxheimer reaction occurred in 11.8% of patients receiving cefuroxime axetil and 11.5% of patients receiving doxycycline. These transient reactions generally last only 1–2 days.

Overgrowth with nonsusceptible organisms (e.g., perianal, oral, or vaginal candidiasis; pseudomembranous colitis; superinfection) has occurred in patients receiving cefuroxime sodium or cefuroxime axetil. (See Cautions: GI Effects and also see Precautions and Contraindications.)

Mild to severe hearing loss has been reported in a few pediatric patients receiving cefuroxime sodium for the treatment of meningitis. Persistence of positive CSF cultures at 18–36 hours has been observed with cefuroxime sodium injection; however, the clinical relevance of this finding is unknown.

Muscle spasm of the neck, muscle cramps or stiffness, chest pain or tightness, shortness of breath, tachycardia, chills, lockjaw-type reaction, viral illness, upper respiratory infection, sinusitis, fever, cough, joint swelling, and arthralgia have been reported in less than 1% of patients receiving oral cefuroxime axetil therapy. Diaper rash has been reported in 3.4% of pediatric patients receiving cefuroxime axetil as the commercially available oral suspension.

■ Precautions and Contraindications Prior to initiation of cefuroxime therapy, careful inquiry should be made concerning previous hypersensitivity reactions to cephalosporins, penicillins, or other drugs. Cefuroxime axetil and cefuroxime sodium are contraindicated in patients who are hypersensitive to cefuroxime or other cephalosporins and should be used with caution in patients with a history of hypersensitivity to penicillins. Use of cephalosporins should be avoided in patients who have had an immediate-type (anaphylactic) hypersensitivity reaction to penicillins. Although it has not been definitely proven that allergic reactions to antibiotics are more frequent in atopic individuals, the manufacturer states that parenteral cefuroxime should be used with caution in patients with a history of allergy, particularly to drugs.

To reduce development of drug-resistant bacteria and maintain effectiveness of cefuroxime and other antibacterials, the drug should be used only for the treatment or prevention of infections proven or strongly suspected to be caused by susceptible bacteria. When selecting or modifying anti-infective therapy, results of culture and in vitro susceptibility testing should be used. In the absence of such data, local epidemiology and susceptibility patterns should be considered when selecting anti-infectives for empiric therapy.

Patients should be advised that antibacterials (including cefuroxime) should only be used to treat bacterial infections and not used to treat viral infections (e.g., the common cold). Patients also should be advised about the importance of completing the full course of therapy, even if feeling better after a few days, and that skipping doses or not completing therapy may decrease effectiveness and increase the likelihood that bacteria will develop resistance and will not be treatable with cefuroxime or other antibacterials in the future.

As with other anti-infectives, prolonged use of cefuroxime axetil or cefuroxime sodium may result in overgrowth of nonsusceptible organisms. Careful observation of the patient during cefuroxime therapy is essential. If suprainfection or superinfection occurs, appropriate therapy should be instituted.

Individuals with phenylketonuria (i.e., homozygous genetic deficiency of phenylalanine hydroxylase) and other individuals who must restrict their intake of phenylalanine should be warned that Ceftin® oral suspensions containing 125 or 250 mg of cefuroxime per 5 mL contains aspartame (NutraSweet®), which is metabolized in the GI tract to provide 11.8 or 25.2 mg of phenylalanine/5 mL, respectively.

Like other dextrose-containing solutions, the commercially available Duplex® drug delivery system containing 750 mg or 1.5 g of cefuroxime and 50 mL of dextrose injection should be used with caution in patients with overt or known subclinical diabetes mellitus or in patients with carbohydrate intolerance for any reason.

Because CDAD has been reported with the use of cefuroxime and other cephalosporins, it should be considered in the differential diagnosis of patients who develop diarrhea during or after cefuroxime therapy. (See Clostridium difficile-associated Diarrhea and Colitis under Cautions: GI Effects.) Patients should be advised that diarrhea is a common problem caused by anti-infectives and usually resolves when the drug is discontinued; however, they should contact a clinician if watery and bloody stools (with or without stomach cramps and fever) occur during or as late as 2 months or longer after the last dose. Cefuroxime should be used with caution in patients with a history of GI disease, particularly colitis. The safety and efficacy of cefuroxime axetil therapy in patients with GI malabsorption have not been established.

Although cefuroxime sodium only rarely causes adverse renal effects, the manufacturers state that renal function should be monitored during therapy with the drug, especially when maximum dosage is used in seriously ill patients.

Safety and efficacy of oral cefuroxime axetil in patients with renal impairment have not been established. Because serum concentrations of cefuroxime are higher and more prolonged in patients with renal impairment than in patients with normal renal function, dose and/or frequency of administration of parenteral cefuroxime sodium should be decreased in patients with transient or persistent renal impairment. (See Dosage in Renal Impairment in Dosage and Administration: Dosage.)

Several cephalosporins (including cefuroxime) have been associated with the development of seizures, particularly in patients with renal impairment, in whom dosage of the drug was not reduced. If seizures associated with cefuroxime develop, the drug should be discontinued and anticonvulsant therapy initiated as clinically indicated.

Because some cephalosporins have been associated with a decrease in prothrombin activity, the manufacturers state that prothrombin time (PT) should be monitored when cefuroxime is used in patients with renal or hepatic impairment, in patients with poor nutritional status, in patients receiving a protracted course of anti-infective therapy, or in those previously stabilized on anticoagulant therapy. Vitamin K should be administered if indicated.

■ Pediatric Precautions Safety and efficacy of oral cefuroxime axetil or parenteral cefuroxime sodium in children younger than 3 months of age have not been established.

In vitro studies indicate that cefuroxime does not appear to displace bilirubin appreciably from albumin binding sites in neonates†.

Cefuroxime Axetil The manufacturers state that safety and efficacy of cefuroxime axetil for the treatment of acute bacterial maxillary sinusitis in pediatric patients 3 months to 12 years of age have been established based on safety and efficacy of the drug in adults. In addition, use of cefuroxime axetil in pediatric patients is supported by pharmacokinetic and safety data in adult and pediatric patients, clinical and microbiologic data from adequate and well-controlled studies of the treatment of acute bacterial maxillary sinusitis in adults and acute otitis media with effusion in pediatric patients, and postmarketing surveillance of adverse effects.

Cefuroxime axetil tablets and oral suspension generally are well tolerated in children aged 3 months to 12 years. Cefuroxime axetil has a strong, persistent, bitter taste and complaints caused by the taste were reported in up to 66% of children who received the drug as crushed tablets and vomiting was induced aversively in some of these children. This bitter taste and/or problems with administering the drug required discontinuance of such cefuroxime axetil therapy in 2–28% of children in clinical trials. Although discontinuance of therapy with the suspension because of its taste or other problems with administration occurred in 1.4% of children receiving the oral suspension, the commercially available oral suspension should be used in children who cannot swallow the tablets whole.

Cefuroxime Sodium To avoid overdosage, the commercially available Duplex® drug delivery system containing 750 mg or 1.5 g of cefuroxime should not be used in pediatric patients only if the entire 750-mg or 1.5-g dose in the container is required.

■ Geriatric Precautions In clinical studies of cefuroxime axetil, 375 patients were 65 years of age or older and 151 were 75 years of age or older. There were no apparent differences in safety or effectiveness between these individuals and younger adults. Although the group of patients aged 65 years or older experienced a lower incidence of some adverse effects (e.g., vaginal candidiasis, GI effects) compared with patients 12–64 years of age, no clinically important differences were observed between geriatric and younger patients and there have been no reports of differences in response in either group.

In clinical studies of cefuroxime sodium involving over 1900 patients, approximately 47% of the patients were 65 years of age or older and 22% were 75 years of age or older. Although no overall differences in efficacy or safety were observed between geriatric and younger patients, and other clinical experience revealed no evidence of age-related differences, the possibility that some geriatric patients may exhibit increased sensitivity to the drug cannot be ruled out.

Cefuroxime is substantially excreted by the kidney, and renal elimination of the drug may be decreased and the risk of severe adverse reactions may be increased in patients with impaired renal function. Limited data indicate that mean serum elimination half-life of cefuroxime is prolonged in geriatric patients (mean age: 83.9 years) who have a mean creatinine clearance of approximately 35 mL/minute. Despite this prolonged elimination, the manufacturers state that age-based dosage adjustment does not appear to be necessary. However, because geriatric patients are more likely to have decreased renal function, dosage should be selected with caution in these patients and monitoring of renal function may be useful.

■ Mutagenicity and Carcinogenicity No evidence of mutagenicity was observed with cefuroxime in various in vitro and in vivo test systems, including the mouse lymphoma assay, micronucleus test, and bacterial mutation tests. Cefuroxime produced positive results in the in vitro chromosome aberration assay. Studies have not been performed to date to evaluate the carcinogenic potential of cefuroxime.

■ Pregnancy, Fertility, and Lactation Reproduction studies in mice and rabbits using cefuroxime sodium in dosages up to 6 and 2 times the usual human dosage based on mg/m², respectively, and reproduction studies in mice and rats using cefuroxime axetil in dosages up to 14 and 9 times, respectively, the usual human dosage based on mg/m² have not revealed evidence of impaired fertility or harm to the fetus. There are no adequate and controlled studies to date using cefuroxime in pregnant women, and cefuroxime axetil and cefuroxime sodium should be used during pregnancy only when clearly needed. Cefuroxime axetil has not been studied for use during labor and delivery.

Because cefuroxime is distributed into milk, cefuroxime axetil and cefuroxime sodium should be used with caution in nursing women.

Drug Interactions

■ Aminoglycosides In vitro studies indicate that the antibacterial activity of cefuroxime and aminoglycosides may be additive or synergistic against some organisms including *Enterobacter*, *Escherichia coli*, *Klebsiella*, *Proteus mirabilis*, and *Serratia marcescens*.

Concurrent use of aminoglycosides and certain cephalosporins reportedly may increase the risk of nephrotoxicity during therapy. Although this effect has not been reported to date with cefuroxime, the possibility that nephrotoxicity may be potentiated should be considered if the drug is used concomitantly with an aminoglycoside.

■ Diuretics The manufacturers state that cefuroxime should be used with caution in patients receiving diuretics because concurrent use of these drugs may increase the risk of adverse renal effects.

■ **Estrogens or Progestins** Cefuroxime axetil may affect gut flora, leading to decreased estrogen reabsorption and reduced efficacy of oral contraceptives containing estrogen and progestin.

■ **Probenecid** Oral probenecid administered shortly before or concomitantly with cefuroxime usually slows the rate of tubular secretion of cefuroxime and produces higher and more prolonged serum concentrations of cefuroxime. This effect has been used to therapeutic advantage in the treatment of gonorrhea. Peak serum concentrations of cefuroxime and the half-life of the drug are reportedly increased by up to 30% when probenecid is administered concomitantly; the area under the concentration-time curve (AUC) of cefuroxime is increased by about 50%. Concomitant administration of probenecid also reportedly decreases the apparent volume of distribution of cefuroxime by about 20%.

Laboratory Test Interferences

■ **Immunohematology Tests** Positive direct antiglobulin (Coombs') test results have been reported in a few patients receiving cefuroxime axetil or cefuroxime sodium. This reaction may interfere with hematologic studies or transfusion cross-matching procedures.

■ **Tests for Glucose** Like most other cephalosporins, cefuroxime reportedly causes false-positive results in urine glucose determinations using cupric sulfate solution (Benedict's reagent, Clinitest®); however, glucose oxidase tests (Clinistix®) are unaffected by the drug.

Cefuroxime may cause false-negative results when ferricyanide methods are used to determine blood glucose concentrations.

■ **Tests for Creatinine** Although some cephalosporins reportedly cause falsely elevated serum or urine creatinine values when the Jaffé reaction is used, cefuroxime does not appear to interfere with this laboratory test.

Acute Toxicity

Limited information is available on the acute toxicity of cefuroxime in humans. Overdosage of cephalosporins can cause CNS irritation leading to seizures. If acute overdosage of cefuroxime occurs, hemodialysis and/or peritoneal dialysis can be used to enhance elimination of the drug from the body.

Mechanism of Action

Cefuroxime is usually bactericidal in action. Like other cephalosporins, the antibacterial activity of the drug results from inhibition of mucopeptide synthesis in the bacterial cell wall. For information on the mechanism of action of cephalosporins, see Mechanism of Action in the Cephalosporins General Statement 8:12.06.

Spectrum

Based on its spectrum of activity, cefuroxime is classified as a second generation cephalosporin. For information on the classification of cephalosporins and closely related β-lactam antibiotics based on spectra of activity, see Spectrum in the Cephalosporins General Statement 8:12.06.

Like other currently available second generation cephalosporins (e.g., cefaclor, cefamandole, cefprozil), cefuroxime generally is more active in vitro against gram-negative bacteria than first generation cephalosporins but has a narrower spectrum of activity against gram-negative bacteria than third generation cephalosporins. The spectrum of activity of cefuroxime resembles that of cefamandole and, to a lesser extent, that of cefoxitin. Cefuroxime is more resistant to hydrolysis by β-lactamases than cefamandole and is active against some strains of gram-negative bacteria (e.g., *Escherichia coli, Enterobacter, Klebsiella, Neisseria*) that are resistant to cefamandole. Cefoxitin is active against several organisms that generally are resistant to cefuroxime (e.g., *Serratia marcescens, Proteus vulgaris, Bacteroides fragilis*).

■ **In Vitro Susceptibility Testing** Results of in vitro cefuroxime susceptibility tests are not generally affected by inoculum size, culture media, presence of serum, or pH. However, results of susceptibility tests for some gram-negative bacilli (e.g., *Morganella morganii, Bacteroides fragilis, Serratia*) may be affected by the size of the inoculum.

Different interpretive criteria are used for defining in vitro susceptibility of certain organisms to cefuroxime axetil and cefuroxime sodium, and the appropriate zone diameter or MIC categories should be used when determining whether or not an isolate is susceptible to the parenteral or oral preparation of the drug.

Strains of staphylococci resistant to penicillinase-resistant penicillins (oxacillin-resistant [methicillin-resistant] staphylococci) should be considered resistant to cefuroxime and cefuroxime axetil, although results of in vitro susceptibility tests may indicate that the organisms are susceptible to the drug. In addition, β-lactamase-negative, ampicillin-resistant (BLNAR) strains of *H. influenzae* should be considered resistant to cefuroxime and cefuroxime axetil despite the fact that results of in vitro susceptibility tests may indicate that the organisms are susceptible to the drug.

For information on interpreting results of in vitro susceptibility testing (disk susceptibility tests, dilution susceptibility tests) when cefuroxime and cefuroxime axetil susceptibility testing is performed according to the standards of the Clinical and Laboratory Standards Institute (CLSI; formerly National Committee for Clinical Laboratory Standards [NCCLS]), see Spectrum: In Vitro Susceptibility Testing, in the Cephalosporins General Statement 8:12.06.

■ **Gram-Positive Aerobic Bacteria** In vitro, cefuroxime concentrations of 0.5–1 mcg/mL inhibit most strains of *Staphylococcus aureus* (including penicillinase-producing and nonpenicillinase-producing strains) and concentrations of 1–2 mcg/mL inhibit most strains of *S. epidermidis*. Most strains of staphylococci resistant to penicillinase-resistant penicillins also are resistant to cefuroxime.

In vitro, α-hemolytic and β-hemolytic streptococci are usually inhibited by cefuroxime concentrations of 0.05–0.5 mcg/mL and *Streptococcus pneumoniae* is usually inhibited by concentrations of 0.01–0.13 mcg/mL. Most strains of enterococci, including *E. faecalis* (formerly *S. faecalis*), are generally resistant to cefuroxime.

Listeria monocytogenes generally is resistant to cefuroxime.

■ **Gram-Negative Aerobic Bacteria** Cefuroxime is active in vitro against most gram-negative aerobic cocci and many gram-negative aerobic bacilli including Enterobacteriaceae. *Pseudomonas aeruginosa* is resistant to cefuroxime. *Acinetobacter calcoaceticus* is also usually resistant to the drug.

Generally, cefuroxime is active in vitro against the following Enterobacteriaceae: *Citrobacter diversus, C. freundii, Enterobacter aerogenes, Escherichia coli, Klebsiella pneumoniae, Proteus mirabilis, Providencia stuartii, Salmonella*, and *Shigella*. Although cefuroxime is active in vitro against some strains of *Morganella morganii* (formerly *Proteus morganii*), *Providencia rettgeri* (formerly *Proteus rettgeri*), and *Proteus vulgaris*, most strains of these organisms are resistant to the drug. In addition, *Enterobacter cloacae, Legionella, Pseudomonas, Campylobacter* spp., *Providencia*, and most strains of *Serratia* are usually resistant to cefuroxime. Most susceptible Enterobacteriaceae are inhibited in vitro by cefuroxime concentrations of 1–12.5 mcg/mL. In vitro on a weight basis, the activity of cefuroxime against susceptible Enterobacteriaceae is approximately equal to that of cefoxitin but less than that of cefotaxime. Cefuroxime may be active in vitro against some strains of *E. aerogenes* that are resistant to cefoxitin; however, cefotaxime and, to a lesser extent, cefoxitin may be active in vitro against some strains of *P. vulgaris* and *Serratia* resistant to cefuroxime.

Cefuroxime is active in vitro against *Haemophilus influenzae* (including ampicillin-resistant strains) and *H. parainfluenzae*. Most susceptible strains of *H. influenzae* are inhibited in vitro by cefuroxime concentrations of 0.1–2 mcg/mL.

Cefuroxime is active in vitro against *Neisseria gonorrhoeae* (including both penicillinase-producing and nonpenicillinase-producing strains) and *N. meningitidis*. The MIC_{90} (minimum inhibitory concentration of the drug at which 90% of strains tested are inhibited) of cefuroxime reported for *N. gonorrhoeae* (including both penicillinase-producing and nonpenicillinase-producing strains) is 0.1–0.5 mcg/mL.

■ **Anaerobic Bacteria** Cefuroxime is active in vitro against some anaerobic bacteria including *Actinomyces, Eubacterium, Fusobacterium, Lactobacillus, Peptococcus, Peptostreptococcus, Propionibacterium*, and *Veillonella*. Cefuroxime is active in vitro against some strains of *Clostridium*; however, *C. difficile* is usually resistant to the drug.

Most susceptible anaerobes are inhibited in vitro by cefuroxime concentrations of 0.5–16 mcg/mL. Although cefuroxime concentrations of 16 mcg/mL inhibit some strains of *Bacteroides fragilis* in vitro, most strains of the organism are resistant to the drug.

■ **Spirochetes** Cefuroxime is active in vitro and in vivo against *Borrelia burgdorferi*, the causative organism of Lyme disease. In vitro, the MIC of cefuroxime for *B. burgdorferi* reportedly is 0.13 mcg/mL and the minimum bactericidal concentration (MBC) is 1 mcg/mL.

Resistance

For information on possible mechanisms of bacterial resistance to cephalosporins, see Resistance in the Cephalosporins General Statement 8:12.06.

Because cefuroxime contains a methoxyimino group that protects the β-lactam ring from hydrolysis by many penicillinases and cephalosporinases, the drug is more resistant to hydrolysis by β-lactamases than are first generation cephalosporins or cefamandole. Cefuroxime is generally resistant to hydrolysis by β-lactamases classified as Richmond-Sykes types I, II, III, IV, and V and most β-lactamases produced by *Neisseria gonorrhoeae, Haemophilus influenzae*, and staphylococci. However, cefuroxime is hydrolyzed by β-lactamases produced by *B. fragilis* and some type I β-lactamases produced by *Serratia, P. vulgaris*, and *P. rettgeri*. Results of one in vitro study indicate that cefuroxime is hydrolyzed more rapidly than cefotaxime by β-lactamases produced by *P. vulgaris* and *B. fragilis*. Although cefuroxime is resistant to hydrolysis by β-lactamases produced by *Ps. aeruginosa*, these organisms are resistant to cefuroxime because the drug cannot penetrate their cell wall.

Pharmacokinetics

In all studies described in the Pharmacokinetics section, cefuroxime was administered orally as the 1-(acetyloxy)ethyl ester (i.e., cefuroxime axetil) and parenterally as the sodium salt; dosages and concentrations of the drug are expressed in terms of cefuroxime. Because cefuroxime axetil is hydrolyzed rapidly ($t_{1/2}$: 3.5 minutes) in vitro in blood or serum, some clinicians recommend that acetonitrile be added immediately to blood or serum samples intended for pharmacokinetic determinations of the drug in order to prevent further hydrolysis and resultant falsely high concentrations of active drug.

■ **Absorption** ***Cefuroxime Axetil*** Following oral administration of cefuroxime axetil, the drug is absorbed as the 1-(acetyloxy)ethyl ester from the GI tract and rapidly hydrolyzed to cefuroxime by nonspecific esterases in the intestinal mucosa and blood. Cefuroxime remaining within the intestinal lumen following hydrolysis of the ester is not absorbed appreciably. The drug has little, if any, microbiologic activity until hydrolyzed in vivo to cefuroxime.

Bioavailability following oral administration of cefuroxime axetil is variable and depends on the formulation used and presence of food in the GI tract. Many published studies on the pharmacokinetics of the drug used various formulations that provided poorer bioavailability than the currently available tablets and cannot be used to provide information on the currently available preparation.

When tested in healthy adults, the bioavailability of cefuroxime axetil oral suspension was found *not* to be equivalent to that of cefuroxime axetil tablets. Mean area under the concentration-time curve (AUC) for the oral suspension was 91% of the AUC for the tablets, and the mean peak plasma concentration of cefuroxime following administration of the cefuroxime axetil oral suspension was 71% of that achieved following administration of cefuroxime axetil tablets. Therefore, cefuroxime axetil oral suspension and tablet formulations are not substitutable on a mg/mg basis. (See Dosage: Pediatric Dosage in Dosage and Administration.)

In adults, bioavailability of cefuroxime following oral administration of commercially available cefuroxime axetil tablets averages about 37% when given in the fasting state and 52% when given with or shortly after food. Absorption of the drug is increased when given with milk or infant formula. In one study, the extent but not the rate of absorption was substantially greater when the drug was administered concomitantly with milk compared with applesauce or fasting.

Following oral administration in adults of a single 125-mg, 250-mg, 500-mg, or 1-g dose of commercially available cefuroxime axetil tablets immediately following a meal, peak serum cefuroxime concentrations are attained approximately 2–3 hours after the dose and average 2.1, 4.1, 7, or 13.6 mcg/mL, respectively; serum concentrations 6 hours after the dose average 0.3, 0.7, 2.2, or 3.4 mcg/mL, respectively. AUC of the drug in these individuals averaged 6.7, 12.9, 27.4, or 50 mcg-h/mL, respectively.

Results of a study in healthy adults indicate that cefuroxime axetil oral suspensions containing 125 mg/5 mL or 250 mg/5 mL are bioequivalent. In healthy adults who received a 250-mg dose of cefuroxime axetil given as a suspension containing 125 mg/5 mL or 250 mg/5 mL with food, peak plasma concentrations of cefuroxime were 2.4 or 2.2 mcg/mL, respectively, and were attained 3 hours after the dose.

In pharmacokinetic studies of cefuroxime axetil oral suspension in children, the drug was administered postprandially or with food; no data are available regarding absorption of the suspension in fasting children. Following oral administration to children 3 months to 12 years of age (mean age: 23 months) of a single 10-, 15-, or 20-mg/kg dose of commercially available cefuroxime axetil oral suspension concomitantly with milk or milk products, peak serum cefuroxime concentrations are attained approximately 3.6, 2.7, or 3.1 hours after the dose, respectively, and average 3.3, 5.1, or 7 mcg/mL, respectively.

Cefuroxime Sodium Cefuroxime sodium is not appreciably absorbed from the GI tract and must be given parenterally. Following IM administration of a single 500-mg, 750-mg, or 1-g dose of cefuroxime in healthy adults with normal renal function, peak serum concentrations of the drug are attained within 15–60 minutes and range from 20.8–25.7, 26–34.9, and 32–40 mcg/mL, respectively. In one study following IM administration of a single 750-mg dose of cefuroxime in healthy adults, serum concentrations of the drug averaged 32.8 mcg/mL 40 minutes after the dose, 19.1 mcg/mL 2 hours after the dose, 6.1 mcg/mL 4 hours after the dose, 1.5 mcg/mL 6 hours after the dose, and 0.7 mcg/mL 8 hours after the dose. IM injection of a single 1.5-g dose of the drug reportedly results in peak serum concentrations averaging 46 mcg/mL. Mean peak serum concentrations of cefuroxime and the areas under the concentration-time curve (AUC) are not substantially different after IM injection of cefuroxime as a suspension or as a solution. The AUC of cefuroxime is proportional to the dose administered and is similar following IM or IV administration of the drug. In one preliminary study in women, serum concentrations of cefuroxime were lower when IM injections of the drug were given into the gluteus maximus than when the same dose was given into the thigh.

In one study in healthy adults with normal renal function, a single 500-mg or 1-g dose of cefuroxime given by IV injection over 3 minutes resulted in serum concentrations of cefuroxime that averaged 66.3 and 99.2 mcg/mL, respectively, immediately after the injection; serum concentrations of the drug averaged 2.1 and 3.6 mcg/mL, respectively, 4 hours after the injection. In another study in healthy adults with normal renal function, IV injection over 2–3 minutes of a single 750-mg dose of cefuroxime resulted in serum concentrations of cefuroxime that averaged 52.6 mcg/mL 15 minutes after the injection, 24 mcg/mL 1 hour after the injection, 9.7 mcg/mL 2 hours after the injection, 3.5 mcg/mL 4 hours after the injection, and 0.5 mcg/mL 8 hours after the injection.

IV infusion over 30 minutes of a single 500- or 750-mg dose of cefuroxime reportedly results in peak serum concentrations of the drug averaging 37.8 and 51.1 mcg/mL, respectively. IV infusion over 1 hour of a single 750-mg or 1-g dose of cefuroxime reportedly results in peak serum concentrations of the drug averaging 38 and 64.4 mcg/mL, respectively.

In one study in neonates, IM administration of a single cefuroxime dose of 25 mg/kg resulted in serum concentrations of the drug that averaged 45 mcg/mL 30 minutes after the injection, 35 mcg/mL 3 hours after the injection, and 10.5 mcg/mL 12 hours after the injection. IM administration of a single cefuroxime dose of 10 mg/kg in neonates younger than 3 weeks of age reportedly resulted in serum concentrations of the drug that ranged from 15–25 mcg/mL 30–60 minutes after injection.

■ **Distribution** The apparent volume of distribution of cefuroxime in healthy adults ranges from 9.3–15.8 L/1.73 m^2.

Following IM or IV administration of usual dosages of cefuroxime, the drug is widely distributed into body tissues and fluids including the kidneys, heart, gallbladder, liver, prostatic adenoma tissue, uterine and ovarian tissue, aqueous humor, saliva, sputum, bronchial secretions, bone, bile, adipose tissue, wound exudates, peritoneal fluid, ascitic fluid, synovial fluid, pericardial fluid, and pleural fluid.

Following oral administration of cefuroxime axetil in pediatric patients with acute otitis media with effusion or with chronic or recurrent otitis media with effusion, cefuroxime is distributed into middle ear effusions. In a study in pediatric patients 1–4 years of age with acute otitis media with effusion who received a single 15 mg/kg dose of cefuroxime as cefuroxime axetil oral suspension, cefuroxime concentrations in middle ear effusions 2–5 hours after a dose ranged from 0.2–3.6 mcg/mL; concurrent serum concentrations were 2.8–7.3 mcg/mL.

Cefuroxime is 33–50% bound to serum proteins.

Cefuroxime concentrations in CSF are low following IV administration of usual dosages of the drug in patients with uninflamed meninges; however, therapeutic concentrations of cefuroxime may be attained following IV administration of the drug in patients with inflamed meninges. In one study in adults receiving 1–2 g of cefuroxime IV every 8 hours, the maximum CSF concentration of cefuroxime in patients with uninflamed or inflamed meninges was 0.1 or 8.28 mcg/mL, respectively. In adults with meningitis receiving 1.5 g of cefuroxime every 6 or 8 hours, mean CSF concentrations of the drug attained within 8 hours after dosing are 6 mcg/mL (range: 1.5–13.5) or 5.2 mcg/mL (range: 2.7–8.9), respectively. In one study in children 1–4 years of age with meningitis receiving rapid IV injection of cefuroxime 50 mg/kg every 6 hours, CSF concentrations of the drug after at least 2 days of therapy ranged from 1.1–9.8 mcg/mL in CSF specimens obtained 2 hours after a dose. In pediatric patients 4 weeks to 6.5 years of age with meningitis receiving 50 mg/kg every 6 hours, mean CSF concentrations of cefuroxime were 6.6 mcg/mL (range: 0.9–17.3). In another study in pediatric patients 7 months to 9 years of age with meningitis receiving 67–77 mg/kg every 8 hours, mean CSF concentrations of cefuroxime were 8.3 mcg/mL (range: less than 2 up to 22.5).

Cefuroxime readily crosses the placenta. Amniotic fluid concentrations of cefuroxime reportedly average 17–18.6 mcg/mL 3–5.5 hours after a single 750-mg IM dose of the drug. Cefuroxime is distributed into milk.

■ **Elimination** In adults, the serum or plasma half-life of cefuroxime following oral administration of commercially available cefuroxime axetil tablets or oral suspension ranges from 1.2–1.6 hours. In adults with normal renal function, the serum half-life of cefuroxime following IM or IV administration reportedly ranges from 1–2 hours. In adults, approximately 50% of an administered dose of cefuroxime axetil is recovered in the urine within 12 hours.

In patients with renal impairment, the serum half-life of the drug is prolonged and generally ranges from 1.9–16.1 hours depending on the degree of impairment. In one study, the serum half-life of cefuroxime was 1 hour in patients with creatinine clearances of 50–79 mL/minute, 2.55 hours in patients with creatinine clearances of 25–46 mL/minute, 5.1 hours in patients with creatinine clearances of 10–24 mL/minute, and 14.8 hours in patients with creatinine clearances less than 10 mL/minute. A serum half-life of 15–22 hours has been reported in anuric patients.

In neonates and children, the serum half-life of cefuroxime is inversely proportional to age. Following oral administration of cefuroxime axetil oral suspension in children 3 months to 12 years of age, the serum half-life of cefuroxime averages 1.4–1.9 hours. The serum half-life of cefuroxime following IM or IV administration is reportedly 5.1–5.8 hours in neonates 3 days of age or younger, 2–4.2 hours in neonates 6–14 days of age, and 1–1.5 hours in neonates 3–4 weeks of age. The manufacturers of cefuroxime axetil state that the urinary pharmacokinetics of cefuroxime axetil have not been determined in children and that the renal pharmacokinetics of oral cefuroxime axetil as established in the adult population should not be extrapolated to children.

Following oral administration, cefuroxime axetil is rapidly hydrolyzed to cefuroxime by nonspecific esterases in the intestinal mucosa and blood; the axetil moiety is metabolized to acetaldehyde and acetic acid. Cefuroxime is not metabolized and is excreted unchanged principally in urine by both glomerular filtration and tubular secretion. In adults with normal renal function, 90–100% of a single IM or IV dose of cefuroxime is excreted unchanged in urine within 24 hours; most of the dose is excreted within the first 6 hours following administration. Following IM administration of a single 750-mg dose of cefuroxime, urinary concentrations of the drug average 1.3 mg/mL in urine collected during the first 8 hours after administration. Urinary concentrations of cefuroxime average 1.15 or 2.5 mg/mL in urine collected over the first 8 hours following IV administration of a single 750-mg or 1.5-g dose of the drug, respectively.

Concomitant administration of probenecid competitively inhibits renal tubular secretion of cefuroxime and produces higher and more prolonged serum concentrations of the drug. (See Drug Interactions: Probenecid.)

Cefuroxime is removed by hemodialysis and by peritoneal dialysis.

Chemistry and Stability

■ **Chemistry** Cefuroxime is a semisynthetic cephalosporin antibiotic. cefuroxime contains a methoxyimino group at position 7 on the β-lactam ring and also contains a carbamate group at position 3 on the ring. The methoxyimino group results in stability against hydrolysis by many β-lactamases and the carbamate group results in metabolic stability.

Cefuroxime is commercially available for parenteral administration as the sodium salt. The drug is commercially available for oral administration as film-coated tablets or as a powder for suspension of cefuroxime axetil, the 1-(acetyloxy)ethyl ester of the drug. Potency of cefuroxime sodium and cefuroxime axetil is expressed in terms of cefuroxime.

Cefuroxime Axetil Cefuroxime axetil is a prodrug of cefuroxime and has little, if any, antibacterial activity until hydrolyzed in vivo to cefuroxime. Esterification of the carboxyl C-4 group of cefuroxime results in a more lipophilic and readily absorbable (from the GI tract) form of the drug. Cefuroxime axetil occurs as a white to cream-colored, amorphous powder.

Cefuroxime Sodium Cefuroxime sodium occurs as a white to off-white powder. The drug has solubilities of about 200 mg/mL in water and 1 mg/mL in alcohol. The drug has a pK_a of 2.45. The sodium salt of cefuroxime contains 2.4 mEq of sodium per gram of cefuroxime.

Following reconstitution, cefuroxime sodium solutions are light yellow to amber in color and have a pH of 6–8.5, depending on the concentration of the drug and the diluent used. Reconstitution of cefuroxime sodium sterile powder for injection to provide a final concentration of 208 mg/mL results in the formation of a suspension; dilution to at least 100 mg/mL effects complete dissolution of the drug.

When the commercially available Duplex® delivery system containing 750 mg or 1.5 g of cefuroxime and 50 mL of dextrose injection in separate chambers is reconstituted (activated) according to the manufacturer's directions, the resultant solution is iso-osmotic and has an osmolality of approximately 290 mOsm/kg.

The commercially available frozen premixed injection of cefuroxime sodium containing 1.5 g of cefuroxime is a sterile, nonpyrogenic, iso-osmotic solution of the drug provided in a plastic container fabricated from specially formulated multilayered plastic PL 2040. The 1.5-g frozen injection contains 600 mg of sodium citrate hydrous as a buffer and 222 mg (9.7 mEq) of sodium, and has an osmolality of approximately 300 mOsm/kg. After thawing, the injection has a pH to 5–7.5.

■ **Stability** ***Cefuroxime Axetil*** Cefuroxime axetil tablets should be stored in tight containers at 20–25°C or 15–30°C, depending on the manufacturer. When cefuroxime axetil tablets are allowed to disintegrate in apple juice, the drug is stable for 24 hours at room temperature.

Commercially available cefuroxime axetil powder for oral suspension should be stored at 2–30°C. Following reconstitution, oral suspensions of cefuroxime axetil containing 125 mg/5 mL or 250 mg/5 mL should be stored immediately at 2–8°C in a refrigerator. Any unused oral suspension should be discarded after 10 days.

Cefuroxime Sodium Commercially available cefuroxime sodium sterile powder for injection should be stored at 15–30°C and protected from light.

Following reconstitution of vials containing 750 mg or 1.5 g of cefuroxime or the pharmacy bulk vial containing 7.5 g of the drug with sterile water for injection according to the manufacturer's directions, solutions for IV administration are stable for 24 hours at room temperature or 48 hours (750-mg and 1.5-g vials) or 7 days (7.5-g pharmacy bulk vial) when refrigerated (5°C). More dilute solutions, such as 750 mg or 1.5 g in 100 mL of sterile water for injection, 5% dextrose injection, or 0.9% sodium chloride injection also are stable for 24 hours at room temperature or 7 days when refrigerated.

Following reconstitution of 750-mg or 1.5-g ADD-Vantage® (TwistVial®) vials of cefuroxime with 5% dextrose injection, 0.9% sodium chloride injection, or 0.45% sodium chloride injection according to the manufacturer's directions, solutions are stable for 24 hours at room temperature or 7 days under refrigeration; joined vials that have not been activated (diluted) may be used within a 14-day period.

IM injections containing 225 mg/mL of cefuroxime prepared using the 750-mg vial and sterile water for injection according to the manufacturer's directions are stable for 24 hours at room temperature or 48 hours when refrigerated (5°C).

Cefuroxime sodium is chemically and physically compatible with the following IV solutions: 0.9% sodium chloride; Ringer's; lactated Ringer's; 5% dextrose; 5% dextrose and 0.2%, 0.45%, or 0.9% sodium chloride; 10% dextrose; 10% invert sugar; or ⅙ *M* sodium lactate. Reconstituted solutions of cefuroxime that have been further diluted to a concentration of 1–30 mg/mL with one of the above IV solutions are stable for 24 hours at room temperature or at least 7 days when refrigerated.

The manufacturer of Zinacef® states that cefuroxime sodium solutions prepared using the 750-mg or 1.5-g vials or the 7.5-g pharmacy bulk vial may be frozen immediately after reconstitution and dilution; the entire contents from the reconstituted 750-mg or 1.5-g vial or 8 or 16 mL from the 7.5-g vial should be immediately withdrawn and added to a Viaflex® minibag containing 50 or 100 mL of 0.9% sodium chloride injection or 5% dextrose injection and frozen. These extemporaneously prepared solutions are stable for 6 months when frozen at −20°C. After thawing at room temperature, these solutions are stable for 24 hours at room temperature or 7 days when refrigerated; these solutions should not be refrozen.

The commercially available Duplex® drug delivery system containing 750 mg or 1.5 g of cefuroxime and 50 mL of dextrose injection should be stored at 20–25°C, but may be exposed to 15–30°C. Following reconstitution (activation), these IV solutions must be used within 24 hours if stored at room temperature or within 7 days if stored in a refrigerator and should not be frozen.

The commercially available frozen premixed cefuroxime sodium injection should be stored at −20°C or lower. The frozen injection should be thawed at room temperature (25°C) or under refrigeration (5°C) and, once thawed, should not be refrozen. Thawed solutions of the commercially available frozen injection are stable for 24 hours at room temperature (25°C) or 28 days under refrigeration (5°C). The commercially available frozen injection of the drug is provided in a plastic container fabricated from specially formulated multilayered plastic PL 2040 (Galaxy® containers). Solutions in contact with PL 2040 can leach out some of its chemical components in very small amounts within the expiration period of the injection; however, safety of the plastic has been confirmed in tests in animals according to USP biological tests for plastic containers as well as by tissue culture toxicity studies.

Cefuroxime sodium sterile powder and solutions of the drug tend to darken, depending on storage conditions; however, this discoloration does not necessarily indicate a change in potency.

Cefuroxime sodium is potentially physically and/or chemically incompatible with some drugs, including aminoglycosides, but the compatibility depends on several factors (e.g., concentrations of the drugs, specific diluents used, resulting pH, temperature). Specialized references should be consulted for specific compatibility information. Admixtures in 0.9% sodium chloride injection containing cefuroxime sodium and heparin (10 or 50 units/mL) or potassium chloride (10 or 40 mEq/L) are stable for 24 hours at room temperature. The manufacturer of Zinacef® states that cefuroxime sodium not be diluted with sodium bicarbonate injection. Because of the potential for incompatibility, the manufacturers state that cefuroxime sodium and aminoglycosides should not be admixed.

For further information on chemistry, mechanism of action, spectrum, resistance, pharmacokinetics, uses, cautions, drug interactions, laboratory test interferences, and dosage and administration of cefuroxime, see the Cephalosporins General Statement 8:12.06.

Preparations

Excipients in commercially available drug preparations may have clinically important effects in some individuals; consult specific product labeling for details.

Cefuroxime Axetil

Oral		
For Suspension	125 mg (of cefuroxime) per 5 mL*	**Ceftin®**, GlaxoSmithKline **Cefuroxime Axetil for Suspension**
	250 mg (of cefuroxime) per 5 mL*	**Ceftin®**, GlaxoSmithKline **Cefuroxime Axetil for Suspension**
Tablets, film-coated	125 mg (of cefuroxime)*	**Cefuroxime Axetil Tablets**
	250 mg (of cefuroxime)*	**Ceftin®**, GlaxoSmithKline **Cefuroxime Axetil Tablets**
	500 mg (of cefuroxime)*	**Ceftin®**, GlaxoSmithKline **Cefuroxime Axetil Tablets**

*available from one or more manufacturer, distributor, and/or repackager by generic (nonproprietary) name

Cefuroxime Sodium

Parenteral		
For injection	750 mg (of cefuroxime)*	**Cefuroxime Sodium for Injection** **Zinacef®**, Covis
	1.5 g (of cefuroxime)*	**Cefuroxime Sodium for Injection** **Zinacef®**, Covis
	7.5 g (of cefuroxime) pharmacy bulk package*	**Cefuroxime Sodium for Injection** **Zinacef®**, Covis
For injection, for IV infusion	750 mg (of cefuroxime)*	**Cefuroxime Sodium for Injection** (available in dual-chambered Duplex® drug delivery system with 4.1% dextrose injection), B Braun **Zinacef® TwistVial®**, Covis
	1.5 g (of cefuroxime)*	**Cefuroxime Sodium for Injection** (available in dual-chambered Duplex® drug delivery system with 2.9% dextrose injection), B Braun **Zinacef® TwistVial®**, Covis

*available from one or more manufacturer, distributor, and/or repackager by generic (nonproprietary) name

Cefuroxime Sodium in Water

Parenteral		
Injection (frozen), for IV infusion	30 mg (of cefuroxime) per mL (1.5 g)	**Zinacef® Iso-osmotic in Sterile Water Injection** (Galaxy® [Baxter]), Covis

†Use is not currently included in the labeling approved by the US Food and Drug Administration

Selected Revisions October 2013, © Copyright, April 1984, American Society of Health-System Pharmacists, Inc.

THIRD GENERATION CEPHALOSPORINS 8:12.06.12

Cefdinir

■ Cefdinir is a semisynthetic, third generation cephalosporin antibiotic.

Uses

Cefdinir is used orally for the treatment of mild to moderate upper and lower respiratory tract infections (i.e., acute maxillary sinusitis, acute exacerbations of chronic bronchitis, community-acquired pneumonia) caused by susceptible bacteria. The drug also is used orally for the treatment of acute bacterial otitis media, streptococcal pharyngitis and tonsillitis, and mild to moderate, uncomplicated skin and skin structure infections caused by susceptible bacteria.

■ **Acute Otitis Media** Oral cefdinir is used in children 6 months of age or older for the treatment of acute otitis media (AOM) caused by *Streptococcus pneumoniae* (penicillin-susceptible strains only), *Haemophilus influenzae* (including β-lactamase-producing strains), or *Moraxella catarrhalis* (including β-lactamase-producing strains).

When anti-infective therapy is indicated for the treatment of AOM, the American Academy of Pediatrics (AAP) recommends high-dose amoxicillin or amoxicillin and clavulanate potassium as the drugs of first choice for initial treatment. These experts recommend certain cephalosporins (cefdinir, cefuroxime, cefpodoxime, ceftriaxone) as alternatives for initial treatment in penicillin-allergic patients who do not have a history of severe and/or recent penicillin-allergic reactions.

In a controlled study in children 6 months to 12 years of age with acute suppurative otitis media, a 10-day regimen of once-daily cefdinir (14 mg/kg as a single daily dose), twice-daily cefdinir (7 mg/kg twice daily), or amoxicillin and clavulanate potassium (13.3 mg/kg of amoxicillin 3 times daily) produced similar clinical and bacteriologic responses.

For additional information regarding treatment of AOM, including information on diagnosis and management strategies, anti-infectives for initial treatment, duration of initial treatment, and anti-infectives after initial treatment failure, see Acute Otitis Media under Uses: Otitis Media, in the Cephalosporins General Statement 8:12.06.

■ **Pharyngitis and Tonsillitis** Oral cefdinir is used for the treatment of pharyngitis and tonsillitis caused by susceptible *S. pyogenes* (group A β-hemolytic streptococci) in adults and children 6 months of age and older. Although cefdinir may effectively eradicate *S. pyogenes* from the nasopharynx, efficacy of the drug in the subsequent prevention of rheumatic fever has not been fully evaluated to date.

Selection of an anti-infective for the treatment of *S. pyogenes* pharyngitis and tonsillitis should be based on the drug's spectrum of activity, bacteriologic and clinical efficacy, potential adverse effects, ease of administration, patient compliance, and cost. No regimen has been found to date that effectively eradicates group A β-hemolytic streptococci in 100% of patients.

Because the drugs have a narrow spectrum of activity, are inexpensive, and generally are effective with a low frequency of adverse effects, the AAP, Infectious Diseases Society of America (IDSA), American Heart Association (AHA), and others recommend a penicillin regimen (i.e., 10 days of oral penicillin V or oral amoxicillin or single dose of IM penicillin G benzathine) as the treatment of choice for *S. pyogenes* pharyngitis and tonsillitis and prevention of initial attacks (primary prevention) of rheumatic fever. Other anti-infectives (e.g., oral cephalosporins, oral macrolides, oral clindamycin) are recommended as alternatives in penicillin-allergic individuals.

If an oral cephalosporin is used for the treatment of *S. pyogenes* pharyngitis and tonsillitis, a 10-day regimen of a first generation cephalosporin (cefadroxil, cephalexin) is preferred instead of other cephalosporins with broader spectrums of activity (e.g., cefaclor, cefdinir, cefixime, cefpodoxime, cefuroxime).

Although there is some evidence that a shorter duration of therapy with certain oral cephalosporins (e.g., a 5-day regimen of cefadroxil, cefdinir, cefixime, or cefpodoxime proxetil or a 4- or 5-day regimen of cefuroxime axetil) achieves bacteriologic and clinical cure rates equal to or greater than those achieved with the traditional 10-day oral penicillin V regimen, the IDSA and AHA state that use of cephalosporin regimens administered for 5 days or less for the treatment of *S. pyogenes* pharyngitis and tonsillitis cannot be recommended at this time.

In double-blind, controlled studies in adults, adolescents, and children with streptococcal pharyngitis, the clinical and microbiologic response to a 10-day regimen of oral cefdinir was superior to that of a 10-day regimen of oral penicillin V and the clinical and microbiologic response to a 5-day regimen of oral cefdinir was similar to that of the 10-day regimen of oral penicillin V. In controlled comparative studies in adults, adolescents, and children, the bacterial eradication rate 4–10 days after completion of therapy was 91–94% in those who received cefdinir for 10 days, 89–90% in those who received cefdinir for 5 days, and 70–83% in those who received penicillin V for 10 days. The clinical cure rate 4–10 days after completion of therapy was about 95–97, 89–91, and 85–90%, respectively. When cefdinir is used in the treatment of pharyngitis and tonsillitis, a once-daily dosing regimen reportedly is as effective as a twice-daily dosing regimen.

■ **Respiratory Tract Infections** ***Acute Exacerbations of Chronic Bronchitis*** Cefdinir is used in adults and adolescents 13 years of age or older for the treatment of acute exacerbations of chronic bronchitis caused by susceptible *S. pneumoniae* (penicillin-susceptible strains only) or β-lactamase- and non-β-lactamase-producing strains of *H. influenzae*, *H. parainfluenzae*, or *M. catarrhalis*. Although co-trimoxazole generally has been considered the drug of choice for the treatment of upper respiratory tract infections and bronchitis caused by susceptible *H. influenzae* or *M. catarrhalis*, second or third generation cephalosporins are considered by many clinicians to be alternative for the treatment of these infections.

Acute Sinusitis Cefdinir is used in adults and adolescents 13 years of age or older for the treatment of acute maxillary sinusitis caused by susceptible *S. pneumoniae* (penicillin-susceptible strains only), *H. influenzae* (including β-lactamase-producing strains), or *M. catarrhalis* (including β-lactamase-producing strains). While efficacy of cefdinir for the treatment of acute maxillary sinusitis in children 6 months through 12 years of age has not been fully established, use of the drug for the treatment of this infection in pediatric patients is supported by evidence from studies in adults and adolescents, the similar pathophysiology of acute sinusitis in adults and children, and data regarding the pharmacokinetics of cefdinir in children.

When anti-infective therapy is indicated for the treatment of acute bacterial sinusitis, the IDSA recommends amoxicillin and clavulanate potassium and the AAP recommends either amoxicillin or amoxicillin and clavulanate potassium as the drug of choice for initial empiric treatment. Because of variable activity against *S. pneumoniae* and *H. influenzae*, the IDSA no longer recommends second or third generation oral cephalosporins for empiric monotherapy of sinusitis in adults or children. If an oral cephalosporin is used as an alternative for empiric treatment of acute bacterial sinusitis in children (e.g., in penicillin-allergic individuals), the IDSA and AAP recommend a combination regimen that includes a third generation cephalosporin (cefixime or cefpodoxime) and clindamycin (or linezolid).

In controlled studies in patients 13 years of age or older with acute maxillary sinusitis, comparable clinical and bacteriologic responses were obtained with once-daily cefdinir (600 mg once daily), twice-daily cefdinir (300 mg twice daily), or amoxicillin and clavulanate potassium (500 mg of amoxicillin 3 times daily). When patients were subdivided based on the causative organism, the bacterial eradication rate in those with *S. pneumoniae* or *M. catarrhalis* infection was 89–100% with either drug; however, in those with *H. influenzae* infection, the eradication rate was 78% in those who received cefdinir and 57% in those who received amoxicillin and clavulanate potassium.

Community-acquired Pneumonia Cefdinir is used in adults and adolescents 13 years of age or older for the treatment of mild to moderate community-acquired pneumonia (CAP) caused by susceptible *S. pneumoniae* (penicillin-susceptible strains only) or β-lactamase- and non-β-lactamase-producing strains of *H. influenzae*, *H. parainfluenzae*, or *M. catarrhalis*.

If an oral cephalosporin is used as an alternative to penicillin G or amoxicillin for treatment of CAP caused by penicillin-susceptible *S. pneumoniae*, the American Thoracic Society (ATS) and IDSA recommend cefdinir, cefditoren, cefpodoxime, cefprozil, or cefuroxime.

Limited data in patients with CAP caused by organisms susceptible to the drugs indicate that the clinical response to cefdinir is similar to that reported with cefaclor, but may be inferior to that reported with amoxicillin and clavulanate potassium. In a double-blind, prospective, randomized study in adults and adolescents 13 years of age or older with CAP, a satisfactory clinical response (cure plus improvement) was achieved 6–14 days after completion of therapy in 89% of those who received cefdinir (300 mg twice daily for 10 days) and in 86% of those who received cefaclor (500 mg 3 times daily for 10 days). In another study conducted principally in Europe, the clinical cure rate 6–14 days after completion of therapy was 80% in those who received cefdinir (300 mg twice daily for 10 days) and 89% in those who received amoxicillin and clavulanate potassium (500 mg of amoxicillin 3 times daily for 10 days). In these studies, the bacteriologic eradication rate 6–14 days following completion of therapy was 89–92% in those who received cefdinir, 93% in those who received cefaclor, and 93% in those who received amoxicillin and clavulanate potassium. When patients were subdivided based on the causative organism, the presumptive bacteriologic eradication 6–14 days after completion of cefdinir therapy was 95–100% in those with *S. pneumoniae* infection, 74–85% in those with *H. influenzae* infection, 91–100% in those with *H. parainfluenzae* infection, and 100% in those with *M. catarrhalis* infection.

For additional information on treatment of CAP, see Community-acquired Pneumonia under Uses: Respiratory Tract Infections, in the Cephalosporins General Statement 8:12.06.

■ **Skin and Skin Structure Infections** Oral cefdinir is used in adults, adolescents, and children 6 months of age or older for the treatment of mild to moderate, uncomplicated skin and skin structure infections caused by *S. aureus* (including β-lactamase-producing strains) or *S. pyogenes*.

In a comparative study in children 6 months to 12 years of age with mild to moderate bacterial skin and skin structure infections (e.g., impetigo, infected dermatitis, wound infection, cellulitis, paronychia, abscess), oral cefdinir (7 mg/kg twice daily for 10 days) was as effective as oral cephalexin (10 mg/kg 4 times daily for 10 days). In a comparative study in adults and adolescents 13 years of age or older, oral cefdinir (300 mg twice daily for 10 days) was as effective as oral cephalexin (500 mg 4 times daily for 10 days) for the treatment of bacterial skin and skin structure infections (e.g., abscess, wound infection, paronychia, infected dermatitis, impetigo, cellulitis).

Dosage and Administration

■ Reconstitution and Administration

Cefdinir is administered orally.

Cefdinir may be given without regard to meals. (See Pharmacokinetics: Absorption.)

Oral iron preparations, including multivitamin and mineral preparations containing iron, may interfere with the absorption of oral cefdinir resulting in decreased plasma concentrations of the cephalosporin. If concomitant use is necessary, cefdinir doses should be given at least 2 hours before or after the oral iron preparation. Cefdinir oral suspension can be administered concomitantly with iron-fortified infant formula since concomitant administration with such formula (2.2 mg elemental iron/180 mL) does not alter absorption of the cephalosporin. The effect of iron-fortified food (e.g., iron-fortified breakfast cereal) on oral absorption of cefdinir has not been studied.

While concomitant administration of antacids containing aluminum or magnesium interferes with the absorption of oral cefdinir, administration of aluminum- or magnesium-containing antacids 2 hours before or after a dose of cefdinir is not associated with clinically important changes in the pharmacokinetics of the cephalosporin. Therefore, doses of cefdinir should be given at least 2 hours before or after a dose of aluminum- or magnesium-containing antacid.

Cefdinir may be administered as a single daily dose or in divided doses every 12 hours. Once- and twice-daily regimens are similarly effective for the treatment of acute bacterial exacerbations of chronic bronchitis, acute maxillary sinusitis, acute bacterial otitis media, and pharyngitis and tonsillitis caused by susceptible organisms and either regimen may be used in these infections. However, pending further study regarding the efficacy of once-daily cefdinir regimens in the treatment of community-acquired pneumonia and uncomplicated skin and skin structure infections, the manufacturer states that a twice-daily regimen should be used for these infections.

Reconstitution Cefdinir powder for oral suspension should be reconstituted at the time of dispensing by adding the amount of water specified on the container to provide a suspension containing 125 or 250 mg of cefdinir per 5 mL. The water should be added in 2 equal portions and the bottle inverted and shaken after each addition.

The oral suspension should be shaken well prior to administration of each dose.

■ Dosage

Adult Dosage **Pharyngitis and Tonsillitis.** For the treatment of pharyngitis and tonsillitis, the usual dosage of cefdinir for adults and adolescents 13 years of age or older is 300 mg every 12 hours for 5–10 days or 600 mg once daily for 10 days.

Cephalosporin regimens administered for 5 days or less are not recommended for the treatment of *S. pyogenes* pharyngitis and tonsillitis. (See Uses: Pharyngitis and Tonsillitis.)

Respiratory Tract Infections. For the treatment of acute exacerbations of chronic bronchitis, the usual dosage of cefdinir in adults and adolescents 13 years of age or older is 300 mg every 12 hours for 5–10 days or 600 mg once daily for 10 days.

For the treatment of acute maxillary sinusitis in adults and adolescents 13 years of age or older, the usual dosage is 300 mg every 12 hours or 600 mg once daily for 10 days.

Adult or adolescents 13 years of age or older should receive cefdinir in a dosage of 300 mg every 12 hours for 10 days for the treatment of community-acquired pneumonia (CAP).

Skin and Skin Structure Infections. For the treatment of uncomplicated skin and skin structure infections caused by susceptible bacteria, the usual dosage of cefdinir for adults and adolescents 13 years of age or older is 300 mg every 12 hours for 10 days.

Pediatric Dosage Children 13 year of age or older or those weighing more than 43 kg may receive the usual adult dosage of cefdinir.

General Pediatric Dosage. For pediatric patients beyond the neonatal period, the American Academy of Pediatrics (AAP) recommends a cefdinir dosage of 14 mg/kg daily in 1 or 2 equally divided doses for the treatment of mild or moderate infections. The AAP states that the drug is inappropriate for the treatment of severe infections.

Acute Otitis Media. For the treatment acute bacterial otitis (AOM), children 6 months through 12 years of age should receive cefdinir in a dosage of 7 mg/kg every 12 hours for 5–10 days or 14 mg/kg once daily for 10 days.

The AAP states that oral anti-infective regimens of less than 10 days' duration are not recommended for the treatment of AOM in children younger than 2 years of age or in patients with severe symptoms.

Pharyngitis and Tonsillitis. For the treatment of pharyngitis and tonsillitis in children 6 months through 12 years of age, the usual dosage of cefdinir is 7 mg/kg every 12 hours for 5–10 days or 14 mg/kg once daily for 10 days.

Cephalosporin regimens administered for 5 days or less are not recommended for the treatment of *S. pyogenes* pharyngitis and tonsillitis. (See Uses: Pharyngitis and Tonsillitis.)

Respiratory Tract Infections. The usual dosage of cefdinir for the treatment of acute maxillary sinusitis in children 6 months through 12 years of age is 7 mg/kg every 12 hours for 10 days or 14 mg/kg once daily for 10 days.

Skin and Skin Structure Infections. For the treatment of mild to moderate, uncomplicated skin and skin structure infections in children 6 months through 12 years of age, the usual dosage of cefdinir is 7 mg/kg every 12 hours for 10 days.

■ Dosage in Renal and Hepatic Impairment

Patients with creatinine clearances of 30 mL/minute or greater may receive the usual dosage of cefdinir.

Adults with creatinine clearances less than 30 mL/minute should receive cefdinir in a dosage of 300 mg once daily and children with creatinine clearances less than 30 mL/minute per 1.73 m^2 should receive the drug in a dosage of 7 mg/kg (up to 300 mg) once daily.

For patients maintained on long-term hemodialysis, the usual initial dosage of cefdinir is 300 mg every 48 hours for adults or 7 mg/kg (up to 300 mg) every 48 hours for children. Because cefdinir is partially removed by hemodialysis, a supplemental dose of cefdinir (300 mg in adults or 7 mg/kg in children) should be given at the end of each dialysis period and subsequent doses administered every 48 hours.

While the pharmacokinetics of cefdinir have not been studied in patients with hepatic impairment, hepatic metabolism of the drug is negligible and the manufacturer states that dosage adjustments are not expected to be necessary in such patients.

Cautions

■ Adverse Effects

Adverse effects reported with cefdinir are similar to those reported with other oral cephalosporins. (See Cautions in the Cephalosporins General Statement 8:12.06.) Cefdinir generally is well tolerated. Diarrhea, the most frequent adverse effect, has been reported in 16% of adult or adolescent patients and in 8% of pediatric patients receiving usual dosages of the drug. Adverse effects usually are transient and mild in severity, but have been severe enough to require discontinuance of the drug in up to 3% of patients.

■ Precautions and Contraindications

Cefdinir shares the toxic potentials of other cephalosporins, and the usual cautions, precautions, and contraindications associated with cephalosporin therapy should be observed. Prior to initiation of cefdinir therapy, careful inquiry should be made concerning previous hypersensitivity reactions to cephalosporins, penicillins, or other drugs. There is clinical and laboratory evidence of partial cross-allergenicity among cephalosporins and other β-lactam antibiotics, including penicillins and cephamycins. Cefdinir is contraindicated in patients who are hypersensitive to the drug or other cephalosporins and should be used with caution in patients with a history of hypersensitivity to penicillins. Use of cephalosporins should be avoided in patients who have had an immediate-type (anaphylactic) hypersensitivity reaction to penicillins. If an allergic reaction occurs during cefdinir therapy, the drug should be discontinued and the patient treated with appropriate therapy (e.g., epinephrine, corticosteroids, and maintenance of an adequate airway and oxygen) as indicated.

To reduce development of drug-resistant bacteria and maintain effectiveness of cefdinir and other antibacterials, the drug should be used only for the treatment or prevention of infections proven or strongly suspected to be caused by susceptible bacteria. When selecting or modifying anti-infective therapy, results of culture and in vitro susceptibility testing should be used. In the absence of such data, local epidemiology and susceptibility patterns should be considered when selecting anti-infectives for empiric therapy.

Patients should be advised that antibacterials (including cefdinir) should only be used to treat bacterial infections and not used to treat viral infections (e.g., the common cold). Patients also should be advised about the importance of completing the full course of therapy, even if feeling better after a few days, and that skipping doses or not completing therapy may decrease effectiveness and increase the likelihood that bacteria will develop resistance and will not be treatable with cefdinir or other antibacterials in the future.

Because *Clostridium difficile* infection (CDI) and *C. difficile*-associated diarrhea and colitis (CDAD; also known as antibiotic-associated diarrhea and colitis or pseudomembranous colitis) have been reported with nearly all anti-infectives, including cephalosporins, it should be considered in the differential diagnosis of patients who develop diarrhea during or after cefdinir therapy. Patients should be advised that diarrhea is a common problem caused by anti-infectives and usually ends when the drug is discontinued; however, they should contact a clinician if watery and bloody stools (with or without stomach cramps and fever) occur during or as late as 2 months or longer after the last dose.

Individuals with diabetes mellitus and/or their caregivers should be informed that cefdinir oral suspension contains sucrose. Depending on the manufacturer, the reconstituted oral suspension contains 1.37–2.86 g of sucrose per 5 mL.

For a more complete discussion of these and other precautions associated with the use of cefdinir, see Cautions: Precautions and Contraindications in the Cephalosporins General Statement 8:12.06.

■ Pediatric Precautions

Safety and efficacy of cefdinir in neonates and infants younger than 6 months of age have not been established.

Although adverse effects reported in pediatric patients receiving cefdinir are similar to those reported in adults, the incidence of diarrhea and rash appears to be higher in pediatric patients 2 years of age or younger than in older pediatric patients. Diarrhea has been reported in 17% of those 2 years of age or younger and 4% of those older than 2 years of age. Rash (principally diaper rash in the younger patients) has been reported in 8% of those 2 years of age or younger and 1% of those older than 2 years of age.

■ **Geriatric Precautions** Cefdinir is well tolerated in geriatric patients, and the incidence of adverse effects (including diarrhea) reported in clinical trials generally has been lower in geriatric patients than in younger adults. Although single-dose studies indicate that peak plasma concentrations and the area under the plasma-concentration time curve (AUC) of cefdinir may be higher in older adults than in younger adults, no adjustments in cefdinir dosage appear to be necessary other than those related to renal impairment. (See Dosage and Administration: Dosage in Renal and Hepatic Impairment.)

■ **Mutagenicity and Carcinogenicity** In vivo and in vitro studies evaluating cefdinir have not shown evidence of mutagenicity. Studies have not been performed to evaluate the carcinogenic potential of the drug.

■ **Pregnancy, Fertility, and Lactation** Reproduction studies in rats or rabbits using oral cefdinir in dosages 70 or 0.7 times, respectively, the usual human dosage (based on mg/kg daily) have not revealed evidence of teratogenicity. There are no adequate and controlled studies using cefdinir in pregnant women or during labor and delivery, and the drug should be used during pregnancy only when clearly needed.

Studies in rats using oral cefdinir in dosages up to 70 times the usual human dosage (based on mg/kg daily) have not revealed evidence of impaired fertility.

Cefdinir was not detected in human milk following a single 600-mg oral dose of the drug.

Spectrum

Based on its spectrum of activity, cefdinir is classified as a third generation cephalosporin. For information on the classification of cephalosporins and closely related β-lactam antibiotics based on spectra of activity, see Spectrum in the Cephalosporins General Statement 8:12.06.

Cefdinir is stable in the presence of a wide variety of β-lactamases produced by gram-negative and gram-positive bacteria but may be hydrolyzed by certain plasmid-mediated extended-spectrum β-lactamases. Like other currently available oral third generation cephalosporins (e.g., cefpodoxime proxetil, ceftibuten), cefdinir has an expanded spectrum of activity against aerobic gram-negative bacteria compared with first and second generation cephalosporins but is inactive against most strains of *Enterobacter* and *Pseudomonas aeruginosa*.

In vitro on a weight basis, cefdinir is more active against susceptible staphylococci and streptococci than other currently available oral third generation cephalosporins (e.g., cefpodoxime proxetil, ceftibuten). Cefdinir is inactive against enterococci (e.g., *Enterococcus faecalis*) and methicillin-resistant (oxacillin-resistant) staphylococci.

■ **In Vitro Susceptibility Testing** Strains of staphylococci resistant to penicillinase-resistant penicillins (methicillin-resistant [oxacillin-resistant] staphylococci) should be considered resistant to cefdinir, although results of in vitro susceptibility tests may indicate that the organisms are susceptible to the drug.

For information on interpreting results of in vitro susceptibility testing (disk susceptibility tests, dilution susceptibility tests) when cefdinir susceptibility testing is performed according to the standards of the Clinical and Laboratory Standards Institute (CLSI; formerly National Committee for Clinical Laboratory Standards [NCCLS]), see Spectrum: In Vitro Susceptibility Testing, in the Cephalosporins General Statement 8:12.06.

Pharmacokinetics

Cefdinir exhibits nonlinear dose-dependent pharmacokinetics. The pharmacokinetics of cefdinir have been studied in adults and pediatric patients 6 months to 12 years of age. There is no evidence of gender- or race-related differences in the pharmacokinetics of the drug. Studies in adults with impaired renal function indicate that the pharmacokinetics of cefdinir are affected by the degree of renal impairment and that decreases in elimination rate, apparent oral clearance, and renal clearance are approximately proportional to reductions in creatinine clearance. Differences in the pharmacokinetics of the drug in geriatric individuals appear to be related to changes in renal function rather than age. Pharmacokinetics of cefdinir have not been studied in patients with hepatic impairment.

■ **Absorption** Following oral administration of cefdinir capsules or oral suspension, peak plasma concentrations are attained 2–4 hours after the dose. Relative bioavailability of cefdinir administered to adults as the commercially available oral suspension is 120% of that achieved following administration of commercially available capsules of the drug. When administered as capsules, estimated oral bioavailability of cefdinir is 21% following a 300-mg dose and 16% following a 600-mg dose; estimated absolute bioavailability is 25% following administration of the oral suspension.

In healthy adults who received a single 300- or 600-mg oral dose of cefdinir as capsules, peak plasma concentrations about 3 hours after the dose were 1.6 or 2.87 mcg/mL, respectively. Results of a study in adults 19–91 years of age given a single 300-mg oral dose of cefdinir indicate that peak plasma concentrations may be 44% higher and the area under the plasma concentration-time curve (AUC) 86% higher in older adults compared with younger adults.

In pediatric patients 6 months to 12 years of age who received a single 7-mg/kg oral dose of cefdinir as the suspension, peak plasma concentrations were attained 2.2 hours after the dose and averaged 2.3 mcg/mL. Single 14-mg/kg oral doses in these patients resulted in peak plasma concentrations averaging 3.86 mcg/mL at 1.8 hours after the dose.

Compared with administration in the fasting state, concomitant administration of cefdinir capsules with a high-fat meal decreases peak plasma concentrations and AUC of oral cefdinir by 16 and 10%, respectively. When studied in adults, concomitant administration of cefdinir oral suspension with a high-fat meal decreased peak plasma concentrations and AUC of the drug by 44 and 33%, respectively.

There is no evidence that cefdinir accumulates in plasma following multiple doses in patients with normal renal function receiving the drug once or twice daily.

■ **Distribution** The volume of distribution of cefdinir averages 0.35 L/kg in adults and 0.67 L/kg in children 6 months to 12 years of age.

Following oral administration, cefdinir is distributed into blister fluid, middle ear fluid, tonsils, sinus tissue, and bronchial mucosa and epithelial lining fluid in concentrations ranging from 15–48% of concurrent plasma concentrations.

In adults undergoing elective tonsillectomy who received single 300- or 600-mg oral doses of cefdinir, median concentrations of the drug in tonsils 4 hours after the dose were 0.25 or 0.36 mcg/g, respectively. In adults undergoing elective maxillary and ethmoid sinus surgery, median sinus tissue concentrations 4 hours after single 300- or 600-mg oral doses of the drug were less than 0.12 or 0.21 mcg/g, respectively. In adults undergoing diagnostic bronchoscopy who received single 300- or 600-mg oral doses of cefdinir, median bronchial mucosa concentrations 4 hours after the dose were 0.78 or 1.14 mcg/mL, respectively, and median epithelial lining fluid concentrations were 0.29 or 0.49 mcg/mL, respectively.

In pediatric patients with acute bacterial otitis media who received single 7- or 14-mg/kg oral doses of cefdinir, median concentrations of the drug in middle ear fluid 3 hours after the dose were 0.21 or 0.72 mcg/mL, respectively.

Median maximal concentrations of cefdinir in blister fluid 4–5 hours after single 300- or 600-mg oral doses of the drug were 0.65 or 1.1 mcg/mL, respectively.

It is not known whether cefdinir is distributed into CSF following oral administration.

Cefdinir was not detected in human milk following oral administration of single 600-mg doses of the drug.

Cefdinir is 60–70% bound to plasma proteins in adults or children; binding is independent of drug concentration.

■ **Elimination** Cefdinir is not appreciably metabolized. The drug is eliminated principally by renal excretion. In adults with normal renal function, the mean plasma elimination half-life of cefdinir is 1.7–1.8 hours and renal clearance is 2 mL/minute per kg. Following oral administration of 300- or 600-mg of cefdinir, apparent oral clearance is 11.6 or 15.5 mL/minute per kg, respectively, and 18.4 or 11.6% of the dose, respectively, is eliminated unchanged in urine.

Clearance of cefdinir is decreased in patients with impaired renal function. In patients with creatinine clearances of 30–60 mL/minute, peak plasma concentrations and plasma elimination half-life of the drug are increased approximately twofold and the AUC is increased approximately threefold. In patients with creatinine clearances less than 30 mL/minute, peak plasma concentrations are increased approximately twofold but plasma elimination half-life and AUC are increased approximately fivefold and sixfold, respectively.

Cefdinir is removed by hemodialysis. A 4-hour period of dialysis removes approximately 63% of the drug and decreases the apparent elimination half-life of cefdinir in patients with substantial renal impairment from 16 to 3.2 hours.

Chemistry and Stability

■ **Chemistry** Cefdinir is a semisynthetic cephalosporin antibiotic. The drug is an oral aminothiazolyl hydroxyimino cephalosporin. Cefdinir is structurally similar to other oral (cefpodoxime proxetil, ceftibuten) or parenteral (cefepime, cefotaxime, ceftazidime, ceftriaxone) cephalosporins that contain an aminothiazolyl side chain at position 7 of the cephalosporin nucleus; however, cefdinir contains an unsubstituted oxime group rather than the methoxyimino group contained in many aminothiazolyl cephalosporins. The oxime group may contribute to improved activity against gram-positive bacteria. Like cefixime, cefdinir contains a vinyl moiety at position 3 of the cephalosporin nucleus which makes the drug suitable for oral administration.

Cefdinir is a white to white to light yellow crystalline powder. Depending on the manufacturer, commercially available cefdinir powder for oral suspension occurs as a white to off-white cherry-flavored powder or cream-colored, strawberry-flavored powder. Following reconstitution, the oral suspension contains 125 or 250 mg of cefdinir per 5 mL.

■ **Stability** Cefdinir capsules and powder for oral suspension should be stored at 20–25°C, but may be exposed to temperatures ranging from 15–30°C.

Following reconstitution, cefdinir oral suspension should be stored in a tight container at controlled room temperature; any unused suspension should be discarded after 10 days.

For further information on chemistry, mechanism of action, spectrum, resistance, uses, cautions, acute toxicity, drug interactions, or laboratory test interferences of cefdinir, see the Cephalosporins General Statement 8:12.06.

Preparations

Excipients in commercially available drug preparations may have clinically important effects in some individuals; consult specific product labeling for details.

Cefdinir

Oral		
Capsules	300 mg*	Cefdinir Capsules
For suspension	125 mg/5 mL*	Cefdinir for Suspension
	250 mg/5 mL*	Cefdinir for Suspension

*available from one or more manufacturer, distributor, and/or repackager by generic (nonproprietary) name

Cefditoren Pivoxil

■ Cefditoren pivoxil is a semisynthetic third generation cephalosporin.

Uses

■ **Pharyngitis and Tonsillitis** Cefditoren pivoxil is used for the treatment of pharyngitis and tonsillitis caused by susceptible *Streptococcus pyogenes* (group A β-hemolytic streptococci). Although cefditoren usually is effective in eradicating *S. pyogenes* from the nasopharynx, efficacy of the drug in the subsequent prevention of rheumatic fever remains to be established.

Selection of an anti-infective for the treatment of *S. pyogenes* pharyngitis and tonsillitis should be based on the drug's spectrum of activity, bacteriologic and clinical efficacy, potential adverse effects, ease of administration, patient compliance, and cost. No regimen has been found to date that effectively eradicates group A β-hemolytic streptococci in 100% of patients.

Because the drugs have a narrow spectrum of activity, are inexpensive, and generally are effective with a low frequency of adverse effects, the American Academy of Pediatrics (AAP), Infectious Diseases Society of America (IDSA), American Heart Association (AHA), and others recommend a penicillin regimen (i.e., 10 days of oral penicillin V or oral amoxicillin or a single dose of IM penicillin G benzathine) as the treatment of choice for *S. pyogenes* pharyngitis and tonsillitis and prevention of initial attacks (primary prevention) of rheumatic fever. Other anti-infectives (e.g., oral cephalosporins, oral macrolides, oral clindamycin) are recommended as alternatives in penicillin-allergic individuals.

If an oral cephalosporin is used for the treatment of *S. pyogenes* pharyngitis and tonsillitis, a 10-day regimen of a first generation cephalosporin (cefadroxil, cephalexin) is preferred instead of other cephalosporins with broader spectrums of activity (e.g., cefaclor, cefdinir, cefixime, cefpodoxime, cefuroxime).

■ **Respiratory Tract Infections** ***Acute Exacerbations of Chronic Bronchitis*** Cefditoren pivoxil is used for the treatment of mild to moderate acute bacterial exacerbations of chronic bronchitis caused by susceptible *Haemophilus influenzae* (including β-lactamase-producing strains), *H. parainfluenzae* (including β-lactamase-producing strains), *Streptococcus pneumoniae* (penicillin-susceptible strains only), or *Moraxella catarrhalis* (including β-lactamase-producing strains).

Community-acquired Pneumonia Cefditoren pivoxil is used for the treatment of community-acquired pneumonia (CAP) caused by susceptible *H. influenzae* (including β-lactamase-producing strains), *H. parainfluenzae* (including β-lactamase-producing strains), *S. pneumoniae* (penicillin-susceptible strains only), or *M. catarrhalis* (including β-lactamase-producing strains).

If an oral cephalosporin is used as an alternative to penicillin G or amoxicillin for treatment of CAP caused by penicillin-susceptible *S. pneumoniae*, the American Thoracic Society (ATS) and IDSA recommend cefpodoxime, cefprozil, cefuroxime, cefdinir, or cefditoren.

For additional information on treatment of CAP, see Community-acquired Pneumonia under Uses: Respiratory Tract Infections, in the Cephalosporins General Statement 8:12.06.

■ **Skin and Skin Structure Infections** Cefditoren pivoxil is used orally for the treatment of uncomplicated skin and skin structure infections caused by susceptible *Staphylococcus aureus* (including β-lactamase-producing strains) or *S. pyogenes*.

For additional information on these and other uses of cephalosporins, see Uses in the Cephalosporins General Statement 8:12.06

Dosage and Administration

■ **Administration** Cefditoren pivoxil is administered orally with meals (to enhance GI absorption).

■ **Dosage** Dosage of cefditoren pivoxil is expressed in terms of cefditoren.

Adult Dosage **Pharyngitis and Tonsillitis.** For the treatment of pharyngitis and tonsillitis, the usual adult dosage of cefditoren is 200 mg twice daily for 10 days.

Respiratory Tract Infections. For the treatment of acute bacterial exacerbations of chronic bronchitis, the usual adult dosage of cefditoren is 400 mg twice daily for 10 days.

For the treatment of community-acquired pneumonia, the usual adult dosage of cefditoren is 400 mg twice daily for 14 days.

Skin and Skin Structure Infections. For the treatment of skin and skin structure infections, the usual adult dosage of cefditoren is 200 mg twice daily for 10 days.

Pediatric Dosage **Pharyngitis and Tonsillitis.** For the treatment of pharyngitis and tonsillitis, the usual dosage of cefditoren in adolescents 12 years of age or older is 200 mg twice daily for 10 days.

Respiratory Tract Infections. For the treatment of acute bacterial exacerbations of chronic bronchitis, the usual dosage of cefditoren in adolescents 12 years of age or older is 400 mg twice daily for 10 days.

For the treatment of community-acquired pneumonia, the usual dosage of cefditoren in adolescents 12 years of age or older is 400 mg twice daily for 14 days.

Skin and Skin Structure Infections. For the treatment of skin and skin structure infections, the usual dosage of cefditoren in adolescents 12 years of age or older is 200 mg twice daily for 10 days.

■ **Special Populations** Patients with mild renal impairment (creatinine clearance of 50–80 mL/min per 1.73 m²) may receive the usual dosage of cefditoren. The manufacturer recommends a maximum dosage of 200 mg twice daily for patients with moderate renal impairment (creatinine clearance of 30–49 mL/min per 1.73 m²) and a maximum dosage of 200 mg once daily for those with severe renal impairment (creatinine clearance less than 30 mL/min per 1.73 m²). The appropriate dosage in patients with end-stage renal disease has not been determined.

The manufacturer states that dosage adjustments are not necessary in patients with mild (Child-Pugh class A) or moderate (Child-Pugh class B) hepatic impairment. The pharmacokinetics of cefditoren have not been studied in patients with severe hepatic impairment (Child-Pugh class C).

No dosage adjustments in geriatric patients except those related to renal impairment. Cautious dosage selection because of age-related decreases in renal function.

Cautions

■ **Contraindications** Known hypersensitivity to cefditoren, other cephalosporins, or any ingredient in the formulation.

Carnitine deficiency or an inborn error of metabolism that may result in clinically important carnitine deficiency.

Milk protein hypersensitivity (not lactose intolerance).

■ **Warnings/Precautions** ***Warnings*** **Superinfection/Clostridium difficile-associated Diarrhea and Colitis.** Use of cefditoren may result in overgrowth of nonsusceptible organism, including fungi. The patient should be carefully monitored and appropriate therapy instituted if a superinfection occurs.

Treatment with anti-infectives alters normal colon flora and may permit overgrowth of *Clostridium difficile*. *C. difficile* infection (CDI) and *C. difficile*-associated diarrhea and colitis (CDAD; also known as antibiotic-associated diarrhea and colitis or pseudomembranous colitis) have been reported with nearly all anti-infectives, including cefditoren, and may range in severity from mild diarrhea to fatal colitis. *C. difficile* produces toxins A and B which contribute to the development of CDAD.

CDAD should be considered in the differential diagnosis in patients who develop diarrhea during or after anti-infective therapy. Careful medical history is necessary since CDAD has been reported to occur as late as 2 months or longer after anti-infective therapy is discontinued.

If CDAD is suspected or confirmed, anti-infective therapy not directed against *C. difficile* should be discontinued whenever possible. Patients should be managed with appropriate supportive therapy (e.g., fluid and electrolyte management, protein supplementation), anti-infective therapy directed against *C. difficile* (e.g., metronidazole, vancomycin), and surgical evaluation as clinically indicated.

Sensitivity Reactions **Hypersensitivity Reactions.** There is clinical and laboratory evidence of partial cross-sensitivity among cephalosporins and other β-lactam antibiotics. Prior to initiation of therapy, make careful inquiry concerning previous hypersensitivity reactions to cephalosporins, penicillins, or other drugs. Cefditoren pivoxil should be used with caution in patients with a history of hypersensitivity to penicillins; the drug should be avoided in patients who have had an immediate-type (anaphylactic) hypersensitivity reaction to penicillins.

Cefditoren tablets contain sodium caseinate, a milk protein, and should not be used in patients with milk protein hypersensitivity (not lactose intolerance).

If hypersensitivity reaction occurs, cefditoren should be discontinued and appropriate therapy initiated as indicated (e.g., epinephrine, corticosteroids, maintenance of an adequate airway and oxygen).

General Precautions **Carnitine Deficiency.** Cefditoren pivoxil should not be used when prolonged anti-infective therapy is required since use of other pivalate-containing compounds over periods of months has caused clinical manifestations of carnitine deficiency.

In individuals receiving short-term treatment with cefditoren pivoxil (200 or 400 mg of cefditoren twice daily for 14 days), a 30–63% decrease in serum carnitine concentrations has occurred; no adverse effects attributable to decreased carnitine concentrations were reported and concentrations returned to normal 7–10 days after the drug was discontinued.

Cefditoren pivoxil should not be used in patients with carnitine deficiency or inborn errors of metabolism that may result in clinically important carnitine deficiency. In addition, the fact that some patients (e.g., those with renal impairment or decreased muscle mass) may be at increased risk for reduced serum carnitine concentrations during cefditoren pivoxil therapy should be considered.

Selection and Use of Anti-infectives. To reduce development of drug-resistant bacteria and maintain effectiveness of cefditoren and other antibacterials, cefditoren should be used only for the treatment of infections proven or strongly suspected to be caused by susceptible bacteria.

When selecting or modifying anti-infective therapy, results of culture and in vitro susceptibility testing should be used. In the absence of such data, local epidemiology and susceptibility patterns should be considered when selecting anti-infectives for empiric therapy.

Hematologic Effects. Reduced prothrombin activity has been reported rarely with cephalosporins. The manufacturer recommends that prothrombin time (PT) be monitored and vitamin K administered as indicated in patients at risk for reduced prothrombin activity (e.g., patients with renal or hepatic impairment or poor nutritional status, patients receiving prolonged antimicrobial therapy or previously stabilized on anticoagulant therapy).

Specific Populations **Pregnancy.** Category B. (See Users Guide.)

Lactation. Cefditoren is distributed into milk in rats; the drug should be used with caution in nursing women.

Pediatric Use. Safety and efficacy, including any effects of altered carnitine concentrations, have not been established in infants and children younger than 12 years of age. The drug is not recommended for use in pediatric patients younger than 12 years of age.

Geriatric Use. No clinically important differences in safety and efficacy have been reported in adults 65 years of age or older compared with younger adults.

Cefditoren is substantially eliminated by the kidneys; the risk of toxicity may be greater in patients with impaired renal function. Dosage should be selected with caution and renal function monitoring should be considered because of age-related decreases in renal function. (See Dosage and Administration: Special Populations.)

■ **Common Adverse Effects** Adverse effects reported in 1–15% of patients receiving cefditoren include diarrhea, nausea, headache, abdominal pain, vaginal moniliasis, dyspepsia, and vomiting.

Drug Interactions

■ **Antacids and H_2-Receptor Antagonists** Pharmacokinetic interaction (decreased absorption of cefditoren); clinical importance not known. The manufacturer recommends that cefditoren not be administered concomitantly with antacids or H_2-receptor antagonists.

■ **Probenecid** Pharmacokinetic interaction (increased plasma concentrations of cefditoren).

■ **Oral Contraceptives** No effect on the pharmacokinetics of ethinyl estradiol observed.

Description

Cefditoren pivoxil is a semisynthetic cephalosporin antibiotic. The drug is an oral aminothiazolyl cephalosporin with a methylthiazolyl group at position 3 of the cephalosporin nucleus. Cefditoren pivoxil is a prodrug and has little, if any, antibacterial activity until hydrolyzed in vivo to cefditoren. Following oral administration of cefditoren pivoxil, the drug is absorbed from the GI tract and hydrolyzed by esterases to cefditoren. Hydrolysis of cefditoren pivoxil also results in the formation of pivalate, which is absorbed and excreted as pivaloylcarnitine in urine. Cefditoren is not appreciably metabolized. The drug is eliminated principally unchanged by renal excretion.

Based on its spectrum of activity, cefditoren is classified as a third generation cephalosporin. Cefditoren is stable in the presence of a variety of β-lactamases (including penicillinases and some cephalosporinases) produced by gram-positive and -negative bacteria. Like other currently available third generation cephalosporins (e.g., cefdinir, cefixime, ceftibuten, cefpodoxime), cefditoren has an expanded spectrum of activity against gram-negative bacteria compared with first and second generation cephalosporins; however, the methylthiazolyl group in cefditoren, which also is found in first generation cephalosporins but not in other currently available third generation cephalosporins, enhances activity of cefditoren against gram-positive bacteria.

Cefditoren is active in vitro and in clinical infections against most strains of *Staphylococcus aureus* (methicillin-susceptible [oxacillin-susceptible] strains, including β-lactamase-producing strains), *Streptococcus pneumoniae* (penicillin-susceptible strains only), *Streptococcus pyogenes* (group A β-hemolytic streptococci), *Haemophilus influenzae* (including β-lactamase-producing strains), *H. parainfluenzae* (including β-lactamase-producing strains), and *Moraxella catarrhalis* (including β-lactamase-producing strains). Cefditoren also has demonstrated in vitro activity against *S. agalactiae* (group B streptococci), groups C and G streptococci, and viridans streptococci (penicillin-susceptible and -intermediate strains); however, the safety and efficacy of cefditoren in treating clinical infections caused by these microorganisms have not been established in adequate and well-controlled clinical trials to date.

Advice to Patients

Advise patients that antibacterials (including cefditoren) should only be used to treat bacterial infections and not used to treat viral infections (e.g., the common cold).

Importance of completing full course of therapy, even if feeling better after a few days.

Advise patients that skipping doses or not completing the full course of therapy may decrease effectiveness and increase the likelihood that bacteria will develop resistance and will not be treatable with cefditoren or other antibacterials in the future.

Advise patients that diarrhea is a common problem caused by anti-infectives and usually ends when the drug is discontinued. Importance of contacting a clinician if watery and bloody stools (with or without stomach cramps and fever) occur during or as late as 2 months or longer after the last dose.

Necessity for patients with milk protein hypersensitivity (not lactose intolerance) to avoid taking cefditoren pivoxil tablets.

Importance of taking cefditoren pivoxil tablets with meals for optimum absorption. Cefditoren may be used concomitantly with oral estrogen-progestin contraceptives.

Importance of monitoring for signs of hypersensitivity. Importance of reporting persistent or worsening symptoms of infection.

Importance of women informing clinicians if they are or plan to become pregnant or plan to breast-feed.

Importance of informing clinicians of existing or contemplated concomitant therapy, including prescription and OTC drugs, as well as any concomitant illnesses.

Importance of informing patients of other important precautionary information. (See Cautions.)

Overview® (see Users Guide). For additional information on this drug until a more detailed monograph is developed and published, the manufacturer's labeling should be consulted. It is *essential* that the manufacturer's labeling be consulted for more detailed information on usual cautions, precautions, contraindications, potential drug interactions, laboratory test interferences, and acute toxicity.

Preparations

Excipients in commercially available drug preparations may have clinically important effects in some individuals; consult specific product labeling for details.

Cefditoren Pivoxil

Oral

Tablets, film-coated	200 mg (of cefditoren)	**Spectracef®**, Vansen
	400 mg (of cefditoren)	**Spectracef®**, Vansen

Cefixime

■ Cefixime is a semisynthetic, third generation cephalosporin antibiotic.

Uses

Cefixime is used orally in adult and pediatric patients for the treatment of acute otitis media caused by susceptible bacteria; pharyngitis and tonsillitis caused by *Streptococcus pyogenes* (group A β-hemolytic streptococci); respiratory tract infections (e.g., acute exacerbations of chronic bronchitis, pneumonia†) caused by susceptible bacteria; and uncomplicated urinary tract infections caused by susceptible bacteria. The drug also has been used for the treatment of gonorrhea and infections caused by susceptible *Salmonella*† or *Shigella*†.

Because cefixime has a long serum half-life and can be administered once or twice daily, some clinicians suggest that the drug may be particularly useful when patient compliance is a concern (e.g., in the treatment of otitis media). Although cefixime is an effective alternative to other anti-infective agents for the treatment of many infections, the drug offers no clear advantage (except for a convenient dosage regimen) over other equally effective, less expensive anti-infectives available for the treatment of uncomplicated urinary tract infections or upper and lower respiratory tract infections. In addition, use of cefixime as empiric therapy in some infections (e.g., urinary tract infections, respiratory tract infections, soft tissue infections) is limited by its spectrum of activity since the drug is inactive against staphylococci, enterococci, and *Pseudomonas aeruginosa*. Because cefixime is inactive against most anaerobic bacteria, the drug is ineffective in and should not be used alone if a mixed aerobic-anaerobic bacterial infection is suspected.

Prior to initiation of cefixime therapy, appropriate specimens should be obtained for identification of the causative organism(s) and in vitro susceptibility tests. Cefixime therapy may be started pending results of susceptibility tests, but should be discontinued and other appropriate anti-infective therapy substituted if the organism is found to be resistant to cefixime.

■ **Acute Otitis Media** Cefixime is used in adults or children for the treatment of acute otitis media (AOM) caused by *Haemophilus influenzae*, *Moraxella catarrhalis*, *Streptococcus pyogenes* (group A β-hemolytic streptococci), or *S. pneumoniae*†.

When anti-infective therapy is indicated for the treatment of AOM, the

American Academy of Pediatrics (AAP) recommends high-dose amoxicillin or amoxicillin and clavulanate potassium as the drug of first choice for initial treatment. These experts recommend certain cephalosporins (cefdinir, cefpodoxime, cefuroxime, ceftriaxone) as alternatives for initial treatment in penicillin-allergic patients who do not have a history of severe and/or recent penicillin-allergic reactions.

In clinical studies in children 6 months to 16 years of age with AOM, a 10-day regimen of oral cefixime produced a favorable clinical response (e.g., clinical cure or improvement with absence of fever, irritability, otalgia, and tympanic membrane erythema with or without middle ear effusion) in 83–100% and a presumptive bacteriologic cure in 60–97% of patients. At 2–4 weeks after cefixime therapy, a clinical cure was still evident in 71–77% of children with *H. influenzae* infections, 84–100% of those with *M. catarrhalis* infections, and 69–82% of those with *S. pneumoniae* infections; persistent effusions were present in 15% of patients and 17% were considered to be treatment failures. In studies in children with AOM, oral cefixime (8 mg/kg once daily or 4 mg/kg twice daily) was as effective as oral amoxicillin (20 or 40 mg/kg daily given in 3 equally divided doses), oral amoxicillin and clavulanate potassium (40 mg of amoxicillin per kg daily in 3 equally divided doses), oral cefpodoxime proxetil (10 mg/kg once daily), or oral cefaclor (40 mg/kg daily given in 3 equally divided doses) for the treatment of infections caused by susceptible β-lactamase-producing *M. catarrhalis* or *H. influenzae*. Both the once- and twice-daily cefixime regimens appear to be equally effective in the treatment of AOM caused by susceptible organisms.

There is some evidence that cefixime is less effective than some other anti-infective agents for the treatment of otitis media caused by *S. pneumoniae*. In some studies where results were stratified according to causative organism, the bacteriologic response reported for cefixime in infections caused by *S. pneumoniae* was lower than that reported for amoxicillin. Because at least one case of pneumococcal bacteremia developed in a child who was receiving cefixime for the treatment of otitis media, some clinicians suggest that cefixime *not* be used for the treatment of otitis media known or suspected of being caused by *S. pneumoniae*. Although the clinical importance is unclear, staphylococci have been isolated from middle-ear fluid after treatment in a few patients receiving cefixime.

For additional information regarding treatment of AOM, including information on diagnosis and management strategies, anti-infectives for initial treatment, duration of initial treatment, and anti-infectives after initial treatment failures, see Acute Otitis Media under Uses: Otitis Media, in the Cephalosporins General Statement 8:12.06.

■ **Pharyngitis and Tonsillitis** Oral cefixime is used in the treatment of pharyngitis and tonsillitis caused by susceptible *S. pyogenes* (group A β-hemolytic streptococci). Although cefixime usually is effective in eradicating *S. pyogenes* from the nasopharynx, efficacy of the drug for prevention of subsequent rheumatic fever has not been established to date.

Selection of an anti-infective for the treatment of *S. pyogenes* pharyngitis and tonsillitis should be based on the drug's spectrum of activity, bacteriologic and clinical efficacy, potential adverse effects, ease of administration, patient compliance, and cost. No regimen has been found to date that effectively eradicates group A β-hemolytic streptococci in 100% of patients.

Because the drugs have a narrow spectrum of activity, are inexpensive, and generally are effective with a low frequency of adverse effects, the AAP, Infectious Diseases Society of America (IDSA), American Heart Association (AHA), and others recommend a penicillin regimen (i.e., 10 days of oral penicillin V or oral amoxicillin or a single dose of IM penicillin G benzathine) as the treatment of choice for *S. pyogenes* pharyngitis and tonsillitis and prevention of initial attacks (primary prevention) of rheumatic fever. Other anti-infectives (e.g., oral cephalosporins, oral macrolides, oral clindamycin) are recommended as alternatives in penicillin-allergic individuals.

If an oral cephalosporin is used for the treatment of *S. pyogenes* pharyngitis and tonsillitis, a 10-day regimen of a first generation cephalosporin (cefadroxil, cephalexin) is preferred instead of other cephalosporins with broader spectrums of activity (e.g., cefaclor, cefdinir, cefixime, cefpodoxime, cefuroxime).

Although there is some evidence that a shorter duration of therapy with certain oral cephalosporins (e.g., a 5-day regimen of cefadroxil, cefdinir, cefixime, or cefpodoxime proxetil or a 4- or 5-day regimen of cefuroxime axetil) achieves bacteriologic and clinical cure rates equal to or greater than those achieved with the traditional 10-day oral penicillin V regimen, the IDSA and AHA state that use of cephalosporin regimens administered for 5 days or less for the treatment of *S. pyogenes* pharyngitis and tonsillitis cannot be recommended at this time.

Results of open-label, randomized studies in pediatric patients with *S. pyogenes* pharyngitis and tonsillitis indicate that a 10-day regimen of oral cefixime is more effective than a 10-day regimen of oral penicillin V and that a 5-day regimen of oral cefixime is at least as effective as the 10-day penicillin V regimen. The bacteriologic eradication rate was 94% in those who received a 10-day regimen of oral cefixime, 82.6% in those who received a 5-day regimen of oral cefixime, and 77–88% in those who received a 10-day regimen of oral penicillin V. Once-daily dosing with cefixime is as effective as twice-daily dosing in the treatment of pharyngitis and tonsillitis.

■ **Respiratory Tract Infections** ***Acute Sinusitis*** Cefixime has been effective in a limited number of adults and children for the treatment of sinusitis† caused by *S. pneumoniae*, *H. influenzae*, *M. catarrhalis*, *Escherichia coli*†, *H. parahaemolyticus*†, or *H. parainfluenzae*†.

When anti-infective therapy is indicated for the treatment of acute bacterial sinusitis, the IDSA recommends amoxicillin and clavulanate potassium and the AAP recommends either amoxicillin or amoxicillin and clavulanate potassium as the drug of choice for initial empiric treatment. Because of variable activity against *S. pneumoniae* and *H. influenzae*, the IDSA no longer recommends second or third generation oral cephalosporins for empiric monotherapy of sinusitis in adults or children. If an oral cephalosporin is used as an alternative for empiric treatment of acute bacterial sinusitis in children (e.g., in penicillin-allergic individuals), the IDSA and AAP recommend a combination regimen that includes a third generation cephalosporin (cefixime or cefpodoxime) and clindamycin (or linezolid).

Acute and Chronic Bronchitis Cefixime is used in adults or children for the treatment of acute exacerbations of chronic bronchitis caused by *S. pneumoniae*, *H. influenzae*, or *M. catarrhalis*†.

There is some evidence that 5- or 10-day regimens of oral cefixime (400 mg once daily) are equally effective in patients with acute exacerbation of chronic bronchitis; in one study, the clinical and bacteriologic response rates reported with a 5-day regimen were 88–91 and 69–74%, respectively, and those reported with the 10-day regimen were 88–91 and 53–82%, respectively (intent-to-treat analysis). In one study in adults, cefixime (400 mg once daily) was as effective as oral amoxicillin (500 mg 3 times daily) for the treatment of lower respiratory tract infections caused by susceptible organisms. Other controlled studies in adults indicate that cefixime (200 mg twice daily or 400 mg once daily) was as effective as oral amoxicillin and clavulanate potassium (500 mg/125 mg 3 times daily), oral cefaclor (500 mg 3 times daily), or oral cephalexin (250 mg 4 times daily) for the treatment of these infections. However, the bacteriologic cure rate reported with cefixime in the treatment of lower respiratory tract infections has ranged from 54–100%, and some clinicians suggest that further study is needed to evaluate the drug's role in the treatment of these infections.

Pneumonia Oral cefixime has been effective when used in adults or children for the treatment of mild to moderate pneumonia, including community-acquired pneumonia†. When used in the treatment of hospitalized patients with community-acquired pneumonia, therapy was initiated with a parenteral third generation cephalosporin (e.g., ceftriaxone, cefotaxime) and then changed to oral cefixime, as appropriate, allowing therapy to be completed on an outpatient basis.

■ **Urinary Tract Infections** ***Uncomplicated Urinary Tract Infections*** Cefixime generally has been effective when used in men, women, or children for the treatment of uncomplicated urinary tract infections (UTIs) caused by susceptible *E. coli* or *Proteus mirabilis*. The drug also has been effective when used in a limited number of adults or children for the treatment of uncomplicated UTIs caused by other gram-negative bacteria, including *Citrobacter spp.*†, *C. diversus*†, *C. freundii*†, *Enterobacter spp.*†, *E. aerogenes*†, *E. agglomerans*†, *Klebsiella spp.*†, *K. pneumoniae*†, *Morganella morganii*†, *Proteus spp.*†, or *Serratia*†. In controlled studies in men and women with uncomplicated UTIs caused by susceptible gram-negative bacteria, oral cefixime (400 mg once daily or 200 mg twice daily) was as effective as oral co-trimoxazole (160 mg of trimethoprim and 800 mg of sulfamethoxazole every 12 hours) or oral amoxicillin (250 mg 3 times daily). The once- and twice-daily cefixime regimens were equally effective and resulted in a bacteriologic cure in about 90–100% of adults with uncomplicated UTIs. In a study in pediatric patients 1–24 months of age with urinary tract infections, a 14-day regimen of oral cefixime (16 mg/kg on day 1 followed by 8 mg/kg once daily) was as effective as a 14-day regimen that included a parenteral drug (IV cefotaxime 200 mg/kg daily given in 4 divided doses for 3 days or until the child is afebrile for 24 hours) followed by oral cefixime (8 mg/kg once daily).

Cefixime has been effective in a few adults for the treatment of uncomplicated UTIs caused by gram-positive bacteria, including *Staphylococcus epidermidis*†, *Staphylococcus spp.*†, *Streptococcus agalactiae*†, nonhemolytic streptococci†, or *Enterococcus faecalis*†. However, treatment failures have occurred when cefixime was used in the treatment of UTIs caused by gram-positive bacteria, and some of these organisms (e.g., staphylococci, *S. agalactiae*, enterococci) have been isolated in urine either during or after therapy with the drug.

Some clinicians suggest that cefixime offers no advantage over other equally effective, less expensive anti-infective agents (e.g., sulfisoxazole, amoxicillin, co-trimoxazole) for the treatment of uncomplicated UTIs. For empiric therapy of acute, uncomplicated UTIs, co-trimoxazole, a fluoroquinolone, fosfomycin, or nitrofurantoin usually is recommended. Because cefixime is inactive in vitro against enterococci and staphylococci, the drug probably should not be used for empiric therapy of nosocomial UTIs. It has been suggested that cefixime be reserved for the treatment of UTIs caused by multidrug-resistant gram-negative bacteria (e.g., *E. coli*) and used as an alternative to co-trimoxazole, amoxicillin and clavulanate potassium, norfloxacin, and ciprofloxacin for these infections.

Complicated Urinary Tract Infections Cefixime has been used with some success in a limited number of adults for the treatment of pyelonephritis and other complicated UTIs† caused by susceptible *Enterobacteriaceae*, including *E. coli*. Response rates in patients with complicated UTIs receiving cefixime are not as good as those reported in patients with uncomplicated UTIs; bacteriologic cure rates in adults with complicated UTIs have been reported to be 67–100%. Further study is needed to evaluate efficacy of cefixime in the treatment of complicated UTIs.

■ **Gonorrhea and Associated Infections** ***Uncomplicated Gonorrhea*** Cefixime is used for the treatment of uncomplicated gonorrhea. However, because of concerns related to recent reports of *Neisseria gonorrhoeae* with reduced susceptibility to cephalosporins, the US Centers for Disease Control and Prevention (CDC) states that cefixime is no longer recommended as first-line treatment for uncomplicated gonorrhea.

For the treatment of uncomplicated urogenital, anorectal, or pharyngeal gonorrhea, the CDC states that a combination regimen that includes a single 250-mg IM dose of ceftriaxone *and* either oral azithromycin (single 1-g dose) or oral doxycycline (100 mg twice daily for 7 days) is the regimen of choice. If ceftriaxone is not available or cannot be used and the patient has urogenital or rectal† gonorrhea, the CDC recommends an alternative combination regimen that includes a single 400-mg dose of oral cefixime *and* either oral azithromycin (single 1-g dose) or oral doxycycline (100 mg twice daily for 7 days). If the patient has severe cephalosporin allergy, an alternative regimen of oral azithromycin (single 2-g dose) alone is recommended. Test-of-cure follow-up (culture or nucleic acid amplification test [NAAT]) should be performed 1 week after treatment in all patients who receive cefixime or other alternative regimens. If there is evidence of treatment failure, the CDC recommends that the patient receive a combination regimen that includes a single 250-mg IM dose of ceftriaxone *and* oral azithromycin (single 2-g dose) and that the case be reported to the CDC through local or state health departments.

Although cefixime has been effective when given as a single 400- or 800-mg oral dose for the treatment of acute uncomplicated endocervical gonorrhea in women and urethral gonorrhea in men caused by penicillinase- and nonpenicillinase-producing *N. gonorrhoeae*, *N. gonorrhoeae* with reduced susceptibility to cefixime, including some treatment failures, have been reported in the US and other countries with increasing frequency during the last decade. Because of the possibility of emergence of resistance and because bactericidal concentrations attained with a 400-mg dose of oral cefixime are lower and not as sustained as those provided by a single 250-mg IM dose of ceftriaxone, cefixime should *only* be used for the treatment of urogenital or rectal† gonococcal infections when ceftriaxone is unavailable or cannot be used and such patients should receive test-of-cure follow-up after treatment. In addition, cefixime is not recommended for the treatment of pharyngeal gonorrhea since it has only limited efficacy for the treatment of these infections.

The CDC recommends that health-care providers treating gonorrhea remain vigilant for treatment failures (evidenced by persistent symptoms or a positive follow-up test despite treatment). If there is evidence of treatment failure, relevant clinical specimens should be cultured and in vitro susceptibility testing performed. In addition, an infectious disease specialist, an STD/HIV Prevention Training Center (http://www.nnptc.org), or the CDC (404-639-8659) should be consulted for treatment advice and the case should be reported to the CDC through local or state health departments within 24 hours of diagnosis. A test-of-cure should be performed 1 week after retreatment. For all patients with gonorrhea, clinicians should ensure that the patient's sexual partners from the preceding 60 days are evaluated promptly using cultures and treated with a recommended regimen if indicated.

For additional information on current recommendations for the treatment of gonorrhea and associated infections, see Uses: Gonorrhea and Associated Infections, in Ceftriaxone 8:12.06.12.

■ **Lyme Disease** Oral cefixime has been used in a limited number of patients for the treatment of Lyme disease†. In an open, randomized study in patients with disseminated Lyme borreliosis, oral cefixime (200 mg daily with oral probenecid 500 mg 3 times daily) given for 100 days was as effective as a regimen of IV ceftriaxone (2 g daily given for 14 days) followed by oral amoxicillin (500 mg 3 times daily with oral probenecid 500 mg 3 times daily) given for 100 days. However, other cephalosporins (ceftriaxone, cefotaxime, cefuroxime axetil) are recommended by the IDSA and others when a cephalosporin is used in the treatment of Lyme disease. (See Uses: Lyme Disease in the Cephalosporins General Statement 8:12.06.)

■ **Shigellosis** Oral cefixime (8 mg/kg daily for 5 days) has been effective when used in children for the treatment of shigellosis† caused by susceptible *Shigella* and, in one study, was more effective than ampicillin and sulbactam sodium for the treatment of these infections. However, in a study in adults with shigellosis who received oral cefixime (400 mg once daily for 5 days), the clinical response rate to the drug was only 53% and the bacteriologic eradication rate was 40%. Anti-infective therapy generally is indicated in addition to fluid and electrolyte replacement for the treatment of severe cases of shigellosis since anti-infectives appear to shorten the duration of diarrhea and the period of fecal excretion of *Shigella*. Multiple-drug resistant strains of *Shigella* have been reported with increasing frequency. For susceptible strains, ampicillin or co-trimoxazole is effective; amoxicillin is less effective. A fluoroquinolone or, alternatively, a parenteral third-generation cephalosporins (e.g., ceftriaxone) are considered the agents of choice for the treatment of shigellosis when the susceptibility of the isolate is unknown or strains resistant to ampicillin and co-trimoxazole are likely. Some clinicians state that the benefits of oral third generation cephalosporins (e.g., cefixime) in the treatment of shigellosis are unclear.

■ **Typhoid Fever and Other Salmonella Infections** Oral cefixime has been used in children for the treatment of typhoid fever (enteric fever) or septicemia caused by multidrug-resistant strains of *Salmonella typhi*†. Multidrug-resistant strains of *S. typhi* (i.e., strains resistant to ampicillin, chloramphenicol, and/or co-trimoxazole) have been reported with increasing frequency, and fluoroquinolones (e.g., ciprofloxacin, ofloxacin) and third generation cephalosporins (e.g., ceftriaxone, cefotaxime) are considered the agents of first choice for the treatment of typhoid fever or other severe infections known or suspected to be caused by these strains. In a study in children 6 months to 13 years of age with typhoid fever caused by multidrug-resistant *S. typhi* who were randomized to receive a 14-day regimen of oral cefixime (5 mg/kg twice daily) or IV ceftriaxone (65 mg/kg once daily), the time to defervescence was 8.3 days in those who received cefixime and 8 days in those who received ceftriaxone; the relapse rate was 5 and 14%, respectively.

Dosage and Administration

■ **Reconstitution and Administration** Cefixime is administered orally as capsules, conventional tablets, chewable tablets, or an oral suspension.

Cefixime capsules and conventional tablets may be administered without regard to meals. Presence of food in the GI tract decreases the rate of absorption of cefixime, but generally does not affect the extent of absorption of the drug. (See Pharmacokinetics: Absorption.)

Cefixime chewable tablets must be chewed or crushed before swallowing.

Reconstitution Cefixime powder for oral suspension should be reconstituted at the time of dispensing by adding the amount of water specified on the container to provide a suspension containing 100, 200, or 500 mg of cefixime per 5 mL. The water should be added to the powder in 2 equal portions and the bottle shaken well after each addition.

The suspension should be shaken well just prior to administration of each dose.

■ **Dosage** Cefixime is commercially available as the trihydrate; potency of the drug is expressed in terms of cefixime (the free acid), calculated on the anhydrous basis.

Cefixime may be administered once or twice daily. Once- and twice-daily regimens reportedly are similarly effective for the treatment of otitis media, tonsillitis, or uncomplicated urinary tract infections. Relative efficacy of the 2 regimens has not been evaluated in other infections, and some clinicians suggest that twice-daily dosing may be preferable for the treatment of some lower respiratory tract infections or for complicated urinary tract infections†. Results of most studies indicate that the incidence of GI effects is similar with once- and twice-daily regimens. (See Cautions: GI Effects.)

Capsules containing 400 mg of cefixime are bioequivalent to conventional tablets containing 400 mg of the drug when administered under fasting conditions.

Cefixime chewable tablets are bioequivalent to cefixime oral suspension.

Cefixime conventional tablets and oral suspension are not bioequivalent. (See Pharmacokinetics: Absorption.)

Adult Dosage **Acute Otitis Media.** The usual adult dosage of cefixime for the treatment of acute otitis media (AOM) is 400 mg once daily or 200 mg every 12 hours for 10–14 days.

Only the chewable tablets or oral suspension should be used for the treatment of AOM; cefixime capsules and conventional tablets should *not* be used for the treatment of AOM.

Pharyngitis and Tonsillitis. The usual adult dosage of cefixime for the treatment of pharyngitis and tonsillitis caused by *Streptococcus pyogenes* (group A β-hemolytic streptococci) is 400 mg once daily or 200 mg every 12 hours for at least 10 days.

Respiratory Tract Infections. The usual adult dosage of cefixime for the treatment of respiratory tract infections (acute exacerbations of chronic bronchitis) is 400 mg once daily or 200 mg every 12 hours. The usual duration of cefixime therapy for the treatment of upper respiratory tract infections is 5–10 days.

Urinary Tract Infections. The usual adult dosage of cefixime for the treatment of urinary tract infections is 400 mg once daily or 200 mg every 12 hours. The usual duration of cefixime therapy for the treatment of uncomplicated urinary tract infectionsis 5–10 days.

Gonorrhea and Associated Infections. A single 400-mg dose of cefixime is recommended for the treatment of uncomplicated urethral, endocervical, or rectal† gonorrhea in adults and adolescents. A single 800-mg dose of cefixime also has been used.

If cefixime is used as an alternative for the treatment of uncomplicated urogenital or rectal† gonorrhea when ceftriaxone is not available or cannot be used, the US Centers for Disease Control and Prevention (CDC) recommends a single 400-mg dose of oral cefixime *and* either oral azithromycin (single 1-g dose) or oral doxycycline (100 mg twice daily for 7 days). Cefixime is not recommended by the CDC as first-line treatment for uncomplicated gonorrhea. (See Uses: Gonorrhea and Associated Infections.)

Lyme Disease. For the treatment of Lyme disease†, adults have received cefixime in a dosage of 200 mg daily for 100 days (administered with oral probenecid 500 mg 3 times daily).

Pediatric Dosage Children older than 12 years of age or those weighing more than 45 kg may receive the usual adult dosage of cefixime.

General Pediatric Dosage. For pediatric patients beyond the neonatal period, the American Academy of Pediatrics (AAP) recommends a cefixime dosage of 8 mg/kg daily given in 1 or 2 divided doses for the treatment of mild to moderate infections. The AAP states that cefixime is inappropriate for the treatment of severe infections.

The oral suspension containing 100 mg of cefixime per 5 mL is the preferred preparation for use in children weighing 5–7.5 kg; oral suspensions containing 100 or 200 mg of cefixime per 5 mL are the preferred preparations in those weighing 7.6–10 kg.

Cefixime chewable tablets are not recommended in children weighing less than 10 kg.

Acute Otitis Media. The usual dosage of cefixime for the treatment of AOM in children 6 months to 12 years of age is 8 mg/kg once daily or 4 mg/kg every 12 hours for 10–14 days.

Only the chewable tablets or oral suspension should be used for the treatment of AOM; cefixime capsules and conventional tablets should *not* be used for the treatment of AOM.

Pharyngitis and Tonsillitis. The usual dosage of cefixime for the treatment of group A β-hemolytic streptococcal pharyngitis and tonsillitis in children 6 months to 12 years of age is 8 mg/kg once daily or 4 mg/kg every 12 hours for at least 10 days.

Respiratory Tract Infections. The usual dosage of cefixime for the treatment of acute exacerbations of chronic bronchitis in children 6 months to 12 years of age is 8 mg/kg once daily or 4 mg/kg every 12 hours. The usual duration of cefixime therapy for the treatment of upper respiratory tract infections is 5–10 days.

For empiric treatment of acute bacterial sinusitis† in children, a cefixime dosage of 8 mg/kg daily given in 2 equally divided doses for 10–14 days has been recommended.

Urinary Tract Infections. The usual dosage of cefixime for the treatment of uncomplicated urinary tract infections in children 6 months to 12 years of age is 8 mg/kg once daily or 4 mg/kg every 12 hours. The usual duration of cefixime therapy for the treatment of uncomplicated urinary tract infections is 5–10 days.

Gonorrhea and Associated Infections. For the treatment of uncomplicated gonorrhea, the AAP recommends a single cefixime dose of 8 mg/kg (up to 400 mg) in prepubertal children weighing less than 45 kg or a single 400-mg dose in children 8 years of age or older weighing 45 kg or more.

Cefixime should be used in conjunction with a single dose of oral azithromycin or a 7-day regimen of oral doxycycline. Cefixime is not recommended by the CDC as first-line treatment for uncomplicated gonorrhea. (See Uses: Gonorrhea and Associated Infections.)

Shigellosis. For the treatment of shigellosis†, children have received cefixime in a dosage of 8 mg/kg daily for 5 days.

Typhoid Fever. For the treatment of typhoid fever†, children 6 months to 16 years of age have received cefixime in a dosage of 5–10 mg/kg twice daily. Treatment usually is continued for 14 days; a high rate of treatment failure occurred when the drug was given for only 7 days.

■ **Dosage in Renal Impairment** In patients with creatinine clearances less than 60 mL/minute, dose and/or frequency of administration of cefixime should be modified in response to the degree of renal impairment. The manufacturer recommends that adults with creatinine clearances of 21–59 mL/minute and those undergoing hemodialysis receive a cefixime dosage of 260 mg daily administered as oral suspension, preferably as oral suspension containing 200 or 500 mg of cefixime per 5 mL; cefixime conventional tablets and chewable tablets are not recommended in these patients. The manufacturer also recommends that adults with creatinine clearances of 20 mL/minute or less and those undergoing continuous peritoneal dialysis receive a cefixime dosage of 200 mg daily as conventional tablets or chewable tablets, 172 mg daily as oral suspension containing 100 mg/5 mL, 176 mg daily as oral suspension containing 200 mg/5 mL, or 180 mg daily as oral suspension containing 500 mg/5 mL. Because cefixime is not substantially removed by hemodialysis or peritoneal dialysis, additional supplemental doses of the drug are not necessary during or after either procedure.

■ **Dosage in Geriatric Patients** Modification of the usual dosage of cefixime is not necessary in geriatric adults based on age, but may be required because of age-related decreases in renal function. (See Dosage and Administration: Dosage in Renal Impairment.)

Cautions

Adverse effects reported with cefixime are similar to those reported with other cephalosporins. Cefixime generally is well tolerated; most adverse effects of the drug are transient and mild to moderate in severity. Adverse effects have been reported in up to 50% of patients receiving the drug but have been severe enough to require discontinuance in about 5% of patients.

■ **GI Effects** The most frequent adverse effects of cefixime involve the GI tract. Adverse GI effects have been reported in up to 30% of adults receiving tablets of the drug and have been mild in 20%, moderate in 5–9%, and severe in 2–3% of patients. Diarrhea or loose, frequent stools have been reported in up to 27% and abdominal pain, anorexia,nausea, vomiting, dyspepsia, flatulence, pruritus ani, and dry mouth have been reported in 1–11% of patients receiving the drug.

Adverse GI effects generally appear during the first or second day of cefixime therapy and probably are direct effects of the drug and not the result of changes in bowel flora. In both adults and children, up to 80% of reported cases of diarrhea or loose stools have occurred within the first 4 days of cefixime therapy. In a few studies, adverse GI effects appeared to be more frequent in patients receiving 400 mg of cefixime once daily than in those receiving 200 mg of the drug twice daily. However, results of most other studies in both adults and children indicate that the incidence of GI effects is similar with both regimens and is not affected by dosing frequency. Adverse GI effects generally respond to symptomatic treatment or resolve when cefixime therapy is discontinued. Rarely, these effects may be severe enough to require discontinuance of the drug.

Severe diarrhea and/or colitis, which required hospitalization in some cases, has been reported rarely in patients receiving cefixime (i.e., in less than 2% of patients). (See Clostridium difficile-associated Diarrhea and Colitis under Cautions: GI Effects.)

Cefixime exerts several effects on normal bowel flora. Cefixime (200 mg twice daily or 400 mg once daily) given for 1–2 weeks reduces total bacterial counts of normal fecal anaerobic bacteria, including *Clostridia*, *Bifidobacterium*, and some *Bacteroides*. The drug also decreases bacterial counts of some normal fecal aerobic bacteria including some Enterobacteriaceae and streptococci. In some patients, however, cefixime therapy results in increased fecal counts of group D streptococci, principally *Enterococcus faecalis* (formerly *Streptococcus faecalis*). Fecal flora generally returns to pretreatment levels within 2 weeks following discontinuance of cefixime.

Clostridium difficile-associated Diarrhea and Colitis Treatment with anti-infectives alters normal colon flora and may permit overgrowth of *Clostridium difficile*.

C. difficile infection (CDI) and *C. difficile*-associated diarrhea and colitis (CDAD; also known as antibiotic-associated diarrhea and colitis or pseudomembranous colitis) have been reported with nearly all anti-infectives, including cefixime, and may range in severity from mild diarrhea to fatal colitis. *C. difficile* produces toxins A and B which contribute to the development of CDAD; hypertoxin-producing strains of *C. difficile* are associated with increased morbidity and mortality since they may be refractory to anti-infectives and colectomy may be required.

CDAD should be considered in the differential diagnosis in patients who develop diarrhea during or after anti-infective therapy and managed accordingly. Careful medical history is necessary since CDAD has been reported to occur as late as 2 months or longer after anti-infective therapy is discontinued.

If CDAD is suspected or confirmed, anti-infectives not directed against *C. difficile* should be discontinued whenever possible. Patients should be managed with appropriate supportive therapy (e.g., fluid and electrolyte management, protein supplementation), anti-infective therapy directed against *C. difficile* (e.g., metronidazole, vancomycin), and surgical evaluation as clinically indicated. (See Cautions: Precautions and Contraindications.)

■ **Nervous System Effects** Headache has been reported in up to 3–16% and dizziness, nervousness, insomnia, somnolence, malaise, and fatigue have been reported in up to 4% of patients receiving cefixime. Seizures have been reported in less than 2% of patients receiving cefixime. Several other cephalosporins also have been implicated in precipitating seizures, particularly in patients with renal impairment in whom the dosage was not reduced. If seizures occur during cefixime therapy, the drug should be discontinued and appropriate anticonvulsant therapy administered as indicated.

■ **Sensitivity Reactions** Hypersensitivity reactions have been reported in up to 7% of patients receiving cefixime and include rash, urticaria, drug fever, pruritus, and arthralgia.

Anaphylaxis, angioedema, facial edema, Stevens-Johnson syndrome, erythema multiforme, toxic epidermal necrolysis, and serum sickness-like reactions have been reported in less than 2% of patients receiving cefixime.

■ **Hematologic Effects** Transient thrombocytopenia, thrombocytosis, leukopenia, leukocytosis, eosinophilia, and decreased hemoglobin concentration and hematocrit have been reported in less than 2% of patients receiving cefixime.

Prolonged prothrombin time and prolonged partial thromboplastin time have been reported rarely. Patients with renal or hepatic impairment, poor nutritional status, prolonged anti-infective therapy, and previous anticoagulant therapy (stabilized) appear to be at risk.

Neutropenia, pancytopenia, agranulocytosis, aplastic anemia, hemolytic anemia, and hemorrhage have been reported with other cephalosporins but have not been reported to date with cefixime.

■ **Hepatic Effects** Transient increases in AST (SGOT), ALT (SGPT), alkaline phosphatase, bilirubin, and LDH have been reported in less than 2% of patients receiving cefixime. Hepatitis and jaundice have been reported in less than 2% of patients receiving cefixime. Hepatic dysfunction, including cholestasis, also has been reported with other cephalosporins.

■ **Renal and Genitourinary Effects** Transient increases in BUN and serum creatinine concentrations and acute renal failure have been reported in less than 2% of patients receiving cefixime. Dysuria and pyuria have been reported rarely.

Genital pruritus, vaginitis, and vaginal candidiasis have been reported in less than 2% of patients receiving cefixime. Renal dysfunction and toxic nephropathy have been reported with other cephalosporins.

■ **Other Adverse Effects** Increased serum amylase concentrations have been reported in 1.5–5% of patients receiving cefixime; however, there was no apparent correlation between increased serum amylase concentrations and adverse GI effects in these patients.

■ Precautions and Contraindications Prior to initiation of cefixime therapy, careful inquiry should be made concerning previous hypersensitivity reactions to cephalosporins, penicillins, or other drugs. There is clinical and laboratory evidence of partial cross-allergenicity among β-lactam antibiotics including penicillins, cephalosporins, and cephamycins. Caution is advised. Cefixime is contraindicated in individuals who are hypersensitive to the drug or other cephalosporins. Use of cephalosporins should be avoided in patients who have had an immediate-type (anaphylactic) hypersensitivity reaction to penicillins.

To reduce development of drug-resistant bacteria and maintain effectiveness of cefixime and other antibacterials, the drug should be used only for the treatment or prevention of infections proven or strongly suspected to be caused by susceptible bacteria. When selecting or modifying anti-infective therapy, results of culture and in vitro susceptibility testing should be used. In the absence of such data, consider local epidemiology and susceptibility patterns should be considered when selecting anti-infectives for empiric therapy.

Patients should be advised that antibacterials (including cefixime) should only be used to treat bacterial infections and not used to treat viral infections (e.g., the common cold). Patients also should be advised about the importance of completing the full course of therapy, even if feeling better after a few days, and that skipping doses or not completing therapy may decrease effectiveness and increase the likelihood that bacteria will develop resistance and will not be treatable with cefixime or other antibacterials in the future.

As with other anti-infectives, prolonged use of cefixime may result in overgrowth of nonsusceptible organisms. Superinfection with gram-positive bacteria (e.g., staphylococci, enterococci) has occurred in patients receiving cefixime for the treatment of otitis media or urinary tract infections. Careful observation of the patient during cefixime therapy is essential. If suprainfection or superinfection occurs, appropriate therapy should be instituted.

Because CDAD has been reported with the use of cefixime or other cephalosporins, it should be considered in the differential diagnosis of patients who develop diarrhea during or after cefixime therapy. (See Cautions: GI Effects.) Patients should be advised that diarrhea is a common problem caused by anti-infectives and usually resolves when the drug is discontinued; however, they should contact a clinician if watery and bloody stools (with or without stomach cramps and fever) occur during or as late as 2 months or longer after the last dose.

Because decreased prothrombin activity has been reported with cephalosporins, prothrombin time should be monitored in patients at risk (see Cautions: Hematologic Effects) and exogenous vitamin K administered as indicated.

Individuals with phenylketonuria should be cautioned that cefixime chewable tablets containing 100, 150, and 200 mg of the drug contain aspartame (NutraSweet®), which is metabolized in the GI tract to provide 3.3, 5, and 6.7 mg of phenylalanine, respectively.

Because serum concentrations of cefixime are higher and more prolonged in patients with renal impairment than in patients with normal renal function, doses and/or frequency of administration of the drug should be decreased in patients with impaired renal function, including those undergoing continuous ambulatory peritoneal dialysis (CAPD) or hemodialysis. Patients undergoing dialysis should be monitored carefully during cefixime therapy. (See Dosage and Administration: Dosage in Renal Impairment.)

■ Pediatric Precautions Safety and efficacy of cefixime in children younger than 6 months of age have not been established.

The frequency of adverse GI effects (e.g., diarrhea, loose stools) reported in pediatric patients receiving cefixime oral suspension is similar to that reported in adults receiving cefixime tablets. Diarrhea or loose stools has been reported in up to 15% of children 6 months to 13 years of age receiving oral cefixime. CDAD has been reported rarely in children receiving cefixime. In 3 reported cases, the onset of symptoms (abdominal pain, diarrhea) occurred 4–14 days after the first dose of cefixime.

■ Geriatric Precautions Clinical studies did not include sufficient numbers of patients 65 years of age or older to determine whether geriatric patients respond differently than younger adults. Other reported clinical experience has not identified differences in responses between geriatric and younger patients.

Some evidence indicates that oral bioavailability of the drug may be increased in geriatric patients, but such increases are not considered clinically important. (See Pharmacokinetics: Absorption.)

Because renal function decreases with age and may be impaired in geriatric patients, the possibility that adjustment of cefixime dosage may be necessary in this age group should be considered. (See Dosage and Administration: Dosage in Renal Impairment.)

■ Mutagenicity and Carcinogenicity Cefixime was not mutagenic when tested in vitro or in vivo in bacteria or mammalian cells for the ability to cause point mutations, induce unscheduled DNA synthesis, or cause chromosome aberrations. The drug did not exhibit clastogenic potential in vivo in the mouse micronucleus test.

Long-term animal carcinogenicity studies using cefixime have not been conducted to date.

■ Pregnancy, Fertility, and Lactation Reproduction studies in mice and rats using oral cefixime dosages up to 40 times the usual human dosage have not revealed evidence of harm to the fetus. There are no adequate and controlled studies to date using cefixime in pregnant women, and the drug should be used during pregnancy only when clearly needed. Use of cefixime during labor and delivery has not been studied to date, and the drug should be used in these circumstances only when clearly needed.

There was no evidence of impaired fertility or adverse effects on reproductive performance in rats receiving cefixime dosages up to 25 times the usual adult dosage.

Cefixime is distributed into milk in rats. Although the drug reportedly was not detected in milk following a single dose in lactating women in one study (see Pharmacokinetics: Distribution), it is not known whether cefixime is distributed into milk in humans. Therefore, consideration should be given to temporarily discontinuing nursing during therapy with the drug.

Drug Interactions

■ Antacids Results of a study in healthy men indicate that administration of an antacid containing aluminum hydroxide and magnesium hydroxide either simultaneously with or 2 hours before or after a single 400-mg oral dose of cefixime has no clinically important effects on the pharmacokinetics of the anti-infective agent.

■ Anticoagulants Increased prothrombin time (with or without bleeding) has been reported following concomitant use of cefixime with an anticoagulant (e.g., warfarin).

■ Carbamazepine Concomitant administration of cefixime and carbamazepine has resulted in increased plasma carbamazepine concentrations. Carbamazepine concentrations should be monitored if the drug is used concomitantly with cefixime.

■ Nifedipine Concomitant administration of cefixime and nifedipine increases oral bioavailability of cefixime as a result of higher peak plasma concentrations and area under the plasma concentration-time curve (AUC).

■ Probenecid Although specific information is unavailable, concomitant administration of probenecid reportedly increases peak serum concentrations and the AUC of cefixime and decreases renal clearance and volume of distribution of the drug.

■ Salicylates In one in vitro study in pooled serum, salicylic acid apparently displaced cefixime from protein binding sites, resulting in more than a 50% increase in concentrations of free cefixime; this effect appeared to be concentration-dependent. Concomitant administration of a 650-mg oral dose of aspirin and a 400-mg oral dose of cefixime in healthy adult men did not appear to affect protein binding, serum half-life, or renal clearance of cefixime but did result in a 20–25% decrease in peak serum concentrations and AUCs of the anti-infective agent. Although the manufacturer states that this effect was not considered clinically important since serum concentrations of cefixime remained higher than the MIC values reported for most susceptible organisms, some clinicians state that this potential interaction may be clinically important in certain infections.

Laboratory Test Interferences

■ Tests for Urinary Glucose or Ketones Like most cephalosporins, cefixime may cause false-positive results in urinary glucose determinations using cupric sulfate (e.g., Benedict's solution, Clinitest®, Fehling's solution); however, glucose oxidase methods (e.g., Clinistix®, Tes-Tape®) are unaffected by the drug.

Cefixime may cause false-positive results for ketones in urine if nitroprusside tests are used; this effect has not been reported with tests using nitroferricyanide.

■ Immunohematology Tests Although not reported to date with cefixime, positive direct antiglobulin (Coombs') test results have been reported in patients receiving other cephalosporins. This reaction may interfere with hematologic studies or transfusion cross-matching procedures and should be considered in patients receiving cefixime.

Acute Toxicity

The oral LD_{50} of cefixime exceeds 10 g/kg in mice, rats, and rabbits. In dogs, LD_{50} determinations have been limited by emesis, which occurred when cefixime doses of 320 mg/kg or greater were used in these animals.

Limited information is available on the acute toxicity of cefixime in humans. In healthy adults who received cefixime in single doses up to 2 g, adverse effects were similar to those seen with usual doses of the drug and included mild to moderate adverse GI effects.

If acute overdosage of cefixime occurs, the stomach should be emptied by gastric lavage. Cefixime is not removed in clinically important quantities by hemodialysis or peritoneal dialysis.

Mechanism of Action

Cefixime is usually bactericidal in action. Like other cephalosporins, the antibacterial activity of the drug results from inhibition of mucopeptide synthesis in the bacterial cell wall. For information on the mechanism of action of cephalosporins, see Mechanism of Action in the Cephalosporins General Statement 8:12.06.

Studies evaluating the binding of cefixime to penicillin-binding proteins (PBPs), the target enzymes of β-lactam antibiotics, indicate that cefixime has a high affinity for PBPs 3, 1a, and 1b of *Escherichia coli*. Since PBP 1b is a killing site for β-lactam anti-infectives, cefixime's high affinity for this site may be a major factor in the drug's potent bactericidal activity against this organism. Cefixime has only low affinity for PBP 2 of staphylococci and little or no affinity for PBP 4 or 5.

In vitro studies indicate that low concentrations of cefixime usually cause the formation of filamentous cells in susceptible *E. coli* or *Klebsiella pneumoniae*. At higher concentrations, direct lysis of the organisms may occur as well as spheroplast formation and rupture. Following in vitro exposure to cefixime, morphologic changes in β-lactamase-producing *E. coli* are the same as those seen in non-β-lactamase-producing strains of the organism. Lysis occurs in susceptible anaerobic bacteria following in vitro exposure to cefixime.

For most susceptible organisms, the minimum bactericidal concentration (MBC) of cefixime is only 1–4 times higher than the minimum inhibitory concentration (MIC). However, for some strains of *Enterobacter*, *Klebsiella*, *Morganella*, *Proteus*, *Providencia*, and *Serratia*, the MBC may be 9–32 times higher than the MIC.

Spectrum

Based on its spectrum of activity, cefixime is classified as a third generation cephalosporin. For information on the classification of cephalosporins and closely related β-lactam antibiotics based on spectra of activity, see Spectrum in the Cephalosporins General Statement 8:12.06.

Like other currently available third generation cephalosporins (e.g., cefdinir, cefoperazone, cefotaxime, cefpodoxime, ceftazidime, ceftibuten, ceftriaxone), cefixime has an expanded spectrum of activity against gram-negative bacteria compared with first and second generation cephalosporins. In vitro on a weight basis, however, cefixime usually is less active than many other currently available third generation cephalosporins against susceptible Enterobacteriaceae and is inactive in vitro against most strains of*Enterobacter* and *Pseudomonas*. Although some other currently available third generation cephalosporins have some activity against staphylococci, cefixime usually is inactive against these organisms.

■ **In Vitro Susceptibility Testing** Results of in vitro cefixime susceptibility tests are not usually affected by the pH of the media or the presence of certain cations (e.g., calcium, magnesium, sodium). There generally is little effect on in vitro susceptibility test results when the pH of the media is within the range of 5–8. In vitro activity of cefixime against Enterobacteriaceae is not affected by the presence of urine or serum.

Inoculum size may affect in vitro susceptibility to cefixime. MICs of most susceptible organisms are not greatly affected when the size of the inoculum is increased from 10^3 to 10^5 colony-forming units (CFU) per mL; however, MICs of some Enterobacteriaceae may be 15–500 times higher when the size of the inoculum is increased from 10^3 to 10^7 CFU.

Strains of staphylococci resistant to penicillinase-resistant penicillins (methicillin-resistant [oxacillin-resistant] staphylococci) should be considered resistant to cefixime, although results of in vitro susceptibility tests may indicate that the organisms are susceptible to the drug.

For information on interpreting results of in vitro susceptibility testing (disk susceptibility tests, dilution susceptibility tests) when cefixime susceptibility testing is performed according to the standards of the Clinical and Laboratory Standards Institute (CLSI; formerly National Committee for Clinical Laboratory Standards [NCCLS]), see Spectrum: In Vitro Susceptibility Testing, in the Cephalosporins General Statement 8:12.06.

■ **Gram-positive Aerobic Bacteria** ***Gram-positive Aerobic Cocci*** Cefixime generally is active in vitro against *Streptococcus pyogenes* (group A β-hemolytic streptococci), *S. agalactiae* (group B streptococci), and groups C, F, and G streptococci. The MIC_{90} (minimum inhibitory concentration of the drug at which 90% of strains tested are inhibited) of cefixime reported for *S. pyogenes* and *S. agalactiae* is 0.1–0.5 mcg/mL, and the MIC_{90} reported for groups C, F, and G streptococci is 0.05–1 mcg/mL. In vitro on a weight basis, cefixime is either equally or more active than most first and second generation cephalosporins (e.g., cephalexin, cefadroxil, cefaclor, cefuroxime) against *S. pyogenes*, but is less active than ampicillin or amoxicillin against these organisms.

Cefixime is active in vitro against some strains of *S. pneumoniae*; however, in vitro on a weight basis, the drug generally is less active against this organism than some other oral cephalosporins (e.g., cefdinir, cefpodoxime, cefprozil, cefuroxime). While penicillin-susceptible *S. pneumoniae* may be inhibited in vitro by cefixime concentrations of 4 mcg/mL or less, the MIC_{90} of cefixime reported for strains of *S. pneumoniae* that have intermediate resistance to penicillin (relatively resistant) and strains that are highly resistant to penicillin is 16–32 mcg/mL and these strains are considered resistant to cefixime.

Nonenterococcal group D streptococci (e.g., *S. bovis*) and viridans streptococci (e.g., *S. mitis*) generally require cefixime concentrations of 1–32 mcg/mL for in vitro inhibition, and most strains are considered resistant to the drug. In one study, the MIC_{50} and MIC_{90} of cefixime for the *S. milleri* group of viridans streptococci (*S. anginosus*, *S. constellatus*, *S. intermedius*) were 4 and 8 mcg/mL, respectively. Enterococci, including*Enterococcus faecalis* (formerly *S. faecalis*) and *E. faecium* (formerly *S. faecium*), are resistant to cefixime.

Unlike other currently available cephalosporins, cefixime is inactive in vitro against penicillinase-producing and nonpenicillinase-producing staphylococci, including *Staphylococcus aureus*, *S. epidermidis*, and *S. saprophyticus*. Although some staphylococci may be inhibited in vitro by cefixime concentrations of 3–16 mcg/mL, most strains require high concentrations of cefixime for in vitro inhibition and are considered resistant to the drug. Like other cephalosporins, cefixime is inactive against methicillin-resistant (oxacillin-resistant) staphylococci.

Gram-positive Aerobic Bacilli *Corynebacterium*, including JK strains of *Corynebacterium JK*, generally are resistant to cefixime and have MIC_{90}s of 32 mcg/mL or greater. *Listeria monocytogenes* generally are resistant to cefixime in vitro.

■ **Gram-negative Aerobic Bacteria** ***Neisseria*** Cefixime is active in vitro against *Neisseria meningitidis*, and most strains of this organism are inhibited by cefixime concentrations of 0.01–0.06 mcg/mL.

Cefixime is active in vitro against penicillinase-producing (PPNG) and nonpenicillinase-producing *N. gonorrhoeae*. The drug also is active in vitro against *N. gonorrhoeae* with chromosomally mediated resistance to penicillin (CMRNG) or plasmid-mediated tetracycline resistance (TRNG). The MIC_{90} of cefixime reported for nonpenicillinase-producing *N. gonorrhoeae*, PPNG, or CMRNG usually has ranged from 0.001–0.06 mcg/mL. However, *N. gonorrhoeae* with reduced susceptibility to cefixime (MICs 0.25 mcg/mL or greater) have been reported in the US and other countries with increasing frequency during the last decade; treatment failures have been reported. (See Uses: Gonorrhea and Associated Infections.)

Haemophilus Cefixime is active in vitro against most β-lactamase-producing and non-β-lactamase-producing strains of *Haemophilus influenzae* and *H. parainfluenzae*. The MIC_{90} reported for β-lactamase-producing and non-β-lactamase-producing *H. influenzae* is 0.015–0.25 mcg/mL.

In vitro on a weight basis, cefixime is more active against β-lactamase-producing *H. influenzae* than is cefaclor, cephalexin, cefuroxime, or amoxicillin and clavulanate potassium, but may be equally or slightly less active than is ciprofloxacin, ceftriaxone, or co-trimoxazole against these organisms. Cefixime is active in vitro against multiple-drug resistant strains of *H. influenzae* that are resistant to ampicillin, chloramphenicol, tetracycline, co-trimoxazole, cefaclor, and/or erythromycin. However, some strains of non-β-lactamase-producing *H. influenzae* that are resistant to ampicillin and second generation cephalosporins also may have reduced susceptibility to cefixime.

Moraxella catarrhalis Cefixime is active in vitro against both β-lactamase- and non-β-lactamase-producing *Moraxella catarrhalis*, and the MIC_{90} of the drug reported for this organism is 0.03–0.4 mcg/mL. Cefixime is active in vitro against strains of *M. catarrhalis* resistant to ampicillin, cephalexin, and cefaclor.

Enterobacteriaceae Cefixime is active in vitro against most clinically important Enterobacteriaceae. With the exception of *Citrobacter freundii*, *Enterobacter*, *Morganella morganii*, and *Serratia*, the MIC_{90} of cefixime for Enterobacteriaceae is generally 2 mcg/mL or less.

In vitro on a weight basis, cefixime is equally or less active than other third generation cephalosporins (e.g., cefotaxime, ceftriaxone) or ciprofloxacin against Enterobacteriaceae. Cefixime is active in vitro against many strains of *E. coli*, *Citrobacter freundii*, *K. pneumoniae*, and *P. mirabilis* resistant to other anti-infectives (e.g., aminoglycosides, tetracycline, ampicillin, amoxicillin, cefaclor, cephalexin). Cefixime is active in vitro against strains of *Salmonella typhi* resistant to ampicillin, chloramphenicol, and/or co-trimoxazole.

Table 1: MIC_{50}s and MIC_{90}s of cefixime reported for Enterobacteriaceae

Organism	MIC_{50} (mcg/mL)	MIC_{90} (mcg/mL)
Citrobacter spp.		
C. amalonaticus	0.25–0.5	1–1.5
C. diversus	0.06–0.25	0.06–0.5
C. freundii	1–3.13	2–128
Enterobacter spp.	3.27–4	20–32
E. aerogenes	0.4–16	8–100
E. agglomerans	0.05–0.5	8–32
E. cloacae	0.1–16	8–128
Escherichia coli	0.1–0.5	0.12–2
Hafnia alvei	0.4–4	2–32
Klebsiella spp.	0.08–0.25	0.25–0.5
K. oxytoca	0.013–0.125	0.05–4
K. pneumoniae	0.025–0.125	0.05–0.5
Morganella morganii	0.39–8	4–32
Proteus spp.		
P. mirabilis	0.01–0.25	0.01–0.25
P. vulgaris	0.01–0.25	0.05–2
Providencia spp.	0.125–0.4	0.5–16
P. rettgeri	0.01–0.25	0.05–2
P. stuartii	0.01–0.25	0.12–2
Serratia spp.	0.5–2	8–64
S. marcescens	0.25–3.13	2–128
Salmonella spp.	0.05–0.1	0.2–0.39
S. enteritidis	0.125–0.25	0.34–0.5
S. typhi	0.02–0.4	0.06
Shigella spp.	0.12–0.25	0.25–0.78
Yersinia enterocolitica	0.25–1	1–4

Pseudomonas Some strains of *Pseudomonas cepacia, Ps. pseudomallei*, and *Ps. stutzeri* are inhibited in vitro by cefixime concentrations of 1.56–8 mcg/mL. However, the MIC_{90} of cefixime for *Ps. aeruginosa* and for most other *Pseudomonas*, including *Ps. fluorescens, Ps. putida, Ps. maltophilia* (*Xanthomonas maltophilia*), and most strains of *Ps. stutzeri*, usually exceeds 16 mcg/mL and these organisms are considered resistant to the drug.

Other Gram-negative Aerobic Bacteria Cefixime has some in vitro activity against *Acinetobacter*; however, the MIC_{90} reported for *A. calcoaceticus* var. *lwoffi* and *A. calcoaceticus* var. *anitratus* generally ranges from 3.1–100 mcg/mL. *Aeromonas hydrophila* generally is inhibited in vitro by cefixime concentrations of 0.01–4 mcg/mL. Some strains of *Alcaligenes* are inhibited in vitro by cefixime concentrations of 8 mcg/mL.

Some strains of *Campylobacter fetus* subsp. *jejuni* are inhibited in vitro by cefixime concentrations of 1.6–8 mcg/mL, but many strains of the organism are resistant to the drug. Cefixime is active against *Helicobacter pylori* (formerly *Campylobacter pylori* or *C. pyloridis*). The MIC_{90} of cefixime for *H. pylori* has been reported as 0.25–0.5 mcg/mL.

Cefixime concentrations of 12.5–16 mcg/mL inhibit some strains of *Bordetella pertussis*; however, *B. bronchiseptica* and *B. parapertussis* are resistant to the drug. *Pasteurella multocida* is inhibited in vitro by cefixime concentrations of 0.012–1 mcg/mL.

Achromobacter xylosoxidans and *Flavobacterium meningosepticum, F. adoratum*, and *F. indologenes* are resistant to cefixime.

■ **Anaerobic Bacteria** Cefixime has only limited in vitro activity against anaerobic bacteria. Some strains (45–91% of those tested) of *Lactobacillus, Peptococcus, Peptostreptococcus, Actinomyces, Propionibacterium, Fusobacterium*, and *Veillonella* are inhibited in vitro by cefixime concentrations of 1–4 mcg/mL. Most strains of *Bacteroides fragilis* and other *Bacteroides*species are resistant to cefixime in vitro. Although some *Clostridium* are inhibited in vitro by cefixime concentrations of 1.56–8 mcg/mL, most strains of *Clostridia* (including *C. difficile*) are considered resistant to the drug.

■ **Chlamydia and Mycoplasma** Cefixime is inactive against *Chlamydia trachomatis* and *Ureaplasma urealyticum*.

■ **Spirochetes** Cefixime has some activity against *Borrelia burgdorferi*, the causative organism of Lyme disease, and concentrations of 0.8 mcg/mL reportedly inhibit the organism in vitro.

Resistance

For information on possible mechanisms of bacterial resistance to cephalosporins, see Resistance in the Cephalosporins General Statement 8:12.06.

Cefixime has a high degree of β-lactamase stability and is stable against hydrolysis by many plasmid- and chromosomally mediated β-lactamases. The drug generally is more stable against inactivation by β-lactamases than are cefaclor, cefoxitin, cefuroxime, and cephalexin. Cefixime generally is not hydrolyzed by β-lactamases classified as Richmond-Sykes types Ia (P99), III (TEM-1, TEM-2, SHV-1), IV (K-1), and V (OXA-2, OXA-3, PSE-1, PSE-4). The drug is hydrolyzed by some β-lactamases produced by *Enterobacter, Klebsiella oxytoca, Proteus vulgaris*, and *Pseudomonas cepacia*. The drug is hydrolyzed by Richmond-Sykes type I produced by*Pseudomonas cepacia* and Ia produced by *Citrobacter freundii* and *Enterobacter cloacae*. The drug also is hydrolyzed by β-lactamases produced by *Flavobacterium* and *Bacteroides fragilis*.

Resistance to cefixime in staphylococci appears to be related to the drug's poor affinity for PBP 2 of these organisms. Resistance in enterococci and *Listeria monocytogenes* may also be related to poor binding of cefixime to the PBPs of these organisms. In vitro studies indicate that resistance to cefixime in *C. freundii* and *Enterobacter* apparently is related to factors that affect permeability of the organisms to the drug and also is related to the production of β-lactamases. Resistance to cefixime in *Pseudomonas* and *Acinetobacter* is related to permeability factors.

Unlike some β-lactam anti-infectives (e.g., cefoxitin, imipenem), cefixime is a weak inducer of β-lactamases and does not derepress inducible, chromosomally mediated enzymes in *C. freundii, E. cloacae, E. aerogenes, Providencia stuartii, Serratia liquefaciens*, or *S. marcescens*. Cefixime does, however, induce β-lactamase production in some strains of *Morganella morganii*, but the drug remains active in vitro against these *M. morganii* strains following derepression of inducible β-lactamases.

Pharmacokinetics

■ **Absorption** Approximately 30–50% of a single dose of cefixime is absorbed following oral administration. Studies in rats indicate that the drug is absorbed from the upper and middle part of the small intestine and probably is transported across the intestinal membrane by a dipeptide carrier system.

Capsules containing 400 mg of cefixime are bioequivalent to conventional tablets containing 400 mg of the drug when administered under fasting conditions. Cefixime chewable tablets are bioequivalent to cefixime oral suspension. Cefixime conventional tablets and oral suspension are not bioequivalent; the oral suspension results in peak serum concentrations 25–50% higher than concentrations attained with the tablets.

When cefixime is administered as conventional tablets or oral suspension, about 40–50% of a dose is absorbed whether the drug is given with or without food; however, the time to peak concentrations is increased approximately 0.8 hours when the drug is given with food. When cefixime is administered as capsules with food, absorption of the drug is decreased by approximately 15% based on area under the concentration-time curve (AUC) or approximately 25% based on peak serum concentrations.

GI absorption of cefixime is not affected by concomitant administration of antacids. (See Drug Interactions: Antacids.)

Following oral administration of a single 200- or 400-mg dose of cefixime as capsules, tablets, or oral suspension, the time to peak serum concentrations averages 3.1–4.4 hours (range: 2–6 hours). In one study in healthy, fasting adults, time to peak serum concentrations of cefixime was dose dependent and averaged 2.7, 3.4, 3.9, and 4.3 hours following a single 50-, 100-, 200-, and 400-mg oral dose, respectively. Following oral administration of a single 200- or 400-mg tablet of cefixime, peak serum concentrations average 2 mcg/mL (range: 1–4 mcg/mL) or 3.7 mcg/mL (range: 1.3–7.7 mcg/mL); serum concentrations average 1.5 or 2.7 mcg/mL, respectively, 6 hours after the dose and average 0.4 or 0.6 mcg/mL, respectively, 12 hours after the dose.

In adults, peak serum concentrations of cefixime are approximately 25–50% higher when the drug is administered as an oral suspension rather than as tablets. When 200- or 400-mg doses of cefixime are administered to adults as an oral suspension, peak serum concentrations average 3 mcg/mL (range: 1–4.5 mcg/mL) or 4.6 mcg/mL (range: 1.9–7.7 mcg/mL), respectively. In the dosage range of 100–400 mg, the AUC in adults is approximately 10–25% higher with the oral suspension than with the tablets.

Studies in healthy adults using cefixime doses of 100 mg to 2 g given as capsules or an oral solution or suspension indicate that peak serum concentrations and AUCs increase with increasing dose but are not directly dose proportional; there is some evidence that decreased GI absorption occurs with increasing dose. Studies in children using cefixime doses of 4–8 mg/kg also indicate that serum concentrations of cefixime are not directly dose proportional.

There is no evidence that cefixime accumulates in serum or urine of patients with normal renal function following multiple doses of the drug given once or twice daily. In one study in healthy adults receiving 400 mg once daily or 200 mg twice daily as cefixime capsules, peak serum concentrations and AUCs determined after 8 and 14–15 days of therapy were similar to those reported on the first day of therapy.

Although the difference was not considered clinically important, one study in geriatric patients older than 64 years of age receiving 400-mg doses of cefixime once daily for 5 days indicated that peak serum concentrations of cefixime were 20–26% higher and AUCs were approximately 40–42% higher in these geriatric adults than in healthy adults 18–35 years of age.

In pediatric patients 6 months to 6 years of age or older receiving a single 4-, 6-, or 8-mg/kg dose of cefixime as an oral suspension, serum concentrations of the drug 3.5–4.5 hours after the dose average 2.18–2.44, 3.55–4.07, and 3.4–3.91 mcg/mL, respectively.

■ **Distribution** Information on distribution of cefixime is limited. Following oral administration, cefixime is distributed into bile, sputum, tonsils, maxillary sinus mucosa, middle ear discharge, blister fluid, and prostatic fluid. Sputum concentrations may be 2–10% of concurrent serum concentrations; in one study, a single 200-mg oral dose of cefixime resulted in sputum concentrations of 0.03–0.12 mcg/mL.

In children 3 months to 5 years of age with acute otitis media with effusion or with otitis media with effusion that required tympanostomy tube placement, a single 8-mg/kg oral dose of cefixime resulted in middle ear fluid concentrations averaging 1.3–1.4 mcg/mL at 3–5 hours after the dose; concurrent serum concentrations of the drug averaged 2.5–3.2 mcg/mL.

In cholecystectomized patients who received a single 100-, 200-, or 400-mg oral dose of cefixime, concentrations of the drug in gallbladder tissue and bile 3.5–12 hours after the dose averaged 8–18.6 mg/kg and 134–190 mg/L, respectively. In one patient with a biliary tract infection who received a single 200-mg dose of cefixime, concentrations of the drug in common duct bile were 0.3 mg/L 1.5 hours after the dose and 99 mg/L 4.5 hours after the dose.

Cefixime concentrations in prostatic fluid are reported to range from less than 0.01 to 0.83 mcg/mL in samples obtained 1–3 hours after a single 200- or 400-mg oral dose of the drug.

It is not known whether cefixime is distributed into CSF following oral administration.

The apparent volume of distribution of cefixime in healthy adults averages 0.1 L/kg (range: 0.095–0.11 L/kg.

Cefixime is approximately 65–70% bound to serum proteins, principally albumin, and such binding is not concentration dependent over the range of 0.5–30 mcg/mL. The fraction of free cefixime in plasma may be slightly greater in patients with impaired renal function than in those with normal renal function, but this generally is not considered clinically important.

Cefixime crosses the placenta and is distributed in low concentrations into amniotic fluid and cord serum; cord serum concentrations may be 15–50% of concurrent maternal plasma concentrations.

In one study in women who received a single 100-mg oral dose of cefixime, the drug reportedly was not detected in milk when samples were obtained 1–6 hours after the dose. In a study in rats receiving cefixime via intraperitoneal infusion, only low concentrations of the drug were attained in the plasma of nursing pups.

■ **Elimination** The serum elimination half-life of cefixime in adults with normal renal function averages 2.4–4 hours. Although not reported in published studies, the manufacturer states that the serum elimination half-life of cefixime may range up to 9 hours in some healthy adults. Serum half-life of cefixime is independent of dosage form and is not dose dependent.

The serum half-life of cefixime is prolonged in patients with impaired renal function. In adults with moderate renal impairment (creatinine clearances of 20–40 mL/minute), serum half-life averages 6.4 hours. In adults with severe renal impairment (creatinine clearances of 5–20 mL/minute), half-life averages 11.5 hours.

Cefixime is not substantially removed by hemodialysis or peritoneal dialysis. In one study in a limited number of adults undergoing hemodialysis and receiving 400-mg oral doses of cefixime, pharmacokinetics of the drug were similar to those reported for patients with creatinine clearances of 21–60 mL/minute. It is not known whether impaired hepatic function has an effect on the pharmacokinetics of cefixime.

There is no evidence that cefixime is metabolized in vivo; no microbiologically active metabolites have been detected in serum or urine following oral administration of the drug.

Cefixime is eliminated by renal and nonrenal mechanisms. Approximately 7–41% of a single oral dose of the drug is excreted unchanged in urine within 24 hours; the drug is excreted principally by glomerular filtration and to a lesser extent by tubular secretion. The remainder of the dose (up to 60%) is eliminated by nonrenal mechanisms. Studies in animals indicate that more than 10% of a single oral dose of cefixime is excreted unchanged in bile. Fecal concentrations of cefixime in healthy adults may range from 0.237–1.55 g/kg following usual oral doses of the drug as capsules or tablets.

Clearance of cefixime from serum averages 0.39–0.45 mL/minute per kg and renal clearance averages 27–43 mL/minute in healthy adults with normal renal function. Urinary concentrations of cefixime generally range from 2.2–103 mcg/mL during the first 2 hours and from 15.7–305 mcg/mL 6–8 hours after a single 200- or 400-mg oral dose of the drug.

Only small amounts of cefixime are removed by hemodialysis or peritoneal dialysis; these amounts are not considered clinically important.

Chemistry and Stability

■ **Chemistry** Cefixime is a semisynthetic cephalosporin antibiotic. The drug is an oral aminothiazolyl methoxyimino cephalosporin. Cefixime is structurally similar to other oral (cefdinir, cefpodoxime proxetil, ceftibuten) or parenteral (cefotaxime, ceftazidime, ceftriaxone) cephalosporins that contain an aminothiazolyl side chain at position 7 of the cephalosporin nucleus. The aminothiazolyl side chain enhances antibacterial activity, particularly against Enterobacteriaceae, and the methoxyimino group imparts stability against hydrolysis by many β-lactamases. Like cefdinir, cefixime contains a vinyl moiety at position 3 of the cephalosporin nucleus. This vinyl moiety, which is a small uncharged group, is partially responsible for the GI absorption characteristics of cefixime. The vinyl moiety also may contribute to cefixime's potent bactericidal activity, although it appears to be partially responsible for the drug's poor in vitro activity against staphylococci.

Cefixime is commercially available as the trihydrate; potency of the drug is expressed in terms of cefixime (the free acid), calculated on the anhydrous basis. Cefixime occurs as a white to slightly yellowish-white, nonhygroscopic, crystalline powder with a slight characteristic odor. The drug has a pK_a of 3.73. The aqueous solubility of cefixime is pH dependent. At room temperature, cefixime has solubilities in water of 0.5 mg/mL at pH 3.2 and 18 mg/mL at pH 4.2. Cefixime has a solubility of 8.3 mg/mL in alcohol at room temperature. Cefixime powder for oral suspension occurs as an off-white to pale yellow, strawberry-flavored powder. Following reconstitution, the suspension has a pH of 2.5–4.5.

■ **Stability** Cefixime capsules, conventional tablets, or chewable tablets should be stored at 20–25°C.

Cefixime powder for oral suspension should be stored in tight containers at 20–25°C. After reconstitution, the oral suspension should be stored in a tight container and is stable for 14 days at room temperature or when refrigerated; any unused suspension should be discarded after 14 days.

Preparations

Excipients in commercially available drug preparations may have clinically important effects in some individuals; consult specific product labeling for details.

Cefixime (Trihydrate)

Oral		
Capsules	400 mg (of cefixime)	Suprax®, Lupin
For suspension	100 mg (of cefixime) per 5 mL	Suprax®, Lupin
	200 mg (of cefixime) per 5 mL	Suprax®, Lupin
	500 mg (of cefixime) per 5 mL	Suprax®, Lupin
Tablets, chewable	100 mg (of cefixime)	Suprax®, Lupin
	150 mg (of cefixime)	Suprax®, Lupin
	200 mg (of cefixime)	Suprax®, Lupin
Tablets, film-coated	400 mg (of cefixime)	Suprax® (scored), Lupin

†Use is not currently included in the labeling approved by the US Food and Drug Administration

Cefotaxime Sodium

■ Cefotaxime is a semisynthetic, third generation cephalosporin antibiotic.

Uses

Cefotaxime is used for the treatment of serious bone and joint infections, serious intra-abdominal and gynecologic infections (including peritonitis, endometritis, pelvic inflammatory disease, pelvic cellulitis), meningitis and other CNS infections, serious lower respiratory tract infections (including pneumonia), bacteremia/septicemia, serious skin and skin structure infections, and serious urinary tract infections caused by susceptible bacteria. The drug also is used in the treatment of gonorrhea, typhoid fever and other infections caused by *Salmonella*†, infections caused by *Vibrio parahaemolyticus*† or *V. vulnificus*†, and Lyme disease†. Cefotaxime also has been used for perioperative prophylaxis.

Prior to initiation of cefotaxime therapy, appropriate specimens should be obtained for identification of the causative organism and in vitro susceptibility tests. If cefotaxime therapy is started pending results of susceptibility tests, it should be discontinued if the causative organism is found to be resistant to the drug. Because resistant strains of some organisms, especially *Enterobacter, Ps. aeruginosa*, and *Serratia*, have developed during cefotaxime therapy, it is important that appropriate specimens be obtained periodically until the infection is eradicated and cefotaxime is discontinued. In certain cases of confirmed or suspected gram-positive or gram-negative sepsis or in the empiric treatment of other serious infections when the causative organism has not been identified, cefotaxime may be used concomitantly with an aminoglycoside pending results of in vitro susceptibility tests. In infections which fail to respond to cefotaxime although in vitro tests indicate that the causative organism is susceptible to the drug, the presence of undrained abscesses or vascular infections should be suspected. The possibility that the organism may be tolerant to cefotaxime should also be considered. (See Resistance.) Use of cefotaxime does not replace surgical procedures such as incision and drainage when indicated.

■ **Gram-positive Aerobic Bacterial Infections** Cefotaxime is used in the treatment of lower respiratory tract infections caused by susceptible *Streptococcus pneumoniae, S. pyogenes* (group A β-hemolytic streptococci), other streptococci (except enterococci), or *Staphylococcus aureus* (penicillinase-producing and nonpenicillinase-producing strains); genitourinary tract infections caused by susceptible *S. aureus, S. epidermidis*, or enterococci; gynecologic infections caused by susceptible *S. epidermidis* or streptococci (including enterococci); skin and skin structure infections caused by susceptible *S. aureus, S. epidermidis*, group A β-hemolytic streptococci, or other streptococci (including enterococci); intra-abdominal infections caused by susceptible streptococci; or bone and joint infections caused by susceptible *S. aureus*, group A β-hemolytic streptococci, or other streptococci. Cefotaxime generally should not be used in the treatment of infections caused by gram-positive bacteria when a penicillin or a first generation cephalosporin could be used. Although cefotaxime has been effective in the treatment of cellulitis, wound infections, septicemia, and lower respiratory tract infections caused by susceptible staphylococci or streptococci, treatment failures have been reported when the drug was used in the treatment of osteomyelitis caused by *S. aureus*.

■ **Gram-negative Aerobic Bacterial Infections** Cefotaxime is used in the treatment of lower respiratory tract infections caused by susceptible *Escherichia coli, Klebsiella, Haemophilus influenzae* (including ampicillin-resistant strains), *H. parainfluenzae, Proteus mirabilis*, indole-positive *Proteus, Serratia marcescens*, or *Enterobacter*; genitourinary tract infections caused by susceptible *Citrobacter, Enterobacter, E. coli, Klebsiella, P. mirabilis, Providencia stuartii* (formerly group B *Proteus inconstans*), *Pseudomonas, Morganella morganii, Providencia rettgeri, P. vulgaris, S. marcescens*, or *Neisseria gonorrhoeae*; intra-abdominal and gynecologic infections caused by susceptible *E. coli, Enterobacter, Klebsiella*, or *P. mirabilis*; bacteremia or septicemia caused by susceptible *E. coli, Klebsiella*, or *S. marcescens*; skin and skin structure infections caused by susceptible *E. coli, Enterobacter, Klebsiella, P. mirabilis, M. morganii, P. rettgeri, P. vulgaris, Pseudomonas*, or *S. marcescens*; or bone and joint infections caused by susceptible *P. mirabilis*.

It has been suggested that certain parenteral cephalosporins (i.e., cefepime, cefotaxime, ceftriaxone, ceftazidime) may be drugs of choice for the treatment of many infections caused by susceptible Enterobacteriaceae, including susceptible *E. coli, K. pneumoniae, P. rettgeri, M. morganii, P. vulgaris, P. stuartii*, or *Serratia*; an aminoglycoside (amikacin, gentamicin, tobramycin) usually is used concomitantly in severe infections.

Although cefotaxime has been effective when used in the treatment of infections caused by susceptible *Ps. aeruginosa*, other anti-infectives generally are preferred for the treatment of pseudomonal infections. Because most strains of *Ps. aeruginosa* require high concentrations of the drug for in vitro inhibition and resistant strains have developed during cefotaxime therapy, an aminoglycoside should be used concomitantly if cefotaxime is used in any infection where *Ps. aeruginosa* may be present.

■ **Anaerobic and Mixed Aerobic-Anaerobic Bacterial Infections** Cefotaxime has been used in the treatment of skin and skin structure infections, intra-abdominal infections, or gynecologic infections caused by susceptible *Bacteroides* (including *B. fragilis*), *Clostridium, Fusobacterium* (including *F. nucleatum*), or anaerobic gram-positive cocci (including *Peptococcus* and *Pep-*

tostreptococcus); however, cefotaxime is not considered a drug of choice for these infections. Cefotaxime has been effective when used in the treatment of mixed aerobic-anaerobic infections, including intra-abdominal and gynecologic infections (see Uses: Pelvic Inflammatory Disease). Because many strains of *B. fragilis*are resistant to cefotaxime, some clinicians recommend that cefotaxime *not* be used alone for the treatment of serious intra-abdominal infections when *B. fragilis* may be present.

■ **Meningitis and Other CNS Infections** Cefotaxime is used in neonates, children, or adults for the treatment of meningitis and ventriculitis caused by susceptible *H. influenzae*, *N. meningitidis*, or *S. pneumoniae*. The drug also has been used for the treatment of meningitis and other CNS infections caused by susceptible Enterobacteriaceae† (e.g., *Escherichia coli*, *Klebsiella pneumoniae*). Cefotaxime is ineffective in and should not be used alone for empiric treatment of meningitis when *Listeria monocytogenes*, enterococci, staphylococci, or *Pseudomonas aeruginosa* may be involved.

Empiric Treatment of Meningitis Pending results of CSF culture and in vitro susceptibility testing, the most appropriate anti-infective regimen for empiric treatment of suspected bacterial meningitis should be selected based on results of CSF Gram stain and antigen tests, age of the patient, the most likely pathogen(s) and source of infection, and current patterns of bacterial resistance within the hospital and local community. When results of culture and susceptibility tests become available and the pathogen is identified, the empiric anti-infective regimen should be modified (if necessary) to ensure that the most effective regimen is being administered. There is some evidence that short-term adjunctive therapy with IV dexamethasone may decrease the incidence of audiologic and/or neurologic sequelae in infants and children with *H. influenzae* meningitis and possibly may provide some benefit in patients with *S. pneumoniae* meningitis. The American Academy of Pediatrics (AAP) and other clinicians suggest that use of adjunctive dexamethasone therapy may be considered during the initial 2–4 days of anti-infective therapy in infants and children 6–8 weeks of age or older with known or suspected bacterial meningitis, especially in those with suspected or proven *H. influenzae* infection. If used, dexamethasone should be initiated before or concurrently with the first dose of anti-infective. (See Uses: Bacterial Meningitis in the Corticosteroids General Statement 68:04 and see Dexamethasone 68:04.)

Bacterial meningitis in neonates usually is caused by *S. agalactiae* (group B streptococci), *L. monocytogenes*, or aerobic gram-negative bacilli (e.g., *E. coli*, *K. pneumoniae*). The AAP and other clinicians recommend that neonates 4 weeks of age or younger with suspected bacterial meningitis receive an empiric regimen of IV ampicillin and an aminoglycoside pending results of CSF culture and susceptibility testing. Alternatively, neonates can receive an empiric regimen of IV ampicillin and IV cefotaxime or IV ceftazidime (with or without gentamicin). Because frequent use of cephalosporins in neonatal units may result in rapid emergence of resistant strains of some gram-negative bacilli (e.g., *Enterobacter cloacae*, *Klebsiella*, *Serratia*), the AAP cautions that cephalosporins should be used for empiric treatment of meningitis in neonates only if gram-negative bacterial meningitis is strongly suspected. Consideration should be given to including IV vancomycin in the initial empiric regimen if *S. pneumoniae*, enterococci, or staphylococci is suspected. Because ceftriaxone should be used with caution in neonates who are hyperbilirubinemic (especially those born prematurely), cefotaxime may be the preferred cephalosporin in neonates. Alternatively, because premature, low-birthweight neonates are at increased risk for nosocomial infection caused by staphylococci or gram-negative bacilli, some clinicians suggest that these neonates receive an empiric regimen of IV ceftazidime and IV vancomycin.

In infants beyond the neonatal stage who are younger than 3 months of age, bacterial meningitis may be caused by *S. agalactiae*, *L. monocytogenes*, *Haemophilus influenzae*, *S. pneumoniae*, *N. meningitidis*, or aerobic gram-negative bacilli (e.g., *E. coli*, *K. pneumoniae*). An empiric regimen recommended for infants in this age group is IV ampicillin and either IV cefotaxime or IV ceftriaxone. Because of the increased prevalence of *S. pneumoniae* resistant to penicillin, cefotaxime, and ceftriaxone, the initial empiric regimen in children 1 month of age or older should include vancomycin and either cefotaxime or ceftriaxone if meningitis is known or suspected to be caused by *S. pneumoniae*.

In children 3 months through 17 years of age, bacterial meningitis usually is caused by *N. meningitidis*, *S. pneumoniae*, or *H. influenzae*, and the most common cause of bacterial meningitis in adults 18–50 years of age is *N. meningitidis* or *S. pneumoniae*. Most clinicians recommend that children 3 months through 17 years of age and adults 18–50 years of age receive IV cefotaxime or IV ceftriaxone for empiric therapy of suspected bacterial meningitis; an alternative regimen in children 3 months through 17 years of age is IV ampicillin and IV chloramphenicol. In addition, because of the increasing incidence of penicillin-resistant *S. pneumoniae* with reduced susceptibility to cephalosporins, the AAP and others suggest that the initial empiric regimen include IV vancomycin (with or without rifampin) pending results of in vitro susceptibility tests; vancomycin and rifampin should be discontinued if the causative organism is found to be susceptible to cephalosporins.. The US Centers for Disease Control and Prevention (CDC) and some clinicians have recommended that vancomycin be added to the empiric regimen in areas where there have been reports of highly penicillin-resistant strains of *S. pneumoniae*, but other clinicians suggest that use of cefotaxime or ceftriaxone in conjunction with vancomycin provides the optimal initial empiric regimen. While *L. monocytogenes* meningitis is relatively rare in this age group, the empiric regimen should include ampicillin if *L. monocytogenes* is suspected.

In adults older than 50 years of age, bacterial meningitis usually is caused by *S. pneumoniae*, *L. monocytogenes*, *N. meningitidis*, or aerobic gram-negative bacilli, and the empiric regimen recommended for this age group is IV ampicillin given in conjunction with IV cefotaxime or IV ceftriaxone. If *S. pneumoniae* is suspected, the empiric regimen also should include IV vancomycin (with or without rifampin); vancomycin and rifampin should be discontinued if the causative organism is found to be susceptible to the cephalosporin.

Meningitis Caused by Streptococcus pneumoniae IV cefotaxime and IV ceftriaxone are considered drugs of choice for the treatment of meningitis caused by *S. pneumoniae*. While cefotaxime and ceftriaxone generally have been considered the drugs of choice for the treatment of meningitis caused by penicillin-resistant *S. pneumoniae*, treatment failures have been reported when the drugs were used alone for the treatment of meningitis caused by strains of *S. pneumoniae* with intermediate or high-level penicillin resistance (i.e., penicillin MIC 0.1 mcg/mL or greater). In addition, strains of *S. pneumoniae* with reduced susceptibility to cephalosporins have been reported with increasing frequency, and use of cefotaxime or ceftriaxone alone may be ineffective for the treatment of meningitis caused by these strains. The prevalence of *S. pneumoniae* with reduced susceptibility to penicillin and/or cephalosporins varies geographically, and clinicians should be aware of the prevalence and pattern of *S. pneumoniae* drug resistance in the local community to optimize empiric regimens and initial therapy for serious pneumococcal infections. Because susceptibility can no longer be assumed, *S. pneumoniae* isolates should be routinely tested for in vitro susceptibility.

If anti-infective therapy in a patient with meningitis is initiated with an empiric regimen of IV cefotaxime and IV vancomycin (with or without rifampin) and results of culture and in vitro susceptibility testing indicate that the pathogen involved is a strain of *S. pneumoniae* susceptible to cefotaxime and susceptible or resistant to penicillin, vancomycin can be discontinued and therapy completed using cefotaxime alone. If the isolate is found to have reduced susceptibility to cefotaxime *and* penicillin, both IV cefotaxime and IV vancomycin (with or without rifampin) usually are continued. If the patient's condition does not improve or worsens or results of a second repeat lumber puncture (performed 24–36 hours after initiation of anti-infective therapy) indicate that the anti-infective regimen has not eradicated or reduced the number of pneumococci in CSF, rifampin probably should be added to the regimen or vancomycin discontinued and replaced with rifampin. If meningitis is caused by *S. pneumoniae* highly resistant to cefotaxime (i.e., MIC 2–4 mcg/mL or greater), consultation with an infectious disease expert is recommended.

Meningitis Caused by Haemophilus influenzae IV cefotaxime and IV ceftriaxone are considered drugs of choice for the treatment of meningitis caused by susceptible *H. influenzae* (including penicillinase-producing strains). The AAP suggests that children with meningitis possibly caused by *H. influenzae* receive an initial treatment regimen of cefotaxime, ceftriaxone, or a regimen of ampicillin given in conjunction with chloramphenicol; some clinicians prefer cefotaxime or ceftriaxone for the initial treatment of meningitis caused by *H. influenzae* since the drugs are active against both β-lactamase-producing and non-β-lactamase-producing strains. The incidence of *H. influenzae* meningitis in the US has decreased considerably since *H. influenzae* type b conjugate vaccines became available for immunization of infants.

Meningitis Caused by Neisseria meningitidis Although IV penicillin G or ampicillin generally are considered the drugs of choice for the treatment of meningitis caused by *N. meningitidis*, IV cefotaxime and IV ceftriaxone are acceptable alternatives.

Meningitis Caused by Enterobacteriaceae Some clinicians recommend that meningitis caused by Enterobacteriaceae (e.g., *E. coli*, *K. pneumoniae*) be treated with a third generation cephalosporins (i.e., cefotaxime, ceftazidime, ceftriaxone) with or without an aminoglycoside. Because ceftazidime or cefepime (but not cefotaxime or ceftriaxone) is effective for the treatment of meningitis caused by *Ps. aeruginosa*, some clinicians suggest that a regimen of ceftazidime or cefepime (with or without an aminoglycoside) may be preferred for the treatment of meningitis caused by gram-negative bacilli pending results of culture and susceptibility testing.

Brain Abscess and Other CNS Infections IV cefotaxime has been effective when used in conjunction with metronidazole for empiric treatment of brain abscess in patients 6 months of age or older. Bacterial brain abscesses and other CNS infections (e.g., subdural empyema, intracranial epidural abscesses) often are polymicrobial and can be caused by gram-positive aerobic cocci, Enterobacteriaceae (e.g., *E. coli*, *Haemophilus*, *Klebsiella*), and/or anaerobic bacteria (e.g., *Bacteroides*, *Fusobacterium*).

The choice of anti-infectives for empiric therapy of these infections should be based on the predisposing condition and site of primary infection. Some clinicians suggest that the empiric anti-infective regimen in patients who develop the CNS infections after respiratory tract infection (e.g., otitis media, mastoiditis, paranasal sinusitis, pyogenic lung disease) should consist of an appropriate IV third generation cephalosporin (e.g., cefotaxime) given in conjunction with metronidazole, employing the cephalosporin rather than a penicillin to extend coverage to *Haemophilus* and facultative anaerobic gram-negative bacteria; if presence of staphylococci is suspected, a penicillinase-resistant penicillin (e.g., nafcillin, oxacillin) or vancomycin should be added to the empiric regimen. In patients who develop brain abscess, subdural empyema, or intracranial epidural abscess after trauma or neurosurgery, the empiric regimen should consist of an appropriate IV third generation cephalosporin (e.g., cefotaxime) given in conjunction with a penicillinase-resistant penicillin or vancomycin. Prolonged anti-infective therapy (e.g., 3–6 weeks or longer) usually is required for these CNS infections.

■ **Gonorrhea and Associated Infections** ***Gonococcal Infections in Adults and Adolescents*** **Uncomplicated Gonorrhea.** Cefotaxime has been used for the treatment of uncomplicated cervical, urethral, or rectal gonorrhea caused by susceptible *Neisseria gonorrhoeae*, including penicillinase-producing *N. gonorrhoeae* (PPNG) in adults and adolescents.

For the treatment of uncomplicated urogenital, anorectal, or pharyngeal gonorrhea, the CDC states that a combination regimen that includes a single 250-mg IM dose of ceftriaxone *and* either oral azithromycin (single 1-g dose) or oral doxycycline (100 mg twice daily for 7 days) is the regimen of choice. Although a single 500-mg dose of IM cefotaxime may be effective for the treatment of uncomplicated urogenital and anorectal gonorrhea, the CDC states that the drug does not offer any advantages over IM ceftriaxone for urogenital infections and its efficacy for pharyngeal infections is less certain.

Disseminated Gonococcal Infections. IV cefotaxime has been used for *initial* treatment of disseminated gonococcal infections† in adults and adolescents.

The CDC recommends that treatment of disseminated gonococcal infections in adults and adolescents be initiated with a multiple-dose regimen of IM or IV ceftriaxone; a multiple-dose regimen of IV cefotaxime is considered an alternative. The initial parenteral regimen should be continued for 24–48 hours after improvement begins; therapy can then be switched to oral cefixime and continued to complete at least 1 week of treatment.

The CDC recommends that the patient be hospitalized for initial treatment, especially when compliance may be a problem, when the diagnosis is uncertain, or when the patient has purulent synovial effusions or other complications. Patients should be examined for clinical evidence of endocarditis and meningitis; the recommended regimen for these infections is IV ceftriaxone.

Gonococcal Infections in Neonates and Infants Cefotaxime is used for the treatment of *N. gonorrhoeae* infections in neonates, including disseminated gonococcal infections and gonococcal scalp abscesses†. The CDC states that IV or IM ceftriaxone or IV or IM cefotaxime are the drugs of choice for these infections in neonates; the AAP states that cefotaxime is preferred in neonates with hyperbilirubinemia. IV or IM ceftriaxone is the drug of choice for the treatment of nondisseminated gonococcal infections in neonates, including gonococcal ophthalmia (ophthalmia neonatorum), and also is the drug of choice for disseminated gonococcal infections (e.g., sepsis, arthritis, meningitis) in children.

Gonococcal infections in neonates usually occur as the result of exposure to the mother's infected cervical exudate and are apparent 2–5 days after birth. The most serious manifestations of *N. gonorrhoeae* infection in neonates are ophthalmia neonatorum and sepsis, arthritis, and meningitis; less serious manifestations include rhinitis, vaginitis, urethritis, and inflammation at sites of fetal monitoring (e.g., scalp). Because a neonate with gonococcal infection usually has acquired the organism from its mother, both the mother and her sexual partner(s) should be evaluated and treated for gonorrhea.

While universal *topical prophylaxis* using 0.5% erythromycin ophthalmic ointment, silver nitrate 1% topical solution (no longer commercially available in the US), or 1% tetracycline ophthalmic ointment (no longer commercially available in the US) is recommended for *all* neonates as soon as possible after birth to prevent gonococcal ophthalmia neonatorum, these topical anti-infectives are inadequate for prophylaxis of gonococcal infections at other sites, and may be ineffective in preventing chlamydial ocular infections. Because neonates born to mothers with untreated gonorrhea are at high risk of infection with *N. gonorrhoeae*, the CDC and AAP recommend that, in addition to *topical prophylaxis*, these neonates should receive *parenteral prophylaxis* against the disease. The CDC and AAP currently recommend that neonates born to mothers with documented peripartum gonococcal infection receive *parenteral prophylaxis* with a single IM or IV dose of ceftriaxone (25–50 mg/kg not to exceed 125 mg).

For additional information on current recommendations for the treatment of gonorrhea and associated infections, see Uses: Gonorrhea and Associated Infections, in Ceftriaxone 8:12.06.12.

■ **GI Infections** Cefotaxime is used for empiric treatment of infectious diarrhea†. For empiric treatment of severe diarrhea in HIV-infected individuals, the CDC, National Institutes of Health (NIH), and Infectious Diseases Society of America (IDSA) state that ciprofloxacin is the drug of choice and ceftriaxone and cefotaxime are reasonable alternatives. (For information on *Salmonella* gastroenteritis, see Salmonella Gastroenteritis under Uses: Typhoid Fever and Other Salmonella Infections.)

Yersinia Infections Although GI infections caused by *Yersinia enterocolitica* or *Y. pseudotuberculosis* usually are self-limited and anti-infective therapy unnecessary, the AAP, IDSA, and others recommend use of anti-infectives in immunocompromised individuals or for the treatment of severe infections or when septicemia or other invasive disease occurs. GI infections caused by *Y. enterocolitica* or *Y. pseudotuberculosis* can occur as the result of ingesting undercooked pork, unpasteurized milk, or contaminated water; infection has occurred in infants whose caregivers handled contaminated chitterlings (raw pork intestines) or tofu. Use of co-trimoxazole, an aminoglycoside (e.g., amikacin, gentamicin, tobramycin), a fluoroquinolone (e.g., ciprofloxacin), doxycycline, or cefotaxime has been recommended when treatment is considered necessary; combination therapy may be necessary. Some clinicians suggest that, while cefotaxime may be effective in the treatment of *Y. enterocolitica* bacteremia, the role of anti-infectives, including oral anti-infectives, in the management of enterocolitis, pseudoappendicitis syndrome, or mesenteric adenitis caused by *Yersinia* needs further evaluation.

■ **Lyme Disease** Cefotaxime is used in the treatment of Lyme disease†. The IDSA and other clinicians recommend IV cefotaxime as a preferred alternative to IV ceftriaxone for the treatment of early neurologic Lyme disease† with acute neurologic manifestations such as meningitis or radiculopathy, Lyme carditis†, Lyme arthritis†, and late neurologic Lyme disease†.

Lyme disease is a tick-borne spirochetal disease. In the US, Lyme disease is caused by the spirochete *Borrelia burgdorferi*, which is transmitted by the bite of *Ixodes scapularis* or *I. pacificus* ticks. For additional information on Lyme disease, see Lyme Disease in Uses: Spirochetal Infections, in the Tetracyclines General Statement 8:12.24.

Early Lyme Disease **Early Neurologic Lyme Disease.** Although oral anti-infectives (doxycycline, amoxicillin, cefuroxime axetil) generally are effective for the treatment of the early localized or early disseminated Lyme disease associated with erythema migrans, in the absence of specific neurologic manifestations or advanced atrioventricular (AV) heart block, parenteral anti-infectives are recommended for the treatment of early Lyme disease when there are acute neurologic manifestations such as meningitis or radiculoneuritis.

The IDSA and other clinicians recommend a 14-day regimen (range: 10–28 days) of IV ceftriaxone as the preferred parenteral regimen for the treatment of acute neurologic Lyme disease manifested by meningitis or radiculopathy; IV cefotaxime and IV penicillin G sodium are the preferred alternatives. In patients with acute neurologic manifestations who are intolerant of cephalosporins and penicillin, there is some evidence that oral doxycycline may be an adequate alternative that can be considered for use in adults and children 8 years of age or older.

Although IV cefotaxime appears to be as effective as IV ceftriaxone for the treatment of acute neurologic Lyme disease and does not cause the biliary complications reported with ceftriaxone, ceftriaxone has the advantage of once-daily dosing. Limited data suggest that IV cefotaxime (6 g daily in divided doses for 10 days) is at least as effective as IV penicillin G (20 million units daily for 10 days) in patients with late complications of Lyme disease (e.g., severe radiculitis and/or meningitis, peripheral neuropathy, arthritis).

Lyme Carditis. Cefotaxime is used as an alternative to ceftriaxone when a parenteral regimen is indicated for the treatment of Lyme carditis†. The IDSA states that patients with AV heart block and/or myopericarditis associated with early Lyme disease may be treated with a 14-day regimen (range: 14–21 days) of oral or parenteral anti-infectives. Although there is no evidence to date to suggest that a parenteral regimen is more effective than an oral regimen for the treatment of Lyme carditis, a parenteral regimen usually is recommended for initial treatment of hospitalized patients; an oral regimen can be used to complete therapy and for the treatment of outpatients. When a parenteral regimen is used, IV ceftriaxone or, alternatively, IV cefotaxime or IV penicillin G sodium is recommended. When an oral regimen is used, oral doxycycline, oral amoxicillin, or oral cefuroxime axetil is recommended.

Because of the potential for life-threatening complications, hospitalization and continuous monitoring is advisable for patients who are symptomatic (syncope, dyspnea, chest pain) and also is recommended for those with second- or third-degree AV block or first-degree heart block when the PR interval is prolonged to 0.3 seconds or longer. Patients with advanced heart block may require a temporary pacemaker and consultation with a cardiologist is recommended.

Late Lyme Disease **Lyme Arthritis.** Cefotaxime is used as an alternative to ceftriaxone when a parenteral regimen is indicated for the treatment of Lyme arthritis†. While patients with uncomplicated Lyme arthritis without clinical evidence of neurologic disease generally can be treated with a 28-day regimen of oral anti-infectives (doxycycline, amoxicillin, cefuroxime axetil), the IDSA and other clinicians state that patients with Lyme arthritis and concomitant neurologic disease should receive a 14-day parenteral regimen (range: 14–28 days) of IV ceftriaxone or, alternatively, IV cefotaxime or IV penicillin G. While oral regimens are easier to administer, associated with fewer serious adverse effects, and less expensive than IV regimens, some patients with Lyme arthritis treated with oral anti-infectives have subsequently developed overt neuroborreliosis, which may require IV therapy for successful resolution. Therefore, additional study is needed to fully evaluate the comparative safety and efficacy of oral versus IV anti-infectives for the treatment of Lyme arthritis.

In patients who have persistent or recurrent joint swelling after a recommended oral regimen, the IDSA and other clinicians recommend retreatment with the oral regimen or a switch to a parenteral regimen. Some clinicians prefer retreatment with an oral regimen for patients whose arthritis substantively improved but did not completely resolve; these clinicians reserve parenteral regimens for those patients whose arthritis failed to improve or worsened. It has been suggested that clinicians should consider allowing several months for joint inflammation to resolve after initial treatment before an additional course of anti-infectives is given.

Late Neurologic Lyme Disease. Cefotaxime is used as an alternative to ceftriaxone for the treatment of late neurologic Lyme disease†. The IDSA and other clinicians state that patients with late neurologic Lyme disease affecting the CNS or peripheral nervous system (e.g., encephalopathy, neuropathy) should receive a 14-day regimen (range: 14–28 days) of IV ceftriaxone or, alternatively, IV cefotaxime or IV penicillin G sodium. Response to anti-infective treatment usually is slow and may be incomplete in patients with late neurologic Lyme disease. The IDSA states that retreatment is not recommended unless relapse is shown by reliable objective measures.

■ Pelvic Inflammatory Disease Cefotaxime has been used for the treatment of pelvic inflammatory disease (PID). Because cefotaxime (like other cephalosporins) has no activity against *Chlamydia trachomatis*, it should be given in conjunction with an anti-infective active against this organism (e.g., doxycycline) whenever it is used in the treatment of PID.

PID is an acute or chronic inflammatory disorder in the upper female genital tract and can include any combination of endometritis, salpingitis, tubo-ovarian abscess, and pelvic peritonitis. PID generally is a polymicrobial infection most frequently caused by *N. gonorrhoeae* and/or *Chlamydia trachomatis*; however, organisms that are part of the normal vaginal flora (e.g., anaerobic bacteria, *Gardnerella vaginalis*, *H. influenzae*, enteric gram-negative bacilli, *S. agalactiae*) or mycoplasma (e.g., *Mycoplasma hominis*, *Ureaplasma urealyticum*) also may be involved. PID is treated with an empiric regimen that provides broad-spectrum coverage. The regimen should be effective against *N. gonorrhoeae* and *C. trachomatis* and also probably should be effective against anaerobes, gram-negative facultative bacteria, and streptococci. The optimum empiric regimen for the treatment of PID has not been identified. A wide variety of parenteral and oral regimens have been shown to achieve clinical and microbiologic cure in randomized studies with short-term follow-up; however, only limited data are available to date regarding elimination of infection in the endometrium and fallopian tubes or intermediate or long-term outcomes, including the impact of these regimens on the incidence of long-term sequelae of PID (e.g., tubal infertility, ectopic pregnancy, pain).

When a parenteral regimen is indicated for the treatment of PID, the CDC recommends a 2-drug regimen of cefoxitin (2 g IV every 6 hours) or cefotetan (2 g IV every 12 hours) given in conjunction with doxycycline (100 mg IV or orally every 12 hours) or a 2-drug regimen of clindamycin (900 mg IV every 8 hours) and gentamicin (usually a 2-mg/kg IV or IM loading dose followed by 1.5 mg/kg every 8 hours). While there is some evidence that other parenteral cephalosporins (e.g., cefotaxime, ceftriaxone) may be effective for the treatment of PID, the CDC states that these drugs are less active than cefoxitin or cefotetan against anaerobic bacteria.

When an oral regimen is used for the outpatient treatment of mild to moderately severe acute PID, the CDC recommends a regimen that consists of a single IM dose of ceftriaxone, cefoxitin (with oral probenecid), or cefotaxime given with oral doxycycline (with or without oral metronidazole). The optimal cephalosporin for the regimen is unclear, although cefoxitin has better anaerobic coverage and ceftriaxone has better coverage against *N. gonorrhoeae*.

For additional information on treatment of PID, including information on follow-up and management of sexual partners, see Uses: Pelvic Inflammatory Disease, in the Cephalosporins General Statement 8:12.06.

■ Respiratory Tract Infections ***Community-acquired Pneumonia*** Cefotaxime is used for the treatment of community-acquired pneumonia (CAP). The American Thoracic Society (ATS) and IDSA recommend cefotaxime as an alternative to penicillin G or amoxicillin for treatment of community-acquired pneumonia (CAP) caused by penicillin-susceptible *S. pneumoniae* and as a preferred drug for treatment of CAP caused by penicillin-resistant *S. pneumoniae*, provided in vitro susceptibility has been demonstrated. IDSA and ATS also recommend use of cefotaxime in certain combination regimens used for empiric treatment of CAP.

Initial treatment of CAP generally involves use of an empiric anti-infective regimen based on the most likely pathogens and local susceptibility patterns; therapy may then be changed (if possible) to provide a more specific regimen (pathogen-directed therapy) based on results of in vitro culture and susceptibility testing. The most appropriate empiric regimen varies depending on the severity of illness at the time of presentation and whether outpatient treatment or hospitalization in or out of an intensive care unit (ICU) is indicated and the presence or absence of cardiopulmonary disease and other modifying factors that increase the risk of certain pathogens (e.g., penicillin- or multidrug-resistant *S. pneumoniae*, enteric gram-negative bacilli, *Ps. aeruginosa*).

Most experts recommend that an empiric regimen for treatment of CAP include an anti-infective active against *S. pneumoniae* since this organism is the most commonly identified cause of bacterial pneumonia and causes more severe disease than many other common CAP pathogens. Pathogens most frequently involved in *outpatient* CAP include *S. pneumoniae*, *M. pneumoniae*, *Chlamydophila pneumoniae* (formerly *Chlamydia pneumoniae*), respiratory viruses, and *H. influenzae*. Pathogens most frequently involved in *inpatient* CAP in non-ICU patients are *S. pneumoniae*, *M. pneumoniae*, *C. pneumoniae*, *H. influenzae*, *Legionella*, and respiratory viruses. Patients with severe CAP admitted into the ICU usually have infections caused by *S. pneumoniae*, *S. aureus*, *Legionella*, gram-negative bacilli, or *H. influenzae*. Coverage against anaerobic bacteria usually is indicated only in classic aspiration pleuropulmonary syndrome in patients who had loss of consciousness as a result of alcohol or drug overdosage after seizures in patients with concomitant gingival disease or esophageal motility disorders.

Inpatient treatment of CAP is initiated with a parenteral regimen, although therapy may be changed to an oral regimen if the patient is improving clinically, is hemodynamically stable, able to ingest drugs, and has a normally functioning GI tract. CAP patients usually have a clinical response within 3–7 days after initiation of therapy and a switch to oral therapy generally can be made during this period.

For empiric *inpatient* treatment of CAP in non-ICU patients, IDSA and ATS recommend monotherapy with a fluoroquinolone (moxifloxacin, gemifloxacin, levofloxacin) or, alternatively, a combination regimen that includes a *β*-lactam (usually cefotaxime, ceftriaxone, or ampicillin) given in conjunction with a macrolide (azithromycin, clarithromycin, erythromycin). For empiric *inpatient* treatment of CAP in ICU patients when *Pseudomonas* and oxacillin-resistant (methicillin-resistant) *S. aureus* are *not* suspected, IDSA and ATS recommend a combination regimen that includes a *β*-lactam (cefotaxime, ceftriaxone, fixed combination of ampicillin and sulbactam) given in conjunction with either azithromycin or fluoroquinolone (gemifloxacin, levofloxacin, moxifloxacin).

For additional information on treatment of CAP, see Community-acquired Pneumonia under Uses: Respiratory Tract Infections, in the Cephalosporins General Statement 8:12.06.

■ Septicemia Cefotaxime is used for the treatment of bacteremia/septicemia caused by *E. coli*, *Klebsiella*, *S. marcescens*, *S. aureus*, and streptococci (including *S. pneumoniae*).

The choice of anti-infective agent for the treatment of sepsis syndrome should be based on the probable source of infection, causative organism, immune status of the patient, and local patterns of bacterial resistance. For initial treatment of life-threatening sepsis in adults, some clinicians recommend that a third or fourth generation cephalosporin (cefepime, cefotaxime, ceftriaxone, ceftazidime), the fixed combination of piperacillin and tazobactam, or a carbapenem (doripenem, imipenem, meropenem) be used in conjunction with vancomycin; some experts also suggest including an aminoglycoside or fluoroquinolone during the initial few days of treatment.

■ Typhoid Fever and Other Salmonella Infections ***Typhoid Fever*** Cefotaxime has been used in adults or children for the treatment of typhoid fever† (enteric fever) or septicemia caused by *Salmonella typhi*† or *S. paratyphi*†, including multidrug-resistant strains. Multidrug-resistant strains of *S. typhi* (i.e., strains resistant to ampicillin, chloramphenicol, and/or co-trimoxazole) have been reported with increasing frequency, and third generation cephalosporins (e.g., cefotaxime, ceftriaxone) and fluoroquinolones (e.g., ciprofloxacin, ofloxacin) are considered the agents of first choice for the treatment of typhoid fever or other severe infections known or suspected to be caused by these strains.

Cefotaxime also has been used in the treatment of infections caused by nontyphi *Salmonella*, including bacteremia, osteomyelitis, and meningitis caused by *S. typhimurium*.

Salmonella Gastroenteritis Anti-infective therapy generally is not indicated in otherwise healthy individuals with uncomplicated (noninvasive) gastroenteritis caused by non-typhi *Salmonella* (e.g., *S. enteritidis*, *S. typhimurium*) since such therapy may prolong the duration of fecal excretion of the organism and there is no evidence that it shortens the duration of the disease; however, the CDC, AAP, IDSA, and others recommend anti-infective therapy in individuals with severe *Salmonella* gastroenteritis and in those who are at increased risk of invasive disease. These individuals at increased risk include infants younger than 3–6 months of age; individuals older than 50 years of age; individuals with hemoglobinopathies, severe atherosclerosis or valvular heart disease, prostheses, uremia, chronic GI disease, or severe colitis; and individuals who are immunocompromised because of malignancy, immunosuppressive therapy, HIV infection, or other immunosuppressive illness.

When an anti-infective agent is considered necessary in an individual with *Salmonella* gastroenteritis, the CDC, AAP, IDSA, and others recommend use of ceftriaxone, cefotaxime, a fluoroquinolone (should be used in children only if the benefits outweigh the risks and no alternative exists), ampicillin, amoxicillin, co-trimoxazole, or chloramphenicol, depending on the susceptibility of the causative organism.

HIV-Infected Individuals Because HIV-infected individuals with *Salmonella* gastroenteritis† are at high risk for bacteremia, the CDC, NIH, and IDSA recommend that such patients receive anti-infective treatment. These experts state that the initial drug of choice for the treatment of *Salmonella* gastroenteritis (with or without bacteremia) in HIV-infected adults is ciprofloxacin; other fluoroquinolones (levofloxacin, moxifloxacin) also are likely to be effective, but clinical data are limited. Depending on results of in vitro susceptibility testing of the causative organism, alternatives for treatment of *Salmonella* gastroenteritis in HIV-infected adults are co-trimoxazole or third generation cephalosporins (ceftriaxone, cefotaxime).

HIV-infected individuals who have been treated for *Salmonella* bacteremia should be monitored for recurrence. The CDC, NIH, and IDSA state that long-term maintenance anti-infective therapy (secondary prophylaxis) to prevent recurrence should be considered for those with recurrent *Salmonella* bacteremia and also may be considered for those with recurrent gastroenteritis (with or without bacteremia) or those who have $CD4^+$ T-cell counts less than 200 cells/mm^3 and severe diarrhea. However, the value of such prophylaxis has not been established and the possible benefits must be weighed against the risks of long-term anti-infective exposure.

■ Capnocytophaga Infections Based on results of in vitro susceptibility tests that indicate that *Capnocytophaga* generally are inhibited by cefotaxime, some clinicians suggest that cefotaxime can be used in the treatment of infections caused by *Capnocytophaga*†. *Capnocytophaga* is a gram-negative bacilli that can cause life-threatening septicemia, meningitis, and/or endocarditis and often is associated with disseminated intravascular coagulation; splenectomized and immunocompromised individuals are at particularly high risk for serious infections caused by the organism. *C. canimorsus* infection usually occurs as the result of a dog bite. The optimum regimen for the treatment of infections caused by *Capnocytophaga* has not been identified but some clinicians recommend use of penicillin G or, alternatively, a third generation cephalosporin (cefotaxime, ceftriaxone), a carbapenem (imipenem, meropenem), vancomycin, a fluoroquinolone, or clindamycin.

■ **Vibrio Infections** ***Vibrio parahaemolyticus Infections*** Cefotaxime is one of several alternatives recommended for the treatment of severe cases of *Vibrio parahaemolyticus*† infection when anti-infective therapy is indicated in addition to supportive care. *V. parahaemolyticus* infection is a relatively rare foodborne illness that can occur as the result of ingestion of undercooked or raw fish or shellfish; the incubation period usually is 2–48 hours. The signs and symptoms of *V. parahaemolyticus* infection are watery diarrhea, abdominal cramps, and nausea and vomiting lasting 2–5 days. Although supportive care usually is sufficient, some clinicians recommend use of tetracycline, doxycycline, gentamicin, or cefotaxime in severe cases.

Vibrio vulnificus Infections Some clinicians suggest that cefotaxime is a drug of choice for the treatment of infections caused by *V. vulnificus*†. *V. vulnificus* can cause potentially fatal septicemia, wound infections, or gastroenteritis and generally is transmitted through ingestion of contaminated raw or undercooked seafood (especially raw oysters) or through contamination of a wound with seawater or seafood drippings. *V. vulnificus* is naturally present in marine environments, thrives in warm ocean water, and frequently is isolated from oysters and other shellfish harvested from the Gulf of Mexico and from US coastal waters along the Pacific and Atlantic ocean. Individuals with preexisting liver disease are at high risk for developing fatal septicemia following ingestion of seafood contaminated with *V. vulnificus* and debilitated or immunocompromised individuals (e.g., those with chronic renal impairment, cancer, diabetes mellitus, steroid-dependent asthma, chronic GI disease) or individuals with iron overload states (e.g., thalassemia, hemochromatosis) also are at increased risk for fatal infections. The incubation period for *V. vulnificus* infection reportedly is 1–7 days and the duration of illness usually is 2–8 days. In immunocompromised individuals, fever, nausea, myalgia, and abdominal cramps may occur as soon as 24–48 hours after ingestion of seafood contaminated with *V. vulnificus* and sepsis and cutaneous bullae may be present within 36 hours of the onset of symptoms.

Because the case fatality rate for *V. vulnificus* septicemia exceeds 50% in immunocompromised individuals and those with preexisting liver disease, these individuals should be informed about the health hazards of ingesting raw or undercooked seafood (especially oysters), the need to avoid contact with seawater during the warm months, and the importance of using protective clothing (e.g., gloves) when handling shellfish. *V. vulnificus* infection should be considered in the differential diagnosis of fever of unknown etiology, and individuals who present with fever (especially when bullae, cellulitis, or wound infection is present) and who have preexisting liver disease or are immunocompromised should be questioned regarding a history of raw oyster ingestion or seawater contact. While optimum anti-infective therapy for the treatment of *V. vulnificus* infections has not been identified, use of a tetracycline or third generation cephalosporin (e.g., cefotaxime, ceftazidime) is recommended. Because of the high fatality rate associated with *V. vulnificus* infections, anti-infective therapy should be initiated promptly if indicated.

■ **Perioperative Prophylaxis** Cefotaxime has been used for perioperative prophylaxis in patients undergoing liver transplantation†, and some experts recommend cefotaxime in conjunction with ampicillin as a regimen of choice for such prophylaxis in patients undergoing this procedure.

Cefotaxime has been used perioperatively to reduce the incidence of infection in patients undergoing contaminated or potentially contaminated surgery, including biliary tract, colorectal, and other intra-abdominal or GI procedures (e.g., appendectomy), genitourinary surgery, or abdominal or vaginal hysterectomy, and in patients undergoing cesarean section. However, other anti-infectives (e.g., cefazolin) usually are recommended for perioperative prophylaxis in patients undergoing these procedures.

A first or second generation cephalosporin (cefazolin, cefoxitin, cefotetan, cefuroxime) generally is preferred when a cephalosporin is used for perioperative prophylaxis. Third generation cephalosporins (cefotaxime, ceftriaxone, ceftazidime) and fourth generation cephalosporins (cefepime) are not usually recommended for perioperative prophylaxis because they are expensive, some are less active than first or second generation cephalosporins against staphylococci, they have spectrums of activity wider than necessary for organisms encountered in elective surgery, and their use for prophylaxis may promote emergence of resistant organisms. (See Uses: Perioperative Prophylaxis in the Cephalosporins General Statement 8:12.06.)

Dosage and Administration

■ **Reconstitution and Administration** Cefotaxime sodium is administered IV or by deep IM injection. The drug should be given IV rather than IM in patients with septicemia, bacteremia, peritonitis, meningitis, or other severe or life-threatening infections or in patients with lowered resistance resulting from debilitating conditions (e.g., malnutrition, trauma, surgery, diabetes, heart failure, malignancy), particularly if shock is present.

Intermittent IV Injection For direct intermittent IV administration, 10 mL of sterile water for injection should be added to a vial labeled as containing 500 mg, 1 g, or 2 g of cefotaxime to provide a solution containing approximately 50, 95, or 180 mg of cefotaxime per mL, respectively. A solution of 1 g of cefotaxime per 14 mL of sterile water for injection is isotonic.

The appropriate dose may then be injected directly into a vein over a 3- to 5-minute period or slowly into the tubing of a freely flowing compatible IV solution. Cefotaxime should *not* be injected IV over less than 3 minutes since rapid (over less than 1 minute) injection was consistently associated with potentially life-threatening arrhythmias during postmarketing surveillance.

Intermittent or Continuous IV Infusion For intermittent or continuous IV infusion, 50 or 100 mL of 0.9% sodium chloride injection or 5% dextrose injection should be added to an infusion bottle labeled as containing 1 or 2 g of cefotaxime or, alternatively, reconstituted solutions of cefotaxime may be further diluted with 50 mL to 1 L of a compatible IV solution. ADD-Vantage® vials or infusion bottles labeled as containing 1 or 2 g of cefotaxime or the 10-g pharmacy bulk package of cefotaxime should be reconstituted according to the manufacturer's directions. The cefotaxime bulk package is *not* intended for direct IV infusion; doses of the drug from the reconstituted bulk package must be further diluted in a compatible IV infusion solution prior to administration.

Thawed solutions of the commercially available frozen premixed cefotaxime sodium injection should be administered only by intermittent or continuous IV infusion. The frozen injections should be thawed at room temperature or under refrigeration (5°C or lower); the injection should not be thawed by warming in a water bath or by exposure to microwave radiation. Precipitates that may have formed in the frozen injection usually will dissolve with little or no agitation when the injection reaches room temperature; potency is not affected. After thawing to room temperature, the injection should be agitated and the container checked for minute leaks by firmly squeezing the bag. The injection should be discarded if container seals or outlet ports are not intact or leaks are found or if the solution is cloudy or contains an insoluble precipitate. Additives should not be introduced into the injection container. The injection should not be used in series connections with other plastic containers, since such use could result in air embolism from residual air being drawn from the primary container before administration of fluid from the secondary container is complete.

Other IV solutions flowing through a common administration tubing or site should be discontinued while cefotaxime is being infused unless the solutions are known to be compatible and the flow-rate is adequately controlled.

Rate of Administration. Intermittent IV infusions of cefotaxime are generally infused over 20–30 minutes; solutions should preferably be infused via butterfly or scalp vein-type needles.

IM Injection IM injections of cefotaxime are prepared by adding 2, 3, or 5 mL of sterile or bacteriostatic water for injection to a vial labeled as containing 500 mg, 1 g, or 2 g of the drug. Resultant solutions contain approximately 230, 300, or 330 mg of cefotaxime per mL, respectively.

IM injections should be made deeply into a large muscle mass such as the upper outer quadrant of the gluteus maximus; aspiration should be performed to avoid inadvertent injection into a blood vessel. The manufacturers state that if an IM dose of 2 g of cefotaxime is indicated, the dose should be divided and administered at 2 different injection sites. However, because large IM doses of cefotaxime may be painful, some clinicians recommend that large doses of the drug be given IV.

■ **Dosage** Dosage of cefotaxime sodium is expressed in terms of cefotaxime and is identical for IM or IV administration.

Adult Dosage The usual adult dosage of cefotaxime for the treatment of uncomplicated infections is 1 g IM or IV every 12 hours. Moderate to severe infections usually respond to 1–2 g IM or IV every 8 hours, but some infections (e.g., septicemia) should be treated with 2 g IV every 6–8 hours. Severe or life-threatening infections may require 2 g IV every 4 hours.

The maximum adult dosage recommended by the manufacturers is 12 g daily.

Meningitis and Other CNS Infections. For the treatment of meningitis or other CNS infections caused by susceptible bacteria, the usual adult dosage of cefotaxime is 2 g IV every 6 hours for 7–21 days. Some clinicians recommend that adults receive 8–12 g daily in divided doses every 4–6 hours for the treatment of meningitis. Other clinicians recommend that patients with meningitis known or suspected to be caused by *S. pneumoniae* receive an initial cefotaxime dosage of 350 mg/kg daily given in 4 divided doses; if results of in vitro susceptibility testing indicate that the organism is susceptible to penicillin, dosage can be reduced to 225 mg/kg daily given in 3 divided doses.

While 7 days of cefotaxime therapy may be adequate for the treatment of uncomplicated meningitis caused by susceptible *Haemophilus influenzae* or *Neisseria meningitidis*, at least 10–14 days of therapy is recommended for complicated cases or meningitis caused by *Streptococcus pneumoniae* and at least 21 days of therapy is recommended for meningitis caused by susceptible Enterobacteriaceae (e.g., *Escherichia coli, Klebsiella*).

Gonorrhea and Associated Infections. For the treatment of uncomplicated urethral, cervical, or rectal gonorrhea caused by susceptible *N. gonorrhoeae*, adults and adolescents should receive a single 500-mg IM dose of cefotaxime. The manufacturers recommend a single 1-g IM dose for the treatment of rectal gonorrhea in males.

For the treatment of disseminated gonorrhea†, adults and adolescents should receive 1 g of cefotaxime IV every 8 hours. Parenteral cefotaxime should be continued for 24–48 hours after improvement begins; therapy can then be switched to oral cefixime to complete at least 1 week of therapy.

GI Infections. If cefotaxime is used as an alternative for empiric treatment of infectious diarrhea† in HIV-infected adults, the US Centers for Disease Control and Prevention (CDC), National Institutes of Health (NIH), and Infectious Diseases Society of America (IDSA) recommend a dosage of 1 g IV every 8 hours. If there is no clinical response after 5–7 days, stool culture and in vitro susceptibility testing should be considered.

If cefotaxime is used as an alternative for the treatment of *Salmonella* gastroenteritis† (with or without bacteremia) in HIV-infected adults, the CDC, NIH, and IDSA recommend a dosage of 1 g IV every 8 hours. The recommended duration of treatment is 7–14 days in those with $CD4^+$ T-cell counts of 200 cells/mm^3 or greater (14 days or longer if the patient is bacteremic or the infection is complicated) or 2–6 weeks in those with $CD4^+$ T-cell counts less than 200 cells/mm^3.

Lyme Disease. If cefotaxime is used for the treatment of early Lyme disease† in adults with acute neurologic disease manifested by meningitis or radiculopathy, the Infectious Diseases Society of America (IDSA) and other clinicians recommend a dosage of 2 g IV every 8 hours for 14 days (range: 10–28 days).

If cefotaxime is used when a parenteral regimen is indicated for the treatment of Lyme carditis† in patients with atrioventricular (AV) heart block and/or myopericarditis associated with early Lyme disease, the IDSA and other clinicians recommend a dosage of 2 g IV every 8 hours for 14 days (range: 14–21 days). Although a parenteral regimen is recommended for initial treatment of hospitalized patients, the parenteral regimen can be switched to an oral regimen (doxycycline, amoxicillin, cefuroxime axetil) to complete therapy and for outpatients.

If cefotaxime is used when a parenteral regimen is indicated for the treatment of Lyme arthritis† in patients with evidence of neurologic disease or when arthritis has not responded to an oral regimen, the IDSA recommends that adults receive 2 g IV every 8 hours for 14 days (range: 14–28 days).

If cefotaxime is used for the treatment of late neurologic Lyme disease† affecting the CNS or peripheral nervous system, the IDSA recommends that adults receive 2 g IV every 8 hours for 14 days (range: 14–28 days).

Respiratory Tract Infections. For the treatment of community-acquired pneumonia (CAP) in adults who are hospitalized for inpatient treatment, cefotaxime usually is given in a dosage of 1 g every 6–8 hours.

If used for empiric treatment of CAP, cefotaxime is used in conjunction with other anti-infectives. (See Community-acquired Pneumonia under Uses: Respiratory Tract Infections.)

Perioperative Prophylaxis. If cefotaxime is used for perioperative prophylaxis in contaminated or potentially contaminated surgery, the manufacturers recommend that adults receive 1 g IM or IV given 30–90 minutes prior to surgery. If cefotaxime is used prophylactically in patients undergoing cesarean section, the manufacturers recommend 1 g given IV as soon as the umbilical cord is clamped, followed by 1 g IM or IV 6 and 12 hours after the first dose.

Although not usually considered a drug of choice for perioperative prophylaxis (see Uses: Perioperative Prophylaxis), if cefotaxime is used for perioperative prophylaxis some experts recommend that adults receive 1 g of cefotaxime (2 g in obese patients) within 60 minutes prior to surgical incision. If the procedure is prolonged (longer than 3–4 hours) or if major blood loss occurs, additional intraoperative doses of cefotaxime may be given every 3 hours. The duration of prophylaxis should be less than 24 hours for most procedures; there is no evidence to support continuing prophylaxis after wound closure or until all indwelling drains and intravascular catheters are removed.

Pediatric Dosage

General Dosage for Neonates. The usual dosage of cefotaxime recommended by the manufacturers for premature or full-term neonates less than 1 week of age is 50 mg/kg every 12 hours and the usual dosage for neonates 1–4 weeks of age is 50 mg/kg every 8 hours.

The American Academy of Pediatrics (AAP) recommends that neonates 7 days of age or younger receive IV or IM cefotaxime in a dosage of 50 mg/kg every 12 hours, regardless of weight. For neonates 8–28 days of age, the AAP recommends a dosage of 50 mg/kg every 8–12 hours for those weighing 2 kg or less and 50 mg/kg every 8 hours for those weighing more than 2 kg.

General Dosage for Infants and Children. Children weighing 50 kg or more should receive the usual daily adult dosage, but dosage should not exceed 12 g daily.

The manufacturers recommend that children 1 month to 12 years of age weighing less than 50 kg receive 50–180 mg/kg daily given in 4–6 equally divided doses; the higher dosages should be used for more severe or serious infections, including meningitis.

The AAP recommends that pediatric patients beyond the neonatal period receive cefotaxime in a dosage of 50–180 mg/kg daily given in 3 or 4 equally divided doses for the treatment of mild to moderate infections or 200–225 mg/kg daily given in 4 or 6 equally divided doses for the treatment of severe infections.

Meningitis and Other CNS Infections. For the treatment of meningitis caused by susceptible bacteria, the manufacturers recommend that children 1 month to 12 years of age who weigh less than 50 kg receive a cefotaxime dosage at the high end of the range of 50–180 mg/kg daily.

Some clinicians recommend that infants and children younger than 18 years of age with meningitis receive cefotaxime in a dosage of 50 mg/kg IV every 6 hours. Other clinicians recommend a cefotaxime dosage of 100–150 mg/kg daily given in divided doses every 8–12 hours in neonates 7 days of age or younger, 150–200 mg/kg daily given in divided doses every 6–8 hours in neonates 8–28 days of age, and 225–300 mg/kg daily given in divided doses every 6–8 hours in older infants and children.

The AAP states that a cefotaxime dosage up to 300 mg/kg daily given in 4 or 6 divided doses can be used for the treatment of meningitis in pediatric patients beyond the neonatal period.

While 7 days of therapy may be adequate for the treatment of uncomplicated meningitis caused by susceptible *H. influenzae* or *N. meningitidis*, at least 10–14 days of therapy is recommended for complicated cases or for meningitis caused by *S. pneumoniae* and at least 21 days is recommended for meningitis caused by susceptible Enterobacteriaceae (e.g., *E. coli*, *Klebsiella*).

Gonorrhea and Associated Infections. The usual dosage of cefotaxime for the treatment of disseminated gonococcal infection† (e.g., sepsis, arthritis, meningitis) or gonococcal scalp abscesses† in neonates is 25 mg/kg IV or IM every 12 hours for 7 days; if meningitis is documented, the drug should be continued for 10–14 days.

Lyme Disease. If cefotaxime is used for the treatment of early Lyme disease† in children with acute neurologic disease manifested by meningitis or radiculopathy, the IDSA and other clinicians recommend a dosage of 150–200 mg/kg daily (up to 6 g daily) given IV in divided doses every 6–8 hours for 14 days (range: 10–28 days).

If cefotaxime is used when a parenteral regimen is indicated for the treatment of Lyme carditis† in patients with atrioventricular (AV) heart block and/or myopericarditis associated with early Lyme disease, the IDSA and other clinicians recommend that children receive a dosage of 150–200 mg/kg daily (up to 6 g daily) given IV in divided doses every 6–8 hours for 14 days (range: 14–21 days). Although a parenteral regimen is recommended for initial treatment of hospitalized patients, the parenteral regimen can be switched to an oral regimen (doxycycline, amoxicillin, cefuroxime axetil) to complete therapy and for outpatients.

If cefotaxime is used when a parenteral regimen is indicated for the treatment of Lyme arthritis† in patients with evidence of neurologic disease or when arthritis has not responded to an oral regimen, the IDSA recommends that children receive a dosage of 150–200 mg/kg daily (up to 6 g daily) given IV in divided doses every 6–8 hours for 14 days (range: 14–28 days).

If cefotaxime is used for the treatment of late neurologic Lyme disease† affecting the CNS or peripheral nervous system, the IDSA recommends that children receive a dosage of 150–200 mg/kg daily (up to 6 g daily) given IV in divided doses every 6–8 hours for 14 days (range: 14–28 days).

Duration of Therapy

The duration of cefotaxime therapy depends on the type of infection but should generally be continued for at least 48–72 hours after the patient becomes afebrile or evidence of eradication of the infection is obtained. Although other drugs generally are preferred, if cefotaxime is used in infections caused by group A β-hemolytic streptococci, therapy should be continued for at least 10 days to decrease the risk of rheumatic fever or glomerulonephritis. Chronic urinary tract infections may require several weeks of therapy, and bacteriologic and clinical assessments should be made frequently during therapy and for several months after therapy is discontinued.

■ Dosage in Renal and Hepatic Impairment

Modification of the usual dosage of cefotaxime is unnecessary in patients with creatinine clearances of 20 mL/minute or greater per 1.73 m^2. However, in patients with creatinine clearances less than 20 mL/minute per 1.73 m^2, doses and/or frequency of administration should be modified in response to the degree of renal impairment. The manufacturers recommend that these patients receive half the usual dose of cefotaxime at the usual time interval.

In patients undergoing hemodialysis, some clinicians recommend that 0.5–2 g be given as single daily doses and that a supplemental dose of cefotaxime be given after each dialysis period.

Although serum half-life and clearance of cefotaxime and its major metabolite may be prolonged in patients with impaired hepatic function, dosage adjustments are not necessary in such patients unless renal function also is impaired.

Cautions

■ Dermatologic and Sensitivity Reactions

Hypersensitivity reactions have been reported to occur in approximately 2% of patients receiving cefotaxime. These reactions include rash (maculopapular or erythematous), pruritus, fever, and eosinophilia. Urticaria, anaphylaxis, erythema multiforme, Stevens-Johnson syndrome, and toxic epidermal necrolysis have occurred rarely. If a severe hypersensitivity reaction occurs during cefotaxime therapy, the drug should be discontinued and the patient given appropriate therapy (e.g., epinephrine, corticosteroids, maintenance of an adequate airway, oxygen) as indicated.

Positive direct antiglobulin (Coombs') test results have also been reported occasionally in patients receiving cefotaxime; however, it is not clear whether the mechanism of this reaction is immunologic in nature.

■ Local Effects

The most frequent adverse reactions to cefotaxime are local reactions at the injection site which occur in approximately 4% of patients. IV administration has caused inflammation, phlebitis, and thrombophlebitis and IM administration has caused pain, induration, and tenderness at the injection site. Extensive perivascular extravasation of cefotaxime may result in tissue damage requiring surgical intervention; however, in most cases, perivascular extravasation responds to changing the infusion site. To minimize the potential for tissue inflammation, the manufacturers recommend that IV infusion sites be monitored regularly and changed appropriately.

■ GI Effects Adverse GI effects including anorexia, diarrhea, nausea, vomiting, abdominal pain, and colitis have occurred in approximately 1% of patients receiving cefotaxime.

Treatment with anti-infectives alters the normal colon flora and may permit overgrowth of *Clostridium difficile*. *C. difficile* infection (CDI) and *C. difficile*-associated diarrhea and colitis (CDAD; also known as antibiotic-associated diarrhea and colitis or pseudomembranous colitis) have been reported with nearly all anti-infectives, including cefotaxime, and may range in severity from mild diarrhea to fatal colitis. *C. difficile* produces toxins A and B which contribute to the development of CDAD; hypertoxin-producing strains of *C. difficile* are associated with increased morbidity and mortality since they may be refractory to anti-infectives and colectomy may be required.

CDAD should be considered in the differential diagnosis in patients who develop diarrhea during or after anti-infective therapy and managed accordingly. Careful medical history is necessary since CDAD has been reported to occur as late as 2 months or longer after anti-infective therapy is discontinued.

If CDAD is suspected or confirmed, anti-infectives not directed against *C. difficile* should be discontinued whenever possible. Patients should be managed with appropriate supportive therapy (e.g., fluid and electrolyte management, protein supplementation), anti-infective therapy directed against *C. difficile* (e.g., metronidazole, vancomycin), and surgical evaluation as clinically indicated.

■ Hematologic Effects Transient neutropenia, granulocytopenia, leukopenia, eosinophilia, or thrombocytopenia have occurred in less than 1% of patients receiving cefotaxime. Agranulocytosis reportedly may occur rarely with cefotaxime treatment, particularly during prolonged therapy; therefore, blood cell counts should be performed in patients receiving treatment courses lasting for more than 10 days. Hemolytic anemia has also been reported rarely. Prolongation of the prothrombin time and hypoprothrombinemia have been reported only rarely in patients receiving cefotaxime.

■ Renal Effects Transient increases in BUN and/or serum creatinine concentrations and interstitial nephritis have been reported in a few patients receiving cefotaxime. A transient increase in urinary concentration of alanine aminopeptidase, which may be an indication of transient tubular damage, has been reported in a few patients receiving the drug. Most studies indicate that cefotaxime is not nephrotoxic and that urine concentrations of alanine aminopeptidase are usually unchanged during therapy with the drug.

■ Other Adverse Effects Transient increases in serum AST (SGOT), ALT (SGPT), LDH, bilirubin, and alkaline phosphatase concentrations have been reported in less than 1% of patients receiving cefotaxime.

Headache, agitation, confusion, fatigue, and nocturnal perspiration have also been reported in less than 1% of patients receiving the drug. Seizures have been reported with some cephalosporins.

During postmarketing surveillance, potentially life-threatening arrhythmias were reported in several patients who received cefotaxime by rapid (less than 1 minute) bolus injection through a central venous catheter.

■ Precautions and Contraindications Prior to initiation of cefotaxime therapy, careful inquiry should be made concerning previous hypersensitivity reactions to cefotaxime, cephalosporins, penicillins, or other drugs. There is clinical and laboratory evidence of partial cross-allergenicity among cephalosporins and other β-lactam antibiotics including penicillins and cephamycins; however, the true incidence of cross-allergenicity among these anti-infectives has not been established. Cefotaxime is contraindicated in patients with a history of allergic reactions to the drug or other cephalosporins and should be used with caution in patients with a history of hypersensitivity to penicillins. Use of cephalosporins should be avoided in patients who have had an immediate-type (anaphylactic) hypersensitivity reaction to penicillins. Although it has not been definitely proven that allergic reactions to antibiotics are more frequent in atopic individuals, the manufacturers state that cefotaxime should be used with caution in patients with a history of allergy, particularly to drugs.

To reduce development of drug-resistant bacteria and maintain effectiveness of cefotaxime and other antibacterials, the drug should be used only for the treatment or prevention of infections proven or strongly suspected to be caused by susceptible bacteria. When selecting or modifying anti-infective therapy, results of culture and in vitro susceptibility testing should be used. In the absence of such data, local epidemiology and susceptibility patterns should be considered when selecting anti-infectives for empiric therapy.

Patients should be advised that antibacterials (including cefotaxime) should only be used to treat bacterial infections and not used to treat viral infections (e.g., the common cold). Patients also should be advised about the importance of completing the full course of therapy, even if feeling better after a few days, and that skipping doses or not completing therapy may decrease effectiveness and increase the likelihood that bacteria will develop resistance and will not be treatable with cefotaxime or other antibacterials in the future.

Like other anti-infectives, prolonged use of cefotaxime may result in overgrowth of nonsusceptible organisms, especially *Candida* and *Pseudomonas*. Vaginitis and moniliasis have occurred in less than 1% of patients receiving cefotaxime. Resistant strains of some organisms, especially *Enterobacter*, *Ps. aeruginosa*, and *Serratia*, have developed during therapy with cefotaxime. Careful observation of the patient during cefotaxime therapy is essential. If suprainfection or superinfection occurs, appropriate therapy should be instituted.

Because CDAD has been reported with the use of cefotaxime or other cephalosporins, it should be considered in the differential diagnosis of patients who develop diarrhea during or after cefotaxime therapy. (See Cautions: GI Effects.) Patients should be advised that diarrhea is a common problem caused by anti-infectives and usually resolves when the drug is discontinued; however, they should contact a clinician if watery and bloody stools (with or without stomach cramps and fever) occur during or as late as 2 months or longer after the last dose. Cefotaxime should be used with caution in patients with a history of GI disease, particularly colitis.

Seizures have been reported with several cephalosporins, particularly in patients with renal impairment in whom dosage of the drug was not reduced. If seizures occur during cephalosporin therapy, the drug should be discontinued and anticonvulsant therapy initiated as clinically indicated.

■ Pediatric Precautions Cefotaxime is well tolerated in pediatric patients, and adverse effects reported in children receiving the drug are similar to those reported in adults. A retrospective review of children 3 months to 18 years of age who received cefotaxime indicates that adverse effects occurred in up to 2.5% of these children and included adverse local reactions, rash, and adverse GI effects such as diarrhea and vomiting.

Safety of the chemical components that may leach out of the plastic containing commercially available frozen cefotaxime sodium injections has not been established in children.

■ Geriatric Precautions In clinical studies of cefotaxime sodium, there were no overall differences in safety or efficacy between geriatric adults 65 years of age or older and younger adults. Other clinical experience revealed no evidence of age-related differences; however, the possibility that some geriatric patients may exhibit increased sensitivity to the drug cannot be ruled out.

Cefotaxime is substantially excreted by the kidney, and the risk of severe adverse reactions may be increased in patients with impaired renal function. Because geriatric patients are more likely to have decreased renal function, dosage should be selected with caution in these patients and renal function monitoring may be useful.

■ Mutagenicity and Carcinogenicity Cefotaxime was not mutagenic in the mouse micronucleus test or the Ames test. Studies have not been performed to date to evaluate the carcinogenic potential of cefotaxime.

■ Pregnancy, Fertility, and Lactation Reproduction studies in mice or rats using IV cefotaxime dosages up to 1.2 g/kg daily (0.4 or 0.8 times, respectively, the usual human dosage based on mg/m^3) have not revealed evidence of embryotoxicity or teratogenicity. However, the offspring of rats that received 1.2 g/kg of cefotaxime weighed less at birth and also remained smaller during 21 days of nursing than offspring of rats that did not receive the drug. There are no adequate and controlled studies to date using cefotaxime in pregnant women, and the drug should be used during pregnancy only when clearly needed.

There was no evidence of impaired fertility in rats given cefotaxime subcutaneously at dosages up to 250 mg/kg daily or in mice given the drug IV at dosages up to 2 g/kg daily (0.2 or 0.7 times, respectively, the recommended human dosage based on mg/m^3).

Because cefotaxime is distributed into milk, the drug should be used with caution in nursing women.

Drug Interactions

■ Aminoglycosides In vitro studies indicate that the antibacterial activity of cefotaxime and aminoglycosides may be additive or synergistic against some organisms including some strains of *Ps. aeruginosa* and *S. marcescens*. However, synergism is unpredictable and antagonism has also occurred in vitro when cefotaxime was used in combination with an aminoglycoside.

Concurrent use of aminoglycosides and cephalosporins may increase the risk of nephrotoxicity during therapy. Although this effect has not been reported to date with cefotaxime, the manufacturers state that the possibility that nephrotoxicity may be potentiated if the drug is used concomitantly with an aminoglycoside should be considered.

■ Other Anti-infective Agents In one in vitro study which used the checkerboard technique to assess synergism, a combination of cefotaxime and ampicillin appeared to be partially additive or synergistic against a few strains of group B streptococci. However, when the killing-curve technique was used to assess synergism, the combination was no more effective than cefotaxime alone against these organisms. In one in vitro study, a combination of cefotaxime and clindamycin was neither synergistic nor antagonistic against Enterobacteriaceae.

Laboratory Test Interferences

■ Immunohematology Tests Positive direct antiglobulin (Coombs') test results have been reported in some patients receiving cefotaxime. This reaction may interfere with hematologic studies or transfusion cross-matching procedures.

■ Tests for Glucose and Creatinine Although other currently available cephalosporins reportedly cause false-positive results in urine glucose determinations using cupric sulfate solution (Benedict's reagent, Clinitest®) and may cause falsely elevated serum or urine creatinine values when the Jaffé reaction is used, cefotaxime does not appear to interfere with these laboratory tests.

Acute Toxicity

In neonatal and adult mice and rats, acute overdosage of cefotaxime resulted in significant mortality at parenteral dosages exceeding 6 g/kg daily. Common toxic signs in those that died included a decrease in spontaneous activity, tonic and clonic convulsions, dyspnea, hypothermia, and cyanosis.

Acute overdosage of cefotaxime in patients has most frequently resulted in increased serum concentrations of BUN and creatinine, but most cases were not associated with overt toxicity. If acute overdosage occurs, the patient should be closely observed and given supportive treatment.

Mechanism of Action

Cefotaxime has a mechanism of action similar to that of other cephalosporins. For information on the mechanism of action of cephalosporins, see Mechanism of Action in the Cephalosporins General Statement 8:12.06.

The target enzymes of β-lactam antibiotics have been classified as penicillin-binding proteins (PBPs) and appear to vary substantially among bacterial species. Studies evaluating the binding of cefotaxime to PBPs indicate that the drug has a high affinity for PBPs 1a, 1b, and 3 of *Escherichia coli* and PBPs 1a, 1b, 3, and 4 of *Pseudomonas aeruginosa*. The affinities of various β-lactam antibiotics for different PBPs appear to explain the differences in morphology which occur in susceptible organisms following exposure to different β-lactam antibiotics and may also explain differences in the spectrum of activity of β-lactam antibiotics which are not due to the presence or absence of β-lactamases.

Spectrum

Based on its spectrum of activity, cefotaxime is classified as a third generation cephalosporin. For information on the classification of cephalosporins and closely related β-lactam antibiotics based on spectra of activity, see Spectrum in the Cephalosporins General Statement 8:12.06.

Like other currently available parenteral third generation cephalosporins (e.g., ceftazidime, ceftriaxone), cefotaxime generally is less active in vitro against susceptible staphylococci than first generation cephalosporins but has an expanded spectrum of activity against gram-negative bacteria compared with first and second generation cephalosporins. The spectrum of activity of cefotaxime closely resembles that of ceftriaxone. In vitro on a weight basis, the activity of cefotaxime against most susceptible Enterobacteriaceae is approximately equal to that of ceftriaxone. Cefotaxime is inactive against *Chlamydia*, fungi, and viruses.

The major metabolite of cefotaxime, desacetylcefotaxime, is also microbiologically active. In vitro, desacetylcefotaxime has only about 10% of the antibacterial activity of cefotaxime. However, desacetylcefotaxime is more active in vitro against susceptible gram-positive aerobic bacteria than is cefazolin or cefoxitin. It has been suggested that the antibacterial activity of desacetylcefotaxime may be clinically important in infections in patients with impaired renal function or in infections in organs or tissues where desacetylcefotaxime accumulates. Preliminary data indicate that the antibacterial activities of cefotaxime and desacetylcefotaxime are additive or synergistic against cefotaxime-susceptible *S. aureus* and Enterobacteriaceae.

■ **In Vitro Susceptibility Testing** For most organisms, inoculum size, pH, test media, and presence of serum do not appear to influence results of in vitro cefotaxime susceptibility tests. However, results of susceptibility tests for some gram-negative bacilli (especially *Proteus, Providencia, Pseudomonas aeruginosa, Klebsiella*, and *Serratia marcescens*) may be greatly affected by the size of the inoculum.

Strains of staphylococci resistant to penicillinase-resistant penicillins (oxacillin-resistant [methicillin-resistant] staphylococci) should be considered resistant to cefotaxime, although results of in vitro susceptibility tests may indicate that the organisms are susceptible to the drug.

For information on interpreting results of in vitro susceptibility testing (disk susceptibility tests, dilution susceptibility tests) when cefotaxime susceptibility testing is performed according to the standards of the Clinical and Laboratory Standards Institute (CLSI; formerly National Committee for Clinical Laboratory Standards [NCCLS]), see Spectrum: In Vitro Susceptibility Testing, in the Cephalosporins General Statement 8:12.06.

■ **Gram-positive Aerobic Bacteria** In vitro, cefotaxime concentrations of 0.5 mcg/mL or less inhibit most strains of *Streptococcus pneumoniae, S. pyogenes* (group A β-hemolytic streptococci), and *S. agalactiae* (group B streptococci). Some strains of viridans streptococci are inhibited in vitro by cefotaxime concentrations of 4 mcg/mL or less. In one study, the MIC_{50} and MIC_{90} of cefotaxime for the *S. milleri* group of viridans streptococci (*S. anginosus, S. constellatus, S. intermedius*) were 0.25 and 0.5 mcg/mL, respectively. Cefotaxime concentrations of 4 mcg/mL or less inhibit most strains of *Staphylococcus aureus* in vitro. Cefotaxime is active in vitro against most strains of penicillinase-producing *S. aureus*; however, almost all strains of staphylococci resistant to penicillinase-resistant penicillins are also resistant to cefotaxime. The MIC_{90} (minimum inhibitory concentration of the drug at which 90% of strains are inhibited) of cefotaxime for *S. epidermidis* generally is 4.8–16 mcg/mL, although lower MIC_{90}s have been reported occasionally; in a few studies, however, the MIC_{90} was 64 mcg/mL or greater. *Listeria monocytogenes* and enterococci, including *E. faecalis* (formerly *S. faecalis*), generally are resistant to the drug. Strains of *S. pneumoniae* with MICs of 2 mcg/mL or greater generally are considered resistant to cefotaxime.

The MIC_{90} of desacetylcefotaxime reported for susceptible *S. pneumoniae* and *S. pyogenes* is 4 mcg/mL or less. *S. aureus* is generally resistant to desacetylcefotaxime.

■ **Gram-negative Aerobic Bacteria** Cefotaxime is active in vitro against a wide variety of gram-negative bacteria including most Enterobacteriaceae and some strains of *Pseudomonas aeruginosa*. Cefotaxime is active against some gram-negative bacteria that are resistant to first and second generation cephalosporins and currently available penicillins and aminoglycosides, especially *Escherichia coli, Klebsiella pneumoniae*, and *Serratia marcescens*.

Enterobacteriaceae Generally, cefotaxime is active in vitro against the following Enterobacteriaceae: *Citrobacter freundii, C. diversus, Enterobacter aerogenes, E. cloacae, Escherichia coli, Klebsiella pneumoniae, K. oxytoca, Morganella morganii* (formerly *Proteus morganii*), *Proteus mirabilis, P. vulgaris, Providencia stuartii* (formerly group B *Proteus inconstans*), *P. rettgeri* (formerly *Proteus rettgeri*), *Salmonella, Serratia marcescens, Shigella*, and *Yersinia enterocolitica*. The MIC_{90} of cefotaxime for many of these gram-negative bacilli is 4 mcg/mL or less. However, the MIC_{90} of cefotaxime for *C. freundii, E. aerogenes, E. cloacae, M. morganii*, and *Serratia* generally ranges from 0.1–32 mcg/mL, although higher MIC_{90}s have been reported. The MIC_{90} of desacetylcefotaxime reported for susceptible *E. coli, K. pneumoniae, P. mirabilis*, and *Providencia stuartii* is 4 mcg/mL or less; *E. aerogenes, E. cloacae, M. morganii, P. vulgaris*, and *S. marcescens* are generally resistant to desacetylcefotaxime.

Pseudomonas The in vitro activity of cefotaxime against *Pseudomonas* is variable. Although some strains of *Ps. aeruginosa* and *Ps. maltophilia* (*Stenotrophomonas maltophilia*) are inhibited in vitro by cefotaxime concentrations of 32 mcg/mL or less, most strains of these organisms require cefotaxime concentrations of 64 mcg/mL or greater for in vitro inhibition and are therefore considered resistant to the drug. Cefotaxime is less active in vitro against susceptible *Ps. aeruginosa* than is ceftazidime or some extended-spectrum penicillins. *Ps. aeruginosa* generally is resistant to desacetylcefotaxime.

Other Gram-negative Aerobic Bacteria Cefotaxime is active in vitro against *Haemophilus influenzae* (including ampicillin-resistant strains) and *H. parainfluenzae*. The MIC_{90}s of cefotaxime reported for *H. influenzae* and *H. parainfluenzae* are 0.01–0.8 and 0.024–4 mcg/mL, respectively, and the MIC_{90} of desacetylcefotaxime reported for *H. influenzae* is 4 mcg/mL or less.

Cefotaxime is active in vitro against *Neisseria meningitidis* and *Neisseria gonorrhoeae*. The MIC_{90} of cefotaxime reported for *N. gonorrhoeae* (including both penicillinase-producing and nonpenicillinase-producing strains) is 0.1–0.4 mcg/mL.

Both β-lactamase- and non-β-lactamase-producing strains of *Moraxella catarrhalis* are inhibited in vitro by cefotaxime concentrations of 0.03–0.5 mcg/mL.

Cefotaxime is active in vitro against *Eikenella corrodens*, and the MIC_{90} of the drug for this organism generally is 0.06–0.5 mcg/mL. *Campylobacter fetus* subsp. *jejuni*, an organism that can be microaerophilic or anaerobic, generally is inhibited in vitro by cefotaxime concentrations of 2–6.25 mcg/mL.

Although cefotaxime has some activity in vitro against *Acinetobacter*, the MIC_{90} of the drug generally ranges from 8–32 mcg/mL for *A. calcoaceticus* var. *lwoffi* and from 16–32 mcg/mL for *A. calcoaceticus* var. *anitratus*; higher MIC_{90}s also have been reported.

In vitro, some strains of *Bartonella bacilliformis* are inhibited by cefotaxime concentrations of 0.03–0.12 mcg/mL.

While some strains of *Burkholderia cepacia* (formerly *Pseudomonas cepacia*) are inhibited in vitro by cefotaxime concentrations of 16 mcg/mL, the MIC_{90} of the drug for this organism is 64 mcg/mL and most strains are resistant to the drug.

Cefotaxime is active in vitro against *Capnocytophaga*. In an in vitro study, the MIC_{90} of cefotaxime for *Capnocytophaga* was 0.25 mcg/mL. Cefotaxime-resistant strains of *C. sputigena* (formerly CDC group DF-1) have been reported.

Vibrio vulnificus may be inhibited in vitro by cefotaxime concentrations of 0.03 mcg/mL. While the clinical importance is unclear, results of an in vitro study and a study in mice indicate that the combination of cefotaxime and minocycline is more active against *V. vulnificus* than either anti-infective alone.

■ **Anaerobic Bacteria** Cefotaxime is active in vitro against *Bacteroides, Eubacterium, Fusobacterium, Peptococcus, Peptostreptococcus, Propionibacterium*, and *Veillonella*. Cefotaxime is also active against some strains of *Clostridium* including *C. perfringens*; however, *C. difficile* is usually resistant to the drug.

Although the MIC_{90} of cefotaxime reported for most susceptible anaerobes is 16 mcg/mL or less, cefotaxime concentrations of 16–64 mcg/mL are generally required in vitro to inhibit *Bacteroides* (including *B. fragilis*). In vitro, cefotaxime is less active than cefoxitin against susceptible *B. fragilis*.

■ **Spirochetes** *Borrelia burgdorferi*, the causative organism of Lyme disease, reportedly may be inhibited in vitro by a cefotaxime concentration of 0.12 mcg/mL.

Resistance

For information on possible mechanisms of bacterial resistance to cephalosporins, see Resistance in the Cephalosporins General Statement 8:12.06.

Because cefotaxime contains an α-*syn*-methoximino group which protects the β-lactam ring from hydrolysis by many penicillinases and cephalosporinases, cefotaxime is more resistant to hydrolysis by most β-lactamases than first and second generation cephalosporins. Cefotaxime is generally resistant to hydrolysis by β-lactamases classified as Richmond-Sykes types I, II, III, IV, and V, and most penicillinases produced by *S. aureus*. However, β-lactamases produced by *B. fragilis* and *P. vulgaris* can slowly hydrolyze cefotaxime.

Resistant strains of some organisms, especially *Enterobacter, Ps. aeruginosa*, or *Serratia*, have developed during therapy with cefotaxime. Strains of *Ps. aeruginosa* which are only moderately susceptible to cefotaxime in vitro at the beginning of therapy appear to be especially likely to become resistant during therapy.

Like most cephalosporins and penicillins, cefotaxime is inactivated by inducible, chromosomally mediated β-lactamases produced by some strains of *Citrobacter, Enterobacter, Pseudomonas*, and *Serratia*. Therefore, organisms that possess inducible β-lactamases are usually resistant to cefotaxime following derepression of the enzymes. Inducible β-lactamases may be derepressed by mutation to a stable derepressed state or may be reversibly derepressed by an enzyme inducer. Cefoxitin and imipenem are potent inducers of these enzymes, and in vitro exposure of organisms possessing these enzymes to these drugs results in resistance to cefotaxime as well as to many other β-lactam antibiotics. Inducible β-lactamases inactivate cephalosporins and penicillins either by hydrolyzing the drugs or by binding to them to prevent access to penicillin-binding proteins (PBPs). The clinical importance of these inducible β-lactamases is unclear, but emergence of cefotaxime resistance in some organisms during therapy with the drug may be related to these enzymes.

Strains of *S. pneumoniae* considered resistant to cefotaxime have been reported with increasing frequency. These strains generally have intermediate- or high-level resistance to penicillin G as well as decreased susceptibility to third generation cephalosporins. Resistance to cefotaxime in *S. pneumoniae* appears to be related to alterations in the PBPs of the organism.

Tolerance to cefotaxime has been reported to occur in some bacteria including some strains of *Enterobacter, Proteus*, and *Ps. aeruginosa*. In vitro, tolerant bacteria have a minimum bactericidal concentration (MBC) of cefotaxime which is much greater than the MIC of the drug. Bacteria which are tolerant to cefotaxime appear to be inhibited but not necessarily killed by the drug. Preliminary studies suggest that tolerant organisms may have decreased concentrations of autolysins or an increased concentration of an unidentified inhibitor of autolysis. Tolerance may be important clinically since infections caused by these organisms may persist during cefotaxime therapy despite in vitro susceptibility tests which indicate that the organisms are susceptible to the drug.

Pharmacokinetics

In all studies described in the Pharmacokinetics section, cefotaxime was administered as the sodium salt; dosages of the drug are expressed in terms of cefotaxime.

The antibacterial activity of both cefotaxime and its major metabolite, desacetylcefotaxime, must be considered when attempting to correlate the pharmacokinetics with the therapeutic effect of the drug. In early published studies on the pharmacokinetics of cefotaxime, microbiologic assays were used to determine body fluid and tissue concentrations of the drug. Microbiologic assays which used test organisms susceptible to cefotaxime but resistant to desacetylcefotaxime accurately reflect concentrations of the parent drug; however, microbiologic assays used in some published pharmacokinetic studies of cefotaxime actually measured total microbiologic activity since both cefotaxime and desacetylcefotaxime were active against the test organism. Information on body fluid and tissue concentrations of cefotaxime obtained from studies that used nonspecific microbiologic assays or from studies that did not identify the test organism used is reported as*microbiologic activity* in the following sections on the pharmacokinetics of the drug. More recent pharmacokinetic studies generally use high-performance liquid chromatography (HPLC) that differentiates between cefotaxime and desacetylcefotaxime and can specifically measure concentrations of cefotaxime and/or its metabolite.

■ Absorption Cefotaxime is not appreciably absorbed from the GI tract and must be given parenterally.

Following IM administration of a single 500-mg or 1-g dose of cefotaxime in healthy adults with normal renal function, peak serum concentrations of the drug are attained within 30 minutes and average 11.7–11.9 mcg/mL and 20.5–25.3 mcg/mL, respectively. Plasma concentrations of cefotaxime are undetectable 8 hours after a single 500-mg IM dose of the drug but average 1 mcg/mL 8 hours after a single 1-g IM dose of the drug. In one multiple-dose study in adults with normal renal function receiving 500-mg doses of cefotaxime by IM injection every 8 hours, steady-state peak serum concentrations of cefotaxime ranged from 9.2–11.9 mcg/mL and steady-state trough serum concentrations of the drug ranged from 0.1–0.6 mcg/mL.

In one study in healthy adults with normal renal function, a single 500-mg, 1-g, or 2-g dose of cefotaxime given by IV injection over 5 minutes resulted in serum concentrations of cefotaxime which averaged 37.9 mcg/mL, 102.4 mcg/mL, and 214.1 mcg/mL, respectively, immediately after the injection; serum concentrations of the drug averaged 1 mcg/mL, 1.9 mcg/mL, and 3.3 mcg/mL, respectively, 4 hours after the injection. In a multiple-dose study in healthy adults with normal renal function receiving 1-g doses of cefotaxime every 6 hours by IV infusion over 30 minutes, steady-state peak serum concentrations of cefotaxime ranged from 40.6–46 mcg/mL and steady-state trough serum concentrations of the drug ranged from 1.1–1.6 mcg/mL.

Following a single cefotaxime dose of 50 mg/kg given by IV infusion over 10 minutes in average birthweight neonates 1–7 days of age, *microbiologic activity* in serum averaged 133 mcg/mL immediately after completion of the infusion, 85 mcg/mL 1 hour later, 52 mcg/mL 4 hours later, and 38 mcg/mL 6 hours later.

In one study in children 1 month to 12 years of age, serum concentrations of cefotaxime averaged 25.3 mcg/mL 30 minutes after a single cefotaxime dose of 25 mg/kg given by IM injection and averaged 53.3 mcg/mL 5 minutes after a single dose of 25 mg/kg of the drug given by IV injection.

■ Distribution Following IM or IV administration of usual dosages of cefotaxime, *microbiologic activity* is widely distributed into body tissues and fluids including the aqueous humor, bronchial secretions, sputum, middle ear effusions, bone, bile, and ascitic, pleural, and prostatic fluids. The apparent volume of distribution of cefotaxime in adults is reported to be 0.22–0.29 L/kg.

Cefotaxime is 13–38% bound to serum proteins in vitro.

Cefotaxime and its major metabolite are distributed into CSF following parenteral administration. Following IV administration of a single 2-g IV dose of cefotaxime in patients with *uninflamed* meninges, low concentrations of cefotaxime (0.14–1.81 mcg/mL) and desacetylcefotaxime (0.06–0.38 mcg/mL) are attained in CSF; however, higher concentrations are attained in patients with *inflamed* meninges. In one study in neonates and children 2 weeks to 2 years of age with inflamed meninges, IV injection or infusion over 30 minutes of cefotaxime doses of 50 mg/kg every 4–6 hours resulted in *microbiologic activity* in CSF which ranged from 1–13.2 mcg/mL 1–4 hours after administration. In another study in children 2 months to 12 years of age with meningitis who received cefotaxime in a dosage of 50 mg/kg IV every 6 hours, CSF concentrations of cefotaxime or its major metabolite averaged 6.2 or 5.6 mcg/mL, respectively, 1 hour after a dose; concurrent serum concentrations were 61.44 and 19.3 mcg/mL, respectively. In a study in adults with bacterial meningitis receiving 2 g of cefotaxime IV every 4 hours, trough CSF cefotaxime and desacetylcefotaxime concentrations ranged from 5.6–44.3 mcg/mL and 3.7–44 mcg/mL, respectively, after 1–3 days of therapy.

Following IM or IV administration of usual dosages of cefotaxime, *microbiologic activity* in hepatic bile is reported to be 15–75% of concurrent *microbiologic activity* in serum and *microbiologic activity* in gallbladder bile is reported to be up to 3 times greater than concurrent *microbiologic activity* in serum. *Microbiologic activity* in ascitic fluid is reported to be 40% of concurrent *microbiologic activity* in serum.

In patients receiving 2-g doses of cefotaxime IV every 6 hours, concentrations of cefotaxime and desacetylcefotaxime in bronchial secretions averaged 1.7 and 5.8 mcg/mL, respectively, and plasma concentrations averaged 23.1 and 9.3 mcg/mL, respectively, in samples obtained 1–2 hours after the fourth dose.

Cefotaxime readily crosses the placenta, and *microbiologic activity* in amniotic fluid is reported to be equal to or greater than concurrent *microbiologic activity* in maternal serum following multiple doses of the drug.

Cefotaxime is distributed into milk. In one study, *microbiologic activity* in milk ranged from 0.25–0.52 mcg/mL 2–3 hours after a single 1-g IV dose of cefotaxime.

■ Elimination Cefotaxime is partially metabolized in the liver to desacetylcefotaxime which has antibacterial activity. (See Spectrum.) Desacetylation of cefotaxime occurs rapidly in vivo and rapidly in vitro in hemolyzed blood. Following IV injection over 5 minutes of a single 500-mg or 2-g dose of cefotaxime in adults with normal renal function, peak plasma concentrations of desacetylcefotaxime are generally attained within 45 minutes and average 2.7 mcg/mL and 9.8 mcg/mL, respectively. Desacetylcefotaxime is partially converted in the liver to desacetylcefotaxime lactone which is inactive and is further degraded to 2 unidentified inactive metabolites currently designated as UP_1 and its optical isomer UP_2.

Serum concentrations of cefotaxime appear to decline in a biphasic manner. In adults with normal renal function, the serum half-life of cefotaxime in the initial phase ($t_{1/2\alpha}$) averages 0.2–0.4 hours and the serum half-life of the drug in the terminal phase ($t_{1/2\beta}$) averages 0.9–1.7 hours. The $t_{1/2\beta}$ of desacetylcefotaxime is longer than that of the parent drug and is reported to be 1.4–1.9 hours in adults with normal renal function. In adults with renal impairment, the $t_{1/2\alpha}$ of cefotaxime is not affected, and the $t_{1/2\beta}$ is only slightly prolonged in patients with creatinine clearances of 20 mL/min or greater per 1.73 m^2. In adults with creatinine clearances of 10 mL/min or less per 1.73 m^2, the $t_{1/2\beta}$ of cefotaxime is reported to range from 1.4–11.5 hours and the $t_{1/2\beta}$ of desacetylcefotaxime is reported to range from 8.2–56.8 hours. The $t_{1/2\beta}$ of both cefotaxime and desacetylcefotaxime may be prolonged in patients with impaired hepatic function. In a study in patients with chronic parenchymal liver disease with or without jaundice, edema, or ascites, the $t_{1/2\beta}$ of the parent drug ranged from 1.49–2.42 hours and the apparent $t_{1/2}$ of the metabolite ranged from 7.1–13.4 hours.

In one study in children 5 months to 1 year of age, the $t_{1/2\alpha}$ of cefotaxime averaged 0.2 hours and the $t_{1/2\beta}$ averaged 1.2 hours. In children 2–12 years of age, the $t_{1/2\alpha}$ averaged 0.3 hours and the $t_{1/2\beta}$ averaged 1.5 hours. In neonates, the half-life of cefotaxime depends principally on gestational and chronologic age. The $t_{1/2\alpha}$ is reported to range from 0.1–0.4 hours in premature or full-term neonates. The $t_{1/2\beta}$ of cefotaxime averages 5–6 hours in premature neonates less than 1 week of age, 3.4–3.5 hours in premature neonates 1–4 weeks of age, 2–3.4 hours in full-term neonates less than 1 week of age, and 2 hours in full-term neonates 1–4 weeks of age.

Cefotaxime and its metabolites are excreted principally in urine; tubular secretion of the drug occurs. In adults with normal renal function, approximately 40–60% of a single IM or IV dose of cefotaxime is excreted in urine as unchanged drug and approximately 24% is excreted as desacetylcefotaxime within 24 hours. The majority of the IM or IV dose is excreted within the first 2 hours following administration. In one study, urine concentrations of cefotaxime ranged from 90–3261 mcg/mL in urine collected over 2 hours following a single 500-mg IM dose of cefotaxime.

The serum clearance of cefotaxime in adults with normal renal function is reported to be 207–342 mL/minute per 1.73 m². In one study, the serum clearance of the drug averaged 23 mL/minute per 1.73 m² in low birthweight neonates 1–7 days of age and 44 mL/minute per 1.73 m² in average birthweight neonates 1–7 days of age.

Oral probenecid administered shortly before or concomitantly with cefotaxime usually slows the rate of excretion of the antibiotic and its metabolites and produces higher and more prolonged serum concentrations of cefotaxime and its metabolites. The volume of distribution of cefotaxime does not appear to be affected by concomitant administration of oral probenecid.

Cefotaxime and its metabolites are removed by hemodialysis. The amount of cefotaxime removed during hemodialysis depends on several factors (e.g., type of coil used, dialysis flow-rate); however, a 4- to 6-hour period of hemodialysis in one study removed into the dialysate 60% of a single 15 mg/kg dose of cefotaxime when the dose was given by IV injection immediately prior to dialysis. Only minimal amounts of cefotaxime are removed by peritoneal dialysis.

Chemistry and Stability

■ **Chemistry** Cefotaxime is a semisynthetic cephalosporin antibiotic. Like cefepime, ceftazidime, and ceftriaxone, cefotaxime is a parenteral aminothiazolyl cephalosporin. Cefotaxime contains an aminothiazolyl-acetyl side chain, with an *α-syn*-methoximino group, at position 7 of the cephalosporin nucleus. The aminothiazolyl side chain enhances antibacterial activity, particularly against Enterobacteriaceae, and generally results in enhanced stability against β-lactamases; the methoximino group contributes to stability against hydrolysis by many β-lactamases.

Cefotaxime is commercially available as the sodium salt. Potency of cefotaxime sodium is expressed in terms of cefotaxime. Cefotaxime sodium occurs as an off-white to pale yellow, crystalline powder. Cefotaxime sodium is sparingly soluble in water, slightly soluble in alcohol, and has a pK_a of 3.4. The sodium salt of cefotaxime contains approximately 50.5 mg (2.2 mEq) of sodium per gram of cefotaxime.

Commercially available frozen premixed cefotaxime sodium injections containing 1 or 2 g of cefotaxime are sterile, nonpyrogenic, iso-osmotic solutions of the drug provided in a plastic container fabricated from specially formulated multilayered plastic (PL 2040). The 1- and 2-g frozen injections of cefotaxime contain approximately 1.7 g and 700 mg of dextrose hydrous, respectively, to adjust osmolality. The injections are buffered with sodium citrate hydrous and may contain hydrochloric acid and/or sodium hydroxide to adjust pH. After thawing, the injections are pale yellow to light amber solutions.

■ **Stability** Cefotaxime sodium powder for injection and solutions of the drug tend to darken, depending on storage conditions, and should be protected from excess heat and light. Discoloration of cefotaxime sodium sterile powder for injection or solutions of the drug may indicate a loss of potency.

Commercially available cefotaxime sodium sterile powder for injection should be stored at 15–30°C.

Following reconstitution as directed by the manufacturer, cefotaxime sodium solutions containing 50–330 mg of cefotaxime per mL have a pH of 4.5–6.5 and are light yellow to amber in color. Following reconstitution with sterile or bacteriostatic water for injection, IM solutions containing 230–330 mg/mL are stable in their original containers for 12 hours at room temperature (22°C or lower) or 7 days when refrigerated (5°C or lower). Following reconstitution with sterile water for injection, IV solutions containing 50 or 95 mg/mL are stable for 24 hours at room temperature (22°C or lower) or 7 days when refrigerated (5°C or lower). When reconstituted as directed in 0.9% sodium chloride injection or 5% dextrose injection, solutions prepared from ADD-Vantage® vials of the drug are stable for 24 hours at a room temperature of 22°C or less; these solutions should not be frozen.

Cefotaxime sodium is physically and chemically compatible with the following IV solutions: 0.9% sodium chloride; 5% or 10% dextrose; 5% dextrose and 0.2%, 0.45%, or 0.9% sodium chloride; lactated Ringer's; ¼ *M* sodium lactate; 10% invert sugar; or Travasol® 8.5%. Reconstituted solutions of cefotaxime sodium which have been further diluted with 50 mL to 1 liter of one of the above IV solutions are physically and chemically stable for 24 hours at room temperature or at least 5 days when refrigerated at 5°C or less. Cefotaxime sodium solutions are most stable at a pH of 5–7 and the drug should not be diluted with IV solutions (e.g., sodium bicarbonate) which have a pH greater than 7.5.

Reconstituted solutions of cefotaxime sodium which have been further diluted with 50 mL to 1 liter of 0.9% sodium chloride injection or 5% dextrose injection may be frozen in Viaflex® containers immediately after preparation and are stable for 13 weeks. Frozen solutions of cefotaxime sodium should be thawed at room temperature. Once thawed, solutions are stable for 24 hours at room temperature or 5 days at less than 5°C and should not be refrozen.

The commercially available frozen premixed cefotaxime sodium injection should be stored at −20°C or lower. Thawed solutions of the commercially available frozen injection are stable for 24 hours at room temperature (22°C or lower) or 10 days when refrigerated at 5°C or lower. The commercially available frozen injection of the drug is provided in a plastic container fabricated from specially formulated multilayered plastic PL 2040 (Galaxy® container). Solutions in contact with PL 2040 can leach out some of its chemical components in very small amounts within the expiration period of the injection; however, safety of the plastic has been confirmed in tests in animals according to USP biological tests for plastic containers as well as by tissue culture toxicity studies.

Cefotaxime sodium is potentially physically and/or chemically incompatible with some drugs, including aminoglycosides, but the compatibility depends on several factors (e.g., concentrations of the drugs, specific diluents used, resulting pH, temperature). Specialized references should be consulted for specific compatibility information. Because of the potential for incompatibility, cefotaxime sodium and aminoglycosides should not be admixed.

Preparations

Excipients in commercially available drug preparations may have clinically important effects in some individuals; consult specific product labeling for details.

Cefotaxime Sodium

Parenteral		
For injection	500 mg (of cefotaxime)*	**Cefotaxime Sodium for Injection**
		Claforan®, Sanofi-Aventis
	1 g (of cefotaxime)*	**Cefotaxime Sodium for Injection**
		Claforan®, Sanofi-Aventis
	2 g (of cefotaxime)*	**Cefotaxime Sodium for Injection**
		Claforan®, Sanofi-Aventis
	10 g (of cefotaxime) pharmacy bulk package*	**Cefotaxime Sodium for Injection**
		Claforan®, Sanofi-Aventis
For injection, for IV infusion	1 g (of cefotaxime)	**Claforan®**, Sanofi-Aventis
		Claforan® ADD-Vantage®, Sanofi-Aventis
	2 g (of cefotaxime)	**Claforan®**, Sanofi-Aventis
		Claforan® ADD-Vantage®, Sanofi-Aventis

*available from one or more manufacturer, distributor, and/or repackager by generic (nonproprietary) name

Cefotaxime Sodium in Dextrose

Parenteral		
Injection (frozen), for IV infusion	20 mg (of cefotaxime) per mL (1 g) in 3.4% Dextrose*	**Cefotaxime Sodium Iso-osmotic in Dextrose Injection** (Galaxy® [Baxter])
	40 mg (of cefotaxime) per mL (2 g) in 1.4% Dextrose*	**Cefotaxime Sodium Iso-osmotic in Dextrose Injection** (Galaxy® [Baxter])

*available from one or more manufacturer, distributor, and/or repackager by generic (nonproprietary) name

†Use is not currently included in the labeling approved by the US Food and Drug Administration

Cefpodoxime Proxetil

■ Cefpodoxime is a semisynthetic, third generation cephalosporin antibiotic.

Uses

Cefpodoxime proxetil is used orally for the treatment of mild to moderate respiratory tract infections (i.e., acute exacerbations of chronic bronchitis, acute maxillary sinusitis, community-acquired pneumonia) caused by susceptible bacteria; the treatment of acute otitis media caused by susceptible bacteria; and the treatment of pharyngitis and tonsillitis caused by *Streptococcus pyogenes* (group A β-hemolytic streptococci). The drug also is used orally for the treatment of uncomplicated gonorrhea and for the treatment of mild to moderate uncomplicated skin and skin structure or uncomplicated urinary tract infections caused by susceptible bacteria.

Prior to initiation of cefpodoxime proxetil therapy, appropriate specimens should be obtained for identification of the causative organism and in vitro susceptibility tests. Cefpodoxime proxetil may be started pending results of susceptibility tests but should be discontinued if the organism is found to be resistant to the drug.

■ **Acute Otitis Media** Oral cefpodoxime proxetil is used for the treatment of acute otitis media (AOM) caused by *Streptococcus pneumoniae* (penicillin-susceptible strains only), *Haemophilus influenzae* (including β-lactamase-producing strains), or *Moraxella catarrhalis* (including β-lactamase-producing strains).

When anti-infective therapy is indicated for the treatment of AOM, the American Academy of Pediatrics (AAP) recommends high-dose amoxicillin or amoxicillin and clavulanate potassium as the drugs of first choice for initial treatment. These experts recommend certain cephalosporins (cefdinir, cefpodoxime, cefuroxime, ceftriaxone) as alternatives for initial treatment in penicillin-allergic patients who do not have a history of severe and/or recent penicillin-allergic reactions.

Results of controlled clinical studies in children 2 months to 18 years of age with AOM indicate that an 8 to 10-day regimen of oral cefpodoxime proxetil is as effective as a 10-day regimen of oral amoxicillin and clavulanate potassium or a 10-day regimen of oral cefixime. In published studies, the overall clinical response rate to a 10-day regimen of oral cefpodoxime proxetil in pediatric patients with AOM has been 83–92% and the bacteriologic eradication rate has been 88–92%.

Cefpodoxime proxetil also has been effective for the treatment of AOM in pediatric patients when administered in a 5-day regimen. In one study in pediatric patients 1 month to 11 years of age with AOM randomized to receive a 5-day regimen of oral cefpodoxime proxetil (5 mg/kg of cefpodoxime every 12 hours) or a 5-day regimen of oral cefaclor (40 mg/kg daily given in 3 divided doses), the clinical response rate (cure or improvement) at the end of treatment was 93.6% in those who received cefpodoxime and 91.6% in those who received cefaclor; the rate of recurrence 30 days after completion of therapy was 6.4 or 7.2%, respectively. The AAP states that oral anti-infective regimens of less than 10 days' duration are not recommended for the treatment of AOM in children younger than 2 years of age or in patients with severe symptoms.

For additional information regarding treatment of AOM, including information on diagnosis and management strategies, anti-infectives for initial treatment, duration of initial treatment, and anti-infectives after initial treatment failure, see Acute Otitis Media under Uses: Otitis Media, in the Cephalosporins General Statement 8:12.06.

■ **Pharyngitis and Tonsillitis** Oral cefpodoxime proxetil is used for the treatment of pharyngitis and tonsillitis caused by susceptible *S. pyogenes* (group A β-hemolytic streptococci). Although cefpodoxime usually is effective in eradicating *S. pyogenes* from the nasopharynx, substantial data to establish efficacy of the drug for prophylaxis of subsequent rheumatic fever are not available to date.

Selection of an anti-infective for the treatment of *S. pyogenes* pharyngitis and tonsillitis should be based on the drug's spectrum of activity, bacteriologic and clinical efficacy, potential adverse effects, ease of administration, patient compliance, and cost. No regimen has been found to date that effectively eradicates group A β-hemolytic streptococci in 100% of patients.

Because the drugs have a narrow spectrum of activity, are inexpensive, and generally are effective with a low incidence of adverse effects, the AAP, Infectious Diseases Society of America (IDSA), American Heart Association (AHA), and others recommend a penicillin regimen (i.e., 10 days of oral penicillin V or oral amoxicillin or a single dose of IM penicillin G benzathine) as the treatment of choice for *S. pyogenes* pharyngitis and tonsillitis and prevention of initial attacks (primary prevention) of rheumatic fever. Other anti-infectives (e.g., oral cephalosporins, oral macrolides, oral clindamycin) are recommended as alternatives in penicillin-allergic individuals.

If an oral cephalosporin is used for the treatment of *S. pyogenes* pharyngitis and tonsillitis, a 10-day regimen of a first generation cephalosporin (cefadroxil, cephalexin) is preferred instead of other cephalosporins with broader spectrums of activity (e.g., cefaclor, cefdinir, cefixime, cefpodoxime, cefuroxime).

Although there is some evidence that a shorter duration of therapy with certain oral cephalosporins (e.g., a 5-day regimen of cefadroxil, cefdinir, cefixime, or cefpodoxime proxetil or a 4- or 5-day regimen of cefuroxime axetil) achieves bacteriologic and clinical cure rates equal to or greater than those achieved with the traditional 10-day oral penicillin V regimen, the IDSA and AHA state that use of cephalosporin regimens administered for 5 days or less for the treatment of *S. pyogenes* pharyngitis and tonsillitis cannot be recommended at this time.

Results of a randomized, multicenter study in pediatric patients 18 months to 18 years of age with *S. pyogenes* pharyngitis and tonsillitis indicate that a 10-day regimen of oral cefpodoxime proxetil (5 mg/kg of cefpodoxime twice daily) is more effective than a 10-day regimen of oral penicillin V (13.4 mg/kg 3 times daily). The clinical response rate (cure plus improvement) was 83.8% in those who received cefpodoxime and 77.5% in those who received penicillin V; the bacteriologic eradication rates were 93.1 or 81.2%, respectively.

Results of controlled comparative studies in adults and children with *S. pyogenes* pharyngitis and tonsillitis indicate that a 5-day regimen of oral cefpodoxime proxetil is at least as effective as a 5-day regimen of oral cefuroxime axetil or a 10-day regimen of oral penicillin V in eradicating the organism. In one study in adults and adolescents 11 years of age or older who were randomized to receive a 5-day regimen of oral cefpodoxime proxetil (100 mg of cefpodoxime twice daily) or a 10-day regimen of oral penicillin V (600 mg 3 times daily), the bacteriologic eradication rates were 96.7 or 94.2%, respectively.

■ **Respiratory Tract Infections** ***Acute Sinusitis*** Oral cefpodoxime proxetil is used for the treatment of acute maxillary sinusitis caused by susceptible *S. pneumoniae*, *H. influenzae* (including β-lactamase-producing strains), or *M. catarrhalis*.

When anti-infective therapy is indicated for the treatment of acute bacterial sinusitis, the IDSA recommends amoxicillin and clavulanate potassium and the AAP recommends either amoxicillin or amoxicillin and clavulanate potassium as the drug of choice for initial empiric treatment. Because of variable activity against *S. pneumoniae* and *H. influenzae*, the IDSA no longer recommends second or third generation oral cephalosporins for empiric monotherapy of sinusitis in adults or children. If an oral cephalosporin is used as an alternative for empiric treatment of acute bacterial sinusitis in children (e.g., in penicillin-allergic individuals), the IDSA and AAP recommend a combination regimen that includes a third generation cephalosporin (cefixime or cefpodoxime) and clindamycin (or linezolid).

In one study in adults with acute sinusitis who were randomized to receive oral cefpodoxime proxetil (200 mg of cefpodoxime twice daily) or oral cefaclor (500 mg 3 times daily), the overall clinical response rate (cure or improvement) was 95% in those who received cefpodoxime and 93% in those who received cefaclor; the bacteriologic eradication rates were 95 and 91%, respectively. Since sinus aspirate cultures are not routinely indicated in patients with acute sinusitis, the infection is treated empirically with an anti-infective regimen active against bacteria commonly involved in sinus infections (e.g., *S. pneumoniae*, *H. influenzae*, *M. catarrhalis*, *S. pyogenes*).

Acute Exacerbations of Chronic Bronchitis Oral cefpodoxime proxetil is used for the treatment of acute exacerbations of chronic bronchitis caused by susceptible *S. pneumoniae*, *H. influenzae* (non-β-lactamase-producing strains only), or *M. catarrhalis*. The manufacturer states that there is insufficient data available to establish efficacy of the drug in the treatment of acute bacterial exacerbations of chronic bronchitis caused by β-lactamase-producing strains of *H. influenzae*.

In one study in adults with acute exacerbations of chronic obstructive pulmonary disease who were randomized to receive a 10-day regimen of oral cefpodoxime proxetil (200 mg of cefpodoxime twice daily) or oral cefaclor (250 mg 3 times daily), the clinical response rate (cure or improvement) was 99% in those who received cefpodoxime and 92% in those who received cefaclor; the bacteriologic eradication rates were 91 and 92%, respectively. When results of patients who received cefpodoxime were stratified according to causative organism, the bacteriologic eradication rate was 91–100% in those with infections caused by *H. influenzae* (including β-lactamase-producing strains), *H. parainfluenzae* (including β-lactamase-producing strains), or non-β-lactamase-producing *M. catarrhalis* and 86% in those with infections caused by β-lactamase-producing *M. catarrhalis* or *S. pneumoniae*.

Community-acquired Pneumonia Oral cefpodoxime proxetil is used for the treatment of mild to moderate community-acquired pneumonia (CAP) caused by susceptible *S. pneumoniae* or *H. influenzae* (including β-lactamase-producing strains). The American Thoracic Society (ATS) and IDSA recommended cefpodoxime as an alternative for treatment of CAP caused by penicillin-susceptible *S. pneumoniae* and as an alternative in certain combination regimens used for empiric treatment of CAP.

Initial treatment of CAP generally involves use of an empiric anti-infective regimen based on the most likely pathogens and local susceptibility patterns; therapy may then be changed (if possible) to provide a more specific regimen (pathogen-directed therapy) based on results of in vitro culture and susceptibility testing. The most appropriate empiric regimen varies depending on the severity of illness at the time of presentation and whether outpatient treatment or hospitalization in or out of an intensive care unit (ICU) is indicated and the presence or absence of cardiopulmonary disease and other modifying factors that increase the risk of certain pathogens (e.g., penicillin- or multidrug-resistant *Streptococcus pneumoniae*, enteric gram-negative bacilli, *Pseudomonas aeruginosa*). Most experts recommend that an empiric regimen for treatment of CAP include an anti-infective active against *S. pneumoniae* since this organism is the most commonly identified cause of bacterial pneumonia and causes more severe disease than many other common CAP pathogens.

For empiric *outpatient* treatment of CAP when risk factors for drug-resistant *S. pneumoniae* are present (e.g., comorbidities such as chronic heart, lung, liver, or renal disease, diabetes, alcoholism, malignancies, asplenia, immunosuppression, use of anti-infectives within the last 3 months), ATS and IDSA recommend monotherapy with a fluoroquinolone active against *S. pneumoniae* (moxifloxacin, gemifloxacin, levofloxacin) or, alternatively, a combination regimen that includes a β-lactam active against *S. pneumoniae* (high-dose amoxicillin or fixed combination of amoxicillin and clavulanic acid or, alternatively, ceftriaxone, cefpodoxime, or cefuroxime) given in conjunction with a macrolide (azithromycin, clarithromycin, erythromycin) or doxycycline. Cefuroxime and cefpodoxime may be less active against *S. pneumoniae* than amoxicillin or ceftriaxone.

If an oral cephalosporin is used as an alternative to penicillin G or amoxicillin for treatment of CAP caused by penicillin-susceptible *S. pneumoniae*, ATS and IDSA recommend cefdinir, cefditoren, cefpodoxime, cefprozil, or cefuroxime.

For additional information on treatment of CAP, see Community-acquired

Pneumonia under Uses: Respiratory Tract Infections, in the Cephalosporins General Statement 8:12.06.

■ **Skin and Skin Structure Infections** Oral cefpodoxime proxetil is used for the treatment of mild to moderate uncomplicated skin and skin structure infections caused by *Staphylococcus aureus* (including penicillinase- and non-penicillinase-producing strains) or *S. pyogenes*. The manufacturer cautions that results of clinical trials indicate that effective treatment of skin and skin structure infections generally requires cefpodoxime dosages higher than those used for the treatment of other infections. (See Dosage and Administration: Dosage.) When cefpodoxime is used in the treatment of skin and skin structure infections, the fact that abscesses usually require surgical drainage should be considered.

■ **Urinary Tract Infections** Oral cefpodoxime proxetil is used for the treatment of uncomplicated urinary tract infections (cystitis) caused by susceptible *Escherichia coli, Klebsiella pneumoniae, Proteus mirabilis*, or *S. saprophyticus*.

In clinical studies in adults with uncomplicated urinary tract infections who received oral cefpodoxime proxetil (100 mg of cefpodoxime twice daily), the bacteriologic eradication rate has been 75–80% for infections caused by *E. coli, P. mirabilis*, or *S. saprophyticus* or 100% for infections caused by *Klebsiella*. However, the manufacturer cautions that cefpodoxime therapy has been associated with a lower clinical cure rate and a lower bacteriologic eradication rate than some other anti-infectives used for the treatment of cystitis, and this fact should be considered when selecting an anti-infective agent for the treatment of these infections.

Some clinicians suggest that certain oral third generation cephalosporins (cefdinir, cefpodoxime, ceftibuten) are one of several alternatives that can be used for the outpatient treatment of recurrent urinary tract infections or urinary tract infections that occur in patients who have indwelling urinary catheters or are acquired in hospitals or nursing homes since these infections are likely to be caused by multidrug-resistant gram-negative bacilli.

■ **Gonorrhea and Associated Infections** ***Uncomplicated Gonorrhea*** Oral cefpodoxime proxetil has been used for the treatment of acute uncomplicated urethral gonorrhea in men and uncomplicated urethral or endocervical gonorrhea in women caused by penicillinase-producing strains of *Neisseria gonorrhoeae* (PPNG) or nonpenicillinase-producing strains of the organism. The drug also has been used for the treatment of anorectal gonococcal infections in women, but efficacy for the treatment of anorectal gonococcal infections in men or pharyngeal gonococcal infections in men or women have not been established.

Because of concerns related to recent reports of *N. gonorrhoeae* with reduced susceptibility to cephalosporins, the US Centers for Disease Control and Prevention (CDC) states that oral cephalosporins are no longer recommended as first-line treatment for uncomplicated gonorrhea. For the treatment of uncomplicated urogenital, anorectal, or pharyngeal gonorrhea, the CDC recommends a combination regimen that includes a single dose of IM ceftriaxone *and* either a single dose of oral azithromycin or a 7-day regimen of oral doxycycline.

For information on current recommendations for the treatment of gonorrhea and associated infections, see Uses: Gonorrhea and Associated Infections in Ceftriaxone 8:12.06.12.

Dosage and Administration

■ **Reconstitution and Administration** Cefpodoxime proxetil is administered orally.

Cefpodoxime proxetil tablets should be administered with food to enhance GI absorption of the drug. (See Pharmacokinetics: Absorption.)

Cefpodoxime proxetil for oral suspension may be administered without regard to meals.

Reconstitution Cefpodoxime proxetil powder for oral suspension should be reconstituted at the time of dispensing by adding the amount of distilled water specified on the container to provide a suspension containing 50 or 100 mg of cefpodoxime per 5 mL. The water should be added in 2 approximately equal portions and the bottle shaken vigorously after each addition.

The oral suspension should be shaken prior to administration of each dose.

■ **Dosage** Cefpodoxime is commercially available as cefpodoxime proxetil; dosage is expressed in terms of cefpodoxime.

Adult Dosage **Pharyngitis and Tonsillitis.** The usual dosage of cefpodoxime for the treatment of pharyngitis and tonsillitis caused by *Streptococcus pyogenes* (group A β-hemolytic streptococci) in adults and adolescents 12 years of age or older is 100 mg every 12 hours for 5–10 days.

Cephalosporin regimens administered for 5 days or less are not recommended for the treatment of group A β-hemolytic streptococcal pharyngitis and tonsillitis. (See Uses: Pharyngitis and Tonsillitis.)

Respiratory Tract Infections. For the treatment of mild to moderate acute maxillary sinusitis, mild to moderate acute exacerbations of chronic bronchitis, or mild to moderate community-acquired pneumonia in adults and adolescents 12 years of age or older, the usual dosage of cefpodoxime is 200 mg every 12 hours for 10, 10, or 14 days, respectively.

Skin and Skin Structure Infections. For mild to moderate uncomplicated skin and skin structure infections in adults and adolescents 12 years of age or older, the usual dosage of cefpodoxime is 400 mg every 12 hours for 7–14 days.

Urinary Tract Infections. For the treatment of mild to moderate uncomplicated urinary tract infections in adults and adolescents 12 years of age or older, the usual dosage of cefpodoxime is 100 mg every 12 hours for 7 days.

Gonorrhea and Associated Infections. In adults and adolescents 12 years of age or older, the manufacturer states that a single 200-mg dose of cefpodoxime can be used for the treatment of uncomplicated urethral gonorrhea in men or uncomplicated urethral, endocervical, or anorectal gonorrhea in women. However, the US Centers for Disease Control and Prevention (CDC) does not recommend oral cephalosporins for first-line treatment of uncomplicated gonorrhea. (See Uses: Gonorrhea and Associated Infections.)

Pediatric Dosage Children 12 years of age or older may receive the usual adult dosage of cefpodoxime.

General Pediatric Dosage. For pediatric patients beyond the neonatal period, the American Academy of Pediatrics (AAP) recommends a cefpodoxime dosage of 10 mg/kg daily given in 2 divided doses for the treatment of mild to moderate infections. The AAP states that cefpodoxime is inappropriate for the treatment of severe infections.

Acute Otitis Media. For the treatment of acute otitis media (AOM) in children 2 months through 12 years of age, the dosage of cefpodoxime recommended by the manufacturer is 5 mg/kg (up to 200 mg) every 12 hours for 5 days.

The AAP states that oral anti-infective regimens of less than 10 days' duration are not recommended for the treatment of AOM in children younger than 2 years of age or in patients with severe symptoms.

Pharyngitis and Tonsillitis. For the treatment of mild to moderate pharyngitis and tonsillitis caused by *S. pyogenes* (group A β-hemolytic streptococci) in children 2 months through 12 years of age, the usual dosage of cefpodoxime is 5 mg/kg (up to 100 mg) every 12 hours for 5–10 days.

Cephalosporin regimens administered for 5 days or less are not recommended for the treatment of group A β-hemolytic streptococcal pharyngitis and tonsillitis. (See Uses: Pharyngitis and Tonsillitis.)

Acute Sinusitis. For the treatment of mild to moderate acute maxillary sinusitis in children 2 months through 12 years of age, the usual dosage of cefpodoxime is 5 mg/kg (up to 200 mg) every 12 hours for 10 days.

■ **Dosage in Renal and Hepatic Impairment** Patients with creatinine clearances of 30 mL/minute or greater may receive the usual dosage of cefpodoxime.

Patients with creatinine clearances less than 30 mL/minute should receive the usual dose of cefpodoxime given once every 24 hours. Patients maintained on hemodialysis should receive the usual dose 3 times weekly following dialysis.

The manufacturer states that modification of the usual dosage of cefpodoxime is not necessary in patients with hepatic impairment.

Cautions

■ **Adverse Effects** Adverse effects reported with cefpodoxime proxetil are similar to those reported with other oral cephalosporins. (See Cautions in the Cephalosporins General Statement 8:12.06.) Cefpodoxime proxetil generally is well tolerated. Most adverse effects are transient and mild to moderate in severity, but have been severe enough to require discontinuance of the drug in up to 2% of patients. GI effects, including diarrhea, loose stools, nausea, and vomiting, are the most frequent adverse reactions reported with cefpodoxime. Adverse GI effects may be dose related. Diarrhea or loose stools have been reported in about 6% of adults receiving a dosage of 200 mg of cefpodoxime daily, but have been reported in up to 11% of those receiving a dosage of 800 mg daily.

■ **Precautions and Contraindications** Cefpodoxime proxetil shares the toxic potentials of other cephalosporins, and the usual cautions, precautions, and contraindications associated with cephalosporin therapy should be observed. Prior to initiation of cefpodoxime proxetil therapy, careful inquiry should be made concerning previous hypersensitivity reactions to cephalosporins, penicillins, or other drugs. There is clinical and laboratory evidence of partial cross-allergenicity among cephalosporins and other β-lactam antibiotics, including penicillins and cephamycins. Cefpodoxime proxetil is contraindicated in patients who are hypersensitive to the drug or other cephalosporins and should be used with caution in patients with a history of hypersensitivity to penicillins. Use of cephalosporins should be avoided in patients who have had an immediate-type (anaphylactic) hypersensitivity reaction to penicillins. If a hypersensitivity reaction occurs during cefpodoxime proxetil therapy, the drug should be discontinued and the patient treated with appropriate therapy (e.g., epinephrine, corticosteroids, and maintenance of an adequate airway and oxygen) as indicated.

To reduce development of drug-resistant bacteria and maintain effectiveness of cefpodoxime and other antibacterials, the drug should be used only for the treatment or prevention of infections proven or strongly suspected to be caused by susceptible bacteria. When selecting or modifying anti-infective therapy, results of culture and in vitro susceptibility testing should be used. In the absence of such data, local epidemiology and susceptibility patterns should be considered when selecting anti-infectives for empiric therapy.

Patients should be advised that antibacterials (including cefpodoxime) should only be used to treat bacterial infections and not used to treat viral infections (e.g., the common cold). Patients also should be advised about the importance of completing the full course of therapy, even if feeling better after a few days, and that skipping doses or not completing therapy may decrease effectiveness and increase the likelihood that bacteria will develop resistance and will not be treatable with cefpodoxime or other antibacterials in the future.

Because *Clostridium difficile* infection (CDI) and *C. difficile*-associated diarrhea and colitis (CDAD; also known as antibiotic-associated diarrhea and colitis or pseudomembranous colitis) have been reported with nearly all anti-infectives, including cephalosporins, it should be considered in the differential diagnosis of patients who develop diarrhea during or after cefpodoxime therapy. Patients should be advised that diarrhea is a common problem caused by anti-infectives and usually ends when the drug is discontinued; however, they should contact a clinician if watery and bloody stools (with or without stomach cramps and fever) occur during or as late as 2 months or longer after the last dose.

Individuals with phenylketonuria should be cautioned that, depending on the manufacturer, cefpodoxime oral suspension may contain aspartame (NutraSweet®) that is metabolized in the GI tract to provide 17 mg of phenylalanine per 5 mL.

For a more complete discussion of these and other precautions associated with the use of cefpodoxime proxetil, see Cautions: Precautions and Contraindications in the Cephalosporins General Statement 8:12.06.

■ Pediatric Precautions Safety and efficacy of cefpodoxime proxetil in neonates and infants younger than 2 months of age have not been established.

Adverse effects reported in pediatric patients receiving oral cefpodoxime proxetil are similar to those reported in adults receiving the drug and include mild to moderate GI effects (diarrhea, vomiting) and dermatologic effects (rash, urticaria, pruritus).

■ Geriatric Precautions Efficacy and safety of cefpodoxime proxetil in geriatric adults are similar to those observed in younger adults. Although the plasma half-life of cefpodoxime may be slightly longer in geriatric adults than in younger adults, other pharmacokinetic parameters are unaffected and no adjustments in cefpodoxime dosage appear to be necessary in geriatric patients other than those related to renal impairment. (See Dosage and Administration: Dosage in Renal and Hepatic Impairment.)

■ Mutagenicity and Carcinogenicity In vivo and in vitro studies evaluating cefpodoxime have not shown evidence of mutagenicity. Long-term animal studies have not been performed to date to evaluate the carcinogenic potential of the drug.

■ Pregnancy, Fertility, and Lactation Reproduction studies in rats or rabbits using cefpodoxime dosages up to 100 mg/kg daily (approximately 2 times the usual human dosage on a mg/m² basis) or 30 mg/kg daily (approximately 1–2 times the usual human dosage on a mg/m² basis), respectively, have not revealed evidence of teratogenicity or harm to the fetus. There are no adequate and controlled studies using cefpodoxime proxetil in pregnant women or during labor and delivery, and the drug should be used during pregnancy only when clearly needed.

Studies in rats using oral cefpodoxime in dosages up to 100 mg/kg daily (approximately 2 times the usual human dosage based on a mg/m² basis) have not revealed evidence of impaired fertility.

Cefpodoxime is distributed into milk in low concentrations following oral administration. Because of the potential for serious adverse effects in nursing infants, a decision should be made whether to discontinue nursing or the drug, taking into account the importance of the drug to the mother.

Spectrum

Based on its spectrum of activity, cefpodoxime is classified as a third generation cephalosporin. For information on the classification of cephalosporins and closely related β-lactam antibiotics based on spectra of activity, see Spectrum in the Cephalosporins General Statement 8:12.06.

Cefpodoxime is stable in the presence of a variety of β-lactamases produced by gram-positive and gram-negative bacteria. Like other currently available oral third generation cephalosporins (e.g., cefdinir, cefixime, ceftibuten), cefpodoxime has an expanded spectrum of activity against aerobic gram-negative bacteria compared with first and second generation cephalosporins.

Cefpodoxime generally is inactive against enterococci (e.g., *Enterococcus faecalis*), methicillin-resistant (oxacillin-resistant) staphylococci, *Pseudomonas*, *Enterobacter*, and anaerobic bacteria.

■ In Vitro Susceptibility Testing Strains of staphylococci resistant to penicillinase-resistant penicillins (methicillin-resistant [oxacillin-resistant] staphylococci) should be considered resistant to cefpodoxime, although results of in vitro susceptibility tests may indicate that the organisms are susceptible to the drug.

For information on interpreting results of in vitro susceptibility testing (disk susceptibility tests, dilution susceptibility tests) when cefpodoxime susceptibility testing is performed according to the standards of the Clinical and Laboratory Standards Institute (CLSI; formerly National Committee for Clinical Laboratory Standards [NCCLS]), see Spectrum: In Vitro Susceptibility Testing, in the Cephalosporins General Statement 8:12.06.

Pharmacokinetics

Cefpodoxime proxetil is a prodrug and is inactive until hydrolyzed in vivo to cefpodoxime. Following oral administration of cefpodoxime proxetil, the drug is almost completely hydrolyzed to cefpodoxime by nonspecific esterases within the intestinal lumen.

In all studies described in the pharmacokinetics section, cefpodoxime was administered orally as cefpodoxime proxetil and dosages and concentrations of the drug are expressed in terms of cefpodoxime. Results of a study in healthy adults who received single 100-mg doses of cefpodoxime as cefpodoxime proxetil film-coated tablets or cefpodoxime proxetil oral suspension indicate that these formulations are bioequivalent.

Cefpodoxime exhibits linear pharmacokinetics over the oral dosage range of 100–400 mg; however, the drug exhibits nonlinear, dose-dependent pharmacokinetics at doses exceeding 400 mg. There is no evidence that cefpodoxime accumulates in plasma following multiple oral doses (up to 400 mg every 12 hours) in adults with normal renal function.

Studies in healthy geriatric adults indicate that the plasma half-life of cefpodoxime is increased slightly compared with the plasma half-life reported in younger adults, but other pharmacokinetic parameters are similar to those reported in younger adults. Studies in adults with impaired renal function indicate that the pharmacokinetics of cefpodoxime are affected by the degree of renal impairment and plasma half-life of the drug increases with decreasing renal impairment. The pharmacokinetics of cefpodoxime generally are unaffected by hepatic impairment, and the presence of ascites does not appear to affect pharmacokinetic parameters of the drug in individuals with cirrhosis.

■ Absorption Following oral administration of a single 100-mg oral dose of cefpodoxime in fasting adults, approximately 50% of the dose is absorbed from the GI tract.

Presence of food in the GI tract affects the bioavailability of cefpodoxime proxetil film-coated tablets, but does not appear to affect the bioavailability of cefpodoxime proxetil oral suspension. Compared with administration in the fasting state, administration of a 200-mg dose of cefpodoxime as cefpodoxime proxetil tablets with a meal results in a 21–33% increase in the area under the concentration-time curve (AUC) and a 15–24% increase in average peak plasma concentrations of the drug; the time to peak plasma concentrations is not affected. While administration of the commercially available oral suspension of cefpodoxime proxetil with food decreases the rate of absorption, the extent of absorption and peak plasma concentrations are not affected.

In healthy fasting adults who receive a single 100-, 200-, or 400-mg oral dose of cefpodoxime as cefpodoxime proxetil film-coated tablets, peak plasma concentrations of cefpodoxime are attained within 2–3 hours and average 1.4, 2.3, or 3.9 mcg/mL, respectively; plasma concentrations 8 hours after the dose average 0.29, 0.62, or 1.3 mcg/mL, respectively.

In pediatric patients 1–17 years of age who receive a single 5-mg/kg dose of cefpodoxime as cefpodoxime proxetil oral suspension, plasma concentrations of cefpodoxime average 1.4, 2.1, 1.7, 0.9, and 0.4 mcg/mL at 1, 2, 4, 6, and 8 hours, respectively, after the dose.

■ Distribution The apparent volume of distribution of cefpodoxime ranges from 0.7–1.15 L/kg in healthy adults with normal renal function.

Following oral administration, cefpodoxime is distributed into blister fluid, interstitial fluid, middle ear fluid, tonsils, maxillary sinus mucosa, bronchial mucosa, pleural fluid, lung tissue, epithelial lining fluid, myometrium, seminal fluid, prostatic adenoma tissue, and bile. In patients receiving cefpodoxime in an oral dosage of 200- or 400-mg every 12 hours for 5 days, peak concentrations of the drug in blister fluid averaged 1.6 or 2.8 mcg/mL, respectively; blister fluid concentrations 12 hours after dosing averaged 0.2 or 0.4 mcg/mL, respectively.

Following a single 100-mg oral dose of cefpodoxime as cefpodoxime proxetil film-coated tablets, peak concentrations of cefpodoxime in tonsillar tissue are attained 4 hours after the dose and average 0.24 mcg/mL; tonsillar tissue concentrations average 0.09 mcg/mL 7 hours after the dose and are undetectable 12 hours after the dose.

Following a single 4-mg/kg dose of cefpodoxime as cefpodoxime proxetil oral suspension in children 5 months to 9 years of age with acute otitis media, peak concentrations of the drug in middle ear fluid average 0.87 mcg/mL 2 hours after the dose.

Following a single 200-mg oral dose of cefpodoxime as cefpodoxime proxetil film-coated tablets, peak concentrations of the drug in lung tissue are attained 3 hours after the dose and average 0.63 mcg/mL; concentrations in lung tissue average 0.52 or 0.19 mcg/mL at 6 or 12 hours, respectively, after the dose.

Information on distribution of cefpodoxime into CSF is not available.

Cefpodoxime is distributed into milk in low concentrations following oral administration. In 3 nursing women who received a single 200-mg oral dose of cefpodoxime, concentrations of the drug in milk 4 hours after the dose were 0, 2, or 6% of concurrent plasma concentrations; milk concentrations 6 hours after the dose were 0, 9, or 16% of concurrent plasma concentrations.

Cefpodoxime is 22–33% bound to serum proteins or 21–29% bound to plasma proteins; binding is independent of drug concentration over the range of 0.1–7.1 mcg/mL.

■ Elimination In adults with normal renal function, the plasma half-life of cefpodoxime ranges from 2.1–2.9 hours.

Studies in healthy adults using radiolabeled cefpodoxime proxetil oral solution indicate that approximately 53% of the radioactivity is eliminated in urine and 43% is eliminated in feces as cefpodoxime. Studies in healthy adults indicate that approximately 29–33% of a single 100- to 400-mg oral dose of cefpodoxime is eliminated in urine within 12 hours.

The plasma half-life of cefpodoxime is prolonged in patients with renal impairment. In patients with mild renal impairment (creatinine clearance of 50–80 mL/minute), plasma half-life of the drug averages 3.5 hours; however, in those with moderate impairment (creatinine clearance of 30–49 mL/minute) or severe impairment (creatinine clearance 5–29 mL/minute), half-life of the drug averages 5.9 or 9.8 hours, respectively.

Cefpodoxime is removed by hemodialysis; approximately 23% of a single oral dose of the drug is removed by a 3-hour period of dialysis.

Chemistry and Stability

■ **Chemistry** Cefpodoxime is a semisynthetic cephalosporin antibiotic. The drug is an oral aminothiazolyl cephalosporin. Cefpodoxime is structurally similar to other oral (cefdinir, cefixime, ceftibuten) and parenteral (cefepime, cefotaxime, ceftazidime, ceftriaxone) cephalosporins that contain an aminothiazolyl side chain at position 7 of the cephalosporin nucleus. The aminothiazolyl group enhances antibacterial activity, particularly against Enterobacteriaceae, and generally results in enhanced stability against β-lactamases.

Cefpodoxime is commercially available for oral administration as cefpodoxime proxetil, the isopropyloxycarbonylethyl ester of cefpodoxime. Cefpodoxime proxetil is a prodrug of cefpodoxime and has little, if any, antibacterial activity until hydrolyzed in vivo to cefpodoxime. Esterification of the carboxy C-4 group of cefpodoxime results in a more lipophilic form of the drug that is more readily absorbed from the GI tract. Potency of cefpodoxime proxetil is expressed in terms of cefpodoxime.

Following reconstitution, cefpodoxime proxetil oral suspension contains 50 or 100 mg of cefpodoxime per 5 mL.

■ **Stability** Cefpodoxime proxetil tablets and powder for oral suspension should be stored at 20–25°C.

Following reconstitution, cefpodoxime proxetil oral suspension should be stored in a tight container at 2–8°C; any unused suspension should be discarded after 14 days.

For further information on chemistry, mechanism of action, spectrum, resistance, uses, cautions, acute toxicity, drug interactions, or laboratory test interferences of cefpodoxime proxetil, see the Cephalosporins General Statement 8:12.06.

Preparations

Excipients in commercially available drug preparations may have clinically important effects in some individuals; consult specific product labeling for details.

Cefpodoxime Proxetil

Oral		
For suspension	50 mg (of cefpodoxime) per 5 mL*	**Cefpodoxime Proxetil for Suspension**
	100 mg (of cefpodoxime) per 5 mL*	**Cefpodoxime Proxetil for Suspension**
Tablets, film-coated	100 mg (of cefpodoxime)*	**Cefpodoxime Proxetil Film-coated Tablets**
	200 mg (of cefpodoxime)*	**Cefpodoxime Proxetil Film-coated Tablets**

*available from one or more manufacturer, distributor, and/or repackager by generic (nonproprietary) name

cefTAZidime

■ Ceftazidime is a semisynthetic, third generation cephalosporin antibiotic.

Uses

Ceftazidime is used for the treatment of bone and joint infections, intra-abdominal and gynecologic infections, meningitis and other CNS infections, lower respiratory tract infections, skin and skin structure infections, septicemia, and complicated or uncomplicated urinary tract infections caused by susceptible bacteria. The drug also is used for empiric anti-infective agent therapy in febrile neutropenic patients† and has been used for perioperative prophylaxis†.

Ceftazidime therapy may be started pending results of susceptibility tests, but should be discontinued if the organism is found to be resistant to the drug. When the causative organism is unknown, concomitant therapy with another anti-infective agent may be indicated pending results of in vitro susceptibility tests. In severe or life-threatening infections or in immunocompromised patients, ceftazidime may be used concomitantly with other anti-infectives such as aminoglycosides, vancomycin, or clindamycin.

■ **Gram-positive Aerobic Bacterial Infections** Like other parenteral third generation cephalosporins (cefotaxime, ceftriaxone), ceftazidime is less active than first and second generation cephalosporins against some gram-positive bacteria (e.g., staphylococci) and generally should not be used in the treatment of infections caused by these organisms when a penicillin or first or second generation cephalosporin could be used. Although ceftazidime has been effective when used alone in adults or children for the treatment of septicemia, cellulitis, urinary tract infections, osteomyelitis, or respiratory tract infections (including pneumonia) caused by susceptible gram-positive cocci (e.g., *Staphylococcus aureus*, *S. epidermidis*, groups A and B streptococci, *Streptococcus pneumoniae*), treatment failures also have been reported in some of these infections, especially in immunocompromised patients or patients with cystic fibrosis. Therefore, ceftazidime is not used alone for empiric therapy in infections where gram-positive bacteria may be involved (e.g., community-acquired pneumonia).

■ **Gram-negative Aerobic Bacterial Infections** Ceftazidime generally has been effective when used alone in adults or children for the treatment of respiratory tract infections (including pneumonia), skin and skin structure infections, osteomyelitis, septicemia, intra-abdominal infections, or urinary tract infections caused by susceptible Enterobacteriaceae (e.g., *Enterobacter*, *Escherichia coli*, *Klebsiella*, *Morganella*, *Proteus*, *Serratia*). A principal use of ceftazidime is for the treatment of infections known or suspected to be caused by multidrug-resistant Enterobacteriaceae (e.g., nosocomial urinary tract infections or pneumonia, suspected septicemia in non-neutropenic patients) and serious gram-negative infections when other anti-infectives are contraindicated or ineffective. It has been suggested that certain parenteral cephalosporins (i.e., cefepime, cefotaxime, ceftriaxone, ceftazidime) may be drugs of choice for the treatment of infections caused by susceptible *E. coli*, *K. pneumoniae*, *P. rettgeri*, *M. morganii*, *P. vulgaris*, *P. stuartii*, or *Serratia*; an aminoglycoside (amikacin, gentamicin, tobramycin) should be used concomitantly in severe infections. There is some evidence that for the treatment of some infections (e.g., pneumonia, bacteremia) caused by susceptible Enterobacteriaceae, ceftazidime used alone can be as effective as a 2-drug regimen of a third generation cephalosporin or an extended-spectrum penicillin used in conjunction with an aminoglycoside.

■ **Mixed Aerobic-Anaerobic Bacterial Infections** Ceftazidime has been used with some success in the treatment of mixed aerobic-anaerobic bacterial infections. The manufacturers indicate that ceftazidime may be used in the treatment of polymicrobial intra-abdominal infections caused by aerobic and anaerobic bacteria, including *Bacteroides*; however, the drug should not be used alone for the treatment of any infection when *B. fragilis* may be present, since it generally is inactive against this organism.

■ **Intra-abdominal and Gynecologic Infections** Ceftazidime is used for the treatment of gynecologic infections (including endometritis, pelvic cellulitis, other infections of the female genital tract) caused by susceptible *E. coli*.

Ceftazidime also is used for the treatment of intra-abdominal infections (including peritonitis) caused by susceptible *S. aureus* (oxacillin-susceptible strains only), *E. coli*, or *Klebsiella*. and polymicrobial infections caused by aerobic and anaerobic bacteria.

For initial empiric treatment of high-risk or severe community-acquired extrabiliary intra-abdominal infections in adults (e.g., those with advanced age, immunocompromise, severe physiologic disturbance), the Infectious Diseases Society of America (IDSA) recommends either monotherapy with a carbapenem (doripenem, imipenem, meropenem) or the fixed combination of piperacillin and tazobactam, or a combination regimen that includes either a cephalosporin (cefepime, ceftazidime) or fluoroquinolone (ciprofloxacin, levofloxacin) in conjunction with metronidazole. IDSA also recommends ceftazidime in conjunction with metronidazole as one of several regimens that can be used for initial empiric treatment of health-care-associated complicated intra-abdominal infections in adults and community-acquired complicated intra-abdominal infections in pediatric patients.

For additional information regarding management of intra-abdominal infections, the current IDSA clinical practice guidelines available at http://www.idsociety.org should be consulted.

■ **Meningitis and Other CNS Infections** Ceftazidime used in conjunction with an aminoglycoside is considered a regimen of choice for the treatment of meningitis caused by susceptible *Pseudomonas aeruginosa* or susceptible Enterobacteriaceae† (e.g., *E. coli*, *P. mirabilis*, *Enterobacter*, *S. marcescens*). While ceftazidime also has been effective when used alone for the treatment of meningitis caused by susceptible *Haemophilus influenzae*, *Neisseria meningitidis*, or *S. pneumoniae*, cefotaxime or ceftriaxone generally is preferred when a cephalosporin is indicated for the treatment of meningitis caused by these organisms. (See Uses: Meningitis and Other CNS Infections in the Cephalosporins General Statement 8:12.06.)

Because preterm, low-birthweight neonates are at increased risk for nosocomial infection caused by staphylococci or gram-negative bacilli, some clinicians suggest that these neonates receive an empiric regimen of IV ceftazidime and IV vancomycin for suspected bacterial meningitis. Immunocompromised individuals, geriatric individuals, and individuals with recent head trauma, neurosurgery, or CSF shunts also are at increased risk for meningitis caused by gram-negative bacilli and some clinicians recommend that IV ceftazidime be use for empiric therapy in these patients. If ceftazidime is used for empiric therapy in individuals with meningitis, concomitant use of IV ampicillin should be considered to provide coverage against *Listeria monocytogenes*, especially in patients who are immunocompromised, infants younger than 3 months of age, or adults older than 50 years of age. In addition, for empiric therapy of meningitis in individuals with recent head trauma, neurosurgery, or CSF shunts, concomitant use of vancomycin should be considered to provide coverage against gram-positive bacteria. When results of culture and in vitro susceptibility tests become available and the pathogen is identified, the empiric anti-infective regimen should be modified (if necessary) to ensure that the most effective regimen is being administered.

In patients with meningitis caused by *Ps. aeruginosa*, many clinicians recommend that therapy be initiated with a regimen of ceftazidime and a parenteral aminoglycoside (amikacin, gentamicin, tobramycin). If the patient fails to respond to this regimen, concomitant use of intrathecal or intraventricular aminoglycoside therapy or use of an alternative parenteral anti-infective (e.g., aztreonam, meropenem, a fluoroquinolone) should be considered based on results of in vitro susceptibility tests.

■ **Septicemia** Ceftazidime is used in adult and pediatric patients for the treatment of septicemia caused by *S. aureus*, *S. pneumoniae*, *E. coli*, *H. influenzae*, *K. pneumoniae*, or *Ps. aeruginosa*. Some clinicians recommend that an aminoglycoside (amikacin, gentamicin, tobramycin) be used concomitantly for the treatment of gram-negative bacteremia in seriously ill patients.

The choice of anti-infective agent for the treatment of sepsis syndrome should be based on the probable source of infection, causative organism, immune status of the patient, and local patterns of bacterial resistance. For initial treatment of life-threatening sepsis in adults, some clinicians recommend that a third or fourth generation cephalosporin (cefepime, cefotaxime, ceftriaxone, ceftazidime), the fixed combination of piperacillin and tazobactam, or a carbapenem (doripenem, imipenem, meropenem) be used in conjunction with vancomycin; some experts also suggest including an aminoglycoside or fluoroquinolone during the initial few days of treatment.

■ **Urinary Tract Infections** Ceftazidime is used in adult and pediatric patients for the treatment of complicated and uncomplicated urinary tract infections caused by *Enterobacter*, *E. coli*, *Klebsiella*, *M. morganii*, *P. mirabilis*, *P. vulgaris*, or *Ps. aeruginosa*. The most appropriate agent for the treatment of urinary tract infections should be selected based on the severity of the infection and results of culture and in vitro susceptibility testing. It has been suggested that certain parenteral cephalosporins (i.e., cefepime, cefotaxime, ceftriaxone, ceftazidime) may be drugs of choice for the treatment of infections caused by susceptible Enterobacteriaceae, including susceptible *E. coli*, *K. pneumoniae*, *P. rettgeri*, *M. morganii*, *P. vulgaris*, *P. stuartii*, or *Serratia*; an aminoglycoside should be used concomitantly in severe infections. However, ceftazidime, like other third generation cephalosporins, generally should not be used in the treatment of uncomplicated urinary tract infections when other anti-infectives with a narrower spectrum of activity could be used.

■ **Pseudomonas aeruginosa Infections** Ceftazidime is used in adult and pediatric patients for the treatment of septicemia, osteomyelitis, respiratory tract, skin and skin structure, or urinary tract infections caused by susceptible *Ps. aeruginosa*. The drug also is used for the treatment of meningitis caused by *Ps. aeruginosa* (see Uses: Meningitis and Other CNS Infections) and has been used for the treatment of malignant otitis externa† caused by *Ps. aeruginosa* (see Otitis Externa under Uses: Otitis, in the Cephalosporins General Statement 8:12.06).

Ceftazidime generally has been considered a drug of choice for the treatment of infections caused by *Ps. aeruginosa* since it is more active in vitro on a weight basis against the organism than most other currently available cephalosporins and is active against some strains resistant to many other cephalosporins, aminoglycosides, and extended-spectrum penicillins. However, ceftazidime-resistant strains of *Ps. aeruginosa* can emerge during therapy with the drug, and superinfection with resistant strains has occurred. In severe infections, especially in immunocompromised patients, concomitant use of ceftazidime and an aminoglycoside (e.g., amikacin, gentamicin, tobramycin) is recommended.

For the treatment of community-acquired pneumonia (CAP) caused by *Ps. aeruginosa*, the American Thoracic Society (ATS) and IDSA recommend a combination regimen that includes an antipseudomonal β-lactam (cefepime, ceftazidime, aztreonam, imipenem, meropenem, piperacillin, ticarcillin) given in conjunction with ciprofloxacin, levofloxacin, or an aminoglycoside. For additional information on treatment of CAP, see Community-Acquired Pneumonia under Uses: Respiratory Tract Infections, in the Cephalosporins General Statement 8:12.06.

Ceftazidime is used alone or in conjunction with an aminoglycoside for the treatment of acute exacerbations of bronchopulmonary *Ps. aeruginosa* infections in children and adults with cystic fibrosis and generally is considered a drug of choice for these infections. In cystic fibrosis patients with acute exacerbations of *Ps. aeruginosa* infection, there is some evidence that an empiric regimen of ceftazidime and an aminoglycoside may be more effective than ceftazidime monotherapy; however, ceftazidime monotherapy appears to be as effective or more effective than monotherapy with aztreonam, ciprofloxacin, or meropenem or combination therapy with ticarcillin and tobramycin. Although anti-infective therapy in patients with cystic fibrosis may result in clinical improvement and *Ps. aeruginosa* may be temporarily cleared from the sputum, a bacteriologic cure is rarely obtained and should not be expected. Continuous IV infusion of ceftazidime has been used effectively for the treatment of *Ps. aeruginosa* infections in some adult and pediatric cystic fibrosis patients, including patients who failed to respond to ceftazidime administered by intermittent IV injection or infusion. Because a ceftazidime dosing regimen that consists of an IV loading dose followed by continuous IV infusion may provide more consistent concentrations of the drug than an intermittent dosing regimen, it has been suggested that such a regimen theoretically would be more effective in suppressing *Ps. aeruginosa* and possibly may decrease emergence of drug-resistant strains of the organism. Ceftazidime has been administered on an outpatient basis for the treatment of acute exacerbations of *Ps. aeruginosa* infections in cystic fibrosis patients; such community-based parenteral therapy generally is used to complete a course of ceftazidime therapy initiated during hospitalization.

■ **Burkholderia Infections** ***Burkholderia cepacia* Infections** Ceftazidime has been used alone or in conjunction with an aminoglycoside for the treatment of septicemia or pulmonary infections caused by *Burkholderia cepacia* (formerly *Ps. cepacia*)†. Patients with cystic fibrosis often are colonized with *B. cepacia* (with or without *Ps. aeruginosa* colonization). In addition, *B. cepacia* has recently been recognized as a cause of nosocomial pneumonia or nosocomial bacteremia in immunocompromised patients (e.g., patients with malignancy) *B. cepacia* is an aerobic, nonfermentative gram-negative bacilli resistant to many anti-infective agents, and no anti-infective regimen has been identified that effectively eradicates the organism in colonized cystic fibrosis patients. The optimum regimen for the treatment of infections caused by *B. cepacia* has not been identified. Some clinicians consider co-trimoxazole the drug of choice and ceftazidime, chloramphenicol, and imipenem alternative agents for the treatment of *B. cepacia* infections. Ceftazidime monotherapy has been used effectively to treat nosocomial *B. cepacia* bacteremia in a limited number of patients with severe underlying disease (e.g., malignancy); many of these patients had indwelling central venous catheters or recent surgery that may have precipitated the infection.

Melioidosis Ceftazidime is considered by many clinicians to be a drug of choice for the treatment of severe melioidosis†, a potentially life-threatening disease caused by *B. pseudomallei* (formerly *Ps. pseudomallei*).

B. pseudomallei is an aerobic, nonfermentative gram-negative bacilli resistant to many anti-infective agents (e.g., penicillins, first and second generation cephalosporins, aminoglycosides). *B. pseudomallei* may cause subclinical illness and localized infections or fulminant septicemia; disseminated infections may include hepatic and splenic abscesses. The incubation period usually is 1–21 days (median 9 days), but can be prolonged (years). In some asymptomatic individuals, the disease has remained dormant and active melioidosis was not evident for more than 20 years, usually at a time when the patient was immunosuppressed. If left untreated, severe septicemic infections can be fatal within 24–48 hours after onset. *B. pseudomallei* is widely distributed in water and soil in many tropical and subtropical countries and melioidosis is endemic in Southeast Asia (e.g., Thailand, Malaysia, Singapore) and northern Australia, and also is found in the Indian subcontinent and South and Central America. The disease occurs only rarely in the US. Person-to-person spread occurs only rarely. *B. pseudomallei* usually is transmitted to humans from contaminated materials (e.g., soil) via contact with nasal, oral, or conjunctival mucous membranes, contact with abraded or lacerated skin, or, rarely, by inhalation. Laboratory workers have become infected via aerosols from *B. pseudomallei* cultures.

Melioidosis, regardless of severity, should be treated with an initial parenteral regimen of ceftazidime, imipenem, or meropenem (some clinicians recommend that co-trimoxazole also be included, especially if the patient is septicemic) followed by a prolonged maintenance regimen of oral anti-infectives (e.g., co-trimoxazole with or without doxycycline). In patients with melioidosis septic shock, adjunctive use of filgrastim (granulocyte colony-stimulating factor; G-CSF) during initial treatment has been suggested. *B. pseudomallei* is difficult to eradicate, and relapse of melioidosis commonly occurs. Therefore, after the maintenance regimen is completed, life-long follow-up is recommended since relapse of melioidosis can occur despite effective anti-infective therapy. The fact that resistant strains of *B. pseudomallei* have developed during ceftazidime therapy should be considered.

B. pseudomallei has been studied for and is considered a potential pathogen for aerosol distribution in the context of biologic warfare or bioterrorism. Acute respiratory or systemic infection probably would occur following high-dose aerosol exposure to *B. pseudomallei*. Some experts (e.g., US Army Medical Research Institute of Infectious Diseases [USAMRIID], European Commission's Task Force on Biological and Chemical Agent Threats [BICHAT]) state that the same treatment regimens recommended for naturally occurring melioidosis should be used if the disease occurs in the context of biologic warfare or bioterrorism.

Ceftazidime monotherapy (40 mg/kg or 2 g IV 3 times daily) has been effective for the treatment of severe septicemic or pulmonary melioidosis, and has been associated with a lower mortality rate than a 3-drug regimen of IV chloramphenicol, oral doxycycline, and oral co-trimoxazole. In an open, prospective study in adults with acute severe melioidosis randomized to receive an initial parenteral regimen of IV ceftazidime or IV imipenem followed by an oral maintenance regimen, the survival rate at 48 hours was similar with both drugs (20.8% of those receiving ceftazidime and 25% of those receiving imipenem died within the first 48 hours), and the choice of initial drug did not appear to influence the final outcome; however, a higher percentage of patients receiving ceftazidime were considered to be treatment failures after 48 hours and had to be switched to an alternative drug because of primary treatment failure.

■ **Vibrio vulnificus Infections** Ceftazidime is considered by some clinicians to be a drug of choice for the treatment of infections caused by *Vibrio vulnificus*†. *V. vulnificus*, a gram-negative aerobic bacteria that can cause potentially fatal septicemia, wound infections, or gastroenteritis, generally is transmitted through ingestion of contaminated raw or undercooked seafood (especially raw oysters) or through contamination of a wound with seawater or seafood drippings. *V. vulnificus* is naturally present in marine environments, thrives in warm ocean water, and frequently is isolated from oysters and other shellfish harvested from the Gulf of Mexico and from US coastal waters along the Pacific and Atlantic ocean. Individuals with preexisting liver disease are at high risk for developing fatal septicemia following ingestion of seafood contaminated with *V. vulnificus* and debilitated or immunocompromised individuals (e.g., those with chronic renal impairment, cancer, diabetes mellitus, steroid-dependent asthma, chronic GI disease) or individuals with iron overload states (e.g., thalassemia and hemochromatosis) also are at increased risk for fatal infections. The incubation period for *V. vulnificus* infection reportedly is 1–7 days and the duration of illness usually is 2–8 days. In immunocompromised individuals, fever, nausea, myalgia, and abdominal cramps may occur as soon as 24–48 hours after ingestion of seafood contaminated with *V. vulnificus* and sepsis and cutaneous bullae may be present within 36 hours of the onset of symptoms.

Because the case fatality rate for *V. vulnificus* septicemia exceeds 50% in immunocompromised individuals or those with preexisting liver disease, these individuals should be informed about the health hazards of ingesting raw or undercooked seafood (especially oysters), the need to avoid contact with seawater during the warm months, and the importance of using protective clothing (e.g., gloves) when handling shellfish. *V. vulnificus* infection should be considered in the differential diagnosis of fever of unknown etiology, and individuals who present with fever (especially when bullae, cellulitis, or wound infection is present) and who have preexisting liver disease or are immunocompromised should be questioned regarding a history of raw oyster ingestion or seawater contact. While optimum anti-infective therapy for the treatment of *V. vulnificus* infections has not been identified, use of a tetracycline or third generation cephalosporin (e.g., cefotaxime, ceftazidime) is recommended. Because the high fatality rate associated with *V. vulnificus* infections, anti-infective therapy should be initiated promptly if indicated.

■ **Empiric Therapy in Febrile Neutropenic Patients** Ceftazidime has been effective when used alone or in conjunction with other anti-infectives for empiric anti-infective therapy of presumed bacterial infections in febrile granulocytopenic adults or children†.

Results of several studies in febrile granulocytopenic patients indicate that ceftazidime used alone may be as effective as combination regimens that include ceftazidime and an aminoglycoside (e.g., amikacin, gentamicin, tobramycin) or combination regimens that include some other β-lactam antibiotic (e.g., cefepime, ceftriaxone, piperacillin) and an aminoglycoside for empiric therapy in these patients. Results of a randomized study in adults indicate that ceftazidime monotherapy (2 g IV every 8 hours) is as effective as meropenem monotherapy (1 g IV every 8 hours) for empiric anti-infective therapy in febrile neutropenic patients; at the end of therapy, a satisfactory response was obtained in 49 or 46% of those receiving ceftazidime or meropenem, respectively. Because gram-positive bacteria are being reported with increasing frequency in febrile granulocytopenic patients and because ceftazidime is less active against these organisms than many other cephalosporins and β-lactam antibiotics, some clinicians suggest that an anti-infective agent active against staphylococci (e.g., vancomycin) probably should be used concomitantly if ceftazidime is used for empiric therapy in these patients. However, unlike ceftazidime, other anti-infectives used for empiric therapy (e.g., cefepime, imipenem, meropenem) have good activity against viridans streptococci and *S. pneumoniae*.

Successful treatment of infections in granulocytopenic patients requires prompt initiation of empiric anti-infective therapy (even when fever is the only sign or symptom of infection) and appropriate modification of the initial regimen if the duration of fever and neutropenia is protracted, if a specific site of infection is identified, or if organisms resistant to the initial regimen are present. The initial empiric regimen should be chosen based on the underlying disease and other host factors that may affect the degree of risk; local epidemiologic data regarding the type, frequency of occurrence, and in vitro susceptibility of bacterial isolates recovered from other patients in the same health-care facility; and the individual patient's pattern of colonization and resistance. No empiric regimen has been identified that would be appropriate for initial treatment of all febrile neutropenic patients. Regardless of the initial regimen selected, patients should be reassessed daily and the anti-infective regimen altered (if indicated) based on the presence or absence of fever, identification of the causative organism, and the clinical condition of the patient.

The fact that gram-positive bacteria have become a predominant pathogen in febrile neutropenic patients should be considered when selecting an empiric anti-infective regimen. The IDSA states that ceftazidime is no longer a reliable agent for empiric monotherapy in febrile neutropenic patients because of decreasing potency against gram-negative bacteria and poor activity against many gram-positive bacteria (e.g., streptococci).

Published protocols for the treatment of infections in febrile neutropenic patients should be consulted for specific recommendations regarding selection of the initial empiric anti-infective regimen, when to change the initial regimen, possible subsequent regimens, and duration of therapy in these patients. In addition, consultation with an infectious disease expert knowledgeable about infections in immunocompromised patients is advised.

■ **Perioperative Prophylaxis** Ceftazidime has been used for perioperative prophylaxis† in patients undergoing vaginal hysterectomy, biliary or intra-abdominal surgery, or transurethral resection of the prostate; however, many clinicians state that ceftazidime should not be used prophylactically.

A first or second generation cephalosporin (cefazolin, cefoxitin, cefotetan, cefuroxime) generally is preferred when a cephalosporin is used for perioperative prophylaxis. Third generation cephalosporins (cefotaxime, ceftriaxone, ceftazidime) and fourth generation cephalosporins (cefepime) are not usually recommended for perioperative prophylaxis because they are expensive, some are less active than first or second generation cephalosporins against staphylococci, they have spectrums of activity wider than necessary for organisms encountered in elective surgery, and their use for prophylaxis may promote emergence of resistant organisms. (See Uses: Perioperative Prophylaxis, in the Cephalosporins General Statement 8:12.06.)

Dosage and Administration

■ **Reconstitution and Administration** Ceftazidime sodium (as commercially available formulations of ceftazidime with sodium carbonate) is administered by intermittent IV injection or infusion or by deep IM injection. Ceftazidime sodium premixed with dextrose injection is administered by continuous or intermittent IV infusion. Ceftazidime sodium also has been administered by continuous IV infusion† and has been administered intraperitoneally in dialysis solutions. *Intra-arterial injection should be avoided since distal necrosis can occur.*

The IV route usually is preferred in patients with septicemia, meningitis, peritonitis, or other severe or life-threatening infections and in patients with lowered resistance resulting from malnutrition, trauma, surgery, diabetes, heart failure, or malignancy, particularly if shock is present or impending.

If an aminoglycoside or vancomycin is administered concomitantly with ceftazidime or ceftazidime sodium, the drugs should be administered at separate sites. Reconstituted and diluted solutions of ceftazidime or ceftazidime sodium should be inspected visually for particulate matter prior to administration whenever solution and container permit.

Intermittent IV Infusion Vials labeled as containing 500 mg, 1 g, or 2 g of ceftazidime with sodium carbonate should be reconstituted with 5.3, 10, or 10 mL, respectively, of sterile water for injection or a compatible IV solution to provide solutions containing approximately 100, 100, or 170 mg/mL, respectively. After adding the diluent to the vial, the vial should be shaken to dissolve the drug. With sodium carbonate formulations of ceftazidime, carbon dioxide is released as the drug dissolves and the solution will become clear within 1–2 minutes. The appropriate dose of the drug should then be added to a compatible IV solution. When withdrawing a dose from reconstituted vials, ensure that the syringe needle opening remains within the solution. The withdrawn solution may contain some carbon dioxide bubbles, which should be expelled from the syringe before injection.

Alternatively, TwistVial® (Fortaz®) or ADD-Vantage® (Tazicef®) vials labeled as containing 1 or 2 g of ceftazidime with sodium carbonate should be reconstituted according to the manufacturer's directions. Carbon dioxide that forms inside the package in sodium carbonate formulations of ceftazidime should be relieved by inserting a vent needle; to preserve sterility, it is important that the vent needle be inserted through the vial closure only after the drug has dissolved. The vent needle should be removed prior to use of the solution.

Alternatively, the commercially available Duplex® drug delivery system containing 1 or 2 g of ceftazidime and 50 mL of 5% dextrose injection in separate chambers should be reconstituted (activated) according to the manufacturer's directions and administered by IV infusion. If stored in the refrigerator after reconstitution (see Chemistry and Stability: Stability), the solution should be allowed to reach room temperature prior to administration.

The 6-g pharmacy bulk vial of ceftazidime as a sodium carbonate formulation should be reconstituted with sterile water for injection according to the manufacturer's directions. The pharmacy bulk vial is *not* intended for direct IV infusion.

Thawed solutions of the commercially available frozen premixed ceftazidime sodium injection in dextrose may be administered by continuous or intermittent IV infusion. The frozen injections should be thawed at room temperature (25°C) or under refrigeration (5°C); the injections should *not* be thawed by warming in a water bath or by exposure to microwave radiation. Precipitates that may have formed in the frozen injections usually will dissolve with little or no agitation when the injections reach room temperature; potency is not affected. After thawing to room temperature, the injection should be agitated and the container checked for minute leaks by firmly squeezing the bag. The injection should be discarded if container seals or outlet ports are not intact or leaks are found or if the solution is cloudy or contains an insoluble precipitate. Additives should not be introduced into the injection container. The injections should not be used in series connections with other plastic containers, since such use could result in air embolism from residual air being drawn from the primary container before administration of fluid from the secondary container is complete.

If a Y-type administration set is used, the other solution flowing through the tubing should be discontinued while ceftazidime or ceftazidime sodium is being infused.

Rate of Administration. Intermittent IV infusions of ceftazidime sodium have generally been infused over 15–30 minutes in adults, neonates, and children.

Intermittent IV Injection For direct intermittent IV injection, vials labeled as containing 500 mg, 1 g, or 2 g of ceftazidime with sodium carbonate should be reconstituted with sterile water for injection as for initial reconstitution for IV infusion to provide solutions containing 100, 100, or 170 mg/mL, respectively. (See Reconstitution and Administration: Intermittent IV Infusion, in Dosage and Administration.) When withdrawing a dose from reconstituted vials of ceftazidime sodium, ensure that the syringe needle opening remains within the solution. Any carbon dioxide bubbles that may be present in the withdrawn solution of ceftazidime sodium should be expelled from the syringe prior to injection.

The appropriate dose of reconstituted ceftazidime sodium should be injected over a period of 3–5 minutes directly into a vein or the tubing of a compatible IV solution.

IM Injection For IM injection, vials labeled as containing 500 mg or 1 g of ceftazidime with sodium carbonate (Fortaz®) are prepared by adding 1.5 or 3 mL of sterile or bacteriostatic water for injection or 0.5 or 1% lidocaine hydrochloride injection, respectively, to provide solutions containing approximately 280 mg/mL. When withdrawing a dose from reconstituted vials of ceftazidime sodium, ensure that the syringe needle opening remains within the solution. Any carbon dioxide bubbles that may be present in the withdrawn solution of ceftazidime sodium should be expelled from the syringe prior to injection.

IM injections should be made deeply into a large muscle mass, such as the upper outer quadrant of the gluteus maximus or lateral part of the thigh, using usual techniques and precautions.

Intraperitoneal Instillation For intraperitoneal instillation, a sodium carbonate formulation of ceftazidime powder for injection can be reconstituted with sterile water for injection as for initial reconstitution for IV infusion. (See Reconstitution and Administration: Intermittent IV Infusion, in Dosage and Administration.) The manufacturers of the sodium carbonate formulations of ceftazidime recommend that the drug then be further diluted in a compatible peritoneal dialysis solution to provide a solution containing 250 mg of ceftazidime in each 2 L of dialysis solution.

■ Dosage

Following reconstitution of the commercially available powders for injection containing a mixture of ceftazidime (as the pentahydrate) and sodium carbonate, solutions contain ceftazidime sodium; dosage of the drug is expressed in terms of anhydrous ceftazidime.

To avoid unintentional overdosage, the commercially available Duplex® drug delivery system containing ceftazidime and dextrose injection should *not* be used in patients who require less than the entire 1- or 2-g dose in the container.

Adult Dosage **General Adult Dosage.** The usual adult dosage of ceftazidime for the treatment of less severe infections caused by susceptible organisms is 1 g given IV or IM every 8 or 12 hours; however, the dosage and route of administration should be determined by the susceptibility of the causative organism, the severity of the infection, and the condition and renal function of the patient. For severe or life-threatening infections, especially in immunocompromised patients, a dosage of 2 g every 8 hours is recommended.

The maximum adult dosage of ceftazidime recommended by the manufacturers is 6 g daily.

Bone and Joint Infections. For the treatment of bone and joint infections, the usual adult dosage is 2 g IV every 12 hours.

Intra-abdominal and Gynecologic Infections. For the treatment of serious gynecologic and intra-abdominal infections, the usual adult dosage of ceftazidime is 2 g IV every 8 hours.

Meningitis. For the treatment of meningitis, the usual dosage of ceftazidime is 2 g IV every 8 hours. Because of a high rate of relapse, anti-infective therapy in patients with meningitis caused by gram-negative bacilli generally should be continued for at least 3 weeks.

Respiratory Tract Infections. The usual adult dosage of the drug for the treatment of uncomplicated pneumonia is 0.5–1 g IV or IM every 8 hours.

Skin and Skin Structure Infections. The usual adult dosage of the drug for the treatment of mild skin and skin structure infections is 0.5–1 g IV or IM every 8 hours.

Urinary Tract Infections. The manufacturers recommend that adults with uncomplicated urinary tract infections receive 250 mg of ceftazidime IV or IM every 12 hours and that adults with complicated urinary tract infections receive 500 mg IV or IM every 8 or 12 hours.

Pseudomonas aeruginosa Infections. For the treatment of pulmonary infections caused by *Pseudomonas aeruginosa* in patients with cystic fibrosis and normal renal function, the usual dosage of ceftazidime is 30–50 mg/kg given IV every 8 hours up to a maximum dosage of 6 g daily. Clinical improvement may occur, but bacteriologic cures should not be expected in patients with chronic respiratory disease and cystic fibrosis.

Burkholderia Infections. For the treatment of melioidosis† caused by *Burkholderia pseudomallei*, the US Army Medical Research Institute of Infectious Diseases (USAMRIID) recommends a ceftazidime dosage of 40 mg/kg every 8 hours. Other clinicians recommend a ceftazidime dosage of 2 g IV every 8 hours (up to 6 g daily) or 50 mg/kg (up to 2 g) IV every 6 hours. Concomitant co-trimoxazole (6–8 mg/kg of trimethoprim daily in 4 divided doses) or doxycycline (100 mg IV twice daily) may be indicated in septicemic or other severe cases. The initial parenteral regimen should be continued for at least 10–14 days and until there is clinical improvement. Although the median time to fever resolution is 9 days, some patients may remain febrile for prolonged periods despite appropriate antimicrobial therapy. When appropriate, treatment may be changed to an oral maintenance regimen (e.g., oral co-trimoxazole with or without oral doxycycline) and continued for at least 3–6 months to prevent recrudence or relapse. More prolonged oral maintenance therapy (up to 12 months) may be necessary, depending on the response to therapy and severity of initial illness.

Although only limited experience is available regarding the treatment of human cases of glanders†, some clinicians suggest that the regimens recommended for the treatment of severe melioidosis also can be used for the treatment of glanders.

Empiric Therapy in Febrile Neutropenic Patients. If ceftazidime is used for empiric anti-infective therapy in febrile neutropenic patients† (see Uses: Empiric Therapy in Febrile Neutropenic Patients), the usual dosage of the drug is 100 mg/kg daily given IV in 3 divided doses or 2 g IV every 8 hours either alone or in conjunction with an aminoglycoside (amikacin, gentamicin, tobramycin).

Pediatric Dosage Children 12 years of age and older may receive the usual adult dosage of ceftazidime.

General Dosage for Neonates. The usual dosage of ceftazidime recommended by the manufacturers for neonates up to 4 weeks of age is 30 mg/kg IV every 12 hours.

The American Academy of Pediatrics (AAP) recommends that neonates 7 days of age or younger receive 50 mg/kg of ceftazidime every 12 hours, regardless of weight. For neonates 8–28 days of age, the AAP recommends a dosage of 50 mg every 8–12 hours for those weighing 2 kg or less and 50 mg/kg every 8 hours for those weighing more than 2 kg.

General Dosage for Infants and Children. The usual dosage of ceftazidime for children 1 month to 12 years of age is 25–50 mg/kg IV every 8 hours, depending on the type and severity of infection. The manufacturers state that the maximum ceftazidime dosage for children 1 month to 12 years of age is 6 g daily, and that the higher dosage (i.e., 50 mg/kg every 8 hours) should be used in immunocompromised children or children with cystic fibrosis or meningitis.

The AAP recommends that children beyond the neonatal period receive ceftazidime in a dosage of 90–150 mg/kg daily in 3 equally divided doses for the treatment of mild to moderate infections or 200–300 mg/kg daily in 3 equally divided doses for the treatment of severe infections.

Meningitis. For the treatment of meningitis, some clinicians recommend a ceftazidime dosage of 100–150 mg/kg daily in 2 or 3 equally divided doses for neonates 7 days of age or younger and 150 mg/kg daily in 3 divided doses in older neonates and children. Because of a high rate of relapse, anti-infective therapy in patients with meningitis caused by gram-negative bacilli generally should be continued for at least 3 weeks. For treatment of meningitis in neonates, some clinicians recommend that anti-infective treatment be continued for 2 weeks beyond the first sterile CSF culture or at least 3 weeks, whichever is longer.

Burkholderia Infections. For the treatment of melioidosis† caused by *B. pseudomallei*, some clinicians recommend a ceftazidime dosage of 60 mg/kg daily given IV in 2 equally divided doses in children younger than 2 months of age or 100 mg/kg daily given IV in 3 equally divided doses in children 2 months of age or older. Concomitant co-trimoxazole (6–8 mg/kg of trimethoprim daily) or doxycycline may be indicated in septicemic or other severe cases. The initial parenteral regimen should be continued for at least 10–14 days and until there is clinical improvement. When appropriate, treatment may be changed to an oral maintenance regimen (e.g., oral co-trimoxazole with or without oral doxycycline) and continued for at least 3–6 months to prevent recrudence or relapse. More prolonged oral maintenance therapy (up to 12 months) may be necessary, depending on the response to therapy and severity of initial illness.

Empiric Therapy in Febrile Neutropenic Patients. For empiric anti-infective therapy in febrile neutropenic patients†, pediatric patients 2 years of age or older have received ceftazidime in a dosage of 50 mg/kg (maximum 2 g) every 8 hours. (See Uses: Empiric Therapy in Febrile Neutropenic Patients.)

Duration of Therapy The duration of ceftazidime therapy depends on the type and severity of infection and should be determined by the clinical and bacteriologic response of the patient. For most infections, therapy generally should be continued for at least 48 hours after the patient becomes asymptomatic or evidence of eradication of the infection has been obtained. Complicated infections may require more prolonged therapy.

■ Dosage in Renal and Hepatic Impairment

In patients with renal impairment, doses and/or frequency of administration of ceftazidime should be modified in response to the degree of renal impairment, severity of the infection, and susceptibility of the causative organism. Excessive dosage and elevated plasma concentrations of the drug in patients with renal impairment can precipitate serious neurotoxicity (e.g., seizures, encephalopathy, coma, asterixis, neuromuscular excitability, myoclonia).

The manufacturers recommend that adults with creatinine clearances of 50 mL/minute or less receive an initial loading dose of 1 g of ceftazidime and a maintenance dosage based on the patient's creatinine clearance. (See Table 1.)

Table 1. Maintenance Dosage for Adults with Renal Impairment

Creatinine Clearance (mL/minute)	Dosage
31–50	1 g every 12 h
16–30	1 g every 24 h
6–15	500 mg every 24 h
<5	500 mg every 48 h

In patients with renal impairment and severe infections who would generally receive a ceftazidime dosage of 6 g daily if their renal function were normal, the manufacturers state that doses in the above table may be increased by 50% or the dosing frequency may be increased appropriately.

Alternatively, some clinicians recommend that adults with creatinine clearances of 30–80 mL/minute receive the usual doses of ceftazidime every 12–24 hours, adults with creatinine clearances of 10–29 mL/minute receive the usual doses every 24–36 hours, and adults with creatinine clearances less than 10 mL/minute receive the usual doses every 36–48 hours.

Because ceftazidime is removed by hemodialysis, a supplemental dose of the drug is generally indicated after each dialysis period. The manufacturers recommend that adults undergoing hemodialysis receive an initial 1-g loading dose of ceftazidime followed by a 1-g dose after each dialysis period.

In adults undergoing intraperitoneal dialysis or continuous ambulatory peritoneal dialysis, the manufacturers recommend that an initial 1-g loading dose of ceftazidime be given followed by a 500-mg dose every 24 hours. Some clinicians recommend that patients undergoing peritoneal dialysis receive 500 mg of ceftazidime every 24 hours and a supplemental 500-mg dose of the drug at the end of each dialysis period. If ceftazidime (as a sodium carbonate formulation) is administered intraperitoneally in the dialysis solution, the manufacturers recommend that 250 mg of the drug be added to each 2 L of dialysis solution.

In children with impaired renal function, the frequency of dosing should be decreased based on the degree of impairment.

Modification of the usual dosage of ceftazidime is generally unnecessary in patients with impaired hepatic function, unless renal function is also impaired.

Cautions

Adverse effects reported with ceftazidime are similar to those reported with other cephalosporins. For information on adverse effects reported with cephalosporins, see Cautions in the Cephalosporins General Statement and other monographs in 8:12.06. Ceftazidime is generally well tolerated; adverse effects have been reported in about 9% of patients receiving the drug and have required discontinuance in about 2% of patients.

■ **Hematologic Effects** Eosinophilia has generally been reported in less than 7% of patients receiving ceftazidime. Thrombocytosis has occurred in about 2% of patients receiving the drug. Transient leukopenia, neutropenia, thrombocytopenia, agranulocytosis, and lymphocytosis have been reported rarely.

Positive direct antiglobulin (Coombs') test results have occurred in about 5% of patients receiving ceftazidime. In most reported cases, there was no clinical or laboratory evidence of hemolysis. However, hemolytic anemia has been reported rarely. In one patient with a positive direct antiglobulin test, mild hemolytic anemia occurred; the serum of this patient reacted with ceftazidime-treated erythrocytes, but did not react with untreated erythrocytes.

Cephalosporins have been reported to cause hypothrombinemia. Patients with renal or hepatic impairment, poor nutritional status, or those receiving a protracted course of anti-infective therapy are at particular risk of cephalosporin-induced hypothrombinemia. Prothrombin time should be monitored and vitamin K administered as indicated in patients who are at risk of developing hypothrombinemia.

■ **GI Effects** Adverse GI effects, including diarrhea, nausea, vomiting, abdominal pain, and a metallic taste, have been reported in less than 2% of patients receiving ceftazidime.

***Clostridium difficile*-associated Diarrhea and Colitis** Treatment with anti-infectives alters the normal flora of the colon and may permit overgrowth of *Clostridium difficile*.

C. difficile infection (CDI) and *C. difficile*-associated diarrhea and colitis (CDAD; also known as antibiotic-associated diarrhea and colitis or pseudomembranous colitis) have been reported with nearly all anti-infectives, including ceftazidime, and may range in severity from mild diarrhea to fatal colitis. *C. difficile* produces toxins A and B which contribute to the development of CDAD; hypertoxin-producing strains cause increased morbidity and mortality since these infections may be refractory to anti-infective therapy and may require colectomy.

CDAD should be considered in the differential diagnosis in patients who develop diarrhea during or after anti-infective therapy and managed accordingly. Careful medical history is necessary since CDAD has been reported to occur as late as 2 months or longer after anti-infective therapy is discontinued.

If CDAD is suspected or confirmed, anti-infectives not directed against *C. difficile* should be discontinued whenever possible. Patients should be managed with appropriate supportive therapy (e.g., fluid and electrolyte management, protein supplementation), anti-infective therapy directed against *C. difficile* (e.g., metronidazole, vancomycin), and surgical evaluation as clinically indicated.

■ **Dermatologic and Sensitivity Reactions** Hypersensitivity reactions have been reported in 1–3% of patients receiving ceftazidime and include pruritus, rash (maculopapular or erythematous), urticaria, photosensitivity, angioedema, and fever.

Immediate hypersensitivity reactions, including anaphylaxis (manifested as bronchospasm and/or hypotension), have occurred rarely with ceftazidime. Toxic epidermal necrolysis, Stevens-Johnson syndrome, and erythema multiforme have been reported with cephalosporins, including ceftazidime.

The manufacturer of the commercially available Duplex® drug delivery system containing ceftazidime and 5% dextrose injection cautions that hypersensitivity reactions, including anaphylaxis, have been reported with administration of dextrose-containing solutions. These reactions have been reported in patients receiving high concentrations of dextrose (i.e., 50% dextrose) and also have been reported when corn-derived dextrose solutions were administered to patients with or without a history of hypersensitivity to corn products.

If a hypersensitivity reaction occurs during ceftazidime therapy, the drug should be discontinued. Severe acute hypersensitivity reactions should be treated with appropriate therapy (e.g., epinephrine, oxygen, antihistamines, corticosteroids, IV fluids, vasopressors, airway management) as indicated.

■ **Hepatic Effects** Transient increases in serum concentrations of AST (SGOT), ALT (SGPT), alkaline phosphatase, LDH, and/or γ-glutamyltransferase (γ-glutamyl transpeptidase, GGT, GGTP) have been reported in 3–9% of patients receiving ceftazidime. Increased serum concentrations of bilirubin have occurred in less than 1% of patients receiving the drug. Jaundice has been reported with ceftazidime.

■ **Renal Effects** Transient increases in BUN and/or serum creatinine concentrations have been reported in less than 2% of patients receiving ceftazidime.

A transient, mild to moderate decrease in glomerular filtration rate has occurred in a few patients receiving ceftazidime. Although excretion of thermophilic aminopeptidase (alanine aminopeptidase), an enzyme originating from renal proximal tubular cells, was increased slightly in some of these patients, serum creatinine and urinary β_2-microglobulin concentrations were generally unaffected, suggesting that ceftazidime did not adversely affect proximal tubular cells. In healthy adults who received 6 g of ceftazidime daily for 3 days, urinary excretion of thermophilic aminopeptidase was unaffected by the drug. It has been suggested that ceftazidime's potential to slightly decrease glomerular filtration rate may be clinically important in patients with preexisting renal impairment if adequate dosage adjustments are not made in these patients. (See Dosage and Administration: Dosage in Renal and Hepatic Impairment.)

Renal failure has been reported in a few patients receiving ceftazidime; however, a causal relationship to the drug has not been established. Like cephaloridine (a cephalosporin known to be nephrotoxic; no longer commercially available in the US), ceftazidime contains a methylpyridinium at position 3 of the cephalosporin nucleus; however, there is no evidence to date that this group is associated with nephrotoxicity, and the manufacturers state that ceftazidime has not been shown to be nephrotoxic. Nephrotoxicity of cephaloridine apparently results from accumulation of the drug in renal proximal tubular cells; there is no evidence to date that ceftazidime accumulates in renal tubular cells.

■ **Nervous System Effects** Coma, encephalopathy, asterixis, hallucinations, neuromuscular excitability, and myoclonia have been reported in patients with renal impairment who received usual dosages of ceftazidime.

■ **Local Effects** Adverse local reactions, including phlebitis and pain or inflammation at the injection site, have been reported in less than 3% of patients receiving ceftazidime. Following IM injection of the drug, pain at the injection site is reportedly mild to moderate for about 2–5 minutes and subsides within 10–20 minutes.

Distal necrosis can occur after inadvertent intra-arterial administration of ceftazidime.

■ **Other Adverse Effects** Other adverse effects that have been reported in less than 1% of patients receiving ceftazidime include candidiasis (e.g., oral thrush) and vaginitis.

■ **Precautions and Contraindications** Ceftazidime shares the toxic potentials of the cephalosporins, and the usual precautions of cephalosporin therapy should be observed. Prior to initiation of therapy with ceftazidime, careful inquiry should be made concerning previous hypersensitivity reactions to cephalosporins, penicillins, or other drugs. There is clinical and laboratory evidence of partial cross-allergenicity among cephalosporins and other β-lactam antibiotics including penicillins and cephamycins. Ceftazidime is contraindicated in patients who are hypersensitive to any cephalosporin and should be used with caution in patients with a history of hypersensitivity reactions to penicillins. Use of cephalosporins should be avoided in patients who have had an immediate-type (anaphylactic) hypersensitivity reaction to penicillins.

To reduce development of drug-resistant bacteria and maintain effectiveness of ceftazidime and other antibacterials, the drug should be used only for the treatment or prevention of infections proven or strongly suspected to be caused by susceptible bacteria. When selecting or modifying anti-infective therapy, results of culture and in vitro susceptibility testing should be used. In the absence of such data, local epidemiology and susceptibility patterns should be considered when selecting anti-infectives for empiric therapy should be considered.

Patients should be advised that antibacterials (including ceftazidime) should only be used to treat bacterial infections and not used to treat viral infections (e.g., the common cold). Patients also should be advised about the importance of completing the full course of therapy, even if feeling better after a few days, and that skipping doses or not completing therapy may decrease effectiveness and increase the likelihood that bacteria will develop resistance and will not be treatable with ceftazidime or other antibacterials in the future.

Like other dextrose-containing solutions, the commercially available Duplex® drug delivery system containing ceftazidime and 5% dextrose injection should be used with caution in patients with overt or known subclinical diabetes mellitus or in patients with carbohydrate intolerance for any reason.

Use of ceftazidime may result in overgrowth of nonsusceptible organisms, especially *Candida*, *Staphylococcus aureus*, enterococci, *Enterobacter*, or *Pseudomonas*. Resistant strains of *Ps. aeruginosa* and*Enterobacter*have developed during therapy with ceftazidime. (See Resistance.) Careful observation of the patient during ceftazidime therapy is essential. If superinfection or suprainfection occurs, appropriate therapy should be instituted.

Because CDAD has been reported with the use of ceftazidime and other cephalosporins, it should be considered in the differential diagnosis of patients who develop diarrhea during or after ceftazidime therapy. (See Cautions: GI Effects.) Patients should be advised that diarrhea is a common problem caused by anti-infectives and usually ends when the drug is discontinued; however, they should contact a clinician if watery and bloody stools (with or without stomach cramps and fever) occur during or as late as 2 months or longer after the last dose. Ceftazidime should be used with caution in patients with a history of GI disease, especially colitis.

As with other extended-spectrum β-lactams, resistance to ceftazidime in some gram-negative bacteria (e.g., *Enterobacter*, *Pseudomonas*) can develop during therapy, leading to clinical failure in some cases. When ceftazidime is used to treat infections caused by these gram-negative bacteria, periodic susceptibility testing should be performed when clinically appropriate. If patients fail to respond to ceftazidime monotherapy, adding an aminoglycoside or similar agent to the regimen should be considered.

High and prolonged serum ceftazidime concentrations may occur if usual dosages of the drug are used in patients with transient or persistent reduction in urinary output because of renal insufficiency. Doses and/or frequency of administration of ceftazidime should be decreased in patients with transient or persistent renal impairment. (See Dosage and Administration: Dosage in Renal and Hepatic Impairment.) Increased serum ceftazidime concentrations can result in serious adverse nervous system effects (e.g., seizures, encephalopathy, coma, asterixis, neuromuscular excitability, myoclonia). (See Cautions: Nervous System Effects.) Continued dosage should be determined by degree of renal impairment, severity of infection, and susceptibility of the causative organisms.

■ **Geriatric Precautions** Clinical studies of ceftazidime did not include sufficient numbers of patients 65 years of age or older to determine whether geriatric patients respond differently than younger patients. Of the 2221 adults who received ceftazidime in clinical studies, 37% were 65 years of age or older, while 18% were 75 years of age or older. Although no overall differences in efficacy or safety were observed between geriatric and younger patients and other clinical experience revealed no age-related differences, the possibility that some older patients may exhibit increased sensitivity to the drug cannot be ruled out.

Ceftazidime is known to be substantially excreted by the kidney, and the risk of ceftazidime-induced toxicity may be greater in patients with renal impairment. Because geriatric patients may have decreased renal function, initial dosage should be selected carefully and it may be useful to monitor renal function. (See Dosage and Administration: Dosage in Renal and Hepatic Impairment.)

■ **Mutagenicity and Carcinogenicity** In vitro studies using microbial (i.e., Ames test) or mammalian cell (i.e., mouse micronucleus) systems have not shown ceftazidime to be mutagenic. Studies have not been performed to date to evaluate the carcinogenic potential of ceftazidime.

■ **Pregnancy, Fertility, and Lactation** Safe use of ceftazidime during pregnancy has not been definitely established. Reproduction studies in mice and rats using ceftazidime dosages up to 40 times the usual human dosage have not revealed evidence of harm to the fetus. There are no adequate or controlled studies using ceftazidime in pregnant women, and the drug should be used during pregnancy only when clearly needed.

Reproduction studies in mice and rats using ceftazidime dosages up to 40 times the usual human dosage have not revealed evidence of impaired fertility.

Because ceftazidime is distributed into milk, sodium carbonate formulations of the drug should be used with caution in nursing women.

Drug Interactions

■ **Probenecid** Concomitant administration of 2 g of oral probenecid does not affect the pharmacokinetics of ceftazidime, presumably because ceftazidime is excreted principally by glomerular filtration.

■ **Anti-infective Agents** ***Aminoglycosides*** In vitro studies indicate that the antibacterial activity of ceftazidime and an aminoglycoside may be additive or synergistic against some strains of Enterobacteriaceae and *Pseudomonas aeruginosa*. Organisms with high-level resistance to both ceftazidime and the aminoglycoside alone are unlikely to be synergistically inhibited by concomitant use of the drugs.

Concomitant use of aminoglycosides and certain cephalosporins reportedly may increase the risk of nephrotoxicity during therapy. Although this effect has not been reported to date with ceftazidime, the manufacturers suggest that renal function be carefully monitored when an aminoglycoside is used concomitantly with ceftazidime, especially if high aminoglycoside dosage is used or if therapy is prolonged.

β-Lactam Antibiotics Although a synergistic or partially synergistic effect has occurred in vitro against a few strains of *Ps. aeruginosa* when ceftazidime and carbenicillin, cefsulodin, mezlocillin, or piperacillin were used concomitantly, use of ceftazidime and another cephalosporin or an extended-spectrum penicillin has generally resulted in an effect that was only slightly additive or indifferent against *Ps. aeruginosa*. In addition, the combination of ceftazidime and cefoxitin has been antagonistic in vitro against *Ps. aeruginosa*.

The clinical importance is unclear, but concomitant use of ceftazidime and ampicillin in vitro has resulted in antagonism against group B streptococci and *Listeria monocytogenes*.

Quinolones Although the clinical importance is unclear, in vitro studies indicate that the combination of ceftazidime and ciprofloxacin exerts a synergistic effect against *Burkholderia cepacia*. In an in vitro study using *B. cepacia* isolates from patients with cystic fibrosis, the combination of ceftazidime and ciprofloxacin resulted in increased killing activity against most isolates (except ciprofloxacin-resistant strains). While a 3-drug combination (ceftazidime, ciprofloxacin, and tobramycin or rifampin) resulted in increased killing activity against *B. cepacia* isolates compared with ceftazidime alone, this effect was not substantially greater than that attained with the 2-drug combination of ceftazidime and ciprofloxacin.

Other Anti-infectives In vitro, the combination of ceftazidime and clindamycin has been reported to be neither synergistic nor antagonistic against *Bacteroides fragilis*.

In vitro results indicate that the combination of ceftazidime and metronidazole may be at least partially synergistic against *Clostridium*, but results against *B. fragilis* are conflicting.

Chloramphenicol has been reported to antagonize the bactericidal activity of β-lactam antibiotics including ceftazidime, in vitro, and the possibility of in vivo antagonism should be considered. Therefore, the manufacturers recommend that combined therapy with chloramphenicol and ceftazidime be avoided, particularly when bactericidal activity is considered important.

■ **Clavulanic Acid** In vitro studies indicate that the combination of ceftazidime and clavulanic acid, a β-lactamase inhibitor, is synergistic against some strains of *B. fragilis* resistant to ceftazidime alone. The combination was not effective against other *Bacteroides*, such as *B. distasonis*, that are not β-lactamase producers. In vitro studies indicate that the combination of ceftazidime and chloramphenicol may be antagonistic against some organisms.

■ **Diuretics** Although concomitant use of cephalosporins and potent diuretics (e.g., furosemide) reportedly may adversely affect renal function, this effect apparently did not occur when furosemide was used concomitantly with ceftazidime in a few patients.

Laboratory Test Interferences

■ **Immunohematology Tests** Positive direct antiglobulin (Coombs') test results have been reported in patients receiving ceftazidime. This reaction may interfere with hematologic studies or transfusion cross-matching procedures.

■ **Tests for Glucose** Like most cephalosporins, ceftazidime interferes with urinary glucose determinations using cupric sulfate (e.g., Benedict's solution, Fehling's solution, Clinitest®). Urinary glucose determinations using glucose oxidase methods (e.g., Clinistix®) are unaffected by the drug. In addition, ceftazidime does not interfere with glucose oxidase or hexokinase methods used to determine serum glucose concentrations.

■ **Tests for Creatinine** Ceftazidime does not appear to interfere with manual or automated methods used to determine serum or urinary creatinine concentrations, including those using the Jaffé reaction.

Acute Toxicity

Limited information is available on the acute toxicity of ceftazidime. Inappropriately large doses of parenteral cephalosporins may cause seizures, especially in patients with renal impairment. Overdosage of ceftazidime in patients with renal failure has produced seizures, encephalopathy, coma, asterixis, neuromuscular excitability, and myoclonia. The drug should be discontinued promptly if seizures occur; anticonvulsant therapy may be administered if indicated. If acute overdosage of ceftazidime occurs, hemodialysis or peritoneal dialysis may be used to enhance elimination of the drug.

Mechanism of Action

Ceftazidime usually is bactericidal in action. Like other cephalosporins, the antibacterial activity of the drug results from inhibition of mucopeptide synthesis in the bacterial cell wall. For information on the mechanism of action of cephalosporins, see Mechanism of Action in the Cephalosporins General Statement 8:12.06.

Studies evaluating the binding of ceftazidime to penicillin-binding proteins (PBPs), the target enzymes of β-lactam antibiotics, indicate that ceftazidime binds principally to PBP 3 of *Escherichia coli* and *Pseudomonas aeruginosa*.

The drug also has some affinity for PBP 1a of these organisms, but has little affinity for PBPs 2, 4, 5, and 6. Ceftazidime binds less well than cefuroxime to PBPs 1, 2, and 3 of *Staphylococcus aureus*.

Spectrum

Based on its spectrum of activity, ceftazidime is classified as a third generation cephalosporin. For information on the classification of cephalosporins and closely related β-lactam antibiotics based on spectra of activity, see Spectrum in the Cephalosporins General Statement 8:12.06.

Like other currently available parenteral third generation cephalosporins (e.g., cefotaxime, ceftriaxone), ceftazidime generally is less active in vitro against susceptible staphylococci than first generation cephalosporins but has an expanded spectrum of activity against gram-negative bacteria compared with first and second generation cephalosporins. The spectrum of activity of ceftazidime resembles that of cefotaxime and ceftriaxone; however, ceftazidime is more active in vitro on a weight basis against *Pseudomonas* than most other currently available parenteral third generation cephalosporins, but less active in vitro on a weight basis against anaerobes and gram-positive aerobic cocci than these drugs.

■ In Vitro Susceptibility Testing Results of in vitro susceptibility tests with ceftazidime for some Enterobacteriaceae, *Pseudomonas aeruginosa*, and *Bacteroides* may be affected by the size of the inoculum. For most organisms there is generally little difference in MICs of ceftazidime when the size of the inoculum is increased from 10^3 to 10^5 colony-forming units (CFU) per mL, but MICs of some organisms (e.g., *Citrobacter freundii, Enterobacter, Morganella morganii, Proteus, Ps. aeruginosa*) may be 8–128 times greater when the size of the inoculum is increased from 10^5 to 10^7 CFU/mL. Results of ceftazidime susceptibility tests are generally unaffected by culture media, pH, or presence of serum.

Strains of staphylococci resistant to penicillinase-resistant penicillins (oxacillin-resistant [methicillin-resistant] staphylococci) should be considered resistant to ceftazidime, although results of in vitro susceptibility tests may indicate that the organisms are susceptible to the drug.

For information on interpreting results of in vitro susceptibility testing (disk susceptibility tests, dilution susceptibility tests) when ceftazidime susceptibility testing is performed according to the standards of the Clinical and Laboratory Standards Institute (CLSI; formerly National Committee for Clinical Laboratory Standards [NCCLS]), see Spectrum: In Vitro Susceptibility Testing, in the Cephalosporins General Statement 8:12.06.

■ Gram-positive Aerobic Bacteria Ceftazidime generally is active in vitro against the following gram-positive aerobic cocci: penicillinase-producing and nonpenicillinase-producing strains of *Staphylococcus aureus* and *S. epidermidis, Streptococcus pneumoniae, S. pyogenes* (group A β-hemolytic streptococci), *S. agalactiae* (group B streptococci), and viridans streptococci. However, in vitro on a weight basis, ceftazidime is slightly less active than most other currently available third generation cephalosporins against these gram-positive bacteria.

Staphylococci resistant to penicillinase-resistant penicillins are resistant to ceftazidime. *Listeria monocytogenes* and enterococci, including *E. faecalis* (formerly *S. faecalis*), also are generally resistant to the drug.

The MIC_{90} (minimum inhibitory concentration of the drug at which 90% of strains tested are inhibited) of ceftazidime for penicillinase-producing and nonpenicillinase-producing *S. aureus* is 8–25 mcg/mL. Although the MIC_{50} of ceftazidime reported for *S. epidermidis* is 8–16 mcg/mL, the MIC_{90} of the drug for *S. epidermidis* or *S. saprophyticus* usually is 8–50 mcg/mL. The MIC_{90} of ceftazidime for group A β-hemolytic streptococci or group B streptococci is 0.06–2 mcg/mL. The MIC_{90} of the drug reported for *Streptococcus pneumoniae* is 0.13–4 mcg/mL, and the MIC_{90} reported for viridans streptococci is 3.1–8 mcg/mL. In one study, the MIC_{50} and MIC_{90} of ceftazidime for the *S. milleri* group of viridans streptococci (*S. anginosus, S. constellatus, S. intermedius*) were 4 and 8 mcg/mL, respectively.

■ Gram-negative Aerobic Bacteria ***Neisseria*** Ceftazidime is active in vitro against *Neisseria meningitidis* and most strains of penicillinase-producing and nonpenicillinase-producing *Neisseria gonorrhoeae*. Ceftazidime concentrations of 0.001–0.06 mcg/mL generally inhibit *N. meningitidis*. The MIC_{90} of ceftazidime is 0.02–0.25 mcg/mL for nonpenicillinase-producing *N. gonorrhoeae* and 0.001–0.03 mcg/mL for penicillinase-producing strains of the organism.

Haemophilus Ceftazidime is active in vitro against most β-lactamase-producing and non-β-lactamase-producing strains of *Haemophilus influenzae, H. parainfluenzae*, and *H. ducreyi*. The MIC_{90} of the drug reported for *H. influenzae* is 0.1–1 mcg/mL. In one study, the MIC_{90} of ceftazidime for *H. ducreyi* was 0.13 mcg/mL.

Enterobacteriaceae Generally, ceftazidime is active in vitro against the following Enterobacteriaceae: *Citrobacter diversus, C. freundii, Enterobacter agglomerans, E. cloacae, E. aerogenes, Escherichia coli, Klebsiella oxytoca, K. pneumoniae, Morganella morganii* (formerly *Proteus morganii*), *Proteus mirabilis, P. vulgaris, Providencia rettgeri* (formerly *Proteus rettgeri*), *P. stuartii, Serratia marcescens, Salmonella, Shigella*, and *Yersinia enterocolitica*.

The MIC_{90} of ceftazidime for *E. coli, Klebsiella* (including *K. pneumoniae*), *M. morganii, Providencia*, and *S. marcescens* is 0.2–6.3 mcg/mL. The MIC_{90} of the drug for *P. mirabilis, P. vulgaris*, and *Y. enterocolitica* is 0.05–0.8 mcg/mL.

The MIC_{90} of ceftazidime reported for *C. diversus* is 0.2–1 mcg/mL. The in vitro activity of ceftazidime against *C. freundii*, however, varies considerably. In some studies the MIC_{90} of ceftazidime for *C. freundii* was 0.2–8 mcg/mL, and in other studies it was 32 mcg/mL or greater. The in vitro activity of ceftazidime against *Enterobacter* also varies considerably. The MIC_{90} of ceftazidime reported for *E. agglomerans* is 0.5–6.3 mcg/mL, and the MIC_{90} of the drug reported for *E. aerogenes* is 0.2–32 mcg/mL. In some studies the MIC_{90} of ceftazidime reported for *E. cloacae* was 0.5–12.5 mcg/mL, but in other studies it was 32–64 mcg/mL or greater.

The MIC_{90} of ceftazidime reported for *Salmonella enteritidis, S. newport*, and *S. typhi* is 0.1–6.5 mcg/mL. In one study, strains of *S. typhi* resistant to ampicillin and chloramphenicol were susceptible in vitro to ceftazidime concentrations of 0.1–0.2 mcg/mL. The MIC_{90} of ceftazidime reported for *Shigella*, including *Sh. flexneri* and *Sh. sonnei*, is 0.12–6.3 mcg/mL.

Pseudomonas Ceftazidime is active in vitro against *Pseudomonas aeruginosa*. In vitro on a weight basis, ceftazidime is more active against *Ps. aeruginosa* than most other cephalosporins. In addition, ceftazidime is active in vitro against some strains of *Ps. aeruginosa* resistant to other third generation cephalosporins, aminoglycosides, and extended-spectrum penicillins. The MIC_{90} of ceftazidime reported for *Ps. aeruginosa* is 0.5–32 mcg/mL.

Ceftazidime is also active against *Pseudomonas* other than *Ps. aeruginosa*. The MIC_{90} of ceftazidime reported for *Ps. acidovorans, Ps. fluorescens, Ps. putida*, and *Ps. stutzeri* is 0.5–16 mcg/mL.

Burkholderia Ceftazidime is active in vitro against some strains of *Burkholderia cepacia* (formerly *Ps. cepacia*). The MIC_{50} and MIC_{90} of ceftazidime reported for some strains of *B. cepacia* are 2–8 and 4–32 mcg/mL, respectively; however, strains of *B. cepacia* isolated from patients with cystic fibrosis generally require higher ceftazidime concentrations for in vitro inhibition than strains isolated from patients who do not have cystic fibrosis and many of these strains have MIC_{90}s of 64 mcg/mL or greater and are resistant to the drug. Although the clinical importance is unclear, in vitro studies indicate that the combination of ceftazidime and amikacin or ciprofloxacin exerts a synergistic effect against *B. cepacia*. (See Quinolones under Drug Interactions: Anti-infective Agents.)

Ceftazidime also has in vitro activity against some strains of *B. pseudomallei* (formerly *Ps. pseudomallei*). Susceptible strains of *B. pseudomallei* are inhibited in vitro by ceftazidime concentrations of 1–8 mcg/mL; other strains are resistant to the drug.

Other Gram-negative Aerobic Bacteria Ceftazidime has some activity in vitro against *Acinetobacter*. The MIC_{90} of ceftazidime reported for *A. calcoaceticus, A. lwoffi*, and *A. baumannii* is 8–32 mcg/mL.

Moraxella catarrhalis generally is inhibited in vitro by ceftazidime concentrations of 0.06–0.13 mcg/mL. Some strains of *M. osloensis* and *M. nonliquefaciens* are inhibited in vitro by ceftazidime concentrations of 8 mcg/mL.

Ceftazidime also is active in vitro against *Eikenella corrodens* and *Pasteurella multocida*. The MIC_{90} of the drug is 16 mcg/mL for *E. corrodens* and 0.13–1.6 mcg/mL for *P. multocida*.

Campylobacter fetus subsp. *jejuni*, an organism that can be microaerophilic or anaerobic, may be inhibited in vitro by ceftazidime concentrations of 3.1–6.25 mcg/mL.

While some strains of *Alcaligenes denitrificans, A. faecalis*, and *A. xylosoxidans* may be inhibited in vitro by ceftazidime concentrations of 1–16 mcg/mL, the MIC_{90} of the drug reported for *Alcaligenes* ranges from 2 to more than 64 mcg/mL.

In vitro, some strains of *Bartonella bacilliformis* are inhibited by ceftazidime concentrations of 0.12–0.25 mcg/mL.

The MIC_{90} of ceftazidime reported for some strains of *Chryseobacterium gleum* (formerly *Flavobacterium gleum*, CDC group IIb) and *C. indologenes* (formerly *F. indologenes*, CDC group IIb) is 8 mcg/mL and the MIC_{90} reported for *Sphingobacterium multivorum* (formerly *F. multivorum*) is 32 mcg/mL. *C. meningosepticum* (formerly *F. meningosepticum*) generally are resistant to ceftazidime.

Rare strains of *Stenotrophomonas maltophilia* (formerly *Ps. maltophilia* or *Xanthomonas maltophilia*) are inhibited in vitro by ceftazidime concentrations of 4–16 mcg/mL; however, most strains require ceftazidime concentrations of 32 mcg/mL or greater for in vitro inhibition and are considered resistant to the drug. Although the clinical importance is unclear, in vitro studies indicate that the combination of ceftazidime and a quinolone (e.g., ciprofloxacin, levofloxacin, trovafloxacin) exerts a synergistic bactericidal activity against some strains of *S. maltophilia*.

■ Anaerobic Bacteria Ceftazidime is active in vitro against some gram-positive anaerobic bacteria including some strains of *Bifidobacterium, Clostridium, Eubacterium, Lactobacillus, Peptococcus, Peptostreptococcus*, and *Propionibacterium*. The MIC_{90} of ceftazidime reported for most of these gram-positive anaerobic bacteria is 4–32 mcg/mL. *C. perfringens* generally is inhibited in vitro by ceftazidime concentrations of 2–16 mcg/mL; however, *C. difficile* is resistant to the drug. The MIC_{50} of ceftazidime for *Actinomyces* is reportedly 6–8 mcg/mL, but the MIC_{90} is 48–64 mcg/mL.

Ceftazidime has little in vitro activity against gram-negative anaerobic bacteria. Although the MIC_{90} of ceftazidime reported for *Bacteroides melaninogenicus* is 4–16 mcg/mL, other *Bacteroides* (including *B. fragilis*) are generally resistant to the drug. The MIC_{50} of ceftazidime reported for *B. fragilis, B. distasonis, B. ovatus*, and *B. thetaiotaomicron* is 8–32 mcg/mL, and the MIC_{90} of the drug reported for these organisms is usually 64 mcg/mL or greater.

Although the MIC_{50} of ceftazidime reported for *Fusobacterium* and *Veillonella* is 4–16 mcg/mL, the MIC_{90} of the drug for these organisms is 32 mcg/mL or greater and many strains are considered resistant to the drug.

Resistance

For information on possible mechanisms of bacterial resistance to cephalosporins, see Resistance in the Cephalosporins General Statement 8:12.06.

Ceftazidime generally is stable against hydrolysis by β-lactamases classified as Richmond-Sykes types I, II, III (TEM type), IV, and V and most PSE types. The drug is hydrolyzed to some extent by chromosomally mediated β-lactamases isolated from *Bacteroides* and *Providencia*. Ceftazidime is more stable than cefotaxime against hydrolysis by β-lactamases, but as stable as or slightly less stable than cefoxitin.

Resistant strains of *Enterobacter* and *Pseudomonas* have developed during therapy with ceftazidime. Resistance to ceftazidime in some Enterobacteriaceae (e.g., *Enterobacter cloacae, Citrobacter freundii*) reportedly results from increased production of chromosomally mediated β-lactamases, nonspecific binding of PBPs, and permeability factors. In vitro studies indicate that resistance to ceftazidime in *Ps. aeruginosa, Acinetobacter*, and some strains of *Serratia* is generally related to permeability factors; however, in a few strains of *Ps. aeruginosa* that developed resistance to ceftazidime during therapy with the drug, resistance appeared to result partly from increased production of chromosomally mediated β-lactamases. *Bacteroides* are generally resistant to ceftazidime because of permeability factors and because the drug has little affinity for the PBPs of this organism.

Ceftazidime-resistant strains of *Klebsiella pneumoniae* have been reported, and these strains have been involved in nosocomial outbreaks in hospitals and chronic care facilities. Resistance in these strains results from acquisition of plasmid-mediated extended-spectrum β-lactamases (TEM- or SHV-derived extended-spectrum β-lactamases).

In vitro studies indicate that ceftazidime can induce β-lactamase production in some strains of *Enterobacter* and *Ps. aeruginosa* that possess these inducible, chromosomally mediated enzymes; however, the drug is not an efficient inducer when compared with cefoxitin.

Pharmacokinetics

In all studies described in the Pharmacokinetics section, ceftazidime was administered as ceftazidime sodium; dosages and concentrations of the drug are expressed in terms of ceftazidime.

■ **Absorption** Ceftazidime is not absorbed from the GI tract and must be given parenterally.

Following IM administration of a single 0.5- or 1-g dose of ceftazidime in healthy adults, peak serum concentrations of the drug are attained approximately 1 hour after the dose and average 17 or 29–39 mcg/mL, respectively. Following IM injection into the gluteus maximus or vastus lateralis, ceftazidime may be absorbed more slowly in women than in men. In women, peak serum concentrations of the drug may be lower following IM injection into the gluteus maximus than into the vastus lateralis.

Following IV infusion over 20–30 minutes of a single 0.5- or 1-g dose of ceftazidime in healthy men, peak serum concentrations of the drug at completion of the infusion average 42 or 69 mcg/mL, respectively. IV infusion over 20–30 minutes of a single 2-g dose in healthy adults results in peak serum ceftazidime concentrations at completion of the infusion that average 159–185.5 mcg/mL and serum concentrations at 0.5, 1, 2, 4, and 6 hours after completion of the infusion that average 87.9, 65.2–70.6, 38.7, 16.7–16.9, and 7.7 mcg/mL, respectively.

Following IV injection over 3–5 minutes of a single 0.5- or 1-g dose of ceftazidime in healthy men, serum concentrations of the drug at 0.25, 0.5, 1, 2, 4, 6, and 8 hours after the dose average 34.1, 24.5, 17.1, 11.2, 5.6, 2.1–2.4, and 0.9–1.3 mcg/mL, respectively, after the 0.5-g dose and 59.9–83.3, 45.3–60.9, 32.1–40.9, 22.9–23.2, 9.7, 4.4–5.3, and 1.9–3.2 mcg/mL, respectively, after the 1-g dose.

In adults with suspected gram-negative infections who received a 2-g IV loading dose of ceftazidime followed by 3 g given by continuous IV infusion over 24 hours, steady-state serum concentrations averaged 29.7 mcg/mL. Serum concentrations averaged 21.3–56.4 mcg/mL in cystic fibrosis patients 9–25 years of age who received a 7.5- or 10-mg/kg IV loading dose of ceftazidime followed by 3.4 or 4.5 mg/kg hourly given by continuous IV infusion over 24 hours.

In neonates 1–15 days of age with infections who received a single 50-mg/kg dose of ceftazidime by IM injection, serum concentrations of the drug averaged 67.2, 68.2, 42.1, 23.7, and 8.9 mcg/mL at 0.5, 1, 3, 6, and 12 hours, respectively, after the dose. In neonates and children with infections who received a single 30-mg/kg dose by IV injection, serum concentrations of ceftazidime averaged 54.1, 31.2, and 18.6 mcg/mL at 3, 6, and 9 hours, respectively, after the dose in those less than 2 months of age and 26.5, 12.3, 6.4, and 3.3 mcg/mL at 3, 5, 7, and 9 hours, respectively, after the dose in those 2–12 months of age. In neonates who received 25-mg/kg doses every 12 hours by IV injection, serum ceftazidime concentrations on the third or fourth day of therapy averaged 81.7, 70, 68, 50, 39.5, and 16.1 mcg/mL at 0.25, 0.5, 1, 3, 5, and 12 hours, respectively, after a dose.

In children 5–14 years of age with cystic fibrosis who received 35-mg/kg doses of ceftazidime every 8 hours by IV injection, serum concentrations averaged 110, 86, 50, 25.5, 8.1, 4.3, and 2.3 mcg/mL at 0.25, 0.5, 1, 2, 4, 6, and 8 hours, respectively, after the eighth dose.

In patients with end-stage chronic renal failure who received a single 1-g dose of ceftazidime via an intraperitoneal catheter, peak serum concentrations were attained 2.75 hours after the dose and averaged 44.7 mcg/mL; serum ceftazidime concentrations at 0.25, 2, and 8 hours after the dose averaged 14.2, 40, and 32 mcg/mL, respectively. Following intraperitoneal administration of a 200-mg dose of ceftazidime in 2 L of dialysis fluid in patients with end-stage chronic renal failure undergoing a 12-hour period of peritoneal dialysis (12 cycles of dialysis, each exchanging 2 L of dialysate for 15–20 minutes), serum ceftazidime concentrations averaged 1.3, 25.3, and 18.7 mcg/mL at 1, 12, and 24 hours, respectively, after the start of dialysis. Concentrations of the drug in the dialysis effluent averaged 42.2 mcg/mL.

■ **Distribution** Following IM or IV administration, ceftazidime is widely distributed into body tissues and fluids including the gallbladder, bone, bile, skeletal muscle, prostatic tissue, endometrium, myometrium, heart, skin, adipose tissue, aqueous humor, and sputum, and pleural, peritoneal, synovial, ascitic, lymphatic, and blister fluids.

The volume of distribution of ceftazidime at steady state (V_{ss}) averages 0.18–0.31 L/kg in healthy adults. In neonates 2–9 days of age, the V_{ss} of ceftazidime averaged 0.42–0.55 L/kg. In patients with cystic fibrosis, the volume of distribution of ceftazidime reportedly averages 0.15–0.19 L/kg in the central compartment and 0.17–0.27 L/kg in the peripheral compartment.

Ceftazidime generally diffuses into CSF following IV administration; however, CSF concentrations of the drug are higher in patients with inflamed meninges than in those with uninflamed meninges. CSF concentrations of ceftazidime do not appear to correlate with CSF leukocyte cell counts or CSF protein concentrations. In adults with meningitis who received 2 g of ceftazidime every 8 hours by IV infusion over 30 minutes, CSF concentrations of the drug on days 2–4 of therapy averaged 9.8 mcg/mL in samples obtained 2 hours after a dose and 9.4 mcg/mL in samples obtained 3 hours after a dose. On days 11–20 of therapy, when the meninges were presumably healed, CSF concentrations of ceftazidime averaged 4.1 and 7.2 mcg/mL in samples obtained 2 and 3 hours, respectively, after a dose. In neonates with meningitis who received IV ceftazidime in a dosage of 90–150 mg/kg daily, CSF concentrations 2–4 hours after a dose were 22–30 mcg/mL.

Ceftazidime generally is distributed into bile, but biliary concentrations of the drug following IM or IV administration may be lower than concurrent serum concentrations. In women 36–70 years of age undergoing cholecystectomy who received a single 2-g dose of ceftazidime by IV infusion over 15 minutes, ceftazidime concentrations in gallbladder bile 25–160 minutes after the dose ranged from 6.6–58 mcg/mL and concurrent serum concentrations of the drug ranged from 51.6–108 mcg/mL. In another study in patients 34–72 years of age also undergoing cholecystectomy who received a single 1-g IV dose of the drug, ceftazidime concentrations in gallbladder and bile duct bile 60 minutes following the dose averaged 3.9 mcg/mL (range: 0.1–15.2 mcg/mL) and 31.8 mcg/mL (range: 12.5–55.4 mcg/mL), respectively, and concurrent serum concentrations of the drug averaged 36.1 mcg/mL (range: 23.6–46.8 mcg/mL).

In cystic fibrosis patients aged 5–32 years who received 35- or 50-mg/kg doses of ceftazidime every 8 hours by IV injection, concentrations of ceftazidime in sputum ranged from 0.7–9.8 mcg/mL; peak sputum concentrations were usually attained 1 hour after a dose.

In patients undergoing cataract surgery who received a single 2-g dose of ceftazidime by IV injection over 3–5 minutes, aqueous humor concentrations of the drug averaged 2.8, 4, 3.2, 3.4, and 1.9 mcg/mL at 0.5, 1, 2, 4, and 6 hours, respectively, after the dose.

Ceftazidime is 5–24% bound to serum proteins. The degree of protein binding is independent of the concentration of the drug.

Ceftazidime crosses the placenta and is distributed into amniotic fluid. Ceftazidime is also distributed into milk. In lactating women with endometritis who received 2 g of ceftazidime IV every 8 hours, concentrations of the drug in milk obtained during days 2–4 of therapy averaged 3.8 mcg/mL immediately prior to a dose and 5.2 and 4.5 mcg/mL at 1 and 3 hours, respectively, after a dose.

■ **Elimination** Plasma concentrations of ceftazidime decline in a biphasic manner. In adults with normal renal and hepatic function, the distribution half-life ($t_{1/2\alpha}$) of ceftazidime is 0.1–0.6 hours and the elimination half-life ($t_{1/2\beta}$) is 1.4–2 hours.

Ceftazidime is not metabolized and is excreted unchanged principally in urine by glomerular filtration. Following IM or IV administration of a single 0.5- or 1-g dose of ceftazidime in adults with normal renal function, 80–90% of the dose is excreted in urine unchanged within 24 hours; approximately 50% of the dose is excreted within 2 hours after the dose.

Serum clearance of ceftazidime averages 98–122 mL/minute in healthy adults. In geriatric patients 63–83 years of age with urinary tract infections, serum clearance of ceftazidime averaged 79 mL/minute and the serum half-life of the drug averaged 2.9 hours. In patients with cystic fibrosis, the serum clearance of ceftazidime ranges from 142–316 mL/minute per 1.73 m^2; the serum half-life of the drug in these patients, however, ranges from 1–2.2 hours and is generally within the same range as that for healthy individuals.

The serum half-life of ceftazidime is longer in neonates than in older children and adults, but does not appear to be related to gestational age or birthweight. The $t_{1/2\beta}$ of ceftazidime in neonates 1–23 days of age reportedly ranges from 2.2–4.7 hours. In a group of children 2–12 months of age, the $t_{1/2\beta}$ of ceftazidime averaged 2 hours.

Serum concentrations of ceftazidime are higher and the serum half-life of the drug is prolonged in patients with impaired renal function. The $t_{1/2\beta}$ of ceftazidime ranged from 3–4.6 hours in patients with creatinine clearances of 39–73 mL/minute and 9.4–10.3 hours in patients with creatinine clearances of 13–27 mL/minute. The $t_{1/2\beta}$ of ceftazidime in patients with creatinine clearances less than 10 mL/minute ranges from 11.9–35 hours.

The serum half-life of ceftazidime is only slightly prolonged in patients with impaired hepatic function and accumulation of the drug does not generally occur in these patients unless renal function is also impaired. In a group of patients who had normal renal function but impaired hepatic function (e.g., alcoholic cirrhosis, chronic active hepatitis B, biliary cirrhosis), the serum half-life of ceftazidime averaged 2.9 hours. In another group of patients with ascites who had normal renal function, the $t_{1/2\alpha}$ of ceftazidime averaged 0.4 hours and the $t_{1/2\beta}$ averaged 5.9 hours.

Ceftazidime is readily removed by hemodialysis. The drug is also removed by peritoneal dialysis.

Chemistry and Stability

■ Chemistry Ceftazidime is a semisynthetic cephalosporin antibiotic. Like cefepime, cefotaxime, and ceftriaxone, ceftazidime is a parenteral aminothiazolyl cephalosporin. Ceftazidime contains an aminothiazolyl side chain at position 7 of the cephalosporin nucleus. The aminothiazolyl side chain enhances antibacterial activity, particularly against Enterobacteriaceae, and generally results in enhanced stability against β-lactamases. However, ceftazidime contains a carboxypropyl oxyimino group in the side chain rather than the methoxyimino group contained in many aminothiazolyl cephalosporins. This difference results in increased stability against hydrolysis by β-lactamases, increased activity against *Pseudomonas*, and decreased activity against gram-positive bacteria. Ceftazidime also contains a pyridine at position 3 of the cephalosporin nucleus.

Ceftazidime is commercially available as sterile powders for injection containing a mixture of ceftazidime (as the pentahydrate) and sodium carbonate. In these formulations, sodium carbonate has been admixed with ceftazidime to facilitate its dissolution; ceftazidime sodium is formed *in situ* following reconstitution of the powdered mixture as directed. These preparations contain 118 mg of sodium carbonate per gram of ceftazidime or 54 mg (2.3 mEq) of sodium per gram of ceftazidime. Potency of ceftazidime sodium is expressed in terms of ceftazidime, calculated on the anhydrous basis.

Ceftazidime occurs as a white to off-white powder. The drug has solubilities of 5 mg/mL in water and less than 1 mg/mL in alcohol. Ceftazidime has pK_as of 1.9, 2.7, and 4.1. When reconstituted as directed, ceftazidime sodium solutions have a pH of 5–8, and are light yellow to amber in color depending on the diluent used, concentration of the drug, and length of storage.

When the commercially available Duplex® drug delivery system containing 1 or 2 g of ceftazidime and 50 mL of 5% dextrose injection in separate chambers is reconstituted (activated) according to the manufacturer's directions, the resultant solution has an osmolality of approximately 340 and 400 mOsm/kg, respectively. The solutions are light yellow to amber in color and have a pH of 5–7.5.

Commercially available frozen premixed injections of ceftazidime sodium in dextrose are sterile, nonpyrogenic, iso-osmotic solutions of the drug provided in a plastic container (Galaxy® container) fabricated from specially formulated multilayered plastic (PL 2040). The 1- and 2-g frozen injections of ceftazidime contain approximately 2.2 or 1.6 g of dextrose, respectively, and have osmolalities of approximately 300 mOsm/kg; The frozen injections also contain hydrochloric acid and/or sodium hydroxide to adjust pH to 5–7.5; sodium hydroxide neutralizes ceftazidime pentahydrate free acid to the sodium salt.

■ Stability Ceftazidime powder and solutions of ceftazidime sodium tend to darken depending on storage conditions; however, color changes do not necessarily indicate loss of potency.

The commercially available vials of Fortaz® sterile powder for injection containing ceftazidime (as the pentahydrate) with sodium carbonate should be stored at 15–30°C and protected from light. Following reconstitution with sterile water for injection according to the manufacturer's directions, Fortaz® solutions for IV administration containing 100, 170, or 200 mg of ceftazidime per mL are stable for 12 hours at room temperature or 3 days when refrigerated. IV solutions prepared according to the manufacturer's directions using Fortaz® TwistVial® vials containing 1 or 2 g of ceftazidime and 0.9 or 0.45% sodium chloride injection or 5% dextrose injection are stable for 12 hours at room temperature or 3 days under refrigeration.

Following reconstitution with sterile water for injection, bacteriostatic water for injection, or 0.5 or 1% lidocaine hydrochloride injection, Fortaz® solutions for IM injection containing 280 mg/mL are stable for 12 hours at room temperature or 3 days when refrigerated.

The manufacturer of Fortaz® states that ceftazidime at concentrations of 1–40 mg/mL is chemically and physically stable for 12 hours at room temperature or for 3 days when refrigerated in the following IV solutions: 0.9% sodium chloride; ⅙*M* sodium lactate; 5 or 10% dextrose; 5% dextrose and 0.225, 0.45, or 0.9% sodium chloride; Ringer's; lactated Ringer's; 10% invert sugar; or Normosol®-M and 5% dextrose. Fortaz® solutions in 5% dextrose or 0.9% sodium chloride are stable for at least 6 hours at room temperature in plastic tubing, drip chambers, and volume control devices of common IV infusion sets.

The commercially available vials of Tazicef® sterile powder for injection containing ceftazidime (as the pentahydrate) with sodium carbonate should be stored at 20–25°C and protected from light. Following reconstitution with sterile water for injection according to the manufacturer's directions, Tazicef® solutions for IV or IM administration containing 95, 180, or 280 mg of ceftazidime per mL are stable for 24 hours at room temperature or 7 days when refrigerated. IV solutions prepared according to the manufacturer's directions using Tazicef® ADD-Vantage® vials containing 1 or 2 g of ceftazidime and 0.45 or 0.9% sodium chloride injection or 5% dextrose injection are stable for 24 hours at room temperature.

The commercially available Duplex® drug delivery system containing 1 or 2 g of ceftazidime and 50 mL of 5% dextrose injection in separate chambers should be stored at 20–25°C, but may be exposed to temperatures ranging from 15–30°C. Following reconstitution (activation), these IV solutions must be used within 12 hours if stored at room temperature or within 3 days if stored in a refrigerator and should not be frozen.

The commercially available frozen premixed injections of ceftazidime sodium in dextrose (Fortaz®) should be stored at −20°C or lower. The frozen injections should be thawed at room temperature (25°C) or under refrigeration (5°C) and, once thawed, should not be refrozen. Thawed solutions of the commercially available frozen injections are stable for 8 hours at room temperature or 7 days when refrigerated. The commercially available frozen injections of the drug are provided in plastic containers fabricated from specially formulated multilayered plastic PL 2040 (Galaxy® containers). Solutions in contact with PL 2040 can leach out some of its chemical components in very small amounts within the expiration period of the injections; however, safety of the plastic has been confirmed in tests in animals according to USP biological tests for plastic containers as well as by tissue culture toxicity studies.

Ceftazidime and ceftazidime sodium are potentially physically and/or chemically incompatible with some drugs, including aminoglycosides and vancomycin, but the compatibility depends on several factors (e.g., concentrations of the drugs, specific diluents used, resulting pH, temperature). Specialized references should be consulted for specific compatibility information. Sodium bicarbonate injection should not be used as a diluent for ceftazidime or ceftazidime sodium since the drug is less stable in sodium bicarbonate than in other IV solutions. Because of the potential for incompatibility, the manufacturers state that ceftazidime or ceftazidime sodium should not be admixed with aminoglycosides or vancomycin.

For further information on chemistry, mechanism of action, spectrum, resistance, pharmacokinetics, uses, cautions, drug interactions, laboratory test interferences, and dosage and administration of ceftazidime, see the Cephalosporins General Statement 8:12.06.

Preparations

Excipients in commercially available drug preparations may have clinically important effects in some individuals; consult specific product labeling for details.

cefTAZidime

Parenteral		
For injection	equivalent to anhydrous ceftazidime 500 mg (with sodium carbonate)*	**cefTAZidime for Injection**
		Fortaz®, Covis
	equivalent to anhydrous ceftazidime 1 g (with sodium carbonate)*	**cefTAZidime for Injection**
		Fortaz®, Covis
		Tazicef®, Hospira
	equivalent to anhydrous ceftazidime 2 g (with sodium carbonate)*	**cefTAZidime for Injection**
		Fortaz®, Covis
		Tazicef®, Hospira
	equivalent to anhydrous ceftazidime 6 g pharmacy bulk package (with sodium carbonate)*	**cefTAZidime for Injection**
		Fortaz®, Covis
		Tazicef®, Hospira
For injection, for IV infusion	equivalent to anhydrous ceftazidime 1 g (with sodium carbonate)	**cefTAZidime for Injection** (available in dual-chambered Duplex® drug delivery system with 5% dextrose injection), B Braun
		Fortaz® TwistVial®, Covis
		Tazicef® ADD-Vantage®, Hospira
	equivalent to anhydrous ceftazidime 2 g (with sodium carbonate)	**cefTAZidime for Injection** (available in dual-chambered Duplex® drug delivery system with 5% dextrose injection), B Braun
		Fortaz® TwistVial®, Covis
		Tazicef® ADD-Vantage®, Hospira

*available from one or more manufacturer, distributor, and/or repackager by generic (nonproprietary) name

cefTAZidime Sodium in Dextrose

Parenteral		
Injection (frozen), for IV infusion	equivalent to 20 mg (of anhydrous ceftazidime) per mL (1 g) in 4.4% Dextrose	**Fortaz® Iso-osmotic in Dextrose Injection** (Galaxy® [Baxter]), Covis
	equivalent to 40 mg (of anhydrous ceftazidime) per mL (2 g) in 3.2% Dextrose	**Fortaz® Iso-osmotic in Dextrose Injection** (Galaxy® [Baxter]), Covis

†Use is not currently included in the labeling approved by the US Food and Drug Administration

cefTAZidime and Avibactam Sodium

Ceftazidime/avibactam, Ceftazidime-avibactam, CAZ-AVI

■ Ceftazidime and avibactam sodium is a fixed combination of ceftazidime (a third generation cephalosporin) and avibactam (a non-β-lactam β-lactamase inhibitor); avibactam inactivates certain bacterial β-lactamases and expands ceftazidime's spectrum of activity against some bacteria that produce these β-lactamases.

Uses

■ **Intra-abdominal Infections** Ceftazidime and avibactam is used in conjunction with metronidazole for the treatment of complicated intra-abdominal infections caused by susceptible *Enterobacter cloacae, Escherichia coli, Klebsiella oxytoca, K. pneumoniae, Proteus mirabilis, Providencia stuartii*, or *Pseudomonas aeruginosa*.

Use of ceftazidime and avibactam for the treatment of complicated intra-abdominal infections should be reserved for patients with limited or no alternative treatment options since only limited data are available regarding safety and efficacy of the drug.

Clinical Experience Efficacy and safety of ceftazidime and avibactam for the treatment of complicated intra-abdominal infections is based on results from a phase 2, randomized, double-blind, active-controlled study in 204 adults with evidence of intra-abdominal infection requiring surgical intervention and anti-infective treatment. Patients were randomized in a 1:1 ratio to receive 5–14 days of treatment with the fixed combination of ceftazidime and avibactam (2.5 g [ceftazidime 2 g and avibactam 0.5 g] given by IV infusion every 8 hours) in conjunction with metronidazole (500 mg given by IV infusion every 8 hours) or treatment with meropenem (1 g given by IV infusion every 8 hours) in conjunction with placebo. Baseline characteristics were generally similar between groups (mean age 43 years, 69–79% male, 55–64% white, 83–87% with peritonitis, 39–44% with visceral perforation, 26–28% with abscess). Clinical response (defined as complete resolution or substantial improvement of signs and symptoms of infection with no requirement for additional antibiotics or surgery at the test-of-cure visit [2 weeks after the last treatment dose]) in the microbiologically evaluable population was achieved by 91.2% of patients treated with ceftazidime and avibactam in conjunction with metronidazole and 93.4% of those treated with meropenem.

■ **Urinary Tract Infections** Ceftazidime and avibactam is used for the treatment of complicated urinary tract infections, including pyelonephritis, caused by susceptible *E. coli, Citrobacter freundii, C. koseri, E. aerogenes, E. cloacae, K. pneumoniae, Proteus*, or *Ps. aeruginosa*.

Use of ceftazidime and avibactam for the treatment of complicated urinary tract infections should be reserved for patients with limited or no alternative treatment options since only limited data are available regarding safety and efficacy of the drug.

Clinical Experience Efficacy and safety of ceftazidime and avibactam for the treatment of complicated urinary tract infections is based on results from a phase 2, randomized, double-blind study in 137 adults with complicated urinary tract infection, including pyelonephritis, caused by gram-negative bacteria and requiring parenteral anti-infective treatment. Patients were randomized in a 1:1 ratio to receive treatment with the fixed combination of ceftazidime and avibactam (625 mg [ceftazidime 500 mg and avibactam 125 mg] given by IV infusion every 8 hours) or the fixed combination of imipenem and cilastatin (500 mg of imipenem given by IV infusion every 6 hours). Dosage of ceftazidime and avibactam used in this study is lower than the usually recommended dosage of the drug. After at least 4 days of IV treatment, patients with clinical improvement (afebrile for at least 24 hours, with resolution of nausea and vomiting and improved signs and symptoms) who had pathogens susceptible to both study anti-infectives were permitted to switch to oral ciprofloxacin (500 mg twice daily). The total duration of IV and/or oral anti-infective treatment was 7–14 days. Baseline characteristics were generally similar between groups (mean age 46–48 years, 25–27% male, 59–61% white, 61–65% diagnosed with acute pyelonephritis). Favorable microbiologic response (defined as eradication of all uropathogens at the test-of-cure visit 5–9 days after the last treatment dose) in the microbiologically evaluable population was achieved by 70.4% of patients treated with ceftazidime and avibactam and 71.4% of those treated with imipenem and cilastatin.

Dosage and Administration

■ **Administration** Ceftazidime and avibactam is administered by IV infusion.

IV Infusion **Reconstitution and Dilution.** Ceftazidime and avibactam powder must be reconstituted and further diluted prior to IV infusion.

Single-dose vials of ceftazidime and avibactam labeled as containing 2.5 g (ceftazidime 2 g and avibactam 0.5 g) should be reconstituted by adding 10 mL of a compatible IV solution (sterile water for injection, 0.9% sodium chloride injection, 5% dextrose injection, 2.5% dextrose and 0.45% sodium chloride injection, lactated Ringer's injection) to the vial and gently mixing. The volume of the reconstituted solution is approximately 12 mL and the approximate concentration is ceftazidime 167 mg/mL and avibactam 42 mg/mL. Reconstituted ceftazidime and avibactam solution may be stored for up to 30 minutes prior to transfer and dilution.

Prior to IV infusion, reconstituted ceftazidime and avibactam solution *must* be further diluted. To prepare the indicated dose, the appropriate volume of reconstituted solution should be withdrawn from the vial and added to a compatible IV solution to achieve a total final volume of 50–250 mL in an IV infusion bag. (See Table 1.) With the exception of sterile water for injection, the same IV solution used for reconstitution should be used for dilution; any other compatible IV solution should be used for dilution if sterile water for injection was used for reconstitution. The diluted solution should be mixed gently to ensure that the drug is completely dissolved.

Table 1. Dilution of Reconstituted Ceftazidime and Avibactam

Recommended Dose of Ceftazidime and Avibactam	Volume to Withdraw from Reconstituted Vial for Further Dilution
2.5 g (ceftazidime 2 g and avibactam 0.5 g)	12 mL (entire contents)
1.25 g (ceftazidime 1 g and avibactam 0.25 g)	6 mL
940 mg (ceftazidime 750 mg and avibactam 190 mg)	4.5 mL

The reconstituted and diluted solution of ceftazidime and avibactam should be inspected visually for particulate matter and discoloration prior to administration; the solution should appear clear and colorless to light yellow.

Following reconstitution and dilution, ceftazidime and avibactam solutions may be stored in the IV infusion bag at room temperature for up to 12 hours. Alternatively, these solutions may be stored at 2–8°C for up to 24 hours and then used within 12 hours after removal from refrigeration to room temperature.

Rate of Administration. IV infusions of ceftazidime and avibactam should be given over 2 hours.

Dispensing and Dosage and Administration Precautions. FDA alerted healthcare professionals about the risk of medication errors with ceftazidime and avibactam. There have been reports of errors occurring during preparation of IV solutions of the drug that resulted in administration of incorrect dosage (higher than intended); the errors were due to confusion about how dosage of ceftazidime and avibactam is expressed (total of the dosage of each of the 2 active components) and how drug strength was displayed on vial labels and carton packaging. To prevent such errors, vial labels and carton packaging have been revised to indicate the strength of the fixed combination as the total of the 2 active components.

Healthcare professionals should be aware that dosage of ceftazidime and avibactam is expressed as the total (sum) of the dosage of each of the 2 active components (i.e., dosage of ceftazidime plus dosage of avibactam). This dosage convention should be considered when prescribing, preparing, and dispensing ceftazidime and avibactam. FDA urges healthcare professionals and patients to report any medication errors and adverse effects involving the drug to the FDA MedWatch program.

■ **Dosage** Ceftazidime and avibactam is a fixed combination containing a 4:1 ratio of ceftazidime to avibactam.

The ceftazidime component is provided as a mixture of ceftazidime pentahydrate and sodium carbonate (dosage of this component is expressed in terms of anhydrous ceftazidime); the avibactam component is provided as avibactam sodium (dosage of this component is expressed in terms of avibactam).

Dosage of the fixed combination of ceftazidime and avibactam is expressed in terms of the total of the ceftazidime and avibactam content.

Each single-dose vial of ceftazidime and avibactam contains a total of 2.5 g (i.e., 2 g of ceftazidime and 0.5 g of avibactam).

Adult Dosage **Intra-abdominal Infections.** The recommended dosage of ceftazidime and avibactam for the treatment of complicated intra-abdominal infections in adults is 2.5 g (ceftazidime 2 g and avibactam 0.5 g) every 8 hours given in conjunction with metronidazole. The duration of treatment is 5–14 days.

Urinary Tract Infections. The recommended dosage of ceftazidime and avibactam for the treatment of complicated urinary tract infections, including pyelonephritis, in adults is 2.5 g (ceftazidime 2 g and avibactam 0.5 g) every 8 hours. The duration of treatment is 7–14 days.

■ **Dosage in Renal Impairment** Dosage of ceftazidime and avibactam must be adjusted in adults with creatinine clearances of 50 mL/minute or less, including those undergoing hemodialysis. (See Table 2.)

Creatinine clearance should be monitored at least once daily in patients with changing renal function and dosage of ceftazidime and avibactam adjusted accordingly.

Table 2. Ceftazidime and Avibactam Dosage for Adults with Renal Impairment

Estimated Creatinine Clearance (mL/minute)	Recommended Dosage
31–50	1.25 g (ceftazidime 1 g and avibactam 0.25 g) every 8 hours
16–30	940 mg (ceftazidime 750 mg and avibactam 190 mg) every 12 hours
6–15[a]	940 mg (ceftazidime 750 mg and avibactam 190 mg) every 24 hours
≤5[a]	940 mg (ceftazidime 750 mg and avibactam 190 mg) every 48 hours

[a] On hemodialysis days, the dose should be administered after dialysis.

■ **Dosage in Hepatic Impairment** Dosage adjustments are not needed when ceftazidime and avibactam is used in adults with hepatic impairment.

■ **Dosage in Geriatric Patients** Dosage adjustments based solely on age are not needed when ceftazidime and avibactam is used in geriatric patients. However, because geriatric patients are more likely to have decreased renal function and because dosage of ceftazidime and avibactam needs to be adjusted based on renal impairment, dosage should be selected with caution and it may be useful to monitor renal function.

Cautions

■ **Adverse Effects** Adverse effects reported in 5% or more of patients receiving ceftazidime and avibactam in phase 2 clinical trials include GI effects (nausea, vomiting, diarrhea, abdominal pain, constipation), pyrexia, increased AST, increased ALT, increased blood alkaline phosphatase, increased leukocyte count, headache, dizziness, chest pain, hypertension, cough, anxiety, insomnia, and infusion site reactions.

■ **Precautions and Contraindications** ***Sensitivity Reactions*** Ceftazidime and avibactam is contraindicated in patients with known serious hypersensitivity to ceftazidime and/or avibactam, avibactam-containing preparations, or other cephalosporins.

Serious and occasionally fatal hypersensitivity (anaphylactic) reactions and serious skin reactions have been reported in patients receiving β-lactam antibacterials. Before initiating therapy with ceftazidime and avibactam, the clinician should carefully inquire about the patient's previous hypersensitivity reactions to other cephalosporins, penicillins, or carbapenems. Ceftazidime and avibactam should be used with caution in patients allergic to penicillins or other β-lactams since cross-sensitivity among β-lactams antibacterials has been established.

Patients should be advised that allergic reactions, including serious allergic reactions, could occur and that serious reactions require immediate treatment.

If an allergic reaction occurs, ceftazidime and avibactam should be discontinued.

Reduced Efficacy in Patients with Moderate Renal Impairment Results of a subgroup analysis of a phase 3 clinical trial in patients with complicated intra-abdominal infections indicated that the clinical cure rate in patients with moderate renal impairment was lower than the clinical cure rate in those with normal renal function or only mild renal impairment, and this difference was more marked in those treated with a regimen of ceftazidime and avibactam in conjunction with metronidazole than in those treated with the comparator drug (meropenem). The clinical cure rate in patients treated with ceftazidime and avibactam in conjunction with metronidazole was 45% in those with baseline creatinine clearances of 30–50 mL/minute compared with 85% in those with baseline creatinine clearances greater than 50 mL/minute. Although the reason for this reduced efficacy is unclear, the dosage of ceftazidime and avibactam used in this study in patients with creatinine clearances of 30–50 mL/minute was 33% lower than the currently recommended dosage of the drug for such patients and it is possible that those with rapidly changing renal function did not receive appropriate dosage.

Creatinine clearance should be monitored at least once daily in patients with changing renal function and dosage of ceftazidime and avibactam adjusted accordingly. (See Other Precautions and Contraindications under Cautions: Precautions and Contraindications.)

Nervous System Effects Seizures, nonconvulsive status epilepticus, encephalopathy, coma, asterixis, neuromuscular excitability, and myoclonia have been reported in patients receiving ceftazidime, particularly in patients with renal impairment. Dosage of ceftazidime and avibactam should be adjusted based on creatinine clearance. (See Dosage and Administration: Dosage in Renal Impairment.)

Patients should be advised that adverse neurologic reactions can occur while receiving ceftazidime and avibactam and that they should immediately inform a clinician if any neurologic signs and symptoms, including encephalopathy (disturbance of consciousness such as confusion, hallucinations, stupor, coma), myoclonus, or seizures, occur since immediate treatment, dosage adjustment, or discontinuance of ceftazidime and avibactam may be necessary.

Hematologic Effects In clinical trials, seroconversion from a negative to a positive direct Coombs' test result occurred in 7.3% of patients receiving ceftazidime and avibactam in conjunction with metronidazole and in 1.9% of patients receiving ceftazidime and avibactam alone. Adverse reactions representing hemolytic anemia were not reported in any treatment group.

Eosinophilia and thrombocytopenia have been reported in less than 5% of patients receiving ceftazidime and avibactam.

Superinfection/Clostridium difficile-associated Diarrhea and Colitis (CDAD) Use of ceftazidime and avibactam may result in emergence and overgrowth of nonsusceptible bacteria or fungi. The patient should be carefully monitored and appropriate therapy instituted if superinfection occurs.

Treatment with anti-infectives alters normal colon flora and may permit overgrowth of *Clostridium difficile*. *C. difficile* infection (CDI) and *C. difficile*-associated diarrhea and colitis (CDAD; also known as antibiotic-associated diarrhea and colitis or pseudomembranous colitis) have been reported in patients receiving nearly all anti-infectives, including ceftazidime and avibactam, and may range in severity from mild diarrhea to fatal colitis. *C. difficile* produces toxins A and B which contribute to development of CDAD; hypertoxin-producing strains of *C. difficile* are associated with increased morbidity and mortality since they may be refractory to anti-infectives and colectomy may be required.

CDAD should be considered in the differential diagnosis of patients who develop diarrhea during or after anti-infective therapy. Careful medical history is necessary since CDAD has been reported to occur as late as 2 months or longer after anti-infective therapy is discontinued.

If CDAD is suspected or confirmed, anti-infective therapy not directed against *C. difficile* should be discontinued whenever possible. Patients should be managed with appropriate supportive therapy (e.g., fluid and electrolyte management, protein supplementation), anti-infective therapy directed against *C. difficile* (e.g., metronidazole, vancomycin), and surgical evaluation as clinically indicated.

Patients should be advised that diarrhea is a common problem caused by anti-infectives and usually resolves when the drug is discontinued; however, they should contact a clinician if watery and bloody stools (with or without stomach cramps and fever) occur during or as late as 2 months or longer after the last dose.

Selection and Use of Anti-infectives To reduce development of drug-resistant bacteria and maintain effectiveness of ceftazidime and avibactam and other antibacterials, the drug should be used only for treatment of infections proven or strongly suspected to be caused by susceptible bacteria.

When selecting or modifying anti-infective therapy, results of culture and in vitro susceptibility testing should be used. In the absence of such data, local epidemiology and susceptibility patterns should be considered when selecting anti-infectives for empiric therapy.

Patients should be advised that antibacterials (including ceftazidime and avibactam) should only be used to treat bacterial infections and not used to treat viral infections (e.g., the common cold). Patients also should be advised about the importance of completing the full course of therapy, even if feeling better after a few days, and that skipping doses or not completing therapy may decrease effectiveness and increase the likelihood that bacteria will develop resistance and will not be treatable with ceftazidime and avibactam or other antibacterials in the future.

Precautions Related to Use of Fixed Combinations When ceftazidime and avibactam is used, the cautions, precautions, contraindications, and drug interactions associated with both drugs in the fixed combination must be considered. Cautionary information applicable to specific populations (e.g., pregnant or nursing women, individuals with hepatic or renal impairment, geriatric patients) should be considered for each drug. (For additional cautionary information on ceftazidime, see Cautions in Ceftazidime 8:12.06.12.)

When prescribing, preparing, and dispensing ceftazidime and avibactam, healthcare professionals should consider that dosage of the fixed combination is expressed as the total (sum) of the dosage of each of the 2 active components (i.e., dosage of ceftazidime plus dosage of avibactam). (See Dispensing and Dosage and Administration Precautions under Administration: IV Infusion, in Dosage and Administration.)

Other Precautions and Contraindications Ceftazidime and avibactam are principally eliminated by the kidneys, and the risk of adverse effects may be greater in patients with renal impairment. In addition, a lower cure rate has been reported in some patients with moderate renal impairment (see Reduced Efficacy in Patients with Moderate Renal Impairment under Cautions: Precautions and Contraindications). Dosage of ceftazidime and avibactam should be adjusted in patients with moderate or severe renal impairment (creatinine clearances of 50 mL/minute or less), including those undergoing hemodialysis. In patients with changing renal function, creatinine clearance should be monitored at least once daily and dosage adjusted accordingly. (See Dosage and Administration: Dosage in Renal Impairment.)

■ **Pediatric Precautions** Safety and efficacy of ceftazidime and avibactam have not been established in patients younger than 18 years of age.

■ **Geriatric Precautions** In phase 2 clinical trials evaluating ceftazidime and avibactam for the treatment of complicated intra-abdominal infections or complicated urinary tract infections, 10.7% of patients were 65 years of age or older. Since only limited data are available, age-related differences in outcomes or specific risks with ceftazidime and avibactam cannot be ruled out.

Ceftazidime and avibactam are eliminated principally by the kidneys, and the risk of adverse effects may be greater in those with impaired renal function. Because geriatric patients are more likely to have reduced renal function, dosage should be selected with caution and renal function monitoring should be considered. Dosage adjustments in geriatric patients should be based on renal function.

■ **Mutagenicity and Carcinogenicity** Ceftazidime was not mutagenic in a microbial (i.e., Ames test) or mammalian cell (i.e., mouse micronucleus) test. Avibactam was not genotoxic in the Ames assay, unscheduled DNA synthesis test, chromosomal aberration assay, or a rat micronucleus study.

■ **Pregnancy, Fertility, and Lactation** ***Pregnancy*** Reproduction studies in mice and rats using ceftazidime dosages up to 40 times the usual human dose have not revealed evidence of harm to the fetus. Avibactam was not teratogenic in rats or rabbits. In rats, there was no evidence of embryofetal toxicity at an avibactam dosage of 1 g/kg daily (approximately 9 times the human dosage based on area under the concentration-time curve [AUC]) and no effects on pup growth and viability at a dosage of 825 mg/kg daily. In rabbits, there was no evidence of embryofetal toxicity at an avibactam dosage of 100 mg/kg, but increased implantation loss, lower mean fetal weights, delayed ossification of bones, and other anomalies were observed at higher dosages.

There are no adequate and controlled studies using ceftazidime and avibactam in pregnant women, and the drug should be used during pregnancy only if clearly needed.

Fertility Avibactam had no adverse effects on fertility in male and female rats using dosages up to 1 g/kg daily (approximately 20 times higher than the recommended human dosage based on body surface area). In female rats, IV avibactam dosages of 0.5 g/kg or higher resulted in dose-related increases in the percentage of pre- and post-implantation loss compared with controls.

Lactation Ceftazidime is distributed into human milk in low concentrations. It is not known whether avibactam is distributed into human milk. (See Pharmacokinetics: Distribution.)

Ceftazidime and avibactam should be used with caution in nursing women.

Drug Interactions

The following drug interactions are based on studies using the fixed combination containing ceftazidime and avibactam, ceftazidime alone, or avibactam alone. When ceftazidime and avibactam is used, interactions associated with both drugs in the fixed combination should be considered.

■ **Drugs Affecting or Metabolized by Hepatic Microsomal Enzymes** Ceftazidime does not induce cytochrome P-450 (CYP) 1A1, 1A2, 2B6, or 3A4/5 when tested in vitro in human hepatocytes.

In vitro, avibactam does not inhibit CYP1A2, 2A6, 2B6, 2C8, 2C9, 2C19, 2D6, 2E1, or 3A4/5 and does not induce CYP1A2, 2B6, 2C9, or 3A4. At concentrations exceeding clinically relevant exposures, avibactam shows some potential to induce CYP2E1.

■ **Drugs Affecting or Affected by Organic Anion Transporters** In vitro, avibactam is a substrate of organic anion transporter (OAT) 1 and OAT3 kidney transporters. In vitro, probenecid (a potent OAT1/OAT3 inhibitor) inhibits uptake of avibactam by 56–70% and has the potential to decrease elimination of avibactam. (See Drug Interactions: Probenecid.)

Ceftazidime and avibactam do not inhibit OAT1 or OAT3 and ceftazidime does not inhibit avibactam transport mediated by OAT1 and OAT3.

■ **Drugs Affecting or Affected by Other Membrane Transporters** In vitro, ceftazidime and avibactam do not inhibit multidrug-resistance transporter (MDR) 1, breast cancer resistance protein (BCRP), organic anion transporting polypeptide (OATP) 1B1, OATP1B3, bile salt export pump (BSEP), multidrug resistance-associated protein (MRP) 4, organic cation transporter (OCT) 1, or OCT2 at clinically relevant concentrations. Avibactam is not a substrate of MDR1, BCRP, MRP4, or OCT2.

■ **Anti-infectives** ***Metronidazole*** In healthy males, administration of ceftazidime and avibactam (2.5 g [ceftazidime 2 g and avibactam 0.5 g] given by IV infusion over 2 hours) following metronidazole (500 mg given by IV infusion over 1 hour every 8 hours for 3 days) had no effect on peak plasma concentrations or area under the plasma concentration-time curve (AUC) of ceftazidime or avibactam compared with use of ceftazidime and avibactam alone. Similarly, administration of metronidazole (500 mg given by IV infusion over 1 hour) followed by ceftazidime and avibactam (2.5 g [ceftazidime 2 g and avibactam 0.5 g] given by IV infusion over 2 hours every 8 hours for 3 days) in healthy males had no effect on peak plasma concentrations and AUC of metronidazole compared with use of metronidazole alone.

There is no in vitro evidence of antagonistic antibacterial effects between ceftazidime and avibactam and metronidazole.

Other Anti-infectives There is no in vitro evidence of antagonistic antibacterial effects between ceftazidime and avibactam and colistin (commercially available in US as colistimethate sodium), levofloxacin, linezolid, tigecycline, tobramycin, or vancomycin.

■ **Probenecid** In vitro studies indicate probenecid (a potent OAT1/OAT3 inhibitor) has the potential to decrease elimination of avibactam by inhibiting renal uptake of the drug. Therefore, concomitant use of probenecid with ceftazidime and avibactam is not recommended.

Laboratory Test Interferences

■ **Tests for Urinary Glucose** Administration of ceftazidime may result in a false-positive reaction for urine glucose when certain testing methods are used. Urine glucose tests based on enzymatic glucose oxidase reactions should be used in patients receiving ceftazidime and avibactam.

Mechanism of Action

Ceftazidime and avibactam is bactericidal in action.

Like other cephalosporins, the antibacterial activity of ceftazidime results from inhibition of mucopeptide synthesis in the bacterial cell wall and is mediated through binding to penicillin-binding proteins (PBPs). (For information on the mechanism of action of cephalosporins, see Mechanism of Action in the Cephalosporins General Statement 8:12.06.)

Avibactam is a non-β-lactam β-lactamase inhibitor that inactivates certain β-lactamases, including some extended-spectrum β-lactamases (ESBLs). Avibactam inactivates many β-lactamases in Ambler class A (e.g., ESBLs, carbapenemases such as *Klebsiella pneumoniae* carbapenemases [KPCs]), class C (e.g., cephalosporinases such as AmpC), and class D (e.g., some oxacillinases [OXAs]). Avibactam binds to the β-lactamase active site serine residue by covalent acylation, which is partially reversible; subsequently, deacylation can occur resulting in release of intact avibactam allowing additional β-lactamase inhibition. This mechanism of action differs from that of some other β-lactamase inhibitors (e.g., clavulanic acid, sulbactam, tazobactam) that can form covalent, irreversible, acyl-enzyme intermediates that may undergo hydrolysis, resulting in decomposition of the β-lactamase inhibitor. Avibactam cannot inactivate Ambler class B metallo-β-lactamases (MBLs) or certain OXA-type carbapenemases.

Because avibactam inactivates certain β-lactamases, concomitant use with ceftazidime can protect ceftazidime from degradation by these β-lactamases and expand the spectrum of activity of the cephalosporin to include many β-lactamase-producing bacteria that are resistant to ceftazidime alone. Avibactam does not decrease the antibacterial activity of ceftazidime against ceftazidime-susceptible bacteria.

Spectrum

Based on its spectrum of activity, ceftazidime and avibactam is classified as a third generation cephalosporin. (For information on the classification of cephalosporins and closely related β-lactam antibiotics based on spectra of activity, see Spectrum in the Cephalosporins General Statement 8:12.06.)

Like other currently available parenteral third generation cephalosporins (e.g., cefotaxime, ceftriaxone), ceftazidime generally is less active against staphylococci but has an expanded spectrum of activity against gram-negative bacteria compared with first and second generation cephalosporins. Ceftazidime is distinguished from many other cephalosporins by its activity against *Pseudomonas aeruginosa*. (For information on the spectrum of activity of ceftazidime used alone, see Spectrum in Ceftazidime 8:12.06.12.)

Ceftazidime and avibactam has a wider spectrum of activity than ceftazidime alone. Ceftazidime and avibactam is active against many β-lactamase-producing gram-negative bacteria that are resistant to ceftazidime alone, including many strains that produce extended-spectrum β-lactamases (ESBLs). The fixed combination is active in vitro against Enterobacteriaceae that produce TEM, SHV, CTX-M, *Klebsiella pneumoniae* carbapenemase (KPC), AmpC, and certain oxacillinase (OXA) β-lactamases and also is active in vitro against *Ps. aeruginosa* that produce certain AmpC β-lactamases.

Ceftazidime and avibactam is active in vitro against some Enterobacteriaceae and *Ps. aeruginosa* that are resistant to carbapenems, other cephalosporins (including ceftazidime alone), or fluoroquinolones.

■ **In Vitro Susceptibility Testing** When in vitro susceptibility testing is performed according to the standards of the Clinical and Laboratory Standards Institute (CLSI; formerly National Committee for Clinical Laboratory Standards [NCCLS]), clinical isolates identified as *susceptible* to ceftazidime and avibactam are inhibited by drug concentrations usually achievable when dosage recommended for the site of infection is used. If results of in vitro susceptibility testing indicate that a clinical isolate is *resistant* to ceftazidime and avibactam, the strain is not likely to be inhibited by drug concentrations generally achievable with usual dosage schedules and other anti-infective therapy should be selected.

Disk Susceptibility Tests When the disk-diffusion procedure is used to test susceptibility to ceftazidime and avibactam, a disk containing 30 mcg of ceftazidime and 20 mcg of avibactam is used.

When disk-diffusion susceptibility testing is performed according to CLSI standardized procedures, Enterobacteriaceae with growth inhibition zones of 21 mm or greater are susceptible to ceftazidime and avibactam and those with zones of 20 mm or less are resistant to the drug. *Ps. aeruginosa* with growth inhibition zones of 18 mm or greater are susceptible to ceftazidime and avibactam and those with zones of 17 mm or less are resistant to the drug.

Dilution Susceptibility Tests When dilution susceptibility testing (agar or broth dilution) is used to test susceptibility to ceftazidime and avibactam, tests should be performed using serial dilutions of ceftazidime combined with a fixed avibactam concentration of 4 mcg/mL. If a broth dilution test is used, results should be read within 18 hours because degradation of ceftazidime activity occurs by 24 hours.

When dilution susceptibility testing is performed according to CLSI standardized procedures, Enterobacteriaceae and *Ps. aeruginosa* with MICs of 8 mcg/mL or less of ceftazidime and 4 mcg/mL or less of avibactam are susceptible to ceftazidime and avibactam and those with MICs of 16 mcg/mL or greater of ceftazidime and 4 mcg/mL or greater of avibactam are resistant to the drug.

■ **Gram-negative Aerobic Bacteria** Ceftazidime and avibactam is active in vitro against many Enterobacteriaceae, including *Citrobacter freundii, C. koseri, Enterobacter aerogenes, E. cloacae, Escherichia coli, K. pneumoniae, K. oxytoca, Morganella morganii, Proteus* (including *P. mirabilis* and *P. vulgaris*), *Providencia rettgeri, P. stuartii*, and *Serratia marcescens*.

Ceftazidime and avibactam is active in vitro against many strains of *Ps. aeruginosa*, including some multidrug-resistant (MDR) and extensively drug-resistant (XDR) *Ps. aeruginosa*.

■ **Anaerobic Bacteria** Although ceftazidime and avibactam has been active in vitro against a few strains of *Bacteroides fragilis, Prevotella*, and *Porphyromonas*, the fixed combination shows only limited in vitro activity against most anaerobic bacteria.

Resistance

Resistance or reduced susceptibility to ceftazidime and avibactam can occur. The mechanism of resistance to the fixed combination may be multifactorial.

Bacteria that produce Ambler class B metallo-β-lactamases (MBLs) are resistant to ceftazidime and avibactam because avibactam does not inhibit this type of β-lactamase. In addition, bacterial strains producing certain oxacillinase (OXA) β-lactamases (e.g., *Acinetobacter, Pseudomonas aeruginosa*) also are resistant to ceftazidime and avibactam. There is some in vitro evidence that point mutations in existing β-lactamases can result in selection of resistant mutants that have β-lactamases with reduced affinity for avibactam or changes that prevent the β-lactamase inhibitor from binding to and inhibiting the enzyme.

Bacteria resistant to ceftazidime because of altered penicillin-binding proteins (PBPs) may also be resistant to ceftazidime and avibactam. Some strains of gram-negative bacteria (e.g., *Ps. aeruginosa, Serratia marcescens*) that overexpress efflux pumps or have porin mutations that result in resistance to ceftazidime may also have reduced susceptibility or resistance to ceftazidime and avibactam.

Cross-resistance between ceftazidime and avibactam and other classes of anti-infectives has not been reported.

Pharmacokinetics

Following IV administration of the fixed combination of ceftazidime and avibactam sodium, pharmacokinetic parameters for ceftazidime and avibactam are similar to those reported when each drug is administered alone. In addition, pharmacokinetic parameters are similar following single or multiple IV doses of the fixed combination.

■ **Absorption** In healthy adult males with normal renal function receiving multiple doses of ceftazidime and avibactam (2.5 g [ceftazidime 2 g and avibactam 0.5 g]) given by IV infusion over 2 hours every 8 hours for 11 days, peak plasma concentrations of ceftazidime were 90.4 mcg/mL and peak plasma concentrations of avibactam were 14.6 mcg/mL.

Peak plasma concentrations and area under the plasma concentration-time curve (AUC) of ceftazidime increase in proportion to the dose; avibactam demonstrated approximately linear pharmacokinetics when single IV doses ranging from 50 mg to 2 g were given alone.

There is no appreciable accumulation of ceftazidime or avibactam in healthy adults with normal renal function following multiple doses of ceftazidime and avibactam (2.5 g [ceftazidime 2 g and avibactam 0.5 g]) given by IV infusion every 8 hours for up to 11 days.

In healthy adults 65 years of age or older who received a single 0.5-g IV dose of avibactam, the AUC of the drug was 17% higher than the AUC reported in healthy adults 18–45 years of age; peak plasma concentrations of avibactam in these adults were not substantially affected by age.

In a study in healthy adults who received a single 0.5-g IV dose of avibactam, peak plasma concentrations of the drug in males were 18% lower than in females; gender did not affect the AUC of avibactam.

■ **Distribution** The steady-state volumes of distribution of ceftazidime and avibactam are 17 and 22.2 L, respectively, in healthy adults following multiple doses of ceftazidime and avibactam (2.5 g [ceftazidime 2 g and avibactam 0.5 g]) given by IV infusion every 8 hours for 11 days.

Ceftazidime is less than 10% protein bound; avibactam is approximately 5.7–8.2% bound to plasma proteins.

Ceftazidime is distributed into human milk in low concentrations. In rats, avibactam is distributed into milk in a dose-dependent manner; it is not known whether avibactam is distributed into human milk.

■ **Elimination** Ceftazidime and avibactam do not undergo clinically important metabolism, and both drugs are principally eliminated unchanged in urine.

There was no evidence of metabolism of avibactam in vitro in human liver preparations (microsomes and hepatocytes), and unchanged avibactam was the major component in human plasma and urine after a single IV dose of 0.5 g of avibactam.

Following an IV dose of ceftazidime, approximately 80–90% of the dose is excreted unchanged by the kidneys over 24 hours. Following an IV dose of avibactam, an average of 97% of the dose is eliminated in urine and 0.2% is eliminated in feces.

The plasma elimination half-lives of ceftazidime and avibactam are 2.8 and 2.7 hours, respectively, in healthy adult males with normal renal function receiving multiple doses of ceftazidime and avibactam (2.5 g [ceftazidime 2 g and avibactam 0.5 g]) given by IV infusion over 2 hours every 8 hours.

The serum half-life of ceftazidime is prolonged in patients with renal impairment. Following a single 100-mg IV dose of avibactam in adults with mild, moderate, or severe renal impairment not requiring hemodialysis, the AUC of avibactam was 2.6-, 3.8-, or 7-fold higher, respectively, compared with the AUC reported in healthy adults with normal renal function. In adults with end-stage renal disease (ESRD) who received a single 100-mg IV dose of avibactam 1 hour after hemodialysis, the AUC of avibactam was 19.5-fold higher than the AUC reported in healthy adults with normal renal function.

Both ceftazidime and avibactam are removed by hemodialysis. In patients with ESRD who received 1 g of ceftazidime or 100 mg of avibactam prior to a 4-hour hemodialysis session, 55% of the ceftazidime dose or 55% of the avibactam dose was recovered in the dialysate.

There was no effect on ceftazidime pharmacokinetics when ceftazidime was given in a dosage of 2 g IV every 8 hours for 5 days in adults with hepatic impairment. Pharmacokinetics of avibactam have not been established in patients with hepatic impairment; however, avibactam does not appear to undergo clinically important hepatic metabolism and systemic clearance of the drug is not expected to be affected by hepatic impairment.

Chemistry and Stability

■ **Chemistry** Ceftazidime and avibactam sodium is a fixed combination of ceftazidime (a third generation cephalosporin antibiotic) and avibactam (a non-β-lactam β-lactamase inhibitor); avibactam inactivates certain bacterial β-lactamases and expands ceftazidime's spectrum of activity against some bacteria that produce these β-lactamases.

Ceftazidime contains an aminothiadiazole ring that enhances antibacterial activity against gram-negative bacteria, a carboxypropyl-oxyimino group that contributes to stability in the presence of β-lactamases, and a methylpyridinium group responsible for the drug's antipseudomonal activity. (For additional information on ceftazidime, see Ceftazidime 8:12.06.12.)

Avibactam is a diazabicyclooctanone derivative non-β-lactam β-lactamase inhibitor that differs structurally and pharmacologically from β-lactam β-lactamase inhibitors (e.g., sulbactam, clavulanic acid, tazobactam). Avibactam does not contain a β-lactam core, but does resemble β-lactams in key areas (i.e., carbonyl at position 7, sulfate at position 6, carboxamide at position 2), which allows binding to and inactivation of certain β-lactamases produced by bacteria.

Ceftazidime and avibactam is commercially available as a white to yellow sterile powder for IV infusion containing a 4:1 ratio of ceftazidime to avibactam. The ceftazidime component is provided as a mixture of ceftazidime (as the pentahydrate) and sodium carbonate (facilitates dissolution of ceftazidime); the avibactam component is provided as avibactam sodium. Drug strength and dosage are expressed as the total of the 2 active components. (See Dispensing and Dosage and Administration Precautions under Administration: IV Infusion, in Dosage and Administration.)

Each single-dose vial of ceftazidime and avibactam contains 2.5 g (2 g of ceftazidime [equivalent to 2.635 g of the ceftazidime pentahydrate and sodium carbonate mixture] and 0.5 g of avibactam [equivalent to 0.551 g of avibactam sodium]). The total sodium content is approximately 146 mg (6.4 mEq) per single-dose vial.

■ **Stability** Ceftazidime and avibactam powder for IV infusion should be stored at 25°C, but may be exposed to temperatures ranging from 15–30°C. Vials should be protected from light.

Following reconstitution and dilution, ceftazidime and avibactam solutions should be used within 12 hours when stored at room temperature. Alternatively, reconstituted and diluted solutions of the drug may be stored for up to 24 hours at 2–8°C and then used within 12 hours after removal from refrigeration to room temperature.

For further information on chemistry, mechanism of action, spectrum, resistance, uses, cautions, acute toxicity, drug interactions, or laboratory test interferences of cephalosporins, see the Cephalosporins General Statement 8:12.06.

Preparations

Excipients in commercially available drug preparations may have clinically important effects in some individuals; consult specific product labeling for details.

cefTAZidime and Avibactam Sodium

Parenteral

For injection, for IV infusion	2.5 g (2 g of ceftazidime and 0.5 g of avibactam)	**Avycaz®**, Forest

Ceftibuten

■ Ceftibuten is a semisynthetic, third generation cephalosporin antibiotic.

Uses

Ceftibuten is used orally for the treatment of mild to moderate respiratory tract infections (i.e., acute exacerbations of chronic bronchitis) caused by susceptible bacteria. The drug also is used orally for the treatment of acute otitis media caused by susceptible bacteria and pharyngitis and tonsillitis caused by *Streptococcus pyogenes* (group A β-hemolytic streptococci). Oral ceftibuten also has been used for the treatment of urinary tract infections† caused by susceptible bacteria.

■ **Acute Otitis Media** Oral ceftibuten is used for the treatment of acute otitis media (AOM) caused by *Haemophilus influenzae* (including β-lactamase-producing strains), *Moraxella catarrhalis* (including β-lactamase-producing strains), or *S. pyogenes*. Ceftibuten is not considered a drug of first choice for treatment of AOM.

Since there is some evidence that ceftibuten may be less effective than some other β-lactam antibiotics for the treatment of otitis media caused by *S. pneumoniae*, the manufacturer cautions that ceftibuten should be used for the empiric treatment of acute bacterial otitis media only when adequate antimicrobial coverage against *S. pneumoniae* has been previously administered.

When anti-infective therapy is indicated for the treatment of AOM, the American Academy of Pediatrics (AAP) recommends high-dose amoxicillin or amoxicillin and clavulanate potassium as the drugs of first choice for initial treatment. These experts recommend certain cephalosporins (cefdinir, cefpodoxime, cefuroxime, ceftriaxone) as alternatives for initial treatment in penicillin-allergic patients who do not have a history of severe and/or recent penicillin-allergic reactions.

Results of controlled clinical studies in children 6 months to 11 years of age with clinically and/or microbiologically confirmed AOM indicate that a 10-day regimen of oral ceftibuten generally is as effective as a 10-day regimen of oral cefaclor, oral amoxicillin and clavulanate potassium, or oral cefprozil. In published studies, the overall clinical response rate to a 10-day regimen of oral ceftibuten in pediatric patients with AOM has been 83.3–93%. In one study when results were stratified according to causative organism, the clinical response rate to ceftibuten in pediatric patients with AOM caused by *Haemophilus* (including *H. influenzae*), *M. catarrhalis*, or *S. pyogenes* was 92–100% and the response rate in those with otitis media caused by *S. pneumoniae* was 80%.

For additional information regarding treatment of AOM, including information on diagnosis and management strategies, anti-infectives for initial treatment, duration of initial treatment, and anti-infectives after initial treatment failure, see Acute Otitis Media under Uses: Otitis Media, in the Cephalosporins General Statement 8:12.06.

■ **Pharyngitis and Tonsillitis** Oral ceftibuten is used for the treatment of pharyngitis and tonsillitis caused by *S. pyogenes* (group A β-hemolytic streptococci). Although ceftibuten usually is effective in eradicating *S. pyogenes* from the nasopharynx, efficacy of the drug in the subsequent prevention of rheumatic fever remains to be established.

Selection of an anti-infective for the treatment of *S. pyogenes* pharyngitis and tonsillitis should be based on the drug's spectrum of activity, bacteriologic and clinical efficacy, potential adverse effects, ease of administration, patient compliance, and cost. No regimen has been found to date that effectively eradicates group A β-hemolytic streptococci in 100% of patients.

Because the drugs have a narrow spectrum of activity, are inexpensive, and generally are effective with a low incidence of adverse effects, the AAP, Infectious Diseases Society of America (IDSA), American Heart Association (AHA), and others recommend a penicillin regimen (i.e., 10 days of oral penicillin V or oral amoxicillin or a single dose of IM penicillin G benzathine) as the treatment of choice for *S. pyogenes* pharyngitis and tonsillitis and prevention of initial attacks (primary prevention) of rheumatic fever. Other anti-infectives (e.g., oral cephalosporins, oral macrolides, oral clindamycin) generally are recommended as alternatives in penicillin-allergic individuals.

If an oral cephalosporin is used for the treatment of *S. pyogenes* pharyngitis and tonsillitis, a 10-day regimen of a first generation cephalosporin (cefadroxil, cephalexin) is preferred instead of other cephalosporins with broader spectrums of activity (e.g., cefaclor, cefdinir, cefixime, cefpodoxime, cefuroxime).

Although there is some evidence that a shorter duration of therapy with certain oral cephalosporins (e.g., a 5-day regimen of cefadroxil, cefdinir, cefixime, or cefpodoxime proxetil or a 4- or 5-day regimen of cefuroxime axetil) achieves bacteriologic and clinical cure rates equal to or greater than those achieved with the traditional 10-day oral penicillin V regimen, the IDSA and AHA state that use of cephalosporin regimens administered for 5 days or less for the treatment of *S. pyogenes* pharyngitis and tonsillitis cannot be recommended at this time.

Results of a randomized, multicenter study in children 3–18 years of age with *S. pyogenes* pharyngitis or tonsillitis indicate that 10 days of therapy with oral ceftibuten (9 mg/kg once daily) is more effective than 10 days of therapy with oral penicillin V (25 mg/kg daily given in 3 divided doses). At early follow-up (i.e., 5–7 days after completion of therapy), 97% of those who received ceftibuten and 89% of those who received penicillin V had clinical cure or improvement and the bacteriologic elimination rate in these groups was 91 and 80%, respectively. At late follow-up (i.e., 2–3 weeks after completion of therapy), the bacteriologic elimination rate was 89% in those who received ceftibuten and 79% in those who received penicillin V and the relapse rate was 4 and 6%, respectively.

■ **Respiratory Tract Infections** ***Acute Sinusitis*** Oral ceftibuten has been effective when used in adults for the treatment of acute maxillary sinusitis† caused by susceptible *S. pneumoniae, H. influenzae*, or *M. catarrhalis*.

When anti-infective therapy is indicated for the treatment of acute bacterial sinusitis, the IDSA recommends amoxicillin and clavulanate potassium and the AAP recommends either amoxicillin or amoxicillin and clavulanate potassium as the drug of choice for initial empiric treatment. Because of variable activity against *S. pneumoniae* and *H. influenzae*, the IDSA no longer recommends second or third generation oral cephalosporins for empiric monotherapy of sinusitis in adults or children. If an oral cephalosporin is used as an alternative for empiric treatment of acute bacterial sinusitis in children (e.g., in penicillin-allergic individuals), the IDSA and AAP recommend a combination regimen that includes a third generation cephalosporin (cefixime or cefpodoxime) and clindamycin (or linezolid).

Acute Exacerbations of Chronic Bronchitis Oral ceftibuten is used for the treatment of acute exacerbations of chronic bronchitis caused by susceptible *S. pneumoniae* (penicillin-susceptible strains only), *H. influenzae* (including β-lactamase-producing strains), or *M. catarrhalis* (including β-lactamase-producing strains.

Results of randomized clinical studies in adults with acute exacerbations of chronic bronchitis indicate that oral ceftibuten is at least as effective as oral amoxicillin and clavulanate potassium, oral cefaclor, oral clarithromycin, or oral ciprofloxacin for the empiric treatment of these infections. The overall clinical success rates reported in these studies were 79.3–84, 79, or 83.7% in those who received ceftibuten, amoxicillin and clavulanate potassium, or ciprofloxacin, respectively. When results were stratified according to the causative organism, the microbiologic eradication rate in patients receiving ceftibuten was 66–100% in those with infections caused by *S. pneumoniae*, 72–100% in those with infections caused by *M. catarrhalis*, and 73–95.2% in those with infections caused by *H. influenzae* or *H. parainfluenzae*. The manufacturer cautions that, while ceftibuten has been clinically equivalent to comparator drugs in clinical studies, ceftibuten was associated with a lower bacteriologic eradication rate than the comparator in some studies when used for the treatment of acute bacterial exacerbations of chronic bronchitis when *M. catarrhalis* was isolated from infected sputum at baseline.

■ **Urinary Tract Infections** Oral ceftibuten has been used effectively for the treatment of acute uncomplicated urinary tract infections† or the treatment of complicated or recurrent urinary tract infections† caused by susceptible *Escherichia coli, Klebsiella, Proteus mirabilis, Enterobacter*, or staphylococci. In one study in adult women with acute uncomplicated urinary tract infections who received a 7-day regimen of oral ceftibuten (400 mg once daily), the clinical cure and bacteriologic eradication rate 5–9 days after completion of therapy was 93%. In pediatric patients 6 months to 12 years of age with complicated, recurrent urinary tract infections randomized to receive a 10-day regimen of oral ceftibuten or oral co-trimoxazole, the clinical response rate (cure plus improvement) was 98% in those who received ceftibuten and 96% in those who received co-trimoxazole; however, the bacteriologic elimination rate was 99 and 88%, respectively.

Some clinicians suggest that certain oral third generation cephalosporins (cefdinir, cefpodoxime proxetil, ceftibuten) are one of several alternatives that can be used for the outpatient treatment of recurrent urinary tract infections or urinary tract infections that occur in patients who have indwelling urinary catheters or acquired their infections in hospitals or nursing homes since these infections are likely to be caused by multidrug-resistant gram-negative bacilli.

Dosage and Administration

■ **Reconstitution and Administration** Ceftibuten dihydrate is administered orally.

Ceftibuten dihydrate capsules may be administered without regard to meals.

Ceftibuten dihydrate oral suspension should be administered at least 2 hours before or 1 hour after meals since bioavailability of the drug from the oral suspension is decreased when administered with food. (See Pharmacokinetics: Absorption.)

Reconstitution Ceftibuten dihydrate powder for oral suspension should be reconstituted at the time of dispensing by adding the amount of water specified on the container to provide a suspension containing 90 mg of ceftibuten per 5 mL. The water should be added in 2 equal portions and the bottle shaken after each addition.

The oral suspension should be shaken prior to administration of each dose.

■ **Dosage** Ceftibuten is commercially available as ceftibuten dihydrate; dosage is expressed in terms of anhydrous ceftibuten.

Adult Dosage For the treatment of acute otitis media, pharyngitis and tonsillitis, or acute exacerbations of chronic bronchitis in adults and adolescents 12 years of age and older, the usual dosage of ceftibuten is 400 mg once daily for 10 days.

Adults have received ceftibuten in a dosage of 400 mg once daily for 7 days for the treatment of uncomplicated urinary tract infections† caused by susceptible bacteria.

Pediatric Dosage Adolescents 12 years of age or older may receive the usual adult dosage of ceftibuten.

The usual dosage of ceftibuten for the treatment of acute otitis media or pharyngitis and tonsillitis in children 6 months of age through 11 years of age is 9 mg/kg (up to 400 mg) once daily for 10 days. When the oral suspension is used, pediatric patients weighing 10, 20, or 40 kg should receive once-daily doses of 90, 180, or 360 mg respectively. Pediatric patients weighing more than 45 kg should receive the maximum dosage of 400 mg daily.

■ **Dosage in Renal and Hepatic Impairment** Patients with creatinine clearances of 50 mL/minute or greater may receive the usual dosage of ceftibuten.

The manufacturer recommends that patients with creatinine clearances of 30–49 mL/minute receive a ceftibuten dosage of 4.5 mg/kg or 200 mg every 24 hours. Patients with creatinine clearances of 5–29 mL/minute should receive a ceftibuten dosage of 2.25 mg/kg or 100 mg every 24 hours.

Since ceftibuten is partially removed by hemodialysis, patients undergoing hemodialysis 2 or 3 times weekly may receive a single dose of 400 mg (given as a capsule) or 9 mg/kg (up to 400 mg; given as the oral suspension) at the end of each dialysis period.

Limited data suggest that chronic hepatic impairment does not affect the pharmacokinetics of ceftibuten; the manufacturer makes no specific recommendations for modification of dosage in patients with hepatic impairment.

Cautions

■ **Adverse Effects** Adverse effects reported with ceftibuten are similar to those reported with other oral cephalosporins. (See Cautions in the Cephalosporins General Statement 8:12.06.) Ceftibuten generally is well tolerated. Most adverse effects are transient and mild to moderate in severity, but have been severe enough to require discontinuance of the drug in up to 2% of patients. GI effects, including nausea, diarrhea, melena, dyspepsia, vomiting, and abdominal pain, are the most frequent adverse reactions reported with ceftibuten and these effects generally have been reported in 1–4% of patients receiving the drug.

■ **Precautions and Contraindications** Ceftibuten shares the toxic potentials of other cephalosporins, and the usual cautions, precautions, and contraindications associated with cephalosporin therapy should be observed. Prior to initiation of ceftibuten therapy, careful inquiry should be made concerning previous hypersensitivity reactions to cephalosporins, penicillins, or other drugs. There is clinical and laboratory evidence of partial cross-allergenicity among cephalosporins and other β-lactam antibiotics, including penicillins and cephamycins. Ceftibuten is contraindicated in patients who are hypersensitive to the drug or other cephalosporins and should be used with caution in patients with a history of hypersensitivity to penicillins. Use of cephalosporins should be avoided in patients who have had an immediate-type (anaphylactic) hypersensitivity reaction to penicillins. If a hypersensitivity reaction occurs during ceftibuten therapy, the drug should be discontinued and the patient treated with appropriate therapy (e.g., epinephrine, corticosteroids, and maintenance of an adequate airway and oxygen) as indicated.

Because *Clostridium difficile* infection (CDI) and *C. difficile*-associated diarrhea and colitis (CDAD; also known as antibiotic-associated diarrhea and colitis or pseudomembranous colitis) have been reported with nearly all anti-infectives, including cephalosporins, it should be considered in the differential diagnosis of patients who develop diarrhea during or after ceftibuten therapy. Patients should be advised that diarrhea is a common problem caused by anti-infectives and usually ends when the drug is discontinued; however, they should contact a clinician if watery and bloody stools (with or without stomach cramps and fever) occur during or as late as 2 months or longer after the last dose.

Individuals with diabetes mellitus should be informed that reconstituted ceftibuten oral suspension contains 1 g of sucrose per 5 mL.

For a more complete discussion of these and other precautions associated with the use of ceftibuten, see Cautions: Precautions and Contraindications in the Cephalosporins General Statement 8:12.06.

■ **Pediatric Precautions** Safety and efficacy of ceftibuten in neonates and infants younger than 6 months of age have not been established.

Adverse effects reported in pediatric patients receiving oral ceftibuten are similar to those reported in adults receiving the drug and include GI effects (diarrhea, vomiting, abdominal pain) and rash. The manufacturer states that diarrhea has been reported more frequently in younger children than in older children and has been reported in 8% of those who were 2 years of age or younger and in 2% of those older than 2 years of age.

■ **Geriatric Precautions** Although pharmacokinetic studies indicate that peak plasma concentrations and half-life of the drug may be higher in geriatric patients than in younger adults, the clinical importance of these effects is not clear since it is not known whether these geriatric individuals had renal impairment. The manufacturer states that adjustments in ceftibuten dosage may be necessary in geriatric patients based on the degree of renal impairment. (See Dosage and Administration: Dosage in Renal and Hepatic Impairment.)

■ **Mutagenicity and Carcinogenicity** In vivo and in vitro studies evaluating ceftibuten have not shown evidence of mutagenicity. Long-term animal studies have not been performed to date to evaluate the carcinogenic potential of the drug.

■ **Pregnancy, Fertility, and Lactation** Reproduction studies in rats or rabbits using oral ceftibuten dosages up to 400 mg/kg daily (approximately 8.6 times the usual human dosage on a mg/m^2 basis) or 40 mg/kg daily (approximately 1.5 times the usual human dosage on a mg/m^2 basis), respectively, have not revealed evidence of teratogenicity or harm to the fetus. There are no adequate and controlled studies using ceftibuten in pregnant women or during labor and delivery, and the drug should be used during pregnancy only when clearly needed.

Studies in rats using oral ceftibuten in dosages up to 2 g/kg daily (approximately 43 times the usual human dosage based on a mg/m^2 basis) have not revealed evidence of impaired fertility.

Since it is not known whether ceftibuten is distributed into milk, the drug should be used with caution in nursing women.

Spectrum

Based on its spectrum of activity, ceftibuten is classified as a third generation cephalosporin. For information on the classification of cephalosporins and closely related β-lactam antibiotics based on spectra of activity, see Spectrum in the Cephalosporins General Statement 8:12.06.

Ceftibuten is stable in the presence of a variety of β-lactamases produced by gram-positive and gram-negative bacteria. Like other currently available oral third generation cephalosporins (e.g., cefixime, cefpodoxime proxetil, cefdinir), ceftibuten has an expanded spectrum of activity against aerobic gram-negative bacteria compared with first and second generation cephalosporins, but is inactive against most strains of *Enterobacter* and *Pseudomonas aeruginosa*. In vitro on a weight basis, ceftibuten is more active than other currently available oral third generation cephalosporins against Enterobacteriaceae that produce plasmid-mediated β-lactamases.

Ceftibuten generally is inactive against enterococci (e.g., *Enterococcus faecalis*, methicillin-resistant [oxacillin-resistant] staphylococci, and anaerobic bacteria.

■ **In Vitro Susceptibility Testing** Strains of staphylococci resistant to penicillinase-resistant penicillins (methicillin-resistant [oxacillin-resistant] staphylococci) should be considered resistant to ceftibuten, although results of in vitro susceptibility tests may indicate that the organisms are susceptible to the drug.

For information on interpreting results of in vitro susceptibility testing (disk susceptibility tests, dilution susceptibility tests) when ceftibuten susceptibility testing is performed according to the standards of the Clinical and Laboratory Standards Institute (CLSI; formerly National Committee for Clinical Laboratory Standards [NCCLS]), see Spectrum: In Vitro Susceptibility Testing, in the Cephalosporins General Statement 8:12.06.

Pharmacokinetics

Ceftibuten exhibits linear dose-dependent pharmacokinetics over the dosage range of 200–400 mg, but exhibits nonlinear pharmacokinetics at higher dosages. In healthy adult males with normal renal function, peak plasma concentrations of ceftibuten at steady state are approximately 20% higher than those after a single oral dose of the drug. Peak plasma concentrations of ceftibuten are slightly higher and the plasma half-life of the drug is more prolonged in geriatric adults than in younger adults; however, these differences appear to be related to changes in renal function rather than age. Studies in adults with impaired renal function indicate that the pharmacokinetics of ceftibuten are affected by the degree of renal impairment and that plasma half-life and total body clearance of the drug decrease in proportion to increases in renal impairment. Limited data suggest that chronic hepatic impairment does not affect the pharmacokinetics of ceftibuten.

■ **Absorption** Ceftibuten is rapidly and almost completely absorbed following oral administration as capsules or oral suspension, and oral bioavailability of the drug ranges from 75–90%. Results of crossover studies in healthy adult males indicate that a 400-mg oral dose of ceftibuten given as the oral suspension is bioequivalent to a 400-mg oral dose of the drug given as 400- or 200-mg capsules.

Food decreases the rate and extent of absorption of oral ceftibuten; however, food has a greater effect on the bioavailability of ceftibuten when the drug is administered as the oral suspension than when it is administered as capsules. Compared with administration in the fasting state, administration of a 400-mg oral dose of ceftibuten as capsules to healthy adult males immediately after a standardized meal (53.8 g fat, 31.6 g protein; 841 calories) delays the time to peak plasma concentrations by 1.75 hours and decreases the peak plasma concentration and area under the plasma concentration-time curve (AUC) by 18 and 8%, respectively. Results of a crossover study in healthy adult males indicate that administration of a single 400-mg oral dose of ceftibuten as the oral suspension with a high-fat, 850-calorie meal decreases the peak plasma concentration and AUC by 26 or 17%, respectively, compared with administration in the fasting state; administration of the same dose with a nonfat, 400-calorie meal decreased the peak plasma concentration and AUC by 17 and 12%, respectively.

In healthy adults who receive a single 400- or 800-mg oral dose of ceftibuten as capsules, peak plasma concentrations of the drug are attained within 2–2.6 hours and average 15–17.6 or 23.3 mcg/mL, respectively. Following oral administration of a single 400-mg dose of ceftibuten as capsules in healthy adult males, plasma concentrations average 6.1, 11.3, 11.2, 3.2, and 1.1 mcg/

mL at 1, 2, 4, 8, and 12 hours, respectively, after the dose. In a study in healthy adults receiving oral ceftibuten in a dosage of 400 mg twice daily, peak plasma concentrations after the first dose averaged 17.6 mcg/mL and steady-state peak plasma concentrations averaged 20.6 mcg/mL.

In children 6 months to 16 years of age who receive a single 9- or 13.5-mg/kg oral dose of ceftibuten as the oral suspension, peak plasma concentrations are attained within 1.9–2.6 hours and average 13.4–16.2 or 23.2 mcg/mL, respectively. In children 6 months to 12 years of age who receive a single 9-mg/kg oral dose of ceftibuten as the oral suspension, plasma concentrations of the drug average 9.3, 11.2, 6.6, 1.6, and 0.5 mcg/mL at 1, 2, 4, 8, and 12 hours, respectively, after the dose.

■ **Distribution** The volume of distribution of ceftibuten averages 0.21 L/kg in healthy adults and 0.5 L/kg in pediatric patients.

Following oral administration, ceftibuten is distributed into blister fluid, bronchial secretions, nasal secretions, sputum, middle ear fluid, tracheal secretions, and tonsillar tissue.

In adults with acute exacerbations of chronic bronchitis who received a single 400-mg oral dose of ceftibuten, peak concentrations of the drug in bronchial secretions were attained 4 hours after the dose and averaged 9.2 mcg/mL; concentrations in bronchial secretions 24 hours after the dose averaged 0.4 mcg/mL. Concentrations of ceftibuten in epithelial lining fluid or bronchial mucosa generally are 15 or 37%, respectively, of concurrent plasma concentrations.

Concentrations of ceftibuten in sputum are approximately 7% of concurrent plasma concentrations. In a study in adults who received oral ceftibuten in a dosage of 200 mg twice daily or 400 mg once daily, peak concentrations were attained in sputum 2 hours after a dose and averaged 1.5 mcg/mL.

In pediatric patients 7 months to 4 years of age with acute otitis media who received oral ceftibuten in a dosage of 9 mg/kg once daily, concentrations of the drug in middle ear fluid on the third day of therapy averaged 4.4, 14.3, 0.8, and 0.9 mcg/mL at 2, 4, 6, and 12 hours, respectively, after a dose; concurrent serum concentrations of the drug were 14.5, 10, 2.72, and 0.28 mcg/mL, respectively.

Information on distribution of ceftibuten into CSF is not available.

It is not known whether ceftibuten crosses the placenta or is distributed into human milk.

Ceftibuten is approximately 65% bound to plasma proteins; binding is independent of plasma concentrations of the drug.

■ **Elimination** The plasma half-life of ceftibuten averages 2–2.6 hours in healthy adults with normal renal function and 1.9–2.5 hours in children 6 months to 16 years of age. In a study in pediatric patients, plasma half-life averaged 1.9–2 hours in those 6 months to 10 years of age and 2.2 hours in those older than 10 years of age.

Ceftibuten is present in plasma and urine principally as *cis*-ceftibuten; however, about 10% of a dose is converted in vivo to *trans*-ceftibuten. The *trans*-isomer has some antibacterial activity, but only about 12% of that of the *cis*-isomer.

Plasma half-life of ceftibuten is prolonged in patients with renal impairment. In one study, plasma half-life of the drug averaged 7.1, 13.4, or 22.3 hours in patients with creatinine clearances of 30–49, 5–29, or less than 5 mL/minute, respectively.

The *cis*- and *trans*-isomers of ceftibuten are eliminated principally in urine. Following oral administration of a single 400-mg oral dose of ceftibuten as capsules in healthy men, approximately 57–70% of the dose is eliminated in urine as unchanged ceftibuten and approximately 7–20% is eliminated in urine as *cis*-ceftibuten. Following oral administration of radiolabeled ceftibuten, approximately 56% of the radioactivity is eliminated in urine and 39% is eliminated in feces within 24 hours.

Ceftibuten is removed by hemodialysis; it is not known whether the drug is removed by peritoneal dialysis. The amount of ceftibuten removed during hemodialysis depends on several factors (e.g., type of coil used, dialysis flow-rate); however, a 2- to 4-hour period of hemodialysis reportedly removes 39–65% of the drug from the body.

Chemistry and Stability

■ **Chemistry** Ceftibuten is a semisynthetic cephalosporin antibiotic. The drug is an oral aminothiazolyl cephalosporin. Ceftibuten is structurally similar to other oral (cefdinir, cefixime, cefpodoxime proxetil) and parenteral (cefepime, cefotaxime, ceftazidime, ceftriaxone) cephalosporins that contain an aminothiazolyl side chain at position 7 of the cephalosporin nucleus. The aminothiazolyl group enhances antibacterial activity, particularly against Enterobacteriaceae, and generally results in enhanced stability against β-lactamases. However, ceftibuten contains a carboxyethylidine group in the side chain rather than the methoxyimino group contained in many aminothiazolyl cephalosporins. The carboxyethylidine group may contribute to oral bioavailability and increased stability against β-lactamases.

Ceftibuten is administered orally as the *cis*-isomer of the drug and is commercially available as ceftibuten dihydrate; potency is expressed on the anhydrous basis. Ceftibuten dihydrate occurs as a white to off-white powder and has a solubility of less than 0.1 mg/mL in water and a solubility of 0.13 mg/mL in alcohol at 20°C. The drug has pK_as of 2.17, 3.67, and 4.07.

Commercially available ceftibuten dihydrate powder for oral suspension occurs as a light yellow to buff, cherry-flavored powder. Following reconstitution, the oral suspension contains 90 mg of ceftibuten per 5 mL and has a pH of 3.5–5.5.

■ **Stability** Ceftibuten capsules and powder for oral suspension should be stored at 2–25°C.

Following reconstitution, ceftibuten oral suspension should be stored in a tight container at 2–8°C; any unused suspension should be discarded after 14 days.

For further information on chemistry, mechanism of action, spectrum, resistance, uses, cautions, acute toxicity, drug interactions, or laboratory test interferences of ceftibuten, see the Cephalosporins General Statement 8:12.06.

Preparations

Excipients in commercially available drug preparations may have clinically important effects in some individuals; consult specific product labeling for details.

Ceftibuten Dihydrate

Oral		
Capsules	400 mg (of anhydrous ceftibuten)	**Cedax®**, Pernix
For suspension	90 mg (of anhydrous ceftibuten) per 5 mL	**Cedax®**, Pernix

†Use is not currently included in the labeling approved by the US Food and Drug Administration

Ceftolozane Sulfate and Tazobactam Sodium

Ceftolozane/tazobactam, Ceftolozane-tazobactam, CXA-TAZ

■ Ceftolozane sulfate and tazobactam sodium is a fixed combination of ceftolozane (a third generation cephalosporin) and tazobactam (a β-lactamase inhibitor); tazobactam inactivates certain bacterial β-lactamases and expands ceftolozane's spectrum of activity against some bacteria that produce these β-lactamases.

Uses

■ **Intra-abdominal Infections** Ceftolozane and tazobactam is used in conjunction with metronidazole for the treatment of complicated intra-abdominal infections caused by susceptible *Enterobacter colacae, Escherichia coli, Klebsiella oxytoca, K. pneumoniae, Proteus mirabilis, Pseudomonas aeruginosa, Bacteroides fragilis, Streptococcus anginosus, S. constellatus,* or *S. salivarius.*

Clinical Experience Efficacy and safety of ceftolozane and tazobactam for the treatment of complicated intra-abdominal infections are based on results from 2 identical phase 3, randomized, double-blind, placebo-controlled studies in 979 hospitalized adults with complicated intra-abdominal infections, including appendicitis, cholecystitis, diverticulitis, gastric or duodenal perforation, intestinal perforation, or other causes of intra-abdominal abscesses and peritonitis. Patients were randomized in a 1:1 ratio to receive 4–14 days of treatment with the fixed combination of ceftolozane and tazobactam (1.5 g [ceftolozane 1 g and tazobactam 0.5 g] given by IV infusion every 8 hours) in conjunction with metronidazole (500 mg given by IV infusion every 8 hours) or treatment with meropenem (1 g given by IV infusion every 8 hours) in conjunction with placebo. Baseline characteristics were similar between groups (mean age 50–51 years, 56–60% male, 93–94% white, 75% from Eastern Europe, 6.3% from the US, 45–49% with diagnosis of appendiceal perforation or abscess). In a pooled analysis of both studies, the clinical cure rate (defined as complete resolution or marked improvement in signs and symptoms of the index infection at the test-of-cure visit [24–32 days after first treatment dose]) in the microbiological intent-to-treat (MITT) population was 83% in patients treated with ceftolozane and tazobactam in conjunction with metronidazole and 87.3% in those treated with meropenem. Based on clinical cure rate in the MITT population at the test-of-cure visit, ceftolozane and tazobactam in conjunction with metronidazole was noninferior to meropenem. When results were stratified according to causative organism, clinical cure rates at the test-of-cure visit in patients treated with ceftolozane and tazobactam in conjunction with metronidazole were 80.8% for *E. cloacae*, 84.7% for *E. coli*, 87.5% for *K. oxytoca*, 75.6% for *K. pneumoniae*, 91.7% for *P. mirabilis*, 79% for *Ps. aeruginosa*, 89.4% for *B. fragilis*, 84.4% for *B. ovatus*, 84% for *B. thetaiotaomicron*, 80% for *B. vulgatus*, 72.2% for *S. anginosus*, 75% for *S. constellatus*, and 81.8% for *S. salivarius*.

■ **Urinary Tract Infections** Ceftolozane and tazobactam is used for the treatment of complicated urinary tract infections, including pyelonephritis, caused by susceptible *E. coli*, *K. pneumoniae*, *P. mirabilis*, or *Ps. aeruginosa*.

Clinical Experience Efficacy of ceftolozane and tazobactam for the treatment of complicated urinary tract infections is based on results from a phase 3 randomized, double-blind clinical trial in 1068 hospitalized adults with complicated urinary tract infections, including pyelonephritis. Patients were randomized to receive 7 days of treatment with the fixed combination of ceftolozane and tazobactam (1.5 g [ceftolozane 1 g and tazobactam 0.5 g] given by IV infusion every 8 hours) or levofloxacin (750 mg given by IV infusion once daily). The MITT population had a median age of 51 years, 74% were female, 82% were diagnosed with pyelonephritis, 76% were enrolled in Eastern Europe, and 1.8% were enrolled in the US. The composite end point of microbiologic and clinical cure rate (defined as complete resolution or marked improvement in signs and symptoms and microbiologic eradication at the test-of-cure visit [approximately 7 days after the last treatment dose]) in the MITT population was 76.9% in patients treated with ceftolozane and tazobactam and 68.4% in those treated with levofloxacin. When results were stratified according to causative organism, the composite end point of microbiologic and clinical cure rates at the test-of-cure visit in patients treated with ceftolozane and tazobactam were 81% for *E. coli*, 66.7% for *K. pneumoniae*, 91.7% for *P. mirabilis*, and 75% for *Ps. aeruginosa*.

Dosage and Administration

■ **Administration** Ceftolozane and tazobactam is administered by IV infusion.

IV Infusion IV solutions of ceftolozane and tazobactam should not be admixed with or added to solutions containing other drugs.

Reconstitution and Dilution. Ceftolozane and tazobactam powder must be reconstituted and further diluted prior to IV infusion.

Single-dose vials of ceftolozane and tazobactam labeled as containing 1.5 g (ceftolozane 1 g and tazobactam 0.5 g) should be reconstituted by adding 10 mL of sterile water for injection or 0.9% sodium chloride injection to the vial and shaking gently until the contents are dissolved. Reconstituted ceftolozane and tazobactam solutions may be stored for up to 1 hour prior to transfer and dilution; reconstituted solutions should not be frozen.

Prior to IV infusion, reconstituted ceftolozane and tazobactam solutions *must* be further diluted. To prepare the indicated dose, the appropriate volume of reconstituted solution should be withdrawn from the vial and added to 100 mL of 0.9% sodium chloride or 5% dextrose injection. (See Table 1.)

Table 1. Dilution of Reconstituted Ceftolozane and Tazobactam

Recommended Dose of Ceftolozane and Tazobactam	Volume to Withdraw from Reconstituted Vial for Further Dilution
1.5 g (ceftolozane 1 g and tazobactam 0.5 g)	11.4 mL (entire contents)
750 mg (ceftolozane 500 mg and tazobactam 250 mg)	5.7 mL
375 mg (ceftolozane 250 mg and tazobactam 125 mg)	2.9 mL
150 mg (ceftolozane 100 mg and tazobactam 50 mg)	1.2 mL

The reconstituted and diluted solution of ceftolozane and tazobactam should be inspected visually for particulate matter and discoloration prior to administration; the solution should appear clear and colorless to slightly yellow.

Following reconstitution and dilution, ceftolozane and tazobactam solutions may be stored at room temperature for up to 24 hours or at 2–8°C for up to 7 days; diluted solutions should not be frozen.

Rate of Administration. IV infusions of ceftolozane and tazobactam should be given over 1 hour.

Dispensing and Dosage and Administration Precautions. FDA alerted healthcare professionals about the risk of medication errors with ceftolozane and tazobactam. There have been reports of errors occurring during preparation of IV solutions of the drug that resulted in administration of incorrect dosage (50% overdosage in some cases); the errors were due to confusion about how dosage of ceftolozane and tazobactam is expressed (total of the dosage of each of the 2 active components) and how drug strength was displayed on vial labels and carton packaging. To prevent such errors, vial labels and carton packaging have been revised to indicate the strength of the fixed combination as the total of the 2 active components.

Healthcare professionals should be aware that dosage of ceftolozane and tazobactam is expressed as the total (sum) of the dosage of each of the 2 active components (i.e., dosage of ceftolozane plus dosage of tazobactam). This dosage convention should be considered when prescribing, preparing, and dispensing ceftolozane and tazobactam. FDA urges healthcare professionals and patients to report any medication errors and adverse effects involving the drug to the FDA MedWatch program.

■ **Dosage** Ceftolozane and tazobactam is a fixed combination containing a 2:1 ratio of ceftolozane to tazobactam.

The ceftolozane component is provided as ceftolozane sulfate (dosage of this component is expressed in terms of ceftolozane); the tazobactam component is provided as tazobactam sodium (dosage of this component is expressed in terms of tazobactam).

Dosage of the fixed combination of ceftolozane and tazobactam is expressed in terms of the total of the ceftolozane and tazobactam content.

Each single-dose vial of ceftolozane and tazobactam contains a total of 1.5 g (i.e., 1 g of ceftolozane and 0.5 g of tazobactam).

Adult Dosage **Intra-abdominal Infections.** The recommended dosage of ceftolozane and tazobactam for the treatment of complicated intra-abdominal infections in adults is 1.5 g (ceftolozane 1 g and tazobactam 0.5 g) every 8 hours in conjunction with metronidazole (500 mg given by IV infusion every 8 hours).

The recommended duration of treatment is 4–14 days. Duration should be guided by the severity and site of infection and the patient's clinical and bacteriologic progress.

Urinary Tract Infections. The recommended dosage of ceftolozane and tazobactam for the treatment of complicated urinary tract infections in adults is 1.5 g (ceftolozane 1 g and tazobactam 0.5 g) every 8 hours.

The recommended duration of treatment is 7 days. Duration should be guided by the severity and site of infection and the patient's clinical and bacteriologic progress.

■ **Dosage in Renal Impairment** Dosage of ceftolozane and tazobactam must be adjusted in adults with creatinine clearances of 50 mL/minute or less, including those undergoing hemodialysis. (See Table 2.)

Creatinine clearance should be monitored at least once daily in patients with changing renal function and dosage of ceftolozane and tazobactam adjusted accordingly.

Table 2. Ceftolozane and Tazobactam Dosage for Adults with Renal Impairment

Estimated Creatinine Clearance (mL/minute)	Recommended Dosage
30–50	750 mg (ceftolozane 500 mg and tazobactam 250 mg) every 8 hours
15–29	375 mg (ceftolozane 250 mg and tazobactam 125 mg) every 8 hours
End-stage renal disease on hemodialysis	Single loading dose of 750 mg (ceftolozane 500 mg and tazobactam 250 mg) followed by maintenance dosage of 150 mg (ceftolozane 100 mg and tazobactam 50 mg) every 8 hours[a]

[a] On hemodialysis days, the dose should be administered as soon as possible after dialysis.

■ **Dosage in Hepatic Impairment** Dosage adjustments are not needed when ceftolozane and tazobactam is used in adults with hepatic impairment.

■ **Dosage in Geriatric Patients** Dosage adjustments based solely on age are not needed when ceftolozane and tazobactam is used in geriatric patients. However, because geriatric patients are more likely to have decreased renal function and because dosage of ceftolozane and tazobactam needs to be adjusted based on renal impairment, dosage should be selected with caution and it may be useful to monitor renal function.

Cautions

■ **Adverse Effects** Adverse effects reported in 5% or more of patients receiving ceftolozane and tazobactam in phase 3 clinical trials include GI effects (nausea, diarrhea), headache, and pyrexia.

■ **Precautions and Contraindications** ***Sensitivity Reactions*** Ceftolozane and tazobactam is contraindicated in patients with known serious hypersensitivity to ceftolozane and/or tazobactam, the fixed combination of piperacillin and tazobactam, or other β-lactams.

Serious and occasionally fatal hypersensitivity (anaphylactic) reactions have been reported in patients receiving β-lactam antibacterials. Before initiating therapy with ceftolozane and tazobactam, the clinician should carefully inquire about the patient's previous hypersensitivity reactions to other cephalosporins, penicillins, or other β-lactams. Ceftolozane and tazobactam should be used with caution in patients allergic to cephalosporins, penicillins, or other β-lactams since cross-sensitivity among β-lactam antibacterials has been established.

Patients should be advised that allergic reactions, including serious allergic reactions, could occur and that serious reactions require immediate treatment.

If an anaphylactic reaction occurs, ceftolozane and tazobactam should be discontinued and appropriate therapy initiated.

Reduced Efficacy in Patients with Moderate Renal Impairment Results of a subgroup analysis of a phase 3 clinical trial in patients with complicated intra-abdominal infections indicated that the clinical cure rate in patients with moderate renal impairment (baseline creatinine clearances of 30–50 mL/minute) was lower than the clinical cure rate in those with normal renal function or only mild renal impairment (creatinine clearances of 50 mL/minute or greater), and this difference was more marked in those treated with ceftolozane and tazobactam in conjunction with metronidazole than in those treated with the comparator drug (meropenem). The clinical cure rate in patients treated with ceftolozane and tazobactam in conjunction with metronidazole was 47.8% in those with baseline creatinine clearances of 30–50 mL/minute compared with 85.2% in those with baseline creatinine clearances of 50 mL/minute or greater. A similar trend also was observed in a clinical trial evaluating ceftolozane and tazobactam for treatment of complicated urinary tract infections.

Creatinine clearance should be monitored at least once daily in patients with changing renal function and dosage of ceftolozane and tazobactam adjusted accordingly. (See Other Precautions and Contraindications under Cautions: Precautions and Contraindications.)

Superinfection/Clostridium difficile-associated Diarrhea and Colitis (CDAD) Use of ceftolozane and tazobactam may result in emergence and overgrowth of nonsusceptible bacteria or fungi. The patient should be carefully monitored and appropriate therapy instituted if superinfection occurs.

Treatment with anti-infectives alters normal colon flora and may permit overgrowth of *Clostridium difficile*. *C. difficile* infection (CDI) and *C. difficile*-associated diarrhea and colitis (CDAD; also known as antibiotic-associated diarrhea and colitis or pseudomembranous colitis) have been reported in patients receiving nearly all anti-infectives, including ceftolozane and tazobactam, and may range in severity from mild diarrhea to fatal colitis. *C. difficile* produces toxins A and B which contribute to development of CDAD; hypertoxin-producing strains of *C. difficile* are associated with increased morbidity and mortality since they may be refractory to anti-infectives and colectomy may be required.

CDAD should be considered in the differential diagnosis of patients who develop diarrhea during or after anti-infective therapy. Careful medical history is necessary since CDAD has been reported to occur as late as 2 months or longer after anti-infective therapy is discontinued.

If CDAD is suspected or confirmed, anti-infective therapy not directed against *C. difficile* should be discontinued whenever possible. Patients should be managed with appropriate supportive therapy (e.g., fluid and electrolyte management, protein supplementation), anti-infective therapy directed against *C. difficile* (e.g., metronidazole, vancomycin), and surgical evaluation as clinically indicated.

Patients should be advised that diarrhea is a common problem caused by anti-infectives and usually resolves when the drug is discontinued; however, they should contact a clinician if watery and bloody stools (with or without stomach cramps and fever) occur during or as late as 2 months or longer after the last dose.

Selection and Use of Anti-infectives To reduce development of drug-resistant bacteria and maintain effectiveness of ceftolozane and tazobactam and other antibacterials, the drug should be used only for treatment of infections proven or strongly suspected to be caused by susceptible bacteria.

When selecting or modifying anti-infective therapy, results of culture and in vitro susceptibility testing should be used. In the absence of such data, local epidemiology and susceptibility patterns should be considered when selecting anti-infectives for empiric therapy.

Patients should be advised that antibacterials (including ceftolozane and tazobactam) should only be used to treat bacterial infections and not used to treat viral infections (e.g., the common cold). Patients also should be advised about the importance of completing the full course of therapy, even if feeling better after a few days, and that skipping doses or not completing therapy may decrease effectiveness and increase the likelihood that bacteria will develop resistance and will not be treatable with ceftolozane and tazobactam or other antibacterials in the future.

Precautions Related to Use of Fixed Combinations When ceftolozane and tazobactam is used, the cautions, precautions, contraindications, and drug interactions associated with both drugs in the fixed combination must be considered. Cautionary information applicable to specific populations (e.g., pregnant or nursing women, individuals with hepatic or renal impairment, geriatric patients) should be considered for each drug.

When prescribing, preparing, and dispensing ceftolozane and tazobactam, healthcare professionals should consider that dosage of the fixed combination is expressed as the total (sum) of the dosage of each of the 2 active components (i.e., dosage of ceftolozane plus dosage of tazobactam). (See Dispensing and Dosage and Administration Precautions under Administration; IV Infusion, in Dosage and Administration.)

Other Precautions and Contraindications Ceftolozane and tazobactam are substantially eliminated by the kidneys, and the risk of adverse reactions may be greater in patients with renal impairment. In addition, a lower cure rate has been reported in some patients with moderate renal impairment (see Reduced Efficacy in Patients with Moderate Renal Impairment under Cautions: Precautions and Contraindications). Dosage of ceftolozane and tazobactam should be adjusted in patients with moderate or severe renal impairment (creatinine clearances of 50 mL/minute or less), including those undergoing hemodialysis. In patients with changing renal function, creatinine clearance should be monitored at least once daily and dosage adjusted accordingly. (See Dosage and Administration: Dosage in Renal Impairment.)

■ Pediatric Precautions Safety and efficacy of ceftolozane and tazobactam have not been established in patients younger than 18 years of age.

■ Geriatric Precautions In phase 3 trials evaluating ceftolozane and tazobactam for the treatment of complicated intra-abdominal infections or complicated urinary tract infections, 24.6% of patients were 65 years of age or older, while about 11% were 75 years of age or older. The incidence of adverse effects reported in geriatric patients treated with ceftolozane and tazobactam was higher than that reported in younger adults treated with the drug. In addition, in adults 65 years of age or older with complicated intra-abdominal infections, the clinical cure rate was 69% in those treated with ceftolozane and tazobactam in conjunction with metronidazole compared with 82.4% in those treated with the comparator drug. A difference in cure rates between the ceftolozane and tazobactam regimen and the comparator regimen was not observed in geriatric patients with complicated urinary tract infections.

Ceftolozane and tazobactam are substantially eliminated by the kidneys, and the risk of adverse effects may be greater in those with impaired renal function. Because geriatric patients are more likely to have reduced renal function, dosage should be selected with caution and renal function monitoring should be considered. Dosage adjustments in geriatric patients should be based on renal function.

■ Mutagenicity and Carcinogenicity Ceftolozane and tazobactam was not genotoxic in an in vitro mouse lymphoma assay or an in vivo rat bone marrow micronucleus assay. There was evidence of structural aberrations when the drug was used in an in vitro chromosomal aberration assay in Chinese hamster ovary cells.

Long-term animal studies have not been performed to date to evaluate the carcinogenic potential of ceftolozane and tazobactam.

■ Pregnancy, Fertility, and Lactation ***Pregnancy*** Embryofetal development studies in mice and rats using ceftolozane dosages associated with exposures approximately 7 and 4 times, respectively, the exposure expected in humans receiving a ceftolozane dosage of 1 g three times daily did not reveal evidence of fetal toxicity. In a study in rats, ceftolozane administered during pregnancy and lactation was associated with decreased auditory startle response in male pups at postnatal day 60.

Embryofetal development studies in rats using tazobactam dosages approximately 19 times the recommended human dosage revealed evidence of maternal toxicity (decreased food consumption and body weight gain), but no evidence of fetal toxicity. In a study in rats, tazobactam administered during pregnancy and lactation in dosages approximately 8 times the recommended human dosage produced decreased maternal food consumption and body weight gain at the end of gestation and an increased incidence of stillbirths. Although pups of dams receiving tazobactam in dosages of 320–1280 mg/kg daily had substantially reduced postnatal body weight at 21 days after delivery, there was no evidence of effects on development, function, learning, or fertility of the pups.

There are no adequate and controlled studies using ceftolozane and tazobactam in pregnant women, and the drug should be used during pregnancy only if potential benefits to the woman justify potential risks to the fetus.

Fertility Ceftolozane showed no evidence of impaired fertility in male or female rats receiving ceftolozane dosages approximately 3 times higher than the recommended human dosage based on mean plasma exposure.

Tazobactam showed no evidence of impaired fertility in male or female rats receiving tazobactam dosages approximately 4 times higher than the recommended human dosage based on body surface area.

Lactation Because it is not known whether ceftolozane or tazobactam is distributed into human milk, the fixed combination of ceftolozane and tazobactam should be used with caution in nursing women.

Drug Interactions

The following drug interactions are based on studies using the fixed combination containing ceftolozane and tazobactam, ceftolozane alone, or tazobactam alone. When ceftolozane and tazobactam is used, interactions associated with both drugs in the fixed combination should be considered.

■ Drugs Affecting or Metabolized by Hepatic Microsomal Enzymes Drug interactions are not expected between ceftolozane and tazobactam and inhibitors or inducers of cytochrome P-450 (CYP) enzymes.

In vivo data indicate ceftolozane and tazobactam is not a substrate for CYP enzymes. In vitro, ceftolozane, tazobactam, and the M1 metabolite of tazobactam do not inhibit CYP1A2, 2B6, 2C8, 2C9, 2C19, 2D6, or 3A4 and do not induce CYP1A2, 2B6, or 3A4 at therapeutic concentrations.

Results from in vitro induction studies show that ceftolozane, tazobactam, and the M1 metabolite of tazobactam decrease CYP1A2 and 2B6 enzyme activity and mRNA levels in human hepatocytes and decrease CYP3A4 mRNA levels at supratherapeutic plasma concentrations. In addition, the M1 metabolite of tazobactam decreased CYP3A4 activity at supratherapeutic plasma concentrations. A clinical drug interaction study showed that drug interactions involving inhibition of CYP1A2 or 3A4 by ceftolozane and tazobactam are not expected.

■ Drugs Affecting or Affected by Organic Anion Transporters Tazobactam is a substrate of organic anion transporter (OAT) 1 and OAT3. Therefore, concomitant use of OAT1 and/or OAT3 inhibitors (e.g., probenecid) with ceftolozane and tazobactam may increase tazobactam plasma concentrations. (See Drug Interactions: Probenecid.)

In vitro, tazobactam inhibits OAT1 and OAT3; ceftolozane does not inhibit OAT1 or OAT3. Clinically important interactions involving OAT1 or OAT3 inhibition by ceftolozane and tazobactam are not expected.

■ Drugs Affecting or Affected by Other Membrane Transporters In vitro, ceftolozane and tazobactam are not substrates or inhibitors of P-glycoprotein (P-gp) or breast cancer resistance protein (BCRP); tazobactam is not a substrate of organic cation transporter (OCT) 2.

In vitro data indicate that ceftolozane and tazobactam do not inhibit organic anion transporting polypeptide (OATP) 1B1 or 1B3, organic cation transporter (OCT) 1 or 2, or bile salt export pump (BSEP) at therapeutic plasma concentrations. In addition, ceftolozane does not inhibit multidrug resistance-associated protein (MRP) or multidrug and toxin extrusion (MATE) 1 or 2-K.

■ Anti-infectives There is no in vitro evidence of antagonistic antibacterial effects between ceftolozane and tazobactam and amikacin, aztreonam, daptomycin, levofloxacin, linezolid, meropenem, metronidazole, rifampin, tigecycline, or vancomycin.

■ Probenecid Concomitant use of probenecid (an OAT1/OAT3 inhibitor) prolongs the half-life of tazobactam by 71%.

Mechanism of Action

Ceftolozane and tazobactam is bactericidal in action.

Like other cephalosporins, the antibacterial activity of ceftolozane results from inhibition of mucopeptide synthesis in the bacterial cell wall and is mediated through binding to penicillin-binding proteins (PBPs). (For information on the mechanism of action of cephalosporins, see Mechanism of Action in the Cephalosporins General Statement 8:12.06.)

Tazobactam is a β-lactam β-lactamase inhibitor that inactivates certain β-lactamases, including some extended-spectrum β-lactamases (ESBLs). Tazobactam binds to and forms covalent, irreversible, acyl-enzyme intermediates with certain β-lactamases. After this complex is formed, functional inhibition of the β-lactamase depends on the relative rates of deacylation, tautomerization, or hydrolysis of the complex. Tazobactam inactivates many β-lactamases in Ambler class A (e.g., penicillinases, ESBLs) and some in class C (e.g., cephalosporinases such as AmpC). Tazobactam cannot inactivate Ambler class A carbapenemases (e.g., *Klebsiella pneumoniae* carbapenemases [KPCs]), Ambler class D β-lactamases, or Ambler class B metallo-β-lactamases (MLBs).

Because tazobactam inactivates certain β-lactamases, concomitant use with ceftolozane can protect ceftolozane from degradation by these β-lactamases and expand the spectrum of activity of the cephalosporin to include some β-lactamase-producing bacteria that are resistant to ceftolozane alone.

Spectrum

Based on its spectrum of activity, ceftolozane and tazobactam is classified as a third generation cephalosporin. (For information on the classification of cephalosporins and closely related β-lactam antibiotics based on spectra of activity, see Spectrum in the Cephalosporins General Statement 8:12.06.)

Like other currently available parenteral third generation cephalosporins (e.g., cefotaxime, ceftazidime, ceftriaxone), ceftolozane generally is less active against staphylococci but has an expanded spectrum of activity against gram-negative bacteria compared with first and second generation cephalosporins. Ceftolozane is distinguished from many other cephalosporins by its activity against *Pseudomonas aeruginosa*.

Ceftolozane and tazobactam has a wider spectrum of activity than ceftolozane alone. Ceftolozane and tazobactam is active against many gram-negative aerobic and anaerobic bacteria and select gram-positive bacteria. Ceftolozane and tazobactam is active in vitro against many β-lactamase-producing gram-negative bacteria that are resistant to ceftolozane alone, including Enterobacteriaceae that produce extended-spectrum β-lactamases (ESBLs).

Some bacteria that are resistant to other cephalosporins and/or other anti-infectives because of β-lactamase production may be susceptible to ceftolozane and tazobactam. The fixed combination also is active in vitro against some bacteria resistant to other β-lactams (e.g., carbapenems) because of loss of outer membrane porin (OprD).

■ In Vitro Susceptibility Testing When in vitro susceptibility testing is performed according to the standards of the Clinical and Laboratory Standards Institute (CLSI; formerly National Committee for Clinical Laboratory Standards [NCCLS]), clinical isolates identified as *susceptible* to ceftolozane and tazobactam are inhibited by drug concentrations usually achievable when dosage recommended for the site of infection is used. A report of *intermediate* should be considered equivocal and, if the isolate is not fully susceptible to alternative anti-infectives, the test should be repeated. The intermediate category implies possible clinical applicability in body sites where the drug is physiologically concentrated and provides a buffer zone which should prevent small, uncontrolled technical factors from causing major discrepancies in interpretation. If results of in vitro susceptibility testing indicate that a clinical isolate is *resistant* to ceftolozane and tazobactam, the strain is not likely to be inhibited by drug concentrations generally achievable with usual dosage schedules and other anti-infective therapy should be selected.

Disk Susceptibility Tests When the disk-diffusion procedure is used to test susceptibility to ceftolozane and tazobactam, a disk containing 30 mcg of ceftolozane and 10 mcg of tazobactam is used.

When disk-diffusion susceptibility testing is performed according to CLSI standardized procedures, *Ps. aeruginosa* with growth inhibition zones of 21 mm or greater are susceptible to ceftolozane and tazobactam, those with zones of 17–20 mm have intermediate susceptibility, and those with zones of 16 mm or less are resistant to the drug.

Dilution Susceptibility Tests When dilution susceptibility testing (agar or broth dilution) is used to test susceptibility to ceftolozane and tazobactam, tests should be performed using serial dilutions of ceftolozane combined with a fixed tazobactam concentration of 4 mcg/mL.

When dilution susceptibility testing is performed according to CLSI standardized procedures, Enterobacteriaceae with ceftolozane MICs of 2 mcg/mL or less in the presence of 4 mcg/mL of tazobactam are susceptible to ceftolozane and tazobactam, isolates with ceftolozane MICs of 4 mcg/mL in the presence of 4 mcg/mL of tazobactam have intermediate resistance, and those with ceftolozane MICs of 8 mcg/mL or greater in the presence of 4 mcg/mL of tazobactam are resistant to the drug.

When susceptibility of *Ps. aeruginosa* is tested using dilution susceptibility testing, those with ceftolozane MICs of 4 mcg/mL or less in the presence of 4 mcg/mL of tazobactam are susceptible to ceftolozane and tazobactam, isolates with ceftolozane MICs of 8 mcg/mL in the presence of 4 mcg/mL of tazobactam have intermediate susceptibility, and those with ceftolozane MICs of 16 mcg/mL or greater in the presence of 4 mcg/mL of tazobactam are resistant to the drug.

When susceptibility of *Bacteroides fragilis, Streptococcus anginosus, S. constellatus*, or *S. salivarius* is tested using dilution susceptibility testing, isolates with ceftolozane MICs of 8 mcg/mL or less in the presence of 4 mcg/mL of tazobactam are susceptible to ceftolozane and tazobactam, those with ceftolozane MICs of 16 mcg/mL in the presence of 4 mcg/mL of tazobactam have intermediate susceptibility, and those with ceftolozane MICs of 32 mcg/mL or greater in the presence of 4 mcg/mL of tazobactam are resistant to the drug.

■ Gram-positive Aerobic Bacteria Ceftolozane and tazobactam is active in vitro against *Streptococcus anginosus, S. constellatus, S. salivarius, S. agalactiae* (group B streptococci, GBS), *S. intermedius, S. pyogenes* (group A β-hemolytic streptococci, GAS), and *S. pneumoniae*.

■ Gram-negative Aerobic Bacteria Ceftolozane and tazobactam is active in vitro against many Enterobacteriaceae, including *Enterobacter aerogenes, E. cloacae, Escherichia coli, Klebsiella oxytoca, K. pneumoniae, Proteus mirabilis, P. vulgaris, Citrobacter freundii, C. koseri, Morganella morganii, Providencia rettgeri, P. stuartii, Serratia liquefacians*, and *S. marcescens*. The fixed combination is active in vitro against some Enterobacteriaceae that produce one or more ESBLs, including certain TEM, SHV, CTX-M, or OXA β-lactamases.

Ceftolozane and tazobactam is active in vitro against *Ps. aeruginosa*, including some multidrug-resistant (MDR) strains. The fixed combination is active in vitro against *Ps. aeruginosa* resistant to some others drugs (e.g., ceftazidime, ciprofloxacin, imipenem, piperacillin and tazobactam, tobramycin) because of chromosomal AmpC β-lactamase, reduction in cell permeability because of loss of OprD, and/or up-regulation of efflux pumps (e.g., MexXY, MexAB).

Ceftolozane and tazobactam is active in vitro against *Acinetobacter baumannii, Burkholderia cepacia, Haemophilus influenzae, Moraxella catarrhalis*, and *Pantoea agglomerans*.

■ Anaerobic Bacteria Ceftolozane and tazobactam is active in vitro against some gram-negative anaerobic bacteria, including some strains of *Bacteroides fragilis, Fusobacterium*, and *Prevotella*.

The fixed combination also is active in vitro against some gram-positive anaerobic bacteria, including *Propionibacterium*.

Resistance

Resistance or reduced susceptibility to ceftolozane and tazobactam can occur.

Bacteria that produce Ambler class B metallo-β-lactamases (MLBs) or serine carbapenemases (such as *Klebsiella pneumoniae* carbapenemase [KPC]) are resistant to ceftolozane and tazobactam because tazobactam does not inhibit these types of β-lactamases. Although some isolates of *Escherichia coli* and *K. pneumoniae* producing β-lactamases in certain enzyme groups (e.g., CTX-M, OXA, TEM, SHV) were susceptible to ceftolozane and tazobactam in vitro, other isolates of *E. coli* and *K. pneumoniae* producing β-lactamases in these enzyme groups were resistant to the drug. *Pseudomonas aeruginosa* with reduced susceptibility or resistance to ceftolozane and tazobactam have been produced in vitro.

Cross-resistance between ceftolozane and tazobactam and other cephalosporins may occur; however, some bacteria resistant to other cephalosporins may be susceptible to ceftolozane and tazobactam.

Pharmacokinetics

Following IV administration of the fixed combination of ceftolozane sulfate and tazobactam sodium, pharmacokinetic parameters for ceftolozane and tazobactam are similar to those reported when each drug is administered alone. In addition, pharmacokinetic parameters are similar following single or multiple IV doses of the fixed combination.

■ Absorption Peak plasma concentrations and areas under the plasma concentration-time curve (AUCs) of both ceftolozane and tazobactam increase in proportion to the dose of ceftolozane and tazobactam.

In healthy adults with normal renal function receiving multiple doses of ceftolozane and tazobactam (1.5 g [ceftolozane 1 g and tazobactam 0.5 g]) given by IV infusion over 1 hour every 8 hours for 10 days, peak plasma concentrations of ceftolozane and tazobactam are 74.4 and 18 mcg/mL, respectively, and are attained at approximately 1 hour.

There is no appreciable accumulation of ceftolozane or tazobactam in adults with normal renal function following multiple doses of ceftolozane and tazobactam given by IV infusion every 8 hours for 10 days.

In a population pharmacokinetic analysis, age, gender, and race did not result in clinically important differences in ceftolozane and tazobactam exposures.

■ Distribution The steady-state volumes of distribution of ceftolozane and tazobactam are 13.5 and 18.2 L, respectively, in healthy adult males following a single IV dose of ceftolozane and tazobactam, suggesting that both drugs distribute into extracellular space.

Ceftolozane and tazobactam were both distributed into pulmonary epithelial lining fluid following IV administration of ceftolozane and tazobactam in healthy adults.

Ceftolozane is approximately 16–21% bound to plasma proteins; tazobactam is 30% bound to plasma proteins.

It is not known whether ceftolozane crosses the placenta. Tazobactam crosses the placenta in rats; fetal concentrations in rats are 10% or less of maternal plasma concentrations.

It is not known whether ceftolozane or tazobactam is distributed into human milk.

■ **Elimination** Ceftolozane does not appear to be metabolized to any appreciable extent. Tazobactam is partially metabolized by hydrolysis of the β-lactam ring to form an inactive metabolite, M1.

Ceftolozane, tazobactam, and the MI metabolite of tazobactam are eliminated by the kidneys. Following a single IV dose of ceftolozane and tazobactam (1.5 g [ceftolozane 1 g and tazobactam 0.5 g]) in healthy adult males, more than 95% of the ceftolozane dose is eliminated in urine unchanged and more than 80% of the tazobactam dose is eliminated in urine unchanged (the remainder is eliminated as the M1 metabolite).

The plasma elimination half-lives of ceftolozane and tazobactam are approximately 3 and 1 hour, respectively, following multiple doses of ceftolozane and tazobactam in healthy adults with normal renal function.

In adults with mild, moderate, or severe renal impairment, the dose-normalized geometric mean AUC of ceftolozane is increased by 1.26-, 2.5-, or 5-fold, respectively, and the dose-normalized geometric mean AUC of tazobactam is increased by 1.3-, 2-, or 4-fold, respectively, compared with AUCs reported in healthy individuals with normal renal function.

Both ceftolozane and tazobactam are removed by hemodialysis. In adults with end-stage renal disease, a 4-hour hemodialysis session decreases the AUC of ceftolozane and tazobactam by approximately 66 and 56%, respectively.

Chemistry and Stability

■ **Chemistry** Ceftolozane sulfate and tazobactam sodium is a fixed combination of ceftolozane (a third generation cephalosporin antibiotic) and tazobactam (a β-lactamase inhibitor); tazobactam inactivates certain bacterial β-lactamases and expands ceftolozane's spectrum of activity against some bacteria that produce these β-lactamases.

Ceftolozane is structurally similar to ceftazidime and contains an aminothiadiazole ring that enhances antibacterial activity against gram-negative bacteria, an oxime group that contributes to stability in the presence of β-lactamases, and a dimethylacetic acid moiety that provides enhanced antipseudomonal activity. Unlike ceftazidime, ceftolozane contains a pyrazole ring at the 3-position of the cephem ring which prevents hydrolysis and improves stability against AmpC β-lactamase-overproducing *Pseudomonas aeruginosa*.

Tazobactam is a penicillanic acid sulfone β-lactamase inhibitor that is structurally similar to sulbactam. Tazobactam contains a β-lactam ring and a triazole group at the C-2 β-methyl position that facilitates binding to β-lactamases.

Ceftolozane and tazobactam is commercially available as a white to yellow powder for IV infusion containing a 2:1 ratio of ceftolozane to tazobactam. The ceftolozane component is provided as ceftolozane sulfate and the tazobactam component is provided as tazobactam sodium. Drug strength and dosage are expressed as the total of the 2 active components. (See Dispensing and Dosage and Administration Precautions under Administration: IV Infusion, in Dosage and Administration.)

Each single-dose vial of ceftolozane and tazobactam contains 1.5 g (1 g of ceftolozane [equivalent to 1.147 g of ceftolozane sulfate] and 0.5 g of tazobactam [equivalent to 0.537 g of tazobactam sulfate]). Each single-dose vial of the drug also contains 487 mg of sodium chloride as a stabilizing agent and 21 mg of citric acid and approximately 600 mg of L-arginine as excipients.

■ **Stability** Ceftolozane and tazobactam powder for IV infusion should be stored at 2–8°C and protected from light.

Following reconstitution and dilution, ceftolozane and tazobactam solutions may be stored for up to 24 hours at room temperature or for up to 7 days when refrigerated at 2–8°C.

For further information on chemistry, mechanism of action, spectrum, resistance, uses, cautions, acute toxicity, drug interactions, or laboratory test interferences of cephalosporins, see the Cephalosporins General Statement 8:12.06.

Preparations

Excipients in commercially available drug preparations may have clinically important effects in some individuals; consult specific product labeling for details.

Ceftolozane Sulfate and Tazobactam Sodium

Parenteral

For injection, for IV infusion	1.5 g (1 g of ceftolozane and 0.5 g of tazobactam)	**Zerbaxa®**, Cubist

cefTRIAXone Sodium

Rocephin

■ Ceftriaxone is a semisynthetic, third generation cephalosporin antibiotic.

Uses

Ceftriaxone is used for the treatment of bone and joint infections, endocarditis†, intra-abdominal infections, meningitis and other CNS infections, otitis media, respiratory tract infections, septicemia, skin and skin structure infections, and urinary tract infections caused by susceptible bacteria. The drug also is used for the treatment of chancroid†, gonorrhea and associated infections, pelvic inflammatory disease, infections caused by *Neisseria meningitidis*†, infections caused by *Shigella*†, and typhoid fever† and other infections caused by *Salmonella*†. In addition, ceftriaxone is used for the treatment of Lyme disease† and has been used for empiric anti-infective therapy in febrile neutropenic patients† and for perioperative prophylaxis.

Ceftriaxone has a wide spectrum of activity and is effective for the treatment of infections caused by a variety of gram-positive and gram-negative bacteria. Like other parenteral third generation cephalosporins (cefotaxime, ceftazidime), ceftriaxone is less active than first and second generation cephalosporins against some gram-positive aerobic bacteria (e.g., staphylococci) and generally should not be used in the treatment of infections caused by these organisms when a penicillin or first or second generation cephalosporin could be used. However, ceftriaxone may be a drug of choice for serious infections caused by certain other gram-positive bacteria, including *Streptococcus pneumoniae*. Ceftriaxone is considered a drug of choice for many infections caused by gram-negative bacteria, and a principal use of the drug is for the treatment of serious gram-negative bacterial infections, especially nosocomial infections, when other anti-infectives are ineffective or contraindicated.

Because ceftriaxone has a long serum half-life and can be administered once daily, the drug has been used for community-based parenteral anti-infective therapy for the treatment of infections that require prolonged therapy (e.g., community-acquired pneumonia, osteomyelitis, endocarditis†). Ceftriaxone has been administered parenterally to adults and children in outpatient settings, including clinicians' office, outpatient clinics, infusion centers, skilled nursing facilities, rehabilitation centers, and the patient's home. Outpatient parenteral anti-infective therapy generally is used to complete a course of ceftriaxone therapy initiated during hospitalization, but ceftriaxone therapy also has been initiated on an outpatient basis in patients who were clinically stable. When considering use of community-based ceftriaxone therapy, the benefits and risks of such therapy should be considered.

Prior to initiation of ceftriaxone therapy, appropriate specimens should be obtained for identification of the causative organism and in vitro susceptibility tests. Ceftriaxone therapy may be started pending results of susceptibility tests, but should be discontinued if the organism is found to be resistant to the drug.

■ **Bone and Joint Infections** Ceftriaxone is used in adults and pediatric patients for the treatment of bone and joint infections (e.g., osteomyelitis, septic arthritis) caused by susceptible *Staphylococcus aureus, Streptococcus pneumoniae, Escherichia coli, Proteus mirabilis, Klebsiella pneumoniae*, or *Enterobacter*.

For the treatment of native vertebral osteomyelitis or prosthetic joint infections caused by oxacillin-susceptible staphylococci, the Infectious Diseases Society of America (IDSA) recommends IV nafcillin (or oxacillin), IV cefazolin, or IV ceftriaxone as the drugs of choice. If native vertebral osteomyelitis or prosthetic joint infections are caused by β-hemolytic streptococci†, IDSA recommends IV penicillin G or IV ceftriaxone. For the treatment of native vertebral osteomyelitis or prosthetic joint infections caused by *Cutibacterium acnes*† (formerly *Propionibacterium acnes*), IDSA recommends IV penicillin G or IV ceftriaxone. These experts also recommend IV ceftriaxone as an alternative to ciprofloxacin for the treatment of native vertebral osteomyelitis caused by susceptible *Salmonella*†.

For additional information on management of bone and joint infections, current clinical practice guidelines from IDSA available at http://www.idsociety.org should be consulted.

■ **Endocarditis** Ceftriaxone is used for the treatment of endocarditis† caused by various streptococci, including viridans group streptococci (e.g., *S. milleri* group, *S. mutans, S. salivarius, S. sanguis*), nonenterococcal group D streptococci (e.g., *S. gallolyticus* [formerly *S. bovis*]), *S. pneumoniae, S. pyogenes* (group A β-hemolytic streptococci; GAS), *S. agalactiae* (group B streptococci; GBS), or streptococci groups C, F, or G. The drug also is used for the treatment of endocarditis† caused by enterococci (e.g., *Enterococcus faecalis, E. faecium*) or fastidious gram-negative bacilli of the HACEK group (i.e., *Haemophilus, Aggregatibacter, Cardiobacterium hominis, Eikenella corrodens, Kingella*). Ceftriaxone has been administered on an outpatient basis for the treatment of endocarditis† caused by susceptible bacteria.

Ceftriaxone also is used for prevention of α-hemolytic (viridans group) streptococcal endocarditis† in individuals undergoing certain dental or upper respiratory tract procedures who have cardiac conditions that put them at highest risk of adverse outcomes from endocarditis. (See Uses: Prevention of Bacterial Endocarditis.)

The American Heart Association (AHA) recommends that treatment of endocarditis be managed in consultation with an infectious disease expert, especially when endocarditis is caused by *S. pneumoniae*, β-hemolytic streptococci, staphylococci, or enterococci.

For additional information on management of endocarditis, current guidelines from AHA should be consulted.

Endocarditis Caused by Viridans Group Streptococci or S. gallolyticus For the treatment of native valve endocarditis† caused by viridans group streptococci or *S. gallolyticus* (formerly *S. bovis*) highly susceptible to penicillin (penicillin MIC 0.12 mcg/mL or less), AHA states that a 4-week regimen of IV penicillin G or IV or IM ceftriaxone is reasonable in adults and pediatric patients. If necessary in those unable to tolerate penicillin G or ceftriaxone, a 4-week regimen of IV vancomycin can be used. In *selected* adults, AHA states that a 2-week regimen that consists of IV penicillin G or IV or IM ceftriaxone in conjunction with IV or IM gentamicin is reasonable. The 2-week regimen should be considered only in adults with uncomplicated native valve endocarditis caused by highly penicillin-susceptible viridans group streptococci or *S. gallolyticus* who are at low risk for gentamicin adverse effects; the 2-week regimen is *not* recommended in those with known cardiac or extracardiac abscess, creatinine clearance less than 20 mL/minute, impaired eighth cranial nerve function, or infections caused by *Abiotrophia*, *Granulicatella*, or *Gemella*. In addition, AHA states that the 2-week regimen is *not* recommended in pediatric patients because of lack of clinical data.

For the treatment of native valve endocarditis† caused by viridans group streptococci or *S. gallolyticus* relatively resistant to penicillin (penicillin MIC greater than 0.12 mcg/mL but less than 0.5 mcg/mL), AHA states that a 4-week regimen of either IV penicillin G (or IV ampicillin) or IV or IM ceftriaxone in conjunction with IV or IM gentamicin given during the initial 2 weeks of treatment is reasonable in adults and pediatric patients. If the isolate is susceptible to ceftriaxone, AHA states that a 4-week regimen of ceftriaxone alone may be considered in adults. A 4-week regimen of vancomycin alone is a reasonable alternative only in adults unable to tolerate β-lactam anti-infectives.

If native valve endocarditis is caused by viridans group streptococci, *Abiotrophia defectiva*, or *Granulicatella* that are resistant to penicillin (penicillin MIC 0.5 mcg/mL or greater), AHA states that a regimen of IV penicillin G (or ampicillin) in conjunction with gentamicin is reasonable in adults. These experts state that a regimen of ceftriaxone in conjunction with gentamicin may be a reasonable alternative in adults for the treatment of native valve endocarditis† caused by viridans group streptococci that are resistant to penicillin but susceptible to ceftriaxone.

For the treatment of endocarditis† involving prosthetic valves or other prosthetic material caused by viridans group streptococci or *S. gallolyticus* highly susceptible to penicillin (penicillin MIC 0.12 mcg/mL or less), AHA states that a 6-week regimen of IV penicillin G or IV or IM ceftriaxone given with or without IV or IM gentamicin during the initial 2 weeks of treatment is reasonable in adults. When highly penicillin-susceptible strains are involved, there is no evidence that use of the combination regimen that includes gentamicin during the first 2 weeks is more effective than use of the β-lactam alone. If endocarditis† involving prosthetic valves or other prosthetic material is caused by viridans group streptococci or *S. gallolyticus* relatively or highly resistant to penicillin (penicillin MIC greater than 0.12 mcg/mL), AHA states that it is reasonable for adults to receive a 6-week regimen of IV penicillin G or IV or IM ceftriaxone given with a 6-week regimen of IV or IM gentamicin. In adults unable to tolerate penicillin G, ceftriaxone, or gentamicin, a 6-week regimen of IV vancomycin can be used.

Endocarditis Caused by S. pneumoniae, S. pyogenes, S. agalactiae, or Groups C, F, and G Streptococci For the treatment of endocarditis† involving native valves or prosthetic valves or other prosthetic material caused by *S. pneumoniae* highly susceptible to penicillin (penicillin MIC 0.1 mcg/mL or less), AHA states that penicillin G, ceftriaxone, or cefazolin are reasonable choices in adults. If endocarditis is caused by *S. pneumoniae* with penicillin resistance (penicillin MIC greater than 0.1 mcg/mL), AHA states that treatment with high-dose penicillin G or a third generation cephalosporin (cefotaxime, ceftriaxone) is reasonable in adults if meningitis is not present; cefotaxime or ceftriaxone is reasonable if meningitis is present. AHA states that use of cefotaxime or ceftriaxone in conjunction with vancomycin and rifampin may be considered in adults if endocarditis is caused by *S. pneumoniae* resistant to cefotaxime (cefotaxime MIC greater than 2 mcg/mL).

For the treatment of endocarditis† caused by *S. pyogenes*, AHA states that penicillin G is a reasonable regimen in adults and ceftriaxone is a reasonable alternative. Vancomycin is a reasonable alternative only for those unable to tolerate β-lactam anti-infectives.

AHA states that penicillin G or ceftriaxone is a reasonable regimen for the treatment of endocarditis† caused by *S. agalactiae* or groups C and G streptococci in adults, but concomitant use of gentamicin during the initial weeks of treatment should be considered.

Enterococcal Endocarditis For the treatment of enterococcal endocarditis†, AHA states that a double-β-lactam regimen of ampicillin and ceftriaxone is a reasonable option in certain adults.

Enterococcus (e.g., *E. faecalis*, *E. faecium*) are relatively resistant to penicillins and vancomycin and a synergistic combination regimen of penicillin, ampicillin, or vancomycin in conjunction with an aminoglycoside (gentamicin or streptomycin) has usually been used for the treatment of enterococcal endocarditis. However, enterococci resistant to aminoglycosides have been reported with increasing frequency and AHA states that all enterococcal isolates should be routinely tested for in vitro susceptibility to penicillin and vancomycin and for high-level resistance to gentamicin to predict synergistic interactions and aid in selection of the most appropriate treatment regimen.

Although there are few therapeutic alternatives to aminoglycoside-containing regimens for the treatment of enterococcal endocarditis, there are some data from in vitro and in vivo studies and limited clinical experience indicating that a double β-lactam regimen of ampicillin and ceftriaxone can be effective for the treatment of endocarditis caused by *E. faecalis*, including gentamicin-resistant strains. The major advantages of the ampicillin and ceftriaxone regimen are the lower risk of nephrotoxicity and the lack of any need to measure aminoglycoside serum concentrations; a potential disadvantage of this regimen is the possibility of hypersensitivity reactions to 2 separate β-lactam anti-infectives.

For the treatment of enterococcal endocarditis† involving native valves, prosthetic valves, or other prosthetic material caused by strains susceptible to penicillin and gentamicin in adults who can tolerate β-lactam anti-infectives, AHA states that either a regimen of IV ampicillin or IV penicillin G given in conjunction with gentamicin for 4–6 weeks or a double β-lactam regimen of IV ampicillin and IV ceftriaxone given for 6 weeks is reasonable. The most appropriate regimen should be selected based on characteristics of the individual patient. The double β-lactam regimen is recommended in adults who should not receive an aminoglycoside (i.e., creatinine clearance less than 50 mL/minute [pretreatment or developed during treatment with a gentamicin-containing regimen], impaired eighth cranial nerve function).

For the treatment of enterococcal endocarditis† involving native valves, prosthetic valves, or other prosthetic material caused by strains susceptible to penicillin but resistant to gentamicin in adults who can tolerate β-lactam anti-infectives, AHA states that a double β-lactam regimen of IV ampicillin and IV ceftriaxone given for 6 weeks is reasonable. If enterococcal endocarditis is caused by penicillin-susceptible strains that are gentamicin-resistant but streptomycin-susceptible, a double β-lactam regimen of IV ampicillin and IV ceftriaxone given for 6 weeks is reasonable in adults; alternatively, a regimen of IV ampicillin or IV penicillin G given in conjunction with IV or IM streptomycin for 4–6 weeks can be considered if the patient has a creatinine clearance of 50 mL/minute or greater and rapid tests for streptomycin serum concentrations are available. A 6-week regimen of vancomycin in conjunction with gentamicin should be considered only when enterococcal endocarditis is caused by strains intrinsically resistant to penicillin or the patient cannot tolerate β-lactam anti-infectives.

Endocarditis Caused by the HACEK Group AHA states that ceftriaxone is a reasonable option for the treatment of endocarditis† caused by the HACEK group in adults and pediatric patients.

The slow-growing fastidious gram-negative bacilli known as the HACEK group (i.e., *Haemophilus*, *Aggregatibacter*, *C. hominis*, *E. corrodens*, *Kingella*) account for approximately 5–10% of cases of community-acquired native valve endocarditis in patients who are not IV drug abusers and also rarely cause prosthetic valve endocarditis. Because β-lactamase-producing strains have been reported with increasing frequency, AHA states that the HACEK group should be considered ampicillin-resistant and penicillin and ampicillin should not be used for the treatment of HACEK endocarditis unless results of in vitro susceptibility testing are available.

AHA states that a 4-week regimen of IV or IM ceftriaxone alone is a reasonable choice for the treatment of native valve endocarditis† caused by the HACEK group and a 6-week regimen of the drug is a reasonable choice for the treatment of endocarditis involving prosthetic valves or other prosthetic material† caused by the HACEK group since most strains are susceptible to ceftriaxone or other third or fourth generation cephalosporins. Although ceftriaxone is preferred in such patients, cefotaxime or another third or fourth generation cephalosporin could be substituted and IV ampicillin is an option if in vitro susceptibility testing is performed and the isolate is susceptible. For the treatment of HACEK endocarditis in adults unable to tolerate ceftriaxone or other appropriate cephalosporin, AHA states that a fluoroquinolone (ciprofloxacin, levofloxacin, moxifloxacin) may be considered as an alternative since the HACEK group usually is susceptible to fluoroquinolones in vitro; however, such patients should be treated in consultation with an infectious disease specialist.

In pediatric patients with endocarditis caused by the HACEK group, AHA recommends a 4-week regimen of ceftriaxone or another third-generation cephalosporin (e.g., cefotaxime) used alone or a regimen of ampicillin in conjunction with gentamicin (or amikacin or tobramycin).

■ **GI Infections** Ceftriaxone has been used for the treatment of gastroenteritis† caused by *Salmonella* or *Shigella*. Ceftriaxone also is recommended as an alternative for empiric treatment of infectious diarrhea† in individuals with human immunodeficiency virus (HIV) infection or for long-term suppressive antibacterial therapy† (secondary prophylaxis) in such individuals.

Salmonella Gastroenteritis Anti-infective therapy generally is not indicated in otherwise healthy individuals with uncomplicated (noninvasive) gastroenteritis caused by nontyphoidal *Salmonella* (e.g., *Salmonella* serovars Enteritidis or Typhimurium) since such therapy may prolong the duration of fecal excretion of the organism and there is no evidence that it shortens the duration of the disease; however, the US Centers for Disease Control and Prevention (CDC), National Institutes of Health (NIH), IDSA, and others recommend anti-infective therapy in individuals with severe *Salmonella* gastroenteritis and in those who are at increased risk for invasive disease. These individuals include infants younger than 3–6 months of age; individuals older than 50 years of age; individuals with hemoglobinopathies, severe atherosclerosis or valvular heart disease, prostheses, uremia, chronic GI disease, or severe colitis; and individuals who are immunocompromised because of malignancy, immunosuppressive therapy, HIV infection, or other immunosuppressive illness.

When an anti-infective agent is considered necessary in an individual with *Salmonella* gastroenteritis, CDC, AAP, IDSA, and others recommend ceftriaxone, cefotaxime, a fluoroquinolone (should be used in children only if benefits outweigh risks and no other alternative exists), ampicillin, amoxicillin, co-trimoxazole, or chloramphenicol, depending on susceptibility of the causative organism. Some experts recommend that patients with presumed or proven nontyphoidal *Salmonella* gastroenteritis receive an initial dose of ceftriaxone followed by oral azithromycin pending results of diagnostic evaluation. The fact that multidrug-resistant *Salmonella* have been reported with increasing frequency in the US should be considered.

Because HIV-infected individuals with *Salmonella* infections are at increased risk for bacteremia and mortality compared with patients without HIV infection, CDC, NIH, and IDSA recommend that *all* HIV-infected patients with salmonellosis receive antibacterial treatment. In addition, some clinicians suggest that long-term suppressive antibacterial therapy (secondary prophylaxis) can be considered in HIV-infected adults and adolescents with recurrent *Salmonella* gastroenteritis (with or without bacteremia) and in those with $CD4^+$ T-cell counts less than 200 cells/mm^3 and severe diarrhea. However, the value of secondary prophylaxis has not been established and possible benefits must be weighed against the risks of long-term antibacterial exposure. CDC, NIH, and IDSA state that ciprofloxacin is the drug of choice for the treatment of *Salmonella* gastroenteritis (with or without bacteremia) and for long-term suppressive therapy in HIV-infected adults and adolescents; other fluoroquinolones (e.g., levofloxacin, moxifloxacin) are likely to be effective, but clinical data are limited. Depending on in vitro susceptibility of the causative organism, these experts recommend co-trimoxazole, ceftriaxone, or cefotaxime as alternatives for such treatment or secondary prophylaxis in HIV-infected adults and adolescents.

For information on the treatment of typhoid and paratyphoid fever (enteric fever) or bacteremia caused by *Salmonella*, see Uses: Typhoid Fever and Other Invasive Salmonella Infections.

Shigella Infections Ceftriaxone has been effective when used for the treatment of shigellosis† caused by susceptible *Shigella sonnei* or *S. flexneri* and has been recommended as an alternative when anti-infectives are indicated for the treatment of shigella infections.

Infections caused by *S. sonnei* usually are self-limited (48–72 hours), and mild cases may not require treatment with anti-infectives. However, since anti-infectives may shorten the duration of diarrhea and period of fecal excretion of *Shigella*, anti-infective treatment generally is recommended in addition to fluid and electrolyte replacement in patients with severe shigellosis, dysentery, or underlying immunosuppression.

Although an empiric regimen can be used initially when anti-infectives are indicated in the treatment of *Shigella* infections, in vitro susceptibility testing of clinical isolates is indicated since resistance to ampicillin and co-trimoxazole is common and strains resistant to ciprofloxacin, ceftriaxone, or azithromycin have been reported with increasing frequency. For infections caused by *Shigella* resistant to ampicillin and co-trimoxazole or when in vitro susceptibility of the isolate is unknown, ceftriaxone, a fluoroquinolone (e.g., ciprofloxacin), or azithromycin is recommended.

For the treatment of *Shigella* infections in HIV-infected adults and adolescents, CDC, NIH, and IDSA state that the drug of choice is ciprofloxacin and alternatives are levofloxacin, moxifloxacin, co-trimoxazole, or azithromycin.

Empiric Treatment of Infectious Diarrhea CDC, NIH, and IDSA recommend that adults and adolescents with advanced HIV disease ($CD4^+$ T-cell counts less than 200 cells/mm^3 or concomitant AIDS-defining illness) who have clinically severe diarrhea (i.e., 6 or more liquid stools per day, bloody stools, or any number of liquid stools per day accompanied by fever or chills) should undergo diagnostic evaluation to determine the etiology of the diarrheal illness and receive appropriate anti-infective treatment. These experts state that ciprofloxacin is preferred and ceftriaxone and cefotaxime are reasonable alternatives when empiric treatment of severe bacterial diarrhea is indicated in HIV-infected adults and adolescents. Treatment should be adjusted if needed when results of diagnostic testing are available. If diarrhea persists for longer than 14 days without other clinical signs of severity (e.g., bloody stool, dehydration), additional evaluation is indicated and pathogen-directed therapy should be initiated after a diagnosis is confirmed.

The possibility of resistant infections should be considered when selecting an empiric anti-infective regimen for treatment of diarrhea in HIV-infected travelers during travel or after return to the US.

■ **Intra-abdominal Infections** Ceftriaxone is used for the treatment of intra-abdominal infections caused by susceptible *E. coli*, *K. pneumoniae*, *Clostridium*, or *Peptostreptococcus*. The drug also has been used for the treatment of various gynecologic infections, including pelvic inflammatory disease. (See Uses: Pelvic Inflammatory Disease.) Although the manufacturers state that ceftriaxone can be used for the treatment of intra-abdominal infections caused by *Bacteroides fragilis*, the drug has been ineffective in the treatment of intra-abdominal infections when *B. fragilis* was present and superinfection with this organism has been reported occasionally.

Although monotherapy with ceftriaxone is an option for initial empiric treatment of mild to moderate community-acquired biliary tract infections (acute cholecystitis or cholangitis), ceftriaxone should be used in conjunction with metronidazole for initial empiric treatment of mild to moderate extrabiliary community-acquired intra-abdominal infections.

For additional information on management of intra-abdominal infections, current clinical practice guidelines from IDSA available at http://www.idsociety.org should be consulted.

■ **Meningitis and Other CNS Infections** Ceftriaxone is used in neonates, children, and adults for the treatment of meningitis caused by susceptible *H. influenzae*, *N. meningitidis*, or *S. pneumoniae*. The drug also has been used for the treatment of meningitis and other CNS infections caused by susceptible Enterobacteriaceae† (e.g., *E. coli*, *Klebsiella*†) or *S. epidermidis*.

IV cefotaxime with or without other anti-infectives (e.g., ampicillin, gentamicin, vancomycin) has been recommended for empiric treatment of meningitis†. Pending results of CSF culture and in vitro susceptibility testing, the most appropriate anti-infective regimen for empiric treatment of suspected bacterial meningitis should be selected based on results of CSF gram stain and antigen tests, age of the patient, the most likely pathogen(s) and source of infection, and current patterns of bacterial resistance within the hospital and local community. When results of culture and susceptibility tests become available and the pathogen is identified, the empiric anti-infective regimen should be modified (if necessary) to ensure that the most effective regimen is being administered. Ceftriaxone should *not* be used alone for empiric treatment of meningitis when *Listeria monocytogenes*, enterococci, staphylococci, or *Pseudomonas aeruginosa* may be involved.

Meningitis Caused by Streptococcus pneumoniae IV ceftriaxone and IV cefotaxime are considered drugs of choice for the treatment of meningitis caused by susceptible *S. pneumoniae*. While cefotaxime and ceftriaxone generally have been considered the drugs of choice when meningitis is caused by penicillin-resistant *S. pneumoniae*, treatment failures have been reported when these cephalosporins were used alone for the treatment of meningitis caused by *S. pneumoniae* with intermediate or high-level penicillin resistance (i.e., penicillin MIC 0.1 mcg/mL or greater). In addition, strains of *S. pneumoniae* with reduced susceptibility to cephalosporins have been reported with increasing frequency and use of cefotaxime or ceftriaxone alone may be ineffective for the treatment of meningitis caused by these strains. The prevalence of *S. pneumoniae* with reduced susceptibility to penicillin and/or cephalosporins varies geographically, and clinicians should be aware of the prevalence and pattern of *S. pneumoniae* drug resistance in the local community to optimize empiric and initial treatment regimens for serious pneumococcal infections. Because susceptibility can no longer be assumed, *S. pneumoniae* isolates should be routinely tested for in vitro susceptibility.

If anti-infective therapy in a patient with meningitis is initiated with an empiric regimen of IV ceftriaxone and IV vancomycin (with or without rifampin) and results of culture and in vitro susceptibility testing indicate that the pathogen involved is a strain of *S. pneumoniae* susceptible to ceftriaxone and susceptible or resistant to penicillin, vancomycin and rifampin can be discontinued and therapy completed using ceftriaxone alone. If the isolate is found to have reduced susceptibility to ceftriaxone *and* penicillin, both IV ceftriaxone and IV vancomycin usually are continued and consideration given to adding rifampin to the regimen. If meningitis is caused by *S. pneumoniae* highly resistant to ceftriaxone (i.e., MIC 4 mcg/mL or greater), consultation with an infectious disease expert is recommended.

Meningitis Caused by Haemophilus influenzae IV ceftriaxone and IV cefotaxime are considered drugs of choice for initial treatment of meningitis caused by susceptible *H. influenzae* (including penicillinase-producing strains). In children, AAP suggests that ampicillin may be substituted if the isolate is susceptible; however, because of the prevalence of ampicillin-resistant *H. influenzae*, ampicillin should not be used alone for empiric treatment of meningitis when *H. influenzae* may be involved. The incidence of *H. influenzae* meningitis in the US has decreased considerably since *H. influenzae* type b (Hib) conjugate vaccines became available for immunization of infants.

Meningitis Caused by Neisseria meningitidis IV ceftriaxone and IV cefotaxime are considered drugs of choice for empiric treatment of meningitis when *N. meningitidis* may be involved. If a diagnosis of *N. meningitidis* meningitis is confirmed, AAP and other clinicians suggest treatment with penicillin G or, alternatively, ampicillin, ceftriaxone, or cefotaxime. Chloramphenicol, if available, is recommended by AAP for the treatment of *N. meningitidis* meningitis in patients with a history of anaphylactoid-type hypersensitivity reactions to penicillin.

Meningitis Caused by Enterobacteriaceae Some clinicians recommend that meningitis caused by Enterobacteriaceae† (e.g., *E. coli*, *K. pneumoniae*†) be treated with a third generation cephalosporins (i.e., cefotaxime, ceftazidime, ceftriaxone) with or without an aminoglycoside. Because ceftazidime (but not cefotaxime or ceftriaxone) is effective for the treatment of meningitis caused by *Ps. aeruginosa*, some clinicians suggest that a regimen of ceftazidime and an aminoglycoside may be preferred for the treatment of meningitis caused by gram-negative bacilli pending results of culture and in vitro susceptibility testing.

Meningitis Caused by Streptococcus agalactiae Third generation cephalosporins (i.e., ceftriaxone, cefotaxime) have been suggested as an alternative for the treatment of meningitis caused by *S. agalactiae*†.

For initial treatment of meningitis or other severe infection caused by *S. agalactiae*, a regimen of IV ampicillin or IV penicillin G given in conjunction with an aminoglycoside is recommended. Some clinicians suggest that IV ampicillin is the drug of choice for the treatment of *S. agalactiae* meningitis and that an aminoglycoside (IV gentamicin) should be used concomitantly during the first 72 hours until in vitro susceptibility testing is completed and a clinical response is observed; thereafter, ampicillin can be given alone if the strain is susceptible to the drug.

Meningitis Caused by Listeria monocytogenes The optimal regimen for the treatment of meningitis caused by *L. monocytogenes* has not been established. Ceftriaxone is ineffective in and should not be used alone for the treatment of meningitis caused by *L. monocytogenes*. AAP and other clinicians generally recommend that meningitis or other severe infection caused by *L. monocytogenes* be treated with a regimen of IV ampicillin with or without an aminoglycoside (usually gentamicin); alternatively, a regimen of penicillin G in conjunction with gentamicin can be used. In patients hypersensitive to penicillin, the preferred alternative regimen for treatment of meningitis caused by *L. monocytogenes* is co-trimoxazole.

Other CNS Infections Ceftriaxone is a drug of choice for the treatment of healthcare-associated ventriculitis and meningitis caused by susceptible β-lactamase-producing *H. influenzae* or susceptible Enterobacteriaceae†. Ceftriaxone also is a drug of choice for the treatment of healthcare-associated ventriculitis and meningitis caused by susceptible *S. pneumoniae* when penicillin G is not the preferred anti-infective (i.e., penicillin MIC 0.12 mcg/mL or greater). Some experts state that ceftriaxone can be used alone if the infection is caused by *S. pneumoniae* with penicillin MIC less than 1 mcg/mL, but should be used in conjunction with vancomycin if the strain has a penicillin MIC 1 mcg/mL or greater and that consideration should be given to also including rifampin in the regimen if the strain has a ceftriaxone MIC greater than 2 mcg/mL.

Although penicillin G usually is the drug of choice, ceftriaxone is recommended as an alternative for the treatment of healthcare-associated ventriculitis and meningitis caused by susceptible *C. acnes*† (formerly *P. acnes*).

■ **Acute Otitis Media** IM ceftriaxone is used for the treatment of acute otitis media (AOM) caused by *S. pneumoniae*, *H. influenzae* (including β-lactamase-producing strains), or *Moraxella catarrhalis* (including β-lactamase-producing strains).

When anti-infective therapy is indicated for the treatment of AOM, AAP recommends high-dose amoxicillin or amoxicillin and clavulanate potassium as the drug of first choice for initial treatment. These experts recommend certain cephalosporins (cefdinir, cefpodoxime, cefuroxime, ceftriaxone) as alternatives for initial treatment in penicillin-allergic patients who do not have a history of severe and/or recent penicillin-allergic reactions.

Ceftriaxone has been shown to be effective for initial or repeat treatment of AOM, and is a good choice when the patient has persistent vomiting or cannot otherwise tolerate an oral regimen. The manufacturers recommend a single-dose regimen of IM ceftriaxone for the treatment of AOM, but caution that the potential advantages of this single-dose parenteral regimen should be balanced against its potentially lower clinical cure rate compared with a 10-day oral anti-infective regimen. AAP states that either a 1- or 3-day regimen† of IM or IV ceftriaxone can be used for initial treatment of AOM, but cautions that there is some evidence that more than a single dose of the drug may be required to prevent recurrence of middle ear infections within 5–7 days after the initial dose. A 3-day regimen† of ceftriaxone is recommended for retreatment in patients who fail to respond to initial treatment with other anti-infectives.

Results of several controlled clinical studies in pediatric patients with AOM indicate that the short-term clinical response rate to a single-dose IM ceftriaxone regimen is similar to that of a 10-day regimen of oral cefaclor (40 mg/kg daily), a 7- or 10-day regimen of oral amoxicillin (40 mg/kg daily), a 10-day regimen of oral co-trimoxazole (8 mg/kg trimethoprim and 40 mg/kg of sulfamethoxazole daily), or a 10-day regimen of oral amoxicillin and clavulanate potassium; however, in one study, the single-dose IM ceftriaxone regimen had a lower clinical cure rate than a 10-day regimen of oral amoxicillin and clavulanate potassium.

A 3-day regimen of IM ceftriaxone has been shown to be more effective than a 1-day regimen for retreatment in patients who fail to respond to initial treatment with another anti-infective. The 3-day ceftriaxone regimen has been effective for the treatment of persistent or relapsing otitis media caused by *H. influenzae*, *M. catarrhalis*, *S. pyogenes*, or penicillin-susceptible *S. pneumoniae*; however, treatment failures have been reported when the causative agent was *S. pneumoniae* with reduced susceptibility to penicillin.

For additional information on diagnosis and management of AOM, current AAP clinical practice guidelines for AOM should be consulted.

■ **Respiratory Tract Infections** Ceftriaxone is used in adults and pediatric patients for the treatment of lower respiratory tract infections (including pneumonia) caused by susceptible gram-positive cocci (e.g., *S. pneumoniae*, *S. aureus*) or gram-negative bacteria (e.g., *H. influenzae*, *H. parainfluenzae*, *K. pneumoniae*, *E. coli*, *Enterobacter aerogenes*, *P. mirabilis*, *Serratia marcescens*). Ceftriaxone generally has been effective in the treatment of pneumonia caused by *S. pneumoniae* with intermediate resistance to penicillin (i.e., penicillin MIC less than 0.1–2 mcg/mL), but treatment failures have been reported when the drug was used alone in the treatment of severe infections (e.g., meningitis) caused by strains with intermediate or high-level penicillin resistance (i.e., penicillin MIC 0.12 mcg/mL or greater). (See Uses: Meningitis and Other CNS Infections.)

Acute Sinusitis Ceftriaxone is used as an alternative for the treatment of acute bacterial sinusitis†.

When anti-infective therapy is indicated for the treatment of acute bacterial sinusitis, IDSA recommends amoxicillin and clavulanate potassium and AAP recommends either amoxicillin or amoxicillin and clavulanate potassium as the drug of choice for initial empiric treatment. Because of variable activity against *S. pneumoniae* and *H. influenzae*, IDSA no longer recommends second or third generation oral cephalosporins for empiric monotherapy of sinusitis in adults or children. If an oral cephalosporin is used as an alternative for empiric treatment of acute bacterial sinusitis in children (e.g., in penicillin-allergic individuals), IDSA and AAP recommend a combination regimen that includes a third generation cephalosporin (cefixime or cefpodoxime) and clindamycin (or linezolid). In children who are vomiting, unable to tolerate oral therapy, or unlikely to adhere to the initial doses, treatment of acute sinusitis can be initiated with a single dose of IV or IM ceftriaxone and then switched to an oral regimen if clinical improvement is observed at 24 hours. IV ceftriaxone also is an alternative for severe sinusitis requiring hospitalization.

Community-acquired Pneumonia IDSA and the American Thoracic Society (ATS) recommend ceftriaxone as an alternative to penicillin G, ampicillin, or amoxicillin for the treatment of community-acquired pneumonia (CAP) caused by penicillin-susceptible *S. pneumoniae* and as a preferred drug for the treatment of CAP caused by penicillin-resistant *S. pneumoniae*, provided in vitro susceptibility has been demonstrated. These experts state that ceftriaxone is a preferred anti-infective for the treatment of CAP caused by β-lactamase-producing *H. influenzae*. IDSA and ATS also recommend use of ceftriaxone in certain combination regimens used for empiric treatment of CAP. The drug has been administered on an outpatient basis for empiric anti-infective therapy in adults with CAP who did not require hospitalization.

Initial treatment of CAP generally involves use of an empiric anti-infective regimen based on the most likely pathogens and local susceptibility patterns; therapy may then be changed (if possible) to provide a more specific regimen (pathogen-directed therapy) based on results of in vitro culture and susceptibility testing. The most appropriate empiric regimen varies depending on the severity of illness at the time of presentation and whether outpatient treatment or hospitalization in or out of an intensive care unit (ICU) is indicated and the presence or absence of cardiopulmonary disease and other modifying factors that increase the risk of certain pathogens (e.g., penicillin- or multidrug-resistant *S. pneumoniae*, enteric gram-negative bacilli, *Ps. aeruginosa*).

Most experts recommend that an empiric regimen for treatment of CAP include an anti-infective active against *S. pneumoniae* since this organism is the most commonly identified cause of bacterial pneumonia and causes more severe disease than many other common CAP pathogens. Pathogens most frequently involved in *outpatient* CAP include *S. pneumoniae*, *M. pneumoniae*, *Chlamydophila pneumoniae* (formerly *Chlamydia pneumoniae*), respiratory viruses, and *H. influenzae*. Pathogens most frequently involved in *inpatient* CAP in non-ICU patients are *S. pneumoniae*, *M. pneumoniae*, *C. pneumoniae*, *H. influenzae*, *Legionella*, and respiratory viruses. Patients with severe CAP admitted into the ICU usually have infections caused by *S. pneumoniae*, *S. aureus*, *Legionella*, gram-negative bacilli, or *H. influenzae*. Coverage against anaerobic bacteria usually is indicated only in classic aspiration pleuropulmonary syndrome in patients who had loss of consciousness as a result of alcohol or drug overdosage or after seizures in patients with concomitant gingival disease or esophageal motility disorders.

Inpatient treatment of CAP is initiated with a parenteral regimen, although therapy may be changed to an oral regimen if the patient is improving clinically, is hemodynamically stable, able to ingest drugs, and has a normally functioning GI tract. CAP patients usually have a clinical response within 3–7 days after initiation of therapy and a switch to oral therapy generally can be made during this period.

For empiric *outpatient* treatment of CAP in adults when risk factors for drug-resistant *S. pneumoniae* are present (e.g., comorbidities such as chronic heart, lung, liver, or renal disease, diabetes, alcoholism, malignancies, asplenia, immunosuppression, use of anti-infectives within the last 3 months), ATS and IDSA recommend monotherapy with a fluoroquinolone active against *S. pneumoniae* (moxifloxacin, gemifloxacin, levofloxacin) or, alternatively, a combination regimen that includes a β-lactam active against *S. pneumoniae* (high-dose amoxicillin or fixed combination of amoxicillin and clavulanic acid or, alternatively, ceftriaxone, cefpodoxime, or cefuroxime) given in conjunction with a macrolide (azithromycin, clarithromycin, erythromycin) or doxycycline.

For empiric *inpatient* treatment of CAP in adult non-ICU patients, IDSA and ATS recommend monotherapy with a fluoroquinolone (moxifloxacin, gemifloxacin, levofloxacin) or, alternatively, a combination regimen that includes a β-lactam (usually cefotaxime, ceftriaxone, or ampicillin) given in conjunction with a macrolide (azithromycin, clarithromycin, erythromycin). For empiric *inpatient* treatment of CAP in adult ICU patients when *Pseudomonas* and methicillin-resistant *S. aureus* (MRSA; also known as oxacillin-resistant *S. aureus* or ORSA) are *not* suspected, IDSA and ATS recommend a combination regimen that includes a β-lactam (cefotaxime, ceftriaxone, fixed combination of ampicillin and sulbactam) given in conjunction with either azithromycin or a fluoroquinolone (gemifloxacin, levofloxacin, moxifloxacin).

For additional information on management of respiratory tract infections, including CAP, current clinical practice guidelines from IDSA available at http://www.idsociety.org should be consulted.

■ **Septicemia** Ceftriaxone is used in adults and pediatric patients for the treatment of septicemia caused by *S. aureus*, *S. pneumoniae*, *H. influenzae*, *E. coli*, or *K. pneumoniae*.

■ **Skin and Skin Structure Infections** Ceftriaxone is used for the treatment of skin and skin structure infections caused by susceptible *S. aureus*, *S. epidermidis*, *S. pyogenes*, viridans group streptococci, *E. cloacae*, *E. coli*, *K. oxytoca*, *K. pneumoniae*, *P. mirabilis*, *Morganella morganii*, *S. marcescens*, *Acinetobacter calcoaceticus*, *B. fragilis*, or *Peptostreptococcus*.

Ceftriaxone has been recommended for use in multiple-drug anti-infective regimens for empiric treatment of necrotizing infections of the skin, fascia, and muscle†. Because necrotizing fasciitis (including Fornier gangrene) may be polymicrobial (e.g., mixed aerobic-anaerobic infections) or monomicrobial (e.g., *S. pyogenes*, *S. aureus*, *Vibrio vulnificus*, *Aeromonas hydrophila*, *Peptostreptococcus*), IDSA recommends that empiric anti-infective regimens be selected to provide broad-spectrum coverage.

Ceftriaxone in conjunction with metronidazole has been recommended as an option for the treatment of surgical site infections that occur following GI or genitourinary surgery. For the treatment of surgical site infections that occur following procedures involving the axilla or perineum, ceftriaxone is recommended as an option; concomitant vancomycin may also be needed for coverage against methicillin-resistant *S. aureus*.

Ceftriaxone also is one of several options recommended for empiric treatment of infected animal bite wounds or for empiric treatment of moderate or severe diabetic foot infections.

Although the manufacturers state that ceftriaxone can be used for the treatment of skin and skin structure infections caused by *Ps. aeruginosa*, treatment failures have been reported when ceftriaxone was used alone in the treatment of urinary tract infections or respiratory tract infections caused by *Ps. aeruginosa*. Some of these failures occurred because superinfection with resistant strains of *Ps. aeruginosa* occurred during treatment with the drug. Because many strains of *Ps. aeruginosa* are only susceptible to high concentrations of ceftriaxone in vitro and because resistant strains of the organism have developed during treatment with the drug, many clinicians state that ceftriaxone should not be used alone in any infection where *Ps. aeruginosa* may be present.

For additional information on management of skin and skin structure infections, current clinical practice guidelines from IDSA available at http://www.idsociety.org should be consulted.

■ **Urinary Tract Infections** Ceftriaxone is used in adult and pediatric patients for the treatment of complicated and uncomplicated urinary tract infections caused by *E. coli*, *K. pneumoniae*, *M. morganii*, *P. mirabilis*, or *P. vulgaris*.

The most appropriate anti-infective for the treatment of urinary tract infections should be selected based on the severity of the infection and results of culture and in vitro susceptibility testing. It has been suggested that certain parenteral cephalosporins (i.e., cefepime, cefotaxime, ceftriaxone, ceftazidime) may be drugs of choice for the treatment of complicated urinary tract infections caused by susceptible Enterobacteriaceae, including susceptible strains of *E. coli*, *K. pneumoniae*, *P. rettgeri*, *M. morganii*, *P. vulgaris*, or *P. stuartii*; an aminoglycoside usually is used concomitantly in severe infections. Ceftriaxone may be particularly useful as initial therapy for the treatment of nosocomial urinary tract infections known or suspected to be caused by multidrug-resistant Enterobacteriaceae. However, ceftriaxone, like other third generation cephalosporins, generally should *not* be used in the treatment of uncomplicated urinary tract infections when other anti-infectives with a narrower spectrum of activity could be used.

■ **Chancroid** A single IM dose of ceftriaxone is used for the treatment of chancroid† (genital ulcers caused by *H. ducreyi*).

CDC and other clinicians state that a single IM dose of ceftriaxone, a single oral dose of azithromycin, a 3-day oral ciprofloxacin regimen (contraindicated in pregnant or lactating women), or a 7-day oral erythromycin regimen are recommended for the treatment of chancroid.

HIV-infected individuals and patients who are uncircumcised may not respond to treatment of chancroid as well as those who are HIV-negative or circumcised. Clinicians should consider that, although treatment failures can occur with any of the recommended regimens, only limited data are available regarding efficacy of the single-dose ceftriaxone and single-dose azithromycin regimens for the treatment of chancroid in HIV-infected individuals. Because treatment failures and slow healing of ulcers are more likely in HIV-infected individuals, such patients should be monitored closely and more prolonged treatment or retreatment may be necessary.

Data are limited regarding the prevalence of *H. ducreyi* resistant to the anti-infectives recommended for treatment. Some treatment failures that have occurred in HIV-infected individuals who received the single-dose ceftriaxone regimen for the treatment of chancroid did not appear to be related to ceftriaxone resistance since isolates of *H. ducreyi* obtained from these individuals were susceptible to ceftriaxone in vitro.

For additional information on management of chancroid, current CDC sexually transmitted diseases treatment guidelines available at http://www.cdc.gov/std should be consulted.

■ **Gonorrhea and Associated Infections** Ceftriaxone is used in adults, adolescents, and pediatric patients for the treatment of uncomplicated gonorrhea, disseminated gonorrhea (including meningitis and endocarditis), and various other gonococcal infections caused by *Neisseria gonorrhoeae*, including infections caused by penicillin-, fluoroquinolone-, and tetracycline-resistant strains. Ceftriaxone in conjunction with azithromycin is the regimen of choice for the treatment of gonococcal infections in most patients. Unlike the majority of other drugs that have been used for the treatment of gonococcal infections, ceftriaxone usually is effective for the treatment of gonorrhea at all sites, including cervical, urethral, rectal, and pharyngeal gonococcal infections.

Recommendations for the treatment of gonorrhea have changed multiple times over the last several decades because of the ability of *N. gonorrhoeae* to develop resistance to anti-infectives. Ceftriaxone has been considered a drug of choice for the treatment of uncomplicated and disseminated gonococcal infections since 1989 when CDC first altered their guidelines to no longer recommend use of penicillins or tetracyclines for these infections because of the widespread prevalence of antibiotic-resistant *N. gonorrhoeae*, including penicillinase-producing *N. gonorrhoeae* resistant to penicillins (PPNG), strains with plasmid-mediated resistance to tetracyclines (TRNG), and strains with chromosomally mediated resistance to multiple anti-infectives (CMRNG).

In 2007, CDC altered their guidelines to no longer recommend use of fluoroquinolones for the treatment of gonococcal infections because quinolone-resistant *N. gonorrhoeae* (QRNG) had become widespread in the US and elsewhere. As a result, cephalosporins became the only remaining class of anti-infectives that could be considered for the treatment of gonococcal infections. However, *N. gonorrhoeae* with reduced susceptibility to ceftriaxone and/or cefixime or other cephalosporins have also been reported with increasing frequency in the US and elsewhere (e.g., Asia, Europe, Canada) and there have been rare reports of *N. gonorrhoeae* with high-level ceftriaxone resistance in some countries (Japan, France, Spain).

In 2012, based on evidence of declining cefixime susceptibility among urethral *N. gonorrhoeae* isolates collected during 2006–2011 in the US and elsewhere and reports of treatment failures with cefixime and other oral cephalosporins in some countries, CDC again altered their guidelines to state that IM ceftriaxone is the cephalosporin of choice for the treatment of uncomplicated urogenital, anorectal, and pharyngeal gonorrhea and that cefixime and other oral cephalosporins should not be used for first-line treatment.

Currently, CDC and other clinicians state that dual combination treatment with ceftriaxone *and* azithromycin is the regimen of choice for gonococcal infections in the US. The theoretical basis of dual combination treatment is that the use of 2 anti-infectives with different mechanisms of action against *N. gonorrhoeae* may improve treatment efficacy and potentially delay emergence and spread of cephalosporin resistance. In addition, because individuals with *N. gonorrhoeae* infection frequently are coinfected with *Chlamydia trachomatis*, a dual regimen that includes azithromycin provides coverage against such infections. Although CDC previously stated that either a single dose of oral azithromycin or a 7-day regimen of oral doxycycline could be used as the second anti-infective in dual treatment regimens, single-dose azithromycin is now preferred because of convenience and compliance advantages and because the prevalence of *N. gonorrhoeae* resistant to tetracyclines is substantially higher than that reported for azithromycin. In patients allergic to azithromycin, multiple-dose doxycycline can be substituted for single-dose azithromycin in recommended or alternative dual treatment regimens. Dual treatment regimens should be used in all adults and adolescents with gonorrhea, regardless of the presence or absence of chlamydial coinfection.

HIV-infected individuals should receive the same treatment regimens recommended for other individuals with gonococcal infections.

CDC recommends that health-care providers treating gonorrhea remain vigilant for treatment failures (evidenced by persistent symptoms or a positive follow-up test despite treatment). If there is evidence of treatment failure and reinfection is unlikely, relevant clinical specimens should be obtained for culture (preferable with simultaneous nucleic acid amplification test [NAAT]) and in vitro susceptibility testing should be performed if *N. gonorrhoeae* is isolated. Whenever treatment failure is suspected, an infectious disease specialist, an STD/HIV Prevention Training Center (http://www.nnptc.org), local or state health department STD program, or CDC (404-639-8659) should be consulted for advice on obtaining cultures, in vitro susceptibility testing, and treatment. Suspected treatment failures should be reported to CDC through local or state health departments within 24 hours of diagnosis and clinical isolates should be sent to CDC and stored at local laboratories for possible further testing.

For additional information on management of gonococcal infections, current CDC sexually transmitted diseases treatment guidelines available at http://www.cdc.gov/std should be consulted.

Gonococcal Infections in Adults and Adolescents **Uncomplicated Cervical, Urethral, and Rectal Gonorrhea.** For the treatment of uncomplicated cervical, urethral, or rectal gonorrhea in adults and adolescents, CDC states that a dual combination regimen that includes a single 250-mg IM dose of ceftriaxone *and* a dose of azithromycin (single 1-g oral dose) is the regimen of choice. In clinical trials, a single 250-mg IM dose of ceftriaxone was associated with a 99.2% cure rate in patients with uncomplicated urogenital and anorectal gonorrhea. There are no clinical data to support a ceftriaxone dose greater than 250 mg for the treatment of uncomplicated gonorrhea. Although other parenteral cephalosporins (e.g., a single 500-mg IM dose of cefotaxime or single 2-g IM dose of cefoxitin) are safe and generally effective for the treatment of uncomplicated urogenital and anorectal gonorrhea, these drugs offer no advantage over ceftriaxone for urogenital infections.

If necessary because ceftriaxone is not available or cannot be used, CDC states that adults and adolescents can receive an alternative dual combination regimen that includes a single 400-mg dose of oral cefixime *and* a dose of azithromycin (single 1-g oral dose) for the treatment of uncomplicated urogenital or anorectal gonorrhea. The oral cefixime regimen does not provide the high, sustained bactericidal blood concentrations provided by IM ceftriaxone and has been associated with a cure rate of 97.5% in patients with uncomplicated urogenital and anorectal gonorrhea.

In adults and adolescents with cephalosporin allergy, CDC states that a dual treatment regimen that includes a single dose of oral gemifloxacin (320 mg) and a single dose of oral azithromycin (2 g) or a dual treatment regimen that includes a single dose of IM gentamicin (240 mg) and a single dose of oral azithromycin (2 g) could be considered for the treatment of uncomplicated urogenital gonorrhea; however, GI effects may limit use of these regimens. If available, spectinomycin (no longer commercially available in the US) is an effective alternative for the treatment of urogenital and anorectal gonorrhea. Although monotherapy with a single 2-g dose of oral azithromycin was previously recommended for the treatment of uncomplicated urogenital gonorrhea in patients with cephalosporin allergy, CDC states that monotherapy is no longer recommended because of concerns related to development of resistance and because there have been documented treatment failures with azithromycin monotherapy.

A test-of-cure follow-up (culture or NAAT) is not usually needed in patients with uncomplicated urogenital or rectal gonorrhea who receive a recommended or alternative dual treatment regimen.

Uncomplicated Pharyngeal Gonorrhea. For the treatment of uncomplicated gonorrhea of the pharynx† in adults and adolescents, CDC states that a dual combination regimen that includes a single 250-mg IM dose of ceftriaxone *and* a dose of azithromycin (single 1-g oral dose) is the regimen of choice.

Pharyngeal gonococcal infections are more difficult to eradicate than cervical, urethral, or rectal infections. Ceftriaxone generally has been effective in the treatment of pharyngeal gonococcal infections; most other anti-infectives, including oral cephalosporins, do not reliably cure such infections. In clinical trials, a single 250-mg IM dose of ceftriaxone was associated with a cure rate of 98.9% in patients with pharyngeal infections.

A test-of-cure follow-up is not usually needed in patients with uncomplicated pharyngeal gonorrhea who receive the recommended ceftriaxone dual treatment regimen; however, if an alternative regimen is used in patients with pharyngeal gonorrhea, a test-of-cure follow-up (culture or NAAT) is recommended 14 days after treatment.

Gonococcal Conjunctivitis. The regimen of choice for the treatment of gonococcal conjunctivitis† in adults and adolescents is a dual combination regimen that includes a single IM dose of ceftriaxone *and* a single dose of oral azithromycin. As an adjunct to anti-infective therapy, the infected eye can be irrigated once with sterile sodium chloride solution. Because only limited data are available regarding treatment of gonococcal conjunctivitis, consultation with an infectious disease specialist should be considered.

Disseminated Gonococcal Infections. For initial treatment of disseminated gonococcal infections that include arthritis and arthritis-dermatitis syndrome†, CDC recommends that adults and adolescents receive a dual combination regimen that includes a multiple-dose regimen of IM or IV ceftriaxone *and* a single dose of oral azithromycin. The alternative for initial treatment is a multiple-dose regimen of IV cefotaxime *and* a single dose of oral azithromycin. The initial parenteral regimen should be continued for 24–48 hours after substantial improvement occurs; treatment can then be switched to an oral regimen that is selected based on in vitro susceptibility testing and continued to complete at least 1 week of treatment.

For the treatment of gonococcal meningitis† or gonococcal endocarditis†, CDC recommends that adults and adolescents receive a dual combination regimen that includes a multiple-dose regimen of IV ceftriaxone *and* a single dose of oral azithromycin. The parenteral regimen should be continued for 10–14 days in patients with meningitis and for at least 4 weeks in patients with endocarditis.

Initial treatment of disseminated gonococcal infections should be undertaken in consultation with an infectious disease specialist, especially if the diagnosis is uncertain, purulent synovial effusions or other complications are present, or adherence to the regimen is uncertain. Evaluation for clinical evidence of endocarditis and meningitis is recommended in all patients with disseminated gonorrhea.

Gonococcal Epididymitis. Ceftriaxone is a drug of choice for the treatment of acute epididymitis†. Although acute epididymitis in sexually active men younger than 35 years of age is most frequently caused by *C. trachomatis* or *N. gonorrhoeae*, epididymitis can also be caused by other organisms (e.g., sexually transmitted enteric bacteria, *Mycoplasma*, *Ureaplasma*). Presumptive treatment is usually initiated prior to availability of all diagnostic laboratory test results and is selected based on the patient's risk for chlamydia, gonorrhea, and/or enteric bacteria (e.g., *E. coli*).

For empiric treatment of acute epididymitis most likely caused by sexually transmitted chlamydia and gonorrhea†, CDC recommends that adults receive a single dose of IM ceftriaxone given in conjunction with a 10-day regimen of oral doxycycline.

For empiric treatment of acute epididymitis most likely caused by sexually transmitted chlamydia, gonorrhea, and enteric bacteria†, CDC recommends that adults receive a single dose of IM ceftriaxone given in conjunction with a 10-day regimen of oral levofloxacin or oral ofloxacin. CDC states that levofloxacin or ofloxacin monotherapy can be considered for empiric treatment of acute epididymitis most likely caused by enteric bacteria if gonorrhea has been ruled out using gram, methylene blue, or gentian violet microscopy stain.

Gonococcal Proctitis. For presumptive treatment of acute proctitis† prior to availability of diagnostic laboratory test results, CDC recommends that adults receive a single dose of IM ceftriaxone given in conjunction with a 7-day regimen of oral doxycycline.

Gonococcal Infections in Neonates Gonococcal infections in neonates usually occur as the result of exposure to the mother's infected cervical exudate and are apparent 2–5 days after birth. The most serious manifestations of *N. gonorrhoeae* infection in neonates are ophthalmia neonatorum and sepsis, arthritis, and meningitis; less serious manifestations include rhinitis, vaginitis, urethritis, and reinfection at sites of fetal monitoring (e.g., scalp). Because a neonate with gonococcal infection usually has acquired the organism from their mother, both the mother and her sexual partner(s) should be evaluated and treated for gonorrhea.

Prophylaxis and Presumptive Treatment of Gonococcal Infections in Neonates. CDC and AAP recommend routine topical prophylaxis using 0.5% erythromycin ophthalmic ointment in *all* neonates as soon as possible after birth to prevent gonococcal ophthalmia neonatorum; however, topical anti-infectives are inadequate for prophylaxis of gonococcal infections at other sites and may be ineffective in preventing chlamydial neonatal conjunctivitis.

Because neonates born to women with untreated gonorrhea are at high risk of infection with *N. gonorrhoeae*, CDC and AAP recommend that such neonates receive a single dose of IM or IV ceftriaxone for *parenteral prophylaxis*† and presumptive treatment of gonorrhea†. The single-dose ceftriaxone regimen also is recommended in other neonates if topical ophthalmic erythromycin is unavailable, especially for neonates born to women who are at risk for gonococcal infection or received no prenatal care. Topical erythromycin prophylaxis is unnecessary in neonates who receive parenteral prophylaxis with ceftriaxone.

CDC states that data are not available regarding the use of dual combination treatment regimens in neonates born to women with gonorrhea.

Gonococcal Ophthalmia Neonatorum. For the *treatment* of ophthalmia neonatorum† caused by *N. gonorrhoeae*, CDC and AAP recommend that neonates receive a single dose of IM or IV ceftriaxone.

As an adjunct to parenteral treatment of gonococcal ophthalmia neonatorum, the neonate's eyes should be irrigated with sterile sodium chloride solution immediately and at frequent intervals until the discharge is eliminated. Topical anti-infectives are inadequate for the treatment of gonococcal ophthalmia neonatorum and are unnecessary when appropriate systemic anti-infective therapy is given.

Infants born to mothers with untreated gonorrhea are at increased risk for gonococcal ophthalmia neonatorum if they do not receive appropriate parenteral prophylaxis at birth. Other neonates at increased risk for gonococcal ophthalmia neonatorum include those with mothers who received no prenatal care or have a history of sexually transmitted diseases or substance abuse. In all cases of neonatal conjunctivitis, conjunctival exudate should be cultured for *N. gonorrhoeae* and tested for anti-infective susceptibility and both mother and infant should be tested for chlamydial infection. Although the single-dose ceftriaxone regimen is adequate for treatment of gonococcal conjunctivitis, infants with ophthalmia neonatorum be hospitalized and evaluated for signs of disseminated infection (e.g., sepsis, arthritis, meningitis). CDC recommends that infants with gonococcal ophthalmia be managed in consultation with an infectious disease specialist.

Disseminated Gonococcal Infections and Gonococcal Scalp Abscesses in Neonates. Neonates with documented gonococcal infection at any site (including the eyes or scalp) should be evaluated for the possibility of disseminated infection (e.g., sepsis, arthritis, meningitis). If disseminated gonococcal infection is present, CDC and AAP recommend a multiple-dose regimen of IV or IM ceftriaxone or IV or IM cefotaxime. While either ceftriaxone or cefotaxime can be used for the treatment of disseminated gonococcal infections in neonates, ceftriaxone is contraindicated in certain neonates (see Cautions: Pediatric Precautions). AAP states that cefotaxime is preferred in infants with hyperbilirubinemia.

CDC states that data are not available regarding the use of dual combination regimens for the treatment of disseminated gonococcal infections or gonococcal scalp abscesses in neonates.

Gonococcal Infections in Infants and Children **Uncomplicated Gonorrhea.** For the treatment of uncomplicated gonococcal vulvovaginitis, cervicitis, epididymitis, urethritis, pharyngitis, or proctitis in infants and children, CDC and AAP recommend a single dose of IM ceftriaxone. AAP states that a dual combination treatment regimen that includes a single dose of IM ceftriaxone *and* a single dose of oral azithromycin can be used for the treatment of uncomplicated gonorrhea in children weighing at least 45 kg. CDC states that data are not available regarding the use of dual combination regimens for the treatment of uncomplicated gonorrhea in children weighing 45 kg or less.

CDC and AAP state that adolescents with uncomplicated gonorrhea should receive a dual combination treatment regimen recommended for adults. (See Gonococcal Infections in Adults and Adolescents under Uses: Gonorrhea.)

Disseminated Gonococcal Infections. For the treatment of disseminated gonococcal infections† (e.g., bacteremia, arthritis) in infants and children, CDC and AAP recommend a multiple-dose regimen of IM or IV ceftriaxone. AAP states that a dual combination treatment regimen that includes IM or IV ceftriaxone *and* oral erythromycin can be used for the treatment of complicated gonococcal infections in children weighing less than 45 kg and a dual combination treatment regimen that includes IM or IV ceftriaxone *and* oral azithromycin can be used in children weighing at least 45 kg. CDC states that data are not available regarding the use of dual combination regimens for the treatment of complicated gonorrhea in children weighing 45 kg or less.

CDC and AAP state that adolescents with disseminated gonococcal infections should receive a dual combination treatment regimen recommended for adults. (See Gonococcal Infections in Adults and Adolescents under Uses: Gonorrhea.)

Prophylaxis in Sexual Assault Victims A single dose of IM ceftriaxone is used in conjunction with a single dose of oral azithromycin and a single dose of either oral metronidazole or oral tinidazole for empiric anti-infective prophylaxis in adult or adolescent victims of sexual assault†. Gonorrhea, genital chlamydial infection, trichomoniasis, and bacteria vaginosis are the sexually transmitted diseases most commonly diagnosed in women following sexual assault; however, the prevalence of these infections is substantial among sexually active women and their presence after assault does not necessarily indicate that the infections were acquired during the assault. Gonococcal and chlamydial infections among females are of special concern because of the possibility of ascending infection.

CDC recommends routine empiric prophylaxis after a sexual assault, and use of such prophylaxis probably benefits most patients since follow-up of assault victims can be difficult and such prophylaxis allays the patient's concerns about possible infections. The 3-drug empiric anti-infective prophylaxis regimen recommended for adults and adolescents (ceftriaxone, azithromycin, and either metronidazole or tinidazole) provides coverage against gonorrhea, chlamydia, trichomoniasis, and bacterial vaginosis, but efficacy in preventing these infections after sexual assault has not been evaluated. Patients should be counseled regarding the potential benefits and toxicities associated with the regimen (e.g., GI effects).

Routine postexposure vaccination with hepatitis B virus (HBV) vaccine also is recommended for adult and adolescent sexual assault victims who have not previously received the vaccine or whose immunity against HBV is uncertain; hepatitis B immune globulin also should be given to previously unvaccinated individuals if the assailant is known to be hepatitis B surface antigen (HBsAg)-positive. In addition, vaccination with human papillomavirus (HPV) vaccine is recommended for previously unvaccinated or incompletely vaccinated female assault victims 9–26 years of age and male assault victims 9–21 years of age. CDC states that a decision to offer antiretroviral postexposure prophylaxis against HIV should be individualized taking into account the probability of HIV transmission (e.g., likelihood of the assailant having HIV, exposure characteristics that might increase the risk for HIV transmission, time elapsed after the event) and potential benefits and risks of such prophylaxis. (See Guidelines for Use of Antiretroviral Agents: Antiretrovirals for Postexposure Prophylaxis following Sexual, Injection Drug Use, or other Nonoccupational Exposures to HIV [nPEP], in the Antiretroviral Agents General Statement 8:18.08.)

■ **Pelvic Inflammatory Disease** Ceftriaxone is used for the treatment of pelvic inflammatory disease (PID) caused by *N. gonorrhoeae*. Ceftriaxone, like other cephalosporins, generally is inactive against *C. trachomatis* and should not be used alone in the treatment of PID.

PID is an acute or chronic inflammatory disorder in the upper female genital tract and can include any combination of endometritis, salpingitis, tubo-ovarian abscess, and pelvic peritonitis. PID generally is a polymicrobial infection most frequently caused by *N. gonorrhoeae* and/or *Chlamydia trachomatis*; however, organisms that can be part of the normal vaginal flora (e.g., anaerobic bacteria, *Gardnerella vaginalis*, *H. influenzae*, enteric gram-negative bacilli, *S. agalactiae*) or mycoplasma (e.g., *Mycoplasma hominis*, *Ureaplasma urealyticum*) also may be involved. PID is treated with an empiric regimen that provides broad-spectrum coverage. The regimen should be effective against *N. gonorrhoeae* and *C. trachomatis* and also probably should be effective against anaerobes. The optimum empiric regimen for the treatment of PID has not been identified. A variety of parenteral and oral regimens have been shown to achieve clinical and microbiologic cure in randomized studies with short-term follow-up.

IV Regimens for PID When a parenteral regimen is indicated for the treatment of PID, CDC and other clinicians generally recommend a 2-drug regimen of cefoxitin (2 g IV every 6 hours) or cefotetan (2 g IV every 12 hours) given in conjunction with doxycycline (100 mg IV or orally every 12 hours) or a 2-drug regimen of clindamycin (900 mg IV every 8 hours) and gentamicin (usually a 2-mg/kg IV or IM loading dose followed by 1.5 mg/kg every 8 hours; regimen of 3–5 mg/kg once daily can be substituted). While certain parenteral cephalosporins (e.g., cefotaxime, ceftriaxone) also have been used and may be effective for the treatment of PID, CDC states that there is less experience with use of these cephalosporins in patients with PID and these drugs may be less active than cefotetan or cefoxitin against anaerobic bacteria.

The parenteral regimen should be continued until 24–48 hours after the patient improves clinically and then, based on clinical experience, a transition to an oral regimen can be considered to complete 14 days of treatment. If tubo-ovarian abscess is present, at least 24 hours of inpatient observation is recommended.

IM and Oral Regimens for PID In women with mild to moderately severe acute PID, CDC states that an IM and oral regimen can be considered since clinical outcomes with these regimens are similar to IV regimens in such patients. However, if there is no response to the IM and oral regimen within 72 hours, the patient should be reevaluated to confirm the diagnosis and an IV regimen initiated.

If an IM and oral regimen is used, CDC recommends a single dose of an IM cephalosporin (e.g., ceftriaxone, cefoxitin with oral probenecid, cefotaxime) given in conjunction with a 14-day regimen of oral doxycycline (with or without oral metronidazole). The optimal cephalosporin is unclear; although cefoxitin usually has better anaerobic coverage, ceftriaxone has better coverage against *N. gonorrhoeae*.

For additional information on management of PID, current CDC sexually transmitted diseases treatment guidelines available at http://www.cdc.gov/std should be consulted.

■ **Actinomycosis** Ceftriaxone has been used in a limited number of patients to treat infections caused by *Actinomyces*†. IV ceftriaxone has been effective when given on an outpatient basis for the treatment of thoracic actinomycosis. However, IV penicillin G generally is the drug of choice for initial treatment of all forms of actinomycosis, including thoracic, abdominal, genitourinary, CNS, and cervicofacial infections. Alternative anti-infectives that can be used for the treatment of actinomycosis include amoxicillin, tetracyclines, erythromycins, chloramphenicol, clindamycin, third generation cephalosporins, and meropenem.

■ **Bartonella Infections** IM or IV ceftriaxone has been used in conjunction with oral erythromycin or oral azithromycin for the treatment of bacteremia caused by *Bartonella quintana*† (formerly *Rochalimaea quintana*). *B. quintana*, a gram-negative bacilli, can cause cutaneous bacillary angiomatosis, trench fever, bacteremia, endocarditis, and chronic lymphadenopathy. *B. quintana* infections have been reported most frequently in immunocompromised patients (e.g., HIV-infected individuals), homeless individuals in urban areas, and chronic alcohol abusers. Optimum anti-infective regimens for the treatment of infections caused by *B. quintana* have not been identified, and various drugs have been used or are recommended to treat these infections, including doxycycline, erythromycin, azithromycin, clarithromycin, chloramphenicol, or cephalosporins. There is evidence that these *B. quintana* infections tend to persist or recur and prolonged therapy (several months or longer) usually is necessary.

The possible role of ceftriaxone in the treatment of infections caused by *Bartonella henselae*† (formerly *Rochalimaea henselae*) (e.g., cat scratch disease, bacillary angiomatosis, peliosis hepatitis) has not been determined. Cat scratch disease generally is a self-limited illness in immunocompetent individuals and may resolve spontaneously in 2–4 months; however, some clinicians suggest that anti-infective therapy be considered for acutely or severely ill patients with systemic symptoms, particularly those with hepatosplenomegaly or painful lymphadenopathy, and such therapy probably is indicated in immunocompromised patients. Anti-infectives also are indicated in patients with *B. henselae* infections who develop bacillary angiomatosis, neuroretinitis, or Parinaud's oculoglandular syndrome. While the optimum anti-infective regimen for the treatment of cat scratch disease or other *B. henselae* infections has not been identified, some clinicians recommend azithromycin, clarithromycin, erythromycin, doxycycline, ciprofloxacin, rifampin, co-trimoxazole, gentamicin, or third generation cephalosporins.

In HIV-infected patients, *Bartonella* infections occur most frequently in those with median $CD4^+$ T-cell counts less than 50 cells/mm^3. CDC, NIH, and IDSA recommend that all HIV-infected adults and adolescents diagnosed with a *Bartonella* infection receive at least 3 months of antibacterial treatment; if relapse occurs, long-term suppressive antibacterial treatment (secondary prophylaxis) may be needed. For initial treatment or long-term suppressive therapy of *Bartonella* infections in HIV-infected adults or adolescents, doxycycline or a macrolide (erythromycin, azithromycin, clarithromycin) is recommended. Although pregnant HIV-infected women should usually receive a macrolide (erythromycin) for treatment of these infections, CDC, NIH, and IDSA state that ceftriaxone may be a possible alternative when macrolides cannot be used.

■ **Capnocytophaga Infections** Based on results of in vitro susceptibility tests that indicate that *Capnocytophaga* generally is inhibited by ceftriaxone, some clinicians suggest that ceftriaxone can be used in the treatment of infections caused by *C. canimorsus*† (formerly CDC group DF-2). *Capnocytophaga* is a gram-negative bacilli that can cause life-threatening septicemia, meningitis, and/or endocarditis and often is associated with disseminated intravascular coagulation; splenectomized and immunocompromised individuals are at particularly high risk for serious *Capnocytophaga* infections. *C. canimorsus* infection usually occurs as the result of a dog bite or other close contact with a dog. The optimum regimen for the treatment of infections caused by *Capnocytophaga* has not been identified, but some clinicians recommend penicillin G or, alternatively, a third generation cephalosporin (cefotaxime, ceftriaxone), a carbapenem (imipenem or meropenem), vancomycin, a fluoroquinolone, or clindamycin.

■ **Leptospirosis** Ceftriaxone is used in the treatment of severe leptospirosis† caused by *Leptospira*. Leptospirosis is a spirochete infection that may range in severity from an asymptomatic or subclinical illness that is self-limited to a severe, life-threatening illness that includes jaundice, renal failure, hemorrhage, cardiac arrhythmias, pneumonitis, and hemodynamic collapse (Weil syndrome).

Penicillin G generally has been considered the drug of choice for the treatment of moderate to severe leptospirosis, and doxycycline has been used in less severe infections. Other anti-infectives recommended for the treatment of severe leptospirosis include cephalosporins (ceftriaxone, cefotaxime), aminopenicillins (ampicillin, amoxicillin), tetracyclines (doxycycline, tetracycline), or macrolides (azithromycin).

In one randomized study in adults, IV ceftriaxone was as effective as IV penicillin G for the treatment of severe leptospirosis. The duration of fever was decreased to 3 days in both treatment groups, and there were comparable improvements in complications associated with the infection (renal failure, respiratory failure, liver impairment, thrombocytopenia).

■ Lyme Disease Ceftriaxone is used in the treatment of Lyme disease†. IDSA, AAP, and other clinicians recommend IV ceftriaxone as a drug of choice for the treatment of early neurologic Lyme disease† with acute neurologic manifestations such as meningitis or radiculopathy, Lyme carditis†, Lyme arthritis†, and late neurologic Lyme disease†.

Lyme disease is a tick-borne spirochetal disease. In the US, Lyme disease is caused by the spirochete *Borrelia burgdorferi*, which is transmitted by the bite of *Ixodes scapularis* or *I. pacificus* ticks. For additional information on Lyme disease, see Lyme Disease in Uses: Spirochetal Infections, in the Tetracyclines General Statement 8:12.24.

Early Lyme Disease **Erythema Migrans.** Oral anti-infectives (doxycycline, amoxicillin, cefuroxime axetil) generally are effective for the treatment of early localized or early disseminated Lyme disease associated with erythema migrans, in the absence of specific neurologic manifestations or advanced atrioventricular (AV) heart block. Although IV ceftriaxone is effective for early Lyme disease manifested as erythema migrans, it is not superior to the recommended oral drugs and is more likely to cause serious adverse effects; therefore, ceftriaxone is not usually recommended for the treatment of early Lyme disease in the absence of neurologic involvement or advanced AV heart block.

Early Neurologic Lyme Disease. Ceftriaxone is a drug of choice for the treatment of early neurologic Lyme disease†. Parenteral anti-infectives are recommended for the treatment of early Lyme disease when there are acute neurologic manifestations such as meningitis or radiculoneuritis.

IDSA and other clinicians recommend a 14-day regimen (range: 10–28 days) of IV ceftriaxone as the preferred parenteral regimen for the treatment of acute neurologic Lyme disease manifested by meningitis or radiculopathy; IV cefotaxime and IV penicillin G sodium are the preferred alternatives. In patients with acute neurologic manifestations who are intolerant of cephalosporins and penicillin, there is some evidence that oral doxycycline may be an adequate alternative that can be considered for use in adults and children 8 years of age or older.

Lyme Carditis. Ceftriaxone is the drug of choice when a parenteral regimen is indicated for the treatment of Lyme carditis†. IDSA states that patients with AV heart block and/or myopericarditis associated with early Lyme disease may be treated with a 14-day regimen (range: 14–21 days) of oral or parenteral anti-infectives. Although there is no evidence to date to suggest that a parenteral regimen is more effective than an oral regimen for the treatment of Lyme carditis, a parenteral regimen usually is recommended for initial treatment of hospitalized patients; an oral regimen can be used to complete therapy and for the treatment of outpatients. When a parenteral regimen is used, IV ceftriaxone or, alternatively, IV cefotaxime or IV penicillin G sodium is recommended. When an oral regimen is used, doxycycline, amoxicillin, or cefuroxime axetil is recommended.

Because of the potential for life-threatening complications, hospitalization and continuous monitoring is advisable for patients who are symptomatic (syncope, dyspnea, chest pain) and also is recommended for those with second- or third-degree AV block or first-degree heart block when the PR interval is prolonged to 0.3 seconds or longer. Patients with advanced heart block may require a temporary pacemaker and consultation with a cardiologist is recommended.

Late Lyme Disease **Lyme Arthritis.** Ceftriaxone is the drug of choice when a parenteral regimen is indicated for the treatment of Lyme arthritis†. While patients with uncomplicated Lyme arthritis without clinical evidence of neurologic disease generally can be treated with a 28-day oral regimen (doxycycline, amoxicillin, or cefuroxime axetil), IDSA and other clinicians state that patients with Lyme arthritis and concomitant neurologic disease should receive a 14-day parenteral regimen (range: 14–28 days) of IV ceftriaxone or, alternatively, IV cefotaxime or IV penicillin G. While oral regimens are easier to administer, associated with fewer serious adverse effects, and less expensive than IV regimens, some patients with Lyme arthritis treated with oral anti-infectives have subsequently developed overt neuroborreliosis, which may require IV therapy for successful resolution. Therefore, additional study is needed to fully evaluate the comparative safety and efficacy of oral versus IV anti-infectives for the treatment of Lyme arthritis.

In patients who have persistent or recurrent joint swelling after a recommended oral regimen, IDSA and other clinicians recommend retreatment with the oral regimen or a switch to a parenteral regimen. Some clinicians prefer retreatment with an oral regimen for patients whose arthritis substantively improved but did not completely resolve; these clinicians reserve parenteral regimens for those patients whose arthritis failed to improve or worsened. It has been suggested that clinicians should consider allowing several months for joint inflammation to resolve after initial treatment before an additional course of anti-infectives is given.

Late Neurologic Lyme Disease. Ceftriaxone is the drug of choice for the treatment of late neurologic Lyme disease†. IDSA and other clinicians state that patients with late neurologic Lyme disease affecting the CNS or peripheral nervous system (e.g., encephalopathy, neuropathy) should receive 2–4 weeks of IV ceftriaxone or, alternatively, IV cefotaxime or IV penicillin G sodium. Response to anti-infective treatment usually is slow and may be incomplete in patients with late neurologic Lyme disease. IDSA states that retreatment is not recommended unless relapse is documented with reliable objective measures.

In a limited number of adults with late complications of Lyme disease (i.e., CNS dysfunction, peripheral neuropathy, and/or arthritis), most of whom failed to respond adequately to other anti-infectives (e.g., penicillin, tetracycline), ceftriaxone therapy (1 or 2 g IM or IV twice daily for 14 days) resulted in clinical improvement, including resolution of arthritis and chronic fatigue. A regimen of IV ceftriaxone (2 g once daily for 30 days) has been used with some success for the treatment of Lyme encephalopathy. Although IV penicillin G therapy can be effective in treating neurologic abnormalities of Lyme disease, central or peripheral neurologic deficits associated with disease progression have been noted in a few patients after such therapy, and some clinicians suggest that therapy with IV ceftriaxone may be preferred for serious manifestations (i.e., involving major organs) of disseminated or late Lyme disease because of its greater in vitro and in vivo activity against *B. burgdorferi* compared with IV penicillin G and the prolonged serum concentrations and excellent CSF penetration achievable with once-daily administration of ceftriaxone.

■ Neisseria meningitidis Infections Ceftriaxone is used in the treatment of invasive infections caused by *N. meningitidis* and also is used to eliminate nasopharyngeal carriage of *N. meningitidis*† and for chemoprophylaxis to prevent meningococcal disease in close contacts of patients with invasive disease†.

For suspected meningococcal disease, including presumptive *N. meningitidis* meningitis, AAP and IDSA recommend a third generation cephalosporin (ceftriaxone or cefotaxime) for initial empiric treatment. If the infection is found to be caused by penicillin-susceptible *N. meningitidis*, IV penicillin G or ampicillin can be substituted or the third generation cephalosporin can be continued. Although IV penicillin G generally has been considered the drug of choice for the treatment of meningitis known to be caused by susceptible *N. meningitidis*, some experts recommend ampicillin, ceftriaxone, or cefotaxime.

Patients with invasive meningococcal disease who have been treated with penicillin G or any anti-infective agent other than ceftriaxone or another third generation cephalosporin may still be carriers of *N. meningitidis* and should receive an anti-infective regimen to eradicate nasopharyngeal carriage of the organism prior to hospital discharge. The treatments of choice to eradicate nasopharyngeal carriage of *N. meningitidis* are ceftriaxone (single IM dose), rifampin (2-day regimen), and ciprofloxacin (single oral dose). These regimens are all 90–95% effective and any of these is an acceptable regimen in appropriate patients.

Chemoprophylaxis in Household and Other Close Contacts of Individuals with Invasive Meningococcal Disease Chemoprophylaxis in close contacts of a patients with invasive meningococcal disease is an important means of preventing secondary cases in household and other close contacts. Recommended regimens for chemoprophylaxis against meningococcal disease include a single dose of IM ceftriaxone, 2-day regimen of oral rifampin (not recommended in pregnant women), or a single dose of oral ciprofloxacin (not recommended in individuals younger than 18 years of age unless no other regimen can be used and not recommended for pregnant or lactating women). These regimens are all 90–95% effective and any of these is an acceptable regimen for chemoprophylaxis. AAP suggests that rifampin may be the drug of choice for chemoprophylaxis in most children.

The attack rate for household contacts who do not receive chemoprophylaxis has been estimated to be 4 cases per 1000 individuals exposed, which is 500–800 times greater than that for the general population. A decision to administer chemoprophylaxis to close contacts of an individual with invasive meningococcal disease is based on the degree of risk. Throat and nasopharyngeal cultures are *not* useful in determining the need for chemoprophylaxis and may unnecessarily delay administration of the regimen.

The USPHS Advisory Committee on Immunization Practices (ACIP), AAP, and others recommend that chemoprophylaxis be administered to contacts of patients with invasive meningococcal disease who are considered at high risk of infection. These high risk individuals include household contacts (especially children younger than 2 years of age) and any individual who has slept or eaten frequently in the same dwelling with the index case; child care and nursery school contacts who were exposed during the 7 days before the onset of disease in the index case; individuals exposed directly to oropharyngeal secretions of the index case (e.g., through kissing or sharing toothbrushes, eating utensils, or drinking containers) during the 7 days before the onset of disease in the index case; and medical personnel and others who had intimate exposure (e.g., through mouth to mouth resuscitation or unprotected contact during endotracheal intubation or suctioning) to the index case during the 7 days before the onset of disease. For travelers, chemoprophylaxis should be considered for any passenger who had direct contact with respiratory secretions from an index case or for anyone seated directly next to an index case on a prolonged flight (i.e., lasting 8 hours or longer).

Chemoprophylaxis is *not* routinely recommended for contacts of patients with invasive meningococcal disease who are considered at low risk of infection. Individuals considered in most circumstances as being at low risk include casual contacts with no history of direct exposure to the index case's oral secretions (e.g., school or work contacts); individuals who had only indirect contact with the index case (only contact was with a high-risk contact of the index case); and medical personnel who had no direct exposure to the index case's oral secretions. Because reports of secondary cases after close contact with patients with noninvasive pneumonia or conjunctivitis caused by *N. men-*

ingitidis are rare, chemoprophylaxis is not recommended for close contacts of patients who only have evidence of *N. meningitidis* in nonsterile sites (e.g., oropharyngeal, conjunctival, endotracheal secretions).

When chemoprophylaxis is indicated in high-risk contacts, it must be administered promptly (ideally within 24 hours after identification of the index case) since the attack rate of secondary disease is greatest in the few days following disease onset in the index case. All high-risk contacts should be informed that even if chemoprophylaxis is taken or started, the development of any suspicious clinical manifestation warrants early, rapid medical attention. Chemoprophylaxis probably is of limited or no value if administered more than 14 days after contact with the index case. If high-risk exposure to a new index case occurs more than 2 weeks after initial chemoprophylaxis, additional chemoprophylaxis is indicated.

Outbreak Control When an outbreak of meningococcal disease occurs in the US and the outbreak is caused by a vaccine-preventable meningococcal strain (e.g., serogroups A, C, Y, or W-135), large-scale vaccination programs with meningococcal polysaccharide vaccine in the appropriate target group may be indicated. (See Uses: Outbreak Control in Meningococcal Polysaccharide Vaccine 80:12.) Mass chemoprophylaxis programs (i.e., administration of ceftriaxone, rifampin, or ciprofloxacin to large population groups) are not recommended to control large outbreaks since the disadvantages of such programs (e.g., costs, difficulty in ensuring simultaneous administration of the anti-infectives to large populations, adverse effects of the drugs, emergence of resistant organisms) probably outweigh any possible benefit in disease prevention. However, when outbreaks involve limited populations (e.g., a single school), administration of chemoprophylaxis to all individuals in the population may be considered, especially if the outbreak involves a meningococcal serogroup not represented in currently available meningococcal vaccines. Other measures, such as restricting travel to areas with a suspected meningococcal outbreak, closing schools or universities, or canceling sporting or social events, are not usually recommended to control meningococcal outbreaks in the US.

While the vast majority of cases of meningococcal disease in the US are sporadic, localized outbreaks of meningococcal disease do occur. When a suspected outbreak of meningococcal disease occurs in the US, public health authorities will then determine whether mass vaccinations (with or without mass chemoprophylaxis) is indicated and delineate the target population based on risk assessment.

■ **Nocardia Infections** Ceftriaxone has been used for the treatment of nocardiosis† caused by *Nocardia*.

Co-trimoxazole (fixed combination of sulfamethoxazole and trimethoprim) usually is considered the drug of choice for the treatment of nocardiosis. Other drugs that have been used alone or in combination regimens for the treatment of nocardiosis include a sulfonamide alone (sulfamethoxazole [not commercially available in the US], sulfadiazine), amikacin, tetracyclines, cephalosporins (ceftriaxone, cefotaxime, cefuroxime), cefoxitin, carbapenems (imipenem, meropenem), fixed combination of amoxicillin and clavulanate, clarithromycin, cycloserine, or linezolid. A regimen of amikacin and ceftriaxone has been effective for the treatment of disseminated *N. asteroides* infection complicated by cerebral abscess.

Ceftriaxone has been recommended as one of several alternatives to co-trimoxazole for the treatment of skin and skin structure infections caused by *Nocardia*† (e.g., *N. farcinica, N. brasiliensis*). Prolonged anti-infective treatment (6–24 months) and/or a multiple-drug anti-infective regimen may be necessary for severe or disseminated infections or in patients with immunosuppression.

In vitro susceptibility testing, if available, is recommended to guide selection of anti-infectives for the treatment of severe nocardiosis or for treatment in patients who cannot tolerate or failed to respond to sulfonamide treatment.

■ **Relapsing Fever** Ceftriaxone may be effective for the treatment of relapsing fever† caused by *Borrelia recurrentis*; however, other drugs (e.g., tetracycline, penicillin G) are considered the drugs of choice for the treatment of the disease.

■ **Syphilis** Ceftriaxone has some activity against *Treponema pallidum* and there is some limited evidence that the drug may be effective for the treatment of syphilis†.

IM penicillin G benzathine is the drug of choice for the treatment of primary syphilis (i.e., ulcer or chancre at infection site), secondary syphilis (i.e., manifestations that include, but are not limited to, rash, mucocutaneous lesions, and lymphadenopathy), and tertiary syphilis (i.e., cardiac, gummatous lesions, tabes dorsalis, and general paresis) in adults, adolescents, and children. IM penicillin G benzathine also is the drug of choice for the treatment of latent syphilis (i.e., detected by serologic testing but lacking clinical manifestations), including both early latent syphilis (latent syphilis acquired within the preceding year) and late latent syphilis (i.e., all other cases of latent syphilis or syphilis of unknown duration) in all age groups. For the treatment of neurosyphilis and otic or ocular syphilis, IV penicillin G potassium or sodium is the drug of choice and IM penicillin G procaine (with oral probenecid) is an alternative if compliance can be ensured.

CDC states that limited clinical studies as well as biologic and pharmacologic evidence suggest that a multiple-dose ceftriaxone regimen may be effective for the treatment of primary and secondary syphilis† and, on the basis of biologic plausibility and pharmacologic properties, may also be effective for the treatment of latent syphilis† in penicillin-allergic patients. However, optimal dosage and duration of ceftriaxone for the treatment of syphilis have not been defined and there is more extensive clinical experience using tetracyclines (doxycycline, tetracycline) as alternatives for the treatment of primary, secondary, or latent syphilis in penicillin-allergic patients.

CDC states that limited data suggest that a multiple-dose ceftriaxone regimen can be used as an alternative for the treatment of neurosyphilis† in penicillin-allergic patients.

Decisions regarding the treatment of syphilis in penicillin-allergic patients should be made in consultation with a specialist. Because of limited experience with penicillin alternatives, close follow-up is essential if ceftriaxone is used for the treatment of syphilis in penicillin-allergic patients and the possibility of cross-sensitivity between penicillin and ceftriaxone should be considered. If compliance with an alternative regimen or follow-up cannot be ensured, CDC recommends desensitization and treatment with the appropriate penicillin G preparation.

Data are insufficient to recommend use of ceftriaxone or other alternatives for the treatment of any stage of syphilis in penicillin-allergic pregnant women or for the treatment of congenital syphilis in neonates, infants, or children with known or suspected penicillin allergy; CDC recommends that such patients be desensitized and treated with the appropriate penicillin G preparation.

In certain circumstance when there is a penicillin shortage and penicillin G is not available, CDC states that a multiple-dose ceftriaxone regimen can be considered for the treatment of congenital syphilis. In such situations, CDC recommends that ceftriaxone be used with close clinical, serologic, and CSF follow-up and in consultation with a specialist in the treatment of infants with congenital syphilis.

For additional information on management of syphilis, current CDC sexually transmitted diseases treatment guidelines available at http://www.cdc.gov/std should be consulted.

■ **Typhoid Fever and Other Invasive Salmonella Infections**

Ceftriaxone has been effective when used in adults or children for the treatment of typhoid fever† or paratyphoid fever† (enteric fever) or septicemia caused by *Salmonella* serovars Typhi or Paratyphi, respectively, including multidrug-resistant strains. Ceftriaxone also has been used and is recommended for the treatment of invasive infections (e.g., bacteremia, osteomyelitis) caused by nontyphoidal *Salmonella*, including *Salmonella* serovar Typhimurium.

Multidrug-resistant strains of *Salmonella* serovar Typhi (i.e., strains resistant to ampicillin, chloramphenicol, and/or co-trimoxazole) have been reported with increasing frequency, and third generation cephalosporins (e.g., ceftriaxone, cefotaxime) and fluoroquinolones (e.g., ciprofloxacin, ofloxacin) are considered the drugs of first choice for the treatment of typhoid fever or other severe infections known or suspected to be caused by these strains. AAP states that ceftriaxone is a drug of choice for empiric treatment of enteric fever pending results of in vitro susceptibility tests. Strains of *S. typhi* resistant to ceftriaxone have been reported rarely in the US.

IV ceftriaxone (3 or 4 g once daily in adults or 75 mg/kg once daily in children) given for 5–7 days has been as effective as a 14-day course of oral or IV chloramphenicol in the treatment of typhoid fever caused by susceptible *S. typhi*. Although bacteremia resolved sooner with ceftriaxone in some patients, the time to defervescence was faster with chloramphenicol.

■ **Whipple's Disease** Ceftriaxone has been effective when used in the treatment of Whipple's disease†, a progressive systemic infection caused by *Tropheryma whipplei* (formerly *Tropheryma whippelii*). Optimal regimens for the treatment of Whipple's disease have not been identified, in part because of difficulties in identifying and cultivating the causative agent and because relapses commonly occur, even after adequate and long-term anti-infective treatment. Some clinicians recommend an initial parenteral regimen (e.g., ceftriaxone or penicillin G used with or without streptomycin) followed by a long-term regimen of oral co-trimoxazole given for 1–2 years.

Ceftriaxone has been effective for the treatment of Whipple's disease when the CNS was involved. For the treatment of encephalitis caused by *T. whipplei*, IDSA recommends initial treatment with ceftriaxone given for 2–4 weeks followed by co-trimoxazole or cefixime for 1–2 years. Some clinicians suggest that ceftriaxone may be a drug of choice for patients who experience cerebral relapse during or after treatment with penicillin G or co-trimoxazole.

■ **Empiric Therapy in Febrile Neutropenic Patients** Ceftriaxone has been used in conjunction with an aminoglycoside for empiric anti-infective therapy of presumed bacterial infections in febrile neutropenic adults or pediatric patients†. While ceftriaxone has been used alone for empiric therapy in some febrile neutropenic patients considered to be at low risk, use of ceftriaxone monotherapy may not provide adequate coverage against some potential pathogens (e.g., *Ps. aeruginosa*) and generally is *not* recommended for empiric anti-infective therapy in febrile neutropenic patients.

In studies in febrile neutropenic cancer patients 1 year of age or older, the overall response rate to a once-daily regimen of IV ceftriaxone (30 mg/kg once daily in adults or 80 mg/kg once daily in children) given in conjunction with IV amikacin (20 mg/kg daily) was similar to that of a regimen of IV ceftazidime (100–150 mg/kg daily given in 3 divided doses) given in conjunction with amikacin (20 mg/kg given once daily or in 3 divided doses).

Published protocols for the treatment of infections in febrile neutropenic patients should be consulted for specific recommendations regarding selection of the initial empiric anti-infective regimen, when to change the initial regimen, possible subsequent regimens, and duration of therapy in these patients. In addition, consultation with an infectious disease expert knowledgeable about infections in immunocompromised patients is advised.

■ **Prevention of Bacterial Endocarditis** Ceftriaxone is used as an alternative for *prevention* of α-hemolytic (viridans group) streptococcal endocarditis† in adults and children undergoing certain dental or upper respiratory tract procedures who have certain cardiac conditions that put them at the highest risk of adverse outcome from endocarditis.

The cardiac conditions identified by AHA as those associated with highest risk of adverse outcomes from endocarditis and for which anti-infective prophylaxis is reasonable are prosthetic cardiac valves or prosthetic material used for cardiac valve repair, previous infective endocarditis, cardiac valvulopathy after cardiac transplantation, and certain forms of congenital heart disease (i.e., unrepaired cyanotic congenital heart disease including palliative shunts and conduits; a completely repaired congenital heart defect where prosthetic material or device was placed by surgery or catheter intervention within the last 6 months; repaired congenital heart disease with residual defects at the site or adjacent to the site of a prosthetic patch or prosthetic device that inhibits endothelialization).

AHA states that anti-infective prophylaxis for prevention of α-hemolytic (viridans group) streptococcal bacterial endocarditis is reasonable for patients with the above cardiac risk factors if they are undergoing any dental procedures that involve manipulation of gingival tissue or the periapical region of teeth or perforation of the oral mucosa (e.g., biopsies, suture removal, placement of orthodontic bands). AHA states that anti-infective prophylaxis is *not* needed for routine anesthetic injections through noninfected tissue, dental radiographs, placement of removable prosthodontic or orthodontic appliances, adjustment of orthodontic appliances, placement of orthodontic brackets, shedding of deciduous teeth, or bleeding from trauma to the lips or oral mucosa.

AHA states that anti-infective prophylaxis for prevention of bacterial endocarditis also is reasonable for patients with the above cardiac risk factors if they are undergoing invasive procedures of the respiratory tract that involve incision or biopsy of respiratory mucosa (e.g., tonsillectomy, adenoidectomy) and may be reasonable for such patients if they are undergoing surgical procedures that involve infected skin, skin structure, or musculoskeletal tissue. However, anti-infective prophylaxis solely to prevent infective endocarditis is no longer recommended by AHA for GI or genitourinary tract procedures.

Oral amoxicillin is the drug of choice when prevention of bacterial endocarditis is indicated in patients undergoing certain dental or upper respiratory tract procedures who have certain cardiac conditions that put them at highest risk of adverse outcomes from endocarditis. If an oral regimen cannot be used in such patients, AHA recommends IM or IV ampicillin or IM or IV cefazolin or ceftriaxone. Alternatives for penicillin-allergic patients include oral cephalexin, oral azithromycin or clarithromycin, oral or parenteral clindamycin, or parenteral cefazolin or ceftriaxone; cephalosporins should not be used for such prophylaxis in individuals with a history of anaphylaxis, angioedema, or urticaria after receiving a penicillin.

For additional information on which cardiac conditions are associated with the highest risk of adverse outcomes from endocarditis and additional information regarding use of prophylaxis to prevent bacterial endocarditis, current recommendations published by AHA should be consulted.

■ **Perioperative Prophylaxis** Ceftriaxone has been used perioperatively to reduce the incidence of infection in patients undergoing certain contaminated or potentially contaminated surgical procedures, including biliary tract procedures (e.g., cholecystectomy), colorectal procedures, intra-abdominal surgery, or vaginal or abdominal hysterectomy, and in those undergoing certain clean surgical procedures in which the development of infection at the surgical site would represent a serious risk, including coronary artery bypass, open heart surgery, thoracic surgery, or orthopedic surgery. The drug also has been used perioperatively in patients undergoing transurethral resection of the prostate† or renal transplantation†.

Ceftriaxone in conjunction with metronidazole is one of several options recommended for perioperative prophylaxis in patients undergoing colorectal surgery. Ceftriaxone also is one of several options recommended for perioperative prophylaxis in patients undergoing biliary tract procedures, but should not be used in those undergoing cholecystectomy for noninfected biliary conditions, including biliary colic or dyskinesia without infection.

A first or second generation cephalosporin (e.g., cefazolin, cefuroxime) generally is preferred when a cephalosporin is used for perioperative prophylaxis. Third generation cephalosporins (e.g., cefotaxime, ceftriaxone, ceftazidime) and fourth generation cephalosporins (e.g., cefepime) are not usually recommended for routine perioperative prophylaxis because they are expensive, some are less active than first or second generation cephalosporins against staphylococci, they have spectrums of activity wider than necessary for organisms encountered in elective surgery, and their use for prophylaxis may promote emergence of resistant organisms. (See Uses: Perioperative Prophylaxis, in the Cephalosporins General Statement 8:12.06.)

Dosage and Administration

■ **Reconstitution and Administration** Ceftriaxone sodium is administered by IV infusion or deep IM injection.

Ceftriaxone should *not* be administered intrathecally.

Ceftriaxone has been administered IM or IV to adults or children in outpatient settings, including clinicians' offices, outpatient clinics, infusion centers, skilled nursing facilities, rehabilitation centers, or the patient's home, for the treatment of certain infections suitable for community-based parenteral anti-infective agent therapy (e.g., community-acquired pneumonia, osteomyelitis, endocarditis†). Outpatient parenteral anti-infective therapy often is used to complete a course of ceftriaxone therapy initiated during hospitalization, but ceftriaxone therapy also has been initiated on an outpatient basis. Ceftriaxone usually is administered in the outpatient setting by a healthcare provider; however, the drug has been self-administered in the patients' home by the patient, family member, or other responsible person.

Ceftriaxone should *not* be reconstituted with or further diluted with diluents containing calcium (e.g., Ringer's/lactated Ringer's solution, Hartmann's solution) because a precipitate can form. (See Interaction with Calcium-containing Products under Cautions: Precautions and Contraindications.)

Because precipitation of ceftriaxone-calcium can occur, ceftriaxone must *not* be admixed with calcium-containing solutions and must *not* be administered *simultaneously* with calcium-containing IV solutions, including continuous infusions of calcium-containing solutions such as parenteral nutrition, even via different infusion lines at different sites in any patient (irrespective of age). In adult and pediatric patients older than 28 days of age, ceftriaxone and calcium-containing solutions may be administered *sequentially* if the infusion lines are thoroughly flushed between infusions with a compatible fluid (e.g., 0.9% sodium chloride injection, 5% dextrose injection).

Ceftriaxone is contraindicated in neonates (28 days of age or younger) if they are receiving (or expected to require) treatment with calcium-containing IV solutions, including continuous calcium-containing infusions such as parenteral nutrition.

Patients receiving ceftriaxone should be adequately hydrated.

Intermittent IV Infusion For intermittent IV infusion, vials labeled as containing 250 mg, 500 mg, 1 g, or 2 g of ceftriaxone should be reconstituted with 2.4, 4.8, 9.6, or 19.2 mL, respectively, of a compatible IV solution to provide solutions containing approximately 100 mg/mL. The reconstituted solution should then be further diluted to the desired concentration by withdrawing the entire contents of the vial and adding it to an appropriate IV diluent. Ceftriaxone solutions for IV infusion containing 10–40 mg/mL are recommended; however, lower concentrations may be used.

Alternatively, ADD-Vantage® vials containing 1 or 2 g of ceftriaxone should be reconstituted with 0.9% sodium chloride or 5% dextrose injection in ADD-Vantage® flexible containers according to the manufacturer's directions and administered by IV infusion.

Alternatively, the commercially available Duplex® drug delivery system containing 1 or 2 g of lyophilized ceftriaxone and 50 mL of dextrose 3.74 or 2.22% injection, respectively, in separate chambers should be reconstituted (activated) according to the manufacturer's directions and administered by IV infusion. If stored in the refrigerator after reconstitution (see Chemistry and Stability: Stability), the solution should be allowed to reach room temperature prior to administration.

The 10-g pharmacy bulk package of ceftriaxone is reconstituted by adding 95 mL of a compatible IV solution to provide a solution containing approximately 100 mg/mL. Reconstituted solutions in the ceftriaxone pharmacy bulk package should *not* be used for direct IV infusion; these reconstituted solutions must be further diluted in a compatible IV infusion solution, generally to a concentration of 10–40 mg/mL, although lower concentrations may be used if desired.

Thawed solutions of the commercially available frozen premixed ceftriaxone sodium injection in dextrose should be administered only by intermittent IV infusion. The commercially available frozen injection should be thawed at room temperature (25°C) or under refrigeration (5°C); the injection should not be thawed by warming in a water bath or by exposure to microwave radiation. The container may be fragile in the frozen state and should be handled with care. Precipitates that may have formed in the frozen injection usually will dissolve with little or no agitation when the injection reaches room temperature; potency is not affected. After thawing at room temperature, the injection should be agitated and the container checked for minute leaks by firmly squeezing the bag. The injection should be discarded if container seals or outlet ports are not intact or leaks are found or if the solution is cloudy or contains an insoluble precipitate. Additives should not be introduced into the injection container. The injection should not be used in series connections with other plastic containers, since such use could result in air embolism from residual air being drawn from the primary container before administration of fluid from the secondary container is complete.

Rate of Administration. The manufacturers recommend that intermittent IV infusions of ceftriaxone sodium be infused over 30 minutes (except in neonates).

In neonates, the manufacturers recommend that intermittent IV infusions of ceftriaxone be given over 60 minutes. (See Cautions: Pediatric Precautions.)

IM Injection IM injections of ceftriaxone sodium should be prepared by adding 0.9, 1.8, 3.6, or 7.2 mL of compatible diluent (e.g., sterile water for injection, 0.9% sodium chloride injection, 5% dextrose injection, bacteriostatic water for injection containing 0.9% benzyl alcohol, 1% lidocaine hydrochloride without epinephrine) to vials labeled as containing 250 mg, 500 mg, 1 g, or 2 g of ceftriaxone, respectively, to provide solutions containing approximately 250 mg/mL or by adding 1, 2.1, or 4.2 mL of one of these diluents to vials labeled as containing 500 mg, 1 g, or 2 g of ceftriaxone, respectively, to provide solutions containing approximately 350 mg/mL. More dilute solutions of the drug may be used for IM injection if required.

Solutions of the drug for IM injection that have been reconstituted with bacteriostatic water containing benzyl alcohol should not be used in neonates. (See Cautions: Pediatric Precautions.)

IM injections of ceftriaxone should be made deeply into a large muscle mass, using usual techniques and precautions.

■ **Dosage** Dosage of ceftriaxone sodium is expressed in terms of ceftriaxone and is identical for IM or IV administration.

To avoid unintentional overdosage, the commercially available Duplex delivery system containing ceftriaxone and dextrose injection should *not* be used in patients who require less than the entire 1- or 2-g dose in the container.

Pediatric Dosage **General Pediatric Dosage.** The American Academy of Pediatrics (AAP) recommends that neonates 28 days of age or younger receive ceftriaxone in a dosage of 50 mg/kg once daily, regardless of weight.

For pediatric patients beyond the neonatal period, AAP recommends a ceftriaxone dosage of 50–75 mg/kg once daily for the treatment of mild to moderate infections or a dosage of 100 mg/kg daily given in 1 or 2 doses for the treatment of severe infections.

The manufacturers state that the usual dosage of ceftriaxone for the treatment of serious infections (other than meningitis) in pediatric patients is 50–75 mg/kg daily given in divided doses every 12 hours. The maximum dosage recommended by the manufacturers for pediatric patients is 2 g daily.

Endocarditis. For the treatment of native valve endocarditis† caused by streptococci highly susceptible to penicillin (penicillin MIC 0.1 mcg/mL or less), including *Streptococcus pyogenes* (group A *β*-hemolytic streptococci; GAS), *S. agalactiae* (group B streptococci; GBS), streptococci groups C or G, most viridans group streptococci, or nonenterococcal group D streptococci (e.g., *S. gallolyticus* [formerly *S. bovis*], *S. equinas*), the American Heart Association (AHA) states that pediatric patients may receive IV ceftriaxone in a dosage of 100 mg/kg daily in divided doses every 12 hours for 4 weeks. Alternatively, AHA states that IV ceftriaxone can be given in a dosage of 80 mg/kg once daily (up to 4 g daily), but doses greater than 2 g should be given in divided doses every 12 hours.

For the treatment of native valve endocarditis† caused by streptococci relatively resistant to penicillin (penicillin MIC greater than 0.1 but less than 0.5 mcg/mL), AHA states that pediatric patients may receive IV ceftriaxone in a dosage of 100 mg/kg daily in divided doses every 12 hours for 4 weeks in conjunction with gentamicin (3–6 mg/kg daily IV in divided doses every 8 hours given concomitantly during the first 2 weeks of ceftriaxone treatment). Alternatively, AHA states that IV ceftriaxone can be given in a dosage of 80 mg/kg once daily (up to 4 g daily) in this regimen.

For the treatment of endocarditis† involving prosthetic valves or other prosthetic material caused by penicillin-susceptible streptococci (penicillin MIC 0.1 mcg/mL or less), AHA states that pediatric patients may receive IV ceftriaxone in a dosage of 100 mg/kg daily in divided doses every 12 hours for 6 weeks in conjunction with gentamicin (3–6 mg/kg daily IV in divided doses every 8 hours given concomitantly during the first 2 weeks of ceftriaxone treatment). Alternatively, AHA states that IV ceftriaxone can be given in a dosage of 80 mg/kg once daily (up to 4 g daily) in this regimen. If endocarditis involving prosthetic valves or other prosthetic material is caused by streptococci with penicillin MIC greater than 0.1 mcg/mL or caused by *Abiotrophia* or *Granulicatella*, AHA recommends that ceftriaxone be given for 6 weeks in conjunction with gentamicin (given concomitantly for the entire 6 weeks of ceftriaxone treatment).

For the treatment of endocarditis† caused by the HACEK group (i.e., *Haemophilus, Aggregatibacter, Cardiobacterium hominis, Eikenella corrodens, Kingella*), AHA states that pediatric patients may receive IV ceftriaxone in a dosage of 100 mg/kg daily in divided doses every 12 hours for 4 weeks. Alternatively, AHA states that IV ceftriaxone can be given in a dosage of 80 mg/kg once daily (up to 4 g daily) for 4 weeks.

GI Infections. If ceftriaxone is used as an alternative for the treatment of *Salmonella* gastroenteritis† (with or without bacteremia) in adolescents with human immunodeficiency virus (HIV) infection, the US Centers for Disease Control and Prevention (CDC), National Institutes of Health (NIH), and Infectious Diseases Society of America (IDSA) recommend a dosage of 1 g IV every 24 hours. The recommended duration of treatment is 7–14 days in those with $CD4^+$ T-cell counts of 200 cells/mm^3 or greater (14 days or longer if bacteremia is present or the infection is complicated) or 2–6 weeks in those with $CD4^+$ T-cell counts less than 200 cells/mm^3.

For the treatment of shigellosis† caused by *Shigella sonnei* or *S. flexneri*, pediatric patients have received ceftriaxone in a dosage of 50 mg/kg once daily for 2–5 days.

If ceftriaxone is used as an alternative for empiric treatment of infectious diarrhea† in HIV-infected adolescents, CDC, NIH, and IDSA recommend a dosage of 1 g IV every 24 hours. If there is no clinical response after 5–7 days, stool culture and in vitro susceptibility testing should be considered.

Intra-abdominal Infections. If ceftriaxone is used for empiric treatment of complicated intra-abdominal infections in pediatric patients, a dosage of 50–75 mg/kg once or twice daily is recommended. Although ceftriaxone may be used alone for initial empiric treatment of community-acquired biliary tract infections (cholecystitis or cholangitis), the drug should be used in conjunction with metronidazole for initial empiric treatment of extrabiliary community-acquired intra-abdominal infections.

Meningitis and Other CNS Infections. For the treatment of meningitis caused by susceptible bacteria, the manufacturers and some clinicians recommend that pediatric patients receive an initial ceftriaxone dosage of 100 mg/kg (up to 4 g) followed by 100 mg/kg daily (up to 4 g daily) given once daily or in equally divided doses every 12 hours for 7–21 days. Other clinicians recommend a dosage of 80–100 mg/kg daily (up to 4 g daily) given once daily or in divided doses every 12 hours. A twice-daily dosing regimen may be preferred for the treatment of meningitis caused by *S. pneumoniae*.

While 7 days of anti-infective therapy may be adequate for the treatment of uncomplicated meningitis caused by susceptible *H. influenzae* or *N. meningitidis*, at least 10–14 days of therapy is suggested for complicated cases or meningitis caused by *S. pneumoniae* and at least 21 days is suggested for meningitis caused by susceptible Enterobacteriaceae† (e.g., *Escherichia coli, Klebsiella*†). In neonates, some experts state that treatment of meningitis should be continued for 2 weeks beyond the first sterile CSF culture or for at least 3 weeks, whichever is longer.

If IV ceftriaxone is used for the treatment of healthcare-associated ventriculitis and meningitis caused by susceptible bacteria (see Uses: Meningitis and Other CNS Infections), IDSA recommends that infants and children receive a dosage of 100 mg/kg daily as a single dose or in divided doses every 12 hours. The duration of treatment depends on the causative organism and patient characteristics. The recommended treatment duration is 10–14 days for infections caused by gram-negative bacilli (with or without significant CSF pleocytosis, CSF hypoglycorrhachia, or clinical symptoms or systemic features); some experts recommend a duration of 21 days.

Respiratory Tract Infections. If ceftriaxone is used in children for the treatment of severe acute bacterial rhinosinusitis† requiring hospitalization, IDSA recommends a dosage of 50 mg/kg daily given IV in divided doses every 12 hours.

For the treatment of community-acquired pneumonia (CAP) caused by *S. pneumoniae* in pediatric patients 3 months of age or older, IDSA recommends that ceftriaxone be given in a dosage of 50–100 mg/kg daily as a single dose or in divided doses every 12 hours if the infection is caused by penicillin-susceptible strains or a dosage of 100 mg/kg daily as a single dose or in divided doses every 12 hours if the infection is caused by penicillin-resistant strains. Treatment usually is continued for 10 days.

For the treatment of CAP caused by susceptible *S. pyogenes* (group A *β*-hemolytic streptococci; GAS) or *H. influenzae* in pediatric patients 3 months of age or older, IDSA recommends that ceftriaxone be given in a dosage of 50–100 mg/kg daily as a single daily dose or in divided doses every 12 hours. Treatment usually is continued for 10 days.

Skin and Skin Structure Infections. The usual dosage of ceftriaxone for the treatment of skin and skin structure infections caused by susceptible organisms in pediatric patients is 50–75 mg/kg daily given as a single daily dose or in equally divided doses every 12 hours.

Acute Otitis Media. For the treatment of acute otitis media (AOM), the manufacturers recommend that pediatric patients receive a single 50-mg/kg IM dose of ceftriaxone (maximum dose 1 g).

For initial treatment of AOM, AAP recommends a ceftriaxone dosage of 50 mg/kg daily given IM or IV for 1 to 3 days†. AAP cautions that more than a single dose may be required to prevent recurrence.

For retreatment in patients with AOM who failed to respond to an initial anti-infective regimen, AAP recommends a ceftriaxone dosage of 50 mg/kg daily given for 3 days†.

Chancroid. When ceftriaxone is used for the treatment of chancroid† (genital ulcers caused by *H. ducreyi*), AAP recommends that infants and children weighing less than 45 kg receive a single 50-mg/kg IM dose (up to 250 mg) and that pediatric patients weighing 45 kg or more receive a single 250-mg IM dose.

Gonococcal Infections in Neonates. When ceftriaxone is used for parenteral *prophylaxis*† or presumptive treatment of gonorrhea† in neonates born to mothers with gonorrhea, CDC and AAP recommend that a single dose of 25–50 mg/kg (maximum 125 mg) of the drug be given IM or IV at birth.

For the *treatment* of gonococcal ophthalmia neonatorum†, CDC and AAP recommend that neonates receive a single IM or IV dose of 25–50 mg/kg (maximum 125 mg) of ceftriaxone.

For the treatment of disseminated gonococcal infections (e.g., sepsis, arthritis, meningitis) or gonococcal scalp abscess in neonates†, the usual dosage of ceftriaxone is 25–50 mg/kg IM or IV once daily for 7 days. If meningitis is documented, ceftriaxone should be continued for 10–14 days.

Gonococcal Infections in Infants and Children. For the treatment of uncomplicated gonorrhea in children beyond the neonatal age (prepubertal), AAP recommends that those weighing less than 45 kg receive a single 125-mg IM dose of ceftriaxone and that those weighing 45 kg or more receive a single 250-mg IM dose of ceftriaxone *and* a dose of azithromycin (single 1-g oral dose). CDC recommends that infants and children with uncomplicated gonococcal infections (vulvovaginitis, cervicitis, urethritis, pharyngitis, proctitis) weighing 45 kg or less receive a single IV or IM ceftriaxone dose of 25–50 mg/kg (up to 125 mg IM) and that those weighing more than 45 kg receive a single 250-mg IM dose of ceftriaxone *and* a dose of azithromycin (single 1-g oral dose).

For the treatment of disseminated or complicated gonococcal infections† (e.g., arthritis-dermatitis syndrome) in children beyond the neonatal period (prepubertal), AAP recommends that those weighing less than 45 kg receive IV or IM ceftriaxone in a dosage of 50 mg/kg once daily (up to 1 g daily) for 7 days in conjunction with erythromycin (30 mg/kg daily given orally in 4 divided doses [up to 2 g daily] for 14 days) and that those weighing 45 kg or more receive IV or IM ceftriaxone in a dosage of 1 g once daily for 7 days in conjunction with a dose of azithromycin (single 1-g oral dose). If meningitis or endocarditis is present, AAP recommends that dosage and duration of ceftriaxone in these regimens be increased to 50 mg/kg IV or IM every 12–24 hours for 10–14 days in those weighing less than 45 kg or 1–2 g IV every 12–24 hours for 10–14 days in those weighing 45 kg or more.

For the treatment of gonococcal bacteremia or arthritis in children, CDC recommends that those weighing 45 kg or less receiving IM or IV ceftriaxone in a dosage of 50 mg/kg daily (maximum 1 g daily) for 7 days and that those weighing more than 45 kg receive an IM or IV ceftriaxone dosage of 1 g once daily for 7 days.

Gonorrhea and Associated Infections in Adolescents. For the treatment of uncomplicated cervical, urethral, rectal, or pharyngeal gonorrhea, CDC recommends that adolescents receive a single 250-mg IM dose of ceftriaxone *and* a dose of azithromycin (single 1-g oral dose).

For the treatment of gonococcal conjunctivitis†, adolescents should receive a single 1-g IM dose of ceftriaxone *and* a dose of azithromycin (single 1-g oral dose).

For the treatment of gonococcal arthritis and arthritis-dermatitis syndrome†, CDC recommends that adolescents receive 1 g of ceftriaxone IV or IM once daily *and* a dose of azithromycin (single 1-g oral dose). Ceftriaxone should be continued until 24–48 hours after substantial clinical improvement; treatment can then be switched to an oral antibacterial selected based on in vitro susceptibility testing and given to complete a total treatment duration of at least 7 days.

For the treatment of gonococcal meningitis† or gonococcal endocarditis†, CDC recommends that adolescents receive 1–2 g of ceftriaxone IV every 12–24 hours *and* a dose of azithromycin (single 1-g oral dose). Ceftriaxone should be continued for 10–14 days in those with meningitis and for at least 4 weeks in those with endocarditis.

Prophylaxis in Sexual Assault Victims. For empiric anti-infective prophylaxis for gonorrhea, chlamydia, and trichomoniasis in adolescent sexual assault victims†, CDC recommends that a single 250-mg IM dose of ceftriaxone be given in conjunction with azithromycin (single 1-g oral dose) and either metronidazole (single 2-g oral dose) or tinidazole (single 2-g oral dose).

Lyme Disease. If IV ceftriaxone is used for the treatment of early Lyme disease† in children with acute neurologic disease manifested by meningitis or radiculopathy, IDSA and AAP recommend a dosage of 50–75 mg/kg (up to 2 g) once daily for 14 days (range: 10–28 days).

When a parenteral regimen is indicated for the treatment of Lyme carditis† in patients with atrioventricular (AV) heart block and/or myopericarditis associated with early Lyme disease, IDSA recommends that children receive IV ceftriaxone in a dosage of 50–75 mg/kg (up to 2 g) once daily for 14 days (range: 14–21 days). Although a parenteral regimen is recommended for initial treatment of hospitalized patients, the parenteral regimen can be switched to an oral regimen (doxycycline, amoxicillin, cefuroxime axetil) to complete therapy and for outpatients.

When a parenteral regimen is indicated for the treatment of Lyme arthritis† in patients with evidence of neurologic disease or when arthritis has not responded to an oral regimen, IDSA and AAP recommend that children receive IV ceftriaxone in a dosage of 50–75 mg/kg (up to 2 g) once daily for 14 days (range: 14–28 days).

For the treatment of late neurologic Lyme disease† affecting the central or peripheral nervous system, IDSA and AAP recommend that children receive IV ceftriaxone in a dosage of 50–75 mg/kg (up to 2 g) once daily for 2–4 weeks.

Neisseria meningitidis Infections. When ceftriaxone is used to eliminate nasopharyngeal carriage of *N. meningitidis*† or for chemoprophylaxis in close contacts of individuals with invasive meningococcal disease†, a single 125-mg IM dose should be used in children and adolescents younger than 15 years of age and a single 250-mg IM dose should be used in adolescents 15 years of age or older.

For dosage recommendations for the treatment of meningitis caused by *N. meningitidis*, see Meningitis and Other CNS Infections under Dosage: Pediatric Dosage, in Dosage and Administration.)

Pelvic Inflammatory Disease. For the treatment of mild to moderately severe acute pelvic inflammatory disease (PID) when an IM and oral regimen is indicated, adolescents may receive a single 250-mg IM dose of ceftriaxone followed by a 14-day regimen of doxycycline (100 mg orally twice daily) with or without metronidazole (500 mg orally twice daily). If there is no clinical response within 72 hours, the patient should be reevaluated to confirm the diagnosis and an IV regimen should be administered if indicated.

Syphilis. If ceftriaxone is used as an alternative in infants or children with clinical evidence of congenital syphilis† when penicillin G is not available, dosage should be based on age and weight. CDC states that infants 30 days of age or older may receive a dosage of 75 mg/kg IV or IM once daily for 10–14 days (dosage adjustments may be needed based on weight) and children may receive 100 mg/kg IV or IM once daily for 10–14 days. Clinicians should consider that ceftriaxone is contraindicated in certain neonates (see Cautions: Pediatric Precautions). Ceftriaxone should be used for the treatment of congenital syphilis *only* when necessary (i.e., during a penicillin shortage) and should be used in consultation with a specialist in the treatment of infants with congenital syphilis and with close clinical, serologic, and CSF follow-up.

If ceftriaxone is used as an alternative to IM penicillin G benzathine for the treatment of primary or secondary syphilis† in penicillin-allergic nonpregnant adolescents, CDC and other clinicians recommend a ceftriaxone dosage of 1–2 g IM or IV once daily for 10–14 days. Some clinicians suggest that this ceftriaxone dosage also can be used as an alternative in penicillin-allergic nonpregnant adolescents with early latent syphilis.

If ceftriaxone is used as an alternative to IV penicillin G for the treatment of neurosyphilis† in penicillin-allergic nonpregnant adolescents, CDC and others suggest a dosage of 2 g IM or IV daily for 10–14 days based on limited data.

CDC cautions that the optimal dosage and duration of ceftriaxone for the treatment of syphilis have not been defined and close follow-up is essential. (See Uses: Syphilis.)

Typhoid Fever and Other Invasive Salmonella Infections. For the treatment of typhoid fever† (enteric fever) or septicemia caused by *Salmonella* serovar Typhi†, including multidrug-resistant strains, pediatric patients have received ceftriaxone in a dosage of 50–75 mg/kg given IM or IV once daily. While ceftriaxone has been effective for the treatment of typhoid fever when administered for 3–7 days, anti-infective therapy for the treatment of typhoid fever usually is continued for at least 14 days to prevent relapse and a duration of at least 4–6 weeks may be necessary for the treatment of immunocompromised individuals (including HIV-infected individuals) or for the treatment of *Salmonella* meningitis.

Empiric Therapy in Febrile Neutropenic Patients. When used for empiric anti-infective therapy in febrile neutropenic patients†, children have received ceftriaxone in a dosage of 80 mg/kg (up to 2 g) once daily in conjunction with amikacin (20 mg/kg IV daily).

Prevention of Bacterial Endocarditis. If ceftriaxone is used as an alternative for prevention of α-hemolytic (viridans group) streptococcal endocarditis† in individuals with certain cardiac conditions who are undergoing certain dental or upper respiratory tract procedures (see Uses: Prevention of Bacterial Endocarditis), AHA recommends that children receive a single dose of 50 mg/kg given IV or IM 30–60 minutes prior to the procedure.

Adult Dosage

General Adult Dosage. The usual adult dosage of ceftriaxone for the treatment of most infections caused by susceptible organisms is 1–2 g given once daily or in equally divided doses twice daily, depending on the type and severity of the infection.

One manufacturer recommends that adults receive ceftriaxone in a dosage of 50–75 mg/kg every 12 hours (maximum 2 g daily) for the treatment of serious infections other than meningitis.

The maximum adult dosage of ceftriaxone recommended by the manufacturers is 4 g daily.

Bone and Joint Infections. For the treatment of native vertebral osteomyelitis caused by susceptible staphylococci, β-hemolytic streptococci†, or *Cutibacterium acnes*† (formerly *Propionibacterium acnes*), IDSA recommends that adults receive ceftriaxone in a dosage of 2 g IV once daily for 6 weeks.

If ceftriaxone is used as an alternative for the treatment of native vertebral osteomyelitis caused by susceptible *Salmonella*† (nalidixic acid-resistant strains), IDSA recommends that adults receive a dosage of 2 g IV once daily for 6–8 weeks.

For the treatment of prosthetic joint infections caused by susceptible staphylococci, IDSA recommends that adults receive ceftriaxone in a dosage of 1–2 g IV once daily for 2–4 weeks in conjunction with rifampin (300–450 mg orally twice daily) and that this regimen be followed by an oral anti-infective regimen (e.g., rifampin and ciprofloxacin or levofloxacin) to complete a total treatment duration of 3 months for infections related to total hip arthroplasty or 6 months for infections related to total knee arthroplasty.

For the treatment of prosthetic joint infections caused by susceptible β-hemolytic streptococci or *C. acnes*†, IDSA recommends that adults receive 2 g IV once daily for 4–6 weeks.

Endocarditis. For the treatment of native valve endocarditis† caused by viridans group streptococci or *S. gallolyticus* highly susceptible to penicillin (penicillin MIC 0.12 mcg/mL or less), AHA recommends that adults receive IV or IM ceftriaxone in a dosage of 2 g once daily for 4 weeks. Alternatively, adults with uncomplicated endocarditis† caused by highly penicillin-susceptible viridans group streptococci or *S. gallolyticus* who are at low risk for adverse effects related to aminoglycoside therapy may receive a 2-week regimen consisting of IV or IM ceftriaxone in a dosage of 2 g once daily in conjunction with gentamicin (3 mg/kg daily IV or IM given as a single daily dose or as 1 mg/kg every 8 hours). The 2-week regimen is not recommended for patients with known cardiac or extracardiac abscesses, creatinine clearance less than 20 mL/minute, impaired eighth cranial nerve function, or infection with *Abiotrophia*, *Granulicatella*, or *Gemella*.

For the treatment of endocarditis† involving prosthetic valves or other prosthetic material caused by viridans group streptococci or *S. gallolyticus* highly susceptible to penicillin (penicillin MIC 0.12 mcg/mL or less), AHA states that adults can receive IV or IM ceftriaxone in a dosage of 2 g once daily for 6 weeks with or without gentamicin (3 mg/kg daily IV or IM as a single daily dose or as 1 mg/kg every 8 hours given concomitantly during the first 2 weeks of ceftriaxone treatment). When endocarditis involving prosthetic valves or other prosthetic material is caused by viridans group streptococci or *S. gallolyticus* relatively or highly resistant to penicillin (penicillin MIC greater than 0.12 mcg/mL), AHA states that it is reasonable to extend the duration of concomitant gentamicin to the entire 6 weeks of ceftriaxone treatment.

When a double β-lactam regimen is used for the treatment of enterococcal endocarditis† involving native valves or prosthetic valves or other prosthetic material (see Enterococcal Endocarditis under Uses: Endocarditis), AHA recommends that adults receive ceftriaxone in a dosage of 2 g IV every 12 hours in conjunction with ampicillin (2 g IV every 4 hours). Both drugs should be continued for 6 weeks.

For the treatment of endocarditis† caused by the HACEK group (i.e., *Haemophilus, Aggregatibacter, C. hominis, E. corrodens, Kingella*), AHA recommends that adults receive IV or IM ceftriaxone in a dosage of 2 g once daily. A duration of 4 weeks is reasonable for the treatment of native valve endocarditis and 6 weeks is reasonable for the treatment of endocarditis involving prosthetic valves or other prosthetic material.

GI Infections. If ceftriaxone is used as an alternative for the treatment of *Salmonella* gastroenteritis† (with or without bacteremia) in HIV-infected adults, CDC, NIH, and IDSA recommend a dosage of 1 g IV every 24 hours. The recommended duration of treatment is 7–14 days in those with $CD4^+$ T-cell counts of 200 cells/mm^3 or greater (14 days or longer if the patient is bacteremic or the infection is complicated) or 2–6 weeks in those with $CD4^+$ T-cell counts less than 200 cells/mm^3.

If ceftriaxone is used as an alternative for empiric treatment of infectious diarrhea† in HIV-infected adults, CDC, NIH, and IDSA recommend a dosage of 1 g IV every 24 hours. If there is no clinical response after 5–7 days, stool culture and in vitro susceptibility testing should be considered.

Intra-abdominal Infections. If ceftriaxone is used for empiric treatment of complicated intra-abdominal infections, a dosage of 1–2 g once or twice daily is recommended. Although ceftriaxone may be used alone for initial empiric treatment of community-acquired biliary tract infections (cholecystitis or cholangitis), the drug should be used in conjunction with metronidazole for initial empiric treatment of extrabiliary community-acquired intra-abdominal infections.

Meningitis and Other CNS Infections. For the treatment of meningitis caused by susceptible bacteria, the usual adult dosage of ceftriaxone is 2 g IV every 12 hours. Some manufacturers and clinicians suggest a ceftriaxone dosage of 50–100 mg/kg (up to 4 g) once daily or in 2 equally divided doses every 12 hours; some clinicians suggest a dosage of 4 g daily given in 1 or 2 equally divided doses.

While 7 days of anti-infective therapy may be adequate for the treatment of uncomplicated meningitis caused by susceptible *H. influenzae* or *N. meningitidis*, at least 10–14 days of therapy is suggested for complicated cases or meningitis caused by *S. pneumoniae* and at least 21 days of therapy is suggested for meningitis caused by susceptible Enterobacteriaceae† (e.g., *E. coli, Klebsiella*†).

If ceftriaxone is used for the treatment of healthcare-associated ventriculitis and meningitis caused by susceptible bacteria (see Uses: Meningitis and Other CNS Infections), IDSA recommends that adults receive a dosage of 4 g daily given in divided doses every 12 hours. The duration of treatment depends on the causative organism and patient characteristics. The recommended treatment duration is 10–14 days for infections caused by gram-negative bacilli (with or without significant CSF pleocytosis, CSF hypoglycorrhachia, or clinical symptoms or systemic features); some experts recommend a duration of 21 days.

Respiratory Tract Infections. If ceftriaxone is used for the treatment of severe acute bacterial rhinosinusitis† requiring hospitalization, IDSA recommends that adults receive a dosage of 1–2 g IV every 12–24 hours.

Skin and Skin Structure Infections. For the treatment of skin and skin structure infections, adults should receive ceftriaxone in a dosage of 50–75 mg/kg once daily or in 2 equally divided doses every 12 hours (maximum 2 g daily).

If ceftriaxone is used for the treatment of necrotizing fasciitis involving *Aeromonas hydrophila*†, IDSA recommends that adults receive a dosage of 1–2 g IV once daily in conjunction with doxycycline (100 mg IV every 12 hours). If necrotizing fasciitis involves *Vibrio vulnificus*†, IDSA recommends that adults receive ceftriaxone in a dosage of 1 g IV once daily in conjunction with doxycycline (100 mg IV every 12 hours).

If ceftriaxone is used for the treatment of surgical site infections following intestinal or genitourinary tract surgery, IDSA recommends a dosage of 1 g once daily in conjunction with metronidazole (500 mg IV every 8 hours). For the treatment of surgical site infections following procedures involving the axilla or perineum, IDSA recommends that ceftriaxone be given in a dosage of 1 g once daily; concomitant vancomycin (15 mg/kg every 12 hours) may also be needed.

If ceftriaxone is used for the treatment of an infected animal bite wound, IDSA recommends a dosage of 1 g IV every 12 hours.

Urinary Tract Infections. For the treatment of acute pyelonephritis (e.g., pending results of in vitro susceptibility testing), a single 1-g IV dose of ceftriaxone has been recommended followed by an appropriate oral anti-infective regimen given for 7–14 days.

Chancroid. If ceftriaxone is used for the treatment of chancroid† (genital ulcers caused by *H. ducreyi*), CDC and other clinicians recommend that adults receive a single 250-mg IM dose of the drug.

Gonorrhea and Associated Infections. For the treatment of uncomplicated cervical, urethral, rectal, or pharyngeal gonorrhea, adults should receive a single 250-mg IM dose of ceftriaxone *and* a dose of azithromycin (single 1-g oral dose). (See Gonococcal Infections in Adults and Adolescents in Uses: Gonorrhea and Associated Infections.)

For the treatment of gonococcal conjunctivitis†, adults should receive a single 1-g IM dose of ceftriaxone *and* a dose of azithromycin (single 1-g oral dose).

For the treatment of gonococcal arthritis and arthritis-dermatitis syndrome†, CDC recommends that adults receive 1 g of ceftriaxone IV or IM once daily *and* a dose of azithromycin (single 1-g oral dose). Ceftriaxone should be continued until 24–48 hours after substantial clinical improvement; treatment can then be switched to an oral antibacterial (selected based on in vitro susceptibility testing) to complete a total treatment duration of at least 7 days.

For the treatment of gonococcal meningitis† or gonococcal endocarditis†, CDC recommends that adults receive 1–2 g of ceftriaxone IV every 12–24 hours in conjunction with a dose of azithromycin (single 1-g oral dose). Ceftriaxone should be continued for 10–14 days in those with meningitis and for at least 4 weeks in those with endocarditis.

For presumptive treatment of acute epididymitis most likely caused by sexually transmitted chlamydia and gonorrhea†, adults should receive a single 250-mg IM dose of ceftriaxone given in conjunction with doxycycline (100 mg orally twice daily for 10 days).

For presumptive treatment of acute epididymitis most likely caused by sexually transmitted chlamydia, gonorrhea, and enteric bacteria† (e.g., *E. coli*), adults should receive a single 250-mg IM dose of ceftriaxone given in conjunction with levofloxacin (500 mg orally once daily for 10 days) or ofloxacin (300 mg orally twice daily for 10 days).

For presumptive treatment of acute proctitis†, adults should receive a single 250-mg IM dose of ceftriaxone given in conjunction with doxycycline (100 mg orally twice daily for 7 days).

Prophylaxis in Sexual Assault Victims. For empiric anti-infective prophylaxis for gonorrhea, chlamydia, and trichomoniasis in adult sexual assault victims†, CDC recommends that a single 250-mg IM dose of ceftriaxone be given in conjunction with azithromycin (single 1-g oral dose) and either metronidazole (single 2-g oral dose) or tinidazole (single 2-g oral dose).

Leptospirosis. For the treatment of severe leptospirosis†, adults have received ceftriaxone in a dosage of 1 g IV once daily for 7 days.

Lyme Disease. If ceftriaxone is used for the treatment of early Lyme disease† in adults with acute neurologic disease manifested by meningitis or radiculopathy, IDSA and other clinicians recommend a dosage of 2 g IV once daily for 14 days (range: 10–28 days).

When a parenteral regimen is indicated for the treatment of Lyme carditis† in adults with AV heart block and/or myopericarditis associated with early Lyme disease, IDSA and other clinicians recommend a ceftriaxone dosage of 2 g IV once daily for 14 days (range: 14–21 days). Although a parenteral regimen is recommended for initial treatment of hospitalized patients, the parenteral regimen can be switched to an oral regimen (doxycycline, amoxicillin, cefuroxime axetil) to complete therapy and for outpatients.

When a parenteral regimen is indicated for the treatment of Lyme arthritis† in patients with evidence of neurologic disease or when arthritis has not responded to an oral regimen, IDSA and other clinicians recommend that adults receive a ceftriaxone dosage of 2 g IV once daily for 14 days (range: 14–28 days).

For the treatment of late neurologic Lyme disease† affecting the central or peripheral nervous system, IDSA and other clinicians recommend that adults receive ceftriaxone in a dosage of 2 g IV once daily for 2–4 weeks.

Neisseria meningitidis Infections. When ceftriaxone is used to eliminate nasopharyngeal carriage of *N. meningitidis*† or for chemoprophylaxis in close contacts of individuals with invasive meningococcal disease†, adults should receive a single 250-mg IM dose.

For dosage recommendations for the treatment of meningitis caused by *N. meningitidis*, see Meningitis and Other CNS Infections under Dosage: Adult Dosage, in Dosage and Administration.)

Pelvic Inflammatory Disease. For the treatment of mild to moderately severe acute pelvic inflammatory disease (PID) when an IM and oral regimen is indicated, adults may receive a single 250-mg IM dose of ceftriaxone followed by a 14-day regimen of doxycycline (100 mg orally twice daily) with or without oral metronidazole (500 mg twice daily). If there is no clinical response within 72 hours, the patient should be reevaluated to confirm the diagnosis and an IV regimen should be administered if indicated.

Syphilis. If ceftriaxone is used as an alternative to IM penicillin G benzathine for the treatment of primary or secondary syphilis† in penicillin-allergic nonpregnant adults, CDC and other clinicians recommend a ceftriaxone dosage of 1–2 g IM or IV once daily for 10–14 days. Some clinicians suggest that this ceftriaxone dosage also can be used as an alternative in penicillin-allergic nonpregnant adults with early latent syphilis.

If ceftriaxone is used as an alternative to IV penicillin G for the treatment of neurosyphilis† in penicillin-allergic nonpregnant adults, a dosage of 2 g IM or IV daily for 10–14 days has been suggested by CDC and others based on limited data.

CDC cautions that the optimal dosage and duration of ceftriaxone for the treatment of syphilis have not been defined and close follow-up is essential. (See Uses: Syphilis.)

Typhoid Fever and Other Invasive Salmonella Infections. For the treatment of typhoid fever† or septicemia caused by *Salmonella* serovars Typhi† or Paratyphi†, including infections caused by multidrug-resistant strains, adults have received ceftriaxone in a dosage of 2–4 g IM or IV once daily for 3–7 days. Alternatively, adults have received a dosage of 1 g once daily for 15 days.

While ceftriaxone has been effective for the treatment of typhoid fever when administered for 3–7 days, anti-infective therapy for the treatment of typhoid fever usually is continued for at least 14 days to prevent relapse and a duration of at least 4–6 weeks may be necessary for the treatment of immunocompromised individuals (including those with HIV infection) or for the treatment of *Salmonella* meningitis.

Whipple's Disease. For the treatment of Whipple's disease† caused by *Tropheryma whipplei* (formerly *Tropheryma whippelii*), some clinicians recommend that ceftriaxone be given in a dosage of 2 g IV once daily for 2–4 weeks followed by oral co-trimoxazole given for 1–2 years. For the treatment of encephalitis caused by *T. whipplei*, IDSA recommends initial treatment with ceftriaxone given for 2–4 weeks followed by co-trimoxazole or cefixime for 1–2 years.

Empiric Therapy in Febrile Neutropenic Patients. When used for empiric anti-infective therapy in febrile neutropenic patients†, adults have received ceftriaxone in a dosage of 30 mg/kg (up to 2 g) given IV once daily in conjunction with amikacin (20 mg/kg IV once daily).

Perioperative Prophylaxis. If ceftriaxone is used for perioperative prophylaxis in adults, the manufacturers and some clinicians recommend that a single 1-g dose be given IV 0.5–2 hours prior to surgery.

For perioperative prophylaxis in patients undergoing cholecystectomy, adults have received a single 1-g dose of ceftriaxone given IV 0.5–2 hours prior to surgery; however, higher doses (e.g., 2 g) also have been used.

For perioperative prophylaxis in adults undergoing colorectal procedures, some experts recommend that a single 2-g dose of ceftriaxone be given IV in conjunction with metronidazole (single 500-mg IV dose) within 1 hour prior to surgery.

Prevention of Bacterial Endocarditis. If ceftriaxone is used as an alternative for prevention of α-hemolytic (viridans group) streptococcal endocarditis† in individuals with certain cardiac conditions who are undergoing certain dental or upper respiratory tract procedures (see Uses: Prevention of Bacterial Endocarditis), AHA recommends that adults receive a single dose of 1 g given IM or IV 30–60 minutes prior to the procedure.

■ Dosage in Renal and Hepatic Impairment

Modification of the usual dosage of ceftriaxone is not usually necessary in adults with impaired renal or hepatic function alone who are receiving the drug in dosages up to 2 g daily. However, if the drug is used in patients with hepatic impairment *and* clinically important renal impairment, caution is advised and dosage should not exceed 2 g daily.

Some clinicians state that serum concentrations of the drug should be monitored when ceftriaxone is used in patients with severe renal impairment (e.g., dialysis patients) or in patients with both hepatic and substantial renal impairment.

Because ceftriaxone is not removed by hemodialysis or peritoneal dialysis, supplemental doses of the drug are unnecessary during or after dialysis.

Cautions

Adverse effects reported with ceftriaxone are similar to those reported with other cephalosporins. For information on adverse effects reported with cephalosporins, see Cautions in the Cephalosporins General Statement 8:12.06. Ceftriaxone generally is well tolerated; adverse effects have been reported in about 10% of patients receiving ceftriaxone and have required discontinuance of the drug in less than 2% of these patients.

■ Hematologic Effects

Hematologic effects are among the most frequent adverse effects reported with ceftriaxone. Eosinophilia has been reported in about 6%, thrombocytosis in about 5%, and leukopenia in about 2% of patients receiving ceftriaxone. Anemia, neutropenia, lymphopenia, and thrombocytopenia have been reported in less than 1% and leukocytosis, lymphocytosis, monocytosis, agranulocytosis, basophilia, and coagulopathy have been reported in less than 0.1% of patients receiving ceftriaxone.

Hypoprothrombinemia or prolongation of prothrombin time (PT), with or without bleeding, has been reported in patients receiving ceftriaxone. (See Other Precautions and Contraindications under Cautions: Precautions and Contraindications.) Although very high concentrations of ceftriaxone (3–4 g/L) inhibited platelet aggregation in an in vitro study, in vivo studies indicate that the drug does not interfere with platelet function.

Immune-mediated hemolytic anemia has been reported in patients receiving ceftriaxone. Severe cases of hemolytic anemia, including fatalities, have occurred in both adults and children. Some cases occurred shortly after administration of a ceftriaxone dose, and some reactions have consisted of severe intravascular hemolysis and anemia, decreased hemoglobin concentrations, reticulocytosis, hemoglobinuria, and cardiac arrest. In at least one case, the direct antiglobulin (Coombs') test was strongly positive and the patient's serum agglutinated washed erythrocytes in the presence of complement and ceftriaxone. (See Other Precautions and Contraindications under Cautions: Precautions and Contraindications.)

■ GI Effects

Diarrhea or loose stools has generally been reported in 2–4% of patients receiving ceftriaxone. However, transient diarrhea was reported in 42–44% of children receiving ceftriaxone in 2 studies and in 28% (10/36) of adults receiving the drug in another study. Nausea, vomiting, and dysgeusia have been reported in less than 1% and abdominal pain, flatulence, dyspepsia, colitis, gallbladder sludge, and biliary lithiasis have been reported in less than 0.1% of patients receiving the drug. Stomatitis and glossitis also have been reported.

Pancreatitis, possibly secondary to biliary obstruction, has been reported in patients treated with ceftriaxone. Most patients presented with risk factors for biliary stasis and biliary sludge (preceding major therapy, severe illness, total parenteral nutrition). A cofactor role of ceftriaxone-related biliary precipitation cannot be ruled out.

Clostridium difficile-associated Diarrhea and Colitis Treatment with anti-infectives alters the normal colon flora and may permit overgrowth of *Clostridium difficile*.

C. difficile infection (CDI) and *C. difficile*-associated diarrhea and colitis (CDAD; also known as antibiotic-associated diarrhea and colitis or pseudomembranous colitis) have been reported with nearly all anti-infectives, including ceftriaxone, and may range in severity from mild diarrhea to fatal colitis. *C. difficile* produces toxins A and B, which contribute to the development of CDAD; hypertoxin-producing strains of *C. difficile* are associated with increased morbidity and mortality since these infections may be refractory to anti-infective therapy and may require colectomy.

CDAD should be considered in the differential diagnosis in patients who develop diarrhea during or after anti-infective therapy. Careful medical history is necessary since CDAD has been reported to occur as late as 2 months or longer after anti-infective therapy is discontinued.

If CDAD is suspected or confirmed, anti-infectives not directed against *C. difficile* should be discontinued as soon as possible. Patients should be managed with appropriate anti-infective therapy directed against *C. difficile* (e.g., vancomycin, fidaxomicin, metronidazole), supportive therapy (e.g., fluid and electrolyte management, protein supplementation), and surgical evaluation as clinically indicated. (See Superinfection/Clostridium difficile-associated Diarrhea and Colitis under Cautions: Precautions and Contraindications.)

Gallbladder Pseudolithiasis Ceftriaxone-calcium precipitates in the gallbladder have been observed in patients receiving ceftriaxone. These precipitates appear on sonography as an echo without acoustical shadowing suggesting sludge or as an echo with acoustical shadowing which may be misinterpreted as gallstones. Although patients may be asymptomatic, symptoms of gallbladder disease (e.g., colic, nausea, vomiting, anorexia) can occur and may be severe enough to require discontinuance of ceftriaxone therapy.

The condition appears to be reversible and generally resolves following discontinuance of the drug and conservative management; surgery may not be necessary. The time to resolution, however, is variable and may range from a few days to several months. Upper abdominal ultrasonography should be considered for patients who develop biliary colic while receiving ceftriaxone therapy; biliary precipitates of ceftriaxone may be detected by ultrasonography after only 4 days of ceftriaxone therapy. The risk of precipitation may depend on the dose and rate of IV administration of ceftriaxone, occurring more frequently with relatively high dosages and rapid (e.g., over several minutes) rates of administration. In some patients with renal impairment or those receiving higher than usual dosages of the drug, precipitates containing traces of ceftriaxone, possibly combined with calcium, have been recovered in surgical specimens.

The probability of gallbladder precipitates associated with ceftriaxone therapy appears to be greatest in pediatric patients. In one study in children with various infections who received IV ceftriaxone in a dosage of 60–100 mg/kg daily, gallbladder precipitates developed in 43% of patients. The typical abnormality observed sonographically in these children was a strikingly hyperechogenic material with postacoustic shadowing; the precipitates differed from typical biliary sludge or cholelithiasis, usually were mobile, and tended to clump in the most dependent part of the gallbladder.

In a retrospective study of more than 1300 patients admitted to the hospital during a 2-year period with a diagnosis of Lyme disease, biliary symptoms (e.g., cholecystitis, cholelithiasis) or cholecystectomy occurred in approximately 2% of patients (84% were female with a median age of 12 years [range: 3–40 years]); 56% of these patients underwent laparoscopic cholecystectomy, mainly for cholelithiasis. Among cases and controls who received anti-infective therapy for treatment of suspected Lyme disease, each patient had received a median of 3 courses of oral and/or IV anti-infectives. All patients with biliary symptoms had received IV ceftriaxone therapy within 90 days prior to the occurrence of biliary disease; daily ceftriaxone dosage at the time of onset of biliary symptoms in these patients averaged 57 mg/kg (range: 27–96 mg/kg), and the median duration of therapy was 28 days (range: 4–170 days). These data suggest an association between biliary complications and the repeated and often prolonged courses of IV ceftriaxone therapy used in these patients, most of whom lacked documented objective clinical or laboratory evidence of Lyme disease. (See Lyme Disease in Uses: Spirochetal Infections.)

In studies in dogs and baboons receiving high dosages of ceftriaxone sodium, concretions consisting of the precipitated calcium salt of ceftriaxone have been found in gallbladder bile. These appeared as gritty sediment in dogs who received ceftriaxone in a dosage of 100 mg/kg daily for 4 weeks but were evident in the baboon only after a daily dosage of 335 mg/kg or more for 6 months. The likelihood of this occurrence in humans has been considered to be low since ceftriaxone has a longer plasma half-life in humans, the calcium salt of ceftriaxone is more soluble in human gallbladder bile, and the calcium content of human gallbladder bile is relatively low.

■ Dermatologic and Sensitivity Reactions

Rash (e.g., erythematous, urticarial) has been reported in about 2% of patients receiving ceftriaxone and pruritus, fever, and chills have been reported in less than 1% of patients receiving the drug.

Serious, occasionally fatal, hypersensitivity reactions (anaphylaxis or anaphylactoid) have been reported in patients receiving ceftriaxone. Bronchospasm and serum sickness have been reported in less than 0.1% of patients receiving the drug.

Exanthema, allergic dermatitis, urticaria, and edema have been reported in patients receiving ceftriaxone. There also have been postmarketing reports of generalized exanthematous pustulosis and isolated reports of severe cutaneous adverse reactions (e.g., erythema multiforme, Stevens-Johnson syndrome, Lyell's syndrome/toxic epidermal necrolysis).

■ Hepatic Effects Increased serum concentrations of AST (SGOT) and ALT (SGPT) have been reported in about 3% of patients and increased serum concentrations of alkaline phosphatase and bilirubin have been reported in less than 1% of patients receiving ceftriaxone. Jaundice has been reported in less than 0.1% of patients receiving the drug and there have been postmarketing reports of hepatitis.

■ Renal Effects Increased concentrations of BUN have been reported in about 1% of patients receiving ceftriaxone and increased concentrations of serum creatinine and the presence of casts in urine have been reported in less than 1% of patients receiving the drug. Glycosuria, hematuria, renal precipitates, and nephrolithiasis have been reported in less than 0.1% of patients receiving the drug. Oliguria, ureteric obstruction, and post-renal acute renal failure also have been reported.

Ceftriaxone-calcium precipitates in the urine have been observed in patients receiving ceftriaxone and may be detected as sonographic abnormalities. The probability of such precipitates appears to be greatest in pediatric patients. Patients may be asymptomatic or may develop symptoms of urolithiasis, ureteral obstruction, and post-renal acute renal failure. The condition appears to be reversible following discontinuance of the drug and conservative management.

■ Pulmonary and Renal Precipitates Fatalities have been reported in some neonates who received ceftriaxone and calcium-containing IV solutions. A crystalline material was observed in the lungs and kidneys of these neonates at autopsy. In some cases, the same IV infusion line had been used for both ceftriaxone and the calcium-containing fluid and, in some, a precipitate was observed in the IV infusion line. At least 1 fatality occurred in a neonate who received ceftriaxone and calcium-containing fluids administered at different times and through different infusion lines; no crystalline material was observed at autopsy in this neonate. (See Interactions with Calcium-containing Products under Cautions: Precautions and Contraindications.) There have been no similar reports in patients other than neonates treated with ceftriaxone and calcium-containing IV solutions.

To date, there have been no reports of an interaction between ceftriaxone and oral calcium-containing preparations or between IM ceftriaxone and calcium-containing preparations (IV or oral).

■ Local Effects Local reactions, including pain, induration, ecchymosis, and tenderness at the injection site have been reported in patients receiving IM ceftriaxone. The overall incidence of pain, induration, and tenderness following IM injection of the drug is 1–2%. The incidence of warmth, tightness, or induration reported following IM injection of ceftriaxone doses of 250 or 350 mg/mL was 5 or 17%, respectively. Local reactions occur less frequently and are less intense when IM injections of ceftriaxone are reconstituted with 1% lidocaine hydrochloride (without epinephrine) rather than sterile water for injection. (See Other Precautions and Contraindications under Cautions: Precautions and Contraindications.)

Results of a cross-over study involving IM injection into the buttock of 1-g doses of ceftriaxone diluted in 2 mL of sterile water for injection, 1% lidocaine, or 1% lidocaine buffered with sodium carbonate indicate that the pharmacokinetics of ceftriaxone are not affected by the diluent; however, use of a lidocaine diluent was associated with a 50–78% reduction in injection pain scores compared with use of sterile water for injection. Buffered lidocaine did not appear to offer any advantages over unbuffered lidocaine.

Phlebitis has been reported in less than 1% of patients receiving IV ceftriaxone.

■ Other Adverse Effects Other adverse effects that have been reported in less than 1% of patients receiving ceftriaxone include diaphoresis and flushing, headache, dizziness, oral candidiasis, and candidal vaginitis. Palpitation and epistaxis have been reported in less than 0.1% of patients receiving the drug.

In at least one patient, inadvertent IV injection over 5 minutes of a 2-g dose of ceftriaxone resulted in a reaction that consisted of restlessness, shivering, diaphoresis with dilated pupils, and palpitations; this reaction did not occur when the drug was administered by IV infusion over 30 minutes as recommended by the manufacturer.

■ Precautions and Contraindications Ceftriaxone is contraindicated in patients with known hypersensitivity to ceftriaxone, any other cephalosporin, or any ingredient in the formulation. Patients with previous hypersensitivity reactions to penicillin and other β-lactam anti-infectives may be at greater risk of hypersensitivity to ceftriaxone. Some manufacturers state that ceftriaxone is contraindicated in patients with a history of anaphylaxis to ceftriaxone, other cephalosporins, penicillins, or other β-lactam anti-infectives. (See Sensitivity Reactions under Cautions: Precautions and Contraindications.)

Ceftriaxone is contraindicated in certain neonates (e.g., premature or hyperbilirubinemic neonates, those requiring calcium-containing IV solutions). (See Cautions: Pediatric Precautions.)

Ceftriaxone shares the toxic potentials of the cephalosporins, and the usual precautions of cephalosporin therapy should be observed.

Sensitivity Reactions Prior to initiation of therapy with ceftriaxone, careful inquiry should be made concerning previous hypersensitivity reactions to ceftriaxone, cephalosporins, penicillins, other β-lactam anti-infectives, or other drugs. There is clinical and laboratory evidence of partial cross-allergenicity among cephalosporins and other β-lactam antibiotics including penicillins and cephamycins.

As with all β-lactam anti-infectives, serious and occasionally fatal hypersensitivity reactions, including anaphylaxis, have been reported with ceftriaxone.

Although it has not been proven that allergic reactions to antibiotics are more frequent in atopic individuals, some manufacturers state that ceftriaxone should be used with caution in patients with a history of allergy, particularly to drugs.

The manufacturer of the commercially available frozen premixed ceftriaxone injection in dextrose states that dextrose-containing solutions may be contraindicated in patients with known allergy to corn or corn products. Hypersensitivity reactions, including anaphylaxis, have been reported with administration of dextrose products. These reactions have been reported in patients receiving high concentrations of dextrose (i.e., 50% dextrose) and also have been reported when corn-derived dextrose solutions were administered to patients with or without a history of hypersensitivity to corn products.

Patients should be advised that allergic reactions, including serious allergic reactions, could occur and that serious reactions require immediate treatment.

If a severe hypersensitivity reaction occurs during ceftriaxone therapy, the drug should be discontinued immediately and the patient treated with appropriate therapy (e.g., epinephrine, corticosteroids, maintenance of an adequate airway, oxygen) as indicated.

Interaction with Calcium-containing Products Because of the risk of precipitation of ceftriaxone-calcium and because fatalities associated with ceftriaxone-calcium precipitates in lungs and kidneys have been reported in neonates (see Cautions: Pulmonary and Renal Precipitates), ceftriaxone is contraindicated in neonates (28 days of age or younger) who are receiving (or are expected to require) treatment with calcium-containing IV solutions, including continuous calcium-containing infusions such as parenteral nutrition.

Intravascular or pulmonary ceftriaxone-calcium precipitates have not been reported to date in patients other than neonates treated with ceftriaxone and calcium-containing IV solutions. There is some evidence that neonates have an increased risk for precipitation of ceftriaxone-calcium. In vitro studies evaluating the combination of ceftriaxone and calcium in adult plasma and neonatal plasma from umbilical cord blood indicate that recovery of ceftriaxone from plasma was reduced in adult plasma when calcium concentrations were 24 mg/dL or greater and was reduced in neonatal plasma when calcium concentrations were 16 mg/dL or greater. This may reflect ceftriaxone-calcium precipitation.

Ceftriaxone must *not* be admixed with calcium-containing IV solutions and must *not* be administered *simultaneously* with calcium-containing IV solutions, including continuous infusions of calcium-containing solutions such as parenteral nutrition, even via different infusion lines or sites in any patient (irrespective of age). In adults or pediatric patients older than 28 days of age, ceftriaxone and calcium-containing solutions may be administered *sequentially* if the IV infusion lines are thoroughly flushed between infusions with a compatible fluid. (See Dosage and Administration: Reconstitution and Administration.)

Selection and Use of Anti-infectives To reduce development of drug-resistant bacteria and maintain effectiveness of ceftriaxone and other antibacterials, the drug should be used only for the treatment or prevention of infections proven or strongly suspected to be caused by susceptible bacteria. When selecting or modifying anti-infective therapy, results of culture and in vitro susceptibility testing should be used. In the absence of such data, local epidemiology and susceptibility patterns should be considered when selecting anti-infectives for empiric therapy.

Patients should be advised that antibacterials (including ceftriaxone) should only be used to treat bacterial infections and not used to treat viral infections (e.g., the common cold). Patients also should be advised about the importance of completing the full course of therapy, even if feeling better after a few days, and that skipping doses or not completing therapy may decrease effectiveness and increase the likelihood that bacteria will develop resistance and will not be treatable with ceftriaxone or other antibacterials in the future.

Superinfection/Clostridium difficile-associated Diarrhea and Colitis Use of ceftriaxone may result in overgrowth of nonsusceptible organisms, especially *Candida*, enterococci, *Bacteroides fragilis*, or *Pseudomonas aeruginosa*. Resistant strains of *Ps. aeruginosa* and *Enterobacter* have developed during therapy with ceftriaxone. (See Resistance.) Careful observation of the patient during ceftriaxone therapy is essential. If superinfection or suprainfection occurs, appropriate therapy should be instituted.

Because CDAD has been reported with the use of ceftriaxone or other cephalosporins, it should be considered in the differential diagnosis of patients who develop diarrhea during or after ceftriaxone therapy. (See Clostridium difficile-associated Diarrhea and Colitis under Cautions: GI Effects.) Patients should be advised that diarrhea is a common problem caused by anti-infectives and usually ends when the drug is discontinued; however, they should contact a clinician if watery and bloody stools (with or without stomach cramps and fever) occur during or as late as 2 months or longer after the last dose.

Some manufacturers state that ceftriaxone should be used with caution in patients with a history of GI disease, particularly colitis.

Other Precautions and Contraindications Because potentially fatal immune-mediated hemolytic anemia has been reported with cephalosporins, including ceftriaxone, the diagnosis of cephalosporin-associated anemia should be considered if anemia occurs in a patient receiving ceftriaxone. The drug should be discontinued until the etiology of the anemia is determined.

Ceftriaxone can precipitate in the gallbladder. (See Cautions: GI Effects.) Some clinicians recommend that ceftriaxone be used with caution in patients with preexisting disease of the gallbladder, biliary tract, liver, or pancreas, and, if the drug is used in such patients, serial abdominal ultrasonography should be performed during therapy. Ceftriaxone should be discontinued and conservative management considered in any patient who develops signs and symptoms suggestive of gallbladder disease, including sonographic abnormalities.

Ceftriaxone can precipitate in the urinary tract. (See Cautions: Renal Effects.) Patients receiving the drug should be adequately hydrated. Ceftriaxone should be discontinued if there are signs and symptoms suggestive of urolithiasis, oliguria, or renal failure and/or if sonographic abnormalities are detected.

Because prolonged PT has been reported in patients receiving ceftriaxone, the manufacturers state that PT should be monitored when the drug is used in patients with impaired vitamin K synthesis or low vitamin K stores (e.g., patients with chronic hepatic disease, malnutrition). The manufacturers state that administration of vitamin K (10 mg weekly) may be necessary if the PT is prolonged before or during ceftriaxone therapy. Concomitant use of ceftriaxone and vitamin K antagonists may increase the risk of bleeding. (See Drug Interactions: Anticoagulants.)

Seizures have been reported with some cephalosporins, including ceftriaxone. Ceftriaxone should be discontinued if seizures occur and anticonvulsant therapy should be administered if clinically indicated. Patients should be advised that adverse neurologic events can occur and to immediately contact a clinician if any neurologic signs and symptoms, including encephalopathy (disturbance of consciousness including confusion, hallucinations, stupor, coma), myoclonus, or seizures, occur since immediate treatment, dosage adjustment, or discontinuance of ceftriaxone therapy is required.

Like other dextrose-containing solutions, the commercially available Duplex® drug delivery system containing 1 or 2 g of lyophilized ceftriaxone and 50 mL of dextrose 3.74 or 2.22% injection should be used with caution in patients with overt or known subclinical diabetes mellitus or in patients with carbohydrate intolerance for any reason.

Although IM injections of ceftriaxone may be prepared using diluents containing 1% lidocaine hydrochloride (see IM Injection under Dosage and Administration: Reconstitution and Administration), all contraindications to lidocaine should be considered before administering such injections. IV administration of ceftriaxone solutions containing lidocaine is contraindicated.

Dosage adjustments are not usually necessary when ceftriaxone is used in patients with renal impairment or hepatic impairment alone. Some clinicians recommend that serum concentrations of the drug be monitored when ceftriaxone is used in patients with severe renal impairment (e.g., dialysis patients) or in patients with hepatic impairment and clinically important renal impairment. (See Dosage and Administration: Dosage in Renal and Hepatic Impairment.)

■ **Pediatric Precautions** Ceftriaxone is contraindicated in premature neonates up to postmenstrual age 41 weeks (i.e., time elapsed since first day of the mother's last menstrual period to birth plus time elapsed after birth).

Ceftriaxone is contraindicated in hyperbilirubinemic neonates, particularly those who are premature. Ceftriaxone, at therapeutic concentrations, has been shown to displace bilirubin from albumin binding sites in vitro. Because ceftriaxone can displace bilirubin from serum albumin, there is a risk that bilirubin encephalopathy could develop if the drug is used in hyperbilirubinemic neonates. Addition of ceftriaxone to blood samples obtained from hyperbilirubinemic neonates resulted in increased free and erythrocyte-bound bilirubin concentrations and decreased unconjugated (albumin-bound) bilirubin concentrations.

Ceftriaxone is contraindicated in neonates (28 days of age or younger) if they are receiving (or expected to require) treatment with calcium-containing IV solutions, including continuous infusions of calcium-containing solutions such as parenteral nutrition, because of the risk of precipitation of a ceftriaxone-calcium salt. Fatalities associated with ceftriaxone-calcium precipitates in lungs and kidneys have been reported in neonates who received ceftriaxone and calcium-containing IV solutions. (See Cautions: Pulmonary and Renal Precipitates and see Interaction with Calcium-containing Products under Cautions: Precautions and Contraindications.)

To reduce the risk of bilirubin encephalopathy, IV infusions of ceftriaxone should be given over 60 minutes in neonates. (See Dosage and Administration: Reconstitution and Administration.)

Ceftriaxone that has been reconstituted for IM use with bacteriostatic water for injection containing benzyl alcohol should *not* be used in neonates. Although a causal relationship has not been established, administration of injections preserved with benzyl alcohol has been associated with toxicity in neonates. Toxicity appears to have resulted from administration of large amounts (i.e., about 100–400 mg/kg daily) of benzyl alcohol in these neonates.

To avoid unintentional overdosage, the commercially available Duplex® drug delivery system containing 1 or 2 g of ceftriaxone and 50 mL of dextrose injection in separate chambers should *not* be used in pediatric patients who require less than the entire 1- or 2-g dose in the container.

■ **Geriatric Precautions** In clinical studies, safety and efficacy of ceftriaxone in geriatric adults 60 years of age or older have been similar to those observed in younger adults. Although other clinical experience has revealed no evidence of age-related differences, the possibility that some older patients may exhibit increased sensitivity to the drug cannot be ruled out.

The pharmacokinetics of ceftriaxone are only minimally altered in geriatric patients compared with healthy younger adults. Dosage adjustments based solely on age are not necessary in geriatric patients receiving ceftriaxone dosages up to 2 g daily, provided they do not have severe renal and hepatic impairment.

Ceftriaxone is substantially eliminated by the kidneys, and the risk of adverse effects may be greater in those with impaired renal function. Because geriatric patients are more likely to have reduced renal function, dosage should be selected with caution and monitoring of renal function should be considered.

■ **Mutagenicity and Carcinogenicity** In vitro studies using microbial (i.e., Ames test) or mammalian cell (i.e., human lymphoblasts) systems have not shown ceftriaxone to be mutagenic. Specific studies to determine the carcinogenic potential of ceftriaxone have not been performed to date, and animal toxicity studies have been performed to a maximum duration of only 6 months.

■ **Pregnancy, Fertility, and Lactation** Reproduction studies in mice, rats, and primates have not revealed evidence of embryotoxicity, fetotoxicity, or teratogenicity. There are no adequate or controlled studies using ceftriaxone in pregnant women, and the drug should be used during pregnancy only when clearly needed.

Studies in rats using IV ceftriaxone have not revealed evidence of impaired fertility.

Because ceftriaxone is distributed into milk, the drug should be used with caution in nursing women.

Drug Interactions

■ **Alcohol** A disulfiram-like reaction reportedly occurred in one patient who ingested alcohol while receiving ceftriaxone. However, this effect generally has been reported only with β-lactam antibiotics that contain an *N*-methylthiotetrazole (NMTT) side chain (e.g., cefamandole, cefoperazone, cefotetan).

■ **Aminoglycosides** In vitro studies indicate that the antibacterial activity of ceftriaxone and aminoglycosides (amikacin, gentamicin, tobramycin) may be additive or synergistic against some strains of Enterobacteriaceae and some strains of *Pseudomonas aeruginosa*. Although the clinical importance has not been determined to date, antagonism has also occurred rarely in vitro when ceftriaxone was used in combination with an aminoglycoside. Organisms with high-level resistance to both the aminoglycoside and the β-lactam antibiotic alone are unlikely to be synergistically inhibited by concomitant use of the drugs.

■ **Anticoagulants** Concomitant use of ceftriaxone and vitamin K antagonists may increase the risk of bleeding. Increased international normalized ratio (INR) has been reported in patients receiving warfarin and ceftriaxone concomitantly. In one patient who had been receiving long-term warfarin therapy with stable INR, administration of a single 1-g IM dose of ceftriaxone for the treatment of a urinary tract infection resulted in a substantially increased INR that was managed by withholding a warfarin dose and administering vitamin K. If ceftriaxone is used in patients receiving a vitamin K antagonist (e.g., warfarin), coagulation parameters should be monitored frequently and dosage of the anticoagulant adjusted as needed, both during and after ceftriaxone treatment.

■ **Chloramphenicol** Antagonism has been reported in vitro when ceftriaxone was used in combination with chloramphenicol.

■ **Probenecid** Concomitant administration of oral probenecid (500 mg daily) does not appear to affect the pharmacokinetics of ceftriaxone, presumably because ceftriaxone is excreted principally by glomerular filtration and nonrenal mechanisms. However, higher dosages of oral probenecid (1 or 2 g daily) administered concomitantly reportedly may partially block biliary secretion of ceftriaxone as well as displace the drug from plasma proteins. As a result, serum clearance of ceftriaxone may be increased by about 30% and elimination half-life of ceftriaxone may be decreased by about 20%.

■ **Quinolones** Although the clinical importance is unclear, results of an in vitro study indicate that the combination of ceftriaxone and trovafloxacin (not commercially available in the US) is synergistic against both penicillin-susceptible and penicillin-resistant *Streptococcus pneumoniae*, including some strains that also were resistant to ceftriaxone alone. There was no evidence of antagonism with the combination of ceftriaxone and trovafloxacin.

Laboratory Test Interferences

■ **Tests for Glucose** False-positive results for urinary glucose may occur in patients receiving ceftriaxone if nonenzymatic glucose test methods are used. Like most cephalosporins, ceftriaxone interferes with urinary glucose determinations using cupric sulfate (e.g., Benedict's solution, Clinitest®); however, glucose oxidase methods (e.g., Clinistix®, Tes-Tape®) are unaffected by the drug. Enzymatic methods should be used to test for urinary glucose in patients receiving ceftriaxone.

The presence of ceftriaxone may result in falsely low estimated blood glucose concentrations measured using some blood glucose monitoring systems. The manufacturer's instructions for the glucose monitoring system should be consulted and alternative testing methods should be used if necessary.

■ **Tests for Creatinine** In one in vitro study, high concentrations of ceftriaxone (50 mcg/mL or greater) caused falsely elevated serum creatinine values when a manual method was used; however, other studies indicate that the drug does not interfere with automated methods for determining serum or urinary creatinine concentrations.

Acute Toxicity

Limited information is available on the acute toxicity of ceftriaxone; there is no specific antidote. If acute overdosage of ceftriaxone occurs, supportive and symptomatic treatment should be initiated. Ceftriaxone is not removed by hemodialysis or peritoneal dialysis, and these procedures would be ineffective in reducing ceftriaxone concentrations following overdosage.

Mechanism of Action

Ceftriaxone usually is bactericidal in action. Like other cephalosporins, the antibacterial activity of the drug results from inhibition of mucopeptide synthesis in the bacterial cell wall. For information on the mechanism of action of cephalosporins, see Mechanism of Action in the Cephalosporins General Statement 8:12.06.

Spectrum

Based on its spectrum of activity, ceftriaxone is classified as a third generation cephalosporin. For information on the classification of cephalosporins and closely related β-lactam antibiotics based on spectra of activity, see Spectrum in the Cephalosporins General Statement 8:12.06.

Like other currently available parenteral third generation cephalosporins (e.g., cefotaxime, ceftazidime), ceftriaxone generally is less active in vitro against susceptible staphylococci than first generation cephalosporins but has an expanded spectrum of activity against gram-negative bacteria compared with first and second generation cephalosporins. The spectrum of activity of ceftriaxone closely resembles that of cefotaxime and ceftazidime. In vitro on a weight basis, the activity of ceftriaxone against most susceptible organisms, including most Enterobacteriaceae, is approximately equal to that of cefotaxime.

■ **In Vitro Susceptibility Testing** Results of in vitro susceptibility tests with ceftriaxone for some bacteria (e.g., *Enterobacter cloacae*, *Klebsiella pneumoniae*, *Proteus*, *Pseudomonas*, *Serratia*, staphylococci) may be affected by the size of the inoculum. Although results of ceftriaxone susceptibility tests do not appear to be affected by culture media, results may be affected by pH or the presence of serum. MICs of ceftriaxone for *Staphylococcus aureus*, *Pseudomonas aeruginosa*, or Enterobacteriaceae may be 4–8 times higher when tested in the presence of serum.

Strains of staphylococci resistant to penicillinase-resistant penicillins (methicillin-resistant [oxacillin-resistant] staphylococci) should be considered resistant to ceftriaxone, although results of in vitro susceptibility tests may indicate that the organisms are susceptible to the drug.

For information on interpreting results of in vitro susceptibility testing (disk susceptibility tests, dilution susceptibility tests) when ceftriaxone susceptibility testing is performed according to the standards of the Clinical and Laboratory Standards Institute (CLSI; formerly National Committee for Clinical Laboratory Standards [NCCLS]), see Spectrum: In Vitro Susceptibility Testing, in the Cephalosporins General Statement 8:12.06.

■ **Gram-positive Aerobic Bacteria** Ceftriaxone is active in vitro against most gram-positive aerobic cocci including penicillinase-producing and nonpenicillinase-producing strains of *Staphylococcus aureus* and *S. epidermidis*; *Streptococcus pneumoniae*; *S. pyogenes* (group A β-hemolytic streptococci; GAS); *S. agalactiae* (group B streptococci; GBS); and viridans streptococci (including the *S. milleri* group [*S. anginosus*, *S. constellatus*, *S. intermedius*]). Staphylococci resistant to penicillinase-resistant penicillins also generally are resistant to ceftriaxone. Group D streptococci and enterococci, including *E. faecalis* (formerly *S. faecalis*), generally are resistant to ceftriaxone.

The MIC_{90} (minimum inhibitory concentration of the drug at which 90% of strains tested are inhibited) of ceftriaxone for penicillinase-producing and nonpenicillinase-producing *S. aureus* is 3–8 mcg/mL. The MIC_{90} of the drug reported for *S. epidermidis* is 16–50 mcg/mL and the MIC_{50} of the drug reported for this organism is 3.1–7.3 mcg/mL.

The MIC_{90} of ceftriaxone for *S. pyogenes* is 0.15–0.25 mcg/mL, and the MIC_{90} of the drug reported for *S. agalactiae* is 0.06–0.78 mcg/mL. The MIC_{90} reported for viridans streptococci is 0.5–4 mcg/mL. In one study, the MIC_{50} and MIC_{90} of ceftriaxone for the *S. milleri* group of viridans streptococci were 0.25 and 0.5 mcg/mL, respectively.

Although the MIC_{90} reported for *S. pneumoniae* generally is 0.15–0.25 mcg/mL, some strains have reduced susceptibility and require ceftriaxone concentrations of 0.5–2 mcg/mL or greater for in vitro inhibition. Strains of *S. pneumoniae* with MICs of 2 mcg/mL or greater generally are considered resistant to ceftriaxone; however, strains with MICs of 0.5–1 mcg/mL that are isolated from patients with meningitis generally also are considered resistant to the drug.

Other Gram-positive Bacteria Although a few strains of *Listeria monocytogenes* may be inhibited in vitro by ceftriaxone concentrations of 0.8–32 mcg/mL, most strains of the organism are resistant to the drug.

Ceftriaxone is active in vitro against some strains of *Nocardia*, including some strains of *N. asteroides* and *N. brasiliensis*. However, resistance to ceftriaxone also has been reported in environmental isolates of *N. asteroides* and clinical isolates of *N. farcinica*.

■ **Gram-negative Aerobic Bacteria** ***Neisseria*** Ceftriaxone is active in vitro against *Neisseria meningitidis*, and most strains of this organism are inhibited by ceftriaxone concentrations of 0.001–0.025 mcg/mL.

Ceftriaxone is active in vitro against penicillinase-producing (PPNG) and nonpenicillinase-producing *Neisseria gonorrhoeae* and those with chromosomally mediated resistance (e.g., to penicillin) (CMRNG) or plasmid-mediated tetracycline resistance (TRNG). The MIC_{90} of ceftriaxone reported for *N. gonorrhoeae* usually is 0.001–0.05 mcg/mL. However, *N. gonorrhoeae* with reduced susceptibility to ceftriaxone (MICs 0.125 mcg/mL or greater), including some ceftriaxone-resistant strains, have been reported with increasing frequency during the last decade; some treatment failures have been reported. (See Resistance.)

Haemophilus Ceftriaxone is active in vitro against most β-lactamase-producing and non-β-lactamase-producing strains of *Haemophilus influenzae*, *H. parainfluenzae*, and *H. ducreyi*. The MIC_{90} of the drug reported for *H. influenzae* is 0.003–0.03 mcg/mL. *H. ducreyi* generally is inhibited in vitro by ceftriaxone concentrations of 0.002–0.06 mcg/mL.

Enterobacteriaceae Generally, ceftriaxone is active in vitro against the following Enterobacteriaceae: *Citrobacter diversus*, *C. freundii*, *Enterobacter cloacae*, *E. aerogenes*, *Escherichia coli*, *Klebsiella pneumoniae*, *Morganella morganii* (formerly *Proteus morganii*), *Proteus mirabilis*, *P. vulgaris*, *Providencia rettgeri* (formerly *Proteus rettgeri*), *P. stuartii*, *Serratia marcescens*, *Salmonella*, *Shigella*, and *Yersinia enterocolitica*.

The MIC_{90} of ceftriaxone for most of these Enterobacteriaceae, including *Citrobacter*, *E. coli*, *Klebsiella*, *M. morganii*, *P. vulgaris*, *Providencia*, and *Yersinia enterocolitica*, is 0.05–4 mcg/mL. The MIC_{90} of the drug for *P. mirabilis* is 0.006–0.1 mcg/mL. Although the MIC_{90} of ceftriaxone reported for *E. aerogenes* generally is 0.12–8 mcg/mL, the MIC_{90} of the drug reported for *E. cloacae* is 0.5–25 mcg/mL. The MIC_{90} of ceftriaxone for *S. marcescens* is 0.25–32 mcg/mL.

The MIC_{90} of ceftriaxone reported for *Salmonella enteritidis*, *S. paratyphi*, *S. sendai*, *S. typhi*, and *S. typhimurium* is 0.04–0.1 mcg/mL. Strains of *Salmonella* resistant to ceftriaxone have been reported rarely. Multidrug-resistant *Salmonella* serotype Newport has been reported with increasing frequency in the US. These strains usually are resistant to ampicillin, amoxicillin clavulanate, cefoxitin, cephalothin, chloramphenicol, streptomycin, sulfamethoxazole, or tetracycline and have either decreased susceptibility or resistance to ceftriaxone.

The MIC_{90} of ceftriaxone reported for *Shigella*, including *Sh. sonnei*, is 0.02–0.5 mcg/mL.

Pseudomonas Although ceftriaxone is active in vitro against some strains of *Ps. aeruginosa*, many strains of the organism require ceftriaxone concentrations of 64 mcg/mL or greater for in vitro inhibition and are therefore considered resistant to the drug. Ceftriaxone generally is less active in vitro against susceptible *Ps. aeruginosa* than ceftazidime or extended-spectrum penicillins (e.g., piperacillin). In some in vitro studies, the MIC_{50} of ceftriaxone for *Ps. aeruginosa* was 4–16 mcg/mL and the MIC_{90} of the drug was 16–32 mcg/mL. However, in other studies, the MIC_{50} was 16–64 mcg/mL and the MIC_{90} was 64 mcg/mL or greater.

Ceftriaxone has some activity against *Pseudomonas* other than *Ps. aeruginosa*. The MIC_{90} of ceftriaxone reported for *Ps. acidovorans* and *Ps. stutzeri* is 2–16 mcg/mL, but *Ps. fluorescens* and *Ps. putida* generally are resistant to the drug.

Other Gram-Negative Aerobic Bacteria Ceftriaxone is active in vitro against *Moraxella* and *Eikenella corrodens*, and the MIC_{90} of the drug reported for these organisms is 1–2 mcg/mL.

While ceftriaxone has some activity in vitro against *Acinetobacter* and the MIC_{90} of ceftriaxone reported for *A. calcoaceticus* and *A. lwoffi* is 8–32 mcg/mL, the MIC_{90} reported for *A. baumannii* is 64 mcg/mL and this organism is considered resistant to the drug.

Alcaligenes faecalis may be inhibited in vitro by ceftriaxone concentrations of 0.5 mcg/mL or less; however, *A. denitrificans* and *A. xylosoxidans* generally are resistant to the drug.

Bartonella henselae and *B. quintana* may be inhibited in vitro by ceftriaxone concentrations of 0.06–0.25 mcg/mL. Some strains of *B. bacilliformis* are inhibited in vitro by ceftriaxone concentrations of 0.003–0.006 mcg/mL.

In one study, all strains of *Burkholderia cepacia* (formerly *Pseudomonas cepacia*) tested were resistant to ceftriaxone.

Ceftriaxone is active in vitro against *Capnocytophaga*, including *C. canimorsus* (formerly CDC group DF-2). The MIC_{90} of ceftriaxone reported for *Capnocytophaga* is 4 mcg/mL.

Stenotrophomonas maltophilia (formerly *Ps. maltophilia* or *Xanthomonas maltophilia*) generally is resistant to ceftriaxone.

Some strains of *Weeksella virosa* are inhibited in vitro by ceftriaxone concentrations of 0.5 mcg/mL or lower.

■ **Anaerobic Bacteria** Ceftriaxone is active in vitro against some anaerobic bacteria including *Actinomyces, Fusobacterium, Lactobacillus, Peptococcus, Peptostreptococcus, Propionibacterium,* and *Veillonella*. The MIC_{90} of ceftriaxone reported for most of these anaerobic bacteria is 0.5–16 mcg/mL.

Some strains of *Clostridium*, including *C. perfringens*, are inhibited in vitro by ceftriaxone concentrations of 0.5–16 mcg/mL; however, *C. difficile* generally is resistant to the drug.

Most strains of *Bacteroides fragilis* are resistant to ceftriaxone. Although the MIC_{50} of ceftriaxone reported for *B. fragilis, B. distasonis, B. ovatus, B. thetaiotaomicron,* and *B. vulgatus* is 2–64 mcg/mL, the MIC_{90} is 32 mcg/mL or greater.

The MIC_{90} of ceftriaxone reported for *Prevotella melaninogenica* (formerly *Bacteroides melaninogenicus*) is 4–16 mcg/mL.

■ **Spirochetes** Studies in rabbits with experimentally induced syphilis indicate that ceftriaxone has some activity against *Treponema pallidum*.

Borrelia burgdorferi, the causative organism of Lyme disease, reportedly may be inhibited in vitro by ceftriaxone concentrations of 0.1–1 mcg/mL; minimum bactericidal concentrations (MBCs) of ceftriaxone for *B. burgdorferi* generally have ranged from 0.02–0.16 mcg/mL.

Ceftriaxone is active in vitro against *Leptospira*. In one study, all strains of *L. interrogans* and *L. weilii* tested were inhibited in vitro by ceftriaxone concentrations of 0.06 mcg/mL or less.

■ **Chlamydia** Studies using a limited number of isolates indicate that some strains of *Chlamydia trachomatis* are inhibited in vitro by ceftriaxone concentrations of 8–32 mcg/mL; however, the clinical importance of this in vitro activity is unclear. Ceftriaxone generally is considered to be inactive against *C. trachomatis*.

Resistance

For information on possible mechanisms of bacterial resistance to cephalosporins, see Resistance in the Cephalosporins General Statement 8:12.06.

Ceftriaxone generally is stable against hydrolysis by β-lactamases classified as Richmond-Sykes types II, III (TEM types), and V; some PSE types; and most β-lactamases produced by *Neisseria gonorrhoeae, Haemophilus influenzae,* and staphylococci. Ceftriaxone may be inactivated by Richmond type IV β-lactamases, and in vitro studies indicate that some β-lactamases produced by *Bacteroides, Citrobacter, Enterobacter, Morganella, Proteus,* and *Pseudomonas* can inactivate the drug. Ceftriaxone generally is as stable as cefotaxime against inactivation by β-lactamases but less stable than cefoxitin.

Resistant strains of some organisms, including *Enterobacter* and *Ps. aeruginosa*, have developed during therapy with ceftriaxone. Although further study is needed, it has been suggested that resistance may develop in many of these organisms because they possess inducible β-lactamases. These inducible enzymes generally are chromosomally mediated cephalosporinases classified as Richmond-Sykes type I. In vitro studies indicate that following exposure to certain β-lactam antibiotics (e.g., cefoxitin), inducible β-lactamases are derepressed. Inducible β-lactamases appear to inactivate β-lactam antibiotics by binding to the drugs, which prevents them from binding to penicillin-binding proteins of the organism. Most β-lactam antibiotics, including second and third generation cephalosporins and extended-spectrum penicillins, are inactivated by inducible β-lactamases.

Strains of *S. pneumoniae* considered resistant to ceftriaxone have been reported with increasing frequency. These strains generally have intermediate- or high-level resistance to penicillin G as well as decreased susceptibility to third generation cephalosporins. Resistance to ceftriaxone in *S. pneumoniae* appears to be related to alterations in the target enzymes, penicillin-binding proteins (PBPs), of the organism.

N. gonorrhoeae with reduced susceptibility to ceftriaxone and/or cefixime or other cephalosporins have been reported with increasing frequency in the US and elsewhere (e.g., Asia, Europe, Canada). Strains with reduced susceptibility to ceftriaxone generally have ceftriaxone MICs of 0.125 mcg/mL or greater. There also have been rare reports of *N. gonorrhoeae* with high-level ceftriaxone resistance (MICs 1–4 mcg/mL) in some countries (Japan, France, Spain), including at least one patient with pharyngeal gonorrhea. Susceptibility of *N. gonorrhoeae* in the US is being monitored by CDC Gonococcal Isolate Surveillance Project (GISP). GISP data from 2000–2010 indicate that the percentage of US *N. gonorrhoeae* isolates with elevated ceftriaxone MICs (MICs 0.125 mcg/mL or greater) increased from 0.1% to 0.3% and the percentage with elevated cefixime MICs (MICs 0.25 mcg/mL or greater) increased from 0.2% to 1.4%. GISP data regarding *N. gonorrhoeae* isolates from men who have sex with men indicate that the percentage of isolates with elevated ceftriaxone MICs increased from 0% in 2006 to 1% in 2011 and the percentage of isolates with elevated cefixime MICs increased from 0.2% in 2006 to 3.8% in 2011.

Pharmacokinetics

In all studies described in the Pharmacokinetics section, ceftriaxone was administered as ceftriaxone sodium; dosages and concentrations of the drug are expressed in terms of ceftriaxone.

Ceftriaxone exhibits nonlinear dose-dependent pharmacokinetics. Serum concentrations, the area under the serum concentration-time curve (AUC), and most pharmacokinetic parameters (except elimination half-life and the fraction excreted unchanged in urine) of total ceftriaxone (both protein-bound and unbound drug) are dose dependent and increase nonlinearly with increases in dosage. However, pharmacokinetic parameters of free (unbound) ceftriaxone are not dose dependent and increase linearly with dosage. Dose-dependent changes in the pharmacokinetic parameters of ceftriaxone apparently occur because the drug exhibits concentration-dependent protein binding. (See Pharmacokinetics: Distribution.) Some clinicians suggest that because of this concentration-dependent protein binding, distribution and clearance parameters calculated with data obtained using concentrations of total ceftriaxone may be invalid and misleading. Other clinicians suggest that concentration-dependent protein binding and dose-related changes in the pharmacokinetic parameters of ceftriaxone over the usual dosage range of the drug are small and not clinically important.

■ **Absorption** Ceftriaxone is not appreciably absorbed from the GI tract and must be given parenterally.

Following IM administration of a single ceftriaxone dose of 0.5–1 g in healthy adults, the drug appears to be completely absorbed, and peak serum concentrations are attained 1.5–4 hours after the dose. In one study in healthy adults who received a single 1-g IM dose of ceftriaxone, serum concentrations of the drug averaged 28.9, 43.7, 62.3, 83.2, 40.6, 35.5, and 7.8 mcg/mL at 0.25, 0.5, 1, 2, 6, 12, and 24 hours, respectively, after the dose.

Following IV infusion over 30 minutes of a single 1-g dose of ceftriaxone in healthy adults, peak serum concentrations of the drug at completion of the infusion average 123.2–150.7 mcg/mL and serum concentrations at 1, 2, 6, 12, and 24 hours after start of the infusion average 109.5–111, 60.8–88.2, 33–52.5, 20.2–28.1, and 4.6–9.3 mcg/mL, respectively. IV infusion over 30 minutes of a single 2-g dose of ceftriaxone in healthy adults results in peak serum concentrations of the drug at completion of the infusion that range from 223–276 mcg/mL and serum concentrations at 1, 2, 6, 12, and 24 hours after start of the infusion that range from 166–209, 135–173, 75–104, 32–58, and 7–22 mcg/mL, respectively.

In one study in healthy adults, a ceftriaxone dosage of 2 g daily was given either as 1 g every 12 hours or 2 g every 24 hours; each dose was administered by IV infusion over 30 minutes. At steady state, peak serum concentrations of the drug ranged from 132–213 mcg/mL in those who received 1 g every 12 hours and from 216–281 mcg/mL in those who received 2 g every 24 hours; trough serum concentrations ranged from 23–58 and 7–27 mcg/mL, respectively. Average steady-state serum concentrations of ceftriaxone were similar for both regimens and were 72 mcg/mL when 1 g was given every 12 hours and 63 mcg/mL when 2 g was given every 24 hours.

In multiple-dose studies in healthy adults who received a ceftriaxone dosage of 0.5–2 g given every 12 or 24 hours by IM injection or IV infusion over 30 minutes, serum concentrations of the drug at steady state on the fourth day of therapy were 15–36% higher than serum concentrations attained with single doses of the drug.

In one study in adults with neoplastic disease, IM administration of a single 500-mg dose of ceftriaxone resulted in serum concentrations of the drug averaging 28, 31.9, 32.9, 28.3, and 25.5 mcg/mL at 0.5, 1, 2, 4, and 6 hours, respectively, after the dose. IV infusion over 5 minutes of a single ceftriaxone dose of 500 mg or 1 g in these patients resulted in serum concentrations of the drug at 0.5, 1, 2, 4, and 8 hours that averaged 54.4, 44.7, 33.5, 25.4, and 16.8 mcg/mL, respectively, after the 500-mg dose and 79.3, 65.7, 52.2, 28.7, and 22.3 mcg/mL, respectively, after the 1-g dose.

In one study in neonates and children 1–45 days of age with meningitis who received a single ceftriaxone dose of 50 mg/kg by IV infusion over 15 minutes, serum concentrations of the drug immediately following the infusion and 1, 2, 4, and 6 hours later averaged 136–173, 91–116, 80–112, 70–86, and 66–74 mcg/mL, respectively. In another study in neonates 1–4 days of age with meningitis who received a single 50-mg/kg dose of ceftriaxone by IV infusion over 5 minutes, serum concentrations of the drug 1, 12, and 24 hours after the dose ranged from 108–141, 43–76, and 20–52 mcg/mL, respectively. Serum concentrations of ceftriaxone in neonates 9–30 days of age with meningitis who received a single 100-mg/kg dose of the drug by IV infusion over 5 minutes ranged from 100–262, 43–140, and 8–33 mcg/mL at 1, 12, and 24 hours, respectively, after the dose.

In one study in children 7–15 months of age who received a single ceftriaxone dose of 50 mg/kg by IV infusion over 5 minutes, serum concentrations of the drug ranged from 139–197, 66.6–99.2, 31.3–58.9, 2.4–14.8, and 0.85–8.4 mcg/mL at 0.5, 4, 8, 24, and 32 hours, respectively, after the dose. When the same dose was administered by IV infusion over 5 minutes to children 2–6 years of age, serum concentrations of the drug at the same time intervals ranged from 180–209, 74.4–108, 32.5–70.2, 5.1–16.1, and 2.4–7.3 mcg/mL, respectively. In another study in children 2 months to 16 years of age with CNS infections who received a single ceftriaxone dose of 50 or 75 mg/kg by IV infusion over 15 minutes, peak serum concentrations of the drug occurred immediately following the infusion and ranged from 162–370 mcg/mL after the 50-mg/kg dose and 218–348 mcg/mL after the 75-mg/kg dose; serum concentrations of the drug 12 hours after the dose ranged from 8–56.7 and 13.4–51.2 mcg/mL, respectively.

■ **Distribution** The volume of distribution of ceftriaxone is dose dependent and ranges from 5.8–13.5 L in healthy adults. The volume of distribution of the drug averages 8.5–9.4 L in healthy adults following a single 500-mg dose of the drug and 10–11.4 L following a single 2-g dose. The volume of distribution of ceftriaxone is 0.497–0.608 L/kg in neonates 1–45 days of age and 0.26–0.54 L/kg in children 1.5 months to 16 years of age following a single ceftriaxone dose of 50–100 mg/kg.

Following IM or IV administration, ceftriaxone is widely distributed into body tissues and fluids including the gallbladder, lungs, bone, heart, bile, prostate adenoma tissue, uterine tissue, atrial appendage,sputum, tears, middle ear fluid, and pleural, peritoneal, synovial, ascitic, and blister fluids.

In pediatric patients with otitis media who received a single 50-mg/kg IM dose of ceftriaxone, peak concentrations of ceftriaxone (both protein-bound and unbound drug) in middle ear fluid were attained 24–30 hours after the dose and averaged 35 mcg/mL; middle ear fluid concentrations 48–52 hours after the dose averaged 19 mcg/mL.

In one study in adults with normal hepatobiliary and renal function who received a single 500-mg IV dose of ceftriaxone, peak concentrations of the drug in bile occurred 1–2 hours after the dose and concentrations in bile were generally 2–5 times higher than concurrent serum concentrations. In another study in patients who received a single 1-g IV dose of ceftriaxone, concentrations of the drug in specimens obtained 1–3 hours after the dose averaged 62.1 mcg/mL in plasma, 78.2 mcg/g in the gallbladder wall, and 581, 788, and 898 mcg/mL in gallbladder, common duct, and cystic duct biles, respectively.

In one study in patients undergoing open heart surgery who received a single 1-g IV dose of ceftriaxone approximately 1 hour prior to surgery, concentrations of the drug in the right atrial appendage ranged from 3.6–10.2 mcg/g in samples obtained 1.5–3 hours after the dose. In a study in patients undergoing abdominal or vaginal hysterectomy who received a single 2-g IV dose of ceftriaxone, peak concentrations of the drug in gynecologic tissue occurred during the first 2 hours after the dose and concentrations of the drug were higher in the salpinges than in myometrium or endometrium. Ceftriaxone concentrations in the salpinges averaged 53.1 and 31.3 mcg/mL at 1–2 and 4–5 hours, respectively, after the dose, and concentrations in myometrium or endometrium averaged 29.8–36.6 and 21.4–24.9 mcg/mL at 1–2 and 4–5 hours, respectively, after the dose.

Only low concentrations of ceftriaxone are distributed into aqueous humor following IV or IM administration of the drug. In one study in patients undergoing cataract surgery who received a single 1- or 2-g dose of ceftriaxone by IV infusion over 10 minutes, peak concentrations of the drug in aqueous humor were attained approximately 2 hours after the dose and averaged 0.93 and 2.47 mcg/mL, respectively. Aqueous humor concentrations averaged 0.88 mcg/mL 12 hours after the 1-g dose and were 2.1 and 2.5 mcg/mL in two patients 12 hours after the 2-g dose.

Ceftriaxone generally diffuses into CSF following IM or IV administration of the drug; however, CSF concentrations of the drug are higher in patients with inflamed meninges than in those with uninflamed meninges. Studies in neonates and children with meningitis indicate that peak CSF concentrations of ceftriaxone generally are attained 3–6 hours after an IV dose of the drug, and CSF concentrations of ceftriaxone may be 1–32% of concurrent serum concentrations. CSF concentrations of ceftriaxone do not generally correlate with CSF leukocyte cell counts or CSF protein or glucose concentrations. In one study in neonates and children with meningitis who received a single 50- or 100-mg/kg dose of ceftriaxone, CSF concentrations of the drug were 5–31.6 and 1.4–4.5 mcg/mL at 4 and 24 hours, respectively, after the dose. In another study in children 2–42 months of age with meningitis who received a single ceftriaxone dose of 50 mg/kg given by IV infusion over 10–15 minutes, CSF concentrations of the drug averaged 1.2–3, 1.4–4.3, and 2.8–7.2 mcg/mL at 1, 4, and 6 hours, respectively, after the dose. In one adult with meningitis who received 2 g of the drug once daily, the concentration in CSF was 8.5 mcg/mL in a specimen obtained 5 hours after the third dose of the drug.

The degree of protein binding of ceftriaxone is concentration dependent and decreases nonlinearly with increasing concentrations of the drug. It has been suggested that ceftriaxone may have more than one concentration-dependent protein binding site. The drug is 93–96% bound to plasma proteins at a concentration less than 70 mcg/mL, 84–87% bound at a concentration of 300 mcg/mL, and 58% or less bound at a concentration of 600 mcg/mL. Ceftriaxone binds mainly to albumin. Protein binding of ceftriaxone is lower in neonates and children than in adults because of decreased plasma albumin concentrations in this age group. In one study in children 7 months to 6 years of age with ceftriaxone plasma concentrations of 118–202 mcg/mL, ceftriaxone was 80–87% bound to plasma proteins. Ceftriaxone also is less protein bound in patients with renal or hepatic impairment as the result of decreased plasma albumin concentrations or displacement from protein binding sites by bilirubin and other endogenous compounds that may accumulate.

Ceftriaxone crosses the placenta and is distributed into amniotic fluid. In one study in women who received a single 2-g dose of ceftriaxone given by IV injection over 2–5 minutes during labor, peak concentrations of the drug in cord blood, amniotic fluid, and the placenta occurred 4–8 hours after the dose; ceftriaxone concentrations in the first voided urine of infants born to these women ranged from 6–92 mcg/mL. Ceftriaxone also is distributed into milk in low concentrations. In one study in lactating women who received a single 1-g IM or IV dose of ceftriaxone, peak concentrations of the drug in milk occurred 4–6 hours after the dose and the AUC for milk was 3–4% of the AUC for serum.

■ **Elimination** Plasma concentrations of ceftriaxone decline in a biphasic manner. In adults with normal renal and hepatic function, the distribution half-life ($t_{1/2\alpha}$) of ceftriaxone is 0.12–0.7 hours and the elimination half-life ($t_{1/2\beta}$) is 5.4–10.9 hours.

Ceftriaxone is excreted both by renal and nonrenal mechanisms. The drug is excreted principally in urine by glomerular filtration and also is excreted in feces via bile. Following IM or IV administration of a single dose of ceftriaxone in adults with normal renal and hepatic function, 33–67% of the dose is excreted in urine as unchanged drug and the remainder of the dose is excreted in feces as unchanged drug and microbiologically inactive metabolites.Ceftriaxone is metabolized to a small extent in the intestines after biliary excretion.

Following IM or IV administration of a single 1-g dose of ceftriaxone in healthy adults, urinary concentrations of the drug average 504–995 mcg/mL in urine collected over the first 2 hours after the dose, 293–418 mcg/mL in urine collected 4–8 hours after the dose, and 132 mcg/mL in urine collected 12–24 hours after the dose.

Serum clearance of ceftriaxone is dose dependent and ranges from 9.7–25 mL/minute in healthy adults. The serum clearance of the drug averages 10.2–16.7 mL/minute in healthy adults following a single 500-mg IV dose and 19.8–21.6 mL/minute following a single 2-g IV dose. In children 2 months to 16 years of age who receive a single ceftriaxone dose of 50–100 mg/kg, the serum clearance of ceftriaxone averages 32–40.8 mL/minute per 1.73 m^2. Preliminary studies in patients with cystic fibrosis suggest that serum clearance of ceftriaxone is higher in these patients than in healthy individuals.

The serum half-life of ceftriaxone is longer in neonates than in older children and adults. In one study, the serum half-life of ceftriaxone was longer in neonates weighing less than 1.5 kg than in heavier neonates. Results of another study in neonates 1–8 days of age weighing 1.8–3.9 kg suggested that there was no correlation between weight and serum half-life of the drug at this weight range. In one study, the serum half-life of the drug averaged 16.2 hours in neonates 1–4 days of age and 9.2 hours in those 9–30 days of age. The serum half-life of ceftriaxone in children is similar to that reported in adults, and the elimination half-life of the drug averages 4–7.7 hours in children 1.5 months to 16 years of age. In one study in children 2–42 months of age, the $t_{1/2\alpha}$ of ceftriaxone averaged 0.25 hours and the $t_{1/2\beta}$ of the drug averaged 4 hours.

The elimination half-life of ceftriaxone is only slightly prolonged in patients with moderately impaired renal function and has been reported to range from 10–16 hours in adults with creatinine clearances of 5–73 mL/minute. In patients with creatinine clearances less than 5 mL/minute, the elimination half-life of ceftriaxone has generally been reported to average 12.2–18.2 hours. However, the elimination half-life of ceftriaxone was 15–57 hours in several uremic patients with creatinine clearances less than 5 mL/minute who had no apparent liver impairment.

Studies in patients with hepatic impairment (e.g., patients with fatty liver, liver fibrosis, compensated liver cirrhosis) indicate that the pharmacokinetics of ceftriaxone are not generally altered in these patients. Although the elimination half-life of ceftriaxone was not prolonged in patients with ascites, the volume of distribution and plasma clearance of the drug were increased slightly compared with healthy individuals and averaged 22 L and 28 mL/minute, respectively.

Ceftriaxone is not removed by hemodialysis or peritoneal dialysis.

Chemistry and Stability

■ **Chemistry** Ceftriaxone is a semisynthetic cephalosporin antibiotic. Like cefepime, cefotaxime, and ceftazidime, ceftriaxone is a parenteral aminothiazolyl cephalosporin. Ceftriaxone contains an aminothiazolyl-acetyl side chain, with a methoxyimino group, at position 7 of the cephalosporin nucleus. The aminothiazolyl side chain enhances antibacterial activity, particularly against Enterobacteriaceae, and generally results in enhanced stability against β-lactamases; the methoxyimino group contributes to stability against hydrolysis by many β-lactamases. Ceftriaxone also has an acidic enol in the triazine moiety at position 3 of the cephalosporin nucleus, which presumably is responsible for the long serum half-life of the drug.

Ceftriaxone is commercially available as the disodium salt; however, the drug is referred to as ceftriaxone sodium. Potency of ceftriaxone sodium is expressed in terms of ceftriaxone. Each mg of ceftriaxone sodium contains not less than 776 mcg of ceftriaxone, calculated on the anhydrous free acid basis.

Ceftriaxone sodium is readily soluble in water, having an aqueous solubility of 400 mg/mL at 25°C. The drug has a solubility of 1 mg/mL in alcohol at 25°C. Ceftriaxone sodium has pK_as of 3, 3.2, and 4.1. Ceftriaxone sodium contains approximately 83 mg (3.6 mEq) of sodium per gram of ceftriaxone.

Commercially available sterile ceftriaxone sodium powder for injection occurs as a white to yellowish or yellowish-orange crystalline powder. When reconstituted as directed, solutions of the drug are light yellow to amber in color depending on the diluent used, concentration of the drug, and length of storage. The pH of an aqueous solution containing 10 mg of ceftriaxone per mL is approximately 6.7.

When the commercially available Duplex® drug delivery system that contains 1 or 2 g of ceftriaxone powder and 50 mL of dextrose injection in separate chambers is reconstituted (activated) according to the manufacturer's directions, the resultant solution is iso-osmotic and has an osmolality of approximately 290 mOsm/kg.

Commercially available frozen premixed ceftriaxone sodium injections in dextrose are sterile, nonpyrogenic, iso-osmotic solutions of the drug provided in a plastic container (Galaxy® containers) fabricated from specially formulated multilayered plastic PL 2040 plastic. The 1- and 2-g frozen injections of ceftriaxone contain approximately 1.9 and 1.2 g of dextrose hydrous, respectively, to adjust osmolality and may contain sodium hydroxide and/or hydrochloric acid to adjust pH. After thawing, the injections are light yellow to amber in color and have a pH of 6–8.

■ **Stability** Commercially available ceftriaxone sodium sterile powder for injection should be stored at 20–25°C and protected from light. It is unnecessary to protect reconstituted solutions of the drug from normal light.

Following reconstitution of ceftriaxone powder for injection with sterile water for injection, 0.9% sodium chloride injection, or 5% dextrose injection, ceftriaxone sodium solutions for IM injection containing approximately 250 or 350 mg of ceftriaxone per mL are stable for 24 hours at room temperature (25°C) or 3 days refrigerated at 4°C and solutions containing approximately 100 mg/mL are stable for 2 days at 25°C or 10 days at 4°C. Following reconstitution with 1% lidocaine hydrochloride injection (without epinephrine) or bacteriostatic water for injection (containing 0.9% benzyl alcohol), solutions of the drug for IM injection containing 250 or 350 mg/mL are stable for 24 hours at 25°C or 3 days at 4°C and solutions containing 100 mg/mL are stable for 24 hours at 25°C or 10 days at 4°C.

Following reconstitution of ceftriaxone powder for injection as directed by the manufacturer and further dilution with sterile water for injection, 0.9% sodium chloride injection, or 5 or 10% dextrose injection, solutions containing 10–40 mg of ceftriaxone per mL are stable in glass or PVC containers for 2 days at room temperature (25°C) or 10 days when refrigerated at 4°C. If 5% dextrose in 0.45 or 0.9% sodium chloride is used for dilution, solutions of the drug containing 10–40 mg/mL are stable for 2 days at room temperature when stored in glass or PVC containers but are unstable at 4°C. Solutions of the drug containing 10–40 mg/mL are stable for 24 hours at room temperature (25°C) in 10% invert sugar, 5% sodium bicarbonate, 5 or 10% mannitol, FreAmine® III, Normosol®-M in 5% dextrose, or Ionosol® B in 5% dextrose when stored in glass containers. The same concentrations of the drug are stable for 24 hours at room temperature in sodium lactate or Normosol®-M in 5% dextrose when stored in PVC containers.

The manufacturers state that following reconstitution with 0.9% sodium chloride injection or 5% dextrose injection, extemporaneously prepared ceftriaxone sodium solutions containing 10–40 mg of ceftriaxone per mL are stable for 26 weeks when frozen at −20°C in PVC or polyolefin containers. Frozen solutions of ceftriaxone sodium should be thawed at room temperature; once thawed, unused portions should be discarded and should not be refrozen.

Commercially available 10-g pharmacy bulk packages of ceftriaxone that have been reconstituted to a concentration of 100 mg/mL with a compatible IV solution should be further diluted in a compatible IV infusion solution without delay; any unused portions of the reconstituted solution should be discarded after 4 hours.

Following reconstitution of ADD-Vantage® vials containing 1 or 2 g of ceftriaxone with 0.9% sodium chloride injection or 5% dextrose injection according to the manufacturer's directions, IV solutions containing 10–40 mg/mL in 0.9% sodium chloride or 5% dextrose in ADD-Vantage® flexible containers are stable for 2 days at room temperature (25°C) or 10 days refrigerated at 4°C.

The commercially available Duplex® drug delivery system that contains 1 or 2 g of lyophilized ceftriaxone and 50 mL of dextrose injection should be stored at 20–25°C, but may be exposed to 15–30°C. Following reconstitution (activation), these IV solutions must be used within 24 hours if stored at room temperature or within 7 days if stored in a refrigerator and should not be frozen.

The commercially available frozen premixed ceftriaxone sodium injection in dextrose should be stored at −20°C or lower. The frozen injection should be thawed at room temperature (25°C) or under refrigeration (5°C) and, once thawed, should not be refrozen. Thawed solutions of the commercially available frozen injection are stable for 48 hours at room temperature (25°C) or 21 days under refrigeration (5°C). The commercially available frozen injection of the drug is provided in a plastic container fabricated from specially formulated multilayered plastic PL 2040 (Galaxy®) . Solutions in contact with PL 2040 can leach out some of its chemical components in very small amounts within the expiration period of the injection; however, safety of the plastic has been confirmed in tests in animals according to USP biological tests for plastic containers as well as by tissue culture toxicity studies.

Ceftriaxone is physically incompatible with aminoglycosides, fluconazole, and vancomycin, and the manufacturers state that ceftriaxone should not be admixed with these drugs. If an aminoglycoside, fluconazole, or vancomycin is to be administered in a patient receiving ceftriaxone by intermittent IV infusion, the drugs should be given sequentially and IV infusion lines should be thoroughly flushed with a compatible infusion fluid before administering the other drug. Admixtures containing ceftriaxone 10 mg/mL and metronidazole hydrochloride 5–7.5 mg/mL in 0.9% sodium chloride injection or 5% dextrose injection are stable for 24 hours at room temperature; however, precipitation will occur if these admixtures are refrigerated or if metronidazole concentrations greater than 8 mg/mL are used.

Ceftriaxone is incompatible with calcium-containing diluents or solutions (e.g. Ringer's/lactated Ringer's solution, Hartmann's solution); particulate formation can result if the drug is admixed with calcium-containing diluents or solutions.

Specialized references should be consulted for specific compatibility information.

Preparations

Excipients in commercially available drug preparations may have clinically important effects in some individuals; consult specific product labeling for details.

cefTRIAXone Sodium

Parenteral

For injection	250 mg (of ceftriaxone)*	**cefTRIAXone for Injection**
	500 mg (of ceftriaxone)*	**cefTRIAXone for Injection**
	1 g (of ceftriaxone)*	**cefTRIAXone for Injection**
	2 g (of ceftriaxone)*	**cefTRIAXone for Injection**
For injection, for IV infusion	1 g (of ceftriaxone)*	**cefTRIAXone ADD-Vantage®**, Hospira
		cefTRIAXone for Injection, for IV Infusion (available in dual-chambered Duplex® drug delivery system with 3.74% dextrose injection), B Braun
		cefTRIAXone for Injection, for IV Infusion
	2 g (of ceftriaxone)*	**cefTRIAXone ADD-Vantage®**, Hospira
		cefTRIAXone for Injection, for IV Infusion (available in dual-chambered Duplex® drug delivery system with 2.22% dextrose injection), B Braun
		cefTRIAXone for Injection for IV Infusion
	10 g (of ceftriaxone) pharmacy bulk package*	**cefTRIAXone for Injection, for IV Infusion**
	100 g (of ceftriaxone) pharmacy bulk package*	**cefTRIAXone for Injection, for IV Infusion**

*available from one or more manufacturer, distributor, and/or repackager by generic (nonproprietary) name

cefTRIAXone Sodium in Dextrose

Parenteral

Injection (frozen), for IV infusion	20 mg (of ceftriaxone) per mL (1 g) in 3.8% Dextrose*	**cefTRIAXone Iso-osmotic in Dextrose Injection** (Galaxy® [Baxter])
	40 mg (of ceftriaxone) per mL (2 g) in 2.4% Dextrose*	**cefTRIAXone Iso-osmotic in Dextrose Injection** (Galaxy® [Baxter])

*available from one or more manufacturer, distributor, and/or repackager by generic (nonproprietary) name

†Use is not currently included in the labeling approved by the US Food and Drug Administration

FOURTH GENERATION CEPHALOSPORINS 8:12.06.16

Cefepime Hydrochloride

■ Cefepime is a semisynthetic, fourth generation cephalosporin antibiotic.

Uses

Cefepime is used for the treatment of uncomplicated and complicated urinary tract infections (including pyelonephritis), uncomplicated skin and skin structure infections, and moderate to severe pneumonia caused by susceptible organisms. For the treatment of complicated intra-abdominal infections, cefepime is used in conjunction with IV metronidazole. In addition, cefepime is used alone or in conjunction with other anti-infectives for empiric anti-infective therapy in febrile neutropenic patients.

■ **Intra-abdominal Infections** IV cefepime is used in conjunction with IV metronidazole for the treatment of complicated intra-abdominal infections caused by *Escherichia coli*, viridans streptococci, *Pseudomonas aeruginosa*, *Klebsiella pneumoniae*, *Enterobacter*, or *Bacteroides fragilis* in adults. Safety and efficacy of cefepime used in conjunction with metronidazole has been evaluated in a randomized, double-blind, multicenter study in adults with surgically confirmed complicated intra-abdominal infections who were randomized to receive cefepime (2 g IV every 12 hours) and metronidazole (7.5 mg/kg or 500 mg IV every 6 hours) or monotherapy with imipenem and cilastatin sodium (500 mg IV every 6 hours). The overall clinical cure rate was 88% in those who received combination therapy with cefepime and metronidazole and 76% in those who received monotherapy with imipenem and cilastatin sodium.

For initial empiric treatment of high-risk or severe community-acquired extrabiliary intra-abdominal infections in adults (e.g., those with advanced age, immunocompromised state, severe physiologic disturbance), the Infectious Diseases Society of America (IDSA) recommends either monotherapy with a carbapenem (doripenem, imipenem, meropenem) or the fixed combination of piperacillin and tazobactam, or a combination regimen that includes either a cephalosporin (cefepime, ceftazidime) or fluoroquinolone (ciprofloxacin, levofloxacin) in conjunction with metronidazole. IDSA also recommends cefepime in conjunction with metronidazole as one of several regimens that can be used for initial empiric treatment of health-care associated complicated intra-abdominal infections in adults and community-acquired complicated intra-abdominal infections in pediatric patients. For additional information regarding management of intra-abdominal infections, the current IDSA clinical practice guidelines available at http://www.idsociety.org should be consulted.

While cefepime has been effective when used alone for the treatment of acute obstetric and gynecologic infections† (e.g., pelvic inflammatory disease, pelvic surgical wound infection, postpartum endometritis), safety and efficacy of the drug for use as monotherapy in the treatment of such infections have not been established.

■ **Respiratory Tract Infections** Cefepime is used in adult and pediatric patients 2 months of age or older for the treatment of moderate to severe pneumonia, including that associated with concurrent bacteremia, caused by susceptible *Streptococcus pneumoniae*. The drug also is used in adult and pediatric patients 2 months of age or older for the treatment of moderate to severe pneumonia caused by susceptible *Ps. aeruginosa*, *K. pneumoniae*, or *Enterobacter*.

Community-acquired Pneumonia Cefepime appears to be at least as effective and as well tolerated as ceftriaxone or ceftazidime for the treatment of community-acquired pneumonia (CAP). In an open-label, randomized study in hospitalized adults who were randomized to receive 5–10 days (14 days maximum) of therapy with either cefepime (2 g IV every 12 hours) or ceftriaxone (1 g IV every 12 hours) for empiric treatment of CAP, a satisfactory clinical response (cure or improvement) was achieved in 95% of those receiving cefepime and 97.8% of those receiving ceftriaxone. When cefepime (1 g IV or IM every 12 hours) was compared with ceftazidime (1 g IV every 8 hours) for empiric therapy in adults 21–90 years of age with community-acquired lower respiratory tract infections, the clinical cure rate was 87% in those who received cefepime and 86% in those who received ceftazidime. The most common pathogens in these studies were *S. pneumoniae*, *Haemophilus influenzae*, *Moraxella catarrhalis*, and/or *Staphylococcal aureus*.

The American Thoracic Society (ATS) and IDSA recommend use of cefepime in the treatment of CAP only when *Ps. aeruginosa* is known or suspected to be involved. Factors that increase the risk of *Ps. aeruginosa* infection in CAP patients include severe CAP requiring treatment in an intensive care unit (ICU), structural lung disease (bronchiectasis), severe chronic obstructive pulmonary disease (COPD), smoking, alcoholism, chronic corticosteroid therapy, and frequent anti-infective therapy. In CAP patients with risk factors for *Ps. aeruginosa*, the ATS and IDSA recommend use of an empiric combination regimen that includes an antipneumococcal, antipseudomonal β-lactam (cefepime, imipenem, meropenem, fixed combination of piperacillin and tazobactam) given in conjunction with a fluoroquinolone (ciprofloxacin, levofloxacin); a combination regimen that includes one of these antipseudomonal β-lactams, an aminoglycoside, and azithromycin; or a combination regimen that includes one of these antipseudomonal β-lactams, an aminoglycoside, and an antipneumococcal fluoroquinolone. The ATS and IDSA state that if *Ps. aeruginosa* has been identified by appropriate microbiologic testing, the preferred treatment regimen is an antipseudomonal β-lactam (cefepime, ceftazidime, aztreonam, imipenem, meropenem, piperacillin, ticarcillin) given in conjunction with ciprofloxacin, levofloxacin, or an aminoglycoside and the preferred alternative regimen is an aminoglycoside given in conjunction with ciprofloxacin or levofloxacin.

For additional information on use of cephalosporins in the treatment of CAP, see Community-acquired Infections under Uses: Respiratory Tract Infections, in the Cephalosporins General Statement 8:12.06.

Nosocomial Infections Cefepime is used in the treatment of nosocomial pneumonia. The ATS, IDSA, and other clinicians recommend use of an antipseudomonal cephalosporin (cefepime, ceftazidime), antipseudomonal penicillin (piperacillin and tazobactam, ticarcillin and clavulanate), or an antipseudomonal carbapenem (imipenem or meropenem) for initial therapy of hospital-acquired pneumonia, ventilator-associated pneumonia, or health-care associated pneumonia because these drugs have a broad spectrum of activity against gram-positive, gram-negative, and anaerobic bacteria. In hospitals where methicillin-resistant *S. aureus*(MRSA; also known as oxacillin-resistant *S. aureus* or ORSA) is common or if there are risk factors for these strains, the initial regimen also should include vancomycin or linezolid.

■ **Skin and Skin Structure Infections** Cefepime is used in adult and pediatric patients 2 months of age or older for the treatment of uncomplicated skin and skin structure infections caused by susceptible *S. aureus* (methicillin-susceptible [oxacillin-susceptible] strains only) or susceptible *Streptococcus pyogenes*.

■ **Urinary Tract Infections** Cefepime is used in adult and pediatric patients 2 months of age or older for the treatment of severe uncomplicated and complicated urinary tract infections (including those associated with pyelonephritis and/or concurrent bacteremia) caused by susceptible *E. coli* or *K. pneumoniae*. Cefepime also is used in adult and pediatric patients 2 months of age or older for the treatment of mild to moderate uncomplicated and complicated urinary tract infections (including those associated with pyelonephritis and/or with concurrent bacteremia) when the causative organism is *E. coli*, *K. pneumoniae*, or *Proteus mirabilis*.

■ **Endocarditis** For empiric treatment of culture-negative endocarditis† in prosthetic valve recipients with early onset endocarditis (within 1 year after prosthetic valve placement), the American Heart Association (AHA) recommends a multiple-drug regimen that includes vancomycin, gentamicin, cefepime, and rifampin. Blood cultures are negative in up to 20% of patients with infective endocarditis because of inadequate microbiologic technique, infection with highly fastidious bacteria or nonbacterial pathogens, or administration of anti-infective agents prior to obtaining blood cultures. Selection of the most appropriate anti-infective regimen for the treatment of culture-negative endocarditis is difficult and should be guided by epidemiologic features and clinical course of the infection. Consultation with an infectious diseases specialist is recommended.

■ **Meningitis and Other CNS Infections** Cefepime has been used in adult and pediatric patients 2 months of age or older for the treatment of meningitis† caused by susceptible gram-negative bacteria (e.g., *H. influenzae*, *Neisseria meningitidis*, *E. coli*, *E. aerogenes*, *Ps. aeruginosa*) or gram-positive bacteria (e.g., *S. pneumoniae*, *S. aureus*, *S. epidermidis*). However, safety and efficacy of cefepime for the treatment of meningitis have not been established, and the manufacturers caution that an alternative anti-infective with demonstrated clinical efficacy in this setting should be used in patients in whom meningeal seeding from a distant infection site or in whom meningitis is suspected or documented.

IDSA states that cefepime is one of several alternatives that can be used for the treatment of meningitis caused by *H. influenzae* or *E. coli* or treatment of meningitis caused by *S. pneumonia* susceptible to penicillins and third generation cephalosporins. For the treatment of meningitis caused by *Ps. aeruginosa*, IDSA and other experts recommend a regimen that consists of an antipseudomonal cephalosporin (cefepime or ceftazidime) or carbapenem (imipenem or meropenem) given with or without an aminoglycoside (amikacin, gentamicin, tobramycin). Treatment of these infections should be guided by results of in vitro susceptibility tests.

IDSA also recommends a regimen of cefepime and vancomycin as one of several regimens that can be used in adult and pediatric patients for empiric treatment of penetrating head trauma or postneurosurgical infections caused by *S. aureus*, coagulase-negative staphylococci (especially *S. epidermidis*), or aerobic gram-negative bacilli (including *Ps. aeruginosa*).

In a prospective, randomized study in infants and children 2 months to 15 years of age, IV cefepime was as effective as IV cefotaxime for the treatment of meningitis caused by susceptible gram-negative or gram-positive bacteria. However, some clinicians suggest that additional study is needed regarding cefepime's efficacy for the treatment of meningitis, particularly for infections caused by penicillin- and/or cefotaxime-resistant *S. pneumoniae*. In addition, it has been suggested that cefepime would not be a good choice for empiric treatment of meningitis if *Acinetobacter* may be involved.

■ **Septicemia** Cefepime is used for the treatment of septicemia† caused by susceptible gram-negative bacteria.

The choice of anti-infective agent for the treatment of sepsis syndrome should be based on the probable source of infection, causative organism, immune status of the patient, and local patterns of bacterial resistance. For initial treatment of life-threatening sepsis in adults, some clinicians recommend that a third or fourth generation cephalosporin (cefepime, cefotaxime, ceftriaxone, ceftazidime), the fixed combination of piperacillin and tazobactam, or a carbapenem (imipenem or meropenem) be used in conjunction with vancomycin; some experts also suggest including an aminoglycoside or fluoroquinolone during the initial few days of treatment.

■ **Empiric Therapy in Febrile Neutropenic Patients** Cefepime is used in adult and pediatric patients 2 months of age or older as monotherapy for empiric anti-infective therapy of presumed bacterial infections in febrile neutropenic patients. The manufacturers caution that use of monotherapy for empiric therapy in patients at high risk for *severe* infection (e.g., those with a history of recent bone marrow transplantation, hypotension on presentation, underlying hematologic malignancy, or severe or prolonged neutropenia) may not be appropriate and data regarding efficacy of cefepime monotherapy in these patients is limited to date.

Safety and efficacy of cefepime monotherapy for empiric therapy in febrile neutropenic patients were initially evaluated in a pilot study that involved 84 granulocytopenic cancer patients who received cefepime (2 g IV every 8 hours) for a minimum of 7 days or until infections resolved; the overall response rate in these patients was 71%. Cefepime also has been used in conjunction with amikacin for empiric therapy in febrile neutropenic patients in an open-label, randomized study in adults with chemotherapy-induced neutropenia who were considered at high risk of infection. Patients were randomized to receive empiric therapy with a combination regimen of cefepime (2 g IV every 12 hours) and amikacin (7.5 mg/kg every 12 hours) or ceftazidime (2 g IV every 8 hours) and amikacin (7.5 mg/kg every 12 hours); both regimens were comparable in terms of clinical response, rates of bacteriologic eradication, incidence of new infection, and survival.

There is evidence from open-label, randomized studies in febrile neutropenic patients that empiric therapy with cefepime monotherapy is as effective as empiric monotherapy with ceftazidime, imipenem, or the fixed combination of piperacillin and tazobactam or empiric treatment with combination regimens that consist of piperacillin sodium and gentamicin sulfate or ceftriaxone and amikacin.

Successful treatment of infections in granulocytopenic patients requires prompt initiation of empiric anti-infective therapy (even when fever is the only sign or symptom of infection) and appropriate modification of the initial regimen if the duration of fever and neutropenia is protracted, if a specific site of infection is identified, or if organisms resistant to the initial regimen are present. The initial empiric regimen should be chosen based on the underlying disease and other host factors that may affect the degree of risk and on local epidemiologic data regarding the type, frequency of occurrence, in vitro susceptibility of bacterial isolates recovered from other patients in the same health-care facility, and the individual patient's pattern of colonization and resistance. The fact that gram-positive bacteria have become a predominant pathogen in febrile neutropenic patients should be considered when selecting an empiric anti-infective regimen. However, although gram-positive bacteria reportedly account for about 60% and gram-negative bacteria account for about 35% of microbiologically documented infections, gram-negative infections are associated with greater mortality.

No empiric regimen has been identified that would be appropriate for initial treatment of all febrile neutropenic patients. The IDSA recommends use of a parenteral empiric regimen in most febrile neutropenic patients; use of an oral regimen (e.g., oral ciprofloxacin and oral amoxicillin and clavulanate potassium) should be considered *only* for selected adults at low risk for complications who have adequate and stable renal and hepatic function, an expected duration of neutropenia less than 7 days, and no active medical comorbidities. All other patients are considered high risk and should receive an initial IV empiric regimen consisting of an antipseudomonal β-lactam (e.g., cefepime, imipenem, meropenem, fixed-combination of piperacillin and tazobactam). Other anti-infectives (e.g., aminoglycosides, fluoroquinolones, and/or vancomycin) may be added to the regimen for the management of complications (e.g., pneumonia) or when antimicrobial resistance is suspected or proven. Vancomycin or other anti-infectives active against aerobic gram-positive cocci are not usually included in the initial empiric regimen except in certain clinical scenarios, including suspected catheter-related infections, skin and soft tissue infections, pneumonia, or hemodynamic instability.

Regardless of the initial regimen selected, patients should be reassessed daily and the anti-infective regimen altered (if indicated) based on the presence or absence of fever, identification of the causative organism, and the clinical condition of the patient; anti-infectives active against gram-positive organisms may be discontinued after 2 days if there is no evidence of such infections.

Published protocols for the treatment of infections in febrile neutropenic patients should be consulted for specific recommendations regarding selection of the initial empiric anti-infective regimen, when to change the initial regimen, possible subsequent regimens, and duration of therapy in these patients. In addition, consultation with an infectious disease expert knowledgeable about infections in immunocompromised patients is advised.

For additional information on the role of parenteral cephalosporins in the treatment of these and other infections, see Uses in the Cephalosporins General Statement 8:12.06.

Dosage and Administration

■ Reconstitution and Administration

Cefepime preferably is administered by IV infusion but also can be given by deep IM injection when indicated depending on the severity of the infection being treated.

The manufacturer states that IM administration of the drug is indicated *only* for the treatment of mild to moderate uncomplicated or complicated urinary tract infections caused by *Escherichia coli* and *only* when this route is considered more appropriate

If an aminoglycoside, ampicillin (at a concentration exceeding 40 mg/mL), metronidazole, vancomycin, or aminophylline is administered concomitantly with cefepime, the drugs should be administered separately.

Reconstituted and diluted solutions of cefepime should be inspected visually for particulate matter prior to administration whenever solution and container permit.

Intermittent IV Infusion

For intermittent IV infusion, vials labeled as containing 500 mg, 1 g, or 2 g of cefepime should be reconstituted with 5, 10, or 10 mL, respectively, of a compatible IV solution to provide solutions containing approximately 100, 100, or 160 mg/mL of the drug, respectively. The appropriate dose of the drug should then be added to a compatible IV solution.

Alternatively, ADD-Vantage® vials containing 1 or 2 g of cefepime should be reconstituted with 50 or 100 mL, respectively, of 0.9% sodium chloride or 5% dextrose injection according to the manufacturer's directions and administered by IV infusion.

Another alternative is the commercially available Duplex® drug delivery system that contains 1 or 2 g of cefepime and 50 mL of 5% dextrose injection in separate chambers, which should be reconstituted (activated) according to the manufacturer's directions and administered by IV infusion. If stored in the refrigerator after reconstitution (see Chemistry and Stability: Stability), the solution should be allowed to reach room temperature prior to administration.

Thawed solutions of the commercially available frozen premixed cefepime injection in dextrose should be administered only by IV infusion. The frozen injection should be thawed at room temperature (25°C) or under refrigeration (5°C); the injection should not be thawed by warming in a water bath or by exposure to microwave radiation. Precipitates that may have formed in the frozen injection usually will dissolve with little or no agitation when the injection reaches room temperature; potency is not affected. After thawing to room temperature, the injection should be agitated and the container checked for minute leaks by firmly squeezing the bag; the container may be fragile and should be handled with care. The injection should be discarded if container seals or outlet ports are not intact or leaks are found or if the solution is cloudy or contains an insoluble precipitate. Additives should not be introduced into the injection container. The injection should not be used in series connections with other plastic containers, since such use could result in air embolism from residual air being drawn from the primary container before administration of fluid from the secondary container is complete.

If a Y-type administration set is used, the other solution flowing through the tubing should be discontinued while cefepime is being infused.

Rate of Administration. The cefepime dose should be administered by IV infusion over approximately 30 minutes.

IM Injection

IM injections of cefepime are prepared by adding 1.3 or 2.4 mL of an appropriate diluent (i.e., sterile water for injection, 0.9% sodium chloride, 5% dextrose, 0.5 or 1% lidocaine hydrochloride, bacteriostatic water for injection with parabens or benzyl alcohol) to a vial labeled as containing 500 mg or 1 g of cefepime, respectively, to provide a solution containing approximately 280 mg/mL.

■ Dosage

Cefepime is commercially available as cefepime hydrochloride, which is monohydrated; dosage is expressed in terms of cefepime, calculated on the anhydrous basis.

Adult Dosage

Intra-abdominal Infections. For the treatment of complicated intra-abdominal infections (in conjunction with IV metronidazole), the usual adult dosage of cefepime is 2 g given IV every 12 hours for 7–10 days.

For the treatment of complicated intra-abdominal infections (in conjunction with IV metronidazole), some experts recommend that adults receive cefepime in a dosage of 2 g every 8–12 hours for 4–7 days. A longer duration of treatment has not been associated with improved outcome and is not recommended unless adequate source control is difficult to achieve.

Respiratory Tract Infections. For the treatment of moderate to severe pneumonia caused by *Streptococcus pneumoniae* (including those with concurrent bacteremia), the usual adult dosage of cefepime is 1–2 g given IV every 12 hours for 10 days.

For initial treatment of hospital-acquired pneumonia, ventilator-associated pneumonia, or health-care associated pneumonia, some clinicians recommend that adults receive a cefepime dosage of 1–2 g every 8–12 hours.

Skin and Skin Structure Infections. For the treatment of moderate to severe uncomplicated skin and skin structure infections caused by *Staphylococcus aureus* or *Streptococcus pyogenes*, the usual adult dosage of cefepime is 2 g IV every 12 hours for 10 days.

Urinary Tract Infections. For the treatment of mild to moderate uncomplicated or complicated urinary tract infections (including those associated with pyelonephritis and/or with concurrent bacteremia), the usual adult dosage of cefepime is 0.5–1 g administered IV or IM every 12 hours for 7–10 days.

For the treatment of severe uncomplicated or complicated urinary tract infections (including those associated with pyelonephritis and/or concurrent bacteremia), adults should received 2 g of cefepime IV every 12 hours for 10 days.

Endocarditis. If cefepime is used in a multiple-drug regimen for empiric treatment of culture-negative endocarditis† in prosthetic valve recipients (see Uses: Endocarditis), the American Heart Association (AHA) recommends that adults receive IV cefepime in a dosage of 6 g daily given in 3 equally divided doses in conjunction with vancomycin (30 mg/kg daily given IV in 2 equally divided doses), gentamicin (3 mg/kg daily given IV or IM in 3 equally divided doses), and rifampin (900 mg daily given orally or IV in 3 equally divided doses). The multiple-drug regimen should be continued for 6 weeks; gentamicin should be discontinued after the first 2 weeks of treatment.

Meningitis and Other CNS Infections. For the treatment of meningitis† in adults, the Infectious Diseases Society of America (IDSA) recommends that IV cefepime be given in a dosage of 2 g every 8 hours.

IDSA states that the duration of therapy should be individualized based on response and recommends a duration of 7 days for infections caused by *Haemophilus influenzae* or *Neisseria meningitidis*, 10–14 days for infections caused by *S. pneumoniae*, or 21 days for infections caused by aerobic gram-negative bacilli.

Empiric Therapy in Febrile Neutropenic Patients. When cefepime is used as monotherapy for empiric anti-infective therapy in febrile neutropenic patients, adults should receive a dosage of 2 g IV every 8 hours for 7 days or until neutropenia resolves. The need for continued anti-infective therapy in patients whose fever resolves but who remain neutropenic for longer than 7 days should be frequently reevaluated.

Pediatric Dosage

General Pediatric Dosage. For the treatment of uncomplicated and complicated urinary tract infections (including pyelonephritis), uncomplicated skin and skin structure infections, or pneumonia, the manufacturers recommend that pediatric patients 2 months to 16 years of age weighing less than 40 kg receive cefepime in a dosage of 50 mg/kg given IV every 12 hours. Pediatric dosage should not exceed the recommended adult dosage.

Although safety and efficacy of cefepime have not been established in neonates or infants younger than 2 months of age, the American Academy of Pediatrics (AAP) states that neonates 28 days of age or younger† may receive IV or IM cefepime in a dosage of 30 mg/kg every 12 hours and that a dosage of 50 mg/kg every 12 hours may be required for *Pseudomonas* infections.

The AAP states that pediatric patients beyond the neonatal period may receive IV or IM cefepime in a dosage of 100 mg/kg daily in 2 equally divided doses for the treatment of mild to moderate infections or a dosage of 100–150 mg/kg daily in 2 or 3 equally divided doses for the treatment of severe infections.

To avoid unintentional overdosage, the manufacturers state that the commercially available Duplex® drug delivery systems containing cefepime and the commercially available frozen premixed cefepime injection should *not* be used in pediatric patients who require less than the entire 1- or 2-g dose in the container.

Intra-abdominal Infections. For the treatment of complicated intra-abdominal infections (in conjunction with IV metronidazole) in pediatric patients, some experts recommend a cefepime dosage of 50 mg/kg every 12 hours for 4–7 days. A longer duration of treatment has not been associated with improved outcome and is not recommended unless adequate source control is difficult to achieve.

Endocarditis. If cefepime is used in a multiple-drug regimen for empiric treatment of culture-negative endocarditis† in prosthetic valve recipients (see Uses: Endocarditis), the AHA recommends that pediatric patients receive IV cefepime in a dosage of 150 mg/kg daily given in 3 equally divided doses in conjunction with vancomycin (40 mg/kg daily given IV in 2 or 3 equally divided doses), gentamicin (3 mg/kg daily given IV or IM in 3 equally divided doses), and rifampin (20 mg/kg daily given orally or IV in 3 equally divided doses). The multiple-drug regimen should be continued for 6 weeks; gentamicin should be discontinued after the first 2 weeks of treatment.

Meningitis and Other CNS Infections. For the treatment of meningitis†, infants and children 2 months to 15 years of age have received IV cefepime in a dosage of 50 mg/kg every 8 hours for 7–10 days.

IDSA states that the duration of therapy should be individualized based on response and recommends a duration of 7 days for infections caused by *H. influenzae* or *N. meningitidis*, 10–14 days for infections caused by *S. pneumoniae*, or 21 days for infections caused by aerobic gram-negative bacilli.

Empiric Therapy in Febrile Neutropenic Patients. When cefepime is used as monotherapy for empiric anti-infective therapy in febrile neutropenic pediatric patients 2 months to 16 years of age who weigh less than 40 kg, the manufacturers recommend a dosage of 50 mg/kg given IV every 8 hours. The need for continued anti-infective therapy in patients whose fever resolves but who remain neutropenic for longer than 7 days should be frequently reevaluated.

■ Dosage in Renal and Hepatic Impairment

In patients with renal impairment (i.e., creatinine clearance of 60 mL/minute or less), doses and/or frequency of administration of cefepime should be modified in response to the degree of renal impairment, severity of the infection, and susceptibility of the causative organism.

The manufacturers recommend that adults with creatinine clearance of 60 mL/minute or less (not receiving hemodialysis) receive the same initial dose of cefepime recommended for patients with normal renal function followed by a maintenance dosage of cefepime based on the patient's measured or estimated creatinine clearance. (See Table 1 and Table 2.)

Table 1. Maintenance Dosage for Treatment of Infections in Adults with Renal Impairment

Creatinine Clearance (mL/minute)	Initial dose: 500 mg	Initial dose: 1 g	Initial dose: 2 g
30–60	500 mg every 24 h	1 g every 24 h	2 g every 24 h
11–29	500 mg every 24 h	500 mg every 24 h	1 g every 24 h
<11	250 mg every 24 h	250 mg every 24 h	500 mg every 24 h

Table 2. Maintenance Dosage for Empiric Therapy in Febrile Neutropenic Adults with Renal Impairment

Creatinine Clearance (mL/minute)	Initial Dose: 2 g
30–60	2 g every 12 h
11–29	2 g every 24 h
<11	1 g every 24 h

The manufacturers recommend that adults undergoing hemodialysis receive an initial 1-g dose of cefepime on day 1, then 500 mg once daily thereafter for the treatment of infections or 1 g once daily for empiric therapy of presumed bacterial infections in febrile neutropenic patients. The manufacturers also recommend that the daily dose be given at the same time of day whenever possible; on hemodialysis days, the dose should be given after the procedure.

Adults undergoing continuous ambulatory peritoneal dialysis (CAPD) should receive the usual cefepime dose every 48 hours.

Data regarding use of cefepime in pediatric patients with impaired renal function are not available. Because the pharmacokinetics of cefepime are similar in pediatric and adult patients, the manufacturers recommend that dosage modifications proportional to those recommended for adults be used in pediatric patients with impaired renal function.

Since pharmacokinetics of cefepime appear not to be altered in patients with hepatic impairment, the manufacturers state that dosage adjustments are not necessary in such patients.

Cautions

■ Adverse Effects

Adverse effects reported with cefepime are similar to those reported with other parenteral cephalosporins. (See Cautions in the Cephalosporins General Statement 8:12.06.) Cefepime generally is well tolerated. Most adverse effects are transient and mild to moderate in severity, but have been severe enough to require discontinuance of the drug in up to 3% of patients. Headache, rash, diarrhea, nausea, and vomiting have been reported in up to 2% and local reactions, including phlebitis, pain and/or inflammation, and rash, have been reported in up to 3% of patients receiving cefepime in a dosage of 0.5–2 g every 12 hours. In patients receiving cefepime in a dosage of 2 g every 8 hours, rash occurred in 4%, diarrhea in 3%, nausea in 2%, and vomiting, headache, pruritus, or fever in 1% of patients. Neutropenia has been reported rarely in patients receiving cefepime.

■ Precautions and Contraindications

Cefepime shares the toxic potentials of other cephalosporins, and the usual cautions, precautions, and contraindications associated with cephalosporin therapy should be observed.

Sensitivity Reactions Prior to initiation of cefepime therapy, careful inquiry should be made concerning previous hypersensitivity reactions to cefepime, cephalosporins, penicillins, or other drugs. There is clinical and laboratory evidence of partial cross-allergenicity among cephalosporins and other β-lactam antibiotics, including penicillins and cephamycins.

Cefepime is contraindicated in patients who are hypersensitive to the drug or other cephalosporins and should be used with caution in patients with a history of hypersensitivity to penicillins. Use of cephalosporins generally should be avoided in patients who have had an immediate-type (anaphylactic) hypersensitivity reaction to penicillins.

The manufacturers of the commercially available Duplex® drug delivery system containing cefepime and dextrose injection and the commercially available frozen premixed cefepime injection in dextrose state that solutions containing dextrose may be contraindicated in patients with known allergy or hypersensitivity to corn or corn products.

Anaphylaxis, including anaphylactic shock, has been reported in a few patients receiving cefepime.

If a hypersensitivity reaction occurs during cefepime therapy, the drug should be discontinued and the patient treated with appropriate therapy (e.g., epinephrine, corticosteroids, and maintenance of an adequate airway and oxygen) as indicated.

Neurotoxicity Serious adverse events, including life-threatening or fatal encephalopathy (disturbance of consciousness including confusion, hallucinations, stupor, and coma), myoclonus, and seizures, have been reported in patients receiving cefepime during postmarketing experience. Nonconvulsive status epilepticus, characterized by alteration of consciousness without convulsions that is associated with continuous epileptiform EEG activity, also has been reported.

Most cases of cefepime-associated neurotoxicity have occurred in patients with renal impairment who received a cefepime dosage that exceeded the recommended dosage for such patients. However, some cases of neurotoxicity occurred in patients who received a dosage appropriately adjusted for renal impairment or in patients with normal renal function. In most reported cases, symptoms of neurotoxicity were reversible and resolved after discontinuance of cefepime and/or after hemodialysis.

If neurotoxicity associated with cefepime therapy occurs, consideration should be given to discontinuing the drug or making appropriate dosage adjustments based on the patient's renal function. (See Dosage and Administration: Dosage in Renal and Hepatic Impairment.)

Patients should be advised that neurologic adverse events can occur and to immediately contact a clinician if any neurologic signs and symptoms, including encephalopathy (disturbance of consciousness including confusion, hallucinations, stupor, coma), myoclonus, seizures, or nonconvulsive status epilepticus, occur since immediate treatment, dosage adjustment, or discontinuance of cefepime therapy is required.

Increased Mortality In November 2007, FDA announced that a safety review of cefepime was initiated after a published meta-analysis described a higher risk of all-cause mortality in patients treated with cefepime compared with patients treated with comparator β-lactams. The published meta-analysis looked at all-cause mortality data from 57 randomized controlled trials that compared cefepime with other β-lactams for various indications and found a risk ratio of 1.26 in those who received cefepime. FDA began working with Bristol-Myers Squibb to further evaluate the findings presented in the published meta-analysis and additional safety data.

On June 17, 2009, FDA announced that, although the safety review is ongoing, it has determined that cefepime remains an appropriate therapy for its approved indications based on results of FDA's additional meta-analyses. FDA performed meta-analyses based on both trial- and patient-level data derived from all available cefepime comparative clinical trials. FDA's trial-level meta-analysis included data from 88 clinical trials (total of 9467 cefepime-treated patients and 8288 comparator-treated patients) and found no statistically significant differences in mortality between cefepime and the comparator drugs. Results of the trial-level meta-analysis indicated that all-cause mortality rates 30 days after treatment were 6.21% for cefepime-treated patients and 6% for comparator-treated patients. FDA's patient-level meta-analysis included data from 35 clinical trials and results indicated that all-cause mortality rates 30 days after treatment were 5.63% for cefepime-treated patients and 5.68% for comparator-treated patients. In addition, in a trial-level meta-analysis of 24 febrile neutropenia trials, there was no statistically significant increase in mortality in cefepime-treated patients compared with comparator-treated patients. A review of deaths reported in 7 of these febrile neutropenia trials indicated that most patients appeared to have died from their underlying malignancies and/or comorbid conditions.

Selection and Use of Anti-infectives To reduce development of drug-resistant bacteria and maintain effectiveness of cefepime and other antibacterials, the drug should be used only for the treatment or prevention of infections proven or strongly suspected to be caused by susceptible bacteria. When selecting or modifying anti-infective therapy, use results of culture and in vitro susceptibility testing. In the absence of such data, consider local epidemiology and susceptibility patterns when selecting anti-infectives for empiric therapy.

Patients should be advised that antibacterials (including cefepime) should only be used to treat bacterial infections and not used to treat viral infections (e.g., the common cold). Patients also should be advised about the importance of completing the full course of therapy, even if feeling better after a few days, and that skipping doses or not completing therapy may decrease effectiveness and increase the likelihood that bacteria will develop resistance and will not be treatable with cefepime or other antibacterials in the future.

Superinfection/Clostridium difficile-associated Diarrhea and Colitis As with other anti-infectives, prolonged cefepime therapy may result in overgrowth of nonsusceptible organisms. Careful observation of the patient is essential. If superinfection occurs, appropriate therapy should be initiated.

Treatment with anti-infectives alters the normal colon flora and may permit overgrowth of *Clostridium difficile*. *C. difficile* infection (CDI) and *C. difficile*-associated diarrhea and colitis (CDAD; also known as antibiotic-associated diarrhea and colitis or pseudomembranous colitis) have been reported with nearly all anti-infectives, including cefepime, and may range in severity from mild diarrhea to fatal colitis. *C. difficile* produces toxins A and B, which contribute to the development of CDAD; hypertoxin-producing strains of *C. difficile* are associated with increased morbidity and mortality since these infections may be refractory to anti-infective therapy and may require colectomy.

CDAD should be considered in the differential diagnosis of patients who develop diarrhea during or after anti-infective therapy. Careful medical history is necessary since CDAD has been reported to occur as late as 2 months or longer after anti-infective therapy is discontinued.

If CDAD is suspected or confirmed, anti-infective therapy not directed against *C. difficile* should be discontinued whenever possible. Patients should be managed with appropriate supportive therapy (e.g., fluid and electrolyte management, protein supplementation), anti-infective therapy directed against *C. difficile* (e.g., metronidazole, vancomycin), and surgical evaluation as clinically needed.

Patients should be advised that diarrhea is a common problem caused by anti-infectives and usually resolves when the drug is discontinued; however, they should contact a clinician if severe watery or bloody diarrhea develops.

Other Precautions and Contraindications Cefepime should be used with caution in patients with a history of GI disease, particularly colitis. (See Superinfection/Clostridium difficile-associated Diarrhea and Colitis under Cautions: Precautions and Contraindications.)

Commercially available cefepime preparations contain L-arginine to adjust pH. (See Chemistry and Stability: Chemistry.) At concentrations 33 times higher than the amount provided by the maximum recommended human cefepime dosage, arginine has been shown to alter glucose metabolism and transiently increase serum potassium concentrations. The effect of lower arginine concentrations is not known.

Like other dextrose-containing solutions, the commercially available Duplex® drug delivery system containing cefepime and 5% dextrose injection should be used with caution in patients with overt or known subclinical diabetes mellitus or in patients with carbohydrate intolerance for any reason.

High or prolonged serum cefepime concentrations can occur if usual dosage is used in patients with renal impairment or other conditions that may compromise renal function. Serious adverse events, including life-threatening or fatal encephalopathy, may occur if inappropriate cefepime dosage is used in patients with impaired renal function. (See Neurotoxicity under Cautions: Precautions and Contraindications.) The maintenance dosage of cefepime should be decreased whenever the drug is used in patients with renal impairment (i.e., creatinine clearance 60 mL/minute or less) and continued dosage should be determined by the degree of renal impairment, severity of the infection, and susceptibility of the causative organisms. (See Dosage and Administration: Dosage in Renal and Hepatic Impairment.)

For a more complete discussion of these and other precautions associated with the use of cefepime, see Cautions: Precautions and Contraindications in the Cephalosporins General Statement 8:12.06.

■ **Pediatric Precautions** Safety and efficacy of cefepime have not been established in neonates or infants younger than 2 months of age.

Safety and efficacy of cefepime have been established for use in pediatric patients 2 months to 16 years of age for the treatment of uncomplicated and complicated urinary tract infections (including pyelonephritis), uncomplicated skin and skin structure infections, and pneumonia and for empiric therapy for febrile neutropenic patients. Use of cefepime in this age group is supported by evidence from adequate and well-controlled studies evaluating the drug in adults and additional pharmacokinetic and safety data from pediatric studies.

Adverse effects reported when cefepime was used in pediatric patients 2 months to 16 years of age have been similar to those reported in adults.

The manufacturers caution that cefepime should not be used in pediatric patients of any age for the treatment of serious infections that are suspected or known to be caused by *Haemophilus influenzae* type b (Hib) and states that pediatric patients in whom meningeal seeding from a distant infection site or in whom meningitis is suspected or documented should receive an alternative anti-infective with demonstrated clinical efficacy in this setting.

Although safety and efficacy for the treatment of meningitis† have not been established, cefepime has been used effectively in a limited number of children 2 months to 15 years of age for the treatment of meningitis caused by susceptible bacteria. (See Uses: Meningitis and Other CNS Infections.) In one study in pediatric patients with meningitis, adverse effects were reported in 18% of patients receiving cefepime and included diarrhea, macular rash, candidal thrush, and eosinophilia.

The manufacturers state that the commercially available Duplex® drug delivery system containing cefepime and the commercially available frozen premixed cefepime injection should be used in pediatric patients *only* if the entire 1- or 2-g dose in the container is required.

■ **Geriatric Precautions** Studies evaluating safety and efficacy of cefepime indicate that there are no age-related differences when the drug is used in geriatric patients or in younger adults.

Cefepime is substantially eliminated by kidneys, and the risk of toxicity may be greater in those with impaired renal function. Serious adverse effects (e.g., life-threatening or fatal encephalopathy, myoclonus, or seizures) have occurred in geriatric patients with renal impairment who received cefepime dosages that were not adjusted based on the degree of renal impairment.

Whenever cefepime is used in geriatric patients, select dosage with caution and monitor renal function because of age-related decreases in renal function. (See Dosage and Administration: Dosage in Renal and Hepatic Impairment.)

■ **Mutagenicity and Carcinogenicity** In vivo and in vitro studies evaluating cefepime have not shown evidence of mutagenicity. Long-term animal studies have not been performed to evaluate the carcinogenic potential of the drug.

■ **Pregnancy, Fertility, and Lactation** Reproduction studies in rats, rabbits, or mice using cefepime dosages approximately 1.6 times or 0.3 times, or equal to the recommended maximum human dosage (calculated on a mg/m^2 basis), respectively, have not revealed evidence of teratogenicity or embryotoxicity. There are no adequate and controlled studies using cefepime in pregnant women or during labor and delivery, and the drug should be used during pregnancy only when clearly needed.

Studies in rats using subcutaneous cefepime dosages 1.6 times the recommended maximum human dosage (calculated on a mg/m^2 basis) have not revealed evidence of impaired fertility.

Cefepime is distributed into milk in low concentrations following parenteral administration, and the drug should be used with caution in nursing women.

Spectrum

Based on its spectrum of activity and decreased susceptibility to certain β-lactamases, cefepime is classified as a fourth generation cephalosporin. For information on the classification of cephalosporins and closely related β-lactam antibiotics based on spectra of activity, see Spectrum in the Cephalosporins General Statement 8:12.06.

Fourth generation cephalosporins (e.g., cefepime) usually have a spectrum of activity against gram-negative bacteria that includes organisms susceptible to most third generation cephalosporins; however, the drugs also are active against some gram-negative bacteria, including *Pseudomonas aeruginosa* and certain Enterobacteriaceae, that generally are resistant to most third generation cephalosporins. The activity of cefepime against *Ps. aeruginosa* is similar to that of ceftazidime. Cefepime is more active in vitro against some gram-positive bacteria (e.g., staphylococci) than some third generation cephalosporins (e.g., ceftazidime).

■ **In Vitro Susceptibility Testing** Strains of staphylococci resistant to penicillinase-resistant penicillins (methicillin-resistant [oxacillin-resistant] staphylococci) should be considered resistant to cefepime, although results of in vitro susceptibility tests may indicate that the organisms are susceptible to the drug.

For information on interpreting results of in vitro susceptibility testing (disk susceptibility tests, dilution susceptibility tests) when cefepime susceptibility testing is performed according to the standards of the Clinical and Laboratory Standards Institute (CLSI; formerly National Committee for Clinical Laboratory Standards [NCCLS]), see Spectrum: In Vitro Susceptibility Testing, in the Cephalosporins General Statement 8:12.06.

Pharmacokinetics

Studies in adults indicate that cefepime exhibits linear dose-dependent pharmacokinetics over the dosage range of 250 mg to 2 g, and there is no evidence of accumulation following multiple doses in healthy adults with normal renal function receiving usual parenteral dosages of the drug. While there is no evidence of accumulation of cefepime in pediatric patients 2 months to 11 years of age when the drug is given in a dosage of 50 mg/kg every 12 hours, steady-state peak plasma concentration, area under the concentration-time curve (AUC), and plasma half-life are increased about 15% when the drug is given in a dosage of 50 mg/kg every 8 hours.

There is no evidence of gender-related differences in the pharmacokinetics of cefepime, and differences in the pharmacokinetics of the drug in geriatric individuals appear to be related to changes in renal function rather than age.

Studies in adults with impaired renal function indicate that the pharmacokinetics of cefepime are affected by the degree of renal impairment and that total body clearance of the drug decreases in proportion to decreases in creatinine clearance. The pharmacokinetics of cefepime do not appear to be affected by hepatic impairment.

■ **Absorption** Cefepime is almost completely absorbed following IM administration. In healthy adult males who received single 500-mg, 1-g, or 2-g IM doses of cefepime, peak plasma concentrations of the drug were attained within 1.4–1.6 hours and averaged 13.9, 29.6, or 57.5 mcg/mL, respectively; plasma concentrations averaged 1.9, 4.5, or 8.7 mcg/mL, respectively, 8 hours after the dose. In children 2 months to 16 years of age who received a single 50-mg/kg dose IM, plasma cefepime concentrations averaged 76, 75.2, 64, and 4.8 mcg/mL at 0.5, 0.75, 1, and 8 hours, respectively, after the dose. The absolute bioavailability of cefepime after a single 50-mg/kg IM dose in pediatric patients has been reported to be 82.3%.

Following IV infusion over 30 minutes of a single 500-mg, 1-g, or 2-g dose of cefepime in healthy adult males, peak plasma concentrations of the drug average 31.6–39.1, 65.9–81.7, or 126–163.9 mcg/mL; plasma concentrations were still detectable 8 hours after the dose and averaged 1.4, 2.4, and 3.9 mcg/mL, respectively, in one study.

In pediatric patients 2 months to 15 years of age with bacterial meningitis who received cefepime dosages of 50 mg/kg every 8 hours given by IV infusion over 15–20 minutes, plasma concentrations averaged 67.1, 44.1, 23.9, 11.7, and 4.9 mcg/mL at 0.5, 1, 2, 4, and 8 hours, respectively, after the third dose. The manufacturers state that IV administration of a single 50-mg/kg dose of cefepime in pediatric patients results in cefepime exposure similar to that reported in adults following IV administration of a single 2-g dose of the drug.

■ **Distribution** The volume of distribution of cefepime at steady state ranges from 13–22 L in healthy adults, and averages 0.3 L/kg in pediatric patients 2 months to 11 years of age.

Following parenteral administration, cefepime is widely distributed into tissues and fluids, including blister fluid, bronchial mucosa, sputum, bile, peritoneal fluid, appendix, gallbladder, and prostate. In adults with acute cholecystitis who received 2 g of cefepime IV every 12 hours, concentrations of the drug in peritoneal fluid, bile, and gallbladder tissue in samples obtained 2–15 hours after a dose averaged 5.66 mcg/mL, 15.51 mcg/mL, and 5.35 mcg/g, respectively; concurrent plasma concentrations averaged 7.6 mcg/mL.

Cefepime is distributed into CSF following IV administration in adult or pediatric patients. In a study in adults who received cefepime in a dosage of 2 g every 12 hours given by IV infusion over 30 minutes, CSF concentrations ranged from 0.34–11.8 mcg/mL and minimum CSF concentrations were 5–58% of minimum serum concentrations. In children 2 months to 15 years of age who received 50-mg/kg doses of cefepime every 8 hours given by IV infusion over 15–20 minutes, CSF concentrations of the drug were 5.7, 4.3, 3.6, 4.2, and 3.3 mcg/mL at 0.5, 1, 2, 4, and 8 hours, respectively, after the third dose. There is evidence from a limited study in neonates with meningitis that cefepime CSF concentrations in premature neonates are higher than those reported in full-term neonates.

Cefepime is distributed into human milk. Following a single 1-g dose of cefepime given by IV infusion over 1 hour, peak concentrations of the drug in milk averaged 1.2 mcg/mL.

Cefepime is approximately 20% bound to serum proteins; binding is independent of drug concentrations.

■ **Elimination** In healthy adults with normal renal function, the plasma half-life of cefepime averages 2–2.3 hours and total body clearance averages 120 mL/minute. In pediatric patients, the plasma half-life of cefepime averages 1.9 hours in those 2 months up to 6 months of age and 1.5–1.7 hours in those 6 months to 16 years of age. Total body clearance reportedly averages 3.3 mL/minute per kg in pediatric patients 2 months to 11 years of age. Limited data from neonates younger than 2 months of age indicate that the mean plasma half-life of cefepime is 4.9 hours in this age group.

The plasma half-life of cefepime is prolonged in patients with renal impairment and averages 4.9, 10.5, and 13.5 hours in adults with creatinine clearances of 31–60, 11–30, or less than 10 mL/minute, respectively. Results of a single-dose study in a limited number of patients with impaired hepatic function indicate that the pharmacokinetics of cefepime are not affected by hepatic impairment.

Cefepime is partially metabolized in vivo to *N*-methylpyrrolidine (NMP) which is rapidly converted to the *N*-oxide (NMP-*N*-oxide). The drug is eliminated principally unchanged in urine by glomerular filtration. In adults with normal renal function, 80–82% of a single dose of cefepime is excreted unchanged in urine; less than 1% of the dose is eliminated as NMP, 6.8% as NMP-*N*-oxide, and 2.5% as an epimer of cefepime. In adults with normal renal function who received single 500-mg, 1-g, or 2-g IV doses of cefepime, urine concentrations of the drug in samples obtained within 4 hours after the dose averaged 292, 926, or 3120 mcg/mL, respectively. In pediatric patients 2 months to 11 years of age who received a single 50-mg/kg IV dose of cefepime, 60% of the dose was excreted unchanged in urine and the average renal clearance was 2 mL/minute per kg.

Cefepime is removed by hemodialysis and peritoneal dialysis. The amount of cefepime removed during hemodialysis depends on several factors (e.g., type of coil used, dialysis flow-rate); however, a 3- to 5-hour period of hemodialysis removes into the dialysate approximately 20–68% of a dose of the drug. In a study in patients with end-stage renal failure undergoing continuous ambulatory peritoneal dialysis (CAPD) who received a single 1- or 2-g IV dose of cefepime given over 30 minutes, approximately 25% of the dose was removed into the peritoneal dialysate over 72 hours; the plasma half-life of the drug in these patients ranged from 15.4–22.6 hours.

Chemistry and Stability

■ **Chemistry** Cefepime is a semisynthetic cephalosporin antibiotic. The drug is a parenteral zwitterionic aminothiazolyl cephalosporin. Cefepime is structurally similar to parenteral third generation cephalosporins that contain an aminothiazolyl side chain at position 7 of the cephalosporin nucleus (e.g., cefotaxime, ceftazidime, ceftriaxone). The aminothiazolyl side chain enhances antibacterial activity, particularly against Enterobacteriaceae, and generally results in enhanced stability against β-lactamases. However, cefepime contains an alkoxyimino group in the side chain rather than the methoxyimino group contained in many aminothiazolyl cephalosporins. The alkoxyimino group results in increased activity against staphylococci. In addition, cefepime contains a quaternary *N*-methylpyrrolidine (NMP) group at the 3-position, resulting in a zwitterion that enhances stability against certain β-lactamases and penetration through the outer membrane of gram-negative bacteria.

Cefepime is commercially available for parenteral use as cefepime hydrochloride, which is monohydrated; potency of cefepime hydrochloride is expressed in terms of cefepime, calculated on the anhydrous basis. Cefepime hydrochloride occurs as a white to pale yellow powder and contains the equivalent of not less than 825 mcg and not more than 911 mcg of cefepime per mg, calculated on the anhydrous basis. The drug is highly soluble in water and has pK_as of 1.5–1.6 and 3.1–3.2.

Cefepime hydrochloride powder for IM injection or IV infusion that is commercially available in vials contains a mixture of the drug and L-arginine; the powder for injection contains 707 mg of L-arginine per g of cefepime. When vials containing 500 mg, 1 g, or 2 g of cefepime are reconstituted as directed, the resultant cefepime hydrochloride solutions have a pH of 4–6 and range in color from pale yellow to amber.

When the commercially available Duplex® delivery system that contains 1 or 2 g of cefepime powder (with approximately 725 mg of L-arginine per g of cefepime) and 50 mL of 5% dextrose injection in separate chambers is reconstituted (activated) according to the manufacturer's directions, the resultant solution has a pH of 4–6 and an osmolality of approximately 431 or 577 mOsm/kg, respectively. The reconstituted solution may range in color from colorless to amber.

Commercially available frozen premixed injections of cefepime hydrochloride in dextrose are sterile, nonpyrogenic, iso-osmotic solutions of the drug provided in a plastic container fabricated from specially formulated multilayered plastic PL 2040 (Galaxy®). The 1- or 2-g frozen injections of cefepime contain 1.03 or 2.06 g of dextrose, respectively, to adjust osmolality. The 1- or 2-g frozen injections also contain 725 mg or 1.45 g of L-arginine, respectively, and may contain hydrochloric acid to adjust pH to 4–6. These premixed injections may range in color from colorless to amber.

■ **Stability** Like some other cephalosporins, cefepime hydrochloride powder for injection and solutions of the drug tend to darken, depending on storage conditions; however, such discoloration does not indicate loss of potency.

Vials containing cefepime hydrochloride powder for IM injection or IV infusion should be stored at 20–25°C and protected from light. Following reconstitution and dilution in 0.9% sodium chloride, 5 or 10% dextrose, ⅙ *M* sodium lactate, 5% dextrose and 0.9% sodium chloride, lactated Ringer's and 5% dextrose, Normosol®-R, or Normosol®-M in 5% dextrose injection, cefepime solutions for IV infusion containing 1–40 mg/mL are stable for 24 hours when stored at a room temperature of 20–25°C or for 7 days when refrigerated at 2–8°C.

Following reconstitution with sterile water for injection, 0.9% sodium chloride, 5% dextrose, 0.5 or 1% lidocaine hydrochloride, sterile bacteriostatic water for injection with parabens or benzyl alcohol, cefepime solutions for IM injection containing 280 mg/mL are stable for 24 hours when stored at a room temperature of 20–25°C or for 7 days when refrigerated at 2–8°C.

Following reconstitution of ADD-Vantage® vials containing 1 or 2 g of cefepime according to the manufacturer's directions, IV solutions containing 10–40 mg/mL in 5% dextrose injection or 0.9% sodium chloride injection are stable for 24 hours at 20–25°C or 7 days at 2–8°C.

The commercially available Duplex® delivery system that contains 1 or 2 g of cefepime and 50 mL of 5% dextrose injection in separate chambers should be stored at 20–25°C, but may be exposed to temperatures ranging from 15–30°C. Following reconstitution (activation), these IV solutions must be used within 12 hours if stored at room temperature or within 5 days if stored in a refrigerator and should not be frozen.

The commercially available frozen premixed cefepime hydrochloride injection in dextrose should be stored at −20°C or lower. The frozen injections should be thawed at room temperature (25°C) or under refrigeration (5°C) and, once thawed, should not be refrozen. Thawed solutions of the commercially available frozen injections are stable for 24 hours at room temperature (25°C) or 7 days under refrigeration (5°C). The commercially available frozen injections of the drug are provided in plastic containers fabricated from specially formulated multilayered plastic PL 2040 (Galaxy®). Solutions in contact with PL 2040 can leach out some of its chemical components in very small amounts within the expiration period of the injection; however, safety of the plastic has been confirmed in tests in animals according to USP biological tests for plastic containers as well as by tissue culture toxicity studies.

For further information on chemistry, mechanism of action, spectrum, resistance, uses, cautions, acute toxicity, drug interactions, or laboratory test interferences of cefepime, see the Cephalosporins General Statement 8:12.06.

Preparations

Excipients in commercially available drug preparations may have clinically important effects in some individuals; consult specific product labeling for details.

Cefepime Hydrochloride

Parenteral		
For injection	500 mg (of anhydrous cefepime)*	**Cefepime Hydrochloride for Injection**
		Maxipime®, Hospira
	1 g (of anhydrous cefepime)*	**Cefepime Hydrochloride for Injection**
		Maxipime®, Hospira
	2 g (of anhydrous cefepime)*	**Cefepime Hydrochloride for Injection**
		Maxipime®, Hospira
For injection, for IV infusion	1 g (of anhydrous cefepime)*	**Cefepime Hydrochloride for Injection** (available in dual-chambered Duplex® drug delivery system with 5% dextrose injection), B Braun
		Maxipime® ADD-Vantage®, Hospira
	2 g (of anhydrous cefepime)*	**Cefepime Hydrochloride for Injection** (available in dual-chambered Duplex® drug delivery system with 5% dextrose injection), B Braun
		Maxipime® ADD-Vantage®, Hospira

*available from one or more manufacturer, distributor, and/or repackager by generic (nonproprietary) name

Cefepime Hydrochloride in Dextrose

Parenteral		
Injection (frozen), for IV infusion	20 mg (of cefepime) per mL (1 g) in 2% Dextrose*	**Cefepime Hydrochloride Iso-osmotic in Dextrose Injection** (Galaxy® [Baxter])
	20 mg (of cefepime) per mL (2 g) in 2% Dextrose*	**Cefepime Hydrochloride Iso-osmotic in Dextrose Injection** (Galaxy® [Baxter])

*available from one or more manufacturer, distributor, and/or repackager by generic (nonproprietary) name

†Use is not currently included in the labeling approved by the US Food and Drug Administration

Selected Revisions August 2013,

FIFTH GENERATION CEPHALOSPORINS 8:12.06.20

Ceftaroline Fosamil

■ Ceftaroline is a semisynthetic, fifth generation cephalosporin antibiotic.

Uses

■ **Community-acquired Pneumonia** Ceftaroline fosamil is used for the treatment of community-acquired bacterial pneumonia (CABP, CAP) caused by susceptible *Streptococcus pneumoniae* (including cases with concurrent bacteremia), *Staphylococcus aureus* (methicillin-susceptible [oxacillin-susceptible] strains only), *Haemophilus influenzae, Klebsiella pneumoniae, K. oxytoca,* or *Escherichia coli* in adults and pediatric patients 2 months of age and older.

Initial treatment of CAP generally involves use of an empiric anti-infective regimen based on the most likely pathogens and local susceptibility patterns; treatment may then be changed (if possible) to provide a more specific regimen

(pathogen-directed therapy) based on results of in vitro culture and susceptibility testing. The most appropriate empiric regimen varies depending on the severity of illness at the time of presentation, whether outpatient treatment or hospitalization in or out of an intensive care unit (ICU) is indicated, and the presence or absence of cardiopulmonary disease and other modifying factors that increase the risk of certain pathogens (e.g., methicillin-resistant *S. aureus* [MRSA; also known as oxacillin-resistant *S. aureus* or ORSA], penicillin-resistant *S. pneumoniae*, multidrug-resistant *S. pneumoniae* [MDRSP], enteric gram-negative bacilli, *Pseudomonas aeruginosa*).

For information regarding the treatment of CAP, including infections caused by MRSA, the current clinical practice guidelines from the Infectious Diseases Society of America (IDSA) available at http://www.idsociety.org should be consulted.

Clinical Experience Efficacy of ceftaroline fosamil for the treatment of CAP in adults is based on results of 2 randomized, double-blind, active-controlled, phase 3 noninferiority trials in 1231 adults with CAP requiring hospitalization (Pneumonia Outcome Research Team [PORT] risk class III or IV and *not* admitted to an intensive care unit). Patients in each trial (Focus 1 and Focus 2) were randomized to receive either ceftaroline fosamil (600 mg given by IV infusion over 1 hour every 12 hours) or ceftriaxone (1 g given by IV infusion over 30 minutes every 24 hours); patients in the first trial also received oral clarithromycin on the initial day of treatment (500 mg every 12 hours for 2 doses). Treatment duration was 5–7 days (maximum 7 days); a switch to oral therapy was not allowed. Patients with CAP known or suspected to be caused by methicillin-resistant *S. aureus* (MRSA; also known as oxacillin-resistant *S. aureus* or ORSA) or caused by an atypical pathogen (e.g., *Chlamydophila pneumoniae, Mycoplasma pneumoniae, Legionella*) alone were excluded from the trials.

In the first trial (Focus 1), clinical cure rates at the test-of-cure visit (8–15 days after treatment ended) in the clinically evaluable population were similar for ceftaroline- and ceftriaxone-treated patients (87 and 78%, respectively). Similarly, clinical cure rates in the second trial (Focus 2) were 82% with ceftaroline and 77% with ceftriaxone. When results from both adult trials were combined, the overall clinical cure rate in the clinically evaluable population was similar in patients treated with ceftaroline fosamil (84%) compared with those receiving ceftriaxone (78%). In addition, when results from both trials were pooled, the 30-day all-cause mortality rate did not differ between treatment groups.

When results from both adult trials were combined and stratified according to causative organism, the clinical cure rates at the test-of-cure visit in the microbiologically evaluable population that received ceftaroline fosamil were 86% for CAP caused by *S. pneumonia*, 72% for methicillin-susceptible *S. aureus*, 83% for *H. influenzae*, 100% for *K. pneumoniae*, 83% for *K. oxytoca*, and 83% for *E. coli*.

■ **Skin and Skin Structure Infections** Ceftaroline fosamil is used for the treatment of acute bacterial skin and skin structure infections (ABSSSI) caused by susceptible *S. aureus* (including MRSA), *S. pyogenes* (group A β-hemolytic streptococci, GAS), *S. agalactiae* (group B streptococci, GBS), *E. coli, K. pneumoniae,* or *K. oxytoca* in adults and children 2 months of age and older.

Ceftaroline fosamil is one of several anti-infectives that have been recommended for treatment of skin and skin structure infections caused by MRSA, including empiric treatment of surgical site infections in patients at high risk for MRSA (e.g., nasal colonization, prior MRSA infection, recent hospitalization, recent anti-infective therapy).

For information regarding the treatment of skin and skin structure infections, including infections caused by MRSA, the current IDSA clinical practice guidelines available at http://www.idsociety.org should be consulted.

Clinical Experience Efficacy of ceftaroline fosamil for the treatment of skin and skin structure infections in adults is based on the results of 2 randomized, double-blind, active-controlled trials in 1396 adults with complicated skin and skin structure infections (e.g., cellulitis, major abscess, infected wound/ulcer/burn). Patients in each trial (Canvas 1 and Canvas 2) were randomized to receive either ceftaroline fosamil with placebo (600 mg of ceftaroline fosamil given by IV infusion over 1 hour followed by placebo given by IV infusion over 1 hour every 12 hours) or a 2-drug regimen of vancomycin and aztreonam (1 g of vancomycin given by IV infusion over 1 hour followed by 1 g of aztreonam given by IV infusion over 1 hour every 12 hours). Treatment duration was 5–14 days (mean approximately 8 days); a switch to oral therapy was not allowed.

In the first trial (Canvas 1), clinical cure rates at the test-of-cure visit in the clinically evaluable population for ceftaroline-treated patients were similar to clinical cure rates for vancomycin- and aztreonam-treated patients (91 and 93%, respectively). Similarly, the clinical cure rate in the second trial (Canvas 2) was 92% in both treatment groups. When results from both adult trials were combined, the overall clinical cure rate in the clinically evaluable population was similar in those treated with ceftaroline fosamil (92%) compared with those treated with vancomycin and aztreonam (93%). Of the 693 patients in the modified intent-to-treat population from both trials, 20 patients had *S. aureus* bacteremia at baseline (11 with methicillin-susceptible strains, 9 with MRSA); 65% of these patients were clinical responders at study day 3 and 90% were considered clinical success at the test-of-cure visit (8–15 days after treatment ended).

When results from both adult trials were combined and stratified according to causative organism, the clinical cure rates in the microbiologically evaluable population that received ceftaroline fosamil were 93% for methicillin-susceptible *S. aureus*, 93% for MRSA, 100% for *S. pyogenes*, 96% for *S. agalactiae*, 95% for *E. coli*, 94% for *K. pneumoniae*, and 83% for *K. oxytoca*.

For additional information on the role of parenteral cephalosporins in the treatment of these and other infections, see Uses in the Cephalosporins General Statement 8:12.06.

Dosage and Administration

■ Administration

Ceftaroline fosamil is administered by IV infusion.

Ceftaroline fosamil solutions should not be admixed with or added to solutions containing other drugs.

Reconstitution and Dilution Ceftaroline fosamil must be reconstituted and further diluted prior to IV infusion. Strict aseptic technique must be observed when preparing IV solutions of the drug.

Single-use vials labeled as containing 400 or 600 mg of ceftaroline fosamil should be reconstituted by adding 20 mL of sterile water for injection, 0.9% sodium chloride injection, 5% dextrose injection, or lactated Ringer's injection, to provide a solution containing approximately 20 or 30 mg/mL, respectively. The vial should be gently mixed; reconstitution should be complete in less than 2 minutes.

Prior to IV administration, the appropriate dose of reconstituted solution must be further diluted in 50–250 mL of an appropriate infusion solution. The same diluent should be used for both reconstitution and further dilution unless the drug was reconstituted with sterile water, in which case the dose should be further diluted using any compatible IV solution (e.g., 0.45 or 0.9% sodium chloride injection, 2.5 or 5% dextrose injection, lactated Ringer's injection).

To prepare a 600-mg dose of ceftaroline fosamil in a 50-mL infusion bag for administration in adults, 20 mL of the diluent should be removed from the infusion bag prior to injecting the entire reconstituted contents of a 600-mg vial of the drug; the concentration of the final infusion solution is approximately 12 mg/mL.

To prepare a 400-mg dose of ceftaroline fosamil in a 50-mL infusion bag for administration in adults or pediatric patients 2 months of age or older weighing more than 33 kg, 20 mL of the diluent should be removed from the infusion bag prior to injecting the entire reconstituted contents of a 400-mg vial of the drug; the concentration of the final infusion solution is approximately 8 mg/mL.

To prepare a dose in a 50-mL infusion bag for administration in pediatric patients 2 months of age or older weighing 33 kg or less, the amount of diluent to be removed from the infusion bag *and* the amount of reconstituted solution of drug to be withdrawn from the vial and added to the diluent vary depending on the age and weight of the child. The concentration of the final infusion solution for these pediatric patients should not exceed 12 mg/mL.

Reconstituted and diluted ceftaroline fosamil solutions should appear clear and light to dark yellow, depending on the concentration and storage conditions. Final ceftaroline fosamil solutions in the IV infusion bag should be used within 6 hours when stored at room temperature or within 24 hours when stored in the refrigerator at 2–8°C. (See Chemistry and Stability: Stability.)

Rate of Administration IV infusions of ceftaroline fosamil should be given over 5–60 minutes.

■ Dosage

Ceftaroline fosamil is commercially available as ceftaroline fosamil monoacetate monohydrate; dosage is expressed in terms of anhydrous ceftaroline fosamil.

Adult Dosage **Community-acquired Pneumonia.** The recommended dosage of ceftaroline fosamil for the treatment of community-acquired bacterial pneumonia (CABP, CAP) in adults is 600 mg every 12 hours for 5–7 days.

The duration of therapy should be guided by the severity and site of infection and the patient's clinical and bacteriologic progress.

Skin and Skin Structure Infections. The recommended dosage of ceftaroline fosamil for the treatment of acute bacterial skin and skin structure infections (ABSSSI) in adults is 600 mg every 12 hours for 5–14 days.

The duration of therapy should be guided by the severity and site of infection and the patient's clinical and bacteriologic progress.

Pediatric Dosage **Community-acquired Pneumonia.** The recommended dosage of ceftaroline fosamil for the treatment of community-acquired bacterial pneumonia in pediatric patients 2 months to less than 2 years of age is 8 mg/kg every 8 hours. Pediatric patients 2 years to less than 18 years of age weighing 33 kg or less should receive 12 mg/kg every 8 hours and those 2 years to less than 18 years of age weighing more than 33 kg should receive 400 mg every 8 hours or 600 mg every 12 hours.

The manufacturer recommends a treatment duration of 5–14 days in pediatric patients; the duration of therapy should be guided by the severity and site of infection and the patient's clinical and bacteriologic progress.

Skin and Skin Structure Infections. The recommended dosage of ceftaroline fosamil for the treatment of acute bacterial skin and skin structure infections in pediatric patients 2 months to less than 2 years of age is 8 mg/kg every 8 hours. Pediatric patients 2 years to less than 18 years of age weighing 33 kg or less should receive 12 mg/kg every 8 hours and those 2 years to less than 18 years of age weighing more than 33 kg should receive 400 mg every 8 hours or 600 mg every 12 hours.

The manufacturer recommends a treatment duration of 5–14 days in pediatric patients; the duration of therapy should be guided by the severity and site of infection and the patient's clinical and bacteriologic progress.

■ Dosage in Renal and Hepatic Impairment

Dosage of ceftaroline fosamil must be modified according to the degree of renal impairment in adults with creatinine clearances of 50 mL/minute or less, including those undergoing hemodialysis. (See Table 1.)

Table 1. Ceftaroline Fosamil Dosage for Adults with Renal Impairment

Estimated Creatinine Clearance (mL/minute)	Recommended Dosage
31–50	400 mg every 12 hours
15–30	300 mg every 12 hours
<15 or receiving hemodialysis	200 mg every 12 hours; on hemodialysis days, give dose after hemodialysis

Dosage adjustments are not necessary if ceftaroline fosamil is used in pediatric patients with creatinine clearances greater than 50 mL/minute per 1.73 m^2. Data are insufficient to make dosage recommendations for pediatric patients with creatinine clearances less than 50 mL/minute per 1.73 m^2.

Pharmacokinetics of ceftaroline fosamil have not been studied in patients with impaired hepatic function, but hepatic impairment is not expected to have a clinically important effect on systemic clearance of the drug.

■ Dosage in Geriatric Patients

Dosage of ceftaroline fosamil should be selected with caution in geriatric patients. Dosage adjustments are not required based on age, but may be required based on age-related changes in renal function. (See Dosage and Administration: Dosage in Renal and Hepatic Impairment.)

Cautions

■ Adverse Effects

Adverse effects reported with ceftaroline fosamil are similar to those reported with other cephalosporins. (See Cautions in the Cephalosporins General Statement 8:12.06.) Ceftaroline fosamil generally is well tolerated; serious adverse effects have been reported in up to 7.5% of adults receiving the drug in phase 3 clinical trials and have required discontinuance of the drug in about 3% of patients.

Adverse effects reported in 2% or more of adults receiving ceftaroline fosamil in phase 3 clinical trials include GI effects (diarrhea, nausea, vomiting, constipation), headache, rash, pruritus, hypokalemia, increased transaminases, and phlebitis.

■ Precautions and Contraindications

Ceftaroline fosamil shares the toxic potentials of the cephalosporins, and the usual precautions of cephalosporin therapy should be observed.

Sensitivity Reactions Serious, sometimes fatal hypersensitivity (anaphylactic) reactions and serious skin reactions have been reported in patients receiving β-lactam antibiotics. Anaphylaxis has been reported in some patients receiving ceftaroline fosamil.

Prior to initiation of ceftaroline fosamil therapy, careful inquiry should be made concerning previous hypersensitivity reactions to ceftaroline, other cephalosporins, penicillins, or carbapenems. There is clinical and laboratory evidence of partial cross-sensitivity among β-lactam antibiotics.

Ceftaroline fosamil is contraindicated in patients with known serious hypersensitivity to the drug or other cephalosporins. If ceftaroline fosamil is used in patients allergic to penicillin or other β-lactams, the patient should be closely monitored.

Patients should be advised that allergic reactions, including serious allergic reactions, could occur and that serious reactions require immediate treatment.

If a hypersensitivity reaction occurs, ceftaroline fosamil should be discontinued and appropriate treatment and supportive measures initiated.

Clostridium difficile-associated Diarrhea and Colitis Treatment with anti-infectives alters normal colon flora and may permit overgrowth of *Clostridium difficile*.

C. difficile infection (CDI) and *C. difficile*-associated diarrhea and colitis (CDAD; also known as antibiotic-associated diarrhea and colitis or pseudomembranous colitis) have been reported with nearly all systemic anti-infectives, including ceftaroline, and may range in severity from mild diarrhea to fatal colitis. *C. difficile* produces toxins A and B which contribute to the development of CDAD; hypertoxin-producing strains of *C. difficile* are associated with increased morbidity and mortality since they may be refractory to anti-infectives and colectomy may be required.

CDAD should be considered in the differential diagnosis in patients who develop diarrhea during or after anti-infective therapy. Careful medical history is necessary since CDAD has been reported to occur as late as 2 months or longer after anti-infective therapy is discontinued.

If CDAD is suspected or confirmed, anti-infective therapy not directed against *C. difficile* should be discontinued whenever possible. Patients should be managed with appropriate supportive therapy (e.g., fluid and electrolyte management, protein supplementation), anti-infective therapy directed against *C. difficile* (e.g., metronidazole, vancomycin), and surgical evaluation as clinically indicated.

Patients should be advised that diarrhea is a common problem caused by anti-infectives and usually resolves when the drug is discontinued; however, they should contact a clinician if severe watery or bloody diarrhea develops.

Hematologic Effects Neutropenia, leukopenia, and agranulocytosis have been reported in patients receiving ceftaroline fosamil during postmarketing experience.

Seroconversion from negative to positive direct antiglobulin (Coombs') test results was reported in about 10–11% of adults receiving ceftaroline fosamil in phase 3 clinical trials compared with about 4–5% of adults receiving comparator anti-infectives. In pediatric trials, seroconversion from negative to positive direct antiglobulin (Coombs') test results was reported in about 18% of those receiving ceftaroline fosamil compared with about 3% of those receiving comparator anti-infectives. There was no evidence of hemolytic anemia in these adult or pediatric patients.

Drug-induced hemolytic anemia should be considered in patients who develop anemia during or after treatment with ceftaroline fosamil. In such patients, diagnostic studies should be performed and should include a direct antiglobulin test. If drug-induced hemolytic anemia is suspected, discontinuance of ceftaroline fosamil should be considered and supportive treatment (e.g., transfusion) should be administered as clinically indicated.

Selection and Use of Anti-infectives To reduce development of drug-resistant bacteria and maintain effectiveness of ceftaroline fosamil and other antibacterials, the drug should be used only for the treatment of infections proven or strongly suspected to be caused by susceptible bacteria.

When selecting or modifying anti-infective therapy, results of culture and in vitro susceptibility testing should be used. In the absence of such data, local epidemiology and susceptibility patterns should be considered when selecting anti-infectives for empiric therapy.

Patients should be advised that antibacterials (including ceftaroline fosamil) should only be used to treat bacterial infections and not used to treat viral infections (e.g., the common cold). Patients also should be advised about the importance of completing the full course of therapy, even if feeling better after a few days, and that skipping doses or not completing therapy may decrease effectiveness and increase the likelihood that bacteria will develop resistance and will not be treatable with ceftaroline fosamil or other antibacterials in the future.

Precautions in Patients with Renal Impairment Because the area under the concentration-time curve (AUC) and plasma half-life of ceftaroline are increased in patients with renal impairment, dosage adjustments are recommended for adults with creatinine clearances less than 50 mL/minute, including those undergoing hemodialysis. Data are insufficient to date to make dosage recommendations for use of ceftaroline fosamil in pediatric patients with creatinine clearances less than 50 mL/minute per 1.73 m². (See Dosage and Administration: Dosage in Renal and Hepatic Impairment.)

■ **Pediatric Precautions** Safety and efficacy of ceftaroline fosamil have not been established in pediatric patients younger than 2 months of age.

Safety and efficacy of ceftaroline fosamil for the treatment of community-acquired bacterial pneumonia and acute bacterial skin and skin structure infections have been established in pediatric patients 2 months to less than 18 years of age. Use of the drug for these indications in this age group is supported by evidence from adequate and well-controlled studies in adults and additional pharmacokinetic and safety data from pediatric trials.

Data indicate that clinical cure rates reported with ceftaroline fosamil for the treatment of community-acquired bacterial pneumonia or acute bacterial skin and skin structure infections in children 2 months to less than 18 years of age are similar to clinical cure rates reported in adults 18 years of age or older. In addition, adverse effects reported with ceftaroline fosamil in pediatric trials are similar to those reported in adult trials. Adverse effects reported in 3% or more of children 2 months to less than 18 years of age receiving ceftaroline fosamil in clinical trials include GI effects (diarrhea, nausea, vomiting), pyrexia, and rash.

■ **Geriatric Precautions** In phase 3 trials evaluating ceftaroline fosamil for the treatment community-acquired bacterial pneumonia or acute bacterial skin and skin structure infections in adults, about 31% of patients were 65 years of age or older and no overall differences in efficacy or safety relative to younger adults were observed.

Ceftaroline is substantially eliminated by the kidneys, and the risk of adverse effects may be greater in those with impaired renal function. Because geriatric patients are more likely to have reduced renal function, dosage should be selected with caution and monitoring of renal function should be considered. Dosage adjustments in geriatric patients should be based on renal function. (See Dosage and Administration: Dosage in Renal and Hepatic Impairment.)

■ **Mutagenicity and Carcinogenicity** In vivo and in vitro studies evaluating ceftaroline fosamil have not shown evidence of mutagenicity. Although ceftaroline fosamil and ceftaroline were clastogenic in the absence of metabolic activation in an in vitro chromosomal aberration assay, this did not occur in the presence of metabolic activation.

Long-term animal studies have not been performed to date to evaluate the carcinogenic potential of ceftaroline fosamil.

■ **Pregnancy, Fertility, and Lactation** ***Pregnancy*** Adequate data are not available regarding use of ceftaroline fosamil in pregnant women.

Animal studies in rats using ceftaroline fosamil dosages up to 4 times the maximum recommended human dosage (MRHD) or in rabbits using dosages up to approximately equal to the MRHD have not revealed evidence of fetal harm.

Fertility There was no evidence of impaired fertility in male or female rats receiving ceftaroline fosamil dosages approximately 4 times higher than the MRHD based on body surface area.

Lactation It is not known whether ceftaroline is distributed into human milk; possible effects of the drug on a breast-fed infant or on milk production are unknown.

Benefits of breast-feeding and the importance of ceftaroline fosamil to the woman should be considered along with the potential adverse effects on the breast-fed infant from the drug or from the underlying maternal condition.

Drug Interactions

No formal drug interaction studies have been performed to date using ceftaroline fosamil. Interactions are unlikely between ceftaroline fosamil and drugs that are cytochrome P-450 (CYP) substrates, inhibitors, or inducers or drugs that undergo active renal secretion or alter renal blood flow.

In vitro, ceftaroline does not inhibit CYP isoenzymes 1A1, 1A2, 2A6, 2B6, 2C8, 2C9, 2C19, 2D6, 2E1, or 3A4 and does not induce CYP isoenzymes 1A2, 2B6, 2C8, 2C9, 2C19, or 3A4/5. Therefore, pharmacokinetic interactions with drugs metabolized by these isoenzymes are unlikely.

■ **Aminoglycosides** In vitro, the antibacterial effects of ceftaroline and amikacin were synergistic against *Escherichia coli* and *Klebsiella pneumoniae* that produce extended-spectrum β-lactamases (ESBL-producing), AmpC-derepressed *Enterobacter cloacae*, and *Pseudomonas aeruginosa*; there was no evidence of antagonism between the drugs.

■ **Aztreonam** In vitro, the antibacterial effects of ceftaroline and aztreonam were indifferent against ESBL-producing *E. coli* and *K. pneumoniae*, AmpC-derepressed *E. cloacae*, and *Ps. aeruginosa*; there was no evidence of synergism or antagonism between the drugs.

■ **Carbapenems** In vitro, the antibacterial effects of ceftaroline and meropenem were synergistic against ESBL-producing *E. coli* and indifferent against ESBL-producing *K. pneumoniae*, AmpC-derepressed *E. cloacae*, and *Ps. aeruginosa*; there was no evidence of antagonism between the drugs.

■ **Other Anti-infectives** To date, there has been no in vitro evidence of antagonism between ceftaroline and azithromycin, daptomycin, levofloxacin, linezolid, tigecycline, or vancomycin.

■ **Warfarin** Increased prothrombin time (PT) and elevated international normalized ratio (INR) have been reported when ceftaroline fosamil was initiated in a patient receiving a stable warfarin dosage.

Mechanism of Action

Ceftaroline usually is bactericidal in action. Like other cephalosporins, the antibacterial activity of the drug results from inhibition of mucopeptide synthesis in the bacterial cell wall. For information on the mechanism of action of cephalosporins, see Mechanism of Action in the Cephalosporins General Statement 8:12.06.

Studies evaluating the binding of ceftaroline to penicillin-binding proteins (PBPs), the target enzymes of β-lactam antibiotics, indicate that ceftaroline has high affinity for PBPs 1, 2, 2a, and 3 of *Staphylococcus aureus*. High affinity for PBP2a appears to be associated with bactericidal activity against methicillin-resistant *S. aureus* (MRSA; also known as oxacillin-resistant *S. aureus*, ORSA). Ceftaroline also has high affinity for PBPs 1a, 1b, 2a, 2b, 2x, and 3 of *Streptococcus pneumoniae*. Penicillin resistance in *S. pneumoniae* appears to involve PBP 2b, 2x, and 1a.

For most susceptible bacteria, the minimum bactericidal concentration (MBC) of ceftaroline is only 1–4 times higher than the minimum inhibitory concentration (MIC).

Spectrum

Based on its spectrum of activity, ceftaroline is classified as a fifth generation cephalosporin. For information on the classification of cephalosporins and closely related β-lactam antibiotics based on spectra of activity, see Spectrum in the Cephalosporins General Statement 8:12.06.

Like third and fourth generation cephalosporins, fifth generation cephalosporins have an expanded spectrum of activity that includes both gram-positive and gram-negative bacteria. However, unlike first, second, third, and fourth generation cephalosporins, fifth generation cephalosporins have activity against methicillin-resistant *Staphylococcus aureus* (MRSA; also known as oxacillin-resistant *S. aureus*, ORSA).

■ **In Vitro Susceptibility Testing** For information on interpreting results of in vitro susceptibility testing (disk susceptibility tests, dilution susceptibility tests) when ceftaroline susceptibility testing is performed according to the standards of the Clinical and Laboratory Standards Institute (CLSI; formerly National Committee for Clinical Laboratory Standards [NCCLS]), see Spectrum: In Vitro Susceptibility Testing, in the Cephalosporins General Statement 8:12.06.

■ **Gram-positive Aerobic Bacteria** Ceftaroline is active in vitro against *S. aureus*, including MRSA, vancomycin-resistant *S. aureus* [VRSA], and daptomycin-nonsusceptible *S. aureus*. The drug also is active in vitro against coagulase-negative staphylococci (e.g., *S. epidermidis*), including methicillin-resistant (oxacillin-resistant) strains. The MIC_{90} of ceftaroline reported for methicillin-susceptible (oxacillin-susceptible) *S. aureus* is 0.25 mcg/mL, and the MIC_{90} of the drug reported for MRSA is 1–2 mcg/mL.

Ceftaroline is active in vitro against *Streptococcus pneumoniae*, including penicillin-resistant *S. pneumoniae* and multidrug-resistant *S. pneumoniae* (MDRSP). The MIC_{90} of the drug is 0.015–0.12 mcg/mL for penicillin-susceptible *S. pneumoniae* and 0.12–0.25 mcg/mL for penicillin-resistant and multidrug-resistant strains.

Ceftaroline is active in vitro against *S. pyogenes* (group A β-hemolytic streptococci, GAS), *S. agalactiae* (group B streptococci, GBS), viridans streptococci, and *S. dysgalactiae*. The MIC_{90} of the drug reported for *S. pyogenes* and *S. agalactiae* is 0.03 mcg/mL or less.

Ceftaroline has only limited activity against *Enterococcus*. Some strains of *Enterococcus faecalis* are inhibited in vitro by ceftaroline concentrations of 2–4 mcg/mL, but *E. faecium* are resistant to the drug.

■ **Gram-negative Aerobic Bacteria** Ceftaroline is active in vitro against many Enterobacteriaceae, including some *Citrobacter freundii*, *C. koseri*, *Enterobacter aerogenes*, *E. cloacae*, *Escherichia coli*, *Klebsiella pneumoniae*, *K. oxytoca*, *Morganella morganii*, and *Proteus mirabilis*. The MIC_{90} of ceftaroline for most susceptible Enterobacteriaceae is 0.25–1 mcg/mL. However, the MIC_{90} of the drug has been reported to be 4 mcg/mL or higher for many Enterobacteriaceae, including *P. mirabilis*, *C. freundii* (ceftazidime-nonsusceptible strains), *M. morganii*, and *Serratia*. *Providencia* and *Acinetobacter* usually are resistant. The activity of ceftaroline against gram-negative bacteria is similar to that reported with third generation cephalosporins. Ceftaroline is not active against Enterobacteriaceae that produce extended-spectrum β-lactamases (ESBL-producing), AmpC cephalosporinases, metallo-β-lactamases, or serine carbapenemases.

Ceftaroline is active in vitro against β-lactamase-producing and non-β-lactamase-producing *Haemophilus influenzae*, *H. parainfluenzae*, and *Moraxella catarrhalis*, and the MIC_{90} reported for most of these organisms is 0.015–0.25 mcg/mL. The MIC_{90} of ceftaroline reported for *Neisseria gonorrhoeae* and *N. meningitidis* is 0.004–0.25 mcg/mL.

The MIC_{90} of ceftaroline reported for *Pasteurella multocida* is 0.06 mcg/mL. In vitro studies indicate that *Acinetobacter* is resistant to ceftaroline.

Ceftaroline is not active against *Pseudomonas aeruginosa*.

■ **Anaerobic Bacteria** Ceftaroline has some in vitro activity against anaerobic bacteria. The MIC_{90} of ceftaroline reported for some gram-positive anaerobic bacteria, including *Actinomyces*, *Eubacterium*, *Lactobacillus*, *Clostridium*, *Peptostreptococcus*, and *Propionibacterium*, has been 0.06–4 mcg/mL. The MIC_{90} of ceftaroline reported for some gram-negative anaerobic bacteria, including *Fusobacterium*, *Porphyromonas*, and *Veillonella*, has been 0.03–0.5 mcg/mL. In vitro studies indicate that *Bacteroides* and *Prevotella* are resistant to ceftaroline.

Resistance

Methicillin-resistant *Staphylococcus aureus* (MRSA; also known as oxacillin-resistant *S. aureus*, ORSA) with reduced susceptibility or resistance to ceftaroline have been produced in vitro and have been reported in clinical isolates. Although resistance to ceftaroline in MRSA generally is associated with modifications in the *mec*A-encoded penicillin-binding protein 2a (PBP2a), other mechanisms of resistance may also be involved.

Gram-negative bacteria that produce extended-spectrum β-lactamases (ESBLs) from the TEM, SHV or CTX-M families, AmpC cephalosporinases, class B metallo-β-lactamases, or serine carbapenemases (such as KPC) are resistant to ceftaroline.

Although cross-resistance may occur between ceftaroline and other cephalosporins, some bacteria resistant to other cephalosporins may be susceptible to ceftaroline.

Pharmacokinetics

■ **Absorption** Ceftaroline is administered as ceftaroline fosamil, a prodrug that is inactive until converted in vivo to ceftaroline by a plasma phosphatase.

Peak plasma concentrations and area under the concentration-time curve (AUC) of ceftaroline in healthy adults increase approximately in proportion to dose following single IV doses of 50–1000 mg of ceftaroline fosamil.

There is no appreciable accumulation of ceftaroline when 600-mg doses of ceftaroline fosamil are given by IV infusion over 1 hour every 12 hours for up to 14 days in adults with normal renal function.

In healthy adults receiving ceftaroline fosamil in a dosage of 600 mg given by IV infusion over 1 hour every 12 hours for 14 days, peak plasma concentrations of ceftaroline average 21.3 mcg/mL and the median time to peak plasma concentrations is 0.9 hours.

When 600-mg doses of ceftaroline fosamil in 50 mL of compatible infusion solution were given by IV infusion over 5 or 60 minutes every 8 hours for 5 days in healthy adults, mean peak plasma concentrations of ceftaroline were 32.5 mcg/mL after the 5-minute infusions and 17.4 mcg/mL after the 60-minute infusion; the time to peak plasma concentrations (about 5 minutes after the end of the infusion) and AUC were similar for both infusion rates.

In healthy adolescents 12–17 years of age, peak plasma concentrations and AUC after a single 8-mg/kg IV dose (600 mg in those weighing more than 75 kg) are 10 and 23% lower, respectively, compared with healthy adults who received a single 600-mg IV dose.

■ **Distribution** The steady-state volume of distribution of ceftaroline in healthy adults following a single 600-mg IV dose of ceftaroline fosamil is 20.3 L and is similar to extracellular fluid volume.

Ceftaroline is approximately 20% bound to plasma proteins. Protein binding decreases slightly with increasing ceftaroline concentrations exceeding 1–50 mcg/mL.

Limited data are available regarding tissue distribution of ceftaroline; animal data indicate that the drug is distributed into kidneys, skin, and lungs.

It is not known whether ceftaroline is distributed into milk.

■ **Elimination** Ceftaroline fosamil is rapidly converted in vivo to ceftaroline by a plasma phosphatase, principally during IV infusion. In addition, the β-lactam ring of ceftaroline is hydrolyzed to an inactive, open-ring metabolite (ceftaroline M-1).

Ceftaroline is not a substrate of cytochrome P-450 (CYP) isoenzymes.

Ceftaroline and its metabolites are principally eliminated in urine by glomerular filtration. Following a single 600-mg IV dose of ceftaroline fosamil, approximately 88% is eliminated in urine (approximately 64% as unchanged drug and 2% as ceftaroline M-1) and 6% is eliminated in feces within 48 hours.

The terminal elimination half-life of ceftaroline is 2.7 hours in healthy adults receiving ceftaroline fosamil in a dosage of 600 mg given by IV infusion over 1 hour every 12 hours for 14 days. When 600-mg doses of ceftaroline fosamil in 50 mL of compatible infusion solution were given by IV infusion over 5 or 60 minutes every 8 hours for 5 days in healthy adults, the terminal elimination half-life of ceftaroline was similar for both infusion rates.

The pharmacokinetics of ceftaroline in pediatric patients 2 months to less than 18 years of age are similar to the pharmacokinetics reported in adults.

The pharmacokinetics of ceftaroline in patients with hepatic impairment have not been established.

In adults with renal impairment, the AUC and plasma half-life of ceftaroline are increased.

Ceftaroline is removed by hemodialysis. In adults with end-stage renal disease who received 400 mg of ceftaroline fosamil, 76.5 mg of the drug (approximately 21.6% of the dose) was recovered in the dialysate following a 4-hour hemodialysis session started 4 hours after the dose.

Chemistry and Stability

■ **Chemistry** Ceftaroline is a semisynthetic cephalosporin antibiotic. Ceftaroline is structurally similar to parenteral third and fourth generation cephalosporins (e.g., cefepime, cefotaxime, ceftazidime, ceftriaxone). Like many third and fourth generation drugs, ceftaroline contains a 1,2,4-thiadiazole ring that enhances antibacterial activity against gram-negative bacteria and an oxime group that contributes to stability in the presence of β-lactamases. Unlike other commercially available cephalosporins, ceftaroline contains a 1,3-thiazole ring linked to the 3-position of the cephem ring by a sulfur which appears to contribute to activity against methicillin-resistant *Staphylococcus aureus* (MRSA; also known as oxacillin-resistant *S. aureus* or ORSA).

Ceftaroline is commercially available for parenteral use as ceftaroline fosamil monoacetate monohydrate; potency is expressed in terms of anhydrous ceftaroline fosamil. Ceftaroline fosamil is a prodrug that is inactive until converted in vivo to ceftaroline by a plasma phosphatase. Commercially available ceftaroline fosamil powder for IV infusion is a pale yellowish-white to light yellow powder. Each vial of the drug also contains L-arginine as an excipient. When reconstituted as directed, ceftaroline fosamil solutions have a pH of 4.8–6.5. Depending on the concentration and storage conditions, ceftaroline fosamil solutions are clear, light to dark yellow.

■ **Stability** Ceftaroline fosamil powder for IV infusion should be stored at 25°C, but may be exposed to temperatures ranging from 15–30°C.

Following reconstitution and dilution, ceftaroline fosamil solutions in IV infusion bags should be used within 6 hours when stored at room temperature or within 24 hours when refrigerated at 2–8°C. Stability testing indicates that ceftaroline fosamil solutions containing 4–12 mg/mL diluted in 50- or 100-mL infusion bags containing 0.9% sodium chloride (Baxter Mini-Bag Plus containers) may be stored for up to 6 hours at room temperature or for up to 24 hours at 2–8°C.

For further information on chemistry, mechanism of action, spectrum, resistance, uses, cautions, acute toxicity, drug interactions, or laboratory test interferences of cephalosporins, see the Cephalosporins General Statement 8:12.06.

Preparations

Excipients in commercially available drug preparations may have clinically important effects in some individuals; consult specific product labeling for details.

Ceftaroline Fosamil

Parenteral

For injection, for IV infusion	400 mg	**Teflaro®**, Forest
	600 mg	**Teflaro®**, Forest

MISCELLANEOUS β-LACTAMS 8:12.07

CARBAPENEMS 8:12.07.08

Doripenem

■ Doripenem is a synthetic carbapenem β-lactam antibiotic structurally and pharmacologically related to other carbapenems (e.g., ertapenem, imipenem, meropenem).

Uses

■ **Intra-abdominal Infections** Doripenem is used as monotherapy for treatment of complicated intra-abdominal infections caused by susceptible *Escherichia coli, Klebsiella pneumoniae, Pseudomonas aeruginosa, Bacteroides fragilis, B. caccae, B. thetaiotaomicron, B. uniformis, B. vulgatus, Streptococcus intermedius, Streptococcus constellatus,* or *Peptostreptococcus micros.*

For initial empiric treatment of high-risk or severe community-acquired, extrabiliary, complicated intra-abdominal infections in adults (e.g., those with advanced age, immunocompromised state, severe physiologic disturbance), the Infectious Diseases Society of America (IDSA) recommends either monotherapy with a carbapenem (doripenem, fixed combination of imipenem and cilastatin, meropenem) or the fixed combination of piperacillin and tazobactam, or a combination regimen that includes either a cephalosporin (cefepime, ceftazidime) or fluoroquinolone (ciprofloxacin, levofloxacin) in conjunction with metronidazole.

For empiric treatment of healthcare-associated complicated intra-abdominal infections in adults, IDSA recommends monotherapy with a carbapenem (doripenem, fixed combination of imipenem and cilastatin, meropenem) or the fixed combination of piperacillin and tazobactam, or a combination regimen that includes a cephalosporin (cefepime, ceftazidime) in conjunction with metronidazole.

For additional information regarding management of intra-abdominal infections, the current IDSA clinical practice guidelines available at http://www.idsociety.org should be consulted.

Clinical Experience Efficacy of doripenem for the treatment of complicated intra-abdominal infections was evaluated in 2 randomized, multicenter, double-blind phase 3 studies that compared doripenem with meropenem. In these studies, 946 hospitalized adults with complicated intra-abdominal infections (including complicated appendicitis, bowel perforation, cholecystitis, intra-abdominal or solid organ abscess, and generalized peritonitis) were randomized to receive either IV doripenem (500 mg by IV infusion over 1 hour every 8 hours) or IV meropenem (1 g by IV injection over 3–5 minutes every 8 hours) with an option to switch to oral amoxicillin and clavulanate potassium (875 mg of amoxicillin and 125 mg of clavulanic acid twice daily) after a minimum of 3 days of IV therapy for a total of 5–14 days of IV and oral treatment. Results indicate that doripenem is noninferior to meropenem in terms of clinical cure rates in microbiologically evaluable (ME) patients (i.e., patients with susceptible pathogens isolated at baseline and no major protocol deviations at test-of-cure visit) and in microbiologic modified intent-to-treat (m-MITT) patients (i.e., patients with baseline pathogens isolated regardless of susceptibility). Clinical cure rates in the ME patients at test-of-cure visit (25–45 days after completion of treatment) were similar in those who received doripenem (82.8 and 81%) or meropenem (85.9 and 82.1%). Clinical cure rates in the mMITT patients at test-of-cure visit (25–45 days after completion of treatment) were similar in those who received doripenem (73.7 and 71.9%) or meropenem (78 and 74.2%).

■ **Urinary Tract Infections** Doripenem is used as monotherapy for treatment of complicated urinary tract infections (including pyelonephritis) caused by susceptible *E. coli* (including cases with concurrent bacteremia) or susceptible *K. pneumoniae, Proteus mirabilis, Ps. aeruginosa,* or *Acinetobacter baumannii.*

Clinical Experience Efficacy of doripenem for the treatment of complicated urinary tract infections (including pyelonephritis) was evaluated in 1171 adults in 2 randomized, multicenter clinical studies. One was a randomized, multicenter, double-blind phase 3 study where adults were randomized to receive doripenem (500 mg by IV infusion over 1 hour every 8 hours) or IV levofloxacin (250 mg every 24 hours). The second study was a noncomparative, open-label phase 3 study. Both studies permitted the option of switching to oral levofloxacin (250 mg every 24 hours) after a minimum of 3 days of IV therapy for a total of 10 days of treatment; patients with confirmed concurrent bacteremia were allowed to receive levofloxacin (500 mg either IV or orally) for a total of 10–14 days of treatment. Results indicate that doripenem is noninferior to levofloxacin in terms of microbiologic eradication rates in the ME patients (i.e., patients with baseline uropathogens isolated, no major protocol deviations, and urine cultures at test-of-cure visit) and in the mMITT patients (i.e., patients with pretreatment urine cultures). In the phase 3 comparative study, microbiologic eradication rates in ME patients at test-of-cure visit 5–11 days after completing therapy were similar following treatment with doripenem (82.1%) or levofloxacin (83.4%). In addition, the microbiologic eradication rates in mMITT patients were similar following treatment with doripenem (79.2%) or levofloxacin (78.2%).

■ **Respiratory Tract Infections** ***Nosocomial Pneumonia*** Doripenem has been used for treatment of nosocomial pneumonia†, including ventilator-associated pneumonia† (VAP). However, doripenem is *not* labeled by the US Food and Drug Administration (FDA) for treatment of any type of pneumonia, including VAP, and results from a randomized, controlled study in patients with VAP showed lower cure rates and higher 28-day all-cause mortality in patients receiving doripenem compared with those receiving the fixed combination of imipenem and cilastatin. (See Increased Mortality in Patients with Ventilator-associated Pneumonia under Cautions: Warnings/Precautions.)

Clinical Experience. Efficacy of doripenem for treatment of nosocomial pneumonia, including early-onset VAP, was evaluated in a randomized, multicenter, comparative, open-label phase 3 study in 448 adults (NCT00211003). Patients were randomized to receive either IV doripenem (500 mg by IV infusion over 1 hour every 8 hours) or IV piperacillin sodium and tazobactam sodium (4.5 g by IV infusion over 30 minutes every 6 hours) with an option to switch to oral levofloxacin (750 mg daily) after at least 72 hours of IV therapy. Pending identification of the causative organisms, patients also received amikacin; if *Ps. aeruginosa* was identified, amikacin was continued in those receiving piperacillin and tazobactam but could be discontinued in those receiving doripenem if the patient had improved clinically and the isolate was susceptible to meropenem. If oxacillin-resistant (methicillin-resistant) *Staphylococcus aureus* (MRSA) was suspected, patients also received vancomycin. In clinically evaluable (CE) patients, clinical cure rates 6–20 days after completion of treatment were 81.3% in those who received doripenem and 79.8% in those who received the fixed combination of piperacillin and tazobactam. In the clinical modified intent-to-treat (cMITT) patients, clinical cure rates were 69.5% in those who received doripenem and 64.1% in those who received piperacillin and tazobactam. In ME patients, the microbiologic cure rates in patients with *Ps. aeruginosa* or *K. pneumoniae* infections were 83.3 or 78.6%, respectively, in those who received doripenem and 70.6 or 63.6%, respectively, in those who received piperacillin and tazobactam.

Efficacy of doripenem in the treatment of VAP was also evaluated in another multicenter, randomized, comparative, open-label phase 3 study in 531 adults. Patients were randomized to receive IV doripenem (500 mg by IV infusion over 4 hours every 8 hours) or IV imipenem and cilastatin sodium (500 mg by IV infusion over 30 minutes every 6 hours or 1 g by IV infusion over 60 minutes every 8 hours) given for 7–14 days. If MRSA or *Ps. aeruginosa* was suspected, clinicians could add vancomycin or an aminoglycoside (e.g., amikacin), respectively, to the study regimen. In CE patients, clinical cure rates 7–14 days after completion of treatment were 68.3% in those who received doripenem and 64.8% in those who received imipenem. In the cMITT patients, clinical cure rates were 59% in those who received doripenem and 57.8% in those who received imipenem.

Efficacy and safety of doripenem for treatment of VAP also were evaluated in a randomized, double-blind study in 227 adults. Patients were randomized to receive doripenem (1 g by IV infusion over 4 hours every 8 hours for 7 days) or the fixed combination of imipenem and cilastatin (1 g [of imipenem] by IV infusion over 1 hour every 8 hours for 10 days). Patients could *not* be switched to oral antibacterial therapy. Vancomycin or linezolid could be added to the regimen if considered necessary for MRSA coverage; amikacin could be added if the patient was considered at risk for carbapenem-resistant gram-negative pathogens. Baseline characteristics were generally balanced between treatment groups (65% male, mean age 56 years, 85% white, 5% black or African-American, 5% with bacteremia). However, a larger proportion of patients receiving doripenem had pneumonia due to *Ps. aeruginosa* or *Acinetobacter* (21.5 or 19%, respectively) compared with those receiving imipenem and cilastatin (11.4 or 11.4%, respectively). At day 10, the clinical cure rate in the microbiologic intent-to-treat (MITT) population was 45.6% in those who received doripenem compared with 56.8% in those who received imipenem and cilastatin. In addition, 28-day all-cause mortality in the intent-to-treat (ITT) population was higher among patients who received doripenem compared with those who received imipenem and cilastatin (23 and 16.7%, respectively).

Pulmonary Infections in Cystic Fibrosis Patients Doripenem has been designated an orphan drug by FDA for treatment of bronchopulmonary infections in patients with cystic fibrosis who are colonized with *Ps. aeruginosa* or *Burkholderia cepacia*†. In vitro studies indicate that the drug is active against some strains of *Ps. aeruginosa* and *B. cepacia* isolated from cystic fibrosis patients, including some multidrug-resistant strains.

Dosage and Administration

■ **Administration** Doripenem is administered by IV infusion.

Doripenem should *not* be administered via inhalation. (See Pneumonitis under Cautions: Warnings/Precautions.)

Reconstitution and Dilution Commercially available doripenem powder for injection for IV infusion in single-use vials must be reconstituted and diluted prior to IV infusion.

Vials labeled as containing 250 or 500 mg of doripenem should be reconstituted by adding 10 mL of sterile water for injection or 0.9% sodium chloride injection and gently shaking the vial to provide suspensions containing 25 or 50 mg/mL, respectively. The reconstituted suspension is not for direct injection and must be further diluted prior to administration. The reconstituted suspension is stable in the original vial for up to 1 hour and should not be frozen.

For a 500-mg dose of doripenem, the contents of a reconstituted 500-mg vial should be withdrawn with a 21-gauge needle and added to an infusion bag containing 100 mL of 0.9% sodium chloride injection or 5% dextrose injection; the bag should be gently shaken until the solution is clear. The final solution contains 500 mg of doripenem (approximately 4.5 mg/mL).

For a 250-mg dose of doripenem, the contents of a reconstituted 250-mg vial should be withdrawn with a 21-gauge needle and added to an infusion bag containing either 50 or 100 mL of 0.9% sodium chloride injection or 5% dextrose injection; the bag should be gently shaken until the solution is clear. The final solution contains 250 mg of doripenem (approximately 4.2 or 2.3 mg/mL in the 50- or 100-mL infusion bag, respectively).

Alternatively, for a 250-mg dose of doripenem, the contents of a reconstituted 500-mg vial should be withdrawn with a 21-gauge needle and added to an infusion bag containing 100 mL of 0.9% sodium chloride injection or 5% dextrose injection; the bag should be gently shaken until the solution is clear. Then, 55 mL of the solution should be removed from the bag and discarded; the remaining solution contains 250 mg of doripenem (approximately 4.5 mg/mL).

Alternatively, if doripenem solutions for IV infusion are prepared in Baxter Minibag Plus® infusion bags, instructions provided by the infusion bag manufacturer should be consulted.

Following reconstitution with sterile water for injection or 0.9% sodium chloride injection and further dilution in 0.9% sodium chloride injection, doripenem solutions are stable for 12 hours at room temperature (including infusion time) or 72 hours at 2–8°C (including infusion time). Following reconstitution with sterile water for injection or 0.9% sodium chloride injection and further dilution in 5% dextrose injection, doripenem solutions are stable for 4 hours at room temperature (including infusion time) or 24 hours at 2–8°C (including infusion time).

Doripenem contains no preservatives; strict aseptic technique must be observed when preparing solutions of the drug. Reconstituted and diluted doripenem solutions should be inspected visually for particulate matter and discoloration. Final solutions of the drug may range in color from clear and colorless to clear and slightly yellow; potency is not affected by color variations within this range.

Doripenem should not be admixed or added to solutions containing other drugs.

Rate of Administration IV infusions of doripenem should be given over 1 hour.

■ **Dosage** Doripenem is commercially available as the monohydrate; dosage is expressed in terms of doripenem.

Intra-abdominal Infections The recommended dosage of doripenem for treatment of complicated intra-abdominal infections in adults is 500 mg every 8 hours for 5–14 days. This duration includes a possible switch to an appropriate oral anti-infective if clinical improvement is demonstrated after at least 3 days of parenteral doripenem.

The Infectious Diseases Society of America (IDSA) recommends a treatment duration of 4–7 days for most complicated intra-abdominal infections in adults; a longer duration of treatment has not been associated with improved outcome and is not recommended unless adequate source control is difficult to achieve.

Urinary Tract Infections The recommended dosage of doripenem for treatment of complicated urinary tract infections in adults is 500 mg every 8 hours for 10 days. This duration includes a possible switch to an appropriate oral anti-infective if clinical improvement is demonstrated after at least 3 days of parenteral doripenem. Duration can be extended to a total of 14 days for patients with concurrent bacteremia.

■ **Special Populations** Because doripenem is eliminated principally by renal excretion, adults with creatinine clearances of 50 mL/minute or less should receive reduced dosage. Adults with creatinine clearances of 30–50 mL/minute should receive a doripenem dosage of 250 mg every 8 hours. Adults with creatinine clearances of 11–29 mL/minute should receive a doripenem dosage of 250 mg every 12 hours.

Doripenem is removed by hemodialysis; data are insufficient to recommend dosage adjustments in patients undergoing hemodialysis.

Pharmacokinetics of doripenem have not been established in patients with hepatic impairment; doripenem does not appear to undergo hepatic metabolism. Hepatic impairment is not expected to affect pharmacokinetics of doripenem.

Dosage adjustment is not necessary in geriatric individuals 65 years of age or older with normal renal function; dosage should be selected with caution since geriatric patients are more likely to have decreased renal function or prerenal azotemia than younger adults.

Dosage adjustments based on gender or race are not necessary.

Cautions

■ **Contraindications** Known hypersensitivity to doripenem or other carbapenems.

History of anaphylactic reaction to β-lactams.

■ **Warnings/Precautions** ***Sensitivity Reactions*** **Hypersensitivity Reactions.** Serious and occasionally fatal hypersensitivity reactions (e.g., anaphylaxis) and serious skin reactions have been reported with β-lactams.

Although causality was not established, there have been postmarketing reports of anaphylaxis, Stevens-Johnson syndrome, and toxic epidermal necrolysis in patients receiving doripenem.

If hypersensitivity occurs, doripenem should be discontinued and appropriate emergency treatment initiated as clinically indicated.

Cross-hypersensitivity. Cross-allergenicity occurs among β-lactam antibiotics, including penicillins and cephalosporins.

Prior to initiation of doripenem therapy, careful inquiry should be made concerning previous hypersensitivity reactions to doripenem, cephalosporins, penicillins, or other drugs. Doripenem should be used with caution in patients allergic to penicillin or other β-lactams, and is contraindicated in those who have had an anaphylactic reaction to β-lactams. (See Cautions: Contraindications.)

■ **Increased Mortality in Patients with Ventilator-associated Pneumonia** In a clinical trial in patients with ventilator-associated pneumonia† (VAP), 28-day all-cause mortality in the intent-to-treat population was higher in patients receiving doripenem (23%) than in those receiving imipenem and cilastatin (16.7%). In addition, the clinical cure rate was lower in patients receiving doripenem (46%) than in those receiving imipenem and cilastatin (57%).

Doripenem is *not* labeled by FDA for treatment of any type of pneumonia, including VAP. Healthcare providers should consider whether benefits of doripenem are likely to exceed potential risks in patients who develop pneumonia while on ventilators.

■ **CNS Effects** Seizures have been reported in patients receiving doripenem. In clinical trials, certain patients appeared to be at greater risk for seizures, including those with preexisting CNS disorders (e.g., stroke, history of seizures), patients with compromised renal function, and patients receiving doripenem dosages exceeding 500 mg every 8 hours.

Seizures and other CNS effects (e.g., confusional states, myoclonic activity) have been reported in patients receiving other carbapenems (e.g., ertapenem, imipenem, meropenem), especially in those with underlying CNS disorders (e.g., brain lesions, history of seizures) and/or compromised renal function. Data obtained from rodent studies suggest that doripenem has less potential for convulsant activity than some other carbapenems (e.g., imipenem).

■ **Interactions** In patients with seizure disorders being controlled with valproic acid or valproate sodium, concomitant use of doripenem increases the risk of breakthrough seizures. There is evidence that concomitant use of valproic acid and doripenem can decrease serum concentrations of valproic acid below therapeutic range (50–100 mcg/mL) by 12 hours after initiation of doripenem. There also are published case reports of similar interactions involving concomitant use of valproic acid and other carbapenems; in some of these reports, increasing the dosage of valproic acid or valproate sodium did not result in higher serum concentrations of valproic acid. (See Drug Interactions: Valproic Acid and Valproate Sodium.)

Alternative antibacterial therapy should be considered in patients receiving valproic acid or valproate sodium. If use of doripenem is necessary, alternative or supplemental anticonvulsant therapy should be considered.

■ **Pneumonitis** Administration of doripenem by inhalation† has resulted in pneumonitis. The drug should *not* be administered by inhalation.

■ **Superinfection/Clostridium difficile-associated Diarrhea and Colitis (CDAD)** Use of doripenem may result in emergence and overgrowth of nonsusceptible bacteria or fungi. The patient should be carefully monitored and appropriate therapy instituted if superinfection occurs.

Treatment with anti-infectives alters normal colon flora and may permit overgrowth of *Clostridium difficile*. *C. difficile* infection (CDI) and *C. difficile*-associated diarrhea and colitis (CDAD; also known as antibiotic-associated diarrhea and colitis or pseudomembranous colitis) have been reported in patients receiving nearly all anti-infectives, including doripenem, and may range in severity from mild diarrhea to fatal colitis. *C. difficile* produces toxins A and B which contribute to development of CDAD; hypertoxin-producing strains of *C. difficile* are associated with increased morbidity and mortality since they may be refractory to anti-infectives and colectomy may be required.

CDAD should be considered in the differential diagnosis of patients who develop diarrhea during or after anti-infective therapy. Careful medical history is necessary since CDAD has been reported to occur as late as 2 months or longer after anti-infective therapy is discontinued.

If CDAD is suspected or confirmed, anti-infective therapy not directed against *C. difficile* should be discontinued whenever possible. Patients should be managed with appropriate supportive therapy (e.g., fluid and electrolyte management, protein supplementation), anti-infective therapy directed against *C. difficile* (e.g., metronidazole, vancomycin), and surgical evaluation as clinically indicated.

■ **Selection and Use of Anti-infectives** To reduce development of drug-resistant bacteria and maintain effectiveness of doripenem and other antibacterials, use only for treatment of infections proven or strongly suspected to be caused by susceptible bacteria.

When selecting or modifying anti-infective therapy, use results of culture and in vitro susceptibility testing. In the absence of such data, consider local epidemiology and susceptibility patterns when selecting anti-infectives for empiric therapy.

Specific Populations **Pregnancy.** Category B. (See Users Guide.)

Lactation. It is not known whether doripenem is distributed into milk in humans. Caution is advised if the drug is used in nursing women.

Pediatric Use. Safety and efficacy of doripenem have not been established in children younger than 18 years of age.

Geriatric Use. No substantial differences in safety relative to younger adults, but increased sensitivity cannot be ruled out.

Doripenem is substantially eliminated by the kidneys; risk of adverse reactions may be greater in patients with impaired renal function or prerenal azotemia. Dosage should be selected with caution and renal function monitoring should be considered since geriatric patients are more likely to have decreased renal function or prerenal azotemia.

Hepatic Impairment. Pharmacokinetics of doripenem have not been established in patients with hepatic impairment. Doripenem does not appear to undergo hepatic metabolism; hepatic impairment is not expected to affect pharmacokinetics of the drug.

Renal Impairment. Pharmacokinetics of doripenem is affected by renal impairment; mean area under the concentration-time curve (AUC) is increased.

Dosage adjustments are recommended in patients with moderate or severe renal impairment (creatinine clearance 50 mL/minute or less). (See Dosage and Administration: Special Populations.) Renal function should be monitored in such patients.

■ **Common Adverse Effects** Adverse effects reported in 5% or more of patients receiving doripenem include anemia, diarrhea, headache, nausea, phlebitis, rash, and elevated hepatic enzymes.

Drug Interactions

■ **Drugs Affecting or Metabolized by Hepatic Microsomal Enzymes** In vitro studies indicate that doripenem does not inhibit cytochrome P-450 (CYP) isoenzymes 1A2, 2A6, 2B6, 2C8, 2C9, 2C19, 2D6, 2E1, 3A4/5, or 4A11. In vitro studies also indicate that the drug is not expected to induce CYP1A2, 2B6, 2C9, 2C19, or 3A4/5. Pharmacokinetic interactions with drugs metabolized by these isoenzymes are unlikely.

■ **Drugs Metabolized by Uridine Diphosphate-glucuronosyltransferase 1A1** In vitro studies indicate that doripenem is not expected to induce uridine diphosphate-glucuronosyltransferase 1A1 (UGT 1A1).

■ **Anti-infective Agents** In vitro studies indicate doripenem has minimal potential to antagonize or be antagonized by other anti-infectives (e.g., amikacin, co-trimoxazole, daptomycin, levofloxacin, linezolid, vancomycin).

■ **Probenecid** Pharmacokinetic interaction (decreased renal tubular secretion of doripenem; increased plasma concentrations, increased area under the concentration-time curve [AUC], and prolonged half-life of doripenem). Concomitant use of probenecid and doripenem is not recommended.

■ **Valproic Acid and Valproate Sodium** Pharmacokinetic interaction with valproic acid (decreased plasma concentrations and AUC of valproic acid; no effect on doripenem pharmacokinetics). Increased risk of breakthrough seizures.

Concomitant use of valproic acid (500 mg every 12 hours for 7 days) and doripenem (500 mg every 8 hours for 4 doses) in healthy individuals resulted in valproic acid peak plasma concentrations, minimum plasma concentrations, and AUC that were about 45, 78, and 63% lower compared with administration of valproic acid alone. Serum valproic acid concentrations decreased below the therapeutic range (50–100 mcg/mL) within 12 hours after initiation of doripenem. Although the mechanism of the interaction is unclear, in vitro and animal studies suggest that doripenem may inhibit hydrolysis of the valproic acid glucuronide metabolite, thereby inhibiting conversion of the metabolite back to valproic acid and decreasing plasma concentrations of valproic acid. The interaction reported with valproic acid and doripenem is consistent with case reports of reduced serum concentrations of valproic acid in patients receiving the drug concomitantly with other carbapenems. In some of these case reports, increasing the dosage of valproic acid or valproate sodium did not result in higher serum concentrations of valproic acid.

Because patients with seizure disorders controlled with valproic acid or valproate sodium will be at increased risk for breakthrough seizures if doripenem is used concomitantly, alternative antibacterial therapy should be considered for patients receiving these drugs. If use of doripenem is necessary, alternative or supplemental anticonvulsant therapy should be considered.

Description

Doripenem is a synthetic carbapenem β-lactam antibiotic structurally and pharmacologically related to other carbapenems (e.g., ertapenem, imipenem, meropenem).

Doripenem is bactericidal in action. Like other β-lactams, doripenem inhibits bacterial cell wall synthesis by inactivating multiple penicillin binding proteins (PBPs) resulting in cell death. Doripenem has a high affinity for PBP 2 and PBP 3 in *Pseudomonas aeruginosa* and PBP 2 in *Escherichia coli*.

Doripenem exhibits linear pharmacokinetics over an IV dosage range of 0.5–1 g. The drug is distributed into intra-abdominal tissues and fluids including retroperitoneal fluid, peritoneal exudate, bile, gallbladder tissue, and urine. The median steady-state volume of distribution is 16.8 L (range: 8.09–55.5 L) in healthy adults. Doripenem is approximately 8.1% bound to plasma proteins.

Doripenem is partially metabolized to an inactive ring-opened metabolite (doripenem M1) primarily via dehydropeptidase-I. In vitro studies indicate the drug is not metabolized by hepatic cytochrome P-450 (CYP) isoenzymes. Doripenem is primarily eliminated unchanged by the kidneys and undergoes both glomerular filtration and active tubular secretion. Following a single 500-mg doripenem dose, approximately 71% of the dose is recovered in urine as unchanged drug and 15% as the inactive metabolite; less than 1% is excreted in feces. Doripenem does not accumulate following multiple doses (500 mg or 1 g administered over 1 hour every 8 hours for 7–10 days) in patients with normal renal function. The plasma elimination half-life is approximately 1 hour in healthy nonelderly adults. The area under the concentration-time curve (AUC) is increased in patients with renal impairment. The drug is removed by hemodialysis. At usual dosage, doripenem does not appear to have an effect on the QT interval corrected for rate (QT_c).

■ **Spectrum** Doripenem has a broad spectrum of activity and is active against many aerobic and anaerobic gram-positive and gram-negative bacteria and some anaerobic bacteria. The spectrum of activity of doripenem resembles that of meropenem and imipenem, but doripenem has been reported to be more active than some other carbapenems against Enterobacteriaceae and *Ps. aeruginosa.*

Doripenem is active in vitro and in clinical infections against facultative gram-positive aerobic bacteria, including *Streptococcus intermedius* and *Streptococcus constellatus*. The drug also is active in vitro against *Staphylococcus aureus* (including oxacillin-susceptible [methicillin-susceptible] strains), *S. epidermidis*, *S. agalactiae* (group B streptococci), and *S. pyogenes* (group A β-hemolytic streptococci).

Doripenem is active in vitro and in clinical infections against some facultative gram-negative aerobic bacteria, including *E. coli*, *Klebsiella pneumoniae*, *Proteus mirabilis*, *Ps. aeruginosa*, and *Acinetobacter baumannii*. The drug also is active in vitro against *Citrobacter freundii*, *Enterobacter cloacae*, *E. aerogenes*, *K. oxytoca*, *Morganella morganii*, and *Serratia marcescens* and some strains of *Burkholderia cepacia*.

Doripenem is active in vitro and in clinical infections against many anaerobic bacteria, including *Bacteroides fragilis*, *B. caccae*, *B. thetaiotaomicron*, *B. uniformis*, *B. vulgatus*, and *Peptostreptococcus micros*.

■ **Resistance** Mechanisms of resistance to doripenem include drug inactivation by carbapenem-hydrolyzing enzymes (e.g., metallo-β-lactamases), mutant or acquired PBPs, decreased outer membrane permeability, and active efflux. Doripenem is resistant to hydrolysis by a variety of β-lactamases (including penicillinases and cephalosporinases), but not carbapenem-hydrolyzing β-lactamases.

Cross-resistance may occur between doripenem and other carbapenems; however, some isolates (e.g., some strains of *Ps. aeruginosa*) resistant to other carbapenems may be susceptible to doripenem.

Advice to Patients

Advise patients that antibacterials (including doripenem) should only be used to treat bacterial infections and not used to treat viral infections (e.g., the common cold).

Importance of completing full course of therapy, even if feeling better after a few days.

Advise patients that skipping doses or not completing the full course of therapy may decrease effectiveness and increase the likelihood that bacteria will develop resistance and will not be treatable with doripenem or other antibacterials in the future.

Importance of informing clinicians of any previous hypersensitivity reactions to doripenem, other carbapenems, β-lactams, or other allergens.

Importance of discontinuing therapy and informing clinician if an allergic or hypersensitivity reaction occurs.

Importance of informing clinicians of existing CNS disorders (e.g., stroke, history of seizures) or treatment with valproic acid or valproate sodium.

Importance of informing clinicians of existing or contemplated concomitant therapy, including prescription and OTC drugs, and any concomitant illnesses.

Importance of women informing clinicians if they are or plan to become pregnant or plan to breast-feed.

Importance of informing patients of other important precautionary information. (See Cautions.)

Overview® (see Users Guide). For additional information on this drug until a more detailed monograph is developed and published, the manufacturer's labeling should be consulted. It is *essential* that the manufacturer's labeling be consulted for more detailed information on usual cautions, precautions, contraindications, potential drug interactions, laboratory test interferences, and acute toxicity.

Preparations

Excipients in commercially available drug preparations may have clinically important effects in some individuals; consult specific product labeling for details.

Doripenem (Monohydrate)

Parenteral		
For injection, for IV infusion	250 mg (of doripenem)	**Doribax®**, Shionogi
	500 mg (of doripenem)	**Doribax®**, Shionogi

†Use is not currently included in the labeling approved by the US Food and Drug Administration

Ertapenem Sodium

■ Ertapenem is a synthetic carbapenem β-lactam antibiotic.

Uses

Ertapenem is used IV in adults for the treatment of moderate to severe infections, including complicated intra-abdominal and acute pelvic infections, complicated skin and skin structure infections, community-acquired pneumonia, and complicated urinary tract infections, caused by susceptible organisms.

■ **Intra-abdominal and Gynecologic Infections** Ertapenem is used IV for the treatment of complicated intra-abdominal infections caused by susceptible strains of *Escherichia coli, Clostridium clostridioforme* (*C. clostridiiforme*), *Eubacterium lentum, Peptostreptococcus* spp., *Bacteroides fragilis, B. distasonis, B. ovatus, B. thetaiotaomicron*, or *B. uniformis*. In a clinical trial in patients with complicated intra-abdominal infections, the combined clinical and microbiologic cure rate at 4–6 weeks following treatment was 84 or 80% in patients receiving ertapenem (1 g IV daily) or piperacillin sodium and tazobactam sodium (3.375 g [3 g of piperacillin and 0.375 g of tazobactam] IV every 6 hours), respectively, for 5–14 days.

Ertapenem is used IV for the treatment of acute pelvic infections, including postpartum endomyometritis, septic abortion, and postsurgical gynecologic infections, caused by susceptible strains of *Streptococcus agalactiae, E. coli, B. fragilis, Porphyromonas asaccharolytica* (*B. asaccharolytica*), *Peptostreptococcus* spp., or *Prevotella bivia*. Clinical success at 2–4 weeks following treatment was achieved in 94% of patients receiving ertapenem (1 g IV daily) and 92% of those receiving piperacillin sodium and tazobactam sodium (3.375 g [3 g of piperacillin and 0.375 g of tazobactam] IV every 6 hours) for 3–10 days.

■ **Skin and Skin Structure Infections** Ertapenem is used IV for the treatment of complicated skin and skin structure infections caused by susceptible strains of *Staphylococcus aureus* (methicillin-susceptible strains only), *Streptococcus pyogenes, E. coli*, or *Peptostreptococcus* spp. In a clinical trial in patients with complicated skin and skin structure infections, clinical success at 10–21 days following treatment was achieved in 84% of patients receiving ertapenem (1 g IV daily) and 85% of those receiving piperacillin sodium and tazobactam sodium (3.375 g [3 g of piperacillin and 0.375 g of tazobactam] IV every 6 hours) for 7–14 days.

■ **Community-acquired Pneumonia** Ertapenem is used IV for the treatment of community-acquired pneumonia caused by susceptible strains of *Streptococcus pneumoniae* (penicillin-susceptible strains only), including cases with concurrent bacteremia, *Haemophilus influenzae* (non-β-lactamase-producing strains only), or *Moraxella* (formerly *Branhamella*) *catarrhalis*. In 2 clinical trials, clinical success rates at 7–14 days following treatment were similar (91–92%) with ertapenem (1 g IV daily) and with ceftriaxone (1 g IV daily). Anti-infective therapy was continued for 10–14 days; each regimen included an option to switch to oral amoxicillin trihydrate and clavulanate potassium to complete the course of therapy.

■ **Urinary Tract Infections** Ertapenem is used IV for the treatment of complicated urinary tract infections, including pyelonephritis, caused by susceptible strains of *E. coli*, including cases with concurrent bacteremia, or *Klebsiella pneumoniae*. Pooled data from 2 clinical trials in patients with complicated urinary tract infections showed a microbiologic cure rate at 5–9 days following treatment of 90 or 91% in patients receiving ertapenem (1 g IV daily) or ceftriaxone (1 g IV daily), respectively. Anti-infective therapy was continued for 10–14 days; each regimen included an option to switch to oral ciprofloxacin to complete the course of therapy.

Dosage and Administration

■ **Reconstitution and Administration** Ertapenem sodium is administered by IV infusion over 30 minutes or by IM injection. The manufacturer states that the drug may be administered once daily by IV infusion for up to 14 days or by IM injection for up to 7 days.

For IV infusion, ertapenem sodium powder for injection must be reconstituted and diluted prior to administration. The manufacturer states that 10 mL of sterile water for injection, 0.9% sodium chloride injection, or bacteriostatic water for injection should be used to reconstitute the powder and then the reconstituted solution should be further diluted with 50 mL of 0.9% sodium chloride. The reconstituted solution may be stored at room temperature and infused IV within 6 hours of reconstitution or refrigerated at 5°C for up to 24 hours and infused IV within 4 hours after removal from the refrigerator. Solutions of ertapenem sodium should not be frozen. Ertapenem sodium should *not* be reconstituted or diluted with dextrose-containing solutions or admixed with other drugs.

For IM injection, ertapenem sodium powder for injection must be reconstituted with 3.2 mL of 1% lidocaine injection (*without epinephrine*) and shaken thoroughly to ensure dissolution; this solution should *not* be administered IV. The entire contents of the vial should be withdrawn, and injected IM deeply into a large muscle mass, such as the gluteus or lateral part of the thigh.

Parenteral ertapenem sodium solutions should be inspected visually for particulate matter and discoloration prior to administration whenever solution and container permit.

■ **Dosage** Dosage of ertapenem sodium is expressed in terms of ertapenem.

The usual adult dosage of ertapenem is 1 g once daily. The duration of ertapenem therapy depends on the type and severity of infection. The manufacturer recommends that anti-infective therapy generally be continued for 5–14 days in patients with complicated intra-abdominal infections, 7–14 days in patients with complicated skin and skin structure infections, 10–14 days in patients with community-acquired pneumonia or complicated urinary tract infections (including pyelonephritis), and 3–10 days in patients with acute pelvic infections including postpartum endomyometritis, septic abortion, and postsurgical gynecologic infections. Patients with community-acquired pneumonia or complicated urinary tract infections who are treated initially with IV ertapenem may be switched to oral therapy after at least 3 days of parenteral therapy, if clinically appropriate.

■ **Special Populations** No dosage adjustment is necessary in adults with creatinine clearances exceeding 30 mL/minute per 1.73 m^2; however, the manufacturer recommends a dosage of 500 mg daily for those with severe renal impairment (creatinine clearance of 30 mL/minute per 1.73 m^2 or less) or end-stage renal disease (creatinine clearance of 10 mL/minute per 1.73 m^2 or less). In adults undergoing hemodialysis, the manufacturer also recommends a dosage of 500 mg daily. If the daily dose is given within 6 hours prior to hemodialysis, a supplemental dose of 150 mg should be administered following the dialysis period; a supplemental dose is not necessary if the daily dose is given at least 6 hours prior to hemodialysis.

Cautions

■ **Contraindications** Known hypersensitivity to ertapenem, other carbapenems, or any ingredient in the formulation; history of anaphylactic reaction to β-lactams. Patients with known hypersensitivity to local anesthetics of the amide type should not receive ertapenem sodium reconstituted with lidocaine hydrochloride for IM injection.

■ **Warnings/Precautions** ***Sensitivity Reactions*** **Hypersensitivity Reactions.** Serious and occasionally fatal hypersensitivity reactions have been reported in patients receiving β-lactams. Ertapenem should be discontinued at the first appearance of a rash or any other sign of hypersensitivity.

Major Toxicities **Clostridium difficile-associated Colitis.** Reported with numerous anti-infectives, including ertapenem; may range in severity from mild to life-threatening. Evaluate and monitor patients who develop diarrhea during therapy.

General Precautions **Seizures.** Reported in patients receiving ertapenem. Caution is advised in patients with known or suspected CNS disorders (e.g., brain lesions, history of seizures) or compromised renal function.

Specific Populations **Pregnancy.** Category B. (See Users Guide.)

Lactation. Ertapenem is distributed into breast milk; caution if used in nursing women.

Pediatric Use. Safety and efficacy not established in children younger than 18 years of age.

Geriatric Use. No substantial differences in safety and efficacy relative to younger adults.

■ **Common Adverse Effects** Adverse effects occurring in 1% or more of patients receiving ertapenem sodium include diarrhea, infused vein complication, nausea, headache, vaginitis, phlebitis or thrombophlebitis, and vomiting.

Drug Interactions

■ **Probenecid** Pharmacokinetic interaction (decreased clearance of ertapenem). Concomitant use of probenecid to prolong the half-life of ertapenem is not recommended.

■ **Drugs Metabolized by Hepatic Microsomal Enzymes** Pharmacokinetic interaction unlikely.

■ **Drugs with *p*-Glycoprotein-mediated Clearance** Pharmacokinetic interaction unlikely for drugs that undergo *p*-glycoprotein-mediated clearance (e.g., digoxin, vinblastine).

Description

Ertapenem is a synthetic carbapenem β-lactam antibiotic that is structurally and pharmacologically related to imipenem and meropenem. Like meropenem but unlike imipenem, ertapenem has a methyl group at position 1 of the 5-membered ring, which confers stability against hydrolysis by dehydropeptidase 1 (DHP 1) present on the brush border of proximal renal tubular cells, and therefore does not require concomitant administration with a DHP-1 inhibitor such as cilastatin.

Ertapenem is almost completely absorbed following IM administration, having a mean bioavailability of 90%. Ertapenem exhibits nonlinear pharmacokinetics and is highly bound to plasma proteins, principally albumin. The drug has a mean plasma half-life of approximately 4 hours and may be administered once daily. (See Dosage and Administration: Reconstitution and Administration.) Ertapenem does not inhibit cytochrome P-450 (CYP) isoenzymes 1A2, 2C9, 2C19, 2D6, 2E1, or 3A4 in vitro and does not inhibit the *p*-glycoprotein transport system or act as a substrate for *p*-glycoprotein-mediated transport. (See Drug Interactions: Drugs with *p*-Glycoprotein-Mediated Clearance.) The drug is eliminated principally by renal excretion.

Ertapenem has in vitro activity against gram-positive and gram-negative aerobic and anaerobic bacteria. The drug is stable in the presence of a variety of *β*-lactamases (including penicillinases, cephalosporinases, and extended-spectrum *β*-lactamases). Ertapenem is active in vitro and in clinical infections against most strains of *Staphylococcus aureus* (methicillin-susceptible strains only), *Streptococcus agalactiae*, *S. pneumoniae* (penicillin-susceptible strains only), *S. pyogenes*, *Escherichia coli*, *Haemophilus influenzae* (non-*β*-lactamase-producing strains only), *Klebsiella pneumoniae*, *Moraxella catarrhalis*, *Bacteroides fragilis*, *B. distasonis*, *B. ovatus*, *B. thetaiotaomicron*, *B. uniformis*, *Clostridium clostridioforme*, *Eubacterium lentum*, *Peptostreptococcus* spp., *Porphyromonas asaccharolytica*, and *Prevotella bivia*. Ertapenem also has demonstrated in vitro activity against *S. pneumoniae* (penicillin-intermediate strains), *Citrobacter freundii*, *C. koseri*, *Enterobacter aerogenes*, *E. cloacae*, *H. influenzae* (*β*-lactamase-producing strains), *H. parainfluenzae*, *Klebsiella oxytoca* (excluding extended-spectrum *β*-lactamase-producing strains), *Morganella morganii*, *Proteus mirabilis*, *P. vulgaris*, *Serratia marcescens*, *C. perfringens*, and *Fusobacterium* spp.; however, the safety and efficacy of ertapenem in treating clinical infections caused by these microorganisms have not been established in adequate and well-controlled clinical trials to date.

Each gram of ertapenem provides approximately 6 mEq (137 mg) of sodium.

Advice to Patients

Importance of informing clinicians of other medical conditions, including any history of seizures. Importance of monitoring for signs of hypersensitivity reaction. Importance of reporting persistent or worsening symptoms of infection. Importance of women informing clinicians if they are or plan to become pregnant or to breast-feed. Importance of informing clinicians of existing or contemplated concomitant therapy, including prescription and OTC drugs.

Overview® (see Users Guide). For additional information on this drug until a more detailed monograph is developed and published, the manufacturer's labeling should be consulted. It is *essential* that the manufacturer's labeling be consulted for more detailed information on usual cautions, precautions, contraindications, potential drug interactions, laboratory test interferences, and acute toxicity.

Preparations

Excipients in commercially available drug preparations may have clinically important effects in some individuals; consult specific product labeling for details.

Ertapenem Sodium

Parenteral

For injection 1 g (of ertapenem) **INVanz®**, Merck

Imipenem and Cilastatin Sodium

Imipemide, N-F-Thienamycin, N-Formimidoylthienamycin

■ Imipenem and cilastatin sodium is a fixed combination of imipenem monohydrate (a semisynthetic carbapenem *β*-lactam antibiotic) and cilastatin sodium, which prevents renal metabolism of imipenem by dehydropeptidase I (DHP I).

Uses

Imipenem and cilastatin sodium solution is used IV in the treatment of serious infections caused by susceptible organisms including lower respiratory tract, skin and skin structure, intra-abdominal, gynecologic, or bone and joint infections. The drug also is used IV in the treatment of serious complicated or uncomplicated urinary tract infections, septicemia, or endocarditis caused by susceptible organisms.

If IM therapy is considered appropriate, imipenem and cilastatin sodium for injectable suspension can be used IM in the treatment of serious but mild to moderately severe infections caused by susceptible organisms including lower respiratory tract, skin and skin structure, intra-abdominal, and gynecologic infections. The drug has been used IM for mild-to-moderate urinary tract infections† (UTIs) caused by susceptible organisms, although recurrences occasionally have occurred, particularly in those with a history of chronic infection. Treatment failures and/or recurrences also have been reported when the drug was administered IM in the treatment of other infections and may have been related to the route of administration in some cases. Therefore, while it is not always possible to predict outcome, patients for whom IM therapy with the drug is being considered should be selected carefully; IM imipenem and cilastatin sodium therapy is *not* intended for use in severe and/or life-threatening infections (e.g., sepsis, endocarditis) or in patients with major physiologic impairment (e.g., shock). IM therapy with the drug also may be useful for prolonged anti-infective therapy after an initial IV course.

Because of its wide spectrum of activity, one of the principal uses of IV imipenem and cilastatin sodium is the treatment of polymicrobial bacterial infections. The drug is especially useful for empiric IV therapy of serious nosocomial infections that may include both gram-positive and gram-negative aerobic bacteria as well as anaerobic bacteria. IV imipenem and cilastatin sodium generally should not be used for the treatment of monobacterial infections when an anti-infective agent with a narrower spectrum of activity would be effective when used alone or for the treatment of most community-acquired infections caused by organisms susceptible to other anti-infective agents. IV imipenem and cilastatin sodium has been effective in the treatment of monobacterial and polymicrobial bacterial infections that failed to respond to other anti-infective agents, including cephalosporins, penicillins, and/or aminoglycosides. Imipenem and cilastatin sodium should *not* be used for perioperative prophylaxis. In addition, the manufacturer states that the drug should not be used in the treatment of CNS infections because safety and efficacy of the drug in these infections have not been definitely established.

Prior to initiation of imipenem and cilastatin sodium therapy, appropriate specimens should be obtained for identification of the causative organism and in vitro susceptibility tests. Imipenem and cilastatin sodium therapy may be started pending results of susceptibility tests, but generally should be discontinued if the organism is found to be resistant to the drug. Because resistant strains of *Pseudomonas aeruginosa* have developed during therapy with imipenem and cilastatin sodium, concomitant therapy with an aminoglycoside is recommended and in vitro susceptibility tests should probably be performed periodically when the drug is used in the treatment of infections caused by this organism.

■ **Gram-positive Aerobic Bacterial Infections** ***Infections Caused by Aerobic Gram-positive Cocci*** Imipenem and cilastatin sodium has been used IV in the treatment of serious lower respiratory tract infections caused by susceptible penicillinase-producing *Staphylococcus aureus*); serious complicated or uncomplicated urinary tract infections or septicemia caused by susceptible enterococci or penicillinase-producing *S. aureus*; serious skin and skin structure, bone and joint, or intra-abdominal infections caused by susceptible *S. epidermidis*, enterococci, or penicillinase-producing *S. aureus*; serious gynecologic infections caused by susceptible *S. epidermidis*, group B streptococci, enterococci, or penicillinase-producing *S. aureus*; or endocarditis caused by penicillinase-producing *S. aureus*. However, imipenem and cilastatin sodium generally is not considered an initial drug of choice for these infections. Imipenem and cilastatin sodium has also been used IV in the treatment of polymicrobial infections in which *Streptococcus pneumoniae*, *S. pyogenes* (group A *β*-hemolytic streptococci), or nonpenicillinase-producing *S. aureus* is one of the causative organisms, but other anti-infective agents with a narrower spectrum of activity (e.g., natural penicillins) are indicated for the treatment of monobacterial infections caused by these gram-positive aerobic cocci.

Imipenem and cilastatin sodium has been used IM in the treatment of serious lower respiratory tract infections of mild to moderate severity caused by susceptible *Streptococcus pneumoniae*; serious intra-abdominal infections of mild to moderate severity caused by susceptible *Enterococcus faecalis* (formerly *Streptococcus faecalis*) or *S. viridans* group organisms; serious skin and skin structure infections of mild to moderate severity caused by susceptible *S. aureus* (including penicillinase-producing *S. aureus*), *S. pyogenes*, or group D streptococci (including *E. faecalis*); or serious gynecologic infections of mild-to-moderate severity caused by susceptible group D streptococci (including *E. faecalis*).

Imipenem and cilastatin sodium usually is effective when used in the treatment of infections caused by penicillinase-producing *S. aureus* and has been effective when used alone IV in a limited number of patients for the treatment of endocarditis caused by penicillinase-producing *S. aureus*. However, penicillinase-resistant penicillins are generally the drugs of choice for the treatment of infections caused by susceptible penicillinase-producing staphylococci. Imipenem and cilastatin sodium has been used IV in the treatment of a limited number of infections caused by methicillin-resistant staphylococci (MRSA); however, the efficacy of the drug in these infections and adequate in vitro methods for determining susceptibility of MRSA to imipenem have not been established.

Although imipenem and cilastatin sodium may be effective in the treatment of some enterococcal infections (e.g., skin and skin structure infections), the drug should not be used in the treatment of enterococcal endocarditis. Imipenem and cilastatin sodium has been effective when used alone IV in a limited number of patients for the treatment of enterococcal endocarditis; however, imipenem is not bactericidal against enterococci and the drug has been less effective than penicillin G used in conjunction with an aminoglycoside in the treatment of *E. faecalis* (formerly *S. faecalis*) endocarditis in animal models.

Bacillus Infections Some clinicians suggest that imipenem and cilastatin sodium can be used for the treatment of invasive infections caused by *Bacillus cereus*†. Individuals with *B. cereus* food poisoning usually require only supportive care (oral rehydration or, occasionally IV fluid and electrolyte replacement for those with severe dehydration); however, patients with invasive disease require anti-infective therapy and prompt removal of potentially infected foreign bodies (e.g., indwelling intravascular catheters, implanted devices). Some clinicians consider vancomycin the drug of choice for invasive *B. cereus* infections and recommend carbapenems (imipenem or meropenem) or clindamycin as alternatives.

Nocardia Infections Imipenem and cilastatin sodium has been effective when used for the treatment of infections caused by *Nocardia*, including pulmonary nocardiosis caused by *N. asteroides* and primary cutaneous nocardiosis. Many clinicians suggest that co-trimoxazole is the drug of first choice for *Nocardia* infections. Other recommended regimens for *Nocardia* include a sulfonamide (e.g., sulfisoxazole) with or without minocycline or amikacin; a tetracycline (e.g., doxycycline, minocycline); a carbapenem (imipenem or meropenem) with or without amikacin; amoxicillin and clavulanate; cycloserine; or linezolid. In patients with CNS or disseminated disease or overwhelming infection, concomitant amikacin may be indicated during the first 4–12 weeks or until the patients improves clinically.

Rhodococcus Infections Imipenem and cilastatin sodium used in conjunction with vancomycin is one of several regimens recommended for the treatment of infections caused by *Rhodococcus equi*. *R. equi* has been identified as a cause of pulmonary infections (e.g., lung abscess) in immunocompromised individuals such as patients with human immunodeficiency virus (HIV) infection and solid organ transplant recipients. While optimum regimens for the treatment of these infections have not been identified, combination regimens usually are recommended. Some clinicians suggest that *R. equi* infections be treated with a regimen of vancomycin given with a fluoroquinolone, rifampin, a carbapenem (imipenem or meropenem), or amikacin.

■ **Gram-negative Aerobic Bacterial Infections** ***Infections Caused by Enterobacteriaceae*** Imipenem and cilastatin sodium is used IV in the treatment of serious lower respiratory tract infections or septicemia caused by susceptible *Enterobacter*, *Escherichia coli*, *Klebsiella*, or *Serratia marcescens*; serious complicated or uncomplicated urinary tract infections caused by susceptible *Enterobacter*, *E. coli*, *Klebsiella*, *Morganella morganii*, *Proteus vulgaris*, or *Providencia rettgeri*; or serious bone and joint infections caused by susceptible *Enterobacter*. The drug is also used IV in the treatment of serious intra-abdominal infections caused by susceptible *Citrobacter*, *Enterobacter*, *E. coli*, *Klebsiella*, *M. morganii*, or*Proteus*; serious gynecologic infections caused by susceptible *Enterobacter*, *E. coli*, *Klebsiella*, or *Proteus*; or serious skin and skin structure infections caused by susceptible *Citrobacter*, *Enterobacter*, *E. coli*, *Klebsiella*, *M. morganii*, *P. vulgaris*, *P. rettgeri*, or *Serratia*.

Imipenem and cilastatin sodium is used IM in the treatment of serious intra-abdominal or gynecologic infections of mild-to-moderate severity caused by susceptible *E. coli* or *K. pneumoniae* or serious skin and skin structure infections of mild-to-moderate severity caused by susceptible *Citrobacter*, *E. coli*, *Enterobacter cloacae*, or *K. pneumoniae*.

Imipenem and cilastatin sodium has generally been effective when used alone IV in the treatment of serious infections caused by susceptible Enterobacteriaceae. Although some clinicians recommend that an aminoglycoside be used concomitantly if the drug is used IV for empiric therapy of nosocomial gram-negative bacteremia in seriously ill patients, other clinicians state that imipenem and cilastatin sodium can generally be used alone IV for these infections unless there is a possibility that *Pseudomonas aeruginosa* may be present.

Pseudomonas aeruginosa Infections Imipenem and cilastatin sodium is used IM or IV in the treatment of intra-abdominal or skin and skin structure infections, and is used IV in the treatment of serious complicated or uncomplicated urinary tract infections, septicemia, or bone and joint infections caused by susceptible *Pseudomonas aeruginosa*. Because resistant strains of *Ps. aeruginosa* have emerged during imipenem and cilastatin sodium therapy, most clinicians state that an aminoglycoside should be used concomitantly whenever the drug is used in the treatment of serious infections known or suspected to be caused by *Ps. aeruginosa*.

Clinical improvement has been observed in some patients when imipenem and cilastatin sodium was used IV for the treatment of acute exacerbations of bronchopulmonary *Ps. aeruginosa* infections in patients with cystic fibrosis; however, as with other anti-infective agents, a bacteriologic cure is rarely obtained and should not be expected in these patients.

Acinetobacter Infections Imipenem and cilastatin sodium is used in the treatment of serious infections caused by *Acinetobacter*; it is administered IV in the treatment of lower respiratory tract infections and IM or IV in the treatment of skin and skin structure infections caused by these organisms. Some clinicians suggest that carbapenems (imipenem or meropenem) are drugs of choice for the treatment of *Acinetobacter* infections and recommend concomitant use of an aminoglycoside (amikacin, gentamicin, tobramycin) in severe infections.

Campylobacter Infections Some clinicians suggest that imipenem and cilastatin sodium is a drug of choice for the treatment of systemic infections caused by *Campylobacter fetus*. *Campylobacter* are spiral or curved, motile, microaerophilic gram-negative bacilli. Most *Campylobacter* infections reported in the US are caused by *C. jejuni* and involve mild to moderate gastroenteritis, although complications can occur as the result of local invasion of the organism (e.g., GI hemorrhage, proctitis, pancreatitis) and systemic infection has been reported. While relatively rare in the US, *C. fetus* infection usually involves systemic disease, including bacteremia, sepsis, and meningitis, especially in neonates and debilitated hosts. Erythromycin or azithromycin usually is considered the drug of choice for the treatment of gastroenteritis or locally invasive infections caused by *C. jejuni* when such therapy is considered necessary; systemic infections caused by *C. jejuni* or *C. fetus* usually require parenteral therapy. Some clinicians suggest that the treatment of choice for *C. fetus* infection is a carbapenem antibiotic (imipenem or meropenem) and that gentamicin can be used as an alternative.

Melioidosis Imipenem and cilastatin sodium has been used effectively for the treatment of localized or septicemic melioidosis†, a potentially life-threatening disease caused by *Burkholderia pseudomallei* (formerly *Ps. pseudomallei*). *B. pseudomallei* is an aerobic, nonfermentative gram-negative bacilli resistant to many anti-infective agents. Some clinicians suggest that drugs of choice for the treatment of melioidosis are imipenem or ceftazidime. Other drugs that have been recommended as alternative agents for the treatment of melioidosis include IV amoxicillin and clavulanate potassium (not commercially available in the US), IV meropenem, oral amoxicillin and clavulanate potassium, or a 3-drug regimen of chloramphenicol, doxycycline, and co-trimoxazole. *B. pseudomallei* is difficult to eradicate, and relapse of melioidosis commonly occurs. Therefore, anti-infective therapy usually is continued for 6 weeks to 6 months or, alternatively, a parenteral anti-infective (e.g., ceftazidime) is given for at least 1–2 weeks followed by an oral anti-infective (e.g., amoxicillin and clavulanate potassium) given for at least 3–6 months.

Actinomycosis Imipenem and cilastatin sodium has been effective when used in a limited number of patients for the treatment of thoracic actinomycosis†. However, IV penicillin G or ampicillin usually are the drugs of choice for the treatment of all forms of actinomycosis, including thoracic, abdominal, CNS, and cervicofacial infections.

Capnocytophaga Infections Some clinicians suggest that imipenem and cilastatin sodium can be used in the treatment of infections caused by *Capnocytophaga canimorsus*† (formerly CDC group DF-2). *C. canimorsus* is a gram-negative bacilli that can cause life-threatening septicemia, meningitis, and/or endocarditis and often is associated with disseminated intravascular coagulation; *Capnocytophaga* infection usually occurs as the result of a dog bite or other close contact with a dog. The optimum regimen for the treatment of infections caused by *Capnocytophaga* has not been identified, but some clinicians recommend use of penicillin G or, alternatively, a third generation cephalosporin (cefotaxime, ceftizoxime, ceftriaxone), a carbapenem (imipenem or meropenem), vancomycin, a fluoroquinolone, or clindamycin.

Legionella Infections Imipenem and cilastatin sodium has been effective when used in a few patients for the treatment of *Legionella pneumophila*† respiratory tract infections. However, other anti-infectives (e.g., a macrolide or a fluoroquinolone with or without rifampin) generally are preferred for *L. pneumophila* infections.

■ **Anaerobic and Mixed Aerobic-Anaerobic Bacterial Infections** Imipenem and cilastatin sodium is used either IM or IV in the treatment of infections caused by gram-positive and gram-negative anaerobic bacteria. The drug has been effective IV in the treatment of serious intra-abdominal infections caused by susceptible *Bifidobacterium*, *Clostridium*, *Peptococcus*, *Peptostreptococcus*, *Eubacterium*, or *Propionibacterium*; serious gynecologic infections caused by susceptible *Bifidobacterium*, *Peptococcus*, *Peptostreptococcus*, or *Propionibacterium*; or serious skin and skin structure infections caused by susceptible *Peptococcus* or *Peptostreptococcus*. IV imipenem and cilastatin sodium has also been effective in the treatment of septicemia or serious intra-abdominal, gynecologic, or skin and skin structure infections caused by susceptible *Bacteroides*, including *B. fragilis*, and in the treatment of serious intra-abdominal tract or skin and skin structure infections caused by susceptible *Fusobacterium*.

Imipenem and cilastatin sodium is used IM or IV in the treatment of serious intra-abdominal infections of mild-to-moderate severity caused by susceptible *Bacteroides* (including *B. fragilis*, *B. distasonis*, *B. thetaiotaomicron*), *Fusobacterium*, *Prevotella intermedia* (formerly *B. intermedius*)†, or *Peptostreptococcus*; serious skin and skin structure infections of mild-to-moderate severity caused by susceptible *Bacteroides*, including *B. fragilis*; or serious gynecologic infections of mild-to-moderate severity caused by susceptible *P. intermedia* or *Peptostreptococcus*.

Imipenem and cilastatin sodium has been effective when used alone IV in the treatment of mixed aerobic-anaerobic infections such as peritonitis, intra-abdominal abscess, and gynecologic infections. In several controlled studies, IV imipenem and cilastatin sodium alone was at least as effective as gentamicin used in conjunction with clindamycin for the treatment of mixed aerobic-anaerobic bacterial infections. However, further study is needed to establish the relative efficacy and safety of therapy with IV imipenem and cilastatin sodium compared with therapy with an aminoglycoside used in conjunction with clindamycin, metronidazole, or cefoxitin or with other regimens used in the treatment of mixed aerobic-anaerobic bacterial infections.

■ **Respiratory Tract Infections** Imipenem and cilastatin sodium has been used IV in the treatment of serious lower respiratory tract infections (including pneumonia) caused by susceptible penicillinase-producing *S. aureus*), *S. pneumoniae*, *Enterobacter*, *E. coli*, *Klebsiella*, or *S. marcescens*.

Community-acquired Pneumonia Although imipenem generally is active against *S. pneumoniae* (including drug-resistant *S. pneumoniae*), the American Thoracic Society (ATS) and the Infectious Diseases Society of America (IDSA) state that the drug is not usually considered a drug of first choice for the empiric treatment of community-acquired pneumonia (CAP). The ATS suggests that use of imipenem in the treatment of CAP be reserved for patients at risk for *Ps. aeruginosa* infections. Factors that increase the risk of *Ps. aeruginosa* infection in CAP patients include severe CAP requiring treatment in an intensive care unit (ICU), structural lung disease (bronchiectasis, cystic fibrosis), corticosteroid therapy (prednisone dosage exceeding 10 mg daily), broad-spectrum anti-infective therapy given for longer than 7 days within the past month, and malnutrition. In CAP patients with risk factors for *Ps. aeruginosa*, the ATS recommends use of an empiric regimen that includes 2 antipseudomonal agents and also provides coverage for drug-resistant *S. pneumoniae* and *Legionella*. These experts suggest that this can be accomplished with a regimen that includes an IV antipseudomonal β-lactam anti-infective (e.g., cefepime, piperacillin and tazobactam, imipenem, meropenem) in conjunction with an IV antipseudomonal fluoroquinolone (e.g., ciprofloxacin) or a regimen that includes one of these IV antipseudomonal β-lactam anti-infectives, an IV aminoglycoside, and either an IV macrolide (e.g., azithromycin) or an IV nonpseudomonal quinolone. If anaerobic bacteria have been identified or are suspected in patients with pulmonary infections, the IDSA recommends use of clindamycin, a β-lactam/β-lactamase inhibitor combination, imipenem, or meropenem.

■ **Empiric Therapy in Febrile Neutropenic Patients** Imipenem and cilastatin sodium has been effective when used alone for empiric anti-infective therapy of presumed bacterial infections in febrile neutropenic adults or pediatric patients†. Imipenem and cilastatin sodium used alone generally is as effective for empiric therapy in these patients as ceftazidime used alone or ceftazidime used in combination with an aminoglycoside or piperacillin.

Successful treatment of infections in granulocytopenic patients requires prompt initiation of empiric anti-infective therapy (even when fever is the only sign or symptom of infection) and appropriate modification of the initial regimen if the duration of fever and neutropenia is protracted, if a specific site of infection is identified, or if organisms resistant to the initial regimen are present. The initial empiric regimen should be chosen based on the underlying disease and other host factors that may affect the degree of risk and on local epidemiologic data regarding usual pathogens in these patients and data regarding their in vitro susceptibility to available anti-infective agents. The fact that gram-positive bacteria have become a predominant pathogen in febrile neutropenic patients should be considered when selecting an empiric anti-infective regimen.

No empiric regimen has been identified that would be appropriate for all patients. Regimens that have been recommended for empiric therapy in febrile neutropenic patients with presumed bacterial infections include *monotherapy* with a third or fourth generation cephalosporin (i.e., ceftazidime, cefepime) or a carbapenem (e.g., imipenem and cilastatin sodium, meropenem); *combination therapy* consisting of a β-lactam antibiotic (e.g., ceftazidime, ceftriaxone), a carbapenem (e.g., imipenem, meropenem), an extended-spectrum penicillin (e.g., mezlocillin, piperacillin, ticarcillin), or a fixed combination of an extended-spectrum penicillin and a β-lactamase inhibitor (e.g., piperacillin sodium and tazobactam sodium, ticarcillin disodium and clavulanate potassium) given in conjunction with an aminoglycoside (e.g., amikacin, gentamicin, tobramycin); or *combination therapy* consisting of 2 β-lactam antibiotics (e.g., ceftazidime given with piperacillin).

The IDSA recommends use of a parenteral empiric regimen in most febrile neutropenic patients; use of an oral regimen (e.g., oral ciprofloxacin and oral amoxicillin and clavulanate) should only be considered in selected adults at low risk for complications who have no focus of bacterial infection and no signs or symptoms of systemic infection other than fever. At health-care facilities where gram-positive bacteria are common causes of serious infection and use of vancomycin in the initial empiric regimen is considered necessary, the IDSA recommends 2- or 3-drug combination therapy that includes vancomycin and either cefepime, ceftazidime, imipenem, or meropenem given with or without an aminoglycoside; vancomycin should be discontinued 24–48 hours later if a susceptible gram-positive bacterial infection is not identified. At health-care facilities where vancomycin is not indicated in the initial empiric regimen, the IDSA recommends monotherapy with a third or fourth generation cephalosporin (ceftazidime, cefepime) or a carbapenem (imipenem, meropenem) for uncomplicated cases; however, for complicated cases or if anti-infective resistance is a problem, combination therapy consisting of an aminoglycoside (amikacin, gentamicin, tobramycin) given in conjunction with an antipseudomonal penicillin (ticarcillin and clavulanate, piperacillin and tazobactam), an antipseudomonal cephalosporin (cefepime, ceftazidime), or a carbapenem (imipenem, meropenem) is recommended. Regardless of the initial regimen selected, patients should be reassessed after 3–5 days of treatment and the anti-infective regimen altered (if indicated) based on the presence or absence of fever, identification of the causative organism, and the clinical condition of the patient.

Published protocols for the treatment of infections in febrile neutropenic patients should be consulted for specific recommendations regarding selection of the initial empiric regimen, when to change the initial regimen, possible subsequent regimens, and duration of therapy in these patients.

Dosage and Administration

■ **Reconstitution and Administration** Imipenem and cilastatin sodium is administered by intermittent IV infusion as a solution and by deep IM injection as a suspension. IM administration of the drug should be limited to mild to moderately severe infections.

Intermittent IV Infusion Piggyback units containing 250 mg of imipenem and 250 mg of cilastatin or those containing 500 mg of imipenem and 500 mg of cilastatin should be reconstituted with 100 mL of a compatible IV solution to provide solutions containing 2.5 or 5 mg/mL of each drug, respectively. ADD-Vantage® vials containing imipenem and cilastatin sodium should be reconstituted according to the manufacturer's directions with the diluent provided. For IV administration, the manufacturer recommends that an imipenem concentration of 5 mg/mL not be exceeded since the physical and chemical stability of solutions of the drug may be adversely affected at higher concentrations. Alternatively, the contents of vials containing 250 mg of imipenem and 250 mg of cilastatin or 500 mg of imipenem and 500 mg of cilastatin may be initially suspended with a portion of a compatible IV solution and then the resulting suspension of drug added to the remaining IV solution to a volume of 100 mL. A suggested procedure for preparing an initial suspension is to add approximately 10 mL from a 100-mL container of the IV solution to the vial of drug. The resulting initial suspension should be shaken well and then transferred to the IV solution container. To ensure complete transfer of the vial contents, an additional 10 mL from the IV solution container should be added to the vial and transferred back to the IV solution container. Initial suspensions of the drug should*not* be infused IV. The resulting solution of imipenem and cilastatin sodium should be agitated until clear, but should *not* be heated to facilitate dissolution.

The rate of IV infusion of imipenem depends on the dose of the drug. Each 125-, 250- or 500-mg dose of imipenem should generally be infused over 20–30 minutes, and each 1-g dose of the drug should generally be infused over 40–60 minutes. If nausea and/or vomiting occur during administration of imipenem, the rate of IV infusion may be decreased.

If an aminoglycoside is administered concomitantly with imipenem and cilastatin sodium, the drugs should not be admixed but may be administered from separate containers through the same IV tubing. Imipenem and cilastatin sodium solutions should be inspected visually for particulate matter prior to administration whenever solution and container permit.

IM Injection Imipenem and cilastatin sodium powder for injectable suspension should be reconstituted with lidocaine hydrochloride 1% injection(without epinephrine). To reconstitute the suspension, 2 or 3 mL of the diluent should be added to the vial labeled as containing 500 or 750 mg of imipenem, respectively. The vial should be agitated well to form a suspension and the entire contents of the vial withdrawn for IM injection.

Imipenem and cilastatin sodium for injectable suspension is administered by deep IM injection into a large muscle mass (such as the gluteal muscle or lateral aspect of the thigh) with a 21-gauge, 2-inch needle. To avoid inadvertent injection of the suspension into a blood vessel, the plunger of the syringe should be drawn back prior to IM administration to ensure that blood is not aspirated. *The IM preparation should not be used IV.*

■ **Dosage** Dosage of imipenem and cilastatin sodium is generally expressed in terms of the imipenem content of the fixed combination; dosage of imipenem monohydrate is expressed in terms of anhydrous imipenem.

The dosage of imipenem should be given in equally divided doses based on type and severity of infection, susceptibility of the causative organism(s), and the patient's renal function and body weight.

Adult Dosage The manufacturer states that recommended usual IV dosages of imipenem and cilastatin sodium are for adults weighing at least 70 kg. Modification of dosage is recommended for patients weighing less than this. (See Dosage and Administration: Dosage in Renal and Hepatic Impairment and Reduced Body Weight.)

For the treatment of mild infections, the usual adult IV dosage of imipenem is 250 mg every 6 hours (1 g daily) for infections caused by fully susceptible gram-positive or -negative aerobic or anaerobic bacteria and 500 mg every 6 hours (2 g daily) for infections caused by moderately susceptible bacteria. Adults with moderately severe infections caused by fully susceptible organisms should receive 500 mg of imipenem IV every 6 (2 g daily) or 8 (1.5 g daily) hours, and adults with moderately severe infections caused by moderately susceptible organisms should receive 500 mg every 6 hours (2 g daily) to 1 g IV every 8 hours (3 g daily).

For the treatment of severe, life-threatening infections, adults should receive 500 mg IV every 6 hours (2 g daily) for infections caused by fully susceptible organisms and 1 g IV every 6 (4 g daily) or 8 (3 g daily) hours for infections caused by moderately susceptible organisms.

The maximum adult IV dosage of imipenem recommended by the manufacturer is 50 mg/kg daily or 4 g daily, whichever is lower. However, patients older than 12 years of age with cystic fibrosis who had normal renal function have received daily dosages up to 90 mg/kg (maximum daily dosage: 4 g), given in divided doses. The manufacturer states that there is no evidence that higher dosages would be more effective.

When IM imipenem is used for treatment of lower respiratory tract, skin and skin structure, or gynecologic infections of mild-to-moderate severity, adults can receive 500 or 750 mg of imipenem IM every 12 hours, depending on the severity of the infection. For the IM treatment of intra-abdominal infections of mild-to-moderate severity, adults can receive 750 mg of imipenem IM every 12 hours. The maximum adult dosage of IM imipenem recommended by the manufacturer is 1.5 g daily. The duration of therapy depends on the type and severity of the infection. Generally, IM imipenem therapy should be continued for at least 2 days after the signs and symptoms of infection have resolved; the safety and efficacy of IM therapy beyond 14 days have not been established.

Urinary Tract Infections. For the treatment of uncomplicated urinary tract infection, the usual adult IV dosage of imipenem is 250 mg every 6 hours (1 g daily) for infections caused by fully susceptible gram-positive or -negative aerobic or anaerobic bacteria or by moderately susceptible bacteria. For the treatment of complicated urinary tract infection, the usual adult IV dosage of imipenem is 500 mg every 6 hours (2 g daily) for infections caused by fully susceptible gram-positive or -negative aerobic or anaerobic bacteria or by moderately susceptible bacteria.

Empiric Therapy in Febrile Neutropenic Patients. For empiric anti-infective therapy in febrile neutropenic patients†, IV imipenem and cilastatin sodium has been given in a dosage of 500 mg every 6 hours.

Pediatric Dosage The usual IV dosage of imipenem and cilastatin sodium for pediatric patients 3 months of age or older for the treatment of infections (other than CNS infections) caused by susceptible bacteria is 15–25 mg/kg every 6 hours. Based on studies in adults, the manufacturer states that the maximum daily dosage of the drug in pediatric patients is 2 g daily in those with infections caused by fully susceptible bacteria or 4 g daily in those with infections caused by moderately susceptible bacteria (e.g., some strains of *Pseudomonas aeruginosa*); however, higher dosage (up to 90 mg/kg daily in older children) has been used in some cystic fibrosis patients.

The recommended dosage of IV imipenem and cilastatin sodium for the treatment of infections (other than CNS infections) in infants 4 weeks to 3 months of age who weigh at least 1.5 kg is 25 mg/kg every 6 hours. Neonates younger than 1 week of age who weigh at least 1.5 kg can receive an IV dosage of 25 mg/kg every 12 hours and neonates 1–4 weeks of age who weigh at least 1.5 kg can receive an IV dosage of 25 mg/kg every 8 hours.

When IV imipenem and cilastatin sodium is used in pediatric patients, doses of 500 mg or less should be given by IV infusion over 15–30 minutes and doses greater than 500 mg should be given by IV infusion over 40–60 minutes.

■ Dosage in Renal Impairment and Reduced Body Weight

Modification of the usual dosage of imipenem generally is unnecessary in patients with creatinine clearances greater than 70 mL/minute per 1.73 m^2 who weigh at least 70 kg. However, modification of dosage is necessary in those with normal renal function weighing less than 70 kg and in any patient with impaired renal function regardless of body weight. Safety and efficacy of IM imipenem and cilastatin sodium therapy in patients with creatinine clearances less than 20 mL/minute per 1.73 m^2 have not been established. In patients with creatinine clearances of 70 mL/minute per 1.73 m^2 or less and in those weighing less than 70 kg, doses and/or frequency of IV administration of imipenem should be modified in response to the degree of renal impairment, body weight, type and severity of the infection, and susceptibility of the causative organisms. Serum creatinine concentrations alone may not be sufficiently accurate to assess the degree of renal impairment; dosage preferably should be based on the patient's measured or estimated creatinine clearance. The patient's creatinine clearance (Ccr) can be estimated by using the following formulas:

$$Ccr\ male = \frac{(140 - age) \times weight}{72 \times serum\ creatinine}$$

$$Ccr\ female = 0.85 \times Ccr\ male$$

where age is in years, weight is in kg, and serum creatinine is in mg/dL.

The manufacturer recommends the following *reduced* IV dosage based on the patient's creatinine clearance and body weight (see Table 1).

The manufacturer recommends that patients with creatinine clearances of 6–20 mL/minute per 1.73 m^2 receive 125 or 250 mg of imipenem every 12 hours for infections caused by most susceptible organisms. When the 500-mg IV dose given twice daily (every 12 hours) is used in these patients, there may be an increased risk of seizures. In patients undergoing hemodialysis, IV imipenem and cilastatin sodium therapy is recommended only when the potential benefit from the drug outweighs the potential risk of drug-induced seizures. *Patients with creatinine clearances of 5 mL/minute or less per 1.73 ² should not receive imipenem and cilastatin sodium IV unless hemodialysis is instituted within 48 hours.* The manufacturer states that IV dosage recommendations and precautions for patients with creatinine clearances of 6–20 mL/minute per 1.73 m^2 also apply when imipenem and cilastatin sodium is used IV in patients with creatinine clearances of 5 mL/minute or less per 1.73 m^2 who are undergoing hemodialysis. If imipenem and cilastatin sodium is used IV in hemodialysis patients, a supplemental dose of the drug should be given after each dialysis period and at 12-hour intervals thereafter. If the drug is used IV in dialysis patients, especially those with CNS disease, the patients should be carefully monitored for adverse CNS effects (e.g., confusion, myoclonic activity, seizures). (See Cautions: Precautions and Contraindications.)

Cautions

Adverse effects reported with imipenem and cilastatin sodium are similar to those reported with other β-lactam antibiotics, and the drug is generally well tolerated. Adverse CNS effects, including seizures and myoclonus, have been reported occasionally with IV imipenem and cilastatin sodium. Although further experience with the drug is needed before the true incidence of these adverse CNS effects can be determined, experience to date indicates that these effects may occur more frequently with IV imipenem and cilastatin sodium than with the IM formulation of the drug or with other currently available β-lactam antibiotics.

■ GI Effects Adverse GI effects are among the most frequent adverse reactions to imipenem and cilastatin sodium. Nausea, diarrhea, and vomiting have been reported in up to 4% of patients receiving the drug. Nausea and vomiting appear to be related to the rate of IV infusion, especially when 1-g doses of the drug are being administered, and have rarely been accompanied by hypotension or hyperventilation. Nausea and vomiting are generally ameliorated by decreasing the IV infusion rate, but may occasionally be severe enough to require discontinuance of the drug.

Clostridium difficile-associated diarrhea and colitis (also known as antibiotic-associated pseudomembranous colitis), caused by toxin-producing clostridia resistant to imipenem, has occurred in less than 0.2% of patients during or following discontinuance of imipenem and cilastatin sodium therapy. *C. difficile* and/or its toxin has been isolated from the feces of patients who developed diarrhea and/or colitis during therapy with the drug. Mild cases of colitis may respond to discontinuance of the drug alone, but diagnosis and management of moderate to severe cases should include appropriate bacteriologic studies and treatment with fluid, electrolyte, and protein supplementation as indicated; rarely, cautious use of sigmoidoscopy (or other appropriate endoscopic examination) may be considered necessary. If colitis is moderate to severe or is not relieved by discontinuance of imipenem and cilastatin sodium,

Table 1. Reduced intravenous dosage of imipenem and cilastatin sodium IV in adult patients with impaired renal function and/or body weight <70 kg.

and Body Weight (kg) is:	If Total Recommended Daily Dose is: 1 g/day and creatinine clearance (mL/min per 1.73 m²) is:				1.5 g/day and creatinine clearance (mL/min per 1.73 m²) is:				2 g/day and creatinine clearance (mL/min per 1.73 m²) is:			
	≥71	41–70	21–40	6–20	≥71	41–70	21–40	6–20	≥71	41–70	21–40	6–20
	then the reduced dosage regimen (mg) is:				then the reduced dosage regimen (mg) is:				then the reduced dosage regimen (mg) is:			
≥70	250 q6h	250 q8h	250 q12h	250 q12h	500 q8h	250 q6h	250 q8h	250 q12h	500 q6h	500 q8h	250 q6h	250 q12h
60	250 q8h	125 q6h	250 q12h	125 q12h	250 q6h	250 q8h	250 q8h	250 q12h	500 q8h	250 q6h	250 q8h	250 q12h
50	125 q6h	125 q6h	125 q8h	125 q12h	250 q6h	250 q8h	250 q12h	250 q12h	250 q6h	250 q6h	250 q8h	250 q12h
40	125 q6h	125 q8h	125 q12h	125 q12h	250 q8h	125 q6h	125 q8h	125 q12h	250 q6h	250 q8h	250 q12h	250 q12h
30	125 q8h	125 q8h	125 q12h	125 q12h	125 q6h	125 q8h	125 q8h	125 q12h	250 q8h	125 q6h	125 q8h	125 q12h

Cilastatin Sodium (Renal Impairment Dosage Continued)

and Body Weight (kg) is:	If Total Recommended Daily Dose is: 3 g/day and creatinine clearance (mL/min per 1.73 m²) is:				4 g/day and creatinine clearance (mL/min per 1.73 m²) is:			
	≥71	41–70	21–40	6–20	≥71	41–70	21–40	6–20
	then the reduced dosage regimen (mg) is:				then the reduced dosage regimen (mg) is:			
≥70	1000 q8h	500 q6h	500 q8h	500 q12h	1000 q6h	750 q8h	500 q6h	500 q12h
60	750 q8h	500 q8h	500 q8h	500 q12h	1000 q8h	750 q8h	500 q8h	500 q12h
50	500 q6h	500 q8h	250 q6h	250 q12h	750 q8h	500 q6h	500 q8h	500 q12h
40	500 q8h	250 q6h	250 q8h	250 q12h	500 q6h	500 q8h	250 q6h	250 q12h
30	250 q6h	250 q8h	250 q8h	250 q12h	500 q8h	250 q6h	250 q8h	250 q12h

appropriate anti-infective therapy (e.g., oral metronidazole or vancomycin) should be administered. Isolation of the patient may be advisable. Other causes of colitis also should be considered.

Other adverse GI effects that have been reported in less than 0.2% of patients receiving IV imipenem and cilastatin sodium include hemorrhagic colitis, gastroenteritis, abdominal pain, glossitis, papillar hypertrophy of the tongue, staining of the teeth and/or tongue, heartburn, pharyngeal pain, taste perversion, and increased salivation.

Imipenem and cilastatin sodium therapy generally has only a minimal effect on normal bowel flora. Either no decrease or only a slight decrease in total bacterial counts of normal aerobic and anaerobic fecal flora occurs during or following therapy with the drug, presumably because only low concentrations of microbiologically active drug are attained in the intestine following IV administration.

■ Hematologic Effects Eosinophilia has been reported in up to 4% of patients receiving imipenem and cilastatin sodium. Transient leukopenia, neutropenia, agranulocytosis, pancytopenia, bone marrow depression, hemolytic anemia, thrombocytopenia, and thrombocytosis have been reported in less than 2% of patients receiving the drug. Leukocytosis, monocytosis, lymphocytosis, and basophilia have also been reported rarely. Although decreased hemoglobin concentration, decreased hematocrit, decreased erythrocyte count, and prolonged prothrombin time have been reported rarely in patients receiving imipenem and cilastatin sodium, a causal relationship to the drug has not been established.

Positive direct antiglobulin (Coombs') test results, without clinical or laboratory evidence of hemolysis, have been reported in about 2% of patients receiving imipenem and cilastatin sodium.

■ CNS Effects Adverse CNS effects have been reported occasionally in patients receiving IV imipenem and cilastatin sodium; however, similar CNS effects have not been reported to date with IM imipenem and cilastatin sodium therapy. Seizures have been reported in up to 1.5% and dizziness, somnolence, encephalopathy, confusion, myoclonus, tremor, paresthesia, vertigo, headache, and psychic disturbances, and hallucinations have been reported in less than 0.3% of patients receiving the drug IV. In most reported cases, seizures or myoclonus occurred in patients with preexisting CNS disorders (e.g., a history of seizures, brain lesions, recent head trauma) and/or who had received relatively high IV dosages of the drug in relation to renal function and body size (e.g., geriatric patients). However, seizures have also occurred during IV imipenem and cilastatin sodium therapy in some patients with no recognized or documented underlying CNS disorder. Generalized seizures developed during concurrent therapy with ganciclovir and subsided in some patients despite continued ganciclovir therapy when imipenem and cilastatin sodium was discontinued. (See Drug Interactions: Ganciclovir.) Further study is needed to identify other factors that may contribute to the development of adverse CNS effects during IV imipenem and cilastatin sodium therapy, but there is some evidence that the drug may potentiate seizure activity or lower the seizure threshold in patients with other predisposing factors. Therefore, if IM or IV imipenem and cilastatin sodium is used in patients with a known seizure disorder, anticonvulsant therapy should be continued during imipenem and cilastatin sodium therapy. If focal tremors, myoclonus, or seizures occur in patients receiving IV or IM imipenem and cilastatin sodium, anticonvulsant therapy should be initiated and dosage of imipenem and cilastatin sodium should be decreased or the drug discontinued.

■ Dermatologic and Hypersensitivity Reactions Hypersensitivity reactions including rash, fever, pruritus, and urticaria have been reported in less than 3% of patients receiving imipenem and cilastatin sodium. Allergic dermatitis, erythema multiforme, facial edema or angioedema, Stevens-Johnson syndrome, toxic epidermal necrolysis, and flushing have also been reported rarely. Hypersensitivity reactions to imipenem and cilastatin sodium have occurred when the drug was administered to patients hypersensitive to penicillins. (See Cautions: Precautions and Contraindications.)If a hypersensitivity reaction occurs during imipenem and cilastatin sodium therapy, the drug should be discontinued. Severe hypersensitivity or anaphylactic reactions should be treated with appropriate therapy (e.g., epinephrine, oxygen, IV corticosteroids, airway management including intubation) as indicated.

■ Renal Effects Transient increases in BUN and/or serum creatinine concentrations have been reported in less than 2% of patients receiving imipenem and cilastatin sodium. Oliguria/anuria, polyuria, proteinuria, discoloration of urine, acute renal failure, and the presence of erythrocytes, leukocytes, bilirubin, urobilinogen, bacteria, or casts in urine have also been reported rarely in patients receiving the drug. The role of imipenem and cilastatin sodium in producing these changes in renal function is difficult to determine, since factors predisposing to prerenal azotemia or to impaired renal function usually have been present.

When given alone, imipenem is nephrotoxic in animals; however, concomitant administration of cilastatin sodium apparently may decrease the nephrotoxic potential of the drug. Acute tubular necrosis occurred in rabbits and monkeys who received imipenem alone in doses greater than 100 mg/kg; nephrotoxicity did not occur when 360-mg/kg doses of cilastatin sodium were administered concomitantly with 360-mg/kg doses of imipenem. Although the mechanism by which cilastatin apparently decreases the nephrotoxic potential of imipenem has not been determined to date, it has been suggested that since cilastatin competes with imipenem for tubular secretion it may protect the kidneys by preventing accumulation of imipenem and/or its metabolites in renal tubular cells. Usual dosages of imipenem and cilastatin sodium do not appear to be nephrotoxic in humans. Urinary β_2-microglobulin concentrations were generally unaffected or increased only slightly in healthy adults who received 1-g doses of the drug IV every 6 hours for 10 days.

■ Local Effects Phlebitis and/or thrombophlebitis have generally been reported in 2–5% of patients receiving imipenem and cilastatin sodium IV. In some studies, however, phlebitis occurred in up to 60% of patients receiving the drug. Phlebitis is generally mild, but may be severe enough to require discontinuance of the drug. Other adverse local reactions, including pain, erythema, induration, or infection at the IV infusion site, have been reported in 1% or less of patients receiving the drug.

Pain at the site of injection has been reported in 1.2% of patients receiving imipenem and cilastatin sodium IM; concomitant injection with lidocaine hydrochloride 1% can minimize but not eliminate the risk of such pain.

■ Hepatic Effects Transient increases in serum concentrations of AST (SGOT), ALT (SGPT), and alkaline phosphatase have been reported in 2–6% of patients receiving imipenem and cilastatin sodium; jaundice has been reported in less than 0.2% of patients receiving the drug. Increases in serum bilirubin and LDH concentrations and hepatitis have also been reported rarely.

■ Other Adverse Effects Hypotension has been reported in less than 1% and chest discomfort, dyspnea, hyperventilation, thoracic spinal pain, palpitation, tachycardia, polyarthralgia, and asthenia and/or weakness have been reported in less than 0.2% of patients receiving imipenem and cilastatin sodium. Other adverse effects that have been reported in less than 0.2% of patients receiving the drug include cyanosis, hyperhidrosis, skin texture changes, candidiasis, pruritus vulvae, decreased serum sodium concentrations, increased serum potassium and chloride concentrations, tinnitus, and hearing loss.

■ Precautions and Contraindications Prior to initiation of therapy with imipenem and cilastatin sodium, careful inquiry should be made concerning previous hypersensitivity reactions to β-lactam antibiotics, including penicillins and cephalosporins, or to other allergens. There is clinical and laboratory evidence of partial cross-allergenicity among penicillins and other β-lactam antibiotics, and hypersensitivity reactions to imipenem and cilastatin sodium have occurred in patients hypersensitive to penicillins. Therefore, imipenem and cilastatin sodium should be used with caution in patients with a history of hypersensitivity reactions to penicillins. Imipenem and cilastatin sodium is contraindicated in patients who are hypersensitive to any ingredient in the formulation.

Imipenem and cilastatin sodium that has been reconstituted with lidocaine hydrochloride for IM injection is contraindicated in patients with a known history of hypersensitivity to local anesthetics of the amide type and in patients with severe shock or heart block. IM imipenem and cilastatin sodium is *not* intended for use in severe and/or life-threatening infections (e.g., sepsis, endocarditis). (See Uses.) Care should be taken to avoid inadvertent injection of IM imipenem and cilastatin sodium into a blood vessel.

Adverse CNS effects such as confusional states, myoclonus, and seizures have been reported with IV imipenem and cilastatin sodium, particularly when administered in dosages exceeding those recommended by the manufacturer. (See Cautions: CNS Effects.) Similar CNS effects have not been reported to date with IM imipenem and cilastatin sodium therapy. Although adverse CNS effects have been reported most frequently in patients with CNS disorders (e.g., a history of seizures, brain lesions, recent head trauma) and/or patients with renal impairment, these effects have also been reported in some patients with no recognized or documented underlying CNS disorders or renal impairment. Patients with renal impairment (i.e., those with creatinine clearances ≤ 20 mL/minute per 1.73 m^2) whether or not undergoing hemodialysis, who received imipenem and cilastatin dosages exceeding those recommended by the manufacturer, had a higher risk of developing seizures than those without renal impairment. Dosage recommendations for imipenem and cilastatin sodium should be adhered to, especially in patients with factors known to predispose to seizures. Anticonvulsant therapy should be continued during IV and IM imipenem and cilastatin sodium therapy if the drug is used in patients with a known seizure disorder. If focal tremors, myoclonus, or seizures occur during imipenem and cilastatin sodium therapy, patients should be evaluated neurologically, anticonvulsant therapy should be initiated in patients who are not already receiving such therapy, and the imipenem and cilastatin sodium dosage should be reassessed to determine whether dosage should be decreased or the drug discontinued. Because safety and efficacy of imipenem and cilastatin sodium in patients with meningitis has not been established, the manufacturer states that the drug should not be used in patients with this condition.

Renal, hepatic, and hematologic systems should be evaluated periodically during prolonged therapy with imipenem and cilastatin sodium.

Because serum concentrations of imipenem are higher and more prolonged in patients with renal impairment than in patients with normal renal function, doses and/or frequency of administration of IV imipenem and cilastatin sodium should be decreased in patients with renal impairment. (See Dosage and Administration: Dosage in Renal Impairment and Reduced Body Weight.) Patients with severe or marked renal impairment, including those undergoing hemodialysis, have a higher risk of imipenem and cilastatin sodium-induced seizures when receiving the maximum recommended dosage of the drug than do patients with normal renal function. Therefore, the maximum recommended dosage of the drug should be used in such patients only when clearly needed. Patients with creatinine clearances of 5 mL/minute or less per 1.73 m^2 should not receive imipenem and cilastatin sodium IV unless hemodialysis is instituted within 48 hours. In patients undergoing hemodialysis, IV imipenem and cilastatin sodium is recommended only when the potential benefit from the drug outweighs the possible risk of drug-induced seizures. If the drug is used IV in dialysis patients, particularly those with CNS disorders, the patients should be carefully monitored.

The safety and efficacy of IM imipenem and cilastatin sodium therapy in patients with creatinine clearances of less than 20 mL/minute per 1.73 m^2 have not been established.

As with other anti-infective agents, prolonged use of imipenem and cilastatin sodium may result in overgrowth of nonsusceptible organisms, especially *Candida*, enterococci, and *Pseudomonas*. Resistant strains of *Ps. aeruginosa* have developed during therapy with the drug. Careful observation of the patient during imipenem and cilastatin sodium therapy is essential. If superinfection occurs, appropriate therapy should be instituted.

Because *Clostridium difficile*-associated diarrhea and colitis has been reported with imipenem and cilastatin sodium, it should be considered in the differential diagnosis of patients who develop diarrhea during or following therapy with the drug.

■ **Pediatric Precautions** The manufacturer states that safety and efficacy of IM imipenem and cilastatin sodium in children younger than 12 years of age have not been established. Safety and efficacy of IV imipenem and cilastatin sodium in neonates and children 16 years of age or younger is supported by evidence from adequate and controlled studies in adults and by pharmacokinetic and clinical efficacy studies in pediatric patients. Adverse effects reported with the drug in neonates and children are similar to those reported in adults and include GI effects (e.g., diarrhea, vomiting, gastroenteritis), rash, urogenital effects (e.g., urine discoloration, oliguria, anuria), and reactions at the site of IV infusion (e.g., phlebitis, IV site irritation). Such adverse effects generally have been reported in 1–4% of pediatric patients receiving imipenem and cilastatin sodium. However, seizures have been reported in neonates and children 3 months of age or younger receiving the drug. In addition, there was a high incidence of seizures in one study in children 3 months to 12 years of age who received imipenem and cilastatin sodium (25 mg/kg IV every 6 hours) for empiric treatment of bacterial meningitis. Therefore, because of the risk of seizures, the manufacturer states that IV imipenem and cilastatin sodium should *not* be used in pediatric patients with CNS infections. The manufacturer also states that because there is insufficient data to date evaluating IV imipenem and cilastatin sodium in pediatric patients with impaired renal function who weigh less than 30 kg, the drug should*not* be used in these patients.

Diluents containing benzyl alcohol should *not* be used to prepare imipenem and cilastatin sodium for IV administration to neonates or children 3 months of age or younger. Although a causal relationship has not been established, administration of injections preserved with benzyl alcohol has been associated with toxicity in neonates. Toxicity appears to have resulted from administration of large amounts (i.e., about 100–400 mg/kg daily) of benzyl alcohol in these neonates. Toxicity has not been demonstrated in pediatric patients older than 3 months of age, although small pediatric patients in this age range may also be at risk for benzyl alcohol toxicity.

■ **Geriatric Precautions** Clinical studies of IM imipenem and cilastatin sodium have not included sufficient numbers of individuals 65 years of age and older to determine whether they respond differently than younger adults. In clinical studies of IV imipenem and cilastatin involving approximately 2800 adults 18 years of age or older, approximately 800 were 65 years of age or older and 300 were 75 years of age or older. There were no apparent differences in safety or effectiveness between these individuals and younger adults and other clinical experience has not revealed evidence of differences in response between these age groups. However, the possibility that some geriatric patients may exhibit increased sensitivity to the drug cannot be ruled out.

Imipenem is substantially excreted by the kidney, and the risk of severe adverse reactions may be increased in patients with impaired renal function. Limited data indicate that the mean serum half-life of imipenem in healthy geriatric adults 65–75 years of age (with renal function normal for their age) is similar to that expected in individuals with slight renal impairment. The manufacturer states that age-based dosage adjustment does not appear to be necessary. However, because geriatric patients are more likely to have decreased renal function, the manufacturer states that dosage should be selected with caution in these patients and monitoring of renal function may be useful. Dosage should be modified in response to the degree of renal impairment. (See Dosage and Administration: Dosage in Renal Impairment and Reduced Body Weight.)

■ **Mutagenicity and Carcinogenicity** In vitro studies using imipenem or cilastatin sodium alone in a microbial system (i.e., Ames test), imipenem or imipenem and cilastatin sodium in a mammalian cell system (i.e., V79 mammalian cell mutation assay), or imipenem and cilastatin sodium in an unscheduled DNA synthesis assay have not shown evidence of mutagenicity. There also was no evidence of mutagenicity when imipenem and cilastatin sodium was used in an in vivo mouse cytogenicity test.

No long-term carcinogenicity studies of imipenem and cilastatin sodium have been performed to date.

■ **Pregnancy, Fertility, and Lactation** Reproduction studies in rabbits and rats using imipenem dosages up to 2 and 30 times the usual human dosage, respectively, and studies in rabbits using dosages equivalent to the usual human dosage have not revealed evidence of harm to the fetus. Similarly, reproduction studies in rabbits or rats using cilastatin sodium dosages 10 or 33 times the usual human dosage, respectively, have not revealed evidence of harm to the fetus. When imipenem and cilastatin sodium was given at dosages up to 11 times the usual human dosage to pregnant mice and rats during the period of major fetal organogenesis, there was no evidence of teratogenicity, nor was there evidence of adverse effects on fetal viability, fetal growth, or postnatal development of pups when pregnant rats were given dosages up to 8 times the usual human dosage. However, when the drug was administered to pregnant rabbits at dosages equivalent to or exceeding the usual human dosage, weight loss, diarrhea, and some abortions and maternal deaths were observed. When comparable doses of the drug were administered to nonpregnant rabbits, weight loss, diarrhea, and deaths also were observed. The manufacturer states that these adverse effects are similar to those observed in this species with other β-lactam antibiotics, and may be related to alteration of GI flora.

Teratogenicity studies in cynomolgus monkeys receiving IV (by direct injection) or subcutaneous imipenem and cilastatin sodium dosages of 40 or 160 mg/kg daily, respectively, revealed maternal toxicity (e.g., emesis, lack of appetite, weight loss, diarrhea, abortion, maternal death). However, no similar toxicity was observed in nonpregnant cynomolgus monkeys receiving dosages up to 180 mg/kg daily subcutaneously. No maternal death or evidence of teratogenicity and only minimal maternal toxicity (consisting of occasional emesis) were observed in pregnant cynomolgus monkeys receiving the combination at an imipenem dosage of about 100 mg/kg daily (approximately 2 or 3 times the maximum recommended human IV or IM dosage, respectively) by IV infusion at a rate similar to that used in humans; however, there was an increase in embryonic loss when compared with control groups. The drug was well tolerated in other studies in pregnant rats and mice using dosages up to 11 times the average human dosage.

Both imipenem and cilastatin sodium cross the placenta and are distributed into cord blood and amniotic fluid in humans. There are no adequate and controlled studies to date using imipenem and cilastatin sodium in pregnant women, and the drug should be used during pregnancy only when the potential benefits justify the possible risks to the fetus.

Reproduction studies in male and female rats using imipenem and cilastatin sodium dosages up to 8 times the usual human dosage have not revealed evidence of impaired fertility or effects on reproductive performance.

Since imipenem is distributed into milk, the drug should be used with caution in nursing women. There was no evidence of adverse effect on lactation in rats administered the drug late in gestation.

Drug Interactions

■ **Probenecid** Concomitant administration of probenecid and imipenem and cilastatin sodium produces higher and prolonged serum concentrations of cilastatin but results in only minimal increases in serum concentrations and half-life of imipenem. Therefore, there is no therapeutic benefit from concomitant use of the drugs and the manufacturer of imipenem and cilastatin sodium states that concomitant use of probenecid and the combination is not recommended.

■ **Aminoglycosides** The antibacterial activity of imipenem and aminoglycosides is additive or synergistic in vitro against some gram-positive bacteria including *Enterococcus faecalis* (formerly *Streptococcus faecalis*), *Staphylococcus aureus*, and *Listeria monocytogenes*. Depending on the method used to determine in vitro synergism, the combination of imipenem and an aminoglycoside is synergistic against 35–98% of *E. faecalis*tested. The combination of imipenem and an aminoglycoside is generally neither synergistic nor antagonistic in vitro against most strains of *Pseudomonas aeruginosa* and Enterobacteriaceae.

■ **β-Lactam Antibiotics** In vitro, imipenem antagonizes the antibacterial activity of other β-lactam antibiotics (including aztreonam and most cephalosporins and extended-spectrum penicillins) against many strains of *Ps. aeruginosa* and some strains of *Citrobacter*, *Enterobacter*, *Klebsiella pneumoniae*, *Morganella morganii*, and *Serratia marcescens*. The antagonism apparently occurs because imipenem, like cefoxitin, is a potent inducer of β-lactamase production and can derepress inducible, chromosomally mediated enzymes in organisms that possess these enzymes. Although inducible β-lactamases have no effect on the antibacterial activity of imipenem, the enzymes inactivate most cephalosporins and penicillins either by hydrolyzing the drugs or by binding to them to prevent access to penicillin-binding proteins. The clinical importance of this in vitro antagonism has not been determined to date, but imipenem and cilastatin sodium probably should not be used in conjunction with other β-lactam antibiotics.

■ **Ganciclovir** Generalized seizures have occurred in several patients who received concomitant therapy with IV imipenem and cilastatin sodium and IV ganciclovir. While the mechanism of this potential interaction currently is not known, the seizures resolved in all but one patient when either both IV imipenem and cilastatin sodium and ganciclovir or just IV imipenem and cilastatin sodium was discontinued. In the patient whose seizures failed to resolve following discontinuance of IV imipenem and cilastatin sodium, continued seizures were attributed to encephalitis rather than the drugs. Because of the risk of seizures, IV imipenem and cilastatin sodium should be used concomitantly with ganciclovir only when the potential benefits are thought to outweigh the possible risks.

■ Other Anti-infectives The clinical importance has not been determined to date, but the antibacterial activity of imipenem and co-trimoxazole has generally been synergistic in vitro against *Nocardia asteroides*.

Results of an in vitro study using *Klebsiella pneumoniae* indicate that chloramphenicol can antagonize the bactericidal activity of imipenem. It has been suggested that if chloramphenicol is used in conjunction with imipenem and cilastatin sodium, chloramphenicol should be administered a few hours after the combination; however, the necessity of this precaution has not been established.

In an in vitro study using strains of *Ps. aeruginosa* resistant to aminoglycosides and carbenicillin, the antibacterial activities of imipenem and norfloxacin were synergistic or partially synergistic against about one-third and indifferent against about two-thirds of strains tested; antagonism did not occur.

Laboratory Test Interferences

■ Tests for Urinary Glucose Like most other currently available β-lactam antibiotics, imipenem and cilastatin sodium interferes with urinary glucose determinations using cupric sulfate (e.g., Benedict's solution, Clinitest®), but does not appear to interfere with glucose oxidase tests (e.g., Diastix®, Tes-Tape®).

Acute Toxicity

The manufacturer states that there is no information to date on overdosage of imipenem and cilastatin sodium in humans. The IV LD_{50} of imipenem and cilastatin sodium when administered concomitantly in a 1:1 ratio in mice and rats is approximately 1 g (of imipenem) per kg daily. The IV LD_{50} of imipenem alone is approximately 1.5 g/kg in mice and greater than 2 g/kg in rats, and the IV LD_{50} of cilastatin sodium alone is approximately 8.7 and 5 g/kg, respectively.

Ataxia, clonic seizures, and death were reported in mice 4–56 minutes following IV administration of 751- to 1359-mg/kg doses of imipenem and cilastatin sodium (administered concomitantly in a 1:1 ratio). In rats, toxicity was observed 5–10 minutes following IV administration of 771- to 1583-mg/kg doses of imipenem and cilastatin sodium. Drug toxicity in female rats was manifested by decreased activity, bradypnea, and death which was preceded by ptosis with clonic seizures; in male rats, ptosis, tremors, and clonic seizures were reported; however, tremors and seizures were not observed in male rats receiving IV administration of 771-mg/kg dose of imipenem and cilastatin sodium. In addition, death occurred 6–88 minutes following IV administration of 771- to 1734-mg/kg doses of imipenem and cilastatin sodium to male rats.

In acute overdosage, the drug should be discontinued and the patient treated symptomatically (including supportive measures). Although imipenem and cilastatin sodium is hemodialyzable, the manufacturer states that the usefulness of this procedure in enhancing the elimination of imipenem and cilastatin sodium is questionable.

Mechanism of Action

Imipenem usually is bactericidal in action. Like other β-lactam antibiotics, the antibacterial activity of imipenem results from inhibition of mucopeptide synthesis in the bacterial cell wall. Imipenem has an affinity for and binds to most penicillin-binding proteins (PBPs) of susceptible organisms, including PBPs 1a, 1b, 2, 4, 5, and 6 of *Escherichia coli*; PBPs 1a, 1b, 2, 4, and 5 of *Pseudomonas aeruginosa*; and PBPs 1, 2, 3, and 4 of *S. aureus*. In susceptible gram-negative bacteria, imipenem has the greatest affinity for PBP 2 and the lowest affinity for PBP 3. This results in the formation of spheroplasts or ellipsoidal cells without filament formation. Because imipenem also has a high affinity for PBPs 1a and 1b of these organisms, the spheroplasts lyse rapidly. Imipenem is able to penetrate the outer membrane of most gram-negative bacteria and gain access to the PBPs more readily than many other currently available β-lactam antibiotics.

In vitro studies indicate that imipenem may have a postantibiotic inhibitory effect against some susceptible organisms. Although the mechanism of this postantibiotic effect has not been determined to date, in vitro studies using *Staphylococcus aureus*, *E. coli*, and *Ps. aeruginosa* indicate that following exposure to bactericidal concentrations of imipenem these organisms do not immediately resume growth after the drug is removed. It is not known whether a postantibiotic effect occurs in vivo, but it has been suggested that this effect would be beneficial since imipenem may be able to prevent regrowth of susceptible organisms although drug concentrations at the site of infection may fall below the MIC during a dosing interval.

Cilastatin sodium reversibly and competitively inhibits dehydropeptidase I (DHP I). Imipenem is hydrolyzed in vivo to a microbiologically inactive metabolite by DHP I present on the brush border of proximal renal tubular cells; concurrent administration of cilastatin prevents this renal metabolism of the antibiotic. The normal physiologic role of DHP I has not been fully elucidated, but the enzyme does not appear to be essential to normal mammalian metabolism. Cilastatin is a specific inhibitor of DHP I and does not inhibit other dipeptidases or bacterial β-lactamases. Cilastatin sodium has no antibacterial activity and does not affect the mechanism of action of imipenem.

Spectrum

Imipenem has a spectrum of activity that is broader than that of most other currently available β-lactam antibiotics. Imipenem is active in vitro against most gram-positive and gram-negative aerobic bacteria as well as most gram-positive and gram-negative anaerobic bacteria. The drug also has some activity in vitro against *Mycobacterium*, but is inactive against *Mycoplasma*, *Chlamydia*, fungi, and viruses. Cilastatin sodium has no antibacterial activity and does not affect the antibacterial activity of imipenem when used concomitantly.

■ In Vitro Susceptibility Testing For most organisms, inoculum size does not appear to affect susceptibility to imipenem. MICs of imipenem for *Pseudomonas aeruginosa* and most Enterobacteriaceae generally are only 2–4 times greater when the size of the inoculum is increased from 10^5 to 10^8 colony-forming units (CFU) per mL, although MICs for some strains of *Enterobacter*, *Klebsiella*, and *Proteus* may be 4–16 times greater when the inoculum is increased to 10^8 CFU/mL. Results of imipenem susceptibility tests generally are unaffected by the presence of serum.

The Clinical and Laboratory Standards Institute (CLSI; formerly National Committee for Clinical Laboratory Standards [NCCLS]) states that, if results of in vitro susceptibility testing indicate that a clinical isolate is *susceptible* to imipenem, then an infection caused by this strain may be appropriately treated with the dosage of the drug recommended for that type of infection and infecting species, unless otherwise contraindicated. If results indicate that a clinical isolate has *intermediate susceptibility* to imipenem, then the strain has a minimum inhibitory concentration (MIC) that approaches usually attainable blood and tissue drug concentrations and response rates may be lower than for strains identified as susceptible. Therefore, the intermediate category implies clinical applicability in body sites where the drug is physiologically concentrated (e.g., urine) or when a high dosage of the drug can be used. This intermediate category also includes a buffer zone which should prevent small, uncontrolled technical factors from causing major discrepancies in interpretation, especially for drugs with narrow pharmacotoxicity margins. If results of in vitro susceptibility testing indicate that a clinical isolate is *resistant* to imipenem, the strain is not inhibited by systemic concentrations of the drug achievable with usual dosage schedules and/or MICs fall in the range where specific microbial resistance mechanisms are likely and efficacy has not been reliably demonstrated in clinical trials.

CLSI states that strains of staphylococci resistant to penicillinase-resistant penicillins should be considered resistant to imipenem, although results of in vitro susceptibility tests may indicate that the organisms are susceptible to the drug.

Disk Susceptibility Tests When the disk-diffusion procedure is used to test susceptibility to imipenem, a disk containing 10 mcg of imipenem should be used.

When disk-diffusion susceptibility testing is performed according to CLSI standardized procedures using CLSI interpretive criteria, *Staphylococcus*, Enterobacteriaceae, *Pseudomonas aeruginosa*, or *Acinetobacter* with growth inhibition zones of 16 mm or greater are susceptible to imipenem, those with zones of 14–15 mm have intermediate susceptibility, and those with zones of 13 mm or less are resistant to the drug.

When disk-diffusion susceptibility testing is performed according to CLSI standardized procedures using *Haemophilus* test medium (HTM), *Haemophilus* with growth inhibition zones of 16 mm or greater are susceptible to imipenem.

Dilution Susceptibility Tests When dilution susceptibility testing (agar or broth dilution) is performed according to CLSI standardized procedures using CLSI interpretive criteria, *Staphylococcus*, Enterobacteriaceae, and *Ps. aeruginosa* and other non-Enterobacteriaceae gram-negative bacilli (e.g., other *Pseudomonas* spp., *Acinetobacter*, *Stenotrophomonas maltophilia*) with MICs of 4 mcg/mL or less are susceptible to imipenem, those with MICs of 8 mcg/mL have intermediate susceptibility, and those with MICs of 16 mcg/mL or greater are resistant to the drug.

When dilution susceptibility testing of *Haemophilus* is performed according to CLSI standardized procedures using HTM, isolates with MICs of 4 mcg/mL or less are considered susceptible to imipenem. Because of limited data on resistant strains, CLSI recommends than any *Haemophilus* isolate that appears to be nonsusceptible to imipenem should be submitted to a reference laboratory for further testing.

When broth dilution susceptibility testing of *S. pneumoniae* is performed according to CLSI standardized procedures using cation-adjusted Mueller-Hinton broth (supplemented with 2–5% lysed horse blood), *S. pneumoniae* with MICs of 0.12 mcg/mL or less are considered susceptible to imipenem, those with MICs of 0.25–0.5 mcg/mL have intermediate susceptibility, and those with MICs of 1 mcg/mL or greater are resistant to the drug.

■ Gram-positive Aerobic Bacteria ***Gram-positive Aerobic Cocci*** Imipenem is generally active in vitro against the following gram-positive aerobic cocci: penicillinase- and nonpenicillinase-producing strains of *Staphylococcus aureus* and *S. epidermidis*, *S. saprophyticus*, *Streptococcus pneumoniae*, *S. pyogenes* (group A β-hemolytic streptococci), group B streptococci (e.g., *S. agalactiae*), viridans streptococci, and groups C, G, and H streptococci. Unlike cephalosporins and many penicillins, imipenem has some activity against enterococci, although the drug is only bacteriostatic against these organisms. Imipenem is active in vitro against many strains of *E. faecalis* (formerly *S. faecalis*) and *S. durans*, but most strains of *S. faecium* are considered resistant to the drug.

The MIC_{90} (minimum inhibitory concentration of the drug at which 90% of strains tested are inhibited) of imipenem for penicillinase- and nonpenicillinase-producing *S. aureus* is 0.01–0.5 mcg/mL. The MIC_{90} of imipenem for *S. epidermidis* is generally 0.1–4 mcg/mL, although in a few studies the MIC_{90}

was 32 mcg/mL. The in vitro activity of imipenem against staphylococci resistant to penicillinase-resistant penicillins is variable, and a wide range of MIC values has been reported depending on the method used to test susceptibility. In some in vitro studies, when cultures were incubated for up to 18 hours at 30–37°C, the MIC_{90} of imipenem for methicillin-resistant *S. aureus* (MRSA) ranged from 0.5–8 mcg/mL. In other in vitro studies when cultures were incubated for 48 hours at 30 or 35°C, the MIC_{90} of imipenem for MRSA was 25 mcg/mL or higher and most strains were considered resistant to the drug. Strains of staphylococci resistant to penicillinase-resistant penicillins should be considered resistant to imipenem.

The MIC_{90} of imipenem for *S. pneumoniae* is 0.01–1 mcg/mL, and the MIC_{90} of the drug for *S. pyogenes*, viridans streptococci, or groups B, C, G, or H streptococci is 0.01–0.125 mcg/mL.

The MIC_{90} of imipenem reported for *E. faecalis* is 0.3–4 mcg/mL. Imipenem is less active in vitro against *S. faecium* than *E. faecalis* or *S. durans*. The MIC_{90} of imipenem reported for *S. faecium* ranges from 0.5–50 mcg/mL, and most strains are considered resistant to the drug. Imipenem is not bactericidal against enterococci. Although results vary depending on the method used to test bactericidal activity, the MBC_{90} (minimum bactericidal concentration of the drug at which 90% of strains tested are killed) of imipenem for most strains of *E. faecalis* is 64 mcg/mL or greater.

Gram-positive Aerobic Bacilli Imipenem is active in vitro against most strains of *Listeria monocytogenes*, but the drug is not generally bactericidal against this organism. The MIC_{90} of imipenem reported for *L. monocytogenes* is 0.015–4 mcg/mL, and the MBC_{90} ranges from 0.25–250 mcg/mL.

Imipenem is active in vitro against *Bacillus*, including *B. cereus*.

Imipenem also is active in vitro against some strains of *Nocardia asteroides*, and the MIC_{90} of the drug reported for this organism is 0.19–8 mcg/mL.

The mean MIC_{90} of imipenem for *Erysipelothrix rhusiopathiae* reportedly is 0.015 mcg/mL. *Corynebacterium* generally are resistant to imipenem and have a mean MIC_{90} of the drug of more than 32 mcg/mL.

■ **Gram-negative Aerobic Bacteria** ***Neisseria*** Imipenem is active in vitro against *Neisseria meningitidis* and most strains of penicillinase- and nonpenicillinase-producing *Neisseria gonorrhoeae*. The MIC_{90} of imipenem is 0.03–0.11 mcg/mL for *N. meningitidis* and 0.12–0.64 mcg/mL for nonpenicillinase- or penicillinase-producing *N. gonorrhoeae*.

Haemophilus Imipenem is active in vitro against most β-lactamase- and non-β-lactamase-producing strains of *Haemophilus influenzae* and *H. parainfluenzae*. The MIC_{90} of the drug reported for *H. influenzae* and *H. parainfluenzae* is 0.25–8 mcg/mL. Imipenem is active in vitro against strains of *H. influenzae* resistant to ampicillin and/or chloramphenicol as well as some strains resistant to ampicillin, chloramphenicol, and co-trimoxazole. *H. ducreyi* also are inhibited in vitro by imipenem.

Enterobacteriaceae Imipenem is active in vitro against most clinically important Enterobacteriaceae, including *Citrobacter diversus, C. freundii, Enterobacter agglomerans, E. cloacae, E. aerogenes, Escherichia coli, Hafnia alvei, Klebsiella oxytoca, K. pneumoniae, Morganella morganii* (formerly *Proteus morganii*), *Proteus mirabilis, P. vulgaris, Providencia rettgeri* (formerly *Proteus rettgeri*), *P. stuartii, Serratia liquefaciens, S. marcescens, Salmonella, Shigella, Yersinia enterocolitica*, and *Y. pseudotuberculosis*.

The MIC_{90} of imipenem for *C. diversus, C. freundii, E. aerogenes, E. agglomerans, E. cloacae, E. coli, K. oxytoca, K. pneumoniae*, and *Y. enterocolitica* is 0.1–4 mcg/mL. The MIC_{90} for *M. morganii, P. mirabilis, P. vulgaris, P. rettgeri, P. stuartii*, and *S. marcescens* is 0.5–8 mcg/mL.

The MIC_{90} of imipenem reported for *Salmonella* is 0.1–2 mcg/mL. In one study, the MIC_{90} of the drug for *S. enteritidis* and *S. typhi* was 0.25–0.5 mcg/mL. The MIC_{90} of imipenem reported for *Shigella* is 0.1–0.5 mcg/mL.

Pseudomonas Imipenem is active in vitro against many strains of *Pseudomonas aeruginosa*. In vitro on a weight basis, the activity of imipenem against *Ps. aeruginosa* appears to be approximately equal to or slightly greater than that of ceftazidime. In addition, imipenem is active in vitro against some strains of *Ps. aeruginosa* resistant to third generation cephalosporins, aminoglycosides, and extended-spectrum penicillins. The MIC_{90} of imipenem reported for *Ps. aeruginosa* is 1.1–16 mcg/mL.

Imipenem is also active against some *Pseudomonas* other than *Ps. aeruginosa*. The MIC_{90} of imipenem reported for *Ps. acidovorans, Ps. fluorescens, Ps. putida*, and *Ps. stutzeri* is 0.5–2.5 mcg/mL.

Other Gram-Negative Aerobic Bacteria Imipenem is active in vitro against *Acinetobacter*. The MIC_{90} of the drug reported for *A. calcoaceticus* var. *anitratus* is 0.25–0.5 mcg/mL, and the MIC_{90} reported for *A. calcoaceticus*var. *lwoffi* is 0.15–0.39 mcg/mL.

Moraxella catarrhalis (formerly *Branhamella catarrhalis*) generally is inhibited in vitro by imipenem concentrations of 0.03–0.12 mcg/mL.

Imipenem is active in vitro against *Bordetella bronchiseptica, Eikenella corrodens*, and *Pasteurella multocida*. The MIC_{90} of the drug reported for *B. bronchiseptica* and *E. corrodens* is 0.25–4 mcg/mL.

Brucella melitensis is inhibited in vitro by imipenem concentrations of 0.33–2 mcg/mL. Imipenem also is active in vitro against *Alcaligenes denitrificans, A. xylosoxidans, Aeromonas hydrophila*, and *Plesiomonas shigelloides*. The MIC_{90} of imipenem reported for *A. xylosoxidans* and *A. denitrificans* is 1.3–8 mcg/mL.

Imipenem has some activity in vitro against *Flavobacterium*, but the MIC_{90} of imipenem reported for *Chryseobacterium meningosepticum* (formerly *F. meningosepticum*) is usually 20–32 mcg/mL and most strains of the organism are considered resistant to the drug.

Imipenem is active in vitro against some strains of *Brevundimonas diminuta* (formerly *Ps. diminuta*). While some strains of *Burkholderia cepacia* (formerly *Ps. cepacia*) are inhibited in vitro by imipenem concentrations of 16 mcg/mL or less, most strains of the organism are resistant to the drug.

Imipenem is active in vitro against *Capnocytophaga*. The MIC_{90} of imipenem reported for *Capnocytophaga* is 0.5 mcg/mL.

Imipenem is active in vitro against *Campylobacter coli, C. fetus* subsp. *fetus*, and *C. jejuni*, including β-lactamase-producing strains. The MIC_{90} of imipenem reported for *C. fetus* subsp. *fetus* is 0.03–0.125 mcg/mL.

The MIC_{90} of imipenem for *Helicobacter pylori* (*C. pylori*) reportedly is 0.13 mcg/mL.

In vitro, *Legionella pneumophila* generally are inhibited by imipenem concentrations of 0.03–0.25 mcg/mL.

Gardnerella vaginalis (formerly *Haemophilus vaginalis*) reportedly are inhibited in vitro by imipenem.

Stenotrophomonas maltophilia (formerly *Ps. maltophilia*) generally is resistant to imipenem.

■ **Anaerobic Bacteria** Imipenem is active in vitro against most gram-positive anaerobic bacteria including *Actinomyces, Bifidobacterium, Clostridium,Eubacterium, Lactobacillus, Peptococcus, Peptostreptococcus*, and *Propionibacterium*. The MIC_{90} of imipenem reported for most of these gram-positive anaerobic bacteria is 0.015–4 mcg/mL. *C. perfringens* are generally inhibited in vitro by imipenem concentrations of 0.015–1.3 mcg/mL. Unlike most other currently available β-lactam antibiotics, imipenem is active in vitro against some strains of *C. difficile*. The MIC_{90} of the drug reported for *C. difficile* is 2–16 mcg/mL.

Imipenem is active in vitro against gram-negative anaerobic bacteria including most strains of *Bacteroides, Fusobacterium, Leptotrichia buccalis, Prevotella*, and *Veillonella*.

The MIC_{90} of imipenem reported for *Bacteroides fragilis, B. distasonis, B. ovatus, B. thetaiotaomicron*, and *B. vulgatus* is 0.03–4 mcg/mL. Imipenem is active in vitro against some strains of *Bacteroides*, including *B. fragilis*, resistant to clindamycin and cefoxitin.

Prevotella bivia, P. disiens, P. melaninogenica, and *P. oralis* (formerly *B. bivius, B. disiens B. melaninogenicus*, and *B. oralis*) are inhibited in vitro by imipenem concentrations of 4 mcg/mL or less.

The MIC_{90} of imipenem reported for *Fusobacterium, L. buccalis*, and *Veillonella* is 0.015–2 mcg/mL.

■ **Other Organisms** The clinical importance has not been determined to date, but imipenem is active in vitro against some *Mycobacterium* including *M. fallax* and *M. fortuitum*. In one study, 1012 isolates of *M. fortuitum* were inhibited in vitro by imipenem concentrations of 6.25 mcg/mL.

Although a few strains of *Chlamydia trachomatis* were inhibited in vitro by imipenem in one study, the mean MIC_{90} of the drug for *C. trachomatis* usually is 32 mcg/mL or higher and the organism is considered resistant to imipenem.

Resistance

Imipenem has a high degree of stability against hydrolysis by bacterial β-lactamases, including both plasmid-mediated and chromosomally mediated enzymes. The drug generally is more stable against inactivation by β-lactamases than are cefoxitin, cefotaxime, or cefuroxime. Imipenem generally is stable against hydrolysis by staphylococcal β-lactamases and β-lactamases classified as Richmond-Sykes types I, II, III (TEM type), IV, or V (PSE and OXA types), but is inactivated by a β-lactamase produced by *Bacteroides fragilis*. Although imipenem is hydrolyzed to some extent by a β-lactamase produced by *Stenotrophomonas maltophilia* (formerly *Pseudomonas maltophilia*), resistance to imipenem in this organism may also be related to other factors since this enzyme has a low affinity for the drug.

Resistance to imipenem in gram-positive bacteria, including *Staphylococcus epidermidis* and methicillin-resistant staphylococci, is generally the result of altered penicillin-binding proteins (PBPs). In vitro exposure of some strains of methicillin-resistant *S. aureus* (MRSA) to imipenem has induced imipenem resistance in strains that were originally susceptible to the drug. Tolerance to the bactericidal effects of imipenem has been reported in enterococci and some strains of *Listeria monocytogenes* and methicillin-resistant staphylococci. Although most susceptible organisms have an MBC of imipenem that is 1–4 times greater than the MIC of the drug, bacteria that are tolerant to imipenem have an MBC that is at least 16 times higher than the MIC.

Resistant strains of *Ps. aeruginosa* have developed during therapy with imipenem and have resulted in treatment failures in some cases. The mechanism of imipenem resistance in these organisms is unclear, but resistance may develop rapidly following initiation of therapy with the drug. Resistance to imipenem in *Ps. aeruginosa* appears to result from chromosomal β-lactamase activity and decreased permeability due to loss of an outer-membrane porin protein (OprD2) or may result from a plasmid-mediated metallo-β-lactamase. Tolerance to the bactericidal effects of imipenem has been reported in some strains of *Ps. aeruginosa*.

In vitro studies indicate that imipenem, like cefoxitin, is a potent inducer of β-lactamases and can reversibly derepress inducible, chromosomally mediated β-lactamases in *Ps. aeruginosa* and Enterobacteriaceae that possess these enzymes. Although these enzymes inactivate aztreonam and most cephalosporins and penicillins either by hydrolyzing the drugs or by binding to them to prevent access to PBPs, these β-lactamases have no effect on the antibacterial activity of imipenem. (See Drug Interactions: β-Lactam Antibiotics.) Imipenem does not appear to select mutants stably derepressed for β-lactamase production.

Cross-resistance generally does not occur between imipenem and other anti-infective agents, including cephalosporins, penicillins, and aminoglycosides. However, strains of *Ps. aeruginosa* resistant to imipenem that also were resistant to meropenem have been reported rarely. There has been at least one report of a strain of metronidazole-resistant *B. fragilis* that was cross-resistant in vitro to imipenem, amoxicillin and clavulanate potassium, and tetracycline; the strain was susceptible to chloramphenicol or clindamycin in vitro.

Pharmacokinetics

Cilastatin prevents metabolism of imipenem by dehydropeptidase I (DHP I) present on the brush border of proximal renal tubular cells and, when administered concomitantly, results in urinary concentrations of active imipenem that are higher than could be obtained following administration of the antibiotic alone. Concomitant cilastatin also results in a slight increase in serum concentrations of imipenem, but does not appreciably affect its serum half-life. Imipenem has no effect on the pharmacokinetics of cilastatin sodium.

Unless specified otherwise, serum and tissue concentrations of imipenem and pharmacokinetic parameters presented for imipenem and cilastatin were obtained from studies where imipenem monohydrate and cilastatin sodium were administered concomitantly in a 1:1 ratio. Imipenem is administered as the monohydrate, but dosages and concentrations of the drug are expressed in terms of anhydrous imipenem. Dosage of imipenem and cilastatin sodium is expressed in terms of the imipenem content of the drug.

■ Absorption

Neither imipenem nor cilastatin is appreciably absorbed from the GI tract and, therefore, imipenem and cilastatin sodium must be given parenterally.

Following IV infusion over 20–30 minutes of a single 250-mg, 500-mg, or 1-g dose of imipenem and cilastatin sodium in healthy adults with normal renal function, peak serum concentrations of imipenem immediately following completion of the infusion range from 14–24, 21–58, and 41–83 mcg/mL, respectively. Serum concentrations 4–6 hours after these doses decline to 1.5 mcg/mL or less. In adults with infections who receive 500-mg or 1-g doses of imipenem and cilastatin sodium by IV infusion over 30–60 minutes every 6 hours, peak serum imipenem concentrations are 19.3–38.3 or 16.7–67.3 mcg/mL, respectively, and trough concentrations average 1 or 3.1 mcg/mL, respectively.

Following IV infusion over 15–20 minutes of a single 25-mg/kg dose of imipenem and cilastatin sodium in children 2–12 years of age with infections, serum imipenem concentrations 0.5 and 6 hours after the dose average 33.5 and 0.79 mcg/mL, respectively. In children 3 months to 13 years of age with infections who received imipenem and cilastatin sodium in a dosage of 60–100 mg/kg daily, peak serum imipenem concentrations at steady state ranged from 12.8–80.8 mcg/mL and trough serum concentrations ranged from 0–0.7 mcg/mL. In neonates 1–8 days of age with infections who received a single 25-mg/kg dose of the drug, serum imipenem concentrations averaged 97.3, 45.5, 30.6, 14.4, 3.1, and 0.9 mcg/mL immediately following completion of the infusion and 1, 2, 4, 8, and 12 hours later, respectively. In a dose-ranging study in premature, low-birthweight neonates (0.7–1.9 kg) 1 week of age or younger who received imipenem and cilastatin sodium in a dosage of 20 mg/kg every 12 hours given IV over 15–30 minutes, mean peak and trough plasma concentrations averaged 43 and 1.7 mcg/mL, respectively. While the clinical importance is unclear, multiple IV doses of imipenem and cilastatin sodium in neonates may result in moderate accumulation of cilastatin.

Imipenem is incompletely absorbed following IM administration of the commercially available suspension, and plasma concentrations of the drug peak later but are more prolonged than those achieved following IV administration. Following IM administration of the commercially available suspension of imipenem and cilastatin sodium, the bioavailabilities of imipenem and cilastatin range from 60–75 and 95–100%, respectively. Following IM administration of a 500- or 750-mg dose of imipenem and cilastatin sodium suspension (diluted with 1% lidocaine hydrochloride injection without epinephrine), peak plasma concentrations of imipenem occur within 2 hours and average 10 or 12 mcg/mL, respectively; peak plasma concentrations of cilastatin occur within 1 hour and average 24 or 33 mcg/mL, respectively. Plasma concentrations of imipenem exceed 2 mcg/mL for at least 6 or 8 hours following IM administration of a 500- or 750-mg dose, respectively. Absorption of imipenem from the IM injection site continues for 6–8 hours; absorption of cilastatin is virtually complete by 4 hours.

Following IV administration of single 500- or 750-mg doses of imipenem and cilastatin sodium solution, plasma imipenem concentrations during the first 2 hours exceeded those attained following IM administration of the same doses given as suspensions (reconstituted with lidocaine hydrochloride 1% without epinephrine); however, plasma imipenem concentrations achieved 4–6 hours after an IM dose exceeded those after an IV dose and they persisted longer. Following IV administration of a single 500- or 750-mg dose of imipenem and cilastatin sodium, peak plasma imipenem concentrations were 45 or 57 mcg/mL, respectively, and occurred at 25 minutes while those following the same IM doses were 10 or 11.4 mcg/mL, respectively, and occurred at 2 hours. Plasma concentrations of imipenem were undetectable 12 hours after IV administration; however, 12 hours after IM administration of a 500- or 750-mg dose, plasma imipenem concentrations were 0.5 or 0.8 mcg/mL, respectively.

■ Distribution

Following IV administration, imipenem is distributed into saliva, sputum, aqueous humor, bone, bile, reproductive organs, myometrium, endometrium, heart valve, intestine, and pleural, peritoneal, interstitial, blister, and wound fluids.

In adults, the apparent volume of distribution of imipenem in the central compartment (V_c) averages 0.16 L/kg and the volume of distribution at steady state (V_{ss}) averages 0.23–0.35 L/kg. In children 2–12 years of age, V_c averages 0.326 L/kg. In neonates 1–8 days of age, V_{ss} ranges from 0.251–0.418 L/kg.

Only low concentrations of imipenem diffuse into CSF following IV administration; CSF concentrations are generally 1–10% of concurrent serum concentrations. Following a single 1-g IV dose of imipenem and cilastatin sodium in patients with uninflamed meninges, CSF concentrations approximately 1 hour after the dose average 0.8 mcg/mL. In children 4 months to 11 years of age with meningitis who received 25-mg/kg IV doses of the drug every 6 hours, CSF imipenem concentrations ranged from 0.27–3.5 mcg/mL in samples obtained 1.5–3.6 hours after a dose; serum concentrations 1.7–3.1 hours after the dose ranged from 2.9–25 mcg/mL. CSF imipenem concentrations in these children did not appear to be affected by the degree of meningeal inflammation.

Imipenem is 13–21% and cilastatin is approximately 40% bound to serum proteins.

Both imipenem and cilastatin sodium cross the placenta and are distributed into cord blood and amniotic fluid. In one study in pregnant women who received a single 500-mg IV dose of imipenem and cilastatin sodium, amniotic fluid concentrations varied greatly. In women in early pregnancy, mean amniotic fluid concentrations in samples taken 3 hours after the dose were 47% of simultaneous maternal plasma concentrations; in women in late pregnancy, mean concentrations were 16% of simultaneous maternal plasma concentrations in samples obtained 30 minutes after the dose. Imipenem is distributed into milk.

■ Elimination

Serum imipenem concentrations appear to decline in a biphasic manner following IV administration of imipenem and cilastatin sodium in adults with normal renal function. In adults with normal renal function, the distribution half-life of IV imipenem averages 0.23–0.31 hours and the elimination half-life averages 0.85–1.3 hours. In healthy geriatric adults 65–75 years of age (with renal function normal for their age) who received a single dose of 500 mg of imipenem and 500 mg of cilastatin given IV over 20 minutes, the mean plasma half-lives of imipenem and cilastatin were 1.5 and 1.1 hours, respectively, and were similar to half-lives expected in individuals with slight renal impairment. Multiple doses have no effect on the pharmacokinetics of imipenem or cilastatin and accumulation does not occur.

The elimination half-life of IV imipenem averages 1–1.3 hours in children 2–12 years of age and 1.5–2.6 hours in neonates 1–10 days of age. IV cilastatin has an elimination half-life of 0.83–1.1 hours in adults with normal renal function and 3.1–8.8 hours in neonates.

The elimination half-life of imipenem following IM administration of imipenem and cilastatin sodium suspension is 2–3 hours. Little accumulation of imipenem and no accumulation of cilastatin appears to occur following repeated (i.e., every 12 hours) IM doses.

If imipenem is administered alone, the drug is partially hydrolyzed in the kidneys by DHP I to a microbiologically inactive metabolite and only 5–43% of the dose is excreted unchanged in urine. However, when cilastatin sodium is administered concurrently with imipenem in a 1:1 ratio as a suspension or solution, approximately 50 or 70% of the imipenem dose, respectively, and approximately 75% of the cilastatin dose are excreted unchanged in urine within 10 hours. In adults, maximal urinary concentrations of active imipenem are obtained with a 4:1 ratio of imipenem to cilastatin; however, a 1:1 ratio of imipenem to cilastatin ensures that DHP I is inhibited for up to 8–10 hours. Urinary imipenem concentrations may be greater than 10 mcg/mL for up to 8 hours following a single 500-mg IV dose of imipenem and cilastatin sodium. Urinary imipenem concentrations exceed 10 mcg/mL for at least 12 hours after IM administration of 500- or 750-mg doses of the commercially available suspension of the drug.

Imipenem is also metabolized to some extent by a nonrenal mechanism unrelated to DHP I. Approximately 20–30% of an imipenem dose is inactivated by nonspecific hydrolysis of the β-lactam ring. Although the microbiologically inactive metabolite is identical to that formed by renal DHP I, this nonspecific hydrolysis is unaffected by concurrent administration of cilastatin.

Cilastatin is partially metabolized in the kidneys to *N*-acetylcilastatin, which is also an effective inhibitor of DHP I. Approximately 70–80% of an IV dose of cilastatin is excreted in urine unchanged and 12% is excreted as *N*-acetylcilastatin. The metabolic fate of the remainder of the dose has not been elucidated to date.

Imipenem, cilastatin, and their metabolites are excreted principally in urine by both glomerular filtration and tubular secretion. Approximately 20–30% of the renal clearance of imipenem occurs by tubular secretion; however, cilastatin competitively inhibits active tubular secretion of imipenem. Less than 1% of an imipenem dose and less than 2% of a cilastatin dose are excreted in feces following IV administration.

In adults with normal renal function, plasma clearance of imipenem and of cilastatin ranges from 165–207 and 207–218 mL/minute per 1.73 m^2, respectively. Plasma clearance of imipenem averages 270 mL/minute per 1.73 m^2 in children 2–12 years of age and 3.4 mL/minute per kg in neonates 1–10 days of age.

The serum half-lives of both imipenem and cilastatin are prolonged in patients with impaired renal function; however, the half-life of cilastatin is prolonged to a greater extent than that of imipenem. The serum half-life of IV imipenem and of cilastatin averages 2.1 and 2.5 hours, respectively, in adults with creatinine clearances of 17–33 mL/minute per 1.73 m^2, and 2.7–3.7 and 7–17 hours, respectively, in adults with creatinine clearances less than 10 mL/minute per 1.73 m^2.

Both imipenem and cilastatin are removed by hemodialysis; however, the amount of the drugs removed during hemodialysis varies considerably depending on several factors (e.g., type of coil used, dialysis flow rate). In patients who received a single 250- or 500-mg dose of imipenem and cilastatin sodium, a 3- to 4-hour period of hemodialysis removed 20–90% of the imipenem dose and 38–82% of the cilastatin dose into the dialysate. Imipenem and cilastatin are removed by peritoneal dialysis.

Chemistry and Stability

■ **Chemistry** Imipenem and cilastatin sodium is a fixed combination of imipenem monohydrate and the sodium salt of cilastatin.

Imipenem is a semisynthetic carbapenem antibiotic and is the crystalline *N*-formimidoyl derivative of thienamycin, a carbapenem antibiotic produced by *Streptomyces cattleya*. Carbapenems are β-lactam antibiotics that contain a fused β-lactam ring and 5-membered ring system similar to that contained in penicillins; however, the 5-membered ring in carbapenems is unsaturated and contains a carbon rather than a sulfur atom. Imipenem has a hydroxyethyl group at position 6 of the β-lactam ring rather than the acylamino group present at this position in penicillins and cephalosporins; the hydroxyethyl group in imipenem has a *trans* configuration unlike the acylamino groups in penicillins and cephalosporins which have a *cis* configuration. These structural differences result in increased antibacterial activity and stability against hydrolysis by most β-lactamases. Imipenem contains a basic alkylthio side chain on the 5-membered ring; this side chain results in antipseudomonal activity.

Cilastatin sodium, the sodium salt of a derivatized heptenoic acid, is a specific and reversible inhibitor of dehydropeptidase I (DHP I). DHP I is a dipeptidase present on the brush border of proximal renal tubular cells which inactivates imipenem by hydrolyzing the β-lactam ring. Concomitant use of cilastatin prevents in vivo metabolism of imipenem by DHP I and results in urinary concentrations of active imipenem that are higher than could be obtained following use of the antibiotic alone. (See Pharmacokinetics.)

Imipenem and cilastatin sodium is commercially available as a sterile powder for injection for IV use and as a sterile powder for injectable suspension for IM use; these powders contain a 1:1 ratio of imipenem to cilastatin. Commercially available imipenem and cilastatin sodium for injection or for injectable suspension contains 3.2 or 2.8 mEq of sodium per gram of imipenem, respectively. Potency of imipenem monohydrate is expressed in terms of imipenem, calculated on the anhydrous basis, and potency of cilastatin sodium is expressed in terms of cilastatin.

Imipenem monohydrate occurs as a white or off-white, nonhygroscopic, crystalline compound and has solubilities of 11 mg/mL in water at room temperature and approximately 0.2 mg/mL in alcohol at 25°C. Cilastatin sodium occurs as an off-white to yellowish-white, hygroscopic, amorphous compound and has solubilities of greater than 2 g/mL in water and approximately 6 mg/mL in alcohol at 25°C.

When reconstituted as directed, solutions of imipenem and cilastatin sodium prepared from the powder for injection for IV use are clear and colorless to yellow, have a pH of 6.5–7.5, and have osmolarities that approximate those of the diluents. Reconstituted suspensions of the drug prepared from the sterile powder for IM use are white to light tan in color; variations of color within this range do not affect potency.

■ **Stability** Commercially available imipenem and cilastatin sodium sterile powders for injection or for injectable suspension should be stored at less than 25°C. Solutions and suspensions of imipenem and cilastatin sodium may darken (i.e., IV solutions may turn deep yellow or IM suspensions may turn light tan) with time; this color change does not indicate loss of potency. However, IV solutions of the drug should be discarded if they become brown.

Imipenem and cilastatin sodium is stable for 4 hours at room temperature or 24 hours when refrigerated at 5°C following reconstitution with 100 mL of one of the following IV solutions: 0.9% sodium chloride injection; 5 or 10% dextrose; 5% dextrose and 0.225, 0.45, or 0.9% sodium chloride; 0.15% potassium chloride in 5% dextrose; or 5, or 10% mannitol. Following reconstitution of ADD-Vantage® vials containing imipenem and cilastatin sodium with the diluent provided by the manufacturer (i.e., 100 mL of 0.9% sodium chloride injection or 5% dextrose injection), solutions of the drug are stable for 4 hours at room temperature.

Following reconstitution of the powder for injectable suspension with lidocaine hydrochloride 1% injection (without epinephrine), the imipenem and cilastatin sodium suspension should be used within 1 hour.

The stability of imipenem is temperature and pH dependent. Solutions of imipenem and cilastatin sodium should not be frozen since freezing at temperatures warmer than −70°C results in decomposition of the drug similar to that observed with ampicillin. The drug is inactivated at alkaline or acidic pH, but is generally stable at neutral pH. Imipenem is unstable in vitro at room temperature, 35–37°C, or −20°C in serum or urine and in certain media used for in vitro susceptibility testing. Serum, urine, and dialysate specimens to be assayed for imipenem should be stabilized immediately following collection by the addition of appropriate buffers and then frozen at −70 to −80°C. The manufacturer should be consulted for specific information on how to stabilize imipenem in serum, urine, or dialysate specimens.

Because of the potential for incompatibility, the manufacturer states that imipenem and cilastatin sodium solution or suspension and other anti-infective agents should not be admixed.

Preparations

Excipients in commercially available drug preparations may have clinically important effects in some individuals; consult specific product labeling for details.

Imipenem and Cilastatin Sodium

Parenteral		
For injectable suspension, for IM use only	500 mg (of anhydrous imipenem) and 500 mg (of cilastatin)	**Primaxin® I.M.**, Merck
	750 mg (of anhydrous imipenem) and 750 mg (of cilastatin)	**Primaxin® I.M.**, Merck
For injection, for IV infusion	250 mg (of anhydrous imipenem) and 250 mg (of cilastatin)	**Primaxin® I.V.** (available in infusion bottles and vials), Merck **Primaxin® ADD-Vantage®**, Merck
	500 mg (of anhydrous imipenem) and 500 mg (of cilastatin)	**Primaxin® I.V.** (available in infusion bottles and vials), Merck **Primaxin® ADD-Vantage®**, Merck

†Use is not currently included in the labeling approved by the US Food and Drug Administration

Selected Revisions September 2016,

Meropenem

■ Meropenem is a synthetic carbapenem β-lactam antibiotic that is structurally and pharmacologically related to imipenem, but does not require concomitant administration with a dehydropeptidase 1 (DHP 1) inhibitor such as cilastatin.

Uses

Meropenem is used for the treatment of intra-abdominal infections, meningitis, and skin and skin structure infections caused by susceptible bacteria. The drug also is used for the treatment of respiratory tract infections†, septicemia†, and urinary tract infections† caused by susceptible bacteria and for empiric anti-infective therapy in febrile neutropenic patients†.

Prior to initiation of meropenem therapy, appropriate specimens should be obtained for identification of the causative organism and in vitro susceptibility tests. Meropenem can be initiated empirically pending completion of susceptibility testing, with continuance or alteration (e.g., substitution of an appropriate alternative anti-infective) determined by the results of culture and susceptibility tests.

■ **Intra-abdominal Infections** Meropenem is used for the treatment of intra-abdominal infections, including complicated appendicitis and peritonitis, caused by susceptible bacteria. The drug may be used as monotherapy for the treatment of intra-abdominal infections caused by susceptible viridans streptococci, *Escherichia coli*, *Klebsiella pneumonia*, *Pseudomonas aeruginosa*, *Bacteroides fragilis*, *B. thetaiotaomicron*, or *Peptostreptococcus*. Because meropenem has a broad spectrum of antibacterial activity, the drug may be used empirically to treat intra-abdominal infections before identification of the causative organism.

The Infectious Diseases Society of America (IDSA) states that patients with community-acquired intra-abdominal infections of mild to moderate severity may receive initial treatment with an empiric regimen that has a narrower spectrum of activity since unnecessary use of broad spectrum agents in such infections may contribute to emergence of resistance. Therefore, IDSA recommends use of the fixed combination of ampicillin and sulbactam, cefazolin or cefuroxime in conjunction with metronidazole, the fixed combination of ticarcillin and clavulanate, ertapenem monotherapy, or a fluoroquinolone (ciprofloxacin, levofloxacin, moxifloxacin, gatifloxacin) in conjunction with metronidazole for treatment of mild to moderate community-acquired intra-abdominal infections. Patients who are immunosuppressed or have more severe community-acquired intra-abdominal infections, however, should receive a regimen that has a broader spectrum of activity. Regimens recommended by IDSA for such individuals include meropenem monotherapy; imipenem and cilastatin monotherapy; a third or fourth generation cephalosporin (cefotaxime, ceftriaxone, ceftizoxime, ceftazidime, cefepime) in conjunction with metronidazole; ciprofloxacin in conjunction with metronidazole; the fixed combination of piperacillin and tazobactam; or aztreonam in conjunction with metronidazole. Other clinicians suggest that severely ill patients and those with prolonged hospitalization should receive an initial regimen that includes an antipseudomonal agent such as an antipseudomonal penicillin (ticarcillin and clavulanate, piperacillin and tazobactam), a carbapenem (imipenem or meropenem), ceftazidime, or cefepime used in conjunction with metronidazole. These clinicians state that an aminoglycoside also could be included in the empiric regimen; however, IDSA states that aminoglycosides should not be used routinely in patients with community-acquired intra-abdominal infections but may be included in empiric regimens for treatment of nosocomial intra-abdominal infections, depending on local patterns of in vitro susceptibility of nosocomial isolates. Postoperative (nosocomial) intra-abdominal infections usually require treatment with multiple-drug regimens and, since these infections often involve resistant organisms, IDSA recommends that empiric regimens be selected based on local nosocomial susceptibility patterns.

In clinical studies in patients with intra-abdominal infections, meropenem monotherapy was similar in efficacy to a 2-drug regimen of tobramycin and clindamycin or monotherapy with imipenem and cilastatin sodium. At follow-up 7 or more days after empiric anti-infective therapy was completed, clinical cure was achieved in 69, 76, or 65% of evaluable patients treated with meropenem, tobramycin combined with clindamycin, or imipenem and cilastatin, respectively, and the respective rate of microbiologic eradication was 67, 76, or 62%. In one study, meropenem monotherapy was less effective than a 2-drug regimen of cefotaxime and metronidazole for empiric treatment of complicated intra-abdominal infections; however, the difference in efficacy may have resulted from uneven assignment of patients with more severe infection to the group that received meropenem.

■ **Meningitis** Meropenem is used for the treatment of bacterial meningitis caused by susceptible *Streptococcus pneumoniae*, *Haemophilus influenzae* (including β-lactamase-producing strains), or *Neisseria meningitidis* in children 3 months of age and older. The drug also is used in the treatment of meningitis in adults†. Efficacy of meropenem for the treatment of meningitis caused by highly penicillin- or cephalosporin-resistant *S. pneumoniae* has not been established.

Meropenem can be used as monotherapy for the treatment of meningitis caused by susceptible bacteria. Although meropenem usually is not considered an initial drug of choice, it is recommended as an alternative agent in children and adults for the treatment of meningitis caused by *S. pneumoniae*, *H. influenzae*, and various other bacteria and may be useful for meningitis caused by susceptible gram-negative bacteria (e.g., *Enterobacter*†, *Citrobacter*†, *Serratia marcescens*†) that are resistant to usually recommended regimens.

IDSA states that meropenem monotherapy is one of several alternatives that can be used for empiric treatment of meningitis in adults† when the causative organism has been presumptively identified by CSF gram stain as *S. pneumoniae*, *H. influenzae*, *Listeria monocytogenes*†, or *E. coli*†, and the regimens of choice cannot be used. In addition, if in vitro susceptibility tests indicate that the causative organism is susceptible to meropenem, IDSA states that the drug can be used as an alternative to penicillin G, ampicillin, or third generation cephalosporins (ceftriaxone or cefotaxime) for the treatment of meningitis caused by *S. pneumoniae* or *N. meningitidis* (only if the strains have penicillin MICs of 1 mcg/mL or less), as an alternative to penicillin G or ampicillin for meningitis caused by *L. monocytogenes*†, as an alternative to third generation cephalosporins (ceftriaxone or cefotaxime) for meningitis caused by *E. coli*† or other Enterobacteriaceae†, as an alternative to cefepime or ceftazidime for meningitis caused by *Ps. aeruginosa*†, or as an alternative to nafcillin or oxacillin for meningitis caused by oxacillin-susceptible (methicillin-susceptible) *S. aureus*. IDSA also recommends meropenem used in conjunction with vancomycin as one of several regimens of choice for empiric therapy in patients with purulent meningitis associated with penetrating head trauma, recent neurosurgery, or a CSF shunt.

In clinical studies that included children who were at least 3 months of age but younger than 17 years of age, clinical cure of bacterial meningitis was achieved in 78% of those receiving meropenem monotherapy (40 mg/kg IV every 8 hours) or 77% of those receiving monotherapy with usual dosages of cefotaxime or ceftriaxone. When results were stratified according to the most frequent causative organisms, the clinical cure rate in those receiving meropenem or a comparator drug was 71 or 63%, respectively, if meningitis was caused by *S. pneumoniae*; 80 or 100%, respectively, if caused by β-lactamase-producing *H. influenzae*; 75 or 73%, respectively, if caused by *H. influenzae* that either did not produce β-lactamase or was not tested for such; and 86 or 90%, respectively, if caused by *N. meningitidis*. Sequelae was the most common reason patients were assessed as clinically not cured; a few patients receiving meropenem were considered not cured because of relapse or continued growth of *Ps. aeruginosa*.

■ **Respiratory Tract Infections** Meropenem is used in the treatment of respiratory tract infections†, including community-acquired pneumonia (CAP) and nosocomial pneumonia, caused by susceptible bacteria.

Community-acquired Pneumonia Although meropenem generally is active against *S. pneumoniae* (including drug-resistant *S. pneumoniae*), the American Thoracic Society (ATS), IDSA, and other clinicians state that the drug usually is considered an alternative, not a drug of first choice, for empiric treatment of CAP† caused by *S. pneumoniae*. ATS and IDSA suggest that use of meropenem in the treatment of CAP be reserved for when the infection may be caused by *Ps. aeruginosa*, *Klebsiella*, or other gram-negative bacteria. Factors that increase the risk of *Ps. aeruginosa* infection in CAP patients include severe CAP requiring treatment in an intensive care unit (ICU), structural lung disease (bronchiectasis, cystic fibrosis), corticosteroid therapy (prednisone dosage exceeding 10 mg daily), broad-spectrum anti-infective therapy given for longer than 7 days within the past month, and malnutrition. In CAP patients with risk factors for *Ps. aeruginosa*, the empiric regimen should include 2 antipseudomonal agents and also provide coverage for drug-resistant *S. pneumoniae* and *Legionella*. The ATS and IDSA suggest that this can be accomplished with a regimen that includes an IV antipseudomonal β-lactam anti-infective (e.g., cefepime, piperacillin and tazobactam, imipenem, meropenem) in conjunction with an IV antipseudomonal fluoroquinolone (e.g., ciprofloxacin) or a regimen that includes one of these IV antipseudomonal β-lactam anti-infectives, an IV aminoglycoside, and either an IV macrolide (e.g., azithromycin) or an IV nonpseudomonal quinolone.

If anaerobic bacteria have been identified or are suspected in patients with pulmonary infections, IDSA recommends use of clindamycin, a β-lactam/β-lactamase inhibitor combination, imipenem, or meropenem.

Nosocomial Pneumonia Meropenem is considered a drug of choice for empiric treatment of nosocomial pneumonia†. ATS, IDSA, and other clinicians recommend use of an antipseudomonal cephalosporin (cefepime, ceftazidime), antipseudomonal penicillin (piperacillin and tazobactam, ticarcillin and clavulanate), or an antipseudomonal carbapenem (imipenem or meropenem) for initial therapy of hospital-acquired pneumonia, ventilator-associated pneumonia, or health-care associated pneumonia because these drugs have a broad spectrum of activity against gram-positive, gram-negative, and anaerobic bacteria. In severely ill patients or in those with late-onset disease or risk factors for multidrug-resistant bacteria, the initial regimen should also include an aminoglycoside (amikacin, gentamicin, tobramycin) or antipseudomonal fluoroquinolone (ciprofloxacin or levofloxacin) to improve coverage against *Pseudomonas*. In hospitals where oxacillin-resistant (methicillin-resistant) *Staphylococcus* are common or if there are risk factors for these strains, the initial regimen also should include vancomycin or linezolid. In hospitals where multidrug-resistant *Ps. aeruginosa* are frequent causes of nosocomial pneumonia, some clinicians suggest that the initial regimen of choice is cefepime or a carbapenem (imipenem or meropenem) in conjunction with an aminoglycoside.

■ **Septicemia** Meropenem has been used for the treatment of septicemia† caused by susceptible bacteria. There is evidence that concurrent bacteremia associated with bacterial meningitis has been eliminated during meropenem meningitis treatment.

The choice of anti-infective agent for the treatment of sepsis syndrome should be based on the probable source of infection, gram-stained smears of appropriate clinical specimens, the immune status of the patient, and current patterns of bacterial resistance within the hospital and local community. For the treatment of gram-negative sepsis, a parenteral third or fourth generation cephalosporin (cefepime, cefotaxime, ceftizoxime, ceftriaxone, ceftazidime), an antipseudomonal penicillin (piperacillin and tazobactam or ticarcillin and clavulanate), a carbapenem (imipenem or meropenem), or aztreonam can be used. The antipseudomonal penicillins or carbapenems offer the advantages of activity against most strains of *Ps. aeruginosa* and activity against anaerobes. For initial treatment of life-threatening sepsis in adults, some clinicians recommend a regimen that includes either a parenteral third or fourth generation cephalosporin (cefepime, cefotaxime, ceftriaxone, ceftazidime), the fixed combination of piperacillin and tazobactam, or a carbapenem (imipenem or meropenem) in conjunction with an aminoglycoside (amikacin, gentamicin, tobramycin). Vancomycin (alone or in conjunction with gentamicin and/or rifampin) may be included in the initial regimen if oxacillin-resistant (methicillin-resistant) *S. epidermidis* is suspected.

■ **Skin and Skin Structure Infections** Meropenem is used for the treatment of complicated skin and skin structure infections caused by susceptible *Staphylococcus aureus* (including β-lactamase-producing strains, but not oxacillin-resistant [methicillin-resistant] strains), *S. pyogenes* (group A β-hemolytic streptococci), *S. agalactiae* (group B streptococci), viridans streptococci, *Enterococcus faecalis* (except vancomycin-resistant strains), *Ps. aeruginosa*, *E. coli*, *Proteus mirabilis*, *B. fragilis*, or *Peptostreptococcus*.

Some clinicians state that reasonable choices for empiric treatment of complicated skin and skin structure infections are imipenem, meropenem, the fixed combination of piperacillin and tazobactam, or the fixed combination of ticarcillin and clavulanate; however, vancomycin or linezolid should be included in the empiric regimen whenever oxacillin-resistant (methicillin-resistant) *S. aureus* may be involved.

Safety and efficacy of meropenem for the treatment of complicated skin and skin structure infections were evaluated in a randomized, double-blind trial in adults with complicated cellulitis, complex abscesses, perirectal abscesses, or infections requiring IV anti-infectives, hospitalization, and surgical intervention (37% had diabetes, 12% had peripheral vascular disease, 67% required surgical intervention). Patients were randomized to receive meropenem (500 mg IV every 8 hours) or imipenem and cilastatin (500 mg of imipenem IV every 8 hours). In clinically evaluable patients, the success rate at follow-up was 86% in those who received meropenem and 83% in those who received imipenem. In the group that received meropenem, the clinical cure rate was 90–93% for infections caused by *S. aureus* (oxacillin-susceptible strains), *S. pyogenes*, or viridans streptococci; 71 or 75% for those caused by *S. agalactiae* or *E. faecalis*, respectively; 80 or 85% for those caused by *E. coli* or *P. mirabilis*, respectively; 73% for those caused by *Ps. aeruginosa*; and 91 or 77% for those caused by *B. fragilis* or *Peptostreptococcus*, respectively.

Urinary Tract Infections Although safety and efficacy have not been established, meropenem has been used for the treatment of complicated urinary tract infections† caused by susceptible bacteria. Some clinicians suggest that urinary tract infections in hospitalized patients should be treated with a third generation cephalosporin, a fluoroquinolone, fixed combination of ticarcillin and clavulanate, fixed combination of piperacillin and tazobactam, imipenem, or meropenem; an aminoglycoside should be used concomitantly, especially in patients with sepsis. (See Uses: Septicemia.)

Acinetobacter Infections Meropenem used alone or in conjunction with an aminoglycoside (amikacin, gentamicin, tobramycin) is a drug of choice for the treatment of infections caused by *Acinetobacter*†.

Anthrax Although data are not available regarding in vivo activity of meropenem against *Bacillus anthracis*, the drug has in vitro activity against the organism, and it has been suggested that meropenem is one of several anti-infectives that can be included in multiple-drug regimens used for the treatment of anthrax†, including inhalational anthrax and anthrax meningitis.

Based on clinical experience from the bioterrorism-related anthrax exposures of 2001 and the possibility that a *B. anthracis* strain resistant to one or more anti-infectives might be used in a future bioterrorism event, CDC and other experts (e.g., US Working Group on Civilian Biodefense) recommend that treatment of clinically apparent inhalational anthrax in adults, adolescents, or children that occurs as the result of exposure to anthrax spores in the context of biologic warfare or bioterrorism be initiated with a multiple-drug parenteral regimen that includes ciprofloxacin or doxycycline and 1 or 2 additional anti-infectives predicted to be effective. Other drugs to be included in the initial treatment regimen with ciprofloxacin or doxycycline should be selected based on in vitro susceptibility, possibility of efficacy, adverse effects, and cost. Based on in vitro data, other drugs that have been suggested as possibilities to augment ciprofloxacin or doxycycline in such multiple-drug regimens include chloramphenicol, clindamycin, rifampin, vancomycin, clarithromycin, imipenem, meropenem, penicillin, or ampicillin. Optimum regimens for treatment of anthrax meningitis are unknown. However, if meningitis is established or suspected, early and aggressive anti-infective treatment is critical. Some clinicians suggest a multiple-drug regimen that includes a fluoroquinolone (e.g., ciprofloxacin) and 2 additional agents with good CSF penetration (e.g., ampicillin or penicillin, meropenem, rifampin, vancomycin).

For information on treatment of anthrax and recommendations for prophylaxis following exposure to anthrax spores, see Uses: Anthrax, in Ciprofloxacin 8:12.18.

Bacillus Infections Meropenem is used for the treatment of infections caused by *Bacillus cereus*†. Although vancomycin is considered the drug of choice, carbapenems (imipenem or meropenem) or clindamycin are alternatives.

Burkholderia Infections ***Melioidosis*** Meropenem is used as an alternative to imipenem or ceftazidime for the treatment of melioidosis† caused by *Burkholderia pseudomallei*.

B. pseudomallei may cause subclinical illness and localized infections or fulminant septicemia; disseminated infections may include hepatic and splenic abscesses. The incubation period usually is 1–21 days; however, in some asymptomatic individuals, the disease has remained dormant for prolonged periods and active melioidosis was not evident for up to 29 years later, usually at a time when the patient was immunosuppressed. If left untreated, severe septicemic infections can be fatal within 24–48 hours after onset. *B. pseudomallei* is widely distributed in water and soil in many tropical and subtropical countries and melioidosis is endemic in Southeast Asia and northern Australia. Person-to-person spread occurs only rarely. *B. pseudomallei* usually is transmitted to humans from contaminated materials (e.g., soil) via contact with nasal, oral, or conjunctival mucous membranes, contact with abraded or lacerated skin, or, rarely, by inhalation. Laboratory workers have become infected via aerosols from *B. pseudomallei* cultures.

Patients with localized or mild disease may be effectively treated with a prolonged regimen of oral anti-infectives (e.g., oral doxycycline in conjunction with oral co-trimoxazole). However, patients with severe illness should receive an initial parenteral regimen of ceftazidime, imipenem, or meropenem (some clinicians recommend that co-trimoxazole also be included, especially if the patient is septicemic) followed by a prolonged maintenance regimen of oral anti-infectives (e.g., co-trimoxazole with or without doxycycline). (See Burkholderia Infections under Dosage and Administration: Adult Dosage.) In patients with melioidosis septic shock, adjunctive use of filgrastim (granulocyte colony-stimulating factor; G-CSF) during initial treatment has been suggested. After the maintenance regimen is completed, life-long follow-up is recommended since relapse of melioidosis can occur despite effective anti-infective therapy.

B. pseudomallei has been studied for and is considered a potential pathogen for aerosol distribution in the context of biologic warfare or bioterrorism. Acute respiratory or systemic infection probably would occur following high-dose aerosol exposure to *B. pseudomallei*. Some experts (e.g., US Army Medical Research Institute of Infectious Diseases [USAMRIID], European Commission's Task Force on Biological and Chemical Agent Threats [BICHAT]) state that the same treatment regimens recommended for naturally occurring melioidosis should be used if the disease occurs in the context of biologic warfare or bioterrorism.

Glanders Meropenem has been recommended for the treatment of glanders† caused by *B. mallei*.

Human infection with *B. mallei* is rare and has occurred principally in veterinarians, horse and donkey caretakers, and abattoir workers exposed to infected animals (usually horses, mules, or donkeys). There have been no naturally acquired cases of human glanders reported in the US for more than 50 years, and the disease currently is reported only sporadically in Asia, Africa, the Middle East, and South America. *B. mallei* occurs only in infected, susceptible hosts, and the transmission rate from infected animals to humans appears to be low. Person-to-person spread occurs only rarely.

Because experience is limited regarding the treatment of human cases of glanders, optimum regimens have not been identified. Some clinicians suggest that streptomycin in conjunction with a tetracycline is the regimen of choice and alternatives are streptomycin in conjunction with chloramphenicol or imipenem monotherapy. Other clinicians suggest that, pending results of in vitro susceptibility tests, regimens recommended for treatment of melioidosis can be used for initial empiric treatment of glanders since these *Burkholderia* species are similar and efficacy data are available regarding use of these regimens in patients with melioidosis.

B. mallei has been studied for and is considered a possible pathogen for aerosol distribution in the context of biologic warfare or bioterrorism. Some experts (e.g., USAMRIID, BICHAT) state that the same treatment regimens recommended for naturally occurring glanders should be used if the disease occurs in the context of biologic warfare or bioterrorism.

Campylobacter Infections Meropenem is used for the treatment of systemic infections caused by *Campylobacter fetus*†. Some clinicians suggest that the drug of choice for these infections is a third generation cephalosporin or gentamicin, and alternatives are ampicillin, imipenem, or meropenem.

Capnocytophaga Infections Meropenem has been recommended for the treatment of infections caused by *Capnocytophaga canimorsus*†.

Optimum regimens for the treatment of infections caused by *Capnocytophaga* have not been identified. Some clinicians recommend use of penicillin G or, alternatively, a third generation cephalosporin (cefotaxime, ceftizoxime, ceftriaxone), a carbapenem (imipenem or meropenem), vancomycin, a fluoroquinolone, or clindamycin.

Clostridium Infections Meropenem is recommended by some clinicians as an alternative to penicillin G for the treatment of infections caused by *Clostridum perfringens*† in individuals with penicillin hypersensitivity or for polymicrobial infections.

Nocardia Infections Meropenem is used for the treatment of infections caused by *Nocardia*†. Co-trimoxazole usually is considered the drug of first choice for *Nocardia* infections; alternatives include sulfisoxazole, a tetracycline (e.g., doxycycline, minocycline), a carbapenem (imipenem or meropenem), amikacin, ceftriaxone, fixed combination of amoxicillin and clavulanate, cycloserine, or linezolid. In vitro susceptibility testing, if available, is recommend for isolates from patients with invasive disease and those unable to tolerate a sulfonamide.

Rhodococcus Infections Meropenem in conjunction with vancomycin is recommended for the treatment of infections caused by *Rhodococcus equi*†. Optimum regimens for these infections have not been identified. Some clinicians suggest that the regimen of choice is vancomycin with or without a fluoroquinolone, rifampin, a carbapenem (imipenem or meropenem), or amikacin.

Empiric Therapy in Febrile Neutropenic Patients Meropenem is used alone or in conjunction with other anti-infectives for empiric anti-infective therapy of presumed bacterial infections in febrile neutropenic patients†.

Successful treatment of infections in granulocytopenic patients requires prompt initiation of empiric anti-infective therapy (even when fever is the only sign or symptom of infection) and appropriate modification of the initial regimen if the duration of fever and neutropenia is protracted, if a specific site of infection is identified, or if organisms resistant to the initial regimen are present. The initial empiric regimen should be chosen based on the underlying disease and other host factors that may affect the degree of risk and on local epidemiologic data regarding usual pathogens in these patients and data regarding their in vitro susceptibility to available anti-infective agents. The fact that gram-positive bacteria have become a predominant pathogen in febrile neutropenic patients should be considered when selecting an empiric anti-infective regimen.

No empiric regimen has been identified that would be appropriate for all patients. Regimens that have been recommended for empiric therapy in febrile neutropenic patients with presumed bacterial infections include *monotherapy* with a third or fourth generation cephalosporin (i.e., ceftazidime, cefepime) or a carbapenem (e.g., imipenem and cilastatin sodium, meropenem) or *combination therapy* consisting of a β-lactam antibiotic (e.g., ceftazidime, ceftriaxone), a carbapenem (e.g., imipenem, meropenem), an extended-spectrum penicillin (e.g., ticarcillin), or a fixed combination of an extended-spectrum penicillin and a β-lactamase inhibitor (e.g., piperacillin and tazobactam, ticarcillin and clavulanate) given in conjunction with an aminoglycoside (e.g., amikacin, gentamicin, tobramycin).

IDSA recommends use of a parenteral empiric regimen in most febrile neutropenic patients; use of an oral regimen (e.g., oral ciprofloxacin and oral amoxicillin and clavulanate) should be considered only in selected adults at low risk for complications who have no focus of bacterial infection and no signs or symptoms of systemic infection other than fever. At health-care facilities where gram-positive bacteria are common causes of serious infection and use of vancomycin in the initial empiric regimen is considered necessary, IDSA recommends 2- or 3-drug combination therapy that includes vancomycin and either cefepime, ceftazidime, imipenem, or meropenem given with or without an aminoglycoside;

vancomycin should be discontinued 24–48 hours later if a susceptible gram-positive bacterial infection is not identified. At health-care facilities where vancomycin is not indicated in the initial empiric regimen, IDSA recommends monotherapy with a third or fourth generation cephalosporin (ceftazidime, cefepime) or a carbapenem (imipenem, meropenem) for uncomplicated cases; however, for complicated cases or if anti-infective resistance is a problem, combination therapy consisting of an aminoglycoside (amikacin, gentamicin, tobramycin) given in conjunction with an antipseudomonal penicillin (ticarcillin and clavulanate, piperacillin and tazobactam), an antipseudomonal cephalosporin (cefepime, ceftazidime), or a carbapenem (imipenem, meropenem) is recommended. Regardless of the initial regimen selected, patients should be reassessed after 3–5 days of treatment and the anti-infective regimen altered (if indicated) based on the presence or absence of fever, identification of the causative organism, and the clinical condition of the patient.

Published protocols for the treatment of infections in febrile neutropenic patients should be consulted for specific recommendations regarding selection of the initial empiric regimen, when to change the initial regimen, possible subsequent regimens, and duration of therapy in these patients.

Dosage and Administration

■ Administration Meropenem is administered by IV injection or IV infusion.

Reconstitution and Dilution For direct intermittent IV injection, 10 or 20 mL of sterile water for injection should be added to a vial labeled as containing 500 mg or 1 g, respectively, of meropenem to provide a solution containing approximately 50 mg/mL. The vial should be shaken until dissolution occurs and then allowed to stand until the solution is clear. Reconstituted solutions should be used promptly, but may be stored for up to 2 hours at 15–25°C or up to 12 hours at 4°C.

For IV infusion, vials labeled as containing 500 mg or 1 g of meropenem should be diluted in a compatible IV solution. Alternatively, vials labeled as containing 500 mg or 1 g may be reconstituted as directed for direct intermittent IV injection and the resulting solution added to an IV container and further diluted with a compatible IV solution.

Rate of Administration IV injections of meropenem should be given over a 3- to 5-minute period.

IV infusions of meropenem should be given over approximately 15–30 minutes.

■ Dosage Meropenem is commercially available as the trihydrate; potency and dosage of the drug are expressed on the anhydrous basis.

To minimize the risk of seizures, recommended meropenem dosage should not be exceeded, especially in patients with factors known to predispose to seizure activity. (See CNS Effects under Warning/Precautions: Warnings, in Cautions.)

Adult Dosage **Intra-abdominal Infections.** The usual adult dosage of meropenem for the treatment of intra-abdominal infections is 1 g every 8 hours.

Meningitis. For the treatment of bacterial meningitis in adults†, some clinicians recommend a dosage of 6 g daily. A dosage of 40 mg/kg every 8 hours daily (up to 6 g daily) has been used in conjunction with ceftriaxone or cefotaxime in adults with meningitis.

Respiratory Tract Infections. If meropenem is used for the treatment of nosocomial pneumonia† (including hospital-acquired, ventilator-associated, or health-care-associated infections), some clinicians recommend that adults receive a dosage of 1 g every 8 hours.

Skin and Skin Structure Infections. The usual adult dosage of meropenem for the treatment of complicated skin and skin structure infections is 500 mg every 8 hours.

Burkholderia Infections. For the treatment of severe melioidosis† caused by *Burkholderia pseudomallei*, the US Army Medical Research Institute of Infectious Diseases (USAMRIID) and other clinicians recommend a meropenem dosage of 25 mg/kg IV every 8 hours (up to 6 g daily); concomitant co-trimoxazole (8 mg/kg of trimethoprim daily given in 4 divided doses) may be indicated in septicemic individuals. Other clinicians recommend a meropenem dosage of 0.5–1 g every 8 hours with or without co-trimoxazole. The initial parenteral regimen should be continued for at least 14 days and until there is clinical improvement. Although the median time to fever resolution is 9 days, some patients may remain febrile for prolonged periods despite appropriate antimicrobial therapy. When appropriate, treatment may be changed to an oral maintenance regimen (e.g., oral co-trimoxazole with or without oral doxycycline) and continued for at least 3–6 months to prevent recrudence or relapse. More prolonged oral maintenance therapy (up to 12 months) may be necessary, depending on the response to therapy and severity of initial illness.

Although only limited experience is available regarding the treatment of human cases of glanders†, some clinicians suggest that the meropenem regimens recommended for the treatment of severe melioidosis also can be used for the treatment of glanders.

Pediatric Dosage Children weighing more than 50 kg should receive the usually recommended adult dosage of meropenem.

Intra-abdominal Infections. For the treatment of intra-abdominal infections, children 3 months of age and older weighing 50 kg or less should receive 20 mg/kg (up to 1 g) every 8 hours.

Meningitis. For the treatment of meningitis, children 3 months of age and older weighing 50 kg or less should receive 40 mg/kg (up to 2 g) every 8 hours.

Skin and Skin Structure Infections. For the treatment of complicated skin and skin structure infections, children 3 months of age and older weighing 50 kg or less should receive 10 mg/kg (up to 500 mg) every 8 hours.

Burkholderia Infections. Some clinicians suggest that children older than 3 months of age can receive meropenem in a dosage of 10–20 mg/kg every 8 hours for the initial treatment of melioidosis† caused by *B. pseudomallei* or glanders† caused by *B. mallei*. Concomitant therapy with co-trimoxazole may be indicated in those with severe illness. These clinicians state that children weighing more than 40 kg may receive the meropenem dosage recommended for adults with these infections. (See Burkholderia Infections under Dosage and Administration: Adult Dosage.)

Geriatric Dosage The manufacturer states that dosage adjustment is not necessary for geriatric patients with creatinine clearances exceeding 50 mL/minute. For geriatric patients with reduced renal function, dosage should be adjusted according to the guidelines for other adults with renal impairment. (See Dosage in Renal and Hepatic Impairment under Dosage and Administration: Dosage.)

■ Dosage in Renal and Hepatic Impairment Dosage of meropenem should be modified according to the degree of renal impairment in adults with creatinine clearances of 50 mL/minute or less. The manufacturer and some clinicians recommend that adults with creatinine clearances of 26–50 mL/minute can receive the usual dose every 12 hours, those with creatinine clearances of 10–25 mL/minute can receive half the usual dose every 12 hours, and those with creatinine clearances less than 10 mL/minute can receive half the usual dose every 24 hours. If a measured creatinine clearance is unavailable, the patient's creatinine clearance (Ccr) can be estimated using the following formulas:

$$Ccr\ male = \frac{(140 - age) \times weight}{72 \times serum\ creatinine}$$

$$Ccr\ female = 0.85 \times Ccr\ male$$

where age is in years, weight is in kg, and serum creatinine is in mg/dL.

Because meropenem is removed by hemodialysis, supplemental doses should be given after each hemodialysis session. Meropenem also is removed by various forms of continuous renal replacement therapy, including continuous venovenous hemodiafiltration (CVVHDF), continuous venovenous hemofiltration (CVVHF), and continuous ambulatory peritoneal dialysis (CAPD). Therefore, to avoid inadequate meropenem concentrations in anuric patients undergoing these procedures, dosage adjustments are necessary and should be based on characteristics of the specific procedure (e.g., filter or membrane type, amount of filtrate produced, dialysate flow rate).

The manufacturer states that there is a lack of experience with use of meropenem in pediatric patients with renal impairment. Some clinicians suggest that pediatric patients undergoing hemodialysis receive meropenem doses after hemodialysis.

Dosage adjustment is not necessary in patients with hepatic impairment.

Cautions

■ Contraindications Known hypersensitivity to meropenem, other carbapenems, or any ingredient in the formulation.

History of anaphylactic reaction to β-lactams.

■ Warnings/Precautions ***Warnings*** **Superinfection/Clostridium difficile-associated Colitis.** Possible emergence and overgrowth of nonsusceptible organism. Careful observation of the patient is essential. Institute appropriate therapy if superinfection occurs.

Treatment with anti-infectives may permit overgrowth of clostridia. Consider *Clostridium difficile*-associated diarrhea and colitis (antibiotic-associated pseudomembranous colitis) if diarrhea develops and manage accordingly.

Some mild cases of *C. difficile*-associated diarrhea and colitis may respond to discontinuance alone. Manage moderate to severe cases with fluid, electrolyte, and protein supplementation; appropriate anti-infective therapy (e.g., oral metronidazole or vancomycin) recommended if colitis is severe.

CNS Effects. Seizures and other adverse CNS effects reported during meropenem therapy, especially in those with underlying CNS disorders (e.g., brain lesions, history of seizures), bacterial meningitis, or compromised renal function.

Do not exceed recommended dosage, especially in those with known factors that predispose to seizures. Anticonvulsant therapy should be continued in those with known seizure disorders.

If focal tremors, myoclonus, or seizures occur, evaluate the patient neurologically, initiate anticonvulsant therapy if necessary, and determine whether meropenem dosage should be decreased or the drug discontinued.

Sensitivity Reactions **Hypersensitivity Reactions.** Serious and occasionally fatal hypersensitivity reactions (e.g., anaphylaxis) reported with β-lactams.

If hypersensitivity occurs, discontinue meropenem and institute appropriate therapy as indicated (e.g., epinephrine, corticosteroids, and maintenance of an adequate airway and oxygen).

Cross-hypersensitivity. Partial cross-allergenicity among β-lactam antibiotics, including penicillins, cephalosporins, and other β-lactams.

Prior to initiation of meropenem therapy, make careful inquiry concerning previous hypersensitivity reactions to meropenem, cephalosporins, penicillins, or other drugs.

General Precautions **Selection and Use of Anti-infectives.** To reduce development of drug-resistant bacteria and maintain effectiveness of meropenem and other antibacterials, use only for treatment or prevention of infections proven or strongly suspected to be caused by susceptible bacteria.

When selecting or modifying anti-infective therapy, use results of culture and in vitro susceptibility testing. In the absence of such data, consider local epidemiology and susceptibility patterns when selecting anti-infectives for empiric therapy.

Laboratory Monitoring. Periodically assess organ system functions, including renal, hepatic, and hematopoietic, during prolonged therapy.

Sodium Content. Each g of meropenem contains 3.92 mEq (90.2 mg) of sodium as sodium carbonate.

Specific Populations **Pregnancy.** Category B. (See Users Guide)

Lactation. Not known whether meropenem is distributed into milk. Use with caution.

Pediatric Use. Safety and efficacy not established in children younger than 3 months of age.

Geriatric Use. No substantial differences in safety and efficacy relative to younger adults, but increased sensitivity cannot be ruled out.

Substantially eliminated by kidneys; risk of toxicity may be greater in patients with impaired renal function. Select dosage with caution and assess renal function periodically since geriatric patients are more likely to have renal impairment.

No dosage adjustments except those related to renal function. (See Dosage in Renal and Hepatic Impairment under Dosage and Administration: Dosage.)

Hepatic Impairment. Pharmacokinetics not affected by hepatic impairment; dosage adjustments not required.

Renal Impairment. Decreased clearance. Dosage adjustments recommended in patients with creatinine clearance less than 50 mL/minute. (See Dosage in Renal and Hepatic Impairment under Dosage and Administration: Dosage.)

■ **Common Adverse Effects** Adverse effects reported in 1% or more of patients receiving meropenem including GI effects (diarrhea, nausea, vomiting, constipation), local reactions (pain and inflammation at injection site, phlebitis/thrombophlebitis), headache, anemia, rash, pruritus, sepsis, apnea, shock, glossitis, and oral candidiasis.

Drug Interactions

■ **Aminoglycosides** Potential pharmacologic interaction (synergistic antibacterial effects against *Pseudomonas aeruginosa*).

■ **Probenecid** Pharmacokinetic interaction (decreased renal tubular secretion of meropenem; increased systemic exposure and prolonged meropenem half-life). Concomitant use not recommended.

■ **Valproic Acid** Pharmacokinetic interaction (valproic acid serum concentrations may be decreased to subtherapeutic concentrations; possible increased risk of seizures). Use concomitantly with caution.

Description

Meropenem is a synthetic carbapenem antibiotic structurally and pharmacologically related to other carbapenems (e.g., imipenem, ertapenem). Unlike imipenem, meropenem has a methyl group at position 1 of the 5-membered ring, which confers stability against hydrolysis by dehydropeptidase 1 (DHP 1) present on the brush border of proximal renal tubular cells and therefore does not require concomitant administration with a DHP-1 inhibitor such as cilastatin.

Meropenem usually is bactericidal in action. Like other β-lactam antibiotics, the antibacterial activity of meropenem results from inhibition of bacterial cell wall synthesis. Meropenem has a broad spectrum of antibacterial activity and is active against many gram-positive and -negative bacteria and some anaerobic bacteria. The spectrum of activity of meropenem resembles that of imipenem; however, meropenem generally is more active in vitro against Enterobacteriaceae and less active against gram-positive bacteria. Like imipenem, meropenem is highly resistant to hydrolysis by a variety of β-lactamases (including penicillinases, cephalosporinases, and extended-spectrum β-lactamases) but appears to be more susceptible to hydrolysis by metallo-β-lactamases.

Meropenem is active in vitro and in clinical infections against many gram-positive aerobic and facultatively aerobic bacteria, including *Streptococcus pneumoniae* (penicillin-susceptible strains only), *S. pyogenes* (group A β-hemolytic streptococci), *S. agalactiae* (group B streptococci), *Staphylococcus aureus* (including β-lactamase-producing strains, but not oxacillin-resistant [methicillin-resistant] strains), *Enterococcus faecalis* (not vancomycin-resistant strains), and viridans streptococci. The drug also is active in vitro against *S. epidermidis* (including β-lactamase-producing strains, but not oxacillin-resistant strains).

Meropenem is active in vitro and in clinical infections against many gram-negative aerobic and facultatively aerobic bacteria, including *Escherichia coli*, *Haemophilus influenzae* (including β-lactamase-producing strains), *Klebsiella pneumoniae*, *Neisseria meningitidis*, *Proteus mirabilis*, and *Pseudomonas aeruginosa*. The drug also is active in vitro against *Acinetobacter*, *Aeromonas hydrophila*, *Campylobacter jejuni*, *Citrobacter diversus*, *C. freundii*, *Enterobacter cloacae*, *H. influenzae* (ampicillin-resistant, non-β-lactamase-producing strains; BLNAR), *Havnia alvei*, *K. oxytoca*, *Moraxella catarrhalis* (including β-lactamase-producing strains), *Morganella morganii*, *Pasteurella multocida*, *P. vulgaris*, *Salmonella*, *Shigella*, *Serratia marcescens*, and *Yersinia enterocolitica*.

Meropenem is active in vitro and in clinical infections against some anaerobic bacteria, including *Bacteroides fragilis*, *B. thetaiotaomicron*, and *Peptostreptococcus*. The drug also is active in vitro against *B. distasonis*, *B. ovatus*, *B. uniformis*, *B. ureolyticus*, *B. vulgatus*, *Clostridium difficile*, *C. perfringens*, *Eubacterium lentum*, *Fusobacterium*, *Prevotella bivia*, *P. intermedia*, *P. melaninogenica*, *Porphyromonas asaccharolytica*, and *Propionibacterium acnes*.

Cross resistance may occur between meropenem and other carbapenems (e.g., imipenem).

Meropenem is distributed into most body tissues and fluids, including bronchial mucosa, lung, bile, gynecologic tissue (endometrium, myometrium, ovary, cervix, fallopian tube), muscle, heart valves, skin, interstitial and peritoneal fluid, and CSF. Plasma protein binding is approximately 2%. The drug is partially metabolized to at least one microbiologically inactive metabolite. About 70% of an IV dose is eliminated in urine as unchanged drug by tubular secretion and glomerular filtration. The plasma half-life of meropenem is approximately 1 hour in adults with normal renal function and 1.5 hours in children 3 months to 2 years of age. Plasma half-life is increased and clearance of the drug is decreased in patients with renal impairment.

Advice to Patients

Advise patients that antibacterials (including meropenem) should only be used to treat bacterial infections and not used to treat viral infections (e.g., the common cold).

Importance of completing full course of therapy, even if feeling better after a few days.

Advise patients that skipping doses or not completing the full course of therapy may decrease effectiveness and increase the likelihood that bacteria will develop resistance and will not be treatable with meropenem or other antibacterials in the future.

Importance of informing clinicians of other medical conditions, including history of seizures.

Importance of discontinuing therapy and informing clinician if an allergic or hypersensitivity reaction occurs.

Importance of informing clinicians of existing or contemplated concomitant therapy, including prescription and OTC drugs, and any concomitant illnesses.

Importance of women informing clinicians if they are or plan to become pregnant or plan to breast-feed.

Importance of informing patients of other important precautionary information. (See Cautions.)

Overview® (see Users Guide). For additional information on this drug until a more detailed monograph is developed and published, the manufacturer's labeling should be consulted. It is *essential* that the manufacturer's labeling be consulted for more detailed information on usual cautions, precautions, contraindications, potential drug interactions, laboratory test interferences, and acute toxicity.

Preparations

Excipients in commercially available drug preparations may have clinically important effects in some individuals; consult specific product labeling for details.

Meropenem (Trihydrate)

Parenteral

For injection, for IV use only	500 mg (of anhydrous meropenem)	**Merrem® I.V.**, AstraZeneca
	1 g (of anhydrous meropenem)	**Merrem® I.V.**, AstraZeneca

†Use is not currently included in the labeling approved by the US Food and Drug Administration

Meropenem and Vaborbactam

■ Meropenem and vaborbactam is a fixed combination of meropenem (a carbapenem β-lactam antibiotic) and vaborbactam (a non-β-lactam β-lactamase inhibitor); vaborbactam inactivates certain bacterial β-lactamases and expands meropenem's spectrum of activity against some bacteria that produce these β-lactamases.

Uses

■ **Urinary Tract Infections** Meropenem and vaborbactam is used for the treatment of complicated urinary tract infections, including pyelonephritis, caused by susceptible *Escherichia coli*, *Klebsiella pneumoniae*, or *Enterobacter cloacae* species complex.

Clinical Experience Efficacy and safety of meropenem and vaborbactam for the treatment of complicated urinary tract infections is based on results from a phase 3, randomized, double-blind, noninferiority study in 545 adults with complicated urinary tract infections, including pyelonephritis. Patients were randomized in a 1:1 ratio to receive treatment with the fixed combination of meropenem and vaborbactam (4 g [meropenem 2 g and vaborbactam 2 g] given by IV infusion every 8 hours) or the fixed combination of piperacillin and tazobactam (4.5 g [piperacillin 4 g and tazobactam 0.5 g] given by IV infusion every 8 hours). After at least 15 doses of IV treatment, patients with clinical improvement (afebrile for at least 24 hours, urinary tract infection symptoms and leukocytosis improved, urine culture at 24 hours with growth less than 10^4 CFU/mL, negative blood culture in those with bacteremia, able to tolerate oral medications) were permitted to switch to an oral antibacterial (e.g., levofloxacin). The planned total duration of IV and oral anti-infective treatment was 10 days; patients with bacteremia could receive up to 14 days of treatment. The primary efficacy end point was overall success at the end of IV treatment visit (defined as the composite end point of successful clinical outcome [investigator judgment of cure or improvement] *and* microbiologic outcome [baseline pathogen(s) reduced to less than 10^4 CFU/mL on urine culture]). Baseline characteristics were generally similar between treatment groups (mean age 54 years, 93% white, 66% female, 17–19% with diabetes mellitus, 6–8% with bacteremia identified at baseline, 59% with pyelonephritis, 40% with complicated urinary tract infection). The mean duration of IV treatment was 8 days and the mean total treatment duration (IV and oral antibacterial treatment) was 10 days in both groups. Overall success at the end of IV treatment visit was achieved by substantially more patients receiving meropenem and vaborbactam compared with those receiving piperacillin and tazobactam (98.4% versus 94.3%, respectively). At the test-of-cure visit 7 days after completion of treatment in a subset of patients that excluded those with baseline pathogens resistant to piperacillin and tazobactam, the overall success rate in patients receiving meropenem and vaborbactam was noninferior to the success rate in those receiving piperacillin and tazobactam (76.5% versus 73.2%, respectively). In the microbiologically modified intent-to-treat population, the rate of clinical and microbiologic response in patients with bacteremia at baseline who received meropenem and vaborbactam was 83.3%.

Dosage and Administration

■ **Administration** Meropenem and vaborbactam is administered by IV infusion.

IV Infusion **Reconstitution and Dilution.** Meropenem and vaborbactam powder for injection must be reconstituted and further diluted prior to IV infusion.

Single-dose vials of meropenem and vaborbactam labeled as containing 2 g (meropenem 1 g and vaborbactam 1 g) should be reconstituted by withdrawing 20 mL of 0.9% sodium chloride injection from an infusion bag and adding that to the vial and gently mixing. The volume of reconstituted solution in the vial is approximately 21.3 mL and the approximate concentration is meropenem 50 mg/mL and vaborbactam 50 mg/mL.

Immediately after reconstitution and prior to IV infusion, the reconstituted meropenem and vaborbactam solution *must* be further diluted. To prepare the indicated dose, the appropriate volume of reconstituted solution should be withdrawn from the vial(s) and added back into the 0.9% sodium chloride injection infusion bag. (See Table 1.) The final concentration of meropenem and of vaborbactam in the infusion solution is approximately 2–8 mg/mL.

Table 1. Dilution of Reconstituted Meropenem and Vaborbactam

Recommended Dose of Meropenem and Vaborbactam	Volume to Withdraw from Reconstituted Vial(s) for Further Dilution	Volume of Infusion Bag
4 g (meropenem 2 g and vaborbactam 2 g)	Entire contents of 2 reconstituted vials (approximately 21 mL from *each* vial)	250–1000 mL
2 g (meropenem 1 g and vaborbactam 1 g)	Entire contents of 1 reconstituted vial (approximately 21 mL)	125–500 mL
1 g (meropenem 0.5 g and vaborbactam 0.5 g)	10.5 mL of reconstituted solution	70–250 mL

The reconstituted and diluted solution of meropenem and vaborbactam should be inspected visually for particulate matter and discoloration prior to administration; the solution should appear colorless to light yellow.

Unused portions of the reconstituted and diluted solution should be discarded.

Following reconstitution and dilution, IV infusion of meropenem and vaborbactam solutions *must* be completed within 4 hours if stored at room temperature. Alternatively, IV infusion of these solutions *must* be completed within 22 hours if stored under refrigeration (2–8°C).

Rate of Administration. IV infusions of meropenem and vaborbactam should be given over 3 hours.

Dispensing and Dosage and Administration Precautions. Healthcare professionals should be aware that dosage of meropenem and vaborbactam is expressed as the total (sum) of the dosage of each of the 2 active components (i.e., dosage of meropenem plus dosage of vaborbactam). This dosage convention should be considered when prescribing, preparing, and dispensing meropenem and vaborbactam.

■ **Dosage** Meropenem and vaborbactam is a fixed combination containing a 1:1 ratio of meropenem to vaborbactam.

The meropenem component is provided as meropenem trihydrate (dosage of this component is expressed in terms of meropenem).

Dosage of the fixed combination of meropenem and vaborbactam is expressed in terms of the total of the meropenem and vaborbactam content.

Each single-dose vial of meropenem and vaborbactam contains a total of 2 g (i.e., 1 g of meropenem and 1 g of vaborbactam).

Adult Dosage **Urinary Tract Infections.** The recommended dosage of meropenem and vaborbactam for the treatment of complicated urinary tract infections, including pyelonephritis, in adults with normal renal function is 4 g (meropenem 2 g and vaborbactam 2 g) every 8 hours for up to 14 days.

■ **Special Populations** ***Renal Impairment*** Dosage adjustments are recommended in adults with an estimated glomerular filtration rate (eGFR) less than 50 mL/minute per 1.73 m². (See Table 2.) The duration of treatment is up to 14 days.

For patients with changing renal function, serum creatinine concentrations and eGFR should be monitored at least daily and dosage of meropenem and vaborbactam should be adjusted accordingly.

Table 2. Dosage of Meropenem and Vaborbactam in Adults with Renal Impairment

eGFR (mL/minute per 1.73 m²)	Recommended Dosage of Meropenem and Vaborbactam
30–49	2 g (meropenem 1 g and vaborbactam 1 g) every 8 hours
15–29	2 g (meropenem 1 g and vaborbactam 1 g) every 12 hours
Less than 15	1 g (meropenem 0.5 g and vaborbactam 0.5 g) every 12 hours

For patients receiving hemodialysis, meropenem and vaborbactam should be administered after a hemodialysis session.

Geriatric Patients Dosage adjustments based solely on age are not needed when meropenem and vaborbactam is used in geriatric patients. However, because geriatric patients are more likely to have decreased renal function and because dosage of meropenem and vaborbactam needs to be adjusted based on renal impairment, dosage should be selected with caution and it may be useful to monitor renal function.

Cautions

■ **Contraindications** Meropenem and vaborbactam is contraindicated in patients with known hypersensitivity to any component of the drug or other drugs in the same class and in patients who have demonstrated anaphylactic reactions to β-lactam antibacterials.

■ **Warnings/Precautions** ***Sensitivity Reactions*** Hypersensitivity reactions were reported in patients receiving meropenem and vaborbactam in clinical trials. Serious and occasionally fatal hypersensitivity (anaphylactic) reactions and serious skin reactions have been reported in patients receiving β-lactam antibacterials. These reactions are more likely to occur in individuals with a history of sensitivity to multiple allergens. There have been reports of individuals with a history of penicillin hypersensitivity who experienced severe hypersensitivity reactions when treated with another β-lactam antibacterial.

Before initiating meropenem and vaborbactam treatment, the clinician should carefully inquire about the patient's previous hypersensitivity reactions to cephalosporins, penicillins, other β-lactams, or other allergens.

If an allergic reaction to meropenem and vaborbactam occurs, the drug should be immediately discontinued.

CNS Effects Seizures and other adverse CNS effects have been reported during treatment with meropenem, a component of meropenem and vaborbactam. These adverse effects have occurred most commonly in patients with underlying CNS disorders (e.g., brain lesions, history of seizures), bacterial meningitis, and/or compromised renal function.

The recommended dosage of meropenem and vaborbactam should be closely followed, especially in patients with known factors that predispose the patient to seizures. Anticonvulsant therapy should be continued in those with known seizure disorders. (See Risk of Breakthrough Seizures under Cautions: Warnings/Precautions.) If focal tremors, myoclonus, or seizures occur, the patient should be evaluated neurologically, anticonvulsant therapy should be initiated, and meropenem and vaborbactam dosage should be reexamined to determine if it should be decreased or if the drug should be discontinued.

Adverse effects, including seizures, delirium, headaches, and/or paresthesias, can occur in patients receiving meropenem and vaborbactam and may interfere with mental alertness and/or cause motor impairment. Patients receiving meropenem and vaborbactam in an outpatient setting should be informed of the potential for such adverse effects and advised not to operate machinery or motorized vehicles until it is reasonably well established that meropenem and vaborbactam is well tolerated.

Risk of Breakthrough Seizures Case reports have shown that concomitant use of carbapenems, including meropenem, in patients receiving valproic acid or divalproex sodium results in reduced valproic acid concentrations. As a result of this interaction, valproic acid concentrations may fall below the therapeutic range and increase the risk of breakthrough seizures. Increased dosages of valproic acid or divalproex sodium may not be sufficient to overcome this interaction.

Concomitant use of meropenem and vaborbactam with valproic acid or divalproex sodium is generally not recommended. (See Drug Interactions: Valproic Acid and Divalproex Sodium.)

Hematologic Effects Thrombocytopenia has been observed in patients with renal impairment receiving meropenem, but clinical bleeding has not been reported.

Superinfection/Clostridium difficile-associated Diarrhea and Colitis (CDAD) Prolonged use of meropenem and vaborbactam may result in emergence and overgrowth of nonsusceptible bacteria or fungi. The patient should be carefully monitored and appropriate therapy instituted if superinfection occurs.

Treatment with anti-infectives alters normal colon flora and may permit overgrowth of *Clostridium difficile*. *C. difficile* infection (CDI) and *C. difficile*-associated diarrhea and colitis (CDAD; also known as antibiotic-associated diarrhea and colitis or pseudomembranous colitis) have been reported in patients receiving nearly all anti-infectives, including meropenem and vaborbactam, and may range in severity from mild diarrhea to fatal colitis. *C. difficile* produces toxins A and B which contribute to development of CDAD; hypertoxin-producing strains of *C. difficile* are associated with increased morbidity and mortality since they may be refractory to anti-infectives and colectomy may be required.

CDAD should be considered in the differential diagnosis of patients who develop diarrhea during or after anti-infective therapy. Careful medical history is necessary since CDAD has been reported to occur as late as 2 months or longer after anti-infective therapy is discontinued.

If CDAD is suspected or confirmed, anti-infective therapy not directed against *C. difficile* should be discontinued whenever possible. Patients should be managed with appropriate supportive therapy (e.g., fluid and electrolyte management, protein supplementation), anti-infective therapy directed against *C. difficile* (e.g., metronidazole, vancomycin), and surgical evaluation as clinically indicated.

Patients should be advised that diarrhea is a common problem caused by anti-infectives and usually resolves when the drug is discontinued; however, they should contact a clinician if watery and bloody stools (with or without stomach cramps and fever) occur during or as late as 2 months or longer after the last dose.

Selection and Use of Anti-infectives To reduce development of drug-resistant bacteria and maintain effectiveness of meropenem and vaborbactam and other antibacterials, the drug should be used only for treatment of infections proven or strongly suspected to be caused by susceptible bacteria.

When selecting or modifying anti-infective therapy, results of culture and in vitro susceptibility testing should be used. In the absence of such data, local epidemiology and susceptibility patterns should be considered when selecting anti-infectives for empiric therapy.

Patients should be advised that antibacterials (including meropenem and vaborbactam) should only be used to treat bacterial infections and not used to treat viral infections (e.g., the common cold). Patients also should be advised about the importance of completing the full course of therapy, even if feeling better after a few days, and that skipping doses or not completing therapy may decrease effectiveness and increase the likelihood that bacteria will develop resistance and will not be treatable with meropenem and vaborbactam or other antibacterials in the future.

Precautions Related to Use of Fixed Combinations When meropenem and vaborbactam is used, the cautions, precautions, contraindications, and drug interactions associated with both drugs in the fixed combination must be considered. Cautionary information applicable to specific populations (e.g., pregnant or nursing women, individuals with hepatic or renal impairment, geriatric patients) should be considered for each drug. (For additional cautionary information on meropenem, see Cautions in Meropenem 8:12.07.08.)

When prescribing, preparing, and dispensing meropenem and vaborbactam, healthcare professionals should consider that dosage of the fixed combination is expressed as the total (sum) of the dosage of each of the 2 active components (i.e., dosage of meropenem plus dosage of vaborbactam). (See Dispensing and Dosage and Administration Precautions under Administration: IV Infusion, in Dosage and Administration.)

Specific Populations **Pregnancy.** Fetal malformations (e.g., supernumerary lung lobes, interventricular septal defect) were observed in rabbits receiving IV vaborbactam during organogenesis at doses approximately equivalent to or greater than the maximum recommended human dose. Similar malformations or fetal toxicity were not observed in offspring from pregnant rats receiving IV vaborbactam during organogenesis or from late pregnancy and through lactation at doses equivalent to approximately 1.6 times the maximum recommended human dose. No fetal toxicity or malformations were observed in pregnant rats or cynomolgus monkeys receiving IV meropenem during organogenesis at doses up to 1.6 or 1.2 times the maximum recommended human dose, respectively.

Human data are insufficient to determine whether there is a drug-associated risk of major birth defects or miscarriages if the fixed combination of meropenem and vaborbactam, meropenem alone, or vaborbactam alone is used in pregnant women.

Lactation. Meropenem has been reported to be distributed into human milk. It is not known whether vaborbactam is distributed into human milk.

The benefits of breast-feeding and the importance of meropenem and vaborbactam to the woman should be considered along with potential adverse effects on the breast-fed child from the drug or from the underlying maternal condition.

Pediatric Use. Safety and efficacy of meropenem and vaborbactam have not been established in pediatric patients younger than 18 years of age.

Geriatric Use. No overall differences in safety and efficacy of meropenem and vaborbactam were observed in patients 65 years of age and older compared with younger adults, but greater sensitivity in some older individuals cannot be ruled out.

Meropenem is substantially eliminated by the kidneys, and the risk of adverse reactions to the drug may be greater in patients with renal impairment. Because geriatric patients are more likely to have decreased renal function, dosage should be selected with caution and renal function monitoring should be considered. Dosage adjustments in geriatric patients should be based on renal function.

Population pharmacokinetic analysis indicates that the pharmacokinetics of meropenem and vaborbactam in geriatric patients is similar to that in younger adults.

Hepatic Impairment. Hepatic impairment does not affect the pharmacokinetics of meropenem; vaborbactam does not undergo hepatic metabolism. Hepatic impairment is not expected to affect the clearance of meropenem and vaborbactam.

Renal Impairment. Plasma exposures of both meropenem and vaborbactam are increased in patients with renal impairment, and dosage adjustments are recommended in those with estimated glomerular filtration rate (eGFR) less than 50 mL/minute per 1.73 m^2. (See Renal Impairment under Dosage and Administration: Special Populations, in Dosage and Administration.)

Following a single dose of meropenem and vaborbactam in patients with mild, moderate, or severe renal impairment, the area under the plasma concentration-time curve (AUC) of meropenem was 1.3-, 2.1-, or 4.6-fold higher, respectively, and the AUC of vaborbactam was 1.2-, 2.3-, and 7.8-fold higher, respectively, compared with AUCs in individuals with normal renal function.

Hemodialysis removes 38% of the meropenem dose and 53% of the vaborbactam dose.

■ **Common Adverse Effects** Adverse effects reported in 1% or more patients receiving meropenem and vaborbactam include headache, phlebitis or infusion site reactions, diarrhea, hypersensitivity, nausea, increased ALT concentrations, increased AST concentrations, pyrexia, and hypokalemia.

Drug Interactions

■ **Drugs Affecting or Metabolized by Hepatic Microsomal Enzymes** Studies evaluating the potential for meropenem to interact with CYP isoenzymes have not been conducted. Carbapenems as a class have not shown potential for inhibition or induction of CYP isoenzymes and clinical experience suggests such effects are unlikely.

Vaborbactam does not inhibit cytochrome P-450 (CYP) isoenzymes 1A2, 2B6, 2C8, 2C9, 2C19, 2D6, or 3A4 in vitro at therapeutic concentrations and does not show potential to induce CYP1A2, 2B6, or 3A4.

■ **Drugs Affecting or Affected by Organic Anion Transporters** Meropenem is a substrate of organic anion transporter (OAT) 1 and OAT3. Therefore, concomitant use of OAT1 and/or OAT3 inhibitors (e.g., probenecid) with meropenem and vaborbactam may increase meropenem plasma concentrations. (See Drug Interactions: Probenecid.)

Vaborbactam is not a substrate or inhibitor of OAT1 or OAT3.

■ **Drugs Affecting or Affected by Other Membrane Transporters** Studies evaluating the potential for meropenem to interact with active transport systems have not been conducted.

In vitro, vaborbactam is not a substrate or inhibitor of P-glycoprotein (P-gp), breast cancer resistance protein (BCRP), or organic cation transporter (OCT) 2. Vaborbactam does not inhibit OCT1, organic anion transporting polypeptide (OATP) 1B1 or 1B3, or bile salt export pump (BSEP).

■ **Anti-infectives** There is no in vitro evidence of antagonistic antibacterial effects between meropenem and vaborbactam and amikacin, azithromycin, daptomycin, levofloxacin, linezolid, polymyxin, tigecycline, or vancomycin.

■ **Probenecid** Probenecid competes with meropenem for active tubular secretion, resulting in a 56% increase in mean systemic exposure and a 38% increase in mean elimination half-life of meropenem.

Concomitant use of probenecid with meropenem and vaborbactam is not recommended.

■ **Valproic Acid and Divalproex Sodium** Concomitant use of carbapenems, including meropenem, and valproic acid or divalproex sodium, has resulted in decreased valproic acid concentrations. Valproic acid concentrations may fall below the therapeutic range and increase the risk of breakthrough seizures. Although the mechanism of this interaction is not known, data from in vitro and animal studies suggest that carbapenems may inhibit the hydrolysis of valproic acid's glucuronide metabolite (VPA-g) back to valproic acid, which decreases serum concentrations of valproic acid.

Concomitant use of meropenem and vaborbactam with valproic acid or divalproex sodium generally is not recommended. In patients whose seizures are well controlled on valproic acid or divalproex sodium, an alternative to carbapenems should be considered. If use of meropenem and vaborbactam is necessary, alternative or supplemental anticonvulsant therapy should be considered.

Description

Meropenem and vaborbactam is a fixed combination of meropenem (a carbapenem) and vaborbactam (a non-β-lactam β-lactamase inhibitor). Vaborbactam inactivates certain bacterial β-lactamases and expands meropenem's spectrum of activity against some bacteria that produce these β-lactamases. Meropenem and vaborbactam is bactericidal in action.

Meropenem is a synthetic carbapenem antibiotic structurally and pharmacologically related to other carbapenems (e.g., doripenem, ertapenem, imipenem). Like other β-lactam antibiotics, the antibacterial activity of meropenem results from inhibition of bacterial cell wall synthesis and is mediated through binding to penicillin-binding proteins (PBPs). Meropenem is stable to hydrolysis by most β-lactamases, including penicillinases and cephalosporinases produced by gram-negative and gram-positive bacteria, but can be hydrolyzed by carbapenemases.

Vaborbactam is a cyclic boronic acid non-β-lactam β-lactamase inhibitor that protects meropenem from degradation by certain β-lactamases, primarily Ambler class A serine carbapenemases (e.g., *Klebsiella pneumoniae* carbapenemase [KPC]) and some class C serine carbapenemases. Vaborbactam's boronate moiety forms a covalent bond with the catalytic serine side chain of the β-lactamase, thereby inhibiting the enzyme from degrading meropenem. This mechanism of action differs from that of β-lactam β-lactamase inhibitors (e.g., clavulanic acid, sulbactam, tazobactam) and some other non-β-lactam β-lactamase inhibitors (e.g., avibactam). In animal models of infection, vaborbactam restored activity of meropenem against some meropenem non-susceptible KPC-producing Enterobacteriaceae. The drug does *not* inhibit class D carbapenemases (e.g., OXA-48) or class B β-lactamases (e.g., metallo β-lactamases [MBLs]). Vaborbactam does not have antibacterial activity and does not decrease the activity of meropenem against meropenem-susceptible organisms.

Each single-dose vial of meropenem and vaborbactam contains 2 g (1 g of meropenem [equivalent to 1.14 g of meropenem trihydrate] and 1 g of vaborbactam) and also contains 575 mg of sodium carbonate. The total sodium content is approximately 250 mg (10.9 mEq) per single-dose vial.

Following IV administration of 4 g of meropenem and vaborbactam (meropenem 2 g and vaborbactam 2 g) given by IV infusion over 3 hours every 8 hours for 7 days in healthy adults with normal renal function, peak plasma concentrations of the drugs were 43.4 and 55.6 mcg/mL, respectively, and there was no accumulation of either drug. Meropenem is partially metabolized by hydrolysis of the β-lactam ring to a microbiologically inactive hydrolysis product; vaborbactam is not metabolized. The plasma protein binding of meropenem is approximately 2% and the plasma protein binding of vaborbactam is approximately 33%. Both drugs are principally eliminated by the kidneys. Approximately 40–60% of a meropenem dose is eliminated unchanged in urine, 22% is eliminated in urine as the microbiologically inactive hydrolysis product, and approximately 2% is eliminated in feces. Approximately 75–95% of a vaborbactam dose is eliminated unchanged in urine. In healthy adults, meropenem has a plasma half-life of 1.2 hours and vaborbactam has a plasma half-life of 1.7 hours.

■ **Spectrum** Meropenem and vaborbactam is active in vitro and in clinical studies against *Enterobacter cloacae* species complex, *Escherichia coli*, and *K. pneumoniae*.

Although the clinical importance is not known, meropenem and vaborbactam is active in vitro against other gram-negative bacteria, including *Citrobacter freundii*, *C. koseri*, *E. aerogenes*, *K. oxytoca*, *Morganella morganii*, *Proteus mirabilis*, *Providencia*, *Pseudomonas aeruginosa*, and *Serratia marcescens*. Efficacy of meropenem and vaborbactam for treatment of clinical infections caused by these bacteria has not been established in adequate and well-controlled clinical studies.

In vitro, meropenem and vaborbactam is active against Enterobacteriaceae in the presence of some β-lactamases and extended-spectrum β-lactamases (ESBLs), including KPC, SME, TEM, SHV, CTX-M, CMY, and ACT. Meropenem and vaborbactam is *not* active against bacteria that produce MBLs or oxacillinases with carbapenemase activity.

■ **Resistance** Resistance or reduced susceptibility to meropenem and vaborbactam can occur. Mechanisms of resistance to carbapenems include production of β-lactamases, modification of PBPs by gene acquisition or target alteration, up-regulation of efflux pumps, and loss of outer membrane porin. Meropenem and vaborbactam may not be active against gram-negative bacteria with porin mutations *and* overexpression of efflux pumps. Clinical isolates may produce multiple β-lactamases, express varying levels of β-lactamases, have amino acid sequence variations, or have other resistance mechanisms that have not been identified.

Some isolates resistant to carbapenems (including meropenem) and to cephalosporins may be susceptible to meropenem and vaborbactam. Cross-resistance with other classes of anti-infectives has not been reported.

Advice to Patients

Advise patients that antibacterials (including meropenem and vaborbactam) should only be used to treat bacterial infections and not used to treat viral infections (e.g., the common cold).

Importance of completing full course of therapy, even if feeling better after a few days.

Advise patients that skipping doses or not completing the full course of therapy may decrease effectiveness and increase the likelihood that bacteria will develop resistance and will not be treatable with meropenem and vaborbactam or other antibacterials in the future.

Advise patients that allergic reactions, including serious allergic reactions, can occur and that serious reactions require immediate treatment. Ask patients about previous hypersensitivity reactions to meropenem and vaborbactam, penicillins, cephalosporins, other β-lactams, or other allergens.

Inform patients receiving meropenem and vaborbactam on an outpatient basis that adverse effects, including seizures, delirium, headaches, and/or paresthesias, can occur and interfere with mental alertness and/or cause motor impairment. Advise patients to not operate machinery or motorized vehicles until it is reasonably established that meropenem and vaborbactam is well tolerated.

Advise patients that diarrhea is a common problem caused by anti-infectives and usually ends when the drug is discontinued. Importance of contacting a clinician if watery and bloody stools (with or without stomach cramps and fever) occur during or as late as 2 months or longer after the last dose.

Importance of informing clinician if currently being treated with valproic acid or divalproex sodium. If meropenem and vaborbactam used concomitantly with these drugs, valproic acid concentrations in the blood may drop below therapeutic range and increase the risk of seizures. (See Drug Interactions: Valproic Acid and Divalproex Sodium.)

Importance of informing clinicians of existing or contemplated concomitant therapy, including prescription and OTC drugs and dietary or herbal supplements, as well as any concomitant illnesses.

Importance of women informing their clinician if they are or plan to become pregnant or plan to breast-feed.

Importance of informing patients of other important precautionary information. (See Cautions.)

Overview® (see Users Guide). For additional information on this drug until a more detailed monograph is developed and published, the manufacturer's labeling should be consulted. It is *essential* that the manufacturer's labeling be consulted for more detailed information on usual cautions, precautions, contraindications, potential drug interactions, laboratory test interferences, and acute toxicity.

Preparations

Excipients in commercially available drug preparations may have clinically important effects in some individuals; consult specific product labeling for details.

Meropenem and Vaborbactam

Parenteral

For injection, for IV infusion	2 g (1 g of meropenem and 1 g of vaborbactam)	**Vabomere®**, Medicines Company

CEPHAMYCINS 8:12.07.12

cefoTEtan Disodium

■ Cefotetan is a semisynthetic cephamycin β-lactam antibiotic.

Uses

Cefotetan is used for treatment of urinary tract, lower respiratory tract, skin and skin structure, bone and joint, gynecologic, and intra-abdominal infections caused by susceptible bacteria and also is used for perioperative prophylaxis. Cefotetan should not be used for treatment of meningitis or other CNS infections.

Prior to initiation of cefotetan therapy, appropriate specimens should be obtained for identification of the causative organism and in vitro susceptibility tests. Cefotetan therapy may be started pending results of susceptibility tests, but should be discontinued if the organism is found to be resistant to the drug. In certain serious infections, including confirmed or suspected gram-positive or gram-negative sepsis, when the causative organism is unknown, cefotetan and concomitant therapy with an aminoglycoside may be indicated initially pending results of susceptibility tests. If an aminoglycoside is used concomitantly with cefotetan, renal function should be monitored. (See Drug Interactions: Aminoglycosides.)

■ **Gram-positive Aerobic Bacterial Infections** Cefotetan is used in adults for treatment of lower respiratory tract infections caused by susceptible *Streptococcus pneumoniae* or *Staphylococcus aureus*; gynecologic infections caused by susceptible *S. aureus*, *S. epidermidis*, streptococci (except enterococci); skin and skin structure infections caused by susceptible *S. aureus*, *S. epidermidis*, *S. pyogenes* (group A β-hemolytic streptococci), other streptococci (except enterococci); intra-abdominal infections caused by susceptible streptococci (except enterococci); and bone and joint infections caused by susceptible *S. aureus*. The drug also has been used effectively in a limited number of adults for treatment of urinary tract infections caused by susceptible *S. aureus*† or *S epidermidis*†.

Cefotetan, like second and third generation cephalosporins, generally is not a drug of choice for treatment of infections caused by gram-positive bacteria and should not be used for treatment of infections caused by these organisms when a penicillin or a first generation cephalosporin could be used.

■ Gram-negative Aerobic Bacterial Infections Cefotetan is used in adults for treatment of urinary tract infections caused by susceptible *Escherichia coli, Klebsiella, Proteus mirabilis, P. vulgaris, Providencia rettgeri*, or *Morganella morganii*; lower respiratory tract infections caused by susceptible *Haemophilus influenzae, E. coli, Klebsiella, P. mirabilis*, or *Serratia marcescens*; and skin and skin structure infections caused by susceptible *E. coli* or *K. pneumoniae*. The drug is also used in adults for treatment of intra-abdominal infections caused by susceptible *E. coli* or *Klebsiella* and for treatment of gynecologic infections caused by susceptible *E. coli, P. mirabilis*, or *N. gonorrhoeae*.

Cefotetan generally has been as effective as cefoxitin or cefotaxime for treatment of urinary tract infections caused by susceptible gram-negative bacteria. Because *Pseudomonas aeruginosa* generally are resistant to cefotetan, the drug should not be used for treatment of any infection where *Ps. aeruginosa* may be the causative organism.

■ Anaerobic and Mixed Aerobic-Anaerobic Bacterial Infections Cefotetan is used for treatment of gynecologic infections caused by susceptible gram-positive anaerobic cocci, including *Peptococcus* and *Peptostreptococcus*, or susceptible *Fusobacterium* and skin and skin structure infections caused by *Peptococcus* and *Peptostreptococcus*. The drug also is used for treatment of gynecologic and intra-abdominal infections caused by susceptible *Bacteroides* or *Clostridium*.

Cefotetan generally has been effective when used for treatment of mixed aerobic-anaerobic bacterial infections, including peritonitis and gynecologic infections (see Uses: Pelvic Inflammatory Disease). Cefotetan has been used effectively for treatment of mild to moderate infections caused by *B. fragilis*; however, other anti-infectives (e.g., metronidazole, clindamycin) usually are preferred, especially for treatment of severe or life-threatening *B. fragilis* infections.

Because of the increasing prevalence of *B. fragilis* resistant to cefotetan, the Infectious Diseases Society of America (IDSA) states that the drug is not recommended for empiric treatment of intra-abdominal infections. In addition, *B. distasonis, B. ovatus*, and *B. thetaiotaomicron* generally are resistant to cefotetan, and the drug is unlikely to be effective in infections caused by these anaerobes.

■ Pelvic Inflammatory Disease Cefotetan is used for treatment of pelvic inflammatory disease (PID). Cefotetan, like cephalosporins, generally is inactive against *C. trachomatis* and should not be used alone for treatment of PID.

PID is an acute or chronic inflammatory disorder in the upper female genital tract and can include any combination of endometritis, salpingitis, tubo-ovarian abscess, and pelvic peritonitis. PID generally is a polymicrobial infection most frequently caused by *N. gonorrhoeae* and/or *Chlamydia trachomatis*; however, organisms that can be part of the normal vaginal flora (e.g., anaerobic bacteria, *Gardnerella vaginalis, H. influenzae*, enteric gram-negative bacilli, *S. agalactiae*) or mycoplasma (e.g., *Mycoplasma hominis, Ureaplasma urealyticum*) also may be involved. PID is treated with an empiric regimen that provides broad spectrum coverage. The regimen should be effective against *N. gonorrhoeae* and *C. trachomatis* and also probably should be effective against anaerobes, gram-negative facultative bacteria, and streptococci. The optimum empiric regimen for treatment of PID has not been identified. A wide variety of parenteral and oral regimens have been shown to achieve clinical and microbiologic cure in randomized studies with short-term follow-up; however, only limited data are available regarding elimination of infection in the endometrium and fallopian tubes or intermediate or long-term outcomes, including the impact of these regimens on the incidence of long-term sequelae of PID (e.g., tubal infertility, ectopic pregnancy, pain).

Parenteral Regimens for PID When a parenteral regimen is indicated for treatment of PID, the US Centers for Disease Control and Prevention (CDC) and other clinicians generally recommend a 2-drug regimen of cefotetan (2 g IV every 12 hours) or cefoxitin (2 g IV every 6 hours) given in conjunction with doxycycline (100 mg IV or orally every 12 hours) or a 2-drug regimen of clindamycin (900 mg IV every 8 hours) and gentamicin (usually a 2-mg/kg IV or IM loading dose followed by 1.5 mg/kg every 8 hours). While certain parenteral cephalosporins (e.g., cefotaxime, ceftriaxone) also have been used and may be effective for treatment of PID, CDC states that there is less experience with use of these cephalosporins in patients with PID and these drugs may be less active than cefotetan or cefoxitin against anaerobic bacteria. CDC states that only limited data are available to support the use of other parenteral regimens for treatment of acute PID, although a regimen of IV ampicillin and sulbactam given with oral or IV doxycycline may be effective against *C. trachomatis, N. gonorrhoeae*, and anaerobes in women with tubo-ovarian abscess.

CDC states that a transition to oral therapy usually can be initiated within 24–48 hours after the patient demonstrates clinical improvement and decisions regarding such a transition should be guided by clinical experience. At least 24 hours of direct inpatient observation is recommended for patients with tubo-ovarian abscesses.

Oral Regimens for PID When acute PID that is mild to moderately severe is treated with an oral regimen, CDC recommends a regimen that consists of a single dose of IM ceftriaxone, IM cefoxitin (with oral probenecid), or IM cefotaxime given in conjunction with a 14-day regimen of oral doxycycline (100 mg twice daily) with or without oral metronidazole (500 mg twice daily). The optimal parenteral cephalosporin or cephamycin for this outpatient regimen is unclear; although cefoxitin has better anaerobic coverage, ceftriaxone has better coverage against *N. gonorrhoeae*.

For additional information regarding treatment of PID, the current CDC sexually transmitted diseases treatment guidelines available at http://www.cdc.gov/std should be consulted.

■ Perioperative Prophylaxis Cefotetan has been effective when used perioperatively to reduce the incidence of infection in patients undergoing cesarean section, abdominal or vaginal hysterectomy, or transurethral, biliary tract, or GI surgery. Perioperative prophylaxis with an appropriate anti-infective agent can decrease the incidence of infection, particularly surgical site infection, after certain procedures.

GI Surgery **Biliary Tract Surgery.** Perioperative prophylaxis is recommended for patients undergoing biliary tract surgery who are at high risk of infection (e.g., those older than 70 years of age or those with acute cholecystitis, a nonfunctioning gallbladder, obstructive jaundice, or common duct stones). In high-risk patients undergoing endoscopic retrograde cholangiopancreatography (ERCP), perioperative prophylaxis is recommended only if complete biliary drainage is unlikely to be achieved. Perioperative prophylaxis is not considered necessary for low-risk patients undergoing elective laparoscopic cholecystectomy.

For perioperative prophylaxis in high-risk patients undergoing open biliary tract surgery, many clinicians recommend IV cefazolin as the drug of choice. Alternatives include IV cefotetan, IV cefoxitin, or IV ampicillin and sulbactam. In patients allergic to penicillins and cephalosporins, a reasonable alternative is clindamycin or vancomycin used in conjunction with an aminoglycoside (gentamicin or tobramycin), a fluoroquinolone (ciprofloxacin or levofloxacin), or aztreonam; some clinicians suggest metronidazole and an aminoglycoside (gentamicin or tobramycin) or fluoroquinolone (ciprofloxacin or levofloxacin) as another alternative.

Colorectal Surgery. There is evidence that perioperative prophylaxis can decrease the incidence of infection after colorectal surgery, and such prophylaxis is recommended.

For perioperative prophylaxis in patients undergoing colorectal surgery, many clinicians recommend a parenteral regimen of IV cefotetan, IV cefoxitin, IV cefazolin (used in conjunction with IV metronidazole), IV ampicillin and sulbactam, or IV ertapenem. In patients allergic to penicillins and cephalosporins, a reasonable alternative is clindamycin or vancomycin used in conjunction with an aminoglycoside (gentamicin or tobramycin), a fluoroquinolone (ciprofloxacin or levofloxacin), or aztreonam; some clinicians suggest metronidazole and an aminoglycoside (gentamicin or tobramycin) or fluoroquinolone (ciprofloxacin or levofloxacin) as another alternative.

Alternatively, an oral regimen of oral neomycin with either oral erythromycin or oral metronidazole can be used in conjunction with mechanical bowel preparation for perioperative prophylaxis in patients undergoing colorectal surgery. Many clinicians recommend using both an oral regimen and a parenteral regimen for perioperative prophylaxis in patients undergoing colorectal surgery, and there is some evidence that use of an oral regimen (with mechanical bowel preparation) in conjunction with a parenteral regimen is more effective than use of a parenteral regimen alone.

In a randomized, prospective study in patients undergoing elective colorectal surgery, the overall incidence of intra-abdominal septic complications in those who received mechanical bowel preparation and an oral regimen (erythromycin and neomycin) alone was similar to that in those who received both the oral regimen and a parenteral regimen (cefoxitin); however, the incidence of abdominal wound infection was higher in those who received the oral regimen alone (14.6%) than in those who received the combined oral and parenteral regimen (5%).

A single dose of cefotetan has been as effective as multiple doses of cefoxitin for perioperative prophylaxis in patients undergoing colorectal surgery.

Appendectomy. There is evidence that perioperative prophylaxis can reduce the incidence of infection after surgery for acute appendicitis, and such prophylaxis is recommended.

For perioperative prophylaxis in patients undergoing uncomplicated (nonperforated) appendectomy, many clinicians recommend IV cefoxitin, IV cefotetan, or IV cefazolin (used in conjunction with IV metronidazole). In patients allergic to penicillins and cephalosporins, a reasonable alternative is clindamycin or vancomycin used in conjunction with an aminoglycoside (gentamicin or tobramycin), a fluoroquinolone (ciprofloxacin or levofloxacin), or aztreonam; some clinicians suggest metronidazole and an aminoglycoside (gentamicin or tobramycin) or fluoroquinolone (ciprofloxacin or levofloxacin) as another alternative.

If perforation has occurred, anti-infectives are continued postoperatively for about 5 days.

Genitourinary Surgery Cefotetan has been used for perioperative prophylaxis in patients undergoing transurethral surgery; however, the drug is not included in recommendations for perioperative prophylaxis in patients undergoing urinary tract surgery.

Gynecologic and Obstetric Surgery Perioperative prophylaxis decreases the incidence of infection after vaginal or abdominal hysterectomy and also is used for laparoscopic hysterectomies. In addition, there is evidence that perioperative prophylaxis can prevent infection after elective and nonelective cesarean section, and also can prevent infection after elective abortions. A pooled analysis of results of randomized, placebo-controlled studies in women who underwent therapeutic abortion before 16 weeks' gestation indicates that perioperative prophylaxis can reduce the overall risk of postabortal infection by 42% compared with placebo.

Many clinicians suggest that the preferred agents for perioperative prophylaxis in women undergoing vaginal, abdominal, or laparoscopic hysterectomy are IV cefoxitin, IV cefotetan, IV cefazolin, or IV ampicillin and sulbactam. In patients allergic to penicillins and cephalosporins, a reasonable alternative is clindamycin or vancomycin used in conjunction with an aminoglycoside (gentamicin or tobramycin), a fluoroquinolone (ciprofloxacin or levofloxacin), or aztreonam; some clinicians suggest metronidazole and an aminoglycoside (gentamicin or tobramycin) or fluoroquinolone (ciprofloxacin or levofloxacin) as another alternative.

IV cefazolin generally is the preferred agent for prophylaxis in women undergoing cesarean section; oral doxycycline is recommended for prophylaxis in those undergoing abortion.

In a limited number of patients, a single dose of cefotetan appeared to be at least as effective as multiple doses of cefoxitin for perioperative prophylaxis in patients undergoing vaginal or abdominal hysterectomy and at least as effective as multiple doses of cefoxitin or cefazolin in patients undergoing cesarean section. Results of a prospective, randomized study indicate that single-dose regimens of cefazolin, cefotetan, or ampicillin sodium and sulbactam sodium are equally effective in decreasing the incidence of postpartum infections in women undergoing high-risk cesarean section; postpartum endomyometritis was reported in 14.3% of those who received cefazolin, 11.1% of those who received cefotetan, and 7.4% of those who received ampicillin sodium and sulbactam sodium.

Timing and Number of Doses When perioperative prophylaxis is indicated in patients undergoing surgery, administration of an appropriate anti-infective should be timed to ensure that bactericidal concentrations of the drug are established in serum and tissues by the time the initial surgical incision is made; therapeutic concentrations of the drug should then be maintained in serum and tissues for the duration of the procedure.

An IV dose of an appropriate anti-infective should be administered within 60 minutes before the initial incision. If cefotetan is used prophylactically, the manufacturers recommend that the drug be given 30–60 minutes before surgery.

A single preoperative dose usually is sufficient for perioperative prophylaxis. However, if surgery is prolonged (more than 3–4 hours), major blood loss occurs, or other factors are present that shorten the half-life of the drug (e.g., extensive burns), additional doses should be administered during the procedure to ensure adequate serum and tissue concentrations of the anti-infective throughout the procedure. For prolonged procedures in patients with normal renal function, some clinicians suggest that intraoperative doses be given during the procedure at intervals that correspond to 1–2 times the half-life of the drug (e.g., every 6 hours for cefotetan, measured from the time the preoperative dose is initiated). Intraoperative doses may not be warranted if there are factors that prolong the half-life of the drug (e.g., renal impairment).

For most procedures, the duration of prophylaxis should be less than 24 hours. There is no evidence to support continuing prophylaxis after wound closure or until all indwelling drains and intravascular catheters are removed.

Dosage and Administration

■ Reconstitution and Administration

Cefotetan disodium is administered by IV injection or infusion or by deep IM injection.

The IV route is the preferred route in patients with bacteremia, septicemia, or other severe or life-threatening infections and in patients with lowered resistance resulting from debilitating conditions (e.g., malnutrition, trauma, surgery, diabetes, heart failure, malignancy), particularly if shock is present or impending.

If an aminoglycoside is administered concomitantly with cefotetan disodium, the drugs should be administered at separately and should not be admixed.

Cefotetan disodium solutions should be inspected visually for particulate matter and discoloration prior to administration whenever solution and container permit.

Intermittent IV Injection For direct intermittent IV injection, the contents of a vial labeled as containing 1 or 2 g of cefotetan should be reconstituted with 10 or 10–20 mL, respectively, of sterile water for injection to provide solutions containing approximately 95 or 95–182 mg/mL, respectively. The vial should be shaken until the drug is dissolved, and then allowed to stand until the solution is clear.

The appropriate dose of reconstituted solution may then be injected directly into a vein over a 3- to 5-minute period.

Intermittent IV Infusion IV infusions of cefotetan disodium solutions should preferably be given using butterfly or scalp vein-type needles. Other IV solutions flowing through a common administration tubing or set should be discontinued while cefotetan disodium is being infused.

For direct intermittent IV infusion, the contents of a vial labeled as containing 1 or 2 g of cefotetan should be reconstituted with 10 or 10–20 mL, respectively, of sterile water for injection to provide solutions containing approximately 95 or 95–182 mg/mL, respectively. The vial should be shaken until the drug is dissolved, and then allowed to stand until the solution is clear.

Commercially available pharmacy bulk package vials containing 10 g of cefotetan should be reconstituted with 50 or 100 mL of sterile water for injection, 5% dextrose injection, or 0.9% sodium chloride injection to provide solutions containing approximately 180 or 95 mg/mL, respectively. The vial should be shaken until the drug is dissolved and allowed to stand until the solution is clear. Reconstituted solutions in pharmacy bulk package vials should *not* be used for direct IV infusion; the reconstituted solution must be further diluted in a compatible IV infusion solution within 4 hours after reconstitution. (See Chemistry and Stability: Stability.) A suitable sterile transfer device or dispensing set should be used to transfer the contents of the reconstituted bulk package vial to a compatible IV solution; a syringe with a needle is not recommended since leakage could occur during transfer. The manufacturer's directions should be consulted for additional information.

Alternatively, the commercially available Duplex® drug delivery system containing 1 or 2 g of cefotetan disodium powder and 50 mL of 3.58 or 2.08% dextrose injection, respectively, in separate chambers should be reconstituted (activated) according to the manufacturer's directions and administered by IV infusion. If stored in the refrigerator after reconstitution (see Chemistry and Stability: Stability), the solution should be allowed to reach room temperature prior to administration.

Rate of Administration. Cefotetan may be administered by IV infusion over 20–60 minutes.

IM Injection For IM injection, vials labeled as containing 1 or 2 g of cefotetan should be reconstituted by adding 2 or 3 mL of sterile or bacteriostatic water for injection, 0.9% sodium chloride injection, or 0.5 or 1% lidocaine hydrochloride injection, respectively, to provide solutions containing approximately 400 or 500 mg/mL, respectively. The vial should be shaken until the drug is dissolved, and then allowed to stand until the solution is clear.

IM injections of cefotetan disodium should be made deeply into a large muscle, such as the upper outer quadrant of the gluteus maximus, using usual techniques and precautions. The plunger of the syringe should be drawn back before IM injection to ensure that the needle is not in a blood vessel.

■ Dosage

Dosage of cefotetan disodium is expressed in terms of cefotetan.

Adult Dosage The usual adult dosage of cefotetan is 1 or 2 g IV or IM every 12 hours; however, the dosage and route of administration should be determined by the type and severity of infection, the susceptibility of the causative organism, and the condition and renal function of the patient. The maximum adult dosage of cefotetan recommended by the manufacturers is 6 g daily.

For treatment of infections at sites other than the urinary tract, skin, or skin structure, the usual adult dosage is 1 or 2 g IV or IM every 12 hours. However, severe infections in adults may require 2 g IV every 12 hours and life-threatening infections may require 3 g IV every 12 hours.

Skin and Skin Structure Infections. For treatment of mild to moderate skin and skin structure infections, the manufacturers recommend that adults receive 2 g of cefotetan IV every 24 hours or 1 g IV or IM every 12 hours. For mild to moderate infections caused by *Klebsiella pneumoniae*, the manufacturers recommend 1 or 2 g IV or IM every 12 hours.

For treatment of severe skin and skin structure infections, the manufacturers recommend 2 g IV every 12 hours.

Urinary Tract Infections. For treatment of urinary tract infections, the manufacturers recommend that adults receive 500 mg of cefotetan IV or IM every 12 hours or 1 or 2 g IV or IM every 12 or every 24 hours.

Pelvic Inflammatory Disease. For treatment of acute pelvic inflammatory disease (PID), adults and adolescents should receive IV cefotetan in a dosage of 2 g every 12 hours given in conjunction with IV or oral doxycycline (100 mg every 12 hours). The initial parenteral regimen may be discontinued 24–48 hours after there is clinical improvement and oral doxycycline (100 mg twice daily) continued to complete 14 days of therapy.

Perioperative Prophylaxis. For perioperative prophylaxis in women undergoing abdominal, vaginal, or laparoscopic hysterectomy or undergoing cesarean section, 1 or 2 g of cefotetan should be given IV within 30–60 minutes prior to incision. For cesarean section, the manufacturers recommend giving the dose as soon as the umbilical cord is clamped; however, there is some evidence that giving the dose prior to incision may be more effective than giving it after clamping.

For perioperative prophylaxis in adults undergoing colorectal surgery, appendectomy (nonperforated), biliary tract, or other GI surgery, 1 or 2 g of cefotetan should be given IV 30–60 minutes prior to incision.

If cefotetan is used for perioperative prophylaxis in adults undergoing transurethral surgery, the manufacturers recommend that 1 or 2 g of the drug be given IV 30–60 minutes prior to surgery.

During prolonged procedures (longer than 3–4 hours), if major blood loss occurs, or if other factors are present that shorten the half-life of the drug, additional doses should be given during the procedure (e.g., every 6 hours, measured from time the preoperative dose is initiated).

The duration of prophylaxis should be less than 24 hours for most procedures; there is no evidence to support continuing prophylaxis after wound closure or until all indwelling drains and intravascular catheters are removed.

Pediatric Dosage **General Pediatric Dosage.** Although safety and efficacy of cefotetan in children have not been established, the American Academy of Pediatrics (AAP) suggests that children beyond the neonatal period† may receive IM or IV cefotetan in a dosage of 60 mg/kg daily given in 2 divided doses for treatment of mild to moderate infections or a dosage of 100 mg/kg daily given in 2 divided doses for treatment of severe infections.

Perioperative Prophylaxis. If cefotetan is used for perioperative prophylaxis in children 1 year of age or older† undergoing colorectal surgery or appendectomy, some clinicians recommend that 40 mg/kg of cefotetan be given within 60 minutes prior to incision.

During prolonged procedures (longer than 3–4 hours), if major blood loss occurs, or if other factors are present that shorten the half-life of the drug, additional doses should be given during the procedure.

The duration of prophylaxis should be less than 24 hours for most procedures; there is no evidence to support continuing prophylaxis after wound closure or until all indwelling drains and intravascular catheters are removed.

■ **Dosage in Renal Impairment** In patients with renal impairment, doses and/or frequency of administration of cefotetan should be modified in response to the degree of renal impairment, type and severity of the infection, and susceptibility of the causative organisms.

The manufacturers and some clinicians recommend that adults with impaired renal function receive the following dosage of cefotetan given at dosage intervals based on the patient's creatinine clearance. (See Table 1.)

Table 1. Dosage of Cefotetan for Adults with Renal Impairment

Creatinine Clearance (mL/minute)	Dosage
>30	Usual dose every 12 hours
10–30	Usual dose every 24 hours or 50% of usual dose every 12 hours
<10	Usual dose every 48 hours or 25% of usual dose every 12 hours
Hemodialysis patients	25% of usual dose every 24 hours on days between dialysis and 50% of usual dose on the day of dialysis

Cautions

Adverse effects reported with cefotetan are similar to those reported with cephalosporins. For information on adverse effects reported with cephalosporins, see Cautions in the Cephalosporins General Statement and other monographs in 8:12.06. Cefotetan generally is well tolerated; adverse effects have been reported in less than 5% of patients receiving the drug and have required discontinuance of the drug in less than 3% of patients.

■ **Hematologic Effects** Adverse hematologic effects, including eosinophilia, thrombocytosis, thrombocytopenia, neutropenia, leukopenia, agranulocytosis, hemolytic anemia, and positive indirect or direct antiglobulin (Coombs') test results, have been reported in up to 1.4% of patients receiving cefotetan.

Severe hemolytic anemia, including some fatalities, have been reported rarely in association with cefotetan therapy. Hemolytic anemia has been reported in a few women undergoing obstetric and gynecologic procedures who received a single dose of cefotetan for perioperative prophylaxis. Similar cases of immune-mediated hemolytic anemia have been reported rarely in patients receiving cephalosporins (e.g., cefotaxime, ceftizoxime [no longer commercially available in the US], ceftriaxone). If a patient develops hemolytic anemia within 2–3 weeks after initiation of cefotetan therapy, the diagnosis of immune-mediated hemolytic anemia should be considered and the drug discontinued until the etiology of the anemia is determined. (See Cautions: Precautions and Contraindications.)

Prolongation of bleeding time or prothrombin time (PT), with or without bleeding, has been reported rarely in patients receiving cefotetan (i.e., in 0.14% of patients). Monitor PT in patients at risk, including geriatric patients and those with renal or hepatic impairment, malnutrition, or cancer. Administer vitamin K when indicated. Hypoprothrombinemia also has been reported with other β-lactam antibiotics that contain an *N*-methylthiotetrazole (NMTT) side chain like that contained in cefotetan (e.g., cefamandole, cefoperazone; drugs no longer commercially available), and it has been suggested that the NMTT side chain may interfere with hepatic synthesis of vitamin K-dependent clotting factors. Cefotetan does not interfere with adenosine diphosphate-induced, collagen-induced, or arachidonic acid- and epinephrine-induced platelet aggregation.

■ **GI Effects** Adverse GI effects, including diarrhea and nausea, have been reported in up to 1.5% of patients receiving cefotetan. Hiccups also have been reported.

Clostridium difficile-associated Diarrhea and Colitis Treatment with anti-infectives alters normal colon flora and may permit overgrowth of *Clostridium difficile*. *C. difficile* infection (CDI) and *C. difficile*-associated diarrhea and colitis (CDAD; also known as antibiotic-associated diarrhea and colitis or pseudomembranous colitis) have been reported with nearly all anti-infectives, including cefotetan, and may range in severity from mild diarrhea to fatal colitis. *C. difficile* produces toxins A and B, which contribute to development of CDAD; hypertoxin producing strains of *C. difficile* are associated with increased morbidity and mortality since they may be refractory to anti-infectives and colectomy may be required.

CDAD should be considered in the differential diagnosis of patients who develop diarrhea during or after anti-infective therapy. Careful medical history is necessary since CDAD has been reported to occur as late as 2 months or longer after anti-infective therapy is discontinued.

If CDAD is suspected or confirmed, anti-infective therapy not directed against *C. difficile* should be discontinued whenever possible. Patients should be managed with appropriate supportive therapy (e.g., fluid and electrolyte management, protein supplementation), anti-infective therapy directed against *C. difficile* (e.g., metronidazole, vancomycin), and surgical evaluation as clinically indicated.

■ **Sensitivity Reactions** Rash, pruritus, anaphylaxis, urticaria, and fever or chills have been reported in up to 1.5% of patients receiving cefotetan. Erythema multiforme (e.g., Stevens-Johnson syndrome) and toxic epidermal necrolysis have been reported in patients receiving cephalosporin therapy. If a hypersensitivity reaction occurs during cefotetan therapy, the drug should be discontinued and the patient treated with appropriate therapy (e.g., IV fluids, IV antihistamines, corticosteroids, vasopressors, and maintenance of an adequate airway and oxygen) as indicated.

■ **Hepatic Effects** Increased serum concentrations of AST (SGOT), ALT (SGPT), alkaline phosphatase, and LDH have been reported in up to 1.2% of patients receiving cefotetan. Hepatic dysfunction, including cholestasis, and increased serum bilirubin concentrations have been reported in patients receiving cephalosporin therapy.

■ **Local Effects** Adverse local effects have been reported in less than 1% of patients receiving cefotetan, and include phlebitis, pain, inflammation, discomfort, and swelling at the site of administration. Swelling of the forearm also has been reported.

■ **Renal Effects** Cefotetan does not appear to be nephrotoxic. Although a transient increase in urinary concentrations of total protein occurred in healthy adults who received usual dosages of cefotetan for 3 days, urinary albumin concentrations and excretion of thermophilic aminopeptidase (alanine aminopeptidase), an enzyme originating from renal proximal tubular cells, were generally unaffected, suggesting that the drug does not adversely affect these cells. Nephrotoxicity and increases in BUN and serum creatinine concentrations have been reported in patients receiving cefotetan. Impairment of renal function and toxic nephropathy have been reported in patients receiving cephalosporin therapy.

Although a causal relationship to cefotetan has not been established, interstitial nephritis manifested by fever, rash, pruritus, eosinophilia, hematuria, proteinuria, and azotemia have been reported in at least one patient receiving cefotetan. The nephritis resembled that reported with other anti-infective agents and appeared to be a hypersensitivity reaction to the drug. For more information on anti-infective-induced acute interstitial nephritis, see Cautions: Renal Effects, in the Penicillinase-Resistant Penicillins General Statement 8:12.16.12.

■ **Other Adverse Effects** Several cephalosporins have been associated with seizures, generally when usual dosages of the drugs were not reduced in patients with renal impairment. If seizures occur during cefotetan therapy, the drug should be discontinued and appropriate anticonvulsant therapy administered as indicated.

Superinfection, vaginitis, and vaginal candidiasis have been reported in patients receiving cephalosporin therapy.

■ **Precautions and Contraindications** Prior to initiation of cefotetan therapy, careful inquiry should be made concerning previous hypersensitivity reactions to β-lactam antibiotics, including cephalosporins and penicillins, or to other drugs. There is clinical and laboratory evidence of partial cross-allergenicity among β-lactam antibiotics including penicillins, cephalosporins, and cephamycins. Cefotetan is contraindicated in patients who are hypersensitive to the drug or to cephalosporins and should be used with caution in patients hypersensitive to penicillins.

Because potentially fatal, severe hemolytic anemia has been reported rarely in association with cefotetan therapy, patients should be monitored periodically for signs and symptoms of hemolytic anemia, including assessment of hematologic parameters, where appropriate. If a patient develops anemia anytime within 2–3 weeks after administration of cefotetan, the diagnosis of cephalosporin-associated anemia should be considered and the drug stopped until the etiology is determined with certainty. Blood transfusions may be considered as needed.Cefotetan is contraindicated in individuals who have experienced cephalosporin-associated hemolytic anemia.

As with other anti-infective agents, prolonged use of cefotetan may result in overgrowth of nonsusceptible organisms (e.g., enterococci, *Pseudomonas*, *Acinetobacter*, *Candida*). Careful observation of the patient during cefotetan therapy is essential. If superinfection occurs, appropriate therapy should be initiated.

Patients should be advised that diarrhea is a common problem caused by anti-infectives and usually ends when the drug is discontinued; however, they should contact a clinician if watery and bloody stools (with or without stomach cramps and fever) occur during or as late as 2 months or longer after the last dose. Cefotetan should be used with caution in patients with a history of GI disease, especially colitis. (See Clostridium difficile-associated Diarrhea and Colitis under Cautions: GI Effects.)

Although prolonged prothrombin time (PT) has been reported rarely in patients receiving cefotetan (see Cautions: Hematologic Effects), the PT should be monitored when the drug is used in patients at increased risk (e.g., patients with renal or hepatic impairment, malnutrition, geriatric patients, patients with cancer), and vitamin K should be administered when indicated.

Patients should be warned to avoid ingestion of alcohol during and for 72 hours after cefotetan therapy because of the possibility that a disulfiram-like reaction may occur. (See Drug Interactions: Alcohol.)

Like other dextrose-containing solutions, the commercially available Duplex® delivery system containing 1 or 2 g of cefotetan powder and 50 mL of 3.58 or 2.08% dextrose injection, respectively, should be used with caution in patients with overt or known subclinical diabetes mellitus or in patients with carbohydrate intolerance for any reason.

To reduce development of drug-resistant bacteria and maintain effectiveness of cefotetan and other antibacterials, the drug should be used only for treatment or prevention of infections proven or strongly suspected to be caused by susceptible bacteria. When selecting or modifying anti-infective therapy, use results of culture and in vitro susceptibility testing. In the absence of such data, consider local epidemiology and susceptibility patterns when selecting anti-infectives for empiric therapy.

Patients should be advised that antibacterials (including cefotetan) should only be used to treat bacterial infections and not used to treat viral infections (e.g., the common cold). Patients also should be advised about the importance of completing the full course of therapy, even if feeling better after a few days, and that skipping doses or not completing therapy may decrease effectiveness and increase the likelihood that bacteria will develop resistance and will not be treatable with cefotetan or other antibacterials in the future.

Because serum concentrations of cefotetan are higher and more prolonged in patients with renal impairment than in patients with normal renal function, doses and/or frequency of administration of the drug should be decreased in patients with impaired renal function. (See Dosage and Administration: Dosage in Renal Impairment.)

■ **Pediatric Precautions** The manufacturer states that the safety and efficacy of cefotetan in children have not been established. However, the American Academy of Pediatrics (AAP) suggests that the drug may be used for treatment of infections in children beyond the neonatal period†. (See Pediatric Dosage under Dosage and Administration: Dosage.)

■ **Geriatric Precautions** In clinical studies, safety and efficacy of cefotetan in geriatric adults 60 years of age or older have been similar to those observed in younger adults. Although other clinical experience has revealed no evidence of age-related differences, the possibility that some older patients may exhibit increased sensitivity to the drug cannot be ruled out.

Cefotetan is substantially eliminated in urine and the risk of toxicity may be increased in patients with impaired renal function. Because geriatric patients are more likely to have decreased renal function, use caution when selecting dosage for such patients and consider monitoring renal function. (See Dosage in Renal Impairment under Dosage and Administration: Dosage.)

■ **Mutagenicity and Carcinogenicity** In vitro studies have not shown cefotetan to be mutagenic. Long-term studies have not been performed to date to evaluate the carcinogenic potential of the drug.

■ **Pregnancy, Fertility, and Lactation** Safe use of cefotetan during pregnancy has not been definitely established. Reproduction studies in rats and monkeys using cefotetan dosages up to 20 times the usual human dosage have not revealed evidence of impaired fertility or harm to the fetus. There are no adequate or controlled studies using cefotetan in pregnant women, and the drug should be used during pregnancy only when clearly needed.

Cefotetan has caused adverse effects on the testes of prepubertal rats at high dosages. Reduced testicular weight and seminiferous tubule degeneration occurred in all rats tested following subcutaneous administration of cefotetan in a dosage of 500 mg/kg daily (8–16 times the usual human adult dosage). The drug was given to the rats on days 6–35 of life, the days thought to be developmentally analogous to late childhood and prepuberty in humans. Spermatogonia and spermatocytes were affected, but Sertoli and Leydig cells were unaffected. The incidence and severity of lesions appeared to be dose dependent since a dosage of 120 mg/kg daily (2–4 times the usual human adult dosage) resulted in only mild degeneration in 1 of 10 rats. Adverse effects on testicular development did not occur in rats 7 weeks of age following subcutaneous administration of cefotetan in a dosage up to 1 g/kg daily for 5 weeks or in dogs 3 weeks of age following IV administration of the drug in a dosage up to 300 mg/kg daily for 5 weeks. Adverse testicular effects (e.g., reduced testicular weight, seminiferous tubule degeneration, delayed maturity of germinal epithelium) have occurred in prepubertal rats receiving other β-lactam antibiotics that contain an *N*-methylthiotetrazole (NMTT) side chain like that contained in cefotetan (e.g., cefamandole, cefoperazone; drugs no longer commercially available). The relevance of these findings to humans is unknown.

Because cefotetan is distributed into milk, the drug should be used with caution in nursing women.

Drug Interactions

■ **Alcohol** Disulfiram-like reactions characterized by flushing, sweating, headache, and tachycardia may occur if alcohol is ingested within 72 hours after administration of cefotetan. These reactions have been reported with other β-lactam antibiotics that contain an *N*-methylthiotetrazole (NMTT) side chain similar to that contained in cefotetan (e.g., cefamandole, cefoperazone; drugs no longer commercially available) and appear to result from accumulation of acetaldehyde.

■ **Aminoglycosides** In vitro studies indicate that the antibacterial activity of cefotetan and an aminoglycoside may be additive or synergistic against *Staphylococcus aureus*, *Citrobacter*, *Klebsiella*, *Enterobacter*, *Escherichia coli*, and *Serratia*. The combination of cefotetan and an aminoglycoside is generally only additive against *Proteus mirabilis* and *P. vulgaris*. The combination of cefotetan and amikacin reportedly does not result in a synergistic effect in vitro against *Pseudomonas aeruginosa*.

Concomitant use of an aminoglycoside and certain cephalosporins reportedly may increase the risk of nephrotoxicity during therapy. Although cefotetan did not potentiate the nephrotoxicity of gentamicin in rats and this effect has not been reported to date in humans, the manufacturers state that nephrotoxicity may be potentiated if the drug is used concomitantly with an aminoglycoside and that renal function should be monitored.

■ **β-Lactam Antibiotics** An additive or synergistic effect has occurred in vitro against some strains of *E. coli*, *E. aerogenes*, and *Proteus mirabilis* when cefotetan was used concomitantly with cefotaxime or piperacillin. The combination of cefotetan and piperacillin reportedly has been antagonistic in vitro against some gram-negative bacteria.

■ **Probenecid** Concomitant administration of oral probenecid does not appear to affect the pharmacokinetics of cefotetan, presumably because cefotetan is eliminated principally by glomerular filtration and nonrenal mechanisms.

Laboratory Test Interferences

■ **Tests for Urinary Glucose** Cefotetan may cause false-positive results in urinary glucose determinations using cupric sulfate solutions (e.g., Benedict's solution, Clinitest®); glucose oxidase methods (e.g., Clinistix®) should be used in patients receiving cefotetan therapy.

■ **Tests for Creatinine** High concentrations of cefotetan may cause falsely elevated serum or urinary creatinine values when the Jaffé reaction is used.

Acute Toxicity

No information is available on acute overdosage of cefotetan in humans. If acute overdosage of cefotetan occurs, symptomatic treatment should be initiated and hemodialysis considered, especially in patients with renal impairment.

Mechanism of Action

Cefotetan usually is bactericidal in action. Like other β-lactam antibiotics, the antibacterial activity of cefotetan results from inhibition of mucopeptide synthesis in the bacterial cell wall. Studies evaluating the binding of cefotetan to penicillin-binding proteins (PBPs), the target enzymes of β-lactam antibiotics, indicate that the drug has an affinity for and binds to most PBPs of gram-positive bacteria. Cefotetan also has an affinity for and binds to most PBPs of gram-negative bacteria, except PBP 2. Because cefotetan has the highest affinity for PBP 3, the drug usually causes the formation of filamentous forms in susceptible gram-negative bacteria. Cell lysis and death then occur since cefotetan also has an affinity for PBPs 1a and 1b.

Spectrum

Although cefotetan is a cephamycin antibiotic, some clinicians classify the drug as a third generation cephalosporin based on its spectrum of activity. Like third generation cephalosporins, cefotetan usually is less active in vitro against susceptible staphylococci than first generation cephalosporins but has an expanded spectrum of activity against gram-negative bacteria compared with first and second generation cephalosporins. However, most clinicians classify cefotetan as a second generation cephalosporin since the drug generally is less active in vitro on a weight basis than many third generation cephalosporins against gram-negative bacteria and, unlike some currently available third generation cephalosporins, cefotetan generally is inactive against *Pseudomonas aeruginosa*. For information on the classification of cephalosporins and closely related β-lactam antibiotics based on spectra of activity, see Spectrum in the Cephalosporins General Statement 8:12.06.

In vitro on a weight basis, cefotetan generally is less active than cefotaxime or ceftriaxone against most susceptible organisms including gram-positive cocci, *Haemophilus*, *Neisseria*, and Enterobacteriaceae. Cefotetan generally is less active in vitro on a weight basis than cefoxitin against susceptible gram-positive cocci, but generally is more active than cefoxitin against Enterobacteriaceae. The in vitro activity of cefotetan against *Bacteroides fragilis* is equal to or slightly less than that of cefoxitin.

■ **In Vitro Susceptibility Testing** Inoculum size does not generally affect susceptibility to cefotetan, and MICs for most organisms are generally only 2–4 times greater when the size of the inoculum is increased from 10^3 to 10^8 colony-forming units (CFU) per mL. However, MICs for some strains of *Morganella*, *Proteus*, and *Providencia* may be 8 times greater when the inoculum is increased from 10^3 to 10^7 CFU/mL. Results of cefotetan in vitro susceptibility tests are generally unaffected by media, pH, or presence of serum.

Strains of staphylococci resistant to penicillinase-resistant penicillins (oxacillin-resistant [methicillin-resistant] staphylococci) should be considered resistant to cefotetan, although routine in vitro susceptibility tests may indicate that the organisms are susceptible to the drug.

For information on interpreting results of in vitro susceptibility testing (disk susceptibility tests, dilution susceptibility tests) when cefotetan susceptibility testing is performed according to the standards of the Clinical and Laboratory Standards Institute (CLSI; formerly National Committee for Clinical Laboratory Standards [NCCLS]), see Spectrum: In Vitro Susceptibility Testing, in the Cephalosporins General Statement 8:12.06.

■ **Gram-positive Aerobic Bacteria** Cefotetan's activity against gram-positive aerobic bacteria generally is similar to that of cefoxitin. Cefotetan generally is active in vitro against penicillinase- and nonpenicillinase-producing strains of *Staphylococcus aureus*. In addition, most strains of *S. pyogenes* (group A β-hemolytic streptococci), group B streptococci (e.g., *S. agalactiae*), and groups C and G streptococci are susceptible to the drug. Cefotetan also is active in vitro against some strains of *S. epidermidis* and *Streptococcus pneumoniae*. Enterococci, including *E. faecalis* (formerly *S. faecalis*), generally are resistant to the drug.

The MIC_{90} (minimum inhibitory concentration of the drug at which 90% of strains tested are inhibited) of cefotetan for penicillinase- and nonpenicillinase-producing *S. aureus* is 7.5–16 mcg/mL. The MIC_{90} of the drug for *S. pyogenes* and groups B, C, or G streptococci is 2–8 mcg/mL. The MIC_{50} of cefotetan for *S. epidermidis* and *S. pneumoniae* is 1–11.2 mcg/mL, but the MIC_{90} of the drug for these organisms ranges from 8–64 mcg/mL or greater and some strains are considered resistant to the drug.

■ **Gram-negative Aerobic Bacteria** ***Neisseria*** Cefotetan is active in vitro against *Neisseria meningitidis* and most strains of penicillinase- and nonpenicillinase-producing *Neisseria gonorrhoeae*. The MIC_{90} of cefotetan for *N. meningitidis* is 0.12 mcg/mL, and the MIC_{90} of the drug for nonpenicillinase- or penicillinase-producing *N. gonorrhoeae* is 0.5–4 mcg/mL.

Haemophilus Cefotetan is active in vitro against most β-lactamase- and non-β-lactamase-producing strains of *Haemophilus influenzae*. Cefotetan generally is more active in vitro than cefamandole against β-lactamase-producing (ampicillin-resistant) strains of *H. influenzae*. The MIC_{90} of cefotetan reported for *H. influenzae* is 1–4 mcg/mL.

Enterobacteriaceae Cefotetan generally is active in vitro against the following Enterobacteriaceae: *Citrobacter diversus*, *C. freundii*, *Escherichia coli*, *Hafnia alvei*, *Klebsiella oxytoca*, *K. ozaenae*, *K. pneumoniae*, *Morganella morganii* (formerly *Proteus morganii*), *Proteus mirabilis*, *P. vulgaris*, *Providencia rettgeri* (formerly *Proteus rettgeri*), *P. stuartii*, *Serratia marcescens*, *Salmonella*, *Shigella*, and *Yersinia enterocolitica*.

The MIC_{90} of cefotetan for *E. coli*, *H. alvei*, *K. oxytoca*, *K. ozaenae*, *K. pneumoniae*, *P. mirabilis*, and *P. vulgaris* is 0.12–4 mcg/mL. The MIC_{90} of cefotetan for *M. morganii*, *P. rettgeri*, *P. stuartii*, and *Y. enterocolitica* is 0.25–12 mcg/mL. Although the MIC_{90} for *C. diversus* is 0.12–0.5 mcg/mL, the MIC_{90} for *C. freundii* is usually 1–32 mcg/mL. The MIC_{50} of the drug for *Serratia*, including *S. marcescens*, is 0.5–4 mcg/mL, but the MIC_{90} ranges from 0.5–32 mcg/mL.

The in vitro activity of cefotetan against *Enterobacter* varies considerably, and many strains (approximately 50% of *E. aerogenes* or *E. cloacae*) are considered resistant to the drug. The MIC_{90} of cefotetan for *E. agglomerans* is 0.5–32 mcg/mL, but the MIC_{90} for *E. aerogenes* or *E. cloacae* is usually 32 mcg/mL or greater.

The MIC_{90} of cefotetan reported for *Salmonella*, including *S. typhi* and *S. enteritidis*, is 0.05–12.5 mcg/mL. The MIC_{90} of cefotetan reported for *Shigella*, including *Sh. sonnei*, is 0.06–0.5 mcg/mL.

Pseudomonas Most strains of *Pseudomonas aeruginosa* are resistant to cefotetan. Cefotetan has some activity in vitro against *Ps. acidovorans*, and *Ps. stutzeri*, and the MIC_{90} of the drug reported for these organisms is 4–32 mcg/mL. Other *Pseudomonas*, including *Ps. fluorescens*, and *Ps. putida* generally are resistant to cefotetan.

Other Gram-negative Aerobic Bacteria Cefotetan is active in vitro against some strains of *Alcaligenes faecalis* (formerly *A. odorans*) and *Moraxella*, but *Acinetobacter*, *Achromobacter*, and *Flavobacterium* generally are resistant to the drug.

Stenotrophomonas maltophilia (formerly *Ps. maltophilia*) generally is resistant to cefotetan.

■ **Anaerobic Bacteria** Cefotetan is active in vitro against some gram-positive anaerobic bacteria including *Actinomyces*, *Clostridium*, *Peptococcus*, *Peptostreptococcus*, and *Propionibacterium*. The MIC_{90} of cefotetan reported for most of these gram-positive anaerobes, including *Clostridium perfringens* and *C. botulinum*, is 0.06–8 mcg/mL. The MIC_{90} reported for *C. difficile* is 16–32 mcg/mL, but many strains of this organism are resistant to the drug.

Cefotetan is active in vitro against gram-negative anaerobic bacteria including some strains of *Bacteroides*, *Fusobacterium*, and *Veillonella*. The MIC_{90} of cefotetan reported for *Fusobacterium* is 0.13–8 mcg/mL, and the MIC_{90} for *Veillonella* is 1–2 mcg/mL. The MIC_{90} for *B. fragilis*, *B. uniformis*, and *B. vulgatus* is 2–32 mcg/mL. Most strains of *B. asaccharolyticus*, *B. distasonis*, *B. ovatus*, and *B. thetaiotaomicron* are resistant to cefotetan.

Prevotella bivia, *P. disiens*, and *P. melaninogenica* (formerly *B. bivius*, *B. disiens*, and *B. melaninogenicus*) may be inhibited in vitro by cefotetan concentrations of 2–32 mcg/mL.

■ **Other Organisms** Cefotetan has some activity in vitro against *Mycobacterium fortuitum*, but the clinical importance of this in vitro activity has not been determined to date. In one study, 1113 isolates of *M. fortuitum* were inhibited in vitro by cefotetan concentrations of 50 mcg/mL.

Resistance

Because cefotetan contains a 7 α-methoxy group on the β-lactam ring, the drug is generally stable against hydrolysis by penicillinases and most cephalosporinases. Cefotetan is stable against hydrolysis by β-lactamases classified as Richmond-Sykes types I, III (TEM types), IV, and V. The drug is hydrolyzed by PSE 2 β-lactamases produced by *Pseudomonas aeruginosa* and by some β-lactamases produced by *Bacteroides fragilis*. Cefotetan is also hydrolyzed by some β-lactamases produced by *Enterobacter* but is generally more stable than cefoxitin against hydrolysis by cephalosporinases produced by *E. coli* and *E. cloacae*.

Resistance to cefotetan in some gram-negative bacteria, including *Citrobacter*, *Enterobacter*, and *Pseudomonas*, apparently is related to permeability factors. Resistance in *Bacteroides* probably results from nonspecific binding of PBPs and permeability factors.

In vitro studies indicate that cefotetan, like cefoxitin, is a potent inducer of β-lactamases and can derepress inducible, chromosomally mediated enzymes in gram-negative bacteria that possess these enzymes. Cefotetan appears to be active against some strains of *Morganella morganii*, *Providencia stuartii*, and *Serratia marcescens* following derepression of inducible β-lactamases, but *Enterobacter* and *Citrobacter* were generally resistant to the drug following derepression.

Pharmacokinetics

In all studies described in the Pharmacokinetics section, cefotetan was administered as cefotetan disodium; dosages and concentrations of the drug are expressed in terms of cefotetan.

Total body clearance and mean volume of distribution of cefotetan in geriatric patients (older than 65 years of age) with normal renal function generally are similar to pharmacokinetics reported in younger healthy adults.

■ **Absorption** Cefotetan disodium is not absorbed from the GI tract and must be given parenterally.

Following IV infusion over 30 minutes of a single 1-g dose of cefotetan in healthy adults with normal renal function, peak plasma cefotetan concentrations immediately following completion of the infusion averaged 126–158 mcg/mL and plasma concentrations 11–12 hours later averaged 6.5–9 mcg/mL.

■ **Distribution** Cefotetan is widely distributed into body tissues and fluids including gallbladder, skin, muscle, fat, myometrium, endometrium, fallopian tube, cervix, ovary, uterus and adnexa, prostatic tissue, kidney, ureter, bladder, maxillary sinus mucosa, tonsils, sputum, bile, and wound, prostatic, and peritoneal fluids.

The apparent volume of distribution of cefotetan is 8–14.8 L in healthy adults. In one study in healthy adults, the volume of distribution of cefotetan in the central compartment was 0.136 L/kg and the volume of distribution at steady state was 0.194 L/kg. The volume of distribution of cefotetan reported for adults with impaired renal function does not differ substantially from that reported for patients with normal renal function.

Information on the distribution of cefotetan into CSF is limited, but only low concentrations of the drug are probably attained in CSF after IV administration.

Cefotetan is generally distributed into bile, and concentrations in common duct bile are 2–21 times higher than concurrent serum concentrations; concentrations of the drug in gallbladder bile depend on the functional state of the gallbladder. In patients with good gallbladder function who received a single 1-g IV dose of cefotetan, concentrations of the drug in gallbladder bile ranged from 1.3–1.96 mcg/mL and concentrations in common duct bile ranged from 548 mcg/mL to 1.59 mg/mL in samples obtained 1–4 hours after the dose. Biliary concentrations of the drug are low in patients with poor or absent gallbladder function. Cefotetan distributes into prostatic fluid in relatively low concentrations, averaging 0.8 mcg/mL after a 1-g IV dose.

Cefotetan is 76–91% bound to serum proteins. The drug is 87.4% bound at a concentration of 50 mcg/mL and 76.3% bound at a concentration of 400 mcg/mL.

Cefotetan crosses the placenta and is distributed into cord blood and amniotic fluid. Peak cefotetan concentrations in umbilical cord serum and amniotic fluid have been reported to be 29 and 8.6 mcg/mL, respectively, following a 1-g IV dose and were attained approximately 3 hours after the dose. The drug is distributed into milk in low concentrations, averaging 0.22, 0.34, and 0.28 mcg/mL 1, 4, and 6 hours, respectively, after a 1-g IV dose.

■ **Elimination** In adults with normal renal function, the distribution half-life of cefotetan ($t_{1/2\alpha}$) is 0.2–1.1 hours and the elimination half-life ($t_{1/2\beta}$) is 2.8–4.6 hours.

Cefotetan does not appear to be metabolized; however, 1–10% of a cefotetan dose is present in plasma and urine as a tautomer of the drug. This tautomer has microbiologic activity and pharmacokinetic properties similar to those of cefotetan.

Following parenteral administration of a single 0.5- to 2-g dose of cefotetan in adults with normal renal function, 49–81% of the dose is excreted unchanged in urine within 18–24 hours. Urinary concentrations of the drug are generally highest during the first 1–4 hours following a dose. Cefotetan concentrations average 1.4–2 or 3.5–4 mg/mL in urine collected over the first hour following a single 1- or 2-g dose of the drug, respectively, in healthy adults with normal renal function. Following a single 0.5- or 1-g dose of cefotetan in healthy adults with normal renal function, concentrations of the drug in urine collected over the 12th to 24th hours after the dose average 36–77 mcg/mL. Cefotetan is excreted in urine principally by glomerular filtration, although some renal tubular secretion also occurs. The principal nonrenal route of elimination of cefotetan is biliary excretion; approximately 20% of a dose is reportedly excreted in bile.

Total body clearance of cefotetan from plasma in adults with normal renal function ranges from 29.2–49.7 mL/minute per 1.73 m^2. Total body clearance and mean volume of distribution of cefotetan in geriatric patients (older than 65 years of age) with normal renal function generally are similar to pharmacokinetics reported in younger healthy adults.

Serum concentrations of cefotetan are higher and the serum half-life of the drug is prolonged in patients with impaired renal function. In patients with creatinine clearances of 31–94 mL/minute per 1.73 m^2, the $t_{1/2\beta}$ of cefotetan is 3.7–9.1 hours and, in patients with creatinine clearances less than 15 mL/minute per 1.73 m^2, the $t_{1/2\beta}$ is 13.1–35.1 hours. Renal elimination of cefotetan is substantially reduced in patients with impaired renal function; only 5, 8, or 65% of a single 500-mg dose is excreted in urine within 24 hours in patients with creatinine clearances of 0–5, 6–14, or 15–50 mL/minute, respectively. Systemic clearance of cefotetan decreases linearly with decreases in creatinine clearance.

Cefotetan is removed by hemodialysis and peritoneal dialysis. In patients with renal failure undergoing continuous ambulatory peritoneal dialysis who received a single 1-g IV dose of cefotetan, 5–9% of the dose was removed into the dialysate over the 24-hour period immediately following the dose.

Chemistry and Stability

■ **Chemistry** Cefotetan is a semisynthetic cephamycin antibiotic derived from oganomycin G, a substance produced by *Streptomyces oganonensis*. Cephamycins are β-lactam antibiotics that contain a methoxy group rather than a hydrogen at the 7α-position on the β-lactam ring of the cephalosporin nucleus. The methoxy group imparts stability against hydrolysis by many penicillinases and some cephalosporinases. Cefotetan also contains an *N*-methylthiotetrazole (NMTT) side chain at position 3 of the cephalosporin nucleus similar to that contained in cefamandole and cefoperazone (drugs no longer commercially available in the US). The NMTT side chain enhances antibacterial activity, helps to prevent metabolism of the drug, and also may be associated with certain adverse effects (e.g., hypoprothrombinemia, disulfiram-like reactions).

Cefotetan is commercially available as the disodium salt. Potency of cefotetan disodium is expressed in terms of cefotetan, calculated on the anhydrous basis. Commercially available cefotetan disodium is a mixture of the *R*- and *S*-epimers of the drug; in vivo and in weakly alkaline solutions, a tautomer may be present. The isomers and tautomer have equivalent antibacterial activity.

Cefotetan disodium occurs as a white to pale yellow powder and is very soluble in water and slightly soluble in alcohol, having solubilities of 769 and 1.4 mg/mL in water and alcohol, respectively, at 20°C. The drug has pK_as of 2.58 and 3.19.

When the commercially available Duplex® delivery system containing 1 or 2 g of cefotetan powder and 50 mL of 3.58 or 2.08% dextrose injection, respectively, in separate chambers is reconstituted (activated) according to the manufacturer's directions, the resultant solution is iso-osmotic and has an osmolality of approximately 290 mOsm/kg.

■ **Stability** Commercially available vials containing 1 or 2 g of cefotetan should be stored at a temperature of 22°C or cooler and protected from light. Commercially available pharmacy bulk package vials containing 10 g of cefotetan should be stored at 20–25°C and protected from light.

Following reconstitution of 1- or 2-g vials of cefotetan with sterile water for injection, IV solutions containing 95–182 mg/mL are colorless to yellow in color and are stable for 24 hours at room temperature (25°C), 96 hours when refrigerated at 5°C, or at least 1 week when frozen at −20°C. Reconstituted solutions have a pH of approximately 4.5–6.5.

Following reconstitution of 1- or 2-g vials of cefotetan with sterile or bacteriostatic water for injection, 0.9% sodium chloride injection, or 0.5 or 1% lidocaine hydrochloride, IM solutions containing 400 or 500 mg/mL are stable for 24 hours at room temperature (25°C), 96 hours when refrigerated at 5°C, or at least 1 week when frozen at −20°C.

Following reconstitution of 10-g pharmacy bulk package vials of cefotetan with sterile water for injection, 5% dextrose injection, or 0.9% sodium chloride injection, doses should be promptly withdrawn from the container and further diluted in a compatible IV solution within 4 hours. Any unused portion of the reconstituted pharmacy bulk package should be discarded 4 hours after the vial was originally entered. Reconstituted and diluted solutions should be used within 24 hours if stored at room temperature, within 96 hours if stored in a refrigerator at 5°C, or within 1 week if frozen.

The commercially available Duplex® drug delivery system containing 1 or 2 g of cefotetan powder and 50 mL of dextrose injection in separate chambers should be stored at 20–25°C, but may be exposed to temperatures ranging from 15–30°C. Following reconstitution (activation), these IV solutions must be used within 12 hours if stored at room temperature or within 5 days if stored in a refrigerator and should not be frozen.

Cefotetan disodium powder and reconstituted solutions may darken to a deeper yellow; however, such discoloration does not indicate loss of potency.

Cefotetan disodium is physically incompatible with aminoglycosides.

Preparations

Excipients in commercially available drug preparations may have clinically important effects in some individuals; consult specific product labeling for details.

cefoTEtan Disodium in Dextrose

Parenteral		
For injection	1 g (of cefotetan)*	**cefoTEtan Disodium for Injection**
	2 g (of cefotetan)*	**cefoTEtan Disodium for Injection**
For injection, for IV infusion	1 g (of cefotetan)*	**cefoTEtan Disodium for Injection** (available in dual-chambered Duplex® drug delivery system with 3.58% dextrose injection), B Braun
	2 g (of cefotetan)*	**cefoTEtan Disodium for Injection** (available in dual-chambered Duplex® drug delivery system with 2.08% dextrose injection), B Braun
	10 g (of cefotetan) pharmacy bulk package*	**cefoTEtan Disodium for Injection**

*available from one or more manufacturer, distributor, and/or repackager by generic (nonproprietary) name

†Use is not currently included in the labeling approved by the US Food and Drug Administration

cefOXitin Sodium

■ Cefoxitin is a semisynthetic cephamycin β-lactam antibiotic.

Uses

Cefoxitin is used for treatment of serious infections of the lower respiratory tract, skin and skin structure, bone and joint, and urinary tract; septicemia; gynecologic infections (including endometritis, pelvic cellulitis, and pelvic inflammatory disease); and intra-abdominal infections (including peritonitis and intra-abdominal abscess) caused by susceptible bacteria. Cefoxitin also is used for perioperative prophylaxis and has been used for treatment of uncomplicated gonorrhea†.

Prior to and during cefoxitin therapy, the causative organism should be cultured and in vitro susceptibility tests conducted. In serious infections, therapy may be initiated pending results of in vitro tests. Use of cefoxitin does not replace surgical procedures such as incision and drainage when indicated.

■ **Gram-positive Aerobic Bacterial Infections** Cefoxitin is used for treatment of lower respiratory tract infections (including pneumonia and lung abscess) caused by susceptible *Staphylococcus aureus*, *Streptococcus pneumoniae*, or other streptococci (except *Enterococcus faecalis* [formerly *S. faecalis*]); septicemia caused by susceptible *S. aureus* or *S. pneumoniae*; skin and skin structure infections caused by susceptible *S. aureus*, *S. epidermidis*, or streptococci (except *E. faecalis*); and bone and joint infections caused by susceptible *S. aureus*.

Cefoxitin generally is not a drug of choice for treatment of infections caused by gram-positive bacteria and should not be used for treatment of infections caused by these organisms when a penicillin or a first generation cephalosporin could be used.

■ **Gram-negative Aerobic Bacterial Infections** Cefoxitin is used for treatment of lower respiratory tract infections (including pneumonia and lung abscess) caused by susceptible *Haemophilus influenzae*, *Escherichia coli*, or *Klebsiella*; urinary tract infections caused by susceptible *E. coli*, *Klebsiella*, *Morganella morganii*, *Proteus mirabilis*, *P. vulgaris*, or *Providencia rettgeri*; septicemia or intra-abdominal infections (including peritonitis and intra-abdominal abscess) caused by susceptible *E. coli* or *Klebsiella*; gynecologic infections (including endometritis, pelvic cellulitis, pelvic inflammatory disease) caused by susceptible *E. coli* or *Neisseria gonorrhoeae*; and skin or skin structure infections caused by susceptible *E. coli*, *Klebsiella*, or *P. mirabilis*.

■ **Mixed Aerobic-Anaerobic Bacterial Infections** Cefoxitin is used for treatment of lower respiratory tract infections or septicemia caused by susceptible *Bacteroides* (including *B. fragilis*); intra-abdominal infections (including peritonitis and intra-abdominal abscess) caused by susceptible *Bacteroides* or *Clostridium*; or gynecologic infections (including endometritis, pelvic cellulitis, and pelvic inflammatory disease) and skin and skin structure infections caused by susceptible *Bacteroides* (including *B. fragilis*), *Clostridium*, *Peptococcus niger*, *Peptostreptococcus*, or *S. agalactiae* (group B streptococci).

Cefoxitin has been effective for treatment of mixed aerobic-anaerobic infections which failed to respond to an aminoglycoside and clindamycin. In clinical studies in patients with intra-abdominal infections caused by *Bacteroides* (i.e., *B. distasonis*, *B. fragilis*, *B. ovatus*, *B. thetaiotaomicron*), eradication rates 1–2 weeks after cefoxitin therapy were 70–80%. However, cefoxitin may no longer provide reliable coverage against *B. fragilis*, and many clinicians recommend that metronidazole be included in the regimen to provide coverage against *B. fragilis* for empiric treatment of intra-abdominal infections.

For initial empiric treatment of mild to moderate community-acquired, extrabiliary, complicated intra-abdominal infections in adults (e.g., perforated or abscessed appendicitis), the Infectious Diseases Society of America (IDSA) recommends either monotherapy with cefoxitin, ertapenem, moxifloxacin, tigecycline, or the fixed combination of ticarcillin and clavulanic acid, or a combination regimen that includes either a cephalosporin (cefazolin, cefotaxime, ceftriaxone, cefuroxime) or fluoroquinolone (ciprofloxacin, levofloxacin) in conjunction with metronidazole.

■ **Gonorrhea and Associated Infections** Cefoxitin has been used for treatment of uncomplicated gonorrhea† in adults and adolescents.

For treatment of uncomplicated urogenital, anorectal, or pharyngeal gonorrhea, CDC states that a combination regimen that includes a single 250-mg IM dose of ceftriaxone *and* either oral azithromycin (single 1-g dose) or oral doxycycline (100 mg twice daily for 7 days) is the regimen of choice. Although a single 2-g dose of IM cefoxitin (with a single 1-g dose of oral probenecid) may be effective for treatment of uncomplicated urogenital and anorectal gonorrhea, CDC states that the drug does not offer any advantages over IM ceftriaxone for urogenital infections and its efficacy for pharyngeal infections is less certain.

For additional information on current recommendations for treatment of gonorrhea and associated infections, see Uses: Gonorrhea and Associated Infections in Ceftriaxone 8:12.06.12.

■ **Pelvic Inflammatory Disease** Cefoxitin is used for treatment of pelvic inflammatory disease (PID). Because cefoxitin, like cephalosporins, is inactive against *Chlamydia*, the drug should not be used alone for treatment of PID.

PID is an acute or chronic inflammatory disorder in the upper female genital tract and can include any combination of endometritis, salpingitis, tubo-ovarian abscess, and pelvic peritonitis. PID generally is a polymicrobial infection most frequently caused by *N. gonorrhoeae* and/or *Chlamydia trachomatis*; however, organisms that can be part of the normal vaginal flora (e.g., anaerobic bacteria, *Gardnerella vaginalis*, *H. influenzae*, enteric gram-negative bacilli, *S. agalactiae*) or mycoplasma (e.g., *Mycoplasma hominis*, *Ureaplasma urealyticum*) also may be involved. PID is treated with an empiric regimen provides broad-spectrum coverage. The regimen should be effective against *N. gonorrhoeae* and *C. trachomatis* and also probably should be effective against anaerobes, gram-negative facultative bacteria, and streptococci. The optimum empiric regimen for treatment of PID has not been identified. A wide variety of parenteral and oral regimens have been shown to achieve clinical and microbiologic cure in randomized studies with short-term follow-up; however, only limited data are available regarding elimination of infection in the endometrium and fallopian tubes or intermediate or long-term outcomes, including the impact of these regimens on the incidence of long-term sequelae of PID (e.g., tubal infertility, ectopic pregnancy, pain).

Parenteral Regimens for PID When a parenteral regimen is indicated for treatment of PID, CDC and other clinicians generally recommend a 2-drug regimen of cefoxitin (2 g IV every 6 hours) or cefotetan (2 g IV every 12 hours) given in conjunction with doxycycline (100 mg IV or orally every 12 hours) or a 2-drug regimen of clindamycin (900 mg IV every 8 hours) and gentamicin (usually a 2-mg/kg IV or IM loading dose followed by 1.5 mg/kg every 8 hours). While certain parenteral cephalosporins (e.g., cefotaxime, ceftriaxone) also have been used and may be effective for treatment of PID, CDC states that there is less experience with use of these cephalosporins in patients with PID and these drugs may be less active than cefoxitin or cefotetan against anaerobic bacteria. CDC states that only limited data are available to support the use of other parenteral regimens for treatment of acute PID, although a regimen of IV ampicillin and sulbactam given with oral or IV doxycycline may be effective against *C. trachomatis*, *N. gonorrhoeae*, and anaerobes in women with tubo-ovarian abscess.

CDC states that a transition to oral therapy usually can be initiated within 24–48 hours after the patient demonstrates clinical improvement and decisions regarding such a transition should be guided by clinical experience. At least 24 hours of direct inpatient observation is recommended for patients with tubo-ovarian abscess.

Oral Regimens for PID When acute PID that is mild to moderately severe is treated with an oral regimen, CDC recommends a regimen that consists of a single dose of IM ceftriaxone, IM cefoxitin (with oral probenecid), or IM cefotaxime given in conjunction with a 14-day regimen of oral doxycycline (100 mg twice daily) with or without oral metronidazole (500 mg twice daily). The optimal parenteral cephalosporin or cephamycin for this outpatient regimen is unclear; although cefoxitin has better anaerobic coverage, ceftriaxone has better coverage against *N. gonorrhoeae*. A single dose of cefoxitin effectively produces a short-term clinical response in women with PID; however, the theoretical limitations in anaerobic coverage might require that metronidazole be included in the regimen. With the addition of metronidazole, the regimen should be effective for treatment of bacterial vaginosis, which is frequently associated with PID.

For additional information regarding treatment of PID, the current CDC sexually transmitted diseases treatment guidelines available at http://www.cdc.gov/std should be consulted.

■ **Mycobacterial Infections** Cefoxitin has been used in conjunction with other antimycobacterial anti-infectives for treatment of infections caused by *Mycobacterium abscessus*† or *M. fortuitum*†.

For serious skin, soft tissue, and bone infections caused by *M. abscessus*†, the American Thoracic Society (ATS) and IDSA recommend a multiple-drug regimen of oral clarithromycin (or azithromycin) used in conjunction with parenteral anti-infectives (e.g., amikacin, cefoxitin, imipenem). This multiple-drug regimen also has been used for treatment of *M. abscessus* lung disease. However, although periodic administration of multiple-drug regimens that include a macrolide and at least one parenteral agent (amikacin, cefoxitin, imipenem) or a multiple-drug regimen of several parenteral agents continued for several months may help control symptoms and disease progression in patients with lung infections, long-term sputum conversion is unlikely. In patients with focal infections and limited lung disease, curative therapy may be possible if surgical resection is used in conjunction with a multiple-drug treatment regimen.

Cefoxitin is one of several anti-infectives recommended for use in multiple-drug regimens used for treatment of infections caused by *M. fortuitum*. Although optimum regimens have not been identified, the ATS and IDSA recommend that *M. fortuitum* pulmonary infections be treated with a regimen consisting of at least 2 anti-infectives selected based on results of in vitro susceptibility testing and tolerability (e.g., amikacin, clarithromycin, cefoxitin, ciprofloxacin or ofloxacin, a sulfonamide, imipenem, doxycycline). At least 4 months of treatment with at least 2 anti-infectives active against the clinical isolate is necessary to provide a high likelihood of cure in patients with serious skin, bone, and soft tissue infections; 6 months of treatment is recommended for bone infections. Surgery usually is indicated for extensive disease, abscess formation, or when drug therapy is difficult.

■ **Perioperative Prophylaxis** Cefoxitin is used perioperatively to reduce the incidence of infections in patients undergoing GI surgery (e.g., colorectal surgery, nonperforated appendectomy) or gynecologic and obstetric surgery (e.g., vaginal, abdominal, or laparoscopic hysterectomy, cesarean section). Perioperative prophylaxis with an appropriate anti-infective agent can decrease the incidence of infection, particularly surgical site infection, after certain procedures.

GI Surgery **Biliary Tract Surgery.** Perioperative prophylaxis is recommended for patients undergoing biliary tract surgery who are at high risk of infection (e.g., those older than 70 years of age or those with acute cholecystitis, a nonfunctioning gallbladder, obstructive jaundice, or common duct stones). In high-risk patients undergoing endoscopic retrograde cholangiopancreatography (ERCP), perioperative prophylaxis is recommended only if complete biliary drainage is unlikely to be achieved. Perioperative prophylaxis is not considered necessary for low-risk patients undergoing elective laparoscopic cholecystectomy.

For perioperative prophylaxis in high-risk patients undergoing open biliary tract surgery, many clinicians recommend IV cefazolin as the drug of choice. Alternatives include IV cefotetan, IV cefoxitin, or IV ampicillin and sulbactam. In patients allergic to penicillins and cephalosporins, a reasonable alternative is clindamycin or vancomycin used in conjunction with an aminoglycoside (gentamicin or tobramycin), a fluoroquinolone (ciprofloxacin or levofloxacin), or aztreonam; some clinicians suggest metronidazole and an aminoglycoside (gentamicin or tobramycin) or fluoroquinolone (ciprofloxacin or levofloxacin) as another alternative.

Colorectal Surgery. There is evidence that perioperative prophylaxis can decrease the incidence of infection after colorectal surgery, and such prophylaxis is recommended.

For perioperative prophylaxis in patients undergoing colorectal surgery, many clinicians recommend a parenteral regimen of IV cefoxitin, IV cefotetan, IV cefazolin (used in conjunction with IV metronidazole), IV ampicillin and sulbactam, or IV ertapenem. In patients allergic to penicillins and cephalosporins, a reasonable alternative is clindamycin or vancomycin used in conjunction with an aminoglycoside (gentamicin or tobramycin), a fluoroquinolone (ciprofloxacin or levofloxacin), or aztreonam; some clinicians suggest metronidazole and an aminoglycoside (gentamicin or tobramycin) or fluoroquinolone (ciprofloxacin or levofloxacin) as another alternative.

Alternatively, an oral regimen of oral neomycin with either oral erythromycin or oral metronidazole can be used in conjunction with mechanical bowel preparation for perioperative prophylaxis in patients undergoing colorectal surgery. Many clinicians recommend using both an oral and a parenteral regimen for perioperative prophylaxis in patients undergoing colorectal surgery, and there is some evidence that use of an oral regimen (with mechanical bowel preparation) in conjunction with a parenteral regimen is more effective than use of a parenteral regimen alone.

Appendectomy. There is evidence that perioperative prophylaxis can reduce the incidence of infection after surgery for acute appendicitis, and such prophylaxis is recommended.

For perioperative prophylaxis in patients undergoing uncomplicated (nonperforated) appendectomy, many clinicians recommend IV cefoxitin, IV cefotetan, or IV cefazolin (used in conjunction with IV metronidazole). In patients allergic to penicillins and cephalosporins, a reasonable alternative is clindamycin or vancomycin used in conjunction with an aminoglycoside (gentamicin or tobramycin), a fluoroquinolone (ciprofloxacin or levofloxacin), or aztreonam; some clinicians suggest metronidazole and an aminoglycoside (gentamicin or tobramycin) or fluoroquinolone (ciprofloxacin or levofloxacin) as another alternative.

If perforation has occurred, anti-infectives are continued postoperatively for about 5 days.

Gynecologic and Obstetric Surgery Perioperative prophylaxis decreases the incidence of infection after vaginal or abdominal hysterectomy and also is used for laparoscopic hysterectomies. In addition, there is evidence that perioperative prophylaxis can prevent infection after elective and nonelective cesarean section, and also can prevent infection after elective abortions. A pooled analysis of results of randomized, placebo-controlled studies in women who underwent therapeutic abortion before 16 weeks' gestation indicates that perioperative prophylaxis can reduce the overall risk of postabortal infection in these women by 42% compared with placebo.

Many clinicians suggest that the preferred agents for perioperative prophylaxis in women undergoing vaginal, abdominal, or laparoscopic hysterectomy are IV cefoxitin, IV cefotetan, IV cefazolin, or IV ampicillin and sulbactam. In patients allergic to penicillins and cephalosporins, a reasonable alternative is clindamycin or vancomycin used in conjunction with an aminoglycoside (gentamicin or tobramycin), a fluoroquinolone (ciprofloxacin or levofloxacin), or aztreonam; some clinicians suggest metronidazole and an aminoglycoside (gentamicin or tobramycin) or fluoroquinolone (ciprofloxacin or levofloxacin) as another alternative.

IV cefazolin generally is the preferred agent for prophylaxis in women undergoing cesarean section; oral doxycycline is recommended for prophylaxis in those undergoing abortion.

Timing and Number of Doses When perioperative prophylaxis is indicated in patients undergoing surgery, administration of an appropriate anti-infective should be timed to ensure that bactericidal concentrations of the drug are established in serum and tissues by the time the initial surgical incision is made; therapeutic concentrations of the drug should then be maintained in serum and tissues for the duration of the procedure.

An IV dose of an appropriate anti-infective should be administered within 60 minutes before the initial incision. If cefoxitin is used prophylactically, the manufacturers recommend that the drug be given 30–60 minutes before the initial incision to ensure adequate cefoxitin tissue concentrations at the time of surgery.

A single preoperative dose usually is sufficient for perioperative prophylaxis. However, if surgery is prolonged (more than 3–4 hours), major blood loss occurs, or other factors are present that shorten the half-life of the drug (e.g., extensive burns), additional doses should be administered during the procedure to ensure adequate serum and tissue concentrations of the anti-infective throughout the procedure. For prolonged procedures in patients with normal renal function, some clinicians suggest that intraoperative doses be given during the procedure at intervals that correspond to 1–2 times the half-life of the drug (e.g., every 2 hours for cefoxitin, measured from the time the preoperative dose is initiated). Intraoperative doses may not be warranted if there are factors that prolong the half-life of the drug (e.g., renal impairment).

For most procedures, the duration of prophylaxis should be less than 24 hours. There is no evidence to support continuing prophylaxis after wound closure or until all indwelling drains and intravascular catheters are removed.

Dosage and Administration

■ Reconstitution and Administration

Cefoxitin sodium is administered by IV injection or infusion. The drug also has been administered by IM injection†.

Cefoxitin should be given IV in patients with septicemia or other severe or life-threatening infections, or in patients with lowered resistance resulting from debilitating conditions (e.g., malnutrition, trauma, surgery, diabetes, heart failure, malignancy), particularly with shock.

Intermittent IV Injection For direct IV injection, the contents of a vial labeled as containing 1 or 2 g of cefoxitin should be reconstituted with 10 mL of sterile water for injection to provide a solution containing approximately 95 or 180 mg/mL, respectively. The vial should be shaken until the drug is dissolved, and then allowed to stand until the solution is clear.

The appropriate dose of reconstituted solution may then be injected directly into a vein over a 3- to 5-minute period or slowly into the tubing of a compatible IV infusion solution.

Intermittent or Continuous IV Infusion For IV infusion, the contents of a vial labeled as containing 1 or 2 g of cefoxitin should be reconstituted with 10 or 10–20 mL, respectively, of sterile or bacteriostatic water for injection, 0.9% sodium chloride injection, or 5% dextrose injection to provide solutions containing approximately 95 or 95–180 mg/mL, respectively. The vial should be shaken until the drug is dissolved, and then allowed to stand until the solution is clear. The reconstituted solution should be further diluted in 50 mL to 1 L of a compatible IV solution.

Commercially available pharmacy bulk packages containing 10 g of cefoxitin should be reconstituted with 43 or 93 mL of sterile or bacteriostatic water for injection, 0.9% sodium chloride injection, or 5% dextrose injection to provide solutions containing approximately 200 or 100 mg/mL, respectively. The vial should be shaken until the drug is dissolved, and then allowed to stand until the solution is clear. Reconstituted solutions in pharmacy bulk packages should *not* be used for direct IV infusion; the reconstituted solution must be further diluted in 50 mL to 1 L of a compatible IV infusion solution within 4 hours after reconstitution. (See Chemistry and Stability: Stability.) A suitable sterile transfer device or dispensing set should be used to transfer the contents of the reconstituted bulk package vial to a compatible IV solution; a syringe with a needle is not recommended since leakage could occur during transfer. The manufacturer's directions should be consulted for additional information.

Alternatively, the commercially available Duplex® drug delivery system containing 1 or 2 g of cefoxitin powder and 50 mL of 4 or 2.2% dextrose injection, respectively, in separate chambers should be reconstituted (activated) according to the manufacturer's directions and administered by IV infusion. If stored in the refrigerator after reconstitution (see Chemistry and Stability: Stability), the solution should be allowed to reach room temperature prior to administration.

Thawed solutions of the commercially available frozen premixed cefoxitin injection in dextrose should be given only by intermittent or continuous IV infusion. The frozen injection should be thawed at room temperature (25°C) or under refrigeration (5°C); the injection should not be thawed by warming in a water bath or by exposure to microwave radiation. Precipitates that may have formed in the frozen injection usually will dissolve with little or no agitation when the injection reaches room temperature; potency is not affected. After thawing to room temperature, the injection should be agitated and the container checked for minute leaks by firmly squeezing the bag. The injection should be discarded if container seals or outlet ports are not intact or leaks are found or if the solution is cloudy or contains an insoluble precipitate. Additives should not be introduced into the injection container. The injection should not be used in series connections with other plastic containers, since such use could result in air embolism from residual air being drawn from the primary container before administration of fluid from the secondary container is complete.

Other IV solutions flowing through a common administration tubing or site be discontinued while cefoxitin is being infused. If an aminoglycoside is administered concomitantly with cefoxitin, the drugs should be administered at separate sites.

IM Injection IM injections† of cefoxitin have been prepared by adding 2 mL of sterile water for injection or 0.5 or 1% lidocaine hydrochloride injection (without epinephrine) to each g of cefoxitin. IM injections of cefoxitin should be made deeply into a large muscle such as the upper outer quadrant of the gluteus maximus, using usual techniques and precautions. The plunger of the syringe should be drawn back before IM injection to ensure that the needle is not in a blood vessel.

■ Dosage

Dosage of cefoxitin sodium is expressed in terms of cefoxitin.

Adult Dosage **General Adult Dosage.** The usual adult dosage of cefoxitin is 1–2 g every 6–8 hours, depending on the severity of the infection and the susceptibility of the causative organism. In severe, life-threatening infections, up to 12 g daily may be required.

The manufacturers suggest that adults with uncomplicated infections (e.g., pneumonia, urinary tract infections, cutaneous infections) receive 1 g IV every 6–8 hours, those with moderately severe or severe infections receive 1 g IV every 4 hours or 2 g IV every 6–8 hours, and those with infections requiring higher dosage receive 2 g IV every 4 hours or 3 g IV every 6 hours.

The duration of cefoxitin therapy depends on the type of infection. In infections caused by group A β-hemolytic streptococci, therapy should be continued for at least 10 days.

Gonorrhea and Associated Infections. If cefoxitin is used for treatment of uncomplicated gonorrhea†, the US Centers for Disease Control and Prevention (CDC) recommends that adults and adolescents receive a single 2-g IM† dose of the drug (with a single 1-g oral dose of probenecid).

Pelvic Inflammatory Disease. For treatment of acute pelvic inflammatory disease (PID) when a parenteral regimen is used, CDC and others recommend that adults and adolescents receive an IV cefoxitin dosage of 2 g 4 times daily (every 6 hours) given in conjunction with IV or oral doxycycline (100 mg twice daily). The initial parenteral regimen may be discontinued 24–48 hours after there is clinical improvement and oral doxycycline (100 mg twice daily) continued to complete 14 days of therapy.

For treatment of PID when an oral regimen is used, CDC recommends that adults and adolescents receive a single 2-g IM dose of cefoxitin and oral probenecid (1 g), followed by oral doxycycline (100 mg twice daily) with or without oral metronidazole (500 mg twice daily) given for 14 days.

Mycobacterial Infections. If cefoxitin is included in initial combination regimens used for treatment of serious skin, soft tissue, and bone infections caused by *Mycobacterium abscessus*† (see Uses: Mycobacterial Infections), the American Thoracic Society (ATS) and Infectious Diseases Society of America (IDSA) recommend an IV cefoxitin dosage up to 12 g daily given in divided doses for at least 2 weeks until clinical improvement. At least 4 months of antimycobacterial treatment is necessary for treatment of serious skin and soft tissue infections; 6 months of antimycobacterial treatment is recommended for bone infections.

Perioperative Prophylaxis. For perioperative prophylaxis in women undergoing abdominal, vaginal, or laparoscopic hysterectomy or undergoing cesarean section, 1 or 2 g of cefoxitin should be given IV within 30–60 minutes prior to incision. For cesarean section, the manufacturers recommend giving the dose as soon as the umbilical cord is clamped; however, there is some evidence that giving the dose prior to incision is more effective than giving it after clamping. Although the manufacturers state that additional 2-g doses should be given every 6 hours (for up to 24 hours) in hysterectomy patients or at 4 and 8 hours after the initial dose in cesarean section patients, postoperative doses are usually unnecessary.

For perioperative prophylaxis in patients undergoing colorectal surgery, appendectomy (nonperforated), or other uncontaminated GI surgery, 1 or 2 g of cefoxitin should be given IV within 30–60 minutes prior to incision. Although the manufacturers state that additional 2-g doses should be given every 6 hours (for up to 24 hours) after the initial dose, postoperative doses are usually unnecessary.

During prolonged procedures (more than 3–4 hours), if major blood loss occurs, or if other factors are present that shorten the half-life of the drug, additional doses of cefoxitin should be given during the procedure (e.g., every 2 hours, measured from the time the preoperative dose is initiated).

The duration of prophylaxis should be less than 24 hours for most procedures; there is no evidence to support continuing prophylaxis after wound closure or until all indwelling drains and intravascular catheters are removed.

Pediatric Dosage **General Pediatric Dosage.** The usual dosage of cefoxitin for pediatric patients 3 months of age or older is 80–160 mg/kg daily given in 4–6 equally divided doses. The maximum dosage is 12 g daily. Safe use of cefoxitin in infants younger than 3 months of age has not been established.

The American Academy of Pediatrics (AAP) recommends that pediatric patients beyond the neonatal period receive cefoxitin in a dosage of 80 mg/kg daily given in 3–4 divided doses for treatment of mild to moderate infections or 160 mg/kg daily given in 4 divided doses for treatment of severe infections.

The duration of cefoxitin therapy depends on the type of infection. In infections caused by group A β-hemolytic streptococci, therapy should be continued for at least 10 days.

Perioperative Prophylaxis. For perioperative prophylaxis in pediatric patients 3 months of age or older, the manufacturers recommend that a cefoxitin dose of 30–40 mg/kg be given 30–60 minutes prior to incision. Although the manufacturers state that additional doses of 30–40 mg/kg may be given every 6 hours (for up to 24 hours) after the initial dose, postoperative doses are usually unnecessary.

If cefoxitin is used for perioperative prophylaxis in children 1 year of age or older undergoing colorectal surgery or uncomplicated appendectomy, some clinicians recommend that 40 mg/kg of cefoxitin be given within 60 minutes prior to incision.

During prolonged procedures (longer than 3–4 hours), if major blood loss occurs, or if other factors are present that shorten the half-life of the drug, additional doses should be given during the procedure.

The duration of prophylaxis should be less than 24 hours for most procedures; there is no evidence to support continuing prophylaxis after wound closure or until all indwelling drains and intravascular catheters are removed.

■ Dosage in Renal Impairment

In patients with impaired renal function, doses and/or frequency of administration must be modified in response to the degree of impairment, severity of the infection, and susceptibility of the causative organism. Dosage adjustments are not necessary in adults with creatinine clearances greater than 50 mL/minute.

Adult Dosage In adults with creatinine clearances of 50 mL/minute or lower, the manufacturers recommend a loading dose of 1–2 g followed by a maintenance dosage based on the patient's creatinine clearance. (See Table 1.)

Table 1. Maintenance Dosage of Cefoxitin for Adults with Renal Impairment

Creatinine Clearance (mL/minute)	Dosage
30–50	1–2 g every 8–12 h
10–29	1–2 g every 12–24 h
5–9	0.5–1 g every 12–24 h
<5	0.5–1 g every 24–48 h

In adults with renal impairment undergoing hemodialysis, a loading dose of 1–2 g should be given after each dialysis period followed by a maintenance dosage based on the patient's creatinine clearance. (See Table 1.)

Pediatric Dosage If cefoxitin is used in pediatric patients with renal impairment, dosage adjustments should be made similar to those recommended for adults.

Cautions

■ Hypersensitivity Reactions

Maculopapular or erythematous rash, exfoliative dermatitis, pruritus, urticaria, eosinophilia, fever, and other hypersensitivity reactions have occurred with cefoxitin. Anaphylaxis and angioedema have been reported rarely in patients who received cefoxitin. If a hypersensitivity reaction occurs during cefoxitin therapy, the drug should be discontinued and the patient given appropriate therapy (e.g., epinephrine, corticosteroids, maintenance of an adequate airway, oxygen) as indicated.

■ Local Effects

Local reactions are the most frequent adverse effects of cefoxitin. Pain, tenderness, and induration have been reported with IM† administration, and thrombophlebitis has occurred with IV administration. The discomfort of IM injections may be minimized by administering the drug in 0.5% or 1% lidocaine hydrochloride solution, and the use of butterfly or scalp vein type needles rather than indwelling polyethylene catheters may decrease the incidence of thrombophlebitis with IV administration.

■ Renal Effects

Elevations in serum creatinine and/or BUN concentrations have been reported with cefoxitin. Rarely, renal toxicity and oliguria have occurred. These effects are most likely to occur in patients older than 50 years of age, patients with prior renal impairment, or patients who are receiving other nephrotoxic drugs. (See Drug Interactions: Nephrotoxic Drugs.)

■ Hematologic Effects

Transient leukopenia, neutropenia, granulocytopenia, thrombocytopenia, and bone marrow depression have been reported rarely in patients receiving cefoxitin. Anemia, including hemolytic anemia, has also been reported. Although a definite causal relationship has not been established, bleeding from the GI tract, surgical wounds, or genitourinary tract, and prolonged prothrombin time (PT) and/or activated partial thromboplastin time (APTT) have been reported rarely in patients receiving cefoxitin. Positive direct antiglobulin (Coombs') test results have been reported during cefoxitin therapy, especially in patients with azotemia.

■ GI Effects

Rarely, adverse GI effects including nausea, vomiting, and diarrhea have been reported in patients receiving cefoxitin.

Treatment with anti-infectives alters normal colon flora and may permit overgrowth of *Clostridium difficile*. *C. difficile* infection (CDI) and *C. difficile*-associated diarrhea and colitis (CDAD; also known as antibiotic-associated diarrhea and colitis or pseudomembranous colitis) have been reported with nearly all anti-infectives, including cefoxitin, and may range in severity from mild diarrhea to fatal colitis. *C. difficile* produces toxins A and B, which contribute to development of CDAD; hypertoxin producing strains of *C. difficile* are associated with increased morbidity and mortality since they may be refractory to anti-infectives and colectomy may be required.

CDAD should be considered in the differential diagnosis of patients who develop diarrhea during or after anti-infective therapy. Careful medical history is necessary since CDAD has been reported to occur as late as 2 months or longer after anti-infective therapy is discontinued.

If CDAD is suspected or confirmed, anti-infective therapy not directed against *C. difficile* should be discontinued whenever possible. Patients should be managed with appropriate supportive therapy (e.g., fluid and electrolyte management, protein supplementation), anti-infective therapy directed against *C. difficile* (e.g., metronidazole, vancomycin), and surgical evaluation as clinically indicated.

■ Other Adverse Effects

Transient increases in serum AST (SGOT), ALT (SGPT), LDH, and alkaline phosphatase concentrations and jaundice have occurred in patients receiving cefoxitin. Hypotension has also been reported.

■ Precautions and Contraindications

Prior to initiation of cefoxitin therapy, careful inquiry should be made concerning previous hypersensitivity reactions to cefoxitin, cephalosporins, penicillins, or other drugs. There is clinical and laboratory evidence of partial cross-allergenicity among cephamycins, cephalosporins, and penicillins. Cefoxitin is contraindicated in patients who are hypersensitive to the drug or to cephalosporins and should be used with caution in patients hypersensitive to penicillins. Although it has not been proven that allergic reactions to antibiotics are more frequent in atopic individuals, the manufacturers state that cefoxitin should be used with caution in individuals with a history of allergy, particularly to drugs.

As with other anti-infective agents, prolonged use of cefoxitin may result in overgrowth of nonsusceptible organisms. If superinfection occurs, appropriate therapy should be instituted.

Patients should be advised that diarrhea is a common problem caused by anti-infectives and usually ends when the drug is discontinued; however, they should contact a clinician if watery and bloody stools (with or without stomach cramps and fever) occur during or as late as 2 months or longer after the last dose. Cefoxitin should be used with caution in patients with a history of GI disease, particularly colitis. (See Cautions: GI Effects.)

As with any potent anti-infective agent, periodic assessment of organ system functions (including renal, hepatic, and hematopoietic) is advisable during prolonged cefoxitin therapy.

Like other dextrose-containing solutions, the commercially available Duplex® drug delivery system containing 1 or 2 g of cefoxitin powder and 50 mL of 4 or 2.2% dextrose injection, respectively, in separate chambers should be used with caution in patients with overt or known subclinical diabetes mellitus or in patients with carbohydrate intolerance for any reason.

To reduce development of drug-resistant bacteria and maintain effectiveness of cefoxitin and other antibacterials, the drug should be used only for treatment or prevention of infections proven or strongly suspected to be caused by susceptible bacteria. When selecting or modifying anti-infective therapy, use results of culture and in vitro susceptibility testing. In the absence of such data, consider local epidemiology and susceptibility patterns when selecting anti-infectives for empiric therapy.

Patients should be advised that antibacterials (including cefoxitin) should only be used to treat bacterial infections and not used to treat viral infections (e.g., the common cold). Patients also should be advised about the importance of completing the full course of therapy, even if feeling better after a few days, and that skipping doses or not completing therapy may decrease effectiveness and increase the likelihood that bacteria will develop resistance and will not be treatable with cefoxitin or other antibacterials in the future.

■ Pediatric Precautions

Safety and efficacy of cefoxitin in infants younger than 3 months of age have not been established. In pediatric patients 3 months of age and older, high doses of cefoxitin have been associated with an increased incidence of eosinophilia and elevation of serum AST concentration.

Cefoxitin that has been reconstituted with bacteriostatic water for injection containing benzyl alcohol should *not* be used in infants. Although a causal relationship has not been established, administration of injections preserved with benzyl alcohol has been associated with toxicity in neonates. Toxicity appears to have resulted from administration of large amounts (i.e., about 100–400 mg/kg daily) of benzyl alcohol in these neonates. The manufacturers of cefoxitin state that while this toxicity has not been demonstrated in infants older than 3 months of age, small infants in this age range may also be at risk for benzyl alcohol toxicity.

■ **Geriatric Precautions** In clinical studies, safety and efficacy of cefoxitin in geriatric adults 65 years of age or older have been similar to those observed in younger adults. Although other clinical experience has revealed no evidence of age-related differences, the possibility that some older patients may exhibit increased sensitivity to the drug cannot be ruled out.

Cefoxitin is substantially eliminated in urine and the risk of toxicity may be increased in patients with impaired renal function. Because geriatric patients are more likely to have decreased renal function, use caution when selecting dosage for such patients and consider monitoring renal function.

■ **Mutagenicity and Carcinogenicity** Long-term studies in animals have not been performed to date to evaluate the mutagenic or carcinogenic potential of cefoxitin.

■ **Pregnancy, Fertility, and Lactation** Reproduction and teratologic studies in mice and rats using parenteral cefoxitin doses 1–7.5 times the maximum recommended human dose have not revealed evidence of impaired fertility or harm to the fetus, although a slight decrease in fetal weight was observed. When used in rabbits, cefoxitin was associated with a high incidence of abortion and maternal death; however, this was considered to be an expected consequence of the rabbit's unusual sensitivity to antibiotic-induced changes in intestinal flora rather than a teratogenic effect. There are no adequate and controlled studies to date using cefoxitin in pregnant women. Because animal reproduction studies are not always predictive of human response, cefoxitin should be used during pregnancy only when clearly needed.

Because cefoxitin is distributed into milk in small amounts, the drug should be used with caution in nursing women.

Drug Interactions

■ **Probenecid** Concomitant administration of oral probenecid competitively inhibits tubular secretion resulting in higher and more prolonged serum concentrations of cefoxitin. The clinical application of this effect is limited mainly to the treatment of gonorrhea.

■ **Nephrotoxic Drugs** Concurrent use of nephrotoxic agents such as aminoglycosides, colistin, polymyxin B, or vancomycin may increase the risk of nephrotoxicity with some cephalosporins. The possibility that this may occur with concurrent use of these nephrotoxic agents and cefoxitin should be considered.

Laboratory Test Interferences

■ **Immunohematology Tests** Positive direct antiglobulin (Coombs') test results have been reported in patients receiving cefoxitin. This reaction may interfere with hematologic studies or transfusion cross-matching procedures.

■ **Tests for Urinary Glucose** Cefoxitin reportedly causes false-positive results in urine glucose determinations using cupric sulfate solution (Benedict's reagent, Clinitest®). Glucose oxidase methods (Clinistix®, Tes-Tape®) are unaffected.

■ **Tests for Creatinine** At concentrations greater than 100 mcg/mL, cefoxitin may cause falsely elevated serum or urine creatinine values when the Jaffe reaction is used. Serum samples should not be tested for creatinine by the Jaffe reaction if drawn within 2 hours after drug administration.

Mechanism of Action

Cefoxitin is usually bactericidal in action. Like other β-lactam antibiotics, the antibacterial activity of cefoxitin results from inhibition of mucopeptide synthesis in the bacterial cell wall.

Spectrum

Although cefoxitin is a cephamycin antibiotic, the spectrum of activity of the drug resembles that of the second generation cephalosporins. Therefore, based on its spectrum of activity, cefoxitin can be classified as a second generation cephalosporin. For information on the classification of cephalosporins and closely related β-lactam antibiotics based on spectra of activity, see Spectrum in the Cephalosporins General Statement 8:12.06.

Cefoxitin generally is less active in vitro on a weight basis against susceptible gram-positive cocci than first generation cephalosporins and some second generation cephalosporins; however, the drug may be active against strains of gram-negative bacteria, especially *Escherichia coli, Klebsiella*, and *Proteus*, that are resistant to first generation cephalosporins. Unlike other currently available second generation cephalosporins, cefoxitin is active in vitro against some strains of *Bacteroides fragilis*. Cefoxitin also is active against some *Mycobacterium*.

■ **In Vitro Susceptibility Testing** Inoculum size, pH, and test media do not usually influence results of cefoxitin in vitro susceptibility tests.

Strains of staphylococci resistant to penicillinase-resistant penicillins (oxacillin-resistant [methicillin-resistant] staphylococci) should be considered resistant to cefoxitin, although results of in vitro susceptibility tests may indicate that the organisms are susceptible to the drug.

For information on interpreting results of in vitro susceptibility testing (disk susceptibility tests, dilution susceptibility tests) when cefoxitin susceptibility testing is performed according to the standards of the Clinical and Laboratory Standards Institute (CLSI; formerly National Committee for Clinical Laboratory Standards [NCCLS]), see Spectrum: In Vitro Susceptibility Testing, in the Cephalosporins General Statement 8:12.06.

■ **Gram-positive Aerobic Bacteria** In vitro, cefoxitin concentrations of 6.25 mcg/mL or less inhibit most strains of α- and β-hemolytic streptococci, *Streptococcus pneumoniae*, and staphylococci. The drug is active against most strains of penicillin G-resistant *Staphylococcus aureus*; however, oxacillin-resistant (methicillin-resistant) staphylococci usually also are resistant to cefoxitin. *Enterococcus faecalis* (formerly *S. faecalis*) is resistant to cefoxitin concentrations obtainable in serum.

■ **Gram-negative Aerobic Bacteria** Cefoxitin is generally active in vitro against the following Enterobacteriaceae: *Escherichia coli, Klebsiella* (including *K. pneumoniae*), *Morganella morganii* (formerly *Proteus morganii*), *Proteus mirabilis, P. vulgaris, Providencia rettgeri* (formerly *Proteus rettgeri*), *Salmonella*, and *Shigella*. The MIC_{90} (minimum inhibitory concentration of the drug at which 90% of strains tested are inhibited) of cefoxitin for most of these Enterobacteriaceae is 4–16 mcg/mL.

Cefoxitin is active in vitro against most strains of *Haemophilus influenzae* and is also active against many strains of *N. gonorrhoeae*, including both penicillinase- and nonpenicillinase-producing strains. However, antibiotic-resistant strains of *N. gonorrhoeae* are being reported with increasing frequency, and decreased susceptibility to cefoxitin has been reported in strains with chromosomally mediated resistance and in those with plasmid-mediated resistance to tetracycline (TRNG).

Pseudomonas aeruginosa is resistant to the drug.

Cefoxitin is active in vitro against β-lactamase-negative strains of *Eikenella corrodens*. In vitro, cefoxitin concentrations of 0.25 mcg/mL or less inhibit most strains of *Legionella pneumophila*; however, in vivo activity has not been demonstrated to date.

■ **Anaerobic Bacteria** Cefoxitin is active in vitro against certain gram-negative anaerobic bacteria, including some strains of *Bacteroides, Fusobacterium*, and *Prevotella*, and certain gram-positive anaerobic bacteria, including some strains of *Clostridium, Peptococcus, Peptostreptococcus*, and *Propionibacterium*.

The MIC_{50} of cefoxitin reported for *B. fragilis, B. distasonis, B. ovatus, B. thetaiotamicron, B. uniformis*, and *B. vulgatus* is 8–32 mcg/mL; however, the MIC_{90} of the drug reported for these *Bacteroides* is 16–64 mcg/mL or greater.

The MIC_{90} of cefoxitin reported for *Prevotella bivia, P. disiens, P. oralis*, and *P. melaninogenica* (formerly *B. bivius, B. disiens, B. oralis*, and *B. melaninogenicus*) is 2–16 mcg/mL.

Fusobacterium nucleatum, F. necrophorum, F. varium, Peptostreptococcus, and *Propionibacterium acnes* generally are inhibited in vitro by cefoxitin concentrations of 1–16 mcg/mL.

While the MIC_{90} of cefoxitin reported for *C. perfringens* is 1 mcg/mL, *C. difficile* is resistant to the drug.

■ **Mycobacteria** Cefoxitin is active in vitro against some mycobacteria, including *Mycobacterium abscessus, M. fortuitum*, and *M. mucogenicum*. Cefoxitin has variable activity against *M. smegmatis*; however, *M. chelonae* and *M. immunogenum* are resistant to the drug.

Resistance

For information on possible mechanisms of bacterial resistance to β-lactam antibiotics, see Resistance in the Cephalosporins General Statement 8:12.06.

Because of the 7α-methoxy group on the β-lactam ring, cefoxitin is generally more resistant than first generation cephalosporins to staphylococcal β-lactamases and most β-lactamases produced by gram-negative aerobic and anaerobic bacteria.

Pharmacokinetics

■ **Absorption** Cefoxitin sodium is not appreciably absorbed from the GI tract and must be given parenterally. Following a single 1-g IM dose of cefoxitin in healthy adults with normal renal function, peak serum cefoxitin concentrations are attained within 20–30 minutes and average 22–24 mcg/mL; serum concentrations of the drug average 6.4 mcg/mL at 2 hours. After a single 1-g IV dose of cefoxitin given over 3 minutes in adults with normal renal function, serum concentrations of the drug average 110–125 mcg/mL at 5 minutes and less than 1–2 mcg/mL at 4 hours. A single 2-g IV dose given over 3 minutes results in average serum cefoxitin concentrations of 221 mcg/mL at 5 minutes and 3.6 mcg/mL at 4 hours.

In a group of children 3 months to 6 years of age, 37.5 mg/kg of cefoxitin administered IV over 5 minutes every 6 hours resulted in average serum drug concentrations of 82 mcg/mL at 15 minutes, 27 mcg/mL at 1 hour, and 1.4 mcg/mL at 4 hours after each dose.

■ **Distribution** Cefoxitin is widely distributed into body tissues and fluids including ascitic, pleural, and synovial fluid. Therapeutic concentrations of the drug may be obtained in bile if biliary obstruction is not present. The drug diffuses poorly into CSF following IM or IV administration, even when meninges are inflamed. Cefoxitin is 50–80% bound to plasma proteins.

Cefoxitin readily crosses the placenta, and fetal serum concentrations may be equal to maternal serum concentrations. Small amounts of the drug are distributed into milk.

■ **Elimination** The serum half-life of cefoxitin is 0.7–1.1 hours in adults with normal renal function. In one study in geriatric patients 64–88 years of age with renal function normal for their age, the half-life of cefoxitin was 0.9–1.5 hours and plasma concentrations of the drug were higher than in younger adults.

Serum concentrations of the drug are higher and the serum half-life is prolonged in patients with renal impairment. Serum half-life is reported to average 6.3 hours and 21.5 hours in adults with creatinine clearances of about 18 mL/minute and 2 mL/minute, respectively.

Approximately 2% or less of a dose of cefoxitin is metabolized to descarbamylcefoxitin which is microbiologically inactive. Cefoxitin is rapidly excreted in urine by both glomerular filtration and tubular secretion. The same system of anion transport is responsible for the tubular secretion of cefoxitin as for other β-lactam antibiotics and probenecid. Oral probenecid administered shortly before, or with cefoxitin usually slows the rate of excretion of cefoxitin and produces higher and more prolonged serum concentrations. In adults with normal renal function, approximately 85% of a single IM or IV dose of cefoxitin is excreted unchanged in the urine within 6 hours. Peak urinary concentrations of the drug may be 3 mg/mL or greater following a single 1-g IM dose in adults.

Cefoxitin is removed by hemodialysis, but not by peritoneal dialysis.

Chemistry and Stability

■ **Chemistry** Cefoxitin is a semisynthetic cephamycin antibiotic derived from cephamycin C, a substance produced by *Streptomyces lactamdurans*. The drug is a β-lactam antibiotic structurally and pharmacologically related to cephalosporins and penicillins. Cephamycins contain a methoxy group rather than a hydrogen at the 7α-position on the β-lactam ring of the cephalosporin nucleus.

Cefoxitin is commercially available as the sodium salt which occurs as a somewhat hygroscopic, white to off-white powder or granules having a slight characteristic odor. Cefoxitin sodium is very soluble in water and slightly soluble in alcohol. Each gram of cefoxitin as the sodium salt contains approximately 53.8 mg (2.3 mEq) of sodium.

Following reconstitution of the commercially available powder for injection with sterile or bacteriostatic water for injection, 0.9% sodium chloride injection, or 5% dextrose injection, cefoxitin sodium solutions have a pH of 4.2–7 and are colorless to light amber.

When the commercially available Duplex® delivery system containing 1 or 2 g of cefoxitin powder and 50 mL of 4 or 2.2% dextrose injection, respectively, in separate chambers is reconstituted (activated) according to the manufacturer's directions, the resultant solution is iso-osmotic and has an osmolality of approximately 290 mOsm/kg.

Commercially available frozen premixed injections of cefoxitin sodium in dextrose are sterile, nonpyrogenic, iso-osmotic solutions of the drug provided in a plastic container fabricated from specially formulated multilayered plastic PL 2040 (Galaxy®). The 1- or 2-g frozen injections of cefoxitin contain approximately 2 or 1.1 g of dextrose, respectively, to adjust osmolality. The 1- or 2-g frozen injections also contain sodium bicarbonate and may contain hydrochloric acid to adjust pH to approximately 6.5.

■ **Stability** Cefoxitin sodium powder for injection should be stored at 2–25°C and should not exposed to temperatures exceeding 50°C.

Following reconstitution with sterile or bacteriostatic water for injection, 0.9% sodium chloride injection, or 5% dextrose injection, cefoxitin sodium IV solutions containing approximately 100 mg of cefoxitin per mL are stable for 6 hours at room temperature or 1 week when refrigerated at less than 5°C. Reconstituted IV solutions that have been further diluted in 50 mL to 1 L of a compatible IV infusion solution are stable for an additional 18 hours at room temperature or an additional 48 hours when refrigerated.

The commercially available Duplex® drug delivery system containing 1 or 2 g of cefoxitin powder and 50 mL of dextrose injection in separate chambers should be stored at 20–25°C, but may be exposed to 15–30°C. Following reconstitution (activation), these IV infusions must be used within 12 hours if stored at room temperature or within 7 days if stored in a refrigerator and should not be frozen.

The commercially available frozen premixed cefoxitin sodium injection in dextrose should be stored at −20°C or lower. The frozen injections should be thawed at room temperature (25°C) or under refrigeration (5°C) and, once thawed, should not be refrozen. Thawed solutions of the commercially available frozen injections are stable for 24 hours at room temperature (25°C) or 21 days under refrigeration (2–8°C); after these periods, any unused solution should be discarded. The commercially available frozen premixed injections of the drug are provided in plastic containers fabricated from specially formulated multilayered plastic PL 2040 (Galaxy® containers). Solutions in contact with PL 2040 can leach out some of its chemical components in very small amounts within the expiration period of the injection; however, safety of the plastic has been confirmed in tests in animals according to USP biological tests for plastic containers as well as by tissue culture toxicity studies.

Cefoxitin sodium powder for injection and solutions of the drug may darken; however, this is not an indication of change in potency. Cefoxitin sodium is most stable at pH 4–8; the free acid may precipitate at pH less than 4, and hydrolysis of the β-lactam ring may occur at pH greater than 8.

Cefoxitin sodium is potentially physically and/or chemically incompatible with some drugs, including aminoglycosides, but the compatibility depends on several factors (e.g., concentrations of the drugs, specific diluents used, resulting pH, temperature). Specialized references should be consulted for specific compatibility information. Because of the potential for incompatibility, the manufacturer states that cefoxitin sodium and aminoglycosides should not be admixed.

Preparations

Excipients in commercially available drug preparations may have clinically important effects in some individuals; consult specific product labeling for details.

cefOXitin Sodium

Parenteral		
For injection	1 g (of cefoxitin)*	**Cefoxitin Sodium for Injection**
	2 g (of cefoxitin)*	**Cefoxitin Sodium for Injection**
For injection, for IV infusion	1 g (of cefoxitin)*	**Cefoxitin Sodium for Injection** (available in dual-chambered Duplex® drug delivery system with 4% dextrose injection), B Braun
	2 g (of cefoxitin)*	**Cefoxitin Sodium for Injection** (available in dual-chambered Duplex® drug delivery system with 2.2% dextrose injection), B Braun
	10 g (of cefoxitin) pharmacy bulk package*	**Cefoxitin Sodium for Injection**

*available from one or more manufacturer, distributor, and/or repackager by generic (nonproprietary) name

cefOXitin Sodium in Dextrose

Parenteral		
Injection (frozen), for IV infusion	20 mg (of cefoxitin) per mL (1 g) in 4% Dextrose*	**Mefoxin® in Dextrose Injection,** Bioniche
	40 mg (of cefoxitin) per mL (2 g) in 2.2% Dextrose*	**Mefoxin® in Dextrose Injection,** Bioniche

*available from one or more manufacturer, distributor, and/or repackager by generic (nonproprietary) name

†Use is not currently included in the labeling approved by the US Food and Drug Administration

MONOBACTAMS 8:12.07.16

Aztreonam

Azthreonam

■ Aztreonam is a synthetic monocyclic β-lactam (i.e., monobactam) antibiotic.

Uses

Aztreonam is used parenterally for the treatment of intra-abdominal infections (including peritonitis), gynecologic infections (including endometritis and pelvic cellulitis), lower respiratory tract infections (including pneumonia and bronchitis), septicemia, skin and skin structure infections (including those associated with postoperative wounds or ulcers and burns), and complicated and uncomplicated urinary tract infections (including pyelonephritis and cystitis) caused by susceptible gram-negative aerobic bacteria.

Aztreonam is used by oral inhalation via nebulization to improve respiratory symptoms in certain cystic fibrosis patients with *Pseudomonas aeruginosa* in the lungs.

Parenteral aztreonam should *not* be used alone for empiric therapy in seriously ill patients if there is a possibility that the infection may be caused by gram-positive bacteria or if a mixed aerobic-anaerobic bacterial infection is suspected. If potential pathogens also include gram-positive or anaerobic bacteria, an anti-infective active against such bacteria should be used concomitantly with aztreonam pending results of in vitro culture and susceptibility testing. Parenteral aztreonam has been used safely and effectively in conjunction with vancomycin, clindamycin, an aminoglycoside, erythromycin, metronidazole, or a penicillin. However, anti-infectives that have been shown to be potent inducers of β-lactamase production in gram-negative aerobes in vitro (e.g., cefoxitin, imipenem) should *not* be used concomitantly with aztreonam since the drugs may antagonize the antibacterial activity of aztreonam. (See β-Lactam Antibiotics under Drug Interactions: Antibacterial Agents.) If an aminoglycoside is used concomitantly with aztreonam, renal function should be monitored, especially if high aminoglycoside dosage is used or if concomitant therapy is prolonged.

■ **Bone and Joint Infections** Aztreonam has been effective when used parenterally in adults for the treatment of bone and joint infections† caused by susceptible aerobic gram-negative bacteria, including osteomyelitis or septic arthritis, caused by susceptible *Enterobacter, Escherichia coli, Klebsiella, Proteus mirabilis, Ps. aeruginosa,* or *Serratia marcescens*. The drug also has been effective when used parenterally in a limited number of children for the treatment of osteomyelitis, osteochondritis, or septic arthritis caused by susceptible *Ps. aeruginosa* or *Haemophilus influenzae*†. An antistaphylococcal anti-infective agent (e.g., a penicillinase-resistant penicillin, vancomycin) should be used concomitantly with aztreonam if gram-positive bacteria are known or suspected to also be involved.

The Infectious Diseases Society of America (IDSA) states that aztreonam can be considered an alternative for the treatment of native vertebral osteomyelitis† caused by *Ps. aeruginosa* when a drug of first choice (i.e., cefepime, meropenem, doripenem) cannot be used because the patient has severe penicillin allergy and when ciprofloxacin cannot be used because the infection is caused by a quinolone-resistant strain.

For additional information on management of osteomyelitis, the current clinical practice guidelines from IDSA available at http://www.idsociety.org should be consulted.

■ **Gynecologic Infections** Aztreonam has been used parenterally for the treatment of gynecologic infections (including endometritis or pelvic cellulitis) caused by susceptible gram-negative aerobic bacteria, including *Enterobacter* (including *E. cloacae*), *E. coli, Klebsiella pneumoniae*, or *P. mirabilis*.

Because gynecologic infections generally are polymicrobial and frequently are mixed aerobic-anaerobic bacterial infections, aztreonam should *not* be used alone for empiric treatment of these infections. If used for initial treatment of gynecologic infections, aztreonam generally is used in conjunction with clindamycin or metronidazole. Aztreonam is not included in US Centers for Disease Control and Prevention guidelines for treatment of acute pelvic inflammatory disease (PID).

■ **Intra-abdominal Infections** Aztreonam is used parenterally for the treatment of intra-abdominal infections (including peritonitis) caused by susceptible gram-negative aerobic bacteria, including *Citrobacter* (including *C. freundii*), *Enterobacter* (including *E. cloacae*), *E. coli, Klebsiella* (including *K. pneumoniae*), *Ps. aeruginosa*, or *Serratia* (including *S. marcescens*).

Because intra-abdominal infections generally are polymicrobial and frequently are mixed aerobic-anaerobic bacterial infections, aztreonam should *not* be used alone for empiric treatment of these infections. Aztreonam generally is used in conjunction with clindamycin or metronidazole for initial treatment of intra-abdominal infections. In controlled studies in patients with intra-abdominal infections (including peritonitis), parenteral aztreonam used in conjunction with clindamycin was as effective as gentamicin or tobramycin used in conjunction with clindamycin for the treatment of these infections.

For initial empiric treatment of high-risk or severe community-acquired, extrabiliary, complicated intra-abdominal infections in adults (e.g., those with advanced age, immunocompromise, severe physiologic disturbance), IDSA recommends either monotherapy with a carbapenem (doripenem, imipenem, meropenem) or the fixed combination of piperacillin and tazobactam (piperacillin/tazobactam), or a combination regimen that includes either a cephalosporin (cefepime, ceftazidime) or fluoroquinolone (ciprofloxacin, levofloxacin) in conjunction with metronidazole. These experts state that aztreonam in conjunction with metronidazole is an alternative regimen for initial empiric treatment in these patients, but an additional anti-infective agent active against gram-positive bacteria is recommended pending results of in vitro culture and susceptibility tests. For additional information on management of intra-abdominal infections, the current clinical practice guidelines from IDSA available at http://www.idsociety.org should be consulted.

For the treatment of peritonitis in patients undergoing continuous ambulatory peritoneal dialysis (CAPD), aztreonam has been administered intraperitoneally†. Some clinicians suggest that intraperitoneal anti-infectives are preferred over IV anti-infectives for empiric treatment of peritonitis in CAPD patients and such regimens should provide coverage against both gram-positive and gram-negative bacteria pending results of in vitro culture and susceptibility testing. Vancomycin or a first generation cephalosporin (e.g., cefazolin) given intraperitoneally can be used for gram-positive coverage; a third generation cephalosporin (e.g., cefepime, ceftazidime) or aminoglycoside given intraperitoneally usually is used for gram-negative coverage. An intraperitoneal regimen of vancomycin and aztreonam has been used for the treatment of peritonitis in CAPD patients, and some clinicians state that intraperitoneal aztreonam is an alternative for empiric gram-negative coverage in CAPD patients allergic to cephalosporins.

■ **Respiratory Tract Infections** Aztreonam is used parenterally for the treatment of lower respiratory tract infections (including pneumonia or bronchitis) caused by susceptible gram-negative aerobic bacteria including *Enterobacter, E. coli, H. influenzae, K. pneumoniae, P. mirabilis, Ps. aeruginosa,* or *S. marcescens*. The drug also has been effective for the treatment of lower respiratory tract infections caused by susceptible *Citrobacter*†, *Hafnia*†, *K. oxytoca*†, *Morganella*†, *P. vulgaris*†, *Providencia stuartii*†, or *Moraxella catarrhalis*†.

Because lower respiratory tract infections frequently are caused by gram-positive and/or anaerobic bacteria, aztreonam should *not* be used alone for empiric treatment of these infections. A combination regimen of clindamycin and aztreonam has been used for initial empiric treatment of lower respiratory tract infections (especially nosocomial infections).

For additional information on management of respiratory tract infections, including community-acquired pneumonia (CAP), the current clinical practice guidelines from IDSA available at http://www.idsociety.org should be consulted.

Cystic Fibrosis Patients Parenteral aztreonam has been used alone or in conjunction with a parenteral aminoglycoside for the treatment of acute exacerbations of bronchopulmonary *Ps. aeruginosa* infections in some patients with cystic fibrosis. As with other anti-infective agents, a bacteriologic cure is rarely obtained and should not be expected in cystic fibrosis patients.

Oral Inhalation via Nebulization. Aztreonam is used by oral inhalation via nebulization to improve respiratory symptoms in cystic fibrosis patients 7 years of age or older with *Ps. aeruginosa* in the lungs. Safety and efficacy of aztreonam oral inhalation therapy have *not* been established in pediatric patients younger than 7 years of age, in patients with forced expiratory volume in 1 second (FEV_1) less than 25% or exceeding 75% of predicted values, or in patients colonized with *Burkholderia cepacia*.

When aztreonam oral inhalation therapy is indicated, solutions for oral inhalation via nebulization should be prepared using *only* the commercially available powder for inhalation solution (see Oral Inhalation via Nebulization under Dosage and Administration: Reconstitution and Administration). Commercially available preparations of the drug for parenteral use should *not* be used to prepare extemporaneous solutions for oral inhalation.

Efficacy of aztreonam oral inhalation therapy in cystic fibrosis patients 7 years of age or older with *Ps. aeruginosa* in the lungs was evaluated in a randomized, double-blind, placebo-controlled, multicenter trial. The trial enrolled 164 adults and pediatric patients 7 years of age or older with FEV_1 of 25–75% of predicted values (mean age 30 years [77% were 18 years of age or older], 43% female, 96% Caucasian, mean baseline FEV_1 55% of predicted values). Patients were randomized in a 1:1 ratio to receive a 28-day regimen of aztreonam (75 mg 3 times daily) or volume-matched placebo (3 times daily) administered by oral inhalation via nebulization. All patients were required to take a dose of an inhaled bronchodilator (β-agonist) prior to each inhaled dose of aztreonam or placebo. Patients were receiving standard care for cystic fibrosis, including drugs for obstructive airway diseases; those who had received an anti-infective within the last 28 days were excluded. The primary efficacy end point was improvement in respiratory symptoms on the last day of oral inhalation treatment with aztreonam or placebo; respiratory symptoms also were assessed 2 weeks after completion of treatment. Changes in respiratory symptoms (e.g., cough, wheezing, sputum production) were assessed using a patient questionnaire.

On the last day of oral inhalation treatment, improvement in respiratory symptoms was noted in aztreonam-treated patients relative to placebo-treated patients. Statistically significant improvements were seen in both adult and pediatric patients, but were substantially smaller in adults. At 2 weeks after completion of treatment, a difference in respiratory symptoms between treatment groups was still present, but the difference was smaller. Pulmonary function, as measured by FEV_1 (L), increased from baseline in patients treated with aztreonam and decreased in those treated with placebo. On the last day of treatment, there was a 10% difference between aztreonam-treated and placebo-treated patients in percent change in FEV_1 (L); improvements in FEV_1 were comparable between adult and pediatric patients. At 2 weeks after completion of treatment, the difference in FEV_1 between aztreonam-treated and placebo-treated patients had decreased to 6%.

■ **Septicemia** Aztreonam is used parenterally for the treatment of septicemia caused by susceptible gram-negative aerobic bacteria, including *Enterobacter, E. coli, K. pneumoniae, Ps. aeruginosa, P. mirabilis,* and *S. marcescens*. The drug also has been effective when used parenterally in a limited number of adults for the treatment of septicemia caused by susceptible *Citrobacter*† or *H. influenzae*†.

Aztreonam has generally been effective in either community-acquired or nosocomial septicemia known to be caused by susceptible gram-negative aerobes, and has been as effective as gentamicin or ceftazidime in the treatment of these infections.

■ **Skin and Skin Structure Infections** Aztreonam is used parenterally for the treatment of skin and skin structure infections, including those associated with postoperative wounds or ulcers and burns, caused by susceptible gram-negative aerobic bacteria, including *Citrobacter, Enterobacter, E. coli, K. pneumoniae, P. mirabilis, Ps. aeruginosa,* or *S. marcescens*.

Aztreonam is used as an adjunct to surgery in the management of abscesses, cutaneous infections, infections complicating hollow viscus perforations, or infections of serous surfaces caused by susceptible gram-negative aerobic bacteria.

When empiric treatment of moderate or severe diabetic foot infections is indicated, IDSA recommends use of a broad-spectrum regimen pending results of in vitro culture and susceptibility testing. When probable pathogens include methicillin-resistant *Staphylococcus aureus* (MRSA; also known as oxacillin-resistant *S. aureus* or ORSA), Enterobacteriaceae, *Pseudomonas*, and obligate anaerobes, IDSA recommends an empiric regimen of vancomycin used in conjunction with ceftazidime, cefepime, piperacillin/tazobactam, aztreonam, or a carbapenem. If aztreonam, ceftazidime, or cefepime is used in conjunction with vancomycin, the empiric regimen should also include an additional anti-infective for anaerobic coverage.

For additional information on management of skin and skin structure infections, the current clinical practice guidelines from IDSA available at http://www.idsociety.org should be consulted.

■ **Urinary Tract Infections** Aztreonam is used parenterally for the treatment of complicated or uncomplicated urinary tract infections (UTIs), including pyelonephritis and initial and recurrent cystitis, caused by susceptible gram-negative aerobes, including *Citrobacter*, *E. cloacae*, *E. coli*, *K. oxytoca*, *K. pneumoniae*, *P. mirabilis*, *Ps. aeruginosa*, and *S. marcescens*. The drug also has been effective when used parenterally in a limited number of adults for the treatment of UTIs caused by susceptible *E. aerogenes*†, *Morganella morganii*†, *P. vulgaris*†, or *Providencia*†. Aztreonam has been effective in the treatment of cystitis or pyelonephritis caused by gram-negative aerobic bacteria resistant to aminopenicillins, first or second generation cephalosporins, and/or aminoglycosides.

In controlled studies in men and women with UTIs, 5–14 days of aztreonam therapy was at least as effective as 5–14 days of therapy with an aminoglycoside (i.e., gentamicin, tobramycin) or a parenteral cephalosporin (i.e., cefotaxime, ceftriaxone). Although aztreonam therapy generally is associated with less toxicity than aminoglycoside therapy, colonization or superinfection with gram-positive bacteria (especially *Enterococcus faecalis* [formerly *Streptococcus faecalis*]) has been reported more frequently with aztreonam than with aminoglycosides.

In a controlled study in women with uncomplicated cystitis caused by *E. coli*, a single 1-g IM dose of aztreonam was as effective as 10 days of therapy with oral amoxicillin (250 mg 3 times daily); however, efficacy of a single dose of aztreonam in the treatment of these infections has not been established.

■ **Perioperative Prophylaxis** Aztreonam has been used parenterally in conjunction with other anti-infectives for perioperative prophylaxis† in patients undergoing certain surgical procedures in which aerobic gram-negative bacteria are common pathogens.

Some clinicians state that a regimen of vancomycin (or clindamycin) in conjunction with aztreonam can be used as an alternative regimen for perioperative prophylaxis in patients undergoing gastroduodenal or biliary tract surgery, hysterectomy (vaginal or abdominal), or certain organ transplant procedures (liver, pancreas, pancreas-kidney). These clinicians state that a regimen of clindamycin and aztreonam can be used as an alternative regimen in patients undergoing appendectomy, colorectal or small intestine surgery, or urologic surgery involving an implanted prosthesis.

Some clinicians recommend that an anti-infective active against enteric gram-negative bacilli (e.g., aztreonam, an aminoglycoside, a fluoroquinolone) be used concomitantly when vancomycin is used for perioperative prophylaxis in patients undergoing neurosurgery or cardiac, orthopedic, or vascular surgery.

■ **Empiric Therapy in Febrile Neutropenic Patients** Aztreonam has been used parenterally in conjunction with vancomycin (with or without amikacin) for empiric anti-infective therapy in febrile granulocytopenic adults†. Because gram-positive bacteria (especially *S. epidermidis*) are being reported with increasing frequency in febrile granulocytopenic patients and because aztreonam is inactive against these organisms, an anti-infective agent active against staphylococci (e.g., vancomycin) should be used in conjunction with aztreonam if the drug is used for empiric therapy in these patients. Some clinicians suggest that a regimen of aztreonam and vancomycin can be used as an alternative empiric regimen in patients with immediate-type penicillin hypersensitivity (see Cautions: Precautions and Contraindications).

Published protocols for the treatment of infections in febrile neutropenic patients should be consulted for specific recommendations regarding selection of the initial empiric regimen, when to change the initial regimen, possible subsequent regimens, and duration of therapy in these patients.

Dosage and Administration

■ **Reconstitution and Administration** Aztreonam is administered by IV injection or infusion or by deep IM injection.

Aztreonam also is administered by oral inhalation via nebulization using the commercially available powder for inhalation solution.

Aztreonam has been administered intraperitoneally† in dialysis fluid.

Parenteral Administration Aztreonam is administered IV or IM depending on the type and severity of infection, susceptibility of the causative organism, and condition of the patient.

The manufacturers recommend that aztreonam be given IV (rather than IM) in patients with septicemia, localized parenchymal abscess (such as intra-abdominal abscess), peritonitis, or other severe systemic or life-threatening infection and when individual doses greater than 1 g are indicated.

Aztreonam solutions for IV or IM administration should be inspected visually for particulate matter and discoloration prior to administration whenever solution and container permit. Any unused solution should be discarded.

When aztreonam is given IV via a common administration tubing used to administer another drug, especially one that is incompatible with aztreonam, the tubing should be flushed before and after aztreonam administration with an IV infusion solution compatible with both drugs; the drugs should not be given simultaneously. When a Y-type IV administration set is used to administer aztreonam, careful attention should be given to the calculated volume of aztreonam solution to ensure that the entire dose is infused.

Intermittent IV Injection. For direct intermittent IV injection, the contents of a single-dose vial labeled as containing 500 mg, 1 g, or 2 g of aztreonam should be reconstituted by adding 6–10 mL of sterile water for injection. The vial should be vigorously shaken immediately after the diluent is added.

The appropriate dose of reconstituted solution should then be injected slowly over a period of 3–5 minutes either directly into a vein or into the tubing of a compatible IV solution.

Intermittent IV Infusion. For intermittent IV infusion, a single-dose vial labeled as containing 500 mg, 1 g, or 2 g of aztreonam should be reconstituted by adding at least 1.5, 3, or 6 mL, respectively, of sterile water for injection. The vial should be vigorously shaken immediately after the diluent is added. The reconstituted solution should then be further diluted in a compatible IV infusion solution to provide a solution with a final concentration not exceeding 20 mg/mL. A volume control IV administration set may be used to add the appropriate dose of reconstituted aztreonam solution to the compatible IV infusion solution during administration; this final dilution should provide a solution with a concentration of 20 mg/mL or less.

Alternatively, thawed solutions of the commercially available frozen premixed aztreonam injection in dextrose in Galaxy plastic containers should be administered by intermittent IV infusion. The frozen premixed aztreonam injections should be thawed at room temperature (25° C) or in a refrigerator (2–8°C); the frozen injections should not be thawed by warming in a water bath or by exposure to microwave radiation. After thawing, the container should be inverted to assure a well-mixed solution and checked for minute leaks by firmly squeezing the bag. Precipitates that may have formed in the frozen solution usually dissolve with little or no agitation when the solution reaches room temperature. The premixed injection should be discarded if the container seal or outlet ports are not intact or leaks are found or if the solution is cloudy, discolored, or contains a precipitate. Additives should not be introduced into the container and other drugs should not be infused simultaneously through the same IV line. The premixed injections should not be used in series connections with other plastic containers since such use could result in air embolism from residual air being drawn from the primary container before administration of fluid from the secondary container is complete. The manufacturer recommends that the IV administration set be replaced every 48 hours.

Intermittent IV infusions of aztreonam should be infused over 20–60 minutes.

IM Injection. For IM administration, a single-dose vial labeled as containing 500 mg, 1 g, or 2 g of aztreonam should be reconstituted by adding at least 1.5, 3, or 6 mL, respectively, of sterile water for injection, 0.9% sodium chloride injection, bacteriostatic water for injection (with benzyl alcohol or parabens), or bacteriostatic sodium chloride injection (with benzyl alcohol). The vial should be vigorously shaken immediately after the diluent is added.

The appropriate dose of reconstituted solution should be given by deep IM injection into a large muscle (e.g., upper outer quadrant of the gluteus maximus, lateral part of the thigh). Aztreonam generally is well tolerated when given IM and should not be admixed with local anesthetic agents.

Oral Inhalation via Nebulization For administration by oral inhalation via nebulization, aztreonam is commercially available in a kit containing single-dose vials of lyophilized aztreonam powder for inhalation solution and single-dose ampuls of 0.17% sodium chloride diluent.

Following reconstitution, aztreonam inhalation solution is administered via nebulization using *only* an Altera® nebulizer system. The manufacturer states that the reconstituted inhalation solution should *not* be administered using any other type of nebulizer and should *not* be administered IV or IM.

Patients receiving aztreonam oral inhalation therapy should use a bronchodilator before aztreonam is administered. Short-acting bronchodilators can be taken between 15 minutes and 4 hours prior to each aztreonam dose. Alternatively, long-acting bronchodilators can be taken 0.5–12 hours prior to administration of aztreonam. For patients taking multiple inhaled therapies, the recommended order of administration is a bronchodilator, mucolytics, and, lastly, aztreonam.

Aztreonam powder for inhalation solution should be reconstituted using *only* the diluent provided in the kit supplied by the manufacturer and should *not* be reconstituted until it is time to administer a dose.

To prepare a dose of aztreonam inhalation solution for oral inhalation via nebulization, the contents of a single-dose ampul of diluent provided by the manufacturer should be added to a single-dose vial of aztreonam powder for inhalation solution. The vial should be gently swirled until the powder has completely dissolved. The inhalation solution should be administered by oral inhalation via nebulization *immediately* after reconstitution.

The reconstituted aztreonam inhalation solution should be poured into the handset of the Altera® nebulizer system and the unit should be turned on. The reconstituted inhalation solution should *not* be mixed with any other drug in the Altera® nebulizer handset.

To administer the dose, the patient should be seated in a relaxed, upright position. The mouthpiece of the nebulizer handset should be placed into the mouth; with lips closed around the mouthpiece, the patient should breathe normally through the mouthpiece.

A period of about 2–3 minutes usually is required to administer the complete dose of reconstituted inhalation solution via the nebulizer. The manufacturer's information should be consulted for additional information on how to administer aztreonam inhalation solution. Instructions on testing nebulizer functionality and cleaning the handset are provided in the instructions for use included with the nebulizer system.

■ **Dosage** Dosage and route of administration of aztreonam should be determined by the type and severity of infection, susceptibility of the causative organism, and the condition of the patient. Dosages lower than the recommended dosage of the drug should not be used.

For most infections, parenteral aztreonam treatment should be continued for at least 48 hours after the patient becomes asymptomatic or evidence of eradication of the infection has been obtained. Persistent infections may require several weeks of treatment.

Parenteral Adult Dosage **General Adult Dosage.** The usual adult IV or IM dosage of aztreonam for the treatment of moderately severe systemic infections in adults is 1 g IV or IM or 2 g IV every 8 or 12 hours. For the treatment of severe systemic or life-threatening infections in adults, including infections caused by *Pseudomonas aeruginosa*, the usual adult dosage of aztreonam is 2 g IV every 6 or 8 hours.

Dosage in geriatric patients should be selected with caution because of the greater frequency of decreased hepatic, renal, and/or cardiac function and of concomitant disease and drug therapy observed in these patients. Aztreonam is substantially eliminated by the kidneys and the risk of adverse reactions may be greater in patients with impaired renal function. Because geriatric patients are more likely to have renal impairment, renal function should be monitored and appropriate dosage modifications made if necessary. (See Renal Impairment under Dosage: Dosage in Renal and Hepatic Impairment, in Dosage and Administration.)

The manufacturers state that the maximum recommended IV or IM dosage of aztreonam for adults is 8 g daily.

Bone and Joint Infections. If aztreonam is used as an alternative for the treatment of osteomyelitis† caused by *Ps. aeruginosa*, the Infectious Diseases Society of America (IDSA) recommends that adults receive 2 g IV every 8 hours for 6 weeks.

Intra-abdominal Infections. If aztreonam is used in the treatment of intra-abdominal infections (see Uses: Intra-abdominal Infections), IDSA recommends that adults receive 1–2 g IV every 6–8 hours. These experts state that the usual duration of anti-infective treatment for complicated intra-abdominal infections is 4–7 days, unless it is difficult to achieve adequate source control.

Urinary Tract Infections. The usual adult IV or IM dosage of aztreonam for the treatment of urinary tract infections is 500 mg or 1 g every 8 or 12 hours.

The usual duration of aztreonam therapy for the treatment of uncomplicated urinary tract infections is 5–10 days; therapy should be continued for at least 10–18 days for the treatment of complicated urinary tract infections.

Perioperative Prophylaxis. If aztreonam is used for perioperative prophylaxis† (see Uses: Perioperative Prophylaxis), some clinicians recommend that adults receive 2 g within 1 hour prior to initial incision. During prolonged procedures (longer than 4 hours) or if major blood loss occurs, additional intraoperative doses of aztreonam should be given every 4 hours. The duration of prophylaxis should be less than 24 hours for most procedures; there is no evidence to support continuing prophylaxis after wound closure or until all indwelling drains and intravascular catheters are removed.

Parenteral Pediatric Dosage **General Pediatric Dosage.** The manufacturers recommend that pediatric patients 9 months of age or older with normal renal function receive aztreonam in a dosage of 30 mg/kg IV every 8 hours for the treatment of mild to moderate infections or 30 mg/kg IV every 6 or 8 hours for the treatment of moderate to severe infections. The manufacturers state that the maximum recommended dosage of aztreonam for pediatric patients is 120 mg/kg daily; however, higher dosage may be warranted in those with cystic fibrosis. A dosage of 50 mg/kg IV every 6 or 8 hours (i.e., 150–200 mg/kg daily) has been suggested by some clinicians for the treatment of infections in children with cystic fibrosis†.

Although safe use of aztreonam in neonates has not been established, the American Academy of Pediatrics (AAP) states that neonates 7 days of age or younger† may receive 30 mg/kg of aztreonam IV or IM every 12 hours if they weigh 2 kg or less or 30 mg/kg IV or IM every 8 hours if they weigh more than 2 kg and that neonates 8–28 days of age† may receive 30 mg/kg IV or IM every 8–12 hours if they weigh 2 kg or less or 30 mg/kg IV or IM every 6 hours if they weigh more than 2 kg. For the treatment of *Pseudomonas* infections in neonates 28 days of age or younger, AAP states that IV or IM doses of 50 mg/kg may be necessary.

For pediatric patients beyond the neonatal period, AAP recommends an aztreonam dosage of 90 mg/kg daily given IV or IM in 3 divided doses for the treatment of mild to moderate infections or a dosage of 90–120 mg/kg daily given IV or IM in 3 or 4 divided doses for the treatment of severe infections.

Intra-abdominal Infections. If aztreonam is used in the treatment of intra-abdominal infections, IDSA recommends that pediatric patients receive 90–120 mg/kg daily given IV in divided doses every 6–8 hours. These experts state that the usual duration of anti-infective treatment for complicated intra-abdominal infections is 4–7 days, unless it is difficult to achieve adequate source control.

Oral Inhalation Dosage **Adult and Pediatric Dosage.** When the commercially available aztreonam powder for inhalation solution for administration by oral inhalation via nebulization is used to improve respiratory symptoms in cystic fibrosis patients with *Ps. aeruginosa* in the lungs, the recommended dosage for adults and pediatric patients 7 years of age or older is 75 mg of aztreonam 3 times daily for 28 days. Oral inhalation doses should be taken at least 4 hours apart (e.g., in the morning, after school, at bedtime). The 28-day oral inhalation regimen should be followed by a 28-day period when the drug is not administered.

In clinical trials, adults and pediatric patients with cystic fibrosis have received up to 9 courses of aztreonam oral inhalation therapy; each course consisted of 28 days of aztreonam oral inhalation therapy (75 mg 3 times daily), followed by 28 days without such therapy.

Intraperitoneal Dosage If aztreonam is administered intraperitoneally† for the treatment of peritonitis in adults undergoing continuous ambulatory peritoneal dialysis (CAPD), some clinicians recommend that a 1-g loading dose of the drug be given IV followed by maintenance doses of 500 mg given intraperitoneally† in 2 L of dialysate every 6 hours. For empiric gram-negative coverage in the treatment of peritonitis in patients undergoing CAPD, some clinicians recommend a continuous aztreonam dosing regimen consisting of a loading dose of 1 g per L of dialysate followed by maintenance doses of 250 mg per L of dialysate.

■ Dosage in Renal and Hepatic Impairment

Renal Impairment In adults with renal impairment, doses and/or frequency of administration of IV or IM aztreonam should be modified in response to the degree of renal impairment.

Data are insufficient to date to make dosage recommendations for parenteral aztreonam in pediatric patients with impaired renal function.

When aztreonam is administered by oral inhalation via nebulization, dosage adjustments are not necessary in adults or pediatric patients 7 years of age or older with mild, moderate, or severe renal impairment.

Because serum creatinine concentrations alone may not be sufficiently accurate to assess the degree of renal impairment, especially in geriatric adults, dosage of IV or IM aztreonam preferably should be based on the patient's measured or estimated creatinine clearance. The patient's creatinine clearance (Ccr) can be estimated by using the following formulas:

$$\textit{Ccr male} = \frac{(140 - \textit{age}) \times \textit{weight}}{72 \times \textit{serum creatinine}}$$

$$\textit{Ccr female} = 0.85 \times \textit{Ccr male}$$

where age is in years, weight is in kg, and serum creatinine is in mg/dL.

Adults with creatinine clearances greater than 30 mL/minute per 1.73 m^2 may receive the usual adult dosage of IV or IM aztreonam.

Adults with creatinine clearances of 10–30 mL/minute per 1.73 m^2 should receive an initial 1- or 2-g IV or IM loading dose of aztreonam followed by maintenance doses equal to one-half the usual dose (i.e., 250 mg, 500 mg, or 1 g) given at the usual dosage intervals.

In adults with severe renal failure (creatinine clearances less than 10 mL/minute per 1.73 m^2) and adults undergoing hemodialysis, an initial IV or IM loading dose equal to the usual dose (i.e., 500 mg, 1 g, or 2 g) should be used followed by maintenance doses equal to one-fourth the usual dose (i.e., 125 mg, 250 mg, or 500 mg) given at the usual dosage intervals.

Because aztreonam is removed by hemodialysis, patients with serious or life-threatening infections undergoing hemodialysis receiving IV or IM aztreonam should receive a supplemental IV or IM dose of the drug equal to one-eighth the initial dose (i.e., 62.5 mg, 125 mg, or 250 mg) immediately after each dialysis period in addition to the recommended maintenance doses.

In adults undergoing CAPD, some clinicians recommend an initial IV loading dose of aztreonam equal to the usual dose (i.e., 500 mg, 1 g, or 2 g) followed by maintenance doses equal to one-fourth the usual dose (i.e., 125 mg, 250 mg, or 500 mg) given at the usual dosage intervals.

Hepatic Impairment The serum half-life of aztreonam is only slightly prolonged in patients with hepatic impairment. Modification of usual IV or IM dosage probably is unnecessary in patients with stable primary biliary cirrhosis or other chronic hepatic disease, unless renal function also is impaired. Although some clinicians recommend that parenteral aztreonam dosage be decreased by 20–25% in patients with alcoholic cirrhosis, especially if long-term therapy with the drug is required, others state that this decrease in dosage is unnecessary unless renal function also is impaired.

Cautions

Adverse effects reported with IV or IM aztreonam are similar to those reported with other β-lactam antibiotics, and the drug generally is well tolerated. Adverse effects have been reported in 7% or less of patients receiving parenteral aztreonam and have required discontinuance in about 2% of patients.

■ GI Effects

Diarrhea, nausea, and vomiting have been reported in about 1–2% and GI bleeding, abdominal cramps, and bloating have been reported in less than 1% of patients receiving parenteral aztreonam. A transient, unusual taste has been reported occasionally during and after IV infusion of aztreonam, and numbness of the tongue, oral ulceration, and halitosis have been reported in less than 1% of patients receiving the drug.

Parenteral aztreonam therapy exerts a selective effect on normal bowel flora. Total bacterial counts of normal fecal aerobic gram-negative bacteria are decreased, but total counts of normal fecal anaerobic bacteria generally are unaffected during or following therapy with IV aztreonam. An increase in total fecal counts of enterococci has occurred in healthy adults receiving IV aztreonam, but total fecal counts of staphylococci and fungi generally are unaffected. Bacterial counts of normal fecal flora generally return to pretreatment levels within 1 week after aztreonam therapy is discontinued.

In clinical trials evaluating aztreonam administered by oral inhalation via nebulization, vomiting and abdominal pain were reported in 6 and 7% of patients, respectively.

***Clostridium difficile*-associated Diarrhea and Colitis** Treatment with anti-infectives alters normal colon flora and may permit overgrowth of *Clostridium difficile.*

C. difficile infection (CDI) and *C. difficile*-associated diarrhea and colitis (CDAD; also known as antibiotic-associated diarrhea and colitis or pseudomembranous colitis) have been reported with nearly all systemic anti-infectives, including aztreonam, and may range in severity from mild diarrhea to fatal colitis. *C. difficile* produces toxins A and B, which contribute to the development of CDAD; hypertoxin-producing strains of *C. difficile* are associated with increased morbidity and mortality since they may be refractory to anti-infectives and colectomy may be required. (See Superinfection/Clostridium difficile-associated Diarrhea and Colitis under Cautions: Precautions and Contraindications.)

■ **Dermatologic and Sensitivity Reactions** Rash (with or without eosinophilia) has been reported in about 1–2% of patients receiving parenteral aztreonam. Rash generally has been mild, transient, pruritic, and erythematous, but rarely has been maculopapular or urticarial. Pruritus, purpura, erythema multiforme, angioedema, toxic epidermal necrolysis, urticaria, exfoliative dermatitis, petechiae, and diaphoresis have been reported in less than 1% of patients receiving the drug. Toxic epidermal necrolysis has been reported in association with aztreonam in a few patients undergoing bone marrow transplant; these patients had multiple risk factors including graft versus host disease, sepsis, and radiation therapy, and were receiving other drugs that have been associated with toxic epidermal necrolysis.

Immediate hypersensitivity reactions, including anaphylaxis, bronchospasm, generalized urticaria with or without palpebral and lingual edema and respiratory impairment, and a severe episode of shock, rash, and eosinophilia, have been reported in less than 1% of patients receiving parenteral aztreonam.

Toxic epidermal necrolysis has been reported rarely when parenteral aztreonam was used in patients undergoing bone marrow transplantation; these patients had multiple risk factors, including sepsis, radiation therapy, and concomitant treatment with drugs associated with toxic epidermal necrolysis.

In clinical trials evaluating aztreonam administered by oral inhalation via nebulization, rash was reported in 2% of patients. Allergic reactions with facial rash, facial swelling, and throat tightness were also reported.

The immunogenic risk of aztreonam has not been fully determined. Administration of aztreonam to individuals with a history of hypersensitivity to penicillins and/or cephalosporins has rarely resulted in possible hypersensitivity reactions to aztreonam (i.e., localized or urticarial rash, pharyngeal edema). Cross-allergenicity between ceftazidime and aztreonam has been reported in some individuals. In a study that included 212 individuals with documented immediate (IgE-mediated) hypersensitivity to penicillins who had positive skin test reactions to at least 1 penicillin reagent, all individuals had negative skin test reactions to aztreonam; there was no reaction to aztreonam in the 211 of these individuals who were willing to receive an IM aztreonam challenge. In another study that included 214 individuals with nonimmediate (T cell-mediated) hypersensitivity to penicillins who had positive patch and/or delayed-reading skin test responses to at least 1 penicillin reagent, all individuals had negative skin test reactions to aztreonam and all tolerated IM aztreonam challenges. Studies in rabbits and humans suggest that antibodies produced in response to penicillin G (including IgE antibodies to major and minor determinants) or to cephalothin (no longer commercially available in the US) show negligible cross-reactivity with aztreonam. Likewise, antibodies produced in response to aztreonam have had negligible cross-reactivity with penicillin G, cephalothin, and cefotaxime. In one study in healthy men who had not previously received aztreonam, no IgE antibody response to aztreonam was detectable after therapy with the drug (500-mg or 1-g doses every 8 hours for 7 days). A few of these individuals did have naturally occurring side-chain-specific IgG antibodies to aztreonam, but only one demonstrated an IgG response to the drug. Although there appears to be little cross-allergenicity between aztreonam and bicyclic β-lactam antibiotics, the possibility that cross-sensitivity to aztreonam may occur in patients with a history of hypersensitivity to other β-lactam antibiotics should be considered. (See Cautions: Precautions and Contraindications.)

■ **Hematologic Effects** Transient eosinophilia has been reported in up to 11% of patients receiving parenteral aztreonam. Leukopenia, neutropenia, thrombocytopenia, pancytopenia, anemia, leukocytosis, and thrombocytosis have been reported in less than 1% of patients receiving the drug. Decreased hemoglobin concentration and hematocrit have been reported rarely. Positive direct antiglobulin (Coombs') test results, without clinical or laboratory evidence of hemolytic anemia, also have been reported rarely.

Slight prolongation of the prothrombin time (up to 1.5 times baseline values) and activated partial thromboplastin time, without evidence of bleeding, has been reported rarely during parenteral aztreonam therapy. Clinically apparent bleeding, possibly related to aztreonam therapy, has been reported in several seriously ill patients who received aztreonam as well as several other drugs. In vitro studies indicate that high concentrations of aztreonam (i.e., greater than 2.7 mg/mL) can inhibit adenosine diphosphate (ADP)-, collagen-, and epinephrine-induced platelet aggregation. Although aztreonam therapy (2 g IV every 6 hours) may cause slight inhibition of ADP-induced platelet aggregation, usual dosages of the drug do not appear to have any clinically important effects on platelet function or blood coagulation in adults with normal renal and hepatic function.

■ **Hepatic Effects** Transient increases in serum AST (SGOT), ALT (SGPT), and alkaline phosphatase concentrations have been reported in 2–40% of patients receiving parenteral aztreonam. In most reported cases, liver enzyme concentrations were increased only up to 3 times normal, were not associated with symptoms of hepatobiliary dysfunction, and returned to pretreatment concentrations shortly after aztreonam therapy was completed. Rarely, serum AST and ALT concentrations have increased to more than 10 times normal during aztreonam therapy; hepatitis and jaundice and other manifestations of hepatotoxicity have been reported in less than 1% of patients receiving the drug.

Transient increases in serum bilirubin, LDH, and γ-glutamyltransferase (γ-glutamyl transpeptidase, GGT, GGTP) have been reported rarely.

■ **Local Effects** Phlebitis and/or thrombophlebitis have been reported in 2–3% of patients receiving IV aztreonam. Phlebitis and thrombophlebitis are usually mild, occur about 1 week after initiation of aztreonam therapy, and generally are relieved by changing administration sites, applying warm packs, and other general measures.

Discomfort, pain, and swelling at the injection site have been reported in up to 2–3% of patients receiving IM aztreonam. The drug generally is well tolerated when administered IM and should not be admixed with local anesthetic agents.

■ **Cardiovascular Effects** Hypotension and transient ECG changes, including ventricular bigeminy and ventricular premature complexes (VPCs, PVCs), have been reported in less than 1% of patients receiving parenteral aztreonam. Bradycardia, flushing, chest pain, lower limb edema, and subclavian vein thrombosis have occurred rarely.

■ **Nervous System Effects** Seizures, confusion, disturbed mental processes, insomnia, dizziness, vertigo, paresthesia, weakness, fatigue, malaise, and headache have occurred in less than 1% of patients receiving parenteral aztreonam.

■ **Renal Effects** Transient increases in BUN and/or serum creatinine concentrations have been reported rarely in patients receiving parenteral aztreonam. Aztreonam does not appear to be nephrotoxic in humans. In at least one patient, acute renal failure associated with rash and eosinophilia occurred within about 9 days after initiating aztreonam therapy. Urinary concentrations of β_2-microglobulin and excretion of thermophilic aminopeptidase (alanine aminopeptidase) and *N*-acetyl-β-glucosaminidase, enzymes that originate from renal proximal tubular cells, generally are unaffected in healthy adults receiving usual dosages of the drug. In addition, urinary excretion of *N*-acetyl-β-glucosaminidase reportedly is unaffected during aztreonam therapy in patients with urinary tract infections and impaired renal function.

■ **Respiratory Effects** Dyspnea, wheezing, sneezing, and nasal congestion have been reported in less than 1% of patients receiving parenteral aztreonam.

In clinical trials evaluating aztreonam administered by oral inhalation via nebulization, cough was reported in 54%, nasal congestion and wheezing were each reported in 16%, and bronchospasm was reported in 3% of patients. (See Oral Inhalation via Nebulization under Cautions: Precautions and Contraindications.)

■ **Other Adverse Effects** Fever, chills, cold sweats, tinnitus, impaired hearing in one ear, diplopia, myalgia, vaginitis, vaginal candidiasis, and breast tenderness have been reported in less than 1% of patients receiving parenteral aztreonam.

In clinical trials evaluating aztreonam administered by oral inhalation via nebulization, pyrexia was reported in 13%, pharyngolaryngeal pain was reported in 12%, and chest discomfort was reported in 8% of patients. In addition, there have been postmarketing reports of arthralgia and joint swelling in patients receiving aztreonam by oral inhalation via nebulization.

■ **Precautions and Contraindications** Aztreonam is contraindicated in individuals with known hypersensitivity to the drug or any component in the formulation.

Prior to initiation of aztreonam, careful inquiry should be made concerning previous hypersensitivity reactions to β-lactam antibiotics, other drugs, or allergens. There is clinical and laboratory evidence of partial cross-allergenicity among bicyclic β-lactam antibiotics (e.g., carbapenems, cephalosporins, cephamycins, penicillins). Although cross-allergenicity between aztreonam and bicyclic β-lactam antibiotics has been reported only rarely, the drug should be used with caution in patients with a history of hypersensitivity to β-lactam antibiotics. Treatment with aztreonam can result in hypersensitivity reactions in patients with or without prior exposure to the drug. In addition, hypersensitivity reactions to aztreonam (e.g., localized or urticarial rash) have occurred rarely when the drug was used in patients with a history of hypersensitivity to penicillins and/or cephalosporins. (See Cautions: Dermatologic and Sensitivity Reactions.)

If a hypersensitivity reaction occurs during aztreonam therapy, the drug should be discontinued and appropriate therapy initiated (e.g., vasopressors, antihistamines, corticosteroids, maintenance of ventilation). Serious hypersensitivity reactions may require epinephrine and other emergency measures.

Parenteral **Superinfection/Clostridium difficile-associated Diarrhea and Colitis.** As with other anti-infective agents, use of parenteral aztreonam may result in overgrowth of nonsusceptible organisms, especially gram-positive bacteria (e.g., enterococci, *Staphylococcus aureus*, *Streptococcus pneumoniae*) or fungi. Colonization or superinfection with aztreonam-resistant organisms has occurred in up to 60% of patients receiving the drug, and superinfections have required treatment with another anti-infective agent in about 4–11% of patients. Use of indwelling catheters or the presence of tracheotomy sites or open, draining wounds appears to contribute to the occurrence of superinfections during aztreonam therapy. Resistant strains of some organisms (e.g., *Pseudomonas aeruginosa*, *Klebsiella pneumoniae*) have developed during parenteral aztreonam therapy. (See Resistance.) If superinfection occurs, appropriate therapy should be instituted.

Because CDAD has been reported with the use of anti-infective agents, including aztreonam, it should be considered in the differential diagnosis of patients who develop diarrhea during or after parenteral aztreonam therapy. Careful medical history is necessary since CDAD has been reported to occur as late as 2 months or longer after anti-infective therapy is discontinued. If CDAD is suspected or confirmed, anti-infective therapy not directed against *C. difficile* should be discontinued whenever possible. Patients should be managed with appropriate supportive therapy (e.g., fluid and electrolyte management, protein supplementation), anti-infective therapy directed against *C. difficile* (e.g., metronidazole, vancomycin), and surgical evaluation as clinically indicated. Other causes of colitis also should be considered.

Patients should be advised that diarrhea is a common problem caused by systemic anti-infectives and usually ends when the drug is discontinued; however, it is important to contact a clinician if watery and bloody stools (with or without stomach cramps and fever) occur during or as late as 2 months or longer after the last dose.

Selection and Use of Anti-infectives. To reduce development of drug-resistant bacteria and maintain effectiveness of parenteral aztreonam and other antibacterials, the drug should be used only for the treatment or prevention of infections proven or strongly suspected to be caused by susceptible bacteria.

When selecting or modifying anti-infective therapy, results of culture and in vitro susceptibility testing should be considered. In the absence of such data, local epidemiology and susceptibility patterns should be considered when selecting anti-infectives for empiric therapy. Culture and susceptibility testing performed periodically during therapy provides information on the therapeutic effect of the anti-infective agent and the possible emergence of bacterial resistance.

Patients should be advised that antibacterials (including aztreonam) should only be used to treat bacterial infections and should not be used to treat viral infections (e.g., the common cold). Patients also should be advised about the importance of completing the full course of therapy, even if feeling better after a few days, and that skipping doses or not completing therapy may decrease effectiveness and increase the likelihood that bacteria will develop resistance and will not be treatable with aztreonam or other antibacterials in the future.

Because aztreonam has little or no activity against gram-positive bacteria and anaerobes, another anti-infective active against such bacteria should be used concomitantly if IV or IM aztreonam is used empirically in infections that may involve gram-positive bacteria or anaerobes (e.g., gynecologic, intra-abdominal, or respiratory tract infections).

Patients with Renal and/or Hepatic Impairment. Appropriate laboratory tests should be monitored when aztreonam is used in patients with impaired renal or hepatic function. Doses and/or frequency of administration of IV or IM aztreonam should be decreased in patients with impaired renal function, since serum concentrations of the drug are higher and prolonged in these patients compared with patients with normal renal function. Some clinicians suggest that liver function tests (i.e., serum hepatic enzyme concentrations) be determined once weekly in patients receiving IV or IM aztreonam; however, the manufacturer and other clinicians question the necessity of this precaution.

Oral Inhalation via Nebulization Aztreonam powder for inhalation solution for administration by oral inhalation via nebulization should *only* be used to treat patients with cystic fibrosis who are known to have *Ps. aeruginosa* in the lungs. Use of aztreonam oral inhalation therapy in the absence of known *Ps. aeruginosa* infection is unlikely to provide benefit and increases the risk of development of drug-resistant bacteria.

Safety and efficacy of aztreonam inhalation solution administered by oral inhalation via nebulization have *not* been established in pediatric patients younger than 7 years of age, in patients with forced expiratory volume in 1 second (FEV_1) less than 25% or exceeding 75% of predicted values, or in patients colonized with *Burkholderia cepacia*.

Bronchospasm. Clinicians should consider that bronchospasm is a known complication associated with nebulized therapies, including aztreonam. In clinical trials in patients pretreated with a bronchodilator, a reduction of 15% or more in FEV_1 was reported in 3% of patients immediately following administration of a dose of aztreonam inhalation solution administered by oral inhalation via nebulization.

Decreased FEV_1. In clinical trials, patients with increases in FEV_1 during a 28-day course of aztreonam oral inhalation therapy were sometimes treated for pulmonary exacerbations when FEV_1 declined after the treatment period. When evaluating whether a change in FEV_1 after treatment is caused by a pulmonary exacerbation, clinicians should consider the patient's baseline FEV_1 measured prior to initiation of aztreonam oral inhalation therapy and the presence of other symptoms.

Administration Precautions. Patients should be advised that aztreonam powder for inhalation solution should be reconstituted using *only* the diluent provided by the manufacturer and should *only* be administered by oral inhalation via nebulization using the Altera® nebulizer system. Patients should be instructed to use a bronchodilator prior to administration of the reconstituted aztreonam inhalation solution. Those being treated with several inhaled drugs should be advised to administer the drugs in the following order: bronchodilator, mucolytics, and, lastly, aztreonam oral inhalation via nebulization. (See Oral Inhalation via Nebulization under Dosage and Administration: Reconstitution and Administration.)

Patients receiving aztreonam oral inhalation therapy should be advised to complete the full 28-day oral inhalation regimen, even if they are feeling better and, if they miss a dose, they should take all 3 daily doses as long as the doses are at least 4 hours apart.

Patients should be advised to inform their clinician if they have new or worsening symptoms and to immediately contact a clinician if they experience a possible allergic reaction to aztreonam inhalation solution administered by oral inhalation via nebulization.

■ **Pediatric Precautions** The manufacturers state that use of IV aztreonam in children 9 months of age or older is supported by evidence from adequate and well-controlled studies in adults and additional efficacy, safety, and pharmacokinetic data from noncomparative clinical studies in pediatric patients. However, data are insufficient to date to determine safety and efficacy of IV aztreonam in pediatric patients 9 months of age or older for the treatment of septicemia or skin and skin structure infections (when skin infection suspected or known to be caused by *Haemophilus influenzae* type b). In addition, the manufacturers state that data are insufficient to date to evaluate IM administration of aztreonam in pediatric patients or use of the drug in pediatric patients with impaired renal function.

In clinical studies evaluating parenteral aztreonam in pediatric patients, discontinuance of the drug because of adverse effects was required in less than 1%. Rash, diarrhea, and fever have been reported in 1–4.3% of pediatric patients. In pediatric patients receiving IV aztreonam, pain was reported in 12% and erythema, induration, or phlebitis were reported in 0.9–2.9% of patients overall; in US patients, pain occurred in 1.5% and other local reactions occurred in about 0.5%. Eosinophilia, neutropenia, or increased platelet count has been reported in 6.3, 3.2, or 3.6% of pediatric patients, respectively, and increased serum AST, ALT, or serum creatinine has been reported in 3.8–6.5%. In US pediatric studies, neutropenia (absolute neutrophil count less than 1000/mm^3) occurred in 11.3% of patients younger than 2 years of age receiving aztreonam in a dosage of 30 mg/kg every 6 hours and increased serum AST and ALT (greater than 3 times the upper limit of normal) occurred in 15–20% of patients 2 years of age or older receiving a dosage of 50 mg/kg every 6 hours. It is unclear whether the increased frequency of these adverse effects was related to increased severity of illness in the patients or aztreonam dosage administered.

Aztreonam has been used IM or IV in a limited number of neonates† and infants as young as 1 month of age† without unusual adverse effects.

Safety and efficacy of aztreonam administered by oral inhalation via nebulization have not been established in pediatric patients younger than 7 years of age. The drug has been used by oral inhalation via nebulization for the treatment of newly acquired *Ps. aeruginosa* respiratory tract infections in a limited number of cystic fibrosis patients 3 months through 6 years of age† without unusual adverse effects. In clinical trials evaluating aztreonam inhalation therapy in cystic fibrosis patients 7 years of age or older, pyrexia was reported more frequently in pediatric patients than in adults.

■ **Geriatric Precautions** Clinical studies evaluating IV or IM aztreonam or aztreonam administered by oral inhalation via nebulization did not include sufficient numbers of patients 65 years of age and older to determine whether they respond differently than younger patients. Other reported clinical experience with parenteral aztreonam has not identified differences in responses between geriatric patients and younger adults.

Aztreonam is substantially eliminated by the kidneys, and the risk of adverse effects may be greater in those with impaired renal function. Because geriatric patients are more likely to have reduced renal function, IV or IM dosage of aztreonam should be selected with caution and renal function should be monitored. (See Dosage and Administration: Dosage.)

■ **Mutagenicity and Carcinogenicity** No evidence of mutagenicity or clastogenic potential was seen at the chromosomal or gene level when aztreonam was evaluated in several in vitro (Ames test, mouse lymphoma forward mutation assay, gene conversion assay, chromosome aberration assay in human lymphocytes) and in vivo (mouse bone marrow cytogenetic assay) test systems.

Studies have not been performed to date to evaluate the carcinogenic potential of IV aztreonam. In a 104-week inhalation toxicology study in rats, there was no evidence of drug-related increases in the incidence of tumors in rats exposed to aerosolized aztreonam (up to 4 hours daily).

■ **Pregnancy, Fertility, and Lactation** ***Pregnancy*** There are no adequate and controlled studies to date using parenteral aztreonam or aztreonam administered by oral inhalation via nebulization in pregnant women. IV or IM aztreonam or aztreonam oral inhalation therapy should be used during pregnancy only when clearly needed. Aztreonam crosses the placenta in pregnant women and enters fetal circulation.

No evidence of embryotoxicity, fetotoxicity, or teratogenicity was found in reproduction studies in pregnant rats and rabbits using parenteral aztreonam dosages up to 1.8 and 1.2 g/kg, respectively; these aztreonam dosages were

2.2- and 2.9-fold greater than the maximum recommended human dosage (MRHD) based on body surface area. There was no evidence of drug-induced changes in any maternal, fetal, or neonatal parameters when parenteral aztreonam was used in a perinatal/postnatal study in rats; the highest dosage used in this study (1.8 g/kg daily) was 2.2 times the MRHD based on body surface area. However, in a 2-generation reproduction study in rats using parenteral aztreonam dosages up to 2.4 g/kg daily (2.9-fold greater than the MRHD), there was a slightly reduced survival rate during the lactation period in offspring of rats that received the highest dosage, but not in offspring of rats that received lower dosages.

Fertility In a 2-generation reproduction study in rats using parenteral aztreonam dosages up to 2.4 g/kg daily (2.9-fold greater than the MRHD), there was no evidence of impaired fertility.

Lactation Because aztreonam is distributed into milk in low concentrations following parenteral administration and because safety of aztreonam in neonates has not been fully evaluated to date, temporary discontinuance of nursing should be considered if parenteral aztreonam is used in lactating women.

The manufacturer states that aztreonam administered by oral inhalation via nebulization in lactating women is unlikely to pose a risk to breast-feeding infants since peak plasma concentrations following a 75-mg dose administered by oral inhalation via nebulization are approximately 1% of peak plasma concentrations reported following a 500-mg IV dose of the drug.

Drug Interactions

Drug interactions reported are based on parenteral aztreonam. Formal drug interaction studies have not been conducted to date using aztreonam administered by oral inhalation via nebulization.

■ **Antibacterial Agents** ***Aminoglycosides*** In a study in healthy adults who received a single 1-g IV dose of aztreonam concomitantly with a single 80-mg IV dose of gentamicin, peak serum concentrations of aztreonam were decreased by about 13%, but other pharmacokinetic parameters of the drugs (e.g., half-lives, areas under the serum concentration-time curves [AUCs]) were not affected by concomitant administration. This was not considered clinically important. Further study using multiple doses of the drugs and/or higher doses is probably needed to confirm that there are no clinically important pharmacokinetic interactions between aztreonam and gentamicin.

The antibacterial activity of aztreonam and aminoglycosides is additive or synergistic in vitro against most strains of *Pseudomonas aeruginosa* and some strains of *Ps. cepacia*, *Ps. fluorescens*, and *Ps. maltophilia*. The combination of aztreonam and an aminoglycoside also is synergistic against some Enterobacteriaceae, including some strains of *Enterobacter*, *Escherichia coli*, *Klebsiella*, and *Serratia*.

In vitro, the combination of aztreonam and an aminoglycoside has occasionally been synergistic against *Acinetobacter*, although the combination more frequently is only additive or indifferent against this organism.

The combination of aztreonam and an aminoglycoside generally is indifferent against gram-positive bacteria, including *Staphylococcus aureus*, *S. epidermidis*, and *Enterococcus faecalis* (formerly *Streptococcus faecalis*).

β-Lactam Antibiotics In a single-dose IV study, there were no clinically important pharmacokinetic interactions between nafcillin sodium and aztreonam.

An additive or synergistic effect has occurred in vitro against some strains of *Ps. aeruginosa* when aztreonam was used concomitantly with piperacillin or cefotaxime. The combination of aztreonam and ampicillin, piperacillin, or cefotaxime generally is indifferent or only slightly additive against Enterobacteriaceae, including *Enterobacter*, *E. coli*, *S. marcescens*, and *Klebsiella*.

In vitro, the combination of aztreonam and cefoxitin has been synergistic against some strains of *Enterobacter*, *E. coli*, *Klebsiella*, *S. marcescens*, *Salmonella*, and *Shigella*. However, antagonism has occurred in vitro when aztreonam was used in combination with cefoxitin against *Enterobacter* or *S. marcescens*. Antagonism also has occurred in vitro when imipenem was used in combination with aztreonam against *Ps. aeruginosa*. Antagonism between aztreonam and these anti-infectives may occur because cefoxitin and imipenem are potent β-lactamase inducers and can derepress inducible, chromosomally mediated β-lactamases in gram-negative bacteria that possess these enzymes (e.g., *Enterobacter*, *Serratia*, *Ps. aeruginosa*). Although aztreonam is relatively stable against hydrolysis by inducible β-lactamases, it has been suggested that the enzymes may inactivate aztreonam by binding to the drug and preventing access to penicillin-binding proteins (PBPs). Because the combinations may be antagonistic, anti-infective agents that are potent inducers of β-lactamase production (e.g., cefoxitin, imipenem) should not be used concomitantly with aztreonam.

Chloramphenicol Results of an in vitro study using *K. pneumoniae* indicate that chloramphenicol can antagonize the bactericidal activity of aztreonam. It has been suggested that if concomitant use of the drugs is indicated, chloramphenicol should be administered a few hours after aztreonam; however, the necessity of this precaution has not been established.

Clindamycin In a study in healthy adults who received a single IV dose of aztreonam concomitantly with a single IV dose of clindamycin, total urinary excretion of aztreonam was increased by about 5%. This was not considered clinically important, and other parameters (e.g., half-lives, AUCs) were not affected by concomitant administration of the drugs. Further study using multiple and/or higher doses of the drugs probably are needed to confirm that there are no clinically important pharmacokinetic interactions between aztreonam and clindamycin.

In vitro, the antibacterial activity of aztreonam and clindamycin has been synergistic against some strains of *E. coli*, *Klebsiella*, and *Enterobacter*, although the combination more frequently is indifferent or additive against these organisms. Indifferent or slightly additive effects also have been reported when aztreonam was used in conjunction with clindamycin against anaerobic bacteria.

Metronidazole In a study in healthy adults who received a single IV dose of aztreonam concomitantly with a single IV dose of metronidazole, peak serum concentrations of aztreonam were decreased by about 10%. This was not considered clinically important, and other parameters (e.g., half-lives, AUCs) were not affected by concomitant administration of the drugs. Further study using multiple and/or higher doses of the drugs probably are needed to confirm that there are no clinically important pharmacokinetic interactions between aztreonam and metronidazole.

In vitro, indifferent or slightly additive effects have been reported when aztreonam was used in conjunction with metronidazole against anaerobic bacteria.

■ **Clavulanic Acid** In vitro studies indicate that the combination of aztreonam and clavulanic acid, a β-lactamase inhibitor, is synergistic against some strains of β-lactamase-producing *Enterobacter*, *Klebsiella*, and *Bacteroides fragilis* resistant to aztreonam alone. The combination of aztreonam and clavulanic acid may also be antagonistic against some organisms. Clavulanic acid can induce production of chromosomally mediated β-lactamases in some gram-negative bacteria (e.g., *Enterobacter*, *Ps. aeruginosa*) and therefore could interfere with the antibacterial activity of aztreonam by a mechanism similar to that seen with cefoxitin or imipenem. Concomitant use of clavulanic acid and aztreonam does not alter the in vitro susceptibility of *S. aureus* to aztreonam since resistance to the drug in these organisms is intrinsic.

■ **Furosemide** Concomitant use of furosemide can increase serum concentrations of aztreonam, but this effect is not considered clinically important.

■ **Probenecid** Concomitant use of probenecid slows the rate of renal tubular secretion of aztreonam and can increase serum concentrations of aztreonam. This effect, however, is not sufficient to be of therapeutic benefit since it produces only a 5% increase in serum aztreonam concentrations and an 11% increase in the serum half-life of the drug. Concomitant probenecid also appears to decrease the binding of aztreonam to plasma proteins by about 13%, presumably by competing with the drug for plasma and tissue protein binding sites, and decreases the steady-state volume of distribution of aztreonam by about 16%.

Laboratory Test Interferences

■ **Tests for Urinary Glucose** Like most other currently available β-lactam antibiotics, aztreonam interferes with urinary glucose determinations using cupric sulfate (e.g., Benedict's solution, Clinitest®), but does not appear to interfere with glucose oxidase tests (e.g., Diastix®, Tes-Tape®).

■ **Tests for Creatinine** Aztreonam does not appear to interfere with serum or urinary creatinine determinations when the Jaffé reaction is used.

Acute Toxicity

Limited information is available on the acute toxicity of aztreonam in humans. The IV LD_{50} of the drug is 3.3 g/kg in mice, and the intraperitoneal LD_{50} is 6.6 g/kg in rats.

If acute overdosage of aztreonam occurs, hemodialysis and/or peritoneal dialysis may enhance elimination of the drug from the body.

Overdosage of aztreonam administered by oral inhalation via nebulization has not been reported to date. Systemic safety issues associated with overdosage of the drug administered by oral inhalation are not anticipated since peak serum concentrations of aztreonam following 75-mg doses of the drug given by oral inhalation via nebulization are approximately 0.6 mcg/mL, compared with peak serum concentrations of 54 mcg/mL attained following parenteral administration of 500 mg of aztreonam. In clinical trials, 225-mg doses of aztreonam given by oral inhalation via nebulization were associated with higher rates of drug-related adverse respiratory reactions, particularly cough.

Mechanism of Action

Like bicyclic β-lactam antibiotics, the antibacterial activity of aztreonam results from inhibition of mucopeptide synthesis in the bacterial cell wall. Aztreonam has a high affinity for and preferentially binds to penicillin-binding protein 3 (PBP 3) of susceptible gram-negative bacteria. The drug also has some affinity for PBP 1a of these bacteria, but little or no affinity for PBPs 1b, 2, 4, 5, or 6. Because PBP 3 is involved in septation, aztreonam causes the formation of abnormally elongated or filamentous forms in susceptible gram-negative bacteria. As a consequence, cell division is inhibited and breakage of the cell wall occurs resulting in lysis and death. Studies using *Staphylococcus aureus* indicate that aztreonam does not bind to the essential PBPs of gram-positive bacteria. Aztreonam also has poor affinity for the PBPs of anaerobic bacteria. The drug, therefore, generally is inactive against these organisms.

Aztreonam usually is bactericidal in action. Since aztreonam has poor affinity for PBPs 1a and 1b of susceptible gram-negative bacteria, it is not as rapidly bactericidal as some other β-lactam antibiotics (e.g., imipenem, cefotaxime, cefoxitin, ceftriaxone) against these organisms. For most susceptible Enterobacteriaceae, the minimum bactericidal concentration (MBC) of aztreonam is equal to or only 2–4 times higher than the minimum inhibitory concentration (MIC) of the drug. For *Pseudomonas aeruginosa*, the MBC of aztreonam is usually only 2 times higher than the MIC, but may be up to 125 times higher than the MIC for some strains of the organism.

Spectrum

Aztreonam has a narrow spectrum of activity. The drug is active in vitro against many gram-negative aerobic bacteria, including most Enterobacteriaceae and *Pseudomonas aeruginosa*, but has little or no activity against gram-positive aerobic bacteria or against anaerobic bacteria. Aztreonam is inactive against *Chlamydia*, *Mycoplasma*, fungi, and viruses.

■ **In Vitro Susceptibility Testing** Results of in vitro susceptibility tests with aztreonam may be affected by the size of the inoculum. MICs of aztreonam for Enterobacteriaceae or *Ps. aeruginosa* are generally only 1–4 times greater when the size of the inoculum is increased from 10^3 or 10^4 to 10^6 colony-forming units (CFU) per mL; however, MICs for these organisms may be 15–500 times greater when the inoculum is increased from 10^4 or 10^5 to 10^7–10^8 CFU/mL. The clinical importance of this inoculum effect has not been determined. It has been suggested that it may occur because aztreonam causes the formation of abnormally elongated or filamentous forms in susceptible gram-negative bacteria, but is not rapidly bactericidal, which may result in an initial increase in bacterial mass. In macrobroth or microbroth dilution susceptibility tests that use turbidity to determine the presence of bacterial growth, this initial increase in bacterial mass could result in a corresponding increase in optical density that could be interpreted as growth or resistance. The increase in bacterial mass may not result in visually detectable turbidity when an inoculum smaller than 10^5 CFU/mL is used.

Although results of aztreonam susceptibility tests generally are unaffected by the presence of serum, the minimum bactericidal concentration (MBC) of the drug for *Ps. aeruginosa* or *Proteus mirabilis* is 2–128 times greater in the presence of 75% serum. MICs and MBCs of aztreonam generally are unaffected by the type of media or pH changes between 6–8. The drug is equally active in vitro when susceptibility tests are performed under aerobic or anaerobic conditions.

When in vitro susceptibility testing is performed according to the standards of the Clinical and Laboratory Standards Institute (CLSI; formerly National Committee for Clinical Laboratory Standards [NCCLS]), clinical isolates identified as *susceptible* to aztreonam are inhibited by drug concentrations usually achievable when the recommended dosage is used for the site of infection. Clinical isolates classified as *intermediate* have minimum inhibitory concentrations (MICs) that approach usually attainable blood and tissue concentrations and response rates may be lower than for strains identified as susceptible. Therefore, the intermediate category implies clinical applicability in body sites where the drug is physiologically concentrated or when a higher than usual dosage can be used. This intermediate category also includes a buffer zone which should prevent small, uncontrolled technical factors from causing major discrepancies in interpretation, especially for drugs with narrow pharmacotoxicity margins. If results of in vitro susceptibility testing indicate that a clinical isolate is *resistant* to aztreonam, the strain is not inhibited by drug concentrations generally achievable with usual dosage schedules and/or MICs fall in the range where specific microbial resistance mechanisms are likely and clinical efficacy of the drug against the isolate has not been reliably demonstrated in clinical studies.

Disk Susceptibility Tests When the disk-diffusion procedure is used to test susceptibility to aztreonam, a disk containing 30 mcg of the drug should be used.

When disk-diffusion susceptibility testing is performed according to CLSI standardized procedures, Enterobacteriaceae with growth inhibition zones of 21 mm or greater are susceptible to aztreonam, those with zones of 18–20 mm have intermediate susceptibility, and those with zones of 17 mm or less are resistant to the drug.

When disk-diffusion susceptibility testing is performed according to CLSI standardized procedures, *Ps. aeruginosa* with growth inhibition zones of 22 mm or greater are susceptible to aztreonam, those with zones of 16–21 mm have intermediate susceptibility, and those with zones of 15 mm or less are resistant to the drug.

When disk-diffusion susceptibility testing is performed according to CLSI standardized procedures using *Haemophilus* test medium (HTM), *H. influenzae* and *H. parainfluenzae* with growth inhibition zones of 26 mm or greater are considered susceptible to aztreonam. Because of limited data on resistant strains, CLSI recommends than *Haemophilus* isolates with growth inhibition zones less than 26 mm should be reported as nonsusceptible to aztreonam.

Dilution Susceptibility Tests When dilution susceptibility testing (agar or broth dilution) is performed according to CLSI standardized procedures, Enterobacteriaceae with MICs of 4 mcg/mL or less are susceptible to aztreonam, those with MICs of 8 mcg/mL have intermediate susceptibility, and those with MICs of 16 mcg/mL or greater are resistant to the drug.

When dilution susceptibility testing (agar or broth dilution) is performed according to CLSI standardized procedures, *Ps. aeruginosa* and other non-Enterobacteriaceae gram-negative bacilli (excluding *Acinetobacter*, *Burkholderia*, *Stenotrophomonas maltophilia*) with MICs of 8 mcg/mL or less are susceptible to aztreonam, those with MICs of 16 mcg/mL have intermediate susceptibility, and those with MICs of 32 mcg/mL or greater are resistant to the drug.

When CLSI standardized procedures for broth dilution are performed using HTM, *H. influenzae* and *H. parainfluenzae* with MICs of 2 mcg/mL or less are considered susceptible to aztreonam. Because of limited data on resistant strains, CLSI recommends than *Haemophilus* isolates with MICs greater than 2 mcg/mL should be reported as nonsusceptible to aztreonam.

■ **Gram-positive Aerobic Bacteria** Aztreonam has little activity against most gram-positive aerobic bacteria. Some strains of *Streptococcus pyogenes* (group A β-hemolytic streptococci, GAS) and groups C and G streptococci may be inhibited in vitro by aztreonam concentrations of 6.25–32 mcg/mL, but the MIC_{90} (minimum inhibitory concentration at which 90% of strains tested are inhibited) of the drug for these organisms is usually 12.5–64 mcg/mL. *S. agalactiae* (group B streptococci, GBS), viridans streptococci, nonenterococcal group D streptococci, and enterococci are resistant to aztreonam. Penicillinase-producing, nonpenicillinase-producing, and methicillin-resistant strains of *Staphylococcus aureus*, *S. epidermidis*, and *S. saprophyticus* are resistant to aztreonam. *Listeria monocytogenes* and *Nocardia* also are resistant to the drug.

■ **Gram-negative Aerobic Bacteria** ***Neisseria*** Aztreonam is active in vitro against *Neisseria meningitidis* and *N. gonorrhoeae*. The MIC_{90} of aztreonam is 0.03–0.06 mcg/mL for *N. meningitidis* and 0.06–0.25 mcg/mL for both penicillinase- and nonpenicillinase-producing *N. gonorrhoeae*.

Haemophilus Aztreonam is active in vitro against both β-lactamase- and non-β-lactamase-producing *Haemophilus influenzae*, and the MIC_{90} of the drug reported for these organisms is 0.06–0.25 mcg/mL. Aztreonam generally is active in vitro against strains of *H. influenzae* resistant to ampicillin and/or chloramphenicol as well as some strains resistant to ampicillin, chloramphenicol, and co-trimoxazole.

Moraxella catarrhalis Both β-lactamase- and non-β-lactamase-producing strains of *Moraxella catarrhalis* generally are inhibited by aztreonam concentrations of 0.5–2 mcg/mL, and the MIC_{90} of the drug for this organism is 2 mcg/mL.

Enterobacteriaceae Aztreonam is active in vitro against many Enterobacteriaceae. *C. diversus*, *E. agglomerans*, *Escherichia coli*, *Hafnia alvei*, *Klebsiella pneumoniae*, *Morganella morganii*, *Proteus mirabilis*, *P. vulgaris*, *Providencia*, *Serratia marcescens*, *Salmonella*, and *Shigella* generally are inhibited in vitro by aztreonam concentrations of 4 mcg/mL or less. The in vitro activity of aztreonam against *Citrobacter freundii*, *Enterobacter aerogenes*, and *E. cloacae* varies considerably, and some strains of these organisms are resistant to the drug. Aztreonam is active in vitro against some, but not all, strains of *Enterobacter*, *Klebsiella*, and *Serratia* resistant to aminoglycosides. Strains of *Enterobacter* resistant to both cefamandole and ticarcillin may also be resistant to aztreonam.

The following table includes MIC_{50}s (minimum inhibitory concentration at which 50% of strains tested are inhibited) and MIC_{90}s of aztreonam reported for Enterobacteriaceae:

Table 1.

Organism	MIC_{50} (mcg/mL)	MIC_{90} (mcg/mL)
Citrobacter spp.	0.06–2	0.7–48
C. diversus	0.03–0.25	0.06–16
C. freundii	0.03–32	0.20–32
Enterobacter spp.	0.06–2	0.12–64
E. aerogenes	0.06–16	0.20–33
E. agglomerans	0.03–0.5	0.06–0.5
E. cloacae	0.06–16	3.10–32
Escherichia coli	0.03–0.25	0.06–4
Hafnia alvei	0.12	0.12
Klebsiella spp.	0.06–0.5	0.12–1
K. oxytoca	0.05–0.5	0.25–12.5
K. pneumoniae	0.03–0.25	0.06–0.5
Morganella morganii	0.01–0.25	0.05–32
Proteus mirabilis	0.01–0.25	0.01–0.5
P. vulgaris	0.01–0.25	0.03–0.25
Providencia spp.	0.03–0.25	0.25–0.5
P. rettgeri	0.01–0.1	0.06–0.8
P. stuartii	0.01–0.1	0.03–0.5
Serratia spp.	0.06–0.5	0.9–8
S. marcescens	0.06–0.5	0.39–6.3
Salmonella spp.	0.03–0.12	0.10–0.3
S. enteritidis	0.05–0.25	0.10–0.25
S. typhi	0.02–0.1	0.05–0.2
Shigella spp.	0.03–0.2	0.06–5.7
Sh. flexneri	0.05	0.10
Sh. sonnei	0.03–0.25	0.06–0.25
Yersinia enterocolitica	0.2–0.78	0.5–3.1

Pseudomonas Aztreonam is active in vitro against most strains of *Pseudomonas aeruginosa*, and the MIC_{50} and MIC_{90} of the drug for the organism are 2–16 and 4–32 mcg/mL, respectively. In vitro on a weight basis, aztreonam is more active than cefotaxime, ceftriaxone, or extended-spectrum penicillins, but less active than ceftazidime or imipenem against *Ps. aerugi-*

nosa. Aztreonam is active in vitro against some, but not all, aminoglycoside-resistant *Ps. aeruginosa*. In studies using amikacin-resistant strains of *Ps. aeruginosa*, the MIC_{90} of aztreonam was 32 mcg/mL for isolates that were resistant to amikacin because of decreased uptake of the aminoglycoside and 32 mcg/mL or greater for isolates that were resistant to amikacin because of aminoglycoside-modifying enzymes.

Aztreonam has some activity in vitro against *Ps. acidovorans* and *Ps. stutzeri*; the MIC_{90} of the drug for these organisms is 4–32 mcg/mL. *Ps. diminuta*, *Ps. fluorescens*, and *Ps. putida* are resistant to aztreonam.

Other Gram-negative Aerobic Bacteria *Pasteurella multocida* generally are inhibited in vitro by aztreonam concentrations of 0.02–0.1 mcg/mL. Some strains of *Moraxella* are inhibited in vitro by aztreonam concentrations of 0.25–4 mcg/mL, but the MIC_{90} of the drug for the organism is greater than 64 mcg/mL.

The MIC_{50} of aztreonam reported for *Acinetobacter calcoaceticus* subsp. *anitratus* and *A. calcoaceticus* subsp. *lwoffi* is 8–25 mcg/mL, but the MIC_{90} is usually 32 mcg/mL or greater and most strains are considered resistant to the drug.

Aeromonas hydrophila and *Plesiomonas shigelloides* generally are inhibited in vitro by aztreonam, and the MIC_{90} of the drug for these organisms is 0.03–3.1 mcg/mL.

Burkholderia, including *B. cepacia*, *B. cenocepacia*, *B. gladioli*, and *B. multivorans*, and *Stenotrophomonas maltophilia* (formerly *Ps. maltophilia*) generally are resistant to aztreonam.

Alcaligenes xylosoxidans (formerly *Achromobacter xylosoxidans*), *Alcaligenes faecalis*, and *A. denitrificans* are resistant to aztreonam. *Bordetella bronchiseptica*, *Brucella melitensis*, *Flavobacterium meningosepticum*, and *Legionella pneumophila* also are resistant to the drug.

■ **Anaerobic Bacteria** Aztreonam generally is inactive against gram-positive and -negative anaerobic bacteria including *Clostridium perfringens*, *C. difficile*, *Eubacterium*, *Peptococcus*, *Peptostreptococcus*, *Fusobacterium*, *Veillonella*, *Bacteroides fragilis*, and *Prevotella melaninogenica* (*Bacteroides melaninogenicus*). The MIC_{90} of aztreonam usually is 64 mcg/mL or greater for anaerobic bacteria.

Resistance

Aztreonam has a high degree of stability against hydrolysis by bacterial β-lactamases, including both plasmid-mediated and chromosomally mediated enzymes, and retains activity in the presence of some penicillinases and cephalosporinases produced by gram-negative and gram-positive bacteria. The drug generally is more stable against inactivation by β-lactamases than cefotaxime. Aztreonam generally is stable against hydrolysis by β-lactamases classified as Richmond-Sykes types I, III (TEM-1, TEM-2, SHV-1), and V (PSE and OXA types). The drug is stable against hydrolysis by most chromosomally mediated Richmond-Sykes type I enzymes produced by *Citrobacter*, *Enterobacter*, *Morganella*, *Proteus*, *Providencia*, *Serratia*, and *Proteus*. The drug also is stable against hydrolysis by staphylococcal β-lactamases and most β-lactamases produced by *Bacteroides*.

Aztreonam is hydrolyzed by a chromosomally mediated Richmond-Sykes type IV enzyme (K-1) produced by some strains of *Klebsiella oxytoca*, and strains that produce this enzyme generally are resistant to the drug. Aztreonam also is hydrolyzed to some extent by PSE 2, a Richmond-Sykes type V plasmid-mediated β-lactamase produced by *Ps. aeruginosa*; the drug generally is stable against hydrolysis by PSE 1, 3, and 4. A chromosomally mediated β-lactamase produced by *Bacteroides* (B1) can also slowly hydrolyze aztreonam.

In vitro studies indicate that aztreonam is a poor inducer of β-lactamase production and generally does not derepress inducible, chromosomally mediated enzymes in gram-negative bacteria that possess these enzymes (e.g., some strains of *Pseudomonas*, *Citrobacter*, *Enterobacter*, and *Serratia*). Although aztreonam is relatively stable against hydrolysis by inducible β-lactamases, it has been suggested that the enzymes may inactivate the drug by binding to it and preventing access to penicillin-binding proteins (PBPs). Therefore, gram-negative bacteria that possess these inducible β-lactamases may be resistant to aztreonam following derepression of the enzymes.

Resistance to aztreonam has been produced in vitro in some strains of *E. cloacae* initially susceptible to the drug, and aztreonam-resistant strains of the organism have emerged during aztreonam therapy. *E. cloacae* resistant to aztreonam may also be resistant to third generation cephalosporins and extended-spectrum penicillins, but may be susceptible to imipenem. Aztreonam resistance in some strains of *E. cloacae* appears to be related to alterations in outer-membrane porin proteins and/or other factors that affect permeability of the organism to the drug.

Pharmacokinetics

Aztreonam exhibits linear, dose-independent pharmacokinetics. The pharmacokinetics of the drug after IV administration are best described by an open, linear, 2-compartment model and pharmacokinetics after IM administration are best described by an open, one-compartment model with first-order absorption and elimination. The pharmacokinetics of aztreonam in pediatric patients 9 months of age or older are similar to those in adults.

■ **Absorption** ***IV or IM*** Aztreonam is rapidly and completely absorbed following IM administration, and peak serum concentrations of the drug generally are attained within 1 hour after an IM dose. Although peak serum concentrations of aztreonam attained with an IM dose are slightly lower than those attained with an equivalent IV dose, serum aztreonam concentrations 1 hour or longer after dosing are similar. Following IM administration of a single 500-mg aztreonam dose in healthy adults, serum concentrations of the drug average 19–23.6, 21–26.7, 17.2–21.4, 8.6–11.2, 3.8–5.9, 1.5–3.3, and 0.1–1.7 mcg/mL at 0.5, 1, 2, 4, 6, 8, and 12 hours, respectively, after the dose. IM administration of a single 1-g IM dose of aztreonam in healthy adults results in serum aztreonam concentrations averaging 46.5, 18.4, 8.2, 3.5, and 0.7 mcg/mL at 1, 4, 6, 8, and 12 hours, respectively, after the dose.

In healthy adults, IV injection over 2–3 minutes of a single 0.5-, 1-, or 2-g dose of aztreonam results in peak serum concentrations of the drug averaging 56.3–67.2, 72.5–125, or 242 mcg/mL, respectively. Serum concentrations 1, 4, 6, 8, and 12 hours after injection average 38–48.6, 11–13.2, 4.9–6, 2.6–2.7, and 0.5–0.8 mcg/mL, respectively, after the 1-g dose and 91, 26, 13, 6, and 1.2 mcg/mL, respectively, after the 2-g dose.

Following IV infusion over 30 minutes of a single 0.5-, 1-, or 2-g dose of aztreonam in healthy adults, peak serum concentrations of the drug immediately following completion of the infusion average 54–65.5, 90–164, or 204–255 mcg/mL, respectively. Serum aztreonam concentrations 1, 2, 4, 8, and 12 hours after completion of the infusion average 48.8, 35.1, 16.2, 3, and 0.9 mcg/mL, respectively, after the 1-g dose and 111, 66.9, 35.5, 6–8.5, and 1.9 mcg/mL, respectively, after the 2-g dose.

Multiple-dose studies in adults with normal renal and hepatic function receiving an IM or IV aztreonam dosage of 0.5–1 g every 8 hours for 7 days indicate that neither peak nor trough serum concentrations of the drug increase after repeated dosing and that the drug does not accumulate. In healthy adults receiving 1- or 2-g doses of aztreonam IM or IV every 8 hours, steady-state trough serum concentrations of the drug average 1–1.8 or 2.5–3.8 mcg/mL, respectively.

In children following IV injection over 3 minutes of a single 30-mg/kg dose of aztreonam, serum concentrations of the drug 15 minutes and 6 hours after the dose average 118.7 and 11.8 mcg/mL, respectively, in those 2–21 months of age and 96.9 and 5.8 mcg/mL, respectively, in those 2–12 years of age. IV infusion over 10 minutes of 30-mg/kg doses of aztreonam every 12 hours in neonates 1–4 days of age weighing 0.5–2 kg results in peak serum aztreonam concentrations averaging 65.2–83.3 mcg/mL. In a study in premature neonates who received a single 30-mg/kg dose of aztreonam given IV over 3 minutes, plasma concentrations of the drug 1 hour after the dose averaged 46.33 mcg/mL in those with a gestational age of less than 30 weeks who weighed less than 1.5 kg and 49.72 mcg/mL in those with a gestational age of more than 30 weeks who weighed more than 1.5 kg; plasma concentrations 8 hours after the dose averaged 14.1 and 14.83 mcg/mL, respectively.

Oral Inhalation via Nebulization Data from adults and pediatric patients with cystic fibrosis indicate that variable concentrations of aztreonam enter systemic circulation when the drug is administered by oral inhalation via nebulization, but accumulation does not occur following multiple doses. When the commercially available aztreonam powder for inhalation solution was administered by oral inhalation via nebulization in a dosage of 75 mg 3 times daily for 28 days, mean plasma concentrations of aztreonam 1 hour after the first dose were 0.59 mcg/mL and mean peak plasma concentrations of the drug on days 0, 14, and 28 were 0.55, 0.67, and 0.65 mcg/mL, respectively.

Intraperitoneal In patients with chronic renal failure undergoing continuous ambulatory peritoneal dialysis (CAPD), intraperitoneal administration of a single 1-g dose of aztreonam in 2 L of dialysis fluid instilled over 10 minutes results in serum aztreonam concentrations averaging 10.9, 30, 4, and 0.4 mcg/mL at 0.5, 6, 24, and 48 hours, respectively, after the dose.

■ **Distribution** ***IV or IM*** Aztreonam is widely distributed into body tissues and fluids following IM or IV administration. The drug is distributed into skeletal muscle, adipose tissue, skin, bone, gallbladder, liver, lungs, kidneys, atrial appendage, intestines, prostatic tissue, myometrium, endometrium, fallopian tubes, ovaries, and cervical and vaginal tissue. Aztreonam also is distributed into saliva, sputum, bronchial secretions, aqueous humor, and bile, and into pericardial, pleural, peritoneal, synovial, and blister fluids.

In healthy adults, the apparent volume of distribution of aztreonam in the central compartment (V_c) averages 0.05–0.13 L/kg and the volume of distribution at steady state (V_{ss}) averages 0.11–0.22 L/kg. The V_c and V_{ss} of aztreonam in adults with mild to moderate renal impairment are similar to those in healthy adults; however, in one study in adults with severe renal impairment (creatinine clearances less than 10 mL/minute), the V_c and V_{ss} of the drug were 0.13–0.38 and 0.24–0.67 L/kg, respectively. The V_{ss} of aztreonam averages 0.26–0.36 L/kg in neonates and 0.2–0.29 L/kg in children 1 month to 12 years of age. The V_{ss} of the drug may be increased in patients with cystic fibrosis.

Aztreonam is distributed into CSF following IV administration. CSF concentrations of aztreonam generally are higher in patients with inflamed meninges than in those with uninflamed meninges; the ratio of CSF/serum concentration is generally 0.03–0.52 in patients with inflamed meninges and 0.02–0.30 in patients with uninflamed meninges. In adults who received a single 2-g dose of aztreonam given by IV injection over 5 minutes, CSF concentrations of the drug 1 and 4 hours after the dose were 2 and 3.2 mcg/mL, respectively, in those with inflamed meninges and 0.5 and 1 mcg/mL, respectively, in those with uninflamed meninges. In a neonate and several children 3 months to 2 years of age with bacterial meningitis who received a single 30-mg/kg dose of aztreonam by IV injection over 3 minutes, CSF aztreonam concentrations ranged from 2.1–20.8 mcg/mL in samples obtained 0.8–4.3 hours after the dose and the CSF/serum ratio ranged from 0.06–0.24.

Aztreonam concentrations in peritoneal fluid are approximately equal to concurrent serum concentrations of the drug. In patients receiving 2-g IV doses of aztreonam, peritoneal fluid concentrations 1–6 hours after a dose ranged from 12–90 mcg/mL. In several patients with abdominal infections, peritoneal fluid concentrations were about 50% lower in those with purulent fluid than in those with clear, serous fluid.

In adults who received a single 2-g dose of aztreonam by IV injection over 5 minutes, aztreonam concentrations approximately 1 hour after the dose averaged 362.5 mcg/mL in common duct bile, 102.8 mcg/mL in gallbladder bile, 27.1 mcg/g in gallbladder, and 89.6 mcg/mL in serum. In patients undergoing cholecystectomy who received a single 1-g IV dose of aztreonam, peak concentrations of the drug in T-tube biliary drainage were attained approximately 2.4 hours after the dose and ranged from 9.7–88.2 mcg/mL; biliary concentrations ranged from 5.4–39.8 mcg/mL at 6 hours after the dose. When a single 1-g IV dose of aztreonam was given to patients with biliary obstruction, peak concentrations of the drug in bile were attained 1 hour after the dose and ranged from 5.6–23.3 mcg/mL.

At serum concentrations of 1–100 mcg/mL, aztreonam is 46–60% bound to serum proteins in healthy adults. In adults with impaired renal function and decreased serum albumin concentrations, aztreonam is 22–49% bound to serum proteins.

Aztreonam crosses the placenta and is distributed into amniotic fluid. Aztreonam concentrations in amniotic fluid have been reported to be 2 mcg/mL 6–8 hours after a single 1-g IV dose.

The drug is distributed into milk in low concentrations. In lactating women who received a single 1-g IM or IV dose of aztreonam, peak milk concentrations were attained 2–6 hours after the dose and averaged 0.2 or 0.3 mcg/mL, respectively, and concurrent serum concentrations averaged 126 or 43 mcg/mL, respectively.

Oral Inhalation via Nebulization When aztreonam is administered by oral inhalation via nebulization in adult and pediatric patients with cystic fibrosis, sputum concentrations of the drug exhibit considerable interindividual variation, but accumulation does not occur following multiple doses. When the commercially available aztreonam powder for inhalation solution was administered by oral inhalation via nebulization in a dosage of 75 mg 3 times daily for 28 days, mean sputum concentrations 10 minutes after the first dose were 726 mcg/g and mean sputum concentrations 10 minutes after a dose on days 0, 14, and 28 were 984, 793, and 715 mcg/g, respectively.

■ **Elimination** Aztreonam is partially metabolized to several microbiologically inactive metabolites; no active metabolites of the drug have been found in serum or urine. The principal metabolite of aztreonam, which is formed by nonspecific hydrolysis of the β-lactam ring, is 2-[[(2-amino-4-thiazolyl)[(1-carboxy-1-methylethoxy) imino]acetyl]amino]-3-(sulfoamino)butanoic acid (SQ 26,992). Other inactive metabolites, which have not been identified, reportedly may be demethylated products of SQ 26,992.

IV or IM Serum concentrations of aztreonam decline in a biphasic manner after IV administration. In adults with normal renal and hepatic function, the distribution half-life ($t_{1/2\alpha}$) of aztreonam averages 0.2–0.7 hours and the elimination half-life ($t_{1/2\beta}$) averages 1.3–2.2 hours. The $t_{1/2\beta}$ of SQ 26,992 is longer than that of aztreonam and is about 26 hours in adults with normal renal and hepatic function.

In geriatric adults, renal clearance of aztreonam is decreased and the $t_{1/2}$ of the drug is prolonged compared with younger adults. The $t_{1/2\beta}$ of aztreonam ranges from 1.7–4.3 hours in adults 64–82 years of age with renal function normal for their age.

The $t_{1/2\beta}$ of aztreonam averages 1.7 hours in children 2 months to 12 years of age. Half-life of the drug is longer in neonates than in older children and adults and is inversely related to age and birthweight. In neonates younger than 7 days of age, $t_{1/2\beta}$ of aztreonam averages 5.5–9.9 hours in those weighing less than 2.5 kg and 2.6 hours in those weighing more than 2.5 kg. In neonates 1 week to 1 month of age, $t_{1/2\beta}$ of the drug averages 2.4 hours.

In patients with renal impairment, serum concentrations of aztreonam are higher and the serum half-life prolonged. In adults with renal impairment, the $t_{1/2\beta}$ of aztreonam averages 3.4–3.6, 5.3–5.9, 7.8–7.9, or 8.4–8.7 hours in adults with creatinine clearances of 30–80, 10–29, 3–9, or less than 2 mL/minute, respectively.

In patients with hepatic impairment, serum half-life of aztreonam is only slightly prolonged since the liver is a minor pathway of elimination for the drug. In a study in patients with cirrhosis but with normal renal function, the $t_{1/2\beta}$ of aztreonam averaged 2.2 hours in those with primary biliary cirrhosis and 3.2 hours in those with alcoholic cirrhosis.

Aztreonam is excreted principally in urine as unchanged drug via both glomerular filtration and tubular secretion. Following IM or IV administration of a single 0.5-, 1-, or 2-g dose of aztreonam in adults with normal renal function, approximately 58–74% of the dose is excreted in urine unchanged, 1–7% is excreted as SQ 26,992, and 3–4% is excreted as unidentified inactive metabolites. Urinary excretion of unchanged aztreonam is essentially complete 8–12 hours after a single dose of the drug, but SQ 26,992 is excreted for up to 48 hours after the dose. Following IM administration of a single 0.5- or 1-g dose of aztreonam in adults with normal renal function, urinary concentrations of the drug average 500 or 1200 mcg/mL, respectively, in urine collected over the first 2 hours after the dose and 180 or 470 mcg/mL, respectively, in urine collected over 6–8 hours after the dose. In adults with normal renal function, urinary concentrations of aztreonam after a single 0.5- or 1-g dose given by IV injection over 3–5 minutes or IV infusion over 30 minutes average 1–1.5 or 3–3.5 mg/mL, respectively, in urine collected over the first 2 hours after the dose and 250–330 or 710–720 mcg/mL, respectively, in urine collected over 4–6 hours after the dose. After a single 2-g IV dose, urinary concentrations of aztreonam average 5.6–6.6 mg/mL in urine collected over the first 2 hours after the dose and 1.8 mg/mL in urine collected over 4–6 hours after the dose.

Aztreonam is partially excreted in feces, presumably via biliary elimination. Approximately 1% of a single 500-mg IV dose of the drug is excreted in feces unchanged, 3% as SQ 26,992, and 7.5–10.8% as unidentified inactive metabolites.

Total body clearance of aztreonam from serum averages 0.91–1.68 mL/minute per kg and renal clearance of the drug averages 0.59–1.03 mL/minute per kg in healthy adults. Total body clearance from serum averages 0.61–1.13 mL/minute per kg in neonates younger than 7 days of age weighing less than 2.5 kg, 1.41–1.68 mL/minute per kg in neonates weighing more than 2.5 kg, 1.87 mL/minute per kg in children 2–21 months of age, and 2.5 mL/minute per kg in children 2–12 years of age. Total body clearance from serum in adults with impaired renal function decreases linearly with decreases in creatinine clearance.

Cystic fibrosis patients may eliminate aztreonam at a faster rate than healthy individuals. Serum half-life of the drug averaged 1–1.3 hours in several patients with cystic fibrosis. Further study is needed to determine if this effect is clinically important since use of usual parenteral dosages of the drug in patients with cystic fibrosis may result in lower serum concentrations than expected.

Aztreonam and SQ 26,992 are removed by hemodialysis. The amount of the drug and its metabolites removed during hemodialysis depends on several factors (e.g., type of coil used, dialysis flow rate). In one group of patients with end-stage renal disease undergoing hemodialysis, the serum half-life of aztreonam averaged 2.7 hours during hemodialysis and 7.9 hours between dialysis sessions. A 4-hour period of hemodialysis generally removes into the dialysate about 27–58% of a single 1-g IV dose of aztreonam when the dose is given 1 hour prior to dialysis.

Aztreonam is removed to a lesser extent by peritoneal dialysis. In patients with chronic renal failure undergoing CAPD with a 6-hour dwell time, about 10% of a single 1-g IV dose of aztreonam is removed into the dialysate within 48 hours after the dose.

Oral Inhalation via Nebulization When the commercially available aztreonam powder for inhalation solution is administered by oral inhalation via nebulization, approximately 10% of the total dose is excreted unchanged in urine; glomerular filtration and tubular secretion are equally involved in elimination of systemically absorbed drug.

In adults with cystic fibrosis receiving aztreonam by oral inhalation via nebulization, the plasma elimination half-life of systemically absorbed drug is approximately 2.1 hours.

Chemistry and Stability

■ **Chemistry** Aztreonam is a synthetic monobactam antibiotic. Unlike other currently available β-lactam antibiotics, which are bicyclic and contain an adjoining ring fused to the β-lactam ring (e.g., carbapenems, cephalosporins, cephamycins, penicillins), monobactams are monocyclic β-lactam antibiotics.

Naturally occurring monobactams are produced by various bacteria found in soil (e.g., *Acetobacter*, *Agrobacterium*, *Chromobacterium*, *Flexibacter*, *Gluconobacter*) and generally have only weak antibacterial activity. Synthetic monobactams, including aztreonam, contain a 3-aminomonobactamic acid (3-AMA) nucleus; addition of various substituents on the 3-AMA nucleus results in monobactam derivatives that differ in spectra of activity, antimicrobial potency, and stability against hydrolysis by β-lactamases. Aztreonam contains a sulfonic acid group on the nitrogen at the 1-position of the 3-AMA nucleus, which activates the β-lactam ring. The drug contains an aminothiazolyl oxime side chain at position 3 of the 3-AMA nucleus, which results in potent activity against gram-negative bacteria; the carboxyl and methyl groups on the side chain result in enhanced activity against *Pseudomonas aeruginosa* and decreased activity against gram-positive bacteria. This aminothiazolyl side chain is similar to that contained in ceftazidime. In addition, aztreonam contains an α-methyl group at position 4 of the 3-AMA nucleus, which results in stability against hydrolysis by many β-lactamases and increased antibacterial potency against gram-negative bacteria, but decreased activity against gram-positive bacteria.

Parenteral Commercially available aztreonam for injection for IV or IM administration is a dry mixture of sterile aztreonam and arginine, and occurs as a white to yellowish-white, lyophilized powder; the injection contains approximately 780 mg of arginine per gram of aztreonam. Aztreonam has solubilities of 10 mg/mL in water and 0.2 mg/mL in alcohol at 25°C. The drug has pK_as of −0.7, 2.75, and 3.91 at 25°C. Aqueous solutions of aztreonam have a pH of 4.5–7.5. Potency of aztreonam powder for injection is calculated on the anhydrous and arginine-free basis. When reconstituted as directed by the manufacturers, solutions of aztreonam are colorless to light straw yellow depending on the concentration of the drug and the diluent used. Aztreonam solutions may turn slightly pink on standing; this color change does not indicate loss of potency.

The commercially available frozen premixed aztreonam injections in dextrose are sterile, nonpyrogenic, iso-osmotic solutions of the drug provided in a plastic container (Galaxy container) fabricated from specially formulated multilayered plastic (PL 2040). The 1- and 2-g frozen premixed injections contain approximately 1.7 or 0.7 g, respectively, of dextrose to adjust osmolality to about 300 mOsm/kg and also contain approximately 0.78 or 1.6 g of arginine, respectively. After thawing, the injections are colorless to yellow in color and have a pH of 4.5–7.5.

Oral Inhalation via Nebulization Aztreonam for oral inhalation via nebulization is commercially available in a kit containing single-dose vials of lyophilized aztreonam powder for inhalation solution and single-dose ampuls of 0.17% sodium chloride diluent. Each vial of lyophilized aztreonam powder for inhalation solution contains 75 mg of aztreonam and 46.7 mg of lysine; the sterile powder is white to off-white and is hygroscopic and light sensitive. The formulation does not contain preservatives.

Following reconstitution with the 0.17% sodium chloride diluent provided by the manufacturer, aztreonam inhalation solutions for oral inhalation via nebulization have a pH of 4.5 to 6.

■ **Stability** Aztreonam is most stable at pH 6. In acidic solutions with pH 2–5, aztreonam is inactivated by isomerization of the oxime side chain and hydrolysis of the β-lactam ring. The drug also is inactivated in solutions with pH less than 1 or greater than 8.

Parenteral Commercially available aztreonam powder for injection for IV or IM administration should be stored at room temperature (20–25°C) and should not be exposed to excessive heat (temperatures warmer than 40°C). The powder for injection also should be protected from moisture. If exposed to strong light, the powder may yellow slightly.

Following reconstitution with sterile water for injection or 0.9% sodium chloride injection, IM injections of aztreonam are stable for 48 hours at 15–30°C or for 7 days when refrigerated at 2–8°C. IM injections of the drug reconstituted with bacteriostatic water for injection (with benzyl alcohol or parabens) or bacteriostatic sodium chloride injection (with benzyl alcohol or parabens) should be used immediately after reconstitution.

At a concentration of 20 mg or less per mL, aztreonam is chemically and physically stable for 48 hours at 15–30°C or for 7 days when refrigerated at 2–8°C in the following IV infusion solutions: 0.9% sodium chloride injection; 5 or 10% dextrose injection; Ringer's; lactated Ringer's; 5% dextrose and 0.2, 0.45, or 0.9% sodium chloride; ⅙ *M* sodium lactate; 5 or 10% mannitol; 5% dextrose with lactated Ringer's; 5% dextrose with Plasma-Lyte® M; Ionosol® B with 5% dextrose; Isolyte® E; Isolyte® E with 5% dextrose; Isolyte® M with 5% dextrose; Normosol®-R; Normosol®-R with 5% dextrose; or Normosol®-M with 5% dextrose. At concentrations greater than 20 mg/mL, aztreonam is stable for 48 hours at 2–8°C in sterile water for injection or 0.9% sodium chloride injection; solutions containing aztreonam concentrations greater than 20 mg/mL prepared using other compatible IV solutions should be used immediately.

The commercially available frozen premixed aztreonam injection in dextrose should be stored at −20°C or lower. The frozen premixed injection should be thawed at room temperature (25°C) or under refrigeration (2–8°C) and, once thawed, should not be refrozen. Thawed solutions of the commercially available frozen premixed injection are stable for 48 hours at room temperature (25°C) or 14 days under refrigeration (2–8°C). The commercially available frozen aztreonam injection is provided in a plastic container fabricated from specially formulated multilayered plastic PL 2040 (Galaxy container). Solutions in contact with PL 2040 can leach out some of its chemical components in very small amounts within the expiration period of the injection; however, safety of the plastic has been confirmed in tests in animals according to USP biological tests for plastic containers as well as by tissue culture toxicity studies.

Admixtures containing aztreonam (10 or 20 mg/mL) and clindamycin phosphate (3, 6, or 9 mg/mL) or cefazolin (5 or 20 mg/mL) in 0.9% sodium chloride injection or 5% dextrose injection are stable for up to 48 hours at room temperature (25°C) or for 7 days when refrigerated at 4–5°C. Admixtures containing aztreonam (10 or 20 mg/mL) and ampicillin (5 or 20 mg/mL) in 0.9% sodium chloride injection are stable for 24 hours at room temperature (25°C) or for 48 hours when refrigerated at 4°C; similar admixtures of these drugs in 5% dextrose injection are stable for only 2 hours at room temperature or for 8 hours when refrigerated at 4°C. Admixtures containing aztreonam (10 or 20 mg/mL) and cefoxitin (10 or 20 mg/mL) in one of these diluents are stable for 12 hours at 25°C or 7 days at 4°C.

Although many bicyclic β-lactam antibiotics (e.g., penicillins) are physically and/or chemically incompatible with aminoglycosides and can inactivate the drugs in vitro, aztreonam appears to be less likely to inactivate aminoglycosides in vitro. Admixtures containing aztreonam (10 or 20 mg/mL) and tobramycin (0.2 or 0.8 mg/mL) in 0.9% sodium chloride injection or 5% dextrose injection are stable for up to 48 hours at room temperature (25°C) or for 7 days at 4°C. The manufacturer states that similar solutions containing gentamicin (0.2 or 0.8 mg/mL) are also stable for up to 48 hours at room temperature or for 7 days when refrigerated. However, there is evidence that loss of gentamicin potency may occur with such admixtures at these storage temperatures and times; therefore, it has been suggested that solutions containing aztreonam (10 or 20 mg/mL) and gentamicin (0.2 or 0.8 mg/mL) be considered stable for only 8 hours at 25°C or for 24 hours at 4°C.

Admixtures containing aztreonam and either cloxacillin sodium (no longer commercially available in the US) or vancomycin hydrochloride in Dianeal® 137 with 4.25% dextrose are stable for up to 24 hours at room temperature.

Aztreonam is physically and/or chemically incompatible with some drugs, but the compatibility depends on several factors (e.g., concentrations of the drugs, specific diluents used, resulting pH, temperature). Specialized references should be consulted for specific compatibility information. Aztreonam is incompatible with nafcillin sodium, cephradine (no longer commercially available in the US), and metronidazole, and these drugs should be administered separately.

Oral Inhalation via Nebulization The commercially available kit containing single-dose vials of lyophilized aztreonam powder for inhalation solution and single-dose ampuls of 0.17% sodium chloride diluent should be stored at 2–8°C. After removal from the refrigerator, the kit may be stored at room temperature (up to 25°C) for up to 28 days.

The lyophilized drug should be protected from light and should not be used if stored at room temperature for longer than 28 days. The diluent should not be used if it is cloudy or contains particles.

Following reconstitution of the powder with the diluent provided in the kit, aztreonam inhalation solution for oral inhalation via nebulization should be used immediately.

Preparations

Excipients in commercially available drug preparations may have clinically important effects in some individuals; consult specific product labeling for details.

Aztreonam

Oral Inhalation		
Kit	Aztreonam 75 mg powder for inhalation solution for nebulization 0.17% sodium chloride diluent	**Cayston®**, Gilead
Parenteral		
For injection	500 mg*	**Aztreonam for Injection**
	1 g*	**Azactam®**, Squibb **Aztreonam for Injection**
	2 g*	**Azactam®**, Squibb **Aztreonam for Injection**

*available from one or more manufacturer, distributor, and/or repackager by generic (nonproprietary) name

Aztreonam in Dextrose

Parenteral		
Injection (frozen), for IV infusion	20 mg/mL (1 g) in 3.4% Dextrose	**Azactam® in Iso-osmotic Dextrose Injection** (Galaxy [Baxter]), Squibb
	40 mg/mL (2 g) in 1.4% Dextrose	**Azactam® in Iso-osmotic Dextrose Injection Galaxy®** (Galaxy [Baxter]), Squibb

†Use is not currently included in the labeling approved by the US Food and Drug Administration

Selected Revisions October 2016, © Copyright, September 1987, American Society of Health-System Pharmacists, Inc.

CHLORAMPHENICOL 8:12.08

Chloramphenicol Sodium Succinate Chloromycetin

■ Chloramphenicol is a broad-spectrum antibacterial agent.

Uses

Chloramphenicol must be used only for the treatment of serious infections caused by susceptible bacteria or *Rickettsia* when potentially less toxic anti-infectives are contraindicated or ineffective. The drug must not be used for the treatment of trivial infections or when it is not indicated (e.g., treatment of colds, influenza, throat infections) and must not be used as a prophylactic agent to prevent bacterial infections.

Prior to initiation of chloramphenicol therapy, appropriate specimens should be collected for identification of the causative organism and in vitro susceptibility tests. Chloramphenicol may be started pending results of in vitro susceptibility testing, but the drug should be discontinued as soon as possible if results indicate that the causative organism is resistant to chloramphenicol or if the organism is found to be susceptible to potentially less toxic anti-infectives. If results of in vitro susceptibility testing indicate that chloramphenicol and another anti-infective are both likely to be effective, a decision to continue use of chloramphenicol rather than switching to the other anti-infective should be based on the severity of the infection, comparative in vitro susceptibility of the drugs, expected efficacy of the drugs in the specific infection, and comparative safety profiles of the drugs.

■ **Meningitis** Chloramphenicol is used as an alternative for the treatment of meningitis caused by susceptible bacteria, including susceptible *Haemophilus influenzae*, *Neisseria meningitidis*, or *Streptococcus pneumoniae*. Chloramphenicol is not considered a drug of first choice for the treatment of meningitis and generally is used only when penicillins and cephalosporins are contraindicated or ineffective. Despite evidence of in vitro activity against *Listeria monocytogenes*, chloramphenicol has been ineffective for the treatment of systemic infections caused by this organism. Chloramphenicol should not be used for the treatment of meningitis caused by gram-negative bacilli.

Pending results of CSF culture and in vitro susceptibility testing, the most appropriate anti-infective regimen for empiric treatment of suspected bacterial meningitis should be selected based on results of CSF gram stain and antigen tests, age of the patient, the most likely pathogen(s) and source of infection, and current patterns of bacterial resistance within the hospital and local community. When results of culture and susceptibility tests become available and the pathogen is identified, the empiric anti-infective regimen should be modified (if necessary) to ensure that the most effective regimen is being administered.

Although chloramphenicol has been recommended as an alternative to penicillins and third generation cephalosporins for the treatment of meningitis caused by susceptible β-lactamase-producing or non-β-lactamase-producing *H. influenzae*, strains of chloramphenicol-resistant *H. influenzae* have been reported in some areas of the world and this limits use of the drug, including for empiric treatment when *H. influenzae* may be involved. There also is some evidence that third generation cephalosporins are as effective or more effective than chloramphenicol for the treatment of meningitis caused by susceptible *H. influenzae*.

IV penicillin G, ampicillin, and third generation cephalosporins usually are considered the drugs of choice for the treatment of meningitis caused by *N. meningitidis*, and chloramphenicol is recommended as one of several alternatives when penicillins and cephalosporins cannot be used. Strains of *N. meningitidis* resistant to chloramphenicol have been reported.

Chloramphenicol has been used as an alternative to penicillins and third generation cephalosporins for the treatment of meningitis caused by penicillin-susceptible *S. pneumoniae*. However, treatment failures have been reported when chloramphenicol was used in the treatment of infections caused by penicillin-resistant *S. pneumoniae*, despite the fact that in vitro susceptibility tests indicated that the clinical isolates were susceptible to chloramphenicol.

■ Rickettsial Infections Chloramphenicol has been used for the treatment of rickettsial infections and has been recommended as a possible alternative to tetracyclines in certain situations. The US Centers for Disease Control and Prevention (CDC) and other experts state that doxycycline is the drug of choice for the treatment of *all* rickettsial infections in *all* age groups (including children younger than 8 years of age). These experts state that empiric treatment with a tetracycline (preferably doxycycline) should be initiated immediately in patients with known or suspected rickettsial disease and should not be delayed while waiting for confirmatory testing since some of these infections can be rapidly progressive and may be fatal or lead to long-term sequelae. If an alternative to doxycycline is being considered for the treatment of a rickettsial infection, CDC recommends consultation with an expert.

Rocky Mountain Spotted Fever and Other Tickborne Spotted Fevers CDC and the American Academy of Pediatrics (AAP) state that doxycycline is the drug of choice for the treatment of *all* tickborne rickettsial infections, including Rocky Mountain spotted fever (RMSF) caused by *Rickettsia rickettsii*, regardless of patient age. Chloramphenicol has been recommended as a possible alternative to doxycycline for the treatment of RMSF in patients who have had potentially life-threatening allergic reactions to the drug (e.g., anaphylaxis, Stevens-Johnson syndrome) and in pregnant women. However, there is some epidemiologic evidence that the risk of death in patients with RMSF is higher in those treated with chloramphenicol than in those treated with a tetracycline and close monitoring is required if chloramphenicol is used. CDC states that the risks and benefits of chloramphenicol versus doxycycline in patients with a history of allergic reactions to tetracyclines should be considered for the individual patient. For those with a history of non-life-threatening reactions to tetracyclines, CDC states that administering doxycycline in an observed setting is a possible option. Although data are limited, CDC states that rapid doxycycline desensitization in consultation with an allergy and immunology specialist may be an option for individuals with a history of life-threatening hypersensitivity reactions to tetracyclines.

CDC states that, although chloramphenicol is a potential alternative to doxycycline for the treatment of RMSF in pregnant women, chloramphenicol must be used with caution during the third trimester of pregnancy because of the theoretical risk of gray syndrome (see Cautions: Gray Syndrome).

Endemic, Epidemic, and Scrub Typhus Chloramphenicol has been recommended as a possible alternative to doxycycline for the treatment of endemic typhus (murine typhus; fleaborne typhus) caused by *R. typhi* or *R. felis*, but may be less effective than doxycycline. Doxycycline is the drug of choice for the treatment of endemic typhus, regardless of patient age.

Chloramphenicol has been recommended as a possible alternative to doxycycline for the treatment of epidemic typhus (louseborne typhus; sylvatic typhus) caused by *R. prowazekii* (e.g., in patients with life-threatening allergic reactions to doxycycline). Doxycycline is the drug of choice for the treatment of epidemic typhus, regardless of patient age.

Although chloramphenicol has been used for the treatment of scrub typhus caused by *Orientia tsutsugamushi* and is recommended as a possible alternative to doxycycline for the treatment of such infections, chloramphenicol resistance and persistence or relapse of the infection has been reported.

Anaplasmosis and Ehrlichiosis Chloramphenicol should *not* be used for the treatment of anaplasmosis caused by *Anaplasma phagocytophilum* (also known as human granulocytic anaplasmosis; HGA) or ehrlichiosis caused by *Ehrlichia chaffeensis* (also known as human monocytic ehrlichiosis; HME). CDC and other experts state that doxycycline is the drug of choice for the treatment of human ehrlichiosis and anaplasmosis, regardless of patient age.

Although chloramphenicol has been used in some patients for the treatment of ehrlichiosis† caused by *E. chaffeensis* or *E. canis* and was recommended in the past as a possible alternative to tetracyclines for these infections, such use is not supported by results of in vitro susceptibility testing for these organisms and the drug is considered ineffective for these infections.

■ Typhoid Fever and Other Severe Salmonella Infections Chloramphenicol has been used for the treatment of typhoid fever (enteric fever) caused by susceptible *Salmonella enterica* serovar Typhi. The drug also has been used for the treatment of paratyphoid fever caused by *S. enterica* serovar Paratyphi.

Various anti-infectives have been used for the treatment of typhoid fever, including ampicillin, amoxicillin, chloramphenicol, co-trimoxazole, cefotaxime, ceftriaxone, fluoroquinolones, and azithromycin. Although chloramphenicol was a drug of choice for the treatment of infections caused by typhoidal *Salmonella* in the past, multidrug-resistant strains of *S. enterica* serovar Typhi (i.e., strains resistant to ampicillin, chloramphenicol, and/or co-trimoxazole) are reported worldwide and are common in many regions of the world. In addition, strains with decreased susceptibility or resistance to other drugs used for the treatment of typhoid fever (e.g., fluoroquinolones, third generation cephalosporins) have been reported. Whenever possible, anti-infectives for the treatment of typhoid fever should be selected based on results of in vitro susceptibility testing. For empiric treatment of typhoid fever known or likely to be caused by multidrug-resistant strains, azithromycin or a parenteral third generation cephalosporin (e.g., ceftriaxone, cefotaxime) has been recommended.

Chloramphenicol should *not* be used for the treatment of typhoid carriers. Depending on susceptibility of the strain, a fluoroquinolone (e.g., ciprofloxacin), ampicillin, amoxicillin, or co-trimoxazole usually is recommended to treat the typhoid carrier state.

Chloramphenicol should *not* be used for the treatment of uncomplicated *Salmonella* gastroenteritis.

■ Anthrax Chloramphenicol has been recommended as an alternative for the *treatment* of anthrax†. Although there is evidence that chloramphenicol has in vitro activity against *Bacillus anthracis*, limited clinical data exist regarding use of the drug in the treatment of anthrax.

Penicillins generally have been considered the drugs of choice for the treatment of anthrax (inhalational, GI, meningitis) caused by penicillin-susceptible *B. anthracis* that occurs as the result of natural or endemic exposures, although a fluoroquinolone (e.g., ciprofloxacin) or doxycycline also has been recommended for the treatment of naturally occurring anthrax. A multiple-drug regimen may be indicated in patients with severe infections. Chloramphenicol has been suggested as an alternative for the treatment of naturally occurring anthrax in patients hypersensitive to penicillins or as one of several options for use in multiple-drug regimens for the treatment of anthrax; however, the World Health Organization (WHO) states that chloramphenicol is no longer recommended as an alternative for the treatment of naturally occurring anthrax because evidence of in vivo efficacy in the treatment of severe anthrax is lacking and the drug is associated with serious adverse effects.

For the treatment of inhalational anthrax that occurs as the result of exposure to *B. anthracis* spores in the context of biologic warfare or bioterrorism, CDC, AAP, and the US Working Group on Civilian Biodefense recommend that treatment be initiated with a multiple-drug parenteral regimen that includes a fluoroquinolone (preferably ciprofloxacin) or doxycycline and 1 or 2 additional anti-infective agents predicted to be effective. Based on in vitro data, drugs that have been suggested as possibilities to augment ciprofloxacin or doxycycline in such multiple-drug regimens include clindamycin, rifampin, a carbapenem (doripenem, imipenem, meropenem), chloramphenicol, vancomycin, penicillin, ampicillin, linezolid, gentamicin, and clarithromycin. IV anti-infective therapy is recommended for initial treatment of clinically apparent GI, inhalational, septicemic, or meningeal anthrax and also is indicated for the treatment of cutaneous anthrax when there are signs of systemic involvement, extensive edema, or head and neck lesions.

For the treatment of systemic anthrax with possible or confirmed meningitis, CDC and AAP recommend a regimen of IV ciprofloxacin with an IV bactericidal anti-infective (preferably meropenem) and an IV protein synthesis inhibitor (preferably linezolid). These experts state that IV chloramphenicol is a possible alternative to linezolid in this regimen, but should be used only if clindamycin and rifampin are not available.

■ Burkholderia Infections *Burkholderia cepacia* Infections Chloramphenicol has been used in patients with cystic fibrosis and has been recommended as an alternative for the treatment of infections caused by *Burkholderia cepacia*† (formerly *Ps. cepacia*). However, *B. cepacia* usually is resistant to chloramphenicol in vitro.

Patients with cystic fibrosis often are chronically infected or colonized with species within the *B. cepacia* complex. In addition, the *B. cepacia* complex has been associated with infections in immunocompromised patients (e.g., those with chronic granulomatous disease, hemoglobinopathies, malignant neoplasms) and in preterm infants. Optimum regimens for the treatment of chronic *B. cepacia* complex infections have not been identified and anti-infectives should be selected based on in vitro susceptibility data and previous clinical responses. Anti-infectives that have been recommended for the treatment of these infections include meropenem, imipenem, co-trimoxazole, ceftazidime, doxycycline, and chloramphenicol; some experts recommend that multiple-drug regimens be used.

Melioidosis Chloramphenicol has been used in conjunction with doxycycline and co-trimoxazole for the treatment of melioidosis†, a life-threatening disease caused by *B. pseudomallei* (formerly *Ps. pseudomallei*); however, chloramphenicol is not usually recommended. *B. pseudomallei* is an aerobic, nonfermentative gram-negative bacilli resistant to many anti-infectives. The drugs of choice for the treatment of melioidosis depend on the type of infection, results of in vitro susceptibility tests, and the presence of comorbidities (e.g., diabetes mellitus, liver or renal disease, malignancies, hemoglobinopathies, cystic fibrosis). Many clinicians recommend ceftazidime or a carbapenem (either meropenem or imipenem) as the drugs of choice for initial treatment of severe melioidosis, followed by long-term treatment with an oral anti-infective (e.g., co-trimoxazole, amoxicillin and clavulanate potassium, doxycycline) given for at least 3 months to reduce the risk of relapse. There is some evidence that ceftazidime monotherapy has been associated with a lower mortality rate than a 3-drug regimen of IV chloramphenicol, oral doxycycline, and oral co-trimoxazole. In addition, there is evidence that a 2-drug oral regimen of co-trimoxazole and doxycycline is as effective and better tolerated for follow-up treatment than a 3-drug oral regimen of co-trimoxazole, doxycycline, and chloramphenicol (oral preparation no longer available in the US). *B. pseudomallei* may be difficult to eradicate, and relapse of melioidosis may occur, especially if there is poor compliance with the follow-up regimen.

■ **Plague** Chloramphenicol is used as an alternative for the treatment of plague† caused by *Yersinia pestis*.

Streptomycin (or gentamicin) historically has been considered the drug of choice for the treatment of plague. Alternatives recommended when these aminoglycosides are not used include fluoroquinolones (ciprofloxacin, levofloxacin, moxifloxacin), doxycycline (or tetracycline), chloramphenicol, or co-trimoxazole (may be less effective than other alternatives). Chloramphenicol is considered a drug of choice for the treatment of plague meningitis.

Anti-infective regimens recommended for the treatment of naturally occurring or endemic bubonic, septicemic, or pneumonic plague also are recommended for the treatment of plague that occurs following exposure to *Y. pestis* in the context of biologic warfare or bioterrorism. Such exposures would most likely result in primary pneumonic plague, and prompt initiation of anti-infective therapy (within 18–24 hours of onset of symptoms) is essential in the treatment of pneumonic plague. Some experts (e.g., the US Working Group on Civilian Biodefense, US Army Medical Research Institute of Infectious Diseases [USAMRIID]) recommend that treatment of plague in the context of biologic warfare or bioterrorism be initiated with a parenteral anti-infective regimen of streptomycin (or gentamicin) or, alternatively, doxycycline, a fluoroquinolone (ciprofloxacin, levofloxacin, moxifloxacin), or chloramphenicol. An oral regimen of doxycycline (or tetracycline) or a fluoroquinolone (ciprofloxacin, levofloxacin, moxifloxacin, ofloxacin) may be substituted when the patient's condition improves or when parenteral therapy is unavailable (e.g., when there are supply or logistic problems because large numbers of individuals require treatment in a mass casualty setting). Although oral chloramphenicol has been recommended as an alternative in these situations, an oral preparation of chloramphenicol is no longer commercially available in the US.

In the context of biologic warfare or bioterrorism, some experts (e.g., the US Working Group on Civilian Biodefense, USAMRIID) recommend that asymptomatic individuals with exposure to plague aerosol or asymptomatic individuals with household, hospital, or other close contact (within about 2 m) with an individual who has pneumonic plague receive an oral anti-infective for postexposure prophylaxis; however, any exposed individual who develops a temperature of 38.5°C or higher or new cough should promptly receive a parenteral anti-infective for treatment of the disease. If postexposure prophylaxis is indicated, these experts recommend an oral regimen of doxycycline (or tetracycline) or a fluoroquinolone (ciprofloxacin, levofloxacin, moxifloxacin, ofloxacin). Although oral chloramphenicol has been recommended as an alternative for postexposure prophylaxis following exposure to *Y. pestis* in the context of biologic warfare or bioterrorism, an oral preparation of chloramphenicol is no longer commercially available in the US.

■ **Tularemia** Chloramphenicol is used as an alternative for the treatment of tularemia† caused by *Francisella tularensis*.

Streptomycin generally has been considered the drug of choice for the treatment of tularemia; however, gentamicin is more readily available and is considered an alternative drug of choice when streptomycin is unavailable. Alternatives recommended for the treatment of tularemia when these aminoglycosides are not used include tetracyclines (doxycycline), chloramphenicol, or ciprofloxacin. Some clinicians state that chloramphenicol should be reserved for the treatment of tularemic meningitis (usually used in conjunction with streptomycin), and should not be used for other forms of tularemia.

Anti-infective regimens recommended for the treatment of naturally occurring or endemic tularemia also are recommended for the treatment of tularemia that occurs following exposure to *F. tularensis* in the context of biologic warfare or bioterrorism. However, the fact that a fully virulent streptomycin-resistant strain of *F. tularensis* was developed in the past for use in biologic warfare should be considered. Exposures to *F. tularensis* in the context of biologic warfare or bioterrorism would most likely result in inhalational tularemia with pleuropneumonitis, although the organism also can infect humans through the skin, mucous membranes, and GI tract.

Dosage and Administration

■ **Reconstitution and Administration** Chloramphenicol sodium succinate is administered IV.

Although chloramphenicol has been administered IM†, plasma concentrations following IM injection are unpredictable. The manufacturer states that chloramphenicol sodium succinate should *not* be given IM since the drug may be ineffective when administered by this route.

Chloramphenicol has been administered orally as the base or as chloramphenicol palmitate; however, oral preparations of the drug are no longer commercially available in the US.

IV Administration Prior to IV administration, chloramphenicol sodium succinate vials labeled as containing 1 g of chloramphenicol should be reconstituted by adding 10 mL of aqueous diluent (e.g., sterile water for injection, 5% dextrose injection) to provide a solution containing 100 mg of chloramphenicol per mL.

Rate of Administration. The appropriate dose of reconstituted chloramphenicol solution should be injected IV over a period of at least 1 minute.

The drug also has been given by intermittent IV infusion† over 15–60 minutes.

■ **Dosage** Dosage of chloramphenicol sodium succinate is expressed in terms of chloramphenicol.

Because the difference between therapeutic and toxic plasma concentrations of chloramphenicol is narrow (i.e., a narrow therapeutic index) and because of interindividual differences in chloramphenicol metabolism and elimination, most clinicians recommend that plasma concentrations of chloramphenicol be monitored in all patients receiving the drug and dosage adjusted accordingly. Blood samples to measure peak plasma concentrations of chloramphenicol usually are obtained 0.5–1.5 hours after an IV dose.

Chloramphenicol dosage generally should be adjusted to maintain plasma concentrations of 5–20 mcg/mL (usually 10–20 mcg/mL). When used in pediatric patients beyond the neonatal period, the American Academy of Pediatrics (AAP) suggests that chloramphenicol dosage be adjusted to maintain target plasma concentrations of 15–25 mcg/mL. Some clinicians suggest that dosage in pediatric patients be adjusted to maintain peak plasma concentrations of 15–25 mcg/mL for the treatment of meningitis or 10–20 mcg/mL for the treatment of other infections. Chloramphenicol plasma concentrations greater than 25 mcg/mL have been associated with toxicity.

Chloramphenicol should be used no longer than is necessary to eradicate the infection with little or no risk of relapse. IV chloramphenicol should be switched to an appropriate oral anti-infective as soon as feasible.

Repeated courses of chloramphenicol should be avoided if possible.

Pediatric Dosage **General Dosage for Neonates.** The manufacturer states that an IV chloramphenicol dosage of 25 mg/kg daily given in 4 equally divided doses every 6 hours usually provides and maintains blood and tissue concentrations of the drug that are adequate for most indications. The manufacturer also states that, after the first 2 weeks of life, full-term neonates usually may receive a dosage up to 50 mg/kg daily given in 4 equally divided doses every 6 hours. If a higher dosage is required for the treatment of severe infections in neonates, the manufacturer recommends that such dosage be given only to maintain blood concentrations within a therapeutically effective range.

Some clinicians recommend that neonates receive an IV loading dose of chloramphenicol of 20 mg/kg followed 12 hours later by maintenance dosage based on age and weight. These clinicians recommend a maintenance dosage of 25 mg/kg once every 24 hours in neonates 7 days of age or younger, 25 mg/kg once every 24 hours in neonates older than 7 days of age weighing 2 kg or less, and 25 mg/kg once every 12 hours in those older than 7 days of age weighing more than 2 kg.

Other clinicians recommend that neonates receive an IV loading dose of 20 mg/kg followed 12 hours later by maintenance dosage based on age and weight. These clinicians recommend that premature neonates weighing 1.2 kg or less receive a maintenance dosage of 22 mg/kg once every 24 hours and that premature neonates 1 week of age or younger weighing 2 kg or less receive a maintenance dosage of 25 mg/kg once every 24 hours. These clinicians recommend that full-term neonates younger than 2 weeks of age receive a maintenance dosage of 25 mg/kg daily in divided doses every 12 hours and that full-term neonates 2–4 weeks of age receive a maintenance dosage of 25–50 mg/kg daily in divided doses every 12 hours.

Chloramphenicol should be used with caution in neonates because immature metabolic processes in this age group may result in excessive plasma concentrations of the drug. (See Cautions: Pediatric Precautions.)

General Dosage for Pediatric Patients Beyond the Neonatal Period. The manufacturer states that an IV chloramphenicol dosage of 50 mg/kg daily given in 4 divided doses every 6 hours provides blood concentrations of the drug that are adequate for most indications in pediatric patients. For the treatment of severe infections (e.g., bacteremia, meningitis), especially when adequate CSF concentrations are desired, the manufacturer states that a dosage up to 100 mg/kg daily may be required; however, this dosage should be reduced to 50 mg/kg daily as soon as possible.

If IV chloramphenicol is used for the treatment of severe infections in pediatric patients beyond the neonatal period, AAP recommends a dosage of 50–100 mg/kg daily given in 4 divided doses.

General Dosage for Pediatric Patients with Immature Metabolic Processes. The manufacturer states that IV chloramphenicol given in a dosage of 25 mg/kg daily will usually produce therapeutic blood concentrations of the drug in young infants and other pediatric patients in whom immature metabolic functions are suspected.

Chloramphenicol plasma concentrations should be carefully monitored in patients with immature metabolic processes because high concentrations of the drug may occur and tend to increase with succeeding doses. (See Cautions: Pediatric Precautions.)

Rickettsial Infections. If IV chloramphenicol is used as an alternative for the treatment of rickettsial infections, including Rocky Mountain spotted fever (RMSF) in children, a dosage of 12.5–25 mg/kg every 6 hours for 5–10 days has been recommended.

In patients with known or suspected RMSF, anti-infective treatment should be initiated promptly and should be continued for at least 3 days after fever subsides and until there is evidence of clinical improvement. The minimum duration of treatment is 5–7 days; a longer duration may be required for severe or complicated disease.

When considering use of chloramphenicol for the treatment of rickettsial infections, consultation with an expert is recommended. (See Uses: Rickettsial Infections.)

Typhoid Fever and other Severe Salmonella Infections. For the treatment of typhoid fever, pediatric patients 14 years of age or older have received IV chloramphenicol in a dosage of 50 mg/kg daily in 4 divided doses (up to 3 g daily) for 14 days. In children 2 years of age or older with typhoid fever, the drug has been given in a dosage of 60 mg/kg daily until defervescence, followed by 40 mg/kg daily to complete 14 days of treatment.

To lessen the possibility of relapse, some clinicians recommend that chloramphenicol dosage be adjusted to provide therapeutic plasma concentrations of the drug and treatment be continued for 8–10 days after the patient becomes afebrile.

Anthrax. If IV chloramphenicol is used as an alternative for the treatment of anthrax† (inhalational, GI, meningitis) that occurs as the result of natural or endemic exposures to *Bacillus anthracis* (see Uses: Anthrax), some clinicians recommend that children receive a dosage of 50–75 mg/kg daily given in divided doses every 6 hours. Treatment of naturally occurring or endemic anthrax generally should be continued for at least 14 days after symptoms abate.

If IV chloramphenicol is used as an alternative in a multiple-drug regimen for initial treatment of severe anthrax† (inhalational, GI, meningitis, or cutaneous with systemic involvement, extensive edema, or head or neck lesions) that occurs in the context of biologic warfare or bioterrorism, AAP recommends that full-term or preterm neonates 7 days of age or younger receive IV chloramphenicol in a dosage of 25 mg/kg once daily and that those 1–4 weeks of age receive 50 mg/kg daily in divided doses every 12 hours. AAP recommends that children 1 month of age or older receive IV chloramphenicol in a dosage of 100 mg/kg daily in divided doses every 6 hours. The multiple-drug parenteral regimen should be continued for at least 2–3 weeks until the patient is clinically stable; treatment can then be switched to appropriate oral anti-infectives.

Plague. If IV chloramphenicol is used as an alternative for the treatment of pneumonic plague† that occurs as the result of exposure to *Yersinia pestis* in the context of biologic warfare or bioterrorism, some experts (e.g., the US Working Group on Civilian Biodefense) recommend that children 2 years of age or older receive a dosage of 25 mg/kg 4 times daily and that dosage be adjusted to maintain plasma chloramphenicol concentrations of 5–20 mcg/mL. Other experts (e.g., US Army Medical Research Institute of Infectious Diseases [USAMRIID]) recommend that children 2 years of age or older receive an IV loading dose of 25 mg/kg followed by 15 mg/kg IV every 6 hours and that dosage be adjusted based on plasma concentrations.

Treatment can be switched to an appropriate oral anti-infective when clinically indicated; the total duration of treatment usually is 10–14 days.

Tularemia. If IV chloramphenicol is used as an alternative for the treatment of tularemia† that occurs as the result of exposure to *Francisella tularensis* in the context of biologic warfare or bioterrorism, some experts (e.g., US Working Group on Civilian Biodefense) recommend that children receive a dosage of 15 mg/kg 4 times daily. Treatment can be switched to an appropriate oral anti-infective when clinically indicated; the total duration of treatment usually is 14–21 days.

If IV chloramphenicol is used in conjunction with streptomycin (or gentamicin) for the treatment of tularemic meningitis in children, some clinicians recommend a dosage of 15 mg/kg every 6 hours (maximum 4 g daily) given for 14–21 days.

Adult Dosage **General Dosage for Adults.** The manufacturer recommends that adults with normal renal and hepatic function receive an IV chloramphenicol dosage of 50 mg/kg daily given in divided doses every 6 hours.

In infections caused by less susceptible organisms, the manufacturer states that an IV chloramphenicol dosage up to 100 mg/kg daily may be required. However, because toxic plasma concentrations of the drug may occur in many patients receiving dosages of 100 mg/kg daily, some clinicians suggest that a dosage of 75 mg/kg daily be used initially for the treatment of such infections. Dosage should be reduced to 50 mg/kg daily as soon as possible.

Rickettsial Infections. If IV chloramphenicol is used as an alternative for the treatment of rickettsial infections, including endemic typhus or epidemic typhus, in adults, a dosage of 60–75 mg/kg daily in 4 divided doses for 5–10 days has been recommended. For the treatment of scrub typhus caused by *Orientia tsutsugamushi*, a dosage of 50–100 mg/kg daily (up to 3 g daily) in divided doses every 6 hours has been recommended.

In patients with known or suspected RMSF, anti-infective treatment should be initiated promptly and should be continued for at least 3 days after fever subsides and until there is evidence of clinical improvement. The minimum duration of treatment is 5–7 days; a longer duration may be required for severe or complicated disease.

When considering use of chloramphenicol for the treatment of a rickettsial infection, consultation with an expert is recommended. (See Uses: Rickettsial Infections.)

Typhoid Fever and Other Salmonella Infections. For the treatment of typhoid fever in adults, IV chloramphenicol has been given in a dosage of 50 mg/kg daily in 4 divided doses for 14 days. The drug also has been given in a dosage of 60 mg/kg daily in 4 divided doses until defervescence followed by 40 mg/kg daily in 4 divided doses to complete 14 days of treatment.

To lessen the possibility of relapse, some clinicians recommend that chloramphenicol be given in a dosage that provides therapeutic plasma concentrations of the drug and treatment be continued for 8–10 days after the patient becomes afebrile.

Anthrax. If IV chloramphenicol is used as an alternative in a multiple-drug regimen for the treatment of anthrax† (inhalational, GI, meningitis) that occurs as the result of natural or endemic exposures to *B. anthracis* (see Uses: Anthrax), some clinicians recommend that adults receive a dosage of 50–100 mg/kg daily given in divided doses every 6 hours. Treatment of naturally occurring or endemic anthrax generally should be continued for at least 14 days after symptoms abate.

If IV chloramphenicol is used as an alternative in a multiple-drug regimen for initial treatment of severe anthrax† (inhalational, GI, meningitis, or cutaneous with systemic involvement, extensive edema, or head or neck lesions) that occurs in the context of biologic warfare or bioterrorism, the US Centers for Disease Control and Prevention (CDC) recommends that adults receive a dosage of 1 g every 6–8 hours. The multiple-drug parenteral regimen should be continued for at least 2–3 weeks until the patient is clinically stable; treatment can then be switched to appropriate oral anti-infectives.

Plague. If IV chloramphenicol is used as an alternative for the treatment of pneumonic plague† that occurs as the result of exposure to *Y. pestis* in the context of biologic warfare or bioterrorism, some experts (e.g., the US Working Group on Civilian Biodefense) recommend that adults receive a dosage of 25 mg/kg 4 times daily and that dosage be adjusted to maintain plasma chloramphenicol concentrations of 5–20 mcg/mL. Other experts (e.g., USAMRIID) recommend an IV loading dose of 25 mg/kg followed by 15 mg/kg IV every 6 hours and that dosage be adjusted based on plasma concentrations.

Treatment can be switched to an appropriate oral anti-infective when clinically indicated; total duration of treatment usually is 10–14 days.

Tularemia. If IV chloramphenicol is used as an alternative for the treatment of tularemia† that occurs as the result of exposure to *F. tularensis* in the context of biologic warfare or bioterrorism, some experts (e.g., the US Working Group on Civilian Biodefense) recommend that adults receive a dosage of 15 mg/kg 4 times daily. Other experts (e.g., USAMRIID) recommend a dosage of 15–25 mg/kg IV every 6 hours. Treatment can be switched to an appropriate oral anti-infective when clinically indicated; the total duration of treatment usually is 14–21 days.

If IV chloramphenicol is used in conjunction with streptomycin (or gentamicin) for the treatment of tularemic meningitis, some clinicians recommend that adults receive a dosage of 15–25 mg/kg every 6 hours (maximum 4 g daily) given for 14–21 days.

■ **Dosage in Renal and Hepatic Impairment** Because patients with renal and/or hepatic impairment may have reduced ability to metabolize and eliminate chloramphenicol, dosage should be based on plasma chloramphenicol concentrations and adjusted accordingly.

Clinicians should consider that pediatric patients with impaired renal or hepatic function may retain excessive amounts of the drug. (See General Dosage for Pediatric Patients with Immature Metabolic Processes under Dosage: Pediatric Dosage, in Dosage and Administration.)

Cautions

■ **Hematologic Effects** Serious and fatal blood dyscrasias (aplastic anemia, hypoplastic anemia, thrombocytopenia, granulocytopenia) have occurred in patients receiving both short-term and prolonged treatment with chloramphenicol. Aplastic anemia attributed to chloramphenicol, which later terminated in leukemia, has been reported.

Two forms of hematologic toxicity may occur with chloramphenicol. The first type is the most common and is a dose-related bone marrow suppression that appears to be a direct pharmacologic effect of chloramphenicol and usually is reversible upon discontinuance of the drug. This type of bone marrow suppression is characterized by anemia, leukopenia, reticulocytopenia, thrombocytopenia, increased concentrations of serum iron, increased serum iron-binding capacity, and vacuolation of erythroid and myeloid precursors. It is more likely to occur in patients receiving a chloramphenicol dosage of 4 g daily or higher and in those with plasma chloramphenicol concentrations greater than 25 mcg/mL.

The second type of hematologic toxicity that can occur in patients receiving chloramphenicol is a rare, but often fatal, irreversible aplastic anemia that does not appear to be dose related. This type of bone marrow effect leading to aplastic anemia has been reported with oral or parenteral chloramphenicol and has been associated with a mortality rate greater than 50%. Bone marrow aplasia or hypoplasia may occur weeks or months after the drug has been discontinued. Pancytopenia is frequently observed peripherally, but in some cases only 1 or 2 of the major cell types (erythrocytes, leukocytes, platelets) may be depressed.

Paroxysmal nocturnal hemoglobinuria has been reported in patients receiving chloramphenicol. Hemolytic anemia has been reported when chloramphenicol was used in patients with glucose-6-phosphate dehydrogenase deficiency.

■ **Gray Syndrome** A type of circulatory collapse, referred to as the gray syndrome, has occurred in neonates and premature infants receiving chloramphenicol. In most cases, chloramphenicol therapy had been instituted within the first 48 hours of life; however, the gray syndrome has occurred in older infants and in infants born to mothers who received chloramphenicol during the late stages of pregnancy or during labor. In addition, a similar syndrome has been reported in older children and adults following chloramphenicol overdosage.

Symptoms of the gray syndrome in infants usually develop 2–9 days after chloramphenicol therapy is initiated and include abdominal distention (with or without vomiting), progressive pallid cyanosis, flaccidity, and vasomotor collapse which may frequently be accompanied by irregular respiration. Gray syndrome can be fatal within a few hours after onset of symptoms. However, if chloramphenicol is discontinued when early evidence of symptoms becomes apparent, the process may be reversible and complete recovery may follow.

The gray syndrome may occur because chloramphenicol impairs myocardial contractility by directly interfering with myocardial tissue respiration and oxidative phosphorylation. It has been attributed to high plasma concentrations of chloramphenicol and is believed to occur more frequently in neonates and young infants because of their inability to conjugate chloramphenicol and excrete the unconjugated drug.

■ **Nervous System Effects** Optic neuritis, rarely resulting in optic atrophy and blindness, has been reported in patients receiving chloramphenicol, usually following long-term therapy with the drug. Although symptoms tend to be reversible, permanent vision loss may occur.

Peripheral neuritis has occurred following long-term chloramphenicol therapy. Headache, ophthalmoplegia, depression, confusion, and delirium have been reported.

■ **GI and Hepatic Effects** Adverse GI effects, including nausea, vomiting, diarrhea, glossitis, stomatitis, and enterocolitis have been reported rarely with chloramphenicol.

■ **Sensitivity Reactions** Hypersensitivity reactions, including anaphylaxis, rash (macular and vesicular), angioedema, urticaria, and fever, have occurred in patients receiving chloramphenicol.

Herxheimer-like reactions have occurred in patients receiving chloramphenicol for the treatment of typhoid fever.

■ **Precautions and Contraindications** Chloramphenicol is contraindicated in patients with a history of hypersensitivity and/or toxic reactions to the drug.

Because serious, sometimes fatal, reactions have been reported in patients who received chloramphenicol, patients should be hospitalized during therapy with the drug so that appropriate laboratory studies and clinical observations can be made. Chloramphenicol *must not* be used for the treatment of trivial infections or when it is not indicated (e.g., treatment of colds, influenza, throat infections) and *must not* be used for prophylaxis. The drug should be administered no longer than is necessary to eradicate the infection with little or no risk of relapse, and repeated courses should be avoided if possible.

Because of the narrow margin between effective therapeutic and toxic dosages of chloramphenicol and because there are interindividual differences in metabolism and elimination of the drug, most clinicians recommend that plasma concentrations of chloramphenicol be monitored in all patients receiving the drug. In general, plasma chloramphenicol concentrations should be maintained at 5–20 mcg/mL to ensure efficacy and avoid toxicity. (See Dosage and Administration: Dosage.)

It is essential that adequate hematologic studies be performed prior to and approximately every 2 days during chloramphenicol therapy. The drug should be discontinued if reticulocytopenia, leukopenia, thrombocytopenia, anemia, or other hematologic abnormalities attributable to chloramphenicol occur. Although peripheral blood studies may detect leukopenia, reticulocytopenia, or granulocytopenia before these become irreversible, such studies cannot be relied on to detect bone marrow depression prior to development of aplastic anemia.

If optic or peripheral neuritis occurs during chloramphenicol therapy (see Cautions: Nervous System Effects), the drug should be discontinued immediately.

Chloramphenicol should be used with caution in patients with impaired renal and/or hepatic function and in neonates and infants or other pediatric patients with immature metabolic processes. Plasma chloramphenicol concentrations should be monitored closely in these patients and dosage should be adjusted accordingly.

When selecting or modifying anti-infective therapy, results of culture and in vitro susceptibility testing should be used. In the absence of such data, local epidemiology and susceptibility patterns should be considered when selecting anti-infectives for empiric therapy.

As with other anti-infectives, use of chloramphenicol may result in overgrowth of nonsusceptible organisms, including fungi. If infection caused by nonsusceptible organisms occurs, appropriate therapy should be instituted.

■ **Pediatric Precautions** Chloramphenicol should be used with caution in premature and full-term neonates and infants to avoid potential toxicity, including a type of circulatory collapse referred to as the gray syndrome. (See Cautions: Gray Syndrome.)

Excessive plasma concentrations of chloramphenicol may occur in neonates and infants or other pediatric patients with immature metabolic processes, even when recommended chloramphenicol dosage is used. Plasma concentration of the drug should be determined at appropriate intervals during chloramphenicol treatment and dosage should be adjusted accordingly. (See Dosage and Administration: Dosage.)

■ **Geriatric Precautions** Clinical studies of chloramphenicol did not include sufficient numbers of patients 65 years of age or older to determine whether geriatric adults respond differently than younger patients. Other reported clinical experience has not identified differences in responses between geriatric and younger adults.

Chloramphenicol is substantially eliminated by the kidneys, and the risk of adverse effects may be greater in those with impaired renal function. Dosage in geriatric patients should be selected with caution, usually starting at the low end of the dosage range, and it may be useful to monitor renal function during chloramphenicol treatment. The greater frequency of decreased renal, hepatic, and/or cardiac function and of concomitant disease and drug therapy observed in geriatric patients should be considered.

■ **Mutagenicity and Carcinogenicity** Animal and human studies have not been performed to evaluate the mutagenic and carcinogenic potential of chloramphenicol.

■ **Pregnancy, Fertility, and Lactation** ***Pregnancy*** There are no adequate and well-controlled studies evaluating use of chloramphenicol in pregnant women. Animal reproduction studies have not been conducted using the drug.

Studies using oral chloramphenicol (no longer commercially available in the US) indicate that the drug crosses the placenta.

Use of chloramphenicol during late pregnancy and during labor has been associated with the gray syndrome and other adverse effects in the fetus or infant. (See Cautions: Gray Syndrome.)

Because of potential toxic effects on the fetus, the manufacturer states that chloramphenicol should be used during pregnancy only if potential benefits justify potentials risks to the fetus.

Fertility Animal and human studies have not been performed to evaluate whether chloramphenicol affects fertility.

Lactation Studies using oral chloramphenicol (no longer commercially available in the US) indicate that the drug is distributed into human milk.

Because chloramphenicol potentially could cause serious adverse effects in breast-fed infants (see Cautions: Gray Syndrome), the manufacturer states that a decision should be made whether to discontinue nursing or chloramphenicol, taking into account the importance of the drug to the woman.

Drug Interactions

■ **Drugs Affecting or Metabolized by Hepatic Microsomal Enzymes** Chloramphenicol inhibits cytochrome P-450 (CYP) isoenzymes 2C9 and 3A4.

■ **Antianemia Drugs** When administered concurrently with iron preparations, vitamin B_{12}, or folic acid, chloramphenicol may delay the response to these drugs.

■ **Anticoagulants** Chloramphenicol may prolong the half-life of warfarin.

■ **Anticonvulsants** Concomitant use of fosphenytoin and chloramphenicol may result in altered (increased or decreased) chloramphenicol concentrations.

Concomitant use of phenobarbital and chloramphenicol has resulted in decreased plasma concentrations of chloramphenicol. Concomitant use of the drugs may increase clearance of chloramphenicol resulting in a 30–40% reduction in plasma concentrations of the drug. In addition, phenobarbital plasma concentrations may be increased by up to 50%.

Concomitant use of phenytoin and chloramphenicol may result in altered (increased or decreased) chloramphenicol concentrations and may result in potentially toxic plasma chloramphenicol concentrations. In addition, concomitant use of the drugs may increase plasma concentrations and prolong the half-life of phenytoin resulting in phenytoin toxicity.

■ **Antidiabetic Agents** Chloramphenicol may decrease metabolism of some sulfonylurea antidiabetic agents (e.g., chlorpropamide, tolbutamide) and may increase plasma half-lives of these drugs.

■ **Anti-infective Agents** Chloramphenicol has been reported to antagonize the bactericidal activity of certain penicillins, cephalosporins, fluoroquinolones, and aminoglycosides in vitro. Although the clinical importance of this in vitro data is unclear, some clinicians recommend that chloramphenicol and these anti-infectives be used concomitantly with caution or that concomitant use be avoided.

Results of an in vitro study using *Klebsiella pneumoniae* indicate that chloramphenicol can antagonize the bactericidal activity of aztreonam. It has been suggested that if concomitant use of the drugs is indicated, chloramphenicol should be administered a few hours after aztreonam; however, the necessity of this precaution has not been established.

Concomitant use of chloramphenicol and rifampin may increase clearance of chloramphenicol resulting in decreased plasma concentrations of the drug.

■ **Cyclophosphamide** Concomitant use of cyclophosphamide and chloramphenicol may prolong the half-life of cyclophosphamide and result in decreased concentrations of the active cyclophosphamide metabolite and reduced effectiveness of the drug.

■ **Immunosuppressive Agents** Concomitant use of cyclosporine and chloramphenicol may result in increased cyclosporine concentrations and increased risk of renal dysfunction, cholestasis, and paresthesias.

Concomitant use of tacrolimus and chloramphenicol may result in increased tacrolimus concentrations.

■ **Myelosuppressive Agents** Because of potential additive effects on bone marrow, concomitant use of chloramphenicol and other drugs associated with bone marrow depression should be avoided.

■ **Typhoid Vaccine** Concomitant use of chloramphenicol and typhoid vaccine live oral Ty21a may decrease efficacy of the live, attenuated vaccine.

Mechanism of Action

Chloramphenicol usually is bacteriostatic in action, but may be bactericidal against some organisms.

Chloramphenicol inhibits protein synthesis in susceptible organisms by reversibly binding to the peptidyl transferase cavity of the 50S ribosomal subunit of the bacterial 70S ribosome. This prevents the aminoacyl-tRNA from binding to the ribosome and terminates polypeptide chain synthesis.

Chloramphenicol also appears to inhibit protein synthesis in rapidly proliferating mammalian cells. It has been suggested that dose-related bone marrow depression due to chloramphenicol is the result of inhibition of protein synthesis in mitochondria of bone marrow cells.

Spectrum

Chloramphenicol has a broad spectrum of activity and is active in vitro against many gram-positive and gram-negative aerobic bacteria, some anaerobic bacteria, and some other organisms, including some *Rickettsia*, *Chlamydia*, and *Mycoplasma*. The drug is inactive against *Mycobacterium* and protozoa.

■ **Gram-positive Bacteria** Chloramphenicol is active in vitro against many gram-positive aerobic cocci, including *Staphylococcus aureus*, *S. epidermidis*, *Streptococcus pneumoniae*, *S. pyogenes* (group A β-hemolytic streptococci; GAS), *S. agalactiae* (group B streptococci; GBS), α-hemolytic streptococci, and *Enterococcus faecalis*. Chloramphenicol may be active in vitro against some methicillin-resistant *S. aureus* (MRSA; also known as oxacillin-resistant *S. aureus* or ORSA) and some *S. aureus* resistant to vancomycin.

Chloramphenicol also is active in vitro against some other gram-positive bacteria, including *Corynebacterium diphtheriae* and *Listeria monocytogenes*. The drug is not active against *Nocardia*.

Chloramphenicol has in vitro activity against *Bacillus anthracis*. Results of in vitro susceptibility testing of 11 *B. anthracis* isolates that were associated with cases of inhalational or cutaneous anthrax that occurred in the US (Florida, New York, District of Columbia) during September and October 2001 in the context of an intentional release of anthrax spores (biologic warfare, bioterrorism) indicate that these strains had chloramphenicol MICs of 4 mcg/mL and were considered susceptible to the drug. Limited clinical data are available to date regarding in vivo activity of chloramphenicol against *B. anthracis* or use of the drug in the treatment of anthrax.

■ **Gram-negative Bacteria** Chloramphenicol is active in vitro against some gram-negative aerobic bacteria, including *Haemophilus influenzae*, *H. parainfluenzae*, *Moraxella catarrhalis*, *Neisseria gonorrhoeae*, and *N. meningitidis*.

Although chloramphenicol is active against some Enterobacteriaceae, including some *Citrobacter*, *Enterobacter*, *Escherichia coli*, *Hafnia*, *Klebsiella*, *Proteus*, *Providencia*, *Salmonella*, and *Shigella*, susceptibility is variable and many strains are resistant to the drug.

Yersinia pestis and *Y. enterocolitica* usually are susceptible to chloramphenicol, but resistant strains have been reported.

Burkholderia pseudomallei generally is susceptible to chloramphenicol. *B. cepacia* and *Pseudomonas aeruginosa* usually are resistant to the drug.

Chloramphenicol usually is active against *Aeromonas*, *Bordetella pertussis*, *Brucella*, *Campylobacter jejuni*, *Francisella tularensis*, *Helicobacter pylori*, *Legionella pneumophila*, *Pasteurella multocida*, and *Vibrio parahaemolyticus*. Although *V. cholerae* usually are susceptible to chloramphenicol, resistance has been reported.

■ **Anaerobic Bacteria** Chloramphenicol is active in vitro against many gram-positive anaerobic bacteria, including *Actinomyces*, *Bifidobacterium*, *Clostridium*, *Eubacterium*, *Lactobacillus*, *Peptococcus*, *Peptostreptococcus*, and *Propionibacterium*.

Chloramphenicol also is active in vitro against some gram-negative anaerobic bacteria, including *Bacteroides fragilis*, *Fusobacterium*, *Prevotella*, and *Veillonella*.

■ **Other Organisms** *Treponema pallidum*, *Chlamydia*, and *Mycoplasma* are susceptible to chloramphenicol.

Chloramphenicol is active against some *Rickettsia*, including *R. rickettsii* and causative agents of various typhus fevers. The drug also is active against *Coxiella burnetii*.

■ **In Vitro Susceptibility Testing** When in vitro susceptibility testing is performed according to the standards of the Clinical and Laboratory Standards Institute (CLSI; formerly National Committee for Clinical Laboratory Standards [NCCLS]), clinical isolates identified as *susceptible* to chloramphenicol are inhibited by drug concentrations usually achievable when the recommended dosage is used for the site of infection. Clinical isolates classified as *intermediate* have minimum inhibitory concentrations (MICs) that approach usually attainable blood and tissue concentrations and response rates may be lower than for strains identified as susceptible. Therefore, the intermediate category implies clinical applicability in body sites where the drug is physiologically concentrated or when a higher than usual dosage can be used. This intermediate category also includes a buffer zone which should prevent small, uncontrolled technical factors from causing major discrepancies in interpretation, especially for drugs with narrow pharmacotoxicity margins. If results of in vitro susceptibility testing indicate that a clinical isolate is *resistant* to chloramphenicol, the strain is not inhibited by drug concentrations generally achievable with usual dosage schedules and/or MICs fall in the range where specific microbial resistance mechanisms are likely and clinical efficacy of the drug against the isolate has not been reliably demonstrated in clinical studies.

Disk Susceptibility Tests When the disk-diffusion procedure is used to test susceptibility to chloramphenicol, a disk containing 30 mcg/mL of the drug should be used.

When disk-diffusion susceptibility testing is performed according to CLSI standardized procedures using CLSI interpretive criteria, *Staphylococcus* or *Enterococcus* with growth inhibition zones of 18 mm or greater are susceptible to chloramphenicol, those with zones of 13–17 mm have intermediate susceptibility, and those with zones of 12 mm or less are resistant to the drug.

When the disk-diffusion procedure is performed according to CLSI standardized procedures, *Haemophilus* with growth inhibition zones of 29 mm or greater are susceptible to chloramphenicol, those with zones of 26–28 mm have intermediate susceptibility, and those with zones of 25 mm or less are resistant to the drug.

When testing susceptibility of *S. pneumoniae* according to CLSI standardized procedures, *S. pneumoniae* with growth inhibition zones of 21 mm or greater are susceptible to chloramphenicol and those with zones of 20 mm or less are resistant to the drug. When testing streptococci other than *S. pneumoniae*, those with zones of 21 mm or greater are susceptible to chloramphenicol, those with zones of 18–20 mm have intermediate susceptibility, and those with zones of 17 mm or less are resistant to the drug.

When the disk-diffusion procedure is performed according to CLSI standardized procedures, *N. meningitidis* with growth inhibition zones of 26 mm or greater are susceptible to chloramphenicol, those with zones of 20–25 mm have intermediate susceptibility, and those with zones of 19 mm or less are resistant to the drug.

Dilution Susceptibility Tests When dilution susceptibility testing (agar or broth dilution) is performed according to CLSI standardized procedures, *Staphylococcus*, *Enterococcus*, Enterobacteriaceae, non-Enterobacteriaceae gram-negative bacilli (e.g., *B. cepacia* complex, *Pseudomonas* spp. other than *Ps. aeruginosa*) with MICs of 8 mcg/mL or less are susceptible to chloramphenicol, those with MICs of 16 mcg/mL have intermediate susceptibility, and those with MICs of 32 mcg/mL or greater are resistant to the drug.

When broth dilution susceptibility testing is performed according to CLSI standardized procedures, *Haemophilus* or *N. meningitidis* with MICs of 2 mcg/mL or less are susceptible to chloramphenicol, those with MICs of 4 mcg/mL have intermediate susceptibility, and those with MICs of 8 mcg/mL or greater are resistant to the drug.

When testing susceptibility of *S. pneumoniae* according to CLSI standardized procedures, *S. pneumoniae* with MICs of 4 mcg/mL or less are susceptible to chloramphenicol and those with MICs of 8 mcg/mL or greater are resistant to the drug. Streptococci other than *S. pneumoniae* with MICs of 4 mcg/mL or less are susceptible to chloramphenicol, those with MICs of 8 mcg/mL have intermediate susceptibility, and those with MICs of 16 mcg/mL or greater are resistant to the drug.

When broth dilution susceptibility testing is performed according to CLSI standardized procedures, anaerobes with MICs of 8 mcg/mL or less are susceptible to chloramphenicol, those with MICs of 16 mcg/mL have intermediate susceptibility, and those with MICs of 32 mcg/mL or greater are resistant to the drug.

Resistance

Resistance to chloramphenicol has been induced in vitro and has been shown to be induced in a stepwise manner. The reported incidence of chloramphenicol resistance in clinical isolates varies considerably worldwide and may be reported more frequently in regions of the world where the drug is still commonly used and has not been reserved for the treatment of serious infections.

Several mechanisms of resistance to chloramphenicol have been reported. A common mechanism of resistance to the drug is enzymatic acetylation and inactivation by chloramphenicol acetyltransferases (CATs). CATs have been identified in many different bacteria and may be readily transmitted to other bacteria. Other mechanisms of resistance to chloramphenicol involve transmembrane efflux pumps, decreased membrane permeability, or alterations in the 50S ribosomal subunit.

Staphylococcus aureus, S. epidermidis, S. hemolyticus, Streptococcus pneumoniae, S. pyogenes, and *Enterococcus faecium* resistant to chloramphenicol have been reported.

Escherichia coli, Salmonella, and *Shigella* resistant to chloramphenicol have been reported with increasing frequency. Chloramphenicol-resistant strains of *Haemophilus influenzae* and *Neisseria meningitidis* have been reported rarely.

Clostridium difficile and *C. perfringens* resistant to chloramphenicol have been reported.

Pharmacokinetics

■ **Absorption** Following IV administration of chloramphenicol sodium succinate, there is considerable interindividual variation in plasma chloramphenicol concentrations attained in adults, children, or neonates. (For information on monitoring plasma chloramphenicol concentrations, see Dosage and Administration: Dosage.) Chloramphenicol sodium succinate is a prodrug and is hydrolyzed in vivo to active chloramphenicol. The rate and extent of hydrolysis of the ester are highly variable. Bioavailability of chloramphenicol following IV administration of chloramphenicol sodium succinate also depends on renal clearance of the unchanged ester, which also is highly variable.

■ **Distribution** Chloramphenicol is widely distributed into body tissues and fluids including ascitic fluid, pleural fluid, synovial fluid, saliva, and aqueous and vitreous humor. Highest concentrations of the drug are found in the liver and kidneys.

Chloramphenicol is distributed into CSF, even in the absence of meningeal inflammation. CSF concentrations of chloramphenicol have been reported to be at least 50% of concurrent plasma concentrations in patients with uninflamed meninges. In 3 neonates 2–6 weeks of age receiving IV chloramphenicol for the treatment of meningitis or ventriculitis, CSF concentrations of the drug were 45–89% of concurrent plasma concentrations.

Chloramphenicol crosses the placenta.

Chloramphenicol is distributed into milk.

Chloramphenicol is approximately 60% bound to plasma proteins.

■ **Elimination** Chloramphenicol sodium succinate is hydrolyzed in vivo, presumably by esterases in the liver, kidneys, and lungs, to form active chloramphenicol. Chloramphenicol is then metabolized primarily in the liver to chloramphenicol glucuronide, an inactive metabolite.

Following IV administration of chloramphenicol sodium succinate in adults with normal renal and hepatic function, approximately 30% of the dose is excreted unchanged in urine; however, the fraction of the dose excreted unchanged in urine varies considerably and may range from 6–80%. Small amounts of the dose (2–3%) are eliminated in bile and about 1% is eliminated in feces.

The plasma half-life of chloramphenicol in adults with normal renal and hepatic function is 1.2–4.1 hours.

Because neonates and premature infants have immature mechanisms for glucuronide conjugation and renal excretion, usual doses of chloramphenicol may produce high and prolonged plasma concentrations of the drug in such neonates and infants. The plasma half-life of chloramphenicol is inversely related to age. In one study, plasma half-life was 10–36 hours in neonates 1–8 days of age and 5.5–15.7 hours in infants 11 days to 8 weeks of age.

The elimination half-life of chloramphenicol is prolonged and clearance of the drug is decreased in patients with reduced hepatic function.

In patients with impaired renal function, the elimination half-life of chloramphenicol is not significantly prolonged, although accumulation of the inactive conjugated metabolite may occur. Following IV administration of chloramphenicol sodium succinate in patients with renal impairment, plasma chloramphenicol concentrations may be increased since renal excretion of the succinate ester is reduced in these patients.

Increased chloramphenicol clearance has been reported in patients undergoing hemodialysis. Plasma half-life of chloramphenicol is not affected by peritoneal dialysis. The drug appears to be readily removed by charcoal hemoperfusion.

Chemistry and Stability

■ **Chemistry** Chloramphenicol is a broad-spectrum antibiotic originally isolated from *Streptomyces venezuelae* and now produced synthetically. Chloramphenicol occurs as fine, white to grayish or yellowish white, needle-like crystals or elongated plates, has a solubility of approximately 2.5 mg/mL in water at 25°C, and is freely soluble in alcohol. The pK_a of the drug is 5.5. Chloramphenicol sodium succinate occurs as a white to light yellow powder and is freely soluble in water and in alcohol.

Chloramphenicol sodium succinate is commercially available as a lyophilized powder that should be reconstituted as directed by the manufacturer to provide an IV solution containing 100 mg of chloramphenicol per mL. Each 1 g of chloramphenicol in the reconstituted solution contains approximately 52 mg (2.25 mEq) of sodium.

■ **Stability** Chloramphenicol sodium succinate powder for injection should be stored at 20–25°C.

Chloramphenicol has been reported to be physically incompatible with some drugs, but the compatibility depends on several factors (e.g., the concentration of the drugs, specific diluents used, resulting pH, temperature). Specialized references should be consulted for specific compatibility information.

Preparations

Excipients in commercially available drug preparations may have clinically important effects in some individuals; consult specific product labeling for details.

Chloramphenicol Sodium Succinate

Parenteral

For injection, for IV use only	1 g (of chloramphenicol)*	**Chloramphenicol Sodium Succinate**

*available from one or more manufacturer, distributor, and/or repackager by generic (nonproprietary) name

†Use is not currently included in the labeling approved by the US Food and Drug Administration

MACROLIDES 8:12.12

ERYTHROMYCINS 8:12.12.04

Erythromycins General Statement

■ Erythromycins are macrolide antibiotics that are active principally against gram-positive cocci and bacilli and to a lesser extent gram-negative cocci and bacilli; the drugs also exhibit activity against chlamydia, mycoplasma, ureaplasma, spirochetes, and mycobacteria.

Uses

Prior to initiation of erythromycin therapy, appropriate specimens should be obtained for identification of the causative organism and in vitro susceptibility tests. Use of erythromycin does not preclude the necessity for surgical procedures (such as incision and drainage) as needed. There does not appear to be a difference in clinical efficacy among the erythromycin derivatives when each is administered in appropriate doses. However, some clinicians believe that the risk of hepatotoxicity from the estolate derivative does not justify its use.

■ **Streptococcal Infections** Erythromycin is used for the treatment of mild to moderately severe infections of the upper and lower respiratory tract, skin, and soft tissue caused by *Streptococcus pyogenes* (group A β-hemolytic streptococci). Erythromycin also is used to treat mild to moderately severe infections of the upper and lower respiratory tract caused by *Streptococcus pneumoniae*. Other macrolides (azithromycin, clarithromycin) generally are used orally as alternatives to first-line therapy with a natural penicillin for the treatment of mild to moderate upper and lower respiratory tract infections caused by susceptible *S. pyogenes* or *S. pneumoniae* when oral therapy of such infections is considered appropriate and when therapy with erythromycin or other less expensive anti-infectives would likely be less effective and/or associated with GI intolerance or noncompliance.

Pharyngitis and Tonsillitis Erythromycin or other macrolides (azithromycin, clarithromycin) are used orally for the treatment of pharyngitis and tonsillitis caused by *S. pyogenes* (group A β-hemolytic streptococci). Although macrolides usually are effective in eradicating *S. pyogenes* from the nasopharynx, efficacy of the drugs in the subsequent prevention of rheumatic fever remains to be established.

Selection of an anti-infective agent for the treatment of *S. pyogenes* pharyngitis or tonsillitis should be based on the drug's spectrum of activity as well as the regimen's bacteriologic and clinical efficacy, potential adverse effects, ease of administration and patient compliance, and cost. No regimen has been found to date that effectively eradicates group A β-hemolytic streptococci in 100% of patients. Because penicillin has a narrow spectrum of activity, is inexpensive, and generally is effective, the US Centers for Disease Control and Prevention (CDC), American Academy of Pediatrics (AAP), American Academy of Family Physicians (AAFP), Infectious Diseases Society of America (IDSA), American Heart Association (AHA), American College of Physicians (ACP), and others consider natural penicillins (i.e., 10 days of oral penicillin V or a single IM dose of penicillin G benzathine) the treatment of choice for streptococcal pharyngitis and tonsillitis and prevention of initial attacks (primary prevention) of rheumatic fever, although oral amoxicillin often is used instead of penicillin V in small children because of a more acceptable taste. Other anti-infectives (e.g., oral cephalosporins, oral macrolides) generally are considered alternative agents.

A 10-day regimen of oral erythromycin usually is considered the preferred alternative for the treatment of streptococcal pharyngitis in patients hypersensitive to penicillin. It has been suggested that oral azithromycin offers an advantage over oral erythromycin in terms of improved GI tolerance and ease of administration (i.e., fewer daily doses and a 5-day regimen). However, because of limited data to date, the IDSA states that use of anti-infective regimens administered for 5 days or less for the treatment of *S. pyogenes* pharyngitis cannot be recommended at this time.

Although strains of *S. pyogenes* resistant to erythromycin and other macrolides have been reported and may be prevalent in some areas of the world (e.g., Japan, Finland) and have resulted in treatment failures, the incidence of these resistant *S. pyogenes* in the US has been relatively low to date. (See Resistance.)

For additional information on treatment of *S. pyogenes* pharyngitis, see Pharyngitis and Tonsillitis under Gram-positive Aerobic Bacterial Infections: Streptococcus pyogenes Infections, in Uses in the Natural Penicillins General Statement 8:12.16.04.

Prophylaxis of Recurrent Rheumatic Fever Oral erythromycin is used as an alternative to IM penicillin G benzathine, oral penicillin V potassium, and oral sulfadiazine or sulfisoxazole for prevention of recurrent attacks of rheumatic fever (secondary prophylaxis) in patients hypersensitive to penicillins and sulfonamides. The AHA and AAP recommend that patients with a well-documented history of rheumatic fever (including cases manifested solely by Sydenham's chorea) and those with evidence of rheumatic heart disease receive continuous antibiotic prophylaxis to prevent recurrent attacks. Continuous prophylaxis should be initiated as soon as the diagnosis of rheumatic fever or rheumatic heart disease is made, although patients with acute rheumatic fever should first receive the usual recommended anti-infective therapy for group A β-hemolytic streptococcal infections. In general, prevention of recurrent rheumatic fever requires long-term, continuous prophylaxis and the recommended duration depends on the presence or absence of residual heart damage The risk of rheumatic fever recurrence decreases with increasing age and as the interval since the most recent attack increases. Patients without rheumatic heart disease are at lower risk of recurrence than patients with cardiac involvement. The AHA recommends that patients who have had rheumatic fever without carditis receive secondary prophylaxis for at least 5 years or until the individual is 21 years of age (whichever is longer) and that those with rheumatic fever and carditis (but no clinical or echocardiographic evidence of residual heart disease) receive secondary prophylaxis for 10 years or well into adulthood (whichever is longer). The AHA recommends that those with rheumatic fever and carditis with residual heart disease (clinical or echocardiographic evidence of persistent valvar disease) receive secondary prophylaxis for at least 10 years since the last episode and at least until 40 years of age; lifelong prophylaxis may be indicated in these patients.

Anti-infective regimens used for the prophylaxis of recurrent rheumatic fever are inadequate for prophylaxis of bacterial endocarditis in adults and children with rheumatic valvular heart dysfunction undergoing certain dental and surgical procedures that put them at increased risk of endocarditis caused by viridans streptococci or certain GI, biliary, or genitourinary procedures that put them at risk of enterococcal endocarditis. Therefore, these individuals should receive short-term prophylaxis for prevention of bacterial endocarditis when indicated (see Uses: Prophylaxis of Bacterial Endocarditis in the Aminopenicillins General Statement 8:12.16.08). Individuals who have had rheumatic fever without evidence of valvar heart disease do not need additional short-term prophylaxis for prevention of bacterial endocarditis.

When selecting anti-infectives for prophylaxis of recurrent rheumatic fever, the current recommendations published by the AHA should be consulted.

Prevention of Perinatal Group B Streptococcal Disease Parenteral erythromycin is used as an alternative to parenteral penicillin G or ampicillin for prevention of perinatal group B streptococcal (GBS) disease† in women who are hypersensitive to penicillin. Pregnant women who are colonized with GBS in the genital or rectal areas can transmit GBS infection to their infants during labor and delivery resulting in invasive neonatal infection that can be associated with substantial morbidity and mortality. Intrapartum anti-infective prophylaxis for prevention of early-onset neonatal GBS disease is administered *selectively* to women at high risk for transmitting GBS infection to their neonates.

When intrapartum prophylaxis is indicated in the mother, penicillin G (5 million units IV initially followed by 2.5 million units IV every 4 hours until delivery) is the regimen of choice and ampicillin (2 g IV initially followed by 1 g IV every 4 hours until delivery) is the preferred alternative. When intrapartum prophylaxis to prevent GBS in the neonate is indicated in women who are hypersensitive to penicillins, the CDC recommends a regimen of IV clindamycin (900 mg IV every 8 hours until delivery) or IV erythromycin (500 mg IV every 6 hours until delivery) for those allergic to penicillins who are at high risk for anaphylaxis (e.g., those with a history of immediate penicillin hypersensitivity, such as anaphylaxis, angioedema, or urticaria; those with a history of asthma or other conditions that would make anaphylaxis more dangerous or difficult to treat, including individuals receiving β-adrenergic blocking agents). For those allergic to penicillins who are *not* at high risk for anaphylaxis, the CDC states that a regimen of IV cefazolin (2 g IV initially followed by 1 g IV every 8 hours until delivery) should be used since this cephalosporin has a narrow spectrum of activity and is associated with high intraamniotic concentrations.

The fact that *S. agalactiae* (group B streptococci) with in vitro resistance to clindamycin and erythromycin have been reported with increasing frequency should be considered when choosing an alternative to penicillins. When use of erythromycin or clindamycin is being considered in a women hypersensitive to penicillin, in vitro susceptibility testing of clinical isolates obtained during GBS prenatal screening should be performed whenever possible to determine if the isolates are susceptible to these drugs. Strains of GBS resistant to erythromycin often are resistant to clindamycin, although this may not be evident in results of in vitro testing. If in vitro susceptibility testing is not possible, results are unknown, or isolates are found to be resistant to erythromycin or clindamycin, a regimen of vancomycin (1 g IV every 12 hours until delivery) should be used for intrapartum prophylaxis in women with penicillin allergy who are at high risk for anaphylaxis.

For additional information on prevention of perinatal GBS disease, see Uses: Prevention of Perinatal Group B Streptococcal Disease, in the Natural Penicillins General Statement 8:12.16.04.

Prevention of Bacterial Endocarditis Some macrolides (azithromycin, clarithromycin) have been recommended for prevention of α-hemolytic (viridans group) streptococcal bacterial endocarditis† in penicillin-allergic adults and children with congenital heart disease, rheumatic or other acquired valvular heart dysfunction (even after valvular surgery), prosthetic heart valves (including bioprosthetic or allograft valves), surgically constructed systemic pulmonary shunts or conduits, hypertrophic cardiomyopathy, mitral valve prolapse with valvular regurgitation and/or thickened leaflets, or previous bacterial endocarditis (even in the absence of heart disease) who undergo dental procedures that are likely to result in gingival or mucosal bleeding (e.g., dental extractions; periodontal procedures such as scaling, root planing, probing, and maintenance; dental implant placement or reimplantation of avulsed teeth; root-filling procedures; subgingival placement of antibiotic fibers or strips; initial placement of orthodontic bands; intraligamentary local anesthetic injections; routine professional cleaning) or minor upper respiratory tract surgery or instrumentation (e.g., tonsillectomy, adenoidectomy, bronchoscopy).

While erythromycin previously was recommended by the AHA as an alternative to penicillins for prevention of bacterial endocarditis in penicillin-allergic patients, the AHA states that it no longer includes erythromycin in its recommendations because of adverse GI effects and the complicated pharmacokinetics of the various erythromycin formulations. However, the AHA states that practitioners who have successfully used an erythromycin (i.e., erythromycin ethylsuccinate, erythromycin stearate) for prophylaxis in individual patients may choose to continue using these agents. The AHA recognizes that its current recommendations for prophylaxis against bacterial endocarditis are empiric, since no controlled efficacy studies have been published, and that prophylaxis of endocarditis is not always effective. However, the AHA, the ADA, and most clinicians generally recommend routine use of prophylactic anti-infectives in patients at risk for bacterial endocarditis. A national registry established by the AHA in the early 1980s analyzed 52 cases of apparent failure of anti-infective prophylaxis against bacterial endocarditis; only 6 (12%) cases had received AHA-recommended prophylactic regimens. Erythromycin is not suitable for prophylaxis against bacterial endocarditis in patients undergoing GI, biliary, or genitourinary tract surgery or instrumentation because causative organisms are likely to be resistant to erythromycin. When selecting anti-infectives for prophylaxis of bacterial endocarditis, the current recommendations published by the AHA should be consulted.

■ **Acute Otitis Media** A fixed-combination preparation containing erythromycin ethylsuccinate and sulfisoxazole acetyl is used in children for the treatment of acute otitis media (AOM) caused by susceptible *Haemophilus influenzae*. Erythromycin is not effective when used alone for the treatment of *H. influenzae* infections.

Macrolides (azithromycin, clarithromycin, the fixed combination of erythromycin ethylsuccinate and sulfisoxazole acetyl) are considered alternative agents and are not drugs of first choice for the treatment of AOM. These macrolides are recommended as alternatives for treatment of AOM in patients with type I penicillin hypersensitivity. The fixed combination of erythromycin ethylsuccinate and sulfisoxazole acetyl may not be effective for the treatment of AOM that fails to respond to amoxicillin since a high incidence of *S. pneumoniae* resistant to the fixed-combination drug has been reported. (For further information on treatment of AOM, see Uses: Otitis Media, in the Cephalosporins General Statement 8:12.06.)

■ **Respiratory Tract Infections** Erythromycin or other macrolides (azithromycin, clarithromycin) are used for the treatment of respiratory tract infections caused by *Mycoplasma pneumoniae*. Erythromycin also is used in the treatment of respiratory tract infections caused by *C. pneumoniae* (see Uses: Chlamydial Infections). Erythromycin or tetracyclines appear to be equally effective in shortening the duration of clinical symptoms and hastening radiographic improvement in adults with mycoplasmal pneumonia, despite failure to eradicate the pathogen from nasopharyngeal or sputum cultures. Although data are limited regarding efficacy for treatment of mycoplasmal pneumonia in children, some clinicians suggest that erythromycin is preferred for treating children with the infection.

Although erythromycin usually is not effective for the treatment of respiratory tract infections caused by *Haemophilus influenzae*, other macrolides (e.g., azithromycin, clarithromycin) are used for the treatment of pneumonia or acute exacerbations of chronic bronchitis caused by this bacterium. Limited evidence suggests that response to these macrolides in such infections is comparable to that observed with second or third generation oral cephalosporins (i.e., cefuroxime axetil, cefaclor, or cefixime).

Community-acquired Pneumonia Erythromycin or other macrolides (azithromycin, clarithromycin) are used in the treatment of community-acquired pneumonia (CAP).

Initial treatment of CAP generally involves use of an empiric anti-infective regimen based on the most likely pathogens; therapy may then be changed (if possible) to a pathogen-specific regimen based on results of in vitro culture and susceptibility testing, especially in hospitalized patients. The most appropriate empiric regimen varies depending on the severity of illness at the time of presentation and whether outpatient treatment or hospitalization in or out of an intensive care unit (ICU) is indicated and the presence or absence of cardiopulmonary disease and other modifying factors that increase the risk of certain pathogens (e.g., penicillin- or multidrug-resistant *S. pneumoniae*, enteric gram-negative bacilli, *Ps. aeruginosa*). For both outpatients and inpatients, most experts recommend that an empiric regimen for the treatment of CAP include an anti-infective active against *S. pneumoniae* since this organism is the most commonly identified cause of bacterial pneumonia and causes more severe disease than many other common CAP pathogens.

The duration of CAP therapy depends on the causative pathogen, illness severity at the onset of anti-infective therapy, response to treatment, comorbid illness, and complications. CAP secondary to *S. pneumoniae* generally can be treated for 7–10 days or 72 hours after the patient becomes afebrile. CAP caused by bacteria that can necrose pulmonary parenchyma generally should be treated for at least 2 weeks. Patients chronically treated with corticosteroids also may require at least 2 weeks of therapy. CAP caused by *M. pneumoniae* or *C. Pneumoniae* should be treated for 10–14 days.

Outpatient Regimens for CAP. Pathogens most frequently involved in *outpatient* CAP include *S. pneumoniae*, *Mycoplasma pneumoniae*, *Chlamydia pneumoniae*, respiratory viruses, and *H. influenzae* (especially in cigarette smokers). Therefore, for empiric outpatient treatment of acute CAP in immunocompetent adults, the IDSA recommends monotherapy with an oral macrolide (azithromycin, clarithromycin, erythromycin), oral doxycycline, or an oral fluoroquinolone active against *S. pneumoniae* (e.g., gatifloxacin, levofloxacin, moxifloxacin) and states that alternative empiric regimens include oral amoxicillin and clavulanate or certain oral cephalosporins (cefpodoxime, cefprozil, cefuroxime axetil). Because erythromycin does not provide coverage for *H. influenzae*, azithromycin or clarithromycin generally is preferred for empiric therapy if this organism is suspected.

For outpatient treatment of CAP in immunocompetent adults without cardiopulmonary disease or other modifying factors that would increase the risk of multidrug-resistant *S. pneumoniae* or gram-negative bacteria, the American Thoracic Society (ATS) recommends an empiric regimen of monotherapy with azithromycin or clarithromycin or, alternatively, doxycycline. If *H. influenzae* are unlikely because the patient is a nonsmoker without cardiopulmonary disease, any macrolide (including erythromycin) could be used for these outpatients; however, azithromycin or clarithromycin are preferred since they have a lower incidence of adverse GI effects than erythromycin and require fewer daily doses which may improve compliance. For the outpatient treatment of immunocompetent adults with cardiopulmonary disease (congestive heart failure or chronic obstructive pulmonary disease [COPD]) and/or other modifying factors that increase the risk for multidrug-resistant *S. pneumoniae* or gram-negative bacteria, the ATS recommends a 2-drug empiric regimen consisting of a *β*-lactam anti-infective (e.g. oral cefpodoxime, oral cefuroxime axetil, high-dose amoxicillin, amoxicillin and clavulanate, parenteral ceftriaxone followed by oral cefpodoxime) and a macrolide or doxycycline or, alternatively, monotherapy with a fluoroquinolone active against *S. pneumoniae* (e.g., ciprofloxacin, ofloxacin, gatifloxacin, levofloxacin, moxifloxacin, sparfloxacin, trovafloxacin [risk of hepatic toxicity should be considered]). The CDC suggests that use of these oral fluoroquinolones in the *outpatient* treatment of CAP be reserved for when other anti-infectives are ineffective or cannot be used or when highly penicillin-resistant *S. pneumoniae* (i.e., penicillin MICs 4 mcg/mL or greater) are identified as the cause of infection. If ampicillin is used in the *β*-lactam and macrolide regimen, it will not provide coverage against *H. influenzae* and use of azithromycin or clarithromycin (rather than erythromycin) is recommended for the macrolide component.

Inpatient Regimens for CAP. In addition to *S. pneumoniae*, other pathogens often involved in *inpatient* CAP are *H. influenzae*, enteric gram-negative bacilli, *S. aureus*, *Legionella*, *M. pneumoniae*, *C. pneumoniae*, and viruses. Patients with severe CAP admitted into the ICU may have *Ps. aeruginosa* infections (especially those with underlying bronchiectasis or cystic fibrosis) and Enterobacteriaceae often are involved. In addition, anaerobic infection should be suspected in patients with aspiration pneumonia or lung abscess.

Inpatient treatment of CAP is initiated with a parenteral regimen, although therapy may be changed to an oral regimen if the patient is improving clinically, is hemodynamically stable, and able to ingest drugs. CAP patients usually have a clinical response within 3–5 days after initiation of therapy and failure to respond to the initial empiric regimen generally indicates an incorrect diagnosis, host failure, inappropriate anti-infective regimen (drug selection, dosage, route), unusual pathogen, adverse drug reaction, or complication (e.g., pulmonary superinfection, empyema).

For empiric inpatient treatment of CAP in immunocompetent adults who require hospitalization in a non-ICU setting, the IDSA recommends a 2-drug regimen consisting of a parenteral *β*-lactam anti-infective (e.g., cefotaxime, ceftriaxone, ampicillin and sulbactam, piperacillin and tazobactam) and a macrolide (e.g., azithromycin, clarithromycin, erythromycin) or monotherapy with a fluoroquinolone active against *S. pneumoniae* (e.g., gatifloxacin, levofloxacin, moxifloxacin). For empiric inpatient treatment of CAP in immunocompetent adults who are hospitalized in a non-ICU setting and have cardiopulmonary disease (congestive heart failure or chronic obstructive pulmonary disease [COPD]) and/or other modifying factors that increase the risk for multidrug-resistant *S. pneumoniae* or gram-negative bacteria, the ATS recommends a 2-drug regimen consisting of a parenteral *β*-lactam anti-infective (cefotaxime, ceftriaxone, ampicillin and sulbactam, high-dose ampicillin) and an oral or IV macrolide (azithromycin or clarithromycin; doxycycline can be used in those with macrolide sensitivity or intolerance) or, alternatively, monotherapy with an IV fluoroquinolone active against *S. pneumoniae*. If anaerobes are documented or lung abscess is present, clindamycin or metronidazole should be added to the regimen. For CAP patients admitted to a non-ICU setting who do not have cardiopulmonary disease or other modifying factors, the ATS suggests an empiric regimen of monotherapy with IV azithromycin; for those with macrolide sensitivity or intolerance, a 2-drug regimen of doxycycline and a *β*-lactam or monotherapy with a fluoroquinolone active against *S. pneumoniae* can be used.

For inpatient treatment of CAP in immunocompetent adults who require hospitalization in an ICU, the IDSA recommends an empiric 2-drug regimen consisting of a *β*-lactam anti-infective (cefotaxime, ceftriaxone, ampicillin and sulbactam, piperacillin and tazobactam) and either a macrolide or a fluoroquinolone. For inpatient treatment of severe CAP in patients hospitalized in an ICU, the ATS recommends that those *not* at risk for *Ps. aeruginosa* infection receive a 2-drug empiric regimen consisting of an IV *β*-lactam anti-infective (cefotaxime, ceftriaxone) and either an IV macrolide (azithromycin) or IV fluoroquinolone. If risk factors for *Ps. aeruginosa* are present in patients with severe CAP admitted to an ICU, the ATS recommends an empiric regimen that includes 2 antipseudomonal agents and provides coverage for multidrug-resistant *S. pneumonia* and *Legionella*. Therefore, the ATS recommends that these patients receive a 2-drug empiric regimen that includes an IV antipseudomonal *β*-lactam anti-infective (e.g., cefepime, piperacillin and tazobactam, imipenem, meropenem) and an IV antipseudomonal fluoroquinolone (e.g., ciprofloxacin) or, alternatively, a 3-drug empiric regimen that includes one of the IV antipseudomonal *β*-lactams, an IV aminoglycoside, and either an IV macrolide (e.g., azithromycin) or an IV nonpseudomonal quinolone. When an IV macrolide is indicated, azithromycin usually is preferred over erythromycin because of ease of administration and lower incidence of adverse effects.

■ **Skin and Skin Structure Infections** Acute mild to moderate infections of the skin and soft tissue caused by *Staphylococcus aureus* have been treated with erythromycins, but resistance may develop during treatment. Azithromycin and clarithromycin also have been used in the treatment of skin and skin structure infections caused by *Staphylococcus aureus* or *Streptococcus pyogenes* and appear to have efficacy comparable to that of erythromycin or an oral cephalosporin.

■ **Acne** Oral erythromycins are used with good results in the treatment of acne†. For information on the topical use of erythromycin in acne, see Erythromycin 84:04.04.

■ **Amebiasis** Although the manufacturers state that oral erythromycin can be used for the treatment of intestinal amebiasis caused by *Entamoeba histolytica*, a regimen of metronidazole or tinidazole followed by a luminal amebicide such as iodoquinol or paromomycin is recommended for the treatment of intestinal amebiasis.

■ **Anthrax** Erythromycin is used as an alternative agent in the *treatment* of anthrax†. Parenteral penicillins generally have been considered the drugs of choice for the treatment of naturally occurring or endemic anthrax caused by susceptible strains of *Bacillus anthracis*, including clinically apparent GI, inhalational, or meningeal anthrax and anthrax septicemia, although IV ciprofloxacin or IV doxycycline also are recommended. Erythromycin is suggested as an alternative to penicillin G for the treatment of naturally occurring or endemic anthrax in patients hypersensitive to penicillins.

For the treatment of inhalational anthrax that occurs as the result of exposure to *B. anthracis* spores in the context of biologic warfare or bioterrorism, the CDC and the US Working Group on Civilian Biodefense recommend that treatment be initiated with a multiple-drug parenteral regimen that includes ciprofloxacin or doxycycline and 1 or 2 other anti-infectives predicted to be effective. Based on in vitro data, drugs that have been suggested as possibilities to augment ciprofloxacin or doxycycline in such multiple-drug regimens include chloramphenicol, clindamycin, rifampin, vancomycin, clarithromycin, imipenem, penicillin, or ampicillin. If meningitis is established or suspected, some clinicians suggest a multiple-drug regimen that includes ciprofloxacin (rather than doxycycline) and chloramphenicol, rifampin, or penicillin. Although there is evidence that erythromycin has in vitro activity against *B. anthracis*, strains of the organism that were associated with cases of inhalational or cutaneous anthrax that occurred in the US (Florida, New York, District of Columbia) during September and October 2001 in the context of an intentional release of anthrax spores (biologic warfare, bioterrorism) had only intermediate susceptibility to erythromycin. Limited or no clinical data are available to date regarding in vivo activity of erythromycin against *B. anthracis* and the drug is not considered a drug of choice for the treatment or prophylaxis of anthrax that occurs as the result of exposure to anthrax spores in the context of biologic warfare or bioterrorism.

IV anti-infective therapy is recommended for the initial treatment of clinically apparent GI, inhalational, or meningeal anthrax and anthrax septicemia and also is indicated for the treatment of cutaneous anthrax when there are signs of systemic involvement, extensive edema, or head and neck lesions; oral therapy may be adequate for mild, uncomplicated cutaneous anthrax.

For additional information on treatment of anthrax and recommendations for prophylaxis following exposure to anthrax spores, see Uses: Anthrax, in Ciprofloxacin 8:12.18.

■ **Bartonella Infections** Oral erythromycin or oral azithromycin has been used in conjunction with IM or IV ceftriaxone for the treatment of bacteremia caused by *Bartonella quintana*† (formerly *Rochalimaea quintana*). *B. quintana*, a gram-negative bacilli, can cause cutaneous bacillary angiomatosis, trench fever, bacteremia, endocarditis, and chronic lymphadenopathy. *B. quintana* infections have been reported most frequently in immunocompromised patients (e.g., individuals with HIV infection), homeless individuals in urban areas, and chronic alcohol abusers. Optimum anti-infective regimens for the treatment of infections caused by *B. quintana* have not been identified, and various drugs have been used to treat these infections, including doxycycline, erythromycin, azithromycin, chloramphenicol, or cephalosporins. There is evidence that these infections tend to persist or recur and prolonged therapy (several months or longer) usually is necessary.

The possible role of macrolides in the treatment of infections caused by *Bartonella henselae* (formerly *Rochalimaea henselae*) (e.g., cat scratch disease, bacillary angiomatosis, peliosis hepatitis) has not been determined. Cat scratch disease generally is a self-limited illness in immunocompetent individuals and may resolve spontaneously in 2–4 months; however, some clinicians suggest that anti-infective therapy be considered for acutely or severely ill patients with systemic symptoms, particularly those with hepatosplenomegaly or painful lymphadenopathy, and probably is indicated in immunocompromised patients. Anti-infectives also are indicated in patients with*B. henselae* infections who develop bacillary angiomatosis, neuroretinitis, or Parinaud's oculoglandular syndrome. While the optimum anti-infective regimen for the treatment of cat scratch disease or other *B. henselae* infections has not been identified, some clinicians recommend use of erythromycin, azithromycin, doxycycline, ciprofloxacin, rifampin, co-trimoxazole, gentamicin, or third generation cephalosporins.

HIV-infected individuals (especially severely immunosuppressed individuals) are at unusually high risk for severe disease caused by *Bartonella* and relapse or reinfection sometimes occurs following initial treatment of these infections. Therefore, although data are insufficient to make firm recommendations, the Prevention of Opportunistic Infections Working Group of the US Public Health Service and the Infectious Diseases Society of America (USPHS/IDSA) suggest that long-term suppression with erythromycin or doxycycline be considered to prevent recurrence of *Bartonella* infection in HIV-infected patients.

■ **Campylobacter Infections** The CDC, IDSA, and AAP consider oral erythromycin a treatment of choice for symptomatic enteric infections caused by *Campylobacter jejuni*†. Azithromycin and fluoroquinolones (e.g., ciprofloxacin) also are recommended for these infections; tetracycline also can be used for patients 8 years of age or older.

When initiated early in the course of the *Campylobacter* infection, erythromycin or azithromycin shortens the duration of illness and prevents relapse. Both of these macrolides usually eradicate the organism from the stool within 2–3 days; in patients with gastroenteritis, the recommended duration of therapy is 5–7 days.

■ **Chancroid** Oral erythromycin is used for the treatment of chancroid† (genital ulcers caused by *H. ducreyi*). While a few erythromycin-resistant isolates of *H. ducreyi* were reported in Asia more than a decade ago, similar isolates have not been reported elsewhere.

The CDC and others state that a single oral dose of azithromycin, a single IM dose of ceftriaxone, a 3-day regimen of oral ciprofloxacin (contraindicated in pregnant or lactating women), or a 7-day regimen of oral erythromycin are the regimens of choice for the treatment of chancroid. All 4 regimens generally are effective for the treatment of chancroid; however, patients with human immunodeficiency virus (HIV) infection and patients who are uncircumcised may not respond to treatment as well as those who are HIV-negative or circumcised. Because data on efficacy of the single-dose azithromycin and ceftriaxone regimens for the treatment of chancroid in patients with HIV infection are limited, the CDC recommends that these regimens be used in HIV patients only if follow-up can be ensured; some experts recommend that HIV-infected individuals with chancroid receive the 7-day erythromycin regimen.

In the US, chancroid usually occurs in discrete outbreaks, but the disease is endemic in some areas. Approximately 10% of patients with chancroid acquired in the US also are coinfected with *Treponema pallidum* or herpes simplex virus (HSV); this percentage is higher in individuals who acquired the infection outside the US. In addition, high rates of HIV infection have been reported in patients with chancroid, and the disease appears to be a cofactor for HIV transmission. Evaluation of the physical features of genital ulcers (without laboratory evaluation and testing) usually is inadequate to provide a differential diagnosis between chancroid, primary syphilis, and genital HSV infection. Ideally, diagnostic evaluation of patients with genital ulcers should include a serologic test for syphilis and either darkfield examination or direct immunofluorescence test for *T. pallidum*, culture for *H. ducreyi*, and culture or antigen test for HSV. A definitive diagnosis of chancroid requires identification of *H. ducreyi* on special culture media that is not widely available. However, a probable diagnosis of chancroid can be made if the patient has one or more painful genital ulcers, there is no evidence of *T. pallidum* infection based on a negative darkfield examination of ulcer exudate or a negative serologic test for syphilis (performed at least 7 days after onset of ulcers), culture or antigen test for HSV is negative, and the clinical presentation, appearance of genital ulcers, and regional lymphadenopathy (if present) are typical for chancroid. While the presence of a painful ulcer and tender inguinal adenopathy occur in about one-third of chancroid patients and suggests a diagnosis of chancroid, the additional presence of suppurative inguinal adenopathy is a clearer indication of the disease.

Patient Follow-up and Management of Sexual Partners The CDC recommends that all patients diagnosed with chancroid be tested for HIV and, if initial tests for syphilis and HIV are negative, the tests repeated 3 months later. Patients with chancroid should be examined 3–7 days after initiation of anti-infective therapy. If the regimen was effective, symptomatic improvement in the ulcers is evident within 3 days and objective improvement is evident within 7 days. If clinical improvement is not evident within 3–7 days, consideration should be given to the possibility that the diagnosis was incorrect, there is coinfection with another sexually transmitted disease, the patient was noncompliant with the regimen, the strain of *H. ducreyi* is resistant to the anti-infective agent used, or the patient is HIV seropositive.

The time required for complete healing is related to the size of the ulcer; large ulcers may require more than 2 weeks to heal. Healing of ulcers may be slower in uncircumcised men who have ulcers under the foreskin. Resolution of fluctuant lymphadenopathy is slower than that of ulcers, and needle aspiration or incisional drainage may be necessary even during otherwise effective anti-infective therapy. While needle aspiration of buboes is a simpler procedure, incision and drainage of buboes may be preferred.

The CDC recommends that any individual who had sexual contact with a patient with chancroid within 10 days before the onset of the patient's symptoms should be examined and treated for the disease, even if no symptoms are present.

■ **Chlamydial Infections** Oral erythromycin is used for the treatment of urethritis caused by *Ureaplasma urealyticum* in adult males and for the treatment of uncomplicated urethral, endocervical, or rectal infections caused by *Chlamydia trachomatis* in adults in whom tetracyclines and azithromycin are contraindicated or not tolerated. Oral erythromycin also is used for the treatment of chlamydial urogenital infections during pregnancy and for the treatment of chlamydial pneumonia in infants. The AAP, CDC, and other clinicians also recommend oral erythromycin for the treatment of initial episodes and recurrences of chlamydial conjunctivitis in neonates.

Although oral erythromycin has not been evaluated extensively in culture-confirmed cases, the drug is used as an alternative to doxycycline for the treatment of genital, inguinal, or anorectal infections caused by lymphogranuloma venereum serotypes of *C. trachomatis*†.

Urogenital Chlamydial Infections in Adults and Adolescents For the treatment of urogenital chlamydial infections in nonpregnant adults and adolescents, the CDC and other clinicians recommend a single dose of oral azithromycin or a 7-day regimen of oral doxycycline. Alternatively, these adults and adolescents can receive a 7-day regimen of oral erythromycin base or ethylsuccinate or a 7-day regimen of oral ofloxacin or levofloxacin. Erythromycin is less effective than either azithromycin or doxycycline and GI effects associated with the drug may discourage patient compliance with the regimen. To maximize compliance with 7-day regimens, the CDC recommends that the drugs be dispensed on site and that the first dose be taken under supervision.

Individuals with HIV infection who also are infected with chlamydia should receive the same treatment regimens recommended for other individuals with chlamydial infections.

Patient Follow-up and Management of Sexual Partners. Since azithromycin and doxycycline regimens are highly effective for the treatment of urogenital chlamydial infections, a test of cure probably is unnecessary in patients who receive one of these regimens unless symptoms persist or reinfection is suspected; however, a test of cure should be considered 3 weeks after completion of an erythromycin regimen.

Patients being treated for chlamydial infection should be instructed to refer their sexual partner(s) for evaluation and treatment, and to abstain from sexual intercourse for 7 days after single-dose therapy or until completion of a 7-day regimen. In addition, to minimize the risk of reinfection, patients should be instructed to abstain from sexual intercourse until after all their sexual partners are cured. Although the CDC acknowledges that the exposure intervals are somewhat arbitrary, they recommend that individuals who had sexual contact with the chlamydia patient within 60 days before the onset of symptoms or diagnosis in the patient should be evaluated and treated. If the patient reports that the last sexual contact occurred more than 60 days prior to the onset of symptoms or diagnosis, their most recent sexual partner should be treated.

Chlamydial Infections during Pregnancy The CDC recommends that urogenital chlamydial infections in pregnant women be treated with a 7-day regimen of oral erythromycin base or oral amoxicillin; alternative regimens recommended by the CDC for the treatment of urogenital chlamydial infection in pregnant women are a 14-day regimen of oral erythromycin base or ethylsuccinate, a 7-day regimen of erythromycin ethylsuccinate, or a single dose of oral azithromycin. Other clinicians recommend that urogenital chlamydial infections in pregnant women be treated with a 7-day regimen of oral amoxicillin or, alternatively, a single oral dose of azithromycin or a 7-day regimen of oral erythromycin. Repeat testing, preferably by culture, 3 weeks after completion of therapy is recommended since none of these regimens is highly effective and since frequent adverse effects associated with erythromycin may discourage compliance.

Chlamydial Infections in Neonates and Infants *C. trachomatis* infection in neonates usually occurs as the result of exposure to the mother's infected cervix. Perinatal *C. trachomatis* infection initially involves mucous membranes of the eye, oropharynx, urogenital tract, and rectum and usually becomes apparent when conjunctivitis develops 5–12 days after birth; however, asymptomatic oropharyngeal, genital tract, and rectal infections can occur in neonates. *C. trachomatis* also is a common cause of subacute, afebrile pneumonia occurring in children 1–3 months of age. Because a neonate with chlamydial infection has acquired the organism from their mother, both the mother and her sexual partner(s) should be evaluated and treated for chlamydia following a diagnosis in the neonate.

If erythromycin is used for the treatment of chlamydial infections in neonates, the risk of infantile hypertrophic pyloric stenosis (IHPS) should be considered and the child's parents or caregivers should be informed about the potential risks of developing IHPS and signs of IHPS.

Chlamydial Ophthalmia Neonatorum. A 14-day regimen of oral erythromycin base or ethylsuccinate is a preferred or alternative regimen of choice for the treatment of ophthalmia neonatorum caused by *C. trachomatis*. The neonate should receive appropriate follow-up to ensure that the infection resolves; a second course of erythromycin may be necessary since the drug is effective in approximately 80% of cases. The AAP suggests that oral sulfonamides be used in neonates who cannot tolerate erythromycin. Although data on use of other macrolides (e.g., azithromycin, clarithromycin) for the treatment of neonatal chlamydial infections are limited, there is some evidence that a 3-day regimen of oral azithromycin may be effective for the treatment of chlamydial ophthalmia neonatorum; some clinicians consider azithromycin the regimen of choice. Topical anti-infectives are inadequate for the treatment of chlamydial ophthalmia neonatorum and are unnecessary when appropriate systemic anti-infective therapy is given.

While universal topical prophylaxis using topical anti-infectives (i.e., 1% tetracycline ophthalmic ointment, 0.5% erythromycin ophthalmic ointment, silver nitrate 1% ophthalmic solution) is recommended for *all* neonates as soon as possible after birth to prevent gonococcal ophthalmia neonatorum, these topical anti-infectives do not prevent perinatal transmission of *C. trachomatis* from mother to infant. Infants born to mothers with untreated chlamydial infection are at high risk for infection; however, parenteral prophylaxis in these infants is not indicated since the efficacy of such prophylaxis is unknown. These infants should be monitored to ensure appropriate treatment if chlamydial infection develops. The possibility of a chlamydial infection should be considered in any infant 30 days of age or younger who develops conjunctivitis; ocular exudate from infants being evaluated for chlamydial conjunctivitis also should be tested for *N. gonorrhoeae*.

Chlamydial Pneumonia in Infants. A 14-day regimen of oral erythromycin base or ethylsuccinate is a preferred or alternative regimen for the treatment of chlamydial pneumonia in infants. The infant should receive appropriate follow-up to ensure that the pneumonia resolves; a second course of erythromycin may be necessary since the drug is effective in approximately 80% of cases. Some clinicians suggest that a 3-day regimen of azithromycin is the regimen of choice for chlamydial pneumonia in neonates.

Urogenital Chlamydial Infections in Children For the treatment of urogenital chlamydial infections in children who weigh less than 45 kg, the CDC recommends a 14-day regimen of oral erythromycin base or ethylsuccinate. For the treatment of urogenital chlamydial infections in children younger than 8 years of age who weigh at least 45 kg, the CDC recommends a single 1-g dose of oral azithromycin; for those 8 years of age or older, the CDC recommends a single-dose azithromycin regimen or a 7-day regimen of oral doxycycline. The AAP recommends that infants younger than 6 months of age with urogenital chlamydial infections receive an erythromycin regimen and that those 6 months to 12 years of age receive either erythromycin or azithromycin. Follow-up cultures are necessary to ensure that treatment has been effective.

Lymphogranuloma Venereum A 21-day regimen of oral erythromycin base is recommended as an alternative regimen for the treatment of lymphogranuloma venereum† caused by invasive serotypes of *C. trachomatis* (serovars L1, L2, L3). A 21-day regimen of oral doxycycline generally is considered the regimen of choice for lymphogranuloma venereum; erythromycin can be used as an alternative and is the preferred regimen for pregnant and lactating women. Although oral azithromycin also may be effective, the CDC states that clinical safety and efficacy data are lacking. Effective treatment cures the infection and prevents ongoing tissue damage, although tissue reaction can result in scarring. Aspiration of buboes or incision and drainage may be necessary to prevent the formation of inguinal/femoral ulcerations.

The CDC recommends that individuals who had sexual contact with the lymphogranuloma venereum patient should be examined, tested for urethral or cervical chlamydial infection, and treated if they had sexual contact with the patient within 30 days prior to onset of symptoms in the patient.

While HIV-infected individuals with lymphogranuloma venereum should receive the same treatment regimens recommended for other patients, there is some evidence that HIV-infected patients may require more prolonged therapy and resolution may be delayed.

Chlamydia psittaci Infections While tetracyclines are the drugs of choice for the treatment of *C. psittaci* infections (psittacosis), erythromycin is an alternative for the treatment of psittacosis when tetracyclines are contraindicated (e.g., in pregnant women, children younger than 9 years of age).

■ **Diphtheria** Erythromycin is used as an adjunct to diphtheria antitoxin in the *treatment* of respiratory tract infection caused by *Corynebacterium diphtheria* (diphtheria). Erythromycin also is used for *prevention* of diphtheria in close contacts of patients with diphtheria and to eliminate the diphtheria carrier state. Although cutaneous diphtheria generally is caused by nontoxigenic strains of *C. diphtheriae*, some clinicians recommend that patients with cutaneous infections receive a 10-day regimen of anti-infective therapy in addition to thorough cleansing of the lesions; use of diphtheria antitoxin in these patients also is recommended by some clinicians since toxic sequelae have occurred in some patients with cutaneous lesions.

Use of diphtheria antitoxin is the most important aspect of treatment of respiratory diphtheria. (See Diphtheria Antitoxin 80:04.) Anti-infective therapy may eliminate *C. diphtheriae* from infected sites, prevent spread of the organism and further toxin production, and prevent or terminate the diphtheria carrier state; however, anti-infectives appear to be of no value in neutralizing diphtheria toxin and should not be considered a substitute for antitoxin therapy. For the adjunctive treatment of diphtheria, erythromycin may be given orally or IV; alternatively, a parenteral regimen of penicillin G or penicillin G procaine can be used. Patients usually are no longer contagious 48 hours after initiation of anti-infective therapy. Eradication of *C. diphtheriae* should be confirmed by 2 consecutive negative cultures following completion of anti-infective therapy. Because diphtheria infection often does not confer immunity, active immunization with a diphtheria toxoid preparation (see 80:08) should be initiated or completed during convalescence.

For *prevention* of diphtheria, the CDC, US Public Health Service Advisory Committee on Immunization Practices (ACIP), and AAP recommend that, irrespective of their immunization status, *all* household or other close contacts of individuals with suspected or proven diphtheria should have samples taken for *C. diphtheriae* culture, receive anti-infective prophylaxis, and be kept under surveillance for evidence of the disease for 7 days. Although efficacy of anti-infectives in preventing secondary disease is presumed and not proven, prophylaxis should be initiated promptly and should not be delayed pending culture results. The CDC, ACIP, and AAP recommend that either a single IM dose of penicillin G benzathine or 7–10 days of oral erythromycin be used for chemoprophylaxis in contacts of patients with diphtheria. Erythromycin may be slightly more effective, but IM penicillin G benzathine may be preferred when there are concerns about compliance. In addition, contacts who are inadequately immunized against diphtheria (i.e., have previously received less than 3 doses of diphtheria toxoid) or whose immunization status is unknown should receive an immediate dose of an age-appropriate diphtheria toxoid preparation and the primary immunization series should be completed according to the recommended schedule. Contacts who are fully immunized should receive an immediate booster dose of an age-appropriate diphtheria toxoid preparation if it has been 5 years or longer since their last booster dose. The ACIP and AAP state that use of diphtheria antitoxin in unimmunized close contacts is not recommended because of the risks associated with the antitoxin and because there is no evidence that such therapy has any additional benefit for contacts who receive recommended prophylaxis with penicillin G benzathine or erythromycin.

Erythromycin can be used to eliminate the diphtheria carrier state in individuals known to carry toxigenic strains of *C. diphtheriae*. The ACIP and AAP recommend that carriers receive prophylaxis with either penicillin G benzathine or erythromycin in the regimen recommended for prophylaxis of close contacts of patients with diphtheria. Follow-up cultures should be obtained at least 2 weeks after completion of the regimen; individuals who continue to harbor *C. diphtheriae* after either penicillin G benzathine or erythromycin therapy should receive an additional 10 day course of oral erythromycin and additional follow-up cultures should be obtained.

■ **Gonorrhea and Associated Infections** Erythromycin has been used as an alternative to the preferred regimens (e.g., a single dose of oral azithromycin or a 7-day regimen of oral doxycycline) for the treatment of coexisting chlamydial infections in adults and adolescents receiving treatment for gonorrhea. Gonorrhea frequently is associated with coexisting chlamydial infection; however, cephalosporins, spectinomycin, and most single-dose quinolone regimens used for the treatment of gonorrhea are ineffective for the treatment of chlamydial infection. Because of the risks associated with untreated coexisting chlamydial infection, the CDC and most clinicians recommend that adults and adolescents being treated for uncomplicated gonorrhea or disseminated gonococcal infection also receive an anti-infective regimen effective for presumptive treatment of uncomplicated urogenital chlamydial infection. The strategy of routine administration of a regimen effective against chlamydia in patients being treated for gonococcal infection has been recommended by the CDC for more than 10 years and appears to have resulted in substantial decreases in the prevalence of urogenital chlamydial infection in some populations. In addition, since most *N. gonorrhoeae* isolated in the US are susceptible to doxycycline and azithromycin, dual therapy may delay the development of resistance in *N. gonorrhoeae*. Since the cost of presumptive treatment of chlamydia is less than the cost of testing for presence of chlamydia, routine dual therapy without chlamydial testing can be cost-effective for populations in which coinfection with chlamydia has been reported in 10–30% of patients with *N. gonorrhoeae* infection. In areas where the rate of coinfection with chlamydia is low and chlamydial testing is widely available, some clinicians may prefer to test for chlamydia rather than treat presumptively; however, presumptive treatment is indicated for patients who may not return for test results.

In the treatment of gonococcal infections in children, routine presumptive treatment of chlamydia with erythromycin or tetracycline therapy is not currently included in the CDC recommendations, but the CDC states that children being treated for gonorrhea should be evaluated for coexisting *Chlamydia trachomatis* infection. The AAP recommends presumptive treatment of chlamydial infections for all children beyond the neonatal period being treated for uncomplicated vulvovaginal, urethral, or pharyngeal gonorrhea, epididymitis, proctitis, or disseminated gonococcal infections, including meningitis and endocarditis. The AAP suggests that children who weigh less than 45 kg receive erythromycin or azithromycin for presumptive treatment of coexisting chlamydial infection and that children who weigh 45 kg or more and are 8 years of age or older receive azithromycin or doxycycline.

While IV erythromycin lactobionate followed by oral erythromycin base or stearate is recommended by some manufacturers for the treatment of acute pelvic inflammatory disease (PID) caused by *N. gonorrhoeae*, erythromycins are not included in current CDC recommendations for the treatment of PID.

Topical erythromycin is used for prophylaxis of ophthalmia neonatorum caused by *N. gonorrhoeae*. (See Uses in Erythromycin 52:04.04.)

■ **Granuloma Inguinale (Donovanosis)** Erythromycin or azithromycin has been used orally in the treatment of donovanosis† caused by *Calymmatobacterium granulomatis*. The CDC recommends that donovanosis be treated with regimen of oral co-trimoxazole or oral doxycycline or, alternatively, a regimen of oral ciprofloxacin , oral erythromycin, or oral azithromycin. Anti-infective treatment of donovanosis should be continued until all lesions have healed completely; a minimum of 3 weeks of treatment usually is necessary. If lesions do not respond within the first few days of therapy, some experts recommend that a parenteral aminoglycoside (e.g., 1 mg/kg of gentamicin IV every 8 hours) be added to the regimen. Erythromycin is recommended for the treatment of donovanosis in pregnant and lactating women; addition of a parenteral aminoglycoside (e.g., gentamicin) to the regimen should be strongly considered in these women. Although azithromycin also may be effective for the treatment of donovanosis in pregnant women, clinical safety and efficacy data are lacking. Anti-infective treatment appears to halt progressive destruction of tissue, although prolonged duration of therapy often is required to enable granulation and re-epithelization of ulcers. Despite effective anti-infective therapy, donovanosis may relapse 6–18 months later.

Individuals with HIV infection should receive the same treatment regimens recommended for other individuals with donovanosis; however, the CDC suggests that addition of a parenteral aminoglycoside to the regimen should be considered in HIV-infected patients.

■ **Legionnaires' Disease** Erythromycin (with or without rifampin) is used for the treatment of Legionnaires' disease caused by *Legionella pneumophila*. Macrolides or fluoroquinolones generally are considered the drugs of choice for the treatment of pneumonia caused by *L. pneumophila* and doxycycline or co-trimoxazole are alternatives. A parenteral regimen usually is necessary for the initial treatment of severe Legionnaires' disease and the addition of oral rifampin is recommended during the first 3–5 days of macrolide or doxycycline therapy in severely ill and/or immunocompromised patients; after a response is obtained, rifampin can be discontinued and therapy changed to an oral regimen. Some clinicians suggest that azithromycin may be the preferred macrolide for the treatment of severe Legionnaires' disease and may also be preferred for empiric therapy in patients with severe community-acquired pneumonia (CAP) that may be caused by *Legionella*. (See Community-acquired Pneumonia under Uses: Respiratory Tract Infections.)

■ **Mycobacterium avium Complex (MAC) Infections** Although erythromycin is not used in the treatment of mycobacterial infections, other macrolides (azithromycin, clarithromycin) are used in the treatment and prevention of *Mycobacterium avium* complex (MAC) infections. For information on the use of azithromycin and clarithromycin in the prevention and/or treatment of MAC infections, including see the individual monographs on these drugs and see Management of Other Mycobacterial Diseases: *Mycobacterium avium* Complex (MAC) Infections, in the Antituberculosis Agents General Statement.

■ **Nongonococcal Urethritis** Oral erythromycin or oral azithromycin is used for the treatment of nongonococcal urethritis. While *C. trachomatis* is a frequent cause of nongonococcal urethritis, these infections can be caused by *Ureaplasma urealyticum* or *Mycoplasma genitalium*; *Trichomonas vaginalis* and HSV also are possible causes of nongonococcal urethritis. The CDC currently considers a single oral dose of azithromycin or a 7-day regimen of oral doxycycline the regimens of choice for the treatment of nongonococcal urethritis. Alternative regimens recommended by the CDC are a 7-day regimen of oral erythromycin base or ethylsuccinate or a 7-day regimen of oral ofloxacin or levofloxacin. Patients with persistent or recurrent urethritis who were not compliant with the treatment regimen or were reexposed to untreated sexual partner(s) should be retreated with the initial regimen. If the patient has recurrent and persistent urethritis, was compliant with the regimen, and reexposure can be excluded, the CDC recommends an additional 7-day regimen of oral erythromycin given in conjunction with a single 2-g dose of oral metronidazole.

■ **Pertussis** Erythromycin is considered the drug of choice for the *treatment* of *Bordetella pertussis* infection (pertussis, whooping cough) and for *prevention* in contacts of patients with pertussis.

According to CDC data, there were an average of 2900 cases of pertussis each year in the US from 1980–1990; however, the incidence of pertussis has been gradually increasing during the last decade. In 2000, there were 7867 reported cases (the largest number since 1967). While pertussis can occur at any age, approximately 43% of reported cases that occurred in the US during 1997 were reported in children younger than 5 years of age and 24% were reported in infants younger that 6 months of age. Susceptible infants and young children who have not been completely immunized against pertussis frequently are infected by older siblings or adult contacts who may have mild or atypical illness. According to CDC surveillance data for 1997–2000, there was about a 60% increase in the incidence rate of pertussis in adolescents and adults compared with incidence rates reported for these age groups in 1994–1996. This may reflect a true increase or may reflect improvements in recognition and diagnosis of pertussis among older individuals. The CDC suggests that healthcare providers consider pertussis in the differential diagnosis when evaluating adults with acute cough that has lasted at least 7 days, particularly if the cough is paroxysmal and associated with posttussive vomiting and/or whooping.

Transmission of pertussis can be reduced by prompt diagnosis and treatment of index cases and administration of prophylaxis to close contacts. Use of erythromycin therapy during the catarrhal stage of pertussis may ameliorate the disease, but usually has no discernible effect on the course of the illness if initiated after paroxysms are established; however, anti-infective treatment even at the paroxysmal stage is recommended to limit the spread of the organism to others. The CDC, AAP, and other clinicians recommend anti-infective prophylaxis for *all* household and other close contacts (e.g., those in childcare) of individuals with pertussis, regardless of age or vaccination status. Prophylaxis should be administered as soon as possible after first contact with the index case; prophylaxis administered 21 days or longer after first contact is considered to be of limited value. In addition to anti-infective prophylaxis, all close contacts younger than 7 years of age who are not fully immunized against pertussis should receive the remaining required doses of a preparation containing pertussis vaccine (using minimal intervals between doses) and those who are fully immunized but have not received a vaccine dose within the last 3 years should receive a booster dose of a pertussis vaccine preparation.

The CDC, ACIP, AAP, and others generally recommend a 14-day regimen of oral erythromycin for the treatment of pertussis or for prevention in susceptible contacts. While nasopharyngeal cultures usually become negative for *B. pertussis* within 5 days of initiation of anti-infective therapy and a 7- or 10-day regimen of erythromycin has been effective for the treatment of pertussis in some patients, prophylaxis failures and bacteriologic relapse of pertussis have been reported with erythromycin regimens shorter than 14 days. There is some limited evidence that 5–7 days of azithromycin or clarithromycin may be effective for the treatment of pertussis; however, additional study is needed.

Some clinicians suggest that erythromycin estolate is the preferred erythromycin for the treatment or prevention of pertussis, since it may be better tolerated and because prophylaxis failures and delays or failures in eradication of *B. pertussis* have been reported with some other forms of erythromycin (e.g., erythromycin ethylsuccinate or stearate). However, other clinicians suggest that these other erythromycin preparations can be used if adequate dosage is administered and patient compliance is ensured. An association between oral erythromycin and infantile hypertrophic pyloric stenosis (IHPS) has been reported in infants younger than 6 weeks of age who received the drug for prophylaxis of pertussis; however, a causal relationship has not been clearly established. Because additional study is needed to determine whether erythromycin contributed to these reported cases of IHPS and because only limited information is available regarding alternatives for prophylaxis and treatment of pertussis (e.g., azithromycin, clarithromycin, co-trimoxazole), the AAP continues to recommend use of erythromycin for prophylaxis or treatment of pertussis when indicated and states that parents of neonates should be informed about the potential risks of developing IHPS and signs of IHPS.

Although the clinical importance is unclear, erythromycin-resistant strains of *B. pertussis* have been reported rarely in the US. If a patient with pertussis does not improve with erythromycin therapy, nasopharyngeal cultures should be obtained and in vitro susceptibility testing performed to determine if the isolate is resistant to the drug.

■ **Spirochetal Infections** ***Lyme Disease*** Erythromycin, azithromycin, or clarithromycin has been used in the treatment of early Lyme disease†, a spirochetal disease caused by tick-borne *Borrelia burgdorferi*. However, some evidence in patients with early Lyme disease suggests that certain macrolides (e.g., azithromycin, erythromycin) may be less effective than penicillins or tetracyclines, and the IDSA, AAP, and other clinicians recommend that macrolide antibiotics *not* be used as first-line therapy for early Lyme disease.

Oral doxycycline or oral amoxicillin is recommended as first-line therapy for the treatment of early localized or early disseminated Lyme disease associated with erythema migrans, in the absence of neurologic involvement or third-degree atrioventricular (AV) heart block; alternatively, oral cefuroxime axetil has been used. Therapy with a macrolide antibiotic generally is recommended for the treatment of early Lyme disease in patients who are allergic to or intolerant of penicillins and cephalosporins and in whom tetracyclines are contraindicated (e.g., pregnant or lactating women and children younger than 8–9 years of age). While therapy with clarithromycin (500 mg twice daily for 21 days) appeared to be effective in resolving manifestations of early Lyme disease in a limited number of patients in an open-label study, the IDSA and other clinicians state that macrolide antibiotics should be reserved for patients who are intolerant of amoxicillin, doxycycline, and cefuroxime axetil and that patients treated with macrolides should be monitored closely.

The IDSA, AAP, and other clinicians recommend that patients with more severe forms or late complications of Lyme disease generally receive a higher dosage, more prolonged therapy, and/or parenteral anti-infectives (e.g., IV ceftriaxone, IV cefotaxime, or IV penicillin G for 2–4 weeks).

For more detailed information on the manifestations of Lyme disease and the efficacy of various anti-infective regimens in early or late Lyme disease, see Lyme Disease in Uses: Spirochetal Infections, in the Tetracyclines General Statement 8:12.24.

Syphilis The manufacturers suggest that oral erythromycin can be used for the treatment of primary syphilis. Although the CDC previously suggested use of oral erythromycin as an alternative agent for the treatment of primary or secondary syphilis in nonpregnant adults and adolescents hypersensitive to penicillins, erythromycin is less effective than other possible penicillin alternatives and is no longer included in CDC recommendations for the treatment of any form of syphilis in adults or adolescents (including primary, secondary, latent, or tertiary syphilis or neurosyphilis). Penicillin G is the drug of choice for the treatment of all stages of syphilis. Although efficacy is not well documented, the CDC states that use of oral doxycycline or oral tetracycline or, possibly, oral azithromycin, can be considered in nonpregnant adults and adolescents with primary, secondary, or early latent syphilis who are hypersensitive to penicillin. However, if compliance and follow-up cannot be ensured, these patients should be desensitized and treated with penicillin G. (For information on skin testing to document penicillin hypersensitivity and desensitization procedures, see Cautions: Hypersensitivity Reactions in the Natural Penicillins General Statement 8:12.16.04.) Use of penicillin alternatives (e.g., doxycycline, ceftriaxone, azithromycin) for the treatment of syphilis in HIV-infected individuals has not been studied and should be undertaken with caution.

Erythromycin is no longer recommended by the CDC, AAP, or other clinicians for the treatment of syphilis in pregnant women who are hypersensitive to penicillin since numerous treatment failures (including in the fetus) have been reported with the drug. There are no proven alternatives to penicillin G for the treatment of syphilis during pregnancy, and pregnant women with a history of penicillin hypersensitivity should be desensitized, if indicated, and treated with penicillin G. Because erythromycin administered during pregnancy cannot be considered a reliable cure for the fetus, neonates born to a woman who received such treatment during pregnancy should be treated with penicillin G for presumed congenital syphilis.

Erythromycin is *not* included in CDC recommendations for the treatment of presumed or documented congenital syphilis in neonates or for congenital syphilis in older infants and children. The CDC and AAP state that data are insufficient regarding efficacy of nonpenicillin regimens (e.g., ceftriaxone) for the treatment of syphilis in pediatric patients. Therefore, if treatment for syphilis is necessary in a neonate or child who has a history of penicillin hypersensitivity or who has developed an allergic reaction presumed to be related to penicillin, they should be desensitized and treated with penicillin G.

■ **Preoperative Intestinal Antisepsis** Oral erythromycin base is used in conjunction with oral neomycin sulfate as an adjunct to mechanical cleansing of the large intestine for intestinal antisepsis prior to elective colorectal surgery. For perioperative prophylaxis in patients undergoing colorectal surgery, many clinicians recommend a regimen of IV cefotetan or IV cefoxitin; a regimen of IV cefazolin and IV metronidazole; or a regimen of oral erythromycin and oral neomycin. It has been suggested that the oral regimen may be as effective as the parenteral regimens for patients undergoing elective colorectal surgery. Many clinicians use both the oral regimen and a parenteral regimen for perioperative prophylaxis in patients undergoing colorectal surgery; however, it is unclear whether this combined regimen is more effective than use of either an oral or parenteral regimen alone. In a randomized, prospective study in patients undergoing elective colorectal surgery, the overall incidence of intra-abdominal septic complications in those who received mechanical bowel preparation and an oral regimen (erythromycin and neomycin) alone was similar to that in those who received both the oral regimen and a parenteral regimen (cefoxitin); however, the incidence of abdominal wound infection was higher in those who received the oral regimen alone (14.6%) than in those who received the combined oral and parenteral regimen (5%).

■ **Other Uses** For more information on the uses of azithromycin and clarithromycin, see the individual monographs in 8:12.12.92. For topical uses of erythromycins, see 52:04.04 and 84:04.04.

Dosage and Administration

■ **Administration** Erythromycin base, stearate, ethylsuccinate, and estolate are administered orally. Erythromycin lactobionate is administered by continuous or intermittent IV infusion. In general, the oral route of administration is preferred and should replace the parenteral route as soon as possible.

■ **Dosage** The duration of erythromycin therapy is dependent on the type of infection. In infections caused by *Streptococcus pyogenes* (β-hemolytic streptococci), therapy should be continued for at least 10 days. When oral erythromycin therapy is used for prophylaxis or treatment of β-hemolytic streptococcal infections, the importance of strict adherence to the prescribed dosage regimen must be stressed to the patient.

■ **Dosage in Renal Impairment** Since renal excretion is not a major route of elimination of erythromycin and prolongation of serum half-life of the drug is not clinically important, dosage modifications are not necessary for patients with impaired renal function.

Cautions

With the exception of the estolate, erythromycins are considered among the least toxic anti-infectives and serious adverse effects are rare.

■ **GI Effects** The most common adverse effects of oral erythromycins are GI and are dose related. Erythromycin stimulates smooth muscle and GI motility. Abdominal pain and cramping occur frequently. Nausea, vomiting, and diarrhea have also occurred, especially after large doses. Occasionally, stomatitis, heartburn, anorexia, melena, pruritus ani, and reversible mild acute pancreatitis have occurred.

Clarithromycin causes less stimulation of GI smooth muscle motility than erythromycin in animals, and adverse GI effects appear to occur less frequently with clarithromycin or azithromycin than with oral erythromycin therapy.

■ **Hepatic Effects** Hepatic dysfunction, with or without jaundice, has occurred in patients receiving oral or parenteral erythromycin. Erythromycin estolate may rarely produce hepatotoxicity in the form of reversible cholestatic hepatitis. Erythromycin estolate-induced hepatotoxicity, which occurs mainly in adults, is most likely to appear in patients who receive the drug for longer than 10 days or in repeated courses of therapy. Therefore, use of the drug in these circumstances should be avoided. Erythromycin estolate-induced hepatotoxicity is generally considered to be a hypersensitivity reaction to the propanoate ester linkage at the 2″ position of the drug. However, reversible cholestatic hepatitis similar to that reported with erythromycin estolate has also been reported rarely with erythromycin ethylsuccinate. Some clinicians suggest that use of erythromycin estolate and erythromycin ethylsuccinate should be avoided in patients with a history of hepatitis associated with erythromycin therapy.

■ **Local Effects** Venous irritation and thrombophlebitis have occurred following IV administration of erythromycin lactobionate. The manufacturer states that pain and vessel trauma can be minimized if dilute solutions of the drug are administered by continuous infusion or by intermittent infusion slowly over 20–60 minutes.

■ **Cardiac Effects** Prolongation of the QT interval and development of ventricular arrhythmias, including atypical ventricular tachycardia (torsades de pointes), have been reported rarely with oral or IV erythromycin. Most reported cases have involved IV administration of the drug; limited data suggest that these adverse cardiac effects may depend on serum concentrations and/or rate of infusion of the drug. Erythromycin has exhibited concentration-dependent, reversible effects on cardiac conduction in electrophysiologic studies in humans and in Purkinje fibers isolated from dogs similar to those exhibited by class IA antiarrhythmic agents such as quinidine. Erythromycin prolongs the QT interval and blocks the potassium channel encoded by the human ether-a-gogo-related gene (HERG).

It has been suggested that erythromycins be used with caution in patients at risk for QT prolongation and/or accumulation of the anti-infective, particularly when the drug is administered IV. Some clinicians suggest that decreasing the rate of IV infusion of erythromycin may reduce the risk of cardiac toxicity; however, decreasing the rate may not eliminate the risk, and discontinuance of the drug may be necessary. Additional study and experience are needed to elucidate further the mechanisms and possible risk factors for the development of this toxicity.

There is some evidence that concomitant use of erythromycin with drugs that inhibit metabolism of the anti-infective may be associated with an increased risk of sudden cardiac death. In a population-based study that evaluated the association between erythromycin and the risk of sudden death from cardiac causes (usually ventricular tachyarrhythmia) using data for deaths occurring in a Tennessee Medicaid cohort from 1988–1993, the incidence of sudden death from cardiac causes was twice as high in those who received oral erythromycin during the study period than in those who received no anti-infectives. Concomitant use of oral erythromycin (a drug metabolized by the cytochrome P-450 [CYP] isoenzyme 3A) with drugs that inhibit CYP3A (e.g., fluconazole, ketoconazole, itraconazole, diltiazem, verapamil) increased the risk of sudden death from cardiac causes by a factor of 5. When the effect of specific CYP3A inhibitors was evaluated, calcium-channel blocking agents (diltiazem, verapamil) accounted for nearly all the person-years of follow-up and all cases of sudden death from cardiac causes. Prior use of erythromycin or prior use of CYP3A inhibitors was not associated with an increased risk. Therefore, it has been suggested that concomitant use of erythromycin and drugs that are potent inhibitors of CYP3A should be avoided. (See Drug Interactions.)

■ **Other Adverse Effects** Mild allergic reactions including urticaria, skin eruptions, and rash have occurred with erythromycin therapy. Serious allergic reactions including anaphylaxis have also been reported. Although a causal relationship was not definitely established, Stevens-Johnson syndrome occurred in at least one patient receiving oral erythromycin.

Ototoxicity consisting of bilateral hearing loss, in at least one case irreversible, has been reported rarely with erythromycin lactobionate, stearate, or ethylsuccinate. Tinnitus, alone or with vertigo, has also been reported rarely. Ototoxicity has generally occurred in patients with impaired renal or hepatic function and/or in those who were receiving high dosages of erythromycin (e.g., 4 g/day or more). Although hearing loss usually has been reversible following dosage reduction or discontinuance of the drug, sensorineural hearing loss that had not resolved after a follow-up period of at least 23 weeks also has been reported in a geriatric patient with underlying hepatic disease who received 2 g of IV erythromycin daily. Hypotension has been reported rarely in patients receiving erythromycin therapy.

Although a causal relationship to erythromycin lactobionate has not been established, nervous system effects including seizures, hallucinations, confusion, and vertigo have occurred rarely during therapy with the drug.

■ Precautions and Contraindications Following prolonged or repeated erythromycin therapy, overgrowth of nonsusceptible bacteria or fungi may occur. Appropriate therapy should be instituted if such infection occurs. Because *Clostridium difficile*-associated diarrhea and colitis (also known as antibiotic-associated pseudomembranous colitis) caused by overgrowth of toxin-producing clostridia has been reported with the use of broad-spectrum anti-infective agents, it should be considered in the differential diagnosis of patients who develop diarrhea during anti-infective therapy. Colitis may range in severity from mild to life-threatening. Mild cases of colitis may respond to discontinuance of the drug alone, but diagnosis and management of moderate to severe cases should include sigmoidoscopy, appropriate bacteriologic studies, and treatment with fluid, electrolyte, and protein supplementation as indicated. If colitis is severe or is not relieved by discontinuance of the drug, appropriate anti-infective therapy (e.g., oral metronidazole or vancomycin) should be administered. Other causes of colitis also should be considered.

Erythromycins are contraindicated in patients with a history of hypersensitivity reactions to the drugs. When astemizole and terfenadine were commercially available in the US, erythromycins were contraindicated in patients receiving these antihistamines. Concomitant administration of other macrolide antibiotics (e.g., clarithromycin) also was contraindicated in patients receiving terfenadine or astemizole since macrolides may impair metabolism of the antihistamines, potentially resulting in serious cardiotoxicity. (See Drug Interactions: Astemizole and Terfenadine.) Concomitant administration of cisapride and erythromycin or clarithromycin is contraindicated since these macrolides are expected to produce substantially increased plasma concentrations of unchanged cisapride and increase the potential for serious adverse effects (e.g., life-threatening cardiac arrhythmias) associated with the drug.

Erythromycin estolate is contraindicated in patients with hepatic dysfunction or preexisting liver disease. Other erythromycins should be used with caution in patients with impaired hepatic function or impaired biliary excretion. In addition, monitoring of serum erythromycin concentrations and modification of dosage when indicated may be advisable in these patients. The manufacturer of erythromycin gluceptate recommends monitoring hepatic function when the patient is receiving high doses or prolonged therapy.

■ Mutagenicity and Carcinogenicity Long-term (2-year) studies in rats using oral erythromycin base or erythromycin ethylsuccinate have not shown any evidence of tumorigenicity. Studies have not been performed to date to evaluate the mutagenic potential of erythromycin.

■ Pregnancy, Fertility, and Lactation Reproduction studies in female rats using oral erythromycin base at levels up to 0.25% of the diet prior to and during mating, during gestation, and through weaning of 2 successive litters have not revealed evidence of teratogenicity. Erythromycin has been reported to cross the placenta in humans; however, fetal plasma concentrations are generally low. There are no adequate and controlled studies to date using erythromycin in pregnant women, and the drug should be used during pregnancy only when clearly needed. However, oral erythromycin is used for the treatment of urogenital chlamydial infections in pregnant women. Erythromycin estolate is *not* recommended for this use because of the potential adverse effects on mother and fetus.

Reproduction studies in male and female rats using oral erythromycin base at levels up to 0.25% of the diet have not revealed evidence of impaired fertility.

Because erythromycin is distributed into milk, the drug should be used with caution in nursing women.

Drug Interactions

■ Drugs Affecting or Metabolized by Hepatic Microsomal Enzymes Erythromycin, apparently through inhibition of cytochrome P-450 (CYP) microsomal enzyme systems, can reduce the hepatic metabolism of some drugs including carbamazepine, cyclosporine, hexobarbital, phenytoin, alfentanil,disopyramide, lovastatin, and bromocriptine, thereby decreasing elimination and increasing serum concentrations of these drugs. In patients receiving concomitant erythromycin, serum concentrations of drugs metabolized by cytochrome P-450 microsomal enzyme systems should be monitored closely and dosage adjusted if necessary.

Erythromycin is metabolized by CYP3A and concomitant use with drugs that inhibit the CYP3A isoenzyme may result in increased erythromycin plasma concentrations. There is some evidence that concomitant use of oral erythromycin with drugs that inhibit CYP3A (i.e., fluconazole, ketoconazole, itraconazole, diltiazem, verapamil) is associated with an increased incidence of sudden death from cardiac causes, presumably because of increased plasma erythromycin concentrations resulting in an increased risk of QT prolongation (a dose-associated effect of erythromycin) and serious ventricular arrhythmias. Therefore, it has been suggested that concomitant use of erythromycin and drugs that are potent inhibitors of CYP3A should be avoided.

■ Anti-infective Agents Although in vitro studies have shown varying degrees of additive or synergistic effects against some organisms when erythromycin was used in conjunction with penicillins, streptomycin, sulfonamides, rifampin, or chloramphenicol, the clinical importance of these reports has not been established. Antagonism of bactericidal activity has been observed between erythromycin and clindamycin in vitro. In addition, antagonism has been reported when a bacteriostatic drug was administered with a bactericidal drug, but antagonism has not been convincingly documented clinically.

Antifungal Agents In a population-based study, concomitant use of oral erythromycin and drugs that inhibit CYP3A (i.e., fluconazole, ketoconazole, itraconazole) was associated with an increased incidence of sudden death from cardiac causes. Concomitant use of erythromycin and these drugs presumably increases plasma erythromycin concentrations resulting in an increased risk of QT prolongation (a dose-associated effect of erythromycin) and serious ventricular arrhythmias. Concomitant use of erythromycin and fluconazole, ketoconazole, or itraconazole should be avoided.

■ Astemizole and Terfenadine Erythromycin may interact with astemizole and terfenadine (both drugs no longer commercially available in the US), resulting in potentially serious adverse cardiovascular effects. Some evidence indicates that erythromycin may alter the metabolism of astemizole and terfenadine, probably via inhibition of the cytochrome P-450 microsomal enzyme system. (See Drug Interactions and Cautions: Cardiovascular Effects and Precautions and Contraindications, in the Antihistamines General Statement 4:00.) While erythromycin has been shown to decrease markedly the clearance of the active carboxylic acid metabolite of terfenadine, the effect of the macrolide on unchanged terfenadine concentrations has not been fully elucidated, but appears to show interindividual variation. In studies in extensive metabolizers of dextromethorphan or debrisoquin, erythromycin markedly impaired clearance of the active metabolite of terfenadine in all such individuals but produced measurable effects on unchanged terfenadine in only one-third of these individuals. In addition, erythromycin is known to inhibit the enzyme system responsible for astemizole's metabolism.

Prolongation of the QT interval and ventricular tachycardia, including torsades de pointes, have been reported in some patients receiving astemizole or terfenadine concomitantly with erythromycin or the structurally related macrolide troleandomycin (no longer commercially available in the US). Rarely, cardiac arrest and death have been reported in patients receiving erythromycin and terfenadine concomitantly. Therefore, when terfenadine and astemizole were commercially available in the US, these antihistamines were contraindicated in patients receiving erythromycin, clarithromycin, or troleandomycin. In addition, concomitant administration of astemizole or terfenadine and azithromycin also was not recommended, although limited data suggested that azithromycin did not alter the metabolism of terfenadine.

■ Carbamazepine Concomitant use of erythromycin and carbamazepine in adults or children has resulted in increased serum concentrations of carbamazepine and subsequent signs of carbamazepine toxicity (e.g., ataxia, dizziness, drowsiness, vomiting). Studies in adults indicate that erythromycin can substantially decrease serum clearance of carbamazepine, presumably by inhibiting hepatic metabolism of the drug. Patients receiving erythromycin and carbamazepine concomitantly should be monitored for evidence of carbamazepine toxicity; carbamazepine dosage should be reduced when necessary. Some clinicians suggest that use of an alternative anti-infective agent, instead of erythromycin, may be necessary in patients receiving carbamazepine.

■ Cardiac Drugs Concomitant use of erythromycin and digoxin has resulted in increased serum concentrations of digoxin, and initiation of erythromycin therapy in several patients receiving disopyramide reportedly has been associated with elevated serum disopyramide concentrations, QT-interval prolongation, and polymorphic ventricular tachycardia.

In at least one patient, concomitant administration of oral quinidine sulfate and IV erythromycin lactobionate resulted in increased serum quinidine concentrations and possible quinidine toxicity including asymptomatic, nonsustained ventricular tachycardia. It has been suggested that quinidine concentrations and ECGs be monitored closely if erythromycin is used concomitantly with quinidine.

Calcium-channel Blocking Agents In a population-based study, concomitant use of oral erythromycin and drugs that inhibit CYP3A (i.e., diltiazem, verapamil) was associated with an increased incidence of sudden death from cardiac causes. There was no increase in sudden cardiac death when oral erythromycin was used with calcium-channel blocking agents that do not inhibit CYP3A to a clinically important extent (e.g., nifedipine). Concomitant use of erythromycin and diltiazem or verapamil presumably increased plasma erythromycin concentrations resulting in an increased risk of QT prolongation (a dose-associated effect of erythromycin) and serious ventricular arrhythmias. In addition, erythromycin (a CYP3A inhibitor) is likely to increase plasma concentrations of diltiazem or verapamil leading to an increased risk of adverse effects associated with these drugs. Concomitant use of erythromycin and diltiazem or verapamil should be avoided.

■ Cisapride Oral or IV erythromycin markedly inhibit cytochrome P450 enzymes that metabolize cisapride (CYP3A4) and increase plasma cisapride concentrations, which may increase the potential for serious adverse effects (e.g., life-threatening cardiac arrhythmias) associated with the drug. (See Cautions: Precautions and Contraindications.)

■ **Clozapine** In one patient stabilized on clozapine (800 mg daily), concomitant administration of oral erythromycin therapy (250 mg 4 times daily) appeared to precipitate a tonic-clonic seizure, possibly by interfering with metabolism of the drug.

■ **Cyclosporine** Concomitant use of erythromycin and cyclosporine may result in substantial increases in blood or plasma concentrations of cyclosporine and subsequent signs of cyclosporine toxicity (e.g., nephrotoxicity). Studies in healthy adults indicate that erythromycin can substantially decrease plasma clearance of cyclosporine, presumably by inhibiting hepatic metabolism of the drug, although the exact mechanism remains to be clearly determined. Erythromycin and cyclosporine should be used concomitantly with caution, and patients should be monitored for evidence of cyclosporine toxicity. Renal function and blood or plasma concentrations of cyclosporine should be monitored when erythromycin therapy is administered or discontinued in patients receiving cyclosporine or vice versa, and cyclosporine dosage adjusted appropriately as necessary.

■ **Ergot Alkaloids** Concomitant administration of erythromycin and ergotamine reportedly may induce ischemic reactions, dysesthesia, and peripheral vasospasm.

■ **Midazolam and Triazolam** Erythromycin may alter pharmacokinetics of midazolam. Following concomitant administration of erythromycin with oral midazolam (an oral dosage form of midazolam currently is not available in the US) in healthy individuals, oral bioavailability of midazolam increased, resulting in substantial increases in peak plasma concentrations and half-life and fourfold increases in the area under the plasma concentration-time curve (AUC) of midazolam. Pharmacokinetics of IV midazolam were not affected to the same extent by concomitant administration of erythromycin as were those of oral midazolam; however, clearance of IV midazolam was decreased by 54% and half-life and volume of distribution of IV midazolam were increased. Although the mechanism of these interactions is unknown, it has been suggested that erythromycin may decrease hepatic metabolism of midazolam. In these individuals, erythromycin potentiated the sedative effect of oral midazolam and, to a lesser extent, that of IV midazolam, and also altered substantially the psychomotor effects of midazolam. Some clinicians suggest that erythromycin not be used in patients receiving oral midazolam or, alternatively, dosage of oral midazolam be reduced by 50–75%. Patients should be observed carefully and dosage of IV midazolam should be adjusted in individuals receiving erythromycin concomitantly.

Concomitant use of erythromycin apparently decreases clearance of triazolam and could increase the pharmacologic effects of the drug. A study in healthy adults indicates that peak serum concentration, elimination half-life, and area under the serum concentration time-curve (AUC) of triazolam are increased by about 50%, clearance of triazolam is decreased by about 50%, and the apparent volume of distribution of the drug is decreased by about 30% when erythromycin is given concomitantly. Patients receiving erythromycin and triazolam concomitantly should be monitored closely; a reduction in triazolam dosage may be necessary.

It is not known whether concomitant administration of erythromycin with other benzodiazepines results in similar alterations of pharmacokinetics of the benzodiazepines.

■ **Theophylline** Concomitant use of erythromycin in patients receiving high dosage of theophylline has resulted in decreased clearance of theophylline, elevated serum theophylline concentrations, and a prolonged serum half-life of the bronchodilator. An interaction may be most likely to occur in patients receiving an erythromycin dosage greater than 1.5 g daily for more than 5 days. Patients receiving theophylline should be closely monitored for signs of theophylline toxicity when erythromycin is administered concomitantly; serum theophylline concentrations should be monitored and dosage of the bronchodilator reduced if indicated.

Although further study is needed and the clinical importance has not been determined to date, there is some evidence that concomitant administration of erythromycin and theophylline can also result in decreased serum erythromycin concentrations and subtherapeutic concentrations of erythromycin may occur.

■ **Warfarin** Initiation of erythromycin therapy in some patients stabilized on warfarin has resulted in prolongation of prothrombin time and bleeding. Increased anticoagulant effect may be more pronounced in geriatric patients. The exact mechanism(s) of this interaction has not been clearly established, but erythromycin may inhibit hepatic metabolism of warfarin. Prothrombin time should be monitored more closely than usual in patients receiving warfarin when erythromycin therapy is initiated, and warfarin dosage should be adjusted as necessary.

Laboratory Test Interferences

Erythromycin may falsely elevate concentrations of urinary catecholamines, 17-hydroxycorticosteroids, and 17-ketosteroids. The drug may interfere with colorimetric assays resulting in falsely increased AST (SGOT) and ALT (SGPT) concentrations. Falsely elevated AST concentrations without liver injury may result due to erroneous measurement of unidentified metabolites of erythromycin in colorimetric determinations.

Erythromycin may decrease serum folate assay results if a microbiologic method is used since the drug can inhibit the growth of *Lactobacillus casei*; results are unaffected if the chromatographic procedure of Landon is used. The presence of erythromycin in the blood may interfere with the etiologic diagnosis of mycoplasmal pneumonia by masking a rise in the titer of the tetrazolium reduction inhibition neutralizing antibody to *Mycoplasma pneumoniae*.

Mechanism of Action

Erythromycin is usually bacteriostatic, but it may be bactericidal in high concentrations or against highly susceptible organisms.

Erythromycin inhibits protein synthesis in susceptible organisms by binding to 50S ribosomal subunits, thereby inhibiting translocation of aminoacyl transfer-RNA and inhibiting polypeptide synthesis. The site of action of erythromycin is the same as that of other macrolides (e.g., azithromycin, clarithromycin) and the same as that of clindamycin, lincomycin, and chloramphenicol.

Erythromycin exerts its effect only against multiplying organisms. Only un-ionized erythromycin is believed to penetrate susceptible bacteria, and penetration increases in an alkaline environment as the pK_a of the drug is approached. Erythromycin generally penetrates the cell wall of gram-positive bacteria more readily than that of gram-negative bacteria, and gram-positive organisms may accumulate 100 times more erythromycin than do gram-negative organisms.

Spectrum

Erythromycin is active in vitro against gram-positive cocci (staphylococci and streptococci) and gram-positive bacilli including *Bacillus anthracis, Corynebacterium, Clostridium, Erysipelothrix,* and *Listeria monocytogenes*. Erythromycin also is active in vitro against some gram-negative cocci (*Neisseria*) and some gram-negative bacilli, including some strains of *Haemophilus influenzae, Legionella pneumophila, Pasteurella,* and *Brucella*. Some strains of *Chlamydia, Actinomyces, Mycoplasma pneumoniae, Ureaplasma urealyticum,* Rickettsia, *Treponema,* and *Entamoeba histolytica* are inhibited by erythromycin. Erythromycin also has some in vitro activity against *Mycobacterium kansasii* and *M. scrofulaceum*. Enterobacteriaceae (e.g., *Escherichia coli, Enterobacter, Klebsiella, Proteus, Salmonella, Shigella*) and *Pseudomonas* usually are resistant to erythromycin, as are viruses and fungi.

There is a wide range of minimal inhibitory concentrations (MICs) reported for erythromycin, but generally in vitro erythromycin concentrations of less than 1 mcg/mL inhibit the majority of strains of susceptible staphylococci, streptococci, *Moraxella catarrhalis* (formerly *Branhamella catarrhalis*), *Clostridium, Erysipelothrix, Listeria, Bacillus, Actinomyces,* and *Mycoplasma pneumoniae*. Higher concentrations may be required to inhibit some strains of *Enterococcus faecalis* (formerly *Streptococcus faecalis*) and certain strains of *Corynebacterium, Neisseria, Haemophilus, Brucella, Pasteurella, Bordetella,* and mycobacteria.

Borrelia burgdorferi, the causative organism of Lyme disease, reportedly may be inhibited in vitro by erythromycin concentrations of 0.01–1 mcg/mL or less. Minimum bactericidal concentrations of erythromycin for *B. burgdorferi* generally have ranged from 0.04–0.16 mcg/mL.

Erythromycin has in vitro activity against *Bacillus anthracis*. Anti-infectives are active against the germinated form of *B. anthracis*, but are not active against the organism while it is still in the spore form. Results of in vitro susceptibility testing of 11 *Bacillus anthracis* isolates that were associated with cases of inhalational or cutaneous anthrax that occurred in the US (Florida, New York, District of Columbia) during September and October 2001 in the context of an intentional release of anthrax spores (biologic warfare, bioterrorism) indicate that these strains had erythromycin MICs of 1 mcg/mL. Based on interpretive criteria established for staphylococci, these strains are considered to have intermediate susceptibility to erythromycin. Limited or no data are available to date regarding in vivo activity of erythromycin against *B. anthracis* or use of the drug in the treatment of inhalational anthrax.

Erythromycin is active in vitro against *Helicobacter pylori* (formerly *Campylobacter pylori* or *C. pyloridis*), an organism associated with the development of duodenal and gastric ulcers. However, in vivo efficacy of the drug against this organism has been poor, possibly as a result of inactivation of the drug by stomach acid and/or the rapid development of resistance when erythromycin is used alone for *H. pylori* infections.

In general, clarithromycin displays in vitro activity similar to or greater than that of erythromycin against erythromycin-sensitive organisms; azithromycin and erythromycin have comparable activity against most gram-positive organisms (e.g., streptococci and staphylococci) but azithromycin is more active against gram-negative organisms (e.g., *M. catarrhalis, Neisseria gonorrhoeae, Hemophilus influenzae*).

For more information on the spectra of activity of azithromycin and clarithromycin, see the individual monographs in 8:12.12.92.

■ **In Vitro Susceptibility Testing** Because there are differences in the spectra of activity and potency of the various macrolides, in vitro susceptibility to these drugs must be tested individually. When the disk-diffusion procedure is used, separate drug-specific disks should be used to test susceptibility to azithromycin, clarithromycin, and erythromycin.

The Clinical and Laboratory Standards Institute (CLSI; formerly National Committee for Clinical Laboratory Standards [NCCLS]) states that, if results of in vitro susceptibility testing indicate that a clinical isolate is *susceptible* to erythromycin, then an infection caused by this strain may be appropriately treated with the dosage of the drug recommended for that type of infection and infecting species, unless otherwise contraindicated. If results indicate that a clinical isolate has *intermediate susceptibility* to erythromycin, then the strain has a minimum inhibitory concentration (MIC) that approaches usually attainable blood and tissue concentrations and response rates may be lower than for strains identified as susceptible. Therefore, the intermediate category implies clinical applicability in body sites where the drug is physiologically concentrated or when a high dosage of the drug can be used. This intermediate category also includes a buffer zone which should prevent small, uncontrolled technical factors from causing major discrepancies in interpretation, especially for drugs with narrow pharmacotoxicity margins. If results of in vitro susceptibility testing indicate that a clinical isolate is *resistant* to erythromycin, the strain is not inhibited by systemic concentrations of the drug achievable with usual dosage schedules and/or MICs fall in the range where specific microbial resistance mechanisms are likely and efficacy has not been reliable in clinical studies.

Disk Susceptibility Tests When the disk-diffusion procedure is used to test susceptibility to erythromycin, a disk containing 15 mcg of the drug should be used.

When disk-diffusion susceptibility testing is performed according to CLSI standardized procedures using CLSI interpretive criteria, *Staphylococcus* or *Enterococcus* with growth inhibition zones of 23 mm or greater are susceptible to erythromycin, those with zones of 14–22 mm have intermediate susceptibility, and those with zones of 13 mm or less are resistant to the drug.

When testing susceptibility of *Streptococcus,* including *S. pneumoniae,* according to CLSI standardized procedures using Mueller-Hinton agar (supplemented with 5% defibrinated sheep blood), those with growth inhibition zones of 21 mm or greater are susceptible to erythromycin, those with zones of 16–20 mm have intermediate susceptibility, and those with zones of 15 mm or less are resistant to the drug.

Dilution Susceptibility Tests When dilution susceptibility testing (agar or broth dilution) is performed according to CLSI standardized procedures using CLSI interpretive criteria, *Staphylococcus* or *Enterococcus* with MICs of 0.5 mcg/mL or less are susceptible to erythromycin, those with MICs of 1–4 mcg/mL have intermediate susceptibility, and those with MICs of 8 mcg/mL or greater are resistant to the drug.

When susceptibility of *Streptococcus,* including *S. pneumoniae,* is tested according to CLSI standardized procedures using cation-adjusted Mueller-Hinton broth (with 2–5% lysed horse blood), those with MICs of 0.25 mcg/mL or less are susceptible to erythromycin, those with MICs of 0.5 mcg/mL have intermediate susceptibility, and those with MICs of 1 mcg/mL or greater are resistant to the drug.

Resistance

Resistant strains of *Haemophilus influenzae, Corynebacterium diphtheriae,* and staphylococci, particularly *S. aureus,* have developed during therapy with erythromycin.

Erythromycin-resistant strains of streptococci, including *Streptococcus pyogenes* (group A β-hemolytic streptococci), group B streptococci, *S. pneumoniae,* and viridans streptococci have been reported. In some areas of the world (e.g., Taiwan, Japan, Spain), a large percentage (up to 14–83%) of streptococcal isolates have been reported to be resistant to erythromycin. In Finland, the incidence of erythromycin resistance in *S. pyogenes* increased from about 13% in 1990 to 19% in 1993; however, by 1996, the incidence had decreased to 8.6% and this decrease was attributed in part to a nationwide effort to restrict use of erythromycin in outpatients with minor respiratory tract or skin infections. The incidence of erythromycin-resistant streptococci in the US has been relatively low to date; analysis of clinical isolates at some US medical centers indicate that up to 7% of *S. pyogenes* and 7–16% of group B streptococci are resistant to erythromycin.

Resistance to erythromycin develops stepwise at a rate less than or equal to that with natural penicillins. Resistance usually is not a major problem in short-term erythromycin therapy, but may be clinically important if erythromycins are used frequently or in large quantities.

Cross-resistance generally occurs among the macrolides, including azithromycin, clarithromycin, and erythromycin. Some cross-resistance occurs between macrolides and clindamycin and lincomycin. Erythromycin exhibits a dissociated type of resistance, characteristic of macrolides, in which the presence of erythromycin can influence in vitro susceptibility testing. For example, strains of organisms that are resistant to erythromycin but susceptible to other macrolides or lincomycin may show resistance to these drugs if erythromycin also is present. This phenomenon may be the result of altered metabolism in the organism induced by erythromycin or of competition between erythromycin and lincomycin for the ribosomal binding site.

Pharmacokinetics

■ Absorption

Absorption of orally administered erythromycins occurs mainly in the duodenum. The bioavailability of the drugs is variable and depends on several factors including the particular erythromycin derivative, the formulation of the dosage form administered, acid stability of the derivative, presence of food in the GI tract, and gastric emptying time.

Gastric acidity causes partial inactivation of some of these drugs, with the degree of inactivation depending on the acid stability of the particular derivative and dosage form. Erythromycin base is highly susceptible to gastric acid inactivation, and commercially available tablets are coated with acid-resistant (enteric) coatings or are buffered to protect the drug from gastric acidity. Results of one in vitro study indicate that the stearate is also highly susceptible to gastric acid inactivation. Erythromycin ethylsuccinate is partially dissociated in the intestine where both erythromycin and the undissociated ester are absorbed; in the blood, the ester is partially hydrolyzed to release free erythromycin. The estolate is acid stable because of the presence of the lauryl sulfate moiety. Erythromycin estolate dissociates in the upper intestine, liberating the inactive propanoate ester which is absorbed and partially hydrolyzed in the blood to release free erythromycin.

Single oral doses of the erythromycins generally produce peak serum concentrations within 1–4 hours. Higher peak serum concentrations are achieved when the drugs are given orally in 4 doses daily than following single doses. In general, oral administration of 250 mg of erythromycin as the base, estolate, or stearate, or 400 mg of erythromycin as the ethylsuccinate, 4 times daily maintains antibacterial serum concentrations of 0.1–2 mcg/mL. Higher serum concentrations have been reported to occur in patients receiving erythromycin estolate than in those receiving other derivatives. However, since as much as 80% of the drug in plasma is the inactive propanoate ester and the assay procedure causes hydrolysis of the ester, the apparently greater plasma concentrations achieved with the estolate are not necessarily indicative of greater antibacterial activity. Mean peak serum concentrations of about 0.6 mcg/mL reportedly occur 1.5–2 hours after a single 50-mg IM dose of erythromycin ethylsuccinate in children, or 1–4 hours after a single 100-mg IM dose in adults. Following IV administration of 200 mg of erythromycin lactobionate, peak serum concentrations of 3–4 mcg/mL have been reported.

■ Distribution

Erythromycin is widely distributed into most body tissues and fluids. Following oral or parenteral administration of the drug, most tissues except the brain have erythromycin concentrations that are higher and persist longer than serum concentrations. Only low concentrations of erythromycin (2–13% of serum concentrations) are distributed into CSF. In patients with otitis media, erythromycin appears in the middle ear exudate in concentrations generally 50% of concurrent serum concentrations; however, these concentrations may not be sufficient to inhibit all strains of *H. influenzae.* Concentrations of erythromycin in prostatic fluid and semen are approximately 33% of concurrent serum concentrations. In patients with normal liver function, erythromycin is concentrated in the liver and bile.

Erythromycin base is 73–81% bound and erythromycin estolate is approximately 96% bound to serum proteins.

Erythromycin crosses the placenta, achieving fetal serum concentrations 5–20% of maternal serum concentrations. Erythromycin is distributed into milk in concentrations about 50% of plasma concentrations.

■ Elimination

The serum half-life of erythromycin in patients with normal renal function is usually 1.5–2 hours, but may range from 0.8–3 hours. In anuric patients, the serum half-life may be prolonged to 6 hours, but this is not considered to be clinically important. Although there are few data on the serum half-life of erythromycin in patients with impaired hepatic function, the possibility that the half-life may be prolonged should be considered. In one single-dose study, the terminal elimination half-life in adults with alcoholic liver disease was similar to that in healthy adults, but the initial distribution half-life was slightly prolonged and average and peak serum concentrations were higher in those with alcoholic liver disease.

Erythromycin is partly metabolized by cytochrome P-450 (CYP) isoenzyme 3A4 in the liver by *N*-demethylation to inactive, unidentified metabolites. Erythromycin is mainly excreted unchanged via bile. Some reabsorption follows biliary excretion. Small amounts of erythromycin are also excreted in urine. Only small amounts of erythromycin are removed by hemodialysis.

Chemistry and Stability

■ Chemistry

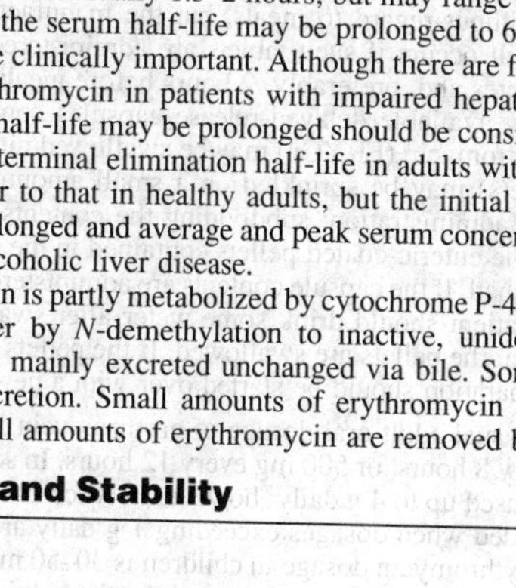

erythromycin

Erythromycin is a macrolide antibiotic produced by *Streptomyces erythreus.* Erythromycin is a weak base that readily forms salts and esters with organic acids. The pK_a of erythromycin base is 8.9. Erythromycin has a bitter taste, and the stearate salt, the ethylsuccinate ester, and the sodium lauryl sulfate salt of the propanoate ester (estolate) have been developed in an attempt to overcome the taste. In addition, many commercially available tablets of the various derivatives are film-coated to mask the taste or enteric-coated to protect the drugs from inactivation by gastric acidity. Erythromycin base, stearate, ethylsuccinate, and estolate are poorly soluble in water; erythromycin lactobionate is freely soluble in water.

Azithromycin and clarithromycin are semisynthetic macrolide antibiotics structurally and pharmacologically related to erythromycin. Azithromycin, an azalide, differs structurally from erythromycin by the addition of a methyl-substituted nitrogen atom into the lactone ring; clarithromycin differs from erythromycin only by the methylation of a hydroxyl group at the 6 position on the lactone ring. These structural modifications in azithromycin and clarithromycin result in improved resistance to acid degradation and enhanced tissue penetration compared with erythromycin.

Tacrolimus is a macrolide antibiotic produced by *Streptomyces tsukubaensis* that exhibits only limited antimicrobial activity; the drug is employed for its immunosuppressive effects (e.g., to prevent rejection in allograft recipients). (See Tacrolimus 92:44.)

■ **Stability** Erythromycin lactobionate is reported to be physically incompatible with many drugs, but the compatibility depends on several factors (e.g., the concentration of the drugs, specific diluents used, temperature). Stability of erythromycin lactobionate solutions is dependent on pH and is optimal at pH 6–8; loss of antibacterial activity occurs rapidly when the pH is less than 5.5. Specialized references should be consulted for specific compatibility information.

For more information on the chemistry and stability of azithromycin and clarithromycin, see the individual monographs in 8:12.12.92.

For specific dosages and additional information on the erythromycins, azithromycin, or clarithromycin, see the individual monographs in 8:12.12.04 and 8:12.12.92.

†Use is not currently included in the labeling approved by the US Food and Drug Administration

Erythromycin

■ Erythromycin is a macrolide antibiotic.

Dosage and Administration

■ **Administration** Erythromycin base is administered orally. The manufacturers of erythromycin delayed-release tablets state that these tablets are well absorbed and may be given without regard to meals. The manufacturers of erythromycin delayed-release capsules (containing enteric-coated pellets) and erythromycin film-coated tablets state that optimal absorption generally occurs when these preparations are administered in the fasting state (at least 30 minutes and, preferably, 2 hours before or after meals). Delayed-release tablets containing enteric-coated particles are well absorbed in most patients and may be given without regard to meals, but the manufacturer states that optimal absorption still occurs if such tablets are administered in the fasting state (at least 30 minutes and, preferably, 2 hours before meals).

The commercially available delayed-release capsules containing enteric-coated pellets of erythromycin (ERYC®) may be swallowed intact or the entire contents of a capsule(s) may be sprinkled on a small amount of applesauce immediately prior to administration; subdividing the contents of a capsule is *not* recommended. The enteric-coated pellets contained in the capsules should *not* be chewed or crushed. If the capsule contents are administered by sprinkling on applesauce, the patient should drink some water after swallowing the applesauce to ensure that the pellets are swallowed. If the pellets are accidentally spilled, the dose preparation should be started over with a new capsule.

■ **Dosage** The usual adult oral dosage of erythromycin is 250 mg every 6 hours, 333 mg every 8 hours, or 500 mg every 12 hours. In severe infections, dosage may be increased up to 4 g daily; however, a twice-daily dosing schedule is not recommended when dosages exceeding 1 g daily are administered.

The usual oral erythromycin dosage in children is 30–50 mg/kg daily given in 2–4 equally divided doses. For more severe infections, this dosage may be doubled but should not exceed 4 g daily. A twice-daily dosing schedule is not recommended when dosages exceeding 1 g daily are administered.

Pharyngitis and Tonsillitis If erythromycin is used for the treatment of pharyngitis and tonsillitis caused by *Streptococcus pyogenes* (group A β-hemolytic streptococci), the drug should be given in the usual dosage for 10 days or longer.

Prophylaxis of Recurrent Rheumatic Fever For continuous prophylaxis to prevent recurrences in patients with a history of rheumatic heart disease, the usual oral dosage of erythromycin is 250 mg twice daily.

When selecting anti-infectives for prophylaxis of recurrent rheumatic fever, the current recommendations published by the American Heart Association (AHA) should be consulted.

Syphilis Although penicillin G is the drug of choice for all stages of syphilis, the manufacturers state that 30–40 g of oral erythromycin has been given in divided doses over 10–15 days for the treatment of primary syphilis. Erythromycin is no longer included in US Centers for Disease Control and Prevention (CDC) recommendations for the treatment of any form of syphilis in adults or adolescents (including primary, secondary, latent, or tertiary syphilis or neurosyphilis) and is *not* recommended for the treatment of congenital syphilis or syphilis in older infants and children. In addition, erythromycin is no longer recommended by the CDC or American Academy of Pediatrics (AAP) for the treatment of syphilis in pregnant women who are hypersensitive to penicillin since numerous treatment failures (including in the fetus) have been reported with the drug.

Lyme Disease For the treatment of early localized or early disseminated Lyme disease† associated with erythema migrans (but without neurologic involvement or third-degree AV heart block) in adults who are allergic to or intolerant of penicillins and cephalosporins and in whom tetracyclines are contraindicated, the Infectious Diseases Society of America (IDSA) suggests an oral erythromycin dosage of 500 mg 4 times daily for 14–21 days. For the treatment of early localized or early disseminated Lyme disease† associated with erythema migrans (but without neurologic involvement or third-degree AV heart block) in children who are allergic to or intolerant of penicillins or cephalosporins and cannot receive a tetracycline (e.g., younger than 8 years of age), the IDSA suggests an oral erythromycin dosage of 12.5 mg/kg (maximum dose: 500 mg) 4 times daily for 14–21 days. Some clinicians suggest that if erythromycin is used in the treatment of early Lyme disease, adults should receive 250 mg 4 times daily for 14–21 days and children should receive 30 mg/kg daily in 3 divided doses (or 250 mg 3 times daily) for 14–21 days. However, erythromycin may not be as effective as other recommended agents (e.g., oral doxycycline, oral amoxicillin) for the treatment of Lyme disease, and patients treated with macrolides should be monitored closely. For additional details on the manifestations of Lyme disease and the efficacy of various anti-infective regimens in early or late Lyme disease, see Lyme Disease in Uses: Spirochetal Infections, in the Tetracyclines General Statement 8:12.24.

Gonorrhea and Associated Infections When an oral erythromycin is indicated for the treatment of coexisting chlamydial infections in conjunction with therapy of uncomplicated or disseminated gonococcal infections, the CDC recommends that adults and adolescents receive 500 mg of erythromycin orally 4 times daily for 7 days. Erythromycins generally are indicated for these infections in pregnant women and in other adults when tetracyclines are contraindicated or not tolerated. (See Uses: Gonorrhea and Associated Infections, in the Erythromycins General Statement 8:12.12.04.)

The AAP currently recommends that all children beyond the neonatal period being treated for uncomplicated vulvovaginal, urethral, or pharyngeal gonorrhea, epididymitis, proctitis, or disseminated gonococcal infections including meningitis or endocarditis receive presumptive treatment for possible coexisting chlamydial infections. If oral erythromycin is used for presumptive treatment of chlamydial infection in children who weigh less than 45 kg, the AAP recommends a dosage of 50 mg/kg daily (maximum 2 g daily) given in 4 divided doses for 7 days.

Although erythromycin is not included in the current CDC recommendations for the treatment of acute pelvic inflammatory disease (PID) caused by *N. gonorrhoeae*, some manufacturers recommend a regimen of 500 mg of erythromycin (as the lactobionate) IV every 6 hours for 3 days followed by an oral regimen of 333 mg of erythromycin (as the base or stearate) every 8 hours for 7 days or 500 mg every 12 hours for 7 days for the treatment of these infections. However, some clinicians believe this oral dosage is inadequate and recommend 500 mg every 6 hours for 7–10 days.

Nongonococcal Urethritis When oral erythromycin is used as an alternative to azithromycin or doxycycline for the treatment of nongonococcal urethritis in adults and adolescents, the CDC and others recommend a regimen of 500 mg of erythromycin 4 times daily for 7 days. Alternatively, a regimen of 666 mg of erythromycin may be given every 8 hours for at least 7 days.

Patients with recurrent and persistent urethritis who were not compliant with the full course of erythromycin therapy or who were reexposed to untreated sexual partner(s) should receive a second course of oral erythromycin. If the patient has recurrent and persistent urethritis, was compliant with the regimen, and reexposure can be excluded, the CDC recommends a regimen of 500 mg of oral erythromycin 4 times daily for 7 days given in conjunction with a single 2-g dose of oral metronidazole.

Chlamydial Infections For the treatment of uncomplicated urethral, endocervical, or rectal infections caused by *Chlamydia trachomatis* in nonpregnant adults and adolescents when azithromycin or doxycycline cannot be used, the CDC and others recommend oral erythromycin in a dosage of 500 mg 4 times daily for 7 days. Alternatively, a dosage of 666 mg every 8 hours for 7 days can be used. The dosage of oral erythromycin recommended by the CDC for the treatment of these infections in children weighing 45 kg or less is 50 mg/kg daily given in 4 divided doses for 14 days.

For the treatment of chlamydial urogenital infections during pregnancy, the recommended dosage of oral erythromycin is 500 mg 4 times daily or 666 mg every 8 hours for at least 7 days. Women who cannot tolerate this regimen may receive a dosage of 500 mg every 12 hours, 333 mg every 8 hours, or 250 mg 4 times daily for at least 14 days.

For the treatment of pneumonia caused by *C. trachomatis* in infants, the recommended dosage of oral erythromycin is 50 mg/kg daily given in 4 divided doses for 14 days; follow-up is recommended and a second course of therapy may be necessary.

For the treatment of ophthalmia neonatorum caused by *C. trachomatis*, the recommended dosage of oral erythromycin is 50 mg/kg daily given in 4 divided doses for 14 days; follow-up is recommended and a second course of therapy may be necessary.

If erythromycin is used as an alternative to doxycycline for the treatment of genital, inguinal, or anorectal infections caused by a lymphogranuloma venereum serotype of *C. trachomatis*†, the CDC and others recommend that adults and adolescents receive an oral dosage of 500 mg 4 times daily for 21 days.

Chancroid For the treatment of chancroid† (genital ulcers caused by *Haemophilus ducreyi*), the CDC and others recommend that adults receive an oral erythromycin dosage of 500 mg 3–4 times daily for 7 days.

The CDC recommends that patients with chancroid be examined 3–7 days after initiation of anti-infective therapy. If the regimen was effective, symptomatic improvement in the ulcers is evident within 3 days and objective improvement is evident within 7 days. The time required for complete healing is related to the size of the ulcer; large ulcers may require more than 2 weeks to heal. Healing of ulcers may be slower in uncircumcised men who have ulcers under the foreskin. Resolution of fluctuant lymphadenopathy is slower than that of ulcers, and needle aspiration or incision and drainage may be necessary even during otherwise effective anti-infective therapy. While needle aspiration of buboes is a simpler procedure, incision and drainage of buboes may be preferred. If clinical improvement is not evident within 3–7 days, consideration should be given to the possibility that the diagnosis was incorrect, there is coinfection with another sexually transmitted disease, the patient was noncompliant with the regimen, the strain of *H. ducreyi* is resistant to the anti-infective agent used, or the patient is HIV seropositive. (See Uses: Chancroid in the Erythromycins General Statement 8:12.12.04.)

Granuloma Inguinale (Donovanosis) When oral erythromycin is used as an alternative to co-trimoxazole or doxycycline for the treatment of granuloma inguinale† (Donovanosis) caused by *Calymmatobacterium granulomatis* (e.g., in pregnant or lactating women), the CDC recommends a dosage of 500 mg orally 4 times daily for at least 3 weeks. If lesions do not respond within the first few days of therapy, some experts recommend that a parenteral aminoglycoside (e.g., 1 mg/kg of gentamicin IV every 8 hours) be added to the regimen. Addition of an aminoglycoside should be strongly considered when treating donovanosis in pregnant or lactating women or in patients with human immunodeficiency virus (HIV) infection. Despite effective anti-infective therapy, donovanosis may relapse 6–18 months later.

Intestinal Amebiasis Although erythromycin is not considered a drug of choice for the treatment of intestinal amebiasis caused by *Entamoeba histolytica*, the manufacturers state that adults may receive 250 mg of erythromycin every 6 hours, 333 mg every 8 hours, or 500 mg every 12 hours for 10–14 days and that children may be given 30–50 mg/kg daily in divided doses for 10–14 days.

Diphtheria **Treatment.** When used as an adjunct to diphtheria antitoxin for the *treatment* of diphtheria, the usual dosage of erythromycin is 40–50 mg/kg daily (maximum 2 g daily) for 14 days. Patients usually are no longer contagious 48 hours after initiation of anti-infective therapy. Eradication of the organism should be confirmed by 2 consecutive negative cultures following completion of therapy.

Prophylaxis. For *prevention* of diphtheria in household or intimate contacts of patients with respiratory or cutaneous diphtheria, the CDC and US Public Health Service Advisory Committee on Immunization Practices (ACIP) recommend that children receive erythromycin in a dosage of 40 mg/kg daily and that adults receive 1 g daily for 7–10 days. The American Academy of Pediatrics (AAP) recommends that these contacts receive an erythromycin dosage of 40–50 mg/kg daily (maximum 2 g daily) for 7 days.

Household or intimate contacts of patients with diphtheria should receive anti-infective *prophylaxis* regardless of their immunization status and should be closely monitored for symptoms of diphtheria for 7 days. In addition, contacts who are inadequately immunized against diphtheria (i.e., have previously received fewer than 3 doses of diphtheria toxoid) or whose immunization status is unknown should receive an immediate dose of an age-appropriate diphtheria toxoid preparation and the primary series should be completed according to the recommended schedule. Contacts who are fully immunized should receive an immediate booster dose of an age-appropriate diphtheria toxoid preparation if it has been 5 years or longer since their last booster dose.

Diphtheria Carrier State. When erythromycin is used to *eliminate the diphtheria carrier state* in identified carriers of toxigenic *Corynebacterium diphtheriae*, the ACIP and AAP recommend that adults and children receive 7–10 days of the drug in the dosages specified above for prevention of diphtheria. Follow-up cultures should be obtained at least 2 weeks after completion of therapy; if cultures are positive, an additional 10-day course of oral erythromycin should be given and additional follow-up cultures obtained.

Pertussis Although the optimum dosage and duration of erythromycin for the *treatment* of pertussis or *prevention* in susceptible contacts have not been established, a dosage of 1 g daily in adults and 40–50 mg/kg daily (maximum 2 g daily) in children given in divided doses for 14 days usually is recommended. While a shorter duration of erythromycin therapy (e.g., 7 or 10 days) may be effective in some patients, prophylaxis failures and bacteriologic relapse of pertussis have been reported with erythromycin regimens shorter than 14 days. Therefore, the CDC, ACIP, AAP, and some clinicians recommend that a 14-day course of erythromycin therapy be used for treatment or prevention of pertussis.

Although data from controlled studies are lacking, the CDC recommends that all household and other close contacts of individuals with pertussis receive a 14-day regimen of prophylaxis (regardless of age and vaccination status) since this may prevent or minimize transmission of the disease. In addition, all close contacts younger than 7 years of age who are not fully immunized against pertussis should receive the remaining required doses of a preparation containing pertussis vaccine (using minimal intervals between doses) and those who are fully immunized but have not received a vaccine dose within the last 3 years should receive a booster dose of a pertussis vaccine preparation.

Legionnaires' Disease Although the optimum dosage and duration of erythromycin for the treatment of Legionnaires' disease have not been established, dosages of 1–4 g daily in divided doses have been given alone or in combination with rifampin. A parenteral regimen usually is necessary for the initial treatment of severe Legionnaires' disease and the addition of rifampin is recommended during the first 3–5 days of therapy in severely ill and/or immunocompromised patients; after a response is obtained, rifampin can be discontinued and therapy changed to oral erythromycin. The duration of therapy in patients with Legionnaires's disease usually is 10–21 days; some clinicians recommend 14 days of therapy for patients with mild disease and 21 days for those who are immunocompromised or have severe disease.

Preoperative Intestinal Antisepsis For preoperative intestinal antisepsis in patients undergoing colorectal surgery, oral erythromycin is usually given in conjunction with oral neomycin sulfate as an adjunct to mechanical cleansing of the large intestine. It is generally recommended that if surgery is scheduled for 8 a.m., 1 g of erythromycin and 1 g of neomycin sulfate should be administered at 1 p.m., 2 p.m., and 11 p.m. on the day preceding surgery.

Chemistry and Stability

■ **Chemistry** Erythromycin occurs as a white or slightly yellow, odorless or practically odorless, bitter, crystalline powder. The drug has a solubility of approximately 1 mg/mL in water and is soluble in alcohol at 25°C.

■ **Stability** Erythromycin delayed-release capsules (containing enteric-coated pellets), delayed-release tablets (containing enteric-coated particles), delayed-release (enteric coated) tablets, and film-coated tablets should be stored at a temperature not exceeding 30°C. The delayed-release capsules should be protected from moisture and excessive heat.

For further information on chemistry, mechanism of action, spectrum, resistance, pharmacokinetics, uses, cautions, drug interactions, laboratory test interferences, and dosage and administration of erythromycin, see the Erythromycins General Statement 8:12.12.04.

Preparations

Excipients in commercially available drug preparations may have clinically important effects in some individuals; consult specific product labeling for details.

Erythromycin

Oral		
Capsules, delayed-release (containing enteric-coated pellets)	250 mg*	ERYC®, Warner Chilcott; Erythromycin Delayed-Release Capsules
Tablets, delayed-release (containing enteric-coated particles)	333 mg	PCE® Dispertab®, Abbott
	500 mg	PCE® Dispertab®, Abbott
Tablets, delayed-release (enteric-coated)	250 mg	Ery-Tab®, Abbott
	333 mg	Ery-Tab®, Abbott
	500 mg	Ery-Tab®, Abbott
Tablets, film-coated	250 mg	Erythromycin Base Filmtab
	500 mg	Erythromycin Base Filmtab

*available from one or more manufacturer, distributor, and/or repackager by generic (nonproprietary) name

†Use is not currently included in the labeling approved by the US Food and Drug Administration

Erythromycin Ethylsuccinate

■ Erythromycin ethylsuccinate is a macrolide antibiotic.

Dosage and Administration

■ **Administration** Erythromycin ethylsuccinate is administered orally. Erythromycin ethylsuccinate oral suspensions, chewable tablets, and film-coated tablets may be administered without regard to meals. Chewable tablets should not be swallowed whole.

The fixed-combination preparation containing erythromycin ethylsuccinate and sulfisoxazole acetyl is administered orally and may be given without regard to meals. Because the fixed-combination preparation contains a sulfonamide, the preparation should not be used in infants younger than 2 months of age, pregnant women at term, or mothers who are nursing infants younger than 2 months of age.

■ **Dosage** Dosage of erythromycin ethylsuccinate is expressed in terms of erythromycin. Since the ethylsuccinate has different absorption characteristics in adults than do other commercially available forms of erythromycin, higher oral doses are needed to achieve therapeutic effects. The manufacturer states that, for adults, 400 mg of erythromycin as the ethylsuccinate provides erythromycin activity similar to that provided by 250 mg of erythromycin as the base, stearate, or estolate.

The usual adult oral dosage of erythromycin as the ethylsuccinate is 400 mg every 6 hours. In severe infections, dosage may be increased up to 4 g daily. The usual oral dosage of erythromycin as the ethylsuccinate in children is 30–50 mg/kg daily in 4 equally divided doses every 6 hours. For more severe infections, this dosage may be doubled. An alternative pediatric dosage of 0.9–3 g/m^2 daily in 4 equally divided doses has been recommended. The manufacturer states that adults and children may receive one-half the total daily dose of erythromycin ethylsuccinate every 12 hours as an alternative dosage schedule, but some clinicians believe this schedule is inadequate for all but minor infections caused by highly susceptible organisms. The manufacturer also states that adults and children may receive one-third the total daily dose every 8 hours as an alternative dosage schedule.

Pharyngitis and Tonsillitis If erythromycin ethylsuccinate is used for the treatment of pharyngitis and tonsillitis caused by *Streptococcus pyogenes* (group A β-hemolytic streptococci), the usual dosage is 40 mg/kg daily given in 2–4 divided doses for 10 days.

Prophylaxis of Recurrent Rheumatic Fever For continuous prophylaxis to prevent recurrences in patients with a history of rheumatic heart disease, the manufacturer recommends oral erythromycin as the ethylsuccinate in a dosage of 400 mg twice daily.

When selecting anti-infectives for prophylaxis of recurrent rheumatic fever, the current recommendations published by the American Heart Association (AHA) should be consulted.

Prevention of Bacterial Endocarditis Because of adverse GI effects and the complicated pharmacokinetics of the various erythromycin formulations, current recommendations of the AHA for prevention of bacterial endocarditis no longer include erythromycins as alternatives to penicillins in penicillin-allergic patients. However, the AHA states that clinicians who have successfully used an erythromycin for prophylaxis in individual patients may choose to continue using these agents. If erythromycin ethylsuccinate is used for prophylaxis of bacterial endocarditis in penicillin-allergic patients at risk who are undergoing certain dental or upper respiratory tract procedures, the AHA recommends that adults receive 800 mg of erythromycin as the ethylsuccinate 2 hours before the procedure and 400 mg 6 hours later and that children receive 20 mg/kg 2 hours before the procedure and 10 mg/kg 6 hours later. Pediatric dosage should not exceed adult dosage.

When selecting anti-infectives for prophylaxis of bacterial endocarditis, the current recommendations published by the AHA should be consulted.

Syphilis Although penicillin G is the drug of choice for all stages of syphilis, the manufacturer states that erythromycin as the ethylsuccinate may be given orally in a dosage of 48–64 g over 10–15 days for the treatment of primary syphilis in adults. Erythromycin is no longer included in US Centers for Disease Control and Prevention (CDC) recommendations for the treatment of any form of syphilis in adults or adolescents (including primary, secondary, latent, or tertiary or neurosyphilis) and is *not* recommended for the treatment of congenital syphilis or syphilis in older infants and children. In addition, erythromycin is no longer recommended by the CDC or American Academy of Pediatrics (AAP) for the treatment of syphilis in pregnant women who are hypersensitive to penicillin since numerous treatment failures (including in the fetus) have been reported with the drug.

Gonorrhea and Associated Infections The AAP currently recommends that all children beyond the neonatal period being treated for uncomplicated vulvovaginal, urethral, or pharyngeal gonorrhea, epididymitis, proctitis, or disseminated gonococcal infections, including meningitis or endocarditis, receive presumptive treatment for possible coexisting chlamydial infections. If oral erythromycin is used for presumptive treatment of chlamydial infection in children who weigh less than 45 kg, the AAP recommends a dosage of 50 mg/kg daily (maximum 2 g daily) given in 4 divided doses for 7 days.

Nongonococcal Urethritis When oral erythromycin ethylsuccinate is used as an alternative to azithromycin or doxycycline for the treatment of nongonococcal urethritis, the CDC and manufacturer recommend a regimen of 800 mg of erythromycin 4 times daily for 7 days.

Patients with recurrent and persistent urethritis who were not compliant with the full course of erythromycin therapy or who were reexposed to untreated sexual partner(s) should receive a second course of oral erythromycin. If the patient has recurrent and persistent urethritis, was compliant with the regimen, and reexposure can be excluded, the CDC recommends that oral erythromycin ethylsuccinate be given in regimen of 800 mg of erythromycin 4 times daily for 7 days in conjunction with a single 2-g dose of oral metronidazole.

Chlamydial Infections For the treatment of uncomplicated urethral, endocervical, or rectal infections caused by *Chlamydia trachomatis* in nonpregnant adults or adolescents when azithromycin or tetracyclines cannot be used, the CDC and others recommend oral erythromycin as the ethylsuccinate in a dosage 800 mg 4 times daily for 7 days. The dosage of erythromycin as the ethylsuccinate recommended by the CDC for the treatment of these infections in children weighing 45 kg or less is 50 mg/kg daily given in 4 divided doses for 14 days.

For the treatment of chlamydial urogenital infections during pregnancy, the recommended dosage of oral erythromycin as the ethylsuccinate is 800 mg 4 times daily for 7 days; for women who cannot tolerate this regimen, a dosage of oral erythromycin as the ethylsuccinate of 400 mg 4 times daily for 14 days may be used.

For the treatment of pneumonia caused by *C. trachomatis* or ophthalmia neonatorum caused by *C. trachomatis* in infants, the recommended dosage of oral erythromycin is 50 mg/kg daily given in 4 divided doses for 14 days; follow-up is recommended and a second course of therapy may be necessary.

For the treatment of trachoma in children, oral erythromycin has been given for 40 days in conjunction with topical anti-infective therapy; however, optimum therapy has not been established, and treatment may be difficult.

Intestinal Amebiasis Although erythromycin is not considered a drug of choice for the treatment of intestinal amebiasis caused by *Entamoeba histolytica*, the manufacturer states that adults may receive 400 mg of erythromycin as the ethylsuccinate orally 4 times daily for 10–14 days, and children may be given 30–50 mg/kg daily in divided doses for 10–14 days.

Pertussis Although the optimum dosage and duration of erythromycin for the *treatment* of pertussis or *prevention* in susceptible contacts have not been established, a dosage of 1 g daily in adults and 40–50 mg/kg daily (maximum 2 g daily) in children given in divided doses for 14 days usually is recommended. While a shorter duration of erythromycin therapy (e.g., 7 or 10 days) may be effective in some patients, prophylaxis failures and bacteriologic relapse of pertussis have been reported with erythromycin regimens shorter than 14 days. Therefore, the CDC, US Public Health Service Advisory Committee on Immunization Practices (ACIP), AAP, and some clinicians recommend that a 14-day course of erythromycin therapy be used for treatment or prevention of pertussis.

Although data from controlled studies are lacking, the CDC recommends that all household and other close contacts of individuals with pertussis receive a 14-day regimen of prophylaxis (regardless of age and vaccination status) since this may prevent or minimize transmission of the disease. In addition, all close contacts younger than 7 years of age who are not fully immunized against pertussis should receive the remaining required doses of a preparation containing pertussis vaccine (using minimal intervals between doses) and those who are fully immunized but have not received a vaccine dose within the last 3 years should receive a booster dose of a pertussis vaccine preparation.

Legionnaires' Disease Although the optimum dosage and duration of erythromycin for the treatment of Legionnaires' disease have not been established, dosages of erythromycin as the ethylsuccinate of 1.6–4 g daily in divided doses have been given alone or in combination with rifampin. A parenteral regimen usually is necessary for the initial treatment of severe Legionnaires' disease and the addition of rifampin is recommended during the first 3–5 days of therapy in severely ill and/or immunocompromised patients; after a response is obtained, rifampin can be discontinued and therapy changed to oral erythromycin. The duration of therapy in patients with Legionnaires's disease usually is 10–21 days; some clinicians recommend 14 days of therapy for patients with mild disease and 21 days for those who are immunocompromised or have severe disease.

Acute Otitis Media For the treatment of acute otitis media caused by susceptible strains of *Haemophilus influenzae* in children 2 months of age or older, a commercially available fixed-combination preparation containing erythromycin ethylsuccinate and sulfisoxazole acetyl is used. Dosage of the combination preparation may be expressed in terms of erythromycin or sulfisoxazole. The usual oral dosage for children 2 months of age or older expressed in terms of erythromycin is 12.5 mg/kg every 6 hours or 17 mg/kg every 8 hours and the usual dosage expressed in terms of sulfisoxazole is 37.5 mg/kg every 6 hours or 50 mg/kg every 8 hours (not to exceed a total daily dose of 6 g). Alternatively, the following approximate dosages, expressed in terms of volumes of erythromycin ethylsuccinate and sulfisoxazole acetyl suspension (200 mg of erythromycin per 5 mL), can be used:

6-Hour Dosing

Weight	Dose (repeated every 6 h for 10 days)
<8 kg	Calculate dose by body weight
8–15.9 kg	2.5 mL
16–23.9 kg	5 mL
24–31.9 kg	7.5 mL
>32 kg	10 mL

8-Hour Dosing

Weight	Dose (repeated every 8 h for 10 days)
<6 kg	Calculate dose by body weight
6–11.9 kg	2.5 mL
12–17.9 kg	5 mL
18–23.9 kg	7.5 mL
24–30 kg	10 mL
>30 kg	12.5 mL

When the fixed-combination preparation is used, the precautions and contraindications of sulfonamides must also be considered. Erythromycin ethylsuccinate and sulfisoxazole acetyl suspension should not be administered to children younger than 2 months of age.

Chemistry and Stability

■ **Chemistry** Erythromycin ethylsuccinate occurs as a white or slightly yellow, odorless or practically odorless, practically tasteless, crystalline powder. The drug is very slightly soluble in water, freely soluble in alcohol, and soluble in polyethylene glycol.

■ **Stability** Erythromycin ethylsuccinate chewable tablets and film-coated tablets should be stored at less than 30°C. The manufacturer of E.E.S.® Liquid recommends that these oral suspensions be stored at 2–8°C until dispensed to preserve taste; once dispensed, these suspensions are stable for 14 days at room temperature. Prior to reconstitution, E.E.S® granules for oral suspension should be stored at less than 30°C; after reconstitution, the oral suspension should be refrigerated and used within 10 days. The manufacturer of EryPed® for oral suspension states that this preparation should be stored at less than 30°C prior to reconstitution; after reconstitution, this oral suspension should be stored at less than 25°C and is stable for 35 days at room temperature. Commercially available suspensions of erythromycin ethylsuccinate have expiration dates of 18 months following the dates of manufacture; commercially available erythromycin ethylsuccinate tablets and powder for oral suspension have expiration dates of 2 years following the dates of manufacture.

The commercially available fixed-combination preparation containing erythromycin ethylsuccinate and sulfisoxazole acetyl should be stored at less than 30°C prior to reconstitution; after reconstitution, the oral suspension should be refrigerated and unused portions discarded after 14 days.

For further information on chemistry, mechanism of action, spectrum, resistance, pharmacokinetics, uses, cautions, drug interactions, laboratory test interferences, and dosage and administration of erythromycin ethylsuccinate, see the Erythromycins General Statement 8:12.12.04.

Preparations

Excipients in commercially available drug preparations may have clinically important effects in some individuals; consult specific product labeling for details.

Erythromycin Ethylsuccinate

Oral		
For suspension	100 mg (of erythromycin) per 2.5 mL	**EryPed® Drops,** Abbott
	200 mg (of erythromycin) per 5 mL	**E.E.S.® Granules,** Abbott
		EryPed®, Abbott
	400 mg (of erythromycin) per 5 mL	**EryPed®,** Abbott
Suspension	200 mg (of erythromycin) per 5 mL*	**E.E.S.® Liquid,** Abbott
		Erythromycin Ethylsuccinate Suspension
	400 mg (of erythromycin) per 5 mL*	**E.E.S.® Liquid,** Abbott
		Erythromycin Ethylsuccinate Suspension
Tablets, chewable	200 mg (of erythromycin)	**EryPed®** (scored), Abbott
Tablets, film-coated	400 mg (of erythromycin)*	**E.E.S.® Filmtab®,** Abbott
		Erythromycin Ethylsuccinate Film-coated Tablets

*available from one or more manufacturer, distributor, and/or repackager by generic (nonproprietary) name

Erythromycin Ethylsuccinate Combinations

Oral		
For suspension	200 mg (of erythromycin) per 5 mL with Sulfisoxazole Acetyl 600 mg (of sulfisoxazole) per 5 mL*	**Erythromycin Ethylsuccinate and Sulfisoxazole Acetyl Suspension**
		Eryzole®, Alra
		Pediazole®, Ross

*available from one or more manufacturer, distributor, and/or repackager by generic (nonproprietary) name

Erythromycin Lactobionate

■ Erythromycin lactobionate is a macrolide antibiotic.

Dosage and Administration

■ **Reconstitution and Administration** Erythromycin lactobionate is administered by continuous or intermittent IV infusion. *Because of the local irritative effects of erythromycin, the drug must not be administered rapidly by direct IV injection (IV push).* The manufacturers state that continuous IV infusion with the drug is preferred to intermittent IV infusion because a slower infusion rate and lower erythromycin concentration is used; however, the drug may be administered by intermittent IV infusion at intervals not greater than every 6 hours. *Oral erythromycin therapy should replace IV erythromycin lactobionate therapy as soon as possible.*

Erythromycin lactobionate vials labeled as containing 500 mg or 1 g of erythromycin are initially reconstituted by adding 10 or 20 mL, respectively, of sterile water for injection *without* preservatives to provide a solution containing 50 mg/mL. No other diluent should be used to prepare this initial solution. (See Chemistry and Stability: Stability.) Prior to administration, the concentrated solution should be further diluted in glass or flexible plastic (Lifecare®) containers of 0.9% sodium chloride injection, lactated Ringer's, or Normosol®-R. Alternatively, IV solutions of 5% dextrose injection, 5% dextrose and lactated Ringer's, or 5% dextrose and 0.9% sodium chloride in glass or flexible plastic containers or Normosol®-M or -R with 5% dextrose in glass containers may also be used if they are first buffered to a pH of 5.5 or higher using 4% sodium bicarbonate (Neut®). (The manufacturers recommend addition of 1 mL of this buffer to every 100 mL of infusion solution.) For continuous IV infusion, the concentrated solution should be diluted to a concentration of 1 mg/mL. For intermittent IV infusion, the appropriate dose (one-fourth of the total daily dose) of the concentrated solution should be diluted to a concentration of 1–5 mg/mL and administered over 20–60 minutes. Not less than 100 mL of diluent should be used for preparing intermittent IV infusion solutions.

ADD-Vantage® vials labeled as containing 500 mg or 1 g of erythromycin should be reconstituted according to the manufacturer's directions. Piggyback vials containing 500 mg of erythromycin are reconstituted by adding 100 mL of 0.9% sodium chloride injection, lactated Ringer's, or Normosol®-R injection to provide a solution containing 5 mg/mL. Alternatively, 100 mL of 5% dextrose injection, 5% dextrose and lactated Ringer's, 5% dextrose and 0.9% sodium chloride, or Normosol®-M or -R with 5% dextrose injection may be used if they are first buffered to a pH of 5.5 or higher using 1 mL of 4% sodium bicarbonate (Neut®). Immediately after the diluent is added, the vial should be shaken well to enhance dissolution; lack of immediate agitation greatly increases the time required for complete dissolution. Solutions reconstituted in piggyback vials or ADD-Vantage® containers are administered by intermittent IV infusion; one-fourth of the total daily dose is administered over 20–60 minutes.

■ **Dosage** Dosage of erythromycin lactobionate is expressed in terms of erythromycin.

The usual dosage of erythromycin as the lactobionate for severe infections in adults and children is 15–20 mg/kg daily, given as a continuous IV infusion or by intermittent IV infusion in divided doses every 6 hours. Alternatively, a pediatric dosage of 300–600 mg/m^2 daily has been recommended. Dosages as high as 4 g daily have been used in very severe infections.

Pelvic Inflammatory Disease Although erythromycin is not included in the current US Centers for Disease Control and Prevention (CDC) recommendations for the treatment of acute pelvic inflammatory disease (PID) caused by *N. gonorrhoeae*, the manufacturers recommend a regimen of 500 mg of IV erythromycin every 6 hours for at least 3 days followed by 250 mg of erythromycin orally every 6 hours for 7 days for the treatment of these infections. However, some clinicians believe this oral dosage is inadequate and recommend 500 mg every 6 hours for 7–10 days.

Legionnaires' Disease Although the optimum dosage and duration of erythromycin for the treatment of Legionnaires' disease have not been established, dosages of 1–4 g daily in divided doses have been given alone or in conjunction with rifampin. A parenteral regimen usually is necessary for the initial treatment of severe Legionnaires' disease and the addition of rifampin is recommended during the first 3–5 days of therapy in severely ill and/or immunocompromised patients; after a response is obtained, rifampin can be discontinued and therapy changed to oral erythromycin. The duration of therapy in patients with Legionnaires' disease usually is 10–21 days.

Anthrax If erythromycin as the lactobionate is used as an alternative agent for the treatment of anthrax† caused by *Bacillus anthracis* susceptible to the drug, some clinicians recommend that adults receive an IV dosage of 15–20 mg/kg (up to 4 g) daily and that children receive 20–40 mg/kg daily given in divided doses every 6 hours. Although erythromycin has been suggested as an alternative to penicillin G for the treatment of naturally occurring or endemic anthrax in patients hypersensitive to penicillin G, limited or no clinical data are available to date regarding in vivo activity of erythromycin against *B. anthracis* and efficacy has not been evaluated in human or animal studies. Erythromycin is not considered a drug of choice for the treatment of anthrax that occurs as the result of exposure to anthrax spores in the context of biologic warfare or bioterrorism. For information on treatment of anthrax and recommendations for prophylaxis following exposure to anthrax spores, see Uses: Anthrax, in Ciprofloxacin 8:12.18.

Prevention of Perinatal Group B Streptococcal Disease If erythromycin is used for intrapartum anti-infective prophylaxis for prevention of perinatal group B streptococcal (GBS) disease† in women with penicillin hypersensitivity who should not receive a β-lactam anti-infective, the CDC recommends that 500 mg of erythromycin be given IV every 6 hours until delivery. When indicated, such prophylaxis is initiated at the time of labor or rupture of membranes. *Streptococcus agalactiae* (group B streptococci) with resistance to erythromycin has been reported with increasing frequency. Therefore, clinical isolates obtained during GBS prenatal screening should be tested for in vitro susceptibility to erythromycin whenever use of the drug is being considered for prevention of perinatal GBS disease in women hypersensitive to penicillin. (See Uses: Prevention of Perinatal Group B Streptococcal Disease, in the Erythromycin General Statement 8:12.12.04.)

Cautions

■ **Pediatric Precautions** Some commercially available formulations of erythromycin lactobionate powder for injection contain benzyl alcohol as a preservative. Although a causal relationship has not been established, administration of injections preserved with benzyl alcohol has been associated with toxicity in neonates. Toxicity appears to have resulted from administration of large amounts (i.e., about 100–400 mg/kg daily) of benzyl alcohol in these neonates. Although use of drugs preserved with benzyl alcohol should be avoided in neonates whenever possible, the American Academy of Pediatrics states that the presence of small amounts of the preservative in a commercially available injection should not proscribe its use when indicated in neonates.

In several neonates with infections caused by *Ureaplasma urealyticum* who received IV administration of erythromycin lactobionate, adverse cardiac effects (e.g., bradycardia, hypotension, cardiac arrest, arrhythmias) requiring cardiopulmonary resuscitation have been reported. Some clinicians state that these adverse effects may depend on serum concentration and/or infusion rate of the drug. (See Cautions: Cardiac Effects, in the Erythromycins General Statement 8:12.12.04.) It has been suggested that prolonged IV infusion of erythromycin lactobionate (e.g., over 60 minutes) may reduce such adverse cardiac effects. However, it has been suggested that certain individuals may be at increased risk of developing erythromycin-induced adverse cardiac effects and that decreasing the rate of IV infusion may decrease but not eliminate the risk of such effects. Further study is needed to determine the pharmacokinetics and safety of erythromycin lactobionate in neonates.

Chemistry and Stability

■ **Chemistry** Erythromycin lactobionate occurs as white or slightly yellow crystals or powder having a faint odor and is freely soluble in water and in alcohol.

■ **Stability** Erythromycin lactobionate powder for injection should be stored at a temperature less than 40°C, preferably between 15–30°C. Erythromycin lactobionate powder for injection has an expiration date of 4 years following the date of manufacture.

Erythromycin lactobionate sterile powder or powder for injection in 500-mg or 1-g vials must be initially reconstituted with sterile water for injection *without* preservatives, as the use of sodium chloride injection or other diluents containing inorganic salts will result in precipitation. The concentrated solution may then be diluted with a compatible IV solution. (See Dosage and Administration: Reconstitution and Administration.) No additional drugs or chemicals should be added to solutions of erythromycin lactobionate unless their effects on the chemical and physical stability of the solution have been determined; specialized references should be consulted for specific compatibility information. The stability of erythromycin lactobionate solutions depends on pH and is optimal at pH 6–8; acidic (pH less than 5.5) solutions of erythromycin lactobionate are unstable and rapidly lose their potency.

Following reconstitution of conventional vials of the drug with sterile water for injection to a concentration of 50 mg/mL, solutions of erythromycin lactobionate have a pH of 7 and are stable for 2 weeks when refrigerated at 2–8°C or for 24 hours at room temperature. Following further dilution of this concentrated solution to 1–5 mg/mL in 0.9% sodium chloride injection, lactated Ringer's, Normosol®-R, 5% dextrose injection, 5% dextrose and 0.9% sodium chloride, 5% dextrose and lactated Ringer's, or Normosol®-M or -R with 5% dextrose, stability of the resultant solutions is variable and depends on several factors, including the IV infusion solution, type of container, resultant pH, and temperature. Because these diluted solutions are not suitable for prolonged storage and because of the variability of specific stability information, the manufacturers state, as a general guide, that the solutions should be completely administered within 8 hours after dilution. Alternatively, the manufacturers can provide more specific stability information. For example, diluted solutions are stable at 22–28°C for 24 hours in glass or flexible plastic (Lifecare®) containers of lactated Ringer's or buffered (see Dosage and Administration: Reconstitution and Administration) 5% dextrose injection.

Piggyback vials of erythromycin lactobionate that have been reconstituted to a concentration of 5 mg of erythromycin per mL with 0.9% sodium chloride injection, lactated Ringer's, or Normosol®-R or with buffered solutions of 5% dextrose injection, 5% dextrose and lactated Ringer's, 5% dextrose and 0.9% sodium chloride, or Normosol®-M or -R with 5% dextrose should be used within 8 hours if stored at room temperature or 24 hours if refrigerated at 2–8°C. Reconstituted erythromycin lactobionate solutions in piggyback vials may be frozen at −20° to −10°C within 4 hours of preparation and stored for 30 days. Frozen solutions of the drug should be thawed in the refrigerator and used within 8 hours after thawing is complete; thawed solutions must not be refrozen.

When reconstituted as directed in 0.9% sodium chloride injection or 5% dextrose injection, solutions prepared from ADD-Vantage® vials of erythromycin lactobionate should be completely administered within 8 or 2 hours, respectively. ADD-Vantage® vials of the drug that have been connected to an ADD-Vantage® diluent container but *not* activated for dissolution can be stored at room temperature for up to 30 days.

For further information on chemistry and stability, mechanism of action, spectrum, resistance, pharmacokinetics, uses, cautions, drug interactions, laboratory test interferences, and dosage and administration of erythromycin lactobionate, see the Erythromycins General Statement 8:12.12.04.

Preparations

Excipients in commercially available drug preparations may have clinically important effects in some individuals; consult specific product labeling for details.

Erythromycin Lactobionate

Parenteral		
For injection, for IV infusion only	500 mg (of erythromycin)	**Erythrocin® Lactobionate-I.V.,** Abbott
		Erythrocin® Lactobionate-I.V. ADD-Vantage®, Abbott
		Erythrocin® Piggyback, Abbott
	1 g (of erythromycin)	**Erythrocin® Lactobionate-I.V.,** Abbott
		Erythrocin® Lactobionate-I.V. ADD-Vantage®, Abbott

†Use is not currently included in the labeling approved by the US Food and Drug Administration

Erythromycin Stearate

■ Erythromycin stearate is a macrolide antibiotic.

Dosage and Administration

■ **Administration** Erythromycin stearate is administered orally. Optimal absorption occurs when the drug is administered in the fasting state or immediately before a meal.

■ **Dosage** Dosage of erythromycin stearate is expressed in terms of erythromycin.

The usual adult dosage of erythromycin as the stearate is 250 mg every 6 hours or 500 mg every 12 hours. In severe infections, dosage in adults may be increased to 4 g or more daily. A twice-daily dosing schedule is not recommended when dosages greater than 1 g daily are administered; some clinicians believe the twice-daily schedule is inadequate for all but minor infections caused by highly susceptible organisms.

The usual erythromycin dosage in children is 30–50 mg/kg daily given in 2–4 equally divided doses. For more severe infections, this dosage may be doubled but should not exceed 4 g daily. An alternative pediatric dosage of 0.9–3 g/m^2 daily given in 4 equally divided doses has been recommended. A twice-daily dosing schedule is not recommended when dosages greater than 1 g daily are administered; some clinicians believe the twice-daily schedule is inadequate for all but minor infections caused by highly susceptible organisms.

Pharyngitis and Tonsillitis If erythromycin stearate is used for the treatment of pharyngitis and tonsillitis caused by *Streptococcus pyogenes* (group A β-hemolytic streptococci), the drug should be given in the usual dosage for 10 days or longer.

Prophylaxis of Recurrent Rheumatic Fever For continuous prophylaxis to prevent recurrences in patients with a history of rheumatic heart disease, the usual oral dosage of erythromycin is 250 mg twice daily.

When selecting anti-infectives for prophylaxis of recurrent rheumatic fever, the current recommendations published by the American Heart Association (AHA) should be consulted.

Prevention of Bacterial Endocarditis Because of adverse GI effects and the complicated pharmacokinetics of the various erythromycin formulations, current recommendations of the AHA for prevention of bacterial endocarditis no longer include erythromycins as alternatives to penicillins in penicillin-allergic patients. However, the AHA states that practitioners who have successfully used an erythromycin for prophylaxis in individual patients may choose to continue using these agents. If erythromycin stearate is used for prophylaxis of bacterial endocarditis in penicillin-allergic patients at risk who are undergoing certain dental or upper respiratory procedures, the AHA recommends that adults receive 1 g of erythromycin as the stearate 2 hours before the procedure and 500 mg 6 hours later and that children receive 20 mg/kg 2 hours before the procedure and 10 mg/kg 6 hours later. Pediatric dosage should not exceed adult dosage.

When selecting anti-infectives for prophylaxis of bacterial endocarditis, the current recommendations published by the AHA should be consulted.

Syphilis Although penicillin G is the drug of choice for all stages of syphilis, the manufacturer states that 30–40 g of oral erythromycin has been given in divided doses over 10–15 days for the treatment of primary syphilis. Erythromycin is no longer included in US Centers for Disease Control and Prevention (CDC) recommendations for the treatment of any form of syphilis in adults or adolescents (including primary, secondary, latent, or tertiary syphilis or neurosyphilis) and is *not* recommended for the treatment of congenital syphilis or syphilis in older infants and children. In addition, erythromycin is no longer recommended by the CDC or American Academy of Pediatrics (AAP) for the treatment of syphilis in pregnant women who are hypersensitive to penicillin since numerous treatment failures (including in the fetus) have been reported with the drug.

Gonorrhea and Associated Infections The AAP currently recommends that all children beyond the neonatal period being treated for uncomplicated vulvovaginal, urethral, or pharyngeal gonorrhea, epididymitis, proctitis, or disseminated gonococcal infections receive presumptive treatment for possible coexisting chlamydial infections. If oral erythromycin is used for presumptive treatment of chlamydial infection in children who weigh less than 45 kg, the AAP recommends a dosage of 50 mg/kg daily (maximum 2 g daily) given in 4 divided doses for 7 days.

Although erythromycin is not included in the current CDC recommendations for the treatment of acute pelvic inflammatory disease (PID) caused by *N. gonorrhoeae*, the manufacturer recommends a regimen of 500 mg of erythromycin (as the lactobionate) IV every 6 hours for 3 days followed by 500 mg of oral erythromycin every 12 hours or 333 mg every 8 hours for 7 days for the treatment of these infections. However, some clinicians believe this oral dosage is inadequate and recommend 500 mg every 6 hours for 7–10 days.

Nongonococcal Urethritis When erythromycin is used as an alternative to azithromycin or doxycycline for the treatment of nongonococcal urethritis† in adults and adolescents, the CDC recommends an oral erythromycin dosage of 500 mg 4 times daily for 7 days.

Patients with recurrent and persistent urethritis who were not compliant with the full course of erythromycin therapy or who were reexposed to untreated sexual partner(s) should receive a second course of oral erythromycin. If the patient has recurrent and persistent urethritis, was compliant with the regimen, and reexposure can be excluded, the CDC recommends a regimen of 500 mg of oral erythromycin 4 times daily for 7 days given in conjunction with a single 2-g dose of oral metronidazole.

Chlamydial Infections For the treatment of uncomplicated urethral, endocervical, or rectal infections caused by *Chlamydia trachomatis* in nonpregnant adults and adolescents, the CDC recommends oral erythromycin in a dosage of 500 mg 4 times daily for 7 days. The dosage of oral erythromycin recommended by CDC for the treatment of these infections in children weighing 45 kg or less is 50 mg/kg daily given in 4 divided doses for 14 days.

For the treatment of chlamydial urogenital infections during pregnancy, the recommended dosage of oral erythromycin is 500 mg 4 times daily for 7 days; for women who cannot tolerate this regimen, a dosage of 250 mg 4 times daily for 14 days may be used.

Intestinal Amebiasis Although erythromycin is not considered a drug of choice for the treatment of intestinal amebiasis caused by *Entamoeba histolytica*, the manufacturers state that adults may receive 250 mg of erythromycin as the stearate 4 times daily for 10–14 days, and children may receive 30–50 mg/kg daily in divided doses for 10–14 days.

Pertussis Although the optimum dosage and duration of erythromycin for the *treatment* of pertussis or *prevention* in susceptible contacts have not been established, a dosage of 1 g daily in adults and 40–50 mg/kg daily (maximum 2 g daily) in children given in divided doses for 14 days usually is recommended. While a shorter duration of erythromycin therapy (e.g., 7 or 10 days) may be effective in some patients, prophylaxis failures and bacteriologic relapse of pertussis have been reported with erythromycin regimens shorter than 14 days. Therefore, the CDC, US Public Health Service Advisory Committee on Immunization Practices (ACIP), AAP, and some clinicians recommend that a 14-day course of erythromycin therapy be used for treatment or prevention of pertussis.

Although data from controlled studies are lacking, the CDC recommends that all household and other close contacts of individuals with pertussis receive a 14-day regimen of prophylaxis (regardless of age and vaccination status) since this may prevent or minimize transmission of the disease. In addition, all close contacts younger than 7 years of age who are not fully immunized against pertussis should receive the remaining required doses of a preparation containing pertussis vaccine (using minimal intervals between doses) and those who are fully immunized but have not received a vaccine dose within the last 3 years should receive a booster dose of a pertussis vaccine preparation.

Legionnaires' Disease Although the optimum dosage and duration of erythromycin for the treatment of Legionnaires' disease have not been established, dosages of 1–4 g daily in divided doses have been given alone or in conjunction with rifampin. A parenteral regimen usually is necessary for the initial treatment of severe Legionnaires' disease and the addition of rifampin is recommended during the first 3–5 days of therapy in severely ill and/or immunocompromised patients; after a response is obtained, rifampin can be discontinued and therapy changed to oral erythromycin. The duration of therapy in patients with Legionnaires' disease usually is 10–21 days; some clinicians recommend 14 days of therapy for patients with mild disease and 21 days for those who are immunocompromised or have severe disease.

Chemistry and Stability

■ **Chemistry** Erythromycin stearate occurs as white or slightly yellow crystals or powder and has a slight bitter taste. The drug is odorless or may have a slight, earthy odor. Erythromycin stearate is practically insoluble in water and soluble in alcohol.

■ **Stability** Commercially available erythromycin stearate film-coated tablets should be stored in tight, light-resistant containers at 30°C or lower. The tablets have expiration dates of 1.5–5 years following the date of manufacture, depending on the manufacturer and packaging.

For further information on chemistry and stability, mechanism of action, spectrum, resistance, pharmacokinetics, uses, cautions, drug interactions, laboratory test interferences, and dosage and administration of erythromycin stearate, see the Erythromycins General Statement 8:12.12.04.

Preparations

Excipients in commercially available drug preparations may have clinically important effects in some individuals; consult specific product labeling for details.

Erythromycin Stearate

Oral		
Tablets, film-coated	250 mg (of erythromycin)*	**Erythrocin® Stearate Filmtab®**, Abbott
		Erythromycin Stearate Tablets
	500 mg (of erythromycin)*	**Erythrocin® Stearate Filmtab®**, Abbott
		Erythromycin Stearate Tablets

*available from one or more manufacturer, distributor, and/or repackager by generic (nonproprietary) name

†Use is not currently included in the labeling approved by the US Food and Drug Administration

OTHER MACROLIDES 8:12.12.92

Azithromycin

■ Azithromycin is an azalide antibiotic, a subclass of macrolide antibiotics.

Uses

Azithromycin is used orally in adults for the treatment of mild to moderate upper and lower respiratory tract infections and uncomplicated skin and skin structure infections caused by susceptible organisms. Oral azithromycin also is used for the treatment of urethritis or cervicitis caused by *Chlamydia trachomatis* or *Neisseria gonorrhoeae*, and for the treatment of chancroid caused by *Haemophilus ducreyi.* Azithromycin is used orally for the treatment of disseminated infections caused by *Mycobacterium avium* complex (MAC) in patients with human immunodeficiency virus (HIV) infection and for prevention of disseminated MAC infection (both primary and secondary prophylaxis) in HIV-infected individuals.

Azithromycin is used orally in children for the treatment of acute otitis media, community-acquired pneumonia, and pharyngitis or tonsillitis caused by susceptible organisms.

IV azithromycin is used for the treatment of community-acquired pneumonia and acute pelvic inflammatory disease (PID) caused by susceptible organisms when initial IV therapy is considered necessary.

Potential advantages of azithromycin compared with erythromycin include improved oral bioavailability and tissue penetration, increased activity against infections caused by gram-negative organisms (e.g., *Haemophilus influenzae*), fewer adverse GI effects, and less frequent and less prolonged dosing (promoting better compliance with therapy). Controlled and uncontrolled clinical studies in patients with community-acquired upper or lower respiratory tract infections suggest that 3–5 days of oral therapy with azithromycin generally is as effective as 7–10 days of oral therapy with other macrolides (erythromycin, clarithromycin), a natural penicillin, amoxicillin (with or without clavulanic acid), or a cephalosporin (e.g., cefaclor). In addition, single-dose therapy with azithromycin for urethritis or cervicitis caused by *Chlamydia trachomatis* may be more cost-effective than longer courses of therapy with another anti-infective (e.g., doxycycline) in populations where noncompliance may be a problem. (See Uses: Chlamydial Infections.) The relative lack of clinically important drug interactions with azithromycin also may be advantageous when oral macrolide therapy is considered for patients in whom multiple-drug therapy is prescribed (e.g., HIV-infected patients, patients receiving theophylline or carbamazepine).

Considering the relative costs of drug therapy, erythromycin generally would be preferred for most infections in which oral macrolide therapy was indicated unless azithromycin would be expected to be more effective than erythromycin, the patient is intolerant of erythromycin (e.g., secondary to GI toxicity), or compliance with 3- or 4-times daily erythromycin dosing is considered a problem.

Prior to initiation of azithromycin therapy, appropriate specimens should be obtained for identification of the causative organism(s) and in vitro susceptibility tests. Azithromycin may be started pending results of susceptibility tests, but should be discontinued and other appropriate anti-infective therapy substituted if the organism is found to be resistant to the drug. (See Spectrum: In Vitro Susceptibility Testing.)

■ **Acute Otitis Media** Azithromycin is used orally in children for the treatment of acute otitis media (AOM) caused by *H. influenzae*, *M. catarrhalis*, or *S. pneumoniae*. Safety and efficacy of azithromycin for the treatment of AOM in children has been established when the drug is given in a single-dose regimen (a single 30-mg/kg dose), a 3-day regimen (10 mg/kg once daily for 3 days), or a 5-day regimen (10 mg/kg on day 1, then 5 mg/kg on days 2–5).

Various anti-infectives, including oral amoxicillin, oral amoxicillin and clavulanate potassium, various oral cephalosporins (cefaclor, cefdinir, cefixime, cefpodoxime proxetil, cefprozil, ceftibuten, cefuroxime axetil, cephalexin), IM ceftriaxone, oral co-trimoxazole, oral erythromycin-sulfisoxazole, oral azithromycin, and oral clarithromycin, have been used in the treatment of AOM. The American Academy of Pediatrics (AAP), Centers for Disease Control and Prevention (CDC), and other clinicians state that, despite the increasing prevalence of multidrug-resistant *S. pneumoniae* and presence of β-lactamase-producing *H. influenzae* or *M. catarrhalis* in many communities, amoxicillin remains the anti-infective of first choice when treatment of uncomplicated AOM is indicated since amoxicillin is highly effective, has a narrow spectrum of activity, is well distributed into middle ear fluid, and is well tolerated and inexpensive.

Azithromycin is not considered a first-line agent for treatment of AOM, but is recommended as an alternative, especially for individuals with type I penicillin hypersensitivity. Because *S. pneumoniae* resistant to amoxicillin also frequently are resistant to co-trimoxazole, clarithromycin, and azithromycin, these drugs may not be effective in patients with AOM who fail to respond to amoxicillin. For additional information regarding treatment of AOM and information regarding prophylaxis of recurrent AOM, treatment of persistent or recurrent AOM, and treatment of otitis media with effusion (OME), see Uses: Otitis Media in the Aminopenicillins General Statement 8:12.16.08.

In a multicenter, randomized, comparative trial in children 1–15 years of age, oral azithromycin therapy (10 mg/kg as a single dose on day 1, followed by 5 mg/kg once daily for 4 days) produced a favorable clinical response (i.e., cure or improvement) in 88 or 73% of patients 11 or 30 days after initiation of therapy, respectively, while therapy with amoxicillin and clavulanate potassium produced a favorable clinical response in 88 or 71% of patients, respectively, at these time points. In another study in children 2–15 years of age with acute otitis media in areas of the US with a high incidence of β-lactamase-producing bacteria, azithromycin therapy produced a favorable clinical response (i.e., cure or improvement) in 84 or 70% of patients 11 or 30 days, respectively, after initiation of therapy. At day 11 or 30, a presumptive bacteriologic/clinical cure was evident in 82 or 71%, respectively, of children with *S. pneumoniae* infections, 80 or 64% of those with *H. influenzae* infections, 80 or 73% of those with *M. catarrhalis* infections, and 100% of those with *S. pyogenes* infections; 14.3% were considered treatment failures. In one open-label comparative study, the overall clinical success rate (i.e., presumed bacteriologic eradication/clinical cure outcomes) 11 or 30 days after initiation of therapy was 88 or 82%, respectively, in azithromycin-treated patients and 82 or 81%, respectively, in patients receiving amoxicillin and clavulanate potassium. In all studies, the adverse effects associated with any of the therapies were principally GI related (e.g., diarrhea), with a substantially lower incidence of adverse effects in the azithromycin-treated group compared with the group receiving amoxicillin and clavulanate potassium.

■ **Pharyngitis and Tonsillitis** Azithromycin is used orally for the treatment of pharyngitis and tonsillitis caused by *Streptococcus pyogenes* (group A β-hemolytic streptococci) in adults and children when first-line therapy (penicillins) cannot be used. Although azithromycin generally is effective in eradicating *S. pyogenes* from the nasopharynx, efficacy of the drug in the subsequent prevention of rheumatic fever has not been established. Strains of *S. pyogenes* resistant to macrolides are common in some areas of the world (e.g., Italy, Japan, Korea, Finland, Spain, Taiwan) and azithromycin-resistant strains have been reported in the US. (See Resistance: Resistance in Gram-positive Bacteria.) Therefore, the manufacturer recommends that in vitro susceptibility tests be performed prior to use of azithromycin in patients with streptococcal pharyngitis.

Because penicillin has a narrow spectrum of activity, is inexpensive, and generally is effective, the CDC, AAP, American Academy of Family Physicians (AAFP), Infectious Diseases Society of America (IDSA), American Heart Association (AHA), American College of Physicians (ACP), and others consider natural penicillins (i.e., 10 days of oral penicillin V or a single IM dose of penicillin G benzathine) the treatment of choice for streptococcal pharyngitis and tonsillitis and prevention of initial attacks (primary prevention) of rheumatic fever, although oral amoxicillin often is used instead of penicillin V in small children because of a more acceptable taste. Other anti-infectives (e.g., oral cephalosporins, oral macrolides) generally are considered alternative agents. A 10-day regimen of oral erythromycin usually is considered the preferred alternative for the treatment of streptococcal pharyngitis in patients hypersensitive to penicillin. It has been suggested that azithromycin offers an advantage over erythromycin in terms of ease of administration (i.e., fewer daily doses and a 5-day regimen) and better GI tolerance. However, because of limited data to date, the IDSA states that use of anti-infective regimens administered for 5 days or less for the treatment of *S. pyogenes* pharyngitis cannot be recommended at this time. Because of lower relative rates of bacteriologic eradication reported in some studies, azithromycin should not be administered in a 3-day regimen for the treatment of streptococcal pharyngitis.

In a controlled comparative study in patients 16 years of age or older with streptococcal pharyngitis, microbiologic and clinical response rates of approximately 91% or greater were achieved with either a 5-day, 5-dose course of azithromycin or a 10-day, 40-dose course of penicillin V. In several double-blind, controlled trials in children 2 years of age or older with streptococcal pharyngitis, clinical and microbiologic response with azithromycin (12 mg/kg once daily for 5 days) was superior to that with penicillin V (250 mg 3 times daily for 10 days). In these trials, bacteriologic eradication at day 14 or 30 occurred in a combined 95 or 77%, respectively, of azithromycin-treated children and 73 or 63%, respectively, of penicillin-treated children; clinical success (i.e., cure or improvement) at day 14 or 30 was achieved in a combined 98 or 94%, respectively, of children given azithromycin and 84 or 74%, respectively, of children given penicillin V. Approximately 1% of azithromycin-susceptible *S. pyogenes* isolates were resistant to the drug following therapy. In another study in children 1.5–14 years of age with streptococcal pharyngitis, oral therapy with azithromycin (10 mg/kg once daily for 3 days) or penicillin V (56 mg/kg daily in 3 divided doses for 10 days) produced clinical success (cure or improvement) in 93 or 89% of patients, respectively. However, bacteriologic eradication was reported in substantially fewer azithromycin-treated patients (65%) than penicillin-treated patients (82%).

■ **GI Infections** ***Campylobacter* Infections** Azithromycin has been used as a first-line agent for the treatment of symptomatic enteric infections caused by *Campylobacter jejuni*†. The CDC, National Institutes of Health (NIH), IDSA, AAP, and other clinicians recommend oral erythromycin or azithromycin or fluoroquinolones (e.g., ciprofloxacin) for empiric treatment of these infections; tetracyclines (doxycycline) also can be used. However, increasing emergence of fluoroquinolone-resistant strains of *Campylobacter* should be considered when selecting a first-line agent.

When initiated early in the course of the *Campylobacter* infection, erythromycin or azithromycin shortens the duration of illness and prevents relapse. Either macrolide usually eradicates the organism from the stool within 2–3 days; however, a longer duration of treatment (5–7 days) is recommended for treatment of gastroenteritis.

Cryptosporidiosis Azithromycin has been used in the treatment of cryptosporidiosis† in HIV-infected adults, adolescents, or children. Oral azithromycin in conjunction with paromomycin was used with some success (i.e., reduction in oocyst excretion, improvement in diarrhea) in a limited number of patients with AIDS-related cryptosporidiosis†. In addition, azithromycin monotherapy may have contributed to resolution of symptoms in a few HIV-infected children with cryptosporidiosis. However, no anti-infective has been found to reliably eradicate *Cryptosporidium*, although several drugs (e.g., paromomycin, azithromycin, nitazoxanide) may improve symptoms or suppress the infection.

HIV-infected individuals at greatest risk for cryptosporidiosis are those with advanced immunosuppression (i.e., CD4$^+$ T-cell counts less than 100/mm^3) and fulminant infections usually have occurred in those with CD4$^+$ T-cell counts less than 50/mm^3. The CDC, NIH, IDSA, and other clinicians state that the most appropriate treatment for cryptosporidiosis in HIV-infected individuals is the use of potent antiretroviral agents and symptomatic treatment of diarrhea. A highly potent antiretroviral regimen can result in immune restoration (CD4$^+$ T-cell counts exceeding 100/mm^3), which usually results in resolution of the infection. Symptomatic treatment of diarrhea in HIV-infected or immunocompetent individuals with cryptosporidiosis should include oral or IV fluids and electrolyte replacement to correct dehydration and nutritional supplementation when necessary; severe diarrhea may require intensive support. Adjunctive use of antimotility agents may be indicated, but these agents are not consistently effective and should be used with caution in young children.

***Escherichia coli* Infections** Azithromycin has been recommended for use in the treatment of GI infections caused by *Escherichia coli*†.

Diarrhea caused by enterotoxigenic *E. coli*† (ETEC) generally is of moderate severity and self-limited, but may be severe. Although anti-infectives are not usually indicated, the AAP, CDC, and others suggest that an anti-infective (e.g., azithromycin, co-trimoxazole, a fluoroquinolone, rifamycin) can be considered in addition to supportive care if diarrhea is severe or intractable and the causative organism is susceptible.

For the treatment of dysentery caused by enteroinvasive *E. coli*† (EIEC), the AAP suggests than an oral anti-infective (e.g., azithromycin, ciprofloxacin, co-trimoxazole) can be used and, whenever possible, the anti-infective should be selected based on results of in vitro tests.

There is some evidence that azithromycin may shorten the course of diarrhea associated with enteroaggregative *E. coli*† (EAEC) in adults and the drug has been recommended as a drug of choice for children with severe or persistent illness caused by this organism.

The role of anti-infectives in patients with hemorrhagic colitis caused by shiga toxin-producing *E. coli*† (STEC; formerly known as enterohemorrhagic *E. coli* [EHEC] or verotoxin-producing *E. coli*) is unclear, and most experts do not recommend use of anti-infectives in the treatment of enteritis caused by *E. coli* 0157:H7 since there is no evidence of benefit from such therapy.

***Shigella* Infections** Azithromycin has been used in adults and children for the treatment of shigellosis† caused by susceptible strains of *Shigella dysenteriae, S. boydii, S. flexneri,* or *S. sonnei.*

Fluoroquinolones (ciprofloxacin, levofloxacin, norfloxacin) usually are considered the drugs of choice for the treatment of shigellosis; alternatives are azithromycin, ampicillin, ceftriaxone, or co-trimoxazole. Because of increasing resistance, the choice of anti-infective should be based on susceptibility patterns of locally circulating *Shigella*. In the US, about 50% of *S. flexneri* and *S. sonnei* isolates are resistant to ampicillin and co-trimoxazole.

Travelers' Diarrhea Oral azithromycin is used as an alternative to fluoroquinolones for the treatment of travelers' diarrhea†.

The most common cause of travelers' diarrhea worldwide is noninvasive enterotoxigenic strains of *E. coli* (ETEC), but travelers' diarrhea also can be caused by various other bacteria including enteroaggregative *E. coli* (EAEC), *Campylobacter jejuni, Shigella, Salmonella, Aeromonas hydrophila, Plesiomonas shigelloides, Yersinia enterocolitica, Vibrio parahaemolyticus*, or non-O-group 1 *Vibrio cholerae*. In some cases, travelers' diarrhea is caused by a parasitic enteric pathogen (e.g., *Giardia duodenalis, Cryptosporidium parvum, Cyclospora cayetanensis, Entamoeba histolytica, Dientamoeba fragilis*) or viral enteric pathogen (e.g., rotavirus, norovirus).

Countries where travelers are at low risk of travelers' diarrhea include the US, Canada, Australia, New Zealand, Japan, and countries in Northern and Western Europe. Travelers are at intermediate risk for travelers' diarrhea in Eastern Europe, South Africa, and some of the Caribbean islands, but are at high risk in Asia, the Middle East, Africa, and Central and South America.

Travelers' diarrhea usually is self-limited and may resolve within 3–4 days without anti-infective treatment. If diarrhea is moderate or severe, persists for longer than 3 days, or is associated with fever or bloody stools, short-term treatment (1–3 days) with an anti-infective may be indicated. A fluoroquinolone (e.g., ciprofloxacin, levofloxacin, norfloxacin, ofloxacin) generally is recommended when treatment, including self-treatment, of travelers' diarrhea is indicated in adults. Azithromycin can be used as a treatment alternative for individuals who should not receive fluoroquinolones (e.g., children, pregnant women) and may be a drug of choice for travelers in areas with a high prevalence of fluoroquinolone-resistant *Campylobacter* (e.g., Thailand, Nepal) or those who have not responded after 48 hours of fluoroquinolone treatment. Rifaximin is another alternative for the treatment of travelers' diarrhea caused by noninvasive *E. coli*. Bismuth subsalicylate or an antimotility agent may be used as an adjunct to anti-infective treatment to provide symptomatic relief; oral rehydration therapy should be used if indicated, especially in young children or geriatric adults. Travelers should consult a physician if diarrhea persists despite treatment.

■ **Respiratory Tract Infections** ***Acute Sinusitis*** Azithromycin is used in adults and children 6 months of age or older for the treatment of acute bacterial sinusitis caused by *H. influenzae, M. catarrhalis*, or *S. pneumoniae*.

In a randomized, controlled study in patients with acute bacterial sinusitis who received azithromycin (500 mg once daily for 3 days) or amoxicillin and clavulanate (500 mg of amoxicillin and 125 mg of clavulanate 3 times daily for 10 days), the clinical cure rate (modified intent-to-treat analysis) at day 10 was 88% in those who received azithromycin and 85% in those who received amoxicillin and clavulanate; the clinical cure rate at day 28 was 71.5% in both groups.

Safety and efficacy of a single-dose azithromycin regimen for the treatment of acute bacterial maxillary sinusitis were evaluated in a randomized, double-blind study in 270 adults. Patients were randomized to receive a single 2-g dose of azithromycin as an extended-release oral suspension (Zmax®) or a 10-day regimen of oral levofloxacin (500 mg once daily). The clinical cure rate was 94.5% in those who received the single-dose azithromycin regimen and 92.9% in those who received the multiple-dose levofloxacin regimen. When patients were stratified according to causative organism, the single-dose azithromycin regimen cured 97.3% of infections caused by *S. pneumoniae*, 96.3% of those caused by *H. influenzae*, and 100% of those caused by *M. catarrhalis*.

Acute Bacterial Exacerbations of Chronic Obstructive Pulmonary Disease Azithromycin is used orally for the treatment of acute bacterial exacerbations of chronic obstructive pulmonary disease (COPD) caused by *Haemophilus influenzae, Streptococcus pneumoniae*, or *Moraxella catarrhalis* when anti-infective therapy is considered appropriate.

Current data from a limited number of randomized, comparative studies suggest similar clinical and microbiologic efficacy for oral azithromycin and oral cefaclor, erythromycin, clarithromycin, or amoxicillin (with or without clavulanic acid) for treatment of acute bacterial exacerbations of COPD. In addition, eradication of *H. influenzae* in patients with chronic bronchitis has occurred more frequently in those receiving azithromycin than in those receiving cefaclor. In these studies, azithromycin generally was administered once daily for 3–5 days, while other anti-infective therapy was given 2 or more times daily for 5–10 days. Although co-trimoxazole generally is considered the drug of choice for the treatment of upper respiratory tract infections and bronchitis caused by *H. influenzae* or *M. catarrhalis*, azithromycin is considered by many clinicians to be alternative therapy for the treatment of these infections.

Azithromycin is used in adults for the treatment of acute bacterial exacerbations of COPD caused by *H. influenzae, M. catarrhalis*, or *S. pneumoniae*. In a randomized, double-blind, controlled study in patients with acute exacerbation of chronic bronchitis who received azithromycin (500 mg once daily for 3 days) or clarithromycin (500 mg twice daily for 10 days), the clinical cure rate (modified intent-to-treat analysis) at day 21–24 was 85% in those who received azithromycin and 82% in those who received clarithromycin. When results from patients who received azithromycin were stratified according to causative organism, the cure rate was 86% for those with *H. influenzae* infections and 91–92% for those with *S. pneumoniae* or *M. catarrhalis* infections.

Community-acquired Pneumonia Azithromycin is used orally for the treatment of mild to moderate community-acquired pneumonia (CAP) caused by susceptible *S. pneumoniae, H. influenzae, Mycoplasma pneumoniae*, or *Chlamydophila pneumoniae* (formerly *Chlamydia pneumoniae*) in adults and children 6 months of age or older when oral therapy is indicated. Limited data in patients with CAP caused by these pathogens suggest that oral azithromycin given for 3†–5 days is as effective as a 10-day regimen of oral cefaclor or clarithromycin. When an oral regimen is appropriate, a single-dose regimen of azithromycin given as an extended-release oral suspension (Zmax®) can be used for the treatment of mild to moderate CAP caused by susceptible *C. pneumoniae, H. influenzae, M. pneumoniae*, or *S. pneumoniae*.

Oral azithromycin should *not* be used in patients who have moderate to severe pneumonia or when there are risk factors that make oral therapy inappropriate (e.g., cystic fibrosis, nosocomial infection, known or suspected bacteremia, illness requiring hospitalization, geriatric or debilitated status, immunodeficiency or functional asplenia or other underlying conditions that may compromise ability to respond to treatment). Although azithromycin is highly distributed into tissues and phagocytes, some clinicians suggest that *oral* azithromycin is unsuitable for the treatment of CAP bacteremia or potentially resistant organisms (e.g., penicillin-resistant *S. pneumoniae*) may be involved because of the relatively low serum concentrations achieved with oral administration of the drug; parenteral therapy with IV azithromycin or another anti-infective agent may be preferred in such situations.

IV azithromycin is used for the treatment of CAP caused by susceptible *C. pneumoniae, H. influenzae, Legionella pneumophila, M. catarrhalis, M. pneumoniae, S. aureus*, or *S. pneumoniae* when initial IV drug therapy is considered necessary. In a comparative study in patients with CAP, clinical success (i.e., cure or improvement) 10–14 days after completion of therapy reportedly occurred in 78% of patients receiving azithromycin (500 mg IV once daily for 2–5 days followed by azithromycin 500 mg orally once daily to complete 7–10 days of therapy) and in 74% of patients receiving cefuroxime (750 mg IV every 8 hours for 2–5 days followed by cefuroxime 500 mg orally every 12 hours to complete 7–10 days of therapy) with or without erythromycin (up to 2 g daily IV or oral). In an uncontrolled study, clinical success (i.e., cure or improvement) was reported in 89% of patients receiving the same regimen of IV and oral azithromycin. In these studies, presumptive bacteriologic eradication (determined according to microbiologic data available at the patient's last completed clinic visit) was evident in 96% of evaluable patients with *S. pneumoniae* infections (including 79% of those with positive blood cultures for *S. pneumoniae*), 95% of those with *H. influenzae* infection, 90% of those with *M. catarrhalis* or *S. aureus* infection. At 10–14 days after azithromycin therapy, presumptive bacteriologic/clinical success was evident in 89% of patients with *M. pneumoniae* infection, 82% of those with *C. pneumoniae* infection, and 81% of those with *L. pneumophila* infection.

Initial treatment of CAP generally involves use of an empiric anti-infective regimen based on the most likely pathogens and local susceptibility patterns, but should be modified to provide more specific therapy (pathogen-directed therapy) based on results of in vitro culture and susceptibility testing, especially in hospitalized patients. The most appropriate empiric regimen varies depending on the severity of illness at the time of presentation and whether outpatient treatment or hospitalization in or out of an intensive care unit (ICU) is indicated and the presence or absence of cardiopulmonary disease and other modifying factors that increase the risk of certain pathogens (e.g., penicillin- or multidrug-resistant *S. pneumoniae*, enteric gram-negative bacilli, *Ps. aeruginosa*). For both outpatients and inpatients, most experts recommend that an empiric regimen for the treatment of CAP include an anti-infective active against *S. pneumoniae* since this organism is the most commonly identified cause of bacterial pneumonia and causes more severe disease than many other common CAP pathogens. Macrolides should *not* be used alone for empiric treatment of CAP in hospitalized patients.

For empiric *outpatient* treatment of CAP in previously healthy adults without risk factors for drug-resistant *S. pneumoniae* (DRSP), IDSA and ATS recommend monotherapy with a macrolide (azithromycin, clarithromycin, erythromycin) or, alternatively, doxycycline. If risk factors for DRSP are present (e.g., chronic heart, lung, liver, or renal disease, diabetes mellitus, alcoholism, malignancy, asplenia, immunosuppression, history of anti-infective treatment within the last 3 months), IDSA and ATS recommend monotherapy with a fluoroquinolone with enhanced activity against *S. pneumoniae* (gemifloxacin, levofloxacin, moxifloxacin) or, alternatively, a combination regimen that includes a β-lactam active against *S. pneumoniae* (high-dose amoxicillin or fixed combination of amoxicillin and clavulanic acid or, alternatively, ceftriaxone, cefpodoxime, or cefuroxime) given in conjunction with a macrolide (azithromycin, clarithromycin, erythromycin) or doxycycline.

For empiric *inpatient* treatment of CAP when treatment in an intensive care unit (ICU) is not necessary, IDSA and ATS recommend adults receive monotherapy with a fluoroquinolone with enhanced activity against *S. pneumoniae* (gemifloxacin, levofloxacin, or moxifloxacin) or, alternatively, a combination regimen that includes a β-lactam (usually cefotaxime, ceftriaxone, or ampicillin) given in conjunction with a macrolide (azithromycin, clarithromycin, erythromycin) or doxycycline. For empiric *inpatient* treatment of CAP in ICU patients when *Pseudomonas* and oxacillin-resistant (methicillin-resistant) *Staphylococcus aureus* are *not* suspected, IDSA and ATS recommend a combination regimen that includes a β-lactam (cefotaxime, ceftriaxone, fixed combination of ampicillin and sulbactam) given in conjunction with either azithromycin or a fluoroquinolone (gemifloxacin, levofloxacin, moxifloxacin).

For empiric treatment of CAP in adults with risk factors for *Ps. aeruginosa*, IDSA and ATS recommend a combination regimen that includes an antipneumococcal, antipseudomonal β-lactam (cefepime, imipenem, meropenem, fixed combination of piperacillin and tazobactam) and ciprofloxacin or levofloxacin; one of these β-lactams, an aminoglycoside, and azithromycin; or one of these β-lactams, an aminoglycoside, and an antipneumococcal fluoroquinolone.

■ Skin and Skin Structure Infections Azithromycin is used in adults for the treatment of uncomplicated skin and skin structure infections caused by susceptible *Staphylococcus aureus*, *S. pyogenes*, or *S. agalactiae* (group B streptococci). Results of comparative studies indicate that oral azithromycin is as effective as oral cloxacillin, oral cephalexin, or oral erythromycin in the treatment of bacterial skin and skin structure infections (e.g., cellulitis, pyoderma, erysipelas, wound infections). However, some clinicians state that azithromycin or any macrolide should not be used for serious staphylococcal infections because of the propensity for development of resistance during therapy. Skin structure infections resulting in abscess formation may require surgical or needle drainage in addition to antibacterial therapy.

■ Babesiosis A combination regimen of atovaquone and azithromycin is recommended as a regimen of choice for the treatment of babesiosis† caused by *Babesia microti*. The other regimen of choice for this infection is clindamycin and quinine. The clindamycin and quinine regimen may be preferred for severe babesiosis; in those with mild or moderate illness, the atovaquone and azithromycin regimen may be as effective and better tolerated than the quinine and clindamycin regimen. Use of exchange transfusions also should be considered in severely ill patients with high levels of parasitemia (at least 10%), substantial hemolysis, or compromised renal, hepatic, or pulmonary function.

Limited data in animals suggest that a regimen of azithromycin and quinine also may be effective in the management of babesiosis.

■ Bartonella Infections Azithromycin has been used for the treatment of infections caused by *Bartonella henselae*† (formerly *Rochalimaea henselae*) (e.g., cat scratch disease, bacillary angiomatosis, peliosis hepatitis). Cat scratch disease generally is a self-limited illness in immunocompetent individuals and may resolve spontaneously in 2–4 months; however, some clinicians suggest that anti-infective therapy be considered for acutely or severely ill patients with systemic symptoms, particularly those with hepatosplenomegaly or painful lymphadenopathy, and such therapy probably is indicated in immunocompromised patients. Anti-infectives also are indicated in patients with *B. henselae* infections who develop bacillary angiomatosis, neuroretinitis, or Parinaud's oculoglandular syndrome. While the optimum anti-infective regimen for the treatment of cat scratch disease or other *B. henselae* infections has not been identified, some clinicians recommend use of azithromycin, ciprofloxacin, erythromycin, doxycycline, rifampin, co-trimoxazole, gentamicin, or third generation cephalosporins.

Azithromycin has been used in conjunction with IM or IV ceftriaxone for the treatment of bacteremia caused by *Bartonella quintana*† (formerly *Rochalimaea quintana*). *B. quintana*, a gram-negative bacilli, can cause cutaneous bacillary angiomatosis, trench fever, bacteremia, endocarditis, and chronic lymphadenopathy. *B. quintana* infections have been reported most frequently in immunocompromised patients (e.g., individuals with HIV infection), homeless individuals in urban areas, and chronic alcohol abusers. Optimum anti-infective regimens for the treatment of infections caused by *B. quintana* have not been identified, and various drugs have been used to treat these infections, including doxycycline, erythromycin, azithromycin, clarithromycin, or chloramphenicol. There is evidence that these infections tend to persist or recur and prolonged therapy (several months or longer) usually is necessary.

■ Chancroid Azithromycin is used orally in the treatment of chancroid (genital ulcers caused by *Haemophilus ducreyi*).

The CDC and others state that a single oral dose of a conventional formulation of azithromycin, a single IM dose of ceftriaxone, a 3-day regimen of oral ciprofloxacin (contraindicated in pregnant or lactating women), or a 7-day regimen of oral erythromycin are the regimens of choice for the treatment of chancroid. The AAP states that a single oral dose of a conventional formulation of azithromycin or a single IM dose of ceftriaxone is the preferred regimen in infants, children, and adolescents. All 4 regimens generally are effective for the treatment of chancroid; however, patients with human immunodeficiency virus (HIV) infection and patients who are uncircumcised may not respond to therapy as well as those who are HIV-negative or circumcised. Because data on the efficacy of the single-dose azithromycin and single-dose ceftriaxone regimens for treatment of chancroid in patients with HIV infection are limited, the CDC recommends that these regimens be used in HIV-infected patients only if follow-up can be ensured; some experts recommend that HIV-infected individuals with chancroid receive the 7-day erythromycin regimen.

Chancroid occurs more frequently in men (90% of infections) than in women and experience with azithromycin treatment of this infection in women is limited. Consequently, efficacy of the drug in the treatment of chancroid in women has not been established to date, and the drug is labeled by the US Food and Drug Administration (FDA) for this use only in men. However, azithromycin has been used successfully for the treatment of chancroid in women†, and chancroid treatment guidelines from CDC, AAP, and other authorities do not provide gender-based recommendations.

In the US, chancroid usually occurs in discrete outbreaks, but the disease is endemic in some areas. Approximately 10% of patients with chancroid acquired in the US also are coinfected with *Treponema pallidum* or herpes simplex virus (HSV); this percentage is higher in individuals who acquired the infection outside the US. In addition, high rates of HIV infection have been reported in patients with chancroid, and the disease appears to be a cofactor for HIV transmission. Evaluation of the physical features of genital ulcers (without laboratory evaluation and testing) usually is inadequate to provide a differential diagnosis between chancroid, primary syphilis, and genital HSV infection. Ideally, diagnostic evaluation of patients with genital ulcers should include a serologic test for syphilis and darkfield examination or direct immunofluorescence test for *T. pallidum*, culture for *H. ducreyi*, and culture or antigen test for HSV. A definitive diagnosis of chancroid requires identification of *H. ducreyi* on special culture media that is not widely available. The presence of a painful ulcer and tender suppurative inguinal adenopathy suggests a diagnosis of chancroid. However, a probable diagnosis of chancroid can be made if the patient has one or more painful genital ulcers, there is no evidence of *T. pallidum* infection based on a negative darkfield examination of ulcer exudate or a negative serologic test for syphilis (performed at least 7 days after onset of ulcers), culture or antigen test for HSV is negative, and the clinical presentation, appearance of genital ulcers, and regional lymphadenopathy (if present) are typical for chancroid.

Patient Follow-up and Management of Sexual Partners The CDC recommends that all patients diagnosed with chancroid be tested for HIV and, if the test is negative, retested for HIV and for syphilis 3 months later. Patients with chancroid should be examined 3–7 days after initiation of anti-infective therapy. If the regimen was effective, symptomatic improvement in the ulcers is evident within 3 days and objective improvement is evident within 7 days. If clinical improvement is not evident within 3–7 days, consideration should be given to the possibility that the diagnosis was incorrect, there is coinfection with another sexually transmitted disease, the patient was noncompliant with the anti-infective regimen, the strain of *H. ducreyi* is resistant to the anti-infective agent used, or the patient is HIV seropositive.

The time required for complete ulcer healing is related to the size of the ulcer; large ulcers may require more than 2 weeks to heal. Healing of ulcers may be slower in uncircumcised men who have ulcers under the foreskin. Resolution of fluctuant lymphadenopathy is slower than that of ulcers, and needle aspiration or incisional drainage may be necessary even during otherwise effective anti-infective therapy. While needle aspiration of buboes is a simpler procedure, incision and drainage of buboes may be preferred.

The CDC recommends that any individual who had sexual contact with a patient with chancroid within 10 days before the onset of the patient's symptoms should be examined and treated for the disease, even if no symptoms are present.

■ Chlamydial Infections ***Urogenital Chlamydial Infections*** Azithromycin is used orally for the treatment of urogenital infections caused by *C. trachomatis*.

Urogenital Chlamydial Infection in Adults and Adolescents. Azithromycin is used orally for the treatment of urethritis and cervicitis caused by *C. trachomatis*.

In the US, urogenital chlamydial infection is the most frequently reported infectious disease and these infections occur most frequently in individuals 25 years of age or younger. Urogenital *C. trachomatis* infection in women can result in serious sequelae, including pelvic inflammatory disease (PID), ectopic pregnancy, and infertility. Asymptomatic infection is common, and some women with uncomplicated cervical infection already have subclinical upper reproductive tract infection. There is evidence that routine screening for chlamydial infection in women can reduce the prevalence of infection and rates of PID. Therefore, the CDC recommends annual screening of all sexually active women 25 years of age or younger and also recommends screening of older women who have risk factors for chlamydial infection (e.g., new or multiple sex partners). Although data are insufficient to date to recommend routine screening for *C. trachomatis* in sexually active young men, the CDC states that screening of such men should be considered in clinical settings with a high prevalence of chlamydial infection (e.g., adolescent clinics, correctional facilities, sexually transmitted disease clinics).

For the treatment of urogenital chlamydial infections in *nonpregnant* adults and adolescents, the CDC, AAP, and other clinicians recommend a single oral dose of a conventional formulation of azithromycin or a 7-day regimen of oral doxycycline. Alternatively, these adults and adolescents can receive a 7-day regimen of oral erythromycin base or ethylsuccinate or a 7-day regimen of oral ofloxacin or levofloxacin. While doxycycline is highly effective and experience with the drug is more extensive than that with azithromycin, azithromycin may be particularly useful and cost-effective when compliance with a multiple-day (e.g., 7-day) anti-infective regimen cannot be ensured. Results from controlled clinical studies in individuals 15 years of age or older indicate that a single 1-g oral dose of a conventional formulation of azithromycin is as effective as a 7-day course of doxycycline in the treatment of uncomplicated chlamydial genital infections.

The CDC, AAP, and others recommend that urogenital chlamydial infections in *pregnant* women be treated with a single-dose regimen of a conventional formulation of azithromycin or a 7-day regimen of oral amoxicillin. Alternative regimens recommended for these infections in pregnant women are a 7- or 14-day regimen of oral erythromycin base or ethylsuccinate. The CDC states that clinical experience and studies suggest that the single-dose azithromycin regimen is safe and effective, and some clinicians suggest that this is the regimen of choice for treatment of urogenital chlamydial infections in pregnant women.

Individuals with HIV infection who also are infected with chlamydia should receive the same treatment regimens recommended for other individuals with chlamydial infections.

When given in the usual dosage for the treatment of uncomplicated sexually transmitted chlamydial infections, azithromycin alone should not be relied on for effective therapy against possible concomitant syphilis and the possibility that the regimen may mask or delay development of the signs and symptoms of incubating syphilis should be considered. Appropriate serologic tests for syphilis and cultures for gonorrhea should be performed prior to initiating azithromycin therapy for chlamydial infection; appropriate anti-infective therapy and follow-up should be initiated if either infection is confirmed.

Urogenital Chlamydial Infection in Infants and Children. For the treatment of uncomplicated urogenital chlamydial infections in children 8 years of age and older, the CDC recommends a single-dose of a conventional formulation of azithromycin or a 7-day regimen of oral doxycycline. For children younger than 8 years of age, the CDC recommends that those weighing at least 45 kg receive a single-dose azithromycin regimen and that those weighing less than 45 kg receive a 14-day regimen of oral erythromycin base or ethylsuccinate. The AAP recommends that infants younger than 6 months of age with urogenital chlamydial infections receive an erythromycin regimen and that those 6 months to 12 years of age receive either azithromycin or erythromycin.

Presumptive Treatment of Chlamydial Infection in Patients with Gonorrhea Because of the risks associated with untreated coexisting chlamydial infection, the CDC and most clinicians recommend that patients being treated for uncomplicated gonorrhea or disseminated gonococcal infection also receive an anti-infective regimen effective for presumptive treatment of uncomplicated urogenital chlamydial infection. For presumptive treatment of chlamydia in adults and adolescents being treated for uncomplicated or disseminated gonococcal infections, the CDC and many clinicians recommend use of a single oral dose of azithromycin or a 7-day regimen of oral doxycycline. The strategy of routine administration of a regimen effective against chlamydia in patients being treated for gonococcal infection has been recommended by the CDC for more than 10 years and appears to have resulted in substantial decreases in the prevalence of genital chlamydial infection in some populations. In addition, since most *N. gonorrhoeae* isolated in the US are susceptible to doxycycline and azithromycin, dual therapy may delay the development of resistance in *N. gonorrhoeae*. Nucleic acid amplification tests (NAAT) for *C. trachomatis* are highly sensitive and patients with a negative chlamydial NAAT result at the time of treatment for gonorrhea do not need to be treated for chlamydia. However, if test results are not available or if a test other than a NAAT was performed and was negative for chlamydia, patients should receive treatment for both gonorrhea and chlamydia.

Lymphogranuloma Venereum Although some clinicians suggest that azithromycin may be effective for the treatment of lymphogranuloma venereum† caused by invasive serotypes of *C. trachomatis* (serovars L1, L2, L3), safety and efficacy of the drug for this use have not been established. The CDC recommends a 21-day regimen of doxycycline as the treatment of choice and a 21-day regimen of erythromycin base as an alternative for the treatment of lymphogranuloma venereum. Although oral azithromycin also may be effective, the CDC states that clinical safety and efficacy data are lacking. Effective treatment cures the infection and prevents ongoing tissue damage, although tissue reaction can result in scarring. Aspiration of buboes through intact skin or incision and drainage may be necessary to prevent the formation of inguinal/femoral ulcerations.

The CDC recommends that individuals who had sexual contact with a lymphogranuloma venereum patient within 60 days before onset of the patient's symptoms should be examined, tested for urethral or cervical chlamydial infection, and treated with a regimen usually recommended for the treatment of urogenital chlamydial infections (a single 1-g dose of azithromycin or 100 mg of doxycycline twice daily for 7 days).

While HIV-infected individuals with lymphogranuloma venereum should receive the same treatment regimens recommended for other patients, there is some evidence that HIV-infected patients may require more prolonged therapy and resolution may be delayed.

Chlamydial Pneumonia in Infants Some clinicians recommend azithromycin for the treatment of chlamydial pneumonia in infants.

Trachoma and Other Ocular Chlamydial Infections Some clinicians recommend azithromycin for the treatment of chlamydial conjunctivitis in neonates.

Azithromycin is used in the treatment of ocular trachoma caused by *C. trachomatis*† and is considered a drug of choice for this infection. Azithromycin is recommended for use in mass treatment programs, usually as a single-dose regimen; however, the optimal number of doses required to minimize reservoirs of infection when mass treatment programs are undertaken in high-prevalence areas is unclear.

Other Chlamydial Infections Azithromycin is used for the treatment of *C. pneumoniae* respiratory tract infections. (See Uses: Respiratory Tract Infections.) IV azithromycin is used for the treatment of pelvic inflammatory disease (PID) caused by *C. trachomatis*. (See Uses: Pelvic Inflammatory Disease.)

Although tetracyclines are the drugs of choice for the treatment of psittacosis† caused by *Chlamydophila psittaci* (formerly *Chlamydia psittaci*), macrolides (erythromycin, azithromycin, clarithromycin) are possible alternatives in children younger than 8 years of age who should not receive tetracyclines.

Azithromycin has been used to treat adults with coronary artery disease (CAD) who have elevated anti-*C. pneumoniae* antibody titers† (a possible risk factor for myocardial infarction [MI] or CAD) in an attempt to reduce recurrent ischemic events. In a randomized, placebo-controlled study in men who had survived an MI and who had elevated anti-*C. pneumoniae* antibody titers, the risk of subsequent adverse cardiovascular events (i.e., MI, unstable angina requiring IV therapy, coronary angioplasty, or coronary artery bypass, cardiovascular death) during a follow-up period averaging 18 months was reduced in individuals who received azithromycin (500 mg daily for 3–6 days) compared with *C. pneumoniae*-seropositive individuals who received placebo and was similar to that in men who were *C. pneumoniae* seronegative. However, these results were not confirmed in other studies. In a large study in stable patients with documented MI (at least 6 weeks previously) and serologic evidence of exposure to *C. pneumoniae*, those who received azithromycin (600 mg daily for 3 days then once weekly for 11 weeks) had a 7% (nonsignificant) reduction in the risk of the primary endpoint (death, MI, coronary revascularization procedure, hospitalization for angina) compared with placebo. Because efficacy has not been proven to date, use of azithromycin for prevention of recurrent CAD is not recommended.

■ **Cholera** Azithromycin has been used in the treatment of cholera† caused by *Vibrio cholerae* O1 or O139.

A tetracycline or, alternatively, a fluoroquinolone or co-trimoxazole generally is used for the treatment of cholera in conjunction with fluid and electrolyte replacement therapy. Although further study is needed, azithromycin may be an alternative, especially for treatment of cholera in children or infections caused by *V. cholerae* resistant to tetracyclines and fluoroquinolones.

■ **Gonorrhea and Associated Infections** Azithromycin is used orally for the treatment of uncomplicated gonorrhea (i.e., urethritis and/or cervices) caused by susceptible *N. gonorrhoeae*.

The CDC and many clinicians currently recommend that uncomplicated gonorrhea in adults and adolescents be treated with a single IM dose of ceftriaxone or a single oral dose of cefixime given in conjunction with an anti-infective regimen effective for presumptive treatment of chlamydia (e.g., a single dose of oral azithromycin or a 7-day regimen of oral doxycycline). Although not recommended for routine use, the CDC and other clinicians state that the single 2-g azithromycin regimen of a conventional preparation can be used as an alternative for the treatment of uncomplicated gonorrhea when preferred drugs cannot be used (e.g., in patients hypersensitive to cephalosporins when spectinomycin is unavailable and desensitization to cephalosporins is not an option).

Limited data suggest that a single 2-g oral dose of a conventional formulation of azithromycin is as effective as a single 250-mg IM dose of ceftriaxone in the treatment of uncomplicated gonorrhea. However, the 2-g azithromycin regimen has been associated with a relatively high incidence of adverse GI effects and does not appear to offer any advantages over IM ceftriaxone for the treatment of uncomplicated gonorrhea.

Although a single 1-g oral dose of a conventional formulation of azithromycin also has been effective in some patients for the treatment of uncomplicated gonorrhea, this lower single-dose regimen has been associated with a substantial incidence of therapeutic failure in some studies. Therefore, the CDC does not recommend use of a 1-g single-dose azithromycin regimen.

The fact that *N. gonorrhoeae* with reduced susceptibility to azithromycin have been isolated in the US should be considered. (See Resistance: Resistance in Neisseria and Treponema.) Because of concerns related to emerging resistance to macrolides, the CDC recommends that azithromycin be used for the treatment of gonorrhea only when considered necessary.

■ **Granuloma Inguinale (Donovanosis)** Oral azithromycin (1 g once weekly) reportedly has been effective in the treatment of granuloma inguinale† (donovanosis), a chronic, progressively destructive sexually transmitted disease caused by *Klebsiella granulomatis* (formerly *Calymmatobacterium granulomatis*).

The CDC and AAP recommend that donovanosis be treated with a regimen of oral doxycycline or, alternatively, an oral regimen of azithromycin, ciprofloxacin, erythromycin, or co-trimoxazole. Anti-infective treatment of donovanosis should be continued until all lesions have healed completely; a minimum of 3 weeks of treatment usually is necessary. If lesions do not respond within the first few days of therapy, the CDC recommends that a parenteral aminoglycoside (e.g., 1 mg/kg of gentamicin IV every 8 hours) be added to the regimen. Anti-infective therapy appears to halt progressive destruction of tissue, although prolonged duration of therapy often is required to enable granulation and re-epithelization of ulcers. Despite effective anti-infective therapy, donovanosis may relapse 6–18 months later.

Individuals with HIV infection should receive the same treatment regimens recommended for other individuals with donovanosis; however, the CDC suggests that addition of a parenteral aminoglycoside to the regimen should be strongly considered in HIV-infected patients.

Any individual who had sexual contact with a patient with donovanosis should be examined and treated if they had sexual contact with the patient during the 60 days preceding the onset of symptoms in the patient and they have clinical signs and symptoms of the disease. The value of empiric therapy in the absence of clinical signs and symptoms has not been established.

■ **Helicobacter pylori Infection and Duodenal Ulcer Disease** Azithromycin has been used in multiple-drug regimens for the treatment of *Helicobacter pylori* infection and peptic ulcer disease†. However, data from a limited number of clinical studies indicate that such combination regimens generally are associated with a high incidence of adverse effects (principally GI effects) or low *H. pylori* eradication rates (i.e., 50–70%). For more information on the treatment of *H. pylori* infection and peptic ulcer disease, see Uses: Helicobacter pylori Infection, in Clarithromycin 8:12.12.92.

■ **Legionella Infections** Oral or IV azithromycin is used for the treatment of Legionnaires' disease† caused by *Legionella pneumophila*. Macrolides (usually azithromycin) or fluoroquinolones are considered the drugs of choice for the treatment of pneumonia caused by *L. pneumophila*; alternatives are doxycycline or co-trimoxazole. An oral regimen (e.g., azithromycin, clarithromycin, doxycycline, erythromycin, a fluoroquinolone) may be effective for patients with mild to moderate Legionnaires' disease. However, a parenteral regimen (e.g., azithromycin, a fluoroquinolone) usually is necessary for the initial treatment of severe Legionnaires' disease and the addition of oral rifampin is recommended during the first 3–5 days therapy in severely ill and/or immunocompromised patients; after a response is obtained, rifampin can be discontinued and therapy changed to an oral regimen.

Some clinicians suggest that azithromycin may be the preferred macrolide for the treatment of severe Legionnaires' disease and may also be preferred for empiric therapy in patients with severe community-acquired pneumonia that may be caused by *Legionella*. (See Community-acquired Pneumonia under Uses: Respiratory Tract Infections.)

■ **Leptospirosis** Azithromycin is considered an alternative for the treatment of leptospirosis† caused by *Leptospira*. Penicillin G is the drug of choice for severe infections; tetracyclines (usually doxycycline) or ceftriaxone are recommended as alternatives for less severe infections. Azithromycin also has been effective.

■ **Malaria** Although further study is needed, azithromycin has been used in conjunction with an antimalarial agent (e.g., chloroquine, quinine, artesunate [not commercially available in the US]) for the treatment of uncomplicated malaria† caused by *Plasmodium falciparum*, including multidrug-resistant strains. Azithromycin should *not* be used alone as monotherapy for the treatment of malaria.

Although further study is needed, azithromycin has been used for the treatment or prevention of *P. vivax* malaria†. When used for treatment of such infections, the rate of resolution of parasitemia reported for azithromycin was considerably slower than that reported for chloroquine.

■ **Mycobacterium avium Complex (MAC) Infections** ***Primary Prevention of Disseminated MAC Infection*** Oral azithromycin is used to prevent *Mycobacterium avium* complex (MAC) bacteremia and disseminated infections (primary prophylaxis) in adults, adolescents, and children with advanced HIV infection. Azithromycin and clarithromycin are the preferred drugs for primary prevention of disseminated MAC infections in adults, adolescents, and children.

In controlled trials, azithromycin monotherapy was more effective than placebo or rifabutin monotherapy in preventing disseminated MAC infection in patients with advanced HIV infection (CD4+ T-cell counts less than 100/mm³) and infrequently resulted in the development of resistant organisms. In a placebo-controlled trial, the cumulative incidence rate of MAC infection at 1 year in patients receiving azithromycin 1.2 g once weekly as a conventional formulation was 10.9% less than that in patients receiving placebo (19.1 versus 8.2% incidence, respectively), while both groups had a comparable incidence of adverse effects. In a randomized, comparative study in patients with advanced HIV infection (CD4+ T-cell counts less than 100/mm³), prophylaxis with rifabutin (300 mg daily), azithromycin (1.2 g once weekly as a conventional formulation), or both drugs concomitantly was associated with a cumulative incidence of MAC infection at 1 year of 15.2, 7.6, or 2.8%, respectively. All patients also received fluconazole (200 mg daily or 400 mg once weekly) for prevention of fungal infections. The risk of MAC infection (after adjustment for baseline CD4+ T-cell counts) in patients receiving azithromycin prophylaxis was 47% lower than that with rifabutin prophylaxis, while prophylaxis with both drugs reduced the risk by 72% compared with rifabutin alone.

The incidences of bacterial infections (e.g., pneumonia, sinusitis) and of manifestations of disseminated MAC infection (e.g., fever, night sweats, weight loss, anemia) in this study were lower with azithromycin or azithromycin-rifabutin prophylaxis than with rifabutin prophylaxis or placebo. Analyses of the occurrence of *Pneumocystis carinii* pneumonia in these patients indicated that prophylaxis with azithromycin (alone or combined with rifabutin) provided additional protection against this opportunistic infection (45% risk reduction) compared with that provided by rifabutin alone in patients without previous *P. carinii* episodes; no additional benefit from azithromycin was observed to enhance when azithromycin was used as secondary prophylaxis (i.e., in patients with prior *P. carinii* episodes). Of patients in whom prophylaxis with azithromycin was unsuccessful, resistance to azithromycin (and clarithromycin) was found in 11%. The overall incidence of adverse effects was similar among the 3 groups (i.e., 76, 88, or 90% of patients receiving rifabutin, azithromycin, or combined rifabutin-azithromycin prophylaxis, respectively), although dose-limiting adverse effects (principally GI effects) occurred more frequently with combined azithromycin-rifabutin prophylaxis (23% of patients) than with rifabutin (16%) or azithromycin (13%) prophylaxis.

Primary prophylaxis against MAC disease is recommended for HIV-infected adults and adolescents (13 years of age or older) who have CD4+ T-cell counts less than 50/mm³. Severely immunocompromised HIV-infected children younger than 13 years of age also should receive primary prophylaxis against MAC according to the following age-specific CD4+ T-cell counts: children 6–13 years of age, less than 50 cells/mm³; children 2–6 years of age, less than 75 cells/mm³; children 1–2 years of age, less than 500 cells/mm³; and children less than 1 year of age, less than 750 cells/mm³.

There is evidence that the combination of azithromycin and rifabutin is more effective than azithromycin alone for primary MAC prophylaxis; however, routine prophylaxis with the combination is not recommended because of additional cost, increased incidence of adverse effects, and absence of a difference in survival in patients receiving the combination compared with azithromycin alone.

Current evidence indicates that primary MAC prophylaxis can be discontinued with minimal risk of developing disseminated MAC disease in HIV-infected adults and adolescents who have responded to highly active antiretroviral therapy (HAART) with an increase in CD4+ T-cell counts to greater than 100/mm³ that has been sustained for at least 3 months. Discontinuance of primary prophylaxis against MAC is recommended in adults and adolescents meeting these criteria because prophylaxis in these individuals appears to add little benefit in terms of disease prevention for MAC or bacterial infections, and discontinuance reduces the medication burden, the potential for toxicity, drug interactions, selection of drug-resistant pathogens, and cost. However, primary MAC prophylaxis should be restarted in adults and adolescents if CD4+ T-cell counts decrease to less than 50–100/mm³. The safety of discontinuing MAC prophylaxis in children whose CD4+ T-cell counts have increased as a result of highly active antiretroviral therapy has not been studied to date.

HIV-infected pregnant women are at risk for MAC disease, and chemoprophylaxis should be given to such women who have T-cell counts less than 50/mm³. However, some clinicians may choose to withhold prophylaxis during the first trimester of pregnancy because of general concerns regarding drug administration during this period. Of the available agents, azithromycin usually is considered the drug of choice for MAC disease prophylaxis in HIV-infected pregnant women because of the drug's safety profile in animal studies and anecdotal information on safety in humans.

HIV-infected patients who develop MAC disease while receiving prophylaxis for the infection require treatment with a multiple-drug regimen since monotherapy results in drug resistance and clinical failure.

Treatment and Prevention of Recurrence of Disseminated MAC Infection Azithromycin is used as part of a multiple-drug regimen for the treatment of disseminated MAC infections and for prevention of recurrence† (secondary prophylaxis or chronic maintenance therapy) of MAC infections in HIV-infected patients.

For the treatment of disseminated MAC infections in HIV-infected adults, adolescents, and children, the ATS, CDC, NIH, IDSA, and other clinicians recommend a regimen of clarithromycin (or azithromycin) and ethambutol and state that consideration may be given to adding a third drug (preferably rifabutin). Some clinicians state that clarithromycin is the preferred macrolide for the initial treatment regimen because of more extensive experience and because it appears to be associated with more rapid clearance of MAC from blood; however, azithromycin can be substituted if clarithromycin cannot be used because of drug interactions or intolerance and is preferred in pregnant women. Rifabutin should be included in the treatment regimen if the patient has advanced immunosuppression (CD4+ T-cell count less than 50/mm³) or high mycobacterial load (exceeding 2 $\log_{10}$ colony forming units/mL of blood) or is not receiving effective antiretroviral therapy because there is an increased risk of mortality and emergence of drug resistance. If a third drug is indicated in the treatment regimen and rifabutin cannot be used (e.g., because of drug interactions or intolerance), use of a fluoroquinolone (ciprofloxacin or levofloxacin) or amikacin may be considered.

To prevent recurrence of MAC disease in HIV-infected adults, adolescents, or children who have previously been treated for an acute episode of MAC infection and in whom macrolide resistance has not been documented, CDC, NIH, and IDSA recommend a regimen consisting of a macrolide (clarithromycin or azithromycin) given with ethambutol (with or without rifabutin). Azithromycin usually is the preferred macrolide for use in conjunction with ethambutol for secondary prophylaxis of disseminated MAC infection in pregnant women. Secondary MAC prophylaxis generally is administered for life in adults and adolescents unless immune recovery has occurred as a result of potent antiretroviral therapy. Limited data indicate that secondary MAC prophylaxis can be discontinued in adults and adolescents who have immune recovery in response to potent antiretroviral therapy. Based on these data and more extensive cumulative data on safety of discontinuing secondary prophylaxis for other opportunistic infections, CDC, NIH, and IDSA state that it may be reasonable to consider discontinuance of secondary MAC prophylaxis in adults and adolescents who have successfully completed at least 12 months of MAC therapy, have remained asymptomatic with respect to MAC, and have CD4+ T-cell counts exceeding 100/mm³ as the result of potent antiretroviral therapy and this increase has been sustained (e.g., for 6 months or longer). Some experts would obtain a blood culture for MAC (even in asymptomatic patients) prior to discontinuing secondary MAC prophylaxis to substantiate that the disease is no longer active. Secondary MAC prophylaxis should be restarted in adults or adolescents if CD4+ T-cell counts decrease to less than 100/mm³. The safety of discontinuing secondary MAC prophylaxis in HIV-infected children receiving potent antiretroviral therapy has not been studied and children with a history of disseminated MAC should receive lifelong secondary prophylaxis.

Treatment of Pulmonary MAC Infections in HIV-negative Adults Azithromycin has been used in multiple-drug regimens for the treatment of pulmonary MAC† infections in patients not infected with HIV.

The ATS recommends that pulmonary MAC infections in HIV-negative adults be treated with a regimen that includes at least 3 drugs, including clarithromycin (500 mg twice daily) or azithromycin (250 mg daily or 500 mg 3 times weekly), rifabutin (300 mg daily) or rifampin (600 mg daily), and ethambutol (25 mg/kg daily for 2 months, then 15 mg/kg daily). For patients with a small body mass and/or who are older than 70 years of age, clarithromycin 250 mg twice daily or azithromycin 250 mg 3 times weekly may be better tolerated. The ATS states that the addition of streptomycin given intermittently (2 or 3 times weekly) for the first 2–3 months may be considered for patients with extensive disease.

A 3-drug regimen of azithromycin (250 mg daily on weekdays) or clarithromycin (500 mg twice daily) with ethambutol (15 mg/kg daily) and clofazimine (100 mg daily) also has been used with some success for the treatment of pulmonary MAC infections in HIV-negative adults.

■ **Mycobacterium abscessus, M. kansasii, and M. marinum Infections** Azithromycin has been recommended for use in combination with other antimycobacterial anti-infectives for the treatment of infections caused by *M. abscessus*†, *M. kansasii*†, and *M. marinum*†.

For serious skin, soft tissue, and bone infections caused by *M. abscessus*, the ATS and IDSA recommend a multiple-drug regimen of clarithromycin (or azithromycin) used in conjunction with a parenteral anti-infective (e.g., amikacin, cefoxitin, imipenem); surgery usually is indicated for extensive disease, abscess formation, and when drug therapy is difficult. This multiple-drug regimen also has been used in the treatment of *M. abscessus* lung disease; anti-infectives may control symptoms and disease progression, but generally cannot produce long-term sputum conversion. Curative therapy may be possible in those with focal infections and limited lung disease if surgical resection is used in conjunction with a multiple-drug treatment regimen.

For the treatment of rifampin-resistant *M. kansasii*† infections, the ATS and IDSA recommend a 3-drug regimen based on results of in vitro susceptibility testing, including clarithromycin (or azithromycin), moxifloxacin, ethambutol, sulfamethoxazole, or streptomycin.

For the treatment of *M. marinum*† infections, a regimen of clarithromycin and ethambutol has been used. Based on experience in other mycobacterial infections, the ATS and IDSA state that a regimen of azithromycin and ethambutol may be an alternative regimen.

■ **Neisseria meningitidis Infections** Azithromycin has been recommended as an alternative for elimination of nasopharyngeal carriage of *N. meningitidis*†.

The CDC and AAP consider rifampin, ceftriaxone, or ciprofloxacin the drugs of choice to eliminate nasopharyngeal carriage of *N. meningitidis* and for postexposure prophylaxis in household or other close contacts of patients with invasive meningococcal disease. Although further study is needed, the CDC suggests that azithromycin can be used as an alternative in areas where ciprofloxacin-resistant *N. meningitidis* have been reported (e.g., Minnesota, North Dakota).

■ **Nongonococcal Urethritis** Azithromycin is used orally for the treatment of nongonococcal urethritis (NGU). CDC currently considers oral azithromycin (a single 1-g dose as a conventional formulation) or oral doxycycline (100 mg twice daily for 7 days) to be the regimens of choice for the treatment of NGU. In a randomized, double-blind, comparative study in men with nongonococcal urethritis, a single 1-g oral dose of azithromycin as a conventional formulation was as effective as a 7-day course of doxycycline; in addition, clinical cure rates were comparable with either regimen regardless of the presence or absence of *Chlamydia* or *Ureaplasma* infection.

■ **Pelvic Inflammatory Disease** IV azithromycin is used for the treatment of acute pelvic inflammatory disease (PID) caused by *C. trachomatis*, *Mycoplasma hominis*, or *N. gonorrhoeae* when initial IV therapy is considered necessary.

Although azithromycin is not included in CDC's recommended or alternative regimens for the treatment of PID, the CDC states that a regimen of azithromycin and metronidazole has demonstrated short-term clinical cure when used in outpatients with PID.

■ **Pertussis** Azithromycin is used for the treatment of pertussis† caused by *Bordetella pertussis* and for postexposure prophylaxis of pertussis in household and other close contacts of an individual with pertussis.

Macrolides (azithromycin, clarithromycin, erythromycin) are the drugs of choice for treatment of pertussis. Although erythromycin traditionally has been considered the drug of choice for treatment and postexposure prophylaxis of pertussis, azithromycin and clarithromycin appear to be as effective and may be associated with better compliance because shorter regimens are required and the drugs are better tolerated than erythromycin.

Treatment For the treatment of pertussis in adults and children 1 month of age or older, the CDC recommends a macrolide (5 days of azithromycin, 7 days of clarithromycin, 14 days of erythromycin). Co-trimoxazole is recommended as an alternative in adults and children 2 months of age or older when a macrolide cannot be used. AAP and CDC state that azithromycin is the preferred macrolide for treatment of pertussis in infants younger than 1 month of age; however, safety and efficacy have not been established in this age group and only limited data are available.

If given during the catarrhal stage of pertussis (approximately 1–2 weeks of nasal congestion, runny nose, mild sore throat, nonproductive cough, minimal or no fever), anti-infectives may reduce the duration and severity of symptoms and lessen the period of communicability. After paroxysmal cough is established, anti-infectives may not affect the course of the illness but are recommended to limit spread of the disease to others.

In a randomized study in children 6 months to 16 years of age with culture-proven *B. pertussis* infection or a cough illness suspected of being pertussis, a 5-day regimen of oral azithromycin (10 mg/kg on day 1 and 5 mg/kg once daily on days 2–5) was as effective and better tolerated than a 10-day regimen of oral erythromycin (40 mg/kg daily).

Prevention All household and other close contacts of an individual with suspected pertussis should receive anti-infective postexposure prophylaxis, regardless of age or vaccination status. Prophylaxis should be initiated within 21 days of exposure; if more than 21 days have elapsed since onset of cough in the index patient, prophylaxis has limited value but should be considered for those in households with high-risk contacts (e.g., young infants, pregnant women, individuals with contact with infants). In addition, all close contacts who are unvaccinated or incompletely vaccinated against pertussis should receive age-appropriate vaccination with a preparation containing pertussis antigens.

■ **Scrub Typhus** Azithromycin is recommended as an alternative for the treatment of scrub typhus caused by *Orientia tsutsugamushi* (formerly *Rickettsia tsutsugamushi*). The usual drug of choice for these infections is doxycycline; alternatives are chloramphenicol or a fluoroquinolone. Some clinicians suggest that azithromycin may be a preferred alternative for treatment of scrub typhus in children or pregnant women or when scrub typhus was acquired in areas where doxycycline-resistant *O. tsutsugamushi* have been reported (e.g., South Korea, Thailand).

■ **Spirochetal Infections** ***Lyme Disease*** Azithromycin has been used in the treatment of early Lyme disease†, a spirochetal infection caused by tick-borne *Borrelia burgdorferi*. However, some evidence in patients with early Lyme disease suggests that azithromycin or erythromycin may be less effective than penicillins or tetracyclines, and the IDSA, AAP, and other clinicians recommend that macrolide antibiotics *not* be used as first-line therapy for early Lyme disease. Results of a randomized, controlled study in patients with erythema migrans (localized skin lesion associated with early Lyme disease) suggest that a 20-day regimen of oral amoxicillin is more effective than a 7-day regimen of oral azithromycin (500 mg daily).

Oral doxycycline or oral amoxicillin is recommended as first-line therapy for the treatment of early localized or early disseminated Lyme disease associated with erythema migrans, in the absence of neurologic involvement or third-degree atrioventricular (AV) heart block; alternatively, oral cefuroxime axetil has been used. The IDSA and other clinicians state that macrolide antibiotics should be reserved for patients who are intolerant of doxycycline, amoxicillin, and cefuroxime axetil and that patients treated with macrolides should be monitored closely. For more detailed information on the manifestations of Lyme disease and the efficacy of various anti-infective regimens in early or late Lyme disease, see Lyme Disease in Uses: Spirochetal Infections, in the Tetracyclines General Statement 8:12.24.

Syphilis Although penicillin G is the drug of choice for the treatment of all stages of syphilis, the CDC, NIH, and IDSA state that oral azithromycin can be considered as a possible alternative for the treatment of primary, secondary, or early latent syphilis† in nonpregnant adults and adolescents who are hypersensitive to penicillin if close follow-up can be ensured.

There is evidence that a single 2-g dose of a conventional formulation of azithromycin can be effective for the treatment of early syphilis in some patients. Single-dose azithromycin regimens are being investigated for treatment of syphilis in disease-control programs, including mass treatment programs. However, efficacy is not well documented (especially in HIV-infected individuals) and resistance and treatment failures have been reported. In addition, a mutation that is associated with in vivo resistance to azithromycin has been identified in some *T. pallidum* isolates. (See Resistance: Resistance in Neisseria and Treponema.) Therefore, azithromycin should be used for the treatment of syphilis with caution and only if close follow-up can be ensured. If compliance and follow-up cannot be ensured, patients with penicillin hypersensitivity should be desensitized and treated with penicillin G.

Azithromycin is *not* included in CDC recommendations for the treatment of any other form of syphilis, including late latent syphilis, latent syphilis of unknown duration, tertiary syphilis, or neurosyphilis. In addition, azithromycin is *not* recommended by the CDC or others for the treatment of syphilis in pregnant women or for the treatment of congenital syphilis in neonates, infants, or older children.

■ **Toxoplasmosis** Azithromycin has been used alone and in conjunction with pyrimethamine and leucovorin for the treatment of infections caused by *Toxoplasma gondii*†, including toxoplasmic encephalitis in HIV-infected patients. Azithromycin also has been used in conjunction with pyrimethamine for the treatment of ocular toxoplasmosis†.

The CDC, NIH, IDSA, and other clinicians usually recommend a regimen of pyrimethamine in conjunction with sulfadiazine and leucovorin for the treatment of toxoplasmosis in adults and children, especially in immunocompromised patients (e.g., HIV-infected individuals). These clinicians state that azithromycin in conjunction with pyrimethamine and leucovorin is one of several alternative regimens that can be considered in adults when the regimen of choice cannot be used; however, the azithromycin regimen has not been evaluated for the treatment of toxoplasmosis in children.

For information on recommendations regarding treatment and prophylaxis of toxoplasmosis, see Toxoplasmosis under Uses: Pyrimethamine, in Pyrimethamine and Sulfadoxine and Pyrimethamine 8:30.08.

■ Typhoid Fever and Other Salmonella Infections Azithromycin has been used in adults or children for the treatment of uncomplicated typhoid fever† caused by susceptible *Salmonella*. Fluoroquinolones (e.g., ciprofloxacin, ofloxacin) usually are considered the drugs of choice for the treatment of typhoid fever or other severe *Salmonella* infections, especially in areas where multidrug-resistant strains (strains resistant to ampicillin, co-trimoxazole, chloramphenicol) are reported; third generation cephalosporins (cefotaxime, ceftriaxone, cefixime) and azithromycin are considered alternatives (e.g., for fluoroquinolone-resistant strains).

When oral azithromycin was used in children 3–17 years of age with uncomplicated typhoid fever, the mean time to defervescence was 4.1–4.5 days and the microbiologic cure rate was 97%.

■ Prevention of Bacterial Endocarditis Azithromycin is recommended for prevention of α-hemolytic (viridans group) streptococcal bacterial endocarditis† in penicillin-allergic adults and children with certain cardiac conditions who are undergoing certain dental procedures (i.e., procedures that involve manipulation of gingival tissue, the periapical region of teeth, or perforation of oral mucosa) or certain invasive respiratory tract procedures (i.e., procedures involving incision or biopsy of respiratory mucosa).

The American Heart Association (AHA) generally recommends routine use of prophylactic anti-infectives prior to certain procedures only in patients with cardiac conditions that are associated with the highest risk of adverse outcome from endocarditis, including congenital heart disease, prosthetic heart valves, cardiac valvulopathy after cardiac transplant, and previous bacterial endocarditis. The AHA no longer recommends prophylaxis against bacterial endocarditis based solely on an increased lifetime risk of acquisition of infective endocarditis. When selecting anti-infectives for prophylaxis of bacterial endocarditis, the current recommendations published by the AHA should be consulted.

■ Prophylaxis in Sexual Assault Victims Azithromycin is used in conjunction with IM ceftriaxone and oral metronidazole for empiric anti-infective prophylaxis in adult or adolescent victims of sexual assault†. The CDC states that trichomoniasis, genital chlamydial infection, gonorrhea, and bacterial vaginosis are the sexually transmitted diseases (STDs) most commonly diagnosed in women following sexual assault; however, the prevalence of these infections is substantial among sexually active women, and their presence after assault does not necessarily indicate that the infections were acquired during the assault. Chlamydial and gonococcal infections among females are of special concern because of the possibility of ascending infection.

Many experts recommend routine empiric prophylactic therapy after a sexual assault, and use of such prophylaxis probably benefits most patients since follow-up of assault victims can be difficult and such prophylaxis allays the patient's concerns about possible infections. When empiric anti-infective prophylaxis is indicated in adult or adolescent sexual assault victims, the CDC recommends administration of a single 125-mg IM dose of ceftriaxone given in conjunction with a single 2-g oral dose of metronidazole and a single 1-g oral dose of a conventional formulation of azithromycin or a 7-day regimen of oral doxycycline (100 mg twice daily). This 3-drug regimen provides coverage against gonorrhea, chlamydia, trichomoniasis, and bacterial vaginosis, but efficacy in preventing these infections after sexual assault has not been specifically evaluated.Because of possible adverse GI effects with the 3-drug regimen, the CDC suggests that the patient be counseled regarding the possible benefits, as well as the possibility of toxicity, of such prophylaxis. Alternative regimens may be required for some patients because of the likelihood of transmission of other STDs from the assailant.

Postexposure hepatitis B vaccination also is recommended for sexual assault victims who have not previously received the vaccine; hepatitis B vaccine (without hepatitis B immune globulin) should be given to susceptible victims at the time of the initial examination. The CDC states that although a definitive recommendation concerning the appropriateness of antiretroviral prophylaxis against HIV cannot be made based on currently available information, such prophylaxis should be considered in cases in which the risk for HIV exposure during the assault is considered high. The decision to offer such prophylaxis should be individualized taking into account the probability of HIV transmission from a single act of intercourse and the nature of the assault (e.g., extent and site of physical trauma and exposure to ejaculate), the potential benefits and risks of prophylaxis, and the time interval between the exposure and initiation of therapy. (See Guidelines for Use of Antiretroviral Agents: Postexposure Prophylaxis following Sexual Assault or Nonoccupational Exposures to HIV, in the Antiretroviral Agents General Statement 8:18.08.)

There are few data available to establish the risk of a child acquiring a sexually transmitted disease as a result of sexual assault or abuse. The risk is believed to be low in most circumstances, although documentation to support this position is inadequate. The CDC currently states that presumptive treatment for children who have been sexually assaulted or abused is not widely recommended because girls appear to be at lower risk for ascending infection than adolescent or adult women and regular follow-up usually can be ensured. Even if the risk is perceived by the health-care provider to be low, some children or their parents or guardians may have concerns about the possibility of the child contracting a sexually transmitted disease as a result of the assault, and these concerns may be an appropriate indication for presumptive treatment in some settings, but only after appropriate specimens for STD testing have been obtained.

Dosage and Administration

■ Reconstitution and Administration Azithromycin is administered orally. or by IV infusion. Azithromycin should *not* be given by direct IV injection or IM.

Oral Administration For oral administration, azithromycin is commercially available as conventional film-coated tablets, conventional powder for oral suspension, and *extended-release* microspheres for oral suspension.

The extended-release oral suspension is *not* bioequivalent to and is *not* interchangeable with conventional oral suspension or tablets.

Reconstituted conventional oral suspension containing 100 or 200 mg of azithromycin per 5 mL and reconstituted single-dose packets of conventional oral suspension containing 1 g of azithromycin can be taken with or without food.

Azithromycin conventional tablets can be taken with or without food; tolerability may be increased when tablets are taken with food.

Reconstituted conventional oral suspension containing 100 or 200 mg of azithromycin per 5 mL may be taken without regard to food. The safety of repeating a dose in children who vomit after receiving 30 mg/kg as a single dose has not been established. The single-dose 1-g packets should *not* be used to administer doses other than 1 g and are *not* for pediatric use.

Reconstituted extended-release oral suspension containing 2 g of azithromycin (Zmax®) should be taken as a single dose on an empty stomach (at least 1 hour before or 2 hours after a meal). Patients should be advised to contact a clinician if they vomit within 1 hour of taking a dose of the extended-release oral suspension. If the patient vomits within 5 minutes of taking the 2-g dose of the extended-release oral suspension, additional anti-infective treatment should be considered because only minimal absorption of the drug would have occurred. If the patient vomits within 5–60 minutes after taking the dose, alternative treatment should be considered because data are insufficient regarding absorption of the drug under these circumstances. If a patient with normal gastric emptying vomits at least 60 minutes after taking the 2-g dose, additional azithromycin doses or alternative treatments are not required.

Although the single-dose extended-release oral suspension of azithromycin (Zmax®) may be taken without regard to antacids containing magnesium hydroxide and/or aluminum hydroxide, conventional oral azithromycin preparations (film-coated tablets, oral suspension) should *not* be taken simultaneously with aluminum- or magnesium-containing antacids.

Reconstitution. For reconstitution of azithromycin for oral suspension in single-dose packets, the contents of a 1-g packet should be mixed thoroughly with 60 mL of water and the entire contents ingested immediately; an additional 60 mL of water should be added, mixed, and the entire contents ingested to ensure complete consumption of the dose. Single-dose packets of azithromycin for oral suspension are *not* for pediatric use and should not be used for administration of azithromycin doses other than 1 g.

Azithromycin for multiple-dose oral suspension should be reconstituted at the time of dispensing by adding 9 mL of water to a bottle labeled as containing 300 mg of azithromycin to obtain a suspension containing 100 mg of azithromycin per 5 mL or by adding 9, 12, or 15 mL of water to a bottle labeled as containing 600 mg, 900 mg, or 1.2 g of azithromycin, respectively, to obtain a suspension containing 200 mg/5 mL. The bottle should be kept tightly closed and should be shaken well before each use.

Azithromycin single-dose extended-release oral suspension (Zmax®) should be reconstituted at the time of dispensing by adding 60 mL of water to the bottle labeled as containing 2 g of azithromycin. The reconstituted suspension should be shaken well at the time of dispensing and immediately prior to consumption; the entire contents of the bottle should be consumed as a single dose. The single-dose extended-release oral suspension is *not* for pediatric use.

IV Infusion Azithromycin for IV infusion must be reconstituted and then further diluted prior to administration.

Other IV substances, additives, or other drugs should not be added to azithromycin IV infusions and should not be infused simultaneously through the same IV line.

Reconstitution and Dilution. For IV infusion, azithromycin for injection should be reconstituted by adding 4.8 mL of sterile water for injection to a vial labeled as containing 500 mg of the drug to provide a solution containing azithromycin 100 mg/mL. Since azithromycin for injection is supplied under vacuum, the manufacturer recommends that a standard 5 mL (non-automated) syringe be used to ensure that exactly 4.8 mL of sterile water for injection is added during reconstitution. Reconstituted solutions should be further diluted prior to administration with 250 or 500 mL of a compatible IV solution to a concentration of 2 or 1 mg/mL.

Prior to administration, azithromycin solutions should be inspected visually for particulate matter; if particulate matter is evident in reconstituted fluids, the solution should be discarded. Azithromycin should not be admixed with other drugs or infused simultaneously through the same tubing with other drugs.

Rate of Administration. IV solutions containing azithromycin in a concentration of 1 mg/mL generally are infused over 3 hours, and solutions containing azithromycin 2 mg/mL generally are infused over 1 hour. The manufacturer states that solutions containing a 500-mg dose of azithromycin should be infused over a period of at least 1 hour.

■ Dosage

Dosage of azithromycin, which is commercially available for oral and IV use as the dihydrate, is expressed in terms of anhydrous azithromycin.

Two 250-mg tablets of azithromycin are bioequivalent to one 500-mg tablet. The extended-release oral suspension is *not* bioequivalent to and is *not* interchangeable with the conventional oral suspension or tablets.

Adult Dosage

Pharyngitis and Tonsillitis. The usual oral dosage of azithromycin in adults for the treatment of pharyngitis or tonsillitis (as second-line therapy) is 500 mg given as a single dose on the first day of therapy, followed by 250 mg once daily on days 2-5 (total cumulative dose: 1.5 g administered over 5 days).

Acute Sinusitis. For the treatment of acute sinusitis, the usual adult oral dosage of azithromycin tablets or conventional oral suspension is 500 mg once daily for 3 days.

If the extended-release oral suspension (Zmax®) is used for the treatment of acute sinusitis, adults should receive a single 2-g dose.

Acute Exacerbations of Chronic Bronchitis. For the treatment of mild to moderate acute bacterial exacerbations of chronic bronchitis, the usual adult dosage of azithromycin is 500 mg once daily for 3 days or, alternatively, 500 mg given as a single dose on the first day of therapy followed by 250 mg once daily on days 2–5 (total cumulative dose: 1.5 g administered over 5 days).

Community-acquired Pneumonia. For the treatment of mild to moderate community-acquired pneumonia (CAP) in adults, the usual dosage of azithromycin is 500 mg given as a single dose on the first day of therapy, followed by 250 mg once daily on days 2–5 (total cumulative dose: 1.5 g administered over 5 days).

If the extended-release oral suspension (Zmax®) is used for the treatment of mild to moderate CAP, adults should receive a single 2-g dose.

For the treatment of CAP in adults or adolescents 16 years of age or older who require initial IV therapy, 500 mg of azithromycin is given IV as a single daily dose for 2 days. IV therapy generally is followed by oral azithromycin given as a single, daily 500-mg dose to complete a 7–10 days of therapy. The timing of the change from IV to oral therapy should be individualized by the clinician, taking into account the clinical response of the patient.

Skin and Skin Structure Infections. The usual oral dosage of azithromycin in adults for the treatment of uncomplicated skin and skin structure infections is 500 mg given as a single dose on the first day of therapy, followed by 250 mg once daily on days 2–5 (total cumulative dose 1.5 g administered over 5 days).

Babesiosis. For the treatment of babesiosis† caused by *Babesia microti*, the Infectious Diseases Society of America (IDSA) recommends an azithromycin dosage of 0.5–1 g once on day 1, then 250 mg once daily for a total of 7–10 days in conjunction with atovaquone (750 mg twice daily for 7–10 days). Higher azithromycin dosage (0.6–1 g daily) may be used in immunocompromised patients.

Other clinicians recommend that adults receive oral azithromycin in a dosage of 600 mg once daily for 7–10 days given in conjunction with atovaquone (750 mg twice daily for 7–10 days).

Bartonella Infections. If oral azithromycin is used for the treatment of cat scratch disease† caused by *Bartonella henselae*† in patients with extensive lymphadenopathy, some clinicians recommend an initial dose of 500 mg on day 1 followed by 250 mg once daily on days 2–5.

If oral azithromycin is used for the treatment of infections caused by *Bartonella*† in HIV-infected adults and adolescents, the US Centers for Disease Control and Prevention (CDC), National Institutes of Health (NIH), and IDSA recommend a dosage of 600 mg once daily for at least 3 months. If relapse occurs, lifelong secondary prophylaxis (chronic maintenance therapy) with erythromycin or doxycycline should be considered.

Campylobacter Infections. If oral azithromycin is used for the treatment of mild to moderate infections caused by *Campylobacter jejuni*† in adults and adolescents, the CDC, NIH, and IDSA recommend a dosage of 500 mg once daily for 7 days. If bacteremia is present, treatment should be continued for at least 2 weeks and use of a second anti-infective (e.g., an aminoglycoside) should be considered.

Chancroid. For the treatment of chancroid, the usual oral dosage of azithromycin in adults or adolescents is 1 g administered as a single dose of a conventional formulation.

Because data on the efficacy of the single-dose azithromycin regimen for treatment of chancroid in patients with HIV infection are limited, the CDC recommends that the single-dose regimen be used in HIV-infected patients only if follow-up can be ensured. (See Uses: Chancroid.)

Chlamydial Infections. For the treatment of uncomplicated chlamydial infections, including nongonococcal urethritis or cervicitis, the usual oral dosage of azithromycin for adults or adolescents is 1 g administered as a single dose of a conventional formulation. The 1-g dose may be administered using one single-dose packet of azithromycin for oral suspension or four 250-mg tablets. Limited evidence indicates that lower doses (e.g., a single 500-mg dose) of azithromycin may be associated with a high failure rate in, and therefore are *not* recommended for the treatment of uncomplicated chlamydial infections.

For the treatment of recurrent or persistent urethritis, the CDC recommends a single 1-g dose of azithromycin in conjunction with a single 2-g dose of oral metronidazole or tinidazole.

For the treatment of ocular trachoma†, the usual dosage of azithromycin for adults is 20 mg/kg (up to 1 g) given as a single dose. Alternatively, a dosage of 1 g once weekly for 3 weeks has been used. The single-dose regimen has been used in mass treatment programs; however, multiple doses (e.g., once yearly for 3 years) may be necessary to minimize reservoirs of infection in high-prevalence areas.

Cholera. For the treatment of cholera caused by *Vibrio cholerae* O1 or O139, adults have received oral azithromycin in a dosage of 1 g given as a single dose.

Cryptosporidiosis. For the symptomatic treatment of cryptosporidiosis† in HIV-infected adults and adolescents, oral azithromycin has been given in a dosage of 600 mg once daily for 4 weeks in conjunction with oral paromomycin (1 g twice daily for 12 weeks).

Gonorrhea and Associated Infections. For the treatment of uncomplicated gonorrhea (urethritis or cervicitis) caused by *Neisseria gonorrhoeae* when the drugs of choice cannot be used, adults may receive a single 2-g dose of azithromycin as a conventional formulation. Because this single-dose regimen has been associated with a relatively high incidence of adverse GI effects, the patient should be observed for at least 30 minutes after ingesting the dose. Taking the dose with food may minimize adverse effects; an antiemetic may be needed.

Because of concerns regarding rapid emergence of macrolide resistance, azithromycin should *not* be given in a lower dosage and should be used for the treatment of gonorrhea only when considered necessary.

Granuloma Inguinale (Donovanosis). For the treatment of granuloma inguinale† (donovanosis), CDC recommends an oral azithromycin dosage of 1 g once weekly for at least 3 weeks or until all lesions have healed completely. Some experts recommend that patients receive an aminoglycoside (e.g., gentamicin 1 mg/kg IV every 8 hours) concomitantly if they are HIV-infected or if improvement is not evident within the first few days of treatment. Despite effective anti-infective therapy, relapse may occur 6–18 months later.

Legionella Infections. For the treatment of Legionnaires' disease†, some clinicians recommend that oral or IV azithromycin be given in a dosage of 500 mg once daily. The usual duration of azithromycin therapy is 3–5 days for the treatment of mild to moderate infections in immunocompetent patients; however, a longer duration of treatment (at least 7–10 days or 3 weeks) may be necessary to prevent relapse in those with more severe infections or with underlying comorbidity or immunodeficiency.

Leptospirosis. For the treatment of leptospirosis† caused by *Leptospira*, adults have received oral azithromycin in a dosage of 1 g as a single dose on day 1 followed by 500 mg once daily for 2 days. Alternatively, a dosage of 15 mg/kg daily in 2 divided doses for 7 days has been used.

Lyme Disease. For the treatment of early localized or early disseminated Lyme disease† associated with erythema migrans, in the absence of neurologic involvement or third-degree AV heart block, when first-line agents (oral doxycycline, amoxicillin, or cefuroxime) cannot be used, the IDSA suggests that adults receive an oral azithromycin dosage of 500 mg once daily for 7–10 days. The patient should be monitored closely to ensure resolution of clinical manifestations since macrolides generally are less effective for treatment of Lyme disease than first-line agents.

Lymphogranuloma Venereum. For the treatment of lymphogranuloma venereum† caused by invasive serotypes of *C. trachomatis* (serovars L1, L2, L3), 1 g of azithromycin orally once weekly for 3 weeks may be effective.

Mycobacterium avium Complex (MAC) Infections (Primary Prophylaxis of Disseminated Infection). For primary prevention of disseminated *Mycobacterium avium* complex (MAC) infection (primary prophylaxis) in adults and adolescents with advanced HIV infection, the usual oral dosage of azithromycin is 1.2 g once weekly. Azithromycin usually is given alone for primary prophylaxis against MAC, but has been given in conjunction with rifabutin. (See Dosage and Administration: Dosage, in Rifabutin 8:16.04.)

The ATS, IDSA, and others recommend primary prophylaxis against disseminated MAC infection in HIV-infected adults and adolescents with CD4+ T-cell counts less than 50/mm³. Although consideration can be given to discontinuing such prophylaxis in adults and adolescents when there is immune recovery in response to potent antiretroviral therapy and an increase in CD4+ T-cell count to greater than 100/mm³ that has been sustained for at least 3 months (see Primary Prevention of Disseminated MAC Infection under Uses: Mycobacterium avium Complex [MAC] Infections), primary MAC prophylaxis should be restarted if the CD4+ T-cell count decreases to less than 50–100/mm³.

Mycobacterium avium Complex (MAC) Infections (Treatment and Prevention of Recurrence of Disseminated Infection). For the treatment of disseminated MAC infection in adults, the manufacturer recommends an azithromycin dosage of 600 mg once daily in conjunction with ethambutol (15 mg/kg daily); additional antimycobacterial drugs may be added to the regimen at the discretion of the clinician. The ATS, CDC, NIH, and IDSA recommend a regimen of 500–600 mg of oral azithromycin once daily in conjunction with ethambutol (15 mg/kg once daily) with or without rifabutin (300 mg once daily) in HIV-infected adults and adolescents.

For prevention of recurrence† (secondary prophylaxis or chronic maintenance therapy) of disseminated MAC in HIV-infected adults or adolescents who responded to treatment, the ATS, CDC, NIH, and IDSA recommend that adults and adolescents receive azithromycin in a dosage of 500–600 mg once daily in conjunction with ethambutol (15 mg/kg once daily) with or without rifabutin (300 mg once daily). Secondary MAC prophylaxis in HIV-infected individuals usually is continued for life. However, consideration may be given to discontinuing secondary MAC prophylaxis in adults and adolescents when there is immune recovery in response to potent antiretroviral therapy (see Treatment and Prevention of Recurrence of Disseminated MAC Infection under Uses: Mycobacterium avium Complex [MAC] Infections), but such prophylaxis should be restarted if $CD4^+$ T-cell counts decrease to less than 100/mm^3.

Mycobacterium avium Complex (MAC) Infections (Treatment of Pulmonary Infections). For initial treatment of pulmonary MAC infections (nodular/bronchiectatic disease) caused by macrolide-susceptible strains, ATS and IDSA recommend an azithromycin dosage of 500–600 mg 3 times weekly in conjunction with ethambutol (25 mg/kg 3 times weekly) and rifampin (600 mg 3 times weekly). The regimen should be continued until the patient has been culture negative on treatment for 1 year. An intermittent (3-times weekly) regimen is not recommended for those with cavitary or moderate or severe disease or those who have been previously treated.

For initial treatment of pulmonary MAC infections (fibrocavitary or severe nodular/bronchiectatic disease) caused by macrolide-susceptible strains, ATS and IDSA recommend an azithromycin regimen of 250–300 mg once daily in conjunction with ethambutol (15 mg/kg once daily) and either rifampin (450–600 mg once daily) or rifabutin (150–300 mg once daily). The regimen should be continued until the patient has been culture negative on treatment for 1 year. Consideration can be given to including amikacin or streptomycin 3-times weekly during the first 2–3 months of treatment for extensive disease, especially fibrocavitary disease, or when previous therapy has failed.

Mycobacterium abscessus Infections. For the treatment of infections caused by *M. abscessus*, azithromycin may be given in a dosage of 250 mg daily in conjunction with parenteral amikacin, cefoxitin, or imipenem. The duration of therapy should be at least 4 months for serious infections; a duration of 6 months is recommended for bone infections.

Neisseria meningitidis Infections. For elimination of nasopharyngeal carriage of *Neisseria meningitidis*, azithromycin may be given in a dosage of 500 mg as a single dose.

Nongonococcal Urethritis. For the treatment of nongonococcal urethritis, the usual oral dosage of azithromycin in men is 1 g administered as a single dose.

Pelvic Inflammatory Disease. For the treatment of acute pelvic inflammatory disease (PID) in patients requiring initial IV therapy, 500 mg of azithromycin is given IV as a single daily dose for 1–2 days. If anaerobic bacteria are suspected, an anti-infective active against anaerobes should also be used. IV therapy generally is followed by oral azithromycin 250 mg once daily to complete a 7-day course of therapy. The timing of the change from IV to oral therapy should be individualized by the clinician, taking into account clinical response of the patient.

Pertussis. For the treatment of pertussis† or for postexposure prophylaxis of pertussis†, the CDC and AAP recommend that adults and adolescents receive an initial azithromycin dose of 500 mg once on day 1 followed by 250 mg once daily on days 2–5.

When postexposure prophylaxis of pertussis is indicated, it should be initiated within 3 weeks of exposure or onset of cough in the index patient.

Scrub Typhus. For the treatment of scrub typhus caused by *Orientia tsutsugamushi* (formerly *Rickettsia tsutsugamushi*), azithromycin has been given in a dosage of 500 mg as a single dose. Alternatively, 1 g has been given as a single dose on day 1 followed by 500 mg once daily for 2 days.

Syphilis. If azithromycin is used as an alternative agent for the treatment of primary, secondary, or early latent syphilis† in nonpregnant adults or adolescents hypersensitive to penicillins, the CDC and others recommend a single 2-g oral dose as a conventional formulation. Close follow-up is essential since efficacy is not well documented.

Shigella Infections. If oral azithromycin is used for the treatment of shigellosis† in adults, an initial dose of 500 mg should be given on day 1 followed by 250 mg once daily on days 2–5. If bacteremia is present, the drug should be continued for 14 days depending on the severity of infection.

Toxoplasmosis. For the treatment of toxoplasmosis† caused by *Toxoplasma gondii*, the CDC, NIH, IDSA, and other clinicians state that adults and adolescents can receive azithromycin in a dosage of 900–1200 mg once daily in conjunction with pyrimethamine and leucovorin given for at least 6 weeks. A longer duration of treatment may be appropriate if the disease is extensive or the response is incomplete at 6 weeks.

Travelers' Diarrhea. If oral azithromycin is used in the empiric treatment of travelers' diarrhea†, some clinicians suggest that adults receive a single 1-g dose as a conventional formulation or, alternatively, 500 mg once daily for 3 days.

Typhoid Fever and Other Salmonella Infections. For the treatment of uncomplicated typhoid fever† caused by susceptible *Salmonella*, adults have received oral azithromycin in a dosage of 1 g once daily for 5 days. A dosage of 8–10 mg/kg (up to 500 mg) once daily for 7 days also has been recommended.

Prevention of Bacterial Endocarditis. When an oral regimen is indicated for the prevention of bacterial endocarditis† in penicillin-allergic adults at risk undergoing certain dental or respiratory tract procedures likely to cause transient bacteremia, the American Heart Association (AHA) states that adults can receive a single azithromycin dose of 500 mg given 30–60 minutes prior to the procedure.

Prophylaxis in Sexual Assault Victims. For empiric anti-infective prophylaxis in adult and adolescent victims of sexual assault†, the usual oral dosage of azithromycin is 1 g administered as a single dose as a conventional formulation given in conjunction with other anti-infectives (e.g., IM ceftriaxone and oral metronidazole).

Pediatric Dosage **Acute Otitis Media.** For the treatment of acute otitis media, children 6 months of age or older can receive a single azithromycin dose of 30 mg/kg or a 3-day regimen of 10 mg/kg once daily. Alternatively, 5-day regimen can be used consisting of 10 mg/kg given once on day 1 followed by 5 mg/kg once daily on days 2–5.

The manufacturer states that the safety of redosing children who vomit after receiving the single 30-mg/kg azithromycin dose has not been established; in clinical studies involving 487 acute otitis media patients, a second 30-mg/kg dose was administered to 8 patients who vomited within 30 minutes of receiving the initial 30-mg/kg dose.

Pharyngitis and Tonsillitis. The usual oral dosage of azithromycin for the treatment of *Streptococcus pyogenes* (group A β-hemolytic streptococci) pharyngitis or tonsillitis in children 2 years of age or older is 12 mg/kg (up to 500 mg) once daily for 5 days.

Acute Sinusitis. The usual oral dosage of azithromycin for the treatment of acute sinusitis in children 6 months of age or older is 10 mg/kg once daily for 3 days.

Community-acquired Pneumonia. The usual oral dosage of azithromycin for the treatment of CAP in children 6 months of age or older is 10 mg/kg dose (maximum 500 mg) given as a single dose on day 1 followed by 5 mg/kg once daily (maximum 250 mg daily) on days 2–5. Efficacy of shorter regimens (e.g., 1-3 days) for the treatment of CAP in children has not been established.

Babesiosis. For the treatment of babesiosis† caused by *Babesia microti*, IDSA recommends that children receive oral azithromycin 10 mg/kg (up to 500 mg) once on day 1, then 5 mg/kg (up to 250 mg) once daily for a total of 7–10 days in conjunction with atovaquone (20 mg/kg [up to 750 mg] twice daily for 7–10 days). Alternatively, some clinicians recommend that pediatric patients receive oral azithromycin in a dosage of 12 mg/kg once daily for 7–10 days given in conjunction with atovaquone (20 mg/kg daily in 2 divided doses for 7–10 days).

Bartonella Infections. If oral azithromycin is used for the treatment of cat scratch disease† caused by *B. henselae*† in children with extensive lymphadenopathy, some clinicians recommend an initial dose of 10 mg/kg on day 1 followed by 5 mg/kg once daily on days 2–5.

Chancroid. For the treatment of chancroid† in infants and children weighing less than 45 kg, the AAP recommends azithromycin 20 mg/kg (maximum 1 g) given as a single oral dose of a conventional formulation. Adolescents and children weighing 45 kg or more should receive 1 g administered as a single dose of a conventional formulation.

Because data on the efficacy of the single-dose azithromycin regimen for treatment of chancroid in patients with HIV infection are limited, the CDC recommends that the single-dose regimen be used in HIV-infected patients only if follow-up can be ensured. (See Uses: Chancroid.)

Chlamydial Infections. When azithromycin is used for the treatment of uncomplicated chlamydial genital tract infection† (urethritis and/or cervicitis), the usual oral dosage for children 8 years of age or older or children younger than 8 years of age who weigh at least 45 kg is a single 1-g dose given as a conventional formulation.

For the treatment of ocular trachoma† in children, oral azithromycin has been given in a dosage of 20 mg/kg (up to 1 g) as a single dose. Alternatively, a dosage of 20 mg/kg once weekly for 3 weeks or 20 mg/kg once every 4 weeks for a total of 6 doses has been used. The single-dose regimen has been used in mass treatment programs; however, multiple doses (e.g., once yearly for 3 years) may be necessary to minimize reservoirs of infection in high-prevalence areas.

Some clinicians suggest that chlamydial pneumonia or ophthalmia neonatorum caused by *C. trachomatis*† can be treated with oral azithromycin given in a dosage of 20 mg/kg once daily for 3 days.

Cryptosporidiosis. For the symptomatic treatment of cryptosporidiosis†, children have received oral azithromycin in a dosage of 10 mg/kg on day 1 followed by 5 mg/kg orally once daily (up to 600 mg daily) on days 2–10. The optimum duration of treatment is unknown; no anti-infective reliably eradicates *Cryptosporidium*.

Escherichia coli Infections. If azithromycin is used for the treatment of severe diarrhea caused by enterotoxigenic *Escherichia coli*† (ETEC) when an anti-infective is considered necessary, some clinicians recommend that children receive oral azithromycin in a dosage of 10 mg/kg once daily for 2 days.

Legionella Infections. For the treatment of legionella infections caused by *Legionella pneumophila*†, AAP recommends that children receive IV azithromycin in a dosage of 10 mg/kg (up to 500 mg) once daily for 5–10 days. If the patient is improving, parenteral therapy may be switched to oral therapy.

Leptospirosis. For the treatment of leptospirosis† caused by *Leptospira*, children 5–18 years of age have received oral azithromycin in a dosage of 15 mg/kg daily in 2 divided doses for 7 days.

Lyme Disease. For the treatment of early localized or early disseminated Lyme disease† associated with erythema migrans, in the absence of neurologic involvement or third-degree AV heart block, when first-line agents (oral doxycycline, amoxicillin, or cefuroxime) cannot be used, the IDSA suggests an oral azithromycin dosage of 10 mg/kg (maximum: 500 mg) once daily for 7–10 days. The patient should be monitored closely to ensure resolution of clinical manifestations since macrolides generally are less effective for treatment of Lyme disease than first-line agents.

Mycobacterium avium Complex (MAC) Infections (Primary Prophylaxis of Disseminated Infection). For primary prevention (primary prophylaxis) of disseminated MAC infections† in infants and children with advanced HIV infection, the usual oral dosage of azithromycin is 20 mg/kg (maximum 1.2 g) once weekly or 5 mg/kg (maximum 250 mg) once daily. In children 6 years of age or older, azithromycin can be given in conjunction with rifabutin (300 mg once daily) for primary prophylaxis against MAC.

Long-term primary prophylaxis against disseminated MAC infection is recommended in severely immunocompromised HIV-infected infants and children (see Primary Prevention of Disseminated MAC Infection under Uses: Mycobacterium avium Complex [MAC] Infections). Primary prophylaxis should be initiated if CD4+ T-cell count is less than 750/mm^3 in those younger than 1 year, less than 500/mm^3 in those 1–2 years, less than 75/mm^3 in those 2–6 years, or less than 50/mm^3 in those 6 years of age or older.

The safety of discontinuing primary MAC prophylaxis in children whose CD4+ T-cell counts have increased as a result of highly active antiretroviral therapy has not been studied to date.

Mycobacterium avium Complex (MAC) Infections (Treatment and Prevention of Recurrence of Disseminated Infection). For treatment of disseminated MAC infections† in HIV-infected children, the CDC, NIH, and IDSA recommend that oral azithromycin be given in a dosage of 10–12 mg/kg once daily (up to 500 mg daily) in conjunction with ethambutol (15–25 mg/kg once daily [up to 1 g daily]) with or without rifabutin (10–20 mg/kg once daily [up to 300 mg daily]).

For prevention of recurrence (secondary prophylaxis or chronic maintenance therapy), an oral azithromycin dosage of 5 mg/kg (maximum 250 mg) once daily in conjunction with ethambutol (15 mg/kg [maximum 900 mg] once daily) with or without rifabutin (5 mg/kg [maximum 300 mg] once daily) is recommended.

The safety of discontinuing secondary MAC prophylaxis in children receiving potent antiretroviral therapy has not been studied to date and HIV-infected children with a history of disseminated MAC should receive lifelong secondary prophylaxis.

Pertussis. For the treatment of pertussis† or for postexposure prophylaxis of pertussis† in children and infants 6 months of age or older, the AAP, CDC, and others recommend an initial azithromycin dose of 10 mg/kg (up to 500 mg) on day 1 followed by 5 mg/kg (up to 250 mg) once daily on days 2–5.

AAP and CDC state that infants 1–5 months of age may receive oral azithromycin in a dosage of 10 mg/kg once daily for 5 days for treatment or postexposure prophylaxis of pertussis. Although only limited data are available in infants younger than 1 month of age, the CDC states that a dosage of 10 mg/kg once daily for 5 days can be used when necessary for treatment or prophylaxis of pertussis in this age group.

When postexposure prophylaxis of pertussis is indicated, it should be initiated within 3 weeks of exposure or onset of cough in the index patient.

Shigella Infections. For the treatment of shigellosis†, children have received oral azithromycin in a dosage of 12 mg/kg (up to 500 mg) on day 1 followed by 6 mg/kg orally once daily (up to 250 mg daily) on days 2–5.

Travelers' Diarrhea. If oral azithromycin is used for empiric treatment of travelers' diarrhea†, some clinicians suggest that children receive 10 mg/kg once daily for 3 days.

Typhoid Fever and Other Salmonella Infections. For the treatment of uncomplicated typhoid fever† caused by susceptible *Salmonella*, children 3–17 years of age have received oral azithromycin in a dosage of 20 mg/kg (up to 1 g) once daily for 5–7 days. An azithromycin dosage of 10 mg/kg (up to 500 mg) once daily for 7 days also has been used.

Prevention of Bacterial Endocarditis. When an oral regimen is indicated for prevention of bacterial endocarditis† in penicillin-allergic children at risk undergoing certain dental or respiratory tract procedures likely to cause transient bacteremia, the AHA states that children can receive a single azithromycin dose of 15 mg/kg (up to 500 mg) given 30–60 minutes prior to the procedure.

■ **Dosage in Renal and Hepatic Impairment** Dosage adjustment is not necessary in patients with renal impairment (glomerular filtration rate 80 mL/minute or less). However, data are limited regarding use of azithromycin in patients with severe renal impairment (glomerular filtration rate less than 10 mL/minute) and the manufacturer states that the drug should be used with caution in these patients.

The pharmacokinetics of azithromycin in patients with hepatic impairment have not been established. The manufacturer states that data are insufficient to make dosage recommendations for patients with hepatic impairment and azithromycin should be used with caution in such patients since the drug is eliminated principally via the liver. Based on results of a limited study in patients with impaired hepatic function, some clinicians state that dosage adjustments are not necessary in patients with class A or B liver cirrhosis.

Cautions

Azithromycin generally is well tolerated. In clinical studies, most adverse effects were mild to moderate in severity and were reversible upon discontinuance of the drug. Limited data from comparative studies suggest that the overall incidence of adverse effects with oral azithromycin therapy is similar to or lower than that with oral erythromycin. As with oral erythromycin, the most common adverse effects of oral azithromycin involve the GI tract.

In addition to effects reported in clinical trials, adverse effects reported in the Cautions section include those reported during postmarketing studies with azithromycin and from case reports for which a causal relationship to the drug may not have been established.

Adverse GI effects (e.g., nausea, vomiting, diarrhea, abdominal pain) and rash are the most frequent adverse effects requiring discontinuance of the drug. The manufacturer states that rate of discontinuance of azithromycin was approximately 0.7% in adults or children receiving a 5-day oral regimen; 0.6% in adults receiving a 3-day oral regimen (500 mg daily); or 1% in children receiving a single 30-mg/kg oral dose or a 3-day oral regimen (10 mg/kg daily). In adults with human immunodeficiency virus (HIV) infection receiving long-term therapy with oral azithromycin (600 mg daily) combined with oral ethambutol for the treatment of *Mycobacterium avium* complex (MAC) infection, the discontinuance rate was 9.1%. The rate of discontinuance of IV azithromycin therapy in adults was 1.2%.

■ **GI Effects** The most frequent adverse effects of azithromycin involve the GI tract (i.e., diarrhea/loose stools, nausea, abdominal pain). While these adverse effects generally are mild to moderate in severity and occur less frequently than with oral erythromycin, adverse GI effects are the most frequent reason for discontinuing azithromycin therapy. Administration of conventional azithromycin tablets or oral suspension with food may improve GI tolerability.

In adults receiving multiple-dose azithromycin regimens, diarrhea/loose stools, nausea, and abdominal pain generally occur in 2–5% of patients. Adverse GI effects have occurred more frequently in patients receiving azithromycin as a single oral dose (1, 1.2, or 2 g) than in those receiving multiple-dose oral regimens. Diarrhea/loose stools or nausea was reported in 7 or 5%, respectively, of adults receiving a single 1-g oral dose of azithromycin and in 12–14 or 4–18%, respectively, of adults receiving a single 2-g oral dose. In adults receiving initial therapy with IV azithromycin followed by oral therapy, diarrhea/loose stools or nausea occurred in 4.3 or 3.9% of those with community-acquired pneumonia, and in 8.5 or 6.6% of those with pelvic inflammatory disease (PID). Diarrhea/loose stools or nausea has been reported in up to 53 or 33%, respectively, of HIV-infected patients receiving the drug for prevention of disseminated MAC infections.

Vomiting was reported in 7 or 2% of adults on the single 2-g dose or single 1-g dose oral regimen, respectively. Vomiting occurred in 1.4% of adults with community-acquired pneumonia who received both IV and oral azithromycin therapy and in 6.7–9% of patients receiving oral azithromycin for prevention of disseminated *M. avium* complex infections. Abdominal pain occurred in 1.9–2.7% of those receiving a regimen that included both IV and oral azithromycin, 5% of those receiving a single 1-g oral dose, 7% of those receiving a single 2-g oral dose, and 27–32.3% of patients receiving azithromycin for prevention of disseminated MAC infections.

Dyspepsia or flatulence occurred in 9 or up to 10.7% of patients receiving azithromycin for prevention of disseminated MAC infections; anorexia was reported in 2.1% of these patients. Anorexia occurred in 1.9% of patients with pelvic inflammatory disease (PID) receiving initial therapy with IV azithromycin followed by oral therapy. Dyspepsia, flatulence, melena, constipation, anorexia, mucositis, enteritis, gastritis, oral candidiasis, pseudomembranous colitis, or vomiting/diarrhea rarely resulting in dehydration has been reported in 1% or less of patients receiving azithromycin for other infections and/or during postmarketing studies. Tongue discoloration has been reported rarely. Taste/smell perversion and/or loss have occurred rarely in patients receiving azithromycin .

In children with otitis media, community-acquired pneumonia, or pharyngitis/tonsillitis receiving oral azithromycin in the recommended regimen, diarrhea/loose stools, vomiting, abdominal pain, or nausea was reported in 2–6, 1–6, 1–3, or 1–2%, respectively.

Treatment with anti-infectives alters normal colon flora and may permit overgrowth of *Clostridium difficile*. *C. difficile*-associated diarrhea and colitis (CDAD; also known as antibiotic-associated diarrhea and colitis or pseudomembranous colitis) has been reported with nearly all anti-infectives, including azithromycin, and may range in severity from mild diarrhea to fatal colitis. Hypertoxin-producing strains of *C. difficile* are associated with increased morbidity and mortality since they may be refractory to anti-infectives and colectomy may be required. (See Cautions: Precautions and Contraindications.)

■ **Dermatologic and Sensitivity Reactions** Serious allergic (i.e., angioedema, anaphylaxis, bronchospasm) and dermatologic (i.e., erythema multiforme, Stevens-Johnson syndrome, toxic epidermal necrolysis) reactions, sometimes resulting in death, have been reported rarely in patients receiving azithromycin. If allergic reactions occur, azithromycin should be discontinued and appropriate therapy initiated. (See Cautions: Precautions and Contraindications.) Allergic symptoms generally resolve following discontinuance of the drug and symptomatic treatment; however, allergic manifestations have reappeared following discontinuance of initial symptomatic treatment in some patients. Patients experiencing serious allergic reactions (i.e., anaphylaxis, angioedema, severe dermatologic reactions) require prolonged periods of observation and symptomatic treatment. The relationship between these prolonged allergic episodes and the long tissue half-life of azithromycin with subsequent prolonged exposure to antigen has not been determined.

Rash, urticaria, pruritus, and photosensitivity have been reported in 1% or less of patients receiving a 5-day regimen of oral azithromycin. Rash or pruritus occurred in 1.9%, and urticaria in 1% or less of adults receiving a regimen that included both IV and oral azithromycin. Pruritus or rash has been reported in up to 4 or 8%, respectively, of patients receiving azithromycin 1.2 g weekly for prevention of disseminated MAC infections. Eczema has been reported rarely during azithromycin therapy.

■ **Local Reactions** Approximately 12% of patients experienced an adverse effect related to IV infusion of azithromycin. Pain at the injection site or local inflammation occurred in 6.5 or 3.1%, respectively, of patients receiving IV azithromycin. The incidence and severity of these local reactions in patients receiving IV azithromycin in 250 mL of fluid (2 mg/mL) infused over 1 hour were essentially the same as those in patients receiving azithromycin in 500 mL of fluid (1 mg/mL) infused over 3 hours.

■ **Hepatic Effects** Elevations in ALT (SGPT), AST (SGOT), or γ-glutamyltransferase (GGT, GGTP) have been reported in 1–2% of adults receiving oral azithromycin; elevations in serum alkaline phosphatase, lactic dehydrogenase (LDH), and/or total bilirubin concentration have been reported in less than 1% of such patients. In patients receiving a regimen that included both IV and oral azithromycin, elevations in ALT or AST were reported in 4–6%, elevations in serum alkaline phosphatase in less than 1%, and elevations in serum bilirubin or LDH concentration in 1–3% of patients. Available follow-up data have revealed that liver function test abnormalities in patients receiving azithromycin therapy generally are reversible. However, azithromycin therapy was discontinued in clinical trials because of treatment-related liver enzyme abnormalities in at least 3 patients receiving a 5-day regimen of oral azithromycin and in less than 2% of patients receiving a regimen that included both IV and oral azithromycin. Elevations in ALT, AST, or serum alkaline phosphatase have been reported in 2–5% of patients receiving azithromycin (1.2 g weekly) for prevention of disseminated MAC infections.

Abnormal liver function, including cholestatic jaundice and hepatitis, and pancreatitis has been reported infrequently in clinical trials or during postmarketing studies with azithromycin. Hepatic necrosis and hepatic failure, sometimes resulting in death, have occurred rarely.

■ **Renal and Genitourinary Effects** Elevation in serum potassium concentration has been reported in 1–2% of adults receiving azithromycin in clinical trials. Elevation in BUN, serum creatinine, or serum phosphate concentration has been reported in less than 1% of adults receiving oral azithromycin, while elevated serum creatinine concentration has been reported in 4–6% of patients receiving IV azithromycin. Available follow-up data revealed that these elevations generally were reversible. Nephritis has been reported in 1% or less of adults receiving azithromycin in clinical studies. Interstitial nephritis and acute renal failure have been reported during postmarketing studies with the drug. Azithromycin was discontinued because of an unspecified renal function abnormality in at least one patient receiving the drug in clinical trials.

Vaginitis has been reported in about 1–2.8% of women receiving azithromycin; candidiasis, including oral moniliasis, has been reported in 1% or less of adults receiving the drug.

■ **Cardiovascular Effects** Palpitations, chest pain, edema hypotension, or syncope has been reported in 1% or less of patients receiving oral azithromycin. While not directly attributed to azithromycin therapy, arrhythmia (including ventricular tachycardia) has been reported in at least one patient receiving the drug. In one patient with a history of arrhythmia, torsades de pointes with subsequent myocardial infarction occurred following completion of azithromycin therapy. FDA states that azithromycin can cause abnormal changes in the electrical activity of the heart that may lead to a potentially fatal irregular heart rhythm. Patients at particular risk for developing this condition include those with known risk factors such as existing QT interval prolongation, low blood concentrations of potassium or magnesium, a slower than normal heart rate, or use of certain drugs used to treat abnormal heart rhythms, or arrhythmias. (See Cautions: Precautions and Contraindications.)

■ **Nervous System Effects** Adverse CNS effects reported in 1% or less of adults receiving azithromycin include dizziness, headache, vertigo, or somnolence, and those reported in 1% or less of children include headache, hyperkinesia, dizziness, agitation, nervousness, fatigue, malaise, and insomnia. Fatigue or malaise has been reported and has occurred in 2–4 or about 1%, respectively, of patients receiving azithromycin 1.2 g weekly. Seizures also have been reported during azithromycin therapy. Dizziness or headache has occurred in about 1–4% of patients receiving azithromycin (1.2 g weekly) for the prevention of disseminated MAC infections. Asthenia, aggressive reaction, anxiety, or paresthesia has been reported during postmarketing studies with azithromycin.

■ **Hematologic Effects** Anemia, leukopenia, neutropenia, neutrophilia, or thrombocytopenia has been reported in less than 1% of adults receiving azithromycin, although a causal relationship to the drug has not been established. In studies in patients receiving azithromycin for prevention of disseminated MAC infections, a hemoglobin concentration less than 8 g/dL was reported in 2% of patients, platelet count less than 50,000/mm^3 in 2%, leukocyte count less than 1000/mm^3 in 3%, or neutrophil count less than 500/mm^3 in 4%.

■ **Otic Effects** While audiometric testing revealed no drug-related hearing abnormalities in a limited number of individuals receiving short-term therapy with oral azithromycin (1.5 g over 5 days or 1 g as a single dose), hearing loss has been reported in some patients receiving long-term high-dose azithromycin therapy (i.e., 500–600 mg daily for up to 9 months). In one study in HIV-infected adults evaluating azithromycin (600 mg daily) in conjunction with ethambutol for the treatment of disseminated MAC infections, reversible hearing loss was reported in 5% of patients. Hearing loss generally develops within 1.5–20 weeks and generally resolves within 5 weeks following discontinuance of azithromycin. Hearing loss, deafness, or tinnitus also has been reported during postmarketing studies.

■ **Other Adverse Effects** Fever or conjunctivitis has been reported in 1% or less of children receiving azithromycin. In patients receiving azithromycin for the prevention of disseminated MAC infections, fever or arthralgia occurred in about 1–3% of patients; fever has been reported in 1% or less of patients receiving the drug for other indications. Arthralgia also has been reported during postmarketing studies with azithromycin. Hypothermia has occurred in a few patients receiving azithromycin.

Increases in serum creatine kinase (CK, creatine phosphokinase, CPK) have occurred in 1–2% of patients receiving oral azithromycin, and increases in blood glucose concentration have been reported in less than 1% of patients.

Hyponatremia and/or the syndrome of inappropriate antidiuretic hormone (SIADH) secretion, has been reported rarely with azithromycin therapy; a causal relationship to the drug has not been established.

■ **Increased Risk of Cancer Relapse with Long-Term Use after Donor Stem Cell Transplant** In August 2018, FDA stated that azithromycin should not be given long-term to prevent bronchiolitis obliterans syndrome in patients with cancers of the blood or lymph nodes who undergo a donor stem cell transplant. Results of a clinical trial found an increased rate of relapse in cancers affecting the blood and lymph nodes, including death, in these patients. Azithromycin is not approved for preventing bronchiolitis obliterans syndrome.

FDA states that health care professionals should not prescribe long-term azithromycin for prophylaxis of bronchiolitis obliterans syndrome to patients who undergo donor stem cell transplants because of the increased potential for cancer relapse and death. Patients who have had a stem cell transplant should not stop taking azithromycin without first consulting with their health care professional. FDA is reviewing additional data and will communicate its conclusions and recommendations when the review is complete.

■ **Effects on Phospholipids** Phospholipidosis (intracellular phospholipid accumulation) has been observed in some tissues of mice, rats, and dogs given multiple doses of azithromycin. Such phospholipid accumulation has been demonstrated in numerous organ systems (e.g., eye, dorsal root ganglia, liver, gallbladder, kidney, spleen, pancreas) in dogs at azithromycin doses approximately equivalent to twice the recommended adult human dose (on a mg/kg basis) and in rats at doses comparable to the recommended adult human dose. Phospholipidosis also has been observed in the tissues of neonatal rats and dogs given azithromycin daily for 10–30 days; the extent of phospholipidosis observed in these neonates was similar to that observed in adult animals. In neonatal rats or dogs given 30 or 10 mg/kg, respectively, of azithromycin, phospholipidosis was observed at a peak plasma azithromycin concentration of 1.3 mcg/mL (6 times greater than the peak plasma concentration of 0.216 mcg/mL observed in children receiving azithromycin 10 mg/kg) or 1.5 mcg/mL (7 times greater than the peak plasma concentration observed in children receiving azithromycin 10 mg/kg), respectively. On a mg/m^2 basis, azithromycin 30 mg/kg in the rat (135 mg/m^2) or 10 mg/kg in the dog (79 mg/m^2) are approximately 0.4 or 0.6 times, respectively, the recommended pediatric dose for a child who weighs 25 kg.

Phospholipidosis in animals has been reversible upon discontinuance of azithromycin treatment, and the clinical importance, if any, of these findings in humans is not known. Ultramicroscopy revealed no azithromycin-related myelin figures (a sensitive indicator of phospholipidosis) in peripheral blood lymphocytes in a limited number of individuals treated for 5 days with oral azithromycin.

■ **Precautions and Contraindications** Azithromycin is contraindicated in patients with known hypersensitivity to azithromycin, erythromycin, or any macrolide or ketolide antibiotic.

Serious hypersensitivity reactions, including angioedema, anaphylaxis, and dermatologic reactions, have occurred rarely in patients receiving azithromycin. Fatalities have been reported. Patients should be advised to discontinue azithromycin therapy immediately and to contact their clinician if any signs of an allergic reaction occur. Severe acute hypersensitivity reactions should be treated with appropriate therapy (e.g., epinephrine, maintenance of an adequate airway, oxygen, IV fluids, maintenance of blood pressure as indicated). In addition, clinicians should be aware that allergic symptoms associated with azithromycin therapy may reappear following discontinuance of initial symptomatic treatment and that patients may require prolonged observation and symptomatic treatment.

The manufacturer warns that oral azithromycin should *not* be used for the treatment of pneumonia that is considered unsuitable for outpatient oral therapy because of the severity of the infection (e.g., moderate to severe) or when risk factors such as nosocomially acquired infection, known or suspected bacteremia, cystic fibrosis, or any clinically important underlying health problem that might compromise the patient's ability to respond adequately (e.g., immunodeficiency, functional asplenia) are present. In addition, the manufacturer warns that the drug should *not* be used for the treatment of pneumonia in patients requiring hospitalization or in geriatric or debilitated patients.

Because azithromycin is eliminated principally via the liver, the drug should be used with caution in patients with impaired hepatic function. In addition, because of limited data regarding use of azithromycin in patients with renal impairment, the drug should be used with caution in patients with glomerular filtration rates less than 10 mL/minute.

Prolonged cardiac repolarization and QT interval with risk of cardiac arrhythmia and torsades de pointes has been reported with macrolides, including azithromycin. There have been reports of arrhythmias, ventricular tachycardia, hypotension, QT prolongation, and torsades de pointes in patients receiving azithromycin during postmarketing surveillance. FDA states that health care professionals should consider the risk of torsades de pointes and fatal heart rhythms with azithromycin when considering treatment options for patients who are already at risk for cardiovascular events. FDA notes that the potential risk of QT prolongation with azithromycin should be placed in appropriate context when choosing an antibacterial drug: Alternative drugs in the macrolide class, or non-macrolides such as the fluoroquinolones, also have the potential for QT prolongation or other clinically significant adverse effects that should be considered when choosing an antibacterial drug.

To reduce development of drug-resistant bacteria and maintain effectiveness of azithromycin and other antibacterials, the drug should be used only for the treatment or prevention of infections proven or strongly suspected to be caused by susceptible bacteria. When selecting or modifying anti-infective therapy, use results of culture and in vitro susceptibility testing. In the absence of such data, consider local epidemiology and susceptibility patterns when selecting anti-infectives for empiric therapy. Patients should be advised that antibacterials (including azithromycin) should only be used to treat bacterial infections and not used to treat viral infections (e.g., the common cold). Patients also should be advised about the importance of completing the full course of therapy, even if feeling better after a few days, and that skipping doses or not completing therapy may decrease effectiveness and increase the likelihood that bacteria will develop resistance and will not be treatable with azithromycin or other antibacterials in the future.

As with other anti-infective agents, use of azithromycin may result in overgrowth of nonsusceptible bacteria or fungi. If superinfection occurs, appropriate therapy should be instituted.

Because *C. difficile*-associated diarrhea and colitis (CDAD; also known as antibiotic-associated diarrhea and colitis or pseudomembranous colitis) has been reported with nearly all anti-infective agents, including macrolides, it should be considered in the differential diagnosis of patients who develop diarrhea during or following azithromycin therapy and managed accordingly. Careful medical history is necessary since CDAD has been reported to occur as late as 2 months or longer after anti-infective therapy is discontinued. If CDAD is suspected or confirmed, azithromycin may need to be discontinued. Some mild cases may respond to discontinuance of the drug alone. Moderate to severe cases should be managed with fluid, electrolyte, and protein supplementation, anti-infective therapy active against *C. difficile* (e.g., oral metronidazole or vancomycin), and surgical evaluation when clinically indicated. Patients should be advised that diarrhea is a common problem caused by anti-infectives and usually ends when the drug is discontinued; however, they should contact a clinician if watery and bloody stools (with or without stomach cramps and fever) occur during or as late as 2 months or longer after the last dose.

■ **Pediatric Precautions** Safety and efficacy of azithromycin extended-release oral suspension (Zmax®) have not been established in pediatric patients.

Safety and efficacy of oral azithromycin for the treatment of acute otitis media (AOM) in children younger than 6 months of age or for the treatment of pharyngitis and tonsillitis in children younger than 2 years of age have not been established.

Safety and efficacy of oral azithromycin for the treatment of acute bacterial sinusitis in children younger than 6 months of age have not been established. Use of the drug for the treatment of acute bacterial sinusitis in children 6 months of age or older is supported by adequate and well-controlled studies in adults, similar pathophysiology of acute sinusitis in adult and pediatric patients, and studies of AOM in pediatric patients.

Safety and efficacy of oral azithromycin for the treatment of community-acquired pneumonia (CAP) in infants younger than 6 months of age have not been established. Safety and efficacy of oral azithromycin for treatment of CAP caused by *Chlamydophila pneumoniae* (*Chlamydia pneumoniae*) or *Mycoplasma pneumoniae* in children 6 months of age or older were documented bacteriologically in pediatric studies, but similar documentation of safety and efficacy is not available for infections caused by *Haemophilus influenzae* or *Streptococcus pneumoniae* because of difficulty in obtaining specimens. However, the manufacturer states that use of oral azithromycin in pediatric patients with CAP caused by *H. influenzae* or *S. pneumoniae* is supported by evidence from adequate, controlled studies in adults.

Safety and efficacy of oral azithromycin for the treatment or prevention of *Mycobacterium avium* complex (MAC) infection in children with human immunodeficiency virus (HIV) infection have not been established. Safety data are available for 72 children 5 months to 18 years of age (mean: 7 years) who received azithromycin for the treatment of opportunistic infections; the mean duration of therapy was 242 days (range: 3–2004 days) and the mean dosage was 12 mg/kg daily (range: from less than 1 to 52 mg/kg daily). Adverse effects were similar to those reported in adults and most involved the GI tract. Treatment-related reversible hearing impairment was reported in 4 children. Azithromycin was discontinued prematurely in 2 children because of adverse effects (back pain or abdominal pain, hot and cold flushes, dizziness, headache, and numbness) and in one child because of eosinophilia.

Safety and efficacy of IV azithromycin in children or adolescents younger than 16 years of age have not been established.

Adverse effects reported in children receiving single- or multiple-doses of azithromycin are similar to those reported in adults, although the incidence rates may differ from those in adults.

■ **Geriatric Precautions** When a 5-day oral azithromycin regimen is used, clinically important differences in the pharmacokinetic profile the drug have not been observed in studies in healthy geriatric individuals (65–85 years of age) compared with younger adults (18–40 years of age). Although azithromycin peak plasma concentrations appear to be higher in geriatric women (but not geriatric men) compared with younger adults, accumulation of the drug has not been reported in these women. Therefore, dosage adjustment on the basis of age in geriatric patients receiving oral azithromycin therapy with conventional or extended-release formulations (Zmax®) generally is not required.

No overall differences in safety and efficacy have been reported with use of conventional or extended-release oral azithromycin formulations in those 65 years of age and older compared with younger adults, but the possibility of increased sensitivity in some geriatric individuals cannot be ruled out. In studies evaluating IV azithromycin in patients with CAP, there were no overall differences in safety in those 65 years of age and older compared with younger adults; similar decreases in clinical response were noted with increasing age in both azithromycin- and comparator-treated patients.

Safety data are available regarding use of azithromycin for the treatment of a variety of opportunistic infections, including MAC, in 30 geriatric patients (65–94 years of age) who received the drug in dosages exceeding 300 mg daily for a mean of 207 days. Adverse effects reported in these geriatric patients generally were similar to those reported in younger adults, although these older patients had a higher incidence of adverse GI effects and reversible hearing impairment.

The pharmacokinetic profile of IV azithromycin in geriatric patients has not been determined to date.

Azithromycin preparations contain sodium. A 2-g dose of azithromycin as the extended-release oral suspension (Zmax®) contains 148 mg (6.43 mEq) of sodium. Patients receiving the usual IV dosage will receive 114 mg (4.96 mEq) of sodium per dose. Geriatric patients may respond to salt loading with blunted natriuresis, and the total sodium content from dietary and nondietary sources may be clinically important with regard to such diseases as congestive heart failure.

■ **Mutagenicity and Carcinogenicity** Azithromycin was not mutagenic in several in vitro tests, including the mouse lymphoma assay, human lymphocyte clastogenic assay, and mouse bone marrow clastogenic assay.

Long-term studies have not been performed to date to evaluate the carcinogenic potential of azithromycin.

■ **Pregnancy, Fertility, and Lactation** Reproduction studies in rats and mice using azithromycin dosages up to 200 mg/kg daily (approximately equivalent on a mg/m^2 basis to 4 and 2 times, respectively, the human daily oral azithromycin dosage of 500 mg; to 2 or 1 times, respectively, the 1.2-g weekly dosage used for prevention of *M. avium* complex infection; or 3.3 or 1.7 times, respectively, the 600-mg daily oral dosage used for the treatment of *M. avium* complex) have not revealed evidence of harm to the fetus. However, there are no adequate and controlled studies to date using azithromycin in pregnant women, and the drug should be used during pregnancy only when clearly needed.

Preliminary data indicate that azithromycin may be safe and effective in the treatment of chlamydial infections in pregnant women; however, there are insufficient data to recommend routine use of the drug during pregnancy. (See Chlamydial Infections: Urogenital Chlamydial Infections, in Uses.) Azithromycin is considered the drug of choice for *Mycobacterium avium* complex (MAC) prophylaxis in HIV-infected pregnant women. (See Mycobacterium Avium Complex (MAC) infections: Prevention of Disseminated MAC Infection, in Uses.)

Reproductive studies with azithromycin have not revealed evidence of impaired fertility.

Azithromycin has been detected in human milk. The drug should be used with caution in nursing women.

Drug Interactions

■ **Drugs Affecting or Metabolized by Hepatic Microsomal Enzymes** Many drug interactions reported in clinical trials with macrolides (e.g., erythromycin, clarithromycin) have not been reported to date with azithromycin. While azithromycin appears to have no effect on the cytochrome P-450 (CYP) enzyme system and interactions mediated by this enzyme system would not be expected to occur, it should be kept in mind that azithromycin and other macrolides have similar pharmacologic effects and the possibility that similar drug interactions may occur cannot be ruled out. The manufacturer recommends careful monitoring in patients receiving digoxin (for elevated serum digoxin concentrations), ergotamine or dihydroergotamine (for ergot toxicity characterized by severe peripheral vasospasm and dysesthesia), or drugs metabolized by CYP isoenzymes, including cyclosporine, hexobarbital, terfenadine (no longer commercially available in the US), or phenytoin (for elevated serum drug concentrations). While interactions with the above agents have not been reported with azithromycin, interactions have occurred with other macrolides.

Prolongation of QT interval and, rarely, serious cardiovascular effects, including ventricular arrhythmias and death, have been reported in patients receiving drugs that inhibit the cytochrome P-450 isoenzyme (e.g., clarithromycin) concomitantly with pimozide. Macrolide antibiotics may inhibit metabolism of pimozide, resulting in increased plasma concentrations of unchanged drug. Because such alterations in pharmacokinetics of pimozide may be associated with prolongation of the QT and QT_c interval, the manufacturer of pimozide states that concomitant administration of pimozide and azithromycin, clarithromycin, or erythromycin is contraindicated.

Unlike some macrolides (i.e., erythromycin, clarithromycin), azithromycin does not appear to alter the metabolism of terfenadine (no longer commercially available in the US).

■ **Albendazole** Increased peak plasma concentration and area under the concentration-time curve (AUC) of azithromycin have been reported when azithromycin was used concomitantly with albendazole and ivermectin. This effect is not considered clinically important. (See Drug Interactions: Ivermectin.)

■ **Antacids** Although the single-dose extended-release oral suspension of azithromycin (Zmax®) may be taken without regard to antacids containing magnesium hydroxide and/or aluminum hydroxide, conventional oral azithromycin preparations (tablets or oral suspension) should not be administered simultaneously with aluminum- or magnesium-containing antacids. A study using azithromycin capsules (no longer commercially available) indicate that administration of oral azithromycin 500 mg with an aluminum- and magnesium hydroxide-containing antacid resulted in a decreased rate of absorption of azithromycin as evidenced by 24% reduction in peak serum azithromycin concentrations; however, the extent of azithromycin absorption (AUC) was unaffected.

■ **Antilipemic Agents** The manufacturer of azithromycin states that concomitant use of atorvastatin and azithromycin results in only a modest effect on the pharmacokinetics of the antilipemic agent and that dosage adjustments are not necessary when azithromycin and atorvastatin are used concomitantly. However, in a patient receiving long-term therapy with lovastatin, administration of oral azithromycin (250 mg daily for 5 days) appeared to precipitate rhabdomyolysis. Rhabdomyolysis has occurred rarely in patients receiving lovastatin, and some evidence suggests that concomitant administration of erythromycin may increase the risk of this adverse effect. While the mechanism of this interaction remains to be determined, the risk of drug-induced rhabdomyolysis should be considered in patients receiving azithromycin, erythromycin, or clarithromycin concomitantly with lovastatin or another hydroxymethylglutaryl-CoA (HMG-CoA) reductase inhibitor.

■ **Antimalarial Agents** ***Chloroquine*** Clinically important pharmacokinetic interactions did not occur when chloroquine and azithromycin were used concomitantly.

There is in vitro evidence of additive to synergistic effects between azithromycin and chloroquine against *P. falciparum*, including multidrug-resistant strains.

Quinine There is in vitro evidence of additive to synergistic effects between azithromycin and quinine against *P. falciparum*, including multidrug-resistant strains.

■ **Antiretroviral Agents** ***HIV Protease Inhibitors*** **Atazanavir.** Clinically important pharmacokinetic interactions between azithromycin and atazanavir are not expected.

Indinavir. Concomitant use of indinavir (800 mg 3 times daily for 5 days) and azithromycin (a single 1.2-g dose on day 5) in healthy adults had only a modest effect on the pharmacokinetics of the HIV protease inhibitor. The manufacturer of azithromycin states that dosage adjustments are not necessary when azithromycin and indinavir are used concomitantly.

Lopinavir. Clinically important pharmacokinetic interactions between azithromycin and lopinavir are not expected.

Nelfinavir. In healthy adults receiving nelfinavir (750 mg 3 times daily), administration of a single 1.2-g oral dose of azithromycin at steady state resulted in a 15% decrease in the mean AUC_{0-8} of nelfinavir and its M8 metabolite, but peak plasma concentrations of nelfinavir and its M8 metabolite were not affected. However, concomitant use of these drugs increases the peak plasma concentration and area under the concentration-time curve (AUC) of azithromycin by about twofold. The manufacturer of azithromycin states that, although dosage adjustments are not necessary when azithromycin and nelfinavir are used concomitantly, patients should be closely monitored for azithromycin adverse effects (e.g., hepatic enzyme abnormalities, hearing impairment).

Nonnucleoside Reverse Transcriptase Inhibitors **Efavirenz.** Concomitant use of efavirenz (400 mg daily for 7 days) and azithromycin (a single 600-mg oral dose on day 7) in healthy adults had no effect on the pharmacokinetics of the antiretroviral agent; peak plasma concentrations of azithromycin were increased about 22% but the AUC was not affected. The manufacturer of azithromycin states that dosage adjustments are not necessary when azithromycin is used concomitantly with efavirenz.

Nucleoside Reverse Transcriptase Inhibitors **Didanosine.** Concomitant administration of oral didanosine (200 mg every 12 hours for 21 days) and oral azithromycin (1.2 g daily on days 8–21) increased the peak plasma concentration and AUC of didanosine by 44 and 14%, respectively. However, these changes were not considered clinically important since similar variability in didanosine pharmacokinetic values occurred in control patients (i.e., patients receiving didanosine and placebo). The manufacturer of azithromycin states that dosage adjustments are not necessary when azithromycin and didanosine are used concomitantly.

Zidovudine. Concomitant use of zidovudine and azithromycin results in a modest effect on the pharmacokinetics of zidovudine, and the manufacturer of azithromycin states that dosage adjustments are not necessary when the drugs are used concomitantly. Concomitant use of oral azithromycin (600 or 1200 mg daily) and oral zidovudine (100 mg every 3 hours, 5 times daily) increased the mean peak plasma concentration, area under the plasma concentration-time curve (AUC), and clearance of zidovudine by 26, 10, and 38%, respectively; increased the mean AUC of phosphorylated zidovudine by 75%, and increased the peak plasma concentration and AUC for zidovudine glucuronide by less than 10%. Limited data in HIV-infected individuals indicate that administration of azithromycin 1 g as a single weekly dose did not produce clinically important changes in plasma concentrations of zidovudine, its glucuronide metabolite, or azithromycin. In HIV-infected patients maintained on zidovudine (10 mg/kg daily), addition of azithromycin 1 g as a single weekly dose increased peak plasma zidovudine concentration and AUC by 25 and 13%, respectively, and increased the peak plasma concentration and AUC of zidovudine glucuronide by 16 and 8%, respectively.

■ **Benzodiazepines** Concomitant use of azithromycin (500 mg on day 1, then 250 mg on day 2) and triazolam (0.125 mg on day 2) or concomitant use of azithromycin (500 mg daily for 3 days) and midazolam (15 mg on day 3) has only a modest effect on the pharmacokinetics of these benzodiazepines. Azithromycin does not appear to alter the effects of oral midazolam on psychomotor performance or subjective feelings of sedation. The manufacturer of azithromycin states that dosage adjustments are not necessary when azithromycin and midazolam or triazolam are used concomitantly.

■ **Carbamazepine** Limited data in healthy adults receiving carbamazepine (200 mg once daily for 2 days, then 200 mg twice daily) suggest that concomitant use of azithromycin (500 mg daily for 3 days) does not alter plasma carbamazepine or carbamazepine 10,11-epoxide concentrations. The manufacturer of azithromycin states that dosage adjustments are not necessary when azithromycin and carbamazepine are used concomitantly.

■ **Cetirizine** Concomitant use of azithromycin and cetirizine has only a modest effect on the pharmacokinetics of cetirizine and the manufacturer of azithromycin states that dosage adjustments are not necessary when the drugs are used concomitantly.

■ **Cimetidine** Administration of cimetidine 800 mg 2 hours prior to azithromycin 500 mg had no effect on absorption or pharmacokinetics of azithromycin.

■ **Co-trimoxazole** Concomitant use of oral co-trimoxazole (160 mg of trimethoprim and 800 mg of sulfamethoxazole for 7 days) and oral azithromycin (a single 1.2-g dose on day 7) in healthy adults had only a modest effect on the pharmacokinetics of azithromycin or either component of co-trimoxazole. The manufacturer of azithromycin states that dosage adjustments are not necessary when azithromycin and co-trimoxazole are used concomitantly.

■ **Cyclosporine** Although specific drug interaction studies have not been performed with azithromycin, concomitant use with other macrolides has resulted in increased cyclosporine concentrations. Therefore, the patient should be carefully monitored if azithromycin and cyclosporine are used concomitantly.

■ **Digoxin** Although specific drug interaction studies have not been performed with azithromycin, concomitant use with other macrolides has resulted in increased digoxin concentrations. Therefore, the patient should be carefully monitored if azithromycin and digoxin are used concomitantly.

■ **Ergot Alkaloids** Although specific drug interaction studies have not been performed with azithromycin, concomitant use with other macrolides has resulted in increased concentrations of ergot alkaloids (ergotamine, dihydroergotamine). Therefore, the patient should be carefully monitored if azithromycin and ergot alkaloids are used concomitantly.

■ **Fluconazole** Concomitant use of a single 1.2-g oral dose of azithromycin and a single 800-mg oral dose of fluconazole in healthy adults did not affect the pharmacokinetics of the antifungal agent; although peak plasma concentrations of azithromycin were decreased by about 18%, the AUC and half-life were not affected. In addition, concomitant use of a single 1.2-g oral dose of azithromycin and a single 200-mg oral dose of fluconazole had only a modest effect on the pharmacokinetics of either drug. The manufacturer of azithromycin states that dosage adjustments are not necessary when azithromycin and fluconazole are used concomitantly.

■ **Ivermectin** Increased peak plasma concentration and AUC of azithromycin and increased peak plasma concentrations and AUC of ivermectin have been reported when azithromycin, ivermectin, and albendazole were used concomitantly. The effect on azithromycin pharmacokinetics is not considered clinically important; additional study is needed to determine the clinical importance of the effect on ivermectin pharmacokinetics.

■ **Phenytoin** Although specific drug interaction studies have not been performed with azithromycin, concomitant use with other macrolides has resulted in increased phenytoin concentrations. Therefore, the patient should be carefully monitored if azithromycin and phenytoin are used concomitantly.

■ **Pimozide** Because concomitant use of pimozide and other macrolides (e.g., clarithromycin) has increased pimozide concentrations and is associated with a risk of prolonged QT interval and serious cardiovascular effects, the manufacturer of pimozide states that concomitant use of pimozide and macrolides (including azithromycin) is contraindicated.

■ **Rifabutin** Concomitant administration of azithromycin and rifabutin does not have a clinically important effect on the pharmacokinetics of rifabutin. In one study, peak plasma concentrations on day 1 in individuals receiving azithromycin (500 mg on day 1, 250 mg daily on days 2–9) with rifabutin (300 mg daily for 10 days) were essentially the same as those in individuals receiving azithromycin alone; mean plasma concentrations for rifabutin one-half day after the last dose were the same as those obtained in individuals receiving rifabutin alone. In addition, plasma concentrations for both drugs obtained 5 days after the last dose were the same as those obtained in individuals receiving either drug alone. The manufacturer of azithromycin states that dosage adjustments are not necessary when azithromycin and rifabutin are used concomitantly.

■ **Sildenafil** Concomitant use of azithromycin and sildenafil has only a modest effect on the pharmacokinetics of sildenafil and the manufacturer of azithromycin states that dosage adjustments are not necessary when the drugs are used concomitantly.

■ **Theophylline** While concurrent use of macrolides (e.g., erythromycin, clarithromycin) and theophylline has been associated with increases in serum theophylline concentrations, current evidence indicates that azithromycin does not induce or activate hepatic cytochrome P-450 (CYP) isoenzymes. The manufacturer of azithromycin states that dosage adjustments are not necessary when azithromycin and IV or oral theophylline are used concomitantly.

Administration of oral azithromycin for 5 days (500 mg on day 1, 250 mg daily on days 2–5) did not affect the plasma concentrations or pharmacokinetics of theophylline administered as a single IV dose. In addition, administration of this 5-day regimen of oral azithromycin reportedly did not affect theophylline plasma concentrations in patients receiving an extended-release theophylline formulation (300 mg twice daily for 15 days).

■ **Warfarin** Azithromycin does not appear to affect the prothrombin time (PT) response to a single dose of warfarin and limited data suggest that oral azithromycin (500 mg on day 1, then 250 mg daily for 4 days) does not affect the PT response in individuals receiving concurrent oral warfarin sodium. However, an increased international normalized ratio (INR) has been reported in one patient maintained on long-term warfarin therapy following completion of a 5-day course of oral azithromycin and concomitant use of warfarin and macrolides has been associated with increased anticoagulant effect in clinical practice. Therefore, the manufacturer of azithromycin states that prudent medical practice dictates careful monitoring of PT or other appropriate test in all patients treated concurrently with azithromycin and warfarin.

Acute Toxicity

Limited information is available on the acute toxicity of azithromycin. The acute lethal dose of the drug in humans is not known. The oral LD_{50} of azithromycin in mice or rats is 3000–4000 mg/kg.

Mechanism of Action

Azithromycin usually is bacteriostatic, although the drug may be bactericidal in high concentrations against selected organisms. Bactericidal activity has been observed in vitro against *Streptococcus pyogenes*, *S. pneumoniae*, and *Haemophilus influenzae*.

Azithromycin inhibits protein synthesis in susceptible organisms by penetrating the cell wall and binding to 50S ribosomal subunits, thereby inhibiting translocation of aminoacyl transfer-RNA and inhibiting polypeptide synthesis. The site of action of azithromycin appears to be the same as that of the macrolides (i.e., erythromycin, clarithromycin), clindamycin, lincomycin, and chloramphenicol. The antimicrobial activity of azithromycin is reduced at low pH. Azithromycin concentrates in phagocytes, including polymorphonuclear leukocytes, monocytes, macrophages, and fibroblasts. (See Pharmacokinetics: Distribution.) Penetration of the drug into phagocytic cells is necessary for activity against intracellular pathogens (e.g., *Staphylococcus aureus*, *Legionella pneumophila*, *Chlamydia trachomatis*, *Salmonella typhi*).

Spectrum

Azithromycin has an expanded spectrum of activity compared with erythromycin and clarithromycin. Azithromycin is active in vitro against many gram-positive and gram-negative aerobic and anaerobic bacteria as well as *Borrelia burgdorferi*, *Chlamydophila pneumoniae* (*Chlamydia pneumoniae*), *C. trachomatis*, *Mycoplasma pneumoniae*, and *Mycobacterium avium* complex (MAC). Azithromycin generally is more active in vitro against gram-negative organisms than erythromycin or clarithromycin and has activity comparable to erythromycin against most gram-positive organisms. Azithromycin has in vitro microbiologic activity similar to clarithromycin or erythromycin against *C. pneumoniae* and *M. pneumoniae*, but clarithromycin is fourfold more active against MAC in vitro than azithromycin. Streptococci and staphylococci that are resistant to erythromycin usually are resistant to azithromycin and clarithromycin. Azithromycin is not inactivated by β-lactamases produced by *H. influenzae* or *M. catarrhalis*.

Azithromycin appears to have a postantibiotic inhibitory effect against susceptible gram-positive and gram-negative aerobic organisms. In in vitro studies, exposure of *S. pyogenes*, *S. pneumoniae*, or *H. influenzae* for 1–2 hours to azithromycin concentrations several times higher than the MIC for the organism resulted in a recovery period of about 3–4, 2.2–5, or 2.5–8 hours, respectively, after the drug was removed before the organism resumed growth.

■ **In Vitro Susceptibility Testing** The in vitro activity of azithromycin is markedly affected by the pH of the microbiologic growth medium during incubation. Incubation in a carbon dioxide atmosphere will result in lowering of media pH (7.2 to 6.6 after 18 hours in 10% carbon dioxide) and an apparent reduction in in vitro susceptibility of gram-positive and gram-negative bacterial isolates to azithromycin. Thus, the initial pH of the growth medium should be 7.2–7.4, and the carbon dioxide content of the incubation atmosphere should be as low as practical.

When in vitro susceptibility testing is performed according to the standards of the Clinical and Laboratory Standards Institute (CLSI; formerly National Committee for Clinical Laboratory Standards [NCCLS]), clinical isolates identified as *susceptible* to azithromycin are inhibited by drug concentrations usually achievable when the recommended dosage is used for the site of infection. Clinical isolates classified as *intermediate* have minimum inhibitory concentrations (MICs) that approach usually attainable blood and tissue concentrations and response rates may be lower than for strains identified as susceptible. Therefore, the intermediate category implies clinical applicability in body sites where the drug is physiologically concentrated or when a higher than usual dosage can be used. This intermediate category also includes a buffer zone which should prevent small, uncontrolled technical factors from causing major discrepancies in interpretation, especially for drugs with narrow pharmacotoxicity margins. If results of in vitro susceptibility testing indicate that a clinical isolate is *resistant* to azithromycin, the strain is not inhibited by drug concentrations generally achievable with usual dosage schedules and/or MICs fall in the range where specific microbial resistance mechanisms are likely and clinical efficacy of the drug against the isolate has not been reliably demonstrated in clinical studies.

The disk diffusion and dilution techniques used to determine susceptibility of gram-positive and gram-negative bacterial isolates should not be used to test susceptibility of MAC isolates to azithromycin. Interpretive criteria for MAC isolates that would represent susceptibility or resistance to azithromycin have not been established. In addition, the clinical relevance of azithromycin in vitro susceptibility tests results for other mycobacteria, including *M. tuberculosis*, using any susceptibility testing method has not been determined.

Disk Susceptibility Tests When the disk-diffusion procedure is used to test susceptibility to azithromycin, a disk containing 15 mcg of the drug should be used.

When disk-diffusion susceptibility testing is performed according to CLSI standardized procedures using CLSI interpretive criteria, *Staphylococcus* with growth inhibition zones of 18 mm or greater are susceptible to azithromycin, those with zones of 14–17 mm have intermediate susceptibility, and those with zones of 13 mm or less are resistant to the drug.

When disk-diffusion susceptibility testing is performed according to CLSI standardized procedures using *Haemophilus* test medium (HTM), *Haemophilus* with growth inhibition zones of 12 mm or greater are considered susceptible to azithromycin. Because of limited data on resistant strains, CLSI recommends that any *Haemophilus* isolate that appears to be nonsusceptible to azithromycin should be retested to confirm results and then submitted to a reference laboratory for further testing.

When disk-diffusion susceptibility testing is performed according to CLSI standardized procedures, *S. pneumoniae* or other streptococci (β-hemolytic streptococci, viridans streptococci) with growth inhibition zones of 18 mm or greater are susceptible to azithromycin, those with zones of 14–17 mm have intermediate susceptibility, and those with zones of 13 mm or less are resistant to the drug.

When testing susceptibility of *Neisseria meningitidis* using CLSI standardized procedures, strains with growth inhibition zones of 20 mm or greater are susceptible to azithromycin. However, these results only pertain to use of the drug for postexposure prophylaxis of meningococcal disease and do not apply to use of the drug for the treatment of invasive meningococcal disease. Because of limited data on resistant strains, CLSI recommends that *N. meningitidis* isolates that appear to be nonsusceptible to azithromycin should be retested to confirm results and then submitted to a reference laboratory for further testing.

Dilution Susceptibility Tests When dilution susceptibility testing (agar or broth dilution) is performed according to CLSI standardized procedures, *Staphylococcus* with MICs of 2 mcg/mL or less are susceptible to azithromycin, those with MICs of 4 mcg/mL have intermediate susceptibility, and those with MICs of 8 mcg/mL or greater are resistant to the drug.

When CLSI standardized procedure for broth dilution is performed using HTM, *Haemophilus* with MICs of 4 mcg/mL or less are considered susceptible to azithromycin. Because of limited data on resistant strains, any *Haemophilus* isolate that appears to be nonsusceptible to azithromycin should be retested to confirm results and then submitted to a reference laboratory for further testing.

When broth dilution susceptibility testing for streptococci is performed according to CLSI standardized procedures, *S. pneumoniae* or other streptococci (β-hemolytic streptococci, viridans streptococci) with MICs of 0.5 mcg/mL or less are susceptible to azithromycin, those with MICs of 1 mcg/mL have intermediate susceptibility, and those with MICs of 2 mcg/mL or greater are resistant to the drug.

When testing susceptibility of *Neisseria meningitidis* using CLSI standardized procedures, strains with MICs of 2 mcg/mL or less are susceptible to azithromycin. However, these results only pertain to use of the drug for post-exposure prophylaxis of meningococcal disease and do not apply to use of the drug for the treatment of invasive meningococcal disease. Because of limited data on resistant strains, CLSI recommends that *N. meningitidis* isolates that appear to be nonsusceptible to azithromycin should be retested to confirm results and then submitted to a reference laboratory for further testing.

■ Gram-positive Aerobic Bacteria Azithromycin is active in vitro and in vivo against *Staphylococcus aureus*, *Streptococcus agalactiae*, *S. pneumoniae*, and *S. pyogenes*. The MIC_{90} (minimum inhibitory concentration of the drug at which 90% of tested strains are inhibited) of azithromycin for erythromycin-susceptible *S. aureus* is 1 mcg/mL; the MIC_{90} for *S. agalactiae* is 0.12 to greater than 12 mcg/mL. The MIC_{90} of azithromycin for *S. pneumoniae* or *S. pyogenes* is 0.12–2 or 0.12–4, respectively. The MIC_{90} of azithromycin for groups C, F, or G streptococci and viridans streptococci is 0.12–0.25 mcg/mL. The MIC of azithromycin for most staphylococci and streptococci generally are similar to or twofold higher than those for erythromycin; azithromycin does not inhibit erythromycin-resistant isolates of these species. Methicillin-resistant staphylococci and coagulase-negative staphylococci (e.g., *Staphylococcus epidermidis*) generally are resistant both to azithromycin and erythromycin. Azithromycin is not active against enterococci (e.g., *Enterococcus faecalis* [formerly *S. faecalis*]).

The MIC_{90} of azithromycin for *Listeria monocytogenes* is 2–4 mcg/mL.

■ Gram-negative Aerobic Bacteria Azithromycin is twofold to eightfold more active than erythromycin against erythromycin-susceptible gram-negative organisms. Azithromycin is active in vitro and in vivo against *Haemophilus influenzae*, *H. ducreyi*, *Moraxella catarrhalis*, *Legionella pneumophila*, and *Neisseria gonorrhoeae*. Azithromycin also is active in vitro against *N. meningitidis* and some strains of *Bordetella pertussis* and *Legionella pneumophila*.

Azithromycin is not inactivated by β-lactamases produced by *H. influenzae* or *M. catarrhalis*. The MIC_{90} of azithromycin for *H. influenzae* or *M. catarrhalis* is 1 or 0.03–0.5 mcg/mL, respectively. The MIC_{90} of azithromycin for *H. ducreyi* is less than 0.125 mcg/mL. The MIC_{90} of azithromycin for *L. pneumophila*, *N. gonorrhoeae*, *Bordetella pertussis*, or *Campylobacter jejuni* ranges from 0.03–2 mcg/mL.

Azithromycin may be more active in vitro than erythromycin against *Escherichia coli*, *Salmonella*, and *Shigella*.

Azithromycin concentrations of 0.006–0.03 inhibit some strains of *Bartonella henselae B. quintana*, *B. bacilliformis*, *B. vinsonii*, and *B. elizabethae* in vitro.

Azithromycin and erythromycin are less active than clarithromycin against *Helicobacter pylori* (formerly *C. pylori*); the MIC_{90} of clarithromycin for *H. pylori* is 0.03 mcg/mL versus 0.25 mcg/mL for azithromycin or erythromycin.

■ Mycobacteria Azithromycin has in vitro and in vivo activity against *Mycobacterium avium* complex (MAC) organisms. MAC represents 2 closely related organisms, *M. avium* and *M. intracellulare*. Although gene probe techniques may be used to distinguish *M. avium* species from *M. intracellulare*, most studies do not distinguish between the organisms and report results on MAC isolates. Azithromycin has activity against phagocytized MAC organisms in mouse and human macrophage cell cultures and in the beige mouse infection model. MAC organisms resistant to clarithromycin also are resistant to azithromycin.

M. tuberculosis, *M. kansasii*, *M. scrofulaceum*, *M. chelonae*, *M. fortuitum* and *M. leprae* are resistant to azithromycin.

■ Anaerobic Bacteria Azithromycin has in vitro activity (i.e., MIC_{90} of 2 mcg/mL or less) against *Clostridium perfringens* and *Peptostreptococcus* spp. Like erythromycin and clarithromycin, azithromycin is active in vitro against *Propionibacterium acnes*, with an MIC_{90} for this organism of 0.03 mcg/mL.

Azithromycin is active in vitro against most *Prevotella* (formerly *Bacteroides*) spp. associated with bacterial vaginosis. The MIC_{90} of azithromycin for *P. bivia*, *P. disiens*, *P. melaninogenica*, or *Bacteroides ureolyticus* is 2 mcg/mL or less. *B. fragilis* spp. generally are resistant to azithromycin.

■ Chlamydiae Azithromycin is active in vitro and in vivo against *Chlamydophila pneumoniae* (*Chlamydia pneumoniae*) and *C. trachomatis*. The MIC_{90} of azithromycin for *C. pneumoniae* is 0.25 mcg/mL and for *C. trachomatis* is 0.06–1 mcg/mL. The reported MIC of azithromycin for *C. psittaci* is 0.125 mcg/mL.

■ Mycoplasma The MIC_{90} of azithromycin for *Mycoplasma pneumoniae* is 0.25 mcg/mL, and the MIC_{90} reported for *Ureaplasma urealyticum* is 0.5–4 mcg/mL. The activity of azithromycin against *M. pneumoniae* generally is comparable to that of erythromycin or clarithromycin, but azithromycin has less activity than clarithromycin against *U. urealyticum*. The MIC_{90} of azithromycin for *M. hominis*reportedly ranges from 4–32 mcg/mL.

■ Spirochetes Azithromycin has exhibited in vitro and in vivo activity against *Borrelia burgdorferi* (the causative agent of Lyme disease). The MIC_{90} of azithromycin for *B. burgdorferi* is 0.015–0.03 mcg/mL.

Azithromycin is active in vitro against *Treponema pallidum*; however, the safety and efficacy of azithromycin in treating infections caused by this organism has not been clearly established.

■ Other Organisms Azithromycin has exhibited in vitro and in vivo activity against *T. gondii*. In addition, synergistic activity against *Toxoplasma gondii* has been reported in in vitro studies employing azithromycin with pyrimethamine. Limited data in animals indicate that azithromycin with either pyrimethamine or sulfadiazine produces enhanced anti-*Toxoplasma* activity (i.e., greater reduction in blood and organ parasite burden, lower incidence of relapse following discontinuation of therapy, reduced mortality rate) compared with administration of azithromycin, pyrimethamine, or sulfadiazine alone.

Azithromycin is active in vitro against *Entamoeba histolytica*.

Azithromycin is active against *Plasmodium falciparum*, *Orientia tsutsugamushi* (formerly *Rickettsia tsutsugamushi*), *Rickettsia conorii*, *R. typhi*, and *Coxiella burnettii*.

Resistance

Resistance to macrolide antibiotics may be natural or acquired. Resistance to macrolide antibiotics may be related to decreased permeability of the cell envelope (e.g., Enterobacteriaceae, *Pseudomonas* spp., *Acinetobacter* spp.), plasmid-mediated active efflux of the antibiotic (e.g., *Staphylococcus epidermidis*), enzymatic inactivation of antibiotic by plasmid-mediated esterases or phosphotransferase (e.g., Enterobacteriaceae), chromosomal-mediated alteration of a single 50S ribosomal protein at the receptor site resulting in decreased macrolide binding affinity (e.g., *Streptococcus pyogenes*, some *Campylobacter* spp., *Escherichia coli*), or alteration of the 23S ribosomal RNA of the 50S ribosomal subunit by methylation of adenine resulting in decreased macrolide binding to the receptor site (e.g., *Staphylococcus aureus*, streptococci, enterococci, *Campylobacter* spp., *Bacteroides fragilis*, *Clostridium perfringens*, *Listeria* spp., *Mycoplasma pneumoniae*, *Legionella* spp.). Resistance as a result of alteration of the 23S ribosomal RNA is referred to as MLS_B phenotype, is usually mediated by plasmids or transposons, may be constitutive or induced, and generally results in resistance to other 14- and 15-membered macrolides.

■ Resistance in Gram-positive Bacteria The overall incidence of macrolide-resistant *Streptococcus pyogenes* (group A β-hemolyte streptococci) in the US is reported to be 3–9%. In one US study, about 7% of *S. pyogenes* isolates (principally pharyngeal isolates) were resistant to azithromycin.

■ Resistance in Neisseria and Treponema In 1999, *Neisseria gonorrhoeae* with reduced susceptibility to azithromycin were isolated from a cluster of 12 men with gonorrhea in Kansas City, MO. These isolates had a median azithromycin MIC of 2 mcg/mL (range: 1–4 mcg/mL) and also were resistant to tetracycline (MIC 1–2 mcg/mL); however, they were susceptible to ceftriaxone, cefixime, spectinomycin, ciprofloxacin, and penicillin.

A mutation in *Treponema pallidum* that confers resistance to macrolides (including azithromycin) has been identified. *T. pallidum* containing this mutation has been isolated from several syphilis patients in San Francisco who failed to respond to azithromycin treatment. The overall prevalence of this mutation in *T. pallidum* has not been determined, but it has been found in specimens obtained in the US (Baltimore, San Francisco, Seattle) and Ireland (Dublin).

■ Resistance in Mycobacteria Macrolide-resistant *Mycobacterium avium* complex (MAC) isolates have been detected in patients with disseminated MAC infections receiving macrolide (i.e., azithromycin, clarithromycin) therapy. In studies evaluating prevention of disseminated MAC disease, drug-resistant isolates were detected in 29–58% of individuals in whom disease developed while receiving clarithromycin and 11% of those receiving azithromycin.

Although the mechanism(s) of resistance or reduced susceptibility of MAC to clarithromycin or azithromycin has not been fully determined to date, base substitution within domain V (the peptidyl transferase region) of the 23S ribosomal RNA gene, resulting in a residue change from adenine to cytosine, guanine, or thymine at position 2274, appears to be the principal mechanism in individuals receiving such therapy. Limited evidence indicates that these changes in the peptidyl transferase loop result in a conformational change in the ribosome at the macrolide binding site.

■ Cross-resistance Streptococci and staphylococci that are resistant to erythromycin also are resistant to azithromycin and clarithromycin.

MAC isolates resistant to azithromycin also are resistant to clarithromycin and complete cross-resistance occurs between these anti-infectives for this organism. Cross-resistance in these isolates appears to be the result of a single point mutation at the position that is homologous to the *Escherichia coli* positions 2058 or 2059 on the 23S rRNA gene. MAC isolates exhibiting cross-resistance generally have an increase in azithromycin MICs to 128 mcg/mL or greater or clarithromycin MICs to 32 mcg/mL or greater (determined using a radiometric broth dilution susceptibility test with Middlebrook 7H12 medium). Although the clinical importance of cross-resistance between azithromycin and clarithromycin is not fully understood, preclinical data suggest that reduced activity to both drugs will occur after MAC isolates produce the 23S rRNA mutation.

Pharmacokinetics

The pharmacokinetic profile of azithromycin is characterized by low plasma drug concentrations but high and persistent tissue concentrations. Although plasma drug concentrations are the traditional predictors of antibiotic activity, the pharmacokinetic characteristics of azithromycin suggest that tissue concentrations may be a more relevant parameter for this drug.

■ Absorption Azithromycin is rapidly absorbed from the GI tract after oral administration; absorption of the drug is incomplete but exceeds that of erythromycin. The absolute oral bioavailability of azithromycin is reported to be approximately 34–52% with single doses of 500 mg to 1.2 g administered as various conventional oral dosage forms (e.g., capsules [no longer commercially available in the US], tablets, oral suspension). Limited evidence indicates that the low bioavailability of azithromycin results from incomplete GI absorption rather than acid degradation of the drug or extensive first-pass metabolism.

Studies evaluating the bioequivalence of oral preparations of azithromycin indicate that peak plasma concentrations and times to peak concentration are similar following administration of 1 g of the drug as a conventional oral suspension or as four 250-mg capsules (no longer commercially available in the US). Limited data also indicate similar pharmacokinetic parameters for azithromycin capsules and tablets. Following oral administration of azithromycin 500 mg as two 250-mg capsules or tablets in fasting healthy men, peak plasma azithromycin concentrations averaged 0.5 mcg/mL at about 2 hours; extent of absorption (AUC_{0-72}) also was similar.

The commercially available extended-release oral suspension of azithromycin (Zmax®) is *not* bioequivalent with the conventional oral suspension or tablets (Zithromax®). Results of a 2-way crossover study in healthy adults who received a single 2-g dose of azithromycin as the extended-release oral suspension or the conventional oral suspension indicate that mean peak serum concentration and AUC of azithromycin are 57 and 17 % lower, respectively, with the extended-release formulation. Bioavailability of the azithromycin extended-release oral solution is approximately 83% of that reported with the conventional oral suspension and, in general, peak serum concentrations are attained approximately 2.5 hours later compared with the conventional oral suspension. However, higher peak serum concentrations and greater systemic exposure (AUC) are achieved with a single 2-g dose as the extended-release suspension relative to that of a 1.5-g dose as conventional tablets given over 3 days (500 mg daily) or 5 days (500 mg on day 1 and 250 mg daily on days 2–5).

After oral administration of a single 500-mg dose of azithromycin (as two 250-mg capsules on day 1 followed by 250 mg daily for the next 4 days in fasting healthy adults 18–40 years of age, peak plasma azithromycin concentrations on days 1 and 5 averaged 0.41 and 0.24 mcg/mL, respectively, at 2.5–3.2 hours. With this dosage regimen, peak and trough plasma azithromycin concentrations remained essentially unchanged from day 2 through day 5; trough concentrations averaged 0.05 mcg/mL. In this study, the disposition of azithromycin in these men and women was similar.

In healthy and asymptomatic HIV-infected adults receiving 1.2 g of azithromycin as two 600-mg tablets, peak plasma drug concentrations averaged 0.66 mcg/mL at 2.5 hours; plasma concentrations averaged 0.074 mcg/mL 24 hours after administration. In asymptomatic HIV-infected adults receiving a single 600-mg tablet of azithromycin once daily for 22 days, steady-state serum azithromycin concentrations were achieved on day 15.

In fasting children 6–15 years of age, administration of azithromycin oral suspension 10 mg/kg as a single dose on day 1 followed by 5 mg/kg daily for the next 4 days produced peak plasma drug concentrations on day 5 averaging 0.383 mcg/mL at 2.4 hours. Administration of this dosage regimen in fasting children 7.5 months to 5 years of age produced peak plasma azithromycin concentrations on day 5 averaging 0.216–0.224 mcg/mL at 1.8–1.9 hours. In fasting children 4 months to 15 years of age, administration of azithromycin 12 mg/kg as a single dose or in multiple daily doses for up to 5 days produced peak plasma drug concentrations averaging 0.318 mcg/mL at 2.4 hours after the dose.

In healthy geriatric men 65–85 years of age who received azithromycin 500 mg as a single oral dose on day 1 followed by 250 mg daily for the next 4 days, pharmacokinetic parameters for azithromycin were similar to those in young adults; peak plasma drug concentrations in geriatric women 60–85 years of age reportedly were 30–50% higher than those in younger adults, although substantial accumulation of azithromycin was not reported.

Pharmacokinetic values for azithromycin following IV administration in patients with community-acquired pneumonia are similar to those in healthy individuals. Following IV infusion of azithromycin 500 mg over 1 hour daily for 2–5 days in patients with community-acquired pneumonia, peak and trough plasma concentrations of azithromycin averaged 3.63 and 0.2 mcg/mL, respectively. In healthy individuals receiving azithromycin 500 mg by IV infusion over 3 hours daily for 5 days, peak and trough plasma concentrations of azithromycin averaged 1.14 and 0.18 mcg/mL, respectively. Compared with values following a single 500-mg IV dose, accumulation of azithromycin occurs when the same dose is given IV daily for 5 days as evidenced by an 8% increase in peak plasma concentration, and a 61% increase in AUC_{0-24}.

Azithromycin plasma concentrations following IV administration of a single 500-mg dose of the drug are substantially higher than those following oral administration of the same dose. In healthy individuals receiving a single 500-mg oral dose of azithromycin, peak plasma concentration, trough concentration, and AUC were 38, 83, and 52% of the values in individuals receiving azithromycin 500 mg IV over 3 hours.

Food Presence of food in the GI tract may affect the extent of absorption of oral azithromycin; however, the effect of food on absorption depends on the dosage form administered.

Food does not have a substantial effect on the extent of absorption (AUC) of azithromycin tablets or conventional oral suspension in adults, although the rate of absorption (as indicated by peak plasma concentrations of the drug) may be increased. In healthy men receiving a single 500-mg dose of azithromycin as the conventional oral suspension with food, peak plasma drug concentration increased by 46% and AUC increased by 14% compared with administration in the fasting state. In another study in healthy men receiving azithromycin conventional oral suspension, peak plasma drug concentration increased by 56% when the suspension was administered with food compared with fasting administration, but food did not affect extent of absorption (AUC). Compared with fasting administration, single-dose administration of azithromycin as two 250-mg tablets with a high-fat meal or as two 600-mg tablets with food was associated with a 23 or 31% increase in peak plasma drug concentrations, respectively, but no change in AUC. Food-associated increases in azithromycin plasma concentration reportedly are short-lived, persisting for less than 4 hours.

When a single 2-g dose of azithromycin was given to adults as the extended-release oral suspension (Zmax®), administration with a high-fat meal (150 kcal proteins, 250 kcal carbohydrates, 500–600 kcal fats) increased the mean peak plasma concentration and mean AUC of the drug by 115 and 23%, respectively, compared with administration in the fasted state. When the same dose was given following a standard meal (56 kcal proteins, 316 kcal carbohydrates, 207 kcal fats), mean peak azithromycin concentrations and mean AUC_{0-72} increased by 119 and 12%, respectively, compared with administration in the fasted state.

■ Distribution Azithromycin appears to be distributed into most body tissues and fluids after oral or IV administration. The extensive tissue uptake of azithromycin has been attributed to cellular uptake of this basic antibiotic into relatively acidic lysosomes as a result of ion trapping and to an energy-dependent pathway associated with the nucleoside transport system.

Results from in vitro studies demonstrate that azithromycin is rapidly concentrated within cells; intracellular to extracellular drug concentration ratios exceed 30 after 1 hour, and ratios of up to 200 have been reported after 24 hours. Azithromycin concentrates in phagocytes, including polymorphonuclear leukocytes, monocytes, macrophages, and fibroblasts, as demonstrated by in vitro incubation techniques. Because azithromycin is released more slowly from phagocytes than is erythromycin, substantial azithromycin concentrations are maintained for prolonged periods within these cells. In asymptomatic HIV-infected adults receiving a single 600-mg tablet of azithromycin once daily, mean peak azithromycin concentrations in peripheral leukocytes was 252 mcg/mL and steady-state trough concentrations in peripheral leukocytes averaged 146 mcg/mL; the mean ratio of peak leukocyte to peak serum concentrations was 456 and the mean AUC ratio was 816. Following oral administration of azithromycin 1.2 g (as two 600-mg tablets), drug concentrations in peripheral leukocytes averaged 140 mcg/mL; azithromycin concentrations in these leukocytes exceeded 32 mcg/mL for about 60 hours following administration. While the clinical importance has not been determined, leukocyte to peak plasma concentrations ratio averaged 258 or 175 in men or women, respectively, and the AUC ratios averaged 804 or 541, respectively. The concentration of azithromycin achieved within phagocytes substantially exceeds that of other antimicrobial agents, including erythromycin. In human polymorphonuclear leukocytes exposed in vitro to azithromycin or erythromycin for 24 hours, intracellular azithromycin concentrations were tenfold higher than those of erythromycin.

In addition to direct tissue uptake, it has been suggested that uptake and release of azithromycin by phagocytic cells contribute to distribution of the drug into inflamed and infected tissues. Spontaneous release of azithromycin from fibroblasts and phagocytes occurs gradually; however, release of the drug from phagocytes may be enhanced by exposure of the cell membrane to bacteria. Although release of azithromycin from fibroblasts is not enhanced by cell membrane exposure to pathogens, fibroblasts may act as drug reservoirs, releasing the drug to phagocytes for subsequent transport to the site of inflammation or infection. The presence of azithromycin within phagocytes does not appear to have clinically important effects on phagocytic function.

Because of rapid distribution into tissues and high intracellular concentrations of azithromycin, tissue concentrations of the drug generally exceed plasma concentrations by 10- to 100-fold following single-dose administration; with multiple dosing, the tissue-to-plasma ratio increases. While extensive distribution of the drug to tissues may be relevant to clinical activity, a quantitative relationship between high tissue concentration and clinical efficacy has not been established. The antimicrobial activity of azithromycin is pH related (i.e., only un-ionized azithromycin has antimicrobial activity). Because lysosomes have a low intraorganelle pH, a substantial portion of azithromycin within the lysosome is ionized (and therefore inactive) drug.

Administration of a single 500-mg oral dose of azithromycin generally produces drug concentrations of 1–9 mcg/g in various tissues, including lung, gastric, prostatic, and gynecologic tissue. Following administration of azithromycin as a single oral 500-mg dose, azithromycin concentrations in sputum averaged 1 or 2.9 mcg/g at 2–4 or 10–12 hours, respectively, and concentrations in lung tissue averaged 4 mcg/g at 73 hours. Following administration of azithromycin 500 mg as a single oral dose in patients with pulmonary infections, peak drug concentrations in sputum, bronchial mucosa, and alveolar macrophages averaged 1.56, 3.48, and 23 mcg/mL, respectively, at 48 hours. Following oral administration of azithromycin 250 mg every 12 hours for 2 doses, drug concentration in tonsillar tissue 9–18 or 180 hours after the second dose averaged 4.5 or 0.9 mcg/g, respectively. While azithromycin concentrations in sinus fluid averaged 1.34 mcg/mL on day 2 and 2.33 mcg/mL on day 6 in patients with acute sinusitis receiving oral azithromycin therapy (i.e., 500 mg on day 1 followed by 250 mg daily for 4 days), drug concentrations in patients with chronic sinusitis receiving this regimen averaged 0.25 and 0.38 mcg/mL on days 2 and 6, respectively, suggesting greater drug delivery to acutely inflamed tissue.

Following administration of azithromycin 500 mg as a single oral dose in patients undergoing gastric resection, drug concentrations in gastric tissue averaged approximately 4 mcg/g within 24 hours and persisted for 96 hours. Azithromycin concentrations in gastric mucosa averaged 0.5 mcg/mL within 24 hours and persisted for 120 hours, while peak drug concentrations of 0.2 mcg/mL in gastric juice were achieved within 73–93 hours.

In patients undergoing prostatectomy who received oral azithromycin 250 mg every 12 hours for 2 doses, drug concentrations in prostatic tissue averaged 2.54, 0.74, or 0.62 mcg/g at 14, 104–122, or 137 hours, respectively, following the second dose. In addition, azithromycin concentrations greater than 1 mcg/g were detected in liver, kidney, bladder wall, adrenal gland, bone, testicle, epididymis, and vas deferens. Distribution of azithromycin into ejaculate also has been reported.

Following administration of azithromycin 500 mg as a single oral dose, drug concentration in the uterine cervix averaged 2.8 mcg/g at 19 hours. In surgical patients receiving a single oral dose of azithromycin 500 mg, drug concentration in ovarian tissue, uterine tissue, and salpinx (fallopian tube) averaged 2.7, 3.5, and 3.3 mcg/g, respectively, at 17 hours. In another study in surgical patients receiving a single 500-mg oral dose of azithromycin, drug concentrations in gynecologic tissue (i.e., uterus, uterine cervix, fallopian tube) averaged 1.44 or 0.78 mcg/g at 24 or 96 hours, respectively.

Following administration of azithromycin as a single 500-mg oral dose, azithromycin concentrations in skin averaged 0.4 mcg/g at 73 hours.

Only very low concentrations of azithromycin (less than 0.01 mcg/mL) have been detected in CSF in the presence of noninflamed meninges.

While tissue levels have not been evaluated following IV administration of azithromycin, extensive tissue uptake would be expected to occur following IV administration of the drug.

The serum protein binding of azithromycin decreases with increasing drug concentration over a concentration range of 0.02–2 mcg/mL. Azithromycin is 51% bound to plasma proteins at drug concentrations of 0.02 mcg/mL and 7% bound at drug concentrations of 2 mcg/mL.

In children 1.6–7.5 years of age receiving oral azithromycin 10 mg/kg daily for 3 days, drug concentrations in tonsillar tissue averaged 10.33, 7.21, 9.3, or 1.49 mg/kg at 1, 2, 4, or 8 days, respectively, after the third dose. In children 1–6 years of age with secretory otitis media who were undergoing insertion of tympanotomy tubes, azithromycin concentrations in ear effusion averaged 1.02, 3.97, or 1.42 mcg/mL at 12, 24, or 48 hours, respectively, following administration of a single oral dose of 10 mg/kg. In children 1–8 years of age with acute otitis media, administration of azithromycin 10 mg/kg on day 1 followed by 5 mg/kg on days 2–5 resulted in azithromycin concentrations in middle ear effusion averaging 8.61 or 9.43 mcg/mL on day 2 or 3, respectively.

Azithromycin crosses the placenta and is distributed into cord blood and amniotic fluid.

Azithromycin is distributed into milk.

■ **Elimination** Plasma azithromycin concentrations following a single 500-mg oral or IV dose decline in a polyphasic manner with a terminal elimination half-life averaging 68 hours. The high values for apparent steady-state volume of distribution (31.3–33.3 L/kg) and plasma clearance (630 mL/minute, 10.18 mL/minute per kg) of azithromycin suggest that the prolonged half-life is related to extensive uptake and subsequent release of the drug from tissues. The average tissue half-life of azithromycin is estimated to be 1–4 days. The half-life of the drug in peripheral leukocytes ranges from 34–57 hours. The recommended azithromycin oral dosing regimen (1.5 g over 5 days) produces drug concentrations in excess of the MIC_{90} for many pathogens at tissue sites of infection for 5 days or longer following completion of therapy.

An elimination half-life of 54.5 hours has been reported in children 4 months to 15 years of age receiving single or multiple oral doses of azithromycin.

Azithromycin is excreted in feces principally as unchanged drug. The principal route of biotransformation involves *N*-demethylation of the desosamine sugar or at the 9a position on the macrolide ring. Other metabolic pathways include *O*-demethylation and hydrolysis and/or hydroxylation of the cladinose and desosamine sugar moieties and the macrolide ring. Up to 10 metabolites of azithromycin have been identified, and all are microbiologically inactive. While short-term administration of azithromycin produces hepatic accumulation of the drug and increases azithromycin demethylase activity, current evidence indicates that hepatic cytochrome P-450 induction or inactivation via cytochrome-metabolite complex formation does not occur. In contrast to erythromycin, azithromycin does not inhibit its own metabolism via this pathway.

Biliary excretion of azithromycin, predominantly as unchanged drug, is a major route of elimination following oral administration. Although the high biliary concentrations of azithromycin relative to serum concentrations suggest biliary excretion as an important route of elimination, transintestinal excretion may be the principal route of excretion for unchanged azithromycin. Only a small portion of each azithromycin dose is excreted in urine. While approximately 6% of a 500-mg oral dose of azithromycin appears in urine as unchanged drug over a 1-week period, 11% of a 500-mg IV dose was recovered over 24 hours on day 1, and 14% was recovered on day 5.

The manufacturer states that azithromycin has not been systematically evaluated in patients with hepatic impairment. In one study, the mean residence time of azithromycin was prolonged in patients with moderate hepatic dysfunction; however, AUC, volume of distribution, and total and renal clearance in these patients were similar to those in healthy individuals.

In a study in adults 21–85 years of age with varying degrees of renal impairment who received a single 1-g oral dose (four 250-mg capsules [no longer commercially available]), peak plasma concentrations and AUC were increased only slightly in patients with mild to moderate renal impairment (glomerular filtration rate 10–80 mL/minute) compared with those with normal renal function; however, peak plasma concentrations were increased 61% and AUC was increased 35% in those with severe renal impairment (glomerular filtration rate less than 10 mL/minute) compared with those with normal renal function.

Chemistry and Stability

■ **Chemistry** Azithromycin is a semisynthetic azalide antibiotic, a subclass of macrolide antibiotics. Azalides are distinguished from other macrolides by the addition of nitrogen at position 9a of the lactone ring. Azithromycin differs structurally from erythromycin by the addition of a methyl-substituted nitrogen atom at the 9a position of the macrolide ring. This structural modification in azithromycin results in resistance to acid degradation, improved tissue-penetration characteristics, improved activity against gram-negative organisms, and a prolonged elimination half-life compared with erythromycin.

Azithromycin is commercially available as the dihydrate; potency is calculated on the anhydrous basis. Azithromycin dihydrate occurs as a white crystalline powder and has solubilities of 39 mg/mL in water (pH 7.4) at 37°C.

For oral administration, azithromycin is commercially available as film-coated tablets, conventional powder for oral suspension, and extended-release microspheres for oral suspension. The extended-release oral suspension contains 148 mg (6.43 mEq) of sodium per 2-g dose.

Azithromycin for injection is a sterile, lyophilized, white to off-white powder; each 500-mg vial of azithromycin for injection contains approximately 413.6 mg of citric acid and 198.3 mg of sodium hydroxide. Intact vials of azithromycin for injection contain a vacuum. Following reconstitution of azithromycin for injection with sterile water for injection, solutions containing 100 mg of azithromycin per mL are clear and colorless and have an a pH of 6.4–6.6.

■ **Stability** Commercially available azithromycin 250- or 500-mg tablets should be stored at 15–30°C.

Azithromycin 600-mg tablets or powder for multiple-dose oral suspension should be stored at temperatures below 30°C. Following reconstitution as directed, the multiple-dose oral suspension of azithromycin should be stored in tight containers at 5–30°C; any unused suspension should be discarded after 10 days.

Azithromycin powder in single-dose packets for oral suspension should be stored at 5–30°C. Following reconstitution, the entire contents of the single-dose packet should be ingested immediately.

Azithromycin powder for extended-release oral suspension (Zmax®) should be stored at 30°C or lower. Following reconstitution, azithromycin single-dose extended-release oral suspension should be stored in the original bottle at 25°C but may be exposed to 15–30°C. The reconstituted suspension should be consumed within 12 hours.

Commercially available azithromycin for injection should be stored at or below 30°C. Following reconstitution with sterile water for injection, solutions containing 100 mg of azithromycin per mL are stable for 24 hours when stored below 30°C. Azithromycin is physically and chemically compatible with the following IV solutions: 0.45% or 0.9% sodium chloride, 5% dextrose, 5% dextrose and 0.3% or 0.45% sodium chloride, 5% dextrose and 0.45% sodium chloride with 20 mEq potassium chloride, 5% dextrose in lactated Ringer's, lactated Ringer's, Normosol®-M in 5% dextrose, and Normosol®-R in 5% dextrose. Reconstituted solutions of azithromycin that have been further diluted with 250–500 mL of one of these IV solutions to provide a solution containing 1–2 mg/mL are physically and chemically stable for 24 hours when stored at or below room temperature (30°C) or 7 days when refrigerated at 5°C.

Preparations

Excipients in commercially available drug preparations may have clinically important effects in some individuals; consult specific product labeling for details.

Azithromycin Dihydrate

Oral

For suspension	100 mg (of anhydrous azithromycin) per 5 mL*	**Azithromycin for Suspension**
		Zithromax®, Pfizer
	200 mg (of anhydrous azithromycin) per 5 mL*	**Azithromycin for Suspension**
		Zithromax®, Pfizer
	1 g (of anhydrous azithromycin) per packet*	**Azithromycin for Suspension**
		Zithromax® Single Dose Packets, Pfizer
For suspension, extended-release	2 g (of anhydrous azithromycin)	**Zmax®**, Pfizer

Tablets, film-coated	250 mg (of anhydrous azithromycin)*	**Azithromycin Tablets**
		Azithromycin Tablets (available as a 5-day mnemonic pack of 6 tablets)
		Zithromax®, Pfizer
		Zithromax® Z-Paks® (available as a 5-day mnemonic pack of 6 tablets), Pfizer
	500 mg (of anhydrous azithromycin)*	**Azithromycin Tablets**
		Azithromycin Tablets (available as a 3-day mnemonic pack of 3 tablets)
		Zithromax®, Pfizer
		Zithromax® Tri-Paks® (available as a 3-day mnemonic pack of 3 tablets), Pfizer
	600 mg (of anhydrous azithromycin)*	**Azithromycin Tablets**
		Zithromax®, Pfizer
Parenteral		
For injection, for IV infusion only	500 mg (of anhydrous azithromycin)*	**Azithromycin for Injection**
		Zithromax®, Pfizer
	2.5 g (of anhydrous azithromycin)*	**Azithromycin for Injection**

*available from one or more manufacturer, distributor, and/or repackager by generic (nonproprietary) name

†Use is not currently included in the labeling approved by the US Food and Drug Administration

Clarithromycin

■ Clarithromycin is a semisynthetic macrolide antibiotic with a broader spectrum than that of erythromycins.

Uses

Clarithromycin is used orally for the treatment of pharyngitis and tonsillitis, mild to moderate respiratory tract infections (acute bacterial exacerbation of chronic bronchitis, acute maxillary sinusitis, community-acquired pneumonia), uncomplicated skin and skin structure infections, and acute otitis media caused by susceptible organisms. Clarithromycin also is used orally in the treatment of disseminated infections caused by *Mycobacterium avium* complex (MAC) in patients with advanced human immunodeficiency virus (HIV) infection and for prevention of disseminated MAC infection (both primary and secondary prophylaxis) in HIV-infected individuals.

Oral clarithromycin is used in combination with amoxicillin and lansoprazole or omeprazole (triple therapy) for the treatment of *Helicobacter pylori* infection and duodenal ulcer disease. Clarithromycin also is used orally in combination with omeprazole (dual therapy) or ranitidine bismuth citrate for the treatment of *H. pylori* infection in patients with an active duodenal ulcer. Clarithromycin also has been used orally in other multiple-drug regimens (with or without amoxicillin, lansoprazole, omeprazole, or ranitidine bismuth citrate) for the treatment of *H. pylori* infection associated with peptic ulcer disease.

Safety and efficacy of clarithromycin extended-release tablets have been established only for the treatment of certain respiratory tract infections in adults (acute bacterial exacerbations of chronic bronchitis, acute maxillary sinusitis, community-acquired pneumonia); safety and efficacy of the extended-release formulation of the drug have not been established for the treatment of other infections that are treated with clarithromycin conventional tablets or oral suspension.

■ **Acute Otitis Media** Clarithromycin (conventional tablets, oral suspension) is used for the treatment of acute otitis media (AOM) caused by *Haemophilus influenzae*, *Moraxella catarrhalis*, or *Streptococcus pneumoniae* in children. Various anti-infectives, including oral amoxicillin, oral amoxicillin and clavulanate potassium, various oral cephalosporins (cefaclor, cefdinir, cefixime, cefpodoxime proxetil, cefprozil, ceftibuten, cefuroxime axetil, cephalexin), IM ceftriaxone, oral co-trimoxazole, oral erythromycin-sulfisoxazole, oral azithromycin, oral clarithromycin, and oral loracarbef, have been used in the treatment of AOM. The American Academy of Pediatrics (AAP), US Centers for Disease Control and Prevention (CDC), and other clinicians state that, despite the increasing prevalence of multidrug-resistant *S. pneumoniae* and presence of β-lactamase-producing *H. influenzae* or *M. catarrhalis* in many communities, amoxicillin remains the anti-infective of first choice when treatment of uncomplicated AOM is indicated since amoxicillin is highly effective, has a narrow spectrum of activity, is well distributed into middle ear fluid, and is well tolerated and inexpensive.

Clarithromycin is not considered a first-line agent for treatment of AOM, but is recommended as an alternative for individuals with type I penicillin hypersensitivity. Because *S. pneumoniae* resistant to amoxicillin also frequently are resistant to co-trimoxazole, clarithromycin, and azithromycin, these drugs may not be effective in patients with AOM who fail to respond to amoxicillin. For additional information regarding treatment of AOM and information regarding prophylaxis of recurrent AOM, treatment of persistent or recurrent AOM, and treatment of otitis media with effusion (OME), see Uses: Otitis Media in the Aminopenicillins General Statement 8:12.16.08.

In controlled clinical trials of therapy for children with otitis media in areas of the US where the rate of β-lactamase-producing bacteria is high, clarithromycin therapy was compared with cephalosporin therapy alone or other antibiotic therapy with a concomitant β-lactamase inhibitor. In these studies, the combined clinical success rate (i.e., cure plus improvement) for clarithromycin therapy ranged from 88–91%, while that for the comparison therapies was 91%. The overall clinical success rate (i.e., presumed bacterial eradication/clinical cure outcomes) for clarithromycin ranged from 81–83%, while that for the comparison agents ranged from 73–97%. In all studies, the adverse effects associated with any therapy were principally GI related (e.g., diarrhea, vomiting), with a similar or lower incidence of effects occurring in the clarithromycin-treated group as compared with group treated with the comparison agent.

■ **Pharyngitis and Tonsillitis** Clarithromycin (conventional tablets, oral suspension) is used for the treatment of pharyngitis and tonsillitis caused by *Streptococcus pyogenes* (group A β-hemolytic streptococci) in adults and children. Although clarithromycin generally is effective in the eradicating *S. pyogenes* from the nasopharynx, efficacy of the drug in the subsequent prevention of rheumatic fever has not been established. Strains of *S. pyogenes* resistant to macrolides are common in some areas of the world (e.g., Italy, Japan, Korea, Finland, Spain, Taiwan) and clarithromycin-resistant strains have been reported in the US. (See Resistance: Resistance in Gram-positive Bacteria.)

Because penicillin has a narrow spectrum of activity, is inexpensive, and generally effective, the CDC, AAP, American Academy of Family Physicians (AAFP), Infectious Diseases Society of America (IDSA), American Heart Association (AHA), American College of Physicians (ACP), and others consider natural penicillins (i.e., 10 days of oral penicillin V or a single IM dose of penicillin G benzathine) the treatment of choice for streptococcal pharyngitis and tonsillitis and prevention of initial attacks (primary prevention) of rheumatic fever, although oral amoxicillin often is used instead of penicillin V in small children because of a more acceptable taste. Other anti-infectives (e.g., oral cephalosporins, oral macrolides) generally are considered alternatives.

In a limited number of controlled, comparative studies, microbiologic and clinical response rates of approximately 90% or greater were achieved in patients 12 years of age or older who received oral therapy with either clarithromycin 250 mg every 12 hours, penicillin V 250 mg every 6 hours, or erythromycin 500 mg every 12 hours; most patients were treated for approximately 7–10 days. Comparable clinical and microbiologic response rates have been reported in children as young as 6 months of age who received clarithromycin 7.5 mg/kg (maximum dose: 250 mg) twice daily or penicillin V 13.3 mg/kg (maximum dose: 500 mg) 3 times daily as oral suspensions.

■ **Respiratory Tract Infections** ***Acute Exacerbations of Chronic Bronchitis*** Clarithromycin (conventional tablets, oral suspension, extended-release tablets) is used for the treatment of acute bacterial exacerbations of chronic bronchitis caused by *H. influenzae*, *H. parainfluenzae*, *M. catarrhalis*, or *S. pneumoniae* in adults. Data from a limited number of studies from which patients with β-lactamase-positive infections generally were excluded suggest similar clinical and microbiologic efficacy for oral clarithromycin and oral ampicillin in these infections.

Acute Sinusitis Clarithromycin (conventional tablets, oral suspension) is used for the treatment of acute maxillary sinusitis caused by *H. influenzae*, *M. catarrhalis*, or *S. pneumoniae* in adults or children; clarithromycin (extended-release tablets) is used for the treatment of these infections in adults.

In one study in patients with acute maxillary sinusitis caused principally by *S. pneumoniae* or *Haemophilus* spp., oral therapy with clarithromycin 500 mg every 12 hours or amoxicillin 500 mg every 8 hours for 9–11 days resulted in clinical response in 91% of patients in each group, with similar microbiologic responses. All microbiologic treatment failures in patients receiving clarithromycin involved *Haemophilus* spp. However, patients with β-lactamase-producing organisms were excluded from this study, and bacteriologic response rates may not be representative of those generally encountered in clinical practice. Limited data from another study in patients with acute maxillary sinusitis suggest that oral clarithromycin 500 mg every 12 hours or amoxicillin and clavulanate potassium 500 mg every 8 hours produce comparable clinical and bacteriologic responses.

Community-acquired Pneumonia Clarithromycin (conventional tablets, oral suspension) is used for the treatment of mild to moderate community-acquired pneumonia (CAP) caused by *Mycoplasma pneumoniae*, *Chlamydophila pneumoniae* (*Chlamydia pneumoniae*), or *S. pneumoniae* in adults and children; clarithromycin (conventional tablets, oral suspension) also is used in adults for the treatment of CAP caused by *H. influenzae*. In addition, clarithromycin (extended-release tablets) is used in adults for the treatment of CAP caused by *H. influenzae*, *H. parainfluenzae*, *M. catarrhalis*, *M. pneumoniae*, *C. pneumoniae*, or *S. pneumoniae*.

Limited data in patients with CAP caused by these pathogens suggest that oral therapy with clarithromycin given twice daily generally is as effective as erythromycin given 2–4 times daily.

Initial treatment of CAP generally involves use of an empiric anti-infective regimen based on the most likely pathogens; therapy may then be changed (if possible) to a pathogen-specific regimen based on results of in vitro culture and susceptibility testing, especially in hospitalized patients. The most appropriate empiric regimen varies depending on the severity of illness at the time of presentation and whether outpatient treatment or hospitalization in or out of an intensive care unit (ICU) is indicated and the presence or absence of cardiopulmonary disease and other modifying factors that increase the risk of certain pathogens (e.g., penicillin- or multidrug-resistant *S. pneumoniae*, enteric gram-negative bacilli, *Ps. aeruginosa*). For both outpatients and inpatients, most experts recommend that an empiric regimen for the treatment of CAP include an anti-infective active against *S. pneumoniae* since this organism is the most commonly identified cause of bacterial pneumonia and causes more severe disease than many other common CAP pathogens.

For information on recommendations of the IDSA and American Thoracic Society (ATS) regarding use of clarithromycin and other macrolides in empiric regimens for the inpatient or outpatient treatment of CAP, see Community-acquired Pneumonia under Uses: Respiratory Tract Infections, in the Erythromycins General Statement 8:12.12.04.

■ Skin and Skin Structure Infections Clarithromycin (conventional tablets, oral suspension) is used in adults and children for the treatment of uncomplicated skin and skin structure infections caused by *Staphylococcus aureus* or *S. pyogenes*. Some data in adults and children suggest that oral clarithromycin has efficacy comparable to that of oral erythromycin or an oral cephalosporin (e.g., cefadroxil) in treating various bacterial skin and skin structure infections (e.g., impetigo, cellulitis). Further comparative studies are needed to determine the relative efficacy of clarithromycin versus other anti-infective agents in treating various skin and skin structure infections, and other drugs (e.g., an oral penicillinase-resistant penicillin or cephalosporin) generally are preferred for the treatment of these infections.

■ Helicobacter pylori Infection and Duodenal Ulcer Disease Clarithromycin (conventional tablets) is used in conjunction with amoxicillin and lansoprazole or omeprazole (triple therapy) for the treatment of *Helicobacter pylori* (formerly *Campylobacter pylori* or *C. pyloridis*) infection in patients with duodenal ulcer disease (active or up to 1-year history of duodenal ulcer). Clarithromycin also is used in conjunction with omeprazole (dual therapy) or ranitidine bismuth citrate for the treatment of *H. pylori* infection in patients with an active duodenal ulcer. Clarithromycin also has been used orally in other multiple-drug regimens (with or without amoxicillin, omeprazole, lansoprazole, or ranitidine bismuth citrate)† for the treatment of *H. pylori* infection associated with peptic ulcer disease. While some evidence indicates that combined therapy with 2 drugs (e.g., clarithromycin-omeprazole, ranitidine bismuth citrate-omeprazole, amoxicillin-omeprazole) can successfully eradicate *H. pylori* infection and prevent recurrence of duodenal ulcer at least in the short term (e.g., at 6 months following completion of anti-*H. pylori* therapy), the American College of Gastroenterology (ACG) and some clinicians currently recommend anti-*H. pylori* regimens consisting of at least 3 drugs (e.g., 2 anti-infective agents plus a proton-pump inhibitor) because of enhanced *H. pylori* eradication rates, decreased treatment failures due to resistance, and shorter treatment periods compared with those apparently required with 2-drug regimens.

Pathogenesis Current epidemiologic and clinical evidence supports a strong association between gastric infection with *H. pylori* and the pathogenesis of duodenal and gastric ulcers; with the exception of ulcers associated with gastrinoma (Zollinger-Ellison syndrome) or use of NSAIAs, almost all cases of duodenal ulcer and most cases of gastric ulcer are associated with *H. pylori* infection.

Although *H. pylori* eradication (generally defined as the absence of *H. pylori* organisms in the stomach documented at least 1 month after completion of anti-*H. pylori* therapy) reduces ulcer relapse rates, other factors appear to be essential for the *development* of peptic ulcer because most individuals with *H. pylori* infection do not develop peptic ulcers, and such ulcers are healed by various other therapies despite the presence of the organism in the stomach. Once acquired, *H. pylori* infection may persist for decades or even for life, causing chronic inflammation, although most infected individuals reportedly are asymptomatic. Since type B active chronic gastritis is caused by *H. pylori* infection and may eventually progress to chronic atrophic gastritis, a well-recognized risk factor for gastric carcinoma, long-term *H. pylori* infection also has been implicated as a risk factor for gastric cancer. However, whether eradication of *H. pylori* ultimately will reduce the incidence of gastric carcinoma remains to be established, and most clinicians currently do not advocate the use of anti-*H. pylori* therapy *solely* as a potential means of lowering the risk of gastric cancer given the prevalence of *H. pylori* infection in the general population and the potential costs and complications of current treatment regimens.

Although *H. pylori* eradication (generally defined as the absence of *H. pylori* organisms in the stomach documented at least 1 month after completion of anti-*H. pylori* therapy) reduces ulcer relapse rates, other factors appear to be essential for the *development* of peptic ulcer because most individuals with *H. pylori* infection do not develop peptic ulcers, and such ulcers are healed by various other therapies despite the presence of the organism in the stomach. Once acquired, *H. pylori* infection may persist for decades or even for life, causing chronic inflammation, although most infected individuals reportedly are asymptomatic. Since type B active chronic gastritis is caused by *H. pylori* infection and may eventually progress to chronic atrophic gastritis, a well-recognized risk factor for gastric carcinoma, long-term *H. pylori* infection also has been implicated as a risk factor for gastric cancer. However, whether eradication of *H. pylori* ultimately will reduce the incidence of gastric carcinoma remains to be established, and most clinicians currently do not advocate the use of anti-*H. pylori* therapy *solely* as a potential means of lowering the risk of gastric cancer given the prevalence of *H. pylori* infection in the general population and the potential costs and complications of current treatment regimens.

Therapeutic Regimens Conventional antiulcer therapy with H_2-receptor antagonists, proton-pump inhibitors, sucralfate, and/or antacids heals ulcers but generally is ineffective in eradicating *H. pylori*, and such therapy is associated with a high rate of ulcer recurrence (e.g., 60–100% per year). Several useful therapeutic regimens for *H. pylori*-associated peptic ulcer disease have been identified, and the ACG, the National Institutes of Health (NIH), and most clinicians currently recommend that *all* patients with initial or recurrent duodenal or gastric ulcer and documented *H. pylori* infection receive anti-infective therapy for treatment of the infection.

The optimum regimen for treatment of *H. pylori* infection has not been established; however, combined therapy with 3 drugs that have activity against *H. pylori* (e.g., a bismuth salt, metronidazole, and tetracycline or amoxicillin) has been effective in eradicating the infection, resolving associated gastritis, healing peptic ulcer, and preventing ulcer recurrence in many patients with *H. pylori*-associated peptic ulcer disease. Although such 3-drug regimens typically have been administered for 10–14 days, current evidence principally from studies in Europe suggests that 1 week of such therapy provides *H. pylori* eradication rates comparable to those of longer treatment periods. Other regimens that combine one or more anti-infective agents (e.g., clarithromycin, amoxicillin) with a bismuth salt and/or an antisecretory agent (e.g., omeprazole, lansoprazole, H_2-receptor antagonist) also have been used successfully for *H. pylori* eradication, and the choice of a particular regimen should be based on the rapidly evolving data on optimal therapy, including consideration of the patient's prior exposure to anti-infective agents, the local prevalence of resistance, patient compliance, and costs of therapy.Current data suggest that eradication of *H. pylori* infection using regimens consisting of 1 or 2 anti-infective agents with a bismuth salt and/or an H_2-receptor antagonist or proton-pump inhibitor (e.g., omeprazole, lansoprazole) is cost effective compared with intermittent or continuous maintenance therapy with an H_2-receptor antagonist (considering the costs associated with ulcer recurrence, including endoscopic or other diagnostic procedures, physician visits, and/or hospitalization).

The ACG and some clinicians currently state that an *H. pylori* eradication rate of approximately 90% with a 1-week treatment period represents a realistic goal of therapy for *H. pylori* infection. However, some clinicians state that results of 1-week anti-*H. pylori* regimens in Europe generally have been superior to those conducted in the US to date and that additional US studies with these regimens are needed to confirm the efficacy of 1-week regimens in the US. Although high eradication rates have been achieved with standard 3-drug, bismuth-based regimens (e.g., bismuth-metronidazole-tetracycline or bismuth-metronidazole-amoxicillin), such regimens typically involve administration of many tablets/capsules and have been associated with a relatively high (although variable) incidence of adverse effects. In addition, the efficacy of these regimens generally is unacceptable in patients with *H. pylori* strains resistant to the imidazole anti-infective (e.g., metronidazole) component.

Current evidence suggests that inclusion of a proton-pump inhibitor (e.g., omeprazole, lansoprazole) in anti-*H. pylori* regimens containing 2 anti-infectives enhances effectiveness, and limited data suggest that such regimens retain good efficacy despite imidazole (e.g., metronidazole) resistance. Therefore, the ACG and many clinicians currently recommend 1 week of therapy with a proton-pump inhibitor and 2 anti-infective agents (usually clarithromycin and amoxicillin or metronidazole), or a 3-drug, bismuth-based regimen (e.g., bismuth-metronidazole-tetracycline) concomitantly with a proton-pump inhibitor, for treatment of *H. pylori* infection. Although few comparative studies have been performed, such regimens appear to provide high (e.g., 85–90%) *H. pylori* eradication rates, are well tolerated, and may be associated with better patient compliance than more prolonged therapy. The ACG states that in a cost-sensitive environment, an alternative regimen consisting of a bismuth salt, metronidazole, and tetracycline for 14 days is a reasonable choice in patients who are compliant and in whom there is a low expectation of metronidazole resistance (no prior exposure to the drug and a low regional prevalence of resistance).

Current data suggest that modification of bismuth-metronidazole-tetracycline regimens by substituting clarithromycin for metronidazole or amoxicillin (but not ampicillin) for tetracycline also results in effective therapy, but the substitution of either amoxicillin or another tetracycline derivative (i.e., doxycycline) for tetracycline hydrochloride in such regimens reduces efficacy. While azithromycin has been used in a limited number of multiple-drug regimens (e.g., with tetracycline, metronidazole, bismuth salts, and/or omeprazole) for the treatment of *Helicobacter pylori* infection and peptic ulcer disease, such combination regimens generally have been associated with a high incidence of adverse effects (principally GI effects) or low *H. pylori* eradication rates (e.g., 50–70%). Additional controlled, comparative studies and long-term follow-up are needed to determine optimal drug regimens for *H. pylori*-associated peptic ulcer and to elucidate the effects of *H. pylori* eradication on potential long-term complications of peptic ulcer disease such as GI bleeding and gastric carcinoma.

Current evidence suggests that eradication of *H. pylori* by anti-infective agents may be facilitated by increased gastric pH, and many clinicians recommend concomitant treatment with antisecretory agents (e.g., omeprazole, lansoprazole, H_2-receptor antagonists) to enhance ulcer healing and symptom relief while allowing relatively short (e.g., 1-week) treatment periods in patients with active peptic ulcer disease. Eradication rates of almost 100% have been reported with addition of omeprazole to a 3-drug anti-*H. pylori* regimen. Therapy with an antisecretory drug and a single anti-infective agent (i.e., "dual therapy") also has been used successfully for treatment of *H. pylori* infection. However, rates of *H. pylori* eradication have varied considerably in some studies using combined therapy with 2 drugs (e.g., amoxicillin and omeprazole) depending on dosage, timing of administration, and possibly the age of the patient. An analysis of pooled data from a number of studies in which combined therapy with omeprazole and either amoxicillin or clarithromycin was used indicate *H. pylori* eradication rates averaging approximately 55–62% with amoxicillin-omeprazole and 67–75% with clarithromycin-omeprazole therapy.

In 4 randomized, controlled trials in patients with active duodenal ulcer, combined therapy with clarithromycin (500 mg 3 times daily for 14 days) and omeprazole (40 mg daily for 14 days followed by either 20 or 40 mg daily for an additional 14 days) was successful in eradicating *H. pylori* (defined as 2 negative tests for *H. pylori* 4 weeks after the end of treatment) in 64–83% of patients compared with 0–1% of patients receiving omeprazole alone or (in 2 trials) 31–39% of patients receiving clarithromycin alone. Ulcer healing rates at 4 weeks averaged 94–100% with clarithromycin-omeprazole treatment, 88– 99% with omeprazole alone, and (in 2 trials) 64–71% with clarithromycin alone. In addition, follow-up evaluations at 6 months in patients whose ulcers were healed demonstrated a reduction in ulcer recurrence in patients in whom *H. pylori* was eradicated. In 2 other randomized, controlled trials in patients with active duodenal ulcer, eradication of *H. pylori* (defined as 2 negative tests for *H. pylori* 4 weeks after the end of anti-*H. pylori* treatment) was achieved in 72 or 71% of patients receiving 2 weeks of combined therapy with clarithromycin (500 mg 2 or 3 times daily, respectively) and ranitidine bismuth citrate (400 mg twice daily) followed by 2 weeks of monotherapy with ranitidine bismuth citrate (400 mg 2 times daily). Follow-up evaluations demonstrated a twofold reduction in the risk of ulcer recurrence within 6 months of completing treatment in patients in whom *H. pylori* was eradicated compared with those in whom the infection was not eradicated. The contribution, if any, of bismuth citrate to the healing effects of ranitidine alone was not evaluated in these studies.

While some studies demonstrate that certain 2-drug anti-*H. pylori* regimens (e.g., clarithromycin-omeprazole, ranitidine bismuth citrate-omeprazole, amoxicillin-omeprazole) can successfully eradicate *H. pylori* infection and prevent recurrence of duodenal ulcer at least in the short term (e.g., at 6 months following completion of anti-*H. pylori* therapy), 3-drug regimens appear to be associated with higher *H. pylori* overall eradication rates than dual-therapy combinations. In 2 randomized, controlled trials in patients with *H. pylori* infection and duodenal ulcer disease (i.e., active ulcer or history of an ulcer within 1 year) who received triple therapy for 14 days with clarithromycin (500 mg twice daily), amoxicillin (1 g twice daily), and lansoprazole (30 mg twice daily), *H. pylori* was eradicated (defined as 2 negative tests for *H. pylori* by culture or histology 4–6 weeks after the end of anti-*H. pylori* treatment) in 92 or 86% of evaluable patients (86 or 83% of patients, respectively, by intent- to-treat analysis); while dual therapy with lansoprazole (30 mg 3 times daily) and amoxicillin (1 g 3 times daily) for 14 days produced *H. pylori* eradication in 77 or 66% of evaluable patients (70 or 61% of patients, respectively, by intent-to-treat analysis). Therapy with the 3-drug combination was more effective than all possible dual-therapy combination regimens with these drugs (i.e., lansoprazole-amoxicillin, lansoprazole-clarithromycin, and amoxicillin-clarithromycin).

In 3 randomized, double-blind trials in patients with *H. pylori* infection and duodenal ulcer disease (active ulcer or a history of duodenal ulcer in the previous 5 years) who were treated for 10 days, triple therapy with clarithromycin (500 mg twice daily), amoxicillin (1 g twice daily), and omeprazole (20 mg twice daily) eradicated *H. pylori* (defined as 2 negative and no positive tests for *H. pylori* as assessed by CLOtest®, histology, and/or culture) in 77, 78, or 90% of evaluable patients (69, 73, or 83% of patients, respectively, by intent-to-treat analysis); dual therapy with clarithromycin and amoxicillin eradicated *H. pylori* infection in 43, 41, or 33% of evaluable patients (37, 36, or 32% of patients, respectively, by intent-to-treat analysis). In 2 of these studies, patients receiving the triple-therapy regimen for eradication of *H. pylori* continued omeprazole 20 mg daily for an additional 18 days.

The ACG and some clinicians currently state that anti-*H. pylori* regimens consisting of at least 3 drugs (e.g., 2 anti-infective agents plus a proton-pump inhibitor) are recommended because of enhanced *H. pylori* eradication rates, decreased failures secondary to resistance, and shorter treatment periods (e.g., 1 week) compared with those apparently required with 2-drug regimens (e.g., 10–14 days). Additional randomized, controlled studies comparing various anti-*H. pylori* regimens are needed to clarify optimum drug combinations, dosages, and duration of treatment for *H. pylori* infection.

Duration of Therapy The minimum duration of therapy required to eradicate *H. pylori* infection in peptic ulcer disease has not been fully established. In a randomized trial in patients with *H. pylori* infection and duodenal ulcer disease, 10 days of therapy with clarithromycin (500 mg twice daily), amoxicillin (1 g twice daily), and lansoprazole (30 mg twice daily) was as effective in eradicating *H. pylori* as 14 days of therapy with this drug regimen; *H. pylori* eradication was achieved in 85% of evaluable patients with the 14-day regimen compared with 84% of those receiving the 10-day regimen (82 versus 81% of patients, respectively, by intent-to-treat analysis). In patients with uncomplicated ulcers who receive a proton-pump inhibitor (e.g., omeprazole) plus 2 anti-infective agents or a proton-pump inhibitor and bismuth-tetracycline-metronidazole, the ACG and many clinicians state that treatment for longer than 1 week probably is not necessary. However, more prolonged anti-infective and/or antisecretory therapy is recommended for patients with complicated, large, or refractory ulcers; therapy in such patients should be continued at least until successful eradication of *H. pylori* has been confirmed.

Resistant and Recurrent Infection The optimum method of treating patients who fail to respond to currently recommended anti-*H. pylori* regimens is unknown. However, clarithromycin or metronidazole should not be used subsequently in patients with *H. pylori* infection who fail therapy that includes these drugs since resistance commonly emerges during such unsuccessful therapy.

Rapid development of resistance by *H. pylori* to certain drugs (e.g., metronidazole, clarithromycin and other macrolides, quinolones) has occurred when these drugs were used as monotherapy or as the only anti-infective agent in anti-*H. pylori* regimens. Resistance commonly emerges during therapy with clarithromycin or metronidazole when eradication of *H. pylori* is not achieved; therefore, prior exposure to these anti-infectives predicts resistance in individual patients and should be considered when selecting anti-*H. pylori* treatment regimens. Clarithromycin-containing regimens should not be used for eradication of *H. pylori* in patients with known or suspected clarithromycin-resistant isolates because of reduced efficacy in such patients. (See Cautions: Precautions and Contraindications.) Some clinicians state that the same anti-infective regimen should not be used for retreatment of *H. pylori* infection even if antibiotic resistance has not developed. In clinical trials in patients who received clarithromycin as the sole anti-infective agent in combination regimens for *H. pylori* infection, some *H. pylori* isolates demonstrated an increase in clarithromycin MICs over time, indicating decreased susceptibility and increasing resistance to the drug. Agents that do not induce resistance in *H. pylori* include amoxicillin, tetracycline, and bismuth; 1 or 2 of these drugs generally are included in regimens that contain metronidazole or clarithromycin. The ACG states that possible regimens for treatment of metronidazole-resistant *H. pylori* infections include bismuth-clarithromycin-tetracycline or omeprazole-amoxicillin-clarithromycin. In patients who develop clarithromycin resistance, the ACG suggests potential alternative therapy consisting of omeprazole, a bismuth salt, metronidazole, and tetracycline; or omeprazole, amoxicillin, and metronidazole. A regimen consisting of amoxicillin (1 g twice daily), rifabutin (300 mg daily), and a proton-pump inhibitor (pantoprazole 40 mg twice daily) for one week reportedly was effective in eradicating *H. pylori* (according to the results of a ^{13}C urea breath test) in about 79% of patients who had failed at least 2 prior courses of anti-*H. pylori* therapy. Some clinicians also suggest that a 3-drug, furazolidone-containing regimen could be used in patients with metronidazole- or clarithromycin-resistant *H. pylori* infection.

The most common cause of ulcer recurrence after anti-infective therapy for *H. pylori* infection is failure to eradicate the organism since reinfection with *H. pylori* in developed countries appears to occur very infrequently. The ACG and some clinicians state that diagnostic confirmation of *H. pylori* eradication is important in patients with complicated, giant, or refractory ulcers but is controversial or generally not needed in those with uncomplicated ulcers who remain asymptomatic after anti-infective therapy. If diagnostic tests for *H. pylori* are used, such tests should be performed at least 1 month or, preferably, longer after discontinuance of anti-*H. pylori* therapy to minimize the potential for false-negative test results attributable to suppression rather than eradication of the organism.

Therapy in Children Combined therapy with 1 or 2 anti-infective agents (e.g., generally amoxicillin with or without metronidazole) and bismuth subsalicylate in children with *H. pylori* infection and associated peptic ulcer disease† appears to promote healing and reduces ulcer recurrence. Although the prevalence of *H. pylori* infection is lower in children than in adults, the organism reportedly has been identified in approximately 50% of children with gastritis or gastric ulcers and in 60% of those with duodenitis or duodenal ulcers. Limited data suggest that therapy with H_2-receptor antagonists or a single antibiotic is associated with a high risk of disease recurrence; in addition, reinfection with *H. pylori* has been reported to be more common in children than in adults. Because the prevalence of *H. pylori* infection and the incidence of *H. pylori*-associated gastroduodenal inflammation are much lower in children than in adults, *H. pylori* is more likely to be associated with peptic ulcer disease when found in a child. Therefore, some clinicians have recommended that children with symptoms suggesting gastroduodenal inflammation that do not respond to antacid therapy should be evaluated for the presence of *H. pylori* and, if the organism is found, given therapy aimed at eradicating the infection. In a study in a limited number of children (mean age: 12.2 years) with *H. pylori*-associated duodenal ulcer, treatment with a 6-week regimen of bismuth subsalicylate and amoxicillin, or these 2 drugs plus metronidazole in cases of initial treatment failure, resulted in endoscopically proved eradication of the organism in 100% of patients at long- term (mean: 6.5 months) follow-up.

Nonulcer Dyspepsia Although it has been suggested that patients with nonulcer dyspepsia and concomitant *H. pylori* infection also may benefit from eradicative therapy for *H. pylori*, evidence from several well-designed clinical trials has been conflicting regarding an association between this organism and nonulcer dyspepsia. Nevertheless, while therapy for *H. pylori* eradication in such patients generally is not routinely recommended, some evidence suggests that initial anti-*H. pylori* therapy may be a cost-effective management strategy compared with initial endoscopy for patients with simple dyspepsia who are *H. pylori*-positive on noninvasive (e.g., serologic) testing.

■ **Bartonella Infections** Clarithromycin has been used in a few patients, including HIV-infected patients, for the treatment of infections caused by *Bartonella henselae*† (formerly *Rochalimaea henselae*) (e.g., cat scratch disease, bacillary angiomatosis, peliosis hepatitis). Cat scratch disease generally is a self-limited illness in immunocompetent individuals and may resolve spontaneously in 2–4 months; however, some clinicians suggest that anti-infective therapy be considered for acutely or severely ill patients with systemic symptoms, particularly those with hepatosplenomegaly or painful lymphadenopathy, and such therapy probably is indicated in immunocompromised patients. Anti-infectives also are indicated in patients with *B. henselae* infections who develop bacillary angiomatosis, neuroretinitis, or Parinaud's oculoglandular syndrome. While the optimum anti-infective regimen for the treatment of cat scratch disease or other *B. henselae* infections has not been identified, some clinicians recommend use of erythromycin, doxycycline, ciprofloxacin, rifampin, co-trimoxazole, gentamicin, azithromycin, clarithromycin, or third generation cephalosporins.

■ **Cryptosporidiosis** It has been reported that use of clarithromycin or rifabutin in HIV-infected adults for prevention of MAC infection may also decrease the incidence of cryptosporidiosis is these patients. No anti-infective agent has been found to reliably eradicate *Cryptosporidium*, although several drugs (e.g., paromomycin, azithromycin, nitazoxanide) may improve symptoms or suppress the infection.

HIV-infected individuals at greatest risk for cryptosporidiosis are those with advanced immunosuppression (i.e., CD4+ T-cell counts less than 100/mm^3) and fulminant infections usually have occurred in those with CD4+ T-cell counts less than 50/ mm^3. The CDC, National Institutes of Health (NIH), IDSA, and other clinicians state that the most appropriate treatment for cryptosporidiosis in HIV-infected individuals is the use of potent antiretroviral agents and symptomatic treatment of diarrhea. A highly potent antiretroviral regimen can result in immune restoration (CD4+ T-cell counts exceeding 100/ mm^3) which usually results in resolution of the infection. Symptomatic treatment of diarrhea in HIV-infected or immunocompetent individuals with cryptosporidiosis should include oral or IV fluids and electrolyte replacement to correct dehydration and nutritional supplementation when necessary; severe diarrhea may require intensive support. Adjunctive use of antimotility agents may be indicated, but these agents are not consistently effective and should be used with caution in young children.

■ **Legionella Infections** Clarithromycin has been used for the treatment of Legionnaires' disease† caused by *Legionella pneumophila*. Macrolides (usually azithromycin) or fluoroquinolones are considered the drugs of choice for the treatment of pneumonia caused by *L. pneumophila* and doxycycline and co-trimoxazole are alternatives. An oral regimen (e.g., azithromycin, erythromycin, doxycycline, clarithromycin, a fluoroquinolone) may be effective for patients with mild to moderate Legionnaires' disease. However, a parenteral regimen (e.g., azithromycin or a fluoroquinolone) usually is necessary for the initial treatment of severe Legionnaires' disease and the addition of oral rifampin is recommended during the first 3–5 days of therapy in severely ill and/or immunocompromised patients; after a response is obtained, rifampin can be discontinued and therapy changed to an oral regimen.

■ **Lyme Disease** Clarithromycin (500 mg twice daily for 21 days) has been used with apparent success (based on a 6-month follow-up period) in a limited number of patients with early Lyme disease†. However, some evidence in patients with early Lyme disease suggests that other macrolides (e.g., azithromycin, erythromycin) may be less effective than penicillins or tetracyclines, and the IDSA, AAP, and other clinicians recommend that macrolide antibiotics *not* be used as first-line therapy for early Lyme disease.

Oral doxycycline or oral amoxicillin is recommended as first-line therapy for the treatment of early localized or early disseminated Lyme disease associated with erythema migrans, in the absence of neurologic involvement or third-degree atrioventricular (AV) heart block; alternatively, oral cefuroxime axetil has been used. The IDSA and other clinicians state that macrolide antibiotics should be reserved for patients who are intolerant of doxycycline, amoxicillin, and cefuroxime axetil and that patients treated with macrolides should be monitored closely. For more detailed information on the manifestations of Lyme disease and the efficacy of various anti-infective regimens in early or late Lyme disease, see Lyme Disease in Uses: Spirochetal Infections, in the Tetracyclines General Statement 8:12.24.

■ **Mycobacterial Infections** ***Mycobacterium avium Complex (MAC) Infections*** **Primary Prevention of Disseminated MAC Infection.** Clarithromycin (conventional tablets, oral suspension) is used to prevent *Mycobacterium avium* complex (MAC) bacteremia and disseminated infections (primary prophylaxis) in patients with advanced HIV infection. The Prevention of Opportunistic Infections Working Group of the US Public Health Service and the Infectious Diseases Society of America (USPHS/IDSA) state that either clarithromycin or azithromycin is the preferred drug for primary prevention of disseminated MAC infection in adults and pediatric patients.

Results of a limited number of controlled studies in patients with HIV infection and absolute helper/inducer (CD4+, T4+) T-cell counts less than 100/ mm^3 indicate that clarithromycin used alone is more effective than placebo in preventing disseminated MAC disease; clarithromycin prophylaxis also has been shown to reduce mortality in at least one placebo-controlled study. In a randomized, double-blind study in patients with acquired immunodeficiency syndrome (AIDS) and baseline median CD4+ counts of 25–30 cells/ mm^3, the risk of MAC infection (defined as at least one positive culture for MAC bacteria from blood or another normally sterile site) was reduced by 69% in patients receiving clarithromycin 500 mg twice daily compared with that in patients receiving placebo (6 versus 16% incidence of MAC infection with clarithromycin or placebo prophylaxis, respectively). On an intent-to-treat basis, the 1-year cumulative incidence of MAC bacteremia was 5% for patients receiving clarithromycin and 19.4% for patients receiving placebo. Clarithromycin-resistant MAC isolates developed in 11 of 19 clarithromycin recipients who developed MAC infection compared with none of the 53 placebo recipients in whom MAC bacteremia developed. Despite this higher incidence of clarithromycin resistance, clarithromycin prophylaxis was associated with reduced mortality compared with placebo, particularly during the first 12 months of the study.

During a follow-up period of about 10 months, the incidence of mortality with clarithromycin prophylaxis was 32% versus 41% with placebo, a 26% reduction. The incidences of hospitalization and of certain complications of HIV infection (e.g., pneumonia, giardiasis) also were reduced in patients receiving clarithromycin prophylaxis. Patients receiving clarithromycin also showed reductions in the manifestations of disseminated MAC disease, including fever, night sweats, weight loss, and anemia. Although the incidence of adverse effects attributed to the study drug was higher in patients receiving clarithromycin (42%) than in those receiving placebo (26%), taste perversion (11 versus 2% with clarithromycin or placebo, respectively) and rectal disorders (8 versus 3%, respectively) were the only adverse effects that occurred more frequently with clarithromycin than with placebo. The incidence of severe adverse effects was similar with clarithromycin (7%) and placebo (6%), and discontinuance of clarithromycin prophylaxis because of adverse events (principally headache, nausea, vomiting, depression and taste perversion) was required in 18% of patients receiving the drug compared with 17% of those receiving placebo.

The USPHS/IDSA recommends primary prophylaxis against MAC disease for HIV-infected adults and adolescents (13 years or older) who have CD4+ T-cell counts less than 50/ mm^3. Severely immunocompromised HIV-infected children younger than 13 years of age also should receive primary prophylaxis against MAC disease according to the following age-specific CD4+ T-cell counts: children 6–13 years of age, less than 50 cells/ mm^3; children 2– 6 years of age, less than 75 cells/ mm^3; children 1–2 years of age, less than 500 cells/ mm^3; and infants younger than 1 year of age, less than 750 cells/ mm^3.

Although either azithromycin or clarithromycin is the preferred drug for primary prophylaxis against MAC, the USPHS/IDSA states that rifabutin may be used if the macrolides cannot be tolerated. There is evidence from placebo-controlled studies that concomitant use of clarithromycin and rifabutin for primary prophylaxis is no more effective than clarithromycin used alone and the combination regimen appears to be associated with an increased incidence of adverse effects. Therefore, the USPHS/IDSA does not recommend concomitant use of clarithromycin and rifabutin for primary MAC prophylaxis. Although the combination of azithromycin and rifabutin is more effective than azithromycin alone for primary MAC prophylaxis, the USPHS/IDSA does not recommend this combination regimen because of additional cost, increased incidence of adverse effects, and absence of a difference in survival in patients receiving the combination compared with azithromycin prophylaxis alone.

Current evidence indicates that primary MAC prophylaxis can be discontinued with minimal risk of developing disseminated MAC disease in HIV-infected adults and adolescents who have responded to highly active antiretroviral therapy (HAART) with an increase in CD4+ T-cell counts to greater than 100/ mm^3 that has been sustained for at least 3 months. The USPHS/IDSA states that discontinuance of primary prophylaxis against MAC is recommended in adults and adolescents meeting these criteria because prophylaxis in these individuals appears to add little benefit in terms of disease prevention for MAC or bacterial infections, and discontinuance reduces the medication burden, the potential for toxicity, drug interactions, selection of drug-resistant pathogens, and cost. However, the USPHS/IDSA states that primary MAC prophylaxis should be restarted in adults and adolescents if CD4+ T-cell counts decrease to less than 50–100/ mm^3. The safety of discontinuing MAC prophylaxis in children whose CD4+ T-cell counts have increased as a result of highly active antiretroviral therapy has not been studied to date.

HIV-infected pregnant women are at risk for MAC disease, and primary prophylaxis against the infection should be given to such women who have T-cell counts less than 50/ mm^3. However, some clinicians may choose to withhold prophylaxis during the first trimester of pregnancy because of general concerns regarding drug administration during this period. Of the available agents, the USPHS/IDSA considers azithromycin the drug of choice for MAC prophylaxis in HIV-infected pregnant women because of the drug's safety profile in animal studies and anecdotal information on safety in humans. Clarithromycin has demonstrated adverse effects on pregnancy outcome and/or embryo-fetal development in animals and should be used during pregnancy only in clinical circumstances where no alternative therapy is appropriate. (See Cautions: Pregnancy, Fertility, and Lactation.).

HIV-infected patients who develop MAC disease while receiving prophylaxis for the infection require treatment with multiple drugs since monotherapy results in drug resistance and clinical failure.

Treatment and Prevention of Recurrence of Disseminated MAC Infection. Clarithromycin (conventional tablets, oral suspension) is used as part of a multiple-drug regimen for the treatment of disseminated MAC infections and for prevention of recurrence (secondary prophylaxis) of MAC infections. Although clarithromycin has been effective when used alone for the treatment of MAC, most authorities recommend the use of multiple-drug regimens for the treatment or secondary prevention of these infections.

For the treatment of disseminated MAC infections in HIV-infected adults, adolescents, and children, the ATS, CDC, NIH, IDSA, and other clinicians recommend a regimen of clarithromycin (or azithromycin) and ethambutol and state that consideration can be given to adding a third drug (preferably rifabutin). Some clinicians state that clarithromycin is the preferred macrolide for the initial treatment regimen because of more extensive experience and because it appears to be associated with more rapid clearance of MAC from blood; however, azithromycin can be substituted if clarithromycin cannot be used because of drug interactions or intolerance and is preferred in pregnant women. Rifabutin should be included in the treatment regimen if the patient has advanced immunosuppression ($CD4^+$ T-cell count less than 50/mm^3) or high mycobacterial load (exceeding 2 log_{10} colony forming units/mL of blood) or is not receiving effective antiretroviral therapy since there is an increased risk of mortality and emergence of drug resistance. If a third drug is indicated in the treatment regimen and rifabutin cannot be used (e.g., because of drug interactions or intolerance), use of a fluoroquinolone (ciprofloxacin or levofloxacin) or amikacin can be considered.

Limited data from comparative trials suggest that concomitant use of ethambutol and clarithromycin may decrease emergence of clarithromycin-resistant MAC; however, inclusion of clofazimine in multiple-drug regimens containing clarithromycin (e.g., with or without ethambutol) does not add to the efficacy (e.g., in terms of prevention of clarithromycin resistance) of such regimens and may even be associated with reduced survival. Therefore, clofazimine should not be used for the treatment of disseminated MAC disease.

Clarithromycin appears to be one of the most active single agents against MAC; however, monotherapy with clarithromycin has been associated with clinical and bacteriologic relapse and the development of clarithromycin-resistant MAC isolates. Randomized studies in adults and children infected with HIV and MAC who had peripheral blood absolute helper/inducer ($CD4^+$, $T4^+$) T-cell counts less than 100/ mm^3 (with most patients having such T-cell counts less than 50/ mm^3), demonstrated that oral monotherapy with clarithromycin (0.5–2 g twice daily in adults, 3.75–15 mg/kg twice daily in children) resulted in clinical and laboratory improvement of the MAC infection. In 52–61% of treated patients in these studies, colony counts of MAC in sequential blood cultures decreased or became absent within 29–54 days; patients also experienced decreases in the incidence of fever, night sweats, weight loss, diarrhea, splenomegaly, and hepatomegaly. However, effects of clarithromycin monotherapy were not sustained; only 8–25% of treated patients maintained negative blood cultures for 12 weeks or longer and median duration of clinical improvement was 2–6 weeks. In addition, development of drug resistance has been reported after 2–7 months of clarithromycin monotherapy.

High clarithromycin dosages (e.g., 1 or 2 g twice daily) for the treatment of disseminated MAC infection have been associated with reduced survival in some studies compared with that in patients receiving clarithromycin 500 mg twice daily; while these findings are not fully understood, dosages exceeding 500 mg twice daily currently are not recommended in HIV-infected patients with disseminated MAC infection. In randomized studies in HIV-infected patients who had peripheral blood absolute helper/inducer ($CD4^+$, $T4^+$) T-cell counts less than 100/ mm^3 (with most patients having such T-cell counts less than 50/ mm^3), median survival was 199–249 or 179–215 days in adults receiving clarithromycin dosages of 0.5 or 1 g twice daily, respectively. Higher dosages (e.g., 1–2 g twice daily) of clarithromycin were associated with better bacteriologic improvement during the first 4 weeks of therapy; median time to achieve negative blood culture was 54, 41, or 29 days in patients receiving 0.5, 1, or 2 g of the drug twice daily, respectively. However, no substantial differences in the time required to achieve negative blood cultures were observed later in therapy.

To prevent recurrence of MAC disease in HIV-infected adults, adolescents, or children who have previously been treated for an acute episode of MAC infection and in whom macrolide resistance has not been documented, the USPHS/IDSA, CDC, NIH, and IDSA recommend a regimen consisting of a macrolide (clarithromycin or azithromycin) given with ethambutol (with or without rifabutin). Azithromycin usually is the preferred macrolide for use in conjunction with ethambutol for secondary prophylaxis of disseminated MAC infection in pregnant women. Secondary MAC prophylaxis generally is administered for life in adults and adolescents unless immune recovery has occurred as a result of potent antiretroviral therapy. Limited data indicate that secondary MAC prophylaxis can be discontinued in adults and adolescents who have immune recovery in response to potent antiretroviral therapy. Based on these data and more extensive cumulative data on safety of discontinuing secondary prophylaxis for other opportunistic infections, the USPHS/IDSA, CDC, NIH, and IDSA state that it may be reasonable to consider discontinuance of secondary MAC prophylaxis in adults and adolescents who have successfully completed at least 12 months of MAC therapy, have remained asymptomatic with respect to MAC, and have $CD4^+$ T-cell counts exceeding 100/ mm^3 as the result of potent antiretroviral therapy and this increase has been sustained (e.g., for 6 months or longer). Some experts would obtain a blood culture for MAC (even in asymptomatic patients) prior to discontinuing secondary MAC prophylaxis to substantiate that the disease is no longer active. Secondary MAC prophylaxis should be restarted in adults or adolescents if $CD4^+$ T-cell counts decrease to less than 100/ mm^3. The safety of discontinuing secondary MAC prophylaxis in HIV-infected children receiving potent antiretroviral therapy has not been studied and children with a history of disseminated MAC should receive lifelong secondary prophylaxis.

Treatment of Pulmonary MAC Infections in HIV-negative Adults. Clarithromycin has been used in multiple-drug regimens for the treatment of pulmonary MAC infections in patients not infected with HIV.

The ATS recommends that pulmonary MAC infections in HIV-negative adults be treated with a regimen that includes at least 3 drugs, including clarithromycin (500 mg twice daily) or azithromycin (250 mg daily or 500 mg 3 times weekly), rifabutin (300 mg daily) or rifampin (600 mg daily), and ethambutol (25 mg/kg daily for 2 months, then 15 mg/kg daily). For patients with a small body mass and/or who are older than 70 years of age, clarithromycin 250 mg twice daily or azithromycin 250 mg 3 times weekly may be better tolerated. The ATS states that the addition of streptomycin given intermittently (2 or 3 times weekly) for the first 2–3 months may be considered for patients with extensive disease.

Other Mycobacterial Infections Clarithromycin has been used with some success in the treatment of various other mycobacterial infections†; however, further experience and study are needed to establish the role of clarithromycin in the treatment of these infections.

The ATS and other clinicians suggest that clarithromycin can be used as an alternative agent for the treatment of infections caused by *M. kansasii*†. Although a regimen of isoniazid, rifampin, and ethambutol usually is recommended for the treatment of pulmonary or extrapulmonary infections caused by *M. kansasii*, the ATS states that clarithromycin is a reasonable alternative in patients who are unable to tolerate one of these drugs or when retreatment is necessary. It also has been suggested that clarithromycin may be substituted for rifampin for the treatment of *M. kansasii* infections in HIV-infected individuals who are receiving indinavir and therefore cannot receive concomitant rifampin. Although *M. kansasii* generally are susceptible to clarithromycin in vitro, clinical experience is limited and efficacy of the drug for the treatment of infections caused by this organism has not been established.

The ATS suggests that use of clarithromycin can be considered for the treatment of cutaneous infections caused by *M. abscessus*† or *M. chelonae*† and states that treatment of these infections should be based on results of in vitro susceptibility testing. Although there is some evidence that clarithromycin monotherapy may be effective for the treatment of cutaneous *M. chelonae* infections in adults, preliminary studies indicate that monotherapy with macrolides is insufficient to produce microbiologic cure for pulmonary *M. abscessus* infection. In an open, noncomparative trial evaluating clarithromycin in cutaneous (disseminated) infection caused by *M. chelonae* in a limited number of patients with immunosuppression secondary to disease (e.g., organ transplant, autoimmune disease) or drug therapy (e.g., corticosteroids, cyclophosphamide), clarithromycin (0.5–1 g twice daily for 6 months) resolved the infection in all patients completing therapy; 82% of patient who completed therapy had complete remission of the infection. Oral clarithromycin has been used in the treatment of an outbreak of cutaneous *M. abscessus* infections involving the hands and feet that occurred in children and one adult as the result of exposure at a public wading pool; however, the benefits of the drug in this infection are unclear since lesions eventually resolved in all patients, including those who did not receive clarithromycin treatment (with or without incision and drainage of lesions).

The ATS and others suggest that clarithromycin monotherapy is one of several acceptable regimens for the treatment of cutaneous infections caused by *M. marinum*†.

Limited in vitro and in vivo studies suggest that clarithromycin has bactericidal activity against *M. leprae*, and the drug has been used with some success in multiple-drug regimens for short periods in a few patients with leprosy†.

■ **Pertussis** Clarithromycin has been effective when used for the treatment of pertussis† caused by *Bordetella pertussis*. In a randomized study in children 1 month to 16 years of age with culture-proven *B. pertussis* infection or a cough illness suspected of being pertussis, a 7-day regimen of oral clarithromycin (7.5 mg/kg twice daily) was as effective and better tolerated than a 14-day regimen of oral erythromycin (13.3 mg/kg 3 times daily).

A 14-day regimen of oral erythromycin usually is considered the drug of choice for the treatment of pertussis and for prevention in contacts of patients with pertussis. However, other macrolides (azithromycin, clarithromycin) appear to be as effective and may be associated with better compliance since they are better tolerated.

■ **Toxoplasmosis** Clarithromycin has been used in conjunction with pyrimethamine for the treatment of encephalitis caused by *Toxoplasma gondii*† in a few patients with AIDS. The USPHS/IDSA states that use of clarithromycin for primary or secondary prophylaxis of toxoplasmosis in HIV-infected individuals cannot be recommended based on current data. The CDC, NIH, IDSA, and other clinicians usually recommend a regimen of pyrimethamine in conjunction with sulfadiazine and leucovorin for the treatment of toxoplasmosis in adults and children, especially immunocompromised patients (e.g., HIV-infected individuals).

For information on recommendations regarding treatment and prophylaxis of toxoplasmosis, see Toxoplasmosis under Uses: Pyrimethamine, in Pyrimethamine and Sulfadoxine and Pyrimethamine 8:30.08.

■ **Prevention of Bacterial Endocarditis** Clarithromycin has been recommended for prevention of α-hemolytic (viridans group) streptococcal endocarditis† in penicillin-allergic adults and children with congenital heart disease, rheumatic or other acquired valvular heart dysfunction (even after valvular surgery), prosthetic heart valves (including bioprosthetic or allograft valves), surgically constructed systemic pulmonary shunts or conduits, hypertrophic cardiomyopathy, mitral valve prolapse with valvular regurgitation and/or thickened leaflets, or previous bacterial endocarditis (even in the absence of heart disease) who undergo dental procedures that are likely to result in gingival or mucosal bleeding (e.g., dental extractions; periodontal procedures such as scaling, root planing, probing, and maintenance; dental implant placement or reimplantation of avulsed teeth; root-filling procedures; subgingival placement of antibiotic fibers or strips; initial placement of orthodontic bands; intraligamentary local anesthetic injections; routine professional cleaning) or minor upper respiratory tract surgery or instrumentation (e.g., tonsillectomy, adenoidectomy, bronchoscopy with a rigid bronchoscope). The AHA recognizes that its current recommendations for prevention of bacterial endocarditis are empiric, since no controlled efficacy studies have been published, and that prophylaxis of endocarditis is not always effective. However, the AHA, the ADA, and most clinicians generally recommend routine use of prophylactic anti-infectives in patients at risk for bacterial endocarditis. When selecting anti-infectives for prophylaxis of recurrent rheumatic fever or prophylaxis of bacterial endocarditis, the current recommendations published by the AHA should be consulted.

Dosage and Administration

■ Reconstitution and Administration Clarithromycin conventional tablets and oral suspension are administered orally and may be given without regard to meals. Clarithromycin oral suspension may be administered with milk. Clarithromycin extended-release tablets should be taken with food.

Clarithromycin granules for oral suspension should be reconstituted at the time of dispensing by adding the amount of water specified on the bottle to provide a suspension containing 125 or 250 mg of clarithromycin per 5 mL of suspension. The water should be added in two portions and the suspension agitated well after each addition. The suspension should be agitated well just prior to each use.

■ Dosage Safety and efficacy of clarithromycin extended-release tablets have been established for the treatment of acute bacterial exacerbations of chronic bronchitis, acute maxillary sinusitis, and community-acquired pneumonia (CAP) in adults; safety and efficacy of the extended-release formulation of the drug have not been established for the treatment of other infections that are treated with clarithromycin conventional tablets or oral suspension.

Adult Dosage **Pharyngitis and Tonsillitis.** The usual oral dosage of clarithromycin conventional tablets or oral suspension for the treatment of pharyngitis and tonsillitis in adults is 250 mg every 12 hours for 10 days.

Acute Exacerbations of Chronic Bronchitis. For the treatment of acute exacerbations of chronic bronchitis caused by *Haemophilus influenzae* or *H. parainfluenzae*, the usual adult dosage of clarithromycin conventional tablets or oral suspension is 500 mg every 12 hours for 7–14 days or 7 days, respectively. The usual adult dosage of clarithromycin conventional tablets or oral suspension for the treatment of acute bacterial exacerbations of chronic bronchitis caused by *Moraxella catarrhalis* or *Streptococcus pneumoniae* is 250 mg every 12 hours for 7–14 days. Lower dosage should not be used (e.g., 250 mg twice daily) since such regimens have failed to eradicate *H. influenzae* in clinical studies.

If clarithromycin *extended-release* tablets are used for the treatment of acute exacerbations of chronic bronchitis caused by *H. influenzae*, *H. parainfluenzae*, *M. catarrhalis*, or *S. pneumoniae*, the usual adult dosage is 1 g (two 500-mg extended-release tablets) once daily for 7 days.

Acute Sinusitis. The usual oral dosage of clarithromycin conventional tablets or oral suspension for the treatment of acute maxillary sinusitis in adults is 500 mg every 12 hours for 14 days.

If clarithromycin *extended-release* tablets are used for the treatment of acute maxillary sinusitis, the usual adult dosage is 1 g (two 500- mg extended-release tablets) once daily for 14 days.

Community-acquired Pneumonia. For the treatment of community-acquired pneumonia (CAP) in adults, the usual dosage of clarithromycin conventional tablets or oral suspension is 250 mg every 12 hours. The usual duration of treatment is 7–14 days for infections caused by *Chlamydophila pneumoniae* (*Chlamydia pneumoniae*), *Mycoplasma pneumoniae*, or *S. pneumoniae* or 7 days for infections caused by *H. influenzae*. The fact that this dosage has failed to eradicate *H. influenzae* in some clinical studies should be considered.

If clarithromycin *extended-release* tablets are used for the treatment of CAP caused by *H. influenzae*, *H. parainfluenzae*, *M. catarrhalis*, *S. pneumoniae*, *C. pneumoniae*, or *M. pneumoniae*, the usual adult dosage is 1 g (two 500 mg extended-release tablets) once daily for 7 days.

Skin and Skin Structure Infections. The usual adult dosage of clarithromycin conventional tablets or oral suspension for the treatment of uncomplicated skin and skin structure infections is 250 mg every 12 hours for 7–14 days.

Helicobacter pylori Infection and Duodenal Ulcer Disease. When used in combination with omeprazole (40 mg daily in the morning for 14 days) for the treatment of *H. pylori* infection in adults with duodenal ulcer disease (active or up to 1-year history), the recommended dosage of clarithromycin (conventional tablets or oral suspension) is 500 mg 3 times daily for 14 days; an additional 14 days of omeprazole monotherapy (20 mg daily in the morning) is recommended for ulcer healing and symptom relief in patients with an active duodenal ulcer at the time treatment is initiated to complete 28 days of therapy.

When used in combination with ranitidine bismuth citrate (400 mg twice daily for 14 days) the recommended dosage of clarithromycin (conventional tablets or oral suspension) for the treatment of *H. pylori* infection and duodenal ulcer is 500 mg 2 or 3 times daily for 14 days; an additional 14 days of ranitidine bismuth citrate monotherapy (400 mg twice daily) is then administered to complete 28 days of therapy.

When used in combination with amoxicillin (1 g twice daily for 10 or 14 days) and lansoprazole (30 mg twice daily for 10 or 14 days), the recommended dosage of clarithromycin (conventional tablets or oral suspension) for the treatment of *H. pylori* infection and duodenal ulcer in adults is 500 mg twice daily for 10 or 14 days.

When used in combination with amoxicillin (1 g twice daily for 10 days) and omeprazole (20 mg twice daily for 10 days), the recommended dosage of clarithromycin (conventional tablets or oral suspension) for the treatment of *H. pylori* infection and duodenal ulcer disease (active or up to 1-year history of duodenal ulcer) in adults is 500 mg twice daily for 10 days. An additional 18 days of omeprazole monotherapy (20 mg daily) is recommended for ulcer healing and symptom relief in patients with an active duodenal ulcer at the time therapy is initiated.

Multiple-drug regimens recommended by the American College of Gastroenterology (ACG) and many clinicians for the treatment of *H. pylori* infection consist of a proton-pump inhibitor (e.g., omeprazole, lansoprazole) and 2 anti-infective agents (e.g., clarithromycin and amoxicillin or metronidazole) or a 3-drug, bismuth-based regimen (e.g., bismuth-metronidazole-tetracycline) concomitantly with a proton-pump inhibitor; when clarithromycin has been used in these regimens, dosages of 250 mg twice daily to 500 mg 3 times daily (generally 500 mg 2 or 3 times daily) have been used.

While the minimum duration of therapy required to eradicate *H. pylori* infection with these 3- or 4-drug regimens has not been fully elucidated, the ACG and many clinicians state that treatment for longer than 1 week probably is not necessary. However, more prolonged therapy is recommended for patients with complicated, large, or refractory ulcers; therapy in such patients should be continued at least until successful eradication of *H. pylori* has been confirmed. (See Helicobacter pylori Infection, in Uses.)

Bartonella Infections. For the treatment of cat scratch disease† caused by *Bartonella henselae*†, clarithromycin has been given in a dosage of 500 mg daily for 4 weeks.

If clarithromycin is used for the treatment of infections caused by *Bartonella*† in HIV-infected adults or adolescents, the CDC, NIH, and IDSA recommend a dosage of 500 mg twice daily for at least 3 months. If relapse occurs, lifelong secondary prophylaxis (chronic maintenance therapy) with erythromycin or doxycycline should be considered.

Legionella Infections. For the treatment of Legionnaires' disease†, some clinicians recommend that clarithromycin be given in a dosage of 500 mg twice daily. The usual duration of clarithromycin therapy is 10 days for the treatment of mild to moderate infections in immunocompetent patients; however, 3 weeks of treatment may be necessary to prevent relapse, especially in those with more severe infections or with underlying comorbidity or immunodeficiency.

Lyme Disease. For the treatment of early localized or early disseminated Lyme disease† associated with erythema migrans (but without neurologic involvement or third-degree AV heart block) in patients who are allergic to or intolerant of amoxicillin, doxycycline, and cefuroxime axetil, the Infectious Diseases Society of America (IDSA) suggests that adults receive oral clarithromycin in a dosage of 500 mg (conventional tablets or oral suspension) twice daily for 14–21 days.

Mycobacterium Avium Complex (MAC) Infections (Primary Prophylaxis). For primary prevention of disseminated *Mycobacterium avium* complex (MAC) infection (primary prophylaxis) in adults and adolescents with human immunodeficiency virus (HIV) infection, the usual dosage of clarithromycin (conventional tablets or oral suspension) is 500 mg every 12 hours.

The Prevention of Opportunistic Infections Working Group of the US Public Health Service and the Infectious Diseases Society of America (USPHS/IDSA) recommends primary prophylaxis against disseminated MAC infection in HIV-infected adults and adolescents with $CD4^+$ T-cell counts less than 50/mm^3. Although consideration can be given to discontinuing such prophylaxis in adults and adolescents when there is immune recovery in response to potent antiretroviral therapy and an increase in $CD4^+$ T-cell count to greater than 100/mm^3 has been sustained for at least 3 months (see Primary Prevention of Disseminated MAC Infection under Mycobacterial Infections: Mycobacterium avium Complex [MAC] Infections under Uses), the USPHS/IDSA states that primary MAC prophylaxis should be restarted if the $CD4^+$ T-cell count decreases to less than 50–100/ mm^3.

Mycobacterium avium Complex (MAC) Infections (Treatment and Prevention of Recurrence). For the treatment of disseminated MAC infection, adults and adolescents should receive 500 mg of clarithromycin (conventional tablets or oral suspension) every 12 hours in conjunction with ethambutol (15 mg/kg daily) with or without a third drug (e.g., rifabutin 300 mg once daily). Clarithromycin dosages higher than 500 mg twice daily are not recommended since such dosages have been associated with reduced survival in clinical studies in patients with disseminated MAC disease.

For prevention of recurrence (secondary prophylaxis or chronic maintenance therapy) of disseminated MAC in HIV-infected adults or adolescents who responded to treatment, the USPHS/IDSA, CDC, NIH, and IDSA recommend that adults and adolescents receive clarithromycin in a dosage of 500 mg twice daily in conjunction with ethambutol (15 mg/kg once daily) with or without rifabutin (300 mg once daily). Secondary MAC prophylaxis in HIV-infected individuals usually is continued for life therapy. However, consideration can be given to discontinuing secondary MAC prophylaxis in adults and adolescents when there is immune recovery in response to potent antiretroviral therapy (see Treatment and Prevention of Recurrence of Disseminated MAC Infection under Mycobacterial Infections: Mycobacterium avium Complex [MAC] Infections in Uses) but such prophylaxis should be restarted if CD4+ T-cell counts decrease to less than 100/ mm³.

Mycobacterium avium Complex (MAC) Infections (Treatment of Pulmonary Infections in HIV-negative Adults). For the treatment of mild to moderately advanced MAC pulmonary infections† in HIV-negative adults, the ATS recommends therapy with clarithromycin 500 mg twice daily in conjunction with rifabutin (300 mg daily) or rifampin (600 mg daily) and ethambutol (25 mg/kg daily for 2 months, then 15 mg/kg daily). A lower dosage of clarithromycin (250 mg twice daily) in this regimen may be better tolerated in patients with a small body mass and/or those who are older than 70 years of age. The ATS states that the addition of streptomycin therapy given intermittently (2 or 3 times weekly) for the first 2–3 months may be considered in patients with extensive disease. The optimal duration of therapy for pulmonary MAC disease has not been established, but patients probably should be treated until they are culture-negative on therapy for 1 year.

Mycobacterium chelonae and M. abscessus Infections. For the treatment of cutaneous infections caused by *Mycobacterium chelonae*† or *M. abscessus*†, adults have received oral clarithromycin in a dosage of 0.5–1 g twice daily for 6 months.

Mycobacterium marinum Infections. For the treatment of cutaneous infections caused by *M. marinum*†, adults have received oral clarithromycin in a dosage of 500 mg twice daily for at least 3 months.

Prevention of Bacterial Endocarditis. For prevention of bacterial endocarditis† in adults undergoing certain dental, oral, respiratory tract, or esophageal procedures, the usual dosage of clarithromycin is 500 mg given as a single dose 1 hour prior to the procedure.

Pediatric Dosage **Acute Otitis Media.** The usual oral dosage of clarithromycin for the treatment of acute otitis media (AOM) in children is 7.5 mg/kg every 12 hours for 10 days.

Pharyngitis and Tonsillitis. The usual oral dosage of clarithromycin conventional tablets or oral suspension for the treatment of pharyngitis and tonsillitis in children is 7.5 mg/kg every 12 hours for 10 days.

Acute Sinusitis. Children receiving clarithromycin conventional tablets or oral suspension for the treatment of acute maxillary sinusitis should receive 7.5 mg/kg every 12 hours for 10 days.

Community-acquired Pneumonia. Children receiving clarithromycin conventional tablets or oral suspension for the treatment of CAP should receive 7.5 mg/kg every 12 hours for 10 days.

Skin and Skin Structure Infections. The usual dosage of clarithromycin conventional tablets or oral suspension for the treatment of uncomplicated skin and skin structure infections in children is 7.5 mg/kg every 12 hours for 10 days.

Lyme Disease. For the treatment of early localized or early disseminated Lyme disease† associated with erythema migrans (but without neurologic involvement or third-degree AV heart block) in patients who are allergic to or intolerant of amoxicillin, doxycycline, and cefuroxime axetil, the IDSA suggests that children receive oral clarithromycin in a dosage 7.5 mg/kg (up to 500 mg) twice daily for 14–21 days.

Mycobacterium avium Complex (MAC) Infections (Primary Prophylaxis). For primary prevention of MAC infection (primary prophylaxis) in HIV-infected children, the usual dosage of clarithromycin (conventional tablets or oral suspension) is 7.5 mg/ kg (maximum 500 mg) every 12 hours. The manufacturer states that no studies evaluating clarithromycin prophylaxis of MAC infection have been conducted in pediatric patients and that clarithromycin dosage recommended for primary prophylaxis in children is derived from studies involving treatment of MAC infections in pediatric patients.

The safety of discontinuing primary MAC prophylaxis in children whose CD4+ T-cell counts have increased as a result of highly active antiretroviral therapy has not been studied to date.

Mycobacterium avium Complex (MAC) Infections (Treatment and Prevention of Recurrence). For the treatment of disseminated MAC infection, the manufacturer recommends that children receive clarithromycin in a dosage of 7.5 mg/kg (maximum 500 mg) every 12 hours in conjunction with other antimycobacterial drugs that have in vitro activity against MAC. The CDC, NIH, and IDSA state that HIV-infected children may receive clarithromycin in a dosage of 7.5–15 mg/kg (maximum 500 mg) twice daily in conjunction with ethambutol (15–25 mg/kg once daily [up to 1 g daily]) with or without rifabutin (10–20 mg/kg once daily [up to 300 mg daily]) for the treatment of MAC infections.

For long-term suppressive or chronic maintenance therapy (secondary prophylaxis) to prevent recurrence of disseminated MAC in HIV-infected infants or children who responded to treatment, the USPHS/IDSA recommends clarithromycin in a dosage of 7.5 mg/kg (maximum 500 mg) twice daily in conjunction with ethambutol (15 mg/kg [maximum 900 mg] once daily) with or without rifabutin (5 mg/kg [maximum 300 mg] once daily).

The safety of discontinuing secondary MAC prophylaxis in children receiving potent antiretroviral therapy has not been studied to date and HIV-infected children with a history of disseminated MAC should receive lifelong secondary prophylaxis.

Mycobacterium abscessus Infections. For the treatment of cutaneous infections caused by *M. abscessus*†, children 1–15 years of age have received oral clarithromycin in a dosage of 15 mg/kg daily (with or without incision and drainage of lesions).

Pertussis. For the treatment of pertussis† in children, oral clarithromycin has been given in a dosage of 15–20 mg/kg in 2 divided doses (up to 1 g daily) for 7 days. In one study in children 1 month to 16 years of age, clarithromycin was effective for the treatment of pertussis when given in a dosage of 7.5 mg/kg twice daily for 7 days.

Prevention of Bacterial Endocarditis. For prevention of bacterial endocarditis† in children undergoing certain dental, oral, respiratory tract, or esophageal procedures, the usual dosage of clarithromycin is 15 mg/kg given as a single dose 1 hour prior to the procedure.

■ **Dosage in Renal and Hepatic Impairment** Clarithromycin generally may be used without dosage adjustment in patients with hepatic impairment and normal renal function. However, in patients with creatinine clearances less than 30 mL/minute with or without hepatic impairment, the dosage should be halved or the dosing interval for clarithromycin doubled. An initial clarithromycin dose of 500 mg (conventional tablets or oral suspension) followed by 250 mg twice daily has been suggested for adults with creatinine clearances less than 30 mL/minute when a usual dosage of 500 mg twice daily would have been used in adults with normal renal function; a dosage of 250 mg (conventional tablets or oral suspension) daily has been suggested for such patients when a usual dosage of 250 mg twice daily would have been used in individuals with normal renal function.

Cautions

Clarithromycin generally is well tolerated. In clinical studies, most adverse effects were mild and transient; only about 1% of reported effects were described as severe. Limited data from comparative studies suggest that the overall incidence of adverse effects with oral clarithromycin therapy is similar to or lower than that with oral erythromycin. As with oral erythromycin, the most common adverse effects of oral clarithromycin involve the GI tract. The manufacturer states that fewer than 3% of patients receiving oral clarithromycin in clinical studies discontinued therapy because of adverse effects. In clinical trials in patients who received combined therapy with clarithromycin and omeprazole for the treatment of *H. pylori* infection and associated duodenal ulcer, most adverse effects reported with such combined therapy were mild to moderate in severity. However, discontinuance of therapy because of adverse effects was required in 3.5% of these patients.

In clinical trials in which dual therapy with clarithromycin and omeprazole or ranitidine bismuth citrate or triple therapy with clarithromycin, amoxicillin, and lansoprazole or omeprazole was used for the treatment of *H. pylori* infection and associated duodenal ulcer, no adverse effects peculiar to these drug combinations were observed. The most frequently reported adverse effects in patients receiving clarithromycin, amoxicillin, and lansoprazole were diarrhea (7% of patients), headache (6% of patients), and taste perversion (5% of patients). The incidence of adverse effects reported with the clarithromycin-amoxicillin-lansoprazole regimen given for 14 days was similar to that reported with the same regimen given for 10 days. The most frequently reported adverse effects in patients receiving triple therapy with clarithromycin, amoxicillin, and omeprazole were diarrhea (14%), taste perversion (10%), and headache (9%). Triple therapy with these drugs was not associated with a higher incidence of adverse effects than dual therapy. The most frequently reported adverse effects in patients receiving clarithromycin and ranitidine bismuth citrate were taste disturbance (8–11%), diarrhea (4–5%), and nausea and vomiting (3–5%).

■ **GI Effects** Diarrhea, nausea, and abnormal taste were reported in 3–6% of patients receiving oral clarithromycin in clinical studies, while dyspepsia and abdominal discomfort occurred in 2% of patients receiving the drug. Oral candidiasis, glossitis, stomatitis, vomiting, flatulence, diaper dermatitis, constipation, tongue discoloration, anorexia, pancreatitis, and laryngismus also have been reported. Tooth discoloration, usually reversible with professional dental cleaning, has been reported in patients receiving clarithromycin.

Results of studies in animals indicate that clarithromycin causes less stimulation of GI smooth muscle motility than erythromycin, and some clinical studies suggest that clarithromycin may cause adverse GI effects less frequently than oral erythromycin. In patients with community-acquired pneumonia, adverse GI effects were reported less frequently in patients receiving clarithromycin (13%) than in those receiving oral erythromycin as the base or stearate salt (32%). In these studies, discontinuance of therapy because of adverse effects (e.g., vomiting, nausea diarrhea, abdominal pain) reportedly was required in 4% of patients receiving clarithromycin versus 17% of those receiving erythromycin as the base or stearate salt. Similar differences in the development of adverse GI effects were seen in comparative studies of clarithromycin versus amoxicillin and clavulanate potassium; 21% of patients receiving clarithromycin and 40% of patients receiving amoxicillin and clavulanate potassium therapy experienced adverse GI effects.

In studies in patients with acute exacerbation of chronic bronchitis or acute maxillary sinusitis, the incidence of GI overall adverse effects in patients receiving clarithromycin extended-release tablets was similar to the incidence in patients receiving clarithromycin conventional tablets; however, those receiving the extended-release tablets reported substantially less severe GI symptoms than those receiving the conventional tablets. In these studies, discontinuance of therapy because of adverse GI effects or abnormal taste was required more frequently in those receiving the conventional tablets than in those receiving the extended-release tablets.

In clinical trials in patients who received combined therapy with clarithromycin and omeprazole for the treatment of *H. pylori* infection and associated duodenal ulcer, taste perversion was reported in 15% of patients (versus 16 or 1% of those receiving clarithromycin or omeprazole alone, respectively). Nausea was reported in 5% of patients receiving clarithromycin-omeprazole therapy (versus 3 or 1% of those receiving clarithromycin or omeprazole alone, respectively), vomiting in 4% (versus 1% or less than 1% of those receiving clarithromycin or omeprazole alone, respectively), diarrhea in 4% (versus 7 or 3% of those receiving clarithromycin or omeprazole alone, respectively), and abdominal pain in 3% of patients (versus 1 or 2% of those receiving clarithromycin or omeprazole alone, respectively). Tongue discoloration was reported in 2% of patients receiving combined clarithromycin-omeprazole therapy in controlled clinical trials.

In clinical trials in patients who received combined therapy with clarithromycin and ranitidine bismuth citrate for the treatment of *H. pylori* infection and associated duodenal ulcer, taste disturbance occurred in 10% (versus 11 or less than 1% of those receiving clarithromycin or ranitidine bismuth citrate alone, respectively). Diarrhea was reported in 8% (versus 5 or 2% of those receiving clarithromycin or ranitidine bismuth citrate alone, respectively), nausea and vomiting in 3% (versus 2 or less than 1% of those receiving clarithromycin or ranitidine bismuth citrate alone, respectively), and constipation in 0% (versus 0 or 1% of those receiving clarithromycin or ranitidine bismuth citrate alone, respectively).

In clinical trials in which combined therapy with clarithromycin, amoxicillin, and lansoprazole was used for the treatment of *H. pylori* infection and associated duodenal ulcer, adverse GI effects reported in less than 3% of patients included abdominal pain, dark stools, dry mouth/thirst, glossitis, rectal itching, nausea, oral candidiasis, stomatitis, tongue discoloration, tongue disorder, and vomiting.

■ **Hepatic Effects** Elevation in serum ALT (SGPT), AST (SGOT), γ-glutamyltransferase (γ- glutamyl transpeptidase, GGT, GGTP), alkaline phosphatase, LDH, and/or total bilirubin concentration has been reported infrequently (e.g., less than 1% of patients) in patients receiving clarithromycin alone or combined with omeprazole therapy. Hepatomegaly and hepatic dysfunction (including cholestasis, with or without jaundice) also have been reported in patients receiving the drug. This hepatic dysfunction may be severe but usually is reversible. However, hepatic failure leading to death has been reported rarely, generally in patients with serious underlying diseases and/or receiving concomitant drug therapy.

In animals, hepatotoxicity occurred in all species tested at clarithromycin dosages comparable to or twice the maximum recommended human dosage (on a mg/m² basis).

■ **Hematologic Effects** Increased prothrombin time has been reported in 1% of adult patients receiving clarithromycin. Decreased white blood cell (WBC) counts have been reported in less than 1% of patients receiving the drug. Thrombocytopenia has been reported in at least one patient receiving clarithromycin therapy.

Lymphoid depletion has occurred in animals at dosages 2–3 times the maximum recommended human dosage (on a mg/m² basis).

■ **Renal Effects** Elevated BUN has been reported in 4% of patients receiving clarithromycin. Elevated serum creatinine concentration has been reported in less than 1% of patients receiving clarithromycin alone or combined with omeprazole therapy. Acute renal failure reportedly has occurred with clarithromycin therapy.

In animals, renal tubular degeneration occurred at dosages 2–12 times (on a mg/m² basis) the maximum recommended human dosage.

■ **CNS Effects** Headache was reported in 2% of patients receiving clarithromycin in clinical studies. Transient adverse CNS effects, including acute psychosis, anxiety, behavioral changes, confusional states, depersonalization, disorientation, hallucinations, insomnia, nightmares, tinnitus, tremor, and vertigo, have been reported during postmarketing experience. These adverse effects usually resolve following discontinuance of clarithromycin therapy.

In clinical trials in patients who received combined therapy with clarithromycin and omeprazole for the treatment of *H. pylori* infection and associated duodenal ulcer, headache was reported in 5% of patients (versus 9 or 6% of those receiving clarithromycin or omeprazole alone, respectively), while infection was reported in 3% of patients receiving combined therapy (versus 2 or 4% of those receiving clarithromycin or omeprazole alone, respectively).

In clinical trials in patients who received combined therapy with clarithromycin and ranitidine bismuth citrate for the treatment of *H. pylori* infection and associated duodenal ulcer, headache occurred in 5% (versus less than 1 or 1% of those receiving clarithromycin or ranitidine bismuth citrate alone, respectively), dizziness in 0% (versus 2 or less than 1% of those receiving clarithromycin or ranitidine bismuth citrate alone, respectively), and sleep disorder in 2% (versus less than 1% each of those receiving clarithromycin or ranitidine bismuth citrate alone, respectively).

In clinical trials in which combined therapy with clarithromycin, amoxicillin, and lansoprazole was used for the treatment of *H. pylori* infection and associated duodenal ulcer, confusion or dizziness was reported in less than 3% of patients.

■ **Dermatologic and Sensitivity Reactions** Allergic reactions ranging from mild urticaria and mild skin eruptions to rare cases of anaphylaxis, leukocytoclastic vasculitis, toxic epidermal necrolysis, and Stevens-Johnson syndrome have been reported in patients receiving clarithromycin. Pruritus and rash (e.g., fixed drug eruption) also have been reported.

■ **Increased Mortality** An increased risk of all-cause mortality and cardiovascular mortality was reported during long-term follow-up of patients enrolled in a randomized, placebo-controlled study designed to evaluate the possible benefits of a 2-week regimen of clarithromycin (500 mg once daily) in patients with stable coronary heart disease (CLARICOR). At a mean follow-up period of 2.6 years, all-cause mortality was 27% higher (as the result of higher cardiovascular mortality) in study participants who had received the 2-week regimen of clarithromycin compared with those who had received placebo. At 10-year follow-up, data indicate that clarithromycin tended to increase all-cause mortality in all study participants and the increased risk was significant in the subset of study participants who were not receiving an HMG-CoA reductase inhibitor (statin) at study entry. Other limited observational studies have shown variable results regarding the effect of clarithromycin on the risk of death or other heart-related adverse effects. A possible mechanism by which clarithromycin may increase the risk of death in patients with heart disease is unknown. It also is unclear whether the follow-up data from patients in the CLARICOR study can be applied to patients without heart disease.

■ **Other Adverse Effects** As with other macrolides, clarithromycin has been associated with QT prolongation and ventricular arrhythmias, including ventricular tachycardia and atypical ventricular tachycardia (torsades de pointes).

Although a causal relationship to the drug has not been demonstrated, reversible hypoacusis (hearing loss) has been reported in a few patients receiving high (e.g., 2 g daily) dosages of clarithromycin for the treatment of *M. avium* complex infections.

Hypoglycemia has been reported rarely with clarithromycin therapy; in some of these cases, patients were receiving concomitant therapy with insulin or oral antidiabetic agents.

In clinical trials in patients who received combined therapy with clarithromycin and ranitidine bismuth citrate for the treatment of *H. pylori* infection and associated duodenal ulcer, gynecologic problems occurred in 3% (versus 6 or less than 1% of those receiving clarithromycin or ranitidine bismuth citrate alone, respectively). Chest symptoms were reported in 2% (versus 0% of those receiving clarithromycin or ranitidine bismuth citrate alone, respectively) and pruritus in 3% (versus 0 or less than 1% of those receiving clarithromycin or ranitidine bismuth citrate alone, respectively).

In clinical trials in which combined therapy with clarithromycin, amoxicillin, and lansoprazole was used for the treatment of *H. pylori* infection and associated duodenal ulcer, other adverse effects reported in less than 3% of patients include myalgia, respiratory disorders, skin reactions, vaginitis, and vaginal candidiasis.

Other adverse effects reported with combined clarithromycin-omeprazole therapy that differed from those reported with omeprazole alone included rhinitis (2% of patients), pharyngitis (1% of patients), and flu syndrome (1% of patients).

Corneal opacities have occurred in animals at clarithromycin dosages 8–12 times the maximum recommended human dosage (on a mg/m² basis).

■ **Precautions and Contraindications** Clarithromycin is contraindicated in patients with known hypersensitivity to clarithromycin, erythromycin, or any other macrolide antibiotic.

Concomitant use of clarithromycin with certain drugs, including terfenadine (no longer commercially available in the US), astemizole (no longer commercially available in the US), cisapride, and pimozide, is contraindicated because such use is likely to produce substantially increased plasma concentrations of the drugs and possibly cause serious and/or life-threatening cardiotoxicity. Concomitant use with ergot alkaloids (ergotamine, dihydroergotamine) also is contraindicated because of potentially serious toxicity. Concomitant use of clarithromycin and ranitidine bismuth citrate is not recommended in patients with creatinine clearance less than 25 mL/minute, and should not be used in patients with a history of acute porphyria. (See Drug Interactions.)

Other Precautions and Contraindications The potential for increased risk of all-cause mortality and cardiovascular mortality in patients with cardiovascular disease (see Cautions: Increased Mortality) should be considered when weighing the risks and potential benefits of clarithromycin in all patients, particularly those with suspected or confirmed cardiovascular disease. Even if only a short course of clarithromycin is indicated, other available anti-infectives should be considered in those with heart disease. Patients should be advised of the importance of informing their clinicians if they have heart disease, especially when an anti-infective is being prescribed, and the importance of seeking immediate medical attention if they experience symptoms of a heart attack or stroke (e.g., chest pain, shortness of breath, pain or weakness in one part or side of the body, slurred speech). Clarithromycin is not indicated for the treatment of coronary artery disease.

To reduce development of drug-resistant bacteria and maintain effectiveness of clarithromycin and other antibacterials, the drug should be used only for the treatment or prevention of infections proven or strongly suspected to be caused by susceptible bacteria. When selecting or modifying anti-infective therapy, use results of culture and in vitro susceptibility testing. In the absence of such data, consider local epidemiology and susceptibility patterns when selecting anti-infectives for empiric therapy. Patients should be advised that antibacterials (including clarithromycin) should only be used to treat bacterial infections and not used to treat viral infections (e.g., the common cold). Patients also should be advised about the importance of completing the full course of therapy, even if feeling better after a few days, and that skipping doses or not completing therapy may decrease effectiveness and increase the likelihood that bacteria will develop resistance and will not be treatable with clarithromycin or other antibacterials in the future.

As with other anti-infective agents, use of clarithromycin may result in overgrowth of nonsusceptible bacteria or fungi. If superinfection occurs, appropriate therapy should be instituted.

Because *Clostridium difficile*-associated diarrhea and colitis (also known as antibiotic-associated pseudomembranous colitis) caused by overgrowth of toxin-producing clostridia has been reported with the use of many anti-infective agents, including macrolides, it should be considered in the differential diagnosis of patients who develop diarrhea during or following anti-infective therapy. Mild cases of colitis may respond to discontinuance of the drug alone, but diagnosis and management of moderate to severe cases should include sigmoidoscopy, appropriate bacteriologic studies, and treatment with fluid, electrolyte, and protein supplementation as indicated. If colitis is severe or is not relieved by discontinuance of the drug, appropriate anti-infective therapy (e.g., oral metronidazole or vancomycin) should be administered. Isolation of the patient may be advisable. Other causes of colitis also should be considered.

If clarithromycin is used as the sole anti-infective agent in regimens used for the treatment of *H. pylori* and duodenal ulcer disease, *H. pylori* with decreased susceptibility or resistance to clarithromycin may emerge. Patients in whom *H. pylori* was not eradicated following therapy with omeprazole/clarithromycin, ranitidine bismuth citrate/clarithromycin, omeprazole/clarithromycin/amoxicillin, or lansoprazole/clarithromycin/amoxicillin are likely to have clarithromycin-resistant *H. pylori* isolates. In vitro susceptibility testing should be performed if possible in patients with *H. pylori* infection who fail therapy (i.e., as determined in clinical trials by a positive result for *H. pylori* on culture or histologic testing 4 weeks following completion of therapy). If clarithromycin resistance is demonstrated or susceptibility testing is not possible, alternative anti-infective therapy (i.e., with a non-clarithromycin-containing regimen) should be instituted. The American College of Gastroenterology (ACG) states that clarithromycin or metronidazole should not be used subsequently in patients with *H. pylori* infection who fail therapy that includes these drugs since resistance commonly emerges during such unsuccessful therapy.

Clarithromycin generally may be used without dosage adjustment in patients with hepatic impairment who have normal renal function. However, in patients who have severe renal impairment with or without hepatic impairment, dosage reduction or prolongation of dosing intervals for clarithromycin may be necessary. (See Dosage and Administration: Dosage.)

■ Pediatric Precautions The manufacturer states that safety and efficacy of clarithromycin in children younger than 6 months of age have not been established, and safety of the drug in children younger than 20 months of age with *M. avium* complex infection has not been established. However, children as young as 6 months of age have received the drug for the treatment of streptococcal pharyngitis or tonsillitis and for skin and skin structure infections without apparent unusual adverse effect.

Safety and efficacy, including associated dosage recommendations, for extended-release tablets of clarithromycin in pediatric patients have not been established.

■ Geriatric Precautions Limited data indicate that peak serum concentrations of clarithromycin and 14-hydroxyclarithromycin and values for area under the concentration-time curve may be increased in healthy geriatric individuals 65–84 years of age relative to those in healthy younger adults; this increase appears to result from age-related decreases in renal function. (See Pharmacokinetics: Absorption.) An increased incidence of adverse effects in geriatric patients has not been reported to date in clinical studies. If clarithromycin is used in geriatric patients with severe renal impairment, use of a reduced dosage of the drug should be considered. (See Dosage and Administration: Dosage in Renal and Hepatic Impairment.)

■ Mutagenicity and Carcinogenicity Clarithromycin failed to exhibit mutagenic potential in several in vitro tests, including the *Salmonella* mammalian microsome test, bacterial induced mutation frequency test, rat hepatocyte DNA synthesis assay, mouse lymphoma assay, mouse dominant lethal test, and mouse micronucleus test. In the in vitro chromosome aberration test, clarithromycin produced weakly positive results in one test and negative results in another. Results of a bacterial reverse-mutation test (Ames test) performed on several clarithromycin metabolites also were negative.

Long-term studies have not been performed to date to evaluate the carcinogenic potential of clarithromycin.

■ Pregnancy, Fertility, and Lactation Although there are no adequate and controlled studies to date in humans, clarithromycin has been associated with adverse effects on pregnancy outcome and/or embryofetal development in animals at dosages that produced plasma drug concentrations 2–17 times those achieved with the maximum recommended human dosage. While the potential risk to the fetus has not been clearly elucidated to date, the manufacturer states that clarithromycin should be used during pregnancy only when safer drugs cannot be used or are ineffective. If clarithromycin is administered during pregnancy or if the patient becomes pregnant while receiving the drug, the patient should be informed of the potential hazard to the fetus.

Teratogenicity studies in rats with oral or IV clarithromycin dosages up to 160 mg/kg daily administered during the period of major organogenesis and in rabbits at oral dosages up to 125 mg/kg daily (approximately twice the maximum recommended human dosage on a mg/m^2 basis) or IV dosages of 30 mg/kg daily administered during days 6–18 of gestation did not demonstrate evidence of teratogenicity. However, other studies in a different rat strain demonstrated a low incidence of cardiovascular anomalies at a clarithromycin dosage of 150 mg/kg daily (resulting in plasma concentrations 2 times those in humans) administered during gestation days 6–15. Studies in mice revealed a variable incidence of cleft palate with oral dosages of 1000 mg/kg daily (resulting in plasma concentrations 17 times those in humans) during gestation days 6–15; cleft palate also was observed at a dosage of 500 mg/kg daily. In monkeys, an oral dosage of 70 mg/kg daily (approximately equivalent to the maximum recommended human dosage on a mg/m^2 basis) produced fetal growth retardation at plasma concentrations twice those attained in humans.

Fertility and reproduction studies in male and female rats using clarithromycin dosages up to 160 mg/kg daily (1.3 times the maximum recommended human dosage on a mg/m^2 basis) have demonstrated no adverse effects of the drug on the estrous cycle, fertility, parturition, or number and viability of offspring. Plasma concentrations in rats following clarithromycin dosages of 150 mg/kg daily were twice those observed in humans. Embryonic loss in monkeys has occurred at an oral clarithromycin dosage of 150 mg/kg daily (2.4 times the maximum recommended dosage in humans on a mg/m^2 basis); this effect has been attributed to marked maternal toxicity at this high dosage. In addition, in utero fetal loss in rabbits has occurred at an IV dosage of 33 mg/m^2, which is 17 times less than the proposed maximum human oral daily dosage of 618 mg/m^2.

Clarithromycin should be used with caution in nursing women. The drug is distributed into milk. In 12 women who received oral clarithromycin in a dosage of 250 mg twice daily for 6 days, mean peak concentrations of clarithromycin and 14-hydroxyclarithromycin in milk were 25 and 75%, respectively, of corresponding serum concentrations. Pre-weaned rats, exposed indirectly via consumption of milk from dams treated with 150 mg/kg daily of clarithromycin for 3 weeks, did not demonstrate adverse effects despite evidence indicating higher drug concentrations in milk than in plasma.

Drug Interactions

■ Drugs Metabolized by Hepatic Microsomal Enzymes Concomitant use of clarithromycin and drugs metabolized by hepatic microsomal enzymes (cytochrome P-450 (CYP) system) may be associated with increased serum concentrations of the latter drugs, and serum concentrations of such concomitantly administered drugs should be monitored closely.

Carbamazepine Clarithromycin should be used with caution in patients receiving carbamazepine; if such concomitant therapy is used, a reduction in carbamazepine dosage and/or monitoring of plasma carbamazepine concentrations is advised.

Limited data in healthy men indicate that clarithromycin may increase area under the serum concentration-time curve (AUC) for carbamazepine and decrease peak serum concentration and AUC for carbamazepine 10,11-epoxide (CBZ-E). In addition, increased plasma concentrations of carbamazepine (but not CBZ-E) and, in some patients, manifestations of carbamazepine toxicity (i.e., drowsiness, dizziness, ataxia) occurred within 3–5 days after initiation of clarithromycin therapy (200 mg twice daily) in several patients receiving carbamazepine (600 mg/day) with or without other drugs; plasma carbamazepine concentrations decreased and toxic manifestations subsided within several days following carbamazepine discontinuation.

Cisapride Concomitant administration of clarithromycin and cisapride is contraindicated.

Coadministration of clarithromycin and/or erythromycin with cisapride has been associated with QT prolongation and serious cardiac arrhythmias (ventricular tachycardia, ventricular fibrillation, torsades de pointes); fatalities have been reported. In 2 patients with chronic renal failure who were receiving cisapride (10 mg 3–4 times daily), QT prolongation and/or torsades de pointes occurred within several days after initiating therapy with clarithromycin (500 mg twice daily). Elevated serum cisapride concentrations observed in one patient decreased following discontinuance of clarithromycin.

Darifenacin The manufacturer of darifenacin states that darifenacin dosage should not exceed 7.5 mg daily in patients receiving the drug concomitantly with potent CYP3A4 inhibitors, including clarithromycin.

Disopyramide If clarithromycin and disopyramide are used concomitantly, ECGs and serum disopyramide concentrations should be monitored. Ventricular fibrillation, prolongation of the QT interval, and a marked increase in disopyramide elimination half-life (40 hours) were reported in a patient maintained on disopyramide (200 mg twice daily) who received clarithromycin (250 mg twice daily), omeprazole (20 mg twice daily), and metronidazole (400 mg twice daily) for the treatment of *H. pylori*-associated chronic duodenal ulceration. QT prolongation, which had not been documented previously during a 7-year period of disopyramide therapy, resolved with a decline in disopyramide plasma concentrations. There have been postmarketing reports of torsades de pointes occurring with concomitant use of clarithromycin and disopyramide.

Erlotinib The manufacturer of erlotinib states that caution is advised if the drug is used concomitantly with potent CYP3A4 inhibitors, including clarithromycin, and a reduction in erlotinib dosage should be considered if severe adverse effects occur.

Eszopiclone The manufacturer of eszopiclone states that eszopiclone dosage should be reduced if the drug is used concomitantly with a potent CYP3A4 inhibitor, including clarithromycin. In such situations, the initial eszopiclone dosage should not exceed 1 mg but may be increased to 2 mg if clinically indicated.

Hydroxymethylglutaryl-CoA (HMG-CoA) Reductase Inhibitors As with other macrolides, clarithromycin has been reported to increase serum concentrations of concomitantly administered HMG-CoA reductase inhibitor (statin) antilipemic agents (e.g., lovastatin, simvastatin) via inhibition of metabolism by cytochrome P-450 isoenzymes. Rhabdomyolysis, sometimes accompanied by acute renal failure secondary to myoglobinuria, has been reported rarely with HMG-CoA reductase inhibitor therapy given alone or concomitantly with macrolide antibiotics (e.g., erythromycin, clarithromycin), immunosuppressive agents (including cyclosporine) in transplant patients, gemfibrozil, niacin (in dosages of at least 1 g daily), or nefazodone. (See Cautions: Musculoskeletal Effects, in Lovastatin 24:06.08.)

Pimozide Concomitant administration of pimozide and macrolide antibiotics, including clarithromycin, is contraindicated. Macrolide antibiotics, including azithromycin, clarithromycin, and erythromycin, inhibit the metabolism of pimozide, resulting in increased plasma pimozide concentrations. Since pimozide prolongs the QT interval, such increased plasma concentrations of the drug may increase the risk of serious cardiovascular effects, including fatal ventricular arrhythmias; at least 2 deaths have been reported in patients following addition of clarithromycin to pimozide therapy. (See Drug Interactions: Drugs Affecting Hepatic Microsomal Enzymes, in Pimozide 28:16.08.92.)

Rifabutin and Rifampin Concomitant administration of clarithromycin and rifabutin or rifampin has been reported to *increase* the metabolism of clarithromycin. In addition, in a randomized study in patients with advanced HIV infection (CD4+ T-cell counts less than 200/mm³), a drug interaction consistent with inhibition of rifabutin metabolism by clarithromycin and induction of clarithromycin metabolism by rifabutin was demonstrated. Four weeks after initiation of therapy with rifabutin (300 mg daily) in HIV-infected patients who had been receiving clarithromycin (500 mg every 12 hours) alone for 2 weeks, clarithromycin AUC had decreased by an average of 44%, AUC for 14-hydroxyclarithromycin had increased by 57%, and peak plasma clarithromycin concentration had decreased by 41%. In the same study, patients who received clarithromycin for 4 weeks after 2 weeks of rifabutin monotherapy had average increases of 99 and 375% in the AUCs of rifabutin and 25-desacetyl rifabutin, respectively, and an increase of 69% in peak plasma rifabutin concentration. It has been suggested that the increased plasma concentrations of rifabutin and/or its 25-desacetyl metabolite associated with concomitant administration of clarithromycin may explain the increased frequency of uveitis observed with such concomitant therapy.

Terfenadine and Astemizole Current evidence indicates that certain macrolide antibiotics (e.g., erythromycin, clarithromycin) alter the metabolism of astemizole and terfenadine; however, these antihistamines are no longer commercially available in the US. (See Drug Interactions and Cautions: Cardiovascular Effects and Precautions and Contraindications in the Antihistamines General Statement 4:00.) Prolongation of the QT interval, ST-U abnormalities, and ventricular tachycardia, including torsades de pointes, have been reported in some patients receiving terfenadine concomitantly with erythromycin. Therefore, terfenadine was contraindicated in patients receiving clarithromycin or erythromycin, especially patients who had preexisting cardiac abnormalities (e.g., arrhythmia, bradycardia, QT interval prolongation, ischemic heart disease, congestive heart failure) or electrolyte disturbances. In addition, QT prolongation and torsades de pointes have been reported in patients receiving concomitant erythromycin and astemizole, and coadministration of these drugs was contraindicated. Because clarithromycin also is metabolized by the cytochrome P-450 system, coadministration of clarithromycin and astemizole also was contraindicated.

Other Drugs Affecting Hepatic Microsomal Enzymes In postmarketing studies, interactions with erythromycin and/or clarithromycin have been reported with a number of other drugs metabolized by the cytochrome P-450 system, including cyclosporine, tacrolimus, hexobarbital, phenytoin, alfentanil, lovastatin, bromocriptine, and valproate. Serum concentrations of drugs metabolized by the cytochrome P-450 system should be monitored closely in patients receiving concomitant therapy with erythromycin or clarithromycin.

■ **Anticoagulants** Postmarketing data suggest that the concomitant administration of clarithromycin and oral anticoagulants may potentiate the effects of the oral anticoagulant. The manufacturer recommends that the prothrombin time be monitored carefully in patients receiving concomitant clarithromycin and oral anticoagulant therapy.

■ **Antiretroviral Agents** ***Amprenavir*** Concomitant use of clarithromycin (500 mg twice daily) and amprenavir (1.2 g twice daily) results in slightly increased amprenavir concentrations and AUC and possible decreased clarithromycin concentrations. Dosage adjustments are not recommended.

Atazanavir Concomitant use of clarithromycin (500 mg twice daily) and atazanavir (400 mg once daily) increased the peak plasma concentration and AUC of clarithromycin, decreased the peak plasma concentration and AUC of 14-hydroclarithromycin, and increased the peak plasma concentration and AUC of atazanavir. Increased concentrations of clarithromycin may result in prolongation of the QT_c interval.

Clarithromycin dosage should be reduced by 50% in patients receiving atazanavir. In addition, alternative anti-infective therapy should be considered for indications other than *Mycobacterium avium* complex (MAC) infections since the decreased plasma concentrations of 14-hydroclarithromycin could adversely affect clarithromycin's efficacy in the treatment of certain infections.

Delavirdine Concomitant use of clarithromycin (500 mg twice daily for 15 days) and delavirdine (300 mg 3 times daily for 30 days) resulted in a 100% increase in the AUC of clarithromycin but had no appreciable effect on the pharmacokinetics of delavirdine.

When clarithromycin is used in patients receiving delavirdine, modification of the usual clarithromycin dosage generally is not necessary in those with normal renal function; however, the clarithromycin dose should be reduced by 50% in patients with creatinine clearances of 30–60 mL/minute and reduced by 75% in patients with creatinine clearances less than 30 mL/minute.

Didanosine Simultaneous administration of clarithromycin tablets and didanosine in a limited number of HIV-infected adults did not alter the pharmacokinetics of didanosine.

Efavirenz Administration of clarithromycin (500 mg every 12 hours) and efavirenz (400 mg daily) for 7 days decreased the peak plasma concentration and AUC of clarithromycin by 26 and 39%, respectively, and increased the peak plasma concentration and AUC of 14-hydroxyclarithromycin by 49 and 34%, respectively. The AUC of efavirenz was not affected. The clinical importance of this pharmacokinetic interaction is not known. Rash developed in 46% of individuals receiving clarithromycin and efavirenz in drug interaction studies. Because of the reported pharmacokinetic interaction between clarithromycin and efavirenz and the high incidence of rash in individuals receiving the drugs concurrently, alternatives to clarithromycin (e.g., azithromycin) should be considered in patients receiving efavirenz. If the drugs are used concomitantly, monitor for macrolide efficacy.

Fosamprenavir Studies using amprenavir indicate that concomitant use of clarithromycin and fosamprenavir may result in increased amprenavir concentrations and AUC. This pharmacokinetic interaction is not considered clinically important and dosage adjustments are not recommended.

Indinavir Concomitant use of clarithromycin (500 mg every 12 hours) and indinavir (800 mg 3 times daily) results in increased indinavir concentrations and increased clarithromycin concentrations. Although some clinicians state that dosage adjustments are not needed if clarithromycin and indinavir are used concomitantly, the manufacturer of indinavir states that appropriate dosages for concomitant use with respect to safety and efficacy have not been established.

Lopinavir Concomitant use of clarithromycin and the fixed combination of lopinavir and ritonavir may result in increased clarithromycin concentrations. The manufacturer of the fixed combination of lopinavir and ritonavir states that when clarithromycin is used in patients receiving lopinavir and ritonavir, modification of the usual dosage of clarithromycin is not necessary in those with normal renal function; however, the clarithromycin dosage should be reduced by 50% in patients with creatinine clearances of 30–60 mL/minute and reduced by 75% in patients with a creatinine clearances less than 30 mL/minute.

Nevirapine Concomitant use of clarithromycin and nevirapine has resulted in decreased plasma concentrations and AUC of clarithromycin, increased plasma concentrations and AUC of its major metabolite (14-hydroxyclarithromycin), and increased nevirapine concentrations. Because the clarithromycin metabolite has reduced activity against *Mycobacterium avium* complex (MAC), overall activity of the drug against this organism may be altered. Therefore, an alternative to clarithromycin (e.g., azithromycin) should be used in patients receiving nevirapine. If the drugs are used concomitantly, monitor for macrolide efficacy.

Ritonavir In a study in healthy individuals, concomitant administration of ritonavir (200 mg every 8 hours) with clarithromycin (500 mg every 12 hours) for 4 days increased the peak plasma concentration and area under the AUC of clarithromycin by 31 and 77%, respectively, and decreased the peak plasma concentration and AUC of 14-hydroxyclarithromycin by 99 and 100%, respectively. The peak plasma concentration and AUC of ritonavir also were increased by 12–15%. Because 14-hydroxyclarithromycin appears to enhance the antimicrobial activity of the parent drug against some pathogens (e.g., *Haemophilus influenzae*), it has been suggested that the decreased plasma concentrations of the metabolite reported with concomitant ritonavir theoretically could adversely affect clarithromycin's efficacy in the treatment of certain infections.

The manufacturer of clarithromycin and ritonavir states that when clarithromycin is used in patients receiving ritonavir, modification of the usual clarithromycin dosage generally is not necessary in those with normal renal function; however, the clarithromycin dosage should be reduced by 50% in patients with creatinine clearances of 30–60 mL/minute and reduced by 75% in patients with creatinine clearances less than 30 mL/minute.

Saquinavir Concomitant use of clarithromycin and saquinavir may result in increased plasma concentrations of both drugs. In healthy individuals receiving clarithromycin (500 mg twice daily) and saquinavir (1.2 g 3 times daily as liquid-filled capsules) for 7 days, AUC or peak plasma concentrations of saquinavir increased 177 or 187%, respectively; AUC or plasma concentrations of clarithromycin increased 45 or 39%, respectively; and AUC and peak plasma concentrations of 14-hydroxyclarithromycin decreased 24 or 34%, respectively. Dosage adjustments may not be needed if clarithromycin and saquinavir are used concomitantly for a limited time at the dosages studied.

For those receiving *ritonavir-boosted* saquinavir, the manufacturer of saquinavir states that modification of dosage is not necessary in those with normal renal function but clarithromycin dosage should be reduced by 50% in those with creatinine clearances of 30–60 mL/minute and reduced by 75% in those with creatinine clearances less than 30 mL/minute.

Zidovudine In one study, simultaneous administration of clarithromycin and zidovudine in HIV-infected adults decreased peak plasma concentrations of zidovudine by about 41% but had no appreciable effect on the pharmacokinetics of clarithromycin. In a limited number of HIV-infected adults, clarithromycin (500 mg twice daily) decreased the steady-state AUC of zidovudine by a mean of 12% (range: from a decrease of 34% to an increase of 14%). When clarithromycin tablets were administered 2–4 hours prior to zidovudine doses, steady-state peak zidovudine serum concentrations were increased twofold but the AUC was unaffected.

■ **Benzodiazepines** Erythromycin has been reported to decrease the clearance of midazolam and triazolam and may increase the pharmacologic effects of these benzodiazepines. CNS effects (e.g., somnolence, confusion) have been reported in postmarketing experience when clarithromycin was used concomitantly with triazolam.

■ **Colchicine** Some clinicians state that colchicine and clarithromycin should not be used concomitantly. There have been postmarketing reports of colchicine toxicity when clarithromycin was used concomitantly with colchicine, especially in elderly patients and/or in patients with renal impairment. In addition, a retrospective analysis of data from hospitalized patients who received colchicine and clarithromycin either concomitantly or sequentially suggests that concomitant use of the drugs increases the risk of fatal colchicine toxicity, especially in patients with renal impairment.

■ **Digoxin** The manufacturer recommends that serum digoxin levels be monitored carefully in patients receiving concomitant clarithromycin and digoxin therapy. Elevated serum concentrations of digoxin have been reported during postmarketing surveillance in patients receiving concomitant digoxin and clarithromycin therapy. Some of these patients exhibited clinical manifestations consistent with digoxin toxicity, including arrhythmias.

■ **Ergot Alkaloids** Concomitant use of clarithromycin and ergot alkaloids (ergotamine, dihydroergotamine) is contraindicated. Concurrent use of clarithromycin and ergotamine or dihydroergotamine has been associated with acute ergot toxicity, characterized by vasospasm and ischemia of the extremities and other tissues, including the CNS.

■ **Fluconazole** In healthy individuals receiving clarithromycin 500 mg twice daily concomitantly with fluconazole 200 mg daily, steady-state trough serum concentrations and area under the serum concentration-time curve (AUC) for clarithromycin reportedly increased by an average of 33 and 18%, respectively; steady-state concentrations of 14-hydroxyclarithromycin were not substantially affected.

■ **Omeprazole** Concomitant administration of clarithromycin and omeprazole alters the pharmacokinetics (e.g., increased concentrations in gastric tissue and/or serum) of clarithromycin, 14-hydroxyclarithromycin, and omeprazole. (See Pharmacokinetics: Absorption.)

■ **Quinidine** Torsades de pointes has been reported rarely in patients receiving clarithromycin and quinidine concomitantly. If clarithromycin and quinidine are used concomitantly, ECGs and serum quinidine concentrations should be monitored.

■ **Ranitidine** Concomitant use of ranitidine bismuth citrate and clarithromycin has resulted in increased plasma ranitidine concentrations (57%), increased plasma bismuth trough concentrations (48%), and increased 14-hydroxy-clarithromycin plasma concentrations (31%). This pharmacokinetic interaction is not considered clinically important. However, clarithromycin should not be used concomitantly with ranitidine bismuth citrate in patients with creatinine clearances less than 25 mL/minute and should not be used in patients with a history of acute porphyria.

■ **Sildenafil** Concomitant erythromycin has been reported to increase the AUC of sildenafil. Because a similar interaction could occur with clarithromycin, a reduction in sildenafil dosage should be considered.

■ **Theophylline** Concomitant use of clarithromycin in patients who are receiving theophylline may be associated with an increase in serum theophylline concentrations, probably as a result of reduced hepatic metabolism and/or clearance of theophylline. Clarithromycin reportedly causes less alteration in serum theophylline concentration than erythromycin, but changes in theophylline dosage have been required in some patients treated concurrently with clarithromycin and theophylline. In 2 studies in healthy individuals who were given an extended-release theophylline preparation (6.5 or 12 mg/kg per dose) concomitantly with clarithromycin (250–500 mg every 12 hours), the peak and trough serum concentrations at steady state and the area under the serum concentration-time curve (AUC) for theophylline reportedly were increased by approximately 20%. However, in at least one of these studies in healthy men, serum theophylline concentrations remained within the therapeutic range, and no clinical toxicity was observed.

The manufacturer states that monitoring of serum theophylline concentrations should be considered for patients receiving clarithromycin concomitantly with high doses of theophylline or in those who have baseline serum theophylline concentrations in the upper therapeutic range. Theophylline dosage should be adjusted if necessary when clarithromycin is added or withdrawn in a patient receiving theophylline.

Mechanism of Action

Clarithromycin usually is bacteriostatic, although it may be bactericidal in high concentrations or against highly susceptible organisms. Bactericidal activity has been observed against *Streptococcus pyogenes*, *S. pneumoniae*, *Haemophilus influenzae*, and *Chlamydia trachomatis*.

Clarithromycin inhibits protein synthesis in susceptible organisms by penetrating the cell wall and binding to 50S ribosomal subunits, thereby inhibiting translocation of aminoacyl transfer-RNA and inhibiting polypeptide synthesis. The site of action of clarithromycin appears to be the same as that of erythromycin, clindamycin, lincomycin, and chloramphenicol.

Spectrum

Clarithromycin generally displays in vitro activity similar to or greater than that of erythromycin against erythromycin-sensitive organisms and also exhibits activity against some organisms (e.g., atypical mycobacteria, *Toxoplasma*) for which therapy currently is limited. The drug's principal metabolite, 14-hydroxyclarithromycin, is as active or only slightly less active in vitro than clarithromycin against most organisms and appears to enhance the antimicrobial activity of the parent drug against selected pathogens (e.g., *Haemophilus influenzae*). However, the activity of 14-hydroxyclarithromycin against *Mycobacterium avium* complex (MAC) isolates was 4–7 times less than that of the parent compound; the clinical importance of this difference in activity is unknown.

■ **In Vitro Susceptibility Testing** The Clinical and Laboratory Standards Institute (CLSI; formerly National Committee for Clinical Laboratory Standards [NCCLS]) states that, if results of in vitro susceptibility testing indicate that a clinical isolate is *susceptible* to clarithromycin, then an infection caused by this strain may be appropriately treated with the dosage of the drug recommended for that type of infection and infecting species, unless otherwise contraindicated. If results indicate that a clinical isolate has *intermediate susceptibility* to clarithromycin, then the strain has a minimum inhibitory concentration (MIC) that approaches usually attainable blood and tissue concentrations and response rates may be lower than for strains identified as susceptible.Therefore, the intermediate category implies clinical applicability in body sites where the drug is physiologically concentrated or when a high dosage of the drug can be used. This intermediate category also includes a buffer zone which should prevent small, uncontrolled technical factors from causing major discrepancies in interpretation, especially for drugs with narrow pharmacotoxicity margins. If results of in vitro susceptibility testing indicate that a clinical isolate is *resistant* to clarithromycin, the strain is not inhibited by systemic concentrations of the drug achievable with usual dosage schedules and/or MICs fall in the range where specific microbial resistance mechanisms are likely and efficacy has not been reliable in clinical studies.

For testing the susceptibility of *M. avium* complex (MAC) isolates to clarithromycin, the usual disk-diffusion procedures or dilution tests used for determining in vitro susceptibility of bacterial isolates should not be used. In vitro susceptibility testing methods and diagnostic products currently available for determining MIC values of clarithromycin against MAC organisms have neither been standardized nor validated. MICs reported for clarithromycin will vary depending on the susceptibility testing method employed, the composition and pH of the media, and use of nutritional supplements. Values representing susceptibility or resistance of MAC isolates to clarithromycin have not been established.

Disk Susceptibility Tests When the disk-diffusion procedure is used to test susceptibility to clarithromycin, a disk containing 15 mcg of clarithromycin should be used.

When the disk-diffusion procedure is performed according to CLSI standardized procedures using CLSI interpretive criteria, *Staphylococcus* with growth inhibition zones of 18 mm or greater are susceptible to clarithromycin, those with zones of 14–17 mm have intermediate susceptibility, and those with zones of 13 mm or less are resistant to the drug.

When the disk-diffusion procedure is performed according to CLSI standardized procedures using *Haemophilus* test medium (HTM), *Haemophilus* with growth inhibition zones of 13 mm or greater are susceptible to clarithromycin, those with zones of 11–12 mm have intermediate susceptibility, and those with zones of 10 mm or less are resistant to the drug.

When susceptibility of *Streptococcus pneumoniae* or other *Streptococcus* spp. is determined according to CLSI standardized procedures using Mueller-Hinton agar (supplemented with 5% sheep blood), those with growth inhibition zones of 21 mm or greater are susceptible to clarithromycin, those with zones of 17–20 mm have intermediate susceptibility, and those with zones of 16 mm or less are resistant to the drug.

Dilution Susceptibility Tests In dilution susceptibility testing procedures (agar or broth dilution), *Staphylococcus* with MICs of 2 mcg/mL or less are susceptible to clarithromycin, those with MICs of 4 mcg/mL have intermediate susceptibility, and those with MICs of 8 mcg/mL or greater are resistant to the drug.

When dilution susceptibility testing is performed according to CLSI standardized procedures using HTM, *Haemophilus* with MICs of 8 mcg/mL or less are susceptible to clarithromycin, those with MICs of 16 mcg/mL have intermediate susceptibility, and those with MICs of 32 mcg/mL or greater are resistant to the drug.

When dilution susceptibility testing of *Helicobacter pylori* is performed according to CLSI standardized procedures using Mueller-Hinton agar with 5% aged sheep blood, *H. pylori* with MICs of 0.25 mcg/mL or less are susceptible to clarithromycin, those with MICs of 0.5 mcg/mL have intermediate susceptibility, and those with MICs of 1 mcg/mL or greater are resistant to the drug. These breakpoints presume that clarithromycin will be used in a regimen that includes a proton-pump inhibitor or an H_2-receptor antagonist.

When dilution susceptibility testing is performed according to CLSI standardized procedures using cation-adjusted Mueller-Hinton broth (supplemented with 2–5% lysed horse blood), *S. pneumoniae* or other streptococci with MICs of 0.25 mcg/mL or less are susceptible to clarithromycin, those with MICs of 0.5 mcg/mL have intermediate susceptibility, and those with MICs of 1 mcg/mL or greater are resistant to the drug.

■ Gram-positive Aerobic Bacteria Clarithromycin is active in vitro against gram-positive cocci (streptococci and staphylococci). Minimum inhibitory concentrations (MICs) of clarithromycin for oxacillin-susceptible *Staphylococcus aureus* (previously known as methicillin-susceptible *S. aureus*) and most streptococci generally are twofold to fourfold lower than those of erythromycin, while oxacillin-resistant staphylococci (previously known as methicillin-resistant staphylococci) and coagulase-negative staphylococci (e.g., *Staphylococcus epidermidis*) generally are resistant to clarithromycin or erythromycin. Most enterococci (e.g., *Enterococcus faecalis* [formerly *Streptococcus faecalis*]) are resistant both to clarithromycin and erythromycin, although the drugs appear to have similar activity against erythromycin-sensitive strains. The in vitro antimicrobial activity (MICs) of clarithromycin against *S. aureus* and *S. epidermidis*, but not *E. faecalis*, appears to decrease when the size of the inoculum is increased.

Clarithromycin is active in vitro against some gram-positive aerobic bacilli such as *Listeria monocytogenes* and some strains of *Corynebacterium*.

Results of in vitro susceptibility testing of 11 *Bacillus anthracis* isolates that were associated with cases of inhalational or cutaneous anthrax that occurred in the US (Florida, New York, District of Columbia) during September and October 2001 in the context of an intentional release of anthrax spores (biologic warfare, bioterrorism) indicate that these strains had clarithromycin MICs of 0.25 mcg/mL. Based on interpretive criteria established for staphylococci, these strains are considered susceptible to clarithromycin. Limited or no data are available to date regarding in vivo activity of clarithromycin against *B. anthracis* or use of the drug in the treatment of anthrax.

■ Gram-negative Aerobic Bacteria Clarithromycin is active in vitro against some gram-negative organisms, including *Neisseria gonorrhoeae* and *Moraxella catarrhalis*. Clarithromycin's activity against *M. catarrhalis* generally exceeds that of erythromycin and reportedly is enhanced by 14-hydroxyclarithromycin. Clarithromycin and erythromycin appear to have similar activity against *Neisseria gonorrhoeae*.

Clarithromycin also is active in vitro against *Haemophilus influenzae*, *H. parainfluenzae*, and *Pasteurella multocida*. Although the in vitro activity of clarithromycin alone against *H. influenzae* generally is similar to or less than that of erythromycin, the 14-hydroxy metabolite of clarithromycin has greater activity against this organism. In in vitro studies, the combination of clarithromycin and 14-hydroxyclarithromycin generally has demonstrated either additive or synergistic activity against *H. influenzae*; however, MICs for this organism vary depending on the method used to determine susceptibility. Limited data from a few studies in which in vitro susceptibilities of β-lactamase-producing strains of *H. influenzae* have been reported separately from those of non-β-lactamase-producing strains suggest no substantial effect of the enzyme on inhibitory or bactericidal activity of clarithromycin. Limited data suggest that high concentrations of and/or prolonged exposure to clarithromycin and its active metabolite may be required for bactericidal activity against some strains of *H. influenzae*.

Clarithromycin has greater activity than erythromycin against *Legionella pneumophila* in vitro and in animals; clarithromycin's activity against *Legionella* spp. also may be enhanced by its 14-hydroxy metabolite.

Clarithromycin also has in vitro activity against *Campylobacter* spp. (e.g., *C. jejuni.*) and *Bordetella pertussis*. Clarithromycin is active against most strains of *Helicobacter pylori* (formerly *Campylobacter pylori* or *C. pyloridis*) in vitro and in clinical infections when used in multiple-drug regimens including omeprazole, omeprazole or lansoprazole and amoxicillin, or ranitidine bismuth citrate. Clarithromycin exhibits greater activity than most other macrolides against *H. pylori*.

■ Mycobacteria Although macrolide antibiotics generally have little activity against *Mycobacterium tuberculosis*, clarithromycin has been shown to inhibit several types of atypical mycobacteria in vitro, including *M. kansasii*, *M. fortuitum*, *M. marinum*,*M. chelonae*, *M. abscessus*, and *M. avium* complex (MAC). MAC represents 2 closely related organisms, *M. avium* and *M. intracellulare*. Although gene probe techniques may be used to distinguish *M. avium* species from *M. intracellulare*, most studies do not distinguish between the organisms and report results on MAC isolates. Clarithromycin has exhibited both in vitro and in vivo activity against *M. leprae*, and reportedly is 8–32 times as active as erythromycin in vitro against MAC. Some in vitro data indicate that clarithromycin is bactericidal against MAC and that this activity is enhanced by ethambutol and/or rifampin. However, resistant strains of MAC have developed during therapy with clarithromycin, both when the drug was used as monotherapy or when used as a component of multiple-drug therapy.

Although the activity of 14-hydroxyclarithromycin against MAC isolates was 4–7 times less than that of clarithromycin, the clinical importance of this difference in activity is unknown.

■ Other Aerobic Bacteria The activity of clarithromycin versus erythromycin against *Mycoplasma pneumoniae* generally is comparable, but clarithromycin has greater activity against *Ureaplasma urealyticum*. Clarithromycin has up to tenfold greater activity in vitro than erythromycin against *Chlamydia trachomatis* and some strains of *C. pneumoniae*.

■ Anaerobic Bacteria Clarithromycin is active in vitro against most strains of *Peptococcus*, *Peptostreptococcus*, *Clostridium perfringens*, and *Propionibacterium acnes*. The activity of clarithromycin against anaerobic gram-positive cocci generally is similar to that of erythromycin, but may be slightly better against *C. perfringens*.

Clarithromycin is active in vitro against most strains of *Prevotella melaninogenica* (formerly *Bacteroides melaninogenicus*); the drug's activity against *Prevotella* spp. and *Bacteroides fragilis* generally is similar to or greater than that of erythromycin but less than that of clindamycin.

■ Other Organisms Clarithromycin reportedly has exhibited in vitro activity against *Toxoplasma gondii*, *Gardnerella vaginalis*, and *Borrelia burgdorferi*, the causative agent of Lyme disease. Limited data in animals also indicate activity of clarithromycin against *Cryptosporidium parvum* and synergism (as determined by reduction in cyst burden in lung tissue) with sulfamethoxazole against *Pneumocystis carinii*. Clarithromycin generally is inactive against Enterobacteriaceae (e.g., *Salmonella enteriditis*, *Yersinia enterocolitica*, *Shigella* and *Vibrio* spp.).

Resistance

Resistance to macrolide antibiotics usually involves an alteration at the antibiotic target site, but resistance caused by modification and/or active efflux of the antibiotic also have been reported. Such resistance may be chromosomally or plasmid mediated and be either constitutive or induced. Bacteria resistant to macrolides produce an enzyme that leads to methylation of adenine residues in ribosomal RNA and subsequent inhibition of binding of the antibiotic to the ribosome. Organisms resistant to erythromycin generally are resistant to all 14- and 15-membered macrolides because all of these drugs induce the methylase enzyme.

■ Resistance in Gram-positive Bacteria The overall incidence of macrolide-resistant *Streptococcus pyogenes* (group A β-hemolytic streptococci) in the US is reported to be 3–9%. In one US study, about 7% of *S. pyogenes* isolates (principally pharyngeal isolates) were resistant to clarithromycin.

■ Resistance in Mycobacteria Strains of *Mycobacterium avium* complex (MAC) with decreased susceptibility or resistance to clarithromycin have been reported in patients who received the drug for treatment or prevention of MAC infection and have developed when the drug was used as monotherapy or as a component of multiple-drug therapy. MAC isolates resistant to clarithromycin are cross-resistant to azithromycin.

■ Resistance in Helicobacter pylori In clinical studies in patients who received clarithromycin as the sole anti- infective agent in combination regimens for *Helicobacter pylori* infection, some *H. pylori* isolates demonstrated an increase in clarithromycin MICs over time, indicating decreased susceptibility and increasing resistance to the drug. In 2 US clinical studies in which clarithromycin and omeprazole were administered concomitantly for the treatment of *H. pylori* infection, 3.5% of patients had *H. pylori* strains resistant to clarithromycin before treatment. In 3 clinical studies in which therapy with clarithromycin, amoxicillin, and omeprazole (triple therapy) was compared with clarithromycin and amoxicillin (dual therapy) for the treatment of *H. pylori* infection, 9.3% of patients (41/439) receiving triple therapy and 3.5% of patients (4/113) receiving dual therapy had clarithromycin-resistant strains of *H. pylori* before treatment. In these studies, 99.3% of patients had pretreatment *H. pylori* isolates that were susceptible to amoxicillin (MIC of 0.25 mcg/mL or less) and 0.7% of patients, all of whom were in the clarithromycin/amoxicillin group, had pretreatment amoxicillin MICs greater than 0.25 mcg/mL. Of the patients who received triple therapy (clarithromycin, amoxicillin, omeprazole) in these studies, *H. pylori* was eradicated in 84.9% (157/185) who had pretreatment amoxicillin-susceptible *H. pylori* isolates (MIC of 0.25 mcg/mL or less). Of the 28 patients who failed therapy, 11 had no posttreatment susceptibility test results and 17 had *H. pylori* isolates that were susceptible to amoxicillin. Clarithromycin-resistant *H. pylori* isolates also were found posttreatment in 11 of the patients who failed triple therapy.

In 5 clinical studies in which therapy with lansoprazole and amoxicillin (dual therapy) or clarithromycin, amoxicillin, and lansoprazole (triple therapy) was given for the treatment of *H. pylori* infection, pretreatment clarithromycin-resistant strains of *H. pylori* were identified in 9.5% of patients using Etest and in 11.3% using agar dilution. In these studies, pretreatment *H. pylori* isolates were susceptible (MIC of 0.25 mcg/mL or less) to amoxicillin in 97.8 or 98% of patients using Etest or agar dilution, respectively. Two patients had an unconfirmed pretreatment amoxicillin MIC exceeding 256 mcg/mL according to Etest. In these studies, *H. pylori* was eradicated in 82.6% who had pretreatment amoxicillin-susceptible*H. pylori* isolates. Of 6 patients who had pretreatment amoxicillin MICs exceeding 0.25 mcg/mL, *H. pylori* was eradicated in 3 patients. Eradication of *H. pylori* was not achieved in 30% of patients (21/70) receiving lansoprazole-amoxicillin and 12.8% of patients (22/172) receiving clarithromycin-amoxicillin-lansoprazole for 10 or 14 days. Clarithromycin-resistant *H. pylori* isolates were found posttreatment in 9 of 11 patients who had amoxicillin posttreatment MICs and who failed triple therapy; 11 patients who failed triple therapy had no posttreatment susceptibility test results.

In a study in which clarithromycin and ranitidine bismuth citrate were given for the treatment of *H. pylori* infection, pretreatment clarithromycin-resistant strains of *H. pylori* were found in 12.6% of patients (44/348).

Pharmacokinetics

■ **Absorption** Clarithromycin is absorbed rapidly from the GI tract after oral administration; GI absorption of the drug exceeds that of erythromycin. The absolute bioavailability of clarithromycin following oral administration of the drug as 250-mg conventional tablets has been reported to be approximately 50–55%, which probably is an underestimate of systemic activity because of the drug's rapid first-pass metabolism to its active metabolite 14-hydroxyclarithromycin. In a study in adults, the bioavailability of 10 mL of 125 mg/5 mL or 250 mg/ 5 mL clarithromycin suspension was similar to that of the 250- or 500-mg conventional tablet, respectively. While the 24-hour area under the plasma concentration-time curves (AUCs) for clarithromycin and 14-hydroxy-clarithromycin following administration of clarithromycin extended-release tablets are equivalent to the 24-hour AUCs following administration of the same total daily dose as conventional tablets, the extended-release tablets result in lower and later steady-state plasma concentrations of clarithromycin and 14-hydroxyclarithromycin compared with conventional tablets.

Food causes a slight delay in the onset of clarithromycin absorption and increases the peak plasma concentration of clarithromycin by 24% when the drug is administered as conventional oral tablets; however, the extent of clarithromycin absorption is unaffected by concomitant ingestion of food. Food does not affect the onset of formation or the peak plasma concentration of 14-hydroxyclarithromycin when the drug is administered as conventional oral tablets; however, the AUC of the metabolite is decreased by about 11% when the conventional tablets are administered with food.

Administration of clarithromycin extended-release tablets under fasting conditions results in a 30% decrease in the AUC of clarithromycin compared with administration with food; the extent of formation of 14-hydroxyclarithromycin is not affected by food when the drug is administered as extended-release tablets .

In a limited number of adults, administration of 250 mg of clarithromycin as the oral suspension with food appeared to decrease the mean peak serum concentration by about 17% and the mean AUC by about 10%, while in a limited number of children, administration of a single 7.5-mg/kg dose of clarithromycin oral suspension with food appeared to increase the mean peak serum concentration of the drug by about 27% and the mean AUC by about 42%.

In fasting healthy adults receiving clarithromycin conventional tablets or oral suspension, peak serum clarithromycin concentrations averaged 0.6 mcg/mL and were attained within 1–4 hours after administration of a single 250-mg dose. Following oral administration of the drug as conventional oral tablets, steady-state peak clarithromycin concentrations were achieved within 3 days and averaged approximately 1–2 or 3–4 mcg/mL following a 250-mg dose of the drug every 12 hours or a 500-mg dose every 8–12 hours, respectively. Following oral administration of clarithromycin as conventional oral tablets, steady-state peak 14-hydroxyclarithromycin concentrations were achieved after 3–4 days and were about 0.6 or up to 1 mcg/mL following a 250-mg dose of the drug every 12 hours or a 500-mg dose every 8–12 hours, respectively. Following oral administration of clarithromycin as extended-release tablets, steady-state peak clarithromycin concentrations of 2–3 mcg/mL were obtained 5–8 hours following a 1-g dose of the drug (two 500-mg extended-release tablets); steady-state peak concentrations were 1–2 mcg/mL and were obtained 5–6 hours following a 500-mg dose. Steady-state peak plasma concentrations of 14-hydroxyclarithromycin of 0.8 or 0.6 mcg/mL were achieved 6–9 hours following a 1- or 500-mg daily dose of clarithromycin extended-release tablets, respectively. Following oral administration of clarithromycin oral suspension in fasting healthy adults, steady-state peak clarithromycin concentrations were achieved after 2–3 days and averaged approximately 2 mcg/mL following a 250- mg dose of the drug every 12 hours. Peak serum concentrations of the principal metabolite, 14-hydroxyclarithromycin, reportedly average about 0.7 mcg/mL and are achieved approximately 2 hours after a 250-mg dose of clarithromycin. Preliminary data from a study in healthy men suggest that the ratio of the AUCs of clarithromycin to 14-hydroxyclarithromycin at steady state is approximately 3:1.

In children receiving therapy with clarithromycin as the oral suspension, administration of 7.5 mg/kg of the drug every 12 hours generally resulted in peak steady-state serum clarithromycin concentrations of 3–7 mcg/mL and peak steady-state serum 14-hydroxyclarithromycin concentrations of 1–2 mcg/mL.

In pharmacokinetic studies of HIV-infected adults receiving 500 mg of clarithromycin orally every 12 hours, steady-state concentrations of the drug and its 14-hydroxy metabolite were similar to those observed in healthy individuals receiving the same dose. Peak plasma concentrations of clarithromycin in HIV-infected adults receiving 0.5- or 1-g doses of the drug orally every 12 hours ranged from 2–4 or 5–10 mcg/mL, respectively. Following oral administration of the drug as the suspension every 12 hours in HIV-infected children, peak steady-state concentrations generally ranged from 6–15 mcg/mL following a dose of 15 mg/kg.

Following IV administration of a 250-mg dose of clarithromycin, peak serum concentrations of the parent drug and 14-hydroxyclarithromycin were 2.8 and 0.5 mcg/mL, respectively.

Plasma concentrations and areas under the concentration-time curve (AUCs) of clarithromycin and 14-hydroxyclarithromycin are increased by concomitant administration of omeprazole. In healthy men receiving clarithromycin 500 mg every 8 hours and omeprazole 40 mg daily, peak and trough plasma concentrations of clarithromycin averaged approximately 10 and 27% higher, respectively, than those following administration of clarithromycin alone, while AUC averaged 15% greater than that with administration of clarithromycin alone. Peak and trough plasma concentrations of 14-hydroxyclarithromycin averaged approximately 45 and 57% higher, respectively, and AUC averaged 45% greater, than those values with clarithromycin alone. In a limited number of healthy men, clarithromycin concentrations 2 hours after administration of clarithromycin alone or with omeprazole averaged 10.5 or 20 mcg/g, respectively, in the gastric antrum; 20.8 or 24.3 mcg/g, respectively, in the gastric fundus; and 4.2 or 39.3 mcg/g, respectively, in gastric mucus.

Concomitant administration of clarithromycin and omeprazole also results in increased steady-state peak plasma concentrations, area under the concentration-time curve (AUC), and elimination half-life of omeprazole compared with omeprazole administration alone. Coadministration of clarithromycin and ranitidine bismuth citrate results in increased plasma ranitidine concentrations, increased plasma bismuth trough concentrations, and increased plasma concentrations of 14- hydroxyclarithromycin. (See Pharmacokinetics: Absorption, in Ranitidine 56:28.12.)

Clarithromycin undergoes extensive first-pass metabolism and exhibits nonlinear, dose-dependent pharmacokinetics, apparently as a result of capacity-limited saturation of metabolic pathways; however, such nonlinearity is slight at the usual dosages of 250–500 mg every 8–12 hours. (See Pharmacokinetics: Elimination.) Disproportionate increases in peak serum concentrations and areas under the concentration-time curve (AUC) of clarithromycin and 14-hydroxyclarithromycin have been reported in patients receiving single high (e.g., 1.2 g) or multiple doses of clarithromycin, although some data indicate that peak serum concentrations of clarithromycin and 14-hydroxyclarithromycin are proportional to dose. In a single-dose study in healthy men, a fivefold increase in clarithromycin dosage (250 mg to 1.2g) resulted in a 13-fold increase in AUC of the parent drug. The AUC of 14-hydroxyclarithromycin following 250-mg oral or IV doses of clarithromycin was higher after oral administration, suggesting that the parent drug undergoes substantial first-pass metabolism in the liver to the 14-hydroxy metabolite.

In healthy geriatric individuals 65–84 years of age who received 500 mg of clarithromycin every 12 hours, peak and trough serum concentrations of clarithromycin and 14-hydroxyclarithromycin at steady state and area under the concentration-time curve (AUC) were increased relative to those in healthy younger adults (18–30 years of age); these increases were attributed to age-related reductions in renal function. (See Pharmacokinetics: Elimination.) Limited data indicate that serum concentrations of clarithromycin at steady state in patients with impaired hepatic function do not differ from those in healthy individuals; however, 14-hydroxyclarithromycin concentrations are lower in patients with hepatic dysfunction. (See Pharmacokinetics: Elimination.)

■ **Distribution** Limited data are available on the distribution of clarithromycin in humans. Clarithromycin and 14-hydroxyclarithromycin appear to be distributed into most body tissues and fluids. Because of high intracellular concentrations of the drug, tissue concentrations are higher than serum concentrations. High concentrations of clarithromycin were present in tissue samples obtained from patients undergoing surgery. In patients who received 250–500 mg of clarithromycin orally every 12 hours for 3 days prior to surgery, peak clarithromycin concentrations in lung, tonsils, and nasal mucosa reportedly were attained 4 hours after administration and averaged 13.5–17.5, 5.3–6.5, and 5.9–8.3 mg/ kg, respectively; however, it has been suggested that these data may represent an overestimate of clarithromycin tissue concentrations because of the microbiologic assay's inability to distinguish between parent drug and its active metabolite. In children receiving clarithromycin suspension for otitis media at a dosage of 7.5 mg/kg every 12 hours for 5 doses, peak clarithromycin and 14- hydroxyclarithromycin concentrations in middle ear fluid were 2.5 and 1.3 mcg/ mL, respectively; concomitant serum concentrations were 1.7 and 0.8 mcg/mL, respectively. Results of studies in animals given radiolabeled clarithromycin or erythromycin indicate higher and more prolonged activity of clarithromycin in various body tissues, particularly the lung.

Clarithromycin is distributed into CSF following oral administration; however, there is no evidence that the drug would be effective in the treatment of meningitis.

Protein binding of clarithromycin in vitro has been reported to range from approximately 42–72% at usual therapeutic concentrations. In one study, protein binding of radiolabeled drug in human serum ranged from approximately 42–50% at clarithromycin concentrations of 0.25–5 mcg/mL. Protein binding of clarithromycin and 14-hydroxyclarithromycin decreases with increasing serum drug concentration.

■ **Elimination** Elimination of clarithromycin appears to follow nonlinear, dose-dependent pharmacokinetics, possibly as a result of capacity-limited metabolism. Following oral administration of single 250-mg or 1.2-g doses of clarithromycin conventional tablets in healthy men, the elimination half-life averaged 4 or 11 hours, respectively. During multiple dosing every 12 hours, the elimination half-life of clarithromycin reportedly increased from 3–4 hours following a 250-mg dose (conventional tablets) every 12 hours to 5–7 hours following a 500-mg dose every 8–12 hours; the half-life of 14-hydroxyclarithromycin increased from 5–6 hours with a 250-mg dose to 7–9 hours with a 500-mg dose. When clarithromycin is administered as the oral suspension, the elimination half-life of the drug and of its 14-hydroxy metabolite appear to be similar to those observed at steady-state following administration of equivalent doses of clarithromycin as tablets.

In a single-dose study in healthy men, average total body clearance of clarithromycin decreased from 1116 mL/minute following a 250-mg dose to 403 mL/minute following a 1.2-g dose. This reduction in total body clearance was attributed principally to a reduction in metabolic (nonrenal) clearance, which declined from 913 mL/minute with the 250-mg dose to 289 mL/minute with the 1.2-g dose. The renal clearance of clarithromycin is relatively independent of dose and approximates the normal glomerular filtration rate.

Total body clearance and renal clearance of clarithromycin in healthy geriatric individuals are decreased compared with those in younger adults, apparently as a result of age-related reductions in renal function. However, since differences in pharmacokinetic values appear to be small and an increase in adverse effects has not been reported in geriatric versus younger adults, dosage adjustment solely on the basis of age generally is not required.

Clarithromycin is eliminated by both renal and nonrenal mechanisms. Clarithromycin is extensively metabolized in the liver, principally by oxidative *N*-demethylation and hydroxylation at the 14 position; hydrolytic cleavage of the cladinose sugar moiety also occurs in the stomach to a minor extent. Although at least 7 metabolites of clarithromycin have been identified, 14-hydroxyclarithromycin is the principal metabolite in serum and the only one with substantial antibacterial activity. (See Spectrum.) While both the *R*- and *S*-epimers of 14-hydroxyclarithromycin are formed in vivo, the *R*-epimer is present in greater amounts and has the greatest antimicrobial activity. Metabolism of clarithromycin appears to be saturable since the amount of 14-hydroxyclarithromycin after an 800-mg dose of the parent drug is only marginally greater than that after a 250-mg dose.

Following oral administration of a single 250-mg dose of radiolabeled clarithromycin in healthy men, approximately 38% of the dose (18% as clarithromycin) was excreted in urine, and 40% in feces (4% as clarithromycin), over 5 days. With oral administration of 250 or 500 mg of clarithromycin as tablets every 12 hours, approximately 20 or 30% of the respective dose is excreted unchanged in urine within 12 hours. After an oral clarithromycin dosage of 250 mg every 12 hours as the suspension, approximately 40% of the administered dose is excreted unchanged in urine. The principal metabolite found in urine is 14-hydroxyclarithromycin, which accounts for approximately 10–15% of the dose following administration of 250 or 500 mg of clarithromycin as tablets.

The serum half-life of clarithromycin is prolonged in patients with impaired renal function. Marked increases in peak serum concentration, AUC, and half-life of clarithromycin and 14-hydroxyclarithromycin have been reported in patients with creatinine clearances less than 30 mL/minute, and reduction of clarithromycin dosage may be required in such patients. (See Dosage and Administration: Dosage in Renal and Hepatic Impairment.) Moderate to severe hepatic impairment reportedly reduces the formation of 14-hydroxyclarithromycin but is accompanied by an increase in the renal clearance of the parent drug; therefore, a decrease in dosage would not be needed in patients with hepatic dysfunction unless renal function also is impaired. In fact, the total concentration of biologically active drug (clarithromycin plus 14-hydroxyclarithromycin) in circulation reportedly is decreased in patients with severe hepatic impairment.

Chemistry and Stability

■ **Chemistry** Clarithromycin is a semisynthetic macrolide antibiotic. The drug differs structurally from erythromycin only by the methylation of a hydroxyl group at position 6 of the lactone ring. The presence of a methyl group at this position minimizes acid-catalyzed degradation of clarithromycin to the inactive 8,9- anhydro-6,9-hemiketal and subsequently the 6,9,9,12-spiroketal products; some erythromycin degradation products (e.g., the anhydrohemiketal form) have been shown to increase GI motility and may contribute to the adverse GI effects of that drug.

Clarithromycin occurs as a white to off-white crystalline powder. The drug is practically insoluble in water and slightly soluble in alcohol, having solubilities of approximately 0.07 mg/mL in water and 5.2 mg/mL in alcohol at room temperature. The solubility of clarithromycin reportedly is pH dependent, increasing with decreasing pH.

■ **Stability** Commercially available clarithromycin 250-mg conventional tablets should be stored in well-closed containers at 15–30°C and should be protected from light. Clarithromycin 500-mg conventional tablets should be stored in well- closed containers at controlled room temperature between 20–25°C. Clarithromycin extended-release tablets should be stored at 20–25°C, but may be exposed to temperatures ranging from 15–30°C. When stored as directed, the commercially available conventional tablets have an expiration date of 2 years following the date of manufacture.

Clarithromycin granules for oral suspension should be stored in well-closed containers at 15–30°C. Following reconstitution as directed, oral suspensions of clarithromycin should be stored at 15–30°C in well-closed containers; the reconstituted suspension should *not* be refrigerated. Any unused suspension should be discarded after 14 days.

The commercially available kit containing clarithromycin, amoxicillin, and lansoprazole (Prevpac®) should be stored at 20–25°C.

Preparations

Excipients in commercially available drug preparations may have clinically important effects in some individuals; consult specific product labeling for details.

Clarithromycin

Oral		
For suspension	125 mg/5 mL*	**Clarithromycin for Suspension**
	250 mg/5 mL*	**Clarithromycin for Suspension**
Tablets, film-coated	250 mg*	**Biaxin® Filmtab®**, AbbVie
		Clarithromycin Tablets
	500 mg*	**Biaxin® Filmtab®**, AbbVie
		Clarithromycin Tablets
Tablets, extended-release, film-coated	500 mg*	**Clarithromycin Tablets Extended-release**

*available from one or more manufacturer, distributor, and/or repackager by generic (nonproprietary) name

Clarithromycin Combinations

Oral		
Kit	4 Capsules, Amoxicillin (trihydrate) 500 mg (of amoxicillin) (Trimox®) 2 Capsules, delayed-release (containing enteric-coated granules), Lansoprazole, 30 mg (Prevacid®) 2 Tablets, film-coated, Clarithromycin, 500 mg (Biaxin® Filmtab®)	**Prevpac®**, Takeda Pharmaceuticals
	4 Capsules, Amoxicillin (trihydrate) 500 mg (of amoxicillin)* 2 Capsules, delayed-release (containing enteric-coated granules), Lansoprazole, 30 mg* 2 Tablets, film-coated, Clarithromycin, 500 mg*	**Amoxicillin, Clarithromycin, and Lansoprazole**

*available from one or more manufacturer, distributor, and/or repackager by generic (nonproprietary) name

†Use is not currently included in the labeling approved by the US Food and Drug Administration

Fidaxomicin

■ Fidaxomicin is a macrocycle antibiotic classified as a macrolide.

Uses

■ **Clostridioides difficile-associated Diarrhea** Fidaxomicin is used for the treatment of diarrhea caused by *Clostridioides difficile* (formerly known as *Clostridium difficile*) infection (CDI; *C. difficile*-associated diarrhea [CDAD]) in adults 18 years of age or older. Although safety and efficacy of fidaxomicin have not been established in children and adolescents, the drug is designated an orphan drug by FDA for the treatment of CDI in pediatric patients†.

C. difficile can cause asymptomatic colonization in the intestinal tract (*C. difficile* carriage) or symptomatic intestinal CDI that can range in severity from mild to moderate diarrhea without colitis to severe diarrhea that may be associated with potentially fatal pseudomembranous colitis requiring colectomy. *C.*

difficile is the most commonly recognized cause of infectious diarrhea in health-care settings. There have been changes in the epidemiology of CDI, including an increased overall incidence of the disease worldwide, increased incidence in community populations previously considered at low risk (e.g., healthy peripartum women), increased morbidity and mortality rates, and reports of hospital outbreaks of severe and recurrent CDI associated with epidemic or hypervirulent strains of *C. difficile* (e.g., PCR ribotype 027, also known as NAP1 or B1). Risk factors for CDI include advanced age, duration of hospitalization, number of comorbidities, severity of underlying disease, immunosuppression as the result of disease or drug therapy, exposure to anti-infectives, and duration and degree of exposure to other patients with CDI. The most important modifiable risk factor for development of CDI is exposure to anti-infectives. Anti-infectives can alter normal intestinal flora and may lead to overgrowth of *C. difficile*. CDI has been reported with nearly all systemic anti-infectives, and should be considered in the differential diagnosis in patients who develop diarrhea during or after anti-infective therapy. The risk of CDI from disruption of intestinal flora is increased during anti-infective therapy and for 3 months after anti-infective therapy is discontinued. If CDI is suspected or confirmed, the inciting anti-infective should be discontinued as soon as possible. Patients should be managed with appropriate supportive therapy (e.g., fluid and electrolyte management, protein supplementation), anti-infective therapy directed against *C. difficile*, and surgical evaluation as clinically indicated.

Vancomycin, fidaxomicin, and metronidazole are considered the anti-infectives of choice for the treatment of CDI. For the treatment of an initial episode of *nonsevere* CDI in adults, the Infectious Diseases Society of America (IDSA) and Society for Healthcare Epidemiology of America (SHEA) recommend a 10-day regimen of oral vancomycin or oral fidaxomicin. These experts state that a 10-day regimen of oral metronidazole is an alternative for an initial episode of *nonsevere* CDI, but is recommended only if vancomycin and fidaxomicin are contraindicated or unavailable. For the treatment of an initial episode of *severe* CDI in adults, IDSA and SHEA state that a 10-day regimen of oral vancomycin or oral fidaxomicin can be used. However, vancomycin is the anti-infective of choice for the treatment of an initial episode of *fulminant* CDI (characterized by hypotension or shock, ileus, or megacolon) in adults and IDSA and SHEA recommend a regimen that includes vancomycin (given orally, by nasogastric tube, and/or rectally as clinically indicated) in conjunction with IV metronidazole for the treatment of such infections, especially if ileus is present. For the treatment of a *first* recurrence of CDI in adults who received a standard 10-day regimen of oral vancomycin initially, IDSA and SHEA recommend a more prolonged oral vancomycin regimen (tapered and pulsed) or a 10-day regimen of oral fidaxomicin. In those who received initial treatment with oral metronidazole and have a *first* recurrence of CDI, these experts recommend a standard 10-day regimen of oral vancomycin. Specialized references should be consulted for additional information on the management of CDI, including diagnosis, infection prevention and control, treatment of CDI in pediatric patients, and additional recommendations for treatment of initial, recurrent, or fulminant CDI in adults.

Fidaxomicin appears to offer some advantages over some other anti-infectives used for the treatment of CDI (e.g., minimal systemic absorption following oral administration, narrow spectrum of activity involving good activity against *C. difficile* and limited activity against normal intestinal flora). There is some evidence that oral fidaxomicin may be as effective or more effective than oral vancomycin in terms of resolution of diarrhea at the end of a 10-day treatment course and may be associated with lower recurrence rates than vancomycin when used for the treatment of initial episodes of CDI in adults. Although there is some evidence from retrospective studies that oral fidaxomicin may be as effective as oral vancomycin for the treatment of recurrent or severe CDI in adults, data are limited and additional study is needed to evaluate the relative efficacy and safety of fidaxomicin and vancomycin for the treatment of recurrent, severe, or fulminant CDI, including severe, life-threatening infections.

Clinical Experience Efficacy of fidaxomicin for treatment of CDAD was evaluated in 2 randomized, double-blind, active-controlled, noninferiority phase 3 trials that compared use of oral fidaxomicin (200 mg twice daily for 10 days) and oral vancomycin (125 mg 4 times daily for 10 days) in more than 1000 adults with CDI. Enrolled patients were 18 years of age or older with a diagnosis of CDAD (defined by a change in bowel habits, with more than 3 unformed bowel movements [or more than 200 mL of unformed stool in those with rectal collection devices] in the 24-hour period before randomization and presence of *C. difficile* toxin A and/or B in a stool specimen obtained within 48 hours before randomization) and had a history of no prior episodes of CDAD or only a single prior episode in the previous 3 months and had received no more than 4 doses of metronidazole or vancomycin in the 24 hours prior to randomization. Patients with life-threatening or fulminant CDI, hypotension, septic shock, peritoneal signs, substantial dehydration, toxic megacolon, previous exposure to fidaxomicin, or history of ulcerative colitis or Crohn's disease were excluded. The demographic profile and baseline CDAD characteristics of enrolled patients were similar in the 2 trials (median age 64 years, 90% white, 58% female, 63% inpatients). The median number of bowel movements per day at baseline was 6, 84% of patients had no prior episodes of CDAD, 45% reported diarrhea symptoms alone, and 37% had severe CDAD (defined as 10 or more unformed bowel movements per day or leukocyte count 15,000/mm^3 or higher).

The primary efficacy end point was the rate of clinical response (clinical cure) at the end of treatment (day 10–11). Clinical response was based on improvement in diarrhea (i.e., frequency of 3 or fewer unformed stools for 2 consecutive days) or other symptoms such that (in the investigator's judgment) further CDAD treatment was not needed; clinical failure was defined by persistence of diarrhea and/or need for additional treatment (according to the investigator's assessment). An additional efficacy end point was sustained clinical response (global cure). Sustained clinical response (defined as clinical response at the end of treatment and survival without proven or suspected CDAD recurrence through 25 days beyond the end of treatment) was evaluated only in patients who had clinical success at the end of treatment. The primary analysis population was the modified intent-to-treat (mITT) population, comprising patients with documented CDAD (more than 3 unformed bowel movements in the 24-hour period prior to randomization and presence of *C. difficile* toxin A and/or B in a stool specimen obtained within 48 hours before randomization) who received at least 1 dose of study drug after randomization.

Results of both phase 3 trials indicated that oral fidaxomicin is noninferior to oral vancomycin for treatment of CDAD in adults and that fidaxomicin is superior to vancomycin in terms of sustained clinical response after treatment. The clinical response rate at the end of treatment in the mITT population was 88% in those who received fidaxomicin compared with 86 or 87% in those who received vancomycin. Mortality rates were similar (approximately 6% in each group). During the follow-up period, substantially fewer patients in the fidaxomicin groups than in the vancomycin groups had recurrences of CDAD. The sustained clinical response rate at 25 days after completion of treatment in the mITT population was 70 or 72% in those who received fidaxomicin compared with 57% in those who received vancomycin. However, when subgroup analysis was performed to evaluate comparative efficacy of fidaxomicin and vancomycin in patients with baseline *C. difficile* isolates identified by restriction endonuclease analysis (REA) as belonging to the BI group (strains associated with increased rates and severity of CDAD), sustained clinical response rates were similar for both drugs (58 or 65% for fidaxomicin and 63 or 52% for vancomycin).

Dosage and Administration

■ **Administration** Fidaxomicin is administered orally without regard to food.

■ **Dosage** ***Clostridioides difficile-associated Diarrhea*** The recommended dosage of fidaxomicin for the treatment of diarrhea caused by *Clostridioides difficile* (formerly known as *Clostridium difficile*) infection (CDI; *C. difficile*-associated diarrhea [CDAD]) in adults 18 years of age or older is 200 mg orally twice daily for 10 days.

■ **Special Populations** ***Hepatic Impairment*** While the manufacturer makes no specific recommendations regarding dosage in adults with hepatic impairment, fidaxomicin pharmacokinetics are not expected to be affected by hepatic impairment. (See Hepatic Impairment under Warnings/Precautions: Specific Populations, in Cautions.)

Renal Impairment Dosage adjustment is not recommended in adults with mild, moderate, or severe renal impairment. (See Renal Impairment under Warnings/Precautions: Specific Populations, in Cautions.)

Geriatric Patients Dosage adjustment is not recommended in geriatric patients 65 years of age and older. (See Geriatric Use under Warnings/Precautions: Specific Populations, in Cautions.)

Cautions

■ **Contraindications** Fidaxomicin is contraindicated in patients hypersensitive to the drug or any ingredient in the formulation.

■ **Warnings/Precautions** ***Hypersensitivity Reactions*** Acute hypersensitivity reactions (e.g., dyspnea, rash, pruritus, angioedema of the mouth, throat, and face) have been reported in patients receiving fidaxomicin. Some patients with such reactions also reported a history of allergy to other macrolides.

Clinicians should consider the possibility of hypersensitivity reactions if fidaxomicin is prescribed for a patient with known macrolide allergy.

If a severe hypersensitivity reaction occurs, fidaxomicin should be discontinued and appropriate therapy administered.

Systemic Infections Fidaxomicin should *only* be used for the treatment of diarrhea caused by *Clostridioides difficile* (formerly known as *Clostridium difficile*). Because only minimal systemic absorption occurs following oral administration of fidaxomicin, the drug is *not* effective for the treatment of other types of infections.

Selection and Use of Anti-infectives To reduce development of drug-resistant bacteria and maintain effectiveness of fidaxomicin and other antibacterials, fidaxomicin should be used *only* for the treatment of infections proven or strongly suspected to be caused by *C. difficile*.

Prescribing fidaxomicin in the absence of proven or strongly suspected *C. difficile* infection (CDI) is unlikely to provide benefit to the patient and increases the risk of development of drug-resistant bacteria.

When selecting or modifying anti-infective therapy, results of culture and in vitro susceptibility testing should be used. In the absence of such data, local epidemiology and susceptibility patterns should be considered when selecting anti-infectives for empiric therapy.

Specific Populations **Pregnancy.** Available data regarding use of fidaxomicin in pregnant women are insufficient to inform any drug-associated risk for major birth defects, miscarriage, or adverse maternal or fetal outcomes.

In embryofetal reproduction studies in rats and rabbits, there was no evidence of harm to the fetus when IV fidaxomicin was administered during organogenesis at dosages resulting in fidaxomicin and OP-1118 (its main metabolite) exposures that were at least 65-fold higher than human exposures reported with the recommended dosage of the drug.

Lactation. It is not known whether fidaxomicin or its main metabolite (OP-1118) is distributed into human milk, affects the breast-fed infant, or affects milk production.

The developmental and health benefits of breast-feeding should be considered along with the mother's clinical need for fidaxomicin and potential adverse effects on the breast-fed infant from the drug or from the underlying maternal condition.

Pediatric Use. The manufacturer states that safety and efficacy of fidaxomicin have not been established in patients younger than 18 years of age. Fidaxomicin is designated an orphan drug by FDA for treatment of CDI in pediatric patients†.

In a phase 2a clinical trial that evaluated the safety and pharmacokinetics of oral fidaxomicin in pediatric patients 6 months of age or older† with *C. difficile*-associated diarrhea, the safety profile of the drug was similar to that reported in adults. The most common adverse effects reported in these pediatric patients were vomiting, fever, upper abdominal pain, and *C. difficile* colitis requiring hospitalization after study enrollment.

Geriatric Use. In controlled trials evaluating safety and efficacy of fidaxomicin, 50% of enrolled patients were 65 years of age and older and 31% were 75 years of age and older. No overall differences in efficacy or safety of fidaxomicin compared with vancomycin were observed in geriatric adults 65 years of age or older compared with younger adults.

Although data from controlled trials indicate that plasma concentrations of fidaxomicin and its main metabolite (OP-1118) are higher in patients 65 years of age or older than in younger adults, concentrations remain in the ng/mL range. This is not considered clinically important and dosage adjustments are not recommended in geriatric patients.

Hepatic Impairment. Although the effect of hepatic impairment on the pharmacokinetics of fidaxomicin has not been formally studied, elimination is not expected to be substantially affected by hepatic impairment since fidaxomicin and its main metabolite (OP-1118) do not appear to undergo substantial hepatic metabolism.

Renal Impairment. In clinical trials in patients with mild, moderate, or severe renal impairment (based on creatinine clearance) receiving fidaxomicin (200 mg orally twice daily for 10 days), plasma concentrations of fidaxomicin and its main metabolite (OP-1118) did not vary by severity of renal impairment. Dosage adjustments are not recommended in patients with renal impairment.

■ **Common Adverse Effects** Adverse effects reported in 2% or more of patients receiving fidaxomicin in clinical trials include nausea (11%), vomiting (7%), abdominal pain (6%), GI hemorrhage (4%), anemia (2%), and neutropenia (2%). Abdominal distension, abdominal tenderness, dyspepsia, dysphagia, flatulence, intestinal obstruction, megacolon, increased blood alkaline phosphatase, decreased blood bicarbonate, increased hepatic enzymes, decreased platelet count, hyperglycemia, metabolic acidosis, drug eruption, pruritus, and rash were reported in less than 2% of patients.

Drug Interactions

■ **Drugs Metabolized by Hepatic Microsomal Enzymes** Metabolism of fidaxomicin and formation of its main metabolite (OP-1118) are not dependent on cytochrome P-450 (CYP) isoenzymes. Drug interaction studies using a CYP3A4 substrate (midazolam), CYP2C9 substrate (warfarin), or CYP2C19 substrate (omeprazole) indicate that fidaxomicin has no clinically important effect on the pharmacokinetics of these drugs. Based on these results, the manufacturer states that dosage adjustments are not warranted if fidaxomicin is used concomitantly with drugs that are CYP isoenzyme substrates.

■ **Drugs Affecting or Affected by P-glycoprotein Transport** Fidaxomicin and its main metabolite (OP-1118) are substrates of the efflux transporter, P-glycoprotein (P-gp), which is expressed in the GI tract.

When cyclosporine (a P-gp inhibitor) was administered 1 hour before fidaxomicin, plasma concentrations of fidaxomicin and OP-1118 were substantially increased but remained in the ng/mL range. Although it is possible that concentrations of fidaxomicin and OP-1118 may be decreased at the site of action (i.e., GI tract) via P-gp inhibition, data from controlled clinical trials indicate that concomitant use of P-gp inhibitors in patients receiving fidaxomicin has no attributable effect on safety or treatment outcome. A drug interaction study using digoxin (a P-gp substrate) indicated that fidaxomicin has no clinically important effect on digoxin pharmacokinetics. Based on these results, the manufacturer states that dosage adjustments are not warranted if fidaxomicin is used concomitantly with P-gp inhibitors or P-gp substrates.

■ **Anti-infectives** In vitro, the antibacterial effects of fidaxomicin and its main metabolite (OP-1118) and the antibacterial effects of rifamycin antibiotics (i.e., rifampin, rifaximin) are synergistic against *Clostridioides difficile* (formerly known as *Clostridium difficile*). Some synergism also was demonstrated in vitro between fidaxomicin and OP-1118 and ampicillin, clindamycin, and metronidazole.

There was no in vitro evidence of antagonism between fidaxomicin and OP-1118 and other anti-infectives (e.g., ampicillin, azithromycin, clindamycin, metronidazole, rifampin, rifaximin, telithromycin, vancomycin).

Description

Fidaxomicin, a macrocycle antibiotic that has been classified as a macrolide, is a fermentation product obtained from the Actinomycete *Dactylosporangium aurantiacum*. While other commercially available macrolides have 14- or 15-member lactone ring structures, fidaxomicin has an 18-member macrocyclic ester structure.

Fidaxomicin has a narrow spectrum of antibacterial activity. The drug is active against certain gram-positive bacteria and has only limited or no activity against gram-negative bacteria and is inactive against *Candida albicans*. Fidaxomicin is active in vitro and in vivo against *Clostridioides difficile* (formerly known as *Clostridium difficile*), a spore-forming, gram-positive anaerobe. The MIC_{90} of fidaxomicin for *C. difficile* generally ranges from 0.125–0.5 mcg/mL. Although the clinical importance is unclear, there is some evidence that PCR ribotype 027 strains of *C. difficile* (also known as NAP1 or B1) may have slightly higher fidaxomicin MICs than non-027 strains. Fidaxomicin appears to have greater in vitro activity against *C. difficile* and may have a more minimal impact in vivo on normal intestinal flora than some other anti-infectives used for treatment of *C. difficile* infection (CDI; *C. difficile*-associated diarrhea [CDAD]); however, additional study is needed to more fully evaluate the effect of fidaxomicin on normal intestinal flora. Although fidaxomicin has in vitro activity against some other gram-positive anaerobes (e.g., *C. perfringens* and other *Clostridium* species, *Peptostreptococcus*) and has limited in vitro activity against certain gram-positive aerobes (e.g., *Staphylococcus aureus*, coagulase-negative staphylococci, *Enterococcus faecalis*, *E. faecium*), the drug is *not* effective for the treatment of systemic infections.

Fidaxomicin and its main metabolite (OP-1118) are bactericidal against *C. difficile* in vitro, and exert a postantibiotic effect against the organism. Although the exact mechanism of action has not been fully determined, the drug acts as an RNA polymerase inhibitor. Fidaxomicin appears to inhibit RNA synthesis in susceptible bacteria by binding to the DNA-RNA polymerase complex prior to formation of the open DNA-RNA polymerase complex needed for initiation of transcription. This mechanism of action is distinct from that of other commercially available macrolides, which interfere with translation in susceptible bacteria by acting at the ribosomal level of protein synthesis.

Although in vitro studies indicate a low frequency of spontaneous resistance to fidaxomicin in *C. difficile*, fidaxomicin-resistant strains of *C. difficile* have been produced in vitro and reduced susceptibility to the drug has been reported rarely in clinical specimens. Point mutations in the gene encoding the β subunit of RNA polymerase, *rpo*B, were identified in *C. difficile* mutants with reduced susceptibility to fidaxomicin that were produced in vitro. A single mutation (Val-1143-Gly) in the β subunit of RNA polymerase was identified in *C. difficile* obtained from a patient who had recurrence of CDAD after fidaxomicin treatment. Although *C. difficile* isolated from this patient at baseline had a fidaxomicin MIC of 0.06 mcg/mL, the MIC was 16 mcg/mL at the time of recurrence. Cross-resistance between fidaxomicin and other anti-infectives has not been reported to date.

Following oral administration of fidaxomicin, only minimal systemic absorption occurs and the drug remains mainly confined to and acts locally in the GI tract. Although plasma concentrations of fidaxomicin and its main metabolite (OP-1118) are approximately 2–6 times higher in patients with CDI than in healthy adults, plasma concentrations remain in the ng/mL range. Administration with a high-fat meal decreases peak plasma concentrations of fidaxomicin and OP-1118 by approximately 22 and 33%, respectively, but AUC is not affected and the effect of food is not considered clinically important. More than 92% of an oral dose is recovered in feces as fidaxomicin and OP-1118; less than 1% of a dose is recovered in urine as OP-1118. In patients treated with fidaxomicin (200 mg twice daily for 10 days), concentrations of fidaxomicin and OP-1118 in feces obtained within 24 hours of the last dose have ranged from 639–2710 mcg/g and 213–1210 mcg/g, respectively. Fidaxomicin is mainly transformed by hydrolysis at the isobutyryl ester to form OP-1118; although OP-1118 has antibacterial activity against *C. difficile*, it is less active than fidaxomicin. Metabolism of fidaxomicin and formation of OP-1118 are not dependent on cytochrome P-450 (CYP) isoenzymes. The plasma elimination half-lives of fidaxomicin and OP-1118 in adults are approximately 12 and 11 hours, respectively.

Advice to Patients

Advise patients that antibacterials (including fidaxomicin) should only be used to treat bacterial infections and not used to treat viral infections (e.g., the common cold). Importance of advising patients that fidaxomicin is used *only* to treat diarrhea associated with *Clostridioides difficile* (formerly known as *Clostridium difficile*) infection (CDI; *C. difficile*-associated diarrhea [CDAD]) and should *not* be used to treat any other infection.

Importance of completing full course of therapy, even if feeling better after a few days.

Advise patients that skipping doses or not completing the full course of therapy may decrease effectiveness and increase the likelihood that bacteria will develop resistance and will not be treatable with fidaxomicin or other antibacterials in the future.

Advise patients that fidaxomicin may be taken with or without food.

Importance of informing clinicians of existing or contemplated concomitant therapy, including prescription and OTC drugs and dietary or herbal supplements, as well as any concomitant illnesses.

Importance of women informing clinicians if they are or plan to become pregnant or plan to breast-feed.

Importance of informing patients of other important precautionary information. (See Cautions.)

Overview® (see Users Guide). For additional information on this drug until a more detailed monograph is developed and published, the manufacturer's labeling should be consulted. It is *essential* that the manufacturer's labeling be consulted for more detailed information on usual cautions, precautions, contraindications, potential drug interactions, laboratory test interferences, and acute toxicity.

Preparations

Excipients in commercially available drug preparations may have clinically important effects in some individuals; consult specific product labeling for details.

Fidaxomicin

Oral		
Tablets, film-coated	200 mg	Dificid®, Merck

†Use is not currently included in the labeling approved by the US Food and Drug Administration

PENICILLINS 8:12.16

Preface to the Penicillins

Classification of Penicillins Based on Spectra of Activity

Penicillins are natural or semisynthetic antibiotics produced by or derived from certain species of the fungus *Penicillium*. The drugs are β-lactam antibiotics structurally and pharmacologically related to other β-lactam antibiotics including cephalosporins and cephamycins. Penicillins contain a 6-aminopenicillanic acid (6-APA) nucleus, which is composed of a β-lactam ring fused to a 5-membered thiazolidine ring. Although the 6-APA nucleus has little antibacterial activity itself, it is a major structural requirement for antibacterial activity of penicillins. In currently available penicillins, cleavage at any point in the penicillin nucleus, including the β-lactam ring, results in complete loss of antibacterial activity. A free carboxyl group in the thiazolidine ring and one or more substituted amino side chains at R are also essential for antibacterial activity.

COOX, CH_3, CH_3, O, N, A, B, S, RCONH

penicillin nucleus; A = β-lactam ring; B = thiazolidine ring

Addition of various side chains at R on the penicillin nucleus results in penicillin derivatives with differences in spectra of activity, stability against hydrolysis by β-lactamases, acid stability, GI absorption, and protein binding.

Currently available penicillins can be divided into 4 groups based principally on their spectra of activity:

- Natural Penicillins
- Penicillinase-Resistant Penicillins
- Aminopenicillins
- Extended-Spectrum Penicillins

NATURAL PENICILLINS

penicillin G   penicillin V

Natural penicillins are produced by fermentation of mutant strains of *Penicillium chrysogenum*. Natural penicillins with different side chains at R are produced by altering the composition of the culture media of *Penicillium*. Although various natural penicillins have been produced (e.g., penicillins F, G, N, O, V, X), only penicillin G and penicillin V currently are used clinically.

Natural penicillins are active in vitro against many gram-positive aerobic cocci including most strains of nonpenicillinase-producing *Staphylococcus aureus* and *S. epidermidis*, *Streptococcus pneumoniae*, groups A, B, C, G, H, K, L, and M streptococci, nonenterococcal group D streptococci, viridans streptococci, and some strains of enterococci. Natural penicillins are readily hydrolyzed by staphylococcal penicillinases and are therefore inactive against penicillinase-producing strains of *S. aureus* and *S. epidermidis*. The drugs are active in vitro against some gram-positive aerobic bacilli including *Corynebacterium diphtheriae*, *Listeria monocytogenes*, and *Bacillus anthracis*.

Natural penicillins also are active in vitro against gram-negative aerobic cocci including *Neisseria meningitidis* and most strains of nonpenicillinase-producing *N. gonorrhoeae*. The drugs are active in vitro against some gram-negative aerobic bacilli including some strains of *Haemophilus influenzae*, *Pasteurella multocida*, *Streptobacillus moniliformis*, and *Spirillum minus*. However, *Pseudomonas* and most Enterobacteriaceae are resistant to natural penicillins.

Natural penicillins are active in vitro against many gram-positive anaerobic bacteria and some gram-negative anaerobic bacteria. The drugs generally are active in vitro against *Actinomyces israelii*, *Peptococcus*, *Peptostreptococcus*, *Fusobacterium*, *Veillonella*, and some strains of *Bacteroides* and *Clostridium*.

The drugs also are active against most spirochetes, including *Treponema pallidum*, *T. pertenue*, *Leptospira*, *Borrelia recurrentis*, and *B. burgdorferi*, the causative agent of Lyme disease.

PENICILLINASE-RESISTANT PENICILLINS

dicloxacillin   oxacillin
nafcillin

Penicillinase-resistant penicillins are semisynthetic derivatives of 6-APA that are stable against hydrolysis by most staphylococcal penicillinases. These penicillins have bulky side chains at R on the 6-APA nucleus that result in steric hindrance and help to prevent attachment of penicillinases to the β-lactam ring.

Because penicillinase-resistant penicillins are not hydrolyzed by most staphylococcal penicillinases, these drugs are active in vitro against many penicillinase-producing strains of *S. aureus* and *S. epidermidis* that are resistant to natural penicillins, aminopenicillins, and extended-spectrum penicillins.

Penicillinase-resistant penicillins also have some in vitro activity against other gram-positive bacteria and some gram-negative bacteria and spirochetes; however, the drugs generally are less active on a weight basis against these organisms than natural penicillins, and use of penicillinase-resistant penicillins generally is limited to the treatment of infections caused by susceptible penicillinase-producing staphylococci.

AMINOPENICILLINS

amoxicillin   ampicillin

Aminopenicillins are semisynthetic derivatives of 6-APA which have a free amino group at the α-position at R on the penicillin nucleus. Partly because of this polar group, aminopenicillins have enhanced activity against gram-negative bacteria compared with natural penicillins and penicillinase-resistant penicillins.

In vitro, aminopenicillins are generally active against gram-positive aerobic cocci and gram-positive aerobic bacilli that are susceptible to natural penicillins. However, with the possible exception of enterococcal infections, natural penicillins are generally the penicillins of choice for the treatment of infections caused by gram-positive cocci that are susceptible to both natural penicillins and aminopenicillins. Like natural penicillins and extended-spectrum penicillins, aminopenicillins are readily hydrolyzed by staphylococcal penicillinases and are therefore inactive against penicillinase-producing strains of *S. aureus* and *S. epidermidis*.

Aminopenicillins are generally active in vitro against gram-negative aerobic cocci, gram-negative aerobic bacilli, and anaerobic bacteria that are susceptible to natural penicillins. In addition, aminopenicillins are active in vitro against some Enterobacteriaceae including some strains of *Escherichia coli*, *Proteus mirabilis*, *Salmonella*, and *Shigella*. Aminopenicillins are generally inactive against other Enterobacteriaceae, *Bacteroides fragilis*, and *Pseudomonas*.

Because clavulanic acid and sulbactam can inhibit certain β-lactamases that generally inactivate aminopenicillins, fixed combinations of amoxicillin and clavulanate potassium (amoxicillin/clavulanate) and fixed combinations of ampicillin sodium and sulbactam sodium (ampicillin/sulbactam) are active in vitro against many β-lactamase-producing organisms that are resistant to the aminopenicillin alone.

EXTENDED-SPECTRUM PENICILLINS

piperacillin   ticarcillin (no longer commercially available in the US)

Extended-spectrum penicillins are semisynthetic derivatives of 6-APA which have a wider spectra of activity than natural penicillins, penicillinase-resistant penicillins, and aminopenicillins.

The group of extended-spectrum penicillins is composed of 2 different subgroups: Acylaminopenicillins (piperacillin) and α-carboxypenicillins (ticarcillin; no longer commercially available in the US). Acylaminopenicillins have basic groups on the side chain at R on the penicillin nucleus and α-carboxypenicillins have a carboxylic acid group at the α-position at R on the penicillin nucleus. Partly because of these polar groups, extended-spectrum penicillins are even more active against gram-negative aerobic and gram-negative anaerobic bacilli than are aminopenicillins, and use of extended-spectrum penicillins is generally limited to the treatment of serious infections caused by susceptible gram-negative bacilli or mixed aerobic-anaerobic bacterial infections.

In vitro, extended-spectrum penicillins are generally active against gram-positive and gram-negative aerobic cocci that are susceptible to natural penicillins and aminopenicillins. Like natural penicillins and aminopenicillins, extended-spectrum penicillins are hydrolyzed by staphylococcal penicillinases and are therefore inactive when used alone against penicillinase-producing strains of *S. aureus* and *S. epidermidis*. Extended-spectrum penicillins have some activity against gram-positive aerobic and gram-positive anaerobic bacilli, but the drugs are generally less active in vitro on a weight basis against these organisms than are natural penicillins and aminopenicillins.

Extended-spectrum penicillins are generally active in vitro against gram-negative bacilli that are susceptible to aminopenicillins. The drugs are also active against many strains of Enterobacteriaceae and some strains of *Pseudomonas* that are resistant to other currently available penicillins. α-Carboxypenicillins are active in vitro against some strains of *E. coli, Morganella morganii* (formerly *Proteus morganii*), *Proteus mirabilis, P. vulgaris, Providencia rettgeri, Salmonella, Shigella*, and *Ps. aeruginosa*. In addition to these organisms, acylaminopenicillins are generally active in vitro against some strains of *Citrobacter,Enterobacter, Klebsiella*, and *Serratia*. Extended-spectrum penicillins are generally more active in vitro against *Bacteroides fragilis* than other currently available penicillins.

The only extended-spectrum penicillin commercially available in the US is piperacillin sodium in fixed combination with tazobactam sodium (piperacillin/tazobactam). Because tazobactam has a high affinity for and irreversibly binds to certain β-lactamases that can inactivate extended-spectrum penicillins, piperacillin/tazobactam is active against many β-lactamase-producing bacteria that would be resistant to piperacillin alone.

For more complete information on the spectra of activity of penicillins and additional information on the drugs, see the General Statements on Natural Penicillins, Aminopenicillins, and Penicillinase-Resistant Penicillins and the individual monographs in 8:12.16.04, 8:12.16.08, 8:12.16.12, and 8:12.16.16.

NATURAL PENICILLINS 8:12.16.04

Penicillin G Benzathine

Benzathine Benzylpenicillin, Benzathine Penicillin G, Benzylpenicillin Benzathine, Dibenzylethylenediamine Benzylpenicillin

■ Penicillin G benzathine, a natural penicillin, is a β-lactam antibiotic. The drug is the benzathine tetrahydrate salt of penicillin G and is a long-acting formulation of penicillin G.

Uses

Penicillin G benzathine is used only for the treatment of mild to moderately severe infections caused by organisms that are susceptible to the low, prolonged concentrations of penicillin G provided by IM penicillin G benzathine and for prophylaxis of certain infections caused by these organisms. When high, sustained concentrations of penicillin G are required for the treatment of severe infections, parenteral penicillin G potassium or sodium should be used.

The fixed combinations of penicillin G benzathine and penicillin G procaine are used for the treatment of moderately severe to severe infections caused by susceptible streptococci (e.g., upper respiratory tract infections, scarlet fever, erysipelas, skin and skin structure infections). The fixed combinations should *not* be used for *initial* treatment of severe pneumococcal infections, including pneumonia, empyema, bacteremia, pericarditis, meningitis, peritonitis, or arthritis. In addition, fixed combinations of penicillin G benzathine and penicillin G procaine should *not* be used for the treatment of syphilis, yaws, bejel, pinta, or gonorrhea.

For additional information on the uses of penicillin G benzathine, see Uses in the Natural Penicillins General Statement 8:12.16.04.

■ **Pharyngitis and Tonsillitis** IM penicillin G benzathine is a drug of choice for the treatment of pharyngitis and tonsillitis caused by *Streptococcus pyogenes* (group A β-hemolytic streptococci; GAS) and prevention of initial attacks (primary prevention) of rheumatic fever.

Selection of an anti-infective for the treatment of *S. pyogenes* pharyngitis and tonsillitis should be based on the drug's spectrum of activity, bacteriologic and clinical efficacy, potential adverse effects, ease of administration, patient compliance, and cost. No regimen has been found to date that effectively eradicates group A β-hemolytic streptococci in 100% of patients.

Because the drugs have a narrow spectrum of activity, are inexpensive, and generally are effective with a low frequency of adverse effects, the American Academy of Pediatrics (AAP), Infectious Diseases Society of America (IDSA), and American Heart Association (AHA) recommend a penicillin regimen (i.e., 10 days of oral penicillin V or oral amoxicillin or a single dose of IM penicillin G benzathine) as the treatment of choice for *S. pyogenes* pharyngitis and tonsillitis. Other anti-infectives (narrow-spectrum oral cephalosporins, oral macrolides, oral clindamycin) are recommended as alternatives in penicillin-allergic patients.

Experts state that the single-dose IM penicillin G benzathine regimen may be the preferred regimen in patients who are unlikely to complete the recommended 10-day regimen of oral penicillin V potassium or amoxicillin and in patients with a personal or family history of rheumatic fever or rheumatic heart disease or with other environmental factors (e.g., crowded living conditions) that place them at increased risk for development of rheumatic fever.

If signs and symptoms of pharyngitis recur shortly after initial treatment and presence of *S. pyogenes* is documented, retreatment with the original or an alternative anti-infective is recommended. Initial treatment failures may occur more frequently with oral penicillins than with IM penicillin G benzathine because of poor adherence to the oral regimen. Alternative regimens recommended for retreatment include a narrow-spectrum oral cephalosporin, oral clindamycin, oral fixed combination of amoxicillin and clavulanate, oral macrolide, or IM penicillin G benzathine.

If there are multiple, recurrent episodes of symptomatic pharyngitis within a period of several months to years, it may be difficult to determine whether these are true episodes of *S. pyogenes* infection or whether the patient is a long-term pharyngeal carrier of *S. pyogenes* who is experiencing repeated episodes of nonstreptococcal (e.g., viral) pharyngitis.

Treatment of asymptomatic chronic pharyngeal carriers of *S. pyogenes* is not usually indicated and these individuals should not receive repeated courses of anti-infective therapy. However, eradication of the carrier state may be desirable in certain situations (e.g., during a community outbreak of acute rheumatic fever, acute poststreptococcal glomerulonephritis, or invasive *S. pyogenes* infections; during an outbreak of *S. pyogenes* pharyngitis in a closed or partially closed community; when multiple episodes of documented symptomatic *S. pyogenes* pharyngitis are occurring within a family for many weeks despite appropriate treatment; when there is a personal or family history of acute rheumatic fever). In such situations, recommended regimens include oral clindamycin, oral fixed combination of amoxicillin and clavulanate, or oral rifampin used in conjunction with either IM penicillin G benzathine or oral penicillin V.

■ **Prevention of Rheumatic Fever Recurrence** IM penicillin G benzathine is used for prevention of recurrent attacks of rheumatic fever (secondary prophylaxis) in individuals who have had a previous attack of rheumatic fever.

IM penicillin G benzathine generally is considered the drug of choice for secondary prophylaxis of rheumatic fever because it ensures compliance; alternatives include oral penicillin V or oral sulfadiazine. Sulfadiazine is recommended when hypersensitivity precludes the use of a penicillin; however, a macrolide (azithromycin, clarithromycin, erythromycin) should be used in patients allergic to penicillins *and* sulfonamides. Even with optimal patient adherence, the risk of recurrence of rheumatic fever is higher in individuals receiving an oral prophylaxis regimen than in those receiving IM penicillin G benzathine.

AHA and AAP recommend long-term (continuous) secondary prophylaxis in patients who have been treated for documented acute rheumatic fever (even if manifested solely by Sydenham chorea) and in those with evidence of rheumatic heart disease (even after prosthetic valve replacement).

Prophylaxis should be initiated as soon as the diagnosis of rheumatic fever or rheumatic heart disease is made, although patients with acute rheumatic fever should first receive the usually recommended anti-infective treatment for *S. pyogenes* pharyngitis and tonsillitis (see Uses: Pharyngitis and Tonsillitis).

■ **Syphilis** IM penicillin G benzathine is used for the treatment of syphilis.

The US Centers for Disease Control and Prevention (CDC) and other experts state that IM penicillin G benzathine is the drug of choice for the treatment of primary syphilis (i.e., ulcer or chancre at infection site), secondary syphilis (i.e., manifestations that include, but are not limited to, rash, mucocutaneous lesions, and lymphadenopathy), and tertiary syphilis (i.e., cardiac syphilis, gummatous lesions, tabes dorsalis, and general paresis) in adults, adolescents, and children.

IM penicillin G benzathine also is the drug of choice for the treatment of latent syphilis (i.e., detected by serologic testing but lacking clinical manifestations), including both early latent syphilis (latent syphilis acquired within the preceding year) and late latent syphilis (i.e., all other cases of latent syphilis or syphilis of unknown duration) in all age groups.

For the treatment of neurosyphilis and otic or ocular syphilis, CDC and other experts state that IV penicillin G potassium or sodium is the drug of choice and IM penicillin G procaine (with oral probenecid) is an alternative if compliance can be ensured.

For the treatment of congenital syphilis, CDC recommends IV penicillin G potassium or sodium or IM penicillin G procaine in neonates with proven or highly probable congenital syphilis (i.e., abnormal physical examination consistent with congenital syphilis, serum quantitative nontreponemal serologic titer fourfold higher than the mother's titer, or positive darkfield test or polymerase chain reaction [PCR] of lesions or body fluids). CDC recommends IV penicillin G potassium or sodium, IM penicillin G procaine, or IM penicillin G benzathine in neonates with possible congenital syphilis (i.e., normal physical examination and serum quantitative nontreponemal serologic titer no more than fourfold higher than the mother's titer and the mother received a recommended treatment regimen less than 4 weeks before delivery; the mother was not treated or was inadequately treated, including treatment with erythromycin or any regimen not included in CDC recommendations; or there is no documentation that the mother received treatment).

Neonates with human immunodeficiency virus (HIV) infection who have congenital syphilis and HIV-infected children, adolescents, and adults who have neurosyphilis or primary, secondary, early latent, late latent, or tertiary syphilis should receive the same treatment regimens as those without HIV infection. Available data indicate that additional treatment doses of IM penicillin G benzathine do not enhance efficacy, including in HIV-infected patients. Because serologic nonresponse and neurologic complications may be more frequent in HIV-infected individuals, close follow-up is essential in those coinfected with syphilis and HIV. In addition, careful neurologic examinations are indicated in all HIV-infected patients coinfected with syphilis.

Limited data support the use of certain alternatives to IM penicillin G benzathine for treatment of primary or secondary syphilis in patients with penicillin hypersensitivity (e.g., doxycycline, tetracycline); however, if compliance with alternative regimens or follow-up cannot be ensured, CDC recommends desensitization and treatment with IM penicillin G benzathine. Some experts state that efficacy of alternatives to IM penicillin G benzathine for the treatment of early syphilis in HIV-infected individuals has not been well studied and use of alternatives in such patients should be undertaken only with close clinical and serologic monitoring.

There are no proven alternatives to penicillin G for the treatment of congenital syphilis in infants and children with known or suspected penicillin hypersensitivity and no proven alternatives to penicillin G for the treatment of any stage of syphilis in pregnant women with penicillin hypersensitivity; therefore, CDC recommends desensitization and treatment with the appropriate penicillin G preparation.

Fixed combinations of penicillin G benzathine and penicillin G procaine (Bicillin® C-R, Bicillin® C-R 900/300) should not be used for the treatment of any form of syphilis; inadvertent use of one of these fixed-combination preparations may not provide the sustained serum concentrations of penicillin G required for treatment of syphilis and could increase the risk of treatment failure and neurosyphilis, especially in HIV-infected patients.

For additional information regarding treatment of syphilis, the current CDC sexually transmitted diseases treatment guidelines available at https://www.cdc.gov/std/syphilis/treatment.htm should be consulted.

Dosage and Administration

■ Administration Penicillin G benzathine and fixed combinations containing penicillin G benzathine and penicillin G procaine are administered *only* by deep IM injection.

Special precaution should be taken to avoid inadvertent intravascular or intra-arterial administration of penicillin G benzathine or fixed combinations of penicillin G benzathine and penicillin G procaine or injection into or near major peripheral nerves or blood vessels because this may result in severe and/or permanent neurovascular damage. (See Cautions: Adverse Effects.)

Penicillin G benzathine and fixed combinations containing penicillin G benzathine and penicillin G procaine must *not* be given IV or admixed with IV solutions because inadvertent IV administration of penicillin G benzathine has been associated with cardiorespiratory arrest and death.

IM Injection Penicillin G benzathine and fixed combinations containing penicillin G benzathine and penicillin G procaine are provided in prefilled syringes and the appropriate dose should be administered undiluted according to the manufacturer's directions.

In adults, IM injections of penicillin G benzathine or fixed combinations of penicillin G benzathine and penicillin G procaine generally should be made deeply into the gluteus maximus (upper outer quadrant of the buttock) or into the midlateral thigh. In neonates, infants, and small children, IM injections of these preparations should be given preferably into the midlateral muscles of the thigh.

To minimize the possibility of damage to the sciatic nerve, one manufacturer of penicillin G benzathine recommends that the periphery of the upper outer quadrant of the gluteal regions be used in infants and small children only when necessary (e.g., in burn patients) and recommends that the deltoid area be used only if well developed, such as in certain adults and older children, and only with caution to avoid radial nerve injury. This manufacturer also suggests that the penicillin G benzathine dose can be divided and administered at 2 separate sites if necessary in children younger than 2 years of age.

IM injections may be less painful if penicillin G benzathine is warmed to room temperature before administration.

IM injections of penicillin G benzathine or fixed combinations of penicillin G benzathine and penicillin G procaine should be made at a slow, steady rate to avoid blockage of the needle.

When the fixed combination of penicillin G benzathine and penicillin G procaine (Bicillin® C-R) is used, the manufacturer states that the dose usually is given at a single session using multiple IM sites; alternatively, if compliance regarding the return visit is ensured, the total dose can be divided and half given on day 1 and half on day 3.

When repeated doses are given, IM injection sites should be rotated. Repeated IM injection into the anterolateral thigh, especially in neonates and infants, should be avoided because quadriceps femoris fibrosis and atrophy have been reported.

■ Dosage Dosage of penicillin G benzathine usually is expressed in terms of penicillin G units, but also has been expressed as mg of penicillin G.

Dosage of the fixed combinations containing penicillin G benzathine and penicillin G procaine (Bicillin® C-R, Bicillin® C-R 900/300) usually is expressed in terms of the total (sum) of penicillin G units of penicillin G benzathine and penicillin G units of penicillin G procaine.

Pediatric Dosage **General Pediatric Dosage.** The American Academy of Pediatrics (AAP) states that the usual dosage of IM penicillin G benzathine for the treatment of mild to moderate infections in pediatric patients beyond the neonatal period is a single dose of 300,000–600,000 units in those weighing less than 27 kg or a single dose of 900,000 units in those weighing 27 kg or more. AAP states that IM penicillin G benzathine is inappropriate for the treatment of severe infections.

If the fixed combination of penicillin G benzathine and penicillin G procaine (Bicillin® C-R) is used in pediatric patients beyond the neonatal period, AAP recommends a single IM dose of 600,000 penicillin G units in those weighing less than 14 kg and a single IM dose of 900,000 to 1.2 million penicillin G units in those weighing 14–27 kg. If this fixed-combination preparation is used in those weighing 27 kg or more, AAP recommends a single dose of 2.4 million penicillin G units.

Pharyngitis and Tonsillitis. For the treatment of pharyngitis or tonsillitis caused by *Streptococcus pyogenes* (group A β-hemolytic streptococci; GAS) and prevention of initial attacks (primary prevention) of rheumatic fever in children, AAP, Infectious Diseases Society of America (IDSA), and American Heart Association (AHA) recommend that IM penicillin G benzathine be given as a single dose of 600,000 units in those weighing less than 27 kg and a single dose of 1.2 million units in those weighing 27 kg or more.

The manufacturers recommend a single IM penicillin G benzathine dose of 300,000–600,000 units in children weighing less than 27 kg and a single dose of 900,000 units in older children for the treatment of *S. pyogenes* pharyngitis.

Although anti-infective treatment is not recommended for most individuals identified as chronic pharyngeal carriers of *S. pyogenes* (see Uses: Pharyngitis and Tonsillitis), IDSA states that a single IM penicillin G benzathine dose of 600,000 units in those weighing less than 27 kg or 1.2 million units in those weighing 27 kg or more given in conjunction with oral rifampin (20 mg/kg daily given in 2 doses [up to 600 mg daily] for 4 days) is an option when eradication of the carrier state is desirable.

Streptococcal Infections. If IM penicillin G benzathine is used for the treatment of mild to moderate infections of the upper respiratory tract caused by susceptible *S. pyogenes*, one manufacturer recommends a single dose of 300,000–600,000 units in children weighing less than 27 kg and 900,000 units in older pediatric patients.

If the fixed combination of penicillin G benzathine and penicillin G procaine (Bicillin® C-R) is used for the treatment of moderately severe to severe infections caused by susceptible *S. pyogenes* (e.g., upper respiratory tract infections, scarlet fever, erysipelas, skin and skin structure infections), the manufacturer recommends that children weighing less than 13.6 kg receive a single IM dose of 600,000 penicillin G units, those weighing 13.6–27.2 kg receive a single IM dose of 900,000 to 1.2 million penicillin G units, and those weighing more than 27.2 kg receive a single IM dose of 2.4 million penicillin G units. If this fixed-combination preparation is used for the treatment of moderately severe infections caused by susceptible *S. pneumoniae* (pneumonia, otitis media), the manufacturer recommends that pediatric patients receive an IM dose of 600,000 penicillin G units once every 2 or 3 days until the patient has been afebrile for 48 hours. Other penicillins are recommended for severe *S. pneumoniae* infections (e.g., pneumonia, empyema, bacteremia, pericarditis, meningitis, peritonitis, arthritis).

If the fixed combination of penicillin G benzathine and penicillin G procaine (Bicillin® C-R 900/300) is used for the treatment of moderately severe to severe infections caused by susceptible *S. pyogenes* (e.g., upper respiratory tract infections, scarlet fever, erysipelas, skin and skin structure infections), the manufacturer states that a single IM dose of 1.2 million penicillin G units usually is sufficient in pediatric patients. If this fixed-combination preparation is used for the treatment of moderately severe infections caused by susceptible *S. pneumoniae* (pneumonia, otitis media), the manufacturer recommends that pediatric patients receive an IM dose of 1.2 million penicillin G units once every 2 or 3 days until the patient has been afebrile for 48 hours. Other penicillins are recommended for severe *S. pneumoniae* infections (e.g., pneumonia, empyema, bacteremia, pericarditis, meningitis, peritonitis, arthritis).

Diphtheria. If IM penicillin G benzathine is used for prevention of diphtheria† in asymptomatic household or close contacts of patients with respiratory or cutaneous diphtheria caused by *Corynebacterium diphtheriae*, the US Centers for Disease Control and Prevention (CDC) and AAP recommend that children younger than 6 years of age or those weighing less than 30 kg receive a single dose of 600,000 units and that children 6 years of age or older or those weighing 30 kg or more receive a single dose of 1.2 million units. Household or close contacts of patients with diphtheria should receive anti-infective prophylaxis regardless of their immunization status and should be closely monitored for symptoms of diphtheria for 7 days. Contacts who are inadequately immunized against diphtheria or whose immunization status is unknown should receive an immediate dose of an age-appropriate preparation containing diphtheria toxoid adsorbed and the primary series should be completed according to the recommended schedule. Contacts who are fully immunized should receive an immediate booster dose of an age-appropriate preparation containing diphtheria toxoid adsorbed if it has been 5 years or longer since their last booster dose.

When IM penicillin G benzathine is used to eliminate the diphtheria carrier state† in identified carriers of toxigenic *C. diphtheriae*, CDC and AAP recommend that children younger than 6 years of age or those weighing less than 30 kg receive a single dose of 600,000 units and that children 6 years of age or older or those weighing 30 kg or more receive a single dose of 1.2 million units. Follow-up cultures should be obtained at least 2 weeks after treatment of diphtheria carriers; if cultures are positive, a 10-day course of oral erythromycin should be given and additional follow-up cultures obtained.

Syphilis. If IM penicillin G benzathine is used for the treatment of possible congenital syphilis or when congenital syphilis is less likely (see Uses: Syphilis), CDC and the manufacturers recommend a single dose of 50,000 units/kg. Neonates with proven or highly probable congenital syphilis (see Uses: Syphilis) should receive a 10-day regimen of IV penicillin G potassium or sodium or IM penicillin G procaine.

In infants and children 1 month of age or older with reactive serologic tests for syphilis but no clinical manifestation of congenital syphilis and a normal evaluation (including CSF examination), CDC states that treatment with IM penicillin G benzathine given in a dosage of 50,000 units/kg (up to 2.4 million units) once weekly for up to 3 weeks can be considered. If a 10-day regimen of IV penicillin G potassium or sodium is used in such patients, a single dose of IM penicillin G benzathine (50,000 units/kg) may be considered after completion of the IV regimen.

For the treatment of primary, secondary, or early latent syphilis in infants and children 1 month of age or older, CDC and others recommend that IM penicillin G benzathine be given as a single dose of 50,000 units/kg (up to 2.4 million units).

For the treatment of late latent syphilis in infants and children 1 month of age or older, CDC and others recommend that IM penicillin G benzathine be given in a dosage of 50,000 units/kg (up to 2.4 million units) administered once weekly for 3 consecutive weeks (up to a maximum total dosage of 7.2 million units).

CDC recommends that treatment of syphilis diagnosed in infants and children 1 month of age or older should be managed by a pediatric infectious disease specialist and that CSF should be examined in those with latent syphilis.

In adolescents 10–19 years of age, some experts state that those with early syphilis (primary, secondary, or early latent syphilis) should receive a single IM penicillin G benzathine dose of 2.4 million units and that those with late latent syphilis or syphilis of unknown duration should receive IM penicillin G benzathine in a dosage of 2.4 million units once weekly for 3 consecutive weeks. The interval between consecutive doses of IM penicillin G benzathine should not exceed 14 days.

Neonates with human immunodeficiency virus (HIV) infection who have congenital syphilis and HIV-infected children and adolescents with any stage of syphilis should receive the same treatment regimens recommended for those without HIV infection.

Fixed combinations of penicillin G benzathine and penicillin G procaine (Bicillin® C-R, Bicillin® C-R 900/300) should not be used for the treatment of any form of syphilis.

Yaws, Pinta, and Bejel. For the treatment of yaws, pinta, and bejel in children, IM penicillin G benzathine has been given as a single dose of 600,000 units in those younger than 10 years of age or 1.2 million units in those 10 years of age or older. A single IM dose of 50,000 units/kg (up to 2.4 million units) also has been used for the treatment of yaws in children.

Fixed combinations of penicillin G benzathine and penicillin G procaine (Bicillin® C-R, Bicillin® C-R 900/300) should not be used for the treatment of yaws, pinta, or bejel.

Prevention of Rheumatic Fever Recurrence. For prevention of recurrent rheumatic fever (secondary prophylaxis), AAP and AHA state that the usual dosage of IM penicillin G benzathine is 600,000 units once every 4 weeks in children weighing 27 kg or less and 1.2 million units once every 4 weeks in those weighing more than 27 kg. The manufacturers recommend that penicillin G benzathine be given in a dosage of 1.2 million units once monthly or 600,000 units once every 2 weeks for such prophylaxis.

AAP and AHA state that an IM penicillin G benzathine regimen that uses a 4-week dosing interval seems adequate and is recommended for most patients in the US, but a 3-week dosing interval may be warranted and is recommended when there is a particularly high risk of rheumatic fever (e.g., recurrent acute rheumatic fever despite adherence to a 4-week regimen). There is some evidence that serum penicillin concentrations may decline to subtherapeutic concentrations before the fourth week in some patients and there is limited evidence of an increased frequency of prophylactic failure with a 4-week interval compared with a 3-week interval in areas with a high risk of rheumatic fever.

Prevention of recurrent rheumatic fever requires long-term, continuous prophylaxis. (See Table 1.) Some clinicians use IM penicillin G benzathine initially and change to oral prophylaxis (usually oral penicillin V) when the patient reaches late adolescence or young adulthood and has remained free of rheumatic attacks for at least 5 years.

Table 1. Recommended Duration of Prophylaxis for Prevention of Rheumatic Fever Recurrence

Patient Category	Duration
Rheumatic fever without carditis	5 years since last episode or until 21 years of age, whichever is longer
Rheumatic fever with carditis but no residual heart disease (no valvular disease)	10 years since last episode or until 21 years of age, whichever is longer
Rheumatic fever with carditis and residual heart disease (persistent valvular disease)	10 years since last episode or until 40 years of age, whichever is longer; sometimes for life

Adult Dosage **Pharyngitis and Tonsillitis.** For the treatment of pharyngitis or tonsillitis caused by *S. pyogenes* (group A β-hemolytic streptococci; GAS) and prevention of initial attacks (primary prevention) of rheumatic fever, the usual adult dosage of penicillin G benzathine is a single IM dose of 1.2 million units.

Although anti-infective treatment is not recommended for most individuals identified as chronic pharyngeal carriers of *S. pyogenes* (see Uses: Pharyngitis and Tonsilitis), IDSA states that a single IM penicillin G benzathine dose of 600,000 units in those weighing less than 27 kg or 1.2 million units in those weighing 27 kg or more given in conjunction with oral rifampin (20 mg/kg daily given in 2 doses [up to 600 mg daily] for 4 days) is an option when eradication of the carrier state is desirable.

Streptococcal Infections. If IM penicillin G benzathine is used for the treatment of mild to moderate upper respiratory tract infections caused by susceptible *S. pyogenes* (group A β-hemolytic streptococci; GAS), adults should receive a single dose of 1.2 million units.

If the fixed combination of penicillin G benzathine and penicillin G procaine (Bicillin® C-R) is used for the treatment of moderately severe to severe infections caused by susceptible *S. pyogenes* (e.g., upper respiratory tract infections, scarlet fever, erysipelas, skin and skin structure infections), the manufacturer recommends that adults receive a single IM dose of 2.4 million penicillin G units. If this fixed-combination preparation is used for the treatment of moderately severe infections caused by susceptible *S. pneumoniae* (pneumonia, otitis media) in adults, the manufacturer recommends an IM dose of 1.2 million penicillin G units once every 2 or 3 days until the patient has been afebrile for 48 hours. Other penicillins are recommended for severe *S. pneumoniae* infections (e.g., pneumonia, empyema, bacteremia, pericarditis, meningitis, peritonitis, arthritis).

Diphtheria. If IM penicillin G benzathine is used for prevention of diphtheria† in asymptomatic household or close contacts of patients with respiratory or cutaneous diphtheria, CDC recommends that adults receive a single dose of 1.2 million units. Household or close contacts of patients with diphtheria should receive anti-infective prophylaxis regardless of their immunization status and should be closely monitored for symptoms of diphtheria for 7 days. Contacts who are inadequately immunized against diphtheria or whose immunization status is unknown should receive an immediate dose of an age-appropriate preparation containing diphtheria toxoid adsorbed and the primary series should be completed according to the recommended schedule. Contacts who are fully immunized should receive an immediate booster dose of an age-appropriate preparation containing diphtheria toxoid adsorbed if it has been 5 years or longer since their last booster dose.

When IM penicillin G benzathine is used to eliminate the diphtheria carrier state† in identified carriers of toxigenic *C. diphtheriae*, adults should receive a single dose of 1.2 million units. Follow-up cultures should be obtained at least 2 weeks after treatment of diphtheria carriers; if cultures are positive, a 10-day course of oral erythromycin should be given and additional follow-up cultures obtained.

Syphilis. For the treatment of primary, secondary, or early latent syphilis in adults, CDC, the manufacturers, and others recommend that IM penicillin G benzathine be given as a single dose of 2.4 million units. For pregnant women with primary, secondary, or early latent syphilis, some clinicians recommend that a second IM penicillin G benzathine dose of 2.4 million units be given 1 week after the initial dose. If retreatment of primary, secondary, or early latent syphilis is necessary and there is no evidence that neurosyphilis is present, CDC and others recommend that adults receive IM penicillin G benzathine in a dosage of 2.4 million units once weekly for 3 consecutive weeks.

For the treatment of late latent syphilis, latent syphilis of unknown duration, or tertiary syphilis, CDC and others recommend that adults receive IM penicillin G benzathine in a dosage of 2.4 million units once weekly for 3 consecutive weeks (total dosage 7.2 million units). The interval between consecutive doses of IM penicillin G benzathine should not exceed 14 days.

Although the manufacturers state that adults can receive 2.4 or 3 million units of penicillin G benzathine IM once weekly for 3 successive weeks for the treatment of neurosyphilis, treatment failures have been reported when penicillin G benzathine was used alone for the treatment of neurosyphilis. CDC and others state that IV penicillin G potassium or sodium is the drug of choice for the treatment of neurosyphilis and IM penicillin G procaine (with oral probenecid) is an alternative if compliance can be ensured. Some clinicians recommend that the IV penicillin G potassium or sodium regimen or IM penicillin G procaine regimen be followed by a regimen of IM penicillin G benzathine (2.4 million units once weekly for up to 3 weeks).

HIV-infected adults with any stage of syphilis should receive the same treatment regimens recommended for those without HIV infection.

Fixed combinations of penicillin G benzathine and penicillin G procaine (Bicillin® C-R, Bicillin® C-R 900/300) should not be used for the treatment of any form of syphilis.

Yaws, Pinta, and Bejel. For the treatment of yaws, pinta, and bejel in adults, IM penicillin G benzathine has been given as a single dose of 1.2 million units. A single IM dose of 2.4 million units also has been used for the treatment of yaws.

Fixed combinations of penicillin G benzathine and penicillin G procaine (Bicillin® C-R, Bicillin® C-R 900/300) should not be used for the treatment of yaws, pinta, or bejel.

Prevention of Rheumatic Fever Recurrence. For prevention of rheumatic fever recurrence (secondary prophylaxis) in adults, AHA states that the usual dosage of IM penicillin G benzathine is 1.2 million units once every 4 weeks. The manufacturers recommend that IM penicillin G benzathine be given in a dosage of 1.2 million units once monthly or 600,000 units once every 2 weeks for such prophylaxis.

AHA and AAP state that an IM penicillin G benzathine regimen that uses a 4-week dosing interval seems adequate and is recommended for most patients in the US, but a 3-week dosing interval may be warranted and is recommended when there is a particularly high risk of rheumatic fever (e.g., recurrent acute rheumatic fever despite adherence to a 4-week regimen). There is some evidence that serum penicillin concentrations may decline to subtherapeutic concentrations before the fourth week in some patients and there is limited evidence of an increased frequency of prophylactic failure with a 4-week interval compared with a 3-week interval in areas with a high risk of rheumatic fever.

Prevention of recurrent rheumatic fever requires long-term, continuous prophylaxis. (See Table 1.)

Table 1. Recommended Duration of Prophylaxis for Prevention of Rheumatic Fever Recurrence

Patient Category	Duration
Rheumatic fever without carditis	5 years since last episode or until 21 years of age, whichever is longer
Rheumatic fever with carditis but no residual heart disease (no valvular disease)	10 years since last episode or until 21 years of age, whichever is longer
Rheumatic fever with carditis and residual heart disease (persistent valvular disease)	10 years since last episode or until 40 years of age, whichever is longer; sometimes for life

Cautions

■ **Adverse Effects** Adverse effects reported with penicillin G benzathine are similar to those reported with other natural penicillins.

Serious and occasionally fatal hypersensitivity reactions, including anaphylaxis, have been reported with penicillins. Rash (maculopapular), exfoliative dermatitis, urticaria, laryngeal edema, fever, eosinophilia, other serum sickness-like reactions (e.g., chills, fever, edema, arthralgia, prostration), and anaphylaxis (including shock and death) have been reported with penicillin G. Fever and eosinophilia may frequently be the only reaction observed.

Inadvertent IV administration of penicillin G benzathine has been associated with cardiorespiratory arrest and death.

Inadvertent intravascular administration (including inadvertent direct intra-arterial injection or injection immediately adjacent to arteries) of penicillin G benzathine or fixed combinations containing penicillin G benzathine and penicillin G procaine has resulted in severe neurovascular damage (e.g., transverse myelitis with permanent paralysis, gangrene requiring amputation of digits and more proximal portions of extremities, necrosis and sloughing at and surrounding the injection site). These severe effects have been reported following injections into the buttock, thigh, and deltoid areas. Other serious complications of suspected intravascular administration include immediate pallor, mottling, or cyanosis of the extremity (both distal and proximal to the injection site), followed by bleb formation or severe edema requiring anterior and/or posterior compartment fasciotomy in the lower extremity. These severe effects and complications have occurred most often in infants and small children.

For additional information on adverse effects reported with natural penicillins, see Cautions in the Natural Penicillins General Statement 8:12.16.04.

■ **Precautions and Contraindications** Penicillin G benzathine and fixed combinations of penicillin G benzathine and penicillin G procaine are contraindicated in patients hypersensitive to any penicillin. The fixed combinations also are contraindicated in patients hypersensitive to procaine.

Penicillin G benzathine shares the toxic potentials of the penicillins, including the risk of hypersensitivity reactions, and the usual precautions of penicillin therapy should be observed.

Prior to administration of penicillin G benzathine or a fixed combination of penicillin G benzathine and penicillin G procaine, careful inquiry should be made concerning previous hypersensitivity reactions to penicillins, cephalosporins, or other allergens. There is clinical and laboratory evidence of partial cross-allergenicity among penicillins and other β-lactam antibiotics, including cephalosporins and cephamycins.

Hypersensitivity reactions to penicillins are more likely to occur in individuals with a history of penicillin hypersensitivity and/or a history of sensitivity to multiple allergens. Penicillin G benzathine and fixed combinations of penicillin G benzathine and penicillin G procaine should be used with caution in individuals with a history of clinically important allergies and/or asthma.

If a hypersensitivity reaction occurs, the drug should be discontinued immediately and appropriate therapy instituted as indicated (e.g., epinephrine, corticosteroids, maintenance of an adequate airway and oxygen).

If use of a fixed combination containing penicillin G benzathine and penicillin G procaine is being considered in a patient with a history of procaine sensitivity, a test dose of procaine (0.1 mL of a 1–2% solution of procaine) should be administered intradermally prior to IM administration of full doses of the fixed combination. Development of erythema or a wheal, flare, or eruption at the intradermal test site indicates procaine sensitivity and the patient should *not* receive a preparation containing penicillin G procaine. If a hypersensitivity reaction to procaine occurs, it should be treated by usual methods; antihistamines may be beneficial and barbiturates may be indicated if seizures occur.

Special precaution should be taken to avoid IV, intravascular, or intra-arterial administration or injection of penicillin G benzathine or fixed combinations containing the drug into or near major peripheral nerves or blood vessels since inadvertent intravascular or intra-arterial injection may produce severe and/or permanent neurovascular damage and inadvertent IV administration has been associated with cardiorespiratory arrest and death. If evidence of compromise of the blood supply occurs at or proximal or distal to the site of injection, an appropriate specialist should be consulted immediately.

Renal and hematologic systems should be evaluated periodically during prolonged therapy with a fixed combination containing penicillin G benzathine and penicillin G procaine, particularly if high dosage is used.

For additional information on precautions associated with the use of penicillin G benzathine, see Cautions: Precautions and Contraindications, in the Natural Penicillins General Statement 8:12.16.04.

■ **Pediatric Precautions** Penicillin G benzathine should be used with caution in neonates and organ system function should be evaluated frequently in such patients.

Renal clearance of penicillin G may be delayed in neonates and young infants because of incompletely developed renal function.

■ **Geriatric Precautions** Clinical studies of penicillin G benzathine or penicillin G procaine did not include sufficient numbers of patients 65 years of age or older to determine whether geriatric patients respond differently than younger patients. Other clinical experience has not identified differences in responses between geriatric and younger patients.

Penicillin G is substantially eliminated by the kidneys and the risk of adverse effects may be greater in those with impaired renal function. Because geriatric patients are more likely to have reduced renal function, dosage should be selected with caution, usually starting at the low end of the dosage range, and renal function monitoring may be useful.

■ **Pregnancy and Lactation** ***Pregnancy*** Reproduction studies evaluating penicillin G in mice, rats, and rabbits have not revealed evidence of impaired fertility or harm to the fetus. Although experience with use of penicillins during pregnancy has not shown any evidence of adverse effects on the fetus, there are no adequate or controlled studies using penicillin G benzathine in pregnant women.

Some clinicians state that IM penicillin G benzathine is considered low risk and safe for use during pregnancy. The drug is included in the US Centers for Disease Control and Prevention (CDC) recommendations for the treatment of syphilis during pregnancy.

The manufacturers state that penicillin G benzathine and fixed combinations containing penicillin G benzathine and penicillin G procaine should be used during pregnancy only when clearly needed.

Lactation Penicillin G is distributed into milk. Some clinicians state that IM penicillin G benzathine usually is considered compatible with breastfeeding. The manufacturers and others state that penicillin G benzathine and fixed combinations of penicillin G benzathine and penicillin G procaine should be used with caution in nursing women.

Spectrum

Based on its spectrum of activity, penicillin G benzathine is classified as a natural penicillin. For information on the classification of penicillins based on spectra of activity, see the Preface to the General Statements on Penicillins 8:12.16.

For specific information on the spectrum of activity of penicillin G and resistance to the drug, see the sections on Spectrum and on Resistance in the Natural Penicillins General Statement 8:12.16.04.

Pharmacokinetics

For additional information on the absorption, distribution, and elimination of penicillin G, see Pharmacokinetics in the Natural Penicillins General Statement 8:12.16.04.

■ **Absorption** Because penicillin G benzathine is relatively insoluble, IM administration of the drug provides a tissue depot from which the drug is slowly absorbed and hydrolyzed to penicillin G. IM administration of penicillin G benzathine results in serum concentrations of penicillin G that are more prolonged, but lower, than those attained with an equivalent IM dose of penicillin G procaine or penicillin G potassium or sodium.

Following IM administration of a single dose of penicillin G benzathine in adults, children, or neonates, peak serum concentrations of penicillin G are attained in 13–24 hours and usually are detectable for 1–4 weeks (depending on the dose).

In adults, a single IM penicillin G benzathine dose of 1.2 million units results in serum penicillin G concentrations of 0.15, 0.03, and 0.003 units/mL at 1, 14, and 32 days, respectively, after the dose. In one study in adults who received IM penicillin G benzathine in a dosage of 2.4 million units administered once weekly for 3 successive weeks, serum penicillin G concentrations ranged from 0.04–0.48 units/mL at 7 days after the first dose, 0.06–0.48 units/mL at 7 days after the second dose, and 0.17–0.52 units/mL at 7 days after the third dose. In adults receiving IM penicillin G benzathine in a dosage of 1.2 million units once every 4 weeks, mean serum penicillin G concentrations were at least 0.02 mcg/mL for 21 days after a dose; however, at 28 days after a dose, the drug was detectable in serum in only 44% of samples and was at least 0.02 mcg/mL in only 36% of samples.

Following a single IM dose of a fixed combination containing 1.2 million penicillin G units (i.e., 600,000 units as penicillin G benzathine and 600,000 units as penicillin G procaine; Bicillin® C-R) in adults, peak blood penicillin G concentrations were 2.1–2.6 units/mL within 3 hours and blood concentrations averaged 0.75 units/mL at 12 hours, 0.28 units/mL at 24 hours, and 0.04 units/mL at 7 days.

Following a single IM dose of a fixed combination containing 1.2 million penicillin G units (i.e., 900,000 units as penicillin G benzathine and 300,000 units as penicillin G procaine; Bicillin® C-R 900/300) in patients weighing 45–64 kg, average blood penicillin G concentrations were 0.24 units/mL at 24 hours, 0.039 units/mL at 7 days, and 0.024 units/mL at 10 days after the dose.

In a study in children 1.8–10.7 years of age who received a single IM penicillin G benzathine dose of 600,000 units if they weighed less than 27 kg or 1.2 million units if they weighed more than 27 kg, peak serum penicillin G concentrations occurred 24 hours after the dose and ranged from 0.11–0.2 mcg/mL. In these children, serum penicillin G concentrations ranged from 0.04–0.19 mcg/mL at 1, 2, and 4 hours after the dose and from 0.03–0.13, 0.02–0.09, and 0–0.02 mcg/mL at 5, 10, and 18 days, respectively, after the dose. In children weighing 11.9–22.6 kg, IM administration of a single dose of a fixed combination containing 1.2 million penicillin G units (900,000 units as penicillin G benzathine and 300,000 units as penicillin G procaine) resulted in peak serum penicillin G concentrations that occurred 1 hour after the dose and averaged 3.9 mcg/mL. Serum penicillin G concentrations in these children ranged from 2.5–5.5, 2.5–5.5, 0.7–3.7, and 0.17–0.48 mcg/mL at 1, 2, 4, and 24 hours, respectively, after the dose and from 0.08–0.12, 0.01–0.09, and 0–0.1 mcg/mL at 5, 10, and 18 days, respectively, after the dose.

In one study in neonates who received a single IM penicillin G benzathine dose of 50,000 units/kg, peak serum penicillin G concentrations occurred 24 hours after the dose and ranged from 0.38–2.1 mg/mL; serum penicillin G concentrations ranged from 0.07–0.09 mcg/mL 12 days after the dose. In another study in neonates, IM administration of a single penicillin G benzathine dose of 100,000 units resulted in serum penicillin G concentrations that ranged from 1.18–3.9 mcg/mL at 24 hours after the dose and were still detectable 5 days after the dose.

■ **Distribution** Following IM administration of penicillin G benzathine, penicillin G is widely distributed throughout the body in varying amounts. Highest concentrations generally are attained in the kidneys, with lower amounts in the liver, skin, and intestines.

Minimal concentrations of penicillin G generally are attained in CSF following IM administration of penicillin G benzathine in patients with inflamed or uninflamed meninges. The minimum treponemicidal concentration of penicillin G is generally defined as 0.03 units/mL or 0.02 mcg/mL. In one study in adults who received IM penicillin G benzathine given in a dosage of 3.6 million units once weekly for up to 4 weeks, penicillin G was undetectable in the CSF of 12/13 patients in specimens obtained following administration of the last dose. In another study in adults who received IM penicillin G benzathine in a dosage of 2.4 or 4.8 million units administered once weekly for 3 successive weeks, CSF penicillin G concentrations were less than 0.03 units/mL in specimens obtained 7 days after the last dose of the drug. In a study in neonates who received a single IM dose of penicillin G benzathine of 100,000 units/kg, peak CSF penicillin G concentrations occurred 12–24 hours after the dose and ranged from 0.012–0.2 mcg/mL; however, CSF penicillin G concentrations were less than 0.01 mcg/mL 48 hours after the dose.

In a study in children who received a single IM dose of penicillin G benzathine of 600,000 units to 1.2 million units, penicillin G concentrations in tonsils were 0.042 mcg/mL or less in specimens obtained 24 hours after the dose; concurrent serum concentrations ranged from 0.03–0.17 mcg/mL.

Penicillin G is about 60% bound to serum proteins.

Penicillin G crosses the placenta and is distributed into milk.

■ **Elimination** Following IM administration of penicillin G benzathine, the drug is slowly absorbed and hydrolyzed to penicillin G and elimination of penicillin G in urine continues over a prolonged period of time. Penicillin G and its metabolites are excreted in urine mainly by tubular secretion.

Penicillin G has been detected in urine for up to 12 weeks after a single IM penicillin G benzathine dose of 1.2 million units. In a study in children 1.8–10.7 years of age who received a single IM dose of penicillin G benzathine of 600,000 units or 1.2 million units, urinary penicillin G concentrations 30 days after the dose ranged from 0.6–12.5 mcg/mL. Following IM administration of a single penicillin G benzathine dose of 50,000 units/kg in neonates, urinary penicillin G concentrations ranged from 4.3–17.2 mcg/mL during the first 4 days after the dose and were 1.4–6 mcg/mL at 12 days after the dose.

The serum half-life of penicillin G may be prolonged in patients with impaired renal function.

Renal clearance of penicillin G is delayed in neonates and young infants.

Renal clearance of penicillin G may be increased in pregnant women during the second and third trimesters.

Chemistry and Stability

■ **Chemistry** Penicillin G benzathine is a natural penicillin. The drug is the benzathine tetrahydrate salt of penicillin G. Penicillin G benzathine is hydrolyzed in vivo to penicillin G and is frequently referred to as a long-acting, depot, or repository form of penicillin G.

Penicillin G benzathine occurs as a white, crystalline powder. The drug is very slightly soluble in water and sparingly soluble in alcohol. Potency of penicillin G benzathine generally is expressed in terms of penicillin G units, but also has been expressed as mg of penicillin G.

Commercially available penicillin G benzathine suspension for IM injection is a viscous, opaque suspension of the drug in sterile water for injection. The IM suspension has a pH of 5–7.5 and is buffered with sodium citrate. The suspension contains methylparaben and propylparaben as preservatives and also contains povidone, lecithin, and carboxymethylcellulose.

Penicillin G benzathine also is commercially available in fixed combination with penicillin G procaine as a viscous, opaque, aqueous suspension for IM injection. Each 2 mL of fixed-combination suspension contains the equivalent of 1.2 million units of penicillin G in a formulation containing the equivalent of 600,000 units of penicillin G as the benzathine salt and 600,000 units of penicillin G as the procaine salt (Bicillin® C-R) *or* a formulation containing the equivalent of 900,000 units of penicillin G as the benzathine salt and 300,000 units of penicillin G as the procaine salt (Bicillin® C-R 900/300).

■ **Stability** Commercially available penicillin G benzathine suspension for IM injection should be stored at 2–8°C; freezing should be avoided.

The fixed combinations of penicillin G benzathine and penicillin G procaine for IM injection should be stored at 2–8°C; freezing should be avoided.

For further information on chemistry and stability, mechanism of action, spectrum, resistance, pharmacokinetics, uses, cautions, drug interactions, laboratory test interferences, and dosage and administration of penicillin G benzathine, see the Natural Penicillins General Statement 8:12.16.04.

Preparations

Excipients in commercially available drug preparations may have clinically important effects in some individuals; consult specific product labeling for details.

Penicillin G Benzathine

Parenteral		
Suspension, for IM Injection	600,000 units (of penicillin G) per mL	**Bicillin® L-A**, Pfizer **Permapen®**, Casper

Penicillin G Benzathine and Penicillin G Procaine

Parenteral		
Suspension, for IM Injection	1.2 million units of penicillin G per 2 mL (600,000 units as penicillin G benzathine and 600,000 units as penicillin G procaine)	**Bicillin® C-R**, Pfizer
	1.2 million units of penicillin G per 2 mL (900,000 units as penicillin G benzathine and 300,000 units as penicillin G procaine)	**Bicillin® C-R 900/300**, Pfizer

†Use is not currently included in the labeling approved by the US Food and Drug Administration

Penicillin G Potassium — Benzylpenicillin Potassium
Penicillin G Sodium — Benzylpenicillin Sodium, Crystalline Penicillin

■ Penicillin G, a natural penicillin, is a *β*-lactam antibiotic.

Uses

Penicillin G potassium and penicillin G sodium are used parenterally when rapid and high concentrations of penicillin G are required, as in the treatment of endocarditis, meningitis, pericarditis, septicemia, severe pneumonia, or other serious infections caused by organisms susceptible to penicillin G.

For additional information on the uses of penicillin G potassium and penicillin G sodium, see Uses in the Natural Penicillins General Statement 8:12.16.04.

■ **Endocarditis** IV penicillin G potassium or sodium is used for the treatment of endocarditis caused by susceptible *Streptococcus pyogenes* (group A *β*-hemolytic streptococci; GAS), other *β*-hemolytic streptococci (including groups C, H, G, L, and M), or *S. pneumoniae*. The American Heart Association (AHA) states that IV penicillin G is a reasonable regimen for the treatment of endocarditis caused by susceptible *S. pyogenes*, *S. agalactiae*† (group B streptococci; GBS), groups C and G streptococci, and highly penicillin-susceptible *S. pneumoniae* (penicillin MIC 0.1 mcg/mL or less), but concomitant use of gentamicin during the initial weeks of penicillin G treatment should be considered if endocarditis is caused by streptococci groups B, C, or G.

For the treatment of endocarditis caused by viridans group streptococci† or nonenterococcal group D streptococci† (including *S. gallolyticus*† [formerly *S. bovis*]) that are highly susceptible to penicillin (penicillin MIC 0.12 mcg/mL or less), AHA states that IV penicillin G (with or without gentamicin) is a regimen of choice. If endocarditis is caused by viridans group streptococci† or *S. gallolyticus*† relatively resistant to penicillin (penicillin MIC greater than 0.12 mcg/mL but less than 0.5 mcg/mL), AHA states that IV penicillin G should be used in conjunction with gentamicin. These recommendations include endocarditis involving native valves or prosthetic valves or other prosthetic material caused by these gram-positive bacteria.

AHA states that IV penicillin G in conjunction with gentamicin is a reasonable regimen for the treatment of native valve endocarditis caused by viridans group streptococci†, *Abiotrophia defectiva*†, or *Granulicatella*† with penicillin MIC 0.5 mcg/mL or greater.

For the treatment of endocarditis involving native valves or prosthetic valves or other prosthetic material caused by *Enterococcus faecalis*†, *E. faecium*†, or other enterococcal species susceptible to both penicillin G *and* gentamicin, AHA states that IV penicillin G in conjunction with gentamicin is a regimen of choice. AHA states that it is reasonable to substitute streptomycin for gentamicin in this regimen if enterococci are susceptible to penicillin *and* streptomycin, but resistant to gentamicin.

IV penicillin G has been used for the treatment of endocarditis caused by nonpenicillinase-producing staphylococci. AHA states that IV penicillin G may be considered for the treatment of native valve endocarditis caused by penicillin-susceptible *S. aureus* or coagulase-negative staphylococci in pediatric patients; however, penicillin G is not included in current AHA recommendations for the treatment of staphylococcal endocarditis in adults.

AHA recommends that treatment of endocarditis should be managed in consultation with an infectious disease expert, especially when endocarditis is caused by *S. pneumoniae*, β-hemolytic streptococci, staphylococci, or enterococci.

For additional information on management of endocarditis, current guidelines from AHA should be consulted.

■ Syphilis IV penicillin G potassium or sodium is used for the treatment of syphilis caused by *Treponema pallidum*.

For the treatment of neurosyphilis and otic or ocular syphilis, the US Centers for Disease Control and Prevention (CDC) and other clinicians state that IV penicillin G potassium or sodium is the drug of choice and IM penicillin G procaine (with oral probenecid) is an alternative if compliance can be ensured.

For the treatment of congenital syphilis, CDC recommends IV penicillin G potassium or sodium or IM penicillin G procaine in neonates with proven or highly probable congenital syphilis (i.e., abnormal physical examination consistent with congenital syphilis, serum quantitative nontreponemal serologic titer fourfold higher than the mother's titer, or positive darkfield test or polymerase chain reaction [PCR] of lesions or body fluids). CDC recommends IV penicillin G potassium or sodium, IM penicillin G procaine, or IM penicillin G benzathine in neonates with possible congenital syphilis (i.e., normal physical examination and serum quantitative nontreponemal serologic titer no more than fourfold higher than the mother's titer and the mother received a recommended treatment regimen less than 4 weeks before delivery; the mother was not treated or was inadequately treated, including treatment with erythromycin or any regimen not included in CDC recommendations; or there is no documentation that the mother received treatment).

CDC and other clinicians state that IM penicillin G benzathine is the drug of choice for the treatment of primary syphilis (i.e., ulcer or chancre at infection site), secondary syphilis (i.e., manifestations that include, but are not limited to, rash, mucocutaneous lesions, and lymphadenopathy), and tertiary syphilis (i.e., cardiac syphilis, gummatous lesions, tabes dorsalis, and general paresis) in adults, adolescents, and children.

IM penicillin G benzathine also is the drug of choice for the treatment of latent syphilis (i.e., detected by serologic testing but lacking clinical manifestations), including both early latent syphilis (latent syphilis acquired within the preceding year) and late latent syphilis (i.e., all other cases of latent syphilis or syphilis of unknown duration) in all age groups.

Neonates with human immunodeficiency virus (HIV) infection who have congenital syphilis and HIV-infected children, adolescents, or adults who have neurosyphilis or primary, secondary, early latent, late latent, or tertiary syphilis should receive the same treatment regimens as those without HIV infection. Because serologic nonresponse and neurologic complications may be more frequent in HIV-infected individuals, close follow-up is essential in those coinfected with syphilis and HIV. In addition, careful neurologic examinations are indicated in all HIV-infected patients coinfected with syphilis.

There are no proven alternatives to penicillin G for the treatment of congenital syphilis in infants and children with known or suspected penicillin hypersensitivity and no proven alternatives to penicillin G for the treatment of any stage of syphilis in pregnant women with penicillin hypersensitivity; therefore, CDC recommends that such patients be desensitized and treated with the appropriate penicillin G preparation.

For additional information on management of syphilis, current CDC sexually transmitted diseases treatment guidelines available at https://www.cdc.gov/std/syphilis/treatment.htm should be consulted.

■ Prevention of Perinatal Group B Streptococcal Disease IV penicillin G potassium or sodium is used in pregnant women during labor (intrapartum) for prevention of early-onset neonatal group B streptococcal (GBS) disease†.

GBS infection is a leading cause of neonatal morbidity and mortality in the US. Pregnant women who are colonized with GBS in the genital or rectal areas can transmit GBS infection to their infants during labor and delivery, resulting in invasive neonatal infection that can be associated with substantial morbidity and mortality.

CDC, AAP, and other experts recommend *routine* universal prenatal screening for GBS colonization (e.g., vaginal and rectal cultures) in *all* pregnant women at 35–37 weeks of gestation, unless GBS bacteriuria is known to be present during the current pregnancy or the woman had a previous infant with invasive GBS disease. These experts state that intrapartum anti-infective prophylaxis for prevention of perinatal GBS is indicated in pregnant women identified as GBS carriers during the routine prenatal GBS screening performed at 35–37 weeks during the current pregnancy, in women with GBS bacteriuria identified at any time during the current pregnancy, and in women who had a previous infant diagnosed with invasive GBS disease. Intrapartum anti-infective prophylaxis also is indicated in women with unknown GBS status at the time of onset of labor (i.e., culture not done, incomplete, or results unknown) if delivery is at less than 37 weeks of gestation, the duration of amniotic membrane rupture is 18 hours or longer, or intrapartum temperature is 38°C or higher. If an intrapartum nucleic acid amplification test (NAAT) is performed in a woman with unknown GBS status at the time of onset of labor (may not be available in all settings) and results are positive for GBS, intrapartum anti-infective prophylaxis is indicated; if an intrapartum NAAT is negative for GBS, anti-infective prophylaxis is indicated if any of the above risk factors for perinatal GBS infection are present.

When intrapartum anti-infective prophylaxis is indicated in the mother for prevention of GBS in the neonate, it should be initiated at the onset of labor or rupture of membranes. If cesarean delivery is performed *before* onset of labor in a woman with intact amniotic membranes, anti-infective prophylaxis is not usually indicated, regardless of the GBS colonization status of the woman or gestational age.

CDC, AAP, and other experts recommend IV penicillin G as the drug of choice and state that IV ampicillin is the preferred alternative for such prophylaxis. Penicillin G is considered the drug of choice because it has a narrower spectrum of activity than ampicillin and is less likely to select for antibiotic-resistant organisms.

Regardless of whether the mother received intrapartum anti-infective prophylaxis, appropriate diagnostic evaluations and anti-infective therapy should be initiated in the neonate if signs or symptoms of active infection develop.

For additional information regarding prevention of perinatal group B streptococcal disease, current guidelines from CDC and AAP should be consulted.

Dosage and Administration

■ Reconstitution and Administration Penicillin G potassium and penicillin G sodium are administered by IM injection or by intermittent IV injection or infusion or continuous IV infusion. Penicillin G has been administered by intrapleural, intraperitoneal, intra-articular, or other local instillations. Although the drug has been administered intrathecally, this route is *not* recommended because of possible neurotoxicity (e.g., seizures).

Vials containing penicillin G potassium or penicillin G sodium powder for injection should be reconstituted to the desired concentration using the amount of diluent specified by the manufacturer. Depending on the specific product and route of administration, the powders generally are reconstituted with sterile water for injection, 0.9% sodium chloride injection, or dextrose injection. The powder should be loosened in the vial and the vial held horizontally and rotated while slowly directing the stream of diluent against the wall of the vial. After the diluent has been added, the vial should be shaken vigorously. Because penicillin G is unstable in solutions at room temperature, reconstituted penicillin G potassium and penicillin G sodium solutions should be used immediately or refrigerated. (See Chemistry and Stability: Stability.)

IM Injection To prepare solutions for IM administration, vials labeled as containing 1 or 5 million units of penicillin G (as penicillin G potassium) or vials labeled as containing 5 million units of penicillin G (as penicillin G sodium) should be reconstituted to the desired concentration using the amount of diluent specified by the manufacturer. If not used immediately, vials reconstituted for IM use should be refrigerated (see Chemistry and Stability: Stability).

Vials labeled as containing 20 million units of penicillin G (as penicillin G potassium) are intended *only* for IV infusion and should *not* be used to prepare solutions for IM injection.

For IM administration, penicillin G potassium solutions containing up to 100,000 penicillin G units/mL may be used with a minimum of discomfort; higher concentrations are physically possible and may be used when needed.

If large doses of penicillin G are required, the drug should be administered IV (not IM).

IV Administration To prepare solutions for IV administration, vials labeled as containing 1, 5, or 20 million units of penicillin G (as penicillin G potassium) or 5 million units of penicillin G (as penicillin G sodium) should be reconstituted according to the manufacturer's directions. If not used immediately, vials reconstituted for IV use should be refrigerated (see Chemistry and Stability: Stability).

For intermittent IV administration, the daily dosage usually is given in equally divided doses every 4–6 hours; however, daily dosage may be given in equally divided doses every 2–3 hours for the treatment of severe infections (e.g., meningitis).

For continuous IV infusion, the volume of IV fluid and rate of administration required by the patient in a 24-hour period should be determined and the appropriate daily dosage of penicillin G should be added to the fluid. For example, if an adult patient requires 2 L of fluid in 24 hours and a dosage of 10 million penicillin G units daily, 5 million units can be added to 1 L of IV solution and the rate of administration adjusted so that the liter of fluid will be infused over 12 hours.

Thawed solutions of the commercially available frozen premixed penicillin G potassium injection in dextrose should be administered *only* by IV infusion. The commercially available frozen injection should be thawed at room temperature (25°C) or under refrigeration (5°C); the injection should not be thawed by warming in a water bath or by exposure to microwave radiation. Precipitates that may have formed in the frozen injection usually will dissolve with little or no agitation when the injection reaches room temperature; potency is not affected. After thawing at room temperature, the injections should be agitated and the container checked for minute leaks by firmly squeezing the bag. The injection should be discarded if the container seals or outlet ports are not intact or leaks are found or if the solution is cloudy or contains a precipitate. Additives should not be introduced into the injection container. The premixed injection should not be used in series connections with other plastic containers since such use could result in air embolism from residual air being drawn from the primary container before administration of fluid from the secondary container is complete.

Rate of Administration. Large IV doses of penicillin G potassium or sodium (greater than 10 million penicillin G units) should be administered slowly because of the potential for serious electrolyte disturbances from the potassium and/or sodium content of these preparations. (See Cautions: Adverse Effects.)

For intermittent IV administration, penicillin G potassium or sodium has been given by IV infusion over 1–2 hours or by IV infusion over 10–30 minutes. Although doses of the drug also have been injected IV over 3–5 minutes, large doses should be administered slowly.

■ Dosage

Dosage of penicillin G potassium and penicillin G sodium usually is expressed in terms of penicillin G units, but also has been expressed as mg of penicillin G.

Pediatric Dosage

General Pediatric Dosage. Dosage of IM or IV penicillin G potassium or sodium for pediatric patients should be individualized and generally is based on weight and the severity of the infection.

The manufacturers state that penicillin G potassium or sodium should *not* be used in pediatric patients requiring less than 1 million penicillin G units per dose.

The American Academy of Pediatrics (AAP) states that the usual dosage of IV or IM penicillin G potassium or sodium in neonates 7 days of age or younger is 25,000–50,000 units/kg every 12 hours. In neonates 8–28 days of age, AAP recommends a dosage of 25,000–50,000 units/kg every 8 hours. Higher dosages may be necessary for the treatment of meningitis in neonates.

In pediatric patients beyond the neonatal period, AAP states that the usual dosage of IV or IM penicillin G potassium or sodium is 100,000–150,000 units/kg daily given in 4 equally divided doses for the treatment of mild to moderate infections or 200,000–300,000 units/kg daily given in 4–6 equally divided doses for the treatment of severe infections. AAP states that the highest dosage recommended for pediatric patients beyond the neonatal period should be used for the treatment of meningitis.

Endocarditis. For the treatment of native valve endocarditis caused by highly penicillin-susceptible streptococci (penicillin MIC 0.1 mcg/mL or less), including *Streptococcus pyogenes* (group A β-hemolytic streptococci; GAS), other β-hemolytic streptococci (e.g., groups C, G), *S. agalactiae*† (group B streptococci; GBS), viridans group streptococci†, or nonenterococcal group D streptococci† (e.g., *S. gallolyticus*† [formerly *S. bovis*], *S. equinus*†), the American Heart Association (AHA) states that pediatric patients may receive IV penicillin G in a dosage of 200,000–300,000 units/kg daily (up to 12–24 million units daily) given in divided doses every 4 hours for 4 weeks.

For the treatment of native valve endocarditis caused by streptococci that are relatively resistant to penicillin† (penicillin MIC greater than 0.1 but less than 0.5 mcg/mL), AHA states that pediatric patients may receive IV penicillin G in a dosage of 200,000–300,000 units/kg daily (up to 12–24 million units daily) given in divided doses every 4 hours for 4 weeks in conjunction with gentamicin (3–6 mg/kg daily IV in divided doses every 8 hours given concomitantly during the first 2 weeks of penicillin G treatment).

For the treatment of native valve endocarditis caused by viridans group streptococci†, *Abiotrophia*†, or *Granulicatella*† with penicillin MIC 0.5 mcg/mL or greater, AHA states that pediatric patients may receive IV penicillin G in a dosage of 200,000–300,000 units/kg daily (up to 12–24 million units daily) given in divided doses every 4 hours for 4–6 weeks in conjunction with gentamicin (3–6 mg/kg IV daily in divided doses every 8 hours given concomitantly during the first 2 weeks of penicillin G treatment).

For the treatment of endocarditis involving prosthetic valves or other prosthetic material caused by penicillin-susceptible viridans group streptococci†, other streptococci, *Abiotrophia*†, or *Granulicatella*† with penicillin MIC 0.1 mcg/mL or greater, AHA states that pediatric patients may receive IV penicillin G in a dosage of 200,000–300,000 units/kg daily (up to 12–24 million units daily) given in divided doses every 4 hours for 6 weeks in conjunction with gentamicin (3–6 mg/kg IV daily in divided doses every 8 hours given concomitantly for the entire 6 weeks of penicillin G treatment).

For the treatment of enterococcal endocarditis† (native valve or prosthetic valve or other prosthetic material), AHA states that pediatric patients may receive IV penicillin G in a dosage of 200,000–300,000 units/kg daily (up to 12–24 million units daily) given in divided doses every 4 hours in conjunction with gentamicin (3–6 mg/kg IV daily in divided doses every 8 hours). The recommended duration of treatment with the 2-drug regimen is 4–6 weeks for native valve enterococcal endocarditis; a longer duration of treatment with both drugs is recommended if prosthetic valves or other prosthetic material is involved.

If IV penicillin G is used for the treatment of endocarditis caused by susceptible *S. aureus* or coagulase-negative staphylococci (penicillin MIC 0.1 mcg/mL or less) in pediatric patients, AHA recommends a dosage of 200,000–300,000 units/kg daily (up to 12–24 million units daily) given in divided doses every 4 hours.

The manufacturers recommend that pediatric patients with endocarditis caused by susceptible streptococci (including *S. pyogenes*, streptococci groups C, H, G, L, and M, or *S. pneumoniae*) receive penicillin G potassium or sodium in a dosage of 150,000–300,000 units/kg daily given in divided doses every 4–6 hours.

Meningitis and Other CNS Infections. For the treatment of meningitis caused by susceptible *Listeria monocytogenes*, the Infectious Diseases Society of America (IDSA) recommends that neonates 7 days of age or younger receive IV penicillin G in a dosage of 150,000 units/kg daily given in divided doses every 8–12 hours and that those 8–28 days of age receive a dosage of 200,000 units/kg daily given in divided doses every 6–8 hours; these experts recommend that treatment in neonates be continued for 2 weeks beyond the first sterile CSF culture or for at least 3 weeks, whichever is longer. In infants and children with *L. monocytogenes* meningitis, IDSA recommends a dosage of 300,000 units/kg daily given in divided doses every 4–6 hours for a duration of at least 21 days. Concomitant use of an aminoglycoside should be considered.

For the treatment of meningitis caused by susceptible *Neisseria meningitidis* (penicillin MIC less than 0.1 mcg/mL), IDSA recommends that neonates 7 days of age or younger receive IV penicillin G in a dosage of 150,000 units/kg daily given in divided doses every 8–12 hours and that those 8–28 days of age receive a dosage of 200,000 units/kg daily given in divided doses every 6–8 hours; these experts recommend that treatment in neonates be continued for 2 weeks beyond the first sterile CSF culture or for at least 3 weeks, whichever is longer. In infants and children with *N. meningitidis* meningitis, a dosage of 300,000 units/kg daily (up to 12 million units daily) given in divided doses every 4–6 hours for a duration of 7 days has been recommended.

For the treatment of meningitis caused by susceptible *S. agalactiae*† (group B streptococci; GBS), AAP recommends that neonates 7 days of age or younger receive IV penicillin G in a dosage of 250,000–450,000 units/kg daily given in 3 divided doses and that those older than 7 days of age receive a dosage of 450,000–500,000 units/kg daily given in 4 divided doses and states that treatment should be continued for at least 14 days. IDSA recommends that neonates 7 days of age or younger receive IV penicillin G in a dosage of 150,000 units/kg daily given in divided doses every 8–12 hours and that those 8–28 days of age receive a dosage of 200,000 units/kg daily given in divided doses every 6–8 hours; these experts recommend that treatment in neonates be continued for 2 weeks beyond the first sterile CSF culture or for at least 3 weeks, whichever is longer. In infants and children with *S. agalactiae* meningitis, IDSA recommends a dosage of 300,000 units/kg daily given in divided doses every 4–6 hours for a duration of 14–21 days. Concomitant use of an aminoglycoside should be considered.

For the treatment of meningitis caused by susceptible *S. pneumoniae*, IDSA recommends that neonates 7 days of age or younger receive IV penicillin G in a dosage of 150,000 units/kg daily given in divided doses every 8–12 hours and that those 8–28 days of age receive a dosage of 200,000 units/kg daily given in divided doses every 6–8 hours; these experts recommend that treatment in neonates be continued for 2 weeks beyond the first sterile CSF culture or for at least 3 weeks, whichever is longer. AAP recommends that infants and children 1 month of age or older with *S. pneumoniae* meningitis receive IV penicillin G in a dosage of 250,000–400,000 units/kg daily given in divided doses every 4–6 hours. IDSA recommends that infants and children receive a dosage of 300,000 units/kg daily given in divided doses every 4–6 hours for a duration of 10–14 days.

For the treatment of healthcare-associated ventriculitis and meningitis caused by susceptible *Cutibacterium acnes*† (formerly *Propionibacterium acnes*), IDSA recommends that pediatric patients receive IV penicillin G in a dosage of 300,000 units/kg daily given in divided doses every 4–6 hours. The recommended treatment duration is 10 days in those with no or minimal CSF pleocytosis, normal CSF glucose, and few clinical symptoms or systemic features or 10–14 days in those with significant CSF pleocytosis, CSF hypoglycorrhachia, or clinical symptoms or systemic features.

The manufacturers recommend that pediatric patients with meningitis caused by susceptible *N. meningitidis* or *S. pneumoniae* receive penicillin G potassium or sodium in a dosage of 250,000 units/kg daily (up to 12–20 million units daily) given in divided doses every 4 hours for 7–14 days.

Respiratory Tract Infections. For the treatment of community-acquired pneumonia (CAP) caused by susceptible *S. pyogenes* (group A β-hemolytic streptococci; GAS) in pediatric patients 3 months of age or older, IDSA recommends that IV penicillin G be given in a dosage of 100,000–200,000 units daily in divided doses every 4–6 hours. For severe infections, 200,000–250,000 units/kg daily may be used.

For the treatment of CAP caused by susceptible *S. pneumoniae* (penicillin MIC 2 mcg/mL or lower) in pediatric patients 3 months of age or older, IDSA recommends that IV penicillin G be given in a dosage of 200,000–250,000 units/kg daily in divided doses every 4–6 hours. AAP recommends that infants and children 1 month of age or older with nonmeningeal infections caused by *S. pneumoniae* receive penicillin G in a dosage of 250,000–400,000 units/kg daily given in divided doses every 4–6 hours. Penicillin G should not be used for empiric treatment of CAP if local epidemiologic data indicate that invasive *S. pneumoniae* have high-level penicillin resistance.

If penicillin G potassium or sodium is used for the treatment of serious respiratory tract infections (e.g., pneumonia) caused by susceptible *S. pyogenes*, streptococci groups C, H, G, L, and M, or *S. pneumoniae*, in pediatric patients, the manufacturers recommend a dosage of 150,000–300,000 units/kg daily in divided doses every 4–6 hours.

Skin and Skin Structure Infections. For the treatment of necrotizing infections of the skin, fascia, and muscle caused by susceptible *S. pyogenes*, IDSA recommends that pediatric patients receive a regimen of IV penicillin G given in a dosage of 60,000–100,000 units/kg every 6 hours in conjunction with clindamycin (10–13 mg/kg IV every 8 hours).

Anthrax. For the treatment of anthrax (inhalational, GI, meningitis) caused by penicillin-susceptible *Bacillus anthracis* that occurs as the result of natural or endemic exposures to anthrax, some clinicians recommend that children receive IV penicillin G in a dosage of 100,000–150,000 units/kg daily given in divided doses every 4–6 hours. For the treatment of severe or life-threatening systemic anthrax (inhalational, GI, meningoencephalitis, sepsis) or the treatment of cutaneous anthrax with signs of systemic involvement, lesions on the head or neck, or extensive edema caused by penicillin-susceptible *B. anthracis* that occurs as the result of natural or endemic anthrax exposure, some experts recommend that children receive IV penicillin G in a dosage of 300,000–400,000 units/kg daily given in divided doses every 4–6 hours. Concomitant use of other anti-infectives (e.g., streptomycin or other aminoglycoside, clindamycin, clarithromycin, rifampin, vancomycin) may also be indicated. Treatment of naturally occurring or endemic anthrax generally should be continued for at least 14 days after symptoms abate.

If IV penicillin G is used in a multiple-drug parenteral regimen for initial treatment of systemic anthrax (inhalational, GI, meningitis, cutaneous anthrax with systemic involvement, lesions on the head or neck, or extensive edema) caused by penicillin-susceptible *B. anthracis* that occurs in the context of biologic warfare or bioterrorism, AAP states that full-term neonates 7 days of age or younger should receive a dosage of 300,000 units/kg daily given in divided doses every 8 hours and those 1–4 weeks of age should receive 400,000 units/kg daily given in divided doses every 6 hours. For the treatment of these systemic anthrax infections in premature neonates, AAP recommends that those with gestational age of 32–34 weeks receive 200,000 units/kg daily given in divided doses every 12 hours from birth until 7 days of age and 300,000 units/kg daily given in divided doses every 8 hours from 1–4 weeks of age; those with gestational age of 34–37 weeks should receive 300,000 units/kg daily given in divided doses every 8 hours from birth until 7 days of age and 400,000 units/kg daily given in divided doses every 6 hours from 1–4 weeks of age. In infants and children 1 month of age or older, AAP recommends that IV penicillin G be given in a dosage of 400,000 units/kg daily in divided doses every 4 hours (up to 4 million units per dose). The multiple-drug parenteral regimen should be continued for at least 2–3 weeks until the patient is clinically stable; treatment can then be switched to an oral regimen. Because of the possible persistence of anthrax spores in lung tissue following an aerosol exposure in the context of biologic warfare or bioterrorism, the US Centers for Disease Control and Prevention (CDC) and other experts state that the total duration of anti-infective treatment should be 60 days.

For additional information on the treatment of anthrax and recommendations for postexposure prophylaxis following exposure to anthrax spores, see Uses: Anthrax, in Ciprofloxacin 8:12.18.

Clostridium Infections. For the treatment of myonecrosis and gas gangrene caused by *Clostridium perfringens* or other clostridium in children, IDSA recommends that IV penicillin G be given in a dosage of 60,000–100,000 units/kg every 6 hours in conjunction with clindamycin (10–13 mg/kg IV every 8 hours). AAP recommends that children with myonecrosis caused by *C. perfringens* receive IV penicillin G in a dosage of 250,000–400,000 units/kg daily and states that concomitant use of clindamycin may be more effective than penicillin G alone. Surgical debridement and/or surgery should be performed as indicated.

If IV penicillin G is used as an adjunct to tetanus immune globulin (TIG) in the management of tetanus caused by *C. tetani*, AAP recommends that children receive a dosage of 100,000 units/kg daily (up to 12 million units daily) given in divided doses every 4–6 hours for 7–10 days. The role of anti-infectives in the adjunctive treatment of tetanus is unclear; metronidazole usually is preferred if an anti-infective is used.

Diphtheria. If penicillin G potassium or sodium is used as an adjunct to diphtheria antitoxin (not commercially available in the US, but may be available from CDC) for the treatment of diphtheria caused by *Corynebacterium diphtheriae* and prevention of the diphtheria carrier state, the manufacturers recommend that pediatric patients receive a dosage of 150,000–250,000 units/kg daily given in divided doses every 6 hours for 7–10 days. CDC recommends a 14-day regimen of IM penicillin G procaine if a penicillin is used for adjunctive treatment of diphtheria. Patients usually are no longer contagious 48 hours after initiation of anti-infective treatment. Eradication of *C. diphtheriae* should be confirmed 24 hours after completion of treatment by 2 consecutive negative cultures taken 24 hours apart.

Lyme Disease. If IV penicillin G is used as an alternative to IV ceftriaxone for the treatment of early Lyme disease† in children with acute neurologic disease manifested as meningitis or radiculopathy, IDSA recommends a dosage of 200,000–400,000 units/kg daily (up to 18–24 million units daily) given in divided doses every 4 hours for 10–28 days.

If IV penicillin G is used as an alternative to IV ceftriaxone or IV cefotaxime for the treatment of late Lyme disease† in children with recurrent Lyme arthritis and objective evidence of neurologic disease, AAP and IDSA recommend a dosage of 200,000–400,000 units/kg daily (up to 18–24 million units daily) given in divided doses every 4 hours for 14–28 days.

For the treatment of late neurologic Lyme disease† affecting the central or peripheral nervous system, IDSA, AAP, and others state that children can receive IV penicillin G in a dosage of 200,000–400,000 units/kg daily (up to 18–24 million units daily) given in divided doses every 4 hours for 14–28 days as an alternative to IV ceftriaxone. IDSA states that retreatment is not recommended unless relapse of neurologic disease is documented with reliable objective measures.

Neisseria meningitidis Infections. For the treatment of serious infections (e.g. endocarditis, pneumonia) caused by susceptible *N. meningitidis*, the manufacturers recommend that pediatric patients receive penicillin G potassium or sodium in a dosage of 150,000–300,000 units/kg daily given in divided doses every 4–6 hours.

For dosage recommendations for the treatment of meningitis caused by *N. meningitidis* in pediatric patients, see Meningitis and Other CNS Infections under Dosage: Pediatric Dosage, in Dosage and Administration.

Rat-Bite Fever. For the treatment of rat-bite fever caused by *Streptobacillus moniliformis* (erythema arthriticum epidemicum, Haverhill fever) or *Spirillum minus* (sodoku), the manufacturers recommend that pediatric patients receive penicillin G potassium or sodium in a dosage of 150,000–250,000 units/kg daily given in divided doses every 4 hours for 4 weeks.

Some clinicians suggest that pediatric patients with rat-bite fever receive IV penicillin G in a dosage of 20,000–50,000 units/kg daily for 5–7 days followed by oral penicillin V (25–50 mg/kg daily [up to 3 g daily] in 4 divided doses for 7 days). For the treatment endocarditis caused by *S. moniliformis* strains that are less susceptible to penicillin G (MIC greater than 0.1 mcg/mL), some clinicians state that pediatric patients should receive IV penicillin G in a dosage of 160,000–240,000 units/kg daily (up to 20 million units daily) for 6 weeks; concomitant use of an aminoglycoside (streptomycin or gentamicin) may be indicated for initial treatment.

Syphilis. For the treatment of proven or highly probable congenital syphilis in neonates (see Uses: Syphilis), CDC recommends an IV penicillin G dosage of 50,000 units/kg every 12 hours during the first 7 days of life and 50,000 units/kg every 8 hours thereafter for a total duration of 10 days. If more than 1 day of treatment is missed in such neonates, the entire course of treatment should be restarted. If IV penicillin G is used in neonates with possible congenital syphilis (see Uses: Syphilis), CDC recommends 50,000 units/kg every 12 hours during the first 7 days of life and 50,000 units/kg every 8 hours thereafter for a total duration 10 days.

In infants and children 1 month of age or older with reactive serologic tests for syphilis, CDC recommends that IV penicillin G be given in a dosage of 200,000–300,000 units/kg daily (50,000 units/kg every 4–6 hours) for 10 days.

CDC, AAP, and the manufacturers recommend that penicillin G potassium or sodium be given in a dosage of 200,000–300,000 units/kg daily (50,000 units every 4–6 hours) for 10–14 days for the treatment of congenital syphilis diagnosed after the neonatal period or for the treatment of neurosyphilis in infants and children 1 month of age or older. Some clinicians recommend that this regimen be followed by a single dose of IM penicillin G benzathine (50,000 units/kg [up to 2.4 million units]).

For the treatment of neurosyphilis and otic or ocular syphilis in adolescents with human immunodeficiency virus (HIV) infection, some clinicians recommend that IV penicillin G be given a dosage of 18–24 million units daily (by continuous IV infusion or given as 3–4 million units every 4 hours) for 10–14 days. Some clinicians recommend that this regimen be followed by a regimen of IM penicillin G benzathine (2.4 million units once weekly for 1–3 weeks).

HIV-infected neonates with congenital syphilis and HIV-infected children and adolescents with any stage of syphilis should receive the same treatment regimens recommended for those without HIV infection.

Adult Dosage **Bone and Joint Infections.** For the treatment of native vertebral osteomyelitis or prosthetic joint infections caused by susceptible β-hemolytic streptococci†, IDSA recommends that adults receive IV penicillin G in a dosage of 20–24 million units daily (by continuous IV infusion or in 6 divided doses). The recommended duration of treatment is 6 weeks in patients with native vertebral osteomyelitis or 4–6 weeks in those with prosthetic joint infections.

For the treatment of native vertebral osteomyelitis or prosthetic joint infections caused by susceptible *Enterococcus*†, IDSA recommends that adults receive IV penicillin G in a dosage of 20–24 million units daily (by continuous IV infusion or in 6 divided doses) for 4–6 weeks. Concomitant treatment with an aminoglycoside given for 4–6 weeks also can be considered and is recommended if infective endocarditis also in present.

For the treatment of native vertebral osteomyelitis or prosthetic joint infections caused by susceptible *C. acnes*† (formerly *P. acnes*), IDSA recommends that adults receive IV penicillin G in a dosage of 20 million units daily (by continuous IV infusion or in 6 divided doses). The recommended duration of treatment is 6 weeks in patients with native vertebral osteomyelitis or 4–6 weeks in those with prosthetic joint infections.

Endocarditis. For the treatment of native valve endocarditis caused by viridans group streptococci† or *S. gallolyticus*† (formerly *S. bovis*) that are highly penicillin-susceptible (penicillin MIC 0.12 mcg/mL or less), AHA recommends that adults receive IV penicillin G in a dosage of 12–18 million units daily (by continuous IV infusion or in 4 or 6 divided doses) given for 4 weeks. Alternatively, adults with uncomplicated endocarditis caused by highly penicillin-susceptible viridans group streptococci† or *S. gallolyticus*† who are at low risk for adverse effects related to aminoglycoside therapy may receive a 2-week regimen consisting of IV penicillin G in a dosage of 12–18 million units daily (by continuous IV infusion or in 6 divided doses) in conjunction with gentamicin (3 mg/kg daily IV or IM given as a single daily dose or as 1 mg/kg every 8 hours). The 2-week regimen is not recommended for patients with known cardiac or extracardiac abscesses, creatinine clearance less than 20 mL/minute, impaired eighth cranial nerve function, or infection with *Abiotrophia*, *Granulicatella*, or *Gemella*.

For the treatment of native valve endocarditis caused by viridans streptococci† or *S. gallolyticus*† that are relatively resistant to penicillin G (penicillin MIC greater than 0.12 mcg/mL but less than 0.5 mcg/mL), AHA recommends that adults receive IV penicillin G in a dosage of 24 million units daily (by continuous IV infusion or in 4–6 divided doses) given for 4 weeks in conjunction with gentamicin (3 mg/kg daily IV or IM given as a single daily dose or as 1 mg/kg every 8 hours during the first 2 weeks of penicillin G treatment).

For the treatment of native valve endocarditis caused by viridans streptococci†, *A. defectiva*†, or *Granulicatella*† with penicillin MIC 0.5 mcg/mL or greater, AHA states that IV penicillin G given in a dosage of 18–30 million units daily (by continuous IV infusion or in 6 divided doses) in conjunction with gentamicin (3 mg/kg daily IV or IM in 2 or 3 divided doses) is a reasonable regimen for adults. AHA states that consultation with an infectious disease expert is recommended to determine the duration of treatment for such infections.

For the treatment of endocarditis involving prosthetic valves or other prosthetic material caused by viridans streptococci† or *S. gallolyticus*† that are highly penicillin-susceptible (penicillin MIC 0.12 mcg/mL or less), AHA states that adults can receive IV penicillin G in a dosage of 24 million units daily (by continuous IV infusion or in 4–6 divided doses) given for 6 weeks with or without gentamicin (3 mg/kg daily IV or IM as a single daily dose or as 1 mg/kg every 8 hours given concomitantly during the first 2 weeks of penicillin G treatment). When endocarditis involving prosthetic valves or other prosthetic material is caused by viridans streptococci† or *S. gallolyticus*† relatively or highly resistant to penicillin G (penicillin MIC greater than 0.12 mcg/mL), AHA states that it is reasonable to extend the duration of concomitant gentamicin to 6 weeks.

For the treatment of enterococcal endocarditis† (native valve or prosthetic valve or other prosthetic material) caused by *Enterococcus* susceptible to penicillin *and* gentamicin, AHA states that adults may receive IV penicillin G in a dosage of 18–30 million units daily (by continuous IV infusion or in 6 divided doses) in conjunction with gentamicin (3 mg/kg daily IV or IM in 2 or 3 divided doses; dose adjusted to achieve gentamicin peak serum concentrations of 3–4 mcg/mL and trough concentrations less than 1 mcg/mL). In patients with native valve enterococcal endocarditis, treatment with both drugs should be continued for 4 weeks in those who had symptoms of infection for less than 3 months prior to treatment or for 6 weeks in those who had symptoms for 3 months or longer prior to treatment. In patients with enterococcal endocarditis involving prosthetic heart valves or other prosthetic material, continuation of both drugs for 6 weeks is reasonable. If endocarditis is caused by enterococci resistant to gentamicin but susceptible to penicillin *and* streptomycin, AHA states that streptomycin (15 mg/kg daily IV or IM in 2 divided doses; dose adjusted to achieve streptomycin peak serum concentrations of 20–35 mcg/mL and trough concentrations less than 10 mcg/mL) can be substituted for gentamicin in recommended regimens. Alternative regimens (e.g., double β-lactam regimens) should be considered in patients with creatinine clearance less than 50 mL/minute.

The manufacturers state that penicillin G potassium or sodium can be given in a dosage of 5–24 million units daily in divided doses every 4–6 hours for the treatment of endocarditis caused by susceptible staphylococci. However, penicillin G is not included in current AHA recommendations for the treatment of staphylococcal endocarditis in adults.

The manufacturers state that penicillin G potassium or sodium can be given in a dosage of 12–24 million units daily in divided doses every 4–6 hours for the treatment of endocarditis caused by susceptible streptococci, including *S. pyogenes*, streptococci groups C, H, G, L, and M, and *S. pneumoniae*.

Meningitis and Other CNS Infections. For the treatment of meningitis caused by susceptible *L. monocytogenes*, IDSA and other clinicians recommend that adults receive IV penicillin G in a dosage of 24 million units daily (4 million units every 4 hours). IDSA recommends a treatment duration of at least 21 days and states that concomitant use of an aminoglycoside should be considered. The manufacturers recommend that adults with meningitis caused by susceptible *L. monocytogenes* receive a penicillin G dosage of 15–20 million units daily given in divided doses every 4–6 hours for 2 weeks.

For the treatment of meningitis caused by susceptible *N. meningitidis*, IDSA recommends that adults receive IV penicillin G in a dosage of 24 million units daily (4 million units every 4 hours) for 7 days. The manufacturers recommend that adults receive a dosage of 24 million units daily (2 million units every 2 hours).

If meningitis is caused by susceptible *S. agalactiae*† (group B streptococci; GBS), IDSA recommends that adults receive IV penicillin G in a dosage of 24 million units daily (4 million units every 4 hours) for 14–21 days. IDSA states that concomitant use of an aminoglycoside should be considered.

For the treatment of meningitis caused by susceptible *S. pneumonia* (penicillin MIC less than 0.1 mcg/mL), IDSA and other clinicians recommend that adults receive IV penicillin G in a dosage of 24 million units daily (4 million units every 4 hours) for 10–14 days. The manufacturers recommend that adults receive a dosage of 12–24 million units daily given in divided doses every 4–6 hours. One manufacturer recommends a dosage of 5–24 million units daily given in divided doses every 4–6 hours.

For the treatment of healthcare-associated ventriculitis and meningitis caused by *C. acnes*† (formerly *P. acnes*), IDSA recommends that adults receive IV penicillin G in a dosage of 24 million units daily given in divided doses every 4 hours. Treatment should be continued for 10 days in those with no or minimal CSF pleocytosis, normal CSF glucose, and few clinical symptoms or systemic features or for 10–14 days in those with significant CSF pleocytosis, CSF hypoglycorrhachia, or clinical symptoms or systemic features.

Respiratory Tract Infections. If penicillin G potassium or sodium is used for the treatment of serious respiratory tract infections (e.g., empyema, pneumonia) caused by susceptible nonpenicillinase-producing staphylococci, the manufacturers recommend that adults receive a dosage of 5–24 million units daily in divided doses every 4–6 hours depending on severity.

If penicillin G potassium is used for the treatment of serious respiratory tract infections (e.g., empyema, pneumonia) caused by susceptible *S. pyogenes*, streptococci groups C, H, G, L, and M, or *S. pneumoniae*, the manufacturers recommend that adults receive a dosage of 12–24 million units daily in divided doses every 4–6 hours depending on severity. If penicillin G sodium is used for the treatment of these infections, the manufacturer recommends a dosage of 5–24 million units daily in divided doses every 4–6 hours depending on severity.

Septicemia. If penicillin G potassium or sodium is used for the treatment of septicemia caused by susceptible nonpenicillinase-producing staphylococci, the manufacturers recommend that adults receive a dosage of 5–24 million units daily in divided doses every 4–6 hours depending on severity.

If penicillin G potassium is used for the treatment of septicemia caused by susceptible *S. pyogenes*, streptococci groups C, H, G, L, and M, or *S. pneumoniae*, the manufacturers recommend that adults receive a dosage of 12–24 million units daily in divided doses every 4–6 hours depending on severity. If penicillin G sodium is used for the treatment of these infections, the manufacturer recommends a dosage of 5–24 million units daily in divided doses every 4–6 hours depending on severity.

Skin and Skin Structure Infections. For the treatment of necrotizing infections of the skin, fascia, and muscle caused by susceptible *S. pyogenes*, IDSA recommends that adults receive a regimen of IV penicillin G given in a dosage of 2–4 million units every 4–6 hours in conjunction with clindamycin (600–900 mg IV every 8 hours).

Actinomycosis. For the treatment of actinomycosis caused by *Actinomyces* in adults, the manufacturers recommend that penicillin G potassium or sodium be given in a dosage of 1–6 million units daily in divided doses every 4–6 hours for cervicofacial disease or 10–20 million units daily in divided doses every 4–6 hours for thoracic or abdominal disease.

Some clinicians state that, although dosage and duration of therapy should be individualized, a reasonable treatment regimen for pulmonary actinomycosis or other severe infections caused by *Actinomyces* is IV penicillin G given in a dosage of 18–24 million units daily (3–4 million units every 4 hours) for at least 2–6 weeks followed by 6–12 additional months of an oral regimen (penicillin V or amoxicillin). A shorter duration of treatment may be sufficient for less extensive disease (e.g., cervicofacial region). Surgical procedures should be performed as indicated.

Anthrax. For the treatment of anthrax (inhalational, GI, meningitis) caused by penicillin-susceptible *B. anthracis* that occurs as the result of naturally occurring or endemic anthrax exposure, some clinicians recommend that adults receive IV penicillin G in a dosage of 8–12 million units daily given in divided doses every 4–6 hours. For the treatment of severe or life-threatening systemic anthrax (inhalational, GI, meningoencephalitis, sepsis) or the treatment of cutaneous anthrax with signs of systemic involvement or extensive edema caused by penicillin-susceptible *B. anthracis* that occurs as the result of natural or endemic anthrax exposure, some clinicians recommend that adults receive IV penicillin G in a dosage of 4 million units every 4–6 hours (16–24 million units daily). Concomitant use of other anti-infectives (e.g., streptomycin or other aminoglycoside, clindamycin, clarithromycin, rifampin, vancomycin) may also be indicated. Treatment of naturally occurring or endemic anthrax generally should be continued for at least 14 days after symptoms abate.

If IV penicillin G is used in a multiple-drug parenteral regimen for initial treatment of systemic anthrax (inhalational, GI, meningitis, cutaneous anthrax with systemic involvement, lesions on the head or neck, or extensive edema) caused by penicillin-susceptible *B. anthracis* that occurs in the context of biologic warfare or bioterrorism, CDC recommends that adults (including pregnant and postpartum women) receive a dosage of 4 million units every 4 hours. The multiple-drug parenteral regimen should be continued for at least 2–3 weeks until the patient is clinically stable; treatment can then be switched to an oral regimen. Because of the possible persistence of anthrax spores in lung tissue following an aerosol exposure in the context of biologic warfare or bioterrorism, CDC and other experts state that the total duration of anti-infective treatment should be 60 days.

The manufacturers state that the minimum dosage of penicillin G potassium or sodium for the treatment of anthrax in adults is 8 million units daily given in divided doses every 6 hours and that higher dosage may be required depending on susceptibility of the organism.

For additional information on the treatment of anthrax and recommendations for postexposure prophylaxis following exposure to anthrax spores, see Uses: Anthrax, in Ciprofloxacin 8:12.18.

Clostridium Infections. For the treatment of myonecrosis and gas gangrene caused by *C. perfringens* or other clostridium, IDSA recommends that adults receive IV penicillin G in a dosage of 2–4 million units every 4–6 hours in conjunction with clindamycin (600–900 mg IV every 8 hours). The manufacturers recommend that adults receive penicillin G potassium or sodium in a dosage of 20 million units daily given in divided doses every 4–6 hours. Surgical debridement and/or surgery should be performed as indicated.

If penicillin G potassium or sodium is used as an adjunct to TIG in the management of tetanus caused by *C. tetani*, the manufacturers recommend that adults receive 20 million units daily given in divided doses every 4–6 hours. The role of anti-infectives in the adjunctive treatment of tetanus is unclear; metronidazole usually is preferred if an anti-infective is used.

If penicillin G potassium or sodium is used as an adjunct in the management of botulism caused by *C. botulinum*, the manufacturers recommend that adults receive 20 million units daily given in divided doses every 4–6 hours. Although the role of anti-infectives is unclear, some clinicians recommend a penicillin G dosage of 10–20 million units daily for adjunctive management of wound botulism. Botulism antitoxin (not commercially available in the US, but may be available from CDC) is the recommended treatment for foodborne and wound botulism and for botulism that occurs in the context of biologic warfare or bioterrorism.

Diphtheria. If penicillin G potassium or sodium is used as an adjunct to diphtheria antitoxin (not commercially available in the US, but may be available from CDC) for the treatment of diphtheria caused by *C. diphtheriae*, the manufacturers recommend that adults receive a dosage of 2–3 million units daily given in divided doses every 4–6 hours for 10–12 days. CDC recommends a 14-day regimen of IM penicillin G procaine if a penicillin is used for adjunctive treatment of diphtheria. Patients usually are no longer contagious 48 hours after initiation of anti-infective treatment. Eradication of *C. diphtheriae* should be confirmed 24 hours after completion of treatment by 2 consecutive negative cultures taken 24 hours apart.

Erysipelothrix Infections. If penicillin G potassium or sodium is used for the treatment of *Erysipelothrix* endocarditis, the manufacturers recommend that adults receive 12–20 million units daily given in divided doses every 4–6 hours for 4–6 weeks.

Fusobacterium Infections. If penicillin G potassium or sodium is used for the treatment of severe *Fusobacterium* infections of the oropharynx (including acute necrotizing ulcerative gingivitis [Vincent's infection], trench mouth, *Fusobacterium* gingivitis or pharyngitis), lower respiratory tract, or genital area, the manufacturers recommend that adults receive 5–10 million units daily in divided doses every 4–6 hours. Penicillin G is not recommended for empiric treatment of such infections because, although the drug may be effective against *Fusobacterium*, other organisms may also be involved (e.g., *Bacteroides fragilis*, *Prevotella*, *Porphyromonas*) that usually are resistant to penicillin G.

Leptospirosis. For the treatment of severe leptospirosis†, IV penicillin G has been given in a dosage of 6 million units daily (1.5 million units every 6 hours) for 7 days. Anti-infective treatment should be initiated as soon as possible after symptom onset; however, the benefits of anti-infective therapy are uncertain, especially if initiated in patients with late and/or severe disease.

Listeria Infections. For the treatment of serious infections caused by susceptible *L. monocytogenes* (e.g., endocarditis, meningitis) in adults, the manufacturers recommend that penicillin G potassium or sodium be given in a dosage of 15–20 million units daily in divided doses every 4–6 hours.

For additional dosage recommendations regarding the treatment of meningitis caused by *L. monocytogenes* in adults, see Meningitis and Other CNS Infections under Dosage: Adult Dosage, in Dosage and Administration.

Lyme Disease. If IV penicillin G is used as an alternative to IV ceftriaxone for the treatment of early Lyme disease† in adults with acute neurologic disease manifested as meningitis or radiculopathy, IDSA recommends a dosage of 18–24 million units daily given in divided doses every 4 hours for 10–28 days.

If IV penicillin G is used as an alternative to IV ceftriaxone for the treatment of late Lyme disease† in adults with recurrent Lyme arthritis and objective evidence of neurologic disease, IDSA recommends a dosage of 18–24 million units daily given in divided doses every 4 hours for 14–28 days.

For the treatment of late neurologic Lyme disease† affecting the central or peripheral nervous system, IDSA and others state that adults can receive IV penicillin G in a dosage of 18–24 million units daily given in divided doses every 4 hours for 14–28 days as an alternative to IV ceftriaxone. IDSA states that retreatment is not recommended unless relapse of neurologic disease is documented with reliable objective measures.

Neisseria meningitidis Infections. For the treatment of septicemia and/or meningitis caused by susceptible *N. meningitidis*, the manufacturers recommend that adults receive penicillin G potassium or sodium in a dosage of 24 million units daily (2 million units every 2 hours).

For additional dosage recommendations regarding the treatment of meningitis caused by *N. meningitidis* in adults, see Meningitis and Other CNS Infections under Dosage: Adult Dosage, in Dosage and Administration.

Pasteurella multocida Infections. For the treatment of serious infections caused by *Pasteurella multocida*, including bacteremia and meningitis, the manufacturers recommend that adults receive penicillin G potassium or sodium in a dosage of 4–6 million units daily given in divided doses every 4–6 hours for 2 weeks.

Rat-Bite Fever. For the treatment of rat-bite fever caused by susceptible *S. moniliformis* (erythema arthriticum epidemicum, Haverhill fever) or *S. minus* (sodoku), the manufacturers recommend that adults receive penicillin G potassium or sodium in a dosage of 12–20 million units daily given in divided doses every 4–6 hours for 3–4 weeks.

CDC recommends that adults with rat-bite fever caused by *S. moniliformis* receive IV penicillin G in a dosage of 1.2 million units daily for 5–7 days; if improvement occurs, treatment can be switched to oral penicillin V or oral ampicillin (500 mg 4 times daily for 7 days). Some clinicians suggest that adults with rat-bite fever can receive IV penicillin G in a dosage of 400,000–600,000 units daily for at least 7 days, but that dosage should be increased to 1.2 million units daily if there is no response to the lower dosage within 2 days.

For the treatment of *S. moniliformis* endocarditis caused by a strain that is less susceptible to penicillin G (MIC greater than 0.1 mcg/mL), some clinicians recommend that adults receive IV penicillin G in a dosage of 20 million units daily for 4 weeks; concomitant use of an aminoglycoside (streptomycin or gentamicin) may be indicated for initial treatment.

Syphilis. For the treatment of neurosyphilis and otic or ocular syphilis, CDC and other clinicians recommend that adults receive IV penicillin G in a dosage of 18–24 million units daily (by continuous IV infusion or given as 3–4 million units every 4 hours) for 10–14 days. Some clinicians recommend that this regimen be followed by a regimen of IM penicillin G benzathine (2.4 million units once weekly for up to 3 weeks).

The manufacturers recommend that adults with neurosyphilis receive penicillin G potassium or sodium in a dosage of 12–24 million units daily (2–4 million units every 4 hours) for 10–14 days; this may be followed by a regimen of IM penicillin G benzathine (2.4 million units once weekly for up to 3 weeks).

HIV-infected adults with any stage of syphilis should receive the same treatment regimens recommended for those without HIV infection.

Whipple's Disease. For initial treatment of Whipple's disease† caused by *Tropheryma whipplei*, some clinicians recommend that IV penicillin G be given in a dosage of 10 million units daily. Others recommend a dosage of 12–24 million units daily (2–4 million units every 4 hours). A regimen of IV penicillin G given in a dosage of 1.2 million units daily in conjunction with parenteral streptomycin (1 g daily) also has been recommended. The initial parenteral regimen usually is continued for 2–4 weeks and should be followed by 1–2 years of treatment with an oral regimen (e.g., co-trimoxazole).

Optimal regimens for treatment of Whipple's disease have not been identified and relapses may occur, even after adequate and long-term anti-infective treatment.

Prevention of Perinatal Group B Streptococcal Disease. When intrapartum anti-infective prophylaxis for prevention of perinatal group B streptococcal (GBS) disease† is indicated in the mother to prevent early-onset GBS disease in her neonate (see Uses: Prevention of Perinatal Group B Streptococcal Disease), CDC and AAP recommend that an initial dose of 5 million units of penicillin G be given IV at the onset of labor or rupture of membranes followed by 2.5–3 million units IV every 4 hours until delivery.

Regardless of whether anti-infective prophylaxis was administered to the mother, appropriate diagnostic evaluations and anti-infective therapy should be initiated in the neonate if signs or symptoms of active infection develop.

■ Dosage in Renal and Hepatic Impairment

In patients with impaired renal function, doses and/or frequency of administration of penicillin G may need to be modified in response to the degree of impairment.

The manufacturers state that dosage of IM or IV penicillin G potassium or sodium should be adjusted in patients with severe renal impairment. These manufacturers and others recommend that patients with creatinine clearance less than 10 mL/minute per 1.73 m^2 receive a loading dose of penicillin G using the usually recommended dose followed by 50% of the usually recommended dose given every 8–10 hours. In uremic patients with creatinine clearance greater than 10 mL/minute per 1.73 m^2, the manufacturers and others recommend a loading dose of penicillin G using the usually recommended dose followed by 50% of the usually recommended dose given every 4–5 hours.

Alternatively, some clinicians suggest that if the usual dosing interval for penicillin G potassium or sodium in patients with normal renal function (creatinine clearance greater than 50 mL/minute) is every 6 or 8 hours, then the usual dose should be given every 8–12 hours in those with creatinine clearance of 10–50 mL/minute or every 12–18 hours in those with creatinine clearance less than 10 mL/minute.

Some clinicians suggest a maximum daily dosage of 4–10 million penicillin G units in adults with severe renal failure.

In patients with impaired hepatic function in addition to impaired renal function, further dosage reductions may be advisable.

Cautions

■ Adverse Effects

Adverse effects reported with penicillin G potassium and penicillin G sodium are similar to those reported with other natural penicillins.

Serious and occasionally fatal hypersensitivity reactions, including anaphylaxis, have been reported with penicillins. Hypersensitivity reactions to penicillins may be immediate reactions (usually occurring within 20 minutes after administration) that range in severity from urticaria and pruritus to angioedema, laryngospasm, bronchospasm, hypotension, vascular collapse, and death; accelerated reactions (usually occurring between 20 minutes and 48 hours after administration) that may include urticaria, pruritus, fever, and, occasionally, laryngeal edema; or delayed reactions (usually occurring within 1–2 weeks after initiation of penicillin therapy) that may include serum sickness-like symptoms (i.e., fever, malaise, urticaria, myalgia, arthralgia, abdominal pain) and rash ranging from maculopapular eruptions to exfoliative dermatitis.

Jarisch-Herxheimer reactions may occur in patients receiving penicillin G potassium or sodium for the treatment of syphilis or other spirochetal infections (e.g., leptospirosis†, Lyme disease†, relapsing fever†).

Because of the potassium and sodium content, penicillin G potassium and penicillin G sodium may cause serious and potentially fatal electrolyte disturbances, particularly if high IV dosage is used. Penicillin G potassium powders for injection contain approximately 66 mg (1.7 mEq) of potassium and approximately 7 mg (0.3 mEq) of sodium in each 1 million units of penicillin G. Frozen premixed penicillin G potassium injections in dextrose contain approximately 1.7 mEq of potassium and approximately 1 mEq of sodium in each 1 million units of penicillin G. Penicillin G sodium powder for injection contains approximately 1.7 mEq of sodium in each 1 million units of penicillin G.

For additional information on adverse effects reported with penicillin G, see Cautions in the Natural Penicillins General Statement 8:12.16.04.

■ **Precautions and Contraindications** Penicillin G potassium and sodium are contraindicated in patients hypersensitive to any penicillin.

The manufacturer of the commercially available frozen premixed penicillin G potassium injections in dextrose states that dextrose-containing solutions may be contraindicated in patients with known allergy to corn or corn products.

Penicillin G potassium and sodium share the toxic potentials of the penicillins, including the risk of hypersensitivity reactions, and the usual precautions of penicillin therapy should be observed.

Prior to initiation of therapy with penicillin G potassium or sodium, careful inquiry should be made concerning previous hypersensitivity reactions to penicillins, cephalosporins, or other drugs. There is clinical and laboratory evidence of partial cross-allergenicity among penicillins and other β-lactam antibiotics including cephalosporins and cephamycins.

Hypersensitivity reactions to penicillins are more likely to occur in individuals with a history of penicillin hypersensitivity and/or a history of sensitivity to multiple allergens. Penicillin G potassium or sodium should be used with caution in individuals with a history of allergies and/or asthma.

If a hypersensitivity reaction occurs, penicillin G should be discontinued immediately and appropriate therapy instituted as indicated (e.g., epinephrine, maintenance of an adequate airway and oxygen, corticosteroids). Desensitization has been used to enable a penicillin to be administered to penicillin-hypersensitive patients who have life-threatening infections for which other effective anti-infective agents are not available (e.g., endocarditis, neurosyphilis or congenital syphilis, syphilis during pregnancy). Such procedures are usually performed in a hospital setting and expert consultation may be indicated. Specialized references should be consulted for specific information on sensitivity testing and desensitization protocols.

During prolonged therapy with high dosage of penicillin G potassium or sodium, the patient's organ system functions should be assessed periodically, including frequent evaluation of hepatic, renal, and hematologic systems, electrolyte balance, and cardiac and vascular status. If any impairment of function is suspected or known to exist, a reduction in total dosage should be considered. (See Dosage and Administration: Dosage in Renal and Hepatic Impairment.)

For a more complete discussion of these and other precautions associated with the use of penicillin G potassium or sodium, see Cautions: Precautions and Contraindications, in the Natural Penicillins General Statement 8:12.16.04.

■ **Pediatric Precautions** Renal clearance of penicillin G may be delayed in neonates and premature or young infants because of incompletely developed renal function. Appropriate reductions in dosage and frequency of administration should be made in such patients.

Neonates receiving penicillin G potassium or sodium should be monitored closely for clinical and laboratory evidence of toxic or adverse effects.

■ **Geriatric Precautions** Clinical studies of penicillin G potassium did not include sufficient numbers of patients 65 years of age or older to determine whether geriatric patients respond differently than younger patients. Other clinical experience has not identified differences in responses between geriatric and younger patients.

Penicillin G is substantially eliminated by the kidneys and the risk of adverse effects may be greater in those with impaired renal function. Because geriatric patients are more likely to have reduced renal function, dosage should be selected with caution, usually starting at the low end of the dosage range, and renal function monitoring may be useful.

The potassium and/or sodium content of penicillin G potassium or sodium preparations and the potential for electrolyte imbalance should be considered. Geriatric patients may respond to salt loading with a blunted natriuresis that may be clinically important in those with certain conditions (e.g., congestive heart failure).

■ **Pregnancy and Lactation** ***Pregnancy*** Reproduction studies evaluating penicillin G in mice, rats, and rabbits have not revealed evidence of impaired fertility or harm to the fetus. Although experience with use of penicillins during pregnancy has not shown any evidence of adverse effects on the fetus, there are no adequate or controlled studies using penicillin G in pregnant women.

Some clinicians state that penicillin G is considered low risk and safe for use during pregnancy. The drug is included in the US Centers for Disease Control and Prevention (CDC) recommendations for the treatment of syphilis during pregnancy.

The manufacturers state that penicillin G potassium or sodium should be used during pregnancy only when clearly needed.

Lactation Penicillin G is distributed into milk. Some clinicians state that penicillin G is usually considered compatible with breast-feeding. The manufacturers and others state that penicillin G potassium or sodium should be used with caution in nursing women.

Spectrum

Based on its spectrum of activity, penicillin G is classified as a natural penicillin. For information on the classification of penicillins based on spectra of activity, see the Preface to the General Statements on Penicillins 8:12.16.

For specific information on the spectrum of activity of penicillin G and resistance to the drug, see the sections on Spectrum and on Resistance in the Natural Penicillins General Statement 8:12.16.04.

Pharmacokinetics

For additional information on the absorption, distribution, and elimination of penicillin G, see Pharmacokinetics in the Natural Penicillins General Statement 8:12.16.04.

■ **Absorption** Penicillin G potassium and penicillin G sodium are rapidly absorbed followed IM administration, and serum concentrations of penicillin G generally are the same following IM administration of equivalent doses of either salt. Following IM administration in adults of a single dose of 600,000 or 1 million units of penicillin G (as either salt), peak serum concentrations of penicillin G generally are attained within 15–30 minutes and average 6–8 or 20 units/mL, respectively. In one study in neonates 6 days of age or younger who received IM penicillin G in a dosage of 25,000 units/kg every 12 hours as the potassium salt, serum penicillin G concentrations ranged from 12.5–36, 7.8–35.1, 4.4–35.1, 0.7–21.9, and 0.3–9.2 mcg/mL at 30 minutes, 1 hour, 2 hours, 4 hours, and 12 hours, respectively, after a dose.

Following IV infusion of penicillin G, peak serum concentrations are attained immediately after completion of the infusion. In a study in 10 patients who received 5 million units of penicillin G given IV over 3–5 minutes, mean serum concentrations were 400, 273, and 3 mcg/mL at 5–6 minutes, 10 minutes, and 4 hours after administration, respectively. In a study in 5 healthy adults who received 1 million units of penicillin G given IV over 4 minutes or 60 minutes, mean serum concentrations 8 minutes after administration were 45 or 14.4 mcg/mL, respectively.

Following intermittent IV infusion of 2 million units of penicillin G every 2 hours or 3 million units of penicillin G every 3 hours (as either salt), serum penicillin G concentrations reportedly average 20 mcg/mL.

Penicillin G potassium or sodium is absorbed from the peritoneal cavity following local instillation and also is absorbed from pleural surfaces, pericardium, and joint cavities.

■ **Distribution** Penicillin G is widely distributed throughout the body in varying amounts following parenteral administration. Penicillin G is distributed into the lungs, liver, kidneys, muscle, bone, and pleural, pericardial, peritoneal, ascitic, synovial, and interstitial fluids. The volume of distribution of penicillin G is reportedly 0.53–0.67 L/kg in adults with normal renal function.

Minimal concentrations of penicillin G generally are attained in CSF following administration of penicillin G potassium or sodium in patients with uninflamed meninges; however, higher penicillin G concentrations are attained in CSF when the meninges are inflamed. Following IV administration of penicillin G sodium, concentrations of penicillin G in CSF reportedly range from 0–10% of concurrent serum concentrations of the drug in patients with normal meninges. In 2 adults with syphilis who received a daily IV dosage of 5 or 10 million units of penicillin G (as the potassium salt) for at least 10 days, penicillin G concentrations in CSF immediately following completion of therapy were 0.3 or 2.4 mcg/mL, respectively. In one study in children 2 weeks to 11 years of age with meningitis who received penicillin G potassium in a dosage of 250,000 units/kg daily given in 6 divided doses by IV infusion over 15 minutes, penicillin G concentrations in CSF specimens obtained between doses averaged 0.8, 0.7, and 0.3 mcg/mL on the first, fifth, and tenth days of therapy, respectively.

Penicillin G is approximately 45–68% bound to serum proteins.

Penicillin G crosses the placenta, although cord blood concentrations of the drug may be less than maternal serum concentrations.

Penicillin G is distributed into milk.

■ **Elimination** The serum half-life of penicillin G in adults with normal renal function is 0.4–0.9 hours.

Approximately 16–30% of an IM dose of penicillin G sodium is metabolized to penicilloic acid which is microbiologically inactive. Small amounts of 6-aminopenicillanic acid (6-APA) have also been found in the urine of patients receiving penicillin G. In addition, the drug appears to be hydroxylated to a small extent to one or more microbiologically active metabolites which also are excreted in urine.

Penicillin G and its metabolites are excreted in urine mainly by tubular secretion. Small amounts of the drug are also excreted in bile. Following IM or IV administration of a single dose of penicillin G in adults with normal renal function, 58–85% of the dose is excreted in urine as unchanged drug and active metabolites within 6 hours.

Serum concentrations of penicillin G may be higher and the serum half-life prolonged in patients with impaired renal function. The serum half-life of the drug is reportedly 1–2 hours in azotemic patients with serum creatinine concentrations less than 3 mg/dL and ranges from 6–20 hours in anuric patients. In anuric patients with hepatic impairment, the serum half-life of penicillin G may be 2–3 times more prolonged than in anuric patients with normal hepatic function.

Renal clearance of penicillin G is delayed in neonates and premature or young infants. The serum half-life of penicillin G varies inversely with age and appears to be independent of birthweight. The serum half-life of the drug is reportedly 3.2–3.4 hours in neonates 6 days of age or younger, 1.2–2.2 hours in neonates 7–13 days of age, and 0.9–1.9 hours in neonates 14 days of age or older.

Renal clearance of penicillin G may be delayed in geriatric patients because of diminished tubular secretion ability.

Renal clearance of penicillin G may be increased in pregnant women during the second and third trimesters.

Penicillin G is removed by hemodialysis and may be removed to a lesser extent by peritoneal dialysis.

Chemistry and Stability

■ **Chemistry** Penicillin G is a natural penicillin produced by fermentation of *Penicillium chrysogenum* in a medium containing phenylacetic acid. Penicillin G potassium and penicillin G sodium are frequently referred to as aqueous, crystalline forms of penicillin G.

Penicillin G potassium occurs as colorless or white crystals or a white, crystalline powder that is odorless or practically odorless and moderately hygroscopic. Penicillin G potassium is very soluble in water. Penicillin G potassium is commercially available as a sterile powder for injection in vials containing the equivalent of 1, 5, or 20 million units of penicillin G. Each 1 million units of penicillin G (as penicillin G potassium) contains approximately 66 mg (1.7 mEq) of potassium and approximately 7 mg (0.3 mEq) of sodium. The sterile powders are buffered with sodium citrate and/or citric acid. Following reconstitution according to the manufacturer's directions, penicillin G potassium solutions have a pH of 6–8.5. Penicillin G potassium also is commercially available as a frozen premixed solution in dextrose.

Penicillin G sodium occurs as a white to almost white, crystalline powder that is almost odorless. Penicillin G sodium is commercially available as a sterile powder for injection in vials containing the equivalent of 5 million units of penicillin G. Each 1 million units of penicillin G (as penicillin G sodium) contains approximately 1.7 mEq of sodium. Following reconstitution according to the manufacturer's directions, penicillin G sodium solutions are colorless and have a pH of 5–7.5.

Commercially available frozen premixed penicillin G potassium injections in dextrose are sterile, iso-osmotic, nonpyrogenic solutions of the drug provided in single-dose plastic containers (Galaxy® containers) fabricated from specially formulated multilayered plastic (PL 2040). The frozen injections containing 1, 2, or 3 million units of penicillin G contain approximately 2, 1.2, or 350 mg of dextrose hydrous, respectively, to adjust osmolality and also contain sodium citrate as a buffer. Hydrochloric acid and/or sodium hydroxide may have been added to adjust pH to 5.5–8. The frozen premixed penicillin G potassium injections in dextrose contain approximately 1.7 mEq of potassium and approximately 1 mEq of sodium in each 1 million units of penicillin G.

Potency of penicillin G potassium and penicillin G sodium generally is expressed in terms of penicillin G units, but also has been expressed as mg of penicillin G. Each mg of penicillin G potassium has a potency of 1440–1680 USP penicillin G units; each mg of penicillin G potassium powder for injection buffered with sodium citrate has a potency of 1355–1595 USP penicillin G units. Each mg of penicillin G sodium has a potency of 1500–1750 USP penicillin G units.

■ **Stability** Commercially available penicillin G potassium sterile powder for injection should be stored at less than 30°C. Following reconstitution, penicillin G potassium solutions should be stored at 2–8°C and are stable for 7 days at this temperature.

Commercially available penicillin G sodium powder for injection should be stored at 20–25°C. Following reconstitution, penicillin G sodium solutions should be stored at 2–8°C and are stable for 3 days at this temperature.

The commercially available frozen premixed penicillin G potassium injections in dextrose should be stored at −20°C or lower. The frozen premixed injections should be thawed at room temperature (25°C) or under refrigeration (5°C) and, once thawed, should not be refrozen. Thawed solutions of the commercially available frozen injections are stable for 24 hours at room temperature (25°C) or 14 days when refrigerated at 5°C. The commercially available frozen injections of the drug are provided in a plastic container fabricated from specially formulated multilayered plastic PL 2040 (Galaxy® containers). Solutions in contact with the polyethylene layer can leach out some of its chemical components in very small amounts within the expiration period of the injection; however, safety of the plastic has been confirmed in tests in animals according to USP biological tests for plastic containers as well as by tissue culture toxicity studies.

Penicillin G is unstable in solution at room temperature and is rapidly inactivated in carbohydrate solutions at alkaline pH. Small amounts of polymer conjugation products reportedly form in solutions of penicillin G during in vitro storage, especially when high concentrations of the drug are stored at room temperature. Penicillin degradation products may be more potent antigens than penicillin G and may play a role in hypersensitivity reactions to the drug. Therefore, reconstituted solutions of penicillin G potassium or penicillin G sodium should be refrigerated as directed by the manufacturer or used shortly following reconstitution.

Penicillin G is potentially physically and/or chemically incompatible with some drugs, including aminoglycosides and tetracyclines, but the compatibility depends on several factors (e.g., concentrations of the drugs, specific diluents used, resulting pH, temperature). Specialized references should be consulted for specific compatibility information.

For further information on chemistry and stability, mechanism of action, spectrum, resistance, pharmacokinetics, uses, cautions, drug interactions, laboratory test interferences, and dosage and administration of penicillin G potassium or sodium, see the Natural Penicillins General Statement 8:12.16.04.

Preparations

Excipients in commercially available drug preparations may have clinically important effects in some individuals; consult specific product labeling for details.

Penicillin G Potassium

Parenteral		
For injection	1 million units (of penicillin G)*	**Penicillin G Potassium for Injection**
	5 million units (of penicillin G)*	**Penicillin G Potassium for Injection**
		Pfizerpen®, Pfizer
	20 million units (of penicillin G)*	**Penicillin G Potassium for Injection**
		Pfizerpen®, Pfizer

*available from one or more manufacturer, distributor, and/or repackager by generic (nonproprietary) name

Penicillin G Potassium in Dextrose

Parenteral		
Injection (frozen), for IV infusion	20,000 units (of penicillin G) per mL (1 million units) in 4% Dextrose*	**Penicillin G Potassium in Iso-osmotic Dextrose Injection Galaxy®**
	40,000 units (of penicillin G) per mL (2 million units) in 2.4% Dextrose*	**Penicillin G Potassium in Iso-osmotic Dextrose Injection Galaxy®**
	60,000 units (of penicillin G) per mL (3 million units) in 0.7% Dextrose*	**Penicillin G Potassium in Iso-osmotic Dextrose Injection Galaxy®**

*available from one or more manufacturer, distributor, and/or repackager by generic (nonproprietary) name

Penicillin G Sodium

Parenteral		
For injection	5 million units (of penicillin G)*	**Penicillin G Sodium for Injection**

*available from one or more manufacturer, distributor, and/or repackager by generic (nonproprietary) name

†Use is not currently included in the labeling approved by the US Food and Drug Administration

Selected Revisions October 2018,

Penicillin G Procaine

Aqueous Procaine Penicillin G, Benzylpenicillin Procaine, Procaine Benzylpenicillin, Procaine Penicillin G

■ Penicillin G procaine, a natural penicillin, is a β-lactam antibiotic. The drug is the procaine monohydrate salt of penicillin G and is a long-acting formulation of penicillin G.

Uses

Penicillin G procaine is used only for the treatment of moderately severe infections caused by organisms that are susceptible to the low, prolonged serum concentrations of penicillin G provided by IM penicillin G procaine. When high, sustained concentrations of penicillin G are required for the treatment of severe infections, parenteral penicillin G potassium or sodium should be used.

The fixed combinations of penicillin G benzathine and penicillin G procaine are used for the treatment of moderately severe to severe infections caused by susceptible streptococci (e.g., upper respiratory tract infections, scarlet fever, erysipelas, skin and skin structure infections). The fixed combinations should *not* be used for *initial* treatment of severe pneumococcal infections, including pneumonia, empyema, bacteremia, pericarditis, meningitis, peritonitis, or arthritis. In addition, fixed combinations of penicillin G benzathine and penicillin G procaine should *not* be used for the treatment of syphilis, yaws, bejel, pinta, or gonorrhea.

For additional information on the uses of penicillin G procaine, see Uses in the Natural Penicillins General Statement 8:12.16.04.

■ **Anthrax** IM penicillin G procaine is used for inhalational anthrax (postexposure) to reduce the incidence or progression of disease following suspected or confirmed exposure to aerosolized *Bacillus anthracis* spores. Ciprofloxacin or doxycycline are the initial drugs of choice for postexposure prophylaxis following suspected or confirmed exposure to aerosolized anthrax spores, including exposures that occur in the context of biologic warfare or bioterrorism. If penicillin susceptibility is confirmed, consideration can be given to changing prophylaxis to a penicillin in infants and children, pregnant or lactating women, or when the drugs of choice are not tolerated or not available; however, oral amoxicillin or penicillin V usually is recommended.

IM penicillin G procaine is used for the treatment of mild, uncomplicated cutaneous anthrax caused by susceptible *B. anthracis* that occurs as the result of naturally occurring or endemic exposure to anthrax. If cutaneous anthrax occurs in the context of biologic warfare or bioterrorism, the initial drugs of choice are ciprofloxacin and doxycycline. If penicillin susceptibility is confirmed, consideration can be given to changing treatment to a penicillin in infants and children, pregnant or lactating women, or when the drugs of choice are not tolerated or not available; however, oral amoxicillin or penicillin V usually is recommended.

For additional information on the treatment of anthrax and recommendations for postexposure prophylaxis following exposure to anthrax spores, see Uses: Anthrax, in Ciprofloxacin 8:12.18.

■ **Syphilis** IM penicillin G procaine is used for the treatment of syphilis.

The US Centers for Disease Control and Prevention (CDC) and other clinicians state that IM penicillin G benzathine is the drug of choice for the treatment of primary syphilis (i.e., ulcer or chancre at infection site), secondary syphilis (i.e., manifestations that include, but are not limited to, rash, mucocutaneous lesions, and lymphadenopathy), and tertiary syphilis (i.e., cardiac syphilis, gummatous lesions, tabes dorsalis, and general paresis) in adults, adolescents, and children.

IM penicillin G benzathine also is the drug of choice for the treatment of latent syphilis (i.e., detected by serologic testing but lacking clinical manifestations), including both early latent syphilis (latent syphilis acquired within the preceding year) and late latent syphilis (i.e., all other cases of latent syphilis or syphilis of unknown duration) in all age groups.

For the treatment of neurosyphilis and otic or ocular syphilis, CDC and other clinicians state that IV penicillin G potassium or sodium is the drug of choice and IM penicillin G procaine (with oral probenecid) is an alternative if compliance can be ensured.

For the treatment of congenital syphilis, CDC recommends IV penicillin G potassium or sodium or IM penicillin G procaine in neonates with proven or highly probable congenital syphilis (i.e., abnormal physical examination consistent with congenital syphilis, serum quantitative nontreponemal serologic titer fourfold higher than the mother's titer, or positive darkfield test or polymerase chain reaction [PCR] of lesions or body fluids). CDC recommends IV penicillin G potassium or sodium, IM penicillin G procaine, or IM penicillin G benzathine in neonates with possible congenital syphilis (i.e., normal physical examination and serum quantitative nontreponemal serologic titer no more than fourfold higher than the mother's titer and the mother received a recommended treatment regimen less than 4 weeks before delivery; the mother was not treated or was inadequately treated, including treatment with erythromycin or any regimen not included in CDC recommendations; or there is no documentation that the mother received treatment).

Neonates with human immunodeficiency virus (HIV) infection who have congenital syphilis and HIV-infected children, adolescents, or adults who have neurosyphilis or primary, secondary, early latent, late latent, or tertiary syphilis should receive the same treatment regimens as those without HIV infection. Because serologic nonresponse and neurologic complications may be more frequent in HIV-infected individuals, close follow-up is essential in those coinfected with syphilis and HIV. In addition, careful neurologic examinations are indicated in all HIV-infected patients coinfected with syphilis.

There are no proven alternatives to penicillin G for the treatment of congenital syphilis in infants and children with known or suspected penicillin hypersensitivity and no proven alternatives to penicillin G for the treatment of any stage of syphilis in pregnant women with penicillin hypersensitivity; therefore, CDC recommends desensitization and treatment with the appropriate penicillin G preparation.

Fixed combinations of penicillin G benzathine and penicillin G procaine (Bicillin® C-R, Bicillin® C-R 900/300) should not be used for the treatment of any form of syphilis; inadvertent use of one of these fixed-combination preparations may not provide the sustained serum concentrations of penicillin G required for treatment of syphilis and could increase the risk of treatment failure and neurosyphilis, especially in HIV-infected patients.

For additional information regarding treatment of syphilis, the current CDC sexually transmitted diseases treatment guidelines available at https://www.cdc.gov/std/syphilis/treatment.htm should be consulted.

Dosage and Administration

■ **Administration** Penicillin G procaine and fixed combinations containing penicillin G benzathine and penicillin G procaine are administered *only* by deep IM injection.

Special precaution should be taken to avoid inadvertent intravascular or intra-arterial administration of penicillin G procaine or fixed combinations of penicillin G benzathine and penicillin G procaine or injection into or near major peripheral nerves or blood vessels because this may result in severe and/or permanent neurovascular damage. (See Cautions: Adverse Effects.)

Fixed combinations containing penicillin G benzathine and penicillin G procaine must *not* be given IV or admixed with IV solutions because inadvertent IV administration of penicillin G benzathine has been associated with cardiorespiratory arrest and death.

IM Injection Penicillin G procaine and fixed combinations containing penicillin G benzathine and penicillin G procaine are provided in prefilled syringes and the appropriate dose should be administered undiluted according to the manufacturer's directions.

In adults, IM injections of penicillin G procaine or fixed combinations of penicillin G benzathine and penicillin G procaine generally should be made deeply into the gluteus maximus (upper outer quadrant of the buttock) or into the midlateral thigh. In neonates, infants, and small children, IM injections of these preparations should be given preferably into the midlateral muscles of the thigh.

IM injections of penicillin G procaine or fixed combinations of penicillin G benzathine and penicillin G procaine should be made at a slow, steady rate to avoid blockage of the needle.

When the fixed combination of penicillin G benzathine and penicillin G procaine (Bicillin® C-R) is used, the manufacturer states that the dose usually is given at a single session using multiple IM sites; alternatively, if compliance regarding the return visit is ensured, the total dose can be divided and half given on day 1 and half on day 3.

When repeated doses are given, IM injection sites should be varied. Repeated IM injection into the anterolateral thigh, especially in neonates and infants, should be avoided since quadriceps femoris fibrosis and atrophy may occur.

■ **Dosage** Dosage of penicillin G procaine usually is expressed in terms of penicillin G units, but also has been expressed as mg of penicillin G.

Dosage of the fixed combinations containing penicillin G benzathine and penicillin G procaine (Bicillin® C-R, Bicillin® C-R 900/300) usually is expressed in terms of the total (sum) of penicillin G units of penicillin G benzathine and penicillin G units of penicillin G procaine.

Pediatric Dosage **General Pediatric Dosage.** The American Academy of Pediatrics (AAP) states that the usual dosage of IM penicillin G procaine in neonates 28 days of age or younger is 50,000 units/kg once every 24 hours.

For the treatment of mild to moderate infections in pediatric patients beyond the neonatal period, AAP states that the usual dosage of IM penicillin G procaine is 50,000 units/kg daily given in 1 or 2 divided doses. AAP states that IM penicillin G procaine is inappropriate for the treatment of severe infections.

If the fixed combination of penicillin G benzathine and penicillin G procaine (Bicillin® C-R) is used in pediatric patients beyond the neonatal period, AAP recommends a single IM dose of 600,000 penicillin G units in those weighing less than 14 kg and a single IM dose of 900,000 to 1.2 million penicillin G units in those weighing 14–27 kg. If this fixed-combination preparation is used in those weighing 27 kg or more, AAP recommends a single dose of 2.4 million penicillin G units.

Staphylococcal Infections. If IM penicillin G procaine is used for the treatment of moderately severe skin and skin structure infections caused by susceptible staphylococci, the manufacturer recommends a dosage of 300,000 units daily in children weighing less than 27 kg and 600,000 to 1 million units daily in others. Because of the high incidence of resistant strains, in vitro culture and susceptibility testing should be performed when treating suspected staphylococcal infections.

Streptococcal Infections. If IM penicillin G procaine is used for the treatment of infections caused by *Streptococcus pyogenes* (group A β-hemolytic streptococci; GAS), such as moderately severe to severe upper respiratory tract infections, tonsillitis, scarlet fever, erysipelas, and skin and skin structure infections, the manufacturer recommends a dosage of 300,000 units daily for at least 10 days in children weighing less than 27 kg and 600,000 to 1 million units daily for at least 10 days in others.

If IM penicillin G procaine is used for the treatment of moderately severe, uncomplicated respiratory tract infections (pneumonia) caused by susceptible *S. pneumoniae*, the manufacturer recommends a dosage of 300,000 units daily in children weighing less than 27 kg and 600,000 to 1 million units daily in others.

If the fixed combination of penicillin G benzathine and penicillin G procaine (Bicillin® C-R) is used for the treatment of moderately severe to severe infections caused by susceptible *S. pyogenes* (e.g., upper respiratory tract infections, scarlet fever, erysipelas, skin and skin structure infections), the manufacturer recommends that children weighing less than 13.6 kg receive a single IM dose of 600,000 penicillin G units, those weighing 13.6–27.2 kg receive a single IM dose of 900,000 to 1.2 million penicillin G units, and those weighing more than 27.2 kg receive a single IM dose of 2.4 million penicillin G units. If this fixed-combination preparation is used for the treatment of moderately severe infections caused by susceptible *S. pneumoniae* (pneumonia, otitis media), the manufacturer recommends that pediatric patients receive an IM dose of 600,000 penicillin G units once every 2 or 3 days until the patient has been afebrile for 48 hours. Other penicillins are recommended for severe *S. pneumoniae* infections (e.g., pneumonia, empyema, bacteremia, pericarditis, meningitis, peritonitis, arthritis).

If the fixed combination of penicillin G benzathine and penicillin G procaine (Bicillin® C-R 900/300) is used for the treatment of moderately severe to severe infections caused by susceptible *S. pyogenes* (e.g., upper respiratory tract infections, scarlet fever, erysipelas, skin and skin structure infections), the manufacturer states that a single IM dose of 1.2 million penicillin G units usually is sufficient in pediatric patients. If this fixed-combination preparation is used for the treatment of moderately severe infections caused by susceptible *S. pneumoniae* (pneumonia, otitis media), the manufacturer recommends that pediatric patients receive an IM dose of 1.2 million penicillin G units once every 2 or 3 days until the patient has been afebrile for 48 hours. Other penicillins are recommended for severe *S. pneumoniae* infections (e.g., pneumonia, empyema, bacteremia, pericarditis, meningitis, peritonitis, arthritis).

Anthrax. If IM penicillin G procaine is used for inhalational anthrax (post-exposure) to reduce the incidence or progression of disease following exposure to aerosolized *Bacillus anthracis* spores, the manufacturer recommends that children receive 25,000 units/kg (up to 1.2 million units) every 12 hours. Because of the possible persistence of anthrax spores in lung tissue following an aerosol exposure, the US Centers for Disease Control and Prevention (CDC) and other experts recommend that the total duration of anti-infective prophylaxis should be at least 60 days. The manufacturer states that safety data for penicillin G procaine administered at the dosage recommended for inhalational anthrax (postexposure) supports a duration of 2 weeks or less, and clinicians must consider the risks versus benefits of administering IM penicillin G procaine for longer than 2 weeks or switching to an appropriate alternative anti-infective.

If IM penicillin G procaine is used for the treatment of mild, uncomplicated cutaneous anthrax caused by susceptible *B. anthracis* that occurs as the result of naturally occurring or endemic anthrax exposure, some experts recommend a dosage of 25,000–50,000 units/kg daily (single or 2 divided doses daily) in children weighing less than 20 kg. Although 3–10 days of anti-infective therapy may be adequate for the treatment of mild, uncomplicated cutaneous anthrax that occurs as the result of naturally occurring or endemic exposures to anthrax, some experts recommend a duration of 7–14 days. CDC and other experts state that anti-infectives should be continued for 60 days if cutaneous anthrax occurred as the result of exposure to aerosolized *B. anthracis* spores in the context of biologic warfare or bioterrorism since the possibility of inhalational anthrax would also exist. Although anti-infective therapy may limit the size of the cutaneous anthrax lesion and it usually becomes sterile within the first 24 hours of treatment, the lesion will still progress through the black eschar stage despite effective treatment.

For additional information on treatment of anthrax and recommendations for postexposure prophylaxis following exposure to anthrax spores, see Uses: Anthrax, in Ciprofloxacin 8:12.18.

Diphtheria. When IM penicillin G procaine is used as an adjunct to diphtheria antitoxin (not commercially available in the US, but may be available from CDC) for the treatment of diphtheria caused by *Corynebacterium diphtheriae*, the manufacturer recommends a dosage of 300,000–600,000 units daily. CDC recommends a 14-day regimen of IM penicillin G procaine given in a dosage of 300,000 units daily in those weighing 10 kg or less and 600,000 units daily in those weighing more than 10 kg for adjunctive treatment of diphtheria. Patients usually are no longer contagious 48 hours after initiation of anti-infective therapy. Eradication of *C. diphtheriae* should be confirmed 24 hours after completion of treatment by 2 consecutive negative cultures taken 24 hours apart.

If IM penicillin G procaine is used to eliminate the diphtheria carrier state in identified carriers of toxigenic *C. diphtheriae*, the manufacturer recommends a dosage of 300,000 units daily for 10 days. CDC and AAP recommend IM penicillin G benzathine if a penicillin G preparation is used for elimination of the diphtheria carrier state. Follow-up cultures should be obtained at least 2 weeks after treatment of diphtheria carriers; if cultures are positive, a 10-day course of oral erythromycin should be given and additional follow-up cultures obtained.

Syphilis. For the treatment of proven or highly probable congenital syphilis in neonates (see Uses: Syphilis), CDC states that IM penicillin G procaine should be given in a dosage of 50,000 units/kg once daily for 10 days. If more than 1 day of treatment is missed in such neonates, the entire course of treatment should be restarted. If IM penicillin G procaine is used in neonates with possible congenital syphilis (see Uses: Syphilis), CDC recommends a dosage of 50,000 units/kg once daily for 10 days.

CDC recommends that treatment of syphilis diagnosed in infants and children 1 month of age or older should be managed by a pediatric infectious disease specialist and that CSF should be examined in those with latent syphilis.

The manufacturer states that children older than 12 years of age with primary, secondary, or latent syphilis with a negative CSF test for syphilis may receive IM penicillin G procaine in a dosage of 600,000 units daily for 8 days (total dosage 4.8 million units) and those with tertiary or latent syphilis with a positive CSF examination or no CSF examination may receive 600,000 units of daily for 10–15 days (total dosage 6–9 million units). CDC and others state that IM penicillin G benzathine is the drug of choice for the treatment of primary, secondary, tertiary, and latent syphilis.

If IM penicillin G procaine is used as an alternative for the treatment of syphilis in adolescents 10–19 years of age, some experts state that those with early syphilis (primary, secondary, or early latent syphilis) can receive a dosage of 1.2 million units once daily for 10–14 days and those with late latent syphilis or syphilis of unknown duration can receive 1.2 million units once daily for 20 days.

Neonates with human immunodeficiency virus (HIV) infection who have congenital syphilis and HIV-infected children and adolescents with any stage of syphilis should receive the same treatment regimens recommended for those without HIV infection.

Fixed combinations of penicillin G benzathine and penicillin G procaine (Bicillin® C-R, Bicillin® C-R 900/300) should not be used for the treatment of any form of syphilis.

Adult Dosage

Staphylococcal Infections. If IM penicillin G procaine is used for the treatment of moderately severe to severe skin and skin structure infections caused by susceptible staphylococci, the manufacturer recommends that adults receive a dosage of 600,000 to 1 million units daily. Because of high incidence of resistant strains, in vitro culture and susceptibility testing should be performed when treating suspected staphylococcal infections.

Streptococcal Infections. If IM penicillin G procaine is used for the treatment of infections caused by susceptible *S. pyogenes* (group A β-hemolytic streptococci; GAS), such as moderately severe to severe upper respiratory tract infections, tonsillitis, pharyngitis, scarlet fever, erysipelas, and skin and skin structure infections, the manufacturer recommends that adults receive a dosage of 600,000 to 1 million units daily for at least 10 days.

The manufacturer states that bacterial endocarditis caused by extremely susceptible *S. pyogenes* may be treated with an IM penicillin G procaine dosage of 600,000 to 1 million units daily. AHA recommends IV penicillin G potassium or sodium if a penicillin G preparation is used for the treatment of endocarditis.

If IM penicillin G procaine is used for the treatment of moderately severe, uncomplicated respiratory tract infections (pneumonia) caused by susceptible *S. pneumoniae*, the manufacturer recommends that adults receive a dosage of 600,000 to 1 million units daily.

If the fixed combination of penicillin G benzathine and penicillin G procaine (Bicillin® C-R) is used for the treatment of moderately severe to severe infections caused by susceptible *S. pyogenes* (e.g., upper respiratory tract infections, scarlet fever, erysipelas, skin and skin structure infections), the manufacturer recommends that adults receive a single IM dose of 2.4 million penicillin G units. If this fixed-combination preparation is used for the treatment of moderately severe infections caused by susceptible *S. pneumoniae* (pneumonia, otitis media) in adults, the manufacturer recommends an IM dosage of 1.2 million penicillin G units given once every 2 or 3 days until the patient has been afebrile for 48 hours. Other penicillins are recommended for severe *S. pneumoniae* infections (e.g., pneumonia, empyema, bacteremia, pericarditis, meningitis, peritonitis, arthritis).

Anthrax. If IM penicillin G procaine is used for inhalational anthrax (post-exposure) to reduce the incidence or progression of disease following exposure to aerosolized *B. anthracis* spores, the manufacturer recommends that adults receive 1.2 million units every 12 hours. Because of the possible persistence of anthrax spores in lung tissue following an aerosol exposure, CDC and other experts recommend that the total duration of anti-infective prophylaxis should be at least 60 days. The manufacturer states that safety data for IM penicillin G procaine administered at the dosage recommended for inhalational anthrax (postexposure) supports a duration of 2 weeks or less, and clinicians must consider the risks versus benefits of administering penicillin G procaine for longer than 2 weeks or switching to an appropriate alternative anti-infective.

If IM penicillin G procaine is used for the treatment of mild, uncomplicated cutaneous anthrax caused by susceptible *B. anthracis* in adults, the manufacturer recommends a dosage of 600,000 to 1 million units daily. Some experts recommend that adults receive a dosage of 600,000 to 1.2 million units every 12–24 hours for the treatment of mild, uncomplicated cutaneous anthrax caused by susceptible *B. anthracis* that occurs as the result of naturally occurring or endemic exposure to anthrax. Although 3–10 days of anti-infective therapy may be adequate for the treatment of mild, uncomplicated cutaneous anthrax that occurs as the result of naturally occurring or endemic exposures to anthrax, some experts recommend a duration of 7–14 days. CDC and other experts state that anti-infectives should be continued for 60 days if cutaneous anthrax occurred as the result of exposure to aerosolized *B. anthracis* spores since the possibility of inhalational anthrax would also exist. Although anti-infective therapy may limit the size of the cutaneous anthrax lesion and it usually becomes sterile within the first 24 hours of treatment, the lesion will still progress through the black eschar stage despite effective treatment.

For additional information on treatment of anthrax and recommendations for postexposure prophylaxis following exposure to anthrax spores, see Uses: Anthrax, in Ciprofloxacin 8:12.18.

Diphtheria. When IM penicillin G procaine is used as an adjunct to diphtheria antitoxin (not commercially available in the US, but may be available from CDC) for the treatment of diphtheria caused by *C. diphtheriae*, the manufacturer recommends a dosage of 300,000–600,000 units daily. CDC recommends a 14-day regimen of IM penicillin G procaine given in a dosage of 600,000 units daily in those weighing more than 10 kg for adjunctive treatment of diphtheria. Patients usually are no longer contagious 48 hours after initiation of anti-infective therapy. Eradication of *C. diphtheriae* should be confirmed 24 hours after completion of treatment by 2 consecutive negative cultures taken 24 hours apart.

If IM penicillin G procaine is used to eliminate the diphtheria carrier state in identified carriers of toxigenic *C. diphtheriae*, the manufacturer recommends a dosage of 300,000 units daily for 10 days. CDC and AAP recommend IM penicillin G benzathine if a penicillin G preparation is used for elimination of the diphtheria carrier state. Follow-up cultures should be obtained at least 2 weeks after treatment of diphtheria carriers; if cultures are positive, a 10-day course of oral erythromycin should be given and additional follow-up cultures obtained.

Erysipeloid. If IM penicillin G procaine is used in the treatment of erysipeloid caused by *Erysipelothrix rhusiopathiae*, the manufacturer recommends a dosage of 600,000 to 1 million units daily.

Necrotizing Ulcerative Gingivitis. If IM penicillin G procaine is used for the treatment of moderately severe infections of the oropharynx caused by *Fusobacterium*, including Vincent's gingivitis and pharyngitis, the manufacturer recommends a dosage of 600,000 to 1 million units daily.

Rat-Bite Fever. For the treatment of rat-bite fever caused by *Streptobacillus moniliformis* (erythema arthriticum epidemicum, Haverhill fever) or *Spirillum minus* (sodoku), the manufacturer recommends that IM penicillin G procaine be given in a dosage of 600,000 to 1 million units daily. Although IM penicillin G procaine has been given in a dosage of 600,000 units every 12 hours for 10–14 days for the treatment of rat-bite fever, CDC and some clinicians state that IV penicillin G potassium or sodium is preferred.

Syphilis. The manufacturer states that adults with primary, secondary, or latent syphilis with a negative CSF test for syphilis may receive IM penicillin G procaine in a dosage of 600,000 units daily for 8 days (total dosage 4.8 million units) and that those with tertiary syphilis or latent syphilis with a positive CSF examination or no CSF examination may receive 600,000 units daily for 10–15 days (total dosage 6–9 million units). CDC and others state that IM penicillin G benzathine is the drug of choice for the treatment of primary, secondary, tertiary, and latent syphilis in adults.

If IM penicillin G procaine is used as an alternative for the treatment of syphilis in adults, some experts state that those with early syphilis (primary, secondary, or early latent syphilis) can receive a dosage of 1.2 million units once daily for 10–14 days and those with late latent syphilis or syphilis of unknown duration can receive 1.2 million units once daily for 20 days.

For the treatment of neurosyphilis in adults when compliance with the regimen can be ensured (see Uses: Syphilis), CDC recommends that IM penicillin G procaine be given in a dosage of 2.4 million units once daily for 10–14 days in conjunction with oral probenecid (500 mg every 6 hours for 10–14 days). Some clinicians recommend that the penicillin G procaine regimen be followed by a regimen of IM penicillin G benzathine (2.4 million units once weekly for up to 3 weeks).

HIV-infected adults with any stage of syphilis should receive the same treatment regimens recommended for those without HIV infection.

Fixed combinations of penicillin G benzathine and penicillin G procaine (Bicillin® C-R, Bicillin® C-R 900/300) should not be used for the treatment of any form of syphilis.

Yaws, Pinta, and Bejel. The manufacturer states that the usual dosage of IM penicillin G procaine for the treatment of yaws, pinta, or bejel is the same as that recommended for the corresponding stage of syphilis.

Fixed combinations of penicillin G benzathine and penicillin G procaine (Bicillin® C-R, Bicillin® C-R 900/300) should not be used for the treatment of yaws, pinta, or bejel.

Cautions

Adverse Effects

Adverse effects reported with penicillin G procaine are similar to those reported with other natural penicillins.

Serious and occasionally fatal hypersensitivity reactions, including anaphylaxis, have been reported with penicillins. Rash (maculopapular), exfoliative dermatitis, urticaria, laryngeal edema, fever, eosinophilia, other serum sickness-like reactions (e.g., chills, fever, edema, arthralgia, prostration), and anaphylaxis (including shock and death) have been reported with penicillin G. Fever and eosinophilia may frequently be the only reaction observed.

Jarisch-Herxheimer reactions have been reported in patients receiving IM penicillin G procaine for the treatment of syphilis.

Immediate toxic reactions to procaine have been reported rarely with IM penicillin G procaine, especially when a large single dose (4.8 million penicillin G units) was administered. These reactions may be manifested by mental disturbances (anxiety, confusion, agitation, depression, weakness, seizures, hallucinations, combativeness, fear of impending death) and usually are transient (lasting about 15–30 minutes). A small percentage of the population is hypersensitive to procaine, and sensitivity reactions to IM penicillin G procaine have been reported. (See Cautions: Precautions and Contraindications.)

Inadvertent intravascular administration (including inadvertent direct intra-arterial injection or injection immediately adjacent to arteries) of penicillin G procaine or fixed combinations of penicillin G benzathine and penicillin G procaine has resulted in severe neurovascular damage (e.g., transverse myelitis with permanent paralysis, gangrene requiring amputation of digits and more proximal portions of extremities, necrosis and sloughing at and surrounding the injection site). These severe effects have been reported following injections into the buttock, thigh, and deltoid areas. Other serious complications of suspected intravascular administration include immediate pallor, mottling, or cyanosis of the extremity (both distal and proximal to the injection site), followed by bleb formation or severe edema requiring anterior and/or posterior compartment fasciotomy in the lower extremity. These severe effects and complications have occurred most often in infants and small children.

For additional information on adverse effects reported with natural penicillins, see Cautions in the Natural Penicillins General Statement 8:12.16.04.

Precautions and Contraindications

Penicillin G procaine and fixed combinations of penicillin G benzathine and penicillin G procaine are contraindicated in patients hypersensitive to any penicillin or to procaine.

Penicillin G procaine shares the toxic potentials of the penicillins, including the risk of hypersensitivity reactions, and the usual precautions of penicillin therapy should be observed.

Prior to administration of penicillin G procaine or a fixed combination of penicillin G benzathine and penicillin G procaine, careful inquiry should be made concerning previous hypersensitivity reactions to penicillins, cephalosporins, or other allergens. There is clinical and laboratory evidence of partial cross-allergenicity among penicillins and other β-lactam antibiotics, including cephalosporins and cephamycins.

Hypersensitivity reactions to penicillins are more likely to occur in individuals with a history of penicillin hypersensitivity and/or a history of sensitivity to multiple allergens. Penicillin G procaine and fixed combinations of penicillin G benzathine and penicillin G procaine should be used with caution in individuals with a history of clinically important allergies and/or asthma.

If a hypersensitivity reaction occurs, the drug should be discontinued immediately and appropriate therapy instituted as indicated (e.g., epinephrine, corticosteroids, maintenance of an adequate airway and oxygen).

If use of penicillin G procaine or a fixed combination containing penicillin G procaine is being considered in a patient with a history of procaine sensitivity, a test dose of procaine (0.1 mL of a 1–2% solution of procaine) should be administered intradermally prior to IM administration of full doses of penicillin G procaine or a fixed combination containing penicillin G procaine. Development of erythema or a wheal, flare, or eruption at the intradermal test site indicates procaine sensitivity and the patient should *not* receive a preparation containing penicillin G procaine. If a hypersensitivity reaction to procaine occurs, it should be treated by usual methods; antihistamines may be beneficial and barbiturates may be indicated if seizures occur.

Special precaution should be taken to avoid IV, intravascular, or intra-arterial administration or injection of penicillin G procaine or fixed combinations containing the drug into or near major peripheral nerves or blood vessels since inadvertent intravascular or intra-arterial injection may produce severe and/or permanent neurovascular damage. In addition, inadvertent IV administration of preparations containing penicillin G benzathine has been associated with cardiorespiratory arrest and death. If evidence of compromise of blood supply occurs at or proximal or distal to the site of injection, an appropriate specialist should be consulted immediately.

Renal and hematologic systems should be evaluated periodically during prolonged therapy with penicillin G procaine or a fixed combination containing penicillin G benzathine and penicillin G procaine, particularly if high dosage is used. In such situations, use of penicillin G procaine for longer than 2 weeks may be associated with an increased risk of neutropenia and an increased incidence of serum sickness-like reactions.

For additional information on precautions associated with the use of penicillin G procaine, see Cautions: Precautions and Contraindications, in the Natural Penicillins General Statement 8:12.16.04.

Pediatric Precautions

Renal clearance of penicillin G may be delayed in neonates and young infants because of incompletely developed renal function.

Geriatric Precautions

Clinical studies of penicillin G procaine or penicillin G benzathine did not include sufficient numbers of patients 65 years of age or older to determine whether geriatric patients respond differently than younger patients. Other clinical experience has not identified differences in responses between geriatric and younger patients.

Penicillin G is substantially eliminated by the kidneys and the risk of adverse effects may be greater in those with impaired renal function. Because geriatric patients are more likely to have reduced renal function, dosage should be selected with caution, usually starting at the low end of the dosage range, and renal function monitoring may be useful.

Pregnancy and Lactation

Pregnancy Reproduction studies evaluating penicillin G in mice, rats, and rabbits have not revealed evidence of impaired fertility or harm to the fetus. Although experience with use of penicillins during pregnancy has not shown any evidence of adverse effects on the fetus, there are no adequate or controlled studies using penicillin G procaine in pregnant women.

Some clinicians state that IM penicillin G procaine is considered low risk and safe for use during pregnancy. The drug is included in the US Centers for Disease Control and Prevention (CDC) recommendations for the treatment of syphilis during pregnancy.

The manufacturers state that penicillin G procaine and fixed combinations containing penicillin G benzathine and penicillin G procaine should be used during pregnancy only when clearly needed.

Lactation Penicillin G is distributed into milk. Some clinicians state that IM penicillin G procaine usually is considered compatible with breast-feeding. The manufacturers and others state that penicillin G procaine and fixed combinations containing penicillin G benzathine and penicillin G procaine should be used with caution in nursing women.

Spectrum

Based on its spectrum of activity, penicillin G procaine is classified as a natural penicillin. For information on the classification of penicillins based on spectra of activity, see the Preface to the General Statements on Penicillins 8:12.16.

For specific information on the spectrum of activity of penicillin G and resistance to the drug, see the sections on Spectrum and on Resistance in the Natural Penicillins General Statement 8:12.16.04.

Pharmacokinetics

For additional information on the absorption, distribution, and elimination of penicillin G, see Pharmacokinetics in the Natural Penicillins General Statement 8:12.16.04.

■ **Absorption** Because penicillin G procaine is relatively insoluble, IM administration of the drug provides a tissue depot from which the drug is slowly absorbed and hydrolyzed to penicillin G. IM administration of penicillin G procaine results in serum concentrations of penicillin G that are generally more prolonged, but lower, than those attained with an equivalent IM dose of penicillin G potassium or sodium.

Following IM administration of a single dose of penicillin G procaine in adults or neonates, peak serum penicillin G concentrations are attained in 1–4 hours and the drug is usually detectable in serum for 1–2 days; however, penicillin G may be detectable in serum for up to 5 days (depending on the dose). In general, increasing the dose of penicillin G procaine to more than 600,000 units tends to prolong the duration of penicillin G serum concentrations rather than increase peak serum concentrations.

Following a single IM dose of a fixed combination containing 1.2 million penicillin G units (i.e., 600,000 units as penicillin G benzathine and 600,000 units as penicillin G procaine; Bicillin® C-R) in adults, peak blood penicillin G concentrations were 2.1–2.6 units/mL within 3 hours and blood concentrations averaged 0.75 units/mL at 12 hours, 0.28 units/mL at 24 hours, and 0.04 units/mL at 7 days.

Following a single IM dose of a fixed combination containing 1.2 million penicillin G units (i.e., 900,000 units as penicillin G benzathine and 300,000 units as penicillin G procaine; Bicillin® C-R 900/300) in patients weighing 45–64 kg, average blood penicillin G concentrations were 0.24 units/mL at 24 hours, 0.039 units/mL at 7 days, and 0.024 units/mL at 10 days after the dose.

In children weighing 11.9–22.6 kg, IM administration of a single dose of a fixed combination containing 1.2 million penicillin G units (900,000 units as penicillin G benzathine and 300,000 units as penicillin G procaine) resulted in peak serum penicillin G concentrations that occurred 1 hour after the dose and averaged 3.9 mcg/mL. Serum penicillin G concentrations in these children ranged from 2.5–5.5, 2.5–5.5, 0.7–3.7, and 0.17–0.48 mcg/mL at 1, 2, 4, and 24 hours, respectively, after the dose and from 0.08–0.12, 0.01–0.09, and 0–0.1 mcg/mL at 5, 10, and 18 days, respectively, after the dose.

In a study in neonates younger than 1 week of age with congenital syphilis who received a penicillin G procaine dosage of 50,000 units/kg IM once daily for 7 days, serum penicillin G concentrations averaged 7.4–8.8 mcg/mL 2–12 hours after a dose and 1.5 mcg/mL 24 hours after a dose in neonates younger than 1 week of age. In neonates older than 1 week of age who received the same dosage of penicillin G procaine, serum penicillin G concentrations averaged 5–6 mcg/mL during the first 4 hours after administration of a dose and 0.4 mcg/mL 24 hours after a dose. In another study in neonates who received a single IM penicillin G procaine dose of 50,000 units/kg, peak serum concentrations of penicillin G occurred 4 hours after the dose and ranged from 7.7–41.9 mcg/mL; serum concentrations of the drug ranged from 0.2–5.8 mcg/mL 24 hours after the dose.

■ **Distribution** Following IM administration of penicillin G procaine, penicillin G is widely distributed throughout the body in varying amounts. Highest concentrations generally are attained in the kidneys, with lower amounts in the liver, skin, and intestines.

Minimal concentrations of penicillin G are generally attained in CSF following IM administration of penicillin G procaine in patients with uninflamed meninges. Higher penicillin G concentrations are attained in CSF when the meninges are inflamed or when oral probenecid is administered concomitantly. The minimum treponemicidal concentration of penicillin G is generally defined as 0.03 units/mL or 0.02 mcg/mL. In one study, CSF concentrations of penicillin G were undetectable to 0.6% of concurrent serum concentrations in patients receiving IM penicillin G procaine in a dosage of 600,000 units once daily without probenecid; however, CSF concentrations of the drug were 2.1–6.6% of concurrent serum concentrations in patients receiving 600,000 units IM once daily with concomitant oral probenecid (500 mg every 6 hours). In a study in adults following IM administration of penicillin G procaine in a dosage of 2.4 million units once daily with oral probenecid (500 mg every 6 hours), CSF concentrations of penicillin G ranged from 0.12–0.6 mcg/mL in specimens obtained 3–3.5 hours after a dose on the third or fourth day of therapy. In another study in adults with syphilis who received IM penicillin G procaine in a dosage of 2.4 million units once daily with oral probenecid (500 mg every 6 hours), CSF penicillin G concentrations ranged from 0.07–1.5 mcg/mL in specimens obtained 2–10 hours after a dose on the second through ninth day of therapy; concurrent serum penicillin G concentrations ranged from 6.3–7.9 mcg/mL.

In a study in neonates younger than 3 days of age who received a single IM penicillin G procaine dose of 10,000 units/kg, penicillin G concentrations in CSF 4 hours after the dose averaged 0.06 mcg/mL and concurrent serum concentrations averaged 6.1 mcg/mL. IM administration of a single penicillin G procaine dose of 50,000 units/kg in these neonates resulted in CSF concentrations averaging 0.14 mcg/mL 4 hours after the dose and concurrent serum concentrations averaging 13.2 mcg/mL. In another study in neonates who received a single penicillin G procaine dose of 50,000 units/kg, peak CSF concentrations of penicillin G occurred 12 hours after the dose and ranged from 0.09–1.98 mcg/mL; CSF concentrations of the drug 24 hours after the dose ranged from 0.03–0.27 mcg/mL.

Penicillin G is about 60% bound to serum proteins.

Penicillin G crosses the placenta and is distributed into milk.

■ **Elimination** Following IM administration of penicillin G procaine, the drug is slowly absorbed and hydrolyzed to penicillin G and elimination of penicillin G in urine continues over a prolonged period of time. Penicillin G and its metabolites are excreted in urine mainly by tubular secretion.

Concurrent administration of oral probenecid increases and prolongs serum penicillin G concentrations by decreasing the apparent volume of distribution and slowing the rate of excretion by competitively inhibiting renal tubular secretion of penicillin.

The serum half-life of penicillin G may be prolonged in patients with impaired renal function.

Renal clearance of penicillin G is delayed in neonates and young infants.

Renal clearance of penicillin G may be increased in pregnant women during the second and third trimesters.

Chemistry and Stability

■ **Chemistry** Penicillin G procaine is a natural penicillin. The drug is the procaine monohydrate salt of penicillin G which is prepared by reacting equimolar amounts of penicillin G sodium or potassium and procaine hydrochloride. Penicillin G procaine is hydrolyzed in vivo to penicillin G and is frequently referred to as a long-acting, depot, or repository form of penicillin G.

Penicillin G procaine occurs as white crystals or a white, microcrystalline powder. The drug is slightly soluble in water. Potency of penicillin G procaine generally is expressed in terms of penicillin G units, but also has been expressed as mg of penicillin G.

Commercially available penicillin G procaine sterile suspension for injection is a viscous, opaque suspension of the drug in sterile water for injection. The IM suspension is buffered with sodium citrate and contains methylparaben and propylparaben as preservatives, povidone, lecithin, and carboxymethylcellulose.

Penicillin G procaine also is commercially available in fixed combination with penicillin G benzathine as a viscous, opaque, aqueous suspension for IM injection. Each 2 mL of fixed-combination suspension contains the equivalent of 1.2 million units of penicillin G in a formulation containing the equivalent of 600,000 units of penicillin G as the benzathine salt and 600,000 units of penicillin G as the procaine salt (Bicillin® C-R) *or* a formulation containing the equivalent of 900,000 units of penicillin G as the benzathine salt and 300,000 units of penicillin G as the procaine salt (Bicillin® C-R 900/300).

■ **Stability** Commercially available penicillin G procaine suspension for IM injection should be stored at 2–8°C; freezing should be avoided.

The fixed combinations of penicillin G benzathine and penicillin G procaine for IM injection should be stored at 2–8°C; freezing should be avoided.

For further information on chemistry and stability, mechanism of action, spectrum, resistance, pharmacokinetics, uses, cautions, drug interactions, laboratory test interferences, and dosage and administration of penicillin G procaine, see the Natural Penicillins General Statement 8:12.16.04.

Preparations

Excipients in commercially available drug preparations may have clinically important effects in some individuals; consult specific product labeling for details.

Penicillin G Procaine

Parenteral

Suspension, for IM Injection	600,000 units (of penicillin G) per mL*	**Penicillin G Procaine Suspension**

*available from one or more manufacturer, distributor, and/or repackager by generic (nonproprietary) name

Penicillin G Benzathine and Penicillin G Procaine

Parenteral

Suspension, for IM Injection	1.2 million units of penicillin G per 2 mL (600,000 units as penicillin G benzathine and 600,000 units as penicillin G procaine)	**Bicillin® C-R,** Pfizer
	1.2 million units of penicillin G per 2 mL (900,000 units as penicillin G benzathine and 300,000 units as penicillin G procaine)	**Bicillin® C-R 900/300,** Pfizer

Penicillin V Potassium

Penicillin Potassium Phenoxymethyl, Phenoxymethylpenicillin Potassium

■ Penicillin V, a natural penicillin, is a β-lactam antibiotic.

Uses

Penicillin V potassium is used for the treatment of mild to moderately severe upper respiratory tract infections caused by susceptible streptococci or mild skin and skin structure infections caused by susceptible streptococci or staphylococci and for prophylaxis of certain streptococcal infections.

For some infections, oral penicillin V is used after an initial response is obtained with parenteral penicillin G. Penicillin V should *not* be used for *initial* treatment of severe infections, including pneumonia, empyema, bacteremia, pericarditis, meningitis, or arthritis. In addition, the high incidence of staphylococci resistant to the drug should be considered.

For additional information on the uses of penicillin V potassium, see Uses in the Natural Penicillins General Statement 8:12.16.04.

■ **Pharyngitis and Tonsillitis** Penicillin V is a drug of choice for the treatment of pharyngitis and tonsillitis caused by *Streptococcus pyogenes* (group A β-hemolytic streptococci; GAS) and prevention of initial attacks (primary prevention) of rheumatic fever.

Selection of an anti-infective for the treatment of *S. pyogenes* pharyngitis and tonsillitis should be based on the drug's spectrum of activity, bacteriologic and clinical efficacy, potential adverse effects, ease of administration, patient compliance, and cost. No regimen has been found to date that effectively eradicates group A β-hemolytic streptococci in 100% of patients.

Because the drugs have a narrow spectrum of activity, are inexpensive, and generally are effective with a low frequency of adverse effects, the American Academy of Pediatrics (AAP), Infectious Diseases Society of America (IDSA), and American Heart Association (AHA) recommend a penicillin regimen (i.e., 10 days of oral penicillin V or oral amoxicillin or a single dose of IM penicillin G benzathine) as the treatment of choice for *S. pyogenes* pharyngitis and tonsillitis. Other anti-infectives (narrow-spectrum oral cephalosporins, oral macrolides, oral clindamycin) are recommended as alternatives in penicillin-allergic patients.

If signs and symptoms of pharyngitis recur shortly after initial treatment and presence of *S. pyogenes* is documented, retreatment with the original or an alternative anti-infective is recommended. Initial treatment failures may occur more frequently with oral penicillins than with IM penicillin G benzathine because of poor adherence to the oral regimen. Alternative regimens recommended for retreatment include a narrow-spectrum oral cephalosporin, oral clindamycin, oral fixed combination of amoxicillin and clavulanate, oral macrolide, or IM penicillin G benzathine.

If there are multiple, recurrent episodes of symptomatic pharyngitis within a period of several months to years, it may be difficult to determine whether these are true episodes of *S. pyogenes* infection or whether the patient is a long-term pharyngeal carrier of *S. pyogenes* who is experiencing repeated episodes of nonstreptococcal (e.g., viral) pharyngitis.

Treatment of asymptomatic chronic pharyngeal carriers of *S. pyogenes* is not usually indicated and these individuals should not receive repeated courses of anti-infective therapy. However, eradication of the carrier state may be desirable in certain situations (e.g., during a community outbreak of acute rheumatic fever, acute poststreptococcal glomerulonephritis, or invasive *S. pyogenes* infections; during an outbreak of *S. pyogenes* pharyngitis in a closed or partially closed community; when multiple episodes of documented symptomatic *S. pyogenes* pharyngitis are occurring within a family for many weeks despite appropriate treatment; when there is a personal or family history of acute rheumatic fever). In such situations, recommended regimens include oral clindamycin, oral fixed combination of amoxicillin and clavulanate, or oral rifampin used in conjunction with either IM penicillin G benzathine or oral penicillin V.

■ **Prevention of Rheumatic Fever Recurrence** Penicillin V is used as an alternative for prevention of recurrent attacks of rheumatic fever (secondary prophylaxis) in individuals who have had a previous attack of rheumatic fever.

IM penicillin G benzathine generally is considered the drug of choice for secondary prophylaxis of rheumatic fever because it ensures compliance; alternatives include oral penicillin V or oral sulfadiazine. Sulfadiazine is recommended when hypersensitivity precludes the use of a penicillin; however, a macrolide (azithromycin, clarithromycin, erythromycin) should be used in patients allergic to penicillins *and* sulfonamides. Even with optimal patient adherence, the risk of recurrence of rheumatic fever is higher in individuals receiving an oral prophylaxis regimen than in those receiving IM penicillin G benzathine.

AHA and AAP recommend long-term (continuous) secondary prophylaxis in patients who have been treated for documented acute rheumatic fever (even if manifested solely by Sydenham chorea) and in those with evidence of rheumatic heart disease (even after prosthetic valve replacement).

Prophylaxis should be initiated as soon as the diagnosis of rheumatic fever or rheumatic heart disease is made, although patients with acute rheumatic fever should first receive the usually recommended anti-infective treatment for *S. pyogenes* pharyngitis and tonsillitis (see Uses: Pharyngitis and Tonsillitis).

■ **Prevention of Invasive Pneumococcal Disease in Asplenic Individuals** Penicillin V is used for prevention of invasive *S. pneumoniae* disease in children with anatomic or functional asplenia† (e.g., congenital asplenia or polysplenia, splenectomy, sickle cell disease, thalassemia). AAP recommends that such prophylaxis be continued until at least 5 years of age in those with sickle cell disease and continued for at least 1 year after splenectomy in all age groups.

Penicillin V also is used for prevention of invasive *S. pneumoniae* disease in certain asplenic adults†. Some clinicians recommend that such prophylaxis be continued for at least 1–2 years after splenectomy in adults.

Asplenic infants, children, adolescents, and adults are at increased risk of fulminant septicemia, most commonly caused by *S. pneumoniae*. Age-appropriate vaccination against pneumococcal disease with pneumococcal 13-valent conjugate vaccine (PCV13) and pneumococcal 23-valent polysaccharide vaccine (PPSV23) is recommended in *all* asplenic individuals. AAP states that anti-infective prophylaxis for prevention of invasive pneumococcal disease is recommended for young children with anatomic or functional asplenia, regardless of vaccination status.

Although penicillin V usually is considered a drug of choice for prevention of pneumococcal infections in asplenic children, some experts recommend amoxicillin.

■ **Anthrax** Penicillin V has been recommended as an alternative for postexposure prophylaxis of anthrax† following exposure to *Bacillus anthracis* spores (inhalational anthrax). Ciprofloxacin or doxycycline are the initial drugs of choice for prophylaxis following suspected or confirmed exposure to aerosolized anthrax spores, including exposures that occur in the context of biologic warfare or bioterrorism. If penicillin susceptibility is confirmed, consideration can be given to changing prophylaxis to a penicillin (oral amoxicillin or penicillin V) in infants and children, pregnant or lactating women, or when the drugs of choice are not tolerated or not available; oral amoxicillin may be preferred, especially in infants and children.

Penicillin V is used for the treatment of mild, uncomplicated cutaneous anthrax† caused by susceptible *B. anthracis* that occurs as the result of naturally occurring or endemic exposure to anthrax. If cutaneous anthrax occurs in the context of biologic warfare or bioterrorism, the initial drugs of choice are ciprofloxacin or doxycycline. If penicillin susceptibility is confirmed, consideration can be given to changing treatment to a penicillin (oral amoxicillin or penicillin V) in infants and children, pregnant or lactating women, or when the drugs of choice are not tolerated or not available; oral amoxicillin may be preferred, especially in infants and children.

For additional information on recommendations for postexposure prophylaxis following exposure to anthrax spores and treatment of anthrax, see Uses: Anthrax, in Ciprofloxacin 8:12.18.

Dosage and Administration

■ **Reconstitution and Administration** Penicillin V potassium is administered orally.

Although the manufacturers state that penicillin V potassium may be given with meals, the drug generally should be administered in the fasting state (preferably 1 hour before meals). Maximum oral absorption is achieved when the drug is administered at least 1 hour before or 2 hours after meals.

Oral penicillin V potassium should *not* be used for initial treatment of severe infections and should *not* be relied on in patients with nausea, vomiting, gastric dilatation, cardiospasm, or intestinal hypermotility.

Penicillin V potassium powder for oral solution should be reconstituted at the time of dispensing by adding the amount of water specified on the bottle to provide a solution containing 125 or 250 mg of penicillin V per 5 mL. The water should be added to the powder for oral solution in 2 portions and the solution agitated vigorously immediately after each addition.

■ **Dosage** Dosage of penicillin V potassium is expressed in terms of penicillin V. Although dosage of the drug is usually expressed as mg of penicillin V, it may be expressed in terms of penicillin V units.

Potency of penicillin V potassium preparations containing 125, 250, or 500 mg of penicillin V is approximately equivalent to 200,000, 400,000, or 800,000 penicillin V units, respectively.

Pediatric Dosage **General Pediatric Dosage.** The American Academy of Pediatrics (AAP) states that the usual dosage of oral penicillin V for the treatment of mild to moderate infections in pediatric patients beyond the neonatal period is 25–75 mg/kg daily given in 3 or 4 divided doses.

Some clinicians recommend that children younger than 5 years of age receive oral penicillin V in a dosage of 125 mg 4 times daily and that those older than 5 years of age receive a dosage of 250–500 mg every 6 hours.

The manufacturers state that pediatric patients 12 years of age or older may receive the usual adult dosage of penicillin V. Some clinicians state that children older than 5 years of age may receive the usual adult dosage of the drug.

Pharyngitis and Tonsillitis. For the treatment of *Streptococcus pyogenes* (group A β-hemolytic streptococci; GAS) pharyngitis and tonsillitis and prevention of initial attacks (primary prevention) of rheumatic fever in children, AAP, American Heart Association (AHA), and Infectious Diseases Society of America (IDSA) recommend that oral penicillin V be given in a dosage of 250 mg 2 or 3 times daily for 10 days. Some experts recommend a dosage of 500 mg 2 or 3 times daily in children weighing more than 27 kg.

When used for the treatment of *S. pyogenes* pharyngitis and tonsillitis and prevention of initial attacks (primary prevention) of rheumatic fever in adolescents, oral penicillin V should be given in a dosage of 500 mg 2 or 3 times daily for 10 days or 250 mg 4 times daily for 10 days.

Although anti-infective treatment is not recommended for most individuals identified as chronic pharyngeal carriers of *S. pyogenes* (see Uses: Pharyngitis and Tonsillitis), IDSA states that a regimen of oral penicillin V given in a dosage of 50 mg/kg daily (up to 2 g daily) in 4 divided doses for 10 days used in conjunction with oral rifampin (20 mg/kg daily as a single dose [up to 600 mg daily] given during the last 4 days of penicillin V treatment) is an option when eradication of the carrier state is desirable.

Respiratory Tract Infections. If oral penicillin V is used for the treatment of mild community-acquired pneumonia (CAP) caused by susceptible *S. pyogenes* or for step-down treatment of CAP caused by *S. pyogenes* after initial parenteral treatment, IDSA recommends that children 3 months of age or older receive 50–75 mg/kg daily in 3 or 4 divided doses.

For the treatment of mild to moderate upper respiratory tract infections (including scarlet fever) caused by susceptible streptococci in adolescents 12 years of age or older, the manufacturers recommend that oral penicillin V be given in a dosage of 125–250 mg every 6–8 hours for 10 days.

For the treatment of mild to moderately severe respiratory tract infections (including otitis media) caused by susceptible *Streptococcus pneumoniae* in adolescents 12 years of age or older, the manufacturers recommend that oral penicillin V be given in a dosage of 250–500 mg every 6 hours until the patient has been afebrile for at least 2 days.

Skin and Skin Structure Infections. For the treatment of mild to moderate erysipelas caused by susceptible streptococci in adolescents 12 years of age or older, the manufacturers recommend that oral penicillin V be given in a dosage of 125–250 mg every 6–8 hours for 10 days.

If oral penicillin V is used for the treatment of mild skin or skin structure infections caused by susceptible non-penicillinase-producing staphylococci in adolescents 12 years of age or older, the manufacturers recommend a dosage of 250–500 mg every 6–8 hours. Because of the high incidence of resistant strains, in vitro culture and susceptibility testing should be performed when treating suspected staphylococcal infections.

Necrotizing Ulcerative Gingivitis. If oral penicillin V is used for the treatment of mild to moderate infections of the oropharynx caused by *Fusobacterium*, including acute necrotizing ulcerative gingivitis (Vincent's infection, trench mouth, *Fusobacterium* gingivitis or pharyngitis), in adolescents 12 years of age or older, the manufacturers recommend a dosage of 250–500 mg every 6–8 hours.

Prevention of Rheumatic Fever Recurrence. For prevention of recurrent rheumatic fever (secondary prophylaxis), AAP and AHA recommend that children receive oral penicillin V in a dosage of 250 mg twice daily. The manufacturers recommend that adolescents 12 years of age or older receive oral penicillin V in a dosage of 125–250 mg twice daily for such prophylaxis.

Prevention of recurrent rheumatic fever requires long-term, continuous prophylaxis. (See Table 1.) Some clinicians use IM penicillin G benzathine initially and change to oral prophylaxis (usually with oral penicillin V) when the patient reaches late adolescence or young adulthood and has remained free of rheumatic attacks for at least 5 years.

Table 1. Recommended Duration of Prophylaxis for Prevention of Rheumatic Fever Recurrence

Patient Category	Duration
Rheumatic fever without carditis	5 years since last episode or until 21 years of age, whichever is longer
Rheumatic fever with carditis but no residual heart disease (no valvular disease)	10 years since last episode or until 21 years of age, whichever is longer
Rheumatic fever with carditis and residual heart disease (persistent valvular disease)	10 years since last episode or until 40 years of age, whichever is longer; sometimes for life

Prevention of Invasive Pneumococcal Disease in Asplenic Individuals. If oral penicillin V is used for prevention of invasive pneumococcal disease† in children with anatomic or functional asplenia, AAP recommends a dosage of 125 mg twice daily in those younger than 3 years of age and 250 mg twice daily in those 3 years of age or older.

In infants with sickle cell anemia, AAP recommends that penicillin V prophylaxis be initiated as soon as the diagnosis is established (preferably by 2 months of age). At 5 years of age, discontinuance of prophylaxis can be considered if the child is receiving regular medical attention, is fully immunized against pneumococcal disease, and has not had a severe pneumococcal infection or surgical splenectomy.

In children with asplenia from causes other than sickle cell anemia, the appropriate duration of prophylaxis is unknown. Some experts recommend that such children receive prophylaxis throughout childhood and into adulthood. AAP recommends that prophylaxis be continued for at least 1 year after splenectomy.

Anthrax. If oral penicillin V is used as an alternative for postexposure prophylaxis of anthrax† following exposure to aerosolized *Bacillus anthracis* spores in the context of biologic warfare or bioterrorism when penicillin-susceptible strains are involved, AAP recommends that infants and children 1 month of age or older receive 50–75 mg/kg daily given in divided doses every 6–8 hours. Because of the possible persistence of anthrax spores in lung tissue following an aerosol exposure, the US Centers for Disease Control and Prevention (CDC), AAP, and other experts recommend that the total duration of anti-infective prophylaxis should be at least 60 days.

If oral penicillin V is used for the treatment of mild, uncomplicated cutaneous anthrax† caused by penicillin-susceptible *B. anthracis* that occurs as the result of naturally occurring or endemic exposure to anthrax and when IV therapy is not considered necessary, the recommended dosage in children is 25–50 mg/kg daily given in 2 or 4 divided doses. For the treatment of cutaneous anthrax without systemic involvement† caused by penicillin-susceptible strains that occurs in the context of biologic warfare or bioterrorism, AAP recommends that infants and children 1 month of age or older receive oral penicillin V in a dosage of 50–75 mg/kg daily given in divided doses every 6–8 hours.

If oral penicillin V is used in full-term neonates as an alternative for post-exposure prophylaxis† following exposure to aerosolized *B. anthracis* spores in the context of biologic warfare or bioterrorism when penicillin-susceptible strains are involved or for the treatment of cutaneous anthrax† without systemic involvement caused by penicillin-susceptible strains that occurred in the context of biologic warfare or bioterrorism, AAP recommends a dosage of 75 mg/kg daily given in divided doses every 6–8 hours in those up to 1 week of age and 75 mg/kg daily given in divided doses every 8 hours in those 1–4 weeks of age. In preterm neonates (gestational age 32–37 weeks), AAP recommends a dosage of 50 mg/kg daily given in divided doses every 12 hours in those up to 1 week of age and 75 mg/kg daily given in divided doses every 8 hours in those 1–4 weeks of age.

Although 3–10 days of anti-infective therapy may be adequate for the treatment of mild, uncomplicated cutaneous anthrax that occurs as the result of naturally occurring or endemic exposures to anthrax, some experts recommend a duration of 7–14 days. CDC and other experts recommend that anti-infectives be continued for 60 days if cutaneous anthrax occurred as the result of exposure to aerosolized *B. anthracis* spores since the possibility of inhalational anthrax would also exist. Although anti-infective therapy may limit the size of the cutaneous anthrax lesion and it usually becomes sterile within the first 24 hours of treatment, the lesion will still progress through the black eschar stage despite effective treatment. It is not known whether infants and young children are at increased risk of disseminated, systemic disease and/or meningoencephalitis after focal anthrax infection. CDC has recommended that initial treatment of cutaneous anthrax in young children (i.e., younger than 2 years of age) in the context of biologic warfare or bioterrorism should be IV (not oral) and combination anti-infective therapy should be considered.

Rat-bite Fever. If oral penicillin V is used in children for the treatment of rat-bite fever† caused by *Streptobacillus moniliformis* after an initial response is obtained with IV penicillin G, a dosage of 25–50 mg/kg daily (up to 3 g daily) in 4 divided doses has been recommended.

Adult Dosage **Pharyngitis and Tonsillitis.** When used for the treatment of *S. pyogenes* (group A β-hemolytic streptococci; GAS) pharyngitis and tonsillitis and prevention of initial attacks (primary prevention) of rheumatic fever in adults, AHA and IDSA recommend that oral penicillin V be given in a dosage of 500 mg 2 or 3 times daily for 10 days or 250 mg 4 times daily for 10 days.

Although anti-infective treatment is not recommended for most individuals identified as chronic pharyngeal carriers of *S. pyogenes* (see Uses: Pharyngitis and Tonsillitis), IDSA states that a regimen of oral penicillin V given in a dosage of 50 mg/kg daily (up to 2 g daily) in 4 divided doses for 10 days used in conjunction with oral rifampin (20 mg/kg daily as a single dose [up to 600 mg daily] given during the last 4 days of penicillin V treatment) is an option when eradication of the carrier state is desirable.

Respiratory Tract Infections. For the treatment of mild to moderate upper respiratory tract infections (including scarlet fever) caused by susceptible streptococci in adults, the manufacturers recommend that oral penicillin V be given in a dosage of 125–250 mg every 6–8 hours for 10 days.

For the treatment of mild to moderately severe respiratory tract infections (including otitis media) caused by susceptible *S. pneumoniae* in adults, the manufacturers recommend that oral penicillin V be given in a dosage of 250–500 mg every 6 hours until the patient has been afebrile for at least 2 days.

Skin and Skin Structure Infections. For the treatment of mild to moderate erysipelas caused by susceptible streptococci in adults, the manufacturers recommend that oral penicillin V be given in a dosage of 125–250 mg every 6–8 hours for 10 days.

For the treatment of nonpurulent skin and skin structure infections (e.g., cellulitis) caused by susceptible streptococci in adults, IDSA recommends that oral penicillin V be given in a dosage of 250–500 mg every 6 hours.

If oral penicillin V is used for the treatment of mild skin or skin structure infections caused by susceptible non-penicillinase-producing staphylococci in adults, the manufacturers recommend a dosage of 250–500 mg every 6–8 hours. Because of the high incidence of resistant strains, in vitro culture and susceptibility tests should be performed when treating suspected staphylococcal infections.

Necrotizing Ulcerative Gingivitis. If oral penicillin V is used in adults for the treatment of mild to moderate infections of the oropharynx caused by *Fusobacterium*, including acute necrotizing ulcerative gingivitis (Vincent's infection, trench mouth, *Fusobacterium* gingivitis or pharyngitis), the manufacturers recommend a dosage of 250–500 mg every 6–8 hours.

Prevention of Rheumatic Fever Recurrence. For prevention of recurrent rheumatic fever (secondary prophylaxis), AHA recommends that oral penicillin

V be given in a dosage of 250 mg twice daily. The manufacturers recommend a dosage of 125–250 mg twice daily for such prophylaxis.

Prevention of recurrent rheumatic fever requires long-term, continuous prophylaxis. (See Table 2.)

Table 2. Recommended Duration of Prophylaxis for Prevention of Rheumatic Fever Recurrence

Patient Category	Duration
Rheumatic fever without carditis	5 years since last episode or until 21 years of age, whichever is longer
Rheumatic fever with carditis but no residual heart disease (no valvular disease)	10 years since last episode or until 21 years of age, whichever is longer
Rheumatic fever with carditis and residual heart disease (persistent valvular disease)	10 years since last episode or until 40 years of age, whichever is longer; sometimes for life

Anthrax. If oral penicillin V is used as an alternative for postexposure prophylaxis of anthrax† following exposure to aerosolized *B. anthracis* spores in the context of biologic warfare or bioterrorism when penicillin-susceptible strains are involved, CDC recommends that adults (including pregnant and postpartum women) receive a dosage of 500 mg every 6 hours. Because of the possible persistence of anthrax spores in lung tissue following an aerosol exposure, CDC and other experts recommend that the total duration of anti-infective prophylaxis should be at least 60 days.

If oral penicillin V is used for the treatment of mild, uncomplicated cutaneous anthrax† caused by penicillin-susceptible *B. anthracis* that occurs as the result of naturally occurring or endemic exposure to anthrax and when IV therapy is not considered necessary, the recommended dosage in adults is 500 mg 4 times daily, although some clinicians recommend 200–500 mg 4 times daily. For the treatment of cutaneous anthrax without systemic involvement† that occurs in the context of biologic warfare or bioterrorism, CDC recommends that adults (including pregnant and postpartum women) receive oral penicillin V in a dosage of 500 mg 4 times daily.

Although 3–10 days of anti-infective therapy may be adequate for the treatment of mild, uncomplicated cutaneous anthrax that occurs as the result of naturally occurring or endemic exposures to anthrax, some experts recommend a duration of 7–14 days. CDC and other experts recommend that anti-infectives be continued for 60 days if cutaneous anthrax occurred as the result of exposure to aerosolized *B. anthracis* spores since the possibility of inhalational anthrax would also exist. Although anti-infective therapy may limit the size of the cutaneous anthrax lesion and it usually becomes sterile within the first 24 hours of treatment, the lesion will still progress through the black eschar stage despite effective treatment.

Actinomycosis. If oral penicillin V is used for the treatment of actinomycosis† in adults after at least 2–6 weeks of initial treatment with IV penicillin G, a dosage of 2–4 g daily given in divided doses every 6 hours for 6–12 months is recommended.

If oral penicillin V is used for the treatment of mild cervicofacial actinomycosis†, a 2-month regimen of the drug may be adequate.

Rat-bite Fever. If oral penicillin V is used for the treatment of rat-bite fever† caused by *S. moniliformis* in adults after an initial response is obtained with IV penicillin G, a dosage of 500 mg every 6 hours has been recommended.

■ Dosage in Renal Impairment

Dosage adjustments are not usually necessary in patients with renal impairment. Some clinicians suggest increasing the dosing interval to every 8 hours in patients with creatinine clearance less than 10 mL/minute.

Cautions

■ Adverse Effects

Adverse effects reported with oral penicillin V potassium are similar to those reported with penicillin G.

The most common adverse effects reported in patients receiving oral penicillins are GI effects (e.g., nausea, vomiting, epigastric distress, diarrhea, black hairy tongue).

Serious and occasionally fatal hypersensitivity reactions, including anaphylaxis, have been reported with penicillins. Hypersensitivity reactions that have been reported with oral penicillins include rash (maculopapular), exfoliative dermatitis, urticaria and other serum sickness-like reactions, laryngeal edema, and anaphylaxis. Fever and eosinophilia may frequently be the only reaction observed.

For additional information on adverse effects reported with penicillin V potassium, see Cautions in the Natural Penicillins General Statement 8:12.16.04.

■ Precautions and Contraindications

Penicillin V potassium is contraindicated in individuals with known hypersensitivity to any penicillin.

Oral penicillin V potassium shares the toxic potentials of the penicillins, including the risk of hypersensitivity reactions, and the usual precautions of penicillin therapy should be observed.

Prior to initiation of therapy with penicillin V potassium, careful inquiry should be made concerning previous hypersensitivity reactions to penicillins, cephalosporins, or other allergens. There is clinical and laboratory evidence of partial cross-allergenicity among penicillins and other β-lactam antibiotics including cephalosporins and cephamycins.

Hypersensitivity reactions are more likely to occur in individuals with a history of penicillin hypersensitivity and/or a history of sensitivity to multiple allergens. Penicillins should be used with caution in individuals with a history of clinically important allergies and/or asthma.

If a hypersensitivity reaction occurs, penicillin V potassium should be discontinued immediately and appropriate therapy instituted as indicated (e.g., epinephrine, corticosteroids, maintenance of an adequate airway and oxygen).

Some penicillin V potassium oral solutions contain aspartame, which is metabolized in the GI tract to phenylalanine following oral administration. These penicillin V potassium oral solutions containing 125 or 250 mg of penicillin V per 5 mL contain 4.5 mg of phenylalanine per 5 mL. The aspartame content should be considered in individuals with phenylketonuria (i.e., homozygous genetic deficiency of phenylalanine hydroxylase) and other individuals who must restrict their intake of phenylalanine.

For additional information on precautions associated with the use of penicillin V potassium, see Cautions: Precautions and Contraindications, in the Natural Penicillins General Statement 8:12.16.04.

■ Pregnancy, Fertility, and Lactation

Pregnancy Available data regarding use of penicillin V in pregnant women, including first-trimester exposures, have not revealed evidence of an association between the drug and congenital defects.

Some clinicians state that penicillin V is considered low risk and safe for use during pregnancy.

Lactation Penicillin V is distributed into milk. Some clinicians state that oral penicillin V usually is considered compatible with breast-feeding; others state that the drug should be used with caution in nursing women.

Spectrum

Based on its spectrum of activity, penicillin V is classified as a natural penicillin. For information on the classification of penicillins based on spectra of activity, see the Preface to the General Statements on Penicillins 8:12.16.

The spectrum of activity of penicillin V is similar to that of penicillin G, but penicillin V is less potent than penicillin G against susceptible bacteria.

For specific information on the spectrum of activity of penicillin V and resistance to the drug, see the sections on Spectrum and on Resistance in the Natural Penicillins General Statement 8:12.16.04.

Pharmacokinetics

For additional information on the absorption, distribution, and elimination of penicillin V, see Pharmacokinetics in the Natural Penicillins General Statement 8:12.16.04.

■ Absorption

Approximately 60–73% of an oral dose of penicillin V (no longer commercially available in the US) or penicillin V potassium is absorbed from the GI tract in healthy, fasting adults. There is considerable interindividual variation in the extent of oral absorption of penicillin V; some patients may not absorb therapeutic concentrations of oral penicillins.

Following oral administration of a single dose of penicillin V or penicillin V potassium in fasting children or adults, peak serum concentrations of penicillin V are generally attained within 30–60 minutes. Peak serum penicillin V concentrations are attained sooner and are slightly higher following administration of the potassium salt than the free acid.

Following oral administration of a single 125-mg tablet of penicillin V potassium in healthy, fasting adults in one study, serum penicillin V concentrations averaged 1.2, 1.2, 0.5, and 0.1 mcg/mL at 30 minutes, 1 hour, 2 hours, and 4 hours, respectively, after the dose. Oral administration of a single 250-mg tablet of penicillin V potassium in healthy, fasting adults results in serum penicillin V concentrations averaging 2.1–2.8, 2.3–2.7, 0.8–0.9, and 0.1–0.2 mcg/mL at 30 minutes, 1 hour, 2 hours, and 4 hours, respectively, after the dose. Following oral administration of a single 500-mg tablet of penicillin V potassium in healthy, fasting adults, serum penicillin V concentrations average 4.7–5, 4.9–6.3, 2.3–3, and 0.04–0.1 mcg/mL at 30 minutes, 1 hour, 2 hours, and 6 hours, respectively, after the dose.

Variable results have been obtained in studies evaluating the effect of food on GI absorption of penicillin V and penicillin V potassium. In most studies, presence of food in the GI tract resulted in lower and delayed peak serum concentrations of penicillin V. If penicillin V is administered 1 hour before a meal, peak serum concentrations may be threefold higher and the total amount absorbed may be twofold higher compared with administration with food.

■ Distribution

Penicillin V is widely distributed into body tissues with highest concentrations attained in the kidneys and lower amounts in the liver, skin, and intestine. Penicillin V also is distributed into bile, tonsils, maxillary sinus secretions, saliva, and ascitic, synovial, pleural, and pericardial fluids.

Minimal concentrations of penicillin V generally distribute into CSF.

Penicillin V is approximately 75–89% bound to serum proteins.

Penicillin V readily crosses the placenta and is distributed into milk.

■ Elimination

The serum half-life of penicillin V in adults with normal renal function is reportedly 0.5 hours.

Approximately 35–70% of an oral dose of penicillin V or penicillin V potassium is metabolized to penicilloic acid which is microbiologically inactive. Small amounts of 6-aminopenicillanic acid (6-APA) have also been found in urine of patients receiving penicillin V. In addition, the drug appears to be hydroxylated to a small extent to one or more microbiologically active metabolites which are also excreted in urine.

Penicillin V and its metabolites are excreted in urine mainly by tubular secretion. Small amounts of the drug are also excreted in feces and bile.

Following oral administration of a single dose of penicillin V or penicillin V potassium in adults with normal renal function, 20–65% of the dose is excreted in urine as unchanged drug and metabolites within 6–8 hours; approximately 32% of the dose is excreted in feces.

Renal clearance of penicillin V is delayed in neonates and young infants and in individuals with impaired renal function.

Renal clearance of penicillin V may be increased in pregnant women during the second and third trimesters.

Chemistry and Stability

■ **Chemistry** Penicillin V is a natural penicillin produced by fermentation of *Penicillium chrysogenum* in a medium containing phenoxyacetic acid. Penicillin V is the phenoxymethyl analog of penicillin G and is commercially available as the potassium salt.

Although potency of penicillin V potassium generally is expressed in terms of mg of penicillin V, potency of the drug may be expressed in terms of penicillin V units. Potency of penicillin V potassium preparations containing 125, 250, or 500 mg of penicillin V is equivalent to 200,000, 400,000, or 800,000 penicillin V units, respectively.

Each tablet containing 250 mg of penicillin V as the potassium salt contains approximately 0.7 mEq (approximately 28 mg) of potassium; each tablet containing 500 mg of penicillin V as the potassium salt contains approximately 1.4 mEq (approximately 56 mg) of potassium. When reconstituted as directed, oral solutions of penicillin V potassium have a pH of 5–7.5.

■ **Stability** Commercially available penicillin V potassium tablets should be stored in a tight container at 20–25°C and protected from moisture.

Penicillin V powder for oral solution should be stored in a tight container at 20–25°C and protected from moisture. Following reconstitution, penicillin V potassium oral solutions should be refrigerated and any unused solution should be discarded after 14 days.

For further information on chemistry and stability, mechanism of action, spectrum, resistance, pharmacokinetics, uses, cautions, drug interactions, laboratory test interferences, and dosage and administration of penicillin V, see the Natural Penicillins General Statement 8:12.16.04.

Preparations

Excipients in commercially available drug preparations may have clinically important effects in some individuals; consult specific product labeling for details.

Penicillin V Potassium

Oral		
For solution	125 mg (of penicillin V) per 5 mL*	**Penicillin V Potassium for Oral Solution**
	250 mg (of penicillin V) per 5 mL*	**Penicillin V Potassium for Oral Solution**
Tablets	250 mg (of penicillin V)*	**Penicillin V Potassium Tablets**
	500 mg (of penicillin V)*	**Penicillin V Potassium Tablets**
Tablets, film-coated	250 mg (of penicillin V)*	**Penicillin V Potassium Tablets**
	500 mg (of penicillin V)*	**Penicillin V Potassium Tablets**

*available from one or more manufacturer, distributor, and/or repackager by generic (nonproprietary) name

†Use is not currently included in the labeling approved by the US Food and Drug Administration

AMINOPENICILLINS 8:12.16.08

Amoxicillin

p-Hydroxyampicillin

■ Amoxicillin is an aminopenicillin antibiotic that is structurally related to ampicillin.

Uses

Amoxicillin shares the uses of other aminopenicillins and is used principally for the treatment of infections caused by susceptible gram-negative bacteria (e.g., *Haemophilus influenzae, Escherichia coli, Proteus mirabilis, Salmonella*). Amoxicillin also is used for the treatment of infections caused by susceptible gram-positive bacteria (e.g., *Streptococcus pneumoniae*, enterococci, nonpenicillinase-producing staphylococci, *Listeria*); however, like other aminopenicillins, amoxicillin generally should not be used for the treatment of streptococcal or staphylococcal infections when a natural penicillin would be effective.

■ **Acute Otitis Media** Amoxicillin is used for the treatment of acute otitis media (AOM) caused by *S. pneumoniae, H. influenzae*, or *M. catarrhalis*. Amoxicillin usually is considered the drug of first choice for initial empiric treatment of AOM, unless the infection is suspected of being caused by β-lactamase-producing bacteria resistant to the drug, in which case the fixed

combination of amoxicillin and clavulanate potassium is recommended. The American Academy of Pediatrics (AAP), American Academy of Family Physicians (AAFP), US Centers for Disease Control and Prevention (CDC), and others state that, despite the increasing prevalence of multidrug-resistant *S. pneumoniae* and presence of β-lactamase-producing *H. influenzae* or *M catarrhalis* in many communities, amoxicillin remains the anti-infective of first choice for treatment of uncomplicated AOM since it is highly effective, has a narrow spectrum of activity, is well distributed into middle ear fluid, is well tolerated, has an acceptable taste, and is inexpensive. Amoxicillin (when given in a dosage of 80–90 mg/kg daily) usually is effective in the treatment of AOM caused by *S. pneumoniae*, including infections involving strains with intermediate resistance to penicillins, and also usually is effective in the treatment of AOM caused by most strains of *H. influenzae*.

AAP, AAFP, and others recommend that patients who fail to respond to an initial amoxicillin regimen (given in a dosage of 80–90 mg/kg daily) should be retreated using a regimen of amoxicillin and clavulanate potassium (90 mg/kg of amoxicillin and 6.4 mg/kg of clavulanate daily).

For additional information regarding treatment of AOM, including information on diagnosis and management strategies, anti-infectives for initial treatment, duration of initial treatment, and anti-infectives for retreatment and for information on current recommendations regarding management of otitis media with effusion (OME), see Uses: Otitis Media, in the Aminopenicillins General Statement 8:12.16.08.

■ **Anthrax** Amoxicillin is used as an alternative for *postexposure prophylaxis of anthrax*† following exposure to *Bacillus anthracis* spores, for the treatment of anthrax† when a parenteral regimen is not available (e.g., when there are supply or logistic problems because large numbers of individuals require treatment in a mass casualty setting), and for the treatment of cutaneous anthrax†. Strains of *B. anthracis* with naturally occurring penicillin resistance have been reported rarely, and there are published reports of *B. anthracis* strains that have been engineered to have penicillin and tetracycline resistance as well as resistance to other anti-infectives (e.g., macrolides, chloramphenicol, rifampin). Therefore, it has been postulated that exposures to *B. anthracis* that occur in the context of biologic warfare or bioterrorism may involve bioengineered resistant strains and this concern should be considered when selecting initial therapy for the treatment of anthrax that occurs as the result of bioterrorism-related exposures or for postexposure prophylaxis following such exposures. For additional information on treatment of anthrax and recommendations for postexposure prophylaxis following exposure to anthrax spores, see Uses: Anthrax, in Ciprofloxacin 8:12.18.

Postexposure Prophylaxis Ciprofloxacin or doxycycline generally are considered the initial drugs of choice for postexposure prophylaxis following suspected or confirmed exposure to aerosolized *B. anthracis* spores that occurs in the context of biologic warfare or bioterrorism. If exposure is confirmed and results of in vitro testing indicate that the organism is susceptible to penicillin, then postexposure prophylaxis may be switched to a penicillin (e.g., oral amoxicillin, oral penicillin V). IM penicillin G procaine also has been recommended as an alternative for postexposure prophylaxis. Although monotherapy with a penicillin is not recommended for the treatment of clinically apparent inhalational anthrax when high concentrations of the organism are likely to be present, penicillins may be considered an option for anti-infective prophylaxis when ciprofloxacin and doxycycline are contraindicated, since the likelihood of β-lactamase induction resulting in an increase in penicillin MICs is lower when only a small number of vegetative cells are present.

Although CDC and other experts recommend that postexposure prophylaxis in children be initiated with ciprofloxacin or doxycycline, if exposure has been confirmed and in vitro tests indicate that the organism is susceptible to penicillin, the postexposure prophylaxis regimen in children may be switched to oral amoxicillin or oral penicillin V.

The possible benefits of postexposure prophylaxis against anthrax should be weighed against the possible risks to the fetus when choosing an anti-infective for postexposure prophylaxis in pregnant women. CDC and other experts state that ciprofloxacin should be considered the drug of choice for initial postexposure prophylaxis in pregnant women exposed to *B. anthracis* spores and that, if in vitro studies indicate that the organism is susceptible to penicillin, then consideration can be given to changing the postexposure regimen to amoxicillin. Women who become pregnant while receiving anti-infective prophylaxis should continue the existing regimen and consult with a healthcare provider or public health official to discuss whether an alternative regimen might be more appropriate.

Cutaneous Anthrax Although natural penicillins (e.g., oral penicillin V, IM penicillin G benzathine, IM penicillin G procaine) generally have been considered drugs of choice for the *treatment* of mild, uncomplicated cutaneous anthrax caused by susceptible strains of *B. anthracis* that occurs as the result of naturally occurring or endemic exposure to anthrax, CDC recommends use of oral ciprofloxacin or oral doxycycline for the treatment of cutaneous anthrax that occurs following exposure to *B. anthracis* spores in the context of biologic warfare or bioterrorism. Therapy may be changed to oral amoxicillin if results of in vitro susceptibility testing indicate that the organism is susceptible to the drug and the patient is improving. Use of a multiple-drug parenteral regimen is recommended for the initial treatment of cutaneous anthrax when there are signs of systemic involvement, extensive edema, or lesions on the head and neck.

For young children (i.e., younger than 2 years of age), CDC recommends that initial therapy for cutaneous anthrax should be IV rather than oral, and combination anti-infective therapy should be considered since it currently is not known whether infants and young children are at increased risk of systemic dissemination of cutaneous anthrax.

For more specific information on the uses of amoxicillin, see Uses in the Aminopenicillins General Statement 8:12.16.08.

For information on the uses of amoxicillin in fixed-ratio combinations with clavulanic acid, see Amoxicillin and Clavulanate Potassium 8:12.16.08.

Dosage and Administration

■ **Reconstitution and Administration** Amoxicillin trihydrate is administered orally. Amoxicillin has also been given IV as the sodium salt, but a parenteral dosage form of amoxicillin is currently not available in the US.

Amoxicillin may be administered orally without regard to meals. However, in studies evaluating the film-coated tablet containing 875 mg of amoxicillin, the tablet was administered at the start of a light meal.

The required dose of reconstituted amoxicillin oral suspension should be placed directly on the child's tongue for swallowing. Alternatively, the required dose of oral suspension may be added to formula, milk, fruit juice, water, or ginger ale and then administered immediately.

Amoxicillin powder for oral suspension should be reconstituted at the time of dispensing by adding the amount of water specified on the bottle to provide a suspension containing 125, 200, 250, or 400 mg of amoxicillin per 5 mL or 50 mg of amoxicillin per mL. After tapping the bottle to thoroughly loosen the powder for oral suspension, the water should be added to the powder in 2 portions and the suspension agitated well after each addition. The suspension should be agitated well just prior to administration of each dose.

■ **Dosage** Dosage of amoxicillin, which is available for oral use as the trihydrate, is expressed in terms of anhydrous amoxicillin.

General Adult Dosage The usual adult dosage of amoxicillin for the treatment of mild to moderate infections of the ear, nose, or throat; skin and skin structure; or genitourinary tract is 500 mg every 12 hours or 250 mg every 8 hours. A dosage of 875 mg every 12 hours or 500 mg every 8 hours should be used for the treatment of severe infections of the ear, nose, or throat; skin and skin structure; or genitourinary tract in adults. The usual adult dosage of amoxicillin for the treatment of mild, moderate, or severe lower respiratory tract infections is 875 mg every 12 hours or 500 mg every 8 hours.

A single 3-g oral dose of amoxicillin has been used effectively for the initial treatment of acute, uncomplicated urinary tract infections in nonpregnant women†.

General Pediatric Dosage When oral amoxicillin is used in neonates and infants 12 weeks of age or younger, the manufacturer states that a dosage up to 30 mg/kg daily can be given in divided doses every 12 hours.

The usual dosage of oral amoxicillin for pediatric patients 3 months of age or older for the treatment of mild to moderate infections of the ear, nose, throat, skin and skin structure, or genitourinary tract is 20 mg/kg daily in divided doses every 8 hours or 25 mg/kg daily in divided doses every 12 hours. The usual dosage of oral amoxicillin for pediatric patients 3 months of age or older for the treatment of mild, moderate, or severe lower respiratory tract infections or for the treatment of severe infections of the ear, nose, throat, skin and skin structure, or genitourinary tract is 40 mg/kg daily in divided doses every 8 hours or 45 mg/kg daily in divided doses every 12 hours.

When oral amoxicillin is used for the treatment of mild to moderate infections in children beyond the neonatal period, the American Academy of Pediatrics (AAP) recommends a dosage of 25–50 mg/kg daily given in 3 divided doses.

When oral amoxicillin is used for step-down therapy in the treatment of severe infections in children beyond the neonatal period, AAP recommends a dosage of 80–100 mg/kg daily given in 3 divided doses. For highly susceptible pathogens, AAP states that a dosage of 90 mg/kg daily given in 2 divided doses can be used.

Acute Otitis Media For the treatment of uncomplicated acute otitis media (AOM), the recommended dosage of oral amoxicillin is 80–90 mg/kg daily given in 2 or 3 divided doses†. The drug usually is given for 10 days, but the optimal duration of therapy is uncertain. AAP recommends that a 10-day regimen be used for the treatment of AOM in children younger than 2 years of age and in those with severe symptoms. For the treatment of mild to moderate AOM in older children, AAP states that 7- and 10-day regimens appear equally effective in those 2–5 years of age and a treatment duration of 5–7 days may be adequate in those 6 years of age or older.

Although amoxicillin has been given in a dosage of 40–45 mg/kg daily for 10 days for the treatment of AOM, AAP, AAFP, US Centers for Disease Control and Prevention (CDC), and others recommend use of the higher amoxicillin dosage. The higher amoxicillin dosage (80–90 mg/kg daily) is especially important in patients with AOM known or suspected of being caused by *Streptococcus pneumoniae* with reduced susceptibility to penicillins and in patients with a history of anti-infective treatment of AOM within the previous few months.

Pharyngitis and Tonsillitis For the treatment of pharyngitis and tonsillitis caused by *Streptococcus pyogenes* (group A β-hemolytic streptococci; GAS), the American Heart Association (AHA) and AAP recommend that oral amoxicillin be given in a dosage of 50 mg/kg (up to 1 g) once daily for 10 days. The Infectious Diseases Society of America (IDSA) recommends that oral amoxicillin be given in a dosage of 50 mg/kg (up to 1 g) once daily for 10 days or 25 mg/kg (up to 500 mg) twice daily for 10 days.

Gonorrhea and Associated Infections Some manufacturers state that adults and children weighing 40 kg or more may receive a single 3-g oral dose of amoxicillin for the treatment of acute, uncomplicated gonorrhea caused by susceptible nonpenicillinase-producing *N. gonorrhoeae.* and that children weighing less than 40 kg who are 2 years of age or older may receive a single 50-mg/kg (maximum 3 g) dose of oral amoxicillin given with a single 25-mg/kg (up to 1 g) oral dose of probenecid. However, penicillins are no longer included in CDC recommendations for the treatment of gonorrhea.

Chlamydial and Mycoplasmal Infections For the treatment of chlamydial urogenital infections during pregnancy, the recommended dosage of oral amoxicillin is 500 mg 3 times daily for 7–10 days.

Lyme Disease IDSA, AAP, and other clinicians consider amoxicillin a drug of choice for the treatment of early localized or early disseminated Lyme disease† associated with erythema migrans, in the absence of neurologic involvement or third-degree atrioventricular (AV) heart block. Amoxicillin is preferred for the treatment of early Lyme disease† in pregnant or lactating women and in children younger than 8 years of age.

For the treatment of mild Lyme carditis† manifested by first- or second-degree AV heart block, amoxicillin 500 mg 3 times daily for 14–21 days is recommended in adults; children younger than 8 years of age should receive amoxicillin 50 mg/kg daily in 3 divided doses (maximum dose: 500 mg).

For the treatment of Lyme arthritis† without associated neurologic disease, amoxicillin 500 mg 3 times daily for 28 days is recommended in adults; children should receive amoxicillin 50 mg/kg daily (maximum: 1.5 g daily). For the treatment of early localized or early disseminated Lyme disease† associated with erythema migrans in adults, amoxicillin 500 mg 3 times daily for 14–21 days is recommended; children younger than 8 years of age should receive amoxicillin 50 mg/kg daily (maximum: 1.5 g daily) in 3 divided doses. (See Lyme Disease in Uses: Spirochetal Infections, in the Aminopenicillins General Statement 8:12.16.08.)

Helicobacter pylori Infection For the treatment of *Helicobacter pylori* (formerly *Campylobacter pylori* or *C. pyloridis*) infection and duodenal ulcer disease (active or 1-year history of duodenal ulcer) in adults, the recommended dosage of amoxicillin is 1 g twice daily in combination with clarithromycin (500 mg twice daily) and lansoprazole (30 mg twice daily) for 14 days (triple therapy). When used in combination with clarithromycin (500 mg twice daily) and omeprazole (20 mg twice daily) for the treatment of *H. pylori* infection and duodenal ulcer disease (active or 1-year history of duodenal ulcer), the recommended dosage of amoxicillin is 1 g twice daily for 10 days (triple therapy). An additional 18 days of omeprazole monotherapy is recommended for ulcer healing and symptom relief in patients with an active duodenal ulcer at the time therapy is initiated.

For the treatment of *H. pylori* infection and duodenal ulcer disease (active or 1-year history of duodenal ulcer) in adults who are either allergic to or intolerant of clarithromycin or in whom resistance to clarithromycin is known or suspected, the recommended dosage of amoxicillin is 1 g 3 times daily in combination with lansoprazole 30 mg 3 times daily for 14 days (dual therapy).

When amoxicillin has been used in other multiple-drug regimens† for the treatment of *H. pylori* infection and peptic ulcer disease in combination with at least one other agent that has activity against *H. pylori*, oral dosages of 500 mg 3 or 4 times daily (or 1 g 2 or 3 times daily) generally have been used; higher dosages of amoxicillin in such regimens reportedly have not been associated with improved results. Studies in which *H. pylori* was eradicated successfully generally have employed regimens consisting of a bismuth salt (e.g., bismuth subsalicylate), a nitroimidazole anti-infective (e.g., metronidazole), and another anti-infective agent (e.g., amoxicillin, tetracycline) or combined therapy with a proton-pump inhibitor (e.g., lansoprazole, omeprazole) and 1 or 2 anti-infective agents (e.g., clarithromycin, amoxicillin).

In a limited number of children with *H. pylori*-associated peptic ulcer disease† (e.g., gastritis, duodenitis/ duodenal ulcer), oral amoxicillin 25–50 mg/kg daily in divided doses (e.g., 250–500 mg 3 times daily) has been administered as part of multiple-drug regimens that included a nitroimidazole anti-infective (e.g., metronidazole) and/or a bismuth salt (e.g., bismuth subsalicylate). Further study is needed to establish an optimal drug regimen for treatment of *H. pylori* infection in children.

Prevention of Bacterial Endocarditis If oral amoxicillin is used for prevention of bacterial endocarditis† in patients with certain cardiac conditions who are undergoing certain dental procedures or certain other procedures (see Prevention of Bacterial Endocarditis under Uses: Prophylaxis, in the Aminopenicillins General Statement 8:12.16.08), AHA recommends that adults receive a single dose of 2 g and that children receive a single dose of 50 mg/kg given 30–60 minutes prior to the procedure.

When selecting anti-infectives for prevention of bacterial endocarditis, the current recommendations published by AHA should be consulted.

Anthrax AAP recommends that infants and children 1 month of age or older receive oral amoxicillin in a dosage of 75 mg/kg daily (up to 1 g daily) given in divided doses every 8 hours if the drug is used as an alternative for postexposure prophylaxis of anthrax† following exposure to aerosolized *Bacillus anthracis* in the context of biologic warfare or bioterrorism when penicillin-susceptible strains are involved or is used as an alternative for treatment of cutaneous anthrax† without systemic involvement or treatment of inhalational anthrax† when these infections are caused by penicillin-susceptible strains.

CDC recommends that adults (including pregnant and postpartum women) receive oral amoxicillin in a dosage of 1 g every 8 hours if the drug is used as an alternative for postexposure prophylaxis of anthrax† in the context of biologic warfare or bioterrorism when penicillin-susceptible *B. anthracis* are involved or is used as an alternative for treatment of cutaneous anthrax† without systemic involvement when the infection is caused by penicillin-susceptible strains.

If oral amoxicillin is used as an alternative for postexposure prophylaxis of anthrax† or for the treatment of anthrax† when a parenteral regimen is not available (e.g., when there are supply or logistic problems because large numbers of individuals require treatment in a mass casualty setting), some experts (e.g., US Working Group on Civilian Biodefense) recommend that adults receive 500 mg 3 times daily and that children receive 80 mg/kg daily (maximum 1.5 mg daily) given in 3 divided doses at 8-hour intervals. Anti-infective postexposure prophylaxis should be continued until exposure to *B. anthracis* has been excluded. If exposure is confirmed, postexposure vaccination with anthrax vaccine (if available) may be indicated in conjunction with prophylaxis. Because of the possible persistence of anthrax spores in lung tissue following an aerosol exposure, CDC and other experts recommend that postexposure prophylaxis be continued for at least 60 days.

If oral amoxicillin is used as an alternative for the treatment of mild, uncomplicated cutaneous anthrax† caused by susceptible *B. anthracis*, some experts (e.g., US Working Group on Civilian Biodefense) recommend that adults receive 500 mg 3 times daily and that children receive 80 mg/kg daily (maximum 1.5 g daily) given in 3 divided doses at 8-hour intervals. CDC has recommended that cutaneous anthrax in infants and children younger than 2 years of age should be treated initially IV. Although 5–10 days of anti-infective therapy may be adequate for the treatment of mild, uncomplicated cutaneous anthrax that occurs as the result of natural or endemic exposures to anthrax, CDC and other experts recommend that therapy be continued for 60 days if the cutaneous infection occurred as the result of exposure to aerosolized anthrax spores since the possibility of inhalational anthrax would also exist. Anti-infective therapy may limit the size of the cutaneous anthrax lesion and it usually becomes sterile within the first 24 hours of treatment, but the lesion will still progress through the black eschar stage despite effective treatment.

■ Duration of Therapy The duration of amoxicillin therapy depends on the type and severity of infection and should be determined by the clinical and bacteriologic response of the patient. For most infections, except gonorrhea, therapy should be continued for at least 48–72 hours after the patient becomes asymptomatic or evidence of eradication of the infection has been obtained. Persistent infections may require several weeks of therapy. Amoxicillin usually is continued for 60 days for postexposure prophylaxis or treatment of inhalational or cutaneous anthrax in the context of biologic warfare or bioterrorism.

If amoxicillin is used in the treatment of infections caused by group A β-hemolytic streptococci, therapy should be continued for at least 10 days to decrease the risk of rheumatic fever and glomerulonephritis.

If amoxicillin is used in the treatment of chronic urinary tract infections, frequent bacteriologic and clinical appraisal is necessary during therapy and may be required for several months after therapy.

■ Dosage in Renal Impairment In patients with renal impairment, doses and/or frequency of administration of amoxicillin should be modified in response to the degree of renal impairment, severity of the infection, and susceptibility of the causative organisms. The manufacturer states that adults with severe renal impairment and creatinine clearances less than 30 mL/minute should not receive the commercially available film-coated tablets containing 875 mg of amoxicillin. The recommended dosage of amoxicillin for adults with creatinine clearances of 10–30 mL/minute is 250 or 500 mg every 12 hours, depending on the severity of the infection, and the recommended dosage for adults with creatinine clearances less than 10 mL/minute is 250 or 500 mg every 24 hours, depending on the severity of the infection.

Patients undergoing hemodialysis should receive 250 or 500 mg of amoxicillin every 24 hours, depending on the severity of the infection, and should receive an additional dose of the drug during and after each dialysis period.

The manufacturer states that data are insufficient to recommend dosage for pediatric patients with renal impairment.

Cautions

■ Adverse Effects Adverse effects reported with amoxicillin are similar to those reported with other aminopenicillins. For information on adverse effects reported with aminopenicillins, see Cautions in the Aminopenicillins General Statement 8:12.16.08.

■ Precautions and Contraindications Amoxicillin shares the toxic potentials of the penicillins, including the risk of hypersensitivity reactions, and the usual precautions of penicillin therapy should be observed. Prior to initiation of therapy with amoxicillin, careful inquiry should be made concerning previous hypersensitivity reactions to penicillins, cephalosporins, or other allergens. There is clinical and laboratory evidence of partial cross-allergenicity among penicillins and other β-lactam antibiotics including cephalosporins and cephamycins. Amoxicillin is contraindicated in patients who are hypersensitive to any penicillin.

Because a high percentage of patients with infectious mononucleosis have developed rash during therapy with aminopenicillins, amoxicillin probably should not be used in patients with the disease.

Individuals with phenylketonuria (i.e., homozygous genetic deficiency of phenylalanine hydroxylase) and other individuals who must restrict their intake of phenylalanine should be warned that the amoxicillin 200- and 400-mg chewable tablets contain aspartame which is metabolized in the GI tract to provide 1.82 or 3.64 mg of phenylalanine, respectively, following oral administration. Amoxicillin powder for oral suspension does not contain aspartame.

Renal, hepatic, and hematologic systems should be evaluated periodically during prolonged therapy with amoxicillin.

For a more complete discussion of these and other precautions associated with the use of amoxicillin, see Cautions: Precautions and Contraindications, in the Aminopenicillins General Statement 8:12.16.08.

■ Pregnancy and Lactation Safe use of amoxicillin during pregnancy has not been definitely established. There are no adequate or controlled studies using aminopenicillins in pregnant women, and amoxicillin should be used during pregnancy only when clearly needed. However, amoxicillin has been administered to pregnant women without evidence of adverse effects to the fetus. In addition, use of the drug is included in the US Centers For Disease Control and Prevention (CDC) recommendations for the treatment of chlamydial infections during pregnancy and CDC recommendations for the treatment of cutaneous anthrax or for postexposure prophylaxis following exposure to *Bacillus anthracis* spores.

Because amoxicillin is distributed into milk and may lead to sensitization of infants, the drug should be used with caution in nursing women. Because of its general safety in infants, CDC states that amoxicillin is an option for anti-infective prophylaxis in breast-feeding women when *B. anthracis* is known to be penicillin susceptible and there is no contraindication to maternal amoxicillin use.

Spectrum

Based on its spectrum of activity, amoxicillin is classified as an aminopenicillin. For information on the classification of penicillins based on spectra of activity, see the Preface to the General Statements on Penicillins 8:12.16.

Amoxicillin generally has the same spectrum of activity and the same level of activity against susceptible organisms as ampicillin; however, amoxicillin is more active in vitro on a weight basis than ampicillin against enterococci and *Salmonella* but less active than ampicillin against *Shigella* and*Enterobacter*. For specific information on the spectrum of activity of amoxicillin and resistance to the drug, see the sections on Spectrum and on Resistance in the Aminopenicillins General Statement 8:12.16.08.

Pharmacokinetics

For additional information on absorption of amoxicillin and for information on distribution and elimination of the drug, see Pharmacokinetics in the Aminopenicillins General Statement 8:12.16.08.

■ Absorption Amoxicillin is generally stable in the presence of acidic gastric secretions, and 74–92% of a single oral dose of the drug is absorbed from the GI tract. Amoxicillin is more completely absorbed from the GI tract than is ampicillin, and peak serum concentrations of amoxicillin are generally 2–2.5 times higher than those attained with an equivalent oral dose of ampicillin. As oral dosage of amoxicillin is increased, the fraction of the dose absorbed from the GI tract decreases only slightly and peak serum concentrations and areas under the serum concentration-time curves (AUCs) increase linearly with increasing dosage.

Peak serum concentrations are usually reached 1–2 hours after oral administration of amoxicillin capsules, film-coated tablets, chewable tablets, or oral suspension in fasting and nonfasting adults. Following oral administration of a single 250- or 500-mg dose of amoxicillin, peak serum concentrations range from 3.5–5 or 5.5–11 mcg/mL, respectively. In one study in healthy, fasting adults who received a single 500-mg oral dose of amoxicillin, serum concentrations of the drug averaged 3.3, 6.7, 9.3, 5.8, and 0.6 mcg/mL at 30 minutes, 1 hour, 2 hours, 3 hours, and 4 hours, respectively, after the dose. The manufacturer states that serum concentrations attained following administration of 125- or 250-mg chewable tablets are similar to those attained when the same dose is given as the oral suspension containing 125 or 250 mg of the drug per 5 mL. In healthy adults who received a single 400-mg dose of amoxicillin given as a 400-mg chewable tablet or the oral suspension containing 400 mg of the drug per 5 mL (dose given at the start of a light meal), peak serum concentrations were attained approximately 1 hour after the dose and averaged 5.18 or 5.92 mcg/mL, respectively, and AUC averaged 17.9 or 17.1 mcg•hr/mL, respectively.

In one study in children 4–45 months of age receiving amoxicillin oral suspension in a dosage of 15 mg/kg daily, serum amoxicillin concentrations ranged from 2.4–8.5, 1.9–11.3, 1.7–6.4, 0.17–1.9, and 0.14–3.3 mcg/mL at 30 minutes, 1 hour, 2 hours, 4 hours, and 6 hours, respectively, after a dose.

Although presence of food in the GI tract reportedly results in lower and delayed peak serum concentrations of amoxicillin, the total amount of drug absorbed does not appear to be affected.

Chemistry and Stability

■ Chemistry Amoxicillin is an aminopenicillin which differs structurally from ampicillin only in the addition of an hydroxyl group on the phenyl ring.

Amoxicillin is commercially available as the trihydrate. Potency of amoxicillin trihydrate is calculated on the anhydrous basis. Amoxicillin occurs as a white, practically odorless, crystalline powder and is sparingly soluble in water.

When reconstituted as directed, amoxicillin oral suspensions have a pH of 5–7.5.

Amoxicillin is commercially available for oral administration as capsules, film-coated tablets, chewable tablets, or powder for oral suspension. Amoxicillin also is commercially available for oral administration in fixed-ratio combinations with clavulanate potassium. (See Amoxicillin and Clavulanate Potassium 8:12.16.08.)

Each 125-, 200-, 250-, or 400-mg amoxicillin chewable tablet contains 0.0019 mEq (0.044 mg), 0.0005 mEq (0.0107 mg), 0.0037 mEq (0.085 mg), or 0.0009 mEq (0.0215 mg) of sodium, respectively. The 200- and 400-mg chewable tablets contain aspartame which is metabolized in the GI tract to provide 1.82 or 3.64 mg of phenylalanine, respectively, following oral administration.

■ **Stability** Amoxicillin capsules, 125- and 250-mg chewable tablets, and powder for oral suspension should be stored in tight containers at 20°C or lower; amoxicillin 200- and 400-mg chewable tablets and amoxicillin film-coated tablets should be stored in tight containers at 25°C or lower.

Following reconstitution, amoxicillin oral suspensions should preferably be refrigerated at 2–8°C, but refrigeration is not necessary and the suspensions are stable for 14 days at room temperature or 2–8°C.

For further information on chemistry and stability, mechanism of action, spectrum, resistance, pharmacokinetics, uses, cautions, drug interactions, laboratory test interferences, and dosage and administration of amoxicillin, see the Aminopenicillins General Statement 8:12.16.08.

Preparations

Excipients in commercially available drug preparations may have clinically important effects in some individuals; consult specific product labeling for details.

Amoxicillin (Trihydrate)

Oral		
Capsules	250 mg (of amoxicillin)*	Amoxicillin Capsules
	500 mg (of amoxicillin)*	Amoxicillin Capsules
For suspension	125 mg (of amoxicillin) per 5 mL*	Amoxicillin for Suspension
	200 mg (of amoxicillin) per 5 mL*	Amoxicillin for Suspension
	250 mg (of amoxicillin) per 5 mL*	Amoxicillin for Suspension
	50 mg (of amoxicillin) per mL*	Amoxicillin for Suspension
	400 mg (of amoxicillin) per 5 mL	Amoxil®, GlaxoSmithKline
Tablets, chewable	125 mg (of amoxicillin)*	Amoxicillin Chewable Tablets
	250 mg (of amoxicillin)*	Amoxicillin Chewable Tablets
Tablets, film-coated	500 mg (of amoxicillin)*	Amoxicillin Tablets
	875 mg (of amoxicillin)*	Amoxicillin Tablets

*available from one or more manufacturer, distributor, and/or repackager by generic (nonproprietary) name

Amoxicillin (Trihydrate) Combinations

4 Capsules, Amoxicillin (trihydrate) 500 mg (of amoxicillin) 2 Capsules, delayed-release (containing enteric-coated granules) Lansoprazole 30 mg (Prevacid®) 2 Tablets, film-coated, Clarithromycin 500 mg (Biaxin®) Filmtab® (with povidone and propylene glycol)	Prevpac®, Takeda

†Use is not currently included in the labeling approved by the US Food and Drug Administration

Selected Revisions September 2018,

Amoxicillin and Clavulanate Potassium

Amoxicillin and Clavulanic Acid, Amoxycillin and Clavulanate Potassium

■ Amoxicillin and clavulanate potassium is a fixed combination of amoxicillin trihydrate (an aminopenicillin antibiotic) and the potassium salt of clavulanic acid (a β-lactamase inhibitor); clavulanic acid synergistically expands amoxicillin's spectrum of activity against many strains of β-lactamase-producing bacteria.

Uses

Amoxicillin and clavulanate potassium is used orally for the treatment of lower respiratory tract infections, otitis media, sinusitis, skin and skin structure infections, and urinary tract infections caused by susceptible organisms. Amoxicillin and clavulanate potassium also has been used orally for the treatment of chancroid† and gonorrhea† caused by susceptible organisms.

Amoxicillin and clavulanate potassium is used principally for the treatment of infections caused by susceptible β-lactamase-producing strains of *Moraxella catarrhalis* (formerly *Branhamella catarrhalis*), *Escherichia coli*, *Haemophilus influenzae*, *Klebsiella*, and *Staphylococcus aureus*. Although amoxicillin and clavulanate potassium also may be effective in the treatment of infections caused by non-β-lactamase-producing organisms susceptible to amoxicillin alone, most clinicians state that an aminopenicillin used alone is preferred to the combination drug for the treatment of these infections and that amoxicillin and clavulanate potassium should be reserved for use in the treatment of infections caused by, or suspected of being caused by, β-lactamase-producing organisms when an aminopenicillin alone would be ineffective.

Prior to initiation of therapy with amoxicillin and clavulanate potassium, appropriate specimens should be obtained for identification of the causative organism and in vitro susceptibility tests. Amoxicillin and clavulanate potassium therapy may be started pending results of susceptibility tests if the infection is believed to be caused by β-lactamase-producing bacteria susceptible to the drug, but should be discontinued if the organism is found to be resistant to the drug. (See Spectrum: In Vitro Susceptibility Testing.) If the infection is found to be caused by non-β-lactamase-producing organisms susceptible to aminopenicillins, some clinicians suggest that therapy generally should be changed to an aminopenicillin alone, unless this is impractical.

■ **Gram-positive Aerobic Bacterial Infections** Amoxicillin and clavulanate potassium has been effective when used orally in adults and children for the treatment of abscesses, cellulitis, and impetigo caused by susceptible penicillinase-producing and nonpenicillinase-producing *Staphylococcus aureus* and *S. epidermidis*, *Streptococcus pyogenes* (group A β-hemolytic streptococci), or *Corynebacterium*. Results of several controlled studies indicate that amoxicillin and clavulanate potassium is as effective as cefaclor in the treatment of these infections. However, natural penicillins are generally the drugs of choice for the treatment of infections caused by nonpenicillinase-producing staphylococci or group A β-hemolytic streptococci and penicillinase-resistant penicillins are generally the drugs of choice for the treatment of infections caused by susceptible penicillinase-producing staphylococci.

Amoxicillin and clavulanate potassium should not be used in the treatment of infections caused by methicillin-resistant staphylococci, even though results of in vitro susceptibility tests may indicate that the organism is susceptible to the drug.

■ **Gram-negative Aerobic Bacterial Infections** ***Haemophilus Infections*** Amoxicillin and clavulanate potassium generally has been effective when used in adults or children for the treatment of otitis media or upper and lower respiratory tract infections such as bronchopneumonia, sinusitis, and acute exacerbations of chronic bronchitis caused by susceptible *H. influenzae*. Amoxicillin and clavulanate potassium usually is the drug of choice for empiric anti-infective therapy of otitis media and sinusitis in communities with a high incidence of ampicillin-resistant *H. influenzae* or *M. catarrhalis* and for infections that fail to respond to other regimens. (See Uses: Acute Otitis Media.)

Chancroid Oral amoxicillin and clavulanate potassium (500 mg of amoxicillin and 125 or 250 mg of clavulanic acid every 8 hours for 7 days) has been effective when used in the treatment of chancroid† (genital ulcers caused by *H. ducreyi*); the mean time to complete healing of ulcers with amoxicillin and clavulanate potassium therapy has been 6.5–11.4 days and buboes have generally resolved within 4 weeks. However, amoxicillin and clavulanate potassium is not included in current US Centers for Disease Control and Prevention (CDC) guidelines for the treatment of chancroid; the CDC states that a single oral dose of azithromycin, a single IM dose of ceftriaxone, a 3-day regimen of oral ciprofloxacin, or a 7-day regimen of oral erythromycin are the regimens of choice for the treatment of chancroid.

Moraxella catarrhalis Infections Infections caused by β-lactamase-producing *M. catarrhalis* have been reported with increasing frequency. This organism recently has been recognized as a common cause of otitis media and maxillary sinusitis in children and of bronchitis and pneumonia in adults, especially those with chronic lung disease. Rarely, septicemia, endocarditis, urethritis, meningitis, neonatal ophthalmia, and conjunctivitis caused by *M. catarrhalis* have been reported. Amoxicillin and clavulanate potassium generally has been effective when used in the treatment of upper and lower respiratory tract infections caused by *M. catarrhalis*, and many clinicians consider it a drug of choice for infections caused by the organism.

Amoxicillin and clavulanate potassium generally has been effective when used for the treatment of acute otitis media or acute maxillary sinusitis caused by *M. catarrhalis*. In several controlled studies, amoxicillin and clavulanate potassium was more effective than cefaclor for the empiric treatment of acute otitis media in children 2 months to 12 years of age. Although adverse GI effects occurred more frequently with amoxicillin and clavulanate potassium than with cefaclor, amoxicillin and clavulanate potassium appears to be more active than cefaclor against β-lactamase-producing *M. catarrhalis*. Some clinicians suggest that amoxicillin and clavulanate potassium is a drug of choice for the empiric treatment of otitis media and sinusitis in communities with a high incidence of β-lactamase-producing *M. catarrhalis*.

Gonorrhea Amoxicillin and clavulanate potassium has been used orally with some success for the treatment of uncomplicated gonorrhea† caused by penicillinase-producing strains of *N. gonorrhoeae* (PPNG) or nonpenicillinase-producing strains of the organism. Regimens consisting of a single oral dose of amoxicillin (3 g) and clavulanic acid (125–500 mg) with or without oral probenecid (1 g) have been effective in some cases for the treatment of uncomplicated gonorrhea caused by PPNG or nonpenicillinase-producing *N. gonorrhoeae*. However, treatment failures have been reported when these single-dose regimens were used in the treatment of infections caused by PPNG, although, in some cases, in vitro tests indicated that the organism was susceptible to the drug. Penicillins, including amoxicillin and clavulanate potassium, are not included in current CDC recommendations for the treatment of gonorrhea.

Urinary Tract Infections Amoxicillin and clavulanate potassium has generally been effective when used orally in adults or children for the treatment of uncomplicated or complicated urinary tract infections (UTIs) caused by susceptible organisms including *E. coli*, *Klebsiella*, *Enterobacter*, or *P. mirabilis*. Although most strains of *Enterobacter* are resistant to amoxicillin and clavulanate potassium in vitro, the drug has been effective in some cases when used in the treatment of UTIs caused by this organism. Because amoxicillin and clavulanate potassium is active in vitro against many urinary pathogens resistant to aminopenicillins, some clinicians suggest that the combination drug may be preferred over ampicillin or amoxicillin alone for the initial treatment of UTIs; however, further studies are needed to evaluate the relative efficacy of amoxicillin and clavulanate potassium and other anti-infectives (e.g., co-trimoxazole) in the treatment of UTIs.

Other Gram-negative Aerobic Bacterial Infections Amoxicillin and clavulanate potassium has been used in the treatment of infections caused by *Eikenella corrodens*† or *Pasteurella multocida*†.

■ **Anaerobic and Mixed Aerobic-Anaerobic Bacterial Infections** Amoxicillin and clavulanate potassium has been used orally with some success in a limited number of patients for the treatment of anaerobic and mixed aerobic-anaerobic bacterial infections† including intra-abdominal and gynecologic infections such as endometritis, salpingitis, pelvic cellulitis, and acute pelvic inflammatory disease. Although oral amoxicillin and clavulanate potassium has been effective in the treatment of these infections, including infections caused by *Bacteroides fragilis*, some clinicians suggest that further study is needed to evaluate efficacy of the drug in the treatment of anaerobic and mixed aerobic-anaerobic bacterial infections and to determine if serum and tissue concentrations of amoxicillin and clavulanic acid obtained following oral administration of the drug are adequate for the treatment of these infections.

■ **Acute Otitis Media** Amoxicillin and clavulanate potassium is used for the treatment of acute otitis media (AOM) caused by *S. pneumoniae*†, *H. influenzae* (including β-lactamase-producing strains), or *M. catarrhalis* (including β-lactamase-producing strains). Amoxicillin usually is considered the drug of first choice for initial treatment of AOM, unless the patient has severe illness (moderate to severe otalgia or fever 39°C or higher) or the infection is suspected of being caused by β-lactamase-producing bacteria resistant to the drug, in which case amoxicillin and clavulanate potassium is recommended for initial treatment. The American Academy of Pediatrics (AAP), American Academy of Family Physicians (AAFP), CDC, and others state that, despite the increasing prevalence of multidrug-resistant *S. pneumoniae* and presence of β-lactamase-producing *H. influenzae* or *M. catarrhalis* in many communities, amoxicillin remains the anti-infective of first choice for treatment of uncomplicated AOM since it is highly effective, has a narrow spectrum of activity, is well distributed into middle ear fluid, is well tolerated, has an acceptable taste, and is inexpensive. Amoxicillin (when given in a dosage of 80–90 mg/kg daily) usually is effective in the treatment of AOM caused by *S. pneumoniae*, including infections involving strains with intermediate resistance to penicillins, and also usually is effective in the treatment of AOM caused by most strains of *H. influenzae*.

Alternatives for initial treatment of AOM in patients with a history of non-type I hypersensitivity reactions to penicillins include oral cephalosporins (cefdinir, cefpodoxime, cefuroxime axetil) or parenteral ceftriaxone. Alternatives for patients with type I penicillin hypersensitivity include oral macrolides (azithromycin, clarithromycin, fixed combination of erythromycin and sulfisoxazole), oral co-trimoxazole, or oral clindamycin (especially in those with infections known or presumed to be caused by penicillin-resistant *S. pneumoniae*).

Amoxicillin and clavulanate potassium (given in a dosage of 80–90 mg/kg of amoxicillin and 6.4 mg/kg of clavulanate daily) is the drug of choice for retreatment in patients who fail to respond to an initial amoxicillin regimen (given in a dosage of 80–90 mg/kg daily). The AAP and AAFP recommend that amoxicillin and clavulanate be substituted if there has been no response to amoxicillin within 48–72 hours. A 3-day regimen of IM or IV ceftriaxone also is recommended for retreatment, especially in those who have severe illness (moderate to severe otalgia or fever 39°C or higher) and in those who are vomiting or cannot otherwise tolerate an oral regimen.

For additional information regarding treatment of AOM, including information on diagnosis and management strategies, anti-infectives for initial treatment, duration of initial treatment, and anti-infectives for retreatment and for information on current recommendations regarding management of otitis media with effusion (OME), see Uses: Otitis Media, in the Aminopenicillins General Statement 8:12.16.08.

■ **Pharyngitis and Tonsillitis** Although not considered a drug of choice for the treatment of pharyngitis and tonsillitis caused by *S. pyogenes*† (group A β-hemolytic streptococci), amoxicillin and clavulanate potassium is recommended as one of several possible alternatives for the treatment of symptomatic patients who have multiple, recurrent episodes of pharyngitis known to caused by *S. pyogenes*†. Natural penicillins (i.e., 10 days of oral penicillin V or a single IM dose of penicillin G benzathine) is the treatment of choice for streptococcal pharyngitis and tonsillitis, although oral amoxicillin often is used instead of penicillin V in small children because of a more acceptable taste.

If there is recurrence of signs and symptoms of pharyngitis shortly after the initial recommended regimen is completed (i.e., within a few weeks) and presence of *S. pyogenes* is detected, retreatment with the original regimen or another regimen of choice is indicated; if compliance with a 10-day oral regimen is a concern, IM penicillin G benzathine should be used for retreatment. Some clinicians suggest use of an alternative agent (e.g., amoxicillin and clavulanate, clindamycin, macrolide) for retreatment. However, if there are multiple, recurrent episodes of symptomatic pharyngitis within a period of months to years, it may be difficult to determine whether these are true episodes of *S. pyogenes* infection or whether the patient is a long-term streptococcal pharyngeal carrier who is experiencing repeated episodes of nonstreptococcal pharyngitis (e.g., viral pharyngitis) in whom treatment is not usually indicated. Continuous anti-infective prophylaxis (secondary prophylaxis) to prevent the recurrence of streptococcal pharyngitis is not recommended in these circumstances, unless the patient has a history of rheumatic fever. Instead, use of an alternative regimen is recommended by some clinicians. Although there are no controlled clinical studies evaluating efficacy, the IDSA suggests that symptomatic individuals with multiple, recurrent episodes of documented *S. pyogenes* pharyngitis receive a regimen of oral amoxicillin clavulanate, oral clindamycin, or IM penicillin G benzathine (with or without oral rifampin).

For additional information on treatment of *S. pyogenes* pharyngitis, see Pharyngitis and Tonsillitis under Gram-positive Aerobic Bacterial Infections: Streptococcus pyogenes Infections in Uses in the Natural Penicillins General Statement 8:12.16.04.

Dosage and Administration

■ **Reconstitution and Administration** Amoxicillin and clavulanate potassium is administered orally. Chewable tablets should be thoroughly chewed before swallowing. Amoxicillin and clavulanate potassium has also been given IV, but a parenteral dosage form of the drug is not currently available in the US.

Because GI absorption of amoxicillin and clavulanate potassium is not affected by food following oral administration of conventional preparations of the drug, these preparations may be administered orally without regard to meals. However, administration of oral amoxicillin and clavulanate potassium with meals reportedly may minimize adverse GI effects. Extended-release tablets of the combination should be administered at the beginning of a meal to enhance GI absorption of amoxicillin and clavulanate and to minimize adverse GI effects; amoxicillin absorption from extended-release tablets is decreased when administered in a fasting state, and clavulanate absorption is decreased when these tablets are administered with a high-fat meal.

Amoxicillin and clavulanate potassium powder for oral suspension should be reconstituted at the time of dispensing by adding the amount of water specified on the bottle to provide a suspension containing 125 mg of amoxicillin and 31.25 mg of clavulanic acid per 5 mL, 200 mg of amoxicillin and 28.5 mg of clavulanic acid per 5 mL, 250 mg of amoxicillin and 62.5 mg of clavulanic acid per 5 mL, or 600 mg of amoxicillin and 42.9 mg of clavulanic acid per 5 mL. After tapping the bottle to thoroughly loosen the powder for oral suspension, the water should be added to the powder in 2 portions and the suspension agitated well after each addition. The suspension should be agitated well just prior to administration of each dose.

■ **Dosage** Dosage of amoxicillin and clavulanate potassium generally is expressed in terms of the amoxicillin content of the fixed combination. Although commercially available amoxicillin and clavulanate potassium contains amoxicillin as the trihydrate and/or the sodium salt and clavulanic acid as the potassium salt, potency of amoxicillin is calculated on the anhydrous basis and potency of clavulanate potassium is expressed in terms of clavulanic acid.

Amoxicillin and clavulanate potassium is commercially available for oral administration as a powder for oral suspension containing a 4:1, 7:1, or 14:1 ratio of amoxicillin to clavulanic acid; as chewable tablets containing a 4:1 or 7:1 ratio of the drugs; as film-coated tablets containing a 2:1 or 4:1 ratio of the drugs; as scored tablets containing a 7:1 ratio of the drugs; and as extended-release tablets containing a 16:1 ratio of the drugs.

Commercially available amoxicillin and clavulanate potassium powders for oral suspension should not be considered interchangeable since they contain different amounts of clavulanic acid. The powder for oral suspension containing 600 mg of amoxicillin and 42.9 mg of clavulanic acid per 5 mL (Augmentin ES-600®) is indicated only for the treatment of persistent or recurrent acute otitis media (AOM) in certain pediatric patients 3 months to 12 years of age; safety and efficacy of this preparation in younger children or in adolescents or adults have not been established. Because commercially available amoxicillin and clavulanate potassium film-coated tablets containing 250 mg of amoxicillin contain 125 mg of clavulanic acid and commercially available chewable tablets containing 250 mg of amoxicillin contain 62.5 mg of clavulanic acid, these preparations should not be considered interchangeable. In addition, since the 250- and 500-mg film-coated tablets of the drug both contain the same amount of clavulanic acid, two 250-mg film-coated tablets are not equivalent to one 500-mg film-coated tablet. Because extended-release tablets of amoxicillin and clavulanate potassium contain different ratios of the drugs, the extended-release tablets are not equivalent to conventional or chewable tablets of the drug.

Children weighing less than 40 kg should *not* receive the 250-mg film-coated tablets since this formulation contains a higher dose of clavulanic acid. (See Dosage: Pediatric Dosage, under Dosage and Administration.) Safety and efficacy of the extended-release tablets have not been established in pediatric patients younger than 16 years of age.

Adult Dosage The usual adult oral dosage of amoxicillin and clavulanate potassium is one 250-mg film-coated tablet (containing 250 mg of amoxicillin and 125 mg of clavulanic acid) every 8 hours or one 500-mg film-coated tablet (containing 500 mg of amoxicillin and 125 mg of clavulanic acid) every 12 hours. For more severe infections and infections of the respiratory tract, the usual adult oral dosage is one 500-mg film-coated tablet (containing 500 mg of amoxicillin and 125 mg of clavulanic acid) every 8 hours or one 875-mg scored tablet (containing 875 mg of amoxicillin and 125 mg of clavulanic acid) every 12 hours. Alternatively, adults who have difficulty swallowing tablets may receive the oral suspension containing 125 or 250 mg of amoxicillin/5 mL instead of the 500-mg film-coated tablet or may receive the oral suspension containing 200 or 400 mg of amoxicillin/5 mL instead of the 875-mg scored tablet.

The usual oral dosage of amoxicillin and clavulanate potassium extended-release tablets for the treatment of acute bacterial sinusitis in patients 16 years of age and older is 2 tablets (containing 1 g of amoxicillin and 62.5 mg of clavulanic acid in each tablet) every 12 hours for 10 days. The usual oral dosage of the extended-release tablets for the treatment of community-acquired pneumonia (CAP) in patients 16 years of age and older is 2 tablets (containing 1 g of amoxicillin and 62.5 mg of clavulanic acid in each tablet) every 12 hours for 7–10 days. Dosage adjustment for extended-release tablets of the combination based solely on age is not necessary in geriatric patients.

Pediatric Dosage Children weighing 40 kg or more may receive the usual adult oral dosage of amoxicillin and clavulanate potassium.

The usual dosage of amoxicillin and clavulanate potassium in neonates and infants younger than 12 weeks of age is 30 mg/kg of amoxicillin daily given in divided doses every 12 hours. Because experience with the oral suspension containing 200 mg of amoxicillin/5 mL is limited in this age group, the manufacturer recommends that the oral suspension containing 125 mg of amoxicillin/5 mL be used in neonates and infants younger than 12 weeks of age.

For the treatment of sinusitis, lower respiratory tract infections, and more severe infections in pediatric patients 12 weeks of age and older, the usual dosage of amoxicillin and clavulanate potassium is 45 mg/kg of amoxicillin daily in divided doses every 12 hours administered as the oral suspension containing 200 or 400 mg of amoxicillin/5 mL or as chewable tablets containing 200 or 400 mg of amoxicillin. Alternatively, these infections in this age group can be treated with a dosage of 40 mg/kg of amoxicillin daily in divided doses every 8 hours administered as the oral suspension containing 125 or 250 mg of amoxicillin/5 mL or as chewable tablets containing 125 or 250 mg of amoxicillin.

For the treatment of less severe infections in pediatric patients 12 weeks of age or older, the usual dosage of amoxicillin and clavulanate potassium is 25 mg/kg of amoxicillin daily in divided doses every 12 hours administered as the oral suspension containing 200 or 400 mg of amoxicillin/5 mL or as chewable tablets containing 200 or 400 mg of amoxicillin. Alternatively, less severe infections in this age group can be treated with a dosage of 20 mg/kg of amoxicillin daily in divided doses every 8 hours administered as the oral suspension containing 125 or 250 mg of amoxicillin/5 mL or as chewable tablets containing 125 or 250 mg of amoxicillin.

Acute Otitis Media For the treatment of acute otitis media (AOM) in pediatric patients, the recommended dosage of amoxicillin and clavulanate potassium is 90 mg/kg of amoxicillin and 6.4 mg/kg of clavulanate daily given in 2 divided doses†. The drug usually is given for 10 days, but the optimal duration of therapy is uncertain. The American Academy of Pediatrics (AAP) and American Academy of Family Physicians (AAFP) recommend that a 10-day regimen be used for treatment of AOM in children younger than 6 years of age and in those with severe disease, but that a duration of 5–7 days may be appropriate in those 6 years of age or older with mild to moderate AOM.

Although amoxicillin and clavulanate potassium can be administered in a dosage of 40–45 mg/kg of amoxicillin daily given in 2 or 3 divided doses for 10 days for the treatment of AOM, the AAP, AAFP, US Centers for Disease Control and Prevention (CDC), and others recommend use of the higher dosage. The higher dosage is especially important in patients with AOM known or suspected of being caused by *Streptococcus pneumoniae* with reduced susceptibility to penicillins, patients with primary treatment failure or persistent or recurrent AOM after treatment with amoxicillin, and in patients who have received anti-infective therapy within the previous few months.

When amoxicillin and clavulanate potassium is administered in the higher dosage for the treatment of AOM in pediatric patients, commercially available formulations containing a 7:1 or 14:1 ratio of amoxicillin to clavulanic acid should be used since these formulations provide a lower daily dosage of clavulanate potassium and minimize the risk of adverse GI effects associated with the clavulanate potassium component. When the oral suspension containing 600 mg of amoxicillin and 42.9 mg of clavulanic acid per 5 mL is used for the treatment of persistent or recurrent AOM in pediatric patients weighing less than 40 kg, the usual dosage is 90 mg/kg of amoxicillin daily given in divided doses every 12 hours for 10 days.

Pharyngitis and Tonsillitis If amoxicillin and clavulanate potassium is used for the treatment of symptomatic patients who have multiple, recurrent episodes of pharyngitis known to be caused by *Streptococcus pyogenes*† (group A β-hemolytic streptococci) (see Uses: Pharyngitis and Tonsillitis), the Infectious Diseases Society of America (IDSA) recommends that children receive 40 mg/kg of amoxicillin daily (maximum 750 mg daily) given in 3 equally divided doses for 10 days. Adults should receive amoxicillin and clavulanate potassium in a dosage of 500 mg of amoxicillin twice daily for 10 days; the IDSA states that this dosage has not been specifically studied in adults and was extrapolated from the pediatric dosage.

■ **Dosage in Renal and Hepatic Impairment** In patients with renal impairment, doses and/or frequency of administration of amoxicillin and clavulanate potassium should be modified in response to the degree of renal impairment. Some clinicians suggest that modification of usual dosage is unnecessary in adults with creatinine clearances greater than 30 mL/minute. These clinicians recommend that adults with creatinine clearances of 15–30 mL/minute receive the usual dose of conventional preparations of the drug every 12–18 hours, adults with creatinine clearances of 5–15 mL/minute receive the usual dose every 20–36 hours, and adults with creatinine clearances less than 5 mL/minute receive the usual dose every 48 hours. However, other clinicians suggest that use of amoxicillin and clavulanate potassium should be avoided in patients with creatinine clearances less than 30 mL/minute until more data are available on use of the drug in these patients.

Some clinicians suggest that adults undergoing hemodialysis receive a 500-mg tablet containing 500 mg of amoxicillin and 125 mg of clavulanic acid halfway through each dialysis period and an additional 500-mg tablet after each dialysis period.

The pharmacokinetics of extended-release tablets of amoxicillin and clavulanate potassium have not been studied in patients with renal impairment, and the manufacturer states that this preparation is contraindicated in patients with severe impairment (creatinine clearance less than 30 mL/minute and those undergoing hemodialysis). The extended-release tablets should be dosed cautiously in patients with hepatic impairment and liver function should be monitored at frequent intervals.

Cautions

■ **Adverse Effects** Adverse effects reported with amoxicillin and clavulanate potassium are generally dose related and are similar to those reported with amoxicillin alone. For information on adverse effects reported with amoxicillin and other aminopenicillins, see Cautions in the Aminopenicillins General Statement 8:12.16.08.

With the exception of adverse GI effects, which have been reported more frequently with amoxicillin and clavulanate potassium than with amoxicillin alone, the frequency and severity of adverse effects reported with the fixed-combination preparations are generally similar to those reported with amoxicillin alone. The manufacturers state that adverse effects reported with oral amoxicillin and clavulanate potassium are generally mild and transient and have required discontinuance of therapy in less than 3% of patients receiving the drug.

GI effects are the most frequent adverse reactions to oral amoxicillin and clavulanate potassium. Diarrhea or loose stools has been reported in about 9% of patients receiving the drug, and nausea and vomiting have been reported in 1–5% of patients. Abdominal discomfort, anorexia, and flatulence, dyspepsia, gastritis, stomatitis, glossitis, black or hairy tongue, and enterocolitis also have been reported. The frequency of nausea and vomiting appears to be related to the dose of clavulanic acid since these effects have been reported in up to 40% of patients when a 250-mg dose of clavulanic acid rather than a 125-mg dose was used in conjunction with amoxicillin. Administration of oral amoxicillin and clavulanate potassium with meals reportedly decreases the frequency and severity of adverse GI effects, and therefore patients should be advised to take the drug with a meal or snack.

Clostridium difficile-associated diarrhea and colitis (also known as antibiotic-associated pseudomembranous colitis) caused by toxin-producing clostridia may occur during or following discontinuance of amoxicillin and clavulanate potassium. Colitis may range in severity from mild to life-threatening. Mild cases of colitis may respond to discontinuance of the drug alone, but diagnosis and management of moderate to severe cases should include appropriate bacteriologic studies and treatment with fluid, electrolyte, and protein supplementation as indicated; rarely, cautious use of sigmoidoscopy (or other appropriate endoscopic examination) may be considered necessary. If colitis is severe or is not relieved by discontinuance of the drug, appropriate anti-infective therapy (e.g., oral metronidazole or vancomycin) should be administered.

Rash and urticaria have been reported in approximately 3% of patients receiving amoxicillin and clavulanate potassium. Other adverse effects that have been reported in 1% or less of patients receiving the drug include candidal vaginitis, dizziness, headache, fever, and slight thrombocytosis.

Moderate increases in serum concentrations of AST (SGOT) and/or ALT (SGPT), alkaline phosphatase, and/or bilirubin have been reported in patients receiving amoxicillin and clavulanate potassium. Hepatic dysfunction has been reported most frequently in geriatric patients, males, or in patients receiving prolonged therapy with the drug. Histologic findings on liver biopsies have consisted of predominantly cholestatic, hepatocellular, or mixed cholestatic-hepatocellular changes. The onset of manifestations of hepatic dysfunction may occur during or several weeks following discontinuance of amoxicillin and clavulanate potassium therapy and usually is reversible. However, fatal cholestatic hepatitis has been reported rarely; these generally have been cases associated with serious underlying diseases or concomitant drug therapy.

Although not reported to date with amoxicillin and clavulanate potassium, positive direct antiglobulin (Coombs') test results have been reported in patients who received therapy with ticarcillin and clavulanic acid. In one study in immunocompromised patients, positive direct antiglobulin test results occurred during 44% of the courses of therapy with ticarcillin and clavulanic acid and concomitant tobramycin. Positive reactions occurred within 48 hours after initiation of therapy and reverted to negative within 2–4 months after completion of therapy. These reactions appear to result from nonimmunologic adsorption of proteins onto erythrocytes in the presence of clavulanic acid; this nonimmunologic mechanism is similar to that observed with cephalosporins. Nonimmunologic adsorption of proteins onto erythrocyte membranes and positive direct antiglobulin test results also occurred in vitro when erythrocytes obtained from healthy individuals were exposed to clavulanic acid; however, exposure of erythrocytes to ticarcillin alone under various conditions did not result in a positive reaction.

■ **Precautions and Contraindications** Amoxicillin and clavulanate potassium shares the toxic potentials of the penicillins, including the risk of hypersensitivity reactions, and the usual precautions of penicillin therapy should be observed. Prior to initiation of therapy with amoxicillin and clavulanate potassium, careful inquiry should be made concerning previous hypersensitivity reactions to penicillins, cephalosporins, or other drugs. There is clinical and laboratory evidence of partial cross-allergenicity among penicillins and other β-lactam antibiotics including cephalosporins and cephamycins.

Renal, hepatic, and hematologic function should be evaluated periodically during prolonged therapy with amoxicillin and clavulanate potassium. Because *C. difficile*-associated diarrhea and colitis has been reported with the use of anti-infective agents including amoxicillin and clavulanate potassium, it should be considered in the differential diagnosis of patients who develop diarrhea during amoxicillin and clavulanate potassium therapy.

Because a high percentage of patients with infectious mononucleosis have developed rash during therapy with aminopenicillins, amoxicillin and clavulanate potassium should not be used in patients with the disease. Amoxicillin and clavulanate potassium is contraindicated in patients who are hypersensitive to any penicillin.

Commercially available amoxicillin and clavulanate potassium chewable tablets containing 200 or 400 mg of amoxicillin and amoxicillin and clavulanate potassium oral suspension containing 200, 400, or 600 mg of amoxicillin per 5 mL contain aspartame, which is metabolized in the GI tract to phenylalanine following oral administration. Individuals with phenylketonuria (i.e., homozygous genetic deficiency of phenylalanine hydroxylase) and other individuals who must restrict their intake of phenylalanine should be warned that each 200- or 400-mg chewable tablet of amoxicillin and clavulanate potassium provides 2.1 or 4.2 mg of phenylalanine, respectively, and each 5 mL of amoxicillin and clavulanate potassium oral suspension containing 200, 400, or 600 mg of amoxicillin provides 7 mg of phenylalanine. While these preparations should not be used in patients with phenylketonuria, other commercially available preparations of amoxicillin and clavulanate potassium do not contain aspartame.

For information on the potassium and sodium content of various amoxicillin and clavulanate potassium preparations, see Chemistry and Stability: Chemistry.

For a more complete discussion of these and other precautions associated with the use of amoxicillin, see Cautions: Precautions and Contraindications in the Aminopenicillins General Statement 8:12.16.08.

■ **Pediatric Precautions** Adverse effects reported in pediatric patients receiving amoxicillin and clavulanate potassium are similar to those reported in adults. In a clinical study in pediatric patients 2 months to 12 years of age with acute otitis media who received amoxicillin and clavulanate potassium oral suspension, the incidence of diarrhea was lower in those who received the drug in a dosage of 45 mg/kg of amoxicillin daily in divided doses every 12 hours than in those who received the drug in a dosage of 40 mg/kg of amoxicillin daily in divided doses every 8 hours. Diarrhea occurred in 14.3% of those receiving the twice-daily regimen and 34.3% of those receiving the 3-times-daily regimen, and 3.1% of those receiving the twice-daily regimen and 7.6% of those receiving the 3-times-daily regimen had severe diarrhea or were withdrawn from the study with diarrhea. It is not known whether a similar difference in the incidence of diarrhea occurs when amoxicillin and clavulanate potassium chewable tablets are administered in a twice-daily or 3-times-daily regimen.

Safety and efficacy of the extended-release tablets of amoxicillin and clavulanate potassium have not been established in pediatric patients younger than 16 years of age.

■ **Mutagenicity and Carcinogenicity** Studies have not been performed to date to evaluate the mutagenic or carcinogenic potential of amoxicillin and clavulanate potassium.

■ **Pregnancy, Fertility, and Lactation** Safe use of amoxicillin and clavulanate potassium during pregnancy has not been definitely established. However, oral amoxicillin and clavulanate potassium has been used in a limited number of pregnant women for the treatment of urinary tract infections or acute pelvic inflammatory disease† (PID) without evidence of adverse effects to the fetus. There are no adequate or controlled studies using amoxicillin and clavulanate potassium in pregnant women, and the drug should be used during pregnancy only when clearly needed.

Aminopenicillins are generally poorly absorbed when given orally during labor. Although the mechanism is unclear and the clinical importance has not been determined to date, studies using oral ampicillin indicate that, when administered during pregnancy, the drug interferes with metabolism and enterohepatic circulation of steroids resulting in decreased urinary concentrations of estrogen metabolites. The manufacturers state that this effect could also occur with amoxicillin and clavulanate potassium. IV administration of ampicillin to guinea pigs has decreased uterine tone and decreased the frequency, height, and duration of uterine contractions; however, it is not known whether use of amoxicillin and clavulanate potassium in humans during labor or delivery could have any immediate or delayed adverse effects on the fetus, prolong the duration of labor, or increase the likelihood of forceps delivery, other obstetrical intervention, or resuscitation of the neonate.

Reproduction studies in mice and rats using doses up to 10 times the usual human dose have not revealed evidence of impaired fertility or harm to the fetus.

Because amoxicillin and clavulanic acid are distributed into milk, amoxicillin and clavulanate potassium should be used with caution in nursing women.

Drug Interactions

■ **Probenecid** Oral probenecid administered shortly before or concomitantly with amoxicillin and clavulanate potassium slows the rate of renal tubular secretion of amoxicillin and produces higher and prolonged serum concentrations of amoxicillin. However, concomitant administration of probenecid with amoxicillin and clavulanate potassium does not affect the area under the serum concentration-time curve (AUC), half-life, or peak serum concentration of clavulanic acid.

■ **Allopurinol** Because an increased incidence of rash reportedly occurs in patients with hyperuricemia who are receiving allopurinol and concomitant amoxicillin or ampicillin compared with those receiving amoxicillin, ampicillin, or allopurinol alone, some clinicians suggest that concomitant use of the drugs should be avoided if possible. The manufacturers state that there are no data to date on concomitant administration of allopurinol and amoxicillin and clavulanate potassium.

■ **Disulfiram** Although the rationale is unclear, the US Food and Drug Administration has required the manufacturers to state in their labeling that amoxicillin and clavulanate potassium should not be used in patients receiving disulfiram. However, there is no evidence to date that concomitant use of the drugs would result in a disulfiram-like reaction, and the need for precaution when concomitant use of the drugs is considered has been questioned.

Laboratory Test Interferences

Ampicillin reportedly interferes with urinary glucose determinations using cupric sulfate (e.g., Benedict's solution, Clinitest®), but does not affect glucose oxidase methods (e.g., Clinistix®, Tes-Tape®). Since this laboratory test interference could also occur with amoxicillin, glucose oxidase methods should be used when urinary glucose determinations are indicated in patients receiving amoxicillin and clavulanate potassium.

Although not reported to date with amoxicillin and clavulanate potassium, positive direct antiglobulin (Coombs') test results have been reported in patients who received ticarcillin and clavulanic acid and appear to be caused by clavulanic acid. (See Cautions: Adverse Effects.) This reaction may interfere with hematologic studies or transfusion cross-matching procedures and should be considered in patients receiving amoxicillin and clavulanate potassium.

Mechanism of Action

Amoxicillin and clavulanate potassium usually is bactericidal in action. Concurrent administration of clavulanic acid does not alter the mechanism of action of amoxicillin. However, because clavulanic acid has a high affinity for and binds to certain β-lactamases that generally inactivate amoxicillin by hydrolyzing its β-lactam ring, concurrent administration of the drug with amoxicillin results in a synergistic bactericidal effect which expands the spectrum of activity of amoxicillin against many strains of β-lactamase-producing bacteria that are resistant to amoxicillin alone. For information on the mechanism of action of amoxicillin, see Mechanism of Action in the Natural Penicillins General Statement 8:12.16.04 and see Aminopenicillins General Statement 8:12.16.08.

In vitro studies indicate that clavulanic acid generally inhibits staphylococcal penicillinases, β-lactamases produced by *Bacteroides fragilis*, β-lactamases produced by *Moraxella catarrhalis* (formerly *Branhamella catarrhalis*), and β-lactamases classified as Richmond-Sykes types II, III (TEM-type), IV, and V. Clavulanic acid can inhibit some cephalosporinases produced by *Proteus vulgaris*, *Bacteroides fragilis*, and *Burkholderia cepacia* (formerly *Pseudomonas cepacia*), but generally does not inhibit inducible, chromosomally mediated cephalosporinases classified as Richmond-Sykes type I.

Clavulanic acid generally acts as an irreversible, competitive inhibitor of β-lactamases. The mechanism by which clavulanic acid binds to and inhibits β-lactamases varies depending on the specific β-lactamase involved. Because clavulanic acid is structurally similar to penicillins and cephalosporins, it initially acts as a competitive inhibitor and binds to the active site on the β-lactamase. An inactive acyl intermediate is then formed but it is only transiently inactive since the intermediate can be hydrolyzed, resulting in restoration of β-lactamase activity and release of clavulanic acid degradation products. With many types of β-lactamases, however, subsequent reactions occur that lead to irreversible inactivation of the β-lactamase.

Synergism does not generally occur between amoxicillin and clavulanic acid if resistance to aminopenicillins is intrinsic (i.e., results from the presence of a permeability barrier in the outer membrane of the organism or alterations in the properties of the penicillin-binding proteins). Synergism between the drugs also does not generally occur against organisms that are susceptible to amoxicillin alone; however, a slight additive effect has been reported in vitro with amoxicillin and clavulanic acid against some non-β-lactamase-producing strains of *Staphylococcus aureus* and *Haemophilus influenzae* and some strains of *Streptococcus pneumoniae* and group A β-hemolytic streptococci. This additive effect may result from clavulanic acid's intrinsic antibacterial activity, but this activity generally is inadequate for the drug to be therapeutically useful alone.

Clavulanic acid, like cefoxitin and imipenem, can induce production of chromosomally mediated type I cephalosporinases in certain gram-negative bacteria that possess these enzymes (e.g., some strains of *Enterobacter*, *Pseudomonas aeruginosa*, *Morganella morganii*). Concomitant use of clavulanic acid with a β-lactam antibiotic that is inactivated by inducible β-lactamases theoretically could result in an antagonistic effect against organisms that possess these enzymes. However, high concentrations of clavulanic acid generally are required to induce production of these β-lactamases and the clinical importance of this effect has not been determined.

Spectrum

Amoxicillin and clavulanate potassium is active in vitro against organisms susceptible to amoxicillin alone. In addition, because clavulanic acid can inhibit certain β-lactamases that generally inactivate amoxicillin, amoxicillin and clavulanate potassium is active in vitro against many β-lactamase-producing organisms that are resistant to amoxicillin alone.

Clavulanic acid alone has some antibacterial activity and is active in vitro against some gram-positive and gram-negative bacteria including *Moraxella catarrhalis* (formerly *Branhamella catarrhalis*), *Bacteroides fragilis*, *Haemophilus influenzae*, *Legionella*, *Neisseria gonorrhoeae*, and *Staphylococcus aureus*. However, high concentrations of clavulanic acid are necessary to inhibit most susceptible organisms and the drug is not therapeutically useful alone.

■ In Vitro Susceptibility Testing

The Clinical and Laboratory Standards Institute (CLSI; formerly National Committee for Clinical Laboratory Standards [NCCLS]) states that, for streptococci (including *Streptococcus pneumoniae*), results of in vitro susceptibility tests using penicillin can be used to predict susceptibility to amoxicillin and clavulanate potassium and, for non-β-lactamase-producing enterococci, results of in vitro susceptibility tests using penicillin or ampicillin can be used to predict susceptibility to amoxicillin and clavulanate potassium. However, to determine susceptibility of staphylococci, Enterobacteriaceae, and *Haemophilus* to amoxicillin and clavulanate potassium, CLSI recommends that disk-diffusion and dilution susceptibility tests be performed using appropriate combinations of amoxicillin and clavulanate potassium. For information on interpretive criteria specified for ampicillin, see Spectrum: In Vitro Susceptibility Testing, in the Aminopenicillins General Statement 8:12.16.08.

To test in vitro susceptibility to amoxicillin and clavulanate potassium, a 2:1 ratio of amoxicillin to clavulanic acid generally is used for both disk-diffusion and agar or broth dilution procedures.

Results of in vitro susceptibility tests with amoxicillin and clavulanate potassium may be affected by inoculum size or test media. However, results of the tests are not generally affected by pH changes between 6 and 8 or the presence of serum.

CLSI, the manufacturers, and most clinicians recommend that strains of staphylococci resistant to penicillinase-resistant penicillins also be considered resistant to amoxicillin and clavulanate potassium, although results of in vitro susceptibility tests may indicate that the organism is susceptible to the drug. In addition, CLSI recommends that non-β-lactamase-producing strains of *Haemophilus influenzae* that are resistant to ampicillin (BLNAR *H. influenzae*) be considered resistant to amoxicillin and clavulanate potassium despite the fact that results of in vitro susceptibility tests may indicate that the organisms are susceptible to the drug.

Disk Susceptibility Tests When disk-diffusion procedures are used to test susceptibility to amoxicillin and clavulanate potassium, a disk containing 20 mcg of amoxicillin and 10 mcg of clavulanic acid is used.

When disk-diffusion susceptibility tests are performed according to CLSI standardized procedures using CLSI interpretive criteria, *Staphylococcus* with growth inhibition zones of 20 mm or greater are considered susceptible to amoxicillin and clavulanate potassium and those with zones of 19 mm or less are resistant to the drug.

When disk-diffusion susceptibility tests are performed according to CLSI standardized procedures, Enterobacteriaceae with growth inhibition zones of 18 mm or greater are susceptible to amoxicillin and clavulanate potassium, those with zones of 14–17 mm have intermediate susceptibility, and those with zones of 13 mm or less are resistant to the drug.

When disk-diffusion susceptibility testing for *Haemophilus* is performed according to CLSI standardized procedures using *Haemophilus* test medium (HTM), *Haemophilus* with growth inhibition zones of 20 mm or greater are considered susceptible to amoxicillin and clavulanate potassium and those with zones of 19 mm or less are resistant to the drug.

Dilution Susceptibility Tests For dilution susceptibility testing (agar or broth dilution), CLSI recommends that a 2:1 ratio of amoxicillin to clavulanic acid be used with each dilution and that the MIC of amoxicillin and clavulanate potassium be reported as mcg/mL of amoxicillin and mcg/mL of clavulanic acid. The MIC of amoxicillin and clavulanate potassium has also been reported as mcg of amoxicillin plus mcg of clavulanic acid per mL (i.e., mcg of "Augmentin" per mL) or in terms of the MIC of amoxicillin in the presence of a specified concentration of clavulanic acid.

When dilution tests are performed using CLSI standardized procedures and a 2:1 ratio of amoxicillin to clavulanic acid with each dilution, *Staphylcoccocus* with MICs of 4 mcg/mL or less of amoxicillin and 2 mcg/mL or less of clavulanic acid are considered susceptible to amoxicillin and clavulanate potassium and those with MICs of 8 mcg/mL or greater of amoxicillin and 4 mcg/mL or greater of clavulanic acid are resistant to the drug.

When broth dilution susceptibility for *S. pneumoniae* (from nonmeningeal sites only) is performed using CLSI standardized procedure and cation-adjusted Mueller-Hinton broth (supplemented with 2–5% lysed horse blood), *S. pneumoniae* with MICs of 2 mcg/mL or less of amoxicillin and 1 mcg/mL or less of clavulanic acid are considered susceptible to amoxicillin and clavulanate potassium, those with MICs of 4 mcg/mL of amoxicillin and 2 mcg/mL of clavulanic acid have intermediate susceptibility, and those with MICs of 8 mcg/mL or greater of amoxicillin and 4 mcg/mL or greater of clavulanic acid are resistant to amoxicillin and clavulanate potassium.

When dilution susceptibility tests are performed according to CLSI standardized procedures using CLSI interpretive criteria, Enterobacteriaceae with MICs of 8 mcg/mL or less of amoxicillin and 4 mcg/mL or less of clavulanic acid are susceptible to amoxicillin and clavulanate potassium, those with MICs of 16 mcg/mL of amoxicillin and 8 mcg/mL of clavulanic acid are considered to have intermediate susceptibility, those with MICs of 16 mcg/mL of amoxicillin and 8 mcg/mL of clavulanic acid have intermediate susceptibility, and those with MICs of 32 mcg/mL or greater of amoxicillin and 16 mcg/mL or greater of clavulanic acid are resistant to the drug.

When susceptibility of *Haemophilus* is tested in a broth dilution procedure according to CLSI standardized procedures using HTM, *Haemophilus* with MICs of 4 mcg/mL or less of amoxicillin and 2 mcg/mL or less of clavulanic acid are susceptible to amoxicillin and clavulanate potassium and those with MICs of 8 mcg/mL or greater of amoxicillin and 4 mcg/mL or greater of clavulanic acid are resistant to the drug.

■ Gram-positive Aerobic Bacteria

Amoxicillin and clavulanate potassium is active in vitro against most gram-positive aerobic cocci including penicillinase-producing and nonpenicillinase-producing strains of *Staphylococcus aureus*, *S. epidermidis*, and *S. saprophyticus*; group A β-hemolytic streptococci; *Streptococcus pneumoniae*; *Enterococcus faecalis* (formerly *S. faecalis*); and viridans streptococci. Amoxicillin and clavulanate potassium is active in vitro against many strains of penicillinase-producing staphylococci that are resistant to amoxicillin alone; however, staphylococci resistant to penicillinase-resistant penicillins are generally also resistant to amoxicillin and clavulanate potassium.

In one in vitro study using dilutions containing a 2:1 ratio of amoxicillin to clavulanic acid, the MIC_{90} (minimum inhibitory concentration of the drug at which 90% of strains tested are inhibited) of amoxicillin and clavulanate potassium for both penicillinase-producing and nonpenicillinase-producing strains of *S. aureus* was 8 mcg/mL of amoxicillin and 4 mcg/mL of clavulanic acid and the MIC_{90} of the drug for group A β-hemolytic streptococci, *S. pneumoniae*, and *E. faecalis* was 0.03–1 mcg/mL of amoxicillin and 0.015–0.5 mcg/mL of clavulanic acid. In a similar in vitro study, the MIC_{90} for penicillinase-producing *S. aureus* was 1.33 mcg/mL of amoxicillin and 0.67 mcg/mL of clavulanic acid.

■ Gram-negative Aerobic Bacteria

Neisseria Amoxicillin and clavulanate potassium is active in vitro against most strains of *Neisseria meningitidis* and penicillinase-producing and nonpenicillinase-producing *N. gonorrhoeae*. Although penicillinase-producing *N. gonorrhoeae* (PPNG) are usually resistant to amoxicillin alone, most strains of the organism are susceptible in vitro to amoxicillin and clavulanate potassium.

The MIC_{90} of amoxicillin and clavulanate potassium for *N. meningitidis* is reportedly 0.12 mcg/mL of amoxicillin and 0.06 mcg/mL of clavulanic acid. In one in vitro study using dilutions containing a 2:1 ratio of amoxicillin to clavulanic acid, the MIC of amoxicillin and clavulanate potassium for nonpenicillinase-producing *N. gonorrhoeae* ranged from 0.08–2.7 mcg/mL of amoxicillin and 0.04–1.3 mcg/mL of clavulanic acid and the MIC for PPNG ranged from 0.67–2.7 mcg/mL of amoxicillin and 0.33–1.3 mcg/mL of clavulanic acid.

Haemophilus Amoxicillin and clavulanate potassium is active in vitro against most β-lactamase-producing and non-β-lactamase-producing strains of *Haemophilus influenzae*, *H. parainfluenzae*, and *H. ducreyi*. However, strains of non-β-lactamase-producing*Haemophilus* that are resistant to aminopenicillins may also be resistant to amoxicillin and clavulanate potassium.

In one in vitro study using dilutions containing a 2:1 ratio of amoxicillin to clavulanate potassium, the MIC of amoxicillin and clavulanate potassium for non-β-lactamase-producing strains of *H. influenzae* was 0.06–0.5 mcg/mL of amoxicillin and 0.03–0.25 mcg/mL of clavulanic acid and the MIC of the drug for β-lactamase-producing strains was 0.5–2 mcg/mL of amoxicillin and 0.25–1 mcg/mL of clavulanic acid. In another in vitro study using β-lactamase-producing *H. influenzae* type b, the MIC of amoxicillin alone ranged from 6.25–12.5 mcg/mL and the MIC of clavulanic acid alone ranged from 12.5–25 mcg/mL, but the MIC of amoxicillin and clavulanate potassium was 0.36 mcg/mL of amoxicillin and 0.36 mcg/mL of clavulanic acid.

Although most strains of *H. ducreyi* produce β-lactamase and are resistant to amoxicillin alone, the MIC of amoxicillin and clavulanate potassium for this organism has been reported to be 4 mcg/mL of amoxicillin and 1 mcg/mL of clavulanic acid.

Moraxella catarrhalis Amoxicillin and clavulanate potassium is active in vitro against both β-lactamase-producing and non-β-lactamase-producing strains of *Moraxella catarrhalis* (formerly *Branhamella catarrhalis*). The MIC_{90} of amoxicillin plus clavulanate acid is 0.005 mcg/mL for non-β-lactamase-producing strains of *M. catarrhalis* and 0.125–0.25 mcg/mL for β-lactamase-producing strains. In an in vitro study of β-lactamase-producing *M. catarrhalis*, the MIC of amoxicillin alone was 25–50 mcg/mL, the MIC of clavulanic acid alone was 2.5–12.5 mcg/mL, and the MIC of amoxicillin plus clavulanate acid was 0.02–0.05 mcg/mL.

Enterobacteriaceae Amoxicillin and clavulanate potassium is active in vitro against Enterobacteriaceae that are susceptible to amoxicillin alone (e.g., some strains of *Escherichia coli, Proteus mirabilis, Salmonella, Shigella*). In addition, amoxicillin and clavulanate potassium is active in vitro against many β-lactamase-producing strains of *Citrobacter diversus, K. pneumoniae, P. mirabilis*, and *P. vulgaris* and some strains of β-lactamase-producing *E. coli* and *Enterobacter* that are resistant to amoxicillin alone.

In one in vitro study using dilutions containing a 2:1 ratio of amoxicillin to clavulanic acid, the MIC_{90} of amoxicillin and clavulanate potassium for *E. coli* was 32 mcg/mL of amoxicillin and 16 mcg/mL of clavulanic acid, the MIC_{90} for *Klebsiella* and *P. vulgaris* was 8 mcg/mL of amoxicillin and 4 mcg/mL of clavulanic acid, and the MIC_{90} for *C. diversus* and *P. mirabilis* was 1–2 mcg/mL of amoxicillin and 0.5–1 mcg/mL of clavulanic acid.

Although rare strains of *C. freundii, Enterobacter cloacae, Morganella morganii* (formerly *Proteus morganii*), *Providencia*, and *Serratia* are inhibited in vitro by high concentrations of amoxicillin and clavulanate potassium, most strains of these organisms are considered resistant to the drug.

Other Gram-negative Aerobic Bacteria Amoxicillin and clavulanate potassium has some in vitro activity against *Legionella*, although the drug may not be effective clinically. In one in vitro study using CYEA media containing 2.5 mcg/mL of clavulanic acid, *L. pneumophila, L. micdadei*, and *L. bozemanii* were inhibited by 0.003 mcg/mL of amoxicillin plus clavulanate potassium. In another in vitro study using *L. pneumophila* and Mueller-Hinton agar, the MIC of amoxicillin alone was 1.95 mcg/mL, the MIC of clavulanic acid alone was 0.2–0.4 mcg/mL, and the MIC of amoxicillin plus clavulanate potassium was 0.61 mcg/mL.

Amoxicillin and clavulanic acid is generally inactive against *Pseudomonas*; however, the drug may be active in vitro against *Burkholderia pseudomallei* (formerly *Pseudomonas pseudomallei*).

■ **Anaerobic Bacteria** Amoxicillin and clavulanate potassium is active in vitro against gram-positive anaerobic bacteria including *Clostridium, Peptococcus*, and *Peptostreptococcus*.

Amoxicillin and clavulanate potassium is active in vitro against *Prevotella melaninogenica* (formerly *Bacteroides melaninogenicus*) and *P. oralis* (formerly *B. oralis*). Although the *Bacteroides fragilis* group (e.g., *B. fragilis, B. distasonis, B. ovatus, B. thetaiotamicron, B. vulgatus*) usually is resistant to amoxicillin alone, amoxicillin and clavulanate potassium is active in vitro against many strains of these organisms. In one in vitro study, the MIC of amoxicillin in the presence of 0.75 mcg/mL of clavulanic acid was 0.5–1 mcg/mL for *B. fragilis, B. ovatus, B. thetaiotamicron*, and *B. vulgatus* and 4 mcg/mL for *B. distasonis*.

■ **Mycobacterium** Although the clinical importance has not been determined to date, amoxicillin and clavulanate potassium is active in vitro against some strains of *Mycobacterium tuberculosis* and *M. fortuitum*. *M. tuberculosis* and *M. fortuitum* are β-lactamase producers and are generally resistant to amoxicillin alone. In one in vitro study using dilutions containing a 2:1 ratio of amoxicillin to clavulanic acid, the MIC of amoxicillin and clavulanate potassium for *M. tuberculosis* was 1–2 mcg/mL of amoxicillin and 0.5–1 mcg/mL of clavulanic acid and the minimum bactericidal concentration (MBC) of the drug was 1–4 mcg/mL of amoxicillin and 0.5–2 mcg/mL of clavulanic acid. In another study using *M. fortuitum*, the MIC of amoxicillin and clavulanate potassium for most strains was 4–16 mcg/mL of amoxicillin and 2–8 mcg/mL of clavulanic acid, although some strains had an MIC of 32 mcg/mL or greater of amoxicillin and 16 mcg/mL or greater of clavulanic acid.

Resistance

Gram-negative aerobic bacilli that produce Richmond-Sykes type I chromosomally mediated β-lactamases (e.g., *Citrobacter freundii, Enterobacter cloacae, Serratia marcescens, Pseudomonas aeruginosa*) are generally resistant to amoxicillin and clavulanate potassium, since clavulanic acid does not inhibit most type I β-lactamases. Strains of *E. coli* with chromosomally mediated β-lactamases are also resistant to amoxicillin and clavulanate potassium.

Strains of *E. cloacae* and *Providencia stuartii* that appear to be resistant to amoxicillin and clavulanate potassium but susceptible to ampicillin in vitro have been reported rarely.

Pharmacokinetics

Crossover studies using fixed combinations of amoxicillin and clavulanate potassium, amoxicillin alone, and clavulanate potassium alone indicate that concomitant administration of clavulanate potassium does not affect the pharmacokinetics of amoxicillin; however, concomitant administration of amoxicillin reportedly may increase GI absorption and renal elimination of clavulanate potassium compared with administration of clavulanate potassium alone.

For additional information on absorption, distribution, and elimination of amoxicillin, see Pharmacokinetics in the Aminopenicillins General Statement 8:12.16.08 and in Amoxicillin 8:12.16.08.

■ **Absorption** Amoxicillin trihydrate and clavulanate potassium are both generally stable in the presence of acidic gastric secretions and are well absorbed following oral administration of amoxicillin and clavulanate potassium. Peak serum concentrations of amoxicillin and of clavulanic acid are generally attained within 1–2.5 hours following oral administration of a single dose of conventional preparations of amoxicillin and clavulanate potassium in fasting adults or a single dose of extended-release tablets in adults fed a standardized meal.

Following oral administration of a single conventional tablet containing 250 mg of amoxicillin and 125 mg of clavulanic acid in healthy, fasting adults, peak serum concentrations of amoxicillin and of clavulanic acid average 3.7–4.8 mcg/mL and 2.2–3.5 mcg/mL, respectively. Following oral administration of a single conventional tablet containing 500 mg of amoxicillin and 125 mg of clavulanic acid in healthy, fasting adults, peak serum concentrations of amoxicillin average 6.5–9.7 mcg/mL and peak serum concentrations of clavulanic acid average 2.1–3.9 mcg/mL. The manufacturer states that serum concentrations of the drugs achieved following oral administration of a single chewable tablet containing 250 mg of amoxicillin and 62.5 mg of clavulanic acid or 2 chewable tablets each containing 125 and 31.25 mg of the drugs, respectively, are similar to those achieved following oral administration of a single equivalent dose of the oral suspension. The manufacturer also states that serum concentrations of amoxicillin achieved following oral administration of conventional preparations or extended-release tablets of amoxicillin and clavulanate potassium are similar to those achieved following oral administration of equivalent doses of amoxicillin alone.

Following oral administration of a single dose of 250 mg of amoxicillin and 62.5 mg of clavulanic acid as an oral suspension, peak serum concentrations of amoxicillin average 6.9 mcg/mL and peak concentrations of clavulanic acid average 1.6 mcg/mL. In one study in children 2–5 years of age with urinary tract infections, oral administration of a single dose of 125 mg of amoxicillin and 31.75 mg of clavulanic acid as an oral suspension resulted in serum concentrations of amoxicillin that averaged 9.4, 9.7, and 6.5 mcg/mL and serum concentrations of clavulanic acid that averaged 2.1, 4.4, and 2.5 mcg/mL at 30, 60, and 90 minutes, respectively, after the dose.

Studies in healthy adults using conventional preparations of amoxicillin and clavulanate potassium indicate that presence of food in the GI tract does not affect oral absorption of either amoxicillin or clavulanic acid following administration of fixed-combination preparations of the drugs. However, amoxicillin and clavulanate are optimally absorbed from extended-release tablets of the combination when administered orally at the beginning of a standardized meal (612 kcal, 89.3 g carbohydrate, 24.9 g fat, and 14 g protein); administration of the extended-release tablets with a high-fat meal is not recommended because clavulanate absorption is decreased, and administration of these tablets in the fasting state is not recommended because amoxicillin absorption is decreased. GI absorption of the drugs from extended-release tablets is not affected by administration simultaneously with or 2 hours before a magnesium and aluminum-containing antacid (Maalox®).

■ **Distribution** Following administration of amoxicillin and clavulanate potassium, amoxicillin and clavulanic acid are both distributed into the lungs, pleural fluid, and peritoneal fluid. Low concentrations (i.e., less than 1 mcg/mL) of each drug are attained in sputum and saliva.

In one study in fasting children who received a single amoxicillin dose of 35 mg/kg given as amoxicillin and clavulanate potassium oral suspension, concentrations of amoxicillin and of clavulanic acid in middle ear effusions averaged 3 and 0.5 mcg/mL, respectively, 2 hours after the dose.

Only minimal concentrations of amoxicillin or clavulanic acid are attained in CSF following oral administration of amoxicillin and clavulanate potassium in patients with uninflamed meninges; higher concentrations may be attained when meninges are inflamed. In one study in patients with uninflamed meninges who received a single 250-mg oral dose of clavulanic acid as the sodium salt, concentrations of clavulanic acid in CSF obtained 1–6 hours after the dose ranged from 0–0.2 mcg/mL. In 2 patients with continuous CSF drainage after neurosurgical procedures who received a similar oral dose of the drug, peak CSF concentrations of clavulanic acid were 2.4 and 0.4 mcg/mL, respectively, and occurred approximately 4 hours after the dose; concurrent serum concentrations of clavulanic acid were 2.3 and 0.3 mcg/mL, respectively.

Amoxicillin is 17–20% bound to serum proteins. In vitro or in vivo following oral administration, clavulanic acid is reportedly 22–30% bound to serum proteins at a concentration of 1–100 mcg/mL.

Amoxicillin and clavulanic acid readily cross the placenta. Amoxicillin and clavulanic acid are distributed into milk in low concentrations.

■ **Elimination** Serum concentrations of amoxicillin and clavulanic acid both decline in a biphasic manner and half-lives of the drugs are similar. Following oral administration of conventional preparations or extended-release tablets of amoxicillin and clavulanate potassium in adults with normal renal function, amoxicillin has an elimination half-life of 1–1.3 hours and clavulanic acid has a distribution half-life of 0.28 hours and an elimination half-life of 0.78–1.2 hours. In one study in children 2–15 years of age, the elimination half-lives of amoxicillin and of clavulanic acid averaged 1.2 and 0.8 hours, respectively.

The metabolic fate of clavulanate potassium has not been fully elucidated; however, the drug appears to be extensively metabolized. In rats and dogs, the major metabolite of clavulanic acid is 1-amino-4-hydroxybutan-2-one; this metabolite has also been found in human urine following administration of clavulanic acid. Clavulanic acid is excreted in urine principally by glomerular filtration. Studies in dogs and rats using radiolabeled clavulanic acid indicate that 34–52, 25–27, and 16–33% of a dose of the drug is excreted in urine, feces, and respired air, respectively.

Following oral administration of a single oral dose of amoxicillin and clavulanate potassium in adults with normal renal function, approximately 50–73 and 25–45% of the amoxicillin and clavulanic acid doses, respectively, are excreted unchanged in urine within 6–8 hours. In one study in healthy adults who received a single oral dose of 250 mg of amoxicillin and 125 mg of clavulanic acid, urinary concentrations of amoxicillin and of clavulanic acid averaged 381 and 118 mcg/mL, respectively, in urine collected over the first 2 hours after the dose.

Serum concentrations of amoxicillin and of clavulanic acid are higher and the serum half-lives prolonged in patients with renal impairment. In one study in patients with creatinine clearances of 9 mL/minute, the serum half-lives of amoxicillin and of clavulanic acid were 7.5 and 4.3 hours, respectively.

Oral probenecid administered shortly before or with amoxicillin and clavulanate potassium competitively inhibits renal tubular secretion of amoxicillin and produces higher and prolonged serum concentrations of the drug; however, probenecid does not appreciably affect the pharmacokinetics of clavulanic acid. (See Drug Interactions: Probenecid.)

Amoxicillin and clavulanic acid are both removed by hemodialysis. The manufacturers state that clavulanic acid is also removed by peritoneal dialysis. Only minimal amounts of amoxicillin appear to be removed by peritoneal dialysis.

Chemistry and Stability

■ **Chemistry** Amoxicillin and clavulanate potassium is a fixed combination of amoxicillin trihydrate and the potassium salt of clavulanic acid. Amoxicillin is an aminopenicillin. (See Amoxicillin 8:12.16.08.) The fixed combination also is commercially available as extended-release tablets containing the sodium salt and the trihydrate of amoxicillin and the potassium salt of clavulanic acid. Clavulanic acid is a β-lactamase inhibitor produced by fermentation of *Streptomyces clavuligerus*. Clavulanic acid contains a β-lactam ring and is structurally similar to penicillins and cephalosporins; however, the β-lactam ring in clavulanic acid is fused with an oxazolidine ring rather than with a thiazolidine ring as in penicillins or a dihydrothiazine ring as in cephalosporins. Although clavulanic acid has only weak antibacterial activity when used alone, the combined use of clavulanic acid and certain penicillins or cephalosporins (e.g., amoxicillin, ampicillin, carbenicillin, cefoperazone, cefotaxime, penicillin G, ticarcillin) results in a synergistic effect that expands the spectrum of activity of the penicillin or cephalosporin against many strains of β-lactamase-producing bacteria. Clavulanic acid and its salts currently are commercially available in the US only in fixed combination with other drugs.

Amoxicillin and clavulanate potassium is commercially available for oral administration as film-coated tablets containing a 2:1 or 4:1 ratio of amoxicillin to clavulanic acid; as scored tablets containing a 7:1 ratio of amoxicillin to clavulanic acid; as chewable tablets containing a 4:1 or 7:1 ratio of amoxicillin to clavulanic acid; as extended-release tablets containing a 16:1 ratio of the drugs; or a powder for oral suspension containing a 4:1, 7:1, or 14:1 ratio of the drugs.

Although commercially available amoxicillin and clavulanate potassium contains amoxicillin as the trihydrate and clavulanic acid as the potassium salt, potency of amoxicillin is calculated on the anhydrous basis and potency of clavulanate potassium is expressed in terms of clavulanic acid.

Amoxicillin occurs as a white, practically odorless, crystalline powder and is sparingly soluble in water. Clavulanate potassium occurs as an off-white, crystalline powder and is very soluble in water and slightly soluble in alcohol at room temperature. Clavulanic acid has a pK_a of 2.7.

Each amoxicillin and clavulanate potassium film-coated tablet containing 250 or 500 mg of amoxicillin and 125 mg of clavulanic acid or each scored tablet containing 875 mg of amoxicillin and 125 mg of clavulanic acid contains 0.63 mEq of potassium. Following reconstitution as directed, each 5 mL of amoxicillin and clavulanate potassium oral suspension containing 125, 200, 250, 400, or 600 mg of amoxicillin contains 0.16, 0.14, 0.32, 0.29, or 0.23 mEq of potassium, respectively. Each amoxicillin and clavulanate potassium chewable tablet containing 125, 200, 250, 400 mg, or 600 of amoxicillin contains 0.16, 0.14, 0.32, or 0.29 mEq of potassium, respectively. Each amoxicillin and clavulanate potassium extended-release tablet containing 1 g of amoxicillin contains 0.32 mEq of potassium and 1.27 mEq of sodium. When reconstituted as directed, the oral suspensions have a pH of 4.8–6.8.

Amoxicillin and clavulanate potassium chewable tables containing 200, 400, or 600 mg of amoxicillin and amoxicillin and clavulanate potassium oral suspension containing 200 or 400 mg of amoxicillin per 5 mL contain aspartame; following metabolism of aspartame in the GI tract, each 200- or 400-mg chewable tablet provides 2.1 or 4.2 mg of phenylalanine, respectively, and each 5 mL of amoxicillin and clavulanate potassium oral suspension containing 200, 400, or 600 mg of amoxicillin provides 7 mg of phenylalanine.

■ **Stability** Commercially available amoxicillin and clavulanate potassium film-coated tablets, scored tablets, chewable tablets, extended-release tablets, and powder for oral suspension should be stored in tight containers at a temperature of 25°C or lower; exposure to excessive humidity should be avoided.

Following reconstitution, oral suspensions of amoxicillin and clavulanate potassium should be stored at 2–8°C, and any unused suspension should be discarded after 10 days.

For further information on chemistry and stability, mechanism of action, spectrum, resistance, pharmacokinetics, uses, cautions, drug interactions, and laboratory test interferences of amoxicillin, see the Aminopenicillins General Statement 8:12.16.08 and see Amoxicillin 8:12.16.08.

Preparations

Excipients in commercially available drug preparations may have clinically important effects in some individuals; consult specific product labeling for details.

Amoxicillin (Trihydrate) and Clavulanate Potassium (Co-amoxiclav)

Oral		
For suspension	125 mg (of amoxicillin) per 5 mL and 31.25 mg (of clavulanic acid) per 5 mL*	**Amoxicillin and Clavulanate Potassium for Oral Suspension** **Augmentin®**, GlaxoSmithKline
	200 mg (of amoxicillin) per 5 mL and 28.5 mg (of clavulanic acid) per 5 mL*	**Amoxicillin and Clavulanate Potassium for Oral Suspension** **Augmentin®**, GlaxoSmithKline
	250 mg (of amoxicillin) per 5 mL and 62.5 mg (of clavulanic acid) per 5 mL	**Augmentin®**, GlaxoSmithKline
	400 mg (of amoxicillin) per 5 mL and 57 mg (of clavulanic acid) per 5 mL*	**Amoxicillin and Clavulanate Potassium for Oral Suspension** **Augmentin®**, GlaxoSmithKline
	600 mg (of amoxicillin) per 5 mL and 42.9 mg (of clavulanic acid) per 5 mL*	**Amoxicillin and Clavulanate Potassium for Oral Suspension** **Augmentin ES-600®**, GlaxoSmithKline
Tablets	875 mg (of amoxicillin) and 125 mg (of clavulanic acid)*	**Amoxicillin and Clavulanate Potassium Tablets** (scored) **Augmentin®** (scored)
Tablets, chewable	125 mg (of amoxicillin) and 31.25 mg (of clavulanic acid)	**Augmentin®**, GlaxoSmithKline
	200 mg (of amoxicillin) and 28.5 mg (of clavulanic acid)*	**Amoxicillin and Clavulanate Potassium Chewable Tablets** **Augmentin®**, GlaxoSmithKline
	250 mg (of amoxicillin) and 62.5 mg (of clavulanic acid)	**Augmentin®**, GlaxoSmithKline
	400 mg (of amoxicillin) and 57 mg (of clavulanic acid)*	**Amoxicillin and Clavulanate Potassium Chewable Tablets** **Augmentin®**, GlaxoSmithKline
Tablets, film-coated	250 mg (of amoxicillin) and 125 mg (of clavulanic acid)*	**Amoxicillin and Clavulanate Potassium Tablets** **Augmentin®**, GlaxoSmithKline
	500 mg (of amoxicillin) and 125 mg (of clavulanic acid)*	**Amoxicillin and Clavulanate Potassium Tablets** **Augmentin®**, GlaxoSmithKline

*available from one or more manufacturer, distributor, and/or repackager by generic (nonproprietary) name

Amoxicillin (Trihydrate), Amoxicillin Sodium, and Clavulanate Potassium

Oral		
Tablets, extended-release	1 g (of amoxicillin) and 62.5 mg (of clavulanic acid)	**Augmentin® XR**, GlaxoSmithKline

†Use is not currently included in the labeling approved by the US Food and Drug Administration

Ampicillin

Aminobenzylpenicillin

■ Ampicillin is an aminopenicillin antibiotic.

Uses

Ampicillin shares the uses of other aminopenicillins and is used principally for the treatment of infections caused by susceptible gram-negative bacteria (e.g., *Haemophilus influenzae*, *Escherichia coli*, *Proteus mirabilis*, *Salmonella*). Ampicillin also is used for the treatment of infections caused by susceptible gram-positive bacteria (e.g., *Streptococcus pneumoniae*, enterococci, nonpenicillinase-producing staphylococci, *Listeria*); however, like other aminopenicillins, ampicillin generally should not be used for the treatment of streptococcal or staphylococcal infections when a natural penicillin would be effective. Orally administered ampicillin should not be used for the initial treatment of severe, life-threatening infections, but may be used as follow-up therapy after parenteral ampicillin therapy. For specific information on the uses of ampicillin, see Uses in the Aminopenicillins General Statement 8:12.16.08.

Dosage and Administration

■ Reconstitution and Administration Ampicillin trihydrate is administered orally. Although ampicillin may be given orally with meals, maximum absorption is achieved when the drug is administered 1 hour before or 2 hours after meals.

Ampicillin sodium may be administered by IM or slow IV injection or by IV infusion.

Parenteral forms of ampicillin should be used only in the treatment of moderately severe or severe infections. Direct IV injections should be made slowly over 10–15 minutes to avoid the possibility of seizures. For intermittent IV infusion, the concentration of ampicillin and rate of infusion should be adjusted so that the total dose of the drug is administered before 10% or more of the drug is inactivated in the IV solution. (See Chemistry and Stability: Stability.)

Ampicillin sodium preparations for parenteral use should be reconstituted according to the manufacturers' instructions. Ampicillin sodium solutions should be inspected visually for particulate matter and discoloration prior to administration whenever solution and container permit.

■ Dosage Dosage of ampicillin sodium and ampicillin trihydrate is expressed in terms of ampicillin.

The manufacturers' dosage recommendations for adults usually are the same for both parenteral and oral routes; however, higher serum concentrations usually are attained parenterally, and this route is used for severe infections.

General Adult Dosage The usual adult dosage of ampicillin for the treatment of respiratory tract or skin and skin structure infections is 250–500 mg every 6 hours. For the treatment of GI or urinary tract infections, the usual adult dosage is 500 mg every 6 hours. For severe infections, larger doses may be required.

The usual adult dosage of ampicillin for the treatment of septicemia or bacterial meningitis is 8–14 g or 150–200 mg/kg daily given parenterally in equally divided doses every 3–4 hours. For the initial treatment of septicemia or meningitis, ampicillin should be given IV for at least 3 days but may then be given IM.

General Pediatric Dosage For oral therapy, most manufacturers state that children weighing more than 20 kg may receive the usual adult dosage of ampicillin. For parenteral therapy, some manufacturers recommend that the usual adult dosage be used in children weighing more than 20 kg, whereas other manufacturers and many clinicians recommend that the usual adult dosage be used in those weighing more than 40 kg. Pediatric dosage should not exceed dosage recommended for similar infections in adults.

For the treatment of respiratory tract or skin and skin structure infections, the usual dosage of ampicillin for children weighing 40 kg or less is 25–50 mg/kg daily administered in equally divided doses every 6 hours. For the treatment of GI or urinary tract infections, the usual dosage for children weighing 40 kg or less is 50–100 mg/kg daily given in equally divided doses every 6 hours.

For the treatment of septicemia or CNS infections, the usual pediatric dosage recommended by the manufacturers is 100–200 mg/kg daily given in divided doses every 3–4 hours, starting with IV administration for 3 days and continuing with IM administration. For empiric treatment of bacterial meningitis in neonates and children younger than 2 months of age, many clinicians recommend that an IV ampicillin dosage of 100–300 mg/kg daily be given in divided doses in conjunction with IM gentamicin pending results of in vitro susceptibility tests. For the empiric treatment of bacterial meningitis in children 2 months to 12 years of age, many clinicians recommend that an IV ampicillin dosage of 200–400 mg/kg daily be given in divided doses every 4–6 hours in conjunction with IV chloramphenicol. If bacterial susceptibility data are not available and clinical and bacteriologic response is unsatisfactory after 24–48 hours, other appropriate anti-infective therapy should be substituted.

When IM or IV ampicillin is used in neonates younger than 7 days of age, the American Academy of Pediatrics (AAP) recommends a dosage of 50 mg/kg every 12 hours in those weighing 2 kg or less or 50 mg/kg every 8 hours in those weighing more than 2 kg. For neonates 8–28 days of age, AAP recommends an IM or IV dosage of 50 mg/kg every 8 hours in those weighing 2 kg or less or 50 mg/kg every 6 hours in those weighing more than 2 kg. AAP states that higher ampicillin dosage may be necessary for the treatment of meningitis in neonates. For the treatment of meningitis caused by *Streptococcus agalactiae* (group B streptococci; GBS), some experts recommend that neonates 28 days of age or younger receive IV ampicillin in a dosage of 75 mg/kg every 6 hours, regardless of weight; others recommend a dosage of 200–300 mg/kg daily given IV in 3 divided doses in neonates 7 days of age or younger or a dosage of 300 mg/kg daily given IV in 4 divided doses in neonates older than 7 days of age. AAP states that a dosage of 100 mg/kg every 12 hours is acceptable for the treatment of early-onset group B streptococcal septicemia *without* meningitis in neonates 7 days of age or younger.

When IM or IV ampicillin is used in pediatric patients beyond the neonatal period, AAP recommends a dosage of 100–150 mg/kg daily given in 4 divided doses for the treatment of mild to moderate infections or a dosage of 200–400 mg/kg daily given in 4 divided doses for the treatment of severe infections. The highest dosage should be used for the treatment of CNS infections. When oral ampicillin is used in pediatric patients beyond the neonatal period, AAP recommends a dosage of 50–100 mg/kg daily in 4 divided doses. AAP states that oral ampicillin is inappropriate for the treatment of severe infections.

Treatment of Enterococcal Endocarditis For the treatment of enterococcal endocarditis, the American Heart Association (AHA) and others recommend that adults receive an ampicillin dosage of 12 g daily (by continuous IV infusion or in 6 equally divided IV doses) in conjunction with gentamicin (1 mg/kg IM or IV every 8 hours). Treatment with both drugs generally should be continued for 4–6 weeks, but patients who had symptoms of infection for more than 3 months before treatment was initiated and patients with prosthetic heart valves require a minimum of 6 weeks of therapy with both drugs.

Gonorrhea and Associated Infections Some manufacturers state that adults and children weighing 45 kg or more may receive a single 3.5-g dose of oral ampicillin (with 1 g of oral probenecid) for the treatment of acute, uncomplicated gonorrhea caused by susceptible nonpenicillinase-producing *Neisseria gonorrhoeae*. However, penicillins are not included in current US Centers for Disease Control and Prevention (CDC) recommendations for the treatment of gonorrhea.

Prevention of Perinatal Group B Streptococcal Disease If IV ampicillin is used as an alternative to IV penicillin G for intrapartum anti-infective prophylaxis for prevention of perinatal group B streptococcal (GBS) disease† (see Prevention of Perinatal Group B Streptococcal Disease under Uses: Prophylaxis, in the Aminopenicillins General Statement 8:12.16.08), CDC and AAP recommend that an initial ampicillin dose of 2 g be given IV at the onset of labor or rupture of membranes followed by 1 g IV every 4 hours until delivery.

Regardless of whether anti-infective prophylaxis was administered to the mother, appropriate diagnostic evaluations and anti-infective therapy should be initiated in the neonate if signs or symptoms of active infection develop.

Prevention of Bacterial Endocarditis If IM or IV ampicillin is used for prevention of bacterial endocarditis† in patients with certain cardiac conditions who are undergoing certain dental procedures or certain other procedures who cannot receive an oral regimen (see Prevention of Bacterial Endocarditis under Uses: Prophylaxis, in the Aminopenicillins General Statement 8:12.16.08), AHA recommends that adults receive a single 2-g dose and that children receive a single 50-mg/kg dose of the drug given 30–60 minutes prior to the procedure.

When selecting anti-infectives for prevention of bacterial endocarditis, the current recommendations published by AHA should be consulted.

Duration of Therapy The duration of ampicillin therapy depends on the type and severity of infection and should be determined by the clinical and bacteriologic response of the patient. For most infections, except gonorrhea, therapy should be continued for at least 48–72 hours after the patient becomes asymptomatic or evidence of eradication of the infection has been obtained. Persistent infections may require several weeks of therapy.

■ Dosage in Renal Impairment In patients with renal impairment, doses and/or frequency of administration of ampicillin should be modified in response to the degree of renal impairment, severity of the infection, and susceptibility of the causative organism. Some clinicians suggest that adults with glomerular filtration rates of 10–50 mL/minute receive the usual dose of ampicillin every 6–12 hours and that adults with glomerular filtration rates less than 10 mL/minute receive the usual dose every 12–16 hours. Alternatively, some clinicians suggest that modification of usual dosage of ampicillin is unnecessary in adults with creatinine clearances of 30 mL/minute or greater, but adults with creatinine clearances of 10 mL/minute or less should receive the usual dose of the drug every 8 hours.

Patients undergoing hemodialysis should receive a supplemental dose of ampicillin after each dialysis period.

Cautions

■ Adverse Effects Adverse effects reported with ampicillin are similar to those reported with other aminopenicillins; however, diarrhea and rash have been reported more frequently with ampicillin than with other currently available aminopenicillins. For information on adverse effects reported with aminopenicillins, see Cautions in the Aminopenicillins General Statement 8:12.16.08.

■ Precautions and Contraindications Ampicillin shares the toxic potentials of the penicillins, including the risk of hypersensitivity reactions, and the usual precautions of penicillin therapy should be observed. Prior to initiation of therapy with ampicillin careful inquiry should be made concerning previous hypersensitivity reactions to penicillins, cephalosporins, or other drugs. There is clinical and laboratory evidence of partial cross-allergenicity among penicillins and other β-lactam antibiotics including cephalosporins, cephamycins, and 1-oxa-β-lactams. Ampicillin is contraindicated in patients who are hypersensitive to any penicillin.

Because a high percentage of patients with infectious mononucleosis have developed rash during therapy with aminopenicillins, ampicillin probably should not be used in patients with this disease.

Renal, hepatic, and hematologic systems should be evaluated periodically during prolonged therapy with ampicillin.

For a more complete discussion of these and other precautions associated with the use of ampicillin, see Cautions: Precautions and Contraindications, in the Aminopenicillins General Statement 8:12.16.08.

■ **Pregnancy and Lactation** Safe use of ampicillin during pregnancy has not been established. There are no adequate or controlled studies using ampicillin in pregnant women, and the drug should be used during pregnancy only when clearly needed. However, ampicillin has been administered to pregnant women, especially in the treatment of urinary tract infections, without evidence of adverse effects to the fetus.

Because ampicillin is distributed into milk, the drug should be used with caution in nursing women.

Spectrum

Based on its spectrum of activity, ampicillin is classified as an aminopenicillin. For information on the classification of penicillins based on spectra of activity, see the Preface to the General Statements on Penicillins 8:12.16.

Ampicillin generally has the same spectrum of activity and the same level of activity against susceptible organisms as amoxicillin; however, ampicillin is less active in vitro on a weight basis than amoxicillin against enterococci and *Salmonella* but more active than amoxicillin against *Shigella* and*Enterobacter*. For specific information on in vitro susceptibility testing and information on the spectrum of activity of ampicillin and resistance to the drug, see the sections on Spectrum and on Resistance in the Aminopenicillins General Statement 8:12.16.08.

Pharmacokinetics

For additional information on absorption and distribution of ampicillin and information on elimination of the drug, see Pharmacokinetics in the Aminopenicillins General Statement 8:12.16.08.

■ **Absorption** Ampicillin trihydrate generally are stable in the presence of acidic gastric secretions, and 30–55% of an oral dose of the drugs is absorbed from the GI tract in fasting adults. Although peak serum concentrations may occur as soon as 1 hour after administration, the maximum serum concentration usually is attained in approximately 2 hours. Two hours after oral administration of 250 mg of ampicillin in fasting individuals, average peak serum concentrations of 1.8–2.9 mcg/mL are attained. A 500-mg oral dose results in average peak serum concentrations of 3–6 mcg/mL. Concentrations of the antibiotic in serum are less than 1 mcg/mL 6 hours after a 500-mg oral dose. Although higher peak serum ampicillin concentrations and larger areas under the serum concentration-time curves (AUCs) have been reported following oral administration of anhydrous ampicillin than following the trihydrate, the differences are generally not considered clinically important. As oral dosage of ampicillin is increased from 500 mg to 2 g, the fraction of the dose absorbed from the GI tract decreases and, there is a nonlinear relationship between dosage and peak serum concentrations or AUCs of ampicillin.

Presence of food in the GI tract generally decreases the rate and extent of absorption of ampicillin.

Following IM administration of ampicillin sodium, peak serum concentrations generally are attained more quickly and are higher than those resulting from equivalent doses of ampicillin given orally. In premature neonates younger than 7 days of age, IM administration of a single ampicillin dose of 50 mg/kg has been reported to produce mean serum concentrations of 104, 87, 60, and 31 mcg/mL at 1, 4, 8, and 12 hours, respectively, after the dose. The same dose in full-term neonates younger than 7 days of age produced mean serum concentrations of 75, 64, 34, and 20 mcg/mL at the same time intervals.

Following IV administration over 20 minutes of a single 2-g dose of ampicillin in healthy adults, serum concentrations of ampicillin averaged 47.6, 23.3, 10.8, and 3.7 mcg/mL at 30 minutes, 1 hour, 2 hours, and 4 hours, respectively, after the infusion.

Serum ampicillin concentrations are higher and the serum half-life is prolonged in patients with impaired renal function. Serum concentrations of the drug also are higher and more prolonged in premature or full-term neonates younger than 6 days of age than in full-term neonates 6 days of age or older.

■ **Distribution** In one study in neonates with meningitis, average ampicillin concentrations in CSF ranged from 1–28 mcg/mL (11–65% of simultaneous serum concentrations) during the 7-hour period following IV administration of 40–70 mg/kg. Highest CSF concentrations occurred at 3–7 hours.

Ampicillin is distributed into bile. Biliary concentrations of ampicillin in patients with normal biliary function may be 1–30 times greater than simultaneous serum concentrations following a single oral dose of ampicillin.

Chemistry and Stability

■ **Chemistry** Ampicillin is an aminopenicillin. Ampicillin differs structurally from penicillin G only in the presence of an amino group at the α-position on the benzene ring at R on the penicillin nucleus.

Ampicillin is commercially available as ampicillin trihydrate for oral administration and as the sodium salt for parenteral administration. Potency of ampicillin trihydrate and ampicillin sodium is expressed in terms of ampicillin and is calculated on the anhydrous basis.

Ampicillin trihydrate occurs as a white, practically odorless, crystalline powder that is slightly soluble in water. Ampicillin trihydrate reportedly has aqueous solubility of about 6 mg/mL at 20°C and about 10 mg/mL at 40°C. Ampicillin sodium occurs as a white to off-white, odorless or practically odorless, crystalline, hygroscopic powder and is very soluble in water, in 0.9% sodium chloride, and in dextrose solutions. Reconstituted solutions of ampicillin sodium containing 10 mg of ampicillin per mL have a pH of 8–10. When reconstituted as directed, ampicillin trihydrate oral suspensions have a pH of 5–7.5.

Commercially available ampicillin sodium powder for injection contains 2.9–3.1 mEq of sodium per g of ampicillin.

■ **Stability** Ampicillin capsules and powder for oral suspension should be stored in tight containers at 15–30°C. Following reconstitution, oral suspension of ampicillin trihydrate preferably should be refrigerated at 2–8°C but is stable for 7 days at room temperature or 14 days at 2–8°C.

Following reconstitution with sterile or bacteriostatic water for injection, ampicillin sodium solutions for IM or direct IV injection should be used within 1 hour after reconstitution and should not be frozen. The stability of ampicillin sodium in solution is concentration dependent and decreases as the concentration of the drug increases. Ampicillin sodium appears to be especially susceptible to inactivation in solutions containing dextrose, which appears to have a catalytic effect on hydrolysis of the drug.

The manufacturers report that when stored at room temperature (25°C), ampicillin sodium solutions containing 30 mg or less of ampicillin per mL in sterile water for injection, 0.9% sodium chloride injection, ⅙ *M* sodium lactate injection, or lactated Ringer's injection lose less than 10% of activity within 8 hours and solutions containing 2 mg or less of ampicillin per mL in 5% dextrose, 5% dextrose and 0.45% sodium chloride, or 10% invert sugar lose less than 10% of activity within 4 hours. At concentrations of 10–20 mg/mL in 5% dextrose, ampicillin loses less than 10% of its activity within 2 hours at room temperature.

When refrigerated at 4°C, ampicillin sodium solutions containing 30 mg of ampicillin per mL are stable for 48 hours in sterile water for injection or 0.9% sodium chloride injection and solutions containing 30 mg or less per mL are stable for 24 hours in lactated Ringer's or 8 hours in ⅙ *M* sodium lactate injection. Solutions of the drug containing 20 mg or less of ampicillin per mL are stable at 4°C for 72 hours in sterile water for injection or 0.9% sodium chloride injection, 4 hours in 5% dextrose, or 3 hours in 10% invert sugar and solutions containing 10 mg or less per mL are stable for 4 hours at 4°C in 5% dextrose and 0.45% sodium chloride.

Following reconstitution of the commercially available 10-g pharmacy bulk package of ampicillin sodium, solutions containing 100 mg of ampicillin per mL should either be used or discarded within 2 hours if stored at room temperature or within 4 hours if refrigerated. If reconstituted solutions of the 10-g bulk unit containing 100 mg/mL are stored for less than 1 hour at room temperature prior to dilution with a compatible IV solution, previously stated stability information associated with the diluents is applicable.

Ampicillin sodium is potentially physically and/or chemically incompatible with some drugs, including aminoglycosides, but the compatibility depends on several factors (e.g., concentrations of the drugs, specific diluents used, resulting pH, temperature). For information on the in vitro and in vivo incompatibility of penicillins and aminoglycosides, see Drug Interactions: Aminoglycosides, in the Aminopenicillins General Statement 8:12.16.08. Specialized references should be consulted for specific compatibility information. Because of the potential for incompatibility, ampicillin sodium and aminoglycosides should not be admixed.

For further information on chemistry and stability, mechanism of action, spectrum, resistance, pharmacokinetics, uses, cautions, drug interactions, laboratory test interferences, and dosage and administration of ampicillin, see the Aminopenicillins General Statement 8:12.16.08.

Preparations

Excipients in commercially available drug preparations may have clinically important effects in some individuals; consult specific product labeling for details.

Ampicillin (Trihydrate)

Oral		
Capsules	250 mg (of ampicillin)*	**Ampicillin Capsules**
	500 mg (of ampicillin)*	**Ampicillin Capsules**
For suspension	125 mg (of ampicillin) per 5 mL*	**Ampicillin for Suspension**
	250 mg (of ampicillin) per 5 mL*	**Ampicillin for Suspension**

*available from one or more manufacturer, distributor, and/or repackager by generic (nonproprietary) name

Ampicillin Sodium

Parenteral		
For injection	125 mg (of ampicillin)*	**Ampicillin Sodium for Injection**
	250 mg (of ampicillin)*	**Ampicillin Sodium for Injection**
	500 mg (of ampicillin)*	**Ampicillin Sodium for Injection**
	1 g (of ampicillin)*	**Ampicillin Sodium for Injection**
	2 g (of ampicillin)*	**Ampicillin Sodium for Injection**
	10 g (of ampicillin) pharmacy bulk package*	**Ampicillin Sodium for Injection**

For injection, for IV infusion	1 g (of ampicillin)*	**Ampicillin Sodium ADD-Vantage®**
		Ampicillin Sodium Piggyback
	2 g (of ampicillin)*	**Ampicillin Sodium ADD-Vantage®**
		Ampicillin Sodium Piggyback

*available from one or more manufacturer, distributor, and/or repackager by generic (nonproprietary) name

†Use is not currently included in the labeling approved by the US Food and Drug Administration

Ampicillin Sodium and Sulbactam Sodium

Ampicillin and Sulbactam

■ Ampicillin sodium and sulbactam sodium is a fixed combination of the sodium salts of ampicillin (an aminopenicillin antibiotic) and sulbactam (a β-lactamase inhibitor); sulbactam synergistically expands ampicillin's spectrum of activity against many strains of β-lactamase-producing bacteria.

Uses

Ampicillin sodium and sulbactam sodium is used parenterally for the treatment of skin and skin structure, intra-abdominal, and gynecologic infections caused by susceptible bacteria. The drug also has been used parenterally for the treatment of other infections, including respiratory tract infections† caused by susceptible bacteria.

Ampicillin sodium and sulbactam sodium is used principally for the treatment of infections caused by, or suspected of being caused by, susceptible β-lactamase-producing strains of staphylococci, Enterobacteriaceae, and/or *Bacteroides*. Although ampicillin sodium and sulbactam sodium also may be effective in the treatment of infections caused by non-β-lactamase-producing bacteria susceptible to ampicillin alone, most clinicians state that an aminopenicillin used alone is preferred to the combination drug for the treatment of these infections and that ampicillin sodium and sulbactam sodium should be reserved for use in the treatment of infections caused by, or suspected of being caused by, β-lactamase-producing bacteria when an aminopenicillin alone would be ineffective. Ampicillin sodium and sulbactam sodium may be particularly useful for the empiric treatment of intra-abdominal or gynecologic infections likely to involve anaerobes (e.g., mixed aerobic-anaerobic infections) or for infections suspected of being caused by both ampicillin-resistant and ampicillin-susceptible bacteria. For most other infections caused by susceptible organisms, including *Staphylococcus aureus* or *S. epidermidis*†, *Bacteroides*, *Klebsiella pneumoniae*, *Escherichia coli*, indole-positive Proteeae (e.g., *Proteus vulgaris*†, *Providencia rettgeri*†, *Morganella morganii*†), *Eikenella corrodens*, or *Pasteurella multocida*†, ampicillin sodium and sulbactam sodium generally is considered an alternative to other anti-infectives. When used for the treatment of infections caused by Enterobacteriaceae in*severely ill* patients, some clinicians recommend combined therapy with ampicillin sodium and sulbactam sodium and an aminoglycoside. Because ampicillin sodium and sulbactam sodium is not active against *Pseudomonas*, the drug should not be used alone in infections known or suspected of being caused by *Ps. aeruginosa*. The relative efficacy of ampicillin sodium and sulbactam sodium compared with other anti-infective combinations that include a β-lactamase inhibitor (e.g., amoxicillin and clavulanate potassium, ticarcillin disodium and clavulanate potassium) remains to be established.

Prior to initiation of therapy with ampicillin sodium and sulbactam sodium, appropriate specimens should be obtained for identification of the causative organism(s) and in vitro susceptibility tests. Ampicillin sodium and sulbactam sodium may be started pending results of susceptibility tests if the infection is believed to be caused by β-lactamase-producing bacteria susceptible to the drug, but should be discontinued and other appropriate anti-infective therapy substituted if the organism is found to be resistant to the drug. (See Spectrum: In Vitro Susceptibility Testing.) If the infection is found to be caused by non-β-lactamase-producing organisms susceptible to ampicillin, some clinicians suggest that therapy should be changed to an aminopenicillin alone, unless this is impractical.

■ **Skin and Skin Structure Infections** Parenteral ampicillin sodium and sulbactam sodium is used in adults and children 1 year of age or older for the treatment of a variety of skin and skin structure infections, including wound infections, cellulitis, ulcers, abscesses, and furunculosis, caused by susceptible β-lactamase-producing strains of *Staphylococcus aureus*, *Escherichia coli*, *Klebsiella* (including *K. pneumoniae*), *Proteus mirabilis*, *Bacteroides* (including *B. fragilis*), or *Acinetobacter*. The drug also has been effective when used in adults for the treatment of skin and skin structure infections caused by other susceptible gram-positive bacteria, including *S. epidermidis*†, *S. warneri*†, or *Enterococcus faecalis* (formerly *Streptococcus faecalis*)†, or other susceptible gram-negative bacteria, including susceptible strains of *Citrobacter*†, *Enterobacter*†, or *Morganella morganii*†.

In controlled studies in adults with serious skin and skin structure infections, parenteral ampicillin sodium and sulbactam sodium was at least as effective as a regimen of clindamycin with or without an aminoglycoside. Parenteral ampicillin sodium and sulbactam sodium therapy generally results in clinical and bacteriologic cure rates of 86–100% in adults with skin and skin structure infections caused by susceptible bacteria. Although parenteral ampicillin sodium and sulbactam sodium appears to be an effective regimen for the treatment of serious skin and skin structure infections, concomitant use of an anti-infective agent that is active against *Pseudomonas* (e.g., an aminoglycoside) may be necessary in some of these infections. In addition, less severe skin and skin structure infections (e.g., cellulitis, impetigo, erysipelas) usually can be treated with other more cost-effective therapies that have a narrower spectrum of activity (e.g., penicillinase-resistant penicillins, erythromycin, cephalosporins).

■ **Intra-abdominal and Gynecologic Infections** Parenteral ampicillin sodium and sulbactam sodium is used effectively in adults for the treatment of a variety of intra-abdominal and gynecologic infections caused by susceptible *E. coli*, *Klebsiella* (including *K. pneumoniae*), *Bacteroides* (including *B. fragilis*), or *Enterobacter*. Most intra-abdominal and gynecologic infections are mixed aerobic-anaerobic infections, and efficacy of ampicillin sodium and sulbactam sodium in these polymicrobial infections is based on the drug's broad spectrum of activity against both gram-positive and gram-negative aerobic and anaerobic bacteria and on its distribution into most tissues and fluids. Depending on suspected organisms and severity of the infection, addition of an aminoglycoside may be considered.

Intra-abdominal Infections Parenteral ampicillin sodium and sulbactam sodium has been effective when used in adults as an adjunct to surgical measures (e.g., drainage) in the treatment of appendicitis, peritonitis, perforated appendix, diverticulitis, postoperative bowel infections, small bowel infarct, intra-abdominal or retroperitoneal abscess, cholecystitis, and secondary liver infections caused by susceptible bacteria.

Use of parenteral ampicillin sodium and sulbactam sodium therapy in adults with intra-abdominal infections has been associated with clinical and bacteriologic cure rates of 78–96%. In a few studies in adults, parenteral ampicillin sodium and sulbactam sodium appeared to be at least as effective as other regimens used in the adjunctive treatment of intra-abdominal infections (e.g., clindamycin or metronidazole and an aminoglycoside, cefoxitin with or without an aminoglycoside, imipenem and cilastatin sodium) and generally was associated with fewer adverse effects than these other regimens. However, in at least one study, parenteral ampicillin sodium and sulbactam sodium was less effective than a regimen of clindamycin and gentamicin in the treatment of patients with perforated or gangrenous appendicitis; most treatment failures in patients receiving ampicillin sodium and sulbactam sodium were the result of overgrowth with *Pseudomonas*. Some clinicians suggest that, although parenteral ampicillin sodium and sulbactam sodium alone may be as effective as multiple-drug regimens for the treatment of less severe intra-abdominal infections, an aminoglycoside probably should be used concomitantly with the drug for empiric therapy in more serious intra-abdominal infections, including hospital-acquired infections, pending results of in vitro susceptibility tests. In addition, some clinicians suggest that other anti-infective agents (e.g., ticarcillin disodium and clavulanate potassium) may be preferred for empiric therapy in serious intra-abdominal infections.

Gynecologic Infections Parenteral ampicillin sodium and sulbactam sodium is used effectively in adults for the treatment of gynecologic infections including endometritis (after abortion or curettage), postpartum endomyometritis, posthysterectomy pelvic cellulitis, vaginal cuff abscess, salpingitis, tubo-ovarian abscess, pelvic peritonitis or abscess, surgical wound sepsis, uncomplicated acute pelvic inflammatory disease (PID), or complicated PID that may include pelvic peritonitis, tubo-ovarian abscesses, endometritis, or posthysterectomy pelvic cellulitis. The clinical and bacteriologic cure rates of parenteral ampicillin sodium and sulbactam in the treatment of these gynecologic infections have been 83–100%.

In several studies in patients with mixed aerobic-anaerobic gynecologic infections, parenteral ampicillin sodium and sulbactam sodium was as effective as cefoxitin or cefotetan or multiple-drug regimens such as clindamycin or metronidazole and an aminoglycoside in the treatment of these infections and generally was associated with fewer adverse effects. The fact that ampicillin sodium and sulbactam sodium generally is considered to be inactive against*Mycoplasma* and to have incomplete inhibitory activity against *Chlamydia* should be considered if the drug is used in the treatment of gynecologic infections, and concomitant tetracycline (e.g., doxycycline) or, alternatively, macrolide therapy probably should be included if there is a possibility that these organisms are involved in the gynecologic infection being treated.

Parenteral ampicillin sodium and sulbactam sodium is effective for the treatment of both gonococcal and nongonococcal PID and appears to be at least as effective in the treatment of these infections as cefoxitin or a regimen of metronidazole or clindamycin given with gentamicin. In the treatment of PID, ampicillin sodium and sulbactam sodium generally has good coverage against *Chlamydia trachomatis*, *N. gonorrhoeae*, and anaerobes and appears to be effective for patients who have tuboovarian abscess. When a parenteral regimen is indicated for the treatment of patients with PID, the US Centers for Disease Control and Prevention (CDC) and other clinicians generally recommend a regimen of cefotetan or cefoxitin given in conjunction with doxycycline or a regimen of clindamycin given in conjunction with gentamicin; however, a regimen of IV ampicillin sodium and sulbactam sodium given in conjunction with doxycycline is one of several alternative parenteral regimens recommended for the treatment of PID. For further information on treatment of PID, see Uses: Pelvic Inflammatory Disease in the Cephalosporins General Statement 8:12.06.

■ **Gonorrhea and Associated Infections** Parenteral ampicillin sodium and sulbactam sodium has been used effectively in the treatment of uncomplicated gonorrhea† caused by penicillinase-producing strains of *Neisseria* *gonorrhoeae* (PPNG) and nonpenicillinase-producing strains of the organism. An oral preparation of ampicillin and sulbactam (sultamicillin; not commercially available in the US) also has been effective when used for the treatment of uncomplicated gonorrhea. However, penicillins, including ampicillin sodium and sulbactam sodium, are not included in current CDC recommendations for the treatment of gonorrhea.

A single 1.5- or 3-g IM dose of ampicillin sodium and sulbactam sodium (1 or 2 g of ampicillin and 0.5 or 1 g of sulbactam) given alone or in conjunction with oral probenecid (1 g) has been effective in men and women for the treatment of uncomplicated urethral and endocervical gonorrhea caused by PPNG or nonpenicillinase-producing *N. gonorrhoeae*. This regimen has been associated with a bacteriologic cure rate of 82–100% in adults with uncomplicated PPNG infections. In one study, more treatment failures were reported in patients with PPNG infections who received IM ampicillin sodium and sulbactam sodium without concomitant oral probenecid; however, in another study, regimens of the drug with or without concomitant oral probenecid appeared to be equally effective. A single 3-g dose of ampicillin sodium and sulbactam sodium (2 g of ampicillin and 1 g of sulbactam) given in conjunction with oral probenecid (1 g) has been effective in the treatment of anorectal gonococcal infections in both men and women and also has been effective for the treatment of pharyngeal gonococcal infections in a few men. Single-dose ampicillin sodium and sulbactam sodium therapy for gonorrhea is ineffective in the treatment of coexisting chlamydial or mycoplasmal infections and generally does not prevent postgonococcal urethritis.

■ **Respiratory Tract Infections** In uncontrolled studies, parenteral ampicillin sodium and sulbactam sodium has been used with some success in adults and children† for the treatment of lower respiratory tract infections†, including pneumonia, bronchitis, acute exacerbations of chronic bronchitis, and bronchiectasis caused by susceptible staphylococci, streptococci, *Haemophilus influenzae, H. parainfluenzae, Moraxella catarrhalis* (formerly *Branhamella catarrhalis*), *E. coli, Klebsiella*, or *Proteus mirabilis*. In most reported cases, parenteral ampicillin sodium and sulbactam sodium therapy resulted in clinical and bacteriologic cure rates of 75–96% in adults with lower respiratory tract infections.

Some clinicians suggest that parenteral ampicillin sodium and sulbactam sodium is an effective alternative for the treatment of lower respiratory tract infections known or suspected of being caused by ampicillin-resistant organisms, including community-acquired or nosocomial pneumonia, chronic obstructive pulmonary disease, and exacerbation of severe chronic bronchitis in hospitalized patients. However, long-term efficacy and rate of relapse associated with use of parenteral ampicillin sodium and sulbactam sodium in the treatment of lower respiratory tract infections remain to be established. In addition, overgrowth with *Ps. aeruginosa* has been reported in some patients receiving parenteral ampicillin sodium and sulbactam sodium alone for the treatment of respiratory infections.

Parenteral ampicillin sodium and sulbactam sodium has been effective in a few patients for the treatment of respiratory tract infections† (e.g., pneumonia, tracheobronchitis) or bacteremia caused by strains of *Acinetobacter baumannii* (*A. calcoaceticus* subsp. *anitratus*)† that were resistant to imipenem and cilastatin sodium as well as most other anti-infective agents tested. However, other anti-infectives (e.g., imipenem and cilastatin sodium or meropenem with or without an aminoglycoside) currently are preferred in the treatment of infections caused by susceptible *Acinetobacter*.

Parenteral ampicillin sodium and sulbactam sodium also has been used in a limited number of adults and children† for the treatment of various ear, nose, and throat infections† including tonsillitis, sinusitis, rhinitis, pharyngitis, acute epiglottitis, and acute and chronic otitis media caused by susceptible staphylococci, streptococci, *Klebsiella, Proteus, M. catarrhalis*, or *H. influenzae*. Although the drug generally was effective in the treatment of these infections and had a clinical cure rate of 98%, other anti-infective agents are considered drugs of choice for these infections.

■ **Bone and Joint Infections** Parenteral ampicillin sodium and sulbactam sodium has been effective when used in a limited number of adults or children† for the treatment of bone and joint infections† including osteomyelitis and/or septic arthritis caused by susceptible β-lactamase-producing organisms. In one pediatric study, an initial phase of parenteral ampicillin sodium and sulbactam sodium therapy (50 mg/kg of ampicillin and 12.5 mg/kg of sulbactam IV every 6 hours) was followed by therapy with an oral formulation of ampicillin and sulbactam (sultamicillin; not commercially available in the US). Although parenteral ampicillin sodium and sulbactam sodium appeared to be effective in the treatment of acute bone and joint infections, further studies are needed to evaluate the long-term efficacy of the drug in these infections.

■ **Perioperative Prophylaxis** Parenteral ampicillin sodium and sulbactam sodium has been used effectively in adults and children† to reduce the incidence of infections in patients undergoing contaminated or potentially contaminated surgery† (e.g., GI or biliary tract surgery, vaginal or abdominal hysterectomy, transurethral prostatectomy). However, less costly anti-infectives, often with narrower spectra of activity (e.g., cephalosporins), generally have been preferred when prophylaxis was indicated in such procedures.

In adults undergoing biliary tract surgery, a single 3-g dose of ampicillin and sulbactam (2 g of ampicillin and 1 g of sulbactam) was as effective as a single dose of cefazolin (1 g) or cefoxitin (2 g) in preventing postoperative wound infection†. A single 1.5-g dose of ampicillin and sulbactam (1 g of ampicillin and 0.5 g of sulbactam) has been used effectively for prophylaxis in various gynecologic procedures†, including abdominal or vaginal hysterectomy and first-trimester vacuum aspiration abortions. When given immediately prior to the procedure in patients undergoing first-trimester abortions, the drug reduced the incidence of early postoperative infections (e.g., endometritis) but not the incidence of late infections. In addition, because the drug generally is considered inactive against chlamydia, it cannot prevent postoperative infections with this organism. In a study in adults, parenteral ampicillin sodium and sulbactam sodium was as effective as cefoxitin for prevention of postoperative infections in patients undergoing colorectal or transurethral surgery†. In a study in children† 5–13 years of age undergoing appendectomy, a single dose of ampicillin and sulbactam (15 mg/kg of ampicillin and 7.5 mg/kg of sulbactam) given IV at the time of anesthesia was as effective as a single dose of metronidazole (7.5 mg/kg) and cefotaxime (25 mg/kg) in the prevention of postoperative sepsis†; therapy with the drug was continued for 72 hours after surgery in patients with gangrenous or perforated appendixes at the time of surgery. Some clinicians suggest that parenteral ampicillin sodium and sulbactam sodium is an effective alternative to other anti-infective regimens used for perioperative prophylaxis in patients undergoing GI or gynecologic surgery. However, further study is needed to evaluate more fully such use of parenteral ampicillin sodium and sulbactam sodium.

Parenteral ampicillin sodium and sulbactam sodium also has been used with some success for perioperative prophylaxis in patients with head and neck cancer undergoing surgery†. Although in one study ampicillin sodium and sulbactam sodium appeared to be as effective as a regimen of clindamycin and amikacin in such patients, patients who received ampicillin and sulbactam had a higher incidence of postoperative infection with anaerobes than patients who received the other regimen.

■ **Meningitis** Parenteral ampicillin sodium and sulbactam sodium has been used effectively in a few adults for the treatment of meningitis† caused by *N. meningitidis* or *S. pneumoniae*. In addition, an IV formulation of the drug containing an 8:1 ratio of ampicillin to sulbactam (not commercially available in the US) has been used effectively in children 1 month to 14 years of age† for the treatment of meningitis† caused by *H. influenzae, S. pneumoniae, N. meningitidis, K. pneumoniae*, or *Listeria*. In one study in infants and children, ampicillin sodium (400 mg/kg daily) and sulbactam sodium (50 mg/kg daily) was as effective as a regimen of IV chloramphenicol (100 mg/kg daily) and IV ampicillin (400 mg/kg daily) for the treatment of meningitis caused by *H. influenzae, S. pneumoniae*, or *N. meningitidis*. Although a few clinicians suggest that parenteral ampicillin sodium and sulbactam sodium therapy may be an effective alternative to therapy with ampicillin and chloramphenicol in infants and children for the treatment of meningitis caused by *H. influenzae, S. pneumoniae*, or*N. meningitidis* and might be especially useful in areas where ampicillin- and chloramphenicol-resistant strains have been reported, other drugs are preferred for the treatment of CNS infections and some clinicians strongly discourage use of ampicillin sodium and sulbactam sodium in these infections. Results of at least one study using animal models suggest that ampicillin sodium and sulbactam sodium may be of limited value for the treatment of meningitis caused by organisms less susceptible to the drug (e.g., *Escherichia coli*), and treatment failures have been reported when the drug was used in patients with meningitis caused by *K. pneumoniae*.

■ **Urinary Tract Infections** Parenteral ampicillin sodium and sulbactam sodium has been used in a limited number of adults or children† for the treatment of uncomplicated urinary tract infections† caused by susceptible bacteria, including *S. epidermidis, E. coli, K. pneumoniae*, or *P. mirabilis*. Although the drug was effective in up to 90% of these infections, treatment failures have been reported and further study is needed to evaluate more fully use of ampicillin sodium and sulbactam sodium in the treatment of complicated urinary tract infections.

Dosage and Administration

■ **Reconstitution and Administration** Ampicillin sodium and sulbactam sodium is administered by IM or slow IV injection or by IV infusion. Ampicillin and sulbactam also have been administered orally as a preparation containing the drugs covalently linked as a double ester in a single molecule (sultamicillin; CP-49,952), but an oral dosage form currently is not commercially available in the US.

IM or IV solutions of ampicillin sodium and sulbactam sodium should be allowed to stand after dissolution to allow any foaming to dissipate in order to permit visual inspection for complete solubilization.

IM Injection For IM injection, vials labeled as containing 1.5 or 3 g of combined ampicillin and sulbactam should be reconstituted with 3.2 or 6.4 mL, respectively, of sterile water for injection or 0.5 or 2% lidocaine hydrochloride injection to provide a solution containing 375 mg of the drug per mL (250 mg of ampicillin and 125 mg of sulbactam per mL). Reconstituting ampicillin sodium and sulbactam sodium with lidocaine hydrochloride can minimize the local pain associated with IM injection of the drug. IM injections should be made deeply into a large muscle mass within 1 hour after reconstitution.

IV Injection or Infusion For IV administration, bottles labeled as containing 1.5 or 3 g of combined ampicillin and sulbactam may be reconstituted directly to the desired concentration with a compatible IV solution (See Chemistry and Stability: Stability.). Vials labeled as containing 1.5 or 3 g of the drug initially should be reconstituted with sterile water for injection to yield solutions containing 375 mg of the drug per mL (250 mg of ampicillin and 125 mg of sulbactam per mL). An appropriate volume of reconstituted drug then should be diluted immediately with a compatible IV solution to yield solutions containing 3–45 mg of the drug per mL (2–30 mg of ampicillin and 1–15 mg of sulbactam per mL). ADD-Vantage® vials labeled as containing 1.5 or 3 g of combined ampicillin and sulbactam should be reconstituted with the 0.9% sodium chloride injection diluent provided according to the manufacturer's directions.

IV injections of ampicillin sodium and sulbactam sodium should be given slowly over at least 10–15 minutes to avoid the possibility of seizures. IV infusions of the drug also should be infused slowly over 15–30 minutes.

■ Dosage Dosage of ampicillin sodium and sulbactam sodium generally is expressed in terms of the total of the ampicillin and sulbactam content of the fixed combination. Potency of both ampicillin sodium and sulbactam sodium are expressed in terms of the bases of the drugs.

Ampicillin sodium and sulbactam sodium is commercially available for parenteral administration as a sterile powder containing a 2:1 ratio of ampicillin to sulbactam. The manufacturer's dosage recommendations for adults are the same for IM and IV administration; however, higher serum concentrations usually are attained with IV administration of the drug, and this route generally is preferred, especially for severe infections.

Adult Dosage The usual adult IM or IV dosage of ampicillin and sulbactam for the treatment of skin and skin structure, intra-abdominal, or gynecologic infections caused by susceptible organisms ranges from 1.5 g (1 of ampicillin and 0.5 g of sulbactam) to 3 g (2 g of ampicillin and 1 g of sulbactam) every 6 hours. The maximum adult dosage of sulbactam recommended by the manufacturer is 4 g (i.e., 8 g of ampicillin and 4 g of sulbactam in fixed combination) daily. While comparative efficacy of various dosages in the usual range have not been established, most patients in clinical studies of these infections received the maximum 3-g (2 g of ampicillin and 1 g of sulbactam) recommended dosage.

For the treatment of acute pelvic inflammatory disease (PID) in adults and adolescents when a parenteral regimen is indicated, IV ampicillin and sulbactam may be given in a dosage of 3 g (2 g of ampicillin and 1 g of sulbactam) every 6 hours in conjunction with doxycycline (100 mg orally or IV every 12 hours). The parenteral regimen may be discontinued 24 hours after clinical improvement; however, oral doxycycline (100 mg twice daily) should be continued to complete 14 days of therapy.

Pediatric Dosage Pediatric patients who weigh 40 kg or more may receive the usual adult dosage of ampicillin sodium and sulbactam sodium.

For the treatment of skin and skin structure infections in pediatric patients 1 year of age or older, the usual dosage of ampicillin and sulbactam is 300 mg/kg daily (200 mg of ampicillin and 100 mg of sulbactam) given by IV infusion in equally divided doses every 6 hours. The manufacturer recommends that the duration of IV ampicillin sodium and sulbactam sodium therapy in pediatric patients not exceed 14 days; in clinical studies, most children received an oral anti-infective after an initial regimen of IV ampicillin sodium and sulbactam sodium.

The American Academy of Pediatrics (AAP) suggests that pediatric patients 1 month of age or older receive ampicillin sodium and sulbactam sodium in a dosage of 100–150 mg/kg of ampicillin daily in 4 divided doses for the treatment of mild to moderate infections or a dosage of 200–300 mg/kg of ampicillin daily in 4 divided doses for the treatment of severe infections.

■ Dosage in Renal Impairment In patients with impaired renal function, doses and/or frequency of administration of ampicillin sodium and sulbactam sodium should be modified in response to the degree of renal impairment, severity of infection, and susceptibility of the causative organism. Because the pharmacokinetics of both ampicillin and sulbactam are affected to the same degree in patients with renal impairment, the recommended 2:1 ratio of the drugs remains the same regardless of the degree of renal impairment.

The manufacturer recommends that patients with renal impairment receive the usually recommended doses of ampicillin and sulbactam but that these doses be given less frequently than usual and that dosing intervals be based on the patient's creatinine clearance. The manufacturer recommends that patients with creatinine clearances of 30 mL/minute per 1.73 m² or greater receive 1.5 g (1 g of ampicillin and 0.5 g of sulbactam) to 3 g (2 g of ampicillin and 1 g of sulbactam) of the drug every 6–8 hours and that patients with creatinine clearances of 15–29 or 5–14 mL/minute per 1.73 m² receive these doses every 12 or 24 hours, respectively.

Because ampicillin and sulbactam are removed by hemodialysis, some clinicians suggest that patients undergoing hemodialysis receive 1.5 g (1 g of ampicillin and 0.5 g of sulbactam) to 3 g (2 g of ampicillin and 1 g of sulbactam) once every 24 hours and that the dose preferably should be given immediately after dialysis.

Cautions

Ampicillin sodium and sulbactam sodium generally is well tolerated. The frequency and severity of adverse effects reported with the commercially available fixed-combination preparation for parenteral administration generally are similar to those reported with parenteral ampicillin alone. With the exception of local reactions at the IM injection site, adverse effects generally have been reported in 10% or less of patients receiving parenteral ampicillin sodium and sulbactam sodium, and have been severe enough to require discontinuance of the drug in less than 1% of patients. The most frequent adverse effects of parenteral ampicillin sodium and sulbactam sodium are pain at the IM or IV injection site, diarrhea, and rash.

Parenteral sulbactam sodium alone is associated with few adverse effects, principally pain at the injection site and diarrhea.

For information on adverse effects reported with ampicillin and other aminopenicillins as well as the usual precautions and contraindications associated with these drugs, see Cautions in the Aminopenicillins General Statement 8:12.16.08.

■ GI Effects Diarrhea, nausea, and vomiting have been reported in up to 4% of patients receiving parenteral ampicillin sodium and sulbactam sodium. Flatulence, abdominal discomfort or distension, rectal bleeding, and glossitis have been reported in less than 1% of patients receiving the drug parenterally. Gastritis, stomatitis, and black or hairy tongue have been reported in patients receiving aminopenicillins, and these reactions may occur with ampicillin sodium and sulbactam sodium.

In one study, parenteral ampicillin sodium and sulbactam sodium therapy decreased total counts of normal anaerobic fecal flora but did not substantially affect total counts of normal aerobic fecal flora. This may have occurred because only low concentrations of ampicillin and sulbactam are excreted in feces. *Clostridium difficile*-associated diarrhea and colitis (also known as antibiotic-associated pseudomembranous colitis) caused by toxin-producing clostridia has been reported with parenteral ampicillin sodium and sulbactam sodium and has also been reported with use of an oral preparation containing ampicillin and sulbactam (sultamicillin; not currently available in the US). Colitis may occur during or following discontinuance of the drug and may range in severity from mild to life-threatening. Mild cases of colitis may respond to discontinuance of ampicillin sodium and sulbactam sodium alone, but diagnosis and management of moderate to severe cases should include appropriate bacteriologic studies and treatment with fluid, electrolyte, and protein supplementation as indicated. If colitis is moderate to severe or is not relieved by discontinuance of the drug, appropriate anti-infective therapy (e.g., oral metronidazole or vancomycin) should be administered.

■ Dermatologic and Sensitivity Reactions Rash has been reported in less than 2% of patients receiving parenteral ampicillin sodium and sulbactam sodium. Urticaria, pruritus, dry skin, and erythema also have been reported with the drug. Erythema multiforme and an occasional case of exfoliative dermatitis have been reported in patients receiving aminopenicillins and these dermatologic reactions may occur with ampicillin sodium and sulbactam sodium. The manufacturer states that such reactions may be controlled with antihistamines and, if necessary, systemic corticosteroids. Whenever such hypersensitivity reactions occur during therapy with ampicillin sodium and sulbactam sodium, the drug should be discontinued, unless the opinion of the physician dictates otherwise.

Serious and occasionally fatal hypersensitivity reactions, including anaphylaxis, can occur during penicillin therapy. (See Cautions: Precautions and Contraindications.) Several patients have developed systemic allergic reactions during parenteral ampicillin sodium and sulbactam sodium therapy that required discontinuance of the drug. In one patient, the reaction consisted of neck tightness, difficulty and pain when breathing, generalized weakness, and hypertension. If a severe hypersensitivity reaction occurs during ampicillin sodium and sulbactam sodium therapy, the drug should be discontinued and the patient given appropriate treatment (e.g., epinephrine, corticosteroids, maintenance of an adequate airway, oxygen) as indicated.

■ Local Reactions The most frequent adverse effect of parenteral ampicillin sodium and sulbactam sodium is pain at the injection site. Pain at the injection site has been reported in 3–16% of patients receiving the drug IM and in up to 3% of patients receiving the drug IV. Pain following IM administration of ampicillin sodium and sulbactam sodium may last for 5–60 minutes and may be minimized or avoided if 0.5 or 2% lidocaine hydrochloride is used as the diluent when preparing IM injections of the drug. Phlebitis, thrombophlebitis, and inflammation at the injection site also have been reported in up to 3% of patients receiving the drug IV.

■ Other Adverse Effects Although a definite causal relationship to the drug has not been established, transient increases in serum concentrations of AST (SGOT) and/or ALT (SGPT), alkaline phosphatase, LDH, creatine kinase (CK, creatine phosphokinase, CPK), bilirubin, and γ-glutamyltransferase (γ-glutamyltranspeptidase, GT, GGTP) have been reported in up to 11% of patients receiving parenteral ampicillin sodium and sulbactam sodium. Decreased concentrations of serum albumin and total protein also have been reported. Increased BUN and serum creatinine concentrations, presence of red blood cells and hyaline casts in urine, urine retention, dysuria, and hematuria have been reported in less than 1% of patients receiving the drug.

Decreased hemoglobin concentration, hematocrit, and erythrocyte, leukocyte, neutrophil, lymphocyte, and platelet counts and increased lymphocyte, monocyte, basophil, eosinophil, and platelet counts have been reported in patients receiving parenteral ampicillin sodium and sulbactam sodium. Although some of these hematologic changes may represent hypersensitivity reactions, many have not been attributed directly to the drug.

Other adverse effects that have been reported in less than 1% of patients receiving parenteral ampicillin sodium and sulbactam sodium include headache, fatigue, malaise, confusion, dizziness, changes in smell or taste perception, chest pain or tightness, edema, facial swelling, chills, throat tightness, substernal pain, epistaxis, and mucosal bleeding.

In at least one patient, acute hyperpyrexia (oral temperatures up to 40°C) occurred approximately 30 minutes after initiation of parenteral ampicillin sodium and sulbactam sodium therapy. Rapid defervescence occurred within 1 hour after completion of the infusion, but the reaction recurred with each subsequent dose. This reaction did not appear to be a hypersensitivity reaction to either drug nor a reaction to some contaminant. Instead, it presumably was caused by the sulbactam sodium component since the patient previously had received ampicillin alone without a similar reaction and the reaction recurred with different lot numbers of the combination but did not occur in other patients.

Reversible glycogenosis has been reported in animals receiving sulbactam. Diffuse hepatocellular glycogen deposits associated with increases in liver enzymes and hepatomegaly have occurred in rats and dogs that received high doses of sulbactam for prolonged periods of time. These adverse effects in animals were dose and time dependent and are not expected to occur in humans with the usually recommended ampicillin sodium and sulbactam sodium dosages and corresponding plasma concentrations of the drug attained during the relatively short periods of therapy. To date, similar glycogen deposits have not been reported in humans receiving ampicillin sodium and sulbactam sodium, although patients with preexisting liver dysfunction, diabetes mellitus, hypoglycemia, or glycogen storage disease were excluded from most early clinical studies of the drug. In subsequent studies in patients with type I or II diabetes mellitus, sulbactam given at the usually recommended dosages did not appear to affect glucose mobilization or regulation.

■ **Precautions and Contraindications** Ampicillin sodium and sulbactam sodium shares the toxic potentials of the penicillins, including the risk of hypersensitivity reactions, and the usual precautions of penicillin therapy should be observed. (See Cautions in the Aminopenicillins General Statement 8:12.16.08.) Prior to initiation of therapy with ampicillin sodium and sulbactam sodium, careful inquiry should be made concerning previous hypersensitivity reactions to penicillins, cephalosporins, or other drugs. There is clinical and laboratory evidence of partial cross-allergenicity among penicillins and other β-lactam antibiotics including cephalosporins and cephamycins.(See Cautions: Hypersensitivity Reactions, in the Natural Penicillins General Statement 8:12.16.04.) Ampicillin sodium and sulbactam sodium is contraindicated in patients who are hypersensitive to any penicillin.

Because *C. difficile*-associated diarrhea and colitis has been reported with the use of anti-infective agents, including ampicillin sodium and sulbactam sodium, it should be considered in the differential diagnosis of patients who develop diarrhea during ampicillin sodium and sulbactam sodium therapy.

Because a high percentage of patients with infectious mononucleosis have developed rash during therapy with aminopenicillins (see Cautions: Ampicillin Rash, in the Aminopenicillins General Statement 8:12.16.08), the manufacturer recommends that ampicillin sodium and sulbactam sodium not be used in patients with the disease.

As with use of other anti-infective agents, use of ampicillin sodium and sulbactam sodium may result in overgrowth of nonsusceptible organisms, especially *Pseudomonas* or *Candida*. Careful monitoring of the patient and periodic in vitro susceptibility tests are essential. If superinfection occurs, the drug should be discontinued and appropriate therapy initiated.

For a more complete discussion of these and other precautions associated with the use of ampicillin, see Cautions: Precautions and Contraindications, in the Aminopenicillins General Statement 8:12.16.08.

■ **Pediatric Precautions** Safety and efficacy of IV ampicillin sodium and sulbactam sodium in children 1 year of age or older have been established for the treatment of skin and skin structure infections. Safety and efficacy of IV ampicillin sodium and sulbactam sodium for the treatment of other infections (e.g., intra-abdominal infections) in pediatric patients have not been established. In addition, safety and efficacy of IM administration of the drug in pediatric patients have not been established.

Various combinations of ampicillin and sulbactam (e.g., 1.3:1, 2:1, 3:1, 4:1, 7:1, and 8:1 ratios of ampicillin to sulbactam) have been administered IM or IV to neonates and children 1 month to 17 years of age without unusual adverse effects. The most frequent adverse effects of parenteral ampicillin sodium and sulbactam sodium in children are transient increases in serum liver enzyme concentrations, diarrhea, and rash. An oral preparation containing ampicillin and sulbactam (sultamicillin; not commercially available in the US) also has been used in children 5 months to 17 years of age. Although the oral preparation generally was well tolerated in children, diarrhea occurred in 42% of children receiving the formulation in one study and was severe enough to require discontinuance of the drug in 14%.

■ **Geriatric Precautions** Although serum half-lives of ampicillin and sulbactam are slightly longer in geriatric adults than in younger adults, dosage of ampicillin sodium and sulbactam sodium does not need to be modified in geriatric patients with renal function normal for their age. In geriatric adults with renal impairment, doses and/or frequency of administration of ampicillin sodium and sulbactam sodium should be modified in response to the degree of renal impairment, severity of infection, and susceptibility of the causative organism. (See Dosage and Administration: Dosage in Renal Impairment.)

■ **Mutagenicity and Carcinogenicity** Studies have not been performed to date to evaluate the mutagenic or carcinogenic potential of ampicillin sodium and sulbactam sodium.

■ **Pregnancy, Fertility, and Lactation** Safe use of ampicillin sodium and sulbactam sodium during pregnancy has not been definitely established. Reproduction studies in mice, rats, and rabbits using ampicillin and sulbactam doses up to 10 times the usual human dose have not revealed evidence of harm to the fetus. Ampicillin alone has been administered to pregnant women, especially in the treatment of urinary tract infections, without evidence of adverse effects to the fetus, and the drug has been recommended by various authorities for the treatment of susceptible infections during pregnancy. However, there are no adequate or controlled studies using ampicillin sodium and sulbactam sodium in pregnant women, and the drug should be used during pregnancy only when clearly needed.

Although the clinical importance is unclear, administration of ampicillin alone to pregnant women has resulted in a transient decrease in plasma concentrations of total conjugated estriol, estriol glucuronide, conjugated estrone, and estradiol; this effect also may occur following administration of ampicillin sodium and sulbactam sodium. IV administration of ampicillin to guinea pigs has resulted in decreased uterine tone and decreased frequency, height, and duration of uterine contractions. While it is not known whether use of ampicillin sodium and sulbactam sodium in humans during labor or delivery could have any immediate or delayed adverse effects on the fetus, prolong the duration of labor, or increase the likelihood of forceps delivery, other obstetrical intervention, or resuscitation of the neonate, ampicillin alone is considered the drug of choice for administration during labor (intrapartum) in the prevention of neonatal group B streptococcal (GBS) infections.

Reproduction studies in mice, rats, and rabbits using ampicillin and sulbactam doses up to 10 times the usual human dose have not revealed evidence of impaired fertility.

Because ampicillin and sulbactam are distributed into milk in low concentrations, ampicillin sodium and sulbactam sodium should be used with caution in nursing women.

Drug Interactions

For further information on these and other drug interactions reported with aminopenicillins, see Drug Interactions in the Aminopenicillins General Statement 8:12.16.08. In addition, while not all drug interactions reported with other penicillins have been reported with aminopenicillins, the possibility that they could occur with these drugs should be considered.

■ **Aminoglycosides** Both ampicillin and sulbactam are potentially physically and/or chemically incompatible with aminoglycosides and can inactivate the drugs in vitro. In one in vitro study, sulbactam concentrations of 25 mcg/mL had no appreciable affect on aminoglycosides in serum at 37°C. However, at concentrations of 75 mcg/mL, sulbactam inactivated tobramycin (but not other aminoglycosides tested) and, at concentrations of 200 mcg/mL or greater (with or without ampicillin), sulbactam inactivated amikacin, gentamicin, netilmicin (no longer commercially available in the US), and tobramycin. Some clinicians suggest that in vivo inactivation of aminoglycosides by sulbactam is unlikely to occur since sulbactam concentrations of 25 mcg/mL usually are not achieved clinically. Although in vivo inactivation of aminoglycosides has not been reported to date with aminopenicillins, including ampicillin, in vivo inactivation of aminoglycosides has been reported in patients receiving concomitant therapy with an extended-spectrum penicillin.

For information on antibacterial synergism between ampicillin and aminoglycosides, see Drug Interactions: Aminoglycosides, in the Aminopenicillins General Statement 8:12.16.08.

■ **Probenecid** Oral probenecid administered shortly before or concomitantly with ampicillin sodium and sulbactam sodium competitively inhibits renal tubular secretion of both ampicillin and sulbactam and produces higher and prolonged serum concentrations of the drugs. The serum half-life of sulbactam may be increased by 18–45% by concomitant probenecid. The effect of probenecid on the pharmacokinetics of the drugs occasionally may be used to therapeutic advantage (e.g., for the treatment of gonorrhea)†.

■ **Allopurinol** An increased incidence of rash reportedly occurs in patients with hyperuricemia who are receiving allopurinol and concomitant ampicillin compared with those receiving either drug alone. It is unclear whether this increased incidence of rash is caused by concomitant use of the drug or the hyperuricemia present in these patients. The manufacturer states that there are no data to date on concomitant use of allopurinol with ampicillin sodium and sulbactam sodium.

Laboratory Test Interferences

For more complete information on these and other laboratory test interferences reported with penicillins, see Laboratory Test Interferences in the Natural Penicillins General Statement 8:12.16.04. Although there is limited information on laboratory test interferences with aminopenicillins and although not all laboratory test interferences reported with other penicillins have been reported with ampicillin, the possibility that these interferences could occur with any of the aminopenicillins should be considered.

Ampicillin reportedly interferes with urinary glucose determinations using cupric sulfate (e.g., Benedict's solution, Clinitest®) but does not affect glucose oxidase methods (e.g., Clinistix®, Tes-Tape®).

Acute Toxicity

Limited information is available on the acute toxicity of ampicillin sodium and sulbactam sodium in humans. Overdosage of the drug would be expected to produce manifestations that principally are extensions of the adverse reactions reported with the drug. The fact that high CSF concentrations of β-lactam antibiotics may cause neurologic effects, including seizures, should be considered. Because ampicillin and sulbactam are both removed from the circulation by hemodialysis, these procedures may enhance elimination of the drug from the body if overdosage occurs in patients with impaired renal function; these procedures probably are unnecessary in patients with normal renal function.

Mechanism of Action

Ampicillin sodium and sulbactam sodium usually is bactericidal in action. Concurrent administration of sulbactam does not alter the mechanism of action of ampicillin. However, because sulbactam has a high affinity for and binds to certain β-lactamases that generally inactivate ampicillin by hydrolyzing the β-lactam ring, concurrent administration of the drug with ampicillin results in a synergistic bactericidal effect which expands the spectrum of activity of ampicillin against many strains of β-lactamase-producing bacteria that are resistant to ampicillin alone. For information on the mechanism of action of ampicillin, see Mechanism of Action in the Natural Penicillins General Statement 8:12.16.04 and in the Aminopenicillins General Statement 8:12.16.08.

Sulbactam generally acts as an irreversible inhibitor and is active against a wide range of bacterial β-lactamases. The drug is considered a "suicide inhibitor" because the interaction between sulbactam and target β-lactamases causes both the drug and the enzyme to be incapable of further action. Sulbactam has a much greater affinity for β-lactamases than does ampicillin or other β-lactam antibiotics, and the drug quickly forms an enzyme-inhibitor complex with target β-lactamases; this complex evolves into one or more irreversibly inactivated proteins. Sulbactam inhibition of β-lactamases is concentration and time dependent. At low sulbactam concentrations, a first-order reaction occurs and at high concentrations a zero-order reaction occurs. Results of in vitro studies indicate that ampicillin to sulbactam ratios of 2:1, 1:1, or 1:2 result in optimal β-lactamase inhibition and antibacterial activity.

Sulbactam inactivates both plasmid- and chromosome-mediated β-lactamases. In vitro studies indicate that sulbactam generally inhibits staphylococcal β-lactamases and β-lactamases classified as Richmond-Sykes types II, III (TEM type, HSV-1), IV, V (PSE and OXA types), and VI. The drug generally does not inhibit inducible, chromosomally mediated cephalosporinases classified as Richmond-Sykes type I, which may be produced by *Pseudomonas aeruginosa*, *Citrobacter*, *Enterobacter*, and *Serratia*.

In addition to its affinity for bacterial β-lactamases, sulbactam has an affinity for and binds to some bacterial penicillin-binding proteins (PBPs). PBPs are the target enzymes of β-lactam antibiotics and this binding may be the mechanism of sulbactam's intrinsic antibacterial activity against some organisms. (see Spectrum.) It also may contribute to the synergistic bactericidal effect that occurs between sulbactam and ampicillin or other β-lactam anti-infective agents. Sulbactam has a strong affinity for PBP 1a of *Proteus mirabilis* and *Escherichia coli* and PBP 2 of *Acinetobacter*. The drug has a lesser affinity for PBPs of *Staphylococcus aureus*, PBP 1a of *E. coli*, and PBP 2 of *E. coli* or *P. mirabilis*.

The minimum bactericidal concentration (MBC) of ampicillin sodium and sulbactam sodium for ampicillin-resistant strains of *S. aureus*, *Haemophilus influenzae*, and *Bacteroides fragilis* generally is only 1–2 times higher than the minimum inhibitory concentration (MIC); however, the MBC may be 8 times higher than the MIC for some strains.

Unlike clavulanic acid, sulbactam generally does not induce production of type I chromosomally mediated cephalosporinases in *Pseudomonas* or Enterobacteriaceae, including *Citrobacter*, *Enterobacter*, *Morganella*, and *Serratia marcescens*.

Spectrum

Ampicillin sodium and sulbactam sodium has a wide spectrum of activity and is active in vitro against many gram-positive and -negative aerobic and anaerobic bacteria. Ampicillin sodium and sulbactam sodium is active in vitro against organisms susceptible to ampicillin alone. In addition, because sulbactam can inhibit certain β-lactamases that generally inactivate ampicillin, ampicillin sodium and sulbactam sodium is active in vitro against many β-lactamase-producing organisms that are resistant to ampicillin alone, including ampicillin-resistant strains of staphylococci, *Haemophilus*, *Neisseria*, and *Bacteroides*.

Sulbactam alone has some intrinsic antibacterial activity against certain organisms. In vitro, sulbactam concentrations of 0.1–4 mcg/mL inhibit many strains of *Neisseria meningitidis*, nonpenicillinase- and penicillinase-producing *N. gonorrhoeae*, non-β-lactamase-producing *Moraxella catarrhalis* (formerly *Branhamella catarrhalis*), and some strains of *Acinetobacter*. In addition, sulbactam concentrations of 8–16 mcg/mL inhibit some strains of *Bacteroides* and *Legionella* in vitro. However, sulbactam concentrations of 25 mcg/mL or greater generally are required for in vitro inhibition of other gram-positive or -negative bacteria, and the drug is not therapeutically useful alone.

■ **In Vitro Susceptibility Testing** The Clinical and Laboratory Standards Institute (CLSI; formerly National Committee for Clinical Laboratory Standards [NCCLS]) states that, for streptococci and non-β-lactamase-producing enterococci, results of in vitro susceptibility tests using ampicillin can be used to predict susceptibility to ampicillin sodium and sulbactam sodium. However, to determine susceptibility of staphylococci and gram-negative enteric bacteria to ampicillin sodium and sulbactam sodium, CLSI recommends that disk-diffusion and dilution susceptibility tests be performed using appropriate combinations of ampicillin sodium and sulbactam sodium. For information on interpretive criteria specified for ampicillin, see Spectrum: In Vitro Susceptibility Testing in the Aminopenicillins General Statement 8:12.16.08.

To test in vitro susceptibility to ampicillin sodium and sulbactam sodium, a 1:1 ratio of ampicillin to sulbactam generally is used for disk-diffusion procedures and a 2:1 ratio of the drugs is used for agar or broth dilution procedures.

Results of in vitro susceptibility tests with ampicillin sodium and sulbactam sodium may be affected by inoculum size. For many ampicillin-resistant bacteria (e.g., *Escherichia coli*, *Klebsiella*, *Proteus*, *Haemophilus influenzae*, *Bacteroides*), MICs of ampicillin sodium and sulbactam sodium may be 2–32 times greater when the size of the inoculum is increased from 10^4 or 10^5 to 10^7 or 10^8 colony-forming units (CFU) per mL. Results of in vitro susceptibility tests generally are unaffected by changes in pH between 6–7.5.

CLSI states that, if results of in vitro susceptibility testing indicate that a clinical isolate is *susceptible* to ampicillin sodium and sulbactam sodium, then an infection caused by this strain may be appropriately treated with the dosage of the drug recommended for that type of infection and infecting species, unless otherwise contraindicated. If results indicate that a clinical isolate has *intermediate susceptibility* to ampicillin sodium and sulbactam sodium, then the strain has a minimum inhibitory concentration (MIC) that approaches usually attainable blood and tissue concentrations and response rates may be lower than for strains identified as susceptible. Therefore, the intermediate category implies clinical applicability in body sites where the drugs are physiologically concentrated (e.g., urine) or when a high dosage of the drug can be used. This intermediate category also includes a buffer zone which should prevent small, uncontrolled technical factors from causing major discrepancies in interpretation, especially for drugs with narrow pharmacotoxicity margins. If results of in vitro susceptibility testing indicate that a clinical isolate is *resistant* to ampicillin sodium and sulbactam sodium, the strain is not inhibited by systemic concentrations of the drug achievable with usual dosage schedules and/or MICs fall in the range where specific microbial resistance mechanisms are likely and efficacy has not been reliably demonstrated in clinical studies.

Strains of staphylococci resistant to penicillinase-resistant penicillins also be considered resistant to ampicillin sodium and sulbactam sodium, although results of in vitro susceptibility tests may indicate that the organisms are susceptible to the drug. In addition, CLSI currently recommends that non-β-lactamase-producing strains of *H. influenzae* that are resistant to ampicillin (BLNAR *H. influenzae*) be considered resistant to ampicillin sodium and sulbactam sodium despite the fact that results of in vitro susceptibility tests may indicate that the organisms are susceptible to the drug.

Disk Susceptibility Tests When the disk-diffusion procedure is used to test susceptibility to ampicillin sodium and sulbactam sodium, a disk containing 20 mcg of the drug (10 mcg of ampicillin and 10 mcg of sulbactam) is used.

When disk-diffusion susceptibility testing is performed according to CLSI standardized procedures using CLSI interpretive criteria, *Staphylococcus*, Enterobacteriaceae, *Pseudomonas aeruginosa*, and *Acinetobacter* with growth inhibition zones of 15 mm or greater are susceptible to ampicillin sodium and sulbactam sodium, those with zones of 12–14 mm have intermediate susceptibility, and those with zones of 11 mm or less are resistant to the drug.

When disk-diffusion susceptibility testing is performed according to CLSI standardized procedures using *Haemophilus* test medium (HTM), *Haemophilus* with growth inhibition zones of 20 mm or greater are considered susceptible to ampicillin sodium and sulbactam sodium and those with zones of 19 mm or less are considered resistant to the drug.

Dilution Susceptibility Tests When dilution susceptibility testing (agar or broth dilution) is performed according to CLSI standardized procedures using CLSI interpretive criteria, *Staphylococcus*, Enterobacteriaceae, and *Ps. aeruginosa* and other non-Enterobacteriaceae gram-negative bacilli (e.g., other *Pseudomonas* spp., *Acinetobacter*, *Stenotrophomona maltophilia*) with MICs of 8 mcg/mL or less of ampicillin in the presence of sulbactam at a constant 2:1 ratio are susceptible to ampicillin sodium and sulbactam sodium, those with MICs of 16 mcg/mL of ampicillin have intermediate susceptibility, and those with MICs of 32 mcg/mL or greater of ampicillin are resistant to the drug.

When susceptibility of *Haemophilus* is tested according to CLSI standardized procedures using HTM, *Haemophilus* with MICs of 2 mcg/mL or less of ampicillin in the presence of sulbactam at a constant 2:1 ratio are susceptible to ampicillin sodium and sulbactam sodium and those with MICs of 4 mcg/mL or greater of ampicillin in the presence of sulbactam at a constant 2:1 ratio are resistant to the drug.

■ **Gram-positive Aerobic Bacteria** ***Gram-positive Aerobic Cocci*** Ampicillin sodium and sulbactam sodium is active in vitro against most gram-positive aerobic cocci including *Streptococcus pneumoniae*, *S. pyogenes* (group A β-hemolytic streptococci), *S. agalactiae* (group B streptococci), viridans streptococci, and penicillinase-producing and nonpenicillinase-producing strains of *Staphylococcus aureus*, *S. epidermidis*, *S. saprophyticus*, and *S. warneri*. The drug is active in vitro against many strains of *Enterococcus faecalis* (formerly *S. faecalis*) and some strains of *E. faecium* (formerly *S. faecium*). Ampicillin sodium and sulbactam sodium is active in vitro against most strains of penicillinase-producing staphylococci that are resistant to ampicillin alone. Ampicillin sodium and sulbactam sodium also is active in vitro against some strains of staphylococci resistant to penicillinase-resistant penicillins including methicillin-resistant *S. aureus* (MRSA) and methicillin-resistant *S. epidermidis*. However, because it is unclear whether in vitro activity against these organisms will correlate with in vivo activity, the manufacturer, CLSI, and most clinicians currently state that strains of staphylococci resistant to penicillinase-resistant penicillins (e.g., nafcillin, oxacillin) should be considered resistant to ampicillin sodium and sulbactam sodium.

In in vitro studies using dilutions containing a 2:1 ratio of ampicillin to sulbactam, the MIC_{90} (minimum inhibitory concentration of the drug at which 90% of strains tested are inhibited) of ampicillin sodium and sulbactam sodium for penicillinase-producing and nonpenicillinase-producing strains of *S. aureus* and *S. epidermidis* is 0.12–8 mcg/mL of ampicillin in the presence of sulbactam at a constant 2:1 ratio of the drugs. The MIC_{90} of ampicillin sodium and sulbactam sodium for group A β- hemolytic streptococci, group B streptococci, *S. pneumoniae*, and *E. faecalis* is 0.03–1 mcg/mL of ampicillin in the presence of sulbactam at a constant 2:1 ratio of the drugs. Although some strains of *E. faecium* are inhibited in vitro by 0.5–8 mcg/mL of ampicillin in the presence of sulbactam at a constant 2:1 ratio of the drugs, many strains of the organism require concentrations of 16 mcg/mL or greater for in vitro inhibition and are considered resistant to the drug. (See Resistance.)

Gram-positive Aerobic Bacilli Ampicillin sodium and sulbactam sodium is active in vitro against *Listeria monocytogenes*. The drug reportedly is inactive against *Nocardia asteroides*.

■ Gram-negative Aerobic Bacteria ***Neisseria*** Ampicillin sodium and sulbactam sodium is active in vitro against most strains of *Neisseria meningitidis* and penicillinase-producing and nonpenicillinase-producing *N. gonorrhoeae*. Although penicillinase-producing *N. gonorrhoeae* (PPNG) usually is resistant to ampicillin alone, most strains of the organism are susceptible in vitro to ampicillin sodium and sulbactam sodium.

In in vitro studies using dilutions containing a 2:1 ratio of ampicillin to sulbactam, the MIC_{90} of ampicillin sodium and sulbactam sodium for *N. meningitidis* is 0.12–2 mcg/mL or less of ampicillin in the presence of sulbactam at a constant 2:1 ratio of the drugs. The MIC_{90} of the drug for PPNG is 4 mcg/mL of ampicillin in the presence of 2 mcg/mL of sulbactam.

Haemophilus Ampicillin sodium and sulbactam sodium is active in vitro against most β-lactamase-producing and non-β-lactamase-producing strains of *Haemophilus influenzae* and *H. ducreyi*. Although some strains of non-β-lactamase-producing *H. influenzae* that are resistant to ampicillin (BLNAR *H. influenzae*) may be susceptible to ampicillin sodium and sulbactam sodium in vitro, CLSI currently recommends that these strains be considered resistant to the drug.

The MIC_{90} of ampicillin sodium and sulbactam sodium reported for non-β-lactamase-producing strains of *H. influenzae* is 0.25–0.5 mcg/mL and the MIC_{90} of the drug for β-lactamase producing strains is 0.78–2 mcg/mL of ampicillin in the presence of sulbactam at a constant 2:1 ratio of the drugs.

Moraxella catarrhalis Ampicillin sodium and sulbactam sodium is active in vitro against both β-lactamase-producing and non-β-lactamase-producing strains of *Moraxella catarrhalis* (formerly *Branhamella catarrhalis*). The MIC_{90} of the drug reported for these organisms is 0.015–0.8 mcg/mL of ampicillin in the presence of sulbactam at a constant 2:1 ratio of the drugs.

Enterobacteriaceae Ampicillin sodium and sulbactam sodium is active in vitro against Enterobacteriaceae that are susceptible to ampicillin alone (e.g., some strains of *Escherichia coli, Proteus mirabilis, Salmonella, Shigella*). In addition, ampicillin sodium and sulbactam sodium is active in vitro against many β-lactamase-producing Enterobacteriaceae that are resistant to ampicillin alone, including many strains of β-lactamase-producing *Citrobacter,Klebsiella, Morganella morganii, Proteus, Providencia*, and *Yersinia enterocolitica* and some strains of β-lactamase-producing *E. coli*. Although ampicillin sodium and sulbactam sodium is active in vitro against some strains of *Enterobacter cloacae, E. aerogenes*, and *E. agglomerans*, many strains of *Enterobacter* as well as most strains of *Serratia* are resistant to the drug. (See Resistance.)

In in vitro studies using dilutions containing a 2:1 ratio of ampicillin to sulbactam, the MIC_{90} of ampicillin sodium and sulbactam sodium for *E. coli*, including multiple-drug resistant strains, generally is 4–16 mcg/mL of ampicillin in the presence of sulbactam at a constant 2:1 ratio of the drugs. However, the MIC_{90} for *E. coli* occasionally has been reported as 16–32 mcg/mL. The MIC_{90} of the drug for*Klebsiella*, including *K. pneumoniae* and *K. oxytoca*, and for *Citrobacter* and *Proteus* is 1–16 mcg/mL of ampicillin in the presence of sulbactam at a constant 2:1 ratio of the drugs. *Serratia marcescens* usually has an MIC_{90} of 16–32 mcg/mL or greater of ampicillin in the presence of sulbactam at a constant 2:1 ratio and generally is considered resistant to the drug. In one study, the MIC_{90} of ampicillin sodium and sulbactam sodium for *Shigella*, including *S. boydii, S. dysenteriae, S. flexneri*, and *S. sonnei*, was 8 mcg/mL of ampicillin in the presence of 4 mcg/mL of sulbactam.

Other Gram-negative Aerobic Bacteria Ampicillin sodium and sulbactam sodium is active in vitro against *Acinetobacter*. The MIC_{90} of the drug reported for *Acinetobacter baumannii* (*A. calcoaceticus* subsp. *anitratus*), *A. lwoffi* (*A. calcoaceticus* subsp. *lwoffi*), and *A. haemolyticus* is 1–8 mcg/mL of ampicillin in the presence of sulbactam at a constant 2:1 ratio of the drugs.

Ampicillin sodium and sulbactam sodium generally is inactive against *Pseudomonas*, including *Ps. aeruginosa*.

Some strains of *Burkholderia pseudomallei* (formerly *Ps. pseudomallei*) and *B. cepacia* (formerly *Ps. cepacia*) may be inhibited in vitro by the drug.

In one study, the MIC_{90} of ampicillin sodium and sulbactam sodium reported for *Legionella*, including *L. pneumophila*, was 2 mcg/mL of ampicillin in the presence of 1 mcg/mL of sulbactam.

Ampicillin sodium and sulbactam sodium has some in vitro activity against *Campylobacter fetus* subsp. *jejuni*.

■ Anaerobic Bacteria Ampicillin sodium and sulbactam sodium is active in vitro against both gram-positive and -negative anaerobic bacteria and is active against some anaerobes that are resistant to many other anti-infective agents, including other β-lactam antibiotics, metronidazole, and clindamycin.

Ampicillin sodium and sulbactam sodium is active in vitro against gram-positive anaerobic bacteria including *Actinomyces, Bifidobacterium, Clostridium, Eubacterium, Lactobacillus, Peptococcus, Peptostreptococcus*, and *Propionibacterium*. The MIC_{90} of ampicillin sodium and sulbactam sodium reported for*Clostridium*, including *C. clostridioforme* (*C. clostridiiforme*), *C. difficile, C. innocuum, C. perfringens, C. ramosum, C. subterminale*, and *C. tertium* is 0.5–8 mcg/mL of ampicillin in the presence of sulbactam in a constant 2:1 ratio of the drugs. Most other susceptible gram-positive anaerobes are inhibited in vitro by ampicillin sodium and sulbactam concentrations of 0.25–2 mcg/mL of ampicillin in the presence of sulbactam at a constant 2:1 ratio of the drugs.

Ampicillin sodium and sulbactam sodium is active in vitro against gram-negative anaerobic bacteria including most strains of *Bacteroides, Porphyromonas, Prevotella*, and *Fusobacterium*. The MIC_{90} of the drug reported for most *Bacteroides* in the *B. fragilis* group (e.g., *B. fragilis, B. caccae, B. distasonis, B. ovatus, B. thetaiotamicron, B. uniformis, B. vulgatus*) is 1.6–16 mcg/mL of ampicillin in the presence of sulbactam at a constant 2:1 ratio of the drugs. The MIC_{90} of the drug reported for *B. capillosus* and *B. ureolyticus* is 0.25–4 mcg/mL of ampicillin in the presence of sulbactam at a constant 2:1 ratio of the drugs. Ampicillin sodium and sulbactam sodium concentrations of 32 mcg/mL of ampicillin in the presence of 16 mcg/mL of sulbactam may be required for in vitro inhibition of *B. gracilis*, and this organism generally is considered resistant to the drug.

The MIC_{90} of ampicillin sodium and sulbactam sodium for *Porphyromonas asaccharolyticus* (*B. asaccharolytica*), *Prevotella bivius* (*B. bivia*), *P. disiens* (*B. disiens*), *P. intermedius* (*B. intermedia*), *P. loescheii* (*B. loescheii*), *P. melaninogenicus* (*B. melaninogenica*), and *P. oralis* (*B. oralis*) is 0.25–4 mcg/mL of ampicillin in the presence of sulbactam at a constant 2:1 ratio of the drugs.

Fusobacterium, including *F. nucleatum*, generally is inhibited in vitro by concentrations of 0.1–8 mcg/mL of ampicillin in the presence of sulbactam at a constant 2:1 ratio of the drugs; however, some strains of *F. necrophorum* may be resistant to ampicillin sodium and sulbactam sodium.

■ Chlamydia and Mycoplasma Ampicillin sodium and sulbactam sodium generally is considered inactive against *Mycoplasma* and *Chlamydia*, including *C. trachomatis*. Like most other penicillins (e.g., amoxicillin, carbenicillin, mezlocillin, penicillin G, piperacillin, ticarcillin), ampicillin reportedly has an incomplete inhibitory effect against *Chlamydia* and may be bacteriostatic but not bactericidal against these organism.

Resistance

Gram-negative aerobic bacilli that produce Richmond-Sykes type I chromosomally mediated β-lactamases (e.g., *Pseudomonas aeruginosa, Citrobacter, Enterobacter, Serratia*) generally are resistant to ampicillin sodium and sulbactam sodium because sulbactam does not inhibit most type I β-lactamases.

Some strains of *Klebsiella, Escherichia coli*, and *Acinetobacter* and rare strains of *Neisseria gonorrhoeae* are resistant to ampicillin sodium and sulbactam sodium. Rarely, strains of *Bacteroides fragilis* resistant to ampicillin sodium and sulbactam sodium have been reported. A few strains of *B. fragilis* resistant to the drug also were resistant to cefoxitin, extended-spectrum penicillins, clindamycin, and/or imipenem and cilastatin sodium.

Results of in vitro studies using ampicillin-resistant strains of *Staphylococcus aureus, Haemophilus influenzae*, and *B. fragilis* indicate that serial passage of these strains in the presence of ampicillin sodium and sulbactam sodium or continuous culture in the presence of subinhibitory concentrations of the drug does not result in resistance to ampicillin sodium and sulbactam sodium.

Enterococcus faecium (formerly *Streptococcus faecium*) generally is resistant to ampicillin sodium and sulbactam sodium. Resistance to aminopenicillins in some enterococci (e.g., *E. faecalis, E. faecium*) can result from β-lactamase production or from decreased binding to and/or increased production of penicillin-binding proteins with a low affinity for the drugs (e.g., PBP 5 or 6). Enterococci that exhibit ampicillin resistance secondary to β-lactamase production may be susceptible in vitro when the aminopenicillin is combined with a β-lactamase inhibitor (e.g., clavulanic acid, sulbactam); however, addition of the β-lactamase inhibitor does not necessarily result in susceptibility to the aminopenicillin in such strains. Some strains of enterococci with relatively high aminopenicillin resistance secondary to β-lactamase production may remain resistant or be only moderately more susceptible to the aminopenicillin combined with a β-lactamase inhibitor. Strains that exhibit ampicillin resistance secondary to alterations in PBPs remain resistant when the drug is combined with a β-lactamase inhibitor such as sulbactam or clavulanic acid, and some evidence suggests that such strains occasionally may emerge secondary to high-dose drug exposure. In addition, enterococci resistant to multiple drugs (e.g., vancomycin, teicoplanin, aminoglycosides, ampicillin, penicillin G, imipenem, tetracyclines, synergistic combinations of β-lactam anti-infectives) have been reported with increasing frequency.

Pharmacokinetics

Cross-over studies using fixed combinations of ampicillin sodium and sulbactam sodium, ampicillin sodium alone, and sulbactam sodium alone indicate that concomitant administration of sulbactam sodium does not appreciably affect the pharmacokinetics of either drug. Dosage of ampicillin sodium and sulbactam sodium generally is expressed in terms of the total of the ampicillin and sulbactam content of the fixed combination.

The pharmacokinetics of ampicillin and sulbactam following parenteral administration are similar and reportedly are best described by an open, 2-compartment model. For additional information on absorption, distribution, and elimination of ampicillin, see Pharmacokinetics in the Aminopenicillins General Statement 8:12.16.08 and in Ampicillin 8:12.16.08.

■ **Absorption** Sulbactam sodium is not absorbed appreciably from the GI tract and must be given parenterally. Although sulbactam is orally bioavailable following administration of an oral formulation containing ampicillin and sulbactam covalently linked as a double ester in a single molecule (sultamicillin; CP-49,952), this formulation currently is not commercially available in the US.

Peak serum concentrations of ampicillin and sulbactam are attained immediately following completion of a 15-minute IV infusion of ampicillin sodium and sulbactam sodium. In adults with normal renal function, peak serum concentrations of ampicillin are 40–71 mcg/mL following administration of a 1.5-g dose of ampicillin and sulbactam (1 g of ampicillin and 0.5 g of sulbactam) or 109–150 mcg/mL following a 3-g dose of the drug (2 g of ampicillin and 1 g of sulbactam); peak serum concentrations of sulbactam following these doses are 21–40 or 48–88 mcg/mL, respectively.

Following IM injection of ampicillin sodium and sulbactam sodium, both drugs are rapidly and almost completely absorbed. Peak serum concentrations of ampicillin and sulbactam generally are attained within 30–40 and 30–52 minutes, respectively. In healthy adults with normal renal function, IM injection of 1.5 g of ampicillin sodium and sulbactam sodium (1 g of ampicillin and 0.5 g of sulbactam) results in peak serum concentrations of ampicillin of 8–37 mcg/mL and of sulbactam of 6–24 mcg/mL.

Peak serum concentrations and areas under the concentration-time curve (AUCs) of ampicillin and sulbactam are slightly higher in geriatric patients than in younger adults; this presumably occurs because of reduced renal clearance in the elderly. In a study in healthy geriatric adults 65–85 years of age, a single 3-g dose of ampicillin and sulbactam (2 g of ampicillin and 1 g of sulbactam) given IV over 30 minutes resulted in peak serum concentrations of ampicillin and sulbactam that averaged 112.4 and 59.1 mcg/mL, respectively; the same dose administered to healthy adults 20–64 years of age resulted in peak serum concentrations of 82.4–99.8 and 42.5–52.2 mcg/mL, respectively.

In a study in neonates who received ampicillin sodium and sulbactam sodium in a 1:1 ratio (50 mg/kg of each drug) given by rapid IV injection every 12 hours, plasma concentrations of ampicillin at 3, 8, and 12 hours after a dose averaged 86.8, 77.3, and 56.8 mcg/mL, respectively, and those of sulbactam at the same intervals averaged 110.2, 72.8, and 38.4 mcg/mL, respectively.

There is no evidence that sulbactam accumulates in serum following IM or IV administration of 0.5-g doses every 6 hours for 3 days in adults with normal renal function.

In a few patients with chronic renal failure undergoing continuous ambulatory peritoneal dialysis, intraperitoneal administration of a single 3-g dose of ampicillin and sulbactam (2 g of ampicillin and 1 g of sulbactam) instilled over 6 hours resulted in peak plasma concentrations of ampicillin and sulbactam of 87.5 and 27.8 mcg/mL, respectively.

■ **Distribution** Following IM or IV administration of ampicillin sodium and sulbactam sodium, both ampicillin and sulbactam are well distributed into fluids and tissues. Although sulbactam reportedly distributes into certain tissues and fluids (e.g., blister fluid, peritoneal fluid, intestinal mucosa) to a greater extent than ampicillin, sulbactam distribution may vary and appears to depend on the degree of local inflammation. Ampicillin and sulbactam distribute into peritoneal fluid, blister fluid, tissue fluid, sputum, middle ear effusion, intestinal mucosa, bronchial wall, alveolar lining fluid, sternum, pericardium, myocardium, endocardium, prostate, gallbladder, bile, myometrium, salpinges, ovaries, and appendix. Concentrations of the drugs in most of these tissues and fluids generally are 53–100% of concurrent serum concentrations.

In adults with normal renal function, the apparent volume of distribution at steady state of ampicillin is 0.28–0.33 L/kg and that of sulbactam is 0.24–0.4 L/kg. The apparent volume of distribution of sulbactam at steady state in infants and children is 0.31–0.38 L/kg.

Both ampicillin and sulbactam are distributed into CSF in low concentrations following IV or IM administration in adults and children. CSF concentrations of the drugs generally are higher in patients with inflamed meninges than in those with uninflamed meninges. In a study in adults receiving 0.8- to 2-g doses of ampicillin IV every 4 hours and 1-g doses of sulbactam IV every 6 hours, ampicillin concentrations in CSF ranged from less than 0.3 to 9.6 mcg/mL in those with mild meningeal inflammation and 1.4–23.8 mcg/mL in those with marked inflammation; sulbactam CSF concentrations in these patients ranged from less than 0.5 to 4.7 mcg/mL and from 1–10.7 mcg/mL, respectively.

In patients undergoing cholecystectomy who received a single 1.5-g IV dose of ampicillin and sulbactam (1 g of ampicillin and 0.5 g of sulbactam), concentrations of ampicillin 0.25–1.5 hours after the dose averaged 15.9 mcg/mL in gallbladder bile, 7.7 mcg/g in gallbladder, and 20.2 mcg/mL in serum; concentrations of sulbactam in these samples averaged 4.3 mcg/mL, 6.3 mcg/g, and 19.9 mcg/mL, respectively.

Ampicillin is approximately 15–28% bound to serum proteins and sulbactam is approximately 38% bound to serum proteins.

Ampicillin and sulbactam both readily cross the placenta and concentrations in umbilical cord blood may be similar to serum concentrations. Ampicillin and sulbactam are distributed into milk in low concentrations. In lactating women who received 500-mg or 1-g doses of sulbactam by IV infusion over 20 minutes every 6 hours, concentrations of the drug in milk averaged 0.52 mcg/mL in samples obtained at random intervals between the first and thirteenth doses.

■ **Elimination** Serum concentrations of ampicillin and sulbactam both decline in a biphasic manner and half-lives of the drugs are similar. In healthy adults with normal renal function, both ampicillin and sulbactam have a distribution half-life ($t_{1/2\alpha}$) of about 15 minutes and an elimination half-life ($t_{1/2\beta}$) of about 1 hour. In some studies, the $t_{1/2\beta}$ of ampicillin ranged from 0.8–1.3 hours and that of sulbactam ranged from 0.97–1.4 hours. The $t_{1/2\beta}$ of ampicillin and sulbactam are slightly longer in geriatric adults than in younger adults. In a study in healthy geriatric adults 65–85 years of age with renal function normal for their age, the elimination half-life of ampicillin averaged 1.4 hours and that of sulbactam averaged 1.6 hours. In other studies in geriatric patients, the $t_{1/2\beta}$ of sulbactam and ampicillin were 2.2 hours compared with 0.8–1.2 hours in young adults.

In infants and children younger than 12 years of age, sulbactam has a $t_{1/2\beta}$ of 0.92–1.9 hours. In neonates, the half-lives of ampicillin and sulbactam vary inversely with age; as renal tubular function matures, the drugs are cleared more rapidly. In a study in premature neonates 6 days of age or younger, the half-life of ampicillin averaged 9.4 hours and the half-life of sulbactam averaged 7.9 hours.

The major route of elimination of both sulbactam and ampicillin is glomerular filtration and tubular secretion. Only small amounts of the drugs are eliminated in feces and bile. Following IM or IV administration of ampicillin sodium and sulbactam sodium in adults with normal renal function, approximately 75–92% of the dose of ampicillin and the dose of sulbactam is excreted unchanged in urine within 8 hours.

Serum concentrations of both ampicillin and sulbactam are higher and the half-lives of the drugs prolonged in patients with renal impairment. The elimination kinetics of both drugs appear to be affected to the same degree by impaired renal function. In one study, the half-lives of ampicillin and sulbactam averaged 1.6 and 1.6 hours, respectively, in adults with creatinine clearances of 30–60 mL/minute and 3.4 and 3.7 hours, respectively, in those with clearances of 7–30 mL/minute. In adults with creatinine clearances less than 7 mL/minute, the $t_{1/2\beta}$ of ampicillin and sulbactam averaged 17.4 and 13.4 hours, respectively.

Oral probenecid administered shortly before or with ampicillin sodium and sulbactam sodium competitively inhibits renal tubular secretion of both ampicillin and sulbactam and produces higher and prolonged serum concentrations of the drugs. (See Drug Interactions: Probenecid.)

Cystic fibrosis patients may eliminate sulbactam at faster rates than healthy individuals. In a study in children with cystic fibrosis, plasma clearance and apparent volume of distribution of sulbactam were about 1.5–2 times higher, peak plasma sulbactam concentrations were about 50% lower, and $t_{1/2\beta}$ of the drug slightly shorter in these children than in children without cystic fibrosis. Further study is needed to determine if this effect is clinically important since use of usual dosages of the drug in patients with cystic fibrosis may result in lower serum concentrations than expected.

In healthy adults with normal renal function, renal clearance of ampicillin is 203–319 mL/minute and that of sulbactam is 169–204 mL/minute.

Ampicillin and sulbactam are both removed by hemodialysis. The amount of the drugs removed during hemodialysis depends on several factors (e.g., type of coil used, dialysis flow rate). In a few patients undergoing chronic dialysis, a 4-hour period of hemodialysis removed into the dialysate about 35% of the ampicillin dose and 45% of the sulbactam dose when a single 3-g dose of ampicillin and sulbactam (2 g of ampicillin and 1 g of sulbactam) was given 2 hours prior to dialysis.

Chemistry and Stability

■ **Chemistry** Ampicillin sodium and sulbactam sodium is a fixed combination of the sodium salts of ampicillin and sulbactam. Ampicillin is an aminopenicillin. (See Ampicillin 8:12.16.08.) Sulbactam, a β-lactamase inhibitor, is a synthetic penicillinate sulfone containing a β-lactam ring and derived from 6-aminopenicillanic acid. Although sulbactam has minimal antibacterial activity when used alone, the combined use of sulbactam sodium and certain penicillins or cephalosporins (e.g., amoxicillin, ampicillin, cefazolin, cefoperazone, ceftizoxime, ceftriaxone, penicillin G) results in a synergistic effect that expands the spectrum of activity of the penicillin or cephalosporin against many strains of β-lactamase-producing bacteria.

Ampicillin sodium and sulbactam sodium is commercially available as a sterile powder for parenteral use containing a 2:1 ratio of ampicillin to sulbactam. Potency of the combination drug is expressed in terms of the total ampicillin content plus the total sulbactam content; each labeled mg of the combination provides not less than 563 mcg of ampicillin and 280 mcg of sulbactam, calculated on the anhydrous basis. Although not currently commercially available in the US, an oral preparation containing ampicillin and sulbactam covalently linked as a double ester in a single molecule (sultamicillin; CP-49,952) has been studied.

Ampicillin sodium and sulbactam sodium for parenteral use occurs as a white to off-white powder that is freely soluble in aqueous diluents. Each 1.5

g of ampicillin and sulbactam (1 g of ampicillin and 0.5 g of sulbactam) contains approximately 5 mEq (115 mg) of sodium; 3 g of the drug (2 g of ampicillin and 1 g of sulbactam) contains approximately 10 mEq (230 mg) of sodium. Following reconstitution, ampicillin sodium and sulbactam sodium solutions containing 375 mg/mL (250 mg of ampicillin and 125 mg of sulbactam per mL) occur as pale yellow to yellow solutions and have a pH of 8–10. Dilute solutions of the drug containing up to 30 mg of ampicillin and 15 mg of sulbactam are essentially colorless to pale yellow and have a pH of 8–10.

■ **Stability** Commercially available ampicillin sodium and sulbactam sodium sterile powder should be stored at 30°C or colder.

The stability of ampicillin sodium in solution is concentration dependent, decreasing as the concentration of the drug increases. Ampicillin sodium appears to be especially susceptible to inactivation in solutions containing dextrose, which appears to have a catalytic effect on hydrolysis of the drug. Sulbactam sodium is much more stable in aqueous solution than ampicillin sodium, but when combined with ampicillin sodium, sulbactam sodium does not substantially improve nor adversely affect the stability of the aminopenicillin. Therefore, the stability of ampicillin sodium and sulbactam sodium solutions is similar to that of ampicillin sodium solutions.

Following reconstitution with sterile water for injection or 0.5 or 2% lidocaine hydrochloride injection, ampicillin sodium and sulbactam sodium solutions for IM injection containing 375 mg/mL (250 mg of ampicillin and 125 mg of sulbactam per mL) are stable for at least 1 hour, and the manufacturer recommends that such solutions be used within this time period.

Following reconstitution with sterile water for injection or 0.9% sodium chloride injection, ampicillin sodium and sulbactam sodium solutions for IV administration containing 45 mg/mL (30 mg of ampicillin and 15 mg of sulbactam per mL) are stable for 8 hours at 25°C or 48 hours at 4°C, and solutions containing 30 mg/mL (20 mg of ampicillin and 10 mg of sulbactam per mL) are stable for 72 hours at 4°C. The manufacturer states that solutions for IV administration containing 45 mg/mL (30 mg of ampicillin and 15 mg of sulbactam per mL) in lactated Ringer's injection or ⅙ *M* sodium lactate injection are stable for 24 or 8 hours, respectively, when refrigerated at 4°C and for 8 hours at 25°C, although some investigators have reported more prolonged stability. Likewise, the manufacturer states that solutions in 5% dextrose injection containing 30 mg/mL (20 mg of ampicillin and 10 mg of sulbactam per mL) are stable for 2 hours at 25°C or 4 hours when refrigerated at 4°C and those containing 3 mg/mL (2 mg of ampicillin and 1 mg of sulbactam per mL) are stable for 4 hours at 25°C, despite some data suggesting more prolonged stability. The manufacturer also states that solutions of the combination in 5% dextrose with 0.45% sodium chloride injection containing 3 mg/mL are stable for 4 hours at 25°C and those containing 15 mg/mL (10 mg of ampicillin and 5 mg of sulbactam per mL) are stable for 4 hours at 4°C, although some investigators also have reported more prolonged stability with such solutions. Similarly, while some data indicate more prolonged stability than that recommended by the manufacturer, the manufacturer states that solutions diluted in 10% invert sugar and containing 3 mg/mL (2 mg of ampicillin and 1 mg of sulbactam per mL) are stable for 4 hours at 25°C and those containing 30 mg/mL (20 mg of ampicillin and 10 mg of sulbactam per mL) are stable for 3 hours when refrigerated.

The manufacturer states that commercially available ampicillin sodium and sulbactam sodium in ADD-Vantage® containers that has been reconstituted with 0.9% sodium chloride injection to a maximum concentration of 30 mg/mL (20 mg of ampicillin and 10 mg of sulbactam per mL) is stable for 8 hours at 25°C. Therefore, it is recommended that such solutions be completely administered within 8 hours to ensure proper potency.

Ampicillin sodium and sulbactam sodium is potentially physically and/or chemically incompatible with some drugs, including aminoglycosides, idarubicin hydrochloride, or ondansetron hydrochloride, but the compatibility depends on several factors (e.g., concentrations of the drugs, specific diluents used, resulting pH, temperature). Specialized references should be consulted for specific compatibility information. Because of the potential for incompatibility, ampicillin sodium and sulbactam sodium and aminoglycosides should not be admixed. For information on the in vitro and in vivo incompatibility of penicillins and aminoglycosides, see Drug Interactions: Aminoglycosides, in the Aminopenicillins General Statement 8:12.16.08.

For further information on chemistry and stability, mechanism of action, spectrum, resistance, pharmacokinetics, uses, cautions, drug interactions, and laboratory test interferences of ampicillin, see the Aminopenicillins General Statement 8:12.16.08 and see Ampicillin 8:12.16.08.

Preparations

Excipients in commercially available drug preparations may have clinically important effects in some individuals; consult specific product labeling for details.

Ampicillin Sodium and Sulbactam Sodium

Parenteral

For injection	1 g (of ampicillin) and 0.5 g (of sulbactam) (labeled as a combined total potency of 1.5 g)*	**Ampicillin and Sulbactam for Injection** **Unasyn®**, Pfizer
	2 g (of ampicillin) and 1 g (of sulbactam) (labeled as a combined total potency of 3 g)*	**Ampicillin and Sulbactam for Injection** **Unasyn®**, Pfizer
	10 g (of ampicillin) and 5 g (of sulbactam) (labeled as a combined total potency of 15 g) pharmacy bulk package*	**Ampicillin and Sulbactam for Injection** **Unasyn®**, Pfizer
For injection, for IV infusion	1 g (of ampicillin) and 0.5 g (of sulbactam) (labeled as a combined total potency of 1.5 g)	**Unasyn®**, Pfizer **Unasyn® ADD-Vantage®**, Pfizer **Unasyn® Piggyback**, Pfizer
	2 g (of ampicillin) and 1 g (of sulbactam) (labeled as a combined total potency of 3 g)	**Unasyn®**, Pfizer **Unasyn® ADD-Vantage®**, Pfizer **Unasyn® Piggyback**, Pfizer

*available from one or more manufacturer, distributor, and/or repackager by generic (nonproprietary) name

†Use is not currently included in the labeling approved by the US Food and Drug Administration

PENICILLINASE-RESISTANT PENICILLINS 8:12.16.12

Dicloxacillin Sodium

Dichlorophenylmethyl Isoxazolyl Penicillin Sodium, Methyldichlorophenyl Isoxazolyl Penicillin Sodium, Sodium Dicloxacillin

■ Dicloxacillin is a semisynthetic penicillinase-resistant penicillin antibiotic.

Uses

Dicloxacillin shares the uses of other penicillinase-resistant penicillins and generally is used only in the treatment of infections caused by, or suspected of being caused by, susceptible penicillinase-resistant staphylococci. Oral dicloxacillin should not be used for the initial treatment of severe, life-threatening infections, including endocarditis, but may be used as follow-up after therapy with a parenteral penicillinase-resistant penicillin (e.g., nafcillin, oxacillin). For specific information on the uses of dicloxacillin, see Uses in the Penicillinase-Resistant Penicillins General Statement 8:12.16.12.

Dosage and Administration

■ **Reconstitution and Administration** Dicloxacillin sodium is administered orally at least 1 hour before or 2 hours after meals. Although the drug also has been given parenterally by slow IV injection or infusion or by IM injection, a parenteral dosage form is no longer commercially available in the US.

Oral dicloxacillin should not be used for the initial treatment of severe infections and should not be relied on in patients with nausea, vomiting, gastric dilatation, cardiospasm, or intestinal hypermotility.

■ **Dosage** Dosage of dicloxacillin sodium is expressed in terms of dicloxacillin. Dosage of the drug should be adjusted according to the type and severity of infection.

Adult Dosage The usual adult oral dosage of dicloxacillin for the treatment of mild to moderate infections caused by susceptible penicillinase-producing staphylococci is 125 mg every 6 hours. For more severe infections, the usual adult oral dosage of dicloxacillin is 250 mg every 6 hours; higher dosage may be necessary depending on the severity of the infection.

Pediatric Dosage Children weighing 40 kg or more may receive the usual adult dosage of dicloxacillin.

In children who weigh less than 40 kg, the usual oral dosage of dicloxacillin for the treatment of mild to moderate infections caused by susceptible penicillinase-producing staphylococci is 12.5 mg/kg daily given in divided doses every 6 hours. The usual oral dosage for the treatment of more severe infections is 25 mg/kg daily given in divided doses every 6 hours; higher dosage may be necessary depending on the severity of the infection. If dicloxacillin is used in neonates, they should be monitored closely for clinical and laboratory evidence of toxic or adverse effects, and serum concentrations of the drug should be determined frequently and appropriate reductions in dosage and frequency of administration made when indicated. (See Cautions: Pediatric Precautions.)

The American Academy of Pediatrics (AAP) suggests that children older than 1 month of age receive oral dicloxacillin in a dosage of 25–50 mg/kg daily in 4 divided doses for the treatment of mild to moderate infections; the AAP states that the oral drug is inappropriate for severe infections.

Some clinicians suggest that, when dicloxacillin is used as follow-up therapy to parenteral penicillinase-resistant penicillin therapy in the treatment of acute or chronic osteomyelitis caused by susceptible staphylococci, children should receive an oral dosage of 50–100 mg/kg daily given in divided doses every 6 hours. If oral anti-infective therapy is used in the treatment of osteomyelitis, compliance must be assured and some clinicians suggest that serum bactericidal titers (SBTs) be used to monitor adequacy of therapy and to adjust dosage. (See Uses: Staphylococcal Infections, in the Penicillinase-Resistant Penicillins General Statement 8:12.16.12.)

Duration of Therapy The duration of dicloxacillin therapy depends on the type and severity of infection and should be determined by the clinical and bacteriologic response of the patient. Dicloxacillin therapy usually should be continued for at least 48 hours after cultures are negative and the patient becomes afebrile and asymptomatic.For severe staphylococcal infections, therapy should be continued for at least 14 days; more prolonged therapy is necessary for the treatment of osteomyelitis, endocarditis, or other metastatic infections. When oral dicloxacillin is used as follow-up therapy to parenteral penicillinase-resistant therapy in the treatment of acute osteomyelitis, the drug generally is given for 3–6 weeks or until the total duration of parenteral and oral therapy is at least 6 weeks; when used as follow-up therapy in the treatment of chronic osteomyelitis, the drug generally is given for at least 1–2 months and has been given for as long as 1–2 years.

■ **Dosage in Renal Impairment** Adjustment of dicloxacillin dosage in patients with renal impairment generally is unnecessary.

Cautions

■ **Adverse Effects** Adverse effects reported with dicloxacillin are similar to those reported with other penicillinase-resistant penicillins. For information on adverse effects reported with penicillinase-resistant penicillins, see Cautions in the Penicillinase-Resistant Penicillins General Statement 8:12.16.12.

■ **Precautions and Contraindications** Dicloxacillin is contraindicated in patients who are hypersensitive to any penicillin.

Dicloxacillin shares the toxic potentials of the penicillins, including the risk of hypersensitivity reactions, and the usual precautions of penicillin therapy should be observed. Prior to initiation of therapy with dicloxacillin, careful inquiry should be made concerning previous hypersensitivity reactions to penicillins, cephalosporins, or other drugs. There is clinical and laboratory evidence of partial cross-allergenicity among penicillins and other β-lactam antibiotics including cephalosporins and cephamycins.

Renal, hepatic, and hematologic systems should be evaluated periodically during prolonged therapy with dicloxacillin. Because adverse hematologic effects have occurred during therapy with penicillinase-resistant penicillins, white blood cell (WBC) count and differential should be performed prior to initiation of therapy and 1–3 times weekly during therapy. In addition, urinalysis should be performed and BUN, serum creatinine, AST (SGOT), and ALT (SGPT) concentrations should be determined prior to and periodically during therapy.

Patients should be advised to discontinue dicloxacillin and notify their clinicians if they develop shortness of breath, wheezing, rash, mouth irritation, black tongue, sore throat, nausea, vomiting, diarrhea, fever, swollen joints, or any unusual bleeding or bruising during therapy with the drug.

For a more complete discussion of these and other precautions associated with the use of dicloxacillin, see Cautions: Precautions and Contraindications, in the Penicillinase-Resistant Penicillins General Statement 8:12.16.12.

■ **Pediatric Precautions** Elimination of penicillins is delayed in neonates because of immature mechanisms for renal excretion, and abnormally high serum concentrations of the drugs may occur in this age group. If dicloxacillin is used in neonates, they should be monitored closely for clinical and laboratory evidence of toxic or adverse effects, and serum concentrations of the drug should be determined frequently and appropriate reductions in dosage and frequency of administration made when indicated.

■ **Pregnancy and Lactation** Safe use of penicillinase-resistant penicillins during pregnancy has not been definitely established. Clinical experience with use of penicillins during pregnancy in humans has not revealed evidence of adverse effects on the fetus. However, there are no adequate and controlled studies using penicillinase-resistant penicillins in pregnant women, and dicloxacillin should be used during pregnancy only when clearly needed.

Because dicloxacillin is distributed into milk, the drug should be used with caution in nursing women.

Spectrum

Based on its spectrum of activity, dicloxacillin is classified as a penicillinase-resistant penicillin. For information on the classification of penicillins based on spectra of activity, see the Preface to the General Statements on Penicillins 8:12.16.

Like other penicillinase-resistant penicillins, dicloxacillin is resistant to inactivation by staphylococcal penicillinases and is active against many penicillinase-producing strains of *Staphylococcus aureus* and *S. epidermidis* that are resistant to other commercially available penicillins. For specific information on the spectrum of activity of dicloxacillin and resistance to the drug, see the sections on Spectrum and on Resistance in the Penicillinase-Resistant Penicillins General Statement 8:12.16.12.

Pharmacokinetics

In all studies described in the Pharmacokinetics section, dicloxacillin was administered as the sodium salt; dosages and concentrations of the drug are expressed in terms of dicloxacillin.

■ **Absorption** Dicloxacillin is resistant to inactivation in the presence of acidic gastric secretions and is rapidly but incompletely absorbed from the GI tract. In healthy, fasting adults, 35–76% of an orally administered dose of dicloxacillin is absorbed from the GI tract and peak serum concentrations of the drug are generally attained within 0.5–2 hours.

Presence of food in the GI tract generally decreases the rate and extent of absorption of dicloxacillin.

Following oral administration of a single 500-mg dose of dicloxacillin in fasting adults, peak serum concentrations of the drug average 10–18 μg/mL; serum concentrations of the drug decline rapidly and are generally low 6 hours after the drug is administered. In fasting adults who receive a single 250-mg oral dose of dicloxacillin as a capsule, serum concentrations of the drug average 2.9–3, 4.6–5.5, 3–5.6, and 1.5–1.7 μg/mL at 30 minutes, 1 hour, 2 hours, and 4 hours, respectively, after the dose.

In one study in children with acute osteomyelitis who received oral dicloxacillin in a dosage of 100 mg/kg daily given in divided doses every 6 hours, serum concentrations of the drug ranged from 12–40 μg/mL 1 hour after dosing and 6.5–20 μg/mL 3 hours after dosing.

■ **Distribution** Dicloxacillin is distributed into bone, bile,pleural fluid, ascitic fluid, and synovial fluid. In one study in children 2–16 years of age with acute osteomyelitis who received dicloxacillin IM in a dosage of 50 mg/kg daily, dicloxacillin concentrations in bone ranged from 1.8–21.6 μg/g and concurrent serum concentrations of the drug ranged from 7–9 μg/mL in samples taken 1–3 hours after a dose. In children 7 months to 14 years of age with suppurative arthritis who received a single oral dicloxacillin dose of 25 mg/kg, dicloxacillin concentrations in synovial fluid obtained 2 hours after the dose were 70% of concurrent serum concentrations; synovial fluid concentrations averaged 9.5 μg/mL and serum concentrations averaged 13.6 μg/mL. Like other penicillins, only minimal concentrations of dicloxacillin are attained in CSF.

Dicloxacillin is 95–99% bound to serum proteins.

Dicloxacillin reportedly distributes into amniotic fluid in therapeutic concentrations following usual dosages. The drug also crosses the placenta and is distributed into milk. Following oral administration of a single 250-mg dose of dicloxacillin in lactating women, milk concentrations of the drug were 0.1–0.3 μg/mL 2 and 4 hours after the dose and undetectable 6 hours after the dose.

■ **Elimination** The serum half-life of dicloxacillin in adults with normal renal function is 0.6–0.8 hours. In one study in children 2–16 years of age, the serum half-life of the drug averaged 1.9 hours.

Dicloxacillin is partially metabolized to active and inactive metabolites. In one study following administration of a single 500-mg oral dose of dicloxacillin, 10% of the absorbed drug was hydrolyzed to penicilloic acids which are microbiologically inactive. Dicloxacillin is also hydroxylated to a small extent to a microbiologically active metabolite which appears to be slightly less active than dicloxacillin.

Dicloxacillin and its metabolites are rapidly excreted in urine mainly by tubular secretion and glomerular filtration. The drug is also partly excreted in feces via biliary elimination. Following oral administration of a single 250-mg, 500-mg, or 1-g dose of dicloxacillin in adults with normal renal function, 31–65% of the dose is excreted in urine as unchanged drug and active metabolites within 6–8 hours; approximately 10–20% of this is the active metabolite.

The serum half-life of dicloxacillin is slightly prolonged in patients with impaired renal function and has been reported to range from 1–2.2 hours in patients with severe renal impairment.

Serum concentrations of dicloxacillin are higher and the serum half-life longer in neonates than in older children.

Patients with cystic fibrosis eliminate dicloxacillin approximately 3 times faster than healthy individuals. In one study following oral administration of a single 6.25-mg/kg dose of the drug, peak serum concentrations and areas under the serum concentration-time curves (AUCs) were, on average, 2.5 times lower in patients with cystic fibrosis than in healthy individuals. Patients with cystic fibrosis had renal clearances of the drug averaging 282 mL/minute per 1.73 m^2 while healthy individuals had renal clearances averaging 95 mL/minute per 1.73 m^2.

Dicloxacillin is only minimally removed by hemodialysis or peritoneal dialysis.

Chemistry and Stability

■ **Chemistry** Dicloxacillin is a semisynthetic penicillinase-resistant penicillin. Dicloxacillin, like cloxacillin (no longer commercially available in the US) and oxacillin, is an isoxazolyl penicillin.

Dicloxacillin is commercially available as the monohydrate sodium salt. Potency of dicloxacillin sodium is expressed in terms of dicloxacillin. Each mg of dicloxacillin sodium contains not less than 850 μg of dicloxacillin. Dicloxacillin sodium occurs as a white to off-white, crystalline powder. The drug is freely soluble in water. Dicloxacillin sodium has a pK_a of 2.7–2.8.

Each 250-mg capsule of dicloxacillin contains approximately 0.6 mEq of sodium.

■ **Stability** Commercially available dicloxacillin sodium capsules should be stored in tight containers at a temperature less than 40°C, preferably between 15–30°C.

For further information on chemistry and stability, mechanism of action, spectrum, resistance, pharmacokinetics, uses, cautions, drug interactions, laboratory test interferences, and dosage and administration of dicloxacillin sodium, see the Penicillinase-Resistant Penicillins General Statement 8:12.16.12.

Preparations

Excipients in commercially available drug preparations may have clinically important effects in some individuals; consult specific product labeling for details.

Dicloxacillin Sodium

Oral		
Capsules	250 mg (of dicloxacillin)*	**Dicloxacillin Sodium**
	500 mg (of dicloxacillin)*	**Dicloxacillin Sodium**

*available from one or more manufacturer, distributor, and/or repackager by generic (nonproprietary) name

Nafcillin Sodium

Ethoxynaphthamido Penicillin Sodium, Sodium Nafcillin

■ Nafcillin is a semisynthetic penicillinase-resistant penicillin antibiotic.

Uses

Nafcillin shares the uses of other parenteral penicillinase-resistant penicillins (e.g., oxacillin) and generally is used only in the treatment of infections caused by, or suspected of being caused by, susceptible penicillinase-producing staphylococci. For specific information on the uses of nafcillin, see Uses in the Penicillinase-Resistant Penicillins General Statement 8:12.16.12.

Dosage and Administration

■ **Reconstitution and Administration** Nafcillin sodium is administered by IM injection or by IV injection or infusion. Although nafcillin also has been administered orally, the drug is poorly absorbed from the GI tract and an oral preparation of the drug is no longer commercially available in the US.

Reconstituted, diluted, and thawed solutions of nafcillin sodium should be inspected visually for particulate matter and discoloration prior to administration whenever solution and container permit.

To reduce the risk of thrombophlebitis and other adverse local reactions associated with IV administration of nafcillin sodium, particularly in geriatric patients, the drug should be administered slowly and care should be taken to avoid extravasation. In addition, the IV route should be used for relatively short periods of time (e.g., 24–48 hours). For additional information, see Cautions: Local Reactions, in the Penicillinase-Resistant Penicillins General Statement 8:12.16.12.

IM Injection For IM injection, nafcillin sodium powder for injection is reconstituted by adding 3.4 or 6.8 mL of sterile water for injection, bacteriostatic water for injection (with benzyl alcohol or parabens), or 0.9% sodium chloride injection to a vial labeled as containing 1 or 2 g of nafcillin, respectively, to provide solutions containing 250 mg/mL.

IM injections of nafcillin sodium should be made deeply into a large muscle (e.g., gluteus maximus) and care should be taken to avoid sciatic nerve injury.

Intermittent IV Injection For direct intermittent IV injection, nafcillin sodium powder for injection should be reconstituted as for IM administration and, when dissolved, the appropriate dose of the drug should be further diluted with 15–30 mL of sterile water for injection or sodium chloride injection.

The appropriate dose of *diluted* nafcillin sodium should then be injected slowly over 5–10 minutes into the tubing of a free-flowing compatible IV solution.

Intermittent IV Infusion For intermittent IV infusion, vials labeled as containing 1 or 2 g of nafcillin should be reconstituted as for IM injection and, when dissolved, should be further diluted with a compatible IV solution according to the manufacturer's directions. Alternatively, ADD-Vantage vials containing 1 or 2 of the drug may be reconstituted according to the manufacturer's directions.

Pharmacy bulk packages containing 10 g of nafcillin should be reconstituted with 93 mL of sterile water for injection or 0.9% sodium chloride injection to provide a solution containing 100 mg/mL. Pharmacy bulk packages of the drug are not intended for direct IV infusion; doses of the drug from the reconstituted pharmacy bulk package must be further diluted in a compatible IV infusion solution prior to administration.

Thawed solutions of the commercially available frozen nafcillin sodium injection are administered by intermittent IV infusion. Commercially available frozen nafcillin sodium injections should not be thawed by warming them in a water bath or by exposure to microwave radiation. A precipitate may form while the commercially available frozen injection in dextrose is frozen; however, this usually will dissolve with little or no agitation upon reaching room temperature, and the potency of the injection is not affected. After thawing at room temperature or under refrigeration, the container should be checked for minute leaks by firmly squeezing the bag. The injection should be discarded if the container seal is not intact or leaks are found or if the solution is cloudy or contains a precipitate. Additives should not be introduced into the injection. The injection should not be used in series connections with other plastic containers, since such use could result in air embolism from residual air being drawn from the primary container before administration of fluid from the secondary container is complete.

Intermittent IV infusions of nafcillin sodium generally are infused over at least 30–60 minutes. (See Chemistry and Stability: Stability.)

■ **Dosage** Dosage of nafcillin sodium is expressed in terms of nafcillin. Dosage of the drug should be adjusted according to the type and severity of infection.

Adult Dosage The usual adult IM dosage of nafcillin for the treatment of infections caused by susceptible penicillinase-producing staphylococci is 500 mg every 4–6 hours; severe infections may require 1 g IM every 4 hours.

The usual adult IV dosage of nafcillin for the treatment of infections caused by susceptible penicillinase-producing staphylococci is 500 mg every 4 hours; severe infections may require 1 g every 4 hours. When nafcillin is used for the treatment of acute or chronic osteomyelitis caused by susceptible penicillinase-producing staphylococci, many clinicians recommend that adults receive 1–2 g of the drug IV every 4 hours. If nafcillin is used for the treatment of staphylococcal infections related to intravascular catheters, some clinicians recommend that adults receive 2 g every 4 hours. Some clinicians recommend that adults receive IV dosages of at least 100–200 mg/kg daily given in equally divided doses every 4–6 hours for the treatment of meningitis.

Staphylococcal Endocarditis. For the treatment of native valve endocarditis caused by staphylococci susceptible to penicillinase-resistant penicillins, the American Heart Association (AHA) recommends that adults receive nafcillin in a dosage of 2 g IV every 4 hours for 4–6 weeks. Although the benefits of concomitant aminoglycoside therapy have not been clearly established in these infections, the AHA states that gentamicin (1 mg/kg IM or IV every 8 hours) may be given concomitantly during the first 3–5 days of nafcillin therapy.

For the treatment of staphylococcal endocarditis in the presence of prosthetic valves or other prosthetic material in patients with infections caused by isolates susceptible to penicillinase-resistant penicillins, the AHA states that adults should receive nafcillin in a dosage of 2 g IV every 4 hours for 6 weeks or longer in conjunction with rifampin (300 mg orally every 8 hours for 6 weeks or longer) and gentamicin (1 mg/kg IM or IV every 8 hours during the first 2 weeks of nafcillin therapy). However, because coagulase-negative staphylococci causing prosthetic valve endocarditis usually are resistant to penicillinase-resistant penicillins (especially when endocarditis develops within 1 year after surgery), coagulase-negative staphylococci involved in prosthetic valve endocarditis should be assumed to be resistant to penicillinase-resistant penicillins unless results of in vitro testing indicate that the isolates are susceptible to the drugs. (See Uses: Endocarditis in the Penicillinase-resistant Penicillins General Statement 8:12.16.12.)

Pediatric Dosage Children weighing 40 kg or more may receive the usual adult dosage of nafcillin.

The manufacturer recommends that pediatric patients weighing less than 40 kg receive IM nafcillin in a dosage of 25 mg/kg twice daily and that neonates receive an IM dosage of 10 mg/kg twice daily.

The American Academy of Pediatrics (AAP) recommends that children 1 month of age or older receive IM or IV nafcillin in a dosage of 50–100 mg/kg daily in 4 equally divided doses for the treatment of mild to moderate infections or 100–150 mg/kg daily in 4 equally divided doses for the treatment of severe infections. Other clinicians recommend that children receive nafcillin in a dosage of 100–200 mg/kg daily given in 4–6 equally divided doses for severe infections.

The AAP and other clinicians recommend that neonates younger than 1 week of age receive IM or IV nafcillin in a dosage of 25 mg/kg every 12 hours if they weigh 2 kg or less or 25 mg/kg every 8 hours if they weigh more than 2 kg. Neonates 1–4 weeks should receive 25 mg/kg every 8 hours if they weigh 2 kg or less (25 mg/kg every 12 hours for those less than 1.2 kg) or 25–35 mg/kg every 6 hours if they weigh more than 2 kg. The higher dosages are recommended for meningitis.

Staphylococcal Endocarditis. For the treatment of native valve endocarditis caused by staphylococci susceptible to penicillinase-resistant penicillins, the AHA recommends that pediatric patients receive nafcillin in a dosage of 200 mg/kg daily given IV in divided doses every 4–6 hours for 6 weeks (maximum daily dosage 12 g). In addition, during the first 3–5 days of oxacillin therapy, gentamicin (3 mg/kg daily given IM or IV in divided doses every 8 hours; dosage adjusted to achieve peak serum gentamicin concentrations approximately 3 mcg/mL and trough concentrations less than 1 mcg/mL) may be given concomitantly if the causative organism is susceptible to the drug.

For the treatment of staphylococcal endocarditis in the presence of prosthetic valves or other prosthetic material in patients with infections caused by isolates susceptible to penicillinase-resistant penicillins, the AHA recommends that pediatric patients receive nafcillin in a dosage of 200 mg/kg daily given IV in divided doses every 4–6 hours for 6 weeks or longer (maximum daily dosage 12 g) in conjunction with rifampin (20 mg/kg daily given orally in divided doses every 8 hours for 6 weeks or longer) and gentamicin (3 mg/kg daily given IM or IV in divided doses every 8 hours during the first 2 weeks of oxacillin therapy; dosage adjusted to achieve peak serum gentamicin concentrations approximately 3 mcg/mL and trough concentrations less than 1 mcg/mL).

Duration of Therapy The duration of nafcillin therapy depends on the type and severity of infection and should be determined by the clinical and bacteriologic response of the patient. In severe staphylococcal infections, therapy should be continued for at least 2 weeks; more prolonged therapy is necessary for the treatment of osteomyelitis, endocarditis, or other metastatic infections.

When nafcillin is used in the treatment of acute or chronic osteomyelitis caused by susceptible penicillinase-producing staphylococci, the drug is generally given for 3–8 weeks; follow-up therapy with an oral penicillinase-resistant penicillin after nafcillin therapy generally is recommended for the treatment of chronic osteomyelitis.

■ **Dosage in Renal and Hepatic Impairment** Modification of nafcillin dosage generally is unnecessary in patients with either renal impairment or hepatic impairment alone; however, modification of dosage may be necessary in patients with both severe renal impairment and hepatic impairment.

Cautions

■ **Adverse Effects** Adverse effects reported with nafcillin are similar to those reported with other penicillinase-resistant penicillins. For information on adverse effects reported with penicillinase-resistant penicillins, see Cautions in the Penicillinase-Resistant Penicillins General Statement 8:12.16.12.

■ **Precautions and Contraindications** Nafcillin is contraindicated in patients who are hypersensitive to any penicillin.

Nafcillin shares the toxic potentials of the penicillins, including the risk of hypersensitivity reactions, and the usual precautions of penicillin therapy should be observed. Prior to initiation of therapy with nafcillin, careful inquiry should be made concerning previous hypersensitivity reactions to penicillins, cephalosporins, or other drugs. There is clinical and laboratory evidence of partial cross-allergenicity among penicillins and other β-lactam antibiotics including cephalosporins and cephamycins.

Renal, hepatic, and hematologic systems should be evaluated periodically during prolonged therapy with nafcillin. Because adverse hematologic effects have occurred during therapy with penicillinase-resistant penicillins, white blood cell (CBC) count and differential should be performed prior to initiation of therapy and 1–3 times weekly during therapy. In addition, urinalysis should be performed and BUN, serum creatinine, AST (SGOT), and ALT (SGPT) concentrations should be determined prior to and periodically during therapy. If eosinophilia, suspected drug fever, rash, arthralgia, hematuria, or unexplained elevations of BUN or serum creatinine occur during penicillinase-resistant penicillin therapy, alternative anti-infective therapy should be considered.

For a more complete discussion of these and other precautions associated with the use of nafcillin, see Cautions: Precautions and Contraindications, in the Penicillinase-Resistant Penicillins General Statement 8:12.16.12.

■ **Pediatric Precautions** If nafcillin is used in neonates, they should be monitored closely for clinical and laboratory evidence of toxic or adverse effects. In addition, serum concentrations of the drug should be determined frequently and appropriate reductions in dosage and frequency of administration made when indicated.

■ **Pregnancy, Fertility, and Lactation** Safe use of nafcillin during pregnancy has not been definitely established. Reproduction studies using nafcillin in rats and rabbits have not revealed evidence of impaired fertility or harm to the fetus. Clinical experience with use of penicillins during pregnancy in humans has not revealed evidence of adverse effects on the fetus. However, there are no adequate and controlled studies using penicillinase-resistant penicillins in pregnant women, and nafcillin should be used during pregnancy only when clearly needed.

Because penicillins are distributed into milk, nafcillin should be used with caution in nursing women.

Spectrum

Based on its spectrum of activity, nafcillin is classified as a penicillinase-resistant penicillin. For information on the classification of penicillins based on spectra of activity, see the Preface to the Penicillins General Statements 8:12.16.

Like other penicillinase-resistant penicillins, nafcillin is resistant to inactivation by most staphylococcal penicillinases and is active against many penicillinase-producing strains of *Staphylococcus aureus* and *S. epidermidis* that are resistant to other commercially available penicillins. For specific information on the spectrum of activity of nafcillin and resistance to the drug, see the sections on Spectrum and on Resistance in the Penicillinase-Resistant Penicillins General Statement 8:12.16.12.

Pharmacokinetics

In all studies described in the Pharmacokinetics section, nafcillin was administered as the sodium salt; dosages and concentrations of the drug are expressed in terms of nafcillin.

■ **Absorption** Nafcillin is poorly absorbed from the GI tract, and oral preparations of the drug are no longer commercially available in the US.

IM injection of a single 1-g dose of nafcillin results in peak serum concentrations of 7.6 mcg/mL at 30–60 minutes after the dose.

Following IV injection over 5 minutes of a single 500-mg dose of nafcillin in healthy adults, serum concentrations of the drug average approximately 40, 10, 4.5, and 1.7 mcg/mL at 5 minutes, 30 minutes, 1 hour, and 2 hours, respectively, after the injection.

In one study in children 1 month to 14 years of age who received nafcillin in a dosage of 150 mg/kg daily in divided doses every 6 hours, serum concentrations of the drug averaged 48.1, 23.6, 6.4, and 1.8 mcg/mL at 30 minutes, 1 hour, 2 hours, and 4 hours, respectively, after a dose.

■ **Distribution** Nafcillin is distributed into synovial, pleural, pericardial, and ascitic fluids. The drug also is distributed into liver, bone, and bile. The volume of distribution of nafcillin reportedly ranges from 0.57–1.55 L/kg in adults, 0.85–0.91 L/kg in children 1 month to 14 years of age, and 0.24–0.53 L/kg in neonates. In one study, the volume of distribution of nafcillin at steady state averaged 27.1 L in adults with normal renal and hepatic function, 19.9 L in adults with cirrhosis, and 15.9 L in adults with extrahepatic biliary obstruction.

Concentrations of nafcillin in bile are generally equal to or greater than concurrent serum concentrations unless biliary obstruction is present.

Like other penicillins, only low concentrations of nafcillin are attained in CSF; however, CSF concentrations of the drug are generally higher when meninges are inflamed than when meninges are uninflamed. In one study following IV administration of 1- or 2-g doses of nafcillin every 4 hours in adults with inflamed or uninflamed meninges, CSF concentrations of the drug ranged from 0.1–58 mcg/mL in specimens obtained approximately 1–2 hours after a dose. In one study in adults with uninflamed meninges who received a single 40-mg/kg dose of nafcillin IV over 30 minutes, CSF concentrations of the drug ranged from 0.02–0.09, 0.03–0.17, 0.06–0.12, and 0–0.07 mcg/mL in specimens obtained 1, 2, 3, and 4 hours, respectively, after the dose. In hydrocephalic children 3 weeks to 8.5 years of age with suspected ventriculoperitoneal shunt infections who received 50 mg/kg of nafcillin every 6 hours given by IV infusion over 30–40 minutes, peak concentrations of the drug in ventricular fluid were generally attained 2–2.5 hours after a dose and ranged from 0.2–10.3 mcg/mL.

Only negligible concentrations of nafcillin are distributed into aqueous humor following parenteral administration. In patients with uninflamed eyes undergoing cataract surgery, IV administration of a single 2-g dose over 10 minutes resulted in serum and aqueous humor concentrations of the drug ranging from 70–120 mcg/mL and unmeasurable to 1.9 mcg/mL, respectively, 30–50 minutes after administration.

Nafcillin is 70–90% bound to serum proteins.

Nafcillin crosses the placenta. Nafcillin, like other penicillins, probably is distributed into milk.

■ **Elimination** The serum half-life of nafcillin in adults with normal renal and hepatic function averages 0.5–1.5 hours. In one study in healthy adults, nafcillin had a distribution half-life ($t_{1/2\alpha}$) of 0.17 hours and an elimination half-life ($t_{1/2\beta}$) of 1.02 hours.

Approximately 60% of a dose of nafcillin is metabolized in the liver to inactive metabolites. Although small amounts of nafcillin are excreted in urine, the drug is eliminated mainly via bile and undergoes enterohepatic circulation. About 27–31% of a single IM or IV dose of nafcillin is excreted in urine as unchanged drug and active metabolites within 12 hours in adults with normal renal and hepatic function.

Serum clearance of nafcillin is reportedly 410–583 mL/minute per 1.73 m^2 in adults with normal renal and hepatic function.

Serum concentrations of nafcillin may be higher and the serum half-life slightly prolonged in patients with impaired renal function. The serum half-life of the drug is reportedly 1.2–1.9 hours in patients with creatinine clearances of 3–59 mL/minute per 1.73 m^2 and 1.8–2.8 hours in patients with creatinine clearances less than 3 mL/minute per 1.73 m^2.

In one study in patients with cirrhosis or extrahepatic biliary obstruction, the $t_{1/2\alpha}$ of nafcillin averaged 0.26 or 0.29 hours, respectively, and the $t_{1/2\beta}$ averaged 1.2 and 1.7 hours, respectively. Serum clearance of the drug in these patients was lower than in patients with normal renal and hepatic function and averaged 291.5 mL/minute in those with cirrhosis and 163.4 mL/minute in those with extrahepatic obstruction.

In children 1 month to 14 years of age, the serum half-life of nafcillin ranges from 0.75–1.9 hours. Serum concentrations of nafcillin are generally higher and the serum half-life is longer in neonates than in older children. In one study, the serum half-life of nafcillin ranged from 2.2–5.5 hours in neonates 3 weeks of age or younger and 1.2–2.3 hours in neonates 4–9 weeks of age.

Nafcillin is only minimally removed by hemodialysis or peritoneal dialysis.

Chemistry and Stability

■ **Chemistry** Nafcillin is a semisynthetic penicillinase-resistant penicillin.

Nafcillin is commercially available as the monohydrate sodium salt. Potency of nafcillin sodium is expressed in terms of nafcillin. Each mg of nafcillin sodium contains not less than 820 mcg of nafcillin. Nafcillin sodium occurs as a white to yellowish white powder which may have a slight characteristic odor. The drug is freely soluble in water and soluble in alcohol. Nafcillin sodium has a pK_a of approximately 2.7.

Commercially available frozen nafcillin sodium in dextrose injections are sterile, nonpyrogenic, iso-osmotic solutions of the drug; about 1.8 or 1 g of dextrose has been added to the 1- or 2-g injections of nafcillin sodium, respectively, to adjust osmolality to about 300 mOsm/kg. Nafcillin sodium in dextrose frozen injections also contain sodium citrate as a buffer and hydrochloric acid and/or sodium hydroxide to adjust pH to 6–8.5.

■ **Stability** Following reconstitution with sterile water for injection, bacteriostatic water for injection, or 0.9% sodium chloride injection, nafcillin sodium solutions containing 250 mg of nafcillin per mL are stable for 3 days at room temperature, 7 days when refrigerated, or 90 days when frozen. The manufacturer states that solutions containing 10–200 mg/mL are stable for 24 hours at room temperature, 7 days when refrigerated, or 90 days when frozen.

The manufacturer states that the stability of the commercially available frozen nafcillin sodium injection may vary. These injections are stable for at least 90 days from the date of shipment when stored at −20°C. The frozen injection should be thawed at room temperature (25°C) or under refrigeration (5°C) and, once thawed, should not be refrozen. Thawed solutions of the commercially available frozen injection are stable for 72 hours at room temperature (25°C) or 21 days when refrigerated at 5°C. The commercially available frozen injection of the drug in dextrose is provided in a plastic container fabricated from specially formulated multilayered plastic PL 2040 (Galaxy®). Solutions in contact with the plastic can leach out some of its chemical components in very small amounts within the expiration period of the injection; however, safety of the plastic has been confirmed in animals according to USP biological tests for plastic containers as well as by tissue culture toxicity studies.

Nafcillin sodium is potentially physically and/or chemically incompatible with some drugs, including aminoglycosides and admixtures resulting in a pH greater than 8 or less than 5, but the compatibility depends on several factors (e.g., concentrations of the drugs, specific diluents used, resulting pH, temperature). For information on the in vitro and in vivo incompatibility of penicillins and aminoglycosides, see Drug Interactions: Aminoglycosides, in the Penicillinase-Resistant Penicillins General Statement 8:12.16.12. Specialized references should be consulted for specific compatibility information. Because of the potential for incompatibility, nafcillin sodium and other drugs should not be admixed.

For further information on chemistry and stability, mechanism of action, spectrum, resistance, pharmacokinetics, uses, cautions, drug interactions, laboratory test interferences, and dosage and administration of nafcillin sodium, see the Penicillinase-Resistant Penicillins General Statement 8:12.16.12.

Preparations

Excipients in commercially available drug preparations may have clinically important effects in some individuals; consult specific product labeling for details.

Nafcillin Sodium in Dextrose

Parenteral		
For injection	1 g (of nafcillin)*	**Nafcillin Sodium for Injection**
	2 g (of nafcillin)*	**Nafcillin Sodium for Injection**
	10 g (of nafcillin) pharmacy bulk package*	**Nafcillin Sodium for Injection**
For injection, for IV infusion	1 g (of nafcillin)*	**Nafcillin Sodium for Injection ADD-Vantage®**, Sandoz
	2 g (of nafcillin)*	**Nafcillin Sodium for Injection ADD-Vantage®**, Sandoz
Injection (frozen), for IV infusion	20 mg (of nafcillin) per mL (1 g) in 3.6% Dextrose*	**Nafcillin Sodium in Iso-osmotic Dextrose Injection Galaxy®**, Baxter
	20 mg (of nafcillin) per mL (2 g) in 3.6% Dextrose*	**Nafcillin Sodium in Iso-osmotic Dextrose Injection Galaxy®**, Baxter

*available from one or more manufacturer, distributor, and/or repackager by generic (nonproprietary) name

Selected Revisions January 2009,

Oxacillin Sodium

Methylphenyl Isoxazolyl Penicillin, Sodium Oxacillin

■ Oxacillin is a semisynthetic penicillinase-resistant penicillin antibiotic.

Uses

Oxacillin shares the uses of other parenteral penicillinase-resistant penicillins (e.g., nafcillin) and generally is used only in the treatment of infections caused by, or suspected of being caused by, susceptible penicillinase-producing staphylococci. For specific information on the uses of oxacillin, see Uses in the Penicillinase-Resistant Penicillins General Statement 8:12.16.12.

Dosage and Administration

■ **Reconstitution and Administration** Oxacillin sodium is administered by IM injection or slow IV injection or infusion. Although oxacillin has been administered orally, an oral preparation of the drug is no longer commercially available in the US.

IM Injection For IM injection, oxacillin sodium powder for injection is reconstituted by adding 5.7 or 11.4 mL of sterile water for injection to a vial containing 1 or 2 g of oxacillin, respectively, to provide solutions containing 167 mg of oxacillin per mL (250 mg/1.5 mL). The vials should be shaken well until a clear solution is obtained.

IM injections of oxacillin sodium should be made deeply into a large muscle (e.g., gluteus maximus) and care should be taken to avoid sciatic nerve injury.

Intermittent IV Injection For direct intermittent IV injection, a solution containing approximately 100 mg/mL may be prepared by adding 10 or 20 mL of sterile water for injection or 0.45 or 0.9% sodium chloride injection to vials containing 1 or 2 g of oxacillin, respectively.

The appropriate dose should then be injected slowly over a period of about 10 minutes. Particular attention to the risk of thrombophlebitis should be given when oxacillin is administered IV to geriatric patients.

Intermittent or Continuous IV Infusion For intermittent IV infusion, vials containing 1 or 2 g of oxacillin should be reconstituted as for direct IV injection and then further diluted with a compatible IV solution to a concentration of 0.5–40 mg/mL. (See Chemistry and Stability: Stability.) Alternatively, ADD-Vantage® vials containing 1 or 2 g of the drug should be reconstituted according to the manufacturer's directions. Pharmacy bulk packages containing 10 g of oxacillin usually are reconstituted by adding 93 mL of sterile water for injection or 0.9% sodium chloride injection to provide a solution containing 100 mg/mL. Pharmacy bulk packages of the drug are *not* intended for direct IV infusion; doses of the drug from the reconstituted pharmacy bulk package must be further diluted in a compatible IV infusion solution prior to administration.

Thawed solutions of the commercially available frozen oxacillin sodium in dextrose injection should be administered by continuous or intermittent IV infusion. These frozen oxacillin sodium injections should not be thawed by warming them in a water bath or by exposure to microwave radiation. A precipitate may form while the commercially available injection in dextrose is frozen; however, this usually will dissolve with little or no agitation upon reaching room temperature, and the potency of the injection is not affected. After thawing at room temperature or under refrigeration, the containers should be checked for minute leaks by firmly squeezing the bag. The injection should be discarded if the container seal is not intact or leaks are found or if the solution is cloudy, discolored, or contains a precipitate. Additives should not be introduced into the injection. The injections should not be used in series connections with other plastic containers, since such use could result in air embolism from residual air being drawn from the primary container before administration of fluid from the secondary container is complete.

For IV infusion of oxacillin, the rate of infusion should be adjusted so that the total dose of oxacillin is administered before the drug is inactivated in the IV solution. (See Chemistry and Stability: Stability.)

■ **Dosage** Dosage of oxacillin sodium is expressed in terms of oxacillin. Dosage of the drug should be adjusted according to the type and severity of infection.

Adult Dosage For the treatment of infections caused by susceptible penicillinase-producing staphylococci, the usual adult IM or IV dosage of oxacillin is 250–500 mg every 4–6 hours for mild to moderate infections or 1 g every 4–6 hours for severe infections. When oxacillin is used for the treatment of acute or chronic osteomyelitis caused by susceptible penicillinase-producing staphylococci, some clinicians recommend that adults receive 1.5–2 g of the drug IV every 4 hours. If oxacillin is used for the treatment of staphylococcal infections related to intravascular catheters, some clinicians recommend that adults receive 2 g every 4 hours.

Staphylococcal Endocarditis. For the treatment of native valve endocarditis caused by staphylococci susceptible to penicillinase-resistant penicillins, the American Heart Association (AHA) recommends that adults receive oxacillin in a dosage of 2 g IV every 4 hours for 4–6 weeks. Although the benefits of concomitant aminoglycoside therapy have not been clearly established in these infections, the AHA states that gentamicin (1 mg/kg IM or IV every 8 hours) may be given concomitantly during the first 3–5 days of oxacillin therapy.

For the treatment of staphylococcal endocarditis in the presence of prosthetic valves or other prosthetic material in patients with infections caused by isolates susceptible to penicillinase-resistant penicillins, the AHA states that adults should receive oxacillin in a dosage of 2 g IV every 4 hours for 6 weeks or longer in conjunction with rifampin (300 mg orally every 8 hours for 6 weeks or longer) and gentamicin (1 mg/kg IM or IV every 8 hours during the first 2 weeks of oxacillin therapy). However, because coagulase-negative staphylococci causing prosthetic valve endocarditis usually are resistant to penicillinase-resistant penicillins (especially when endocarditis develops within 1 year after surgery), coagulase-negative staphylococci involved in prosthetic valve endocarditis should be assumed to be resistant to penicillinase-resistant penicillins unless results of in vitro testing indicate that the isolates are susceptible to the drugs. (See Uses: Endocarditis in the Penicillinase-resistant Penicillins General Statement 8:12.16.12.)

Pediatric Dosage Children weighing 40 kg or more may receive the usual adult dosage of oxacillin.

The usual IM or IV dosage of oxacillin for the treatment of mild to moderate infections caused by susceptible penicillinase-producing staphylococci in children weighing less than 40 kg is 50 mg/kg daily given in equally divided doses every 6 hours. For severe infections, the usual IM or IV dosage in children weighing less than 40 kg is 100–200 mg/kg daily given in equally divided doses every 4–6 hours. The American Academy of Pediatrics (AAP) recommends that children 1 month of age or older receive IM or IV oxacillin in a dosage of 100–150 mg/kg daily in 4 divided doses for the treatment of mild to moderate infections or 150–200 mg/kg daily in 4 divided doses for the treatment of severe infections.

The manufacturer recommends that neonates receive IM or IV oxacillin in a dosage of 25 mg/kg daily. The AAP and other clinicians recommend that neonates younger than 1 week of age receive IM or IV oxacillin in a dosage of 25–50 mg/kg every 12 hours if they weigh 2 kg or less (25 mg/kg every 12 hours for those less than 1.2 kg) or 25–50 mg/kg every 8 hours if they weigh more than 2 kg. Neonates 1–4 weeks should receive 25–50 mg/kg every 8 hours if they weigh 2 kg or less (25 mg/kg every 12 hours for those less than 1.2 kg) or 25–50 mg/kg every 6 hours if they weigh more than 2 kg. The higher dosages are recommended for meningitis.

Staphylococcal Endocarditis. For the treatment of native valve endocarditis caused by staphylococci susceptible to penicillinase-resistant penicillins, the AHA recommends that pediatric patients receive oxacillin in a dosage of 200 mg/kg daily given IV in divided doses every 4–6 hours for 6 weeks (maximum daily dosage 12 g). In addition, during the first 3–5 days of oxacillin therapy, gentamicin (3 mg/kg daily given IM or IV in divided doses every 8 hours; dosage adjusted to achieve peak serum gentamicin concentrations approximately 3 mcg/mL and trough concentrations less than 1 mcg/mL) may be given concomitantly if the causative organism is susceptible to the drug.

For the treatment of staphylococcal endocarditis in the presence of prosthetic valves or other prosthetic material in patients with infections caused by isolates susceptible to penicillinase-resistant penicillins, the AHA recommends that pediatric patients receive oxacillin in a dosage of 200 mg/kg daily given IV in divided doses every 4–6 hours for 6 weeks or longer (maximum daily dosage 12 g) in conjunction with rifampin (20 mg/kg daily given orally in divided doses every 8 hours for 6 weeks or longer) and gentamicin (3 mg/kg daily given IM or IV in divided doses every 8 hours during the first 2 weeks of oxacillin therapy; dosage adjusted to achieve peak serum gentamicin concentrations approximately 3 mcg/mL and trough concentrations less than 1 mcg/mL).

Duration of Therapy The duration of oxacillin therapy depends on the type and severity of infection and should be determined by the clinical and bacteriologic response of the patient. In serious staphylococcal infections, therapy should be continued for at least 1–2 weeks; more prolonged therapy is necessary for the treatment of osteomyelitis or endocarditis.

When oxacillin is used parenterally in the treatment of acute or chronic osteomyelitis caused by susceptible penicillinase-producing staphylococci, the drug generally is given for 3–8 weeks; follow-up therapy with an oral penicillinase-resistant penicillin (e.g., dicloxacillin) generally is recommended for the treatment of osteomyelitis. In the treatment of acute osteomyelitis, a shorter course of parenteral penicillinase-resistant therapy (5–28 days) followed by 3–6 weeks of oral penicillinase-resistant penicillin therapy also has been effective.

■ **Dosage in Renal Impairment** Modification of dosage generally is unnecessary when oxacillin is used in patients with renal impairment; however, some clinicians suggest that the lower range of the usual dosage (1 g IM or IV every 4–6 hours) be used in adults with creatinine clearances less than 10 mL/minute.

Cautions

■ **Adverse Effects** Adverse effects reported with oxacillin are similar to those reported with other penicillinase-resistant penicillins. However, adverse hepatic effects have been reported more frequently with IV oxacillin than with other commercially available penicillinase-resistant penicillins. For information on adverse effects reported with penicillinase-resistant penicillins, see Cautions in the Penicillinase-Resistant Penicillins General Statement 8:12.16.12.

■ **Precautions and Contraindications** Oxacillin is contraindicated in patients who are hypersensitive to any penicillin.

Oxacillin shares the toxic potentials of the penicillins, including the risk of hypersensitivity reactions, and the usual precautions of penicillin therapy should be observed. Prior to initiation of therapy with oxacillin, careful inquiry should be made concerning previous hypersensitivity reactions to penicillins, cephalosporins, or other drugs. There is clinical and laboratory evidence of partial cross-allergenicity among penicillins and other β-lactam antibiotics including cephalosporins and cephamycins.

Renal, hepatic, and hematologic systems should be evaluated periodically during prolonged therapy with oxacillin. Because adverse hematologic effects have occurred during therapy with penicillinase-resistant penicillins, CBCs and differential should be performed prior to initiation of therapy and 1–3 times weekly during therapy. In addition, urinalysis should be performed and BUN and serum creatinine, AST (SGOT), and ALT (SGPT) concentrations should be determined prior to and periodically during therapy.

For a more complete discussion of these and other precautions associated with the use of oxacillin, see Cautions: Precautions and Contraindications, in the Penicillinase-Resistant Penicillins General Statement 8:12.16.12.

■ **Pediatric Precautions** Elimination of penicillins is delayed in neonates because of immature mechanisms for renal excretion, and abnormally high serum concentrations of the drugs may occur in this age group. If oxacillin is used in neonates, they should be monitored closely for clinical and laboratory evidence of toxic or adverse effects including renal impairment; organ systems and serum concentrations of the drug should be monitored frequently and appropriate reductions in dosage and frequency of administration made when indicated.

■ **Pregnancy and Lactation** Safe use of penicillinase-resistant penicillins during pregnancy has not been definitely established. Clinical experience with use of penicillins during pregnancy in humans has not revealed evidence of adverse effects on the fetus. However, there are no adequate and controlled studies using penicillinase-resistant penicillins in pregnant women, and oxacillin should be used during pregnancy only when clearly needed.

Because oxacillin is distributed into milk, the drug should be used with caution in nursing women.

Spectrum

Based on its spectrum of activity, oxacillin is classified as a penicillinase-resistant penicillin. For information on the classification of penicillins based on spectra of activity, see the Preface to the General Statements on Penicillins 8:12.16.

Like other penicillinase-resistant penicillins, oxacillin is resistant to inactivation by most staphylococcal penicillinases and is active against many penicillinase-producing strains of *Staphylococcus aureus* and *S. epidermidis* that are resistant to other commercially available penicillins. For specific information on the spectrum of activity of oxacillin and resistance to the drug, see the sections on Spectrum and on Resistance in the Penicillinase-Resistant Penicillins General Statement 8:12.16.12.

Pharmacokinetics

In all studies described in the Pharmacokinetics section, oxacillin was administered as the sodium salt; dosages and concentrations of the drug are expressed in terms of oxacillin.

■ **Absorption** Oxacillin is resistant to inactivation in the presence of acidic gastric secretions and is rapidly but incompletely absorbed from the GI tract. In healthy, fasting adults, 30–35% of an orally administered dose of oxacillin is absorbed from the GI tract and peak serum concentrations of the drug are generally attained within 0.5–2 hours. Presence of food in the GI tract generally decreases the rate and extent of absorption of oxacillin.

Following oral administration of a single 250- or 500-mg dose of oxacillin as capsules (no longer commercially available in the US) in healthy, fasting adults, peak serum concentrations of the drug average 1.65 or 2.6–3.9 mcg/mL, respectively. Following oral administration of oxacillin as an oral solution (no longer commercially available in the US), peak serum concentrations occur about 30 minutes after the dose and average 1.9 mcg/mL after a single 250-mg dose and 4.8 mcg/mL after a single 500-mg dose.

Oxacillin is rapidly absorbed from IM injection sites. Following IM injection of a single 250- or 500-mg dose of oxacillin in healthy adults with normal renal function, peak serum concentrations of the drug are generally attained within 30 minutes and average 5.3 and 10.9 mcg/mL, respectively. Following IM administration of a single 500-mg dose of oxacillin in healthy adults, serum concentrations of the drug averaged 7.4, 7.4, 4.3, and 0.8 mcg/mL at 30 minutes, 1 hour, 2 hours, and 4 hours, respectively, after the dose.

Following rapid IV injection of a single 500-mg dose of oxacillin in healthy adults, peak serum concentrations of the drug average 52–63 mcg/mL.

In one study in children 1 week to 2 years of age with staphylococcal infections who received an IM oxacillin dosage of 100 mg/kg daily in divided doses every 6 hours, peak serum concentrations of the drug occurred 30 minutes after a dose and ranged from 45–86 mcg/mL; trough serum concentrations ranged from 2.5–7.5 mcg/mL. Following IM injection of a single 20-mg/kg dose of oxacillin in neonates, peak serum concentrations of the drug reportedly average 51.5 mcg/mL in those 8–15 days of age and 47 mcg/mL in those 20–21 days of age.

■ **Distribution** Oxacillin is distributed into synovial, pleural, pericardial, and ascitic fluids. The drug is also distributed into bone, lungs, sputum, and bile. The volume of distribution of oxacillin is reportedly 0.39–0.43 L/kg in healthy adults.

Following IM or IV administration, oxacillin concentrations in bone may be 5–20% of concurrent serum concentrations. In one study in adults who received a single 2-g IV dose of oxacillin, concentrations of the drug in bone ranged from 1.1–18.5 mcg/g.

Like other penicillins, only low concentrations of oxacillin are attained in CSF. Following IM administration, oxacillin does not appear to distribute into aqueous humor in measurable concentrations; in animals, the drug is not distributed into aqueous humor even in the presence of inflammation. In rabbits, subconjunctival injection of a 100-mg dose of oxacillin produced aqueous humor concentrations of 145 mcg/mL 1 hour after the injection and 70 mcg/mL 2 hours after the injection.

Oxacillin is 89–94% bound to serum proteins.

Oxacillin is distributed into cord serum and amniotic fluid and crosses the placenta Oral administration of a single 500-mg dose of oxacillin to pregnant women in labor has resulted in fetal serum concentrations of the drug of 1.4 mcg/mL and amniotic fluid concentrations of 3.2 mcg/mL. Oxacillin is distributed into milk. Following IM administration of a single 500-mg dose of oxacillin in lactating women, milk concentrations of the drug were 0.2–0.7 mcg/mL 1 and 2 hours after the dose and 0.2–0.4 mcg/mL 4 hours after the dose.

■ **Elimination** The serum half-life of oxacillin in adults with normal renal function is 0.3–0.8 hours.

Oxacillin is partially metabolized to active and inactive metabolites. In one study following a single 500-mg oral dose of oxacillin (no longer commercially available in the US), 49% of the absorbed dose was hydrolyzed to penicilloic acids which are microbiologically inactive. Oxacillin is also hydroxylated to a small extent to a microbiologically active metabolite which appears to be slightly less active than oxacillin.

Oxacillin and its metabolites are rapidly excreted in urine mainly by tubular secretion and glomerular filtration. Following oral administration of a single 500-mg dose of oxacillin in adults with normal renal function, 17–24% of the dose is excreted in urine as unchanged drug and active metabolites within 6 hours; approximately 21% of the antibacterial activity in urine is represented by the active metabolite. Following IM administration of a single 500-mg or 1-g dose of oxacillin in adults with normal renal function, 40–70% of the dose is excreted in urine as unchanged drug and active metabolites within 6 hours.

In one study, serum clearance of oxacillin averaged 380 mL/minute per 1.73 m^2 in adults with normal renal function.

Serum concentrations of oxacillin may be higher and the serum half-life slightly prolonged in patients with impaired renal function. The serum half-life of the drug is reportedly 0.5–2 hours in patients with creatinine clearances less than 10 mL/minute per 1.73 m^2.

In one study in children 1 week to 2 years of age, the elimination half-life of oxacillin ranged from 0.9–1.8 hours. Serum concentrations of oxacillin are generally higher and the serum half-life is longer in neonates than in older children. The serum half-life of oxacillin reportedly is 1.6 hours in neonates 8–15 days of age and 1.2 hours in neonates 20–21 days of age.

Oxacillin is only minimally removed by hemodialysis or peritoneal dialysis.

Chemistry and Stability

■ **Chemistry** Oxacillin is a semisynthetic penicillinase-resistant penicillin. Oxacillin, like cloxacillin (no longer commercially available in the US) and dicloxacillin, is an isoxazolyl penicillin.

Oxacillin is commercially available as the monohydrate sodium salt. Potency of oxacillin sodium is expressed in terms of oxacillin. Each mg of oxacillin sodium contains 815–950 mcg of oxacillin. Oxacillin sodium occurs as a fine, white, crystalline powder which is odorless or may have a slight odor. The drug is freely soluble in water. Oxacillin sodium has a pK_a of approximately 2.8.

Each gram of commercially available oxacillin sodium powder for injection contains approximately 2.5 mEq of sodium and is buffered with 20 mg of dibasic sodium phosphate.

Commercially available frozen oxacillin sodium in dextrose injection are sterile, nonpyrogenic, iso-osmotic solutions of the drug; about 1.5 or 0.3 g of dextrose has been added to the 1- or 2-g injection of oxacillin sodium, respectively, to adjust osmolality to about 300 mOsm/kg. Frozen oxacillin sodium in dextrose injection also contains sodium citrate as a buffer and hydrochloric acid and/or sodium hydroxide to adjust pH to 6–8.5.

■ **Stability** Commercially available oxacillin sodium powder for IM or IV injection should be stored at controlled room temperature; the pharmacy bulk package containing 10 g of the drug should be stored at 15–30°C.

When oxacillin sodium powder for injection is reconstituted with sterile water for injection, solutions for IM injection containing 167 mg of oxacillin per mL (250 mg/1.5 mL) are stable for 3 days at room temperature or 7 days when refrigerated. When reconstituted as directed in 0.9% sodium chloride injection or 5% dextrose injection, solutions prepared from ADD-Vantage® vials of the drug are stable for 4 days or 6 hours, respectively, at room temperature.

At concentrations of 0.5–4 mg/mL, oxacillin loses less than 10% of its activity within 6 hours at room temperature in the following IV solutions: 5% dextrose and 0.9% sodium chloride; 10% fructose or 10% fructose and 0.9% sodium chloride; 10% invert sugar and 0.9% sodium chloride or 0.3% potassium chloride; or 10% invert sugar with electrolytes (Travert® 10% with Electrolytes No. 1, 2, or 3).

The commercially available preparations of frozen oxacillin sodium in dextrose injection should be stored at −20°C or lower and are stable for at least 90 days from the date of shipment when stored at −20°C. The frozen injection should be thawed at room temperature (25°C) or under refrigeration (5°C) and, once thawed, should not be refrozen. Thawed solutions of the commercially available frozen injection are stable for 48 hours at room temperature (25°C) or 21 days when refrigerated at 5°C. The commercially available frozen injections of the drug are provided in a plastic container fabricated from specially formulated multilayered plastic PL 2040 (Galaxy®). Solutions in contact with the plastic can leach out some of its chemical components in very small amounts within the expiration period of the injection; however, safety of the plastic has been confirmed in tests in animals according to USP biological tests for plastic containers as well as by tissue culture toxicity studies.

Oxacillin sodium is potentially physically and/or chemically incompatible with some drugs, including aminoglycosides and tetracyclines, but the compatibility depends on several factors (e.g., concentrations of the drugs, specific diluents used, resulting pH, temperature). For information on the in vitro and in vivo incompatibility of penicillins and aminoglycosides, see Drug Interactions: Aminoglycosides, in the Penicillinase-Resistant Penicillins General Statement 8:12.16.12. Specialized references should be consulted for specific compatibility information.

For further information on chemistry and stability, mechanism of action, spectrum, resistance, pharmacokinetics, uses, cautions, drug interactions, laboratory test interferences, and dosage and administration of oxacillin sodium, see the Penicillinase-Resistant Penicillins General Statement 8:12.16.12.

Preparations

Excipients in commercially available drug preparations may have clinically important effects in some individuals; consult specific product labeling for details.

Oxacillin Sodium

Parenteral		
For injection	1 g (of oxacillin)*	**Oxacillin Sodium for Injection**
	2 g (of oxacillin)*	**Oxacillin Sodium for Injection**
	10 g (of oxacillin) pharmacy bulk package*	**Oxacillin Sodium for Injection**
For injection, for IV infusion	1 g (of oxacillin)*	**Oxacillin Sodium ADD-Vantage®**, Sandoz
	2 g (of oxacillin)*	**Oxacillin Sodium ADD-Vantage®**, Sandoz

*available from one or more manufacturer, distributor, and/or repackager by generic (nonproprietary) name

Oxacillin Sodium in Dextrose

Parenteral		
Injection (frozen), for IV infusion	20 mg (of oxacillin) per mL (1 g) in 3% Dextrose*	**Oxacillin Sodium® in Iso-osmotic Dextrose Injection**, Baxter
	40 mg (of oxacillin) per mL (2 g) in 0.6% Dextrose*	**Oxacillin Sodium® in Iso-osmotic Dextrose Injection**, Baxter

*available from one or more manufacturer, distributor, and/or repackager by generic (nonproprietary) name

Selected Revisions January 2009,

EXTENDED-SPECTRUM PENICILLINS 8:12.16.16

Piperacillin Sodium and Tazobactam Sodium

Piperacillin/tazobactam, Piperacillin-tazobactam PIP/TAZ TZP

■ Piperacillin sodium and tazobactam sodium (piperacillin/tazobactam) is a fixed combination of the sodium salts of piperacillin (an extended-spectrum penicillin antibiotic) and tazobactam (a β-lactamase inhibitor); tazobactam inactivates certain bacterial β-lactamases and expands piperacillin's spectrum of activity against some bacteria that produce these β-lactamases.

Uses

The fixed combination of piperacillin sodium and tazobactam sodium (piperacillin/tazobactam) is used for the treatment of moderate to severe infections caused by susceptible β-lactamase-producing bacteria and certain other gram-negative or anaerobic bacteria. Piperacillin/tazobactam is used principally for the treatment of infections caused by susceptible gram-negative bacteria and for empiric treatment of polymicrobial infections such as mixed aerobic-anaerobic infections.

When piperacillin/tazobactam is used for the treatment of infections known or suspected of being caused by *Pseudomonas aeruginosa*, the drug usually is used in conjunction with another anti-infective with antipseudomonal activity (e.g., antipseudomonal fluoroquinolone, aminoglycoside).

■ **Gynecologic and Obstetric Infections** Piperacillin/tazobactam is used for the treatment of postpartum endometritis or pelvic inflammatory disease (PID) caused by susceptible β-lactamase-producing *Escherichia coli*.

Piperacillin/tazobactam is not included in US Centers for Disease Control and Prevention (CDC) recommendations for the treatment of PID. If a penicillin is used for empiric treatment of PID, CDC and other clinicians recommend a parenteral regimen that includes the fixed combination of ampicillin sodium and sulbactam sodium (ampicillin/sulbactam) in conjunction with doxycycline.

■ **Intra-abdominal Infections** Piperacillin/tazobactam is used for the treatment of appendicitis (complicated by rupture or abscess) and peritonitis caused by susceptible β-lactamase-producing *E. coli*, *Bacteroides fragilis*, *B. ovatus*, *B. thetaiotaomicron*, or *B. vulgatus*.

Piperacillin/tazobactam has been used for the treatment of various intra-abdominal infections, and has been recommended as one of several options for initial empiric treatment of high-risk or severe community-acquired extrabiliary intra-abdominal infections (e.g., in patients with advanced age, immunocompromise, severe physiologic disturbance), community-acquired biliary tract infections (e.g., acute cholecystitis), and complicated healthcare-associated intra-abdominal infections.

■ **Respiratory Tract Infections** ***Community-acquired Pneumonia*** Piperacillin/tazobactam is used for the treatment of moderately severe community-acquired pneumonia (CAP) caused by susceptible β-lactamase-producing *Haemophilus influenzae*. The drug also is used for the treatment of CAP caused by susceptible Enterobacteriaceae† or anaerobic bacteria†.

Piperacillin/tazobactam has been recommended as one of several options for empiric treatment of CAP in hospitalized patients requiring treatment in an intensive care unit (ICU). If *Ps. aeruginosa* is known or suspected to be involved, the Infectious Diseases Society of America (IDSA) and American Thoracic Society (ATS) state that piperacillin/tazobactam should be used in conjunction with a fluoroquinolone with antipseudomonal activity (ciprofloxacin, levofloxacin) with or without an aminoglycoside or in conjunction with an aminoglycoside and azithromycin. Factors that increase the risk of *Ps. aeruginosa* infection in CAP patients include severe CAP requiring treatment in an ICU, structural lung disease (e.g., bronchiectasis), repeated exacerbations of severe chronic obstructive pulmonary disease (COPD), alcoholism, chronic corticosteroid therapy, and frequent anti-infective therapy.

Nosocomial Pneumonia Piperacillin/tazobactam is used for the treatment of moderate to severe nosocomial pneumonia caused by susceptible β-lactamase-producing *Staphylococcus aureus* or susceptible *Acinetobacter baumannii, H. influenzae, Klebsiella pneumoniae,* or *Ps. aeruginosa.* If *Ps. aeruginosa* is involved, piperacillin/tazobactam should be used in conjunction with an aminoglycoside or a fluoroquinolone with antipseudomonal activity (e.g., ciprofloxacin, levofloxacin).

IDSA and ATS state that piperacillin/tazobactam is one of several options for initial empiric treatment of hospital-acquired pneumonia (HAP) not associated with mechanical ventilation and initial empiric treatment of ventilator-associated bacterial pneumonia (VAP).

In adults with HAP (not associated with mechanical ventilation) who are not at high risk of mortality, IDSA and ATS state that use of piperacillin/tazobactam alone (monotherapy) can be considered for initial empiric treatment if no factors are present that increase the likelihood of methicillin-resistant *S. aureus* (MRSA; also known as oxacillin-resistant *S. aureus* or ORSA); however, these experts state that piperacillin/tazobactam should be used in conjunction with an antibacterial active against MRSA (vancomycin, linezolid) if such factors are present or if the patient is at high risk of mortality or has received IV anti-infectives during the prior 90 days.

In adults with clinically suspected VAP, IDSA and ATS state that use of piperacillin/tazobactam alone (monotherapy) can be considered for initial empiric treatment in those not at increased risk for MRSA. However, in patients with factors that increase the risk of MRSA or multidrug-resistant gram-negative bacteria, these experts state that piperacillin/tazobactam should be used in conjunction with an anti-infective active against MRSA (vancomycin, linezolid) plus an antipseudomonal fluoroquinolone (ciprofloxacin, levofloxacin), aminoglycoside (amikacin, gentamicin, tobramycin), or polymyxin B.

■ **Septicemia** Piperacillin/tazobactam has been used for the treatment of septicemia†. The drug has been recommended as one of several options for initial empiric treatment of sepsis and bacteremia.

■ **Skin and Skin Structure Infections** Piperacillin/tazobactam is used for the treatment of uncomplicated and complicated skin and skin structure infections (including cellulitis, cutaneous abscesses, ischemic/diabetic foot infections) caused by susceptible β-lactamase-producing *S. aureus.* Piperacillin/tazobactam has been recommended as a possible option for empiric monotherapy of complicated skin and skin structure infections that could be polymicrobial and are unlikely to involve MRSA; the drug should not be used alone in infections that may be caused by MRSA.

Although the fixed combination of amoxicillin and clavulanate potassium (amoxicillin/clavulanate) usually is the drug of choice, piperacillin/tazobactam has been suggested as an alternative for the treatment of infected human or animal (e.g., dog, cat, reptile) bite wounds† when a parenteral anti-infective is used. Purulent bite wounds are likely to be polymicrobial and broad-spectrum anti-infective coverage is recommended. Nonpurulent infected bite wounds usually are caused by staphylococci and streptococci, but can be polymicrobial.

Piperacillin/tazobactam used in conjunction with vancomycin is considered one of several possible regimens for empiric treatment of severe cellulitis or treatment of clostridial myonecrosis† (gas gangrene).

Piperacillin/tazobactam used in conjunction with vancomycin or linezolid also is one of several possible regimens for empiric treatment of necrotizing fasciitis†.

■ **Urinary Tract Infections** Piperacillin/tazobactam has been used with or without an aminoglycoside for the treatment of urinary tract infections† in hospitalized patients.

■ **Empiric Therapy in Febrile Neutropenic Patients** Piperacillin/tazobactam has been used alone (monotherapy) or in conjunction with other anti-infectives (e.g., an aminoglycoside) for empiric anti-infective therapy in febrile neutropenic patients†.

Piperacillin/tazobactam has been recommended as one of several options for initial outpatient management of febrile neutropenia in adults receiving treatment for malignancy.

■ **Perioperative Prophylaxis** Piperacillin/tazobactam has been used for perioperative prophylaxis† to decrease postoperative infections in patients undergoing various urologic procedures (e.g., prostate biopsy), gastroduodenal procedures (e.g., pancreatic duodenectomy), or liver transplantation. However, piperacillin/tazobactam generally is not recommended for perioperative prophylaxis.

Dosage and Administration

■ **Administration** The fixed combination of piperacillin sodium and tazobactam sodium (piperacillin/tazobactam) is administered by IV infusion.

Piperacillin/tazobactam usually is administered by intermittent IV infusion, but also has been administered by continuous IV infusion†.

The drug should not be given by rapid IV injection.

IV Infusion Piperacillin/tazobactam should *not* be admixed with other drugs in a syringe or infusion bottle and should *not* be added to blood products or albumin hydrolysates.

If concomitant use of an aminoglycoside is indicated (e.g., treatment of nosocomial pneumonia), the drugs should be reconstituted, diluted, and administered separately. (See Concomitant Use with Aminoglycosides under Administration: IV Infusion, in Dosage and Administration.)

Piperacillin/tazobactam (Zosyn®) and generic preparations of piperacillin/tazobactam commercially available in the US are *not* identical. Piperacillin/tazobactam (Zosyn®) is formulated with edetate disodium dihydrate (EDTA) and sodium citrate; the generic preparations do not contain EDTA or sodium citrate. Because EDTA acts as a metal-chelating agent and sodium citrate acts as a buffer, certain aspects of chemical degradation and particulate formation are inhibited and there is a lower risk of particulate matter formation and accumulation following reconstitution of Zosyn® with commonly used diluents or storage of solutions of the drug. In addition, the presence of EDTA and sodium citrate allows coadministration of Zosyn® and lactated Ringer's injection via Y-site infusion.

Reconstitution and Dilution. Single-dose vials of piperacillin/tazobactam (Zosyn®, generic) labeled as containing 2.25 g (2 g of piperacillin and 0.25 g of tazobactam), 3.375 g (3 g of piperacillin and 0.375 g of tazobactam), or 4.5 g (4 g of piperacillin and 0.5 g of tazobactam) should be reconstituted with 10, 15, or 20 mL, respectively, of compatible diluent and swirled until the contents are dissolved. Diluents that can be used for reconstitution include 0.9% sodium chloride injection, sterile water for injection, 5% dextrose injection, bacteriostatic water for injection (with parabens or benzyl alcohol), or bacteriostatic sodium chloride injection (with parabens or benzyl alcohol). Reconstituted solutions prepared from single-dose vials of piperacillin/tazobactam should be further diluted and any unused reconstituted solution should be discarded after 24 hours if stored at room temperature (20–25°C) or after 48 hours if refrigerated at 2–8°C. Prior to IV infusion, reconstituted piperacillin/tazobactam solutions should be diluted to the desired volume (usually 50–150 mL) with a compatible diluent (0.9% sodium chloride injection, sterile water for injection [maximum recommended volume is 50 mL], 5% dextrose injection, or 6% dextran in sodium chloride injection). Lactated Ringer's injection is compatible *only* with piperacillin/sodium solutions prepared using piperacillin/tazobactam formulated with EDTA (i.e., Zosyn®) for coadministration via Y-site infusion; lactated Ringer's injection is incompatible with and cannot be used with generic piperacillin/tazobactam preparations that do not contain EDTA.

Single-dose ADD-Vantage® vials of piperacillin/tazobactam (generic) should be reconstituted and diluted according to the manufacturer's labeling. When reconstituted as directed in 0.9% sodium chloride injection or 5% dextrose injection, piperacillin/tazobactam solutions prepared from ADD-Vantage® vials are stable for 24 hours at room temperature; these reconstituted solutions should not be refrigerated or frozen.

Pharmacy bulk vials or bottles of piperacillin/tazobactam (Zosyn®, generic) containing 40.5 g (36 g of piperacillin and 4.5 g of tazobactam) should be reconstituted by adding 152 mL of a compatible IV solution to the vial to provide a solution containing 200 mg/mL of piperacillin and 25 mg/mL of tazobactam. Pharmacy bulk vials or bottles of the drug are not intended for direct IV infusion; prior to administration, solutions reconstituted in the pharmacy bulk package must be further diluted with a compatible IV solution.

The commercially available single-dose frozen premixed injections of piperacillin/tazobactam in dextrose (Zosyn® in Galaxy® containers) should be thawed at room temperature (20–25°C) or under refrigeration (2–8°C); frozen injections should not be thawed by immersion in water baths or by microwave irradiation. Precipitates that may have formed in the frozen injection usually will dissolve with little or no agitation when the injection reaches room temperature; potency is not affected. After thawing at room temperature, the injection should be agitated and the container checked for minute leaks by firmly squeezing the bag. The injection should be discarded if container seals or outlet ports are not intact or leaks are found or if the solution is cloudy or contains an insoluble precipitate. The injection should not be used in series connections with other plastic containers, since such use could result in air embolism from residual air being drawn from the primary container before administration of fluid from the secondary container is complete. Once thawed, the solutions are stable for 24 hours at a room temperature of 20–25°C or 14 days when refrigerated at 2–8°C and should not be refrozen.

Rate of Administration. IV infusions of piperacillin/tazobactam usually are given over 30 minutes.

Piperacillin/tazobactam has been administered by IV infusion over 3–4 hours† and by continuous IV infusion†. Some clinicians suggest that 4-hour intermittent IV infusions or continuous IV infusion of piperacillin/tazobactam may be beneficial in certain clinical situations (e.g., critically ill patients, pathogen with high piperacillin/tazobactam minimum inhibitory concentration [MIC]); there is some evidence that lengthening the duration of piperacillin/tazobactam infusions may maximize the pharmacokinetic/pharmacodynamic properties of the drug.

Concomitant Use with Aminoglycosides. Because piperacillin/tazobactam and aminoglycosides are physically and/or chemically incompatible in vitro, the drugs should be reconstituted, diluted, and administered separately if concomitant use is indicated (e.g., treatment of nosocomial pneumonia).

In certain situations when coadministration of piperacillin/tazobactam and an aminoglycoside via Y-site infusion is considered necessary, this can be accomplished using *only* certain dosages of amikacin or gentamicin and *only* certain acceptable diluents. (See Tables 1 and 2.) For Y-site coadministration, tobramycin or any aminoglycoside other than amikacin or gentamicin should *not* be used. Coadministration via Y-site infusion in any manner other than that specified in the tables may result in inactivation of the aminoglycoside.

Table 1. Y-site Compatibility of Piperacillin/tazobactam in Single-dose Vials and Bulk Vials or Bottles (Zosyn®, generics) with Aminoglycosides

Aminoglycoside	Piperacillin/tazobactam Dose (g)	Piperacillin/tazobactam Diluent (mL)	Aminoglycoside Concentration Range (mg/mL)[a]	Acceptable Diluents
Amikacin	2.25	50	1.75–7.5	0.9% sodium chloride injection or 5% dextrose injection
	3.375	100		
	4.5	150		
Gentamicin	2.25	50	0.7–3.32	0.9% sodium chloride injection or 5% dextrose injection
	3.375	100		
	4.5	150		

[a] Based on amikacin dosage of 10–15 mg/kg daily given in 2 divided doses or gentamicin dosage of 3–5 mg/kg daily given in 3 divided doses; higher dosage or once-daily dosage has not been evaluated for Y-site compatibility.

Table 2. Y-site Compatibility of Piperacillin/tazobactam (Frozen) Premixed Injections in Dextrose (Zosyn® in Galaxy® Containers) with Aminoglycosides

Aminoglycoside	Zosyn® Dose (g)	Aminoglycoside Concentration Range (mg/mL)[a]	Acceptable Diluents
Amikacin	2.25, 3.375, or 4.5	1.75–7.5	0.9% sodium chloride injection or 5% dextrose injection
Gentamicin	2.25 or 4.5 [b]	0.7–3.32	0.9% sodium chloride injection or 5% dextrose injection

[a] Based on amikacin dosage of 10–15 mg/kg daily given in 2 divided doses or gentamicin dosage of 3–5 mg/kg daily given in 3 divided doses; higher dosage or once-daily dosage has not been evaluated for Y-site compatibility.

[b] Frozen premixed Zosyn® injections in Galaxy® containers that contain 3.375 g/50 mL are *not* compatible with gentamicin and should *not* be used for Y-site coadministration with gentamicin.

■ Dosage

Piperacillin/tazobactam is a fixed combination of piperacillin sodium and tazobactam sodium; potency of each component is expressed in terms of the base. The commercially available fixed combination contains an 8:1 ratio of piperacillin to tazobactam.

Dosage of piperacillin/tazobactam usually is expressed as the total (sum) of the dosage of each of the 2 components (i.e., dosage of piperacillin plus dosage of tazobactam). However, dosage of piperacillin/tazobactam for pediatric patients often is expressed in terms of the piperacillin component.

Pediatric Dosage

General Neonatal Dosage. The American Academy of Pediatrics (AAP) recommends that dosage of IV piperacillin/tazobactam in neonates 28 days of age or younger† should be based on postmenstrual age (i.e., gestational age plus chronologic age). AAP recommends that neonates with postmenstrual age of 30 weeks or less receive IV piperacillin/tazobactam in a dosage of 100 mg/kg (of piperacillin) every 8 hours and that those with postmenstrual age greater than 30 weeks receive a dosage of 80 mg/kg (of piperacillin) every 6 hours.

In neonates weighing less than 1 kg†, some clinicians recommend that those 14 days of age or younger receive IV piperacillin/tazobactam in a dosage of 100 mg/kg (of piperacillin) every 12 hours and that those 15–28 days of age receive 100 mg/kg (of piperacillin) every 8 hours. These clinicians recommend that neonates weighing 1 kg or greater† receive a dosage of 100 mg/kg (of piperacillin) every 12 hours if they are 7 days of age or younger or 100 mg/kg (of piperacillin) every 8 hours if they are 8–28 days of age.

For the treatment of severe infections in neonates and infants younger than 2 months of age†, some clinicians suggest that IV piperacillin/tazobactam be given in a dosage of 80 mg/kg (of piperacillin) every 6 hours and others recommend a dosage of 80 mg/kg (of piperacillin) every 4 hours. Some clinicians suggest that shortening the dosing interval to every 6 hours and prolonging the duration of the IV infusion to 4 hours will maximize the pharmacokinetic/pharmacodynamic properties of the drug.

General Pediatric Dosage. AAP states that the usual dosage of IV piperacillin/tazobactam in pediatric patients beyond the neonatal period is 240–300 mg/kg (of piperacillin) daily in 3 or 4 divided doses. These experts state that a dosage of 400–600 mg/kg (of piperacillin) daily in 6 divided doses may be appropriate in some cystic fibrosis patients.

For the treatment of severe infections, some clinicians suggest that pediatric patients 2–9 months of age receive IV piperacillin/tazobactam in a dosage of 80 mg/kg (of piperacillin) every 6–8 hours and that those older than 9 months of age receive a dosage of 100 mg/kg (of piperacillin) every 6–8 hours.

AAP and some other clinicians state that the maximum recommended dosage of IV piperacillin/tazobactam in most pediatric patients is 16 g (of piperacillin) daily; however, AAP states that a maximum dosage of 24 g (of piperacillin) daily may be appropriate in some cystic fibrosis patients.

Intra-abdominal Infections. For the treatment of appendicitis and/or peritonitis in pediatric patients 2–9 months of age, the manufacturer recommends that IV piperacillin/tazobactam be given in a dosage of 80 mg/kg (of piperacillin) and 10 mg/kg (of tazobactam) every 8 hours.

For the treatment of appendicitis and/or peritonitis in pediatric patients 9 months of age or older weighing 40 kg or less with normal renal function, the manufacturer recommends that IV piperacillin/tazobactam be given in a dosage of 100 mg/kg (of piperacillin) and 12.5 mg/kg (of tazobactam) every 8 hours. The manufacturer states that pediatric patients with normal renal function weighing more than 40 kg should receive the usual adult dosage of piperacillin/tazobactam.

For the treatment of complicated intra-abdominal infections in pediatric patients, some clinicians recommend that IV piperacillin/tazobactam be given in a dosage of 200–300 mg/kg (of piperacillin) daily in divided doses every 6–8 hours.

Some clinicians state that the usual duration of treatment for intra-abdominal infections is 4–7 days, unless it is difficult to achieve adequate source control. These clinicians state that longer treatment durations have not been associated with improved outcomes.

Skin and Skin Structure Infections. If IV piperacillin/tazobactam is used for the treatment of necrotizing infections of the skin, fascia, and muscle†, some clinicians recommend that pediatric patients receive a dosage of 60–75 mg/kg (of piperacillin) every 6 hours in conjunction with vancomycin.

Adult Dosage

General Adult Dosage. The manufacturer states that the usual dosage of IV piperacillin/tazobactam for adults is 3.375 g (3 g of piperacillin and 0.375 g of tazobactam) every 6 hours for 7–10 days.

The maximum dosage of IV piperacillin/tazobactam recommended in adults usually is 3.375 g (3 g of piperacillin and 0.375 g of tazobactam) every 4 hours or 4.5 g (4 g of piperacillin and 0.5 g of tazobactam) every 6 hours. The manufacturer recommends a maximum dosage of 18 g (16 g of piperacillin and 2 g of tazobactam) daily.

Gynecologic and Obstetric Infections. For the treatment of postpartum endometritis or pelvic inflammatory disease (PID), the manufacturer states that the usual dosage of IV piperacillin/tazobactam in adults is 3.375 g (3 g of piperacillin and 0.375 g of tazobactam) every 6 hours for 7–10 days.

Intra-abdominal Infections. For the treatment of appendicitis and/or peritonitis, the manufacturer states that the usual dosage of IV piperacillin/tazobactam in adults is 3.375 g (3 g of piperacillin and 0.375 g of tazobactam) every 6 hours for 7–10 days.

For the treatment of complicated intra-abdominal infections in adults, some clinicians recommend that IV piperacillin/tazobactam be given in a dosage of 3.375 g (3 g of piperacillin and 0.375 g of tazobactam) every 6 hours; however, if *Pseudomonas aeruginosa* is identified, these clinicians state that dosage of the drug may be increased to 3.375 g (3 g of piperacillin and 0.375 g of tazobactam) every 4 hours or 4.5 g (4 g of piperacillin and 0.5 g of tazobactam) every 6 hours.

Some clinicians state that the usual duration of treatment for intra-abdominal infections is 4–7 days, unless it is difficult to achieve adequate source control. These clinicians state that longer treatment durations have not been associated with improved outcomes.

Community-acquired Pneumonia. For the treatment of moderately severe community-acquired pneumonia (CAP), the manufacturer states that the usual dosage of IV piperacillin/tazobactam in adults is 3.375 g (3 g of piperacillin and 0.375 g of tazobactam) every 6 hours for 7–10 days.

Nosocomial Pneumonia. For initial empiric treatment of nosocomial pneumonia in adults, the manufacturer recommends that IV piperacillin/tazobactam be given in a dosage of 4.5 g (4 g of piperacillin and 0.5 g of tazobactam) every 6 hours in conjunction with an aminoglycoside. The manufacturer states that the recommended duration of piperacillin/tazobactam therapy for the treatment of nosocomial pneumonia is 7–14 days; if *Ps. aeruginosa* is identified, the aminoglycoside should be continued concomitantly for the full duration of piperacillin/tazobactam treatment.

When IV piperacillin/tazobactam is used with or without other anti-infectives for initial empiric treatment of hospital-acquired pneumonia (HAP) not associated with mechanical ventilation or initial empiric treatment of ventilator-associated pneumonia (VAP), some clinicians recommend that adults receive a dosage of 4.5 g (4 g of piperacillin and 0.5 g of tazobactam) every 6 hours. These experts recommend a treatment duration of 7 days; however, depending on clinical response, a longer or shorter duration may be indicated.

Skin and Skin Structure Infections. For the treatment of skin and skin structure infections in adults, the manufacturer states that the usual dosage of IV piperacillin/tazobactam is 3.375 g (3 g of piperacillin and 0.375 g of tazobactam) every 6 hours for 7–10 days.

For the treatment of incisional surgical site infections†, some clinicians recommended that adults receive IV piperacillin/tazobactam in a dosage of 3.375 g (3 g of piperacillin and 0.375 g of tazobactam) every 6 hours or 4.5 g (4 g of piperacillin and 0.5 g of tazobactam) every 8 hours.

If IV piperacillin/tazobactam is used for the treatment of infected human or animal bite wounds†, a dosage of 3.375 g (3 g of piperacillin and 0.375 g of tazobactam) every 6–8 hours has been recommended.

If IV piperacillin/tazobactam is used for the treatment of necrotizing infections of the skin, fascia, and muscle†, some clinicians recommend that adults receive a dosage of 3.375 g (3 g of piperacillin and 0.375 g of tazobactam) every 6–8 hours in conjunction with vancomycin.

■ **Dosage in Renal and Hepatic Impairment** ***Renal Impairment*** Because serum concentrations of piperacillin and tazobactam are higher and prolonged in patients with renal impairment than in patients with normal renal function, doses and/or frequency of administration of piperacillin/tazobactam should be decreased in patients with renal impairment.

In adults with creatinine clearances of 40 mL/minute or less, including patients undergoing hemodialysis or continuous ambulatory peritoneal dialysis (CAPD), dosage of piperacillin/tazobactam should be decreased based on the degree of renal impairment. (See Table 3.)

The manufacturer makes no dosage recommendations for pediatric patients with impaired renal function.

Table 3. Dosage of Piperacillin/tazobactam for Adults with Renal Impairment

Creatinine Clearance (mL/minute)	Daily Dosage (Except Nosocomial Pneumonia)	Daily Dosage (Nosocomial Pneumonia)
20–40	2.25 g every 6 hours	3.375 g every 6 hours
<20	2.25 g every 8 hours	2.25 g every 6 hours
Hemodialysis Patients[a]	2.25 g every 12 hours; also give 0.75 g after each hemodialysis session	2.25 g every 8 hours; also give 0.75 g after each hemodialysis session
CAPD Patients[b]	2.25 g every 12 hours	2.25 g every 8 hours

[a] Hemodialysis removes approximately 30–40% of a dose of piperacillin/tazobactam (see Pharmacokinetics: Elimination); a supplemental dose of the drug is necessary after each hemodialysis session.

[b] Supplemental doses of piperacillin/tazobactam are not necessary in CAPD patients.

Hepatic Impairment Although serum half-lives of piperacillin and tazobactam are prolonged in patients with hepatic cirrhosis compared with healthy patients, this effect is not clinically important and does not necessitate a change in dosage of piperacillin/tazobactam when the drug is used in patients with hepatic cirrhosis.

Cautions

Adverse effects reported with the fixed combination of piperacillin sodium and tazobactam sodium (piperacillin/tazobactam) are similar to those reported with piperacillin alone and generally are transient and mild to moderate in severity. Adverse effects have been severe enough to require discontinuance of piperacillin/tazobactam in 3% or less of patients receiving the drug. The most frequent adverse effects (reported in more than 5% of patients receiving piperacillin/tazobactam) include GI effects (diarrhea, nausea, constipation), headache, and insomnia.

■ **GI Effects** Diarrhea, nausea, and constipation have been reported in up to 11% of patients receiving IV piperacillin/tazobactam. Vomiting, dyspepsia, and abdominal pain have been reported in up to 3%.

C. difficile-associated Diarrhea and Colitis Treatment with anti-infectives alters normal colon flora and may permit overgrowth of *Clostridioides difficile* (formerly known as *Clostridium difficile*).

C. difficile infection (CDI) and *C. difficile*-associated diarrhea and colitis (CDAD; also known as antibiotic-associated diarrhea and colitis or pseudomembranous colitis) have been reported with nearly all anti-infectives, including piperacillin/tazobactam, and may range in severity from mild diarrhea to fatal colitis. *C. difficile* produces toxins A and B, which contribute to the development of CDAD; hypertoxin-producing strains cause increased morbidity and mortality since these infections may be refractory to anti-infective therapy and may require colectomy. CDAD should be considered if diarrhea develops during or after therapy and managed accordingly. (See Precautions Related to C. difficile-associated Diarrhea and Colitis under Cautions: Precautions and Contraindications.)

■ **Dermatologic and Sensitivity Reactions** Rash (maculopapular, bullous, urticarial), pruritus, and fever have been reported in up to 4% of patients receiving piperacillin/tazobactam. There also have been postmarketing reports of erythema multiforme, Stevens-Johnson syndrome, toxic epidermal necrolysis, drug reaction with eosinophilia and systemic symptoms (DRESS), acute generalized exanthematous pustulosis, and exfoliative dermatitis in patients receiving the drug. (See Precautions Related to Dermatologic and Sensitivity Reactions under Cautions: Precautions and Contraindications.)

Serious and occasionally fatal hypersensitivity reactions, including anaphylaxis or anaphylactoid reactions, have been reported in patients receiving piperacillin/tazobactam. Such reactions are more likely to occur in individuals with a history of penicillin, cephalosporin, or carbapenem hypersensitivity or a history of sensitivity to multiple allergens. (See Precautions Related to Dermatologic and Sensitivity Reactions under Cautions: Precautions and Contraindications.)

■ **Hematologic Effects** Decreased hemoglobin and hematocrit, anemia, thrombocytopenia, increased platelet count, transient eosinophilia, transient leukopenia, and neutropenia have been reported in patients receiving piperacillin/tazobactam. In most reported cases, leukopenia and neutropenia occurred after prolonged therapy with the drug (e.g., 21 days or longer) and generally were reversible; systemic symptoms (e.g., fever, rigors, chills) also occurred in some patients. There have been postmarketing reports of hemolytic anemia, agranulocytosis, and pancytopenia in patients receiving the drug.

Positive direct antiglobulin (Coombs') test results, prolonged prothrombin time, and prolonged partial thromboplastin time have been reported in patients receiving piperacillin/tazobactam.

Epistaxis and purpura have been reported in 1% or less of patients receiving the drug. Manifestations of bleeding, occasionally associated with abnormal results in coagulation tests (e.g., clotting time, platelet aggregation, prothrombin time), have occurred in some patients receiving β-lactam anti-infectives, including piperacillin. Bleeding manifestations are more likely to occur in patients with renal failure than in patients with normal renal function. (See Precautions Related to Hematologic Effects under Cautions: Precautions and Contraindications.)

■ **Nervous System Effects** Headache and insomnia have been reported in up to 8% of patients receiving piperacillin/tazobactam. There have been postmarketing reports of delirium in patients receiving the drug.

As with other penicillins, neuromuscular excitability or seizures could occur if higher than recommended doses of IV piperacillin/tazobactam are given, especially in patients with renal failure.

■ **Renal and Electrolyte Effects** Increased concentrations of serum creatinine and BUN have been reported in patients receiving piperacillin/tazobactam. Renal failure has been reported rarely and there have been postmarketing reports of interstitial nephritis in patients receiving the drug.

When used in critically ill patients, piperacillin/tazobactam has been found to be an independent risk factor for renal failure and was associated with delayed recovery of renal function compared with other β-lactam anti-infectives in such patients. In addition, concomitant use of vancomycin with piperacillin/tazobactam in critically ill patients has been associated with an increased incidence of acute kidney injury. (See Drug Interactions: Vancomycin.)

Changes in serum electrolytes, including increased and decreased serum sodium, potassium, and calcium concentrations, have occurred in patients receiving piperacillin/tazobactam. (See Precautions Related to Renal and Electrolyte Effects under Cautions: Precautions and Contraindications.)

■ **Local Reactions** Adverse reactions at the IV infusion site, including phlebitis and thrombophlebitis, have been reported in 1% or less of patients receiving piperacillin/tazobactam.

■ **Hepatic Effects** Transient increases in AST, ALT, alkaline phosphatase, and bilirubin have been reported in patients receiving piperacillin/tazobactam. There have been postmarketing reports of hepatitis and jaundice.

■ **Other Adverse Effects** Candidiasis, including oral candidiasis, has been reported in 2–4% of patients receiving piperacillin/tazobactam. Stomatitis has been reported in 1% or less of patients receiving the drug.

Hypotension, rigors, myalgia, arthralgia, hypoglycemia, and flushing have been reported in 1% or less of patients receiving piperacillin/tazobactam. There have been postmarketing reports of eosinophilic pneumonia in patients receiving the drug.

■ **Precautions and Contraindications** Piperacillin/tazobactam is contraindicated in patients hypersensitive to any penicillin, cephalosporin, or β-lactamase inhibitor.

Precautions Related to Dermatologic and Sensitivity Reactions Piperacillin/tazobactam shares the toxic potentials of the penicillins, including the risk of hypersensitivity reactions, and the usual precautions of penicillin therapy should be observed. (See Cautions: Hypersensitivity Reactions, in the Natural Penicillins General Statement 8:12.16.04.) Serious hypersensitivity reactions are more likely to occur in individuals with a history of penicillin, cephalosporin, or carbapenem hypersensitivity.

Prior to initiation of piperacillin/tazobactam, careful inquiry should be made concerning previous hypersensitivity reactions to the drug, other β-lactams (including cephalosporins), or other allergens.

Patients should be advised that serious hypersensitivity reactions, including serious allergic cutaneous reactions, could occur that require immediate treatment.

If a severe hypersensitivity reaction occurs during piperacillin/tazobactam therapy, the drug should be discontinued and the patient given appropriate treatment as indicated.

Precautions Related to Hematologic Effects Because manifestations of bleeding have been reported with some β-lactam anti-infectives, including piperacillin, the possibility of bleeding complications should be considered in patients receiving piperacillin/tazobactam, especially when the drug is used in patients with renal impairment. If bleeding manifestations occur, piperacillin/tazobactam should be discontinued and appropriate therapy instituted.

Hematologic function should be evaluated periodically during piperacillin/

tazobactam therapy, especially in patients receiving prolonged therapy with the drug (i.e., 21 days or longer).

Precautions Related to Renal and Electrolyte Effects Renal systems should be evaluated periodically during prolonged therapy with piperacillin/tazobactam.

Because there is evidence that piperacillin/tazobactam is an independent risk factor for renal failure and has been associated with delayed recovery of renal function compared with other β-lactam anti-infectives when used in critically ill patients, the manufacturer states that alternatives to piperacillin/tazobactam should be considered in such patients. If use of piperacillin/tazobactam is considered necessary in critically ill patients because alternative treatment options are inadequate or unavailable, renal function should be monitored during treatment with the drug.

Serum electrolytes should be determined periodically when piperacillin/tazobactam is used in patients with low potassium reserves, and the possibility of hypokalemia should be considered when the drug is used in those with potentially low potassium reserves who are receiving cytotoxic therapy or diuretics.

The sodium content of piperacillin/tazobactam should be considered when the drug is used in geriatric patients or patients whose sodium intake is restricted. Piperacillin/tazobactam (Zosyn®) contains 2.84 mEq (65 mg) of sodium per gram of piperacillin. Most generic preparations of piperacillin/tazobactam contain 2.35 mEq (54 mg) of sodium per gram of piperacillin; some contain 2.43 mEq (56 mg) of sodium per gram of piperacillin.

Precautions Related to C. difficile-associated Diarrhea and Colitis Because CDAD has been reported with the use of nearly all anti-infectives, including piperacillin/tazobactam, it should be considered in the differential diagnosis of patients who develop diarrhea during or after anti-infective therapy. Careful medical history is necessary since CDAD has been reported to occur as late as 2 months or longer after anti-infective therapy is discontinued.

If CDAD is suspected or confirmed, anti-infective therapy not directed against *C. difficile* should be discontinued as soon as possible. Patients should be managed with appropriate anti-infective therapy directed against *C. difficile* (e.g., vancomycin, fidaxomicin, metronidazole), supportive therapy (e.g., fluid and electrolyte management, protein supplementation), and surgical evaluation as clinically indicated.

Patients should be advised that diarrhea is a common problem caused by anti-infectives and usually resolves when the drug is discontinued; however, they should contact a clinician if watery and bloody stools (with or without stomach cramps and fever) occur during or as late as 2 months or longer after the last dose.

Selection and Use of Anti-infectives To reduce development of drug-resistant bacteria and maintain effectiveness of piperacillin/tazobactam and other antibacterials, the drug should be used only for the treatment of infections proven or strongly suspected to be caused by bacteria.

When selecting or modifying anti-infective therapy, results of culture and in vitro susceptibility testing should be used. In the absence of such data, local epidemiology and susceptibility patterns when selecting anti-infectives for empiric therapy patterns should be considered.

Patients should be advised that antibacterials (including piperacillin/tazobactam) should only be used to treat bacterial infections and not used to treat viral infections (e.g., the common cold). Patients also should be advised about the importance of completing the full course of therapy, even if feeling better after a few days, and that skipping doses or not completing therapy may decrease effectiveness and increase the likelihood that bacteria will develop resistance and will not be treatable with piperacillin/tazobactam or other antibacterials in the future.

Information on test methods and quality control standards for in vitro susceptibility testing of antibacterial agents and specific interpretive criteria for such testing recognized by FDA is available at https://www.fda.gov/STIC.

■ **Pediatric Precautions** Safety and efficacy of piperacillin/tazobactam in children younger than 2 months of age have not been established.

The manufacturer states that use of piperacillin/tazobactam for the treatment of appendicitis and/or peritonitis in pediatric patients 2 months of age or older is supported by evidence from well-controlled studies and pharmacokinetic studies in adults and pediatric patients.

Adverse effects reported when piperacillin/tazobactam was used in pediatric patients 2–12 years of age with severe intra-abdominal infections (including appendicitis and/or peritonitis) have been similar to those reported in adults.

■ **Geriatric Precautions** Geriatric patients older than 65 years of age receiving piperacillin/tazobactam are not at increased risk of developing adverse effects based solely on their age. However, geriatric patients are more likely to have decreased renal function compared with younger adults and the risk of toxic reactions to the drug may be greater in patients with impaired renal function.

Because of the greater frequency of decreased hepatic, renal, or cardiac function and of concomitant disease and drug therapy in geriatric patients, dosage of piperacillin/tazobactam generally should be selected cautiously in these patients, usually initiating therapy at the low end of the dosage range, and it may be useful to monitor renal function. In geriatric patients with renal impairment, dosage should be modified in response to the degree of renal impairment. (See Renal Impairment under Dosage and Administration: Dosage in Renal and Hepatic Impairment.)

When piperacillin/tazobactam is used in geriatric patients, the sodium content of the specific preparation used should be considered. Geriatric patients may respond to salt loading with a blunted natriuresis and this may be clinically important in patients with diseases such as heart failure. Piperacillin/tazobactam (Zosyn®) contains 65 mg (2.84 mEq) of sodium per gram of piperacillin; patients would receive 780–1040 mg (34.1–45.5 mEq) of sodium daily with usually recommended dosages of this preparation. The sodium content of commercially available generic preparations of piperacillin/tazobactam differs depending on the manufacturer. (See Precautions Related to Renal and Electrolyte Effects under Cautions: Precautions and Contraindications.)

■ **Mutagenicity and Carcinogenicity** The mutagenic potential of piperacillin/tazobactam has been evaluated in vitro and in vivo. There was no in vitro evidence of mutagenicity when the fixed combination was used in microbial mutagenicity assays, unscheduled DNA synthesis tests, mammalian point mutation assays in Chinese hamster ovary cell HPRT, or mammalian cell (BALB/c-3T3) transformation assays. In addition, in vivo studies in rats using piperacillin/tazobactam indicated that the drug did not induce chromosomal aberrations.

Long-term studies have not been performed to evaluate the carcinogenic potential of piperacillin, tazobactam, or piperacillin/tazobactam.

■ **Pregnancy, Fertility, and Lactation** ***Pregnancy*** Available human data regarding use of piperacillin/tazobactam during pregnancy are inadequate to inform a drug-associated risk for major birth defects and miscarriage. Piperacillin and tazobactam both cross the human placenta.

Reproduction studies in pregnant mice and rats using IV piperacillin/tazobactam (up to 1–2 times the human dosage of piperacillin and 2–3 times the human dosage of tazobactam based on body surface area) did not reveal evidence of teratogenicity or fetal structural abnormalities; however, intraperitoneal administration in rats at doses less than the maximum recommended human daily dosage based on body surface area given prior to mating and throughout gestation or from gestation day 17 through lactation day 21 resulted in maternal toxicity, reduced litter size, and effects on peri- and postnatal development (e.g., reduced pup weights, increased stillbirths, increased pup mortality, ossification delays, rib variations).

Fertility There was no evidence of impaired fertility in reproduction studies in rats using IV piperacillin/tazobactam in dosages similar to the maximum recommended human daily dosage based on body surface area.

Lactation Piperacillin is distributed into human milk; it is not known whether tazobactam is distributed into human milk. Effects of the drugs on breast-fed infants or milk production are not known.

The developmental and health benefits of breast-feeding should be considered along with the woman's clinical need for piperacillin/tazobactam and potential adverse effects on the breast-fed infant from the drug or from the underlying maternal condition.

Drug Interactions

■ **Aminoglycosides** The antibacterial activities of piperacillin and aminoglycosides (e.g., amikacin, gentamicin, tobramycin) have been synergistic in vitro against some strains of Enterobacteriaceae and *Pseudomonas aeruginosa.*

The fixed combination of piperacillin sodium and tazobactam sodium (piperacillin/tazobactam) is physically and/or chemically incompatible with aminoglycosides and can inactivate aminoglycosides in vitro if the drugs are admixed or administered using the same IV infusion line. If concomitant therapy with piperacillin/tazobactam and an aminoglycoside is indicated, the drugs should be reconstituted, diluted, and administered separately. Piperacillin/tazobactam can be coadministered with amikacin or gentamicin (but not tobramycin or other aminoglycosides) via Y-site infusion *only* under certain specific conditions. (See Concomitant Use with Aminoglycosides under Administration: IV Infusion, in Dosage and Administration.)

Piperacillin also can inactivate aminoglycosides in vivo. Decreased aminoglycoside serum concentrations and half-lives have been reported in patients receiving concomitant piperacillin therapy, usually when high piperacillin dosage was used or the patient had impaired renal function. Although *sequential* administration of piperacillin/tazobactam and tobramycin in patients with normal renal function or mild to moderate renal impairment has resulted in modestly decreased serum tobramycin concentrations, the manufacturer of piperacillin/tazobactam states that dosage adjustments are not needed.

Because concomitant use of piperacillin and an aminoglycoside in patients with end-stage renal disease (ESRD) requiring hemodialysis may result in substantially decreased serum concentrations of the aminoglycoside (especially tobramycin), aminoglycoside serum concentrations should be monitored closely in patients receiving piperacillin/tazobactam and an aminoglycoside.

■ **Anticoagulants** Coagulation parameters should be monitored more frequently if piperacillin/tazobactam is used concomitantly with oral anticoagulants, high doses of heparin, or other drugs that affect blood coagulation or thrombocyte function.

■ **Methotrexate** Concomitant use of methotrexate and piperacillin may result in decreased renal clearance of methotrexate due to competition for renal secretion; the effect of tazobactam on methotrexate elimination has not been evaluated.

If concurrent therapy with methotrexate and piperacillin/tazobactam is necessary, serum methotrexate concentrations should be evaluated frequently and the patient should be monitored for signs and symptoms of methotrexate toxicity.

■ Neuromuscular Blocking Agents Prolonged neuromuscular blockade has been reported when vecuronium was used concomitantly with piperacillin, and this also could occur if vecuronium is used concomitantly with piperacillin/tazobactam. Because other nondepolarizing muscle relaxants have similar mechanisms of action, a similar effect could occur if piperacillin/tazobactam is used concomitantly with any of these drugs.

If piperacillin/tazobactam is used concomitantly with a neuromuscular blocking agent, the patient should be monitored for adverse effects related to neuromuscular blockade.

■ Probenecid Probenecid inhibits tubular renal secretion of both piperacillin and tazobactam and prolongs their half-lives by 21 and 71%, respectively.

Concomitant use of probenecid and piperacillin/tazobactam is not recommended unless benefits outweigh risks.

■ Vancomycin Concomitant use of vancomycin and piperacillin/tazobactam in critically ill patients has been associated with an increased incidence of acute kidney injury compared with use of vancomycin alone.

If vancomycin and piperacillin/tazobactam are used concomitantly, renal function should be monitored. In addition, because vancomycin and some piperacillin/tazobactam preparations may be physically and/or chemically incompatible, it has been recommended that the drugs should be administered separately.

Pharmacokinetic interactions between vancomycin and piperacillin/tazobactam have not been reported.

Laboratory Test Interferences

■ Tests for Aspergillus False-positive test results for *Aspergillus* were reported when the Bio-Rad Laboratories Platelia *Aspergillus* EIA test was performed in patients receiving the fixed combination of piperacillin sodium and tazobactam sodium (piperacillin/tazobactam). Cross reactions with non-*Aspergillus* polysaccharides and polyfuranoses have been reported with the Bio-Rad Laboratories Platelia *Aspergillus* EIA test. Positive Platelia *Aspergillus* EIA test results in patients receiving piperacillin/tazobactam should be interpreted with caution and confirmed using other diagnostic methods.

■ Tests for Urinary Glucose As with other penicillins, piperacillin/tazobactam may result in false-positive urinary glucose determinations with tests that use copper reduction (e.g., Clinitest®). Glucose tests based on enzymatic glucose oxidase reactions should be used.

Acute Toxicity

There have been postmarketing reports of overdosage of the fixed combination of piperacillin sodium and tazobactam sodium (piperacillin/tazobactam). Adverse effects reported with such overdosages have included adverse effects reported with usual dosages of the drug (e.g., nausea, vomiting, diarrhea). Neuromuscular excitability or convulsions may occur if higher than recommended dosages of IV piperacillin/tazobactam are given, especially in patients with renal failure.

If acute overdosage of piperacillin/tazobactam occurs, supportive and symptomatic treatment should be initiated as indicated. Because piperacillin and tazobactam are removed by hemodialysis (see Pharmacokinetics: Elimination), this procedure may be effective in reducing excessive serum concentrations of the drugs.

Mechanism of Action

The fixed combination of piperacillin sodium and tazobactam sodium (piperacillin/tazobactam) is bactericidal in action.

Like other penicillins, piperacillin inhibits bacterial septum formation and cell wall synthesis in susceptible bacteria. The mechanism of action of penicillins is mediated through binding to penicillin-binding proteins (PBPs).

Tazobactam alone has only limited intrinsic antibacterial activity because of reduced affinity for PBPs. However, tazobactam is a β-lactamase inhibitor that generally acts as an irreversible inhibitor and can inactivate both plasmid- and chromosome-mediated β-lactamases. In vitro studies indicate that tazobactam can inhibit staphylococcal β-lactamases and β-lactamases classified as Richmond-Sykes types II, III (TEM type, HSV-1), IV, and V (PSE and OXA types). Tazobactam is effective against some type I β-lactamases, including type IC, and may be slightly more active against type I enzymes than some other β-lactamase inhibitors (e.g., clavulanic acid, sulbactam). Unlike clavulanic acid, tazobactam generally does not induce production of type I chromosomally mediated cephalosporins in *Pseudomonas* or Enterobacteriaceae.

Because tazobactam inactivates certain β-lactamases, concomitant use with piperacillin can protect the penicillin from degradation by these β-lactamases and expand its spectrum of activity to include some β-lactamase-producing bacteria that are resistant to piperacillin alone.

Spectrum

Based on its spectrum of activity, the fixed combination of piperacillin sodium and tazobactam sodium (piperacillin/tazobactam) is classified as an extended-spectrum penicillin. For information on the classification of penicillins based on spectrum of activity, see the Preface to the Penicillins 8:12.16.

Piperacillin/tazobactam has a wide spectrum of activity and is active in vitro against various gram-positive and -negative aerobic and anaerobic bacteria. The fixed combination is active against bacteria susceptible to piperacillin alone. In addition, because tazobactam has a high affinity for and binds to certain β-lactamases that generally inactivate piperacillin, piperacillin/tazobactam is active against many β-lactamase-producing bacteria that are resistant to piperacillin alone, including piperacillin-resistant strains of staphylococci, *Haemophilus*, Enterobacteriaceae, and *Bacteroides*.

Piperacillin/tazobactam is not active against *Mycoplasma* and *Chlamydia*.

■ Gram-positive Aerobic Bacteria Piperacillin/tazobactam is active in vitro and in clinical infections against *Staphylococcus aureus* (methicillin-susceptible strains only).

Piperacillin/tazobactam also is active in vitro against *S. epidermidis* (methicillin-susceptible strains only), *Streptococcus pyogenes* (group A β-hemolytic streptococci; GAS), *S. agalactiae* (group B streptococci; GBS), *S. pneumoniae* (penicillin-susceptible strains only), viridans group streptococci, and *Enterococcus faecalis* (ampicillin- or penicillin-susceptible strains only).

Although piperacillin/tazobactam is active against β-lactamase-producing *S. aureus* and *S. epidermidis*, the fixed combination is not active against methicillin-resistant *S. aureus* (MRSA; also known as oxacillin-resistant *S. aureus* or ORSA) or methicillin-resistant *S. epidermidis*.

■ Gram-negative Aerobic Bacteria ***Enterobacteriaceae*** Piperacillin/tazobactam is active in vitro and in clinical infections against *Escherichia coli* and *Klebsiella pneumoniae*.

Piperacillin/tazobactam also is active in vitro against *Citrobacter koseri*, *Enterobacter*, *Morganella morganii*, *Proteus mirabilis*, *P. vulgaris*, *Providencia stuartii*, *P. rettgeri*, *Salmonella*, *Shigella*, and *Serratia marcescens*.

Pseudomonas Piperacillin/tazobactam is active in vitro and in clinical infections against *Pseudomonas aeruginosa*.

Other Gram-negative Aerobic Bacteria Piperacillin/tazobactam is active in vitro and in clinical infections against *Acinetobacter* (including *A. baumannii*) and *Haemophilus influenzae* (except β-lactamase negative, ampicillin-resistant strains; BLNAR). The drug also is active in vitro against *Moraxella catarrhalis* and *Neisseria*.

Piperacillin/tazobactam has some in vitro activity against *Legionella*; however, the drug is not effective against intracellular *Legionella* and is unlikely to be effective for the treatment of *Legionella* infections.

■ Anaerobic Bacteria Piperacillin/tazobactam is active in vitro and in clinical infections against some gram-negative anaerobic bacteria, including *Bacteroides fragilis*, *B. ovatus*, *B. thetaiotaomicron*, and *B. vulgatus*. The drug also is active in vitro against *B. distasonis*, *Fusobacterium*, and *Prevotella melaninogenica*.

Piperacillin/tazobactam is active in vitro against some gram-positive anaerobic bacteria, including *Bacillus*, *Clostridium perfringens*, *Cutibacterium acnes* (formerly *Propionibacterium acnes*), and *Peptostreptococcus*.

Resistance

Resistance or reduced susceptibility to the fixed combination of piperacillin sodium and tazobactam sodium (piperacillin/tazobactam) can occur.

The major mechanism of resistance to piperacillin/tazobactam in gram-positive bacteria is alteration in penicillin-binding proteins (PBPs). Methicillin-resistant *Staphylococcus aureus* (MRSA; also known as oxacillin-resistant *S. aureus* or ORSA) and *Enterococcus faecium* are intrinsically resistant to piperacillin/tazobactam because of low affinity of PBPs.

Resistance to piperacillin/tazobactam in gram-negative bacteria may be multifactorial and may involve β-lactamases, transferable multidrug-resistance genes, alterations in outer membrane porins, and antibiotic efflux. Piperacillin/tazobactam may be active against some Enterobacteriaceae that produce extended-spectrum β-lactamases (ESBLs), but strains that produce multiple ESBLs or have additional mechanisms of resistance (e.g., AmpC β-lactamases) may have reduced susceptibility or resistance to the drug. *Pseudomonas* resistant to piperacillin generally also are resistant to piperacillin/tazobactam.

β-Lactamase-negative, ampicillin-resistant *Haemophilus influenzae* (BLNAR *H. influenzae*) are resistant to piperacillin/tazobactam.

Pharmacokinetics

■ Absorption Following IV infusion of the fixed combination of piperacillin sodium and tazobactam sodium (piperacillin/tazobactam), peak plasma concentrations of piperacillin and tazobactam are attained immediately or 1–2 hours after completion of the infusion. Studies in adults indicate that piperacillin plasma concentrations attained following IV infusion of piperacillin/tazobactam over 30 minutes are similar to those attained with equivalent doses of piperacillin administered alone.

■ Distribution Both piperacillin and tazobactam are widely distributed into tissues and body fluids, including intestinal mucosa, gallbladder, female reproductive tissues (uterus, ovary, fallopian tube), lung, skin, bone, interstitial fluid, synovial fluid, and bile. Mean tissue concentrations generally are 50–100% of plasma concentrations.

Only low concentrations of piperacillin and tazobactam are distributed into CSF in patients with uninflamed meninges.

Both piperacillin and tazobactam cross the placenta.

Piperacillin is distributed into milk; it is not known whether tazobactam is distributed into milk.

The mean volume of distribution of piperacillin is 0.243 L/kg and is independent of age.

Both piperacillin and tazobactam are approximately 30% bound to plasma proteins.

■ **Elimination** Piperacillin is metabolized to a minor microbiologically active desethyl metabolite and an inactive metabolite.

Tazobactam is metabolized to a single metabolite that lacks pharmacologic and antibacterial activity.

Both piperacillin and tazobactam are eliminated in urine by glomerular filtration and tubular secretion. In addition, piperacillin, desethylpiperacillin, and tazobactam are eliminated in bile.

Following IV administration, 68 and 80% of the piperacillin and tazobactam doses, respectively, are eliminated unchanged in urine.

Plasma half-lives of piperacillin and tazobactam range from 0.7–1.2 hours in healthy adults.

In adults with cirrhosis, the half-lives of piperacillin and tazobactam are increased by approximately 25 and 18%, respectively, compared with adults with normal hepatic function.

In adults with renal impairment, the half-lives of piperacillin and tazobactam increase with decreasing creatinine clearance. In adults with creatinine clearances less than 20 mL/minute, the half-life of piperacillin is twofold higher and the half-life of tazobactam is fourfold higher compared with adults with normal renal function.

In geriatric adults 65–80 years of age, the mean half-lives of piperacillin and tazobactam are increased by 32 and 55%, respectively, compared with adults 18–35 years of age; this increase may be the result of age-related changes in creatinine clearance.

In children 9 months to 12 years of age, clearance of piperacillin and tazobactam is comparable to that reported in adults; piperacillin clearance in children 2–9 months of age is estimated to be 80% of that value. Clearance is slower in patients younger than 2 months of age compared with older children.

Both piperacillin and tazobactam are removed by hemodialysis and, to a lesser extent, by peritoneal dialysis. Hemodialysis removes approximately 31 and 39% of the piperacillin and tazobactam dose, respectively; an additional 5% of the tazobactam dose is removed as the tazobactam metabolite. Peritoneal dialysis removes approximately 6 and 21% of the piperacillin and tazobactam dose, respectively; up to 16% of the tazobactam dose is removed as the tazobactam metabolite.

Chemistry and Stability

■ **Chemistry** Piperacillin sodium and tazobactam sodium (piperacillin/tazobactam) is a fixed combination of the sodium salts of piperacillin and tazobactam.

Piperacillin, a piperazine derivative of ampicillin, is an extended-spectrum penicillin. Piperacillin is commercially available in the US only in fixed combination with tazobactam.

Tazobactam, a β-lactamase inhibitor, is a synthetic penicillanic acid sulfone that is structurally similar to sulbactam. Although tazobactam has only limited intrinsic antibacterial activity alone, the combined use of tazobactam and certain penicillins or cephalosporins (e.g., amoxicillin, ampicillin, ceftazidime, ceftolozane, piperacillin) results in a synergistic effect that expands the spectrum of activity of the penicillin or cephalosporin against many strains of β-lactamase-producing bacteria.

Piperacillin/tazobactam contains an 8:1 ratio of piperacillin to tazobactam; potency of the fixed combination is expressed in terms of the piperacillin content plus the tazobactam content.

Piperacillin/tazobactam (Zosyn®) and generic preparations of piperacillin/tazobactam commercially available in the US are *not* identical. Piperacillin/tazobactam (Zosyn®) is formulated with edetate disodium dihydrate (EDTA) and sodium citrate; the generic preparations do not contain EDTA or sodium citrate. Because EDTA acts as a metal-chelating agent and sodium citrate acts as a buffer, certain aspects of chemical degradation and particulate formation are inhibited and there is a lower risk of particulate matter formation and accumulation following reconstitution of Zosyn® with commonly used diluents or storage of solutions of the drug. In addition, the presence of EDTA and sodium citrate allows coadministration of Zosyn® and lactated Ringer's injection via Y-site infusion. (See IV Infusion under Dosage and Administration: Administration.)

Each single-dose vial of piperacillin/tazobactam sterile powder (Zosyn®) contains 2.84 mEq (65 mg) of sodium and 0.25 mg of EDTA per gram of piperacillin.

Commercially available piperacillin/tazobactam sterile powder (generic) in single-dose ADD-Vantage® vials contains 2.35 mEq (54 mg) of sodium per gram of piperacillin.

Bulk vials of piperacillin/tazobactam (Zosyn®) containing 40.5 g (36 g of piperacillin and 4.5 g of tazobactam) contain 100.4 mEq (2304 mg) of sodium and 9 mg of EDTA. Bulk bottles of piperacillin/tazobactam (generic) containing 40.5 g (36 g of piperacillin and 4.5 g of tazobactam) contain 84.6 mEq (1945 mg) of sodium and do not contain EDTA.

Commercially available single-dose frozen premixed piperacillin/tazobactam injections in dextrose (Zosyn® in Galaxy® containers) are sterile, nonpyrogenic, iso-osmotic solutions of the drug formulated with EDTA. The single-dose frozen injection contains 2.79 mEq (64 mg) of sodium and 0.25 mg of EDTA per gram of piperacillin. Sodium bicarbonate and/or hydrochloric acid may have been added to adjust the pH of the injections to 5.5–6.8.

■ **Stability** Piperacillin/tazobactam powder for injection provided in single-dose vials (Zosyn®, generic) should be stored at 20–25°C. Following reconstitution, the solutions should be used immediately; any unused portions should be discarded after 24 hours if stored at 20–25°C or after 48 hours if refrigerated at 2–8°C. These reconstituted solutions should not be frozen.

Single-dose ADD-Vantage® vials of piperacillin/tazobactam (generic) should be stored at 20–25°C. Following reconstitution with 0.9% sodium chloride injection or 5% dextrose injection according to the manufacturer's directions, these IV solutions are stable for 24 hours at room temperature and should not be refrigerated or frozen.

Piperacillin/tazobactam powder for injection provided in bulk vials or bottles (Zosyn®, generic) should be stored at 20–25°C. Following reconstitution, the solutions should be used promptly; any unused portions should be discarded after 24 hours if stored at 20–25°C or after 48 hours if refrigerated at 2–8°C. These reconstituted solutions should not be frozen.

The commercially available single-dose frozen premixed piperacillin/tazobactam injections in dextrose (Zosyn® in Galaxy® containers) should be stored at −20°C or lower. The frozen premixed injections should be thawed at room temperature (20–25°C) or under refrigeration (2–8°C) and, once thawed, should not be refrozen. Thawed solutions of the commercially available frozen injection are stable for 24 hours at room temperature (20–25°C) or 14 days at 2–8°C.

Piperacillin/tazobactam is potentially physically and/or chemically incompatible with some drugs, including aminoglycosides, but the compatibility depends on several factors (e.g., concentration of the drugs, specific diluents used, resulting pH, temperature). Specialized references should be consulted for specific compatibility information.

Preparations

Excipients in commercially available drug preparations may have clinically important effects in some individuals; consult specific product labeling for details.

Piperacillin Sodium and Tazobactam Sodium

Parenteral

For injection, for IV infusion	2.25 g (2 g of piperacillin and 0.25 g of tazobactam)*	**Piperacillin Sodium and Tazobactam Sodium for Injection**
		Piperacillin Sodium and Tazobactam Sodium for Injection ADD-Vantage®, Hospira
		Zosyn®, Wyeth
	3.375 g (3 g of piperacillin and 0.375 g of tazobactam)*	**Piperacillin Sodium and Tazobactam Sodium for Injection**
		Piperacillin Sodium and Tazobactam Sodium for Injection ADD-Vantage®, Hospira
		Zosyn®, Wyeth
	4.5 g (4 g of piperacillin and 0.5 g of tazobactam)*	**Piperacillin Sodium and Tazobactam Sodium for Injection**
		Piperacillin Sodium and Tazobactam Sodium for Injection ADD-Vantage®, Hospira
		Zosyn®, Wyeth
	40.5 g (36 g of piperacillin and 4.5 g of tazobactam) pharmacy bulk package*	**Piperacillin Sodium and Tazobactam Sodium for Injection**
		Zosyn®, Wyeth

*available from one or more manufacturer, distributor, and/or repackager by generic (nonproprietary) name

Piperacillin Sodium and Tazobactam Sodium in Dextrose

Parenteral

Injection (frozen), for IV infusion	2.25 g (40 mg of piperacillin per mL [2 g] and 5 mg of tazobactam per mL [0.25 g]) in 2% Dextrose	**Zosyn® Iso-osmotic in Dextrose Injection** (Galaxy®), Wyeth
	3.375 g (60 mg of piperacillin per mL [3 g] and 7.5 mg of tazobactam per mL [0.375 g]) in 0.7% Dextrose	**Zosyn® Iso-osmotic in Dextrose Injection** (Galaxy®), Wyeth
	4.5 g (40 mg of piperacillin per mL [4 g] and 5 mg of tazobactam per mL [0.5 g]) in 2% Dextrose	**Zosyn® Iso-osmotic in Dextrose Injection** (Galaxy®), Wyeth

†Use is not currently included in the labeling approved by the US Food and Drug Administration

QUINOLONES 8:12.18

Ciprofloxacin
Ciprofloxacin Hydrochloride

■ Ciprofloxacin is a fluoroquinolone anti-infective agent.

Uses

Ciprofloxacin is used orally or IV for the treatment of urinary tract infections (UTIs), chronic bacterial prostatitis, acute sinusitis, lower respiratory tract infections (including nosocomial pneumonia and acute exacerbations of chronic bronchitis), GI infections, skin and skin structure infections, or bone and joint infections caused by susceptible gram-negative and gram-positive aerobic bacteria. Ciprofloxacin is used orally or IV for inhalational anthrax (postexposure) following suspected or confirmed exposure to aerosolized *Bacillus anthracis* spores and also is used for prophylaxis following ingestion of *B. anthracis* spores† and for the treatment of inhalational anthrax†, cutaneous anthrax†, or GI and oropharyngeal anthrax†. Ciprofloxacin is used orally or IV for the treatment or prophylaxis of plague. In addition, ciprofloxacin is used orally or IV in conjunction with metronidazole for the treatment of complicated intra-abdominal infections caused by *Escherichia coli*, *Pseudomonas aeruginosa*, *Proteus mirabilis*, *Klebsiella pneumoniae*, or *Bacteroides fragilis*. Because ciprofloxacin is inactive against most anaerobic bacteria, the drug is ineffective in and should not be used alone if a mixed aerobic-anaerobic bacterial infection is suspected. Ciprofloxacin has been used in conjunction with other anti-infectives for empiric anti-infective therapy in febrile neutropenic patients.

Ciprofloxacin extended-release tablets containing both the hydrochloride and the base are used in adults for the treatment of uncomplicated UTIs (acute cystitis), complicated UTIs, or acute uncomplicated pyelonephritis. Safety and efficacy of ciprofloxacin extended-release tablets have been established *only* for infections involving the urinary tract; the extended-release tablets should *not* be used for the treatment of infections at other sites (e.g., respiratory tract, skin and skin structure, bone and joint, GI tract, intra-abdominal) that are treated with ciprofloxacin conventional tablets or oral suspension or with IV ciprofloxacin.

Prior to initiation of ciprofloxacin therapy, appropriate specimens should be obtained for identification of the causative organism(s) and in vitro susceptibility tests. Ciprofloxacin therapy may be started pending results of susceptibility tests, but should be discontinued and other appropriate anti-infective therapy substituted if the organism is found to be resistant to ciprofloxacin. Because resistant strains of *Pseudomonas aeruginosa* have developed during ciprofloxacin therapy, in vitro susceptibility tests should be performed periodically when the drug is used in the treatment of infections caused by this organism. Because staphylococci may develop resistance to ciprofloxacin during prolonged therapy with the drug, in vitro susceptibility tests should be repeated during therapy, especially when infections are caused by methicillin-resistant strains of *Staphylococcus aureus* (MRSA; also known as oxacillin-resistant *S. aureus* or ORSA).

■ **Bone and Joint Infections** Ciprofloxacin (IV, conventional tablets, oral suspension) is used in adults for the treatment of bone and joint infections, including osteomyelitis, caused by susceptible *E. aerogenes*†, *E. cloacae*, *E. coli*†, *K. pneumoniae*†, *M. morganii*†, *P. mirabilis*†, *Ps. aeruginosa*, or *S. marcescens*.

For the treatment of native vertebral osteomyelitis caused by Enterobacteriaceae or *Ps. aeruginosa*, the Infectious Diseases Society of America (IDSA) recommends ciprofloxacin as an alternative to the drugs of choice (cefepime, carbapenems). For the treatment of native vertebral osteomyelitis caused by *Salmonella*†, these experts recommend ciprofloxacin as the drug of choice and ceftriaxone as an alternative.

For the treatment of prosthetic joint infections caused by *Enterobacter* or *Ps. aeruginosa*, IDSA states that cefepime or a carbapenem is preferred and ciprofloxacin is recommended as an alternative. These experts state that ciprofloxacin may be a preferred drug for the treatment of prosthetic joint infections caused by other Enterobacteriaceae.

For additional information on management of bone and joint infections, current clinical practice guidelines from IDSA available at http://www.idsociety.org should be consulted.

Clinical Experience Clinical response has been reported in 61–86% and bacteriologic cure has been reported in 75–81% of patients with bone and joint infections (caused principally by gram-negative aerobes) who received oral ciprofloxacin. Treatment failures have been reported most frequently in patients with an underlying metal appliance at the site of infection and in patients with ciprofloxacin-resistant *Ps. aeruginosa* or *S. aureus*. However, there is evidence from a randomized, controlled study in patients with culture-proven staphylococcal infections associated with stable orthopedic implants that a long-term regimen (3–6 weeks) of ciprofloxacin and rifampin given after initial debridement and a 2-week IV regimen of flucloxacillin (not commercially available in the US) or vancomycin with rifampin or placebo can result in cure of the infection without removal of the implant.

■ **Endocarditis** ***Endocarditis Caused by the HACEK Group*** Ciprofloxacin is used as an alternative for the treatment of endocarditis† (native or prosthetic valve or other prosthetic material) caused by fastidious gram-negative bacilli known as the HACEK group (*Haemophilus*, *Aggregatibacter*, *Cardiobacterium hominis*, *Eikenella corrodens*, *Kingella*). The HACEK group accounts for up to 10% of cases of community-acquired native valve endocarditis in patients who are not IV drug abusers. These organisms should be considered ampicillin-resistant, but may be susceptible to third or fourth generation cephalosporins or fluoroquinolones.

The American Heart Association (AHA) and IDSA recommend ceftriaxone (or other third or fourth generation cephalosporin) for the treatment of endocarditis caused by the HACEK group, but state that a fluoroquinolone (ciprofloxacin, levofloxacin, moxifloxacin) may be considered in patients who cannot tolerate cephalosporins. Because only limited data are available regarding use of fluoroquinolones for the treatment of HACEK endocarditis, an infectious disease specialist should be consulted when treating such infections in patients who cannot tolerate cephalosporins.

■ **GI Infections** ***Infectious Diarrhea*** Ciprofloxacin is used in adults for the treatment of infectious diarrhea caused by susceptible enterotoxigenic *E. coli*, *Campylobacter*, *Salmonella*†, *Shigella* (*S. flexneri*, *S. boydii*, *S. sonnei*, *S. dysenteriae*), or *Vibrio*† (see Uses: Vibrio Infections).

Because ciprofloxacin is active in vitro against many pathogens associated with infectious diarrhea, including some strains of *Campylobacter*, *E. coli*, *Shigella*, *Salmonella*, *Aeromonas*, *Vibrio*, and *Yersinia enterocolitica*, some clinicians suggest that it may be a drug of choice for empiric treatment of the disease in adults. However, because of concerns about increasing emergence of fluoroquinolone-resistant strains in some enteric pathogens (e.g., *Campylobacter*, *Salmonella*, *Shigella*) secondary to widespread use of the drugs, a decision to use a fluoroquinolone for empiric treatment of infectious diarrhea should be based on local susceptibility patterns.

Campylobacter Infections Ciprofloxacin is used for the treatment of campylobacteriosis caused by susceptible *Campylobacter*.

Optimal treatment of campylobacteriosis in patients with human immunodeficiency virus (HIV) infection has not been identified. Some clinicians withhold anti-infective treatment in HIV-infected patients with CD4$^+$ T-cell counts exceeding 200 cells/mm^3 if they have only mild campylobacteriosis, but initiate treatment if symptoms persist for more than several days. In HIV-infected patients with mild to moderate campylobacteriosis, treatment with a fluoroquinolone (preferably ciprofloxacin or, alternatively, levofloxacin or moxifloxacin) or azithromycin is reasonable. Anti-infective therapy should be modified based on results of in vitro susceptibility testing. In the US, resistance to fluoroquinolones has been reported in 22% of *C. jejuni* and 35% of *C. coli* isolates tested. To limit emergence of resistance, some clinicians suggest that it may be prudent to use an aminoglycoside concomitantly in patients with bacteremic infections.

Cyclospora Infections Ciprofloxacin is recommended by some clinicians as an alternative to co-trimoxazole for the treatment of cyclosporiasis† caused by *Cyclospora cayetanensis*.

Cystoisospora Infections Ciprofloxacin has been used for the treatment of cystoisosporiasis† (formerly isosporiasis) caused by *Cystoisospora belli* (formerly *Isospora belli*).

Although co-trimoxazole is the drug of choice for the treatment of cystoisosporiasis, pyrimethamine, ciprofloxacin, and nitazoxanide are recommended as alternatives. Ciprofloxacin may not be as effective as co-trimoxazole, but may be useful for the treatment of cystoisosporiasis in patients who cannot tolerate co-trimoxazole.

In HIV-infected patients, ciprofloxacin is recommended as an alternative to co-trimoxazole for treatment and chronic maintenance therapy (secondary prophylaxis) of cystoisosporiasis.

Salmonella Gastroenteritis Ciprofloxacin is used for the treatment of *Salmonella* gastroenteritis† (with or without bacteremia).

Anti-infective therapy is not usually indicated in otherwise healthy individuals with uncomplicated (noninvasive) gastroenteritis caused by *Salmonella* since such therapy may prolong the duration of fecal excretion of the organism and there is no evidence that it shortens the duration of the disease; however, the US Centers for Disease Control and Prevention (CDC), American Academy of Pediatrics (AAP), IDSA, and others recommend anti-infective therapy in individuals with severe *Salmonella* gastroenteritis and in those who are at increased risk of invasive disease. These individuals include infants younger than 3–6 months of age; individuals older than 50 years of age; individuals with hemoglobinopathies, severe atherosclerosis or valvular heart disease, prostheses, uremia, chronic GI disease, or severe colitis; and individuals who are immunocompromised because of malignancy, immunosuppressive therapy, HIV infection, or other immunosuppressive illness. When an anti-infective agent is considered necessary in an individual with *Salmonella* gastroenteritis, CDC, AAP, IDSA, and others recommend ceftriaxone, cefotaxime, ciprofloxacin, ampicillin, amoxicillin, co-trimoxazole, chloramphenicol, or azithromycin depending on the susceptibility of the causative organism. If invasive disease is suspected or confirmed, IDSA recommends ceftriaxone over ciprofloxacin because of the increasing incidence of resistance to fluoroquinolones.

Because HIV-infected individuals with *Salmonella* gastroenteritis are at high risk for bacteremia, CDC, National Institutes of Health (NIH), and the

HIV Medicine Association of IDSA recommend that such patients receive anti-infective treatment. These experts state that the initial drug of choice for the treatment of salmonella gastroenteritis (with or without bacteremia) in HIV-infected adults is ciprofloxacin; other fluoroquinolones (levofloxacin, moxifloxacin) also are likely to be effective in these patients, but clinical data are limited. Depending on results of in vitro susceptibility testing of the causative organism, alternatives for treatment of *Salmonella* gastroenteritis in HIV-infected adults are co-trimoxazole or third generation cephalosporins (ceftriaxone, cefotaxime).

The role of long-term treatment (secondary prophylaxis) against *Salmonella* in HIV-infected individuals is not well established, and possible benefits of such prophylaxis should be weighed against the risks of long-term anti-infective exposure. CDC, NIH, and IDSA state that secondary prophylaxis should be considered in those with recurrent bacteremia and may also be considered in those with recurrent gastroenteritis (with or without bacteremia) and in those with $CD4^+$ T-cell counts less than 200 cells/mm^3 and severe diarrhea. These experts state that secondary prophylaxis should be discontinued if the *Salmonella* infection resolves and there has been a sustained response to antiretroviral therapy with $CD4^+$ T-cell counts greater than 200 cells/mm^3.

For information on the treatment of typhoid and paratyphoid fever (enteric fever) or bacteremia caused by *Salmonella*, see Uses: Typhoid Fever and Other Invasive Salmonella Infections.

Shigella Infections Ciprofloxacin is used for the treatment of shigellosis caused by susceptible *Shigella*.

Infections caused by *S. sonnei* usually are self-limited (48–72 hours), and mild cases may not require treatment with anti-infectives. However, because there is some evidence that anti-infectives may shorten the duration of diarrhea and the period of fecal excretion of *Shigella*, anti-infective treatment generally is recommended in addition to fluid and electrolyte replacement in patients with severe shigellosis, dysentery, or underlying immunosuppression. An empiric treatment regimen can be used initially, but in vitro susceptibility testing of clinical isolates is indicated since resistance is common. A fluoroquinolone (preferably ciprofloxacin or, alternatively, levofloxacin or moxifloxacin) generally has been recommended for the treatment of shigellosis. However, fluoroquinolone-resistant *Shigella* have been reported in the US, especially in international travelers, the homeless, and men who have sex with men (MSM). Depending on in vitro susceptibility, other drugs recommended for the treatment of shigellosis include co-trimoxazole, ceftriaxone, azithromycin (not recommended in those with bacteremia), or ampicillin.

Yersinia Infections Although GI infections caused by *Y. enterocolitica* or *Y. pseudotuberculosis* usually are self-limited and anti-infective therapy is unnecessary, some experts recommend use of anti-infectives in immunocompromised individuals or for the treatment of severe infections or when septicemia or other invasive disease occurs. GI infections caused by *Y. enterocolitica* or *Y. pseudotuberculosis* can occur as the result of ingesting undercooked pork, unpasteurized milk, or contaminated water; infection has occurred in infants whose caregivers handled contaminated chitterlings (raw pork intestines) or tofu. When treatment is considered necessary, some clinicians recommend co-trimoxazole as the drug of choice and cefotaxime and ciprofloxacin as alternatives.

Travelers' Diarrhea Ciprofloxacin is used for the short-term treatment of travelers' diarrhea† and has been used for the prevention of travelers' diarrhea† in adults traveling for relatively short periods of time to high-risk areas.

The most common cause of travelers' diarrhea worldwide is noninvasive enterotoxigenic strains of *E. coli* (ETEC), but travelers' diarrhea also can be caused by various other bacteria including enteroaggregative and other *E. coli* pathotypes, *C. jejuni*, *Shigella*, *Salmonella*, *Aeromonas*, *Plesiomonas*, *Y. enterocolitica*, or *V. parahaemolyticus* or non-O-group 1 *V. cholerae*, and, possibly, *Acrobacter*, *Larobacter*, and enterotoxigenic *Bacteroides fragilis*. In some cases, travelers' diarrhea is caused by parasitic enteric pathogens (e.g., *Giardia*, *Cryptosporidium*, *Entamoeba histolytica*) or viral enteric pathogens (e.g., rotavirus, norovirus, astrovirus).

Countries where travelers are at low risk of travelers' diarrhea include the US, Canada, Australia, New Zealand, Japan, and countries in Northern and Western Europe. Travelers are at intermediate risk for travelers' diarrhea in Eastern Europe, South Africa, and some of the Caribbean islands, but are at high risk in most of Asia, the Middle East, Africa, Mexico, and Central and South America.

Treatment. Travelers' diarrhea caused by bacteria may be self-limited and often resolves within 3–7 days without anti-infective treatment. CDC states that anti-infective treatment is *not* recommended in patients with mild travelers' diarrhea. However, CDC and other clinicians state that empiric short-term anti-infective treatment (single dose or up to 3 days) may be used if diarrhea is moderate or severe, associated with high fever or bloody stools, or extremely disruptive to travel plans. Since bacteria are the most common cause of travelers' diarrhea (80–90% of cases), an anti-infective directed against enteric bacterial pathogens usually is used. Fluoroquinolones (e.g., ciprofloxacin, levofloxacin) generally have been considered the anti-infectives of choice for empiric treatment, including self-treatment, of travelers' diarrhea in adults; alternatives include azithromycin and rifaximin.

If the causative pathogen is susceptible to the anti-infective chosen for empiric treatment, the duration of illness may be reduced by about a day. However, the increasing incidence of enteric bacteria resistant to fluoroquinolones and other anti-infectives may limit the usefulness of empiric treatment in individuals traveling in certain geographic areas, and the possible adverse effects of the anti-infective and adverse consequences of such treatment (e.g., development of resistance, effect on normal gut microflora) should be considered.

Prophylaxis. CDC and most experts do *not* recommend anti-infective prophylaxis to prevent travelers' diarrhea in most individuals traveling to areas of risk. However, anti-infective prophylaxis may be considered for short-term travelers who are high-risk individuals (e.g., HIV-infected or other immunocompromised individuals, travelers with poorly controlled diabetes mellitus or chronic renal failure) and those who are taking critical trips during which even a short period of diarrhea could adversely affect the purpose of the trip.

The risks of use of anti-infective prophylaxis in travelers should be weighed against the use of prompt, early self-treatment with an empiric anti-infective if moderate to severe travelers' diarrhea occurs. If anti-infective prophylaxis is used, fluoroquinolones (e.g., ciprofloxacin, levofloxacin) usually have been recommended; alternatives include azithromycin and rifaximin. The increasing incidence of fluoroquinolone resistance in pathogens that cause travelers' diarrhea (e.g., *Campylobacter*, *Salmonella*, *Shigella*) should be considered and may limit their potential usefulness.

■ **Intra-abdominal Infections** Ciprofloxacin (IV, conventional tablets, oral suspension) is used in conjunction with metronidazole for the treatment of complicated intra-abdominal infections caused by *E. coli*, *Ps. aeruginosa*, *P. mirabilis*, *K. pneumoniae*, or *Bacteroides fragilis*.

For additional information on management of intra-abdominal infections, the current clinical practice guidelines from IDSA available at http://www.idsociety.org should be consulted.

■ **Meningitis and Other CNS Infections** IV ciprofloxacin has been used for the treatment of meningitis† caused by gram-negative bacteria.

Ciprofloxacin has been effective when used alone or in conjunction with other drugs (e.g., antipseudomonal aminoglycosides) to treat meningitis and other CNS infections† caused by susceptible *Ps. aeruginosa*. Some clinicians suggest that a regimen of ciprofloxacin (with or without an aminoglycoside) can be used as an alternative for the treatment of *Ps. aeruginosa* meningitis when cefepime or ceftazidime cannot be used.

Ciprofloxacin has been recommended as a preferred alternative for the treatment of healthcare-associated ventriculitis and meningitis† caused by Enterobacteriaceae or *Ps. aeruginosa* when the drugs of choice cannot be used.

Ciprofloxacin also has been used for the treatment of meningitis and other CNS infections† caused by susceptible *Salmonella*. Some clinicians suggest that ciprofloxacin alone or in conjunction with a third generation cephalosporin (cefotaxime, ceftriaxone) may be a drug of choice for the treatment of *Salmonella* meningitis in pediatric patients†, especially when the causative organism is resistant to other drugs.

Because only low concentrations of ciprofloxacin are distributed into CSF and because efficacy and safety of the drug for the treatment of CNS infections have not been established, fluoroquinolones (including ciprofloxacin) should be considered for the treatment of meningitis *only* when the infection is caused by multidrug-resistant gram-negative bacilli or when the usually recommended anti-infectives cannot be used or have been ineffective.

For additional information on management of meningitis and other CNS infections, the current clinical practice guidelines from IDSA available at http://www.idsociety.org should be consulted.

■ **Ophthalmic and Otic Infections** Oral or IV ciprofloxacin is used in the treatment of malignant otitis externa† caused by *Ps. aeruginosa*. Bacterial otitis externa usually is caused by *Ps. aeruginosa* or *S. aureus*. Although acute bacterial otitis externa localized in the external auditory canal may be effectively treated using topical anti-infectives (e.g., ciprofloxacin otic suspension, ofloxacin otic solution), malignant otitis externa is an invasive, potentially life-threatening infection, especially in immunocompromised patients such as those with diabetes mellitus or HIV infection, and requires prompt diagnosis and long-term treatment with systemic anti-infectives. The treatment of choice for malignant otitis externa usually is ciprofloxacin or an antipseudomonal β-lactam (e.g., ceftazidime, imipenem). Because ciprofloxacin-resistant *Ps. aeruginosa* have been reported with increasing frequency in patients with malignant otitis externa and has been associated with treatment failure, clinical isolates should be tested for in vitro susceptibility, especially if there is an inadequate response to treatment.

For use of ciprofloxacin hydrochloride in the topical treatment of ophthalmic and otic infections caused by susceptible bacteria, see Ciprofloxacin 52:04.12.

■ **Respiratory Tract Infections** Ciprofloxacin (IV, conventional tablets, oral suspension) is used in adults for the treatment of respiratory tract infections, including acute sinusitis, acute exacerbations of chronic bronchitis), bronchiectasis, lung abscess, and pneumonia, caused by susceptible *E. aerogenes*†, *E. cloacae*, *E. coli*, *Haemophilus influenzae*, *H. parainfluenzae*, *K. oxytoca*†, *K. pneumoniae*, *P. mirabilis*, *Ps. aeruginosa*, *S. aureus*†, or *S. pneumoniae* (penicillin-susceptible strains). The drug also is used for the treatment of respiratory tract infections caused by susceptible *Moraxella catarrhalis*.

IV ciprofloxacin is used for the treatment of nosocomial pneumonia caused by susceptible *H. influenzae* or *K. pneumoniae* and for the treatment of acute bacterial sinusitis caused by *H. influenzae*, *S. pneumoniae* (penicillin-susceptible strains), or *M. catarrhalis*.

Ciprofloxacin should be used for the treatment of acute bacterial sinusitis or acute bacterial exacerbations of chronic bronchitis only when there are no other treatment options. Because systemic fluoroquinolones, including ciprofloxacin, have been associated with disabling and potentially irreversible serious adverse reactions (e.g., tendinitis and tendon rupture, peripheral neuropathy, CNS effects) that can occur together in the same patient (see Cautions) *and because acute bacterial sinusitis and acute bacterial exacerbations of chronic bronchitis may be self-limiting in some patients, the risks of serious adverse reactions outweigh the benefits of fluoroquinolones for patients with these infections.*

In controlled studies in adults with respiratory tract infections, oral ciprofloxacin therapy was as effective as therapy with oral amoxicillin, oral ampicillin, IV cefamandole, oral doxycycline, or IV imipenem and cilastatin sodium. Oral ciprofloxacin therapy generally resulted in a bacteriologic cure rate of 80–98% in adults with respiratory tract infections. Oral ciprofloxacin has been most effective in the treatment of respiratory tract infections caused by *H. influenzae* or *M. catarrhalis*; treatment failures have occurred when the drug was used in the treatment of infections caused by *S. pneumoniae* or *Ps. aeruginosa*. Treatment failure of *S. pneumoniae* respiratory tract infections may be related to the moderate in vitro susceptibility of this organism to ciprofloxacin. Although ciprofloxacin may be effective, it is not a drug of first choice for the treatment of presumed or confirmed pneumonia secondary to *S. pneumoniae*, and some clinicians suggest that ciprofloxacin generally *not* be used for empiric treatment of community-acquired pneumonia when *S. pneumoniae* is likely or suspected as the causative organism. A β-lactam antibiotic generally is preferred for empiric treatment of these infections and also is preferred in other respiratory tract infections known or suspected to be caused by pneumococci or streptococci. Ciprofloxacin probably should not be used in the treatment of aspiration pneumonia because these infections generally involve anaerobic bacteria.

Acute Exacerbations of Chronic Bronchitis Clinical improvement has occurred when oral ciprofloxacin was used alone for the treatment of acute exacerbations of bronchopulmonary *Ps. aeruginosa* infections in adults with cystic fibrosis. As with other anti-infectives, *Ps. aeruginosa* may be cleared temporarily from the sputum, but a bacteriologic cure rarely is obtained and should not be expected in these patients.

Resistant strains of *Ps. aeruginosa* have developed during ciprofloxacin therapy; in one study, up to 45% of cystic fibrosis patients developed resistance after 2 weeks of therapy with the drug. Clinical improvement occurred in some patients despite the emergence of resistant *Ps. aeruginosa*; in some cases, the resistant organisms reverted to being susceptible after ciprofloxacin therapy was discontinued. Further study is necessary to determine if emergence of resistance will limit use of ciprofloxacin in the treatment of *Ps. aeruginosa* infections in cystic fibrosis patients. Some clinicians caution against long-term use of ciprofloxacin in these patients and recommend that the drug be used in short courses (e.g., 14 days), alternated with other anti-infectives active against *Ps. aeruginosa* (e.g., aztreonam, extended-spectrum penicillins, third generation cephalosporins) and/or used in conjunction with one of these agents. If ciprofloxacin is used, it is important that susceptibility of isolates be tested carefully in subsequent exacerbations.

Nosocomial Pneumonia IV ciprofloxacin is used for the treatment of nosocomial pneumonia, including hospital-acquired pneumonia (HAP) not associated with mechanical ventilation and ventilator-associated pneumonia (VAP).

Local susceptibility data should be used when selecting initial empiric regimens for the treatment of nosocomial pneumonia, including HAP and VAP.

For initial empiric treatment of HAP in adults, IDSA states that ciprofloxacin should be used in conjunction with an anti-infective active against MRSA (vancomycin, linezolid) if factors that increase the likelihood of MRSA are present or if the patient is at high risk of mortality or has received IV anti-infectives during the prior 90 days.

For initial empiric treatment in adults with clinically suspected VAP and factors that increase the risk of MRSA or multidrug-resistant gram-negative bacteria, IDSA states that ciprofloxacin should be used in conjunction with an anti-infective active against MRSA (vancomycin, linezolid) plus an antipseudomonal β-lactam (fixed combination of piperacillin and tazobactam [piperacillin/tazobactam], cefepime, ceftazidime, imipenem, meropenem, aztreonam).

For additional information on management of nosocomial pneumonia, the current clinical practice guidelines from IDSA available at http://www.idsociety.org should be consulted.

■ **Skin and Skin Structure Infections** Ciprofloxacin (IV, conventional tablets, oral suspension) is used in adults for the treatment of skin and skin structure infections caused by susceptible *C. freundii, E. cloacae, E. coli, K. oxytoca*†, *K. pneumoniae, M. morganii, P. mirabilis, P. vulgaris, P. stuartii, Ps. aeruginosa, Serratia marcescens*†, *S. aureus* (methicillin-susceptible strains), *S. epidermidis* (methicillin-susceptible strains), or *S. pyogenes* (group A β-hemolytic streptococci). The drug has been effective in the treatment of cellulitis, abscesses, folliculitis, furunculosis, pyoderma, postoperative wound infections, and infected ulcers, burns, or wounds.

Ciprofloxacin may be particularly useful as an oral agent for the treatment of skin and skin structure infections caused by susceptible gram-negative bacteria. Because staphylococci, streptococci, and anaerobes are only moderately susceptible to ciprofloxacin, ciprofloxacin generally should not be used alone and other anti-infectives remain the drugs of choice for skin and skin structure infections caused by these bacteria. Treatment failures have been reported in patients with skin or skin structure infections caused by *S. aureus* and the increasing emergence of strains of staphylococci resistant to quinolones limits the usefulness of the drugs in the treatment of these infections. Some clinicians suggest that ciprofloxacin therapy may be particularly useful for the treatment of hospital-acquired decubitus ulcers when anti-infective therapy is indicated.

In several controlled studies, oral ciprofloxacin was at least as effective as IV cefotaxime in the treatment of skin and skin structure infections caused by susceptible organisms. Oral ciprofloxacin resulted in a bacteriologic cure rate of 80–92% in patients with skin and skin structure infections.

Although ciprofloxacin is active in vitro against most common aerobic pathogens isolated from animal and human bite wounds, including *Flavobacterium*† and *Eikenella corrodens*†, the in vitro activity of the drug against streptococci, which frequently are isolated from such wounds (usually in mixed cultures), and against anaerobes generally is poor. Therefore, use of the drug as monotherapy in these infections is not recommended pending accumulation of additional efficacy data.

For additional information on management of skin and skin structure infections, the current clinical practice guidelines from IDSA available at http://www.idsociety.org should be consulted.

■ **Urinary Tract Infections and Prostatitis** ***Uncomplicated and Complicated Urinary Tract Infections*** Ciprofloxacin extended-release tablets containing both the hydrochloride and the base are used *only* for the treatment of uncomplicated UTIs (acute cystitis) caused by susceptible *E. faecalis, E. coli, P. mirabilis*, or *S. saprophyticus*, complicated UTIs caused by susceptible *E. coli, K. pneumoniae, P. mirabilis, Ps. aeruginosa*, or *E. faecalis*, or acute uncomplicated pyelonephritis caused by *E. coli* in adults.

Ciprofloxacin (IV, conventional tablets, oral suspension) is used in adults for the treatment of complicated or uncomplicated UTIs caused by susceptible *Citrobacter koseri* (formerly *C. diversus*), *C. freundii, Enterobacter cloacae, E. aerogenes*†, *E. coli, Klebsiella oxytoca*†, *K. pneumoniae, Morganella morganii, Proteus mirabilis, Providencia rettgeri, P. stuartii*†, *Pseudomonas aeruginosa*, or *Serratia marcescens*. The drug also is used in adults for the treatment of UTIs caused by susceptible gram-positive bacteria, including *Staphylococcus aureus*†, *S. epidermidis* (methicillin-susceptible strains), *S. saprophyticus*, or *E. faecalis*.

Ciprofloxacin (IV, conventional tablets, oral suspension) is used in pediatric patients 1 year of age or older for the treatment of complicated UTIs and pyelonephritis caused by susceptible *E. coli*. Although effective in UTIs, ciprofloxacin is not a drug of first choice for these infections in pediatric patients because of the risk of adverse effects (e.g., musculoskeletal effects) reported in this patient population. (See Cautions: Pediatric Precautions.)

Ciprofloxacin should be used for the treatment of uncomplicated UTIs only when there are no other treatment options. Because systemic fluoroquinolones, including ciprofloxacin, have been associated with disabling and potentially irreversible serious adverse reactions (e.g., tendinitis and tendon rupture, peripheral neuropathy, CNS effects) that can occur together in the same patient (see Cautions) *and because uncomplicated UTIs may be self-limiting in some patients, the risk of serious adverse reactions outweigh the benefits of fluoroquinolones for patients with uncomplicated UTIs.*

Some clinicians suggest that ciprofloxacin be reserved for the treatment of complicated UTIs, especially those caused by multidrug-resistant bacteria. IDSA and other experts state that fluoroquinolones (ciprofloxacin, levofloxacin, ofloxacin) generally should be considered alternatives for the treatment of uncomplicated UTIs (e.g., acute cystitis) and should be used in these infections only when other urinary anti-infectives are likely to be ineffective or are contraindicated or not tolerated.

Clinical Experience. In controlled studies in men and women, oral ciprofloxacin therapy was as effective as therapy with oral co-trimoxazole in the treatment of uncomplicated UTIs; bacteriologic cure rates and rate of relapse and/or reinfection were similar with both drugs. Oral ciprofloxacin therapy generally results in a bacteriologic cure in 80–100% of patients with UTIs. Oral ciprofloxacin is more effective in the treatment of uncomplicated UTIs than in complicated infections, and most treatment failures occur in patients with underlying structural abnormalities of the urinary tract (e.g., obstructions, neurogenic bladder) or indwelling catheters.

Oral ciprofloxacin has been as effective as oral co-trimoxazole in the treatment of complicated UTIs, and has been effective in the treatment of UTIs caused by organisms resistant to co-trimoxazole. Prolonged, high-dose oral ciprofloxacin therapy (500–750 mg every 12 hours) has been effective in the treatment of complicated UTIs caused by multidrug-resistant *Ps. aeruginosa*.

A 3-day regimen of oral ciprofloxacin (conventional tablets) generally is effective for the treatment of acute, uncomplicated cystitis caused by susceptible *E. coli, E. faecalis, P. mirabilis*, or *S. saprophyticus* (bacteriologic eradication rate 81–100%). Oral ciprofloxacin (conventional tablets) has been effective in women for the treatment of uncomplicated UTIs when given as a single 100- or 250-mg dose†. However, efficacy of a single dose of the drug for the treatment of these infections has not been clearly established; single-dose therapy was less effective in the treatment of UTIs caused by gram-positive bacteria than in those caused by gram-negative bacteria.

Safety and efficacy of ciprofloxacin extended-release tablets for the treatment of uncomplicated UTIs (acute cystitis) have been evaluated in a randomized, double-blind, controlled study in adults. In this study, adults were randomized to receive ciprofloxacin extended-release tablets (500 mg once daily for 3 days) or conventional ciprofloxacin tablets (250 mg twice daily for 3 days). The bacteriologic eradication rate with no new infections or superinfections at the time of test of cure (post-therapy day 4–11) was 94.5% in those who received the extended-release tablets and 93.7% in those who received conventional tablets. Safety and efficacy of ciprofloxacin extended-release tablets for the treatment of complicated UTIs or acute uncomplicated pyelonephritis also have been evaluated in a randomized, double-blind study. In this study, adults were randomized to receive ciprofloxacin extended-release tablets (1 g once daily for 7–14 days) or conventional ciprofloxacin tablets (500 mg twice daily for 7–14 days). In the per-protocol population, the bacteriologic eradication rate with no new infections or superinfections at the time of test of cure (post-therapy day 5–11) in those who received the extended-release tablets was 89.2 or 87.5% in those with complicated UTIs or uncomplicated pyelonephritis, respectively; in those who received the conventional tablets, the rates were 81.4 or 98.1%, respectively.

In clinical studies evaluating IV or oral ciprofloxacin for the treatment of complicated UTIs and pyelonephritis in pediatric patients 1–17 years of age, the bacteriologic eradication rate was about 84% in those receiving ciprofloxacin compared with about 78% in those receiving a cephalosporin.

Prostatitis Ciprofloxacin (IV, conventional tablets, oral suspension) is used in men for the treatment of recurrent UTIs and chronic prostatitis caused by *E. coli* or *P. mirabilis*. Ciprofloxacin has been most effective in the treatment of prostatitis caused by *E. coli* or other Enterobacteriaceae, and has been effective in infections that did not respond to co-trimoxazole therapy. Prostatitis caused by *Ps. aeruginosa*, enterococci, or staphylococci may respond poorly to the drug. Because high concentrations of ciprofloxacin are attained in prostatic tissues, the drug may become a drug of choice for the treatment of recurrent UTIs associated with prostatitis; however, further study is needed to compare efficacy of ciprofloxacin with that of other anti-infectives used in the treatment of these infections.

■ **Anthrax** Ciprofloxacin (conventional tablets, oral suspension) is used for inhalational anthrax (postexposure) to reduce the incidence or progression of disease following suspected or confirmed exposure to aerosolized *Bacillus anthracis* spores in adults and pediatric patients. Ciprofloxacin (IV, conventional tablets, oral suspension) is used for the treatment of clinically apparent inhalational anthrax†, other systemic anthrax infections (GI, meningitis, or cutaneous with systemic involvement, head or neck lesions, or extensive edema), or uncomplicated cutaneous anthrax†, and for prophylaxis following ingestion of *B. anthracis* spores in contaminated meat†.

Naturally occurring or endemic cutaneous anthrax in humans can occur after exposure to *B. anthracis* spores following contact with contaminated soil or infected animals (e.g., goats, sheep, cattle, swine, horses, buffalo, deer) or animal by-products (e.g., hides, hair, wool, carcasses, bone meal); GI or oropharyngeal anthrax can occur after ingestion of anthrax spores (e.g., in contaminated, raw or undercooked meat); and inhalational anthrax can occur after exposure to *B. anthracis* spores aerosolized during industrial processing of contaminated animal by-products or in the laboratory. Inhalational or cutaneous anthrax also may occur as the result of exposure to aerosolized *B. anthracis* spores in the context of biologic warfare or bioterrorism, including exposure to mail or other fomites contaminated with anthrax spores.

Following exposure to aerosolized *B. anthracis* spores, inhalational anthrax may develop if spore-containing particles are deposited into alveolar spaces. Macrophages ingest the spores and some undergo lysis and destruction. Surviving spores are transported via the lymph system to mediastinal lymph nodes where germination and vegetative growth may occur after a period of spore dormancy. Monkey studies have demonstrated that viable spores can persist in a dormant state in alveolar surface epithelium and mediastinal lymph nodes for up to 100 days after inhalation. The process responsible for the delayed transformation of spores to vegetative cells remains to be elucidated. Once germination occurs, disease follows rapidly. Replicating *B. anthracis* release toxins that can result in hemorrhage, edema, and necrosis. Cutaneous anthrax may occur if *B. anthracis* spores are introduced into a cut or abrasion (e.g., on the face, neck, or arms). Septicemia and meningeal anthrax result from hematogenous spread of the organism from the primary cutaneous, GI, or inhalation site. Although discharge from cutaneous lesions might be infectious, the risk for person-to-person transmission of cutaneous anthrax is low. Person-to-person transmission and secondary cases of anthrax (e.g., in medical personnel) have not been documented to date.

For the treatment of clinically apparent inhalational, GI, or meningeal anthrax and anthrax septicemia that occurs as the result of natural or endemic exposures to *B. anthracis*, parenteral penicillin historically has been considered the drug of choice and IV ciprofloxacin or IV doxycycline have been suggested as alternatives. However, it has been postulated that exposures to *B. anthracis* that occur in the context of biologic warfare or bioterrorism may involve bioengineered resistant strains and this concern should be considered when selecting initial anti-infective regimens for the treatment of anthrax that occurs as the result of bioterrorism-related exposures or when selecting anti-infectives for postexposure prophylaxis following such exposures. *B. anthracis* with natural resistance to penicillins have been reported and there are published reports of *B. anthracis* strains that have been engineered to have tetracycline and penicillin resistance as well as resistance to other anti-infectives (e.g., macrolides, chloramphenicol, rifampin). In addition, reduced susceptibility to ofloxacin (4-fold increase in MICs from baseline) has been produced in vitro following sequential subculture of the Sterne strain of *B. anthracis* in subinhibitory concentrations of the fluoroquinolone.

Recommendations for the treatment and prophylaxis of anthrax have evolved based on experience gained in treating US patients who developed inhalational or cutaneous anthrax during September and October 2001 following bioterrorism-related exposures to *B. anthracis* spores as well results of animal studies and concerns related to treating large numbers of individuals in a mass casualty setting.

For additional information on management of anthrax, including postexposure prophylaxis of anthrax, the current guidelines from CDC and AAP should be consulted.

Postexposure Prophylaxis of Anthrax Ciprofloxacin is used for inhalational anthrax (postexposure) to reduce the incidence or progression of disease following suspected or confirmed exposure to aerosolized *B. anthracis* spores in adults and pediatric patients. CDC, AAP, US Working Group on Civilian Biodefense, and US Army Medical Research Institute of Infectious Diseases (USAMRIID) recommend oral ciprofloxacin and oral doxycycline as the initial drugs of choice for postexposure prophylaxis following exposure to aerosolized anthrax spores, including exposures that occur in the context of biologic warfare or bioterrorism. Other oral fluoroquinolones (levofloxacin, moxifloxacin, ofloxacin) are alternatives for postexposure prophylaxis when ciprofloxacin or doxycycline cannot be used.

Following natural, occupational, or bioterrorism-related exposures to aerosolized *B. anthracis* spores, anti-infective postexposure prophylaxis should be initiated immediately or as soon as possible. Postexposure vaccination with anthrax vaccine (if available) may be indicated in conjunction with anti-infective postexposure prophylaxis in some individuals. Vaccine-induced immunity provides protection if there are issues related to the anti-infective postexposure prophylaxis regimen (e.g., poor adherence, early discontinuance because of adverse effects) or if there are residual spores that germinate after the anti-infective regimen has been completed.

Because of the possible persistence of anthrax spores in lung tissue following an aerosol exposure, prolonged postexposure prophylaxis usually is required. Based on a competing-risks model, some clinicians suggest that the optimum duration of prophylaxis depends on the dose of inhaled spores. These clinicians state that a duration of 60 days may be adequate for a low-dose exposure, but that a duration exceeding 4 months may be necessary to reduce the risk following a high-dose exposure. CDC, AAP, US Working Group on Civilian Biodefense, and USAMRIID recommend that postexposure prophylaxis following a confirmed exposure (including in laboratory workers with confirmed exposures to *B. anthracis* cultures) should be continued for 60 days.

Postexposure anti-infective prophylaxis may be indicated in laboratory workers and other individuals who work in occupations that result in exposure to *B. anthracis* and may also be considered following a naturally occurring GI exposure to *B. anthracis* (e.g., ingestion of meat from an undercooked carcass of an anthrax-infected animal).

Pediatric Patients. Ciprofloxacin (IV, conventional tablets, oral suspension) is labeled by FDA for inhalational anthrax (postexposure) in neonates, infants, and children 17 years of age or younger. Although ciprofloxacin generally is not recommended for use in infants and children (see Cautions: Pediatric Precautions), the benefits of ciprofloxacin in reducing the incidence or progression of disease following exposure to aerosolized *B. anthracis* spores outweigh the risks in pediatric patients.

For initial anti-infective prophylaxis following a suspected exposure to *B. anthracis* spores that occurs in the context of biologic warfare or bioterrorism, AAP states that oral ciprofloxacin is the drug of choice in neonates 4 weeks of age or younger and oral ciprofloxacin or oral doxycycline are the drugs of choice in pediatric patients 1 month of age or older (prior to susceptibility testing and when penicillin-resistant strains have been identified). If exposure has been confirmed and in vitro tests indicate that the organism is susceptible to penicillin, the postexposure prophylaxis regimen in pediatric patients may be switched to oral amoxicillin or, alternatively, oral penicillin V.

Pregnant and Breast-feeding Women. If anti-infective postexposure prophylaxis following a suspected exposure to aerosolized *B. anthracis* spores in the context of biologic warfare or bioterrorism is indicated in pregnant women, postpartum women, and women who are breast-feeding, CDC states that oral ciprofloxacin is preferred over oral doxycycline, unless oral ciprofloxacin is unavailable. If in vitro studies indicate that the organism is susceptible to penicillin, consideration can be given to changing the postexposure regimen to oral amoxicillin or oral penicillin V.

Individuals at Contaminated Sites. For the bioterrorism-related exposures to *B. anthracis* spores that occurred in the US during the fall of 2001, CDC recommended that anti-infective prophylaxis be initiated (pending additional information) in individuals exposed to an air space where a suspicious material may have been aerosolized (e.g., near a suspicious powder-containing letter during opening) and in individuals who shared the air spaces likely to be the source of an inhalational anthrax case. While culture of nasal swabs can occasionally document exposure and provide clues to help assess the exposure circumstances, these nasal swabs are investigative tools only and results cannot be used to rule out exposure to *B. anthracis*. Following confirmation of the presence of *B. anthracis* spores, CDC recommended that a full 60-day postexposure regimen be completed in individuals exposed to an air space known to be contaminated with aerosolized *B. anthracis*, in individuals exposed to an air space known to be the source of an inhalational anthrax case, and in individuals along the transit path of an envelope or other vehicle containing *B. anthracis* that may have been aerosolized (e.g., a postal sorting facility in which an envelope containing *B. anthracis* was processed).

Remediation workers with repeated entries into contaminated sites over a prolonged period of time may require anti-infective prophylaxis for considerably longer than the 60 days recommended for individuals with a single exposure. Some remediation workers exposed during the bioterrorism-related events that occurred in the US during the fall of 2001 received anti-infective prophylaxis for more than 6 months. At that time, CDC recommended that anti-infective prophylaxis be continued throughout the period of risk and for 60 days after the risk of exposure ended, unless a 6-dose series of anthrax vaccine had been completed and annual boosters were up to date.

Laboratory Workers and Other Individuals. Laboratory workers and other individuals who work in occupations that might result in repeated exposure to aerosolized *B. anthracis* spores should receive preexposure vaccination with anthrax vaccine adsorbed. ACIP states that anti-infective postexposure prophylaxis is not necessary in fully vaccinated workers who wear appropriate personal protective equipment (PPE) while working in environments contaminated with *B. anthracis* spores, unless PPE is disrupted. If there is any type of disruption of PPE in a worker who is fully or partially vaccinated against anthrax, ACIP recommends that anti-infective postexposure prophylaxis be given for at least 30 days in conjunction with any remaining indicated doses of anthrax vaccine. Following an occupational exposure to *B. anthracis* spores in previously unvaccinated workers, ACIP recommends that anti-infective postexposure prophylaxis be given for 60 days in conjunction with postexposure vaccination and states that the anti-infective prophylaxis regimen should be continued for 14 days after the third vaccine dose (even if this results in more than 60 days of anti-infective prophylaxis).

Following a bioterrorism-related event, use of anti-infective prophylaxis in asymptomatic individuals in the general population is *not* indicated unless appropriate public health or law-enforcement agencies have ascertained that a risk of exposure to *B. anthracis* spores exists. In addition, CDC states that postexposure prophylaxis is *not* indicated for the prevention of cutaneous anthrax, for autopsy personnel examining bodies infected with anthrax when appropriate isolation precautions and procedures are followed, for hospital personnel caring for patients with anthrax, or for individuals who routinely open or handle mail in the absence of a suspicious letter or credible threat.

Clinical Experience. Although controlled studies evaluating ciprofloxacin for aerosolized anthrax exposure in humans have not been conducted for ethical reasons, the indication for use of ciprofloxacin is based on serum concentrations of the drug achieved in humans, a surrogate end point reasonably likely to predict clinical benefit. Efficacy of ciprofloxacin has been evaluated in a rhesus monkey model of inhalational anthrax. In this study, rhesus monkeys were exposed to an inhaled mean dose of 11 LD_{50} (approximately 5.5 x 10^5) spores (range: 5–30 LD_{50}) of *B. anthracis* and then received a 30-day regimen of placebo or oral ciprofloxacin beginning 24 hours after exposure. Mortality due to anthrax was significantly lower in monkeys that received ciprofloxacin (1/9) compared with those that received placebo (9/10); the one ciprofloxacin-treated monkey that died of anthrax did so following the 30-day drug administration period. In the monkeys studied, mean serum concentrations of ciprofloxacin 1 hour after dosing (at the expected time of peak serum concentrations) following oral dosing to steady state ranged from 0.98–1.69 mcg/mL; mean steady-state trough concentrations at 12 hours after dosing ranged from 0.12–0.19 mcg/mL. The mean serum concentrations of ciprofloxacin associated with a statistically significant improvement in survival in this rhesus monkey model of inhalational anthrax are reached or exceeded in adult and pediatric patients receiving oral or IV ciprofloxacin.

Some data regarding efficacy of ciprofloxacin for postexposure prophylaxis in humans following exposure to aerosolized *B. anthracis* spores is available since the drug was used for postexposure prophylaxis in individuals in the US who were exposed to *B. anthracis* spores in bioterrorism-related incidences that occurred during September and October 2001. Approximately 300 postal or other facilities were tested for *B. anthracis* spores and anti-infective prophylaxis with ciprofloxacin or other anti-infectives was initiated in approximately 32,000 individuals in Florida, New Jersey, New York, and the District of Columbia who had potential exposures. A full 60-day postexposure prophylaxis regimen was recommended for approximately 8424 of these individuals. To date, no individual who received anti-infective prophylaxis following these bioterrorism-related exposures developed microbiologically confirmed anthrax. Although ciprofloxacin postexposure prophylaxis generally was well tolerated, the incidence of adverse effects was higher than that reported previously in controlled clinical trials evaluating the drug for other indications. (See Cautions.)

Treatment of Systemic Anthrax The rapid course of symptomatic inhalational anthrax and high mortality rate make early initiation of anti-infective therapy essential. Because of the difficulty in making a rapid microbiologic diagnosis of anthrax, high-risk individuals who develop fever or other evidence of systemic infection should promptly receive therapy for possible anthrax infection while waiting for results of laboratory studies.

Based on clinical experience from the bioterrorism-related anthrax exposures of 2001 and the possibility that a *B. anthracis* strain resistant to one or more anti-infectives might be used in a future bioterrorism event, CDC, AAP, and other experts (e.g., US Working Group on Civilian Biodefense, USAMRIID) state that treatment of clinically apparent systemic anthrax (inhalational, GI, meningitis, or cutaneous with systemic involvement, head or neck lesions, or extensive edema) in adults and pediatric patients that occurs as the result of exposure to anthrax spores in the context of biologic warfare or bioterrorism should be initiated with a multiple-drug parenteral regimen that includes ciprofloxacin or doxycycline and 1 or 2 additional anti-infectives predicted to be effective. Other drugs to be included in the initial treatment regimen with ciprofloxacin or doxycycline should be selected based on in vitro susceptibility, possibility of efficacy, adverse effects, and cost. Based on in vitro data, other drugs that have been suggested as possibilities to augment ciprofloxacin or doxycycline in such multiple-drug regimens include carbapenems (doripenem, imipenem, meropenem), penicillin G, ampicillin, linezolid, clindamycin, rifampin, chloramphenicol, vancomycin, macrolides (azithromycin, clarithromycin, erythromycin), daptomycin, quinupristin and dalfopristin, and aminoglycosides (gentamicin).

For initial empiric treatment of systemic anthrax (with possible or confirmed meningitis), CDC and AAP recommend use of a multiple-drug parenteral regimen that includes at least 3 anti-infectives with activity against *B. anthracis* and good CNS penetration, including at least one drug that has bactericidal activity against the organism and at least one drug classified as a protein synthesis inhibitor. These experts state that IV ciprofloxacin is recommended as the primary bactericidal component of these regimens. The preferred multiple-drug regimen for the treatment of systemic anthrax (with possible or confirmed meningitis) in adults and pediatric patients (including neonates) is IV ciprofloxacin in conjunction with another IV bactericidal anti-infective (preferably meropenem) and an IV protein synthesis inhibitor (preferably linezolid).

For initial empiric treatment of systemic anthrax when meningitis has been excluded, CDC and AAP recommend use of a multiple-drug parenteral regimen that includes at least 2 anti-infectives with activity against *B. anthracis*, including at least one drug with bactericidal activity against the organism and at least one drug classified as a protein synthesis inhibitor. The preferred multiple-drug regimen for the treatment of systemic anthrax in adults and pediatric patients (including neonates) when meningitis has been excluded is IV ciprofloxacin in conjunction with an IV protein synthesis inhibitor (preferably clindamycin or linezolid in adults or clindamycin in pediatric patients).

If the *B. anthracis* strain is tested and found to be susceptible to penicillin, CDC and AAP state that IV penicillin G and IV ampicillin are acceptable alternatives for the second bactericidal agent (i.e., the carbapenem) used in multiple-drug regimens for the treatment of systemic anthrax (with possible or confirmed meningitis) or the bactericidal agent used in multiple-drug regimens for the treatment of systemic anthrax when meningitis has been excluded.

Some experts suggest that oral ciprofloxacin or other oral fluoroquinolones (levofloxacin, moxifloxacin, ofloxacin) can be considered for the treatment of inhalational anthrax† when a parenteral regimen is not available. Although a multiple-drug parenteral regimen should be used for the treatment of inhalational anthrax that occurs as the result of exposure to *B. anthracis* spores in the context of biologic warfare or bioterrorism, use of these parenteral regimens may not be possible if large numbers of individuals require treatment in a mass casualty setting and it may be necessary to use an oral regimen.

Because of the possible persistence of anthrax spores in lung tissue, anti-infective therapy for the treatment of systemic anthrax that occurs as the result of exposure to aerosolized *B. anthracis* spores in the context of biologic warfare or bioterrorism should be continued for 60 days. The initial multiple-drug parenteral regimen should be continued for at least 2–3 weeks until the patient is clinically stable and can be switched to an appropriate oral anti-infective.

Clinical Experience. A multiple-drug parenteral regimen that was used in 2 patients who survived inhalational anthrax following the bioterrorism-related exposures in 2001 was a 3-drug regimen of ciprofloxacin (400 mg every 8 hours), rifampin (300 mg every 12 hours), and clindamycin (900 mg every 8 hours). Other multiple-drug regimens that were used for the initial treatment of patients who survived inhalational anthrax following these bioterrorism-related anthrax exposures were ciprofloxacin/cefotaxime/azithromycin (1 patient); levofloxacin/rifampin initially then ciprofloxacin rifampin/vancomycin (1 patient); and oral levofloxacin (prior to diagnosis), then ciprofloxacin/azithromycin, then clindamycin/ceftriaxone/azithromycin, then doxycycline (1 patient). Although it is unclear whether the deaths were related to ineffective regimens and/or delays in initiation of therapy, the regimens used in patients who died of inhalational anthrax following these exposures were levofloxacin/clindamycin/penicillin G (1 patient, initiated on the second day of hospitalization after various anti-infectives, died 3 days after admission); levofloxacin monotherapy (1 patient, died day of admission); levofloxacin/rifampin/penicillin G/ceftriaxone (1 patient, died day of admission); levofloxacin monotherapy, then levofloxacin/rifampin/gentamicin/nafcillin, then ciprofloxacin/rifampin/clindamycin/ceftazidime (1 patient, died 3 days after admission); ampicillin-sulbactam/ciprofloxacin/clindamycin (1 patient, initiated on the third day of hospitalization after various other regimens, died 4 days after admission) and ampicillin-sulbactam/ciprofloxacin (1 patient, initiated on the day of hospitalization and clindamycin added on the third day, died 4 days after admission).

Results of in vitro susceptibility testing of strains of *B. anthracis* that were associated with cases of inhalational or cutaneous anthrax that occurred in the US (Florida, New York, District of Columbia) during September and October 2001 in the context of bioterrorism-related exposures to anthrax spores indicated that these strains were susceptible to ciprofloxacin, doxycycline, tetracycline, rifampin, clindamycin, vancomycin, and chloramphenicol. Isolates were susceptible to clarithromycin, azithromycin (borderline susceptibility), and imipenem, but had only intermediate susceptibility to erythromycin. Although these *B. anthracis* strains were susceptible to penicillin and amoxicillin in vitro, additional tests indicated that some of these strains had constitutive and inducible β-lactamases and there is in vitro evidence that exposure of some penicillin-susceptible *B. anthracis* strains to penicillins can induce β-lactamases. Therefore, CDC states that use of a penicillin *alone* is not recommended for the treatment of anthrax that occurs as the result of biologic warfare or bioterrorism when high concentrations of the organism are likely to be present, although penicillin can be included in appropriate combination regimens. *B. anthracis* strains resistant to sulfamethoxazole, trimethoprim, cephalosporins (i.e., cefuroxime, cefotaxime, ceftazidime), or aztreonam have been reported, and these anti-infectives should *not* be used in the treatment of anthrax.

Treatment of Uncomplicated Cutaneous Anthrax Natural penicillins (e.g., oral penicillin V, IM penicillin G benzathine, IM penicillin G procaine) generally have been considered drugs of choice for the treatment of mild, uncomplicated cutaneous anthrax caused by susceptible *B. anthracis* that occurs as the result of naturally occurring or endemic exposure to anthrax, although some clinicians suggest use of oral fluoroquinolones (ciprofloxacin, levofloxacin, ofloxacin), oral amoxicillin, or oral doxycycline if in vitro tests indicate susceptibility.

For the treatment of uncomplicated cutaneous anthrax† (without systemic involvement) that occurs following exposure to *B. anthracis* spores in the context of biologic warfare or bioterrorism, CDC recommends that adults receive an oral regimen of ciprofloxacin, doxycycline, levofloxacin, or moxifloxacin; alternatives include oral amoxicillin or penicillin V (if penicillin susceptibility is confirmed) or oral clindamycin.

For the treatment of uncomplicated cutaneous anthrax† (without systemic involvement) that occurs following exposure to *B. anthracis* spores in the context of biologic warfare or bioterrorism, AAP recommends that pediatric patients (including neonates) receive an oral regimen of ciprofloxacin; alternatives include oral amoxicillin or penicillin V (if penicillin susceptibility is confirmed) or oral doxycycline, clindamycin, or levofloxacin.

CDC, AAP, and other experts recommend that anti-infective treatment be continued for 60 days if the cutaneous infection occurred as the result of exposure to aerosolized anthrax spores since the possibility of inhalational anthrax would also exist. For the treatment of mild, uncomplicated cutaneous anthrax that occurs as the result of natural or endemic exposures to anthrax (e.g., known exposure to infected livestock or their products), a treatment duration of 3–10 days may be sufficient. Anti-infective therapy may limit the size of the cutaneous anthrax lesion and it usually becomes sterile within the first 24 hours of treatment, but the lesion will still progress through the black eschar stage despite effective treatment.

Treatment of GI and Oropharyngeal Anthrax Following Natural or Endemic Exposures Although penicillin usually is considered the drug of choice for the treatment of GI anthrax† that occurs as the result of ingesting contaminated, undercooked meat, ciprofloxacin is considered an alternative for the treatment of these infections. Ciprofloxacin has been used for prophylaxis following ingestion of *B. anthracis* spores† in contaminated meat.

■ **Brucellosis** Ciprofloxacin has been used in the treatment of brucellosis† caused by *Brucella melitensis*, and some clinicians suggest that a regimen of ciprofloxacin and rifampin can be used as an alternative regimen for the treatment of the disease. Most experts recommend a regimen of doxycycline and streptomycin (or gentamicin) or a regimen of doxycycline and rifampin; alternative regimens include co-trimoxazole with or without gentamicin or rifampin; ciprofloxacin (or ofloxacin) and rifampin; or chloramphenicol with or without streptomycin. Monotherapy with any drug usually is associated with a high relapse rate and is not recommended.

In a study in adults with brucellosis, a 30-day regimen of oral ciprofloxacin (500 mg twice daily) and rifampin (600 mg once daily) was as effective as a regimen of oral doxycycline (100 mg twice daily) and rifampin (600 mg once daily). Oral ciprofloxacin has been used in patients with acute brucellosis or acute brucella arthritis-diskitis†. Although oral ciprofloxacin therapy resulted in an initial apparent response in most patients and defervescence within 7 days, at least one patient was considered a treatment failure because blood cultures remained positive and about 25% of patients (generally those with arthritis-diskitis) had relapse or reinfection within 8–32 weeks after the drug was discontinued.

■ **Chancroid** Ciprofloxacin (conventional tablets, oral suspension) has been effective in men for the treatment of chancroid†, genital ulcers caused by *Haemophilus ducreyi*. Although a single 500-mg oral dose of the drug was effective in some men for the treatment of chancroid, multiple-dose regimens generally have been associated with fewer treatment failures.

CDC states that a single IM dose of ceftriaxone, a single oral dose of azithromycin, a 3-day regimen of oral ciprofloxacin (not recommended in pregnant or lactating women), or a 7-day regimen of oral erythromycin are the regimens of choice for the treatment of chancroid.

HIV-infected patients and patients who are uncircumcised may not respond to treatment as well as those who are HIV-negative or circumcised. Clinicians should consider that, although treatment failures can occur with any of these recommended regimens, only limited data are available regarding efficacy of the single-dose ceftriaxone and single-dose azithromycin regimens in HIV-infected patients. Because treatment failures and slow healing of ulcers are more likely in HIV-infected individuals, such patients should be monitored closely and more prolonged treatment or retreatment may be necessary.

Data are limited regarding the prevalence of *H. ducreyi* resistant to the anti-infectives recommended for treatment. Isolates of *H. ducreyi* with intermediate resistance to ciprofloxacin have been reported rarely.

For additional information on management of chancroid, current CDC sexually transmitted diseases treatment guidelines available at http://www.cdc.gov/std should be consulted.

■ **Chlamydial and Mycoplasmal Infections** Multiple-dose oral ciprofloxacin therapy has been used for the treatment of nongonococcal urethritis†, but results have been conflicting. Although 7–10 days of oral ciprofloxacin appeared to be effective for the treatment of nongonococcal urethritis in some men, efficacy of the drug was unpredictable when *Chlamydia* was present, and the rate of relapse was high. If a fluoroquinolone is used as an alternative for the treatment of nongonococcal urethritis when the regimens of choice (azithromycin, doxycycline) are not used, CDC recommends a 7-day regimen of oral ofloxacin or oral levofloxacin.

Oral ciprofloxacin was used with some success in a limited number of women for the treatment of urethral and cervical infections caused by *C. trachomatis* or *Mycoplasma hominis*†. The drug generally has been ineffective in both men and women for the treatment of urogenital infections caused by *Ureaplasma urealyticum*†. If a fluoroquinolone is used as an alternative for the treatment of *C. trachomatis* urogenital infections, CDC recommends a 7-day regimen of oral levofloxacin or oral ofloxacin.

■ **Crohn's Disease** Oral ciprofloxacin (administered with or without metronidazole) has been used for induction of remission of mildly to moderately active Crohn's disease†; the drug also has been used for refractory perianal Crohn's disease. Because intestinal flora appear to have an association with intestinal inflammation, and because ciprofloxacin appears to have immunosuppressive effects, the drug may be useful in the management of Crohn's disease as an adjunct to conventional therapies. However, there currently is no established standard therapy with ciprofloxacin for the management of active Crohn's disease, and further larger studies are needed to confirm study results to date and to establish management criteria and safety considerations for the disease.

Results of several open-label, comparative, retrospective, and at least 1 placebo-controlled study indicate that ciprofloxacin (with or without metronidazole) can result in clinical response (e.g., improvement of clinical condition, clinical remission) in patients with mildly to moderately active Crohn's disease. It appears that the combination of ciprofloxacin and metronidazole is more effective than ciprofloxacin alone. Safety and efficacy of ciprofloxacin in the management of active Crohn's disease were evaluated in a small 6-month preliminary, placebo-controlled, randomized study that included 47 adults with moderately active Crohn's disease who had an inadequate response to conventional therapies (e.g., prednisone, mesalamine, mercaptopurine). To be included in the study, patients had to have had symptomatic disease and a Crohn's Disease Activity Index [CDAI]) greater than 150 at the time of study entry. The CDAI score is based on subjective observations by the patient (e.g., the daily number of liquid or very soft stools, severity of abdominal pain, general well-being) and objective evidence (e.g., number of extraintestinal manifestations, presence of an abdominal mass, use or nonuse of antidiarrheal drugs, the hematocrit, body weight). Patients were randomized to receive ciprofloxacin 500 mg twice daily or placebo while they continued to receive conventional therapy for the disease. Clinical response was described as achievement of a CDAI score of less than 150. Only 37 patients completed the study; 25 of those were receiving ciprofloxacin and 12 were receiving placebo. Mean CDAI score at the end of 6 months was 112 or 205 in those receiving ciprofloxacin or placebo, respectively.

Results of a small, randomized, comparator-drug (ciprofloxacin versus mesalamine) controlled study (patients having a median CDAI score of 217 [range:160–305]) indicate that clinical improvement in patients receiving ciprofloxacin in a dosage of 1 g daily was similar to that in those receiving mesalamine controlled-release capsules in a dosage of 4 g daily. At 6 weeks of therapy, complete remission (defined as a CDAI score of 150 or less, associated with a reduction from baseline CDAI of more than 75 points) was reported in 56 or 55% of patients receiving ciprofloxacin or mesalamine, respectively, while partial remission (defined as a CDAI score of 150 or less, associated with a reduction from baseline CDAI of greater than 50 but less than 70 points) was reported in 17 (3 out of 18 patients) or 4.5% (1 out of 22) patients receiving ciprofloxacin or mesalamine, respectively.

In addition, safety and efficacy of concomitant use of ciprofloxacin and metronidazole have been evaluated in a 12-week comparative (versus methylprednisolone) study in 41 patients with active Crohn's disease (CDAI of more than 200 at the time of study entry). Patients were randomized to receive ciprofloxacin 500 mg twice daily in conjunction with metronidazole 250 mg 4 times daily (22 patients) or methylprednisolone (0.7–1 mg/kg daily initially, followed by variable tapering to 40 mg, and subsequent tapering of 4 mg weekly; 19 patients). At 12 weeks of therapy, clinical remission (defined as a CDAI of 150 points or less) was reported in 63 or 46% of patients receiving the corticosteroid or the combination therapy, respectively. It has been suggested that combination therapy with ciprofloxacin and metronidazole could be an alternative to corticosteroids, although a high incidence of adverse effects (27% discontinued therapy because of such effects) was associated with the anti-infectives.

Limited data indicate that ciprofloxacin may be more effective in patients with ileitis than in those with colitis. It has been suggested that reduced efficacy of ciprofloxacin in colitis may be associated with the low activity of the drug against anaerobic bacteria.

Ciprofloxacin has been used in the management of refractory perianal

Crohn's disease†. Anecdotal reports suggest that ciprofloxacin may be useful in the long-term treatment of active perianal Crohn's disease; however, the drug generally is used for short-term administration for this condition. Relapse usually occurs when the anti-infective is discontinued. Limited data indicate that short-term (8 weeks) combination therapy with ciprofloxacin and metronidazole given with, or followed by, azathioprine (up to about 20 weeks) in patients with perianal Crohn's disease may result in rapid reduction of fistula drainage (induced by the anti-infectives) and beneficial maintenance (associated with the azathioprine).

■ **Gonorrhea and Associated Infections** Although oral ciprofloxacin (conventional tablets, oral suspension) was used in the past for the treatment of uncomplicated urethral, endocervical, rectal†, or pharyngeal† gonorrhea caused by susceptible *Neisseria gonorrhoeae*, quinolone-resistant *N. gonorrhoeae* (QRNG) is widely disseminated throughout the world, including in the US. (See Resistance: Resistance in Neisseria gonorrhoeae.) Therefore, CDC states that fluoroquinolones are no longer recommended for the treatment of gonorrhea and should not be used routinely for any associated infections that may involve *N. gonorrhoeae* (e.g., pelvic inflammatory disease [PID], epididymitis).

From 1993–2000, CDC recommended fluoroquinolones as drugs of choice for the treatment of uncomplicated gonorrhea in the US; however, because of reports of QRNG, subsequent CDC recommendations regarding use of the drugs for the treatment of gonorrhea became more restrictive. Beginning in 2000, CDC no longer recommended use of fluoroquinolones for the treatment of gonorrhea in individuals who acquired their infections in Asia or the Pacific Islands (including Hawaii) because of the high incidence QRNG in these areas. In 2002, this restriction was broadened to include individuals who acquired gonorrhea in California. In 2004, CDC recommended that fluoroquinolones not be used to treat gonorrhea in men who have sex with men because of the increased prevalence of QRNG in this population. Beginning in April 2007, CDC stated that fluoroquinolones should *not* be used for the treatment of gonorrhea or any associated infections that may involve *N. gonorrhoeae* (e.g., PID, epididymitis).

For information on current recommendations for the treatment of gonorrhea and associated infections, see Uses: Gonorrhea and Associated Infections, in Ceftriaxone 8:12.06.12.

■ **Granuloma Inguinale (Donovanosis)** Oral ciprofloxacin is considered an alternative for the treatment of granuloma inguinale (donovanosis)† caused by *Klebsiella granulomatis* (formerly *Calymmatobacterium granulomatis*).

CDC recommends that granuloma inguinale be treated with a regimen of oral azithromycin or, alternatively, a regimen of oral doxycycline, oral ciprofloxacin, oral erythromycin, or oral co-trimoxazole. Anti-infective treatment should be continued until all lesions have healed completely; a minimum duration of 3 weeks usually is necessary. If improvement is not evident within the first few days of treatment, CDC states that consideration can be given to adding a parenteral aminoglycoside (e.g., IV gentamicin) to the regimen. Anti-infective therapy appears to halt progression of lesions, although prolonged duration of therapy often is required to enable granulation and re-epithelization of ulcers. Despite effective anti-infective therapy, granuloma inguinale may relapse 6–18 months later.

Individuals with HIV infection should receive the same treatment regimens recommended for other individuals with granuloma inguinale; however, CDC suggests that addition of a parenteral aminoglycoside to the regimen can be considered if improvement is not evident within the first few days of treatment.

For additional information on management of granuloma inguinale, current CDC sexually transmitted diseases treatment guidelines available at http://www.cdc.gov/std should be consulted.

■ **Legionnaires' Disease** Ciprofloxacin has been used for the treatment of Legionnaires' Disease† caused by *Legionella pneumophila*, including in immunocompromised patients (e.g., transplant recipients).

■ **Malaria** Although ciprofloxacin reportedly has some activity in vitro against *Plasmodium falciparum*, oral ciprofloxacin (750 mg every 12 hours) has been ineffective when used alone in the treatment of uncomplicated malaria caused by chloroquine-resistant *P. falciparum*†.

■ **Mycobacterial Infections** ***Treatment of Active Tuberculosis*** Ciprofloxacin has been used in multiple-drug regimens for the treatment of active tuberculosis† caused by *Mycobacterium tuberculosis*.

Although the potential role of fluoroquinolones and the optimal length of therapy have not been fully defined, the American Thoracic Society (ATS), CDC, IDSA, and others state that use of fluoroquinolones as alternative (second-line) agents can be considered for the treatment of active tuberculosis in patients intolerant of certain first-line agents and in those with relapse, treatment failure, or *M. tuberculosis* resistant to certain first-line agents. If a fluoroquinolone is used in multiple-drug regimens for the treatment of active tuberculosis, ATS, CDC, IDSA, and others recommend levofloxacin or moxifloxacin. Some experts state that ciprofloxacin is no longer recommended for treatment of tuberculosis.

The most recent ATS, CDC, and IDSA recommendations for the treatment of tuberculosis should be consulted for more specific information.

Other Mycobacterial Infections Ciprofloxacin has been used alone or in conjunction with amikacin for the treatment of cutaneous infections caused by *M. fortuitum*†. Although ciprofloxacin appeared to be effective in a few patients with *M. fortuitum* infections, ciprofloxacin-resistant strains of the organism have developed when the drug was used alone or in conjunction with amikacin in the treatment of these infections. Although optimum regimens have not been identified, ATS and IDSA recommend that *M. fortuitum* pulmonary infections be treated with a regimen consisting of at least 2 anti-infectives selected based on results of in vitro susceptibility testing and tolerability (e.g., amikacin, ciprofloxacin or ofloxacin, a sulfonamide, cefoxitin, imipenem, doxycycline).

Ciprofloxacin has been used in multiple-drug regimens for the treatment of pulmonary and extrapulmonary (localized or disseminated) *M. avium* complex† (MAC) infections. However, ATS and IDSA state that the role of fluoroquinolones in the treatment of MAC infections has not been established. If a fluoroquinolone is included in a treatment regimen (e.g., for macrolide-resistant MAC infections), moxifloxacin may be preferred, although many strains are resistant in vitro.

Based on results of in vitro susceptibility testing, ciprofloxacin may be considered for use in combination antimycobacterial regimens used for the treatment of infections caused by *M. chelonae*†, *M. haemophilum*†, or *M. terrae*†. Optimal treatment regimens for these infections have not been identified. Because of considerations related to resistance, ciprofloxacin is not recommended for treatment of *M. marinum* infections.

The most recent ATS, CDC, and IDSA recommendations for the treatment of other mycobacterial infections should be consulted for more specific information.

■ **Neisseria meningitidis Infections** Ciprofloxacin (conventional tablets, oral suspension) is used in adults to eliminate nasopharyngeal carriage of *Neisseria meningitidis*† and for chemoprophylaxis to prevent meningococcal disease in household or other close contacts of patients with invasive disease†.

Patients with invasive meningococcal disease who have been treated with penicillin G or any anti-infective other than ceftriaxone or another third generation cephalosporin may still be carriers of *N. meningitidis* and should receive an anti-infective regimen to eradicate nasopharyngeal carriage of the organism prior to hospital discharge. The treatments of choice to eradicate nasopharyngeal carriage of *N. meningitidis* are ceftriaxone (single IM dose), rifampin (2-day regimen), and ciprofloxacin (single oral dose). These regimens are all 90–95% effective and any of these is an acceptable regimen in appropriate patients.

Chemoprophylaxis in close contacts of a patients with invasive meningococcal disease is an important means of preventing secondary cases in household and other close contacts. Recommended regimens for chemoprophylaxis against meningococcal disease include a single dose of IM ceftriaxone, 2-day regimen of oral rifampin (not recommended in pregnant women), or a single dose of oral ciprofloxacin (not recommended in individuals younger than 18 years of age unless no other regimen can be used and not recommended for pregnant or lactating women). These regimens are all 90–95% effective and any of these is an acceptable regimen for chemoprophylaxis. AAP suggests that rifampin may be the drug of choice for chemoprophylaxis in most children.

The attack rate for household contacts who do not receive chemoprophylaxis has been estimated to be 4 cases per 1000 individuals exposed, which is 500–800 times greater than that for the general population. A decision to administer chemoprophylaxis to close contacts of an individual with invasive meningococcal disease is based on the degree of risk. Throat and nasopharyngeal cultures are not useful in determining the need for chemoprophylaxis and may unnecessarily delay administration of the regimen.

When chemoprophylaxis is indicated in high-risk contacts, it must be administered promptly (ideally within 24 hours after identification of the index case) since the attack rate of secondary disease is greatest in the few days following disease onset in the index case. All high-risk contacts should be informed that even if chemoprophylaxis is taken or started, the development of any suspicious clinical manifestation warrants early, rapid medical attention. Chemoprophylaxis probably is of limited or no value if administered more than 14 days after contact with the index case. If high-risk exposure to a new index case occurs more than 2 weeks after initial chemoprophylaxis, additional chemoprophylaxis is indicated.

Fluoroquinolone-resistant *N. meningitidis* has been reported rarely in the US and elsewhere (e.g., India). Ciprofloxacin should not be used for prophylaxis in close contacts of individuals with meningococcal disease in areas where fluoroquinolone-resistant strains have been reported (e.g., selected counties of North Dakota and Minnesota).

For information on current recommendations regarding chemoprophylaxis in contacts of individuals with invasive meningococcal disease, including information on high-risk individuals, see Uses: Neisseria meningitidis Infections, in Ceftriaxone 8:12.06.12.

■ **Plague** Ciprofloxacin (IV, conventional tablets, oral suspension) is used for the treatment of plague, including pneumonic and septicemic plague, caused by *Yersinia pestis* and for postexposure prophylaxis of plague in adults and children. Based on results of in vitro and animal testing, fluoroquinolones (ciprofloxacin, levofloxacin, moxifloxacin, ofloxacin) are recommended as alternatives for the treatment of plague and for postexposure prophylaxis following a high-risk exposure to *Y. pestis*, including exposures that occur in the context of biologic warfare or bioterrorism.

Efficacy of ciprofloxacin for treatment or prophylaxis of plague has not be evaluated in clinical trials in humans for ethical and feasibility reasons. The drug is labeled by FDA for this indication based on an efficacy study in animals that demonstrated a survival benefit. In a placebo-controlled study, African green monkeys were exposed to an inhaled dose of *Y. pestis* (mean dose of 110 LD_{50} [range 92–127 LD_{50}]) and then randomized to receive either ciprofloxacin (15 mg/kg IV for 10 days) or placebo initiated when fever started or 76 hours post-challenge, whichever occurred first. In vitro testing indicated that the *Y. pestis* strain used in this study (CO92 strain) had a ciprofloxacin MIC of 0.015 mcg/mL. Pharmacokinetic data indicated that mean peak serum concentrations of ciprofloxacin attained in the monkeys at the end of a single 60-minute IV infusion of the drug were approximately 3.5, 3.9, and 4 mcg/mL on days 2, 6, and 10 of treatment, respectively; trough concentrations on these days were all less than 0.5 mcg/mL. Study results indicated that mortality in the ciprofloxacin treatment group was significantly lower (1 out of 10) compared with the placebo group (2 out of 2). The single ciprofloxacin-treated monkey that died had not received the protocol-directed ciprofloxacin dosage because of a failure of the administration catheter; ciprofloxacin serum concentrations in this monkey were less than 0.5 mcg/mL at all time points tested. Although this monkey became culture negative on day 2 of treatment and terminal blood cultures were negative, the animal had a resurgence of low grade bacteremia on day 6 after initiation of ciprofloxacin.

Treatment of Plague For the treatment of plague, IM streptomycin (or IM or IV gentamicin) historically has been considered the regimen of choice. Alternatives recommended for the treatment of plague when aminoglycosides are not used include IV doxycycline (or IV tetracycline), IV chloramphenicol (a drug of choice for plague meningitis), an IV fluoroquinolone (ciprofloxacin [a drug of choice for plague meningitis], levofloxacin, moxifloxacin), or co-trimoxazole (may be less effective than other alternatives).

Anti-infective regimens recommended for the treatment of naturally occurring or endemic bubonic, septicemic, or pneumonic plague also are recommended for the treatment of plague that occurs following exposure to *Y. pestis* in the context of biologic warfare or bioterrorism. Such exposures would most likely result in primary pneumonic plague, and prompt initiation of anti-infective therapy (within 18–24 hours of onset of symptoms) is essential in the treatment of pneumonic plague. Some experts (e.g., US Working Group on Civilian Biodefense, USAMRIID) recommend that treatment of plague in the context of biologic warfare or bioterrorism be initiated with a parenteral anti-infective regimen of streptomycin (or gentamicin) or, alternatively, doxycycline, a fluoroquinolone (ciprofloxacin, levofloxacin, moxifloxacin) or chloramphenicol. However, an oral regimen of doxycycline (or tetracycline) or a fluoroquinolone (ciprofloxacin, levofloxacin, moxifloxacin, ofloxacin) may be substituted when the patient's condition improves or when a parenteral regimen is unavailable (e.g., when there are supply or logistic problems because large numbers of individuals require treatment in a mass casualty setting); oral chloramphenicol is considered an alternative in these situations.

Postexposure Prophylaxis of Plague In the context of biologic warfare or bioterrorism, some experts (e.g., US Working Group on Civilian Biodefense, USAMRIID) recommend that asymptomatic individuals with exposure to plague aerosol or asymptomatic individuals with household, hospital, or other close contact (within about 2 m) with an individual who has pneumonic plague receive an oral anti-infective regimen for postexposure prophylaxis; however, any exposed individual who develops a temperature of 38.5°C or higher or new cough should promptly receive a parenteral anti-infective for treatment of the disease. If postexposure prophylaxis is indicated, these experts recommend a regimen of oral doxycycline (or tetracycline) or an oral fluoroquinolone (ciprofloxacin, levofloxacin, moxifloxacin, ofloxacin).

Although plague vaccine (no longer commercially available in the US) was previously recommended to provide protection against *Y. pestis* infection, the vaccine was effective for preventing or ameliorating bubonic plague but was not effective for prophylaxis against exposure to aerosolized *Y. pestis* and therefore did not provide protection against pneumonic plague.

■ Rickettsial Infections Ciprofloxacin has been used with some success in a limited number of patients for the treatment of various rickettsial infections†, including Mediterranean spotted fever† caused by *Rickettsia conorii*. CDC and other clinicians state that doxycycline is the drug of choice for the treatment of all tickborne rickettsial diseases. Although some fluoroquinolones have in vitro activity against Rickettsiae and some clinicians have suggested that fluoroquinolones (e.g., ciprofloxacin, ofloxacin) may be considered alternatives for the treatment of some rickettsial infections (e.g., Rocky Mountain spotted fever caused by *R. rickettsii*) when doxycycline cannot be used, CDC states that fluoroquinolones are *not* recommended for the treatment of Rocky Mountain spotted fever.

Ciprofloxacin has been used for the long-term treatment of Q fever endocarditis caused by *Coxiella burnetii*†. However, CDC states that doxycycline is the drug of choice when treatment of acute Q fever is indicated and doxycycline in conjunction with hydroxychloroquine is the regimen of choice for the treatment of chronic Q fever, including endocarditis.

■ Tularemia ***Treatment of Tularemia*** Ciprofloxacin (IV, conventional tablets, oral suspension) is recommended as an alternative to aminoglycosides (streptomycin or gentamicin) for the treatment of tularemia† caused by *Francisella tularensis*. Streptomycin generally has been considered the drug of choice for the treatment of tularemia; however, gentamicin is more readily available and is considered an alternative drug of choice when streptomycin is unavailable. Other alternatives for the treatment of tularemia include tetracyclines (doxycycline), chloramphenicol, or ciprofloxacin. Anti-infective regimens recommended for the treatment of naturally occurring or endemic tularemia also are recommended for the treatment of tularemia that occurs following exposure to *F. tularensis* in the context of biologic warfare or bioterrorism. However, the fact that a fully virulent streptomycin-resistant strain of *F. tularensis* was developed in the past for use in biologic warfare should be considered. Exposures to *F. tularensis* in the context of biologic warfare or bioterrorism would most likely result in inhalational tularemia with pleuropneumonitis, although the organism also can infect humans through the skin, mucous membranes, and GI tract.

Postexposure Prophylaxis of Tularemia Postexposure prophylaxis with anti-infectives usually is not recommended after possible exposure to natural or endemic tularemia (e.g., tick bite, rabbit or other animal exposure) and is unnecessary in close contacts of tularemia patients since human-to-human transmission of the disease is not known to occur. However, postexposure prophylaxis is recommended following a high-risk laboratory exposure to *F. tularensis* (e.g., spill, centrifuge accident, needlestick injury). In the context of biologic warfare or bioterrorism, some experts (e.g., US Working Group on Civilian Biodefense, USAMRIID) recommend that asymptomatic individuals with exposure to *F. tularensis* receive postexposure anti-infective prophylaxis; however, any individual who develops an otherwise unexplained fever or flu-like illness within 14 days of presumed exposure should promptly receive a parenteral anti-infective for treatment of the disease. Oral ciprofloxacin or oral doxycycline (or oral tetracycline) usually is recommended for postexposure prophylaxis of tularemia† following such exposures.

■ Typhoid Fever and Other Invasive Salmonella Infections Ciprofloxacin (conventional tablets, oral suspension) is used in adults for the treatment of typhoid fever (enteric fever) or paratyphoid fever† caused by susceptible *Salmonella enterica* serovars Typhi or Paratyphi, respectively. Although fluoroquinolones have been recommended for empiric treatment of *Salmonella* enteric fever in adults, resistance to fluoroquinolones has been reported in more than 80% of such infections in travelers to South and Southeast Asia and treatment failures will occur.

Oral ciprofloxacin has been effective when used to treat chronic typhoid carriers†; however, the manufacturer of ciprofloxacin cautions that efficacy of the drug in the eradication of the chronic typhoid carrier state has not been demonstrated.

Ciprofloxacin is recommended as a drug of choice for the treatment of native vertebral osteomyelitis caused by *Salmonella*†. (See Uses: Bone and Joint Infections.)

Ciprofloxacin has been used to treat meningitis caused by susceptible *Salmonella*†. (See Uses: Meningitis and Other CNS Infections.)

■ Vibrio Infections ***Cholera*** Ciprofloxacin has been used for the treatment of cholera† caused by *Vibrio cholerae* 01 or 0139 in adults or children†. Doxycycline generally is considered the drug of choice when anti-infective therapy is indicated as an adjunct to fluid and electrolyte replacement in patients with cholera; alternatives include azithromycin, co-trimoxazole, ciprofloxacin, or ceftriaxone.

In a controlled study in adults, a 1-g oral dose of oral ciprofloxacin (given as a single dose or in 2 divided doses 12 hours apart) was at least as effective as a 3-day regimen of oral doxycycline (100 mg twice daily for 3 days) for the treatment of cholera. In another study in adults, a single 1-g dose of oral ciprofloxacin was more effective than a single 300-mg oral dose of doxycycline in eradicating *V. cholerae* from stool; although there was no difference between the regimens in terms of duration of diarrhea in those with *V. cholerae* 0139 infections, the duration of diarrhea was shorter in those with *V. cholerae* 01 infections who received ciprofloxacin.

Although further study is needed to evaluate safety and efficacy in children, a single dose of oral ciprofloxacin (20 mg/kg) was as effective as a 3-day regimen of oral erythromycin (12.5 mg/kg every 6 hours) for the treatment of *V. cholerae* 01 or 0139 in children 2–15 years of age. The overall clinical success rate was 60% for ciprofloxacin and 55% for erythromycin; although the bacteriologic eradication rate was lower with ciprofloxacin (42%) than with erythromycin (70%) and erythromycin was associated with a more rapid clearance of *V. cholerae*, there was no difference in duration of diarrhea.

Other Vibrio Infections Some clinicians suggest that fluoroquinolones (e.g., ciprofloxacin) may be an alternative to tetracyclines for the treatment of other *Vibrio* infections, including gastroenteritis or wound infections caused by *V. parahaemolyticus*† or *V. vulnificus*†.

Although optimum anti-infective therapy for *V. vulnificus* infections has not been identified, a tetracycline or third generation cephalosporin (e.g., cefotaxime, ceftazidime), a fluoroquinolone, or aminoglycoside has been recommended. Because the case fatality rate associated with *V. vulnificus* is high, anti-infective therapy should be initiated promptly if indicated.

■ Perioperative Prophylaxis Ciprofloxacin is used for perioperative prophylaxis† to reduce the risk of postoperative infections in patients undergoing certain genitourinary surgery.

Perioperative prophylaxis is not recommended for patients with sterile urine undergoing cystoscopy without manipulation. However, if the patient has positive (or unavailable) urine cultures or an indwelling urinary catheter or is undergoing cystoscopy with manipulation (dilation, biopsy, fulguration, resection, or ureteral instrumentation), some clinicians recommend pretreatment to sterilize the urine before surgery or perioperative prophylaxis with a single preoperative dose of an anti-infective (e.g., ciprofloxacin) active against the most likely urologic pathogens.

Perioperative prophylaxis using an appropriate anti-infective (e.g., ciprofloxacin) is recommended in patients undergoing transurethral prostatectomy, transrectal prostatic biopsies, ureteroscopy, shock wave lithotripsy, percutaneous renal surgery, open laparoscopic procedures, or procedures that involve placement of a urologic prosthesis (e.g., penile implant, artificial sphincter, synthetic pubovaginal sling, bone anchors for pelvic floor reconstruction). Because of increasing resistance of *E. coli* to fluoroquinolones, local susceptibility patterns should be considered when selecting an anti-infective for prophylaxis in patients undergoing genitourinary surgery.

■ Empiric Therapy in Febrile Neutropenic Patients Ciprofloxacin is used for empiric therapy of presumed bacterial infections in febrile neutropenic patients.

IV ciprofloxacin has been used in conjunction with IV piperacillin sodium (no longer commercially available in the US as a single-entity preparation) for empiric anti-infective therapy in febrile neutropenic patients. Safety and efficacy of combination therapy with ciprofloxacin and piperacillin sodium for empiric therapy in febrile neutropenic patients have been evaluated in a multicenter, randomized study in adults. Patients were randomized to receive a regimen of ciprofloxacin (400 mg IV every 8 hours) and piperacillin sodium (50 mg/kg IV every 4 hours) or a regimen of tobramycin (2 mg/kg IV every 8 hours) and piperacillin sodium (50 mg/kg IV every 4 hours). There was clinical resolution of the initial febrile episode (resolution of fever, microbiologic eradication of infection if such infection was microbiologically documented, resolution of signs and symptoms of infection) without modification of the empiric regimen in 27% of those who received ciprofloxacin and piperacillin and in 21.9% of those who received tobramycin and piperacillin; the overall survival rate was 96.1 or 94.1%, respectively.

Anti-infective prophylaxis with a fluoroquinolone during periods of expected neutropenia is recommended by some experts in patients who are at high risk for febrile neutropenia or profound, protracted neutropenia (e.g., most patients with acute myeloid leukemia/myelodysplastic syndromes [AML/MDS] or hematopoietic stem-cell transplantation [HSCT] treated with myeloablative conditioning regimens). These experts state that prophylaxis with a fluoroquinolone is not routinely recommended in patients with solid tumors because the benefits do not outweigh risks in these patients, but may be considered for some patients with solid tumors or lymphoma who are expected to experience profound neutropenia for at least 7 days and are not receiving granulocyte colony-stimulating factor (G-CSF).

An empiric regimen that includes a fluoroquinolone (ciprofloxacin or levofloxacin) in conjunction with the fixed combination of amoxicillin and clavulanate potassium (or clindamycin in those with penicillin allergy) has been recommended for outpatient management of febrile neutropenic adults receiving treatment for malignancy. Use of a fluoroquinolone alone is not recommended for initial empiric therapy for outpatient management in febrile neutropenic patients; however, some studies have shown that monotherapy may be effective in low-risk outpatients.

Published protocols on anti-infective prophylaxis in febrile neutropenic patients should be consulted for specific recommendations regarding when anti-infective prophylaxis is appropriate for immunosuppressed patients with cancer and options for such prophylaxis.

Dosage and Administration

■ Administration Ciprofloxacin is administered orally as conventional tablets containing the hydrochloride, as a conventional oral suspension containing the base, and as extended-release tablets containing both the hydrochloride and the base. Ciprofloxacin is given by IV infusion as the base.

Patients receiving initial therapy with IV ciprofloxacin may be switched to oral ciprofloxacin (conventional tablets, oral suspension) when clinically appropriate.

Ciprofloxacin extended-release tablets are used *only* for the treatment of certain urinary tract infections (UTIs) in adults and should *not* be used for any indication in pediatric patients. The extended-release tablets are *not* interchangeable with other oral ciprofloxacin preparations (conventional tablets, oral suspension).

Patients receiving oral or IV ciprofloxacin should be adequately hydrated and should be instructed to drink fluids liberally to prevent highly concentrated urine and formation of crystals in urine. (See Cautions: Genitourinary Effects.)

Oral Administration Ciprofloxacin conventional tablets, extended-release tablets, or oral suspension may be given without regard to meals. (See Pharmacokinetics.)

Ciprofloxacin conventional tablets, extended-release tablets, or oral suspension should *not* be administered concurrently with dairy products (e.g., milk, yogurt) or calcium-fortified products (e.g., juices) alone (without a meal) since absorption of the drug may be substantially reduced. Doses should preferably be taken 2 hours before or after these calcium-fortified products or substantial calcium intake (greater than 800 mg).

Conventional tablets and extended-release tablets should be swallowed whole and should *not* be split, crushed, or chewed.

Following reconstitution, ciprofloxacin oral suspension containing 250 or 500 mg of ciprofloxacin per 5 mL should be administered using the graduated spoon provided by the manufacturer that has markings for 2.5 and 5 mL. The microcapsules contained in the reconstituted oral suspensions should be swallowed whole and should not be chewed. Water may be ingested after the oral suspension is swallowed.

Reconstitution. Ciprofloxacin microcapsules for oral suspension are provided in a kit that contains a bottle of microcapsules, a bottle of oral suspension diluent, and a graduated dosing spoon. At the time of dispensing, the bottle containing the microcapsules (either 5 or 10 g of ciprofloxacin) should be added to the bottle of diluent according to the manufacturer's directions and shaken vigorously for about 15 seconds to provide a suspension containing 250 or 500 mg of ciprofloxacin per 5 mL, respectively. Only the diluent supplied in the kit should be used; water should *not* be added to the oral suspension.

Prior to administration of each dose, the reconstituted oral suspension should be shaken vigorously for about 15 seconds.

IV Infusion Prior to IV infusion, commercially available ciprofloxacin concentrate for injection containing 10 mg/mL must be diluted with a compatible IV solution (e.g., sterile water for injection, 5% or 10% dextrose injection, 0.9% sodium chloride injection, 5% dextrose and 0.225 or 0.45% sodium chloride injection, or lactated Ringer's injection) to provide a solution containing 1–2 mg/mL.

Alternatively, commercially available premixed ciprofloxacin injection for IV infusion containing 2 mg/mL in 5% dextrose injection may be used without further dilution.

IV infusions should be given into a large vein to minimize discomfort and reduce the risk of venous irritation. If a Y-type administration set is used, the other IV solution flowing through the tubing should be discontinued while ciprofloxacin is being infused. If concomitant use of IV ciprofloxacin and another parenteral drug is necessary, each drug should be given separately.

Rate of Administration. IV infusions of ciprofloxacin should be infused over 1 hour.

Because local reactions (e.g., thrombophlebitis, burning, pain, pruritus, paresthesia, erythema, swelling) at the site of IV infusion are more frequent when the drug is administered rapidly (e.g., over 30 minutes or less) or via a small vein, ciprofloxacin should be infused IV *slowly* over a period of 1 hour as a dilute solution (1–2 mg of ciprofloxacin per mL) via a large vein. If such reactions occur despite these precautions, they generally resolve rapidly following completion of the infusion; the manufacturers state that subsequent IV administration of ciprofloxacin is not contraindicated unless the reaction recurs or worsens.

■ Dosage Dosage of ciprofloxacin hydrochloride and ciprofloxacin is expressed in terms of ciprofloxacin.

Unless otherwise specified, oral ciprofloxacin dosage is for the conventional tablets or oral suspension of the drug.

The extended-release tablets are *not* interchangeable with the conventional tablets or oral suspension.

Dosage of oral and IV ciprofloxacin is *not* identical. Based on pharmacokinetic parameters (i.e., area under the plasma concentration-time curve [AUC]), the following oral and IV ciprofloxacin regimens are considered equivalent: 250 mg orally every 12 hours (conventional tablets) is equivalent to 200 mg IV every 12 hours; 500 mg orally every 12 hours (conventional tablets) is equivalent to 400 mg IV every 12 hours; and 750 mg orally every 12 hours (conventional tablets) is equivalent to 400 mg IV every 8 hours.

The duration of ciprofloxacin therapy depends on the type and severity of infection, and should be determined by the clinical and bacteriologic response of the patient.

Pediatric Dosage **Complicated Urinary Tract Infections and Pyelonephritis.** If ciprofloxacin is used for the treatment of complicated UTIs or pyelonephritis in pediatric patients 1–17 years of age, dosage and route of administration should be based on infection severity. The manufacturers recommend a total treatment duration of 10–21 days; the mean total duration of treatment (IV and/or oral) in clinical trials was 11 days (range 10–21 days).

If IV ciprofloxacin is used for the treatment of complicated UTIs or pyelonephritis in pediatric patients 1–17 years of age, the manufacturer recommends a dosage of 6–10 mg/kg (up to 400 mg) every 8 hours.

If oral ciprofloxacin is used for the treatment of complicated UTIs or pyelonephritis in pediatric patients 1–17 years of age, the manufacturer recommends a dosage of 10–20 mg/kg (up to 750 mg) every 12 hours.

If ciprofloxacin oral suspension containing 250 mg/5 mL is used for the treatment of complicated UTIs or pyelonephritis in pediatric patients 1–17 years of age, the manufacturer recommends a dosage of 125 mg every 12 hours in those weighing 9–12 kg, 250 mg every 12 hours in those weighing 13–18 kg, 250–375 mg every 12 hours in those weighing 19–24 kg, 375–500 mg every 12 hours in those weighing 25–31 kg, 375–625 mg every 12 hours in those weighing 32–37 kg, and 500–750 mg every 12 hours in those weighing 38 kg or more.

If ciprofloxacin oral suspension containing 500 mg/5 mL is used for the treatment of complicated UTIs or pyelonephritis in pediatric patients 1–17 years of age, the manufacturer recommends a dosage of 250 mg every 12 hours in those weighing 13–24 kg, 250–500 mg every 12 hours in those weighing 25 kg, 500 mg every 12 hours in those weighing 26–37 kg, and 500–750 mg every 12 hours in those weighing 38 kg or more.

Postexposure Prophylaxis of Anthrax. If oral ciprofloxacin is used for inhalational anthrax (postexposure) to reduce the incidence or progression of disease following exposure to aerosolized *Bacillus anthracis* spores in the context of biologic warfare or bioterrorism, the manufacturer recommends that neonates, infants, and children 17 years of age or younger receive 15 mg/kg (up to 500 mg) every 12 hours.

If ciprofloxacin oral suspension containing 250 mg/5 mL is used for inhalational anthrax (postexposure) in neonates, infants, and children 17 years of age or younger, the manufacturer recommends a dosage of 125 mg every 12 hours in those weighing 9–12 kg, 250 mg every 12 hours in those weighing

13–18 kg, 250–375 mg every 12 hours in those weighing 19–24 kg, and 500 mg every 12 hours in those weighing 25 kg or more.

If ciprofloxacin oral suspension containing 500 mg/5 mL is used for inhalational anthrax (postexposure) in neonates, infants, and children 17 years of age or younger, the manufacturer recommends a dosage of 250 mg every 12 hours in those weighing 13–24 kg and 500 mg every 12 hours in those weighing 25 kg or more.

If IV ciprofloxacin is used for inhalational anthrax (postexposure) in neonates, infants, and children 17 years of age or younger, the manufacturer recommends a dosage of 10 mg/kg (up to 400 mg) every 12 hours.

For postexposure prophylaxis of anthrax in neonates up to 4 weeks of age following an exposure that occurred in the context of biologic warfare or bioterrorism, the American Academy of Pediatrics (AAP) recommends that oral ciprofloxacin be given in a dosage of 10 mg/kg every 12 hours in preterm neonates (gestational age 32–37 weeks) and 15 mg/kg every 12 hours in full-term neonates. AAP recommends that pediatric patients 1 month of age or older receive oral ciprofloxacin in a dosage of 15 mg/kg (up to 500 mg) every 12 hours for such postexposure prophylaxis.

Postexposure anti-infective prophylaxis should be initiated as soon as possible following suspected or confirmed anthrax exposure.

Because of possible persistence of *B. anthracis* spores in lung tissue following an aerosol exposure, the US Centers for Disease Control and Prevention (CDC), AAP, and others recommend that anti-infective prophylaxis be continued for 60 days following a confirmed exposure (see Postexposure Prophylaxis of Anthrax under Uses: Anthrax).

Treatment of Systemic Anthrax. If IV ciprofloxacin is used in neonates up to 4 weeks of age as part of a multiple-drug parenteral regimen for initial treatment of systemic anthrax† (inhalational, GI, meningitis, or cutaneous with systemic involvement, extensive edema, or head or neck lesions) that occurs in the context of biologic warfare or bioterrorism, AAP recommends a dosage of 10 mg/kg every 12 hours in preterm neonates (gestational age 32–37 weeks) and 15 mg/kg every 12 hours in full-term neonates.

If IV ciprofloxacin is used in pediatric patients 1 month of age or older as part of a multiple-drug parenteral regimen for initial treatment of systemic anthrax† (inhalational, GI, meningitis, or cutaneous with systemic involvement, lesions on the head or neck, or extensive edema) that occurs in the context of biologic warfare or bioterrorism, AAP recommends a dosage of 10 mg/kg (up to 400 mg) every 8 hours.

The multiple-drug parenteral regimen should be continued for at least 2–3 weeks until the patient is clinically stable and treatment can be switched to an appropriate oral anti-infective. If systemic anthrax occurred as the result of exposure to aerosolized *B. anthracis* spores (e.g., in the context of biologic warfare or bioterrorism), the oral follow-up regimen should be continued until 60 days after onset of the illness.

When oral ciprofloxacin is used for follow-up treatment of systemic anthrax after an initial parenteral regimen in neonates up to 4 weeks of age, AAP recommends a dosage of 10 mg/kg every 12 hours in preterm neonates (gestational age 32–37 weeks) and 15 mg/kg every 12 hours in full-term neonates. AAP recommends a dosage of 15 mg/kg (up to 500 mg) every 12 hours when oral ciprofloxacin is used for such follow-up treatment in pediatric patients 1 months of age or older.

Treatment of Uncomplicated Cutaneous Anthrax. If oral ciprofloxacin is used in neonates up to 4 weeks of age for the treatment of uncomplicated cutaneous anthrax† (without systemic involvement) that occurs in the context of biologic warfare or bioterrorism, AAP recommends a dosage of 10 mg/kg every 12 hours in preterm neonates (gestational age 32–37 weeks) and 15 mg/kg every 12 hours in full-term neonates.

If oral ciprofloxacin is used in pediatric patients 1 month of age or older for the treatment of uncomplicated cutaneous anthrax† (without systemic involvement) that occurs in the context of biologic warfare or bioterrorism, AAP recommends a dosage of 15 mg/kg (up to 500 mg) every 12 hours.

If uncomplicated cutaneous anthrax occurred after exposure to aerosolized *B. anthracis* spores in the context of biologic warfare or bioterrorism, anti-infective treatment should be continued for 60 days after onset of the illness. A treatment duration of 7–10 days may be sufficient if uncomplicated cutaneous anthrax occurred as the result of naturally occurring or endemic exposures.

Treatment of Plague. When IV ciprofloxacin is used for the treatment of plague (including pneumonic and septicemic plague) caused by *Yersinia pestis*, the manufacturer recommends that neonates, infants, and children 17 years of age or younger receive a dosage of 10 mg/kg (up to 400 mg) every 8–12 hours.

If oral ciprofloxacin is used for the treatment of plague, the manufacturer recommends that neonates, infants, and children 17 years of age or younger receive a dosage of 15 mg/kg (up to 500 mg) every 8–12 hours.

If ciprofloxacin oral suspension containing 250 mg/5 mL is used for the treatment of plague in neonates, infants, and children 17 years of age or younger, the manufacturer recommends a dosage of 125 mg every 12 hours in those weighing 9–12 kg, 250 mg every 12 hours in those weighing 13–18 kg, 250–375 mg every 12 hours in those weighing 19–24 kg, 375–500 mg every 12 hours in those weighing 25–31 kg, 375–625 mg every 12 hours in those weighing 32–37 kg, and 500–750 mg every 12 hours in those weighing 38 kg or more.

If ciprofloxacin oral suspension containing 500 mg/5 mL is used for the treatment of plague in neonates, infants, and children 17 years of age or younger, the manufacturer recommends a dosage of 250 mg every 12 hours in those weighing 13–24 kg, 250–500 mg every 12 hours in those weighing 25 kg, 500 mg every 12 hours in those weighing 26–37 kg, and 500–750 mg every 12 hours in those weighing 38 kg or more.

Some experts (e.g., US Working Group on Civilian Biodefense, US Army Medical Research Institute of Infectious Diseases [USAMRIID]) recommend that children receive IV ciprofloxacin in a dosage of 15 mg/kg every 12 hours (up to 1 g daily) for the treatment of pneumonic plague that occurs as the result of exposure to *Y. pestis* in the context of biologic warfare or bioterrorism. If oral ciprofloxacin is used for the treatment of plague when the patient's clinical condition improves or when a parenteral regimen is not available (e.g., in mass casualty settings), some experts (e.g., US Working Group on Civilian Biodefense) recommend that children receive 20 mg/kg twice daily (up to 1 g daily).

A parenteral regimen is preferred for initial treatment of plague; an oral regimen can be used after clinical improvement occurs or when a parenteral regimen is not available (e.g., mass casualty setting).

The manufacturer recommends a total treatment duration (IV and oral) of 10–21 days in pediatric patients; some experts state that the total treatment duration should be 10–14 days.

Postexposure Prophylaxis of Plague. When oral ciprofloxacin is used for prophylaxis of plague, the manufacturer recommends that neonates, infants, and children 17 years of age or younger receive a dosage of 15 mg/kg (up to 500 mg) every 8–12 hours for 10–21 days.

If ciprofloxacin oral suspension containing 250 mg/5 mL is used for prophylaxis of plague in neonates, infants, and children 17 years of age or younger, the manufacturer recommends a dosage of 125 mg every 12 hours in those weighing 9–12 kg, 250 mg every 12 hours in those weighing 13–18 kg, 250–375 mg every 12 hours in those weighing 19–24 kg, 375–500 mg every 12 hours in those weighing 25–31 kg, 375–625 mg every 12 hours in those weighing 32–37 kg, and 500–750 mg every 12 hours in those weighing 38 kg or more.

If ciprofloxacin oral suspension containing 500 mg/5 mL is used for the prophylaxis of plague in neonates, infants, and children 17 years of age or younger, the manufacturer recommends a dosage of 250 mg every 12 hours in those weighing 13–24 kg, 250–500 mg every 12 hours in those weighing 25 kg, 500 mg every 12 hours in those weighing 26–37 kg, and 500–750 mg every 12 hours in those weighing 38 kg or more.

If IV ciprofloxacin is used for prophylaxis of plague, the manufacturer recommends that neonates, infants, and children 17 years of age or younger receive a dosage of 10 mg/kg (up to 400 mg) every 8–2 hours for 10–21 days.

Some experts (e.g., US Working Group on Civilian Biodefense, USAMRIID) recommend that children receive oral ciprofloxacin in a dosage of 20 mg/kg twice daily (up to 1 g daily) for postexposure prophylaxis following exposure to *Y. pestis* in the context of biologic warfare or bioterrorism.

Postexposure prophylaxis of plague should be initiated as soon as possible after a suspected or confirmed exposure to *Y. pestis*.

In close contacts of patients with pneumonic plague or individuals exposed to plague aerosol (e.g., in the context of biologic warfare or bioterrorism), prophylaxis should be continued for 7 days or for the duration of the risk of exposure plus 7 days. If fever or cough develops during prophylaxis, the regimen should be switch to that used for treatment of plague.

Treatment of Tularemia. If IV ciprofloxacin is used for the treatment of tularemia† that occurs as the result of exposure to *Francisella tularensis* in the context of biologic warfare or bioterrorism, some experts (e.g., US Working Group on Civilian Biodefense, USAMRIID) recommend that children receive 15 mg/kg every 12 hours (up to 1 g daily) for at least 10–14 days. Oral therapy may be substituted when the patient's condition improves.

If oral ciprofloxacin is used for the treatment of tularemia when the patient's clinical condition improves or if a parenteral regimen is not available, experts recommend that children receive 15 mg/kg twice daily (up to 1 g daily) for a total treatment duration of at least 10–14 days.

Postexposure Prophylaxis of Tularemia. If oral ciprofloxacin is used for postexposure prophylaxis of tularemia† following exposure to *F. tularensis* that occurs in the context of biologic warfare or bioterrorism, some experts (e.g., US Working Group on Civilian Biodefense, USAMRIID) recommend that children receive 15 mg/kg orally twice daily (up to 1 g daily).

Postexposure prophylaxis of tularemia ideally should be initiated within 24 hours of exposure and continued for at least 14 days.

Cystoisospora Infections. If oral ciprofloxacin is used as an alternative for the treatment of infections caused by *Cystoisospora belli*† (formerly *Isospora belli*) in pediatric patients with human immunodeficiency virus (HIV) infection, the recommended dosage is 10–20 mg/kg (up to 500 mg) twice daily for 7 days.

If oral ciprofloxacin is used for chronic maintenance therapy (secondary prophylaxis) of cystoisosporiasis in HIV-infected pediatric patients†, a dosage of 10–20 mg/kg (up to 500 mg) 3 times weekly is recommended. Consideration can be given to discontinuing such prophylaxis in pediatric patients if there is no evidence of active *Cystoisospora* infection and there has been sustained improvement in immunologic status (CDC immunologic category 1 or 2) for more than 6 months in response to antiretroviral therapy.

Meningitis and Other CNS Infections. Although safety and efficacy have not been established, if use of IV ciprofloxacin is considered necessary for the treatment of healthcare-associated ventriculitis and meningitis† caused by susceptible gram-negative bacteria when the drugs of choice cannot be used (see

Cautions: Pediatric Precautions), the Infectious Diseases Society of America (IDSA) recommends that pediatric patients receive a dosage of 30 mg/kg daily given in divided doses every 8–12 hours.

Neisseria meningitidis Infections. If use of ciprofloxacin is considered necessary in children and infants 1 month of age or older to eliminate nasopharyngeal carriage of *Neisseria meningitidis*† or for chemoprophylaxis in household or other close contacts of individuals with invasive meningococcal disease† when other anti-infectives (e.g., rifampin, ceftriaxone) cannot be used (see Cautions: Pediatric Precautions), AAP recommends a single oral dose of 20 mg/kg (up to 500 mg). Ciprofloxacin should be used only if fluoroquinolone-resistant *N. meningitis* have not been identified in the community.

Vibrio Infections. If use of ciprofloxacin is considered necessary in pediatric patients for the treatment of cholera† (see Cautions: Pediatric Precautions), AAP recommends a dosage of 15 mg/kg (up to 500 mg) twice daily for 3 days. Children 2–12 years of age have received a single oral ciprofloxacin dose of 20 mg/kg (up to 750 mg) for the treatment of cholera caused by *V. cholerae* 01 or 0139.

Adult Dosage **Bone and Joint Infections.** If IV ciprofloxacin is used for the treatment of bone and joint infections in adults, the manufacturer recommends a dosage of 400 mg every 8 to 12 hours for 4–8 weeks.

If oral ciprofloxacin is used for the treatment of bone and joint infections in adults, the manufacturer recommends a dosage of 500–750 mg every 12 hours for 4–8 weeks.

For the treatment of native vertebral osteomyelitis, IDSA recommends that IV ciprofloxacin be given in a dosage of 400 mg every 8 hours for 6 weeks for infections caused by *Ps. aeruginosa* or a dosage of 400 mg every 12 hours for the treatment of infections caused by Enterobacteriaceae. If oral ciprofloxacin is used for the treatment of native vertebral osteomyelitis, IDSA recommends a dosage of 750 mg every 12 hours for 6 weeks for infections caused by *Ps. aeruginosa*, 500 mg every 12 hours for 6–8 weeks for infections caused by *Salmonella*, and 500–750 mg every 12 hours for 6 weeks for infections caused by other Enterobacteriaceae.

For the treatment of prosthetic joint infections, IDSA recommends that IV ciprofloxacin be given in a dosage of 400 mg every 12 hours for 4–6 weeks for infections caused by *Ps. aeruginosa* or *Enterobacter*. If oral ciprofloxacin is used for the treatment of prosthetic joint infections, IDSA recommends a dosage of 750 mg twice daily for 4–6 weeks for infections caused by *Ps. aeruginosa* and for infections caused by *Enterobacter* or other Enterobacteriaceae.

Endocarditis. For the treatment of endocarditis† (native or prosthetic valve or other prosthetic material) caused by fastidious gram-negative bacilli of the HACEK group when ceftriaxone (or other third or fourth generation cephalosporin) cannot be used (see Endocarditis Caused by the HACEK Group under Uses: Endocarditis), the American Heart Association (AHA) and IDSA suggest that adults receive IV ciprofloxacin in a dosage of 800 mg daily given in 2 equally divided doses or oral ciprofloxacin in a dosage of 1 g daily given in 2 equally divided doses.

Treatment should be continued for 4 weeks in those with native valve endocarditis or for 6 weeks in those with endocarditis involving prosthetic cardiac valves or other prosthetic cardiac material. Because only limited data are available regarding use of ciprofloxacin for the treatment of these infections, AHA and IDSA recommend that patients with HACEK endocarditis who cannot receive ceftriaxone be treated in consultation with an infectious disease specialist.

Infectious Diarrhea. The usual oral dosage of ciprofloxacin for the treatment of infectious diarrhea in adults is 500 mg every 12 hours for 5–7 days.

Campylobacter Infections. For the treatment of campylobacteriosis caused by susceptible *Campylobacter* in HIV-infected adults, the recommended dosage of oral ciprofloxacin is 500–750 mg every 12 hours. If IV ciprofloxacin is used, the recommended dosage is 400 mg every 12 hours.

The recommended duration of treatment in HIV-infected adults is 7–10 days for gastroenteritis or at least 14 days for bacteremic infections. A duration of 2–6 weeks is recommended for recurrent infections.

Cyclospora Infections. If oral ciprofloxacin is used for the treatment of infections caused by *Cyclospora cayetanensis*†, some clinicians recommend that adults receive 500 mg twice daily for 7 days.

Cystoisospora Infections. If oral ciprofloxacin is used as an alternative for the treatment of infections caused by *C. belli*† (formerly *I. belli*) in HIV-infected adults, the recommended dosage is 500 mg twice daily for 7 days.

If oral ciprofloxacin is used as an alternative for chronic maintenance therapy (secondary prophylaxis) of cystoisosporiasis† in HIV-infected adults with $CD4^+$ T-cell counts less than 200 cells/mm^3, a dosage of 500 mg 3 times weekly is recommended based on limited data. Consideration can be given to discontinuing such prophylaxis if $CD4^+$ T-cell counts exceed 200 cells/mm^3 for more than 6 months in response to antiretroviral therapy.

Salmonella Gastroenteritis. For the treatment of *Salmonella* gastroenteritis† (with or without bacteremia) in HIV-infected adults, the recommended dosage of oral ciprofloxacin is 500–750 mg every 12 hours. Alternatively, 400 mg can be given IV every 12 hours.

The recommended duration of treatment in HIV-infected adults is 7–14 days in those with $CD4^+$ T-cell counts of 200 cells/mm^3 or greater (14 days or longer if the patient is bacteremic or the infection is complicated) or 2–6 weeks in those with $CD4^+$ T-cell counts less than 200 cells/mm^3.

Shigella Infections. For the treatment of shigellosis caused by susceptible *Shigella* in HIV-infected adults, the recommended dosage of oral ciprofloxacin is 500–750 mg every 12 hours. Alternatively, 400 mg can be given IV every 12 hours.

The recommended duration of treatment in HIV-infected adults is 7–10 days for gastroenteritis or at least 14 days for bacteremic infections. Recurrent infections, especially in patients with $CD4^+$ T-cell counts less than 200 cells/mm^3, may require up to 6 weeks of treatment.

Travelers' Diarrhea. If oral ciprofloxacin (conventional tablets or oral suspension) is used for the treatment of travelers' diarrhea† in adults, some clinicians recommend a dosage of 500 once or twice daily for 1–3 days or 750 mg once daily for 1–3 days. Alternatively, if ciprofloxacin extended-release tablets are used, some clinicians recommend a dosage of 500 mg or 1 g once daily for 1–3 days.

If ciprofloxacin is used for empiric treatment of travelers' diarrhea† in HIV-infected adults, an oral dosage of 500–750 mg every 12 hours or IV dosage of 400 mg every 12 hours is recommended. If there is no clinical response after 3–4 days of treatment, stool culture and in vitro susceptibility testing should be considered.

Although the use of anti-infectives for prophylaxis of travelers' diarrhea† generally is discouraged (see Travelers' Diarrhea under Uses: GI Infections), if oral ciprofloxacin (conventional tablets or oral suspension) is used, the recommended adult dosage is 500 mg once daily during the period of risk (not exceeding 2–3 weeks) beginning the day of travel and continuing for 1 or 2 days after leaving the area of risk.

Intra-abdominal Infections. When IV ciprofloxacin is used for the treatment of complicated intra-abdominal infections, the recommended dosage for adults is 400 mg every 12 hours given in conjunction with metronidazole. If oral ciprofloxacin is used for the treatment of complicated intra-abdominal infections, the recommended dosage for adults is 500 mg every 12 hours in conjunction with metronidazole.

The manufacturers recommend a total treatment duration of 7–14 days. IDSA states that the usual duration of treatment for intra-abdominal infections is 4–7 days. A longer duration of treatment has not been associated with improved outcome and is not recommended unless adequate source control is difficult to achieve.

Meningitis and Other CNS Infections. Although efficacy and safety have not been established, some clinicians suggest that adults can receive IV ciprofloxacin in a dosage of 400 mg every 8 hours for the treatment of meningitis† caused by susceptible gram-negative bacteria. Other clinicians recommend a dosage of 800–1200 mg daily for the treatment of meningitis in adults.

If IV ciprofloxacin is used for the treatment of healthcare-associated ventriculitis and meningitis† caused by susceptible gram-negative bacteria when the drugs of choice cannot be used, IDSA recommends that adults receive a dosage of 800–1200 mg daily given in divided doses every 8–12 hours.

Malignant Otitis Externa. If oral ciprofloxacin is used for the treatment of malignant otitis externa†, some clinicians recommend a dosage of 750 mg twice daily. Although there may be rapid relief of symptoms (pain, otorrhea), treatment should be continued for 6–8 weeks.

Because ciprofloxacin-resistant *Pseudomonas aeruginosa* have been isolated from patients with malignant otitis externa with increasing frequency, in vitro susceptibility testing is indicated, especially if there is an inadequate response to treatment.

Acute Sinusitis. If oral ciprofloxacin is used for the treatment of acute sinusitis (see Uses: Respiratory Tract Infections), dosage in adults is 500 mg every 12 hours for 10 days.

The usual IV dosage of ciprofloxacin for the treatment of acute sinusitis in adults is 400 mg every 12 hours for 10 days.

Lower Respiratory Tract Infections. The usual dosage of oral ciprofloxacin for the treatment of lower respiratory tract infections in adults is 500–750 mg every 12 hours for 7–14 days.

The usual IV dosage of ciprofloxacin for the treatment of lower respiratory tract infections in adults is 400 mg every 8 to 12 hours; severe or complicated lower respiratory tract infections should be treated with 400 mg IV every 8 hours. The usual duration of treatment is 7–14 days.

Nosocomial Pneumonia. The usual dosage of IV ciprofloxacin for the treatment of nosocomial pneumonia in adults, including hospital-acquired pneumonia (HAP) not associated with mechanical ventilation and ventilator-associated pneumonia (VAP), is 400 mg every 8 hours.

The manufacturer recommends a treatment duration of 10–14 days. IDSA states that a treatment duration of 7 days is recommended in patients with HAP or VAP; however, a longer or shorter duration may be indicated depending on clinical response.

Skin and Skin Structure Infections. For the treatment of skin and skin structure infections, the usual dosage of oral ciprofloxacin for adults is 500–750 mg every 12 hours for 7–14 days.

The usual IV dosage of ciprofloxacin for the treatment of skin and skin structure infections in adults is 400 mg every 8 to 12 hours for 7–14 days.

Acute, Uncomplicated Cystitis. If ciprofloxacin (conventional tablets or oral suspension) is used for the treatment of acute, uncomplicated cystitis (see Uncomplicated and Complicated Urinary Tract Infections under Uses: Urinary Tract Infections and Prostatitis), dosage in adults is 250 mg every 12 hours for 3 days.

If ciprofloxacin extended-release tablets are used for the treatment of uncomplicated UTIs (acute cystitis) caused by susceptible *E. faecalis*, *Escherichia coli*, *Proteus mirabilis*, or *Staphylococcus saprophyticus* (see Uncomplicated and Complicated Urinary Tract Infections under Uses: Urinary Tract Infections and Prostatitis), the recommended dosage in adults is 500 mg once every 24 hours for 3 days.

Complicated Urinary Tract Infections and Pyelonephritis. The usual oral dosage of ciprofloxacin (conventional tablets or oral suspension) for the treatment of UTIs in adults is 250–500 mg every 12 hours for 7–14 days.

If ciprofloxacin extended-release tablets are used for the treatment of complicated UTIs or acute, uncomplicated pyelonephritis caused by susceptible bacteria, the usual adult dosage is 1 g once every 24 hours for 7–14 days.

The usual IV dosage of ciprofloxacin for the treatment of UTIs in adults is 200–400 mg every 8 to 12 hours for 7–14 days.

Prostatitis. For the treatment of chronic bacterial prostatitis in men, the usual oral dosage of ciprofloxacin (conventional tablets or oral suspension) is 500 mg every 12 hours for 28 days.

The usual IV dosage of ciprofloxacin for the treatment of chronic bacterial prostatitis is 400 mg every 12 hours for 28 days.

Postexposure Prophylaxis of Anthrax. When oral ciprofloxacin is used for inhalational anthrax (postexposure) to reduce the incidence or progression of disease following exposure to aerosolized *B. anthracis* spores in the context of biologic warfare or bioterrorism, adults should receive 500 mg every 12 hours. If IV ciprofloxacin is used for inhalational anthrax (postexposure), adults should receive 400 mg IV every 12 hours.

CDC recommends that adults (including pregnant and postpartum women) receive oral ciprofloxacin in a dosage of 500 mg every 12 hours for postexposure prophylaxis of anthrax.

Postexposure anti-infective prophylaxis should be initiated as soon as possible following suspected or confirmed anthrax exposure.

Because of possible persistence of *B. anthracis* spores in lung tissue following an aerosol exposure, CDC and other experts recommend that anti-infective prophylaxis be continued for 60 days following a confirmed exposure (see Postexposure Prophylaxis of Anthrax under Uses: Anthrax).

For prophylaxis following ingestion of *B. anthracis* spores† in contaminated meat, a ciprofloxacin dosage of 500 mg orally twice daily has been recommended for adults.

If anti-infective prophylaxis is used following a naturally occurring GI exposure to *B. anthracis* (e.g., ingestion of meat from an undercooked carcass of an anthrax-infected animal), ACIP states that a duration of 7–14 days can be considered.

Treatment of Systemic Anthrax. When IV ciprofloxacin is used in a multiple-drug parenteral regimen for initial treatment of systemic anthrax† (inhalational, GI, meningitis, or cutaneous anthrax with systemic involvement, lesions on the head or neck, or extensive edema) that occurs in the context of biologic warfare or bioterrorism, CDC recommends that adults (including pregnant and postpartum women) receive a dosage of 400 mg every 8 hours.

The multiple-drug parenteral regimen should be continued for at least 2–3 weeks until the patient is clinically stable and treatment can be switched to an oral anti-infective. If systemic anthrax occurred as the result of exposure to aerosolized *B. anthracis* spores (e.g., in the context of biologic warfare or bioterrorism), the oral follow-up regimen should be continued until 60 days after onset of the illness.

If oral ciprofloxacin is used for follow-up after an initial parenteral regimen or as an alternative for the treatment of inhalational anthrax† when a parenteral regimen is not available (e.g., when there are supply or logistic problems because large numbers of individuals require treatment in a mass casualty setting), some experts (US Working Group on Civilian Biodefense, USAMRIID) recommend that adults receive an oral dosage of 500 mg every 12 hours.

Treatment of Uncomplicated Cutaneous Anthrax. For the treatment of uncomplicated cutaneous anthrax† (without systemic involvement) that occurs in the context of biologic warfare or bioterrorism, CDC recommends that adults (including pregnant and postpartum women) receive oral ciprofloxacin in a dosage of 500 mg every 12 hours.

If uncomplicated cutaneous anthrax occurred after exposure to aerosolized *B. anthracis* spores in the context of biologic warfare or bioterrorism, anti-infective treatment should be continued for 60 days after onset of the illness. A treatment duration of 3–10 days may be sufficient if uncomplicated cutaneous anthrax occurred as the result of naturally occurring or endemic exposures.

Treatment of GI or Oropharyngeal Anthrax. For treatment of GI and oropharyngeal anthrax† that occurs in the context of biologic warfare or bioterrorism, CDC and other experts (US Working Group on Civilian Biodefense, USAMRIID) recommend that therapy be initiated with the same parenteral multiple-drug regimen recommended for treatment of inhalational anthrax. (See Treatment of Systemic Anthrax under Dosage: Adult Dosage, in Dosage and Administration.)

Brucellosis. For the treatment of brucellosis† caused by *Brucella melitensis*, some clinicians recommend that oral ciprofloxacin be given in a dosage of 500 mg twice daily in conjunction with oral rifampin (600 mg once daily). Oral ciprofloxacin also has been given in a dosage of 500 mg 2 or 3 times daily for 6–12 weeks or 750 mg 3 times daily for 6–8 weeks for the treatment of brucellosis or acute brucella arthritis-diskitis†. Monotherapy or treatment regimens shorter than 4–6 weeks are not recommended.

Chancroid. When oral ciprofloxacin is used in the treatment of chancroid†, CDC recommends that adults receive 500 mg twice daily for 3 days.

Crohn's Disease. Oral ciprofloxacin has been given in a dosage of 500 mg twice daily (with or without metronidazole) for induction of remission of mildly to moderately active Crohn's disease†.

Gonorrhea and Associated Infections. Although ciprofloxacin is no longer recommended for the treatment of gonorrhea (see Uses: Gonorrhea and Associated Infections), the manufacturer recommends a single 250-mg dose of oral ciprofloxacin for the treatment of uncomplicated urethral or endocervical gonorrhea caused by susceptible *Neisseria gonorrhoeae*.

Granuloma Inguinale (Donovanosis). For the treatment of granuloma inguinale† (donovanosis) caused by *Klebsiella granulomatis* (formerly *Calymmatobacterium granulomatis*), 750 mg of oral ciprofloxacin should be given twice daily for at least 3 weeks and until all lesions have completely healed. Consideration can be given to adding a parenteral aminoglycoside (e.g., gentamicin 1 mg/kg IV every 8 hours) if improvement is not evident within the first few days of treatment.

Legionnaires' Disease. For the treatment of Legionnaires' disease†, some clinicians recommend that 500 mg of ciprofloxacin be given orally every 12 hours or 400 mg be given IV every 12 hours for 2–3 weeks.

Mycobacterial Infections. When used in multiple-drug regimens for the treatment of *Mycobacterium avium* complex (MAC) infections†, oral ciprofloxacin has been given to adults in a dosage of 750 mg twice daily.

Neisseria meningitidis Infections. When ciprofloxacin is used to eliminate nasopharyngeal carriage of *N. meningitidis*† or for chemoprophylaxis in household or other close contacts of individuals with invasive meningococcal disease†, adults should receive a single 500-mg oral dose.

Treatment of Plague. When IV ciprofloxacin is used for the treatment of plague caused by *Y. pestis*, the manufacturer recommends that adults receive a dosage of 400 mg every 8 to 12 hours for 14 days.

If oral ciprofloxacin is used for the treatment of plague, the manufacturer recommends that adults receive a dosage of 500–750 mg orally every 12 hours for 14 days.

Some experts (e.g., US Working Group on Civilian Biodefense, USAMRIID) recommend that adults receive a dosage of 400 mg every 12 hours if IV ciprofloxacin is used for as an alternative for the treatment of pneumonic plague that occurs as the result of exposure to *Y. pestis* in the context of biologic warfare or bioterrorism. If oral ciprofloxacin is used for the treatment of plague when the patient's clinical condition improves or when a parenteral regimen is not available (e.g., in mass casualty settings), these experts recommend that adults receive 500–750 mg orally twice daily.

A parenteral regimen is preferred for initial treatment of plague; an oral regimen can be used after clinical improvement occurs or when a parenteral regimen is not available (e.g., mass casualty setting).

The manufacturer recommends a total treatment duration (IV and oral) of 14 days in adults; some experts state that the total treatment duration should be 10–14 days.

Postexposure Prophylaxis of Plague. When oral ciprofloxacin is used for prophylaxis of plague, the manufacturer recommends that adults receive a dosage of 500–750 mg orally every 12 hours for 14 days.

If IV ciprofloxacin is used for prophylaxis of plague, the manufacturer recommends that adults receive a dosage of 400 mg every 8 to 12 hours for 14 days.

Some experts (e.g., US Working Group on Civilian Biodefense, USAMRIID) recommend that oral ciprofloxacin be given in a dosage of 500 mg twice daily if the drug is used for postexposure prophylaxis following exposure to *Y. pestis* in the context of biologic warfare or bioterrorism.

Postexposure prophylaxis of plague should be initiated as soon as possible after a suspected or confirmed exposure to *Y. pestis*.

In close contacts of patients with pneumonic plague or individuals exposed to plague aerosol (e.g., in the context of biologic warfare or bioterrorism), prophylaxis should be continued for 7 days or for the duration of the risk of exposure plus 7 days. If fever or cough develops during prophylaxis, the regimen should be switch to that used for treatment of plague.

Treatment of Tularemia. If IV ciprofloxacin is used for the treatment of tularemia† that occurs as the result of exposure to *F. tularensis* in the context of biologic warfare or bioterrorism, some experts (e.g., US Working Group on Civilian Biodefense, USAMRIID) recommend that adults receive a dosage of 400 mg every 12 hours. Oral therapy may be substituted when the patient's condition improves.

If oral ciprofloxacin is used for the treatment of tularemia when the patient's clinical condition improves or if a parenteral regimen is not available, adults should receive 500 mg orally twice daily.

Postexposure Prophylaxis of Tularemia. If oral ciprofloxacin is used for postexposure prophylaxis of tularemia† following exposure to *F. tularensis* that occurs in the context of biologic warfare or bioterrorism, some experts (e.g., US Working Group on Civilian Biodefense, USAMRIID) recommend that adults receive 500 mg orally every 12 hours.

Postexposure prophylaxis ideally should be initiated within 24 hours of exposure and continued for at least 14 days.

Typhoid Fever and Other Invasive Salmonella Infections. The usual adult oral dosage of ciprofloxacin for the treatment of mild to moderate typhoid fever is 500 mg every 12 hours for 10 days.

Although the optimum dosage and duration of therapy have not been established, oral ciprofloxacin dosages of 750 mg twice daily for 28 days have been used in adults for the treatment of chronic typhoid carriers†.

Vibrio Infections. For the treatment of cholera† caused by *Vibrio cholerae* 01 or 0139, adults have received oral ciprofloxacin in a dosage of 1 g given either as a single dose or in 2 divided doses 12 hours apart.

Perioperative Prophylaxis. If ciprofloxacin is used for perioperative prophylaxis† in high risk patients undergoing genitourinary procedures (see Uses: Perioperative Prophylaxis), some clinicians recommend that a single 500-mg oral dose or a single 400-mg IV dose of ciprofloxacin be given prior to the procedure. If IV ciprofloxacin is used, the dose should be given within 1–2 hours prior to the procedure or initial incision. Postoperative doses generally are unnecessary and should not be used.

Empiric Therapy in Febrile Neutropenic Patients. For empiric anti-infective therapy in febrile neutropenic patients, the manufacturer recommends that adults receive ciprofloxacin in a dosage of 400 mg IV every 8 hours for 7–14 days given in conjunction with piperacillin sodium (50 mg/kg IV every 4 hours, not to exceed 24 g/daily or 300 mg/kg daily; no longer commercially available in the US as a single-entity preparation).

■ Dosage in Renal and Hepatic Impairment

Renal Impairment Dosage adjustments may be necessary when ciprofloxacin is used in adults with renal impairment, especially those with severe impairment.

Dosage recommendations are not available for use of ciprofloxacin in pediatric patients with impaired renal function (creatinine clearances less than 50 mL/minute).

When ciprofloxacin conventional tablets or oral suspension is used in adults, modification of the usual dosage is unnecessary in patients with creatinine clearances exceeding 50 mL/minute. However, dosage should be decreased in adults with creatinine clearances of 50 mL/minute or less. (See Table 1.) The manufacturer states that a dosage of 750 mg administered at the intervals noted in Table 1 may be used with close monitoring in adults with severe infections and severe renal impairment.

Table 1. Dosage of Ciprofloxacin Conventional Tablets or Oral Suspension in Adults with Renal Impairment

Creatinine Clearance (mL/minute)	Dosage
>50	No dosage adjustment
30–50	250–500 mg every 12 hours
5–29	250–500 mg every 18 hours
Hemodialysis or peritoneal dialysis patients	250–500 mg once every 24 hours; give dose after dialysis

Dosage adjustments are not needed when ciprofloxacin 500-mg extended-release tablets are used for the treatment of uncomplicated UTIs (acute cystitis) in adults with renal impairment. However, a decreased dosage of 500 mg once daily is recommended when extended-release tablets are used for the treatment of complicated UTIs or acute uncomplicated pyelonephritis in adults with creatinine clearances of 30 mL/minute or less. (See Table 2.) The maximum dosage of ciprofloxacin extended-release tablets in adults undergoing hemodialysis or peritoneal dialysis (including continuous ambulatory peritoneal dialysis) is 500 mg once daily. The manufacturers state that the 1-g extended-release tablets are *not* recommended in adults who have creatinine clearances of 30 mL/minute or less or are undergoing hemodialysis or peritoneal dialysis.

Table 2. Dosage of Ciprofloxacin Extended-release Tablets in Adults with Renal Impairment

Creatinine Clearance (mL/minute)	Dosage
≤30 (complicated UTIs or acute uncomplicated pyelonephritis)	500 mg once daily
Hemodialysis or peritoneal dialysis patients	Give dose after dialysis period (maximum 500 mg once daily)
Continuous ambulatory peritoneal dialysis	Maximum 500 mg once daily

Dosage adjustments are not needed when IV ciprofloxacin is used in adults with creatinine clearances exceeding 30 mL/minute. However, dosage should be decreased in those with creatinine clearances less than 30 mL/minute. (See Table 3.)

Table 3. Dosage of IV Ciprofloxacin in Adults with Renal Impairment

Creatinine Clearance (mL/minute)	Dosage
>30	No dosage adjustment
5–29	200–400 mg every 18–24 hours

Hepatic Impairment The manufacturers make no specific dosage recommendations for patients with impaired hepatic function. Patients with both hepatic and renal impairment should be carefully monitored. (See Renal Impairment under Dosage and Administration: Dosage in Renal and Hepatic Impairment.)

In preliminary studies in patients with stable chronic liver cirrhosis, no clinically important changes in ciprofloxacin pharmacokinetics were observed; however, the pharmacokinetics of the drug in patients with acute hepatic insufficiency have not been fully studied.

Cautions

Adverse effects reported with ciprofloxacin are similar to those reported with other fluoroquinolone anti-infectives (e.g., gemifloxacin, levofloxacin, moxifloxacin, ofloxacin). Adverse effects have been reported in 5–14% of patients receiving ciprofloxacin, and have been severe enough to require discontinuance in up to 3.5% of patients. The most frequent adverse effects of the drug include nausea, diarrhea, vomiting, abnormal liver function test results and rash.

Systemic fluoroquinolones, including ciprofloxacin, have been associated with disabling and potentially irreversible serious adverse reactions (e.g., tendinitis and tendon rupture, peripheral neuropathy, CNS effects) that can occur together in the same patient. These serious reactions may occur within hours to weeks after a systemic fluoroquinolone is initiated and have occurred in all age groups and in patients without preexisting risk factors for such adverse reactions. (See Cautions: Precautions and Contraindications.)

■ Tendinitis and Tendon Rupture

Systemic fluoroquinolones, including ciprofloxacin, are associated with an increased risk of tendinitis and tendon rupture in all age groups.

The risk of developing fluoroquinolone-associated tendinitis and tendon rupture is increased in older adults (usually those older than 60 years of age), individuals receiving concomitant corticosteroids, and kidney, heart, or lung transplant recipients. Other factors that may independently increase the risk of tendon rupture include strenuous physical activity, renal failure, and previous tendon disorders such as rheumatoid arthritis. However, tendinitis and tendon rupture have been reported in patients receiving fluoroquinolones who did not have any risk factors for such adverse effects.

Fluoroquinolone-associated tendinitis and tendon rupture most frequently involve the Achilles tendon and have also been reported in the rotator cuff (shoulder), hand, biceps, thumb, and other tendon sites. Tendinitis or tendon rupture can occur within hours or days after ciprofloxacin is initiated or as long as several months after completion of therapy and can occur bilaterally.

Ciprofloxacin should be discontinued immediately if pain, swelling, inflammation, or rupture of a tendon occurs. (See Cautions: Precautions and Contraindications.)

■ Peripheral Neuropathy

Systemic fluoroquinolones, including ciprofloxacin, have been associated with an increased risk of peripheral neuropathy.

Sensory or sensorimotor axonal polyneuropathy affecting small and/or large axons resulting in paresthesias, hypoesthesias, dysesthesias, and weakness has been reported in patients receiving systemic fluoroquinolones, including ciprofloxacin. Symptoms may occur soon after initiation of ciprofloxacin and, in some patients, may be irreversible.

Ciprofloxacin should be discontinued immediately if symptoms of peripheral neuropathy (e.g., pain, burning, tingling, numbness, and/or weakness) occur or if there are other alterations in sensations (e.g., light touch, pain, temperature, position sense, vibratory sensation). (See Cautions: Precautions and Contraindications.)

■ CNS Effects

Systemic fluoroquinolones, including ciprofloxacin, have been associated with an increased risk of adverse psychiatric effects, including toxic psychosis, psychotic reactions progressing to suicidal ideations/thoughts, hallucinations, paranoia, depression, self-injurious behavior such as attempted or completed suicide, anxiety, agitation, delirium, confusion, disorientation, disturbances in attention, nervousness, insomnia, nightmares, and memory impairment. These adverse effects may occur after the first dose.

Systemic fluoroquinolones, including ciprofloxacin, have been associated with an increased risk of seizures (convulsions), increased intracranial pressure (including pseudotumor cerebri), dizziness, and tremors. Ciprofloxacin, like other fluoroquinolones, is known to trigger seizures or lower the seizure threshold. Status epilepticus has been reported.

Headache, dizziness, and restlessness have been reported in 1–3% or more of patients receiving ciprofloxacin. Lightheadedness, insomnia, nightmares, hallucinations, paranoia, manic reaction, toxic psychosis, irritability, tremor, ataxia, seizures, lethargy, drowsiness, vertigo, anxiety, nervousness, agitation, confusion, weakness, malaise, phobia, depersonalization, depression, psychotic reactions, suicidal thoughts or acts, paresthesia, and increased intracranial pressure (including pseudotumor cerebri) have also been reported.

Some adverse nervous system effects of ciprofloxacin may be related to the fact that the drug, like other fluoroquinolones, is a γ-aminobutyric acid (GABA) inhibitor. In addition, it has been suggested that some CNS stimulant effects reported in patients receiving the drug may have resulted from ciprofloxacin-induced alterations in caffeine pharmacokinetics. (See Drug Interactions: Xanthine Derivatives.)

If psychiatric or other CNS effects occur during ciprofloxacin therapy, the drug should be discontinued immediately and appropriate measures instituted. (See Cautions: Precautions and Contraindications.)

■ Exacerbation of Myasthenia Gravis

Fluoroquinolones, including ciprofloxacin, have neuromuscular blocking activity and may exacerbate muscle weakness in individuals with myasthenia gravis. Use of fluoroquinolones in myasthenia gravis patients has resulted in requirements for ventilatory support and in death. (See Cautions: Precautions and Contraindications.)

■ Dermatologic and Sensitivity Reactions

Mild, transient rash has been reported in 1–4% and eosinophilia, pruritus, urticaria, cutaneous candidiasis, hyperpigmentation, erythema nodosum, angioedema, and edema of the face, neck, lips, conjunctivae, or hands have been reported in less than 1% of patients. Flushing, fever, and chills also have been reported in less than 1% of patients receiving the drug.

Hypersensitivity Reactions Severe hypersensitivity reactions characterized by rash, fever, eosinophilia, jaundice, and hepatic necrosis and that were fatal have been reported rarely in patients receiving ciprofloxacin and other drugs concomitantly. Toxic epidermal necrolysis (Lyell's syndrome) also has been reported rarely in patients receiving ciprofloxacin. The possibility that these reactions were related to ciprofloxacin therapy could not be excluded. Other serious and occasionally fatal hypersensitivity (anaphylactic and anaphylactoid) reactions have occurred, some with the initial dose, in patients receiving quinolone therapy, including ciprofloxacin.

Some hypersensitivity reactions reported in patients receiving fluoroquinolones, including ciprofloxacin, have been accompanied by cardiovascular collapse, loss of consciousness, paresthesia, pharyngeal or facial edema, dyspnea, urticaria, and/or pruritus.

Other serious and sometimes fatal adverse reactions that have been reported with fluoroquinolones, including ciprofloxacin, and that may or may not be related to hypersensitivity reactions include one of more of the following: fever, rash or severe dermatologic reaction (e.g., toxic epidermal necrolysis, Stevens-Johnson syndrome); vasculitis, arthralgia, myalgia, serum sickness; allergic pneumonitis; interstitial nephritis, acute renal insufficiency or failure; hepatitis, jaundice, acute hepatic necrosis or failure; anemia (including hemolytic and aplastic anemia), thrombocytopenia (including thrombotic thrombocytopenic purpura), leukopenia, agranulocytosis, pancytopenia, and/or other hematologic abnormalities.

Ciprofloxacin should be discontinued immediately at the first appearance of rash, jaundice, or any other sign of hypersensitivity. Appropriate therapy (e.g., epinephrine, corticosteroids, maintenance of an adequate airway, oxygen, maintenance of blood pressure) should be initiated as indicated.

Photosensitivity Reactions Moderate to severe photosensitivity/phototoxicity reactions have been reported in patients receiving fluoroquinolones, including ciprofloxacin.

Phototoxicity may manifest as exaggerated sunburn reactions (e.g., burning, erythema, exudation, vesicles, blistering, edema) on areas exposed to sun or artificial ultraviolet (UV) light (usually the face, neck, extensor surfaces of forearms, dorsa of hands).

Ciprofloxacin should be discontinued if photosensitivity or phototoxicity (sunburn-like reaction, skin eruption) occurs. (See Cautions: Precautions and Contraindications.)

■ Hepatotoxicity

Severe hepatotoxicity, including hepatic necrosis, life-threatening hepatic failure, and fatal events, has been reported in patients receiving ciprofloxacin. Most fatalities have occurred in adults older than 55 years of age.

Acute liver injury has a rapid onset (range 1–39 days) and is often associated with hypersensitivity. The pattern of injury can be hepatocellular, cholestatic, or mixed. Temporary increase in aminotransferase or alkaline phosphatase concentrations or cholestatic jaundice may occur, especially in patients with previous liver damage.

Increased serum concentrations of AST (SGOT) and ALT (SGPT) have been reported in about 2% and increased serum concentrations of alkaline phosphatase, LDH, bilirubin, and γ-glutamyltransferase (GGT, γ-glutamyl transpeptidase, GGTP) have been reported in less than 1% of patients receiving the drug. In addition, fulminant and occasionally fatal hepatic failure has occurred rarely in patients receiving ciprofloxacin.

Ciprofloxacin should be discontinued immediately if any signs or symptoms of hepatitis (e.g., anorexia, jaundice, dark urine, pruritus, tender abdomen) occur. (See Cautions: Precautions and Contraindications.)

■ Aortic Aneurysm and Dissection

Rupture or dissection of aortic aneurysms has been reported in patients receiving systemic fluoroquinolones. Epidemiologic studies indicate an increased risk of aortic aneurysm and dissection within 2 months following use of systemic fluoroquinolones, particularly in elderly patients. The cause for this increased risk has not been identified.

If a patient reports adverse effects suggestive of aortic aneurysm or dissection, fluoroquinolone treatment should be discontinued immediately. (See Cautions: Precautions and Contraindications.)

■ Cardiovascular Effects

Prolonged QT interval leading to ventricular arrhythmias, including torsades de pointes, has been reported with some fluoroquinolones, including ciprofloxacin. Patients with known prolongation of the QT interval or with risk factors for QT interval prolongation or torsades de pointes, patients receiving drugs known to prolong the QT interval (e.g., class IA or III antiarrhythmic agents, tricyclic antidepressants, macrolides, antipsychotics), and geriatric patients may be more susceptible to drug-associated effects on the QT interval. (See Cautions: Precautions and Contraindications.)

Palpitation, atrial flutter, ventricular ectopy, syncope, hypertension, angina pectoris, chest pain, myocardial infarction, cardiopulmonary arrest, and cerebral thrombosis have been reported in less than 1% of patients receiving ciprofloxacin.

■ Hypoglycemia or Hyperglycemia

Systemic fluoroquinolones, including ciprofloxacin, have been associated with alterations in blood glucose concentrations, including symptomatic hypoglycemia and hyperglycemia. Blood glucose disturbances during fluoroquinolone therapy usually have occurred in patients with diabetes mellitus receiving an oral antidiabetic agent (e.g., glyburide) or insulin.

Severe cases of hypoglycemia resulting in coma or death have been reported with some systemic fluoroquinolones. Although most reported cases of hypoglycemic coma have involved patients with risk factors for hypoglycemia,(e.g., older age, diabetes mellitus, renal insufficiency, concomitant use of antidiabetic agents [especially sulfonylureas]), some cases have occurred in patients receiving a fluoroquinolone who were not diabetic and were not reported to be receiving an oral antidiabetic agent or insulin.

If a hypoglycemic reaction occurs, ciprofloxacin should be discontinued and appropriate therapy initiated immediately. (See Cautions: Precautions and Contraindications.)

■ GI Effects

Nausea, diarrhea, vomiting, and abdominal pain/discomfort have been reported in 1–10% of patients receiving ciprofloxacin. These effects generally are mild and transient and occur most frequently in geriatric patients and/or when high dosage is used. Anorexia, dyspepsia, flatulence, GI erosion and bleeding, dysphagia, bad taste, intestinal perforation, painful oral mucosa, and oral candidiasis have been reported in less than 1% of patients receiving the drug.

Effects on Fecal Flora Ciprofloxacin exerts a selective effect on normal bowel flora.

Total bacterial counts of normal anaerobic fecal flora generally are unaffected during or following ciprofloxacin therapy. However, total bacterial counts of normal aerobic fecal flora are decreased within 2–5 days following initiation of therapy with the drug and generally return to pretreatment levels within 1–4 weeks after the drug is discontinued. Ciprofloxacin therapy generally markedly reduces or completely eradicates normal fecal Enterobacteriaceae; the drug reduces fecal aerobic gram-positive bacteria to a lesser extent. Ciprofloxacin therapy does not appear to affect total bacterial counts of normal salivary flora, including streptococci, staphylococci, and anaerobic bacteria.

C. difficile-associated Diarrhea and Colitis Treatment with anti-infectives alters normal colon flora and may permit overgrowth of *Clostridioides difficile* (formerly known as *Clostridium difficile*.

C. difficile infection (CDI) and *C. difficile*-associated diarrhea and colitis (CDAD; also known as antibiotic-associated diarrhea and colitis or pseudomembranous colitis) have been reported with nearly all anti-infectives, including ciprofloxacin, and may range in severity from mild diarrhea to fatal colitis. *C. difficile* produces toxins A and B, which contribute to the development of CDAD; hypertoxin-producing strains of *C. difficile* are associated with increased morbidity and mortality since they may be refractory to anti-infectives and colectomy may be required. (See Superinfection/C. difficile-associated Diarrhea and Colitis under Cautions: Precautions and Contraindications.)

C. difficile generally is resistant to ciprofloxacin. When fluoroquinolones were first marketed, there appeared to be a relative lack of association between use of the drugs and CDAD and the risk of CDAD appeared to be lower than that reported with some other anti-infectives. However, there now is some evidence that increasing use of the drugs may have resulted in emergence of *C. difficile* that are more resistant and/or more virulent than previous strains. Outbreaks of severe CDAD caused by fluoroquinolone-resistant *C. difficile* have been reported in US health-care facilities with increasing frequency over the last several years. Many of these CDAD cases occurred in patients who had received a fluoroquinolone (ciprofloxacin, gatifloxacin [no longer commercially available in the US], levofloxacin, moxifloxacin) or cephalosporin within the prior 4–6 weeks.

■ Genitourinary Effects

Increased serum creatinine and BUN concentrations have occurred in about 1% of patients receiving ciprofloxacin. Interstitial nephritis, nephritis, renal failure, dysuria, polyuria, urinary retention, albuminuria, urethral bleeding, vaginitis, and acidosis have been reported in less than 1% of patients receiving the drug. In at least one patient, acute renal failure associated with interstitial nephritis occurred within about 2 weeks after initiating ciprofloxacin and appeared to be a hypersensitivity reaction to ciprofloxacin; renal biopsy showed marked interstitial edema, with extensive lymphocytic infiltrations and occasional eosinophils.

Crystalluria, cylindruria, and hematuria have been reported rarely in patients receiving ciprofloxacin. Crystalluria generally occurs in patients with alkaline urine who receive high dosage of the drug, and has not been associated with changes in renal function. The risk of crystal formation and crystalluria in patients receiving usual recommended dosages of the drug (250–750 mg) is low if urine pH is within the usual range (i.e., less than 6.8). Patients receiving the drug, particularly at relatively high dosages, should maintain adequate fluid intake; in addition, alkaline urine should be avoided. (See Other Precautions and Contraindications under Cautions: Precautions and Contraindications.) Crystalluria, sometimes associated with nephropathy, occurs in animals receiving ciprofloxacin. This may be related to the fact that ciprofloxacin has reduced solubility under alkaline conditions and the urine of test animals (e.g., rats, monkeys) is predominantly alkaline. In studies in rhesus monkeys, crystalluria (without evidence of nephropathy) has occurred after a single oral ciprofloxacin dose as low as 5 mg/kg (approximately 0.07 times the highest recommended therapeutic dosage based on body surface area [BSA]). Nephropathy did not occur when these monkeys received 6 months of IV ciprofloxacin at a dosage of 10 mg/kg daily; however, nephropathy occurred after 6 months of therapy at a dosage of 20 mg/kg daily (approximately 0.2 times the highest recommended therapeutic dosage based on BSA).

■ Musculoskeletal Effects

Arthralgia, joint or back pain, joint inflammation, joint stiffness, achiness, vasculitis, neck or chest pain, and flare-up of gout have been reported in less than 1% of patients receiving ciprofloxacin.

An increased incidence of musculoskeletal disorders related to joints and/

or surrounding tissues (e.g., arthralgia, abnormal gait, abnormal joint exam, joint sprains, leg pain, back pain, arthrosis, bone pain, myalgia, arm pain, decreased range of motion in a joint) has been reported in pediatric patients receiving ciprofloxacin. These events usually were mild to moderate in intensity and those that occurred by week 6 usually resolved (clinical resolution of signs and symptoms) within 30 days after treatment ended.

Fluoroquinolones, including ciprofloxacin, cause arthropathies (arthrosis) in immature animals of various species. (See Cautions: Pediatric Precautions.) In young beagles, ciprofloxacin given in a dosage of 100 mg/kg daily for 4 weeks caused degenerative articular changes of the knee joint; in a daily dosage of 30 mg/kg, effects on the joint were minimal, although some damage to weight-bearing joints was observed even at the lower dosage. In another study, removal of weight bearing from the joint reduced the lesions, but did not totally prevent them. In a subsequent study in young beagle dogs, oral ciprofloxacin in a dosage of 30 mg/kg or 90 mg/kg daily for 2 weeks (approximately 1.3 or 3.5 times the pediatric dosage based on comparative plasma AUCs) caused articular changes that were still evident on histologic evaluation after a treatment-free period of 5 months. However, a dosage of 10 mg/kg (approximately 0.6 times the pediatric dosage based on comparative plasma AUCs) had no effects on joints and was not associated with arthrotoxicity after an additional treatment-free period of 5 months.

Morphologic changes observed in animals with quinolone-induced arthropathies include erosions in joint cartilage accompanied by noninflammatory, cell-free effusion of the joint space; the cartilage is incapable of regeneration and may serve as a site for the development of arthropathy deformans. In addition, breakdown products of the cartilage may irritate the synovia. The relationship of these effects in animals and the rheumatologic symptoms associated with use of ciprofloxacin in humans is unknown.

■ Hematologic Effects Eosinophilia, leukopenia, neutropenia, increased or decreased platelet count, and pancytopenia have been reported in less than 1% of patients receiving ciprofloxacin.Anemia, decreased hemoglobin, increased monocytes, leukocytosis, and bleeding diathesis have been reported in less than 1% of patients receiving the drug. In at least one patient, decreased hemoglobin was associated with GI bleeding, although there was no evidence of such bleeding in some other patients with hemoglobin reductions. In addition, transient acquired von Willebrand's disease has been reported rarely in patients receiving ciprofloxacin; factor VIII concentration returned to normal values several months (i.e., 5–6 months) following discontinuance of the drug in these patients.

■ Local Effects Local adverse effects have been reported at the site of infusion following IV administration of ciprofloxacin. These reactions generally resolve rapidly after completion of the infusion and have been reported most frequently when IV infusions of the drug were given over 30 minutes or less. The manufacturers state that adverse local reactions to IV ciprofloxacin do not contraindicate subsequent IV administration of the drug, unless the reactions recur or worsen.

■ Other Adverse Effects Epistaxis, laryngeal or pulmonary edema, hiccups, hemoptysis, dyspnea, bronchospasm, and pulmonary embolism have been reported in less than 1% of patients receiving ciprofloxacin.

Blurred vision, disturbed vision (e.g., change in color perception, overbrightness of lights), decreased visual acuity, diplopia, and eye pain have been reported in less than 1% of patients receiving ciprofloxacin. Although reported with some other quinolones, there has been no evidence of ocular toxicity in animal studies using ciprofloxacin. Tinnitus, increased serum amylase, and increased serum uric acid concentrations have been reported rarely (i.e., in less than 0.1% of patients).

■ Adverse Effects Reported when Used for Inhalational Anthrax (Postexposure) Some information regarding the safety of ciprofloxacin for long-term postexposure prophylaxis of anthrax are available based on use of the drug in the fall of 2001 following bioterrorism-related exposures to *Bacillus anthracis* spores. Among individuals surveyed by the US Centers for Disease Control and Prevention (CDC), adverse GI effects (nausea, vomiting, diarrhea, stomach pain), neurologic effects (problems sleeping, nightmares, headache, dizziness, lightheadedness), and musculoskeletal effects (muscle or tendon pain and joint swelling or pain) were reported more frequently than in controlled clinical studies evaluating the drug for other indications. This higher incidence in the absence of a control group could be the result of report bias, concurrent medical conditions, other concomitant drug therapy, emotional stress or other confounding factors, and/or the long duration of ciprofloxacin treatment required for prophylaxis. In response to a questionnaire given to 490 such individuals in Florida on approximately day 7 or 14 of anti-infective prophylaxis, 19% sought medical attention for any anti-infective related adverse effect or reported one or more of the following: pruritus, breathing problems, or swelling of the face, neck, or throat. Although the percentage of patients in this subgroup who received ciprofloxacin versus other anti-infectives was not reported, 86% of all patients (i.e., those who did or did not answer the questionnaire) received ciprofloxacin and 80% continued to receive prophylaxis beyond 14 days.

In an epidemiologic evaluation in 8424 postal workers who were offered 60 days of prophylaxis for anthrax and given a questionnaire in New Jersey, New York City, and the District of Columbia on days 7–10 of anti-infective prophylaxis, 5819 completed or were administered the questionnaire, of whom 3863 had initiated prophylaxis (3428 with ciprofloxacin). Of the ciprofloxacin-treated individuals, 19% reported severe nausea, vomiting, diarrhea, and/or abdominal pain; 14% reported fainting, lightheadedness, and/or dizziness; 7% reported heartburn or acid reflux; 6% reported rash, urticaria, and/or pruritus; and 8% discontinued therapy with the drug (3% for adverse effects, 1% for fear of developing an adverse effect, and 1% because they were confused about the need). Only 2% of those on any anti-infective sought medical attention for possible manifestations of anaphylaxis, none of whom required hospitalization.

■ Precautions and Contraindications Ciprofloxacin is contraindicated in patients with a history of hypersensitivity to the drug, other quinolones, or any ingredient in the formulation.

Systemic fluoroquinolones, including ciprofloxacin, have been associated with disabling and potentially irreversible serious adverse reactions (e.g., tendinitis and tendon rupture, peripheral neuropathy, CNS effects) that can occur together in the same patient. These serious reactions may occur within hours to weeks after a systemic fluoroquinolone is initiated and have occurred in all age groups and in patients without preexisting risk factors for such adverse reactions. Patients receiving ciprofloxacin should be informed about these serious adverse reactions and advised to immediately discontinue ciprofloxacin and contact a clinician if they experience any signs or symptoms of serious adverse effects (e.g., unusual joint or tendon pain, muscle weakness, a "pins and needles" tingling or pricking sensation, numbness of the arms or legs, confusion, hallucinations) while taking the drug. Systemic fluoroquinolones, including ciprofloxacin, should be avoided in patients who have experienced any of the serious adverse reactions associated with fluoroquinolones.

Because fluoroquinolones, including ciprofloxacin, are associated with an increased risk of tendinitis and tendon rupture in all age groups (see Cautions: Tendinitis and Tendon Rupture), patients receiving ciprofloxacin should be informed of this potentially irreversible adverse effect and the drug should be discontinued immediately if pain, swelling, inflammation, or rupture of a tendon occurs. The risk of developing fluoroquinolone-associated tendinitis and tendon rupture is increased in adults older than 60 years of age, individuals receiving concomitant corticosteroids, and kidney, heart, or lung transplant recipients. (See Cautions: Geriatric Precautions and see Drug Interactions: Corticosteroids.) Patients should be advised to rest and refrain from exercise at the first sign of tendinitis or tendon rupture (e.g., pain, swelling, or inflammation of a tendon or weakness or inability to use a joint) and advised to immediately discontinue the drug and contact a clinician. Systemic fluoroquinolones, including ciprofloxacin, should be avoided in patients who have a history of tendon disorders or have experienced tendinitis or tendon rupture.

Because fluoroquinolones, including ciprofloxacin, are associated with an increased risk of peripheral neuropathy (see Cautions: Peripheral Neuropathy), ciprofloxacin should be discontinued immediately if symptoms of peripheral neuropathy (e.g., pain, burning, tingling, numbness, and/or weakness) occur or if there are other alterations in sensations (e.g., light touch, pain, temperature, position sense, vibratory sensation) and/or motor strength since this may minimize development of an irreversible condition. Patients receiving ciprofloxacin should be advised that peripheral neuropathies have been reported in patients receiving systemic fluoroquinolones, including ciprofloxacin, and that symptoms may occur soon after initiation of therapy and, in some patients, may be irreversible. Patients should be advised of the importance of immediately discontinuing the drug and contacting a clinician if such symptoms occur. Systemic fluoroquinolones, including ciprofloxacin, should be avoided in patients who have experienced peripheral neuropathy.

Because fluoroquinolones, including ciprofloxacin, have been associated with an increased risk of adverse CNS effects (see Cautions: CNS Effects), ciprofloxacin should be used with caution in epileptic patients, in patients with known or suspected CNS disorders that predispose to seizures or lower the seizure threshold (e.g., severe cerebral arteriosclerosis, history of convulsions, reduced cerebral blood flow, altered brain structure, stroke), and in the presence of other risk factors that predispose to seizures or lower the seizure threshold (e.g., certain drug therapies, renal dysfunction). Patients should be informed that seizures have been reported in patients receiving ciprofloxacin and advised to inform their clinician of any history of seizures before initiating therapy with the drug. Because increased intracranial pressure has been reported, patients receiving ciprofloxacin should be advised to notify their clinician if persistent headache (with or without blurred vision) occurs. Patients receiving ciprofloxacin also should be advised that ciprofloxacin may cause dizziness or lightheadedness and cautioned not to engage in activities requiring mental alertness and motor coordination (e.g., driving or operating machinery) until they experience how the drug affects them. If seizures or other CNS effects occur, ciprofloxacin should be discontinued immediately and appropriate measures instituted. Systemic fluoroquinolones, including ciprofloxacin, should be avoided in patients who have experienced CNS effects associated with fluoroquinolones.

Ciprofloxacin should be avoided in patients with a known history of myasthenia gravis since fluoroquinolones may exacerbate myasthenia gravis symptoms. Patients should be advised of the importance of informing their clinician of any history of myasthenia gravis. Patients also should be advised to immediately contact a clinician if any symptoms of muscle weakness, including respiratory difficulties, occur.

Because severe hepatotoxicity, including acute hepatitis and fatalities, has been reported in patients receiving ciprofloxacin, the drug should be discontinued immediately if any sign or symptom of hepatitis (e.g., anorexia, jaundice, dark urine, pruritus, tender abdomen) occurs. Patients should be advised to contact their clinician if any sign or symptom of hepatotoxicity (e.g., loss of appetite, nausea, vomiting, fever, weakness, tiredness, right upper quadrant tenderness, itching, yellowing of skin or eyes, light colored bowel movements, dark colored urine) occurs.

Because an increased risk of aortic aneurysm and dissection has been reported with systemic fluoroquinolones, ciprofloxacin should not be used in patients who have an aortic aneurysm or are at increased risk for an aortic aneurysm unless there are no other treatment options. This includes elderly patients and patients with peripheral atherosclerotic vascular disease, hypertension, or certain genetic conditions (e.g., Marfan syndrome, Ehlers-Danlos syndrome). Patients should be informed that systemic fluoroquinolones may increase the risk of aortic aneurysm and dissection and of the importance of informing their clinician of any history of aneurysms, blockages or hardening of the arteries, high blood pressure, or genetic conditions such as Marfan syndrome or Ehlers-Danlos syndrome. Patients receiving ciprofloxacin should be advised to seek immediate medical treatment if they experience sudden, severe, and constant pain in the stomach, chest, or back.

Because prolongation of the QT interval has been reported in patients receiving ciprofloxacin, the drug should be avoided in patients with known prolongation of the QT interval or with risk factors for QT interval prolongation or torsades de pointes (e.g., congenital long QT syndrome, uncorrected electrolyte imbalance such as hypokalemia or hypomagnesemia, cardiac disease such as heart failure, myocardial infarction, or bradycardia). Ciprofloxacin also should be avoided in patients receiving drugs known to prolong the QT interval, including class IA antiarrhythmic agents (quinidine, procainamide), class III antiarrhythmic agents (amiodarone, sotalol), tricyclic antidepressants, macrolides, and antipsychotics. (See Drug Interactions: Drugs that Prolong the QT Interval.) Patients should be advised of the importance of informing their clinician of a personal or family history of QT interval prolongation or proarrhythmic conditions (e.g., hypokalemia, bradycardia, recent myocardial ischemia) or current therapy with any class IA (e.g., quinidine, procainamide) or class III (amiodarone, sotalol) antiarrhythmic agents; patients should be advised to contact their clinician if any symptoms of prolongation of QT interval, including prolonged heart palpitations or loss of consciousness, occur.

Blood glucose concentrations should be carefully monitored when systemic fluoroquinolones, including ciprofloxacin, are used in patients with diabetes mellitus receiving antidiabetic agents. Patients should be informed that hypoglycemia has been reported when systemic fluoroquinolones were used in some patients receiving antidiabetic agents. Patients with diabetes mellitus receiving oral antidiabetic agents or insulin should be advised to discontinue ciprofloxacin and contact a clinician if they experience hypoglycemia or symptoms of hypoglycemia. Appropriate therapy should be initiated immediately.

Ciprofloxacin inhibits cytochrome P-450 (CYP) isoenzyme 1A2, and concomitant use with drugs metabolized by this enzyme (e.g., clozapine, methylxanthines [e.g., caffeine, theophylline], olanzapine, ropinirole, tizanidine) may result in increased plasma concentrations of the concomitant drug and could lead to clinically important adverse effects. Because of an increased risk of adverse effects, ciprofloxacin is contraindicated in patients receiving tizanidine. Concomitant use with theophylline should be avoided since serious and sometimes fatal reactions (e.g., cardiac arrest, seizures, status epilepticus, respiratory failure) have occurred in patients receiving the drugs concomitantly. In addition, concomitant use of ciprofloxacin and other drugs metabolized by CYP1A2 should be avoided or requires particular caution. (See Drug Interactions.)

Sensitivity Reactions Ciprofloxacin, like other quinolones, can cause serious, potentially fatal hypersensitivity reactions, occasionally following the initial dose. (See Cautions: Dermatologic and Sensitivity Reactions.) Patients receiving ciprofloxacin should be advised of this possibility and instructed to immediately discontinue the drug and contact a clinician at the first sign of rash, hives, other skin reaction, jaundice, rapid heartbeat, difficulty swallowing or breathing, any swelling suggesting angioedema (e.g., swelling of lips, tongue, or face; tightness of throat; hoarseness), or any other sign of hypersensitivity. Serious anaphylactic reactions require immediate emergency treatment with epinephrine and other resuscitation measures (e.g., oxygen, IV fluids, IV antihistamines, corticosteroids, pressor amines, airway management such as intubation) as indicated.

Because photosensitivity/phototoxicity reactions have been reported with fluoroquinolones, unnecessary or excessive exposure to sunlight or artificial UV light (sunlamps, tanning beds, UVA/UVB treatment) should be avoided during ciprofloxacin therapy. If the patient needs to be outdoors, they should use sunscreen and wear a hat and clothing that protects skin from sun exposure. Patients should be advised to discontinue ciprofloxacin and contact a clinician if photosensitivity or phototoxicity (sunburn-like reaction, skin eruption) occurs.

Selection and Use of Anti-infectives Ciprofloxacin should be used for the treatment of acute bacterial sinusitis, acute bacterial exacerbations of chronic bronchitis, or uncomplicated urinary tract infections (UTIs) *only* when no other treatment options are available. Because ciprofloxacin, like other systemic fluoroquinolones, has been associated with disabling and potentially irreversible serious adverse reactions (e.g., tendinitis and tendon rupture, peripheral neuropathy, CNS effects) that can occur together in the same patient, the risks of serious adverse reactions outweigh the benefits of ciprofloxacin for patients with these infections.

To reduce development of drug-resistant bacteria and maintain effectiveness of ciprofloxacin and other antibacterials, the drug should be used only for the treatment or prevention of infections proven or strongly suspected to be caused by susceptible bacteria.

Patients should be advised that antibacterials (including ciprofloxacin) should only be used to treat bacterial infections and not used to treat viral infections (e.g., the common cold). Patients also should be advised about the importance of completing the full course of therapy, even if feeling better after a few days, and that skipping doses or not completing therapy may decrease effectiveness and increase the likelihood that bacteria will develop resistance and will not be treatable with ciprofloxacin or other antibacterials in the future.

When selecting or modifying anti-infective therapy, use results of culture and in vitro susceptibility testing. In the absence of such data, consider local epidemiology and susceptibility patterns when selecting anti-infectives for empiric therapy. Culture and susceptibility testing performed periodically during therapy provides information on the therapeutic effect of the anti-infective agent and the possible emergence of bacterial resistance.

Information on test methods and quality control standards for in vitro susceptibility testing of antibacterial agents and specific interpretive criteria for such testing recognized by FDA is available at https://www.fda.gov/STIC.

Superinfection/C. difficile-associated Diarrhea and Colitis As with other anti-infectives, use of ciprofloxacin may result in overgrowth of nonsusceptible organisms, especially enterococci or *Candida*. Resistant strains of some organisms (e.g., *Pseudomonas aeruginosa*, staphylococci) have developed during ciprofloxacin therapy. Careful monitoring of the patient and periodic in vitro susceptibility tests are essential.

Because CDAD has been reported with the use of nearly all anti-infectives, including ciprofloxacin, it should be considered in the differential diagnosis in patients who develop diarrhea during or after ciprofloxacin therapy. Careful medical history is necessary since CDAD has been reported to occur as late as 2 months or longer after anti-infective therapy is discontinued.

If CDAD is suspected or confirmed, anti-infective therapy not directed against *C. difficile* should be discontinued as soon as possible. Patients should be managed with appropriate anti-infective therapy directed against *C. difficile* (e.g., vancomycin, fidaxomicin, metronidazole), supportive therapy (e.g., fluid and electrolyte management, protein supplementation), and surgical evaluation as clinically indicated.

Patients should be advised that diarrhea is a common problem caused by anti-infectives and usually ends when the drug is discontinued; however, it is important to contact a clinician if watery and bloody stools (with or without stomach cramps and fever) occur during or as late as 2 months or longer after the last dose.

Other Precautions and Contraindications Crystalluria has been reported rarely in patients receiving ciprofloxacin. Although crystalluria is not expected to occur under usual conditions with the usual recommended dosages of the drug, patients should be instructed to drink sufficient quantities of fluids to ensure proper hydration and adequate urinary output during ciprofloxacin therapy. Measures also should be taken to avoid alkaline urine.

Ciprofloxacin has *not* been shown to be effective in the treatment of syphilis. Because use of anti-infectives given in high dosage for short periods of time to treat gonorrhea may mask or delay symptoms of incubating syphilis, serologic tests for syphilis should be performed at the time of diagnosis of gonorrhea. If ciprofloxacin is used for the treatment of gonorrhea (see Uses: Gonorrhea and Associated Infections), follow-up serologic tests for syphilis should be performed 3 months after gonorrhea treatment is completed.

Doses and/or frequency of administration of ciprofloxacin should be decreased in patients with severe renal impairment since serum concentrations of the drug are higher and prolonged in these patients compared with patients with normal renal function. (See Dosage and Administration: Dosage in Renal and Hepatic Impairment.)

■ **Pediatric Precautions** Ciprofloxacin, like other fluoroquinolones, is associated with arthropathy and histopathologic changes in weight-bearing joints of juvenile animals. Oral ciprofloxacin caused lameness in immature dogs; histologic evaluation of the weight-bearing joints of these dogs revealed permanent lesions of the cartilage. When used in pediatric patients younger than 18 years of age, ciprofloxacin has been associated with an increased rate of adverse effects involving joints and/or surrounding tissue (e.g., tendons) compared with comparator anti-infectives. (See Cautions: Musculoskeletal Effects.)

The manufacturers state that ciprofloxacin (IV, conventional tablets, oral suspension) should be used in pediatric patients younger than 18 years of age *only* for the treatment of complicated UTIs and pyelonephritis caused by susceptible *Escherichia coli*, inhalational anthrax (postexposure), and treatment and prophylaxis of plague. However, the American Academy of Pediatrics (AAP) and other experts (e.g., the American Heart Association [AHA], Infectious Diseases Society of America [IDSA]) state that use of fluoroquinolones in pediatric patients younger than 18 years of age also may be justified in certain other infections (e.g., endocarditis, multidrug-resistant gram-negative infections). (See Other Infections under Cautions: Pediatric Precautions.) Parents should be advised to inform their child's clinician if the child has a history of joint-related problems present before ciprofloxacin is initiated or if such problems occur during or after therapy with the drug.

Ciprofloxacin extended-release tablets should *not* be used in children and adolescents younger than 18 years of age since safety and efficacy of the extended-release preparation have *not* been established for any indication in pediatric patients.

Urinary Tract Infections Ciprofloxacin (IV, conventional tablets, oral suspension) is labeled by FDA for the treatment of complicated UTIs and pyelonephritis caused by susceptible *E. coli* in pediatric patients 1–17 years of age. However, ciprofloxacin is not considered a drug of first choice for these infections in pediatric patients because an increased incidence of adverse effects has been reported in such patients. In clinical studies evaluating IV or oral ciprofloxacin for the treatment of complicated UTIs and pyelonephritis in pediatric patients 1–17 years of age, the rate of adverse effects (including events related to joints and/or surrounding tissues) occurring during 6 weeks of follow-up was 9.3% in those receiving ciprofloxacin compared with 6% in those receiving a cephalosporin. The rate of adverse effects occurring at any time up to 1 year was 13.7% or 9.5%, respectively and the rate of all adverse effects (regardless of drug relationship) at 6 weeks was 41 or 31%, respectively.

Anthrax Ciprofloxacin (IV, conventional tablets, oral suspension) is labeled by FDA for inhalational anthrax (postexposure) to reduce the incidence or progression of disease following exposure to aerosolized *Bacillus anthracis* spores in pediatric patients from birth to 17 years of age. The manufacturers state that risk-benefit assessment indicates that use of ciprofloxacin is appropriate for this indication in pediatric patients. AAP states that ciprofloxacin is a drug of choice for postexposure prophylaxis of anthrax in pediatric patients. Because of potential adverse effects from prolonged use of ciprofloxacin in pediatric patients and because postexposure prophylaxis should be continued for 60 days following exposures to aerosolized *B. anthracis* spores that occur in the context of biologic warfare or bioterrorism, the postexposure prophylaxis regimen can be changed to oral amoxicillin or oral penicillin V if penicillin susceptibility is confirmed.

AAP states that oral ciprofloxacin is a drug of choice for the treatment of cutaneous anthrax without systemic involvement† in pediatric patients. Because of potential adverse effects from prolonged use of ciprofloxacin in pediatric patients and because a treatment duration of 60 days is recommended when cutaneous anthrax occurs following exposures to aerosolized *B. anthracis* spores that occur in the context of biologic warfare or bioterrorism, the treatment regimen can be changed to oral amoxicillin or oral penicillin V if penicillin susceptibility is confirmed.

IV ciprofloxacin also is considered a drug of choice for use in multiple-drug parenteral regimens for initial treatment of systemic anthrax† (inhalational, GI, meningitis, or cutaneous with systemic involvement, extensive edema, or head or neck lesions) that occurs in the context of biologic warfare or bioterrorism. Because of potential adverse effects from prolonged use of ciprofloxacin in pediatric patients, IV penicillin G or IV ampicillin can replace IV ciprofloxacin in the multiple-drug regimen if penicillin susceptibility is confirmed.

Plague Ciprofloxacin (IV, conventional tablets, oral suspension) is labeled by FDA for treatment of plague, including pneumonic and septicemic plague, and for prophylaxis of plague in pediatric patients from birth to 17 years of age. The manufacturers state that risk-benefit assessment indicates that use of ciprofloxacin is appropriate for this indication in pediatric patients.

Other Infections Some clinicians suggest that quinolones may be used cautiously in adolescents if skeletal growth is complete, and that the potential benefits of ciprofloxacin therapy may outweigh the possible risks in certain children 9–18 years of age with serious infections when the causative organism is resistant to other available anti-infectives.

AAP states that use of a systemic fluoroquinolone may be justified in children younger than 18 years of age in certain specific circumstances when there are no safe and effective alternatives and the drug is known to be effective. AAP states that use of fluoroquinolones may be justified in pediatric patients when parenteral therapy is not practical and no other safe and effective oral agent is available or when the pediatric patient has an infection caused by a multidrug-resistant organism (e.g., *Pseudomonas*, *Mycobacterium*) for which there is no safe and effective alternative. Therefore, in addition to use after exposure to aerosolized *B. anthracis* (to decrease the incidence or progression of the disease), other possible uses of fluoroquinolones in pediatric patients include the treatment of urinary tract infections caused by *Ps. aeruginosa* or other multidrug-resistant gram-negative bacteria, infections caused by multidrug-resistant *Streptococcus pneumoniae*, chronic suppurative otitis media or malignant otitis externa caused by *Ps. aeruginosa*, chronic or acute osteomyelitis or osteochondritis caused by *Ps. aeruginosa* or other multidrug-resistant gram-negative bacteria known to be susceptible to fluoroquinolones and resistant to other alternatives, mycobacterial infections caused by isolates known to be susceptible to fluoroquinolones, gram-negative bacterial infections in immunocompromised patients when oral therapy is desired or when the causative agent is resistant to other alternatives, GI infections known or suspected to be caused by multidrug-resistant *Shigella*, *Salmonella*, *Vibrio cholerae*, or *Campylobacter*, or serious infections caused by fluoroquinolone-susceptible pathogens in pediatric patients with severe allergy to alternative anti-infectives.

■ Geriatric Precautions

Retrospective analysis of 23 multiple-dose controlled clinical studies evaluating ciprofloxacin in over 3500 patients revealed that 25% of patients included in these studies were 65 years of age or older and 10% were 75 years of age or older. In a large, prospective, randomized study evaluating use of ciprofloxacin extended-release tablets for treatment of complicated UTIs, 49% of patients were 65 years of age or older and 30% were 75 years of age or older. Although no overall differences in safety or efficacy were observed between geriatric individuals and younger adults in these studies and other clinical experience revealed no evidence of age-related differences, the possibility that some older patients may exhibit increased sensitivity to the drug cannot be ruled out.

The risk of fluoroquinolone-associated tendon disorders, including tendon rupture, is increased in geriatric adults older than 60 years of age. This risk is further increased in those receiving concomitant corticosteroids. (See Cautions: Precautions and Contraindications.) Ciprofloxacin should be used with caution in geriatric adults, especially those receiving concomitant corticosteroids.

The risk of prolonged QT interval leading to ventricular arrhythmias may be increased in geriatric patients. Ciprofloxacin should be used with caution in those receiving concurrent therapy with drugs that can prolong the QT interval (e.g., class IA or III antiarrhythmic agents) or those with risk factors for torsades de pointes (e.g., known QT prolongation, uncorrected hypokalemia).

The risk of fluoroquinolone-associated aortic aneurysm and dissection may be increased in geriatric patients. (See Cautions: Aortic Aneurysm and Dissection.)

Ciprofloxacin is substantially eliminated by the kidney, and the risk of adverse reactions may be greater in patients with impaired renal function. Although dosage of ciprofloxacin does not need to be modified in individuals older than 65 years of age with normal renal function, the greater frequency of decreased renal function observed in the elderly should be considered and dosage carefully selected in geriatric patients; monitoring renal function may be useful in these patients.

■ Mutagenicity and Carcinogenicity

Ciprofloxacin was not mutagenic in vivo in the rat hepatocyte DNA repair assay or dominant lethal or micronucleus tests in mice. Although ciprofloxacin was positive for mutagenicity in vitro in the mouse lymphoma cell forward mutation assay and rat hepatocyte DNA repair assay, the drug was not mutagenic in other in vitro studies, including the *Salmonella* microsome test, mouse lymphoma cell forward mutation assay, *Escherichia coli* DNA repair assay, Chinese hamster V-79 cell HGPRT test, Syrian hamster embryo cell transformation assay, *Saccharomyces cerevisiae* point mutation assay, and *S. cerevisiae* mitotic crossover and gene conversion assay.

In 2-year carcinogenicity studies in rats or mice, there was no evidence of carcinogenic or tumorigenic potential with oral ciprofloxacin in a dosage of 250 or 750 mg/kg daily (equivalent to approximately 2 or 3 times, respectively, a human dosage of 1 g daily based on BSA).

■ Pregnancy, Fertility, and Lactation

Pregnancy There are no adequate and controlled studies to date using ciprofloxacin in pregnant women. Because ciprofloxacin, like most other fluoroquinolones, causes arthropathy in immature animals, the drug should *not* be used in pregnant women unless potential benefits justify potential risks to the fetus and mother.

CDC states that oral ciprofloxacin is the preferred drug for initial anti-infective postexposure prophylaxis in pregnant and postpartum women following a suspected or confirmed exposure to aerosolized *B. anthracis* spores in the context of biologic warfare or bioterrorism. CDC also states that oral ciprofloxacin is the preferred drug for treatment of uncomplicated cutaneous anthrax and IV ciprofloxacin is the preferred bactericidal component of a multiple-drug regimen for treatment of systemic anthrax in pregnant and postpartum women when such infections occur in the context of biologic warfare or bioterrorism.

An expert review of published data regarding clinical experience with use of ciprofloxacin during pregnancy concluded that therapeutic doses of the drug during pregnancy are unlikely to pose a substantial teratogenic risk, but that data are insufficient to state that there is no risk. Although some safety data are available from several postmarketing epidemiology studies involving short-term, first-trimester exposures to ciprofloxacin, these studies are insufficient to evaluate the risk for less common defects or to permit reliable and definitive conclusions regarding the safety of ciprofloxacin in pregnant women and their developing fetuses. In one controlled prospective observational study of 200 women exposed to fluoroquinolones during pregnancy (68% were first-trimester exposures, 52.5% of exposures involved ciprofloxacin), in utero exposure to fluoroquinolones during embryogenesis did not appear to be associated with an increased risk of major congenital malformations (incidence was 2.2% in the fluoroquinolone group and 2.6% in the control group; background incidence is 1–5%). There also was no evidence of increases in the rates of spontaneous abortion, prematurity, or low birthweight and no clinically important increase in musculoskeletal dysfunction in the ciprofloxacin-exposed children followed to 1 year of age. In another prospective follow-up study that included 549 pregnancies with fluoroquinolone exposure (93% were first-trimester exposures, 70 first-trimester exposures involved ciprofloxacin), there was no increase in the rates of spontaneous abortion, prematurity, or low birthweight, and the malformation rate was similar to the background incidence rate with no evidence of any specific patterns of congenital abnormalities.

Reproduction studies in rats and mice using oral ciprofloxacin dosages up to 100 mg/kg (0.6 and 0.3 times, respectively, the maximum daily human dosage of 1 g based on BSA) have not revealed evidence of harm to the fetus. In rabbits, oral ciprofloxacin dosages of 30 and 100 mg/kg (approximately 0.4 and 1.3 times, respectively, the highest recommended therapeutic dosage based on BSA) caused GI toxicity resulting in maternal weight loss and an increased incidence of abortion, but there was no evidence of teratogenicity. IV ciprofloxacin given to rabbits at dosages up to 20 mg/kg (approximately 0.3 times the highest recommended therapeutic dosage based on BSA) has not resulted in maternal toxicity, embryotoxicity, or teratogenicity.

Fertility Fertility studies in rats using oral ciprofloxacin dosages up to 100 mg/kg (equivalent to the highest recommended daily human dose of 1 g based on BSA) did not reveal evidence of impaired fertility.

Administration of high dosages (100 mg/kg daily) of some quinolones (e.g., norfloxacin [no longer commercially available in the US], pefloxacin [not commercially available in the US] and pipemidic acid [not commercially available in the US]) has been associated with impaired spermatogenesis and/or testicular damage (atrophy in rats and dogs) in chronic (for 3 months or longer) toxicity studies.

Lactation Ciprofloxacin is distributed into milk, but the amount of the drug absorbed by a nursing infant is unknown. Because of the potential for serious adverse effects of ciprofloxacin (including articular damage) in nursing infants, a decision should be made whether to discontinue nursing or the drug, taking into account the importance of the drug to the woman.

AAP considers ciprofloxacin to be usually compatible with breast-feeding since the amount of the fluoroquinolone potentially absorbed by nursing infants would be small and no observable change in infants associated with such exposure has been reported to date.

CDC states that recommendations for use of ciprofloxacin in breast-feeding women for postexposure prophylaxis following a suspected or confirmed exposure to aerosolized *B. anthracis* spores in the context of biologic warfare or bioterrorism and for treatment of uncomplicated cutaneous anthrax or systemic anthrax in such situations are the same as those for other adults.

Drug Interactions

■ **Drugs Metabolized by Hepatic Microsomal Enzymes** Ciprofloxacin inhibits cytochrome P-450 (CYP) isoenzyme 1A2. Concomitant use with CYP1A2 substrates (e.g., clozapine, methylxanthines [e.g., caffeine, theophylline], olanzapine, ropinirole, tizanidine) may result in increased plasma concentrations and increased pharmacologic or adverse effects of the concomitant drug.

■ **Drugs that Prolong the QT Interval** Concomitant use of ciprofloxacin and drugs known to prolong the QT interval, including class IA antiarrhythmics (e.g., quinidine, procainamide), class III antiarrhythmics (e.g., amiodarone, sotalol), tricyclic antidepressants, macrolides, and antipsychotics, may result in additive effects on QT interval prolongation. Concomitant use with these drugs should be avoided; if concomitant use is necessary, caution is advised.

■ **Antacids** Antacids containing magnesium, aluminum, or calcium decrease absorption of oral ciprofloxacin, resulting in decreased serum and urine concentrations of the anti-infective agent. Ciprofloxacin bioavailability may be decreased by as much as 90% and serum ciprofloxacin concentrations generally are decreased by 14–50% in patients receiving an antacid concomitantly; anti-infective treatment failure may occur as a result of reduced quinolone absorption in these patients. The mechanism of this interaction has not been fully elucidated to date, but magnesium, aluminum, and other divalent ions may bind to, and form insoluble complexes with, quinolones in the GI tract.

The manufacturers state that ciprofloxacin conventional tablets, extended-release tablets, or oral suspension should be administered at least 2 hours before or 6 hours after antacids containing magnesium or aluminum. Some clinicians suggest that patients be instructed not to ingest antacids containing magnesium, aluminum, or calcium concomitantly with or within 2–4 hours of a ciprofloxacin dose; however, other clinicians state that these antacids should *not* be used in patients receiving ciprofloxacin and that ciprofloxacin probably should not be used in patients with renal failure who require aluminum hydroxide or aluminum carbonate for intestinal binding of phosphate.

■ **Aminoglycosides** The antibacterial activities of ciprofloxacin and aminoglycosides have been additive or synergistic in vitro against some strains of Enterobacteriaceae and *Pseudomonas aeruginosa*. However, synergism between the drugs is unpredictable, and indifference generally occurs when ciprofloxacin is used in conjunction with amikacin, gentamicin, or tobramycin against *Ps. aeruginosa* or Enterobacteriaceae. Indifference also generally occurs when the drug is used in conjunction with tobramycin against *Acinetobacter*.

■ **Antiarrhythmic Agents** Use ciprofloxacin with caution in those receiving concurrent therapy with drugs that can prolong the QT interval (e.g., class IA or III antiarrhythmic agents). (See Cautions: Geriatric Precautions.)

■ **Anticoagulants** Initiation of oral ciprofloxacin therapy in patients stabilized on warfarin has resulted in prolongation of the prothrombin time; hematemesis occurred in at least 1 patient. The mechanism of this interaction has not been determined to date, but ciprofloxacin may displace the anticoagulant from serum albumin binding sites. The risk may vary with the underlying infection, age, and general status of the patient so that the contribution of ciprofloxacin to the increase in international normalized ratio (INR) is difficult to assess.

Ciprofloxacin should be used with caution in patients receiving warfarin, and prothrombin time and international normalized ratio (INR) should be monitored frequently during and shortly after concomitant therapy.

■ **Antidiabetic Agents** Concomitant use of ciprofloxacin and oral antidiabetic agents (e.g., sulfonylurea agents such as glimepiride or glyburide) has resulted in hypoglycemia, presumably by potentiating the glucose-lowering effect of the antidiabetic agent. Severe hypoglycemia and some fatalities have been reported.

Ciprofloxacin should be used with caution in patients receiving oral antidiabetic agents, and blood glucose concentrations should be monitored. Patients receiving an oral antidiabetic agent and ciprofloxacin concomitantly should be advised to contact their clinician if low blood glucose occurs during ciprofloxacin therapy so that the clinician can determine whether the anti-infective should be changed.

■ **Antimuscarinics** Although the clinical importance has not been determined and further study is needed to evaluate the interactions, concomitant administration of antimuscarinics (e.g., pirenzepine, scopolamine) delays GI absorption of the anti-infective.

■ **Bismuth Subsalicylate** Concomitant administration of a single dose of oral bismuth subsalicylate (428 mg) and a single dose of oral ciprofloxacin (750 mg) results in a slight decrease in peak plasma concentrations and area under the concentration-time curve (AUC) of ciprofloxacin, but this is not considered clinically important.

■ **Clindamycin** The combination of ciprofloxacin and clindamycin has been synergistic in vitro against many strains of *Peptostreptococcus*, *Lactobacillus*, and *B. fragilis* tested.

■ **Corticosteroids** Concomitant use of corticosteroids increases the risk of severe tendon disorders (e.g., tendinitis, tendon rupture), especially in geriatric patients older than 60 years of age. (See Cautions: Tendinitis and Tendon Rupture.)

■ **Clozapine** Concomitant use of ciprofloxacin (250 mg) and clozapine (304 mg) for 7 days increased serum concentrations of clozapine and *N*-desmethylclozapine by 29 and 31%, respectively, potentially resulting in adverse effects.

Clozapine and ciprofloxacin should be used concomitantly with caution; patients should be carefully monitored for clozapine adverse effects during and shortly after concomitant therapy and appropriate clozapine dosage adjustments made.

■ **Cyclosporine** Concomitant use of cyclosporine and ciprofloxacin may result in transient increases in serum creatinine. Acute renal failure occurred within 4 days after initiation of ciprofloxacin in a patient receiving cyclosporine maintenance therapy. The mechanism of this potential interaction has not been elucidated, but could involve synergistic nephrotoxic effects of the drugs and/or interference of cyclosporine metabolism by ciprofloxacin.

Cyclosporine and ciprofloxacin should be used concomitantly with caution and renal function (especially serum creatinine concentrations) should be monitored.

■ **Didanosine** Concomitant use of oral ciprofloxacin and buffered didanosine preparations (pediatric oral solution admixed with antacid) may decrease absorption of ciprofloxacin resulting in decreased serum and urine concentrations of the quinolone.

The manufacturers state that ciprofloxacin conventional tablets, extended-release tablets, or oral suspension should be administered at least 2 hours before or 6 hours after buffered didanosine preparations.

■ **Duloxetine** Concomitant use of duloxetine and potent CYP1A2 inhibitors may result in increased mean peak concentrations and AUC of duloxetine. Although clinical data are not available regarding a possible interaction between duloxetine and ciprofloxacin, similar effects on duloxetine exposure can be expected if duloxetine and ciprofloxacin are administered concomitantly.

Concomitant use of duloxetine and ciprofloxacin should be avoided. If concomitant use cannot be avoided, patients should be monitored for duloxetine toxicity.

■ **Histamine H_2-receptor Antagonists** Histamine H_2-receptor antagonists do not appear to have a clinically important effect on bioavailability of ciprofloxacin. Concomitant cimetidine or ranitidine does not appear to alter GI absorption of ciprofloxacin.

■ **Iron, Multivitamins, and Mineral Supplements** Oral multivitamin and mineral supplements containing divalent or trivalent cations such as calcium, iron, or zinc may interfere with oral absorption of ciprofloxacin resulting in decreased serum and urine concentrations of the quinolone. Therefore, these multivitamins and/or mineral supplements should not be ingested concomitantly with ciprofloxacin.

The manufacturers state that ciprofloxacin conventional tablets, extended-release tablets, or oral suspension should be administered at least 2 hours before or 6 hours after preparations containing calcium, iron, or zinc.

■ **β-Lactam Antibiotics** An additive or synergistic effect has occurred occasionally in vitro against some strains of *Ps. aeruginosa* and *Ps. maltophilia* when ciprofloxacin was used concomitantly with an extended-spectrum penicillin (e.g., mezlocillin [not commercially available], piperacillin). Indifference generally occurs when ciprofloxacin is used in conjunction with an extended-spectrum penicillin against Enterobacteriaceae.

Ciprofloxacin used in conjunction with imipenem, cefoxitin, or a cephalosporin (e.g., cefotaxime, ceftazidime) has been reported to be additive or synergistic against some strains of *Ps. aeruginosa* or Enterobacteriaceae; however, these combinations generally are indifferent rather than additive or synergistic against these bacteria. Although the clinical importance has not been determined, ciprofloxacin used in conjunction with cefotaxime in vitro resulted in a synergistic effect against many strains of *Bacteroides fragilis* tested; antagonism did not occur.

■ **Lanthanum Carbonate** Concomitant administration of lanthanum carbonate may decrease GI absorption of ciprofloxacin and result in a substantial decrease in serum and urine concentrations of the anti-infective agent.

The manufacturers state that ciprofloxacin conventional tablets, extended-release tablets, or oral suspension should be administered at least 2 hours before or 6 hours after lanthanum carbonate.

■ **Lidocaine** Concomitant use of IV lidocaine hydrochloride (1.5 mg/kg) and ciprofloxacin (500 mg twice daily) increased the peak concentrations and AUC of lidocaine by 12 and 26%, respectively. Although lidocaine treatment was well tolerated at this elevated exposure, a possible interaction with ciprofloxacin and increase in lidocaine-associated adverse effects should be considered if the drugs are used concomitantly.

■ **Methotrexate** Concomitant use of ciprofloxacin and methotrexate may result in increased plasma concentrations of methotrexate (as the result of renal tubular transport inhibition) and may increase the risk of methotrexate-associated toxic reactions.

Methotrexate and ciprofloxacin should be used concomitantly with caution; patients should be carefully monitored.

■ **Metoclopramide** Although bioavailability of ciprofloxacin does not appear to be affected, concomitant use of metoclopramide reportedly accelerates the rate of GI absorption of ciprofloxacin resulting in a shorter time to peak plasma concentrations of the drug.

■ **Metronidazole** Concomitant use of metronidazole and ciprofloxacin does not affect serum concentrations of either drug.

■ **Nonsteroidal Anti-inflammatory Agents** Concomitant use of ciprofloxacin and a nonsteroidal anti-inflammatory agent (NSAIA) could increase the risk of CNS stimulation (e.g., seizures). In preclinical studies and during postmarketing experience, concomitant use of ciprofloxacin and very high doses of an NSAIA (except aspirin) provoked seizures. Animal studies suggest that the risk may vary depending on the specific NSAIA.

NSAIAs and ciprofloxacin should be used concomitantly with caution.

■ **Omeprazole** Concomitant administration of a single 500-mg conventional tablet of ciprofloxacin and omeprazole (20 mg once daily for 4 days) resulted in a 16% decrease in mean peak concentration and AUC of ciprofloxacin. Concomitant administration of ciprofloxacin extended-release tablets (single 1-g dose) and omeprazole (40 mg once daily for 3 days) in healthy individuals reduced peak plasma concentrations and AUC of ciprofloxacin by 23 and 20%, respectively. The clinical importance of this interaction has not been determined.

■ **Phenytoin** Concomitant use of ciprofloxacin and phenytoin has resulted in altered serum concentrations of phenytoin (increased or decreased).

Phenytoin and ciprofloxacin should be used concomitantly with caution. To avoid loss of seizure control and prevent adverse effects associated with phenytoin overdosage, phenytoin serum concentrations should be monitored during and shortly after concomitant therapy with ciprofloxacin.

■ **Phosphodiesterase Type 5 Inhibitors** Concomitant use of a single oral dose of sildenafil (50 mg) with ciprofloxacin (500 mg) in healthy individuals increased the mean peak concentration and AUC of sildenafil approximately twofold.

Sildenafil and ciprofloxacin should be used concomitantly with caution; patients should be monitored for sildenafil toxicity.

■ **Probenecid** Concomitant administration of probenecid interferes with renal tubular secretion of ciprofloxacin, resulting in a 50% decrease in renal clearance of ciprofloxacin, a 50% increase in systemic ciprofloxacin concentrations, and a prolonged serum half-life of the drug. This effect may potentiate ciprofloxacin toxicity.

Probenecid and ciprofloxacin should be used concomitantly with caution.

■ **Rifampin** Concomitant use of oral ciprofloxacin (750 mg twice daily) and oral rifampin (300 mg twice daily) does not appear to affect the pharmacokinetics of either drug.

In vitro, the combination of ciprofloxacin and rifampin generally is indifferent against *S. aureus*; however, antagonism also has been reported rarely.

■ **Ropinirole** Concomitant use of oral ciprofloxacin (500 mg twice daily) and oral ropinirole (6 mg daily) has resulted in 60 and 84% increases in peak concentrations and AUC of ropinirole, respectively.

Ropinirole and ciprofloxacin should be used concomitantly with caution; patients should be monitored for ropinirole-associated adverse effects during and shortly after concomitant therapy and ropinirole dosage adjustments should be made as necessary.

■ **Sevelamer** Concomitant administration of sevelamer may decrease GI absorption of ciprofloxacin and result in a substantial decrease in serum and urine concentrations of the anti-infective agent.

The manufacturers state that ciprofloxacin conventional tablets, extended-release tablets, or oral suspension should be administered at least 2 hours before or 6 hours after sevelamer.

■ **Sucralfate** Concomitant sucralfate, presumably because of its aluminum content, decreases GI absorption of ciprofloxacin and may result in a substantial (50–90%) decrease in serum concentrations of the anti-infective agent.

The manufacturers state that ciprofloxacin extended-release tablets, conventional tablets, or oral suspension should be administered at least 2 hours before or 6 hours after sucralfate.

■ **Tizanidine** Concomitant use of tizanidine (single dose of 4 mg) and ciprofloxacin (500 mg twice daily for 3 days) increased peak serum concentrations and AUC of tizanidine by sevenfold and tenfold, respectively.

Concomitant use of ciprofloxacin and tizanidine is contraindicated because the hypotensive and sedative effects of tizanidine are potentiated.

■ **Vancomycin** Synergism does *not* occur in vitro when ciprofloxacin is used in conjunction with vancomycin against *Staphylococcus epidermidis*, *S. aureus* (including methicillin-resistant *S. aureus*), *Corynebacterium*, or *Listeria monocytogenes*.

■ **Xanthine Derivatives** ***Theophyllines*** Concomitant administration of ciprofloxacin in patients receiving a theophylline derivative may result in higher and prolonged serum theophylline concentrations and may increase the risk of theophylline-related adverse effects. Alterations in theophylline pharmacokinetics have shown considerable interindividual variation, with serum theophylline concentrations reportedly increasing by 17–254% and theophylline clearance decreasing by 18–112% following initiation of ciprofloxacin. Generally, however, reductions in theophylline clearance induced by ciprofloxacin have averaged 20–35%. Alterations in theophylline pharmacokinetics may be related to inhibition of metabolism in the liver by the 4-oxo metabolites of these quinolones. However, the potential contribution of the 4-oxo metabolites to this interaction has not been fully elucidated, and there is some evidence that, while formation of these metabolites may correlate with inhibition of theophylline metabolism, the 4-oxo metabolites themselves may not be responsible for the observed inhibition. Theophyllines do not appear to affect the pharmacokinetics of quinolones. However, there is limited in vitro evidence that theophyllines may potentiate quinolone-induced inhibition of γ-aminobutyric acid (GABA), thus possibly potentiating CNS stimulation.

Serious and sometimes fatal reactions (e.g., cardiac arrest, seizures, status epilepticus, respiratory failure) have occurred in patients receiving ciprofloxacin and theophylline concomitantly. Death in at least one patient was associated with seizures and atrial fibrillation during concomitant therapy with the drugs. Other adverse reactions reported during concomitant therapy with the drugs include nausea, vomiting, dizziness, headache, tremor, restlessness, agitation, irritability, confusion, hallucinations, tachycardia, and palpitations. These adverse effects apparently occurred as the result of increased serum theophylline concentrations. While similar effects also have been reported in theophylline-treated patients who were not receiving ciprofloxacin concomitantly, the possibility that such toxicity may have been potentiated by ciprofloxacin cannot be excluded.

Concomitant use of ciprofloxacin and a theophylline derivative should be avoided, if possible, because of the risk of toxicity (e.g., CNS or other adverse effects) associated with increased plasma concentrations of theophylline. If concomitant use of theophylline and ciprofloxacin cannot be avoided, plasma theophylline concentrations should be monitored, the patient observed for manifestations of theophylline toxicity, and appropriate theophylline dosage adjustments made as needed, especially in geriatric patients. The need for theophylline dosage adjustment also should be considered when ciprofloxacin is discontinued since subtherapeutic concentrations may occur.

Caffeine Ciprofloxacin inhibits formation of paraxanthine after caffeine administration, resulting in increased serum concentrations, reduced clearance, and prolonged elimination half-life of caffeine.

Caffeine and ciprofloxacin should be used concomitantly with caution. Patients receiving ciprofloxacin should be advised that regular consumption of large quantities of coffee, tea, or caffeine-containing soft drinks or drugs during therapy with the anti-infective may result in exaggerated or prolonged effects of caffeine. If excessive cardiac or CNS stimulation (e.g., nervousness, insomnia, anxiety, tachycardia) occurs, caffeine intake should be restricted. In addition, caffeine intake should be restricted during ciprofloxacin therapy in patients at risk of adverse effects from CNS or cardiac stimulation.

Pentoxifylline Concomitant use of pentoxifylline and ciprofloxacin results in increased serum concentrations, reduced clearance, and prolonged elimination half-life of pentoxifylline. Ciprofloxacin and pentoxifylline should be used concomitantly with caution; patients should be monitored for xanthine toxicity and dosage adjusted as necessary.

■ **Zolpidem** Concomitant use of zolpidem and ciprofloxacin may increase serum concentrations of zolpidem and is not recommended.

Laboratory Test Interferences

■ **Tests for Urinary Glucose** Ciprofloxacin hydrochloride does not interfere with urinary glucose determinations using cupric sulfate solution (e.g., Benedict's solution, Clinitest®) or with glucose oxidase tests (e.g., Diastix®, Tes-Tape®).

Acute Toxicity

The oral LD_{50} of the drug is greater than 5 g/kg in mice and rats and approximately 2.5 g/kg in rabbits. In mice, rats, rabbits, and dogs, substantial toxicity (including tonic/clonic convulsions) was observed with IV ciprofloxacin doses between 125 and 300 mg/kg.

Reversible renal toxicity has been reported in some cases of acute overdosage of ciprofloxacin. If acute oral overdosage of the drug occurs, the stomach should be emptied by inducing emesis or by gastric lavage; administration of antacids containing magnesium, aluminum, or calcium may reduce oral absorption of ciprofloxacin. If the patient is comatose, having seizures, or lacks the gag reflex, gastric lavage may be performed if an endotracheal tube with cuff inflated is in place to prevent aspiration of gastric contents. Supportive and symptomatic treatment should be initiated. The patient should be observed carefully; renal function and urinary pH should be monitored and the urine acidified if needed. Adequate hydration must be maintained to minimize the risk of crystalluria.

Only a small amount of ciprofloxacin (less than 10%) is removed by hemodialysis or peritoneal dialysis. Some clinicians suggest that the risks associated with hemodialysis or peritoneal dialysis do not justify their possible benefits in ciprofloxacin overdosage.

Mechanism of Action

Ciprofloxacin usually is bactericidal in action. Like other fluoroquinolone anti-infectives, ciprofloxacin inhibits DNA synthesis in susceptible organisms via inhibition of the enzymatic activities of 2 members of the DNA topoisomerase class of enzymes, DNA gyrase and topoisomerase IV. DNA gyrase and topoisomerase IV have distinct essential roles in bacterial DNA replication. DNA gyrase, a type II DNA topoisomerase, was the first identified quinolone target; DNA gyrase is a tetramer composed of 2 GyrA and 2 GyrB subunits. DNA gyrase introduces negative superhelical twists in DNA, an activity important for initiation of DNA replication. DNA gyrase also facilitates DNA replication by removing positive super helical twists. Topoisomerase IV, another type II DNA topoisomerase, is composed of 2 ParC and 2 ParE subunits. DNA gyrase and topoisomerase IV are structurally related; ParC is homologous to GyrA and ParE is homologous to GyrB. Topoisomerase IV acts at the terminal states of DNA replication by allowing for separation of interlinked daughter chromosomes so that segregation into daughter cells can occur. Fluoroquinolones inhibit these topoisomerase enzymes by stabilizing either the DNA—DNA gyrase complex or the DNA—topoisomerase IV complex; these stabilized complexes block movement of the DNA replication fork and thereby inhibit DNA replication resulting in cell death.

Although all fluoroquinolones generally are active against both DNA gyrase and topoisomerase IV, the drugs differ in their relative activities against these enzymes. For many gram-negative bacteria, DNA gyrase is the primary quinolone target and for many gram-positive bacteria, topoisomerase IV is the primary target; the other enzyme is the secondary target in both cases. However, there are exceptions to this pattern. For certain bacteria (e.g., *Streptococcus pneumoniae*), the principal target depends on the specific fluoroquinolone.

The mechanism by which ciprofloxacin's inhibition of DNA gyrase or topoisomerase IV results in death in susceptible organisms has not been fully determined. Unlike β-lactam anti-infectives, which are most active against susceptible bacteria when they are in the logarithmic phase of growth, studies using *Escherichia coli* and *Pseudomonas aeruginosa* indicate that ciprofloxacin can be bactericidal during both logarithmic and stationary phases of growth; this effect does not appear to occur with gram-positive bacteria (e.g., *Staphylococcus aureus*). In vitro studies indicate that ciprofloxacin concentrations that approximate the minimum inhibitory concentration (MIC) of the drug induce filamentation in susceptible organisms; high concentrations of the drug result in enlarged or elongated cells that may not be extensively filamented. Although the bactericidal effect of some fluoroquinolones evidently requires competent RNA and protein synthesis in the bacterial cell, and concurrent use of anti-infectives that affect protein synthesis (e.g., chloramphenicol, tetracyclines) or RNA synthesis (e.g., rifampin) inhibit the in vitro bactericidal activity of these drugs, the bactericidal effect of ciprofloxacin is only partially reduced in the presence of these anti-infectives. This suggests that ciprofloxacin has an additional mechanism of action that is independent of RNA and protein synthesis.

For most susceptible organisms, the minimum bactericidal concentration (MBC) of ciprofloxacin is 1–4 times higher than the minimum inhibitory concentration (MIC), although the MBC occasionally may be 8 times higher.

Mammalian cells contain type II topoisomerase similar to that contained in bacteria. At concentrations attained during therapy, quinolones do not appear to affect the mammalian enzyme, presumably because it functions differently than bacterial DNA gyrase and does not cause supercoiling of DNA.

Although the clinical importance has not been determined, ciprofloxacin appears to have a postantibiotic inhibitory effect against most susceptible aerobic organisms. The duration of the postantibiotic inhibitory effect and the ciprofloxacin concentration required to produce the effect vary depending on the organism; the duration of this effect also varies according to length of exposure to the drug, increasing with increased exposure. In vitro studies in Mueller-Hinton broth using *S. aureus*, Enterobacteriaceae, and *Ps. aeruginosa* exposed for 1–2 hours to ciprofloxacin concentrations several times higher than the MIC indicate that there is a recovery period of about 1–6 hours before these organisms resume growth after the drug is removed. Equivocal results have been observed following in vitro exposure of *Enterococcus faecalis* (formerly *Streptococcus faecalis*) to the drug, and it is unclear whether the drug exerts a postantibiotic inhibitory effect against this organism.

In vitro studies, particularly those involving in vitro susceptibility tests, indicate that the antibacterial activity of ciprofloxacin is decreased in the presence of urine, especially acidic urine. (See Spectrum: Susceptibility Testing.) The clinical importance of this in vitro effect has not been determined to date; however, because ciprofloxacin concentrations attained in urine are usually substantially higher than ciprofloxacin MICs for most urinary tract pathogens, the effect probably is not clinically important. The antibacterial activity of ciprofloxacin also is decreased slightly in unbuffered peritoneal dialysis fluid with a pH of 5.5 compared with its activity in dialysis fluid buffered to a pH of 7.4.

Spectrum

Ciprofloxacin has a spectrum of activity similar to that of some other fluoroquinolones (e.g., ofloxacin). In vitro on a weight basis, the activity of ciprofloxacin is approximately equal to or slightly greater than that of ofloxacin against most susceptible organisms.

Ciprofloxacin is active in vitro against most gram-negative aerobic bacteria, including Enterobacteriaceae and *Pseudomonas aeruginosa*. Ciprofloxacin also is active in vitro against many gram-positive aerobic bacteria, including penicillinase-producing, nonpenicillinase-producing, and methicillin-resistant staphylococci (also known as oxacillin-resistant staphylococci), although many strains of streptococci are relatively resistant to the drug. The drug generally is less active against gram-positive than gram-negative bacteria. Ciprofloxacin has some activity in vitro against obligately anaerobic bacteria, but many of these organisms are considered resistant to the drug. The drug also has some activity in vitro against *Chlamydia, Mycoplasma, Mycobacterium, Plasmodium,* and *Rickettsia*. Ciprofloxacin is inactive against fungi.

■ **In Vitro Susceptibility Testing** Like those of other fluoroquinolones, results of ciprofloxacin in vitro susceptibility tests are affected by the pH of the media and the presence of certain cations (e.g., magnesium). There generally is little effect when the pH of the media is 6–8; however, minimum inhibitory concentrations (MICs) are at least 4–16 times greater when the pH of the media is less than 6. It has been suggested that ionization of the 7-piperazine group as pH decreases may interfere with access or binding to the drug's target enzyme.

Ciprofloxacin MICs also are increased when high concentrations of magnesium are present in the media. The mechanism by which magnesium interferes with the antibacterial activity of ciprofloxacin is unclear, but it has been suggested that this cation may form complexes with the drug which may prevent access or binding to its target enzyme. Presence of calcium or zinc does not appear to affect results of ciprofloxacin susceptibility tests.

Inoculum size generally does not affect in vitro susceptibility to ciprofloxacin. MICs for most organisms are only 2–4 times greater when the size of the inoculum is increased from 10^2 to 10^8 colony-forming units (CFU) per mL; however, in some studies, an inoculum effect did occur with some strains of Enterobacteriaceae or *Pseudomonas aeruginosa* and MIC and minimum bactericidal concentration (MBC) of the drug appeared to be equally affected by increased inoculum size. Presence of serum generally has no effect on results of ciprofloxacin in vitro susceptibility tests, but reportedly may slightly decrease MICs of the drug for some organisms.

MICs of ciprofloxacin are higher when susceptibility tests are performed in pooled urine or urine agar rather than in nutrient broth or Mueller-Hinton media. The MIC of ciprofloxacin for *Escherichia coli* is less than 0.01 mcg/mL in Mueller-Hinton broth at pH 7.4, but is 1.6 mcg/mL in urine at pH 7.5 or 6.5 and 3.1 mcg/mL in urine at pH 5.5. The decreased antibacterial activity in the presence of urine probably occurs because of low pH and because urine contains a higher concentration of magnesium ions than nutrient broth or Mueller-Hinton media.

MICs of ciprofloxacin are increased when activated charcoal is present in the media.

When in vitro susceptibility testing is performed according to the standards of the Clinical and Laboratory Standards Institute (CLSI; formerly National Committee for Clinical Laboratory Standards [NCCLS]), clinical isolates identified as *susceptible* to ciprofloxacin are inhibited by drug concentrations usually achievable when the recommended dosage is used for the site of infection. Clinical isolates classified as *intermediate* have minimum inhibitory concentrations (MICs) that approach usually attainable blood and tissue concentrations and response rates may be lower than for strains identified as susceptible. Therefore, the intermediate category implies clinical applicability in body sites where the drug is physiologically concentrated or when a higher than usual dosage can be used. This intermediate category also includes a buffer zone that should prevent small, uncontrolled technical factors from causing major discrepancies in interpretation, especially for drugs with narrow pharmacotoxicity margins. If results of in vitro susceptibility testing indicate that a clinical isolate is *resistant* to ciprofloxacin, the strain is not inhibited by drug concentrations generally achievable with usual dosage schedules and/or MICs fall in the range where specific microbial resistance mechanisms are likely and clinical efficacy of the drug against the isolate has not been reliably demonstrated in clinical studies.

Results of ciprofloxacin susceptibility tests should not be used to predict susceptibility to other fluoroquinolones.

Disk Susceptibility When the disk-diffusion procedure is used to test susceptibility to ciprofloxacin, a disk containing 5 mcg of ciprofloxacin should be used.

Table 4. Interpretation of Disk Diffusion Zone Diameters (nearest whole mm) for Disk Susceptibility Tests Performed According to CLSI Standardized Procedures

	Susceptible	Intermediate	Resistance
Enterobacteriaceae			
(Note: In vitro susceptibility testing using fluoroquinolones can predict susceptibility of fecal isolates of *Salmonella*, but test isolates from patients with extraintestinal salmonellosis using both the fluoroquinolone and nalidixic acid [no longer commercially available in the US]. Strains that test susceptible to the fluoroquinolone but resistant to nalidixic acid may not be eradicated by the fluoroquinolone and consultation with an infectious disease expert is recommended.)			
Ciprofloxacin	≥21	16–20	≤15
Pseudomonas aeruginosa			
Ciprofloxacin	≥21	16–20	≤15
Acinetobacter			
Ciprofloxacin	≥21	16–20	≤15
Staphylococcus			
(Note: *Staphylococcus* may develop resistance during prolonged fluoroquinolone therapy; initially susceptible isolates may become resistant within 3–4 days after initiation of therapy. Testing of repeat isolates may be warranted.)			
Ciprofloxacin	≥21	16–20	≤15
Enterococcus			
Ciprofloxacin (urinary isolates)	≥21	16–20	≤15
Haemophilus influenzae and Haemophilus parainfluenzae			
(Note: If results for *Haemophilus* indicate nonsusceptible, confirm organism identification and susceptibility testing.)			
Ciprofloxacin	≥21	–	–
Neisseria gonorrhoeae			
Ciprofloxacin	≥41	28–40	≤27
Neisseria meningitidis			
(Note: Breakpoints may be appropriate only for postexposure prophylaxis of meningococcal disease and do not apply to use of the drug for treatment of invasive meningococcal disease.)			
Ciprofloxacin	≥35	33–34	≤32

Dilution Susceptibility Tests

Table 5. Interpretation of MICs (mcg/mL) For Diffusion Susceptibility Tests Performed According to CLSI Standardized Procedures

	Susceptible	Intermediate	Resistant
Enterobacteriaceae			
(Note: In vitro susceptibility testing using fluoroquinolones can predict susceptibility of fecal isolates of *Salmonella*, but test isolates from patients with extraintestinal salmonellosis using both the fluoroquinolone and nalidixic acid [no longer commercially available in the US]. Strains that test susceptible to the fluoroquinolone but resistant to nalidixic acid may not be eradicated by the fluoroquinolone and consultation with an infectious disease expert is recommended.)			
Ciprofloxacin	≤1	2	≥4
Pseudomonas aeruginosa			
Ciprofloxacin	≤1	2	≥4
Acinetobacter			
Ciprofloxacin	≤1	2	≥4
Staphylococcus			
(Note: *Staphylococcus* may develop resistance during prolonged fluoroquinolone therapy; initially susceptible isolates may become resistant within 3–4 days after initiation of therapy. Testing of repeat isolates may be warranted.)			
Ciprofloxacin	≤1	2	≥4
Enterococcus			
Ciprofloxacin (urinary isolates)	≤1	2	≥4
Haemophilus influenzae and Haemophilus parainfluenzae			
(Note: If results for *Haemophilus* indicate nonsusceptible, confirm organism identification and susceptibility testing.)			
Ciprofloxacin	≤1	–	–
Neisseria gonorrhoeae			
Ciprofloxacin	≤0.06	0.12–0.5	≥1
Neisseria meningitidis			
(Note: Breakpoints may be appropriate only for postexposure prophylaxis of meningococcal disease and do not apply to use of the drug for treatment of invasive meningococcal disease.)			
Ciprofloxacin	≤0.03	0.06	0.12

■ Gram-positive Aerobic Bacteria

Gram-positive Aerobic Cocci Ciprofloxacin is active in vitro against most strains of *Staphylococcus aureus*, *S. epidermidis*, *S. saprophyticus*, and *S. hemolyticus*. The drug is active against both penicillinase-producing and nonpenicillinase-producing staphylococci, and also is active in vitro against some methicillin-resistant strains, although to a lesser degree than against methicillin-susceptible strains. Ciprofloxacin is less active in vitro on a weight basis against streptococci than against staphylococci. *Streptococcus pneumoniae*, *S. pyogenes* (group A β-hemolytic streptococci), *S. agalactiae* (group B streptococci), and viridans streptococci generally are inhibited in vitro by ciprofloxacin concentrations of 4 mcg/mL or less. Groups C, F, and G streptococci and nonenterococcal group D streptococci are inhibited in vitro by ciprofloxacin concentrations of 16 mcg/mL or less. Ciprofloxacin is active in vitro against some strains of enterococci, including *Enterococcus faecalis* (formerly *S. faecalis*). The drug is more active in vitro against *E. faecalis* than against *E. faecium* or *E. durans* (formerly *S. faecium* and *S. durans*, respectively). Ciprofloxacin is bactericidal in vitro against enterococci and is active against some strains of *E. faecalis* resistant to penicillin combined with an aminoglycoside.

Table 6 includes MIC_{50}s (minimum inhibitory concentrations of the drug at which 50% of strains tested are inhibited) and MIC_{90}s (minimum inhibitory concentrations of the drug at which 90% of strains tested are inhibited) of ciprofloxacin reported for gram-positive aerobic cocci.

Table 6. MIC_{50}s and MIC_{90}s of ciprofloxacin reported for gram-positive aerobic cocci.

Organism	MIC_{50} (mcg/mL)	MIC_{90} (mcg/mL)
Staphylococcus aureus	0.06–0.5	0.12–2
S. epidermidis	0.06–0.25	0.125–1
S. saprophyticus	0.13–0.25	0.25–0.5
Oxacillin-resistant *S. aureus*	0.12–0.78	0.13–4
Streptococcus pneumoniae	0.5–2	1–4
S. pyogenes (group A β-hemolytic streptococci)	0.5–1	1–4
S. agalactiae (Group B streptococci)	0.5–1	0.8–4
Groups C, F, and G streptococci	0.05–2	0.4–16
Viridans streptococci	0.5–2	0.5–4
Nonenterococcal group D streptococci	1–2	1–6.3
Enterococci	0.5–4	0.5–8

Gram-positive Aerobic Bacilli Ciprofloxacin is active in vitro against *Bacillus anthracis*, and naturally occurring isolates have been inhibited in vitro by ciprofloxacin concentrations of 0.03–0.25 mcg/mL. The MIC of the drug reported for the strain of *B. anthracis* used in a study in the rhesus monkey model of inhalational anthrax was 0.08 mcg/mL. Results of in vitro susceptibility testing of 11 *B. anthracis* isolates that were associated with cases of inhalational or cutaneous anthrax that occurred in the US (Florida, New York, District of Columbia) during September and October 2001 in the context of an intentional release of anthrax spores (biologic warfare, bioterrorism) indicate that these strains had ciprofloxacin MICs of 0.06 mcg/mL or less. Based on interpretive criteria established for staphylococci, these strains are considered susceptible to ciprofloxacin. Anti-infectives are active against the germinated form of *B. anthracis* but are not active against the organism while it is still in the spore form. Strains of *B. anthracis* with naturally occurring resistance to ciprofloxacin have not been reported to date. However, reduced susceptibility to ofloxacin (4-fold increase in MICs from baseline) has been produced in vitro following sequential subculture of the Sterne strain of *B. anthracis* in subinhibitory concentrations of the fluoroquinolone. There are published reports of *B. anthracis* strains that have been engineered to have tetracycline and penicillin resistance as well as resistance to other anti-infectives (e.g., macrolides, chloramphenicol, rifampin).

Ciprofloxacin is active in vitro against *Corynebacterium*. The MIC_{90} of the drug reported for JK strains of *Corynebacterium* and *Corynebacterium* D2 is 0.5–1 mcg/mL.

Ciprofloxacin is active in vitro against *Listeria monocytogenes*, and the MIC_{90} of the drug reported for this organism is 0.25–2 mcg/mL.

The MIC_{90} of ciprofloxacin for *Nocardia asteroides* is 8–16 mcg/mL; these organisms generally are considered resistant to the drug.

■ Gram-negative Aerobic Bacteria

Neisseria Ciprofloxacin is active in vitro against some strains of penicillinase- and nonpenicillinase-producing *Neisseria gonorrhoeae* and *N. gonorrhoeae* with chromosomally mediated resistance to penicillin (CMRNG) or plasmid-mediated tetracycline resistance (TRNG). The MIC_{90} of ciprofloxacin is 0.002–0.05 mcg/mL for most penicillinase- or nonpenicillinase-producing *N. gonorrhoeae*, CMRNG, and TRNG. However, strains of *N. gonorrhoeae* with decreased susceptibility to ciprofloxacin and other fluoroquinolones have been reported with increasing frequency. (See Resistance: Resistance in Neisseria gonorrhoeae.)

Ciprofloxacin is active in vitro against *N. meningitidis*, and the MIC_{90} of the drug for this organism usually is 0.004–0.06 mcg/mL.

Haemophilus Ciprofloxacin is active in vitro against β-lactamase- and non-β-lactamase-producing *Haemophilus influenzae*, and the MIC_{90} of the drug for these organisms is 0.008–0.05 mcg/mL. Ciprofloxacin is active in vitro against strains of β-lactamase-producing *H. influenzae* that are resistant to chloramphenicol. The MIC_{90} of ciprofloxacin for *H. parainfluenzae* and *H. ducreyi* is 0.03 mcg/mL.

Moraxella catarrhalis Ciprofloxacin is active in vitro against both β-lactamase- and non-β-lactamase-producing strains of *Moraxella catarrhalis*, and the MIC_{90} of the drug reported for this organism is 0.015–0.64 mcg/mL.

Enterobacteriaceae Ciprofloxacin is active in vitro against most clinically important Enterobacteriaceae, and the MIC_{90} of the drug for most of these organisms is 1 mcg/mL or less. While ciprofloxacin is active against *Shigella dysenteriae* type 1, the MIC of the drug for this strain generally is several-fold higher than for other *Shigella* strains. Ciprofloxacin is active in vitro against some Enterobacteriaceae resistant to aminoglycosides and/or β-lactam antibiotics.

Table 7 includes MIC_{50}s and MIC_{90}s of ciprofloxacin reported for Enterobacteriaceae.

Table 7. MIC_{50}s and MIC_{90}s of ciprofloxacin reported for Enterobacteriaceae.

Organism	MIC_{50} (mcg/mL)	MIC_{90} (mcg/mL)
Citrobacter spp.	0.01–0.03	0.01–0.13
C. koseri	0.01–0.06	0.01–0.25
C. freundii	0.01–0.13	0.03–1
Edwardsiella tarda	0.06	0.06
Enterobacter spp.	0.01–0.06	0.02–0.5
E. agglomerans	0.01–0.03	0.02–0.13
E. cloacae	0.01–0.06	0.03–1.6
E. aerogenes	0.01–0.06	0.03–0.13
Escherichia coli	0.01–0.16	0.02–0.13
Hafnia alvei	0.01–0.03	0.01–0.13
Klebsiella spp.	0.01–0.12	0.06–1
K. oxytoca	0.01–0.06	0.03–0.13
K. pneumoniae	0.01–0.08	0.06–0.5
Morganella morganii	0.01–0.06	0.02–0.13
Proteus mirabilis	0.02–0.06	0.02–0.125
P. vulgaris	0.02–0.06	0.02–0.5
Providencia rettgeri	0.02–0.5	0.06–2
P. stuartii	0.03–2	0.13–8
Serratia spp.	0.03–0.25	0.06–2
S. marcescens	0.03–0.78	0.06–6.25
Salmonella spp.	0.01–0.03	0.01–0.13
S. enteritidis	0.01	0.02
S. typhi	0.01–0.1	0.02–0.1
Shigella spp.	0.01–0.02	0.01–0.06
Yersinia enterocolitica	0.01–0.1	0.01–0.1

Pseudomonas Ciprofloxacin is active in vitro against most strains of *Ps. aeruginosa* and also has some activity against some other *Pseudomonas*. The MIC_{50} and MIC_{90} of ciprofloxacin for *Ps. aeruginosa* are 0.06–1 and 0.03–4 mcg/mL, respectively. Ciprofloxacin is active in vitro against some strains of *Ps. aeruginosa* that are resistant to aminoglycosides, extended-spectrum penicillins, and cephalosporins. The MIC_{90} of the drug for *Ps. fluorescens* and *Ps. putida* is 0.25–4 mcg/mL; however, the MIC_{90} for *Ps. cepacia* (*Burkholderia cepacia*), *Stenotrophomonas maltophilia* (formerly *Xanthomonas* or *Ps. maltophilia*), and *Ps. pseudomallei* is 0.05–16 mcg/mL and many of these organisms are considered resistant to the drug.

Vibrio Ciprofloxacin is active in vitro against *Vibrio cholerae* (*V. cholerae* 01 and 0139), *V. parahaemolyticus*, and *V. vulnificus*. The MIC_{90} of the drug reported for *Vibrio* is 0.003–0.25 mcg/mL.

Other Gram-negative Aerobic Bacteria The MIC_{90} of ciprofloxacin for *Acinetobacter lwoffi* (*A. calcoaceticus* subsp. *lwoffi*) and *A. baumannii* (*A. calcoaceticus* subsp. *anitratus*) is 0.125–4 mcg/mL.

Aeromonas hydrophila, A. caviae, A. sobria, and *Plesiomonas shigelloides* generally are inhibited in vitro by ciprofloxacin concentrations of 0.1 mcg/mL or less. The MIC_{90} of ciprofloxacin reported for *Alcaligenes*, including *A. faecalis*, is 1.4–12.5 mcg/mL.

Ciprofloxacin is active in vitro against strains of *Campylobacter coli, C. fetus*, and *Helicobacter pylori*. The MIC_{90} of the drug for some strains of *Campylobacter fetus* subsp. *jejuni*, an organism that can be microaerophilic or anaerobic, is 0.12–0.62 mcg/mL. The MIC_{90} of the drug reported for *H. pylori* is 0.25–0.5 mcg/mL, and the MIC_{90} for *C. coli* is 0.39 mcg/mL. However, fluoroquinolone-resistant strains of *Campylobacter* have been reported in areas with widespread use or prolonged therapy with the drugs. (See Resistance.)

Brucella melitensis, Pasteurella multocida, Eikenella corrodens, and *Flavobacterium* generally are inhibited by ciprofloxacin concentrations of 0.01–1 mcg/mL.

Ciprofloxacin has in vitro activity against *Francisella tularensis*. In one study evaluating susceptibility of *F. tularensis* isolated from humans and animals, the MIC of ciprofloxacin for this organism was 0.016 mcg/mL.

Ciprofloxacin has in vitro activity against *Yersinia pestis*. In a study of *Y. pestis* isolates obtained from plague patients, rats, or fleas from Vietnam, the organism was inhibited in vitro by ciprofloxacin concentrations of 0.008–0.062 mcg/mL. In one in vitro study, the MBC of ciprofloxacin against intracellular *Y. pestis* was similar to or slightly higher than the MBC of the drug against extracellular *Y. pestis*. Ciprofloxacin has been shown to have in vivo activity against *Y. pestis* in murine plague infections. However, mutant strains of *Y. pestis* resistant to ciprofloxacin have been selected in vitro.

Some strains of *Gardnerella vaginalis* (formerly *Haemophilus vaginalis*) are inhibited in vitro by ciprofloxacin concentrations of 0.5–8 mcg/mL.

The MIC_{90} of ciprofloxacin reported for *Legionella pneumophila, L. bozemanii, L. dumoffii, L. gormanii, L. jordanis, L. longbeachae, L. micdadei* (the Pittsburgh pneumonia agent), and *L. wadsworthii* is 0.01–0.5 mcg/mL.

■ **Anaerobic Bacteria** Ciprofloxacin has some activity against gram-positive and gram-negative anaerobic bacteria; however, high concentrations of the drug generally are required for in vitro inhibition and many of these organisms are considered resistant to the drug. The MIC_{90} of ciprofloxacin for *Actinomyces, Bifidobacterium, Peptococcus*, and *Peptostreptococcus* is 0.5–8 mcg/mL. Some strains of *Clostridium perfringens* may be inhibited in vitro by ciprofloxacin concentrations of 0.5–1 mcg/mL, but most other *Clostridium* require ciprofloxacin concentrations of 4–32 mcg/mL or greater for in vitro inhibition and are considered resistant to the drug. The MIC_{90} for *Eubacterium* is 1–16 mcg/mL.

The MIC_{90} of ciprofloxacin for *Propionibacterium acnes* and *Veillonella* is 0.12–4 mcg/mL, and the MIC_{90} for *Fusobacterium* is 2–16 mcg/mL. Although some strains of *Bacteroides* are susceptible to ciprofloxacin, most strains are considered resistant to the drug. The MIC_{90} of ciprofloxacin for *Bacteroides fragilis* is 0.8–32 mcg/mL. The MIC_{90} of ciprofloxacin for *B. melaninogenicus, B. ovatus, B. uniformis*, and *B. ureolyticus* is 0.25–16 mcg/mL and the MIC_{90} of the drug for *B. distasonis, B. oralis* (*Prevotella oralis*), *B. thetaiotaomicron*, and *B. vulgatus* generally is 16–64 mcg/mL.

■ **Chlamydia and Mycoplasma** Ciprofloxacin has some in vitro activity against *Chlamydophila pneumoniae* (formerly *Chlamydia pneumoniae*), *Chlamydia trachomatis*, and *C. psittaci*, and these organisms generally are inhibited in vitro by concentrations of 0.5–5 mcg/mL. The MBC of ciprofloxacin reported for *C. trachomatis* is 1–10 mcg/mL.

The MIC_{90} of ciprofloxacin reported for *Mycoplasma hominis* and *M. pneumoniae* is 0.5–2 mcg/mL. In some studies, the MIC_{90} of ciprofloxacin for *Ureaplasma urealyticum* was 2–6.3 mcg/mL; however, in other studies, this organism was resistant to the drug since the MIC_{90} was 32 mcg/mL and the MBC was greater than 64 mcg/mL.

■ **Mycobacterium** Ciprofloxacin is active in vitro against some *Mycobacterium*. In vitro on a weight basis, ciprofloxacin is less active than levofloxacin or moxifloxacin against these organisms. The MIC_{90} of ciprofloxacin for *M. tuberculosis* is 0.1–3.1 mcg/mL.

Other mycobacteria usually are less susceptible to ciprofloxacin. The MIC_{90} for *M. fortuitum, M. kansasii, M. smegmatis*, and *M. xenopi* is 0.05–8 mcg/mL. The MIC_{90} for *M. avium* complex, *M. abscessus*, and *M. chelonae* generally is 1–16 mcg/mL; most strains of *M. abscessus* and *M. chelonae* are considered resistant to ciprofloxacin.

Ciprofloxacin exhibited weak activity against *M. leprae* in an in vitro metabolic screen for potential antileprosy agents that measured intracellular ATP of the bacteria, and no more than a limited bacteriostatic effect in an in vivo mouse footpad study in mice receiving up to 150 mg/kg of the drug daily.

■ **Other Organisms** Ciprofloxacin has some activity in vitro against *Plasmodium falciparum*. In some studies, the drug appeared to be active against both chloroquine-susceptible and -resistant strains of the organism. However, in other studies, chloroquine-resistant strains required high concentrations of the drug for in vitro inhibition. When in vitro activity of ciprofloxacin was assessed using incorporation of radiolabeled hypoxanthine by the organism, the ID_{50} (concentration of the drug required to inhibit hypoxanthine uptake by 50%) of ciprofloxacin for chloroquine-susceptible *P. falciparum* was 3.2 mcg/mL and the ID_{50} of the drug for chloroquine-resistant strains was 6.6 mcg/mL.

Ciprofloxacin reportedly has some activity in vitro against *Rickettsia conorii*, the causative organism of Mediterranean spotted fever. In one study, the MIC of the drug for this organism was 0.5 mcg/mL.

Although further study is needed, results of one study indicate that ciprofloxacin may have some activity in vitro against *Leptospira interrogans*.

Resistance

Resistance to ciprofloxacin can be produced in vitro in some organisms, including some strains of Enterobacteriaceae, *Pseudomonas aeruginosa, Staphylococcus aureus*, and *Enterococcus faecalis* (formerly *Streptococcus faecalis*), by serial passage in the presence of increasing concentrations of the drug. Ciprofloxacin resistance resulting from spontaneous mutation occurs rarely in vitro (i.e., with a frequency of 10^{-9} to 10^{-7}).

The mechanism(s) of resistance to fluoroquinolones, including ciprofloxacin, has not been fully elucidated but appears to involve mutations in the target DNA type II topoisomerase enzymes and mutations that result in alterations in membrane permeability and/or efflux pumps. Current evidence suggests that resistance to ciprofloxacin or other fluoroquinolones usually is chromosomally rather than plasmid mediated.

Resistant strains of *Ps. aeruginosa* have emerged occasionally during therapy with the drug.

Ciprofloxacin-resistant strains of *S. aureus*, including methicillin-resistant strains of *S. aureus* (MRSA; also known as oxacillin-resistant *S. aureus* or ORSA), and *S. epidermidis* also have emerged during therapy with the drug. Strains of *S. aureus*, especially oxacillin-resistant *S. aureus* resistant to ciprofloxacin and other fluoroquinolones have been reported with increasing frequency, and such strains can emerge at relatively rapid rates (e.g., increasing within an institution from 0% of isolates prior to introduction of the drug to 80% 1 year later for oxacillin-resistant *S. aureus*).

Rapid emergence of resistance to fluoroquinolones in *Campylobacter* also has been reported and appears to be associated with widespread use or prolonged therapy with the drugs. Over a 10- to 12-year period in Finland, fluoroquinolone-resistant strains of *C. jejuni* and *C. coli* increased from 0–4% to 9–11%. A similar increase was observed over a 7-year period in *Campylobacter* isolates obtained from poultry and humans in the Netherlands; this increase in resistance was attributed to use of enrofloxacin in the poultry industry. In the US, fluoroquinolone-resistant isolates of *Campylobacter* have been obtained from raw turkey or chicken products in the retail market.

S. typhi and *S. paratyphi* with reduced susceptibility to ciprofloxacin have been reported. *Salmonella* resistant to fluoroquinolones are common in India and southeast Asia.

■ Resistance in Mycobacterium Ciprofloxacin-resistant *Mycobacterium tuberculosis* have been reported and some multidrug-resistant strains (i.e., strains resistant to rifampin and isoniazid) also are resistant to ciprofloxacin or other fluoroquinolones. Extensively drug-resistant tuberculosis (XDR tuberculosis) caused by strains resistant to rifampin and isoniazid (multiple-drug resistant strains) and also resistant to a fluoroquinolone and at least one parenteral second-line antimycobacterial (capreomycin, kanamycin, amikacin) has been reported with increasing frequency.

Ciprofloxacin-resistant strains of initially susceptible *M. fortuitum* have developed in a few patients who received ciprofloxacin alone or in conjunction with amikacin. Many strains of *M. kansasii* are resistant to ciprofloxacin.

■ Resistance in Neisseria gonorrhoeae *Neisseria gonorrhoeae* with decreased susceptibility to ciprofloxacin and other fluoroquinolones (quinolone-resistant *N. gonorrhoeae*; QRNG) are widely disseminated throughout the world, including in the US. QRNG have ciprofloxacin MICs of 1 mcg/mL or greater; isolates with intermediate resistance to fluoroquinolones have ciprofloxacin MICs of 0.12–0.5 mcg/mL. Strains of *N. gonorrhoeae* with decreased susceptibility to ciprofloxacin also have decreased susceptibility to other fluoroquinolones (e.g., levofloxacin, ofloxacin), but may be susceptible to ceftriaxone, cefixime, and spectinomycin (currently not commercially available in the US). A few strains with decreased susceptibility to ciprofloxacin also were resistant to tetracycline.

Until 1992, virtually all strains of *N. gonorrhoeae* tested were susceptible to ciprofloxacin in vitro, but susceptibility of this organism to fluoroquinolones changed. QRNG are endemic in many Asian countries and have been reported sporadically in other parts of the world, including North America, Australia, Africa, Great Britain, and Israel. QRNG have been isolated from all regions of the US. The prevalence of these strains has been particularly high in Hawaii, Ohio, Oregon, California, and Washington and there have been substantial increases in QRNG prevalence reported over the last several years in some other areas of the US, including Philadelphia and Miami. In some cases, QRNG isolates appeared to have been introduced into the US by travelers returning from the Philippines; however, increases in QRNG in Hawaii and Ohio during 1992–1999 appeared to have been the result of endemic spread.

The prevalence of QRNG in the US is being monitored by the Centers for Disease Control and Prevention (CDC) Gonococcal Isolate Surveillance Project (GISP). During 1990–2001, QRNG prevalence in the US remained at less than 1%, but increased to 2.2% in 2002, 4.1% in 2003, 6.8% in 2004, and 9.4% in 2005. GISP data for the first 6 months of 2006 indicated that 13.3% of isolates collected by GISP were resistant to ciprofloxacin; when isolates from Hawaii and California were excluded (areas that discontinued use of fluoroquinolones for gonorrhea treatment in 2000 and 2002, respectively), 6.1 and 8.6% of GISP isolates were QRNG in 2005 and 2006, respectively. The prevalence of QRNG isolates decreased from 14.8% in 2007 to 9.6% in 2009 and then increased to 19.2% by 2014. The 2014 GISP data for the US indicated that QRNG were identified in 27.3% of isolates from the West, 21.4% of isolates from the Northeast, 14.3% from the South, and 10.2% from the Midwest.

QRNG strains are more common in men who have sex with men (MSM) than among heterosexual men, but prevalence has increased in both groups. QRNG prevalence in MSM was 1.6% in 2001, 7.2% in 2002, 15% in 2003, 23.8% in 2004, and 29% in 2005. QRNG prevalence increased more slowly in heterosexual men and was 0.6% in 2001, 0.9% in 2002, 1.5% in 2003, 2.9% in 2004, and 3.8% in 2005. The 2014 GISP data indicate that QRNG were identified in approximately 30% of isolates from MSM and men who have sex with both women and men and in 12.7% of isolates from men who have sex with women.

Beginning in April 2007, based on GISP data for the first 6 months of 2006 indicating that QRNG prevalence had increased among isolates obtained from MSM and heterosexual men and because QRNG was identified in all regions of the US, CDC recommended fluoroquinolones should no longer be used for the treatment of gonorrhea or any associated infections that may involve *N. gonorrhoeae* (e.g., pelvic inflammatory disease [PID], epididymitis). (See Uses: Gonorrhea and Associated Infections.)

■ Resistance in Bacillus anthracis Strains of *Bacillus anthracis* with natural resistance to ciprofloxacin have not been reported to date. There are published reports of *B. anthracis* strains that have been engineered to have tetracycline and penicillin resistance as well as resistance to other anti-infectives (e.g., macrolides, chloramphenicol, rifampin). In addition, reduced susceptibility to ofloxacin (4-fold increase in MICs from baseline) has been produced in vitro following sequential subculture of the Sterne strain of *B. anthracis* in subinhibitory concentrations of the fluoroquinolone.

■ Cross-resistance Cross-resistance can occur among the fluoroquinolones.

Cross-resistance generally does not occur between ciprofloxacin and other anti-infectives, including aminoglycosides, β-lactam antibiotics, sulfonamides (including co-trimoxazole), macrolides, and tetracyclines. However, rare strains of Enterobacteriaceae and *Ps. aeruginosa* resistant to ciprofloxacin have also been resistant to aminoglycosides, β-lactam antibiotics, chloramphenicol, trimethoprim, and/or tetracyclines. Resistance in these organisms appears to be related to decreased permeability of the organism to the drug, principally because of alterations in outer-membrane porin proteins; however, other mechanisms that affect permeability may also be involved.

Pharmacokinetics

In studies in the Pharmacokinetics section, ciprofloxacin was administered orally as conventional tablets containing the monohydrochloride monohydrate salt (i.e., ciprofloxacin hydrochloride), as extended-release tablets containing both ciprofloxacin hydrochloride and ciprofloxacin (base), or as an oral suspension containing the base; ciprofloxacin also was administered parenterally. Dosages and concentrations of the drug are expressed in terms of ciprofloxacin.

Body fluid and tissue concentrations of ciprofloxacin were measured with either a high-pressure liquid chromatographic (HPLC) assay or a microbiologic assay. HPLC assays are more specific for ciprofloxacin than microbiologic assays since the latter method measures the antibacterial activity of the parent drug as well as its microbiologically active metabolites. Controlled studies using HPLC and microbiologic assays indicate that there is good correlation between both methods for serum ciprofloxacin concentrations and pharmacokinetic parameters determined using these serum concentrations. However, mean ciprofloxacin concentrations in urine or bile generally are 30–40% higher when a microbiologic assay is used than when an HPLC assay is used.

The pharmacokinetics of ciprofloxacin after oral administration (as the hydrochloride) are best described by a 2-compartment model assuming zero-order absorption, and pharmacokinetics after IV administration are best described by an open, 3-compartment model.

The manufacturer states that a 500-mg dose of ciprofloxacin administered as ciprofloxacin oral suspension containing 250 mg/5 mL is bioequivalent to a 500-mg conventional tablet and that 10 mL of the ciprofloxacin oral suspension containing 250 mg/5 mL is bioequivalent to 5 mL of the oral suspension containing 500 mg/5 mL.

Ciprofloxacin conventional tablets are *not* bioequivalent to ciprofloxacin extended-release tablets.

■ Absorption ***Oral Administration*** Ciprofloxacin hydrochloride is rapidly and well absorbed from the GI tract following oral administration, and undergoes minimal first-pass metabolism.

The oral bioavailability of ciprofloxacin administered as conventional tablets is 50–85% in healthy, fasting adults, and peak serum concentrations of the drug generally are attained within 0.5–2.3 hours. Peak serum concentrations and area under the serum concentration-time curve (AUC) increase in proportion to the dose over the oral dosage range of 250–1000 mg and are unaffected by gender. Following oral administration of a single 250-, 500-, 750-, or 1000-mg dose of ciprofloxacin as conventional tablets or oral suspension in healthy, fasting adults, peak serum concentrations average 0.76–1.5, 1.6–2.9, 2.5–4.3, or 3.4–5.4 mcg/mL, respectively; serum concentrations 12 hours after the dose average 0.1, 0.2, 0.4, or 0.6 mcg/mL, respectively. In adults, oral administration of 500 mg of ciprofloxacin as conventional tablets every 12 hours results in mean peak or trough serum concentrations at steady-state of 2.97 or 0.2 mcg/mL, respectively.

Following oral administration of extended-release tablets containing ciprofloxacin hydrochloride and base, peak plasma concentrations of ciprofloxacin are attained within 1–4 hours. Ciprofloxacin extended-release tablets contain approximately 35% of the dose within an immediate-release component; the remaining 65% of the dose is contained in a slow-release matrix. Oral administration of ciprofloxacin 500 mg once daily as ciprofloxacin extended-release tablets or 250 mg twice daily as conventional tablets results in steady-state mean peak plasma concentrations of 1.59 or 1.14 mcg/mL, respectively; however, the area under the concentration-time curve (AUC) is similar with both regimens. Oral administration of 1 g once daily as ciprofloxacin extended-release tablets or 500 mg twice daily as conventional tablets results in steady-state mean peak plasma concentrations of 3.11 or 2.06 mcg/mL, respectively; the AUC is similar with both regimens.

Data indicate that peak serum concentrations and AUCs of ciprofloxacin are slightly higher in geriatric patients than in younger adults; this may occur because of increased bioavailability, reduced volume of distribution, and/or reduced renal clearance in these patients. Single-dose oral studies using ciprofloxacin conventional tablets and single- and multiple-dose IV studies indicate that, compared with younger adults, peak plasma concentrations are 16–40% higher, mean AUC is approximately 30% higher, and elimination half-life is prolonged approximately 20% in individuals older than 65 years of age. These differences can be at least partially attributed to decreased renal clearance in this age group and are not clinically important.

Based on population pharmacokinetics, bioavailability of ciprofloxacin oral suspension in children is approximately 60%. Following a single oral dose of 10 mg/kg of ciprofloxacin given as the oral suspension to children 4 months to 7 years of age, the mean peak plasma concentration was 2.4 mcg/mL. There was no apparent age dependence and no increase in peak plasma concentrations following multiple doses.

In one study, GI absorption of ciprofloxacin was slower and the elimination half-life of the drug was shorter in cystic fibrosis patients 18 years of age or older than in healthy adults. Several other studies, however, indicate that the pharmacokinetics of ciprofloxacin are not appreciably altered in cystic fibrosis patients 18 years of age or older compared with healthy adults.

Although peak serum concentrations of ciprofloxacin and the AUC increased slightly after repeated oral doses in a few studies in fasting, healthy adults, most multiple-dose studies in fasting, healthy adults with normal renal function indicate that neither peak nor trough serum concentrations of ciprofloxacin increase after repeated oral doses and that the drug does not accumulate.

Magnesium-, aluminum-, and/or calcium-containing antacids or products containing calcium, iron, or zinc decrease the oral bioavailability of ciprofloxacin hydrochloride. (See Drug Interactions: Antacids.)

Food or Milk. The effect of food and/or milk on GI absorption of ciprofloxacin varies depending on the specific ciprofloxacin preparation (conventional tablets, extended-release tablets, oral solution) and situation.

When ciprofloxacin conventional tablets are administered concomitantly with food, there is a delay in absorption of the drug, but overall absorption is not substantially affected.

The manufacturer states that food does not affect the rate or extent of absorption of ciprofloxacin administered as the oral suspension.

The manufacturers state that, based on pharmacokinetic studies, ciprofloxacin extended-release tablets can be administered with or without food (e.g., with a high- or low-fat meal or under fasting conditions).

Concomitant administration of oral ciprofloxacin with dairy products (e.g., milk, yogurt) or calcium-fortified juices alone (i.e., without a meal) or with substantial calcium intake (greater than 800 mg) can reduce GI absorption of ciprofloxacin. In one study, administration of a 500-mg dose of ciprofloxacin (conventional tablet) with 300 mL of whole milk (360 mg calcium, 33 mg magnesium) or unflavored yogurt (450 mg calcium, 40 mg magnesium) decreased the AUC by 33 or 36%, respectively, and decreased peak plasma concentrations by 36 or 47%, respectively, compared with administration with water. The manufacturers state that oral ciprofloxacin can be taken with dairy products or calcium-fortified juices that are part of a meal.

Concomitant administration with nutritional supplements or enteral feedings may affect GI absorption of ciprofloxacin. When a 750-mg conventional ciprofloxacin tablet was crushed, mixed with 120 mL of enteral premixed liquid (Ensure), and swallowed, the AUC was 28% lower and peak plasma concentrations were 47% lower compared with results attained when the tablet was crushed and mixed with water before swallowing. In another crossover study in healthy adults, the AUC of the drug was 25% lower when a 750-mg conventional ciprofloxacin tablet was administered with 240 mL of a nutritional supplement containing calcium, magnesium, iron, and zinc (Resource) compared with administration with water.

IV Administration Following IV infusion over 60 minutes of a single 200- or 400-mg dose of ciprofloxacin in healthy adults, peak serum concentrations average 2.1 and 4.6 mcg/mL, respectively, immediately following the infusion; serum concentrations 6 hours after the start of infusion (i.e., 5 hours after completion) average 0.3 and 0.7 mcg/mL and those 12 hours after the start of infusion average 0.1 and 0.2 mcg/mL, respectively. In adults receiving 400 mg of ciprofloxacin IV every 12 hours, mean peak or trough serum concentrations at steady-state are 4.56 or 0.2 mcg/mL, respectively.

Following IV injection over 15 minutes of a single 100-mg dose of ciprofloxacin in healthy adults, serum concentrations of the drug average 2.8 mcg/mL immediately following the injection and 0.32, 0.14, and 0.07 mcg/mL at 1, 6, and 12 hours, respectively, after the dose. In healthy adults who receive a single 200-mg dose of ciprofloxacin by IV injection over 10 minutes, serum concentrations of the drug immediately following the injection average 6.3–6.5 mcg/mL and serum concentrations 1 and 12 hours later average 0.87 and 0.1 mcg/mL, respectively.

In a limited number of pediatric patients with severe sepsis who received ciprofloxacin 10 mg/kg given by IV infusion over 1 hour, mean peak plasma concentrations were 6.1 mcg/mL in those younger than 1 year of age and 7.2 mcg/mL in those 1–5 years of age.

■ Distribution Ciprofloxacin is widely distributed into body tissues and fluids following oral or IV administration. Highest concentrations of the drug generally are attained in bile, lungs, kidney, liver, gallbladder, uterus, seminal fluid, prostatic tissue and fluid, tonsils, endometrium, fallopian tubes, and ovaries. Concentrations of the drug achieved in most of these tissues and fluids substantially exceed those in serum. The drug also is distributed into adipose tissue, aqueous humor, bone, cartilage, heart tissue (heart valves, myocardia), muscle, nasal secretions, saliva, skin, sputum, and pleural, peritoneal, ascitic, blister, lymphatic, and renal cyst fluid. Ciprofloxacin is concentrated within neutrophils, achieving concentrations in these cells that may be 2–7 times greater than extracellular concentrations.

In healthy adults, the apparent volume of distribution of ciprofloxacin is 2–3.5 L/kg and the apparent volume of distribution at steady state is 1.7–2.7 L/kg. The apparent volume of distribution of ciprofloxacin in geriatric patients 64–91 years of age averages 3.5–3.6 L/kg.

Only low concentrations of ciprofloxacin are distributed into CSF; peak CSF concentrations may be 6–10% of peak serum concentrations. In adults with meningitis who received 200-mg doses of ciprofloxacin every 12 hours by IV infusion over 30 minutes, the ratio of CSF/serum concentrations in samples obtained 1–2 hours after a dose was 0.11–0.46 during the first 2–4 days of therapy when meninges were inflamed and 0.04–0.3 during days 10–14 when meninges were uninflamed. In one patient with meningitis caused by *Ps. aeruginosa* who received IV ciprofloxacin in a dosage of 400 mg every 8 hours, CSF concentrations of the drug were about 1 mg/mL and drug accumulation in CSF did not occur.

Following oral or IV administration of the drug, biliary ciprofloxacin concentrations are several fold higher than simultaneous serum concentrations of the drug. In adults undergoing cholecystectomy who received a single 750-mg oral dose of ciprofloxacin, peak concentrations of the drug and active metabolites ranged from 68–225 mcg/mL in gallbladder bile, 16–17 mcg/mL in common duct bile, 3.6–32.4 mcg/g in liver, 0.8–14.1 mcg/g in gallbladder, and 1.5–7.8 mcg/mL in serum.

Following oral administration, ciprofloxacin concentrations in prostatic tissue and fluid generally exceed concurrent serum concentrations of the drug. In a study in men undergoing transurethral resection for prostatic hyperplasia or cancer who received 500 mg of the drug orally every 12 hours, ciprofloxacin concentrations in prostatic tissue obtained 75–120 minutes after a dose averaged 3 mg/kg and the ratio of prostate/serum concentrations ranged from 1–7.

Ciprofloxacin is 16–43% bound to serum proteins in vitro.

Ciprofloxacin crosses the placenta and is distributed into amniotic fluid in humans.

Ciprofloxacin is distributed into milk. In lactating women who received 750 mg of ciprofloxacin every 12 hours for 3 doses, concentrations of the drug in milk obtained 2–4 hours after a dose averaged 2.26–3.79 mcg/mL; milk concentrations were higher than concomitant serum concentrations for up to 12 hours after a dose.

■ Elimination The serum elimination half-life of ciprofloxacin in adults with normal renal function is 3–7 hours. Following IV administration in healthy adults, the distribution half-life of ciprofloxacin averages 0.18–0.37 hours and the elimination half-life averages 3–4.8 hours.

The elimination half-life of the drug is slightly longer in geriatric adults than in younger adults, and ranges from 3.3–6.8 hours in adults 60–91 years of age with renal function normal for their age.

Based on population pharmacokinetic analysis of pediatric patients with various infections, the predicted mean half-life of ciprofloxacin in children is approximately 4–5 hours.

In patients with impaired renal function, serum concentrations of ciprofloxacin are higher and the half-life prolonged. In adults with creatinine clearances of 30 mL/minute or less, half-life of the drug ranges from 4.4–12.6 hours.

Further study is needed to evaluate that pharmacokinetics in patients with hepatic impairment. In one study in patients with stable chronic liver cirrhosis, there was no clinically important change in ciprofloxacin pharmacokinetics; however, slightly prolonged half-life has been reported in some other patients with hepatic impairment.

Ciprofloxacin is eliminated by renal and nonrenal mechanisms. The drug is partially metabolized in the liver by modification of the piperazinyl group to at least 4 metabolites. These metabolites, which have been identified as desethyleneciprofloxacin (M1), sulfociprofloxacin (M2), oxociprofloxacin (M3), and *N*-formylciprofloxacin (M4), have microbiologic activity that is less than that of the parent drug.

Ciprofloxacin and its metabolites are excreted in urine and feces. Unchanged ciprofloxacin is excreted in urine by both glomerular filtration and tubular secretion. Following oral administration of a single 250-, 500-, or 750-mg dose in adults with normal renal function, 15–50% of the dose is excreted in urine as unchanged drug and 10–15% as metabolites within 24 hours; 20–40% of the dose is excreted in feces as unchanged drug and metabolites within 5 days. Most, but not all, of unchanged ciprofloxacin in feces appears to result from biliary excretion.

Renal clearance of ciprofloxacin averages 300–479 mL/minute in adults with normal renal function. Urinary concentrations of ciprofloxacin generally exceed 200 mcg/mL during the first 2 hours and average about 30 mcg/mL 8–12 hours after a single 250-mg oral dose of the drug. Following oral administration of a single 500-mg dose in adults with normal renal function, urinary concentrations of ciprofloxacin and active metabolites average 350, 162, and 105 mcg/mL in urine collected over 1–3, 3–6, and 6–12 hours, respectively, after the dose.Concentrations of unchanged drug and active metabolites in feces range from 185–2220 mcg/g after 7 days of therapy with the drug in a dosage of 500 mg every 12 hours.

Small amounts of ciprofloxacin are removed by hemodialysis. The amount of the drug removed during hemodialysis depends on several factors (e.g., type of coil used, dialysis flow rate). In patients with end-stage renal disease undergoing hemodialysis, the serum half-life of ciprofloxacin averaged 3.2 hours during hemodialysis and 5.8 hours between dialysis sessions. A 4-hour period of hemodialysis generally removes into the dialysate 2–30% of a single 250- or 500-mg oral dose of the drug. Only small amounts of ciprofloxacin appear to be removed by peritoneal dialysis.

Chemistry and Stability

■ Chemistry Ciprofloxacin is a fluoroquinolone anti-infective agent. Like all other commercially available fluoroquinolones, ciprofloxacin contains a fluorine at the C-6 position of the quinolone nucleus. Like some other fluoroquinolones (levofloxacin, ofloxacin), ciprofloxacin contains a piperazinyl group at position 7 of the quinolone nucleus. The piperazinyl group in ciprofloxacin results in antipseudomonal activity. The drug also contains a cyclopropyl group at position 1, which enhances antimicrobial activity.

Ciprofloxacin is commercially available for oral administration as conventional tablets containing ciprofloxacin hydrochloride, which is the monohydrochloride monohydrate of the drug. Ciprofloxacin hydrochloride occurs as a faintly yellowish to yellow crystalline powder. Ciprofloxacin hydrochloride has a solubility of approximately 36 mg/mL in water at 25°C. The pK_as of the drug are 6 and 8.8.

Ciprofloxacin also is commercially available for oral administration as extended-release tablets containing ciprofloxacin hydrochloride and ciprofloxacin (base). Ciprofloxacin extended-release tablets contain approximately 35% of the dose within an immediate-release component; the remaining 65% of the dose is contained in a slow-release matrix. Ciprofloxacin (base) occurs as a pale yellowing to light yellow crystalline powder.

In addition, ciprofloxacin is commercially available for oral administration as microcapsules for oral suspension. Following mixture with the diluent provided by the manufacturer, ciprofloxacin oral suspensions containing 250 or 500 mg of the drug per 5 mL occur as a strawberry-flavored, white to slightly yellowish suspension and may contain yellow-orange droplets.

For IV administration, ciprofloxacin is commercially available as the base. Ciprofloxacin concentrate for IV infusion contains 10 mg of ciprofloxacin per mL in an aqueous solution and is provided in glass vials. The commercially available premixed injection for IV infusion contains 2 mg or ciprofloxacin per mL in 5% dextrose. The concentrate and premixed injection in 5% dextrose occur as clear, colorless to slightly yellow solutions. The concentrate for IV infusion has a pH of 3.3–3.9; the commercially available premixed injection in 5% dextrose has a pH of 3.5–4.6. The concentrate and commercially available premixed injection for IV infusion contain lactic acid as a solubilizing agent and may contain hydrochloric acid to adjust pH.

■ **Stability** Ciprofloxacin hydrochloride conventional tablets should be stored at 20–25°C, but may be exposed to temperatures ranging from 15–30°C.

Extended-release tablets containing ciprofloxacin hydrochloride and base should be stored at 20–25°C, in a tight, light-resistant container.

Ciprofloxacin microcapsules for oral suspension and the diluent provided by the manufacturer should be stored at less than 25°C, but may be exposed to temperatures ranging from 15–30°C. Following reconstitution with the diluent, ciprofloxacin oral suspension should be stored at 25°C, but may be exposed to temperatures ranging from 15–30°C, and is stable for 14 days. The microcapsules, diluent, and reconstituted oral suspension should be protected from freezing.

Ciprofloxacin concentrate for IV infusion (10 mg/mL) provided in vials should be stored at 5–30°C and protected from light, excessive heat, and freezing. Following dilution of the ciprofloxacin concentrate for IV infusion in sterile water for injection, 5% or 10% dextrose injection, 0.9% sodium chloride injection, 5% dextrose and 0.225 or 0.45% sodium chloride injection, or lactated Ringer's injection to a final concentration of 0.5–2 mg/mL, the resultant solutions are stable for up to 14 days when refrigerated or stored at room temperature.

The commercially available premixed injection for IV infusion containing 2 mg/mL in 5% dextrose should be stored at 5–25°C and protected from light, excessive heat, and freezing. The premixed injection for IV infusion is provided in single-dose flexible plastic containers. Solutions in contact with the plastic can leach out some of the chemical components in very small amounts (e.g., bis(2-ethylhexyl)phthalate [BEHP, DEHP] in up to 5 ppm) within the expiration period of the injection; however, safety of the plastic has been confirmed in tests in animals according to USP biological tests for plastic containers as well as by tissue culture toxicity studies.

Preparations

Excipients in commercially available drug preparations may have clinically important effects in some individuals; consult specific product labeling for details.

Ciprofloxacin

Oral		
For suspension	250 mg/5 mL*	**Cipro®**, Bayer
		Ciprofloxacin for Oral Suspension
	500 mg/5 mL*	**Cipro®**, Bayer
		Ciprofloxacin for Oral Suspension
Parenteral		
For injection concentrate, for IV infusion	10 mg (of ciprofloxacin) per mL (200 or 400 mg)*	**Ciprofloxacin for Injection Concentrate**

*available from one or more manufacturer, distributor, and/or repackager by generic (nonproprietary) name

Ciprofloxacin and Ciprofloxacin Hydrochloride

Oral		
Tablets, extended-release, film-coated	500 mg total ciprofloxacin (with ciprofloxacin 212.6 mg [of anhydrous ciprofloxacin] and ciprofloxacin hydrochloride 287.5 mg [of anhydrous ciprofloxacin])*	**Ciprofloxacin Extended-release Tablets**
	1 g total ciprofloxacin (with ciprofloxacin 425.2 mg [of anhydrous ciprofloxacin] and ciprofloxacin hydrochloride 574.9 mg [of anhydrous ciprofloxacin])*	**Ciprofloxacin Extended-release Tablets**

*available from one or more manufacturer, distributor, and/or repackager by generic (nonproprietary) name

Ciprofloxacin Hydrochloride

Oral		
Tablets, film-coated	100 mg (of ciprofloxacin)*	**Ciprofloxacin Tablets**
	250 mg (of ciprofloxacin)*	**Cipro®**, Bayer
		Ciprofloxacin Tablets
	500 mg (of ciprofloxacin)*	**Cipro®**, Bayer
		Ciprofloxacin Tablets
	750 mg (of ciprofloxacin)*	**Ciprofloxacin Tablets**

*available from one or more manufacturer, distributor, and/or repackager by generic (nonproprietary) name

Ciprofloxacin in Dextrose

Parenteral		
Injection, for IV infusion	2 mg (of ciprofloxacin) per mL (200 or 400 mg) in 5% dextrose*	**Ciprofloxacin in 5% Dextrose Injection**

*available from one or more manufacturer, distributor, and/or repackager by generic (nonproprietary) name

†Use is not currently included in the labeling approved by the US Food and Drug Administration

Selected Revisions September 2019, © Copyright, November 1988, American Society of Health-System Pharmacists, Inc.

Delafloxacin Meglumine

■ Delafloxacin is a fluoroquinolone anti-infective agent.

Uses

■ **Skin and Skin Structure Infections** Delafloxacin meglumine is used for the treatment of acute bacterial skin and skin structure infections (ABSSSI) caused by susceptible *Staphylococcus aureus* (including methicillin-resistant *S. aureus* [MRSA; also known as oxacillin-resistant *S. aureus* or ORSA] and methicillin-susceptible *S. aureus*), *S. haemolyticus*, *S. lugdunensis*, *Streptococcus pyogenes* (group A β-hemolytic streptococci, GAS), *S. agalactiae* (group B streptococci, GBS), *S. anginosus* group (includes *S. anginosus*, *S. intermedius*, and *S. constellatus*), *Enterococcus faecalis*, *Escherichia coli*, *Enterobacter cloacae*, *Klebsiella pneumoniae*, or *Pseudomonas aeruginosa*.

Clinical Experience Efficacy and safety of delafloxacin were evaluated in 2 randomized, multicenter, multinational, double-blind, double-dummy, noninferiority, phase 3 studies in adults with acute bacterial skin and skin structure infections (e.g., cellulitis/erysipelas, wound infection, major cutaneous abscess, burn infection).

In the first study (Trial 1; NCT01811732), 660 patients (average age 46 years [range: 18–94 years of age], 63% male, 91% white, 9% with diabetes mellitus, 55% reported recent drug abuse [including IV drug abuse], 39% with cellulitis/erysipelas, 35% with wound infection, 25% with major cutaneous abscess, 1% with burn infection, 2% with documented bacteremia at baseline) were randomized to receive delafloxacin (300 mg IV every 12 hours) or a regimen of vancomycin (15 mg/kg IV every 12 hours) in conjunction with aztreonam (2 g IV every 12 hours) for a duration of 5–14 days. Aztreonam was discontinued if baseline cultures did not reveal gram-negative bacteria. Clinical response (i.e., at least 20% decrease in lesion size determined by digital planimetry of the leading edge of erythema) at 48–72 hours after initiation of treatment was achieved in 78.2% of those receiving delafloxacin and 80.9% of those receiving the vancomycin regimen. At a follow-up visit approximately 14 days (range: 13–15 days) after initiation of treatment, investigator-assessed treatment success (defined as complete resolution [cure] *or* clinical improvement with complete or nearly complete resolution of signs and symptoms with no further antibacterial treatment) was achieved by 81.6 or 83.3% of the intent-to-treat population receiving delafloxacin or the vancomycin regimen, respectively; in the subset of patients who were clinically evaluable at the 14-day follow-up visit, treatment success was achieved in 96.7 or 97.5% of patients, respectively.

In the second study (Trial 2; NCT01984684), 850 patients (average age 51 years [range: 18–93 years of age], 63% male, 83% white, 13% with diabetes mellitus, 30% reported recent drug abuse [including IV drug abuse], 48% with cellulitis/erysipelas, 26% with wound infection, 25% with major cutaneous abscess, 1% with burn infection, 2% with documented bacteremia at baseline) were randomized to receive delafloxacin (300 mg IV every 12 hours for 6 doses, then oral delafloxacin 450 mg every 12 hours) or a regimen of IV vancomycin (15 mg/kg every 12 hours) in conjunction with IV aztreonam (2 g every 12 hours) for a duration of 5–14 days. Aztreonam was discontinued if baseline cultures did not reveal gram-negative bacteria. Clinical response (i.e., at least 20% decrease in lesion size determined by digital planimetry of the leading edge of erythema) at 48–72 hours after initiation of treatment was achieved in 83.7% of those receiving delafloxacin and 80.6% of those receiving the vancomycin regimen. At a follow-up visit approximately 14 days (range: 13–15 days) after initiation of treatment, investigator-assessed treatment success (defined as complete resolution [cure] *or* nearly complete resolution of signs and symptoms with no further antibacterial treatment) was achieved by 87.2 or 84.8% of the intent-to-treat population receiving delafloxacin or the vancomycin regimen, respectively; in the subset of patients who were clinically evaluable at the 14-day follow-up visit, treatment success was achieved in 96 or 97% of patients, respectively.

In a pooled subset of microbiologically evaluable patients from both studies that were stratified according to the infecting pathogen, clinical response at 48–72 hours in those with infections caused by MRSA or methicillin-susceptible *S. aureus* was 86.8 or 84.2%%, respectively, in those treated with delafloxacin and 85.8 or 80.9%, respectively, in those treated with the vancomycin regimen. The clinical response in those with infections caused by *S. agalactiae*, *S. pyogenes*, or *S. anginosus* group was 71.4, 73.9, or 92.2%, respectively, in those treated with delafloxacin and 75, 50, or 90.2%, respectively, in those treated with the vancomycin regimen. The clinical response in those with infections caused by *S. haemolyticus*, *S. lugdunensis*, or *E. faecalis* was 73.3, 72.7, or 100%, respectively, in those treated with delafloxacin and 87.5, 66.7, or 75%, respectively, in those treated with the vancomycin regimen. The clinical response in those with infections caused by *E. coli*, *E. cloacae*, *K. pneumoniae*, or *Ps. aeruginosa* was 85.7, 71.4, 86.4, or 81.8%, respectively, in those treated with delafloxacin and 80, 72.7, 95.7, or 91.7%, respectively, in those treated with the vancomycin regimen.

Dosage and Administration

■ **Administration** Delafloxacin meglumine is administered orally or by IV infusion.

Oral Administration Delafloxacin tablets may be given without regard to food.

Delafloxacin tablets should be administered orally at least 2 hours before or 6 hours after antacids containing magnesium or aluminum, metal cations (e.g., iron), sucralfate, multivitamins or dietary supplements containing iron or zinc, or buffered didanosine preparations. These drugs may substantially interfere with oral absorption of delafloxacin, resulting in systemic concentrations lower than desired. (See Drug Interactions.)

IV Infusion Delafloxacin solutions should *not* be infused simultaneously through the same tubing with other drugs and should *not* be administered with any solution containing multivalent cations (e.g., calcium, magnesium).

If a common IV line is used to administer delafloxacin and other drugs, the line should be flushed with 0.9% sodium chloride injection or 5% dextrose injection before and after each delafloxacin infusion.

Vials of delafloxacin lyophilized powder for injection are for single use only.

Reconstitution and Dilution. Delafloxacin meglumine for injection must be reconstituted and further diluted prior to IV infusion.

Vials labeled as containing 300 mg of delafloxacin should be reconstituted by adding 10.5 mL of 0.9% sodium chloride injection or 5% dextrose injection to provide a solution containing 25 mg/mL. The vial should be shaken vigorously until the contents are completely dissolved. The reconstituted solution should appear clear yellow to amber in color.

To prepare a 300-mg dose of delafloxacin in a 250-mL infusion bag containing 0.9% sodium chloride injection or 5% dextrose injection, 12 mL of the diluent should be removed from the infusion bag prior to injecting 12 mL of reconstituted delafloxacin solution into the bag; the concentration of the final infusion solution is 1.2 mg/mL.

To prepare a 200-mg dose of delafloxacin in a 250-mL infusion bag containing 0.9% sodium chloride injection or 5% dextrose injection, 8 mL of the diluent should be removed from the infusion bag prior to injecting 8 mL of reconstituted delafloxacin solution into the bag; the concentration of the final infusion solution is 0.8 mg/mL.

Reconstituted delafloxacin or reconstituted and further diluted solutions of delafloxacin may be stored under refrigeration (2–8°C) or at controlled room temperature (20–25°C) for up to 24 hours, but should not be frozen.

Delafloxacin solutions should be inspected visually for particulate matter and discoloration prior to administration.

Rate of Administration. IV infusions of delafloxacin should be given over 60 minutes.

■ **Dosage** Dosage of delafloxacin meglumine is expressed in terms of delafloxacin.

Adult Dosage **Skin and Skin Structure Infections.** When delafloxacin tablets are used, the recommended dosage of the drug for the treatment of acute bacterial skin and skin structure infections (ABSSSI) in adults is 450 mg orally every 12 hours for a duration of 5–14 days.

When IV delafloxacin is used, the recommended dosage of the drug for the treatment of acute bacterial skin and skin structure infections in adults is 300 mg IV every 12 hours for a duration of 5–14 days.

Alternatively, when IV delafloxacin is used initially in a dosage of 300 mg every 12 hours, therapy may be switched at the discretion of the clinician to delafloxacin tablets given in a dosage of 450 mg orally every 12 hours. The total duration of therapy should be 5–14 days.

■ **Special Populations** ***Hepatic Impairment*** Dosage adjustments are not necessary when delafloxacin is used in adults with mild, moderate, or severe hepatic impairment (Child-Pugh class A, B, or C).

Renal Impairment Dosage adjustments are not necessary when delafloxacin is used in adults with mild or moderate renal impairment (estimated glomerular filtration rate [eGFR] of 30–89 mL/minute per 1.73 m^2).

If delafloxacin tablets are used for the treatment of acute bacterial skin and skin structure infections in adults with severe renal impairment (eGFR of 15–29 mL/minute per 1.73 m^2), dosage adjustments are not necessary.

If IV delafloxacin is used for the treatment of acute bacterial skin and skin structure infections in adults with severe renal impairment (eGFR of 15–29 mL/minute per 1.73 m^2), the recommended dosage is 200 mg IV every 12 hours for a duration of 5–14 days. Alternatively, such patients may receive IV delafloxacin initially given in a dosage of 200 mg every 12 hours and therapy may then be switched to delafloxacin tablets given in a dosage of 450 mg orally every 12 hours. The total duration of therapy should be 5–14 days.

Delafloxacin (oral or IV) is *not* recommended in adults with end-stage renal disease (eGFR less than 15 mL/minute per 1.73 m^2) since data are insufficient to provide dosage recommendations for such patients. (See Renal Impairment under Warnings/Precautions: Specific Populations, in Cautions.)

Cautions

■ **Contraindications** Delafloxacin meglumine is contraindicated in patients with known hypersensitivity to delafloxacin, any component of the preparation, or other fluoroquinolones.

■ **Warnings/Precautions** ***Warnings*** **Disabling and Potentially Irreversible Serious Adverse Reactions.** Systemic fluoroquinolones have been associated with disabling and potentially irreversible serious adverse reactions (e.g., tendinitis and tendon rupture, arthralgia, myalgia, peripheral neuropathy, CNS effects) that can occur together in the same patient. These serious reactions may occur within hours to weeks after a systemic fluoroquinolone is initiated and have occurred in all age groups and in patients without preexisting risk factors for such adverse reactions.

Delafloxacin should be discontinued immediately at the first signs or symptoms of any serious adverse reactions.

Systemic fluoroquinolones, including delafloxacin, should be avoided in patients who have experienced any of the serious adverse reactions associated with fluoroquinolones.

Tendinitis and Tendon Rupture. Systemic fluoroquinolones are associated with an increased risk of tendinitis and tendon rupture in all age groups.

The risk of developing fluoroquinolone-associated tendinitis and tendon rupture is increased in older adults (usually those older than 60 years of age), individuals receiving concomitant corticosteroids, and kidney, heart, or lung transplant recipients. (See Geriatric Use under Warnings/Precautions: Specific Populations, in Cautions.)

Other factors that may independently increase the risk of tendon rupture include strenuous physical activity, renal failure, and previous tendon disorders such as rheumatoid arthritis. Tendinitis and tendon rupture have been reported in patients receiving fluoroquinolones who did not have any risk factors for such adverse effects.

Fluoroquinolone-associated tendinitis and tendon rupture most frequently involve the Achilles tendon and also have been reported in the rotator cuff (shoulder), hand, biceps, thumb, and other tendon sites. Tendinitis or tendon rupture can occur within hours or days after a fluoroquinolone is initiated or as long as several months after completion of therapy and can occur bilaterally.

Delafloxacin should be discontinued immediately if pain, swelling, inflammation, or rupture of a tendon occurs. (See Advice to Patients.)

Systemic fluoroquinolones, including delafloxacin, should be avoided in patients who have a history of tendon disorders or have experienced tendinitis or tendon rupture.

Peripheral Neuropathy. Systemic fluoroquinolones have been associated with an increased risk of peripheral neuropathy.

Sensory or sensorimotor axonal polyneuropathy affecting small and/or large axons resulting in paresthesias, hypoesthesias, dysesthesias, and weakness has been reported in patients receiving systemic fluoroquinolones, including delafloxacin. Symptoms may occur soon after initiation of a fluoroquinolone and, in some patients, may be irreversible.

Delafloxacin should be discontinued immediately if symptoms of peripheral neuropathy (e.g., pain, burning, tingling, numbness, and/or weakness) occur or if there are other alterations in sensations (e.g., light touch, pain, temperature, position sense, vibratory sensation, and/or motor strength). (See Advice to Patients.)

Systemic fluoroquinolones, including delafloxacin, should be avoided in patients who have experienced peripheral neuropathy.

CNS Effects. Systemic fluoroquinolones have been associated with an increased risk of adverse psychiatric effects, including toxic psychosis, hallucinations, paranoia, depression, suicidal thoughts or acts, delirium, disorientation, confusion, disturbances in attention, anxiety, agitation, nervousness, insomnia, nightmares, and memory impairment. These adverse effects may occur after the first dose.

Systemic fluoroquinolones have been associated with an increased risk of convulsions (seizures), increased intracranial pressure (including pseudotumor cerebri), dizziness, and tremors. Delafloxacin, like other fluoroquinolones, should be used in patients with known or suspected CNS disorders (e.g., severe cerebral arteriosclerosis, epilepsy) or other risk factors that predispose to seizures or lower seizure threshold *only* if potential benefits of the drug outweigh risks.

If psychiatric or other CNS effects occur, delafloxacin should be discontinued immediately and appropriate measures initiated. (See Advice to Patients.)

Exacerbation of Myasthenia Gravis. Fluoroquinolones have neuromuscular blocking activity and may exacerbate muscle weakness in individuals with myasthenia gravis. In postmarketing experience, use of fluoroquinolones in myasthenia gravis patients has resulted in requirements for ventilatory support and in death.

Delafloxacin should be avoided in patients with a known history of myasthenia gravis. Patients should be advised to immediately contact a clinician if they have any symptoms of muscle weakness, including respiratory difficulties. (See Advice to Patients.)

Sensitivity Reactions

Hypersensitivity Reactions. Serious and occasionally fatal hypersensitivity and/or anaphylactic reactions have been reported in patients receiving fluoroquinolones. These reactions may occur with the first dose or subsequent doses.

Some hypersensitivity reactions reported in patients receiving fluoroquinolones have been accompanied by cardiovascular collapse, loss of consciousness, tingling, edema (pharyngeal or facial), dyspnea, urticaria, or pruritus.

Hypersensitivity and urticaria have been reported in patients receiving delafloxacin.

Delafloxacin should be discontinued immediately at the first appearance of rash or any other sign of hypersensitivity. (See Advice to Patients.)

Photosensitivity Reactions. There was no evidence of phototoxic potential when oral delafloxacin (200 or 400 mg daily) was administered to healthy individuals exposed to ultraviolet (UVA and UVB) and visible radiation wavelengths ranging from 295–430 nm, including solar simulation.

Other Warnings and Precautions

Risk of Aortic Aneurysm and Dissection. Rupture or dissection of aortic aneurysms has been reported in patients receiving systemic fluoroquinolones. Epidemiologic studies indicate an increased risk of aortic aneurysm and dissection within 2 months following use of systemic fluoroquinolones, particularly in elderly patients. The cause for this increased risk has not been identified.

Unless there are no other treatment options, systemic fluoroquinolones, including delafloxacin, should not be used in patients who have an aortic aneurysm or are at increased risk for an aortic aneurysm. This includes elderly patients and patients with peripheral atherosclerotic vascular disease, hypertension, or certain genetic conditions (e.g., Marfan syndrome, Ehlers-Danlos syndrome).

If a patient reports adverse effects suggestive of aortic aneurysm or dissection, fluoroquinolone treatment should be discontinued immediately. (See Advice to Patients.)

Hypoglycemia or Hyperglycemia. Systemic fluoroquinolones have been associated with alterations in blood glucose concentrations, including symptomatic hypoglycemia and hyperglycemia. Blood glucose disturbances during fluoroquinolone therapy usually have occurred in patients with diabetes mellitus receiving an oral antidiabetic agent (e.g., glyburide) or insulin.

Severe cases of hypoglycemia resulting in coma or death have been reported with some systemic fluoroquinolones. Although most reported cases of hypoglycemic coma have involved patients with risk factors for hypoglycemia (e.g., older age, diabetes mellitus, renal insufficiency, concomitant use of antidiabetic agents [especially sulfonylureas]), some cases have occurred in patients receiving a fluoroquinolone who were not diabetic and were not reported to be receiving an oral antidiabetic agent or insulin.

Blood glucose concentrations should be carefully monitored when systemic fluoroquinolones, including delafloxacin, are used in patients with diabetes mellitus receiving antidiabetic agents.

If a hypoglycemic reaction occurs, fluoroquinolone treatment should be discontinued and appropriate therapy initiated immediately. (See Advice to Patients.)

C. difficile-associated Diarrhea and Colitis. Treatment with anti-infectives alters normal colon flora and may permit overgrowth of *Clostridioides difficile* (formerly known as *Clostridium difficile*). *C. difficile* infection (CDI) and *C. difficile*-associated diarrhea and colitis (CDAD; also known as antibiotic-associated diarrhea and colitis or pseudomembranous colitis) have been reported in patients receiving nearly all anti-infectives, including delafloxacin, and may range in severity from mild diarrhea to fatal colitis. *C. difficile* produces toxins A and B which contribute to development of CDAD; hypertoxin-producing strains of *C. difficile* are associated with increased morbidity and mortality since they may be refractory to anti-infectives and colectomy may be required.

CDAD should be considered in the differential diagnosis of patients who develop diarrhea during or after anti-infective therapy. Careful medical history is necessary since CDAD has been reported to occur as late as 2 months or longer after anti-infective therapy is discontinued.

If CDAD is suspected or confirmed, anti-infective therapy not directed against *C. difficile* should be discontinued as soon as possible. Patients should be managed with appropriate anti-infective therapy directed against *C. difficile* (e.g., vancomycin, fidaxomicin, metronidazole), supportive therapy (e.g., fluid and electrolyte management, protein supplementation), and surgical evaluation as clinically indicated.

Selection and Use of Anti-infectives. To reduce development of drug-resistant bacteria and maintain effectiveness of delafloxacin and other antibacterials, the drug should be used only for treatment of infections proven or strongly suspected to be caused by susceptible bacteria.

When selecting or modifying anti-infective therapy, results of culture and in vitro susceptibility testing should be used. In the absence of such data, local epidemiology and susceptibility patterns should be considered when selecting anti-infectives for empiric therapy.

Information on test methods and quality control standards for in vitro susceptibility testing of antibacterial agents and specific interpretive criteria for such testing recognized by FDA is available at https://www.fda.gov/STIC.

Specific Populations

Pregnancy. Available data regarding use of delafloxacin in pregnant women are insufficient to inform any drug-associated risk for miscarriages or major birth defects.

When delafloxacin (as the N-methyl glucamine salt) was administered orally to pregnant rats during organogenesis, no malformations or fetal deaths were observed at delafloxacin concentrations up to 7 times the estimated clinical exposure. Maternal toxicity and reduced fetal body weight were observed at the highest dosage (1.6 g/kg daily); fetal ossification delays were observed at all doses. When IV delafloxacin was administered to rats in late pregnancy through lactation, no adverse effects on offspring were observed at clinically relevant concentrations.

Lactation. It is not known whether delafloxacin is distributed into human milk, affects the breast-fed infant, or affects milk production. Delafloxacin is distributed into milk in lactating rats.

The developmental and health benefits of breast-feeding should be considered along with the mother's clinical need for delafloxacin and potential adverse effects on the breast-fed infant from the drug or from the underlying maternal condition.

Pediatric Use. Safety and efficacy of delafloxacin have not been established in pediatric patients younger than 18 years of age, and use of the drug in pediatric patients is not recommended.

Fluoroquinolones cause arthropathy in juvenile animals.

The manufacturer states that clinical trials evaluating delafloxacin for the treatment of bacterial skin and skin structure infections did not include patients younger than 18 years of age because the risks versus benefits of the drug do not support use for the treatment of such infections in this age group.

The American Academy of Pediatrics (AAP) states that use of a systemic fluoroquinolone may be justified in children younger than 18 years of age in certain specific circumstances when there are no safe and effective alternatives and the drug is known to be effective. For information regarding when fluoroquinolones may be a preferred option in children, see Cautions: Pediatric Precautions in Ciprofloxacin 8:12.18.

Geriatric Use. Approximately 15% of patients receiving delafloxacin in clinical studies were 65 years of age or older. The clinical response rate at 48–72 hours after initiation of delafloxacin was 75.7% in patients 65 years of age or older compared with 82.3% in those younger than 65 years of age. In the comparator group, the clinical response rate in patients 65 years of age or older was 71.3% compared with 82.1% in those younger than 65 years of age.

The risk of developing severe tendon disorders, including tendon rupture, is increased in older adults (usually those older than 60 years of age). This risk is further increased in those receiving concomitant corticosteroids. (See Tendinitis and Tendon Rupture under Warnings/Precautions: Warnings, in Cautions.) Caution is advised if delafloxacin is used in geriatric adults, especially those receiving concomitant corticosteroids.

The risk of aortic aneurysm and dissection may be increased in geriatric patients. (See Risk of Aortic Aneurysm and Dissection under Warnings/Precautions: Other Warnings and Precautions, in Cautions.)

Pharmacokinetic data indicate that mean peak plasma concentration and area under the plasma concentration-time curve (AUC) of delafloxacin reported in geriatric individuals 65 years of age or older are about 35% higher than those reported in younger adults (18–40 years of age); this difference is not considered clinically important.

Hepatic Impairment. Pharmacokinetics of delafloxacin in adults with mild, moderate, or severe hepatic impairment (Child-Pugh class A, B, or C) are similar to those in adults with normal hepatic function. Dosage adjustments are not necessary in patients with hepatic impairment.

Renal Impairment. Substantial accumulation of the IV delafloxacin vehicle, sulfobutylether-β-cyclodextrin (SBECD), occurs in patients with severe renal impairment (estimated glomerular filtration rate [eGFR] of 15–29 mL/minute per 1.73 m^2) or end-stage renal disease (eGFR less than 15 mL/minute per 1.73 m^2).

If IV delafloxacin is used in patients with severe renal impairment, dosage reduction is recommended (see Renal Impairment under Dosage and Administration: Special Populations) and serum creatinine concentrations and eGFR should be closely monitored. Consideration should be given to switching to oral delafloxacin if serum creatinine concentrations increase during treatment with IV delafloxacin. If eGFR decreases to less than 15 mL/minute per 1.73 m^2, delafloxacin should be discontinued.

Delafloxacin (oral or IV) is not recommended in patients with end-stage renal disease.

■ Common Adverse Effects

Adverse effects occurring in 2% or more of patients receiving delafloxacin include GI effects (nausea, diarrhea, vomiting), headache, and elevated aminotransferase concentrations.

Drug Interactions

■ **Drugs Metabolized by Hepatic Microsomal Enzymes** Delafloxacin meglumine does not inhibit cytochrome P-450 (CYP) isoenzymes 1A2, 2A6, 2B6, 2C8, 2C9, 2C19, 2D6, 2E1, or 3A4/5 in vitro at clinically relevant concentrations and shows no potential for induction of CYP1A2, 2B6, 2C19, or 2C8. In vitro, mild induction of CYP2C9 and 3A4 was observed.

■ **Drugs Affecting or Affected by Membrane Transporters** In vitro, delafloxacin is a substrate of P-glycoprotein (P-gp) transport and breast cancer resistance protein (BCRP); however, the clinical importance of concomitant use of delafloxacin and P-gp inhibitors and/or BCRP inhibitors is not known.

Delafloxacin does not inhibit multidrug-resistance gene (MDR) 1, BCRP, organic anion transporter (OAT) 1, OAT3, organic anion transporting polypeptide (OATP) 1B1, OATP1B3, bile salt export pump (BSEP), organic cation transporter (OCT) 1, or OCT2 at clinically relevant concentrations.

Delafloxacin is not a substrate of OAT1, OAT3, OCT1, OCT2, OATP1B1, or OATP1B3.

■ **Antacids** Pharmacokinetic interaction with delafloxacin tablets if administered concomitantly with aluminum- or magnesium-containing antacids (possible decreased absorption and decreased systemic concentrations of delafloxacin). Delafloxacin tablets should be administered at least 2 hours before or 6 hours after antacids containing aluminum or magnesium.

It is not known if an interaction exists between IV delafloxacin and oral antacids.

■ **Antibacterials** In vitro, there was no evidence of synergistic or antagonistic antibacterial effects when delafloxacin was used with aztreonam, ceftazidime, colistin (commercially available in the US as colistimethate sodium), co-trimoxazole, daptomycin, linezolid, meropenem, tigecycline, or vancomycin.

■ **Didanosine** Pharmacokinetic interaction if delafloxacin tablets are administered concomitantly with buffered didanosine (pediatric powder for oral solution) (possible decreased absorption and decreased systemic concentrations of delafloxacin). Delafloxacin tablets should be administered at least 2 hours before or 6 hours after buffered didanosine.

It is not known if an interaction exists between IV delafloxacin and buffered didanosine.

■ **Iron, Multivitamins, and Mineral Supplements** Pharmacokinetic interaction with delafloxacin tablets if administered concomitantly with oral iron preparations or multivitamins containing iron or zinc (possible decreased absorption and decreased systemic concentrations of delafloxacin). Delafloxacin tablets should be administered at least 2 hours before or 6 hours after such preparations.

It is not known if an interaction exists between IV delafloxacin and oral iron preparations or multivitamins containing iron or zinc. However, IV delafloxacin should not be administered through the same IV line with any solution containing multivalent cations.

■ **Midazolam** Concomitant use of delafloxacin tablets (450 mg every 12 hours for 5 days) and a single 5-mg dose of midazolam (a CYP3A substrate) in healthy individuals did not have a substantial effect on peak plasma concentrations or area under the plasma concentration-time curve (AUC) of midazolam or its metabolite, 1-hydroxymidazolam, compared with administration of midazolam alone.

■ **Sucralfate** Pharmacokinetic interaction if delafloxacin tablets are administered concomitantly with sucralfate (possible decreased absorption and decreased systemic concentrations of delafloxacin). Delafloxacin tablets should be taken at least 2 hours before or 6 hours after sucralfate.

It is not known if an interaction exists between IV delafloxacin and sucralfate.

Description

Delafloxacin meglumine is a fluoroquinolone anti-infective agent. Like other fluoroquinolones, delafloxacin contains a fluorine at the C-6 position of the quinolone nucleus. However, the molecular structure of delafloxacin differs from those of other commercially available fluoroquinolones in 3 notable areas: delafloxacin does not have a strong base at the C-7 position, which allows the drug to be anionic in neutral environments and uncharged in slightly acidic environments; it has a chlorine atom at the C-8 position, which acts as an electron-withdrawing group and reduces the reactivity of the heterocycle; and it has an aromatic ring attached to N1, which increases the molecular surface area compared with other fluoroquinolones. The anionic characteristics of delafloxacin appear to contribute to increased potency of the drug against susceptible bacteria compared with other fluoroquinolones, especially in environments with acidic pH.

Like other fluoroquinolone anti-infectives, the antibacterial activity of delafloxacin is due to inhibition of bacterial topoisomerase IV and DNA gyrase (i.e., topoisomerase II) enzymes, which are required for bacterial DNA replication, transcription, repair, and recombination. Delafloxacin demonstrates similar affinity for both topoisomerase IV and DNA gyrase.

In vitro, delafloxacin exhibits concentration-dependent bactericidal activity against gram-positive and gram-negative bacteria.

■ **Spectrum** Delafloxacin is active in vitro and in clinical infections against many gram-positive aerobic bacteria, including *Staphylococcus aureus* (including methicillin-resistant *S. aureus* [MRSA; also known as oxacillin-resistant *S. aureus* or ORSA] and methicillin-susceptible *S. aureus*), *S. haemolyticus*, *S. lugdunensis*, *Streptococcus pyogenes* (group A β-hemolytic streptococci, GAS), *S. agalactiae* (group B streptococci, GBS), *S. anginosus* group (including *S. anginosus*, *S. intermedius*, and *S. constellatus*), and *Enterococcus faecalis*. Delafloxacin has been active in vitro against some staphylococci (including MRSA), streptococci, and enterococci that were resistant to some other fluoroquinolones.

Delafloxacin is active in vitro and in clinical infections against some gram-negative aerobic bacteria, including *Escherichia coli*, *Enterobacter cloacae*, *Klebsiella pneumoniae*, and *Pseudomonas aeruginosa*.

Although the clinical importance is unknown, delafloxacin also has in vitro activity against some other gram-positive aerobic bacteria, including *S. dysgalactiae*, *S. epidermidis*, *S. pneumoniae*, *E. faecium*, and *Listeria monocytogenes*, and some other gram-negative aerobic bacteria, including *Citrobacter freundii*, *C. koseri*, *Eikenella corrodens*, *E. aerogenes*, *Haemophilus influenzae*, *H. parainfluenzae*, *Helicobacter pylori*, *K. oxytoca*, *Legionella*, *Moraxella catarrhalis*, *Neisseria gonorrhoeae*, *Proteus mirabilis*, *Serratia marcescens*, *Salmonella*, and *Shigella*.

Delafloxacin has some in vitro activity against some anaerobic bacteria, including *Bacteroides fragilis*, *Clostridium perfringens*, and *Clostridioides difficile* (formerly known as *Clostridium difficile*); however, the clinical importance of these in vitro data is unknown.

■ **Resistance** Resistance to fluoroquinolones, including delafloxacin, can occur due to mutations in target regions of topoisomerase IV and/or DNA gyrase (i.e., quinolone-resistance determining regions [QRDRs]) or through altered efflux. In vitro, resistance to delafloxacin develops by multiple step mutations in QRDRs of gram-positive and gram-negative bacteria (e.g., double mutations in *gyr*A and *par*C).

Cross-resistance between delafloxacin and other fluoroquinolones has been observed; however, some gram-positive and gram-negative bacteria resistant to other fluoroquinolones may be susceptible to delafloxacin.

Advice to Patients

Advise patients to read the manufacturer's patient information (medication guide).

Advise patients that antibacterials (including delafloxacin) should only be used to treat bacterial infections and not used to treat viral infections (e.g., the common cold).

Advise patients that delafloxacin tablets may be taken without regard to food.

Importance of taking delafloxacin tablets at least 2 hours before or 6 hours after magnesium- or aluminum-containing antacids; sucralfate; multivitamins or dietary supplements containing iron or zinc; or buffered didanosine (pediatric powder for oral solution).

Importance of completing full course of therapy, even if feeling better after a few days. Advise patients that skipping doses or not completing the full course of therapy may decrease effectiveness and increase the likelihood that bacteria will develop resistance and will not be treatable with delafloxacin or other antibacterials in the future.

If a dose of delafloxacin is missed and remembered within 8 hours after the scheduled time, the dose should be taken as soon as possible and the next dose taken at the regularly scheduled time. If a dose is missed and remembered more than 8 hours after the scheduled time, the dose should be skipped and the next dose taken at the regularly scheduled time.

Inform patients that systemic fluoroquinolones have been associated with disabling and potentially irreversible serious adverse reactions (e.g., tendinitis and tendon rupture, peripheral neuropathy, CNS effects) that may occur together in the same patient. Advise patients to immediately discontinue delafloxacin and contact a clinician if they experience any signs or symptoms of serious adverse effects (e.g., unusual joint or tendon pain, muscle weakness, a "pins and needles" tingling or pricking sensation, numbness of the arms or legs, confusion, hallucinations) while taking the drug. Advise patients to talk with a clinician if they have any questions or concerns.

Inform patients that systemic fluoroquinolones are associated with an increased risk of tendinitis and tendon rupture in all age groups and that this risk is increased in adults older than 60 years of age, individuals receiving corticosteroids, and kidney, heart, or lung transplant recipients. Symptoms may be irreversible. Importance of resting and refraining from exercise at the first sign of tendinitis or tendon rupture (e.g., pain, swelling, or inflammation of a tendon or weakness or inability to use a joint) and importance of immediately discontinuing the drug and contacting a clinician. (See Tendinitis and Tendon Rupture under Warnings/Precautions: Warnings, in Cautions.)

Inform patients that peripheral neuropathies have been reported in patients receiving systemic fluoroquinolones and that symptoms may occur soon after initiation of the drug and may be irreversible. Importance of immediately discontinuing delafloxacin and contacting a clinician if symptoms of peripheral neuropathy (e.g., pain, burning, tingling, numbness, and/or weakness) occur.

Inform patients that systemic fluoroquinolones have been associated with CNS effects (e.g., convulsions, dizziness, lightheadedness, increased intracranial pressure). Importance of informing clinician of any history of convulsions before initiating therapy with the drug. Importance of contacting a clinician if persistent headache with or without blurred vision occurs.

Because fluoroquinolones may cause dizziness and lightheadedness, caution patients that they should not engage in activities requiring mental alertness and motor coordination (e.g., driving a vehicle, operating machinery) until the effects of delafloxacin on the individual are known.

Advise patients that systemic fluoroquinolones may worsen myasthenia gravis symptoms; importance of informing clinician of any history of myasthenia gravis. Importance of immediately contacting a clinician if any symptoms of muscle weakness, including respiratory difficulties, occur.

Inform patients that delafloxacin may be associated with hypersensitivity reactions (including anaphylactic reactions), even after the first dose. Importance of immediately discontinuing delafloxacin and contacting a clinician at first sign of rash, hives or other skin reaction, rapid heartbeat, difficulty swallowing or breathing, any swelling suggesting angioedema (e.g., swelling of lips, tongue, or face; throat tightness; hoarseness), jaundice, or any other sign of hypersensitivity.

Inform patients that systemic fluoroquinolones may increase the risk of aortic aneurysm and dissection; importance of informing clinician of any history of aneurysms, blockages or hardening of the arteries, high blood pressure, or genetic conditions such as Marfan syndrome or Ehlers-Danlos syndrome. Advise patients to seek immediate medical treatment if they experience sudden, severe, and constant pain in the stomach, chest, or back.

Inform patients that hypoglycemia has been reported when systemic fluoroquinolones were used in some patients receiving antidiabetic agents. Advise patients with diabetes mellitus receiving oral antidiabetic agents or insulin to discontinue fluoroquinolone treatment and contact a clinician if they experience hypoglycemia or symptoms of hypoglycemia.

Advise patients that diarrhea is a common problem caused by anti-infectives and usually ends when the drug is discontinued. Importance of contacting a clinician if watery and bloody stools (with or without stomach cramps and fever) occur during or as late as 2 months or longer after the last dose.

Importance of informing clinician of existing or contemplated concomitant therapy, including prescription and OTC drugs, as well as any concomitant illnesses.

Importance of women informing clinicians if they are or plan to become pregnant or plan to breast-feed.

Importance of advising patients of other important precautionary information. (See Cautions.)

Overview® (see Users Guide). For additional information on this drug until a more detailed monograph is developed and published, the manufacturer's labeling should be consulted. It is *essential* that the manufacturer's labeling be consulted for more detailed information on usual cautions, precautions, contraindications, potential drug interactions, laboratory test interferences, and acute toxicity.

Preparations

Excipients in commercially available drug preparations may have clinically important effects in some individuals; consult specific product labeling for details.

Delafloxacin Meglumine

Oral		
Tablets	450 mg (of delafloxacin)	**Baxdela®**, Melinta
Parenteral		
For injection, for IV infusion	300 mg (of delafloxacin)	**Baxdela®**, Melinta

levoFLOXacin

■ Levofloxacin is a fluoroquinolone anti-infective agent.

Uses

■ Respiratory Tract Infections ***Acute Sinusitis*** Levofloxacin is used for the treatment of acute bacterial sinusitis caused by susceptible *Streptococcus pneumoniae*, *Haemophilus influenzae*, or *Moraxella catarrhalis.*

Levofloxacin should be used for the treatment of acute bacterial sinusitis only when there are no other treatment options. Because systemic fluoroquinolones, including levofloxacin, have been associated with disabling and potentially irreversible serious adverse reactions (e.g., tendinitis and tendon rupture, peripheral neuropathy, CNS effects) that can occur together in the same patient (see Cautions) *and because acute bacterial sinusitis may be self-limiting in some patients, the risks of serious adverse reactions outweigh the benefits of fluoroquinolones for patients with acute sinusitis.*

Clinical Experience. In one open study in adults with acute bacterial sinusitis, therapy with oral levofloxacin (500 mg once daily) or oral amoxicillin and clavulanate potassium (500 mg of amoxicillin 3 times daily) resulted in success rates of 88 or 87%, respectively.

In a double-blind, prospective study in adults with acute bacterial sinusitis randomized to receive levofloxacin in a dosage of 500 mg once daily for 10 days or a dosage of 750 mg once daily for 5 days, safety and efficacy of both regimens were similar. The clinical success rate (defined as complete or partial resolution of pretreatment signs and symptoms of sinusitis to such an extent that no further anti-infective treatment was indicated) in the microbiologically evaluable patient population at the test-of-cure visit was 88.6% in those who received the 10-day regimen compared with 91.4% in those who received the 5-day regimen. When results were stratified according to pathogen, the clinical success rate was 96.3 or 92.6% in those with *S. pneumoniae*, 92.6 or 90.5% in those with *H. influenzae*, and 100 or 90.9% in those with *M. catarrhalis.*

Acute Exacerbations of Chronic Bronchitis Levofloxacin is used for the treatment of acute bacterial exacerbations of chronic bronchitis caused by susceptible *Staphylococcus aureus* (methicillin-susceptible [oxacillin-susceptible] strains), *S. pneumoniae*, *H. influenzae*, *H. parainfluenzae*, or *M. catarrhalis.*

Levofloxacin should be used for the treatment of acute bacterial exacerbations of chronic bronchitis only when there are no other treatment options. Because systemic fluoroquinolones, including levofloxacin, have been associated with disabling and potentially irreversible serious adverse reactions (e.g., tendinitis and tendon rupture, peripheral neuropathy, CNS effects) that can occur together in the same patient (see Cautions) *and because acute bacterial exacerbations of chronic bronchitis may be self-limiting is some patients, the risks of serious adverse reactions outweigh the benefits of fluoroquinolones for patients with these infections.*

Clinical Experience. In controlled clinical studies in adults with acute bacterial exacerbations of chronic bronchitis, levofloxacin was as effective as therapy with cefaclor or cefuroxime. Levofloxacin therapy generally resulted in bacterial cure rates of 95–97% in patients with acute bacterial exacerbations of chronic bronchitis. The most prevalent pathogens in these studies were *H. influenzae*, *H. parainfluenzae*, *M. catarrhalis*, and *S. pneumoniae.*

Community-acquired Pneumonia Levofloxacin is used for the treatment of community-acquired pneumonia (CAP) caused by susceptible *S. aureus* (methicillin-susceptible [oxacillin-susceptible] strains), *S. pneumoniae* (including multidrug-resistant *S. pneumoniae* [MDRSP]), *H. influenzae*, *H. parainfluenzae*, *Klebsiella pneumoniae*, *Legionella pneumophila*, *M. catarrhalis*, *Chlamydophila pneumoniae* (formerly *Chlamydia pneumoniae*), or *Mycoplasma pneumoniae.*

Initial treatment of CAP generally involves use of an empiric anti-infective regimen based on the most likely pathogens and local susceptibility patterns; treatment may then be changed (if possible) to provide a more specific regimen (pathogen-directed therapy) based on results of in vitro culture and susceptibility testing. The most appropriate empiric regimen varies depending on the severity of illness at the time of presentation, whether outpatient treatment or hospitalization in or out of an intensive care unit (ICU) is indicated, and the presence or absence of cardiopulmonary disease and other modifying factors that increase the risk of certain pathogens (e.g., methicillin-resistant *S. aureus* [MRSA; also known as oxacillin-resistant *S. aureus* or ORSA], penicillin-resistant *S. pneumoniae*, MDRSP, enteric gram-negative bacilli, *Ps. aeruginosa*).

For additional information on management of CAP, the current clinical practice guidelines from the Infectious Diseases Society of America (IDSA) available at http://www.idsociety.org should be consulted.

Clinical Experience. In one controlled clinical study in adults with CAP, a 7- to 14-day regimen that included IV and/or oral levofloxacin was as effective as a regimen that included IV ceftriaxone and/or oral cefuroxime. Levofloxacin generally resulted in clinical success (cure or improvement) 5–7 days following completion of therapy in 93–95% of adults with CAP. In a randomized study in CAP patients 65 years of age or older (mean age 77.9 years), the clinical cure rate at the test-of-cure visit (5–21 days after end of treatment) was 92.9% in those who received moxifloxacin and 87.9% in those who received levofloxacin; the bacteriologic success rate was 81% in those who received moxifloxacin and 75% in those who received levofloxacin.

In controlled clinical studies, presumptive bacteriologic eradication 5–7 days following completion of therapy was evident in 98% of patients with *H. influenzae* infection, 95% of those with *H. parainfluenzae* infection, 100% of those with *K. pneumoniae* infection, 94% of those with *M. catarrhalis* infection, 88% of those with *S. aureus* infection, and 95% of those with *S. pneumoniae* infection. Clinical success rate 5–7 days following completion of therapy in patients with atypical pneumonia caused by *C. pneumoniae*, *M. pneumoniae*, or *L. pneumoniae* was 96, 96, or 70%, respectively.

Safety and efficacy of a 5-day regimen of levofloxacin (750 mg IV or orally once daily for 5 days) was compared with that of a 10-day regimen of the drug (500 mg IV or orally once daily for 10 days) in a double-blind, randomized, prospective study in adults with clinically or radiologically confirmed mild to severe CAP. The clinical success rate (cure and improvement) was about 91% in both groups.

A clinical and bacteriologic success rate of 95% has been reported when levofloxacin was used in adults for the treatment of CAP caused by multidrug-resistant *S. pneumoniae.*

Nosocomial Pneumonia Levofloxacin is used for the treatment of nosocomial pneumonia caused by susceptible *S. aureus* (methicillin-susceptible [oxacillin-susceptible] strains), *S. pneumoniae*, *H. influenzae*, *Escherichia coli*, *K. pneumoniae*, *Ps. aeruginosa*, or *Serratia marcescens.* Adjunctive therapy should be used as clinically indicated. If the infection is known or suspected of being caused by *Ps. aeruginosa*, concomitant therapy with an antipseudomonal β-lactam anti-infective is recommended.

Local susceptibility data should be used when selecting initial empiric regimens for the treatment of hospital-acquired pneumonia (HAP) not associated with mechanical ventilation or the treatment of ventilator-associated pneumonia (VAP).

For initial empiric treatment of HAP in adults who are not at high risk of mortality and have no factors that increase the likelihood of MRSA, IDSA and the American Thoracic Society (ATS) state that levofloxacin is one of several options that can be considered. However, these experts state that levofloxacin should be used in conjunction with an antibacterial active against MRSA (vancomycin, linezolid) if factors that increase the likelihood of MRSA are present or if the patient is at high risk of mortality or has received IV anti-infectives during the prior 90 days.

In adults with clinically suspected VAP, IDSA and ATS state that levofloxacin is one option that can be considered for initial empiric treatment in those not at increased risk for MRSA. However, in patients with factors that increase the risk of MRSA or multidrug-resistant gram-negative bacteria, these experts state that levofloxacin should be used in conjunction with an anti-infective active against MRSA (vancomycin, linezolid) plus an antipseudomonal β-lactam (fixed combination of piperacillin and tazobactam [piperacillin/tazobactam], cefepime, ceftazidime, imipenem, meropenem, aztreonam).

For additional information on management of nosocomial pneumonia, the current clinical practice guidelines from IDSA available at http://www.idsociety.org should be consulted.

Clinical Experience. In a multicenter, randomized, open-label study in adults with clinical and radiologically documented nosocomial pneumonia, patients were randomized to receive a 7- to 15-day regimen of IV levofloxacin (750 mg once daily) following by oral levofloxacin (750 mg once daily) or IV imipenem and cilastatin sodium (500–1000 mg every 6–8 hours) followed by oral ciprofloxacin (750 mg every 12 hours). Patients with documented *Ps. aeruginosa* infections received adjunctive therapy with ceftazidime or piperacillin and tazobactam sodium (for those receiving levofloxacin) or an aminoglycoside (for those receiving the comparator regimen); those with suspected MRSA received concomitant vancomycin. The overall clinical success rate 3–15 days after completion of therapy was 58.1% for those receiving levofloxacin and 60.6% for those receiving the comparator regimen; the overall microbiologic eradication rate was 66.7 and 60.6%, respectively.

■ **Skin and Skin Structure Infections** Levofloxacin is used for the treatment of mild to moderate uncomplicated skin and skin structure infections caused by susceptible *S. aureus* (methicillin-susceptible [oxacillin-susceptible] strains) or *S. pyogenes* (group A β-hemolytic streptococci) and for the treatment of complicated skin and skin structure infections caused by susceptible *S. aureus* (methicillin-susceptible [oxacillin-susceptible] strains), *Enterococcus faecalis*, *S. pyogenes*, or *Proteus mirabilis*.

For additional information on management of skin and skin structure infections, the current clinical practice guidelines from IDSA available at http://www.idsociety.org should be consulted.

Clinical Experience Levofloxacin has been effective for the treatment of uncomplicated abscesses, cellulitis, erysipelas, furuncles, impetigo, pyoderma, and wound or surgical infections caused by susceptible bacteria. In 2 controlled studies, oral levofloxacin was as effective as oral ciprofloxacin in the treatment of mild to moderate skin infections caused by susceptible bacteria, mainly *S. aureus* and *S. pyogenes*. Levofloxacin resulted in a bacteriologic cure rate of 93–97.5% in patients with mild to moderate skin and skin structure infections.

In an open-label, randomized study in patients with complicated skin and skin structure infections, the overall success rate (improved or cured) in clinically evaluable patients at 2–5 days after completion of treatment was 84.1% in those randomized to receive levofloxacin (750 mg once daily for 7–14 days given IV and/or orally as indicated) and 80.3% in those randomized to the comparator regimen (fixed combination of IV ticarcillin and clavulanate [no longer commercially available in the US] followed by oral amoxicillin and clavulanate for a total duration of 7–14 days). Success rates varied depending on the diagnosis, ranging from 69% in those with infected diabetic ulcers to 90% in those with infected abscesses. In the microbiologically evaluable population, the overall rate of eradication was 83.7% in those who received levofloxacin and 71.4% in those who received the comparator regimen.

■ **Urinary Tract Infections and Prostatitis** ***Uncomplicated Urinary Tract Infections*** Levofloxacin is used for the treatment of mild to moderate uncomplicated urinary tract infections (UTIs) caused by susceptible *E. coli*, *K. pneumoniae*, or *S. saprophyticus*.

Levofloxacin should be used for the treatment of uncomplicated UTIs only when there are no other treatment options. Because systemic fluoroquinolones, including levofloxacin, have been associated with disabling and potentially irreversible serious adverse reactions (e.g., tendinitis and tendon rupture, peripheral neuropathy, CNS effects) that can occur together in the same patient (see Cautions) *and because uncomplicated UTIs may be self-limiting in some patients, the risks of serious adverse reactions outweigh the benefits of fluoroquinolones for patients with uncomplicated UTIs.*

IDSA and other experts state that fluoroquinolones (ciprofloxacin, levofloxacin, ofloxacin) should be considered alternative agents for the treatment of uncomplicated UTIs (e.g., acute cystitis) and should be used in these infections *only* when other urinary anti-infectives are likely to be ineffective or are contraindicated or not tolerated.

Complicated Urinary Tract Infections Levofloxacin is used for the treatment of mild to moderate complicated UTIs caused by susceptible *E. faecalis*, *Enterobacter cloacae*, *E. coli*, *K. pneumoniae*, *P. mirabilis*, or *Ps. aeruginosa* and acute pyelonephritis caused by susceptible *E. coli*, including cases with concurrent bacteremia.

In controlled clinical studies, levofloxacin therapy was as effective as ciprofloxacin in the treatment of complicated UTIs or pyelonephritis. In one study in adults with complicated UTIs, bacterial eradication 5–9 days following completion of therapy was evident in 93% of patients with *E. coli* infection, 97% of those with *K. pneumoniae* infection, and 90% of those with *P. mirabilis* infection.

Prostatitis Levofloxacin is used for the treatment of chronic prostatitis caused by susceptible *E. coli*, *E. faecalis*, or *S. epidermidis* (methicillin-susceptible [oxacillin-susceptible] strains).

In one double-blind controlled study, adults with prostatitis were randomized to receive a 28-day regimen of oral levofloxacin (500 mg once daily) or ciprofloxacin (500 mg twice daily). The overall microbiologic eradication rate 5–18 days after completion of treatment was 75% in those who received levofloxacin and 76.8% in those who received ciprofloxacin. In those with infections caused by *E. coli*, *E. faecalis*, or *S. epidermidis*, the eradication rate was 93.3, 72.2, or 81.8%, respectively, in those who received levofloxacin and 81.8, 75, or 78.6%, respectively, in those who received ciprofloxacin.

■ **Endocarditis** Levofloxacin is used as an alternative for the treatment of endocarditis† (native or prosthetic valve or other prosthetic material) caused by fastidious gram-negative bacilli known as the HACEK group (*Haemophilus*, *Aggregatibacter*, *Cardiobacterium hominis*, *Eikenella corrodens*, *Kingella*).

The American Heart Association (AHA) and IDSA recommend ceftriaxone (or other third or fourth generation cephalosporin) for the treatment of endocarditis caused by the HACEK group, but state that a fluoroquinolone (ciprofloxacin, levofloxacin, moxifloxacin) may be considered in patients who cannot tolerate cephalosporins. Because only limited data are available regarding use of fluoroquinolones for the treatment of HACEK endocarditis, an infectious disease specialist should be consulted when treating such infections in patients who cannot tolerate cephalosporins.

■ **GI Infections** ***Campylobacter Infections*** Levofloxacin has been recommended as an alternative for the treatment of campylobacteriosis† caused by susceptible *Campylobacter*.

Optimal treatment of campylobacteriosis in patients with human immunodeficiency virus (HIV) infection has not been identified. Some clinicians withhold anti-infective treatment in HIV-infected patients with CD4$^+$ T-cell counts exceeding 200 cells/mm^3 if they have only mild campylobacteriosis and initiate treatment if symptoms persist for more than several days. In HIV-infected patients with mild to moderate campylobacteriosis, treatment with a fluoroquinolone (preferably ciprofloxacin or, alternatively, levofloxacin or moxifloxacin) or azithromycin is reasonable. Anti-infective therapy should be modified based on results of in vitro susceptibility testing. In the US, resistance to fluoroquinolones has been reported in 22% of *C. jejuni* and 35% of *C. coli* isolates tested. To limit emergence of resistance, some clinicians suggest that it may be prudent to use an aminoglycoside concomitantly in patients with bacteremic infections.

Salmonella Gastroenteritis Levofloxacin is used for the treatment of *Salmonella* gastroenteritis† (with or without bacteremia).

Anti-infective therapy is not usually indicated in otherwise healthy individuals with uncomplicated (noninvasive) gastroenteritis caused by *Salmonella* since such therapy may prolong the duration of fecal excretion of the organism and there is no evidence that it shortens the duration of the disease; however, the US Centers for Disease Control and Prevention (CDC), American Academy of Pediatrics (AAP), IDSA, and others recommend anti-infective therapy in individuals with severe *Salmonella* gastroenteritis and in those who are at increased risk of invasive disease. These individuals include infants younger than 3–6 months of age; individuals older than 50 years of age; individuals with hemoglobinopathies, severe atherosclerosis or valvular heart disease, prostheses, uremia, chronic GI disease, or severe colitis; and individuals who are immunocompromised because of malignancy, immunosuppressive therapy, HIV infection, or other immunosuppressive illness.

Because HIV-infected individuals with *Salmonella* gastroenteritis are at high risk for bacteremia, CDC, National Institutes of Health (NIH), and HIV Medicine Association of IDSA recommend that such patients receive anti-infective treatment. These experts state that the initial drug of choice for the treatment of salmonella gastroenteritis (with or without bacteremia) in HIV-infected adults is ciprofloxacin; other fluoroquinolones (levofloxacin, moxifloxacin) also are likely to be effective in these patients, but clinical data are limited. Depending on results of in vitro susceptibility testing of the causative organism, alternatives for treatment of *Salmonella* gastroenteritis in HIV-infected adults are co-trimoxazole or third generation cephalosporins (ceftriaxone, cefotaxime).

The role of long-term treatment (secondary prophylaxis) against *Salmonella* in HIV-infected individuals is not well established, and possible benefits of such prophylaxis should be weighed against the risks of long-term anti-infective exposure. CDC, NIH, and IDSA state that secondary prophylaxis should be considered in those with recurrent bacteremia and may also be considered in those with recurrent gastroenteritis (with or without bacteremia) and in those with CD4$^+$ T-cell counts less than 200 cells/mm^3 and severe diarrhea. These experts state that secondary prophylaxis should be discontinued if the *Salmonella* infection resolves and there has been a sustained response to antiretroviral therapy with CD4$^+$ T-cell counts greater than 200 cells/mm^3.

Shigella Infections Levofloxacin is used as an alternative for the treatment of shigellosis† caused by susceptible *Shigella.*

Infections caused by *S. sonnei* usually are self-limited (48–72 hours), and mild cases may not require treatment with anti-infectives. However, because there is some evidence that anti-infectives may shorten the duration of diarrhea and the period of fecal excretion of *Shigella*, anti-infective treatment generally is recommended in addition to fluid and electrolyte replacement in patients with severe shigellosis, dysentery, or underlying immunosuppression. An empiric treatment regimen can be used initially, but in vitro susceptibility testing of clinical isolates is indicated since resistance is common. A fluoroquinolone (preferably ciprofloxacin or, alternatively, levofloxacin or moxifloxacin) generally has been recommended for the treatment of shigellosis. However, fluoroquinolone-resistant *Shigella* have been reported in the US, especially in international travelers, the homeless, and men who have sex with men (MSM). Depending on in vitro susceptibility, other drugs recommended for the treatment of shigellosis include co-trimoxazole, ceftriaxone, azithromycin (not recommended in those with bacteremia), or ampicillin.

Travelers' Diarrhea Oral levofloxacin has been used for the short-term treatment of travelers' diarrhea† and has been used for the prevention of travelers' diarrhea† in adults traveling for relatively short periods of time to high-risk areas.

The most common cause of travelers' diarrhea worldwide is noninvasive enterotoxigenic strains of *E. coli* (ETEC), but travelers' diarrhea also can be caused by various other bacteria, including enteroaggregative and other *E. coli* pathotypes, *C. jejuni*, *Shigella*, *Salmonella*, *Aeromonas*, *Plesiomonas*, and, possibly, *Acrobacter*, *Larobacter*, and enterotoxigenic *Bacteroides fragilis.* In some cases, travelers' diarrhea is caused by parasitic enteric pathogens (e.g., *Giardia*, *Cryptosporidium*, *Entamoeba histolytica*) or viral enteric pathogens (e.g., norovirus, rotavirus, astrovirus).

Countries where travelers are at low risk of travelers' diarrhea include the US, Canada, Australia, New Zealand, Japan, and countries in Northern and Western Europe. Travelers are at intermediate risk for travelers' diarrhea in Eastern Europe, South Africa, and some of the Caribbean islands, but are at high risk in most of Asia, the Middle East, Africa, Mexico, and Central and South America.

Treatment. Travelers' diarrhea caused by bacteria may be self-limited and often resolves within 3–7 days without anti-infective treatment. CDC states that anti-infective treatment is *not* recommended in patients with mild travelers' diarrhea. However, CDC and other clinicians state that empiric short-term anti-infective treatment (single dose or up to 3 days) may be used if diarrhea is moderate or severe, associated with fever or bloody stools, or extremely disruptive to travel plans. Since bacteria are the most common cause of travelers' diarrhea (80–90% of cases), an anti-infective directed against enteric bacterial pathogens usually is used. Fluoroquinolones (e.g., ciprofloxacin, levofloxacin) generally have been considered the anti-infectives of choice for empiric treatment, including self-treatment, of travelers' diarrhea in adults; alternatives include azithromycin and rifaximin.

If the causative pathogen is susceptible to the anti-infective chosen for empiric therapy, the duration of illness may be reduced by about a day. However, the increasing incidence of enteric bacteria resistant to fluoroquinolones and other anti-infectives may limit the usefulness of empiric treatment in individuals traveling in certain geographic areas, and the possible adverse effects of the anti-infective and adverse consequences of such treatment (e.g., development of resistance, effect on normal gut microflora) should be considered.

Prophylaxis. CDC and most experts do *not* recommend prophylactic use of anti-infectives to prevent travelers' diarrhea in most individuals traveling to areas of risk. However, anti-infective prophylaxis may be considered for short-term travelers who are high-risk individuals (e.g., HIV-infected or other immunocompromised individuals, travelers with poorly controlled diabetes mellitus or chronic renal failure) and those who are taking critical trips during which even a short period of diarrhea could adversely affect the purpose of the trip.

The use of anti-infective prophylaxis in travelers should be weighed against the use of prompt, early self-treatment with an empiric anti-infective if moderate to severe travelers' diarrhea occurs. If anti-infective prophylaxis is used, fluoroquinolones (e.g., ciprofloxacin, levofloxacin) usually have been recommended; alternatives include azithromycin and rifaximin. The increasing incidence of fluoroquinolone resistance in pathogens that cause travelers' diarrhea (e.g., *Campylobacter*, *Salmonella*, *Shigella*) should be considered and may limit their potential usefulness.

Helicobacter pylori Infection Levofloxacin has been used as a component of various multiple-drug regimens for the treatment of infections caused by *Helicobacter pylori*†.

Although safety and efficacy of levofloxacin-containing regimens have not been established, a 3-drug regimen that includes a proton-pump inhibitor (PPI), levofloxacin, and amoxicillin has been suggested as a first-line option for the treatment of *H. pylori* infection. In addition, a 4-drug regimen that includes a PPI, levofloxacin, nitazoxanide, and doxycycline and a sequential regimen that includes initial treatment with a PPI and amoxicillin followed by treatment with a PPI, levofloxacin, and a nitroimidazole (either tinidazole or metronidazole) have been suggested as other possible first-line options. Levofloxacin-containing regimens also have been recommended for second-line or salvage therapy in patients with persistent *H. pylori* infection. Data are limited regarding the prevalence of fluoroquinolone-resistant *H. pylori* in the US; the possible impact of such resistance on the efficacy of fluoroquinolone-containing regimens used for the treatment of *H. pylori* infections is not known.

■ **Anthrax** Levofloxacin is used for inhalational anthrax (postexposure) to reduce the incidence or progression of disease following suspected or confirmed exposure to aerosolized *Bacillus anthracis* spores in adults and pediatric patients. Although efficacy of levofloxacin for postexposure prophylaxis to prevent inhalational anthrax has not been evaluated in human clinical trials, the drug is labeled by FDA for this indication based on a surrogate end point derived from a primate model of inhalational anthrax that predicts clinical benefit based on plasma levofloxacin concentrations achievable in humans with recommended oral or IV dosages.

CDC, AAP, US Working Group on Civilian Biodefense, and US Army Medical Research Institute of Infectious Diseases (USAMRIID) recommend oral ciprofloxacin and oral doxycycline as the initial drugs of choice for postexposure prophylaxis following exposure to aerosolized anthrax spores, including exposures that occur in the context of biologic warfare or bioterrorism. Other oral fluoroquinolones (levofloxacin, moxifloxacin, ofloxacin) are alternatives for postexposure prophylaxis when ciprofloxacin or doxycycline cannot be used.

Oral levofloxacin is one of several options recommended for the treatment of uncomplicated cutaneous anthrax† (without systemic involvement) that occurs in the context of biologic warfare or bioterrorism. CDC recommends that adults receive an oral regimen of ciprofloxacin, doxycycline, levofloxacin, or moxifloxacin for the treatment of such infections. AAP recommends that pediatric patients receive oral ciprofloxacin for the treatment of such infections and states that oral amoxicillin or penicillin V (if penicillin susceptibility is confirmed) or oral doxycycline, clindamycin, or levofloxacin are alternatives.

IV levofloxacin is recommended as an alternative to IV ciprofloxacin for use in multiple-drug parenteral regimens for initial treatment of systemic anthrax† (inhalational, GI, meningitis, or cutaneous with systemic involvement, extensive edema, or head or neck lesions) that occurs in the context of biologic warfare or bioterrorism. CDC, AAP, US Working Group on Civilian Biodefense, and USAMRIID recommend that treatment be initiated with a multiple-drug parenteral regimen that includes a fluoroquinolone (preferably ciprofloxacin) or doxycycline and 1 or 2 additional anti-infective agents predicted to be effective; after the patient is clinically stable, treatment can be changed to an oral anti-infective. For initial treatment of systemic anthrax with possible or confirmed meningitis, CDC and AAP recommend a regimen of IV ciprofloxacin in conjunction with another IV bactericidal anti-infective (preferably meropenem) and an IV protein synthesis inhibitor (preferably linezolid). If meningitis has been excluded, these experts recommend an initial regimen of IV ciprofloxacin in conjunction with an IV protein synthesis inhibitor (preferably clindamycin or linezolid).

Some experts suggest that oral ciprofloxacin or other oral fluoroquinolones (levofloxacin, moxifloxacin, ofloxacin) can be considered for the treatment of inhalational anthrax† when a parenteral regimen is not available. Although a multiple-drug parenteral regimen should be used for the treatment of inhalational anthrax, use of these parenteral regimens may not be possible if large numbers of individuals require treatment in a mass casualty setting and it may be necessary to use an oral regimen.

For additional information on postexposure prophylaxis and treatment of anthrax, see Uses: Anthrax in Ciprofloxacin 8:12.18.

■ **Chlamydial Infections** Levofloxacin is considered an alternative for the treatment of urogenital infections caused by *Chlamydia trachomatis*†. CDC states that a single oral dose of azithromycin or a 7-day regimen of oral doxycycline are the recommended regimens for the treatment of *C. trachomatis* urogenital infections in adults and adolescents; a 7-day regimen of oral erythromycin base or ethylsuccinate or a 7-day regimen of oral levofloxacin or ofloxacin are alternative regimens.

Individuals with HIV infection should receive the same treatment regimens recommended for other individuals with *C. trachomatis* urogenital infections.

Any individual who had sexual contact with a patient with *C. trachomatis* urogenital infection during the 60 days preceding the patient's onset of symptoms or diagnosis should be referred for evaluation, testing, and presumptive treatment with a regimen effective against *Chlamydia.* To minimize transmission and avoid reinfection, individuals treated for *C. trachomatis* urogenital infections should abstain from sexual intercourse until they and their partner(s) have been adequately treated (i.e., for 7 days after a single-dose regimen or after completion of a 7-day regimen) and symptoms have resolved.

■ **Gonorrhea and Associated Infections** Although levofloxacin was used in the past for the treatment of uncomplicated gonorrhea† caused by susceptible *Neisseria gonorrhoeae*, quinolone-resistant *N. gonorrhoeae* (QRNG) is widely disseminated throughout the world, including in the US. Therefore, CDC states that fluoroquinolones are no longer recommended for the treatment of gonorrhea and should not be used routinely for any associated infections that may involve *N. gonorrhoeae* (e.g., pelvic inflammatory disease [PID], epididymitis).

Levofloxacin is considered an alternative agent for the treatment of PID†. (See Uses: Pelvic Inflammatory Disease.)

Levofloxacin is considered an alternative agent for the treatment of acute epididymitis†. Although acute epididymitis in sexually active men younger than 35 years of age is most frequently caused by *C. trachomatis* or *N. gonorrhoeae*, epididymitis can also be caused by other organisms (e.g., sexually transmitted enteric bacteria, *Mycoplasma*, *Ureaplasma*, mycobacteria, fungi).

Presumptive treatment is usually initiated prior to availability of all diagnostic laboratory test results, and the anti-infective regimen is selected based on the patient's risk for chlamydia, gonorrhea, and/or sexually transmitted enteric bacteria (e.g., *E. coli*). For treatment of acute epididymitis most likely caused by sexually transmitted chlamydia and gonorrhea, CDC recommends a single IM dose of ceftriaxone used in conjunction with a 10-day regimen of oral doxycycline. For treatment of acute epididymitis most likely caused by sexually transmitted chlamydia and gonorrhea and enteric bacteria (e.g., in men who practice insertive anal sex), CDC recommends a single IM dose of ceftriaxone given in conjunction with a 10-day regimen of oral levofloxacin or ofloxacin. If acute epididymitis is most likely caused by enteric bacteria (e.g., in men who have undergone prostate biopsy, vasectomy, or other urinary tract instrumentation procedure) and gonorrhea has been ruled out (e.g., by gram, methylene blue, or gentian violet stain), CDC states that a 10-day regimen of oral levofloxacin or ofloxacin can be used alone.

For information on current recommendations for the treatment of gonorrhea and associated infections, see Uses: Gonorrhea and Associated Infections in Ceftriaxone 8:12.06.12. For additional information on quinolone-resistant *N. gonorrhoeae* (QRNG), see Uses: Gonorrhea and Associated Infections in Ciprofloxacin 8:12.18.

■ **Mycobacterial Infections** ***Treatment of Active Tuberculosis*** Levofloxacin is used in multiple-drug regimens for the treatment of active tuberculosis† caused by *Mycobacterium tuberculosis*.

Although the potential role of fluoroquinolones and the optimal length of therapy have not been fully defined, ATS, CDC, IDSA, and others state that use of fluoroquinolones as alternative (second-line) agents can be considered for the treatment of active tuberculosis in patients intolerant of certain first-line agents and in those with relapse, treatment failure, or *M. tuberculosis* resistant to certain first-line agents. If a fluoroquinolone is used in multiple-drug regimens for the treatment of active tuberculosis, ATS, CDC, IDSA, and others recommend levofloxacin or moxifloxacin.

Although levofloxacin (or moxifloxacin) has been used instead of ethambutol during the intensive phase of treatment in adults who could not receive ethambutol and has been used instead of isoniazid throughout the course of treatment in adults who could not receive isoniazid, ATS, CDC, and IDSA state that there is no evidence that levofloxacin (or moxifloxacin) can be used to replace a rifamycin or pyrazinamide while maintaining a 6-month treatment regimen.

The fact that there are reports of fluoroquinolone-resistant *M. tuberculosis* and increasing reports of extensively drug-resistant tuberculosis (XDR tuberculosis) should be considered. XDR tuberculosis is caused by strains that are resistant to rifampin and isoniazid (multiple-drug resistant strains) and also are resistant to a fluoroquinolone and at least one parenteral second-line antimycobacterial (capreomycin, kanamycin, amikacin).

The most recent ATS, CDC, and IDSA recommendations for the treatment of tuberculosis should be consulted for more specific information.

Other Mycobacterial Infections Levofloxacin has been used in multiple-drug regimens for the treatment of disseminated *M. avium* complex† (MAC) infections.

ATS and IDSA state that the role of fluoroquinolones in the treatment of MAC infections has not been established. If a fluoroquinolone is included in a multiple-drug treatment regimen (e.g., for macrolide-resistant MAC infections), levofloxacin or moxifloxacin may be preferred, although many strains are resistant in vitro.

The most recent ATS, CDC, and IDSA recommendations for the treatment of other mycobacterial infections should be consulted for more specific information.

■ **Nongonococcal Urethritis** Levofloxacin is considered as an alternative agent for the treatment of nongonococcal urethritis† (NGU). NGU can be caused by various organisms (e.g., *Chlamydia*, *M. genitalium*, *Trichomonas vaginalis*, *Ureaplasma*, enteric bacteria) and is treated presumptively at the time of diagnosis. CDC states that a single dose of oral azithromycin or a 7-day regimen of oral doxycycline are the recommended regimens for the treatment of NGU; a 7-day regimen of oral erythromycin base or ethylsuccinate or a 7-day regimen of oral levofloxacin or ofloxacin are alternative regimens.

CDC states that men with persistent or recurrent NGU who were not compliant with the treatment regimen or were reexposed to untreated sexual partner(s) can be retreated with the initial regimen. In other patients, symptoms alone (without documentation of signs or laboratory evidence of urethral inflammation) are not a sufficient basis for retreatment and an objective diagnosis of persistent or recurrent NGU should be made before considering additional treatment. Because there is some evidence that *M. genitalium* is the most frequent cause of persistent or recurrent NGU, CDC states that those initially treated with doxycycline should receive retreatment with a single dose of oral azithromycin and those initially treated with azithromycin should receive retreatment with a 7-day regimen of oral moxifloxacin. However, if the patient with persistent or recurrent urethritis has sex with women and is in an area where *T. vaginalis* is prevalent, CDC recommends presumptive retreatment with a single 2-g dose of oral metronidazole or tinidazole and referral of their partner(s) for evaluation and appropriate treatment.

NGU may facilitate transmission of HIV and men diagnosed with NGU should be tested for HIV. Individuals with HIV infection should receive the same treatment regimens recommended for other individuals with NGU.

Any individual who had sexual contact with a patient with NGU within the preceding 60 days should be referred for evaluation, testing, and presumptive treatment with a regimen effective against *Chlamydia*. To minimize transmission and avoid reinfection, men treated for NGU should abstain from sexual intercourse until they and their sexual partner(s) have been adequately treated.

■ **Pelvic Inflammatory Disease** Levofloxacin is considered an alternative agent for the treatment of acute pelvic inflammatory disease† (PID), but should *not* be used routinely for treatment of PID or any infections that may involve *N. gonorrhoeae*.

When a combined IM and oral regimen is used for the treatment of mild to moderately severe acute PID, CDC recommends a single IM dose of ceftriaxone, cefoxitin (with oral probenecid), or cefotaxime given in conjunction with a 14-day regimen of oral doxycycline (with or without a 14-day regimen of oral metronidazole). If parenteral cephalosporins are not feasible (e.g., because of cephalosporin allergy), CDC states that a 14-day regimen of oral levofloxacin, ofloxacin, or moxifloxacin given in conjunction with a 14-day regimen of oral metronidazole can be considered if the community prevalence and individual risk of gonorrhea are low and diagnostic testing for gonorrhea is performed. If culture results are positive for *N. gonorrhoeae*, the PID treatment regimen should be selected based on results of in vitro susceptibility testing. If QRNG are identified or if in vitro susceptibility cannot be determined (e.g., only nucleic acid amplification test [NAAT] for gonorrhea is available), consultation with an infectious disease specialist is recommended.

For further information on the treatment of PID, see Uses: Pelvic Inflammatory Disease in the Cephalosporins General Statement 8:12.06.

■ **Plague** Levofloxacin is used for the treatment of plague, including pneumonic and septicemic plague, caused by *Yersinia pestis* and for postexposure prophylaxis of plague in adults and children 6 months of age or older. Based on results of in vitro and animal testing, fluoroquinolones (ciprofloxacin, levofloxacin, moxifloxacin, ofloxacin) are recommended as alternatives for the treatment of plague and for postexposure prophylaxis following a high-risk exposure to *Y. pestis*, including exposures that occur in the context of biologic warfare or bioterrorism.

Efficacy of levofloxacin for treatment or prophylaxis of plague has not been evaluated in clinical trials in humans for ethical and feasibility reasons. The drug is labeled by FDA for this indication based on an efficacy study in animals that demonstrated a survival benefit. In a placebo-controlled study, African green monkeys were exposed to an inhaled dose of *Y. pestis* (mean dose of 65 LD_{50} [range 3–145 LD_{50}]) and then randomized to receive a 10-day regimen of levofloxacin or placebo initiated within 6 hours after the onset of fever. In vitro testing indicated that the *Y. pestis* strain used in this study had a levofloxacin MIC of 0.03 mcg/mL. Pharmacokinetic data from the monkeys indicated that mean levofloxacin plasma concentrations at the end of a single 30-minute IV infusion of the drug ranged from 2.84–3.5 mcg/mL and trough concentrations 24 hours after the dose ranged from less than 0.03 to 0.06 mcg/mL. Study results indicated that mortality in the levofloxacin treatment group (1 out of 17) was significantly lower compared with mortality in the placebo group (7 out of 7). One of the levofloxacin-treated monkeys was euthanized on day 9 after exposure to *Y. pestis* because of a gastric complication; blood cultures in this monkey were positive for *Y. pestis* on day 3, but all subsequent daily blood cultures from days 4 through 7 were negative.

For the treatment of plague, IM streptomycin (or IM or IV gentamicin) historically has been considered the drug of choice. Alternatives recommended for the treatment of plague when aminoglycosides are not used include an IV fluoroquinolone (ciprofloxacin [a drug of choice for plague meningitis], levofloxacin, moxifloxacin), IV doxycycline (or IV tetracycline), IV chloramphenicol (a drug of choice for plague meningitis), or co-trimoxazole (may be less effective than other alternatives).

Anti-infective regimens recommended for treatment of naturally occurring or endemic bubonic, septicemic, or pneumonic plague also are recommended for treatment of plague that occurs following exposure to *Y. pestis* in the context of biologic warfare or bioterrorism. Such exposures would most likely result in primary pneumonic plague, and prompt initiation of anti-infective therapy (within 18–24 hours of onset of symptoms) is essential in the treatment of pneumonic plague. Some experts (e.g., US Working Group on Civilian Biodefense, USAMRIID) recommend that treatment of plague in the context of biologic warfare or bioterrorism be initiated with a parenteral anti-infective regimen of streptomycin (or gentamicin) or, alternatively, a fluoroquinolone (ciprofloxacin, levofloxacin, moxifloxacin), doxycycline, or chloramphenicol. However, an oral regimen of doxycycline (or tetracycline) or a fluoroquinolone (ciprofloxacin, levofloxacin, moxifloxacin, ofloxacin) may be substituted when the patient's condition improves or when a parenteral regimen is unavailable (e.g., when there are supply or logistic problems because large numbers of individuals require treatment in a mass casualty setting).

In the context of biologic warfare or bioterrorism, some experts (e.g., US Working Group on Civilian Biodefense, USAMRIID) recommend that asymptomatic individuals with exposure to plague aerosol or asymptomatic individuals with household, hospital, or other close contact (within about 2 m) with an individual who has pneumonic plague receive an oral anti-infective regimen for postexposure prophylaxis; however, any exposed individual who develops a temperature of 38.5°C or higher or new cough should promptly receive a parenteral anti-infective for treatment of the disease. If postexposure prophylaxis is indicated, these experts recommend a regimen of oral doxycycline (or tetracycline) or an oral fluoroquinolone (ciprofloxacin, levofloxacin, moxifloxacin, ofloxacin).

For additional information on use of fluoroquinolones for treatment or prophylaxis of plague, see Uses: Plague in Ciprofloxacin 8:12.18.

■ **Ophthalmic Infections** **For use of levofloxacin in the topical treatment of ophthalmic infections caused by susceptible organisms, see Levofloxacin 52:04.12.**

Dosage and Administration

■ **Administration** Levofloxacin is administered orally or by IV infusion. The drug should *not* be given IM, subcutaneously, intrathecally, or intraperitoneally.

IV administration of levofloxacin generally is reserved for patients who do not tolerate or are unable to take the drug orally and in other patients in whom the IV route offers a clinical advantage. Because the pharmacokinetics of levofloxacin are similar following oral and IV administration, these routes of administration are considered interchangeable.

Patients receiving oral or IV levofloxacin should be well hydrated and instructed to drink fluids liberally to prevent highly concentrated urine and formation of crystals in urine.

Oral Administration Levofloxacin tablets and oral solution are bioequivalent.

Levofloxacin tablets may be given without regard to meals; however, levofloxacin oral solution should be given 1 hour before or 2 hours after meals.

When levofloxacin tablets are given with a standard high-fat breakfast (e.g., 2 eggs fried in butter, 2 strips of bacon, hash brown potatoes, 2 slices of toast with butter, 180 mL of milk), peak serum levofloxacin concentrations are decreased approximately 14% (not considered clinically important). When given with calcium-fortified orange juice, peak serum concentrations are decreased 18%; when given with a breakfast of calcium-fortified orange juice and whole grain, fortified, ready-to-eat cereal with skim milk, peak concentrations are decreased 24% and the time to peak concentrations is increased 46%. When levofloxacin is given as an oral solution, food decreases peak serum concentrations of the drug by approximately 25%.

Levofloxacin (tablets or oral solution) should be administered orally at least 2 hours before or 2 hours after antacids containing magnesium or aluminum, metal cations (e.g., iron), sucralfate, multivitamins or dietary supplements containing iron or zinc, or buffered didanosine (pediatric oral solution admixed with antacid). These drugs may interfere with oral absorption of levofloxacin, resulting in subtherapeutic systemic concentrations of the quinolone. (See Drug Interactions.)

The manufacturer states that levofloxacin tablets should not be used in pediatric patients weighing less than 30 kg.

IV Infusion Commercially available levofloxacin premixed injection for IV infusion containing 5 mg/mL in 5% dextrose injection in single-use flexible containers is used without further dilution.

Alternatively, if commercially available levofloxacin concentrate for injection containing 25 mg/mL in single-use vials is used, the concentrate *must be diluted* prior to IV infusion with a compatible IV solution (e.g., 0.9% sodium chloride injection, 5% dextrose injection, 5% dextrose in lactated Ringer's injection or 0.9% sodium chloride injection, Plasma-Lyte 56 and 5% dextrose injection) to provide a solution containing 5 mg/mL.

Levofloxacin should not be admixed with other drugs or infused simultaneously through the same tubing with other drugs. Fluoroquinolones, including levofloxacin, should not be infused through the same tubing with any solution containing multivalent cations (e.g., magnesium). If the same administration set is used for sequential infusion of several different drugs, the tubing should be flushed before and after administration of levofloxacin with an IV solution that is compatible with both levofloxacin and the other drug(s).

Levofloxacin solutions should be inspected visually for particulate matter prior to administration whenever solution and container permit; the solutions should be discarded if they are cloudy or contain precipitates.

Levofloxacin premixed injection for IV infusion in 5% dextrose and levofloxacin concentrate for injection for IV infusion contain no preservatives; any unused portions of the solutions should be discarded.

Rate of Administration. Levofloxacin doses of 250 or 500 mg should be administered by IV infusion over a period of 60 minutes; doses of 750 mg should be administered by IV infusion over a period of 90 minutes.

Rapid IV infusion or injection has been associated with hypotension and must be avoided.

■ **Dosage** Dosage of oral and IV levofloxacin is identical.

When IV levofloxacin is used initially, therapy may be changed to oral levofloxacin (when appropriate) using the same dosage to complete therapy.

Safety of levofloxacin for treatment durations longer than 28 days in adults and longer than 14 days in pediatric patients has not been studied; therefore, the manufacturers state that the drug should be given for prolonged periods only when potential benefits outweigh risks.

Pediatric Dosage **Postexposure Prophylaxis of Anthrax.** If levofloxacin is used for inhalational anthrax (postexposure) to reduce the incidence or progression of disease following suspected or confirmed exposure to aerosolized *Bacillus anthracis* spores, including exposures in the context of biologic warfare or bioterrorism, the manufacturers recommend that pediatric patients 6 months of age or older weighing less than 50 kg receive 8 mg/kg (up to 250 mg) every 12 hours and that pediatric patients 6 months of age or older weighing more than 50 kg receive a dosage of 500 mg once daily for 60 days.

If oral levofloxacin is used for postexposure prophylaxis of anthrax in the context of biologic warfare or bioterrorism, the American Academy of Pediatrics (AAP) suggests that pediatric patients as young as 1 month of age† can receive a dosage of 8 mg/kg (up to 250 mg) every 12 hours if they weigh less than 50 kg or 500 mg once daily if they weigh more than 50 kg.

Postexposure prophylaxis should be initiated as soon as possible following suspected or confirmed exposure to aerosolized *B. anthracis*.

Because of possible persistence of *B anthracis* spores in lung tissue following an aerosol exposure, the US Centers for Disease Control and Prevention (CDC), AAP, and others recommend that anti-infective postexposure prophylaxis be continued for 60 days following a confirmed exposure.

Treatment of Uncomplicated Cutaneous Anthrax. If oral levofloxacin is used for the treatment of uncomplicated cutaneous anthrax without systemic involvement† that occurs in the context of biologic warfare or bioterrorism, AAP recommends that pediatric patients 1 month of age or older† receive a dosage of 8 mg/kg (up to 250 mg) every 12 hours if they weigh less than 50 kg or 500 mg once daily if they weigh more than 50 kg.

If uncomplicated cutaneous anthrax occurred after exposure to aerosolized *B. anthracis* spores in the context of biologic warfare or bioterrorism, anti-infective treatment should be continued for 60 days after onset of the illness.

Treatment of Systemic Anthrax. If IV levofloxacin is used in a multiple-drug parenteral regimen for initial treatment of systemic anthrax† (inhalational, GI, meningitis, or cutaneous with systemic involvement, lesions on the head or neck, or extensive edema) that occurs in the context of biologic warfare or bioterrorism (see Uses: Anthrax), AAP recommends that pediatric patients 1 month of age or older† receive a dosage of 8 mg/kg (up to 250 mg) every 12 hours if they weigh less than 50 kg or 500 mg once daily if they weigh more than 50 kg. If meningitis has been excluded, these experts recommend that IV levofloxacin be given in a dosage of 10 mg/kg (up to 250 mg) every 12 hours in those weighing less than 50 kg or 500 mg once daily in those weighing more than 50 kg.

The multiple-drug parenteral regimen should be continued for at least 2–3 weeks until the patient is clinically stable and treatment can be switched to an appropriate oral anti-infective. If systemic anthrax occurred as the result of exposure to aerosolized *B. anthracis* spores in the context of biologic warfare or bioterrorism, the oral follow-up regimen should be continued until 60 days after onset of the illness.

If oral levofloxacin is used for follow-up therapy of systemic anthrax after completion of the initial multiple-drug parenteral regimen, AAP recommends that pediatric patients 1 month of age or older† receive a dosage of 8 mg/kg (up to 250 mg) every 12 hours if they weigh less than 50 kg or 500 mg once daily if they weigh 50 kg or more.

Plague. For the treatment or prophylaxis of plague caused by *Yersinia pestis* in pediatric patients 6 months of age or older weighing less than 50 kg, the manufacturers recommend a dosage of 8 mg/kg (up to 250 mg) every 12 hours for 10–14 days.

For the treatment or prophylaxis of plague in pediatric patients 6 months of age or older weighing more than 50 kg, the manufacturers recommend a dosage of 500 mg once daily for 10–14 days and state that these individuals can receive a higher dosage (i.e., 750 mg once daily) if clinically indicated.

The drug should be initiated as soon as possible after suspected or known exposure to *Y. pestis*.

Adult Dosage **Acute Sinusitis.** If levofloxacin is used for the treatment of acute bacterial sinusitis, the usual adult dosage is 500 mg once every 24 hours for 10–14 days. Alternatively, adults can receive a dosage of 750 mg once every 24 hours for 5 days. (See Acute Sinusitis under Uses: Respiratory Tract Infections.)

Acute Exacerbations of Chronic Bronchitis. If levofloxacin is used for the treatment of acute bacterial exacerbations of chronic bronchitis, the usual adult dosage of levofloxacin is 500 mg once every 24 hours for 7 days. (See Acute Exacerbations of Chronic Bronchitis under Uses: Respiratory Tract Infections.)

Community-acquired Pneumonia. For the treatment of community-acquired pneumonia (CAP) caused by *Staphylococcus aureus*, *Streptococcus pneumoniae* (including multidrug-resistant *S. pneumoniae* [MDRSP]), *Haemophilus influenzae*, *H. parainfluenzae*, *Klebsiella pneumoniae*, *Legionella pneumophila*, *Moraxella catarrhalis*, *Chlamydophila pneumoniae*, or *Mycoplasma pneumoniae*, the usual adult dosage of levofloxacin is 500 mg once every 24 hours for 7–14 days. Alternatively, adults with CAP caused by *S. pneumoniae* (except MDRSP), *H. influenzae*, *H. parainfluenzae*, *C. pneumoniae*, or *M. pneumoniae* can receive a dosage of 750 mg once every 24 hours for 5 days.

When used in empiric regimens for the treatment of CAP or for treatment of CAP caused by *Pseudomonas aeruginosa*, the Infectious Diseases Society of America (IDSA) and American Thoracic Society (ATS) recommend that levofloxacin be given in a dosage of 750 mg once daily.

IDSA and ATS state that CAP should be treated for a minimum of 5 days and patients should be afebrile for 48–72 hours before discontinuing anti-infective therapy.

Nosocomial Pneumonia. For the treatment of nosocomial pneumonia, the usual adult dosage of levofloxacin is 750 mg once every 24 hours for 7–14 days.

Skin and Skin Structure Infections. For the treatment of uncomplicated skin and skin structure infections, the usual adult dosage of levofloxacin is 500 mg once every 24 hours for 7–10 days.

For the treatment of complicated skin and skin structure infections, the usual adult dosage of levofloxacin is 750 mg once every 24 hours for 7–14 days.

Urinary Tract Infections and Prostatitis. If levofloxacin is used for the treatment of *uncomplicated* urinary tract infections (UTIs), the usual adult dosage is 250 mg once every 24 hours for 3 days. (See Uncomplicated Urinary Tract Infections under Uses: Urinary Tract Infections and Prostatitis.)

For the treatment of *complicated* UTIs caused by *Enterococcus faecalis*, *E. cloacae*, *Escherichia coli*, *K. pneumoniae*, *Proteus mirabilis*, or *Ps. aeruginosa* or the treatment of acute pyelonephritis caused by *E. coli*, the usual adult dosage of levofloxacin is 250 mg once every 24 hours for 10 days. Alternatively, adults with *complicated* UTIs caused by *E. coli*, *K. pneumoniae*, or *P. mirabilis* or acute pyelonephritis caused by *E. coli* can receive 750 mg once every 24 hours for 5 days.

The usual adult dosage of levofloxacin for the treatment of chronic prostatitis is 500 mg once every 24 hours for 28 days.

Campylobacter Infections. For the treatment of campylobacteriosis† caused by susceptible *Campylobacter* in adults with human immunodeficiency virus (HIV) infection, the recommended dosage of oral or IV levofloxacin is 750 mg once daily.

The recommended duration of fluoroquinolone treatment in HIV-infected patients is 7–10 days for gastroenteritis or at least 14 days for bacteremic infections. A duration of 2–6 weeks is recommended for recurrent infections.

Salmonella Gastroenteritis. For the treatment of *Salmonella* gastroenteritis† (with or without bacteremia) in HIV-infected adults, the recommended dosage of oral or IV levofloxacin is 750 mg once daily.

The recommended duration of treatment in HIV-infected adults is 7–14 days in those with CD4$^+$ T-cell counts of 200 cells/mm^3 or greater (14 days or longer if the patient is bacteremic or the infection is complicated) or 2–6 weeks in those with CD4$^+$ T-cell counts less than 200 cells/mm^3.

Shigella Infections. For the treatment of shigellosis† caused by susceptible *Shigella* in HIV-infected adults, the recommended dosage of oral or IV levofloxacin is 750 mg once daily.

The recommended duration of fluoroquinolone treatment in these patients is 7–10 days for gastroenteritis or at least 14 days for bacteremic infections. Recurrent infections, especially in patients with CD4$^+$ T-cell counts less than 200 cells/mm^3, may require up to 6 weeks of treatment.

Travelers' Diarrhea. If oral levofloxacin is used for the treatment of travelers' diarrhea† (see Travelers' Diarrhea under Uses: GI Infections), some clinicians recommend adults receive 500 mg once daily for 1–3 days.

Although the use of anti-infectives for prophylaxis of travelers' diarrhea† generally is discouraged (see Travelers' Diarrhea under Uses: GI Infections), if oral levofloxacin is used, the recommended adult dosage is 500 mg once daily during the period of risk (not exceeding 2–3 weeks) beginning the day of travel and continuing for 1 or 2 days after leaving the area of risk.

Helicobacter pylori Infection. When used as a component of various multiple-drug regimens for the treatment of infections caused by *Helicobacter pylori*† (see Helicobacter pylori Infection under Uses: GI Infections), levofloxacin usually has been given in a dosage of 500 mg once daily. A dosage of 250 mg once daily has been used in some regimens.

Postexposure Prophylaxis of Anthrax. If levofloxacin is used for inhalational anthrax (postexposure) to reduce the incidence or progression of disease following suspected or confirmed exposure to aerosolized *B. anthracis* spores, including exposures in the context of biologic warfare or bioterrorism, the manufacturers recommend that adults receive a dosage of 500 mg once daily.

CDC recommends that adults (including pregnant and postpartum women) receive oral levofloxacin in a dosage of 750 mg once daily for postexposure prophylaxis of anthrax in the context of biologic warfare or bioterrorism.

Anti-infective prophylaxis should be initiated as soon as possible following suspected or confirmed exposure to aerosolized *B. anthracis*.

Because of possible persistence of *B. anthracis* spores in lung tissue following an aerosol exposure, CDC and other experts recommend that anti-infective prophylaxis be continued for 60 days following a confirmed exposure.

Treatment of Uncomplicated Cutaneous Anthrax. If oral levofloxacin is used for the treatment of uncomplicated cutaneous anthrax without systemic involvement†, CDC recommends that adults (including pregnant and postpartum women) receive a dosage of 750 mg once daily.

If uncomplicated cutaneous anthrax occurred after exposure to aerosolized *B. anthracis* spores in the context of biologic warfare or bioterrorism, anti-infective treatment should be continued for 60 days after onset of illness.

Treatment of Systemic Anthrax. If IV levofloxacin is used as an alternative to IV ciprofloxacin in a multiple-drug parenteral regimen for initial treatment of systemic anthrax† (inhalational, GI, meningitis, or cutaneous with systemic involvement, lesions on the head or neck, or extensive edema) that occurs in the context of biologic warfare or bioterrorism, CDC recommends that adults (including pregnant and postpartum women) receive a dosage of 750 mg once daily.

The multiple-drug parenteral regimen should be continued for at least 2–3 weeks until the patient is clinically stable and treatment can be switched to an oral regimen. The oral follow-up regimen should be continued until 60 days after onset of the illness.

Chlamydial Infections. If oral levofloxacin is used as an alternative for the treatment of urogenital infections caused by *Chlamydia trachomatis*† in adults and adolescents, CDC recommends a dosage of 500 mg once daily for 7 days.

Epididymitis. For the treatment of acute epididymitis† most likely caused by sexually transmitted enteric bacteria (e.g., *E. coli*) and when *Neisseria gonorrhoeae* has been ruled out, CDC recommends that oral levofloxacin be given a dosage of 500 mg once daily for 10 days.

Levofloxacin should *not* be used alone for treatment of epididymitis unless *N. gonorrhoeae* has been ruled out. (See Uses: Gonorrhea and Associated Infections.)

Treatment of Active Tuberculosis. If levofloxacin is used as an alternative (second-line) agent in multiple-drug regimens for the treatment of active tuberculosis†, ATS, CDC, and IDSA recommend that adults receive 0.5–1 g daily. These experts state that data are insufficient to support intermittent regimens of levofloxacin for the treatment of tuberculosis.

Treatment of Other Mycobacterial Infections. If oral levofloxacin is used as an alternative in multiple-drug regimens for the treatment of disseminated infections caused by *Mycobacterium avium* complex† (MAC) in HIV-infected adults, CDC, National Institutes of Health (NIH), and IDSA recommend a dosage of 500 mg once daily.

Nongonococcal Urethritis. If oral levofloxacin is used as an alternative for the treatment of nongonococcal urethritis† (NGU), CDC recommends a dosage of 500 mg once daily for 7 days. (See Uses: Nongonococcal Urethritis.)

Pelvic Inflammatory Disease. If oral levofloxacin is used as an alternative for the treatment of mild to moderately severe acute pelvic inflammatory disease (PID), CDC recommends a dosage of 500 mg once daily for 14 days given in conjunction with oral metronidazole (500 mg twice daily for 14 days).

Levofloxacin should be used for the treatment of PID only when parenteral cephalosporins are not feasible, the community prevalence and individual risk of gonorrhea are low, and in vitro susceptibility has been confirmed. (See Uses: Pelvic Inflammatory Disease.)

Plague. If levofloxacin is used for the treatment or prophylaxis of plague caused by *Y. pestis* in adults, the manufacturers recommend a dosage of 500 mg once daily for 10–14 days and state that these individuals can receive a higher dosage (i.e., 750 mg once daily) if clinically indicated.

The drug should be initiated as soon as possible after suspected or known exposure to *Y. pestis*.

■ Special Populations

Hepatic Impairment Adjustment of levofloxacin dosage is not be expected to be necessary in patients with hepatic impairment because most of the drug is excreted unchanged in urine.

Renal Impairment Dosage of levofloxacin should be modified according to the degree of renal impairment when the drug is used in adults with creatinine clearances less than 50 mL/minute. The only exception is when levofloxacin is used for the treatment of uncomplicated UTIs. (See Table 1.)

The manufacturers make no dosage recommendations for pediatric patients with renal insufficiency.

Table 1. Levofloxacin Dosage for Adults with Renal Impairment

Usual Daily Dosage for Normal Renal Function (Creatinine Clearance ≥50 mL/minute or greater)	Creatinine Clearance (mL/minute)	Dosage for Renal Impairment
250 mg	20–49	Dosage adjustment not required
250 mg	10–19	Uncomplicated UTIs: Dosage adjustment not required
		Other infections: 250 mg once every 48 hours
250 mg	Hemodialysis or CAPD patients	Information not available
500 mg	20–49	Initial 500-mg dose, then 250 mg once every 24 hours
500 mg	10–19	Initial 500-mg dose, then 250 mg once every 48 hours
500 mg	Hemodialysis or CAPD patients	Initial 500-mg dose, then 250 mg once every 48 hours; supplemental doses not required after dialysis
750 mg	20–49	750 mg once every 48 hours
750 mg	10–19	Initial 750-mg dose, then 500 mg once every 48 hours
750 mg	Hemodialysis or CAPD patients	Initial 750-mg dose, then 500 mg once every 48 hours; supplemental doses not required after dialysis

Geriatric Patients Adjustment of levofloxacin dosage based solely on age is not necessary in geriatric patients. However, dosage of the drug should be selected carefully since geriatric patients are more likely to have decreased renal function than younger adults. (See Geriatric Use under Warnings/Precautions: Specific Populations, in Cautions.)

Cautions

■ Contraindications

Levofloxacin is contraindicated in patients with known hypersensitivity to levofloxacin or other quinolones.

■ **Warnings/Precautions** ***Warnings*** **Disabling and Potentially Irreversible Serious Adverse Reactions.** Systemic fluoroquinolones, including levofloxacin, have been associated with disabling and potentially irreversible serious adverse reactions (e.g., tendinitis and tendon rupture, peripheral neuropathy, CNS effects) that can occur together in the same patient. These serious reactions may occur within hours to weeks after a systemic fluoroquinolone is initiated and have occurred in all age groups and in patients without preexisting risk factors for such adverse reactions.

Levofloxacin should be discontinued immediately at the first signs or symptoms of any serious adverse reactions.

Systemic fluoroquinolones, including levofloxacin, should be avoided in patients who have experienced any of the serious adverse reactions associated with fluoroquinolones.

Tendinitis and Tendon Rupture. Systemic fluoroquinolones, including levofloxacin, are associated with an increased risk of tendinitis and tendon rupture in all age groups.

The risk of developing fluoroquinolone-associated tendinitis and tendon rupture is increased in older adults (usually those over 60 years of age), individuals receiving concomitant corticosteroids, and kidney, heart, or lung transplant recipients. (See Geriatric Use under Warnings/Precautions: Specific Populations, in Cautions.)

Other factors that may independently increase the risk of tendon rupture include strenuous physical activity, renal failure, and previous tendon disorders such as rheumatoid arthritis. Tendinitis and tendon rupture have been reported in patients receiving fluoroquinolones who did not have any risk factors for such adverse reactions.

Fluoroquinolone-associated tendinitis and tendon rupture most frequently involve the Achilles tendon and have also been reported in the rotator cuff (shoulder), hand, biceps, thumb, and other tendon sites. Tendinitis or tendon rupture can occur within hours or days after levofloxacin is initiated or as long as several months after completion of therapy and can occur bilaterally.

Levofloxacin should be discontinued immediately if pain, swelling, inflammation, or rupture of a tendon occurs.

Systemic fluoroquinolones, including levofloxacin, should be avoided in patients who have a history of tendon disorders or have experienced tendinitis or tendon rupture.

Peripheral Neuropathy. Systemic fluoroquinolones, including levofloxacin, have been associated with an increased risk of peripheral neuropathy.

Sensory or sensorimotor axonal polyneuropathy affecting small and/or large axons resulting in paresthesias, hypoesthesias, dysesthesias, and weakness has been reported in patients receiving systemic fluoroquinolones, including levofloxacin. Symptoms may occur soon after initiation of levofloxacin and, in some patients, may be irreversible.

Levofloxacin should be discontinued immediately if symptoms of peripheral neuropathy (e.g., pain, burning, tingling, numbness, and/or weakness) occur or if there are other alterations in sensations (e.g., light touch, pain, temperature, position sense, vibratory sensation). (See Advice to Patients.)

Systemic fluoroquinolones, including levofloxacin, should be avoided in patients who have experienced peripheral neuropathy.

CNS Effects. Systemic fluoroquinolones, including levofloxacin, have been associated with an increased risk of psychiatric adverse effects, including toxic psychosis, hallucinations, paranoia, depression, suicidal thoughts or acts, anxiety, agitation, restlessness, nervousness, confusion, delirium, disorientation, disturbances in attention, insomnia, nightmares, and memory impairment. Attempted or completed suicides have been reported, especially in patients with a history of depression or an underlying risk factor for depression. These adverse effects may occur after the first dose.

System fluoroquinolones, including levofloxacin, have been associated with an increased risk of seizures (convulsions), increased intracranial pressure (including pseudotumor cerebri), dizziness, and tremors.

Levofloxacin, like other fluoroquinolones, should be used with caution in patients with known or suspected CNS disorders that predispose to seizures or lower the seizure threshold (e.g., severe cerebral arteriosclerosis, epilepsy) or with other risk factors that predispose to seizures or lower the seizure threshold (e.g., certain drugs, renal impairment).

If psychiatric or other CNS effects occur, levofloxacin should be discontinued immediately and appropriate measures initiated. (See Advice to Patients.)

Exacerbation of Myasthenia Gravis. Fluoroquinolones, including levofloxacin, have neuromuscular blocking activity and may exacerbate muscle weakness in individuals with myasthenia gravis. Use of fluoroquinolones in myasthenia gravis patients has resulted in requirements for ventilatory support and in death.

Levofloxacin should be avoided in patients with a known history myasthenia gravis. Patients should be advised to immediately contact a clinician if they experience any symptoms of muscle weakness, including respiratory difficulties. (See Advice to Patients.)

Sensitivity Reactions **Hypersensitivity Reactions.** Serious and occasionally fatal hypersensitivity and/or anaphylactic reactions have been reported in patients receiving fluoroquinolones, including levofloxacin. These reactions often occur with the first dose.

Some hypersensitivity reactions have been accompanied by cardiovascular collapse, hypotension or shock, seizures, loss of consciousness, tingling, angioedema (e.g., edema or swelling of the tongue, larynx, throat, or face), airway obstruction (e.g., bronchospasm, shortness of breath, acute respiratory distress), dyspnea, urticaria, pruritus, and other severe skin reactions.

Other serious and sometimes fatal adverse reactions that have been reported with fluoroquinolones, including levofloxacin, and that may or may not be related to hypersensitivity reactions include one or more of the following: fever, rash or other severe dermatologic reactions (e.g., toxic epidermal necrolysis, Stevens-Johnson syndrome); vasculitis, arthralgia, myalgia, serum sickness; allergic pneumonitis; interstitial nephritis, acute renal insufficiency or failure; hepatitis, jaundice, acute hepatic necrosis or failure; anemia (including hemolytic and aplastic anemia), thrombocytopenia (including thrombotic thrombocytopenic purpura), leukopenia, agranulocytosis, pancytopenia and/or other hematologic effects.

Levofloxacin should be discontinued immediately at the first appearance of rash, jaundice, or any other sign of hypersensitivity. Appropriate therapy should be initiated as indicated. (See Advice to Patients.)

Photosensitivity Reactions. Moderate to severe photosensitivity/phototoxicity reactions have been reported with fluoroquinolones, including levofloxacin.

Phototoxicity may manifest as exaggerated sunburn reactions (e.g., burning, erythema, exudation, vesicles, blistering, edema) on areas exposed to sun or artificial ultraviolet (UV) light (usually the face, neck, extensor surfaces of forearms, dorsa of hands).

As with other fluoroquinolones, patients should be advised to avoid unnecessary or excessive exposure to sunlight or artificial UV light (e.g., tanning beds, UVA/UVB treatment) while receiving levofloxacin. If a patient needs to be outdoors, they should wear loose-fitting clothing that protects skin from sun exposure and use other sun protection measures (sunscreen).

Levofloxacin should be discontinued if photosensitivity or phototoxicity (sunburn-like reaction, skin eruption) occurs.

Other Warnings/Precautions **Hepatotoxicity.** Severe hepatotoxicity, including acute hepatitis, has occurred in patients receiving levofloxacin and sometimes resulted in death. Most cases of severe hepatotoxicity occurred within 6–14 days of initiation of levofloxacin therapy and were not associated with hypersensitivity reactions. The majority of fatal cases of hepatotoxicity were in geriatric patients 65 years of age or older. (See Geriatric Use under Warnings/Precautions: Specific Populations, in Cautions.)

Levofloxacin should be discontinued immediately in any patient who develops signs or symptoms of hepatitis (e.g., loss of appetite, nausea, vomiting, fever, weakness, tiredness, right upper quadrant tenderness, itching, yellowing of the skin or eyes, light colored bowel movements, or dark colored urine).

Prolongation of QT Interval. Prolonged QT interval leading to ventricular arrhythmias, including torsades de pointes, has been reported with some fluoroquinolones, including levofloxacin.

Levofloxacin should be avoided in patients with a history of prolonged QT interval, in those with uncorrected electrolyte disorders (e.g., hypokalemia), and in those receiving class IA (e.g., quinidine, procainamide) or class III (e.g., amiodarone, sotalol) antiarrhythmic agents.

The risk of prolonged QT interval may be increased in geriatric patients. (See Geriatric Use under Warnings/Precautions: Specific Populations, in Cautions.)

Risk of Aortic Aneurysm and Dissection. Rupture or dissection of aortic aneurysms has been reported in patients receiving systemic fluoroquinolones. Epidemiologic studies indicate an increased risk of aortic aneurysm and dissection within 2 months following use of systemic fluoroquinolones, particularly in geriatric patients. The cause for this increased risk has not been identified.

Unless there are no other treatment options, systemic fluoroquinolones, including levofloxacin, should not be used in patients who have an aortic aneurysm or are at increased risk for an aortic aneurysm. This includes geriatric patients and patients with peripheral atherosclerotic vascular disease, hypertension, or certain genetic conditions (e.g., Marfan syndrome, Ehlers-Danlos syndrome).

If a patient reports adverse effects suggestive of aortic aneurysm or dissection, fluoroquinolone treatment should be discontinued immediately. (See Advice to Patients.)

Hypoglycemia or Hyperglycemia. Systemic fluoroquinolones, including levofloxacin, have been associated with alterations in blood glucose concentrations, including symptomatic hypoglycemia and hyperglycemia. Blood glucose disturbances during fluoroquinolone therapy usually have occurred in patients with diabetes mellitus receiving an oral antidiabetic agent (e.g., glyburide) or insulin.

Severe cases of hypoglycemia resulting in coma or death have been reported with some systemic fluoroquinolones. Although most reported cases of hypoglycemic coma have involved patients with risk factors for hypoglycemia (e.g., older age, diabetes mellitus, renal insufficiency, concomitant use of antidiabetic agents [especially sulfonylureas]), some cases have occurred in patients receiving a fluoroquinolone who were not diabetic and were not reported to be receiving an oral antidiabetic agent or insulin.

Blood glucose concentrations should be carefully monitored when systemic fluoroquinolones, including levofloxacin, are used in patients with diabetes mellitus receiving antidiabetic agents.

If a hypoglycemic reaction occurs, levofloxacin should be discontinued and appropriate therapy initiated immediately. (See Advice to Patients.)

Musculoskeletal Disorders. An increased incidence of musculoskeletal disorders (arthralgia, arthritis, tendinopathy, gait abnormality) has been reported in pediatric patients receiving levofloxacin. The manufacturers state that levofloxacin should be used in pediatric patients *only* for inhalational anthrax (postexposure) or treatment or prophylaxis of plague and *only* in those 6 months of age or older. (See Pediatric Use under Warnings/Precautions: Specific Populations, in Cautions.)

Fluoroquinolones, including levofloxacin, cause arthropathy and osteochondrosis in immature animals of various species. Persistent lesions in cartilage reported in levofloxacin studies in immature dogs; similar erosions in weight-bearing joints and other signs of arthropathy have been reported with other fluoroquinolones.

C. difficile-associated Diarrhea and Colitis. Treatment with anti-infectives alters normal colon flora and may permit overgrowth of *Clostridioides difficile* (formerly known as *Clostridium difficile*). *C. difficile* infection (CDI) and *C. difficile*-associated diarrhea and colitis (CDAD; also known as antibiotic-associated diarrhea and colitis or pseudomembranous colitis) have been reported with nearly all anti-infectives, including levofloxacin, and may range in severity from mild diarrhea to fatal colitis. *C. difficile* produces toxins A and B which contribute to development of CDAD; hypertoxin-producing strains of *C. difficile* are associated with increased morbidity and mortality since they may be refractory to anti-infectives and colectomy may be required.

CDAD should be considered if diarrhea develops during or after therapy and managed accordingly. Careful medical history is necessary since CDAD has been reported to occur as late as 2 months or longer after anti-infective therapy is discontinued.

If CDAD is suspected or confirmed, anti-infective therapy not directed against *C. difficile* should be discontinued as soon as possible. Patients should be managed with appropriate anti-infective therapy directed against *C. difficile* (e.g., vancomycin, fidaxomicin, metronidazole), supportive therapy (e.g., fluid and electrolyte management, protein supplementation), and surgical evaluation as clinically indicated.

Selection and Use of Anti-infectives. Levofloxacin should be used for the treatment of acute bacterial sinusitis, acute bacterial exacerbations of chronic bronchitis, or uncomplicated urinary tract infections (UTIs) *only* when no other treatment options are available. Because levofloxacin, like other systemic fluoroquinolones, has been associated with disabling and potentially irreversible serious adverse reactions (e.g., tendinitis and tendon rupture, peripheral neuropathy, CNS effects) that can occur together in the same patient, the risks of serious adverse reactions outweigh the benefits of levofloxacin for patients with these infections.

To reduce development of drug-resistant bacteria and maintain effectiveness of levofloxacin and other antibacterials, use only for treatment or prevention of infections proven or strongly suspected to be caused by susceptible bacteria.

When selecting or modifying anti-infective therapy, use results of culture and in vitro susceptibility testing. In the absence of such data, consider local epidemiology and susceptibility patterns when selecting anti-infectives for empiric therapy.

Information on test methods and quality control standards for in vitro susceptibility testing of antibacterial agents and specific interpretive criteria for such testing recognized by FDA is available at https://www.fda.gov/STIC.

Specific Populations **Pregnancy.** There are no adequate and well-controlled studies of levofloxacin in pregnant women, and the drug should be used during pregnancy only if potential benefits justify potential risks to the fetus.

Reproduction studies in rats or rabbits have not revealed evidence of teratogenicity at oral doses 9.4 or 1.1 times the maximum recommended human dose, respectively, or IV doses 1.9 or 0.5 times the maximum human dose, respectively, based on relative body surface area.

Lactation. Levofloxacin is distributed into milk following oral or IV administration.

Because of the potential for serious adverse reactions in the infant, a decision should be made whether to discontinue nursing or the drug, taking into account the importance of the drug to the woman.

Pediatric Use. Safety and efficacy of levofloxacin have not been established for any indication in infants younger than 6 months of age.

Levofloxacin is labeled by FDA for inhalational anthrax (postexposure) or for treatment or prophylaxis of plague in adolescents and children 6 months of age or older. Safety and efficacy of the drug have not been established for any other indication in this age group.

Quinolones, including levofloxacin, cause arthropathy and osteochondrosis in juvenile animals of various species. (See Musculoskeletal Disorders under Warnings/Precautions: Other Warnings/Precautions, in Cautions.)

The American Academy of Pediatrics (AAP) states that use of a systemic fluoroquinolone may be justified in children younger than 18 years of age in certain specific circumstances when there are no safe and effective alternatives and the drug is known to be effective. For information regarding when fluoroquinolones may be a preferred option in children, see Cautions: Pediatric Precautions in Ciprofloxacin 8:12.18.

Geriatric Use. No overall differences in safety and efficacy were observed between geriatric patients and younger adults in clinical trials, but increased sensitivity in some older individuals cannot be ruled out.

The risk of fluoroquinolone-associated tendon disorders, including tendon rupture, is increased in older adults (usually those older than 60 years of age). This risk is further increased in those receiving concomitant corticosteroids. (See Tendinitis and Tendon Rupture under Warnings/Precautions: Warnings, in Cautions.) Caution is advised if levofloxacin is used in geriatric adults, especially those receiving concomitant corticosteroids.

Severe and sometimes fatal hepatotoxicity has been reported in patients receiving levofloxacin, and the majority of fatalities have occurred in geriatric patients 65 years of age or older. (See Hepatotoxicity under Warnings/Precautions: Other Warnings/Precautions, in Cautions.)

The risk of prolonged QT interval leading to ventricular arrhythmias may be increased in geriatric patients, especially those receiving concurrent therapy with other drugs that can prolong QT interval (e.g., class IA or III antiarrhythmic agents) or with risk factors for torsades de pointes (e.g., known QT prolongation, uncorrected hypokalemia). (See Prolongation of QT Interval under Warnings/Precautions: Other Warnings/Precautions, in Cautions.)

The risk of fluoroquinolone-associated aortic aneurysm and dissection may be increased in geriatric patients. (See Risk of Aortic Aneurysm and Dissection under Warnings/Precautions: Other Warnings/Precautions, in Cautions.)

Because levofloxacin is substantially eliminated by the kidneys, age-related decreases in renal function should be considered when selecting dosage for geriatric patients and it may be useful to monitor renal function. (See Geriatric Patients under Dosage and Administration: Special Populations.)

Hepatic Impairment. Pharmacokinetics of levofloxacin have not been studied in patients with hepatic impairment, but pharmacokinetic alterations are unlikely.

Renal Impairment. Levofloxacin clearance is substantially reduced and plasma elimination half-life of the drug is substantially prolonged in patients with impaired renal function (creatinine clearance less than 50 mL/minute).

Levofloxacin should be used with caution in patients with renal impairment. Appropriate renal function tests should be performed prior to and during levofloxacin therapy and dosage adjusted as needed. (See Renal Impairment under Dosage and Administration: Special Populations.)

■ **Common Adverse Effects** Adverse effected reported in 3% or more of patients receiving levofloxacin include GI effects (nausea, diarrhea, constipation), headache, insomnia, and dizziness.

Drug Interactions

■ **Drugs That Prolong QT Interval** Potential pharmacologic interaction between levofloxacin and drugs that prolong the QT interval (additive effects on QT interval prolongation). Concomitant use of levofloxacin and class IA (e.g., quinidine, procainamide) or class III (e.g., amiodarone, sotalol) antiarrhythmic agents should be avoided. (See Prolongation of QT Interval under Warnings/Precautions: Other Warnings/Precautions, in Cautions.)

■ **Antacids** Potential pharmacokinetic interaction between levofloxacin (tablets or oral solution) and antacids containing magnesium or aluminum (decreased absorption of oral levofloxacin). Data are not available regarding concomitant use of IV levofloxacin and antacids.

Levofloxacin tablets or oral solution should be administered at least 2 hours before or 2 hours after such antacids.

■ **Antiarrhythmic Agents** Potential pharmacologic interaction between levofloxacin and antiarrhythmic agents (additive effect on QT interval prolongation). Levofloxacin should be avoided in patients receiving class IA (e.g., quinidine, procainamide) or class III (e.g., amiodarone, sotalol) antiarrhythmic agents. (See Prolongation of QT Interval under Warnings/Precautions: Other Warnings/Precautions, in Cautions.)

Pharmacokinetic interaction between levofloxacin and procainamide (increased half-life and decreased clearance of procainamide).

■ **Antidepressants** Potential pharmacologic interaction between levofloxacin and fluoxetine or imipramine (additive effect on QT interval prolongation).

■ **Antidiabetic Agents** Potential pharmacodynamic interaction (altered blood glucose concentrations and symptomatic hyperglycemia or hypoglycemia) in diabetic patients receiving levofloxacin concomitantly with antidiabetic agents (e.g., insulin, glyburide). (See Hypoglycemia or Hyperglycemia under Warnings/Precautions: Other Warnings/Precautions, in Cautions.)

Careful monitoring of blood glucose concentrations is recommended; levofloxacin should be discontinued if a hypoglycemic reaction occurs.

■ **Cimetidine** Pharmacokinetic interaction between levofloxacin and cimetidine (slightly increased levofloxacin area under the plasma concentration-time curve [AUC] and half-life). This interaction is not considered clinically important, and levofloxacin dosage adjustments are not warranted.

■ **Corticosteroids** Concomitant use of levofloxacin and corticosteroids increases the risk of severe tendon disorders (e.g., tendinitis, tendon rupture), especially in geriatric patients older than 60 years of age. Levofloxacin and corticosteroids should be used concomitantly with caution. (See Tendinitis and Tendon Rupture under Warnings/Precautions: Warnings, in Cautions.)

■ **Cyclosporine and Tacrolimus** Possible pharmacokinetic interactions between levofloxacin and cyclosporine or tacrolimus (increased AUC of the immunosuppressive agent).

The manufacturers of levofloxacin state that concomitant use of cyclosporine and levofloxacin did not have a clinically important effect on the pharmacokinetics of the immunosuppressive agent and dosage adjustments are not required for either drug. Some clinicians suggest that plasma concentrations of cyclosporine or tacrolimus should be monitored if used concomitantly with levofloxacin.

■ **Didanosine** Potential pharmacokinetic interaction between levofloxacin (tablets and oral solution) and buffered didanosine preparations (decreased GI absorption of oral levofloxacin). Data are not available regarding concomitant use of IV levofloxacin and buffered didanosine preparations.

Levofloxacin tablets or oral solution should be administered at least 2 hours before or 2 hours after buffered didanosine (pediatric oral solution admixed with antacid).

■ **Digoxin** Concomitant use of levofloxacin and digoxin did not result in any clinically important effects on the pharmacokinetics of either drug. Dosage adjustments are not necessary for either drug if levofloxacin and digoxin are used concomitantly.

■ **Iron, Multivitamins, and Mineral Supplements** Potential pharmacokinetic interaction between levofloxacin (tablets and oral solution) and iron, multivitamins, or mineral supplements (decreased absorption of oral levofloxacin). Data are not available regarding concomitant use of IV levofloxacin and such preparations.

Levofloxacin tablets or oral solution should be administered at least 2 hours before or 2 hours after iron preparations or multivitamins or dietary supplements containing zinc, calcium, magnesium, or iron.

■ **Nonsteroidal Anti-inflammatory Agents** Potential pharmacologic interaction between levofloxacin and nonsteroidal anti-inflammatory agents (NSAIAs) (possible increased risk of CNS stimulation and seizures). Animal studies suggest the risk may be less than that associated with some other fluoroquinolones and that risk varies depending on the specific NSAIA.

■ **Probenecid** Pharmacokinetic interaction between levofloxacin and probenecid (slightly increased levofloxacin AUC and half-life). This interaction is not considered clinically important; levofloxacin dosage adjustments are not warranted.

■ **Sucralfate** Potential pharmacokinetic interaction between levofloxacin (tablets or oral solution) and sucralfate (decreased absorption of oral levofloxacin); no pharmacokinetic interaction if given 2 hours apart. Data are not available regarding concomitant use of IV levofloxacin and sucralfate.

Levofloxacin tablets or oral solution should be administered at least 2 hours before or 2 hours after sucralfate.

■ **Theophylline** Concomitant use of levofloxacin and theophylline did not have a clinically important effect on the pharmacokinetics of either drug. However, pharmacokinetic interactions (increased theophylline half-life and increased risk of theophylline-related adverse effects) have been reported with some other quinolones.

If levofloxacin and theophylline are used concomitantly, serum theophylline concentrations should be closely monitored and theophylline dosage adjusted accordingly; clinicians should consider that adverse theophylline effects (e.g., seizures) may occur with or without elevated theophylline concentrations.

■ **Warfarin** Concomitant use of levofloxacin in patients receiving warfarin has resulted in increased prothrombin time (PT); clinical episodes of bleeding have been reported. Patients receiving the drugs concomitantly should be monitored for evidence of bleeding and PT and international normalized ratio (INR) should be monitored.

Description

Levofloxacin is a fluoroquinolone anti-infective agent. Like other commercially available fluoroquinolones, levofloxacin contains a fluorine at the C-6 position of the quinolone nucleus. Like some other fluoroquinolones (ciprofloxacin, ofloxacin), levofloxacin contains a piperazinyl group at C-7. The piperazinyl group in levofloxacin results in increased activity against gram-negative bacteria. Levofloxacin is the levorotatory isomer of ofloxacin and is 8–128 times as active against susceptible gram-positive and gram-negative bacteria as the dextrorotatory isomer and approximately twice as active as racemic ofloxacin.

Like other fluoroquinolone anti-infectives, levofloxacin inhibits DNA synthesis in susceptible organisms via inhibition of type II DNA topoisomerases (DNA gyrase, topoisomerase IV). In susceptible *S. pneumoniae*, levofloxacin principally targets topoisomerase IV.

■ **Spectrum** Levofloxacin is more active in vitro against gram-positive bacteria (including *Streptococcus pneumoniae*) and anaerobes than some other currently available fluoroquinolones (e.g., ciprofloxacin, ofloxacin), but is less active in vitro than ciprofloxacin against *Pseudomonas aeruginosa*.

Levofloxacin is active in vitro and in clinical infections against *Staphylococcus aureus* (methicillin-susceptible [oxacillin-susceptible] strains only), *S. epidermidis* (oxacillin-susceptible strains only), *S. saprophyticus*, *S. pneumoniae* (including multidrug-resistant strains [MDRSP]), *S. pyogenes* (group A β-hemolytic streptococci, GAS), and *Enterococcus faecalis* (many strains only moderately susceptible). The drug also is active in vitro against some other gram-positive bacteria, including *S. haemolyticus*, *S. agalactiae* (group B streptococci, GBS), groups C, G, and F streptococci, *S. milleri*, and viridans streptococci. Levofloxacin is active against *Bacillus anthracis* in vitro and in a primate infection model.

Levofloxacin is active in vitro and in clinical infections against *Haemophilus influenzae*, *H. parainfluenzae*, *Klebsiella pneumoniae*, *Moraxella catarrhalis*, *Enterobacter cloacae*, *Escherichia coli*, *Proteus mirabilis*, *Serratia marcescens*, *Ps. aeruginosa* (some may develop resistance during therapy), and *Legionella pneumophila*. The drug also is active in vitro against some other gram-negative bacteria, including *Acinetobacter*, *Bordetella pertussis*, *Citrobacter koseri*, *C. freundii*, *E. aerogenes*, *E. sakazakii*, *K. oxytoca*, *Morganella morganii*, *Pantoea agglomerans*, *Proteus vulgaris*, *Providencia*, and *Ps. fluorescens*. Levofloxacin is active against *Yersinia pestis* in vitro and in a primate infection model.

Although levofloxacin has in vitro activity against *Helicobacter pylori*, resistance to the drug can occur and the prevalence of levofloxacin-resistant strains may be high in some geographic areas.

Levofloxacin also is active against some other organisms, including *Chlamydophila pneumoniae* (formerly *Chlamydia pneumoniae*), *Mycoplasma pneumoniae*, and *Clostridium perfringens*.

Levofloxacin is active in vitro against some mycobacteria, including *Mycobacterium tuberculosis*, and *M. fortuitum*. Although levofloxacin is active against some strains of *M. tuberculosis* resistant to isoniazid and/or rifampin, levofloxacin-resistant *M. tuberculosis* have been reported and some multidrug-resistant *M. tuberculosis* (i.e., strains resistant to rifampin and isoniazid) also are resistant to levofloxacin or other fluoroquinolones. Extensively drug-resistant tuberculosis (XDR tuberculosis) is caused by strains that are resistant to rifampin and isoniazid (multiple-drug resistant strains) and also resistant to a fluoroquinolone and at least one parenteral second-line antimycobacterial (capreomycin, kanamycin, amikacin).

■ **Resistance** Resistance to fluoroquinolones can occur as the result of mutations in defined regions of DNA gyrase or topoisomerase IV (i.e., quinolone-resistance determining regions [QRDRs]) or altered efflux.

Cross-resistance can occur between levofloxacin and other fluoroquinolones, but some bacteria resistant to other fluoroquinolones may be susceptible to levofloxacin.

Advice to Patients

Advise patients to read the manufacturer's patient information (medication guide) prior to initiating levofloxacin therapy and each time the prescription is refilled.

Advise patients that antibacterials (including levofloxacin) should only be used to treat bacterial infections and not used to treat viral infections (e.g., the common cold).

Importance of completing full course of therapy, even if feeling better after a few days.

Advise patients that skipping doses or not completing the full course of therapy may decrease effectiveness and increase the likelihood that bacteria will develop resistance and will not be treatable with levofloxacin or other antibacterials in the future.

Advise patients that the oral solution should be taken 1 hour before or 2 hours after meals; tablets may be taken without regard to meals.

Levofloxacin should be taken at the same time each day and with liberal amounts of fluids.

Importance of taking oral levofloxacin at least 2 hours before or 2 hours after aluminum- or magnesium-containing antacids, metal cations (e.g., iron), sucralfate, multivitamins containing iron or zinc, or buffered didanosine (pediatric oral solution prepared admixed with antacid).

Inform patients that systemic fluoroquinolones, including levofloxacin, have been associated with disabling and potentially irreversible serious adverse reactions (e.g., tendinitis and tendon rupture, peripheral neuropathy, CNS effects) that may occur together in the same patient. Advise patients to immediately discontinue levofloxacin and contact a clinician if they experience any signs or symptoms of serious adverse effects (e.g., unusual joint or tendon pain, muscle weakness, a "pins and needles" tingling or pricking sensation, numbness of the arms or legs, confusion, hallucinations) while taking the drug. Advise patients to talk with a clinician if they have any questions or concerns.

Inform patients that systemic fluoroquinolones, including levofloxacin, are associated with an increased risk of tendinitis and tendon rupture in all age groups and that this risk is increased in adults older than 60 years of age, individuals receiving corticosteroids, and kidney, heart, or lung transplant recipients. Symptoms may be irreversible. Importance of resting and refraining from exercise at the first sign of tendinitis or tendon rupture (e.g., pain, swelling, or inflammation of a tendon or weakness or inability to use a joint) and importance of immediately discontinuing the drug and contacting a clinician. (See Tendinitis and Tendon Rupture under Warnings/Precautions: Warnings, in Cautions.)

Inform patients that peripheral neuropathies have been reported in patients receiving systemic fluoroquinolones, including levofloxacin, and that symptoms may occur soon after initiation of the drug and may be irreversible. Importance of immediately discontinuing levofloxacin and contacting a clinician if symptoms of peripheral neuropathy (e.g., pain, burning, tingling, numbness, and/or weakness) occur.

Inform patients that systemic fluoroquinolones, including levofloxacin, have been associated with CNS effects (e.g., convulsions, dizziness, lightheadedness, increased intracranial pressure). Importance of informing clinician of any history of convulsions before initiating therapy with the drug. Importance of contacting a clinician if persistent headache with or without blurred vision occurs.

Advise patients that levofloxacin may cause dizziness and lightheadedness; caution patients that they should not engage in activities requiring mental alertness and motor coordination (e.g., driving a vehicle, operating machinery) until the effects of the drug on the individual are known.

Advise patients that systemic fluoroquinolones, including levofloxacin, may worsen myasthenia gravis symptoms; importance of informing clinician of any history of myasthenia gravis. Importance of immediately contacting a clinician if any symptoms of muscle weakness, including respiratory difficulties, occur.

Inform patients that levofloxacin may be associated with hypersensitivity reactions (including anaphylactic reactions), even after the first dose. Importance of immediately discontinuing levofloxacin and contacting a clinician at first sign of rash or any symptom of hypersensitivity (e.g., hives, other skin reaction, rapid heartbeat, difficulty swallowing or breathing, throat tightness, hoarseness, swelling of lips, tongue, or face).

Inform patients that photosensitivity/phototoxicity reactions have been reported following exposure to sun or UV light in patients receiving fluoroquinolones. Importance of avoiding or minimizing exposure to sunlight or artificial UV light (e.g., tanning beds, UVA/UVB treatment) and using protective measures (e.g., wearing loose-fitting clothes, sunscreen) if outdoors during levofloxacin therapy. Importance of discontinuing levofloxacin and contacting a clinician if a sunburn-like reaction or skin eruption occurs.

Importance of informing clinician of personal or family history of QT interval prolongation or proarrhythmic conditions (e.g., hypokalemia, bradycardia, recent myocardial ischemia) and of concurrent therapy with any drugs that may affect QT interval (e.g., class IA [quinidine, procainamide] or class III [e.g., amiodarone, sotalol] antiarrhythmic agents). Importance of contacting a clinician if symptoms of prolonged QT interval (e.g., prolonged heart palpitations, loss of consciousness) occur.

Inform patients that systemic fluoroquinolones may increase the risk of aortic aneurysm and dissection; importance of informing clinician of any history of aneurysms, blockages or hardening of the arteries, high blood pressure, or genetic conditions such as Marfan syndrome or Ehlers-Danlos syndrome. Advise patients to seek immediate medical treatment if they experience sudden, severe, and constant pain in the stomach, chest, or back.

Inform patients that hypoglycemia has been reported when systemic fluoroquinolones were used in some patients receiving antidiabetic agents. Advise patients with diabetes mellitus receiving an oral antidiabetic agent or insulin to discontinue levofloxacin and contact a clinician if they experience hypoglycemia or symptoms of hypoglycemia.

Inform patients that severe hepatotoxicity (including acute hepatitis and fatal events) has been reported in patients receiving levofloxacin. Importance of immediately discontinuing levofloxacin and informing clinician if any signs or symptoms of liver injury (e.g., loss of appetite, nausea, vomiting, fever, weakness, tiredness, right upper quadrant tenderness, itching, yellowing of the skin and eyes, light colored bowel movements, dark colored urine) occur.

Advise patients that diarrhea is a common problem caused by anti-infectives and usually ends when the drug is discontinued. Importance of contacting a clinician if watery and bloody stools (with or without stomach cramps and fever) occur during or as late as 2 months or longer after the last dose.

If considering levofloxacin for a pediatric patient (see Pediatric Use under Warnings/Precautions: Specific Populations, in Cautions), importance of parent informing clinician if the child has a history of joint-related problems. Importance of parent contacting a clinician if the child develops any joint-related problems during or following levofloxacin therapy.

Advise patients receiving levofloxacin for inhalational anthrax (postexposure) or for treatment or prophylaxis of plague that human efficacy studies have not been performed for ethical and feasibility reasons and that use in these conditions is based on animal efficacy studies.

Importance of informing clinician of existing or contemplated concomitant therapy, including prescription and OTC drugs (e.g., drugs that may affect QT interval, antidiabetic agents, warfarin), as well as any concomitant illnesses.

Importance of women informing clinicians if they are or plan to become pregnant or plan to breast-feed.

Importance of advising patients of other important precautionary information. (See Cautions.)

Overview® (see Users Guide). For additional information on this drug until a more detailed monograph is developed and published, the manufacturer's labeling should be consulted. It is *essential* that the manufacturer's labeling be consulted for more detailed information on usual cautions, precautions, contraindications, potential drug interactions, laboratory test interferences, and acute toxicity.

Preparations

Excipients in commercially available drug preparations may have clinically important effects in some individuals; consult specific product labeling for details.

levoFLOXacin

Oral		
Solution	125 mg/5 mL*	levoFLOXacin Solution
Tablets, film-coated	250 mg (of anhydrous levofloxacin)*	Levaquin®, Janssen levoFLOXacin Tablets
	500 mg (of anhydrous levofloxacin)*	Levaquin®, Janssen levoFLOXacin Tablets
	750 mg (of anhydrous levofloxacin)*	Levaquin®, Janssen levoFLOXacin Tablets

Parenteral		
For injection, concentrate, for IV infusion	equivalent to levofloxacin 25 mg/mL (500 mg)*	levoFLOXacin Concentrate, for IV Infusion

*available from one or more manufacturer, distributor, and/or repackager by generic (nonproprietary) name

levoFLOXacin in Dextrose

Parenteral		
Injection, for IV infusion	equivalent to levofloxacin 5 mg/mL (250, 500, or 750 mg) in 5% Dextrose*	levoFLOXacin in Dextrose Injection

*available from one or more manufacturer, distributor, and/or repackager by generic (nonproprietary) name

†Use is not currently included in the labeling approved by the US Food and Drug Administration

Moxifloxacin Hydrochloride

■ Moxifloxacin is a fluoroquinolone anti-infective agent.

Uses

■ **Respiratory Tract Infections** ***Acute Sinusitis*** Moxifloxacin is used for the treatment of acute bacterial sinusitis caused by susceptible *Streptococcus pneumoniae*, *Haemophilus influenzae*, or *Moraxella catarrhalis*.

Moxifloxacin should be used for the treatment of acute bacterial sinusitis only when there are no other treatment options. Because systemic fluoroquinolones, including moxifloxacin, have been associated with disabling and potentially irreversible serious adverse reactions (e.g., tendinitis and tendon rupture, peripheral neuropathy, CNS effects) that can occur together in the same patient (see Cautions) *and because acute bacterial sinusitis may be self-limiting in some patients, the risks of serious adverse reactions outweigh the benefits of fluoroquinolones for patients with acute sinusitis.*

Clinical Experience. In a controlled, double-blind study in 457 patients with acute bacterial sinusitis, the clinical success rate (cure plus improvement) at the test-of-cure visit 7–21 days after treatment was 90% in those who received moxifloxacin (400 mg once daily for 10 days) and 89% in those who received cefuroxime axetil (250 mg twice daily for 10 days). In a noncomparative study, the clinical success and eradication/presumed eradication rate at 21–37 days after moxifloxacin treatment (400 mg once daily for 7 days) was 97, 83, or 80% for infections caused by *S. pneumoniae*, *M. catarrhalis*, or *H. influenzae*, respectively.

Acute Exacerbations of Chronic Bronchitis Moxifloxacin is used for the treatment of acute bacterial exacerbations of chronic bronchitis caused by susceptible *S. pneumoniae*, *H. influenzae*, *H. parainfluenzae*, *Klebsiella pneumoniae*, *Staphylococcus aureus* (methicillin-susceptible [oxacillin-susceptible] strains), or *M. catarrhalis*.

Moxifloxacin should be used for the treatment of acute bacterial exacerbations of chronic bronchitis only when there are no other treatment options. Because systemic fluoroquinolones, including moxifloxacin, have been associated with disabling and potentially irreversible serious adverse reactions (e.g., tendinitis and tendon rupture, peripheral neuropathy, CNS effects) that can occur together in the same patient (see Cautions) *and because acute bacterial exacerbations of chronic bronchitis may be self-limiting in some patients, the risks of serious adverse reactions outweigh the benefits of fluoroquinolones for patients with these infections.*

Clinical Experience. In a randomized, double-blind, controlled trial in 629 patients with acute bacterial exacerbations of chronic bronchitis, the clinical success rate 7–17 days after treatment was 89% in those who received moxifloxacin (400 mg once daily for 5 days) and also was 89% in those who received clarithromycin (500 mg twice daily for 10 days). The microbiologic eradication rate (eradication plus presumed eradication) in those who received moxifloxacin was 100% for *S. pneumoniae*, 89% for *H. influenzae*, 100% for *H. parainfluenzae*, 85% for *M. catarrhalis*, 94% for *S. aureus*, and 85% for *K. pneumoniae*.

Community-acquired Pneumonia Moxifloxacin is used for the treatment of community-acquired pneumonia (CAP) caused by susceptible *S. pneumoniae* (including multidrug-resistant strains [MDRSP]), *S. aureus* (methicillin-susceptible [oxacillin-susceptible] strains), *K. pneumoniae*, *H. influenzae*, *Mycoplasma pneumoniae*, *Chlamydophila pneumoniae* (formerly *Chlamydia pneumoniae*), or *M. catarrhalis*.

Initial treatment of CAP generally involves use of an empiric anti-infective regimen based on the most likely pathogens and local susceptibility patterns; treatment may then be changed (if possible) to provide a more specific regimen (pathogen-directed therapy) based on results of in vitro culture and susceptibility testing. The most appropriate empiric regimen varies depending on the severity of illness at the time of presentation, whether outpatient treatment or hospitalization in or out of an intensive care unit (ICU) is indicated, and the presence or absence of cardiopulmonary disease and other modifying factors that increase the risk of certain pathogens (e.g., methicillin-resistant *S. aureus*

[MRSA; also known as oxacillin-resistant *S. aureus* or ORSA], penicillin-resistant *S. pneumoniae*, MDRSP, enteric gram-negative bacilli, *Pseudomonas aeruginosa*).

For additional information on management of CAP, the current clinical practice guidelines from the Infectious Diseases Society of America (IDSA) available at http://www.idsociety.org should be consulted.

Clinical Experience. In randomized studies in patients with clinically and radiologically documented CAP, the rate of clinical success with a sequential regimen of IV moxifloxacin followed by oral moxifloxacin (400 mg daily for 7–14 days) was similar to that achieved with 7–14 days of therapy with similar regimens using other fluoroquinolones (levofloxacin) or a regimen of ceftriaxone with or without erythromycin. In a randomized study in CAP patients 65 years of age or older (mean age 77.9 years), the clinical cure rate at the test-of-cure visit (5–21 days after end of treatment) was 92.9% in those who received moxifloxacin and 87.9% in those who received levofloxacin; the bacteriologic success rate was 81% in those who received moxifloxacin and 75% in those who received levofloxacin.

Data on efficacy of moxifloxacin for the treatment of CAP caused by *S. pneumoniae* in adults have been obtained from various clinical studies. In these studies, moxifloxacin resulted in clinical cure in about 95% of patients with CAP caused by *S. pneumoniae*. In those patients with documented infections caused by penicillin-resistant *S. pneumoniae* (penicillin MICs of 2 mcg/mL or greater), the bacteriologic cure rate was 100%. In 37 patients with CAP caused by multidrug-resistant strains, the clinical cure rate with moxifloxacin was 95%. Moxifloxacin has been effective for the treatment of infections caused by *S. pneumoniae* resistant to penicillin, second generation cephalosporins (e.g., cefuroxime), macrolides, tetracyclines, and/or co-trimoxazole.

Nosocomial Pneumonia Moxifloxacin has been used for the treatment of nosocomial pneumonia†.

Local susceptibility data should be used when selecting initial empiric regimens for the treatment of hospital-acquired pneumonia (HAP) not associated with mechanical ventilation or the treatment of ventilator-associated pneumonia (VAP). If a fluoroquinolone is used for initial empiric treatment of HAP or VAP, IDSA and the American Thoracic Society (ATS) recommend ciprofloxacin or levofloxacin.

For additional information on management of nosocomial pneumonia, the current clinical practice guidelines from IDSA available at http://www.idsociety.org should be consulted.

■ **Skin and Skin Structure Infections** Moxifloxacin is used for the treatment of uncomplicated skin and skin structure infections caused by susceptible *S. aureus* (methicillin-susceptible [oxacillin-susceptible] strains) or *Streptococcus pyogenes* (group A β-hemolytic streptococci) and for the treatment of complicated skin and skin structure infections caused by susceptible *S. aureus* (methicillin-susceptible [oxacillin-susceptible] strains), *Escherichia coli*, *K. pneumoniae*, or *Enterobacter cloacae*.

For additional information on management of skin and skin structure infections, the current clinical practice guidelines from IDSA available at http://www.idsociety.org should be consulted.

Clinical Experience Moxifloxacin has been effective for the treatment of uncomplicated abscesses, furuncles, cellulitis, impetigo, and other skin infections. In a randomized double-blind study, moxifloxacin (400 mg once daily for 7 days) was as effective as cephalexin (500 mg 3 times daily for 7 days) in the treatment of uncomplicated skin and skin structure infections caused by susceptible bacteria; clinical success (resolution or improvement) occurred in 89 or 91% of those receiving moxifloxacin or cephalexin, respectively (intent-to-treat analysis).

In 2 randomized, comparator-controlled studies in adults with complicated skin and skin structure infections, the clinical success rate in those receiving a sequential regimen of IV moxifloxacin followed by oral moxifloxacin (400 mg once daily for 7–14 days) was similar to that in those who received a sequential IV then oral regimen of a fixed-combination preparation containing a β-lactam antibiotic and a β-lactamase inhibitor (77–81% for moxifloxacin versus 82–85% for the comparator agent). When data were stratified by the causative agent, the clinical success rate in patients who received moxifloxacin was about 82% in those with infections caused by *S. aureus* infections (methicillin-susceptible [oxacillin-susceptible] strains), *E. coli*, or *E. cloacae* and 92% in those with infections caused by *K. pneumoniae*.

■ **Intra-abdominal Infections** Moxifloxacin is used for the treatment of complicated intra-abdominal infections, including polymicrobial infections such as abscess caused by susceptible *Bacteroides fragilis*, *B. thetaiotaomicron*, *Clostridium perfringens*, *Enterococcus faecalis*, *E. coli*, *Proteus mirabilis*, *S. anginosus*, *S. constellatus*, or *Peptostreptococcus*.

Moxifloxacin has been recommended as one of several options for initial empiric treatment of mild to moderate, community-acquired intra-abdominal infections. IDSA states that use of moxifloxacin should be avoided in patients who received a quinolone within the past 3 months and are likely to harbor *B. fragilis* since such strains are likely to be resistant to the drug.

For additional information on management of intra-abdominal infections, the current clinical practice guidelines from IDSA available at http://www.idsociety.org should be consulted.

Clinical Experience Safety and efficacy of moxifloxacin monotherapy for the treatment of surgically confirmed complicated intra-abdominal infections (including peritonitis, abscess, appendicitis with perforation, bowel perforation) were established in 2 randomized, active-controlled studies in adults. In one double-blind study, patients were randomized to receive a sequential regimen of IV moxifloxacin followed by oral moxifloxacin (400 mg once daily for 5–14 days) or a sequential regimen of the IV fixed-combination preparation of piperacillin and tazobactam followed by the oral fixed-combination preparation of amoxicillin and clavulanate potassium. At the test-of-cure visit (day 25–50 after initiation of study), the clinical cure rate in the efficacy-valid population was 80% in those who received moxifloxacin and 78% in those who received the comparator regimen. The bacteriologic success rate (eradication or presumed eradication) at the test-of-cure visit was 78% in those who received moxifloxacin (83% of those with hospital-acquired or 77% of those with community-acquired infections) and 77% in those who received the comparator regimen (55% of those with hospital-acquired or 82% of those with community-acquired infections). Similar results were obtained in an open-label study in which patients were randomized to receive 400 mg of moxifloxacin daily for 5–14 days or a sequential regimen of IV ceftriaxone in conjunction with IV metronidazole followed by the oral fixed-combination preparation of amoxicillin and clavulanate potassium. In this open-label study, the clinical success rate at the test-of-cure visit (day 25–50 after initiation of study) was 81% in those who received moxifloxacin and 82% in those who received the comparator regimen.

■ **Endocarditis** Moxifloxacin is used as an alternative for the treatment of endocarditis† (native or prosthetic valve or other prosthetic material) caused by fastidious gram-negative bacilli known as the HACEK group (*Haemophilus*, *Aggregatibacter*, *Cardiobacterium hominis*, *Eikenella corrodens*, *Kingella*).

The American Heart Association (AHA) and IDSA recommend ceftriaxone (or other third or fourth generation cephalosporin) for the treatment of endocarditis caused by the HACEK group, but state that a fluoroquinolone (ciprofloxacin, levofloxacin, moxifloxacin) may be considered in patients who cannot tolerate cephalosporins. Because only limited data are available regarding use of fluoroquinolones for the treatment of HACEK endocarditis, an infectious disease specialist should be consulted when treating such infections in patients who cannot tolerate cephalosporins.

■ **GI Infections** ***Campylobacter Infections*** Moxifloxacin has been recommended as an alternative for the treatment of campylobacteriosis† caused by susceptible *Campylobacter*.

Optimal treatment of campylobacteriosis in patients with human immunodeficiency virus (HIV) infection has not been identified. Some clinicians withhold anti-infective treatment in HIV-infected patients with CD4+ T-cell counts exceeding 200 cells/mm³ if they have only mild campylobacteriosis and initiate treatment if symptoms persist for more than several days. In HIV-infected patients with mild to moderate campylobacteriosis, treatment with a fluoroquinolone (preferably ciprofloxacin or, alternatively, levofloxacin or moxifloxacin) or azithromycin is reasonable. Anti-infective therapy should be modified based on results of in vitro susceptibility testing. In the US, resistance to fluoroquinolones has been reported in 22% of *C. jejuni* and 35% of *C. coli* isolates tested. To limit emergence of resistance, some clinicians suggest that it may be prudent to use an aminoglycoside concomitantly in patients with bacteremic infections.

Salmonella Gastroenteritis Moxifloxacin is used for the treatment of *Salmonella* gastroenteritis† (with or without bacteremia).

Anti-infective therapy is not usually indicated in otherwise healthy individuals with uncomplicated (noninvasive) gastroenteritis caused by *Salmonella* since such therapy may prolong the duration of fecal excretion of the organism and there is no evidence that it shortens the duration of the disease; however, the US Centers for Disease Control and Prevention (CDC), American Academy of Pediatrics (AAP), IDSA, and others recommend anti-infective therapy in individuals with severe *Salmonella* gastroenteritis and in those who are at increased risk of invasive disease. These individuals include infants younger than 3–6 months of age; individuals older than 50 years of age; individuals with hemoglobinopathies, severe atherosclerosis or valvular heart disease, prostheses, uremia, chronic GI disease, or severe colitis; and individuals who are immunocompromised because of malignancy, immunosuppressive therapy, HIV infection, or other immunosuppressive illness.

Because HIV-infected individuals with *Salmonella* gastroenteritis are at high risk for bacteremia, CDC, National Institutes of Health (NIH), and HIV Medicine Association of IDSA recommend that such patients receive anti-infective treatment. These experts state that the initial drug of choice for the treatment of salmonella gastroenteritis (with or without bacteremia) in HIV-infected adults is ciprofloxacin; other fluoroquinolones (levofloxacin, moxifloxacin) also are likely to be effective in these patients, but clinical data are limited. Depending on results of in vitro susceptibility testing of the causative organism, alternatives for treatment of *Salmonella* gastroenteritis in HIV-infected adults are co-trimoxazole or third generation cephalosporins (ceftriaxone, cefotaxime).

The role of long-term treatment (secondary prophylaxis) against *Salmonella* in HIV-infected individuals is not well established, and possible benefits of such prophylaxis should be weighed against the risks of long-term anti-infective exposure. CDC, NIH, and IDSA state that secondary prophylaxis should be considered in those with recurrent bacteremia and may also be considered in those with recurrent gastroenteritis (with or without bacteremia) and in those with CD4+ T-cell counts less than 200 cells/mm³ and severe diarrhea. These experts state that secondary prophylaxis should be discontinued if the *Salmo-*

nella infection resolves and there has been a sustained response to antiretroviral therapy with CD4+ T-cell counts greater than 200 cells/mm³.

Shigella Infections Moxifloxacin is used as an alternative for the treatment of shigellosis† caused by susceptible *Shigella*.

Infections caused by *S. sonnei* usually are self-limited (48–72 hours), and mild cases may not require treatment with anti-infectives. However, because there is some evidence that anti-infectives may shorten the duration of diarrhea and the period of fecal excretion of *Shigella*, anti-infective treatment generally is recommended in addition to fluid and electrolyte replacement in patients with severe shigellosis, dysentery, or underlying immunosuppression. An empiric treatment regimen can be used initially, but in vitro susceptibility testing of clinical isolates is indicated since resistance is common. A fluoroquinolone (preferably ciprofloxacin or, alternatively, levofloxacin or moxifloxacin) generally has been recommended for the treatment of shigellosis. However, fluoroquinolone-resistant *Shigella* have been reported in the US, especially in international travelers, the homeless, and men who have sex with men (MSM). Depending on in vitro susceptibility, other drugs recommended for the treatment of shigellosis include co-trimoxazole, ceftriaxone, azithromycin (not recommended in those with bacteremia), or ampicillin.

■ **Anthrax** Oral moxifloxacin is recommended as an alternative for postexposure prophylaxis of anthrax† following suspected or confirmed exposure to aerosolized *Bacillus anthracis* spores (inhalational anthrax). CDC, AAP, US Working Group on Civilian Biodefense, and US Army Medical Research Institute of Infectious Diseases (USAMRIID) recommend oral ciprofloxacin and oral doxycycline as the initial drugs of choice for postexposure prophylaxis following exposure to aerosolized anthrax spores, including exposures that occur in the context of biologic warfare or bioterrorism. Other oral fluoroquinolones (levofloxacin, moxifloxacin, ofloxacin) are alternatives for postexposure prophylaxis when ciprofloxacin or doxycycline cannot be used.

Oral moxifloxacin is one of several options recommended for the treatment of uncomplicated cutaneous anthrax† (without systemic involvement) that occurs in the context of biologic warfare or bioterrorism. CDC recommends that adults receive an oral regimen of ciprofloxacin, doxycycline, levofloxacin, or moxifloxacin for treatment of such infections.

IV moxifloxacin is recommended as an alternative to IV ciprofloxacin for use in multiple-drug parenteral regimens for initial treatment of systemic anthrax† (inhalational, GI, meningitis, or cutaneous with systemic involvement, extensive edema, or head or neck lesions) that occurs in the context of biologic warfare or bioterrorism. CDC, AAP, US Working Group on Civilian Biodefense, and USAMRIID recommend that treatment be initiated with a multiple-drug parenteral regimen that includes a fluoroquinolone (preferably ciprofloxacin) or doxycycline and 1 or 2 additional anti-infective agents predicted to be effective; after the patient is clinically stable, treatment can be changed to an oral anti-infective. For initial treatment of systemic anthrax with possible or confirmed meningitis, CDC and AAP recommend a regimen of IV ciprofloxacin in conjunction with another IV bactericidal anti-infective (preferably meropenem) and an IV protein synthesis inhibitor (preferably linezolid). If meningitis has been excluded, these experts recommend an initial regimen of IV ciprofloxacin in conjunction with an IV protein synthesis inhibitor (preferably clindamycin or linezolid).

Some experts suggest that oral ciprofloxacin or other oral fluoroquinolones (levofloxacin, moxifloxacin, ofloxacin) can be considered for the treatment of inhalational anthrax† when a parenteral regimen is not available. Although a multiple-drug parenteral regimen should be used for the treatment of inhalational anthrax, use of these parenteral regimens may not be possible if large numbers of individuals require treatment in a mass casualty setting and it may be necessary to use an oral regimen.

For additional information on postexposure prophylaxis or treatment of anthrax, see Uses: Anthrax in Ciprofloxacin 8:12.18.

■ **Meningitis and Other CNS Infections** Moxifloxacin is recommended as an alternative for the treatment of meningitis† caused by certain susceptible gram-positive bacteria (e.g., *S. pneumoniae*). Fluoroquinolones also have been recommended as alternatives for the treatment of meningitis† caused by some gram-negative bacteria (e.g., *Neisseria meningitidis*, *H. influenzae*, *E. coli*, *Ps. aeruginosa*).

Limited data from animal studies indicate that moxifloxacin is distributed into CSF to some extent, and the drug has been effective for the treatment of experimental meningitis caused by *S. pneumoniae* or *E. coli*. Some experts state that fluoroquinolones (e.g., ciprofloxacin, moxifloxacin) should be considered for the treatment of meningitis *only* when the infection is caused by susceptible bacteria and the usually recommended anti-infectives cannot be used or have been ineffective.

■ **Mycobacterial Infections** ***Treatment of Active Tuberculosis*** Moxifloxacin is used in multiple-drug regimens for the treatment of active tuberculosis† caused by *Mycobacterium tuberculosis*.

Although the potential role of fluoroquinolones and the optimal length of therapy have not been fully defined, ATS, CDC, IDSA, and others state that use of fluoroquinolones as alternative (second-line) agents can be considered for the treatment of active tuberculosis in patients intolerant of certain first-line agents and in those with relapse, treatment failure, or *M. tuberculosis* resistant to certain first-line agents. If a fluoroquinolone is used in multiple-drug regimens for the treatment of active tuberculosis, ATS, CDC, IDSA, and others recommend levofloxacin or moxifloxacin.

Although levofloxacin (or moxifloxacin) has been used instead of ethambutol during the intensive phase of treatment in adults who could not receive ethambutol and has been used instead of isoniazid throughout the course of treatment in adults who could not receive isoniazid, ATS, CDC, and IDSA state that there is no evidence that levofloxacin (or moxifloxacin) can be used to replace a rifamycin or pyrazinamide while maintaining a 6-month treatment regimen.

The fact that there are reports of fluoroquinolone-resistant *M. tuberculosis* and increasing reports of extensively drug-resistant tuberculosis (XDR tuberculosis) should be considered. XDR tuberculosis is caused by strains of *M. tuberculosis* that are resistant to rifampin and isoniazid (multiple-drug resistant strains) and also are resistant to a fluoroquinolone and at least one parenteral second-line antimycobacterial (capreomycin, kanamycin, amikacin).

The most recent ATS, CDC, and IDSA recommendations for treatment of tuberculosis should be consulted for more specific information.

Other Mycobacterial Infections Moxifloxacin is used in the treatment of *M. kansasii* infections† in conjunction with other antimycobacterials. ATS and IDSA recommend a multiple-drug regimen of isoniazid, rifampin, and ethambutol for treatment of pulmonary or disseminated infections caused by *M. kansasii*. If rifampin-resistant *M. kansasii* are involved, ATS and IDSA recommend a 3-drug regimen based on results of in vitro susceptibility testing, including clarithromycin (or azithromycin), moxifloxacin, ethambutol, sulfamethoxazole, or streptomycin.

Moxifloxacin has been used in multiple-drug regimens for the treatment of *M. avium* complex† (MAC) infections. ATS and IDSA state that the role of fluoroquinolones in the treatment of MAC infections has not been established. If a fluoroquinolone is included in a treatment regimen (e.g., for macrolide-resistant MAC infections), moxifloxacin or levofloxacin may be preferred, although many strains are resistant in vitro.

The most recent ATS, CDC, and IDSA recommendations for treatment of other mycobacterial infections should be consulted for more specific information.

■ **Nongonococcal Urethritis** Moxifloxacin is considered as an alternative agent for the treatment of nongonococcal urethritis† (NGU). NGU can be caused by various organisms (e.g., *Chlamydia*, *M. genitalium*, *Trichomonas vaginalis*, *Ureaplasma*, enteric bacteria) and is treated presumptively at the time of diagnosis. CDC states that a single dose of oral azithromycin or a 7-day regimen of oral doxycycline are the recommended regimens for the treatment of NGU; a 7-day regimen of oral erythromycin base or ethylsuccinate or a 7-day regimen of oral levofloxacin or ofloxacin are alternative regimens.

CDC states that men with persistent or recurrent NGU who were not compliant with the treatment regimen or were reexposed to untreated sexual partner(s) can be retreated with the initial regimen. In other patients, symptoms alone (without documentation of signs or laboratory evidence of urethral inflammation) are not a sufficient basis for retreatment and an objective diagnosis of persistent or recurrent NGU should be made before considering additional treatment. Because there is some evidence that *M. genitalium* is the most frequent cause of persistent or recurrent NGU, CDC states that those initially treated with doxycycline should receive retreatment with a single dose of oral azithromycin and those initially treated with azithromycin should receive retreatment with a 7-day regimen of oral moxifloxacin. However, if the patient with persistent or recurrent urethritis has sex with women and is in an area where *T. vaginalis* is prevalent, CDC recommends presumptive retreatment with a single 2-g dose of oral metronidazole or tinidazole and referral of their partner(s) for evaluation and appropriate treatment.

NGU may facilitate transmission of HIV and men diagnosed with NGU should be tested for HIV. Individuals with HIV infection should receive the same treatment regimens recommended for other individuals with NGU.

Any individual who had sexual contact with a patient with NGU within the preceding 60 days should be referred for evaluation, testing, and presumptive treatment with a regimen effective against *Chlamydia*. To minimize transmission and avoid reinfection, men treated for NGU should abstain from sexual intercourse until they and their sexual partner(s) have been adequately treated.

■ **Plague** Moxifloxacin is used for the treatment of plague, including pneumonic and septicemic plague, caused by susceptible *Yersinia pestis* and for prophylaxis of plague. Based on results of in vitro and animal testing, fluoroquinolones (e.g., ciprofloxacin, levofloxacin, moxifloxacin, ofloxacin) are recommended as alternatives for the treatment of plague and for postexposure prophylaxis following a high risk exposure to *Y. pestis*, including exposure in the context of biologic warfare or bioterrorism.

Efficacy of moxifloxacin for treatment or prophylaxis of plague has not been evaluated in clinical trials in humans for ethical and feasibility reasons. The drug is labeled by the FDA for this indication based on an efficacy study in animals that demonstrated a survival benefit and supportive animal and human pharmacokinetic data. In a randomized, blinded, placebo-controlled study, African green monkeys were exposed to an inhaled dose of *Y. pestis* (mean dose of 100 LD_{50} [range 92–127 LD_{50}]) and then randomized to receive a 10-day regimen of moxifloxacin or placebo initiated after fever developed and was sustained for at least 4 hours. All study monkeys were febrile and bacteremic with *Y. pestis* prior to initiation of study treatment. In vitro testing indicated that the *Y. pestis* strain (CO92 strain) used in this study had a moxifloxacin MIC of 0.06 mcg/mL. Pharmacokinetic data indicated that mean plasma concentrations of moxifloxacin attained in the study monkeys (4.4 mcg/mL) were similar to mean peak plasma concentrations attained in adults receiving 400 mg of moxifloxacin IV (3.9 mcg/mL). Study results indicated that all monkeys in the moxifloxacin treatment group survived for the 30-day period after treatment (10 out of 10), but all monkeys in the placebo group succumbed to the disease within 83–139 hours (10 out of 10).

For the treatment of plague, IM streptomycin (or IM or IV gentamicin) historically has been considered the drug of choice. Alternatives recommended for the treatment of plague when aminoglycosides are not used include an IV fluoroquinolone (ciprofloxacin [a drug of choice for plague meningitis], levofloxacin, moxifloxacin), IV doxycycline (or IV tetracycline), IV chloramphenicol (a drug of choice for plague meningitis), or co-trimoxazole (may be less effective than other alternatives).

Anti-infective regimens recommended for treatment of naturally occurring or endemic bubonic, septicemic, or pneumonic plague also are recommended for the treatment of plague that occurs following exposure to *Y. pestis* in the context of biologic warfare or bioterrorism. Such exposures would most likely result in primary pneumonic plague, and prompt initiation of anti-infective therapy (within 18–24 hours of onset of symptoms) is essential in the treatment of pneumonic plague. Some experts (e.g., US Working Group on Civilian Biodefense, USAMRIID) recommend that treatment of plague in the context of biologic warfare or bioterrorism be initiated with a parenteral anti-infective regimen of streptomycin (or gentamicin) or, alternatively, a fluoroquinolone (ciprofloxacin, levofloxacin, moxifloxacin), doxycycline, or chloramphenicol. However, an oral regimen of doxycycline (or tetracycline) or a fluoroquinolone (ciprofloxacin, levofloxacin, moxifloxacin, ofloxacin) may be substituted when the patient's condition improves or when a parenteral regimen is unavailable (e.g., when there are supply or logistic problems because large numbers of individuals require treatment in a mass casualty setting).

In the context of biologic warfare or bioterrorism, some experts (e.g., US Working Group on Civilian Biodefense, USAMRIID) recommend that asymptomatic individuals with exposure to plague aerosol or asymptomatic individuals with household, hospital, or other close contact (within about 2 m) with an individual who has pneumonic plague receive an oral anti-infective regimen for postexposure prophylaxis; however, any exposed individual who develops a temperature of 38.5°C or higher or new cough should promptly receive a parenteral anti-infective for treatment of the disease. If postexposure prophylaxis is indicated, these experts recommend a an oral regimen of doxycycline (or tetracycline) or a fluoroquinolone (ciprofloxacin, levofloxacin, moxifloxacin, ofloxacin).

For additional information on use of fluoroquinolones for treatment or prophylaxis of plague, see Uses: Plague in Ciprofloxacin 8:12.18.

■ **Ophthalmic Infections** **For use of moxifloxacin in the topical treatment of ophthalmic infections caused by susceptible organisms, see Moxifloxacin Hydrochloride 52:04.12.**

Dosage and Administration

■ **Administration** Moxifloxacin hydrochloride is administered orally or by IV infusion. The drug should *not* be given IM, subcutaneously, intrathecally, or intraperitoneally.

IV administration of moxifloxacin is indicated in patients who do not tolerate or are unable to take the drug orally and in other patients in whom the IV route offers a clinical advantage.

Patients receiving oral or IV moxifloxacin should be well hydrated and instructed to drink fluids liberally.

Oral Administration Moxifloxacin tablets may be given without regard to meals.

Administration of a 400-mg moxifloxacin tablet with a high-fat breakfast or with yogurt does not have a clinically important effect on absorption of the drug.

Moxifloxacin should be administered orally at least 4 hours before or 8 hours after antacids containing magnesium or aluminum, metal cations (e.g., iron), sucralfate, multivitamins or dietary supplements containing iron or zinc, or buffered didanosine (pediatric oral solution admixed with antacid). These drugs may substantially interfere with absorption of moxifloxacin, resulting in systemic concentrations considerably lower than desired. (See Drug Interactions.)

IV Infusion Commercially available injection for IV infusion containing 400 mg of moxifloxacin in 0.8% sodium chloride injection in single-use flexible containers may be used without further dilution.

Moxifloxacin should not be admixed with other drugs or infused simultaneously through the same tubing with other drugs. If the same IV line or a Y-type line is used for sequential infusion of other drugs or if the piggyback method of administration is used, the tubing should be flushed before and after infusion of moxifloxacin using an IV solution compatible with both moxifloxacin and the other drug(s).

Moxifloxacin IV solutions should be inspected visually for particulate matter prior to administration; the premixed solution should appear yellow.

Because commercially available moxifloxacin premixed injection for IV infusion contains no preservatives, any unused portions of the solution should be discarded.

Rate of Administration. Moxifloxacin solutions should be administered by IV infusion over 1 hour.

Rapid IV infusion of the drug should be avoided.

■ **Dosage** Dosage of moxifloxacin hydrochloride is expressed in terms of moxifloxacin.

Dosage of oral and IV moxifloxacin is identical.

When IV moxifloxacin is used initially, therapy may be changed to oral moxifloxacin (when appropriate) using the same dosage to complete therapy.

Pediatric Dosage **Treatment of Systemic Anthrax.** If IV moxifloxacin is used in a multiple-drug parenteral regimen for initial treatment of systemic anthrax† (inhalational, GI, meningitis, or cutaneous with systemic involvement, extensive edema, or head or neck lesions) that occurs in the context of biologic warfare or bioterrorism (see Uses: Anthrax), the American Academy of Pediatrics (AAP) recommends that preterm neonates† (gestational age 32–37 weeks) up to 4 weeks of age receive a dosage of 5 mg/kg once daily and that full-term neonates† up to 4 weeks of age receive a dosage of 10 mg/kg once daily.

If IV moxifloxacin is used in a multiple-drug parenteral regimen for initial treatment of systemic anthrax† (inhalational, GI, meningitis, or cutaneous with systemic involvement, lesions on the head or neck, or extensive edema) that occurs in the context of biologic warfare or bioterrorism (see Uses: Anthrax) in infants 3 months to less than 2 years of age†, AAP recommends a dosage of 6 mg/kg (up to 200 mg) every 12 hours. AAP recommends an IV dosage of 5 mg/kg (up to 200 mg) every 12 hours in children 2–5 years of age† and 4 mg/kg (up to 200 mg) every 12 hours in those 6–11 years of age†. In adolescents 12–17 years of age†, AAP recommends that those weighing less than 45 kg receive an IV moxifloxacin dosage of 4 mg/kg (up to 200 mg) every 12 hours and that those weighing 45 kg or more receive a dosage of 400 mg once daily.

The multiple-drug parenteral regimen should be continued for at least 2–3 weeks until the patient is clinically stable and treatment can be switched to an appropriate oral anti-infective. If systemic anthrax occurred as the result of exposure to aerosolized *Bacillus anthracis* spores (e.g., in the context of biologic warfare or bioterrorism), the oral follow-up regimen should be continued until 60 days after onset of the illness.

Adult Dosage **Acute Sinusitis.** If moxifloxacin is used for the treatment of acute bacterial sinusitis, the usual adult dosage is 400 mg once daily for 10 days. (See Acute Sinusitis under Uses: Respiratory Tract Infections.)

Acute Exacerbations of Chronic Bronchitis. If moxifloxacin is used for the treatment of acute bacterial exacerbations of chronic bronchitis, the usual adult dosage is 400 mg once daily for 5 days. (See Acute Exacerbations of Chronic Bronchitis under Uses: Respiratory Tract Infections.)

Community-acquired Pneumonia. For the treatment of community-acquired pneumonia (CAP), the usual adult dosage of moxifloxacin is 400 mg once daily for 7–14 days.

Skin and Skin Structure Infections. For the treatment of uncomplicated skin and skin structure infections, the usual adult dosage of moxifloxacin is 400 mg once daily for 7 days.

For the treatment of complicated skin and skin structure infections, the usual adult dosage of moxifloxacin is 400 mg once daily for 7–21 days.

Intra-abdominal Infections. For the treatment of complicated intra-abdominal infections, the usual adult dosage of moxifloxacin is 400 mg once daily. The drug should be administered IV initially, but therapy may be changed to oral administration when clinically appropriate.

The manufacturer recommends a total duration of therapy of 5–14 days for the treatment of complicated intra-abdominal infections. The Infectious Diseases Society of America (IDSA) states that the usual duration of treatment for these infections is 4–7 day; a longer duration of treatment has not been associated with improved outcome and is not recommended unless adequate source control is difficult to achieve.

Campylobacter Infections. For the treatment of campylobacteriosis† caused by susceptible *Campylobacter* in adults with human immunodeficiency virus (HIV) infection, the recommended dosage of oral or IV moxifloxacin is 400 mg once daily.

The recommended duration of fluoroquinolone treatment in HIV-infected patients is 7–10 days for gastroenteritis or at least 14 days for bacteremic infections. A duration of 2–6 weeks is recommended for recurrent infections.

Salmonella Gastroenteritis. For the treatment of *Salmonella* gastroenteritis† (with or without bacteremia) in HIV-infected adults, the recommended dosage of oral or IV moxifloxacin is 400 mg once daily.

The recommended duration of treatment in HIV-infected patients is 7–14 days in those with $CD4^+$ T-cell counts of 200 cells/mm^3 or greater (14 days or longer if the patient is bacteremic or the infection is complicated) or 2–6 weeks in those with $CD4^+$ T-cell counts less than 200 cells/mm^3.

Shigella Infections. For the treatment of shigellosis† caused by susceptible *Shigella* in HIV-infected adults, the recommended dosage of oral or IV moxifloxacin is 400 mg once daily.

The recommended duration of fluoroquinolone treatment in HIV-infected patients is 7–10 days for gastroenteritis or at least 14 days for bacteremic infections. Recurrent infections, especially in those with $CD4^+$ T-cell counts less than 200 cells/mm^3, may require up to 6 weeks of treatment.

Postexposure Prophylaxis of Anthrax. If oral moxifloxacin is used as an alternative for postexposure prophylaxis of anthrax† following exposure to aerosolized *B. anthracis* spores in the context of biologic warfare or bioterrorism, CDC recommends that adults (including pregnant and postpartum women) receive a dosage of 400 mg once daily.

Anti-infective prophylaxis should be initiated as soon as possible following suspected or confirmed exposure to aerosolized *B. anthracis*.

Because of possible persistence of *B. anthracis* spores in lung tissue following an aerosol exposure, CDC and other experts recommend that anti-infective postexposure prophylaxis be continued for 60 days following a confirmed exposure.

Treatment of Uncomplicated Cutaneous Anthrax. If oral moxifloxacin is used for the treatment of uncomplicated cutaneous anthrax without systemic involvement†, CDC recommends that adults (including pregnant and postpartum women) receive a dosage of 400 mg once daily.

If uncomplicated cutaneous anthrax occurred after exposure to aerosolized *B. anthracis* spores in the context of biologic warfare or bioterrorism, anti-infective treatment should be continued for 60 days.

Treatment of Systemic Anthrax. If IV moxifloxacin is used as an alternative to IV ciprofloxacin in a multiple-drug parenteral regimen for initial treatment of systemic anthrax† (inhalational, GI, meningitis, or cutaneous with systemic involvement, lesions on the head or neck, or extensive edema) that occurs in the context of biologic warfare or bioterrorism, CDC recommends that adults (including pregnant and postpartum women) receive a dosage of 400 mg once daily.

The multiple-drug parenteral regimen should be continued for at least 2–3 weeks until the patient is clinically stable and treatment can be switched to an oral anti-infective. If systemic anthrax occurred as the result of exposure to aerosolized *B. anthracis* spores in the context of biologic warfare or bioterrorism, the oral follow-up regimen should be continued until 60 days after onset of the illness.

If oral moxifloxacin is used as an alternative for the treatment of inhalational anthrax† when a parenteral regimen is not available (see Uses: Anthrax), US Working Group on Civilian Biodefense suggests that adults can receive a dosage of 400 mg once daily for 60 days.

Treatment of Active Tuberculosis. If moxifloxacin is used as an alternative (second-line) agent in multiple-drug regimens for the treatment of active tuberculosis†, the American Thoracic Society (ATS), CDC, and IDSA recommend that adults receive 400 mg once daily. These experts state that data are insufficient to support intermittent regimens of moxifloxacin for the treatment of tuberculosis.

Other Mycobacterial Infections. If oral moxifloxacin is used as an alternative in multiple-drug regimens for the treatment of disseminated infections caused by *Mycobacterium avium* complex† (MAC) in HIV-infected adults, CDC, National Institutes of Health (NIH), and IDSA recommend a dosage of 400 mg once daily.

Nongonococcal Urethritis. If oral moxifloxacin is used as an alternative for the treatment of persistent or recurrent nongonococcal urethritis† (NGU) in patients initially treated with azithromycin (see Uses: Nongonococcal Urethritis), CDC recommends a dosage of 400 mg once daily for 7 days.

Plague. If moxifloxacin is used for the treatment or prophylaxis of plague caused by *Yersinia pestis* in adults, the manufacturer recommends a dosage of 400 mg once daily for 10–14 days. The drug should be initiated as soon as possible after suspected or known exposure to *Y. pestis*.

■ Special Populations

Hepatic Impairment Adjustment of moxifloxacin dosage is not necessary in adults with mild, moderate, or severe hepatic impairment (Child-Pugh class A, B, or C). However, moxifloxacin should be used with caution in patients with hepatic impairment. (See Hepatic Impairment under Warning/Precautions: Specific Populations, in Cautions.)

Renal Impairment Adjustment of moxifloxacin dosage is not necessary in adults with renal impairment, including those receiving hemodialysis or continuous ambulatory peritoneal dialysis (CAPD).

Geriatric Patients Adjustment of moxifloxacin dosage based solely on age is not necessary in geriatric patients 65 years of age and older.

Cautions

■ Contraindications

Moxifloxacin is contraindicated in patients with a history of hypersensitivity to moxifloxacin or other quinolones.

■ Warnings/Precautions

Warnings **Disabling and Potentially Irreversible Serious Adverse Reactions.** Systemic fluoroquinolones, including moxifloxacin, have been associated with disabling and potentially irreversible serious adverse reactions (e.g., tendinitis and tendon rupture, peripheral neuropathy, CNS effects) that can occur together in the same patient. These serious reactions may occur within hours to weeks after a systemic fluoroquinolone is initiated and have occurred in all age groups and in patients without preexisting risk factors for such adverse reactions.

Moxifloxacin should be discontinued immediately at the first signs or symptoms of any serious adverse reactions.

Systemic fluoroquinolones, including moxifloxacin, should be avoided in patients who have experienced any of the serious adverse reactions associated with fluoroquinolones.

Tendinitis and Tendon Rupture. Systemic fluoroquinolones, including moxifloxacin, are associated with an increased risk of tendinitis and tendon rupture in all age groups.

The risk of developing fluoroquinolone-associated tendinitis and tendon rupture is increased in older adults (usually those older than 60 years of age), individuals receiving concomitant corticosteroids, and kidney, heart, or lung transplant recipients. (See Geriatric Use under Warnings/Precautions: Specific Populations, in Cautions.)

Other factors that may independently increase the risk of tendon rupture include strenuous physical activity, renal failure, and previous tendon disorders such as rheumatoid arthritis. Tendinitis and tendon rupture have been reported in patients receiving fluoroquinolones who did not have any risk factors for such adverse effects.

Fluoroquinolone-associated tendinitis and tendon rupture most frequently involve the Achilles tendon and have also been reported in the rotator cuff (shoulder), hand, biceps, thumb, and other tendon sites. Tendinitis or tendon rupture can occur within hours or days after moxifloxacin is initiated or as long as several months after completion of therapy and can occur bilaterally.

Moxifloxacin should be discontinued immediately if pain, swelling, inflammation, or rupture of a tendon occurs. (See Advice to Patients.)

Systemic fluoroquinolones, including moxifloxacin, should be avoided in patients who have a history of tendon disorders or have experienced tendinitis or tendon rupture.

Peripheral Neuropathy. Systemic fluoroquinolones, including moxifloxacin, have been associated with an increased risk of peripheral neuropathy.

Sensory or sensorimotor axonal polyneuropathy affecting small and/or large axons resulting in paresthesias, hypoesthesias, dysesthesias, and weakness has been reported in patients receiving systemic fluoroquinolones, including moxifloxacin. Symptoms may occur soon after initiation of moxifloxacin and, in some patients, may be irreversible.

Moxifloxacin should be discontinued immediately if symptoms of peripheral neuropathy (e.g., pain, burning, tingling, numbness, and/or weakness) occur or if there are other alterations in sensations (e.g., light touch, pain, temperature, position sense, vibratory sensation). (See Advice to Patients.)

Systemic fluoroquinolones, including moxifloxacin, should be avoided in patients who have experienced peripheral neuropathy.

CNS Effects. Systemic fluoroquinolones, including moxifloxacin, have been associated with an increased risk of psychiatric adverse effects, including toxic psychosis, hallucinations, paranoia, depression, suicidal thoughts or acts, agitation, nervousness, confusion, delirium, disorientation, disturbances in attention, insomnia, nightmares, and memory impairment. These adverse effects may occur after the first dose.

System fluoroquinolones, including moxifloxacin, have been associated with an increased risk of seizures (convulsions), increased intracranial pressure (including pseudotumor cerebri), dizziness, and tremors. These CNS effects may occur after the first dose.

Moxifloxacin, like other fluoroquinolones, should be used with caution in patients with known or suspected CNS disorders (e.g., severe cerebral arteriosclerosis, epilepsy) or with other risk factors that predispose to seizures or lower seizure threshold.

If psychiatric or other CNS effects occur, moxifloxacin should be discontinued immediately and appropriate measures initiated. (See Advice to Patients.)

Exacerbation of Myasthenia Gravis. Fluoroquinolones, including moxifloxacin, have neuromuscular blocking activity and may exacerbate muscle weakness in individuals with myasthenia gravis. Use of fluoroquinolones in myasthenia gravis patients has resulted in requirements for ventilatory support and in death.

Moxifloxacin should be avoided in patients with a known history of myasthenia gravis. Patients should be advised to immediately contact a clinician if they have any symptoms of muscle weakness, including respiratory difficulties. (See Advice to Patients.)

Sensitivity Reactions **Hypersensitivity Reactions.** Serious and occasionally fatal hypersensitivity and/or anaphylactic reactions have been reported in patients receiving fluoroquinolones, including moxifloxacin. Although generally reported after multiple doses, these reactions may occur with first dose.

Some hypersensitivity reactions have been accompanied by cardiovascular collapse, loss of consciousness, tingling, edema (pharyngeal or facial), dyspnea, urticaria, or pruritus.

Other serious and sometimes fatal adverse reactions that have been reported with fluoroquinolones, including moxifloxacin, and that may or may not be related to hypersensitivity reactions include one or more of the following: fever, rash or severe dermatologic reactions (e.g., toxic epidermal necrolysis, Stevens-Johnson syndrome); vasculitis, arthralgia, myalgia, serum sickness; allergic pneumonitis; interstitial nephritis, acute renal insufficiency or failure; hepatitis, jaundice, acute hepatic necrosis or failure; anemia (including hemolytic and aplastic), thrombocytopenia (including thrombotic thrombocytopenic purpura), leukopenia, agranulocytosis, pancytopenia, and/or other hematologic effects.

Moxifloxacin should be discontinued immediately at the first appearance of rash, jaundice, or any other sign of hypersensitivity. Appropriate therapy should be initiated as indicated (e.g., epinephrine, corticosteroids, maintenance of an adequate airway and oxygen). (See Advice to Patients.)

Photosensitivity Reactions. Moderate to severe photosensitivity/phototoxicity reactions have been reported with fluoroquinolones, including moxifloxacin.

Phototoxicity may manifest as exaggerated sunburn reactions (e.g., burning, erythema, exudation, vesicles, blistering, edema) on areas exposed to sun or artificial ultraviolet (UV) light (usually the face, neck, extensor surfaces of forearms, dorsa of hands).

As with other fluoroquinolones, patients should be advised to avoid unnecessary or excessive exposure to sunlight or artificial UV light (e.g., tanning beds, UVA/UVB treatment) while receiving moxifloxacin. If a patient needs to be outdoors, they should wear loose-fitting clothing that protects skin from sun exposure and use other sun protection measures (sunscreen).

Moxifloxacin should be discontinued if photosensitivity or phototoxicity (sunburn-like reaction, skin eruption) occurs.

Other Warnings/Precautions **Prolongation of QT Interval.** Prolonged QT interval leading to ventricular arrhythmias, including torsades de pointes, has been reported with some fluoroquinolones, including moxifloxacin.

Following an oral dose of 400 mg of moxifloxacin, the mean change in QT interval corrected for rate (QT_c) from baseline was 6 msec. When moxifloxacin was given IV in a dosage of 400 mg once daily by IV infusion over 1 hour, the mean change in QT_c from baseline was 10 msec on day 1 and 7 msec on day 3.

The recommended moxifloxacin dosage and IV infusion rate should not be exceeded since this may increase the risk of QT interval prolongation.

Moxifloxacin should be avoided in patients with known prolongation of the QT interval, ventricular arrhythmias (including torsades de pointes), any ongoing proarrhythmic conditions (including clinically important bradycardia and acute myocardial ischemia), or uncorrected hypokalemia or hypomagnesemia.

Moxifloxacin also should be avoided in patients receiving class IA (e.g., quinidine, procainamide) or III (e.g., amiodarone, sotalol) antiarrhythmic agents or other drugs that prolong the QT interval (e.g., cisapride [commercially available under a limited-access protocol only], erythromycin, antipsychotic agents, tricyclic antidepressants). (See Drug Interactions: Drugs that Prolong QT Interval.)

In addition, moxifloxacin should be used with caution in patients with mild, moderate, or severe liver cirrhosis since metabolic disturbances associated with hepatic insufficiency may lead to QT prolongation. (See Hepatic Impairment under Warnings/Precautions: Specific Populations, in Cautions.)

The risk of prolonged QT interval may be increased in geriatric patients. (See Geriatric Use under Warnings/Precautions: Specific Populations, in Cautions.)

Risk of Aortic Aneurysm and Dissection. Rupture or dissection of aortic aneurysms has been reported in patients receiving systemic fluoroquinolones. Epidemiologic studies indicate an increased risk of aortic aneurysm and dissection within 2 months following use of systemic fluoroquinolones, particularly in geriatric patients. The cause for this increased risk has not been identified.

Unless there are no other treatment options, systemic fluoroquinolones, including moxifloxacin, should not be used in patients who have an aortic aneurysm or are at increased risk for an aortic aneurysm. This includes geriatric patients and patients with peripheral atherosclerotic vascular disease, hypertension, or certain genetic conditions (e.g., Marfan syndrome, Ehlers-Danlos syndrome).

If a patient reports adverse effects suggestive of aortic aneurysm or dissection, fluoroquinolone treatment should be discontinued immediately. (See Advice to Patients.)

Hypoglycemia or Hyperglycemia. Systemic fluoroquinolones, including moxifloxacin, have been associated with alterations in blood glucose concentrations, including symptomatic hypoglycemia and hyperglycemia. Blood glucose disturbances during fluoroquinolone therapy usually have occurred in patients with diabetes mellitus receiving an oral antidiabetic agent (e.g., glyburide) or insulin.

Severe cases of hypoglycemia resulting in coma or death have been reported with some systemic fluoroquinolones. Although most reported cases of hypoglycemic coma have involved patients with risk factors for hypoglycemia (e.g., older age, diabetes mellitus, renal insufficiency, concomitant use of antidiabetic agents [especially sulfonylureas]), some cases have occurred in patients receiving a fluoroquinolone who were not diabetic and were not reported to be receiving an oral antidiabetic agent or insulin.

Blood glucose concentrations should be carefully monitored when systemic fluoroquinolones, including moxifloxacin, are used in patients with diabetes mellitus receiving antidiabetic agents.

If a hypoglycemic reaction occurs, moxifloxacin should be discontinued and appropriate therapy initiated immediately. (See Advice to Patients.)

Hepatotoxicity. Severe hepatotoxicity, including acute hepatitis, has occurred in patients receiving moxifloxacin and sometimes resulted in death.

Musculoskeletal Effects. Fluoroquinolones, including moxifloxacin, cause arthropathy and osteochondrosis in immature animals of various species. The relevance of these adverse effects in immature animals to use in humans is unknown. Safety and efficacy of moxifloxacin have not been established in children younger than 18 years of age. (See Pediatric Use under Warnings/Precautions: Specific Populations, in Cautions.)

***C. difficile*-associated Diarrhea and Colitis.** Treatment with anti-infectives alters normal colon flora and may permit overgrowth of *Clostridioides difficile* (formerly known as *Clostridium difficile*). *C. difficile* infection (CDI) and *C. difficile*-associated diarrhea and colitis (CDAD; also known as antibiotic-associated diarrhea and colitis or pseudomembranous colitis) have been reported in patients receiving fluoroquinolones, including moxifloxacin, and may range in severity from mild diarrhea to fatal colitis. *C. difficile* produces toxins A and B which contribute to development of CDAD; hypertoxin-producing strains of *C. difficile* are associated with increased morbidity and mortality since they may be refractory to anti-infectives and colectomy may be required.

CDAD should be considered in the differential diagnosis of patients who develop diarrhea during or after anti-infective therapy. Careful medical history is necessary since CDAD has been reported to occur as late as 2 months or longer after anti-infective therapy is discontinued.

If CDAD is suspected or confirmed, anti-infective therapy not directed against *C. difficile* should be discontinued as soon as possible. Patients should be managed with appropriate anti-infective therapy directed against *C. difficile* (e.g., vancomycin, fidaxomicin, metronidazole), supportive therapy (e.g., fluid and electrolyte management, protein supplementation), and surgical evaluation as clinically indicated.

Selection and Use of Anti-infectives. Moxifloxacin should be used for the treatment of acute sinusitis or acute bacterial exacerbations of chronic bronchitis *only* when no other treatment options are available. Because moxifloxacin, like other systemic fluoroquinolones, has been associated with disabling and potentially irreversible serious adverse reactions (e.g., tendinitis and tendon rupture, peripheral neuropathy, CNS effects) that can occur together in the same patient, the risks of serious adverse reactions outweigh the benefits of moxifloxacin for patients with these infections.

To reduce development of drug-resistant bacteria and maintain effectiveness of moxifloxacin and other antibacterials, use only for treatment or prevention of infections proven or strongly suspected to be caused by susceptible bacteria.

When selecting or modifying anti-infective therapy, use results of culture and in vitro susceptibility testing. In the absence of such data, consider local epidemiology and susceptibility patterns when selecting anti-infectives for empiric therapy.

Information on test methods and quality control standards for in vitro susceptibility testing of antibacterial agents and specific interpretive criteria for such testing recognized by FDA is available at https://www.fda.gov/STIC.

Specific Populations **Pregnancy.** Human data for moxifloxacin are insufficient to inform any drug-associated risk regarding use of the drug during pregnancy.

Based on animal studies, moxifloxacin may cause fetal harm. Although moxifloxacin was not teratogenic when administered to pregnant rats, rabbits, and monkeys at exposures up to 2.5 times higher than human exposures reported with the usual dosage of the drug, embryofetal toxicity (e.g., decreased neonatal body weights, increased incidence of skeletal variations [rib and vertebra combined], increased fetal loss) was observed when moxifloxacin was administered to pregnant rats or rabbits at dosages associated with maternal toxicity.

Pregnant women should be advised of the potential risk to the fetus.

Lactation. It is not known whether moxifloxacin is distributed into human milk; the drug is distributed into milk in rats.

The developmental and health benefits of breast-feeding should be considered along with the mother's clinical need for moxifloxacin and potential adverse effects on the breast-fed infant from the drug or from the underlying maternal condition.

Pediatric Use. Efficacy of moxifloxacin has not been established for any indication in pediatric patients younger than 18 years of age.

Limited data available from a clinical study in pediatric patients 3 months of age or older indicate that the overall safety profile of moxifloxacin in pediatric patients is comparable to that reported in adults. The most frequently reported adverse effects in pediatric patients were QT interval prolongation, vomiting, diarrhea, arthralgia, and phlebitis.

Fluoroquinolones, including moxifloxacin, cause arthropathy in juvenile animals. (See Musculoskeletal Effects under Warnings/Precautions: Warnings, in Cautions.)

The American Academy of Pediatrics (AAP) states that use of a systemic fluoroquinolone may be justified in children younger than 18 years of age in certain specific circumstances when there are no safe and effective alternatives and the drug is known to be effective. For information regarding when fluoroquinolones may be a preferred option in children, see Cautions: Pediatric Precautions in Ciprofloxacin 8:12.18.

Geriatric Use. Approximately 23 or 42% of patients were 65 years of age or older and 9 or 23% of patients were 75 years of age or older in clinical studies of oral or IV moxifloxacin, respectively. No overall differences in safety or efficacy were observed between geriatric individuals and younger adults.

The risk of developing severe tendon disorders, including tendon rupture, is increased in older adults (usually those older than 60 years of age). This risk is further increased in those receiving concomitant corticosteroids. (See Tendinitis and Tendon Rupture under Warnings/Precautions: Warnings, in Cautions.) Caution is advised if moxifloxacin is used in geriatric adults, especially those receiving concomitant corticosteroids.

The risk of QT interval prolongation may be increased in geriatric patients. Concomitant use of moxifloxacin and class IA (e.g., quinidine, procainamide) or class III (e.g., amiodarone, sotalol) antiarrhythmic agents and use in patients with risk factors for torsades de pointes (e.g., known QT prolongation, uncorrected hypokalemia) should be avoided. (See Prolongation of QT Interval under Warnings/Precautions: Warnings, in Cautions.)

The risk of aortic aneurysm and dissection may be increased in geriatric patients. (See Risk of Aortic Aneurysm and Dissection under Warnings/Precautions: Other Warnings/Precautions, in Cautions.)

Hepatic Impairment. Although dosage adjustments are not necessary in patients with mild, moderate, or severe hepatic impairment (Child-Pugh class A, B, or C), metabolic disturbances associated with hepatic insufficiency may lead to QT interval prolongation. Therefore, moxifloxacin should be used with caution in patients with any degree of hepatic impairment. ECGs should be monitored in patients with liver cirrhosis.

Renal Impairment. Pharmacokinetics of moxifloxacin are not substantially affected by mild, moderate, or severe renal impairment. Dosage adjustments are not necessary in patients with renal impairment.

■ **Common Adverse Effects** Adverse effects occurring in 3% or more of patients receiving moxifloxacin include nausea (7%), diarrhea (6%), headache (4%), and dizziness (3%).

Drug Interactions

■ **Drugs That Prolong QT Interval** Potential pharmacologic interaction (additive effects on QT interval prolongation). Concomitant use of moxifloxacin and class IA (e.g., quinidine, procainamide) or class III (e.g., amiodarone, sotalol) antiarrhythmic agents should be avoided. Moxifloxacin should be used with caution in patients receiving other drugs that prolong the QT interval (e.g., cisapride [currently commercially available under a limited-access protocol only], erythromycin, antipsychotic agents, tricyclic antidepressants). (See Prolongation of QT Interval under Warnings/Precautions: Warnings, in Cautions.)

■ **Drugs Metabolized by Hepatic Microsomal Enzymes** Moxifloxacin is not metabolized by cytochrome P-450 (CYP) isoenzymes and does not inhibit CYP3A4, 2D6, 2C9, 2C19, or 1A2; pharmacokinetic interactions with drugs metabolized by CYP isoenzymes are unlikely.

■ **Antacids** Pharmacokinetic interaction with aluminum- or magnesium-containing antacids (decreased absorption and decreased bioavailability of oral moxifloxacin).

Oral moxifloxacin should be administered at least 4 hours before or 8 hours after antacids that contain aluminum or magnesium.

■ **Antidiabetic Agents** Concomitant use of moxifloxacin and oral antidiabetic agents (e.g., sulfonylurea agents) or insulin has resulted in alterations in blood glucose concentrations, including hypoglycemia and hyperglycemia. (See Hypoglycemia or Hyperglycemia under Warnings/Precautions: Other Warnings/Precautions, in Cautions.)

If moxifloxacin is used in patients with diabetes mellitus receiving an oral antidiabetic agent or insulin, blood glucose concentrations should be carefully monitored. If a hypoglycemic reaction occurs, moxifloxacin should be discontinued and appropriate therapy initiated immediately.

Glyburide When moxifloxacin (40 mg once daily for 5 days) was used in patients with diabetes mellitus receiving glyburide (2.5 mg once daily beginning 2 weeks before initiation of moxifloxacin), mean peak plasma concentrations and area under the plasma concentration-time curve (AUC) of glyburide were decreased 21 and 12%, respectively. Although blood glucose concentrations were decreased slightly in patients receiving glyburide and moxifloxacin concurrently compared with glyburide alone, the manufacturer states that the pharmacokinetic interaction between the drugs was not considered clinically important and that interference by moxifloxacin on the activity of glyburide was not suggested.

■ **Antifungal Agents** No clinically important pharmacokinetic interactions between itraconazole and moxifloxacin.

■ **Atenolol** Moxifloxacin does not have a clinically important effect on the pharmacokinetics of atenolol.

■ **Corticosteroids** Concomitant use of corticosteroids increases the risk of severe tendon disorders (e.g., tendinitis, tendon rupture), especially in geriatric patients older than 60 years of age. (See Tendinitis and Tendon Rupture under Warnings/Precautions: Warnings, in Cautions.)

■ **Cyclosporine** No clinically important pharmacokinetic interactions between cyclosporine and moxifloxacin.

■ **Didanosine** Pharmacokinetic interaction (decreased absorption of oral moxifloxacin).

Oral moxifloxacin should be given at least 4 hours before or 8 hours after buffered didanosine (pediatric oral solution admixed with antacid).

■ **Digoxin** No clinically important pharmacokinetic interactions between digoxin and moxifloxacin. Although a transient increase in digoxin concentrations may occur, this is not considered clinically important. Dosage adjustments are not necessary for either drug.

■ **Estrogens and Progestins** Moxifloxacin does not have a clinically important effect on the pharmacokinetics of oral contraceptives containing ethinyl estradiol and levonorgestrel.

■ **Iron, Multivitamins, and Mineral Supplements** Pharmacokinetic interaction (decreased absorption and decreased bioavailability of oral moxifloxacin) if given concomitantly with iron preparations or multivitamins or dietary supplements containing iron or zinc. Oral moxifloxacin should be taken at least 4 hours before or 8 hours after these preparations.

Calcium dietary supplements do not have any clinically important effects on the pharmacokinetics of moxifloxacin.

■ **Morphine** Morphine does not have a clinically important effect on the pharmacokinetics of moxifloxacin.

■ **Nonsteroidal Anti-inflammatory Agents** Concomitant use of moxifloxacin and nonsteroidal anti-inflammatory agents (NSAIAs) may increase the risk of CNS stimulation and seizures. Animal studies using other fluoroquinolones suggest the risk varies depending on the specific NSAIA.

■ **Probenecid** Probenecid does not have a clinically important effect on the pharmacokinetics of moxifloxacin.

■ **Ranitidine** Ranitidine does not have a clinically important effect on the pharmacokinetics of moxifloxacin.

■ **Sucralfate** Pharmacokinetic interaction (decreased absorption of oral moxifloxacin). Oral moxifloxacin should be taken at least 4 hours before or 8 hours after sucralfate.

■ **Theophylline** No clinically important pharmacokinetic interactions between theophylline and moxifloxacin.

■ **Warfarin** Although clinically important pharmacokinetic interactions have not been reported when warfarin and moxifloxacin were used concomitantly, fluoroquinolones, including moxifloxacin, have been reported to enhance the anticoagulant effects of warfarin or its derivatives. In addition, infectious disease and its accompanying inflammatory process, age, and general status of the patient also are risk factors for increased anticoagulation activity. The prothrombin time (PT), international normalized ratio (INR), or other suitable coagulation tests should be monitored in patients receiving moxifloxacin concomitantly with warfarin.

Description

Moxifloxacin is a fluoroquinolone anti-infective agent. Like other commercially available fluoroquinolones, moxifloxacin contains a fluorine at the C-6 position of the quinolone nucleus. Moxifloxacin, like gatifloxacin (no longer commercially available in the US), contains an 8-methoxy group and has been termed an 8-methoxy fluoroquinolone. The 8-methoxy and 7-diazabicyclo moieties on the quinolone nucleus of moxifloxacin appear to enhance activity against gram-positive bacteria and decrease selection of resistant mutants in gram-positive bacteria.

Like other fluoroquinolone anti-infectives, moxifloxacin inhibits DNA synthesis in susceptible organisms via inhibition of type II DNA topoisomerases (DNA gyrase, topoisomerase IV). In susceptible *S. pneumoniae*, moxifloxacin principally targets DNA gyrase.

Moxifloxacin is well absorbed following oral administration, and has an absolute bioavailability of approximately 90%. The drug has a mean serum elimination half-life of 11.5–15.6 or 8.2–15.4 hours following oral or IV administration, respectively, allowing once-daily dosing. Moxifloxacin is metabolized principally via sulfate and glucuronide conjugation; the drug is not metabolized by and does not appear to affect the cytochrome P-450 (CYP) enzyme system. (See Drug Interactions.)

■ **Spectrum** Moxifloxacin is active in vitro and in clinical infections against most strains of *Staphylococcus aureus* (methicillin-susceptible [oxacillin-susceptible] strains only), *Streptococcus pneumoniae* (including multidrug-resistant strains), *S. anginosus*, *S. constellatus*, *S. pyogenes* (group A β- hemolytic streptococci), *Haemophilus influenzae*, *H. parainfluenzae*, *Enterobacter cloacae*, *Escherichia coli*, *Klebsiella pneumoniae*, *Proteus mirabilis*, *Moraxella catarrhalis*, *Chlamydophila pneumoniae* (formerly *Chlamydia pneumoniae*), *Enterococcus faecalis*, *Bacteroides fragilis*, *B. thetaiotaomicron*, *Clostridium perfringens*, *Peptostreptococcus*, and *Mycoplasma pneumoniae*. Moxifloxacin is active against *Yersinia pestis* in vitro and in a primate infection model. The drug also has in vitro activity against *S. epidermidis* (methicillin-susceptible [oxacillin-susceptible] strains only), *S. agalactiae* (group B streptococci), viridans streptococci, *Citrobacter freundii*, *K. oxytoca*, *Legionella pneumophila*, *Actinomyces*, *Bilophila wadsworthia*, *Eubacterium*, *Fusobacterium* species, *Lactobacillus*, *Porphyromonas*, and *Prevotella* species; however, the clinical importance of this in vitro data is unknown.

Moxifloxacin is active in vitro against some mycobacteria, including *Mycobacterium tuberculosis*, *M. avium complex* (MAC), *M. kansasii*, and *M. fortuitum*. Although moxifloxacin is active against some strains of *M. tuberculosis* resistant to isoniazid, rifampin, or streptomycin, moxifloxacin-resistant *M. tuberculosis* have been reported and some multidrug-resistant strains (i.e., strains resistant to rifampin and isoniazid) also are resistant to moxifloxacin or other fluoroquinolones.

Moxifloxacin has greater activity in vitro against *S. pneumoniae* (including penicillin-resistant strains) than many other fluoroquinolones (e.g., ciprofloxacin, levofloxacin, ofloxacin) while generally retaining the in vitro activity of these drugs against gram-negative bacteria and etiologic agents of atypical pneumonia (e.g., *C. pneumoniae*, *M. pneumoniae*, *Legionella*). The relevance of these in vitro data to the treatment of clinical infections remains to be determined.

■ **Resistance** Resistance to fluoroquinolones can occur as the result of mutations in topoisomerase II (DNA gyrase) or topoisomerase IV genes, decreased outer membrane permeability, or drug efflux. In vitro, resistance to moxifloxacin develops slowly by multiple-step mutations.

Cross-resistance can occur between moxifloxacin and other fluoroquinolones, but some gram-positive bacteria resistant to other fluoroquinolones may be susceptible to moxifloxacin.

Advice to Patients

Advise patients to read the manufacturer's patient information (medication guide) prior to initiating moxifloxacin therapy and each time the prescription is refilled.

Advise patients that antibacterials (including moxifloxacin) should only be used to treat bacterial infections and not used to treat viral infections (e.g., the common cold).

Importance of completing full course of therapy, even if feeling better after a few days.

Advise patients that skipping doses or not completing the full course of therapy may decrease effectiveness and increase the likelihood that bacteria will develop resistance and will not be treatable with moxifloxacin or other antibacterials in the future.

Advise patients that moxifloxacin may be taken without regard to meals, but should be taken with liberal amounts of fluids.

Importance of taking moxifloxacin at least 4 hours before or 8 hours after multivitamins or dietary supplements containing iron or zinc; magnesium- or aluminum- containing antacids; sucralfate; or buffered didanosine (pediatric oral solution admixed with antacid).

Inform patients that systemic fluoroquinolones, including moxifloxacin, have been associated with disabling and potentially irreversible serious adverse reactions (e.g., tendinitis and tendon rupture, peripheral neuropathy, CNS effects) that may occur together in the same patient. Advise patients to immediately discontinue moxifloxacin and contact a clinician if they experience any signs or symptoms of serious adverse effects (e.g., unusual joint or tendon pain, muscle weakness, a "pins and needles" tingling or pricking sensation, numbness of the arms or legs, confusion, hallucinations) while taking the drug. Advise patients to talk with a clinician if they have any questions or concerns.

Inform patients that systemic fluoroquinolones, including moxifloxacin, are associated with an increased risk of tendinitis and tendon rupture in all age groups and that this risk is increased in adults older than 60 years of age, individuals receiving corticosteroids, and kidney, heart, or lung transplant recipients. Symptoms may be irreversible. Importance of resting and refraining from exercise at the first sign of tendinitis or tendon rupture (e.g., pain, swelling, or inflammation of a tendon or weakness or inability to use a joint) and importance of immediately discontinuing the drug and contacting a clinician. (See Tendinitis and Tendon Rupture under Warnings/Precautions: Warnings, in Cautions.)

Inform patients that peripheral neuropathies have been reported in patients receiving systemic fluoroquinolones, including moxifloxacin, and that symptoms may occur soon after initiation of the drug and may be irreversible. Importance of immediately discontinuing moxifloxacin and contacting a clinician if symptoms of peripheral neuropathy (e.g., pain, burning, tingling, numbness, and/or weakness) occur.

Inform patients that systemic fluoroquinolones, including moxifloxacin, have been associated with CNS effects (e.g., convulsions, dizziness, lightheadedness, increased intracranial pressure). Importance of informing clinician of any history of convulsions before initiating therapy with the drug. Importance of contacting a clinician if persistent headache with or without blurred vision occurs.

Advise patients that moxifloxacin may cause dizziness and lightheadedness; caution patients that they should not engage in activities requiring mental alertness and motor coordination (e.g., driving a vehicle, operating machinery) until the effects of the drug on the individual are known.

Advise patients that systemic fluoroquinolones, including moxifloxacin, may worsen myasthenia gravis symptoms; importance of informing clinician of any history of myasthenia gravis. Importance of immediately contacting a clinician if any symptoms of muscle weakness, including respiratory difficulties, occur.

Inform patients that moxifloxacin may be associated with hypersensitivity reactions (including anaphylactic reactions), even after the first dose. Importance of immediately discontinuing moxifloxacin and contacting a clinician at first sign of rash, hives or other skin reaction, rapid heartbeat, difficulty swallowing or breathing, any swelling suggesting angioedema (e.g., swelling of lips, tongue, or face; throat tightness; hoarseness), jaundice, or any other sign of hypersensitivity.

Inform patients that photosensitivity/phototoxicity reactions have been reported following exposure to sun or UV light in patients receiving fluoroquinolones. Importance of avoiding or minimizing exposure to sunlight or artificial UV light (e.g., tanning beds, UVA/UVB treatment) and using protective measures (e.g., wearing loose-fitting clothes, sunscreen) if outdoors during moxifloxacin therapy. Importance of discontinuing moxifloxacin and contacting a clinician if a sunburn-like reaction or skin eruption occurs.

Importance of informing clinician of personal or family history of QT interval prolongation or proarrhythmic conditions (e.g., hypokalemia, bradycardia, recent myocardial ischemia) and of concurrent therapy with any drugs that may affect QT interval (e.g., class IA [quinidine, procainamide] or class III [e.g., amiodarone, sotalol] antiarrhythmic agents). Importance of contacting clinician if symptoms of prolonged QT interval (e.g., prolonged heart palpitations, loss of consciousness) occur.

Inform patients that systemic fluoroquinolones may increase the risk of aortic aneurysm and dissection; importance of informing clinician of any history of aneurysms, blockages or hardening of the arteries, high blood pressure, or genetic conditions such as Marfan syndrome or Ehlers-Danlos syndrome. Advise patients to seek immediate medical treatment if they experience sudden, severe, and constant pain in the stomach, chest, or back.

Inform patients that hypoglycemia has been reported when systemic fluoroquinolones were used in some patients receiving antidiabetic agents. Advise patients with diabetes mellitus receiving an oral antidiabetic agent or insulin to discontinue moxifloxacin and contact a clinician if they experience hypoglycemia or symptoms of hypoglycemia.

Inform patients that severe hepatotoxicity (including acute hepatitis and fatal events) has been reported in patients receiving moxifloxacin. Importance of informing clinician if any signs or symptoms of liver injury (e.g., loss of appetite, nausea, vomiting, fever, weakness, tiredness, right upper quadrant tenderness, itching, yellowing of the skin and eyes, light colored bowel movements, dark colored urine) occur.

Advise patients that diarrhea is a common problem caused by anti-infectives and usually ends when the drug is discontinued. Importance of contacting a clinician if watery and bloody stools (with or without stomach cramps and fever) occur during or as late as 2 months or longer after the last dose.

Importance of informing clinician of existing or contemplated concomitant therapy, including prescription and OTC drugs (e.g., drugs that may affect QT interval), as well as any concomitant illnesses.

Importance of women informing clinicians if they are or plan to become pregnant or plan to breast-feed.

Importance of advising patients of other important precautionary information. (See Cautions.)

Overview® (see Users Guide). For additional information until a more detailed monograph is developed and published, the manufacturer's labeling should be consulted. It is *essential* that the manufacturer's labeling be consulted for more detailed information on usual cautions, precautions, contraindications, potential drug interactions, laboratory test interferences, and acute toxicity.

Preparations

Excipients in commercially available drug preparations may have clinically important effects in some individuals; consult specific product labeling for details.

Moxifloxacin Hydrochloride

Oral		
Tablets, film-coated	400 mg of (of moxifloxacin)*	**Avelox®**, Bayer **Moxifloxacin Hydrochloride Tablets**
Parenteral		
Injection, for IV infusion	400 mg (of moxifloxacin) in 0.8% sodium chloride*	**Avelox®**, Bayer **Moxifloxacin Hydrochloride Injection for IV Infusion**

*available from one or more manufacturer, distributor, and/or repackager by generic (nonproprietary) name

†Use is not currently included in the labeling approved by the US Food and Drug Administration

Ofloxacin

■ Ofloxacin is a synthetic fluoroquinolone anti-infective agent.

Uses

■ **Respiratory Tract Infections** Ofloxacin is used for the treatment of lower respiratory tract infections, including acute exacerbations of chronic bronchitis or community-acquired pneumonia (CAP) caused by susceptible *Haemophilus influenzae* or *Streptococcus pneumoniae*. Ofloxacin also has been used for the treatment of lower respiratory tract infections caused by susceptible *Moraxella catarrhalis*†, *S. aureus*†, viridans streptococci†, Enterobacteriaceae†, or *Ps. aeruginosa*†.

Ofloxacin should be used for the treatment of acute bacterial exacerbations of chronic bronchitis only when there are no other treatment options. Because systemic fluoroquinolones, including ofloxacin, have been associated with disabling and potentially irreversible serious adverse reactions (e.g., tendinitis and tendon rupture, peripheral neuropathy, CNS effects) that can occur together in the same patient (see Cautions) *and because acute bacterial exacerbations of chronic bronchitis may be self-limiting in some patients, the risks of serious adverse reactions outweigh the benefits of fluoroquinolones for patients with these infections.*

In controlled studies in adults with lower respiratory tract infections, oral ofloxacin therapy was at least as effective as oral therapy with amoxicillin, co-trimoxazole, erythromycin, cefazolin, or doxycycline, and more effective than cefaclor. For most susceptible bacteria, ofloxacin therapy resulted in clinical and bacteriologic cure rates of 60–100% in adults with lower respiratory tract infections. However, ofloxacin, like most fluoroquinolones, is less effective in the treatment of *S. pneumoniae* or *Ps. aeruginosa* infections; the bacteriologic cure rates in adults with infections caused by these bacteria were 55–79%.

■ **Skin and Skin Structure Infections** Ofloxacin is used for the treatment of mild to moderate skin and skin structure infections caused by susceptible *S. aureus* (oxacillin-susceptible [methicillin-susceptible] strains), *S. epidermidis*†, *S. pyogenes* (group A β-hemolytic streptococci; GAS), or *P. mirabilis*. However, the increasing emergence of strains of staphylococci resistant to fluoroquinolones limits the usefulness of the drugs in the treatment of these infections. Ofloxacin also has been effective when used in the treatment of skin and skin structure infections caused by other susceptible gram-negative bacteria, including *E. coli*† or *Ps. aeruginosa*†. The drug has been effective when used in the treatment of cellulitis, subcutaneous abscesses, surgical wound infections, furunculosis, and folliculitis, and has been used effectively for the treatment of skin and skin structure infections in patients with diabetes mellitus. Oral ofloxacin resulted in a clinical and bacteriologic cure rate of 76–96% in adults with skin and skin structure infections.

■ **Urinary Tract Infections and Prostatitis** ***Uncomplicated Urinary Tract Infections*** Ofloxacin is used for the treatment of uncomplicated urinary tract infections (UTIs) (cystitis) caused by susceptible gram-negative bacteria, including *Citrobacter diversus*, *C. freundii*†, *Enterobacter aerogenes*, *E. cloacae*†, *Escherichia coli*, *Klebsiella pneumoniae*, *Morganella morganii*†, *Proteus mirabilis*, or *Pseudomonas aeruginosa*.

The drug also has been effective in a limited number of adults when used orally for the treatment of uncomplicated UTIs caused by susceptible gram-positive bacteria, including *Staphylococcus aureus*†, *S. epidermidis*†, *S. saprophyticus*†, *Enterococcus faecalis* (formerly *Streptococcus faecalis*)†, viridans streptococci†, or *Streptococcus agalactiae*† (group B streptococci; GBS). However, because of concerns about emergence of resistant strains of certain gram-positive bacteria (e.g., staphylococci) secondary to widespread use of fluoroquinolones, such use should be selective.

Ofloxacin should be used for the treatment of uncomplicated UTIs only when there are no other treatment options. Because systemic fluoroquinolones, including ofloxacin, have been associated with disabling and potentially irreversible serious adverse reactions (e.g., tendinitis and tendon rupture, peripheral neuropathy, CNS effects) that can occur together in the same patient (see Cautions) *and because uncomplicated UTIs may be self-limiting in some patients, the risks of serious adverse reactions outweigh the benefits of fluoroquinolones for patients with uncomplicated UTIs.*

In the treatment of uncomplicated UTIs in adults, the bacteriologic cure rate reported with 3–7 days of oral ofloxacin therapy has been 81–100%. In several controlled studies in men and women with uncomplicated UTIs, 3–7 days of oral ofloxacin therapy was as effective as 7 days of oral co-trimoxazole therapy. Although a single 100- or 400-mg oral dose† of ofloxacin has been effective in some adults for the treatment of acute cystitis caused by susceptible organisms, efficacy of a single dose of the drug for the treatment of these infections has not been established. In one controlled study, a single 400-mg oral dose of ofloxacin was less effective for the treatment of acute cystitis in women than 3 days of oral ofloxacin therapy (200 mg once daily) or 7 days of oral co-trimoxazole therapy; in another controlled study in adults with uncomplicated UTIs, a single 100-mg oral dose of ofloxacin was as effective as a 3-day regimen (100 mg twice daily) of the drug.

Complicated Urinary Tract Infections Ofloxacin is used for the treatment of pyelonephritis and other complicated UTIs caused by susceptible gram-negative bacteria, including *C. diversus*, *C. freundii*†, *Enterobacter*†, *E. coli*, *K. pneumoniae*, *M. morganii*†, *P. mirabilis*, *P. rettgeri*†, or *Ps. aeruginosa*.

As with other anti-infectives, ofloxacin is more effective in the treatment of uncomplicated UTIs than in complicated infections. In adults with complicated UTIs caused by susceptible organisms, the bacteriologic cure rate reported for 7–10 days of oral ofloxacin therapy has been 63–100%. In controlled studies in adults with complicated UTIs, oral ofloxacin therapy was as effective as therapy with oral co-trimoxazole and slightly more effective than therapy with oral carbenicillin indanyl sodium. In controlled studies in adults with complicated UTIs, 7 days of oral ofloxacin (100 mg twice daily) was as effective as 7 days of oral ciprofloxacin (250 mg twice daily). Oral ofloxacin has been used effectively in renal transplant recipients for the treatment of complicated UTIs.

Prostatitis Ofloxacin is used in men for the treatment of recurrent UTIs and chronic prostatitis caused by susceptible *E. coli*.

Oral ofloxacin therapy given for 6 weeks or longer reportedly has resulted in a bacteriologic cure of 79–100% in men with prostatitis.

■ **GI Infections** ***Shigella Infections*** Oral ofloxacin has been used for the treatment of shigellosis† caused by susceptible *Shigella*.

Infections caused by *S. sonnei* usually are self-limited (48–72 hours), and mild cases may not require treatment with anti-infectives. However, because there is some evidence that anti-infectives may shorten the duration of diarrhea and the period of fecal excretion of *Shigella*, anti-infective treatment generally is recommended in addition to fluid and electrolyte replacement in patients with severe shigellosis, dysentery, or underlying immunosuppression. An empiric treatment regimen can be used initially, but in vitro susceptibility testing of clinical isolates is indicated since resistance is common. A fluoroquinolone (preferably ciprofloxacin or, alternatively, levofloxacin or moxifloxacin) generally has been recommended for the treatment of shigellosis. However, fluoroquinolone-resistant *Shigella* have been reported in the US, especially in international travelers, the homeless, and men who have sex with men (MSM). Depending on in vitro susceptibility, other drugs recommended for the treatment of shigellosis include co-trimoxazole, ceftriaxone, azithromycin (not recommended in those with bacteremia), or ampicillin.

Travelers' Diarrhea Oral ofloxacin has been used for the short-term treatment of travelers' diarrhea† and has been used for the prevention of travelers' diarrhea† in adults traveling for relatively short periods of time to high-risk areas.

Treatment. Travelers' diarrhea caused by bacteria may be self-limited and often resolves within 3–7 days without anti-infective treatment. The US Centers for Disease Control and Prevention (CDC) states that anti-infective treatment is *not* recommended in patients with mild travelers' diarrhea. However, CDC and other clinicians state that empiric short-term anti-infective treatment (single dose or up to 3 days) may be used if diarrhea is moderate or severe, associated with fever or bloody stools, or extremely disruptive to travel plans. Since bacteria are the most common cause of travelers' diarrhea (80–90% of cases), an anti-infective directed against enteric bacterial pathogens usually is used. Fluoroquinolones (e.g., ciprofloxacin, levofloxacin) generally have been considered the anti-infectives of choice for empiric treatment, including self-treatment, of travelers' diarrhea in adults; alternatives include azithromycin and rifaximin.

If the causative pathogen is susceptible to the anti-infective chosen for empiric therapy, the duration of illness may be reduced by about a day. However, the increasing incidence of enteric bacteria resistant to fluoroquinolones and other anti-infectives may limit the usefulness of empiric treatment in individuals traveling in certain geographic areas, and the possible adverse effects of the anti-infective and adverse consequences of such treatment (e.g., development of resistance, effect on normal gut microflora) should be considered.

Prophylaxis. CDC and most experts do *not* recommend anti-infective prophylaxis to prevent travelers' diarrhea in most individuals traveling to areas of risk. However, anti-infective prophylaxis may be considered for short-term travelers who are high-risk individuals (e.g., human immunodeficiency virus [HIV]-infected or other immunocompromised individuals, travelers with poorly controlled diabetes mellitus or chronic renal failure) and those who are taking critical trips during which even a short period of diarrhea could adversely affect the purpose of the trip.

The use of anti-infective prophylaxis in travelers should be weighed against the use of prompt, early self-treatment with an empiric anti-infective if moderate to severe travelers' diarrhea occurs. If anti-infective prophylaxis is used, fluoroquinolones (e.g., ciprofloxacin, levofloxacin) usually have been recommended; alternatives include azithromycin and rifaximin. The increasing incidence of fluoroquinolone resistance in pathogens that cause travelers' diarrhea (e.g., *Campylobacter*, *Salmonella*, *Shigella*) should be considered and may limit their potential usefulness.

Helicobacter pylori Infection Oral ofloxacin has been used in conjunction with other drugs for the treatment of infections caused by *Helicobacter pylori*†.

Multiple-drug regimens that include ofloxacin, azithromycin, omeprazole, and a bismuth salt or ofloxacin, tetracycline, metronidazole, omeprazole, and a bismuth salt have effectively eradicated *H. pylori* in some patients with infections that failed to respond to other treatment regimens. Levofloxacin usually is the fluoroquinolone included in multiple-drug regimens used for first- or second-line and salvage therapy of *H. pylori* infections. Data are limited regarding the prevalence of fluoroquinolone-resistant *H. pylori* in the US; the possible impact of such resistance on the efficacy of fluoroquinolone-containing regimens used for the treatment of *H. pylori* infection is not known.

■ **Anthrax** Oral ofloxacin has been recommended as an alternative for postexposure prophylaxis following suspected or confirmed exposure to aerosolized *Bacillus anthracis* spores (inhalational anthrax)† and for treatment of inhalational anthrax†.

CDC, American Academy of Pediatrics (AAP), US Working Group on Civilian Biodefense, and US Army Medical Research Institute of Infectious Diseases (USAMRIID) recommend oral ciprofloxacin and oral doxycycline as the initial drugs of choice for postexposure prophylaxis following exposure to aerosolized anthrax spores, including exposures that occur in the context of biologic warfare or bioterrorism. Other oral fluoroquinolones (levofloxacin, moxifloxacin, ofloxacin) are alternatives for postexposure prophylaxis when ciprofloxacin or doxycycline cannot be used.

Some experts suggest that oral ciprofloxacin or other oral fluoroquinolones (levofloxacin, moxifloxacin, ofloxacin) can be considered for the treatment of inhalational anthrax† when a parenteral regimen is not available. Although a multiple-drug parenteral regimen should be used for the treatment of inhalational anthrax that occurs as the result of exposure to anthrax spores in the context of biologic warfare or bioterrorism, use of these parenteral regimens may not be possible if large numbers of individuals require treatment in a mass casualty setting and it may be necessary to use an oral regimen.

For additional information on postexposure prophylaxis and treatment of anthrax, see Uses: Anthrax in Ciprofloxacin 8:12.18.

■ **Brucellosis** Ofloxacin has been used in conjunction with other anti-infectives for the treatment of brucellosis† caused by *Brucella melitensis*. Some experts recommend a multiple-drug regimen that includes a tetracycline (doxycycline) and streptomycin (or gentamicin) or a regimen that includes a tetracycline (doxycycline) and rifampin for the treatment of brucellosis; alternative regimens include co-trimoxazole with or without gentamicin or rifampin; ciprofloxacin (or ofloxacin) and rifampin; or chloramphenicol with or without streptomycin. Monotherapy with any drug usually is associated with a high relapse rate and is not recommended.

In one study in patients with brucellosis caused by *B. melitensis*, 6 weeks of a regimen of ofloxacin (400 mg once daily) given in conjunction with rifampin (600 mg once daily) was as effective as a regimen of doxycycline (200 mg once daily) given in conjunction with rifampin (600 mg once daily). The mean time to defervescence was 5.1 days for patients receiving doxycycline and rifampin and 6.3 days for those receiving ofloxacin and rifampin; the relapse rate 1 year after the drugs were discontinued was about 3% in both groups.

■ **Chlamydial Infections** Ofloxacin is used for the treatment of urethral and cervical infections caused by *Chlamydia trachomatis* and is considered an alternative for the treatment of these infections. A bacteriologic cure rate of 67–100% has been reported in men and women who received a 7–10 day regimen of oral ofloxacin (200- or 300-mg twice daily) for the treatment of urogenital chlamydial infections. In several controlled studies, a 7-day regimen of oral ofloxacin (300 mg twice daily) is at least as effective as a 7-day regimen of oral doxycycline (100 mg twice daily) for the treatment of these infections.

CDC states that a single oral dose of azithromycin or a 7-day regimen of oral doxycycline are the recommended regimens for the treatment of *C. trachomatis* urogenital infections in adults and adolescents; a 7-day regimen of oral erythromycin base or ethylsuccinate or a 7-day regimen of oral levofloxacin or ofloxacin are alternative regimens.

Individuals with HIV infection should receive the same treatment regimens recommended for other individuals with *C. trachomatis* urogenital infections.

Any individual who had sexual contact with a patient with *C. trachomatis* urogenital infection during the 60 days preceding the patient's onset of symptoms or diagnosis should be referred for evaluation, testing, and presumptive treatment with a regimen effective against *Chlamydia*. To minimize transmission and avoid reinfection, individuals treated for *C. trachomatis* urogenital infections should abstain from sexual intercourse until they and their partner(s) have been adequately treated (i.e., for 7 days after a single-dose regimen or after completion of a 7-day regimen) and symptoms have resolved.

Ofloxacin is considered an alternative for the treatment of acute epididymitis† that may involve *C. trachomatis*. (See Uses: Gonorrhea and Associated Infections.)

■ **Gonorrhea and Associated Infections** Although ofloxacin was used in the past for the treatment of uncomplicated gonorrhea caused by susceptible *Neisseria gonorrhoeae*, quinolone-resistant *N. gonorrhoeae* (QRNG) is widely disseminated throughout the world, including in the US. (See Resistance: Resistance in Neisseria gonorrhoeae.) Therefore, CDC states that fluoroquinolones are no longer recommended for the treatment of gonorrhea and should not be used routinely for any associated infections that may involve *N. gonorrhoeae* (e.g., pelvic inflammatory disease [PID], epididymitis).

Ofloxacin is considered an alternative for the treatment of acute PID. (See Uses: Pelvic Inflammatory Disease.)

Ofloxacin is considered an alternative for the treatment of acute epididymitis†. Although acute epididymitis in sexually active men younger than 35 years of age is most frequently caused by *C. trachomatis* or *N. gonorrhoeae*, epididymitis can also be caused by other organisms (e.g., sexually transmitted enteric bacteria, *Mycoplasma*, *Ureaplasma*, mycobacteria, fungi). Presumptive treatment is usually initiated prior to availability of all diagnostic laboratory test results, and the anti-infective regimen is selected based on the patient's risk for chlamydia, gonorrhea, and/or sexually transmitted enteric bacteria (e.g., *E. coli*). For treatment of acute epididymitis most likely caused by sexually transmitted chlamydia and gonorrhea, CDC recommends a single IM dose of ceftriaxone used in conjunction with a 10-day regimen of oral doxycycline. For treatment of acute epididymitis most likely caused by sexually transmitted chlamydia and gonorrhea and enteric bacteria (e.g., in men who practice insertive anal sex), CDC recommends a single IM dose of ceftriaxone given in conjunction with a 10-day regimen of oral levofloxacin or ofloxacin. If acute epididymitis is most likely caused by enteric bacteria (e.g., in men who have undergone prostate biopsy, vasectomy, or other urinary tract instrumentation procedure) and gonorrhea has been ruled out (e.g., by gram, methylene blue, or gentian violet stain), CDC states that a 10-day regimen of oral levofloxacin or ofloxacin can be used alone.

For information on current recommendations for the treatment of gonorrhea and associated infections, see Uses: Gonorrhea and Associated Infections in Ceftriaxone 8:12.06.12. For additional information on quinolone-resistant N. gonorrhoeae (QRNG), see Uses: Gonorrhea and Associated Infections in Ciprofloxacin 8:12.18.

■ **Mycobacterial Infections** ***Treatment of Active Tuberculosis*** Ofloxacin has been used in multiple-drug regimens for the treatment of active tuberculosis† caused by *Mycobacterium tuberculosis*.

Although the potential role of fluoroquinolones and the optimal length of therapy have not been fully defined, the American Thoracic Society (ATS), CDC, Infectious Diseases Society of America (IDSA), and others state that use of fluoroquinolones as alternative (second-line) agents can be considered for the treatment of active tuberculosis in patients intolerant of certain first-line agents and in those with relapse, treatment failure, or *M. tuberculosis* resistant to certain first-line agents. If a fluoroquinolone is used in multiple-drug regimens for the treatment of active tuberculosis, ATS, CDC, IDSA, and others recommend levofloxacin or moxifloxacin.

The most recent ATS, CDC, and IDSA recommendations for the treatment of tuberculosis should be consulted for more specific information.

Leprosy Ofloxacin is used as an alternative in multiple-drug therapy (MDT) for treatment of multibacillary leprosy† (Hansen's disease); the drug also is used as a component of a single-dose MDT regimen that has been used for treatment of single-lesion paucibacillary leprosy†.

The World Health Organization (WHO) and US National Hansen's Disease Program (NHDP) recommend that MDT regimens that include rifampin be used for the treatment of all forms of leprosy. MDT can rapidly kill *M. leprae* and render patients noninfectious after only a few days of treatment; however, clearance of dead *M. leprae* from the body may take several years. MDT regimens recommended by NHDP for US patients differ from those recommended by WHO.

For treatment of multibacillary leprosy (i.e., 6 or more lesions or skin smear positive) in adults, WHO recommends a 12-month MDT regimen of dapsone (once daily), rifampin (once monthly), and clofazimine (once daily and once monthly). For treatment of paucibacillary leprosy (i.e., 1–5 lesions) in adults, WHO recommends a 6-month MDT regimen of dapsone (once daily) and rifampin (once monthly). A single-dose rifampin-based MDT regimen that includes a single dose of rifampin, a single dose of ofloxacin, and a single dose of minocycline (ROM) has been used for treatment of paucibacillary leprosy in patients with only a single lesion (i.e., single-lesion paucibacillary leprosy).

For US patients, NHDP recommends more prolonged treatment. NHDP recommends that adults with multibacillary leprosy (i.e., those who are skin smear positive and/or have a biopsy indicating more advanced disease) receive a 24-month MDT regimen of dapsone (once daily), rifampin (once daily), and clofazimine (once daily); NHDP recommends that adults with paucibacillary leprosy (i.e., those who are skin smear negative without evidence of more advanced disease on biopsy) receive a 12-month MDT regimen of dapsone (once daily) and rifampin (once daily). Clofazimine is no longer commercially available in the US, but may be obtained from NHDP under an investigational new drug (IND) protocol for treatment of leprosy. (See Clofazimine 8:16.92.) Data indicate that leprosy is rare in the US (total of approximately 6500 living patients, about 3300 requiring active medical management), although about 150–200 new cases are reported each year.

Both WHO and NHDP recommend ofloxacin as an alternative that can be used instead of clofazimine in MDT regimens in adults who will not accept or cannot tolerate clofazimine.

Treatment of leprosy is complicated and should be undertaken in consultation with a specialist familiar with the disease. In the US, clinicians should contact NHDP at 800-642-2477 on weekdays from 9:00 a.m. to 5:30 p.m. Eastern Standard Time or via email at nhdped@hrsa.gov for assistance with diagnosis or treatment of leprosy or assistance obtaining clofazimine for treatment of leprosy.

Mycobacterium fortuitum Infections Oral ofloxacin has been effective when used alone or in conjunction with amikacin for the treatment of postoperative sternotomy wound or soft tissue infections caused by *M. fortuitum*†. The drug also has been used effectively in a few patients for the treatment of *M. fortuitum* pulmonary or urinary tract infections.

Although optimum regimens have not been identified, ATS and IDSA recommend that *M. fortuitum* pulmonary infections be treated with a regimen consisting of at least 2 anti-infectives selected based on results of in vitro susceptibility testing and tolerability (e.g., amikacin, ciprofloxacin or ofloxacin, a sulfonamide, cefoxitin, imipenem, doxycycline).

■ **Nongonococcal Urethritis** Ofloxacin is used in adults for the treatment of nongonococcal urethritis (NGU). NGU can be caused by various organisms (e.g., *Chlamydia*, *M. genitalium*, *Trichomonas vaginalis*, *Ureaplasma*, enteric bacteria) and is treated presumptively at the time of diagnosis.

CDC states that a single dose of oral azithromycin or a 7-day regimen of oral doxycycline are the recommended regimens for the treatment of NGU; a 7-day regimen of oral erythromycin base or ethylsuccinate or a 7-day regimen of oral levofloxacin or ofloxacin are alternative regimens.

CDC states that men with persistent or recurrent NGU who were not compliant with the treatment regimen or were reexposed to untreated sexual partner(s) can be retreated with the initial regimen. In other patients, symptoms alone (without documentation of signs or laboratory evidence of urethral inflammation) are not a sufficient basis for retreatment and an objective diagnosis of persistent or recurrent NGU should be made before considering additional treatment. Because there is some evidence that *M. genitalium* is the most frequent cause of persistent or recurrent NGU, CDC states that those initially treated with doxycycline should receive retreatment with a single dose of oral azithromycin and those initially treated with azithromycin should receive retreatment with a 7-day regimen of oral moxifloxacin. However, if the patient with persistent or recurrent urethritis has sex with women and is in an area where *T. vaginalis* is prevalent, CDC recommends presumptive retreatment with a single dose of oral metronidazole or tinidazole and referral of their partner(s) for evaluation and appropriate treatment.

NGU may facilitate transmission of HIV and men diagnosed with NGU should be tested for HIV. Individuals with HIV infection should receive the same treatment regimens recommended for other individuals with NGU.

Any individual who had sexual contact with a patient with NGU within the preceding 60 days should be referred for evaluation, testing, and presumptive treatment with a regimen effective against *Chlamydia*. To minimize transmission and avoid reinfection, men treated for NGU should abstain from sexual intercourse until they and their sexual partner(s) have been adequately treated.

■ **Pelvic Inflammatory Disease** Ofloxacin has been used in the treatment of acute pelvic inflammatory disease (PID) caused by susceptible *C. trachomatis*. Ofloxacin is considered an alternative for the treatment of PID, but should *not* be used routinely for treatment of PID or any infections that may involve *N. gonorrhoeae*.

When a combined IM and oral regimen is used for the treatment of mild to moderately severe acute PID, CDC recommends a single IM dose of ceftriaxone, cefoxitin (with oral probenecid), or cefotaxime given in conjunction with a 14-day regimen of oral doxycycline (with or without a 14-day regimen of oral metronidazole). If parenteral cephalosporins are not feasible (e.g., because of cephalosporin allergy), CDC states that a 14-day regimen of oral levofloxacin, ofloxacin, or moxifloxacin given in conjunction with a 14-day regimen of oral metronidazole can be considered if the community prevalence and individual risk of gonorrhea are low and diagnostic testing for gonorrhea is performed. If culture results are positive for *N. gonorrhoeae*, the PID treatment regimen should be selected based on results of in vitro susceptibility testing. If QRNG are identified or if in vitro susceptibility cannot be determined (e.g., only nucleic acid amplification test [NAAT] for gonorrhea is available), consultation with an infectious disease specialist is recommended.

For further information on the treatment of PID, see Uses: Pelvic Inflammatory Disease in the Cephalosporins General Statement 8:12.06.

■ **Plague** Fluoroquinolones (e.g., ciprofloxacin, levofloxacin, moxifloxacin, ofloxacin) have been suggested as alternatives for the treatment of plague† caused by *Yersinia pestis* and also have been recommended for postexposure prophylaxis† following a high risk exposure to *Y. pestis*, including exposure in the context of biologic warfare or bioterrorism. The recommendation for use of fluoroquinolones for treatment or prophylaxis of plague is based on results of in vitro and animal testing. Although human studies are not available, results of in vitro studies indicate that ofloxacin is active against *Y. pestis* and the drug has been effective for the treatment of murine plague infections.

For the treatment of plague, IM streptomycin (or IM or IV gentamicin) historically has been considered the drug of choice. Alternatives recommended for the treatment of plague when aminoglycosides are not used include an IV fluoroquinolone (ciprofloxacin [a drug of choice for plague meningitis], levofloxacin, moxifloxacin), IV doxycycline (or IV tetracycline), IV chloramphenicol (drug of choice for plague meningitis), or co-trimoxazole (may be less effective than other alternatives).

Anti-infective regimens recommended for treatment of naturally occurring or endemic bubonic, septicemic, or pneumonic plague also are recommended for treatment of plague that occurs following exposure to *Y. pestis* in the context of biologic warfare or bioterrorism. Such exposures would most likely result in primary pneumonic plague, and prompt initiation of anti-infective therapy (within 18–24 hours of onset of symptoms) is essential in the treatment of pneumonic plague. Some experts (e.g., US Working Group on Civilian Biodefense, USAMRIID) recommend that treatment of plague in the context of biologic warfare or bioterrorism be initiated with a parenteral anti-infective regimen of streptomycin (or gentamicin) or, alternatively, a fluoroquinolone (ciprofloxacin, levofloxacin, moxifloxacin), doxycycline, or chloramphenicol. However, an oral regimen of doxycycline (or tetracycline) or a fluoroquinolone (e.g., ciprofloxacin, levofloxacin, moxifloxacin, ofloxacin) may be substituted when the patient's condition improves or if a parenteral regimen is unavailable (e.g., when there are supply or logistic problems because large numbers of individuals require treatment in a mass casualty setting).

In the context of biologic warfare or bioterrorism, some experts (e.g., the US Working Group on Civilian Biodefense, USAMRIID) recommend that asymptomatic individuals with exposure to plague aerosol or asymptomatic individuals with household, hospital, or other close contact (within about 2 m) with an individual who has pneumonic plague receive an oral anti-infective regimen for postexposure prophylaxis; however, any exposed individual who develops a temperature of 38.5°C or higher or new cough should promptly receive a parenteral anti-infective for treatment of the disease. If postexposure prophylaxis is indicated, these experts recommend a regimen of oral doxycycline (or tetracycline) or an oral fluoroquinolone (e.g., ciprofloxacin, levofloxacin, moxifloxacin, ofloxacin).

For additional information on use of fluoroquinolones for treatment or prophylaxis of plague, see Uses: Plague in Ciprofloxacin 8:12.18.

■ **Rickettsial Infections** Ofloxacin has been used in a limited number of patients for the treatment of various rickettsial infections†, including Mediterranean spotted fever† (boutonneuse fever) caused by *Rickettsia conorii*. CDC and other clinicians state that doxycycline is the drug of choice for the treatment of all tickborne rickettsial diseases. Although some fluoroquinolones have in vitro activity against Rickettsiae and some clinicians have suggested that fluoroquinolones (e.g., ciprofloxacin, ofloxacin) may be considered alternatives for the treatment of some rickettsial infections (e.g., Rocky Mountain spotted fever caused by *R. rickettsii*) when doxycycline cannot be used, CDC states that fluoroquinolones are *not* recommended for the treatment of Rocky Mountain spotted fever.

Ofloxacin has been used in a few patients for the treatment of acute Q fever pneumonia caused by *Coxiella burnetii*†; the drug produced apyrexia and clinical improvement within the first 2–4 days. However, Q fever pneumonia usually resolves within 15 days without treatment, and clinical evaluation of the efficacy of anti-infective regimens in the treatment of acute infections is difficult. Ofloxacin may be effective for the treatment of Q fever endocarditis†, and has been used in conjunction with doxycycline for the long-term treatment of Q fever endocarditis. However, in one limited study in patients with confirmed *C. burnetii* infection and chronic endocarditis, a regimen of doxycycline and ofloxacin was associated with a higher relapse rate than a regimen of doxycycline and hydroxychloroquine.

■ **Typhoid Fever** Oral ofloxacin has been used for the treatment of typhoid fever† (enteric fever) caused by susceptible *Salmonella enterica* serovar Typhi, including chloramphenicol-resistant strains. Although fluoroquinolones have been recommended for empiric treatment of *Salmonella* enteric fever in adults, resistance to fluoroquinolones has been reported in more than 80% of such infections in travelers to South and Southeast Asia and treatment failures will occur.

■ **Ophthalmic Infections** **For use of ofloxacin in the topical treatment of ophthalmic infections caused by susceptible organisms, see Ofloxacin 52:04.12.**

Dosage and Administration

■ **Administration** Ofloxacin is administered orally. Although ofloxacin also has been administered IV, a parenteral preparation of the drug is no longer commercially available in the US.

While presence of food in the GI tract can decrease the rate and/or extent of absorption of ofloxacin, this is not usually considered clinically important and the manufacturer states that the drug can be given without regard to meals. Milk and yogurt do not appear to affect GI absorption of ofloxacin. (See Pharmacokinetics: Absorption.)

To minimize the possibility of interference with the GI absorption of ofloxacin, patients should be instructed not to ingest antacids containing calcium, magnesium, or aluminum, sucralfate, metal cations such as iron or zinc (including multivitamin preparations containing zinc), or buffered didanosine preparations concomitantly with or within 2 hours of an ofloxacin dose. (See Drug Interactions.)

Patients receiving ofloxacin should be well hydrated and should be instructed to drink fluids liberally. (See Cautions: Precautions and Contraindications.)

■ **Dosage** The usual adult oral dosage of ofloxacin is 200–400 mg every 12 hours.

Respiratory Tract Infections If ofloxacin is used for the treatment of acute exacerbations of chronic bronchitis, the usual adult dosage is 400 mg every 12 hours given for 10 days. (See Uses: Respiratory Tract Infections.)

For the treatment of community-acquired pneumonia (CAP), the usual adult dosage of oral ofloxacin is 400 mg every 12 hours given for 10 days.

Skin and Skin Structure Infections For the treatment of uncomplicated skin and skin structure infections, the usual adult dosage of oral ofloxacin is 400 mg every 12 hours given for 10 days.

Urinary Tract Infections and Prostatitis If ofloxacin is used for the treatment of uncomplicated urinary tract infections (UTIs), the usual adult dosage is 200 mg every 12 hours. Although 3 days of ofloxacin therapy may be adequate for cystitis caused by susceptible *Escherichia coli* or *Klebsiella pneumoniae*, 7 days of therapy usually is required for the treatment of cystitis caused by other susceptible organisms. Various other oral dosage regimens have been used in the treatment of uncomplicated UTIs, including 100-mg doses given twice daily or 100- or 200-mg doses given once daily†; however, efficacy of these regimens has not been definitely established. (See Uncomplicated Urinary Tract Infections under Uses: Urinary Tract Infections and Prostatitis.)

For the treatment of complicated UTIs caused by susceptible organisms, the usual adult dosage of oral ofloxacin is 200 mg every 12 hours for 10 days. Some clinicians suggest that an oral dosage of 400 mg twice daily may be necessary for some complicated UTIs.

The usual adult dosage of oral ofloxacin for the treatment of prostatitis caused by *E. coli* is 300 mg every 12 hours given for 6 weeks or longer.

GI Infections **Travelers' Diarrhea.** For the treatment of travelers' diarrhea†, ofloxacin has been given in a dosage of 300 mg twice daily. If anti-infectives are used in patients with travelers' diarrhea, a treatment duration of 1–3 days is recommended.

Although the use of anti-infectives for prophylaxis of travelers' diarrhea† generally is discouraged (see Travelers' Diarrhea under Uses: GI Infections), if oral ofloxacin is used for such prophylaxis, some clinicians recommend a dosage of 300 mg once daily. If anti-infective prophylaxis is used in travelers, it should be given during the period of risk (not exceeding 2–3 weeks) beginning the day of travel and continuing for 1 or 2 days after leaving the area of risk.

Helicobacter pylori Infection. When used as a component of multiple-drug regimens for the treatment of infections caused by *Helicobacter pylori*†, oral ofloxacin has been given in a dosage of 200 mg twice daily for 7–14 days.

Anthrax **Postexposure Prophylaxis of Anthrax.** If oral ofloxacin is used as an alternative for postexposure prophylaxis following suspected or confirmed exposure to aerosolized *Bacillus anthracis* spores (inhalational anthrax)† (see Uses: Anthrax), the US Working Group on Civilian Biodefense suggests that adults can receive a dosage of 400 mg twice daily.

Anti-infective prophylaxis should be initiated as soon as possible following suspected or confirmed exposure to aerosolized *B. anthracis*.

Because of possible persistence of *B. anthracis* spores in lung tissue following an aerosol exposure, the US Centers for Disease Control and Prevention (CDC) and other experts recommend that anti-infective prophylaxis be continued for 60 days following a confirmed exposure.

Treatment of Anthrax. If oral ofloxacin is used as an alternative for treatment of inhalational anthrax† when a parenteral regimen is not available (see

Uses: Anthrax), US Working Group on Civilian Biodefense suggests that adults can receive a dosage of 400 mg twice daily.

Because of possible persistence of *B. anthracis* spores in lung tissue following an aerosol exposure, the total duration of anti-infective therapy of inhalational anthrax that occurs as the result of exposure to *B. anthracis* in the context of biologic warfare or bioterrorism should be 60 days.

Brucellosis For the treatment of brucellosis†, a 6-week regimen of oral ofloxacin in a dosage of 400 mg once daily in conjunction with oral rifampin (600 mg once daily) has been effective in some patients. Alternatively, an oral ofloxacin dosage of 400 mg twice daily for 6 weeks has been used in multiple-drug regimens for the treatment of brucellosis.

Chlamydial Infections For the treatment of urethritis and/or cervicitis caused by *Chlamydia trachomatis* or uncomplicated urethral, endocervical, or rectal† chlamydial infections, the usual adult dosage of oral ofloxacin is 300 mg twice daily for 7 days.

Gonorrhea and Associated Infections Although fluoroquinolones are no longer recommended for the treatment of gonorrhea or any associated infections that may involve *Neisseria gonorrhoeae* (see Uses: Gonorrhea and Associated Infections), the manufacturer recommends a single 400-mg oral dose of ofloxacin for the treatment of acute, uncomplicated urethral and cervical gonorrhea caused by susceptible *N. gonorrhoeae*.

Epididymitis. For the treatment of acute epididymitis† most likely caused by sexually transmitted enteric bacteria (e.g., *E. coli*) and when *N. gonorrhoeae* has been ruled out, CDC recommends that oral ofloxacin be given in a dosage of 300 mg twice daily for 10 days.

Ofloxacin should *not* be used alone for treatment of epididymitis unless *N. gonorrhoeae* has been ruled out. (See Uses: Gonorrhea and Associated Infections.)

Mycobacterial Infections **Leprosy.** For the treatment of multibacillary leprosy† in adults who will not accept or cannot tolerate clofazimine, the World Health Organization (WHO) recommends a regimen of oral ofloxacin (400 mg once daily), oral rifampin (600 mg once monthly), and oral dapsone (100 mg once daily) given for 12 months. For US patients with multibacillary leprosy who will not accept or cannot tolerate clofazimine, the National Hansen's Disease Program (NHDP) recommends that adults receive oral ofloxacin (400 mg once daily), oral rifampin (600 mg once daily), and oral dapsone (100 mg once daily) given for 24 months.

For the treatment of single-lesion paucibacillary leprosy†, adults have received a single-dose multiple-drug regimen (ROM) that includes a single 600-mg dose of oral rifampin, a single 400-mg dose of oral ofloxacin, and a single 100-mg dose of oral minocycline.

Mycobacterium fortuitum Infections. For the treatment of postoperative sternotomy wound or soft tissue infections caused by *M. fortuitum*†, ofloxacin has been given in a dosage of 300 mg once daily or 1.2 g daily in 3 or 4 divided doses for 3–6 months in conjunction with amikacin (usually 250 mg IM or IV twice daily for 4–8 weeks).

For pulmonary infections, ATS and IDSA recommend that a regimen consisting of at least 2 anti-infectives be used (see Mycobacterium fortuitum Infections under Uses: Mycobacterial Infections) and that treatment be continued for at least 12 months after negative sputum cultures are attained. These experts also recommend that a regimen consisting of at least 2 anti-infectives be given for at least 4 months for the treatment of serious skin or soft tissue infections or for 6 months for bone infections.

Nongonococcal Urethritis For the treatment of nongonococcal urethritis, the usual adult dosage of oral ofloxacin is 300 mg twice daily for 7 days. (See Uses: Nongonococcal Urethritis.)

Pelvic Inflammatory Disease For the treatment of acute pelvic inflammatory disease (PID), the manufacturer recommends an oral ofloxacin dosage of 400 mg every 12 hours given for 10–14 days.

If oral ofloxacin is used as an alternative for the treatment of mild to moderately severe acute PID, CDC recommends a dosage of 400 mg twice daily for 14 days given in conjunction with oral metronidazole (500 mg twice daily for 14 days).

Ofloxacin should be used for the treatment of PID only when parenteral cephalosporins are not feasible, the community prevalence and individual risk of gonorrhea are low, and in vitro susceptibility has been confirmed. (See Uses: Pelvic Inflammatory Disease.)

Rickettsial Infections **Mediterranean Spotted Fever.** For the treatment of Mediterranean spotted fever† (boutonneuse fever) caused by *Rickettsia conorii*, an oral ofloxacin dosage of 200 mg every 12 hours given for 7 days was effective in some patients.

Q Fever. For the treatment of acute Q fever† pneumonia caused by *Coxiella burnetii*, ofloxacin has been given in a dosage of 600 mg daily for up to 16 days. For the treatment of Q fever endocarditis, ofloxacin has been given in a dosage of 200 mg 3 times daily in conjunction with oral doxycycline (100 mg twice daily); long-term treatment (at least 4 years) may be required.

Typhoid Fever For the treatment of typhoid fever† (enteric fever) caused by susceptible *Salmonella*, oral ofloxacin has been given to adults in a dosage of 200–400 mg every 12 hours for 7–14 days. (See Uses: Typhoid Fever.)

■ Dosage in Renal and Hepatic Impairment

Renal Impairment Modification of usual dosage of ofloxacin generally is unnecessary in patients with creatinine clearances greater than 50 mL/minute. In patients with creatinine clearances of 50 mL/minute or less, doses and/or frequency of administration of ofloxacin should be modified in response to the degree of renal impairment.

The manufacturer recommends that adults with creatinine clearances of 50 mL/minute or less receive an initial ofloxacin dose equal to the usually recommended dose and that subsequent dosage be modified according to creatinine clearance. Adults with creatinine clearances of 20–50 mL/minute should receive the usual oral dose of ofloxacin every 24 hours and those with creatinine clearances less than 20 mL/minute should receive half the usually recommended oral dose every 24 hours.

For adults undergoing hemodialysis, some clinicians recommend that a 200-mg loading dose of oral ofloxacin be given followed by 100-mg oral doses once daily. For most patients, additional supplemental doses of the drug are unnecessary following each hemodialysis procedure; however, some clinicians suggest that a single 100-mg supplemental oral dose of the drug be given after the first hemodialysis procedure.

Hepatic Impairment Because excretion of ofloxacin may be reduced in patients with severe hepatic impairment (e.g., cirrhosis with or without ascites), the maximum ofloxacin dosage in these patients is 400 mg daily.

Cautions

Adverse effects reported with ofloxacin are similar to those reported with other fluoroquinolone anti-infectives (e.g., ciprofloxacin). Adverse effects have been reported in 2–12% of patients receiving ofloxacin, and have been severe enough to require discontinuance in 1–4% of patients. The most frequent adverse effects of the drug involve the GI tract or CNS.

Systemic fluoroquinolones, including ofloxacin, have been associated with disabling and potentially irreversible serious adverse reactions (e.g., tendinitis and tendon rupture, peripheral neuropathy, CNS effects) that can occur together in the same patient. These serious reactions may occur within hours to weeks after a systemic fluoroquinolone is initiated and have occurred in all age groups and in patients without preexisting risk factors for such adverse reactions. (See Cautions: Precautions and Contraindications.)

■ Tendinitis and Tendon Rupture

Systemic fluoroquinolones, including ofloxacin, are associated with an increased risk of tendinitis and tendon rupture in all age groups.

The risk of developing fluoroquinolone-associated tendinitis and tendon rupture is increased in older adults (usually those older than 60 years of age), individuals receiving concomitant corticosteroids, and kidney, heart, or lung transplant recipients. Other factors that may independently increase the risk of tendon rupture include strenuous physical activity, renal failure, and previous tendon disorders such as rheumatoid arthritis. However, tendinitis and tendon rupture have been reported in patients receiving fluoroquinolones who did not have any risk factors for such adverse reactions.

Fluoroquinolone-associated tendinitis and tendon rupture most frequently involve the Achilles tendon and have also been reported in the rotator cuff (shoulder), hand, biceps, thumb, and other tendon sites. Tendinitis or tendon rupture can occur within hours or days after ofloxacin is initiated or as long as several months after completion of therapy and can occur bilaterally.

Ofloxacin should be discontinued immediately if pain, swelling, inflammation, or rupture of a tendon occurs. (See Cautions: Precautions and Contraindications.)

■ Peripheral Neuropathy

Systemic fluoroquinolones, including ofloxacin, have been associated with an increased risk of peripheral neuropathy.

Sensory or sensorimotor axonal polyneuropathy affecting small and/or large axons resulting in paresthesias, hypoesthesias, dysesthesias, and weakness has been reported in patients receiving systemic fluoroquinolones, including ofloxacin. Symptoms may occur soon after initiation of ofloxacin and, in some patients, may be irreversible.

Ofloxacin should be discontinued immediately if symptoms of peripheral neuropathy (e.g., pain, burning, tingling, numbness, and/or weakness) occur or if there are other alterations in sensations (e.g., light touch, pain, temperature, position sense, vibratory sensation). (See Cautions: Precautions and Contraindications.)

■ CNS Effects

Systemic fluoroquinolones, including ofloxacin, have been associated with an increased risk of psychiatric adverse effects, including toxic psychosis, hallucinations, agitation, delirium, confusion, disorientation, disturbances in attention, nervousness, restlessness, and memory impairment. These adverse effects may occur after the first dose.

Systemic fluoroquinolones have been associated with an increased risk of convulsions (seizures), increased intracranial pressure (pseudotumor cerebri), lightheadedness, and tremors.

Headache, insomnia, and dizziness are the most frequently reported adverse CNS effects of ofloxacin. These effects have been reported in 1–9% of patients receiving the drug, generally become apparent during the first few days of therapy, and frequently subside during continued therapy with the drug. Fatigue, somnolence, sleep disorders, and nervousness have been reported in 1–3% and asthenia, malaise, anxiety, cognitive changes, depression, dream abnormality, euphoria, hallucinations, agitation, confusion, ataxia, tremor, paresthesia, seizures, myasthenia, syncope, and vertigo have been reported in less than 1% of patients receiving ofloxacin. Increased intracranial pressure, toxic psychosis, paranoia, and suicidal ideation or acts also have been reported. In most reported cases, hallucinations or psychotic reactions generally began within the first 3 days of therapy; these reactions subsided when the drug was discontinued.

Some adverse nervous system effects of ofloxacin may be related to the fact that the drug, like other fluoroquinolones, is an γ-aminobutyric acid (GABA) inhibitor. However, further study is needed to elucidate the mechanism(s) of these adverse CNS effects during fluoroquinolone therapy. In addition, while it also has been suggested that some CNS stimulant effects reported in patients receiving fluoroquinolones may result from quinolone-induced alterations in caffeine pharmacokinetics, ofloxacin is less likely than many other fluoroquinolones to induce such pharmacokinetic alterations. (See Drug Interactions: Xanthine Derivatives.)

If psychiatric or other CNS effects occur during ofloxacin therapy, the drug should be discontinued immediately and appropriate measures instituted. (See Cautions: Precautions and Contraindications.)

■ Exacerbation of Myasthenia Gravis Fluoroquinolones, including ofloxacin, have neuromuscular blocking activity and may exacerbate muscle weakness in individuals with myasthenia gravis. Use of fluoroquinolones in myasthenia gravis patients has resulted in requirements for ventilatory support and in death. (See Cautions: Precautions and Contraindications.)

■ Dermatologic and Sensitivity Reactions Rash and pruritus have been reported in 1–3% and eosinophilia, angioedema, urticaria, and vasculitis have been reported in up to 1% of patients receiving ofloxacin. Although a causal relationship was not definitely established, fatal vasculitis occurred in at least one patient receiving ofloxacin. Fever, chills, and diaphoresis have been reported in less than 3% of patients receiving the drug.

Hypersensitivity Reactions Although most hypersensitivity reactions to ofloxacin are mild cutaneous reactions, serious and occasionally fatal hypersensitivity and/or anaphylactic reactions, sometimes occurring following the first dose, have been reported in patients receiving the drug. Severe hypersensitivity reactions, characterized by rash, fever, jaundice, and hepatic necrosis with a fatal outcome, also have been reported with other fluoroquinolones.

Some hypersensitivity reactions reported in patients receiving fluoroquinolones, including ofloxacin, have been accompanied by cardiovascular collapse, hypotension or shock, seizures, loss of consciousness, tingling, angioedema (including tongue, laryngeal, pharyngeal, or facial edema), airway obstruction (including bronchospasm, shortness of breath, and acute respiratory distress), dyspnea, urticaria, pruritus, and other serious skin reactions.

Other serious and sometimes fatal adverse reactions that have been reported with fluoroquinolones, including ofloxacin, and that may or may not be related to hypersensitivity reactions include one of more of the following: fever, rash or severe dermatologic reaction (e.g., toxic epidermal necrolysis, Stevens-Johnson syndrome); vasculitis, arthralgia, myalgia, serum sickness; allergic pneumonitis; interstitial nephritis, acute renal insufficiency or failure; hepatitis, jaundice, acute hepatic necrosis or failure; anemia (including hemolytic and aplastic anemia), thrombocytopenia (including thrombotic thrombocytopenic purpura), leukopenia, agranulocytosis, pancytopenia, and/or other hematologic abnormalities.

Ofloxacin should be discontinued immediately at the first appearance of rash, jaundice, or any other sign of hypersensitivity. Appropriate therapy (e.g., epinephrine, corticosteroids, maintenance of an adequate airway, oxygen, IV fluids, antihistamines, maintenance of blood pressure) should be initiated as indicated.

Because of a high percentage of false-positive results, skin testing with ofloxacin has not been useful in evaluating hypersensitivity to the drug and is not recommended.

Photosensitivity Reactions Moderate to severe photosensitivity/phototoxicity reactions have been reported in patients receiving fluoroquinolones, including ofloxacin.

Phototoxicity may manifest as exaggerated sunburn reactions (e.g., burning, erythema, exudation, vesicles, blistering, edema) on areas exposed to sun or artificial ultraviolet (UV) light (usually the face, neck, extensor surfaces of forearms, dorsa of hands).

Although studies using topical ofloxacin in guinea pigs have not revealed evidence of phototoxicity, photoallergenicity, or contact allergy, in vitro studies indicate the drug is phototoxic.

Ofloxacin should be discontinued if photosensitivity or phototoxicity (sunburn-like reaction, skin eruption) occurs. (See Cautions: Precautions and Contraindications.)

■ Aortic Aneurysm and Dissection Rupture or dissection of aortic aneurysms has been reported in patients receiving systemic fluoroquinolones. Epidemiologic studies indicate an increased risk of aortic aneurysm and dissection within 2 months following use of systemic fluoroquinolones, particularly in geriatric patients. The cause for this increased risk has not been identified.

If a patient reports adverse effects suggestive of aortic aneurysm or dissection, fluoroquinolone treatment should be discontinued immediately. (See Cautions: Precautions and Contraindications.)

■ Hypoglycemia or Hyperglycemia Systemic fluoroquinolones, including ofloxacin, have been associated with alterations in blood glucose concentrations, including symptomatic hypoglycemia and hyperglycemia. Blood glucose disturbances during fluoroquinolone therapy usually have occurred in patients with diabetes mellitus receiving an oral antidiabetic agent (e.g., glyburide) or insulin.

Severe cases of hypoglycemia resulting in coma or death have been reported with some systemic fluoroquinolones. Although most reported cases of hypoglycemic coma have involved patients with risk factors for hypoglycemia (e.g., older age, diabetes mellitus, renal insufficiency, concomitant use of antidiabetic agents [especially sulfonylureas]), some cases have occurred in patients receiving a fluoroquinolone who were not diabetic and were not reported to be receiving an oral antidiabetic agent or insulin.

If a hypoglycemic reaction occurs, ofloxacin should be discontinued and appropriate therapy initiated immediately. (See Cautions: Precautions and Contraindications.)

■ GI Effects Nausea has been reported in 3–10% and diarrhea, vomiting, abdominal pain/discomfort, abdominal cramps, flatulence, constipation, dyspepsia, heartburn, dry mouth, dysgeusia, decreased appetite, and anorexia have been reported in 5% or less of patients receiving ofloxacin. Adverse GI effects generally are mild and transient and only rarely require discontinuance of ofloxacin.

Effects on GI Flora Ofloxacin therapy has only a minimal effect on normal salivary flora. Following oral administration of a single 400-mg dose of ofloxacin, total bacterial counts of *Branhamella* in saliva were reduced and did not return to pretreatment levels until 4 weeks after the dose; total bacterial counts of salivary streptococci, micrococci, and corynebacteria were unaffected by the drug.

Ofloxacin exerts a selective effect on normal bowel flora. Total bacterial counts of normal anaerobic fecal flora generally are unaffected during or following ofloxacin therapy. However, ofloxacin therapy generally markedly reduces or completely eradicates normal fecal Enterobacteriaceae within 2–6 days and may reduce, but not eliminate, total bacterial counts of fecal aerobic gram-positive bacteria (e.g., *Streptococcus faecalis*). Total bacterial counts of normal fecal flora generally return to pretreatment levels within 1–4 weeks following discontinuance of ofloxacin. In studies evaluating the effects of ofloxacin on physiological and/or biochemical intestinal characteristics that depend on intestinal flora, the drug had no discernible effect on conversion of cholesterol to coprostanol, conversion of bilirubin to urobilinogen, breakdown of mucin, inactivation of tryptic activity, formation of short chain fatty acids, or presence of β-aspartylglycine.

C. difficile-associated Diarrhea and Colitis Treatment with anti-infectives alters normal colon flora and may permit overgrowth of *Clostridioides difficile* (formerly known as *Clostridium difficile*).

C. difficile infection (CDI) and *C. difficile*-associated diarrhea and colitis (CDAD; also known as antibiotic-associated diarrhea and colitis or pseudomembranous colitis) have been reported in patients receiving fluoroquinolones, including ofloxacin, and may range in severity from mild diarrhea to fatal colitis. *C. difficile* produces toxins A and B which contribute to development of CDAD; hypertoxin-producing strains of *C. difficile* are associated with increased morbidity and mortality since they may be refractory to anti-infectives and colectomy may be required. (See Superinfection/C. difficile-associated Diarrhea and Colitis under Cautions: Precautions and Contraindications.)

When fluoroquinolones were first marketed, there appeared to be a relative lack of association between use of the drugs and CDAD and the risk of CDAD appeared to be lower than that reported with some other anti-infectives. However, there now is some evidence that increasing use of the drugs may have resulted in emergence of *C. difficile* that are more resistant and/or more virulent than previous strains.

■ Genitourinary Effects In women receiving ofloxacin, external genital pruritus, candidal vaginitis, and vaginal discharge have been reported in 1–6% and burning, irritation, pain and rash of the genitalia, dysmenorrhea, menorrhagia, and metrorrhagia have been reported in less than 1%.

Ofloxacin does not appear to be nephrotoxic. Increased serum creatinine and BUN concentrations have been reported only rarely and dysuria, urinary retention, increased urinary frequency, and elevated urinary pH have been reported in less than 1% of patients receiving the drug. Glucosuria, proteinuria, hematuria, and pyuria, have been reported in at least 1% of patients receiving the drug. Although crystalluria and cylindruria have not been reported to date with ofloxacin, these adverse effects have been reported rarely in patients receiving some other fluoroquinolones (e.g., ciprofloxacin), generally occurring in patients with alkaline urine who received high dosages of the drugs; these effects were not associated with renal toxicity. Crystalluria, sometimes associated with nephropathy, has occurred in animals receiving other fluoroquinolones (e.g., ciprofloxacin) but has not been observed to date in animal studies using ofloxacin.

■ Musculoskeletal Effects Fluoroquinolones, including ofloxacin, cause arthropathies (arthrosis) in immature animals of various species. In various studies in immature animals, oral ofloxacin has caused blisters and/or erosions in articular cartilage and increased synovial fluid and lesion formation of diarthric joints; in one study in immature rats, adverse effects were detected as soon as 5 hours after a single 1- or 3-g/kg oral dose of the drug. The severity of these adverse effects appears to be species-specific, being more evident in dogs than in rats, rabbits, or mice, and also appears to depend on the age of the animal and dosage and duration of therapy. Morphologic changes observed in animals with quinolone-induced arthropathies include erosions in joint cartilage accompanied by noninflammatory, cell-free effusions of the joint space; the cartilage is incapable of regeneration and may serve as a site for the development of arthropathy deformans. Although arthropathies have been detected in adult dogs receiving some quinolones (e.g., pefloxacin [not commercially available in the US]), there has been no evidence of arthropathies in fully mature dogs or rats when ofloxacin was given in doses up to 5 times the usual human dosage. (See Cautions: Pediatric Precautions.)

Chest or trunk pain has been reported in 1–3% and transient arthralgia, myalgia, or pain in the extremities or body as a whole have been reported in less than 1% of patients receiving ofloxacin.

■ **Hepatic Effects** Transient, mild increases in serum concentrations of AST (SGOT) and/or ALT (SGPT) have been reported in 1–2% and increased serum concentrations of alkaline phosphatase, LDH, bilirubin, and γ-glutamyltransferase (γ-glutamyl transpeptidase, GGT, GGTP) have been reported in less than 1% of patients receiving ofloxacin.

Severe hepatotoxicity, including acute hepatitis and fatalities, has been reported in patients receiving ofloxacin. In some cases, substantial elevations in serum liver enzyme concentrations and other manifestations of hepatitis resolved following discontinuance of the drug.

■ **Hematologic Effects** Eosinophilia, lymphocytopenia, lymphocytosis, leukocytosis, neutropenia, neutrophilia, thrombocytosis, thrombocytopenia, leukopenia, anemia, and elevated erythrocyte sedimentation rate (ESR) have been reported in at least 1% of patients receiving ofloxacin; however, it is not clear in all cases whether these effects were caused by the drug or underlying conditions of the patients.

■ **Cardiovascular Effects** Prolonged QT interval leading to ventricular arrhythmias, including torsades de pointes, has been reported with some fluoroquinolones, including ofloxacin. Geriatric patients may be at increased risk for drug-associated effects on the QT interval. (See Cautions: Geriatric Precautions.)

Edema, hypertension, hypotension, palpitations, tachycardia, vasodilation, and cardiac arrest have been reported in less than 1% of patients receiving ofloxacin.

Rupture or dissection of aortic aneurysms has been reported in patients receiving systemic fluoroquinolones. (See Cautions: Aortic Aneurysm and Dissection.)

■ **Ocular Effects** Transient visual disturbances, including diplopia or changes in visual acuity or color perception, have been reported in 1–3% of patients receiving ofloxacin. Photophobia has been reported in less than 1% of patients receiving the drug. Although ophthalmologic abnormalities, including cataracts and multiple punctate lenticular opacities, have been reported with some other quinolones (e.g., pefloxacin [not commercially available in the US]) in both multiple-dose studies in humans and long-term, high dosage studies in animals, there has been no evidence of ofloxacin-induced ocular toxicity in humans or in animal studies. Although the clinical importance in unclear, in vitro studies using rabbit corneal epithelial cultures indicate that topical ofloxacin at concentrations exceeding 0.05 mg/mL delayed corneal epithelial wound healing.

■ **Other Adverse Effects** Cough, respiratory arrest, rhinorrhea, thirst, and weight loss have been reported in less than 1% of patients receiving ofloxacin.

Decreased hearing acuity and tinnitus have been reported in less than 1% of patients receiving ofloxacin.

■ **Precautions and Contraindications** Ofloxacin is contraindicated in patients with a history of hypersensitivity to the drug or to other quinolones.

Systemic fluoroquinolones, including ofloxacin, have been associated with disabling and potentially irreversible serious adverse reactions (e.g., tendinitis and tendon rupture, peripheral neuropathy, CNS effects) that can occur together in the same patient. These serious reactions may occur within hours to weeks after a systemic fluoroquinolone is initiated and have occurred in all age groups and in patients without preexisting risk factors for such adverse reactions. Patients receiving ofloxacin should be informed about these serious adverse reactions and advised to immediately discontinue ofloxacin and contact a clinician if they experience any signs or symptoms of serious adverse effects (e.g., unusual joint or tendon pain, muscle weakness, a "pins and needles" tingling or pricking sensation, numbness of the arms or legs, confusion, hallucinations) while taking the drug. Systemic fluoroquinolones, including ofloxacin, should be avoided in patients who have experienced any of the serious adverse reactions associated with fluoroquinolones.

Because fluoroquinolones, including ofloxacin, are associated with an increased risk of tendinitis and tendon rupture in all age groups (see Cautions: Tendinitis and Tendon Rupture), patients receiving ofloxacin should be informed of this potentially irreversible adverse effect and the drug should be discontinued immediately if pain, swelling, inflammation, or rupture of a tendon occurs. The risk of developing fluoroquinolone-associated tendinitis and tendon rupture is increased in adults older than 60 years of age, patients receiving concomitant corticosteroids, and kidney, heart, or lung transplant recipients. (See Cautions: Geriatric Precautions and see Drug Interactions: Corticosteroids.) Patients should be advised to rest and refrain from exercise at the first sign of tendinitis or tendon rupture (e.g., pain, swelling, or inflammation of a tendon or weakness or inability to use a joint) and advised to immediately discontinue the drug and contact a clinician. Systemic fluoroquinolones, including ofloxacin, should be avoided in patients who have a history of tendon disorders or have experienced tendinitis or tendon rupture.

Because fluoroquinolones, including ofloxacin, are associated with an increased risk of peripheral neuropathy (see Cautions: Peripheral Neuropathy), ofloxacin should be discontinued immediately if symptoms of peripheral neuropathy (e.g., pain, burning, tingling, numbness, and/or weakness) occur or if there are other alterations in sensations (e.g., light touch, pain, temperature, position sense, vibratory sensation). Patients receiving ofloxacin should be advised that peripheral neuropathies have been reported in patients receiving systemic fluoroquinolones, including ofloxacin, and that symptoms may occur soon after initiation of the drug and, in some patients, may be irreversible. Patients should be advised of the importance of immediately discontinuing the drug and contacting a clinician if such symptoms occur. Systemic fluoroquinolones, including ofloxacin, should be avoided in patients who have experienced peripheral neuropathy.

Because fluoroquinolones, including ofloxacin, have been associated with an increased risk of adverse CNS effects (see Cautions: CNS Effects), ofloxacin should be used with caution in patients with known or suspected CNS disorders (e.g., severe cerebral arteriosclerosis, epilepsy) or other risk factors (e.g., certain drugs, renal impairment) that predispose to seizures or lower the seizure threshold. Patients should be informed that seizures have been reported in patients receiving ofloxacin and advised to inform their clinician of any history of seizures before initiating therapy with the drug. Patients receiving ofloxacin should be advised to notify their clinician if persistent headache (with or without blurred vision) occurs. Patients also should be cautioned not to operate a motor vehicle or machinery or engage in activities requiring mental alertness and coordination until they experience how the drug affects them. Systemic fluoroquinolones, including ofloxacin, should be avoided in patients who have experienced CNS effects associated with fluoroquinolones.

Ofloxacin should be avoided in patients with myasthenia gravis since fluoroquinolones, including ofloxacin, may exacerbate myasthenia gravis symptoms. Patients should be advised to immediately contact their clinician if they have any worsening muscle weakness or breathing problems.

Because an increased risk of aortic aneurysm and dissection has been reported with systemic fluoroquinolones, ofloxacin should not be used in patients who have an aortic aneurysm or are at increased risk for an aortic aneurysm unless there are no other treatment options. This includes geriatric patients and patients with peripheral atherosclerotic vascular disease, hypertension, or certain genetic conditions (e.g., Marfan syndrome, Ehlers-Danlos syndrome). Patients should be informed that systemic fluoroquinolones may increase the risk of aortic aneurysm and dissection and advised of the importance of informing their clinician of any history of aneurysms, blockages or hardening of the arteries, high blood pressure, or genetic conditions such as Marfan syndrome or Ehlers-Danlos syndrome. Patients receiving ofloxacin should be advised to seek immediate medical treatment if they experience sudden, severe, and constant pain in the stomach, chest, or back.

Blood glucose concentrations should be carefully monitored when systemic fluoroquinolones, including ofloxacin, are used in patients with diabetes mellitus receiving antidiabetic agents. Patients should be informed that hypoglycemia has been reported when systemic fluoroquinolones were used in some patients receiving antidiabetic agents. Patients with diabetes mellitus receiving oral antidiabetic agents or insulin should be advised to discontinue ofloxacin and contact a clinician if they experience hypoglycemia or symptoms of hypoglycemia. Appropriate therapy should be initiated immediately.

Because severe hepatotoxicity, including acute hepatitis and fatalities, has been reported in patients receiving ofloxacin, the drug should be discontinued immediately if any sign or symptom of hepatitis (e.g., anorexia, jaundice, dark urine, pruritus, tender abdomen) occurs. Patients should be advised to contact a clinician if any sign or symptom of hepatotoxicity (e.g., loss of appetite, nausea, vomiting, fever, weakness, tiredness, right upper quadrant tenderness, itching, yellowing of skin or eyes, light colored bowel movements, dark colored urine) occurs.

Use of ofloxacin should be avoided in patients with a history of QT interval prolongation, in those with uncorrected electrolyte disorders (e.g., hypokalemia), and in those receiving class IA (e.g., quinidine, procainamide) or class III (e.g., amiodarone, sotalol) antiarrhythmic agents. (See Drug Interactions.) The risk of drug-associated effects on the QT interval may be increased in geriatric patients. (See Cautions: Geriatric Precautions.)

Sensitivity Reactions Ofloxacin, like other quinolones, can cause serious, potentially fatal hypersensitivity reactions, occasionally following the initial dose. (See Cautions: Dermatologic and Sensitivity Reactions.) Patients receiving ofloxacin should be advised of this possibility and instructed to immediately discontinue the drug and contact a clinician at the first sign of rash, urticaria, or other skin reactions, jaundice, or any other sign of hypersensitivity such as rapid heartbeat, difficulty in swallowing or breathing, or any swelling indicative of angioedema (e.g., swelling of the lips, tongue, face; tightness of the throat; hoarseness). Serious anaphylactic reactions require immediate emergency treatment with epinephrine and other resuscitation measures (e.g., oxygen, IV fluids, IV antihistamines, corticosteroids, pressor amines, airway management such as intubation) as indicated.

Because photosensitivity/phototoxicity reactions have been reported following exposure to direct sunlight in patients receiving fluoroquinolones, including ofloxacin, patients receiving ofloxacin should be cautioned to avoid excessive exposure to direct sunlight or artificial UV light (sunlamps, solariums) while receiving the drug. Ofloxacin should be discontinued if photosensitivity or phototoxicity (sunburn-like reaction, skin eruption) occurs.

Selection and Use of Anti-infectives Ofloxacin should be used for the treatment of acute bacterial exacerbations of chronic bronchitis or uncomplicated urinary tract infections *only* when no other treatment options are available. Because ofloxacin, like other systemic fluoroquinolones, has been associated with disabling and potentially irreversible serious adverse reactions (e.g., tendinitis and tendon rupture, peripheral neuropathy, CNS effects) that can occur together in the same patient, the risks of serious adverse reactions outweigh the benefits of ofloxacin for patients with these infections.

To reduce development of drug-resistant bacteria and maintain effectiveness of ofloxacin and other antibacterials, the drug should be used only for the treatment or prevention of infections proven or strongly suspected to be caused by susceptible bacteria. When selecting or modifying anti-infective therapy, results of culture and in vitro susceptibility testing should be used. In the absence of such data, local epidemiology and susceptibility patterns should be considered when selecting anti-infectives for empiric therapy.

Patients should be advised that antibacterials (including ofloxacin) should only be used to treat bacterial infections and not used to treat viral infections (e.g., the common cold). Patients also should be advised about the importance of completing the full course of therapy, even if feeling better after a few days, and that skipping doses or not completing therapy may decrease effectiveness and increase the likelihood that bacteria will develop resistance and will not be treatable with ofloxacin or other antibacterials in the future.

Superinfection/C. difficile-associated Diarrhea and Colitis As with other anti-infectives, use of ofloxacin may result in emergence and overgrowth of nonsusceptible bacteria or fungi, especially enterococci or *Candida*. Resistant strains of some organisms (e.g., *Pseudomonas aeruginosa*, staphylococci) have developed during ofloxacin therapy. Careful monitoring of the patient and periodic in vitro susceptibility tests are essential.

Because CDAD has been reported with the use of nearly all anti-infectives, including ofloxacin, it should be considered in the differential diagnosis in patients who develop diarrhea during or after ofloxacin therapy. Careful medical history is necessary since CDAD has been reported to occur as late as 2 months or longer after anti-infective therapy is discontinued.

If CDAD is suspected or confirmed, anti-infective therapy not directed against *C. difficile* should be discontinued as soon as possible. Patients should be managed with appropriate anti-infective therapy directed against *C. difficile* (e.g., vancomycin, fidaxomicin, metronidazole), supportive therapy (e.g., fluid and electrolyte management, protein supplementation), and surgical evaluation as clinically indicated.

Patients should be advised that diarrhea is a common problem caused by anti-infectives and usually ends when the drug is discontinued; however, it is important to contact a clinician if watery and bloody stools (with or without stomach cramps and fever) occur during or as late as 2 months or longer after the last dose.

Other Precautions and Contraindications Renal, hepatic, and hematologic systems should be evaluated periodically during prolonged ofloxacin therapy.

Crystalluria, cylindruria, and hematuria have been reported with some other fluoroquinolones (e.g., ciprofloxacin). Although crystalluria is not expected to occur under usual conditions with the usual recommended dosages of ofloxacin, patients should be instructed to drink sufficient quantities of fluids to ensure proper hydration and adequate urinary output during therapy with the drug.

Ofloxacin should be used with caution in patients with impaired renal or hepatic function since elimination of the drug may be reduced in these patients. When ofloxacin is used in patients with known or suspected renal or hepatic impairment, the patient should be monitored carefully and appropriate laboratory studies should be performed prior to and during therapy with the drug.

Doses and/or frequency of administration of ofloxacin should be decreased in patients with creatinine clearances of 50 mL/minute or less. (See Dosage and Administration: Dosage in Renal and Hepatic Impairment.)

■ **Pediatric Precautions** Safety and efficacy of ofloxacin have not been established in children younger than 18 years of age. Because ofloxacin, like most other fluoroquinolones, causes arthropathy (arthrosis) in immature animals of several species, some clinicians state that the drug should not be used in children younger than 16–18 years of age. Other clinicians suggest that ofloxacin may be used cautiously in adolescents if skeletal growth is complete and suggest that the potential benefits of therapy with the drug may outweigh the possible risks in certain children 9–18 years of age with serious infections (e.g., cystic fibrosis patients) when the causative organism is resistant to other available anti-infectives.

The American Academy of Pediatrics (AAP) states that use of a systemic fluoroquinolone may be justified in children younger than 18 years of age in certain specific circumstances when there are no safe and effective alternatives and the drug is known to be effective. For information regarding when fluoroquinolones may be a preferred option in children, see Cautions: Pediatric Precautions in Ciprofloxacin 8:12.18.

In immature rats, oral ofloxacin in dosages 5–16 times the usual human oral dosage increased the incidence and severity of osteochondrosis; the lesions were still present and had not regressed 13 weeks after the drug was discontinued. Ofloxacin and most other fluoroquinolones (e.g., ciprofloxacin,) have caused erosions of the cartilage in weight-bearing joints and other signs of arthropathies (arthrosis) in immature animals of various species. (See Cautions: Musculoskeletal Effects.)

■ **Geriatric Precautions** When the total number of patients studied in phase II/III clinical studies of ofloxacin is considered, 14.2 % (688 patients) were 65 years of age or older, while 5.2% (252 patients) were 75 years of age and older. Ofloxacin generally is well tolerated in geriatric patients; the frequency and severity of adverse effects reported in patients older than 65 years of age generally are similar to those reported in younger adults.

Pharmacokinetic parameters in geriatric patients receiving ofloxacin generally are similar to those in younger adults. Results of pharmacokinetic studies in geriatric individuals 65–81 years of age indicate that the rate of absorption, volume of distribution, and route of elimination of ofloxacin in geriatric individuals are similar to those reported in younger adults. However, mean peak plasma concentrations of ofloxacin are 9–21% higher and the plasma elimination half-life more prolonged in geriatric individuals compared with younger adults. (See Pharmacokinetics.) The slower elimination of ofloxacin in geriatric individuals presumably is secondary to reduced renal function and clearance observed in geriatric individuals. Because ofloxacin is excreted by the kidneys and geriatric individuals are more likely to have decreased renal function than younger individuals, dosage adjustment may be necessary in geriatric patients with renal impairment as recommended for all patients with renal impairment. Dosage of ofloxacin does not need to be modified in geriatric patients with creatinine clearances greater than 50 mL/minute. (See Dosage and Administration: Dosage in Renal and Hepatic Impairment.)

The risk of fluoroquinolone-associated tendon disorders, including tendon rupture, is increased in geriatric adults older than 60 years of age. This risk is further increased in those receiving concomitant corticosteroids. (See Cautions: Precautions and Contraindications.) Ofloxacin should be used with caution in geriatric adults, especially those receiving concomitant corticosteroids.

The risk of QT interval prolongation, leading to ventricular arrhythmias may be increased in geriatric patients, especially those receiving concurrent therapy with other drugs that can prolong QT interval (e.g., class IA or III antiarrhythmic agents) or with risk factors for torsades de pointes (e.g., known QT prolongation, uncorrected hypokalemia). (See Cautions: Cardiovascular Effects.)

The risk of fluoroquinolone-associated aortic aneurysm and dissection may be increased in geriatric patients. (See Cautions: Aortic Aneurysm and Dissection.)

■ **Mutagenicity and Carcinogenicity** Ofloxacin was not mutagenic in the Ames microbial (*Salmonella*) mutagen test or in in vitro and in vivo cytogenic assays, including the sister chromatid exchange (Chinese hamster and human cell lines) assay, unscheduled DNA repair assay using human fibroblasts, dominant lethal assay, or mouse micronucleus assay. When ofloxacin was tested in the in vitro rat hepatocyte DNA repair assay, mouse lymphoma assay, and Rec-assay for DNA repair, results were positive, which may indicate a potential for primary DNA damage. However, other more sensitive tests, such as the V-79 mammalian cell assay, have not shown evidence of mutagenicity.

Studies have not been performed to date to evaluate the carcinogenic potential of ofloxacin.

■ **Pregnancy, Fertility, and Lactation** ***Pregnancy*** There are no adequate and controlled studies to date using ofloxacin in pregnant women. Since the drug, like most other fluoroquinolones, causes arthropathy in immature animals, ofloxacin should not be used in pregnant women unless the potential benefits justify the possible risks to the fetus.

Reproduction studies in rats and rabbits using oral ofloxacin in dosages up to 810 and 160 mg/kg daily, respectively, have not revealed evidence of teratogenicity. However, fetotoxicity (decreased fetal body weight and increased fetal mortality) did occur in rats and rabbits receiving oral ofloxacin dosages equivalent to 50 and 10 times the usual human dosage, respectively. In rats receiving ofloxacin dosages of 810 mg/kg daily (more than 50 times the maximum human dosage), retardation in the degree of ossification and minor skeletal variations such as cervical ribs and shortened or absent 13th ribs occurred. Perinatal and postnatal studies in rats using oral dosages up to 360 mg/kg daily revealed a decrease in food intake during gestation and an increase in food and water intake during lactation, but did not reveal evidence of adverse effects on late fetal development, labor, delivery, lactation, neonatal viability, or growth of the offspring.

Fertility Studies in male and female rats using ofloxacin doses up to 360 mg/kg indicate that the drug does not have an appreciable effect on fertility or reproductive performance. Although administration of high dosages of some other quinolones (e.g., norfloxacin [no longer commercially available in the US]) has been associated with impaired spermatogenesis and/or testicular damage (atrophy in rats and dogs) in chronic (for 3 months or longer) toxicity studies, similar studies using ofloxacin have not revealed evidence of these adverse effects.

Lactation Ofloxacin is distributed into milk. Because of the potential for serious adverse effects of ofloxacin in nursing infants, a decision should be made whether to discontinue nursing or the drug, taking into account the importance of the drug to the woman.

Drug Interactions

■ **Drugs That Prolong QT Interval** Ofloxacin, like some other fluoroquinolones, can prolong the QT interval and should be avoided in patients receiving class IA (e.g., quinidine, procainamide) or class III (e.g., amiodarone, sotalol) antiarrhythmic agents.

■ **Antacids** Antacids containing magnesium, aluminum, or calcium may decrease absorption of oral quinolones resulting in decreased serum and urine concentrations of the anti-infectives. The extent of this interaction appears to vary depending on the specific quinolone and antacid involved. In patients receiving ofloxacin and an antacid concomitantly, peak serum ofloxacin concentrations may be decreased by 20–77% and areas under the plasma concentration-time curve (AUCs) decreased by 60–70%. The mechanism of this interaction has not been fully elucidated to date, but magnesium and aluminum ions may bind to and form insoluble complexes with quinolones. To minimize the possibility of an interaction, patients should be instructed not to ingest antacids concomitantly with or within 2 hours of an ofloxacin dose.

■ **Antiarrhythmic Agents** Concomitant use of antiarrhythmic agents may increase the risk of QT interval prolongation during ofloxacin therapy. Concomitant use of class IA (e.g., quinidine, procainamide) or class III (e.g., amiodarone, sotalol) antiarrhythmic agents should be avoided.

■ **Aminoglycosides** The antibacterial activities of ofloxacin and aminoglycosides (e.g., amikacin, gentamicin, tobramycin) may be additive or partially synergistic in vitro against susceptible strains of *Pseudomonas aeruginosa* or *Escherichia coli*. However, synergism between the drugs appears to be unpredictable, and indifference or antagonism has been reported more frequently.

■ **Antimycobacterial Agents** In vitro, the combination of ofloxacin and aminosalicylic acid, ethambutol, ethionamide, isoniazid, kanamycin, rifampin, or streptomycin is neither synergistic nor antagonistic against *Mycobacterium tuberculosis*. Although the clinical importance has not been determined, ofloxacin used in conjunction with ethambutol results in a synergistic effect in vitro against *M. avium* complex (MAC).

Adverse neurologic effects, including insomnia and seizures, have been reported in a few patients with multidrug-resistant pulmonary tuberculosis† who received concomitant oral ofloxacin (600 or 800 mg once daily) and cycloserine (500 or 750 mg once daily or a 2-dose regimen of 500 mg in the morning and 250 mg in the evening). Some clinicians suggest that, pending accumulation of additional information on this possible drug interaction, ofloxacin and cycloserine should be used concomitantly with caution.

In vitro, the combination of ofloxacin and rifampin generally is indifferent or antagonistic against *S. aureus*.

■ ***β*-Lactam Antibiotics** An additive or synergistic effect has occurred in vitro against some strains of *Staphylococcus epidermidis* and methicillin-resistant *Staphylococcus aureus* (MRSA; also known as oxacillin-resistant *S. aureus* or ORSA) when ofloxacin was used concomitantly with oxacillin; this combination generally was indifferent against ORSA. Synergism was demonstrated more readily at 30°C than at 35°C and did not appear to depend on the ofloxacin susceptibility of the organisms since it occurred in some cases even when the strain was resistant to ofloxacin alone. The clinical importance of this in vitro effect is unclear since many strains of staphylococci, principally ORSA, are resistant to ofloxacin.

Indifference generally occurred in vitro when ofloxacin was used in combination with ampicillin or nafcillin against Enterobacteriaceae or *Ps. aeruginosa*.

In vitro, the combination of ofloxacin and cefotaxime was neither synergistic nor antagonistic against Enterobacteriaceae, including *Klebsiella pneumoniae* and *E. coli* that were slightly susceptible or resistant to cefotaxime.

Ofloxacin used in conjunction with imipenem has been additive or synergistic in vitro against some strains of staphylococci, streptococci, *Ps. aeruginosa*, and Enterobacteriaceae; however, synergism appears to be unpredictable and this combination may be indifferent or antagonistic against these organisms.

■ **Antiretroviral Agents** ***Didanosine*** Buffered didanosine preparations (pediatric oral solution admixed with antacid) may interfere with oral absorption of ofloxacin. To minimize the possibility of interaction, patients should be instructed not to ingest buffered didanosine preparations concomitantly with or within 2 hours of an ofloxacin dose.

Zidovudine In vitro studies using ofloxacin and zidovudine indicate that the antiviral agent does not antagonize ofloxacin's antibacterial activity against susceptible *S. aureus*, *S. epidermidis*, *E. coli*, *Salmonella typhimurium*, or *Ps. aeruginosa*. Although the clinical importance in unclear, the combination of ofloxacin and zidovudine resulted in a slightly additive antibacterial effect in vitro against *E. coli* and *S. typhimurium*.

■ **Other Anti-infectives** In one in vitro study, the combination of ofloxacin and bismuth subcitrate was not synergistic against *Helicobacter pylori*.

In vitro, the antibacterial activity of ofloxacin and metronidazole is additive or indifferent against anaerobic bacteria; neither synergism nor antagonism occurs with this combination.

■ **Antidiabetic Agents** Alterations in blood glucose concentrations resulting in hypoglycemia have been reported in diabetic patients receiving ofloxacin and concomitant antidiabetic agents (e.g., insulin, glyburide). If ofloxacin is used in a diabetic patient receiving insulin or an oral antidiabetic agent, blood glucose and concentrations should be monitored carefully. Ofloxacin should be discontinued immediately and a clinician consulted if a hypoglycemic reaction occurs.

■ **Cimetidine, Ranitidine, and Sucralfate** Concomitant administration of cimetidine reportedly may interfere with the elimination of some quinolones resulting in prolonged serum half-lives and AUCs of the drugs. It is not known if this occurs with ofloxacin.

Concomitant administration of ranitidine does not appear to alter oral absorption of ofloxacin.

Concomitant administration of sucralfate reportedly may interfere with GI absorption of ofloxacin, and some clinicians state that concomitant use of ofloxacin with sucralfate is not recommended. If concomitant use of ofloxacin and sucralfate is necessary, the manufacturer and some clinicians recommend that patients be instructed not to ingest sucralfate concomitantly with or within 2 hours of an ofloxacin dose.

■ **Corticosteroids** Concomitant use of corticosteroids increases the risk of severe tendon disorders (e.g., tendinitis, tendon rupture), especially in geriatric patients older than 60 years of age. (See Cautions: Tendinitis and Tendon Rupture.)

■ **Coumarin Anticoagulants** In some patients stabilized on warfarin, prolongation of the prothrombin time occurred following initiation of ofloxacin therapy. Concomitant administration of some other quinolones (e.g., ciprofloxacin) in patients receiving coumarin anticoagulants also has resulted in increased prothrombin times. The mechanism of this interaction has not been determined to date; these drugs may displace the anticoagulants from serum albumin binding sites or may suppress vitamin K production by intestinal bacteria. Ofloxacin should be administered with caution in patients receiving a coumarin anticoagulant, and prothrombin times should be monitored in patients receiving concomitant therapy.

■ **Cyclosporine** Concomitant use of some quinolones in patients receiving cyclosporine reportedly may result in increased cyclosporine serum concentrations. It is not known if this occurs with ofloxacin.

■ **Iron, Multivitamins, and Mineral Supplements** Oral multivitamin and mineral supplements containing divalent or trivalent cations such as iron or zinc may decrease oral absorption of ofloxacin resulting in decreased serum concentrations of the quinolone; therefore, these multivitamins and/or mineral supplements should not be ingested concomitantly with or within 2 hours of an ofloxacin dose.

In a crossover study, concomitant administration of a single dose of oral ferrous sulfate complex and ofloxacin decreased the AUC of the anti-infective by 36%.

■ **Nonsteroidal Anti-inflammatory Agents** Concomitant administration of a fluoroquinolone (i.e., ofloxacin) and fenbufen (a nonsteroidal anti-inflammatory agent [NSAIA]) reportedly resulted in an increased incidence of seizures. Concomitant use of a fluoroquinolone with an NSAIA could increase the risk of CNS stimulation (e.g., seizures). Animal studies using other fluoroquinolones suggest that the risk may vary depending on the specific NSAIA.

■ **Probenecid** Studies using other fluoroquinolones (e.g., ciprofloxacin) indicate that concomitant administration of probenecid interferes with renal tubular secretion of the drugs. The effect of concomitant administration of probenecid and ofloxacin has not been studied to date.

■ **Xanthine Derivatives** Concomitant administration of some fluoroquinolone anti-infectives (e.g., ciprofloxacin, ofloxacin) in patients receiving theophylline has resulted in higher and prolonged serum theophylline concentrations and may increase the risk of theophylline-related adverse effects. The extent of this interaction varies considerably among the commercially available fluoroquinolones; the effect is less pronounced with ofloxacin than with ciprofloxacin. While it has been suggested that the 4-oxo metabolites of these quinolones may inhibit metabolism of theophylline in the liver, and there is some evidence that the degree to which the various quinolones are metabolized to 4-oxo metabolites may correlate with the extent of alteration in theophylline pharmacokinetics when the drugs are administered concomitantly, the potential contribution, if any, of the 4-oxo metabolites to this interaction has not been fully elucidated. In addition, other evidence indicates that, while formation of these metabolites may correlate with inhibition of theophylline metabolism, the 4-oxo metabolites themselves are not responsible for the observed effect.

In some controlled studies in patients receiving ofloxacin and theophylline concomitantly, the pharmacokinetics of theophylline were not altered substantially; in other studies, serum theophylline concentrations were increased by 9-10%, the AUC of the drug increased by 10–13%, and theophylline clearance decreased by 0–16%. Concomitant theophylline does not affect the pharmacokinetics of ofloxacin.

Although the risk of serious adverse effects resulting from theophylline toxicity appears to be low when usual dosages of ofloxacin are used, most studies to date evaluating concomitant therapy have been done in healthy adults; experience with concomitant use of the drugs in patients considered at higher risk for adverse effects (e.g., geriatric patients with chronic obstructive pulmonary disease, patients with impaired renal or hepatic function) is limited. Therefore, the manufacturer and some clinicians recommend that plasma theophylline concentrations be monitored and the patient observed for manifestations of theophylline toxicity whenever ofloxacin is given concomitantly; appropriate theophylline dosage adjustments should be made if needed.

Although some quinolones (e.g., ciprofloxacin) have been reported to alter the pharmacokinetics of caffeine, results of several studies in healthy adults indicate that ofloxacin does not have a clinically important effect on the elimination half-life, total body clearance, or volume of distribution of caffeine. Therefore, although precautions relating to caffeine intake may be necessary in patients receiving these other quinolones, these precautions do not appear to be necessary in patients receiving ofloxacin.

Laboratory Test Interferences

■ **Tests for Opiates** Some quinolones, including ofloxacin, may cause false-positive results for opiates when commercially available immunoassay kits for urine screening are used. It may be necessary to confirm positive opiate screening test results using more specific methods.

Acute Toxicity

The oral LD_{50} of ofloxacin is 3.6–5.5 g/kg in mice and rats and exceeds 200 mg/kg in dogs. The IV LD_{50} of the drug is 208–276 mg/kg in mice and rats and exceeds 70 mg/kg in dogs.

■ **Manifestations** In animals receiving oral ofloxacin, acute toxicity is manifested as ptosis, hypoactivity, sedation, prostration, hypopnea, dyspnea, and seizures. Limited information is available on the acute toxicity of ofloxacin in humans. Overdosage of ofloxacin would be expected to produce manifestations that principally are extensions of the adverse reactions reported with the drug, and may include nausea, vomiting, seizures, vertigo, dysgeusia, and psychosis.

A 23-year-old woman who inadvertently received approximately 3 g of ofloxacin IV over 45 minutes (a parenteral preparation is no longer commercially available in the US) developed drowsiness, nausea, hot and cold flashes, facial flushing and edema, slurred speech, dizziness, and disorientation during the infusion; all manifestations except dizziness, which was exacerbated on standing, and nausea resolved within 1 hour after discontinuance of the infusion, with the latter effects resolving several hours later. Serum ofloxacin concentration 15 minutes after completion of the infusion in this woman was approximately 40 mcg/mL. In a 14-year-old who ingested an unknown quantity of ofloxacin along with therapeutic doses of diphenhydramine and chlormezanone (no longer commercially available in the US), confusion, delirium, agitation, hallucinations, extreme mydriasis, and dry and warm skin occurred within a few hours; plasma concentrations of ofloxacin 12 hours after ingestion were 15 mcg/mL. Although activated charcoal was administered and forced diuresis was initiated, symptoms persisted for the next several days until IV physostigmine salicylate was given. It was suggested that the anticholinergic and psychotic manifestations observed in this patient may have resulted from a drug interaction between ofloxacin and diphenhydramine and/or chlormezanone.

■ **Treatment** If acute overdosage of ofloxacin occurs, the stomach should be emptied by inducing emesis or by gastric lavage. Supportive and symptomatic treatment should be initiated, and the patient should be observed carefully; adequate hydration should be maintained. Because ofloxacin is not efficiently removed by hemodialysis or peritoneal dialysis, these procedures should not be relied on to enhance elimination of the drug from the body.

Mechanism of Action

Ofloxacin usually is bactericidal in action. Like other fluoroquinolone anti-infectives, ofloxacin inhibits DNA synthesis in susceptible organisms via inhibition of the enzymatic activities of 2 members of the DNA topoisomerase class of enzymes, DNA gyrase and topoisomerase IV. DNA gyrase and topoisomerase IV have distinct essential roles in bacterial DNA replication. DNA gyrase, a type II DNA topoisomerase, was the first identified quinolone target; DNA gyrase is a tetramer composed of 2 GyrA and 2 GyrB subunits. DNA gyrase introduces negative superhelical twists in DNA, an activity important for initiation of DNA replication. DNA gyrase also facilitates DNA replication by removing positive super helical twists. Topoisomerase IV, another type II DNA topoisomerase, is composed of 2 ParC and 2 ParE subunits. DNA gyrase and topoisomerase IV are structurally related; ParC is homologous to GyrA and ParE is homologous to GyrB. Topoisomerase IV acts at the terminal states of DNA replication by allowing for separation of interlinked daughter chromosomes so that segregation into daughter cells can occur. Fluoroquinolones inhibit these topoisomerase enzymes by stabilizing either the DNA–DNA gyrase complex or the DNA–topoismerase IV complex; these stabilized complexes block movement of the DNA replication fork and thereby inhibit DNA replication resulting in cell death.

Although all fluoroquinolones generally are active against both DNA gyrase and topoisomerase IV, the drugs differ in their relative activities against these enzymes. For many gram-negative bacteria, DNA gyrase is the primary quinolone target and for many gram-positive bacteria, topoisomerase IV is the primary target. The other enzyme is the secondary target in both cases. However, there are exceptions to this pattern. For certain bacteria (e.g., *Streptococcus pneumoniae*), the principal target depends on the specific fluoroquinolone.

The mechanism by which ofloxacin's inhibition of DNA gyrase or topoisomerase IV results in death in susceptible organisms has not been fully determined. Unlike β-lactam anti-infectives, which are most active against susceptible bacteria when they are in the logarithmic phase of growth, studies using *Escherichia coli* and *Pseudomonas aeruginosa* indicate that ofloxacin can be bactericidal during both logarithmic and stationary phases of growth. In vitro studies indicate that ofloxacin concentrations that approximate the minimum inhibitory concentration (MIC) of the drug induce filamentation in susceptible organisms and lysis; high concentrations of the drug result in enlarged or elongated cells that may not be extensively filamented and may not lyse. Although the bactericidal effect of some fluoroquinolones evidently requires competent RNA and protein synthesis in the bacterial cell, and concurrent use of anti-infectives that affect protein synthesis (e.g., chloramphenicol, tetracyclines) or RNA synthesis (e.g., rifampin) inhibit the in vitro bactericidal activity of these drugs, the bactericidal effect of ofloxacin, like that of ciprofloxacin, is only partially reduced in the presence of these anti-infectives. This suggests that ofloxacin, like ciprofloxacin, has an additional mechanism of action that is independent of RNA and protein synthesis.

For most susceptible organisms, the minimum bactericidal concentration (MBC) of ofloxacin is 1–4 times higher than the MIC.

Mammalian cells contain type II topoisomerase similar to that contained in bacteria. At concentrations attained during therapy, quinolones do not appear to appreciably affect the mammalian enzyme.

Results of in vitro studies indicate that exposure of some plasmid-containing bacteria (e.g., *E. coli*) to ofloxacin or other fluoroquinolones may result in loss of plasmid DNA. This effect is unpredictable and depends on the specific plasmid and concentration of drug. It is unclear whether this effect is related to inhibition of DNA gyrase or some other mechanism of action of the drugs.

In vitro studies, particularly those involving in vitro susceptibility tests, indicate that the antibacterial activity of ofloxacin, like that of ciprofloxacin, is decreased in the presence of urine, especially acidic urine. The clinical importance of this in vitro effect has not been determined to date; however, because ofloxacin concentrations attained in urine are usually substantially higher than ofloxacin MICs for most urinary tract pathogens, the effect probably is not clinically important.

Spectrum

Ofloxacin has a spectrum of activity similar to that of some other fluoroquinolones (e.g., ciprofloxacin). In vitro on a weight basis, the activity of ofloxacin against susceptible gram-positive bacteria is approximately equal to that of ciprofloxacin. The activity of ofloxacin against susceptible gram-negative bacteria is slightly less than that of ciprofloxacin.

Ofloxacin is active in vitro against many gram-positive aerobic bacteria, including penicillinase-producing, nonpenicillinase-producing, and some oxacillin-resistant staphylococci (previously known as methicillin-resistant staphylococci). Ofloxacin is active in vitro against most gram-negative aerobic bacteria, including Enterobacteriaceae and *Pseudomonas aeruginosa*. Like other fluoroquinolones, ofloxacin generally is less active against gram-positive than gram-negative bacteria. Ofloxacin has some activity in vitro against obligately anaerobic bacteria, but most of these organisms, including *Bacteroides fragilis*, are considered resistant to the drug. The drug also has some activity in vitro against *Chlamydia*, *Mycoplasma*, *Mycobacterium*, *Plasmodium*, and *Rickettsia*. Ofloxacin is inactive against fungi.

■ **Gram-positive Aerobic Bacteria** ***Gram-positive Aerobic Cocci*** Ofloxacin is active in vitro against most strains of *Staphylococcus aureus*, *S. epidermidis*, and *S. saprophyticus*. The drug is active against both penicillinase-producing and nonpenicillinase-producing staphylococci and also is active in vitro against some oxacillin-resistant *S. aureus* (ORSA). However, *S. aureus*, including ORSA, that are resistant to ofloxacin and other fluoroquinolones have been reported with increasing frequency. (See: Resistance.)

Ofloxacin is less active in vitro on a weight basis against streptococci than against staphylococci. *Streptococcus pneumoniae*, *S. pyogenes* (group A β-hemolytic streptococci; GAS), and group B streptococci (*S. agalactiae*; GBS), viridans streptococci (e.g., *S. mitis*), Groups C, F, and G streptococci, and nonenterococcal group D streptococci (e.g., *S. bovis*) generally are inhibited in vitro by ofloxacin concentrations of 4 mcg/mL or less. Ofloxacin is equally active against both penicillin-susceptible and -resistant strains of *S. pneumoniae*. Ofloxacin is active in vitro against some strains of enterococci, including *Enterococcus faecalis* (formerly *S. faecalis*).

Table 1 includes MIC_{50}s (minimum inhibitory concentrations of the drug at which 50% of strains tested are inhibited) and MIC_{90}s (minimum inhibitory concentrations of the drug at which 90% of strains tested are inhibited) of ofloxacin reported for gram-positive aerobic cocci:

Table 1.

Organism	MIC_{50} (mcg/mL)	MIC_{90} (mcg/mL)
Staphylococcus aureus	0.2–0.5	0.2–1.6
S. epidermidis	0.2–0.5	0.125–1
S. saprophyticus	0.5–2	0.5–2
Oxacillin-resistant *S. aureus*	0.25–2	0.25–4
Streptococcus pneumoniae	1–3.1	1–6.25
Group A streptococci	1–2	1–4
Group B streptococci	1–4	1–6.3
Groups C, F, and G streptococci	1–2	2–4
Viridans streptococci	1–2	2–4
Nonenterococcal group D streptococci	1.2–2	2.5–4
Enterococci	0.8–4	1.6–6.3

Gram-positive Aerobic Bacilli Ofloxacin is active against *Bacillus anthracis* in vitro. In several in vitro studies, *B. anthracis* isolates had ofloxacin MICs of 0.03–0.25 mcg/mL. Anti-infectives are active against the germinated form of *B. anthracis*, but are not active against the organism when it is still in the spore form. Strains of *B. anthracis* with naturally occurring resistance to fluoroquinolones have not been reported to date. However, reduced susceptibility to ofloxacin (fourfold increase in MICs from baseline) was produced in vitro following sequential subculture of the Sterne strain of *B. anthracis* in subinhibitory concentrations of the fluoroquinolone.

Ofloxacin is active in vitro against *Corynebacterium*. The MIC_{90} of the drug reported for *C. diphtheria*, JK strains of *Corynebacterium*, *Corynebacterium* D2, and *C. jeikeium* is 0.5–1 mcg/mL.

Ofloxacin is active in vitro against *Listeria monocytogenes*, and the MIC_{90} of the drug reported for this organism is 1–8 mcg/mL.

Although some strains of *Nocardia asteroides* are inhibited in vitro by ofloxacin concentrations of 4–8 mcg/mL, this organism generally is considered resistant to the drug.

■ **Gram-negative Aerobic Bacteria** ***Neisseria*** Ofloxacin is active in vitro against some strains of penicillinase- and nonpenicillinase-producing *Neisseria gonorrhoeae* and *N. gonorrhoeae* with chromosomally mediated resistance to penicillin (CMRNG) or plasmid-mediated tetracycline resistance (TRNG). The MIC_{90} of ofloxacin is 0.007–0.1 mcg/mL for most penicillinase- or nonpenicillinase-producing *N. gonorrhoeae*, CMRNG, and TRNG. However, *N. gonorrhoeae* with decreased susceptibility to fluoroquinolones (quinolone-resistant *N. gonorrhoeae*; QRNG) have been reported with increasing frequency. To date, most strains of *N. gonorrhoeae* with reduced susceptibility have ofloxacin MICs of 0.13–0.5 mcg/mL; however, strains with ofloxacin MICs of 2 mcg/mL also have been reported. (See Resistance: Resistance in Neisseria gonorrhoeae.)

Ofloxacin is active in vitro against *N. meningitidis*, and the MIC_{90} of the drug for this organisms usually is 0.015–0.03 mcg/mL.

Haemophilus Ofloxacin is active in vitro against β-lactamase- and non-β-lactamase-producing *Haemophilus influenzae*, and the MIC_{90} of the drug for these organisms is 0.02–0.13. *H. parainfluenzae* generally are inhibited in vitro by ofloxacin concentrations of 0.25 mcg/mL. The MIC_{90} of ofloxacin for *H. ducreyi* is 0.03–2 mcg/mL. Ofloxacin is active against β-lactamase-producing *H. ducreyi* and is active against strains resistant to tetracycline, ampicillin, and sulfamethoxazole.

Moraxella catarrhalis Ofloxacin is active in vitro against both β-lactamase- and non-β-lactamase-producing strains of *Moraxella catarrhalis* (formerly *Branhamella catarrhalis*), and the MIC_{90} of the drug reported for this organism is 0.06–1 mcg/mL.

Enterobacteriaceae Ofloxacin is active in vitro against most clinically important Enterobacteriaceae. With the exception of *Providencia* and *Serratia*, the MIC_{90} of ofloxacin for Enterobacteriaceae generally is 2.5 mcg/mL or less. Ofloxacin is active against some Enterobacteriaceae resistant to aminoglycosides and/or β-lactam antibiotics.

Table 2 includes MIC_{50}s and MIC_{90}s of ofloxacin reported for Enterobacteriaceae:

Table 2.

Organism	MIC_{50} (mcg/mL)	MIC_{90} (mcg/mL)
Citrobacter spp.	0.03–0.1	0.06–0.6
C. diversus	0.03–0.13	0.06–1
C. freundii	0.06–0.4	0.12–0.8
Enterobacter spp.	0.03–0.1	0.06–2.5
E. aerogenes	0.06–0.13	0.125–1.6
E. agglomerans	0.06–0.2	0.25–2
E. cloacae	0.05–0.13	0.25–3.1
Escherichia coli	0.015–0.06	0.05–0.2
Hafnia alvei	0.03–0.125	0.06–0.25
Klebsiella spp.	0.03–0.125	0.06–0.25
K. oxytoca	0.06–0.25	0.06–0.5
K. pneumoniae	0.06–0.25	0.12–0.5
Morganella morganii	0.03–0.15	0.06–0.5
Proteus mirabilis	0.06–0.3	0.12–0.5
P. vulgaris	0.03–0.125	0.06–1.6
Providencia rettgeri	0.12–1	0.5–8
P. stuartii	0.12–1	0.25–6.25
Serratia spp.	0.25–0.3	0.5–2.5
S. marcescens	0.25–1.6	0.5–6.3
Salmonella spp.	0.04–0.13	0.06–0.25
S. enteritidis	0.06	0.125
S. typhi	0.03	0.06–0.12
Shigella spp.	0.03–0.125	0.03–0.25
Yersinia enterocolitica	0.06–0.125	0.06–0.25

Ofloxacin is active in vitro against most strains of *Ps. aeruginosa* and also has some activity against other *Pseudomonas*. The MIC_{50} and MIC_{90} of ofloxacin for *Ps. aeruginosa* are 0.25–3.2 and 1–6.3 mcg/mL, respectively. The MIC_{90} of the drug for *Ps. acidovorans*, *Ps. fluorescens*, and *Ps. putida* is 0.4–1.6 mcg/mL and the MIC_{90} for *Xanthomonas maltophilia* (*Ps. maltophilia*) is 1.6–8 mcg/mL. Although some strains of *Burkholderia cepacia* (formerly *Ps. cepacia*), *Brevundimonas diminuta* (formerly *Ps. diminuta*, *Ps. paucimobilis*, and *B. pseudomallei* (formerly *Ps. pseudomallei*) are inhibited by ofloxacin concentrations of 8 mcg/mL or less, many of these organisms require concentrations of 16–32 mcg/mL for in vitro inhibition and are considered resistant to the drug.

Vibrio Ofloxacin is active in vitro against *Vibrio cholerae* and *V. parahaemolyticus*, and the MIC_{90} of the drug reported for these organisms is 0.008–0.13 mcg/mL.

Other Gram-negative Aerobic Bacteria The MIC_{90} of ofloxacin for *Acinetobacter lwoffi* (*A. calcoaceticus* subsp. *lwoffi*) and *A. baumannii* (*A. calcoaceticus* subsp. *anitratus*) is 0.25–2 mcg/mL.

Aeromonas hydrophila, *A. caviae*, and *A. sobria* generally are inhibited in vitro by ofloxacin concentrations of 0.03–0.1 mcg/mL. The MIC_{90} of ofloxacin reported for *Plesiomonas shigelloides* is 0.015–0.06 mcg/mL. *Alcaligenes xylosoxidans* (*Achromobacter xylosoxidans*) and *Alcaligenes faecalis* may require ofloxacin concentrations of 1.6–32 mcg/mL for in vitro inhibition.

Ofloxacin is active in vitro against some strains of *Campylobacter fetus* subsp. *jejuni*, and the MIC_{90} of the drug for this organism is 0.25–1.25 mcg/mL. The MIC_{90} of ofloxacin reported for *Helicobacter pylori* is 0.25 mcg/mL. However, emergence of strains of *Campylobacter* resistant to fluoroquinolones has been reported in areas with widespread use of the drugs. (See Resistance.)

Bordetella pertussis and *B. parapertussis* generally are inhibited by ofloxacin concentrations of 0.03–0.125 mcg/mL. *B. bronchiseptica* may be inhibited by ofloxacin concentrations of 1.6–8 mcg/mL.

The MIC_{90} of ofloxacin reported for *Brucella melitensis*, *B. abortus*, and *Flavobacterium* is 0.5–4 mcg/mL, and the MIC_{90} reported for *Pasteurella multocida* and *Eikenella corrodens* is 0.03–0.125 mcg/mL.

Ofloxacin has in vitro activity against *Francisella tularensis*.

Ofloxacin has in vitro activity against *Yersinia pestis*. In a study evaluating in vitro susceptibility of 100 *Y. pestis* isolates obtained from plague patients in Africa, all isolates were inhibited by ofloxacin concentrations of 0.12 mcg/mL or less. In another study, isolates obtained from plague patients, rats, or fleas from Vietnam were inhibited by ofloxacin concentrations of 0.03–0.25 mcg/mL. Ofloxacin also has been shown to have in vivo activity against *Y. pestis* in murine plague infections. However, mutant strains of *Y. pestis* resistant to fluoroquinolones (e.g., ciprofloxacin) have been selected in vitro.

Some strains of *Gardnerella vaginalis* (formerly *Haemophilus vaginalis*) are inhibited in vitro by ofloxacin concentrations of 1–2 mcg/mL; other strains require concentrations of 16–32 mcg/mL for in vitro inhibition and are considered resistant to the drug.

Ofloxacin is active in vitro against *Legionella pneumophila*, *L. bozemanii*, *L. dumoffii*, *L. gormanii*, *L. jordanis*, *L. longbeachae*, *L. micdadei* (the Pittsburgh pneumonia agent), and *L. wadsworthii*, and the MIC of the drug reported for these organisms is 0.03–0.25 mcg/mL.

■ **Anaerobic Bacteria** Ofloxacin has some activity against gram-positive and -negative anaerobic bacteria; however, high concentrations of the drug generally are required for in vitro inhibition and most of these organisms are considered resistant to the drug. The MIC_{90} of ofloxacin for *Peptococcus* and *Peptostreptococcus* is 2–8 mcg/mL. Some strains of *Clostridium perfringens* and *C. welchii* may be inhibited in vitro by ofloxacin concentrations of 0.5–1 mcg/mL, but most clostridia require ofloxacin concentrations of 8 mcg/mL or greater for in vitro inhibition and are considered resistant to the drug.

The MIC_{90} of ofloxacin reported for *Bacteroides fragilis* is 2–8 mcg/mL. Ofloxacin concentrations of 0.02–2 mcg/mL may inhibit some strains of *Prevotella melaninogenica* and *B. ureolyticus*. The MIC_{90} of ofloxacin for *B. distasonis*, *B. ovatus*, *B. thetaiotaomicron*, *B. uniformis*, and *B. vulgatus* is 8–32 mcg/mL, and these organisms are considered resistant to the drug. Some strains of *Eubacterium*, *Fusobacterium*, and *Veillonella* may be inhibited in vitro by ofloxacin concentrations of 0.5–4 mcg/mL.

■ **Chlamydia and Mycoplasma** Ofloxacin is active in vitro against *Chlamydia trachomatis*, *C. pneumoniae*, and *C. psittaci*, and these organisms generally are inhibited in vitro by concentrations of 0.5–4 mcg/mL. The minimum lethal concentration (MLC) of ofloxacin reported for *C. trachomatis* is similar to the MIC and ranges from 0.5–8 mcg/mL. Both urogenital and ocular isolates of *C. trachomatis* are inhibited in vitro by ofloxacin.

Ofloxacin also is active in vitro against *Mycoplasma hominis*, *M. pneumoniae*, and *Ureaplasma urealyticum*. The MIC_{90} of ofloxacin reported for *M. hominis* and *M. pneumoniae* is 1–2 mcg/mL and the MIC_{90} for *U. urealyticum* is 1.6–8 mcg/mL.

■ **Mycobacterium** Ofloxacin is active in vitro against some *Mycobacterium*. In vitro on a weight basis, ofloxacin is slightly less active than ciprofloxacin or levofloxacin against these organisms. The MIC_{90} of ofloxacin for *M. tuberculosis* and *M. kansasii* is 0.6–2.4 mcg/mL. The MIC_{90} for *M. bovis*, *M. fortuitum*, *M. gordonae*, and *M. xenopi* is 0.03–2.5 mcg/mL. The MIC_{90} of the drug for *M. avium* complex generally is 2–16 mcg/mL; ofloxacin concentrations greater than 8 mcg/mL are required for in vitro inhibition of *M. chelonae* and *M. scrofulaceum*.

Ofloxacin is active in vitro against *M. leprae* and is bactericidal in vivo against *M. leprae* in mouse footpad studies.

■ **Other Organisms** Although the clinical importance in unclear, ofloxacin has some activity in vitro against *Plasmodium falciparum*. Results of in vitro tests indicate that ofloxacin is active against both chloroquine-susceptible and -resistant *P. falciparum*, but is less active against these organisms than ciprofloxacin.

Ofloxacin has some activity in vitro against *Rickettsia conorii*, the causative organism of Mediterranean spotted fever, and *Coxiella burnetii*, the causative organism of Q fever.

Although the clinical importance has not been determined, ofloxacin has some activity against the Lister strain of vaccinia virus in vitro in mammalian cell cultures and in vivo in mice. In similar tests, the drug had only weak antiviral effects against herpes simplex virus (HSV) and no appreciable effects against influenza virus.

Ofloxacin has some activity against *Trypanosoma cruzi*, the causative organism of Chagas' disease. The drug is inactive against *Treponema pallidum*. Ofloxacin also is inactive against *Trichomonas vaginalis*.

Resistance

Resistance to ofloxacin can be produced easily in vitro in some strains of Enterobacteriaceae, *Pseudomonas aeruginosa*, streptococci, and *Staphylococcus aureus*, including methicillin-resistant *Staphylococcus aureus* (MRSA; also known as oxacillin-resistant *S. aureus* or ORSA), by serial passage in the presence of increasing concentrations of the drug. Ofloxacin resistance resulting from spontaneous mutation occurs only rarely in vitro (i.e., with a frequency of 10^{-11} to 10^{-9}). Spontaneous mutation occurs in a single step and results in low-level resistance to the drug.

Resistant strains of *Ps. aeruginosa* have emerged rarely during therapy with the drug, especially in patients with cystic fibrosis; in some cases, the development of resistance was not associated with clinical failure of ofloxacin therapy. Resistant strains of *Escherichia coli* also have emerged rarely during therapy with the drug. Although the clinical importance is unclear, ofloxacin-resistant strains of *Ps. aeruginosa* and *Bacteroides fragilis* have been reported with increasing frequency since the drug was introduced.

Strains of *S. aureus*, especially ORSA resistant to fluoroquinolones, have been reported with increasing frequency. Emergence of fluoroquinolone resistance in staphylococci has been alarmingly rapid. In one hospital in Georgia, high-level resistance to ciprofloxacin (MIC_{90} 64 mcg/mL or greater) was apparent within 3 months of availability of the drug and increased from a baseline of 0% to 79% of ORSA isolates over a 1-year period; such resistance also increased to 14% of isolates in oxacillin-susceptible strains over the same period. In some countries (e.g., Israel, France, Canada), approximately 30–90% of clinical isolates of ORSA reportedly are resistant to fluoroquinolones; less than 10% of oxacillin-susceptible strains in these countries are resistant to the drugs. Results of resistance surveys indicate that fluoroquinolone resistance has emerged in multiple strains of ORSA; however, at some institutions, resistance occurred principally in a single ORSA strain which was then nosocomially transmitted to other patients.

Rapid emergence of resistance to fluoroquinolones in *Campylobacter* also has been reported and appears to be associated with widespread use or prolonged therapy with the drugs. In several patients with chronic active gastritis and duodenal ulcers, MICs of ofloxacin for *H. pylori* (formerly *C. pylori*) increased from 0.25–1 mcg/mL prior to ofloxacin therapy to 16–32 mcg/mL after 4 weeks of therapy. Over a 10- to 12-year period in Finland, fluoroquinolone-resistant strains of *C. jejuni* and *C. coli* increased from 0–4% to 9–11%. A similar increase was observed over a 7-year period in *Campylobacter* isolates obtained from poultry and humans in the Netherlands; this increase in resistance was attributed to use of enrofloxacin in the poultry industry. In the US, fluoroquinolone-resistant isolates of *Campylobacter* have been obtained from raw turkey or chicken products in the retail market.

■ **Resistance in Neisseria gonorrhoeae** *Neisseria gonorrhoeae* with decreased susceptibility to ofloxacin and other fluoroquinolones (quinolone-resistant *N. gonorrhoeae*; QRNG) are widely disseminated throughout the world, including in the US. *N. gonorrhoeae* with decreased susceptibility to one fluoroquinolone also have decreased susceptibility to other fluoroquinolones (e.g., ciprofloxacin, ofloxacin), but may be susceptible to ceftriaxone, cefixime, and spectinomycin (currently not commercially available in the US).

■ **Resistance in Mycobacterium** Ofloxacin-resistant strains of *Mycobacterium tuberculosis* have been reported. Resistance has developed in initially susceptible *M. tuberculosis* in some patients with pulmonary tuberculosis receiving ofloxacin in conjunction with antituberculosis agents. Some multidrug-resistant strains of *M. tuberculosis* (i.e., strains resistant to rifampin and isoniazid) also are resistant to ofloxacin or other fluoroquinolones. Extensively drug-resistant tuberculosis (XDR tuberculosis) caused by strains resistant to rifampin and isoniazid (multiple-drug resistant strains) and also resistant to a fluoroquinolone and at least one parenteral second-line antimycobacterial (capreomycin, kanamycin, amikacin) has been reported with increasing frequency.

Some strains of *M. kansasii* are resistant to ofloxacin.

■ **Mechanisms of Fluoroquinolone Resistance** The mechanism(s) of resistance to fluoroquinolones, including ofloxacin, has not been fully elucidated but appears to involve mutations in the target DNA type II topoisomerase enzymes and mutations that result in alterations in membrane permeability and/or efflux pumps.

Resistance to fluoroquinolones generally occurs as a result of mutational amino acid substitutions in the subunits (i.e., Gyr A, Gyr B, Par C, Par E) of the more sensitive (i.e., the primary target) topoisomerase enzyme (i.e., DNA gyrase or topoisomerase IV). Mutations in the primary target precede those in the secondary target, in a stepwise selection for resistance; mutations in both targets produce high level resistance. A single mutational event in the more sensitive primary target can result in an increase in the MIC of the drug. If the altered primary-target enzyme remains more sensitive to the quinolone than does the secondary target, the altered primary target will continue to determine the MIC. If the altered primary target becomes less sensitive than the secondary target, the MIC will be determined by the inhibitory activity of the quinolone against the secondary target. If both DNA gyrase and topoisomerase IV are equally sensitive to the quinolone, a single mutational alteration in either enzyme will not result in an increase in MIC.

Resistance to ofloxacin in gram-negative organisms (e.g., Enterobacteriaceae, *Ps. aeruginosa*) appears to result from mutations that alter the A subunits. Resistance in some gram-negative organisms also may be related to alterations in outer-membrane porin proteins and/or other factors that affect permeability of the organism to the drug. The mechanism of resistance in gram-positive bacteria has not been studied as extensively, but results of in vitro studies using *S. aureus* indicate that resistance to fluoroquinolones in some gram-positive bacteria also results from alterations in one of the subunits of topoisomerase IV and DNA gyrase. In addition, resistance in some *S. aureus* appears to be related to the *nor*A gene located in the D fragment of the organism's chromosome. The *nor*A gene apparently encodes a hydrophobic membrane protein that results in decreased membrane permeability by hydrophilic quinolones such as ofloxacin. A third possible mechanism of resistance in *S. aureus* also has been suggested and appears to be related to mutations(s) in the *flq* locus of the A fragment of the chromosome; further study is needed to determine whether mutation(s) in this fragment alters a second topoisomerase or another gene controlling supercoiling or whether it affects permeability. Although further study is needed, it appears that *S. aureus* can have either low-level or high-level resistance to fluoroquinolones that results from one or more alterations in topoisomerase IV and DNA gyrase. Current evidence suggests that resistance to ofloxacin or other fluoroquinolones in either gram-negative or -positive bacteria is chromosomally rather than plasmid mediated.

■ **Cross-resistance** Cross-resistance can occurs between ofloxacin and other fluoroquinolones.

Cross-resistance generally does not occur between ofloxacin and other anti-infectives, including aminoglycosides, β-lactam antibiotics, sulfonamides (including co-trimoxazole), macrolides, and tetracyclines. However, rare strains of Enterobacteriaceae and *Ps. aeruginosa* resistant to fluoroquinolones also are resistant to aminoglycosides, β-lactam antibiotics, chloramphenicol, trimethoprim, and/or tetracyclines. Resistance in these organisms appears to be related to alterations in outer-membrane porin proteins. Rarely, strains of *E. coli* or *Ps. aeruginosa* that were originally susceptible to fluoroquinolones and resistant to aminoglycosides and β-lactam antibiotics developed resistance to fluoroquinolones and reverted to being susceptible to aminoglycosides and β-lactams. It has been suggested that this may occur because exposure of some plasmid-containing bacteria to ofloxacin and other fluoroquinolones can result in loss of plasmid DNA in these organisms. (See Mechanism of Action.) In addition, fluoroquinolone-resistant ORSA frequently also are resistant to aminoglycosides.

Pharmacokinetics

In studies described in the Pharmacokinetics section, body fluid and tissue concentrations of ofloxacin were measured with either a high-pressure liquid chromatographic (HPLC) assay or a microbiologic assay. HPLC assays presumably would be more specific for ofloxacin than microbiologic assays since the latter method measures the antibacterial activity of the parent drug as well as its microbiologically active metabolite(s). However, controlled studies comparing results obtained using HPLC and microbiologic assays indicate that these methods provide essentially equivalent results for serum, urine, and CSF ofloxacin concentrations and pharmacokinetic parameters determined using these concentrations. This apparently occurs because ofloxacin is not extensively metabolized and only low concentrations of active ofloxacin metabolite(s) are attained in serum or urine.

The pharmacokinetics of ofloxacin after oral administration are best described by a 2-compartment open model. There is some evidence that disposition of the commercially available racemic mixture of ofloxacin (see Chemistry and Stability: Chemistry) is stereoselective principally as a result of differences in renal excretion of the enantiomers; however, such differences appear to be small.

■ **Absorption** Ofloxacin is rapidly and almost completely absorbed from the GI tract following oral administration. The drug does not undergo appreciable first-pass metabolism.

Although presence of food in the GI tract can decrease the rate and/or extent of absorption of ofloxacin to some extent, this effect is not usually considered clinically important. In an open, randomized, cross-over study in healthy adult men receiving a single 300-mg oral dose of ofloxacin with or without a standard breakfast, maximum serum concentrations and area under the concentration-time curves (AUCs) were slightly lower when the dose was given with food, but the time to peak serum concentrations, terminal elimination half-life, and urinary concentrations of the drug did not differ substantially between fasted and nonfasting conditions. When a 400-mg ofloxacin tablet was crushed and mixed with 120 mL of enteral premixed liquid (Ensure) and swallowed, the AUC was 10% lower and peak plasma concentrations were 36% lower compared with results attained when the tablet was crushed and mixed with water before swallowing. Milk and yogurt do not appear to affect GI absorption of ofloxacin.

Antacids may decrease the oral bioavailability of ofloxacin. (See Drug Interactions: Antacids.)

The oral bioavailability of ofloxacin is 85–100% in healthy, fasting adults, and peak serum concentrations of the drug generally are attained within 0.5–2 hours. In patients with normal renal and hepatic function, peak serum concentrations and AUCs increase in proportion to the dose over the oral dosage range of 100–600 mg and generally are unaffected by age.

Following oral administration of a single 100-, 200-, 300-, or 400-mg dose of ofloxacin in healthy, fasting adults, peak serum concentrations average 1–1.3, 1.5–2.7, 2.4–4.6, or 2.9–5.6 mcg/mL, respectively. Some accumulation occurs following multiple doses. Steady-state serum concentrations of ofloxacin are achieved after 4 doses of the drug and are approximately 40% higher than concentrations achieved following single oral doses.

Pharmacokinetic parameters in geriatric patients receiving ofloxacin generally are similar to those in younger adults. Although results of pharmacokinetic studies in geriatric individuals 65–81 years of age indicate that the rate of absorption, volume of distribution, and route of excretion in geriatric individuals are similar to those in younger adults, peak serum concentrations are slightly higher (9–21% higher) and half-life more prolonged in geriatric patients than in younger adults. There also is evidence that peak plasma concentration are higher in geriatric women than geriatric men (114% higher following single doses or 54% higher following multiple doses).

Following oral administration of usual dosage of ofloxacin in patients with cystic fibrosis, peak serum concentrations and AUCs are similar to those reported in healthy adults.

■ **Distribution** Ofloxacin is widely distributed into body tissues and fluids following oral administration. In healthy adults, the apparent volume of distribution of ofloxacin averages 1–2.5 L/kg. Impaired renal function does not appear to affect the volume of distribution of ofloxacin; the apparent volume of distribution of the drug averages 1.1–2 L/kg in patients with impaired renal function, including those with severe renal failure undergoing hemodialysis.

Ofloxacin is distributed into bone, cartilage, bile, skin, sputum, bronchial secretions, pleural effusions, tonsils,saliva, gingival mucosa, nasal secretions, aqueous humor, tears, sweat, lung, blister fluid, pancreatic fluid, ascitic fluid, peritoneal fluid, gynecologic tissue, vaginal fluid, cervix, ovary, semen, prostatic fluid, and prostatic tissue. For most of these tissues and fluids, ofloxacin concentrations are approximately 0.5–1.7 times concurrent serum concentrations. Ofloxacin is concentrated within neutrophils, achieving concentrations in these cells that may be up to 8 times greater than extracellular concentrations.

In cholecystectomy patients who received oral ofloxacin in a dosage of 200 mg every 12 hours, concentrations of the drug in samples obtained during surgery (6 hours after the 7th dose) ranged from 1.7–9.9 mcg/g in gallbladder wall, 2.1–79.2 mcg/mL in gallbladder bile, and 3.2–19.6 mcg/mL in common duct bile; concomitant serum concentrations ranged from 1–4.2 mcg/mL.

Following a single 400-mg oral dose of ofloxacin in geriatric men 65–81 years of age, prostatic fluid concentrations ranged from 2.5–5.6 mcg/mL and prostatic adenoma tissue concentrations ranged from 2.4–5.6 mcg/g.

Ofloxacin is distributed into CSF following oral administration. Peak concentrations of ofloxacin in CSF generally are attained within 2–6 hours and exhibit considerable interindividual variation, depending in part on the degree of meningeal inflammation. Peak CSF concentrations may be 28–87% of concurrent serum concentrations. In adults with meningitis, a single 300-mg oral dose of ofloxacin resulted in CSF concentrations ranging from 0.1–2.8 or 0.1–2.2 mcg/mL in samples obtained 3 or 6 hours, respectively, after the dose.

Ofloxacin is 20–32% bound to serum proteins.

Ofloxacin crosses the placenta and is distributed into cord blood and amniotic fluid. The drug is distributed into milk following oral administration. In one study in lactating women who received 400-mg oral doses of ofloxacin every 12 hours, drug concentrations averaged 0.29–2.4 mcg/mL in milk and 0.26–2.5 mcg/mL in serum 2–12 hours after a dose; the drug still was detectable in milk 24 hours after a dose.

■ **Elimination** In healthy adults with normal renal function, the elimination half-life of ofloxacin in the distribution phase ($t_{1/2\alpha}$) averages 0.5–0.6 hours and the elimination half-life in the terminal phase ($t_{1/2\beta}$) averages 4–8 hours. In healthy geriatric adults 64–86 years of age with renal function normal for their age, half-life of the drug averages 6.4–8.5 hours. The slower elimination of ofloxacin in geriatric individuals presumably is due to reduced renal function and clearance observed in geriatric individuals.

In adults with impaired renal function, serum concentrations of ofloxacin are higher and the half-life prolonged. In adults with creatinine clearances of 10–50 mL/minute, half-life of the drug averages 16.4 hours (range: 11–33.5 hours); in adults with creatinine clearances less than 10 mL/minute, half-life averages 21.7 hours (range: 16.9–28.4 hours). In patients with end-stage renal failure, half-life of the drug may range from 25–48 hours. Further study is needed to determine whether hepatic impairment effects the pharmacokinetics of ofloxacin. In one study in cirrhotic adults with ascites and creatinine clearances of 47–123 mL/minute who received a single 200-mg oral dose of ofloxacin, peak serum concentrations of the drug averaged 3.6 mcg/mL and half-life averaged 11.6 hours; however, these alterations in pharmacokinetics appeared to result from renal (tubular) rather than hepatic effects.

Less than 10% of a single dose of ofloxacin is metabolized; approximately 3–6% of the dose is metabolized to desmethyl ofloxacin and 1–5% is metabolized to ofloxacin *N*-oxide. Desmethyl ofloxacin is microbiologically active, but is less active against susceptible organisms than is ofloxacin; ofloxacin *N*-oxide has only minimal antibacterial activity. Ofloxacin and its metabolites are excreted in both urine and feces. Following a single 100- to 600-mg oral dose of ofloxacin, 65–90% of the dose is excreted unchanged in urine within 48 hours; less than 5% of the dose is excreted in urine as metabolites. Approximately 4–8% of the dose is excreted in feces. Following oral administration of a single 200-mg oral dose of ofloxacin, urine concentrations average 220 mcg/mL in urine collected over 0–6 hours after the dose; concentrations in urine collected over 12–24 hours after the dose average 34 mcg/mL. In healthy adults receiving 200-mg oral doses of ofloxacin every 12 hours, fecal concentrations of the drug have been reported to average 38–44 mcg/g (range: 30–65 mcg/g). However, other limited data suggest that this dosage produces fecal concentrations of approximately 300 mcg/g.

Renal clearance of ofloxacin averages 133–200 mL/minute in adults with normal renal function.

Small amounts of ofloxacin and desmethyl ofloxacin are removed by hemodialysis. The amount of drug removed during hemodialysis depends on several factors (e.g., type of coil used, dialysis flow rate). In patients with end-stage renal disease undergoing hemodialysis, the serum half-life of ofloxacin averages 8–12 hours during hemodialysis and 13–48 hours between dialysis sessions. Approximately 10–21% of a single 100- or 200-mg oral dose of ofloxacin is removed by hemodialysis, and approximately 10% of a single 200-mg oral dose is removed by peritoneal dialysis. In a study in patients with end-stage renal failure who were maintained on continuous ambulatory peritoneal dialysis (CAPD), less than 2% of a 400-mg oral dose of ofloxacin was removed by the procedure.

Chemistry and Stability

■ **Chemistry** Ofloxacin is a fluoroquinolone anti-infective agent. Like all other commercially available fluoroquinolones, ofloxacin contains a fluorine at the C-6 position of the quinolone nucleus. Like some other fluoroquinolones (ciprofloxacin, levofloxacin), ofloxacin contains a piperazinyl group at position 7 of the quinolone nucleus. The piperazinyl group in ofloxacin results in antipseudomonal activity. The piperazinyl group contained in ofloxacin is methylated, unlike the piperazinyl group contained in ciprofloxacin, and this may contribute to the greater oral bioavailability of ofloxacin compared with that of these other fluoroquinolones. Ofloxacin also contains an oxazine ring linking the nitrogen at position 1 and the carbon at position 8 of the quinolone nucleus. This fused ring results in increased activity against gram-positive and anaerobic bacteria and also contributes to ofloxacin's low degree of in vivo metabolism. The methyl group at the C-3 position in the oxazine ring results in the formation of isoenantiomers; ofloxacin occurs as a racemic mixture of the two isomers. The *S*-(-)isomer is 8–128 times as active against susceptible gram-positive and gram-negative organisms as the *R*-(+)isomer and approximately twice as active as racemic ofloxacin.

Ofloxacin occurs as an off-white to pale yellow crystalline powder. At room temperature, ofloxacin is soluble in aqueous solutions with pH 2–5, sparingly to slightly soluble (4 mg/mL) in aqueous solutions with pH 7, and freely soluble in aqueous solutions with pH greater than 9. The pK_as of the drug are 5.74 and 7.9.

■ **Stability** Ofloxacin tablets should be stored at 20–25°C in tight, light-resistant containers.

Preparations

Excipients in commercially available drug preparations may have clinically important effects in some individuals; consult specific product labeling for details.

Ofloxacin

Oral		
Tablets, film-coated	200 mg*	**Ofloxacin Tablets**
	300 mg*	**Ofloxacin Tablets**
	400 mg*	**Ofloxacin Tablets**

*available from one or more manufacturer, distributor, and/or repackager by generic (nonproprietary) name

†Use is not currently included in the labeling approved by the US Food and Drug Administration

Selected Revisions September 2019,

SULFONAMIDES 8:12.20

Sulfonamides General Statement

■ Sulfonamides, synthetic derivatives of *p*-aminobenzenesulfonamide (sulfanilamide), are classified as anti-infectives if they possess antibacterial activity that is antagonized by *p*-aminobenzoic acid or *p*-aminobenzoyl glutamic acid.

Uses

Although at one time sulfonamides were widely used in the treatment and prophylaxis of infections, the development of resistance in formerly susceptible organisms has greatly limited the clinical usefulness of the drugs. Whenever possible, sulfonamide therapy should be justified by bacteriologic diagnosis.

■ **Acute Otitis Media** Oral sulfonamides have been used for the treatment of acute otitis media (AOM). The fixed combination containing sulfisoxazole acetyl and erythromycin ethylsuccinate (see Erythromycin Ethylsuccinate 8:12.12.04) has been used for the treatment of AOM caused by susceptible *Haemophilus influenzae*. The fixed combination containing sulfamethoxazole and trimethoprim (co-trimoxazole) has been used for the treatment of AOM caused by susceptible *H. influenzae* or *Streptococcus pneumoniae* when the fixed combination offered some advantage over other anti-infectives usually used for the treatment of AOM. The manufacturers state that the fixed combination of sulfamethoxazole and trimethoprim (co-trimoxazole) should not be used for prolonged periods or for prophylaxis in patients with AOM.

When anti-infective therapy is indicated for the treatment of AOM, the American Academy of Pediatrics (AAP) recommends high-dose amoxicillin or the fixed combination of amoxicillin and clavulanate potassium as the drugs of first choice for initial treatment and certain cephalosporins (cefdinir, cefpodoxime, cefuroxime, ceftriaxone) as alternatives for initial treatment in penicillin-allergic patients who do not have a history of severe and/or recent penicillin-allergic reactions. Because substantial resistance to the drugs has been reported in *S. pneumoniae*, AAP states that the fixed combination of sulfisoxazole acetyl and erythromycin ethylsuccinate and the fixed combination of sulfamethoxazole and trimethoprim (co-trimoxazole) should not be used as alternatives in patients who do not respond to amoxicillin.

■ **GI Infections** ***Cyclospora and Cystoisospora Infections*** The fixed combination of sulfamethoxazole and trimethoprim (co-trimoxazole) is considered the drug of choice for the treatment of GI infections caused by *Cyclospora cayetanensis*† or *Cystoisospora belli*† (formerly *Isospora belli*). The fixed combination also has been recommended for long-term suppressive or chronic maintenance therapy (secondary prophylaxis) to prevent recurrence of cystoisosporiasis in adults and adolescents with human immunodeficiency virus (HIV) infection who have CD4+ T-cell counts less than 200/mm^3 and in HIV-infected children with severe immunosuppression.

Shigella Infections The fixed combination of sulfamethoxazole and trimethoprim (co-trimoxazole) is used for the treatment of enteritis caused by susceptible *Shigella flexneri* or *Sh. sonnei* when anti-infective therapy is indicated. However, data from 2012 indicated that approximately 43% of *Shigella* isolates tested were resistant to the fixed combination.

Infections caused by *Sh. sonnei* usually are self-limited (48–72 hours), and mild cases may not require treatment with anti-infectives. Because there is some evidence that anti-infectives may shorten the duration of diarrhea and the period of fecal excretion of *Shigella*, anti-infective treatment generally is recommended in addition to fluid and electrolyte replacement in patients with severe shigellosis, dysentery, or underlying immunosuppression (e.g., HIV infection). An empiric treatment regimen can be used initially, but in vitro susceptibility testing of clinical isolates is indicated since resistance is common. A fluoroquinolone (e.g., ciprofloxacin, levofloxacin, moxifloxacin), ceftriaxone, or azithromycin (not recommended in those with bacteremia) are considered drugs of choice for the treatment of shigellosis when the susceptibility of the isolate is unknown or when ampicillin- or co-trimoxazole-resistant strains are involved.

Travelers' Diarrhea Although the fixed combination of sulfamethoxazole and trimethoprim (co-trimoxazole) has been used for the treatment of travelers' diarrhea caused by susceptible enterotoxigenic *Escherichia coli*, the fixed combination is no longer considered effective against enteric bacterial pathogens and is not recommended for empiric treatment of travelers' diarrhea.

The most common cause of travelers' diarrhea worldwide is noninvasive enterotoxigenic strains of *E. coli* (ETEC), but travelers' diarrhea also can be caused by various other bacteria, including enteroaggregative *E. coli* (EAEC), *Campylobacter jejuni*, *Shigella*, *Salmonella*, *Aeromonas hydrophila*, *Plesiomonas shigelloides*, *Yersinia enterocolitica*, *V. parahaemolyticus*, or non-O-group 1 *V. cholerae*. In some cases, travelers' diarrhea is caused by parasitic enteric pathogens (e.g., *Giardia duodenalis* [also known as *G. lamblia* or *G. intestinalis*], *Cryptosporidium parvum*, *C. cayetanensis*, *Entamoeba histolytica*, *Dientamoeba fragilis*) or viral enteric pathogens (e.g., rotavirus, norovirus, astrovirus).

For information on treatment and prophylaxis of travelers' diarrhea, see Travelers' Diarrhea under Uses: GI Infections, in Ciprofloxacin 8:12.18.

■ **Respiratory Infections** The fixed combination of sulfamethoxazole and trimethoprim (co-trimoxazole) is used for the treatment of acute exacerbations of chronic bronchitis caused by susceptible *S. pneumoniae* or *H. influenzae* when the fixed combination offers some advantage over single-entity anti-infectives. Some clinicians consider co-trimoxazole the drug of choice for the treatment of upper respiratory tract infections and bronchitis caused by *H. influenzae* and an alternative for the treatment of infections caused by *S. pneumoniae*.

The fixed combination of sulfamethoxazole and trimethoprim (co-trimoxazole) has been recommended as an alternative for the treatment of infections caused by *Legionella*†.

■ **Urinary Tract Infections** Sulfonamides have been used for the treatment of urinary tract infections (UTIs).

Oral sulfadiazine has been used for the treatment of pyelonephritis, pyelitis, and cystitis caused by susceptible *E. coli*, *Klebsiella*, *Enterobacter*, *Staphylococcus aureus*, *Proteus mirabilis*, or *P. vulgaris*. The fixed combination of sulfamethoxazole and trimethoprim (co-trimoxazole) is used orally for the treatment of UTIs caused by susceptible *E. coli*, *Klebsiella*, *Enterobacter*, *Morganella morganii*, *P. mirabilis*, or *P. vulgaris* when the fixed combination offers some advantage over single-entity anti-infectives usually used for the treatment of UTIs. The fixed combination of sulfamethoxazole and trimethoprim (co-trimoxazole) is used IV for the treatment of severe or complicated UTIs caused by susceptible *E. coli*, *Klebsiella*, *Enterobacter*, *M. morganii*, or *Proteus* when oral administration of the drug is not feasible and the causative organism is not susceptible to single-entity anti-infectives usually effective for the treatment of UTIs. Although some experts no longer recommend the fixed combination of sulfamethoxazole and trimethoprim (co-trimoxazole) as a drug of first choice for the treatment of uncomplicated cystitis because of high rates of resistance to the drug, other experts suggest that the fixed combination may be a good choice for empiric treatment of acute, uncomplicated UTIs when the causative agent is known to be susceptible or when local in vitro susceptibility patterns for uropathogens indicate that the rate of resistance to the drug does not exceed 20%.

■ **Chancroid** Oral sulfonamides (e.g., sulfadiazine) have been used for the treatment of chancroid (genital ulcers caused by *Haemophilus ducreyi*). However, sulfonamides are not included in US Centers for Disease Control and Prevention (CDC) recommendations for treatment of chancroid; these experts recommend azithromycin, ceftriaxone, ciprofloxacin, or erythromycin as the drugs of choice.

■ **Chlamydial Infections** Oral sulfonamides (e.g., sulfadiazine) have been used for the treatment of infections caused by *Chlamydia trachomatis* (e.g., inclusion conjunctivitis, trachoma). However, other anti-infectives (e.g., azithromycin, erythromycin) usually are the drugs of choice for treatment of these infections.

■ **Crohn's Disease and Ulcerative Colitis** Sulfasalazine is used in the treatment of mild to moderate ulcerative colitis, as adjunctive therapy in the treatment of severe ulcerative colitis, and for the prolongation of the remission period between acute attacks of ulcerative colitis.

Sulfasalazine also has been used for the management of mildly to moderately active Crohn's disease†, but its role in the management of this condition is not as well defined as in the symptomatic treatment of ulcerative colitis.

■ **Granuloma Inguinale (Donovanosis)** The fixed combination of sulfamethoxazole and trimethoprim (co-trimoxazole) is used for the treatment of granuloma inguinale (donovanosis) caused by *Calymmatobacterium granulomatis*†. CDC recommends that granuloma inguinale be treated with a regimen of azithromycin or, alternatively, a regimen of doxycycline, ciprofloxacin, erythromycin, or the fixed combination of sulfamethoxazole and trimethoprim (co-trimoxazole).

■ **Neisseria meningitidis Infections** Oral sulfonamides (e.g., sulfadiazine) have been used for chemoprophylaxis in close contacts of individuals with invasive meningococcal disease caused by sulfonamide-susceptible *Neisseria meningitidis* serogroup A. However, strains of *N. meningitidis* resistant to sulfonamides are prevalent, and sulfonamides are no longer recommended. CDC and AAP recommend rifampin, ciprofloxacin, or ceftriaxone for chemoprophylaxis in close contacts of patients with invasive meningococcal disease.

Although sulfonamides have been used for the treatment of infections caused by susceptible *N. meningitidis* (including meningitis), other anti-infectives (e.g., ceftriaxone, cefotaxime, penicillin G, ampicillin, chloramphenicol, fluoroquinolones, aztreonam) are recommended for the treatment of these infections.

■ **Nocardia Infections** Sulfonamides have been used for the treatment of nocardiosis caused by *Nocardia*.

The fixed combination of sulfamethoxazole and trimethoprim (co-trimoxazole) usually is considered the drug of choice for the treatment of nocardiosis†. Other sulfonamides (e.g., sulfadiazine, sulfamethoxazole [not commercially available as a single-entity preparation in the US]) also have been used; however, some experts suggest that sulfonamides that are less urine soluble (e.g., sulfadiazine) should be avoided. Multiple-drug regimens may be necessary in patients who are immunocompromised or have severe or disseminated infections. Other drugs that have been used alone or in multiple-drug regimens for the treatment of nocardiosis include amikacin, tetracyclines, cephalosporins (ceftriaxone), carbapenems (imipenem, meropenem), fixed combination of amoxicillin and clavulanate potassium, clarithromycin, cycloserine, or linezolid. In vitro susceptibility testing, if available, is recommended to guide selection of anti-infectives for the treatment of severe nocardiosis or for treatment in patients who cannot tolerate or failed to respond to sulfonamide treatment.

■ **Plague** Sulfonamides (e.g., sulfadiazine, fixed combination of sulfamethoxazole and trimethoprim [co-trimoxazole]) have been used in the treatment of plague† caused by *Yersinia pestis*, but appear to be less effective than other anti-infectives used for treatment of the disease (e.g., streptomycin, gentamicin, tetracycline, doxycycline, chloramphenicol). Because of lack of efficacy, some experts state that the fixed combination of sulfamethoxazole and trimethoprim (co-trimoxazole) should not be used alone for the treatment of pneumonic or septicemic plague.

The fixed combination of sulfamethoxazole and trimethoprim (co-trimoxazole) has been used for postexposure prophylaxis of plague†, especially in infants and children younger than 8 years of age. However, because efficacy of the drug for prevention of plague is unknown, other anti-infectives (e.g., doxycycline, ciprofloxacin, chloramphenicol) are recommended for such prophylaxis.

■ **Pneumocystis jirovecii Pneumonia** The fixed combination of sulfamethoxazole and trimethoprim (co-trimoxazole) is used for the treatment of *Pneumocystis jirovecii* (formerly *Pneumocystis carinii*) pneumonia (PCP) and for prevention of *P. jirovecii* infections.

Treatment of Pneumocystis jirovecii Pneumonia The fixed combination of sulfamethoxazole and trimethoprim (co-trimoxazole) is the drug of choice for the treatment of mild, moderate, or severe PCP, including PCP in HIV-infected adults, adolescents, and children.

CDC, National Institutes of Health (NIH), and Infectious Diseases Society of America (IDSA) state that alternatives for treatment of moderate to severe PCP in HIV-infected adults and adolescents who cannot tolerate or have not responded to the fixed combination of sulfamethoxazole and trimethoprim (co-trimoxazole) include IV pentamidine or a regimen of primaquine in conjunction with clindamycin. For the treatment of PCP in HIV-infected children who cannot tolerate or have not responded after 5–7 days of treatment with the fixed combination of sulfamethoxazole and trimethoprim (co-trimoxazole), CDC, NIH, IDSA, and AAP recommend IV pentamidine; these experts state that treatment in such children can be switched to an appropriate oral regimen (e.g., atovaquone) after an initial response is obtained with IV pentamidine.

Prevention of Pneumocystis jirovecii Infections The fixed combination of sulfamethoxazole and trimethoprim (co-trimoxazole) is the drug of choice for prevention of initial episodes (primary prophylaxis) of PCP in HIV-infected adults, adolescents, and children. CDC, NIH, and IDSA recommend that primary prophylaxis to prevent initial episodes of PCP be initiated in HIV-infected adults and adolescents with $CD4^+$ T-cell counts less than 200/mm^3 or a history of oropharyngeal candidiasis. These experts state that primary PCP prophylaxis also should be considered in HIV-infected adults and adolescents with $CD4^+$ T-cell percentages less than 14% or a history of an AIDS-defining illness who would not otherwise qualify for prophylaxis and also should be considered in those with $CD4^+$ T-cell counts greater than 200/mm^3 but less than 250/mm^3 if frequent monitoring of $CD4^+$ T-cell counts (e.g., every 3 months) is not possible. CDC, NIH, IDSA, and AAP recommend that primary prophylaxis to prevent initial episodes of PCP be initiated in HIV-infected children 1 to less than 6 years of age with $CD4^+$ T-cell counts less than 500/mm^3 or $CD4^+$ T-cell percentages less than 15% and in HIV-infected children 6 years of age or older with $CD4^+$ T-cell counts less than 200/mm^3 or $CD4^+$ T-cell percentages less than 15%. These experts recommend that all HIV-infected infants younger than 1 year of age (regardless of $CD4^+$ T-cell count or percentage) receive primary PCP prophylaxis. In addition, infants born to HIV-infected mothers should be considered for primary PCP prophylaxis beginning at 4–6 weeks of age and those with indeterminate HIV status should continue to receive prophylaxis until they are determined to be non-HIV-infected or presumptively non-HIV-infected.

CDC, NIH, IDSA, and AAP also recommend that HIV-infected adults, adolescents, and children who have a history of PCP receive long-term suppressive or chronic maintenance therapy (secondary prophylaxis) to prevent recurrence. The fixed combination of sulfamethoxazole and trimethoprim (co-trimoxazole) is the drug of choice for secondary PCP prophylaxis in HIV-infected adults, adolescents, and children.

CDC, NIH, IDSA, and AAP recommend that primary or secondary prophylaxis with the fixed combination of sulfamethoxazole and trimethoprim (co-trimoxazole) be continued, if clinically feasible, in individuals who experience adverse reactions to the drug that are not life-threatening; however, prophylaxis with the fixed combination should be permanently discontinued and an alternative used in those with life-threatening adverse reactions to the drug.

For additional information on recommendations regarding treatment and prevention of PCP, see Uses: Pneumocystis jirovecii Pneumonia, in Pentamidine 8:30.92.

■ **Rheumatoid Arthritis** Sulfasalazine is used in the management of rheumatoid arthritis in adults who have had an inadequate response to nonsteroidal anti-inflammatory agents (NSAIAs) and for the management of polyarticular course juvenile rheumatoid arthritis in pediatric patients who have had an inadequate response to NSAIAs.

■ **Toxoplasmosis** Sulfonamides are used for the treatment and prevention of toxoplasmosis caused by *Toxoplasmosis gondii.*

Sulfadiazine is used in conjunction with pyrimethamine (and leucovorin) or, alternatively, in conjunction with atovaquone for the treatment of toxoplasmosis. The fixed combination of sulfamethoxazole and trimethoprim (co-trimoxazole) is used for primary prophylaxis against toxoplasmosis† in HIV-infected adults, adolescents, and children. In addition, sulfadiazine is used in conjunction with pyrimethamine (and leucovorin) for chronic maintenance therapy to prevent relapse of toxoplasmosis (secondary prophylaxis)† in HIV-infected individuals.

Treatment of Toxoplasmosis CDC, NIH, IDSA, AAP, and others state that a regimen of sulfadiazine in conjunction with pyrimethamine (and leucovorin) is the regimen of choice for initial treatment of toxoplasmosis, including toxoplasmosis in HIV-infected adults, adolescents, and children. These experts also recommend a regimen of sulfadiazine in conjunction with atovaquone or a regimen of the fixed combination of sulfamethoxazole and trimethoprim (co-trimoxazole) as alternatives for the treatment of toxoplasmosis in HIV-infected adults and adolescents who are unable to tolerate or who failed to respond to or relapsed with the regimen of choice. When a parenteral regimen is required for initial treatment of toxoplasmosis in severely ill adults or adolescents, some experts suggest that parenteral co-trimoxazole can be used.

Sulfadiazine in conjunction with pyrimethamine (and leucovorin) also is the regimen of choice for treatment of acquired CNS, ocular, or systemic toxoplasmosis in HIV-infected children and for treatment of congenital toxoplasmosis. Empiric treatment of congenital toxoplasmosis should be strongly considered in infants born to HIV-infected women who had symptomatic or asymptomatic toxoplasmosis during pregnancy, regardless of whether the mother received toxoplasmosis treatment during the pregnancy.

Prevention of Toxoplasmosis The fixed combination of sulfamethoxazole and trimethoprim (co-trimoxazole) is the drug of choice for prevention of initial episodes (primary prophylaxis) of toxoplasmosis† in HIV-infected adults, adolescents, and children. CDC, NIH, and IDSA recommend primary prophylaxis against *T. gondii* encephalitis in all HIV-infected adults and adolescents who are seropositive for *Toxoplasma* IgG antibody and have $CD4^+$ T-cell counts less than 100/mm^3. Although specific levels of immunosuppression that increase the risk for *T. gondii* encephalitis in HIV-infected children are less well defined, CDC, NIH, IDSA, and AAP recommend primary prophylaxis against *Toxoplasma* encephalitis in toxoplasma-seropositive children younger than 6 years of age who have $CD4^+$ T-cell percentages less than 15% and in HIV-infected children 6 years of age or older who have $CD4^+$ T-cell counts less than 100/mm^3.

CDC, NIH, IDSA, and AAP also recommend that HIV-infected adults, adolescents, and children who have completed initial treatment of *T. gondii* encephalitis receive chronic maintenance therapy (secondary prophylaxis) to prevent relapse. A regimen of sulfadiazine in conjunction with pyrimethamine (and leucovorin) usually is the regimen of choice for secondary prophylaxis of toxoplasmosis† in HIV-infected adults, adolescents, and children since it provides coverage against both toxoplasmosis and PCP. Limited data indicate that the fixed combination of sulfamethoxazole and trimethoprim (co-trimoxazole) may be an effective alternative for secondary toxoplasmosis prophylaxis in HIV-infected individuals, but is recommended in children only when pyrimethamine regimens are not tolerated.

For additional information on recommendations regarding treatment and prevention of toxoplasmosis, see Uses: Toxoplasmosis, in Pyrimethamine 8:30.08.

■ **Prevention of Rheumatic Fever Recurrence** Sulfadiazine is used as an alternative for prevention of recurrent attacks of rheumatic fever (secondary prophylaxis). IM penicillin G benzathine generally is considered the drug of choice for secondary prophylaxis of rheumatic fever; alternatives include oral penicillin V potassium, oral sulfadiazine, and oral sulfisoxazole (only available in the US in fixed combination with erythromycin ethylsuccinate). A sulfonamide is recommended when hypersensitivity precludes the use of a penicillin; however, a macrolide (azithromycin, clarithromycin, erythromycin) should be used in patients allergic to penicillins and sulfonamides.

The American Heart Association (AHA) and AAP recommend long-term (continuous) secondary prophylaxis in patients who have been treated for documented acute rheumatic fever (even if manifested solely by Sydenham chorea) and in those with documented rheumatic heart disease (even after prosthetic valve replacement).

Sulfonamides, including sulfadiazine and the fixed combination of sulfamethoxazole and trimethoprim (co-trimoxazole), should *not* be used for the *treatment* of *S. pyogenes* (group A β-hemolytic streptococci, GAS) infections (e.g., pharyngitis and tonsillitis) because the drugs will not eradicate *S. pyogenes* and, therefore, will not prevent sequelae such as rheumatic fever and glomerulonephritis.

Dosage and Administration

■ **Administration** Sulfonamides are administered orally.

■ **Dosage** Sulfonamide dosage should be adjusted individually according to the severity of the infection, the pharmacokinetics of the individual sulfonamide being used, and the response and tolerance of the patient. The short-acting sulfonamides must usually be given at 4- to 6-hour intervals; an initial loading dose usually is recommended.

Cautions

Adverse effects of the sulfonamides are numerous and may involve nearly all organ systems. Although serious, in some cases fatal, reactions have been reported, they occur infrequently.

■ **Sensitivity Reactions** Many of the adverse effects that have been attributed to the sulfonamides appear to be hypersensitivity reactions. The incidence of hypersensitivity reactions appears to increase with increased sulfonamide dosage. Although cross-sensitization has been reported to occur between the various anti-infective sulfonamides, some diuretics such as acetazolamide and the thiazides, some goitrogens, and sulfonylurea antidiabetic agents, the association between hypersensitivity to sulfonamide anti-infectives and subsequent sensitivity reactions to non-anti-infective sulfonamides (e.g., thiazides, sulfonylurea antidiabetic agents, furosemide, dapsone, probenecid) appears to result from a predisposition to allergic reactions in general rather than to cross-sensitivity to the sulfa moiety per se. The mechanism of sulfonamide sensitivity is poorly understood, and the contribution of allergens, haptens, and/or other immune mechanisms remains to be established. For additional information on cross-sensitivity, see Cautions: Dermatologic and Sensitivity Reactions in the Thiazides General Statement 40:28.20.

Various dermatologic reactions, including rash, pruritus, urticaria, erythema nodosum, erythema multiforme (Stevens-Johnson syndrome), Lyell's syndrome (may be associated with corneal damage), Behcet's syndrome, toxic epidermal necrolysis, and exfoliative dermatitis, have been reported in patients receiving sulfonamides. Because photosensitivity may also occur, patients should be cautioned against exposure to UV light or prolonged exposure to sunlight. A relatively high proportion of fatalities has occurred as a result of the Stevens-Johnson syndrome, especially in children. Although long-acting sulfonamides (no longer commercially available in the US) have been associated most often with the Stevens-Johnson syndrome, other sulfonamides also have been reported to cause this reaction. Clinicians should be alert to the signs, including high fever, severe headache, stomatitis, conjunctivitis, rhinitis, urethritis, and balanitis, which may precede the onset of the cutaneous lesions of the Stevens-Johnson syndrome. If a rash develops during sulfonamide therapy, the sulfonamide should be discontinued at once. In rare instances, a skin rash may precede a more serious reaction such as Stevens-Johnson syndrome, toxic epidermal necrolysis, hepatic necrosis, and/or serious blood disorders.

Fever, which may develop 7–10 days after the initial sulfonamide dose, is a common adverse effect of sulfonamide therapy. Serum sickness syndrome or serum sickness-like reactions (e.g., fever, chills, rigors, flushing, joint pain, urticarial eruptions, conjunctivitis, bronchospasm, leukopenia), have been reported; rarely, anaphylactoid reactions and anaphylaxis may occur. Lupus erythematosus-like syndrome, disseminated lupus erythematosus, angioedema, vasculitis, vascular lesions including periarteritis nodosa and arteritis, cough, shortness of breath, chills, pulmonary infiltrates, pneumonitis (which may be associated with eosinophilia), fibrosing alveolitis, pleuritis, pericarditis with or without tamponade, allergic myocarditis, hepatitis, hepatic necrosis with or without immune complexes, parapsoriasis varioliformis acuta, alopecia, conjunctival and scleral injection, periorbital edema, and arthralgia have also been reported.

If a hypersensitivity reaction occurs during sulfonamide therapy, the drug should be discontinued immediately. Desensitization to sulfasalazine has been used when reinstitution of therapy with the drug was considered necessary in patients with inflammatory bowel disease who had hypersensitivity reactions to the drug. (See Cautions: Sensitivity Reactions, in Sulfasalazine 8:12.20.) Desensitization to sulfadiazine has also been used in several patients with acquired immunodeficiency syndrome (AIDS) when use of sulfadiazine for the treatment of toxoplasmosis was considered necessary in patients who had hypersensitivity reactions to the drug. Specialized references should be consulted for specific information on desensitization procedures and dosage.

■ **Hematologic Effects** Adverse hematologic effects, including methemoglobinemia, sulfhemoglobinemia, granulocytopenia, leukopenia, congenital neutropenia, eosinophilia, hemolytic anemia, agranulocytosis, aplastic anemia, purpura, clotting disorder, thrombocytopenia, myelodysplastic syndrome, hypofibrinogenemia, and hypoprothrombinemia, rarely resulting in death, have been associated with sulfonamide therapy. Acute hemolytic anemia may occur during the first week of therapy as a result of sensitization or glucose-6-phosphate dehydrogenase (G-6-PD) deficiency. This reaction may also occur in the fetus or premature infant in whom G-6-PD is normally deficient. Mild, chronic hemolytic anemia may occur during prolonged sulfonamide therapy. Agranulocytosis may rarely occur 10–14 days after initiation of therapy. Complete blood cell counts should be performed regularly in patients receiving sulfonamides for longer than 2 weeks. If signs of adverse hematologic effects such as sore throat, fever, pallor, purpura, jaundice, or weakness occur, sulfonamide therapy should be discontinued until the possibility of a blood disorder is eliminated.

■ **Hepatic Effects** Functional and morphologic hepatic changes, possibly causing jaundice, may appear within 3–5 days after initiation of sulfonamide therapy. Focal or diffuse necrosis of the liver has been reported rarely.

■ **Renal Effects** Renal damage, manifested by renal colic, nephritis, urolithiasis, toxic nephrosis with anuria and oliguria, hematuria, proteinuria, kidney stone formation, and elevation of BUN and creatinine concentrations, is usually a result of crystalluria caused by precipitation of the sulfonamide and/or its N^4-acetyl derivative in the urinary tract. The occurrence of crystalluria is related to the urinary concentration and the solubility characteristics of the sulfonamide and its metabolites. The risk of crystalluria may be decreased by maintaining an adequate urinary output and by increasing urinary pH. Unless the urine is highly acidic and/or the drug is relatively insoluble, alkalinization of the urine is usually not necessary if the urinary output is maintained at a minimum of 1500 mL daily. Urinary alkalinization may be achieved by administering 2.5–4 g of sodium bicarbonate orally every 4 hours. Urinalysis and kidney function tests should be performed weekly to detect any renal complications. If persistent, heavy crystalluria, hematuria, or oliguria occurs, sulfonamide therapy should be discontinued and alkali therapy maintained. Nephritis and hemolytic-uremic syndrome also have been reported.

■ **GI Effects** Nausea and vomiting occur frequently in patients receiving sulfonamides. Abdominal pain, anorexia, glossitis, stomatitis, pancreatitis, gastroenteritis, diarrhea, neutropenic enterocolitis, GI hemorrhage, melena, flatulence, and salivary gland enlargement also have been reported.

Treatment with anti-infectives alters normal colon flora and may permit overgrowth of *Clostridium difficile*. *C. difficile* infection (CDI) and *C. difficile*-associated diarrhea and colitis (CDAD; also known as antibiotic-associated diarrhea and colitis or pseudomembranous colitis) have been reported with nearly all anti-infectives, including the fixed combination of sulfamethoxazole and trimethoprim (co-trimoxazole), and may range in severity from mild diarrhea to fatal colitis. *C. difficile* produces toxins A and B, which contribute to the development of CDAD; hypertoxin-producing strains of *C. difficile* are associated with increased morbidity and mortality since they may be refractory to anti-infectives and colectomy may be required. (See Cautions: Precautions and Contraindications.)

■ **Nervous System Effects** Headache occurs frequently in patients receiving sulfonamides. Dizziness, vertigo, peripheral neuritis, ataxia, mental depression, hallucinations, disorientation, confusion, seizures, intracranial hypertension, tinnitus, hearing loss, anxiety, apathy, and acute psychosis, occur less frequently. Peripheral neuropathy, paresthesia, weakness, fatigue, drowsiness, lassitude, restlessness, insomnia, meningitis, cauda equina syndrome, and Guillain-Barré syndrome also have been reported.

■ **Other Adverse Effects** Other reported adverse effects of sulfonamides include goiter production, hypothyroidism, hypoglycemia, diuresis, pharyngitis, arthralgia, acidosis, and cyanosis. The nonabsorbable sulfonamides reportedly decrease bacterial synthesis of vitamin K_1, which may result in hypoprothrombinemia and hemorrhage; these sulfonamides may also reduce fecal output of thiamine.

■ **Precautions and Contraindications** Sulfonamides are contraindicated in patients with a history of hypersensitivity to sulfonamides or other chemically related drugs (e.g., sulfonylureas, thiazides). The drugs are also contraindicated in patients with marked renal or hepatic impairment. Sulfonamides are contraindicated in patients with porphyria, since the drugs may precipitate an acute attack. Sulfasalazine (but not other sulfonamides) is contraindicated in patients hypersensitive to salicylates and in patients with intestinal or urinary obstruction.

Sulfonamides should be used with caution and in reduced dosage in patients with impaired hepatic function, impaired renal function, or urinary obstruction, since excessive accumulation of the drugs may occur in these patients. The drugs should also be administered with caution in patients with blood dyscrasia, severe allergies or asthma, or G-6-PD deficiency. The development of sore throat, fever, rash, pallor, arthralgia, cough, shortness of breath, purpura, or jaundice during sulfonamide therapy may be an early sign of a serious adverse reaction. Renal function tests and complete blood cell counts should be performed frequently during sulfonamide therapy, especially during prolonged therapy with the drugs. Microscopic urinalyses should be done weekly when patients are treated with a sulfonamide for longer than 2 weeks.

Because CDAD has been reported with the use of nearly all anti-infectives, including the fixed combination of sulfamethoxazole and trimethoprim (co-trimoxazole), it should be considered in the differential diagnosis in patients who develop diarrhea during or after sulfonamide therapy. Careful medical history is necessary since CDAD has been reported to occur as late as 2 months or longer after anti-infective therapy is discontinued. If CDAD is suspected or confirmed, anti-infective therapy not directed against *C. difficile* should be discontinued whenever possible. Patients should be managed with appropriate supportive therapy (e.g., fluid and electrolyte management, protein supplementation), anti-infective therapy directed against *C. difficile* (e.g., metronidazole, vancomycin), and surgical evaluation as clinically indicated. Other causes of colitis also should be considered. Patients should be advised that diarrhea is a common problem caused by anti-infectives and usually ends when the drug is discontinued; however, it is important to contact a clinician if watery and bloody stools (with or without stomach cramps and fever) occur during or as late as 2 months or longer after the last dose.

The frequency of resistant organisms limits the usefulness of sulfonamides as sole therapy in the treatment of urinary tract infections, especially for recurrent and complicated urinary tract infections. Since sulfonamides are bacteriostatic and not bactericidal, a complete course of therapy is needed to prevent immediate regrowth and the development of resistant urinary pathogens.

■ **Pediatric Precautions** Kernicterus, caused by displacement of bilirubin from protein-binding sites, has occurred in neonates treated with sulfonamides. Unless indicated for the treatment of congenital toxoplasmosis, sulfonamides are generally contraindicated in children younger than 2 months of age.

■ **Pregnancy and Lactation** Safe use of sulfonamides during pregnancy has not been established. The teratogenic potential of most sulfonamides has not been adequately studied in humans or animals; however, an increase in the incidence of cleft palate and other bony abnormalities has been reported when some sulfonamides were administered orally in doses 7–25 times the usual human dose to pregnant rats and mice. Sulfonamides are contraindicated in pregnant women at term or whenever the possibility of premature birth exists, since the drugs cross the placenta and may cause kernicterus.

Because sulfonamides are distributed into milk, and because of the potential for serious adverse reactions from the drugs in nursing infants, a decision should be made whether to discontinue nursing or to discontinue the drug, taking into account the importance of the drug to the woman. Because of the risk of kernicterus in infants younger than 2 months of age, use of sulfonamides is contraindicated in lactating women who are nursing such infants.

Drug Interactions

■ **Folic Acid Antagonists** Because pyrimethamine and trimethoprim also interfere with folic acid synthesis in susceptible organisms, but at different stages, these drugs act synergistically with sulfonamides against some organisms. This synergism is used to therapeutic advantage in the treatment of toxoplasmosis and malaria.

Sulfonamides may increase concentrations and potentiate the effects of methotrexate by displacing methotrexate from its protein-binding sites or inhibiting renal transport of the antineoplastic agent. Sulfonamides should be administered with caution to patients receiving methotrexate.

■ **p-Aminobenzoic Acid and its Derivatives** Because the antibacterial activity of sulfonamides involves competitive inhibition of *p*-aminobenzoic acid (PABA), the concomitant use of PABA or local anesthetics which are derivatives of PABA (e.g., chloroprocaine, procaine [no longer commercially available in the US], propoxycaine [no longer commercially available in the US], tetracaine) reportedly may antagonize the antibacterial activity of sulfonamides. Although the clinical importance of this effect is unclear, PABA and local anesthetics derived from PABA probably should not be used in patients receiving a sulfonamide.

■ **Anticoagulants** Sulfonamides may potentiate the effects of warfarin by displacing the anticoagulant from protein-binding sites. Patients receiving a sulfonamide and warfarin concomitantly should be monitored closely.

■ **Antidiabetic Agents** Sulfonamides may potentiate the hypoglycemic effects of oral hypoglycemic agents, including sulfonylurea hypoglycemic agents. The fixed combination of sulfamethoxazole and trimethoprim (co-trimoxazole) potentiates the effects of oral antidiabetic agents metabolized by cytochrome P-450 (CYP) 2C8 (e.g., pioglitazone, repaglinide, rosiglitazone), metabolized by CYP2C9 (e.g., glipizide, glyburide), or eliminated renally via organic cation transporter (OCT) 2 (e.g., metformin). Increased glucose monitoring may be warranted in patients receiving a sulfonamide and oral antidiabetic agent concomitantly.

■ **Digoxin** Increased serum digoxin concentrations can occur in patients receiving the fixed combination of sulfamethoxazole and trimethoprim (co-trimoxazole), especially in elderly patients. Sulfasalazine reportedly may reduce GI absorption of digoxin. Serum digoxin concentrations should be monitored in patients receiving sulfonamides.

■ **Methenamine** Since methenamine requires acidic urine for its antibacterial effect, the drug should not be used concomitantly with less soluble sulfonamides (e.g., sulfadiazine, sulfapyridine [no longer commercially available in the US]) which may crystallize in acidic urine. In addition, an insoluble precipitate forms between formaldehyde and sulfamethizole (no longer commercially available in the US) in acidic urine.

■ **Nonsteroidal Anti-inflammatory Agents** Since salicylates and other nonsteroidal anti-inflammatory agents (e.g., fenoprofen, indomethacin, meclofenamate) are highly protein bound, these drugs theoretically could be displaced from binding sites by sulfonamides, or could displace sulfonamides from binding sites. Patients receiving sulfonamides concomitantly with nonsteroidal anti-inflammatory agents should be observed for adverse effects.

Mechanism of Action

Sulfonamides are usually bacteriostatic in action. Sulfonamides interfere with the utilization of *p*-aminobenzoic acid (PABA) in the biosynthesis of tetrahydrofolic acid (the reduced form of folic acid) cofactors in susceptible bacteria. Sulfonamides are structural analogs of PABA and appear to interfere with PABA utilization by competitively inhibiting the enzyme dihydropteroate synthase, which catalyzes the formation of dihydropteroic acid (a precursor of tetrahydrofolic acid) from PABA and pteridine; however, other mechanism(s) affecting the biosynthetic pathway also may be involved. Compounds such as pyrimethamine and trimethoprim, which block later stages in the synthesis of folic acid, act synergistically with sulfonamides. (See Drug Interactions.) Only microorganisms that synthesize their own folic acid are inhibited by sulfonamides; animal cells and bacteria which are capable of utilizing folic acid precursors or preformed folic acid are not affected by these drugs. The antibacterial activity of the sulfonamides is reportedly decreased in the presence of blood or purulent body exudates.

Spectrum

Sulfonamides were originally active against a wide range of gram-positive and gram-negative bacteria; however, the increasing incidence of resistance in bacteria formerly susceptible to sulfonamides has decreased the clinical usefulness of the drugs. Sulfonamides are active in vitro against gram-positive bacteria including some strains of staphylococci, streptococci, *Bacillus anthracis*, *Clostridium tetani*, and *C. perfringens* and many strains of *Nocardia asteroides* and *N. brasiliensis*. Although resistance to sulfonamides has been reported with increasing frequency in gram-negative bacteria, the drugs are active in vitro against many Enterobacteriaceae including *Enterobacter*, *Escherichia coli*, *Klebsiella*, *Proteus mirabilis*, *P. vulgaris*, *Salmonella*, and *Shigella*. Sulfonamides are active in vitro against some strains of *Neisseria gonorrhoeae* and *N. meningitidis*; however, many strains of these organisms are resistant to the drugs.

Sulfonamides are active in vitro against *Chlamydia trachomatis*, but are generally inactive against *Chlamydia psittaci*. Sulfonamides also have some activity against *Toxoplasma gondii* and *Plasmodium*.

■ **In Vitro Susceptibility Testing** Results of in vitro susceptibility tests with sulfonamides vary depending on the specific methods and media used; therefore, results of the tests should be carefully correlated with the bacteriologic and clinical response of the patient.

When the disk-diffusion procedure is used to test susceptibility to sulfonamides, the Clinical and Laboratory Standards Institute (CLSI; formerly National Committee for Clinical Laboratory Standards [NCCLS]) recommends that a disk containing 250 or 300 mcg of sulfisoxazole be used and results can be applied to other sulfonamides. When the disk-diffusion procedure is performed according to CLSI standardized procedures using the sulfisoxazole disk, *Staphylococcus* or Enterobacteriaceae with growth inhibition zones of 17 mm or greater are susceptible to sulfonamides, those with zones of 13–16 mm have intermediate susceptibility, and those with zones of 12 mm or less are resistant to the drugs.

When dilution susceptibility testing (agar or broth dilution) is performed according to CLSI standardized procedures using sulfisoxazole, *Staphylococcus* or Enterobacteriaceae with MICs of 256 mcg/mL or less are susceptible to sulfonamides and those with MICs of 512 mcg/mL or greater are resistant to the drugs.

Resistance

Organisms initially sensitive to sulfonamides may develop resistance both in vitro and in vivo; sulfonamide-resistant strains emerge frequently when therapy is continued for 15 days or longer. Organisms made resistant to one sulfonamide, either in the laboratory or in clinical use, are usually cross-resistant to other sulfonamides. Organisms which are highly resistant to sulfonamides are usually permanently resistant; however, a slight or moderate degree of resistance may be reversible.

Pharmacokinetics

■ **Absorption** Individual sulfonamides differ markedly in their absorption, distribution, and elimination. With the exception of sulfapyridine (no longer commercially available in the US) and sulfasalazine, which are only slightly absorbed, sulfonamides are generally well absorbed from the GI tract. Approximately 70–90% of an oral dose of the absorbable sulfonamides is reportedly absorbed from the small intestine; small amounts may also be absorbed from the stomach. Sulfamethizole (no longer commercially available in the US) and sulfisoxazole (commercially available in the US only in fixed combination with erythromycin ethylsuccinate) are absorbed rapidly; peak blood concentrations are usually obtained within 2–4 hours. Sulfadiazine and sulfapyridine are absorbed at a slower rate with peak blood concentrations occurring within 3–7 hours. Administration of oral sulfonamides with food appears to delay, but not reduce, absorption of the drugs.

Absorption of sulfonamides from the vagina, respiratory tract, or abraded skin is variable and unreliable; however, enough drug may be absorbed to induce sensitization or toxicity.

Although only free (unmetabolized and unbound) sulfonamides are microbiologically active, blood concentrations are often determined on the basis of total sulfonamide concentration. Generally, sulfonamide plasma concentrations are approximately twice the blood concentrations. Wide variations in blood concentrations have been reported in different individuals receiving identical doses of the same sulfonamide. Blood total sulfonamide concentrations of 12–15 mg/dL have been reported to be optimal; blood concentrations greater than 20 mg/dL have been associated with an increased incidence of adverse reactions.

■ **Distribution** Absorbable sulfonamides are widely distributed in the body. Although most sulfonamides appear to cross cell membranes, sulfisoxazole appears to be distributed only in extracellular fluid. Sulfonamides may appear in pleural, peritoneal, synovial, amniotic, prostatic, and seminal vesicular fluid, and aqueous humor. Concentrations of some sulfonamides in the CSF may reach 35–80% of blood concentrations. Small amounts of sulfonamides are also distributed into sweat, tears, saliva, and bile.

Sulfonamides readily cross the placenta; fetal plasma concentrations may exceed 50% of maternal plasma concentrations. Sulfonamides are distributed into milk.

Sulfonamides are bound in varying degrees to plasma proteins. Sulfadiazine and sulfapyridine (no longer commercially available in the US) are reportedly 32–70% bound to plasma proteins and sulfamethizole and sulfisoxazole are reportedly 85–90% bound to plasma proteins. All sulfonamides are loosely bound, mainly to albumin, but small amounts of the drugs may be bound by serum globulin. Protein-bound sulfonamides do not have antibacterial activity and there is evidence that the concentration of sulfonamide in tissues is related to the concentration of unbound sulfonamide in serum.

■ **Elimination** Sulfonamides are generally classified as short-acting, intermediate-acting, or long-acting depending on the rate at which they are absorbed and eliminated. Sulfamethizole (no longer commercially available in the US), sulfasalazine, and sulfisoxazole (commercially available in the US only in fixed combination with erythromycin ethylsuccinate) are considered to be short-acting sulfonamides and have plasma half-lives of about 4–8 hours. Sulfadiazine, sulfamethoxazole (commercially available in the US only in fixed combination with trimethoprim [co-trimoxazole]), and sulfapyridine (no longer commercially available in the US) are considered to be intermediate-acting sulfonamides and have plasma half-lives of about 7–17 hours.

Although the liver is the major site of metabolism, sulfonamides may also be metabolized in other body tissues. Most sulfonamides are metabolized mainly by N^4-acetylation. The degree of acetylation, which is a function of time, varies from less than 5% for sulfamethizole to up to 40% for sulfadiazine. The N^4-acetyl metabolites, which do not possess antibacterial activity, have greater affinity for plasma albumin than does the nonacetylated drug and are usually less soluble than the parent sulfonamide, particularly in acidic urine. Like acetyl derivatives, glucuronide derivatives do not possess antibacterial activity; however, glucuronide derivatives are water soluble, appear to resemble the nonacetylated sulfonamide in plasma binding capacity, and have not been associated with adverse effects.

Sulfonamides and their metabolites are excreted mainly by the kidneys via glomerular filtration, but the drugs vary widely in their rates of excretion and solubility characteristics at various urinary pH values. Although alkalinization of urine generally increases the solubility of sulfonamides and their metabolites, alkalinization decreases tubular reabsorption, resulting in increases renal excretion of the drugs and decreased sulfonamide blood concentrations. The metabolites do not appear to be reabsorbed by the tubules and their concentration in urine is greater than in blood. Protein-bound sulfonamides cannot be filtered by the glomeruli. Except for the poorly absorbed sulfonamides (sulfapyridine, sulfasalazine) only small amounts of sulfonamides are excreted in feces.

Chemistry and Stability

■ Chemistry

H_2N–⟨benzene ring⟩–SO_2NH_2

sulfanilamide

Sulfonamides are synthetic derivatives of *p*-aminobenzenesulfonamide (sulfanilamide). Compounds are classified as anti-infective sulfonamides if they possess antibacterial activity that is antagonized by *p*-aminobenzoic acid or *p*-aminobenzoyl glutamic acid and if they exhibit cross-resistance with sulfanilamide.

A benzene ring with a sulfonamido group and a primary amino group (N^4) *para* to the sulfur side-chain are essential for antibacterial activity of sulfonamides. If the N^4-amino group is replaced with radicals that can be converted to a free amino group in the body, the compound retains antibacterial activity. Substitution in the N^1-amide group produces compounds varying in solubility, protein binding, tissue distribution, and rate and mode of metabolism and excretion. The most active sulfonamides have been obtained by substitution of heterocyclic groups in the N^1 position.

Sulfonamides generally are insoluble in water. The drugs are weak acids and form salts with bases; their sodium salts are very soluble in water.

■ Stability Solutions of the sodium salts of most sulfonamides are strongly basic and deteriorate rapidly. Most sulfonamides slowly darken on exposure to light and should be stored in tight, light-resistant containers.

For specific dosages and further information on chemistry and stability, pharmacokinetics, uses, and cautions of the sulfonamides, see the individual monographs in 8:12.20. For information on the fixed combination containing sulfamethoxazole and trimethoprim, see Co-trimoxazole 8:12.20.

†Use is not currently included in the labeling approved by the US Food and Drug Administration

Selected Revisions October 2015,

Co-trimoxazole

Sulfamethoxazole-Trimethoprim, SMX-TMP

■ Co-trimoxazole is a synergistic fixed combination of sulfamethoxazole (an intermediate-acting antibacterial sulfonamide), and trimethoprim; both sulfamethoxazole and trimethoprim are synthetic folate-antagonist anti-infectives.

Uses

■ Acute Otitis Media Co-trimoxazole is used in adults† and children for the treatment of acute otitis media (AOM) caused by susceptible strains of *Streptococcus pneumoniae* or *Haemophilus influenzae* when the clinician makes the judgment that the drug offers some advantage over use of a single anti-infective. Data are limited to date regarding safety of repeated use of co-trimoxazole in pediatric patients younger than 2 years of age; the drug should not be administered prophylactically or for prolonged periods for the treatment of otitis media in any age group.

Various anti-infectives, including oral amoxicillin, oral amoxicillin and clavulanate potassium, various oral cephalosporins (cefaclor, cefdinir, cefixime, cefpodoxime proxetil, cefprozil, ceftibuten, cefuroxime axetil, cephalexin), IM ceftriaxone, oral co-trimoxazole, oral erythromycin-sulfisoxazole, oral azithromycin, oral clarithromycin, and oral loracarbef, have been used in the treatment of AOM. The AAP, CDC, and other clinicians state that, despite the increasing prevalence of multidrug-resistant *S. pneumoniae* and presence of β-lactamase-producing *H. influenzae* or *M. catarrhalis* in many communities, amoxicillin remains the anti-infective of first choice for treatment of uncomplicated AOM since amoxicillin is highly effective, has a narrow spectrum of activity, is well distributed into middle ear fluid, and is well tolerated and inexpensive.

Co-trimoxazole is not considered a first-line agent for treatment of AOM, but is recommended as an alternative for individuals with type I penicillin hypersensitivity. Because *S. pneumoniae* resistant to amoxicillin also frequently are resistant to co-trimoxazole, clarithromycin, and azithromycin, these drugs may not be effective in patients with AOM who fail to respond to amoxicillin. For additional information regarding treatment of AOM and information regarding prophylaxis of recurrent AOM, treatment of persistent or recurrent AOM, and treatment of otitis media with effusion (OME), see Uses: Otitis Media in the Aminopenicillins General Statement 8:12.16.08.

■ GI Infections ***Travelers' Diarrhea*** Oral co-trimoxazole is used in adults and children† for the treatment of enteritis caused by enterotoxigenic *Escherichia coli* that occurs during or soon after travel to developing countries or other areas where hygiene is poor (travelers' diarrhea). Travelers' diarrhea is a condition characterized by a twofold or greater increase in the frequency of unformed bowel movements; other manifestations may include abdominal cramps, nausea, bloating, urgency, fever, and malaise. The principal cause of travelers' diarrhea is infection with enterotoxigenic *E. coli*, but other infectious agents (e.g., *Shigella, Salmonella, Campylobacter* spp.) have also been associated with the disease.

Treatment of the condition depends on severity of the illness; travelers' diarrhea is usually a mild, self-limited disorder. In individuals with mild to moderate disease, replacement therapy with oral fluids and electrolytes may be sufficient, although therapy with nonspecific or antimotility agents (e.g., bismuth subsalicylate, loperamide) may be useful for temporary relief of associated symptoms (e.g., abdominal cramps and diarrhea). Travelers who develop diarrhea with at least 3 loose stools in an 8-hour period, especially if associated with nausea, vomiting, abdominal cramps, fever, or blood in the stools, may benefit from short-term treatment with an anti-infective agent. Fluoroquinolones (ciprofloxacin, levofloxacin, norfloxacin ofloxacin) usually are considered the drugs of choice when treatment of travelers' diarrhea is indicated. Co-trimoxazole can be used as an alternative in children who cannot receive fluoroquinolones; however, resistance to co-trimoxazole has been reported in many areas.

Efficacy of anti-infective therapy may depend on the etiologic agent and its susceptibility to antibiotics. In several controlled studies, therapy for 3–5 days with oral co-trimoxazole or trimethoprim alone substantially reduced the duration of abdominal pain and nausea and the number of unformed stools in individuals with the disease; mild rash occurred infrequently with both therapies. In another controlled study, concomitant therapy with co-trimoxazole and loperamide for 3 days provided more rapid relief of travelers' diarrhea than therapy with either drug alone, and co-trimoxazole given alone as a single dose† (320 mg of trimethoprim given as co-trimoxazole) was also more effective than placebo in treating the condition. However, because of the development of resistance to co-trimoxazole in many areas, other anti-infective agents (e.g., ciprofloxacin, levofloxacin, ofloxacin), which also have been used with success in the treatment of travelers' diarrhea, may be considered first. Nausea and vomiting without diarrhea should not be treated with anti-infectives. Individuals with persistent diarrhea and severe fluid loss, fever, and blood or mucus in the stools should seek medical attention.

Oral co-trimoxazole also has been used effectively to prevent travelers' diarrhea† in individuals traveling for relatively short periods to areas where enterotoxigenic *E. coli* and other causative bacterial pathogens (e.g., *Shigella*) are known to be susceptible to the drug. Because travelers' diarrhea is a relatively nonthreatening illness that is usually mild and self-limiting and can be effectively treated and because of the risks of widespread use of anti-infective agents prophylactically (i.e., potential adverse drug reactions, selection of resistant organisms and increased susceptibility to infections caused by these or other organisms), the US Centers for Disease Control and Prevention (CDC) and most experts recommend that anti-infectives *not* be used prophylactically by most individuals traveling to areas of risk. In addition, although controlled studies have indicated that various anti-infectives when taken prophylactically have been 52–95% effective in preventing travelers' diarrhea in several developing areas of the world, efficacy depends on resistance patterns of pathogenic bacteria in each travel area, and such information seldom is available. While fluoroquinolone resistance for bacteria causing travelers' diarrhea currently is least common, this could change as use of these drugs increases worldwide. The CDC states that although use of anti-infective agents for prophylaxis of travelers' diarrhea in certain high-risk groups, such as travelers with immunosuppression or immunodeficiency, may seem reasonable, there currently are no specific data to support such prevention in these populations. (For information on prophylaxis of travelers' diarrhea in HIV-infected individuals, see Travelers' Diarrhea under Uses: GI Infections, in Ciprofloxacin 8:12.18.) Anti-infectives that have been used for prophylaxis of travelers' diarrhea are not effective in preventing diarrhea caused by viral or parasitic infections, and use of such prophylaxis may give a false sense of security to the traveler about the risk associated with consuming certain local foods and beverages. The principal preventive measure is prudent dietary practices. If prophylaxis is used, ciprofloxacin, levofloxacin, ofloxacin, or norfloxacin can be given for a maximum of 3 weeks.

Shigella Infections Co-trimoxazole is used IV or orally for the treatment of enteritis caused by susceptible strains of *Shigella flexneri* or *S. sonnei*. Choice of anti-infective therapy should be based on drug susceptibility of the isolated organism. Although therapy may be initiated based on local susceptibility patterns pending results of susceptibility testing, some clinicians currently state that, when the susceptibility of the isolate is unknown, fluoroquinolones are the anti-infectives of choice with co-trimoxazole as an alternate, especially in areas where ampicillin-resistant strains of *Shigella* have been reported. Fluoroquinolones are the drugs of choice and co-trimoxazole an alternate for the treatment of shigellosis when the organism is resistant to ampicillin or the patient is allergic to ampicillin.

***Escherichia coli* Infections** Co-trimoxazole has been used in the treatment of GI infections caused by *Escherichia coli*†.

Optimal therapy for diarrhea caused by enterotoxigenic *E. coli*† (ETEC) is not established and resistance is common. AAP states that if diarrhea caused by ETEC is suspected in a traveler to a resource-limited country, use of co-trimoxazole, azithromycin, or ciprofloxacin should be considered if diarrhea is severe or intractable and if in vitro testing indicates that the causative organism is susceptible. A parenteral regimen should be used if systemic infection is suspected.

For the treatment of dysentery caused by enteroinvasive *E. coli*† (EIEC), the AAP suggests than an oral anti-infective (e.g., co-trimoxazole, azithromycin, ciprofloxacin) can be used if in vitro tests indicate the causative organism is susceptible.

The role of anti-infectives in patients with hemorrhagic colitis caused by shiga toxin-producing *Escherichia coli* (STEC; formerly known as enterohemorrhagic *E. coli*†) is unclear and most experts do not recommend use of anti-infectives for treatment of children with enteritis caused by *E. coli* 0157:H7.

■ **Respiratory Infections** Co-trimoxazole is used in adults for treatment of acute exacerbation of chronic bronchitis caused by susceptible strains of *Streptococcus pneumoniae* or *Haemophilus influenzae* when the clinician makes the judgment that the drug offers some advantage over use of a single anti-infective. Co-trimoxazole is considered by many clinicians to be the drug of choice for the treatment of upper respiratory tract infections and bronchitis caused by *H. influenzae*. The drug also is used as an alternative to penicillin G or penicillin V for the treatment of respiratory tract infections caused by *Streptococcus pneumoniae*. Co-trimoxazole is as effective as amoxicillin, ampicillin, erythromycin, or tetracycline in the treatment of acute exacerbations of chronic bronchitis.

Many clinicians consider co-trimoxazole an alternative for the treatment of infections caused by *Legionella micdadei*† (*L. pittsburgensis*) or *L. pneumophila*†.

Co-trimoxazole should *not* be used in the treatment of pharyngitis caused by *S. pyogenes* (group A β-hemolytic streptococci); results of clinical studies indicate that co-trimoxazole therapy is associated with a higher bacteriologic failure rate (as evidenced by failure to eradicate *S. pyogenes* from the tonsillopharyngeal area) than penicillin therapy.

■ **Urinary Tract Infections** Co-trimoxazole is used for the treatment of urinary tract infections (UTIs) caused by susceptible strains of *E. coli, Proteus* (indole-positive or -negative), *Klebsiella, Morganella morganii*, or *Enterobacter*.

Co-trimoxazole, given in single doses, as 3-day therapy, or for 7–10 days, is effective in the treatment of acute uncomplicated UTIs. Some clinicians consider a 3-day regimen of co-trimoxazole the treatment of choice for the empiric treatment of acute uncomplicated UTIs. Co-trimoxazole also is used for the treatment of acute complicated UTIs (e.g., UTIs associated with abnormalities of the urinary tract or neurogenic bladder), but other anti-infectives are preferred by most clinicians. For the treatment of acute pyelonephritis, some clinicians recommend anti-infective treatment for 7–14 days. Mild cases of pyelonephritis in women can be treated with an oral fluoroquinolone or with co-trimoxazole (if the causative organism in known to be susceptible). If the infection is likely to be caused by gram-positive bacteria, amoxicillin or amoxicillin and clavulanate potassium may be used. Patients with more severe infections should be hospitalized and therapy should be initiated using a parenteral regimen. Some clinicians recommend that acute pyelonephritis be treated with a parenteral fluoroquinolone or, alternatively, an aminoglycoside with or without ampicillin or an extended-spectrum cephalosporin; an aminoglycoside with or without ampicillin sodium and sulbactam sodium is recommended if the infection is likely to be caused by gram-positive bacteria. When treating acute uncomplicated UTI, the causative organism should be cultured and susceptibility tests conducted prior to initiation of co-trimoxazole therapy; co-trimoxazole may be initiated, however, before obtaining the results of these tests. Some clinicians also recommend obtaining follow-up urine cultures after discontinuance of anti-infective therapy to determine whether the bacteria have been eliminated.

Most clinicians reserve co-trimoxazole for the treatment of chronic or recurrent UTIs. In chronic or recurrent UTIs, the drug suppresses fecal and vaginal flora and usually does not select out resistant coliforms. For the treatment of chronic or recurrent UTIs resulting from reinfection or relapse in women, low doses of co-trimoxazole (e.g., 40 mg of trimethoprim and 200 mg of sulfamethoxazole given nightly or 3 times weekly) are as effective as other anti-infectives (e.g., methenamine mandelate, nalidixic acid, nitrofurantoin) and are preferred by many clinicians. Men with prostatitis-associated recurrent UTIs usually respond poorly to anti-infectives. Although 14-day courses of co-trimoxazole in such patients reportedly are associated with failure rates of greater than 60%, efficacy of the drug appears to be increased markedly with treatment courses of 3–6 months.

■ **Brucellosis** Oral co-trimoxazole is considered an alternative to tetracyclines for the treatment of brucellosis† when tetracyclines are contraindicated, including brucellosis in pediatric patients. To decrease the incidence of relapse, many clinicians recommend that rifampin be used in conjunction with co-trimoxazole or a tetracycline. For treatment of serious brucellosis or when there are complications, including endocarditis, meningitis, or osteomyelitis, some clinicians recommend that an aminoglycoside (streptomycin or gentamicin) be used concomitantly with co-trimoxazole or a tetracycline for the first 7–14 days of therapy; rifampin can also be included in the regimen to reduce the risk of relapse.

■ **Burkholderia Infections** Co-trimoxazole is used for the treatment of infections caused by *Burkholderia cepacia*†. Co-trimoxazole is considered the drug of choice and ceftazidime, chloramphenicol, or imipenem are alternatives for these infections.

Co-trimoxaozle is used for the treatment of melioidosis† caused by susceptible *B. pseudomallei*, usually in a multiple-drug regimen with chloramphenicol and doxycycline. Ceftazidime or imipenem monotherapy is recommended as the drug of choice for these infections. *B. pseudomallei* is difficult to eradicate and relapse of melioidosis is common.

■ **Cholera** Co-trimoxazole is used in the treatment of cholera† when anti-infective therapy is indicated as an adjunct to fluid and electrolyte replacement. Tetracyclines usually are considered the drugs of choice for the treatment of cholera, and co-trimoxazole, a fluoroquinolone, erythromycin, or furazolidone (no longer commercially available in the US) is recommended when tetracyclines are contraindicated or when the infection is caused by tetracycline-resistant *Vibrio cholerae*. *V. cholerae* serogroup 0139 Bengal may not be susceptible to co-trimoxazole or furazolidone.

■ **Cyclospora Infections** The CDC and others consider co-trimoxazole the treatment of choice for cyclosporiasis infection† caused by *Cyclospora cayetanensis*, a coccidian parasite that causes severe, generally self-limiting, diarrhea.

■ **Granuloma Inguinale (Donovanosis)** Co-trimoxazole is used for the treatment of granuloma inguinale (donovanosis) caused by *Calymmatobacterium granulomatis*†. The CDC recommends that donovanosis be treated with a regimen of oral co-trimoxazole or oral doxycycline or, alternatively, a regimen of oral ciprofloxacin, oral erythromycin, or oral azithromycin. Anti-infective treatment of donovanosis should be continued until all lesions have healed completely; a minimum of 3 weeks of treatment usually is necessary. If lesions do not respond within the first few days of therapy, the CDC recommends that addition of a parenteral aminoglycoside (e.g., 1 mg/kg of gentamicin IV every 8 hours) to the regimen be considered. Erythromycin should be used to treat donovanosis in pregnant and lactating women; addition of a parenteral aminoglycoside (e.g., gentamicin) to the regimen should be strongly considered in these women. Anti-infective treatment appears to halt progressive destruction of tissue, although prolonged duration of therapy often is required to enable granulation and reepithelialization of ulcers. Despite effective anti-infective therapy, donovanosis may relapse 6–18 months later.

Individuals with HIV infection should receive the same treatment regimens recommended for other individuals with donovanosis; however, the CDC suggests that addition of a parenteral aminoglycoside (e.g., gentamicin) to the regimen should be strongly considered in HIV-infected patients.

Any individual who had sexual contact with a patient with donovanosis should be examined and treated if they had sexual contact with the patient during the 60 days preceding the onset of symptoms in the patient and they have clinical signs and symptoms of the disease.

■ **Isosporiasis** Many clinicians consider co-trimoxazole the drug of choice for the treatment of isosporiasis† caused by *Isospora belli*.

■ **Listeria Infections** Co-trimoxazole has been used successfully in the treatment of meningitis caused by *Listeria monocytogenes*†, and some clinicians consider the drug the preferred alternative for the treatment of listeria infections (except endocarditis) in penicillin-allergic patients.

■ **Mycobacterial Infections** Co-trimoxazole has been used in the treatment of cutaneous infections caused by *Mycobacterium marinum*† and is considered an alternative to minocycline.

■ **Nocardia Infections** Co-trimoxazole has been used in the treatment of infections caused by *Nocardia*†, including *N. asteroides, N. brasiliensis*, and *N. caviae*.Co-trimoxazole or a sulfonamide alone (e.g., sulfisoxazole, sulfamethoxazole) are considered drugs of choice for the treatment of nocardiosis. Alternative anti-infectives for the treatment of nocardiosis include a tetracycline (should not be used in pregnant women or children younger than 8 years of age), amoxicillin and clavulanate potassium, imipenem, meropenem, amikacin, cycloserine, or linezolid. Amikacin and cycloserine generally should be reserved for use in the treatment of severe infections when other drugs are ineffective. Some clinicians suggest that in patients with nocardiosis involving the CNS or when the infection is disseminated or overwhelming, amikacin be included during the first 4–12 weeks of therapy or until there is clinical improvement. In vitro susceptibility testing, if available, is recommended to guide selection of an anti-infective agent for the treatment of severe nocardiosis or for the treatment of patients unable to tolerate a sulfonamide.

Nocardiosis in immunocompetent patients with lymphocutaneous disease usually responds after 6–12 weeks of appropriate anti-infective therapy. Immunocompromised patients and those with invasive disease require 6–12 months of anti-infective therapy and, because of the possibility of relapse, therapy should be continued for at least 3 months after apparent cure; nocardiosis in patients with human immunodeficiency virus (HIV) infection may require even longer therapy. Drainage of abscesses may be beneficial, especially in immunocompromised patients.

■ **Pertussis** Although efficacy of the drug remains to be fully determined, the CDC and other experts currently consider co-trimoxazole an alternative to erythromycin for the treatment of the catarrhal stage of pertussis† to potentially ameliorate the disease and reduce its communicability. Co-trimoxazole also is considered an alternative to erythromycin for the prevention of pertussis† in household and other close contacts (e.g., day-care facility attendees) of patients with the disease.

■ **Plague** Co-trimoxazole has been used for *postexposure prophylaxis* of plague†. Although recommended by the CDC and other clinicians as an alternative agent for such prophylaxis in infants and children younger than 8 years of age, efficacy of the drug for prevention of plague is unknown. Most experts (e.g., CDC, AAP, US Working Group on Civilian Biodefense, US Army Medical Research Institute of Infectious Diseases) recommend oral ciprofloxacin or doxycycline for postexposure prophylaxis in adults and most children. Postexposure prophylaxis with anti-infectives is recommended after high-risk exposures to plague, including close exposure to individuals with naturally occurring plague, during unprotected travel in active epizootic or epidemic areas, or laboratory exposure to viable *Yersinia pestis*.

Co-trimoxazole also has been used in the *treatment* of plague†, but appears to be less effective than other anti-infectives used for treatment of the disease (e.g., streptomycin, gentamicin). Because of lack of efficacy, some experts state that co-trimoxazole should not be used for the treatment of pneumonic plague.

For more information on the management of plague exposure, see Uses: Plague, in Streptomycin 8:12.02.

■ **Pneumocystis jiroveci (Pneumocystis carinii) Pneumonia**

Treatment Co-trimoxazole is used for the treatment of *Pneumocystis jiroveci* (formerly *Pneumocystis carinii*) pneumonia (PCP). When given IV or orally, the drug has a cure rate of 70–80% in patients with PCP. Because co-trimoxazole has excellent tissue penetration and therapy with the agent is associated with rapid clinical response (i.e., 3–5 days in patients with mild to moderate infection), co-trimoxazole currently is considered the initial drug of choice for most patients with this infection. Co-trimoxazole also is considered the drug of choice for the treatment of PCP in patients with acquired immunodeficiency syndrome (AIDS); however, in patients with AIDS, co-trimoxazole is associated with an increased incidence of adverse reactions (especially fever and adverse dermatologic and hematologic reactions). In patients who are intolerant of co-trimoxazole, treatment alternatives include pentamidine isethionate (IV), trimetrexate glucuronate, trimethoprim and dapsone, clindamycin and primaquine, or atovaquone.

Prevention Co-trimoxazole is used for the prophylaxis of PCP, both for the prevention of initial episodes (*primary prevention*) and for the prevention of recurrence (*secondary prevention* or chronic maintenance therapy) following an initial episode, in immunosuppressed individuals considered to be at increased risk of developing PCP. Some clinicians consider HIV-infected patients, patients with cancer (especially children with acute lymphocytic leukemia receiving maintenance chemotherapy), or renal transplant recipients with active cytomegalovirus infections to be candidates for co-trimoxazole prophylaxis.

Co-trimoxazole is used for prophylaxis of PCP in patients with HIV infection, although an increased risk of toxicity in these patients has been reported. Some evidence indicates that co-trimoxazole may be better tolerated in HIV-infected children than adults. In addition, patients receiving the drug for prophylaxis of PCP appear to tolerate the drug better than those patients receiving it for treatment of PCP. In a placebo-controlled study in adults with AIDS and newly diagnosed Kaposi's sarcoma but no history of opportunistic infections, no cases of PCP were observed in patients receiving co-trimoxazole (*primary prevention*) for a mean survival period of about 2 years; such pneumonia occurred in 53% of patients receiving placebo and developed within 5 months in 80% of patients who discontinued co-trimoxazole because of toxicity.

Data from a study of 2 cohorts of HIV-positive men whose cases were followed for more than 9 years demonstrated that the largest increase in survival time from the development of a helper/inducer ($CD4^+$, $T4^+$) T-cell count of 200 cells/ mm^3 was in patients diagnosed with PCP, suggesting that the combination of prophylaxis and antiretroviral therapy was a more important factor than antiretroviral therapy alone in prolonging survival. In another cohort of HIV-infected men, such prophylaxis was associated with a decreased incidence of PCP as the initial AIDS-related illness and, because of this beneficial effect and resultant delays in the onset of initial AIDS-related illness, was associated with increases in the rates of other less common opportunistic infections as the initial AIDS-related illness, including *Mycobacterium avium*complex, wasting syndrome, esophageal candidiasis, and cytomegalovirus infection. It was suggested that PCP prophylaxis may delay the development of the first AIDS-defining illness by 6–12 months. Although the generalizability of these data to other HIV-positive populations (e.g., women) is unclear, they suggest that PCP prophylaxis may have a role in prolonging survival and/or in delaying the development of AIDS-related illness in HIV-infected patients.

Primary Prophylaxis. The Prevention of Opportunistic Working Group of the US Public Health Service and the Infectious Diseases Society of America (USPHS/IDSA) recommends primary prophylaxis against PCP in HIV-infected adults and adolescents with $CD4^+$ T-cell counts less than 200/ mm^3 or a history of oropharyngeal candidiasis. HIV-infected adults and adolescents with a $CD4^+$ T-cell percentage of less than 14% or a history of an AIDS-defining illness who do not otherwise qualify for prophylaxis also should be considered for primary prophylaxis. If $CD4^+$ T-cell counts are monitored less frequently than every 3 months, individuals with $CD4^+$ T-cell counts of greater than 200 but less than 250/ mm^3 also should be considered for primary prophylaxis.

The USPHS/IDSA recommends oral co-trimoxazole as the drug of choice for primary prophylaxis of PCP in HIV-infected individuals. When co-trimoxazole is used for the primary prevention of PCP in adults and adolescents, the preferred dosage regimen is 160 mg of trimethoprim (as co-trimoxazole) daily. This regimen also provides prophylaxis against *Toxoplasma gondii* and some common respiratory bacterial infections. Alternatively, 80 mg of trimethoprim (as co-trimoxazole) daily or 160 mg of trimethoprim (as co-trimoxazole) 3 times a week can be used. For individuals who experience an adverse reaction to co-trimoxazole that is not life-threatening, the USPHS/IDSA recommends that the drug be continued if feasible; for individuals who have discontinued the drug because of an adverse effect, reinstitution of co-trimoxazole should be considered once the adverse effect has resolved. Patients who have experienced adverse effects, especially fever and rash, may tolerate reintroduction of co-trimoxazole better with a gradual increase in dose (desensitization) or reintroduction of the drug at a reduced dose or frequency of administration. Alternative regimens that can be used in patients who cannot tolerate co-trimoxazole include dapsone, dapsone with pyrimethamine and leucovorin, aerosolized pentamidine, or atovaquone.

Current evidence indicates that primary PCP prophylaxis can be discontinued in adults and adolescents responding to potent antiretroviral therapy who have a sustained (3 months or longer) increase in $CD4^+$ T-cell counts from less than 200/ mm^3 to greater than 200/ mm^3. Patients included in studies evaluating discontinuance of prophylaxis generally were receiving primary prophylaxis and antiretroviral regimens that included HIV protease inhibitors; median follow-up ranged from 6–16 months and median $CD4^+$ T-cell count at the time prophylaxis was discontinued exceeded 300/ mm^3. In addition, at the time prophylaxis was discontinued, most patients had $CD4^+$ T-cell counts exceeding 200/ mm^3 for at least 3 months and many patients had sustained plasma HIV-1 RNA levels below the detection limits of the available assays. The USPHS/IDSA states that discontinuance of primary PCP prophylaxis is recommended in patients who have sustained a $CD4^+$ T-cell count exceeding 200/ mm^3 for at least 3 months because such prophylaxis appears to add little benefit in terms of disease prevention (PCP, toxoplasmosis, bacterial infections) and discontinuance reduces the medication burden, the potential for toxicity, drug interactions, selection of drug-resistant pathogens, and cost. However, the USPHS/IDSA states that primary PCP prophylaxis should be restarted if the $CD4^+$ T-cell count decreases to less than 200/ mm^3.

Prevention of Recurrence. The USPHS/IDSA recommends long-term suppressive therapy or chronic maintenance therapy (secondary prophylaxis) in HIV-infected adults and adolescents who have a history of PCP to prevent recurrence. The same regimens recommended for primary prophylaxis are used for suppressive therapy. Secondary prophylaxis generally is administered for life, unless immune recovery has occurred as a result of potent antiretroviral therapy.

Current evidence indicates that secondary PCP prophylaxis can be discontinued in HIV-infected adults and adolescents responding to potent antiretroviral therapy who have a sustained (3 months or longer) increase in $CD4^+$ T-cell counts from less than 200/ mm^3 to greater than 200/ mm^3. Patients in studies evaluating discontinuance of secondary prophylaxis had responded to potent antiretroviral therapy with an increase in $CD4^+$ T-cell count to greater than 200/ mm^3 for at least 3 months. Most patients were receiving an antiretroviral regimen that included HIV protease inhibitors; the median $CD4^+$ T-cell count at the time prophylaxis was discontinued was greater than 300/ mm^3 and most patients had sustained plasma HIV-1 RNA levels below the detection limits of the available assays. The longest follow-up was 13 months. The USPHS/IDSA states that discontinuance of secondary PCP prophylaxis in adults and adolescents who have a sustained (3 months or longer) increase in $CD4^+$ T-cell counts to greater than 200/ mm^3 is recommended because such prophylaxis appears to add little benefit in terms of disease prevention (PCP, toxoplasmosis, bacterial infections) and discontinuance reduces the medication burden, the potential for toxicity, drug interactions, selection of drug-resistant pathogens, and cost. However, in patients who had PCP episodes when they had $CD4^+$ T-cell counts exceeding 200/ mm^3, it probably is prudent to continue secondary PCP prophylaxis for life regardless of how high the $CD4^+$ T-cell count increases in response to potent antiretroviral therapy.

If secondary PCP prophylaxis is discontinued in HIV-infected adults or adolescents meeting the recommended criteria, the USPHS/IDSA recommends that it be restarted if the $CD4^+$ T-cell count decreases to less than 200/ mm^3 or if PCP recurs at a $CD4^+$ T-cell count exceeding 200/ mm^3.

Prophylaxis in HIV-Infected Children. The CDC, American Academy of Pediatrics (AAP), USPHS/IDSA, and most clinicians recommend antimicrobial prophylaxis for PCP in selected HIV-infected children. This recommendation is based on the high mortality rate associated with PCP in infants and children and the established efficacy of prophylaxis in HIV-infected adults; it is unlikely that placebo-controlled studies will ever be performed in HIV-infected children. PCP is the most common serious HIV-associated opportunistic infection among children, occurring in more than 50% of those with perinatally acquired HIV infection that progresses to AIDS within the first year of life, and in about 40% of pediatric AIDS cases overall. In children with perinatally acquired HIV infection, PCP occurs most often at 3–6 months of age. Despite the availability of effective anti-infectives for the treatment of *P. jiroveci* infections, the median survival from the first episode in infants and children is 1–4 months; among AIDS cases reported to CDC, 35% of children with PCP died within 2 months of diagnosis. Overall, about 90% of children with PCP died and 70% survived for less than 6 months in one retrospective study despite active treatment with co-trimoxazole and/or pentamidine. Therefore, current strategies should be aimed at preventing initial and subsequent infection with the protozoa in children at high risk for HIV infection by initiating early prophylactic therapy.

The CDC, USPHS/IDSA, AAP, and other experts recommend that all infants born to HIV-infected women receive primary PCP prophylaxis starting at 4–6 weeks of age, regardless of their $CD4^+$ T-cell count. Infants who are first identified as being HIV-exposed after 6 weeks of age should receive prophylaxis beginning at the time of identification. Because of the potential for adverse drug effects in neonates and the low incidence of *P. jiroveci* infection in this age group, *primary* but not *secondary* prophylaxis should be delayed until 1 month of age. Prophylaxis can be discontinued in children who are found not to be infected with HIV. All HIV-infected infants and infants whose infection status has not yet been determined should continue prophylaxis until 12 months of age.

The need for subsequent prophylaxis should be based on age-specific $CD4^+$ T-cell count thresholds. In HIV-infected children 1–5 years of age, primary prophylaxis against PCP should be initiated if $CD4^+$ T-cell counts are less than 500/ mm^3 or the $CD4^+$ percentage is less than 15%. In HIV-infected children 6–12 years of age, primary prophylaxis against PCP should be initiated if $CD4^+$ T-cell counts are less than 200/ mm^3 or the $CD4^+$ percentage is less than 15%.

The USPHS/IDSA recommends oral co-trimoxazole as the drug of choice for the primary and secondary (suppressive or chronic maintenance therapy) prevention of PCP in HIV-infected infants and children. When co-trimoxazole is used for the primary or secondary prevention of PCP, the preferred dosage regimen is 150 mg/m^2 of trimethoprim (as co-trimoxazole) daily in 2 divided doses for 3 consecutive days each week. Alternatively, this dose can be administered as a single dose for 3 consecutive days each week, in 2 divided doses daily, or in 2 divided doses 3 times a week on alternate days. Alternative regimens that can be used in HIV-infected infants and children include dapsone, aerosolized pentamidine, or atovaquone.

The safety of discontinuing primary or secondary PCP prophylaxis in HIV-infected children receiving potent antiretroviral therapy has not been extensively studied. Children who have a history PCP should receive life-long suppressive therapy to prevent recurrence.

■ **Toxoplasmosis** ***Prevention*** **Primary Prophylaxis.** The USPHS/IDSA recommends that, shortly after being diagnosed with HIV infection, all HIV-infected individuals be tested for IgG antibody to *Toxoplasma* to detect latent infection with *T. gondii*. HIV-infected individuals (particularly those seronegative for *Toxoplasma* antibody) should be counseled concerning the various sources of toxoplasmic infection and how best to avoid these sources, including avoiding raw or undercooked meat, washing raw vegetables, hand washing after contact with raw meat or soil, and hand washing after changing cat litter boxes. The USPHS/IDSA recommends that all HIV-infected adults and adolescents who are seropositive for *Toxoplasma* IgG antibody and who have $CD4^+$ T-cell counts less than 100/ mm^3 receive *primary* prophylaxis against toxoplasmic encephalitis. Primary prophylaxis against toxoplasmosis encephalitis generally is recommended for HIV-infected infants and children with severe immunosuppression who are seropositive for *Toxoplasma* IgG antibody. Co-trimoxazole is the drug of choice for primary prophylaxis against toxoplasmosis encephalitis and dosages of the drug recommended for prophylaxis against PCP appear to be effective against toxoplasmosis encephalitis. When co-trimoxazole is used for primary prevention of toxoplasmosis encephalitis in adults and adolescents, the preferred dosage regimen is 160 mg of trimethoprim (as co-trimoxazole) daily. In patients who cannot tolerate co-trimoxazole, regimens used for primary prophylaxis of PCP that consist of dapsone with pyrimethamine and leucovorin also provide protection against toxoplasmosis encephalitis. Atovaquone with or without pyrimethamine and leucovorin also can be used for primary prophylaxis against toxoplasmosis-encephalitis. However, aerosolized pentamidine does not provide protection against toxoplasmosis encephalitis and regimens consisting of dapsone, pyrimethamine, azithromycin, or clarithromycin used alone cannot be recommended for prophylaxis against toxoplasmosis encephalitis based on current data.

HIV-infected individuals who are seronegative for *Toxoplasma* antibody and who are not currently receiving primary PCP prophylaxis with a regimen known to be active against toxoplasmosis encephalitis should be retested for *Toxoplasma* antibody if their $CD4^+$ T-cell count falls below 100/ mm^3 to determine whether they have seroconverted, are now at risk for toxoplasmosis encephalitis, and have become candidates for primary prophylaxis against the infection.

Current evidence indicates that primary prophylaxis can be discontinued with minimal risk of developing toxoplasmic encephalitis in HIV-infected adults and adolescents responding to potent antiretroviral therapy who have a sustained (3 months or longer) increase in $CD4^+$ T-cell counts from less than 200/ mm^3 to greater than 200/ mm^3. Patients included in these studies generally were receiving primary prophylaxis and antiretroviral regimens that included HIV-protease inhibitors; median follow-up ranged from 7–22 months and median $CD4^+$ T-cell count at the time prophylaxis was discontinued exceeded 300/ mm^3. At the time prophylaxis was discontinued, many patients had sustained plasma HIV-1 RNA levels below the detection limits of the available assays. While patients with $CD4^+$ T-cell counts below 100/ mm^3 are at greatest risk for toxoplasmic encephalitis, the risk in patients whose $CD4^+$ T-cell counts have increased to 100–200/ mm^3 has not been studied as extensively as in those whose $CD4^+$ T-cell counts have increased to greater than 200/ mm^3. Therefore, the recommendation to discontinue primary toxoplasmosis prophylaxis specifies that prophylaxis can be discontinued when the $CD4^+$ T-cell count exceeds 200/ mm^3. The USPHS/IDSA states that discontinuation of primary toxoplasmosis prophylaxis is recommended in adults and adolescents who have a sustained (3 months or longer) increase in $CD4^+$ T-cell counts to greater than 200/ mm^3 because such prophylaxis appears to add little benefit in terms of disease prevention for toxoplasmosis, and discontinuance reduces the pill burden, the potential for toxicity, drug interactions, selection of drug-resistant pathogens, and cost.

If primary toxoplasmosis prophylaxis is discontinued in adults and adolescents meeting the recommended criteria, the USPHS/IDSA states that it should be restarted if the $CD4^+$ T-cell count decreases to less than 100–200/ mm^3.

The safety of discontinuing primary toxoplasmosis prophylaxis in HIV-infected children receiving potent antiretroviral therapy has not been extensively studied.

Prevention of Recurrence. The USPHS/IDSA recommends that HIV-infected individuals who have had toxoplasmic encephalitis receive long-term suppressive or chronic maintenance therapy (secondary prophylaxis) to prevent relapse. Secondary toxoplasmosis prophylaxis generally is administered for life, unless immune recovery has occurred as a result of potent antiretroviral therapy.

The USPHS/IDSA states that the regimen of choice for secondary prophylaxis to prevent relapse of toxoplasmosis in HIV-infected adults, adolescents, infants, and children is a regimen of sulfadiazine and pyrimethamine (with leucovorin). In patients who cannot tolerate sulfonamides, a regimen of clindamycin and pyrimethamine (with leucovorin) is recommended; a regimen of atovaquone with or without pyrimethamine (with leucovorin) also is an alternative in adults and adolescents; Co-trimoxazole is not recommended for secondary toxoplasmosis prophylaxis.

For information on USPHS/IDSA recommendations regarding secondary prophylaxis of toxoplasmosis in HIV-infected individuals, including when to initiate or discontinue such prophylaxis, see Uses: Toxoplasmosis, in Pyrimethamine 8:30.08.

■ **Wegener's Granulomatosis** Co-trimoxazole has reportedly produced beneficial responses in a limited number of patients with Wegener's granulomatosis†, but further study is needed. Prolonged remissions have been observed in many of these patients, including some whose disease relapsed while receiving conventional therapy (e.g., cyclophosphamide), and co-trimoxazole therapy may reduce or eliminate the need for cytotoxic (e.g., cyclophosphamide) and corticosteroid therapy. Relapse has occurred occasionally during co-trimoxazole therapy but may respond to supplemental dosages of trimethoprim or the addition of small dosages of cytotoxic therapy. The precise role of co-trimoxazole in the management of Wegener's granulomatosis and the drug's effect on long-term morbidity and mortality remain to be determined, but the drug appears to be a useful alternative to more toxic drugs (e.g., cyclophosphamide) in some patients.

■ **Whipple's Disease** Co-trimoxazole is used in the treatment of Whipple's disease† caused by *Tropheryma whippelii*.

Dosage and Administration

■ **Reconstitution and Administration** Co-trimoxazole is administered orally or by IV infusion. When oral therapy is not feasible or for severe infections, the drug may be administered IV. The drug should *not* be injected IM.

Co-trimoxazole for injection concentrate *must* be diluted prior to IV infusion. For IV infusion, each 5 mL of the concentrate for injection containing 80 mg of trimethoprim is usually diluted with 125 mL of 5% dextrose. In patients in whom fluid intake is restricted, each 5 mL of the concentrate may be diluted in 75 mL of 5% dextrose.

■ **Dosage** Dosage of co-trimoxazole is expressed in terms of the trimethoprim content of the fixed combination containing 5 mg of sulfamethoxazole to 1 mg of trimethoprim.

Acute Otitis Media For the treatment of acute otitis media in children 2 months of age or older, the usual oral dosage of co-trimoxazole is 8 mg/kg of trimethoprim (as co-trimoxazole) daily in 2 divided doses every 12 hours. The usual duration of treatment is 10 days.

GI Infections **Shigella Infections.** For the treatment of enteritis caused by *S. flexneri* or *S. sonnei*, the usual adult oral dosage of co-trimoxazole is 160 mg of trimethoprim (as co-trimoxazole) administered every 12 hours. The usual oral dosage for children 2 months of age or older is 8 mg/kg daily of trimethoprim (as co-trimoxazole), administered in 2 divided doses every 12 hours for 5 days.

For enteritis caused by *S. flexneri* or *S. sonnei* in children 2 months of age or older and in adults, the usual IV dosage of co-trimoxazole is 8–10 mg/kg of trimethoprim (as co-trimoxazole) daily, administered in 2–4 equally divided doses every 6, 8, or 12 hours for 5 days.

Travelers' Diarrhea. For the treatment of travelers' diarrhea in adults, co-trimoxazole has been given in a dosage of 160 mg of trimethoprim (as co-trimoxazole) every 12 hours for 3–5 days. A single oral dose of 320 mg of trimethoprim (as co-trimoxazole) has also been used for the treatment of travelers' diarrhea.

Although the use of anti-infectives for prophylaxis of travelers' diarrhea† generally is discouraged, an adult oral dosage of trimethoprim 160 mg (as co-trimoxazole) once daily during the period of risk has been used.

Respiratory Tract Infections For the treatment of bronchitis, the usual adult oral dosage of co-trimoxazole is 160 mg of trimethoprim (as co-trimoxazole) administered every 12 hours for 14 days.

Urinary Tract Infections For the treatment of chronic or recurrent urinary tract infections (UTIs) or prostatitis†, the usual adult oral dosage of co-trimoxazole is 160 mg of trimethoprim (as co-trimoxazole) administered every 12 hours. Most clinicians recommend continuing co-trimoxazole treatment for 10–14 days for chronic or recurrent UTIs or for 3–6 months in men with prostatitis†. For the prophylaxis† of chronic or recurrent UTIs, co-trimoxazole doses of 40–80 mg of trimethoprim (as co-trimoxazole) have been administered daily or 3 times weekly for 3–6 months. For the treatment of chronic or recurrent UTIs in children 2 months of age or older, the usual oral dosage is 8 mg/kg daily of trimethoprim (as co-trimoxazole), administered in 2 divided doses every 12 hour for 10 days.

For severe UTIs in children 2 months of age or older and in adults, the usual IV dosage of trimethoprim is 8–10 mg/kg (as co-trimoxazole) daily, administered in 2–4 equally divided doses every 6, 8, or 12 hours for up to 14 days.

Brucellosis For the treatment of brucellosis†, some clinicians recommend that pediatric patients receive a dosage of oral trimethoprim (as co-trimoxazole) of 10 mg/kg daily (maximum 480 mg/daily) in 2 divided doses for 4–6 weeks.

Cholera For the treatment of cholera†, the usual oral dosage of trimethoprim (as co-trimoxazole) is 4–5 mg/kg twice daily for 3 days in children or 160 mg twice daily for 3 days in adults, in conjunction with fluid and electrolyte replacement.

Cyclospora Infections For the treatment of cyclosporiasis†, the usual oral dosage of co-trimoxazole is 160 mg of trimethoprim (as co-trimoxazole) twice daily for 7–10 days in adults or 5 mg/kg twice daily for 7–10 days in children. However, HIV-infected patients may require higher dosage and more prolonged therapy.

Granuloma Inguinale (Donovanosis) For the treatment of granuloma inguinale (donovanosis) caused by *Calymmatobacterium granulomatis*†, the CDC recommends that oral trimethoprim (as co-trimoxazole) be given in a dosage of 160 mg twice daily for at least 3 weeks. If lesions do not respond within the first few days, addition of a parenteral aminoglycoside (1 mg/kg of gentamicin IV every 8 hours) to the regimen should be considered; addition of the aminoglycoside should be strongly considered when treating donovanosis in patients with human immunodeficiency virus (HIV) infection and in pregnant and lactating women. Despite effective anti-infective therapy, donovanosis may relapse 6–18 months later.

Isosporiasis For the treatment of isosporiasis†, some clinicians recommend that adults receive an oral co-trimoxazole dosage of 160 mg of trimethoprim (as co-trimoxazole) twice daily for 10 days and that children receive an oral co-trimoxazole dosage of trimethoprim (as co-trimoxazole) of 5 mg/kg twice daily for 10 days. However, immunocompromised patients may require higher dosage and more prolonged therapy.

Nocardia Infections For the treatment of nfections caused by *Nocardia*†, an average adult oral dosage of trimethoprim (as co-trimoxazole) of 640 mg daily has been administered for an average of 7 months.

Pertussis Although the optimum dosage and duration of co-trimoxazole for the treatment or prevention of pertussis† have not been established, an oral dosage of 8 mg/kg of trimethoprim and 40 mg/kg of sulfamethoxazole daily in 2 divided doses has been recommended for children and a dosage of 320 mg daily in 2 divided doses has been recommended for adults. Because of reports of prophylaxis failures and delays or failure in eradication with shorter courses of anti-infective therapy in this infection, the US Public Health Service Advisory Committee on Immunization Practices (ACIP), American Academy of Pediatrics (AAP), and some clinicians recommend that a 14-day course of therapy be employed for the treatment or prevention of pertussis.

Plague For anti-infective prophylaxis of individuals with close exposure to pneumonic plague or an exceptionally high risk of exposure to plague, the CDC recommends an oral trimethoprim (as co-trimoxazole) dosage of 320–640 mg daily in 2 equally divided doses for 7 days or a dosage of 8 mg/kg daily in 2 equally divided doses for 7 days in children at least 2 months of age.

Pneumocystis jiroveci (Pneumocystis carinii) Pneumonia For the *treatment* of *Pneumocystis jiroveci* (formerly *Pneumocystis carinii*) pneumonia (PCP) in adults and children older than 2 months of age, the usual oral or IV dosage of trimethoprim (as co-trimoxazole) is 15–20 mg/kg daily, given in 3 or 4 equally divided doses. An IV dosage of 10–15 mg/kg daily has also been suggested for the treatment of PCP in adults with normal renal function. The usual duration of co-trimoxazole for treatment of PCP is 14–21 days.

For both *primary* and *secondary* prevention of PCP in HIV-infected adults and adolescents, the Prevention and Opportunistic Infections Working Group of the US Public Health Service and the Infectious Disease Society of America (USPHS/IDSA) and other experts recommend an oral trimethoprim (as co-trimoxazole) dosage of 160 mg once daily; alternatively, an oral trimethoprim (as co-trimoxazole) dosage of 80 mg once daily also is recommended. In patients with acute lymphocytic leukemia undergoing induction and maintenance chemotherapy, co-trimoxazole therapy given on 3 consecutive days (e.g., Monday, Tuesday, and Wednesday) weekly appears to be as effective as daily therapy for the prevention of PCP and may be associated with a lower frequency of systemic fungal infections.

For primary or secondary prophylaxis of PCP in children, including HIV-infected children, the USPHS/IDSA and other clinicians recommend an intermittent regimen of trimethoprim 150 mg/m^2 daily (as co-trimoxazole) in 2 divided doses for 3 consecutive days each week is recommended. Alternatively, the USPHS/IDSA and AAP state that 150 mg/m^2 can be administered as a single daily dose for 3 consecutive days each week, in 2 divided doses daily 7 days each week, or in 2 divided daily doses given 3 times each week on alternate days. AAP states that these dosages can be used in children 4 weeks of age† or older.

Toxoplasmosis For primary prophylaxis against toxoplasmosis† in HIV-infected adults and adolescents, the USPHS/IDSA recommends an oral trimethoprim dosage of 160 mg (as co-trimoxazole) once daily. Alternatively, an oral dosage of trimethoprim of 80 mg once daily (as co-trimoxazole) may be used. For primary prophylaxis against toxoplasmosis in HIV-infected children, the dosage recommended by USPHS/IDSA is trimethoprim 150 mg/m^2 (as co-trimoxazole) daily in 2 divided doses.

■ **Dosage in Renal Impairment** In patients with impaired renal function, doses and/or frequency of administration of co-trimoxazole must be modified in response to the degree of renal impairment, severity of the infection, susceptibility of the causative organism, and serum concentrations of the drug. The manufacturers recommend that the usual adult daily dosage of co-trimoxazole be reduced 50% in patients with creatinine clearances of 15–30 mL/minute. Although the manufacturers recommend not using the drug in patients with creatinine clearances less than 15 mL/minute, some clinicians suggest using the drug in reduced dosages in these patients.

Cautions

The most frequent adverse effects of co-trimoxazole are adverse GI effects (nausea, vomiting, anorexia) and sensitivity skin reactions (e.g., rash, urticaria), each reportedly occurring in about 3.5% of patients. The incidence and severity of these adverse reactions are generally dose related, and adverse reactions may occasionally be obviated by a reduction in dosage. Hypersensitivity and hematologic reactions are the most serious adverse effects of co-trimoxazole, reportedly occurring in less than 0.5% of patients. Fatal hypersensitivity reactions, including Stevens-Johnson syndrome and erythema multiforme, have occurred in several children who received co-trimoxazole. Deaths associated with hypersensitivity reactions, fulminant hepatocellular necrosis, agranulocytosis, aplastic anemia, and other blood dyscrasias have occurred with the administration of sulfonamides.

The frequency of some co-trimoxazole-induced adverse effects, including rash (usually diffuse, erythematous, and maculopapular), fever, leukopenia (neutropenia), thrombocytopenia, hyperkalemia, hyponatremia, and increased serum aminotransferase concentrations, is substantially higher in patients with acquired immunodeficiency syndrome (AIDS) than in other patients. Such adverse effects have occurred in up to 80% of AIDS patients receiving the drug, usually during the second week of therapy, but generally have been reversible following discontinuance of co-trimoxazole therapy. The exact mechanism(s) of this increased risk of co-trimoxazole toxicity has not been determined, but may be immunologically based. While it has been suggested that glutathione deficiency in HIV-infected patients and resultant accumulation of reactive hydroxylamine metabolites of sulfamethoxazole may be involved in this increased risk, this hypothesis requires confirmation. These adverse effects usually recur following rechallenge with the drug, although cautious desensitization has been performed successfully in some patients in whom continued co-trimoxazole therapy was considered necessary. Limited evidence suggests that white AIDS patients may be at greater risk of these adverse effects than black AIDS patients, indicating that genetic factors may also be important. Some evidence also indicates that co-trimoxazole may be better tolerated in HIV-infected children than adults. Adverse effects usually are less severe in patients receiving the drug for prophylaxis of *Pneumocystis jiroveci* (formerly *Pneumocystis carinii*) pneumonia compared with those receiving co-trimoxazole for treatment of the disease.

■ **Sensitivity Reactions** Epidermal necrolysis, exfoliative dermatitis, Stevens-Johnson syndrome, serum sickness, and allergic myocarditis are the most severe allergic reactions reported with sulfonamides alone or co-trimoxazole. Other reported allergic and anaphylactoid reactions include anaphylaxis, arthralgia, erythema multiforme, Schönlein-Henoch purpura, pruritus, urticaria, periorbital edema, corneal ring infiltrates, conjunctival and scleral injection, and photosensitivity. Mild to moderate rashes, when they occur, usually appear within 7–14 days after initiation of co-trimoxazole. Rashes are generally erythematous, maculopapular, morbilliform, and/or pruritic. Generalized pustular dermatosis and fixed drug eruption also have been reported. Patients with AIDS appear to be at particular risk of developing rash (usually diffuse, erythematous, and maculopapular) during co-trimoxazole therapy. (See the opening discussion in Cautions.)

■ **Hematologic Effects** Co-trimoxazole-induced hematologic toxicity has resulted rarely in aplastic anemia, agranulocytosis, leukopenia, neutropenia, thrombocytopenia, eosinophilia, megaloblastic and/or hemolytic anemia, methemoglobinemia, pancytopenia, hypoprothrombinemia, and/or purpura. Hematologic toxicity may occur with increased frequency in folate-depleted patients including geriatric, malnourished, alcoholic, pregnant, or debilitated patients; in patients receiving folate antimetabolites (e.g., phenytoin) or diuretics; in patients with hemolysis or impaired renal function; and in patients receiving co-trimoxazole in high dosages and/or for prolonged periods (e.g., longer than 6 months). In geriatric patients receiving some diuretics (principally thiazides) and co-trimoxazole concomitantly, an increased incidence of thrombocytopenia with purpura has been reported. The risk of leukopenia, neutropenia, and thrombocytopenia also appear to be increased in patients with AIDS.

Folic acid may be administered during co-trimoxazole therapy and will not interfere with the drug's antibacterial effect. Megaloblastic anemia and occasionally neutropenia and thrombocytopenia can be reversed by administration of leucovorin (folinic acid). If signs of bone marrow suppression occur in patients receiving co-trimoxazole, leucovorin should be administered; some clinicians recommend a leucovorin dosage of 5–15 mg daily until normal hematopoiesis is restored.

■ **GI Effects** Nausea, vomiting, and anorexia are the most frequent GI reactions to co-trimoxazole, but glossitis, stomatitis, abdominal pain, pancreatitis (sometimes fatal), pseudomembranous enterocolitis, and diarrhea also have been reported.

■ **Local Effects** Pain, local irritation, inflammation, and rarely thrombophlebitis may occur with IV co-trimoxazole, especially if extravascular infiltration of the drug occurs.

■ **Nervous System Effects** Adverse nervous system effects of co-trimoxazole include headache, insomnia, fatigue, apathy, nervousness, muscle weakness, ataxia, vertigo, tinnitus, peripheral neuritis, mental depression, aseptic meningitis, seizures, and hallucinations. Tremor and other neurologic manifestations (e.g., ataxia, ankle clonus, apathy) developed during co-trimoxazole therapy in several patients with AIDS; although such manifestations also have been associated with the underlying disease process, they resolved in these patients within 2–3 days after discontinuing the drug.

■ **Other Adverse Effects** Other adverse effects reported with co-trimoxazole therapy include drug fever, chills, myalgia, hepatitis (including cholestatic jaundice and hepatic necrosis), increased serum aminotransferase and bilirubin concentrations, renal failure, interstitial nephritis, increased BUN and serum creatinine concentrations, crystalluria and stone formation, toxic nephrosis with oliguria and anuria, pulmonary infiltrates, cough, shortness of breath, hypotension, periarteritis nodosa, and a positive lupus erythematosus phenomenon. Rhabdomyolysis has been reported rarely in patients receiving co-trimoxazole, mainly in HIV-infected patients. Sulfonamides chemically resemble some goitrogens, diuretics (acetazolamide, thiazides), and oral hypoglycemic agents, and cross-sensitivity may exist with these agents. Diuresis and hypoglycemia have been reported rarely in patients receiving sulfonamides.

■ **Precautions and Contraindications** Co-trimoxazole shares the toxic potentials of sulfonamides and trimethoprim, and the usual precautions associated with therapy with these drugs should be observed. (See Cautions in the Sulfonamides General Statement 8:12.20 and see Cautions in Trimethoprim 8:36.) Fatalities, although rare, have occurred in patients receiving sulfonamides, secondary to severe reactions induced by the drugs, including Stevens-Johnson syndrome, toxic epidermal necrolysis, fulminant hepatic necrosis, agranulocytosis, aplastic anemia, and other blood dyscrasias. Such fatal reactions also have been reported when sulfonamides were used in fixed combination with other drugs (e.g., with trimethoprim or erythromycin). Although probably rare, the precise incidence of severe dermatologic, hematologic, and hepatic effects with these combinations, including co-trimoxazole, is not known. Patients receiving co-trimoxazole should be monitored appropriately for the possible occurrence of such potentially severe reactions, and the drug should be discontinued at the first sign of such a reaction. The development of rash, sore throat, fever, pallor, arthralgia, cough, shortness of breath, purpura, or jaundice may be an early sign of a serious adverse reaction.

Co-trimoxazole should be used with caution in patients with impaired renal or hepatic function, possible folate deficiency (e.g., geriatric individuals, chronic alcoholics, patients receiving anticonvulsants, malnourished patients, those with malabsorption syndrome), with severe allergy or bronchial asthma, or with possible folate or glucose-6-phosphate-dehydrogenase (G-6-PD) deficiency. Patients should be warned to report any early signs and symptoms of a serious hematologic disorder, including fever, sore throat, pallor, jaundice, or purpura. The manufacturers recommend that a complete blood count be obtained frequently in patients receiving co-trimoxazole, especially if signs and symptoms of blood disorders occur. The drug should be discontinued at the first appearance of rash or if any reduction in formed blood elements occurs. Leucovorin (folinic acid) should be administered if bone marrow depression occurs, especially if megaloblastic anemia, neutropenia, or thrombocytopenia occurs. Patients with acquired immunodeficiency syndrome (AIDS) who receive co-trimoxazole should be carefully monitored, since they appear to have a particularly high incidence of adverse reactions to the drug (especially fever and adverse dermatologic and hematologic reactions).

Urinalysis and careful microscopic examination of the urine should be performed in patients receiving co-trimoxazole, especially patients with impaired renal function. Patients receiving co-trimoxazole should be cautioned to maintain adequate fluid intake to prevent crystalluria and stone formation.

Co-trimoxazole should be used with caution in geriatric patients, particularly when complicating conditions (e.g., impaired renal and/or hepatic function, concomitant use of other drugs) are present, since these patients may have an increased risk of severe adverse reactions to the drug. Severe adverse dermatologic reactions, generalized bone marrow suppression, and a specific decrease in platelets (with or without purpura) are the most frequently reported severe adverse effects of the drug in geriatric patients. Co-trimoxazole also should be used with caution in patients with a history of hypersensitivity to sulfonamide-derivative drugs (e.g., acetazolamide, thiazides, tolbutamide), since cross-sensitivity may exist with these agents.

Commercially available formulations of co-trimoxazole for injection concentrate contain sodium metabisulfite, a sulfite that may cause allergic-type reactions, including anaphylaxis and life-threatening or less severe asthmatic episodes, in certain susceptible individuals. The overall prevalence of sulfite sensitivity in the general population is unknown and probably low; such sensitivity appears to occur more frequently in asthmatic than in nonasthmatic individuals.

Co-trimoxazole is contraindicated in patients with known hypersensitivity to trimethoprim or sulfonamides, with marked hepatic damage or severe renal impairment when renal function status cannot be monitored, or with documented megaloblastic anemia secondary to folate deficiency. However, cautious desensitization has been performed in some hypersensitive patients in whom co-trimoxazole therapy was considered necessary. The manufacturers recommend that the drug not be used in patients with creatinine clearances less than 15 mL/minute.

■ **Pediatric Precautions** The manufacturers of co-trimoxazole recommend that the drug *not* be used in infants younger than 2 months of age. Commercially available co-trimoxazole injections contain benzyl alcohol as a preservative. Although a causal relationship has not been established, administration of injections preserved with benzyl alcohol has been associated with toxicity in neonates. Toxicity appears to have resulted from administration of large amounts (i.e., about 100-400 mg/kg daily) of benzyl alcohol in these neonates. Safety and efficacy of repeated courses of co-trimoxazole therapy in children younger than 2 years of age, except those with documented *Pneumocystis* infections, have not been fully evaluated. Co-trimoxazole should be used with caution in children who have the fragile X chromosome associated with mental retardation, because folate depletion may worsen the psychomotor regression associated with the disorder.

■ **Mutagenicity and Carcinogenicity** Bacterial mutagenic studies have not been performed with co-trimoxazole. Trimethoprim did not exhibit mutagenic activity in the Ames test. No chromosomal damage was observed in cultured Chinese hamster ovary cells at concentrations approximately 500 times human plasma concentrations, but a low level of chromosomal damage was observed in some studies at concentrations approximately 1000 times human plasma concentrations. No chromosomal abnormalities were observed in human leukocytes cultured in vitro at trimethoprim concentrations up to 20 times human steady-state plasma concentrations. In addition, no chromosomal abnormalities were found in peripheral lymphocytes of patients receiving 320 mg of trimethoprim in combination with up to 1600 mg of sulfamethoxazole daily for as long as 112 weeks.

Long-term studies in animals to evaluate the carcinogenic potential of co-trimoxazole have not been performed.

■ **Pregnancy, Fertility, and Lactation** Trimethoprim and sulfamethoxazole, alone and in combination, have produced teratogenic effects, manifested principally as cleft palate, in some (but not all) studies in rats receiving dosages exceeding the usual human dosages. In addition, in some rabbit studies, an overall increase in fetal loss was associated with trimethoprim doses 6 times the usual human dose. Although there are no adequate and controlled studies to date in humans, studies in pregnant women suggest that the incidence of congenital abnormalities in those who received co-trimoxazole was similar to that in those who received a placebo; there were no abnormalities in 10 children whose mothers had received the drug during the first trimester. In one report, there were no congenital abnormalities in 35 children whose mothers had received co-trimoxazole at the time of conception or shortly thereafter. Because co-trimoxazole crosses the placenta and may interfere with folic acid metabolism, the drug should be used during pregnancy only when the potential benefits justify the possible risks to the fetus. Because sulfonamides may cause kernicterus in neonates, the manufacturers state that use of co-trimoxazole in pregnant women is contraindicated.

The effect of co-trimoxazole on fertility in humans is not known. Reproduction studies in rats using oral trimethoprim (as co-trimoxazole) dosages up to 70 mg/kg daily have not revealed evidence of impaired fertility.

Co-trimoxazole is distributed into milk. Because co-trimoxazole may interfere with folic acid metabolism, the drug should be used in nursing women only if the potential benefits justify the possible risks to the infant. Because sulfonamides may cause kernicterus in infants younger than 2 months of age, a decision should be made whether to discontinue nursing or co-trimoxazole or to use an alternative drug, taking into account the importance of co-trimoxazole to the woman.

Drug Interactions

■ **Warfarin** Co-trimoxazole may prolong the prothrombin time (PT) of patients receiving concomitant warfarin by inhibiting metabolic clearance of warfarin. If co-trimoxazole is used with warfarin, dosage of warfarin and PT must be monitored carefully.

■ **Other Drugs** Because co-trimoxazole possesses anti-folate properties, the drug could theoretically increase the incidence of folate deficiencies induced by other drugs such as phenytoin when used concomitantly. Co-trimoxazole inhibits the metabolism of phenytoin. Concomitant administration of usual dosages of co-trimoxazole and phenytoin can increase the half-life of phenytoin by 39% and decrease metabolic clearance rate of phenytoin by 27%. If the drugs are administered concomitantly, the possibility of an increase in effects associated with phenytoin should be considered.

Co-trimoxazole should be used with caution in patients receiving methotrexate, since sulfonamides can displace methotrexate from plasma protein-binding sites resulting in increased free methotrexate concentrations.

Marked but reversible nephrotoxicity has been reported in renal transplant recipients receiving co-trimoxazole together with cyclosporine.

Increases in serum digoxin concentrations can occur in patients receiving co-trimoxazole; this interaction is more likely to occur in geriatric patients. Serum digoxin concentrations should be monitored in patients receiving digoxin and co-trimoxazole.

Increased plasma sulfamethoxazole concentration may occur in patients receiving indomethacin.

Megaloblastic anemia has been reported in patients receiving co-trimoxazole and pyrimethamine dosages exceeding 25 mg weekly (for malaria prophylaxis).

Concomitant administration of tricyclic antidepressants and co-trimoxazole may decrease the efficacy of the antidepressant.

Like other sulfonamides, co-trimoxazole potentiates the effect of oral hypoglycemic agents.

Toxic delirium has been reported in one individual following administration of co-trimoxazole and amantadine.

Acute Toxicity

■ **Manifestations** Overdosage with co-trimoxazole may produce symptoms of nausea, vomiting, diarrhea, mental depression, confusion, facial swelling, headache, bone marrow depression, and slight elevations of serum aminotransferases (transaminases).

■ **Treatment** In acute overdosage with oral co-trimoxazole, the stomach should be emptied immediately by inducing emesis or by lavage. Supportive and symptomatic treatment should be initiated. Patients should be monitored with blood counts and other appropriate laboratory studies (e.g., serum electrolyte concentrations). Hemodialysis may remove only moderate amounts of the drug; peritoneal dialysis is not effective in enhancing the elimination of co-trimoxazole.

Mechanism of Action

Co-trimoxazole usually is bactericidal. Of its components, sulfamethoxazole is bacteriostatic and trimethoprim usually is bactericidal. Co-trimoxazole acts by sequentially inhibiting enzymes of the folic acid pathway; sulfamethoxazole inhibits the formation of dihydrofolic acid from *p*-aminobenzoic acid and, by inhibiting dihydrofolate reductase, trimethoprim inhibits the formation of tetrahydrofolic acid from dihydrofolic acid. By inhibiting synthesis of tetrahydrofolic acid, the metabolically active form of folic acid, co-trimoxazole inhibits bacterial thymidine synthesis.

Sequential inhibition by co-trimoxazole of two steps in the folic acid pathway appears to be responsible for the antibacterial synergism of the trimethoprim-sulfamethoxazole combination. For most organisms, optimum synergistic antibacterial action occurs in vitro at a trimethoprim:sulfamethoxazole ratio of about 1:20, which is also the approximate peak serum concentration ratio of the 2 drugs achieved following oral or IV administration of co-trimoxazole. Synergistic activity also has been observed in vitro at trimethoprim:sulfamethoxazole ratios of 1:1–1:40.

Susceptibility of organisms to trimethoprim usually is more critical to the efficacy of co-trimoxazole than is susceptibility to sulfamethoxazole. Many organisms that are resistant to sulfamethoxazole but susceptible or only moderately susceptible to trimethoprim will show synergistic antibacterial response to co-trimoxazole. However, for *Neisseria gonorrhoeae*, susceptibility to sulfamethoxazole is required for antibacterial response to co-trimoxazole.

Spectrum

■ **In Vitro Susceptibility Testing** For most organisms, inoculum size may influence the result of in vitro co-trimoxazole susceptibility tests. Accurate in vitro susceptibility testing requires that thymidine *not* be present in the growth medium or that the medium be supplemented with thymidine phosphorylase to inactivate any thymidine that might be present.

The Clinical and Laboratory Standards Institute (CLSI; formerly National Committee for Clinical Laboratory Standards [NCCLS]) states that, if results of in vitro susceptibility testing indicate that a clinical isolate is *susceptible* to co-trimoxazole, then an infection caused by this strain may be appropriately treated with the dosage of the drug recommended for that type of infection and infecting species, unless otherwise contraindicated. If results indicate that a clinical isolate has *intermediate susceptibility* to co-trimoxazole, then the strain has a minimum inhibitory concentration (MIC) that approaches usually attainable blood and tissue concentrations and response rates may be lower than for strains identified as susceptible. Therefore, the intermediate category implies clinical applicability in body sites where the drug is physiologically concentrated or when a high dosage of the drug can be used. This intermediate category also includes a buffer zone which should prevent small, uncontrolled technical factors from causing major discrepancies in interpretation, especially for drugs with narrow pharmacotoxicity margins. If results of in vitro susceptibility testing indicate that a clinical isolate is *resistant* to co-trimoxazole, the strain is not inhibited by systemic concentrations of the drug achievable with normal dosage schedules and/or MICs fall in the range where specific microbial resistance mechanisms are likely and efficacy has not been reliable in clinical studies.

Disk Susceptibility Tests When the disk-diffusion procedure is used for susceptibility testing, a 1.25-mcg trimethoprim/23.75-mcg sulfamethoxazole disk should be used.

When the disk-diffusion susceptibility test is performed according to CLSI standardized procedures, Enterobacteriaceae, *Pseudomonas aeruginosa*, *Acinetobacter*, or *Staphylococci* with growth inhibition zones of 16 mm or greater are susceptible to co-trimoxazole, those with zones of 11–15 mm have intermediate susceptibility, and those with zones of 10 mm or less are resistant to the drug.

When disk-diffusion susceptibility testing is performed according to CLSI standardized procedures using *Haemophilus* test medium (HTM), *Haemophilus* with growth inhibition zones of 16 mm or greater are susceptible to co-trimoxazole, those with zones of 11–15 mm have intermediate susceptibility, and those with zones of 10 mm or less are resistant to the drug.

When testing susceptibility of *S. pneumoniae* according to CLSI standardized procedures using Mueller-Hinton agar (supplemented with 5% defibrinated sheep blood), *S. pneumoniae* with growth inhibition zones of 19 mm or greater are susceptible to co-trimoxazole, those with zones of 16–18 mm have intermediate susceptibility, and those with zones of 15 mm or less are resistant to the drug.

When the disk diffusion procedure is performed according to CLSI standardized procedures, *Vibrio cholerae* with growth inhibition zones of 16 mm or greater are susceptible to co-trimoxazole, those with zones of 11–15 mm have intermediate susceptibility, and those with zones of 10 mm or less are resistant to the drug.

Dilution Susceptibility Tests When dilution susceptibility testing (agar or broth dilution) is performed according to CLSI standardized procedures, Enterobacteriaceae, *Ps. aeruginosa*, other non-Enterobacteriaceae gram-negative bacilli (e.g., *Acinetobacter*, *Stenotrophomonas maltophilia*, other *Pseudomonas* spp), or *Staphylococcus* with MICs equal to or less than 2 mcg/mL of trimethoprim and 38 mcg/mL of sulfamethoxazole are susceptible to co-trimoxazole and those with MICs equal to or greater than 4 mcg/mL of trimethoprim and 76 mcg/mL of sulfamethoxazole are resistant to the drug.

When dilution susceptibility testing for *Haemophilus* is performed according to CLSI standardized procedures using HTM, *Haemophilus* with MICs equal to or less than 0.5 mcg/mL of trimethoprim and 9.5 mcg/mL of sulfamethoxazole are susceptible to co-trimoxazole and those with MICs equal to or greater than 4 mcg/mL of trimethoprim and 76 mcg/mL of sulfamethoxazole are resistant to the drug. *Haemophilus* with an MIC of 1–2 mcg/mL of trimethoprim and 19–38 mcg/mL of sulfamethoxazole have intermediate susceptibility to co-trimoxazole. These same interpretive criteria are used when dilution susceptibility testing for *S. pneumoniae* is performed according to CLSI standardized procedures using cation-adjusted Mueller-Hinton broth (with 2–5% lysed horse blood).

When dilution susceptibility testing is performed according to CLSI standardized procedures, *V. cholerae* with MICs equal to or less than 2 mcg/mL of trimethoprim and 38 mcg/mL of sulfamethoxazole are susceptible to co-trimoxazole and those with MICs of 4 mcg/mL or greater of trimethoprim and 76 mcg/mL or greater are resistant to the drug.

■ **Gram-positive Aerobic Bacteria** In vitro, when the optimum 1:20 synergistic ratio of trimethoprim:sulfamethoxazole is used, trimethoprim concentrations of 0.05–0.15 mcg/mL and sulfamethoxazole concentrations of 0.95–2.85 mcg/mL inhibit most strains of *Streptococcus pneumoniae*. Many strains of *Staphylococcus aureus*, group A β-hemolytic streptococci (*Streptococcus pyogenes*), and *Nocardia* also are susceptible to co-trimoxazole. Some strains of enterococci, including some *E. faecalis* (formerly *Streptococcus faecalis*), are not susceptible to the drug; to accurately determine susceptibility of enterococci to co-trimoxazole, the growth medium must be free of thymidine and other sources of exogenous folate. Some group A β-hemolytic streptococci may not respond to co-trimoxazole in tonsillopharyngeal infections, possibly because of inadequate concentrations of the drug in this area.

Bacillus anthracis strains with in vitro resistance to sulfamethoxazole or trimethoprim have been reported, and these anti-infectives should not be used in the treatment of *B. anthracis* infections (i.e., anthrax).

■ **Gram-negative Aerobic Bacteria** Co-trimoxazole is active in vitro against common gram-negative bacteria associated with urinary tract infections, including most Enterobacteriaceae. The drug is not active against *Pseudomonas aeruginosa*.

Generally, co-trimoxazole is active in vitro against most of the following Enterobacteriaceae: *Acinetobacter*, *Enterobacter*, *Escherichia coli*, *Klebsiella pneumoniae*, *Proteus mirabilis*, *Salmonella*, and *Shigella*. When the optimum 1:20 synergistic ratio of trimethoprim:sulfamethoxazole is used in vitro, the MIC for most of these organisms is 1.5 mcg/mL or less of trimethoprim; for sulfamethoxazole, MICs for *P. mirabilis, Shigella,* and *Salmonella* generally are 2.85 mcg/mL or less, for *E. coli* are 9.5 mcg/mL or less, and for *Klebsiella* and *Enterobacter* are 28.5 mcg/mL or less. Co-trimoxazole also is active in vitro against *Haemophilus influenzae* (including ampicillin-resistant strains), *H. ducreyi*, and *Neisseria gonorrhoeae*.Approximately 70% of indole-positive *Proteus* and 50% of *Providencia* and *Serratia* strains are susceptible to co-trimoxazole.

■ **Anaerobic Bacteria** Co-trimoxazole generally is considered inactive against most strains of *Bacteroides*, and appears to have no activity against strict anaerobes (e.g., *Clostridium*).

■ **Protozoa** Co-trimoxazole is active in vitro and in vivo against *Pneumocystis jiroveci* (formerly *Pneumocystis carinii*).

Resistance

In vitro, resistance develops more slowly to co-trimoxazole than to trimethoprim or sulfamethoxazole alone.

Use of sulfamethoxazole alone results in rapid selection of sulfonamide-resistant fecal coliforms. As many as 50% of hospital-isolated and 20% of community-isolated *Escherichia coli* are resistant to sulfonamides, including sulfamethoxazole. Resistance to sulfamethoxazole in gram-negative bacteria is usually plasmid mediated. In many organisms (e.g., *E. coli, Neisseria meningitis, Streptococcus pneumoniae, Plasmodium falciparum*), point mutations in conserved regions of dihydropteroate synthase (DHPS), an essential enzyme for folate biosynthesis, confer sulfonamide resistance. Mutations in DHPS also have been identified in *Pneumocystis carinii* isolates obtained from HIV-infected patients, including some patients who had not previously received a sulfonamide, and these mutations are being reported with increasing frequency in this organism. It is unclear whether DHPS mutations in *P. carinii* are associated with resistance to co-trimoxazole since *P. carinii* pneumonia has been effectively treated with co-trimoxazole in some patients despite the presence of DHPS mutants. However, there is some evidence from a study in HIV-infected patients with *P. carinii* pneumonia that presence of strains with DHPS mutations may be associated with decreased survival. Resistance to trimethoprim has been shown to occur by several mechanisms, most often chromosomally mediated, but also rarely involving mutation of bacteria to thymidine-dependent strains or plasmid-mediated resistance involving altered production or sensitivity of bacterial dihydrofolate reductase. Plasmid-mediated resistance to trimethoprim has been shown to be transferable among some bacterial strains; plasmid-mediated resistance to trimethoprim usually results in concomitant coding for sulfonamide resistance. Thymidine-dependent strains account for less than 1% of trimethoprim resistance, and chromosomal- and plasmid-mediated resistance accounts for approximately 90% and 10% of reported resistant strains, respectively.

Resistant strains of Enterobacteriaceae, especially *E. coli, Klebsiella,* and *Proteus,* have occurred during therapy with co-trimoxazole. Strains of *Klebsiella* and *Proteus* that are only moderately susceptible to co-trimoxazole in vitro at the beginning of therapy appear to be especially likely to develop resistance during therapy. The incidence of trimethoprim resistance among Enterobacteriaceae in fecal flora and associated with urinary tract infections has been reported to range from 8–38% in some hospitals and to range from 30–100% among fecal Enterobacteriaceae following 2 weeks of co-trimoxazole therapy. In a study in Mexico, more than 95% of fecal *E. coli* resistant to trimethoprim also were resistant to sulfamethoxazole, but the resistant strains were not associated with clinical infection. Strains of Enterobacteriaceae and *S. pneumoniae* resistant to trimethoprim, but sensitive to sulfonamides and penicillin, respectively, have been reported.

Although co-trimoxazole previously was considered nearly uniformly active against *H. influenzae*, resistant strains have been reported rarely. In a national collaborative study of *H. influenzae* isolates from 1986, the incidence of co-trimoxazole resistance was about 1%, including several strains that also were resistant to ampicillin (β-lactamase mediated), chloramphenicol, and tetracycline.

Pharmacokinetics

■ **Absorption** The fixed-combination preparation containing trimethoprim and sulfamethoxazole (co-trimoxazole) is rapidly and well absorbed from the GI tract. Peak serum concentrations of 1–2 mcg/mL of trimethoprim and 40–60 mcg/mL of unbound sulfamethoxazole are reached 1–4 hours after a single oral dose of co-trimoxazole containing 160 mg of trimethoprim and 800 mg of sulfamethoxazole. Following multiple-dose oral administration, steady-state peak serum concentrations usually are 50% greater than those obtained after single-dose administration of the drug. Following oral administration of the fixed-ratio combination preparation, the trimethoprim:sulfamethoxazole ratio of mean steady-state serum concentrations usually is about 1:20.

Mean peak steady-state serum concentrations of approximately 9 and 105 mcg/mL of trimethoprim and sulfamethoxazole, respectively, are reached after IV infusion of 160 mg of trimethoprim and 800 mg of sulfamethoxazole every 8 hours in adults with normal renal function. Steady-state trough concentrations reached with this IV dose are approximately 6 mcg/mL of trimethoprim and 70 mcg/mL of sulfamethoxazole.

■ **Distribution** Both trimethoprim and sulfamethoxazole are widely distributed into body tissues and fluids, including sputum, aqueous humor, middle ear fluid, prostatic fluid, vaginal fluid, bile, and CSF; trimethoprim also distributes into bronchial secretions. Trimethoprim has a larger volume of distribution (V_d) than does sulfamethoxazole. In adults, apparent V_ds of 100–120 and 12–18 L have been reported for trimethoprim and sulfamethoxazole, respectively. In patients with uninflamed meninges, trimethoprim and sulfamethoxazole concentrations in CSF are about 50 and 40%, respectively, of concurrent serum concentrations of the drugs. Trimethoprim and sulfamethoxazole concentrations in middle ear fluid are approximately 75 and 20%, respectively, and in prostatic fluid are approximately 200 and 35%, respectively, of concurrent serum concentrations of the drugs.

Trimethoprim is approximately 44% and sulfamethoxazole is approximately 70% bound to plasma proteins.

Both trimethoprim and sulfamethoxazole readily crosses the placenta. Amniotic fluid concentrations of trimethoprim and sulfamethoxazole are reported to be 80 and 50%, respectively, of concurrent maternal serum concentrations. Both trimethoprim and sulfamethoxazole is distributed into milk. Trimethoprim and sulfamethoxazole concentrations in milk are approximately 125 and 10%, respectively, of concurrent maternal serum concentrations.

■ **Elimination** Trimethoprim and sulfamethoxazole have serum half-lives of approximately 8–11 and 10–13 hours, respectively, in adults with normal renal function. In adults with creatinine clearances of 10–30 and 0–10 mL/minute, serum half-life of trimethoprim may increase to 15 and greater than 26 hours, respectively. In adults with chronic renal failure, sulfamethoxazole half-life may be 3 times that in patients with normal renal function. Trimethoprim serum half-lives of about 7.7 and 5.5 hours have been reported in children less than 1 year of age and between 1 and 10 years of age, respectively.

Both trimethoprim and sulfamethoxazole are metabolized in the liver. Trimethoprim is metabolized to oxide and hydroxylated metabolites and sulfamethoxazole is principally *N*-acetylated and also conjugated with glucuronic acid. Both drugs are rapidly excreted in urine via glomerular filtration and tubular secretion. In adults with normal renal function, approximately 50–60% of a trimethoprim and 45–70% of a sulfamethoxazole oral dose are excreted in urine within 24 hours. Approximately 80% of the amount of trimethoprim and 20% of the amount of sulfamethoxazole recovered in urine are unchanged drug. In adults with normal renal function, urinary concentrations of active trimethoprim are approximately equal to those of active sulfamethoxazole. Urinary concentrations of both active drugs are decreased in patients with impaired renal function.

Only small amounts of trimethoprim are excreted in feces via biliary elimination. Trimethoprim and active sulfamethoxazole are moderately removed by hemodialysis.

Chemistry and Stability

■ **Chemistry** Co-trimoxazole is a fixed combination of sulfamethoxazole and trimethoprim. Sulfamethoxazole is an intermediate-acting antibacterial sulfonamide. Both sulfamethoxazole and trimethoprim are synthetic folate-antagonist anti-infectives. Co-trimoxazole contains a 5:1 ratio of sulfamethoxazole to trimethoprim. Potency of co-trimoxazole is expressed in terms of the trimethoprim content.

Trimethoprim occurs as white to cream-colored, bitter-tasting, odorless crystals or crystalline powder and sulfamethoxazole occurs as a white to off-white, practically odorless, crystalline powder. Sodium hydroxide is added during manufacture of co-trimoxazole for injection concentrate to adjust pH to 10. Co-trimoxazole oral suspension has a pH of 5–6.5.

■ **Stability** Co-trimoxazole for injection concentrate should be stored at 15–25°C or 15–30°C, depending on the formulation (the manufacturers' recommendations should be followed) and should *not* be refrigerated. Oral suspensions of the drug should be stored in tight, light-resistant containers at 15–25 or 15–30°C, depending on the formulation (the manufacturers' recommendations should be followed), and the tablets should be stored in well-closed, light-resistant containers at 15–30°C.

Co-trimoxazole for injection concentrate is physically and chemically compatible with IV solutions of 5% dextrose; admixed solutions of co-trimoxazole in 5% dextrose that are cloudy or contain a precipitate should be discarded. Because of the potential for incompatibility, the manufacturers state that co-trimoxazole IV solutions should not be admixed with other drugs or solutions other than 5% dextrose. Specialized references should be consulted for specific compatibility information.

Co-trimoxazole solutions containing 0.64 mg of trimethoprim and 3.2 mg of sulfamethoxazole per mL of 5% dextrose (1:25 dilution) are stable for 6 hours at room temperature. Co-trimoxazole solutions containing 0.64–0.8 mg of trimethoprim and 3.2–4 mg of sulfamethoxazole per mL of 5% dextrose (1:20 dilution) are stable for 4 hours at room temperature. Co-trimoxazole solutions containing 0.8–1.1 mg of trimethoprim and 4–5.3 mg of sulfamethoxazole per mL of 5% dextrose (1:15 dilution) are stable for 2 hours at room temperature. Co-trimoxazole solutions in 5% dextrose should not be refrigerated. Prior to infusion, solutions of the drug should be inspected visually and discarded if there is evidence of crystallization or cloudiness.

Following initial entry into a multiple-dose vial of co-trimoxazole for injection concentrate, the manufacturers recommend that the contents be used within 48 hours.

Preparations

Excipients in commercially available drug preparations may have clinically important effects in some individuals; consult specific product labeling for details.

Co-trimoxazole

Oral		
Suspension	Trimethoprim 40 mg/5 mL and Sulfamethoxazole 200 mg/5 mL*	**Septra® Suspension,** Monarch
		Septra® Grape Suspension, Monarch
		Sulfatrim® Pediatric Suspension, Actavis
		Sulfatrim® Suspension, Actavis, United Research
Tablets	Trimethoprim 80 mg and Sulfamethoxazole 400 mg*	**Bactrim®** (scored), Women First HealthCare
		Septra®, Monarch
		Sulfamethoxazole and Trimethoprim Tablets
	Trimethoprim 160 mg and Sulfamethoxazole 800 mg*	**Bactrim® DS,** Women First HealthCare
		Septra® DS, Monarch
Parenteral		
For injection concentrate, for IV infusion	Trimethoprim 16 mg/mL and Sulfamethoxazole 80 mg/mL	**Sulfamethoxazole and Trimethoprim Concentrate for Injection**

*available from one or more manufacturer, distributor, and/or repackager by generic (nonproprietary) name

†Use is not currently included in the labeling approved by the US Food and Drug Administration

TETRACYCLINES 8:12.24

Tetracyclines General Statement

■ Tetracyclines are antibiotics and semisynthetic antibiotic derivatives obtained from cultures of *Streptomyces*.

Uses

Tetracyclines are used principally in the treatment of infections caused by susceptible *Rickettsia*, *Chlamydia*, *Mycoplasma*, and a variety of *uncommon* gram-negative and gram-positive bacteria. Because of the development of resistance, tetracyclines are rarely used for the treatment of infections caused by *common* gram-negative or gram-positive bacteria unless other appropriate anti-infectives are contraindicated or are ineffective and in vitro susceptibility tests indicate that the causative organisms are susceptible to the drugs.

Generally, given a susceptible organism, the currently available tetracyclines are all equally effective when administered in appropriate dosages. Because minocycline and, to a lesser extent, doxycycline penetrate most body tissues and fluids better than do other currently available tetracyclines, some clinicians prefer these derivatives in the treatment of infections of the CNS, eye, or prostate. Because of poor CNS penetration, none of the currently available tetracyclines should be used in the treatment of meningitis. Doxycycline generally is the preferred derivative when a tetracycline is indicated in patients with impaired renal function. Because of its low renal clearance, doxycycline may not be as effective as other currently available tetracyclines for the treatment of urinary tract infections in patients with normal or impaired renal function.

■ **Rickettsial Infections** Tetracyclines are used for the treatment of rickettsial infections. The US Centers for Disease Control and Prevention (CDC) and other clinicians state that doxycycline is the preferred tetracycline for the treatment of most rickettsial infections, including spotted fevers (Rocky Mountain spotted fever [RMSF], Mediterranean spotted fever, African tick-bite fever, Queensland tick typhus, North Asian tick fever, oriental spotted fever, rickettsialpox, cat flea typhus), typhus fever (e.g., epidemic typhus, murine typhus) and the typhus group, Q fever, rickettsialpox, ehrlichiosis, Sennetsu fever, and other tick fevers caused by rickettsiae. Although tetracyclines are not usually used in children younger than 8 years of age, doxycycline is recommended by the CDC and American Academy of Pediatrics (AAP) as the drug of choice for presumed or confirmed Rickettsial infections (including RMSF) in children of any age. (See Cautions: Pediatric Precautions.)

Because a delay in treatment can result in severe disease and fatal outcome, treatment of patients with suspected rickettsial disease should be initiated promptly based on clinical and epidemiologic evidence pending laboratory confirmation. An infectious disease or tropical medicine specialist should be consulted. IV therapy generally is indicated for hospitalized patients and oral therapy generally is appropriate for those with early disease, outpatients, or hospitalized patients who are not vomiting or obtunded. Treatment usually is continued for at least 5–10 days and until the patient is afebrile for 3 days or more and clinically improved. Severe illness may require a longer duration of therapy.

Q Fever Although doxycycline alone usually is the drug of choice for the treatment of acute Q fever caused by *Coxiella burnetii*, doxycycline has been used in conjunction with hydroxychloroquine or a fluoroquinolone (e.g., levofloxacin, ofloxacin) for the treatment of Q fever endocarditis. In one limited study in patients with confirmed *C. burnetii* infection and chronic endocarditis, a regimen of doxycycline and hydroxychloroquine was associated with a lower relapse rate than a regimen of doxycycline and ofloxacin. Although both regimens require long-term therapy, the mean duration of therapy for cured patients was 55 months for those who received the doxycycline/quinolone regimen compared with 31 months for those who received the doxycycline/hydroxychloroquine regimen. Prolonged therapy (at least 18 months) with the doxycycline and hydroxychloroquine regimen is necessary to prevent relapse. The CDC recommends a 2- to 3-week regimen of doxycycline for the treatment of acute Q fever, a 1-year regimen of doxycycline and hydroxychloroquine for the treatment of acute Q fever in patients with preexisting valvular heart disease (to prevent progression of acute disease to endocarditis), and a 1.5- to 3-year regimen of doxycycline and hydroxychloroquine for the treatment of chronic Q fever.

It has been suggested that tetracycline may be effective as prophylaxis against Q fever† and may prevent clinical disease if initiated 8–12 days after exposure; however, such prophylaxis is not effective and may only prolong the onset of disease if given immediately (1–7 days) after exposure.

■ **Chlamydial Infections** Tetracyclines are highly effective in the treatment of most chlamydial infections, including urogenital infections caused by *Chlamydia trachomatis*, respiratory tract infections caused by *Chlamydophila pneumoniae* (formerly *Chlamydia pneumoniae*), respiratory tract infections caused by *C. psittaci* (psittacosis), and lymphogranuloma venereum caused by invasive serovars of *C. trachomatis*.

Urogenital Chlamydial Infections in Adults and Adolescents For the treatment of urogenital chlamydial infections in adults and adolescents, the CDC and other clinicians recommend a single dose of oral azithromycin or a 7-day regimen of oral doxycycline. Alternatively, adults and adolescents with urogenital chlamydial infections can receive a 7-day oral regimen of tetracycline, erythromycin base, erythromycin ethylsuccinate, ofloxacin, levofloxacin, or amoxicillin. Results of clinical studies indicate that the single-dose azithromycin and multi-dose doxycycline regimen are equally effective for the treatment of urogenital chlamydial infections when patients are compliant and follow-up encouraged; however, if poor compliance or inability to provide follow-up are a concern, azithromycin may be more cost-effective since the single-dose regimen can be administered under direct supervision. Erythromycin is less effective than either azithromycin or doxycycline and GI effects associated with the drug may discourage patient compliance with the regimen. To maximize compliance with 7-day regimens, the CDC recommends that the drugs be dispensed on site and that the first dose be taken under supervision. Since the azithromycin and doxycycline regimens are highly effective, a test of cure probably is unnecessary in patients who receive one of these regimens unless symptoms persist or reinfection is suspected; however, a test of cure should be considered 3 weeks after completion of an erythromycin regimen. Some studies have demonstrated high rates of infection among women retested for chlamydia after treatment, presumably because of reinfection. In some populations (e.g., adolescents), rescreening women several months after treatment might be effective for detecting further morbidity.

Patients being treated for chlamydial infection should be instructed to refer their sexual partner(s) for evaluation and treatment, and to abstain from sexual intercourse for 7 days after single-dose therapy or until completion of a 7-day regimen. In addition, to minimize the risk of reinfection, patients should be instructed to abstain from sexual intercourse until after all their sexual partners are cured. Although the CDC acknowledges that the exposure intervals are somewhat arbitrary, they recommend that individuals who had sexual contact with the chlamydia patient within 60 days before the onset of symptoms or diagnosis in the patient should be evaluated and treated. If the patient reports that the last sexual contact occurred more than 60 days prior to the onset of symptoms or diagnosis, their most recent sexual partner should be treated.

Individuals with HIV infection who also are infected with chlamydia should receive the same treatment regimens recommended for other individuals with chlamydial infections.

Urogenital Chlamydial Infections in Children For the treatment of urogenital chlamydial infections in children who weigh less than 45 kg, the CDC recommends a 14-day regimen of oral erythromycin base or ethylsuccinate. For the treatment of urogenital chlamydial infections in children younger than 8 years of age who weigh at least 45 kg, the CDC recommends a single dose of oral azithromycin; for those 8 years of age and older, the CDC recommends either a single dose of azithromycin or a 7-day regimen of oral doxycycline.

Presumptive Treatment of Chlamydial Infections in Patients with Gonorrhea Patients infected with *N. gonorrhoeae* frequently also have coexisting chlamydial and mycoplasmal infection; however, cephalosporins, spectinomycin, and most quinolone regimens used for the treatment of gonorrhea are ineffective for the treatment of these infections. Because of the risks associated with untreated coexisting chlamydial infection, the CDC and most clinicians recommend that patients being treated for uncomplicated gonorrhea or disseminated gonococcal infection also receive an anti-infective regimen effective for presumptive treatment of uncomplicated urogenital chlamydial infection. For presumptive treatment of chlamydia in adults and adolescents being treated for uncomplicated or disseminated gonococcal infections, the CDC and others recommend use of a single dose of oral azithromycin or a 7-day regimen of oral doxycycline.

The strategy of routine administration of a regimen effective against chlamydia in patients being treated for gonococcal infection has been recommended by the CDC for more than 10 years and appears to have resulted in substantial decreases in the prevalence of urogenital chlamydial infection in some populations. In addition, since most *N. gonorrhoeae* isolated in the US are susceptible to doxycycline and azithromycin, dual therapy possible may delay the development of resistance in *N. gonorrhoeae*. Since the cost of presumptive treatment of chlamydia is less than the cost of testing for presence of chlamydia, routine dual therapy without chlamydial testing can be cost-effective for populations in which coinfection with chlamydia has been reported in 10–30% of patients with *N. gonorrhoeae* infection. In areas where the rate of coinfection with chlamydia is low and chlamydial testing is widely available, some clinicians may prefer to test for chlamydia rather than treat presumptively; however, presumptive treatment is indicated for patients who may not return for test results.

Trachoma and Inclusion Conjunctivitis An oral tetracycline (with or without a topical tetracycline, topical erythromycin, or topical sulfacetamide) is used for the treatment of trachoma and inclusion conjunctivitis caused by *C. trachomatis* in adults and children older than 8 years of age; however, anti-infective therapy may not eliminate *C. trachomatis* in all cases of chronic trachoma. Inclusion conjunctivitis and trachoma in younger children and neonates and chlamydial infections in pregnant women generally are treated with oral or IV erythromycin.

Lymphogranuloma Venereum Doxycycline generally is considered the drug of choice for the treatment of lymphogranuloma venereum caused by invasive serotypes of *C. trachomatis* (serovars L1, L2, L3), and oral erythromycin is considered an alternative regimen for the treatment of the disease. Some clinicians suggest that tetracycline can be used as an alternative to doxycycline. Erythromycin is the preferred regimen for the treatment of lymphogranuloma venereum in pregnant and lactating women. Effective treatment cures the infection and prevents ongoing tissue damage, although tissue reaction can result in scarring. Aspiration of buboes or incision and drainage may be necessary to prevent the formation of inguinal/femoral ulcerations.

The CDC recommends that individuals who had sexual contact with the lymphogranuloma venereum patient should be examined, tested for urethral or cervical chlamydial infection, and treated with a standard chlamydia regimen (single 1-g dose of azithromycin or 7-day regimen of oral doxycycline 100 mg twice daily) if they had sexual contact with the patient within 60 days prior to onset of symptoms in the patient.

While HIV-infected individuals with lymphogranuloma venereum should receive the same treatment regimens recommended for other patients, there is some evidence that HIV-infected patients may require more prolonged therapy and resolution may be delayed.

Psittacosis Tetracyclines are the drugs of choice for the treatment of *C. psittaci* infections (psittacosis, ornithosis); erythromycin or chloramphenicol is recommended for the treatment of psittacosis when tetracyclines are contraindicated. The CDC states that most individuals with psittacosis respond to an oral regimen of doxycycline or tetracycline hydrochloride. A regimen of IV doxycycline hyclate may be indicated for initial treatment of severely ill patients. Remission of symptoms usually is evident within 48–72 hours, but treatment should be continued for at least 10–14 days after fever abates since relapse can occur.

■ **Nongonococcal Urethritis** While *C. trachomatis* is a frequent cause of nongonococcal urethritis, these infections can be caused by *Ureaplasma urealyticum* or *Mycoplasma genitalium*; *Trichomonas vaginalis* and herpes simplex virus (HSV) also are possible causes of nongonococcal urethritis. The CDC currently considers a single oral dose of azithromycin or a 7-day regimen of oral doxycycline the regimens of choice for the treatment of nongonococcal urethritis. Alternative regimens recommended by the CDC are a 7-day regimen of oral erythromycin base or ethylsuccinate or a 7-day regimen of oral ofloxacin or levofloxacin. Patients with persistent or recurrent urethritis who were not compliant with the treatment regimen or were reexposed to untreated sexual partner(s) should be retreated with the initial regimen. If the patient has recurrent and persistent urethritis, was compliant with the anti-infective regimen, and reexposure can be excluded, the CDC recommends retreatment with a single 1-g dose of oral azithromycin and a 2-g dose of oral metronidazole or oral tinidazole.

■ **Granuloma Inguinale (Donovanosis)** Tetracyclines are drugs of choice for the treatment of granuloma inguinale (donovanosis), caused by *Klebsiella granulomatis* (formerly *Calymmatobacterium granulomatis*). The CDC recommends that donovanosis be treated with a regimen of oral doxycycline or, alternatively, a regimen of oral azithromycin, oral ciprofloxacin, oral erythromycin, or oral co-trimoxazole. Anti-infective treatment of donovanosis should be continued until all lesions have healed completely; a minimum of 3 weeks of treatment usually is necessary. If lesions do not respond within the first few days of therapy, the CDC recommends that a parenteral aminoglycoside (e.g., 1 mg/kg of gentamicin IV every 8 hours) be added to the regimen. Erythromycin is recommended for the treatment of donovanosis in pregnant and lactating women; addition of a parenteral aminoglycoside (e.g., gentamicin) to the regimen should be strongly considered in these women. Anti-infective treatment appears to halt progressive destruction of tissue, although prolonged duration of therapy often is required to enable granulation and re-epithelization of ulcers. Despite effective anti-infective therapy, donovanosis may relapse 6–18 months later.

Individuals with HIV infection should receive the same treatment regimens recommended for other individuals with donovanosis; however, the CDC suggests that addition of a parenteral aminoglycoside to the regimen should be strongly considered in HIV-infected patients.

■ **Pelvic Inflammatory Disease** Doxycycline is used in conjunction with other anti-infectives for the treatment of acute pelvic inflammatory disease† (PID).

One parenteral regimen recommended by the CDC and other clinicians for the treatment of PID in adults and adolescents is a 2-drug regimen of IV cefoxitin or IV cefotetan given in conjunction with oral or IV doxycycline. The parenteral regimen may be discontinued 24 hours after there is clinical improvement and oral doxycycline is then continued to complete 14 days of therapy. Because oral and IV doxycycline have similar bioavailabilities, the CDC states that either may be used for the initial phase of treatment. When tubo-ovarian abscess is present, some clinicians use clindamycin or metronidazole in addition to oral doxycycline to complete 14 days of therapy since this provides more effective anaerobic coverage.

In another parenteral regimen recommended by the CDC and others for the treatment of PID, an initial regimen of IV clindamycin and IV or IM gentamicin is given. The parenteral regimen is discontinued 24 hours after there is clinical improvement and oral doxycycline is used to complete 14 days of therapy; however, if tubo-ovarian abscess is present, some clinicians substitute oral clindamycin instead of oral doxycycline for follow-up after the initial parenteral regimen. An alternative parenteral regimen recommended by the CDC for the treatment of PID is IV ampicillin and sulbactam given in conjunction with oral or IV doxycycline; this regimen has good coverage against *C. trachomatis*, *N. gonorrhoeae*, and anaerobes and is effective for patients with tubo-ovarian abscess.

When an oral regimen is used for the treatment of PID in adults or adolescents, the CDC and many clinicians recommend use of a single IM dose of ceftriaxone, cefoxitin (with oral probenecid), or an equivalent second or third generation cephalosporin (e.g., cefotaxime) followed by a 14-day regimen of oral doxycycline with or without a 14-day regimen of oral metronidazole. The addition of metronidazole to this regimen provides coverage against bacterial vaginosis, which is frequently associated with PID.

For further information on the treatment of PID, see Uses: Pelvic Inflammatory Disease, in the Cephalosporins General Statement 8:12.06.

■ **Gram-Negative Bacterial Infections** Tetracyclines are the drugs of first or second choice for the treatment of many infections caused by *uncommon* gram-negative bacteria.

Bartonella Infections Doxycycline is used in the treatment of infections caused by *Bartonella quintana*† (formerly *Rochalimaea quintana*). *B. quintana*, a gram-negative bacilli, can cause cutaneous bacillary angiomatosis, trench fever, bacteremia, endocarditis, and chronic lymphadenopathy. *B. quintana* infections have been reported most frequently in immunocompromised patients (e.g., individuals with HIV infection), homeless individuals in urban areas, and chronic alcohol abusers. Optimum anti-infective regimens for the treatment of infections caused by *B. quintana* have not been identified, and various drugs have been used to treat these infections, including doxycycline, erythromycin, azithromycin, chloramphenicol, or cephalosporins. There is evidence that these infections tend to persist or recur and prolonged therapy (several months or longer) usually is necessary.

Doxycycline has been used in the treatment of infections caused by *Bartonella henselae* (formerly *Rochalimaea henselae*) (e.g., cat scratch disease, bacillary angiomatosis, peliosis hepatitis); however, the possible role of tetracyclines in the treatment of these infections has not been determined. Cat scratch disease generally is a self-limited illness in immunocompetent individuals and may resolve spontaneously in 2–4 months; however, some clinicians suggest that anti-infective therapy be considered for acutely or severely ill patients with systemic symptoms, particularly those with hepatosplenomegaly or painful lymphadenopathy, and probably is indicated in immunocompromised patients. Anti-infectives also are indicated in patients with *B. henselae* infections who develop bacillary angiomatosis, neuroretinitis, or Parinaud's oculoglandular syndrome. While the optimum anti-infective regimen for the treatment of cat scratch disease or other *B. henselae* infections has not been identified, some clinicians recommend use of erythromycin, azithromycin, doxycycline, ciprofloxacin, rifampin, co-trimoxazole, gentamicin, or third generation cephalosporins.

HIV-infected individuals (especially severely immunosuppressed individuals) are at unusually high risk for severe disease caused by *Bartonella* and relapse or reinfection sometimes occurs following initial treatment of these infections. The CDC, NIH, and Infectious Diseases Society of America (IDSA) suggest that the drug of choice for treatment of bartonellosis in HIV-infected patients is erythromycin or doxycycline, but that doxycycline is preferred for CNS bartonellosis. In addition, although data are insufficient to make firm recommendations, these experts and the Prevention of Opportunistic Infections Working Group of the US Public Health Service and the Infectious Diseases Society of America (USPHS/IDSA) suggest that use of doxycycline or erythromycin for long-term suppressive therapy (secondary prophylaxis) to prevent recurrence of *Bartonella* infection be considered in HIV-infected adults or adolescents with relapse or reinfection.

Brucellosis Tetracyclines (doxycycline, tetracycline hydrochloride) generally are considered the drugs of choice for brucellosis. Limited data suggest that combined anti-infective therapy may reduce the likelihood of disease relapse, and some clinicians recommend that another anti-infective (e.g., streptomycin or gentamicin and/or rifampin) be used in conjunction with a tetracycline for the treatment of brucellosis. For treatment of serious brucellosis or when there are complications, including endocarditis, meningitis, or osteomyelitis, some clinicians recommend that an aminoglycoside (streptomycin or gentamicin) be used concomitantly with the tetracycline for the first 7–14 days of therapy; rifampin can also be used in the regimen to reduce the risk of relapse. Some experts recommend a 3-drug regimen that includes a tetracycline, an aminoglycoside, and rifampin for the treatment of brucellosis in patients with meningoencephalitis or endocarditis. Although data are limited, alternative regimens that have been suggested for the treatment of brucellosis include co-trimoxazole with or without gentamicin or rifampin (recommended for use in children when tetracyclines are contraindicated); ciprofloxacin (or ofloxacin) and rifampin; and chloramphenicol with or without streptomycin.

Postexposure prophylaxis with anti-infectives is not generally recommended after possible exposure to endemic brucellosis; however, use of an anti-infective regimen recommended for the treatment of brucellosis (e.g., doxycycline and rifampin) should be considered following a high-risk exposure to *Brucella*. These high-risk exposures include needle-stick injuries involving the brucella vaccine available for veterinary use (a brucella vaccine for use in humans is not available); inadvertent laboratory exposure to the organism; or confirmed exposure in the context of biologic warfare or bioterrorism.

Burkholderia Infections Tetracyclines (usually doxycycline) are used in the treatment of melioidosis† caused by *Burkholderia pseudomallei*. Doxycycline alone or in conjunction with co-trimoxazole may be effective for the treatment of localized or mild melioidosis. However, severe illness requires an initial parenteral regimen of ceftazidime, imipenem, or meropenem (with or without concomitant co-trimoxazole or doxycycline), followed by a prolonged maintenance regimen of oral anti-infectives (e.g., co-trimoxazole with or without doxycycline).

Although only limited experience is available regarding the treatment of human cases of glanders† caused by *B. mallei*, some clinicians suggest that, pending results of in vitro susceptibility tests, regimens used for the treatment of severe melioidosis also can be used for initial empiric treatment of glanders.

Some experts (e.g., US Army Medical Research Institute of Infectious Diseases [USAMRIID], European Commission's Task Force on Biological and Chemical Agent Threats [BICHAT]) state that the same treatment regimens recommended for naturally occurring melioidosis or glanders should be used if these *Burkholderia* infections occur in the context of biologic warfare or bioterrorism. Although the benefits of postexposure prophylaxis† are unknown, USAMRIID states that adults can receive oral doxycycline in conjunction with oral rifampin for postexposure prophylaxis if exposure occurs in the context of biologic warfare or bioterrorism. The CDC recommends that laboratory workers with high-risk exposure to melioidosis be offered postexposure prophylaxis with oral doxycycline. The optimum duration of postexposure prophylaxis is unknown, but a duration of at least 10 days is recommended.

Gonorrhea and Associated Infections Some manufacturers state that oral doxycycline or oral tetracycline hydrochloride can be used as alternatives for the treatment of uncomplicated gonorrhea. However, tetracyclines are considered inadequate therapy for the treatment of gonorrhea and are not recommended by the CDC for the treatment of uncomplicated or disseminated gonorrhea. The CDC and many clinicians currently recommend use of tetracyclines for presumptive treatment of coexisting chlamydial infections in patients being treated for gonococcal infections. (See Presumptive Treatment of Chlamydial Infections in Patients with Gonorrhea under Uses: Chlamydial Infections.)

For the treatment of epididymitis most likely caused by gonococcal or chlamydial infection, the CDC recommends a single 250-mg IM dose of ceftriaxone given in conjunction with a 10-day regimen of oral doxycycline (100 mg twice daily). For epididymitis most likely to be caused by enteric bacteria (e.g., *Escherichia coli*), for those allergic to tetracyclines and/or cephalosporins, or for patients older than 35 years of age, the CDC recommends a 10-day regimen of oral ofloxacin or oral levofloxacin. Empiric treatment of epididymitis is indicated before in vitro culture results are available. As an adjunct to therapy, bed rest, scrotal elevation, and analgesics are recommended until fever and local inflammation have subsided. Although most patients can be treated as outpatients, hospitalization should be considered when severe pain suggests other diagnoses (e.g., torsion, testicular infarction, abscess) or when patients are febrile or might be noncompliant.

For the treatment of proctitis likely to be caused by *N. gonorrhoeae* or *C. trachomatis*, the CDC recommends a single 125-mg IM dose of ceftriaxone (or another anti-infective effective against rectal and genital gonorrhea) given in conjunction with a 7-day regimen of oral doxycycline (100 mg twice daily).

Plague **Treatment.** Tetracyclines (doxycycline, tetracycline) are used for the treatment of plague caused by *Yersinia pestis*. Streptomycin (or gentamicin) with or without a tetracycline generally is considered the drug of choice for the treatment of plague. Alternative drugs recommended when aminoglycosides are not used include doxycycline (or tetracycline), chloramphenicol, or co-trimoxazole (may be less effective than other alternatives). Based on results of in vitro and animal testing, ciprofloxacin (or other fluoroquinolones) also is recommended as an alternative for the treatment of plague. Chloramphenicol generally is considered the drug of choice for the treatment of plague meningitis or other conditions that require high anti-infective tissue concentrations (e.g., plague pleuritis, endophthalmitis, or myocarditis). An infectious diseases specialist should be consulted regarding management of patients with plague.

Anti-infective regimens recommended for the treatment of naturally occurring or endemic bubonic, septicemic, or pneumonic plague also are recommended for the treatment of plague that occurs following exposure to *Y. pestis* in the context of biologic warfare or bioterrorism. These exposures would most likely result in primary pneumonic plague. Prompt initiation of anti-infective therapy (within 18–24 hours of onset of symptoms) is essential in the treatment of pneumonic plague. Some experts (e.g., the US Working Group on Civilian Biodefense, USAMRIID) recommend that treatment of plague in the context of biologic warfare or bioterrorism should be initiated with a parenteral anti-infective regimen of streptomycin (or gentamicin) or, alternatively, doxycycline, ciprofloxacin, or chloramphenicol, although an oral regimen (doxycycline, ciprofloxacin) may be substituted when the patient's condition improves or if parenteral therapy is unavailable.

Postexposure Prophylaxis. Postexposure prophylaxis† with anti-infectives is recommended after high-risk exposures to plague, including close exposure to individuals with naturally occurring plague or laboratory exposure to viable *Y. pestis*. In the context of biologic warfare or bioterrorism, some experts (e.g., the US Working Group on Civilian Biodefense, USAMRIID) recommend that asymptomatic individuals with exposure to plague aerosol or asymptomatic individuals with household, hospital, or other close contact (within about 2 m) with an individual who has pneumonic plague should receive postexposure anti-infective prophylaxis; however, any exposed individual who develops a temperature of 38.5°C or higher or new cough should promptly receive a parenteral anti-infective for treatment of the disease. An oral regimen of doxycycline or ciprofloxacin usually is recommended for such prophylaxis. Alternatives suggested for postexposure prophylaxis include oral tetracycline, co-trimoxazole, or oral chloramphenicol (an oral preparation is not commercially available in the US). Although plague vaccine (no longer commercially available in the US) was previously recommended to provide protection against *Y. pestis* infection, the vaccine was effective for preventing or ameliorating bubonic plague but was not effective for prophylaxis against exposure to aerosolized *Y. pestis* and therefore did not provide protection against pneumonic plague.

Individuals with unavoidable exposures to plague in active epizootic or epidemic areas (e.g., mainly in rural mountainous or upland areas of most countries in Africa, Asia, and the Americas) during travel are at high risk for plague and should be advised to consider chemoprophylaxis during periods of exposure. CDC recommends tetracycline or doxycycline for prophylaxis against plague† in such travelers; co-trimoxazole is an acceptable alternative for infants and children younger than 8 years of age who should not receive tetracyclines. In addition, personal protective measures should be employed, including using insect repellents containing DEET on skin and clothing, avoiding sick or dead animals or rodent nests and burrows, and avoiding areas where recent plague epidemics or epizootics have been reported. Individuals staying in modern accommodations while in active plague epizootic or epidemic areas are unlikely to be at high risk of exposure.

Tularemia **Treatment.** Tetracyclines (usually doxycycline) are used as alternative agents for the treatment of tularemia caused by *Francisella tularensis*. Streptomycin (or gentamicin) generally are considered the drugs of choice for this infection. Alternatives for the treatment of tularemia include tetracyclines (doxycycline), chloramphenicol, or ciprofloxacin. Anti-infective regimens recommended for the treatment of naturally occurring or endemic tularemia also are recommended for the treatment of tularemia that occurs following exposure to *F. tularensis* in the context of biologic warfare or bioterrorism. However, the fact that a fully virulent streptomycin-resistant strain of *F. tularensis* was developed in the past for use in biologic warfare should be considered. Exposures to*F. tularensis* in the context of biologic warfare or bioterrorism would most likely result in inhalational tularemia with pleuropneumonitis, although the organism also can infect humans through the skin, mucous membranes, and GI tract.

Postexposure Prophylaxis. Postexposure prophylaxis† with anti-infectives usually is not recommended after possible exposure to natural or endemic tularemia (e.g., tick bite, rabbit or other animal exposure) and is unnecessary in close contacts of tularemia patients since human-to-human transmission of the disease is not known to occur. However, postexposure prophylaxis is recommended following a high-risk laboratory exposure to *F. tularensis* (e.g., spill, centrifuge accident, needlestick injury). In the context of biologic warfare or bioterrorism, some experts (e.g., the US Working Group on Civilian Biodefense, US Army Medical Research Institute of Infectious Diseases) recommend that asymptomatic individuals with exposure to *F. tularensis* receive postexposure anti-infective prophylaxis; however, any individual who develops an otherwise unexplained fever or flu-like illness within 14 days of presumed exposure should promptly receive a parenteral anti-infective for treatment of the disease. Oral doxycycline (or oral tetracycline) or oral ciprofloxacin usually is recommended for postexposure prophylaxis following such exposures.

Other Gram-Negative Bacterial Infections When the drugs of choice are contraindicated or are ineffective, tetracyclines are used as *alternatives* to erythromycins, ceftriaxone, or co-trimoxazole in the treatment of *Campylobacter fetus* infections.

Tetracyclines are used as *alternatives* to penicillin G in the treatment of infections caused by *Leptotrichia buccalis* (Vincent's infection).

Although doxycycline has been used for the treatment of chancroid caused by *Haemophilus ducreyi*, tetracyclines are not included in current CDC recommendations for the treatment of chancroid. (For information on treatment of chancroid, see Uses: Chancroid in Ceftriaxone 8:12.06.12.)

Tetracyclines have been effective in the treatment of rat-bite fever† caused by *Spirillum minus* and Haverhill fever† caused by *Streptobacillus moniliformis*; however, penicillin G generally is preferred for the treatment of these infections.

Tetracyclines are considered alternatives to penicillin G for the treatment of infections caused by *Pasteurella multocida*†.

Some clinicians recommend minocycline as an alternative to co-trimoxazole for the treatment of infections caused by *Stenotrophomonas maltophilia*.

Tetracyclines, with or without rifampin, have been used in the treatment of Legionnaires' disease† caused by *Legionella pneumophila*. Macrolides or fluoroquinolones generally are considered the drugs of choice for the treatment of pneumonia caused by *L. pneumophila* and doxycycline and co-trimoxazole are alternatives. A parenteral regimen usually is necessary for the initial treatment of severe Legionnaires' disease and the addition of oral rifampin is recommended during the first 3–5 days of macrolide or doxycycline therapy in severely ill and/or immunocompromised patients; after a response is obtained, rifampin can be discontinued and therapy changed to an oral regimen.

Although minocycline has been used to eliminate meningococci from the nasopharynx of asymptomatic *N. meningitidis* carriers in situations in which the risk of meningococcal meningitis is high, adverse CNS effects (e.g., vestibular symptoms) are reported occasionally with minocycline and the CDC and AAP currently recommend other anti-infective agents (i.e., rifampin, ceftriaxone, ciprofloxacin) for the treatment of carriers of *N. meningitidis*. Minocycline is *not* indicated for the *treatment* of infections caused by *N. meningitidis*.

Tetracyclines have been used for the treatment of infections caused by susceptible *Acinetobacter*, *Bacteroides*, *Enterobacter aerogenes*, *Escherichia coli*, and *Shigella*; respiratory tract infections caused by *H. influenzae*; and respiratory tract and urinary tract infections caused by *K. pneumoniae*. However, many strains of these gram-negative bacteria have been shown to be resistant to tetracyclines and the drugs generally should not be used empirically in infections suspected to be caused by these organisms. Tetracyclines should be used in the treatment of infections caused by *common* gram-negative bacteria only when other appropriate anti-infectives (e.g., aminoglycosides) are contraindicated or are ineffective and when results of in vitro susceptibility tests indicate that the organisms are susceptible.

■ **Gram-Positive Bacterial Infections** ***Anthrax*** Doxycycline and tetracycline hydrochloride are used in the *treatment* of anthrax and for *postexposure prophylaxis* following a suspected or confirmed exposure to aerosolized anthrax spores (inhalational anthrax). Doxycycline is the preferred tetracycline for inhalational anthrax based on efficacy data in monkey studies and ease of administration.

Parenteral penicillin generally has been considered the drug of choice for the treatment of naturally occurring or endemic anthrax caused by susceptible strains of *Bacillus anthracis*, including clinically apparent inhalational, GI, or meningeal anthrax and anthrax septicemia, although IV ciprofloxacin or IV doxycycline also are recommended. However, *B. anthracis* strains with natural resistance to penicillins have been reported and there are published reports of *B. anthracis* strains that have been engineered to have tetracycline and penicillin resistance as well as resistance to other anti-infectives (e.g., macrolides, chloramphenicol, rifampin). Therefore, it has been postulated that exposures to *B. anthracis* that occur in the context of biologic warfare or bioterrorism may involve bioengineered resistant strains and this concern should be considered when selecting initial therapy for treatment of anthrax that occurs as the result of bioterrorism-related exposures or when selecting anti-infective agents for postexposure prophylaxis following such exposures. For additional information on treatment of anthrax and recommendations for postexposure prophylaxis following exposure to anthrax spores, see Uses: Anthrax in Ciprofloxacin 8:12.18.

Postexposure Prophylaxis. Doxycycline is used for inhalational anthrax (postexposure) to reduce the incidence or progression of disease following suspected or confirmed exposure to aerosolized *B. anthracis* spores. Ciprofloxacin or doxycycline are considered initial drugs of choice for postexposure prophylaxis following exposure to aerosolized anthrax spores that occurs in the context of biologic warfare or bioterrorism. There is no evidence to date that ciprofloxacin is more or less effective than doxycycline for such postexposure prophylaxis. During the bioterrorism-related exposures to *B. anthracis* spores during September and October 2001, the CDC initially recommended postexposure prophylaxis with either ciprofloxacin or doxycycline, but later revised these recommendations because of the large number of exposed individuals. At that time, the CDC suggested that use of doxycycline for postexposure prophylaxis was preferable since widespread use of any anti-infective agent can promote resistance to that drug and because many common pathogens already are resistant to tetracycline but still susceptible to fluoroquinolone and this tactic might preserve effectiveness of ciprofloxacin against these common pathogens. The US Working Group on Civilian Biodefense currently recommends use of ciprofloxacin as the initial drug of choice for postexposure prophylaxis and recommend use of doxycycline as an alternative if the organism is found to be susceptible. These experts also state that in vitro studies suggest that oral tetracycline hydrochloride could be substituted for doxycycline, if necessary. Ultimately, selection of an anti-infective agent for postexposure prophylaxis should be based on the clinical setting, susceptibility of the strain involved, and reported adverse effects associated with the drugs and either doxycycline or ciprofloxacin may be preferable for an individual patient.

Anti-infective prophylaxis should be continued until exposure to *B. anthracis* has been excluded. If exposure is confirmed, postexposure vaccination with anthrax vaccine (if available) may be indicated in conjunction with prophylaxis. Because of the possible persistence of anthrax spores in lung tissue following an aerosol exposure, the CDC and other experts recommend that postexposure prophylaxis be continued for at least 60 days after exposure. Because of potential adverse effects from prolonged use of doxycycline in infants and children, amoxicillin is an alternative to complete the postexposure prophylaxis regimen when susceptibility to penicillin is known.

The CDC states that anti-infective prophylaxis is not necessary for workers in contaminated environments who wear appropriate personal protective equipment and who have received the complete vaccine series, unless a breach of respiratory protection occurs. However, remediation workers involved in clean up and decontamination of *B. anthracis*-contaminated sites who have not been vaccinated with the complete 6-dose recommended regimen of anthrax vaccine should receive anti-infective prophylaxis, regardless of other methods being used to protect these individuals from exposure. This recommendation also applies to workers entering areas that already have been remediated but have not yet been cleared for general occupancy. Unvaccinated or incompletely vaccinated remediation workers should begin anti-infective prophylaxis at the time of first entry into the contaminated area, and such prophylaxis should be continued until at least 60 days after last entry into the area for unvaccinated workers. Remediation workers who have received all or part of the 6-dose vaccine regimen should continue anti-infective prophylaxis for at least 30 days and should complete the vaccination regimen. In addition, it might be prudent to continue anti-infective prophylaxis until 7–14 days after the third vaccine dose is administered.

Remediation workers with repeated entries into contaminated sites over a prolonged period of time could require anti-infective prophylaxis for considerably longer than the 60 days recommended for individuals with a single exposure. To date, some remediation workers have received anti-infective prophylaxis for more than 6 months. If anthrax vaccine is administered to an individual while their risk of exposure to anthrax spores continues, the CDC recommends concomitant anti-infective prophylaxis throughout the period of risk and for 60 days after the risk of exposure has ended, unless the 6-dose series of anthrax vaccine has been completed and annual boosters are up-to-date.

Although controlled studies evaluating doxycycline for aerosolized anthrax exposure have not been conducted for ethical reasons, the drug has been evaluated in a rhesus monkey model of inhalational anthrax. In this study, mortality due to anthrax was significantly lower in monkeys that received doxycycline compared with those that received placebo. Peak serum concentrations of doxycycline associated with survival in this rhesus monkey model were within the range usually observed with usual dosages of the drug.

Treatment of Inhalational Anthrax. The rapid course of symptomatic inhalational anthrax and high mortality rate make early initiation of anti-infective therapy essential. While monotherapy with IV penicillin G, ciprofloxacin, or doxycycline has been recommended for the treatment of anthrax that occurs as the result of natural or endemic exposures, the CDC and other experts (e.g., US Working Group on Civilian Biodefense) recommend that treatment of clinically apparent inhalational anthrax that occurs as the result of exposure to anthrax spores in the context of biologic warfare or bioterrorism should be initiated with a multiple-drug parenteral regimen that includes ciprofloxacin or doxycycline and 1 or 2 other anti-infectives predicted to be effective. Drugs to be included in the initial treatment regimen with ciprofloxacin or doxycycline should be selected based on in vitro susceptibility, possibility of efficacy, adverse effects, and cost. Based on in vitro data, drugs that have been suggested as possibilities to augment ciprofloxacin and doxycycline in such multiple-drug regimens include chloramphenicol, clindamycin, rifampin, vancomycin, clarithromycin, imipenem, penicillin, or ampicillin. If meningitis is established or suspected, some clinicians suggest a multiple-drug regimen that includes ciprofloxacin (rather than doxycycline) and chloramphenicol, rifampin, or penicillin.

Because of the difficulty in making a rapid microbiologic diagnosis of anthrax, high-risk individuals who develop fever or other evidence of systemic infection should promptly receive therapy for possible anthrax infection while waiting for results of laboratory studies. If large numbers of individuals require treatment in mass casualty settings, IV therapy with a multiple-drug parenteral regimen may not be possible. In these circumstances, oral therapy with a regimen recommended for postexposure prophylaxis of inhalational anthrax is an option.

Because of the possible persistence of anthrax spores in lung tissue, anti-infective therapy for the treatment of inhalational anthrax that occurs as the result of exposure to aerosolized spores in the context of biologic warfare or bioterrorism should be continued for at least 60 days. Oral anti-infective therapy can be substituted for IV therapy as soon as the patient's clinical condition improves.

Although tetracyclines are not usually used in children younger than 8 years of age, doxycycline can be used in infants and children for the initial treatment of anthrax if considered necessary. (See Cautions: Pediatric Precautions.) If infants and children with inhalational anthrax have clinical improvement while receiving the initial parenteral regimen, an oral regimen of 1 or 2 anti-infectives (including either doxycycline or ciprofloxacin) may be used to complete the first 14–21 days of therapy. Because of potential adverse effects from prolonged use of doxycycline in infants and children, amoxicillin is an option for completion of therapy but is *not* recommended for initial therapy.

For the treatment of inhalational anthrax in pregnant women, the benefits of doxycycline therapy outweigh the risks and the CDC and other experts (e.g., US Working Group on Civilian Biodefense) state that doxycycline can be used when necessary for the treatment of inhalational anthrax. (See Cautions: Pregnancy, Fertility, and Lactation.)

Recommendations for the treatment of anthrax in immunocompromised patients are the same as those for patients who are immunocompetent.

Treatment of Cutaneous Anthrax. Natural penicillins (e.g., oral penicillin V, IM penicillin G benzathine, IM penicillin G procaine) generally have been considered drugs of choice for the treatment of mild, uncomplicated cutaneous anthrax caused by susceptible strains of *B. anthracis* that occurs as the result of naturally occurring or endemic exposure to anthrax, although some clinicians suggest use of oral fluoroquinolones (ciprofloxacin, ofloxacin, levofloxacin), oral amoxicillin, or oral doxycycline if in vitro tests indicate susceptibility. For the treatment of cutaneous anthrax† that occurs following exposure to *B. anthracis* spores in the context of biologic warfare or bioterrorism, the CDC and other experts (e.g., US Working Group on Civilian Biodefense) recommend use of oral ciprofloxacin or oral doxycycline for initial therapy. Therapy may be changed to oral amoxicillin if results of in vitro testing indicate that the organism is susceptible to the drug and the patient is improving. Recommendations for treatment of cutaneous anthrax in immunocompromised patients are the same as those for patients who are immunocompetent. Use of a multiple-drug parenteral anti-infective regimen is recommended for the initial treatment of cutaneous anthrax when there are signs of systemic involvement, extensive edema, or lesions on the head and neck.

Whether infants and young children are at increased risk for systemic dissemination of cutaneous anthrax infections is not known; however, a child 7 months of age infected following a bioterrorism-related exposure developed systemic illness after onset of cutaneous anthrax. Therefore, the CDC recommends that a parenteral regimen be used for the initial treatment of cutaneous anthrax in children younger than 2 years of age and use of a combination regimen should be considered. If a parenteral regimen is indicated for the treatment of cutaneous anthrax and if infants and children have clinical improvement while receiving the parenteral regimen, an oral regimen of 1 or 2 anti-infectives (including either doxycycline or ciprofloxacin) may be used to complete the first 7–10 days of therapy. Because of potential adverse effects from prolonged use of doxycycline in infants and children, amoxicillin is an option for completion of therapy, but is *not* recommended for initial therapy.

Although 5–10 days of anti-infective therapy usually is recommended for the treatment of mild, uncomplicated cutaneous anthrax that occurs as the result of natural or endemic exposures to anthrax, the CDC and other experts recommend that therapy be continued for at least 60 days if the cutaneous infection occurred as the result of exposure to aerosolized anthrax spores since the possibility of inhalational anthrax would also exist. Anti-infective therapy may limit the size of the cutaneous anthrax lesion and it usually becomes sterile within the first 24 hours of treatment, but the lesion will still progress through the black eschar stage despite effective treatment.

Other Gram-Positive Bacterial Infections Tetracyclines are used as alternatives to penicillin G or metronidazole for the treatment of *Clostridium tetani* infections.

When penicillin G is ineffective or is contraindicated, tetracyclines are used in the treatment of actinomycosis caused by *Actinomyces israelii*. Some clinicians recommend that long-term tetracycline hydrochloride therapy be used as follow-up treatment after penicillin G in severe cases of the disease.

Tetracyclines are considered alternatives to co-trimoxazole for the treatment of nocardiosis†. Some clinicians recommend a regimen of a sulfonamide and either minocycline or amikacin as an alternative to co-trimoxazole; although doxycycline or minocycline are also recommended alone as alternative regimens for the treatment of nocardiosis.

Because of increasing resistance, tetracyclines are not considered drugs of choice for infections caused by gram-positive cocci (e.g., *Staphylococcus* or *Streptococcus* and should *not* be used empirically in infections suspected to be caused by these organisms. Tetracyclines should be used in the treatment of infections caused by *Staphylococcus* or *Streptococcus* only when other appropriate anti-infectives (e.g., penicillins, cephalosporins, erythromycin, clindamycin, vancomycin) are ineffective or are contraindicated and when results of in vitro susceptibility tests indicate that the organisms are susceptible to the drugs. If tetracyclines are used in infections caused by β-hemolytic streptococci, therapy should be continued for at least 10 days.

■ **Acne** Tetracyclines are used orally in the treatment of moderate to severe inflammatory acne vulgaris. The drugs are not indicated in the treatment of noninflammatory acne. Therapy of acne vulgaris must be individualized and frequently modified depending on the types of acne lesions that predominate and the response to therapy. Oral minocycline may be effective in patients with inflammatory acne unresponsive to oral tetracycline hydrochloride or oral erythromycin. Although it has been suggested that failure to respond to anti-infective therapy may be caused by the development of resistance by *P. acnes* to the drug being administered, resistance is rare in this organism and failure to respond to anti-infective therapy appears to be more frequently caused by other factors (e.g., poor patient compliance, emotional or psychological factors, use of comedogenic cosmetic products, the presence of deep nodular or cystic lesions, sinus tract formation).

Preliminary studies using topical clindamycin, topical erythromycin, and topical tetracycline hydrochloride (a topical solution is no longer commercially available in the US) indicate that topical anti-infectives are as effective as oral tetracycline hydrochloride or oral erythromycin in the treatment of mild to moderate inflammatory acne. Some clinicians recommend that oral anti-infective therapy be used initially in the treatment of moderate to severe inflammatory acne vulgaris since the response to topical therapy may be delayed. A topical anti-infective is then used concomitantly after a few weeks, and the oral anti-infective is slowly discontinued. However, further controlled studies are needed to determine when each route of administration is preferred and when combined topical and oral administration of anti-infectives is indicated in the treatment of inflammatory acne vulgaris. For information on the topical use of tetracyclines in acne, see Tetracyclines 84:04.04.

■ **Respiratory Tract Infections** Tetracyclines are used in the treatment of respiratory tract infections caused by *M. pneumoniae*, *Haemophilus influenzae*, *Klebsiella*, and *Streptococcus pneumoniae*. Tetracycline should only be used for treatment of infections caused by these bacteria when in vitro susceptibility tests indicate the organism is susceptible.

Tetracyclines are used in the treatment of atypical pneumonia caused by *Mycoplasma pneumoniae*. Available data suggest that erythromycin and tetracycline are equally effective in shortening the duration of clinical symptoms and hastening radiographic improvement in adults with mycoplasma pneumonia, despite failure to eradicate the pathogen from nasopharyngeal or sputum cultures. Although conflicting data regarding the efficacy of antibiotic therapy of mycoplasma pneumonia in children have been reported, some clinicians suggest that erythromycin is preferred for treating children with the disease. The optimal duration of antibiotic therapy for mycoplasma pneumonia has not been established; however, because of the persistence of the pathogen, some clinicians recommend that such therapy be continued for 2–4 weeks to minimize the possibility of relapse.

Community-Acquired Pneumonia Tetracyclines are used in the treatment of community-acquired pneumonia (CAP).

Initial treatment of CAP generally involves use of an empiric anti-infective regimen based on the most likely pathogens; therapy may then be changed (if possible) to a pathogen-specific regimen based on results of in vitro culture and susceptibility testing, especially in hospitalized patients. The most appropriate empiric regimen varies depending on the severity of illness at the time of presentation and whether outpatient treatment or hospitalization in or out of an intensive care unit (ICU) is indicated and the presence or absence of cardiopulmonary disease and other modifying factors that increase the risk of certain pathogens (e.g., penicillin- or multidrug-resistant *S. pneumoniae*, enteric gram-negative bacilli, *Ps. aeruginosa*). For both outpatients and inpatients, most experts recommend that an empiric regimen for the treatment of CAP include an anti-infective active against *S. pneumoniae* since this organism is the most commonly identified cause of bacterial pneumonia and causes more severe disease than many other common CAP pathogens.

When used in empiric regimens for the treatment of CAP, tetracyclines provide coverage against *C. pneumoniae*, *M. pneumoniae*, *Haemophilus influenzae*, and *Legionella*. Although tetracyclines may also provide some coverage for *S. pneumoniae*, many isolates of this organisms are resistant to tetracyclines. Doxycycline generally is the tetracycline recommended for empiric treatment of CAP because of good oral bioavailability, convenient twice-daily regimen, and tolerability. In most situations, either doxycycline or a macrolide is included in outpatient empiric CAP regimens. Although the IDSA doesn't make a distinction between macrolides and doxycycline, the ATS states that use of a macrolide is preferred (rather than doxycycline) because *S. pneumoniae* may be resistant to tetracyclines and recommends use of doxycycline as an alternative in patients hypersensitive or intolerant of macrolides. Tetracyclines are not usually recommended for empiric CAP regimens in patients with severe infections admitted to an intensive care unit (ICU), but doxycycline may be used as an alternative to macrolides in inpatient CAP regimens in patients hospitalized in a non-ICU setting.

The duration of CAP therapy depends on the causative pathogen, illness severity at the onset of anti-infective therapy, response to treatment, comorbid illness, and complications. CAP secondary to *S. pneumoniae* generally can be treated for 7–10 days or 72 hours after the patient becomes afebrile. CAP caused by bacteria that can necrose pulmonary parenchyma generally should be treated for at least 2 weeks. Patients chronically treated with corticosteroids also may require at least 2 weeks of therapy. CAP caused by *M. pneumoniae* or *C. pneumoniae* probably should be treated for at least 10–14 days. CAP caused by *Legionella* in immunocompetent patients also probably should be treated for at least 10–14 days, although some clinicians recommend 21 days.

Outpatient Regimens for CAP. Pathogens most frequently involved in *outpatient* CAP include *S. pneumoniae*, *M. pneumoniae*, *C. pneumoniae*, respiratory viruses, and *H. influenzae* (especially in cigarette smokers). Therefore, for empiric outpatient treatment of acute CAP in immunocompetent adults, the IDSA recommends monotherapy with an oral macrolide (azithromycin, clarithromycin, erythromycin), oral doxycycline, or an oral fluoroquinolone active against *S. pneumoniae* (e.g., gatifloxacin, levofloxacin, moxifloxacin). Some experts prefer macrolides or doxycycline in patients younger than 50 years of age who have no comorbidities and fluoroquinolones for other individuals. The IDSA states that alternative empiric outpatient regimens include oral amoxicillin and clavulanate or certain oral cephalosporins (cefpodoxime, cefprozil, cefuroxime axetil).

For outpatient treatment of CAP in immunocompetent adults without cardiopulmonary disease or other modifying factors that would increase the risk of multidrug-resistant *S. pneumoniae* or gram-negative bacteria, the American Thoracic Society (ATS) recommends an empiric regimen of monotherapy with azithromycin or clarithromycin or, alternatively, doxycycline. However, for the outpatient treatment of immunocompetent adults with cardiopulmonary disease (congestive heart failure or chronic obstructive pulmonary disease [COPD]) and/or other modifying factors that increase the risk for multidrug-resistant *S. pneumoniae* or gram-negative bacteria, the ATS recommends a 2-drug empiric regimen consisting of a β-lactam anti-infective (e.g., oral cefpodoxime, oral cefuroxime axetil, high-dose amoxicillin, amoxicillin and clavulanate, parenteral ceftriaxone followed by oral cefpodoxime) and a macrolide or doxycycline or, alternatively, monotherapy with a fluoroquinolone active against *S. pneumoniae* (e.g., ciprofloxacin, ofloxacin, gatifloxacin, levofloxacin, moxifloxacin). The CDC suggests that use of these oral fluoroquinolones in the *outpatient* treatment of CAP be reserved for when other anti-infectives are ineffective or cannot be used or when highly penicillin-resistant *S. pneumoniae* (i.e., penicillin MICs 4 mcg/mL or greater) are identified as the cause of infection.

Inpatient Regimens for CAP. In addition to *S. pneumoniae*, other pathogens often involved in *inpatient* CAP are *H. influenzae*, enteric gram-negative bacilli, *S. aureus*, *Legionella*, *M. pneumoniae*, *C. pneumoniae*, and viruses. Patients with severe CAP admitted into the ICU may have *Ps. aeruginosa* infections (especially those with underlying bronchiectasis or cystic fibrosis) and Enterobacteriaceae often are involved. In addition, anaerobic infection should be suspected in patients with aspiration pneumonia or lung abscess.

Inpatient treatment of CAP is initiated with a parenteral regimen, although therapy may be changed to an oral regimen if the patient is improving clinically, is hemodynamically stable, and is able to ingest drugs. CAP patients usually have a clinical response within 3–5 days after initiation of therapy and failure to respond to the initial empiric regimen generally indicates an incorrect diagnosis, host failure, inappropriate anti-infective regimen (drug selection, dosage, route), unusual pathogen, adverse drug reaction, or complication (e.g., pulmonary superinfection, empyema).

For empiric inpatient treatment of CAP in immunocompetent adults who require hospitalization in a non-ICU setting, the IDSA recommends a 2-drug regimen consisting of a parenteral β-lactam anti-infective (e.g., cefotaxime, ceftriaxone, ampicillin and sulbactam, piperacillin and tazobactam) and a macrolide (e.g., azithromycin, clarithromycin, erythromycin) or monotherapy with a fluoroquinolone active against *S. pneumoniae* (e.g., gatifloxacin, levofloxacin, moxifloxacin). The IDSA does not recommend use of doxycycline for inpatient empiric regimens.

For empiric inpatient treatment of CAP in immunocompetent adults who are hospitalized in a non-ICU setting and have cardiopulmonary disease (congestive heart failure or chronic obstructive pulmonary disease [COPD]) and/or other modifying factors that increase the risk for multidrug-resistant *S. pneumoniae* or gram-negative bacteria, the ATS recommends a 2-drug regimen consisting of a parenteral β-lactam anti-infective (cefotaxime, ceftriaxone, ampicillin and sulbactam, high-dose ampicillin) and an oral or IV macrolide (azithromycin or clarithromycin; doxycycline can be used in those with macrolide sensitivity or intolerance) or, alternatively, monotherapy with an IV fluoroquinolone active against *S. pneumoniae*. If anaerobes are documented or lung abscess is present, clindamycin or metronidazole should be added to the regimen. For CAP patients admitted to a non-ICU setting who do not have cardiopulmonary disease or other modifying factors, the ATS suggests an empiric regimen of monotherapy with IV azithromycin; for those with macrolide sensitivity or intolerance, a 2-drug regimen of doxycycline and a β-lactam or monotherapy with a fluoroquinolone active against *S. pneumoniae* can be used.

For information on empiric regimens for the inpatient treatment of CAP in patients who require hospitalization in an ICU, see Inpatient Regimens for CAP under Respiratory Tract Infections: Community-Acquired Pneumonia, in Uses in the Erythromycin General Statement 8:12.12.04.

■ Spirochetal Infections

Syphilis Tetracyclines (doxycycline, tetracycline hydrochloride) are used as alternative agents for the treatment of syphilis caused by *Treponema pallidum*. Parenteral penicillin G is the treatment of choice for all stages of syphilis. Although efficacy is not well documented, the CDC and others state that use of oral doxycycline or tetracycline hydrochloride can be considered to treat primary, secondary, latent, or tertiary syphilis (not neurosyphilis) in nonpregnant adults and adolescents hypersensitive to penicillin if compliance and follow-up serologic testing can be ensured. Although there is less clinical experience with doxycycline than tetracycline hydrochloride for the treatment of syphilis, compliance probably is better with doxycycline since it may be better tolerated. If compliance and follow-up with nonpenicillin regimens cannot be ensured, patients with primary, secondary, latent, or tertiary syphilis who are hypersensitive to penicillin should be desensitized, if necessary, and treated with penicillin.

Patients with neurosyphilis who are hypersensitive to penicillin should be desensitized, if necessary, and treated with penicillin or, alternatively, treated in consultation with the CDC or other clinicians who have expertise in the treatment of neurosyphilis.

Although the AAP states that doxycycline or tetracycline hydrochloride can be used to treat primary, secondary, or latent syphilis (not tertiary or neurosyphilis) in children 8 years of age or older with penicillin hypersensitivity, the CDC states that infants and children with syphilis who are hypersensitive to penicillin should be desensitized, if necessary, and treated with penicillin.

Tetracyclines should *not* be used to treat syphilis in pregnant women hypersensitive to penicillin. There are no proven alternatives to penicillin for the treatment of syphilis during pregnancy, and pregnant women with a history of penicillin hypersensitivity should be desensitized, if indicated, and treated with penicillin.

There is little information on use of penicillin alternatives for the treatment of syphilis in HIV-infected patients. The CDC states that HIV-infected patients with primary or secondary syphilis should be managed according to the recommendations for HIV-negative, penicillin-hypersensitive patients. However, if compliance and follow-up cannot be assured, HIV-infected individuals with latent syphilis who are hypersensitive to penicillin should be desensitized and treated with penicillin.

For information on current recommendations regarding treatment and follow-up for all stages and forms of syphilis, see Spirochetal Infections: Syphilis, under Uses in the Natural Penicillins General Statement 8:12.16.04.

Lyme Disease Doxycycline is considered a drug of choice in the treatment of early Lyme disease†.

Lyme disease (Lyme borreliosis) is a spirochetal disease caused by *Borrelia burgdorferi* and currently is the most common tick-borne infection in the US, although the disease has a worldwide distribution. In the US, Lyme disease is transmitted by the bite of *Ixodes scapularis* (also called *I. dammini*) and *I. pacificus* ticks. In addition to *B. burgdorferi*, *I. scapularis* may be simultaneously infected with and transmit *Anaplasma phagocytophilum* (causative agent of human granulocytotropic anaplasmosis [HGA, formerly known as human granulocytic ehrlichiosis]) and/or *Babesia microti* (causative agent of babesiosis). Because coinfection with *A. phagocytophilum* and/or *B. microti* can occur in patients with Lyme disease in geographic areas where these other pathogens are endemic, these diseases should be considered in the differential diagnosis of patients being evaluated for Lyme disease. Concurrent infection with *A. phagocytophilum* and *B. burgdorferi* has been reported, and diagnosing such a mixed infection is critical to ensure appropriate anti-infective therapy. In areas where both Lyme disease and HGA are reported, discerning between the diseases in the early stages of illness may be difficult. Although doxycycline may be effective for the treatment of HGA (see Uses: Ehrlichiosis and Anaplasmosis), other anti-infectives used in the treatment of Lyme disease are ineffective for the treatment of HGA and babesiosis. Therefore, diagnosing such coinfections is critical to ensure that appropriate anti-infectives are used for treatment.

Lyme disease generally occurs in 3 stages that typically occur in sequence, with different clinical manifestations at each stage. However, the disease, like syphilis, can have a variable presentation, and in individual patients the 3 stages can occur alone or may overlap. The 3 stages of Lyme disease usually are early localized, early disseminated, and late disease).

Early localized (stage 1) Lyme disease, which may appear days to weeks after transfer of the spirochete to the human host, usually is manifested by a characteristic skin lesion, erythema migrans (erythema chronicum migrans). Current data suggest that erythema migrans develops in at least 80–90% of patients and typically begins as an erythematous macule or papule at the site of the tick bite that expands circularly to form a large (e.g., up to 70 cm in diameter) annular lesion, sometimes with partial central clearing. Some patients with Lyme disease develop secondary multiple skin lesions, which may resemble the primary lesion somewhat but generally are smaller and migrate less. Erythema migrans often is accompanied by fever, flu-like constitutional symptoms (e.g., chills, malaise, fatigue, headache), or regional lymphadenopathy.

Early disseminated (stage 2) infection, which may be manifested days to months after the initial infection, is associated with hematogenous and lymphatic dissemination of the infection and characteristic symptoms in various organ systems, principally the skin, nervous system, musculoskeletal system, and/or heart. Severe headache and neck stiffness, generally transient, and meningitis with cranial (e.g., facial nerve [Bell's] palsy) or peripheral (e.g., radiculoneuropathy of the limbs or trunk) neuropathy are nervous system manifestations that can occur in the early stages of the disease. Optic nerve involvement, which may occur as a result of inflammation or increased intracranial pressure, has been reported principally in children and may lead to blindness. Manifestations of acute neuroborreliosis may develop in about 15% of untreated patients within weeks after the period of early disseminated infection. Acute neurologic abnormalities typically resolve or improve within weeks or months even in untreated patients, although a small percentage (5%) of untreated patients may exhibit chronic neurologic manifestations. Symptoms of musculoskeletal involvement, which generally are variable and intermittent and occur in about 60% of untreated patients in the US, may include migratory pain in the joints, bursae, tendons, muscle, and bone and, rarely, a deep myositis; brief episodes of arthritis, principally involving one or only a few large joints (particularly the knee), also may occur during the early stages of the disease. Cardiac involvement appears to occur in approximately 4–10% of untreated patients with Lyme disease, usually within 1–3 months after infection. The most frequently occurring cardiac abnormality is AV block of varying degrees (first-degree, Wenckebach, or complete heart block), which is usually of short duration but potentially may require temporary insertion of a pacemaker.

Late Lyme disease (stage 3), which occurs months to years following the tick bite, generally is manifested by intermittent episodes of arthritis, which may become chronic (defined as continuous joint inflammation for 1 year or longer) but eventually resolves even in untreated patients (i.e., the number of patients with recurrent episodes of arthritis decreases by approximately 10–20% each year). Some evidence suggests that chronic arthritis, which occurs in a small percentage of patients despite recommended anti-infective treatment for Lyme disease, may be related to certain immunogenetic or immune factors (e.g., presence of HLA-DR4 haplotype). Other manifestations of late Lyme disease include subtle central or peripheral neurologic abnormalities such as mild subacute encephalopathy (e.g., characterized by memory loss, behavioral changes, somnolence) and/or polyneuropathy (e.g., characterized by intermittent paresthesias, radicular pain). Resolution of late neurologic manifestations of Lyme disease may occur very slowly and, in some patients, may be incomplete.Acrodermatitis chronica atrophicans, a chronic skin lesion characterized by inflammation and subsequent atrophy, is a late manifestation of Lyme disease that has been reported in Europe but only rarely in the United States.

Diagnosis of Lyme disease is based principally on clinical findings, and treating patients with early disease solely on the basis of objective signs and a known exposure often is appropriate. The IDSA states that clinical findings are sufficient for the diagnosis of erythema migrans, but clinical findings alone are not sufficient for diagnosis of extracutaneous manifestations of Lyme disease or for diagnosis of HGA or babesiosis. Individuals with known endemic exposure to *B. burgdorferi* and physician-diagnosed erythema migrans can receive treatment for Lyme disease without serologic testing; however, erythema migrans should be clinically differentiated from similar rashes that are not caused by *B. burgdorferi* infection. In areas of low or no endemic risk, the likelihood of Lyme disease in a patient with a rash resembling erythema migrans is low. Serologic testing can provide valuable supportive diagnostic information in patients with endemic exposure and objective clinical findings that indicate later stage disseminated Lyme disease. Negative test results are useful in ruling out Lyme disease in patients with clinical findings compatible with disseminated or late-stage infection. Since the proportion of false-positive test results increases when the pretest probability of Lyme disease is low, the use of testing to make a diagnosis of Lyme disease in individuals without endemic exposure is not recommended.

When serologic testing is indicated to aid in diagnosis, the CDC, Association of State, Territorial, and Public Health Laboratory Directors (ASTPHLD), and other clinicians recommend initial testing with a sensitive screening test, either an enzyme-linked immunosorbent assay (ELISA) or an indirect fluorescent antibody (IFA) test, followed by testing with the more specific Western blot (immunoblot) test to corroborate equivocal or positive results obtained with the initial test. Although anti-infective treatment in early localized disease may blunt or abrogate the antibody response, patients with early disseminated or late-stage disease usually have strong serologic reactivity and demonstrate expanded IgG Western blot banding patterns to diagnostic *B. burgdorferi* antigens. Antibodies often persist for months or years following successfully treated or untreated infection. Therefore, seroreactivity alone cannot be used as a marker of active disease. Repeated infection with *B. burgdorferi* has been reported, and neither a positive serologic test result and/or a history of prior Lyme disease ensures that an individual has protective immunity.

The CDC, IDSA, and National Institute of Allergy and Infectious Diseases (NIAID) state that clinicians should be familiar with current recommendations for diagnosis and treatment of Lyme disease and should be alert for and know how to minimize potential complications associated with therapy for the disease.

Postexposure Prophylaxis after Tick Bite. There is some evidence from a controlled study in adults that a single dose of oral doxycycline may be effective in preventing Lyme disease when given within 72 hours after a documented *I. scapularis* tick bite. Some clinicians suggest that this single-dose antibiotic regimen may be useful for individuals in Lyme-disease endemic areas who are bitten by an *I. scapularis* tick (particularly a nymphal tick) that is at least partially engorged with blood. However, the accurate and timely identification of tick species or stage of development and infection status of the tick as well as assessment of the degree of tick engorgement are often difficult, and postexposure antibiotic prophylaxis appears unlikely to have a substantial effect on disease incidence since most ticks that are recognized are removed within 48 hours (i.e., usually before transmission of infection). In addition, *I. scapularis* ticks may transmit other infections such as babesiosis (*B. microti*) for which doxycycline may not be appropriate therapy.

The CDC, IDSA, AAP, and other clinicians currently do not recommend *routine* anti-infective prophylaxis or serologic testing for individuals after a tick bite. However, the IDSA states that postexposure prophylaxis with a single oral dose of doxycycline (200 mg in adults or 4 mg/kg in children 8 years of age or older) can be offered to individuals in Lyme disease-endemic areas who are bitten by an *I. scapularis* tick when *all* of the following circumstances exist: the attached tick can be reliably identified as an adult or nymphal *I. scapularis* tick, the estimated duration of tick attachment has been at least 36 hours based on the degree of engorgement of the tick or certainty about the time of exposure to the tick, the doxycycline dose can be given within 72 hours of tick removal, the local rate of infection of *I. scapularis* with *B. burgdorferi* is 20% or greater, and doxycycline is not contraindicated. Prophylaxis after *I. pacificus* bites generally is not necessary since rates of infection with *B. burgdorferi* in these ticks is low.

The best currently available method for preventing *B. burgdorferi* infection and other *Ixodes*-transmitted infections is avoidance of tick exposure; if exposure is unavoidable, the risk of infection can be reduced through use of protective clothing and tick repellents, daily checking of the entire body for ticks, and prompt removal of attached ticks before transmission of *B. burgdorferi* infection. Individuals from whom attached ticks are removed should be closely monitored for 30 days; those who develop a skin lesion at the site of the tick bite, a temperature exceeding 38°C, or other illness within 1 month after removal of an attached tick should receive a prompt assessment for tick-borne diseases, including Lyme disease, HGA, or babesiosis. Current evidence suggests that the infected tick usually must be attached for at least 24–48 hours to transmit *B. burgdorferi*. Patients who have received Lyme disease vaccine (no longer commercially available in the US) have a reduced risk of developing the disease but should be assessed in a similar manner as those who have not been vaccinated against the disease.

In a double-blind, placebo-controlled study, individuals 12–82 years of age who resided in a hyperendemic area and who had within the previous 72 hours removed an attached tick that was entomologist-verified as *I. scapularis* were randomized to receive a single oral dose of doxycycline 200 mg or placebo. At baseline and at 3 and 6 weeks, these individuals were examined for manifestations of *B. burgdorferi* infection, including erythema migrans; serum antibody levels and blood cultures also were obtained at these time points. Erythema migrans at the site of the tick bite (the primary end point) occurred in 1 of 235 individuals (0.4%) who had received doxycycline versus 8 of 247 individuals (3.2%) who received placebo, representing 87% efficacy for this prophylactic regimen. However, extrapolation of the findings of this study to other clinical settings should take into account that this efficacy rate is based on a relatively small number of individuals who developed Lyme disease and that identification of *I. scapularis* ticks by patients and/or clinicians may not be presumed to be as accurate as that by the medical entomologists in this study.

Treatment of Early Localized or Disseminated Lyme Disease. Anti-infective therapy usually is effective in all stages of Lyme disease, and appropriate treatment of early disease shortens the duration of symptoms and generally prevents the development of late sequelae. The IDSA, AAP, and other clinicians currently recommend oral doxycycline, oral amoxicillin, or oral cefuroxime axetil as first-line therapy for the treatment of early localized or early disseminated Lyme disease associated with erythema migrans, in the absence of neurologic involvement or third-degree atrioventricular (AV) heart block. Although the optimal duration of therapy has not been established, most clinicians treat early Lyme disease for 14–21 days. The IDSA states that a 14-day regimen (range 14–21 days) of any of these oral anti-infectives (doxycycline, amoxicillin, cefuroxime axetil) may be used for initial treatment of early Lyme disease since all 3 drugs have been shown to be effective for the treatment of erythema migrans and associated symptoms in prospective clinical studies. Oral doxycycline, amoxicillin, or cefuroxime axetil usually are preferred to other drugs such as oral tetracycline hydrochloride, oral penicillin G, or oral penicillin V, particularly in patients with early disseminated infection, because of improved microbiologic activity, better GI absorption and tolerance, and/or higher CSF drug concentrations. Macrolide antibiotics (e.g., erythromycin, azithromycin, clarithromycin) also have been used for the treatment of early Lyme disease, although limited evidence suggests that erythromycin or azithromycin may not be as effective as other recommended agents. (See Lyme Disease in Uses: Spirochetal Infections, in the Erythromycins General Statement 8:12.12.04.) The IDSA and other clinicians state that macrolide antibiotics are not recommended as first-line therapy for early Lyme disease; these agents should be reserved for patients who are intolerant of amoxicillin, doxycycline, and cefuroxime axetil, and patients treated with macrolides should be monitored closely.

Most patients with erythema migrans who received oral doxycycline, amoxicillin, or cefuroxime axetil in multicenter studies had satisfactory outcomes; although subjective symptoms persisted in some patients after treatment, objective evidence of persistent infection or relapse was rare and retreatment usually was unnecessary. In a randomized, controlled study, doxycycline 100 mg twice daily or amoxicillin 500 mg 3 times daily (plus probenecid 500 mg 3 times daily) for 21 days showed similar efficacy in preventing late complications (e.g., meningitis, myocarditis, arthritis) in patients with early Lyme disease (erythema migrans); mild fatigue or arthralgia occurred infrequently following antibiotic therapy but resolved in all cases within the 6-month follow-up period. In a multicenter study, oral therapy with doxycycline 100 mg 3 times daily or cefuroxime 500 mg twice daily for 20 days resulted in cure or improvement in about 90% of patients, and even those considered to have failed therapy did not show objective evidence of continuing infection. Although effective, ceftriaxone is not superior to recommended oral drugs for the treatment of early Lyme disease and is not a recommended first-line agent in the absence of neurologic manifestations or third-degree atrioventricular block.

While doxycycline has the advantage of also being effective for the treatment of HGA (see Uses: Ehrlichiosis and Anaplasmosis), which may occur concurrently in patients with early Lyme disease, tetracyclines are not usually recommended for pregnant or lactating women or for children younger than 8 years of age. However, the CDC, IDSA, and AAP state that the use of tetracyclines (e.g., doxycycline) may be warranted in pregnant women with presumed or confirmed Rickettsial infections (including RMSF) or ehrlichiosis (including HGA and HME) or other life-threatening illness. Transplacental transmission of *B. burgdorferi* appears to occur rarely, if at all, and epidemiologic studies in pregnant women have not documented an association between exposure to Lyme disease prior to conception or during pregnancy and subsequent fetal death, congenital malformations, or prematurity. The IDSA, AAP, and other clinicians state that pregnant or nursing women need not be treated differently than other patients with Lyme disease, except that they should not receive tetracyclines (unless coinfection with *A. phagocytophilum* is suspected).

Limited evidence in patients with early disseminated Lyme disease (e.g., multiple erythema migrans lesions and/or objective evidence of organ involvement [e.g., arthritis, heart block, facial nerve palsy]) who did not have meningitis suggests that oral doxycycline is a cost-effective alternative to ceftriaxone for preventing late manifestations of the disease. In a randomized, comparative study, clinical cure (resolution of objective clinical findings of Lyme disease) was reported in 88 or 85% of patients receiving oral doxycycline (100 mg twice daily for 21 days) or ceftriaxone (2 g IV or IM daily for 14 days), respectively, and both regimens were well tolerated. Although further study is needed to determine the relative safety and efficacy of oral versus IV antibiotic therapy in the treatment of Lyme disease, oral therapy is easier to administer than IV therapy, is associated with fewer serious complications, and is more economical. Patients with facial nerve palsy alone or uncomplicated Lyme arthritis usually respond adequately to prolonged therapy (e.g., 28 days) with oral anti-infectives (e.g., oral doxycycline, oral amoxicillin, oral cefuroxime axetil). However, more severe or late complications of Lyme disease generally require higher dosages and more prolonged therapy and/or parenteral anti-infectives (e.g., ceftriaxone or alternatively, cefotaxime or IV penicillin G for 14–28 days). (See Lyme Disease in Uses: Spirochetal Infections, in the Natural Penicillins General Statement 8:12.16.04 and see Lyme Disease in Uses: Spirochetal Infections, in Ceftriaxone 8:12.06.12.)

Treatment of Late or Persistent Manifestations of Lyme Disease.

• *Neurologic Manifestations.* Patients with early Lyme disease who have acute neurologic involvement manifested by facial nerve palsy alone should receive antibiotic therapy to prevent further sequelae; antibiotic therapy has not been shown to accelerate resolution of palsy. Neurologic examination, including lumbar puncture, should be performed in patients in whom neurologic disease is strongly suspected on clinical grounds.

The IDSA states that patients with negative CSF examinations may be treated with the same antibiotic regimens recommended for patients with erythema migrans (i.e., oral doxycycline, oral amoxicillin, or oral cefuroxime axetil); those with clinical and laboratory evidence of CNS involvement should be treated with regimens effective against meningitis. The IDSA states that while evidence from studies in Europe suggests that IV penicillin G and ceftriaxone or cefotaxime have similar efficacy in treating acute neurologic manifestations of Lyme disease, ceftriaxone often is used because its once-daily administration schedule allows outpatient management of therapy.

For adults with acute neurologic disease manifested by meningitis or radiculopathy, the IDSA and other clinicians recommend ceftriaxone for 14–28 days; alternatively, IV penicillin G or cefotaxime may be used. Some clinicians suggest that oral or IV doxycycline for 14–28 days may be adequate therapy in adults with acute neurologic manifestations who are intolerant of cephalosporins and penicillin, although experience in the US with such a regimen for Lyme meningitis is limited. Children younger than 8 years of age with acute neurologic manifestations of meningitis or radiculopathy should receive ceftriaxone or cefotaxime for 14–28 days; IV penicillin G may be used as an alternative in such children.

• *Cardiac Manifestations.* Cardiac involvement in Lyme disease usually manifests as atrioventricular (AV) heart block and generally occurs during the first few weeks of infection in conjunction with erythema migrans. The IDSA states that patients with first- or second-degree AV heart block associated with early Lyme disease should be treated with the same antibiotic regimens (i.e., oral doxycycline, amoxicillin, or cefuroxime axetil) as patients with erythema migrans who do not have carditis. However, some clinicians recommend use of IV regimens (e.g., ceftriaxone, cefotaxime, or penicillin G) in patients with first-degree AV block and a PR-interval exceeding 0.3 seconds. The IDSA and other clinicians recommend that patients with third-degree AV heart block be hospitalized for cardiac monitoring because of the potential for life-threatening complications. While evidence supporting the superiority of IV versus oral therapy currently is unavailable, most clinicians recommend that patients with severe cardiac involvement receive ceftriaxone, penicillin G, or cefotaxime IV for 14–28 days. Patients with third-degree AV block may require a temporary pacemaker.

• *Lyme Arthritis.* Patients with uncomplicated Lyme arthritis generally can be treated with a prolonged course (e.g., 28 days) of oral anti-infectives (i.e., doxycycline, amoxicillin, or cefuroxime axetil). While oral regimens are easier to administer, associated with fewer serious adverse effects, and less expensive than IV regimens, some patients with Lyme arthritis treated with oral regimens have subsequently developed overt neuroborreliosis, which may require IV therapy for successful treatment. When Lyme arthritis is accompanied by neurologic disease documented by CSF analysis, the IDSA and other clinicians recommend that adults receive ceftriaxone for 14–28 days; alternative therapy is cefotaxime or IV penicillin G. Ceftriaxone or cefotaxime is recommended in children with coexisting Lyme arthritis and neurologic manifestations; alternatively, IV penicillin G may be given. Long-acting penicillin G benzathine preparations are *not* recommended for treatment of these patients because of the low serum penicillin G concentrations attained after administration of such preparations.

• *Treatment of Late or Persistent Manifestations of Lyme Disease.* Late manifestations of Lyme disease may include oligoarticular arthritis, encephalopathy (principally memory deficit, irritability, and somnolence), and neuropathy (principally distal paresthesias or radicular pain). Comparative studies evaluating different antibiotic regimens in patients with late Lyme disease generally are lacking. Response to therapy for late manifestations of Lyme disease may be slow and improvement may take weeks or months, although most appropriately treated patients eventually recover.

• *Persistent Arthritis.* In patients who have persistent or recurrent joint swelling after receiving recommended antibiotic regimens, the IDSA and other clinicians recommend another 28-day course of a recommended oral antibiotic or 14–28 days of ceftriaxone, cefotaxime, or IV penicillin G. However, the IDSA states that clinicians should consider allowing several months for joint inflammation to resolve after initial treatment before an additional course of antibiotic therapy is given. Many clinicians also suggest that the initial diagnosis of Lyme disease be reevaluated in patients who appear not to respond to recommended anti-infective therapy (e.g., 21–28 days of oral and/or IV antibiotics). Patients with persistent arthritis who have received 2 courses of recommended oral antibiotic therapy or a single course of IV antibiotics should receive symptomatic treatment with a nonsteroidal anti-inflammatory agent (NSAIA); treatment with intra-articular corticosteroids also may be considered. Arthroscopic synovectomy may be indicated and may decrease time to recovery in patients with persistent synovitis who report substantial pain or limited function.

• *Late Neuroborreliosis Affecting the CNS or Peripheral Nervous System.* Patients with late neurologic disease affecting the CNS or peripheral nervous system (e.g., encephalopathy, neuropathy) should receive 14–28 days of ceftriaxone; alternative therapy is cefotaxime or IV penicillin G. Clinical response to these regimens is typically gradual and may be incomplete. However, additional courses of antibiotic therapy are not recommended unless reliable objective measures substantiate relapse of neurologic disease. For children with late CNS or peripheral nervous system manifestations, ceftriaxone for 14–28 days is recommended; alternatively, cefotaxime or IV penicillin G may be given.

Chronic Lyme Disease or Post-Lyme Disease Syndrome. After receiving recommended antibiotic therapy for Lyme disease, some patients manifest a post-infectious syndrome, which some clinicians have referred to as chronic Lyme disease or post- Lyme disease syndrome. Some evidence suggests that this syndrome occurs more frequently in patients who have symptoms of early dissemination of the infection, particularly if there is a delay in treatment. Patients with this syndrome are a diverse group and report various persistent subjective complaints including arthralgia, fatigue, and/or myalgia; some clinicians categorize such symptoms as chronic Lyme disease or a post- Lyme disease syndrome similar to chronic fatigue syndrome or fibromyalgia. Patients with residual *B. burgdorferi* infection (or possibly reinfection) have been reported rarely in Europe; however, residual infection has not been reliably documented to date in a large series of patients in Europe or North America who received appropriate treatment for Lyme disease. The IDSA states that currently available evidence is insufficient to consider chronic Lyme disease a separate diagnostic entity.

Although case reports and uncontrolled studies have reported benefit from prolonged antibiotic therapy in patients with chronic Lyme disease, symptom recurrence after discontinuance of therapy is common; in addition, the prevalence of fatigue and/or arthralgias in the general population reportedly is greater than 10%. In a small percentage of patients appropriately treated for Lyme disease, persistent symptoms may be explained by coinfection with *A. phagocytophilum* or *B. microti*. Although studies of treatment of patients with Lyme disease who remain unwell after standard courses of antibiotic therapy currently are in progress, the IDSA states that no controlled clinical studies currently support the efficacy of repeated or prolonged courses of oral and/or IV antibiotics in such patients. In addition, serious complications (e.g., biliary disease leading to cholecystectomy), including at least one death, have been reported in patients receiving such empiric therapy. (See Lyme Disease in Uses: Spirochetal Infections, in Ceftriaxone 8:12.06.12.) The American College of Rheumatology and IDSA state that the risks and costs of treating suspected Lyme disease empirically with IV antibiotics (e.g., ceftriaxone) exceed the benefits in patients with a positive antibody titer for *B. burgdorferi* and only nonspecific complaints of myalgia or fatigue; such patients are best managed symptomatically rather than with prolonged courses of antibiotics.

Two double-blind, placebo-controlled studies evaluating prolonged antibiotic therapy (IV ceftriaxone followed by oral doxycycline for a total of 90 days) in patients with persistent symptoms of Lyme disease after appropriate initial therapy were discontinued after interim analysis revealed no difference in clinical benefit between prolonged antibiotic therapy and placebo. In these 2 studies, patients were randomized to receive IV ceftriaxone 2 g daily for 30 days followed by oral doxycycline 100 mg twice daily for 60 days, or matching IV and oral placebos. Patients were enrolled in the 2 studies based on their seropositivity or seronegativity for antibodies to *B. burgdorferi* antigen on Western blot assay.All patients included in the studies had one or more of the following diagnoses: a history of single or multiple erythema migrans skin lesions, early neurologic or cardiac symptoms attributed to Lyme disease, radiculoneuropathy, or Lyme arthritis; seronegative patients were required to have a documented history of erythema migrans by an experienced clinician. These patients were experiencing profound fatigue, widespread musculoskeletal pain, cognitive impairment, radicular pain, paresthesias, and/or dysesthesias that had begun within 6 months of the initial documented diagnosis of US-acquired acute Lyme disease and had persisted for at least 6 months but less than 12 years.

Most patients in these studies previously had received oral antibiotic therapy for a median of 50 days; 33% had received IV antibiotic therapy for an average of 30 days. Baseline evaluation included a complete review of patient medical history, physical examination, neuropsychologic testing, CSF analysis, and phlebotomy; cultures and molecular analysis by polymerase chain reaction (PCR) of blood and CSF at baseline or during the studies did not detect any evidence of persistent infection by *B. burgdorferi* in these patients. A planned interim analysis of data from the combined studies at 180 days did not reveal a significant difference in the efficacy of prolonged antibiotic therapy compared with that of placebo based on summary scores for the mental and physical components of a health-related quality of life survey instrument (Medical Outcomes Study 36-item Short-Form General Health Survey); separate analysis of data from the seropositive and the seronegative studies also failed to show any benefit of the prolonged antibiotic regimen compared to placebo.

In an observational study of patients diagnosed as having chronic Lyme disease (i.e., manifesting symptoms for greater than 3 months from at least 2 out of the following 3 groups of symptoms: fatigue, neurologic complaints [e.g., paresthesias, cognitive dysfunction, radicular pain], musculoskeletal complaints [e.g., arthralgias, myalgias, weakness]), 70% of patients reported improvement and 20% reported resolution of symptoms following long-term therapy (generally 3–6 months) with tetracycline hydrochloride (500 mg 3 times daily). In this study, patients with a longer duration of Lyme disease symptoms prior to receiving tetracycline therapy had a slower onset of improvement following initiation of therapy. Additional study is needed to establish the value of prolonged (e.g., 3–6 months) anti-infective therapy in patients with persistent manifestations of Lyme disease.

Leptospirosis Tetracyclines are used in the treatment of leptospirosis† caused by *Leptospira.* Some clinicians state that penicillin G is the drug of choice for treatment of leptospirosis and tetracyclines and ceftriaxone are alternatives. The CDC recommends that leptospirosis be treated with penicillin, amoxicillin, ampicillin, or doxycycline; IV penicillin G or ampicillin is indicated in patients with severe disease.

Doxycycline has been recommended for chemoprophylaxis in individuals exposed to *Leptospira*†. Travelers participating in recreational water activities (e.g., whitewater rafting, adventure racing, or kayaking) in areas where leptospirosis is endemic or epidemic may be at increased risk for the disease, especially during periods of flooding. Individuals considered at an increased risk for leptospirosis should practice personal preventive measures including wearing protective clothing and minimizing contact with potentially contaminated water. Based on limited data, the CDC recommends that travelers at increased risk for leptospirosis be advised to consider doxycycline chemoprophylaxis initiated 1–2 days before exposure and continued through the period of exposure. Travelers who may be at increased risk for leptospirosis and who are also in need of malaria chemoprophylaxis may consider using doxycycline for both indications. (See Prevention of Malaria under Malaria, in Uses.)

Other Spirochetal Infections Tetracyclines are considered the drugs of choice for the treatment of tick-borne (endemic) or louse-borne (epidemic) relapsing fever caused by *Borrelia.* The drugs also appear to be effective in the treatment of yaws, pinta, and bejel and are used as alternatives to penicillin G for the treatment of these diseases.

■ GI Infections ***Helicobacter pylori Infection and Duodenal Ulcer Disease*** Tetracycline hydrochloride is used in combination with metronidazole, bismuth subsalicylate, and an H_2-receptor antagonist for the treatment of *Helicobacter pylori* (formerly *Campylobacter pylori* or *C. pyloridis*) infection in patients with an active duodenal ulcer. Tetracycline hydrochloride also has been used successfully in other multiple-drug regimens (with or without bismuth salts, metronidazole, and/or an H_2-receptor antagonist) for the treatment of *H. pylori* infection† in patients with peptic ulcer disease. Current epidemiologic and clinical evidence supports a strong association between gastric infection with *H. pylori* and the pathogenesis of duodenal and gastric ulcers; long-term *H. pylori* infection also has been implicated as a risk factor for gastric cancer. For additional information on the association of this infection with these and other GI conditions, see *Helicobacter pylori* Infection, under Uses, in Clarithromycin 8:12.12.92.

Conventional antiulcer therapy with H_2-receptor antagonists, proton-pump inhibitors, sucralfate, and/or antacids heals ulcers but generally is ineffective in eradicating *H. pylori*, and such therapy is associated with a high rate of ulcer recurrence (e.g., 60–100% per year). Several useful therapeutic regimens for *H. pylori*-associated peptic ulcer disease have been identified, and the American College of Gastroenterology (ACG), the National Institutes of Health (NIH), and most clinicians currently recommend that *all* patients with initial or recurrent duodenal or gastric ulcer and documented *H. pylori* infection receive anti-infective therapy for treatment of the infection.

The optimum regimen for treatment of *H. pylori* infection has not been established; however, combined therapy with 3 drugs that have activity against *H. pylori* (generally a bismuth salt, metronidazole, and tetracycline or amoxicillin) has been effective in eradicating the infection, resolving associated gastritis, healing peptic ulcer, and preventing ulcer recurrence in many patients with *H. pylori*-associated peptic ulcer disease. Although such 3-drug regimens typically have been administered for 10–14 days, current evidence principally from studies in Europe suggests that 1 week of such therapy provides *H. pylori* eradication rates comparable to those of longer treatment periods. Other regimens that combine one or more anti-infective agents (e.g., clarithromycin, amoxicillin) with a bismuth salt and/or an antisecretory agent (e.g., omeprazole, H_2-receptor antagonist) also have been used successfully for *H. pylori* eradication, and the choice of a particular regimen should be based on the rapidly evolving data on optimal therapy, including consideration of the patient's prior exposure to anti-infective agents, the local prevalence of resistance, patient compliance, and costs of therapy. Current data suggest that eradication of *H. pylori* infection using regimens consisting of 1 or 2 anti-infective agents with a bismuth salt and/or an H_2-receptor antagonist or proton-pump inhibitor (e.g., omeprazole, lansoprazole) is cost effective compared with intermittent or continuous maintenance therapy with an H_2-receptor antagonist (considering the costs associated with ulcer recurrence, including endoscopic or other diagnostic procedures, physician visits, and/or hospitalization).

Although high eradication rates have been achieved with standard 3-drug, bismuth-based regimens (e.g., bismuth-metronidazole-tetracycline or bismuth-metronidazole-amoxicillin), such regimens typically involve administration of many tablets/capsules and have been associated with a relatively high (although variable) incidence of adverse effects. In addition, the efficacy of these regimens generally is unacceptable in patients with *H. pylori* strains resistant to the imidazole anti-infective (e.g., metronidazole) component. Current evidence suggests that inclusion of a proton-pump inhibitor (e.g., omeprazole, lansoprazole) in anti-*H. pylori* regimens containing 2 anti-infectives enhances effectiveness, and limited data suggest that such regimens retain good efficacy despite imidazole (e.g., metronidazole) resistance. Therefore, the ACG and many clinicians currently recommend 1 week of therapy with a proton-pump inhibitor and 2 anti-infective agents (usually clarithromycin and amoxicillin or metronidazole), or a 3-drug, bismuth-based regimen (e.g., bismuth-metronidazole-tetracycline) concomitantly with a proton-pump inhibitor, for treatment of *H. pylori* infection. Although few comparative studies have been performed, such regimens appear to provide high (e.g., 85–90%) *H. pylori* eradication rates, are well tolerated, and may be associated with better patient compliance than more prolonged therapy. The ACG states that in a cost-sensitive environment, an alternative regimen consisting of a bismuth salt, metronidazole, and tetracycline for 14 days is a reasonable choice in patients who are compliant and in whom there is a low expectation of metronidazole resistance (no prior exposure to the drug and a low regional prevalence of resistance).

Rapid development of resistance by *H. pylori* to certain drugs (e.g., metronidazole, clarithromycin and other macrolides, quinolones) has occurred when these drugs were used as monotherapy or as the only anti-infective agent in anti-*H. pylori* regimens. Resistance commonly emerges during therapy with clarithromycin or metronidazole when eradication of *H. pylori* is not achieved; therefore, prior exposure to these anti-infectives predicts resistance in individual patients and should be considered when selecting anti-*H. pylori* treatment regimens. Regimens containing metronidazole or clarithromycin should not be used to treat *H. pylori* infection in patients with known or suspected metronidazole- or clarithromycin-resistant isolates because of reduced efficacy in such patients.

For additional discussion of *H. pylori* infection, including details about the efficacy of various regimens and rationale for drug selection, see *Helicobacter pylori* Infection, under Uses, in Clarithromycin 8:12.12.92.

Vibrio Infections **Cholera.** Tetracyclines (doxycycline, tetracycline hydrochloride) usually are considered the drugs of choice when anti-infective therapy is indicated as an adjunct to fluid and electrolyte replacement in patients with cholera caused by *Vibrio cholerae.* Although some clinicians recommend use of co-trimoxazole for the treatment of cholera in children younger than 8 years of age, the AAP states that in cases of severe cholera, the benefits of tetracyclines may outweigh the risks in this age group. Tetracycline therapy reduces the duration of excretion of *Vibrio cholerae* and, since it decreases the volume and duration of diarrhea, may decrease requirements for fluid replacement. Adjunctive anti-infective therapy should be considered in patients with moderately to severe disease. When the infection is caused by strains of *V. cholerae* resistant to tetracyclines, alternative agents include co-trimoxazole, fluoroquinolones, or furazolidone.

Vibrio parahaemolyticus Infections. Tetracyclines (doxycycline, tetracycline hydrochloride) are one of several alternatives recommended for the treatment of severe cases of *Vibrio parahaemolyticus*† infection when anti-infective therapy is indicated in addition to supportive care. *V. parahaemolyticus* infection is a relatively rare foodborne illness than can occur as the result of ingestion of contaminated, undercooked or raw fish or shellfish; the incubation period usually is 2–48 hours. The signs and symptoms of *V. parahaemolyticus* infection are watery diarrhea, abdominal cramps, and nausea and vomiting lasting 2–5 days. Although supportive care usually is sufficient, some clinicians recommend use of tetracycline, doxycycline, gentamicin, or cefotaxime in severe cases.

Vibrio vulnificus Infections. Although optimum anti-infective therapy has not been identified, a tetracycline or third generation cephalosporin (e.g., cefotaxime, ceftazidime) is recommended for the treatment of infections caused by *Vibrio vulnificus*†. *V. vulnificus*, a gram-negative aerobic bacteria that can cause potentially fatal septicemia, wound infections, or gastroenteritis, generally is transmitted through ingestion of contaminated raw or undercooked seafood (especially raw oysters) or through contamination of a wound with seawater or seafood drippings. *V. vulnificus* is naturally present in marine environments, thrives in warm ocean water, and frequently is isolated from oysters and other shellfish harvested from the Gulf of Mexico and from US coastal waters along the Pacific and Atlantic ocean. Individuals with preexisting liver disease are at high risk for developing fatal septicemia following ingestion of seafood contaminated with *V. vulnificus* and debilitated or immunocompromised individuals (e.g., those with chronic renal impairment, cancer, diabetes mellitus, steroid-dependent asthma, chronic GI disease) or individuals with iron overload states (e.g., thalassemia and hemochromatosis) also are at increased risk for fatal infections. In immunocompromised individuals, fever, nausea, myalgia, and abdominal cramps may occur as soon as 24–48 hours after ingestion of seafood contaminated with *V. vulnificus* and sepsis and cutaneous bullae may be present within 36 hours of the onset of symptoms.

Because the case fatality rate for *V. vulnificus* septicemia exceeds 50% in immunocompromised individuals or those with preexisting liver disease, these individuals should be informed about the health hazards of ingesting raw or undercooked seafood (especially oysters), the need to avoid contact with seawater during the warm months, and the importance of using protective clothing (e.g., gloves) when handling shellfish. *V. vulnificus* should be considered in the differential diagnosis of fever of unknown etiology, and individuals who present with fever (especially when bullae, cellulitis, or wound infection is present) and who have preexisting liver disease or are immunocompromised should be questioned regarding a history of raw oyster ingestion or seawater contact. Because the high fatality rate associated with *V. vulnificus* infections, anti-infective therapy should be initiated promptly if indicated.

Yersinia Infections Tetracyclines (usually doxycycline) are suggested as possible choices for the treatment of GI infections caused by *Yersinia enterocolitica* or *Y. pseudotuberculosis*. (For information on treatment of *Y. pestis* infections, see Plague under Uses: Gram-Negative Bacterial Infections.) *Y. enterocolitica* and *Y. pseudotuberculosis* GI infections usually are self-limited and anti-infective therapy unnecessary; however, the AAP, IDSA, and others recommend use of anti-infectives in immunocompromised individuals or for the treatment of severe infections or when septicemia or other invasive disease occurs. GI infections caused by *Y. enterocolitica* or *Y. pseudotuberculosis* can occur as the result of ingesting undercooked pork, unpasteurized milk, or contaminated water; infection has occurred in infants whose caregivers handled contaminated chitterlings (raw pork intestines) or tofu. Use of co-trimoxazole, an aminoglycoside (amikacin, gentamicin, tobramycin), a fluoroquinolone (e.g., ciprofloxacin), doxycycline, cefotaxime, or ceftizoxime has been recommended when treatment is considered necessary; combination therapy may be necessary. Some clinicians suggest that the role of oral anti-infectives in the management of enterocolitis, pseudoappendicitis syndrome, or mesenteric adenitis caused by *Yersinia* needs further evaluation.

Travelers' Diarrhea Although doxycycline has been used in the past for the treatment of travelers' diarrhea†, other anti-infective agents (i.e., ciprofloxacin, levofloxacin, norfloxacin, ofloxacin, azithromycin) are preferred if anti-infective therapy is indicated in individuals whose diarrhea is severe or associated with fever or bloody stools. The CDC and other experts no longer recommend use of anti-infectives for prophylaxis of travelers' diarrhea in most individuals traveling to areas of risk.

Other GI Infections Tetracycline hydrochloride is considered the treatment of choice for balantidiasis† caused by *Balantidium coli*; metronidazole and iodoquinol are considered alternative agents.

Although the manufacturers state that tetracyclines may be useful as an adjunct to amebicides in the treatment of acute intestinal amebiasis, tetracyclines are not generally recommended for the treatment of amebiasis caused by *Entamoeba*.

Tetracycline is considered a drug of choice for the treatment of infections caused by *Dientamoeba fragilis*†. Many clinicians recommend iodoquinol, paromomycin, tetracycline, or metronidazole for the treatment of *D. fragilis* infections

Tetracycline hydrochloride is used in conjunction with folic acid in the treatment of tropical sprue† (postinfectious tropical malabsorption). Although treatment with folic acid alone can improve symptoms of tropical sprue, it does not cure the diarrhea; combination therapy appears to be most effective in resolving symptoms (including diarrhea) and promoting weight gain.

For the treatment of Whipple's disease† caused by *Tropheryma whippelii*, some clinicians suggest that co-trimoxazole is the drug of choice and penicillin G and tetracyclines are alternatives.

■ **Malaria** ***Prevention of Malaria*** Doxycycline is used for prevention of malaria in individuals traveling to areas where chloroquine-resistant *Plasmodium falciparum* has been reported. The CDC and many clinicians recommend use of the fixed combination of atovaquone and proguanil hydrochloride (Malarone®), doxycycline, or mefloquine for prevention of malaria in individuals traveling to malarious areas where chloroquine-resistant *P. falciparum* has been reported. Doxycycline (unless contraindicated) or the fixed combination of atovaquone and proguanil can be used for prophylaxis in individuals traveling to areas of risk where mefloquine resistance has been confirmed.

Although chloroquine is the drug of choice for travelers to areas where chloroquine-resistant *P. falciparum* malaria has *not* been reported, the CDC states that doxycycline, mefloquine, or the fixed combination of atovaquone and proguanil can be used as alternatives for prophylaxis in individuals traveling to these areas who are unable to take chloroquine or hydroxychloroquine.

Doxycycline is the preferred tetracycline for prevention of malaria. Efficacy of other tetracyclines (e.g., minocycline) for prevention of malaria has not been fully determined. Therefore, CDC recommends that individuals receiving long-term minocycline therapy (e.g., for acne) who also require doxycycline malaria prophylaxis should discontinue minocycline 1–2 days prior to travel and initiate doxycycline for such prophylaxis; minocycline therapy can be reinitiated after doxycycline prophylaxis is finished.

Because doxycycline is active only against the asexual erythrocytic forms of plasmodia, the drug provides substantial, but not complete, suppressive action for *P. falciparum*. In addition, doxycycline cannot prevent delayed primary attacks or relapse of *P. ovale* or *P. vivax* malaria and cannot provide a radical cure in malaria caused by these species since they have exoerythrocytic stages. Therefore, terminal prophylaxis with primaquine phosphate may be indicated in addition to doxycycline prophylaxis if exposure occurred in areas where *P. ovale* or *P. vivax* are endemic. For additional information on the treatment and prevention of *P. ovale* or *P. vivax*, see Primaquine Phosphate 8:30.08.

Specific references, including those most recently published by the CDC and World Health Organization (WHO), should be consulted to determine in which countries a risk of acquiring malaria exists, to determine whether prophylaxis against malaria is indicated in these countries, and to aid in selecting the appropriate antimalarial agent(s). The choice of an antimalarial agent(s) for suppression or chemoprophylaxis depends on the specific malarious area as well as the duration of exposure. Detailed recommendations for prevention of malaria are available from CDC 24 hours a day from the voice information service (877-394-8747) or at http://www.cdc.gov/travel.

No drug regimen is completely effective in preventing malaria, and travelers should be informed that, regardless of the prophylactic regimen used, it is still possible to contract malaria. Travelers should be advised of the importance of taking measures to reduce contact with mosquitoes (e.g., using appropriate insect repellents, wearing clothes that cover most of the body, remaining in air-conditioned or well-screened areas, using mosquito nets [e.g., bed nets] between dusk and dawn, using aerosolized insecticides in rooms where mosquitoes are found). For information on protective measures, see http://www.cdc.gov/travel.

Travelers to countries with malaria should be instructed to seek prompt medical attention *as soon as possible* if they develop symptoms of malaria, including fever with chills and headache or other influenza-like illness, while traveling or after return (especially during the first 2 months). Malaria symptoms can develop as early as 6 days after initial exposure or can appear months after departure from a malarious area, after chemoprophylaxis is discontinued. Travelers should understand that malaria can be effectively treated early in the course of the disease, but that delays before initiation of therapy can have serious or even fatal consequences.

Presumptive Self-treatment of Malaria CDC and other experts recommend use of malaria prophylaxis for travel to malarious areas. However, travelers who elect not to take prophylaxis and travelers who require or choose to use a prophylaxis regimen that may not have optimal efficacy (e.g., chloroquine prophylaxis in areas with chloroquine-resistant *P. falciparum*) are at greater risk of acquiring malaria and may need prompt treatment. In addition, long-term travelers who are taking effective prophylaxis but who will be in very remote areas may decide, in consultation with their health-care provider, to take along an appropriate antimalarial for presumptive self-treatment. The antimalarial regimen provided for presumptive self-treatment should be different than the regimen that the traveler uses for prophylaxis. Travelers should be advised to initiate self-treatment promptly in the event of an influenza-like illness (e.g., fever, chills) if professional medical care will not be available within 24 hours. Use of presumptive self-treatment is only a temporary measure and these travelers should be advised to seek medical advice as soon as possible.

CDC recommends the fixed combination of atovaquone and proguanil (Malarone®) for presumptive self-treatment of malaria in travelers not taking the drug for prophylaxis and states that the CDC Malaria Hotline (770-488-7788) should be consulted regarding other potential options for self-treatment if atovaquone and proguanil cannot be used. There have been several reports of *P. falciparum* resistant to atovaquone and proguanil in isolated locations in Africa. Some clinicians also suggest that a regimen of oral doxycycline in conjunction with oral quinine sulfate or, alternatively, mefloquine alone may be used for presumptive self-treatment of malaria† in travelers.

Treatment of Malaria **Treatment of Uncomplicated Malaria.** Doxycycline or tetracycline hydrochloride is used in conjunction with quinine sulfate for the treatment of uncomplicated malaria caused by chloroquine-resistant *P. falciparum*†. For the treatment of uncomplicated malaria caused by chloroquine-resistant *P. falciparum* and for the treatment of uncomplicated malaria when the plasmodial species has not been identified, CDC recommends the fixed combination of oral atovaquone and proguanil (Malarone®); the fixed combination of oral artemether and lumefantrine (Coartem®); or a regimen that includes oral quinine sulfate in conjunction with oral doxycycline, tetracycline, or clindamycin. Although mefloquine is an alternative, it has been associated with adverse effects (e.g., severe neuropsychiatric reactions) and the CDC recommends that it be used only if the recommended treatment regimens cannot be used.

When a quinine sulfate regimen is used for treatment of uncomplicated, chloroquine-resistant *P. falciparum* malaria, concomitant use with doxycycline or tetracycline generally is preferable to use with clindamycin because more efficacy data exist regarding regimens that include tetracyclines. However, for pregnant women with uncomplicated malaria caused by chloroquine-resistant *P. falciparum*, prompt treatment with quinine sulfate and clindamycin is recommended. Although tetracyclines generally are contraindicated in pregnant women, in rare circumstances (e.g., if other treatment options are not available or not tolerated) quinine sulfate may be used in conjunction with doxycycline or tetracycline if the benefits outweigh the risks.

Doxycycline is used in conjunction with quinine sulfate and primaquine for the treatment of uncomplicated, chloroquine-resistant *P. vivax* malaria†. For the treatment of uncomplicated malaria caused by chloroquine-resistant *P. vivax*, the CDC recommends a regimen of oral quinine sulfate in conjunction with oral doxycycline or tetracycline; the fixed-combination of oral atovaquone and proguanil; or a regimen of oral mefloquine. Because all of these regimens are active only against asexual erythrocytic forms of plasmodia (not exoerythrocytic stages) and cannot prevent delayed primary attacks or relapse of *P. vivax* malaria or provide a radical cure, a 14-day regimen of oral primaquine is indicated in addition to these regimens to eradicate hypnozoites and prevent relapse in patients treated for *P. vivax* malaria.

For additional information on treatment of uncomplicated malaria, see Uses: Malaria, in Quinine Sulfate 8:30.08.

Treatment of Severe Malaria. Doxycycline or tetracycline hydrochloride is used in conjunction with IV quinidine gluconate (followed by oral quinine sulfate) for the treatment of severe *P. falciparum* malaria†. The CDC recommends that severe *P. falciparum* malaria be treated with IV quinidine gluconate therapy in conjunction with a 7-day regimen of doxycycline, tetracycline, or clindamycin administered orally or IV as tolerated. After parasitemia is reduced to less than 1% and the patient can tolerate oral therapy, IV quinidine gluconate therapy can be discontinued and oral quinine sulfate therapy initiated to complete 3 or 7 days of total quinidine and quinine therapy as determined by the geographic origin of the infecting parasite (3 days if malaria was acquired in Africa or South America or 7 days if acquired in Southeast Asia).

Clinicians who desire assistance with diagnosis and treatment of malaria may consult with experts at the CDC Malaria Epidemiology Branch by calling the CDC Malaria Hotline at 770-488-7788from 8:00 a.m. to 4:30 p.m. Eastern Standard Time or the CDC Emergency Operation Center at 770-488-7100 after hours, on weekends, and holidays and request that the individual on call for the Malaria Epidemiology Branch be paged.

For additional information on treatment of severe malaria, see Uses: Malaria, in Quinidine 24:04.04.04.

■ Mycobacterial Infections

Leprosy Minocycline is used as an alternative agent in multiple-drug regimens used for the treatment of multibacillary leprosy† and also is used in a single-dose rifampin-based multiple-drug regimen for the treatment of single-lesion paucibacillary leprosy†.

For the treatment of multibacillary leprosy (i.e., more than 5 lesions or skin smear positive for acid-fast bacteria), the World Health Organization (WHO) currently recommends a multiple-drug regimen that includes rifampin, clofazimine, and dapsone. Minocycline is recommended as an alternative for use in antileprosy regimens in patients with multibacillary leprosy who will not accept or cannot tolerate clofazimine, or when rifampin cannot be used because of adverse effects, intercurrent disease (e.g., chronic hepatitis), or infection with rifampin-resistant *Mycobacterium leprae*.

For the treatment of paucibacillary leprosy (i.e., 2–5 skin lesions), the WHO usually recommends a 6-month multiple-drug regimen that includes rifampin and dapsone. However, patients with single-lesion paucibacillary leprosy (i.e., a single skin lesion with definite loss of sensation but without nerve trunk involvement) have been effectively treated with a single-dose rifampin-based multiple-drug regimen (ROM) that includes a single dose of rifampin, a single dose of ofloxacin, and single dose of minocycline. The single-dose ROM regimen may be an acceptable and cost-effective alternative regimen in antileprosy programs that have detected a large number of patients (e.g., more than 1000 annually) with single-lesion paucibacillary leprosy; however, the WHO states that the single-dose ROM regimen should not be used in antileprosy programs that have detected few single-lesion paucibacillary leprosy patients since it involves additional logistic and informational problems for these programs.

For additional information on the treatment of leprosy, see Rifampin 8:16.04, Dapsone 8:16.92, and Clofazimine 8:16.92.

Other Mycobacterial Infections Minocycline or doxycycline are considered drugs of choice for the treatment of cutaneous infections caused by *Mycobacterium marinum*.

■ Ehrlichiosis and Anaplasmosis

Doxycycline is considered the drug of choice in adults for the treatment of human granulocytotropic anaplasmosis† (HGA; formerly human granulocytic ehrlichiosis [HGE]) caused by *Anaplasma phagocytophilum* (formerly *Ehrlichia phagocytophila*, *E. equi*, agent of HGE), human monocytotropic (or monocytic) ehrlichiosis† (HME) caused by *E. chaffeensis*, and ehrlichiosis† caused by *E. ewingii* or *E. canis*. Doxycycline is recommended by the CDC and AAP as the drug of choice for presumed or confirmed rickettsial infections (including RMSF) or ehrlichiosis† (including HGA and HME) in children of any age.

Treatment of suspected ehrlichiosis,† should be initiated promptly since a delay in treatment while awaiting laboratory confirmation of the diagnosis may increase the risk for severe disease and fatal outcomes. IV therapy generally is indicated for hospitalized patients, and oral therapy generally is appropriate for patients with early disease, outpatients, or hospitalized patients who are not vomiting or obtunded. The optimum duration of therapy has not been established; however, therapy is usually continued at least 5–10 days and until the patient is afebrile for 3 days or longer and clinically improved. A longer duration of therapy may be required for severe illness. The CDC recommends a treatment duration of 10–14 days in those with HGA since this provides an appropriate duration of therapy for adequate treatment of possible concurrent early Lyme disease. (See Lyme Disease under Uses: Spirochetal Infections.)

As alternatives to doxycycline, some clinicians suggest chloramphenicol for the treatment of infections caused by *E. chaffeensis* and rifampin as an alternative for the treatment of infections caused by *A. phagocytophilum*.

■ Periodontitis

Oral doxycycline (administered as 20-mg tablets) is used as an adjunct to scaling and root planing to promote attachment level gain and to reduce pocket depth in adults with periodontitis. Doxycycline (administered subgingivally as a controlled-release preparation) or minocycline (administered subgingivally as sustained-release microspheres) is used in conjunction with scaling and root planing for the reduction of pocket depth in adults with periodontitis. (See Doxycycline Hyclate 52:04.04 and see Minocycline Hydrochloride 52:04.04.)

■ Rheumatoid Arthritis

Minocycline is used in the treatment of rheumatoid arthritis†. Results of one study indicate that minocycline is at least as effective as hydroxychloroquine in the management of rheumatoid arthritis in adults. Minocycline is one of several disease-modifying antirheumatic drugs (DMARDs) that can be used when DMARD therapy is appropriate. (For further information on the treatment of arthritis, see Uses: Rheumatoid Arthritis, in Methotrexate 10:00.)

■ Syndrome of Inappropriate Antidiuretic Hormone Secretion

Demeclocycline (but not other currently available tetracyclines) has been effective when used in the treatment of the syndrome of inappropriate antidiuretic hormone secretion† (SIADH). Because it takes several days for diuresis to occur after initiation of demeclocycline therapy, the drug is of limited value in patients with acute water intoxication caused by excess ADH secretion. However, demeclocycline is effective in inhibiting the action of ADH in patients with the chronic form of the disease, and most clinicians advocate the use of the drug instead of lithium. Further studies are needed to compare the safety and efficacy of demeclocycline and other forms of therapy for SIADH. Demeclocycline has also been used to treat hyponatremia and water retention† in patients with congestive heart failure or cirrhosis. However, use of demeclocycline in these conditions has been associated with a high incidence of renal failure, and the drug probably should not be used in these patients.

■ Pericardial and Pleural Effusions

Tetracycline hydrochloride (no longer commercially available as a parenteral formulation in the US) has been used by intracavitary injection as a sclerosing agent to control pleural effusions† caused by metastatic tumors. Doxycycline also has been administered in a limited number of patients by intracavitary injection† or via lavage drainage† for the management of malignant pleural effusions, and minocycline has been administered by intracavitary injection† for malignant pleural effusions and concurrent postoperative air leaks in a few patients.

Patients with malignant pleural effusions frequently have symptoms of dyspnea, cough, and chest pain and heaviness. Although thoracentesis may provide temporary relief of such symptoms, the effusion often reaccumulates rapidly, and surgical insertion of a thoracostomy tube with subsequent intrapleural instillation of a sclerosing agent generally is considered the treatment of choice for such effusions in patients with neoplasms unresponsive to systemic antineoplastic or radiation therapy. When instilled into the pleural space, tetracyclines and other effective sclerosing agents cause inflammation that results in fibrosis and adherence of serosal surfaces (pleurodesis), thereby obliterating the pleural space and reducing the chance of fluid reaccumulation; however, most current pleurodesis procedures for malignant pleural effusion appear to be associated with a substantial risk of recurrence. Some clinicians recommend removal of the sclerosing fluid after 0.5–4 hours, although it has been suggested that dispersal of the sclerosing agent and pleurodesis may occur within minutes after instillation of tetracycline. Further studies are needed to elucidate fully the optimum length of time that the drug should remain in the pleural cavity. Pleurodesis appears to be most effective when drainage from the thoracostomy tube does not exceed 100 mL/hour and is unlikely to be successful if the patient's underlying disease prevents complete expansion of the lung following drainage of the effusion.

The most common adverse effects reported with intracavitary administration of tetracyclines into the pleural space are chest pain and fever. Opiate analgesics may be administered prior to the procedure to relieve pain associated with pleurodesis; lidocaine also has been instilled into the chest tube prior to pleurodesis to help alleviate discomfort. Although adverse effects attributable to systemic absorption of doxycycline or minocycline appear to be minimal with currently used intrapleural doses of these drugs, therapeutic serum concentrations of tetracycline and lidocaine have been achieved in some patients following intrapleural administration.

Doxycycline or minocycline has been suggested as an alternative to tetracycline hydrochloride for the management of malignant pleural effusions when intrapleural therapy is indicated. Data in a limited number of patients suggest that intrapleural doxycycline prevents pleural fluid reaccumulation in most patients with metastatic pleural effusions, at least in the short term (e.g., 1 month) and appears to be associated with relatively few adverse effects (e.g., chest pain, fever). Another agent, bleomycin, has been reported in at least one controlled study to be more effective and possibly better tolerated but more expensive than tetracycline hydrochloride for the management of such effusions. The efficacy and safety of intrapleural doxycycline or minocycline compared with intrapleural administration of bleomycin or other potentially more toxic and/or complicated therapies (e.g., thoracostomy, talc insufflation, nitrogen mustard) for the management of malignant pleural effusions remains to be determined.

Tetracycline hydrochloride and doxycycline also have been administered by intrapericardial injection† in a limited number of patients with malignant pericardial effusions and associated cardiac tamponade†.

■ **Diagnostic Uses** Because tetracyclines have an affinity for and localize in tumors and necrotic or ischemic tissue, the drugs have been used to detect malignant cells† in gastric washings, pleural fluid, and ascitic fluid. After several days of oral tetracycline therapy, appropriate specimens are obtained and examined under ultraviolet light; malignant cells in the samples exhibit a bright yellow-gold fluorescence. In addition, radiolabeled tetracycline hydrochloride has been used to detect tumors†, especially in the chest, and to detect and measure the extent of ischemia following myocardial infarcts†.

■ **Prophylaxis in Victims of Sexual Assault** Oral doxycycline is used in conjunction with oral metronidazole and IM ceftriaxone for empiric anti-infective prophylaxis in adult or adolescent victims of sexual assault†; postexposure hepatitis B vaccination also is recommended for susceptible victims. Many experts recommend routine empiric prophylactic therapy after a sexual assault, and use of such prophylaxis probably benefits most patients since follow-up of assault victims can be difficult and such prophylaxis allays the patient's concerns about possible infection. Trichomoniasis, genital chlamydial infection, gonorrhea, and bacterial vaginosis are the sexually transmitted diseases most commonly diagnosed in women following sexual assault; however, the prevalence of these infections is substantial among sexually active women and their presence after assault does not necessarily indicate that the infections were acquired during the assault. Chlamydial and gonococcal infections among females are of special concern because of the possibility of ascending infection. When empiric anti-infective prophylaxis is indicated in adult or adolescent sexual assault victims, the CDC recommends administration of a single 125-mg IM dose of ceftriaxone given in conjunction with a single 2-g oral dose of metronidazole and a single 1-g oral dose of azithromycin or a 7-day regimen of oral doxycycline (100 mg twice daily). This 3-drug regimen provides coverage against gonorrhea, chlamydia, trichomoniasis, and bacterial vaginosis, but efficacy in preventing these infections after sexual assault has not been specifically evaluated. Because of possible adverse GI effects with the 3-drug regimen, the CDC suggests that the patient be counseled regarding the possible benefits, as well as the possibility of toxicity of such prophylaxis. Alternative regimens may be required for some patients because of the likelihood of transmission of other sexually transmitted diseases from the assailant. CDC states that a recommendation concerning the appropriateness of antiretroviral prophylaxis against HIV cannot be made based on currently available information, and the decision to offer such prophylaxis should be individualized taking into account the probability of HIV transmission from a single act of intercourse and the nature of the assault (e.g., extent of physical trauma and exposure to ejaculate). (See Guidelines for Use of Antiretroviral Agents: Antiretroviral Agents for Postexposure Prophylaxis following Sexual Assault or Nonoccupational Exposure to HIV, in the Antiretroviral Agents General Statement 8:18.08.)

There are few data available to establish the risk of a child acquiring a sexually transmitted disease as a result of sexual assault or abuse. The risk is believed to be low in most circumstances, although documentation to support this position is inadequate. The CDC currently states that presumptive treatment for children who have been sexually assaulted or abused is not widely recommended because girls appear to be at lower risk for ascending infection than adolescent or adult women and regular follow-up usually can be ensured. Even if the risk is perceived by the health-care provider to be low, some children or their parents or guardians may have concerns about the possibility of the child contracting a sexually transmitted disease as a result of the assault and these concerns may be an appropriate indication for presumptive treatment in some settings.

For topical uses of tetracyclines, see Minocycline Hydrochloride 52:04.04 and Tetracyclines 84:04.04.

Dosage and Administration

■ **Administration** Tetracyclines, in appropriate dosage forms, are administered orally, IV, or by deep IM injection. IV or IM administration should be used only when the oral route is not feasible, and oral therapy should replace parenteral therapy as soon as possible. IM administration of tetracyclines is rarely indicated because this route of administration is painful and, in the usual dosage, produces lower serum concentrations than does oral administration. If the drugs are given IV, the risk of thrombophlebitis should be considered.

Food and/or milk may reduce GI absorption of tetracyclines. This effect appears to vary among the currently available tetracycline derivatives; the effect is most marked with demeclocycline and is less with doxycycline than other derivatives. Demeclocycline, minocycline, and tetracycline hydrochloride should be administered orally at least 1 hour before or 2 hours after meals and/or milk. Although a few manufacturers state that absorption of doxycycline is not markedly influenced by simultaneous ingestion of food or milk and the drug may be taken with food or milk, this effect appears to be variable and concomitant administration with food or milk can decrease the rate and extent of absorption of doxycycline. (See Effect of Food or Milk under Pharmacokinetics: Absorption in Doxycycline 8:12.24.)

■ **Dosage** The duration of tetracycline therapy depends on the type of infection. Generally, therapy should be continued for a minimum of 24–48 hours after the patient becomes asymptomatic or evidence of eradication of the infection has been obtained. For specific dosages and duration of therapy, see the individual monographs in 8:12.24.

■ **Dosage in Renal Impairment** With the exception of doxycycline, doses and/or frequency of administration of tetracyclines must generally be modified in response to the degree of renal impairment.

Cautions

■ **GI Effects** The most frequent adverse reactions to tetracyclines are dose-related GI effects including nausea, vomiting, diarrhea, bulky loose stools, anorexia, flatulence, abdominal discomfort, and epigastric burning and distress. Stomatitis, glossitis, dysphagia, sore throat, hoarseness, black hairy tongue, pancreatitis, and inflammatory lesions in the anogenital region with candidal overgrowth have also been reported occasionally. GI effects occur most frequently when tetracyclines are administered orally, but may also occur when the drugs are administered IM or IV.

Because *Clostridium difficile*-associated diarrhea and colitis (also known as antibiotic-associated pseudomembranous colitis) caused by overgrowth of toxin-producing clostridia has been reported with the use of many anti-infective agents, it should be considered in the differential diagnosis of patients who develop diarrhea during anti-infective therapy. *Clostridium difficile*-associated diarrhea and colitis may range in severity from mild to life-threatening. Mild cases of colitis may respond to discontinuance of the drug alone, but management of moderate to severe cases should include treatment with fluid, electrolyte, protein supplementation, and appropriate anti-infective therapy.

Staphylococcal enterocolitis with severe, fulminating diarrhea, dehydration, and circulatory collapse has also been reported rarely with oral or parenteral tetracycline therapy and is presumably caused by tetracycline- and penicillin-resistant *Staphylococcus aureus*. Although doxycycline and minocycline produce fewer alterations in the intestinal flora than do other tetracyclines following oral administration, there is no evidence that these 2 drugs produce fewer GI-related adverse effects.

In clinical trials in which combined therapy with tetracycline hydrochloride, metronidazole, and bismuth subsalicylate was used for the treatment of *H. pylori* infection and associated duodenal ulcer, adverse effects generally were related to the GI tract, were reversible, and infrequently led to discontinuance of therapy. Adverse GI effects reported in at least 1% of patients receiving combined therapy with tetracycline hydrochloride, metronidazole, and bismuth subsalicylate (generally in conjunction with acid-suppression therapy) were nausea (10.2%), diarrhea (5.1%), abdominal pain (3%), melena (2.5%), anal discomfort (1.5%), anorexia (1.5%), vomiting (1.5%), and constipation (1%). Adverse GI effects reported in less than 1% of patients receiving combined therapy with tetracycline hydrochloride-metronidazole-bismuth subsalicylate in clinical trials were dry mouth, dyspepsia, dysphagia, flatulence, GI hemorrhage, glossitis, and stomatitis.

Rarely, doxycycline hyclate, minocycline hydrochloride, and tetracycline hydrochloride capsules or tablets have caused esophagitis and esophageal ulceration which were local in origin. In most reported cases, capsules of the drugs had been administered at bedtime, with insufficient quantities of fluid, or to patients with hiatal hernia.

Oral candidiasis occurs occasionally during oral, IM, or IV tetracycline therapy and is presumably the result of alterations in the normal microbial flora caused by the anti-infectives. Candidal suprainfections have been reported more frequently with tetracyclines than with penicillins, and occur most frequently during prolonged therapy and/or in debilitated patients.

■ **Sensitivity Reactions** Hypersensitivity reactions have been reported rarely with tetracyclines and include maculopapular, morbilliform, or erythematous rash; exfoliative dermatitis; erythema multiforme; Stevens-Johnson syndrome; pruritus; urticaria; angioedema; pulmonary infiltrates and/or eosinophilia; asthma; anaphylaxis; anaphylactoid purpura; fixed drug eruptions of the genitalia (including balanitis) and other areas; pericarditis; exacerbation of systemic lupus erythematosus; and serum sickness-like reactions with fever, rash, headache, and arthralgia. Patients hypersensitive to one tetracycline derivative are likely to be hypersensitive to all tetracyclines.

■ **Dermatologic Effects** Photosensitivity, manifested as an exaggerated sunburn reaction on sun-exposed areas of the body, has occurred with tetracyclines. Photosensitivity reactions occur most frequently and are most severe with demeclocycline; occur less frequently with doxycycline, oxytetracycline (no longer commercially available in the US), and tetracycline; and very rarely occur with minocycline. Photosensitivity reactions, if they occur, develop within a few minutes to several hours after sun exposure and usually persist 1–2 days after discontinuance of the tetracycline. Although in most cases photosensitivity reactions appear to result from accumulation of the drugs in skin and are phototoxic in nature, photoallergic reactions may also occur. Paresthesia, consisting mainly of tingling and burning of the hands, feet, and nose, may be an early indication of photosensitivity. The CDC states that the risk of such a reaction may be minimized by avoiding prolonged, direct exposure to the sun and by using sunscreens that absorb long-wave UVA radiation; however, some clinicians suggest that sunscreens provide, at most, only limited protection in patients susceptible to these reactions. The manufacturers state that severe photosensitivity reactions may require treatment with antihistamines and corticosteroids.

Onycholysis and discoloration of the nails, alone or associated with photosensitivity reactions, have been reported during tetracycline therapy. Maculopapular and erythematous rash and, rarely, exfoliative dermatitis, also have been reported in patients receiving tetracyclines.

Photosensitivity reaction or rash was reported in less than 1% of patients receiving combined therapy with tetracycline hydrochloride, metronidazole, and bismuth subsalicylate (generally in conjunction with acid-suppression therapy) in clinical trials.

Blue-gray pigmentation at areas of cutaneous inflammation has been reported in a few patients receiving oral minocycline. The pigmentation is presumably caused by a minocycline degradation product or a drug-hemosiderin complex. A generalized muddy-brown pigmentation of the skin, accentuated in sun-exposed areas of the skin, has also been reported in a few patients receiving oral minocycline for the treatment of acne vulgaris.

Rarely, long-term therapy of inflammatory acne with oral tetracycline hydrochloride has resulted in gram-negative folliculitis caused by tetracycline-resistant organisms.

■ **Renal Effects** Increased urinary excretion of nitrogen and increased BUN concentrations, with or without increased serum creatinine concentrations, have been reported rarely during tetracycline therapy. These effects are not usually clinically important in patients with normal renal function or in patients with impaired renal function receiving usual dosages of doxycycline or minocycline. However, if the usual dosage of demeclocycline or tetracycline is used in patients with impaired renal function, progressive azotemia, hyperphosphatemia, and acidosis may occur.

Administration of outdated or deteriorated tetracyclines has caused a reversible Fanconi-like syndrome characterized by nausea, vomiting, lethargy, polydipsia, polyuria, glycosuria, aminoaciduria, phosphaturia, proteinuria, acidosis, and hypokalemia. In most cases, the outdated tetracycline preparation administered contained citric acid (an excipient no longer used in tetracycline preparations) which accelerated deterioration of the antibiotic during storage. Therefore, this reaction is unlikely with currently available tetracycline preparations. In at least 1 patient, use of outdated tetracycline hydrochloride resulted in lactic acidosis in addition to the Fanconi-like syndrome.

Demeclocycline has caused a reversible, dose-related diabetes insipidus syndrome (polyuria, polydipsia, weakness) in some patients who received long-term therapy with the drug. This syndrome has been shown to be nephrogenic, dose-dependent, and reversible when demeclocycline is discontinued. When demeclocycline is used in dosages of 600 mg to 1.2 g daily, this effect reportedly occurs within 5 days after initiation of therapy and reverses within 2–6 days after discontinuance of the drug. This diabetes insipidus syndrome has not been reported with other currently available tetracyclines.

■ **Hepatic Effects** Hepatotoxicity, characterized histologically as fatty metamorphosis of the liver without necrosis or inflammatory reactions and sometimes associated with pancreatitis, has been reported rarely with tetracyclines. Elevations in liver function test results also have been reported. Fatalities have occurred because of irreversible deterioration of pancreatic, hepatic, and renal function. Liver toxicity has been reported most frequently following IV administration of large doses (more than 2 g daily) of tetracycline hydrochloride (no longer commercially available as a parenteral formulation in the US) to pregnant women with pyelonephritis but has also occurred following oral administration of large doses of the drugs to nonpregnant individuals. Liver toxicity is most likely to occur in patients receiving other hepatotoxic drugs or in patients with preexisting hepatic or renal impairment. A syndrome consisting of a severe exfoliative dermatitis followed by acute hepatitis, which progressed to hepatic coma and death in at least one patient, has been reported rarely with minocycline therapy.

■ **Hematologic Effects** Leukocytosis, neutropenia, leukopenia, atypical lymphocytes, toxic granulation of granulocytes, hemolytic anemia, thrombocytopenia, and thrombocytopenic purpura have occurred rarely with long-term tetracycline therapy. Increased urinary excretion of ascorbic acid and decreased leukocyte ascorbic acid concentrations have been reported during tetracycline therapy; although the clinical importance of these effects is unclear, they presumably may interfere with leukocyte migration and phagocytic activity.

■ **Jarisch-Herxheimer Reaction** A Jarisch-Herxheimer reaction has occurred occasionally when tetracyclines were used to treat brucellosis or spirochetal infections, including louse-borne relapsing fever caused by *Borrelia recurrentis*, leptospirosis, and syphilis. This reaction also have been observed in patients with Lyme disease treated with tetracyclines or certain other antibiotics (e.g., penicillins, cephalosporins). The reaction, consisting of headache, fever, chills, malaise, muscular aches, exacerbation of cutaneous lesions, and leukocytosis, is presumably caused by the release of pyrogen and/or endotoxin from phagocytized organisms and generally occurs 12–24 hours after initiation of tetracycline therapy. If tetracyclines are used in the treatment of brucellosis or spirochetal infections, patients should be warned to expect the reaction and should be treated with bedrest and aspirin or other nonsteroidal anti-inflammatory agents (NSAIAs) if necessary.

■ **Nervous System Effects** Adverse CNS effects including lightheadedness, dizziness, vertigo, ataxia, drowsiness, headache, and fatigue occur with minocycline and are often associated with nausea and vomiting. The true incidence of these adverse effects has not been determined. Although vestibular symptoms were previously reported to occur in up to 21% of patients treated with minocycline, these reactions may occur in 30–90% of patients treated with usual dosages of minocycline. Vestibular symptoms appear to be dose related and occur more frequently in women than in men. These symptoms may disappear during continued therapy with minocycline, and rapidly disappear when the drug is discontinued. Tinnitus, hearing loss, and visual disturbances also have been reported with tetracycline therapy.

Dizziness or paresthesia was reported in 1.5% of patients receiving combined therapy with tetracycline hydrochloride, metronidazole, and bismuth subsalicylate (generally in conjunction with acid-suppression therapy) in clinical trials; asthenia or insomnia was reported in 1% of such patients. Nervousness, malaise, or syncope was reported in less than 1% of patients receiving tetracycline hydrochloride-metronidazole-bismuth subsalicylate therapy in clinical trials.

Increased intracranial pressure and bulging fontanels (pseudotumor cerebri; benign intracranial hypertension) have been reported rarely when tetracyclines were used in infants. Pseudotumor cerebri, usually manifested by headache and blurred vision, also has been reported rarely in adults receiving tetracyclines. Although this condition and related symptoms usually resolve following discontinuance of the tetracycline, the possibility of permanent sequelae exists.

Animal studies indicate that tetracyclines may potentiate neuromuscular blockade produced by neuromuscular blocking agents. An increase in muscular weakness (myasthenic syndrome) has been reported in a few patients with myasthenia gravis following IV administration of oxytetracycline hydrochloride (no longer commercially available in the US), but a causal relationship has not been established.

■ **Local Effects** IV administration of tetracyclines frequently causes thrombophlebitis, especially when IV therapy is prolonged or when a single vein is used for repeated infusions. IM administration of tetracyclines is painful. To minimize pain associated with IM administration of the drug, injections should be given deeply into a relatively large muscle, inadvertent intraneural injection or injection into blood vessels or subcutaneous or fat layers should be avoided, and injection sites should be alternated. Pain and induration may be relieved by applying ice packs.

■ **Other Adverse Effects** Prolonged administration of tetracyclines has produced a microscopic brown-black discoloration of the thyroid in animals and humans, and goiter accompanied by elevated radioactive iodine uptake and evidence of thyroid tumors has occurred in rats during long-term treatment with minocycline (See Cautions: Mutagenicity and Carcinogenicity.) However, abnormalities in thyroid function studies have not been reported to date in humans.

Vaginal candidiasis occurs occasionally and systemic candidiasis occurs rarely following oral or parenteral use of tetracyclines. For further discussion of candidiasis, see Cautions: GI Effects In addition to causing a Fanconi-like syndrome (see Cautions: Renal Effects), use of outdated tetracyclines has also caused a lupus erythematosus-like syndrome.

While tooth discoloration has been reported most frequently in children with developing teeth (see Cautions: Pregnancy, Fertility, and Lactation, and see Pediatric Precautions), such discoloration also has been reported rarely in adults receiving tetracyclines.

Pain or upper respiratory infection was reported in 1% of patients receiving combined therapy with tetracycline hydrochloride, metronidazole, and bismuth subsalicylate (generally in conjunction with acid-suppression therapy) in clinical trials, while hypertension, myocardial infarction, or rheumatoid arthritis was reported in less than 1% of such patients.

■ **Precautions and Contraindications** Tetracyclines are contraindicated in patients hypersensitive to any of the tetracyclines.

To reduce development of drug-resistant bacteria and maintain effectiveness of tetracyclines and other antibacterials, the drugs should be used only for the treatment or prevention of infections proven or strongly suspected to be caused by susceptible bacteria. When selecting or modifying anti-infective therapy, use results of culture and in vitro susceptibility testing. In the absence of such data, consider local epidemiology and susceptibility patterns when selecting anti-infectives for empiric therapy.

Patients should be advised that antibacterials (including tetracyclines) should only be used to treat bacterial infections and not used to treat viral infections (e.g., the common cold). Patients also should be advised about the importance of completing the full course of therapy, even if feeling better after a few days, and that skipping doses or not completing therapy may decrease effectiveness and increase the likelihood that bacteria will develop resistance and will not be treatable with tetracyclines or other antibacterials in the future.

Use of tetracyclines may result in overgrowth of nonsusceptible organisms, including fungi. If suprainfection or superinfection occurs, tetracyclines should be discontinued and appropriate therapy instituted.

Capsules or tablets containing tetracyclines should be given with adequate amounts of fluid and probably should not be given at bedtime or to patients with esophageal obstruction or compression.

The manufacturers state that patients receiving tetracyclines who are apt to be exposed to direct sunlight or ultraviolet light (e.g., sun lamps) should be advised that photosensitivity may occur, and the drugs should be discontinued at the first sign of erythema.

Renal, hepatic, and hematologic systems should be evaluated periodically during prolonged therapy with tetracyclines. The manufacturers state that if tetracyclines are indicated in patients with preexisting hepatic or renal impairment, lower than usual dosage should be used, liver and renal function tests should be performed prior to and during therapy, and other potentially hepatotoxic drugs should not be administered concomitantly. In addition, if tetracyclines are used in these patients, serum concentrations of the drugs should be monitored if therapy is prolonged; serum concentrations of tetracycline hydrochloride should not exceed 15 mcg/mL.

Patients who experience CNS symptoms while receiving minocycline should be cautioned about driving vehicles or operating hazardous machinery during therapy. Dizziness, headache, and vertigo have also been reported rarely with other tetracycline derivatives.

Some commercially available tetracycline preparations (e.g., doxycycline calcium oral suspension, tetracycline oral suspension) contain sulfites that may cause allergic-type reactions, including anaphylaxis and life-threatening or less severe asthmatic episodes, in certain susceptible individuals. The overall prevalence of sulfite sensitivity in the general population is unknown but probably low; such sensitivity appears to occur more frequently in asthmatic than in nonasthmatic individuals.

Although a causal relationship has not been definitely established, an increase in muscular weakness has been reported in a few patients with myasthenia gravis following IV administration of oxytetracycline hydrochloride (no longer commercially available in the US). Therefore, parenteral tetracyclines probably should be used with caution in patients with this condition.

When the commercially available combination preparation containing tetracycline hydrochloride, metronidazole, and bismuth subsalicylate (Helidac® Therapy) is used for the treatment of *Helicobacter pylori* infection and associated duodenal ulcer disease, the cautions, precautions, and contraindications associated with metronidazole and bismuth subsalicylate must be considered in addition to those associated with tetracycline hydrochloride.

■ **Pediatric Precautions** Tetracyclines should *not* be used in children younger than 8 years of age unless other appropriate drugs are ineffective or are contraindicated. However, the manufacturers, American Academy of Pediatrics (AAP), US Centers for Disease Control and Prevention (CDC), and Infectious Diseases Society of America (IDSA) state that use of tetracyclines (e.g., doxycycline) in children younger than 8 years of age can be considered in certain circumstances when the benefits outweigh the risks. These circumstances include the treatment or prophylaxis of anthrax (including inhalational anthrax [post-exposure]), treatment of severe cholera, and treatment of presumed or confirmed rickettsial infections, including Rocky Mountain spotted fever (RMSF), Q fever, ehrlichiosis, and anaplasmosis. In addition, the CDC states that children less than 8 years of age with uncomplicated chloroquine-resistant *P. falciparum* malaria, uncomplicated *P. vivax* malaria, or severe *P. falciparum* malaria may receive a regimen that includes doxycycline (or tetracycline) if other treatment options are not available or not tolerated and the potential benefits outweigh risks. However, because of concerns regarding long-term use of tetracyclines in infants and children, the treatment duration should be limited whenever possible if use of a tetracycline is considered necessary in children younger than 8 years of age.

Tetracyclines form a stable calcium complex in any bone-forming tissue. A reversible decrease in fibula growth rate has been observed in premature infants receiving oral tetracycline. Because tetracyclines localize in the dentin and enamel of developing teeth, use of the drugs during tooth development may cause enamel hypoplasia and permanent yellow-gray to brown discoloration of the teeth. Use of tetracyclines may result in discoloration of the deciduous teeth of children if the drugs are used during pregnancy or in children up to 4–6 months of age. Discoloration of the permanent teeth may result if the drugs are used in children 4 months to 8 years of age. Discoloration of the permanent teeth has also occurred in older children and young adults in whom minocycline had been used. These effects are most common following long-term use of tetracyclines but have occurred following repeated short-term use of the drugs.

■ **Mutagenicity and Carcinogenicity** Some tetracyclines (tetracycline, oxytetracycline [no longer commercially available in the US]) reportedly have demonstrated mutagenic potential in in vitro mammalian cell (e.g., mouse lymphoma, Chinese hamster lung cell) assays.

Administration of certain tetracycline antibiotics reportedly has been associated with tumor production in animals. Long-term dietary administration of minocycline has resulted in evidence of thyroid tumors in rats, and adrenal and pituitary tumors have been reported in rats receiving oxytetracycline. However, in studies conducted in mice and rats, tetracycline hydrochloride did not demonstrate evidence of carcinogenicity.

■ **Pregnancy, Fertility, and Lactation** Tetracyclines can cause fetal toxicity when administered to pregnant women;, but potential benefits from use of the drugs may be acceptable in certain conditions despite the possible risks to the fetus.

The CDC states that the use of tetracyclines (e.g., doxycycline) may be warranted in pregnant women with presumed or confirmed rickettsial infections (including Rocky Mountain spotted fever [RMSF]) or ehrlichiosis (including HGA and HME).

Because the benefits of doxycycline outweigh the risks in the treatment of inhalational anthrax, the CDC and other experts (e.g., US Working Group on Civilian Biodefense) state that recommendations for use of doxycycline in pregnant women with anthrax are the same as those for women who are not pregnant. Since adverse effects on developing teeth and bones are dose-related, the CDC suggests that doxycycline might be used for a short period (7–14 days) before 6 months of gestation when necessary.

Malaria infection in pregnant women is associated with high risks of maternal and perinatal morbidity and mortality (e.g., miscarriage, premature delivery, low birth weight, congenital infection and/or perinatal death). CDC states a regimen of quinine in conjunction with doxycycline (or tetracycline) may be used for the treatment of uncomplicated malaria in pregnant women in rare circumstances (e.g., if other treatment options are not available or not tolerated) if benefits outweigh risks.

Results of studies in animals indicate that tetracyclines cross the placenta, are found in fetal tissues, and can have toxic effects on the developing fetus (e.g., retardation of skeletal development). Evidence of embryotoxicity also has been found in animals treated with these drugs early in pregnancy. When tetracyclines are administered during pregnancy or if the patient becomes pregnant while receiving a tetracycline, the patient should be informed of the potential hazard to the fetus.

Liver toxicity has occurred following IV administration of tetracyclines to pregnant women. (See Cautions: Hepatic Effects.) If doxycycline is used in pregnant women, some clinicians recommend that periodic liver function testing be performed.

Reproduction studies in male rats have demonstrated that minocycline impairs fertility. Tetracycline hydrochloride had no effect on fertility when administered in the diet to male and female rats at a daily intake of 25 times the human dosage.

Tetracyclines are distributed into milk. Some manufacturers state that because of the potential for serious adverse reactions from tetracyclines in nursing infants, a decision should be made whether to discontinue nursing or the drug, taking into account the importance of the drug to the woman. However, available limited data suggest that absorption of tetracycline by a nursing infant is negligible because of inhibition of the drug's absorption by calcium in milk and that a short course of tetracycline therapy (e.g., 7–10 days) may be used in nursing women.

Some clinicians recommend that tetracyclines not be used in nursing women, if possible, because of the potential for dental staining in the infant. The AAP considers tetracyclines to be usually compatible with breast-feeding since the amount of the drugs potentially absorbed by nursing infants would be small and no observable change in infants associated with such exposure has been reported to date. The CDC states that although data are very limited regarding the use of doxycycline as an antimalarial agent in nursing women, most experts consider the theoretical risk to nursing infants to be remote. However, because the long-term safety of prolonged exposure of nursing infants to breast milk from doxycycline-treated women currently is not known, the CDC recommends that lactating women who are concerned about the use of doxycycline during anthrax prophylaxis consider expressing and then discarding their breast milk so that breast-feeding can be resumed once anti-infective prophylaxis is complete. Decisions about anti-infective choice and continuation of breast-feeding should be made by the woman and her and the infant's clinicians, taking into consideration the efficacy of the anti-infective, safety for the infant, and benefits of breast-feeding.

Minocycline-induced black pigmentation of milk has been reported in a woman with phenothiazine-induced galactorrhea.

Drug Interactions

Because tetracyclines readily chelate divalent or trivalent cations (see Chemistry and Stability: Stability), concurrent oral administration of other drugs containing these cations may decrease absorption of oral tetracyclines and vice versa. Antacids containing aluminum, calcium, or magnesium and laxatives containing magnesium impair the absorption of oral tetracyclines and should be given 1–2 hours before or after the anti-infective. Oral iron preparations also interfere with GI absorption of tetracyclines, leading to decreased serum concentrations of both the anti-infective and iron. Concurrent administration of an oral iron preparation and an oral tetracycline reportedly results in a 30–90% decrease in absorption of the tetracycline. In one study, oral ferrous sulfate also reportedly decreased the serum half-life of a single IV dose of doxycycline as the hyclate, presumably by interfering with intestinal reabsorption of the anti-infective. If simultaneous administration of an oral iron preparation and a tetracycline is necessary, the tetracycline should be given 3 hours after or 2 hours before the oral iron preparation. In one study, concomitant administration of oral zinc sulfate impaired absorption of oral tetracycline hydrochloride but had no effect on the absorption of oral doxycycline.

■ **Drugs Affecting GI pH** In one study, oral sodium bicarbonate decreased absorption of oral tetracycline hydrochloride when the anti-infective was administered as capsules but had no appreciable effect on absorption when tetracycline hydrochloride was dissolved in water prior to oral administration. In another study, concurrent administration of sodium bicarbonate had no effect on the rate or extent of absorption of tetracycline hydrochloride administered as capsules.

Although concurrent administration of oral cimetidine and tetracycline hydrochloride capsules resulted in slightly decreased serum concentrations of the anti-infective in one study, other studies have shown that serum concentrations of tetracycline hydrochloride are not appreciably affected by concurrent administration of oral cimetidine.

■ **Anti-infective Agents** Tetracyclines have been reported to antagonize the bactericidal activity of aminoglycosides and penicillins in vitro, and the manufacturers and some clinicians recommend that the drugs not be used concomitantly. There have been rare reports of in vivo antagonism when IV tetracyclines were used with IM penicillin in the treatment of pneumococcal meningitis; however, oral tetracyclines have been administered in conjunction with penicillin or streptomycin for other indications with no apparent decrease in activity.

Concomitant use of tetracycline and atovaquone decreases plasma concentrations of atovaquone. Parasitemia should be closely monitored in patients receiving both drugs.

Concomitant use of tetracycline and buffered didanosine preparations may result in decreased tetracycline concentrations, and caution is advised if the drugs are used concomitantly.

■ **Methoxyflurane** Preoperative or postoperative administration of tetracyclines to patients undergoing methoxyflurane anesthesia (no longer commercially available in the US) may produce fatal nephrotoxicity, and concurrent use of the drugs should be avoided.

■ **Oral Anticoagulants** Oral, IM, or IV tetracyclines reportedly may potentiate the effects of oral anticoagulants either by impairing utilization of prothrombin or by decreasing vitamin K production by intestinal bacteria. Prothrombin times should be monitored more frequently than usual in patients receiving concomitant tetracycline and oral anticoagulant therapy, and dosage of the anticoagulant should be adjusted as required. Tetracyclines have also been reported to interfere with the anticoagulant effect of heparin; however, this interaction has not been substantiated and special precautions are probably unnecessary.

■ **Oral Contraceptives** Concurrent use of tetracyclines can reduce the effectiveness of oral contraceptives. When administered concurrently with an oral contraceptive containing estrogen, tetracycline hydrochloride apparently decreased the effectiveness of the contraceptive in one patient resulting in pregnancy and caused breakthrough bleeding in another. Patients should be advised to use a different or additional form of contraception during tetracycline therapy. (See Pregnancy, Fertility, and Lactation.)

■ **Other Drugs** Antidiarrhea agents containing kaolin and pectin or bismuth subsalicylate reportedly impair absorption of oral tetracyclines, and concurrent use probably should be avoided if possible. In patients receiving tetracycline hydrochloride in multiple-drug regimens including bismuth subsalicylate for the treatment of *Helicobacter pylori* infection and associated duodenal ulcer, the clinical importance of an anticipated reduction in tetracycline systemic absorption is unknown as the relative contribution of systemic versus local antimicrobial activity against *H. pylori* has not been determined.

Barbiturates, phenytoin, and carbamazepine decrease the serum half-life of doxycycline. Serum concentrations of demeclocycline and tetracycline are not affected by concomitant administration of barbiturates, phenytoin, or carbamazepine and are preferred when a tetracycline is indicated in a patient receiving one of these drugs.

In one patient stabilized on lithium carbonate, concurrent administration of oral tetracycline hydrochloride resulted in increased serum concentrations of lithium and lithium toxicity.

■ **Live Vaccines** There are theoretical concerns that anti-infectives with antibacterial activity against Ty21a (the live, attenuated strain of *Salmonella typhi* contained in typhoid vaccine live oral) may interfere with the immunogenicity of the vaccine. Administration of typhoid vaccine live oral containing live, attenuated *Salmonella typhi* of the Ty21a strain should be delayed for at least 24 hours after a dose of any anti-infective with antibacterial activity, including doxycycline.

Laboratory Test Interferences

■ **Tests for Urinary Glucose** Although tetracyclines have reportedly caused false-positive results in urine glucose determinations using the cupric sulfate method (Benedict's reagent, Clinitest®), this effect may have been caused by ascorbic acid which is included in parenteral preparations of tetracyclines. Tetracyclines also reportedly cause false-negative results in urine glucose determinations using glucose oxidase reagent (e.g., Clinistix®, Tes-Tape®).

■ **Other Laboratory Tests** Tetracyclines generally interfere with fluorometric determinations of urine catecholamines resulting in falsely increased values.

Mechanism of Action

■ **Antibacterial Effects** Tetracyclines are usually bacteriostatic in action, but may be bactericidal in high concentrations or against highly susceptible organisms.

Tetracyclines appear to inhibit protein synthesis in susceptible organisms mainly by reversibly binding to 30S ribosomal subunits, thereby inhibiting binding of aminoacyl transfer-RNA to those ribosomes. In addition, tetracyclines appear to reversibly bind to 50S ribosomal subunits. There is preliminary evidence that tetracyclines also alter cytoplasmic membranes of susceptible organisms resulting in leakage of nucleotides and other intracellular components from the cell. At high concentrations, tetracyclines also inhibit mammalian protein synthesis.

■ **Effects on Acne** The exact mechanisms by which tetracyclines reduce lesions of acne vulgaris have not been fully elucidated; however, the effect appears to result in part from the antibacterial activity of the drugs. Following oral administration, the drugs inhibit the growth of susceptible organisms (mainly *Propionibacterium acnes*) on the surface of the skin and reduce the concentration of free fatty acids in sebum. The reduction in free fatty acids in sebum may be an indirect result of the inhibition of lipase-producing organisms which convert triglycerides into free fatty acids or may be a direct result of interference with lipase production in these organisms. Free fatty acids are comedogenic and are believed to be a possible cause of the inflammatory lesions (e.g., papules, pustules, nodules, cysts) of acne. However, other mechanisms also appear to be involved because clinical improvement of acne vulgaris with oral tetracycline therapy does not necessarily correspond with a reduction in the bacterial flora of the skin or a decrease in the free fatty acid content of sebum.

In an in vivo study, oral administration of demeclocycline or tetracycline hydrochloride suppressed the local inflammatory response (e.g., erythema, pustules) to patch tests with 40% potassium iodide. Tetracycline hydrochloride also inhibited leukocyte chemotaxis in an in vitro study. It has been hypothesized that these effects could be other mechanisms by which tetracyclines suppress the inflammatory lesions of acne vulgaris.

Spectrum

Tetracyclines have a broad spectrum of activity and are active against most *Rickettsia, Chlamydia, Mycoplasma*, spirochetes, and many gram-negative and gram-positive bacteria. The drugs are inactive against fungi and viruses.

In general, susceptible *Rickettsia*, *Chlamydia*, *Mycoplasma*, and bacteria are inhibited in vitro by demeclocycline, doxycycline, minocycline, or tetracycline concentrations of 0.1–5 mcg/mL. Minocycline and, to a lesser extent, doxycycline are more active in vitro against most susceptible organisms than are other currently available tetracyclines and slightly lower concentrations of these derivatives may be required to inhibit most susceptible organisms. In addition, minocycline is active against some bacteria including *Acinetobacter*, *Enterobacteriaceae*, and *Staphylococcus aureus* resistant to other currently available tetracyclines.

■ **In Vitro Susceptibility Testing** Many factors such as inoculum size, pH, and test media can influence results of in vitro susceptibility tests of the tetracyclines. Results of in vitro susceptibility testing with tetracycline generally can be applied to all currently available tetracyclines, including demeclocycline, doxycycline, and minocycline. However, some organisms (e.g., some staphylococci, *Acinetobacter*) may be more susceptible to doxycycline or minocycline than to tetracycline.

When in vitro susceptibility testing is performed according to the standards of the Clinical and Laboratory Standards Institute (CLSI; formerly National Committee for Clinical Laboratory Standards [NCCLS]), clinical isolates identified as *susceptible* to tetracyclines are inhibited by drug concentrations usually achievable when the recommended dosage is used for the site of infection. Clinical isolates classified as *intermediate* have minimum inhibitory concentrations (MICs) that approach usually attainable blood and tissue concentrations and response rates may be lower than for strains identified as susceptible. Therefore, the intermediate category implies clinical applicability in body sites where the drug is physiologically concentrated or when a higher than usual dosage can be used. This intermediate category also includes a buffer zone that should prevent small, uncontrolled technical factors from causing major discrepancies in interpretation, especially for drugs with narrow pharmacotoxicity margins. If results of in vitro susceptibility testing indicate that a clinical isolate is *resistant* to tetracyclines, the strain is not inhibited by drug concentrations generally achievable with usual dosage schedules and/or MICs fall in the range where specific microbial resistance mechanisms are likely and clinical efficacy of the drug against the isolate has not been reliably demonstrated in clinical studies.

Disk Susceptibility Tests When the disk-diffusion procedure is used for in vitro susceptibility testing, a tetracycline class disk containing 30 mcg of tetracycline hydrochloride may be used and results can generally be applied to all currently available tetracyclines. However, some organisms that are intermediate or resistant to tetracycline may be susceptible to doxycycline and/or minocycline. Additional in vitro testing using disks containing 30 mcg of minocycline or 30 mcg of doxycycline instead of or in addition to tetracycline may be necessary.

Table 1. Interpretation of Disk Diffusion Zone Diameters (nearest whole mm) for Disk Susceptibility Tests Performed According to CLSI Standardized Procedures

	Resistant	Intermediate	Susceptible
Enterobacteriaceae			
Tetracycline	≤14	15–18	≥19
Doxycycline	≤12	13–15	≥16
Minocycline	≤14	15–18	≥19
Pseudomonas aeruginosa			
Tetracycline	≤14	15–18	≥19
Doxycycline	≤12	13–15	≥16
Minocycline	≤14	15–18	≥19
Acinetobacter			
Tetracycline	≤14	15–18	≥19
Doxycycline	≤12	13–15	≥16
Minocycline	≤14	15–18	≥19
Burkholderia			
Minocycline	≤14	15–18	≥19
Stenotrophomonas maltophilia			
Minocycline	≤14	15–18	≥19
Vibrio cholerae			
Tetracycline	≤14	15–18	≥19

Table 2. Interpretation of Disk Diffusion Zone Diameters (nearest whole mm) for Disk Susceptibility Tests Performed According to CLSI Standardized Procedures

	Resistant	Intermediate	Susceptible
Staphylococcus			
Tetracycline	≤14	15–18	≥19
Doxycycline	≤12	13–15	≥16
Minocycline	≤14	15–18	≥19
Enterococcus			
Tetracycline	≤14	15–18	≥19
Doxycycline	≤12	13–15	≥16
Minocycline	≤14	15–18	≥19
Streptococcus pneumoniae			
Tetracycline	≤18	19–22	≥23
Streptococcus (other than S. pneumoniae)			
Tetracycline	≤18	19–22	≥23

Table 3. Interpretation of Disk Diffusion Zone Diameters (nearest whole mm) for Disk Susceptibility Tests Performed According to CLSI Standardized Procedures

	Resistant	Intermediate	Susceptible
Haemophilus influenzae and H. parainfluenzae			
Tetracycline	≤25	26–28	≥29
Neisseria gonorrhoeae			
Tetracycline	≤30	31–37	≥38
Neisseria meningitidis			
Minocycline	—	—	≥26

Dilution Susceptibility Tests When broth or agar dilution susceptibility tests are used to test in vitro susceptibility to tetracyclines, organisms that are susceptible to tetracycline also are considered susceptible to doxycycline and minocycline. However, some organisms that are intermediate or resistant to tetracycline may be susceptible to doxycycline and/or minocycline.

Table 4. Interpretation of MICs (mcg/mL) For Diffusion Susceptibility Tests Performed According to CLSI Standardized Procedures

	Susceptible	Intermediate	Resistant
Enterobacteriaceae			
Tetracycline	≤4	8	≥16
Doxycycline	≤4	8	≥16
Minocycline	≤4	8	≥16
Pseudomonas aeruginosa and Other Non-Enterobacteriaceae (except Acinetobacter, Burkholderia, Stenotrophomonas)			
Tetracycline	≤4	8	≥16
Doxycycline	≤4	8	≥16
Minocycline	≤4	8	≥16
Acinetobacter			
Tetracycline	≤4	8	≥16
Doxycycline	≤4	8	≥16
Minocycline	≤4	8	≥16
Burkholderia cepacia			
Minocycline	≤4	8	≥16
Burkholderia mallei			
Tetracycline	≤4	8	≥16
Burkholderia pseudomallei			
Doxycycline	≤4	8	≥16
Stenotrophomonas maltophilia			
Minocycline	≤4	8	≥16
Vibrio cholerae			
Tetracycline	≤4	8	≥16
Doxycycline	≤4	8	≥16

Table 5. Interpretation of MICs (mcg/mL) For Diffusion Susceptibility Tests Performed According to CLSI Standardized Procedures

	Susceptible	Intermediate	Resistant
Staphylococcus			
Tetracycline	≤4	8	≥16
Doxycycline	≤4	8	≥16
Minocycline	≤4	8	≥16
Enterococcus			
Tetracycline	≤4	8	≥16
Doxycycline	≤4	8	≥16
Minocycline	≤4	8	≥16
Streptococcus pneumoniae			
Tetracycline	≤2	4	≥8
Streptococcus (other than S. pneumoniae)			
Tetracycline	≤2	4	8

Table 6. Interpretation of MICs (mcg/mL) For Diffusion Susceptibility Tests Performed According to CLSI Standardized Procedures

	Susceptible	Intermediate	Resistant
Haemophilus influenzae and H. parainfluenzae			
Tetracycline	≤2	4	≥8
Neisseria gonorrhoeae			
Tetracyclines	≤0.25	0.5–1	≥2
Bacillus anthracis			
Tetracycline	≤1	–	–
Brucella			
Doxycycline	≤1	–	–
Yersinia pestis			
Doxycycline	≤4	8	≥16
Francisella tularensis			
Tetracycline	≤4	–	–
Doxycycline	≤4	–	–

■ **Gram-Negative Bacteria** Tetracyclines generally are active in vitro and in vivo against the following gram-negative bacteria: *Bartonella bacilliformis, Bordetella pertussis, Brucella, Calymmatobacterium granulomatis, Campylobacter fetus, Francisella tularensis, Haemophilus ducreyi, H. influenzae, Legionella pneumophila, Leptotrichia buccalis, Neisseria gonorrhoeae, N. meningitidis, Pasteurella multocida, Burkholderia pseudomallei* (formerly *Pseudomonas pseudomallei*), *B. mallei* (formerly *Ps. mallei, Shigella, Spirillum minus, Streptobacillus moniliformis, Yersinia enterocolitica*, and *Y. pestis*.

Although tetracyclines are active in vitro against some strains of *Acinetobacter, Bacteroides, Enterobacter aerogenes, Escherichia coli*, and *Klebsiella*, most strains of these organisms are resistant to the drugs. Nearly all strains of *Proteus* and *Pseudomonas aeruginosa* are resistant to tetracyclines.

In one study evaluating susceptibility of *F. tularensis* isolated from humans and animals, the MIC of tetracycline for this organism was 0.38 mcg/mL.

In a study evaluating in vitro susceptibility of 100 *Y. pestis* isolates obtained from plague patients in Africa, all isolates were inhibited by doxycycline concentrations of 4 mcg/mL or less or tetracycline concentrations of 2 mcg/mL or less; the MIC_{90} for these drugs was 1 or 2 mcg/mL, respectively. In another study of *Y. pestis* isolates obtained from plague patients, rats, or fleas from Vietnam, these strains were inhibited in vitro by doxycycline concentrations of 0.25–1 mcg/mL and tetracycline concentrations of 0.5–4 mcg/mL. In addition, doxycycline has been shown to have in vivo activity against *Y. pestis* in murine plague infections.

Tetracyclines usually are active in vitro and in vivo against Vibrio cholerae and V. parahaemolyticus. *V. vulnificus* may be inhibited in vitro by minocycline concentrations of 0.06–0.25 mcg/mL. While the clinical importance is unclear, results of an in vitro study and a study in mice indicate that the combination of cefotaxime and minocycline is more active against *V. vulnificus* than either anti-infective alone.

■ **Gram-Positive Bacteria** Tetracyclines are active in vitro and in vivo against some gram-positive bacteria including *Bacillus anthracis, Actinomyces israelii, Arachnia propionica, Clostridium perfringens, C. tetani, Listeria monocytogenes, Nocardia*, and *Propionibacterium acnes*.

Results of in vitro susceptibility testing of 11 *B. anthracis* isolates that were associated with cases of inhalational or cutaneous anthrax that occurred in the US (Florida, New York, District of Columbia) during September and October 2001 in the context of an intentional release of anthrax spores (biologic warfare, bioterrorism) indicate that these strains had tetracycline MICs of 0.06 mcg/mL and doxycycline MICs of 0.03 mcg/mL. Based on interpretive criteria established for staphylococci, these strains are considered susceptible to tetracyclines. Although strains of *B. anthracis* with naturally occurring resistance to tetracycline have not been reported to date, there are published reports of strains that have been engineered to have tetracycline and penicillin resistance as well as resistance to other anti-infectives (e.g., macrolides, chloramphenicol, rifampin). Anti-infectives are effective against the germinated form of *B. anthracis*, but are not effective against the spore form of the organism.

Although tetracyclines also are active in vitro and in vivo against some strains of staphylococci and streptococci, tetracycline resistance has been reported in these organisms with increasing frequency.

■ **Spirochetes** Spirochetes, including *Borrelia recurrentis*, *Leptospira*, *Treponema pallidum*, and *T. pertenue*, generally are inhibited in vivo by tetracyclines. *Borrelia burgdorferi*, the causative organism of Lyme disease, reportedly may be inhibited in vitro by tetracycline, doxycycline, or minocycline concentrations of 0.01–2 mcg/mL. Minimum bactericidal concentrations for *B. burgdorferi* generally have ranged from 0.8 to 3.2 mcg/mL for tetracycline and from 0.4 to 6.4 mcg/mL for doxycycline.

■ **Other Organisms** Tetracyclines generally are active in vitro and in vivo against *Rickettsia akari*, *R. prowazeki*, *R. rickettsii*, *R. tsutsugamushi*, *R. typhi*, and *Coxiella burnetii*.

Tetracyclines are active in vitro and in vivo against *Chlamydia trachomatis* and *C. psittaci*. *Mycoplasma hominis*, *M. pneumoniae*, and *Ureaplasma urealyticum* (formerly T-strain mycoplasma) also are generally inhibited in vitro and in vivo by tetracyclines although some strains are naturally resistant.

Tetracycline has demonstrated activity in vitro against most strains of *Helicobacter pylori* (formerly *Campylobacter pylori* or *C. pyloridis*).

Doxycycline and tetracycline hydrochloride have demonstrated activity in vitro against *Mycobacterium fortuitum*, and tetracycline hydrochloride and minocycline have demonstrated activity in vitro and in vivo against *M. marinum*.

Tetracyclines are active against *Balantidium coli* in vitro and in vivo.

Doxycycline is a blood schizonticidal agent and is active against the asexual erythrocytic forms of *P. falciparum*; however, the drug is not gametocyticidal for *P. falciparum*. Doxycycline usually is not active against exoerythrocytic forms of *P. falciparum*, but the drug may interfere, irregularly, with the early hepatic exoerythrocytic stage of development of the plasmodium.

Resistance

Resistance to tetracyclines may be natural or acquired. Resistance is usually caused by decreased permeability of the cell surface as the result of mutation or the presence of an inducible plasmid-mediated resistance factor which is acquired via conjugation. Plasmid-mediated resistance can be transferred between organisms of the same or different species, and resistance to other tetracyclines and several other anti-infectives (e.g., aminoglycosides, chloramphenicol, sulfonamides) may be transferred on the same plasmid.

N. gonorrhoeae resistant to tetracyclines were reported with increasing frequency in the US beginning in the 1980s. Although some strains of *N. gonorrhoeae* with plasmid-mediated, high-level resistance to tetracyclines (TRNG) may be susceptible to cephalosporins (e.g., ceftriaxone) and/or spectinomycin, strains of penicillinase-producing *N. gonorrhoeae* (PPNG) (which is plasmid mediated) that also have plasmid or chromosomally mediated resistance to tetracyclines have been reported in the US. *N. gonorrhoeae* with chromosomally mediated resistance (CMRNG) to penicillins frequently also exhibit chromosomally mediated resistance to tetracyclines. Rarely, CMRNG may be resistant to penicillins, tetracyclines, and cephalosporins.

Complete cross-resistance usually occurs between demeclocycline, doxycycline, and tetracycline; however, only partial cross-resistance occurs between these derivatives and minocycline, and some organisms resistant to other currently available tetracyclines may be susceptible to minocycline.

Pharmacokinetics

■ **Absorption** Demeclocycline hydrochloride, tetracycline, and tetracycline hydrochloride are approximately 60–80% absorbed from the GI tract in fasting adults. Doxycycline salts and minocycline hydrochloride are 90–100% absorbed from the GI tract in fasting adults. Absorption occurs mainly from the stomach and upper small intestine.

Following oral administration of tetracyclines in fasting adults with normal renal function, peak serum concentrations of the drugs are usually attained within 1.5–4 hours. There is considerable interindividual variation in serum concentrations achieved with a specific oral dose of a tetracycline derivative, presumably because of interindividual differences in GI absorption rates.

Tetracyclines are poorly and erratically absorbed following IM administration.

Effect of Food or Milk Food and/or milk can reduce GI absorption of tetracyclines. This effect appears to vary among the currently available tetracycline derivatives; the effect is most marked with demeclocycline and is less with doxycycline than other derivatives. (See Dosage and Administration: Administration.)

In one study in healthy adults, administration of a single 250-mg dose of tetracycline hydrochloride with food or milk resulted in a 46 or 65% decrease, respectively, in the area under the plasma concentration-time curve (AUC) of the drug compared with administration with water. When a single 100-mg dose of minocycline was administered with food or milk, there was a 13 or 27% decrease, respectively, in the AUC of the drug compared with administration with water. In some studies, administration of doxycycline with food or milk decreased the AUC by up to 20–30%.

■ **Distribution** Tetracyclines are widely distributed into body tissues and fluids including pleural fluid, bronchial secretions, sputum, saliva, ascitic fluid, synovial fluid, aqueous and vitreous humor, and prostatic and seminal fluids. The degree of protein binding for the tetracyclines has been reported as follows:

Table 7.

Drug	% Bound to Serum Proteins
Demeclocycline	36–91
Doxycycline	25–93
Minocycline	55–88
Tetracycline	20–67

Tetracyclines are readily taken up by the reticuloendothelial cells of the liver, spleen, and bone marrow. Only small amounts of tetracyclines generally diffuse into CSF following oral, IM, or IV administration. Minocycline and, to a lesser extent, doxycycline are more lipid soluble than other currently available tetracyclines and penetrate most body tissues and fluids better than do the other tetracyclines.

All the tetracyclines are distributed into bile and undergo enterohepatic circulation in varying degrees. In the absence of biliary obstruction, concentrations of the drugs in bile may be 2–32 times higher than concurrent serum concentrations.

Tetracyclines have an affinity for and localize in tumors and necrotic or ischemic tissue where the drugs may persist for several weeks or months. The drugs also localize in and form stable tetracycline-calcium orthophosphate complexes at sites of new bone formation and calcification and in the dentin and enamel of developing teeth; these complexes have no antimicrobial activity.

Tetracyclines readily cross the placenta and are distributed into milk in concentrations that may be equal to maternal serum concentrations.

■ **Elimination** In adults with normal renal function, the serum half-lives of the tetracyclines (includes data from single and, when available, multiple-dose studies) have been reported as follows:

Table 8.

Drug	Serum half-life (in hours)
Demeclocycline	10–17
Doxycycline	14–24
Minocycline	11–26
Tetracycline	6–12

The half-lives of the drugs increase slightly following multiple doses. Serum concentrations of tetracyclines may be higher and the half-lives slightly prolonged in patients with severe hepatic impairment or obstruction of the common bile duct. Serum concentrations of demeclocycline, minocycline, and tetracycline are higher and the half-lives prolonged in patients with impaired renal function. Serum concentrations of doxycycline are not substantially increased and the half-life of the drug is only slightly prolonged in patients with severe renal impairment.

Demeclocycline and tetracycline do not appear to be metabolized and are excreted unchanged mainly in urine by glomerular filtration. Both doxycycline and minocycline are excreted mainly by nonrenal routes. Although it was previously suggested that doxycycline is partially metabolized in the liver, the drug probably is not metabolized in the liver but is partially inactivated in the intestine by chelate formation. Preliminary studies indicate that minocycline, unlike other currently available tetracyclines, is partially metabolized to at least 6 metabolites.

Tetracyclines are excreted into the GI tract via bile and by nonbiliary routes where they may become bound to fecal materials as inactive salts or complexes. Most tetracyclines are only minimally removed by hemodialysis or peritoneal dialysis.

Chemistry and Stability

■ **Chemistry**

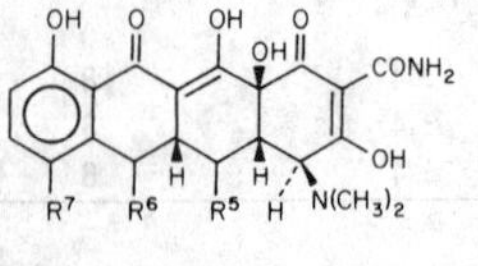

tetracycline nucleus

Tetracyclines are antibiotics and semisynthetic antibiotic derivatives obtained from cultures of *Streptomyces*. All commercially available tetracyclines contain the tetracycline nucleus.

Addition of various groups at R^5, R^6, and R^7 of the tetracycline nucleus results in derivatives with different degrees of antibacterial activity, GI absorption, affinity for divalent and trivalent cations, and protein binding.

Tetracyclines and salts of the drugs generally occur as yellow, crystalline powders. Tetracycline bases are amphoteric and very slightly soluble in water while tetracycline salts are generally sparingly soluble to freely soluble in water.

■ Stability In general, tetracyclines are stable in acid solutions with a pH greater than 2, but the drugs are rapidly inactivated in neutral and alkaline solutions. Tetracyclines, except minocycline, generally exhibit a brilliant yellow fluorescence under ultraviolet light.

Tetracyclines readily chelate divalent and trivalent cations including aluminum, calcium, iron, magnesium, and zinc to form insoluble complexes. Of the currently available tetracyclines, demeclocycline has the greatest affinity and doxycycline has the least affinity for calcium ions. Tetracyclines are potentially physically and/or chemically incompatible with some drugs and IV infusion solutions, but the compatibility depends on the specific drug and several other factors (e.g., concentration of the drugs, specific diluents used, resulting pH, temperature). Specialized references should be consulted for specific compatibility information.

For additional information on chemistry and stability and pharmacokinetics of the tetracyclines, see the individual monographs in 8:12.24.

†Use is not currently included in the labeling approved by the US Food and Drug Administration

Selected Revisions November 2009,

Doxycycline Calcium
Doxycycline Hyclate
Doxycycline Monohydrate

■ Doxycycline is a semisynthetic tetracycline antibiotic derived from oxytetracycline.

Dosage and Administration

■ Reconstitution and Administration Doxycycline calcium, doxycycline hyclate, and doxycycline monohydrate are administered orally.

When oral therapy is not feasible, doxycycline hyclate may be administered by slow IV infusion; however, oral therapy should replace IV therapy as soon as possible. If doxycycline is given IV, the risk of thrombophlebitis should be considered.

Like other tetracyclines, doxycycline should *not* be used in children younger than 8 years of age unless other appropriate drugs would be ineffective or are contraindicated. (See Cautions: Pediatric Precautions in the Tetracyclines General Statement 8:12.24.) However, the manufacturers, American Academy of Pediatrics (AAP), US Centers for Disease Control and Prevention (CDC), and Infectious Diseases Society of America (IDSA) state that use of doxycycline in children younger than 8 years of age can be considered in certain circumstances when the potential benefits outweigh the risks. These circumstances include the treatment or prophylaxis of anthrax (including inhalational anthrax [postexposure]), treatment of severe cholera, and treatment of presumed or confirmed rickettsial infections, including Rocky Mountain spotted fever (RMSF), Q fever, ehrlichiosis†, and anaplasmosis†. In addition, the CDC states that children younger than 8 years of age with uncomplicated chloroquine-resistant *Plasmodium falciparum* malaria, uncomplicated *P. vivax* malaria, or severe *P. falciparum* malaria may receive a regimen that includes doxycycline if other treatment options are not available or not tolerated and the potential benefits outweigh risks. Because of concerns regarding long-term doxycycline therapy in infants and children, the treatment duration should be limited whenever possible if use of doxycycline is considered necessary in children younger than 8 years of age.

Oral Administration Doxycycline calcium is administered orally as a conventional oral suspension. Doxycycline hyclate is administered orally as conventional capsules, conventional film-coated tablets, delayed-release capsules, and delayed-release tablets. Doxycycline monohydrate is administered orally as a conventional oral suspension, conventional capsules, or conventional film-coated tablets.

To reduce the risk of esophageal irritation and ulceration, capsules or tablets containing doxycycline hyclate or doxycycline monohydrate should be administered with adequate amounts of fluid and probably should not be given at bedtime or to patients with esophageal obstruction or compression. Most cases of esophagitis or esophageal ulceration reported with oral doxycycline occurred in patients who took the drug immediately before going to bed.

Some manufacturers and some clinicians suggest that doxycycline may be taken with food or milk to minimize nausea and vomiting or if gastric irritation occurs. However, it has been suggested that doxycycline, like some other tetracyclines, should not be administered with milk. Although a few manufacturers state that absorption of doxycycline is not markedly influenced by simultaneous ingestion of food or milk, this effect appears to be variable and concomitant administration with food or milk can decrease the rate and extent of absorption of the drug. In some studies, administration of doxycycline with food or milk decreased peak plasma concentrations and/or the area under the plasma-concentration time curve (AUC) by up to 20–35%. (See Effect of Food or Milk under Pharmacokinetics: Absorption.)

It has been suggested that individuals receiving doxycycline for prevention of malaria should take the drug in the evening (but not at bedtime), avoid prolonged, direct exposure to the sun, and use sunscreens that absorb long-wave UVA radiation to minimize the risk of doxycycline-induced photosensitivity.

Reconstitution. The commercially available powder for oral suspension containing doxycycline monohydrate should be reconstituted at the time of dispensing according to the manufacturer's instructions. When reconstituted as directed, the oral suspension contains 25 mg of doxycycline per 5 mL.

The commercially available oral suspension containing doxycycline calcium is administered as provided without further dilution and contains 50 mg of doxycycline per 5 mL.

The manufacturer of the delayed-release capsules containing partially enteric-coated pellets of doxycycline hyclate states that the capsules may be administered, if necessary, by carefully opening the capsules and sprinkling the contents on a spoonful of applesauce. The prepared dose of applesauce with doxycycline hyclate pellets should be swallowed immediately without chewing, and the patient should drink a full glass of water to ensure that the dose is completely swallowed. The applesauce should not be hot, and should be soft enough to be swallowed without chewing. The applesauce should be discarded if any loss of doxycycline hyclate pellets occurs during the transfer. In addition, if a prepared dose of applesauce with doxycycline hyclate delayed-release pellets cannot be taken immediately, the mixture should be discarded and not stored for future use.

If necessary because the powder for oral suspension and oral suspensions are not available, it has been suggested that conventional doxycycline film-coated tablets can be ground and mixed with appropriate food or drinks. (See Chemistry and Stability: Stability.) Results of a limited study in adults indicate that ground doxycycline tablets are most palatable when mixed with chocolate pudding, regular or low-fat chocolate milk, simple syrup with sour apple flavor, apple juice with table sugar, or low-fat milk; the bitterness of the drug is not masked with grape or strawberry jellies or cherry yogurt. The possibility that concomitant administration with food or milk may decrease the rate and extent of absorption of doxycycline should be considered. (See Effect of Food or Milk under Pharmacokinetics: Absorption.)

IV Infusion IV solutions of doxycycline hyclate should *not* be given IM or subcutaneously, and extravasation should be avoided.

Reconstitution and Dilution. Doxycycline hyclate powder for IV administration is reconstituted by adding 10 or 20 mL of sterile water for injection or other compatible IV infusion solution to a vial labeled as containing 100 or 200 mg of doxycycline, respectively; resultant solutions contain 10 mg of doxycycline per mL. Prior to administration, each 100 mg of the drug must be further diluted with 100 mL to 1 liter of compatible IV infusion fluid or each 200 mg diluted with 200 mL to 2 liter of compatible IV infusion fluid to provide solutions containing approximately 0.1–1 mg of doxycycline per mL. IV solutions containing doxycycline concentrations lower than 0.1 mg/mL or higher than 1 mg/mL are not recommended.

Rate of Administration. Depending on the dose, IV infusions of doxycycline hyclate usually are given over 1–4 hours. The manufacturer states that 1 hour is the minimum recommended time for infusion of 100 mg of doxycycline in a solution containing 0.5 mg of the drug per mL.

■ Dosage Dosage of doxycycline calcium, doxycycline hyclate, and doxycycline monohydrate is expressed in terms of doxycycline.

General Oral Dosage The usual oral dosage of doxycycline for adults is 100 mg every 12 hours on the first day of treatment, followed by 100 mg daily given in 1 or 2 divided doses. For severe infections, adults should receive 100 mg every 12 hours.

The usual oral dosage of doxycycline for children older than 8 years of age weighing more than 45 kg is 100 mg every 12 hours on the first day of treatment, followed by 100 mg daily given in 1 or 2 divided doses. Children older than 8 years of age weighing 45 kg or less should receive 4.4 mg/kg given in 2 divided doses on the first day of treatment, followed by 2.2 mg/kg daily given in 1 or 2 divided doses. For severe infections, children 8 years of age or older weighing more than 45 kg may receive 100 mg every 12 hours and those weighing 45 kg or less may receive up to 4.4 mg/kg daily. The AAP states that oral doxycycline in inappropriate for severe infections.

General IV Dosage The usual IV dosage of doxycycline for adults is 200 mg on the first day of treatment given in 1 or 2 infusions, followed by 100–200 mg daily. If a dosage of 200 mg daily is used, dosage should be given in 1 or 2 infusions.

The usual IV dosage of doxycycline for children older than 8 years of age weighing more than 45 kg is 200 mg on the first day of treatment given in 1 or 2 infusions, followed by 100–200 mg daily. If a dosage of 200 mg daily is used, dosage should be given in 1 or 2 infusions. The usual IV dosage for children older than 8 years of age weighing 45 kg or less is 4.4 mg/kg on the first day of treatment given in 1 or 2 infusions, followed by 2.2–4.4 mg/kg daily given in 1 or 2 infusions.

Anthrax **Postexposure Prophylaxis.** If doxycycline is used for *postexposure prophylaxis* following suspected or confirmed exposure to aerosolized anthrax spores in the context of biologic warfare or bioterrorism, the CDC and other experts (e.g., US Working Group on Civilian Biodefense, US Army Medical Research Institute of Infectious Diseases [USAMRIID]) recommends that adults and children older than 8 years of age and weighing more than 45 kg receive a dosage of 100 mg orally twice daily and children 8 years of age or younger and children weighing 45 kg or less receive a dosage of 2.2 mg/kg (up to 100 mg) orally twice daily for at least 60 days. Because of concerns regarding long-term doxycycline use in infants and children, consider changing (after 10–14 days) to amoxicillin to complete the prophylaxis regimen in children younger than 8 years of age if penicillin susceptibility is confirmed.

Although the optimum duration of postexposure prophylaxis after an inhalation exposure to *B. anthracis* spores is unclear, prolonged postexposure prophylaxis generally is recommended because of the possible persistence of anthrax spores in lung tissue following aerosol exposure. A duration of 60 days may be adequate for a low-dose exposure, but a duration longer than 4 months may be necessary to reduce the risk following a high-dose exposure. The US Working Group on Civilian Biodefense recommends that postexposure prophylaxis following a confirmed exposure (including in laboratory workers with confirmed exposures to *B. anthracis* cultures and individuals exposed to anthrax spores in the context of biologic warfare or bioterrorism) be continued for at least 60 days. USAMRIID recommends that postexposure prophylaxis be continued for at least 60 days in individuals who are not fully immunized against anthrax and when anthrax vaccine is unavailable or cannot be used for postexposure vaccination.

Treatment of Inhalational Anthrax. For the initial *treatment* of inhalational anthrax, the usual dosage of doxycycline for adults and children weighing more than 45 kg is 100 mg IV every 12 hours and the usual dosage for children weighing 45 kg or less is 2.2 mg/kg (up to 100 mg) IV every 12 hours. If meningitis is suspected, IV doxycycline may be less optimal than IV ciprofloxacin because of poor distribution into CSF.

The CDC and other experts (e.g., US Working Group on Civilian Biodefense, USAMRIID) recommend that treatment of inhalational anthrax be initiated with a multiple-drug regimen that includes ciprofloxacin or doxycycline and 1 or 2 other anti-infectives predicted to be effective. Oral therapy should be substituted for IV therapy as soon as the patient's clinical condition improves. Because of the possible persistence of anthrax spores in lung tissue following an aerosol exposure, the total duration of anti-infective therapy of inhalational anthrax that occurs as the result of exposure to anthrax spores in the context of biologic warfare or bioterrorism should be at least 60 days. Because of concerns regarding long-term doxycycline use in infants and children, consider changing (after 10–14 days) to amoxicillin to complete the treatment regimen in children younger than 8 years of age if penicillin susceptibility is confirmed.

IV therapy with a multiple-drug parenteral regimen may not be possible if large numbers of individuals require treatment in a mass casualty setting; in these circumstances, some experts state that treatment with an oral regimen recommended for postexposure prophylaxis is an option. If oral doxycycline is used for initial treatment of inhalational anthrax when a parenteral regimen is not available (e.g., when there are supply or logistic problems because large numbers of individuals require treatment in a mass casualty setting) or is used to complete a treatment regimen initiated with IV doxycycline, the usual oral dosage for adults and children weighing more than 45 kg is 100 mg twice daily and the usual oral dosage for children weighing 45 kg or less is 2.2 mg/kg (up to 100 mg) twice daily.

Treatment of Cutaneous Anthrax. For the *treatment* of cutaneous anthrax that occurs as the result of exposure to anthrax spores in the context of biologic warfare or bioterrorism, the CDC and other experts (e.g., US Working Group on Civilian Biodefense, USAMRIID) recommend that adults and children older than 8 years of age weighing more than 45 kg receive doxycycline in a dosage of 100 mg orally every 12 hours and that children 8 years of age or younger and children weighing 45 kg or less receive 2.2 mg/kg (up to 100 mg) orally every 12 hours. Although 5–10 days of anti-infective therapy has been recommended for the treatment of mild, uncomplicated cutaneous anthrax that occurs as the result of natural or endemic exposures to anthrax, treatment should be continued for at least 60 days if the cutaneous infection occurred as the result of exposure to aerosolized anthrax spores since the possibility of inhalational anthrax would also exist. Anti-infective therapy may limit the size of the cutaneous anthrax lesion and the lesion usually becomes sterile within the first 24 hours of treatment, but it will still progress through the black eschar stage despite effective treatment.

Although oral therapy may be adequate for the treatment of mild, uncomplicated cutaneous anthrax, a multiple-drug parenteral regimen is recommended for initial treatment of cutaneous anthrax when there are signs of systemic involvement, extensive edema, or head and neck lesions. Cutaneous anthrax in infants and children younger than 2 years of age should be treated IV initially. When a parenteral regimen is indicated for the treatment of cutaneous anthrax, IV dosages recommended for the treatment of inhalational anthrax should be used. If infants and children have clinical improvement while receiving the initial parenteral regimen, an oral regimen of 1 or 2 anti-infectives (including either doxycycline or ciprofloxacin) may be used to complete the first 7–10 days of therapy. Because of concerns regarding long-term doxycycline use in infants and children, consider changing (after 10–14 days) to amoxicillin to complete the treatment regimen in children younger than 8 years of age if penicillin susceptibility is confirmed.

Treatment of GI and Oropharyngeal Anthrax. The CDC and other experts (e.g., US Working Group on Civilian Biodefense) state that doxycycline dosage regimens recommended for the treatment of inhalational anthrax also are recommended for the treatment of GI and oropharyngeal anthrax.

Bartonella Infections For the treatment of *Bartonella* infections, an oral or IV doxycycline dosage of 100 mg twice daily usually is recommended. For the treatment of complicated cat scratch disease (e.g., retinitis) caused by *B. henselae*, some clinicians recommend oral doxycycline in a dosage of 100 mg twice daily in conjunction with oral rifampin (300 mg twice weekly) given for 4–6 weeks. For the treatment of bacillary angiomatosis (BA) or peliosis hepatitis (PH), oral doxycycline has been given in a dosage of 100 mg twice weekly for 3 or 4 months; concomitant oral rifampin (300 mg twice daily) also is recommended in immunocompromised patients with acute, life-threatening *Bartonella* infections. For documented *Bartonella* endocarditis, a regimen of doxycycline 100 mg twice daily for 6 weeks in conjunction with IV gentamicin (3 mg/kg daily) for 2 weeks has been recommended. A doxycycline regimen of 200 mg once daily or 100 mg twice daily for 4 weeks in conjunction with IV gentamicin (3 mg/kg once daily for 2 weeks) has been used for the treatment of trench fever or chronic bacteremia caused by *B. quintana*.

For the treatment of bartonellosis (including CNS infections) in adults and adolescents with human immunodeficiency virus (HIV) infection, the CDC, IDSA, and other clinicians recommend that doxycycline be given orally or IV in a dosage of 100 mg every 12 hours for at least 3 months. In addition, long-term suppressive therapy (secondary prophylaxis) with doxycycline should be considered to prevent relapse.

Brucellosis For the treatment of brucellosis, some clinicians recommend that adults receive 100 mg of oral doxycycline twice daily. The AAP recommends that children 8 years of age or older receive doxycycline in a dosage of 2–4 mg/kg daily in 2 divided doses (up to 200 mg daily). Other clinicians recommend 2.2 mg/kg twice daily (up to 200 mg daily) for children 8 years of age or older.

Doxycycline usually is used in conjunction with another anti-infective (e.g., streptomycin or gentamicin and/or rifampin) to reduce the likelihood of relapse, especially for severe infections and when there are complications such as meningitis, endocarditis, or osteomyelitis. Monotherapy is no longer recommended for the treatment of brucellosis since such therapy is associated with a high relapse rate.

The usual duration of doxycycline treatment is at least 4–6 weeks; streptomycin or gentamicin usually is given concomitantly for up to 2–3 weeks and/or rifampin is given for the full duration of treatment. More prolonged therapy may be required for complicated disease (e.g., hepatitis, splenitis, meningoencephalitis, endocarditis, osteomyelitis). Meningoencephalitis and endocarditis should be treated for at least 90 days and may require a treatment duration of 6 months or more.

Burkholderia Infections For the treatment of localized or mild melioidosis† caused by *Burkholderia pseudomallei*, oral doxycycline given in a dosage of 100 mg twice daily for 60–150 days may be effective. Alternatively, for the treatment of localized disease without toxicity, 100 mg of oral doxycycline twice daily for 20 weeks given in conjunction with oral co-trimoxazole has been recommended. Severe illness requires an initial parenteral regimen of ceftazidime, imipenem, or meropenem (with or without concomitant co-trimoxazole or doxycycline), followed by a prolonged maintenance regimen of oral anti-infectives (e.g., co-trimoxazole with or without doxycycline).

For the initial treatment of severe melioidosis† caused by *B. pseudomallei*, some clinicians recommend that adults and children 8 years of age or older or weighing 45 kg or more may receive 100 mg of IV doxycycline twice daily and children younger than 8 years of age or weighing less than 45 kg may receive 2.2 mg/kg of IV doxycycline twice daily (up to 200 mg daily) in conjunction with IV ceftazidime, imipenem, or meropenem. The initial IV regimen should be continued for at least 14 days and until there is clinical improvement. When appropriate, treatment may be changed to an oral maintenance regimen (e.g., oral co-trimoxazole with or without oral doxycycline) and continued for at least 3–6 months to prevent recrudence or relapse. More prolonged oral maintenance therapy (up to 12 months) may be necessary, depending on the response to therapy and severity of initial illness. Lifelong follow-up is recommended for all patients to identify relapse of melioidosis.

If doxycycline is used for follow-up after the initial parenteral regimen, some clinicians recommend that adults and children 8 years of age or older or those weighing 45 kg or more receive a prolonged maintenance regimen of 2 mg/kg (up to 100 mg) of doxycycline orally twice daily with or without oral co-trimoxazole.

Some experts (e.g., USAMRIID, European Commission's Task Force on Biological and Chemical Agent Threats [BICHAT]) state that the same treatment regimens recommended for naturally occurring melioidosis or glanders should be used if these *Burkholderia* infections occur in the context of biologic warfare or bioterrorism. Although the benefits of postexposure prophylaxis† are unknown, USAMRIID states that adults can receive 200 mg of doxycycline once daily in conjunction with oral rifampin for postexposure prophylaxis if exposure occurs in the context of biologic warfare or bioterrorism. The CDC recommends that laboratory workers with high-risk exposure to melioidosis be offered postexposure prophylaxis with oral doxycycline in a dosage of 2 mg/kg (up to 100 mg) twice daily. The optimum duration of postexposure prophylaxis is unknown, but a duration of at least 10 days is recommended.

Although only limited experience is available regarding the treatment of human cases of glanders† caused by *B. mallei*, some clinicians suggest that, pending results of in vitro susceptibility tests, regimens used for the treatment of severe melioidosis also can be used for initial empiric treatment of glanders.

Chlamydial Infections **Uncomplicated Urethral, Endocervical, or Rectal Infections.** For the treatment of uncomplicated urethral, endocervical, or rectal infections caused by *Chlamydia trachomatis* in adults, adolescents, or children

8 years of age or older, the recommended dosage of oral doxycycline is 100 mg twice daily for 7 days.

For the treatment of nongonococcal urethritis caused by *C. trachomatis* or *Ureaplasma urealyticum* in adults, the recommended dosage of oral doxycycline is 100 mg twice daily for 7 days.

Presumptive Treatment of Chlamydial Infections in Gonorrhea Patients. When oral doxycycline is used for the presumptive treatment of coexisting urogenital chlamydial infections in patients being treated for uncomplicated gonorrhea or disseminated gonococcal infections, the usual dosage for adults and children 8 years of age or older is 100 mg twice daily for 7 days.

Lymphogranuloma venereum. For the treatment of genital, inguinal, or anorectal infections caused by a lymphogranuloma venereum serotype of *C. trachomatis* in adults, the CDC and some clinicians recommend an oral doxycycline dosage of 100 mg twice daily for 21 days.

Psittacosis. The CDC states that individuals with *Chlamydophila psittaci* (formerly *Chlamydia psittaci)* infection (psittacosis, ornithosis) usually respond to oral doxycycline given in a dosage of 100 mg twice daily. Although fever and symptoms usually are controlled within 48–72 hours, therapy should be continued for at least 10–14 days after defervescence to prevent relapse. For initial treatment of severely ill patients, an IV regimen of doxycycline in a dosage of 4.4 mg/kg daily given in 2 divided doses (maximum 100 mg per dose) may be indicated.

Ehrlichiosis and Anaplasmosis For the treatment of human granulocytotropic anaplasmosis† (HGA; formerly human granulocytic ehrlichiosis [HGE]) caused by *Anaplasma phagocytophilum* (formerly *Ehrlichia phagocytophila*, *E. equi*, agent of HGE), the treatment of human monocytotropic ehrlichiosis† (HME) caused by *E. chaffeensis*, or the treatment of ehrlichiosis† caused by *E. ewingii* or *E. canis*, the CDC, AAP, and other experts recommend that adults receive oral or IV doxycycline in a dosage of 100 mg twice daily and that children receive oral or IV doxycycline in a dosage of 2–2.2 mg/kg (up to 100 mg) twice daily.

Treatment should be initiated promptly since a delay can result in severe disease and a fatal outcome. IV therapy generally is indicated for hospitalized patients; oral therapy generally is appropriate for patients with early disease, outpatients, or hospitalized patients who are not vomiting or obtunded. The optimum duration of treatment has not been established; however, treatment usually is continued at least 5–10 days and until the patient is afebrile for 3 days or longer and clinically improved. A longer duration of treatment may be required for severe illness. For the treatment of HGA, the CDC and IDSA recommend a treatment duration of 10–14 days since this provides an adequate duration of treatment for possible coexisting *Borrelia burgdorferi* infection and early Lyme disease. (See Lyme Disease under Dosage and Administration: Dosage.) If fever persists for longer than 48 hours after initiation of doxycycline treatment, the diagnosis of HGA may be incorrect and the remote possibility that the patient may be coinfected with *Babesis microti* (causative agent of babesiosis) should be considered.

Gonorrhea and Associated Infections **Uncomplicated Gonorrhea.** If oral doxycycline is used as an alternative for the treatment of uncomplicated gonorrhea, the manufacturers recommend that adults receive 100 mg twice daily for 7 days or, alternatively, an initial 300-mg dose of the drug can be given followed by a second 300-mg dose 1 hour later.

Tetracyclines are *not* included in current CDC recommendations for the treatment of uncomplicated or disseminated gonorrhea; however, the CDC and many clinicians recommend use of doxycycline for presumptive treatment of coexisting chlamydial infections in patients being treated for gonococcal infections. (See Chlamydial Infections under Dosage and Administration: Dosage.)

Epididymitis. For the treatment of acute, sexually transmitted epididymitis caused by *Neisseria gonorrhoeae* and/or *C. trachomatis* in adults, adolescents, and children 8 years of age and older, the CDC, AAP, and other clinicians recommend that oral doxycycline be given in a dosage of 100 mg twice daily for 10 days as follow-up to a single 250-mg dose of IM ceftriaxone.

Proctitis. For the treatment of proctitis† likely to be caused by *N. gonorrhoeae* and/or *C. trachomatis*, adults and adolescents should receive 100 mg of oral doxycycline twice daily for 7 days after a single 125-mg dose of IM ceftriaxone.

Granuloma Inguinale (Donovanosis) For the treatment of granuloma inguinale (donovanosis) caused by *Klebsiella granulomatis* (formerly *Calymmatobacterium granulomatis*), the CDC recommends that adults and adolescents receive oral doxycycline in a dosage of 100 mg twice daily. The drug should be continued until all lesions have healed completely; a minimum of 3 weeks of treatment usually is necessary. If lesions do not respond within the first few days of therapy, some experts recommend that a parenteral aminoglycoside (e.g., 1 mg/kg of gentamicin IV every 8 hours) be added to the regimen. Use of a parenteral aminoglycoside in addition to doxycycline should be strongly considered when treating donovanosis in HIV-infected patients.

Legionella Infections In the treatment of *Legionella pneumophila* infections† when erythromycin was contraindicated or ineffective, the usual oral dosage of doxycycline has been given either alone or in conjunction with rifampin.

Leptospirosis For the treatment of leptospirosis†, oral doxycycline has been given in a dosage of 100 mg twice daily for 7 days.

If doxycycline is used for prophylaxis in individuals at risk for leptospirosis†, such as those participating in recreational water activities (e.g., whitewater rafting, adventure racing, kayaking) in areas where leptospirosis is endemic or epidemic, the CDC and others recommend that oral doxycycline be given in a dosage of 200 mg once every 7 days. Such prophylaxis should be initiated 1–2 days before exposure and continued through the period of exposure.

Lyme Disease **Prophylaxis of Lyme Disease.** For the prevention of Lyme disease† in individuals in Lyme disease-endemic areas who are bitten by an *Ixodes scapularis* tick, the IDSA states that adults can receive a single 200-mg dose of oral doxycycline and children 8 years of age or older can receive a single 4-mg/kg oral dose (up to 200 mg). The IDSA states that *routine* use of such prophylaxis is not recommended. However, doxycycline prophylaxis can be offered when *all* of the following circumstances exist: the attached tick can be reliably identified as an adult or nymphal *I. scapularis* tick, the estimated duration of tick attachment has been at least 36 hours based on the degree of engorgement of the tick or certainty about the time of exposure to the tick, the doxycycline dose can be given within 72 hours of tick removal, the local rate of infection of *I. scapularis* with *B. burgdorferi* is 20% or greater, and doxycycline is not contraindicated. Prophylaxis after *I. pacificus* bites generally is not necessary since rates of infection with *B. burgdorferi* in these ticks are low.

Accurate and timely identification of tick species or stage of development and determination of the infection status of the tick as well as assessment of the degree of tick engorgement are often difficult. The best method for preventing infection with *B. burgdorferi* and other infections transmitted by *Ixodes* ticks is avoidance of tick-infested areas. If exposure to *Ixodes* ticks is unavoidable, measures should be taken to reduce the risk of infection, including use of protective clothing and tick repellants, daily body checks for ticks, and prompt removal of attached ticks before transmission can occur. (See Postexposure Prophylaxis after Tick Bite under Spirochetal Infections: Lyme Disease, in Uses in the Tetracyclines General Statement 8:12.24.)

Erythema Migrans. For the treatment of early localized or early disseminated Lyme disease† manifested as erythema migrans, in the absence of specific neurologic involvement or advanced atrioventricular (AV) heart block, the IDSA, AAP, and other clinicians recommend that adults receive oral doxycycline in a dosage of 100 mg twice daily for 14 days (range 14–21 days). The IDSA recommends that children 8 years of age or older receive oral doxycycline in a dosage of 4 mg/kg daily in 2 divided doses (up to 100 mg per dose) for 14 days (range 14–21 days) for the treatment of early localized or early disseminated Lyme disease. Other clinicians have recommended that these children receive oral doxycycline in a dosage of 1–2 mg/kg twice daily (up to 100 mg per dose).

Early Neurologic Lyme Disease, Lyme Carditis, or Borrelial Lymphocytoma. If an oral regimen is used for the treatment of early neurologic Lyme disease† in patients with cranial nerve palsy alone without clinical evidence of meningitis, the treatment of Lyme carditis†, or the treatment of borrelial lymphocytoma†, the IDSA recommends that adults receive oral doxycycline in a dosage of 100 mg twice daily and that children 8 years of age or older receive 4 mg/kg daily in 2 divided doses (up to 100 mg per dose) for 14 days (range 14–21 days).

Lyme Arthritis. For the treatment of uncomplicated Lyme arthritis† in patients without clinical evidence of neurologic disease, the IDSA and other clinicians recommend that adults receive oral doxycycline in a dosage of 100 mg twice daily and that children 8 years of age or older receive 4 mg/kg daily in 2 divided doses (up to 100 mg per dose) for 28 days.

Malaria **Prevention of Malaria.** For prevention of malaria in individuals traveling to areas with chloroquine-resistant *Plasmodium falciparum*, the CDC, WHO, and the manufacturers recommend that adults receive 100 mg of doxycycline once daily and that children 8 years of age or older receive 2 mg/kg (maximum 100 mg) once daily. If necessary (e.g., because the individuals is unable to take chloroquine or hydroxychloroquine), this doxycycline regimen also can be used to prevent malaria in travelers to areas where chloroquine-resistant *P. falciparum* has not been reported.

Doxycycline prophylaxis should be initiated 1–2 days prior to entering a malarious area and continued for 4 weeks after leaving the area. If concerns exist regarding tolerance or drug interactions in an individual patient, it may be advisable to initiate doxycycline prophylaxis 3–4 weeks prior to departure to ensure that the drug or combination of drugs (in individuals receiving other drugs) is well tolerated and to allow ample time to switch to another antimalarial agent if required.

Because doxycycline cannot prevent delayed primary attacks or relapse of *P. ovale* or *P. vivax* malaria and cannot provide a radical cure in malaria caused by these species, terminal prophylaxis with primaquine may be indicated during the last 2 weeks of doxycycline prophylaxis if exposure occurred in areas where *P. ovale* or *P. vivax* are endemic. (See Primaquine Phosphate 8:30.08.)

Presumptive Self-treatment of Malaria. If doxycycline is used in conjunction with quinine sulfate for presumptive self-treatment of malaria† in the event of an influenza-like illness (e.g., fever, chills) during travel, some clinicians recommend that adults receive 100 mg orally twice daily for 7 days given in conjunction with quinine sulfate (650 mg 3 times daily given for 3 days if malaria was acquired in Africa or South America or for 7 days if acquired in Southeast Asia). For presumptive self-treatment of malaria in children 8 years of age or older, these clinicians recommend that oral doxycycline be given in a dosage of 4 mg/kg daily in 2 equally divided doses for 7 days given in conjunction with oral quinine sulfate (10 mg/kg 3 times daily given for 3 days if malaria was acquired in Africa or South America or for 7 days if acquired in Southeast Asia).

Travelers should be advised to keep an amount of doxycycline and quinine sufficient for self-treatment in their possession during travel and to take it promptly in the event of a febrile illness during or after their travel if professional medical care is not readily available. It must be emphasized that such presumptive self-treatment of a possible malarial infection is only a temporary measure and that professional medical follow-up care should be obtained as soon as possible.

Treatment of Uncomplicated Malaria. When oral doxycycline is used in conjunction with oral quinine sulfate for the treatment of uncomplicated malaria† caused by chloroquine-resistant *P. falciparum*, the CDC and other clinicians recommend that adults receive 100 mg twice daily for 7 days given in conjunction with quinine sulfate (650 mg 3 times daily given for 3 days if malaria was acquired in Africa or South America or for 7 days if acquired in Southeast Asia). These experts recommend that children 8 years of age or older receive oral doxycycline in a dosage of 4 mg/kg daily in 2 equally divided doses (maximum 200 mg daily) for 7 days given in conjunction with oral quinine sulfate (10 mg/kg 3 times daily given for 3 days if infection was acquired in Africa or South America or for 7 days if acquired in Southeast Asia).

When oral doxycycline is used in conjunction with quinine sulfate and primaquine phosphate for the treatment of uncomplicated chloroquine-resistant *P. vivax* malaria†, the CDC and other clinicians recommend that adults receive 100 mg twice daily for 7 days given in conjunction with oral quinine sulfate (650 mg 3 times daily given for 3 days if malaria was acquired in Africa or South America or for 7 days if acquired in Southeast Asia). These experts recommend that children 8 years of age or older receive oral doxycycline in a dosage of 4 mg/kg daily in 2 equally divided doses for 7 days (maximum 200 mg daily) given in conjunction with oral quinine sulfate (10 mg/kg 3 times daily given for 3 days if infection was acquired in Africa or South America or for 7 days if acquired in Southeast Asia). In addition, a 14-day regimen of oral primaquine (30 mg once daily in adults or 0.6 mg/kg once daily in children) should be given with the quinine sulfate and tetracycline hydrochloride regimen to provide a radical cure and prevent delayed attacks or relapse of *P. vivax* malaria.

For additional information on treatment of uncomplicated malaria, see Uses: Malaria, in Quinine Sulfate 8:30.08.

Treatment of Severe P. falciparum Malaria. When doxycycline is used in conjunction with IV quinidine gluconate (followed by oral quinine sulfate) for the treatment of severe malaria caused by *P. falciparum*†, the drug should be administered orally or IV for a total duration of 7 days; IV doxycycline should be switched to oral doxycycline as soon as it is tolerated to complete the 7-day regimen. In patients who cannot tolerate oral therapy, adults should receive doxycycline in a dosage 100 mg IV every 12 hours. Children older than 8 years of age who are intolerant of oral therapy and who weigh less than 45 kg should receive 4 mg/kg IV daily in 2 equally divided doses and those weighing 45 kg or more may receive 100 mg IV every 12 hours. In patients able to tolerate oral therapy, adults should receive doxycycline in a dosage of 100 mg twice daily and children older than 8 years of age should receive 4 mg/kg daily in 2 equally divided doses. Pediatric dosage should not exceed the recommended adult oral dosage.

For additional information on treatment of severe malaria, see Uses: Malaria, in Quinidine 24:04.04.04.

Mycobacterial Infections **Mycobacterium marinum Infections.** The American Thoracic Society (ATS) has recommended that oral doxycycline be given in a dosage of 100 mg twice daily for at least 3 months for the treatment of cutaneous *Mycobacterium marinum* infections† and states that a minimum of 4–6 weeks of therapy is necessary to determine whether or not the infection is responding.

Pelvic Inflammatory Disease **Parenteral Regimens.** For the treatment of acute pelvic inflammatory disease† (PID) in adults or adolescents when *N. gonorrhoeae* or *C. trachomatis* is suspected as the primary pathogen and a parenteral regimen is indicated, the CDC and many clinicians suggest the use of an IV or oral doxycycline dosage of 100 mg twice daily (every 12 hours) in conjunction with either cefoxitin (2 g IV every 6 hours) or cefotetan (2 g IV every 12 hours). This initial regimen may be discontinued 24 hours after there is clinical improvement and oral doxycycline is then given in a dosage of 100 mg twice daily to complete 14 days of therapy. If tubo-ovarian abscess is present, many clinicians would include clindamycin or metronidazole with oral doxycycline to provide more effective coverage against anaerobes.

Another parenteral regimen recommended by the CDC and many clinicians for the treatment of PID includes parenteral clindamycin (900 mg IV every 8 hours) and gentamicin (loading dose of 2 mg/kg IV or IM followed by 1.5 mg/kg every 8 hours or, alternatively, single daily dosing) for the initial phase, followed by oral doxycycline in a dosage of 100 mg twice daily to complete a total of 14 days of therapy. If tubo-ovarian abscess is present, many clinicians substitute oral clindamycin (450 mg 4 times daily) for oral doxycycline in the second phase of therapy.

An alternative parenteral regimen recommended by the CDC and others for the treatment of PID is ampicillin and sulbactam (3 g IV every 6 hours) and oral or IV doxycycline given in a dosage of 100 mg every 12 hours; this regimen has good coverage against *C. trachomatis*, *N. gonorrhoeae*, and anaerobes and is effective for patients with tubo-ovarian abscess.

Oral Regimens. When an oral regimen is indicated for the treatment of acute PID† in adults or adolescents, the CDC and many clinicians recommend a single IM dose of ceftriaxone, IM cefoxitin (with oral probenecid), or other parenteral third generation cephalosporin (e.g., cefotaxime) and oral doxycycline given in a dosage of 100 mg twice daily for 14 days with or without oral metronidazole (500 mg twice daily for 14 days).

The CDC states that clinical trials of outpatient regimens have provided little information regarding intermediate and long-term outcomes, and patients who do not respond to an oral regimen within 72 hours should be reevaluated to confirm the diagnosis and treated with a parenteral regimen on either an outpatient or inpatient basis.

Plague **Treatment.** If doxycycline is used for the treatment of pneumonic plague that occurs as the result of exposure to *Yersinia pestis* in the context of biologic warfare or bioterrorism, some experts (e.g., the US Working Group on Civilian Biodefense, USAMRIID) recommend that adults and children weighing 45 kg or more receive a dosage of 100 mg IV every 12 hours or 200 mg IV once daily and that children weighing less than 45 kg receive doxycycline in a dosage of 2.2 mg/kg IV every 12 hours (up to 200 mg daily).

Prompt initiation of anti-infective therapy (within 18–24 hours of symptom onset) is essential in the treatment of pneumonic plague. Treatment of pneumonic plague should be initiated with a parenteral regimen, although an oral regimen may be substituted when the patient's condition improves or if parenteral therapy is unavailable. Anti-infective therapy usually is continued for 10 days; some experts recommend a duration of at least 10–14 days.

Postexposure Prophylaxis. For postexposure prophylaxis following a high-risk exposure to *Y. pestis*, including exposure that occurs in the context of biologic warfare or bioterrorism, some experts recommend that adults and children weighing 45 kg or more receive doxycycline in a dosage of 100 mg orally every 12 hours and that children weighing less than 45 kg receive 2.2 mg/kg orally every 12 hours (up to 200 mg daily). For high-risk exposures to pneumonic plague, the Advisory Committee on Immunization Practices (ACIP) has recommended that adults 18 years of age and older receive 100–200 mg daily in 2 equally divided doses and that children 9–17 years of age receive 2–4 mg/kg daily in 2 equally divided doses.

The recommended duration of prophylaxis following exposure to plague aerosol or a patient with suspected pneumonic plague is 7 days or the duration of exposure risk plus 7 days. Some experts recommend that postexposure anti-infective prophylaxis be given to all asymptomatic individuals with exposure to plague aerosol and all asymptomatic individuals who have had household, hospital, or other close contact (within about 2 m) with an individual who has pneumonic plague; however, any exposed individual who develops a temperature of 38.5°C or higher or new cough should promptly receive a parenteral anti-infective for treatment of the disease.

Pleural Effusions When used as a sclerosing agent to control pleural effusions associated with metastatic tumors†, 500 mg of doxycycline has been diluted with 25–30 mL of 0.9% sodium chloride injection and instilled into the pleural space through a thoracostomy tube following drainage of the accumulated pleural fluid; the tube is then clamped and the fluid subsequently removed. The pleurodesis procedure has been repeated in some patients to achieve control of the effusion, although repeated administration may have limited effects.

Prior to instillation of doxycycline in patients with effusions, the pleural cavity is drained by thoracentesis (needle aspiration) or via the thoracostomy tube by gravity or suction (i.e., closed chest tube drainage). Efficacy of the procedure may be reduced if the sclerosing agent is introduced into the pleural cavity when fluid drainage from the chest tube exceeds 100 mL per 24 hours. To achieve pleurodesis in patients who have recurrent malignant pleural effusions†, doxycycline also has been administered as a less concentrated solution (500 mg diluted with 250 mL of 0.9% sodium chloride injection) via chest tube lavage and drainage†. For this procedure, the tube has been clamped for 24 hours and the entire procedure repeated daily until the drainage volume approximates the amount of solution instilled.

Rickettsial Infections For the treatment of most rickettsial infections, including Rocky Mountain spotted fever (RMSF), typhus fever and the typhus group, Q fever, rickettsialpox, and tick fever caused by rickettsiae, the CDC and others recommend that adults receive 100 mg of oral or IV doxycycline twice daily. For the treatment of most rickettsial infections in children, the CDC and AAP recommend 2.2 mg/kg of oral or IV doxycycline (up to 100 mg) twice daily. Treatment should be initiated promptly since a delay can result in severe disease and a fatal outcome. Treatment usually is continued for at least 5–7 days and until the patient is afebrile for 3 days or more and clinically improved. Severe illness may require a longer duration of treatment.

IV treatment generally is indicated for hospitalized patients and oral therapy generally is appropriate for patients with early disease, outpatients, or hospitalized patients who are not vomiting or obtunded.

Q Fever. For the treatment of acute Q fever†, the CDC and other clinicians recommend that adults receive doxycycline in a dosage of 100 mg twice daily for 2–3 weeks and that children receive 2.2 mg/kg (up to 100 mg) twice daily for at least 14 days. For the treatment of acute Q fever in patients with preexisting valvular heart disease, the CDC recommends a doxycycline dosage of 200 mg daily given in conjunction with hydroxychloroquine (465 mg [600 mg of hydroxychloroquine sulfate] daily; dosage adjusted to maintain plasma concentrations at 1 ± 0.2 mcg/mL); the recommended duration of treatment is 1 year to prevent progression of acute disease to endocarditis. For the treatment of chronic Q fever endocarditis, the same regimen of doxycycline and hydroxychloroquine should be given for 1.5–3 years.

It has been suggested that oral doxycycline given for 5–7 days in a dosage of 100 mg every 12 hours in adults or 2.2 mg/kg twice daily in children may be effective as prophylaxis against Q fever† and may prevent clinical disease if initiated 8–12 days after exposure; however, such prophylaxis is *not* effective and may only prolong the onset of disease if given immediately (1–7 days) after exposure.

Syphilis While parenteral penicillin G is the drug of choice for all stages of syphilis, the CDC, other clinicians, and some manufacturers state that nonpregnant adults or adolescents with primary or secondary syphilis who are hypersensitive to penicillin can receive 100 mg of doxycycline orally twice daily for 14 days. In addition, nonpregnant adults or adolescents with early latent syphilis (syphilis of less than 1-year duration) can receive 100 mg of oral doxycycline twice daily for 14 days and those with late latent syphilis, syphilis of unknown duration, or tertiary syphilis (except neurosyphilis) can receive 100 mg twice daily for 4 weeks. Some manufacturers state that the recommended dosage for the treatment of primary or secondary syphilis is 300 mg daily given for at least 10 days.

Care should be taken to ensure optimal compliance with these regimens since patient compliance with multiple-day tetracycline regimens may be poor. If compliance with the doxycycline regimen and serologic follow-up cannot be ensured, adults and adolescents with a history of penicillin hypersensitivity should be desensitized, if necessary, and treated with penicillin. The CDC states that infants and children with syphilis who are hypersensitive to penicillin should be desensitized, if necessary, and treated with penicillin. For information on recommendations regarding treatment and follow-up for all stages and forms of syphilis, see Spirochetal Infections: Syphilis, under Uses in the Natural Penicillins General Statement 8:12.16.04.

Tularemia **Treatment.** If doxycycline is used for the treatment of tularemia that occurs as the result of exposure to *Francisella tularensis* in the context of biologic warfare or bioterrorism, or naturally occurring or endemic tularemia, some experts (e.g., US Working Group on Civilian Biodefense, USAMRIID) recommend that adults and children weighing 45 kg or more receive 100 mg IV twice daily and that children weighing less than 45 kg receive 2.2 mg/kg (up to 100 mg) IV twice daily. Treatment should be continued for at least 14–21 days. Although therapy should be initiated with IV doxycycline, oral doxycycline can be substituted when the patient's condition improves or if parenteral doxycycline is unavailable.

Postexposure Prophylaxis. If doxycycline is used for postexposure prophylaxis following a high-risk laboratory exposure to *F. tularensis* (e.g., spill, centrifuge accident, needlestick injury) or in individuals exposed to the organism in the context of biologic warfare or bioterrorism, some experts (e.g., the US Working Group on Civilian Biodefense, USAMRIID) recommend that adults and children weighing 45 kg or more receive a dosage of 100 mg orally twice daily and that children weighing less than 45 kg receive a dosage of 2.2 mg/kg (up to 100 mg) orally twice daily. Postexposure prophylaxis should be initiated within 24 hours of exposure and continued for at least 14 days. Drugs of choice for *postexposure prophylaxis* following a high-risk laboratory exposure to *F. tularensis* are doxycycline, tetracycline, or ciprofloxacin.

Postexposure prophylaxis usually is *not* recommended after exposure to natural or endemic tularemia (e.g., tick bite, rabbit or other animal exposure) and is unnecessary in close contacts of tularemia patients since human-to-human transmission does not occur.

Vibrio Infections **Cholera.** For the treatment of cholera caused by *Vibrio cholerae*, the usual oral dosage of doxycycline has been given for 3 days in conjunction with fluid and electrolyte replacement. Some clinicians suggest that doxycycline can be given as a single 300-mg dose for the treatment of cholera.

Prophylaxis in Sexual Assault Victims The CDC currently states that if empiric anti-infective prophylaxis is indicated in adult or adolescent victims of sexual assault†, a single 2-g dose of oral metronidazole is given in conjunction with a single 125-mg dose of IM ceftriaxone, followed by oral doxycycline given in a dosage of 100 mg twice daily for 7 days.

■ Dosage in Renal Impairment

Unlike other currently available tetracycline derivatives, usual dosage of doxycycline may be used in patients with impaired renal function.

Pharmacokinetics

■ Absorption

Approximately 90–100% of an oral dose of doxycycline hyclate is absorbed from the GI tract in fasting adults. Absorption takes place principally in the stomach and upper small intestine. Commercially available doxycycline hyclate extended-release tablets contain coated doxycycline hyclate pellets with a pH-dependent coating designed to delay release of the drug until the pellets reach the higher pH environment of the small intestine.

Following oral administration of capsules containing doxycycline hyclate in fasting adults with normal renal function, peak serum concentrations of doxycycline are attained within 1.5–4 hours and average 1.5–2.1 mcg/mL following a single 100-mg dose and 2.6–3 mcg/mL following a single 200-mg dose.

Following oral administration of a single 200-mg dose of doxycycline monohydrate in healthy adults, peak serum concentrations of doxycycline are attained within approximately 2.5 hours and average about 3.6 mcg/mL.

In healthy fasting adults, mean peak serum concentrations of 1.1 mcg/mL are attained at a mean of 2.6 hours after a single 100-mg dose of doxycycline as extended-release tablets containing doxycycline hyclate pellets.

Following IV infusion over 1 hour of 100 mg of doxycycline as the hyclate (in a concentration of 0.4 mg/mL), peak serum concentrations of the drug average 2.5 mcg/mL. Following IV infusion over 2 hours of 200 mg of doxycycline as the hyclate (in a concentration of 0.4 mg/mL), peak serum concentrations of the drug average 3.6 mcg/mL.

Excessive accumulation of doxycycline does not appear to occur when usually recommended dosages of the drug are used in patients with normal or impairment renal function.

Because tetracyclines readily chelate divalent or trivalent cations including aluminum, calcium, iron, and magnesium, concurrent oral administration of antacids and other drugs containing these cations may decrease oral absorption of doxycycline preparations. Of the currently available tetracyclines, doxycycline has the least affinity for calcium ions. (See Drug Interactions in the Tetracyclines General Statement 8:12.24.)

Effect of Food or Milk The effect of food or milk on GI absorption of doxycycline appears to be variable, and further study is needed to clarify whether this variability depends on the specific salt (doxycycline calcium, doxycycline hyclate, doxycycline monohydrate) or dosage form (conventional capsules, tablets, or oral suspension; extended-release capsules or tablets) and/or the food parameters (food with or without milk, high- or low-fat meal, whole or skim milk). There is evidence that administration with food or milk can decrease the rate and extent of absorption of oral doxycycline; however, a slight increase in the extent of absorption also has been reported in some individuals who received the drug with food. Although a few manufacturers and clinicians suggest that the effect of simultaneous ingestion of food or milk is not likely to be clinically important and doxycycline may be administered with food or milk, other manufacturers state the clinical importance of this effect is unclear, and some clinicians suggest that doxycycline, like some other tetracyclines, should not be administered with milk.

In one study evaluating doxycycline (unspecified preparation) in a limited number of healthy adults, concomitant administration of the drug with food increased the time to peak serum concentrations from 2 hours to 4 hours, but did not reduce peak serum doxycycline concentrations. In a study using doxycycline hyclate conventional capsules (Vibramycin®) in a limited number of healthy adults, concomitant administration of a single 200-mg dose of doxycycline with a high-fat or high-protein meal decreased serum doxycycline concentrations by approximately 20% compared with administration in the fasting state.

In a cross-over study in healthy adult males, concomitant administration of a single 100-mg dose of doxycycline as an extended-release tablet containing doxycycline hyclate pellets (Doryx®) with a high-fat, high-calorie meal resulted in a 24% decrease in mean peak serum doxycycline concentrations and a 13% decrease in the mean area under the plasma concentration-time curve (AUC) of the drug compared with administration in the fasting state. Although mean peak serum concentrations were 1.1 mcg/mL when the dose was given in the fasting state, mean peak serum concentrations were 0.87 mcg/mL when the dose was given with a high-fat, high-calorie meal. The clinical importance of this effect is unclear.

Studies evaluating the effect of concomitant administration of doxycycline and milk have given inconsistent results. In an early study evaluating doxycycline (unspecified preparation) in a limited number of healthy adults, administration with milk (without food) reduced the peak serum concentration by about 20%, but did not affect the time to peak concentrations. In a study evaluating single 200-mg doses of doxycycline as doxycycline hyclate conventional capsules (Vibramycin®), there was no difference in mean serum doxycycline concentrations attained (over the first 24 hours after the dose) when the dose was given with either 150 mL of milk or water. Conversely, in another study in healthy adults, peak serum concentrations were 24% lower and the AUC was 30–35% lower when a 200-mg dose of doxycycline (soft gelatin capsules) was given with 300 mL of milk compared with administration with the same amount of water. In a study using single 100-mg doses of doxycycline conventional capsules containing the monohydrate (Vibramycin®), absorption of the drug was only slightly impaired by ingestion with a glass of skim milk (peak serum concentrations 1.45 mcg/mL) compared with administration in the fasting state (peak serum concentrations 1.79 mcg/mL). However, when administered with both food and milk, peak serum doxycycline concentrations were only 1.18 mcg/mL and were not attained until 4 hours after the dose.

The effect of food and milk on GI absorption of doxycycline is less than that reported with some other tetracyclines (e.g., demeclocycline, tetracycline hydrochloride). It has been suggested that milk may have a lesser effect on GI absorption of doxycycline because the drug has higher lipophilicity and a lower affinity for calcium than these other tetracycline derivatives.

■ Elimination

The serum half-life of doxycycline is about 15–16 hours after a single dose and about 22 hours after multiple doses in patients with normal renal function. In patients with severe renal impairment, the serum half-life of doxycycline is reported to be 18–26 hours after a single dose, and 20–30 hours after multiple doses. The serum half-life of doxycycline is not altered in patients undergoing hemodialysis.

In patients with normal renal function, approximately 20–26% of a single oral or IV dose of doxycycline is excreted in urine and 20–40% is excreted in feces within 48 hours as active drug. In patients with creatinine clearances less than 10 mL/minute, the fraction of doxycycline excreted in urine within 72 hours may decrease to about 1–5%. Although it was previously suggested that doxycycline is partially metabolized in the liver, the drug does not appear to be metabolized but is partially deactivated in the intestine by chelate formation.

Chemistry and Stability

■ **Chemistry** Doxycycline is a semisynthetic tetracycline antibiotic derived from oxytetracycline. Doxycycline is commercially available as the calcium, the hyclate, and the monohydrate salts. Doxycycline hyclate and doxycycline monohydrate occur as yellow, crystalline powders. The hyclate is soluble in water and slightly soluble in alcohol; the monohydrate is very slightly soluble in water and sparingly soluble in alcohol. Doxycycline calcium is formed *in situ* during the manufacturing process. Following reconstitution of doxycycline hyclate powder for IV administration with sterile water for injection, solutions have a pH of 1.8–3.3.

■ **Stability** Depending on the manufacturer, doxycycline hyclate and doxycycline monohydrate conventional capsules and conventional film-coated tablets should be stored at 15–30°C or at less than 30°C in tight, light-resistant containers.

Doxycycline delayed-release capsules containing partially enteric-coated pellets of doxycycline hyclate should be stored at 20–25°C.

Doxycycline delayed-release tablets containing partially enteric-coated pellets of doxycycline hyclate should be stored at 25°C, but may be exposed to temperatures ranging from 15–30°C.

Doxycycline calcium oral suspension and doxycycline monohydrate powder for oral suspension should be stored at less than 30°C in tight, light-resistant containers. Following reconstitution with water, doxycycline monohydrate oral suspensions are stable for 2 weeks at room temperature.

Limited data indicate that doxycycline tablets that have been crushed and mixed with food or drinks (chocolate pudding, regular or low-fat chocolate milk, apple juice with table sugar, low-fat milk) are stable for 24 hours at room temperature (22–26°C) or when refrigerated at 2–8°C; crushed doxycycline tablets mixed with low-fat chocolate milk were stable when refrigerated for 1 week. In addition, crushed doxycycline tablets were stable for at least 6 days when wrapped in aluminum foil and stored at room temperature.

When reconstituted and diluted with 0.9% sodium chloride or 5% dextrose, doxycycline hyclate IV solutions containing 0.1–1 mg of doxycycline per mL are stable for 48 hours at 25°C; when reconstituted and diluted with Ringer's, 10% invert sugar, Normosol-M® in D5W, Normosol-R® in D5W, Plasma-Lyte® 56 in 5% dextrose, or Plasma-Lyte® 148 in 5% dextrose, doxycycline hyclate IV solutions containing 0.1–1 mg/mL are stable for 12 hours at room temperature. The manufacturer states that doxycycline hyclate solutions prepared with any of these infusion solutions are stable for 72 hours at 2–8°C when protected from direct sunlight and artificial light; however, after storage in this manner, infusion of these solutions must be completed within 12 hours. Doxycycline hyclate IV solutions diluted to a concentration of 0.1–1 mg/mL with lactated Ringer's injection or 5% dextrose in lactated Ringer's injection must be infused within 6 hours to ensure stability. During infusion, all doxycycline hyclate IV solutions must be protected from direct sunlight.

Solutions of doxycycline hyclate containing 10 mg of doxycycline per mL may be frozen immediately after reconstitution with sterile water for injection and are stable for 8 weeks when stored at −20°C. If the solutions are warmed to facilitate thawing, care should be taken to avoid heating after thawing is completed. Once thawed, solutions should not be refrozen.

For further information on chemistry and stability, mechanism of action, spectrum, resistance, pharmacokinetics, uses, cautions, drug interactions, laboratory test interferences, and dosage and administration of doxycycline, see the Tetracyclines General Statement 8:12.24.

Preparations

Excipients in commercially available drug preparations may have clinically important effects in some individuals; consult specific product labeling for details.

Doxycycline Calcium

Oral		
Suspension	50 mg (of doxycycline) per 5 mL	**Vibramycin® Calcium Syrup,** Pfizer

Doxycycline Hyclate

Oral		
Capsules	50 mg (of doxycycline)*	**Doxycycline Hyclate Capsules**
		Vibramycin® Hyclate, Pfizer
	100 mg (of doxycycline)*	**Doxycycline Hyclate Capsules**
		Vibramycin® Hyclate, Pfizer
Capsules, delayed-release (containing partially enteric-coated pellets)	75 mg (of doxycycline)*	**Doxycycline Hyclate Delayed-release Capsules**
	100 mg (of doxycycline)*	**Doxycycline Hyclate Delayed-release Capsules**
Tablets, delayed-release (containing partially enteric-coated pellets)	75 mg (of doxycycline)	**Doryx®**
	100 mg (of doxycycline)	**Doryx®**
Tablets, film-coated	100 mg (of doxycycline)*	**Doxycycline Film-coated Tablets**
		Vibra-Tabs®
Parenteral		
For injection, for IV use only	100 mg (of doxycycline)*	**Doxy 100®**
		Vibramycin® Hyclate Intravenous
	200 mg (of doxycycline)*	**Vibramycin® Hyclate Intravenous**

*available from one or more manufacturer, distributor, and/or repackager by generic (nonproprietary) name

Doxycycline Monohydrate

Oral		
Capsules	50 mg (of doxycycline)*	**Doxycycline Monohydrate Capsules**
		Monodox®, Oclassen
	100 mg (of doxycycline)*	**Doxycycline Monohydrate Capsules**
		Monodox®, Aqua Pharmaceuticals
For suspension	25 mg (of doxycycline) per 5 mL	**Vibramycin® Monohydrate,** Pfizer
Tablets, film-coated	50 mg (of doxycycline)*	**Doxycycline Monohydrate Film-coated Tablets**
	100 mg (of doxycycline)*	**Doxycycline Monohydrate Film-coated Tablets**

*available from one or more manufacturer, distributor, and/or repackager by generic (nonproprietary) name

†Use is not currently included in the labeling approved by the US Food and Drug Administration

Minocycline Hydrochloride

■ Minocycline is a semisynthetic tetracycline antibiotic derived from tetracycline.

Dosage and Administration

■ **Reconstitution and Administration** Minocycline hydrochloride is administered orally. Minocycline has been administered IV, but a parenteral preparation no longer is commercially available in the US.

Minocycline hydrochloride capsules, pellet-filled capsules, or film-coated tablets should be administered at least 1 hour before or 2 hours after meals. The manufacturer of Dynacin® capsules states that the capsules may be taken with or without food. Although the effect appears to be variable, concomitant administration with food and/or milk can decrease the rate and extent of absorption of minocycline by up to about 27%. (See Effect of Food or Milk under Pharmacokinetics: Absorption.)

To reduce the risk of esophageal irritation and ulceration, minocycline hydrochloride capsules and film-coated tablets should be administered with adequate amounts of fluid and probably should not be given at bedtime or to patients with esophageal obstruction or compression. The pellet-filled capsules should be swallowed whole.

■ **Dosage** Dosage of minocycline hydrochloride is expressed in terms of minocycline.

General Adult Dosage The usual adult oral dosage of minocycline is 200 mg initially, followed by 100 mg every 12 hours. Alternatively, if more frequent doses are preferred, adults may receive 100–200 mg of minocycline initially, followed by 50 mg 4 times daily.

General Pediatric Dosage The usual oral dosage of minocycline for children older than 8 years of age is 4 mg/kg initially, followed by 2 mg/kg every 12 hours.

For information on the use of minocycline hydrochloride for the treatment of periodontitis, see Minocycline 52:04.04.

Acne In the adjunctive treatment of inflammatory acne vulgaris unresponsive to other oral anti-infectives (tetracycline hydrochloride, erythromycin), 50 mg of minocycline has been given orally 1–3 times daily.

Chlamydial Infections For the treatment of nongonococcal urethritis caused by *Chlamydia trachomatis* or *Ureaplasma urealyticum*, the manufacturers state that adults can receive oral minocycline in a dosage of 100 mg every 12 hours for at least 7 days.

Doxycycline is the tetracycline recommended by the US Centers for Disease Control and Prevention (CDC) for the treatment of nongonococcal urethritis and also is the preferred tetracycline for the presumptive treatment of coexisting chlamydial infections in patients with gonorrhea.

Gonorrhea and Associated Infections The manufacturers state that uncomplicated gonorrhea (other than urethritis and anorectal infections in men) may be treated with 200 mg of oral minocycline initially, followed by 100 mg every 12 hours for a minimum of 4 days; follow-up cultures should be done within 2–3 days after completion of therapy. For the treatment of uncomplicated gonococcal urethritis in adult males, the manufacturers state that the recommended dosage of oral minocycline is 100 mg every 12 hours for 5 days.

Tetracyclines are *not* included in current CDC guidelines for the treatment of gonorrhea, and doxycycline is the preferred tetracycline for presumptive treatment of coexisting chlamydial infections in patients with gonorrhea.

Mycobacterial Infections **Leprosy.** For the treatment of multibacillary leprosy† in adults who cannot receive rifampin because of adverse effects, intercurrent disease (e.g., chronic hepatitis), or infection with rifampin-resistant *Mycobacterium leprae*, the World Health Organization (WHO) recommends supervised administration of a regimen of clofazimine (50 mg daily), ofloxacin (400 mg daily), and minocycline (100 mg daily) given for 6 months, followed by a regimen of clofazimine (50 mg daily) and minocycline (100 mg daily) given for at least an additional 18 months.

For the treatment of multibacillary leprosy in adults who will not accept or cannot tolerate clofazimine, the WHO recommends supervised administration of a once-monthly rifampin-based multiple-drug regimen (ROM) that includes rifampin (600 mg once monthly), ofloxacin (400 mg once monthly), and minocycline (100 mg once monthly) given for 24 months.

For the treatment of single-lesion paucibacillary leprosy† in certain patient groups, the WHO currently states that adults may receive a single-dose rifampin-based multiple-drug regimen (ROM) that includes a single 600-mg dose of rifampin, a single 400-mg dose of ofloxacin, and a single 100-mg dose of minocycline.

For the treatment of single-lesion paucibacillary leprosy in pediatric patients, the WHO recommends that children 5–14 years of age receive a single 300-mg dose of rifampin, a single 200-mg dose of ofloxacin, and a single 50-mg dose of minocycline. Children younger than 5 years of age should receive an appropriately adjusted dose of each drug.

For additional information on the treatment of leprosy, see Rifampin 8:16.04, Dapsone 8:16.92, and Clofazimine 8:16.92.

Mycobacterium marinum Infections. The manufacturers state that optimum dosage has not been established, but granulomas of the skin caused by *Mycobacterium marinum* have been successfully treated with 100 mg of oral minocycline every 12 hours for 6–8 weeks. The American Thoracic Society (ATS) recommends that oral minocycline be given in a dosage of 100 mg twice daily for at least 3 months for the treatment of cutaneous *M. marinum* infections and states that a minimum of 4–6 weeks of therapy is necessary to determine whether or not the infection is responding.

Neisseria meningitidis Infections **N. meningitidis Carriers.** To eliminate meningococci from the nasopharynx of asymptomatic *Neisseria meningitidis* carriers in situations in which the risk of meningococcal meningitis is high, the manufacturers state that 100 mg of oral minocycline may be given every 12 hours for 5 days.

The CDC and the American Academy of Pediatrics (AAP) currently recommend other anti-infective agents (i.e., rifampin, ceftriaxone, ciprofloxacin) for chemoprophylaxis in close contacts of individuals with invasive meningococcal disease.

Nocardiosis For the treatment of nocardiosis†, the usual dosage of oral minocycline has been given in conjunction with a sulfonamide for 12–18 months.

Pleural Effusions When used intrapleurally† as a sclerosing agent to control pleural effusions associated with metastatic tumors†, 300 mg of minocycline reportedly has been diluted with 40–50 mL of 0.9% sodium chloride injection and instilled into the pleural space through a thoracostomy tube, followed by clamping of the tube and subsequent removal of the fluid.

Rheumatoid Arthritis When used in the management of rheumatoid arthritis†, adults have received oral minocycline in a dosage of 100 mg twice daily. A benefit may be evident 1–3 months after initiation of minocycline therapy.

Syphilis The manufacturers state that the usual dosage of oral minocycline may be given for 10–15 days for the treatment of syphilis; close follow-up and laboratory tests are recommended.

Parenteral penicillin G is the drug of choice for all stages of syphilis and doxycycline or tetracycline hydrochloride are the tetracyclines recommended by the CDC for the treatment of primary, secondary, latent, or tertiary syphilis in nonpregnant adults, adolescents, and children 8 years of age or older who are hypersensitive to penicillin.

Vibrio Infections **Cholera.** For the treatment of cholera in conjunction with fluid and electrolyte replacement, an initial 200-mg oral dose of minocycline has been given followed by 100-mg oral doses every 12 hours for 48–72 hours.

■ **Dosage in Renal Impairment** In patients with renal impairment, doses and/or frequency of administration of minocycline should be decreased in response to the degree of impairment. Some manufacturers state that dosage of oral minocycline should not exceed 200 mg daily in patients with impaired renal function.

Cautions

Adverse CNS effects (e.g., vestibular reactions) occur more frequently with minocycline than with other currently available tetracyclines. The true incidence of these adverse effects has not been determined. Previously, vestibular symptoms were reported to occur in up to 21% of patients treated with minocycline. However, recent studies indicate that these reactions may occur in 30–90% of patients treated with usual dosages of minocycline. For a more complete discussion of these and other cautions associated with the use of minocycline, see Cautions in the Tetracyclines General Statement 8:12.24.

Pharmacokinetics

In all studies described in the Pharmacokinetics section, minocycline was administered as the hydrochloride salt.

■ **Absorption** Approximately 90–100% of an oral dose of minocycline hydrochloride is absorbed from the GI tract in fasting adults. Peak serum concentrations usually are attained within 1–4 hours.

Following oral administration of a single 200-mg dose of minocycline powder- or pellet-filled capsules in fasting adults with normal renal function, peak serum concentrations of the drug are attained within 1–4 hours (average 2.1 hours) and range from 2.1–5.1 mcg/mL (average 3.5 mcg/mL). In one study in adults with normal renal function given an initial 200-mg oral dose of minocycline as powder-filled capsules followed by 100-mg oral doses every 12 hours, steady-state serum concentrations of minocycline averaged 2.3–3.5 mcg/mL.

Following oral administration of a single 100-mg dose of minocycline as tablets in healthy, fasting adults, peak serum concentrations were attained in 1–3 hours (average 1.7 hours) and ranged from 0.5–1.3 mcg/mL (average 0.8 mcg/mL).

Because tetracyclines readily chelate divalent or trivalent cations including aluminum, calcium, iron, and magnesium, concurrent oral administration of antacids or other drugs containing these cations may decrease oral absorption of minocycline hydrochloride. (See Drug Interactions in the Tetracyclines General Statement 8:12.24.)

Effect of Food or Milk Food and/or milk can decrease the rate and extent of absorption of oral minocycline hydrochloride.

In one study in healthy adults, administration of a single 100-mg dose of minocycline with food resulted in a 13% decrease in the area under the plasma concentration-time curve (AUC) of the drug compared with administration with water. When the same dose was administered with milk, there was a 27% decrease in the AUC compared with administration with water.

When healthy adults received pellet-filled capsules of minocycline following a standardized meal containing dairy products, peak plasma minocycline concentrations were decreased 11.2% and delayed by approximately 1 hour compared with administration in the fasting state; however, the extent of absorption (as represented by the AUC) was similar in fed and fasting individuals.

When minocycline hydrochloride tablets were given concomitantly with a meal containing dairy products, there was a 12% decrease in peak plasma concentrations, a 1-hour delay in peak concentrations, and a 6% decrease in the extent of absorption of the drug.

■ **Elimination** The serum half-life of minocycline is 11–26 hours in adults with normal renal function. In one study, the half-life was reported to be about 17 hours after a single dose and 21 hours after multiple doses.

In a limited number of patients with hepatic dysfunction, the serum half-life of minocycline reportedly ranged from 11–16 hours. Although results of studies using minocycline in patients with renal impairment are conflicting, most studies indicate that the serum half-life of the drug is not significantly affected by alterations in renal function. In patients with severe renal impairment, the serum half-life of minocycline is generally reported to be 12–30 hours following single or multiple doses.

In patients with normal renal function, approximately 4–19% of a single oral dose of minocycline is excreted in urine and 20–34% is excreted in feces within 72 hours as active drug. Some studies indicate that minocycline, unlike other currently available tetracyclines, is partially metabolized to at least 6 metabolites.

Chemistry and Stability

■ **Chemistry** Minocycline is a semisynthetic tetracycline antibiotic derived from tetracycline. Minocycline is commercially available as the hydrochloride salt in capsules, pellet-filled capsules, or film-coated tablets. Minocycline hydrochloride occurs as a yellow, crystalline powder and is soluble in water and slightly soluble in alcohol.

■ **Stability** Minocycline hydrochloride capsules, pellet-filled capsules, or film-coated tablets, should be stored at a controlled room temperature of 20–25°C. These preparations should be protected from light, moisture, and excessive heat.

For further information on chemistry and stability, mechanism of action, spectrum, resistance, pharmacokinetics, uses, cautions, drug interactions, laboratory test interferences, and dosage and administration of minocycline hydrochloride, see the Tetracyclines General Statement 8:12.24.

Preparations

Excipients in commercially available drug preparations may have clinically important effects in some individuals; consult specific product labeling for details.

Minocycline Hydrochloride

Oral		
Capsules	50 mg (of minocycline)*	**Minocycline Hydrochloride Capsules**
	75 mg (of minocycline)*	**Dynacin®**, Medicis
		Minocycline Hydrochloride Capsules
	100 mg (of minocycline)*	**Dynacin®**, Medicis
		Minocycline Hydrochloride Capsules
Capsules, pellet-filled	50 mg (of minocycline)	**Minocin®**, Triax
	100 mg (of minocycline)	**Minocin®**, Triax
Tablets, film coated	50 mg (of minocycline)*	**Dynacin®**, Medicis
		Minocycline Hydrochloride Tablets
		Myrac®, Glades
	75 mg (of minocycline)*	**Dynacin®**, Medicis
		Minocycline Hydrochloride Tablets
		Myrac®, Glades
	100 mg (of minocycline)*	**Dynacin®**, Medicis
		Minocycline Hydrochloride Tablets
		Myrac®, Glades

*available from one or more manufacturer, distributor, and/or repackager by generic (nonproprietary) name

†Use is not currently included in the labeling approved by the US Food and Drug Administration

Tetracycline
Tetracycline Hydrochloride

■ Tetracycline is an antibiotic derived from *Streptomyces aureofaciens* or produced semisynthetically from oxytetracycline.

Dosage and Administration

■ **Reconstitution and Administration** Tetracycline and tetracycline hydrochloride are administered orally. Although tetracycline hydrochloride has been administered by IM and IV injection, parenteral preparations of the drug are no longer commercially available in the US.

To reduce the risk of esophageal irritation and ulceration, tetracycline capsules or tablets should be administered with adequate amounts of fluid and probably should not be given at bedtime or to patients with esophageal obstruction or compression.

Because food and/or milk reduce GI absorption of tetracycline and tetracycline hydrochloride, oral preparations of the drugs should be given 1 hour before or 2 hours after meals and/or milk.

■ **Dosage** Dosage of tetracycline and tetracycline hydrochloride is expressed in terms of tetracycline hydrochloride.

General Adult Dosage The usual adult oral dosage of tetracycline hydrochloride is 1–2 g daily given in 2–4 divided doses. A dosage of 500 mg twice daily or 250 mg 4 times daily may be adequate for mild to moderate infections; a dosage of 500 mg 4 times daily may be required for severe infections.

General Pediatric Dosage The usual oral dosage of tetracycline hydrochloride for children older than 8 years of age is 25–50 mg/kg daily given in 4 divided doses. The American Academy of Pediatrics (AAP) states that oral tetracycline is inappropriate for severe infections.

Acne For the adjunctive treatment of inflammatory acne, 500 mg to 1 g of tetracycline hydrochloride is given orally in 4 divided doses daily for 1–2 weeks or until clinical improvement occurs. Dosage is then decreased slowly to 125–500 mg daily or the lowest dosage which suppresses lesions. This dosage is then continued until clinical improvement allows discontinuation of the drug. Prolonged maintenance therapy may be necessary.

For information on the topical use of tetracyclines in acne, see Tetracyclines 84:04.04.

Actinomycosis In severe cases of actinomycosis, the usual dosage of tetracycline hydrochloride has been given orally for 12–18 months after 3–4 weeks of penicillin G.

Anthrax **Postexposure Prophylaxis.** Although doxycycline generally is the tetracycline recommended for postexposure prophylaxis following suspected or confirmed exposure to aerosolized anthrax spores in the context of biologic warfare or bioterrorism, some experts state that in vitro studies suggest that adults can receive oral tetracycline hydrochloride in a dosage of 500 mg every 6 hours for *postexposure prophylaxis* following exposure to anthrax spores† if necessary as an alternative to doxycycline. Although the optimum duration of postexposure prophylaxis after an inhalation exposure to *B. anthracis* spores is unclear, prolonged postexposure prophylaxis is generally recommended because of the possible persistence of anthrax spores in lung tissue following aerosol exposure. A duration of 60 days may be adequate for a low-dose exposure, but a duration longer than 4 months may be necessary to reduce the risk following a high-dose exposure. The US Working Group on Civilian Biodefense and the US Army Medical Research Institute of Infectious Diseases (USAMRIID) recommend that postexposure prophylaxis be continued for *at least* 60 days in individuals who are not fully immunized against anthrax and when anthrax vaccine is unavailable or cannot be used for postexposure vaccination.

Treatment of Inhalational Anthrax. Although doxycycline generally is the tetracycline recommended for treatment of inhalational anthrax, some experts state that in vitro studies suggest that adults can receive oral tetracycline hydrochloride in a dosage of 500 mg every 6 hours if necessary as an alternative to oral doxycycline.

The US Centers for Disease Control and Prevention (CDC) and other experts (e.g., US Working Group on Civilian Biodefense, USAMRIID) recommend that treatment of inhalational anthrax be initiated with a multiple-drug regimen that includes ciprofloxacin or doxycycline and 1 or 2 other anti-infectives predicted to be effective. IV therapy with a multiple-drug parenteral regimen may not be possible if large numbers of individuals require treatment in a mass casualty setting; in these circumstances, some experts recommend that treatment with an oral regimen recommended for postexposure prophylaxis is an option. (See Anthrax under Dosage and Administration: Dosage in Doxycycline 8:12.24.)

Balantidiasis For the treatment of balantidiasis† caused by *Balantidium coli*, the usual dosage of oral tetracycline hydrochloride is 500 mg 4 times daily for 10 days in adults and 40 mg/kg in 4 divided doses daily (up to 2 g daily) for 10 days in children 8 years of age or older.

Brucellosis For the treatment of brucellosis, the manufacturers recommend that tetracycline hydrochloride be given in a dosage of 500 mg orally 4 times daily for 3 weeks in conjunction with IM streptomycin (1 g twice daily during the first week and once daily during the second week of treatment). The AAP recommends an oral tetracycline dosage of 30–40 mg/kg daily (up to 2 g daily) in 4 divided doses given for at least 6 weeks.

A tetracycline (usually doxycycline) generally is used in conjunction with another anti-infective (e.g., streptomycin or gentamicin and/or rifampin) to reduce the likelihood of relapse, especially for severe infections and when there are complications such as meningitis, endocarditis, or osteomyelitis. Monotherapy is no longer recommended for the treatment of brucellosis since such therapy is associated with a high relapse rate.

The usual duration of treatment of brucellosis is at least 4–6 weeks; streptomycin or gentamicin usually is given concomitantly for up to 2–3 weeks and/or rifampin is given for the full duration of treatment. More prolonged therapy may be required for complicated disease (e.g., hepatitis, splenitis, meningoencephalitis, endocarditis, osteomyelitis). Meningoencephalitis and endocarditis should be treated for at least 90 days and may require a treatment duration of 6 months or more.

Burkholderia Infections For the treatment of melioidosis† caused by *Burkholderia pseudomallei*, oral tetracycline has been given in a dosage of 2–3 g for 1–3 months. However, doxycycline is the preferred tetracycline for the treatment of melioidosis and other infections caused by *Burkholderia*. (See Burkholderia Infections under Dosage and Administration: Dosage in Doxycycline 8:12.24.)

Campylobacter Infections If tetracycline hydrochloride is used in the treatment of *Campylobacter fetus* infections, some clinicians recommend that the usual dosage of the drug be given for 10 days.

Chancroid When tetracycline hydrochloride is used as an alternative to the drugs of choice for the treatment of chancroid (genital ulcers caused by *Haemophilus ducreyi*), some clinicians recommend that the usual oral dosage of the drug be given for 2–4 weeks.

Chlamydial and Mycoplasmal Infections **Uncomplicated Urethral, Endocervical, or Rectal Infections.** For the treatment of uncomplicated urethral, endocervical, or rectal infections caused by *Chlamydia trachomatis*, the manufacturers and some clinicians suggest that adults can receive oral tetracycline hydrochloride in a dosage of 500 mg 4 times daily for at least 7 days. However, doxycycline is the tetracycline recommended by the CDC for the treatment of these urogenital infections, including presumptive treatment of chlamydial infections in patients with gonorrhea.

Mycoplasma pneumoniae Infections. Atypical pneumonia caused by *Mycoplasma pneumoniae* has been treated with the usual oral dosage of tetracycline hydrochloride given for 1–4 weeks.

Psittacosis. The CDC states that psittacosis (ornithosis) caused by *Chlamydophila psittaci* (formerly *Chlamydia psittaci*) usually responds to oral tetracycline hydrochloride given in a dosage of 500 mg 4 times daily. Doxycycline and tetracycline are the drugs of choice. Although fever and symptoms usually are controlled within 48–72 hours, therapy should be continued for at least 10–14 days after defervescence to prevent relapse. For initial treatment of severely ill patients, an IV regimen of doxycycline hyclate may be indicated.

***Dientamoeba fragilis* Infections** For the treatment of infections caused by *Dientamoeba fragilis*†, oral tetracycline hydrochloride is given in a dosage of 500 mg 4 times daily for 10 days in adults and 40 mg/kg in 4 divided doses daily (up to 2 g daily) for 10 days in children 8 years of age or older.

Gonorrhea and Associated Infections The manufacturers state that uncomplicated gonorrhea in adults may be treated with oral tetracycline hydrochloride in a dosage of 500 mg 4 times daily for 7 days. However, tetracyclines are not included in current CDC guidelines for the treatment of gonorrhea and doxycycline is the preferred tetracycline for presumptive treatment of coexisting chlamydial infections in patients being treated for gonococcal infections.

For the treatment of acute, sexually transmitted epididymitis† caused by *N. gonorrhoeae* and/or *C. trachomatis* in adults and children 8 years of age and older, some clinicians suggest that oral tetracycline hydrochloride can be given in dosage of 500 mg 4 times daily for 10 days in conjunction with a single 250-mg IM dose of ceftriaxone. However, the CDC recommends oral doxycycline in conjunction with a single IM dose of ceftriaxone for treatment of these infections.

Granuloma Inguinale (Donovanosis) The usual oral dosage of tetracycline hydrochloride has been given for 2–4 weeks for the treatment of granuloma inguinale (donovanosis) caused by *Klebsiella granulomatis* (formerly *Calymmatobacterium granulomatis*). However, doxycycline is the tetracycline recommended by the CDC for the treatment of donovanosis.

Helicobacter pylori Infection and Duodenal Ulcer Disease For the treatment of *Helicobacter pylori* (formerly *Campylobacter pylori* or *C. pyloridis*) infection in adults with an active duodenal ulcer, the FDA-labeled dosage of tetracycline hydrochloride is 500 mg in combination with metronidazole (250 mg) and bismuth subsalicylate (525 mg) 4 times daily (at meals and at bedtime) for 14 days; these drugs should be given concomitantly with an H_2-receptor antagonist in recommended dosage. Tetracycline hydrochloride (generally in a dosage of 500 mg 4 times daily) also has been used in other multiple-drug regimens† with at least 2 other agents that have activity against *H. pylori*. If an initial 14-day regimen does not eradicate *H. pylori*, a retreatment regimen that does not include metronidazole should be used.

The minimum duration of therapy required to eradicate *H. pylori* infection in peptic ulcer disease has not been fully established. The ACG and many clinicians currently recommend 1 week of therapy with a proton-pump inhibitor and 2 anti-infective agents (usually clarithromycin and amoxicillin or metronidazole), or a 3-drug, bismuth-based regimen (e.g., bismuth-metronidazole-tetracycline) concomitantly with a proton-pump inhibitor, for treatment of *H. pylori* infection. However, the ACG states that in a cost-sensitive environment, an alternative regimen consisting of a bismuth salt, metronidazole, and tetracycline for 14 days is a reasonable choice in patients who are compliant and in whom there is a low expectation of metronidazole resistance (no prior exposure to the drug and a low regional prevalence of resistance). (See Helicobacter pylori Infection in Uses: GI Infections, in the Tetracyclines General Statement 8:12.24.)

Leptospirosis When penicillin G was contraindicated or was ineffective for the treatment of leptospirosis†, tetracycline hydrochloride daily has been given for 5–7 days in a dosage of 1–2 g daily. Doxycycline is the preferred tetracycline for treatment or prevention of these infections.

Lyme Disease For the treatment of early Lyme disease†, an oral tetracycline hydrochloride dosage of 250–500 mg (preferably 500 mg in adults) 4 times daily for 10–30 days has been used in adults. However, the Infectious Diseases Society of America (IDSA) and other clinicians recommend doxycycline when a tetracycline is used in the treatment of Lyme disease. (See Lyme Disease in Uses: Spirochetal Infections, in the Tetracyclines General Statement 8:12.24 and see Lyme Disease under Dosage and Administration: Dosage in Doxycycline 8:12.24.)

Malaria **Treatment of Uncomplicated Malaria.** When oral tetracycline hydrochloride is used in conjunction with oral quinine sulfate for the treatment of uncomplicated chloroquine-resistant *Plasmodium falciparum* malaria†, the CDC and other clinicians recommend that adults receive 250 mg of tetracycline hydrochloride 4 times daily for 7 days given in conjunction with quinine sulfate (650 mg 3 times daily given for 3 days if malaria was acquired in Africa or South America or for 7 days if acquired in Southeast Asia). These experts recommend that children 8 years of age or older receive oral tetracycline hydrochloride in a dosage of 6.25 mg/kg 4 times daily for 7 days given in conjunction with oral quinine sulfate (10 mg/kg 3 times daily given for 3 days if infection was acquired in Africa or South America or for 7 days if acquired in Southeast Asia).

When oral tetracycline hydrochloride is used in conjunction with quinine sulfate and primaquine phosphate for the treatment of uncomplicated chloroquine-resistant *P. vivax* malaria†, the CDC and other clinicians recommend that adults receive 250 mg of tetracycline hydrochloride 4 times daily for 7 days given in conjunction with oral quinine sulfate (650 mg 3 times daily given for 3 days if malaria was acquired in Africa or South America or for 7 days if acquired in Southeast Asia). These experts recommend that children 8 years of age or older receive tetracycline hydrochloride in a dosage of 6.25 mg/kg 4 times daily for 7 days given in conjunction with oral quinine sulfate (10 mg/kg 3 times daily given for 3 days if infection was acquired in Africa or South America or for 7 days if acquired in Southeast Asia). In addition, a 14-day regimen of oral primaquine (30 mg once daily in adults or 0.6 mg/kg once daily in children) should be given with the quinine sulfate and tetracycline hydrochloride regimen to provide a radical cure and prevent delayed attacks or relapse of *P. vivax* malaria.

For additional information on treatment of uncomplicated malaria, see Uses: Malaria, in Quinine Sulfate 8:30.08.

Treatment of Severe Malaria. When tetracycline hydrochloride is used in conjunction with IV quinidine gluconate (followed by oral quinine sulfate) for the treatment of severe malaria caused by *P. falciparum*†, adults who can tolerate oral therapy may receive 250 mg of tetracycline hydrochloride 4 times daily for 7 days. Children 8 years of age or older who can tolerate oral therapy may receive oral tetracycline hydrochloride in a dosage of 6.25 mg/kg 4 times daily for 7 days. Pediatric dosage should not exceed the recommended adult oral dosage. Patients intolerant of oral therapy may receive IV doxycycline hyclate or IV clindamycin for initial therapy in conjunction with IV quinidine gluconate until they can be switched to oral therapy.

For additional information on treatment of severe malaria, see Uses: Malaria, in Quinidine 24:04.04.04.

Plague **Treatment.** If oral tetracycline hydrochloride is used for the treatment of plague caused by *Yersinia pestis*, adults should receive 2–4 g daily in 4 divided doses and children 8 years of age or older should receive 25–50 mg/kg daily in 4 divided doses.

Prompt initiation of anti-infective therapy (within 18–24 hours of symptom onset) is essential in the treatment of pneumonic plague. Treatment of pneumonic plague should be initiated with a parenteral regimen (e.g., IV doxycycline, IM streptomycin, IM or IV gentamicin), although an oral regimen may be substituted when the patient's condition improves or if parenteral therapy is unavailable. Anti-infective therapy usually is continued for 10 days; some experts recommend a duration of at least 10–14 days.

Postexposure Prophylaxis. For postexposure prophylaxis following high-risk exposure to *Y. pestis*†, including exposure that occurs in the context of biologic warfare or bioterrorism, some experts recommend that adults receive tetracycline hydrochloride 1–2 g daily in 2 or 4 divided doses and children 8 years of age or older receive 25–50 mg/kg daily in 2 or 4 divided doses.

The recommended duration of prophylaxis following exposure to plague aerosol or a patient with suspected pneumonic plague is 7 days or the duration of exposure risk plus 7 days. Some experts recommend that postexposure anti-infective prophylaxis be given to all asymptomatic individuals with exposure to plague aerosol and all asymptomatic individuals who have had household, hospital, or other close contact (within about 2 m) with an individual who has pneumonic plague; however, any exposed individual who develops a temperature of 38.5°C or higher or new cough should promptly receive a parenteral anti-infective for treatment of the disease.

Relapsing Fever For the treatment of louse-borne relapsing fever caused by *Borrelia recurrentis*, the usual oral dosage of tetracycline hydrochloride has been given until the patient is afebrile for 7 days. A single 500-mg oral dose of the drug has also been effective in some patients.

Rickettsial Infections For the treatment of Rocky Mountain spotted fever, louse-borne (epidemic) typhus, Brill-Zinsser disease, endemic (murine) typhus, Q fever, and rickettsialpox, the usual adult dosage of oral tetracycline hydrochloride generally is given for at least 3–7 days or until the patient has been afebrile for approximately 2–3 days. Doxycycline is the drug of choice for most rickettsial infections.

Q Fever. For the treatment of acute Q fever caused by *Coxiella burnetii*, some clinicians recommend that oral tetracycline hydrochloride be given in a dosage of 500 mg every 6 hours for at least 14 days.

It has been suggested that tetracycline hydrochloride given in a dosage of 500 mg every 6 hours for 5–7 days may be effective as prophylaxis against Q fever† and may prevent clinical disease if initiated 8–12 days after exposure; however, such prophylaxis is not effective and may only prolong the onset of disease if given immediately (1–7 days) after exposure.

Syphilis While parenteral penicillin G is the drug of choice for all stages of syphilis, the CDC and AAP state that nonpregnant adults or adolescents with primary or secondary syphilis who are hypersensitive to penicillin can receive 500 mg of oral tetracycline hydrochloride 4 times daily for 14 days. In addition, nonpregnant adults or adolescents with early latent syphilis (syphilis of less than 1-year duration) who are hypersensitive to penicillin can receive 500 mg of oral tetracycline hydrochloride 4 times daily for 14 days and those with late latent syphilis, latent syphilis of unknown duration, or tertiary syphilis (except neurosyphilis) can receive 500 mg 4 times daily for 28 days. For the treatment of syphilis, some manufacturers state that a total of 30–40 g should be given in equally divided doses over a period of 10–15 days.

Care should be taken to encourage optimal compliance with these regimens, since patient compliance with multiple-day tetracycline regimens may be poor. If compliance with the tetracycline regimen and serologic follow-up cannot be ensured, patients with a history of penicillin hypersensitivity should be desensitized and treated with penicillin G. The CDC states that infants and children with syphilis who are hypersensitive to penicillin should be desensitized, if necessary, and treated with penicillin. For information on recommendations regarding treatment and follow-up for all stages and forms of syphilis, see Spirochetal Infections: Syphilis, under Uses in the Natural Penicillins General Statement 8:12.16.04.

Tularemia **Treatment.** If tetracycline hydrochloride is used for the treatment of tularemia that occurs as the result of exposure to *Francisella tularensis* in the context of biologic warfare or bioterrorism or naturally occurring or endemic tularemia, some experts recommend that adults receive 500 mg orally 4 times daily for at least 14–21 days. Relapse may occur as long as 6 months after treatment with tetracycline; however, retreatment with the same dosage usually is curative.

Postexposure Prophylaxis. If tetracycline hydrochloride is used for postexposure prophylaxis following a high-risk laboratory exposure to *F. tularensis* (e.g., spill, centrifuge accident, needlestick injury) or in individuals exposed to the organism in the context of biologic warfare or bioterrorism, some experts (e.g., USAMRIID) state that adults can receive 500 mg orally 4 times daily. Postexposure prophylaxis should be initiated within 24 hours of exposure and continued for at least 14 days.

Postexposure prophylaxis usually is *not* recommended after exposure to natural or endemic tularemia (e.g., tick bite, rabbit or other animal exposure) and is unnecessary in close contacts of tularemia patients since human-to-human transmission does not occur.

Vibrio Infections **Cholera.** For the treatment of cholera in conjunction with fluid and electrolyte replacement, some clinicians recommend a tetracycline hydrochloride dosage of 500 mg 4 times daily for 3 days.

Yaws and Pinta When penicillin G was contraindicated or was ineffective, 1–2 g of tetracycline hydrochloride daily has been given for 10–14 days for the treatment of yaws caused by *Treponema pertenue* or the treatment of pinta caused by *T. carateum.* Doxycycline is the preferred tetracycline for treatment or prevention of these spirochetal infections.

Pleural and Pericardial Effusions When used as a sclerosing agent to control pleural effusions† caused by metastatic tumors, 500 mg of tetracycline hydrochloride (a parenteral formulation of tetracycline hydrochloride no longer is commercially available in the US) has been diluted with 30–50 mL of 0.9% sodium chloride injection and instilled into the chest through a thoracostomy tube followed by instillation of 50 mL of 0.9% sodium chloride injection.

To control pericardial effusions† caused by metastatic tumors, 500 mg to 1 g of tetracycline hydrochloride has been diluted with 20 mL of 0.9% sodium chloride injection and instilled intrapericardially through an indwelling pericardial cannula.

■ **Dosage in Renal Impairment** If tetracycline is used in patients with impaired renal function, doses and/or frequency of administration must be modified in response to the degree of renal impairment.

Pharmacokinetics

■ **Absorption** Approximately 75–80% of an oral dose of tetracycline or tetracycline hydrochloride is absorbed from the GI tract in fasting adults.

Following oral administration of tetracycline hydrochloride as capsules or tablets in fasting adults with normal renal function, peak serum concentrations of tetracycline are attained within 2–4 hours and average 1.5–2.2 mcg/mL following a single 250-mg dose and 3–4.3 mcg/mL following a single 500-mg dose. In adults with normal renal function receiving 250 or 500 mg of tetracycline hydrochloride as capsules or tablets every 6 hours, steady-state serum concentrations of tetracycline average 1–3 mcg/mL and 2–5 mcg/mL, respectively. In one study in adults with normal renal function, a single 250-mg dose of tetracycline hydrochloride oral suspension resulted in average peak serum concentrations of the drug of 2.4 mcg/mL at 3 hours; serum concentrations averaged 1.0 mcg/mL at 12 hours.

Because tetracyclines readily chelate divalent or trivalent cations including aluminum, calcium, iron, magnesium, and zinc, concurrent oral administration of antacids or other drugs containing these cations may also decrease oral absorption of tetracycline preparations.

Effect of Food or Milk Food and/or milk reduce GI absorption of tetracycline and tetracycline hydrochloride by 50% or more.

In one study in healthy adults, administration of a single 250-mg dose of tetracycline hydrochloride with food resulted in a 42% decrease in peak serum concentrations and a 46% decrease in the area under the plasma concentration-time curve (AUC) of the drug compared with administration with water. When the same dose was administered with milk, there was a 58% decrease in peak serum concentrations and a 65% decrease in the AUC compared with administration with water.

■ **Elimination** The serum half-life of tetracycline is 6–12 hours in adults with normal renal function and is reported to be 57–120 hours in patients with severe renal impairment. In patients with normal renal function, 48–60% of a single oral dose of tetracycline hydrochloride is excreted in urine as active drug within 72 hours.

Chemistry and Stability

■ **Chemistry** Tetracycline is an antibiotic derived from *Streptomyces aureofaciens* or produced semisynthetically from oxytetracycline. Tetracycline is commercially available as the base and the hydrochloride salt. The drugs occur as yellow, crystalline powders. Tetracycline has solubilities of approximately 0.4 mg/mL in water and 20 mg/mL in alcohol at 25°C. Tetracycline hydrochloride is moderately hygroscopic and has solubilities of approximately 100 mg/mL in water and 10 mg/mL in alcohol at 25°C.

■ **Stability** Tetracycline and tetracycline hydrochloride are stable in air, but darken on exposure to strong sunlight in moist air.

Tetracycline hydrochloride capsules and tablets should be stored in tight, light-resistant containers at 15–30°C.

Tetracycline oral suspension should be stored in tight, light-resistant containers at less than 30°C.

For further information on chemistry and stability, mechanism of action, spectrum, resistance, pharmacokinetics, uses, cautions, drug interactions, laboratory test interferences, and dosage and administration of tetracycline, see the Tetracyclines General Statement 8:12.24. For topical uses of tetracycline, see Tetracyclines 52:04.04 and 84:04.04.

Preparations

Excipients in commercially available drug preparations may have clinically important effects in some individuals; consult specific product labeling for details.

Tetracycline

Oral		
Suspension	equivalent to 125 mg tetracycline hydrochloride per 5 mL	**Sumycin® Syrup**, Par

Tetracycline Hydrochloride

Oral		
Capsules	250 mg*	**Tetracycline Hydrochloride Capsules**
	500 mg*	**Tetracycline Hydrochloride Capsules**
Tablets, film-coated	250 mg	**Sumycin®**, Par
	500 mg	**Sumycin®**, Par

*available from one or more manufacturer, distributor, and/or repackager by generic (nonproprietary) name

Tetracycline Hydrochloride Combinations

4 Capsules, Tetracycline Hydrochloride 500 mg 4 Tablets, Metronidazole 250 mg 8 Tablets, chewable Bismuth Subsalicylate	**Helidac Therapy®** (available as 14 dose cards/carton), Prometheus

†Use is not currently included in the labeling approved by the US Food and Drug Administration

AMINOMETHYLCYCLINES 8:12.24.04

Sarecycline Hydrochloride

■ Sarecycline hydrochloride is a tetracycline anti-infective agent.

Uses

■ **Acne Vulgaris** Sarecycline hydrochloride is used for the treatment of inflammatory lesions of non-nodular moderate to severe acne vulgaris in adults and pediatric patients 9 years of age and older.

Therapy of acne vulgaris must be individualized and modified as needed depending on the types of acne lesions that predominate and the response to therapy. Tetracyclines (e.g., doxycycline, minocycline, tetracycline) are considered first-line therapy when a systemic anti-infective is indicated in the adjunctive treatment of moderate to severe inflammatory acne, unless contraindicated. Data are not available to date regarding the comparative efficacy and safety of oral sarecycline and other oral tetracyclines used for the treatment of acne.

Sarecycline has *not* been evaluated for the treatment of infections.

Clinical Experience The safety and efficacy of sarecycline for the treatment of inflammatory lesions of non-nodular moderate to severe acne have been evaluated in two 12-week multicenter, randomized, double-blind, placebo-controlled, phase 3 studies that included a total of 2002 adult and pediatric patients 9–45 years of age (57% female, 78% white, 51% adults 18–45 years of age) with facial acne (NCT02320149 [study 1] and NCT02322866 [study 2]). Patients had baseline investigator's global assessment (IGA) scores of moderate (3) or severe (4) with 20–50 inflammatory lesions, no more than 100 noninflammatory lesions, and no more than 2 nodules and were randomized to receive a 12-week regimen of oral sarecycline (60, 100, or 150 mg once daily based on weight [1.5 mg/kg daily]) or placebo once daily. The 2 primary efficacy end points were the percentage of patients with IGA success (i.e., IGA scores of clear [0] or almost clear [1] with a 2-point decrease in IGA from baseline to week 12) and the absolute reduction from baseline in inflammatory lesion count at week 12. IGA success percentage at week 12 in patients in study

1 or 2 treated with sarecycline was 21.9 or 22.6%, respectively, compared with 10.5 or 15.3%, respectively, in those treated with placebo. The mean absolute reduction in inflammatory lesions at week 12 in patients in study 1 or 2 treated with sarecycline was 15.3 or 15.5, respectively, compared with 10.2 or 11.1, respectively, in those treated with placebo. In both studies, the mean absolute and percent reduction in inflammatory lesions at weeks 3, 6, and 9 were greater in the sarecycline group compared with the placebo group. Onset of efficacy in improvement in inflammatory lesions occurred by week 3 and the mean percentage reduction in inflammatory lesions at week 12 in study 1 or 2 was 51.8 or 49.9%, respectively, in those treated with sarecycline compared with 35.1 or 35.4%, respectively, in those treated with placebo.

Dosage and Administration

■ **Administration** Sarecycline hydrochloride is administered orally once daily with or without food.

Sarecycline tablets should be taken with adequate amounts of fluid to reduce the risk of esophageal irritation and ulceration.

■ **Dosage** Dosage of sarecycline hydrochloride is expressed in terms of sarecycline.

Acne Vulgaris For the treatment of inflammatory lesions of non-nodular moderate to severe acne vulgaris in adults and pediatric patients 9 years of age or older, the recommended dosage of sarecycline is based on weight. (See Table 1.)

If there is no improvement after 12 weeks of sarecycline treatment, use of the drug should be reassessed. The manufacturer states that efficacy of sarecycline for longer than 12 weeks and safety of the drug for longer than 12 months have not been established.

Table 1: Sarecycline Dosage in Adults and Pediatric Patients 9 years of Age and Older

Body Weight (kg)	Dosage
33–54 kg	60-mg tablet once daily
55–84 kg	100-mg tablet once daily
85–136 kg	150-mg tablet once daily

■ **Special Populations** ***Hepatic Impairment*** Dosage adjustments are not necessary in patients with mild to moderate hepatic impairment (Child-Pugh class A or B). Data are not available regarding use of sarecycline in patients with severe hepatic impairment (Child-Pugh class C).

Renal Impairment Dosage adjustments are not necessary in patients with mild, moderate, or severe renal impairment. Data are not available regarding use of sarecycline in patients with end-stage renal disease.

Cautions

■ **Contraindications** Sarecycline hydrochloride is contraindicated in patients hypersensitive to any tetracycline.

■ **Warnings/Precautions** ***Sensitivity Reactions*** **Photosensitivity Reactions.** Photosensitivity, manifested by an exaggerated sunburn reaction, has been reported in patients receiving tetracyclines.

Exposure to natural or artificial sunlight (tanning beds or UVA/B treatment) should be minimized or avoided during sarecycline treatment. If a patient needs to be outdoors, they should be advised to wear loose-fitting clothes that protect skin from sun exposure and to consider other sun protection measures.

Dental and Bone Effects The use of tetracyclines during tooth development (e.g., during second and third trimesters of pregnancy, infancy, childhood up to 8 years of age) may cause permanent yellow-gray to brown discoloration of teeth and enamel hypoplasia. These dental effects are most common following long-term use of tetracyclines, but have been reported following repeated short-term use of the drugs.

Tetracyclines form a stable calcium complex in any bone-forming tissue. A reversible decrease in fibula growth rate has occurred in premature infants given oral tetracycline in a dosage of 25 mg/kg every 6 hours.

Fetal/Neonatal Morbidity Animal studies indicate that tetracyclines cross the placenta, are found in fetal tissue, and can cause fetal toxicity (e.g., retardation of skeletal development) and embryotoxicity. If sarecycline is used during pregnancy or if the patient becomes pregnant while taking sarecycline, the patient should be apprised of the potential hazard to the fetus. (See Pregnancy under Warnings/Precautions: Specific Populations, in Cautions.)

CNS Effects Adverse CNS effects (e.g., lightheadedness, dizziness, vertigo) have been reported with tetracyclines and may impair the patient's ability to drive vehicles or operate hazardous machinery. These symptoms may disappear during tetracycline therapy or when the drug is discontinued.

Intracranial hypertension has been reported in adults and adolescents receiving tetracyclines; clinical manifestations include headache, blurred vision, and papilledema. Although signs and symptoms of intracranial hypertension usually resolve after the tetracycline is discontinued, there is a possibility that sequelae (e.g., visual loss) may be permanent or severe. Women of childbearing age who are overweight have a greater risk for developing intracranial hypertension.

Because systemic retinoids are also known to cause intracranial hypertension, sarecycline should not be used concomitantly with oral retinoids. (See Drug Interactions: Retinoids.)

Patients should be questioned about the presence of visual disturbances prior to initiation of treatment with tetracyclines. If visual disturbances occur during treatment, the patient should be checked for papilledema.

Superinfection/Clostridium difficile-associated Colitis Use of sarecycline may result in overgrowth of nonsusceptible organisms, including fungi. The drug should be discontinued and appropriate therapy instituted if superinfection occurs.

Treatment with anti-infectives alters normal colon flora and may permit overgrowth of *Clostridium difficile*. *C. difficile* infection (CDI) and *C. difficile*-associated diarrhea and colitis (CDAD; also known as antibiotic-associated diarrhea and colitis or pseudomembranous colitis) have been reported in patients receiving nearly all systemic anti-infectives and may range in severity from mild diarrhea to fatal colitis. *C. difficile* produces toxins A and B which contribute to development of CDAD; hypertoxin-producing strains of *C. difficile* are associated with increased morbidity and mortality since they may be refractory to anti-infectives and colectomy may be required.

CDAD should be considered in the differential diagnosis of patients who develop diarrhea during or after anti-infective therapy. Careful medical history is necessary since CDAD has been reported to occur as late as 2 months or longer after anti-infective therapy is discontinued.

If CDAD is suspected or confirmed, anti-infective therapy not directed against *C. difficile* should be discontinued whenever possible. Patients should be managed with appropriate anti-infective therapy directed against *C. difficile* (e.g., vancomycin, fidaxomicin, metronidazole), appropriate supportive therapy (e.g., fluid and electrolyte management, protein supplementation), and surgical evaluation as clinically indicated.

Selection and Use of Anti-infectives Use of sarecycline for the treatment of acne vulgaris may result in emergence of bacteria resistant to tetracyclines.

To reduce development of drug-resistant bacteria and maintain effectiveness of other antibacterials, sarecycline should be used only when indicated.

Specific Populations **Pregnancy.** Like other tetracyclines, sarecycline may cause fetal harm, permanent discoloration of teeth, and reversible inhibition of bone growth if administered during pregnancy. Human data are insufficient to inform a drug-associated risk for birth defects or miscarriage with sarecycline; however, tetracyclines are known to cross the placenta.

If sarecycline is used during pregnancy or if the patient becomes pregnant while taking sarecycline, the patient should be apprised of the potential hazard to the fetus.

Because potential risks to the fetus outweigh potential benefits to the mother, pregnant patients should discontinue sarecycline as soon as pregnancy is recognized.

In an embryofetal developmental study in rats, sarecycline administered to pregnant rats at oral dosages up to 500 mg/kg daily (7 times the maximum recommended human dosage [MRHD] based on area under the plasma concentration-time curve [AUC] comparison) during organogenesis was associated with decreased maternal body weight, fetal body weight, and litter size and increased numbers of resorption and postimplantation losses. Skeletal malformations (bent forelimb, hind limb, and scapula) were also reported at all dosage levels tested (50 mg/kg daily or higher; 1.4 or more times the MRHD based on AUC comparison). In an embryofetal developmental study in rabbits, sarecycline was administered to pregnant rabbits at oral dosages up to 150 mg/kg daily during the period of organogenesis. Excessive maternal toxicity (mortality/moribundity/abortion) occurred at 150 mg/kg daily (5 times the MRHD based on AUC comparison) and this dosage group was terminated early. Maternal moribundity also occurred at 100 mg/kg daily (0.6 times the MRHD based on AUC comparison); no significant embryofetal toxicity or malformations were observed at dosages up to 100 mg/kg daily.

In a prenatal and postnatal developmental study in rats, sarecycline was administered to maternal rats at oral dosages up to 400 mg/kg daily during the period of organogenesis through lactation. Excessive litter toxicity (litter loss and stillbirth) occurred at 400 mg/kg daily (8 times the MRHD based on AUC comparison), which led to early termination of dams at parturition. Decreases in body weight and food consumption of dams during the lactation period occurred at 150 mg/kg daily (3 times the MRHD based on AUC comparison). Decreases in offspring survival and offspring body weight during the pre-weaning and growth period, and decreases in implantation sites and viable embryos in female offspring occurred at 150 mg/kg daily (3 times the MRHD based on AUC comparison). However, no significant maternal or developmental toxicity was observed at 50 mg/kg daily (1.4 times the MRHD based on AUC comparison).

Lactation. Tetracyclines are distributed into human milk. Because of the potential for serious adverse effects on bone and tooth development in nursing infants from tetracycline anti-infectives, women should be advised that breast-feeding is not recommended during sarecycline treatment.

Fertility. The manufacturer states that sarecycline should be avoided in males attempting to conceive a child.

In an animal fertility study in male and female rats, sarecycline adversely affected spermatogenesis (decreased sperm motility, decreased sperm count and concentration, increased percentage of abnormal sperm) when given orally to male rats at a dosage 8 times higher than the MRHD based on AUC comparison. This dosage did not affect fertility in the female rats.

Pediatric Use. Safety and efficacy of sarecycline have not been established in pediatric patients younger than 9 years of age. The use of tetracyclines in pediatric patients younger than 8 years of age is not recommended due to potential for tooth discoloration. (See Dental and Bone Effects under Cautions: Warnings/Precautions.)

The safety and efficacy of sarecycline for the treatment of inflammatory lesions of non-nodular moderate to severe acne vulgaris in pediatric patients 9 years of age and older have been established by controlled clinical studies that included children in this age group.

Geriatric Use. There is insufficient experience in geriatric patients 65 years of age and older to determine whether they respond differently than younger adults.

Clinically important age-related differences in the pharmacokinetics of sarecycline have not been reported when the drug was used in adults up to 73 years of age.

Hepatic Impairment. Mild to moderate hepatic impairment (Child-Pugh class A or B) does not have a clinically important effect on the pharmacokinetics of sarecycline; however, the effects of severe hepatic impairment (Child-Pugh class C) on the pharmacokinetics of the drug have not been studied.

Renal Impairment. Mild, moderate, or severe renal impairment does not have a clinically important effect on the pharmacokinetics of sarecycline; however, the effects of end-stage renal disease on the pharmacokinetics of the drug have not been studied.

■ **Common Adverse Effects** The most common adverse effect of sarecycline is nausea, which was reported in 3–5% of patients in clinical trials.

Drug Interactions

■ **Drugs Metabolized by Hepatic Microsomal Enzymes** In vitro studies indicate that sarecycline does not inhibit cytochrome P-450 (CYP) isoenzymes 1A2, 2A6, 2B6, 2C8, 2C9, 2C19, 2D6, 2E1, or 3A4/5 and does not induce CYP1A2, 2B6, or 3A4/5.

In vitro studies indicate that sarecycline is minimally metabolized by hepatic microsomal enzymes.

■ **Drugs Affected by P-glycoprotein Transport System** In vitro studies indicate that sarecycline inhibits P-glycoprotein (P-gp). Sarecycline is not a substrate of P-gp.

Concomitant use of sarecycline with P-gp substrates (e.g., digoxin) may increase concentrations of the P-gp substrate. If sarecycline is used concomitantly with a P-gp substrate, patients should be monitored for toxicities associated with the P-gp substrate and dosage of the P-gp substrate may need to be reduced.

■ **Drugs Affected by Other Membrane Transporters** In vitro studies indicate that sarecycline does not inhibit breast cancer resistance protein (BCRP), organic anion transporter (OAT) 1, OAT3, organic anion transporting polypeptide (OATP) 1B1, or OATP1B3.

Sarecycline is not a substrate of BCRP, OATP1B1, or OATP1B3.

■ **Antacids** Antacids containing aluminum, bismuth, calcium, or magnesium may impair sarecycline absorption and decrease efficacy of the drug. Sarecycline should not be administered concomitantly with antacids containing aluminum, bismuth, calcium, or magnesium.

■ **Anticoagulants** Sarecycline may depress plasma prothrombin activity, which may increase the risk of bleeding in patients receiving anticoagulants. If sarecycline is used concomitantly with an anticoagulant, dosage of the anticoagulant should be adjusted as needed.

■ **Digoxin** Concomitant use of sarecycline (single 150-mg dose) and digoxin resulted in a 26% increase in peak plasma concentrations of digoxin. If sarecycline is used concomitantly with digoxin, patients should be monitored for digoxin toxicity and dosage of the drug may need to be reduced.

■ **Estrogens and Progestins** Concomitant use of sarecycline and a fixed-combination oral contraceptive containing ethinyl estradiol (20 mcg) and norethindrone acetate (1 mg) increased peak plasma concentrations and area under the plasma concentration-time curve (AUC) of ethinyl estradiol by 14 and 11%, respective, and increased peak plasma concentrations and AUC of norethindrone by 18 and 23%, respectively. This interaction is not considered clinically important.

■ **Iron-containing Preparations** Iron-containing preparations may impair sarecycline absorption and decrease efficacy of the drug. Sarecycline should not be administered concomitantly with iron-containing preparations.

■ **Penicillins** Similar to other tetracyclines, sarecycline may interfere with the bactericidal action of penicillin. Concomitant use of sarecycline and penicillin should be avoided.

■ **Retinoids** Because systemic retinoids (e.g., acitretin, isotretinoin) and tetracyclines have both been reported to cause intracranial hypertension and increased intracranial pressure, sarecycline should not be used concomitantly with oral retinoids.

Description

Sarecycline is an aminomethylcycline tetracycline anti-infective agent. Although the exact mechanisms of action of sarecycline in the treatment of acne vulgaris is not known, the mechanism of action may result from a combination of anti-infective and anti-inflammatory effects similar to that reported with other tetracyclines. Sarecycline has a narrower spectrum of activity compared with other commercially available tetracyclines. Like other tetracyclines used in the treatment of acne vulgaris (e.g., doxycycline, minocycline, tetracycline), sarecycline is active in vitro against *Cutibacterium acnes* (formerly *Propionibacterium acnes*), a gram-positive anaerobe that is a factor in the etiology of acne; however, sarecycline is less active in vitro than these other tetracyclines against enteric gram-negative bacteria or other anaerobic bacteria.

Following oral administration, peak plasma concentrations of sarecycline are attained in 1.5–2 hours. When the drug is given in dosages ranging from 60–150 mg once daily, steady-state concentrations are attained by day 7; steady-state peak plasma concentrations and area under the plasma concentration-time curve (AUC) are slightly less than dose proportional. Administration with a high-fat, high-caloric meal that included milk delayed the time to peak plasma concentrations of sarecycline by approximately 0.53 hours and decreased peak plasma concentrations and AUC of the drug by 31 and 27%, respectively; this effect is not considered clinically important. Sarecycline is about 63–75% bound to plasma proteins. In vitro studies indicate that sarecycline is minimally metabolized by hepatic microsomal enzymes. Minor metabolites resulting from nonenzymic epimerization, *O*/*N*-demethylation, hydroxylation, and desaturation have been identified. After a single 100-mg oral dose of radiolabeled sarecycline, approximately 43% of the dose was recovered in feces (14.9% as unchanged drug) and 44% was recovered in urine (24.7% as unchanged drug). The mean elimination half-life of sarecycline is 21–22 hours.

Advice to Patients

Advise patients to read the manufacturer's patient information.

Importance of drinking sufficient quantities of fluids when taking sarecycline tablets to reduce the risk of esophageal irritation and ulceration.

Importance of taking as directed because of the potential for development of drug-resistant bacteria. Advise patients that skipping doses or not completing the full course of therapy may decrease effectiveness and increase the likelihood that bacteria will develop resistance and will not be treatable with other anti-infectives in the future.

Inform patients that photosensitivity manifested by an exaggerated sunburn reaction has been reported in some individuals taking tetracyclines. Advise patients to minimize or avoid sunlight or artificial UV light (e.g., tanning beds, UVA/B treatment) during sarecycline treatment and to discontinue the drug at the first sign of skin erythema. If a patient needs to be outdoors, advise them to wear loose-fitting clothes that protect skin from sun exposure and also consider other sun protection measures.

Inform patients that intracranial hypertension can occur with tetracyclines. Importance of seeking medical attention if headache or blurred vision occurs.

Advise patients to use caution when driving vehicles or using hazardous machinery if they experience CNS effects (lightheadedness, dizziness, vertigo) during sarecycline treatment. Importance of seeking medical attention if these CNS effects persist.

Advise patients that *Clostridium difficile* colitis can occur with anti-infective therapy. Importance of seeking medical attention if watery or bloody stools occur.

Importance of informing clinicians of existing or contemplated concomitant therapy, including prescription and OTC drugs, and any concomitant illnesses.

Importance of women informing clinicians if they are or plan to become pregnant or plan to breast-feed. Advise patients that sarecycline should not be taken by pregnant women or by women or men attempting to conceive a child. (See Pregnancy and see Fertility under Warnings/Precautions: Specific Populations, in Cautions.) Advise women that breast-feeding is not recommended during sarecycline treatment.

Importance of advising patients of other important precautionary information. (See Cautions.)

Overview® (see Users Guide). For additional information on this drug until a more detailed monograph is developed and published, the manufacturer's labeling should be consulted. It is *essential* that the manufacturer's labeling be consulted for more detailed information on usual cautions, precautions, contraindications, potential drug interactions, laboratory test interferences, and acute toxicity.

Preparations

Excipients in commercially available drug preparations may have clinically important effects in some individuals; consult specific product labeling for details.

Sarecycline Hydrochloride

Oral		
Tablets, film-coated	60 mg (of sarecycline)	**Seysara®**, Almirall
	100 mg (of sarecycline)	**Seysara®**, Almirall
	150 mg (of sarecycline)	**Seysara®**, Almirall

GLYCYLCYCLINES 8:12.24.12

Tigecycline

■ Tigecycline, a synthetic derivative of minocycline, is a glycylcycline antibiotic.

Uses

Tigecycline is used for the treatment of complicated intra-abdominal infections, community-acquired pneumonia, and complicated skin and skin structure infections caused by certain susceptible gram-positive and gram-negative bacteria.

Because a higher incidence of all-cause mortality has been reported in patients receiving tigecycline compared with those receiving comparator anti-infectives, tigecycline should be reserved for use in situations when alternative anti-infectives are not suitable. (See Increased Mortality under Warnings/Precautions: Warnings, in Cautions.)

Prior to initiation of tigecycline, appropriate specimens should be obtained for identification of the causative organism and in vitro susceptibility testing. Tigecycline may be initiated as empiric monotherapy pending results of these tests.

■ **Intra-abdominal Infections** Tigecycline is used for the treatment of complicated intra-abdominal infections caused by *Citrobacter freundii*, *Enterobacter cloacae*, *Escherichia coli*, *Klebsiella oxytoca*, *K. pneumoniae*, *Enterococcus faecalis* (vancomycin-susceptible strains only), *Staphylococcus aureus* (including methicillin-resistant *S. aureus* [MRSA; also known as oxacillin-resistant *S. aureus* or ORSA]), *Streptococcus anginosus* group (*S. anginosus*, *S. intermedius*, *S. constellatus*), *Bacteroides fragilis*, *B. thetaiotaomicron*, *B. uniformis*, *B. vulgatus*, *Clostridium perfringens*, or *Peptostreptococcus micros*.

For initial empiric treatment of mild to moderate community-acquired, extrabiliary, complicated intra-abdominal infections in adults (e.g., perforated or abscessed appendicitis), the Infectious Diseases Society of America (IDSA) recommends either monotherapy with cefoxitin, ertapenem, moxifloxacin, tigecycline, or the fixed combination of ticarcillin and clavulanic acid, or a combination regimen that includes either a cephalosporin (cefazolin, ceftriaxone, cefotaxime, cefuroxime) or fluoroquinolone (ciprofloxacin, levofloxacin) in conjunction with metronidazole.

For additional information regarding management of intra-abdominal infections, the current IDSA clinical practice guidelines available at http://www.idsociety.org should be consulted.

Clinical Experience Safety and efficacy of tigecycline were established in 2 randomized, double-blind, active-controlled phase 3 studies in adults with complicated intra-abdominal infections, including appendicitis, cholecystitis, diverticulitis, gastric/duodenal perforation, intra-abdominal abscess, intestinal perforation, and peritonitis. In these studies, patients were randomized to receive tigecycline (100 mg IV initially, followed by 50 mg IV every 12 hours) or imipenem and cilastatin sodium (500 mg of imipenem IV every 6 hours) for 5–14 days. In a pooled analysis of both studies, the clinical cure rate in the clinically evaluable population was similar in patients treated with tigecycline (87%) and in those treated with imipenem and cilastatin (87%). In the subset of microbiologically evaluable patients from these clinical studies and 2 additional resistant-pathogen studies, the clinical cure rate in those who received tigecycline ranged from 71–95%, depending on the pathogen. When stratified according to causative organism, the clinical cure rate was 85% in infections caused by *E. coli*, 85% in infections caused by *S. anginosus*, 89% in infections caused by *K. pneumoniae*, and 77% in infections caused by the *B. fragilis* group.

In 2 randomized, open-label, multicenter, phase 3b/4 studies, tigecycline was compared with a combination regimen of ceftriaxone in conjunction with metronidazole for the treatment of complicated intra-abdominal infections in adults. In both studies, patients were randomized to receive either tigecycline (100 mg IV initially, followed by 50 mg IV every 12 hours) or a 2-drug regimen of ceftriaxone (2 g IV once daily) and metronidazole (1–2 g daily in divided doses) for 4–14 days. In the first open-label study, demographic characteristics were balanced between groups (mean age 48 years, 64.7% male, 65.3% Caucasian, 52% with primary diagnosis of complicated appendicitis). Clinical cure rate in the clinically evaluable population (376 patients) was 70% in the tigecycline group compared with 74% in the ceftriaxone and metronidazole group. In the subset of microbiologically evaluable patients (275 patients), the clinical cure rate in those who received tigecycline was 66% compared with 70% in the ceftriaxone and metronidazole group. When stratified according to causative organism, the clinical cure rate in the tigecycline group was 70% for infections caused by *E. coli*, 79% for infections caused by *S. anginosus*, 40% for infections caused by *Klebsiella*, and 64% for infections caused by the *B. fragilis* group.

In the second open-label study, demographic characteristics were balanced between groups (mean age 47–49 years, 66–69% male, 38–47% with primary diagnosis of complicated appendicitis). The mean Acute Physiologic Assessment and Chronic Health Evaluation (APACHE) II score was 6–7 and the mean duration of treatment was 7 days in both groups. Clinical cure rate in the clinically evaluable population (387 patients) was 82% in the tigecycline group compared with 79% in the ceftriaxone and metronidazole group. In the subset of microbiologically evaluable patients (227 patients), the clinical cure rate in those who received tigecycline was 82% compared with 80% in the ceftriaxone and metronidazole group. When stratified according to causative organism, the clinical cure rate in the tigecycline group was 83% for infections caused by *E. coli*, 94% for infections caused by the *S. anginosus* group, 77% for infections caused by *K. pneumoniae*, and 67% for infections caused by the *B. fragilis* group.

■ **Respiratory Tract Infections** ***Community-acquired Pneumonia*** Tigecycline is used for the treatment of community-acquired pneumonia caused by *S. pneumoniae* (penicillin-susceptible strains only), including cases with concurrent bacteremia, or caused by *Haemophilus influenzae* (β-lactamase-negative strains only) or *Legionella pneumophila*.

Clinical Experience. Safety and efficacy of tigecycline were established in 2 randomized, double-blind, active-controlled studies in adults with community-acquired pneumonia requiring hospitalization. Patients were randomized to receive tigecycline (100 mg IV initially, followed by 50 mg IV every 12 hours) or levofloxacin (500 mg IV every 12 or 24 hours) for 7–14 days. Clinical cure rates in the clinically evaluable population from the first study were similar in tigecycline-treated patients (89%) and levofloxacin-treated patients (85%). In the second study, patients in both treatment arms could be switched to oral levofloxacin (500 mg daily) after at least 3 days of IV treatment, and the clinical cure rates in the clinically evaluable population were 91% for tigecycline-treated patients and 87% for levofloxacin-treated patients. In the subset of microbiologically evaluable patients from both studies, the clinical cure rate in patients who received tigecycline was 96% in infections caused by *S. pneumoniae* (penicillin-susceptible strains only), 82% in infections caused by *H. influenzae*, and 100% in infections caused by *L. pneumophila*.

Hospital-acquired Pneumonia Tigecycline has *not* been shown to be effective and is *not* labeled by the US Food and Drug Administration (FDA) for the treatment of hospital-acquired pneumonia†, including ventilator-associated pneumonia†. Results of a randomized, comparator-controlled trial evaluating tigecycline in patients with hospital-acquired pneumonia† failed to show efficacy. The subgroup of patients with ventilator-associated pneumonia† who received tigecycline demonstrated lower cure rates (47.9% in those treated with tigecycline versus 70.1% in those treated with a comparator anti-infective) and a higher incidence of death (19.1% in those treated with tigecycline versus 12.3% in those treated with a comparator anti-infective). (See Increased Mortality under Warnings/Precautions: Warnings, in Cautions.)

■ **Skin and Skin Structure Infections** Tigecycline is used for the treatment of complicated skin and skin structure infections caused by *S. aureus* (including MRSA), *Streptococcus agalactiae* (group B streptococci), *S. anginosus* group (*S. anginosus*, *S. intermedius*, *S. constellatus*), *S. pyogenes* (group A β-hemolytic streptococci), *E. faecalis* (vancomycin-susceptible strains only), *E. cloacae*, *E. coli*, *K. pneumoniae*, or *B. fragilis*.

Tigecycline has *not* been shown to be effective and is *not* labeled by FDA for the treatment of diabetic foot infections†. In a phase 3, randomized, double-blind study that included 813 clinically evaluable adults with diabetic foot infection, tigecycline (150 mg IV once daily) did not meet the primary end point of noninferiority to ertapenem (1g IV once daily with or without vancomycin). In addition, a higher incidence of death has been observed in patients with diabetic foot infections receiving tigecycline (1.3%) compared with those receiving comparator anti-infectives (0.6%). (See Increased Mortality under Warnings/Precautions: Warnings, in Cautions.)

Clinical Experience Safety and efficacy of tigecycline were established in 2 randomized, double-blind, active-controlled studies in adults with complicated deep soft tissue infections, including wound infections and cellulitis (10 cm or larger, requiring surgery or drainage, or with complicated underlying disease), major abscesses, infected ulcers, and burns. In these studies, patients were randomized to receive tigecycline (100 mg IV initially, followed by 50 mg IV every 12 hours) or a combination regimen of vancomycin (1 g IV every 12 hours) and aztreonam (2 g IV every 12 hours) for 5–14 days. In a pooled analysis of both studies, the clinical cure rate in the clinically evaluable population was 87% in patients treated with tigecycline and 89% in those treated with the 2-drug regimen of vancomycin and aztreonam. In the subset of microbiologically evaluable patients from these clinical studies and 2 additional resistant-pathogen studies, clinical cure rates ranged from 71–100%, depending on the pathogen. This included clinical cure rates of 91% in those with infections caused by methicillin-susceptible (oxacillin-susceptible) *S. aureus*, 83% in those with infections caused by MRSA, 97% in those with infections caused by *S. pyogenes*, and 81% in those with infections caused by *E. coli*.

In a phase 3b/4 randomized, open-label, multicenter study, the safety and efficacy of tigecycline for the treatment of complicated skin and skin structure infections (e.g., deep soft tissue infection, major abscess, infected ulcers, burns covering less than 5% of body surface area) were evaluated in 405 adults. Patients were randomized to receive tigecycline (100 mg IV initially, followed by 50 mg IV every 12 hours) or a comparator anti-infective regimen (i.e., fixed combination of ampicillin and sulbactam [1.5–3 g IV every 6 hours] or fixed combination of amoxicillin and clavulanate [1.2 g IV every 6–8 hours]) for 4–14 days. Baseline characteristics were balanced between groups (mean age 51–52 years, 61–64% male, 53–56% white). Clinical cure was achieved in 77.5% of patients in the tigecycline group compared with 77.6% of patients in the comparator group. In the subset of microbiologically evaluable patients (219 patients), the eradication rate at the test-of-cure assessment was 79 and 77% in the tigecycline and comparator groups, respectively. When stratified according to causative organism, the clinical cure rate in the tigecycline group was 83% in those with infections caused by methicillin-susceptible (oxacillin-susceptible) *S. aureus*, 69% in those with infections caused by MRSA, 73% in those with infections caused by *S. pyogenes*, and 77% in those with infections caused by *E. coli*.

Dosage and Administration

■ **Administration** Tigecycline is administered by IV infusion.

Tigecycline may be administered through a dedicated line or through a Y-site. If the same IV line is used for sequential infusion of several drugs, the line should be flushed before and after infusion of tigecycline with 0.9% sodium chloride, 5% dextrose, or lactated Ringer's injection. Tigecycline should *not* be administered simultaneously through the same Y-site with amphotericin B, amphotericin B lipid complex, diazepam, esomeprazole, or omeprazole.

Reconstitution and Dilution Tigecycline powder for injection must be reconstituted and diluted before IV infusion. The final tigecycline solution should have a maximum concentration of 1 mg/mL.

Tigecycline powder for injection should be reconstituted by adding 5.3 mL of 0.9% sodium chloride, 5% dextrose, or lactated Ringer's injection to the vial labeled as containing 50 mg of tigecycline to provide a solution containing 10 mg/mL. The vial should be swirled gently until the drug dissolves. The reconstituted solution should be yellow or orange in color; if not, the solution should be discarded.

For preparation of a 50-mg dose, 5 mL of the reconstituted solution should be withdrawn from the vial and diluted in 100 mL of 0.9% sodium chloride or 5% dextrose injection. For preparation of a 100-mg dose, *two* 50-mg vials of tigecycline should be reconstituted, and 10 mL of the reconstituted solution should be diluted in 100 mL of 0.9% sodium chloride or 5% dextrose injection.

Following reconstitution with 0.9% sodium chloride injection, 5% dextrose injection, or lactated Ringer's injection, tigecycline solutions may be stored at room temperature (not to exceed 25°C) for up to a total of 24 hours (up to 6 hours in original vial, remaining time after dose is diluted in an IV bag containing 0.9% sodium chloride or 5% dextrose injection). If storage conditions after reconstitution exceed 25°C, tigecycline should be used immediately. Alternatively, if the dose of reconstituted tigecycline is immediately diluted in an IV bag containing 0.9% sodium chloride or 5% dextrose, the solution may be stored at 2–8°C for up to 48 hours.

Parenteral tigecycline solutions should be inspected visually for particulate matter and discoloration (e.g., green, black) prior to administration.

Rate of Administration Tigecycline should be administered by IV infusion over approximately 30–60 minutes.

■ **Dosage** ***Adult Dosage*** **Intra-abdominal Infections.** The recommended dosage of tigecycline for the treatment of complicated intra-abdominal infections in adults 18 years of age and older is an initial dose of 100 mg, followed by 50 mg every 12 hours. Duration of therapy should be guided by the severity and site of infection and the patient's clinical and bacteriologic progress; the usual duration of therapy is 5–14 days.

Community-acquired Pneumonia. The recommended dosage of tigecycline for the treatment of community-acquired pneumonia in adults 18 years of age and older is an initial dose of 100 mg, followed by 50 mg every 12 hours. Duration of therapy should be guided by the severity and site of infection and the patient's clinical and bacteriologic progress; the usual duration of therapy is 7–14 days.

Skin and Skin Structure Infections. The recommended dosage of tigecycline for the treatment of complicated skin and skin structure infections in adults 18 years of age and older is an initial dose of 100 mg, followed by 50 mg every 12 hours. Duration of therapy should be guided by the severity and site of infection and the patient's clinical and bacteriologic progress; the usual duration of therapy is 5–14 days.

Pediatric Dosage **General Pediatric Dosage.** Safety and efficacy of tigecycline have *not* been established in pediatric patients and the drug should *not* be used in patients younger than 18 years of age unless no alternative anti-infectives are available. If no alternative anti-infectives are available, the manufacturer recommends the following tigecycline dosage for patients 8 years of age or older based on pharmacokinetic studies that included limited numbers of pediatric patients. (See Pediatric Use under Warnings/Precautions: Specific Populations, in Cautions.)

When use of the drug is considered necessary, the manufacturer states that children 8–11 years of age can receive tigecycline in a dosage of 1.2 mg/kg IV every 12 hours (maximum 50 mg IV every 12 hours) and children and adolescents 12–17 years of age can receive a dosage of 50 mg IV every 12 hours.

■ **Special Populations** Dosage adjustments are not required in patients with mild to moderate hepatic impairment (Child-Pugh class A or B). If tigecycline is used in adults with severe hepatic impairment (Child-Pugh class C), an initial dose of 100 mg should be given followed by a maintenance dosage of 25 mg every 12 hours. (See Hepatic Impairment under Warnings/Precautions: Specific Populations, in Cautions.)

Dosage adjustments are not necessary in patients with renal impairment or in those undergoing hemodialysis.

Dosage adjustments based on age are not necessary in geriatric patients.

Dosage adjustments based on gender or race are not necessary.

Cautions

■ **Contraindications** Known hypersensitivity to tigecycline or any ingredient in the formulation.

■ **Warnings/Precautions** ***Warnings*** **Increased Mortality.** Meta-analyses of phase 3 and 4 clinical trials indicate that all-cause mortality was higher in patients treated with tigecycline than in those treated with comparator anti-infectives. Tigecycline should be reserved for use in situations when alternative treatments are not suitable.

Based on meta-analyses of data from clinical trials, there was an increased risk of death when tigecycline was used for FDA-labeled or unlabeled uses. The reason for the increased mortality risk has not been established. In general, deaths resulted from worsening infections, complications of infection, or other underlying medical conditions.

In a pooled analysis of over 7400 patients from 13 phase 3 and 4, active-controlled clinical trials evaluating tigecycline for the treatment of serious infections, the mortality rate was 4% in tigecycline-treated patients versus 3% in patients treated with comparator anti-infectives. Overall, the adjusted risk difference in all-cause mortality between patients receiving tigecycline and those receiving comparator anti-infectives was 0.6%.

Data from 10 clinical trials evaluating tigecycline for FDA-labeled indications (i.e., complicated skin and skin structure infections, complicated intra-abdominal infections, community-acquired pneumonia) indicate an adjusted mortality rate of 2.5% for tigecycline-treated patients versus 1.8% for patients treated with comparator anti-infectives. The adjusted risk difference in mortality stratified by trial weight was 0.6%.

Data indicate that the mortality risk has been greatest when tigecycline was used for the treatment of hospital-acquired pneumonia†, particularly ventilator-associated pneumonia†, a use not included in FDA-approved labeling. (See Patients with Hospital-acquired Pneumonia under Warnings/Precautions: Other Warnings/Precautions, in Cautions.)

Sensitivity Reactions **Hypersensitivity Reactions.** Potentially life-threatening anaphylaxis/anaphylactoid reactions have been reported with tigecycline.

There have been postmarketing reports of severe skin reactions, including Stevens-Johnson syndrome.

Tigecycline should be used with caution in patients with known hypersensitivity to tetracyclines.

Other Warnings/Precautions **Hepatic Effects.** Elevated total bilirubin and aminotransferase concentrations and prolonged prothrombin time have been reported in tigecycline-treated patients. Clinically important hepatic dysfunction and hepatic failure have been reported rarely, and there have been postmarketing reports of hepatic cholestasis and jaundice in patients receiving tigecycline. Adverse hepatic effects may occur after the drug is discontinued.

Patients who develop abnormal liver function tests during tigecycline therapy should be monitored for evidence of worsening hepatic function, and the risks and benefits of continuing tigecycline treatment should be evaluated.

Patients with Hospital-acquired Pneumonia. Tigecycline has *not* been shown to be effective and is *not* labeled by FDA for the treatment of hospital-acquired pneumonia†, including ventilator-associated pneumonia†.

Results of a randomized, comparator-controlled trial evaluating tigecycline in patients with hospital-acquired pneumonia† failed to show efficacy. In the subgroup of patients with ventilator-associated pneumonia†, the mortality rate was 19.1% in those treated with tigecycline compared with 12.3% in those treated with comparator anti-infectives. Mortality was particularly high in tigecycline-treated patients with ventilator-associated pneumonia† who had bacteremia at baseline (mortality rate 50% in those treated with tigecycline versus 7.7% in those treated with a comparator anti-infective). (See Increased Mortality under Warnings/Precautions: Warnings, in Cautions.)

Pancreatitis. Acute pancreatitis, including fatalities, has been reported in patients receiving tigecycline. Some cases have been reported in patients with no known risk factors for pancreatitis. Improvement usually occurs after the drug is discontinued.

A diagnosis of pancreatitis should be considered in any patient receiving tigecycline who develops symptoms, signs, or laboratory abnormalities suggestive of acute pancreatitis. In suspected cases of pancreatitis, consideration should be given to discontinuing tigecycline.

Fetal/Neonatal Morbidity and Mortality. Tigecycline may cause fetal harm; teratogenicity and embryolethality have been demonstrated in animals. Pregnancy should be avoided during tigecycline therapy. If a patient becomes pregnant while receiving tigecycline, she should be apprised of the potential fetal hazard.

Superinfection/Clostridium difficile-associated Diarrhea and Colitis (CDAD). Use of tigecycline may result in emergence and overgrowth of nonsusceptible bacteria or fungi. The patient should be carefully monitored and appropriate therapy instituted if a superinfection occurs.

Treatment with anti-infectives alters normal colon flora and may permit overgrowth of *Clostridium difficile*. *C. difficile* infection (CDI) and *C. difficile*-associated diarrhea and colitis (CDAD; also known as antibiotic-associated diarrhea and colitis or pseudomembranous colitis) have been reported with nearly all anti-infectives, including tigecycline, and may range in severity from mild diarrhea to fatal colitis. *C. difficile* produces toxins A and B which contribute to development of CDAD; hypertoxin-producing strains of *C. difficile* are associated with increased morbidity and mortality since these infections may be refractory to anti-infectives and colectomy may be required.

CDAD should be considered in the differential diagnosis of patients who develop diarrhea during or after anti-infective therapy. Careful medical history is necessary since CDAD has been reported to occur as late as 2 months or longer after anti-infective therapy is discontinued.

If CDAD is suspected or confirmed, anti-infective therapy not directed against *C. difficile* should be discontinued whenever possible. Patients should be managed with appropriate supportive therapy (e.g., fluid and electrolyte management, protein supplementation), anti-infective therapy directed against *C. difficile* (e.g., metronidazole, vancomycin), and surgical evaluation as clinically indicated.

Patients with Intestinal Perforation. Tigecycline should be used with caution in patients with complicated intra-abdominal infections secondary to clinically apparent intestinal perforation. Although a causal relationship has not been established, sepsis or septic shock has been reported in several patients who received tigecycline for the treatment of complicated intra-abdominal infections secondary to intestinal perforation.

Tetracycline-class Effects. Because tigecycline is structurally related to conventional tetracyclines, adverse effects reported with tetracyclines (e.g., photosensitivity, pseudotumor cerebri, antianabolic activity that may result in increased BUN, azotemia, acidosis, and hypophosphatemia) may occur. (See Cautions in the Tetracyclines General Statement 8:12.24.) Pancreatitis has been associated with conventional tetracyclines and has been reported in patients receiving tigecycline. (See Pancreatitis under Warnings/Precautions: Other Warnings/Precautions, in Cautions.)

Endocrine Effects. Symptomatic hypoglycemia has been reported during postmarketing experience in patients with and without diabetes receiving tigecycline.

Selection and Use of Anti-infectives. To reduce development of drug-resistant bacteria and maintain effectiveness of tigecycline and other antibacterials, the drug should be used only for treatment of infections proven or strongly suspected to be caused by susceptible bacteria.

When selecting or modifying anti-infective therapy, results of culture and in vitro susceptibility testing should be used. In the absence of such data, local epidemiology and susceptibility patterns should be considered when selecting anti-infectives for empiric therapy.

Specific Populations

Pregnancy. Category D. (See Users Guide.) Tigecycline crosses the placenta and is found in fetal tissues. (See Fetal/Neonatal Morbidity and Mortality under Warnings/Precautions: Other Warnings/Precautions, in Cautions.)

Use of tigecycline during tooth development (last half of pregnancy) may cause permanent discoloration (yellow-gray-brown) of the teeth. (See Cautions: Pediatric Precautions in the Tetracyclines General Statement 8:12.24.)

Lactation. Tigecycline is distributed into milk in rats. It is not known whether tigecycline is distributed into human milk; caution is advised if the drug is administered in nursing women.

Pediatric Use. Safety and efficacy of tigecycline have *not* been established in patients younger than 18 years of age and use in this age group is *not* recommended. Because of the increased mortality observed in adults receiving tigecycline, clinical trials evaluating safety and efficacy of tigecycline in pediatric patients have not been conducted.

For circumstances when there are no alternative anti-infectives, pediatric dosage has been proposed based on data from pharmacokinetic studies that included limited numbers of pediatric patients. For children 8–11 years of age, a pharmacokinetic simulation showed that a tigecycline dosage of 1.2 mg/kg in this age group would likely result in an area under the plasma concentration-time curve (AUC) similar to that reported in adults receiving the recommended adult dosage. For children and adolescents 12–16 years of age, a tigecycline dosage of 50 mg twice daily would likely result in exposures comparable to those observed in adults receiving the recommended adult dosage. (See Pediatric Dosage under Dosage and Administration: Dosage.)

Because use of tigecycline during tooth development (i.e., in infants and children younger than 8 years of age) may cause permanent discoloration (yellow-gray-brown) of the teeth, the drug should not be used in this age group unless other anti-infectives cannot be used. (See Cautions: Pediatric Precautions in the Tetracyclines General Statement 8:12.24.)

Geriatric Use. There are no substantial differences in safety and efficacy in patients 65 years of age or older relative to younger adults, but increased sensitivity cannot be ruled out.

Hepatic Impairment. Tigecycline should be used with caution and at a reduced dosage in patients with severe hepatic impairment (Child-Pugh class C); such patients should be monitored for treatment response. (See Dosage and Administration: Special Populations.)

In adults with mild hepatic impairment (Child-Pugh class A), tigecycline pharmacokinetics were similar to those in healthy adults. In those with moderate hepatic impairment (Child-Pugh class B), systemic clearance of tigecycline was reduced by 25%, AUC was increased by 50%, and half-life was prolonged by 23%. In those with severe hepatic impairment (Child-Pugh class C), systemic clearance was reduced by 55%, AUC was increased by 105%, and half-life was prolonged by 43%.

Renal Impairment. In a small study, the pharmacokinetic profile of tigecycline in adults with severe renal impairment (creatinine clearance less than 30 mL/minute) or end-stage renal impairment was not substantially altered. Tigecycline is not removed by hemodialysis. Dosage adjustments are not necessary in patients with renal impairment or in those undergoing hemodialysis.

Obese Patients. In otherwise healthy adults with class III obesity (body mass index [BMI] 40 kg/m^2 or higher), a single 100-mg IV dose of tigecycline resulted in serum and urine concentrations of the drug that were similar to concentrations in healthy adults with normal weight (BMI 18.5–24.99 kg/m^2).

■ Common Adverse Effects

Nausea, vomiting, and diarrhea are the most common adverse effects reported with tigecycline and have been reported in up to 35% of patients in clinical studies.

Adverse effects reported in 2–8% of patients receiving tigecycline include abdominal pain, abnormal healing, abscess, anemia, asthenia, bilirubinemia, dizziness, dyspepsia, headache, hypoproteinemia, increased ALT or AST concentrations, increased alkaline phosphatase concentrations, increased amylase concentrations, increased BUN, infection, phlebitis, and rash.

Drug Interactions

■ Drugs Affecting or Metabolized by Hepatic Microsomal Enzymes

Pharmacokinetic interactions are unlikely with drugs metabolized by or affecting cytochrome P-450 (CYP) isoenzymes 1A2, 2C8, 2C9, 2C19, 2D6, or 3A4. Tigecycline is not metabolized by these CYP isoenzymes and does not inhibit these isoenzymes in vitro.

■ Antibacterials

Although the clinical importance is unknown, in vitro studies indicate that tigecycline and colistin (commercially available as colistimethate sodium) are synergistic against some strains of *Escherichia coli, Klebsiella pneumoniae*, *Enterobacter*, and *Acinetobacter baumannii*, including some carbapenem-resistant strains; however, indifference or only an additive effect has also been reported. There also is some evidence of in vitro synergism between tigecycline and levofloxacin, amikacin, or imipenem against some multidrug-resistant (MDR) *A. baumanii*.

Although in vitro antagonism between tigecycline and colistin against *Serratia marcescens* was reported in one study, in vitro antagonism between tigecycline and other commonly used anti-infectives has not been confirmed.

■ Digoxin

Potential pharmacokinetic interaction (slight decrease in peak plasma concentrations of digoxin, but no change in area under the concentration time curve [AUC]); no effect on digoxin pharmacodynamics (as measured by changes in ECG parameters). No effect on tigecycline pharmacokinetics. Dosage adjustment are not needed for either drug.

■ Oral Contraceptives

Potential pharmacologic interaction (decreased effectiveness of oral contraceptives).

■ Warfarin

Potential pharmacokinetic interaction (decreased clearance of warfarin, resulting in increased warfarin concentrations and AUC); pharmacologic interaction (altered international normalized ratio [INR]) unlikely. No effect on tigecycline pharmacokinetics. Monitor prothrombin time (PT) or other suitable coagulation tests if tigecycline is used concomitantly with warfarin.

Description

Tigecycline, a synthetic derivative of minocycline, is a glycylcycline antibiotic. Tigecycline is structurally related to tetracyclines, differing mainly in the addition of a glycylamido moiety at position 9 of the tetracycline nucleus. Like tetracyclines, tigecycline inhibits protein synthesis in susceptible organisms mainly by reversibly binding to 30S ribosomal subunits, thereby inhibiting binding of aminoacyl transfer-RNA to those ribosomes.

Tigecycline has a broad spectrum of antibacterial activity and usually is bacteriostatic in action. Tigecycline is active in vitro and in clinical infections against various gram-positive aerobic and facultatively aerobic bacteria, including *Staphylococcus aureus* (including methicillin-resistant [oxacillin-resistant] strains), *Streptococcus agalactiae* (group B streptococci), *S. anginosus* group (*S. anginosus*, *S. intermedius*, *S. constellatus*), *S. pneumoniae*(penicillin-susceptible strains), *S. pyogenes* (group A β-hemolytic streptococci), and *Enterococcus faecalis* (vancomycin-susceptible strains only). The drug also is active in vitro and in clinical infections against various gram-negative aerobic and facultatively aerobic bacteria, including *Citrobacter freundii*, *Enterobacter cloacae*, *Escherichia coli*, *Haemophilus influenzae* (β-lactamase-negative strains), *Klebsiella oxytoca*, *K. pneumoniae*, and *Legionella pneumophila*, and some anaerobic bacteria, including *Bacteroides fragilis*, *B. thetaiotaomicron*, *B. uniformis*, *B. vulgatus*, *Clostridium perfringens*, and *Peptostreptococcus micros*.

Tigecycline may be active against some bacteria resistant to conventional tetracyclines since susceptibility to the drug is not affected by the 2 major tetracycline resistance mechanisms (i.e., ribosomal protection, efflux). In addition, susceptibility to tigecycline is not affected by many other common resistance mechanisms, including β-lactamases (e.g., extended-spectrum β-lactamases [ESBLs]), target site modifications, macrolide efflux pumps, or enzyme target (e.g., gyrase, topoisomerase) changes. Tigecycline resistance in some bacteria (e.g., *Acinetobacter calcoaceticus-baumannii* complex) is attributed to multidrug-resistant (MDR) efflux pumps. In vitro studies have demonstrated synergism between tigecycline and some other antibacterials (e.g., colistin) against some Enterobacteriaceae. (See Drug Interactions: Antibacterials.)

Tigecycline is extensively distributed into various tissues, including alveolar cells, epithelial lining fluid, skin blister fluid, gall bladder, lung, colon, synovial fluid, and bone. Tigecycline concentrations in certain tissues (i.e., alveolar cells, gallbladder, lung, colon, epithelial fluid) are substantially higher than concentrations in serum. Animal studies indicate that tigecycline crosses the placenta and is found in fetal tissues. The drug is approximately 71–89% bound to plasma proteins. Tigecycline is not extensively metabolized; each of the recovered metabolites (a glucuronide, an *N*-acetyl metabolite, and a tigecycline epimer) constitutes less than 10% of the administered dose. The half-life of tigecycline is 27.1 or 42.4 hours following single or multiple dosing, respectively. Tigecycline is principally eliminated by biliary and fecal excretion as unchanged tigecycline and metabolites. About 59% of a dose is eliminated by biliary and fecal excretion; 33% is eliminated in urine (22% as unchanged drug).

Advice to Patients

Advise patients that antibacterials (including tigecycline) should only be used to treat bacterial infections and not used to treat viral infections (e.g., the common cold).

Importance of completing full course of therapy, even if feeling better after a few days.

Advise patients that skipping doses or not completing the full course of therapy may decrease effectiveness and increase the likelihood that bacteria will develop resistance and will not be treatable with tigecycline or other antibacterials in the future.

Advise patients that diarrhea is a common problem caused by anti-infectives and usually ends when the drug is discontinued. Importance of contacting a clinician if watery and bloody stools (with or without stomach cramps and fever) occur during or as late as 2 months or longer after the last dose.

Importance of informing clinicians of existing or contemplated concomitant therapy, including prescription and OTC drugs, as well as any concomitant illnesses.

Importance of women informing clinicians if they are or plan to become pregnant or plan to breast-feed. Advise pregnant women of risk to the fetus.

Importance of informing patients of other important precautionary information. (See Cautions.)

Overview® (see Users Guide). For additional information on this drug until a more detailed monograph is developed and published, the manufacturer's labeling should be consulted. It is *essential* that the manufacturer's labeling be consulted for more detailed information on usual cautions, precautions, contraindications, potential drug interactions, laboratory test interferences, and acute toxicity.

Preparations

Excipients in commercially available drug preparations may have clinically important effects in some individuals; consult specific product labeling for details.

Tigecycline		
Parenteral		
For injection, for IV infusion	50 mg	**Tygacil®**, Pfizer

†Use is not currently included in the labeling approved by the US Food and Drug Administration

Selected Revisions August 2014,

Miscellaneous Antibacterials 8:12.28

Cyclic Lipopeptides 8:12.28.12

Daptomycin

■ Daptomycin is a cyclic lipopeptide antibiotic.

Uses

Daptomycin is used for the treatment of complicated skin and skin structure infections or bacteremia caused by certain susceptible gram-positive bacteria. The drug should *not* be used in the treatment of pneumonia.

■ **Skin and Skin Structure Infections** Daptomycin is used for the treatment of complicated skin and skin structure infections caused by susceptible *Staphylococcus aureus* (including methicillin-resistant *S. aureus* [MRSA; also known as oxacillin-resistant *S. aureus* or ORSA]), *Streptococcus pyogenes* (group A *β*-hemolytic streptococci, GAS), *S. agalactiae* (group B streptococci, GBS), *S. dysgalactiae* subsp. *equisimilis*, and *Enterococcus faecalis* (vancomycin-susceptible strains only).

For information on management of skin and skin structure infections, the current clinical practice guidelines from the Infectious Diseases Society of America (IDSA) available at http://www.idsociety.org should be consulted.

Clinical Experience In 2 randomized, multicenter, comparative studies in adults with complicated skin and skin structure infections (e.g., wound infection, major abscess, ulcer infection, complicated cellulitis), clinical success rates reported with daptomycin (4 mg/kg IV once every 24 hours) were similar to those reported with vancomycin (1 g IV every 12 hours) or a penicillinase-resistant penicillin (4–12 g IV daily of nafcillin, oxacillin, or cloxacillin [no longer commercially available in the US], or flucloxacillin [not commercially available in the US]). After a minimum of 4 days of IV treatment, patients could be switched to oral anti-infective therapy if clinical improvement was observed; however, most patients (approximately 90%) received IV therapy exclusively. In the intent-to-treat population, clinical success was achieved in 63–80% of patients receiving daptomycin and 61–81% of those receiving comparator anti-infectives.

In a subset of patients who were microbiologically evaluable and stratified according to the infecting pathogen, the daptomycin clinical success rate was 73% in those with infections caused by *E. faecalis* (vancomycin-susceptible strains only), 75% in those with MRSA, 86% in those with methicillin-susceptible *S. aureus*, 85% in those with *S. agalactiae*, 94% in those with *S. pyogenes*, and 100% in those with *S. dysgalactiae* subsp. *equisimilis*.

■ **Bacteremia and Endocarditis** Daptomycin is used for the treatment of bacteremia (blood stream infection) caused by susceptible *S. aureus* (including MRSA).

Daptomycin also is used for the treatment of *S. aureus* bacteremia in patients with right-sided infective endocarditis. However, efficacy of the drug has not been established in patients with left-sided infective endocarditis caused by *S. aureus*; limited data suggest that such patients have a poor outcome despite daptomycin treatment.

Safety and efficacy of daptomycin have not been studied in patients with prosthetic valve endocarditis.

Infective endocarditis usually is treated empirically until results of blood cultures are available and a pathogen is identified. The empiric regimen is selected based on various patient characteristics (e.g., history of injection drug use, presence of indwelling cardiovascular devices, immunocompromising medical conditions, prior infections and anti-infective treatment); consultation with an infectious disease specialist is recommended for assistance in selecting the optimal regimen. For the treatment of native valve infective endocarditis caused by methicillin-susceptible *S. aureus*, the American Heart Association (AHA) recommends a parenteral *β*-lactam (nafcillin or oxacillin; cefazolin for those with nonanaphylactoid reactions to penicillins) and states that daptomycin is a reasonable alternative to vancomycin for the treatment of these infections in patients with anaphylactoid-type hypersensitivity to *β*-lactams. Although these experts also state that daptomycin may be a reasonable alternative to vancomycin for the treatment of left-sided native valve infective endocarditis† caused by MRSA, optimal daptomycin dosage for these infections has not been identified and consultation with an infectious disease expert is recommended.

For information on diagnosis and management of infective endocarditis and its complications, including anti-infective treatment of staphylococcal bacteremia and endocarditis, the current AHA guidelines available at http://my.americanheart.org/statements should be consulted.

Clinical Experience Efficacy of daptomycin for the treatment of *S. aureus* bacteremia with or without endocarditis was evaluated in a randomized, multicenter, controlled, open-label study in 246 adults with at least one positive blood culture for *S. aureus* (obtained within 2 days prior to the first dose of the study drug). At study entry, 16% of patients had a definite diagnosis of endocarditis and 61% had a possible diagnosis of endocarditis based on the modified Duke criteria. Patients were randomized to receive daptomycin (6 mg/kg IV once every 24 hours) or a comparator anti-infective regimen of vancomycin (1 g IV every 12 hours) or a penicillinase-resistant penicillin (2 g IV every 4 hours of nafcillin, oxacillin, or flucloxacillin [not commercially available in the US]). Less than 1% of patients in the daptomycin group also received gentamicin (1 mg/kg IV every 8 hours for the first 4 days of treatment), whereas 93% of those in the comparator group also received gentamicin. Patients with prosthetic heart valves, intravascular foreign material that was not planned for removal within 4 days after the first anti-infective dose, severe neutropenia, known osteomyelitis, polymicrobial bloodstream infections, creatinine clearance less than 30 mL/minute, and pneumonia were excluded from the study.

The clinical success rate in the intent-to-treat population 6 weeks after the last treatment dose was 44% in patients who received daptomycin and 42% in those who received a comparator anti-infective. There was no overall difference in time to clearance of *S. aureus* bacteremia between the 2 groups; the median time to clearance of methicillin-susceptible *S. aureus* was 4 days and the median time to clearance of MRSA was 8 days.

There were some persisting or relapsing infections, including some deaths, during the study. Most patients who failed treatment due to persisting or relapsing *S. aureus* infection had deep-seated infections and did not receive necessary surgical intervention. Among patients with persisting or relapsing *S. aureus* infections, there were 8 deaths in those who had been randomized to receive daptomycin and 7 deaths in those randomized to receive a comparator anti-infective. (See Persisting or Relapsing Staphylococcus aureus Bacteremia/Endocarditis under Cautions: Warnings/Precautions.)

Dosage and Administration

■ **Reconstitution and Administration** Daptomycin is administered by IV injection or infusion.

Daptomycin is commercially available for IV use as 2 different formulations: a lyophilized powder for solution that does not contain sucrose (Cubicin®

or generics) and a lyophilized powder for solution that contains 713 mg of sucrose per vial (Cubicin® RF). Instructions for storage, reconstitution, and dilution differ for the 2 daptomycin formulations and recommendations for the specific formulation used should be followed.

Additives and other drugs should not be added to daptomycin solutions or infused simultaneously through the same IV line. If the same IV line is used for sequential infusion of different drugs, the line should be flushed with a compatible infusion solution before and after infusion of daptomycin. Daptomycin is *not* compatible with dextrose-containing diluents (e.g., 5% dextrose injection).

Daptomycin should not be used in conjunction with ReadyMed® elastomeric infusion pumps since stability studies identified an impurity (i.e., 2-mercaptobenzothiazole) leaching from this pump system into the daptomycin solution.

Strict aseptic technique must be observed in preparing daptomycin solutions since the drug contains no preservative. Daptomycin solutions should be inspected visually for particulate matter prior to administration. Reconstituted daptomycin solutions range in color from pale yellow to light brown.

Daptomycin (Cubicin® or generics): The lyophilized powder should be stored at 2–8°C. The reconstituted daptomycin solution (in the original vial) and reconstituted and further diluted solutions (in an IV infusion bag) are stable for 12 hours at room temperature or up to 48 hours when refrigerated at 2–8°C; the combined storage time (vial and infusion bag) at room temperature or under refrigeration should not exceed 12 or 48 hours, respectively.

Daptomycin (Cubicin® RF): The lyophilized powder should be stored at 20–25°C, but may be exposed to 15–30°C. The stability of reconstituted daptomycin solution and reconstituted and further diluted solutions varies based on the specific diluent and container used. (See Table 1.)

Table 1: Stability of Daptomycin (Cubicin® RF) After Reconstitution

Container	Diluent	Stability at 20–25°C	Stability at 2–8°C
Vial	Sterile water for injection	1 day	3 days
	Bacteriostatic water for injection	2 days	3 days
Syringe[a]	Sterile water for injection	1 day	3 days
	Bacteriostatic water for injection	2 days	5 days
Infusion bag	Reconstituted with sterile water for injection and immediate dilution in 0.9% sodium chloride injection	19 hours	3 days
	Reconstituted with bacteriostatic water for injection and immediate dilution in 0.9% sodium chloride injection	2 days	5 days

[a] Polypropylene syringe with elastomeric plunger stopper.

IV Injection **Reconstitution.** Daptomycin (Cubicin® or generics): Single-dose vials labeled as containing 500 mg of daptomycin should be reconstituted by slowly adding 10 mL of 0.9% sodium chloride injection to provide a solution containing 50 mg/mL. The diluent should be added to the vial using a beveled sterile transfer needle (21 gauge or smaller) or a needleless device, and the diluent should be directed toward the wall of the vial. The vial should be gently rotated to ensure that the entire lyophilized powder is wetted. The vial should be allowed to remain undisturbed for 10 minutes, and then should be rotated or swirled for a few minutes (as needed) to obtain a completely reconstituted solution. To minimize foaming, vigorous agitation or shaking of the vial should be avoided during and after reconstitution. For IV injection, the appropriate volume of reconstituted daptomycin solution containing 50 mg/mL should be slowly removed from the vial using a beveled sterile needle (21 gauge or smaller) and administered without further dilution. Any unused portion of the reconstituted solution should be discarded.

Daptomycin (Cubicin® RF): Sodium chloride solutions should *not* be used for reconstitution of this formulation since this would result in a hyperosmotic solution. Single-dose vials labeled as containing 500 mg of daptomycin should be reconstituted by slowly adding 10 mL of sterile water for injection or bacteriostatic water for injection to provide a solution containing 50 mg/mL. The diluent should be added to the vial using a beveled sterile transfer needle (21 gauge or smaller), and the diluent should be directed toward the wall of the vial. The vial should be rotated or swirled for a few minutes (as needed) to obtain a completely reconstituted solution. For IV injection, the appropriate volume of reconstituted daptomycin solution containing 50 mg/mL should be slowly removed from the vial using a beveled sterile needle (21 gauge or smaller) and administered without further dilution. Any unused portion of the reconstituted solution should be discarded.

Rate of Administration. IV injections of daptomycin (Cubicin® or generics; Cubicin® RF) should be given over 2 minutes.

IV Infusion **Reconstitution and Dilution.** Daptomycin (Cubicin® or generics): Single-dose vials labeled as containing 500 mg of daptomycin should be reconstituted by slowly adding 10 mL of 0.9% sodium chloride injection to provide a solution containing 50 mg/mL. The diluent should be added to the vial using a beveled sterile transfer needle (21 gauge or smaller) or a needleless device, and the diluent should be directed toward the wall of the vial. The vial should be gently rotated to ensure that the entire lyophilized powder is wetted. The vial should be allowed to remain undisturbed for 10 minutes, and then should be rotated or swirled for a few minutes (as needed) to obtain a completely reconstituted solution. To minimize foaming, vigorous agitation or shaking of the vial should be avoided during and after reconstitution. For IV infusion, the appropriate volume of reconstituted daptomycin solution containing 50 mg/mL should be slowly removed from the vial using a beveled sterile needle (21 gauge or smaller) and added to 50 mL of 0.9% sodium chloride injection in an IV infusion bag. The final concentration of the diluted solution should not exceed 20 mg/mL. Any unused portion of the reconstituted solution should be discarded.

Daptomycin (Cubicin® RF): Sodium chloride solutions should *not* be used for reconstitution of this formulation since this would result in a hyperosmotic solution. Single-dose vials labeled as containing 500 mg of daptomycin should be reconstituted by slowly adding 10 mL of sterile water for injection or bacteriostatic water for injection to provide a solution containing 50 mg/mL. The diluent should be added to the vial using a beveled sterile transfer needle (21 gauge or smaller), and the diluent should be directed toward the wall of the vial. The vial should be rotated or swirled for a few minutes (as needed) to obtain a completely reconstituted solution. For IV infusion, the appropriate volume of reconstituted daptomycin solution containing 50 mg/mL should be slowly removed from the vial using a beveled sterile needle (21 gauge or smaller) and added to 50 mL of 0.9% sodium chloride injection in an IV infusion bag. Any unused portion of the reconstituted solution should be discarded.

Rate of Administration. IV infusions of daptomycin (Cubicin® or generics; Cubicin® RF) should be given over 30 minutes.

■ Dosage

Skin and Skin Structure Infections For the treatment of complicated skin and skin structure infections in adults, the usual dosage of daptomycin is 4 mg/kg IV once every 24 hours for 7–14 days.

Daptomycin should not be administered more frequently than once daily. (See Musculoskeletal Effects under Cautions: Warnings/Precautions.)

Bacteremia and Endocarditis For the treatment of bacteremia (blood stream infections) and right-sided infective endocarditis in adults, the usual dosage of daptomycin is 6 mg/kg IV once every 24 hours for 2–6 weeks. Limited safety data are available regarding use of daptomycin for longer than 28 days; in a phase 3 clinical study, only 14 patients received daptomycin for more than 28 days.

Daptomycin should not be administered more frequently than once daily. (See Musculoskeletal Effects under Cautions: Warnings/Precautions.)

■ Special Populations

Because daptomycin is eliminated principally by renal excretion, patients with creatinine clearances less than 30 mL/minute, including those requiring hemodialysis or continuous ambulatory peritoneal dialysis (CAPD), should receive reduced daptomycin dosage. The recommended dosage of daptomycin for adults with creatinine clearances less than 30 mL/minute is 4 mg/kg IV once every 48 hours for the treatment of complicated skin and skin structure infections or 6 mg/kg IV once every 48 hours for the treatment of bacteremia and right-sided infective endocarditis. In hemodialysis patients, dosing of the drug should be timed so that the daily dose given on hemodialysis days is administered following the procedure, whenever possible.

Dosage adjustments are not necessary when daptomycin is used in patients with mild to moderate hepatic impairment; pharmacokinetics of the drug have not been evaluated in patients with severe hepatic impairment.

Dosage adjustments based solely on age are not necessary when daptomycin is used in geriatric patients, but dosage adjustments are indicated in those with renal impairment.

Dosage adjustments are not necessary based on gender or weight.

Cautions

■ Contraindications

Daptomycin is contraindicated in patients with known hypersensitivity to the drug.

■ Warnings/Precautions

Sensitivity Reactions Hypersensitivity reactions, including anaphylaxis and other reactions that may be life-threatening, have been reported in patients receiving daptomycin.

Angioedema, drug rash with eosinophilia and systemic symptoms (DRESS), pruritus, urticaria, shortness of breath, difficulty swallowing, truncal erythema, and pulmonary eosinophilia (see Eosinophilic Pneumonia under Cautions: Warnings/Precautions) have been reported during postmarketing experience in patients receiving daptomycin.

If a hypersensitivity reaction occurs, daptomycin should be discontinued and appropriate therapy initiated.

Musculoskeletal Effects Myopathy, defined as muscle aching or muscle weakness, in conjunction with serum creatine kinase (CK, creatine phosphokinase, CPK) concentrations increased up to 10 times the upper limit of normal (ULN) have been reported in patients receiving daptomycin. Rhabdomyolysis, with or without renal failure, also has been reported.

In a phase 3 study evaluating daptomycin (4 mg/kg IV once daily) for the treatment of complicated skin and skin structure infections, elevated CK concentrations were reported in 2.8% of patients receiving daptomycin and 1.8% of those receiving a comparator anti-infective. In a study evaluating daptomycin (6 mg/kg IV once daily) for the treatment of bacteremia, elevated CK concentrations were reported in 9.2% of those receiving daptomycin and less than 1% of those receiving a comparator anti-infective. Some patients who developed increased CK concentrations were previously or concomitantly treated with an hydroxymethylglutaryl-CoA (HMG-CoA) reductase inhibitor (statin).

Because there is evidence from phase 1 and 2 studies that elevated serum CK concentrations occurred more frequently when daptomycin was given more than once daily, the drug should not be administered more frequently than once daily.

Patients receiving daptomycin should be monitored for the development of muscle pain or weakness, particularly of the distal extremities. Serum CK concentrations should be monitored weekly in patients receiving daptomycin; however, these concentrations should be monitored more frequently than once weekly in patients who develop increases in serum CK concentrations during daptomycin therapy and in those who recently received or are currently receiving treatment with an HMG-CoA reductase inhibitor. Serum CK concentrations and renal function also should be monitored more frequently than once weekly in patients with renal insufficiency.

Daptomycin should be discontinued in patients with unexplained signs and symptoms of myopathy in conjunction with increases in CK greater than 1000 U/L (i.e., approximately 5 times the ULN) or in patients without reported symptoms who have substantial increases in serum CK concentrations (i.e., at least 2000 U/L [10 times the ULN]).

Consideration should be given to temporarily discontinuing drugs associated with rhabdomyolysis (e.g., HMG-CoA reductase inhibitors) in patients receiving daptomycin. (See Drug Interactions: HMG-CoA Reductase Inhibitors.)

Eosinophilic Pneumonia Eosinophilic pneumonia has been reported in some patients receiving daptomycin. In most reported cases, patients developed fever, dyspnea with hypoxic respiratory insufficiency, and diffuse pulmonary infiltrates, usually 2–4 weeks after daptomycin therapy was initiated. Improvement or resolution of symptoms generally occurred following discontinuance of the drug; most patient received treatment with systemic corticosteroids. When daptomycin was reinitiated in a few of these patients, eosinophilic pneumonia recurred.

Based on a review of postmarketing reports of possible cases of eosinophilic pneumonia in patients who received daptomycin, FDA determined that there appears to be a temporal association between use of the drug and the development of eosinophilic pneumonia. Some cases were reported in patients receiving daptomycin for uses that are not FDA labeled. Clinicians should consider that eosinophilic pneumonia can progress to respiratory failure and is potentially fatal if not recognized quickly and managed appropriately.

Patients receiving daptomycin should be closely monitored for signs and symptoms of eosinophilic pneumonia (e.g., new onset or worsening fever, dyspnea, difficulty breathing, new pulmonary infiltrates).

Daptomycin should be discontinued immediately if there are any signs or symptoms of eosinophilic pneumonia. Prompt medical evaluation is indicated, and treatment with systemic corticosteroids is recommended.

Nervous System Effects There have been postmarketing reports of peripheral neuropathy in patients receiving daptomycin. Clinicians should be alert to possible manifestations of neuropathy in patients receiving daptomycin.

Persisting or Relapsing Staphylococcus aureus Bacteremia/Endocarditis Treatment failure due to persisting or relapsing *Staphylococcus aureus* infection can occur. *S. aureus* with reduced susceptibility or resistance to daptomycin have been reported and have emerged during treatment with the drug.

In a clinical study evaluating daptomycin for the treatment of bacteremia, 16% of daptomycin-treated patients and 10% of patients treated with a comparator anti-infective (vancomycin or a penicillinase-resistant penicillin) had persisting or relapsing *S. aureus* infections; some fatalities occurred. In vitro studies indicated that isolates from some of these patients developed reduced susceptibility to the anti-infective during or following treatment. Most patients with persistent or relapsing infections had deep-seated infections and did not receive necessary surgical intervention.

Repeat blood cultures should be performed in patients with persisting or relapsing infection or with poor clinical response. If cultures are positive for *S. aureus*, in vitro susceptibility testing of the isolate should be performed using standardized MIC procedures. In addition, a diagnostic evaluation should be performed to rule out sequestered foci of infection. Surgical intervention (e.g., debridement, removal of prosthetic devices, valve replacement surgery) and/or a change in anti-infective regimen may be required.

Reduced Efficacy in Patients with Moderate Renal Impairment Results of a subgroup analysis of a phase 3 study in patients with *S. aureus* bacteremia/endocarditis indicated that the clinical success rate in daptomycin-treated patients with baseline creatinine clearances of 30 to less than 50 mL/minute was only 14% and was lower than clinical success rates observed in those with baseline creatinine clearances of 50–80 mL/minute or greater than 80 mL/minute (46 or 60%, respectively). Decreased clinical success rates to this extent were not observed in patients receiving comparator anti-infectives.

Although only limited data are available from phase 3 studies in patients with complicated skin and skin structure infections, the clinical success rate in daptomycin-treated patients with creatinine clearances of 30 to less than 50 mL/minute was 47% compared with a clinical success rate of 66% in those with creatinine clearances of 50–70 mL/minute.

Clinicians should consider these data regarding reduced efficacy when selecting anti-infective treatment for patients with baseline moderate to severe renal impairment.

Tests Used to Monitor Coagulation Daptomycin causes concentration-dependent false prolongation of the prothrombin time (PT) and elevated international normalized ratio (INR) if certain recombinant thromboplastin reagents are used for these tests. Interference with PT/INR testing may be minimized by drawing blood specimens for coagulation tests near the time of trough plasma daptomycin concentrations; however, the possibility that trough plasma concentrations still may be high enough to interfere with such tests should be considered.

If abnormally elevated PT/INR tests are reported in a patient receiving daptomycin, coagulation testing should be repeated using blood specimens drawn just prior to the next daptomycin dose (i.e., at trough concentrations). If results using these blood specimens remain substantially elevated over what would otherwise be expected, alternative methods of measuring PT/INR should be considered. In addition, the patient should be evaluated for other causes of abnormally elevated PT/INR.

Superinfection/Clostridium difficile-associated Diarrhea and Colitis (CDAD) Use of daptomycin may result in emergence and overgrowth of nonsusceptible bacteria or fungi. The patient should be carefully monitored and appropriate therapy instituted if superinfection occurs.

Treatment with anti-infectives alters normal colon flora and may permit overgrowth of *Clostridium difficile*. *C. difficile* infection (CDI) and *C. difficile*-associated diarrhea and colitis (CDAD; also known as antibiotic-associated diarrhea and colitis or pseudomembranous colitis) have been reported with nearly all anti-infectives, including daptomycin, and may range in severity from mild diarrhea to fatal colitis. *C. difficile* produces toxins A and B which contribute to development of CDAD; hypertoxin-producing strains of *C. difficile* are associated with increased morbidity and mortality since they may be refractory to anti-infectives and colectomy may be required.

CDAD should be considered in the differential diagnosis of patients who develop diarrhea during or after anti-infective therapy. Careful medical history is necessary since CDAD has been reported to occur as late as 2 months or longer after anti-infective therapy is discontinued.

If CDAD is suspected or confirmed, anti-infective therapy not directed against *C. difficile* should be discontinued whenever possible. Patients should be managed with appropriate supportive therapy (e.g., fluid and electrolyte management, protein supplementation), anti-infective therapy directed against *C. difficile* (e.g., metronidazole, vancomycin), and surgical evaluation as clinically indicated.

Selection and Use of Anti-infectives To reduce development of drug-resistant bacteria and maintain effectiveness of daptomycin and other antibacterials, the drug should be used only for the treatment of infections proven or strongly suspected to be caused by susceptible bacteria.

When selecting or modifying anti-infective therapy, results of culture and in vitro susceptibility testing should be used. In the absence of such data, local epidemiology and susceptibility patterns should be considered when selecting anti-infectives for empiric therapy.

Daptomycin should not be used for the treatment of pneumonia.

Safety and efficacy of daptomycin have not been studied in patients with prosthetic valve endocarditis .

Specific Populations **Pregnancy.** Category B. (See Users Guide.)

There are no adequate and well-controlled studies evaluating daptomycin in pregnant women. Daptomycin should be used during pregnancy only if potential benefits to the woman outweigh possible risks to the fetus.

Lactation. Daptomycin is distributed into human milk, but has poor oral bioavailability. In a case study involving a nursing woman receiving daptomycin (6.7 mg/kg IV once daily for 28 days), the highest daptomycin concentration measured in breast milk was 45 ng/mL and the calculated maximum daily daptomycin dose for a nursing infant (assuming mean milk consumption of 150 mL/kg daily) was 0.1% of the maternal dose.

Daptomycin should be used with caution in nursing women.

Pediatric Use. Safety and efficacy of daptomycin have not been established in pediatric patients.

Use of daptomycin should be avoided in children younger than 12 months of age because of the potential risk of adverse muscular, neuromuscular, peripheral nervous system, and CNS effects; such adverse effects have been observed in neonatal dogs receiving IV daptomycin.

Geriatric Use. When the total number of patients studied in phase 3 clinical trials of daptomycin for the treatment of complicated skin and skin structure infections are considered, 27% were 65 years of age or older and 12% were 75 years of age or older. In a phase 3 clinical trial of daptomycin for the treatment of bacteremia and endocarditis, 25% of patients were 65 years of age or older and 16% were 75 years of age or older. There was some evidence from these studies that clinical success rates were lower and treatment-emergent adverse effects were more common in geriatric patients 65 years of age or older compared with younger adults.

Although daptomycin exposures are higher in healthy geriatric adults than in healthy young adults, adjustment of daptomycin dosage is not necessary in geriatric patients based solely on age. However, age-related decreases in renal function should be considered when selecting dosage in geriatric patients. (See Dosage and Administration: Special Populations.)

Hepatic Impairment. The pharmacokinetics of daptomycin were not altered in patients with moderate hepatic impairment (Child-Pugh class B) compared with healthy individuals without liver disease. Daptomycin has not been studied in patients with severe hepatic impairment.

Renal Impairment. Daptomycin is eliminated principally by the kidneys, and plasma clearance of the drug is decreased and area under the concentration-time curve (AUC) and half-life are increased in patients with impaired renal function.

Renal function and serum CK concentrations should be monitored more frequently than once weekly in patients with renal impairment.

Dosage adjustments are recommended in adults with creatinine clearances less than 30 mL/minute. (See Dosage and Administration: Special Populations and also see Musculoskeletal Effects under Cautions: Warnings/Precautions.)

■ **Common Adverse Effects** Adverse effects occurring in 2% or more of patients receiving daptomycin for the treatment of complicated skin and skin structure infections in clinical trials and reported as frequently or more frequently than with comparator anti-infectives include diarrhea, nervous system effects (headache, dizziness), rash, abnormal liver function test results, elevated serum creatine kinase (CK, creatine phosphokinase, CPK) concentrations, urinary tract infections, hypotension, and dyspnea.

Adverse effects occurring in 5% or more of patients receiving daptomycin for the treatment of bacteremia and endocarditis in a clinical trial and reported as frequently or more frequently than with comparator anti-infectives include abdominal pain, insomnia, pharyngolaryngeal pain, infections (sepsis, bacteremia), chest pain, edema, pruritus, increased sweating, elevated CK concentrations, and hypertension.

Drug Interactions

■ **Drugs Metabolized by Hepatic Microsomal Enzymes** Daptomycin does not inhibit or induce cytochrome P-450 (CYP) isoenzymes 1A2, 2A6, 2C9, 2C19, 2D6, 2E1, and 3A4; pharmacokinetic interactions with drugs metabolized by these isoenzymes is unlikely.

■ **Aminoglycosides** In vitro studies using gentamicin and tobramycin indicate that daptomycin and aminoglycosides may exert synergistic antibacterial effects against staphylococci and enterococci. Additive or indifferent antibacterial effects also were reported, but antagonism did not occur.

Tobramycin Concomitant use of tobramycin (1 mg/kg IV) and daptomycin (2 mg/kg IV) increased the mean peak plasma concentration and area under the plasma concentration-time curve (AUC) of daptomycin by approximately 13 and 9%, respectively, and decreased the mean peak plasma concentration and AUC of tobramycin by approximately 11 and 7%, respectively. These differences were not statistically significant; however, the extent of possible interaction between daptomycin and tobramycin when the recommended daptomycin dosages are used is not known.

■ **β-Lactam Anti-infectives** In vitro studies using penicillins (ampicillin, oxacillin, ampicillin and sulbactam, piperacillin and tazobactam, ticarcillin and clavulanate), cephalosporins (cefepime, ceftriaxone), aztreonam, or imipenem indicate that daptomycin and β-lactam anti-infectives may exert synergistic antibacterial effects against staphylococci and enterococci. Additive or indifferent antibacterial effects also were reported, but antagonism generally did not occur.

Aztreonam Concomitant use of daptomycin (6 mg/kg IV) and aztreonam (1 g IV) did not have a clinically important effect on the mean peak plasma concentration and AUC of daptomycin.

■ **HMG-CoA Reductase Inhibitors** Concomitant use of hydroxy-methylglutaryl-CoA (HMG-CoA) reductase inhibitors (statins) and daptomycin may increase the risk of myopathy, manifested as muscle pain or weakness in association with increased serum creatine kinase (CK, creatine phosphokinase, CPK). In a phase 3 study evaluating daptomycin in adults with *Staphylococcus aureus* bacteremia/endocarditis, elevated serum CK concentrations were reported in some patients who received prior or concurrent treatment with an HMG-CoA reductase inhibitor.

In a study in healthy adults receiving a stable simvastatin dosage of 40 mg daily, concurrent use of daptomycin (4 mg/kg IV once daily for 14 days) did not affect plasma trough concentrations of simvastatin and was not associated with a higher incidence of adverse effects (including skeletal myopathy) compared with patients receiving placebo.

The manufacturer of daptomycin states that experience with concurrent use of HMG-CoA reductase inhibitors and daptomycin is limited, and temporary discontinuance of HMG-CoA reductase inhibitors should be considered in patients receiving daptomycin. (See Musculoskeletal Effects under Cautions: Warnings/Precautions.)

■ **Probenecid** Concurrent use of probenecid (500 mg 4 times daily) and a single daptomycin dose (4 mg/kg IV) did not substantially alter the peak plasma concentration or AUC of daptomycin.

■ **Rifampin** In vitro studies indicate that daptomycin and rifampin may exert synergistic antibacterial effects against staphylococci and enterococci, including vancomycin-resistant enterococci. Additive or indifferent antibacterial effects also were reported, but antagonism did not occur.

■ **Warfarin** Concurrent use of daptomycin (6 mg/kg IV once every 24 hours for 5 days) and warfarin (single 25-mg oral dose) did not result in substantial effects on the pharmacokinetics of either drug or substantial alterations of the international normalized ratio (INR). However, if warfarin and daptomycin are used concomitantly, the possibility that daptomycin may cause concentration-dependent false prolongation of the prothrombin time (PT) and elevated INR when certain testing methods are used should be considered. (See Tests Used to Monitor Coagulation under Cautions: Warnings/Precautions.)

Description

Daptomycin is a cyclic lipopeptide antibiotic produced by fermentation of *Streptomyces roseosporus*. The drug differs structurally and pharmacologically from other currently available anti-infective agents. In vitro studies indicate that daptomycin exhibits rapid concentration-dependent bactericidal effects against susceptible gram-positive bacteria. Daptomycin binds to bacterial cell membranes and causes rapid membrane depolarization in susceptible bacteria, which leads to inhibition of protein, DNA, and RNA synthesis and results in cell death.

Daptomycin is active against many gram-positive bacteria, but is inactive against gram-negative bacteria. The drug is active in vitro and in clinical infections against *Staphylococcus aureus* (including methicillin-resistant *S. aureus* [MRSA; also known as oxacillin-resistant *S. aureus* or ORSA]), *Streptococcus pyogenes* (group A β-hemolytic streptococci, GAS), *S. agalactiae* (group B streptococci, GBS), *S. dysgalactiae* subsp. *equisimilis*, and *Enterococcus faecalis* (vancomycin-susceptible strains only). Daptomycin also has in vitro activity against some strains of *Corynebacterium jeikeium*, *E. faecalis* (vancomycin-resistant strains), *E. faecium* (including vancomycin-resistant strains), *S. epidermidis* (including methicillin-resistant strains), and *S. haemolyticus*; however, the safety and efficacy of daptomycin in treating clinical infections caused by these bacteria have not been established in adequate and well-controlled studies to date.

S. aureus and *E. faecalis* with reduced susceptibility or resistance to daptomycin have been reported. The mechanism of resistance or transferable elements that might confer resistance to daptomycin have not been identified to date. Reduced susceptibility to daptomycin (8- to 32-fold increase in MIC) has been produced in vitro by serial passage of *S. aureus* in the presence of increasing concentrations of the drug. In addition, daptomycin-resistant strains of *S. aureus* have emerged in patients treated with the drug. In a clinical study in patients with complicated skin and skin structure infections, *S. aureus* resistant to daptomycin was isolated from a patient who received the drug at less than the protocol-specified dosage during the first 5 days of therapy.

Although further study is needed, there is evidence that cross-resistance can occur between daptomycin and vancomycin. Some strains of MRSA that develop resistance to daptomycin also may develop resistance or reduced susceptibility to vancomycin and daptomycin-resistant MRSA may emerge during daptomycin therapy in some patients with prior exposure to vancomycin.

Daptomycin exhibits nearly linear and time-independent pharmacokinetics at dosages up to 4–12 mg/kg once daily administered by IV infusion over 30 minutes. Steady-state concentrations are achieved by the third daily dose. Daptomycin has a mean elimination half-life of 7.7–8.3 hours at steady state in adults. The drug is eliminated principally by renal excretion, with approximately 78 and 6% of an administered dose recovered in urine and feces, respectively. In vitro studies indicate that daptomycin is not metabolized by cytochrome P-450 (CYP) isoenzymes. In vitro studies using human hepatocytes indicate that daptomycin does not inhibit or induce CYP1A2, 2A6, 2C9, 2C19, 2D6, 2E1, or 3A4.

Advice to Patients

Advise patients that antibacterials (including daptomycin) should only be used to treat bacterial infections and not used to treat viral infections (e.g., the common cold).

Importance of completing full course of therapy, even if feeling better after a few days.

Advise patients that skipping doses or not completing the full course of therapy may decrease effectiveness and increase the likelihood that bacteria will develop resistance and will not be treatable with daptomycin or other antibacterials in the future.

Advise patients that allergic reactions, including serious allergic reactions, could occur and that serious reactions require immediate treatment. Importance of informing clinician of any previous allergic reactions to daptomycin.

Importance of patients immediately informing their clinician if they develop new or worsening fever, cough, shortness of breath, or difficulty breathing.

Importance of contacting a clinician if muscle pain, weakness, tingling, or numbness occurs, particularly in the forearms or lower legs.

Advise patients that diarrhea is a common problem caused by anti-infectives and usually ends when the drug is discontinued. Importance of contacting a clinician if watery and bloody stools (with or without stomach cramps and fever) occur during or as late as 2 months or longer after the last dose.

Importance of women informing clinicians if they are or plan to become pregnant or plan to breast-feed.

Importance of informing clinicians of existing or contemplated concomitant therapy, including prescription and OTC drugs.

Importance of informing patients of other important precautionary information. (See Cautions.)

Overview® (see Users Guide). For additional information on this drug until a more detailed monograph is developed and published, the manufacturer's labeling should be consulted. It is *essential* that the manufacturer's labeling be consulted for more detailed information on usual cautions, precautions, contraindications, potential drug interactions, laboratory test interferences, and acute toxicity.

Preparations

Excipients in commercially available drug preparations may have clinically important effects in some individuals; consult specific product labeling for details.

Daptomycin

Parenteral		
For injection	500 mg*	**Cubicin®, Merck**
		Cubicin® RF, Merck
		Daptomycin for Injection

*available from one or more manufacturer, distributor, and/or repackager by generic (nonproprietary) name
†Use is not currently included in the labeling approved by the US Food and Drug Administration

GLYCOPEPTIDES 8:12.28.16

Dalbavancin Hydrochloride

■ Dalbavancin hydrochloride, a lipoglycopeptide antibacterial, is a semisynthetic derivative of a naturally occurring glycopeptide.

Uses

■ **Skin and Skin Structure Infections** Dalbavancin hydrochloride is used for the treatment of acute bacterial skin and skin structure infections (ABSSSI) caused by susceptible *Staphylococcus aureus* (including methicillin-resistant *S. aureus* [MRSA; also known as oxacillin-resistant *S. aureus* or ORSA] and methicillin-susceptible *S. aureus*), *Streptococcus pyogenes* (group A *β*-hemolytic streptococci, GAS), *S. agalactiae* (group B streptococci, GBS), or *S. anginosus* group (includes *S. anginosus*, *S. intermedius*, and *S. constellatus*).

Clinical Experience Efficacy and safety of dalbavancin were evaluated in 2 randomized, multicenter, double-blind, noninferiority, phase 3 studies (DISCOVER 1 and DISCOVER 2) in adults with acute bacterial skin and skin structure infections (e.g., cellulitis, major abscess, or wound infection, each associated with at least 75 cm² of erythema). Patients had at least 2 local signs of infection (e.g., purulent drainage or discharge, fluctuance, localized warmth, tenderness, swelling or induration) and were thought to require at least 3 days of IV therapy or had least 1 sign of systemic infection at baseline (e.g., temperature 38°C or higher, leukocyte count greater than 12,000 cells/mm³, 10% or more band forms on leukocyte differential). Over 1300 patients (mean age 50 years, 57–60% male, 12–14% with diabetes mellitus, 14–16% IV drug users, 53–54% with cellulitis, 25–27% with major abscess, 20–21% with wound or surgical site infection, median baseline lesion area 341 cm²) were randomized to receive a 2-dose regimen of dalbavancin (1 g IV on day 1 followed by 500 mg IV on day 8; those with creatinine clearance less than 30 mL/minute received 750 mg IV on day 1 followed by 375 mg on day 8) or a 10–14 day regimen of vancomycin (1 g or 15 mg/kg IV every 12 hours) with the option to switch to oral linezolid (600 mg every 12 hours) after 3 days of vancomycin. Protocol-specified empiric gram-negative coverage with aztreonam could be used concomitantly. In a pooled analysis of both studies using data at 48–72 hours after initiation of treatment, the dalbavancin regimen was noninferior to the vancomycin regimen. Clinical response (i.e., no increase in lesion area from baseline, temperature consistently 37.6°C or less) was achieved in 79.7% of those receiving dalbavancin and 79.8% of those receiving the vancomycin regimen. A similar proportion of patients receiving dalbavancin or the vancomycin regimen (88.6 or 88.1%, respectively) achieved a 20% or greater reduction in lesion area from baseline at 48–72 hours. In the subset of patients who were microbiologically evaluable and stratified according to the infecting pathogen, the clinical success rate (defined as decrease in lesion size, temperature of 37.6° C or less, and meeting pre-specified criteria for local signs of infection) on day 26–30 in those with infections caused by MRSA or methicillin-susceptible *S. aureus* was 83 or 85%, respectively, in those treated with dalbavancin and 85 or 91%, respectively, in those treated with the vancomycin regimen. The clinical success rate in those with infections caused by *S. agalactiae*, *S. pyogenes*, or *S. anginosus* group was 83, 89, or 96%, respectively, in those treated with dalbavancin and 79, 89, or 92%, respectively, in those treated with the vancomycin regimen.

Dalbavancin was evaluated in a randomized, double-blind, phase 3 study in 854 adults with complicated skin and skin structure infections (e.g., major abscess, major burn, traumatic or surgical wound infection, extensive or ulcerating cellulitis, infection suspected to be caused by MRSA) with at least 2 signs of local infection and at least 1 sign of systemic infection. Patients were randomized in a 2:1 ratio to receive dalbavancin (1 g IV on day 1 followed by 500 mg IV on day 8) or a 14-day regimen of linezolid (600 mg IV every 12 hours) with the option to switch to oral linezolid. Empiric coverage with aztreonam and/or metronidazole could be used concomitantly. Baseline characteristics were balanced between groups (61–62% male, 30–33% major abscess, 27–30% cellulitis); however, there was a higher proportion of patients with vascular disease in the dalbavancin group than in the linezolid group (11 and 6%, respectively). Of the clinically evaluable patients at the test-of-cure visit (approximately 14 days after completion of treatment), 88.9% of patients in the dalbavancin group and 91.2% of patients in the linezolid group achieved clinical success (i.e., improvement of signs and symptoms of infection such that no further antibacterial therapy was needed). In the subset of patients who were microbiologically evaluable, the microbiologic success rate at the test-of-cure visit was 90% in those treated with dalbavancin and 88% in those treated with linezolid; MRSA eradication rates at the test-of-cure visit were 91 or 89% in the dalbavancin or linezolid groups, respectively.

Dosage and Administration

■ **Administration** Dalbavancin hydrochloride is administered by IV infusion.

IV Administration If the same IV line is used for sequential infusion of dalbavancin and other drugs, the IV line should be flushed with 5% dextrose injection before and after the dalbavancin infusion.

Dalbavancin solutions should *not* be infused with other drugs or electrolytes. Dalbavancin solutions are compatible with 5% dextrose injection, but compatibility with other IV solutions, drugs, additives, or substances has not been established.

Vials of dalbavancin lyophilized powder for injection contain no preservatives and are intended for single use only.

Reconstitution and Dilution. Dalbavancin hydrochloride for injection must be reconstituted and further diluted prior to IV infusion. Strict aseptic technique must be observed when preparing IV solutions of the drug.

Vials labeled as containing 500 mg of dalbavancin should be reconstituted by adding 25 mL of sterile water for injection to provide a solution containing 20 mg/mL. To avoid foaming, the vial should be alternately swirled and inverted until vial contents are completely dissolved; the vial should not be shaken. The reconstituted solution should appear clear and colorless to yellow.

Reconstituted dalbavancin must then be further diluted by withdrawing the correct dose of the drug from the reconstituted vial(s) and adding it to an IV bag or bottle containing 5% dextrose injection. The final diluted solution *must* have a dalbavancin concentration of 1–5 mg/mL. Any unused portion of reconstituted solution should be discarded.

Reconstituted or further diluted solutions of dalbavancin may be stored under refrigeration (2–8°C) or at controlled room temperature (i.e., 20–25°C), but should not be frozen. Total storage time from the time of reconstitution to administration should not exceed 48 hours whether refrigerated at 2–8°C or stored at room temperature.

Dalbavancin solutions should be inspected visually for particulate matter prior to administration.

Rate of Administration. Dalbavancin solutions should be administered by IV infusion over 30 minutes.

■ **Dosage** Dosage of dalbavancin hydrochloride is expressed in terms of dalbavancin.

Adult Dosage **Skin and Skin Structure Infections.** The recommended dosage of dalbavancin for the treatment of acute bacterial skin and skin structure infections (ABSSSI) in adults is a 2-dose regimen of 1 g given by IV infusion followed 1 week later by 500 mg given by IV infusion.

■ **Special Populations** ***Renal Impairment*** Dosage adjustments are not needed in adults with mild (creatinine clearance 50–79 mL/minute) or moderate (creatinine clearance 30–49 mL/minute) renal impairment.

Adults with severe renal impairment (creatinine clearances less than 30 mL/minute) *not* receiving regularly scheduled hemodialysis should receive a 2-dose regimen of 750 mg of dalbavancin given by IV infusion followed 1 week later by 375 mg given by IV infusion.

Dosage adjustments are not recommended for adults with renal impairment receiving regularly scheduled hemodialysis; dalbavancin may be administered in such patients without regard to hemodialysis timing. (See Renal Impairment under Warnings/Precautions: Specific Populations, in Cautions.)

Hepatic Impairment Dosage adjustments are not needed in adults with mild hepatic impairment (Child-Pugh class A).

Dosage recommendations for those with moderate or severe hepatic impairment (Child-Pugh class B or C) are not available; the drug should be used with caution in such individuals. (See Hepatic Impairment under Warnings/Precautions: Specific Populations, in Cautions.)

Geriatric Patients Dosage adjustments are not needed in geriatric patients based solely on age. Dosage should be selected with caution since geriatric patients are more likely to have decreased renal function than younger adults. (See Geriatric Use under Warnings/Precautions: Specific Populations, in Cautions.)

Cautions

■ **Contraindications** Dalbavancin is contraindicated in patients with known hypersensitivity to the drug.

■ **Warnings/Precautions** ***Sensitivity Reactions*** Serious hypersensitivity (anaphylactic) and skin reactions have been reported in patients receiving dalbavancin.

Data are not available to date regarding cross-reactivity between dalbavancin and other glycopeptides (e.g., oritavancin, telavancin, vancomycin). Because of the possibility of cross-sensitivity, patients should be questioned about previous hypersensitivity reactions to glycopeptides and dalbavancin should be used with caution in those with a history of glycopeptide allergy.

If an allergic reaction occurs, dalbavancin should be discontinued.

Infusion Reactions Rapid IV infusion of dalbavancin can cause a reaction referred to as "red-man syndrome" (i.e., flushing of the upper body, urticaria, pruritus, rash).

To reduce the risk of infusion-related reactions, IV infusions of dalbavancin should be given over 30 minutes. If an infusion-related reaction occurs, stopping or decreasing the infusion rate may result in cessation of symptoms.

Hepatic Effects In patients with normal baseline aminotransferase concentrations in phase 2 and phase 3 clinical trials, more dalbavancin-treated patients developed ALT elevations greater than 3 times the upper limit of normal (ULN) compared with patients receiving a comparator treatment (0.8 or 0.2%, respectively). Overall, the frequency of liver laboratory test abnormalities (e.g., ALT, AST, bilirubin) was similar in patients receiving dalbavancin or a comparator treatment.

Superinfection/Clostridium difficile-associated Diarrhea and Colitis (CDAD) Use of dalbavancin may result in emergence and overgrowth of nonsusceptible bacteria or fungi. The patient should be carefully monitored and appropriate therapy instituted if superinfection occurs.

Treatment with anti-infectives alters normal colon flora and may permit overgrowth of *Clostridium difficile*. *C. difficile* infection (CDI) and *C. difficile*-associated diarrhea and colitis (CDAD; also known as antibiotic-associated diarrhea and colitis or pseudomembranous colitis) have been reported in patients receiving nearly all anti-infectives, including dalbavancin, and may range in severity from mild diarrhea to fatal colitis. *C. difficile* produces toxins A and B which contribute to development of CDAD; hypertoxin-producing strains of *C. difficile* are associated with increased morbidity and mortality since they may be refractory to anti-infectives and colectomy may be required.

CDAD should be considered in the differential diagnosis of patients who develop diarrhea during or after anti-infective therapy. Careful medical history is necessary since CDAD has been reported to occur as late as 2 months or longer after anti-infective therapy is discontinued.

If CDAD is suspected or confirmed, anti-infective therapy not directed against *C. difficile* should be discontinued whenever possible. Patients should be managed with appropriate supportive therapy (e.g., fluid and electrolyte management, protein supplementation), anti-infective therapy directed against *C. difficile* (e.g., metronidazole, vancomycin), and surgical evaluation as clinically indicated.

Selection and Use of Anti-infectives To reduce development of drug-resistant bacteria and maintain effectiveness of dalbavancin and other antibacterials, the drug should be used only for treatment of infections proven or strongly suspected to be caused by susceptible bacteria.

When selecting or modifying anti-infective therapy, results of culture and in vitro susceptibility testing should be used. In the absence of such data, local epidemiology and susceptibility patterns should be considered when selecting anti-infectives for empiric therapy.

Specific Populations **Pregnancy.** Category C. (See Users Guide.)

There are no adequate and well-controlled studies of dalbavancin in pregnant women, and the drug should be used during pregnancy only if potential benefits justify potential risks to the fetus.

In an embryofetal study in rats, delayed fetal maturation was observed at a dosage of 45 mg/kg daily (3.5 times the human dosage on an exposure basis). In a prenatal and postnatal development study in rats, increased embryolethality and increased offspring deaths during the first week postpartum were observed at a dosage of 45 mg/kg daily.

Lactation. Dalbavancin is distributed into milk in lactating rats; it is not known whether the drug is distributed into human milk.

Dalbavancin should be used with caution in nursing women.

Pediatric Use. Safety and efficacy of dalbavancin have not been established in pediatric patients.

Geriatric Use. In clinical studies evaluating dalbavancin for the treatment of acute bacterial skin and skin structure infections, efficacy and tolerability were similar to comparator treatments regardless of age.

There were no substantial differences in the pharmacokinetics of dalbavancin according to age; therefore, dosage adjustments are not needed based solely on age.

Dalbavancin is substantially eliminated by the kidneys; the risk of adverse effects may be greater in patients with impaired renal function. Dosage should be selected with caution since geriatric patients are more likely to have decreased renal function.

Hepatic Impairment. Dalbavancin should be used with caution in patients with moderate or severe hepatic impairment (Child-Pugh class B or C); there are no data available to determine an appropriate dosage of the drug in such patients. The mean area under the plasma concentration-time curve (AUC) of dalbavancin is decreased by 28 or 31% in patients with moderate or severe hepatic impairment (Child-Pugh class B or C); however, the clinical importance of decreased AUC in such patients has not been established.

Dalbavancin pharmacokinetics are not altered in patients with mild hepatic impairment (Child-Pugh class A).

Renal Impairment. In patients with mild, moderate, or severe renal impairment, mean plasma clearance of dalbavancin is decreased by 11, 35, or 47%, respectively, and AUC is increased compared with patients with normal renal function. Dalbavancin pharmacokinetics in patients with end-stage renal disease receiving regularly scheduled hemodialysis are similar to those in patients with mild to moderate renal impairment.

Patients with creatinine clearance less than 30 mL/minute who are *not* receiving regularly scheduled hemodialysis should receive reduced dalbavancin dosage. (See Renal Impairment under Dosage and Administration: Special Populations.)

■ **Common Adverse Effects** Adverse effects reported in 2% or more of patients receiving dalbavancin include nausea, vomiting, diarrhea, headache, rash, and pruritus.

Drug Interactions

Formal drug interaction studies have not been conducted with dalbavancin to date.

■ **Drugs Affecting or Metabolized by Hepatic Microsomal Enzymes** Based on in vitro studies, dalbavancin is not a substrate, inhibitor, or inducer of cytochrome P-450 (CYP) isoenzymes, and there is minimal potential that the drug will interact with substrates, inhibitors, or inducers of CYP isoenzymes. Results of a population pharmacokinetic analysis indicate that dalbavancin pharmacokinetics are not affected when the drug is used concomitantly with known CYP isoenzyme substrates, inducers, inhibitors, or other tested drugs (e.g., acetaminophen, aztreonam, fentanyl, metronidazole, furosemide, proton-pump inhibitors [omeprazole, esomeprazole, pantoprazole, lansoprazole], midazolam, simvastatin).

■ **Antibacterial Agents** Dalbavancin pharmacokinetics do not appear to be affected by concomitant use of aztreonam or metronidazole.

In vitro studies indicate that the antibacterial effects of dalbavancin and oxacillin are synergistic against some gram-positive bacteria (methicillin-resistant *Staphylococcus aureus* [MRSA; also known as oxacillin-resistant *S. aureus* or ORSA]).

In vitro studies indicate that the antibacterial effects of dalbavancin and aztreonam, clindamycin, daptomycin, gentamicin, levofloxacin, linezolid, quinupristin and dalfopristin, rifampin, or vancomycin are not synergistic or antagonistic.

Description

Dalbavancin hydrochloride is a semisynthetic lipoglycopeptide antibacterial derived from a naturally occurring glycopeptide produced by *Nonomuraea*, an actinomycete. The drug is a teicoplanin-type lipoglycopeptide and contains a heptapeptide core structure that differs from that of vancomycin. Dalbavancin is a mixture of 5 closely related homologs (i.e., A_0, A_1, B_0, B_1, B_2), each sharing the same core structure. Of the 5 homologs, B_0 is the major component of dalbavancin.

The mechanism of action of dalbavancin is similar to that of other glycopeptides (e.g., oritavancin, telavancin, vancomycin). Dalbavancin binds to the D-alanyl-D-alanine terminus of growing peptidoglycan chains, thereby inhibiting bacterial cell wall synthesis. The drug also appears to dimerize and anchor in the bacterial membranes.

In vitro, dalbavancin is bactericidal in action against certain gram-positive bacteria, including staphylococci, streptococci, and enterococci. The drug is active in vitro and in clinical infections against *S. aureus* (including methicillin-resistant *S. aureus* [MRSA; also known as oxacillin-resistant *S. aureus* or ORSA]), *S. pyogenes* (group A β-hemolytic streptococci, GAS), *S. agalactiae* (group B streptococci, GBS), and *S. anginosus* group (includes *S. anginosus*, *S. intermedius*, and *S. constellatus*). Dalbavancin also is active in vitro against some vancomycin-susceptible *Enterococcus faecium* and *E. faecalis*; however, safety and efficacy of the drug in treating clinical infections caused by these bacteria have not been established. Dalbavancin is active in vitro against some vancomycin-intermediate *S. aureus* (VISA) and VanB and VanC phenotypes of vancomycin-resistant enterococci (VRE), but VRE with the VanA phenotype have reduced in vitro susceptibility or resistance to dalbavancin.

Reduced susceptibility or resistance to dalbavancin was not produced in vitro by serial passage of *S. aureus* in the presence of increasing concentrations of the drug. Certain intrinsically glycopeptide-resistant bacteria and those expressing the VanA phenotype of acquired resistance to vancomycin also may be resistant to dalbavancin. Cross-resistance between dalbavancin and nonglycopeptide anti-infectives is unlikely.

Dalbavancin exhibits linear, dose-dependent pharmacokinetics following IV administration, and there is no apparent accumulation following multiple IV doses of the drug. In adults with skin and skin structure infections, a single 1-g IV dose of dalbavancin given on day 1 followed by a single 500-mg IV dose on day 8 resulted in mean plasma dalbavancin concentrations of 30 mg/L immediately before the second dose and mean plasma concentrations of 21 mg/mL (range 8–40 mg/L) 20 days after the initial dose. Dalbavancin is distributed into skin blister fluid following IV administration, and mean blister fluid concentrations are at least 30 mg/L for up to 7 days following a single 1-g IV dose. The drug is approximately 93% bound to plasma proteins, mainly albumin. Dalbavancin is not a substrate, inhibitor, or inducer of cytochrome P-

450 (CYP) isoenzymes; a minor metabolite, hydroxydalbavancin, has been detected in urine. Based on population pharmacokinetic analyses, the effective half-life of dalbavancin is approximately 8.5 days (204 hours). Following a single 1-g dose of dalbavancin, 20% of a dose is eliminated in feces by day 70 after the dose. An average of 33% of the dose is eliminated in urine as unchanged drug and approximately 12% is eliminated in urine as the metabolite by day 42 after the dose. Less than 6% of an administered dose of dalbavancin is removed after 3 hours of hemodialysis.

Advice to Patients

Advise patients that antibacterials (including dalbavancin) should only be used to treat bacterial infections and not used to treat viral infections (e.g., the common cold).

Importance of completing full course of therapy, even if feeling better after a few days.

Advise patients that skipping doses or not completing the full course of therapy may decrease effectiveness and increase the likelihood that bacteria will develop resistance and will not be treatable with dalbavancin or other antibacterials in the future.

Advise patients that allergic reactions, including serious allergic reactions, could occur and require immediate treatment. Importance of informing clinician about any previous hypersensitivity reactions to dalbavancin or other glycopeptides (e.g., oritavancin, telavancin, vancomycin).

Advise patients that diarrhea is a common problem caused by anti-infectives and usually ends when the drug is discontinued. Importance of contacting a clinician if watery and bloody stools (with or without stomach cramps and fever) occur during or as late as 2 months or longer after the last dose.

Importance of informing clinicians of existing or contemplated concomitant therapy, including prescription and OTC drugs and dietary or herbal supplements, as well as any concomitant illnesses.

Importance of women informing clinicians if they are or plan to become pregnant or plan to breast-feed.

Importance of informing patients of other important precautionary information. (See Cautions.)

Overview® (see Users Guide). For additional information on this drug until a more detailed monograph is developed and published, the manufacturer's labeling should be consulted. It is *essential* that the manufacturer's labeling be consulted for more detailed information on usual cautions, precautions, contraindications, potential drug interactions, laboratory test interferences, and acute toxicity.

Preparations

Excipients in commercially available drug preparations may have clinically important effects in some individuals; consult specific product labeling for details.

Dalbavancin Hydrochloride

Parenteral		
For injection, for IV infusion	500 mg (of dalbavancin)	**Dalvance®**, Durata Therapeutics

Oritavancin Diphosphate

■ Oritavancin diphosphate, a lipoglycopeptide antibacterial, is a semisynthetic derivative of a naturally occurring glycopeptide.

Uses

■ **Skin and Skin Structure Infections** Oritavancin diphosphate is used for the treatment of acute bacterial skin and skin structure infections (ABSSSI) caused by susceptible *Staphylococcus aureus* (including methicillin-resistant *S. aureus* [MRSA; also known as oxacillin-resistant *S. aureus* or ORSA] and methicillin-susceptible *S. aureus*), *Streptococcus pyogenes* (group A β-hemolytic streptococci, GAS), *S. agalactiae* (group B streptococci, GBS), *S. dysgalactiae*, *S. anginosus* group (includes *S. anginosus*, *S. intermedius*, and *S. constellatus*), or vancomycin-susceptible *Enterococcus faecalis*.

Clinical Experience Efficacy and safety of oritavancin were evaluated in 2 randomized, multicenter, double-blind, noninferiority, phase 3 studies (SOLO I and SOLO II) in 1987 adults with acute bacterial skin and skin structure infections (e.g., cellulitis, major abscess, wound infection, erysipelas) suspected or proven to be caused by a gram-positive pathogen. Eligible patients exhibited at least 2 local signs of infection (e.g., purulent drainage or discharge, fluctuance, localized warmth, tenderness, swelling or induration), at least 1 sign of systemic inflammation at baseline (e.g., proximal lymph node swelling, temperature 38°C or higher or less than 36°C, leukocyte count greater than 10,000 cells/mm^3, greater than 10% bandemia, increased C-reactive protein), and were thought to require at least 7 days of IV therapy. Patients were randomized in a 1:1 ratio to receive oritavancin (single 1.2-g IV dose) or vancomycin (1 g or 15 mg/kg IV every 12 hours for 7–10 days). Aztreonam or metronidazole could be used concomitantly for gram-negative or anaerobic coverage, respectively.

In SOLO I, baseline demographic characteristics were similar between groups (mean age 44–46 years, 63% male, 20% with diabetes mellitus, 49–51% with cellulitis, 29–30% with abscess, 19–22% with wound infection, median baseline lesion area 226–248 cm^2). At 48–72 hours after initiation of treatment, 82.3% of patients receiving oritavancin and 78.9% of patients receiving vancomycin achieved the primary efficacy end point of early clinical response (i.e., no increase in lesion area from baseline, absence of fever, and no rescue antibacterial drugs needed). Decrease in lesion size of 20% or more at 48–72 hours after initiation of treatment was achieved by 86.9 or 82.9% of patients receiving oritavancin or vancomycin, respectively, and investigator-assessed clinical success at 7–14 days after the end of therapy was achieved by 79.6 or 80% of patients, respectively.

In SOLO II, baseline demographic characteristics were similar between groups (mean age 44–45 years, 67–68% male, 9% with diabetes mellitus, 29–33% with cellulitis, 32–33% with abscess, 35–38% with wound infection, median baseline lesion area 288–309 cm^2). At 48–72 hours after initiation of treatment, 80.1% of patients receiving oritavancin and 82.9% of patients receiving vancomycin achieved the primary efficacy end point of early clinical response (i.e., no increase in lesion area from baseline, absence of fever, and no rescue antibacterial drugs needed). Decrease in lesion size of 20% or more at 48–72 hours after initiation of treatment was achieved by 85.9 or 85.3% of patients receiving oritavancin or vancomycin, respectively, and investigator-assessed clinical success at 7–10 days after the end of therapy was achieved by 82.7 or 80.5% of patients, respectively.

In a pooled analysis (SOLO I and SOLO II) of the subset of patients who were microbiologically evaluable and stratified according to the infecting pathogen, the clinical success rate (defined as complete or nearly complete resolution of baseline signs and symptoms) on day 14–24 in those with infections caused by MRSA or methicillin-susceptible *S. aureus* was 83 or 82%, respectively, in those treated with oritavancin and 84 or 84%, respectively, in those treated with vancomycin. The clinical success rate in those with infections caused by *S. agalactiae*, *S. pyogenes*, *S. anginosus* group, *S. dysgalactiae*, or *E. faecalis* was 88, 81, 76, 78, or 62%, respectively, in those treated with oritavancin and 92, 72, 84, 50, or 75%, respectively, in those treated with vancomycin.

Dosage and Administration

■ **Administration** Oritavancin diphosphate is administered by IV infusion.

IV Administration Oritavancin should *not* be administered simultaneously with commonly used IV drugs through a common port.

If the same IV line or port is used for sequential infusion of oritavancin and other drugs, the IV line should be flushed with 5% dextrose injection before and after the oritavancin infusion.

Sodium chloride 0.9% is incompatible with oritavancin diphosphate and may cause precipitation. Sodium chloride 0.9% should *not* be used to dilute oritavancin. Other IV solutions, additives, or drugs mixed in 0.9% sodium chloride injection should *not* be added to oritavancin vials or infused simultaneously through the same IV line or port.

Drugs formulated at an alkaline or neutral pH may be incompatible with oritavancin.

Vials of oritavancin lyophilized powder for injection contain no preservatives and are intended for single use only.

Reconstitution and Dilution. Oritavancin diphosphate for injection must be reconstituted and further diluted prior to IV infusion. Strict aseptic technique must be observed when preparing IV solutions of the drug.

Vials labeled as containing 400 mg of oritavancin should be reconstituted by adding 40 mL of sterile water for injection to provide a solution containing 10 mg/mL. A total of 3 vials is required to prepare a single 1.2-g dose. To avoid foaming, vials should be gently swirled until contents are completely dissolved. The reconstituted solution should appear clear and colorless to pale yellow.

Reconstituted oritavancin must then be further diluted in 5% dextrose injection. Before adding oritavancin to a 1-L IV bag of 5% dextrose injection, 120 mL of the dextrose injection should be withdrawn and discarded. Then, 40 mL of reconstituted oritavancin should be withdrawn from each of the 3 reconstituted vials and added to the 5% dextrose IV bag bringing the bag volume to 1 L. The final diluted oritavancin solution has a concentration of 1.2 mg/mL.

Following reconstitution and further dilution, oritavancin solutions should be used within 6 hours when stored at room temperature or within 12 hours when refrigerated at 2–8°C. The combined total storage time and 3-hour infusion time should not exceed 6 hours at room temperature or 12 hours at 2–8°C.

Oritavancin solutions should be inspected visually for particulate matter prior to administration.

Rate of Administration. Oritavancin solutions should be administered by IV infusion over 3 hours.

■ **Dosage** Dosage of oritavancin diphosphate is expressed in terms of oritavancin.

Adult Dosage **Skin and Skin Structure Infections.** The recommended dosage of oritavancin for the treatment of acute bacterial skin and skin structure infections (ABSSSI) in adults is a single 1.2-g dose given by IV infusion.

■ **Special Populations** ***Renal Impairment*** Dosage adjustments are not needed in patients with mild or moderate renal impairment. Pharmacokinetics of oritavancin have not been studied in patients with severe renal impairment. (See Renal Impairment under Warnings/Precautions: Specific Populations, in Cautions.)

Hepatic Impairment Dosage adjustments are not needed in patients with mild or moderate hepatic impairment. Pharmacokinetics of oritavancin have not been studied in patients with severe hepatic impairment. (See Hepatic Impairment under Warning/Precautions: Specific Populations, in Cautions.)

Cautions

■ **Contraindications** Oritavancin is contraindicated in patients with known hypersensitivity to the drug.

Unfractionated heparin sodium is contraindicated for 48 hours after oritavancin because activated partial thromboplastin time (aPTT) is expected to remain falsely elevated for this period of time after administration of the anti-infective. (See Tests Used to Monitor Coagulation under Cautions: Warnings/Precautions.)

■ **Warnings/Precautions** ***Sensitivity Reactions*** Serious hypersensitivity reactions have been reported in patients receiving oritavancin. In phase 3 clinical trials, the median onset of hypersensitivity reactions in patients receiving oritavancin was 1.2 days and the median duration of the reactions was 2.4 days.

Because of the possibility of cross-sensitivity, patients should be questioned about previous hypersensitivity reactions to glycopeptides (e.g., dalbavancin, telavancin, vancomycin). Individuals with a history of glycopeptide allergy should be carefully monitored for signs of hypersensitivity during oritavancin infusion.

If an acute hypersensitivity reaction occurs during the oritavancin infusion, the drug should be discontinued immediately and appropriate supportive care initiated.

Infusion Reactions Infusion-related reactions (e.g., pruritus, urticaria, flushing) have been reported in patients receiving oritavancin.

If an infusion-related reaction occurs, slowing or interrupting the oritavancin infusion should be considered.

Tests Used to Monitor Coagulation Oritavancin has been shown to artificially prolong certain tests used to monitor coagulation, including prothrombin time (PT), international normalized ratio (INR), and aPTT, and also is expected to prolong activated clotting time (ACT). This occurs because oritavancin binds to phospholipid reagents and prevents activation of coagulation in commonly used laboratory coagulation tests. Oritavancin does *not* have an effect on the coagulation system.

PT and INR have been shown to be artificially prolonged for 24 hours after oritavancin administration and aPTT has been shown to be artificially prolonged for 48 hours after oritavancin administration. These effects may complicate laboratory monitoring in patients receiving certain anticoagulants (e.g., heparin, warfarin).

For patients requiring aPTT monitoring within 48 hours of oritavancin administration, a non-phospholipid-dependent coagulation test (e.g., factor Xa [chromogenic] assay) should be used or an alternative anticoagulant not requiring aPTT monitoring considered.

Concomitant Use with Warfarin Concomitant use of oritavancin and warfarin may increase warfarin exposure and may increase the risk of bleeding. (See Drug Interactions: Warfarin.)

Oritavancin and chronic warfarin therapy should be used concomitantly *only* when the benefits are expected to outweigh the risk of bleeding. If the drugs are used concomitantly, the patient should be frequently monitored for signs of bleeding. Clinicians should consider that laboratory monitoring of the anticoagulant effects of warfarin is unreliable for 24 hours after oritavancin administration because the anti-infective artificially prolongs certain coagulation tests. (See Tests Used to Monitor Coagulation under Cautions: Warnings/Precautions.)

Osteomyelitis In clinical trials, osteomyelitis was reported more frequently in patients receiving oritavancin than in those receiving vancomycin.

Patients receiving oritavancin should be monitored for signs and symptoms of osteomyelitis. If osteomyelitis is suspected or diagnosed, appropriate alternative antibacterial therapy should be initiated.

Superinfection/Clostridium difficile-associated Diarrhea and Colitis (CDAD) Use of oritavancin may result in emergence and overgrowth of nonsusceptible bacteria or fungi. The patient should be carefully monitored and appropriate therapy instituted if superinfection occurs.

Treatment with anti-infectives alters normal colon flora and may permit overgrowth of *Clostridium difficile*. *C. difficile* infection (CDI) and *C. difficile*-associated diarrhea and colitis (CDAD; also known as antibiotic-associated diarrhea and colitis or pseudomembranous colitis) have been reported in patients receiving nearly all anti-infectives, including oritavancin, and may range in severity from mild diarrhea to fatal colitis. *C. difficile* produces toxins A and B which contribute to development of CDAD; hypertoxin-producing strains of *C. difficile* are associated with increased morbidity and mortality since they may be refractory to anti-infectives and colectomy may be required.

CDAD should be considered in the differential diagnosis of patients who develop diarrhea during or after anti-infective therapy. Careful medical history is necessary since CDAD has been reported to occur as late as 2 months or longer after anti-infective therapy is discontinued.

If CDAD is suspected or confirmed, anti-infective therapy not directed against *C. difficile* should be discontinued whenever possible. Patients should be managed with appropriate supportive therapy (e.g., fluid and electrolyte management, protein supplementation), anti-infective therapy directed against *C. difficile* (e.g., metronidazole, vancomycin), and surgical evaluation as clinically indicated.

Selection and Use of Anti-infectives To reduce development of drug-resistant bacteria and maintain effectiveness of oritavancin and other antibacterials, the drug should be used only for treatment of infections proven or strongly suspected to be caused by susceptible bacteria.

When selecting or modifying anti-infective therapy, results of culture and in vitro susceptibility testing should be used. In the absence of such data, local epidemiology and susceptibility patterns should be considered when selecting anti-infectives for empiric therapy.

Specific Populations **Pregnancy.** Category C. (See Users Guide.)

There are no adequate and well-controlled studies of oritavancin in pregnant women, and the drug should be used during pregnancy only if potential benefits justify potential risks to the fetus.

Reproduction studies in rats or rabbits have not revealed evidence of harm to the fetus at dosages equivalent to a human dose of 300 mg (25% of the recommend 1.2-g single dose); higher doses have not been evaluated.

Lactation. Oritavancin is distributed into milk in lactating rats; it is not known whether the drug is distributed into human milk.

Oritavancin should be used with caution in nursing women.

Pediatric Use. Safety and efficacy of oritavancin have not been established in pediatric patients younger than 18 years of age.

Geriatric Use. Clinical trials of oritavancin did not include sufficient numbers of patients 65 years of age and older to determine whether they respond differently than younger adults. Other clinical experience has not revealed age-related differences in response, but the possibility of greater sensitivity in some older patients cannot be ruled out.

Hepatic Impairment. The pharmacokinetics of oritavancin have not been studied in patients with severe hepatic impairment. There were no clinically important differences in pharmacokinetics of oritavancin in patients with moderate hepatic impairment (Child-Pugh class B) compared with healthy adults.

Renal Impairment. The pharmacokinetics of oritavancin have not been studied in patients with severe renal impairment or in those receiving dialysis. There were no clinically important differences in pharmacokinetics of oritavancin in patients with mild or moderate renal impairment compared with those with normal renal function.

■ **Common Adverse Effects** Adverse effects reported in 1.5% or more of patients receiving oritavancin include GI effects (i.e., diarrhea, nausea, vomiting, constipation), dizziness, headache, infusion site reactions (including phlebitis and extravasation), pruritus, urticaria, pyrexia, chills, abscess (limb or subcutaneous), cellulitis, increased AST and ALT concentrations, tachycardia, insomnia, and fatigue.

Drug Interactions

■ **Drugs Affecting or Metabolized by Hepatic Microsomal Enzymes** Oritavancin is a weak inhibitor of cytochrome P-450 (CYP) 2C9 and CYP2C19 and a weak inducer of CYP3A4 and CYP2D6. Oritavancin and drugs that are metabolized by these CYP isoenzymes and have a narrow therapeutic index should be used concomitantly with caution and patients closely monitored for signs of toxicity or lack of efficacy.

■ **Drugs Affecting or Affected by P-glycoprotein Transport System** Oritavancin is not a substrate or inhibitor of the P-glycoprotein (P-gp) efflux transporter.

■ **Antibacterial Agents** In vitro, the antibacterial effects of oritavancin and gentamicin, moxifloxacin, or rifampin are synergistic against methicillin-susceptible *Staphylococcus aureus*. In vitro studies indicate that the antibacterial effects of oritavancin and gentamicin or linezolid are synergistic against vancomycin-intermediate *S. aureus* (VISA), heterogeneous VISA (hVISA), and vancomycin-resistant *S. aureus* (VRSA). In addition, the antibacterial effects of oritavancin and rifampin are synergistic in vitro against VRSA.

In vitro, the antibacterial effects of oritavancin and ciprofloxacin or gentamicin are synergistic against some vancomycin-resistant enterococci (VRE).

There is no in vitro evidence of antagonistic antibacterial effects between oritavancin and ciprofloxacin, gentamicin, moxifloxacin, linezolid, or rifampin.

■ **Dextromethorphan** Concomitant use of oritavancin (single 1.2-g dose) and dextromethorphan results in a 31% decrease in the ratio of dextromethorphan to dextrorphan concentrations in urine.

■ **Heparin** Because the activated partial thromboplastin time (aPTT) is expected to be falsely elevated for approximately 48 hours after oritavancin administration, unfractionated heparin sodium is contraindicated for 48 hours after oritavancin. (See Tests Used to Monitor Coagulation under Cautions: Warnings/Precautions.)

■ **Midazolam** Concomitant use of oritavancin (single 1.2-g dose) and midazolam results in an 18% decrease in the mean area under the plasma concentration-time curve (AUC) of midazolam.

■ **Omeprazole** Concomitant use of oritavancin (single 1.2-g dose) and omeprazole results in a 15% increase in the ratio of omeprazole to 5-hydroxyomeprazole concentrations in plasma.

■ **Warfarin** Concomitant use of oritavancin (single 1.2-g dose) and warfarin results in a 31% increase in the mean AUC of warfarin and may increase the risk of bleeding. Oritavancin and chronic warfarin therapy should be used concomitantly *only* when the benefits are expected to outweigh the risk of bleeding.

If oritavancin and warfarin are used concomitantly, the patient should be frequently monitored for signs of bleeding. Because prothrombin time (PT) and international normalized ratio (INR) are expected to be falsely elevated for approximately 24 hours after oritavancin administration, monitoring the anticoagulation effects of warfarin is unreliable for 24 hours after oritavancin. (See Tests Used to Monitor Coagulation under Cautions: Warnings/Precautions.)

Description

Oritavancin diphosphate is a semisynthetic lipoglycopeptide antibacterial derived from chloroeremomycin, a naturally occurring glycopeptide. Oritavancin contains a heptapeptide core structure similar to that of vancomycin, but has side chains that enhance antibacterial activity.

The mechanism of action of oritavancin is similar to that of other glycopeptides (e.g., dalbavancin, vancomycin). Oritavancin binds to the D-alanyl-D-alanine terminus of growing peptidoglycan chains, thereby inhibiting bacterial cell wall, synthesis. In addition, the drug binds to the peptide bridging segments of the cell wall, thereby inhibiting the transpeptidation (crosslinking) step of cell wall biosynthesis, and can dimerize and anchor into the bacterial cell membrane, which improves its ability to bind to its target.

In vitro, oritavancin is bactericidal in action against certain gram-positive bacteria, including staphylococci, streptococci, and enterococci. In vitro and in clinical studies, oritavancin is active against *Staphylococcus aureus* (including methicillin-resistant *S. aureus* [MRSA; also known as oxacillin-resistant *S. aureus* or ORSA]), *Streptococcus pyogenes* (group A β-hemolytic streptococci, GAS), *S. agalactiae* (group B streptococci, GBS), *S. dysgalactiae*, *S. anginosus* group (includes *S. anginosus*, *S. intermedius*, and *S. constellatus*), and vancomycin-susceptible *Enterococcus faecalis*.

Oritavancin also is active in vitro against vancomycin-susceptible *E. faecium*, *Clostridium perfringens*, *C. difficile*, *Peptostreptococcus*, *Propionibacterium acnes*, *S. pneumoniae*, vancomycin-intermediate *S. aureus* (VISA), vancomycin-resistant *S. aureus* (VRSA), and daptomycin-nonsusceptible *S. aureus* (DNSSA). However, safety and efficacy of oritavancin in treating clinical infections caused by these bacteria have not been established.

Reduced susceptibility or resistance to oritavancin has been produced in vitro by serial passage of *S. aureus* or *E. faecalis* in the presence of increasing concentrations of the drug.

Oritavancin exhibits linear, dose-dependent pharmacokinetics following IV administration. Oritavancin is extensively distributed into tissues, including skin blister fluid, extracellular lung fluid, and alveolar macrophages. Mean oritavancin concentrations in skin blister fluid are approximately 20% of those in plasma after a single 800-mg dose in healthy individuals. The drug is approximately 85% bound to plasma proteins. Oritavancin is not metabolized. Based on population pharmacokinetic analyses, the terminal half-life of oritavancin is approximately 10 days (245 hours). The drug is slowly eliminated unchanged in feces and urine; less than 1 and 5% of a single IV dose is recovered in feces and urine, respectively, by 2 weeks after the dose. The drug is not removed by hemodialysis or continuous renal replacement therapy (CRRT).

Advice to Patients

Advise patients that antibacterials (including oritavancin) should only be used to treat bacterial infections and not used to treat viral infections (e.g., the common cold).

Importance of completing full course of therapy, even if feeling better after a few days.

Advise patients that skipping doses or not completing the full course of therapy may decrease effectiveness and increase the likelihood that bacteria will develop resistance and will not be treatable with oritavancin or other antibacterials in the future.

Advise patients that allergic reactions, including serious allergic reactions, could occur and require immediate treatment. Importance of informing clinician about any previous hypersensitivity reactions to oritavancin or other glycopeptides (e.g., dalbavancin, telavancin, vancomycin).

Advise patients that diarrhea is a common problem caused by anti-infectives and usually ends when the drug is discontinued. Importance of contacting a clinician if watery and bloody stools (with or without stomach cramps and fever) occur during or as late as 2 months or longer after the last dose.

Importance of informing clinicians of existing or contemplated concomitant therapy, including prescription and OTC drugs and dietary or herbal supplements, as well as any concomitant illnesses.

Importance of women informing clinicians if they are or plan to become pregnant or plan to breast-feed.

Importance of informing patients of other important precautionary information. (See Cautions.)

Overview® (see Users Guide). For additional information on this drug until a more detailed monograph is developed and published, the manufacturer's labeling should be consulted. It is *essential* that the manufacturer's labeling be consulted for more detailed information on usual cautions, precautions, contraindications, potential drug interactions, laboratory test interferences, and acute toxicity.

Preparations

Excipients in commercially available drug preparations may have clinically important effects in some individuals; consult specific product labeling for details.

Oritavancin Diphosphate

Parenteral

For injection, for IV infusion	400 mg (of oritavancin)	**Orbactiv®**, Medicines Company

Telavancin Hydrochloride

■ Telavancin, a lipoglycopeptide antibacterial, is a semisynthetic derivative of vancomycin.

Uses

■ **Respiratory Tract Infections** ***Nosocomial Pneumonia*** Telavancin hydrochloride is used for the treatment of nosocomial pneumonia, including hospital-acquired and ventilator-associated pneumonia, caused by susceptible *Staphylococcus aureus* (including methicillin-resistant *S. aureus* [MRSA; also known as oxacillin-resistant *S. aureus* or ORSA]). If documented or presumed pathogens also include gram-negative or anaerobic bacteria, concomitant use of an anti-infective active against such bacteria may be clinically indicated.

The manufacturer states that telavancin should be reserved for use when alternative treatments for hospital-acquired or ventilator-associated bacterial pneumonia are not suitable.

Clinical Experience. Telavancin was evaluated in 2 identical, randomized, double-blind, parallel-group, phase 3 studies in adults with hospital-acquired or ventilator-associated pneumonia known or suspected to be caused by *S. aureus*. The mean age of study patients was 63 years, 64% were male, 70% were white, more than 50% were admitted to an intensive care unit, 23% had chronic obstructive pulmonary disease, 29% had ventilator-associated pneumonia, and 6% had bacteremia. Patients were randomized to receive 7–21 days of treatment with telavancin (10 mg/kg IV once every 24 hours) or vancomycin (1 g IV every 12 hours with dosage individualized and adjusted according to standard practices at the site). Other appropriate anti-infectives (e.g., aztreonam and/or metronidazole) were used concomitantly if documented or presumed pathogens also included gram-negative or anaerobic bacteria; the fixed combination of piperacillin sodium and tazobactam sodium could be used concomitantly for gram-negative coverage if aztreonam resistance was confirmed or suspected. The primary end point was clinical response (i.e., resolution of signs and symptoms, no further antibacterial therapy after completion of treatment, improvement or no progression of baseline radiographic findings) at the test-of-cure visit 7–14 days after completion of treatment; 28-day all-cause mortality was a prespecified secondary end point. In both studies, clinical response rates in telavancin-treated patients were similar to those reported in vancomycin-treated patients. In clinically evaluable patients (CE population), clinical response was achieved in 83.7 or 81.3% of those who received telavancin and in 80 or 81% of those who received vancomycin. In a subset of patients who were microbiologically evaluable and stratified according to the infecting pathogen, the clinical cure rate in those with infections caused by methicillin-susceptible *S. aureus* or MRSA was 78% in those treated with telavancin and 75% in those treated with vancomycin. The overall 28-day all-cause mortality in patients with at least one baseline gram-positive respiratory pathogen was 29 or 24% in telavancin-treated patients and 24 or 22% in vancomycin-treated patients. All-cause mortality in patients treated with telavancin was higher in those with baseline creatinine clearances of 50 mL/minute or lower (41 or 44%) compared with those with baseline creatinine clearances exceeding 50 mL/minute (22 or 18%).

■ **Skin and Skin Structure Infections** Telavancin hydrochloride is used for the treatment of complicated skin and skin structure infections caused by susceptible *S. aureus* (including MRSA), *Streptococcus pyogenes* (group A β-hemolytic streptococci, GAS), *S. agalactiae* (group B streptococci, GBS), *S. anginosus* group (includes *S. anginosus*, *S. intermedius*, and *S. constellatus*), or *Enterococcus faecalis* (vancomycin-susceptible strains only). If documented or presumed pathogens also include gram-negative or anaerobic bacteria, concomitant use of an anti-infective active against such bacteria may be clinically indicated.

For information on diagnosis and management of skin and skin structure infections, the current clinical practice guidelines from the Infectious Diseases Society of America (IDSA) available at http://www.idsociety.org should be consulted.

Clinical Experience Telavancin was evaluated in 2 randomized, multicenter, active-controlled phase 3 studies in adults with complicated skin and skin structure infections (e.g., major abscess, deep/extensive cellulitis, wound infection, infected ulcer, infected burn) with MRSA as the suspected or confirmed primary cause of infection (studies 0017 and 0018; ATLAS 1 and 2). Patients were randomized to receive 7–14 days of treatment with telavancin

(10 mg/kg IV once every 24 hours) or vancomycin (1 g IV every 12 hours with dosage individualized and adjusted according to standard practices at the site). Other appropriate anti-infectives (e.g., aztreonam and/or metronidazole) were used concomitantly if documented or presumptive pathogens also included gram-negative or anaerobic bacteria. The primary end point was clinical cure rates 7–14 days after completion of treatment. Clinical cure rates reported with telavancin were similar to those reported with vancomycin. In clinically evaluable patients (CE population), clinical cure was achieved in 84.3 or 83.9% of those who received telavancin and 82.8 or 87.7% of those who received vancomycin. In a subset of patients who were microbiologically evaluable and stratified according to the infecting pathogen, the clinical cure rate in those with infections caused by methicillin-susceptible *S. aureus* or MRSA was 82 or 87%, respectively, in those treated with telavancin and 85.1 or 85.9%, respectively, in those treated with vancomycin. The clinical cure rate in those with infections caused by *S. pyogenes*, *S. agalactiae*, *S. anginosus* group, or *E. faecalis* was 84.2, 73.7, 76.5, or 95.6%, respectively, in those treated with telavancin and 90.5, 86.7, 100, or 80%, respectively, in those treated with vancomycin. There was evidence that the clinical cure rate with telavancin was lower in patients in the CE population who were 65 years of age or older (72%) compared with those younger than 65 years of age (87%). In addition, the clinical cure rate with telavancin was lower in those with baseline creatinine clearances of 50 mL/minute or lower compared with those with baseline creatinine clearances exceeding 50 mL/minute.

Dosage and Administration

■ Administration Telavancin hydrochloride is administered by IV infusion.

Telavancin solutions should not be admixed or added to solutions containing other drugs.

If the same IV line is used for sequential infusion of other drugs, the IV line should be flushed with 0.9% sodium chloride injection, 5% dextrose injection, or lactated Ringer's injection before and after the telavancin infusion.

IV Infusion **Reconstitution and Dilution.** Commercially available telavancin hydrochloride for injection must be reconstituted and then further diluted prior to IV infusion. Strict aseptic technique must be observed when preparing IV solutions of telavancin since the drug contains no preservative.

Single-dose vials labeled as containing 250 or 750 mg of telavancin should be reconstituted by adding 15 or 45 mL, respectively, of 5% dextrose injection, sterile water for injection, or 0.9% sodium chloride injection to provide a solution containing 15 mg/mL. To minimize foaming during reconstitution, the vial vacuum should be allowed to pull the diluent from the syringe into the vial; the diluent should not be forcefully injected into the vial. The vial should be discarded if the vacuum is insufficient to pull the diluent into the vial. The reconstituted solution should be mixed thoroughly without forcefully shaking the vial and inspected to ensure complete dissolution. Reconstitution usually takes less than 2 minutes, but may take up to 20 minutes.

For telavancin doses of 150–800 mg, the correct dose should be withdrawn from the reconstituted vial and added to 100–250 mL of appropriate IV infusion solution (i.e., 0.9% sodium chloride injection, 5% dextrose injection, lactated Ringer's injection).

For telavancin doses less than 150 mg or greater than 800 mg, the correct dose should be withdrawn from the reconstituted vial and added to a volume of appropriate IV infusion solution (i.e., 0.9% sodium chloride injection, 5% dextrose injection, or lactated Ringer's injection) that results in a final concentration of 0.6–8 mg/mL.

Reconstituted telavancin solutions (in the original vial) and reconstituted and diluted telavancin solutions (in an IV infusion bag) are stable for 12 hours at room temperature or 7 days when refrigerated at 2–8°C. The total storage time (vial plus IV infusion bag) should not exceed 12 hours at room temperature or 7 days at 2–8°C. Final telavancin IV infusion solutions also can be stored in the infusion bag for up to 32 days at −30 to −10°C.

IV infusion solutions of telavancin should not be shaken. Telavancin solutions should be inspected visually for particulate matter prior to administration.

Rate of Administration. Telavancin solutions should be administered by IV infusion over 1 hour.

Rapid IV infusions should be avoided. (See Infusion Reactions under Warnings/Precautions: Other Warnings/Precautions, in Cautions.)

■ Dosage Dosage of telavancin hydrochloride is expressed in terms of telavancin.

Respiratory Tract Infections **Nosocomial Pneumonia.** The recommended dosage of telavancin for the treatment of hospital-acquired or ventilator-associated bacterial pneumonia in adults 18 years of age or older is 10 mg/kg given by IV infusion once every 24 hours for 7–21 days.

The duration of therapy should be guided by the severity of the infection and the patient's clinical response.

Skin and Skin Structure Infections The recommended dosage of telavancin for the treatment of complicated skin and skin structure infections in adults 18 years of age or older is 10 mg/kg given by IV infusion once every 24 hours for 7–14 days.

The duration of therapy should be guided by the severity and location of the infection and the patient's clinical response.

■ Special Populations ***Renal Impairment*** Because telavancin is eliminated principally by renal excretion, dosage of the drug should be reduced in adults with creatinine clearances of 10–50 mL/minute. (See Table 1.)

Data are insufficient to make dosage recommendations for adults with end-stage renal disease (creatinine clearance less than 10 mL/minute), including those undergoing hemodialysis.

Use of telavancin in patients with preexisting moderate or severe renal impairment (creatinine clearances of 50 mL/minute or lower) should be considered only when anticipated benefits outweigh potential risks. (See Increased Mortality in Patients with Renal Impairment under Warnings/Precautions: Warnings, in Cautions.)

Table 1. Telavancin Dosage for Adults with Renal Impairment

Creatinine Clearance (mL/minute)[a]	Telavancin Dosage
>50	10 mg/kg once every 24 hours
30–50	7.5 mg/kg once every 24 hours
10–<30	10 mg/kg once every 48 hours

[a] Calculate using Cockcroft-Gault formula and ideal body weight; use actual body weight if it is less than ideal body weight.

Hepatic Impairment Dosage adjustments are not needed in adults with mild or moderate hepatic impairment. Pharmacokinetics of telavancin have not been studied in adults with severe hepatic impairment. (See Hepatic Impairment under Warnings/Precautions: Specific Populations, in Cautions.)

Geriatric Patients Dosage adjustments based solely on age are not needed when telavancin is used in geriatric patients, but dosage should be adjusted based on renal function. Because geriatric patients are more likely to have decreased renal function than younger adults, dosage should be selected with caution. (See Geriatric Use under Warnings/Precautions: Specific Populations, in Cautions.)

Cautions

■ Contraindications Telavancin is contraindicated in patients with known hypersensitivity to the drug.

IV unfractionated heparin sodium is contraindicated in patients receiving telavancin. Activated partial thromboplastin time (aPTT) is expected to be artificially prolonged for up to 18 hours after telavancin administration. (See Tests Used to Monitor Coagulation under Cautions: Other Warnings/Precautions.)

■ Warnings/Precautions ***Warnings*** **Increased Mortality in Patients with Renal Impairment.** Increased mortality was observed in patients with preexisting moderate or severe renal impairment (creatinine clearances of 50 mL/minute or lower) receiving telavancin for the treatment of hospital-acquired or ventilator-associated bacterial pneumonia compared with those receiving vancomycin. In an analysis of 2 phase 3 clinical studies evaluating telavancin for the treatment of hospital-acquired or ventilator-associated bacterial pneumonia, all-cause mortality within 28 days of starting treatment in patients with baseline moderate or severe renal impairment was 39% in those treated with telavancin compared with 30% in those treated with vancomycin. In patients with baseline creatinine clearances exceeding 50 mL/minute, all-cause mortality was 17% in those treated with telavancin and 18% in those treated with vancomycin.

Use of telavancin in patients with preexisting moderate or severe renal impairment (creatinine clearances of 50 mL/minute or lower) should be considered only when anticipated benefits outweigh potential risks.

Nephrotoxicity. New-onset or worsening renal impairment has been reported in patients receiving telavancin for the treatment of hospital-acquired or ventilator-associated bacterial pneumonia or complicated skin and skin structure infections. In patients with normal baseline serum creatinine concentrations in clinical studies, increased serum creatinine (1.5 times baseline) was reported more frequently in telavancin-treated patients than in vancomycin-treated patients.

Adverse renal effects are more likely to occur in patients with conditions known to increase the risk of renal impairment (e.g., preexisting renal disease, diabetes mellitus, congestive heart failure, hypertension) and in those receiving concomitant therapy with a drug that affects renal function (e.g., nonsteroidal anti-inflammatory agents [NSAIAs], certain diuretics, angiotensin-converting enzyme [ACE] inhibitors).

Renal function (i.e., serum creatinine, creatinine clearance) should be monitored in all patients receiving telavancin. Renal function tests should be performed prior to initiation of telavancin, every 48–72 hours during treatment (more frequently if indicated), and at the end of treatment.

If renal function decreases, the benefits of continuing telavancin treatment should be weighed against discontinuing the drug and initiating an alternative anti-infective.

Fetal/Neonatal Morbidity. Adverse developmental outcomes have been observed in 3 animal species given telavancin at clinically relevant doses during the period of organogenesis. Because these animal studies have raised concerns about potential adverse developmental outcomes in humans, telavancin should be avoided during pregnancy unless the potential benefits to the woman outweigh potential risks to the fetus. (See Pregnancy under Warnings/Precautions: Specific Populations, in Cautions.)

Women of childbearing potential (i.e., those who have not had complete absence of menses for at least 24 months, medically confirmed menopause or primary ovarian failure, history of hysterectomy, bilateral oophorectomy, or tubal ligation) should have a serum pregnancy test to exclude pregnancy before initiating telavancin. In addition, women of childbearing potential should use effective contraception to prevent pregnancy while receiving telavancin.

Sensitivity Reactions Serious and potentially fatal hypersensitivity reactions, including anaphylactic reactions, have been reported after the first dose or subsequent doses of telavancin.

Telavancin should be discontinued at the first sign of rash or any other sign of hypersensitivity.

Telavancin is a semisynthetic derivative of vancomycin; however, it is not known if patients with hypersensitivity reactions to vancomycin will experience cross-reactivity to telavancin. Telavancin should be used with caution in patients with known hypersensitivity to vancomycin.

Although data are not available regarding cross-reactivity with other glycopeptides (e.g., dalbavancin, oritavancin), the possibility of cross-sensitivity among the glycopeptides should be considered.

Other Warnings/Precautions **Infusion Reactions.** Rapid IV infusion of glycopeptide anti-infectives (including telavancin) can result in a reaction referred to as the "red-man syndrome". Flushing of the upper body, urticaria, pruritus, or rash may occur.

To reduce the risk of infusion-related reactions, IV infusions of telavancin should be given over 1 hour. If an infusion reaction occurs, such reactions may cease if the infusion is discontinued or the rate of infusion slowed.

Cardiovascular Effects. Prolongation of the corrected QT (QT_c) interval has been reported in individuals receiving telavancin.

Caution is advised if telavancin is used concomitantly with drugs known to prolong the QT interval.

Telavancin should be avoided in patients with congenital long QT syndrome, known prolongation of the QT_c interval, uncompensated heart failure, or severe left ventricular hypertrophy since such individuals were not included in telavancin clinical trials.

Hematologic Effects. Telavancin does not interfere with coagulation and has no effect on platelet aggregation. Increased risk of bleeding was not observed in clinical trials of the drug. Evidence of hypercoagulability has not been observed, and healthy adults receiving telavancin have normal levels of D-dimer and fibrin degradation products.

Reduced Efficacy in Patients with Moderate or Severe Renal Impairment. Results of a subgroup analysis of phase 3 clinical trials in patients with skin and skin structure infections indicated that the clinical cure rate in telavancin-treated patients with baseline moderate or severe renal impairment (creatinine clearances of 50 mL/minute or lower) was 67% and was lower than the clinical cure rate in those with baseline creatinine clearances exceeding 50 mL/minute (87%). Reductions in clinical cure rates of this magnitude were not observed in patients receiving the comparator anti-infective (vancomycin).

Clinicians should consider such data regarding reduced efficacy when selecting anti-infectives for treatment of complicated skin and skin structure infections in patients with baseline moderate or severe renal impairment (creatinine clearances of 50 mL/minute or lower).

Tests Used to Monitor Coagulation. Telavancin interferes with certain tests used to monitor coagulation, including prothrombin time (PT), international normalized ratio (INR), activated partial thromboplastin time (aPTT), activated clotting time, and tests based on factor X activity assay, if blood for these tests is drawn 0–18 hours after a telavancin dose. This occurs because telavancin binds to the artificial phospholipid surfaces added to the anticoagulation tests and interferes with the ability of the coagulation complexes to assemble on the surface of the phospholipids and promote in vitro clotting. The manufacturer recommends that blood specimens for such tests be drawn just before a dose of telavancin.

Telavancin does not affect the results of other coagulation tests, including thrombin time, whole blood (Lee-White) clotting time, platelet aggregation study, chromogenic anti-factor Xa assay, functional (chromogenic) factor X activity assay, bleeding time, and tests for D-dimer and fibrin degradation products. Blood specimens for these coagulation tests may be collected at any time in patients receiving telavancin.

In patients requiring aPTT monitoring while receiving telavancin, a non-phospholipid-dependent coagulation test (e.g., factor Xa chromogenic assay) should be used or an alternative anticoagulant not requiring aPTT monitoring may be considered.

Tests Used to Monitor Urine Protein. Telavancin interferes with urine qualitative dipstick protein assays and quantitative dye methods (e.g., pyrogallol red-molybdate) used to measure urine protein. Microalbumin assays are not affected by telavancin and can be used to monitor urinary protein excretion in patients receiving telavancin.

Superinfection/Clostridium difficile-associated Diarrhea and Colitis (CDAD). Use of telavancin may result in overgrowth of nonsusceptible organisms, including fungi. The patient should be carefully monitored and appropriate therapy should be instituted if a superinfection occurs.

Treatment with anti-infectives alters normal colon flora and may permit overgrowth of *Clostridium difficile*. *C. difficile* infection (CDI) and *C. difficile*-associated diarrhea and colitis (CDAD; also known as antibiotic-associated diarrhea and colitis or pseudomembranous colitis) have been reported with nearly all anti-infectives and may range in severity from mild diarrhea to fatal colitis. *C. difficile* produces toxins A and B which contribute to development of CDAD; hypertoxin-producing strains of *C. difficile* are associated with increased morbidity and mortality since these infections may be refractory to anti-infective therapy and may require colectomy.

CDAD should be considered in the differential diagnosis of patients who develop diarrhea during or after anti-infective therapy. Careful medical history is necessary since CDAD has been reported to occur as late as 2 months or longer after anti-infective therapy is discontinued.

If CDAD is suspected or confirmed, anti-infective therapy not directed against *C. difficile* should be discontinued whenever possible. Patients should be managed with appropriate supportive therapy (fluid and electrolyte management, protein supplementation), anti-infective therapy directed against *C. difficile* (e.g., metronidazole, vancomycin), and surgical evaluation as clinically indicated.

Selection and Use of Anti-infectives. To reduce development of drug-resistant bacteria and maintain effectiveness of telavancin and other antibacterials, the drug should be used only for treatment of infections proven or strongly suspected to be caused by susceptible bacteria.

When selecting or modifying anti-infective therapy, results of culture and in vitro susceptibility testing should be used. In the absence of such data, local epidemiology and susceptibility patterns should be considered when selecting anti-infectives for empiric therapy.

If documented or presumed pathogens include gram-negative or anaerobic bacteria, concomitant use of an anti-infective active against such bacteria may be clinically indicated. (See Uses.)

Specific Populations **Pregnancy.** Category C. (See Users Guide.)

A pregnancy registry has been established to monitor maternal-fetal outcomes in pregnant women exposed to telavancin. Clinicians are encouraged to contact the registry at 855-633-8479 to report cases of prenatal exposure to telavancin; alternatively, pregnant women may enroll.

In reproduction studies in rats, rabbits, and minipigs that received telavancin during the period of organogenesis at doses that resulted in exposure levels approximately onefold to twofold the human exposure (area under the plasma concentration-time curve [AUC]) at the maximum recommended human dosage, there was evidence that telavancin has the potential to cause limb and skeletal malformations and reduced fetal weight. Malformations included brachymelia (rats, rabbits), syndactyly (rats, minipigs), adactyly (rabbits), and polydactyly (minipigs).

Although telavancin has not been evaluated in pregnant women, the animal data raise concerns about potential adverse developmental outcomes in humans. Telavancin should be avoided during pregnancy unless the potential benefits to the woman outweigh the potential risks to the fetus. (See Fetal/Neonatal Morbidity under Warnings/Precautions: Warnings, in Cautions.)

Lactation. Not known whether telavancin is distributed into milk in humans. Telavancin should be used with caution in nursing women.

Pediatric Use. Safety and efficacy of telavancin have not been evaluated in patients younger than 18 years of age.

Geriatric Use. In clinical studies evaluating telavancin for the treatment of complicated skin and skin structure infections, the drug appeared to be less effective in adults 65 years of age or older relative to adults younger than 65 years of age. Although there were no overall differences in frequency of treatment-emergent adverse events in geriatric adults compared with younger adults in these studies, the incidence of adverse events indicating renal impairment was higher in geriatric adults treated with telavancin than in younger adults treated with the drug.

In clinical studies evaluating telavancin for the treatment of hospital-acquired or ventilator-associated bacterial pneumonia, treatment-emergent adverse events as well as deaths and other serious adverse events occurred more often in patients 65 years of age or older than in those younger than 65 years of age in both the telavancin treatment group and comparator treatment group.

Telavancin is substantially eliminated by the kidneys, and the risk of adverse effects may be greater in patients with impaired renal function. Dosage should be selected with caution since geriatric patients are more likely to have decreased renal function. Dosage adjustments in geriatric patients should be based on renal function.

Hepatic Impairment. Telavancin pharmacokinetics are not altered in adults with moderate hepatic impairment (Child-Pugh class B); pharmacokinetics of the drug have not been evaluated in those with severe hepatic impairment (Child-Pugh class C). Dosage adjustment is not needed in adults with mild or moderate hepatic impairment.

Renal Impairment. In clinical studies evaluating telavancin for the treatment of hospital-acquired or ventilator-associated bacterial pneumonia, mortality rates in adults with creatinine clearances of 50 mL/minute or lower were higher in telavancin-treated patients compared with those receiving the comparator anti-infective (vancomycin). In clinical studies evaluating telavancin for the treatment of complicated skin and skin structure infections, the clinical cure rate with telavancin was lower in adults with creatinine clearances of 50 mL/minute or lower compared with those with creatinine clearances exceeding 50 mL/minute. Such data should be considered when selecting an anti-infective for adults with baseline moderate or severe renal impairment (creatinine clearances of 50 mL/minute or lower), and telavancin should be considered for such patients only when the anticipated benefits outweigh the potential risks.

Patients with preexisting renal impairment or risk factors for renal dysfunction may be at greater risk for adverse renal effects during telavancin therapy than individuals with normal renal function. (See Nephrotoxicity under Warnings/Precautions: Other Warnings/Precautions, in Cautions.)

Patients with creatinine clearances of 10–50 mL/minute should receive a reduced telavancin dosage. (See Dosage and Administration: Special Populations.)

Hydroxypropyl-β-cyclodextrin (an inactive ingredient in the formulation) may accumulate in individuals with renal impairment. If renal toxicity is suspected, an alternative anti-infective should be considered.

■ Common Adverse Effects Adverse effects reported in 5% or more of patients receiving telavancin for the treatment of hospital-acquired or ventilator-associated bacterial pneumonia include GI effects (nausea, vomiting, diarrhea, constipation), anemia, hypokalemia, hypotension, decubitus ulcer, insomnia, peripheral edema, and renal effects (renal impairment or insufficiency, acute renal failure, chronic renal failure, increased serum creatinine).

Adverse effects reported in 7% or more of patients receiving telavancin for the treatment of complicated skin and skin structure infections include GI effects (taste disturbance, nausea, vomiting, diarrhea, constipation), headache, insomnia, and foamy urine.

Drug Interactions

■ Drugs Affecting or Metabolized by Hepatic Microsomal Enzymes In vitro studies indicate that telavancin inhibits the cytochrome P-450 (CYP) isoenzyme 3A4/5.

■ Anti-infective Agents In vitro, the antibacterial effects of telavancin and cefepime, ceftriaxone, ciprofloxacin, gentamicin, meropenem, or rifampin are synergistic against methicillin-resistant *Staphylococcus aureus* (MRSA; also known as oxacillin-resistant *S. aureus* or ORSA).

In vitro studies indicate that the antibacterial effects of telavancin and amikacin, aztreonam, cefepime, ceftriaxone, ciprofloxacin, co-trimoxazole, gentamicin, imipenem, meropenem, oxacillin, fixed combination of piperacillin sodium and tazobactam sodium (piperacillin and tazobactam), or rifampin are not antagonistic against telavancin-susceptible staphylococci, streptococci, or enterococci.

Aztreonam Concomitant use of aztreonam and telavancin does not affect the pharmacokinetics of either drug.

Dosage adjustments are not needed if aztreonam and telavancin are used concomitantly.

Piperacillin and Tazobactam Concomitant use of piperacillin and tazobactam and telavancin does not affect the pharmacokinetics of either drug.

Dosage adjustments are not needed if piperacillin and tazobactam is used concomitantly with telavancin.

■ Heparin Because activated partial thromboplastin time (aPTT) is expected to be artificially prolonged for up to 18 hours after telavancin administration, IV unfractionated heparin sodium is contraindicated in patients receiving telavancin. (See Tests Used to Monitor Coagulation under Warnings/Precautions: Other Warnings/Precautions, in Cautions.)

■ Midazolam Concomitant use of midazolam and telavancin does not affect the pharmacokinetics of either drug.

Description

Telavancin is a lipoglycopeptide antibacterial and is a semisynthetic derivative of vancomycin.

In vitro, telavancin is bactericidal in action against susceptible gram-positive bacteria. Telavancin inhibits bacterial cell wall synthesis by inhibiting peptidoglycan synthesis and blocking the transglycosylation step. Telavancin binds to the bacterial membrane and disrupts membrane barrier function.

Telavancin is active in vitro and in clinical infections against *Staphylococcus aureus* (including methicillin-resistant *S. aureus* [MRSA; also known as oxacillin-resistant *S. aureus* or ORSA]), *Streptococcus pyogenes* (group A β-hemolytic streptococci, GAS), *S. agalactiae* (group B streptococci, GBS), *S. anginosus* group (includes *S. anginosus*, *S. intermedius*, and *S. constellatus*), and *Enterococcus faecalis* (vancomycin-susceptible strains only).

Telavancin also is active in vitro against *E. faecium* (vancomycin-susceptible strains only), *S. haemolyticus*, *S. dysgalactiae* subsp. *equisimilis*, and *S. epidermidis*; however, safety and efficacy of the drug in treating clinical infections caused by these bacteria have not been established.

Some vancomycin-resistant enterococci have reduced susceptibility to telavancin. Cross-resistance between telavancin and other anti-infectives has not been reported to date.

Advice to Patients

Telavancin medication guide must be provided to the patient each time the drug is dispensed; importance of patient reading the medication guide prior to initiating telavancin therapy and each time the prescription is refilled.

Advise patients that antibacterials (including telavancin) should only be used to treat bacterial infections and not used to treat viral infections (e.g., the common cold).

Importance of completing full course of therapy, even if feeling better after a few days.

Advise patients that skipping doses or not completing the full course of therapy may decrease effectiveness and increase the likelihood that bacteria will develop resistance and will not be treatable with telavancin or other antibacterials in the future.

Advise patients that diarrhea is a common problem caused by anti-infectives and usually ends when the drug is discontinued. Importance of contacting a clinician if watery and bloody stools (with or without stomach cramps and fever) occur during or as late as 2 months or longer after the last dose.

Advise patients about the common adverse effects reported with telavancin (e.g., taste disturbance, nausea, vomiting, headache, foamy urine) and importance of informing a clinician if they develop any unusual symptom or if any known symptom persists or worsens.

Importance of informing clinicians of existing or contemplated concomitant therapy, including prescription and OTC drugs, and any concomitant illnesses.

Importance of women informing clinicians if they are or plan to become pregnant or plan to breast-feed. Advise women of childbearing potential about potential risk of fetal harm if telavancin is used during pregnancy. (See Pregnancy under Warnings/Precautions: Specific Populations, in Cautions.)

Importance of excluding pregnancy with a serum pregnancy test before starting telavancin. Advise women of childbearing potential to use effective contraception to prevent pregnancy during telavancin therapy and to notify a clinician if pregnancy occurs during telavancin therapy. (See Pregnancy under Warnings/Precautions: Specific Populations, in Cautions.)

Importance of informing patients of other important precautionary information. (See Cautions.)

Overview® (see Users Guide). For additional information on this drug until a more detailed monograph is developed and published, the manufacturer's labeling should be consulted. It is *essential* that the manufacturer's labeling be consulted for more detailed information on usual cautions, precautions, contraindications, potential drug interactions, laboratory test interferences, and acute toxicity.

Preparations

Excipients in commercially available drug preparations may have clinically important effects in some individuals; consult specific product labeling for details.

Telavancin Hydrochloride

Parenteral

For injection, for IV infusion	250 mg (of telavancin)	**Vibativ®**, Theravance
	750 mg (of telavancin)	**Vibativ®**, Theravance

Vancomycin Hydrochloride

■ Vancomycin is a tricyclic glycopeptide antibiotic that is unrelated to other commercially available antibiotics.

Uses

IV vancomycin hydrochloride is used in the treatment of potentially life-threatening infections caused by susceptible bacteria when other less toxic anti-infectives cannot be used or would be ineffective. Vancomycin is used principally for the treatment of severe infections caused by gram-positive bacteria in patients who cannot receive or who have failed to respond to penicillins and cephalosporins or for the treatment of gram-positive bacterial infections that are resistant to β-lactams and other anti-infectives.

■ Drug Use Guidelines for the Prevention of Vancomycin Resistance Use of, and exposure to, anti-infectives are major risk factors for the emergence of anti-infective–resistant pathogens, and anti-infective resistance results in increased morbidity, mortality, and healthcare costs. Prevention of the emergence of drug resistance, its dissemination among pathogens, and the spread of such pathogens has become an increasingly important public health problem. Medical, pharmacy, and other staff and individuals responsible for drug-use policy and formulary decisions should review and restrict the use of certain anti-infectives, including vancomycin, and ensure that their use is appropriate. Clinicians should recognize that unnecessary and inappropriate use of anti-infectives has important, far-reaching implications for human health globally.

Because of the rapidly increasing prevalence of vancomycin-resistant enterococci in the US and concerns regarding the possibility of vancomycin-resistant strains of other gram-positive bacteria (e.g., *Staphylococcus aureus*) (see Resistance), a subcommittee of the US Centers for Disease Control and Prevention (CDC) Hospital Infection Control Practices Advisory Committee and others have made recommendations designed to prevent the spread of vancomycin resistance. The CDC recommends that hospitals in collaboration with quality improvement and infection control programs, pharmacy and therapeutics committees, and clinical, microbiology, nursing, administrative, and housekeeping departments develop comprehensive, institution-specific strategic plans for the detection, prevention, and control of infection and colonization with vancomycin-resistant enterococci and other bacterial pathogens. Since vancomycin use has consistently been reported to be a risk factor for colonization and infection with vancomycin-resistant enterococci, these strategic plans should include recommendations for the prudent use of vancomycin. In addition, all hospitals and other health-care delivery services (even those that have not had reports of vancomycin-resistant enterococci) should develop a comprehensive antimicrobial-utilization plan to provide education for their medical staff and medical students, oversee surgical prophylaxis, and develop guidelines for the appropriate use of vancomycin as applicable to their particular institution. Continuing education programs for hospital staff (e.g., attending and consulting physicians, medical students and residents, personnel in pharmacy, nursing, and laboratory departments) should include information on the epidemiology of vancomycin-resistant enterococci and the potential impact on cost and outcome of patient care. Enterococcal isolates obtained from blood, sterile body sites (with the possible exception of sterile urine), and other sites as clinically indicated should be evaluated for vancomycin resistance and high-level resistance to penicillin (or ampicillin) and aminoglycosides. If resources permit, laboratories may choose to routinely test wound and urine isolates for resistance to vancomycin, penicillin, and ampicillin.

Patients with vancomycin-resistant *Enterococcus faecium* (VREF) or staphylococcal infections that have not responded to appropriate anti-infective therapy or in whom vancomycin-resistant strains are suspected or documented may be candidates for treatment with linezolid (Zyvox®) or the fixed combination of quinupristin and dalfopristin (Synercid®). (See Uses in Quinupristin and Dalfopristin 8:12.28.32 and in Linezolid 8:12.28.24). Linezolid may be active against vancomycin-resistant *E. faecalis*, but quinupristin and dalfopristin is *not* active against *E. faecalis*, and enterococcal species differentiation is important to avoid misidentification of this organism.

Based on recent reports of staphylococci, including oxacillin-resistant staphylococci, with reduced susceptibility to vancomycin and concerns about the possible appearance of staphylococci highly resistant to vancomycin,the CDC Hospital Infection Control Practices Advisory Committee also has issued interim guidelines designed to prevent and control the spread of infection caused by such strains. The interim guidelines include steps to decrease the likelihood of emergence of staphylococci with reduced susceptibility to vancomycin (e.g., limiting overuse and misuse of vancomycin), information on how to identify strains with reduced susceptibility to vancomycin (see Spectrum: In Vitro Susceptibility Testing), information on how to obtain an investigational antistaphylococcal anti-infective agent if use of such an agent is considered necessary (see Uses: Staphylococcal Infections), and information on infection control measures that should be used to prevent the spread of such strains within and between facilities and minimize the potential for the organism to become endemic.

The CDC recommends that vancomycin be reserved for use in the treatment of serious infections caused by gram-positive bacteria resistant to β-lactam anti-infectives; treatment of gram-positive bacterial infections in patients with severe hypersensitivity to β-lactam anti-infectives; prophylaxis in certain patients at high risk for bacterial endocarditis as recommended by the American Heart Association (AHA); treatment of antibiotic-associated pseudomembranous colitis that is severe or potentially life-threatening or that fails to respond to oral metronidazole; and for perioperative prophylaxis for major surgical procedures involving implantation of prosthetic materials or devices (e.g., cardiac and vascular procedures and total hip replacement) at institutions with a high rate of oxacillin-resistant (methicillin-resistant) *S. aureus* (ORSA; MRSA) or *S. epidermidis*. The CDC suggests that use of the drug in other situations be discouraged. Situation in which the use of vancomycin should be discouraged include: treatment of antibiotic-associated colitis when metronidazole would be effective; *routine* empiric therapy for febrile neutropenic patients, unless there is strong evidence that the infection is caused by gram-positive organisms (e.g., inflamed exit site of Hickman catheter) and the prevalence of ORSA in the hospital is substantial; continued use after results of in vitro tests indicate that an infection is not caused by gram-positive organisms resistant to β-lactam anti-infectives; selective decontamination of the GI tract; eradication of colonization with ORSA; *routine* prophylaxis in patients undergoing surgery, except in patients with life-threatening allergy to β-lactam anti-infectives; routine prophylaxis in patients undergoing continuous ambulatory peritoneal dialysis or hemodialysis; systemic or local (e.g., antibiotic lock) prophylaxis for infection or colonization of indwelling central or peripheral intravascular catheters; routine prophylaxis in very low birthweight neonates; use for topical application or irrigation; use for treatment of infections caused by gram-positive organisms susceptible to β-lactam anti-infectives; and use in response to a single blood culture positive for coagulase-negative staphylococci if other blood cultures drawn in the same time frame are negative (i.e., contamination of the blood culture with skin flora is likely).

■ **Staphylococcal Infections** Although vancomycin hydrochloride is not effective by the oral route for the treatment of systemic infections, the drug is used orally for the treatment of enterocolitis caused by *S. aureus* (including oxacillin-resistant strains). Some clinicians consider vancomycin the drug of choice for staphylococcal enterocolitis because it does not affect the normal coliform bacteria present in the GI tract.

IV vancomycin has been used effective when used alone in the treatment of endocarditis, osteomyelitis, pneumonia, septicemia, and soft-tissue infections caused by *S. aureus* or *S. epidermidis*, including oxacillin-resistant strains.

IV vancomycin, alone or in conjunction with other anti-infectives, generally is considered the treatment of choice for infections caused by oxacillin-resistant staphylococci. Because oxacillin-resistant staphylococci are being reported with increasing frequency, initial therapy for suspected staphylococcal infections should include vancomycin if oxacillin-resistant strains are prevalent in the community or hospital. Patients with diabetes mellitus, peripheral vascular disease, or burn wounds appear to be at particularly high risk of acquiring oxacillin-resistant *S. aureus* or *S. epidermidis* has been reported frequently in patients with prosthetic valve endocarditis or infected CSF shunts and in granulocytopenic children with cancer. However, in a study of empiric therapy in a limited number of febrile, neutropenic cancer patients, addition of vancomycin to a regimen of ceftazidime and amikacin did not improve outcome and was associated with more frequent nephrotoxicity; it has been suggested that such vancomycin use generally be limited to patients with likely or documented gram-positive bacteremia or in institutions where gram-positive bacteremia (especially if caused by oxacillin-resistant staphylococci) is common. In addition, if empiric therapy initially includes vancomycin, it generally is recommended that the drug be discontinued 3–4 days later if a fulminant gram-positive infection is not confirmed. (See Uses: Empiric Therapy in Febrile Neutropenic Patients.)

Infections caused by oxacillin-resistant *S. epidermidis* generally are treated with vancomycin alone or vancomycin in conjunction with rifampin and/or an aminoglycoside. When ORSA is suspected in patients with bacteremia or sepsis, vancomycin (with or without gentamicin and/or rifampin) often is added to the empiric regimen. Vancomycin has been effective when given by instillation via the arteriovenous shunt† for the treatment and prophylaxis of staphylococcal infections in hemodialysis patients. The drug also has been effective when given IV for the treatment of peritonitis caused by susceptible staphylococci or other gram-positive bacteria in peritoneal dialysis patients.

Vancomycin does not replace appropriate surgical measures when staphylococcal infections are localized and purulent.

IV vancomycin is considered the drug of choice for the treatment of endocarditis caused by oxacillin-resistant staphylococci. While a regimen of vancomycin administered alone is recommended for oxacillin-resistant staphylococcal endocarditis in patients with native cardiac valves, patients with a prosthetic valve or other prosthetic material should receive a combination regimen of IV vancomycin, oral or IV rifampin, and IV or IM gentamicin. Patients with endocarditis caused by oxacillin-susceptible staphylococci generally should receive a regimen that consists of a penicillinase-resistant penicillin (i.e., IV nafcillin or IV oxacillin) with or without IM or IV gentamicin; oral or IV rifampin is added if a prosthetic valve or other prosthetic material is present. Penicillin- allergic patients with oxacillin-susceptible staphylococcal endocarditis who have native cardiac valves usually can receive IV cefazolin with or without IM or IV gentamicin unless they have a history of immediate-type penicillin hypersensitivity; IV vancomycin usually is reserved for use as an alternative agent for the treatment of patients with a history of immediate-type hypersensitivity to penicillin. Patients with a prosthetic valve or other prosthetic materials who have staphylococcal endocarditis caused by oxacillin-susceptible strains should receive a regimen of a penicillinase-resistant penicillin (i.e., IV nafcillin or IV oxacillin) with oral or IV rifampin and IM or IV gentamicin; IV cefazolin or IV vancomycin should be substituted for the penicillin in those with penicillin hypersensitivity.

Because staphylococcal isolates with reduced susceptibility to vancomycin have recently been reported in patients who received the drug, staphylococci from patients who fail to respond to vancomycin therapy should be tested to determine if resistance to the drug has developed. Patients with staphylococcal infections that have not responded to appropriate anti-infective therapy may be candidates for treatment with quinupristin and dalfopristin (Synercid®) if the causative organism is found to have reduced susceptibility to vancomycin. (See Uses in Quinupristin and Dalfopristin 8:12.28.32.)

■ **Streptococcal Infections** While a regimen of IV penicillin G (with or without IM or IV gentamicin) or a regimen of IV or IM ceftriaxone usually is recommended for the treatment of endocarditis caused by viridans streptococci or *S. bovis*, IV vancomycin is the regimen of choice for patients with a history of immediate-type hypersensitivity to penicillin. For the treatment of enterococcal endocarditis, a regimen of either IV penicillin G or IV ampicillin with IM or IV gentamicin is preferred for most patients; however, a regimen of IV vancomycin with IM or IV gentamicin is considered the regimen of choice for the treatment of enterococcal endocarditis in patients with a history of immediate-type hypersensitivity to penicillins.

Vancomycin is used alone or in conjunction with a third generation cephalosporin (ceftriaxone, cefotaxime) with or without rifampin for the treatment of infections caused by *Streptococcus pneumoniae* that are highly resistant to penicillins. Highly penicillin-resistant *S. pneumoniae* also may have reduced susceptibility to third generation cephalosporins (e.g., cefotaxime, ceftriaxone). In areas where there have been reports of highly penicillin-resistant*S. pneumoniae* that also have reduced susceptibility to third generation cephalosporins, the CDC and many clinicians recommend use of vancomycin (with or without rifampin) in conjunction with a third generation cephalosporin (e.g., cefotaxime, ceftriaxone) for empiric treatment of severe, life-threatening infections (e.g., meningitis) pending results of in vitro susceptibility tests. Vancomycin should be discontinued if the causative organism is found to be susceptible to the cephalosporin. Vancomycin has been used in conjunction with rifampin for the treatment of pneumococcal meningitis in patients hypersensitive to penicillins. There is evidence that vancomycin used alone may not achieve effective CSF concentrations in some patients, and the drug should not be used alone for the treatment of pneumococcal meningitis. Although vancomycin has been administered intrathecally† for the treatment of meningitis caused by susceptible organisms, the manufacturers state that safety and efficacy of intrathecal (intralumbar or intraventricular) administration have not been determined.

■ **Endocarditis** IV vancomycin is used for the treatment of bacterial endocarditis and for prevention of bacterial endocarditis.

Treatment IV vancomycin is used for the treatment of endocarditis caused by *S. aureus* or *S. epidermidis*, including oxacillin-resistant strains, and is considered the drug of choice for the treatment of endocarditis caused by oxacillin-resistant staphylococci. (See Uses: Staphylococcal Infections.) IV vancomycin also is used for the treatment of endocarditis caused by viridans streptococci or *S. bovis* in patients with a history of immediate-type hypersensitivity to penicillin. (See Uses: Enterococcal Infections.) Vancomycin also has been reported to be effective for the treatment of diphtheroid endocarditis.

Prevention IV vancomycin is used as an alternative agent for prevention of enterococcal endocarditis in penicillin-allergic adults and children with congenital heart disease, rheumatic or other acquired valvular heart dysfunction (even after valvular surgery), prosthetic heart valves (including bioprosthetic and allograft valves), surgically constructed systemic pulmonary shunts or conduits, hypertrophic cardiomyopathy, mitral valve prolapse with valvular regurgitation and/or thickened leaflets, or previous bacterial endocarditis (even in the absence of heart disease), who undergo certain GI, biliary tract, or genitourinary surgery or instrumentation likely to cause transient bacteremia and increase the risk of endocarditis. These procedures include sclerotherapy for esophageal varices; esophageal structure dilation; endoscopic retrograde cholangiography with biliary obstruction, biliary tract surgery; surgical operations that involve intestinal mucosa; prostatic surgery, cystoscopy; and urethral dilation.

The AHA recognizes that its current recommendations for prophylaxis against bacterial endocarditis are empiric, since no controlled efficacy studies have been published, and that prophylaxis of endocarditis is not always effective. However, the AHA generally recommends routine use of prophylactic anti-infectives in patients with the cardiac conditions described above since these are associated with a high or moderate risk for bacterial endocarditis.

Prophylaxis against bacterial endocarditis is not considered necessary for adults or children with cardiac conditions considered to be associated with a negligible risk for endocarditis since these individuals are at no greater risk than the general population. Therefore, prophylaxis against bacterial endocarditis is not considered necessary for individuals with a history of isolated secundum atrial septal defect; surgical repair of atrial septal defect, ventricular septal defect, or patent ductus arteriosus (without residua beyond 6 months); previous coronary artery bypass graft surgery; mitral valve prolapse without valvar regurgitation; physiologic, functional, or innocent heart murmurs; previous Kawasaki disease without valvar dysfunction; previous rheumatic fever without valvar dysfunction; or cardiac pacemaker (intravascular and epicardial) and implanted defibrillators. When selecting anti-infectives for prophylaxis of bacterial endocarditis, the current recommendations of the AHA should be consulted.

■ **Clostridium difficile-associated Diarrhea and Colitis** Although vancomycin hydrochloride is not effective by the oral route for the treatment of systemic infections, the drug is used orally for the treatment of *Clostridium difficile*-associated diarrhea and colitis (CDAD; also known as antibiotic-associated diarrhea and colitis, *C. difficile* diarrhea, *C. difficile* colitis, and pseudomembranous colitis) in seriously ill patients (i.e., with severe or potentially life-threatening colitis) or those who cannot tolerate or do not respond to oral metronidazole.

Oral metronidazole appears to be as effective as oral vancomycin for the treatment of pseudomembranous colitis caused by *C. difficile*. Therefore, because of cost considerations and concerns about increasing enterococcal and other (e.g., staphylococcal) resistance to vancomycin (see Resistance) and the risk of selection of such strains secondary to widespread and/or injudicious use of the drug, most experts and clinicians state that oral metronidazole therapy is preferred (unless a resistant strain of *C. difficile* is suspected or therapy with metronidazole is contraindicated or not tolerated) when anti-infective therapy is indicated for most cases of antibiotic-associated colitis and diarrhea. The relative efficacy of oral metronidazole for *severe, potentially life-threatening* cases of pseudomembranous colitis remains unclear, and some clinicians continue to consider vancomycin the drug of choice when anti-infective therapy is indicated for such cases (e.g., in critically ill patients). Most clinicians currently recommend that oral vancomycin only be used for the treatment of *C. difficile*-associated colitis in seriously ill patients (i.e., with severe or potentially life-threatening colitis) or those who cannot tolerate or do not respond to oral metronidazole.

After oral vancomycin therapy is initiated, fever may resolve within 24–48 hours and diarrhea generally remits gradually over about 3–5 days; however, resolution of fever and diarrhea occasionally may take a week or longer, probably because of persistent inflammation despite cessation of toxin production. Relapse, which usually is apparent within several weeks (occasionally up to several months) and probably is secondary to persistent germinating *C. difficile* spores or reinfection with the same or different strains, occurs in about 10–35% of patients treated with an effective anti-infective but generally responds to additional therapy with the same or an alternative anti-infective; true treatment failures (i.e., secondary to resistant strains) are rare. Although oral vancomycin also has been used in combination with oral rifampin for possible synergistic or other combined activity against *C. difficile* and/or its spores, the role, if any, of this approach in the treatment of multiple relapses remains to be established.

Oral vancomycin or oral metronidazole also has been used to *prevent* nosocomial outbreaks of *C. difficile* diarrhea and colitis† in institutionalized patients who asymptomatically harbor the organism. However, current evidence suggests that the risks of such prophylactic therapy (e.g., in selecting potentially resistant organisms such as enterococci), particularly with vancomycin, outweigh any possible benefit. Most experts currently recommend that appropriate enteric and barrier precautions (e.g., isolation of patients, private bathroom facilities, strict hygiene) rather than prophylactic anti-infective therapy be implemented to prevent nosocomial transmission of the organisms.

For additional information on the management of this infection, see Uses: *Clostridium difficile*-associated Diarrhea and Colitis in Metronidazole 8:30.04, and also see Cautions: GI Effects in Clindamycin 8:12.28.20.

■ **Respiratory Tract Infections** Although not considered a drug of choice for the treatment of community-acquired pneumonia† (CAP), there may be some situations when IV vancomycin is included in anti-infective regimen used for empiric therapy of severe CAP that may be caused by *S. aureus* (e.g., in patients from a nursing home known to harbor this organism). In addition, use of IV vancomycin may be considered for the initial treatment of pneumonia caused by highly penicillin-resistant *S. pneumoniae*, especially when cephalosporins (e.g., ceftriaxone, cefotaxime) cannot be used. (See Uses: Streptococcal Infections.)

■ **Bacillus Infections** Vancomycin is recommended by some clinicians as a drug of choice for the treatment of infections caused by *Bacillus cereus*† or *B. subtilis*†.

■ **Capnocytophaga Infections** Vancomycin is used for the treatment of infections caused by *Capnocytophaga*†. Optimum regimens for the treatment of infections caused by *Capnocytophaga* have not been identified; however, some clinicians recommend use of penicillin G or, alternatively, a third generation cephalosporin (cefotaxime, ceftizoxime, ceftriaxone), a carbapenem (imipenem and cilastatin sodium, meropenem), vancomycin, a fluoroquinolone, or clindamycin.

■ **Corynebacterium Infections** Vancomycin is recommended by some clinicians as a drug of choice for the treatment of infections caused by *Corynebacterium jeikeium* (JK group). The drug has been used concomitantly with rifampin and/or an aminoglycoside for the treatment of early-onset prosthetic valve endocarditis caused by diphtheroids (e.g., *C. jeikeium*).

■ **Rhodococcus Infections** Some clinicians suggest that infections caused by *Rhodococcus equi*† be treated with a regimen of vancomycin used in conjunction with a fluoroquinolone, rifampin, imipenem (or meropenem), or amikacin. In at least one HIV-infected patient, vancomycin used in conjunction with imipenem was effective for the treatment of pulmonary infection caused by *R. equi*. *R. equi* has been identified as a cause of pulmonary infections (e.g., lung abscess) in immunocompromised individuals, including HIV-infected patients and solid organ transplant recipients. Although optimum regimens for the treatment of these infections have not been identified, combination regimens usually are recommended.

■ **Prevention of Perinatal Group B Streptococcal Disease** IV vancomycin is used as an alternative to parenteral penicillin G or ampicillin for prevention of perinatal group B streptococcal (GBS) disease† in certain women who are hypersensitive to penicillin. Pregnant women who are colonized with GBS in the genital or rectal areas can transmit GBS infection to their infants during labor and delivery resulting in invasive neonatal infection that can be associated with substantial morbidity and mortality. Intrapartum anti-infective prophylaxis for prevention of early-onset neonatal GBS disease is administered *selectively* to women at high risk for transmitting GBS infection to their neonates.

When intrapartum prophylaxis is indicated in the mother, penicillin G is the regimen of choice and ampicillin is the preferred alternative. When intrapartum prophylaxis to prevent GBS in the neonate is indicated in women who are hypersensitive to penicillins, the CDC recommends a regimen of IV cefazolin for those allergic to penicillins who are *not* at high risk for anaphylaxis. For those allergic to penicillins who are at high risk for anaphylaxis (e.g., those with a history of immediate penicillin hypersensitivity, such as anaphylaxis, angioedema, or urticaria; those with a history of asthma or other conditions that would make anaphylaxis more dangerous or difficult to treat, including individuals receiving β-adrenergic blocking agents), the CDC recommends a regimen of IV clindamycin or IV erythromycin. However, the fact that *S. agalactiae* (group B streptococci) with in vitro resistance to clindamycin and erythromycin have been reported with increasing frequency should be considered when choosing an alternative to penicillins for these patients. In addition, strains of GBS resistant to erythromycin often are resistant to clindamycin, although this may not be evident in results of in vitro testing. When use of erythromycin or clindamycin is being considered in a women hypersensitive to penicillin, in vitro susceptibility testing of clinical isolates obtained during GBS prenatal screening should be performed whenever possible to determine if the isolates are susceptible to these drugs. If in vitro susceptibility testing is not possible, results are unknown, or isolates are found to be resistant to erythromycin or clindamycin, a regimen of vancomycin should be used for intrapartum prophylaxis in women with penicillin allergy who are at high risk for anaphylaxis.

For additional information on prevention of perinatal GBS disease, see Uses: Prevention of Perinatal Group B Streptococcal Disease, in the Natural Penicillins General Statement 8:12.16.04.

■ **Perioperative Prophylaxis** IV vancomycin is used for perioperative prophylaxis† to reduce the risk of infection in patients undergoing cardiac surgery (e.g., placement of electrophysiologic devices, ventricular assist devices, ventriculoatrial shunts, arterial patches), neurosurgery (e.g., craniotomy, spinal surgery), orthopedic surgery (e.g., joint replacement, internal fixation of compound or open fractures with nails, plates, screws, or wires), thoracic (noncardiac) surgery (pulmonary resection, closed-tube thoracostomy for chest trauma with hemothorax or pneumothorax), or vascular surgery (arterial reconstructive surgery involving the abdominal aorta, leg procedures that include a groin incision, lower extremity amputation for ischemia) at institutions where oxacillin-resistant *S. epidermidis* are frequent causes of postoperative wound infection. Vancomycin also is used for perioperative prophylaxis in patients undergoing these procedures when the drugs of first choice (cefazolin, cefuroxime) cannot be used because the patient is hypersensitive to β-lactam anti-infectives. However, *routine* use of vancomycin for perioperative prophylaxis is not recommended since such use may promote emergence of vancomycin-resistant enterococci or staphylococci.

■ **Empiric Therapy in Febrile Neutropenic Patients** IV vancomycin is used in conjunction with 1 or 2 other anti-infectives for empiric anti-infective therapy of presumed bacterial infections in febrile neutropenic patients. Vancomycin should never be used alone for empiric therapy in febrile neutropenic patients. Some clinicians suggest that it may be prudent to include vancomycin in an initial empiric regimen in selected patients with clinically suspected serious catheter-related infections (e.g., bacteremia, cellulitis); known colonization with penicillin- and cephalosporin-resistant *S. pneumoniae* or oxacillin-resistant *S. aureus*; initial blood culture results indicating presence of gram-positive bacteria; or hypotension or other evidence of cardiovascular impairment. However, if vancomycin is included in an initial empiric regimen, it should be discontinued within 24–48 hours if results of cultures do not identify gram-positive bacteria susceptible to the drug.

Successful treatment of infections in granulocytopenic patients requires prompt initiation of empiric anti-infective therapy (even when fever is the only sign or symptom of infection) and appropriate modification of the initial regimen if the duration of fever and neutropenia is protracted, if a specific site of infection is identified, or if organisms resistant to the initial regimen are present. No empiric regimen has been identified that would be appropriate for initial treatment of all febrile neutropenic patients. The initial empiric regimen should be chosen based on the underlying disease and other host factors that may affect the degree of risk and on local epidemiologic data regarding usual pathogens in these patients and data regarding their in vitro susceptibility to available anti-infective agents. The fact that gram-positive bacteria have become a predominant pathogen in febrile neutropenic patients should be considered when selecting an empiric anti-infective regimen.

The Infectious Diseases Society of America (IDSA) recommends use of a parenteral empiric regimen in most febrile neutropenic patients; use of an oral regimen (e.g., oral ciprofloxacin and oral amoxicillin and clavulanate) should only be considered in selected adults at low risk for complications who have no focus of bacterial infection and no signs or symptoms of systemic infection other than fever. At health-care facilities where gram-positive bacteria are common causes of serious infection and use of vancomycin in the initial empiric regimen is considered necessary, the IDSA recommends 2- or 3-drug combination therapy that includes vancomycin and either cefepime, ceftazidime, imipenem, or meropenem given with or without an aminoglycoside; vancomycin should be discontinued 24–48 hours later if a susceptible gram-positive bacterial infection is not identified. At health-care facilities where vancomycin is not indicated in the initial empiric regimen, the IDSA recommends monotherapy with a third or fourth generation cephalosporin (ceftazidime, cefepime) or a carbapenem (imipenem, meropenem) for uncomplicated cases; however, for complicated cases or if anti-infective resistance is a problem, combination therapy consisting of an aminoglycoside (amikacin, gentamicin, tobramycin) given in conjunction with an antipseudomonal penicillin (ticarcillin and clavulanate, piperacillin and tazobactam), an antipseudomonal cephalosporin (cefepime, ceftazidime), or a carbapenem (imipenem, meropenem) is recommended. Regardless of the initial regimen selected, patients should be reassessed after 3–5 days of treatment and the anti-infective regimen altered (if indicated) based on the presence or absence of fever, identification of the causative organism, and the clinical condition of the patient.

Published protocols for the treatment of infections in febrile neutropenic patients should be consulted for specific recommendations regarding selection of the initial empiric regimen, when to change the initial regimen, possible subsequent regimens, and duration of therapy in these patients. In addition, consultation with an infectious diseases expert knowledgeable about infections in immunocompromised patients is advised.

Dosage and Administration

■ **Reconstitution and Administration** Vancomycin hydrochloride is administered by slow IV infusion for the treatment of systemic infections. Vancomycin hydrochloride is given orally as capsules for the treatment of enterocolitis caused by *Staphylococcus aureus* (including oxacillin-resistant [methicillin-resistant] strains) or for antibiotic-associated pseudomembranous colitis caused by *Clostridium difficile*; if necessary, the parenteral form of vancomycin hydrochloride may be diluted and administered orally or by nasogastric tube for the treatment of these infections.

Vancomycin is very irritating to tissue and must *not* be given IM. (See Cautions: Local Effects.) Safety and efficacy of intrathecal (intralumbar or intraventricular) or intraperitoneal administration of vancomycin have not been determined.

Oral Administration Commercially available vancomycin hydrochloride capsules or the powder for IV administration can be used for oral administration.

When necessary, an oral solution for administration via a nasogastric tube can be prepared by diluting the appropriate dose of vancomycin hydrochloride powder for IV infusion in 30 mL of water. The 500-mg single-use vial should be used to prepare these oral solutions; ADD-Vantage® vials should not be used. For patients who are too ill to receive oral therapy, administration via a long intestinal tube†, via enema†, or by direct instillation via a colostomy or ileostomy† has been suggested.

IV Infusion Vancomycin hydrochloride usually is administered by intermittent IV infusion, but has been administered by continuous IV infusion when intermittent infusions were not feasible.

Vancomycin hydrochloride powder for injection is reconstituted by adding 10 or 20 mL of sterile water for injection to a vial labeled as containing 500 mg or 1 g of vancomycin, respectively, to provide solutions containing 50 mg of the drug per mL. For intermittent IV infusion, the reconstituted solutions containing 500 mg or 1 g must be diluted further with at least 100 mL or at least 200 mL, respectively, of a compatible IV solution and administered over a period of at least 1 hour.

Alternatively, ADD-Vantage® vials labeled as containing 500 mg or 1 g of vancomycin may be reconstituted according to the manufacturer's directions using 5% dextrose injection or 0.9% sodium chloride injection. ADD-Vantage® vials of the drug should be used only when actual doses of 500 mg or 1 g are appropriate and should *not* be used in neonates, infants, or young children who require doses less than 500 mg.

The pharmacy bulk package is *not* intended for direct IV infusion; doses of the drug from the reconstituted bulk package must be further diluted in a compatible IV infusion solution prior to administration.

Thawed solutions of the commercially available frozen vancomycin hydrochloride injection in 5% dextrose should be administered *only* by IV infusion. The commercially available frozen vancomycin hydrochloride in 5% dextrose injection should be thawed at room temperature (25°C) or under refrigeration (5°C) and should *not* be thawed by immersion in a water bath or by exposure to microwave radiation. A precipitate may form while the commercially available injection in 5% dextrose is frozen; however, this usually will dissolve with little or no agitation upon reaching room temperature, and the potency of vancomycin hydrochloride frozen injection is not affected. After thawing at room temperature or under refrigeration, the container should be checked for minute leaks by firmly squeezing the bag. The injection should be discarded if the container seal or outlet ports are not intact or leaks are found or if the solution is discolored, cloudy, or contains a precipitate. The thawed injection should not be used in series connections with other plastic containers, since such use could result in air embolism from residual air being drawn from the primary container before administration of fluid from the secondary container is complete.

For continuous IV infusion when intermittent infusions are not feasible, 1–2 g of reconstituted vancomycin may be added to a sufficient volume of 0.9% sodium chloride or 5% dextrose injection to permit administration of the desired daily dosage over a 24-hour period.

The frequency and severity of thrombophlebitis can be minimized if vancomycin is administered slowly as a dilute solution (2.5–5 mg/mL) and administration sites are frequently rotated. Pretreatment with antihistamines (e.g., diphenhydramine hydrochloride 1 mg/kg IV and cimetidine 4 mg/kg IV) may attenuate but not eliminate the risk of certain adverse effects (e.g., red-man syndrome) associated with rapid IV infusion of vancomycin. (See Cautions: Dermatologic and Sensitivity Reactions.)

Rate of Administration. Intermittent IV infusions of vancomycin should be given over a period of at least 1 hour.

Rapid IV infusion (e.g., over several minutes) should be avoided, and patients should be monitored closely during infusion of the drug to detect a hypotensive reaction if it occurs. (See Dermatologic and Sensitivity Reactions: Red-man Syndrome, in Cautions.) To minimize adverse effects, vancomycin should be administered IV at a rate not exceeding 10 mg/minute; however, the possibility that adverse effects associated with vancomycin infusion could occur at any infusion rate should be considered.

■ **Dosage** Dosage of vancomycin hydrochloride is expressed in terms of vancomycin.

Oral Dosage Orally administered vancomycin is *not* effective for and should *not* be used for the treatment of systemic infections.

Adult Dosage. For the treatment of enterocolitis caused by *S. aureus* (including oxacillin-resistant strains), the usual adult oral dosage of vancomycin is 0.5–2 g daily given in 3 or 4 divided doses for 7–10 days.

For the treatment of *C. difficile*-associated diarrhea and colitis (CDAD; also known as antibiotic-associated diarrhea and colitis, *C. difficile* diarrhea, *C. difficile* colitis, and pseudomembranous colitis), the usual adult oral dosage of vancomycin is 0.5–2 g daily given in 3 or 4 divided doses for 7–10 days. Because clinical and bacteriologic responses in *C. difficile*-associated diarrhea and colitis generally appear to be similar for the low and high dosages in this range, most clinicians recommend using the lower dosage for cost considerations, unless ileus is impending or the infection is severe (e.g., in critically ill patients). Many clinicians recommend that oral vancomycin be given in a dosage of 125 mg 4 times daily for 7–10 days.

Pediatric Dosage. For the treatment of staphylococcal enterocolitis or antibiotic-associated pseudomembranous colitis in children, the usual oral dosage of vancomycin is 40 mg/kg daily given in 3 or 4 divided doses for 7–10 days. Dosage of oral vancomycin in children should not exceed 2 g daily.

IV Dosage **General Adult Dosage.** For the treatment of potentially life-threatening systemic infections in adults with normal renal function, the usual IV dosage of vancomycin is 500 mg every 6 hours or 1 g every 12 hours.

General Pediatric Dosage. Numerous vancomycin dosage regimens have been suggested for pediatric patients, particularly neonates and young infants. The American Academy of Pediatrics (AAP) states that optimal vancomycin dosage in neonates should be based on serum concentrations of the drug, especially in those with low birthweight (i.e., less than 1.5 kg).

For neonates and young infants with normal renal function, the manufacturers recommend an initial IV dose of 15 mg/kg, followed by 10 mg/kg every 12 hours in neonates younger than 1 week of age and 10 mg/kg every 8 hours for infants 1 week to 1 month of age; close monitoring of serum vancomycin concentrations may be warranted in these patients. AAP recommends that neonates younger than 1 week of age receive 15 mg/kg every 24 hours if they weigh less than 1.2 kg, 10–15 mg/kg of vancomycin every 12–18 hours if they weigh 1.2–2 kg, or 10–15 mg/kg every 8–12 hours if they weigh more than 2 kg. For neonates 1 week of age or older, the AAP recommends 15 mg/kg every 24 hours in those weighing less than 1.2 kg, 10–15 mg/kg given every 8–12 hours in those weighing 1.2–2 kg, or 10–15 mg/kg every 6–8 hours in those weighing more than 2 kg.

For older children with normal renal function, the manufacturers recommend an IV dosage of 10 mg/kg every 6 hours. Alternatively, for older children, some clinicians suggest an IV dosage of 1.2 g/m^2 daily given in divided doses. AAP suggests that children 1 month of age or older with mild to moderate infections receive IV vancomycin in a dosage of 40 mg/kg daily given in 3–4 divided doses and that those with severe infections receive 40–60 mg/kg daily given in 4 divided doses. For the treatment of meningitis in children 1 month of age or older, the AAP and other clinicians recommend that vancomycin be given in a dosage of 60 mg/kg daily (maximum 2 g daily) given in divided doses every 6 hours.

For specific information on other pediatric dosage regimens, published protocols and specialized references should be consulted.

Treatment of Endocarditis. For the *treatment* of native valve endocarditis caused by oxacillin-resistant staphylococci, the American Heart Association (AHA) and Infectious Diseases Society of America (IDSA) recommend that adults receive IV vancomycin in a dosage of 30 mg/kg daily given in 2 equally divided doses (maximum dose 2 g daily unless serum concentrations are inappropriately low) and that pediatric patients receive 40 mg/kg daily given in 2 or 3 equally divided doses for 6 weeks.

Adults with oxacillin-resistant staphylococcal endocarditis who have a prosthetic valve or other prosthetic material should receive IV vancomycin in a dosage of 30 mg/kg daily given in 2 equally divided doses (maximum dose 2 g daily unless serum concentrations are inappropriately low) given for at least 6 weeks in conjunction with oral or IV rifampin (300 mg every 8 hours given for at least 6 weeks) and IM or IV gentamicin (3 mg/kg daily in 2 or 3 equally divided doses during the first 2 weeks of vancomycin therapy). Pediatric patients with oxacillin-resistant staphylococcal endocarditis who have a prosthetic valve or other prosthetic material should receive IV vancomycin in a dosage of 40 mg/kg daily given in 2 or 3 equally divided doses for at least 6 weeks in conjunction with oral or IV rifampin (20 mg/kg daily in 3 equally divided doses given for at least 6 weeks) and IM or IV gentamicin (3 mg/kg daily in 3 equally divided doses during the first 2 weeks of vancomycin therapy).

For the *treatment* of endocarditis caused by viridans streptococci or *Streptococcus bovis* when penicillin G or ceftriaxone cannot be used, the AHA and IDSA recommend that adults receive IV vancomycin in a dosage of 30 mg/kg daily given in 2 equally divided doses (maximum dose 2 g daily unless serum concentrations are inappropriately low) and that pediatric patients receive 40 mg/kg daily given in 2–3 equally divided doses. Vancomycin should be given for 4 weeks for the treatment of native valve endocarditis or for 6 weeks for endocarditis that involves prosthetic valves or other prosthetic materials.

For the *treatment* of enterococcal endocarditis when penicillin G or ampicillin cannot be used, the AHA and IDSA recommend that adults receive IV vancomycin in a dosage of 30 mg/kg daily given in 2 equally divided doses for 6 weeks given in conjunction with IM or IV gentamicin (3 mg/kg daily given in 3 equally divided doses for 6 weeks). Pediatric patients with enterococcal endocarditis who cannot receive penicillin G or ampicillin should receive IV vancomycin in a dosage of 40 mg/kg daily given in 2 or 3 equally divided doses for 6 weeks in conjunction with IM or IV gentamicin (3 mg/kg daily in 3 equally divided doses given for 6 weeks).

If vancomycin is used in a multiple-drug regimen for the empiric treatment of culture-negative endocarditis† involving native valves when the fixed combination of ampicillin and sulbactam cannot be used, the AHA and IDSA recommend that adults receive IV vancomycin in a dosage of 30 mg/kg daily given in 2 equally divided doses in conjunction with IM or IV gentamicin (3 mg/kg daily given in 3 equally divided doses) and ciprofloxacin (1 g daily given orally in 2 equally divided doses or 800 mg daily given IV in 2 equally divided doses). Pediatric patients should receive IV vancomycin in a dosage of 40 mg/kg daily given in 2 or 3 equally divided doses in conjunction with gentamicin (3 mg/kg daily given IM or IV in 3 equally divided doses) and ciprofloxacin (20–30 mg/kg daily given orally or IV in 2 equally divided doses). All 3 drugs should be given for 4–6 weeks.

Prevention of Bacterial Endocarditis. For *prevention* of enterococcal endocarditis in penicillin-allergic patients at high or moderate risk who are undergoing certain GI, biliary tract, or genitourinary tract surgery or instrumentation (see Uses: Endocarditis), the AHA recommends that adults receive a single 1-g dose of vancomycin and that pediatric patients receive a single 20-mg/kg dose of vancomycin given IV over 1–2 hours with the infusion completed within 30 minutes of the start of the procedure. While patients with cardiac conditions that put them at moderate risk of enterococcal endocarditis may receive vancomycin alone for prophylaxis, adults and pediatric patients with cardiac conditions that put them at high risk also should receive a single 1. 5-mg/kg dose of gentamicin (maximum dose 120 mg) given IM or IV within 30 minutes prior to the start of the procedure. When selecting anti-infectives for the prevention of bacterial endocarditis, the current recommendations published by the AHA should be consulted.

Prevention of Neonatal Group B Streptococcal Disease. If IV vancomycin is used for intrapartum anti-infective prophylaxis for prevention of perinatal group B streptococcal (GBS) disease† in women with penicillin hypersensitivity who should not receive a β-lactam anti-infective and should not receive clindamycin and erythromycin because of known or suspected resistance, the CDC recommends that 1 g of vancomycin be given IV every 12 hours until delivery. When indicated, such prophylaxis is initiated at the time of labor or rupture of membranes.

Perioperative Prophylaxis. For perioperative prophylaxis† in adults undergoing certain cardiac, neurosurgical, orthopedic, thoracic (noncardiac), or vascular surgical procedures when use of vancomycin is considered necessary because of a high incidence of oxacillin-resistant staphylococci at the institution or when cephalosporins (cefazolin, cefuroxime) cannot be used, a single 1-g dose of vancomycin should be given IV prior to the procedure.

The vancomycin infusion should be started 1–2 hours prior to the time of incision to minimize the risk of an adverse reaction occurring at the time of induction of anesthesia and to ensure adequate tissue concentrations of the drug at the time of incision. (See Drug Interactions: Anesthetics.) If surgery is prolonged (more than 4 hours), additional intraoperative doses of vancomycin may be given every 6–12 hours for the duration of the procedure. Additional doses may also be indicated if substantial blood loss occurs. However, postoperative doses generally are unnecessary and should not be used.

■ **Dosage in Renal Impairment** In patients with impaired renal function, including premature infants and geriatric patients, doses and/or frequency of administration of vancomycin must be modified in response to the degree of impairment, severity of the infection, susceptibility of the causative organism, and serum concentrations of the drug. Several methods of calculating vancomycin dosage for patients with impaired renal function have been proposed; however, in these patients or patients undergoing hemodialysis or peritoneal dialysis, dosage should generally be based on actual serum concentrations of the drug.

In patients with impaired renal function, including geriatric and functionally anephric patients, an initial IV dose of 15 mg/kg should be given. Subsequent dosage must be based mainly on renal function and serum concentrations of the drug. Clinicians should consult published protocols and specialized references for information on specific methods of dosage adjustment. Some clinicians have recommended that 1 g of vancomycin be administered at 12-hour intervals in patients with serum creatinine concentrations less than 1.5 mg/dL, at 3- to 6-day intervals in patients with serum creatinine of 1.5–5 mg/dL, and at 10- to 14-day intervals in patients with serum creatinine greater than 5 mg/dL. Others have recommended that the usual individual dose be administered every 3–10 days in patients with glomerular filtration rates of 10–50 mL/minute and every 10 days in patients with glomerular filtration rates less than 10 mL/minute.

Cautions

■ **Otic and Renal Effects** Ototoxicity and nephrotoxicity are the most serious adverse effects of parenteral vancomycin therapy. The incidences of ototoxicity and nephrotoxicity have not been well established, but clinical experience to date suggests that these adverse effects occur relatively infrequently.

Ototoxicity and nephrotoxicity are most likely to occur in patients with renal impairment, patients receiving IV vancomycin in high doses or for prolonged periods, or patients receiving other ototoxic and/or nephrotoxic drugs. (See Drug Interactions: Ototoxic and Nephrotoxic Drugs.) Although ototoxicity and nephrotoxicity have been associated with serum or blood vancomycin concentrations of 80–100 mcg/mL, these reactions have occurred with concentrations as low as 25 mcg/mL. Correlations between serum vancomycin concentrations and ototoxicity and nephrotoxicity still remain to be clarified.

Ototoxicity may be transient or permanent. Vancomycin may cause damage to the auditory branch of the eighth cranial nerve and permanent deafness has occurred. Vertigo, dizziness, and tinnitus have been reported rarely. Tinnitus may precede the onset of deafness and necessitates discontinuance of the drug. Deafness may progress despite cessation of vancomycin therapy.

Vancomycin-induced nephrotoxicity may be manifested by transient elevations in BUN or serum creatinine concentrations, and the presence of hyaline and granular casts and albumin in the urine. Fatal uremia has occurred. Rarely, the drug has been associated with acute interstitial nephritis.

■ **Local Effects** Vancomycin hydrochloride is very irritating to tissue and causes necrosis when given IM; therefore, it must be administered IV and care must be taken to avoid extravasation. Pain and thrombophlebitis occur after IV administration in many patients, and occasionally may be severe.

■ Dermatologic and Sensitivity Reactions Urticaria, exfoliative dermatitis, macular rashes, eosinophilia, vasculitis, a shock-like state, transient anaphylaxis, and, occasionally, vascular collapse have been reported in patients receiving vancomycin. The drug also has been associated with Stevens-Johnson syndrome in at least one patient.

Hypersensitivity reactions reportedly occur in 5–10% of patients receiving vancomycin. Successful desensitization was reported in some patients who had experienced severe systemic allergic reactions to vancomycin but required further therapy with the drug.

Red-man Syndrome Rapid IV administration of vancomycin has resulted in a hypotensive reaction frequently referred to as the "red-man syndrome" or "red-neck syndrome". The reaction is characterized by a sudden decrease in blood pressure which can be severe and may be accompanied by flushing and/or a maculopapular or erythematous rash on the face, neck, chest, and upper extremities; the latter manifestations may also occur in the absence of hypotension. Wheezing, dyspnea, angioedema, urticaria, and pruritus may also occur. Rarely, cardiac arrest or seizures have occurred.

Vancomycin-induced hypotension appears to result from a negative inotropic and vasodilating action produced in part by a release of histamine, which is directly related to the rate of infusion; the release of histamine also appears to be responsible for the usual manifestations (e.g., erythema, rash, pruritus) of the "red" characterization. The reaction usually begins a few minutes after the vancomycin infusion is started, but may not occur until after the infusion is completed, and usually resolves spontaneously over one to several hours after discontinuance of the infusion. If the hypotensive reaction is severe, the use of antihistamines, corticosteroids, or IV fluids may be necessary. The hypotensive reaction is related to the rate of infusion of vancomycin and has been reported most frequently when the drug was administered over a period of 10 minutes or less; however, the reaction may also occur rarely when the drug is infused over a period of 1 hour or longer.

To minimize the risk of a hypotensive reaction, vancomycin should be infused over a period of at least 1 hour and the patient's blood pressure should be monitored during the infusion. In patients who have had the reaction, subsequent doses of vancomycin can usually be given without adverse effect if administered at a slow rate (e.g., over several hours). Pretreatment with antihistamines may be of benefit. If attempts to minimize the reaction fail, use of another anti-infective agent may be necessary. The reaction reportedly has occurred in more than 50% of healthy individuals given vancomycin but less frequently when the drug is used therapeutically.

In one study, intradermal skin tests with vancomycin were used to assess the possibility of predicting the *severity* of vancomycin-associated anaphylactoid reactions (i.e., "red-man syndrome" or "red-neck syndrome"). Although the intradermal tests were positive (wheal and flare) in all patients and all patients subsequently experienced anaphylactoid reactions following an IV dose of the drug, the magnitude of cutaneous response was of little value in predicting the severity of "red-man syndrome". Desensitization, employing sequential incremental concentration and dose increases (in a manner typical for drug desensitization procedures) and pretreatment with an antihistamine and corticosteroid, has been performed successfully in a few patients in whom vancomycin therapy was considered necessary.

In at least one patient, *oral* administration of vancomycin resulted in the "red-man syndrome". This reaction was characterized by intense pruritus on the arms, scalp, and face; flushing on the face and neck; and erythema on the face, neck, chest, and arms. Administration of a parenteral antihistamine provided some relief.

Evidence from at least one patient suggests possible cross-sensitivity between teicoplanin administration and vancomycin-induced red-man syndrome.

■ Hematologic Effects Adverse hematologic effects reported in patients receiving vancomycin include neutropenia, eosinophilia, and, rarely, thrombocytopenia. Neutropenia, which appears to be rapidly reversible following discontinuance of the drug, usually has occurred beginning 7 or more days after initiation of vancomycin therapy or after a total dose of more than 25 g of the drug.

Although a causal relationship to vancomycin has not been established, reversible agranulocytosis (granulocytes less than 500/mm^3) has been reported rarely in patients receiving vancomycin.

■ GI Effects Antibiotic-associated pseudomembranous colitis, caused by toxin-producing clostridia (e.g., *C. difficile*), has been reported with the use of nearly all anti-infectives, including IV vancomycin, and should be considered in the differential diagnosis of patients who present with diarrhea subsequent to administration of anti-infectives. Pseudomembranous colitis may occur during or following discontinuance of anti-infective therapy and ranges in severity from mild to life-threatening. Mild cases of colitis may respond to discontinuance of the drug alone, but diagnosis and management of moderate to severe cases should include appropriate bacteriologic studies and treatment with fluid, electrolyte, and protein supplementation as indicated. If colitis is moderate to severe and is not relieved by discontinuance of the drug, appropriate anti-infective therapy (e.g., metronidazole) should be administered.

Nausea also has been reported in patients receiving vancomycin therapy.

■ Other Adverse Effects A throbbing pain in the muscles of the back and neck has been reported with vancomycin and can usually be minimized or avoided by slower administration of the drug. In patients undergoing continuous ambulatory peritoneal dialysis (CAPD), intraperitoneal administration of vancomycin has been associated with chemical peritonitis, a syndrome consisting of a cloudy dialysate, which may be accompanied by abdominal pain and fever. Chemical peritonitis usually disappears shortly after discontinuance of intraperitoneal vancomycin.

Other adverse effects of vancomycin include chills and fever. Priapism after a second IV dose of vancomycin, with recurrence on inadvertent rechallenge, occurred in a 37-year-old man with severe underlying diabetes mellitus; bilateral phlebotomy of the corpus cavernosum resulted in resolution of the priapism.

■ Precautions and Contraindications Vancomycin is contraindicated in patients with known hypersensitivity to the drug. The manufacturer of the commercially available frozen vancomycin hydrochloride injection in 5% dextrose states that solutions containing dextrose may be contraindicated in patients with known allergy to corn or corn products.

Because vancomycin is ototoxic and nephrotoxic, the drug should be used with caution in patients with impaired renal function and should be avoided in patients with previous hearing loss. If it is necessary to use vancomycin in such patients, dosage should be reduced. Patients with borderline renal function and those older than 60 years of age should be given serial tests of auditory function, and serum or blood vancomycin concentrations should be determined regularly during treatment with the drug. All patients receiving vancomycin should have periodic urinalysis and renal function tests. The manufacturers also recommend periodic monitoring of the leukocyte count in patients receiving prolonged vancomycin therapy and in those receiving concomitant therapy with drugs that may cause neutropenia.

The possibility that infusion reactions, including potentially severe hypotension, may occur with IV vancomycin should be considered. (See Dermatologic and Sensitivity Reactions: Red-man Syndrome, in Cautions.) Rapid IV administration (e.g., over several minutes) of the drug should be avoided since it may be associated with exaggerated hypotension, including shock, and may rarely be with associated with cardiac arrest.

Because reversible neutropenia has been reported in patients receiving vancomycin, leukocyte counts should be monitored periodically in patients receiving prolonged vancomycin therapy and in those who are receiving concomitant therapy with drugs that may cause neutropenia.

To reduce development of drug-resistant bacteria and maintain effectiveness of vancomycin and other antibacterials, the drug should be used only for the treatment or prevention of infections proven or strongly suspected to be caused by susceptible bacteria. When selecting or modifying anti-infective therapy, use results of culture and in vitro susceptibility testing. In the absence of such data, consider local epidemiology and susceptibility patterns when selecting anti-infectives for empiric therapy. Patients should be advised that antibacterials (including vancomycin) should only be used to treat bacterial infections and not used to treat viral infections (e.g., the common cold). Patients also should be advised about the importance of completing the full course of therapy, even if feeling better after a few days, and that skipping doses or not completing therapy may decrease effectiveness and increase the likelihood that bacteria will develop resistance and will not be treatable with vancomycin or other antibacterials in the future.

Prolonged use of vancomycin hydrochloride may result in overgrowth of nonsusceptible organisms. The patient should be carefully monitored and appropriate therapy should be instituted if a superinfection occurs. Because antibiotic-associated pseudomembranous colitis has been reported with the use of anti-infective agents, including IV vancomycin, it should be considered in the differential diagnosis of patients who develop diarrhea during therapy with the drug.

■ Pediatric Precautions Safety and efficacy of oral vancomycin have not been established in pediatric patients.

IV vancomycin should be used with caution in premature neonates and young infants because of the renal immaturity of these patients and the potential for increased serum concentrations of the drug. Close monitoring of serum vancomycin concentrations may be warranted in pediatric patients, especially neonates and young infants.

Concomitant administration of vancomycin and anesthetic agents in children has been associated with erythema and histamine-like flushing. The occurrence of infusion-related adverse effects may be minimized by infusing vancomycin over a period of at least 1 hour prior to induction of anesthesia.

Safety of the chemical components that may leach out of the plastic container for commercially available frozen vancomycin injections has not been established in children.

■ Geriatric Precautions Clinical studies of oral vancomycin hydrochloride did not include sufficient numbers of patients 65 years of age or older to determine whether they respond differently than younger adults. Other reported clinical experience has not identified any differences in response between geriatric and younger adults.

Vancomycin dosage for geriatric patients should be selected with caution, usually starting at the low end of the dosing range, because of age-related decreases in hepatic, renal, and/or cardiac function and potential for concomitant disease and drug therapy.

Vancomycin dosage in geriatric patients should be adjusted based on the degree of renal impairment. (See Dosage: Dosage in Renal Impairment.) Because geriatric adults may have decreasing glomerular filtration with increasing age, increased serum vancomycin concentrations may occur if dosage is not adjusted in these patients.

■ **Mutagenicity and Carcinogenicity** Vancomycin was not mutagenic in vitro in the mouse lymphoma forward mutation assay or the primary rat hepatocyte unscheduled DNA synthesis assay or in vivo in the Chinese hamster sister chromatid exchange assay or the mouse micronucleus assay.

No long-term animal carcinogenicity studies have been performed.

■ **Pregnancy, Fertility, and Lactation** There was no evidence of teratogenicity when vancomycin was administered IV to rats in dosages up to 200 mg/kg daily (1180 mg/m^2 or equivalent to the recommended maximum human dosage based on mg/m^2) or to rabbits in dosage up to 120 mg/kg daily (1320 mg/m^2 or 1.1 times the recommended maximum human dosage based on mg/m^2). There were no effects on fetal weight or development in rats at the highest dosage tested or in rabbits given 80 mg/kg daily (880 mg/m^2 or 0.74 times the maximum recommended human dosage based on mg/m^2).

In one study, no sensorineural hearing loss or nephrotoxicity was reported in neonates born to women who received IV vancomycin for severe staphylococcal infections associated with IV drug abuse during pregnancy. In one infant whose mother received IV vancomycin in the third trimester of pregnancy, conductive hearing loss was reported; however, a causal relationship to vancomycin has not been established. Because the number of pregnant women in this study was limited and vancomycin was only administered during the second and third trimester of pregnancy, it is not known whether the drug can cause fetal harm when administered to pregnant women. Vancomycin should be used during pregnancy only when clearly needed.

Vancomycin is distributed into milk following IV administration. Systemic absorption of oral vancomycin is very low and it is not known whether the drug distributes into human milk following oral administration. However, IV and oral vancomycin should be used with caution in nursing women. Because of the potential for serious adverse reactions from the drug in nursing infants, a decision should be made whether to discontinue nursing or the drug, taking into account the importance of vancomycin to the woman.

Drug Interactions

■ **Ototoxic and Nephrotoxic Drugs** Because of the possibility of additive toxicities, the concurrent or sequential systemic or topical use of other ototoxic and/or nephrotoxic drugs (e.g., aminoglycosides, amphotericin B, bacitracin, cisplatin, colistin, polymyxin B) and vancomycin requires careful serial monitoring of renal and auditory function. These drugs should be used with caution in patients receiving vancomycin therapy.

■ **Aminoglycosides** In vitro, the antibacterial effects of vancomycin and aminoglycosides are synergistic against many strains of *Staphylococcus aureus*, nonenterococcal group D streptococci (*Streptococcus bovis*), enterococci (*Enterococcus faecalis*), and viridans streptococci. However, concomitant use of vancomycin and aminoglycosides is associated with an increased risk of ototoxicity and/or nephrotoxicity. (See Drug Interactions: Ototoxic and Nephrotoxic Drugs.)

■ **Anesthetics** Concomitant use of vancomycin and anesthetic agents has been associated with anaphylactoid reactions and an increased frequency of infusion reactions (e.g., hypotension, flushing, erythema, urticaria, pruritus). Erythema and histamine-like flushing has occurred in pediatric patients receiving vancomycin and anesthetic agents concomitantly. The risk of infusion-related adverse effects may be minimized if vancomycin is given as a 1-hour IV infusion prior to induction of anesthesia.

Acute Toxicity

Limited information is available on the acute toxicity of vancomycin. The IV LD_{50} of the drug in rats or mice is 319 or 400 mg/kg, respectively. Treatment of vancomycin overdosage is mainly supportive with maintenance of glomerular filtration. The drug is not appreciably removed by dialysis; however, hemofiltration and hemoperfusion using polysulfone resin reportedly has been of limited value.

Mechanism of Action

Vancomycin is bactericidal and appears to bind to the bacterial cell wall causing blockage of glycopeptide polymerization. This effect, which occurs at a site different from that affected by the penicillins, produces immediate inhibition of cell wall synthesis and secondary damage to the cytoplasmic membrane. Magnesium, manganese, calcium, and ferrous ions reduce the degree of adsorption of vancomycin to the cell wall, but the in vivo importance of this interaction is unknown.

Spectrum

Vancomycin is active in vitro and in vivo against many gram-positive bacteria, including *Staphylococcus aureus* (including oxacillin-resistant [methicillin-resistant] strains), *S. epidermidis* (including oxacillin-resistant strains), nonenterococcal group D streptococci (*Streptococcus bovis*), enterococci (*Enterococcus faecalis*), viridans streptococci, *Corynebacterium*, and *Clostridium* (including *C. difficile*). The drug also is active in vitro against *S. pyogenes* (group A β-hemolytic streptococci), *S. agalactiae* (group B streptococci), *S. pneumoniae* (including penicillin-resistant strains), *Listeria monocytogenes*, *Actinomyces*, and *Lactobacillus*.

In vitro, vancomycin is bactericidal for most gram-positive organisms at a concentration less than 5 mcg/mL. Most strains of *S. aureus* are susceptible to vancomycin concentrations of 1.6 mcg/mL or less, although a few strains have been found to be naturally resistant to clinically achievable concentrations of the drug.

Vancomycin is not active against gram-negative bacteria, fungi, or yeast.

■ **In Vitro Susceptibility Testing** The Clinical and Laboratory Standards Institute (CLSI; formerly National Committee for Clinical Laboratory Standards [NCCLS]) states that, if results of in vitro susceptibility testing indicate that a clinical isolate is *susceptible* to vancomycin, then an infection caused by this strain may be appropriately treated with the dosage of the drug recommended for that type of infection and infecting species, unless otherwise contraindicated. If results indicate that a clinical isolate has *intermediate susceptibility* to vancomycin, then the strain has a minimum inhibitory concentration (MIC) that approaches usually attainable blood and tissue drug concentrations and response rates may be lower than for strains identified as susceptible. Therefore, the intermediate category implies clinical applicability in body sites where the drug is physiologically concentrated (e.g., urine) or when a high dosage of the drug can be used. This intermediate category also includes a buffer zone which should prevent small, uncontrolled technical factors from causing major discrepancies in interpretation, especially for drugs with narrow pharmacotoxicity margins. If results of in vitro susceptibility testing indicate that a clinical isolate is *resistant* to vancomycin, the strain is not inhibited by systemic concentrations of the drug achievable with usual dosage schedules and/or MICs fall in the range where specific microbial resistance mechanisms are likely and efficacy has not been reliably demonstrated in clinical trials.

Strains of staphylococci with reduced susceptibility to vancomycin may not be reliably detected with current disk-diffusion procedures, and it has been recommended that a quantitative method (broth or agar dilution, agar gradient diffusion) be used to evaluate susceptibility of staphylococci to vancomycin.

Disk Susceptibility Tests When the disk-diffusion procedure is used to test susceptibility to vancomycin, a disk containing 30 mcg/ of vancomycin should be used.

When disk-diffusion susceptibility testing is performed according to CLSI standardized procedures and CLSI interpretive criteria, *Staphylococcus* with growth inhibition zones of 15 mm or greater are considered susceptible to vancomycin. All *Staphylococcus* with growth inhibition zones of 14 mm or less should be tested using a dilution susceptibility test.

When the disk-diffusion test is performed according to CLSI standardized procedures, *Enterococcus* with growth inhibition zones of 17 mm or greater are susceptible to vancomycin, those with zones of 15–16 mm have intermediate susceptibility, and those with zones of 14 mm or less are resistant to the drug. Accurate detection of vancomycin-resistant enterococci requires that plates be incubated for a full 24 hours and that growth inhibition zones be examined carefully with transmitted light for evidence of small colonies or a light film growing within the zone. Enterococci isolated from patients with serious infections that are identified as having intermediate susceptibility in the disk-diffusion procedure should then be tested using a dilution susceptibility method.

When testing susceptibility of *Streptococcus* (including *S. pneumoniae*) according to CLSI standardized procedures using Mueller-Hinton agar (supplemented with 5% sheep blood) incubated in 5% CO_2, *Streptococcus* with growth inhibition zones of 17 mm or greater are susceptible to vancomycin. Because of limited data on resistant strains of these organisms, CLSI recommends that streptococcal isolates that appear to be nonsusceptible to vancomycin should be submitted to a reference laboratory for further testing.

Dilution Susceptibility Tests When dilution susceptibility testing (agar or broth dilution) is performed according to CLSI standardized procedures using CLSI interpretive criteria, *Staphylococcus* with MICs of 4 mcg/mL or less are susceptible to vancomycin, those with MICs of 8–16 mcg/mL have intermediate susceptibility, and those with MICs of 32 mcg/mL or greater are resistant to the drug. Because of limited data on resistant strains, CLSI recommends that any *Staphylococcus* isolate that has an MIC of 4 mcg/mL or greater should be send to a reference laboratory. The US Centers for Disease Control and Prevention (CDC) has recommended that, after retesting to confirm species identification and susceptibility results, *Staphylococcus* with vancomycin MICs of 4 mcg/mL or greater should be reported to the state health department and the CDC Hospital Infections Program, National Center for Infectious Disease (404-639-6413) and sent to the CDC for microbiologic and epidemiologic evaluation.

When broth dilution is performed according to CLSI standardized procedures using CLSI interpretive criteria, *Enterococcus* with MICs of 4 mcg/mL or less are susceptible to vancomycin, those with MICs of 8–16 mcg/mL have intermediate susceptibility, and those with MICs of 32 mcg/mL or greater are resistant to the drug. Accurate identification of resistant strains of *Enterococcus* requires that vancomycin plates be held for a full 24-hour incubation period and that isolates with MICs of 8–16 mcg/mL be tested further using specific biochemical tests.

When broth dilution susceptibility testing of *Streptococcus*, including *S. pneumoniae* is performed according to CLSI standardized procedures using cation-adjusted Mueller-Hinton broth (supplemented with 2–5% lysed horse blood), streptococci with MICs of 1 mcg/mL or less are considered susceptible to vancomycin. Any streptococcal isolate that appears to be nonsusceptible to vancomycin should be submitted to a reference laboratory for further testing.

Resistance

■ Resistance in Enterococci Resistance to vancomycin has been reported in *Enterococcus faecalis* (formerly *Streptococcus faecalis*), *E. faecium* (VREF; formerly *S. faecium*), and *E. gallinarum*, and strains of enterococci resistant to vancomycin have been reported with increasing frequency. According to US Centers for Disease Control and Prevention (CDC) surveillance data, since 1989 there has been a 20-fold increase in the percentage of vancomycin-resistant enterococci associated with nosocomial infections in the US and a 34-fold increase in the percentage of resistant strains associated with infections in hospital intensive-care units. Approximately 0.3% of enterococci isolated from nosocomial infections in the US in 1989 were resistant to vancomycin; in 1993, this percentage was 7.9%. Vancomycin-resistant strains of enterococci have been isolated most frequently from GI/intra-abdominal and urinary tract infections, but also have been isolated from skin and soft tissue, bloodstream, and other infections.

Several different forms of vancomycin resistance have been identified in enterococci, including high-level resistance and low-level resistance. Strains of enterococci with high-level resistance generally require vancomycin concentrations of 128 mcg/mL or more and strains with low-level resistance generally require concentrations of 16–64 mcg/mL for in vitro inhibition. High-level vancomycin resistance has been reported in *E. faecium* and *E. faecalis*, appears to be plasmid mediated, and can be induced by exposure to vancomycin and, to a lesser extent, exposure to teicoplanin. Low-level vancomycin resistance has been reported in *E. faecium*, *E. faecalis*, and *E. gallinarum* and may also be induced by exposure to vancomycin, but may or may not be induced by exposure to teicoplanin.

The mechanisms of vancomycin resistance in enterococci have not been fully elucidated. High-level vancomycin resistance most frequently has been associated with the presence of a certain protein and a phenotype termed VanA; low-level resistance usually has been associated with the presence of a different phenotype, termed VanB. Two other phenotypes, VanC and VanD, also have been identified. In general, VanA resistance is high level, transferable, and accompanied by high-level teicoplanin resistance. VanB resistance is widely variable in level, transferable, and *not* accompanied by teicoplanin resistance; VanC resistance is low level, *not* transferable, and *not* associated with teicoplanin resistance; and VanD resistance is intermediate level and associated with low-level teicoplanin resistance. Presence of vancomycin resistance in enterococci, especially low-level resistance, may be difficult to detect with standard in vitro susceptibility tests.

Some strains of *E. faecium* resistant to vancomycin may be susceptible in vitro to linezolid or the fixed combination of quinupristin and dalfopristin; some strains of *E. faecalis* resistant to vancomycin may be susceptible to linezolid in vitro but these strains are resistant to quinupristin and dalfopristin. Although strains of enterococci with high-level, plasmid-mediated vancomycin resistance generally are cross-resistant to other glycopeptides, including teicoplanin, ristocetin, and actaplanin, some strains of *E. faecalis*, *E. faecium*, *E. casseliflavus*, *E. flavascens*, and *E. gallinarum* with low-level vancomycin resistance may be susceptible to teicoplanin in vitro. Strains of vancomycin-resistant enterococci may also be resistant to other drugs (e.g., aminoglycosides, ampicillin, penicillin G, imipenem, tetracyclines, synergistic combinations of β-lactam anti-infectives). These multidrug-resistant strains of enterococci have been reported with increasing frequency.

■ Resistance in Staphylococci Until recently, clinical isolates of *Staphylococcus*, including oxacillin-resistant [oxacillin-resistant] *S. aureus*, have consistently been susceptible to vancomycin in vitro. However, in vitro exposure of staphylococci to increasing concentrations of glycopeptide anti-infectives can produce strains with decreased susceptibility and emergence of vancomycin-resistant strains of *S. haemolyticus* and *S. epidermidis* have been reported rarely in patients receiving the drug. A strain of oxacillin-resistant *S. aureus* with reduced susceptibility to vancomycin (MIC of 8 mcg/mL) was first identified in 1996 in a Japanese child receiving the drug for a nosocomial surgical site infection. In 1997, the first oxacillin-resistant *S. aureus* isolate with reduced (intermediate) susceptibility to vancomycin was identified in the US in a patient who had received multiple courses of intraperitoneal and IV vancomycin therapy for repeated episodes of oxacillin-resistant *S. aureus*-associated peritonitis. A second isolate with reduced (intermediate) susceptibility to vancomycin was identified in the US in a patient with diabetes mellitus after 18 weeks of IV vancomycin therapy for oxacillin-resistant bacteremia. In vitro testing indicated that these isolates had a vancomycin MIC of 8 mcg/mL but were susceptible to rifampin, chloramphenicol, co-trimoxazole, and tetracycline.

Epidemiologic and laboratory investigations are under way to assess the risk for person-to-person transmission of staphylococci with reduced susceptibility to vancomycin and to determine the mechanism of resistance in these strains. In vitro studies indicate that the VanA gene associated with vancomycin resistance in enterococci may be transferable to other gram-positive bacteria, including *S. aureus*, and can result in vancomycin-resistant strains of this organism. However, polymerase chain reaction testing of at least one isolate of oxacillin-resistant *S. aureus* with reduced susceptibility to vancomycin did not detect the VanA or VanB gene.

Pharmacokinetics

■ Absorption Vancomycin hydrochloride is not appreciably absorbed from the GI tract in most patients and must be given parenterally for the treatment of systemic infections. Oral bioavailability usually is less than 5%; however, limited data suggest that clinically important serum concentrations of the drug may result following enteral or oral administration of vancomycin in some patients with colitis and/or in those with renal impairment.

In adults with normal renal function who received multiple 1-g doses of vancomycin (15 mg/kg) given by IV infusion over 1 hour, mean plasma concentrations immediately after completion of the infusion are approximately 63 mcg/mL and mean plasma concentrations 2 and 11 hours later are approximately 23 or 8 mcg/mL, respectively. When multiple 500-mg doses are given by IV infusion over 30 minutes, mean plasma concentrations are about 49 mcg/mL immediately following the infusion and about 10 mcg/mL 6 hours after infusion.

Serum vancomycin concentrations are higher in patients with renal dysfunction than in those with normal renal function, and toxic serum concentrations may result.

■ Distribution Following IV administration, vancomycin is widely distributed in body tissues and diffuses readily into pericardial, pleural, ascitic, and synovial fluids. Small amounts of the drug are distributed into bile.

Vancomycin does *not* readily distribute into CSF in the absence of inflammation unless serum concentrations are exceedingly high. Low concentrations of the drug may be present in CSF if meninges are inflamed, but negligible amounts are detected in the CSF of most patients with uninflamed meninges. In a limited number of adults and children with meningitis who received IV vancomycin in a dosage of 10–15 mg/kg daily, average CSF concentrations 1–3 hours after a dose were 3.3–3.8 mcg/mL and were 21–22% of concurrent serum concentrations. However, the relationship between CSF concentrations and clinical efficacy of vancomycin in the treatment of meningitis is unclear.

Vancomycin is 30–60% bound to serum proteins. Protein binding may be lower (19–29%) in patients with hypoalbuminemia (e.g., burn patients, those with end-stage renal disease).

Vancomycin readily crosses the placenta and is distributed into cord blood. Vancomycin is distributed into milk.

■ Elimination The serum elimination half-life of vancomycin in adults with normal renal function has been reported to average 4–7 hours; accumulation tends to occur after 2–3 days of IV administration at 6- or 12-hour intervals. In geriatric adults 65 years of age older, the mean half-life of the drug has been reported to be 12.1 hours.

The mean half-life of vancomycin is 6.7 hours in full-term neonates and 4.1 hours in infants 1 month of age or older but younger than 1 year of age. In children 2.5–11 years of age, half-life of the drug is reported to be 5.6 hours.

The serum elimination half-life of vancomycin is increased in patients with renal dysfunction. In one study, the elimination half-life averaged 32.3 hours (range: 10.1–75.1 hours) in patients with creatinine clearances of 10–60 mL/minute and 146.7 hours (range: 44.1–406.4 hours) in those with creatinine clearances less than 10 mL/minute. However, because of increased clearance, half-life of vancomycin averages 4 hours in burn patients.

Vancomycin does not appear to be metabolized. Following oral administration, the drug is excreted mainly in feces. Following IV administration, about 75–90% of a dose is eliminated unchanged in urine by glomerular filtration and only small amounts are excreted in bile.

Vancomycin is only minimally removed by hemodialysis or peritoneal dialysis, including continuous ambulatory peritoneal dialysis. The drug is substantially removed by hemofiltration.

Chemistry and Stability

■ Chemistry Vancomycin is a tricyclic glycopeptide antibiotic obtained from cultures of *Amycolatopsis orientalis* (formerly *Nocardia orientalis*).

Vancomycin is structurally unrelated to other commercially available antibiotics. Vancomycin is commercially available as the hydrochloride salt; potency of commercially available vancomycin hydrochloride is expressed in terms of vancomycin. Vancomycin hydrochloride occurs as an amphoteric, tan to brown, free-flowing powder with a bitter taste. The drug is freely soluble in water and insoluble in alcohol. A 5% aqueous solution of vancomycin hydrochloride has a pH of 2.5–4.5.

The commercially available frozen vancomycin hydrochloride injections containing 500 mg of vancomycin in approximately 5% dextrose injection are frozen, nonpyrogenic, sterile, iso-osmotic solutions of the drug; hydrochloric acid and, possibly, sodium hydroxide have been added to adjust pH to 3–5.

■ Stability Commercially available vancomycin hydrochloride capsules and powder for IV administration should be stored at 15–30°C.

When reconstituted with sterile water for injection, vancomycin hydrochloride injection is stable for 2 weeks at room temperature; the manufacturers state that reconstituted injections may be stored for 96 hours at 2–8°C without substantial loss of potency. When reconstituted as directed in 0.9% sodium chloride injection or 5% dextrose injection, solutions prepared from ADD-Vantage® vials of the drug are stable for 24 hours at room temperature. Vancomycin solutions containing 5 mg/mL in 0.9% sodium chloride injection or 5% dextrose injection are reportedly stable for at least 17 days when stored at 24°C in glass or PVC containers and for at least 63 days when stored at 5°C or −10°C in glass containers. Following reconstitution with sterile water for injection as directed, vancomycin solutions that have been further diluted to a concentration of 5 mg/mL in 5–30% dextrose injection are stable when stored in plastic syringes for 24 hours at 4°C and then subsequently for 2 hours at room temperature.

The commercially available frozen injection of vancomycin hydrochloride in 5% dextrose should be stored at a temperature not greater than −20°C. The manufacturer states that the stability of the commercially available frozen vancomycin hydrochloride injection in dextrose may vary; these injections are stable for at least 90 days from the date of shipment when stored as directed. The commercially available frozen injection in 5% dextrose should be thawed at room temperature (25°C) or under refrigeration (5°C) and, once thawed, should not be refrozen. Thawed solutions are stable for 72 hours at room temperature (25°C) or 30 days when refrigerated at 5°C. The commercially available frozen injection of the drug in dextrose is provided in a plastic container fabricated from specially formulated multilayered plastic PL 2040 (Galaxy®). Solutions in contact with the plastic can leach out some of its chemical components in very small amounts within the expiration period of the injection; however, safety of the plastic has been confirmed in tests in animals according to USP biological tests for plastic containers as well as by tissue culture toxicity studies.

Vancomycin hydrochloride injection has been reported to be physically incompatible with many drugs (especially alkaline injections), but the compatibility depends on several factors (e.g., concentrations of the drugs, specific diluents used, resulting pH, temperature). Specialized references should be consulted for specific compatibility information.

Ophthalmic solutions that have been prepared extemporaneously by diluting vancomycin hydrochloride sterile powder with artificial tears (i.e., Liquifilm® Tears, Tears Naturale®) to a final vancomycin concentration of 31–50 mg/mL have been reported to have variable pH and stability. In one study in which the drug was diluted with 10 mL of artificial tears to provide a resultant concentration of 50 mg/mL, recommendations concerning stability and storage were not possible since pH of the resultant ophthalmic solution decreased rapidly to less than 3.5 by the seventh day, a pH that would not be tolerated by the eye. In another study in which the sterile powder initially was diluted with 5 mL of sterile water for injection to a concentration of 100 mg/mL and then further diluted to a concentration of 31 mg/mL by withdrawing 4.6 mL of this solution and diluting it in approximately 10.4 mL of artificial tears, no substantial change in pH occurred (3.7–5) over time, but the final solution had a pH of 5 and would likely be irritating to the eye. In this study, vancomycin was stable for 45 days at −10°C, 10 days at 4°C, and 7 days at 25°C.

Preparations

Excipients in commercially available drug preparations may have clinically important effects in some individuals; consult specific product labeling for details.

Vancomycin Hydrochloride

Oral		
Capsules	125 mg (of vancomycin)	**Vancocin® HCl Pulvules®**, ViroPharma
	250 mg (of vancomycin)	**Vancocin® HCl Pulvules®**, ViroPharma
Parenteral		
For injection	5 g (of vancomycin) pharmacy bulk package*	**Vancomycin Hydrochloride for Injection**
	10 g (of vancomycin) pharmacy bulk package*	**Vancomycin Hydrochloride for Injection**
For injection, for IV infusion	500 mg (of vancomycin)*	**Vancomycin Hydrochloride for Injection**
		Vancomycin Hydrochloride Sterile ADD-Vantage®, Hospira
	1 g (of vancomycin)*	**Vancomycin Hydrochloride for Injection**
		Vancomycin Hydrochloride for Injection ADD-Vantage®, Hospira

*available from one or more manufacturer, distributor, and/or repackager by generic (nonproprietary) name

Vancomycin Hydrochloride in Dextrose

Parenteral		
Injection (frozen), for IV infusion	5 mg (of vancomycin) per ml (500 mg) in 5% Dextrose	**Vancocin® HCl in Iso-osmotic Dextrose Injection** (Galaxy® [Baxter]), Lilly

†Use is not currently included in the labeling approved by the US Food and Drug Administration

LINCOMYCINS 8:12.28.20

Clindamycin Hydrochloride
Clindamycin Palmitate Hydrochloride
Clindamycin Phosphate

■ Clindamycin, a lincosamide antibiotic, is a derivative of lincomycin.

Uses

Clindamycin is used for the treatment of certain serious infections caused by susceptible aerobic gram-positive bacteria (staphylococci, streptococci, pneumococci) and for the treatment of certain serious infections caused by susceptible anaerobic bacteria. Use of clindamycin generally should be reserved for the treatment of serious infections when less toxic anti-infectives cannot be used (e.g., penicillin-allergic patients or other patients for whom a penicillin is inappropriate). Because clindamycin has been associated with potentially fatal colitis (see Cautions: GI Effects), the manufacturer recommends that clinicians consider the nature of the infection and the suitability of less toxic alternatives (e.g., erythromycin).

Certain infections may require incision and drainage or other indicated surgical procedures in addition to anti-infective treatment. Use of clindamycin does not eliminate the need for surgical procedures when indicated.

Because clindamycin does not distribute adequately into the CNS, the drug should *not* be used for the treatment of meningitis.

■ **Gram-positive Aerobic Bacterial Infections** Clindamycin is used orally or parenterally for the treatment of serious respiratory tract infections caused by susceptible staphylococci, *Streptococcus pneumoniae*, or other streptococci or serious skin and skin structure infections caused by susceptible staphylococci, *S. pneumoniae*, or *S. pyogenes* (group A β-hemolytic streptococci; GAS). Clindamycin also is used parenterally for the treatment of septicemia caused by susceptible *Staphylococcus aureus* or streptococci, treatment of serious bone and joint infections (including acute hematogenous osteomyelitis) caused by susceptible *S. aureus*, and as adjunctive therapy in the surgical treatment of chronic bone and joint infections caused by susceptible bacteria. However, clindamycin generally should be reserved for use in penicillin-allergic or other patients when less toxic alternatives cannot be used.

■ **Anaerobic Bacterial Infections** Clindamycin is used orally or parenterally for the treatment of serious lower respiratory tract infections (e.g., empyema, pneumonia, lung abscess), serious skin and skin structure infections, septicemia, intra-abdominal infections (e.g., peritonitis, intra-abdominal abscess), and gynecologic infections (e.g., endometritis, nongonococcal tubo-ovarian abscess, pelvic cellulitis, postsurgical vaginal cuff infections) caused by susceptible anaerobic bacteria. Parenteral clindamycin also is used for the treatment of serious bone and joint infections (including acute hematogenous osteomyelitis) caused by susceptible anaerobes and as adjunctive therapy in the surgical treatment of chronic bone and joint infections caused by susceptible bacteria. Although previously considered a drug of choice for the treatment of infections caused by *Bacteroides*, clindamycin is no longer *routinely* recommended for the treatment of intra-abdominal infections because of the increasing incidence of *B. fragilis* resistant to the drug. In the treatment of mixed aerobic-anaerobic bacterial infections (e.g., pelvic inflammatory disease), clindamycin has been used in conjunction with an IM or IV aminoglycoside.

■ **Acute Otitis Media** Oral clindamycin is used as an alternative for the treatment of acute otitis media† (AOM).

When anti-infective therapy is indicated for the treatment of AOM, the American Academy of Pediatrics (AAP) recommends high-dose amoxicillin or amoxicillin and clavulanate as the drug of first choice for initial treatment. These experts recommend certain cephalosporins (cefdinir, cefpodoxime, cefuroxime, ceftriaxone) as alternatives for initial treatment in penicillin-allergic patients who do not have a history of severe and/or recent penicillin-allergic reactions.

AAP states that clindamycin (with or without a third generation cephalosporin) is a possible alternative for the treatment of AOM in patients who fail to respond to initial treatment with first-line or preferred alternatives. When retreatment of AOM is indicated after failure of initial treatment, high-dose amoxicillin and clavulanate or IM ceftriaxone usually is recommended. Although clindamycin may be effective in infections caused by penicillin-resistant *S. pneumoniae*, the drug may not be effective against multidrug-resistant *S. pneumoniae* and usually is inactive against *Haemophilus influenzae*. If clindamycin is used for retreatment of AOM, concomitant use of an anti-infective active against *H. influenzae* and *Moraxella catarrhalis* (e.g., cefdinir, cefixime, cefuroxime) should be considered.

For additional information regarding treatment of AOM, including information on diagnosis and management strategies, anti-infectives for initial treatment, duration of initial treatment, and anti-infectives after initial treatment failure, see Acute Otitis Media under Uses: Otitis Media, in the Cephalosporins General Statement 8:12.06.

■ **Pharyngitis and Tonsillitis** Oral clindamycin is used as an alternative for the treatment of pharyngitis and tonsillitis† caused by *S. pyogenes* (group A β-hemolytic streptococci; GAS). Although clindamycin usually is effective in eradicating *S. pyogenes* from the nasopharynx, it is reserved for use as an alternative in patients who cannot receive β-lactam anti-infectives. In addition, clindamycin is recommended as one of several possible alternatives for the treatment of symptomatic patients who failed to respond to initial penicillin treatment or have multiple, recurrent episodes of pharyngitis known to be caused by *S. pyogenes*.

Selection of an anti-infective for the treatment of *S. pyogenes* pharyngitis and tonsillitis should be based on the drug's spectrum of activity, bacteriologic and clinical efficacy, potential adverse effects, ease of administration, patient compliance, and cost. No regimen has been found to date that effectively eradicates group A β-hemolytic streptococci in 100% of patients.

Because the drugs have a narrow spectrum of activity, are inexpensive, and generally are effective with a low frequency of adverse effects, AAP, Infectious Diseases Society of America (IDSA), and American Heart Association (AHA) recommend a penicillin regimen (i.e., 10 days of oral penicillin V or oral amoxicillin or a single dose of IM penicillin G benzathine) as the treatment of choice for *S. pyogenes* pharyngitis and tonsillitis and prevention of initial attacks (primary prevention) of rheumatic fever. Other anti-infectives (e.g., oral cephalosporins, oral macrolides, oral clindamycin) are recommended as alternatives in penicillin-allergic patients.

■ **Respiratory Tract Infections** Clindamycin is used for the treatment of serious respiratory tract infections (e.g., pneumonia, empyema, lung abscess) caused by susceptible *S. aureus*, *S. pneumoniae*, other streptococci, or anaerobes.

IDSA and American Thoracic Society (ATS) consider clindamycin an alternative agent for the treatment of community-acquired pneumonia (CAP) caused by *S. pneumoniae* or *S. aureus* (methicillin-susceptible strains) in adults. IDSA also considers clindamycin an alternative for the treatment of CAP caused by *S. pneumoniae*, *S. pyogenes*, or *S. aureus* in pediatric patients. For the treatment of pneumonia caused by methicillin-resistant *S. aureus* (MRSA; also known as oxacillin-resistant *S. aureus* or ORSA), IDSA states that clindamycin is one of several options, unless the strain is resistant to clindamycin.

For information regarding the treatment of CAP, including infections caused by MRSA, the current clinical practice guidelines from IDSA available at http://www.idsociety.org should be consulted.

■ **Skin and Skin Structure Infections** Clindamycin is used for the treatment of serious skin and skin structure infections caused by susceptible staphylococci, *S. pneumoniae*, other streptococci, or anaerobes. Clindamycin is recommended as one of several options for the treatment of staphylococcal and streptococcal skin and skin structure infections, including those known or suspected to be caused by susceptible MRSA.

Clindamycin is used in conjunction with or as an alternative to penicillin G for the treatment of clostridial myonecrosis† (gas gangrene) caused by *Clostridium perfringens* or other *Clostridium*.

Although the fixed combination of amoxicillin and clavulanate usually is the drug of choice for the treatment of infected human or animal (e.g., dog, cat, reptile) bite wounds, alternative regimens include clindamycin in conjunction with either an extended-spectrum cephalosporin or co-trimoxazole. Purulent bite wounds usually are polymicrobial and broad-spectrum anti-infective coverage is recommended. Nonpurulent infected bite wounds usually are caused by staphylococci and streptococci, but can be polymicrobial.

For information regarding the treatment of skin and skin structure infections, including infections caused by MRSA, the current clinical practice guidelines from IDSA available at http://www.idsociety.org should be consulted.

■ **Actinomycosis** Clindamycin has been recommended as an alternative to penicillin G or ampicillin for the treatment of actinomycosis†, including infections caused by *Actinomyces israelii*.

■ **Anthrax** Although limited clinical data are available regarding use of clindamycin in the treatment of anthrax†, clindamycin was included in a multiple-drug regimen that was effective for the treatment of several patients in the US who developed anthrax during September and October 2001 following exposure to an intentional release of anthrax spores (biologic warfare, bioterrorism). At least 2 patients were treated with a parenteral regimen of ciprofloxacin (400 mg every 8 hours), rifampin (300 mg every 12 hours), and clindamycin (900 mg every 8 hours).

Because of the rapid course of symptomatic inhalational anthrax and high mortality rate, prompt recognition of symptoms and early initiation of anti-infective therapy is essential. The US Centers for Disease Control and Prevention (CDC) and other experts (e.g., US Working Group on Civilian Biodefense) recommend that treatment of inhalational anthrax that occurs as the result of exposure to anthrax spores in the context of biologic warfare or bioterrorism should be initiated with a multiple-drug parenteral regimen that includes ciprofloxacin or doxycycline and 1 or 2 additional anti-infective agents predicted to be effective. Multiple-drug parenteral regimens also are recommended for the treatment of cutaneous anthrax if there are signs of systemic involvement, extensive edema, or lesions on the head and neck. Based on in vitro data, drugs that have been suggested as possibilities to augment ciprofloxacin or doxycycline in such multiple-drug regimens include chloramphenicol, clindamycin, rifampin, vancomycin, clarithromycin, imipenem, penicillin, or ampicillin. Strains of *Bacillus anthracis* that were associated with cases of inhalational or cutaneous anthrax† that occurred in the US (Florida, New York, District of Columbia) during September and October 2001 following bioterrorism-related anthrax exposures were susceptible to clindamycin in vitro.

Based on in vitro data, clindamycin also has been suggested as a possible alternative for postexposure prophylaxis following a suspected or confirmed exposure to aerosolized anthrax spores† (inhalational anthrax) when the drugs of choice (ciprofloxacin, doxycycline) are not tolerated or cannot be used.

For information on treatment of anthrax and recommendations for prophylaxis following exposure to anthrax spores, see Uses: Anthrax, in Ciprofloxacin 8:12.18.

■ **Babesiosis** Oral or IV clindamycin is used in conjunction with oral quinine sulfate for the treatment of babesiosis† caused by *Babesia microti* or other *Babesia*.

Although several species of *Babesia* can infect humans (e.g., *B. microti*, *B. divergens*, *B. duncani*, *B. venatorum*), *B. microti* is the most common cause of babesiosis in the US. *B. microti* is transmitted by *Ixodes scapularis* ticks, which also may be simultaneously infected with and transmit *Borrelia burgdorferi* (causative agent of Lyme disease) and *Anaplasma phagocytophilum* (causative agent of human granulocytotropic anaplasmosis [HGA, formerly known as human granulocytic ehrlichiosis]). Therefore, the possibility of coinfection with *B. burgdorferi* and/or *A. phagocytophilum* should be considered in patients who have severe or persistent symptoms despite appropriate anti-infective treatment for babesiosis.

IDSA states that all patients with active babesiosis (i.e., symptoms of viral-like infection and identification of babesial parasites in blood smears or by polymerase chain reaction [PCR] amplification of babesial DNA) should receive anti-infective treatment because of the risk of complications; however, symptomatic patients whose serum contains antibody to babesia but whose blood lacks identifiable babesial parasites on smear or babesial DNA by PCR should not receive treatment. In addition, these experts state that treatment is not generally recommended initially for asymptomatic individuals, regardless of the results of serologic examination, blood smears, or PCR, but should be considered if parasitemia persists for longer than 3 months.

When anti-infective treatment of babesiosis is indicated, IDSA and other clinicians recommend that either a regimen of clindamycin and quinine or a regimen of atovaquone and azithromycin be used. There is some evidence that, in patients with mild or moderate illness, the atovaquone and azithromycin regimen may be as effective and better tolerated than the clindamycin and quinine regimen. However, the clindamycin and quinine regimen generally is preferred for the treatment of severe babesiosis caused by *M. microti* and infections caused by *M. divergens*, *B. duncani*, *B. divergens*-like organisms, or *B. venatorum*. Patients with moderate to severe babesiosis should be monitored closely during treatment to ensure clinical improvement. Exchange transfusions have been used successfully in asplenic patients with life-threatening babesiosis and should be considered, especially in severely ill patients with high levels of parasitemia (10% or more), significant hemolysis, or compromised renal, hepatic, or pulmonary function.

■ **Bacterial Vaginosis** Oral clindamycin is used in the treatment of bacterial vaginosis† (formerly called *Haemophilus* vaginitis, *Gardnerella* vaginitis, nonspecific vaginitis, *Corynebacterium* vaginitis, or anaerobic vaginosis). The drug also is used intravaginally as a vaginal cream or vaginal suppository for the treatment of bacterial vaginosis (see Clindamycin Phosphate 84:04.04).

Bacterial vaginosis is a polymicrobial syndrome that can occur when normal hydrogen peroxide-producing *Lactobacillus* in the vagina are replaced by overgrowth of various anaerobic bacteria (e.g., *Prevotella*, *Mobiluncus*), *Gardnerella vaginalis*, *Ureaplasma urealyticum*, *Mycoplasma hominis*, *Atopobium vaginae*, or other bacteria. Treatment of bacterial vaginosis usually is recommended to relieve signs and symptoms of infection, regardless of pregnancy status.

For the treatment of bacterial vaginosis, CDC and other experts recommend a 7-day regimen of oral metronidazole (500 mg twice daily); a 5-day regimen of intravaginal metronidazole 0.75% gel; or a 7-day regimen of intravaginal clindamycin 2% cream. Alternative regimens include a 2-day regimen of oral tinidazole (2 g once daily); a 5-day regimen of oral tinidazole (1 g once daily); a 7-day regimen of oral clindamycin (300 mg twice daily); or a 3-day regimen of intravaginal clindamycin 100-mg suppositories. CDC and other clinicians state that the oral or intravaginal metronidazole or clindamycin regimens can be used to treat symptomatic bacterial vaginosis in pregnant women.

Regardless of the treatment regimen used, relapse or recurrence of bacterial vaginosis is common. Retreatment with the same regimen or an alternative regimen (e.g., oral therapy when topical therapy was used initially) can be effective for treating persistent or recurrent bacterial vaginosis after the first occurrence. Maintenance suppressive therapy with intravaginal metronidazole (0.75% gel twice weekly for 4–6 months) may reduce recurrences, but this benefit may not persist after suppressive therapy is discontinued.

■ **Malaria** ***Treatment of Uncomplicated Malaria*** Oral clindamycin is used in conjunction with oral quinine sulfate for the *treatment* of uncomplicated chloroquine-resistant *Plasmodium falciparum* malaria† or when the plasmodial species has not been identified. Clindamycin is *not* effective when used alone for the treatment of malaria.

For the treatment of uncomplicated malaria caused by chloroquine-resistant *P. falciparum* or the treatment of uncomplicated malaria when the plasmodial species has not been identified, CDC and other clinicians recommend the fixed combination of atovaquone and proguanil hydrochloride (atovaquone/proguanil), the fixed combination of artemether and lumefantrine (artemether/lumefantrine), or a regimen that includes quinine sulfate in conjunction with doxycycline, tetracycline, or clindamycin. Although mefloquine is another option for treatment in these patients, CDC states that mefloquine should only be considered when other options cannot be used and is not recommended if malaria was acquired in Southeast Asia.

When a quinine sulfate regimen is used, concomitant doxycycline or tetracycline generally is preferable to concomitant clindamycin because more efficacy data exist regarding regimens that include tetracyclines. However, for pregnant women with uncomplicated malaria caused by chloroquine-resistant *P. falciparum*, a regimen of quinine sulfate and clindamycin is recommended. Although tetracyclines generally are contraindicated in pregnant women, in rare circumstances (e.g., if other treatment options are not available or are not tolerated) quinine sulfate may be used in conjunction with doxycycline or tetracycline if the benefits outweigh the risks.

Pediatric patients with uncomplicated malaria generally can receive the same treatment regimens recommended for adults using age- and weight-appropriate drugs and dosages. However, because doxycycline and tetracycline generally are contraindicated in children younger than 8 years of age, children in this age group with uncomplicated chloroquine-resistant *P. falciparum* malaria or when the plasmodial species has not been identified may receive a regimen of oral quinine sulfate *alone* for a full 7 days (regardless of geographic area where infection was acquired) or atovaquone/proguanil, artemether/lumefantrine, or a regimen of oral quinine sulfate in conjunction with oral clindamycin. Mefloquine should only be considered in these children when other options cannot be used and is not recommended if malaria was acquired in Southeast Asia. In rare circumstances when other treatment options are unavailable or are not tolerated, CDC states that doxycycline or tetracycline may be used in conjunction with quinine sulfate in children younger than 8 years of age if the benefits of tetracycline therapy outweigh the risks.

Treatment of Severe Malaria Oral or IV clindamycin is used in conjunction with IV quinidine gluconate for the *treatment* of severe *P. falciparum* malaria† in adults and children.

Patients with severe malaria require aggressive antimalarial treatment initiated as soon as possible after the diagnosis using a parenteral regimen. CDC recommends that severe malaria be treated with IV quinidine gluconate therapy in conjunction with a 7-day course of doxycycline, tetracycline, or clindamycin administered orally or IV as tolerated. After parasitemia is reduced to less than 1% and the patient can tolerate oral therapy, IV quinidine gluconate can be discontinued and oral quinine sulfate initiated to complete 3 or 7 days of total quinidine and quinine therapy as determined by the geographic origin of the infecting parasite (7 days if acquired in Southeast Asia or 3 days if acquired elsewhere).

Assistance with diagnosis or treatment of malaria is available by contacting the CDC Malaria Hotline at 770-488-7788 or 855-856-4713 from 9:00 a.m. to 5:00 p.m. Eastern Standard Time or the CDC Emergency Operation Center at 770-488-7100 after hours and on weekends and holidays.

■ **Pelvic Inflammatory Disease** IV clindamycin used in conjunction with IV or IM gentamicin is one of several possible parenteral regimens for the treatment of acute pelvic inflammatory disease (PID) in adults and adolescents. PID is a polymicrobial infection most frequently caused by *Neisseria gonorrhoeae* and/or *Chlamydia trachomatis*; however, organisms that can be part of the normal vaginal flora (e.g., anaerobic bacteria, *G. vaginalis*, *H. influenzae*, enteric gram-negative bacilli, *S. agalactiae*) or mycoplasma (e.g., *M. hominis*, *U. urealyticum*) also may be involved. PID is treated with an empiric regimen that provides broad-spectrum coverage. The regimen should be effective against *N. gonorrhoeae* and *C. trachomatis* and also probably should be effective against anaerobes. In addition, women with PID often have bacterial vaginosis concurrently, a polymicrobial infection that can include anaerobes. (See Uses: Bacterial Vaginosis.)

The optimum regimen for the treatment of PID has not been identified. A variety of parenteral and oral regimens have been recommended by CDC and other clinicians. When a parenteral regimen is used, these experts recommend a regimen of IV cefotetan in conjunction with oral or IV doxycycline; IV cefoxitin in conjunction with oral or IV doxycycline; or IV clindamycin in conjunction with IM or IV gentamicin. The parenteral regimen should be continued until 24–48 hours after the patient improves clinically and then an oral regimen of either doxycycline (100 mg twice daily) or clindamycin (450 mg 4 times daily) is used to complete 14 days of therapy. If tubo-ovarian abscess is present, at least 24 hours of inpatient observation is recommended and use of oral clindamycin or oral metronidazole in addition to oral doxycycline is preferred for follow-up oral therapy since this provides more effective coverage against anaerobes than doxycycline alone.

■ **Pneumocystis jirovecii Pneumonia** ***Treatment of Pneumocystis jirovecii Pneumonia*** Clindamycin is used in conjunction with primaquine for the treatment of *Pneumocystis jirovecii* (formerly *Pneumocystis carinii*) pneumonia† (PCP) in individuals with human immunodeficiency virus (HIV) infection. Clindamycin is designated an orphan drug by FDA for the treatment of PCP associated with acquired immunodeficiency syndrome (AIDS).

Co-trimoxazole is the drug of choice for the treatment of mild, moderate, or severe PCP, including PCP in HIV-infected adults, adolescents, and children. CDC, National Institutes of Health (NIH), and IDSA state that a regimen of primaquine and clindamycin is an alternative for the treatment of mild, moderate, or severe PCP in HIV-infected adults and adolescents who have had an inadequate response to co-trimoxazole or when co-trimoxazole is contraindicated or not tolerated. Although data are not available regarding use in children, CDC, NIH, IDSA, and AAP state that a regimen of primaquine and clindamycin also can be considered an alternative to co-trimoxazole for the treatment of PCP in HIV-infected children based on data in adults.

Results of clinical studies indicate that clindamycin administered IV (1.8–3.6 g given in 3 or 4 divided doses daily) or orally (1.2–3.6 g in 3 or 4 divided doses daily [in some cases oral clindamycin was administered after initial IV administration]) in conjunction with oral primaquine (15 or 30 mg daily) for a total 21 days of therapy is effective for the treatment of PCP in HIV-infected adults. Most patients exhibit clinical improvement within 2–7 days, and the combination generally appears to be well tolerated.

Prevention of Pneumocystis jirovecii Pneumonia Co-trimoxazole is the drug of choice for prevention of initial episodes (primary prophylaxis) of PCP in HIV-infected adults, adolescents, and children. CDC, NIH, and IDSA state that a regimen of primaquine and clindamycin is *not* recommended for primary PCP prophylaxis because data are insufficient to determine efficacy of the regimen for such prophylaxis.

Although a regimen of clindamycin and primaquine has been used as an alternative to co-trimoxazole for long-term suppressive or chronic maintenance therapy (secondary prophylaxis) of PCP† in a limited number of AIDS patients, this regimen is *not* included in CDC, NIH, IDSA, and AAP recommendations for secondary prophylaxis of PCP in HIV-infected adults, adolescents, or children. Co-trimoxazole is the drug of choice for secondary PCP prophylaxis in HIV-infected adults, adolescents, and children.

■ **Toxoplasmosis** ***Treatment of Toxoplasmosis*** Clindamycin is used in conjunction with pyrimethamine (and leucovorin) as an alternative for the treatment of toxoplasmosis caused by *Toxoplasma gondii*.

Pyrimethamine (and leucovorin) in conjunction with sulfadiazine is the regimen of choice for initial treatment of toxoplasmosis, including toxoplasmic encephalitis in HIV-infected adults, adolescents, and children. A regimen of pyrimethamine (and leucovorin) in conjunction with clindamycin is the preferred alternative in HIV-infected adults and adolescents who are unable to tolerate sulfadiazine or who failed to respond to an initial regimen of pyrimethamine and sulfadiazine. When a parenteral regimen is required for initial treatment of toxoplasmosis in severely ill adults or adolescents, some experts suggest parenteral co-trimoxazole or a regimen of oral pyrimethamine (and leucovorin) in conjunction with parenteral clindamycin.

Pyrimethamine (and leucovorin) in conjunction with sulfadiazine also is the regimen of choice for the treatment of congenital toxoplasmosis and the treatment of acquired CNS, ocular, or systemic toxoplasmosis in HIV-infected children. The preferred alternative for the treatment of toxoplasmosis in neonates or HIV-infected children with sulfonamide sensitivity is pyrimethamine (and leucovorin) in conjunction with clindamycin. Empiric treatment of congenital toxoplasmosis should be strongly considered in infants born to HIV-infected women who had symptomatic or asymptomatic toxoplasmosis during pregnancy, regardless of whether the mother received toxoplasmosis treatment during the pregnancy. Pregnant women with suspected or confirmed primary toxoplasmosis and neonates with possible or documented congenital toxoplasmosis should be managed in consultation with an appropriate infectious disease specialist.

Prevention of Recurrence of Toxoplasmosis CDC, NIH, IDSA, and AAP state that HIV-infected adults, adolescents, and children who have completed initial treatment of *T. gondii* encephalitis should receive chronic maintenance therapy (secondary prophylaxis) to prevent relapse.

Pyrimethamine (and leucovorin) in conjunction with sulfadiazine is the regimen of choice for long-term suppressive or chronic maintenance therapy (secondary prophylaxis) of toxoplasmosis in HIV-infected adults, adolescents, and children. A regimen of pyrimethamine (and leucovorin) in conjunction with clindamycin is one of several alternatives for secondary prophylaxis of toxoplasmosis in HIV-infected adults, adolescents, and children who cannot tolerate sulfonamides.

CDC, NIH, and IDSA state that secondary prophylaxis against toxoplasmosis generally can be discontinued in HIV-infected adults and adolescents who have successfully completed initial therapy for toxoplasmic encephalitis, remain asymptomatic with respect to toxoplasmic encephalitis, and have $CD4^+$ T-cell counts that have remained greater than 200/mm^3 for more than 6 months in response to antiretroviral therapy. Some experts recommend obtaining a magnetic resonance image (MRI) of the brain as part of the evaluation to determine whether discontinuance of secondary prophylaxis is appropriate. Secondary prophylaxis against toxoplasmosis should be reinitiated in HIV-infected adults and adolescents if $CD4^+$ T-cell counts decrease to less than 200/mm^3, regardless of plasma HIV viral load.

The safety of discontinuing secondary toxoplasmosis prophylaxis in HIV-infected children receiving potent antiretroviral therapy has not been extensively studied. However, based on data from adults, CDC, NIH, IDSA, and AAP state that discontinuance of secondary prophylaxis against toxoplasmosis can be considered in HIV-infected children 1 to less than 6 years of age who have completed toxoplasmosis treatment, have received more than 6 months of stable antiretroviral therapy, are asymptomatic with respect to toxoplasmosis, and have $CD4^+$ T-cell percentages that have remained greater than 15% for more than 6 consecutive months. In HIV-infected children 6 years of age or older who have received more than 6 months of antiretroviral therapy, consideration can be given to discontinuing secondary prophylaxis against toxoplasmosis if $CD4^+$ T-cell counts have remained greater than 200/mm^3 for more than 6 consecutive months. Prophylaxis should be reinitiated in HIV-infected children if these parameters are not met.

■ **Perioperative Prophylaxis** IV clindamycin is recommended as an alternative for perioperative prophylaxis† to reduce the incidence of infections in patients undergoing certain clean, contaminated surgeries when the drugs of choice (e.g., cefazolin, cefuroxime, cefoxitin, cefotetan) cannot be used because the patient is hypersensitive to β-lactam anti-infectives.

Some experts state that clindamycin or vancomycin is a reasonable alternative for perioperative prophylaxis in patients allergic to β-lactam anti-infectives who are undergoing cardiac surgery (e.g., coronary artery bypass grafting, valve repairs, cardiac device implantation), neurosurgery (e.g., craniotomy, spinal and CSF-shunting procedures, intrathecal pump placement), orthopedic surgery (e.g., spinal procedures, hip fracture, internal fixation, total joint replacement), non-cardiac thoracic surgery (e.g., lobectomy, pneumonectomy, lung resection, thoracotomy), vascular surgery (e.g., arterial procedures involving a prosthesis, the abdominal aorta, or a groin incision), lower extremity amputation for ischemia, or certain transplant procedures (e.g., heart and/or lung). These experts state that clindamycin also is a reasonable alternative for perioperative prophylaxis in patients allergic to β-lactam anti-infectives who are undergoing head and neck surgery (e.g., incisions through oral or pharyngeal mucosa).

For procedures that might involve exposure to enteric gram-negative bacteria, some experts state that clindamycin or vancomycin used in conjunction with an aminoglycoside (e.g., amikacin, gentamicin, tobramycin), aztreonam, or a fluoroquinolone is a reasonable alternative in patients allergic to β-lactam anti-infectives. These procedures include certain GI and biliary tract procedures (e.g., esophageal or gastroduodenal procedures, appendectomy for uncomplicated appendicitis, surgery involving unobstructed small intestine, colorectal procedures), gynecologic and obstetric surgery (e.g., cesarean section, hysterectomy), urologic procedures involving an implanted prosthesis, and certain transplant procedures (e.g., liver, pancreas and/or kidney).

■ **Prevention of Bacterial Endocarditis** Clindamycin is used as an alternative to amoxicillin or ampicillin for prevention of α-hemolytic (viridans group) streptococcal bacterial endocarditis† in penicillin-allergic adults and children undergoing certain dental or upper respiratory tract procedures who have cardiac conditions that put them at highest risk of adverse outcomes from endocarditis.

The cardiac conditions identified by AHA as those associated with highest risk and for which endocarditis prophylaxis is reasonable are prosthetic cardiac valves or prosthetic material used for cardiac valve repair, previous infective endocarditis, cardiac valvulopathy after cardiac transplantation, and certain forms of congenital heart disease (i.e., unrepaired cyanotic congenital heart disease including palliative shunts and conduits; a completely repaired congenital heart defect where prosthetic material or device was placed by surgery or catheter intervention within the last 6 months; repaired congenital heart disease with residual defects at the site or adjacent to the site of a prosthetic patch or prosthetic device that inhibit endothelialization).

AHA states that anti-infective prophylaxis for prevention of α-hemolytic (viridans group) streptococcal bacterial endocarditis is reasonable for patients with the above cardiac risk factors if they are undergoing any dental procedures that involve manipulation of gingival tissue or the periapical region of teeth or perforation of the oral mucosa (e.g., biopsies, suture removal, placement of orthodontic bands). AHA states that anti-infective prophylaxis is not needed for routine anesthetic injections through noninfected tissue, dental radiographs, placement of removable prosthodontic or orthodontic appliances, adjustment of orthodontic appliances, placement of orthodontic brackets, shedding of deciduous teeth, or bleeding from trauma to the lips or oral mucosa.

AHA states that anti-infective prophylaxis for prevention of bacterial endocarditis also is reasonable for patients with these cardiac risk factors if they are undergoing invasive procedures of the respiratory tract that involve incision or biopsy of respiratory mucosa (e.g., tonsillectomy, adenoidectomy) and may be reasonable for such patients if they are undergoing surgical procedures that involve infected skin, skin structure, or musculoskeletal tissue. However, anti-infective prophylaxis solely to prevent infective endocarditis is no longer recommended by AHA for GI or genitourinary tract procedures.

For additional information on which cardiac conditions are associated with the highest risk of adverse outcomes from endocarditis and more specific information regarding use of prophylaxis to prevent endocarditis in these patients, the current recommendations published by AHA should be consulted.

■ **Prevention of Perinatal Group B Streptococcal Disease** IV clindamycin is used as an alternative to parenteral penicillin G or ampicillin for prevention of perinatal group B streptococcal (GBS) disease† in certain women who are hypersensitive to penicillins.

Pregnant women who are colonized with GBS in the genital or rectal areas can transmit GBS infection to their infants during labor and delivery, resulting in invasive neonatal infection that can be associated with substantial morbidity and mortality. Intrapartum anti-infective prophylaxis for prevention of early-onset neonatal GBS disease is administered *selectively* to women at high risk for transmitting GBS infection to their neonates. CDC and AAP recommend *routine* universal prenatal screening for GBS colonization (e.g., vaginal and rectal cultures) in *all* pregnant women at 35–37 weeks of gestation, unless GBS bacteriuria is known to be present during the current pregnancy or the woman had a previous infant with invasive GBS disease. Intrapartum anti-infective prophylaxis for prevention of perinatal GBS is indicated in pregnant women identified as GBS carriers during the routine prenatal GBS screening performed at 35–37 weeks during the current pregnancy, in women with GBS bacteriuria identified at any time during the current pregnancy, and in women who had a previous infant diagnosed with invasive GBS disease. Intrapartum anti-infective prophylaxis also is indicated in women with unknown GBS status at the time of onset of labor (i.e., culture not done, incomplete, or results unknown), if delivery is at less than 37 weeks of gestation, the duration of amniotic membrane rupture is 18 hours or longer, intrapartum temperature is 38°C or higher, or an intrapartum nucleic acid amplification test (NAAT) was positive for GBS.

When intrapartum anti-infective prophylaxis is indicated in the mother for prevention of GBS in the neonate, it should be initiated at the onset of labor or rupture of membranes. CDC, AAP, and others recommend penicillin G as the drug of choice and ampicillin as the preferred alternative for such prophylaxis. If intrapartum prophylaxis is indicated in a penicillin-allergic woman who is *not* at high risk for anaphylaxis (i.e., does not have a history of anaphylaxis, angioedema, respiratory distress, or urticaria after receiving a penicillin or cephalosporin), CDC, AAP, and others recommend IV cefazolin. If intrapartum prophylaxis is indicated in a penicillin-allergic woman who is at high risk for anaphylaxis (e.g., history of anaphylaxis, angioedema, respiratory distress, or urticaria after receiving a penicillin or cephalosporin), IV clindamycin is recommended if the GBS isolate is tested and found to be susceptible to clindamycin *and* erythromycin. GBS isolates susceptible to clindamycin but resistant to erythromycin in vitro should be evaluated for inducible clindamycin resistance. IV vancomycin can be used as an alternative in penicillin-allergic women if the GBS isolate is intrinsically resistant to clindamycin, demonstrates inducible resistance to clindamycin, or if susceptibility to clindamycin and erythromycin is unknown.

For additional information regarding prevention of perinatal group B streptococcal disease, the current guidelines from CDC or AAP should be consulted.

■ **Topical Uses** For topical uses of clindamycin, see Clindamycin Phosphate 84:04.04.

Dosage and Administration

■ **Reconstitution and Administration** Clindamycin hydrochloride and clindamycin palmitate hydrochloride are administered orally.

Clindamycin phosphate is administered by IM injection or by intermittent or continuous IV infusion. Clindamycin phosphate should *not* be administered by rapid IV injection.

In the treatment of serious anaerobic infections, the parenteral route is usually used initially but may be switched to the oral route when warranted by the patient's condition. In clinically appropriate circumstances, the oral route may be used initially.

Oral Administration Clindamycin hydrochloride capsules and clindamycin palmitate hydrochloride oral solution can be administered without regard to food.

Capsules. Clindamycin hydrochloride capsules should be administered orally with a full glass of water to avoid the possibility of esophageal irritation. The capsules should be swallowed whole and are not suitable for use in pediatric patients who are unable to swallow capsules.

Oral Solution. Clindamycin palmitate hydrochloride powder (granules) for oral solution must be reconstituted by adding 75 mL of water to the 100-mL bottle. A large portion of the 75 mL should be added initially and the bottle shaken vigorously; the remainder of the water should then be added and the bottle shaken until the solution is uniform.

The reconstituted oral solution contains 75 mg of clindamycin per 5 mL.

IM Injection For IM injection, commercially available clindamycin phosphate solution containing 150 mg of clindamycin per mL is administered undiluted.

Single IM doses should not exceed 600 mg.

IV Infusion Prior to IV infusion, commercially available clindamycin phosphate solution (including solutions provided in ADD-Vantage® vials) must be diluted with a compatible IV solution to a concentration not exceeding 18 mg/mL.

Clindamycin phosphate usually is administered by intermittent IV infusion. As an alternative, clindamycin phosphate may be given by continuous IV infusion *after* the first dose of the drug has been given by rapid IV infusion. (See Table 1.)

Commercially available premixed solutions of clindamycin phosphate in 5% dextrose are administered *only* by IV infusion. Clindamycin phosphate in 5% dextrose injection should be inspected visually for particulate matter and discoloration before administration whenever solution and container permit. Premixed solutions provided in flexible containers should be checked for minute leaks by firmly squeezing the bag. Premixed solutions should be discarded if the container seal is not intact or leaks are found or if the solution is not clear. Additives should not be introduced into containers of premixed solutions of clindamycin phosphate in 5% dextrose. Flexible containers should not be used in series connections with other plastic containers, since such use could result in air embolism from residual air being drawn from the primary container before administration of the fluid from the secondary container is complete.

Dilution. When commercially available clindamycin phosphate solution containing 150 mg of clindamycin per mL is used for IV infusion, the appropriate dose should be diluted in a compatible IV infusion solution and administered using the recommended rate of administration. (See Rate of Administration under Reconstitution and Administration: IV Infusion, in Dosage and Administration.)

Clindamycin phosphate solution provided in ADD-Vantage® vials must be diluted prior to IV infusion according to the directions provided by the manufacturer. The ADD-Vantage® vials are for IV infusion only.

Commercially available clindamycin phosphate pharmacy bulk packages are *not* intended for direct IV infusion; doses of the drug from the bulk package must be further diluted in a compatible IV infusion solution. The bulk package is intended for use only in a laminar flow hood. Entry into the bulk pharmacy vial should be made using a sterile transfer set or other sterile dispensing device, and the contents dispensed in aliquots using appropriate technique; multiple entries with a syringe and needle are not recommended. After entry into a pharmacy bulk package vial, the entire contents of the vial should be used promptly; any unused portion should be discarded within 24 hours after initial entry into the pharmacy bulk package vial.

Rate of Administration. Intermittent IV infusions of clindamycin phosphate solutions should be given over a period of at least 10–60 minutes and at a rate less than 30 mg/minute. No more than 1.2 g should be given by IV infusion in a single 1-hour period.

The manufacturer recommends that 300-mg doses should be diluted in 50 mL of compatible diluent and infused over 10 minutes; 600-mg doses should be diluted in 50 mL of diluent and infused over 20 minutes; 900-mg doses should be diluted in 50–100 mL of diluent and infused over 30 minutes; and 1.2-g doses should be diluted in 100 mL of diluent and infused over 40 minutes.

As an alternative to intermittent IV infusions, the manufacturer states that the drug can be given by continuous IV infusion in adults *after* an initial dose is given by IV infusion over 30 minutes. (See Table 1.)

Table 1. Infusion Rates for Continuous IV Infusion of Clindamycin Phosphate in Adults

Target Serum Clindamycin Concentrations	Infusion Rate for Initial Dose	Maintenance Infusion Rate
Greater than 4 mcg/mL	10 mg/minute for 30 minutes	0.75 mg/minute
Greater than 5 mcg/mL	15 mg/minute for 30 minutes	1 mg/minute
Greater than 6 mcg/mL	20 mg/minute for 30 minutes	1.25 mg/minute

■ Dosage

Dosage of clindamycin hydrochloride, clindamycin palmitate hydrochloride, and clindamycin phosphate is expressed in terms of clindamycin.

Dosage and duration of treatment depend on the severity of the infection. If clindamycin is used in infections caused by *Streptococcus pyogenes* (group A β-hemolytic streptococci; GAS), therapy should be continued for at least 10 days. At least 6 weeks of therapy may be required for certain serious infections (e.g., osteomyelitis).

Oral Dosage

General Dosage for Neonates. When clindamycin oral solution is used in pediatric patients, the manufacturer recommends 8–12 mg/kg daily for the treatment of serious infections, 13–16 mg/kg daily for severe infections, and 17–25 mg/kg daily for more severe infections; daily dosage is given in 3 or 4 equally divided doses. In pediatric patients weighing 10 kg or less, the manufacturer recommends a minimum clindamycin dosage of 37.5 mg 3 times daily.

When oral clindamycin is used in neonates 7 days of age or younger, the American Academy of Pediatrics (AAP) recommends a dosage of 5 mg/kg every 12 hours in those weighing 2 kg or less or 5 mg/kg every 8 hours in those weighing more than 2 kg.

In neonates 8–28 days of age, AAP recommends an oral clindamycin dosage of 5 mg/kg every 8 hours in those weighing 2 kg or less or 5 mg/kg every 6 hours in those weighing more than 2 kg. In extremely low-birthweight neonates (less than 1 kg), a dosage of 5 mg/kg every 12 hours can be considered until 2 weeks of age.

General Dosage for Infants and Children. When clindamycin capsules are used in pediatric patients able to swallow capsules, the manufacturer recommends 8–16 mg/kg daily given in 3 or 4 equally divided doses for the treatment of serious infections or 16–20 mg/kg daily given in 3 or 4 equally divided doses for more severe infections.

When the oral solution is used in pediatric patients, the manufacturer recommends 8–12 mg/kg daily for the treatment of serious infections, 13–16 mg/kg daily for severe infections, and 17–25 mg/kg daily for more severe infections; daily dosage is given in 3 or 4 equally divided doses. In pediatric patients weighing 10 kg or less, the manufacturer recommends a minimum dosage of 37.5 mg 3 times daily.

When oral clindamycin is used in pediatric patients beyond the neonatal period, AAP recommends a dosage of 10–25 mg/kg daily given in 3 equally divided doses for the treatment of mild to moderate infections or 30–40 mg/kg daily given in 3 or 4 equally divided doses for the treatment of severe infections.

General Adult Dosage. The usual adult dosage of oral clindamycin is 150–300 mg every 6 hours for the treatment of serious infections or 300–450 mg every 6 hours for the treatment of more severe infections.

Acute Otitis Media. If oral clindamycin is used as an alternative for the treatment of acute otitis media† (AOM) in children 6 months through 12 years of age, AAP recommends a dosage of 30–40 mg/kg daily given in 3 divided doses (with or without a third generation cephalosporin). (See Uses: Acute Otitis Media.)

Pharyngitis and Tonsillitis. If oral clindamycin is used as an alternative for the treatment of pharyngitis and tonsillitis caused by *S. pyogenes*† (group A β-hemolytic streptococci; GAS) (see Uses: Pharyngitis and Tonsillitis), AAP recommends a dosage of 10 mg/kg 3 times daily (up to 900 mg daily) for 10 days. The Infectious Diseases Society of America (IDSA) recommends a dosage of 7 mg/kg (up to 300 mg) 3 times daily for 10 days. The American Heart Association (AHA) recommends a dosage of 20 mg/kg daily (up to 1.8 g daily) given in 3 divided doses for 10 days.

Although anti-infective treatment is not recommended for most individuals identified as chronic pharyngeal GAS carriers, AAP and IDSA state that oral clindamycin can be given in a dosage of 20–30 mg/kg daily in 3 equally divided doses (up to 300 mg per dose or up to 900 mg daily) for 10 days when treatment is indicated in such patients.

Respiratory Tract Infections. If oral clindamycin is used in adults for the treatment of healthcare-associated or community-acquired pneumonia (CAP) caused by susceptible methicillin-resistant *Staphylococcus aureus* (MRSA; also known as oxacillin-resistant *S. aureus* or ORSA), IDSA recommends a dosage of 600 mg 3 times daily for 7–21 days.

If oral clindamycin is used for the treatment of CAP caused by susceptible gram-positive bacteria (e.g., *S. pneumoniae*, *S. pyogenes*, *S. aureus*) in children older than 3 months of age, IDSA recommends a dosage of 30–40 mg/kg daily given in 3 or 4 divided doses.

Babesiosis. For the treatment of babesiosis† caused by *Babesia microti* or other *Babesia* species, IDSA and other experts recommend that adults receive clindamycin in a dosage of 600 mg orally every 8 hours (or 300–600 mg IV every 6 hours) in conjunction with oral quinine sulfate (650 mg every 6 or 8 hours) given for 7–10 days.

For the treatment of babesiosis in pediatric patients, IDSA recommends an oral (or IV) clindamycin dosage of 7–10 mg/kg (up to 600 mg) every 6–8 hours in conjunction with oral quinine sulfate (8 mg/kg [up to 650 mg] every 8 hours) given for 7–10 days. Other clinicians recommend an oral (or IV) clindamycin dosage of 20–40 mg/kg (up to 600 mg) daily given in 3 or 4 divided doses for 7–10 days in conjunction with oral quinine sulfate (24 mg/kg daily given in 3 divided doses for 7–10 days).

Patients with mild to moderate babesiosis should have clinical improvement within 48 hours after treatment is initiated; symptoms should resolve completely within 3 months. Patients with severe babesiosis should receive IV clindamycin rather than oral clindamycin. Some patients may have persistent low-grade parasitemia for months after anti-infective treatment. Some experts suggest that anti-infective treatment in immunosuppressed patients should be continued for a minimum of 6 weeks and at least 2 weeks after the last positive smear. Regardless of the presence or absence of symptoms, IDSA suggests that retreatment be considered if babesial parasites or amplifiable babesial DNA is detected in blood 3 months or longer after initial treatment.

Bacterial Vaginosis. When oral clindamycin is used as an alternative for the treatment of bacterial vaginosis† in symptomatic women, the US Centers for Disease Control and Prevention (CDC) and other clinicians recommend a dosage of 300 mg twice daily for 7 days.

Malaria. If clindamycin is used in conjunction with quinine sulfate for the treatment of uncomplicated malaria caused by chloroquine-resistant *Plasmodium falciparum*† or when the plasmodial species has not been identified, CDC and other clinicians recommend that adults receive oral clindamycin in a dosage of 20 mg/kg daily in 3 equally divided doses given for 7 days in conjunction with oral quinine sulfate (650 mg 3 times daily given for 7 days if acquired in Southeast Asia or for 3 days if acquired elsewhere). Children with uncomplicated chloroquine-resistant *P. falciparum* malaria can receive oral clindamycin in a dosage of 20 mg/kg daily in 3 equally divided doses given for 7 days in conjunction with oral quinine sulfate (10 mg/kg 3 times daily given for 7 days if acquired in Southeast Asia or 3 days if acquired elsewhere).

If clindamycin is used in conjunction with IV quinidine gluconate (followed by oral quinine sulfate) for the treatment of severe malaria caused by *P. falciparum*† and if the patient is intolerant of oral therapy, treatment may be initiated in adults and children with a 10-mg/kg loading dose of IV clindamycin followed by 5 mg/kg IV every 8 hours continued until treatment can be switched to oral clindamycin (given in dosages recommended for uncomplicated malaria). The total duration of clindamycin therapy should be 7 days.

Pneumocystis jirovecii Pneumonia. If a regimen of oral clindamycin and primaquine is used as an alternative for the treatment of mild to moderate *Pneumocystis jirovecii* pneumonia† (PCP), CDC, National Institutes of Health (NIH), and IDSA recommend that adults and adolescents receive oral clindamycin in a dosage of 450 mg every 6 hours or 600 mg every 8 hours for 21 days in conjunction with oral primaquine (30 mg once daily for 21 days).

If a regimen of oral clindamycin and primaquine is used as an alternative for the treatment of moderate to severe PCP†, CDC, NIH, and IDSA recommend that adults and adolescents receive oral clindamycin in a dosage of 450 mg every 6 hours or 600 mg every 8 hours for 21 days in conjunction with oral primaquine (30 mg once daily for 21 days).

Although data regarding use in children are not available, if a regimen of oral clindamycin and primaquine is used as an alternative for the treatment of PCP in pediatric patients, some clinicians recommend that oral clindamycin be given in a dosage of 10 mg/kg (up to 300–450 mg) every 6 hours for 21 days in conjunction with oral primaquine (0.3 mg/kg once daily [up to 30 mg daily] for 21 days).

Toxoplasmosis. For the treatment of toxoplasmosis† caused by *Toxoplasma gondii* in HIV-infected adults and adolescents who cannot receive sulfadiazine or did not respond to an initial regimen, CDC, NIH, and IDSA recommend an oral (or IV) clindamycin dosage of 600 mg every 6 hours in conjunction with oral pyrimethamine (200-mg loading dose followed by 50 mg once daily in those weighing less than 60 kg or 75 mg once daily in those weighing 60 kg or more) and oral leucovorin (10–25 mg once daily; may be increased to 50 mg once or twice daily). Treatment should be continued for at least 6 weeks; a longer duration may be appropriate if disease is extensive or there is an incomplete response at 6 weeks.

For the treatment of congenital toxoplasmosis† or the treatment of acquired CNS, ocular, or systemic toxoplasmosis† in HIV-infected children who cannot receive sulfadiazine, CDC, NIH, and IDSA recommend an oral (or IV) clindamycin dosage of 5–7.5 mg/kg (up to 600 mg) 4 times daily in conjunction with oral pyrimethamine (2 mg/kg once daily for 2 days followed by 1 mg/kg once daily) and oral or IM leucovorin (10 mg with each pyrimethamine dose). Although optimal duration of treatment of congenital toxoplasmosis has not been determined, some clinicians recommend that the treatment regimen be continued for 12 months. In HIV-infected children with acquired CNS, ocular, or systemic toxoplasmosis, the treatment regimen should be continued for at least 6 weeks; a longer duration may be appropriate if disease is extensive or there is an incomplete response at 6 weeks.

For long-term suppressive therapy or chronic maintenance therapy† (secondary prophylaxis) to prevent relapse of toxoplasmosis in HIV-infected patients when the regimen of first choice (pyrimethamine and sulfadiazine) cannot be used, CDC, NIH, and IDSA recommend that adults and adolescents receive oral clindamycin in a dosage of 600 mg every 8 hours with pyrimethamine (25–50 mg once daily) and leucovorin (10–25 mg once daily). For secondary prophylaxis in HIV-infected infants and children, CDC, NIH, IDSA, and AAP recommend an oral clindamycin dosage of 7–10 mg/kg 3 times daily with oral pyrimethamine (1 mg/kg or 15 mg/m^2 [up to 25 mg] once daily) and oral leucovorin (5 mg once every 3 days). Long-term suppressive therapy for prophylaxis against relapse of toxoplasmosis in HIV-infected individuals generally can be discontinued if immune recovery has occurred as the result of potent antiretroviral therapy. (See Prevention of Recurrence of Toxoplasmosis under Uses: Toxoplasmosis.)

Prevention of Bacterial Endocarditis. When oral clindamycin is used as an alternative for prevention of bacterial endocarditis† in penicillin-allergic patients with certain cardiac conditions who are undergoing certain dental procedures or certain other procedures (see Uses: Prevention of Bacterial Endocarditis), AHA recommends that adults receive a single 600-mg dose and that children receive a single 20-mg/kg dose of the drug 30–60 minutes before the procedure.

Parenteral Dosage **General Dosage for Neonates.** The manufacturer recommends that neonates younger than 1 month of age receive IM or IV clindamycin in a dosage of 15–20 mg/kg daily given in 3 or 4 equally divided doses. The lower dosage may be adequate for small, premature neonates.

When IM or IV clindamycin is used in neonates 7 days of age or younger, AAP recommends 5 mg/kg every 12 hours in those weighing 2 kg or less or 5 mg/kg every 8 hours in those weighing more than 2 kg.

In neonates 8–28 days of age, AAP recommends an IM or IV clindamycin dosage of 5 mg/kg every 8 hours in those weighing 2 kg or less or 5 mg/kg every 6 hours in those weighing more than 2 kg. In extremely low-birthweight neonates (less than 1 kg), a dosage of 5 mg/kg every 12 hours can be considered until 2 weeks of age.

General Dosage for Infants and Children. The IM or IV dosage of clindamycin recommended by the manufacturer for infants and children 1 month of age or older is 20–40 mg/kg daily administered in 3 or 4 equally divided doses; the higher dosage should be used for more severe infections. Alternatively, the manufacturer states that these infants and children may receive 350 mg/m^2 daily for the treatment of serious infections or 450 mg/m^2 daily for the treatment of more severe infections.

In pediatric patients beyond the neonatal period, AAP recommends an IM or IV clindamycin dosage of 20–30 mg/kg daily given in 3 equally divided doses for the treatment of mild to moderate infections or 40 mg/kg daily given in 3 or 4 equally divided doses for the treatment of severe infections.

General Adult Dosage. The recommended adult dosage of IM or IV clindamycin is 600 mg to 1.2 g daily given in 2–4 equally divided doses for the treatment of serious infections or 1.2–2.7 g daily given in 2–4 equally divided doses for the treatment of more severe infections. In the treatment of life-threatening infections, adult IV dosage may be increased to a maximum of 4.8 g daily.

If continuous IV infusion of clindamycin is used to maintain serum clindamycin concentrations above 4–6 mcg/mL in adults, an initial dose is given by rapid IV infusion prior to continuous IV infusion. (See Table 1.)

Respiratory Tract Infections. If IV clindamycin is used in adults for the treatment of healthcare-associated pneumonia or CAP caused by susceptible methicillin-resistant *S. aureus* (MRSA), IDSA recommends a dosage of 600 mg 3 times daily for 7–21 days.

If parenteral clindamycin is used for the treatment of CAP caused by susceptible gram-positive bacteria (e.g., *S. pneumoniae*, *S. pyogenes*, *S. aureus*) in children older than 3 months of age, IDSA recommends a dosage of 40 mg/kg daily given in divided doses every 6–8 hours.

Anthrax. Although the optimum regimen for the treatment of inhalational anthrax† remains to be established, several patients who developed inhalational anthrax in the context of an intentional release of anthrax spores (biologic warfare, bioterrorism) were treated successfully with a multiple-drug regimen that included IV clindamycin (900 mg every 8 hours), IV ciprofloxacin (400 mg every 8 hours), and IV rifampin (300 mg every 12 hours). (See Uses: Anthrax.)

Duration of treatment is 60 days if anthrax occurred as the result of exposure to anthrax spores in the context of biologic warfare or bioterrorism.

Babesiosis. For the treatment of babesiosis† caused by *B. microti* or other *Babesia* species, IDSA and other experts recommend that adults receive clindamycin in a dosage of 300–600 mg IV every 6 hours (or 600 mg orally every 8 hours) in conjunction with oral quinine sulfate (650 mg every 6 or 8 hours) given for 7–10 days.

For the treatment of babesiosis in pediatric patients, IDSA recommends an IV (or oral) clindamycin dosage of 7–10 mg/kg (up to 600 mg) every 6–8 hours in conjunction with oral quinine sulfate (8 mg/kg [up to 650 mg] every 8 hours) given for 7–10 days. Other clinicians recommend an IV (or oral) clindamycin dosage of 20–40 mg/kg (up to 600 mg) daily given in 3 or 4 divided doses for 7–10 days in conjunction with oral quinine sulfate (24 mg/kg daily given in 3 divided doses for 7–10 days).

Patients with mild to moderate babesiosis should have clinical improvement within 48 hours after treatment is initiated; symptoms should resolve completely within 3 months. Patients with severe babesiosis should receive IV clindamycin rather than oral clindamycin. Some patients may have persistent low-grade parasitemia for months after anti-infective treatment. Some experts suggest that anti-infective treatment in immunosuppressed patients should be continued for a minimum of 6 weeks and at least 2 weeks after the last positive smear. Regardless of the presence or absence of symptoms, IDSA suggests that retreatment be considered if babesial parasites or amplifiable babesial DNA is detected in blood 3 months or longer after initial treatment.

Pelvic Inflammatory Disease. For the treatment of acute pelvic inflammatory disease (PID) when a parenteral regimen is indicated, adults and adolescents may receive 900 mg of clindamycin IV every 8 hours. Gentamicin sulfate should be administered concomitantly (initial IM or IV gentamicin dose of 2 mg/kg followed by 1.5 mg/kg every 8 hours; alternatively, 3–5 mg/kg of gentamicin can be given as a single daily dose). Both parenteral drugs can be discontinued 24–48 hours after there is clinical improvement and therapy continued with oral clindamycin in a dosage of 450 mg 4 times daily to complete 14 days of therapy. Alternatively, oral doxycycline (100 mg twice daily) can be given to complete 14 days of therapy. (See Uses: Pelvic Inflammatory Disease.)

Patients with PID who do not demonstrate substantial clinical improvement (e.g., defervescence; reduction in direct or rebound abdominal tenderness; reduction in uterine, adnexal, and cervical motion tenderness) within 72 hours of initiating parenteral or oral therapy usually require additional diagnostic tests and/or surgical intervention.

Pneumocystis jirovecii Pneumonia. If a regimen of IV clindamycin and oral primaquine is used as an alternative for the treatment of moderate to severe PCP†, CDC, NIH, and IDSA recommend that adults and adolescents receive IV clindamycin in a dosage of 600 mg every 6 hours or 900 mg every 8 hours for 21 days in conjunction with oral primaquine (30 mg once daily for 21 days).

Although data regarding use in children are not available, if a regimen of IV clindamycin and oral primaquine is used as an alternative for the treatment of PCP in pediatric patients, some clinicians recommend that IV clindamycin be given in a dosage of 10 mg/kg (up to 600 mg) every 6 hours for 21 days in conjunction with oral primaquine (0.3 mg/kg once daily [up to 30 mg daily] for 21 days).

Toxoplasmosis. For the treatment of toxoplasmosis† in HIV-infected adults and adolescents who cannot receive sulfadiazine or did not respond to an initial regimen, CDC, NIH, and IDSA recommend that adults and adolescents receive IV (or oral) clindamycin in a dosage of 600 mg every 6 hours in conjunction with oral pyrimethamine (200-mg loading dose followed by 50 mg once daily in those weighing less than 60 kg or 75 mg once daily in those weighing 60 kg or more) and oral leucovorin (10–25 mg once daily; may be increased to 50 mg once or twice daily).

For the treatment of congenital toxoplasmosis† or the treatment of acquired CNS, ocular, or systemic toxoplasmosis† in HIV-infected children, CDC, NIH, and IDSA recommend an IV (or oral) clindamycin dosage of 5–7.5 mg/kg (up to 600 mg) 4 times daily in conjunction with oral pyrimethamine (2 mg/kg once daily for 2 days followed by 1 mg/kg once daily) and oral or IM leucovorin (10 mg with each pyrimethamine dose). Although optimal duration of treatment has not been determined, some experts recommend that treatment of congenital toxoplasmosis be continued for 12 months. The treatment regimen should be continued for at least 6 weeks in HIV-infected children with acquired CNS, ocular, or systemic toxoplasmosis; a longer duration may be appropriate for extensive disease or if there is an incomplete response at 6 weeks.

Perioperative Prophylaxis. If clindamycin is used alone or in conjunction with another anti-infective for perioperative prophylaxis in patients undergoing certain surgeries when the drugs of choice cannot be used (see Uses: Perioperative Prophylaxis), some clinicians recommend that adults receive 900 mg of the drug and that pediatric patients receive 10 mg/kg of the drug given IV within 60 minutes prior to the initial incision.

During prolonged procedures, some clinicians suggest that additional intraoperative doses of clindamycin can be given every 6 hours for the duration of the procedure in patients with normal renal function. Postoperative doses of prophylactic anti-infectives generally are not recommended.

Prevention of Bacterial Endocarditis. When IM or IV clindamycin is used as an alternative for prevention of bacterial endocarditis† in penicillin-allergic patients (or patients unable to take oral medication) with certain cardiac conditions who are undergoing certain dental procedures or certain other procedures (see Uses: Prevention of Bacterial Endocarditis), AHA recommends that adults receive a single 600-mg dose and that children receive a single 20-mg/kg dose of the drug given 30–60 minutes before the procedure.

Prevention of Perinatal Group B Streptococcal Disease. If clindamycin is used for intrapartum anti-infective prophylaxis for prevention of perinatal group B streptococcal (GBS) disease† in women with penicillin hypersensitivity who should not receive a β-lactam anti-infective, CDC and AAP recommend that 900 mg of clindamycin be given IV at the time of onset of labor or rupture of membranes followed by 900 mg IV every 8 hours until delivery. Because *S. agalactiae* (group B streptococci; GBS) with resistance to clindamycin has been reported with increasing frequency, clinical isolates obtained during GBS prenatal screening should be tested for in vitro susceptibility to clindamycin whenever use of the drug is being considered for prevention of perinatal GBS disease. (See Uses: Prevention of Perinatal Group B Streptococcal Disease.)

■ Dosage in Renal and Hepatic Impairment

Renal Impairment Dosage adjustments are not usually necessary in patients with renal impairment.

Hepatic Impairment Dosage adjustments are not usually necessary in patients with hepatic impairment. However, because the plasma half-life of clindamycin may be prolonged, hepatic function should be monitored if the drug is used in those with severe hepatic impairment.

Cautions

■ GI Effects

Adverse GI effects frequently occur with oral, IM, or IV clindamycin and may be severe enough to necessitate discontinuance of the drug. Adverse GI effects reported in patients receiving clindamycin include nausea, vomiting, diarrhea, abdominal pain, and esophagitis. In addition, tenesmus, flatulence, bloating, anorexia, and weight loss have been reported.

An unpleasant or metallic taste has been reported in patients receiving oral clindamycin and also has been reported following IV administration of high doses of the drug.

Clostridium difficile-associated Diarrhea and Colitis Treatment with anti-infectives alters normal colon flora and may permit overgrowth of *Clostridium difficile*.

C. difficile infection (CDI) and *C. difficile*-associated diarrhea and colitis (CDAD; also known as antibiotic-associated diarrhea and colitis or pseudomembranous colitis) have been reported with nearly all anti-infectives, including clindamycin, and may range in severity from mild diarrhea to fatal colitis. *C. difficile* produces toxins A and B, which contribute to the development of CDAD; hypertoxin-producing strains of *C. difficile* are associated with increased morbidity and mortality since they may be refractory to anti-infectives and colectomy may be required. (See Superinfection/Clostridium difficile-associated Diarrhea and Colitis under Cautions: Precautions and Contraindications.)

■ Sensitivity and Dermatologic Reactions

Anaphylactic shock and anaphylactoid reactions with hypersensitivity have been reported in patients receiving clindamycin.

Other severe hypersensitivity reactions, including severe skin reactions such as toxic epidermal necrolysis, drug reaction with eosinophilia and systemic symptoms (DRESS), and Stevens-Johnson syndrome, have been reported and have been fatal in some cases. Acute generalized exanthematous pustulosis and erythema multiforme also have been reported.

Generalized mild to moderate morbilliform-like (maculopapular) rash is the most frequently reported adverse reaction to clindamycin. Vesiculobullous rash, urticaria, pruritus, angioedema, and rare instances of exfoliative dermatitis also have been reported.

■ Local Effects

Thrombophlebitis, erythema, pain, and swelling have occurred with IV administration of clindamycin.

IM administration of clindamycin has caused pain, induration, and sterile abscess at the injection site. Reversible increases in serum creatine kinase (CK, creatine phosphokinase, CPK) concentrations have been reported.

Local reactions can be minimized by giving deep IM injections or avoiding prolonged use of indwelling IV catheters.

■ Other Adverse Effects

Cardiopulmonary arrest and hypotension have been reported when IV clindamycin was administered too rapidly.

Although renal damage has not been directly attributed to clindamycin, renal dysfunction manifested as azotemia, oliguria, and/or proteinuria has been observed in patients receiving clindamycin.

Transient neutropenia (leukopenia) and eosinophilia, agranulocytosis, and thrombocytopenia have been reported in patients receiving clindamycin; however, a causal relationship was not established.

Jaundice, abnormal liver function tests, polyarthritis, and vaginitis also have been reported.

■ Precautions and Contraindications

Clindamycin is contraindicated in patients hypersensitive to clindamycin or lincomycin.

Prior to initiation of clindamycin, the patient should be questioned regarding prior hypersensitivity to drugs and other allergens. Clindamycin should be used with caution in atopic individuals.

If an anaphylactic or severe hypersensitivity reaction occurs during clindamycin therapy, the drug should be permanently discontinued and appropriate therapy instituted as necessary.

Superinfection/Clostridium difficile-associated Diarrhea and Colitis As with other anti-infectives, use of clindamycin may result in overgrowth of nonsusceptible organisms, especially yeasts. If superinfection occurs, appropriate therapy should be instituted.

Because CDAD has been reported with the use of nearly all anti-infectives, including clindamycin, it should be considered in the differential diagnosis in patients who develop diarrhea during or after clindamycin therapy. Careful medical history is necessary since CDAD has been reported to occur as late as 2 months or longer after anti-infective therapy is discontinued. If CDAD is suspected or confirmed, anti-infective therapy not directed against *C. difficile* should be discontinued whenever possible. Patients should be managed with appropriate supportive therapy (e.g., fluid and electrolyte management, protein supplementation), anti-infective therapy directed against *C. difficile* (e.g., metronidazole, vancomycin), and surgical evaluation as clinically indicated.

Patients should be advised that diarrhea is a common problem caused by anti-infectives and usually ends when the drug is discontinued; however, it is important to contact a clinician if watery and bloody stools (with or without stomach cramps and fever) occur during or as late as 2 months or longer after the last dose.

Clindamycin should always be discontinued if clinically important diarrhea occurs. The drug should be used with caution in patients with a history of GI disease, particularly colitis.

Selection and Use of Anti-infectives To reduce development of drug-resistant bacteria and maintain effectiveness of clindamycin and other antibacterials, the drug should be used only for the treatment or prevention of infections proven or strongly suspected to be caused by susceptible bacteria. When selecting or modifying anti-infective therapy, results of culture and in vitro susceptibility testing should be used. In the absence of such data, local epidemiology and susceptibility patterns should be considered when selecting anti-infectives for empiric therapy. Culture and susceptibility testing performed periodically during therapy provides information on the therapeutic effect of the anti-infective agent and the possible emergence of bacterial resistance.

Patients should be advised that antibacterials (including clindamycin) should only be used to treat bacterial infections and not used to treat viral infections (e.g., the common cold). Patients also should be advised about the importance of completing the full course of therapy, even if feeling better after a few days, and that skipping doses or not completing therapy may decrease effectiveness and increase the likelihood that bacteria will develop resistance and will not be treatable with clindamycin or other antibacterials in the future.

Other Precautions and Contraindications Some commercially available capsules of clindamycin hydrochloride (e.g., Cleocin HCl® 75- and 150-mg capsules) contain the dye tartrazine (FD&C yellow No. 5), which may cause allergic reactions, including bronchial asthma, in susceptible individuals. Although the incidence of tartrazine sensitivity is low, it frequently occurs in patients who are sensitive to aspirin.

Because clindamycin does not distribute adequately into the CNS, the drug should *not* be used for the treatment of CNS infections.

During prolonged clindamycin therapy, liver and renal function tests and blood cell counts should be performed periodically.

If clindamycin is used in patients with hepatic impairment, dosage adjustments may not be necessary; however, liver enzymes should be monitored periodically when the drug is used in those with severe hepatic impairment.

■ Pediatric Precautions

When clindamycin is used in pediatric patients (birth to 16 years of age), organ system functions should be monitored.

Each mL of clindamycin phosphate injection contains 9.45 mg of benzyl alcohol. Although a causal relationship has not been established, administration of injections preserved with benzyl alcohol has been associated with toxicity in neonates, including potentially fatal "gasping syndrome." Toxicity appears to have resulted from administration of large amounts (i.e., about 100–400 mg/kg daily) of benzyl alcohol in these neonates. Although the amounts of benzyl alcohol in recommended dosages of IM or IV clindamycin are substantially lower than amounts reported in association with "gasping syndrome," the minimum amount of benzyl alcohol at which toxicity may occur is unknown. The risk of benzyl alcohol toxicity depends on the quantity administered and capacity of the liver and kidneys to detoxify the chemical. Premature and low-birthweight infants may be more likely to develop toxicity. Although use of drugs preserved with benzyl alcohol should be avoided in neonates whenever possible, the American Academy of Pediatrics (AAP) states that the presence of small amounts of the preservative in a commercially available injection should not proscribe its use when indicated in an infant.

■ Geriatric Precautions

Clinical studies of clindamycin did not include sufficient numbers of patients 65 years of age or older to determine whether geriatric patients respond differently than younger patients. Clinical experience indicates that *C. difficile*-associated diarrhea and colitis (see Cautions: GI Effects) seen in association with most anti-infectives may occur more frequently and be more severe in patients older than 60 years of age. Therefore, geriatric patients receiving clindamycin should be carefully monitored for the development of diarrhea (e.g., changes in bowel frequency).

Studies to date have not revealed any clinically important differences in the pharmacokinetics of oral or parenteral clindamycin between younger adults and geriatric patients with normal hepatic function and normal (age-adjusted) renal function. Dosage adjustments are not usually necessary if clindamycin is used in geriatric patients with normal hepatic function and normal (age-adjusted) renal function.

■ **Mutagenicity and Carcinogenicity** Clindamycin was not mutagenic in a rat micronucleus test or the Ames *Salmonella* reversion test.

Long-term studies in animals have not been performed to date to evaluate the carcinogenic potential of clindamycin.

■ **Pregnancy, Fertility, and Lactation** ***Pregnancy*** Reproduction studies in rats and mice using oral or parenteral dosages of clindamycin up to 600 mg/kg daily (3.2 and 1.6 times, respectively, the maximum recommended human oral dosage or 2.1 and 1.1 times, respectively, the maximum recommended human parenteral dosage on a mg/m^2 basis) have not revealed evidence of teratogenicity.

In clinical trials that included pregnant women, systemic clindamycin administered during the second and third trimesters was not associated with an increased frequency of congenital abnormalities. There are no adequate and well-controlled studies to date using clindamycin in pregnant women during the first trimester of pregnancy. Because animal reproduction studies are not always predictive of human response, clindamycin should be used during pregnancy only when clearly needed.

Clindamycin phosphate injection contains benzyl alcohol as a preservative; benzyl alcohol can cross the placenta. (See Cautions: Pediatric Precautions.)

Fertility Fertility studies in rats treated with oral clindamycin doses up to 300 mg/kg daily (about 1.1–1.6 times the maximum recommended human dose on a mg/m^2 basis) have not revealed evidence of impaired fertility or mating ability.

Lactation Clindamycin is distributed into milk (see Pharmacokinetics: Distribution), and has the potential to cause adverse effects on the GI flora of breast-fed infants.

The manufacturer states that use of oral or IV clindamycin in the mother is not a reason to discontinue breast-feeding; however, it may be preferable to use an alternate anti-infective. If clindamycin is used in a breast-feeding mother, the infant should be monitored for possible adverse effects on GI flora, including diarrhea and candidiasis (thrush, diaper rash) or, rarely, blood in the stool indicating possible antibiotic-associated colitis. The benefits of breast-feeding and the importance of clindamycin to the woman should be considered along with potential adverse effects on the breast-fed child from the drug or from the underlying maternal condition.

Drug Interactions

■ **Drugs Affecting or Metabolized by Hepatic Microsomal Enzymes** In vitro studies indicate that clindamycin is a moderate inhibitor of cytochrome P-450 (CYP) isoenzyme 3A4 and does not inhibit CYP1A2, 2C9, 2C19, 2E1, or 2D6.

Clindamycin is a substrate of CYP3A4 and, to a lesser extent, CYP3A5. Concomitant use with CYP3A4 or 3A5 inhibitors may result in increased plasma concentrations of clindamycin, and concomitant use with CYP3A4 or 3A5 inducers may result in decreased plasma concentrations of clindamycin. If clindamycin is used concomitantly with a potent CYP3A4 inhibitor, the patient should be monitored for adverse effects. If clindamycin is used concomitantly with a potent CYP3A4 inducer (e.g., rifampin), the patient should be monitored for loss of clindamycin effectiveness.

■ **Neuromuscular Blocking Agents** Clindamycin has been shown to have neuromuscular blocking properties that may enhance the neuromuscular blocking action of other agents (e.g., ether, tubocurarine, pancuronium). Clindamycin should be used with caution in patients receiving such agents, and such patients should be observed for prolongation of neuromuscular blockade.

Acute Toxicity

Convulsions, depression, and death have been reported in mice receiving IV clindamycin doses of 855 mg/kg; death has been reported in rats receiving oral or subcutaneous clindamycin doses of 2.6 mg/kg.

Clindamycin is not removed by hemodialysis or peritoneal dialysis.

Mechanism of Action

Clindamycin palmitate hydrochloride and clindamycin phosphate are inactive until hydrolyzed to free clindamycin. This hydrolysis occurs rapidly in vivo.

Clindamycin usually is bacteriostatic in action, but may be bactericidal depending on the concentration of the drug attained at the site of infection and the susceptibility of the infecting organism.

Clindamycin inhibits protein synthesis in susceptible bacteria by binding to the 23S RNA of the 50S ribosomal subunits; the primary effect is inhibition of peptide bond formation. The site of action appears to be the same as that of erythromycin, chloramphenicol, and lincomycin.

Spectrum

Clindamycin is active in vitro against many gram-positive aerobic and anaerobic bacteria and some gram-negative anaerobic bacteria. Clindamycin generally is inactive against most gram-negative aerobic bacteria.

Clindamycin is active in vitro against *Staphylococcus aureus* (methicillin-susceptible strains), *S. epidermidis* (methicillin-susceptible strains), *Streptococcus pneumoniae* (penicillin-susceptible strains), *S. pyogenes* (group A β-hemolytic streptococci; GAS), *S. agalactiae* (group B streptococci; GBS), *S. anginosus*, *S. mitis*, and *S. oralis*. The drug is not active against *Enterococcus faecalis* or *E. faecium*.

Clindamycin is active in vitro against some anaerobic and microaerophilic organisms including *Actinomyces israelii*, *Clostridium clostridioforme*, *C. perfringens*, *Eggerthella lenta* (previously known as *Eubacterium lentum*), *Finegoldia anaerobius*, *Finegoldia magna*, *Fusobacterium necrophorum*, *F. nucleatum*, *Micromonas micros*, *Mobiluncus*, *Prevotella* (*P. disiens*, *P. intermedia*, *P. melaninogenica*, *P. vivia*), *Porphyromonas*, and *Propionibacterium acnes*.

Clindamycin is active in vitro and in vivo against *Gardnerella vaginalis*.

Clindamycin has in vitro activity against *Toxoplasma gondii* in infected human fibroblasts. The drug has been reported to have some activity against *Plasmodium falciparum* in vitro.

Clindamycin generally is inactive against gram-negative aerobic bacteria, including Enterobacteriaceae, *Pseudomonas*, *Acinetobacter*, and most strains of *Haemophilus influenzae* and *Neisseria*.

■ **In Vitro Susceptibility Testing** When in vitro susceptibility testing is performed according to the standards of the Clinical and Laboratory Standards Institute (CLSI; formerly National Committee for Clinical Laboratory Standards [NCCLS]), clinical isolates identified as *susceptible* to clindamycin are inhibited by drug concentrations usually achievable when the recommended dosage is used for the site of infection. Clinical isolates classified as *intermediate* have minimum inhibitory concentrations (MICs) that approach usually attainable blood and tissue concentrations and response rates may be lower than for strains identified as susceptible. Therefore, the intermediate category implies clinical applicability in body sites where the drug is physiologically concentrated or when a higher than usual dosage can be used. This intermediate category also includes a buffer zone which should prevent small, uncontrolled technical factors from causing major discrepancies in interpretation, especially for drugs with narrow pharmacotoxicity margins. If results of in vitro susceptibility testing indicate that a clinical isolate is *resistant* to clindamycin, the strain is not inhibited by drug concentrations generally achievable with usual dosage schedules and/or MICs fall in the range where specific microbial resistance mechanisms are likely and clinical efficacy of the drug against the isolate has not been reliably demonstrated in clinical studies.

Disk Susceptibility Tests When the disk-diffusion procedure is used to test susceptibility to clindamycin, a disk containing 2 mcg of the drug should be used.

When disk susceptibility testing is performed according to CLSI standardized procedures, *Staphylococcus* with growth inhibition zones of 21 mm or greater are susceptible to clindamycin, those with zones of 15–20 mm have intermediate susceptibility, and those with zones of 14 mm or less are resistant to the drug.

When susceptibility of *Streptococcus* is evaluated according to CLSI standardized procedures, *Streptococcus* (including *S. pneumoniae*) with growth inhibition zones of 19 mm or greater are susceptible to clindamycin, those with zones of 16–18 mm have intermediate susceptibility, and those with zones of 15 mm or less are resistant to the drug.

Dilution Susceptibility Tests When dilution susceptibility testing (agar or broth dilution) is performed according to CLSI standardized procedures, *Staphylococcus* with MICs of 0.5 mcg/mL or less are susceptible to clindamycin, those with MICs of 1–2 mcg/mL have intermediate susceptibility, and those with MICs of 4 mcg/mL or greater are resistant to the drug.

When broth dilution susceptibility testing is performed according to CLSI standardized procedures, *Streptococcus* (including *S. pneumoniae*) with MICs of 0.25 mcg/mL or less are susceptible to clindamycin, those with MICs of 0.5 mcg/mL have intermediate susceptibility, and those with MICs of 1 mcg/mL or greater are resistant to the drug.

When broth dilution susceptibility testing is performed according to CLSI standardized procedures, anaerobic bacteria with MICs of 2 mcg/mL or less are susceptible to clindamycin, those with MICs of 4 mcg/mL have intermediate susceptibility, and those with MICs of 8 mcg/mL or greater are resistant to the drug.

Resistance

Resistance to clindamycin has been induced in vitro in staphylococci and has been shown to be acquired in a stepwise manner. Clindamycin resistance has been reported in clinical isolates of *Staphylococcus aureus*, especially methicillin-resistant *S. aureus* (MRSA; also known as oxacillin-resistant *S. aureus* or ORSA).

S. agalactiae (group B streptococci; GBS) clinical isolates resistant to clindamycin have been reported with increasing frequency. Data from 2006–2011 indicated that 13–30% of GBS clinical isolates in the US were resistant to clindamycin. Because GBS isolates that appear susceptible to clindamycin but resistant to erythromycin in vitro may have inducible resistance to clindamycin, appropriate in vitro susceptibility testing methods should be used whenever in vitro susceptibility of GBS to clindamycin is being evaluated.

Clinical isolates of *Bacteroides fragilis* with resistance or reduced susceptibility to clindamycin have been reported with increasing frequency.

Resistance to clindamycin is most frequently caused by modification of specific bases of the 23S ribosomal RNA.

Complete cross-resistance occurs between clindamycin and lincomycin. Because of overlapping binding sites, partial cross-resistance has been reported between clindamycin and macrolides (e.g., erythromycin) and streptogramin B. In vitro, bacteria resistant to erythromycin and susceptible to clindamycin may exhibit a dissociated type of resistance to clindamycin during susceptibility testing if erythromycin is also present. This phenomenon may be the result of competition between erythromycin and clindamycin for the ribosomal binding site.

Pharmacokinetics

■ **Absorption** Following oral administration of clindamycin hydrochloride, approximately 90% of the dose is rapidly absorbed from the GI tract. Following oral administration of a single 150-mg dose of clindamycin hydrochloride to healthy fasting adults, peak serum concentrations of clindamycin average 1.9–3.9 mcg/mL and are attained within 45–60 minutes; serum concentrations of clindamycin average 1.5 mcg/mL at 3 hours and 0.7 mcg/mL at 6 hours. Serum concentrations of clindamycin appear to be predictable, increasing linearly with increased doses.

Following oral administration of clindamycin palmitate hydrochloride oral solution, the drug is rapidly hydrolyzed in the GI tract to active clindamycin. Oral doses of clindamycin palmitate hydrochloride produce serum concentrations of clindamycin similar to those achieved with oral clindamycin hydrochloride. In a study in healthy children receiving 2, 3, or 4 mg/kg of clindamycin every 6 hours as the clindamycin palmitate hydrochloride oral solution, mean peak serum clindamycin concentrations were 1.24, 2.25, or 2.44 mcg/mL, respectively, 1 hour after the first dose. After the fifth dose, peak serum concentrations of the drug averaged 2.46, 2.98, or 3.79 mcg/mL, respectively.

Clindamycin is not inactivated by gastric acidity. Administration of clindamycin hydrochloride capsules or clindamycin palmitate hydrochloride oral solution with food does not appreciably affect absorption or serum concentrations of the drug. Accumulation in plasma does not occur following multiple oral doses, including in neonates and infants up to 6 months of age.

Following IM or IV administration, clindamycin phosphate is rapidly hydrolyzed in plasma to active clindamycin. Following IM administration of clindamycin phosphate, peak serum concentrations occur within 3 hours in adults and 1 hour in children. In healthy adult males, IM doses of 600 mg of clindamycin every 12 hours resulted in average peak serum clindamycin concentrations of 9 mcg/mL. IV doses of 600 mg of clindamycin infused over 30 minutes every 6 or 8 hours in healthy adult males resulted in average peak serum clindamycin concentrations of 11 mcg/mL and IV doses of 900 mg infused over 30 minutes every 8 hours resulted in average peak serum clindamycin concentrations of 14 mcg/mL. In a study in pediatric patients with infections, a single IM dose of 3–5 mg/kg resulted in average peak serum clindamycin concentrations of 4 mcg/mL and single IV or IM doses of 5–7 mg/kg resulted in average peak serum clindamycin concentrations of 10 or 8 mcg/mL, respectively.

■ **Distribution** Clindamycin is widely distributed into body tissues and fluids, including saliva, ascites fluid, peritoneal fluid, pleural fluid, synovial fluid, bone, and bile. The concentration of clindamycin in synovial fluid and bone is reported to be 60–80% of concurrent serum concentrations of the drug; the degree of penetration does not appear to be affected by joint inflammation.

Clinically important concentrations of clindamycin are not attained in CSF, even in the presence of inflamed meninges.

Clindamycin readily crosses the placenta, and cord blood concentrations of the drug have been reported to be up to 50% of concurrent maternal blood concentrations.

Clindamycin is distributed into milk. Breast milk concentrations of 0.7–3.8 mcg/mL have been reported following clindamycin dosages of 150 mg orally to 600 mg IV. In one study in women who received oral clindamycin in a dosage of 150 mg 3 times daily, breast milk concentrations of the drug ranged from less than 0.5 to 3.1 mcg/mL.

At a concentration of 1 mcg/mL, clindamycin is approximately 93% bound to serum proteins.

■ **Elimination** Clindamycin is partially metabolized to bioactive and inactive metabolites. In vitro studies indicate that clindamycin is predominantly metabolized by cytochrome P-450 (CYP) isoenzyme 3A4 and, to a lesser extent, by CYP3A5 to the major bioactive metabolite clindamycin sulfoxide and minor metabolite *N*-desmethylclindamycin.

The serum half-life of clindamycin is 2–3 hours in adults and children. In neonates, the serum half-life of clindamycin depends on gestational and chronologic age and body weight. Half-life of the drug reportedly averages 8.7 or 3.6 hours in premature or full-term neonates, respectively, and about 3 hours in infants 4 weeks to 1 year of age; serum half-life was longer in infants weighing less than 3.5 kg than in heavier infants.

Pharmacokinetic studies using IV clindamycin phosphate in healthy older adults (61–79 years of age) and younger adults (18–39 years of age) indicate that age alone does not alter clindamycin pharmacokinetics (clearance, elimination half-life, volume of distribution, area under the serum concentration-time curve [AUC]). Following oral administration of clindamycin hydrochloride, elimination half-life increased to approximately 4 hours (range: 3.4–5.1 hours) in geriatric patients compared with 3.2 hours (range: 2.1–4.2 hours) in younger adults. Following oral administration of clindamycin palmitate, the elimination half-life in geriatric adults was 4.5 hours.

The serum half-life of clindamycin is increased slightly in patients with markedly reduced renal or hepatic function.

Clindamycin sulfoxide and *N*-desmethylclindamycin are excreted in urine, bile, and feces. Approximately 10% of an oral dose of clindamycin is excreted in urine and 3.6% is excreted in feces as active drug and metabolites; the remainder is excreted as inactive metabolites.

Clindamycin is not appreciably removed by hemodialysis or peritoneal dialysis.

Chemistry and Stability

■ **Chemistry** Clindamycin is a semisynthetic derivative of lincomycin that differs structurally from lincomycin by the presence of a methoxy group instead of the hydroxyl group at position 7 on the molecule.

Clindamycin is commercially available as the hydrochloride hydrate, the palmitate hydrochloride, and the phosphate ester. Potency of clindamycin hydrochloride, clindamycin palmitate hydrochloride, and clindamycin phosphate is expressed in terms of clindamycin. Each mg of the hydrochloride hydrate, palmitate hydrochloride, or phosphate has a potency of not less than 800, 540, or 758 mcg of clindamycin, respectively; potency of the phosphate is calculated on the anhydrous basis. The hydrochloride, palmitate hydrochloride, and phosphate occur as a white or practically white crystalline powder, a white to off-white amorphous powder, and a white to off-white hygroscopic crystalline powder, respectively, which may have faint, characteristic odors and are freely soluble in water. Clindamycin phosphate reportedly has a solubility of about 400 mg/mL in water at 25°C. The pK_a of clindamycin is 7.45.

Clindamycin hydrochloride is commercially available for oral administration as capsules. Clindamycin palmitate hydrochloride is commercially available as a powder (granules) for oral solution; when reconstituted as directed, each 5 mL of oral solution contains 75 mg of clindamycin.

Clindamycin phosphate is commercially available as a sterile solution containing 150 mg of clindamycin that must be diluted prior to IV administration; each mL of the solution also contains 0.5 mg of disodium edetate per mL and 9.45 mg of benzyl alcohol as a preservative. Clindamycin phosphate also is commercially available as a premixed solution for IV infusion containing 300, 600, or 900 mg of clindamycin in 5% dextrose. The premixed solutions contain 0.04 mg of disodium edetate per mL and sodium hydroxide and/or hydrochloric acid may have been added to adjust pH.

■ **Stability** Clindamycin hydrochloride capsules should be stored at 20–25°C.

Clindamycin palmitate hydrochloride powder (granules) for oral solution should be stored at 20–25°C. Following reconstitution with water, clindamycin palmitate hydrochloride oral solution is stable for 2 weeks at room temperature. The reconstituted oral solution should *not* be refrigerated since it will thicken if chilled and become difficult to pour.

Clindamycin phosphate solutions containing 150 mg of clindamycin per mL (including ADD-Vantage® vials) should be stored at a controlled room temperature of 20–25°C.

Premixed solutions containing clindamycin phosphate in 5% dextrose injection should be stored at room temperature (25°C), and exposure to temperatures warmer than 30°C should be avoided. Some premixed solutions of clindamycin phosphate in 5% dextrose are provided in plastic containers fabricated from specially formulated multilayered plastic PL 2501. Solutions in contact with the plastic can leach out some of the chemical components in very small amounts within the expiration period of the injection; however, safety of the plastic has been confirmed in tests in animals as well as by tissue culture studies.

At a concentration of 6, 9, or 12 mg of clindamycin per mL, clindamycin phosphate is physically and chemically compatible for at least 16 days at 25°C or at least 32 days when refrigerated at 4°C in glass or polyvinyl chloride (PVC) containers, or for at least 8 weeks when frozen at −10°C in PVC containers of the following IV solutions: 5% dextrose, 0.9% sodium chloride, or lactated Ringer's. At a concentration of 18 mg of clindamycin per mL, clindamycin phosphate is physically and chemically compatible for at least 16 days at 25°C in PVC containers of 5% dextrose.

Clindamycin phosphate is physically and microbiologically compatible for 24 hours at room temperature in IV solutions containing sodium chloride, dextrose, potassium, or vitamin B complex in concentrations used clinically. However, certain concentrations or admixtures of calcium salts may result in physical incompatibility. Clindamycin phosphate has been reported to be incompatible with various drugs (e.g., aminophylline, barbiturates, ceftriaxone, ciprofloxacin, magnesium sulfate, phenytoin sodium); however, the compatibility depends on several factors (e.g., concentration of the drugs, specific diluents used, resulting pH, temperature). Specialized references should be consulted for specific compatibility information.

Preparations

Excipients in commercially available drug preparations may have clinically important effects in some individuals; consult specific product labeling for details.

Clindamycin Hydrochloride

Oral		
Capsules	75 mg (of clindamycin)*	**Cleocin HCl®**, Pfizer
		Clindamycin Hydrochloride Capsules
	150 mg (of clindamycin)*	**Cleocin HCl®**, Pfizer
		Clindamycin Hydrochloride Capsules
	300 mg (of clindamycin)*	**Cleocin HCl®**, Pfizer
		Clindamycin Hydrochloride Capsules

*available from one or more manufacturer, distributor, and/or repackager by generic (nonproprietary) name

Clindamycin Palmitate Hydrochloride

Oral		
For solution	75 mg (of clindamycin) per 5 mL*	**Cleocin Pediatric®**, Pfizer
		Clindamycin Palmitate Hydrochloride for Oral Solution

*available from one or more manufacturer, distributor, and/or repackager by generic (nonproprietary) name

Clindamycin Phosphate

Parenteral		
Injection	150 mg (of clindamycin) per mL*	**Cleocin Phosphate®**, Pfizer
		Clindamycin Phosphate Injection
	9 g (150 mg/mL) (of clindamycin) pharmacy bulk package	**Cleocin Phosphate®**, Pfizer
Injection, for IV infusion only	150 mg (of clindamycin) per mL (300 mg)*	**Cleocin Phosphate® ADD-Vantage®**, Pfizer
		Clindamycin Phosphate ADD-Vantage®
	150 mg (of clindamycin) per mL (600 and 900 mg)*	**Cleocin Phosphate® ADD-Vantage®**, Pfizer
		Clindamycin Phosphate ADD-Vantage®

*available from one or more manufacturer, distributor, and/or repackager by generic (nonproprietary) name

Clindamycin Phosphate in Dextrose

Parenteral		
Injection, for IV infusion	6 mg (of clindamycin) per mL (300 mg) in 5% Dextrose*	**Cleocin Phosphate® IV**, Pfizer
		Clindamycin Phosphate in 5% Dextrose
	12 mg (of clindamycin) per mL (600 mg) in 5% Dextrose*	**Cleocin Phosphate® IV**, Pfizer
		Clindamycin Phosphate in 5% Dextrose
	18 mg (of clindamycin) per mL (900 mg) in 5% Dextrose*	**Cleocin Phosphate® IV**, Pfizer
		Clindamycin Phosphate in 5% Dextrose

*available from one or more manufacturer, distributor, and/or repackager by generic (nonproprietary) name

†Use is not currently included in the labeling approved by the US Food and Drug Administration

OXAZOLIDINONES 8:12.28.24

Linezolid

■ Linezolid is an oxazolidinone anti-infective agent.

Uses

Linezolid is used for the treatment of community-acquired pneumonia, nosocomial pneumonia, and uncomplicated or complicated skin and skin structure infections caused by certain susceptible staphylococci or streptococci. Linezolid also is used for the treatment of infections caused by vancomycin-resistant *Enterococcus faecium*.

Linezolid is *not* indicated for the treatment of infections caused by gram-negative bacteria. It is imperative that an anti-infective active against gram-negative bacteria be used concomitantly if documented or presumed pathogens include gram-negative bacteria.

■ **Respiratory Tract Infections** ***Community-acquired Pneumonia*** Linezolid is used for the treatment of community-acquired pneumonia (CAP), including infections associated with concurrent bacteremia, caused by susceptible *Staphylococcus aureus* (methicillin-susceptible [oxacillin-susceptible] strains only) or *Streptococcus pneumoniae*). Although not labeled by FDA for the treatment of CAP caused by methicillin-resistant *S. aureus*† (MRSA; also known as oxacillin-resistant *S. aureus* or ORSA), linezolid is one of several anti-infectives that have been recommended for the treatment of these infections.

Initial treatment of CAP generally involves use of an empiric anti-infective regimen based on the most likely pathogens and local susceptibility patterns; treatment may then be changed (if possible) to provide a more specific regimen (pathogen-directed therapy) based on results of in vitro culture and susceptibility testing. The most appropriate empiric regimen varies depending on the severity of illness at the time of presentation, whether outpatient treatment or hospitalization in or out of an intensive care unit (ICU) is indicated, and the presence or absence of cardiopulmonary disease and other modifying factors that increase the risk of certain pathogens (e.g., MRSA, penicillin-resistant *S. pneumoniae*, multidrug-resistant *S. pneumoniae* [MDRSP], enteric gram-negative bacilli, *Pseudomonas aeruginosa*).

For information regarding the treatment of CAP, including infections caused by MRSA, the current clinical practice guidelines from the Infectious Diseases Society of America (IDSA) available at http://www.idsociety.org should be consulted.

Clinical Experience. In 2 randomized clinical studies in patients 13 years of age or older with CAP, cure rates with linezolid (600 mg every 12 hours for 7–14 days given IV or orally initially, then orally) were approximately 90% and were similar to those achieved with oral cefpodoxime proxetil (200 mg every 12 hours for 10–14 days) or IV ceftriaxone (1 g every 12 hours) followed by oral cefpodoxime proxetil (200 mg every 12 hours) for 7–14 days. In a subset of hospitalized patients with CAP and associated *S. pneumoniae* bacteremia, linezolid was substantially more effective than a regimen of IV ceftriaxone (cure rate of 93 versus 70%, respectively).

Efficacy and safety of linezolid for the treatment of CAP in pediatric patients is supported by evidence from adequate and well-controlled studies in adults, pharmacokinetic studies in pediatric patients, an uncontrolled study in pediatric patients 8 months through 12 years of age, and additional data from a randomized, open-label, comparator-controlled study of documented or suspected gram-positive bacterial infections in neonates and pediatric patients through 11 years of age.

Nosocomial Pneumonia Linezolid is used for the treatment of nosocomial pneumonia caused by susceptible *S. aureus* (including MRSA) or *S. pneumoniae*.

For empiric treatment of hospital-acquired bacterial pneumonia, including healthcare-associated and ventilator-associated pneumonia in patients with risk factors for multidrug-resistant bacteria, the American Thoracic Society (ATS) and IDSA recommend use of anti-infectives that have a broad spectrum of activity against gram-positive, gram-negative, and anaerobic bacteria. An anti-infective active against MRSA (e.g., vancomycin, linezolid) should be included in the initial empiric regimen in hospitals where MRSA is common or if there are other factors that increase the risk for these strains.

For information regarding the diagnosis and management of nosocomial pneumonia, including infections caused by MRSA, the current IDSA clinical practice guidelines available at http://www.idsociety.org should be consulted.

Clinical Experience. In a randomized, double-blind study in adults with nosocomial bacterial pneumonia, the cure rate in clinically evaluable patients was 57% in those treated with linezolid (600 mg every 12 hours IV for 7–21 days) compared with 60% in those treated with vancomycin (1 g every 12 hours IV for 7–21 days). Both treatment groups also received concomitant therapy with aztreonam (1–2 g every 8 hours IV) for gram-negative coverage. In clinically evaluable patients with ventilator-associated pneumonia, the cure rate was 47% in those who received linezolid and 40% in those who received vancomycin. When results were stratified according to causative organism, linezolid was effective in 59% of infections caused by MRSA and 100% of infections caused by *S. pneumoniae*.

Efficacy and safety of linezolid for the treatment of nosocomial bacterial pneumonia in pediatric patients is supported by evidence from adequate and well-controlled studies in adults, pharmacokinetic studies in pediatric patients, and additional data from a randomized, open-label, comparator-controlled study of documented or suspected gram-positive bacterial infections in neonates and pediatric patients through 11 years of age. In the comparator-controlled study in pediatric patients with documented or suspected gram-positive infections, the cure rate in pediatric patients with nosocomial pneumonia (intent-to-treat analysis) was 72% in those treated with linezolid and 92% in those treated with vancomycin; the cure rate in clinically evaluable pediatric patients with nosocomial pneumonia was 100% in both groups.

■ **Skin and Skin Structure Infections** Linezolid is used for the treatment of uncomplicated skin and skin structure infections caused by susceptible *S. aureus* (methicillin-susceptible strains only) or *S. pyogenes* (group A β-hemolytic streptococci, GAS). The drug also is used for the treatment of complicated skin and skin structure infections (including diabetic foot infections), without concurrent osteomyelitis, caused by susceptible *S. aureus* (including MRSA), *S. pyogenes*, or *S. agalactiae* (group B streptococci, GBS). The use of linezolid in the treatment of decubitus ulcers has not been studied.

Pending results of in vitro culture and susceptibility testing, coverage against MRSA is recommended for empiric treatment of purulent cellulitis in outpatients or nonpurulent cellulitis in outpatients who do not respond to β-lactam treatment and should be considered for empiric treatment of complicated skin and skin structure infections in hospitalized patients. Linezolid is one of several anti-infectives that have been recommended for the treatment of purulent or nonpurulent cellulitis and for the treatment of complicated skin and skin structure infections caused by MRSA.

For information regarding the treatment of skin and skin structure infections, including infections caused by MRSA, the current IDSA clinical practice guidelines available at http://www.idsociety.org should be consulted.

Clinical Experience In a randomized, double-blind clinical study in adults with complicated skin and skin structure infections, the efficacy rates (clinical, microbiologic, and overall outcomes) were similar for linezolid (600 mg every 12 hours IV initially, with an option to convert to oral administration) or oxacillin (2 g every 6 hours IV) with an option to switch to oral dicloxacillin (500 mg every 6 hours) for 10–21 days. Patients in both treatment groups received concomitant aztreonam (1–2 g every 6–8 hours IV) if empiric gram-negative coverage was considered necessary. The cure rate in clinically evaluable patients was 90% in those treated with linezolid and 85% in those treated with oxacillin. When results for treatment of these complicated skin and skin structure infections were stratified according to causative organism, linezolid was effective in 88% of infections caused by *S. aureus*, 67% of infections caused by MRSA, 69% of infections caused by *S. pyogenes*, and 100% of infections caused by *S. agalactiae*.

In a randomized clinical study in patients 13 years of age or older with known or suspected MRSA skin and skin structure infections, efficacy (clinical, microbiologic, and overall outcomes) was similar for therapy with linezolid (600 mg every 12 hours IV initially, with an option to convert to oral administration) or vancomycin (1 g every 12 hours IV) for 14–28 days. In an open-label, randomized study in hospitalized adults with documented or suspected MRSA skin and skin structure infections who received 7–28 days of treatment with linezolid (600 mg every 12 hours given IV initially, then orally) or vancomycin (1 g every 12 hours IV) given with or without concomitant aztreonam or gentamicin if clinically indicated, the cure rate in microbiologically evaluable patients was 79% in those treated with linezolid and 73% in those treated with vancomycin.

In a randomized, multicenter open-label comparative study in adults with diabetic foot infections, efficacy rates (clinical and microbiologic outcomes) were similar in patients receiving linezolid (600 mg every 12 hours IV or orally) or an aminopenicillin (ampicillin sodium and sulbactam sodium 1.5–3 g every 6 hours IV, amoxicillin and clavulanate potassium 500–875 mg every 8–12 hours orally, or amoxicillin and clavulanate potassium 0.5–2 g every 6 hours IV [IV preparation not commercially available in the US]) for 14–28 days. Patients in both treatment groups received concomitant aztreonam (1–2 g every 8–12 hours IV) if gram-negative pathogens were isolated from the infection site and patients receiving an aminopenicillin also were treated with vancomycin (1 g every 12 hours IV) if MRSA was isolated from the foot infection. Most patients also received appropriate adjunctive treatment usually required for the treatment of diabetic foot infections (e.g., debridement). When results for treatment of these diabetic foot infections were stratified according to causative organism, linezolid was effective in 78% of infections caused by *S. aureus*, 71% of infections caused by MRSA, and 86% of infections caused by *S. agalactiae*.

Efficacy and safety of linezolid for the treatment of complicated skin and skin structure infections in pediatric patients is supported by evidence from adequate and well-controlled studies in adults, pharmacokinetic studies in pediatric patients, and additional data from a randomized, comparator-controlled study of documented or suspected gram-positive bacterial infections in neonates and pediatric patients through 11 years of age. In the comparator-controlled study in pediatric patients with documented or suspected gram-positive infections, the cure rate in pediatric patients with complicated skin and skin structure infections (intent-to-treat analysis) was 85% in those treated with linezolid and 91% in those treated with vancomycin; the cure rate in clinically evaluable pediatric patients with complicated skin and skin structure infections was 94 and 96%, respectively.

Efficacy and safety of linezolid for the treatment of uncomplicated skin and skin structure infections in pediatric patients caused by *S. aureus* (methicillin-susceptible [oxacillin-susceptible] strains only) or *S. pyogenes* is supported by data from a comparator-controlled study in pediatric patients 5–17 years of age.

■ Vancomycin-resistant Enterococcus faecium Infections Linezolid is used for the treatment of vancomycin-resistant *E. faecium* infections, including infections associated with concurrent bacteremia.

Linezolid has been used in some patients for the treatment of native valve or prosthetic valve infective endocarditis† caused by vancomycin-resistant or multidrug-resistant *E. faecium*. The American Heart Association (AHA) states that patients with infective endocarditis attributable to enterococci resistant to penicillins, aminoglycosides, and vancomycin should be managed by a team of specialists in infectious disease, cardiology, cardiovascular surgery, clinical pharmacy, and, if necessary, pediatrics.

For information on diagnosis and management of infective endocarditis and its complications, including anti-infective treatment of enterococcal endocarditis, the current AHA guidelines available at http://my.americanheart.org/statements should be consulted.

Clinical Experience In a randomized, double-blind study in adults comparing high-dose linezolid (600 mg every 12 hours IV or orally) with low-dose linezolid (200 mg every 12 hours IV or orally) for 7–28 days, cure rates for patients with documented vancomycin-resistant *E. faecium* at any infection site were 67 or 52% for those treated with high- or low-dose linezolid, respectively, based on intent-to-treat analysis. Some patients received concomitant therapy with aztreonam or aminoglycosides. Compared with patients in the high-dose group, there were more adverse events and more deaths among patients in the low-dose group.

Efficacy and safety of linezolid for the treatment of vancomycin-resistant *E. faecium* infections in pediatric patients is supported by evidence from adequate and well-controlled studies in adults, pharmacokinetic studies in pediatric patients, and additional data from a randomized, open-label, comparator-controlled study of documented or suspected gram-positive bacterial infections in neonates and pediatric patients through 11 years of age. Data from the open-label, comparator-controlled study indicate that the cure rate was 75% in the 8 microbiologically evaluable pediatric patients with vancomycin-resistant *E. faecium* infections who received linezolid.

■ Catheter-related Bloodstream Infections Although linezolid has been investigated for the treatment of intravascular catheter-related bloodstream infections†, linezolid is *not* labeled by FDA for the treatment of catheter-related bacteremia or catheter-site infections and is *not* indicated for the treatment of gram-negative bacterial infections.

Data from an open-label, randomized study in patients with intravascular catheter-related bloodstream infections indicated that mortality was higher in patients receiving linezolid than in patients receiving comparator anti-infectives. In this study, seriously ill patients with intravascular catheter-related bloodstream infections were randomized to receive linezolid or vancomycin (patients randomized to vancomycin were switched to dicloxacillin or oxacillin if the pathogen was oxacillin-susceptible); patients could receive concomitant therapy for gram-negative infection. Although there was no difference in mortality between linezolid and the comparator regimens in patients with only gram-positive bacteria identified in the baseline culture, mortality was higher in linezolid-treated patients who had gram-negative bacterial infections, mixed gram-negative and gram-positive bacterial infections, or no pathogen identified at baseline.

■ CNS Infections Linezolid has been recommended as an alternative to vancomycin for the treatment of CNS infections caused by MRSA† (e.g., meningitis†, brain abscess†, subdural empyema†, spinal epidural abscess†). The manufacturer states that linezolid is *not* recommended for empiric treatment of CNS infections in pediatric patients (see Pediatric Use under Warnings/Precautions: Specific Populations, in Cautions).

For information regarding the treatment of CNS infections caused by MRSA, the current IDSA clinical practice guidelines available at http://www.idsociety.org should be consulted.

Dosage and Administration

■ Reconstitution and Administration Linezolid is administered orally or by IV infusion.

Oral Administration Orally administered linezolid may be given without regard to meals. However, large quantities of foods or beverages with high tyramine content should be avoided during linezolid treatment. (See Monoamine Oxidase Inhibition under Warnings/Precautions: Warnings, in Cautions.)

Linezolid powder for oral suspension should be reconstituted at the time of dispensing with the amount of water specified on the bottle to provide a suspension containing 100 mg/5 mL. After tapping the bottle gently to loosen the powder, the water should be added in 2 portions and the suspension agitated well after each addition.

The reconstituted oral suspension should be stored at room temperature and used within 21 days. Prior to administration of each dose, the suspension should be *gently* mixed by inverting the bottle 3–5 times but should not be shaken.

IV Administration Linezolid premixed injection for IV administration in single-use flexible containers is administered by IV infusion without further dilution.

Linezolid premixed solutions should be inspected visually for particulate matter prior to administration and should not be used if visible particles are evident. The solution may exhibit a yellow color that can intensify over time without adversely affecting potency. The bags should be squeezed firmly to check for minute leaks. If leaks are detected, the solution should be discarded since sterility may be impaired.

Linezolid premixed injection for IV administration in single-use flexible infusion bags should not be used in series connections, and additives should not be introduced into the solution.

Linezolid is compatible with 5% dextrose, 0.9% sodium chloride, and lactated Ringer's injection.

During simulated Y-site administration, linezolid was physically incompatible with amphotericin B, chlorpromazine hydrochloride, co-trimoxazole, diazepam, erythromycin lactobionate, pentamidine isethionate, and phenytoin sodium. In addition, linezolid is chemically incompatible with ceftriaxone sodium.

Rate of Administration. Linezolid premixed injection for IV administration in single-use flexible containers should be administered by IV infusion over 30–120 minutes.

■ **Dosage** When clinically appropriate, patients treated initially with IV linezolid may be switched to oral linezolid without dosage adjustment.

Safety and efficacy of more than 28 days of linezolid treatment have not been evaluated in controlled clinical trials.

Adult Dosage **Respiratory Tract Infections.** The usual adult oral or IV dosage of linezolid for the treatment of community-acquired pneumonia (CAP) caused by susceptible *Staphylococcus aureus* (methicillin-susceptible [oxacillin-susceptible] strains only) or *Streptococcus pneumoniae* is 600 mg every 12 hours for 10–14 days. If linezolid is used for the treatment of CAP caused by susceptible methicillin-resistant *S. aureus*† (MRSA; also known as oxacillin-resistant *S. aureus* or ORSA), an oral or IV dosage of 600 mg twice daily for 7–21 days has been recommended.

The usual adult oral or IV dosage of linezolid for the treatment of nosocomial pneumonia caused by susceptible *S. aureus* (including MRSA) or *S. pneumoniae* is 600 mg every 12 hours for 10–14 days. IDSA recommends a duration of 7–21 days for the treatment of healthcare-associated pneumonia caused by MRSA.

Skin and Skin Structure Infections. For the treatment of uncomplicated skin and skin structure infections caused by susceptible *S. aureus* (methicillin-susceptible [oxacillin-susceptible] strains only) or *S. pyogenes* (group A *β*-hemolytic streptococci, GAS), the usual adult oral dosage of linezolid is 400 mg every 12 hours for 10–14 days. For purulent or nonpurulent cellulitis caused by MRSA, IDSA recommends that outpatients receive an oral dosage of 600 mg twice daily for 5–10 days; treatment duration should be based on clinical response.

The usual adult oral or IV dosage of linezolid for the treatment of complicated skin and skin structure infections, including diabetic foot infections, without concomitant osteomyelitis, caused by susceptible *S. aureus* (including MRSA), *S. pyogenes* (group A *β*-hemolytic streptococci), or *S. agalactiae* (group B streptococci, GBS) is 600 mg every 12 hours for 10–14 days. IDSA recommends a duration of 7–14 days for the treatment of complicated skin and skin structure infections caused by MRSA; treatment duration should be based on clinical response.

Vancomycin-resistant Enterococcus faecium Infections. The usual adult oral or IV dosage of linezolid for the treatment of vancomycin-resistant *Enterococcus faecium* infections, including infections with concurrent bacteremia, is 600 mg every 12 hours for 14–28 days.

CNS Infections. If linezolid is used in adults for the treatment of CNS infections caused by MRSA† (See Uses: CNS Infections), IDSA recommends an oral or IV dosage of 600 mg twice daily.

Pediatric Dosage **General Dosage for Neonates.** In premature neonates younger than 7 days of age, the manufacturer recommends an initial linezolid dosage of 10 mg/kg every 12 hours; a dosage of 10 mg/kg every 8 hours may be considered in those with an inadequate response to the lower dosage. The manufacturer recommends that all neonates 7 days of age or older receive a linezolid dosage of 10 mg/kg every 8 hours.

When linezolid is used in neonates 7 days of age or younger, the American Academy of Pediatrics (AAP) recommends an IV dosage of 10 mg/kg every 12 hours in those weighing 2 kg or less and 10 mg/kg every 8 hours in those weighing more than 2 kg. For neonates 8–28 days of age, AAP recommends an IV dosage of 10 mg/kg every 8 hours, regardless of weight.

General Dosage for Infants and Children. The manufacturer usually recommends that infants and children through 11 years of age receive oral or IV linezolid in a dosage of 10 mg/kg every 8 hours and that adolescents 12 years of age or older receive 600 mg every 12 hours.

When linezolid is used in pediatric patients beyond the neonatal period, AAP recommends an oral or IV dosage of 10 mg/kg 3 times daily in children younger than 12 years of age and a dosage of 600 mg twice daily in adolescents 12 years of age or older.

Respiratory Tract Infections. The usual oral or IV dosage of linezolid for the treatment of CAP caused by susceptible *S. aureus* (methicillin-susceptible [oxacillin-susceptible] strains only) or *S. pneumoniae* is 10 mg/kg every 8 hours in pediatric patients 7 days of age through 11 years of age and 600 mg every 12 hours in adolescents 12 years of age or older. The recommended duration of treatment is 10–14 days.

The usual oral or IV dosage of linezolid for the treatment of nosocomial pneumonia caused by susceptible *S. aureus* (including MRSA) or *S. pneumoniae* is 10 mg/kg every 8 hours in pediatric patients 7 days through 11 years of age and 600 mg every 12 hours in adolescents 12 years of age or older. The recommended duration of treatment is 10–14 days.

IDSA recommends a duration of 7–21 days for the treatment of CAP or healthcare-associated pneumonia caused by MRSA.

Skin and Skin Structure Infections. For the treatment of uncomplicated skin and skin structure infections caused by susceptible *S. aureus* (methicillin-susceptible [oxacillin-susceptible] strains only) or *S. pyogenes* in pediatric patients, the usual oral dosage of linezolid is 10 mg/kg every 8 hours in those younger than 5 years of age, 10 mg/kg every 12 hours in those 5 through 11 years of age, and 600 mg every 12 hours in adolescents 12 years of age or older. The recommended duration of treatment is 10–14 days.

The usual oral or IV dosage of linezolid for the treatment of complicated skin and skin structure infections caused by susceptible *S. aureus* (including MRSA), *S. pyogenes*, or *S. agalactiae* is 10 mg/kg every 8 hours in pediatric patients 7 days of age through 11 years of age and 600 mg every 12 hours in adolescents 12 years of age or older. The recommended duration of treatment is 10–14 days.

Vancomycin-resistant Enterococcus faecium Infections. The usual oral or IV dosage of linezolid for the treatment of vancomycin-resistant *E. faecium* infections is 10 mg/kg every 8 hours in pediatric patients 7 days of age through 11 years of age and 600 mg every 12 hours in adolescents 12 years of age or older. The recommended duration of treatment is 14–28 days.

CNS Infections. If linezolid is used in pediatric patients for the treatment of CNS infections caused by MRSA† (See Uses: CNS Infections), IDSA recommends an oral or IV dosage of 10 mg/kg (up to 600 mg) every 8 hours.

■ **Special Populations** ***Hepatic Impairment*** Dosage adjustments are not necessary in patients with mild to moderate hepatic impairment (Child-Pugh class A or B). Data are not available regarding the pharmacokinetics of linezolid in patients with severe hepatic impairment.

Renal Impairment Dosage adjustments are not necessary in patients with renal impairment. However, the 2 principal metabolites of linezolid may accumulate in patients with renal impairment and the clinical importance of accumulation of these metabolites has not been determined. (See Renal Impairment under Cautions: Specific Populations.)

Because linezolid is removed by hemodialysis, patients undergoing hemodialysis should receive linezolid doses after the dialysis session.

Geriatric Patients Dosage adjustments are not necessary in geriatric patients.

Cautions

■ **Contraindications** Linezolid is contraindicated in patients with known hypersensitivity to linezolid or any ingredient in the formulation.

Linezolid should not be used in patients who are receiving (or have received within the last 2 weeks) drugs that inhibit monoamine oxidase (MAO) A or B, including MAO inhibitor antidepressants (e.g., isocarboxazid, phenelzine). (See Drug Interactions: Monoamine Oxidase Inhibitors.)

■ **Warnings/Precautions** ***Hematologic Effects*** Myelosuppression (e.g., anemia, leukopenia, pancytopenia, thrombocytopenia) has been reported in patients receiving linezolid.

Toxicity studies in adult and juvenile dogs and rats indicate myelosuppression (bone marrow hypocellularity/decreased hematopoiesis; decreased extramedullary hematopoiesis in spleen and liver; decreased levels of circulating erythrocytes, leukocytes, and platelets) and lymphoid depletion in thymus, lymph nodes, and spleen.

Complete blood cell counts (CBCs) should be monitored weekly during linezolid treatment, especially in patients receiving the drug for more than 2 weeks and in those who have preexisting myelosuppression, are receiving concomitant drugs that produce bone marrow suppression, or have a chronic infection that was or is being treated with concomitant anti-infective therapy.

Discontinuance of linezolid should be considered if myelosuppression develops or worsens. Hematologic parameters generally have increased toward pretreatment values following discontinuance of the drug.

Peripheral and Optic Neuropathy Peripheral and optic neuropathies have been reported in adults and children receiving linezolid; these events have occurred principally in patients receiving the drug for longer than the maximum recommended duration of treatment (28 days). Optic neuropathy sometimes progressed to loss of vision when linezolid was used for longer than 28 days. Blurred vision has been reported in some patients who received the drug for less than 28 days.

If a patient experiences symptoms of visual impairment (e.g., changes in visual acuity or color vision, blurred vision, or visual field defect), an ophthalmic evaluation should be performed promptly. All patients receiving linezolid for extended periods of time (i.e., 3 months or longer) should have their visual function monitored. In addition, all patients reporting a new visual symptom, regardless of the length of linezolid treatment, should have their visual function monitored.

If peripheral or optic neuropathy occurs, the potential benefits of linezolid should be weighed against the potential risks of continued treatment with the drug.

Serotonin Syndrome Serotonin syndrome (including some fatalities) has been reported in patients receiving linezolid concomitantly with serotonergic drugs. Signs and symptoms of serotonin syndrome include mental changes (confusion, hyperactivity, memory problems), muscle twitching, excessive sweating, shivering, shaking, diarrhea, loss of coordination, and/or fever.

Most reported cases of serotonin syndrome have occurred in patients receiving linezolid concomitantly with selective serotonin-reuptake inhibitors (SSRIs) or selective serotonin- and norepinephrine-reuptake inhibitors (SNRIs). FDA has not concluded whether concomitant use of linezolid and other drugs with lesser degrees of serotonergic activity (e.g., tricyclic antidepressants, MAO inhibitors) is associated with a risk comparable to that reported with concomitant use of linezolid and SSRIs or SNRIs.

Linezolid should not be used in patients with carcinoid syndrome or in patients receiving SSRIs, tricyclic antidepressants, serotonin 5-HT_1 receptor agonists (triptans), meperidine, bupropion, or buspirone unless concomitant therapy is considered clinically appropriate and patients can be carefully monitored for signs and/or symptoms of serotonin syndrome or neuroleptic malignant syndrome-like (NMS-like) reactions. (See Drug Interactions: Monoamine Oxidase Inhibitors and see Drug Interactions: Serotonergic Drugs.)

Mortality In a study in seriously ill patients with intravascular catheter-related infections†, mortality was higher in linezolid-treated patients than in those treated with a comparator anti-infective (vancomycin, dicloxacillin, oxacillin). (See Uses: Catheter-related Bloodstream Infections.)

Monoamine Oxidase Inhibition Linezolid is a weak, nonselective, reversible inhibitor of monoamine oxidase (MAO). The drug potentially may interact with MAO inhibitors and adrenergic and serotonergic agents. (See Drug Interactions: Monoamine Oxidase Inhibitors, Drug Interactions: Sympathomimetic Agents, and Drug Interactions: Serotonergic Drugs.)

A significant pressor response has been reported when tyramine doses exceeding 100 mg were used in adults receiving linezolid. Patients should be instructed to avoid large quantities of foods or beverages with high tyramine content during linezolid treatment. Foods high in tyramine include those that may have undergone protein changes by aging, fermentation, pickling, or smoking to improve flavor (e.g., aged cheeses, fermented or air-dried meat, sauerkraut, soy sauce, tap beer, red wine). Tyramine content of any protein-rich food may be increased if stored for long periods or improperly refrigerated. For additional information on interactions in patients receiving MAO inhibitors and foods containing large amounts of tyramine, see Food under Drug Interactions: Food and Drugs Associated with Hypertensive Crisis, in the Monoamine Oxidase Inhibitors General Statement 28:16.04.12.

Risk of Hypertension Unless patients are monitored for potential increases in blood pressure, linezolid should not be used in patients with uncontrolled hypertension, pheochromocytoma, or thyrotoxicosis or in patients receiving direct- or indirect-acting sympathomimetic agents (e.g., pseudoephedrine), vasopressor agents (e.g., epinephrine, norepinephrine), or dopaminergic agents (e.g., dopamine, dobutamine). (See Drug Interactions: Sympathomimetic Agents.)

Lactic Acidosis Lactic acidosis, characterized by recurrent nausea and vomiting, has been reported in patients receiving linezolid. Patients who develop recurrent nausea and vomiting, unexplained acidosis, or a low bicarbonate concentration while receiving linezolid should undergo immediate medical evaluation.

Seizures Seizures have been reported in patients receiving linezolid. Some cases were reported in patients with a history of seizures or risk factors for seizures.

Hypoglycemia Symptomatic hypoglycemia has been reported in patients with diabetes mellitus receiving linezolid concomitantly with insulin or oral antidiabetic agents. (See Drug Interactions: Antidiabetic Agents.)

Although a causal relationship between linezolid and hypoglycemia has not been established, patients with diabetes mellitus should be cautioned about the potential for hypoglycemia during linezolid treatment.

If hypoglycemia occurs, dosage reduction of insulin or oral antidiabetic agents or discontinuance of linezolid, insulin, or oral antidiabetic agents may be necessary.

Sensitivity Reactions Anaphylaxis, angioedema, and bullous skin disorders, such as those described as Stevens-Johnson syndrome, reported.

Tooth Discoloration Superficial tooth discoloration and tongue discoloration have been reported in patients receiving linezolid. In cases with known outcome, tooth discoloration was removable with professional dental cleaning (manual descaling).

Phenylketonuria Individuals who must restrict their intake of phenylalanine should be warned that linezolid for oral suspension contains aspartame, which is metabolized in the GI tract following oral administration, to provide 20 mg of phenylalanine per 5 mL of suspension.

Linezolid tablets do not contain aspartame and should be used in individuals with phenylketonuria (i.e., homozygous genetic deficiency of phenylalanine hydroxylase) and other individuals who must restrict their intake of phenylalanine.

Superinfection/Clostridium difficile-associated Diarrhea and Colitis Use of linezolid may result in emergence and overgrowth of nonsusceptible organisms. Appropriate therapy should be instituted if superinfection occurs.

Treatment with anti-infectives alters normal colon flora and may permit overgrowth of *Clostridium difficile*. *C. difficile* infection (CDI) and *C. difficile*-associated diarrhea and colitis (CDAD; also known as antibiotic-associated diarrhea and colitis or pseudomembranous colitis) have been reported with nearly all anti-infectives, including linezolid, and may range in severity from mild diarrhea to fatal colitis. *C. difficile* produces toxins A and B which contribute to the development of CDAD; hypertoxin-producing strains of *C. difficile* are associated with increased morbidity and mortality since they may be refractory to anti-infectives and colectomy may be required.

CDAD should be considered in the differential diagnosis of patients who develop diarrhea during or after anti-infective therapy. Careful medical history is necessary since CDAD has been reported to occur as late as 2 months or longer after anti-infective therapy is discontinued.

If CDAD is suspected or confirmed, anti-infective therapy not directed against *C. difficile* should be discontinued whenever possible. Patients should be managed with appropriate supportive therapy (e.g., fluid and electrolyte management, protein supplementation), anti-infective therapy directed against *C. difficile* (e.g., metronidazole, vancomycin), and surgical evaluation as clinically indicated.

Selection and Use of Anti-infectives Linezolid is indicated only for the treatment of certain infections caused by certain gram-positive bacteria. The drug has no clinical activity against gram-negative bacteria and is *not* indicated for the treatment of infections caused by gram-negative bacteria.

It is imperative that an anti-infective active against gram-negative bacteria be used concomitantly if documented or presumed pathogens include gram-negative bacteria. (See Uses.)

Safety and efficacy of linezolid given for longer than 28 days have not been evaluated in controlled clinical trials. (See Dosage and Administration: Dosage.)

To reduce development of drug-resistant bacteria and maintain effectiveness of linezolid and other antibacterials, the drug should be used only for treatment of infections proven or strongly suspected to be caused by susceptible bacteria.

When selecting or modifying anti-infective therapy, results of culture and in vitro susceptibility testing should be used. In the absence of such data, local epidemiology and susceptibility patterns should be considered when selecting anti-infectives for empiric therapy.

Specific Populations **Pregnancy.** Category C. (See Users Guide)

In studies in mice, rats, and rabbits, linezolid was not teratogenic; however, embryo and fetal toxicities were reported. These nonteratogenic effects included increased postimplantational embryo death, decreased fetal body weights, and increased incidence of costal cartilage fusion in mice; decreased fetal body weights, reduced ossification of sternebrae, and decreased survival of pups in rats; and reduced fetal body weight in rabbits. Linezolid should be used during pregnancy only if potential benefits justify potential risk to the fetus.

Lactation. Linezolid and its metabolites are distributed into milk in rats; it is not known whether the drug and metabolites are distributed into human milk.

Linezolid should be used with caution in nursing women.

Pediatric Use. Safety and efficacy of linezolid for the treatment of community-acquired pneumonia (CAP), nosocomial pneumonia, complicated skin and skin structure infections, or vancomycin-resistant *Enterococcus faecium* infections in pediatric patients are supported by adequate and well-controlled studies in adults, pharmacokinetic studies in pediatric patients, and additional data from a comparator-controlled study of gram-positive infections in neonates and children through 11 years of age. Safety and efficacy of the drug for the treatment of CAP in pediatric patients also is supported by evidence from an uncontrolled study in patients 8 months through 12 years of age.

Safety and efficacy of linezolid for the treatment of uncomplicated skin and skin structure infections in pediatric patients have been established in a comparator-controlled study in pediatric patients 5–17 years of age.

While some pharmacokinetic parameters (i.e., peak plasma concentration, volume of distribution) are similar in children of all ages, linezolid clearance varies with age. Excluding neonates younger than 1 week of age, clearance is most rapid in the youngest age groups (i.e., those 7 days to 11 years of age); as children age, the clearance of linezolid decreases and clearance values in adolescents approach those observed in adults. Systemic exposure (mean daily area under the plasma concentration-time curve [AUC]) in pediatric patients younger than 12 years of age receiving linezolid every 8 hours generally is similar to that in adults and adolescents receiving the drug every 12 hours. There is wider intraindividual variability in linezolid clearance and in systemic drug exposure in all pediatric age groups relative to adults.

The manufacturer states that linezolid is not recommended for empiric treatment of CNS infections in pediatric patients; therapeutic concentrations of the drug were not consistently achieved or maintained in CSF of pediatric patients with ventriculoperitoneal shunts.

Inadequate systemic exposure, site and severity of infection, and underlying medical conditions should be considered in children with a suboptimal response to linezolid, especially those with infections caused by gram-positive bacteria that have minimum inhibitory concentrations (MICs) of 4 mcg/mL.

Geriatric Use. No overall differences in safety, efficacy, or pharmacokinetics have been observed in geriatric adults 65 years of age or older compared with younger adults. Other clinical experience has not revealed age-related differences in response, but the possibility of greater sensitivity in some older patients cannot be ruled out.

Renal Impairment. Linezolid pharmacokinetics are not altered in patients with renal impairment. However, the 2 principal metabolites of linezolid may accumulate in patients with impaired renal function and the amount of accumulation increases with the severity of renal impairment. Because the clinical importance of accumulation of linezolid metabolites has not been determined, the potential benefits of linezolid in patients with renal impairment should be weighed against the potential risks of accumulation of the metabolites. (See Renal Impairment under Dosage and Administration: Special Populations.)

Hepatic Impairment. Linezolid pharmacokinetics are not altered in patients with mild or moderate hepatic impairment (Child-Pugh class A or B); pharmacokinetics of the drug have not been evaluated in patients with severe hepatic impairment.

■ **Common Adverse Effects** Adverse effects occurring in 2% or more of adults receiving linezolid include GI effects (diarrhea, nausea, vomiting), headache, anemia, rash, and dizziness. Adverse effects reported in 2% or more of pediatric patients receiving linezolid in clinical studies include GI effects (diarrhea, nausea, vomiting, localized or generalized abdominal pain, loose stools), headache, anemia, and thrombocytopenia.

Drug Interactions

■ **Drugs Affecting or Metabolized by Hepatic Microsomal Enzymes** Linezolid is minimally metabolized (possibly mediated by cytochrome P-450 [CYP] enzymes), does not induce CYP enzymes, and does not inhibit CYP isoenzymes 1A2, 2C9, 2C19, 2D6, 2E1, or 3A4.

Linezolid is not expected to affect the pharmacokinetics of other drugs metabolized by CYP isoenzymes.

Although the mechanism of the interaction is unknown and may be related to induction of hepatic enzymes, concomitant use of rifampin and linezolid has resulted in decreased linezolid concentrations. It is possible that concomitant use of other potent inducers of hepatic enzymes (e.g., carbamazepine, phenytoin, phenobarbital) could result in decreased linezolid exposures.

■ **Antidiabetic Agents** Hypoglycemia has been reported in patients with diabetes mellitus receiving linezolid concomitantly with insulin or oral antidiabetic agents. Although a causal relationship has not been established, linezolid is a nonselective, reversible monoamine oxidase (MAO) inhibitor and some MAO inhibitors have been associated with hypoglycemic episodes in patients with diabetes mellitus who were also receiving insulin or oral antidiabetic agents. Patients should be warned of the potential for hypoglycemia. If hypoglycemia occurs, dosage reduction of the antidiabetic agent or discontinuance of linezolid or the antidiabetic agent may be necessary.

■ **Anti-infective Agents** ***Aminoglycosides*** Concomitant use of linezolid and gentamicin does not affect the pharmacokinetics of either drug.

In vitro studies indicate the antibacterial effects of linezolid and gentamicin or streptomycin may be additive or indifferent.

Ampicillin In vitro studies indicate the antibacterial effects of linezolid and ampicillin may be additive or indifferent.

Aztreonam Concomitant use of linezolid and aztreonam does not result in clinically important effects on the pharmacokinetics of either drug.

In vitro studies indicate the antibacterial effects of linezolid and aztreonam may be additive or indifferent.

Carbapenems In vitro studies indicate the antibacterial effects of linezolid and imipenem may be additive or indifferent.

Rifampin Concomitant use of linezolid (600 mg twice daily for 2.5 days) and rifampin (600 mg once daily for 8 days) resulted in a 21% decrease in peak plasma concentrations of linezolid and a 32% decrease in the area under the plasma concentration-time curve (AUC) of linezolid. The mechanism and clinical importance of this pharmacokinetic interaction are unknown, although the interaction may be related to induction of hepatic enzymes.

In vitro studies indicate the antibacterial effects of linezolid and rifampin may be additive or indifferent.

Vancomycin In vitro studies indicate the antibacterial effects of linezolid and vancomycin may be additive or indifferent.

■ **Monoamine Oxidase Inhibitors** Linezolid is a weak, nonselective, reversible MAO inhibitor and there is potential for pharmacologic interactions with other MAO inhibitors. Because of the potential for interaction, linezolid should not be used in patients who are receiving (or have received within the last 2 weeks) a drug that inhibits MAO-A or MAO-B (e.g., isocarboxazid, phenelzine, selegiline, tranylcypromine).

Although FDA has not concluded whether the risk of serotonin syndrome associated with concomitant use of linezolid and MAO inhibitors is comparable to that reported when linezolid is used concomitantly with selective serotonin-reuptake inhibitors (SSRIs) or selective serotonin- and norepinephrine-reuptake inhibitors (SNRIs), linezolid generally should not be used in patients receiving serotonergic drugs, including MAO inhibitors (e.g., isocarboxazid, phenelzine, selegiline, tranylcypromine). (See Drug Interactions: Serotonergic Drugs.)

■ **Phenytoin** Concomitant use of linezolid and phenytoin is not expected to affect the pharmacokinetics of phenytoin, but may possibly result in decreased linezolid exposures. Dosage adjustments are not required if linezolid and phenytoin are used concomitantly.

■ **Serotonergic Drugs** Concomitant use of linezolid and serotonergic drugs is associated with a risk of serotonin syndrome. There have been postmarketing reports of serotonin syndrome, including some fatalities, in patients who received linezolid concurrently with or shortly after discontinuance of serotonergic agents, particularly SSRIs (e.g., citalopram, escitalopram, fluoxetine, fluvoxamine, paroxetine, sertraline) or SNRIs (e.g., desvenlafaxine, duloxetine, venlafaxine). While FDA has not received reports of serotonin syndrome with concomitant use of linezolid and vilazodone, the risk is considered comparable to that with SSRIs. It is unclear whether concomitant use of linezolid and other drugs with lesser degrees of serotonergic activity, including tricyclic antidepressants (amitriptyline, clomipramine, desipramine, doxepin, imipramine, nortriptyline, protriptyline, trimipramine), MAO inhibitors (isocarboxazid, phenelzine, transdermal selegiline, tranylcypromine), amoxapine, bupropion, buspirone, maprotiline, mirtazapine, nefazodone, and trazodone, is associated with a risk of serotonin syndrome comparable to that reported when linezolid is used concomitantly with SSRIs or SNRIs.

Because of the risk of serotonin syndrome, linezolid should not be used in patients receiving serotonergic drugs, including SSRIs, tricyclic antidepressants, serotonin 5-HT_1 receptor agonists (triptans), meperidine, bupropion, or buspirone, unless concomitant therapy is considered clinically appropriate and patients can be carefully monitored for signs and/or symptoms of serotonin syndrome or neuroleptic malignant syndrome-like (NMS-like) reactions.

There may be some cases when a patient is already receiving a serotonergic antidepressant or buspirone and requires urgent treatment with linezolid (e.g., life-threatening infections caused by methicillin-resistant *Staphylococcus aureus* [MRSA; also known as oxacillin-resistant *S. aureus* or ORSA] or vancomycin-resistant *Enterococcus faecium*). In these situations, if alternatives to linezolid are not available and the potential benefits of linezolid outweigh the risks of serotonin syndrome or NMS-like reactions, the serotonergic antidepressant should be stopped promptly and linezolid administered. The patient should be monitored for manifestations of serotonin syndrome or NMS-like reactions (e.g., hyperthermia, rigidity, myoclonus, autonomic instability, mental status changes that include extreme agitation progressing to delirium and coma) for 2 weeks (5 weeks if fluoxetine was taken) or until 24 hours after the last dose of linezolid, whichever comes first. The patient also should be monitored for symptoms associated with discontinuance of the antidepressant.

Treatment with serotonergic drugs should not be initiated in a patient receiving linezolid; when necessary, the serotonergic drug may be started or reinitiated 24 hours after the last linezolid dose.

For further information on serotonin syndrome, including manifestations and treatment, see Drug Interactions: Serotonergic Drugs, in Fluoxetine Hydrochloride 28:16.04.20.

■ **Sympathomimetic Agents** Concomitant use of linezolid and indirect-acting sympathomimetic agents (e.g., phenylpropanolamine, pseudoephedrine), vasopressor agents (e.g., epinephrine, norepinephrine), or dopaminergic agents (e.g., dopamine, dobutamine) may result in a reversible enhancement of the pressor response to these agents.

Unless patients are monitored for potential increases in blood pressure, linezolid should not be used in patients receiving direct- or indirect-acting sympathomimetic agents (e.g., pseudoephedrine), vasopressor agents (e.g., epinephrine, norepinephrine), or dopaminergic agents (e.g., dopamine, dobutamine).

If an adrenergic agent (e.g., dopamine, epinephrine) is initiated in a patient receiving linezolid, lower initial doses of the adrenergic agent should be used and dosage titrated to achieve the desired response.

■ **Vitamins** Concomitant use of linezolid (600 mg orally on day 1 and day 8) and ascorbic acid (1 g daily on days 2–9) or vitamin E (800 units daily on days 2–9) increased the AUC of linezolid by 2.3 or 10.9%, respectively.

Adjustment of linezolid dosage is not needed if the drug is used concomitantly with ascorbic acid or vitamin E.

■ **Warfarin** Linezolid does not have a substantial effect on the pharmacokinetics of warfarin; dosage adjustments are not required if linezolid and warfarin are used concomitantly.

Description

Linezolid is an oxazolidinone anti-infective agent. The mechanism of action of linezolid involves binding to a site on the bacterial 23S ribosomal RNA of the 50S subunit and prevention of formation of a functional 70S initiation complex, which is an essential component of the bacterial translation process.

In vitro, linezolid is bacteriostatic against susceptible enterococci and staphylococci and bactericidal against susceptible streptococci. Linezolid is active in vitro against most strains of *Staphylococcus aureus* (including methicillin-resistant *S. aureus* [MRSA; also known as oxacillin-resistant *S. aureus* or ORSA]), *Streptococcus agalactiae* (group B streptococci, GBS), *S. pneumoniae*, *S. pyogenes* (group A β-hemolytic streptococci, GAS), and vancomycin-resistant *Enterococcus faecium*. Linezolid also has in vitro activity against *E. faecalis* (including vancomycin-resistant strains), *E. faecium* (vancomycin-susceptible strains), *S. epidermidis* (including methicillin-resistant strains [oxacillin-resistant strains]), *S. haemolyticus*, viridans group streptococci, group G streptococci, *Corynebacterium*, and *Pasteurella multocida*; however, safety and efficacy of linezolid in treating clinical infections caused by these bacteria have not been established in adequate and well-controlled clinical studies to date.

Linezolid is active in vitro against *Mycobacterium tuberculosis*, including some multiple-drug resistant (MDR) and extensively drug-resistant (XDR) strains. Linezolid also has activity in vitro against some strains of *M. chelonaei*, *M. fortuitum*, *M. gilvum*, *M. gordonae*, *M. kansasii*, *M. mucgenicum*, and *M. simiae*.

Resistance to linezolid has been produced in vitro by serial passage of MRSA or enterococci (i.e., *E. faecalis*, *E. faecium*) in the presence of increasing concentrations of the drug, and resistance to linezolid has emerged in patients receiving the drug for the treatment of infections caused by MRSA or enterococci. Linezolid resistance generally is associated with point mutations in the 23S rRNA gene. However, linezolid resistance in staphylococci mediated by the chloramphenicol-florfenicol (*cfr*) gene located on a plasmid has been reported and such resistance is transferable between staphylococci.

Cross-resistance between linezolid and other oxazolidinones (e.g., tedizolid) has been reported. Bacteria resistant to linezolid because of mutations in chromosomal genes encoding the 23S rRNA or ribosomal proteins (L3 and L4) usually are cross-resistant to other oxazolidinones (e.g., tedizolid) and vice versa. However, in vitro data indicate that the presence of the *cfr* gene in *S. aureus* that results in resistance to linezolid does not necessarily result in cross-resistance to tedizolid in the absence of chromosomal mutations. Cross-resistance between linezolid and non-oxazolidinone anti-infectives is unlikely.

Linezolid is well absorbed following oral administration (absolute bioavailability approximately 100%) and is readily distributed to well-perfused tissues. The drug is metabolized principally via oxidation to 2 inactive metabolites: an aminoethoxyacetic acid metabolite and a hydroxyethyl glycine metabolite. Linezolid is minimally metabolized and metabolism may be mediated by the cytochrome P-450 (CYP) enzyme system. Linezolid does not inhibit CYP isoenzymes 1A2, 2C9, 2C19, 2D6, 2E1, or 3A4 and is not an enzyme inducer, suggesting that the drug is unlikely to alter the pharmacokinetics of drugs metabolized by these enzymes.

Advice to Patients

Advise patients that antibacterials (including linezolid) should only be used to treat bacterial infections and not used to treat viral infections (e.g., the common cold).

Importance of completing full course of treatment, even if feeling better after a few days.

Advise patients that skipping doses or not completing the full course of treatment may decrease effectiveness and increase the likelihood that bacteria will develop resistance and will not be treatable with linezolid or other antibacterials in the future.

Advise patients that linezolid may be taken orally without regard to meals. If using the oral suspension, importance of not shaking the bottle vigorously and gently inverting the bottle 3–5 times to resuspend the drug prior to administration of each dose.

Advise patients of the potential risk of serotonin syndrome, particularly if linezolid is used concomitantly with monoamine oxidase (MAO) inhibitors, selective serotonin-reuptake inhibitors (SSRIs), selective serotonin- and norepinephrine-reuptake inhibitors (SNRIs), tricyclic antidepressants, or other serotonergic drugs. Importance of immediately contacting clinician if signs and symptoms of serotonin syndrome develop (e.g., confusion, hyperactivity, memory problems, muscle twitching, excessive sweating, shivering, shaking, diarrhea, loss of coordination, fever). Importance of not discontinuing serotonergic drugs without first consulting clinician.

Advise patients, particularly those with diabetes mellitus, that hypoglycemic reactions (diaphoresis and tremulousness) and low blood glucose concentrations may occur during linezolid treatment. Importance of contacting a clinician to obtain proper treatment if such reactions occur.

Importance of avoiding large quantities of foods or beverages with high tyramine content during linezolid treatment; this includes foods or beverages that have been aged, fermented, pickled, or smoked to improve flavor (e.g., aged cheeses, fermented or air-dried meats, sauerkraut, soy sauce, tap beer, red wine). Consider that tyramine content of any protein-rich food may be increased if stored for long periods or improperly refrigerated.

Advise individuals with phenylketonuria that the oral suspension contains aspartame, which is metabolized in the GI tract to provide 20 mg of phenylalanine per 5 mL of suspension.

Importance of notifying clinicians of any history of hypertension or seizures.

Importance of notifying clinician if any change in vision occurs.

Advise patients that diarrhea is a common problem caused by anti-infectives and usually ends when the drug is discontinued. Importance of contacting a clinician if watery and bloody stools (with or without stomach cramps and fever) occur during or as late as 2 months or longer after the last dose.

Importance of informing clinicians of existing or contemplated concomitant therapy, including prescription drugs (e.g., antidepressants) and OTC drugs (e.g., pseudoephedrine), as well as any concomitant illnesses.

Importance of women informing clinicians if they are or plan to become pregnant or plan to breast-feed.

Importance of informing patients of other important precautionary information. (See Cautions.)

Overview (see Users Guide). For additional information until a more detailed monograph is developed and published, the manufacturer's labeling should be consulted. It is *essential* that the manufacturer's labeling be consulted for more detailed information on usual cautions, precautions, contraindications, potential drug interactions, laboratory test interferences, and acute toxicity.

Preparations

Excipients in commercially available drug preparations may have clinically important effects in some individuals; consult specific product labeling for details.

Linezolid

Oral		
For suspension	100 mg/5 mL*	**Linezolid for Suspension** **Zyvox®**, Pfizer
Tablets, film-coated	600 mg*	**Linezolid Tablets** **Zyvox®**, Pfizer
Parenteral		
Injection, for IV infusion	2 mg/mL (200, 400, and 600 mg) in sterile isotonic solution*	**Linezolid Injection** **Zyvox® Injection** (in flexible containers), Pfizer

*available from one or more manufacturer, distributor, and/or repackager by generic (nonproprietary) name

†Use is not currently included in the labeling approved by the US Food and Drug Administration

Selected Revisions March 2016, © Copyright, June 2000, American Society of Health-System Pharmacists, Inc.

Tedizolid Phosphate

■ Tedizolid phosphate is an oxazolidinone antibacterial agent.

Uses

■ **Skin and Skin Structure Infections** Tedizolid phosphate is used for the treatment of acute bacterial skin and skin structure infections (ABSSSI) caused by susceptible *Staphylococcus aureus* (including methicillin-resistant *S. aureus* [MRSA; also known as oxacillin-resistant *S. aureus* or ORSA] and methicillin-susceptible *S. aureus*), *Streptococcus pyogenes* (group A β-hemolytic streptococci, GAS), *S. agalactiae* (group B streptococci, GBS), *S. anginosus* group (includes *S. anginosus*, *S. intermedius*, and *S. constellatus*), or *Enterococcus faecalis*.

Clinical Experience Efficacy and safety of tedizolid were evaluated in 2 randomized, multicenter, double-blind, noninferiority, phase 3 studies (ESTABLISH-1 and ESTABLISH-2) in adults with acute bacterial skin and skin structure infections (e.g., cellulitis, erysipelas, major cutaneous abscess, wound infection) with local signs and symptoms of infection and at least 1 regional or systemic sign of infection at baseline (i.e., lymphadenopathy, temperature 38°C or greater, leukocyte count greater than 10,000 cells/mm³ or less than 4000 cells/mm³, or 10% or greater band forms on leukocyte differential).

In ESTABLISH-1, 649 patients (median age 43 years, 61% male, 7% with diabetes mellitus, 36% current or recent IV drug users, 40% with cellulitis/erysipelas, 30% with major cutaneous abscess, 30% with wound infection, overall median baseline lesion surface area 190 cm²) were randomized to receive oral tedizolid (200 mg of tedizolid phosphate once daily for 6 days) or oral linezolid (600 mg twice daily for 10 days). In patients with wound infections, adjunctive use of aztreonam and/or metronidazole for coverage against gram-negative bacteria was permitted. After 48–72 hours of treatment, 79.3 or 79.1% of patients in the intent-to-treat (ITT) population who received tedizolid or linezolid, respectively, achieved early clinical response (i.e., no increase in lesion surface area from baseline, oral temperature 37.6°C or less), and 78 or 75.5%, respectively, achieved a 20% or greater reduction in lesion surface area from baseline. At 7–14 days after the end of treatment, 85.8% of patients receiving tedizolid and 85.6% of patients receiving linezolid achieved clinical success (i.e., resolution or near resolution of most disease-specific signs and symptoms, absence or near resolution of systemic signs of infection, and no new signs, symptoms, or complications attributable to the infection requiring further treatment of the primary lesion).

In ESTABLISH-2, 666 patients (median age 46 years, 68% male, 10% with diabetes mellitus, 20% current or recent IV drug users, 50% with cellulitis/erysipelas, 20% with major cutaneous abscess, 30% with wound infection, overall median baseline lesion surface area 231 cm²) were randomized to receive tedizolid (200 mg of tedizolid phosphate IV once daily for 6 days) or linezolid (600 mg IV twice daily for 10 days). All patients received at least 2 IV doses with the option to switch to oral therapy if the patient met study criteria. In patients with wound infections, adjunctive use of aztreonam and/or metronidazole for coverage against gram-negative bacteria was permitted. After 48–72 hours of treatment, 86.1 or 84.1% of patients in the ITT population who received tedizolid or linezolid, respectively, achieved early clinical response (i.e., no increase in lesion surface area from baseline, oral temperature 37.6°C or less), and 85.2 or 82.6%, respectively, achieved a 20% or greater reduction in lesion surface area from baseline. At 7–14 days after the end of treatment, 88% of patients receiving tedizolid and 87.7% of patients receiving linezolid achieved clinical success (i.e., resolution or near resolution of most disease-specific signs and symptoms, absence or near resolution of systemic signs of infection, and no new signs, symptoms, or complications attributable to the infection requiring further treatment of the primary lesion).

In a pooled analysis of the subset of patients who were microbiologically evaluable and stratified according to the infecting pathogen (ESTABLISH-1 and ESTABLISH-2), the clinical success rate on day 7–14 in those with infections caused by MRSA or methicillin-susceptible *S. aureus* was 84 or 92%, respectively, in those treated with tedizolid and 81 or 94%, respectively, in those treated with linezolid. The clinical success rate in those with infections caused by *S. agalactiae*, *S. pyogenes*, *S. anginosus* group, or *E. faecalis* was 89, 91, 70, or 70%, respectively, in those treated with tedizolid and 80, 95, 89, or 100%, respectively, in those treated with linezolid.

Dosage and Administration

■ **Administration** Tedizolid phosphate is administered orally or by IV infusion.

Oral Administration Tedizolid phosphate tablets may be given orally without regard to meals.

IV Administration Tedizolid phosphate for injection should be administered *only* by IV infusion. The drug should *not* be administered by rapid or direct IV injection, and is *not* intended for IM, intra-arterial, intrathecal, intraperitoneal, or subcutaneous administration.

Other IV substances, additives, or drugs should *not* be added to tedizolid phosphate vials or infused simultaneously.

If the same IV line is used for sequential infusion of several different drugs, the line should be flushed with 0.9% sodium chloride injection before and after infusion of tedizolid phosphate.

Tedizolid phosphate is incompatible with solutions containing divalent cations (e.g., calcium, magnesium), including lactated Ringer's injection and Hartmann's solution.

Vials of tedizolid phosphate lyophilized powder for injection contain no preservatives and are intended for single use only.

Reconstitution and Dilution. Tedizolid phosphate for injection must be reconstituted and further diluted prior to IV infusion. Strict aseptic technique must be observed when preparing IV solutions of the drug.

Vials labeled as containing 200 mg of tedizolid phosphate should be reconstituted by adding 4 mL of sterile water for injection. The vial should be gently swirled, then left standing until the lyophilized powder or cake dissolves and foam disperses; vigorous agitation or shaking of the vial should be avoided to minimize foaming. Reconstituted solutions should be inspected to ensure that no particulate matter, powder, or cake is attached to the sides of the vial. If needed, the vial may be inverted and gently swirled to dissolve any remaining powder. The reconstituted solution should appear clear and colorless to pale yellow in color.

Reconstituted tedizolid phosphate must then be further diluted in 250 mL of 0.9% sodium chloride injection. The vial containing the reconstituted solution should be tilted and 4 mL of the solution withdrawn from the bottom corner of the vial using a syringe; inverting the vial while withdrawing the solution should be avoided. The 4 mL of reconstituted solution should be slowly added to an infusion bag containing 250 mL of 0.9% sodium chloride injection; the bag should be gently inverted to mix and should not be shaken. The reconstituted and diluted IV solution should appear clear and colorless to pale yellow in color. The solution should be inspected visually for particulate matter prior to administration and should be discarded if particles are observed.

Reconstituted or further diluted solutions of tedizolid phosphate may be stored under refrigeration (2–8°C) or at room temperature. Total storage time from reconstitution to administration should not exceed 24 hours whether stored at 2–8°C or room temperature.

Rate of Administration. Tedizolid phosphate solutions should be administered by IV infusion over 1 hour.

■ **Dosage** Tedizolid phosphate is a prodrug that is inactive until metabolized in vivo to tedizolid (see Description); dosage of the drug is expressed in terms of the prodrug (i.e., tedizolid phosphate).

Dosage adjustments of tedizolid phosphate are not needed when switching from IV to oral administration.

Adult Dosage **Skin and Skin Structure Infections.** The recommended oral or IV dosage of tedizolid phosphate for the treatment of acute bacterial skin and skin structure infections (ABSSSI) in adults is 200 mg once daily for 6 days.

■ **Special Populations** Dosage adjustments are not needed in adults with hepatic impairment or renal impairment, including those undergoing hemodialysis.

Dosage adjustments are not needed based on age, gender, race, body weight, or body mass index (BMI).

Cautions

■ **Contraindications** The manufacturer states there are no contraindications to use of tedizolid phosphate.

■ **Warnings/Precautions** ***Patients with Neutropenia*** Safety and efficacy of tedizolid in patients with neutropenia (i.e., neutrophil counts less than 1000 cells/mm^3) have not been evaluated. In an animal model of infection, the antibacterial activity of tedizolid was reduced in the absence of granulocytes.

Alternative therapies should be considered for the treatment of acute bacterial skin and skin structure infections in patients with neutropenia.

Hematologic Effects In phase 1 studies in healthy adults who received tedizolid for 21 days, there was evidence of a possible dose and duration effect on hematologic parameters after day 6. In phase 3 studies in patients with acute bacterial skin and skin structure infections, the rate of clinically important changes in neutrophil count, platelet count, and hemoglobin concentration generally were similar in those treated with a 6-day regimen of tedizolid or a 10-day regimen of linezolid.

Neuropathy Peripheral and optic neuropathies have been reported in patients who received more than 28 days of treatment with an oxazolidinone anti-infective (not tedizolid). In phase 3 studies evaluating tedizolid in patients with acute bacterial skin and skin structure infections, peripheral neuropathy or optic nerve disorders were reported in 1.2 or 0.3%, respectively, of patients receiving tedizolid compared with 0.6 or 0.2%, respectively, of patients receiving linezolid. Data are not available for patients exposed to tedizolid for longer than 6 days.

Superinfection/Clostridium difficile-associated Diarrhea and Colitis (CDAD) Use of tedizolid may result in emergence and overgrowth of nonsusceptible bacteria or fungi. The patient should be carefully monitored and appropriate therapy instituted if superinfection occurs.

Treatment with anti-infectives alters normal colon flora and may permit overgrowth of *Clostridium difficile*. *C. difficile* infection (CDI) and *C. difficile*-associated diarrhea and colitis (CDAD; also known as antibiotic-associated diarrhea and colitis or pseudomembranous colitis) have been reported in patients receiving nearly all anti-infectives, including tedizolid, and may range in severity from mild diarrhea to fatal colitis. *C. difficile* produces toxins A and B which contribute to development of CDAD; hypertoxin-producing strains of *C. difficile* are associated with increased morbidity and mortality since they may be refractory to anti-infectives and colectomy may be required.

CDAD should be considered in the differential diagnosis of patients who develop diarrhea during or after anti-infective therapy. Careful medical history is necessary since CDAD has been reported to occur as late as 2 months or longer after anti-infective therapy is discontinued.

If CDAD is suspected or confirmed, anti-infective therapy not directed against *C. difficile* should be discontinued whenever possible. Patients should be managed with appropriate supportive therapy (e.g., fluid and electrolyte management, protein supplementation), anti-infective therapy directed against *C. difficile* (e.g., metronidazole, vancomycin), and surgical evaluation as clinically indicated.

Selection and Use of Anti-infectives To reduce development of drug-resistant bacteria and maintain effectiveness of tedizolid and other antibacterials, the drug should be used only for treatment of infections proven or strongly suspected to be caused by susceptible bacteria.

When selecting or modifying anti-infective therapy, results of culture and in vitro susceptibility testing should be used. In the absence of such data, local epidemiology and susceptibility patterns should be considered when selecting anti-infectives for empiric therapy.

Specific Populations **Pregnancy.** Category C. (See Users Guide.)

There are no adequate and well-controlled studies of tedizolid in pregnant women, and the drug should be used during pregnancy only if potential benefits justify potential risks to the fetus.

In embryofetal studies, tedizolid was shown to produce fetal developmental toxicities in mice, rats, and rabbits. In mice, reduced fetal weight and increased incidence of costal cartilage anomalies were observed at a dosage of 25 mg/kg daily (4 times the estimated human exposure level based on area under the plasma concentration-time curve [AUC]). In rats, decreased fetal weight and increased skeletal variations (e.g., reduced ossification of the sternebrae, vertebrae, and skull) were observed at a dosage of 15 mg/kg daily (6 times the estimated human exposure based on AUC) and were associated with maternal toxicity (reduced maternal body weight). In rabbits, reduced fetal weights, but no malformations or variations, were observed at dosages associated with maternal toxicity.

Lactation. Tedizolid is distributed into milk in rats; it is not known whether the drug is distributed into human milk.

Tedizolid phosphate should be used with caution in nursing women.

Pediatric Use. Safety and efficacy of tedizolid phosphate have not been established in pediatric patients younger than 18 years of age.

Geriatric Use. Clinical studies did not include sufficient numbers of patients 65 years of age or older to determine whether they respond differently than younger adults. Differences in tedizolid pharmacokinetics were not observed between geriatric and younger patients. Dosage adjustments are not needed in geriatric patients.

Hepatic Impairment. Clinically important changes in tedizolid pharmacokinetics (peak plasma concentrations, AUC) were not observed in adults with moderate or severe hepatic impairment (Child-Pugh class B or C); dosage adjustments are not needed.

Renal Impairment. Clinically important changes in tedizolid pharmacokinetics (peak plasma concentrations, AUC) were not observed in adults with severe renal impairment (creatinine clearance less than 30 mL/minute per 1.73 m^2). Hemodialysis does not result in clinically important removal of tedizolid from systemic circulation. Dosage adjustments are not needed in patients with renal impairment or undergoing hemodialysis.

■ **Common Adverse Effects** Adverse effects reported in 2% or more of patients receiving tedizolid phosphate include nausea, headache, diarrhea, vomiting, dizziness, and fatigue.

Drug Interactions

■ **Drugs Affecting or Metabolized by Hepatic Microsomal Enzymes** In vitro, tedizolid phosphate and tedizolid do not appear to be substrates for and do not inhibit or induce cytochrome P-450 (CYP) isoenzymes, including CYP1A2, 2B6, 2D6, 2C8, 2C9, 2C19, and 3A4. Drug interactions involving oxidative metabolism and CYP isoenzymes are unlikely.

■ **Drugs Affecting or Affected by Membrane Transporters** In vitro, tedizolid phosphate and tedizolid do not have clinically important effects on drug uptake or drug efflux membrane transporters (e.g., organic anion transporter [OAT] 1, OAT3, organic anion transporting polypeptide [OATP] 1B1, OATP1B3, organic cation transporter [OCT] 1, OCT2, P-glycoprotein [P-gp], breast cancer resistance protein [BCRP]).

■ **Antibacterial Agents** In vitro studies indicate that the antibacterial effects of tedizolid and aztreonam, ceftazidime, ceftriaxone, ciprofloxacin, clindamycin, co-trimoxazole, daptomycin, gentamicin, imipenem, minocycline, rifampin, or vancomycin are not synergistic or antagonistic against gram-positive bacteria (methicillin-resistant *Staphylococcus aureus*, *Streptococcus pneumoniae*, *S. pyogenes*, *Enterococcus faecalis*) or gram-negative bacteria (*Escherichia coli*).

■ **Antifungal Agents** In vitro studies indicate that tedizolid and amphotericin B, ketoconazole, or terbinafine are not synergistic or antagonistic against gram-positive bacteria (methicillin-resistant *S. aureus*, *S. pneumoniae*, *S. pyogenes*, *E. faecalis*).

■ **Monoamine Oxidase Inhibitors** In vitro, tedizolid is a weak reversible inhibitor of monoamine oxidase (MAO). Patients receiving MAO inhibitors were excluded during phase 2 and 3 clinical trials evaluating tedizolid phosphate; interactions between tedizolid and MAO inhibitors have not been evaluated.

■ **Pseudoephedrine** Concomitant use of oral tedizolid (200 mg of tedizolid phosphate once daily for 5 days) and pseudoephedrine (single 60-mg dose on day 5) in healthy adults did not result in substantial increases in maximum blood pressure or heart rate when compared with increases observed in those receiving pseudoephedrine concomitantly with placebo. Concomitant use of tedizolid and pseudoephedrine did not affect the pharmacokinetics of either drug.

■ **Serotonergic Drugs** When studied in a mouse model that predicts serotonergic activity, the serotonergic effects of tedizolid phosphate dosages up to 30-fold higher than the equivalent human dosages were similar to those seen with a vehicle control. Patients receiving serotonergic agents (e.g., selective serotonin-reuptake inhibitors [SSRIs], tricyclic antidepressants, serotonin type 1 [5-hydroxytryptamine type 1; 5-HT_1] receptor agonists ["triptans"], meperidine, buspirone) were excluded from phase 3 trials evaluating tedizolid phosphate.

■ **Tyramine-containing Foods** In healthy adults receiving tedizolid (200 mg of tedizolid phosphate once daily), the median tyramine dose required to increase systolic blood pressure by 30 mm Hg or more from baseline within 2 hours of tyramine administration was 325 mg compared with a dose of 425 mg when tyramine was used concomitantly with placebo. Palpitations were reported in 72.4% of those receiving tedizolid concomitantly with tyramine compared with 46.4% of those receiving tyramine and placebo.

Recommended dosage of tedizolid phosphate (200 mg daily) is not expected to exert a clinically important pressor response in patients receiving a tyramine-rich meal; restriction of foods with high tyramine content is not necessary.

Description

Tedizolid phosphate is an oxazolidinone anti-infective agent. Tedizolid phosphate is a prodrug that is inactive until hydrolyzed in vivo to tedizolid. The phosphate prodrug is highly water soluble, which facilitates oral absorption and enhances bioavailability of tedizolid. The mechanism of activity of tedizolid is mediated by binding to the 50S subunit of bacterial ribosomes resulting in inhibition of bacterial translation and inhibition of protein synthesis. Although the binding site for tedizolid is similar to the binding site for other oxazolidinones (e.g., linezolid), tedizolid may engage additional ribosomal sites compared with linezolid.

In vitro, tedizolid is bacteriostatic against certain gram-positive bacteria, including staphylococci, streptococci, and enterococci. The drug is active in vitro and in clinical infections against *Staphylococcus aureus* (including methicillin-resistant *S. aureus* [MRSA; also known as oxacillin-resistant *S. aureus*]), *S. pyogenes* (group A β-hemolytic streptococci, GAS), *Streptococcus agalactiae* (group B streptococci, GBS), *S. anginosus* group (includes *S. anginosus*, *S. intermedius*, and *S. constellatus*), and *Enterococcus faecalis*. There is some evidence from in vitro studies that tedizolid may be more potent than linezolid against susceptible bacteria, and tedizolid has been active against some strains of *S. aureus* resistant to linezolid. Tedizolid also has in vitro activity against *E. faecium*, *S. epidermidis* (including methicillin-resistant strains [oxacillin-resistant strains]), *S. haemolyticus*, and *S. lugdunensis;* however, safety and efficacy of the drug in treating clinical infections caused by these bacteria have not been established in adequate and well-controlled clinical studies to date. Although further study is needed, there is some in vitro evidence that tedizolid has activity against *Mycobacterium tuberculosis*.

Reduced susceptibility or resistance to tedizolid has been produced in vitro by serial passage of *S. aureus* or *E. faecium* in the presence of increasing concentrations of the drug. In vitro, spontaneous mutations conferring reduced susceptibility to tedizolid have occurred at a frequency rate of approximately 10^{-10}.

Cross-resistance between tedizolid and linezolid has been reported. Bacteria resistant to oxazolidinones (e.g., linezolid) because of mutations in chromosomal genes encoding the 23S rRNA or ribosomal proteins (L3 and L4) usually are cross-resistant to tedizolid. However, in vitro date indicate that the presence of the chloramphenicol-florfenicol resistance (*cfr*) gene in *S. aureus* that results in resistance to linezolid may not result in resistance to tedizolid in the absence of chromosomal mutations. Cross-resistance between tedizolid and non-oxazolidinone anti-infectives is unlikely.

Tedizolid phosphate is rapidly converted in vivo by phosphatases to the active moiety, tedizolid. The drug is well absorbed following oral administration (absolute bioavailability approximately 91%); systemic exposure is similar whether the drug is given orally in the fasted state or with a high-fat, high-calorie meal. Peak plasma concentrations of tedizolid are achieved approximately 3 hours after oral administration of tedizolid phosphate in the fasted state or at the end of a 1-hour IV infusion. Steady-state concentrations are achieved within approximately 3 days with oral or IV administration; accumulation is approximately 30% after 7 or more days of once-daily dosing. Tedizolid has a half-life of approximately 12 hours. The drug is distributed into the interstitial space fluid of adipose and skeletal muscle tissue at concentrations similar to plasma concentrations; the drug also has been shown to distribute into epithelial lining fluid of pulmonary tissue in concentrations higher than those found in plasma. Tedizolid is 70–90% bound to plasma proteins. Tedizolid phosphate and tedizolid do not appear to be substrates of cytochrome P-450 (CYP) enzymes. A major metabolite (tedizolid sulfate) and several minor metabolites have been identified in feces and urine. Following a single oral dose of tedizolid phosphate, tedizolid is excreted in feces (82%) and urine (18%), principally as the noncirculating sulfate conjugate; less than 3% of the tedizolid phosphate dose is eliminated in feces and urine as unchanged tedizolid. Approximately 10% of a dose is removed by hemodialysis.

Advice to Patients

Advise patients that antibacterials (including tedizolid) should only be used to treat bacterial infections and not used to treat viral infections (e.g., the common cold).

Importance of completing full course of therapy, even if feeling better after a few days.

Advise patients that skipping doses or not completing the full course of therapy may decrease effectiveness and increase the likelihood that bacteria will develop resistance and will not be treatable with tedizolid or other antibacterials in the future.

Advise patients that tedizolid may be taken orally without regard to meals and without any dietary restriction.

Importance of informing patients that if they miss a dose and it is remembered within 8 hours after the scheduled time, they should take the dose as soon as possible and then take their next scheduled dose at the usual time. If less than 8 hours remain before the next scheduled dose, the patient should skip the dose and wait until their next scheduled dose.

Advise patients that diarrhea is a common problem caused by anti-infectives and usually ends when the drug is discontinued. Importance of contacting a clinician if watery and bloody stools (with or without stomach cramps and fever) occur during or as late as 2 months or longer after the last dose.

Importance of informing clinicians of existing or contemplated concomitant therapy, including prescription and OTC drugs and dietary or herbal supplements, as well as any concomitant illnesses.

Importance of women informing clinicians if they are or plan to become pregnant or plan to breast-feed.

Importance of informing patients of other important precautionary information. (See Cautions.)

Overview® (see Users Guide). For additional information on this drug until a more detailed monograph is developed and published, the manufacturer's labeling should be consulted. It is *essential* that the manufacturer's labeling be consulted for more detailed information on usual cautions, precautions, contraindications, potential drug interactions, laboratory test interferences, and acute toxicity.

Preparations

Excipients in commercially available drug preparations may have clinically important effects in some individuals; consult specific product labeling for details.

Tedizolid Phosphate

Oral		
Tablets, film-coated	200 mg	**Sivextro®**, Cubist
Parenteral		
For injection, for IV infusion only	200 mg	**Sivextro®**, Cubist

POLYMYXINS 8:12.28.28

Colistimethate Sodium

Sodium Colistinmethanesulfonate, CMS

■ Colistimethate sodium is a prodrug of colistin. Colistin (also known as polymyxin E) is a polymyxin antibiotic structurally and pharmacologically related to polymyxin B.

Uses

■ **Gram-negative Aerobic Bacterial Infections** Colistimethate sodium is used parenterally for the treatment of acute or chronic infections caused by certain susceptible gram-negative bacteria (e.g., *Enterobacter aerogenes, Escherichia coli, Klebsiella pneumoniae, Pseudomonas aeruginosa*). Other more effective and less toxic anti-infectives (e.g., fluoroquinolones, aminoglycosides, third generation cephalosporins, extended-spectrum penicillins, carbapenems) usually are drugs of choice for most gram-negative bacterial infections. Colistimethate sodium should be used in the treatment of infections caused by susceptible gram-negative bacteria only when other more effective and less toxic anti-infectives are contraindicated or are ineffective. However, colistimethate sodium may be useful alone or in conjunction with other anti-infectives for the treatment of infections caused by multiple-drug resistant gram-negative bacteria, such as respiratory tract infections in cystic fibrosis patients caused by multiple-drug resistant *Ps. aeruginosa*. Colistimethate sodium is not indicated for infections caused by *Proteus* or *Neisseria*.

Colistin sulfate (no longer commercially available in the US) has been used orally for the treatment of gastroenteritis caused by susceptible *Shigella*; however, substantial evidence of effectiveness is lacking and other anti-infectives (e.g., fluoroquinolones, azithromycin, ampicillin, co-trimoxazole) generally are preferred if anti-infective therapy is indicated in the treatment of these infections. Colistin sulfate also has been used orally for the treatment of diarrhea caused by susceptible strains of enteropathogenic *E. coli*; however, use of anti-infectives for treatment of diarrhea caused by enteropathogenic *E. coli* is controversial and management usually involves replacement of fluids and electrolytes.

■ **Respiratory Tract Infections** ***Cystic Fibrosis Patients*** **Oral Inhalation.** Colistimethate sodium has been administered by oral inhalation via nebulization† for early treatment of *Ps. aeruginosa* respiratory tract infections in adult and pediatric cystic fibrosis patients and for suppressive therapy in cystic fibrosis patients colonized with *Ps. aeruginosa*. Safety and efficacy of such treatment have not been established, and colistimethate sodium is not labeled by the US Food and Drug Administration (FDA) for administration via nebulization. Adverse respiratory effects (e.g., bronchoconstriction) have occurred with this route, and there has been at least one fatality in a patient who self-administered a nebulizer treatment using a premixed solution of the drug. (See Cautions: Respiratory Effects.)

There is some evidence from a randomized study and observational studies that early initiation of a treatment regimen that includes colistimethate sodium administered by oral inhalation† (usually given in conjunction with oral ciprofloxacin) in addition to standard therapy for cystic fibrosis may prevent or delay chronic colonization in some adult and pediatric cystic fibrosis patients with *Ps. aeruginosa* respiratory tract infections. A review of anti-infective strategies for eradicating *Ps. aeruginosa* in patients with cystic fibrosis that analyzed results of studies involving tobramycin or colistimethate sodium administered by oral inhalation concluded that there is some evidence that such anti-infective treatment of early *Ps. aeruginosa* infection in cystic fibrosis patients results in short-term eradication, but it remains uncertain whether there is an associated clinical benefit.

Results of a randomized study of colistimethate sodium or tobramycin administered by oral inhalation in adult and pediatric cystic fibrosis patients chronically infected with *Ps. aeruginosa* indicate that either treatment reduced the bacterial load, but only nebulized tobramycin significantly improved lung function as measured by FEV_1. Results of a randomized study of colistimethate sodium administered by oral inhalation in adult and pediatric cystic fibrosis patients with chronic *Ps. aeruginosa* lung infections indicate that such therapy may be a useful supplement to IV antipseudomonal anti-infectives. A review of use of nebulized antipseudomonal anti-infectives in patients with cystic fibrosis concluded that such treatment may have a beneficial effect on lung function and may reduce exacerbations of respiratory infections, but that more research is needed to determine the duration of benefit, risk of emergence of resistant *Ps. aeruginosa*, and optimal drug and dosage regimens.

Dosage and Administration

■ **Reconstitution and Administration** Colistimethate sodium is administered by IM injection, IV injection, or continuous IV infusion. The drug also has been administered by oral inhalation via nebulization†.

Dispensing and Dosage and Administration Precautions The Institute for Safe Medication Practices (ISMP) alerted healthcare professionals about the risk of serious and potentially fatal medication errors related to dosage of colistimethate sodium.

Colistimethate sodium is a prodrug of colistin and is inactive until hydrolyzed in vivo to colistin. In the US, vials and carton packaging of colistimethate sulfate are labeled as colistimethate for injection; however, strength and dosage of the drug are expressed in terms of colistin base activity (colistin). This dosage convention *must* be considered when prescribing, preparing, and dispensing colistimethate sodium.

Healthcare professionals should be aware that, in the US, colistimethate sodium must *only* be prescribed in terms of colistin. If the drug is prescribed as colistimethate or colistimethate sodium, the prescriber should be contacted to verify the dosage in terms of colistin. At least 1 fatality related to acute renal failure and other complications occurred when colistimethate sodium was prescribed in terms of the prodrug (instead of colistin), resulting in administration of a dosage approximately 2.5 times greater than it should have been.

Healthcare professionals also should be aware that strength and dosage of colistimethate sodium preparations commercially available in some other countries may be expressed in terms of colistimethate sodium, in terms of colistin, or as international units. (See Dosage and Administration: Dosage.)

Any medication errors involving colistimethate sodium should be reported to the ISMP National Medication Error Reporting Program and the FDA MedWatch program.

Parenteral Administration Colistimethate sodium sterile powder is reconstituted by adding 2 mL of sterile water for injection to a vial labeled as containing 150 mg of colistin; the vial should be swirled gently to avoid frothing. The resultant solution contains 75 mg of colistin per mL.

Reconstituted solutions of colistimethate sodium should be used within 7 days, but final solutions for continuous IV infusion should be freshly prepared and used within 24 hours. (See Chemistry and Stability: Stability)

IM Administration. For IM injection, the appropriate dose (as reconstituted solution) should be given by deep IM injection into a large muscle mass (e.g., gluteal muscle or lateral part of the thigh).

IV Injection. For direct intermittent IV administration, one-half of the total daily dose (as reconstituted solution) should be injected directly into a vein over a 3- to 5-minute period every 12 hours.

IV Infusion. For continuous IV infusion, one-half of the total daily dose (as reconstituted solution) should be injected directly into a vein over a 3- to 5-minute period; the remaining one-half of the total daily dose (as reconstituted solution) should be added to a compatible IV solution (see Chemistry and Stability: Stability) and administered 1–2 hours later (over the next 22–23 hours) by slow IV infusion.

The specific IV solution and volume of the solution used should be based on the patient's fluid and electrolyte requirements.

Oral Inhalation For oral inhalation via nebulization†, an isotonic solution of colistimethate sodium has been prepared by diluting the appropriate dose in 2–4 mL of preservative-free 0.9% sodium chloride injection, sterile water, or a mixture of 0.9% sodium chloride injection and sterile water.

Solutions of colistimethate sodium for oral inhalation via nebulization† should be used promptly after being prepared. A fatality has been reported in a cystic fibrosis patient who self-administered a nebulizer treatment using a premixed solution of the drug. (See Cautions: Respiratory Effects.)

■ **Dosage** Dosage of colistimethate sodium commercially available in the US is expressed in terms of colistin.

Dosage of colistimethate sodium preparations commercially available in some other countries (e.g., United Kingdom, Greece) may be expressed in terms of colistimethate sodium, in terms of colistin, or as international units. *The fact that dosages reported in published clinical studies or case reports may vary depending on the country of origin and the preparation used should be considered.*

Although not the dosage convention in the US, it has been suggested that dosage of colistimethate sodium should preferably be expressed in terms of international units to avoid confusion. When expressed in terms of international units, each mg of colistin base has a potency of 30,000 international units and each mg of colistimethate sodium has a potency of 12,500 international units.

Parenteral Dosage The usual IM or IV dosage of colistimethate sodium for adults and children with normal renal function is 2.5–5 mg/kg of colistin daily given in 2–4 divided doses, depending on the severity of the infection.

The maximum IM or IV dosage of colistimethate sodium recommended by the manufacturer for patients with normal renal function is 5 mg/kg of colistin daily.

The manufacturer recommends that dosage for obese patients should be based on an estimate of ideal body weight.

Oral Inhalation Dosage For early treatment of *Pseudomonas aeruginosa* respiratory tract infections in adult and pediatric cystic fibrosis patients or for suppressive therapy in adult or pediatric cystic fibrosis patients colonized with *Ps. aeruginosa*, colistimethate sodium has been given by oral inhalation via nebulization† in a dosage of 33.33–66.66 mg of colistin 2 or 3 times daily. This corresponds to a dosage of 1–2 million international units 2 or 3 times daily.

■ **Dosage in Renal Impairment** In patients with renal impairment, dosage of colistimethate sodium should be decreased in proportion to the degree of renal impairment.

Dosage for Adults with Renal Impairment

Creatinine Clearance (mL/minute)	IM or IV Dosage (of Colistin)
80 or greater	2.5–5 mg/kg daily given in 2–4 divided doses
50–79	2.5–3.8 mg/kg daily given in 2 divided doses
30–49	2.5 mg/kg daily given as a single dose or in 2 divided doses
10–29	1.5 mg/kg given once every 36 hours

Cautions

Adverse effects reported with colistimethate sodium are similar to those reported with polymyxin B sulfate. Nephrotoxicity and neurotoxicity are the most serious adverse effects of colistimethate sodium and are most likely to occur when the drug is used in higher than recommended dosages or in patients with impaired renal function.

■ Renal Effects Nephrotoxicity, manifested as decreased urine output, increased serum concentrations of BUN and creatinine, proteinuria, hematuria, and casts in the urine, has been reported in patients receiving usual dosage of colistimethate sodium. Acute tubular necrosis has been reported with colistimethate sodium and was not necessarily preceded by progressive renal impairment.

Nephrotoxicity is generally reversible when colistimethate sodium is discontinued; however, additional increases in concentrations of serum creatinine have frequently occurred for 1–2 weeks following discontinuance of the drug. Administration of colistimethate sodium in doses that exceed the renal excretory capacity will lead to high serum concentrations of the drug which can result in further impairment of renal function. (See Cautions: Precautions and Contraindications.)

■ GI Effects GI disturbance has been reported in patients receiving colistimethate sodium.

Clostridium difficile-associated diarrhea and colitis (CDAD; also known as antibiotic-associated diarrhea and colitis or pseudomembranous colitis) has been reported with nearly all anti-infectives, including colistimethate sodium, and may range in severity from mild diarrhea to fatal colitis. CDAD should be considered in the differential diagnosis of patients who develop diarrhea during or after anti-infective therapy. Mild cases of colitis may respond to discontinuance of the drug alone, but management of moderate to severe cases should include treatment with fluid, electrolyte, protein supplementation, appropriate anti-infective therapy (e.g., oral metronidazole or vancomycin), and surgical evaluation when clinically indicated. Careful medical history is necessary since CDAD has been reported to occur as late as 2 months or longer after anti-infective therapy is discontinued.

■ Nervous System Effects Transient nervous system effects, including circumoral or peripheral paresthesia or numbness, tingling or formication of the extremities or tongue, dizziness, vertigo, giddiness, ataxia, blurred vision, and slurred speech, have been reported in patients receiving colistimethate sodium. If these adverse nervous system effects occur, they generally appear within the first 4 days of therapy and disappear when the drug is discontinued. If adverse nervous system effects occur, colistimethate sodium therapy does not necessarily have to be discontinued, but the patient should be monitored closely; some of these adverse nervous system effects may be alleviated by reducing dosage of the drug.

More severe neurotoxic effects including mental confusion, coma, psychosis, and seizures also have been reported with colistimethate sodium, especially in patients receiving high dosage or in patients with renal impairment.

Neuromuscular blockade, which may result in respiratory arrest, can occur in patients receiving colistimethate sodium, especially when the drug is used in patients with neuromuscular disease such as myasthenia gravis or in patients who are receiving neuromuscular blocking agents, general anesthetics, or other drugs with neuromuscular blocking potential. (See Drug Interactions.) Apnea and neuromuscular blockade have been reported most frequently when colistimethate sodium was used in patients with impaired renal function and dosage of the drug was not reduced in proportion to the degree of renal impairment. If apnea occurs during therapy with colistimethate sodium, respiration should be assisted and calcium chloride injections and oxygen should be administered if appropriate. Neuromuscular blockade induced by colistimethate sodium is noncompetitive and is not reversed by neostigmine.

■ Respiratory Effects Bronchoconstriction has been reported in adult and pediatric cystic fibrosis patients who received colistimethate sodium by oral inhalation via nebulization†. Bronchoconstriction has occurred almost immediately after initiation of nebulization and can last for more than 30 minutes in some patients. It has been suggested that premedication with bronchodilators may reduce the potential for development of bronchoconstriction in patients receiving the drug by nebulization. Pre- and post-treatment pulmonary function tests have been recommended to identify patients who may be predisposed to bronchoconstriction. In young children who are unable to perform pulmonary function tests, bronchodilator premedication has been recommended.

Respiratory distress that progressed over several days to acute respiratory failure, multi-organ system failure, and death has been reported in a patient who received colistimethate sodium by oral inhalation via nebulization†. This patient self-administered the nebulizer treatment using a solution of colistimethate sodium that had been prepared by a pharmacy and dispensed in premixed unit dose ready-to-use vials. The patient developed respiratory distress within hours of the nebulization treatment and died about 19 days later. It has been suggested that this fatality may have been related to the fact that a premixed solution of colistimethate sodium was used in the nebulizer. After colistimethate sodium is mixed with water and buffer, it undergoes spontaneous hydrolysis to colistin. A component of colistin (polymyxin E1) has been shown to cause pulmonary inflammatory reactions in animals and may contribute to such local toxicity in humans. (See Cautions: Precautions and Contraindications.)

■ Other Adverse Effects Generalized pruritus, urticaria, rash, and fever have been reported in patients receiving colistimethate sodium. Anaphylaxis has also been reported.

Although a causal relationship has not been definitely established, leukopenia, granulocytopenia, and hepatotoxicity have been reported rarely with colistimethate sodium.

■ Precautions and Contraindications Colistimethate sodium is contraindicated in individuals who are hypersensitive to the drug or any ingredient in its formulation.

Because transient neurologic disturbances may occur during therapy with colistimethate sodium (see Cautions: Nervous System Effects), patients should be warned that the drug may impair their ability to perform hazardous activities requiring mental alertness or physical coordination (e.g., operating machinery, driving a motor vehicle).

Renal function should be monitored in patients receiving colistimethate sodium, since adverse renal effects may occur regardless of the dosage of the drug. If diminishing urine output or increasing concentrations of BUN or serum creatinine occur, colistimethate sodium should be discontinued immediately.

Colistimethate sodium should be used with caution in patients in whom the possibility of renal impairment exists (e.g., geriatric patients). Administration of colistimethate sodium in dosages in excess of renal excretory capacity will lead to high serum concentrations of the drug which can result in further impairment of renal function and possibly acute renal insufficiency, renal shutdown, and neuromuscular blockade. If colistimethate sodium is used in patients with renal impairment, extreme caution should be exercised and dosage and frequency of administration reduced in proportion to the degree of impairment.

Adults and children who receive colistimethate sodium by oral inhalation via nebulization† may be at risk of bronchoconstriction. Premedication with bronchodilators may reduce the potential for development of bronchoconstriction in patients receiving the drug by nebulization. The FDA states that health-care providers who choose to prescribe colistimethate sodium for administration by oral inhalation via nebulization† should be familiar with the chemistry of the drug and aware of the potential for serious and life-threatening side effects from inhalation of premixed, ready-to-use liquid preparations of the drug. If colistimethate sodium is administered via a nebulizer, the solution should be used promptly after being mixed. Premixing colistimethate sodium into an aqueous solution and storing it for longer than 24 hours results in increased concentrations of colistin in the solution and increases the potential for lung toxicity if the premixed solution is administered via nebulization. Patients should be advised not to use any premixed, ready-to-use liquid preparations of colistimethate sodium for nebulization and to discard any unused vials of premixed, ready-to-use liquid preparations of the drug that they may have in their possession.

Prolonged use of colistimethate sodium may result in overgrowth of nonsusceptible organisms (e.g., *Proteus*). If suprainfection or superinfection occurs during therapy with colistimethate sodium, appropriate anti-infective therapy should be instituted.

To reduce development of drug-resistant bacteria and maintain effectiveness of colistimethate sodium and other antibacterials, the drug should be used only for the treatment or prevention of infections proven or strongly suspected to be caused by susceptible bacteria. When selecting or modifying anti-infective therapy, use results of culture and in vitro susceptibility testing. In the absence of such data, consider local epidemiology and susceptibility patterns when selecting anti-infectives for empiric therapy.

Because *Clostridium difficile*-associated diarrhea and colitis has been reported with colistimethate sodium, it should be considered in the differential diagnosis of patients who develop diarrhea during or after therapy. Patients should be advised that diarrhea is a common problem caused by anti-infectives and usually ends when the drug is discontinued; however, they should contact a clinician if watery and bloody stools (with or without stomach cramps and fever) occur during or as late as 2 months or longer after the last dose.

Patients should be advised that antibacterials (including colistimethate sodium) should only be used to treat bacterial infections and not used to treat viral infections (e.g., the common cold). Patients also should be advised about the importance of completing the full course of therapy, even if feeling better after a few days, and that skipping doses or not completing therapy may decrease effectiveness and increase the likelihood that bacteria will develop resistance and will not be treatable with colistimethate or other antibacterials in the future.

■ Pediatric Precautions Colistimethate sodium has been used in neonates, infants, children, and adolescents. The adverse effect profile in pediatric patients appears to be similar to that in adults; however, subjective symptoms of toxicity may not be reported by pediatric patients and close monitoring of these patients is recommended.

■ **Geriatric Precautions** Clinical studies of colistimethate sodium did not include sufficient numbers of patients 65 years of age and older to determine whether geriatric patients respond differently than younger patients. While other clinical experience has not revealed age-related differences in response, dosage generally should be selected carefully for geriatric patients, usually initiating therapy at the low end of the dosage range. The greater frequency of decreased hepatic, renal, and/or cardiac function and of concomitant disease and drug therapy observed in the elderly also should be considered.

Since the drug is substantially eliminated by the kidney, the risk of adverse effects may be greater in patient with impaired renal function. The greater frequency of decreased renal function observed in the elderly should be considered and dosage should be selected carefully in geriatric patients; monitoring renal function may be useful in these patients.

■ **Mutagenicity and Carcinogenicity** Long-term studies in animals have not been performed to date to evaluate the carcinogenic potential of colistimethate sodium.

■ **Pregnancy, Fertility, and Lactation** Safe use of colistimethate sodium during pregnancy has not been established. When colistimethate sodium was given to rabbits during organogenesis in an IM dosage of 4.15 or 9.3 mg/kg (0.25 or 0.55 times, respectively, the maximum daily human dosage based on mg/m^2), talipes varus occurred in 2.6 or 2.9% of fetuses, respectively. In addition, increased resorption occurred at the 9.3 mg/kg dosage. The drug was not teratogenic when the same dosages were used in rats (0.13 or 0.3 times the maximum daily human dosage, respectively, based on mg/mm^2). There are no adequate and controlled studies to date using colistimethate sodium in pregnant women, and the drug should be used during pregnancy only when the potential benefits justify the possible risks to the fetus.

There was no evidence of adverse effects on fertility or reproduction when colistimethate sodium was given to rats at dosages of 9.3 mg/kg daily (0.3 times the maximum daily dosage based on mg/m^2).

It is not known whether colistimethate sodium is distributed into milk, but colistin sulfate has been detected in milk. Therefore, colistimethate sodium should be used with caution in nursing women.

Drug Interactions

Since nephrotoxic and/or neurotoxic effects may be additive, concurrent or sequential use of colistimethate sodium and other drugs with similar toxic potentials (e.g., aminoglycosides, amphotericin B, capreomycin, methoxyflurane [no longer commercially available in the US], polymyxin B sulfate, vancomycin) should be avoided, if possible.

Neuromuscular blocking agents (e.g., tubocurarine, succinylcholine, ether, decamethonium [no longer commercially available in the US], gallamine [no longer commercially available in the US], decamethonium) and other drugs (e.g., sodium citrate) potentiate neuromuscular blockade induced by colistimethate sodium and these drugs should be used with extreme caution in patients receiving colistimethate sodium.

Acute Toxicity

Overdosage of colistimethate sodium can cause neuromuscular blockade characterized by paresthesia, lethargy, confusion, dizziness, ataxia, nystagmus, disorders of speech, and apnea. Respiratory muscle paralysis may lead to apnea, respiratory arrest, and death. Overdosage of the drug may also cause acute renal failure, manifested as decreased urine output and increases in serum concentrations of BUN and creatinine.

If overdosage of colistimethate sodium occurs, the drug should be discontinued and general supportive measures initiated. Colistimethate sodium may be removed by hemodialysis and, to a lesser extent, by peritoneal dialysis.

Mechanism of Action

Colistimethate sodium is a prodrug and is inactive until hydrolyzed to colistin; this hydrolysis occurs in vivo and in vitro in aqueous solutions of the drug.

Colistin is usually bactericidal in action. The mechanism of action of colistin is similar to that of polymyxin B. Colistin acts like a cationic detergent and binds to and damages the bacterial cytoplasmic membrane of susceptible bacteria. Damage to the bacterial cytoplasmic membrane alters the osmotic barrier of the membrane and causes leakage of essential intracellular metabolites and nucleosides.

Spectrum

Colistin (the active metabolite of colistimethate sodium) has a spectrum of activity that is similar to that of polymyxin B. Colistin is active in vitro against many gram-negative bacteria; however, the drug is inactive against gram-positive bacteria, fungi, and viruses.

■ **Gram-negative Bacteria** Colistin is active in vitro against many strains of *Acinetobacter, Citrobacter, Escherichia coli, Enterobacter, Haemophilus influenzae, Klebsiella pneumoniae, Pseudomonas aeruginosa, Salmonella, Shigella,* and some strains of *Bordetella* and *Vibrio.* Most strains of *Proteus, Providencia, Serratia, Neisseria gonorrhoeae, N. meningitidis,* and *Bacteroides fragilis* are resistant to colistin.

In vitro, colistin concentrations of 0.01–4 mcg/mL inhibit most susceptible strains of *E. coli, E. aerogenes, H. influenzae, K. pneumoniae, Salmonella,* and *Shigella* and concentrations of 0.8–8 mcg/mL inhibit most susceptible strains of *Ps. aeruginosa.*

Resistance

Resistance to colistin (the active metabolite of colistimethate sodium) has been induced in vitro in strains originally susceptible to the drug; in some cases, resistance may be reversible when the antibiotic is withdrawn. Resistance to colistin has developed rarely during therapy with colistimethate sodium or colistin sulfate.

Pseudomonas aeruginosa resistant to colistin have been reported rarely, including in some patients who received long-term treatment with colistimethate sodium administered by oral inhalation via nebulization†. *Acinetobacter baumannii Enterobacter cloacae,* and *Klebsiella pneumoniae* resistant to colistin also have been reported rarely.

Complete cross-resistance occurs between colistin and polymyxin B; however, cross-resistance with other anti-infectives has not been reported to date.

Pharmacokinetics

■ **Absorption** Colistimethate sodium, a prodrug of colistin, is not absorbed from the GI tract and must be given parenterally. Colistimethate sodium does not appear to be absorbed from mucous membranes or intact or denuded skin.

Following IM administration of colistimethate sodium in a dosage of 150 mg of colistin, peak serum concentrations of antimicrobial activity are attained within 2 hours and average 5–7.5 mcg/mL; serum concentrations of antimicrobial activity may be detectable 12 hours after the dose.

Following IV administration of colistimethate sodium in a dosage of 5–7 mg/kg of colistin daily given in 3 equally divided doses (maximum 70–100 mg every 8 hours) in cystic fibrosis patients 14–53 years of age, mean peak serum concentrations were 21.4 mcg/mL after the first dose and 23 mcg/mL at steady state. Mean 8-hour trough concentrations were 2.8 mcg/mL after the first dose and 4.5 mcg/mL at steady state. Peak serum concentrations of antimicrobial activity are higher, but decline more rapidly than those achieved with IM administration of the drug.

Following oral inhalation via nebulization† of colistimethate sodium in a dosage of 66.66 mg of colistin (2 million international units) in cystic fibrosis patients 12–48 years of age, mean peak serum concentrations were 0.17 mcg/mL and were attained in 1.5 hours.

■ **Distribution** Following IM or IV administration of colistimethate sodium, the drug is widely distributed into body tissues, but only negligible concentrations of antimicrobial activity are attained in synovial, pleural, or pericardial fluids. Animal studies indicate that colistin, like polymyxin B sulfate, reversibly binds to and persists in body tissues such as the liver, kidneys, lung, heart, and muscle.

In cystic fibrosis patients 14–53 years of age receiving IV colistimethate sodium in a dosage of 5–7 mg/kg of colistin daily given in 3 equally divided doses, the volume of distribution at steady state was 0.09 L/kg.

Following oral inhalation via nebulization† of colistimethate sodium in a dosage of 66.66 mg of colistin (2 million international units) in cystic fibrosis patients 12–48 years of age, sputum concentrations peaked 1 hour after inhalation and remained greater than 4 mcg/mL for up to 12 hours in most patients.

Colistin is reportedly more than 50% bound to serum proteins.

Only minimal concentrations of antimicrobial activity are attained in CSF following IM or IV administration of colistimethate sodium in patients with normal or inflamed meninges.

Colistin crosses the placenta and is distributed into milk.

■ **Elimination** Colistimethate sodium is hydrolyzed in vivo to colistin and possibly other metabolites with fewer substituted amino groups. The rate and extent of hydrolysis as well as the specific metabolites and their antibacterial activities have not been determined to date.

The plasma half-life of antimicrobial activity following IM or IV administration of colistimethate sodium is 1.5–8 hours in adults with normal renal function. Serum concentrations of antimicrobial activity following administration of colistimethate sodium appear to decline more rapidly in children than in adults.

Serum concentrations are higher and the half-life is prolonged in patients with impaired renal function. In patients with creatinine clearances less than 20 mL/minute, the half-life of colistin ranges from 10–20 hours. Following administration of colistimethate sodium in a few anuric patients, half-life of antimicrobial activity reportedly ranged up to 2–3 days.

The mean plasma half-life in cystic fibrosis patients 14–53 years of age who received IV colistimethate sodium in a dosage of 5–7 mg/kg of colistin daily given in 3 equally divided doses was 3.4 hours after the first dose and 3.5 hours at steady state.

The plasma half-life following oral inhalation via nebulization† of colistimethate sodium in a dosage of 66.66 mg of colistin (2 million international units) in cystic fibrosis patients 12–48 years of age was 4.1–4.5 hours.

Colistimethate sodium and metabolites of the drug are excreted mainly by the kidneys via glomerular filtration. Antimicrobial activity in urine is generally higher than antimicrobial activity in serum. Following IM or IV administration of a single 150-mg dose of colistin as colistimethate sodium in patients with normal renal function, antimicrobial concentrations in urine are 200–270 mcg/mL at 2 hours after the dose and 15–25 mcg/mL at 8 hours after the dose.

Colistimethate sodium may be removed by hemodialysis and, to a lesser extent, by peritoneal dialysis.

Chemistry and Stability

■ **Chemistry** Colistimethate sodium is the sulfamethyl derivative (methane sulfonate) of colistin. Colistimethate sodium is a prodrug that is inactive until hydrolyzed in vivo and in vitro to colistin. Colistin (also known as polymyxin E) is a polymyxin antibiotic obtained from cultures of *Bacillus polymyxa* var. *colistinus* and is structurally and pharmacologically related to polymyxin B.

Colistin may be commercially available as colistin sulfate for oral administration in other countries; however, oral colistin sulfate is no longer commercially available in the US.

Colistimethate sodium occurs as a white to slightly yellow, fine powder and is freely soluble in water. Following reconstitution with sterile water for injection, colistimethate sodium solutions have a pH of 7–8.

■ **Stability** Colistimethate sodium powder for injection should be stored at 20–25°C.

Following reconstitution with sterile water for injection, colistimethate sodium solutions containing 75 mg of colistin per mL should be stored at 2–8°C or 20–25°C and used within 7 days. However, reconstituted solutions that have been further diluted with a compatible IV solution should be used within 24 hours.

Solutions of colistimethate sodium prepared extemporaneously for oral inhalation via nebulization† should be used promptly after being mixed. (See Cautions: Respiratory Effects.)

Colistimethate sodium is physically and chemically compatible with the following IV solutions: 0.9% sodium chloride, 5% dextrose, 5% dextrose and 0.225%, 0.45%, or 0.9% sodium chloride, lactated Ringer's, or 10% invert sugar.

Colistimethate sodium is potentially physically and/or chemically incompatible with some drugs, but the compatibility depends on several factors (e.g., concentrations of the drugs, specific diluents used, resulting pH, temperature). Specialized references should be consulted for specific compatibility information.

Preparations

Excipients in commercially available drug preparations may have clinically important effects in some individuals; consult specific product labeling for details.

Colistimethate Sodium

Parenteral		
For injection	150 mg (of colistin)*	**Colistimethate Sodium for Injection**
		Coly-Mycin® M Parenteral, Par

*available from one or more manufacturer, distributor, and/or repackager by generic (nonproprietary) name

†Use is not currently included in the labeling approved by the US Food and Drug Administration

Polymyxin B Sulfate

■ Polymyxin B is a polymyxin antibiotic that is structurally and pharmacologically related to colistin.

Uses

Polymyxin B sulfate is used for the treatment of serious infections, including infections of the urinary tract, meninges, or bloodstream, caused by susceptible gram-negative bacteria (e.g., *Pseudomonas aeruginosa, Escherichia coli, Enterobacter aerogenes, Klebsiella pneumoniae, Haemophilus influenzae*). The drug also is used in the treatment of respiratory tract infections† caused by susceptible gram-negative bacteria (e.g., *Ps. aeruginosa, Acinetobacter baumannii*†). Although other less toxic anti-infectives (e.g., fluoroquinolones, aminoglycosides, third generation cephalosporins, extended-spectrum penicillins, carbapenems) usually are the drugs of choice for most gram-negative bacterial infections, polymyxin B may be indicated when these drugs are ineffective or contraindicated, especially for serious infections caused by multidrug-resistant *Ps. aeruginosa* or *A. baumannii*.

■ **Meningitis and Other CNS Infections** Polymyxin B sulfate is used intrathecally or intraventricularly† for the treatment of meningeal infections caused by susceptible gram-negative bacteria, including *Ps. aeruginosa, E. coli*†, *K. pneumoniae*†, and *H. influenzae*. In some cases, intrathecal polymyxin B has been effective when used alone for the treatment of these infections; however, intrathecal or intraventricular polymyxin B usually has been used in conjunction with a parenteral anti-infective (e.g., IV or IM polymyxin B, IV meropenem, IV penicillin, IV cephalosporin). Because polymyxin B penetrates poorly into CSF following IM or IV administration, parenteral therapy with the drug should not be used alone for the treatment of meningitis or other CNS infections.

Treatment of meningitis caused by *Ps. aeruginosa* should be guided by results of in vitro susceptibility tests. The usual regimen of choice for these infections is parenteral therapy with an antipseudomonal cephalosporin (ceftazidime, cefepime) or carbapenem (meropenem) with or without an aminoglycoside (amikacin, gentamicin, tobramycin). Intrathecal or intraventricular polymyxin B may be indicated for infections caused by multidrug-resistant *Ps. aeruginosa* that are resistant to or do not respond to the usual regimens of choice.

Polymyxin B has been used intraventricularly† in conjunction with IV meropenem for the treatment of ventriculitis caused by ceftazidime-resistant *K. pneumoniae*†.

Intrathecal polymyxin B is considered an alternative for the treatment of meningitis caused by susceptible *H. influenzae*. The usual drug of choice for the treatment of these infections is a parenteral third-generation cephalosporin (e.g., cefotaxime, ceftriaxone), although parenteral ampicillin can be used if the infection is caused by β-lactamase-negative strains.

■ **Respiratory Tract Infections** IV polymyxin B sulfate is used as an alternative for the treatment of respiratory tract infections†, including nosocomial pneumonia, ventilator-associated pneumonia, or healthcare-associated pneumonia, caused by multidrug-resistant gram-negative bacteria (e.g., *Ps. aeruginosa, A. baumannii*). Polymyxin B is not usually considered a drug of choice for *initial* empiric therapy of respiratory tract infections, and generally is used in these infections only when other less toxic anti-infectives are ineffective or contraindicated.

In some patients, IV polymyxin B has been used alone or in conjunction with IV aztreonam for the treatment of nosocomial pneumonia caused by multidrug-resistant *Ps. aeruginosa* that produce metallo-β-lactamases. Nosocomial infections caused by metallo-β-lactamase-producing *Ps. aeruginosa* have a high mortality rate and fatalities may occur despite appropriate anti-infective therapy. Optimal regimens for treatment of these infections have not been identified to date.

Polymyxin B has been administered by oral inhalation via nebulization† for the treatment of respiratory tract infections† caused by susceptible gram-negative bacteria (e.g., *Ps. aeruginosa, A. baumannii*). In patients with pneumonia, polymyxin B administered by oral inhalation generally has been used in conjunction with a parenteral anti-infective (e.g., IV polymyxin B); however, the drug has been effective when given by oral inhalation alone in some patients with infections caused by susceptible gram-negative bacteria. Although safety and efficacy have not been established and additional study is needed, the American Thoracic Society (ATS) and the Infectious Diseases Society of America (IDSA) and other clinicians suggest that adjunctive use of aerosolized polymyxin B can be considered for the treatment of serious respiratory tract infections (e.g., ventilator-associated pneumonia) caused by multidrug-resistant gram-negative bacteria that have not responded to treatment with parenteral anti-infectives alone.

Polymyxin B also has been administered by oral inhalation for prophylaxis in an attempt to prevent nosocomial pneumonia† in seriously ill patients; however, such prophylaxis appears to promote development of polymyxin B-resistant bacteria.

■ **Septicemia** IV or IM polymyxin B sulfate is used for the treatment of septicemia or bacteremia caused by susceptible *Ps. aeruginosa, E. aerogenes*, or *K. pneumoniae*. The drug also has been used IV for the treatment of bloodstream infections caused by multidrug-resistant *A. baumannii*†. Polymyxin B generally is used in the treatment of septicemia or bacteremia only when other less toxic anti-infectives are ineffective or contraindicated.

Polymyxin B may be a drug of choice for the treatment of septicemia or bacteremia caused by *Ps. aeruginosa* and has been used alone or in conjunction with other anti-infectives (e.g., aztreonam) for infections caused by multidrug-resistant *Ps. aeruginosa*, including those that produce metallo-β-lactamases. Nosocomial blood stream infections caused by metallo-β-lactamase-producing *Ps. aeruginosa* have a high presence of mortality rate, and fatalities may occur despite appropriate anti-infective therapy. Optimal regimens for treatment of these infections have not been identified to date.

■ **Urinary Tract Infections** IV or IM polymyxin B sulfate is used for the treatment of serious urinary tract infections caused by susceptible *Ps. aeruginosa* or *E. coli*. Polymyxin B generally is used in these infections only when other less toxic anti-infectives are ineffective or contraindicated.

■ **Bacteriuria and Bacteremia Associated with Indwelling Catheters** The fixed-combination solution for irrigation containing polymyxin B sulfate and neomycin sulfate is used in abacteriuric patients for short-term (up to 10 days) irrigation or rinse of the urinary bladder to help prevent bacteriuria and gram-negative rod septicemia associated with the use of indwelling catheters.

Bacteria can gain entrance to the bladder by way of, through, and around indwelling catheters and clinically significant bacteriuria may be induced by bacterial multiplication in bladder urine, the mucoid film that may be present between the catheter and urethra, and in other sites. Urinary tract infection may result from the repeated presence of large numbers of pathogenic bacteria in the urine, and the use of closed systems with indwelling catheters has been shown to reduce the risk of infection. The manufacturers state that use of a 3-way closed catheter system and bladder rinse with the fixed-combination solution for irrigation containing polymyxin B sulfate and neomycin sulfate may help prevent development of infection in patients with indwelling catheters. However, some clinicians state that irrigation or rinse of the urinary bladder with anti-infective solutions is unlikely to be of benefit while the catheter is in place and such a strategy is not recommended.

In a randomized, double-blind study in adults 19–82 years of age with spinal cord injury and neurogenic bladder dysfunction who had indwelling urinary catheters and existing bacteriuria (at least 100,000 colony-forming units per mL [cfu/mL]), bladder irrigation (30 mL twice daily for 8 weeks) with neomycin sulfate and polymyxin B sulfate solution for irrigation, 0.25% acetic acid, or normal saline did not reduce the degree of bacteriuria or inflammation. Culture data obtained prior to, during, and after the 8-week irrigation regimen indicated no substantial change in colony count (counts remained at least 100,000 cfu/mL in almost all individuals). Although there was an increase in the number of patients harboring *Enterococcus*, the variety of other bacteria present in the urine generally remained the same. In addition, there was no evidence of an increased incidence of resistant bacteria, including multidrug-resistant strains.

For information on use of topical fixed-combination preparations containing polymyxin B sulfate and other anti-infectives for the prevention or treatment of superficial skin infections, see Bacitracin 84:04.04 and see Neomycin Sulfate 84:04.04.

For information on use of topical or subconjunctival polymyxin B sulfate for the treatment of ophthalmic infections or use of topical fixed-combination preparations containing polymyxin B sulfate and other anti-infectives for the treatment of ophthalmic or otic infections, see Polymyxin B Sulfate 52:04.04.

Dosage and Administration

■ Reconstitution and Administration

Polymyxin B sulfate usually is administered IV. Although polymyxin B sulfate may also be given by IM injection, IM administration of the drug is not routinely recommended because severe pain occurs at the injection site, especially in infants and children.

For the treatment of meningitis, polymyxin B sulfate is administered intrathecally or intraventricularly†. Polymyxin B should *not* be given IV or IM alone for the treatment of meningitis or other CNS infections since distribution of the drug into CNS is expected to be low following these routes.

Although safety and efficacy have not been established, polymyxin B sulfate has been administered by oral inhalation via nebulization† for the adjunctive treatment of respiratory tract infections†. (See Uses: Respiratory Tract Infections.)

The fixed-combination solution for irrigation containing polymyxin B sulfate and neomycin sulfate is administered by continuous irrigation of the urinary bladder.

IV Administration For IV administration, polymyxin B sulfate powder for injection is reconstituted by dissolving 500,000 units of the drug in 300–500 mL of 5% dextrose injection to provide solutions containing approximately 1000–1667 units/mL.

IV infusions of polymyxin B usually are given over a period of 60–90 minutes. An infusion period less than 30 minutes should *not* be used. Because of the risk of neuromuscular blockade, rapid IV injections should be avoided.

IM Administration For IM administration, polymyxin B sulfate powder for injection is reconstituted by adding 2 mL of sterile water for injection, 0.9% sodium chloride injection, or 1% procaine hydrochloride injection to a vial labeled as containing 500,000 units of polymyxin B to provide a solution containing approximately 250,000 units/mL.

IM injections should be given deeply into the upper outer quadrant of the gluteal muscle and injection sites should be alternated. The fact that IM injections may cause severe injection site pain should be considered.

Intrathecal Administration For intrathecal administration, polymyxin B sulfate powder for injection is reconstituted by adding 10 mL of 0.9% sodium chloride injection to a vial labeled as containing 500,000 units of the drug to provide a solution containing approximately 50,000 units/mL. Procaine hydrochloride solutions should *not* be used to prepare intrathecal injections of polymyxin B.

Oral Inhalation For oral inhalation via nebulization†, 0.5% solutions of polymyxin B sulfate have been prepared using 0.9% sodium chloride. Polymyxin B concentrations higher than 10 mg/mL should not be used for administration by oral inhalation since the drug may cause bronchial irritation.

Urinary Bladder Irrigation For continuous irrigation of the urinary bladder, the commercially available fixed-combination solution for irrigation containing 200,000 units of polymyxin B and 40 mg of neomycin should be diluted by adding the contents of the 1-mL ampul containing the irrigation solution to 1 L of 0.9% sodium chloride solution.

The diluted solution for irrigation should be administered via a 3-way catheter at a rate of 1 L every 24 hours (approximately 40 mL/hour). If the patient's urine output exceeds 2 L/day, the inflow rate should be adjusted to deliver 2 L every 24 hours. If not used immediately, the diluted solution should be stored at 4°C and used within 48 hours.

It is important that the bladder irrigation be given continuously for up to 10 days; the inflow or rinse solution should not be interrupted for more than a few minutes.

■ Dosage

Dosage of polymyxin B sulfate usually is expressed in terms of polymyxin B activity (units of polymyxin B). Dosage of the drug also may be expressed as mg of polymyxin B base. Each mg of polymyxin B is equivalent to 10,000 units of polymyxin B.

Adult Dosage **Meningitis and Other CNS Infections.** For the treatment of meningitis caused by susceptible gram-negative bacteria, the manufacturers recommend that adults receive an intrathecal dosage of polymyxin B of 50,000 units once daily for 3 or 4 days, followed by 50,000 units once every other day given for at least 2 weeks after CSF cultures are negative and CSF glucose content is normal.

For the treatment of ventriculitis† in an adult caused by ceftazidime-resistant *Klebsiella pneumoniae*, polymyxin B has been given intraventricularly† in a dosage of 50,000 units once daily for 7 days in conjunction with IV meropenem continued for 21 days after the first negative CSF culture.

Although safety and efficacy have not been established, a variety of other dosage regimens of intrathecal or intraventricular† polymyxin B (with or without concomitant parenteral therapy with IV or IM polymyxin B or other anti-infectives) have been used for the treatment of meningitis caused by susceptible gram-negative bacteria.

Respiratory Tract Infections. Although safety and efficacy of polymyxin B administered by oral inhalation via nebulization† have not been established, adults have received the drug by oral inhalation in a dosage of 2.5 mg/kg daily in divided doses every 6 hours for adjunctive treatment of respiratory tract infections caused by susceptible *Pseudomonas aeruginosa*.' If a 0.5% solution of the drug is prepared using 0.9% sodium chloride and this dosage regimen is used, the average 70-kg patient would receive 6 mL of solution per dose.

In a study in adults who had respiratory tract infections caused by multi-drug-resistant gram-negative bacilli that had not responded to parenteral anti-infectives alone, polymyxin B was given by oral inhalation in a dosage of 500,000 units twice daily given approximately 20 minutes after an oral inhalation dose of a β_2-adrenergic agonist. Patients with pneumonia received polymyxin B administered by oral inhalation in conjunction with IV polymyxin B therapy; those with tracheobronchitis caused by *Ps. adrenergic* received the drug by oral inhalation alone. Treatment was continued for an average of 14 days (range: 4–25 days).

The total daily dosage administered by oral inhalation should not exceed that recommended for parenteral administration.

Septicemia or Urinary Tract Infections. The usual IV dosage of polymyxin B for the treatment of septicemia or urinary tract infections caused by susceptible gram-negative bacteria in adults with normal renal function is 15,000–25,000 units/kg daily (1.5–2.5 mg/kg daily). Daily dosage may be given in 2 divided doses every 12 hours. The total daily IV dosage in these patients should not exceed 25,000 units/kg.

The usual IM dosage of polymyxin B for the treatment of septicemia or urinary tract infections caused by susceptible gram-negative bacteria in adults with normal renal function is 25,000–30,000 units/kg daily (2.5–3 mg/kg daily); the daily dosage may be divided and given at 4- to 6-hour intervals. The total daily IM dosage in these patients should not exceed 30,000 units/kg.

Bacteriuria and Bacteremia Associated with Indwelling Catheters. For continuous irrigation of the urinary bladder, the diluted solution of neomycin sulfate and polymyxin B sulfate irrigation solution should be administered via a 3-way catheter at a rate of 1 L every 24 hours (approximately 40 mL/hour). The solution should be administered at a rate of 2 L every 24 hours if the patient's urine output exceeds 2 L/day.

The duration of irrigation therapy should not exceed 10 days.

Pediatric Dosage **Meningitis and Other CNS Infections.** For the treatment of meningitis caused by susceptible gram-negative bacteria in children younger than 2 years of age, the manufacturers recommend an initial intrathecal dosage of polymyxin B of 20,000 units once daily for 3 or 4 days or 25,000 units once every other day. With either regimen, treatment should be continued with 25,000 units once every other day given for at least 2 weeks after CSF cultures are negative and CSF glucose content is normal.

For the treatment of meningitis caused by susceptible gram-negative bacteria in children older than 2 years of age, the manufacturers recommend an intrathecal dosage of polymyxin B of 50,000 units once daily for 3 or 4 days, followed by 50,000 units once every other day given for at least 2 weeks after CSF cultures are negative and CSF glucose content is normal.

Although safety and efficacy have not been established, a variety of other dosage regimens of intrathecal or intraventricular† polymyxin B (with or without concomitant parenteral therapy with IV or IM polymyxin B or other anti-infectives) have been used for the treatment of meningitis caused by susceptible gram-negative bacteria.

Septicemia or Urinary Tract Infections. The usual IV dosage of polymyxin B for the treatment of septicemia or urinary tract infections caused by susceptible gram-negative bacteria in children with normal renal function is 15,000–25,000 units/kg daily (1.5–2.5 mg/kg daily). Daily dosage may be administered in 2 divided doses every 12 hours. The manufacturers state that the total daily IV dosage in children should not exceed 25,000 units/kg, but that infants with normal renal function may receive an IV dosage of up to 40,000 units/kg daily (4 mg/kg daily) without adverse effects.

Clinicians should consider that IM administration of polymyxin B is not routinely recommended in children and infants because severe pain occurs at the injection site. If the drug is given IM for the treatment of septicemia or urinary tract infections caused by susceptible gram-negative bacteria in children with normal renal function, the usual IM dosage is 25,000–30,000 units/kg daily (2.5–3 mg/kg daily); daily dosage may be divided and given at 4- to 6-hour intervals. The manufacturers state that the total daily IM dosage in children should not exceed 30,000 units/kg, but that infants with normal renal function may receive an IM dosage of up to 40,000 units/kg daily (4 mg/kg daily) without adverse effects. A dosage as high as 45,000 units/kg daily (4.5 mg/kg daily) has been used in limited clinical studies in premature and full-term neonates for the treatment of sepsis caused by *Ps. aeruginosa*.

■ **Dosage in Renal Impairment** Dosage of polymyxin B should be decreased in patients with renal impairment. Serum polymyxin B concentrations should be monitored and IV or IM dosage adjusted to maintain desired serum concentrations of the drug.

Various dosage regimens have been recommended for use of polymyxin B in patients with renal impairment; however, these regimens are *not* well established and are *not* based on pharmacokinetic data from patients with renal impairment.

It has been recommended that patients with creatinine clearances of 30–80 mL/minute receive an IV loading dose of polymyxin B of 2.5 mg/kg on the first day of treatment followed by 1–1.5 mg/kg daily and that those with creatinine clearances less than 25–30 mL/minute receive these doses once every 2–3 days. For anuric patients, some clinicians have recommended an IV loading dose of 2.5 mg/kg followed by 1–1.5 mg/kg given once every 5–7 days.

Alternatively, it has been suggested that patients with creatinine clearances greater than 20 mL/minute receive 75–100% of the usual daily dose in 2 divided doses every 12 hours, those with creatinine clearances of 5–20 mL/minute receive 50% of the usual daily dose in 2 divided doses every 12 hours, and those with creatinine clearances less than 5 mL/minute receive 30% of the usual daily dose every 12–18 hours. Some clinicians have used 75% of the usual daily dose in those with creatinine clearances 20–50 mL/minute and 33% of the usual daily dose in those with creatinine clearances less than 20 mL/minute.

Cautions

Adverse effects reported with polymyxin B sulfate are similar to those reported with colistimethate sodium and colistin sulfate (not commercially available in the US). Nephrotoxicity and neurotoxicity are the most serious adverse effects of polymyxin B and are most likely to occur when the drug is used in higher than recommended dosages or in patients with renal impairment.

■ **Nephrotoxicity** Polymyxin B can cause nephrotoxicity. Polymyxin B-associated nephrotoxicity is considered to be dose-dependent and has been reported in 6–25% of patients receiving usual dosages of the drug. Nephrotoxicity generally is reversible after the drug is discontinued.

Nephrotoxicity usually is manifested by albuminuria or proteinuria, cylindruria, azotemia, increasing blood concentrations of the drug (not related to an increase in dosage), and an increase in serum creatinine concentration and decrease in creatinine clearance. Acute tubular necrosis, oliguria, hematuria, leukocyturia, and excessive excretion of electrolytes may occur.

Renal function should be assessed prior to initiation of polymyxin B therapy and monitored frequently during therapy. If signs of renal impairment develop, the drug should be discontinued. (See Cautions: Precautions and Contraindications.)

■ **Neurotoxicity** Polymyxin B can cause neurotoxicity. Neurotoxicity is considered to be dose-dependent and may manifest as facial flushing, dizziness that may progress to ataxia, altered mental status or mental confusion, irritability, nystagmus, muscle weakness, drowsiness, giddiness, and peripheral paresthesia (circumoral and stocking glove). Numbness, blurring of vision or vision disturbances, slurred speech, coma, or seizures also can occur. These adverse effects generally subside after the drug is discontinued.

Respiratory paralysis resulting in respiratory failure or apnea may occur as a result of neuromuscular blockade, especially in patients with neuromuscular disease such as myasthenia gravis or in patients who are receiving neuromuscular blocking agents or general anesthetics. (See Drug Interactions.) Polymyxin B-induced neuromuscular blockade is not easily reversed and is resistant to neostigmine and edrophonium; calcium chloride has been used successfully in some cases. Neuromuscular blockade usually improves within 24 hours after polymyxin B is discontinued.

Intrathecal administration of polymyxin B sulfate may cause meningeal irritation, such as headache, fever, stiff neck, and increased leukocytes and protein in the CSF. In addition, nerve root irritation may occur causing neuritic pain and urine retention. High doses given intrathecally or intraventricularly† may lead to seizures and signs of meningismus.

■ **Other Adverse Effects** Fever, rash, pruritus, urticaria, skin exanthemata, eosinophilia, and anaphylactoid reactions with dyspnea and tachycardia have been reported rarely during parenteral polymyxin B therapy.

Cough, bronchospasm, and acute airway obstruction have been reported when polymyxin B was administered by oral inhalation via nebulization†. Bronchospasm may have been the result of an allergic reaction or bronchial irritation.

Severe pain may occur at IM injection sites, especially in infants and children. Thrombophlebitis has been reported at IV injection sites.

■ **Precautions and Contraindications** Polymyxin B sulfate is contraindicated in individuals with a history of hypersensitivity to polymyxins.

Polymyxin B can cause potentially serious nephrotoxicity and/or neurotoxicity. The drug should be given IV, IM, and/or intrathecally only to hospitalized patients who are under constant supervision by a clinician.

Baseline renal function should be determined prior to initiation of polymyxin B therapy and renal function should be monitored frequently during therapy using blood tests and urinalysis. The manufacturers also recommend that serum concentrations of the drug be monitored frequently during therapy. Dosage of polymyxin B should be reduced in patients with impaired renal function or renal damage and nitrogen retention. (See Dosage and Administration: Dosage in Renal Impairment.) If urine output diminishes or BUN concentration increases during polymyxin B therapy, the drug should be discontinued.

Polymyxin B-associated neurotoxicity may be manifested by irritability, weakness, drowsiness, ataxia, perioral paresthesia, numbness of the extremities, and blurred vision. These symptoms usually are associated with high serum polymyxin B concentrations found in patients with impaired renal function and/or nephrotoxicity. Neurotoxicity can result in respiratory paralysis from neuromuscular blockade, especially if polymyxin B is given soon after anesthesia and/or muscle relaxants. (See Drug Interactions.) If signs of respiratory paralysis occur, respiration should be assisted as required and the drug discontinued.

Concurrent or sequential use of other nephrotoxic and/or neurotoxic drugs should be avoided. (See Drug Interactions.)

To reduce development of drug-resistant bacteria and maintain effectiveness of polymyxin B and other antibacterials, the drug should be used only for the treatment or prevention of infections proven or strongly suspected to be caused by susceptible bacteria. When selecting or modifying anti-infective therapy, results of culture and in vitro susceptibility testing should be used. In the absence of such data, local epidemiology and susceptibility patterns should be considered when selecting anti-infectives for empiric therapy.

Patients should be advised that antibacterials (including polymyxin B) should only be used to treat bacterial infections and not used to treat viral infections (e.g., the common cold). Patients also should be advised about the importance of completing the full course of therapy, even if feeling better after a few days, and that skipping doses or not completing therapy may decrease effectiveness and increase the likelihood that bacteria will develop resistance and will not be treatable with polymyxin B or other antibacterials in the future.

As with other anti-infectives, use of polymyxin B may result in overgrowth of nonsusceptible organisms, including fungi. Appropriate therapy should be instituted if superinfection occurs.

Precautions Related to Fixed-combination Solution for Bladder Irrigation When the fixed-combination solution for bladder irrigation containing polymyxin B sulfate and neomycin sulfate solution is used, the precautions and contraindications related to both polymyxin B and neomycin should be considered.

The fixed-combination solution for irrigation is contraindicated in individuals hypersensitive to polymyxins, neomycin, or any ingredient in the solution. Because cross-sensitivity can occur among aminoglycosides, a history of hypersensitivity or serious toxic reaction to an aminoglycoside may also contraindicate use of any other aminoglycoside.

The fixed-combination solution for irrigation should be used *only* for irrigation of the bladder and should *not* be used for irrigation of other areas.

The fixed-combination solution for irrigation should not be used for prophylactic bladder care if there is a possibility of systemic absorption. The likelihood of toxicity following topical irrigation of the intact urinary bladder with the fixed-combination solution is low since appreciable amounts of polymyxin B or neomycin do not enter systemic circulation if the duration of irrigation does not exceed 10 days. However, absorption of neomycin from the denuded bladder surface has been reported. Systemic absorption after topical application of neomycin to open wounds, burns, and granulating surfaces is clinically significant, and serum concentrations comparable to and often higher than those attained following oral and parenteral therapy have been reported.

The fixed-combination solution for irrigation is intended for continuous prophylactic irrigation (maximum of 10 days) of the lumen of the intact urinary bladder of patients with indwelling catheters who are under constant supervision by a clinician. Because of the risk of toxicity due to systemic absorption following diffusion into absorptive tissues and spaces, irrigation should be avoided in patients with defects in bladder mucosa or bladder wall, such as vesical rupture, or in association with operative procedures on the bladder wall.

If absorption occurs, the fact that both polymyxin B and neomycin are nephrotoxic and neurotoxic and that the effects of these drugs may be additive should be considered.

Irrigation of the bladder with the fixed-combination solution containing polymyxin B and neomycin may result in overgrowth of nonsusceptible organisms, including fungi, and appropriate measures should be taken if this occurs.

Urine specimens for urinalysis, culture, and susceptibility testing should be collected during prophylactic bladder care. Positive cultures suggest the presence of organisms resistant to polymyxin B and neomycin.

■ **Pediatric Precautions** IV polymyxin B sulfate is used in infants and children. IM polymyxin B sulfate is not routinely recommended in infants and children because severe pain occurs at the injection site, especially in this age group.

Safety and efficacy of the fixed-combination solution for irrigation containing polymyxin B sulfate and neomycin sulfate have not been established in children.

■ **Pregnancy** The safety of polymyxin B sulfate in pregnant women has not been established.

Some clinicians state that polymyxin B should not be used during pregnancy, except in rare situations when other appropriate anti-infectives cannot be used.

If use of the fixed-combination solution for irrigation containing polymyxin B sulfate and neomycin sulfate is being considered for a pregnant woman, the woman should be informed of the potential hazard to the fetus. Aminoglycosides cross the placenta and there have been reports of complete, irreversible, bilateral congenital deafness in children whose mothers received an aminoglycoside (i.e., streptomycin) during pregnancy.

Drug Interactions

■ **Nephrotoxic and Neurotoxic Drugs** Since nephrotoxic and neurotoxic effects may be additive, concurrent or sequential use of polymyxin B sulfate and other nephrotoxic and/or neurotoxic drugs, particularly aminoglycosides (amikacin, gentamicin, kanamycin, neomycin, paromomycin, streptomycin, tobramycin), bacitracin, colistimethate/colistin, and viomycin (not commercially available in the US) should be avoided.

■ **Anti-infectives** ***Carbapenems*** In vitro, the antibacterial effects of polymyxin B and imipenem have been synergistic against some strains of *Pseudomonas aeruginosa*, but were indifferent against other strains. In one study, the combination of polymyxin B and meropenem was indifferent against *Ps. aeruginosa.*

In vitro studies evaluating the antibacterial effects of combinations of polymyxin B and imipenem or meropenem against *Acinetobacter baumannii* have provided conflicting results. In some in vitro studies, these combinations had synergistic, partially synergistic, or additive antibacterial effects against *A. baumannii*; however, there was no evidence of synergism in other in vitro studies.

The clinical importance of in vitro studies evaluating combinations of polymyxin B and carbapenems against gram-negative bacteria is unclear.

Rifampin In an in vitro study, the antibacterial effects of polymyxin B and rifampin were synergistic against only 1 out of 10 strains of multidrug-resistant *Ps. aeruginosa*; however, a 3-drug combination of polymyxin B, rifampin, and imipenem was bactericidal against all strains.

In some in vitro studies, the combination of polymyxin B and rifampin (with or without imipenem) was synergistic or additive against *A. baumannii.*

The combination of polymyxin B and rifampin has been synergistic in vitro against *Klebsiella pneumoniae.*

The clinical importance of in vitro studies evaluating combinations of polymyxin B and rifampin against gram-negative bacteria is unclear.

Other Anti-infectives A synergistic antibacterial effect has been reported between polymyxin B and some other anti-infectives (e.g., tetracyclines, chloramphenicol, azithromycin, erythromycin, sulfonamides).

In an in vitro study, the antibacterial effects of polymyxin B and azithromycin were synergistic against 6 out of 10 strains of multidrug-resistant *Ps. aeruginosa*; the combination was bactericidal against some strains, but bacteriostatic against other strains. The clinical importance of in vitro studies evaluating combinations of polymyxin B and azithromycin against gram-negative bacteria is unclear.

■ **Neuromuscular Blocking Agents and Anesthetics** Polymyxin B can cause respiratory paralysis from neuromuscular blockade, especially if the drug is given soon after anesthesia and/or muscle relaxants. Concurrent use of polymyxin B and neuromuscular blocking agents (e.g., succinylcholine, ether, gallamine [not commercially available in the US], tubocurarine [not commercially available in the US], decamethonium [not commercially available in the US]) and other neurotoxic drugs (e.g., sodium citrate) should be avoided since these agents may precipitate respiratory paralysis. If signs of respiratory paralysis occur, respiration should be assisted as required and the drug discontinued.

Mechanism of Action

Polymyxin B usually is bactericidal in action. The bactericidal activity of the drug is concentration dependent.

Polymyxin B binds to phosphate groups in the lipids of the bacterial cytoplasmic membrane of susceptible bacteria and acts as a cationic detergent, thereby altering the osmotic barrier of the membrane and causing leakage of essential intracellular components.

Spectrum

Polymyxin B has a spectrum of activity that is similar to that of colistin. Polymyxin B is active in vitro against many gram-negative aerobic bacteria; however, the drug is inactive against gram-positive bacteria, anaerobic bacteria, fungi, and viruses.

■ **Gram-negative Bacteria** Polymyxin B generally is active in vitro against *Pseudomonas aeruginosa* and is active against many multidrug-resistant strains, including metallo-β-lactamase-producing *Ps. aeruginosa.* The drug also is active against many strains of *Acinetobacter baumannii*, including multidrug-resistant strains. Although polymyxin B is active against some strains of *Stenotrophomonas maltophilia*, it is inactive against *Burkholderia cepacia* (formerly *Ps. cepacia*).

Polymyxin B is active in vitro against most Enterobacteriaceae, including most strains of *Citrobacter*, *Escherichia coli*, *Klebsiella pneumoniae*, *Salmonella*, and *Shigella*, and some strains of *Enterobacter*. Polymyxin B generally is inactive against *Proteus*, *Providencia*, *Morganella*, and *Serratia marcescens.*

Polymyxin B has some activity against *Haemophilus influenzae*, *Bordetella pertussis*, and *Legionella pneumophila*, but is inactive against *Moraxella catarrhalis*, *Neisseria*, and *Brucella.*

■ **In Vitro Susceptibility Tests** When broth or agar dilution susceptibility tests are used to test in vitro susceptibility of *Ps. aeruginosa* to polymyxin B, the Clinical and Laboratory Standards Institute (CLSI; formerly National Committee for Clinical Laboratory Standards [NCCLS]) states that strains with minimum inhibitory concentrations (MICs) of 2 mcg/mL or less are susceptible to polymyxin B, those with MICs of 4 mcg/mL have intermediate susceptibility, and those with MICs of 8 mcg/mL or greater are resistant to the drug.

When broth or agar dilution susceptibility tests are used to test in vitro susceptibility of *Acinetobacter* to polymyxin B, CLSI states that strains with MICs of 2 mcg/mL or less are susceptible to polymyxin B and those with MICs of 4 mcg/mL or greater are resistant to the drug.

If a disk diffusion procedure is used to test susceptibility to polymyxin B, a 300-unit polymyxin B disk is used and organisms with growth inhibition zones 12 mm or greater are considered susceptible to polymyxin B. However, the disk diffusion method usually is not recommended for testing susceptibility to polymyxin B since the drug diffuses poorly in agar and false-susceptible results may occur. If a disk diffusion procedure is used, results indicating susceptibility to polymyxin B should be confirmed using a broth or agar dilution method.

Resistance

Resistance to polymyxin B has been reported rarely in *Pseudomonas aeruginosa* and *Acinetobacter baumannii*. Surveillance data based on clinical isolates obtained from North America, Latin America, Europe, and the Asia-Pacific region during 2001–2004 indicated that 1.1–2.9% of *Ps. aeruginosa* isolates and 1.7–2.7% of *Acinetobacter* isolates were resistant to polymyxin B.

Two types of resistance to polymyxin B have been identified in *Ps. aeruginosa*, including low-level, transmissible mutations and high-level, stepwise resistance.

Complete cross-resistance occurs between polymyxin B and colistin, but there is no evidence to date of cross-resistance between these polymyxins and other anti-infectives.

Pharmacokinetics

■ **Absorption** Polymyxin B sulfate is not absorbed from the GI tract.

After IM administration of a single polymyxin B dose of 20,000–40,000 units/kg (2–4 mg/kg) in adults, peak serum concentrations of 1–8 mcg/mL are obtained within approximately 2 hours. Serum concentrations are higher in infants and children. Following IM administration of polymyxin B to adults with normal renal function, detectable amounts of the drug are present in serum for up to 12 hours.

In a study in critically ill adults who received polymyxin B doses of 0.5–1.5 mg/kg by IV infusion over 60 minutes, peak plasma concentrations at completion of the infusion ranged from 2.38–13.9 mcg/mL, and concentrations of polymyxin B_1 were fourfold higher than concentrations of polymyxin B_2. (See Chemistry.)

Serum concentrations are higher and more prolonged in patients with renal impairment.

Polymyxin B does not appear to be absorbed to an appreciable extent from mucous membranes or intact or denuded skin.

■ **Distribution** In a study in critically ill adults, the volume of distribution of polymyxin B ranged from 71–194 mL/kg.

Polymyxin B diffuses poorly in tissues.

Following IV or IM administration, polymyxin B is not distributed into CSF (even when meninges are inflamed) or synovial fluid. Systemically administered polymyxin B does not penetrate into the aqueous humor of the eye, even in the presence of inflammation.

Polymyxin B does not cross the placenta.

Animal studies indicate that following IV or IM administration, approximately 50% of a dose is reversibly bound to phospholipids of cell membranes in the liver, kidneys, heart, muscle, brain, and probably other tissues.

In an in vitro study using plasma from critically ill adults receiving polymyxin B, the drug was 78.5–92.4% bound to plasma proteins; however, mean protein binding was only 55.9% when testing was done using pooled plasma from healthy individuals.

■ **Elimination** The serum half-life of polymyxin B is reported to be 4.3–6 hours in adults with normal renal function. In patients with creatinine clearances less than 10 mL/minute, the serum half-life of polymyxin B has been reported to be 2–3 days.

Polymyxin B is eliminated in urine principally by glomerular filtration. Some studies indicate only low amounts of the dose are eliminated in urine within the first 12 hours after a dose, but eventually approximately 60% of a dose of polymyxin B is excreted in urine. Other studies suggest that less than 1% of a dose is eliminated unchanged in urine over 3 days. In adults, there is a 12- to 24-hour time lag following the initial dose during which very little polymyxin B appears in the urine, possibly as a result of binding of the drug to phospholipids of kidney cell membranes. Excretion continues for 24–72 hours after the final dose is administered. In adults with normal renal function, urinary drug concentrations have averaged 20–100 mcg/mL following usual

IM doses at 6-hour intervals over a period of a few days. Infants excrete polymyxin B faster than do adults; 40–60% of an administered dose is excreted within 8 hours in the urine.

In a study in critically ill adults who received polymyxin B doses by IV infusion over 60 minutes, total body clearance ranged from 0.27–0.81 mL/minute per kg and less than 1% of a dose was eliminated unchanged in urine.

Polymyxin B is not removed to an appreciable extent by hemodialysis or peritoneal dialysis.

Chemistry and Stability

■ **Chemistry** Polymyxin B is a polymyxin antibiotic derived from *Bacillus polymyxa*. Polymyxin B is structurally and pharmacologically related to colistin. Commercially available polymyxin B sulfate is a mixture of the sulfate salts of polymyxins B_1 and B_2.

Polymyxin B sulfate occurs as a white to buff-colored, hygroscopic powder that is odorless or has a faint odor. The drug is freely soluble in water and in 0.9% sodium chloride injection and slightly soluble in alcohol. Each mg of pure polymyxin B is equivalent to 10,000 units of polymyxin B activity. Aqueous solutions of polymyxin B sulfate have a pH of 5–7.5.

■ **Stability** Polymyxin B sulfate powder for injection should be stored at 15–30°C or 20–25°C, depending on the manufacturer, and should be protected from light. Following reconstitution, polymyxin B solutions should be stored at 2–8°C; any unused portions should be discarded after 72 hours.

The commercially available fixed-combination solution for irrigation containing polymyxin B sulfate and neomycin sulfate should be stored at 2–8°C. Following dilution in 0.9% sodium chloride solution, the solution for irrigation should be stored at 4°C and used within 48 hours.

Polymyxin B is inactivated by strong acidic or alkaline solutions. The drug is chemically incompatible with many drugs including amphotericin B, ampicillin, cefazolin, chloramphenicol sodium succinate, chlorothiazide sodium, and heparin sodium. Polymyxin B in solution is also incompatible with the salts of calcium and magnesium.

Preparations

Excipients in commercially available drug preparations may have clinically important effects in some individuals; consult specific product labeling for details.

Polymyxin B Sulfate

Powder	100 million units (of polymyxin B)*	**Poly-Rx®**, X-Gen
Parenteral		
For injection	500,000 units (of polymyxin B)*	**Polymyxin B Sulfate For Injection**

*available from one or more manufacturer, distributor, and/or repackager by generic (nonproprietary) name

Neomycin and Polymyxin B Sulfates

Urogenital		
Solution, for irrigation	Neosporin Sulfate (40 mg of neomycin) per mL and Polymyxin B Sulfate 200,000 units (of polymyxin B) per mL	**Neomycin and Polymyxin B Sulfates Solution for Irrigation** **Neosporin® G.U. Irrigant,** Monarch

†Use is not currently included in the labeling approved by the US Food and Drug Administration

RIFAMYCINS 8:12.28.30

rifAXIMin

■ Rifaximin, a structural analog of rifampin, is a rifamycin antibiotic.

Uses

■ **Hepatic Encephalopathy** ***Reduction of Risk of Recurrence*** Rifaximin is used for reduction of risk of recurrence of overt hepatic encephalopathy in adults.

The comparative efficacy of rifaximin used alone or in conjunction with lactulose for prevention of overt hepatic encephalopathy recurrence has not been established. Some experts recommend that rifaximin be used as an adjunct to lactulose for prevention of hepatic encephalopathy recurrence in patients who have had at least 1 episode of overt hepatic encephalopathy while receiving lactulose alone. Rifaximin has not been studied for reduction of risk of recurrence of overt hepatic encephalopathy in patients with scores exceeding 25 on the model for end-stage liver disease (MELD).

Efficacy and safety of rifaximin for reduction of risk of recurrence of overt hepatic encephalopathy were evaluated in a randomized, placebo-controlled, double-blind study in adults who were in remission from hepatic encephalopathy (Conn score of 0 or 1) after having 2 or more episodes of hepatic encephalopathy associated with chronic liver disease during the previous 6 months. A total of 299 adults (mean age 56 years [81% younger than 65 years of age], 61% male, 86% white, 67% with Conn score of 0, 68% with asterixis grade 0, 27% with MELD score 10 or less, 64% with MELD score 11–18, 9% Child-Pugh class C) were randomized to receive rifaximin 550 mg or placebo twice daily for 6 months or until the drug was discontinued because of a breakthrough episode of hepatic encephalopathy or another reason (e.g., adverse effects, request to withdraw). Concomitant use of lactulose was permitted (91.4% of those receiving rifaximin and 91.2% of those receiving placebo also received lactulose). The primary end point was time to first breakthrough episode of overt hepatic encephalopathy (defined as a marked deterioration in neurologic function and an increase from a baseline Conn score of 0 or 1 to a score of 2 or more or an increase from a baseline Conn score of 0 to a score of 1 plus a 1-unit increase in asterixis grade). Comparison of Kaplan-Meier estimates of event-free curves showed that rifaximin reduced the risk of hepatic encephalopathy episodes by 58% compared with placebo during the 6-month treatment period; 22% of patients in the rifaximin treatment group and 46% of patients in the placebo group experienced breakthrough episodes of overt hepatic encephalopathy. Efficacy of rifaximin was consistent regardless of gender, baseline Conn score, duration of current remission, and presence or absence of diabetes mellitus. During the 6-month treatment period, rifaximin also reduced the risk of hepatic encephalopathy-associated hospitalizations by 50% compared with placebo; hepatic encephalopathy-associated hospitalizations were reported in 14 and 23% of patients in the rifaximin and placebo groups, respectively.

Treatment Although safety and efficacy have not been established, rifaximin also has been used for the treatment of hepatic encephalopathy† and is designated an orphan drug by FDA for treatment of this condition.

Efficacy of rifaximin for the treatment of hepatic encephalopathy has been evaluated in several controlled studies and adjunctive use of the drug appears to be effective in reducing blood ammonia concentrations and decreasing the severity of neurologic manifestations. In one double-blind, dose-ranging study, 54 adults with cirrhosis and mild to moderate hepatic encephalopathy were randomized to receive 600, 1200, or 2400 mg of rifaximin daily in 3 divided doses for 7 days. Rifaximin treatment at the 2 higher dosages (1200 or 2400 mg daily) was associated with an improvement in the portal-systemic encephalopathy index (based on mental state, asterixis, number connection test time, EEG mean cycle frequency, and blood ammonia concentrations). In another double-blind study, 58 adults with cirrhosis and portosystemic encephalopathy were randomized to receive 1200 mg of rifaximin daily for 15 days or 30 g of lactulose daily for 15 days. Although clinical improvement in manifestations of portosystemic encephalopathy was reported for both drugs and correlated with reductions in serum ammonia concentrations, data suggested that rifaximin may be better tolerated than lactulose. Clinical improvement was also reported in a case series of 55 adults with cirrhosis and grade 1, 2, and 3 portosystemic encephalopathy treated with rifaximin (1200 mg daily in 3 divided doses) in conjunction with lactulose therapy at a dosage sufficient to induce 2 or 3 evacuations daily.

A meta-analysis of 12 randomized, controlled trials comparing rifaximin to nonabsorbable disaccharides (e.g., lactulose, lactitol) or to other oral anti-infectives (e.g., neomycin, paromomycin) was conducted to assess the efficacy and safety of rifaximin for the treatment of hepatic encephalopathy in adults. Results from an analysis of the 7 studies that compared rifaximin to nonabsorbable disaccharides indicated that resolution or clinical improvement of hepatic encephalopathy occurred with both types of treatment; analysis of the 5 studies that compared rifaximin to other anti-infectives indicated that efficacy of rifaximin was similar to that of neomycin or paromomycin. A combined analysis of all 12 studies indicated that rifaximin was associated with fewer adverse effects than the other treatments.

Information from the American Association for the Study of Liver Diseases (AASLD) and European Association for the Study of the Liver (EASL) regarding the management of hepatic encephalopathy, including recommendations for treatment and prevention of recurrence, is available at http://www.aasld.org.

■ **Irritable Bowel Syndrome with Diarrhea** Rifaximin is used for the treatment of irritable bowel syndrome (IBS) with diarrhea in adults.

Efficacy and safety of rifaximin for the treatment of IBS with diarrhea have been evaluated in 3 randomized, double-blind, placebo-controlled, phase 3 studies.

TARGET 1 (NCT00731679) and TARGET 2 (NCT00724126) were identically designed studies that included a total of 1258 adults who met Rome II criteria for diarrhea-predominant IBS (mean age 46 years, 24–30% male, 89–94% white, 4–10% black); patients with constipation-predominant IBS (according to Rome II criteria) were excluded. After a screening phase of 7–13 days, patients were randomized in a 1:1 ratio to receive rifaximin 550 mg or placebo 3 times daily for 14 days followed by a 10-week treatment-free evaluation period. The primary end point was the proportion of patients who had adequate relief of global IBS symptoms for at least 2 of the 4 weeks during the first month of the treatment-free evaluation period (primary evaluation period). This end point (adequate relief) was defined as a "yes" by the patient to a once-weekly subject global assessment question: "In regard to all your symptoms of IBS, as compared with the way you felt before you started the study medication, have you, in the past 7 days, had adequate relief of your IBS symptoms?". During the primary evaluation period, adequate relief was experienced by 41% of patients treated with rifaximin and 31–32% of patients treated with placebo. Substantially more patients in the rifaximin group experienced continued relief through 3 months compared with those in the placebo group. In addition, an exploratory, composite end point (defined as at least 30% improvement from baseline in abdominal pain *and* weekly mean stool consistency score less than 4 for at least 2 of the 4 weeks during the primary evaluation period) was achieved in 47% of patients treated with rifaximin compared with 36–39% of those treated with placebo.

TARGET 3 evaluated efficacy and safety of repeat courses of rifaximin for the treatment of diarrhea-predominant IBS. A total of 2579 adults received open-label rifaximin for 14 days followed by a 4-week treatment-free evaluation period. Of the 2438 evaluable patients, 1074 (44%) responded to initial rifaximin treatment (defined as the composite end point of at least a 30% improvement from baseline in abdominal pain *and* at least a 50% reduction in the number of days per week with a daily stool consistency of Bristol Stool Scale type 6 or 7). These responders were then followed for recurrence for up to an additional 20-week treatment-free period. A total of 636 initial responders subsequently had recurrence of IBS symptoms (return of abdominal pain or lack of stool consistency for at least 3 weeks during a 4-week follow-up period); the median time to recurrence was 10 weeks (range 6–24 weeks). Patients who experienced recurrence were then enrolled in a double-blind, placebo-controlled, repeat treatment phase and randomized in a 1:1 ratio to receive rifaximin 550 mg or placebo 3 times daily for 2 additional 14-day repeat treatment courses separated by 10 weeks. The primary end point of this randomized portion of the study was the proportion of patients who were responders to repeat treatment in the composite outcome of at least a 30% improvement from baseline in IBS-related abdominal pain *and* at least a 50% reduction in the number of days per week with a daily stool consistency of Bristol Stool Scale type 6 or 7 during the 4 weeks following the first 14-day repeat treatment course. Response at 4 weeks after completion of the first repeat treatment course was achieved by 38% of patients treated with rifaximin and 31% of those treated with placebo. During the 10-week treatment free follow up period, 17.1 or 11.7% of patients treated with rifaximin or placebo, respectively, had no recurrence of signs and symptoms of IBS.

■ **Travelers' Diarrhea** Rifaximin is used for the treatment of travelers' diarrhea caused by noninvasive strains of *Escherichia coli* in adults and adolescents 12 years of age and older.

Rifaximin is *not* effective in and should *not* be used for the treatment of diarrhea complicated by fever or bloody stools or for the treatment of diarrhea caused by pathogens other than *E. coli*. Rifaximin is *not* effective in and should *not* be used for the treatment of travelers' diarrhea caused by *Campylobacter jejuni*. In addition, efficacy of the drug has *not* been established for the treatment of travelers' diarrhea caused by *Shigella* or *Salmonella*. (See Precautions Related to Treatment of Travelers' Diarrhea under Cautions: Warnings/Precautions.)

In a multicenter, randomized, double-blind, placebo-controlled study in 380 adults with travelers' diarrhea, including 43 cases caused by enteroaggregative *E. coli*, treatment with rifaximin (200 mg 3 times daily for 3 days) was associated with a more rapid resolution of diarrhea and an increased rate of clinical cure (defined as 48 hours without unformed stools and without fever or 24 hours without watery stools, no more than 2 soft stools, and absence of other clinical symptoms) compared with placebo. The primary study end point was the median elapsed time after initiating therapy to the passage of the last unformed stool (time to the last unformed stool [TLUS]) and was 32.5 hours in patients treated with rifaximin and 59–60 hours in those treated with placebo. The rate of clinical cure within 5 days (120 hours) of initiating therapy was 79% in those treated with rifaximin and 60–61% in those treated with placebo. Treatment with a higher rifaximin dosage (400 mg 3 times daily) did not provide additional clinical benefit. In this study, the overall rate of microbiological cure (i.e., the absence of *E. coli* or other pathogen in stool cultured after 72 hours of therapy) in those treated with rifaximin (69%) was similar to the microbiologic cure rate in those treated with placebo (67%).

The most common cause of travelers' diarrhea worldwide is noninvasive enterotoxigenic strains of *E. coli*, but travelers' diarrhea may be caused by various other bacteria, including enteroadherent and other *E. coli* pathotypes, *C. jejuni*, *Shigella*, *Salmonella*, *Aeromonas*, or *Plesiomonas*. In some cases, travelers' diarrhea is caused by parasitic enteric pathogens (e.g., *Giardia duodenalis* [also known as *G. lamblia* or *G. intestinalis*], *Cryptosporidium*, *Cyclospora*, *Entamoeba histolytica*, *Dientamoeba fragilis*) or viral enteric pathogens (e.g., norovirus, rotavirus, astrovirus).

Travelers' diarrhea caused by bacteria may be self-limited and often resolves within 3–7 days without anti-infective treatment. If diarrhea is moderate or severe, associated with fever or bloody stools, persisting longer than 3 days, or extremely disruptive to travel plans, short-term (1–3 days) treatment with an anti-infective usually is recommended. Since bacteria are the most common cause of travelers' diarrhea (80–90% of cases), an anti-infective directed against enteric bacterial pathogens is used for empiric treatment. The US Centers for Disease Control and Prevention (CDC) and other experts state that a fluoroquinolone (e.g., ciprofloxacin, levofloxacin) generally is considered the anti-infective of choice for empiric treatment, including self-treatment, of travelers' diarrhea in adults. Azithromycin can be used as a treatment alternative for individuals who should not receive fluoroquinolones (e.g., children, pregnant women) and is a drug of choice for travelers in areas with a high prevalence of fluoroquinolone-resistant *Campylobacter* (e.g., South and Southeast Asia) or those who have not responded after 48 hours of fluoroquinolone treatment. Rifaximin can be considered an alternative when the causative organism is enterotoxigenic *E. coli*; however, since it may be difficult for travelers to distinguish between invasive and noninvasive diarrhea and since travelers would have to carry a back-up anti-infective, the overall usefulness of rifaximin for empiric self-treatment of travelers' diarrhea remains to be determined.

Although safety and efficacy have not been established, rifaximin has been used in some adults for prevention of travelers' diarrhea†. Because travelers' diarrhea is a relatively nonthreatening illness that usually is mild and self-limiting and can be effectively treated and because of the risks of widespread use of prophylactic anti-infectives (i.e., potential adverse drug reactions, selection of resistant organisms, increased susceptibility to infections caused by these or other organisms), CDC and other experts state that anti-infective prophylaxis for prevention of travelers' diarrhea is not recommended for most travelers.

For additional information on treatment and prevention of travelers' diarrhea, see Travelers' Diarrhea under Uses: GI Infections, in Ciprofloxacin 8:12.18.

Dosage and Administration

■ **Administration** Rifaximin is administered orally without regard to meals.

■ **Dosage** ***Hepatic Encephalopathy*** For reduction of risk of recurrence of overt hepatic encephalopathy in adults, the recommended dosage of rifaximin is 550 mg twice daily.

For the treatment of hepatic encephalopathy† in adults, rifaximin has been given in a dosage of 600–1200 mg daily (usually in 3 divided doses) for 7–21 days.

Irritable Bowel Syndrome with Diarrhea For the treatment of irritable bowel syndrome (IBS) with diarrhea in adults, the recommended dosage of rifaximin is 550 mg 3 times daily for 14 days. If symptoms recur, up to 2 additional courses of rifaximin may be given using the same 14-day regimen.

Travelers' Diarrhea For the treatment of travelers' diarrhea caused by noninvasive strains of *Escherichia coli* in adults and adolescents 12 years of age or older, the recommended dosage of rifaximin is 200 mg 3 times daily for 3 days. If diarrhea worsens or persists for more than 24–48 hours after initiating rifaximin, the drug should be discontinued and an alternative anti-infective considered.

■ **Special Populations** ***Hepatic Impairment*** Rifaximin dosage adjustment is not necessary in patients with hepatic impairment; however, the drug should be used with caution in patients with severe hepatic impairment (Child-Pugh class C). (See Hepatic Impairment under Warnings/Precautions: Specific Populations, in Cautions.)

Renal Impairment The pharmacokinetics of rifaximin have not been specifically studied in patients with renal impairment; however, clinically important changes in rifaximin elimination are not expected in those with renal impairment since the drug is poorly absorbed from the GI tract and is almost entirely excreted in feces as unchanged drug.

Geriatric Patients The pharmacokinetics of rifaximin have not been specifically studied in geriatric patients 65 years of age or older. (See Geriatric Use under Warnings/Precautions: Specific Populations, in Cautions.)

Cautions

■ **Contraindications** Rifaximin is contraindicated in patients with known hypersensitivity to rifaximin, other rifamycin anti-infectives, or any ingredient in the formulation.

■ **Warnings/Precautions** ***Sensitivity Reactions*** Hypersensitivity reactions, including exfoliative dermatitis, rash, angioedema (swelling of face and tongue and difficulty swallowing), urticaria, flushing, pruritus, and anaphylaxis, have been reported during postmarketing experience. Such reactions have occurred as soon as 15 minutes after a dose of rifaximin.

Precautions Related to Treatment of Travelers' Diarrhea Rifaximin should *not* be used for the treatment of diarrhea complicated by fever or bloody stools or for the treatment of diarrhea known or suspected to be caused by pathogens other than *Escherichia coli* (e.g., *Campylobacter jejuni*, *Salmonella*, *Shigella*).

If diarrhea worsens or persists for more than 24–48 hours after initiating rifaximin, the drug should be discontinued and treatment with another anti-infective considered.

Interactions Concomitant use of rifaximin with drugs that are P-glycoprotein (P-gp) transport inhibitors (e.g., cyclosporine) may substantially increase rifaximin systemic exposure. In patients with hepatic impairment, a potential additive effect of reduced hepatic metabolism and concomitant use with P-gp inhibitors may further increase rifaximin exposures. Caution is advised if concomitant use of rifaximin and a P-gp inhibitor is necessary. (See Drug Interactions.)

Superinfection/Clostridium difficile-associated Diarrhea and Colitis (CDAD) Treatment with anti-infectives alters normal colon flora and may permit overgrowth of *Clostridium difficile*. *C. difficile* infection (CDI) and *C. difficile*-associated diarrhea and colitis (CDAD; also known as antibiotic-associated diarrhea and colitis or pseudomembranous colitis) have been reported in patients receiving nearly all anti-infectives, including rifaximin, and may range in severity from mild diarrhea to fatal colitis. *C. difficile* produces toxins A and B which contribute to development of CDAD; hypertoxin-producing strains of *C. difficile* are associated with increased morbidity and mortality since they may be refractory to anti-infectives and colectomy may be required.

CDAD should be considered in the differential diagnosis of patients who develop diarrhea during or after anti-infective therapy. Careful medical history is necessary since CDAD has been reported to occur as late as 2 months or longer after anti-infective therapy is discontinued.

If CDAD is suspected or confirmed, anti-infective therapy not directed against *C. difficile* should be discontinued whenever possible. Patients should be managed with appropriate supportive therapy (e.g., fluid and electrolyte management, protein supplementation), anti-infective therapy directed against *C. difficile* (e.g., metronidazole, vancomycin), and surgical evaluation as clinically indicated.

Selection and Use of Anti-infectives Rifaximin is *not* suitable for the treatment of systemic bacterial infections because plasma concentrations of the drug are low and variable following oral administration. (See Description.)

To reduce development of drug-resistant bacteria and maintain effectiveness of rifaximin and other antibacterials, the drug should be used only for treatment of infections proven or strongly suspected to be caused by susceptible bacteria.

When selecting or modifying anti-infective therapy, results of culture and in vitro susceptibility testing should be used. In the absence of such data, local epidemiology and susceptibility patterns should be considered when selecting anti-infectives for empiric therapy.

Specific Populations **Pregnancy.** Data are not available regarding the use of rifaximin in pregnant women. In animal reproduction studies, teratogenic effects (e.g., ocular, oral and maxillofacial, cardiac, and lumbar spine malformations) were observed in rats and rabbits at rifaximin dosages approximately 0.9–5 times and 0.7–33 times, respectively, the recommended human dosage (600–1650 mg daily).

Lactation. It is not known whether rifaximin is distributed into human milk, affects human milk production, or affects the breast-fed infant.

Benefits of breast-feeding and the importance of rifaximin to the woman should be considered along with the potential adverse effects on the breast-fed child from the drug or from the underlying maternal condition.

Pediatric Use. Hepatic encephalopathy: Safety and efficacy of rifaximin have not been established in children and adolescents younger than 18 years of age.

Irritable bowel syndrome (IBS) with diarrhea: Safety and efficacy of rifaximin have not been established in children and adolescents younger than 18 years of age.

Travelers' diarrhea: Safety and efficacy of rifaximin have not been established in children younger than 12 years of age.

Geriatric Use. Hepatic encephalopathy: There were no overall differences in safety or efficacy between patients 65 years of age and older and younger adults in clinical studies (19% of patients were 65 years of age or older); other reported clinical experience has not identified differences in response between geriatric and younger patients, but greater sensitivity in some older individuals cannot be ruled out.

IBS with diarrhea: There were no overall differences in safety or efficacy between patients 65 years of age and older and younger adults in clinical studies (11% of patients were 65 years of age or older); other reported clinical experience has not identified differences in response between geriatric and younger patients, but greater sensitivity in some older individuals cannot be ruled out.

Travelers' diarrhea: Experience in those 65 years of age or older is insufficient to determine whether they respond differently than younger patients.

Hepatic Impairment. Rifaximin should be used with caution in patients with severe hepatic impairment (Child-Pugh class C). Although dosage adjustments are not necessary in patients with hepatic impairment, severe hepatic impairment results in increased rifaximin systemic exposure.

In patients with a history of hepatic encephalopathy, mean rifaximin exposure (area under the plasma concentration-time curve [AUC]) is higher than that reported in healthy individuals. When rifaximin dosage of 550 mg twice daily was evaluated in patients with a history of hepatic encephalopathy, mean systemic exposure in those with mild, moderate, or severe hepatic impairment was approximately 10-, 14-, or 21-fold higher, respectively, than systemic exposure reported in healthy individuals. Clinical trials evaluating rifaximin in patients with a history of hepatic encephalopathy did not include patients with scores exceeding 25 on the model for end-stage liver disease (MELD).

Renal Impairment. The pharmacokinetics of rifaximin have not been specifically studied in patients with renal impairment. Clinically important changes in rifaximin elimination are not expected since the drug is poorly absorbed from the GI tract and is almost entirely excreted in feces.

■ **Common Adverse Effects** Hepatic encephalopathy: Adverse effects occurring in 5% or more of patients receiving rifaximin and at a higher rate than that reported with placebo in clinical trials include peripheral edema, nausea, dizziness, fatigue, ascites, muscle spasms, pruritus, abdominal pain, anemia, depression, nasopharyngitis, upper abdominal pain, arthralgia, dyspnea, pyrexia, and rash.

IBS with diarrhea: Adverse effects occurring in 2% or more of patients receiving rifaximin and at a higher rate than that reported with placebo in clinical trials include nausea and increased ALT concentrations.

Travelers' diarrhea: Adverse effects occurring in 2% or more of patients receiving rifaximin and at a higher rate than that reported with placebo in clinical trials include headache.

Drug Interactions

■ **Drugs Metabolized by Hepatic Microsomal Enzymes** Rifaximin is a substrate of cytochrome P-450 (CYP) isoenzyme 3A4. Based on in vitro studies, rifaximin is not expected to inhibit CYP1A2, 2A6, 2B6, 2C9, 2C19, 2D6, 2E1, or 3A4.

Although in vitro studies indicate that rifaximin induces CYP3A4, drug interaction studies with midazolam (a CYP3A4 substrate) indicate that therapeutic dosages of rifaximin do not have clinically important effects on the activity of intestinal or hepatic CYP3A4. In patients with normal hepatic function, pharmacokinetic interactions between rifaximin and drugs metabolized by CYP3A4 are not expected. However, it is not known whether rifaximin can have a clinically important effect on the pharmacokinetics of such drugs in patients with hepatic impairment who have increased plasma concentrations of rifaximin.

■ **Drugs Affecting or Affected by P-glycoprotein Transport** Rifaximin is a substrate of P-glycoprotein (P-gp) transport in vitro. Concomitant use of rifaximin and a P-gp inhibitor (e.g., cyclosporine) may result in substantially increased rifaximin exposures.

Although in vitro studies indicate that rifaximin inhibits P-gp transport, the effect of the drug on P-gp transport in vivo is unknown.

■ **Drugs Affecting or Affected by Organic Anion Transport Polypeptides** Rifaximin is a substrate of organic anion transporting polypeptides (OATP) 1A2, 1B1, and 1B3 in vitro; the drug is not a substrate of OATP2B1.

Although in vitro studies indicate that rifaximin inhibits OATP1B1, 1A2, and 1B3, the effect of the drug on these transporters in vivo is unknown.

■ **Cyclosporine** In healthy individuals, concomitant use of rifaximin (single 550-mg dose) and cyclosporine (single 600-mg dose) results in an 83- and 124-fold increase in rifaximin peak plasma concentrations and area under the plasma concentration-time curve (AUC), respectively. Because cyclosporine inhibits P-gp and OATPs and is a weak inhibitor of CYP3A4, the relative contributions of these effects on rifaximin pharmacokinetics are unknown. In addition, the clinical importance of increased rifaximin systemic exposures in patients receiving cyclosporine is unknown.

■ **Midazolam** Concurrent use of rifaximin (200 mg orally 3 times daily for 3 or 7 days) and a single dose of midazolam (2 mg IV or 6 mg orally) did not substantially alter systemic exposure or elimination of midazolam or its major metabolite (1′-hydroxymidazolam). Concurrent use of rifaximin (550 mg orally 3 times daily for 7 or 14 days) and midazolam (single 2-mg IV dose) resulted in slightly decreased midazolam peak plasma concentrations and AUC; this effect is not considered clinically important.

Dosage adjustment is not necessary if midazolam and rifaximin are used concomitantly.

■ **Hormonal Contraceptives** Concurrent use of rifaximin (200 mg orally 3 times daily for 3 days) and a single dose of an oral estrogen-progestin combination contraceptive (ethinyl estradiol 70 mcg in fixed combination with norgestimate 500 mcg) did not substantially alter the disposition of ethinyl estradiol and norgestimate. Concurrent use of rifaximin (550 mg 3 times daily for 7 days) and a single dose of an oral estrogen-progestin combination contraceptive (ethinyl estradiol 25 mcg in fixed combination with norgestimate 250 mcg) resulted in a 25 and 13% decrease in peak plasma concentrations of ethinyl estradiol and norgestimate, respectively; the mean AUCs of norgestimate metabolites were decreased by 7–11% but the AUC of ethinyl estradiol was not affected. The clinical importance of these effects on estrogen-progestin combination contraceptives is not known.

Description

Rifaximin is a semisynthetic rifamycin antibiotic. Unlike other commercially available rifamycins (e.g., rifampin, rifabutin, rimactane), rifaximin contains an additional pyridoimidazole ring that makes the drug relatively nonabsorbable following oral administration.

Like other rifamycins, rifaximin inhibits RNA synthesis in susceptible bacteria by binding to the β subunit of bacterial DNA-dependent RNA polymerase.

Rifaximin is active in vitro and in clinical infections (i.e., infectious diarrhea) against enterotoxigenic *Escherichia coli* (ETEC) and enteroaggregative *E. coli* (EAEC). Although the clinical importance is unclear, rifaximin also is active in vitro against some other *E. coli* strains (including enterohemorrhagic, enteroinvasive, enteropathogenic, and Hep-2 adherent strains) and has some in vitro activity against *Aeromonas, Bacillus, Bacteroides, Bifidobacterium, Campylobacter jejuni, Enterobacter cloacae, Fusobacterium, Helicobacter, Klebsiella pneumoniae, Plesiomonas shigelloides, Peptostreptococcus, Prevotella, Salmonella, Shigella* (including *S. dysenteriae, S. flexneri, S. sonnei*), *Vibrio*, and *Yersinia enterocolitica*.

Resistance to rifaximin has been produced in vitro in *E. coli* (ETEC and EAEC strains). Resistance to rifaximin also has been reported in various *E. coli* clinical isolates from patients with travelers' diarrhea or inflammatory bowel disease, including some patients who previously received the drug. Clinical isolates of *Campylobacter, Salmonella,* and *Shigella* with in vitro resistance to rifaximin also have been reported. Although some strains of *Clostridium difficile* are susceptible to rifaximin in vitro, clinical isolates resistant to rifaximin (some with high-level resistance) have been reported.

Resistance to rifaximin generally is associated with mutations in the *rpo*B gene that change the binding site on DNA-dependent RNA polymerase and decrease rifaximin binding affinity. Presence of efflux pumps also appears to cause or contribute to development of rifaximin resistance in some organisms. Cross-resistance between rifaximin and other classes of anti-infectives has not been observed.

Rifaximin is poorly absorbed from the GI tract; less than 0.4% of an oral dose is absorbed. Following oral administration of rifaximin (single or multiple doses of 550 mg) in healthy individuals, mean peak plasma concentrations are attained about 1 hour after dosing and range from 2.4–4 ng/mL. In patients treated with oral rifaximin (200 mg 3 times daily for 3 days), plasma concentrations and systemic exposure (area under the plasma concentration-time curve [AUC]) are low and variable and accumulation of the drug does not occur. In patients with a history of hepatic encephalopathy receiving rifaximin (550 mg twice daily), the mean AUC of rifaximin is approximately 12-fold higher than that reported in healthy individuals. In patients with irritable bowel syndrome (IBS) with diarrhea receiving rifaximin (550 mg 3 times daily for 14 days), the time to peak plasma concentrations, mean peak plasma concentrations, and AUC of rifaximin are similar to those reported in healthy individuals. When rifaximin was administered 30 minutes after a high-fat meal in healthy individuals, peak plasma concentrations of the drug were not affected; however, the time to peak plasma concentrations was delayed from 0.75 to 1.5 hours after the dose and the AUC was increased twofold. Rifaximin is moderately bound to human plasma proteins (67.5 or 62% in healthy individuals or patients with hepatic impairment, respectively). Systemically absorbed rifaximin undergoes extensive metabolism, principally by cytochrome P-450 (CYP) isoenzyme 3A4. Following a 400-mg oral dose of rifaximin, 96.6% of the dose is excreted in feces (mostly as unchanged drug) and 0.3% is excreted in urine (mostly as metabolites). The mean half-life of rifaximin at steady-state is 5.6 hours in healthy individuals and 6 hours in patients with IBS with diarrhea.

Advice to Patients

Advise patients that antibacterials (including rifaximin) should only be used to treat bacterial infections and not used to treat viral infections (e.g., the common cold).

Importance of completing full course of therapy, even if feeling better after a few days.

Advise patients that skipping doses or not completing the full course of therapy may decrease effectiveness and increase the likelihood that bacteria will develop resistance and will not be treatable with rifaximin or other antibacterials in the future.

Advise patients and/or their caregivers that rifaximin may be taken with or without food.

If used for the treatment of travelers' diarrhea, advise patients of the importance of discontinuing rifaximin and seeking medical care if diarrhea worsens or persists for more than 24–48 hours after the drug is initiated or if fever and/or bloody diarrhea develop.

If used in patients with severe hepatic impairment (Child-Pugh class C), advise patients that rifaximin systemic exposure is increased. (See Hepatic Impairment under Warnings/Precautions: Specific Populations, in Cautions.)

Advise patients that diarrhea is a common problem caused by anti-infectives and usually ends when the drug is discontinued. Importance of contacting a clinician if watery and bloody stools (with or without stomach cramps and fever) occur during or as late as 2 months or longer after the last dose.

Importance of informing clinicians of existing or contemplated concomitant therapy, including prescription and OTC drugs, as well as any concomitant illnesses.

Importance of women informing clinicians if they are or plan to become pregnant or plan to breast-feed.

Importance of informing patients of other important precautionary information. (See Cautions.)

Overview® (see Users Guide). For additional information on this drug until a more detailed monograph is developed and published, the manufacturer's labeling should be consulted. It is *essential* that the manufacturer's labeling be consulted for more detailed information on usual cautions, precautions, contraindications, potential drug interactions, laboratory test interferences, and acute toxicity.

Preparations

Excipients in commercially available drug preparations may have clinically important effects in some individuals; consult specific product labeling for details.

rifAXIMin

Oral

Tablets	200 mg	**Xifaxan®**, Salix
	550 mg	**Xifaxan®**, Salix

†Use is not currently included in the labeling approved by the US Food and Drug Administration

STREPTOGRAMINS 8:12.28.32

Quinupristin and Dalfopristin quinupristin/dalfopristin

■ Quinupristin and dalfopristin (quinupristin/dalfopristin) is a fixed combination containing 2 semisynthetic streptogramin antibiotics; quinupristin and dalfopristin act synergistically against susceptible bacteria, resulting in increased antibacterial activity compared with either drug alone.

Uses

■ **Skin and Skin Structure Infections** Quinupristin and dalfopristin (quinupristin/dalfopristin) is used IV for the treatment of complicated skin and skin structure infections caused by *Staphylococcus aureus* (methicillin-susceptible [oxacillin-susceptible] strains) or *Streptococcus pyogenes* (group A β-hemolytic streptococci, GAS).

In 2 randomized, open-label, phase 3, comparator-controlled studies in adults with complicated skin and skin structure infections (e.g., erysipelas, postoperative infections, traumatic wound infections), efficacy and safety of quinupristin/dalfopristin (7.5 mg/kg given IV every 12 hours) was compared with oxacillin (2 g given IV every 6 hours) or cefazolin (1 g given IV every 8 hours). In the comparator groups, vancomycin (1 g given IV every 12 hours) could be substituted for the comparator drug if necessary (e.g., β-lactam hypersensitivity, suspected or confirmed methicillin-resistant *S. aureus* [MRSA; also known as oxacillin-resistant *S. aureus* or ORSA]). The clinical success rate (defined as cure or improvement) in the clinically evaluable population in these 2 studies was 50 or 66% in those treated with quinupristin/dalfopristin versus 52 or 64% in those treated with the comparator anti-infective. Drug discontinuance because of adverse effects occurred more than 4 times as often in the quinupristin/dalfopristin treatment groups than in the comparator treatment groups; approximately 50% of those who discontinued quinupristin/dalfopristin did so because of adverse effects at the IV infusion site. (See Administration Precautions under Warnings/Precautions: Other Warnings and Precautions, in Cautions.)

For information on diagnosis and management of skin and skin structure infections, the current clinical practice guidelines from the Infectious Diseases Society of America (IDSA) available at http://www.idsociety.org should be consulted.

■ **Methicillin-resistant Staphylococcus aureus Infections** Quinupristin/dalfopristin has been used IV as salvage therapy in critically ill patients for the treatment of severe infections (e.g., bacteremia, infective endocarditis) caused by methicillin-resistant *S. aureus*† (MRSA; also known as oxacillin-resistant *S. aureus* or ORSA) when vancomycin was ineffective.

Although safety and efficacy of quinupristin/dalfopristin for the treatment of MRSA infections has not been established, some clinicians state that the drug is one of several options for the treatment of persistent MRSA bacteremia in adults who fail to respond to vancomycin or when the infection is known to be caused by MRSA with reduced susceptibility to vancomycin and daptomycin.

For information regarding the treatment of infections caused by MRSA, the current clinical practice guidelines from IDSA available at http://www.idsociety.org should be consulted. For information on diagnosis and management of infective endocarditis caused by MRSA, the current AHA guidelines available at http://my.americanheart.org/statements should be consulted.

■ **Vancomycin-resistant Enterococcus faecium Infections** Quinupristin/dalfopristin has been used IV for the treatment of serious or life-threatening infections caused by susceptible vancomycin-resistant *Enterococcus faecium*†, including bacteremia, infective endocarditis, intra-abdominal infections, skin and skin structure infections, and urinary tract infections. Although quinupristin/dalfopristin has been effective in some patients for the treatment of infections caused by vancomycin-resistant *E. faecium*, this indication is no longer included in FDA-approved labeling for the drug because data submitted to FDA failed to confirm clinical benefit. Some clinicians suggest that use of quinupristin/dalfopristin for the treatment of infections caused by vancomycin-resistant *E. faecium* should be reserved for refractory infections that fail to respond to other anti-infectives.

Efficacy of quinupristin/dalfopristin for the treatment of serious infections caused by vancomycin-resistant *S. faecium* varies depending on the site of infection. Data from 2 prospective emergency-use studies indicated lower success rates when the drug was used for the treatment of bacteremia of unknown origin (52%) or intra-abdominal infections (59%) caused by vancomycin-resistant *S. faecium* and higher success rates when the drug was used for the treatment of skin and skin structure infections (72%), central catheter-related bacteremia (83%), or urinary tract infections (89%) caused by vancomycin-resistant *S. faecium*.

Dosage and Administration

■ **Administration** Quinupristin and dalfopristin (quinupristin/dalfopristin) is administered by IV infusion over 60 minutes.

Quinupristin/dalfopristin should *not* be given by rapid IV infusion or injection. An infusion pump or device may be used to control the rate of infusion.

Following completion of peripheral infusions of quinupristin/dalfopristin, the vein should be flushed with 5% dextrose injection to decrease the incidence of venous irritation. If necessary, a peripherally inserted central catheter (PICC) or central venous catheter can be used to administer quinupristin/dalfopristin. (See Administration Precautions under Warnings/Precautions: Other Warnings and Precautions, in Cautions.)

Other drugs should not be added to quinupristin/dalfopristin solutions.

If the same IV line is used for sequential infusion of different drugs, the IV line should be flushed with 5% dextrose injection before and after infusion of quinupristin/dalfopristin. Because of incompatibilities, sodium chloride injections or heparin solutions should *not* be used to flush the IV line.

IV Infusion **Reconstitution and Dilution.** Quinupristin/dalfopristin powder for injection must be reconstituted and then further diluted prior to IV infusion. Strict aseptic technique must be observed when preparing IV solutions of quinupristin/dalfopristin since the drug contains no preservatives.

The manufacturer states that *only* 5% dextrose injection or sterile water for injection should be used to reconstitute quinupristin/dalfopristin powder for injection and *only* 5% dextrose injection should be used to dilute the reconstituted drug. Because of incompatibility, sodium chloride injections should *not* be used.

Single-dose vials labeled as containing 500 mg (150 mg of quinupristin and 350 mg of dalfopristin) should be reconstituted by slowly adding 5 mL of 5% dextrose injection or sterile water for injection to provide a solution containing 100 mg/mL. The vial should be gently swirled by manual rotation to ensure dissolution; shaking should be avoided to limit foaming. The vial should then be allowed to sit for a few minutes until all the foam has disappeared; the resulting solution should be clear.

Reconstituted solutions of quinupristin/dalfopristin *must* be further diluted in 5% dextrose injection within 30 minutes. The appropriate dose of reconstituted solution should be diluted in 250 mL of 5% dextrose injection. For infusion via a central line, the appropriate dose of reconstituted solution may be diluted in 100 mL of 5% dextrose injection.

If moderate or severe venous irritation occurs (see Administration Precautions under Warnings/Precautions: Other Warnings and Precautions, in Cautions), consideration should be given to increasing the infusion volume to 500 or 750 mL, changing the infusion site, or infusing the drug via a PICC or central venous catheter.

Reconstituted and diluted solutions of quinupristin/dalfopristin should be used as soon as possible. The manufacturer states that diluted solutions of the drug are stable for up to 5 hours at room temperature or up to 54 hours when refrigerated at 2–8°C. Quinupristin/dalfopristin solutions should not be frozen.

Reconstituted and diluted solutions of quinupristin/dalfopristin should be inspected visually for particulate matter prior to administration.

Rate of Administration. Quinupristin/dalfopristin solutions should be administered by IV infusion over 60 minutes.

Rapid IV infusion should be avoided. (See Administration Precautions under Warnings/Precautions: Other Warnings and Precautions, in Cautions.)

■ **Dosage** Quinupristin/dalfopristin is a fixed combination containing a 30:70 (w/w) ratio of quinupristin to dalfopristin.

Dosage of the fixed combination quinupristin/dalfopristin is expressed in terms of the total dosage of the 2 components (i.e., dosage of quinupristin plus dosage of dalfopristin).

Each single-dose vial of quinupristin/dalfopristin contains a total of 500 mg (i.e., 150 mg of quinupristin and 350 mg of dalfopristin).

Skin and Skin Structure Infections The recommended dosage of quinupristin/dalfopristin for the treatment of complicated skin and skin structure infections caused by susceptible *Staphylococcus aureus* (methicillin-susceptible [oxacillin-susceptible] strains) or *Streptococcus pyogenes* (group A β-hemolytic streptococci, GAS) in adults is 7.5 mg/kg every 12 hours. The minimum recommended treatment duration for complicated skin and skin structure infections is 7 days.

Although safety and efficacy of quinupristin/dalfopristin have not been established in pediatric patients younger than 16 years of age (see Pediatric Use under Warnings/Precautions: Specific Populations, in Cautions), the manufacturer states that the recommended dosage of the drug for children 12 years of age or older is 7.5 mg/kg every 12 hours. Dosage recommendations are not available for pediatric patients younger than 12 years of age.

Methicillin-resistant Staphylococcus aureus Infections Quinupristin/dalfopristin has been given in a dosage of 7.5 mg/kg every 8 hours for salvage therapy in the treatment of severe infections caused by methicillin-resistant *S. aureus*† (MRSA; also known as oxacillin-resistant *S. aureus* or ORSA) when vancomycin was ineffective.

Vancomycin-resistant Enterococcus faecium Infections Quinupristin/dalfopristin has been given in a dosage of 7.5 mg/kg every 8 hours for the treatment of vancomycin-resistant *Enterococcus faecium* infections†.

■ **Special Populations** ***Hepatic Impairment*** Although quinupristin/dalfopristin pharmacokinetic data in patients with hepatic cirrhosis (Child-Pugh class A and B) suggest that dosage reductions may be necessary in patients with hepatic impairment, the manufacturer states that data are insufficient to make specific recommendations for dosage modifications in such patients. (See Hepatic Impairment under Warnings/Precautions: Specific Populations, in Cautions.)

Renal Impairment Dosage adjustments are not necessary when quinupristin/dalfopristin is used in patients with renal impairment or in those undergoing peritoneal dialysis. (See Renal Impairment under Warnings/Precautions: Specific Populations, in Cautions.)

Geriatric Patients Dosage adjustments are not necessary when quinupristin/dalfopristin is used in geriatric patients.

Cautions

■ **Contraindications** Quinupristin and dalfopristin (quinupristin/dalfopristin) is contraindicated in patients with known hypersensitivity to quinupristin/dalfopristin or other streptogramins (e.g., pristinamycin, virginiamycin).

■ **Warnings/Precautions** ***Warnings*** **Interactions.** Concomitant use of quinupristin/dalfopristin and drugs that are metabolized by cytochrome P-450 (CYP) 3A4 and have a narrow therapeutic index requires caution and monitoring (e.g., cyclosporine) or should be avoided (e.g., drugs that prolong the QT interval corrected for rate [QT_c]). (See Drug Interactions.)

Sensitivity Reactions Anaphylactic shock and angioedema have been reported in patients receiving quinupristin/dalfopristin.

Rash, urticaria, and pruritus also have been reported.

Other Warnings and Precautions **Administration Precautions.** Adverse effects at the quinupristin/dalfopristin IV infusion site often occur, especially with peripheral infusions. In comparative clinical trials, inflammation or pain was reported in 38–45%, edema in 17–18%, and thrombophlebitis in 2% of patients receiving quinupristin/dalfopristin. Concomitant use of hydrocortisone or diphenhydramine in clinical trials did not appear to alleviate venous inflammation or pain associated with quinupristin/dalfopristin.

To minimize venous irritation, IV infusion lines should be flushed with 5% dextrose injection following completion of peripheral infusions of quinupristin/dalfopristin. Because of possible incompatibilities, IV infusion lines should *not* be flushed with sodium chloride injections or heparin solutions.

If moderate to severe venous irritation occurs following IV infusion of quinupristin/dalfopristin that has been diluted in 250 mL of 5% dextrose injection, consideration should be given to increasing the infusion volume to 500 or 750 mL, changing the infusion site, or establishing central venous access.

Rapid IV administration of quinupristin/dalfopristin in animals was associated with greater toxicity than slow IV infusion of the drug. Because safety of rapid IV injection of the drug has not been studied in humans and because clinical trial experience has exclusively involved IV infusion over 60 minutes, the manufacturer states that more rapid IV infusion rates cannot be recommended.

Musculoskeletal Effects. Arthralgia and myalgia, severe in some cases, have been reported in patients receiving quinupristin/dalfopristin. In some patients receiving the drug every 8 hours, symptoms improved when frequency was changed to every 12 hours. In those available for follow-up, symptoms resolved after the drug was discontinued. The etiology of these myalgias and arthralgias is unknown.

Hepatic Effects. Hyperbilirubinemia, with total bilirubin concentrations exceeding 5 times the upper limit of normal, occurred in approximately 25% of patients receiving quinupristin/dalfopristin in noncomparative clinical studies. In some patients, isolated hyperbilirubinemia (principally increased conjugated bilirubin) can occur during treatment, possibly as the result of competition between bilirubin and quinupristin/dalfopristin for excretion.

In comparative clinical studies, AST and ALT elevations occurred with similar frequency in those receiving quinupristin/dalfopristin or comparator therapy.

Precautions Related to Use of Fixed Combinations. When quinupristin/dalfopristin is used, the cautions, precautions, contraindications, and drug interactions associated with both drugs in the fixed combination must be considered. Cautionary information applicable to specific populations (e.g., pregnant or nursing women, individuals with hepatic or renal impairment, geriatric patients) should be considered for each drug.

When prescribing, preparing, and dispensing quinupristin/dalfopristin, healthcare professionals should consider that dosage of the fixed combination is expressed as the total (sum) of the dosage of each of the 2 active components (i.e., dosage of quinupristin plus dosage of dalfopristin). (See Dosage and Administration: Dosage.)

Superinfection/Clostridium difficile-associated Diarrhea and Colitis. Use of quinupristin/dalfopristin may result in overgrowth of nonsusceptible organisms. If superinfection occurs, appropriate therapy should be instituted.

Treatment with anti-infectives alters normal colon flora and may permit overgrowth of *Clostridium difficile*. *C. difficile* infection (CDI) and *C. difficile*-associated diarrhea and colitis (CDAD; also known as antibiotic-associated diarrhea and colitis or pseudomembranous colitis) have been reported with nearly all anti-infectives, including quinupristin/dalfopristin, and may range in severity from mild diarrhea to fatal colitis. *C. difficile* produces toxins A and B which contribute to the development of CDAD; hypertoxin-producing strains of *C. difficile* are associated with increased morbidity and mortality since they may be refractory to anti-infectives and colectomy may be required.

CDAD should be considered in the differential diagnosis of patients who develop diarrhea during or after anti-infective therapy. Careful medical history is necessary since CDAD has been reported to occur as late as 2 months or longer after anti-infective therapy is discontinued.

If CDAD is suspected or confirmed, anti-infective therapy not directed against *C. difficile* should be discontinued whenever possible. Patients should be managed with appropriate supportive therapy (e.g., fluid and electrolyte management, protein supplementation), anti-infective therapy directed against *C. difficile* (e.g., metronidazole, vancomycin), and surgical evaluation as clinically indicated.

Specific Populations **Pregnancy.** Category B. (See Users Guide.)

There are no adequate and well-controlled studies evaluating quinupristin/dalfopristin in pregnant women; the drug should be used during pregnancy only if clearly needed.

Lactation. Quinupristin and dalfopristin are distributed into milk in rats; it is not known whether the drugs are distributed into human milk.

Quinupristin/dalfopristin should be used with caution in nursing women.

Pediatric Use. Safety and efficacy of quinupristin/dalfopristin have not been established in pediatric patients younger than 16 years of age. In addition, pharmacokinetics of the drug have not been studied in pediatric patients younger than 16 years of age. Quinupristin/dalfopristin has been given in a dosage of 7.5 mg/kg every 8 or 12 hours in a limited number of pediatric patients under emergency-use conditions. (See Skin and Skin Structure Infections under Dosage and Administration: Dosage.)

Geriatric Use. No overall differences in frequency, type, or severity of adverse effects, including cardiovascular effects, have been observed in geriatric adults 65 years of age or older compared with younger adults. Results of a study in adults 69–74 years of age indicate that the pharmacokinetics of quinupristin/dalfopristin in geriatric adults are similar to pharmacokinetics reported in younger adults.

Hepatic Impairment. In patients with hepatic impairment (Child-Pugh class A and B), the areas under the plasma concentration-time curves (AUCs) of quinupristin and dalfopristin and their major metabolites are increased. However, because the effect of reducing the dose or increasing the dosing interval on the pharmacokinetics of quinupristin and dalfopristin has not been studied, the manufacturer states that specific recommendations for dosage modifications in patients with hepatic impairment cannot be made.

Clinical studies suggest that the incidence of adverse effects in patients with chronic hepatic disease or cirrhosis is comparable to that in patients without hepatic impairment.

Renal Impairment. Although the AUCs of quinupristin and dalfopristin and their major metabolites are increased in patients with creatinine clearances of 6–28 mL/minute, the manufacturer states that dosage adjustments are not necessary in patients with renal impairment or in those undergoing peritoneal dialysis.

Only negligible amounts of quinupristin, dalfopristin, and their metabolites are removed by continuous ambulatory peritoneal dialysis (CAPD); it is unlikely that the drugs would be removed by hemodialysis.

■ **Common Adverse Effects** Adverse effects at the IV infusion site (pain, burning, inflammation, edema) occur in a large percentage of patients, particularly when quinupristin/dalfopristin is given by peripheral infusion. (See Administration Precautions under Warnings/Precautions: Other Warnings and Precautions, in Cautions.) Other adverse effects occurring in 1% or more of patients include GI effects (nausea, vomiting, diarrhea, anorexia), arthralgia and myalgia, hyperbilirubinemia, headache, thrombophlebitis, pain, asthenia, rash, or pruritus.

Drug Interactions

■ **Drugs Metabolized by Hepatic Microsomal Enzymes** Quinupristin and dalfopristin (quinupristin/dalfopristin) inhibits cytochrome P-450 (CYP) isoenzyme 3A4 and may increase plasma concentrations of drugs metabolized by this hepatic enzyme, resulting in increased or prolonged therapeutic effects and/or increased adverse effects associated with the drugs. Caution is advised if quinupristin/dalfopristin is used concomitantly with drugs that are CYP3A4 substrates and have a narrow therapeutic index.

Quinupristin/dalfopristin does not have a clinically important effect on CYP isoenzymes 1A2, 2A6, 2C9, 2C19, 2D6, or 2E1; drug interactions with drugs metabolized by these CYP isoenzymes are not expected.

■ **Drugs That Prolong QT Interval** Concomitant use with drugs that are CYP3A4 substrates and are known to prolong the QT interval corrected for rate (QT_c) should be avoided.

■ **Antiarrhythmic Agents** Possible pharmacokinetic interactions between antiarrhythmic agents metabolized by CYP3A4 (e.g., disopyramide, lidocaine, quinidine) and quinupristin/dalfopristin (increased plasma concentrations of the antiarrhythmic agent). Caution is advised if quinupristin/dalfopristin is used concomitantly with an antiarrhythmic agent metabolized by CYP3A4.

■ **Antibacterial Agents** There is some in vitro evidence that the antibacterial effects of vancomycin and quinupristin/dalfopristin are synergistic against vancomycin-resistant *Enterococcus faecium*.

In vitro studies indicate that the antibacterial effects of quinupristin/dalfopristin and certain aminoglycosides (gentamicin), β-lactams (amoxicillin, ampicillin, cefepime), glycopeptides (vancomycin), quinolones (ciprofloxacin), tetracyclines (doxycycline), or chloramphenicol are not antagonistic against staphylococci or enterococci.

In vitro studies indicate that the antibacterial effects of quinupristin/dalfopristin and certain aminoglycosides (gentamicin), β-lactams (aztreonam, cefotaxime), or quinolones (ciprofloxacin) are not antagonistic against Enterobacteriaceae or *Pseudomonas aeruginosa*.

■ **Antineoplastic Agents** Possible pharmacokinetic interactions between vinca alkaloids (e.g., vinblastine), docetaxel, or paclitaxel and quinupristin/dalfopristin (increased plasma concentrations of the antineoplastic agent). Caution is advised if quinupristin/dalfopristin is used concomitantly with any of these antineoplastic agents.

■ **Antiretroviral Agents** Possible pharmacokinetic interactions between quinupristin/dalfopristin and certain antiretrovirals metabolized by CYP3A4, including some HIV nonnucleoside reverse transcriptase inhibitors such as delavirdine and nevirapine and some HIV protease inhibitors such as indinavir and ritonavir (increased plasma concentrations of the antiretroviral). Caution is advised if quinupristin/dalfopristin is used concomitantly with antiretroviral agents metabolized by CYP3A4.

■ **Benzodiazepines** Concomitant use of midazolam (single dose) and quinupristin/dalfopristin in healthy individuals increased the peak plasma concentration and area under the plasma concentration-time curve (AUC) of midazolam by 14 and 33%, respectively.

Possible pharmacokinetic interactions between other benzodiazepines metabolized by CYP3A4 (e.g., diazepam) and quinupristin/dalfopristin (increased plasma concentrations of the benzodiazepine).

Caution is advised if quinupristin/dalfopristin is used concomitantly with benzodiazepines metabolized by CYP3A4.

■ **Calcium-channel Blocking Agents** Concomitant use of nifedipine and quinupristin/dalfopristin in healthy individuals increased the peak plasma concentration and AUC of nifedipine by 18 and 44%, respectively.

Possible pharmacokinetic interactions between other calcium-channel blocking agents metabolized by CYP3A4 (e.g., diltiazem, verapamil) and quinupristin/dalfopristin (increased plasma concentrations of the calcium-channel blocker).

Caution is advised if quinupristin/dalfopristin is used concomitantly with calcium-channel blocking agents metabolized by CYP3A4.

■ **Carbamazepine** Possible pharmacokinetic interactions between carbamazepine and quinupristin/dalfopristin (increased plasma concentrations of the anticonvulsant). Caution is advised if carbamazepine and quinupristin/dalfopristin are used concomitantly.

■ **Cisapride** Possible pharmacokinetic interactions between cisapride and quinupristin/dalfopristin (increased plasma concentrations of cisapride). Caution is advised if cisapride and quinupristin/dalfopristin are used concomitantly.

■ **Corticosteroids** Possible pharmacokinetic interactions between methylprednisolone and quinupristin/dalfopristin (increased plasma concentrations of the corticosteroid). Caution is advised if methylprednisolone and quinupristin/dalfopristin are used concomitantly.

■ **Digoxin** Pharmacokinetic interactions between digoxin and quinupristin/dalfopristin based on CYP3A4 inhibition are unlikely. However, in vitro data indicate that quinupristin/dalfopristin inhibits *Eubacterium lentum*; therefore, the drug possibly may interfere with GI metabolism of digoxin that occurs via intestinal bacteria.

■ **HMG-CoA Reductase Inhibitors** Possible pharmacokinetic interactions between HMG-CoA reductase inhibitors (statins) metabolized by CYP3A4 (e.g., lovastatin) and quinupristin/dalfopristin (increased plasma concentrations of the statin). Caution is advised if quinupristin/dalfopristin is used concomitantly with statins metabolized by CYP3A4.

■ **Immunosuppressive Agents** ***Cyclosporine*** Concomitant use of cyclosporine and quinupristin/dalfopristin affects the pharmacokinetics of cyclosporine and has resulted in a 30% increase in peak plasma concentrations, 63% increase in AUC, 77% increase in plasma half-life, and 34% decrease in clearance of the immunosuppressive agent.

If cyclosporine and quinupristin/dalfopristin must be used concomitantly, caution is advised and cyclosporine plasma concentrations should be monitored.

Tacrolimus Possible pharmacokinetic interactions between tacrolimus and quinupristin/dalfopristin (increased plasma concentrations of tacrolimus). Tacrolimus and quinupristin/dalfopristin should be used concomitantly with caution.

Description

Quinupristin and dalfopristin (quinupristin/dalfopristin) is a fixed combination containing 2 semisynthetic streptogramin antibiotics. Naturally occurring streptogramin antibiotics (e.g., pristinamycin, virginiamycin) are produced by certain *Streptomyces* bacteria and contain 2 macrocyclic lactone peptolide components (i.e., streptogramin type A and streptogramin type B) that act synergistically against susceptible bacteria. Quinupristin is derived from pristinamycin I and is a type B streptogramin; dalfopristin is derived from pristinamycin II_A and is a type A streptogramin.

Quinupristin/dalfopristin is commercially available as a lyophilized powder containing a 30:70 (w/w) ratio of quinupristin to dalfopristin. Unlike pristinamycin, quinupristin and dalfopristin are both water-soluble and therefore suitable for IV administration. In vitro studies indicate that metabolism of quinupristin and dalfopristin is not dependent on cytochrome P-450 (CYP) isoenzymes or glutathione transferase enzymes.

Quinupristin and dalfopristin act synergistically against susceptible bacteria, and the in vitro activity of the fixed combination is greater than that of each individual component. In addition, quinupristin is partially converted in vivo to 2 major active metabolites (a glutathione conjugate and a cysteine conjugate) and quinupristin is partially converted in vivo to a major active metabolite formed by hydrolysis. These major active metabolites contribute to the antibacterial activity of quinupristin/dalfopristin since they have antibacterial activity and act synergistically with the parent drugs.

The mechanism of action of quinupristin/dalfopristin, like other streptogramins, involves inhibition of protein synthesis. The 2 components of quinupristin/dalfopristin bind to different sites on the 50S subunit of the bacterial ribosome. Dalfopristin (a type A streptogramin) affects an early phase of protein synthesis and inhibits peptidyl transferase activity; quinupristin (a type B streptogramin) affects a later phase of protein synthesis and inhibits peptide chain elongation. Synergy results in part because quinupristin's affinity for the 50S subunit is enhanced by the conformational change produced when dalfopristin binds to the 50S subunit.

Quinupristin/dalfopristin usually is bactericidal against susceptible staphylococci and streptococci, but bacteriostatic against susceptible enterococci.

■ **Spectrum** Quinupristin/dalfopristin is active in vitro and in clinical infections caused by methicillin-susceptible (oxacillin-susceptible) *Staphylococcus aureus* and *Streptococcus pyogenes* (group A β-hemolytic streptococci, GAS). Although the clinical importance in unknown, quinupristin also has in vitro activity against methicillin-resistant *S. aureus* (MRSA; also known as oxacillin-resistant *S. aureus* or ORSA), *S. epidermidis* (including methicillin-resistant strains), *S. pneumoniae*, *S. agalactiae* (group B streptococci, GBS), groups C and G streptococci, viridans streptococci, *Listeria monocytogenes*, and *Corynebacterium jeikeium*. The MIC_{90} of quinupristin/dalfopristin for most susceptible staphylococci and streptococci is 1 mcg/mL or less.

Quinupristin/dalfopristin is active in vitro against *Enterococcus faecium*, including vancomycin-resistant *E. faecium* and multidrug-resistant *E. faecium*. The drug appears to be equally active in vitro against VanA and VanB phenotypes of vancomycin-resistant *E. faecium*. Susceptible *E. faecium*, including vancomycin-resistant strains, are usually inhibited in vitro by quinupristin/dalfopristin concentrations of 2 mcg/mL or less. However, *E. faecalis* generally require high concentrations of quinupristin/dalfopristin for in vitro inhibition and most strains are intrinsically resistant to the drug.

Although the clinical importance is unclear, quinupristin/dalfopristin has in vitro activity against some aerobic gram-negative bacteria, including *Haemophilus influenzae*, *Legionella*, *Moraxella catarrhalis*, and *Neisseria*, and some anaerobic bacteria, including *Clostridium* and *Lactobacillus*. Quinupristin/dalfopristin is inactive against Enterobacteriaceae, *Pseudomonas aeruginosa*, and *Acinetobacter*.

■ **Resistance** Resistance to quinupristin/dalfopristin has been reported and has emerged during treatment with the drug. Resistance to streptogramins, including quinupristin/dalfopristin, can occur as the result of alterations in the ribosomal target site, enzymatic inactivation, or efflux systems that actively transport the drugs out of the bacterial cell.

Resistance to quinupristin/dalfopristin has been reported only rarely in staphylococci or *S. pyogenes*.

Reduced susceptibility or resistance to quinupristin/dalfopristin has emerged in vancomycin-resistant *E. faecium* during treatment with quinupristin/dalfopristin.

The manufacturer states that cross-resistance between quinupristin/dalfopristin and aminoglycosides, β-lactams, glycopeptides, quinolones, macrolides, lincomycins, and tetracyclines has not been reported.

Advice to Patients

Advise patients that diarrhea is a common problem caused by anti-infectives and usually ends when the drug is discontinued. Importance of contacting a clinician if watery and bloody stools (with or without stomach cramps and fever) occur during or as late as 2 months or longer after the last dose.

Importance of informing clinicians of existing or contemplated concomitant therapy, including prescription and OTC drugs, as well as any concomitant illnesses.

Importance of women informing clinicians if they are or plan to become pregnant or plan to breast-feed.

Importance of informing patients of other important precautionary information. (See Cautions.)

Overview (see Users Guide). For additional information until a more detailed monograph is developed and published, the manufacturer's labeling should be consulted. It is *essential* that the manufacturer's labeling be consulted for more detailed information on usual cautions, precautions, contraindications, potential drug interactions, laboratory test interferences, and acute toxicity.

Preparations

Excipients in commercially available drug preparations may have clinically important effects in some individuals; consult specific product labeling for details.

Quinupristin and Dalfopristin

Parenteral

For injection, for IV infusion	500 mg (150 mg of quinupristin and 350 mg of dalfopristin)	**Synercid**®, Pfizer

†Use is not currently included in the labeling approved by the US Food and Drug Administration

ANTIFUNGALS 8:14

AZOLES 8:14.08

Fluconazole

■ Fluconazole, a synthetic triazole derivative, is an azole antifungal agent.

Uses

Fluconazole is used in the treatment of various infections caused by *Candida*, including candidemia and disseminated candidiasis, oropharyngeal candidiasis, esophageal candidiasis, and vulvovaginal candidiasis.

Fluconazole also is used for the treatment of cryptococcal meningitis and for the treatment of blastomycosis†, coccidioidomycosis†, and histoplasmosis†. Fluconazole has been used for the treatment of superficial fungal infections, dermatophytoses†, onychomycosis†, and pityriasis (tinea) versicolor. In addition, the drug is used for prevention of serious fungal infections (e.g., coccidioidomycosis, cryptococcosis, mucocutaneous candidiasis) in patients with human immunodeficiency virus (HIV) infection†, and for prevention of *Candida* infections in other immunocompromised individuals (e.g., cancer patients and bone marrow, hematopoietic stem cell†, and solid organ transplant recipients†).

Prior to initiation of fluconazole therapy, appropriate specimens for fungal culture and other relevant laboratory studies (e.g., serology, histopathology) should be obtained in order to isolate and identify the causative organism(s). Fluconazole therapy may be started pending results of these in vitro tests; however, once results are available, therapy should be adjusted accordingly. If fluconazole in vitro susceptibility tests are performed, results should be interpreted cautiously since in vitro tests may not accurately reflect fluconazole's in vivo activity.

■ **Candida Infections** ***Candidemia and Disseminated Candida Infections*** Fluconazole is used for the treatment of candidemia, disseminated candidiasis (e.g., chronic disseminated hepatosplenic infections), and other serious *Candida* infections, including urinary tract infections, peritonitis, meningitis, osteoarticular infections (e.g., osteomyelitis, septic arthritis), intravascular infections (e.g., endocarditis, implantable cardiac device infections), pneumonia, endophthalmitis, and neonatal candidiasis† (including CNS infections). The drug has been effective in the treatment of some *Candida* infections that did not respond to IV amphotericin B.

While fluconazole may be better tolerated and easier to administer than IV amphotericin B, fluconazole-resistant strains of *C. albicans* are being isolated with increasing frequency from patients who have received prior fluconazole therapy (especially in HIV-infected patients) and some *Candida* infections (e.g., candidemia) are increasingly caused by strains that are intrinsically resistant to fluconazole (e.g., *C. krusei*) or likely to be resistant or have reduced susceptibility to fluconazole (e.g., *C. glabrata*). The choice of an antifungal for the treatment of candidemia or invasive *Candida* infections should take into consideration any history of recent exposure to azole or echinocandin antifungals or intolerance to antifungals, local and/or institutional epidemiologic data regarding prevalence of the various *Candida* strains and their patterns of resistance, severity of illness, relevant comorbidities, presence and duration of neutropenia or immunosuppression, and evidence of involvement of the CNS, cardiac valves, and/or visceral organs.

For the treatment of candidemia in *nonneutropenic* patients or for empiric treatment of suspected invasive candidiasis† in *nonneutropenic* patients in intensive care units (ICUs), the Infectious Diseases Society of America (IDSA) recommends an IV echinocandin (anidulafungin, caspofungin, micafungin) for *initial* therapy. IDSA states that fluconazole (IV or oral) is an acceptable alternative for *initial* therapy in selected patients, including those who are not critically ill and are unlikely to have infections caused by fluconazole-resistant *Candida*. If echinocandin- and azole-resistant *Candida* are suspected, IV amphotericin B is recommended; IV amphotericin B also is a reasonable alternative when echinocandins and fluconazole cannot be used because of intolerance, limited availability, or resistance. IDSA states that transition from the echinocandin (or amphotericin B) to fluconazole can be considered (usually within 5–7 days) in patients who are clinically stable, have isolates susceptible to fluconazole (e.g., *C. albicans*), and have negative repeat blood cultures after initial antifungal treatment. Although fluconazole has been considered the drug of choice for the treatment of infections caused by *C. parapsilosis* in nonneutropenic patients (based in part on concerns related to decreased in vitro susceptibility and resistance to echinocandins), IDSA states that there are no clinical studies to date indicating superiority of fluconazole over echinocandins for the treatment of *C. parapsilosis* infections.

For the treatment of candidemia in *neutropenic* patients, IDSA recommends an IV echinocandin (anidulafungin, caspofungin, micafungin) or, alternatively, IV amphotericin B for *initial* therapy. Fluconazole is an alternative for *initial* therapy in those who are not critically ill and have had no prior exposure to azole antifungals and also can be used for step-down therapy during neutropenia in clinically stable patients who have fluconazole-susceptible isolates and documented bloodstream clearance. Voriconazole can be used as an alternative for *initial* therapy when broader antifungal coverage is required and also can be used as step-down therapy during neutropenia in clinically stable patients who have voriconazole-susceptible isolates and documented bloodstream clearance. For infections known to be caused by *C. krusei*, an echinocandin, amphotericin B, or voriconazole is recommended.

For the treatment of disseminated candidiasis in neonates† (neonatal candidiasis), IV amphotericin B usually is the drug of choice. IDSA states that fluconazole is a reasonable alternative in those who have not been receiving fluconazole prophylaxis, and the American Academy of Pediatrics (AAP) states that fluconazole can be considered for step-down treatment after an initial response has been obtained with IV amphotericin B. Fluconazole also has been used for prophylaxis to reduce the incidence of invasive candidiasis in low birthweight neonates at high risk†. (See Uses: Prevention of Candidiasis in Transplant Recipients, Cancer Patients, or Other Patients at High Risk.)

For the treatment of CNS candidiasis, IDSA recommends initial treatment with IV amphotericin B (with or without oral flucytosine) and follow-up (step-down) treatment with fluconazole.

IDSA states that antifungal treatment is not recommended in patients with asymptomatic candiduria, unless there is a high risk of disseminated candidiasis (e.g., neutropenic patients, low birthweight infants [less than 1.5 kg], patients who will undergo urologic manipulations). These experts state that asymptomatic candiduria in neutropenic patients and low birthweight infants should be treated using regimens recommended for patients with candidemia and that patients undergoing urologic procedures who have asymptomatic candiduria should be treated with oral fluconazole or IV amphotericin B for several days before and after the procedures. For the treatment of symptomatic candiduria (e.g., cystitis, pyelonephritis, fungus balls) caused by fluconazole-susceptible *Candida*, fluconazole is the drug of choice. When fluconazole-resistant *Candida* (e.g., *C. glabrata, C. krusei*) are likely, IV amphotericin B or oral flucytosine is recommended for symptomatic cystitis, and IV amphotericin B (with or without oral flucytosine) or oral flucytosine alone is recommended for pyelonephritis and fungus balls.

For the treatment of osteoarticular infections (e.g., osteomyelitis, septic arthritis) caused by *Candida*, IDSA recommends *initial* treatment with fluconazole or an IV echinocandin (anidulafungin, caspofungin, micafungin) and follow-up treatment with fluconazole. If septic arthritis involved a prosthetic device that cannot be removed, long-term suppressive or maintenance therapy (secondary prophylaxis)† with fluconazole is recommended if the isolate is susceptible.

For the treatment of endocarditis (native or prosthetic valve) or implantable cardiac device infections caused by *Candida*, IDSA recommends *initial* treatment with IV amphotericin B (with or without oral flucytosine) or an IV echinocandin (anidulafungin, caspofungin, micafungin) and follow-up treatment with fluconazole. If the isolate is susceptible, long-term suppressive or maintenance therapy (secondary prophylaxis)† with fluconazole is recommended to prevent recurrence in those with native valve endocarditis who cannot undergo valve replacement and in those with prosthetic valve endocarditis.

Fluconazole has been used with good results in some patients with endophthalmitis† caused by *Candida*, but treatment failures have been reported. Studies in rabbits indicate that fluconazole is distributed into the eye and that the drug inhibits growth of *C. albicans* in rabbit choroid-retina tissue and vitreous body when IV therapy is initiated within 24 hours postinoculation; the drug did not effectively inhibit growth of the organism when IV therapy was initiated 7 days postinoculation when the infection was well established. For the treatment of chorioretinitis (with or without vitritis) caused by *Candida*, IDSA recommends fluconazole or voriconazole when isolates are susceptible and amphotericin B (with or without oral flucytosine) when isolates are resistant to fluconazole and voriconazole; intravitreal amphotericin B or voriconazole may also be indicated.

Fluconazole is used prophylactically to reduce the incidence of candidiasis in bone marrow or hematopoietic stem cell transplant recipients† who are receiving chemotherapy or radiation therapy. The drug also has been used for primary prophylaxis of candidiasis in other patients considered at high risk for developing such infections (e.g., high-risk patients undergoing urologic procedures†, solid organ transplant recipients†, high-risk patients in ICUs†). (See Uses: Prevention of Candidiasis in Transplant Recipients, Cancer Patients, or Other Patients at High Risk.)

For additional information on management of candidemia and disseminated candidiasis, the current clinical practice guidelines from IDSA available at http://www.idsociety.org should be consulted.

Oropharyngeal Candidiasis Oral or IV fluconazole is used for the treatment of oropharyngeal candidiasis in immunocompromised adults with acquired immunodeficiency syndrome (AIDS), advanced AIDS-related complex (ARC), malignancy, or other serious underlying disease.

Fluconazole appears to be at least as effective as and, in some cases, more effective than other antifungals used for initial treatment of oropharyngeal *Candida* infections and is considered a drug of choice for the treatment of moderate to severe disease. Fluconazole has produced clinical resolution of signs and symptoms of the infection in 79–100% of patients with oropharyngeal candidiasis; however, microbiologic cures generally have been obtained in 44–87% of patients and the rate of relapse may be high, especially in neutropenic patients. In a study in HIV-infected adults with oropharyngeal candidiasis, the response rate and mycologic eradication rate after 14 days of therapy were 100 and 75%, respectively, in those who received oral fluconazole (100 mg once daily) and were 65 and 20%, respectively, in those who received topical clotrimazole (10-mg oral lozenge 5 times daily). In another study, 14 days of therapy with oral fluconazole (100 mg once daily as an oral suspension) was more effective than 14 days of therapy with topical nystatin (500,000 units as an oral suspension 4 times daily). The mycologic cure rate was 60% in the fluconazole group and 6% in the nystatin group and the rate of relapse at day 42 was 27 and 11%, respectively.

For the treatment of mild oropharyngeal candidiasis, IDSA recommends topical treatment with clotrimazole lozenges or miconazole buccal tablets; nystatin (oral suspension or tablets) is the recommended alternative. For moderate to severe disease, IDSA recommends oral fluconazole. For fluconazole-refractory oropharyngeal candidiasis, IDSA recommends itraconazole oral solution or posaconazole oral suspension; oral voriconazole or amphotericin B oral suspension (not commercially available in US) are recommended as alternatives. Other alternatives for refractory oropharyngeal candidiasis are IV echinocandins (anidulafungin, caspofungin, micafungin) or IV amphotericin B.

For the treatment of oropharyngeal candidiasis in HIV-infected adults and adolescents, the US Centers for Disease Control and Prevention (CDC), National Institutes of Health (NIH), and IDSA recommend oral fluconazole as the preferred drug of choice for initial episodes. If topical therapy is used for the treatment of oropharyngeal candidiasis (e.g., mild to moderate episodes), these experts recommend clotrimazole lozenges or miconazole buccal tablets. Alternatives for systemic treatment of oropharyngeal candidiasis in HIV-infected adults and adolescents are itraconazole oral solution or posaconazole oral suspension; nystatin oral suspension is an alternative if topical treatment is used. For fluconazole-refractory oropharyngeal infections in HIV-infected adults and adolescents, posaconazole oral suspension is preferred; itraconazole oral solution is an alternative.

Routine long-term suppressive or maintenance therapy (secondary prophylaxis)† to prevent relapse or recurrence is not usually recommended in patients adequately treated for oropharyngeal candidiasis (including HIV-infected individuals), unless the patient has frequent or severe recurrences of oropharyngeal candidiasis. If secondary prophylaxis of oropharyngeal candidiasis is indicated, oral fluconazole is recommended; however, the potential for development of azole resistance should be considered.

For additional information on management of oropharyngeal candidiasis, the current clinical practice guidelines from IDSA available at http://www.idsociety.org and the current clinical practice guidelines from CDC, NIH, and IDSA on the prevention and treatment of opportunistic infections in HIV-infected individuals available at http://www.aidsinfo.nih.gov should be consulted.

Esophageal Candidiasis Oral or IV fluconazole is used for the treatment of esophageal candidiasis in adults with AIDS, malignancy, or other serious underlying disease, including progressive systemic sclerosis. Fluconazole appears to be at least as effective as and, in some cases, more effective than other antifungals used for initial treatment of esophageal *Candida* infections and is considered a drug of choice.

In adults with esophageal candidiasis documented by endoscopy, fluconazole has produced clinical resolution of signs and symptoms of the infection in about 61–93% of patients. In one study in adults with esophageal candidiasis and progressive systemic sclerosis, fluconazole therapy produced mycologic cures in about 93% of patients within 2–4 weeks, but the relapse rate was almost 100% within 3 months after fluconazole therapy was discontinued.

Esophageal candidiasis requires treatment with a systemic antifungal (not a topical antifungal).

IDSA recommends oral fluconazole as the preferred drug of choice for the treatment of esophageal candidiasis; if oral therapy is not tolerated, IV fluconazole or an IV echinocandin (anidulafungin, caspofungin, micafungin) is recommended; IV amphotericin B is another alternative. For fluconazole-refractory esophageal candidiasis, IDSA recommends itraconazole oral solution or oral or IV voriconazole; alternatives for fluconazole-refractory disease are IV echinocandins (anidulafungin, caspofungin, micafungin) or IV amphotericin B. IDSA states that oral posaconazole (oral suspension or delayed-release tablets) could be considered another alternative for the treatment of fluconazole-refractory esophageal candidiasis.

For the treatment of esophageal candidiasis in HIV-infected adults and adolescents, CDC, NIH, and IDSA recommend oral or IV fluconazole or itraconazole oral solution. Alternatives include oral or IV voriconazole, an IV echinocandin (anidulafungin, caspofungin, micafungin), or IV amphotericin B. For refractory esophageal candidiasis in HIV-infected adults and adolescents, including fluconazole-refractory infections, these experts recommend posaconazole oral suspension or itraconazole oral solution; alternatives include an IV echinocandin (anidulafungin, caspofungin, micafungin), oral or IV voriconazole, or IV amphotericin B.

Routine long-term suppressive or maintenance therapy (secondary prophylaxis)† to prevent relapse or recurrence is not usually recommended in patients adequately treated for esophageal candidiasis (including HIV-infected individuals) unless the patient has frequent or severe recurrences of esophageal candidiasis. If secondary prophylaxis of esophageal candidiasis is indicated, oral fluconazole is recommended and posaconazole oral suspension is a possible alternative; however, the potential for development of azole resistance should be considered.

For additional information on management of esophageal candidiasis, the current clinical practice guidelines from IDSA available at http://www.idsociety.org and the current clinical practice guidelines from CDC, NIH, and IDSA on the prevention and treatment of opportunistic infections in HIV-infected individuals available at http://www.aidsinfo.nih.gov should be consulted.

Vulvovaginal Candidiasis Oral fluconazole is used for the treatment of uncomplicated vulvovaginal candidiasis and for the treatment of complicated vulvovaginal candidiasis† in *nonpregnant* women.

Vulvovaginal candidiasis frequently occurs during pregnancy. CDC states that topical (intravaginal) azole antifungals (not oral fluconazole) should be used for the treatment of vulvovaginal candidiasis during pregnancy. (See Pregnancy under Cautions: Pregnancy, Fertility, and Lactation.)

Uncomplicated Vulvovaginal Candidiasis. Oral fluconazole is effective for the treatment of uncomplicated vulvovaginal candidiasis when given as a single dose. A single 150-mg oral dose of fluconazole produces clinical cures (i.e., absence of vulvovaginal burning, itching, swelling, erythema, excoriation, dyspareunia, and/or ulceration and substantial decreases in vaginal discharge) 5–16 days after the dose in approximately 90–100% and mycologic cures in approximately 77–100% of *nonpregnant* women with uncomplicated vulvovaginal candidiasis. At 27–62 days after the single dose, clinical and mycologic cure rates are 61–90%, and the rate of relapse, reinfection, or recolonization is about 23%. Results of several studies in patients with uncomplicated vulvovaginal candidiasis suggest that a single 150-mg dose of oral fluconazole is as effective for this condition as multiple dose regimens of intravaginal clotrimazole, econazole, miconazole, or terconazole. In addition, the single-dose oral fluconazole regimen appears to be as effective for uncomplicated vulvovaginal candidiasis as oral itraconazole or oral ketoconazole.

In controlled studies in patients with vulvovaginal candidiasis, clinical and mycologic cure rates at 14 and 30–35 days were similar in patients receiving oral fluconazole (given as a single 150-mg dose) compared with patients receiving intravaginal clotrimazole (given as a 100-mg vaginal tablet once daily for 7 days) or miconazole (given as a 100-mg vaginal cream once daily for 7 days). At 14 days, the clinical cure rate was reported to be about 95–96% with fluconazole and 95–97% with intravaginal clotrimazole or miconazole and the mycologic cure rate was reported to be 77–80% with fluconazole and 72–82% with intravaginal clotrimazole or miconazole. At 30–35 days, the clinical cure rate was reported to be about 69–75% with fluconazole and 72–80% with intravaginal clotrimazole or miconazole and the mycologic cure rate was reported to be 61–63% with fluconazole and 57–63% with intravaginal clotrimazole or miconazole.

CDC, IDSA, and other clinicians recommend that uncomplicated vulvovaginal candidiasis (defined as vulvovaginal candidiasis that is mild to moderate, sporadic or infrequent, most likely caused by *C. albicans*, and occurring in immunocompetent women) in *nonpregnant* women should be treated with a topical (intravaginal) azole antifungal (e.g., butoconazole, clotrimazole, miconazole, terconazole, tioconazole) given in appropriate single-dose or short-course (1–3 days) regimens or, alternatively, oral fluconazole given in a single-dose regimen. These regimens generally have been associated with clinical and mycologic cure rates of 80–90% in otherwise healthy, *nonpregnant* women with uncomplicated infections. Some clinicians suggest that a single oral dose of fluconazole may offer some advantage over conventional intravaginal antifungal therapy since it ensures compliance and may reduce or eliminate concurrent rectal infections that may serve as a source of reinfection. In weighing the potential risks and benefits of oral versus intravaginal therapy, the potential for toxicity (e.g., hepatotoxicity) and drug interactions (see Drug Interactions) associated with oral therapy should be considered. The incidence of adverse effects is higher in patients receiving single oral doses of fluconazole compared with those receiving intravaginal antifungal therapy; and this also should be weighed carefully.

Complicated and Recurrent Vulvovaginal Candidiasis. Oral fluconazole is used for the treatment of complicated vulvovaginal candidiasis†, including recurrent and severe infections. Complicated vulvovaginal candidiasis is defined as infections that are recurrent or severe, caused by *Candida* other than *C. albicans*, or occurring in women with underlying disease such as diabetes mellitus, debilitation, or immunocompromising conditions (e.g., HIV infection), or those receiving immunosuppressive therapy (e.g., corticosteroids). CDC recommends that vaginal cultures be obtained from women with complicated vulvovaginal candidiasis to confirm the clinical diagnosis and identify unusual species (e.g., *C. glabrata*).

Recurrent vulvovaginal candidiasis (usually defined as 4 or more episodes of symptomatic vulvovaginal candidiasis within a year) affects a small percentage of women (less than 5%). Although each individual episode caused by *C. albicans* may respond to a short course of intravaginal azole antifungal or oral fluconazole, some experts recommend a longer duration of initial therapy (e.g., 7–14 days of an intravaginal azole antifungal or a 3-dose regimen of oral fluconazole [100, 150, or 200 mg given every third day for a total of 3 doses]) to attempt mycologic remission before initiating a maintenance antifungal regimen. For the maintenance regimen, CDC and IDSA recommend oral fluconazole (100, 150, or 200 mg once weekly) for 6 months. If this regimen cannot be used, intermittent use of intravaginal treatments can be considered. These maintenance regimens can be effective in reducing recurrent infections; however, 30–50% of women will have recurrent disease once maintenance therapy is discontinued. Women with recurrent infections who are symptomatic and remain culture-positive despite maintenance antifungal therapy should be managed in consultation with a specialist.

Severe vulvovaginal candidiasis (i.e., extensive vulvar erythema, edema, excoriation, and fissure formation) usually has a lower clinical response rate to short courses of intravaginal or oral antifungal therapy. CDC and IDSA recommend that severe vulvovaginal candidiasis be treated with either 7–14 days of an intravaginal azole antifungal or a 2-dose regimen of oral fluconazole (150 mg repeated 3 days later).

HIV-infected women have higher rates of vaginal *Candida* colonization, and symptomatic vulvovaginal candidiasis may occur more frequently and be more severe than in women without HIV infection. However, because there is no evidence to date that HIV-infected women have a lower response rate to intravaginal or oral antifungal regimens than other women, CDC, IDSA, and other clinicians recommend that treatment of vulvovaginal candidiasis in HIV-infected women should be the same as that in women without HIV infection. Routine long-term suppressive or maintenance therapy (secondary prophylaxis) to prevent relapse or recurrence of vulvovaginal candidiasis is not usually recommended in HIV-infected or other women unless the patient has recurrent or severe infections. If secondary prophylaxis or maintenance therapy of vulvovaginal candidiasis is indicated, oral fluconazole (150 or 200 mg once weekly or 100 mg 3 times weekly) is recommended.

Recurrent vulvovaginal candidiasis rarely may be caused by resistant strains of *C. albicans* or, more commonly, by other *Candida* with reduced susceptibility to azole antifungals (e.g., *C. glabrata*). It has been suggested that repeated treatment of recurrent vulvovaginal candidiasis with intravaginal azole antifungals and widespread and/or injudicious use of these agents for *self-medication* of vulvovaginal candidiasis may favor the selection of *Candida* that are resistant to azole antifungals. Optimum therapy for the treatment of vulvovaginal candidiasis caused by *Candida* other than *C. albicans* has not been determined. CDC recommends 7–14 days of therapy with an antifungal (oral or intravaginal) other than fluconazole. If recurrence occurs, alternatives include topical (intravaginal) boric acid (600-mg gelatin capsule once daily for 14 days; no FDA-labeled preparation commercially available in the US). Referral to a specialist is advised.

For additional information on management of vulvovaginal candidiasis, the current CDC guidelines available at http://www.cdc.gov/std, the current clinical practice guidelines from IDSA available at http://www.idsociety.org, and the current clinical practice guidelines from CDC, NIH, and IDSA on the prevention and treatment of opportunistic infections in HIV-infected individuals available at http://www.aidsinfo.nih.gov should be consulted.

■ **Coccidioidomycosis** Oral fluconazole is used for the treatment and prevention of coccidioidomycosis† caused by *Coccidioides immitis* or *C. posadasii*.

Treatment of Coccidioidomycosis Fluconazole is used for the treatment of coccidioidal pulmonary infections, meningitis, and disseminated (extrapulmonary) infections involving soft tissue or bones and joints.

Antifungal treatment may not be necessary in patients with mild, uncomplicated coccidioidal pneumonia since such infections often are self-limited and may resolve spontaneously. However, antifungal treatment is recommended for patients with more severe or rapidly progressing coccidioidal infections, those with chronic pulmonary or disseminated infections, and immunocompromised or debilitated individuals (e.g., HIV-infected individuals, organ transplant recipients, those receiving immunosuppressive therapy, those with diabetes or cardiopulmonary disease).

IDSA and others state that an oral azole (fluconazole or itraconazole) usually is recommended for initial treatment of symptomatic pulmonary coccidioidomycosis and chronic fibrocavitary or disseminated (extrapulmonary) coccidioidomycosis. However, IV amphotericin B is recommended as an alternative and is preferred for initial treatment of severely ill patients (e.g., those with hypoxia or rapidly progressing disease), for immunocompromised individuals, or when azole antifungals cannot be used (e.g., pregnant women).

For the treatment of clinically mild coccidioidomycosis (e.g., focal pneumonia) in HIV-infected adults and adolescents, CDC, NIH, and IDSA recommend initial therapy with oral fluconazole or oral itraconazole. For the treatment of diffuse pulmonary or extrathoracic disseminated coccidioidomycosis (nonmeningeal) in HIV-infected adults and adolescents, CDC, NIH, and IDSA recommend initial therapy with IV amphotericin B followed by oral azole therapy. Alternatively, some experts recommend initial therapy with IV amphotericin B used in conjunction with an oral azole (e.g., fluconazole or itraconazole) followed by an oral azole alone.

For the treatment of diffuse pulmonary or disseminated coccidioidomycosis (nonmeningeal) in HIV-infected infants and children, CDC, NIH, and IDSA recommend initial treatment with IV amphotericin B followed by oral fluconazole or oral itraconazole. In those with severe disseminated coccidioidomycosis, some experts recommend initial therapy with IV amphotericin B used in conjunction with an oral azole (e.g., fluconazole) followed by an oral azole alone. Use of fluconazole or itraconazole alone may be sufficient for the treatment of coccidioidomycosis in HIV-infected infants and children with only mild disease (e.g., focal pneumonia) and also can be considered an alternative for those with stable pulmonary or disseminated coccidioidomycosis (nonmeningeal).

For the treatment of coccidioidal meningitis in HIV-infected adults, adolescents, and children or other individuals, IV or oral fluconazole (with or without intrathecal amphotericin B) is considered the regimen of choice. Oral itraconazole, oral posaconazole, and oral voriconazole are recommended as alternatives for the treatment of coccidioidal meningitis in adults and adolescents. Patients who do not respond to an azole antifungal alone may be candidates for intrathecal amphotericin B (with or without continued azole therapy) or IV amphotericin B used in conjunction with intrathecal amphotericin B; however, consultation with an expert who has experience in treating coccidioidal meningitis is recommended. Fluconazole has produced clinical and/or laboratory evidence of improvement when used alone or in conjunction with IV amphotericin B in adults with coccidioidal meningitis and has been used for the treatment of coccidioidal meningitis in both HIV-infected and HIV-negative individuals. Because fluconazole generally is well tolerated and exhibits favorable pharmacokinetics (e.g., is distributed into CSF in high concentrations following oral or IV administration), the drug is considered a good option for the treatment of coccidioidal meningitis.

Primary Prophylaxis to Prevent First Episode of Coccidioidomycosis Oral fluconazole is used in certain HIV-infected adults and adolescents for primary prophylaxis against coccidioidomycosis†.

CDC, NIH, and IDSA recommend that HIV-infected adults and adolescents living in areas in the US where coccidioidomycosis is endemic (e.g., lower San Joaquin Valley in California, much of Arizona, southern regions of Utah, Nevada, and New Mexico, western Texas) be tested annually for the disease using IgM or IgG serologic tests. Those with a newly positive IgM or IgG serologic test and $CD4^+$ T-cell counts less than 250/mm^3 should receive oral fluconazole for primary prophylaxis against coccidioidomycosis† (preemptive antifungal therapy) since they are at increased risk of developing active coccidioidomycosis. Routine primary prophylaxis against coccidioidomycosis is not recommended in other HIV-infected adults and adolescents (e.g., those who reside in coccidioidomycosis endemic areas but do not have positive IgM or IgG serologic tests, those who reside in areas where the disease is not endemic) and is not recommended in HIV-infected infants and children.

Prevention of Recurrence (Secondary Prophylaxis) of Coccidioidomycosis Oral fluconazole is used for long-term suppressive or maintenance therapy (secondary prophylaxis) to prevent recurrence or relapse of coccidioidomycosis†.

Because of the risk of relapse, individuals who were treated for coccidioidal meningitis generally should receive long-term (life-long) secondary prophylaxis with oral fluconazole or oral itraconazole.

CDC, NIH, and IDSA recommend that all HIV-infected adults, adolescents, and children who have been adequately treated for coccidioidomycosis should receive long-term secondary prophylaxis with oral fluconazole or oral itraconazole to prevent recurrence or relapse. Because HIV-infected adults and adolescents who had focal coccidioidal pneumonia and responded clinically to antifungal treatment may be at low risk for recurrence if their $CD4^+$ T-cell count increases to greater than 250/mm^3 in response to antiretroviral therapy, it may be reasonable to consider discontinuing secondary prophylaxis against coccidioidomycosis after 12 months, provided such individuals are monitored for recurrence (e.g., serial chest radiographs, coccidioidal serology). However, secondary prophylaxis should be continued indefinitely in HIV-infected adults and adolescents who were treated for more extensive coccidioidomycosis and in all HIV-infected children, regardless of the immune response to antiretroviral therapy. Consultation with an expert is recommended when making decisions regarding discontinuance of secondary prophylaxis against coccidioidomycosis.

For additional information on management of coccidioidomycosis, the current clinical practice guidelines from IDSA available at http://www.idsociety.org and the current clinical practice guidelines from CDC, NIH, and IDSA on the prevention and treatment of opportunistic infections in HIV-infected individuals available at http://www.aidsinfo.nih.gov should be consulted.

■ **Cryptococcosis** ***Treatment of Cryptococcosis*** Oral or IV fluconazole is used in immunocompetent or immunocompromised adults for the treatment of meningitis caused by *Cryptococcus neoformans*. Fluconazole is considered an alternative for initial (induction) therapy of cryptococcal infections involving the CNS, but is the drug of choice for follow-up (consolidation) therapy of these infections. Fluconazole also is used for the treatment of pulmonary cryptococcosis†, cryptococcemia†, and disseminated cryptococcal infections†.

For the treatment of cryptococcal meningitis in HIV-infected adults, adolescents, and children, CDC, NIH, IDSA, and other clinicians state that the preferred regimen is initial (induction) therapy with IV amphotericin B (conventional or lipid formulation) given in conjunction with oral flucytosine for at least 2 weeks until there is evidence of clinical improvement and negative CSF culture after repeat lumbar puncture, then follow-up (consolidation) therapy with oral fluconazole administered for at least 8 weeks.

If an alternative regimen is necessary for the treatment of cryptococcal meningitis in HIV-infected adults, adolescents, and children who cannot receive the preferred regimen, some experts recommend initial (induction) and follow-up (consolidation) therapy with IV amphotericin B (conventional or lipid formulation) alone; induction therapy with IV amphotericin B (conventional or lipid formulation) given in conjunction with oral fluconazole, then consolidation therapy with oral fluconazole; induction therapy with oral or IV fluconazole used in conjunction with oral flucytosine, then consolidation therapy with oral fluconazole; or induction and consolidation therapy with oral fluconazole given alone. These alternative regimens may be less effective and are recommended only in patients who cannot tolerate or have not responded to the preferred regimen.

For the treatment of cryptococcal CNS infections in organ transplant recipients, IDSA recommends initial (induction) therapy with IV amphotericin B liposomal or amphotericin B lipid complex given in conjunction with oral flucytosine for at least 2 weeks, then follow-up (consolidation) therapy with oral fluconazole given for 8 weeks. If the induction regimen does not include flucytosine, it should be continued for at least 4–6 weeks. For organ transplant recipients with mild to moderate pulmonary cryptococcosis (without diffuse pulmonary infiltrates) or other mild to moderate cryptococcal infections not involving the CNS, IDSA recommends fluconazole given for 6–12 months.

In adults and children who do not have HIV infection and are not transplant recipients, IDSA states that the preferred regimen for the treatment of cryptococcal meningitis is initial (induction) therapy with IV amphotericin B (conventional formulation) given in conjunction with oral flucytosine for at least 4 weeks (a 2-week period of induction therapy can be considered in those who are immunocompetent, are without uncontrolled underlying disease, and are at low risk for therapeutic failure), then follow-up (consolidation) therapy with oral fluconazole administered for an additional 8 weeks or longer. IDSA states that data are insufficient to date to recommend fluconazole used alone or in conjunction with flucytosine for induction therapy in non-HIV-infected individuals with cryptococcal meningitis.

For the treatment of mild to moderate pulmonary cryptococcosis† (nonmeningeal) in immunocompetent or immunosuppressed adults or children, IDSA states that the regimen of choice is oral fluconazole given for 6–12 months. A regimen of oral fluconazole given for 6–12 months also can be considered for the treatment of nonmeningeal, nonpulmonary cryptococcosis† in immunocompetent individuals if the infection occurs at a single site and fungemia is not present.

Severe pulmonary cryptococcosis†, cryptococcemia†, and disseminated cryptococcal infections† in immunocompetent or immunosuppressed individuals should be treated using regimens recommended for cryptococcal meningitis.

Clinical Experience. The relative efficacy of initial therapy with conventional IV amphotericin B (0.7 mg/kg daily) given with oral flucytosine (100 mg/kg daily) or placebo for 2 weeks followed by oral fluconazole (800 mg daily for 2 days, then 400 mg daily for 8 weeks) or oral itraconazole (600 mg daily for 3 days, then 400 mg daily for 8 weeks) has been evaluated in a double-blind multicenter trial in patients with AIDS-associated cryptococcal meningitis. At 2 weeks, CSF cultures were negative in 60% of those who received amphotericin B with flucytosine compared with 51% of those who received amphotericin B alone. The clinical response to oral fluconazole or oral itraconazole for follow-up therapy was similar, but the rate of CSF sterilization at 10 weeks was higher in those who received fluconazole (72%) compared with those who received itraconazole (60%).

Fluconazole has been effective in the treatment of acute cryptococcal meningitis in some patients who failed to respond to amphotericin B therapy. However, there is some evidence that fluconazole may be less effective than amphotericin B during early therapy of acute cryptococcal meningitis in patients with AIDS and may produce slower sterilization of CSF. In a randomized, multicenter study comparing IV amphotericin B (mean dosage of 0.4–0.5 mg/kg daily for 10 weeks with or without concomitant oral flucytosine) with oral fluconazole (400 mg in the first day and 200–400 mg thereafter for 10 weeks) in AIDS patients with cryptococcal meningitis, therapy was effective in 40% of patients receiving amphotericin B and in 34% of those receiving fluconazole. Although overall mortality between patients receiving amphotericin B and patients receiving fluconazole was similar (14% in patients receiving amphotericin B versus 18% in patients receiving fluconazole), mortality was higher during the first 2 weeks of therapy in patients receiving fluconazole (15% versus 8% in those receiving amphotericin B). CSF cultures were positive for an average of about 42 or 64 days in patients receiving amphotericin B or fluconazole, respectively. In another study comparing amphotericin B (0.7 mg/kg daily for 1 week, followed by this dose 3 times weekly for 9 weeks combined with flucytosine 150 mg/kg daily) with oral fluconazole (400 mg daily for 10 weeks) in a limited number of AIDS patients with cryptococcal meningitis, initial therapy was effective in all patients receiving amphotericin B but in only 43% of patients receiving fluconazole; CSF cultures were positive for an average of about 16 and 41 days in patients receiving these respective therapies. While patient groups in this study were similar with respect to severity of cryptococcal infection, the helper/inducer ($CD4^+$, $T4^+$) T-cell count was lower in the fluconazole group, confounding interpretation.

Primary Prophylaxis to Prevent First Episode of Cryptococcosis Although there is some evidence that primary prophylaxis with fluconazole or itraconazole can reduce the frequency of cryptococcal disease in HIV-infected adults who have $CD4^+$ T-cell counts less than 100/mm^3, primary prophylaxis against cryptococcal disease in HIV-infected adults, adolescents, and children is not recommended in the US because of the relative infrequency of cryptococcal disease, lack of survival benefits associated with such prophylaxis, possibility of drug interactions, potential antifungal resistance, and cost.

Some experts recommend routine testing for cryptococcal antigen (CrAg) in all newly diagnosed HIV-infected individuals if they have $CD4^+$ T-cell counts of 100/mm^3 or lower.

Prevention of Recurrence (Secondary Prophylaxis) of Cryptococcosis Oral fluconazole is used for long-term suppressive or maintenance therapy (secondary prophylaxis) to prevent recurrence or relapse of cryptococcosis†.

CDC, NIH, and IDSA recommend that all HIV-infected adults, adolescents, and children who have been adequately treated for cryptococcus should receive secondary prophylaxis to prevent recurrence. Oral fluconazole is the drug of choice for secondary prophylaxis of cryptococcosis in HIV-infected adults, adolescents, and children; some experts suggest that oral itraconazole is an alternative in those who cannot tolerate fluconazole, but the drug may be less effective than fluconazole in preventing relapse of cryptococcosis. Conventional IV amphotericin B can be used for secondary prophylaxis if necessary in individuals who cannot receive azole antifungals, but is less effective and not generally recommended.

There is some evidence that the risk for recurrence of cryptococcosis is low in HIV-infected individuals who have been treated successfully with antifungal therapy, remain asymptomatic with regard to signs and symptoms of cryptococcosis, and have a sustained increase in $CD4^+$ T-cell counts in response to antiretroviral therapy. CDC, NIH, and IDSA state that consideration can be given to discontinuing secondary prophylaxis against cryptococcosis in HIV-infected adults, adolescents, and children 6 years of age or older who are asymptomatic for cryptococcosis and have received secondary antifungal prophylaxis (maintenance therapy) for at least 1 year, are receiving antiretroviral therapy, have had undetectable or low plasma HIV RNA levels for at least 3 months, and have $CD4^+$ T-cell counts of $100/mm^3$ or greater. If secondary prophylaxis against cryptococcosis is discontinued, the patient should be followed closely and serial cryptococcal serum antigen tests performed. These experts state that secondary prophylaxis against cryptococcosis should be reinitiated if the $CD4^+$ T-cell count decreases to less than $100/mm^3$ and/or the serum cryptococcal antigen titer increases.

Maintenance therapy (secondary prophylaxis) with oral fluconazole also is recommended in non-HIV-infected adults and children who have been adequately treated for cryptococcal meningitis, including organ transplant recipients who have been adequately treated for CNS cryptococcosis.

For additional information on management of cryptococcosis, the current clinical practice guidelines from IDSA available at http://www.idsociety.org and the current clinical practice guidelines from CDC, NIH, and IDSA on the prevention and treatment of opportunistic infections in HIV-infected individuals available at http://www.aidsinfo.nih.gov should be consulted.

***Cryptococcus gattii* Infections** Although data are limited, CDC, NIH, and IDSA state that recommendations for the treatment of CNS, pulmonary, or disseminated infections caused by *Cryptococcus gattii* and recommendations for maintenance therapy (secondary prophylaxis) of *C. gattii* infections are the same as the recommendations for *C. neoformans* infections. IDSA states that single, small cryptococcoma may be treated with oral fluconazole; however, induction therapy with a regimen of IV amphotericin B (conventional formulation) and oral flucytosine given for 4–6 weeks, followed by consolidation therapy with fluconazole given for 6–18 months should be considered for very large or multiple cryptococcomas caused by *C. gattii*. Regimens that include IV amphotericin B (conventional or liposomal formulations), oral flucytosine, and fluconazole have been effective in a few patients with CNS infections known to be caused by *C. gattii*.

There is some in vitro evidence that fluconazole may be less active against *C. gattii* than some other azole antifungals (e.g., itraconazole, posaconazole, voriconazole). (See Spectrum.)

■ Blastomycosis Oral fluconazole has been used in the treatment of blastomycosis† caused by *Blastomyces dermatitidis*. Oral itraconazole and IV amphotericin B are the drugs of choice for the treatment of blastomycosis. Although oral fluconazole is considered an alternative for the treatment of blastomycosis, it may be less effective and should be used only when the drugs of choice are contraindicated or cannot be used.

IV amphotericin B generally is the drug of choice for initial treatment of severe blastomycosis, especially infections involving the CNS, and for initial treatment of presumptive blastomycosis in immunocompromised patients, including HIV-infected individuals. Oral itraconazole is the preferred azole antifungal for the treatment of mild to moderate pulmonary blastomycosis or mild to moderate disseminated blastomycosis (without CNS involvement) and also is the preferred azole antifungal for follow-up therapy in patients with more severe infections after an initial response has been obtained with IV amphotericin B.

For the treatment of CNS blastomycosis, IDSA recommends initial treatment with IV amphotericin B, followed by an oral azole antifungal. Although oral fluconazole, oral itraconazole, or oral voriconazole can be used for follow-up treatment of CNS blastomycosis, the most appropriate azole for such treatment is unclear. Azole antifungals should not be relied on for initial treatment of CNS blastomycosis. The fact that treatment failures have been reported when an oral antifungal (e.g., ketoconazole) was used in the treatment of cutaneous or pulmonary blastomycosis in patients who had asymptomatic or subclinical CNS involvement at the time of the initial diagnosis should be considered when selecting an antifungal for patients with blastomycosis.

For additional information on management of blastomycosis, the current clinical practice guidelines from IDSA available at http://www.idsociety.org should be consulted.

■ Histoplasmosis Although oral fluconazole has been used with some success for the treatment of histoplasmosis† caused by *Histoplasma capsulatum*, it may be less effective than itraconazole and fluconazole-resistant *H. capsulatum* have developed in some HIV-infected patients who failed to respond to the drug.

The drugs of choice for the treatment of histoplasmosis, including histoplasmosis in HIV-infected individuals, are IV amphotericin B or oral itraconazole. IV amphotericin B is preferred for initial treatment of severe, life-threatening histoplasmosis, especially in immunocompromised patients such as those with HIV infection. Oral itraconazole generally is used for initial treatment of less severe disease (e.g., mild to moderate acute pulmonary histoplasmosis, chronic cavitary pulmonary histoplasmosis) and as follow-up therapy in the treatment of severe infections after a response has been obtained with IV amphotericin B. Other azole antifungals (fluconazole, ketoconazole, posaconazole, voriconazole) are considered second-line alternatives to itraconazole, but can be considered in patients who have less severe disease and cannot tolerate itraconazole.

In HIV-infected adults and adolescents, oral itraconazole is the drug of choice when primary prophylaxis is indicated to prevent initial episodes of histoplasmosis and also is the drug of choice for long-term suppressive or maintenance therapy (secondary prophylaxis) to prevent recurrence or relapse of histoplasmosis in HIV-infected adults, adolescents, and children. Although fluconazole may be less effective, some experts state that it can be considered an alternative for secondary prophylaxis against histoplasmosis in HIV-infected adults, adolescents, and children when itraconazole cannot be used.

For additional information on management of histoplasmosis, the current clinical practice guidelines from IDSA available at http://www.idsociety.org and the current clinical practice guidelines from CDC, NIH, and IDSA on the prevention and treatment of opportunistic infections in HIV-infected individuals available at http://www.aidsinfo.nih.gov should be consulted.

■ Sporotrichosis Fluconazole has been used as an alternative agent for the treatment of lymphocutaneous and cutaneous sporotrichosis† caused by *Sporothrix schenckii*.

IV amphotericin B usually is the drug of choice for initial treatment of severe, life-threatening sporotrichosis and whenever sporotrichosis is disseminated or has CNS involvement. Oral itraconazole is the drug of choice for the treatment of cutaneous, lymphocutaneous, or mild pulmonary or osteoarticular sporotrichosis and for follow-up treatment of severe infections after a response has been obtained with IV amphotericin B.

Although fluconazole can be used as an alternative for the treatment of cutaneous and lymphocutaneous sporotrichosis, it may be less effective than itraconazole and should be used only if the patient cannot tolerate itraconazole or other alternatives (oral terbinafine, oral potassium iodide, local hyperthermia).

Fluconazole should *not* be used for the treatment of pulmonary, osteoarticular, or meningeal sporotrichosis.

For additional information on management of sporotrichosis, the current clinical practice guidelines from IDSA available at http://www.idsociety.org should be consulted.

■ Dermatophytoses Oral fluconazole has been used in the treatment of certain dermatophytoses† (e.g., tinea capitis, tinea corporis, tinea cruris, tinea pedis) caused by *Epidermophyton*, *Microsporum*, or *Trichophyton*.

Oral fluconazole (3–6 mg/kg daily for 2–6 weeks) has been effective for the treatment of tinea capitis† in children 1.5–16 years of age, and has resulted in a clinical and mycologic cure in about 88–90% of patients. For the treatment of tinea corporis†, tinea cruris†, or tinea pedis† in adults, oral fluconazole has been effective when given in a once-weekly regimen (150 mg once weekly for 2–6 weeks), and there is evidence that this once-weekly regimen is as effective as a once-daily regimen of the drug (50 mg once daily) for the treatment of these infections. Results of a randomized study indicate that the eradication rate at the end of treatment in patients with tinea corporis or tinea cruris is 82–88% in those receiving the once-weekly regimen or 94–100% in those receiving the once-daily regimen; at 1-month follow-up, the overall eradication rates were 91–100 or 91–94%, respectively.

Tinea corporis and tinea cruris generally can be effectively treated using a topical antifungal; however, an oral antifungal regimen may be necessary if the disease is extensive, dermatophyte folliculitis is present, the infection is chronic or does not respond to topical therapy, or the patient is immunocompromised or has coexisting disease. Tinea capitis and tinea barbae generally are treated using an oral antifungal regimen. While topical antifungals usually are effective for the treatment of uncomplicated tinea manuum and tinea pedis, an oral antifungal usually is necessary for treatment of severe, chronic, or recalcitrant tinea pedis and for treatment of chronic moccasin-type (dry-type) tinea pedis.

■ Onychomycosis Oral fluconazole has been used for the treatment of onychomycosis†.

Selection of the most appropriate regimen for treatment of onychomycosis depends on the severity and extent of nail involvement, organisms involved, reported cure rates, adverse effects, drug interactions, cost, and patient and clinician preference. Onychomycosis generally is treated using an oral antifungal (e.g., terbinafine, itraconazole, fluconazole) and adjunctive physical modalities (nail trimming, aggressive debridement, nail avulsion) with or without a topical antifungal. Oral fluconazole has been recommended as an alternative in patients those who cannot tolerate terbinafine or itraconazole, but may be less effective than the other oral antifungals.

■ Pityriasis (Tinea) Versicolor Oral fluconazole has been used in the treatment of pityriasis (tinea) versicolor† caused by *Malassezia furfur* (*Pityrosporum orbiculare* or *P. ovale*).

Pityriasis (tinea) versicolor generally can be treated topically with an azole antifungal (e.g., clotrimazole, econazole, ketoconazole, miconazole, oxiconazole, sulconazole), an allylamine antifungal (e.g., naftifine, terbinafine), ciclopirox olamine, or certain other topical therapies (e.g., selenium sulfide 2.5%).

An oral antifungal (e.g., fluconazole, itraconazole, ketoconazole) may be indicated, with or without a topical agent, in patients who have extensive or severe infections or who fail to respond to or have frequent relapses with topical therapy.

■ Prevention of Candidiasis in Transplant Recipients, Cancer Patients, or Other Patients at High Risk Fluconazole is used prophylactically to reduce the incidence of candidiasis in patients at high risk, including those undergoing bone marrow transplantation (BMT), hematopoietic stem cell transplantation† (HSCT), or solid organ transplantation† and neutropenic patients undergoing chemotherapy or radiation therapy†. Fluconazole also is used to prevent *Candida* infections in high-risk patients undergoing urologic procedures† and for prevention of invasive candidiasis in high-risk patients in ICUs† and in low birthweight neonates† at high risk.

There is some evidence that fluconazole prophylaxis in transplant and cancer patients can reduce the frequency of oropharyngeal and/or systemic candidiasis during the period prior to neutrophil recovery. In addition, fluconazole prophylaxis may reduce the need for empiric antifungal therapy in such patients. Efficacy of oral fluconazole (400 mg once daily) for prophylaxis against fungal infections in neutropenic patients has been evaluated in a randomized, placebo-controlled study involving 274 cancer patients 18–80 years of age receiving cytotoxic chemotherapy or conditioning therapy for BMT. While the percentage of patients not requiring empiric therapy with IV amphotericin B therapy was similar in both groups (57% of those receiving fluconazole and 50% of those receiving placebo required no such therapy), complete success without fungal colonization was achieved in 37% of those receiving fluconazole and 20% of those receiving placebo. In addition, there was a lower incidence of superficial fungal infections in those receiving fluconazole (7%) than in those receiving placebo (18%), and only 3% of those receiving fluconazole developed definite invasive fungal infections compared with 17% of those receiving placebo. While fluconazole prophylaxis did not affect the overall mortality rate, intent-to-treat analysis indicates that the number of deaths attributable to definite invasive fungal infection was lower in the fluconazole group (1 of 15) than in the placebo group (6 of 15).

Use of primary antifungal prophylaxis in cancer patients undergoing myelosuppressive therapy or patients undergoing BMT or solid organ transplantation has been controversial, particularly since such prophylaxis may predispose the patient to colonization with resistant fungi and/or result in the emergence of highly resistant organisms. Some retrospective studies have shown an increased risk of colonization with *C. krusei* in BMT recipients and in neutropenic patients who received fluconazole prophylaxis; in one study, about 41% of patients receiving fluconazole had colonization with *C. krusei* compared with 17% of those not receiving fluconazole.

IDSA and other experts recommend primary prophylaxis against *Candida* infections in neutropenic patients when the risk of invasive candida infection is substantial (e.g., allogeneic HSCT recipients, patients with acute leukemia undergoing intensive remission-induction or salvage-induction chemotherapy) and states that an azole antifungal (fluconazole, itraconazole, posaconazole, voriconazole) or IV echinocandin (caspofungin or micafungin) can be used. These experts state that antifungal prophylaxis is not recommended if the anticipated duration of neutropenia is less than 7 days. If primary prophylaxis is used to prevent invasive candidiasis in high-risk adults in ICUs, IDSA recommends fluconazole as the drug of choice and IV echinocandins (anidulafungin, caspofungin, micafungin) as alternatives.

Fluconazole has been used for prophylaxis to reduce the incidence of invasive candidiasis in low birthweight neonates† at high risk. Although such prophylaxis has been controversial since there is concern that it may be associated with emergence of resistant fungi or increased colonization with fluconazole-resistant *Candida*, there is some evidence from retrospective and randomized controlled trials that fluconazole prophylaxis in low birthweight neonates can prevent colonization and reduce the incidence of invasive candidiasis. IDSA and AAP state that use of fluconazole prophylaxis can be considered for very low birthweight neonates (less than 1 kg) in nurseries that have high rates of neonatal invasive candidiasis.

For additional information on prevention of fungal infections in neutropenic patients, the current clinical practice guidelines from IDSA available at http://www.idsociety.org should be consulted.

Dosage and Administration

■ Administration Fluconazole is administered orally or by IV infusion.

Since absorption of fluconazole from the GI tract is rapid and almost complete, IV therapy with the drug generally is reserved for patients who do not tolerate or are unable to take the drug orally.

Oral Administration Fluconazole may be given orally without regard to meals.

Fluconazole powder for oral suspension should be reconstituted at the time of dispensing by adding 24 mL of distilled or purified water to the container labeled as containing 0.35 or 1.4 g of the drug to provide a suspension containing 50 or 200 mg/5 mL, respectively. The bottle should be shaken vigorously to suspend the powder; in addition, the suspension should be shaken well just prior to administration.

IV Administration IV infusions of fluconazole should be administered once daily at a rate not exceeding 200 mg/hour. Fluconazole injections for IV infusion should be inspected visually for discoloration and particulate matter prior to administration whenever solution and container permit. The injection for IV infusion should be discarded if the solution is cloudy or precipitated or if the seal is not intact.

Viaflex® Plus containers of fluconazole should be checked for minute leaks by firmly squeezing the bag. The injection should be discarded if the container seal is not intact or leaks are found or if the solution is cloudy or contains a precipitate. Additives should not be introduced into the plastic injection container. The injection in plastic containers should not be used in series connections with other plastic containers, since such use could result in air embolism from residual air being drawn from the primary container before administration from the secondary container is complete.

■ Dosage Oral and IV dosage of fluconazole are identical.

Use of a fluconazole loading dose that is twice the daily dosage generally is recommended on the first day of treatment since this results in fluconazole plasma concentrations on the second day of treatment that are close to steady-state concentrations.

Dosage of the drug should be based on the type and severity of the infection, identity of the causative organism, and the patient's renal function and response to therapy. Fluconazole therapy should be continued until clinical parameters and/or laboratory tests indicate that active fungal infection has subsided; an inadequate period of treatment may lead to recurrence of active infection.

Adult Dosage **Candidemia and Disseminated Candida Infections.** For the treatment of systemic candidiasis (candidemia, disseminated candidiasis, pneumonia), the manufacturer states that adults have received fluconazole in a dosage of 400 mg daily.

For the treatment of urinary tract infections or peritonitis, the manufacturer states that fluconazole has been given in a dosage of 50–200 mg daily.

For the treatment of candidemia in *nonneutropenic* or *neutropenic* adults, the Infectious Diseases Society of America (IDSA) recommends a loading dose of 800 mg (12 mg/kg) of fluconazole on the first day of therapy, followed by 400 mg (6 mg/kg) daily with treatment continued for 2 weeks after documented clearance of *Candida* from the bloodstream, resolution of candidemia symptoms, and resolution of neutropenia.

For the treatment of chronic disseminated candidiasis (hepatosplenic) in adults who are clinically stable, IDSA recommends that fluconazole be given in a dosage of 400 mg (6 mg/kg) daily. These experts recommend that severely ill patients receive IV amphotericin B initially for several weeks, then follow-up therapy with fluconazole in a dosage of 400 mg (6 mg/kg) daily. Antifungal treatment should be continued until lesions resolve (usually several months) and should be continued through periods of immunosuppression.

For the treatment of CNS candidiasis, IDSA recommends an initial regimen of IV amphotericin B (with or without oral flucytosine) for several weeks, then follow-up therapy with fluconazole in a dosage of 400–800 mg (6–12 mg/kg) daily. Antifungal treatment should be continued until signs and symptoms, CSF abnormalities, and radiologic abnormalities have resolved.

When fluconazole is used for the treatment of urinary tract infections caused by fluconazole-susceptible *Candida*, IDSA recommends that adults receive fluconazole in a dosage of 200 mg (3 mg/kg) daily for 2 weeks for the treatment of symptomatic cystitis or 200–400 mg (3–6 mg/kg) daily for 2 weeks for the treatment of pyelonephritis.

For the treatment of osteoarticular infections caused by *Candida*, IDSA recommends that adults receive fluconazole in a dosage of 400 mg (6 mg/kg) daily given for 6–12 months in those with osteomyelitis or for 6 weeks in those with septic arthritis. If septic arthritis involved a prosthetic device that cannot be removed, long-term suppressive or maintenance therapy (secondary prophylaxis)† with fluconazole given in a dosage of 400 mg (6 mg/kg) daily is recommended to prevent recurrence.

For the treatment of endocarditis (native or prosthetic valve) or implantable cardiac device infections caused by *Candida*, IDSA recommends an initial regimen of IV amphotericin B (with or without oral flucytosine) or an IV echinocandin (anidulafungin, caspofungin, micafungin), then follow-up treatment with fluconazole in a dosage of 400–800 mg (6–12 mg/kg) daily. Antifungal treatment should be continued for at least 6 weeks after valve replacement surgery. Long-term suppressive or maintenance therapy (secondary prophylaxis)† with fluconazole given in dosage of 400–800 mg (6–12 mg/kg) daily is recommended to prevent recurrence in those with native valve endocarditis who cannot undergo valve replacement and in those with prosthetic valve endocarditis.

For the treatment of chorioretinitis (with or without vitritis) caused by *Candida*, IDSA recommends a loading dose of 800 mg (12 mg/kg) of fluconazole on the first day of therapy, followed by 400–800 mg (6–12 mg/kg) daily for at least 4–6 weeks. If there is macular involvement, intravitreal amphotericin B or voriconazole may also be indicated.

Oropharyngeal Candidiasis. For the treatment of oropharyngeal candidiasis, the manufacturer recommends that fluconazole be given in a dosage of 200 mg as a single dose on day 1, then 100 mg once daily. Although clinical evidence of oropharyngeal candidiasis generally resolves within several days following initiation of fluconazole therapy, the manufacturer recommends that the drug be continued for at least 2 weeks to decrease the likelihood of relapse.

For the treatment of moderate to severe oropharyngeal candidiasis, IDSA recommends that adults receive fluconazole in a dosage of 100–200 mg daily for 7–14 days.

For the treatment of oropharyngeal candidiasis in adults and adolescents with human immunodeficiency virus (HIV) infection, the US Centers for Disease Control and Prevention (CDC), National Institutes of Health (NIH), and IDSA recommend that fluconazole be given in a dosage of 100 mg daily for 7–14 days.

If long-term suppressive or maintenance therapy (secondary prophylaxis)† with fluconazole is used in HIV-infected adults and adolescents with frequent or severe recurrences of oropharyngeal candidiasis, a dosage of 100 mg once daily or 3 times weekly is recommended. Although only limited data are available regarding the safety of discontinuing secondary prophylaxis against oropharyngeal candidiasis in HIV-infected individuals, consideration can be given to discontinuing such prophylaxis in HIV-infected adults if the CD4+ T-cell count increases to greater than 200/mm^3 in response to antiretroviral therapy.

Esophageal Candidiasis. For the treatment of esophageal candidiasis, the manufacturer recommends that adults receive fluconazole in a dosage of 200 mg as a single dose on day 1, followed by 100 mg once daily. Dosages up to 400 mg once daily may be used depending on the patient's response. The manufacturer recommends that fluconazole therapy be continued for a minimum of 3 weeks and for at least 2 weeks after symptoms have resolved.

For the treatment of esophageal candidiasis, IDSA recommends that adults receive fluconazole in a dosage of 200–400 mg (3–6 mg/kg) daily for 14–21 days.

For the treatment of esophageal candidiasis in HIV-infected adults and adolescents, CDC, NIH, and IDSA recommend that adults receive fluconazole in a dosage of 100 mg (up to 400 mg) once daily for 14–21 days.

If long-term suppressive or maintenance therapy (secondary prophylaxis)† with fluconazole is used in HIV-infected adults and adolescents with frequent or severe recurrences of esophageal candidiasis, a dosage of 100–200 mg daily or, alternatively, 100–200 mg 3 times weekly is recommended. Although only limited data are available regarding the safety of discontinuing secondary prophylaxis against esophageal candidiasis in HIV-infected individuals, consideration can be given to discontinuing such prophylaxis in these HIV-infected adults if the CD4+ T-cell count increases to greater than 200/mm^3 in response to antiretroviral therapy.

Vulvovaginal Candidiasis. For the treatment of uncomplicated vulvovaginal candidiasis in *nonpregnant* women, the usual dosage of oral fluconazole is a single (1 day only) 150-mg oral dose.

For the treatment of recurrent vulvovaginal candidiasis† in *nonpregnant* women, CDC recommends that 100, 150, or 200 mg of oral fluconazole be given every third day for 3 doses (i.e., days 1, 4, and 7) to attempt mycologic remission. Then, to prevent recurrence, a maintenance regimen of 100, 150, or 200 mg of oral fluconazole should be given once weekly for 6 months. IDSA recommends a maintenance regimen of 150 mg of oral fluconazole given once weekly for 6 months.

For the treatment of severe vulvovaginal candidiasis† in *nonpregnant* women, CDC recommends a 2-dose regimen of oral fluconazole (two 150-mg doses given 72 hours [3 days] apart). IDSA recommends that 150 mg of oral fluconazole be given once every 72 hours for a total of 2 or 3 doses.

For the treatment of uncomplicated vulvovaginal candidiasis or recurrent or severe vulvovaginal candidiasis† in *nonpregnant* HIV-infected women, CDC, NIH, and IDSA recommend the same regimens used for the treatment of these infections in women without HIV infection.

Blastomycosis. If oral fluconazole is used as an alternative for the treatment of mild to moderate pulmonary or mild to moderate disseminated blastomycosis† without CNS involvement in adults, IDSA recommends a dosage of 400–800 mg daily.

If oral fluconazole is used for follow-up therapy in the treatment of CNS blastomycosis† in adults after an initial regimen of IV amphotericin B given for 4–6 weeks, IDSA recommends that fluconazole be given in a dosage of 800 mg daily for at least 12 months and until CSF abnormalities have resolved.

Coccidioidomycosis. For the treatment of coccidioidomycosis†, IDSA and others recommend that adults receive oral or IV fluconazole in a dosage of 400–800 mg once daily. For diffuse pneumonia or disseminated coccidioidomycosis (nonmeningeal), fluconazole usually is used in conjunction with IV amphotericin B or as follow-up after an initial regimen of IV amphotericin B. The duration of treatment for uncomplicated coccidioidal pneumonia usually is 3–6 months; the total duration of treatment for diffuse pneumonia and chronic progressive fibrocavitary pneumonia usually is at least 1 year.

For the treatment of mild coccidioidomycosis (e.g., focal pneumonia) in HIV-infected adults and adolescents, CDC, NIH, and IDSA recommend that oral fluconazole be given in a dosage of 400 mg once daily. This dosage also is recommended for the treatment of severe, nonmeningeal coccidioidomycosis (e.g., diffuse pulmonary infection) in HIV-infected adults and adolescents, but the drug usually is used in conjunction with IV amphotericin B or as follow-up after an initial regimen of IV amphotericin B.

For the treatment of coccidioidal meningitis† in HIV-infected adults and adolescents or other individuals, a fluconazole dosage of 400–800 mg once daily has been recommended. Concomitant intracisternal, intraventricular, or intrathecal amphotericin B therapy has been used in some patients. Consultation with an expert who has experience in treating coccidioidal meningitis is recommended.

When primary prophylaxis against coccidioidomycosis† is indicated in HIV-infected adults and adolescents who live in areas endemic for coccidioidomycosis, have a newly positive IgM or IgG serologic test suggesting imminent active disease, and have CD4+ T-cell counts less than 250/mm^3, CDC, NIH, and IDSA recommend that fluconazole be given in a dosage of 400 mg once daily.

For long-term suppressive or maintenance therapy (secondary prophylaxis) to prevent recurrence or relapse of coccidioidomycosis† in HIV-infected adults and adolescents who have been adequately treated for the disease, CDC, NIH, and IDSA recommend that fluconazole be given in a dosage of 400 mg once daily. In HIV-infected adults and adolescents with a history of adequately treated focal coccidioidal pneumonia, discontinuance of secondary prophylaxis against coccidioidomycosis can be considered after 12 months if they are receiving antiretroviral therapy and have CD4+ T-cell counts of 250/mm^3 or greater. Such patients should be monitored for recurrence (e.g., serial chest radiographs, coccidioidal serology). In HIV-infected adults and adolescents with a history of adequately treated diffuse pulmonary or disseminated coccidioidomycosis (including meningeal infections), secondary prophylaxis against coccidioidomycosis should be continued lifelong, regardless of antiretroviral therapy or immune reconstitution.

Cryptococcosis. For the treatment of cryptococcal meningitis, the manufacturer recommends that adults receive fluconazole in a dosage of 400 mg as a single dose on day 1, followed by 200–400 mg once daily for 10–12 weeks after the CSF is sterile. Some evidence suggests that the 400-mg dosage is more effective than lower dosage in the treatment of this infection.

For the treatment of cryptococcal meningitis in HIV-infected adults and adolescents, CDC, NIH, and IDSA recommend a regimen than includes initial (induction) therapy with IV amphotericin B and oral flucytosine given for at least 2 weeks, then follow-up (consolidation) therapy with oral fluconazole given in a dosage of 400 mg (6 mg/kg) once daily and continued for at least 8 weeks.

For the treatment of cryptococcal meningitis in HIV-infected adults who cannot receive flucytosine, IDSA recommends induction therapy with IV amphotericin B given in conjunction with oral or IV fluconazole 800 mg daily for at least 2 weeks, then consolidation therapy with oral fluconazole given in a dosage of 800 mg daily and continued for at least 8 weeks. For the treatment of cryptococcal meningitis in HIV-infected adults who cannot receive IV amphotericin B or oral flucytosine, IDSA states that fluconazole can be given as monotherapy in a dosage of 800 mg daily or higher (preferably 1.2 g daily or higher) and continued for 10–12 weeks. Although fluconazole dosage as high as 2 g daily has been used, this dosage may be associated with toxicity. If high fluconazole dosage is used, the daily dosage should be given in divided doses to minimize GI toxicity.

For the treatment of cryptococcal meningitis in HIV-infected adults and adolescents who cannot receive amphotericin B, CDC, NIH, and IDSA recommend induction therapy with oral or IV fluconazole given in a dosage of 400 or 800 mg daily in conjunction with oral flucytosine for at least 2 weeks, then consolidation therapy with oral fluconazole given in a dosage of 400 mg daily and continued for at least 8 weeks. Alternatively, if oral or IV fluconazole is used alone for induction therapy, these experts recommend that the drug be given in a dosage of 1.2 g daily for at least 2 weeks, then consolidation therapy with oral fluconazole be given in a dosage of 400 mg daily and continued for at least 8 weeks.

For the treatment of CNS cryptococcosis in adult organ transplant recipients, IDSA recommends induction therapy with IV amphotericin B liposomal or IV amphotericin B lipid complex and oral flucytosine given for at least 2 weeks, then consolidation therapy with oral fluconazole 400–800 mg (6–12 mg/kg) daily given for 8 weeks. For the treatment of mild to moderate pulmonary cryptococcosis (without pulmonary infiltrates) or other mild to moderate non-CNS disease, IDSA recommends fluconazole in a dosage of 400 mg (6 mg/kg) daily for 6–12 months.

For the treatment of cryptococcal meningitis in immunocompetent adults *without* HIV infection who are not transplant recipients, IDSA recommends induction therapy with IV amphotericin B in conjunction with oral flucytosine given for at least 4 weeks, then consolidation therapy with oral fluconazole given in a dosage of 400 mg daily and continued for 8 weeks. If the patient is immunocompetent without uncontrolled, underlying disease and is at low risk for therapeutic failure, IDSA states that this induction regimen can be given for only 2 weeks, then consolidation therapy with oral fluconazole administered in a dosage of 800 mg (12 mg/kg) daily should be given for 8 weeks.

For the treatment of mild to moderate pulmonary cryptococcosis† (nonmeningeal) in immunocompetent or immunocompromised adults, IDSA recommends that fluconazole be given in a dosage of 400 mg (6 mg/kg) daily for 6–12 months. This same dosage can be used for the treatment of nonpulmonary cryptococcosis at a single site† (nonmeningeal).

Severe pulmonary cryptococcosis†, cryptococcemia†, or disseminated cryptococcosis† in immunocompetent or immunocompromised adults should be treated using a regimen recommended for adults with cryptococcal meningitis.

For long-term suppressive or maintenance therapy (secondary prophylaxis) to prevent recurrence or relapse of cryptococcosis† in adult organ transplant recipients or immunocompetent adults *without* HIV infection who are not transplant recipients who have been adequately treated for CNS cryptococcosis, the usual dosage of oral fluconazole is 200–400 mg once daily for 6–12 months.

For long-term suppressive or maintenance therapy (secondary prophylaxis) to prevent recurrence or relapse of cryptococcosis† in HIV-infected adults and adolescents or other adults and adolescents who have had documented, adequately treated cryptococcal meningitis, the usual dosage of oral fluconazole is 200 mg once daily. Secondary prophylaxis should be initiated after the primary infection has been adequately treated and usually is continued for at least 1 year. Consideration can be given to discontinuing secondary prophylaxis against cryptococcosis in HIV-infected adults who are asymptomatic for cryptococcosis and have received secondary antifungal prophylaxis for at least 1 year, are receiving antiretroviral therapy, have had undetectable or low plasma HIV RNA levels for at least 3 months, and have CD4+ T-cell counts of 100/mm^3 or greater. Secondary prophylaxis against cryptococcosis should be reinitiated if the CD4+ T-cell count decreases to less than 100/mm^3 and/or the serum cryptococcal antigen titer increases.

Histoplasmosis. If fluconazole is used for the treatment of histoplasmosis†, a dosage of 400–800 mg once daily is recommended. A fluconazole regimen of 800 mg daily given for 12 weeks, then 400 mg daily has been used.

If fluconazole is used as an alternative for treatment of less severe histoplasmosis† in HIV-infected adults and adolescents, CDC, NIH, and IDSA recommend a dosage of 800 mg daily.

If fluconazole is used as an alternative for long-term suppressive or maintenance therapy (secondary prophylaxis) to prevent recurrence or relapse of histoplasmosis† in HIV-infected adults and adolescents, CDC, NIH, and IDSA recommend a dosage of 400 mg daily. Consideration can be given to discontinuing secondary prophylaxis against histoplasmosis in HIV-infected adults and adolescents who have received secondary antifungal prophylaxis for at least 1 year, have negative fungal blood cultures and serum histoplasma antigen levels less than 2 ng/mL, have been receiving antiretroviral therapy for at least 6 months, and have CD4+ T-cell counts of 150/mm^3 or greater. Secondary prophylaxis against histoplasmosis should be reinitiated if the CD4+ T-cell count decreases to less than 150/mm^3.

Sporotrichosis. If oral fluconazole is used for the treatment of lymphocutaneous and cutaneous sporotrichosis†, a dosage of 400–800 mg once daily is recommended in adults when other drugs cannot be used.

Dermatophytoses. For the treatment of dermatophytoses†, oral fluconazole has been given in a dosage of 150 mg once weekly for 2–6 weeks. For the treatment of tinea corporis that involves small, well-defined lesions, some clinicians recommend that oral fluconazole be given in a dosage of 250 mg once weekly for 2–4 weeks.

For the treatment of tinea pedis†, some clinicians recommend that oral fluconazole be given in a dosage of 150–200 mg once weekly for 1–8 weeks.

Onychomycosis. For the treatment of onychomycosis†, oral fluconazole has been given in a dosage of 100–450 mg once weekly for 2–12 months. Some clinicians recommend that oral fluconazole be given in a dosage of 150–300 mg once weekly for 3–6 months for fingernail infections or for 6–12 months for toenail infections.

Pityriasis (Tinea) Versicolor. For the treatment of pityriasis (tinea) versicolor†, adults have received oral fluconazole as a single 400-mg dose. Alternatively, 150 mg has been given once weekly for 2 or 4 weeks or 300 mg has been given once weekly for 2 weeks.

Prevention of Candidiasis in Transplant Recipients, Cancer Patients, or Other Patients at High Risk. For the prevention of candidiasis in bone marrow transplant (BMT) recipients, the recommended dosage of fluconazole is 400 mg once daily. In patients in whom severe granulocytopenia (neutrophil count less than 500/ mm^3) is anticipated, fluconazole therapy should be initiated several days before expected onset of neutropenia and should be continued for 7 days after the neutrophil count exceeds 1000/mm^3. Antifungal prophylaxis is not usually recommended if the anticipated duration of neutropenia is less than 7 days.

For the prevention of *Candida* infections in hematopoietic stem cell transplant (HSCT) recipients†, adults and adolescents should receive oral or IV fluconazole in a dosage of 400 mg once daily. Fluconazole prophylaxis should be initiated on the day of transplantation (i.e., day 0) and continued until engraftment occurs (i.e., approximately 30 days after HSCT) or until 7 days after the neutrophil count exceeds 1000/mm^3.

If fluconazole is used for prophylaxis against candidiasis in high-risk patients in intensive care units (ICUs)† with a known high incidence of invasive candidiasis, IDSA states that the drug should be given in a dosage of 400 mg (6 mg/kg) once daily.

Pediatric Dosage The usual oral or IV dosage of fluconazole in pediatric patients ranges from 3–12 mg/kg once daily; dosages exceeding 600 mg daily are not recommended. The manufacturer states that a dosage of 3, 6, or 12 mg/kg daily in pediatric patients is equivalent to a dosage of 100, 200, or 400 mg daily, respectively, in adults. Some older children may have clearances similar to those of adults.

Based on limited pharmacokinetic data, the manufacturer recommends that premature neonates (gestational age 26–29 weeks) receive the usual pediatric dosage once every 72 hours during the first 2 weeks of life and then the usual pediatric dosage once daily thereafter.

Candidemia and Disseminated Candida Infections. The usual dosage of fluconazole for the treatment of systemic *Candida* infections in pediatric patients is 6–12 mg/kg daily.

For the treatment of meningitis or septicemia caused by susceptible *Candida*, neonates and infants 3 months of age or younger† have received fluconazole in a dosage of 5–6 mg/kg once daily given orally or by IV infusion over 1 hour. In some neonates and infants with septicemia, an initial loading dose of 10 mg/kg was administered followed by 5 mg/kg once daily.

If fluconazole is used as an alternative for the treatment of neonatal candidiasis†, IDSA and the American Academy of Pediatrics (AAP) recommend a dosage of 12 mg/kg daily for at least 3 weeks.

Oropharyngeal Candidiasis. For the treatment of oropharyngeal candidiasis in pediatric patients, the recommended dosage of fluconazole is 6 mg/kg on day 1, followed by 3 mg/kg once daily. The manufacturer recommends that treatment be continued for a minimum of 2 weeks to decrease the likelihood of relapse.

For the treatment of oropharyngeal candidiasis in HIV-infected infants and children, CDC, NIH, and IDSA recommend that fluconazole be given in a dosage of 6–12 mg/kg (up to 400 mg) once daily for 7–14 days.

If long-term suppressive or maintenance therapy (secondary prophylaxis)† with fluconazole is used in HIV-infected infants and children with frequent or severe recurrences of oropharyngeal candidiasis, a dosage of 3–6 mg/kg (up to 200 mg) once daily is recommended. Limited data are available regarding the safety of discontinuing secondary prophylaxis against oropharyngeal candidiasis in HIV-infected individuals. In HIV-infected infants and children, consideration can be given to discontinuing such prophylaxis when the CD4+ T-cell count or percentage increases to CDC immunologic category 2 or 1.

Esophageal Candidiasis. For the treatment of esophageal candidiasis in pediatric patients, the manufacturer recommends 6 mg/kg of fluconazole on day 1, followed by 3 mg/kg once daily. Dosage may be increased up to 12 mg/kg daily if necessary, based on the condition of the patient and the response to the drug. The manufacturer recommends that treatment be continued for a minimum of 3 weeks and for at least 2 weeks after symptoms have resolved.

For the treatment of esophageal candidiasis in HIV-infected infants and children, CDC, NIH, and IDSA recommend that fluconazole be given in a dosage of 6–12 mg/kg (up to 600 mg) once daily for a minimum of 3 weeks and for at least 2 weeks after symptoms resolve.

If long-term suppressive or maintenance therapy (secondary prophylaxis)† with fluconazole is used in HIV-infected infants and children with frequent or severe recurrences of esophageal candidiasis, a dosage of 3–6 mg/kg (up to 200 mg) once daily is recommended. Limited data are available regarding the safety of discontinuing secondary prophylaxis against esophageal candidiasis in HIV-infected individuals. In HIV-infected infants and children, consideration can be given to discontinuing such prophylaxis when the CD4+ T-cell count or percentage increases to CDC immunologic category 2 or 1.

Coccidioidomycosis. For the treatment of mild to moderate coccidioidomycosis (nonmeningeal)† (e.g., focal pneumonia) in HIV-infected infants and children, CDC, NIH, and IDSA recommend that oral or IV fluconazole be given in a dosage of 6–12 mg/kg (up to 400 mg) once daily. If oral or IV fluconazole is used for the treatment of diffuse pulmonary or disseminated coccidioidomycosis (nonmeningeal)† in HIV-infected infants and children who cannot receive IV amphotericin B, these experts recommend a dosage of 12 mg/kg (up to 800 mg) once daily.

For the treatment of coccidioidal meningitis† in HIV-infected infants and children, CDC, NIH, and IDSA recommend that oral or IV fluconazole be given in a dosage of 12 mg/kg (up to 800 mg) once daily. Consultation with an expert in treating coccidioidal meningitis is recommended.

For prevention of recurrence (secondary prophylaxis) of coccidioidomycosis† in HIV-infected infants and children, CDC, NIH, and IDSA recommend that fluconazole be given in a dosage of 6 mg/kg (up to 400 mg) once daily. Secondary prophylaxis should be initiated after the primary infection has been adequately treated and continued indefinitely in HIV-infected infants and children, regardless of antiretroviral therapy or immune reconstitution.

Cryptococcosis. The manufacturer recommends that cryptococcal meningitis in pediatric patients be treated with an initial 12-mg/kg dose on day 1, followed by 6 mg/kg once daily for 10–12 weeks after the CSF becomes culture negative. Dosage may be increased to 12 mg/kg daily if necessary based on the condition of the patient and the response to the drug.

For the treatment of cryptococcal meningitis in HIV-infected infants and children, CDC, NIH, and IDSA recommend a regimen that includes induction therapy with IV amphotericin B given in conjunction with oral flucytosine for at least 2 weeks, then consolidation therapy with oral or IV fluconazole given in a dosage of 12 mg/kg on day 1 and then 10–12 mg/kg (up to 800 mg) once daily for at least 8 weeks.

For the treatment of cryptococcal meningitis in HIV-infected infants and children who cannot receive IV amphotericin B, CDC, NIH, and IDSA recommend induction therapy with oral or IV fluconazole given in a dosage of 12 mg/kg on day 1 and then 10–12 mg/kg (up to 800 mg) once daily given in conjunction with oral flucytosine (25 mg/kg 4 times daily) for at least 2 weeks, then consolidation therapy with oral or IV fluconazole given in a dosage of 10–12 mg/kg (up to 800 mg) once daily for at least 8 weeks.

For the treatment of localized cryptococcosis without CNS involvement† (e.g., isolated pulmonary disease), CDC, NIH, and IDSA recommend that HIV-infected infants and children receive fluconazole in a dosage of 12 mg/kg on day 1 and then 6–12 mg/kg (up to 600 mg) once daily. The duration of treatment depends on the clinical response and site and severity of infection. A duration of 6–12 months has been recommended.

For the treatment of disseminated or severe pulmonary cryptococcosis without CNS involvement† in HIV-infected infants and children who cannot receive amphotericin B, CDC, NIH, and IDSA recommend that fluconazole be given in a dosage of 12 mg/kg on day 1 and then 6–12 mg/kg (up to 600 mg) once daily. The duration of treatment depends on the clinical response and site and severity of infection. A duration of 6–12 months has been recommended.

For long-term suppressive or maintenance therapy (secondary prophylaxis) to prevent recurrence or relapse of cryptococcosis† in HIV-infected infants and children who have been treated for cryptococcal meningitis, fluconazole is given in a dosage of 6 mg/kg (up to 200 mg) once daily. Secondary prophylaxis should be initiated after the primary infection has been adequately treated and usually is continued for at least 1 year. Consideration can be given to discontinuing secondary prophylaxis against cryptococcosis in HIV-infected children 6 years of age or older who are asymptomatic for cryptococcosis, have received secondary prophylaxis for at least 1 year, are receiving antiretroviral therapy, have had undetectable or low plasma HIV RNA levels for at least 3 months, and have $CD4^+$ T-cell counts of 100/mm^3 or higher. Secondary prophylaxis against cryptococcosis should be reinitiated if the $CD4^+$ T-cell count decreases to less than 100/mm^3.

Histoplasmosis. If oral fluconazole is used as an alternative for treatment of less severe histoplasmosis† in HIV-infected infants and children, CDC, NIH, and IDSA recommend a dosage of 3–6 mg/kg (up to 200 mg) once daily for acute primary pulmonary histoplasmosis.

If oral fluconazole is used as an alternative for long-term suppressive or maintenance therapy (secondary prophylaxis) to prevent recurrence or relapse of histoplasmosis† in HIV-infected infants and children, CDC, NIH, and IDSA recommend a dosage of 3–6 mg/kg (up to 200 mg) once daily. Consideration can be given to discontinuing secondary prophylaxis against histoplasmosis in HIV-infected infants and children who have received secondary prophylaxis for at least 1 year, have negative fungal blood cultures and serum histoplasma antigen levels less than 2 ng/mL, have been receiving antiretroviral therapy for at least 6 months, and have $CD4^+$ T-cell percentage greater than 15% ($CD4^+$ T-cell counts exceeding 150/mm^3 in those 6 years of age or older). Secondary prophylaxis against histoplasmosis should be reinitiated if these parameters are not met.

Dermatophytoses. For the treatment of tinea capitis† in children 1.5–16 years of age, oral fluconazole has been given in a dosage of 3–6 mg/kg daily for 2–6 weeks. AAP recommends a dosage of 6 mg/kg daily for 3–6 weeks.

For the treatment of tinea corporis† or tinea cruris† in children, some clinicians recommend that oral fluconazole be given in a dosage of 150 mg once weekly for 2–6 weeks.

For the treatment of tinea manuum† or tinea pedis† in children, some clinicians recommend that oral fluconazole be given in a dosage of 150 mg once weekly for 4–6 weeks.

Onychomycosis. For the treatment of onychomycosis† in children, some clinicians recommend that oral fluconazole be given in a dosage of 3–6 mg/kg once weekly for 12–16 weeks for fingernail infections or 3–6 mg/kg once weekly for 18–26 weeks for toenail infections. Others recommend 150 mg once weekly for 4–6 months for fingernail infections or 150 mg once weekly for 9–12 months for toenail infections.

Pityriasis (Tinea) Versicolor. For the treatment of pityriasis (tinea) versicolor†, children 11 years of age or older have received oral fluconazole as a single 400-mg dose. Alternatively, 150 mg has been given once weekly for 4 weeks.

Prevention of Candida Infections in Hematopoietic Stem Cell Transplant Recipients. For the prevention of *Candida* infections in HSCT recipients†, children 6 months to 13 years of age should receive oral or IV fluconazole in a dosage of 3–6 mg/kg daily (maximum 600 mg daily). Fluconazole prophylaxis should be initiated on the day of transplantation (i.e., day 0) and continued until engraftment occurs (i.e., approximately 30 days after HSCT) or until 7 days after the neutrophil count exceeds 1000/mm^3.

Prevention of Candida Infections in Low Birthweight Neonates. For prophylaxis to reduce the incidence of invasive candidiasis in low birthweight neonates† at high risk, oral or IV fluconazole has been given in a variety of dosage regimens. If fluconazole prophylaxis is used in neonates at high risk, antifungal resistance, toxicity, and neurodevelopmental outcomes should be monitored.

IDSA states that fluconazole given in a dosage of 3 or 6 mg/kg twice weekly reduces the rate of invasive candidiasis in premature neonates in nurseries that have a high incidence of *Candida* infections.

For prophylaxis in low birthweight neonates (less than 1 kg) at high risk, AAP recommends that fluconazole be initiated with a dose of 3 mg/kg given IV during the first 48–72 hours after birth, followed by 3 mg/kg IV twice weekly for 4–6 weeks or until IV access is no longer required for care.

■ **Dosage in Renal Impairment** In patients with impaired renal function receiving multiple doses, fluconazole dosage must be modified in response to the degree of impairment and should be based on the patient's measured or estimated creatinine clearance. The patient's creatinine clearance (Cl_{cr}) can be estimated by using the following formula:

$$Ccr\ male = \frac{(140 - age) \times weight}{72 \times serum\ creatinine}$$

$$Ccr\ female = 0.85 \times Ccr\ male$$

where age is in years, weight is in kg, and serum creatinine is in mg/dL.

The manufacturer recommends that adults with impaired renal function receive an initial loading dose of 50–400 mg of fluconazole (based on the type of infection being treated), then patients with creatinine clearances exceeding 50 mL/minute should receive 100% of the usual daily dose and those with creatinine clearances of 50 mL/minute or less should receive 50% of the usual daily dose. Patients who are undergoing regular dialysis should receive 100% of the usual daily dose after each dialysis period; on days the patient is not receiving dialysis, reduced dosage based on creatinine clearance should be used. These dosage recommendations are based on the pharmacokinetics of the drug following multiple doses; further dosage adjustments may be necessary depending on the condition of the patient.

The manufacturer states that modification of the recommended single-dose regimen of oral fluconazole for the treatment of vulvovaginal candidiasis is not necessary in patients with impaired renal function.

The manufacturer states that the pharmacokinetics of fluconazole have not been studied in children with impaired renal function; recommendations for dosage reduction in such children should parallel those recommended for adults.

Cautions

Although fluconazole generally is well tolerated, there have been rare reports of serious hepatotoxicity (including some fatalities) in patients receiving the drug. Adverse effects have been reported in about 5–30% of patients receiving fluconazole for 7 days or longer and have been severe enough to require discontinuance of the drug in about 1–2.8% of patients. In addition, adverse effects have been reported in 26–31% of women receiving a single 150-mg oral dose of fluconazole for the treatment of vulvovaginal candidiasis.

Evaluation of some adverse effects and establishment of a causal relationship to fluconazole have been difficult since the drug has been used in many patients with serious underlying diseases, including leukemia, cancer, and acquired immunodeficiency syndrome (AIDS), who were receiving multiple drugs concomitantly. In some cases, the underlying fungal infection being treated (e.g., meningitis) may have caused or contributed to the reported effect (e.g., nervous system effects). In some patients, particularly those with serious underlying diseases such as AIDS and cancer, changes in renal and hematologic function and hepatic abnormalities have been observed during treatment with fluconazole or comparative agents, but the clinical importance and relation to treatment is uncertain. The manufacturer states that adverse effects have been reported more frequently in patients with human immunodeficiency virus (HIV) infection than in patients without HIV infection; however, the proportion of patients requiring discontinuance of fluconazole because of severe adverse effects is similar in both groups.

■ **GI Effects** Mild to moderate nausea, vomiting, abdominal pain, and diarrhea have been reported in about 1.5–8.5% of patients receiving fluconazole. Only rarely were such adverse GI effects severe enough to require discontinuance of the drug. Flatus, bloating, dry mouth, hiccups, heartburn, and anorexia have been reported rarely. Adverse GI effects have been reported in about 15% of women receiving a single dose of fluconazole for the treatment of vulvovaginal candidiasis; abdominal pain, nausea, diarrhea, dyspepsia, and dysgeusia occurred in about 6, 7, 3, 1, and 1% of such women, respectively.

■ **Dermatologic and Sensitivity Reactions** Rash, including diffuse rash accompanied by eosinophilia, and pruritus have been reported in up to about 5% of patients receiving fluconazole. Exfoliative skin disorders have been reported rarely in patients with serious underlying disease (principally AIDS or malignancy) receiving fluconazole; fatalities have been reported. Stevens-Johnson syndrome, which can be fatal, also has been reported in patients receiving fluconazole. However, a definite causal relationship between exfoliative skin eruptions and the drug has not been established, since most patients were receiving multiple drugs concomitantly with fluconazole. Acute generalized exanthematous pustulosis and increased sweating also have been reported during postmarketing experience.

Anaphylaxis has been reported rarely in patients receiving fluconazole. Angioedema and anaphylactic reactions have been reported rarely in women who received a single 150-mg oral dose of fluconazole for the treatment of vulvovaginal candidiasis.

■ **Hepatic Effects** Serious hepatic reactions (e.g., necrosis, clinical hepatitis, cholestasis, fulminant hepatic failure) have been reported rarely in patients receiving fluconazole therapy. The manufacturer states that a clear relationship between these hepatic effects and daily dosage, duration of therapy, gender, or age has not been demonstrated. While hepatotoxicity usually has been reversible, fatalities have been reported. Fatalities principally have occurred in patients with serious underlying disease (e.g., AIDS, malignancy) who were receiving fluconazole concomitantly with other drugs; however, at least one fatality involved an immunocompetent geriatric individual with renal impairment who developed fulminant hepatic necrosis within 10 days after fluconazole therapy was initiated.

Mild, transient increases (1.5–3 times the upper limit of normal) in serum concentrations of AST (SGOT), ALT (SGPT), alkaline phosphatase, γ-glutamyltransferase (GGT, γ-glutamyl transpeptidase, GGTP), and bilirubin have been reported in about 5–7% of patients receiving fluconazole. In most reported cases, concentrations returned to pretreatment levels either during or after fluconazole therapy and were not associated with hepatotoxicity. However, higher increases in serum transaminase concentrations (8 or more times the upper limit of normal), which required discontinuance of the drug, have been reported in about 1% of patients receiving fluconazole. Any patient who develops abnormal liver function test results while receiving fluconazole should be closely monitored for the development of more severe hepatic injury. (See Cautions: Precautions and Contraindications.)

■ **Cardiovascular Effects** Prolonged QT interval has occurred in patients receiving azole antifungals. Prolonged QT interval and torsades de pointes have been reported rarely during postmarketing surveillance in patients receiving fluconazole. Most reported cases involved seriously ill patients with multiple confounding risk factors (e.g., structural heart disease, electrolyte abnormalities, concomitant drugs) that may have contributed to these events.

■ **Nervous System Effects** Dizziness and headache have been reported in up to about 2% of patients receiving fluconazole. Somnolence, insomnia, delirium/coma, dysesthesia, psychiatric disturbances, malaise, asthenia, paresthesia of hands and feet, tremor, and fatigue have been reported rarely. Seizures also have been reported and have occurred in at least one AIDS patient immediately following administration of a single 100-mg oral dose of the drug. Adverse nervous system effects have been reported in about 14–20% of women receiving a single dose of fluconazole for the treatment of vulvovaginal candidiasis; headache and dizziness occurred in about 13 and 1% of such women, respectively.

■ **Hematologic Effects** Eosinophilia has been reported in some patients receiving fluconazole. Anemia, leukopenia, neutropenia, and thrombocytopenia also have been reported. In at least one AIDS patient, thrombocytopenia occurred during fluconazole therapy and resolved following discontinuance of the drug. Severe thrombocytopenia that required treatment and necessitated discontinuance of fluconazole therapy also has been reported.

■ **Endocrine Effects** Studies using usual dosages of fluconazole have not shown evidence of adverse effects related to possible inhibition of testosterone or steroid synthesis. In one study in healthy premenopausal women receiving fluconazole, there was no effect on serum estradiol concentrations or on serum cortisol stimulation response. Results of studies in men receiving oral fluconazole dosages of 25–400 mg once daily for up to 30 days indicate that serum testosterone concentrations are unaffected by the drug. The manufacturer states that in healthy adults who receive fluconazole dosages of 200–400 mg once daily for up to 14 days, there are only small and inconsistent effects on testosterone concentrations, endogenous corticosteroid concentrations, or ACTH-stimulated cortisol response.

■ **Other Adverse Effects** Fever, edema, pleural effusion, oliguria, hypotension, arthralgia/myalgia, and finger stiffness have been reported rarely in patients receiving fluconazole.

Hypokalemia, which required potassium replacement therapy and/or discontinuance of fluconazole, has occurred occasionally, including in several neutropenic patients with acute myeloid leukemia. Increased serum creatinine and BUN concentrations also have been reported. Mild (1.5–2 times the upper limit of normal) increases in serum concentrations of creatine kinase (CK, creatine phosphokinase, CPK) have been reported in at least one patient with coccidioidal meningitis who received fluconazole concomitantly with intrathecal amphotericin B.

Alopecia has been reported in patients receiving fluconazole. In a retrospective study of patients who received fluconazole (100–800 mg daily) for the treatment of systemic fungal infections, alopecia was reported in up to 20% of patients. Alopecia occurred in both men and women, usually was evident at about 3 months (range: 2 weeks to 7 months) after initiation of fluconazole therapy, and resolved in most patients within about 6 months after discontinuance of the drug or dosage reduction. Alopecia involved varying degrees of loss of scalp hair in all patients, but about 30% of patients also reported substantial loss of facial, axillary, pubic, leg, or chest hair.

■ **Precautions and Contraindications** Fluconazole is contraindicated in patients with known hypersensitivity to the drug or any ingredient in the formulation. Although information concerning cross-sensitivity between fluconazole and other triazole or imidazole antifungals is not available, the manufacturer states that fluconazole should be used with caution in individuals hypersensitive to other azoles.

Fluconazole should be used with caution in patients with hepatic impairment. Although serious adverse hepatic effects have been reported only rarely with fluconazole, the possibility that these effects may occur during fluconazole therapy should be considered. (See Cautions: Hepatic Effects.) Fluconazole should be discontinued if signs and symptoms consistent with liver disease develop. If abnormal liver function test results occur during fluconazole therapy, the patient should be monitored for the development of more severe hepatic injury.

Fluconazole should be used with caution in patients with renal impairment. (See Dosage and Administration: Dosage in Renal Impairment.)

Patients receiving fluconazole who drive or operative machinery should be cautioned to take into account that dizziness or seizures may occur occasionally.

Diflucan® powder for oral suspension contains sucrose and should not be used in patients with hereditary fructose, glucose-galactose malabsorption, and sucrase-isomaltase deficiency.

Use of fluconazole may result in overgrowth of nonsusceptible strains of *Candida* other than *C. albicans*, including *C. krusei*. Superinfection caused by nonsusceptible strains of *Candida* has been reported in some patients receiving fluconazole; these patients may require alternative antifungal therapy.

Because prolonged QT interval and torsades de pointes have occurred in patients receiving fluconazole, the drug should be used with caution in patients with potentially proarrhythmic conditions and risk factors for QT prolongation. (See Cautions: Cardiovascular Effects.) Concomitant use of fluconazole and drugs that are metabolized by the cytochrome P450 (CYP) isoenzyme 3A4 and are known to prolong the QT interval (e.g., astemizole [no longer commercially available in the US], cisapride, pimozide, quinidine) is contraindicated. (See Drug Interactions: Drugs that Prolong the QT Interval.)

Because potentially fatal exfoliative skin disorders have been reported rarely in patients with a serious underlying disease receiving fluconazole, the possibility that these effects can occur should be considered. (See Cautions: Dermatologic and Sensitivity Reactions.) If a patient with deep-seated fungal infection develops rash during fluconazole therapy, the patient should be monitored closely and the drug discontinued if the lesions progress. If rash that may be attributable to fluconazole develops in a patient with superficial fungal infections, the drug should be discontinued.

■ **Pediatric Precautions** The manufacturer states that efficacy of fluconazole in children younger than 6 months has not been established; however, the drug has been used safely and effectively in neonates and children younger than 6 months of age (including neonates as young as 1 day of age).

Adverse effects reported in children receiving fluconazole generally have been similar to those reported in adults. In phase II/III trials in pediatric patients 1 day to 17 years of age who received fluconazole in dosages up to 15 mg/kg daily, adverse effects occurred in 13% and were severe enough to require discontinuance of the drug in 2.3% of patients. GI effect, including vomiting, abdominal pain, nausea, and diarrhea, occurred in 2–5% of these pediatric patients. Adverse effects reported when oral or IV fluconazole has been used in neonates and infants (3–6 mg/kg daily) have included transient increases in serum transaminase concentrations, vomiting, and eosinophilia; severe thrombophlebitis was reported in at least one neonate.

■ **Geriatric Precautions** Rash, vomiting, and diarrhea have been reported more frequently in geriatric adults than in younger adults. Although anemia and acute renal failure occurred more frequently in patients 65 years of age and older than in those 12–65 years of age during postmarketing surveillance, the relationship of these events to fluconazole is unknown.

Clinical studies of fluconazole did not include a sufficient number of patients 65 years of age or older to determine whether geriatric patients respond differently for each indication than younger individuals. Other reported clinical experience has not identified differences in response between geriatric and younger patients.

Fluconazole is primarily excreted by the kidneys as unchanged drug. Because geriatric patients may have decreased renal function, careful dosage selection and monitoring of renal function are advised.

■ **Mutagenicity and Carcinogenicity** There was no evidence of mutagenicity when fluconazole was tested with or without metabolic inactivation in 4 strains of *Salmonella typhimurium* or in the mouse lymphoma L5178Y system. In addition, there was no evidence of chromosomal mutations in vivo on murine bone marrow cells following administration of fluconazole or in vitro on human lymphocytes exposed to fluconazole concentrations of 1 mg/mL.

There was no evidence of carcinogenicity in studies in mice and rats receiving oral fluconazole dosages of 2.5–10 mg/kg daily (approximately 2–7 times the usual human dosage) for 24 months. However, there was an increased incidence of hepatocellular adenomas in male rats receiving an oral fluconazole dosage of 5 or 10 mg/kg daily.

■ **Pregnancy, Fertility, and Lactation** ***Pregnancy*** FDA alerted clinicians in April 2016 that it is reviewing safety data regarding use of oral fluconazole during pregnancy and advised cautious prescribing of the drug until the review is completed.

There are no adequate and controlled studies to date using fluconazole in pregnant women.

Congenital abnormalities have been reported in infants born to women who received high-dose fluconazole (400–800 mg daily) for the treatment of serious, life-threatening fungal infections during most or all of the first trimester. These reports have involved a rare and distinct pattern of birth defects that includes brachycephaly, abnormal facies, abnormal calvarial development, cleft palate, femoral bowing, thin ribs and long bones, arthrogryposis, and congenital heart disease and are similar to those reported in animal reproduction studies. Based on these data, FDA reclassified high-dose fluconazole (400–800 mg daily) as pregnancy category D (i.e., there is positive evidence of human fetal risk based on human data, but potential benefits of the drug in pregnant women with serious or life-threatening conditions may be acceptable despite its risks).

Because human data available at that time did not identify an increased risk of congenital anomalies with the use of fluconazole administered as a single 150-mg oral dose for the treatment of vulvovaginal candidiasis, the single-dose oral fluconazole regimen was classified by FDA as pregnancy category C (see Users Guide). Data from a recent Danish study designed to assess the association between use of oral fluconazole during pregnancy and risk of spontaneous abortion and stillbirth indicate an increased risk of spontaneous abortion (i.e., miscarriage during gestational weeks 7 through 22) in pregnant women treated with oral fluconazole (most women received a total cumulative dose of 150–300 mg) compared with matched control pregnancies not exposed to oral fluconazole. Therefore, FDA alerted clinicians that it is reviewing data from the Danish study and additional data and, after completing the review, will communicate its conclusions and updated recommendations regarding use of the single-dose 150-mg oral fluconazole regimen during pregnancy.

The US Centers for Disease Control and Prevention (CDC) states that topical (intravaginal) azole antifungals (not oral fluconazole) should be used for the treatment of vulvovaginal candidiasis during pregnancy.

The Infectious Diseases Society of America (IDSA) states that use of fluconazole for the treatment of serious fungal infections (e.g., blastomycosis†, candidiasis, histoplasmosis†, coccidioidomycosis†, cryptococcosis) should be avoided during pregnancy.

Patients who are pregnant or actively trying to become pregnant should talk to their clinician about alternatives for treatment of vulvovaginal candidiasis.

If fluconazole is used during pregnancy or if the patient becomes pregnant while receiving the drug, the patient should be informed of the potential hazard to the fetus.

In several reproduction studies in pregnant rabbits receiving oral fluconazole dosages of 5, 10, 20, 25, or 75 mg/kg once daily during organogenesis, maternal weight gain was impaired at all dosage levels and abortions occurred with the 75-mg/kg dosage (approximately 20–60 times the usual human dosage); no adverse fetal effects were detected. In studies in pregnant rats receiving oral fluconazole during organogenesis, maternal weight gain was impaired and placental weights were increased at dosages of 25 mg/kg once daily. Although there were no fetal effects in rats receiving oral fluconazole in a dosage of 5 or 10 mg/kg once daily, increases in fetal anatomical variants (supernumerary ribs, renal pelvis dilation) and delays in ossification occurred in those receiving oral dosages of 25 mg/kg or greater once daily. When oral fluconazole dosages of 80 mg/kg once daily (approximately 20–60 times the usual human dosage) to 320 mg/kg once daily were used in these rats, there was an increase in embryolethality and fetal abnormalities (i.e., wavy ribs, cleft palate, abnormal craniofacial ossification). These adverse effects in rats may be attributed to a species-specific effect of fluconazole on estrogen synthesis since lowered estrogen is known to cause effects on pregnancy, organogenesis, and parturition. There is no evidence to date that estrogen concentrations are decreased in women receiving fluconazole. (See Cautions: Other Adverse Effects.)

Fertility Reproduction studies in male and female rats receiving fluconazole in an oral dosage of 5, 10, or 20 mg/kg once daily or an IV dosage of 5, 25, or 75 mg/kg once daily did not reveal evidence of impaired fertility; however, onset of parturition was delayed slightly with the 20-mg/kg oral dosage. In one study in rats receiving an IV fluconazole dosage of 5, 20, or 40 mg/kg once daily, dystocia and prolongation of parturition occurred in a few dams with the 20-mg/kg (approximately 5–15 times the usual human dosage) and 40-mg/kg dosages but not with the 5-mg/kg dosage. Disturbances in parturition in rats were reflected by a slight increase in the number of stillborn pups and a decrease in neonatal survival; these effects presumably are related to a species-specific estrogen-lowering effect caused by high doses of fluconazole.

Lactation Fluconazole is distributed into human milk in concentrations similar to those achieved in plasma. Administration of a single 150-mg oral dose to several nursing women resulted in peak plasma fluconazole concentrations of 2.61 mcg/mL (range: 1.57–3.65 mcg/mL). Fluconazole should be used with caution in nursing woman.

Drug Interactions

While fluconazole can alter the pharmacokinetics of certain drugs that undergo hepatic metabolism, the magnitude of such alterations appears to be less than those associated with ketoconazole; however, comparative studies have not been performed to date. In addition, the possibility that the risk of developing such interactions may be increased at relatively high fluconazole dosages (e.g., 200 mg daily or more) should be considered.

■ **Drugs Metabolized by Hepatic Microsomal Enzymes** Fluconazole is a potent inhibitor of cytochrome P450 (CYP) isoenzyme 2C9 and a moderate inhibitor of CYP3A4. Because fluconazole has a long half-life, its enzyme-inhibiting effects persist for 4–5 days following discontinuance. Concomitant use of fluconazole and drugs metabolized by CYP2C9 or 3A4 may result in increased plasma concentrations of the concomitant drug. When fluconazole is used concomitantly with drugs metabolized by these enzymes, caution should be used and the patient carefully monitored.

■ **Drugs Affecting Gastric Acidity** Studies in fasting, healthy adults indicate that GI absorption of fluconazole is not affected substantially by concomitant use of drugs that decrease gastric acid output or increase gastric pH. When a single 100-mg oral dose of fluconazole was administered 2 hours after a single 400-mg oral dose of cimetidine, the area under the plasma concentration-time curve (AUC) of fluconazole was decreased 13% and peak plasma fluconazole concentrations were decreased by 21%; these effects were *not* considered clinically important. Administration of antacids containing aluminum hydroxide or magnesium hydroxide either with or immediately prior to a single 100-mg oral dose of fluconazole had no effect on absorption or elimination of the antifungal.

■ **Drugs that Prolong the QT Interval** Concomitant use of fluconazole with drugs that are metabolized by CYP3A4 and known to prolong the QT interval (e.g., cisapride, astemizole, pimozide, quinidine) is contraindicated. Concomitant use with erythromycin should be avoided (see Erythromycin under Drugs Interactions: Macrolides).

Prolongation of the QT interval and QT interval corrected for rate (QT_c) and, rarely, serious cardiovascular effects, including arrhythmias (e.g., ventricular tachycardia, atypical ventricular tachycardia [torsades de pointes, ventricular fibrillation]), cardiac arrest, palpitations, hypotension, dizziness, syncope, and death, have been reported in patients receiving recommended dosages of terfenadine or astemizole (neither antihistamine currently is commercially available in the US) concomitantly with another azole antifungal, ketoconazole. Ketoconazole can markedly inhibit the metabolism of astemizole or terfenadine, probably via inhibition of the cytochrome P-450 microsomal enzyme system, resulting in increased plasma concentrations of unchanged drug (to measurable levels) and reduced clearance of the active desmethyl or carboxylic acid metabolite, respectively. Such alterations in the pharmacokinetics of these antihistamines may be associated with prolongation of the QT and QT_c intervals. Similar alterations in the pharmacokinetics of these antihistamines and/or adverse cardiac effects also have been reported in patients receiving the drugs concomitantly with itraconazole, although in vitro data suggest that itraconazole may have a less pronounced effect than ketoconazole on the pharmacokinetics of astemizole. Studies have been performed to determine whether similar interactions occur with concomitant use of terfenadine and fluconazole. In one study, concomitant use of terfenadine and fluconazole (at a dosage of 200 mg daily) did not result in prolongation of QT interval; however, use of higher fluconazole dosages (400 or 800 mg daily) in another study resulted in increased plasma concentrations of terfenadine. The manufacturer of fluconazole has stated that concomitant use of terfenadine and fluconazole in a daily dosage of 400 mg or greater has been contraindicated and it was recommended that patients be carefully monitored if lower fluconazole dosages (i.e., less than 400 mg daily) were administered in patients receiving terfenadine.

Concomitant use of fluconazole and cisapride (currently commercially available in the US only under a limited-access protocol) may result in increased plasma cisapride concentrations and has rarely been associated with adverse cardiac events including torsades de pointes. In a placebo-controlled, randomized, multiple-dose study in individuals receiving fluconazole (200 mg daily), initiation of cisapride (20 mg 4 times daily) after 7 days of fluconazole therapy resulted in a 102–192% increase in the AUC and a 92–153% increase in peak plasma concentrations of cisapride. In addition, administration of fluconazole to individuals receiving cisapride (20 mg 4 times daily for 5 days) resulted in a significant increase in the QT interval corrected for rate. The manufacturer of fluconazole states that concomitant use of fluconazole and cisapride is contraindicated.

Concomitant use of erythromycin and fluconazole may increase the risk of QT interval prolongation and torsades de pointes and subsequent sudden cardiac death. Concomitant use of erythromycin and fluconazole should be avoided.

■ **Anticoagulants** Increased prothrombin time has been reported in patients receiving fluconazole concomitantly with a coumarin anticoagulant (e.g., warfarin). In one study in healthy adults receiving 200 mg of fluconazole daily or placebo, area under the prothrombin time versus time (for a 7-day post-warfarin period) curve for a single 15-mg warfarin dose increased by about 12% when concomitant fluconazole versus placebo were compared. Increased prothrombin times also have been reported when lower dosages of fluconazole (100 mg once daily) were administered concomitantly with warfarin sodium. Concomitant use of fluconazole with nicoumalone (a coumarin anticoagulant not commercially available in the US) resulted in increased prothrombin time and intracranial hemorrhage in at least one patient. Prothrombin times should be monitored carefully when fluconazole is used concomitantly with a coumarin anticoagulant.

■ **Antidiabetic Agents** Administration of fluconazole in individuals receiving tolbutamide, glyburide, or glipizide has resulted in increased AUCs and peak plasma concentrations and reduced metabolism of the antidiabetic agent. The mean increase in AUC or peak plasma concentrations of tolbutamide, glyburide, or glipizide reported in healthy adults receiving concomitant fluconazole is 26–49 or 11–19%, respectively. Clinically important hypoglycemia may be precipitated by concomitant use of oral hypoglycemic agents and fluconazole, and at least one fatality has been reported from hypoglycemia in a patient receiving glyburide and fluconazole concomitantly. In several individuals, symptoms consistent with hypoglycemia occurred; oral glucose therapy was necessary in a few cases.

If fluconazole is used concomitantly with tolbutamide, glyburide, glipizide, or any other oral sulfonylurea antidiabetic agent, blood glucose concentrations should be monitored carefully and dosage of the antidiabetic agent adjusted as necessary.

■ **Antifungal Agents** ***Amphotericin B*** Although the clinical importance is unclear, results of in vitro studies evaluating the antifungal effects of amphotericin B used concomitantly with fluconazole or other azole antifungals (e.g., clotrimazole, itraconazole, ketoconazole) against *Candida albicans*, *C. pseudotropicalis*, *C. glabrata*, or *Aspergillus fumigatus* indicate that antagonism can occur with these combinations. Since amphotericin B exerts its antifungal activity by binding to sterols in the fungal cell membrane and azole antifungals act by altering the cell membrane, antagonism is theoretically possible; however, it is unclear whether such antagonism actually would occur in vivo. Results of studies evaluating combined use of fluconazole and amphotericin B in animal models of aspergillosis, candidiasis, or cryptococcosis have been conflicting. While antagonism occurred in some models (*A. fumigatus* infection in mice, rabbits, or rats treated with amphotericin B and fluconazole), the combination resulted in additive or indifferent effects in other models (e.g., *C. albicans* or *Cryptococcus neoformans* infection in mice or rabbits treated with amphotericin B and fluconazole). In a few studies evaluating the drugs in murine cryptococcosis or candidiasis, sequential use of an initial large dose of amphotericin B followed by an azole antifungal (e.g., fluconazole) was uniformly effective in prolonging survival and decreasing fungal burden. Because further study is needed regarding the interaction between azole antifungals and amphotericin B, it has been suggested that fluconazole and amphotericin B be used concomitantly with caution and close monitoring, particularly in immunocompromised patients.

Results of an in vitro study indicate that the combination of amphotericin B and fluconazole may be synergistic, additive, or indifferent against *Pseudallescheria boydii*; there was no evidence of antagonism.

Flucytosine In an in vitro study, the combination of fluconazole and flucytosine was synergistic, additive, or indifferent against *Cryptococcus neoformans*; there was no evidence of antagonism. Synergism generally did not occur if the *C. neoformans* isolates had fluconazole MICs of 8 mcg/mL or greater. It has been suggested that synergism between the drugs may occur because fluconazole damages the fungal cell membrane allowing greater intracellular penetration of flucytosine.

Voriconazole In healthy men, concomitant use of oral voriconazole (400 mg every 12 hours for 1 day, then 200 mg every 12 hours for 2.5 days) and oral fluconazole (400 mg on day 1, then 200 mg once daily for 4 days) resulted in a 79 and 57% increase in AUC and peak plasma concentration of voriconazole, respectively. Reduced dosage or dosing frequency of voriconazole and fluconazole did not overcome this pharmacokinetic interaction. Concomitant use of voriconazole and fluconazole is not recommended and should be avoided. If voriconazole is used sequentially after fluconazole, the patient should be monitored closely for voriconazole-associated adverse events, particularly during the first 24 hours after the last fluconazole dose.

■ **Antimycobacterial Agents** ***Rifabutin*** Concomitant use of fluconazole (200 mg daily) and rifabutin (300 mg daily) in individuals with human immunodeficiency virus (HIV) infection results in substantially increased plasma concentrations and AUCs of rifabutin and its major metabolite (LM565). This effect presumably occurs via inhibition of CYP isoenzymes involved in metabolism of rifabutin and may account in part for the increased incidence of certain adverse effects (e.g., uveitis) reported with concomitant rifabutin and fluconazole therapy.

Rifabutin and fluconazole should be used concomitantly with caution and close monitoring.

Rifampin Concomitant use of fluconazole and rifampin may affect the pharmacokinetics of both drugs. Administration of a single 200-mg oral dose of fluconazole in healthy adults receiving rifampin (600 mg daily) resulted in approximately a 25% decrease in the AUC and a 20% decrease in the plasma half-life of fluconazole. There also is some evidence that concomitant use of fluconazole and rifampin results in increased rifampin plasma concentrations compared with administration of rifampin alone. The clinical importance of this possible pharmacokinetic interaction between fluconazole and rifampin is unclear; however, it has been suggested that such an interaction may have contributed to relapse of cryptococcal meningitis in a few patients who were receiving fluconazole concomitantly with rifampin.

Rifampin and fluconazole should be used concomitantly with caution and close monitoring. The manufacturer of fluconazole states that, depending on clinical circumstances, consideration can be given to increasing fluconazole dosage when the drug is administered concomitantly with rifampin.

■ **Antiretroviral Agents** ***HIV Nonnucleoside Reverse Transcriptase Inhibitors (NNRTIs)*** **Delavirdine.** Concomitant use of delavirdine (300 mg every 8 hours) and fluconazole (400 mg daily) for 2 weeks in HIV-infected patients was well tolerated and did not appear to affect the pharmacokinetics of either drug. Dosage adjustments are not necessary in patients receiving delavirdine and fluconazole concomitantly.

Efavirenz. Concomitant use of efavirenz (400 mg daily) and fluconazole (200 mg daily) for 7 days in healthy individuals did not result in clinically important changes in the pharmacokinetics of either drug; dosage adjustments are not necessary in patients receiving the drugs concomitantly.

Etravirine. Concomitant use of etravirine and fluconazole results in substantial increases in etravirine plasma concentrations and AUC, but does not have a clinically important effect on fluconazole concentrations. Although dosage adjustments are not needed for either drug if etravirine is used concomitantly with fluconazole, these drugs should be used concomitantly with caution because only limited data are available regarding the safety of increased etravirine concentrations.

Nevirapine. Concomitant use of nevirapine and fluconazole may result in increased nevirapine concentrations, but has no effect on fluconazole concentrations. If nevirapine and fluconazole are used concomitantly, the patient should be monitored for nevirapine toxicity since the risk of hepatotoxicity may be increased. Alternatively, a different antiretroviral agent can be used.

Rilpivirine. Concomitant use of fluconazole and rilpivirine may result in increased rilpivirine plasma concentrations. If rilpivirine is used concomitantly with fluconazole, rilpivirine dosage adjustments are not needed; however, the patient should be monitored for breakthrough fungal infections.

HIV Nucleoside Reverse Transcriptase Inhibitors (NRTIs) Concomitant use of fluconazole appears to interfere with the metabolism and clearance of zidovudine. In one study in men with HIV infection who received zidovudine (200 mg every 8 hours) alone or in conjunction with fluconazole (400 mg daily), the AUC of zidovudine was increased 74% (range: 20–173%), peak serum zidovudine concentrations were increased 84% (range: −1 to 227%), and the terminal elimination half-life of the drug was increased 128% (range: −4 to 189%) in patients receiving concomitant fluconazole. Zidovudine and fluconazole should be used concomitantly with caution and close monitoring. Patients should be monitored closely for zidovudine-associated adverse effects, and zidovudine dosage reductions may be considered.

In one limited study in patients with HIV infection receiving oral didanosine (3.2–7.8 mg/kg daily), concomitant use of oral fluconazole (200 mg every 12 hours for 2 doses, then 200 mg once daily for 6 days) did not result in any clinically important differences in the AUC of didanosine, peak serum didanosine concentrations, or time to peak concentrations.

Concomitant use of fluconazole and stavudine does not result in a clinically important alteration in the pharmacokinetics of either drug.

HIV Protease Inhibitors (PIs) **Atazanavir.** Pharmacokinetic interactions have not been observed and are unlikely if atazanavir (unboosted, *ritonavir-boosted*, or *cobicistat-boosted*) is used concomitantly with fluconazole. Dosage adjustments are not necessary if *ritonavir-boosted* or *cobicistat-boosted* atazanavir is used concomitantly with fluconazole.

Indinavir. Concomitant use of indinavir (1 g every 8 hours) and fluconazole (400 mg once daily) for 1 week resulted in a slight decrease in the AUC of indinavir and no change in the AUC of fluconazole. This pharmacokinetic interaction is not considered clinically important; dosage adjustments are not necessary in patients receiving indinavir concomitantly with fluconazole.

Lopinavir. Clinically important pharmacokinetic interactions between the fixed combination of lopinavir and ritonavir (lopinavir/ritonavir) and fluconazole are not expected.

Ritonavir. Concomitant use of ritonavir (200 mg every 6 hours for 4 days) and fluconazole (400 mg on day 1, then 200 mg daily for 4 days) resulted in a 12 and 15% increase in the AUC and peak plasma concentration of ritonavir, respectively. Dosage adjustments are not needed.

Saquinavir. Concomitant use of saquinavir (1200 mg as Invirase® 3 times daily) and fluconazole (single 400-mg dose on day 2, then 200 mg daily) has resulted in approximate increases of 50 and 56% in saquinavir AUC and peak plasma concentrations, respectively. This interaction is a result of inhibition of CYP3A4 with decreased metabolism of saquinavir and inhibition of P-glycoprotein. Saquinavir and fluconazole should be used concomitantly with caution and close monitoring; saquinavir dosage may need to be adjusted.

Data are not available regarding concomitant use of *ritonavir-boosted* saquinavir and fluconazole; some experts state that dosage adjustments are not needed.

Tipranavir. Concomitant use of *ritonavir-boosted* tipranavir and fluconazole results in increased tipranavir peak plasma concentrations and AUC, but does not affect the pharmacokinetics of fluconazole.

Although dosage adjustments are not needed, fluconazole dosage should not exceed 200 mg daily in patients receiving *ritonavir-boosted* tipranavir. If high-dose fluconazole is indicated, an alternative antiretroviral should be considered.

■ **Calcium-channel Blocking Agents** Fluconazole has the potential to increase systemic exposure to certain dihydropyridine calcium channel blocking agents (amlodipine, felodipine, isradipine, nifedipine, verapamil) that are metabolized by CYP3A4. Calcium channel blocking agents and fluconazole should be used concomitantly with caution and close monitoring; patients should be monitored frequently for adverse events.

■ **CNS Agents** ***Anticonvulsants*** Concomitant use of carbamazepine and fluconazole has resulted in a 30% increase in carbamazepine concentrations and has increased carbamazepine-associated toxicity, presumably as the result of fluconazole inhibiting CYP isoenzymes involved in metabolism of the anticonvulsant. Carbamazepine and fluconazole should be used concomitantly with caution and close monitoring; carbamazepine dosage adjustment may be necessary based on plasma carbamazepine concentrations and clinical effect.

Concomitant use of fluconazole and phenytoin has resulted in increased plasma phenytoin concentrations and AUC and has resulted in phenytoin toxicity. In one study in healthy adults, minimum plasma phenytoin concentrations increased 128% and the AUC of the drug increased 75% during concomitant fluconazole administration; fluconazole pharmacokinetics were not affected. It has been suggested that such alterations in phenytoin pharmacokinetics result from fluconazole-induced inhibition of metabolism of the anticonvulsant. Phenytoin and fluconazole should be used concomitantly with caution and close monitoring. Plasma phenytoin concentrations should be monitored carefully, and dosage of the anticonvulsant adjusted as needed whenever fluconazole is initiated or discontinued.

Antipsychotics Although data are lacking, concomitant use of fluconazole and pimozide may result in increased plasma pimozide concentrations with the potential for QT interval prolongation and, rarely, torsades de pointes. Concomitant use of fluconazole and pimozide is contraindicated.

Benzodiazepines Concomitant use of oral or IV fluconazole and midazolam results in substantial increases in the peak plasma concentration and AUC of midazolam (AUC increased 244–272%) and can increase the psychomotor effects of the benzodiazepine; peak plasma concentration and AUC of fluconazole are not affected. This pharmacokinetic interaction appears to be more pronounced with oral fluconazole than with IV fluconazole. In mechanically ventilated patients sedated with IV midazolam, concomitant use of IV fluconazole resulted in a 20–300% increase in plasma midazolam concentrations in some patients within 18–48 hours after the first dose of fluconazole. In addition, administration of oral fluconazole to healthy individuals receiving IV midazolam reportedly results in a 50% decrease in clearance of the benzodiazepine. Administration of fluconazole to healthy individuals receiving oral midazolam resulted in a 3.5-fold increase in midazolam AUC, a 2.5-fold increase in peak plasma midazolam concentrations, and prolonged midazolam half-life. If a short-acting benzodiazepine metabolized by CYP isoenzymes is used in a patient receiving fluconazole, the patient should be carefully monitored and a decrease in benzodiazepine dosage considered. Because of concerns that prolonged sedation may occur if fluconazole is administered to patients sedated with IV midazolam, some clinicians suggest that a decrease in the midazolam dosage be considered if there is evidence of increased sedation during concomitant fluconazole therapy.

Concomitant use of fluconazole and a single dose of triazolam has resulted in a 50% increase in the AUC of triazolam and a 20–32% increase in peak plasma triazolam concentrations and has prolonged the half-life of triazolam by 25–50%. Triazolam and fluconazole should be used concomitantly with caution and close monitoring; adjustment of triazolam dosage may be necessary.

Nonsteroidal Anti-inflammatory Agents Concomitant use of fluconazole (200 mg daily) and celecoxib (200 mg) has increased the peak plasma concentration and AUC of celecoxib by 68 and 134%, respectively.

Concomitant use of flurbiprofen and fluconazole has increased the peak plasma concentration and AUC of flurbiprofen by 23 and 81%, respectively.

When ibuprofen (single 400-mg dose) was administered to healthy individuals receiving oral fluconazole (400 mg on day 1 and 200 mg on day 2), the peak plasma concentration and AUC of the pharmacologically active S-isomer of ibuprofen were increased by about 15 and 82%, respectively.

Although data are lacking, fluconazole has the potential to increase systemic exposure to other nonsteroidal anti-inflammatory agents (NSAIAs) that are metabolized by CYP2C9 (e.g., diclofenac, lornoxicam [not commercially available in the US], meloxicam, naproxen).

NSAIAs and fluconazole should be used concomitantly with caution and close monitoring. Patients should be monitored frequently for NSAIA-associated adverse events; NSAIA dosage adjustment may be needed.

Opiate Agonists Concomitant use of alfentanil and oral or IV fluconazole in healthy individuals reduced alfentanil clearance by 55%, reduced alfentanil volume of distribution by 19%, and nearly doubled the mean elimination half-life of the drug. This interaction may be a result of inhibition of CYP3A4 by fluconazole. Alfentanil and fluconazole should be used concomitantly with caution and close monitoring; adjustment of alfentanil dosage may be necessary.

Concomitant use of a single IV dose of fentanyl in healthy adults receiving oral fluconazole resulted in substantially delayed fentanyl elimination. Elevated fentanyl concentrations may lead to respiratory depression. A fatality possibly related to fentanyl intoxication has been reported in a patient who received concomitant fluconazole and transdermal fentanyl. Fentanyl and fluconazole should be used concomitantly with caution and close monitoring.

When fluconazole (200 mg daily) was administered for 14 days to individuals receiving stable doses of methadone, mean methadone AUC and peak plasma concentration were increased 35 and 27%, respectively, and methadone clearance was reduced 24%. Methadone and fluconazole should be used concomitantly with caution and close monitoring; methadone dosage adjustment may be necessary.

Tricyclic Antidepressants Concomitant use of amitriptyline or nortriptyline and fluconazole has resulted in increased serum concentrations of the tricyclic antidepressant and may increase adverse effects of the antidepressants. CNS toxicity has been reported in a few patients receiving amitriptyline and fluconazole concomitantly. It has been suggested that fluconazole may interfere with metabolism of amitriptyline by inhibition of CYP isoenzymes involved in metabolism of the antidepressant. Fluconazole and amitriptyline or nortriptyline should be used concomitantly with caution and close monitoring. The manufacturer of fluconazole states that S-amitriptyline and/or 5-nortriptyline may be measured when concomitant therapy is initiated and after 1 week of concomitant use; dosage of amitriptyline or nortriptyline should be adjusted if necessary.

■ **Corticosteroids** In a liver transplant recipient receiving prednisone who received a 3-month course of fluconazole, acute adrenal cortex insufficiency occurred when fluconazole was discontinued. This may be a consequence of increased CYP3A4 activity and enhanced metabolism of prednisone as a result of fluconazole discontinuance. Prednisone and fluconazole should be used concomitantly with caution and close monitoring; if the drugs are used concomitantly for a prolonged period of time, the patient should be monitored carefully for adrenal cortex insufficiency when fluconazole is discontinued.

■ **Cyclophosphamide** Concomitant use of cyclophosphamide and fluconazole results in increased concentrations of serum bilirubin and serum creatinine. Cyclophosphamide and fluconazole should be used concomitantly with caution and close monitoring; the risk of increased serum bilirubin and serum creatinine should be considered.

■ **Estrogens and Progestins** Concomitant use of oral fluconazole and oral estrogen-progestin contraceptives may affect the pharmacokinetics of the contraceptives. Although limited data indicate that fluconazole may inhibit metabolism of ethinyl estradiol, levonorgestrel, and norethindrone, there is no evidence that fluconazole induces metabolism of these hormones. When fluconazole is used in the dosage range of 50–200 mg daily concomitantly with combined oral contraceptives, interference with oral contraceptive efficacy is unlikely.

In healthy premenopausal women who received a single dose of oral contraceptive before and after receiving oral fluconazole given in a low dosage (50 mg once daily for 10 days), the mean increase in AUCs of ethinyl estradiol and levonorgestrel were 6% (range: −47 to 108%) and 17% (range: −33 to 141%), respectively. Although some women had ethinyl estradiol and levonorgestrel concentrations that were decreased 47 and 33%, respectively, the manufacturer suggests that this may have been the result of random variation. In a controlled study in healthy women who received a single dose of oral contraceptive following a 10-day regimen of placebo or oral fluconazole (200 mg once daily), AUCs of both levonorgestrel and ethinyl estradiol were increased substantially in those who received oral fluconazole compared with placebo; mean increases in AUCs of ethinyl estradiol and levonorgestrel were 38% (range: −11 to 101%) and 25% (range: −12 to 82%), respectively.

In another placebo-controlled study, women who had received a full cycle of an oral contraceptive preparation containing ethinyl estradiol and norethindrone received a once-weekly fluconazole regimen (300 mg once weekly) or placebo during the second and third cycles of contraceptive use. During fluconazole treatment, the mean AUCs of ethinyl estradiol and norethindrone were increased by 24 and 13%, respectively, compared with placebo. Fluconazole did not cause a decrease in the ethinyl estradiol AUC in any individual and caused only a slight (less than 5%) decrease in the AUC of norethindrone.

■ **Halofantrine** Concomitant use of fluconazole and halofantrine (not commercially available in the US) may result in increased halofantrine concentrations because of CYP3A4 inhibition by fluconazole. Halofantrine and fluconazole should be used concomitantly with caution and close monitoring.

■ **HCV Antivirals** ***HCV Protease Inhibitor*** **Simeprevir.** Concomitant use of simeprevir and fluconazole may result in increased plasma concentrations of simeprevir.

Concomitant use of fluconazole and simeprevir is not recommended.

HCV Replication Complex Inhibitor **Daclatasvir.** If fluconazole and daclatasvir are used concomitantly, daclatasvir dosage adjustments are not needed.

■ **HMG-CoA Reductase Inhibitors** When fluconazole is used concomitantly with a hydroxymethylglutaryl-CoA (HMG-CoA) reductase inhibitor (i.e., statin) that is metabolized by CYP3A4 (e.g., atorvastatin, simvastatin) or 2C9 (e.g., fluvastatin), the risk of myopathy and rhabdomyolysis is increased. If concomitant therapy is necessary, creatinine kinase (CK, creatine phosphokinase, CPK) should be monitored and the patient assessed for symptoms of myopathy and rhabdomyolysis. If a substantial increase in CK occurs or myopathy or rhabdomyolysis is diagnosed or suspected, the statin should be discontinued.

In a placebo-controlled crossover study, a single dose of fluvastatin (40 mg on day 4) administered to healthy individuals receiving oral fluconazole (400 mg on day 1, then 200 mg daily on days 2-4) resulted in an 84% increase in fluvastatin AUC, a 44% increase in fluvastatin peak plasma concentration, and an 80% prolongation of fluvastatin half-life, but did not affect the AUC of fluconazole.

Fluconazole had no clinically important effect on pravastatin pharmacokinetics in a placebo-controlled crossover study in healthy individuals.

■ **Immunosuppressive Agents** ***Cyclosporine*** Concomitant use of fluconazole and cyclosporine may result in increased plasma cyclosporine concentrations, especially when the drugs are used in renal transplant recipients. In several studies in bone marrow transplant recipients receiving cyclosporine maintenance therapy, administration of 100- or 200-mg oral doses of fluconazole once daily for 14 days resulted in only slight increases in plasma cyclosporine concentrations, which were not considered clinically important. However, administration of usual oral dosages of fluconazole to renal transplant recipients (with or without impaired renal function) receiving cyclosporine has resulted in increases in the AUC and peak plasma concentrations of the immunosuppressive agent. In one study in renal transplant patients who had received at least 6 months of cyclosporine therapy and had been receiving a stable cyclosporine dosage for at least 6 weeks, administration of fluconazole 200 mg daily for 14 days resulted in a mean increase of 60 or 157% in peak or minimum cyclosporine plasma concentrations, respectively, and a mean decrease of 45% in the apparent oral clearance of the drug. In addition, increased serum creatinine concentrations, which returned to pretreatment levels with dosage reduction of both drugs, have been reported in patients receiving fluconazole and cyclosporine concomitantly. While the mechanism of this possible interaction is not known, displacement of cyclosporine from protein-binding sites is unlikely since fluconazole is only minimally protein bound.

Fluconazole and cyclosporine should be used concomitantly with caution and close monitoring. Plasma cyclosporine concentrations and serum creatinine should be monitored carefully; cyclosporine dosage should be decreased based on plasma concentrations of the immunosuppressive agent.

Tacrolimus Concomitant use of oral tacrolimus and fluconazole has resulted in a fivefold increase in serum concentrations of tacrolimus as the result of inhibition of intestinal CYP3A4; clinically important alterations in pharmacokinetics were not observed with IV tacrolimus. Increased tacrolimus concentrations have been associated with nephrotoxicity.

Tacrolimus and fluconazole should be used concomitantly with caution and close monitoring. Tacrolimus dosage should be decreased based on tacrolimus concentrations.

Sirolimus Concomitant use of sirolimus and fluconazole results in increased plasma concentrations of the immunosuppressive agent, probably as a result of decreased sirolimus metabolism secondary to inhibition of CYP3A4 and P-glycoprotein.

Sirolimus and fluconazole should be used concomitantly with caution and close monitoring. Sirolimus dosage should be adjusted based on sirolimus concentrations and clinical effects.

■ **Losartan** When a single dose of losartan (50 mg on day 4) was administered to healthy individuals receiving fluconazole (400 mg on day 1, then 200 mg on days 2-4), the AUC and mean peak plasma concentration of the active losartan metabolite (E-3174) were decreased 30 and 47%, respectively, and the half-life of E-3174 was increased by 167%.

Losartan and fluconazole should be used concomitantly with caution and close monitoring. Because fluconazole inhibits metabolism of losartan to its active metabolite (E-3174) and the metabolite is principally responsible for angiotensin II receptor antagonism during losartan therapy, the possibility of decreased therapeutic effect should be considered and blood pressure closely monitored.

■ **Macrolides** ***Azithromycin*** Concomitant use of a single 1.2-g dose of azithromycin and a single 800-mg dose of fluconazole did not alter the pharmacokinetics of either drug.

Erythromycin Concomitant use of erythromycin and fluconazole should be avoided because of the potential for an increased risk of adverse cardiovascular effects (prolonged QT interval, torsades de pointes) and subsequent sudden cardiac death.

■ **Quinidine** Concomitant use of quinidine and fluconazole may result in inhibition of quinidine metabolism. Quinidine has been associated with QT interval prolongation and rare occurrences of torsades de pointes. (See Drug Interactions: Drugs that Prolong the QT Interval.)

Concomitant use of quinidine and fluconazole is contraindicated.

■ **Theophylline** Concomitant use of theophylline and fluconazole increases serum theophylline concentrations. In a study in healthy adults, administration of a single dose of IV aminophylline (6 mg/kg) after 14 days of oral fluconazole (200 mg daily) resulted in a 21 or 13% increase in the mean AUC or peak plasma concentration of theophylline, respectively, and a mean decrease of 16% in theophylline clearance; the half-life of theophylline increased from 6.6 to 7.9 hours.

Theophylline and fluconazole should be used concomitantly with caution and close monitoring. Serum theophylline concentrations should be monitored carefully in patients receiving fluconazole.

■ **Thiazide Diuretics** In healthy adults receiving 100-mg doses of fluconazole, concomitant administration of 50-mg doses of hydrochlorothiazide resulted in a 43% increase in peak plasma fluconazole concentrations and a 45% increase in the AUC of fluconazole compared with results obtained when the antifungal was given alone. These changes are attributed to a 30% decrease in renal clearance of fluconazole. Fluconazole and hydrochlorothiazide should be used concomitantly with caution and close monitoring; adjustment of fluconazole dosage probably is not necessary.

■ **Tofacitinib** Concomitant use of fluconazole (400 mg on day 1, then 200 mg once daily for 6 days) and tofacitinib (single 30-mg dose on day 5) in healthy individuals increased the mean peak plasma concentration and AUC of tofacitinib by 27 and 79%, respectively, compared with administration of tofacitinib alone.

If tofacitinib and fluconazole are used concomitantly, tofacitinib dosage should be reduced from 5 mg twice daily to 5 mg once daily.

■ **Tretinoin** Pseudotumor cerebri has been reported in a patient who received tretinoin (all-trans retinoic acid) and fluconazole concomitantly; this adverse CNS effect resolved after discontinuance of fluconazole. Tretinoin and fluconazole should be used concomitantly with caution and close monitoring; the possibility of adverse CNS effects should be considered.

■ **Vinca Alkaloids** Although data are not available, inhibition of CYP3A4 by fluconazole may result in increased plasma levels of concomitant vinca alkaloids (e.g., vinblastine, vincristine) and possible neurotoxicity. Vinca alkaloids and fluconazole should be used concomitantly with caution and close monitoring.

Acute Toxicity

■ **Manifestations** Limited information is available on the acute toxicity of fluconazole in humans. In mice and rats receiving very high dosages of fluconazole, decreased motility and respiration, ptosis, lacrimation, salivation, urinary incontinence, loss of righting reflex, and cyanosis occurred. There were no fatalities in mice and rats receiving fluconazole doses of 1 g/kg or less. At higher doses (1–2 g/kg), death occurred 1.5 hours to 3 days after the dose; in some cases, death was preceded by clonic seizures. There have been reports of fluconazole overdosage accompanied by hallucination and paranoid behavior in humans.

■ **Treatment** If acute overdosage of fluconazole occurs, supportive and symptomatic treatment should be initiated. If indicated, the stomach should be emptied by gastric lavage. Elimination of fluconazole can be facilitated by hemodialysis; plasma concentrations of the drug generally are decreased 50% by a 3-hour period of hemodialysis.

Mechanism of Action

Fluconazole usually is fungistatic in action. Fluconazole and other triazole-derivative antifungals (e.g., itraconazole, terconazole) appear to have a mechanism of action similar to that of the imidazole-derivative antifungals (e.g., butoconazole, clotrimazole, econazole, ketoconazole, miconazole, oxiconazole). Like imidazoles, fluconazole presumably exerts its antifungal activity by altering cellular membranes resulting in increased membrane permeability, leakage of essential elements (e.g., amino acids, potassium), and impaired uptake of precursor molecules (e.g., purine and pyrimidine precursors to DNA). Although the exact mechanism of action of fluconazole and other triazoles has not been fully determined, the drugs inhibit cytochrome P-450 14-α-desmethylase in susceptible fungi, which leads to accumulation of C-14 methylated sterols (e.g., lanosterol) and decreased concentrations of ergosterol. It appears that this may occur because a nitrogen atom (-4) in the triazole molecule binds to the heme iron of cytochrome P-450 14-α-desmethylase in susceptible fungi. Unlike some imidazoles (e.g., clotrimazole, econazole, miconazole, oxiconazole) that suppress ATP concentrations in intact cells and spheroplasts of *C. albicans*, fluconazole does not appear to have an appreciable effect on ATP concentrations in the organism. It is unclear whether this effect is related to the in vivo antifungal effects of the drugs. Fluconazole generally is fungistatic against *Candida albicans* when the organism is in either the stationary or early logarithmic phase of growth.

Fluconazole and other triazoles (e.g., itraconazole) have a high affinity for fungal P-450 enzymes and only a weak affinity for mammalian P-450 enzymes and are more specific inhibitors of fungal cytochrome P-450 systems than many imidazoles (e.g., ketoconazole). The drug does not appear to have any effect on cholesterol synthesis in mammalian liver homogenates. In an in vitro study using rat Leydig cells, fluconazole concentrations of 10 mcg/mL caused less than a 30% inhibition of basal testosterone production whereas the same concentration of ketoconazole caused a 95% inhibition. Further study is needed to fully evaluate whether fluconazole affects P-450 enzyme systems and steroid synthesis in humans. While there is some evidence that fluconazole has only a minimal inhibitory effect on microsomal cytochrome P-450 systems, other evidence suggests that the drug may have a potent inhibitory effect. Results of an in vitro study using rat liver indicate that fluconazole may act as a potent inducer of some hepatic cytochrome P-450 enzymes systems involved in drug metabolism, acting as an enzyme inhibitor at low concentrations and an inducer at high concentrations. Unlike most imidazoles (e.g., ketoconazole), fluconazole appears to have only minimal, if any, effects on human steroid synthesis, including production of cholesterol, testosterone, and estrogen in dosages up to 400 mg daily.

Results of in vitro studies using human polymorphonuclear leukocytes (PMNs) obtained from healthy individuals indicate that exposure of PMNs to fluconazole concentrations of 1–50 mcg/mL does not appreciably affect PMN function, including chemotaxis, phagocytosis, and oxidative metabolism, and does not interfere with intracellular killing of *C. albicans* blastoconidia. The drug also does not affect lymphocyte proliferation in vitro.

Spectrum

Fluconazole is active against many fungi, including yeasts and dermatophytes. Fluconazole does not appear to have antibacterial activity.

■ **In Vitro Susceptibility Testing** Like imidazole derivatives and other triazole derivatives, results of in vitro fluconazole susceptibility tests are method dependent, and MIC values vary depending on the culture medium used, incubation temperature, pH, and inoculum size. In addition, currently available in vitro tests do not necessarily reflect the in vivo susceptibility of many fungi (especially *Candida*). Consequently, in vivo animal models of fungal infections may provide a more accurate assessment of the antifungal effectiveness of fluconazole than currently available in vitro susceptibility tests. While fluconazole is less active on a weight basis in vitro than many other antifungals (e.g., itraconazole, ketoconazole, miconazole), the drug often is as or more active than these agents in vivo. The reasons for the current lack of correlation between results of in vitro and in vivo tests are unclear. It has been suggested that substances contained in media used for in vitro susceptibility testing, especially complex media, may antagonize fluconazole. Other factors also probably contribute to the apparent poor correlation between in vitro and in vivo results.

■ **Fungi** When results of in vitro susceptibility tests are compared, fluconazole appears to be less active than ketoconazole against most susceptible organisms since MICs of fluconazole reported for *C. albicans*, *C. neoformans*, and *H. capsulatum* generally are 4–16 times higher than those reported for ketoconazole. However, results of studies using the drugs in various animal models of fungal infections indicate that, despite higher MIC values in vitro, the in vivo effectiveness of fluconazole is equal to or, in many cases, greater than the in vivo effectiveness of ketoconazole. This difference may occur because results of fluconazole in vitro susceptibility tests are affected to a greater extent than those of ketoconazole and/or because pharmacologic differences between the drugs (e.g., fluconazole's higher oral bioavailability and lower protein binding) affect the in vivo effectiveness of the drugs.

Candida In vitro, fluconazole is active against some strains of *Candida*, including some strains of *C. albicans*, *C. dubliniensis*, *C. guilliermondii*, *C. kefyr*, *C. glabrata*, *C. parapsilosis*, *C. lusitaniae*, and *C. tropicalis*. In vitro, susceptible strains of *C. albicans*, *C. guilliermondii*, *C. parapsilosis*, and *C. tropicalis* usually are inhibited by fluconazole concentrations of 0.03–8 mcg/mL. In one study evaluating in vitro susceptibility of clinical isolates of *C. dubliniensis* obtained from patients with or without human immunodeficiency virus (HIV) infection, most strains were inhibited by fluconazole concentrations of 0.125–1 mcg/mL, but some strains had reduced susceptibility to the drug and required fluconazole concentrations of 8–32 mcg/mL for in vitro inhibition.

C. krusei are intrinsically resistant to fluconazole and many strains of *C. glabrata* also are resistant or have reduced susceptibility to the drug. (See Resistance.)

In vitro, some strains of *C. duobushaemulonii* have been inhibited by fluconazole concentrations of 1–16 mcg/mL. *C. haemulonii* and *C. auris* (often misidentified as *C. haemulonii*, *C. famata*, or *Rhodotorula glutinis*) generally are resistant to fluconazole in vitro.

Other Fungi Fluconazole has in vitro activity against some strains of *Cryptococcus neoformans*. In vitro, some strains of *C. neoformans* are inhibited by fluconazole concentrations of 0.125–12.8 mcg/mL. Although fluconazole may be active in vitro against some strains of *C. gattii*, there is in vitro evidence that fluconazole may be less active against *C. gattii* than some other azoles (e.g., itraconazole, posaconazole, voriconazole).

Coccidioides immitis and *C. posadasii* are inhibited in vitro by fluconazole. In one study, the mean MIC of fluconazole for these organisms was 8 mcg/mL.

Fluconazole is active in vitro against some strains of *Histoplasma capsulatum*. A wide range of fluconazole MICs has been reported for this organism. In some in vitro studies, MICs of fluconazole reported for *H. capsulatum* were 0.125–4 mcg/mL; however, in other studies, MICs ranged from 16–250 mcg/mL. In addition, some amphotericin B-susceptible strains of *H. capsulatum* with fluconazole MICs exceeding 1000 mcg/mL have been reported.

Some strains of *Blastomyces dermatitidis* are inhibited in vitro by fluconazole concentrations of 2.5–10 mcg/mL, but other strains require concentrations of 20–80 mcg/mL for in vitro inhibition.

Fluconazole is inactive against *Malassezia pachydermatis* in vitro. The drug generally is inactive against *Aspergillus* in vitro.

Although a few strains of *Penicillium marneffei* may be inhibited in vitro by fluconazole concentrations of 4–8 mcg/mL, most strains tested are resistant to the drug. In vitro, fluconazole is considerably less active than itraconazole or ketoconazole against *P. marneffei*.

Scopulariopsis, including *S. acremonium* and *S. brevicaulis*, generally are resistant to fluconazole in vitro.

■ **In Vivo Susceptibility Testing** In vivo studies using various animal models (e.g., mice, rats, rabbits) and standard laboratory strains of fungi indicate that oral or IV fluconazole has fungistatic activity against a variety of fungal infections. Activity of the drug against fungi in these in vivo studies was generally evaluated based on increased survival rate and reduction of fungal burden in the animals' organs. Fluconazole has been active in vivo in both normal and immunosuppressed mice, rats, and rabbits against systemic and local infections caused by *C. albicans*, including endophthalmitis, endocarditis, pyelonephritis, and intestinal, vaginal, and disseminated candidiasis; in several studies, fluconazole was at least as effective as amphotericin B (alone or combined with flucytosine) and more effective than ketoconazole in vivo against these infections. Fluconazole also has been effective in vivo in animals against systemic *C. parapsilosis* infections. Although fluconazole was active in vivo in mice against infections caused by *C. tropicalis* or *C. glabrata*, the drug was less effective against these infections than amphotericin B; neither fluconazole nor amphotericin B were effective in reducing tissue concentrations of *C. krusei* in these mice.

Fluconazole has been effective in vivo in mice and rabbits against infections caused by *C. neoformans*, including meningitis and pulmonary infections. The drug generally has been effective against systemic infections, including pulmonary infections, caused by *H. capsulatum* in normal and immunosuppressed mice, and was as effective as or less effective than amphotericin B. Fluconazole also generally has been effective in mice against systemic infections, including intracranial infections, caused by *C. immitis*; pulmonary infections in mice caused by *Blastomyces dermatitidis*; and infections in mice caused by *Paracoccidioides brasiliensis*. Results of in vivo testing of fluconazole activity against *Aspergillus* have been conflicting. In some in vivo studies in normal or immunosuppressed mice or rabbits, high dosages of the drug (60–120 mg/kg daily) were effective against infections caused by *A. flavus* and *A. fumigatus*. However, in at least one in vivo study in mice, fluconazole was ineffective against experimental aspergillosis.

In in vivo models of dermatomycoses, fluconazole has been effective against pityriasis (tinea) versicolor caused by *Malassezia furfur* (*Pityrosporum orbiculare* or *P. ovale*) and infections caused by *Trichophyton* or *Microsporum canis*.

Resistance

Resistance to fluconazole can be produced in vitro by serial passage of *Candida albicans* in the presence of increasing concentrations of the drug. Some *Candida* species are intrinsically resistant to fluconazole (e.g., *C. krusei*), and many strains of *C. glabrata* are resistant or have reduced susceptibility to the drug. In addition, strains of *Candida* with decreased in vitro susceptibility to fluconazole have been isolated with increasing frequency. Fluconazole-resistant strains of *C. albicans*, *C. glabrata*, *C. lusitaniae*, *C. norvegensis*, *C. parapsilosis*, and *C. tropicalis* have been isolated from patients receiving fluconazole. Strains of *Cryptococcus neoformans* with decreased susceptibility to fluconazole also have been isolated from patients receiving the drug. Prolonged or intermittent use of oral fluconazole in immunocompromised patients has been suggested as a major contributing factor to the emergence of fluconazole resistance in *Candida*. In one study evaluating the in vitro susceptibility of *Candida* isolates obtained from patients with candidemia, 72% of the isolates obtained from patients who had received prior fluconazole therapy had decreased in vitro susceptibility to fluconazole (MIC greater than 8 mcg/mL) compared with only 12% of isolates obtained from patients who had not previously received fluconazole. There is evidence that decreased in vitro susceptibility to fluconazole may correlate with clinical failure in the treatment of *Candida* infections (e.g., esophageal candidiasis) in HIV-infected patients. Emergence of fluconazole-resistant strains of *C. albicans* also have been reported rarely in immunocompetent patients receiving the drug.

Several mechanisms for decreased susceptibility to fluconazole have been suggested, including reduced intracellular accumulation of the drug as the result of defective lipids or sterols in the fungal cell membrane or active efflux of the drug or mutation of fungal 14-α-desmethylase leading to diminished affinity for the enzyme. In one in vitro study, fluconazole-resistant strains of *C. albicans* reverted to susceptible phenotypes when grown without the presence of fluconazole.

Fluconazole-resistant fungi also may be cross-resistant to other azole antifungals (e.g., itraconazole, ketoconazole, posaconazole, voriconazole).

While the clinical importance is unclear, fluconazole-resistant strains of *C. albicans* that were cross-resistant to amphotericin B have been isolated from a few immunocompromised individuals, including leukemia patients and HIV-infected individuals. In addition, a few isolates of *Cryptococcus neoformans* with decreased susceptibility to fluconazole have shown cross resistance to amphotericin B.

Pharmacokinetics

■ **Absorption** The pharmacokinetics of fluconazole are similar following IV or oral administration. The drug is rapidly and almost completely absorbed from the GI tract, and there is no evidence of first-pass metabolism.

Oral bioavailability of fluconazole exceeds 90% in healthy, fasting adults; peak plasma concentrations of the drug generally are attained within 1–2 hours after oral administration. Results of a few limited studies indicate that oral bioavailability of fluconazole in adults with human immunodeficiency virus (HIV) infection appears to be similar to that reported for healthy adults.

The manufacturer states that the commercially available fluconazole suspensions are bioequivalent to the 100-mg fluconazole tablets.

Unlike some imidazole-derivative antifungals (e.g., ketoconazole), GI absorption of fluconazole does not appear to be affected by gastric pH. In one patient with achlorhydria who received 100-mg oral doses of fluconazole once daily, plasma concentrations of the drug 2 hours after a dose were similar to those reported at the same time interval in healthy adults. Studies in healthy, fasting adults indicate that peak plasma concentrations, areas under the concentration-time curves (AUCs), time to peak plasma concentrations, and elimination half-life of fluconazole are not affected substantially by concurrent administration of drugs that increase gastric pH. (See Drug Interactions: Drugs Affecting Gastric Acidity.)

Peak plasma fluconazole concentrations and AUCs increase in proportion to the dose over the oral dosage range of 50–400 mg. Steady-state plasma concentrations of fluconazole are attained within 5–10 days following oral doses of 50–400 mg given once daily. The manufacturer states that when fluconazole therapy is initiated with a single loading dose equal to twice the usual daily dosage and followed by the usual dosage given once daily thereafter, plasma concentrations of the drug reportedly approach steady state by the second day of therapy.

In healthy, fasting adults who received a single 1-mg/kg oral dose of fluconazole, peak plasma concentrations of the drug averaged 1.4 mcg/mL. Following oral administration of a single 400-mg dose of fluconazole in healthy, fasting adults, peak plasma concentrations average 6.72 mcg/mL (range: 4.12–8.1 mcg/mL). In adults with coccidioidal meningitis who received oral fluconazole in a dosage of 50 or 100 mg daily, peak serum concentrations of the drug ranged from 2.5–3.5 or 4.5–8 mcg/mL, respectively, and were attained in 2–6 hours; serum concentrations averaged 1.2 or 3.1 mcg/mL, respectively, at 24–27 hours after a dose.

In healthy adults receiving 50- or 100-mg doses of fluconazole given once daily by IV infusion over 30 minutes, serum concentrations of the drug 1 hour after dosing on the sixth or seventh day of therapy ranged from 2.14–2.81 or 3.86–4.96 mcg/mL, respectively.

In children 9 months to 13 years of age, oral administration of a single 2- or 8-mg/kg dose of fluconazole resulted in mean peak plasma concentrations of 2.9 or 9.8 mcg/mL, respectively. In a multiple-dose study in children 5–15 years of age, IV administration of 2-, 4-, or 8-mg/kg doses of fluconazole resulted in mean peak plasma concentrations of 5.5, 11.4, or 14.1 mcg/mL, respectively. In a limited study in premature neonates who received 6-mg/kg doses of fluconazole IV every 72 hours, peak serum concentrations of the drug ranged from 3.7–10.2 mcg/mL after the first dose and from 6–17.8 mcg/mL after the third dose (day 7).

Food Data from a pharmacokinetic study in healthy individuals indicate that administration with a high-fat meal does not affect peak plasma concentrations or AUC of fluconazole compared with administration in the fasting state.

■ **Distribution** Fluconazole is widely distributed into body tissues and fluids following oral or IV administration. Studies in mice using IV doses of radiolabeled fluconazole indicate that the drug is evenly distributed throughout body tissues. In adult humans with normal renal function, concentrations of the drug attained in urine and skin may be 10 times higher than concurrent plasma concentrations; concentrations attained in saliva, sputum, nails, blister fluid, blister skin, and vaginal tissue are approximately equal to concurrent plasma concentrations. Concentrations attained in vaginal secretions following administration of a single 150-mg oral dose reportedly are about 40–86% of concurrent plasma concentrations. Fluconazole concentrations in prostatic tissue reportedly average about 30% of concurrent plasma concentrations. In adults with bronchiectasis who received a single 150-mg oral dose of fluconazole, sputum concentrations of the drug in samples obtained at 4 and 24 hours after the dose averaged 3.7 and 2.23 mcg/mL, respectively, and were approximately equal to concurrent plasma concentrations. Studies in rabbits indicate that high concentrations of fluconazole are attained in the cornea, aqueous humor, and vitreous body following IV administration; these concentrations were higher in inflamed than uninflamed eyes.

Fluconazole, unlike some azole-derivative antifungals (e.g., itraconazole, ketoconazole), distributes readily into CSF following oral or IV administration; CSF concentrations of fluconazole may be 50–94% of concurrent plasma concentrations regardless of the degree of meningeal inflammation. In adults with coccidioidal meningitis who received an oral fluconazole dosage of 50 or 100 mg daily, CSF concentrations of the drug in samples obtained 0.5–8 hours after a dose averaged 0.7–2.1 or 3.5–5.3 mcg/mL, respectively.

The apparent volume of distribution of fluconazole approximates that of total body water and has been reported to be 0.7–1 L/kg. In a limited study, the estimated volume of distribution at steady state of fluconazole was slightly lower in HIV-infected adults than in healthy adults.

Unlike some azole-derivative antifungals (e.g., itraconazole, ketoconazole, miconazole), which are highly protein bound, fluconazole is only 11–12% bound to plasma proteins.

It is not known whether fluconazole crosses the placenta in humans. The drug crosses the placenta in rats, and concentrations in amniotic fluid, placenta, fetus, and fetal liver are approximately equal to maternal plasma concentrations. Fluconazole is distributed into human milk in concentrations similar to those attained in plasma. Following administration of a single 150-mg oral dose in nursing women, peak plasma fluconazole concentrations were 2.61 mcg/mL (range: 1.57–3.65 mcg/mL)

■ **Elimination** The plasma elimination half-life of fluconazole in adults with normal renal function is approximately 30 hours (range: 20–50 hours). In one study, plasma elimination half-life of the drug was 22 hours after the first day of therapy and 23.8 and 28.6 hours after 7 and 26 days of therapy, respectively. In a limited, single-dose study in HIV-infected adults, the plasma elimination half-life of fluconazole averaged 32 hours (range: 25–42 hours) in those with absolute helper/inducer ($CD4^+$, $T4^+$) T-cell counts greater than $200mm^3$ and 50 hours (range: 32–69 hours) in those with $CD4^+$ T-cell counts less than $200mm^3$. In other single-dose studies in a limited number of HIV-infected adults with $CD4^+$ T-cell counts less than $200mm^3$, the plasma elimination half-life of the drug averaged 35–40 hours (range 22–75 hours).

The mean plasma half-life of fluconazole in children 9 months to 15 years of age has ranged from about 15–25 hours. In a limited study in premature neonates who received IV fluconazole once every 72 hours, the plasma half-life decreased over time, averaging 88 hours after the first dose and 55 hours after the fifth dose (day 13).

In patients with impaired renal function, plasma concentrations of fluconazole are higher and the half-life prolonged; elimination half-life of the drug is inversely proportional to the patient's creatinine clearance. In addition, elimination of the drug may be impaired in geriatric patients because of decreased kidney function in this age group. The elimination half-life of fluconazole reportedly is not affected by impaired hepatic function.

In healthy adults, fluconazole is eliminated principally by renal excretion. Renal clearance of the drug averages 0.27 mL/minute per kg in adults with normal renal function. In a limited, single-dose study, renal clearance of fluconazole averaged 0.79 L/hour in healthy adults, 0.58 L/hour in HIV-infected adults with $CD4^+$ T-cell counts greater than $200mm^3$, and 0.2 L/hour in those with $CD4^+$ T-cell counts less than $200mm^3$. Approximately 60–80% of a single oral or IV dose of fluconazole is excreted in urine unchanged, and about 11% is excreted in urine as metabolites. Small amounts of the drug are excreted in feces.

Fluconazole is removed by hemodialysis and peritoneal dialysis. The amount of the drug removed during hemodialysis depends on several factors (e.g., type of coil used, dialysis flow rate). A 3-hour period of hemodialysis generally decreases plasma concentrations of the drug by 50%. In 2 adults with fungal peritonitis undergoing continuous ambulatory peritoneal dialysis (CAPD) and receiving an oral fluconazole dosage of 100 mg/kg daily, concentrations of the drug in peritoneal dialysis fluid ranged from 2.3–9 mcg/mL and concurrent plasma concentrations ranged from 3.2–9 mcg/mL.

Chemistry and Stability

■ **Chemistry** Fluconazole, a synthetic triazole derivative, is an azole antifungal agent. The drug is structurally related to imidazole-derivative azole antifungals (e.g., butoconazole, clotrimazole, econazole, ketoconazole, miconazole, oxiconazole) since it contains a 5-membered azole ring attached by a carbon-nitrogen bond to other aromatic rings. However, imidazoles have 2 nitrogens in the azole ring (imidazole ring) and fluconazole and other triazoles (e.g., itraconazole, terconazole) have 3 nitrogens in the ring (triazole ring).

Replacement of the imidazole ring with a triazole ring apparently results in increased antifungal activity and an expanded antifungal spectrum of activity. In addition to this triazole ring, fluconazole contains a second triazole ring and thus is a bistriazole derivative. Presence of these triazole rings may contribute to fluconazole's resistance to first-pass metabolism and the drug's low lipophilicity and protein binding. However, other structural modifications to bistriazole derivatives also affect these characteristics since itraconazole, which also is a bistriazole, is highly lipophilic and protein bound and undergoes extensive hepatic metabolism. Presence of a halogenated phenyl ring increases antifungal activity of bistriazole derivatives and the 2,4-difluorophenyl derivative (fluconazole) has an aqueous solubility suitable for IV formulation.

Fluconazole occurs as a white crystalline powder and is slightly soluble in water, having an aqueous solubility of 8 mg/mL at 37°C. The drug has a solubility of 25 mg/mL in alcohol at room temperature. Fluconazole has a pK_a of 1.76 at 24°C in 0.1 *M* sodium chloride. Fluconazole injections are sterile, iso-osmotic solutions of the drug in a sodium chloride or dextrose diluent; each mL contains 2 mg of fluconazole and either 9 mg of sodium chloride or 56 mg of dextrose. The injections have an osmolarity of 300–315 mOsm/L; the pH ranges from 4–8 in the sodium chloride diluent and from 3.5–6.5 in the dextrose diluent.

■ **Stability** Fluconazole tablets should be stored in tight containers at a temperature less than 30°C; fluconazole powder for oral suspension should be stored at a temperature less than 30°C. After reconstitution, refrigeration of fluconazole oral suspension is not necessary and freezing of the suspension should be avoided. The manufacturer states that the reconstituted suspension is stable for 14 days when stored at 5–30°C and any unused suspension should be discarded after this period.

Commercially available fluconazole injection provided in glass bottles should be stored at 5–30°C and protected from freezing. Fluconazole injection provided in Viaflex® Plus plastic containers should be stored at 5–25°C and protected from freezing; brief exposure of the drug in Viaflex® Plus containers to temperatures up to 40°C will not adversely affect the injection. Commercially available fluconazole injection in glass or plastic containers is stable for 24 or 18 months, respectively, following the date of manufacture. The Viaflex® Plus plastic containers are fabricated from specially formulated polyvinyl chloride (PVC). The amount of water that can permeate from inside the container into the overwrap is insufficient to substantially affect the solution. Solutions in contact with the plastic can leach out some of its chemical components in very small amounts (e.g., bis(2-ethylhexyl)phthalate BEHP, DEHP in up to 5 ppm) within the expiration period of the injection; however, safety of the plastic has been confirmed in tests in animals according to USP biological tests for plastic containers as well as by tissue culture toxicity studies. Additives should not be introduced into the glass or Viaflex® Plus containers of commercially available fluconazole injection.

Preparations

Excipients in commercially available drug preparations may have clinically important effects in some individuals; consult specific product labeling for details.

Fluconazole

Oral		
For suspension	50 mg/5 mL*	Diflucan®, Pfizer Fluconazole for Oral Suspension
	200 mg/5 mL	Diflucan®, Pfizer Fluconazole for Oral Suspension
Tablets	50 mg*	Diflucan®, Pfizer Fluconazole Tablets
	100 mg*	Diflucan® Fluconazole Tablets
	150 mg*	Diflucan®, Pfizer Fluconazole Tablets
	200 mg*	Diflucan®, Pfizer Fluconazole Tablets

*available from one or more manufacturer, distributor, and/or repackager by generic (nonproprietary) name

Fluconazole in Dextrose

Parenteral		
Injection, for IV infusion only	2 mg/mL (200 or 400 mg) in 5.6% Dextrose*	Diflucan® in Iso-osmotic Dextrose Injection (in Viaflex® Plus [Baxter]), Pfizer Fluconazole in Iso-osmotic Dextrose Injection

*available from one or more manufacturer, distributor, and/or repackager by generic (nonproprietary) name

Fluconazole in Sodium Chloride

Parenteral		
Injection, for IV infusion only	2 mg/mL (200 or 400 mg) in 0.9% Sodium Chloride*	Diflucan® in Iso-osmotic Sodium Chloride Injection (in glass and Viaflex® Plus [Baxter]), Pfizer Fluconazole in Iso-osmotic Sodium Chloride Injection

*available from one or more manufacturer, distributor, and/or repackager by generic (nonproprietary) name

†Use is not currently included in the labeling approved by the US Food and Drug Administration

Isavuconazonium Sulfate

■ Isavuconazonium sulfate, a prodrug of isavuconazole, is a triazole antifungal agent; after in vivo conversion to isavuconazole, the drug is active against certain fungi.

Uses

■ **Aspergillosis** Isavuconazonium sulfate is used for the treatment of invasive aspergillosis, and has been designated an orphan drug by the US Food and Drug Administration (FDA) for this indication.

The Infectious Diseases Society of America (IDSA) considers IV voriconazole the drug of choice for primary treatment of invasive aspergillosis; amphotericin B and isavuconazonium sulfate are the recommended alternatives for primary treatment of such infections. For salvage therapy in patients refractory to or intolerant of primary antifungal therapy, IDSA recommends IV amphotericin B, an IV echinocandin (caspofungin, micafungin), oral or IV posaconazole, or itraconazole oral suspension.

For additional information on the management of aspergillosis, the current clinical practice guidelines from IDSA available at http://www.idsociety.org can be consulted.

Clinical Experience Safety and efficacy of isavuconazonium sulfate were evaluated in a randomized, double-blind, active-controlled, noninferiority, phase 3 trial in 516 adults (mean age 51 years, 60% male, 78% white, 66% neutropenic, 84% with hematologic malignancy, 95% with pulmonary involvement) for the treatment of proven, probable, or possible primary invasive fungal disease caused by *Aspergillus* or other filamentous fungi (SECURE; NCT00412893). Patients were randomized to receive IV isavuconazonium sulfate (loading dosage of 372 mg [equivalent to 200 mg of isavuconazole] every 8 hours for the first 48 hours) or IV voriconazole (loading dosage of 6 mg/kg every 12 hours for the first 24 hours, followed by 4 mg/kg every 12 hours for the next 24 hours). After 48 hours, patients in the isavuconazonium group received IV or oral isavuconazonium sulfate (maintenance dosage of 372 mg [equivalent to 200 mg of isavuconazole] once every 24 hours) and patients in the voriconazole group continued IV therapy (maintenance dosage of 4 mg/kg every 12 hours) or were switched to oral voriconazole (maintenance dose of 200 mg every 12 hours) for a maximum total treatment duration of 84 days. At least one *Aspergillus* species was identified in 30% of patients; the most commonly identified pathogens were *A. fumigatus* and *A. flavus*. The all-cause mortality rate through day 42 in the intent-to-treat population (the primary end point) was 19% in the isavuconazonium group and 20% in the voriconazole group; similar results were observed in the subgroup of patients with proven or probable invasive aspergillosis confirmed by serology, culture, or histology. Based on prespecified clinical, mycologic, and radiologic criteria in this subgroup, overall success rate at the end of treatment was 35% in the isavuconazonium group and 38.9% in the voriconazole group. These data indicate that isavuconazonium sulfate is noninferior to voriconazole for the treatment of invasive aspergillosis.

■ **Mucormycosis** Isavuconazonium sulfate is used for the treatment of invasive mucormycosis, and has been designated an orphan drug by FDA for this indication.

Clinical Experience Safety and efficacy of isavuconazonium sulfate for the treatment of mucormycosis were evaluated in a single-arm, open-label, phase 3 trial in a subset of 37 adults (mean age 49 years, 81% male, 68% white, 27% neutropenic, 60% with hematologic malignancy, 59% with pulmonary involvement) with proven or probable invasive mucormycosis (VITAL; NCT00634049). Patients received IV or oral isavuconazonium sulfate (loading dosage of 372 mg [equivalent to 200 mg of isavuconazole] every 8 hours for the first 48 hours followed by a maintenance dosage of 372 mg [equivalent to 200 mg of isavuconazole] once every 24 hours). Patients were stratified by treatment status into 3 groups: those receiving isavuconazonium for initial treatment (primary treatment group), those with disease refractory to other antifungal therapy (refractory treatment group), and those with intolerance to other antifungal therapy (intolerant treatment group). The most commonly identified pathogens were *Rhizopus oryzae*, *Mucor*, and Mucormycetes (not otherwise specified). The all-cause mortality rate through day 42 (the primary end point) was 38% overall and 33, 45–46, and 40% in the primary, refractory, and intolerant treatment groups, respectively. Median treatment duration in these treatment groups was 102, 33, and 85 days, respectively. The response success rate at the end of treatment was 31% overall and 32, 36, and 20% in the primary, refractory, and intolerant treatment groups, respectively. These data provide evidence that isavuconazonium sulfate is effective for the treatment of mucormycosis when historical data for untreated mucormycosis are used as the basis for comparison; invasive mucormycosis has a mortality rate approaching 100% if left untreated. Efficacy of isavuconazonium sulfate for the treatment of invasive mucormycosis has not been evaluated to date in controlled, comparative clinical trials.

■ **Candida Infections** ***Esophageal Candidiasis*** Isavuconazonium sulfate has been used in some patients for the treatment of esophageal candidiasis†, and is recommended as an alternative for the treatment of such infections.

Esophageal candidiasis requires treatment with a systemic antifungal (not a topical antifungal).

IDSA recommends oral fluconazole as the preferred drug of choice for the treatment of esophageal candidiasis; if oral therapy is not tolerated, these experts recommend IV fluconazole or an IV echinocandin (anidulafungin, caspofungin, micafungin) and state that IV amphotericin B is another alternative. For fluconazole-refractory esophageal candidiasis, IDSA recommends itraconazole oral solution or oral or IV voriconazole; alternatives are an IV echinocandin (anidulafungin, caspofungin, micafungin), IV amphotericin B, or oral posaconazole (oral suspension or delayed-release tablets).

For the treatment of esophageal candidiasis in adults with human immunodeficiency virus (HIV) infection, the US Centers for Disease Control and Prevention (CDC), National Institutes of Health (NIH), and HIV Medicine Association of IDSA recommend IV or oral fluconazole or itraconazole oral solution. Alternatives recommended for such patients include oral or IV voriconazole, oral isavuconazonium sulfate, an IV echinocandin (anidulafungin, caspofungin, micafungin), or IV amphotericin B.

For additional information on the management of esophageal candidiasis, the current clinical practice guidelines from IDSA available at http://www.idsociety.org and the current clinical practice guidelines from CDC, NIH, and IDSA on the prevention and treatment of opportunistic infections in HIV-infected individuals available at http://www.aidsinfo.nih.gov should be consulted.

Clinical Experience. Safety and efficacy of isavuconazonium sulfate for the treatment of uncomplicated esophageal candidiasis† were evaluated in a phase 2, randomized, double-blind, parallel-group, noninferiority trial in adults that compared 3 different dosage regimens of oral isavuconazonium sulfate with a regimen of oral fluconazole. A total of 160 eligible adults 18–65 years of age (37% had HIV infection) were randomized to receive 372 mg of oral isavuconazonium sulfate (equivalent to 200 mg of isavuconazole) on day 1 followed by 93 mg of oral isavuconazonium sulfate (equivalent to 50 mg of isavuconazole) once daily (arm A); 744 mg of oral isavuconazonium sulfate (equivalent to 400 mg of isavuconazole) on day 1 followed by 744 mg of oral isavuconazonium sulfate (equivalent to 400 mg of isavuconazole) once weekly given on days 7, 14, and 21 (arm B); 744 mg of oral isavuconazonium sulfate (equivalent to 400 mg of isavuconazole) on day 1 followed by 186 mg of oral isavuconazonium sulfate (equivalent to 100 mg of isavuconazole) once daily (arm C); or 200 mg of oral fluconazole on day 1 followed by 100 mg of oral fluconazole once daily (arm D). The duration of treatment was based on disease severity and clinical response with a minimum duration of 14 days and a maximum duration of 21 days. The primary efficacy end point was endoscopically confirmed clinical response at the end of treatment. Overall, 95.4% of patients in the per-protocol population achieved endoscopically confirmed clinical success at the end of treatment and each of the oral isavuconazonium sulfate regimens (arms A, B, and C) were noninferior to the oral fluconazole regimen (arm D). The oral isavuconazonium sulfate regimens were generally well tolerated; however, adverse GI effects (diarrhea, nausea, vomiting, gastritis) occurred more frequently in patients in arm C than in those treated with the other isavuconazonium sulfate regimens or the fluconazole regimen.

Candidemia and Other Invasive Candida Infections Isavuconazonium sulfate has been used is some patients for the treatment of candidemia and other invasive infections caused by *Candida*†, and has been designated an orphan drug by FDA for the treatment of invasive candidiasis/candidemia.

Clinical Experience. Safety and efficacy of isavuconazonium sulfate for the treatment of candidemia and other invasive *Candida* infections† were evaluated in a phase 3, randomized, double-blind, noninferiority trial (ACTIVE; NCT00413218). A total of 450 adults were randomized to receive treatment with IV isavuconazonium sulfate (loading dosage of 372 mg of isavuconazonium sulfate [equivalent to 200 mg of isavuconazole] 3 times daily on days 1 and 2 followed by a maintenance dosage of 372 mg of isavuconazonium sulfate [equivalent to 200 mg of isavuconazole] once daily) or IV caspofungin (single dose of 70 mg on day 1 followed by 50 mg [70 mg in those weighing more than 80 kg] once daily). After 10 days of the IV regimen, patients who were not neutropenic could be switched to an oral regimen at the discretion of the investigator; those receiving IV isavuconazonium sulfate could be switched to 372 mg of oral isavuconazonium sulfate (equivalent to 200 mg of isavuconazole) once daily and those receiving IV caspofungin could be switched to oral voriconazole (400 mg twice daily on day 1 of oral dosing followed by 200 mg twice daily). Treatment was continued until at least 14 days after the last positive blood culture (up to a maximum total duration of 56 days). Results for the primary end point of overall response at the end of IV therapy (EOIVT) failed to demonstrate noninferiority of isavuconazonium sulfate relative to caspofungin based on the prespecified noninferiority margin; the overall response at EOIVT in the modified intent-to-treat population was 60.3% in patients treated with isavuconazonium sulfate and 71.1% in those treated with caspofungin. The overall response rates at the secondary end point (2 weeks after the end of treatment) were similar in both treatment groups (54.8% in the isavuconazonium sulfate group and 57.2% in the caspofungin group) and all-cause mortality rates on days 14 and 56 were comparable in both treatment groups.

Dosage and Administration

■ **Administration** Isavuconazonium sulfate is administered orally or by IV infusion.

Oral Administration Isavuconazonium sulfate capsules may be given orally without regard to meals.

Capsules should be swallowed whole and should *not* be chewed, crushed, dissolved, or opened.

IV Infusion Isavuconazonium sulfate for injection should be administered *only* by IV infusion. The drug should *not* be administered by rapid or direct IV injection.

Other IV drugs should not be infused simultaneously with isavuconazonium sulfate.

The IV line to be used for infusion of isavuconazonium sulfate solutions should be flushed with 0.9% sodium chloride injection or 5% dextrose injection before and after infusion of the drug.

Reconstituted and diluted isavuconazonium sulfate solutions *must* be administered using an IV infusion set with an inline membrane filter that has a pore size of 0.2–1.2 μm.

Vials of isavuconazonium sulfate lyophilized powder for injection contain no preservatives and are intended for single use only.

Reconstitution and Dilution. Isavuconazonium sulfate for injection must be reconstituted and further diluted prior to IV infusion. Strict aseptic technique must be observed when preparing IV solutions of the drug.

Vials labeled as containing 372 mg of isavuconazonium sulfate should be reconstituted by adding 5 mL of sterile water for injection. The vial should be gently shaken to completely dissolve the lyophilized powder. Reconstituted solutions should be visually inspected for particulate matter and discoloration; the reconstituted solution should appear clear and free of visible particulates. The reconstituted solution should be immediately diluted, but may be stored at less than 25°C for a maximum of 1 hour prior to dilution.

Reconstituted isavuconazonium sulfate must then be further diluted by removing 5 mL of the reconstituted solution from the vial and adding it to an IV infusion bag containing 250 mL of 0.9% sodium chloride injection or 5% dextrose injection to yield a solution containing approximately 1.5 mg of isavuconazonium sulfate per mL. Translucent to white particulates of isavuconazole may be visible in the diluted solution; the IV bag should be gently mixed or rolled to minimize the formation of particulates. Any unnecessary vibration or vigorous shaking of the solution should be avoided; a pneumatic transport system should *not* be used to transport the diluted solution.

Because reconstituted and diluted isavuconazonium sulfate solutions *must* be administered using an infusion set with an inline membrane filter that has a pore size of 0.2–1.2 μm, a reminder sticker for the use of the inline filter should be applied to the IV bag.

IV infusion of isavuconazonium sulfate solutions should be completed within 6 hours after dilution when stored at room temperature. Alternatively, the solution may be refrigerated at 2–8°C immediately after dilution and the IV infusion completed within 24 hours after dilution. The solution should *not* be frozen.

Rate of Administration. Isavuconazonium sulfate solutions should be administered by IV infusion over at least 1 hour.

■ Dosage

Isavuconazonium sulfate is a prodrug that is inactive until metabolized in vivo to isavuconazole (see Description). Dosage of the drug usually is expressed in terms of the prodrug (i.e., isavuconazonium sulfate), but also has been expressed in terms of isavuconazole.

Each 186 mg of isavuconazonium sulfate is equivalent to 100 mg of isavuconazole.

Oral and IV dosages of isavuconazonium sulfate are identical. Switching between the oral and IV routes is acceptable; a loading dosage is not needed when switching between the oral and IV preparations.

Adult Dosage **Aspergillosis.** For the treatment of invasive aspergillosis in adults, an oral or IV loading dosage of 372 mg of isavuconazonium sulfate (equivalent to 200 mg of isavuconazole) should be given every 8 hours for 6 doses; beginning 12–24 hours after the final loading dose, therapy should be continued using a maintenance dosage of 372 mg of isavuconazonium sulfate (equivalent to 200 mg of isavuconazole) once every 24 hours.

The total duration of IV and oral therapy should be based on the severity of the patient's underlying disease, recovery from immunosuppression, and response to the drug. In a clinical study in adults with invasive aspergillosis, the mean duration of isavuconazonium sulfate therapy was 45 days and the protocol-defined maximum treatment duration was 84 days. The Infectious Diseases Society of America (IDSA) recommends that treatment of invasive pulmonary aspergillosis be continued for at least 6–12 weeks.

Mucormycosis. For the treatment of invasive mucormycosis in adults, an oral or IV loading dosage of 372 mg of isavuconazonium sulfate (equivalent to 200 mg of isavuconazole) should be given every 8 hours for 6 doses; beginning 12–24 hours after the final loading dose, therapy should be continued using a maintenance dosage of 372 mg of isavuconazonium sulfate (equivalent to 200 mg of isavuconazole) once every 24 hours.

The total duration of IV and oral therapy should be based on the severity of the patient's underlying disease, recovery from immunosuppression, and response to the drug. In a clinical study in adults with invasive mucormycosis, the median treatment duration of isavuconazonium sulfate therapy was 102, 33, or 85 days in those receiving the drug for initial treatment (primary treatment), disease refractory to other antifungal therapy, or intolerance to other antifungal therapy, respectively.

Esophageal Candidiasis. If oral isavuconazonium sulfate is used as an alternative for the treatment of esophageal candidiasis† in adults with human immunodeficiency virus (HIV) infection, the US Centers for Disease Control and Prevention (CDC), National Institutes of Health (NIH), and HIV Medicine Association of IDSA state that 3 different dosage regimens of the drug can be considered. A loading dose of 372 mg of isavuconazonium sulfate (equivalent to 200 mg of isavuconazole) can be given followed by 93 mg of isavuconazonium sulfate (equivalent to 50 mg of isavuconazole) once daily or a loading dose of 744 mg of isavuconazonium sulfate (equivalent to 400 mg of isavuconazole) can be given followed by 186 mg of isavuconazonium sulfate (equivalent to 100 mg of isavuconazole) once daily. Alternatively, a once-weekly regimen of 744 mg of isavuconazonium sulfate (equivalent to 400 mg of isavuconazole) can be used.

CDC, NIH, and IDSA recommend that treatment of esophageal candidiasis be continued for 14–21 days.

■ Special Populations

Hepatic Impairment The manufacturer states that dosage adjustments are not needed when isavuconazonium sulfate is used in adults with mild or moderate hepatic impairment (Child-Pugh class A or B). Some clinicians suggest that reduced dosage should be considered in such patients.

Dosage recommendations for those with severe hepatic impairment (Child-Pugh class C) are not available. The drug has not been studied in patients with severe hepatic impairment and should be used in such patients only when benefits outweigh risks. (See Hepatic Impairment under Warnings/Precautions: Specific Populations, in Cautions.)

Renal Impairment Dosage adjustments are not needed when isavuconazonium sulfate is used in adults with mild, moderate, or severe renal impairment, including those with end-stage renal disease. (See Renal Impairment under Warnings/Precautions: Specific Populations, in Cautions.)

Geriatric Patients Dosage adjustments based on age or gender are not needed when isavuconazonium sulfate is used in geriatric patients. (See Geriatric Use under Warnings/Precautions: Specific Populations, in Cautions.)

Cautions

■ Contraindications

Isavuconazonium sulfate is contraindicated in patients with known hypersensitivity to isavuconazole (active metabolite of isavuconazonium sulfate).

Isavuconazonium sulfate is contraindicated in patients with familial short QT syndrome. (See Cardiovascular Effects under Cautions: Warnings/Precautions.)

Concomitant use of isavuconazonium sulfate with drugs that are potent cytochrome P-450 (CYP) 3A4 inhibitors (e.g., ketoconazole, high-dose ritonavir) or inducers (e.g., rifampin, carbamazepine, St. John's wort [*Hypericum perforatum*], long-acting barbiturates) is contraindicated since such use may substantially increase or decrease isavuconazole plasma concentrations, respectively. (See Drug Interactions.)

■ Warnings/Precautions

Sensitivity Reactions Serious hypersensitivity (e.g., anaphylaxis) and severe skin reactions (e.g., Stevens-Johnson syndrome) have occurred in patients receiving other azole antifungals.

Data regarding cross-sensitivity between isavuconazonium sulfate and other azole antifungals are not available. The drug should be used with caution in patients hypersensitive to other azoles.

If a severe adverse cutaneous reaction occurs during isavuconazonium therapy, the drug should be discontinued.

Hepatic Effects Serious hepatic effects, including hepatitis, cholestasis, and hepatic failure (sometimes fatal), have been reported in patients with serious underlying medical conditions (e.g., hematologic malignancy) receiving an azole antifungal, including isavuconazonium sulfate.

Less severe hepatic effects (e.g., increased ALT, AST, alkaline phosphatase, total bilirubin concentrations) have been reported in clinical trials of isavuconazonium sulfate. In one study, 4.4% of patients receiving the drug had elevated liver aminotransferase (ALT or AST) concentrations exceeding 3 times the upper limit of normal (ULN) at the end of study treatment; 1.2% had elevations exceeding 10 times the ULN. Liver function test elevations generally were reversible and discontinuance of isavuconazonium was not required.

Liver function should be evaluated prior to and monitored during isavuconazonium sulfate therapy. If abnormal liver function test results occur during therapy with the drug, the patient should be monitored for the development of more severe hepatic injury. If signs and symptoms consistent with liver disease develop, isavuconazonium sulfate should be discontinued.

Infusion Reactions Infusion reactions, including hypotension, dyspnea, chills, dizziness, paresthesia, and hypoesthesia, have occurred during IV infusion of isavuconazonium sulfate. To reduce the risk of infusion reactions, reconstituted isavuconazonium sulfate should be diluted in 250 mL of a compatible diluent and infused over at least 1 hour. (See IV Infusion under Dosage and Administration: Administration.) If an infusion reaction occurs, the IV infusion should be discontinued.

Fetal/Neonatal Morbidity and Mortality Isavuconazonium sulfate may cause fetal harm if administered to pregnant women.

Isavuconazonium has been shown to cause increased perinatal mortality and skeletal abnormalities when given orally to pregnant rats and rabbits; these effects were observed at dosages associated with clinically relevant plasma exposures. Skeletal abnormalities also have been observed in animal studies evaluating other azole antifungals. (See Pregnancy under Warnings/Precautions: Specific Populations, in Cautions.)

Cardiovascular Effects Isavuconazonium sulfate shortens the corrected QT (QT_c) interval in a dose-related manner. In a randomized, placebo- and active-controlled study in healthy adults, oral administration of isavuconazonium sulfate in a dosage of 372 mg (equivalent to 200 mg of isavuconazole) 3 times daily for 2 days followed by either 372 or 1116 mg (equivalent to 200 or 600 mg, respectively, of isavuconazole) once daily for 13 days resulted in shortening of the QT_c interval compared with placebo (least-squares mean difference at 2 hours postdose of −13.1 or −24.6 msec, respectively). Because of this effect, isavuconazonium sulfate is contraindicated in patients with familial short QT syndrome (see Cautions: Contraindications). Concomitant use with other drugs that shorten the QT_c interval was not evaluated. (See Drug Interactions: Drugs that Shorten the QT Interval.)

Other cardiovascular effects reported in patients receiving isavuconazonium sulfate include atrial fibrillation, atrial flutter, bradycardia, palpitations, supraventricular extrasystoles, supraventricular tachycardia, ventricular extrasystoles, and cardiac arrest.

Interactions Concomitant use of isavuconazonium sulfate with drugs that are potent cytochrome P-450 (CYP) 3A4 inhibitors (e.g., ketoconazole, high-dose ritonavir) or inducers (e.g., rifampin, carbamazepine, St. John's wort, long-acting barbiturates) is contraindicated. (See Drug Interactions.)

Administration Precautions IV solutions of isavuconazonium sulfate *must* be administered by IV infusion through an inline filter to remove any insoluble particulates of isavuconazole that may be present. (See IV Infusion under Dosage and Administration: Administration.)

Selection and Use of Antifungals Prior to initiation of isavuconazonium sulfate therapy, appropriate specimens for fungal culture and other relevant laboratory studies (including histopathology) should be obtained to isolate and identify the causative organism(s). The drug may be started pending availability of results, but antifungal therapy should be adjusted as needed when results become available.

Information on test methods and quality control standards for in vitro susceptibility testing of antifungal agents and specific interpretive criteria for such testing recognized by FDA is available at https://www.fda.gov/STIC.

Specific Populations **Pregnancy.** Category C. (See Users Guide.)

There are no adequate and well-controlled studies to date evaluating isavuconazonium sulfate in pregnant women. Based on data from animal reproduction studies, the drug is predicted to have the potential to increase the risk of adverse developmental outcomes above background risk.

Increased perinatal mortality occurred in rats given oral isavuconazonium sulfate at a dosage corresponding to less than half the human maintenance dosage (based on area under the concentration-time curve [AUC] comparisons). In addition, dose-related increases in the incidences of skeletal abnormalities (e.g., rudimentary and/or supernumerary ribs, zygomatic arch fusion) occurred in rats and rabbits given isavuconazonium chloride at dosages corresponding to about 10–20% of human exposure (based on AUC comparisons).

Isavuconazonium sulfate should be used during pregnancy only if potential benefits to the woman outweigh potential risks to the fetus. Women who become pregnant while receiving the drug are encouraged to contact their clinician.

Lactation. Isavuconazole is distributed into milk in rats. Women receiving isavuconazonium sulfate should not breast-feed.

Pediatric Use. Safety and efficacy of isavuconazonium sulfate have not been established in patients younger than 18 years of age.

Geriatric Use. In phase 2 and 3 trials of isavuconazonium sulfate, 16% of patients were older than 65 years of age and 4% were older than 75 years of age. No substantial differences in pharmacokinetics were observed between geriatric and younger adults.

Hepatic Impairment. Isavuconazonium sulfate has not been studied in patients with severe hepatic impairment (Child-Pugh class C). The drug should be used in patients with severe hepatic impairment only if benefits outweigh risks; if the drug is used in such patients, they should be monitored for adverse effects.

Although hepatic impairment does not affect the extent of in vivo conversion of isavuconazonium sulfate to isavuconazole (the active drug), increased peak plasma concentrations and AUC, reduced clearance, and increased half-life of isavuconazole have been reported in individuals with hepatic impairment. Data from patients with mild or moderate hepatic impairment (Child-Pugh class A or B) indicate that mean peak plasma concentrations of isavuconazole are decreased by 2 or 30%, respectively, and mean AUC of isavuconazole is increased by 64 or 84%, respectively, relative to healthy individuals with normal hepatic function. After IV administration, systemic clearance is decreased by 29 or 48% in individuals with mild or moderate hepatic impairment, respectively, relative to healthy individuals and elimination half-life is increased to 224 or 302 hours, respectively, compared with 123 hours in healthy individuals. Similarly, in a population pharmacokinetic evaluation, isavuconazole clearance was decreased by 40 or 48% in those with mild or moderate hepatic impairment, respectively, relative to the healthy population. The clinical importance of such effects is unknown. The manufacturer states that dosage adjustments are not necessary in patients with mild or moderate hepatic impairment.

Renal Impairment. Clinically important changes in isavuconazole pharmacokinetics (peak plasma concentrations, AUC) were not observed in adults with mild, moderate, or severe renal impairment. Hemodialysis does not remove isavuconazole from the circulation. Dosage adjustments are not needed in patients with renal impairment or in those with end-stage renal disease.

■ **Common Adverse Effects** Adverse effects reported in 5% or more of patients receiving isavuconazonium sulfate include GI effects (nausea, vomiting, diarrhea, abdominal pain, constipation, dyspepsia, decreased appetite), elevated bilirubin and liver enzymes (e.g., ALT, AST, alkaline phosphatase, γ-glutamyltransferase), metabolic effects (hypokalemia, hypomagnesemia), respiratory effects (dyspnea, cough, acute respiratory failure), headache, fatigue, insomnia, back pain, chest pain, peripheral edema, hypotension, renal failure, delirium (e.g., agitation, confusional state, disorientation, mental status changes), anxiety, rash, pruritus, and administration site reactions.

Drug Interactions

Because isavuconazonium sulfate is rapidly metabolized to isavuconazole in vivo, drug interactions are reported for isavuconazole.

■ **Drugs Affecting or Metabolized by Hepatic Microsomal Enzymes** Isavuconazole is a substrate of cytochrome P-450 (CYP) 3A4 and inhibitors or inducers of CYP3A4 may increase or decrease plasma concentrations of isavuconazole, respectively. Concomitant use of isavuconazonium sulfate with potent CYP3A4 inhibitors (e.g., ketoconazole, high-dose ritonavir) or inducers (e.g., rifampin, carbamazepine, St. John's wort [*Hypericum perforatum*], long-acting barbiturates) is contraindicated.

Isavuconazole also is a substrate of CYP3A5. Isavuconazole is a moderate inhibitor of CYP3A4. In vitro, isavuconazole inhibits CYP isoenzymes 2C8, 2C9, 2C19, and 2D6 and induces CYP isoenzymes 3A4, 2B6, 2C8, and 2C9.

■ **Drugs Affecting or Affected by Membrane Transporters** Isavuconazole is a weak inhibitor of the P-glycoprotein (P-gp) transport system. Concomitant use of isavuconazonium sulfate with P-gp substrates that have a narrow therapeutic index (e.g., digoxin) may require dosage adjustment of the P-gp substrate.

Isavuconazole is a weak inhibitor of organic cation transporter (OCT) 2. The drug also is an inhibitor of breast cancer resistance protein (BCRP).

Isavuconazole does not inhibit organic anion transporting polypeptide (OATP) 1B1 or OATP1B3.

■ **Drugs that Shorten the QT Interval** Concomitant use of isavuconazonium sulfate with other drugs that shorten the corrected QT (QT_c) interval has not been evaluated in formal ECG studies; the additive effects of such use are unknown. (See Cardiovascular Effects under Cautions: Warnings/Precautions.)

■ **Anticonvulsants** ***Carbamazepine*** Potential pharmacokinetic interactions with carbamazepine (decreased isavuconazole concentrations).

Concomitant use of carbamazepine and isavuconazonium sulfate is contraindicated.

■ **Antifungal Agents** ***Ketoconazole*** Pharmacokinetic interactions with ketoconazole (9% increase in isavuconazole peak plasma concentration and greater than fivefold increase in isavuconazole area under the concentration-time curve [AUC]).

Concomitant use of ketoconazole and isavuconazonium sulfate is contraindicated.

■ **Antimycobacterial Agents** ***Rifampin*** Pharmacokinetic interactions with rifampin (75% decrease in isavuconazole peak plasma concentration and 97% decrease in isavuconazole AUC).

Concomitant use of rifampin and isavuconazonium sulfate is contraindicated.

■ **Antiretroviral Agents** ***HIV Entry and Fusion Inhibitors*** **Maraviroc.** Potential pharmacokinetic interactions with maraviroc (increased maraviroc concentrations).

If maraviroc and isavuconazonium sulfate are used concomitantly, a maraviroc dosage of 150 mg twice daily should be considered.

HIV Integrase Inhibitors (INSTIs) **Bictegravir.** Potential pharmacokinetic interactions with bictegravir (increased bictegravir concentrations).

Some experts state that dosage adjustments are not necessary if bictegravir is used concomitantly with isavuconazonium sulfate.

Elvitegravir. Potential pharmacokinetic interactions with *cobicistat-boosted* elvitegravir (increased isavuconazole concentrations expected; increased elvitegravir and cobicistat concentrations possible).

If isavuconazonium sulfate is used concomitantly with *cobicistat-boosted* elvitegravir, some experts state that consideration should be given to monitoring isavuconazole concentrations and assessing virologic response.

HIV Nonnucleoside Reverse Transcriptase Inhibitors (NNRTIs) **Doravirine and Rilpivirine.** Possible pharmacokinetic interactions with doravirine or rilpivirine (increased concentrations of the NNRTI).

Some experts state that dosage adjustments are not necessary if isavuconazonium sulfate is used concomitantly with doravirine or rilpivirine.

Efavirenz, Etravirine, and Nevirapine. Possible pharmacokinetic interactions with efavirenz, etravirine, or nevirapine (decreased isavuconazole concentrations).

If isavuconazonium sulfate is used concomitantly with efavirenz, etravirine, or nevirapine, some experts state that dosage of the antifungal may need to be adjusted and consideration should be given to monitoring isavuconazole concentrations and antifungal response.

HIV Protease Inhibitors (PIs) **Lopinavir.** Pharmacokinetic interactions with the fixed combination of lopinavir and ritonavir (lopinavir/ritonavir) (74% increase in isavuconazole peak plasma concentration and 96%

increase in isavuconazole AUC; mean decrease of 27 and 31% in AUC of lopinavir and ritonavir, respectively). Decreased lopinavir and ritonavir exposures may result in loss of antiretroviral efficacy.

Caution is advised if lopinavir/ritonavir and isavuconazonium sulfate are used concomitantly. Some experts state that consideration should be given to monitoring isavuconazole concentrations and toxicities and assessing virologic response.

Ritonavir. Potential pharmacokinetic interactions (increased isavuconazole exposure) with high-dose ritonavir (400 mg twice daily).

Concomitant use of high-dose ritonavir and isavuconazonium sulfate is contraindicated.

Other HIV PIs. Potential pharmacokinetic interactions with other HIV PIs (increased isavuconazole concentrations and altered HIV PI concentrations).

If isavuconazonium sulfate is used concomitantly with an HIV PI, some experts state that consideration should be given to monitoring isavuconazole concentrations and toxicities and monitoring HIV PI toxicities and virologic response.

■ **Barbiturates** Potential pharmacokinetic interactions with long-acting barbiturates (decreased isavuconazole concentrations).

Concomitant use of long-acting barbiturates and isavuconazonium sulfate is contraindicated.

■ **Bupropion** Pharmacokinetic interactions with bupropion (decreased bupropion exposure).

Bupropion and isavuconazonium sulfate should be used concomitantly with caution; increased bupropion dosage may be necessary but dosage should not exceed the maximum recommended dosage.

■ **Caffeine** No clinically important effects on caffeine pharmacokinetics.

■ **Corticosteroids** No clinically important effects on prednisone pharmacokinetics.

■ **Cyclophosphamide** Cyclophosphamide and isavuconazonium sulfate should be used concomitantly with caution.

■ **Dextromethorphan** No clinically important effects on dextromethorphan pharmacokinetics.

■ **Digoxin** Pharmacokinetic interactions with digoxin (increased digoxin exposure).

Digoxin and isavuconazonium sulfate should be used concomitantly with caution; digoxin serum concentrations should be monitored and digoxin dosage adjusted accordingly.

■ **Estrogens and Progestins** No clinically important effects on the pharmacokinetics of oral contraceptives containing ethinyl estradiol or norethindrone.

■ **HMG-CoA Reductase Inhibitors** ***Atorvastatin*** Potential pharmacokinetic interactions with atorvastatin (increased atorvastatin exposure).

Atorvastatin and isavuconazonium sulfate should be used concomitantly with caution and patients monitored for atorvastatin-related adverse effects.

■ **Immunosuppressive Agents** ***Cyclosporine*** Pharmacokinetic interactions with cyclosporine (increased cyclosporine exposure).

Isavuconazonium sulfate and cyclosporine should be used concomitantly with caution; cyclosporine concentrations should be monitored and cyclosporine dosage adjusted accordingly.

Mycophenolate Mofetil Pharmacokinetic interactions with mycophenolate mofetil (increased mycophenolic acid exposure).

Mycophenolate mofetil and isavuconazonium sulfate should be used concomitantly with caution; patients should be monitored for mycophenolic acid-related toxicities.

Sirolimus Pharmacokinetic interactions with sirolimus (approximately twofold increase in sirolimus exposure).

Sirolimus and isavuconazonium sulfate should be used concomitantly with caution; sirolimus plasma concentrations should be monitored and sirolimus dosage adjusted accordingly.

Tacrolimus Pharmacokinetic interactions with tacrolimus (approximately twofold increase in tacrolimus exposure).

Tacrolimus and isavuconazonium sulfate should be used concomitantly with caution; tacrolimus concentrations should be monitored and tacrolimus dosage adjusted accordingly.

■ **Metformin** No clinically important effects on metformin pharmacokinetics.

■ **Methadone** No clinically important effects on methadone pharmacokinetics.

■ **Methotrexate** No clinically important effects on methotrexate pharmacokinetics.

■ **Midazolam** Pharmacokinetic interactions with midazolam (approximately twofold increase in midazolam exposure).

Midazolam and isavuconazonium sulfate should be used concomitantly with caution; consideration should be given to reducing midazolam dosage.

■ **Proton-pump Inhibitors** ***Esomeprazole*** No clinically important effects on isavuconazole pharmacokinetics.

Omeprazole No clinically important effects on omeprazole pharmacokinetics.

■ **Repaglinide** No clinically important effects on repaglinide pharmacokinetics.

■ **St. John's Wort** Potential pharmacokinetic interactions with St. John's wort (*Hypericum perforatum*) (decreased isavuconazole concentrations).

Concomitant use of St. John's wort and isavuconazonium sulfate is contraindicated.

■ **Warfarin** No clinically important effects on warfarin pharmacokinetics.

Description

Isavuconazonium sulfate, a prodrug of isavuconazole, is a triazole antifungal agent structurally similar to fluconazole and voriconazole. Isavuconazonium is inactive until converted in vivo to isavuconazole.

Like other triazole antifungals, isavuconazole inhibits 14-α-demethylase, which leads to accumulation of methylated sterols (e.g., 14-α-methylated lanosterol, 4,14-dimethylzymosterol, 24-methylenedihydrolanosterol) and decreased concentrations of ergosterol in fungal cell membranes. Depletion of ergosterol affects cell membrane integrity and function and can lead to fungal cell death.

Following oral or IV administration of isavuconazonium sulfate, the drug is rapidly and almost completely (greater than 98%) hydrolyzed by esterases (principally butylcholinesterase) in the blood to yield the active moiety, isavuconazole, and an inactive cleavage product. Peak plasma concentrations of isavuconazole are achieved in approximately 2–4 hours after oral administration and 0.7–1 hour after the start of IV infusion of isavuconazonium sulfate. It has been estimated that steady-state concentrations of isavuconazole are not achieved until after 2 weeks. The absolute bioavailability of isavuconazole following oral administration of isavuconazonium sulfate is 98%. Oral administration of a 744-mg dose of isavuconazonium sulfate with a high-fat meal resulted in a 9% decrease in isavuconazole peak plasma concentrations and a 9% increase in isavuconazole area under the plasma concentration-time curve (AUC); these effects were not considered clinically important. Isavuconazole is greater than 99% bound to plasma proteins, mainly albumin. In vivo studies indicate that isavuconazole is metabolized by cytochrome P-450 (CYP) isoenzymes 3A4 and 3A5 and, subsequently, by uridine diphosphate-glucuronosyltransferase (UGT). In a single-dose study in adults using oral or IV isavuconazonium sulfate, the mean distribution half-life of isavuconazole was 1.7–2.1 or 0.42–1.6 hours, respectively, and the mean terminal elimination half-life of isavuconazole was 56–77 or 76–104 hours, respectively. Following oral administration of radiolabeled isavuconazonium sulfate, 46% of the total radioactive dose was recovered in feces (approximately 33% as isavuconazole) and 46% was recovered in urine (principally as metabolites of isavuconazole and metabolites of the inactive cleavage product). Less than 1% of a dose of isavuconazonium sulfate is eliminated in urine as active isavuconazole.

■ **Spectrum** Isavuconazole is active in vitro and in clinical infections against *Aspergillus flavus*, *A. fumigatus*, and *A. niger*, and also has in vitro activity against *A. lentulus*, *A. nidulans*, *A. sydowii*, *A. terreus*, *A. versicolor*, and *A. welsitschiae*.

Isavuconazole is active in vitro and in clinical infections against fungi in the order Mucorales, including *Rhizopus* (*R. oryzae*, *R. azygosporus*, *R. microsporus*), *Mucor* (*M. amphibiorum*, *M. circinelloides*), *Lichtheimia* (*L. corymbifera*; formerly *Absidia corymbifera*), and *Rhizomucor* (*R. pusillus*). In vitro studies indicate that isavuconazole is less active against Mucorales compared with *Aspergillus*.

Isavuconazole is active in vitro against *Candida*, including *C. albicans*, *C. dubliniensis*, *C. glabrata*, *C. guilliermondii*, *C. kefyr*, *C. krusei*, *C. lusitaniae*, *C. orthopsilosis*, *C. parapsilosis*, and *C. tropicalis*. Some strains of *C. auris* (often misidentified as *C. haemulonii*, *C. famata*, or *Rhodotorula glutinis*) have been inhibited in vitro by isavuconazole concentrations of 0.004–0.25 mcg/mL. Isavuconazole has in vitro activity against some *Candida* that have reduced susceptibility or resistance to fluconazole.

Although the clinical importance is unclear, isavuconazole also has in vitro activity against *Blastomyces dermatitidis*, *Coccidioides posadasii*, *Cryptococcus gattii*, *C. neoformans*, *Geotrichum capitatum*, *Histoplasma capsulatum*, *Penicillium*, *Pichia*, *Rhodotorula*, *Saccharomyces cerevisiae*, *Scedosporium*, *Trichosporon*, and dermatophytes (*Trichophyton rubrum*, *T. mentagrophytes*, *T. tonsurans*, *Epidermophyton floccosum*, *Microsporum canis*).

■ **Resistance** Resistance or reduced susceptibility to isavuconazole may occur. *Aspergillus* and *Candida* with reduced susceptibility or resistance to isavuconazole have been reported.

Like other azole antifungals, resistance to isavuconazole is likely conferred by multiple mechanisms involving substitutions in the target gene. Resistance to azole antifungals can result from altered cellular accumulation of the drug, increased levels of and/or decreased affinity for the target enzyme, and modifications of the ergosterol biosynthesis pathway. Changes in sterol profile and elevated efflux pump activity have been observed; however, the clinical relevance of such findings is unclear.

Cross-resistance can occur between isavuconazole and other azoles (e.g., itraconazole, voriconazole). Although the relevance of cross-resistance to clinical outcomes has not been fully characterized, alternative antifungal therapy may be required in patients in whom prior azole therapy has failed.

Advice to Patients

Isavuconazonium sulfate can be taken with or without food.

Importance of swallowing capsules whole, without crushing, chewing, dissolving, or opening.

Importance of informing clinicians of existing or contemplated concomitant therapy, including prescription and OTC drugs, and any concomitant illnesses (e.g., liver disease, familial short QT syndrome).

Importance of women informing clinicians if they are or plan to become pregnant or plan to breast-feed. (See Fetal/Neonatal Morbidity and Mortality under Cautions: Warnings/Precautions.)

Importance of advising patients of other important precautionary information. (See Cautions.)

Overview® (see Users Guide). For additional information on this drug until a more detailed monograph is developed and published, the manufacturer's labeling should be consulted. It is *essential* that the manufacturer's labeling be consulted for more detailed information on usual cautions, precautions, contraindications, potential drug interactions, laboratory test interferences, and acute toxicity.

Preparations

Excipients in commercially available drug preparations may have clinically important effects in some individuals; consult specific product labeling for details.

Isavuconazonium Sulfate

Oral		
Capsules	186 mg (equivalent to 100 mg isavuconazole)	**Cresemba®**, Astellas
Parenteral		
For injection, for IV infusion	372 mg (equivalent to 200 mg isavuconazole)	**Cresemba®**, Astellas

†Use is not currently included in the labeling approved by the US Food and Drug Administration

Itraconazole

■ Itraconazole, a synthetic triazole derivative, is an azole antifungal agent.

Uses

Oral itraconazole capsules are used in immunocompromised and immunocompetent patients for the treatment of systemic fungal infections, including blastomycosis (pulmonary and extrapulmonary), histoplasmosis (including chronic cavitary pulmonary disease and disseminated, nonmeningeal disease), and aspergillosis (pulmonary and extrapulmonary). Itraconazole oral solution (but not itraconazole capsules) is used for the treatment of oropharyngeal and esophageal candidiasis. Itraconazole (given IV initially [IV preparation no longer commercially available in the US] followed by itraconazole oral solution) has been used for empiric antifungal therapy in febrile neutropenic patients. Oral itraconazole capsules are used in immunocompetent individuals for the treatment of tinea unguium (onychomycosis) of the toenail and/or fingernail caused by dermatophytes. Itraconazole also is used orally for prevention of serious fungal infections (e.g., coccidioidomycosis, cryptococcosis, histoplasmosis, mucocutaneous candidiasis) in patients with human immunodeficiency virus (HIV) infection†.

Prior to initiation of oral itraconazole capsules for the treatment of systemic fungal infections, appropriate specimens for fungal culture and other relevant laboratory studies (wet mount, histopathology, serology) should be obtained in order to isolate and identify the causative organism(s). Itraconazole therapy may be started pending results of these in vitro tests; however, once results are available, therapy should be adjusted accordingly.

■ **Aspergillosis** Itraconazole is used in the treatment of pulmonary and extrapulmonary aspergillosis in patients who are intolerant of or who are refractory to IV amphotericin B.

The Infectious Diseases Society of America (IDSA) considers voriconazole the drug of choice for primary treatment of invasive aspergillosis in most patients and IV amphotericin B the preferred alternative. For salvage therapy in patients refractory to or intolerant of primary antifungal therapy, IDSA recommends amphotericin B, caspofungin, micafungin, posaconazole, or itraconazole. For empiric or preemptive therapy of presumed aspergillosis, IDSA recommends IV amphotericin B, caspofungin, itraconazole, or voriconazole.

Itraconazole is not considered a drug of choice or preferred alternative for the treatment of invasive aspergillosis in HIV-infected individuals. For the treatment of invasive aspergillosis in adults and adolescents with human immunodeficiency virus (HIV) infection, the US Centers for Disease Control and Prevention (CDC), National Institutes of Health (NIH), and IDSA recommend voriconazole as the drug of choice; amphotericin B, caspofungin, and posaconazole are recommended as alternatives. Voriconazole also is considered the drug of choice for treatment of invasive aspergillosis in HIV-infected children†; amphotericin B and caspofungin are alternatives. Because the drugs have similar mechanisms of action and cross-resistance may occur, itraconazole is not recommended for the treatment of aspergillosis refractory to voriconazole.

Itraconazole is recommended as an alternative for primary prophylaxis of aspergillosis in immunocompromised individuals at high risk of invasive aspergillosis. The IDSA considers posaconazole the drug of choice for primary prophylaxis of aspergillosis in neutropenic patients with acute myelogenous leukemia (AML) or myelodysplastic syndrome (MDS) and in hematopoietic stem cell transplant (HSCT) recipients with graft-versus-host disease (GVHD); itraconazole and micafungin are alternatives for prophylaxis in these individuals.

Clinical Experience In a limited number of patients with invasive aspergillosis who did not respond to or could not tolerate IV amphotericin B, oral itraconazole capsules (200–400 mg daily given for a median duration of therapy of 3–4 months) have been effective as second-line therapy. In an open, multicenter study in adults with active invasive pulmonary aspergillosis (61% had received antifungal prophylaxis and some had received prior empiric antifungal therapy prior to study entry), itraconazole was given in a regimen that included IV itraconazole therapy initially (200 mg twice daily for 2 days then 200 mg once daily for 12 days; IV preparation no longer commercially available in the US) followed by oral itraconazole capsules (200 mg twice daily) for 12 weeks. At the end of itraconazole therapy, 39% had a complete or partial clinical response (intent-to-treat analysis) and the median time to response was 55 days. In a multicenter open study in patients with invasive aspergillosis who received oral itraconazole capsules (200 mg 3 times daily for 4 days, followed by 200 mg twice daily for at least 4 months; some patients received drug therapy for more than 12 months), therapy was effective in about 39% of patients.

■ **Blastomycosis** Itraconazole is used for the treatment of pulmonary and extrapulmonary blastomycosis caused by *Blastomyces dermatitidis*.

The drugs of choice for the treatment of blastomycosis are oral itraconazole and IV amphotericin B. IV amphotericin B is preferred for initial treatment of severe infections, especially infections involving the CNS, and for initial treatment of presumptive blastomycosis in immunocompromised patients, including HIV-infected individuals.

Oral itraconazole is the drug of choice for the treatment of nonmeningeal, non-life-threatening blastomycosis, including mild to moderate pulmonary blastomycosis or mild to moderate disseminated blastomycosis (without CNS involvement), and also is recommended for follow-up therapy in patients with more severe infections after an initial response has been obtained with IV amphotericin B.

For the treatment of CNS blastomycosis, the IDSA recommends initial treatment with IV amphotericin B, followed by an oral azole antifungal. Although oral fluconazole, oral itraconazole, or oral voriconazole can be used for follow-up treatment of CNS blastomycosis, the most appropriate azole for such treatment is unclear. Azole antifungals should not be relied on for initial treatment of CNS blastomycosis. The fact that treatment failures have been reported when an oral antifungal(e.g., ketoconazole) was used in the treatment of cutaneous or pulmonary blastomycosis in patients who had asymptomatic or subclinical CNS involvement at the time of the initial diagnosis should be considered when selecting an antifungalfor patients with blastomycosis.

The IDSA states that long-term suppressive or maintenance therapy (secondary prophylaxis)† with oral itraconazole may be required to prevent relapse or recurrence of blastomycosis in immunocompromised patients and in other patients who experience relapse despite appropriate therapy. Such prophylaxis is not addressed in current CDC, NIH, and IDSA guidelines for the prevention of opportunistic infections in individuals infected with HIV.

■ **Candida Infections** ***Candidemia and Other Invasive Candida Infections*** Itraconazole is not a drug of choice or a preferred alternative for the treatment of candidemia† or other invasive *Candida* infections†. Fluconazole or voriconazole usually is recommended when an azole antifungal is used for the treatment of candidemia.

Itraconazole has been used and is recommended as an alternative for initial empiric treatment of suspected invasive candidiasis in neutropenic patients†. IV amphotericin B, caspofungin, or voriconazole are considered the drugs of choice in these patients; alternatives are fluconazole or itraconazole. An azole antifungal should not be used for empiric treatment of candidemia in patients who previously received an azole for prophylaxis.

Oropharyngeal Candidiasis Itraconazole oral solution is used for the treatment of oropharyngeal candidiasis. Because topical effects and drug exposure may be greater with itraconazole oral solution than with itraconazole capsules, only itraconazole oral solution should be used for the treatment of oropharyngeal candidiasis.

For the treatment of mild oropharyngeal candidiasis, the IDSA recommends topical treatment with clotrimazole lozenges or nystatin oral suspension; oral fluconazole is recommended for moderate to severe disease. For refractory oropharyngeal candidiasis, including fluconazole-refractory infections, the IDSA recommends itraconazole oral solution, oral posaconazole, or oral voriconazole. Other alternatives for refractory infections are an IV echinocandin (caspofungin, micafungin, anidulafungin) or IV amphotericin B.

For the treatment of oropharyngeal candidiasis in HIV-infected adults and adolescents, the CDC, NIH, and IDSA recommend oral fluconazole as the preferred drug of choice for initial episodes; other drugs of choice are clotrimazole lozenges or nystatin oral suspension. Alternatives for initial episodes are itraconazole oral solution or oral posaconazole. For fluconazole-refractory infections in HIV-infected adults and adolescents, itraconazole oral solution or oral posaconazole is preferred; alternatives include IV amphotericin B, an IV echinocandin (caspofungin, micafungin, anidulafungin), or oral or IV voriconazole.

Although routine long-term suppressive or maintenance therapy (secondary prophylaxis)† to prevent relapse or recurrence is not usually recommended in patients adequately treated for oropharyngeal candidiasis, patients with frequent or severe recurrences (including HIV-infected adults, adolescents, and children) may benefit from secondary prophylaxis with oral fluconazole or itraconazole oral solution; however, the potential for azole resistance should be considered. Patients with fluconazole-refractory oropharyngeal candidiasis who responded to an echinocandin should receive voriconazole or posaconazole for secondary prophylaxis until antiretroviral therapy produces immune reconstitution.

Clinical Experience. In 2 controlled studies in patients with oropharyngeal candidiasis (92% were HIV-infected), a clinical response (defined as cured or improved) was attained in 71–84% of patients receiving itraconazole oral solution. There is some evidence that itraconazole oral solution is at least as effective as oral fluconazole tablets and may be more effective than oral clotrimazole lozenges for the treatment of oropharyngeal candidiasis. Itraconazole oral solution has been effective for the treatment of oropharyngeal candidiasis in some patients, including some HIV-infected individuals, who failed to respond to oral fluconazole.

Esophageal Candidiasis Itraconazole oral solution is used for the treatment of esophageal candidiasis. Because topical effects and drug exposure may be greater with itraconazole oral solution than with itraconazole capsules, only itraconazole oral solution should be used for the treatment of esophageal candidiasis.

Esophageal candidiasis requires treatment with a systemic antifungal (not a topical antifungal).

The IDSA recommends oral fluconazole as the preferred drug of choice for treatment of esophageal candidiasis; if oral therapy is not tolerated, IV fluconazole, IV amphotericin B, or an IV echinocandin (caspofungin, micafungin, anidulafungin) is recommended. For fluconazole-refractory infections, preferred alternatives are itraconazole oral solution, oral posaconazole, or oral or IV voriconazole; other alternatives are an IV echinocandin (caspofungin, micafungin, anidulafungin) or IV amphotericin B.

For the treatment of esophageal candidiasis in HIV-infected adults and adolescents, the CDC, NIH, and IDSA recommend oral or IV fluconazole as the preferred drug of choice and itraconazole oral solution as the preferred alternative. Other alternatives include an IV echinocandin (caspofungin, micafungin, anidulafungin), oral or IV voriconazole, oral posaconazole, or IV amphotericin B. For refractory esophageal candidiasis, including fluconazole-refractory infections, in HIV-infected adults and adolescents itraconazole oral solution or oral posaconazole is preferred; alternatives include IV amphotericin B, an IV echinocandin (caspofungin, micafungin, anidulafungin), or oral or IV voriconazole.

Although routine long-term suppressive or maintenance therapy (secondary prophylaxis)† to prevent relapse or recurrence is not usually recommended in patients adequately treated for esophageal candidiasis, patients with frequent or severe recurrences, including HIV-infected adults, adolescents, or children, may benefit from secondary prophylaxis with oral fluconazole or oral posaconazole; however, the potential for azole resistance should be considered. Itraconazole is not included in current recommendations for secondary prophylaxis of esophageal candidiasis.

Clinical Experience. In a double-blind, randomized study in immunocompromised patients with esophageal candidiasis (93% were HIV-infected), a clinical response (defined as cured or improved) was attained in 94% of those who received itraconazole oral solution and 91% of those who received fluconazole tablets. The median time to response was similar in both groups (27 or 28 days). Follow-up of a group of patients who had a clinical response to the drug indicated that 18% of those who had received itraconazole and 27% of those who had received fluconazole had relapse of esophageal candidiasis within 30 days after treatment was discontinued.

Vulvovaginal Candidiasis Oral itraconazole has been used for the treatment of uncomplicated vulvovaginal candidiasis†.

Vulvovaginal candidiasis is usually treated with an intravaginal azole antifungal (e.g., butoconazole, clotrimazole, miconazole, terconazole, tioconazole) or a single-dose oral fluconazole regimen. Although some clinicians suggest that oral itraconazole or oral ketoconazole can be used as alternatives for the treatment of vulvovaginal candidiasis, fluconazole is the only oral antifungal included in CDC recommendations for the treatment of uncomplicated or complicated vulvovaginal candidiasis.

■ **Chromomycosis** Oral itraconazole has been used with some success for the treatment of chromomycosis† (chromoblastomycosis) caused by various dematiaceous fungi (e.g., *Cladosporium, Exophiala, Fonsecaea, Phialophora*).

■ **Coccidioidomycosis** Oral itraconazole is used for the treatment and prevention of coccidioidomycosis† caused by *Coccidioides immitis* or *C. posadasii*.

Treatment of Coccidioidomycosis Oral itraconazole is used for the treatment of coccidioidomycosis†.

Antifungal treatment may not be necessary in patients with mild, uncomplicated coccidioidal pneumonia since such infections often are self-limited and may resolve spontaneously. However, antifungal treatment is recommended for patients with more severe or rapidly progressing coccidioidal infections, those with chronic pulmonary or disseminated infections, and immunocompromised or debilitated individuals (e.g., HIV-infected individuals, organ transplant recipients, those receiving immunosuppressive therapy, those with diabetes or cardiopulmonary disease).

The IDSA states that an oral azole (fluconazole or itraconazole) usually is recommended for initial treatment of symptomatic pulmonary coccidioidomycosis and chronic fibrocavitary or disseminated (extrapulmonary) coccidioidomycosis. However, IV amphotericin B is recommended as an alternative and is preferred for initial treatment of severely ill patients who have hypoxia or rapidly progressing disease, for immunocompromised individuals, or when azole antifungals cannot be used (e.g., pregnant women).

For the treatment of clinically mild coccidioidomycosis (e.g., focal pneumonia or a positive coccidioidal serologic test alone) in HIV-infected adults and adolescents, the CDC, NIH, and IDSA recommend initial therapy with oral fluconazole or oral itraconazole. For the treatment of diffuse pulmonary or extrathoracic disseminated coccidioidomycosis (nonmeningeal) in HIV-infected adults and adolescents, the CDC, NIH, and IDSA recommend initial therapy with IV amphotericin B followed by oral azole therapy. Alternatively, some experts recommend initial therapy with IV amphotericin B used in conjunction with an oral azole (e.g., fluconazole) followed by an oral azole alone.

For the treatment of diffuse pulmonary or disseminated coccidioidomycosis (nonmeningeal) in HIV-infected infants and children, the CDC, NIH, and IDSA recommend initial treatment with IV amphotericin B followed by oral fluconazole or oral itraconazole. In those with severe disseminated coccidioidomycosis, some experts recommend initial therapy with IV amphotericin B used in conjunction with an oral azole (e.g., fluconazole) followed by an oral azole alone. Use of fluconazole or itraconazole alone may be sufficient for the treatment of coccidioidomycosis in HIV-infected infants and children with only mild disease (e.g., focal pneumonia) and also can be considered an alternative for those with stable pulmonary or disseminated coccidioidomycosis (nonmeningeal).

For the treatment of coccidioidal meningitis in HIV-infected adults, adolescents, or children or other individuals, IV or oral fluconazole (with or without intrathecal amphotericin B) is considered the regimen of choice. Oral itraconazole has been recommended as an alternative to fluconazole in adults and adolescents. Consultation with an expert who has experience in treating coccidioidal meningitis is recommended.

Primary Prophylaxis to Prevent First Episode of Coccidioidomycosis Itraconazole is used in certain HIV-infected adults and adolescents for primary prophylaxis against coccidioidomycosis†.

The CDC, NIH, and IDSA recommend that HIV-infected adults and adolescents living in areas where coccidioidomycosis is endemic (e.g., Southwestern US, parts of Central and South America) be tested annually for the disease using IgM or IgG serologic tests. Those with positive IgM or IgG serologic tests and $CD4^+$ T-cell counts less than 250/mm^3 should receive oral fluconazole or oral itraconazole for primary prophylaxis against coccidioidomycosis† since they are at increased risk of developing active coccidioidomycosis. Primary prophylaxis against coccidioidomycosis is not recommended in other HIV-infected adults and adolescents (e.g., those who reside in coccidioidomycosis endemic areas but do not have positive IgM or IgG serologic tests, those who reside in areas where the disease is not endemic) and is not recommended in HIV-infected infants and children.

Prevention of Recurrence (Secondary Prophylaxis) of Coccidioidomycosis Itraconazole is used for long-term suppressive or maintenance therapy (secondary prophylaxis) to prevent recurrence or relapse of coccidioidomycosis†.

Because of the risk of relapse, any individual who was treated for coccidioidal meningitis should receive long-term (life-long) secondary prophylaxis with oral fluconazole or oral itraconazole.

The CDC, NIH, and IDSA recommend that all HIV-infected adults, adolescents, or children who have been adequately treated for coccidioidomycosis should receive long-term secondary prophylaxis with oral fluconazole or oral itraconazole to prevent recurrence or relapse. Because HIV-infected adults and adolescents who had focal coccidioidal pneumonia and responded to antifungal treatment may be at low risk for recurrence if their $CD4^+$ T-cell count increases to greater than 250/mm^3 in response to antiretroviral therapy, it may be reasonable to consider discontinuing secondary prophylaxis against coccidioidomycosis after 12 months provided such individuals are monitored for recurrence (e.g., serial chest radiographs, coccidioidal serology). However, secondary prophylaxis should be continued indefinitely in HIV-infected adults and adolescents who were treated for more extensive coccidioidomycosis and in all HIV-infected children, regardless of the immune response to antiretroviral therapy.

■ **Cryptococcosis** Although not considered a drug of choice or a preferred alternative, oral itraconazole has been used for the treatment of cryptococcosis†.

For the treatment of cryptococcal meningitis in HIV-infected adults, adolescents, and children, the CDC, NIH, and IDSA state that the preferred regimen is initial (induction) therapy with IV amphotericin B (conventional formulation) given in conjunction with oral flucytosine, then follow-up (consolidation) therapy with oral fluconazole. Although data are limited and use of the drug is discouraged, the IDSA and others state that itraconazole can be considered an alternative for induction and consolidation therapy of cryptococcosis if all other alternative regimens have failed or are not available.

For the treatment of mild to moderate pulmonary cryptococcosis in immunocompetent individuals, the regimen of choice is oral fluconazole. Although data are limited, the IDSA states that oral itraconazole, oral voriconazole, and oral posaconazole are acceptable alternatives in immunocompetent individuals if fluconazole is unavailable or contraindicated.

Severe pulmonary cryptococcosis†, cryptococcemia†, and disseminated cryptococcal infections† in immunocompetent or immunosuppressed individuals should be treated using regimens recommended for cryptococcal meningitis.

HIV-infected adults, adolescents, and children who have been adequately treated for cryptococcus should receive long-term suppressive or maintenance therapy (secondary prophylaxis) to prevent recurrence or relapse†. The CDC, NIH, and IDSA recommend oral fluconazole as the drug of choice for secondary prophylaxis of cryptococcosis in HIV-infected adults, adolescents, and children; oral itraconazole is considered an alternative in those who cannot tolerate fluconazole, but may be less effective than fluconazole.

Although data are limited, the IDSA states that recommendations for treatment of CNS or disseminated infections caused by *Cryptococcus gattii* and recommendations for secondary prophylaxis of *C. gattii* infections are the same as the recommendations for *C. neoformans* infections.

For more complete information on the treatment and prevention of cryptococcosis, see Uses: Cryptococcosis, in Fluconazole 8:14.08.

■ **Histoplasmosis** Itraconazole is used for the treatment and prevention† of histoplasmosis caused by *Histoplasma capsulatum*.

Treatment of Histoplasmosis Itraconazole is used for the treatment of histoplasmosis, including chronic cavitary pulmonary disease and disseminated nonmeningeal disease.

The drugs of choice for the treatment of histoplasmosis are IV amphotericin B and oral itraconazole; oral ketoconazole and oral fluconazole are considered alternatives. IV amphotericin B is preferred for initial treatment of severe, life-threatening histoplasmosis, especially in immunocompromised patients such as those with HIV infection. Oral itraconazole generally is used for initial treatment of less severe disease (e.g., mild to moderate acute pulmonary histoplasmosis, chronic cavitary pulmonary histoplasmosis) and as follow-up therapy in the treatment of severe infections after a response has been obtained with IV amphotericin B.

For the treatment of moderately severe to severe acute pulmonary histoplasmosis or progressive disseminated histoplasmosis in HIV-infected adults and adolescents and other adults, the CDC, NIH, and IDSA recommend initial treatment with IV amphotericin B and follow-up treatment with oral itraconazole. Itraconazole has been used alone for the treatment of disseminated histoplasmosis in patients with HIV infection, and the manufacturer states that data from a limited number of patients indicate that the response rate of histoplasmosis to itraconazole therapy in HIV-infected individuals is similar to that in patients not infected with the virus. However, the clinical course of histoplasmosis in HIV-infected individuals generally is more severe and usually requires long-term maintenance therapy to prevent relapse.

For the treatment of progressive disseminated histoplasmosis in children, the IDSA states that IV amphotericin B or an initial regimen of IV amphotericin B and follow-up treatment with oral itraconazole can be used. For the treatment of moderately severe to severe disseminated histoplasmosis in HIV-infected infants and children, the CDC, NIH, and IDSA recommend initial treatment with IV amphotericin B and follow-up treatment with oral itraconazole. Although oral itraconazole may be used alone for the treatment of mild to moderate disseminated histoplasmosis in children, including HIV-infected infants and children, this regimen is not recommended for more severe infections.

For the treatment of meningitis caused by *H. capsulatum* in HIV-infected adults, adolescents, or children and other individuals, the CDC, NIH, and IDSA recommend initial treatment with IV amphotericin B and follow-up treatment with oral itraconazole.

For more complete information on the treatment of histoplasmosis, see Uses: Histoplasmosis, in Amphotericin B 8:14.28.

Primary Prophylaxis to Prevent First Episode of Histoplasmosis HIV-infected adults and adolescents with CD4⁺ T-cell counts less than 150/mm³ who are at high risk because they reside in areas where histoplasmosis is highly endemic should receive primary prophylaxis† against initial episodes of histoplasmosis. Itraconazole is the drug of choice for primary prophylaxis against histoplasmosis in these HIV-infected adults and adolescents. Primary prophylaxis against histoplasmosis is not recommended in HIV-infected children.

Prevention of Recurrence (Secondary Prophylaxis) of Histoplasmosis HIV-infected adults, adolescents, and children and other immunosuppressed individuals who have been adequately treated for histoplasmosis should receive long-term suppressive or maintenance therapy (secondary prophylaxis) to prevent recurrence or relapse†. Itraconazole is the drug of choice for secondary prophylaxis against histoplasmosis.

■ **Microsporidiosis** Itraconazole has been used in the treatment of microsporidiosis†.

Itraconazole has been effective in a few cases of keratoconjunctivitis or sinusitis caused by *Encephalitozoon*. The regimen of choice for ocular microsporidiosis is fumagillin (not commercially available in the US) used in conjunction with albendazole.

Although albendazole usually is the drug of choice for the treatment of intestinal or disseminated microsporidiosis (except infections caused by *Enterocytozoon bienuesi* or *Vittaforma corneae*), some clinicians suggest that itraconazole used in conjunction with albendazole is a possible alternative for disseminated microsporidiosis, especially infections caused by *Trachipleistophora* or *Anncaliia*.

■ **Onychomycosis** Oral itraconazole capsules are used in immunocompetent individuals for the treatment of onychomycosis of the toenails (with or without fingernail involvement) and onychomycosis of the fingernails caused by dermatophytes (tinea unguium). Prior to administration of itraconazole capsules for the treatment of onychomycosis, appropriate nail specimens should be obtained for microbiologic studies (e.g., potassium hydroxide [KOH] preparation, fungal culture, nail biopsy) to confirm the diagnosis. (See Cautions: Precautions and Contraindications.)

Clinical Experience In double-blind, placebo-controlled studies in patients with onychomycosis of the toenails, oral itraconazole (200 mg as capsules given once daily for 12 consecutive weeks) resulted in a mycologic cure in 54% of patients; 35% were considered an overall success (mycologic cure plus clear or minimal nail involvement with significantly decreased signs) and 14% had mycologic cure plus clinical cure (clearance of all signs, with or without residual nail deformity). The mean time to overall success was approximately 10 months; however, 21% of those considered an overall success had relapse of onychomycosis.

In a double-blind, placebo-controlled study in patients with onychomycosis of the fingernails, oral itraconazole given in a pulse-dosing regimen (200 mg as capsules twice daily for the first week, no itraconazole during weeks 2–4, and 200 mg as capsules twice daily during the fifth week) resulted in a mycologic cure in 61% of patients; 56% were considered an overall success and 47% had mycologic cure plus clinical cure. The mean time to overall success was approximately 5 months; there were no relapses in those who were considered an overall success.

■ **Paracoccidioidomycosis** Oral itraconazole is used in the treatment of paracoccidioidomycosis† (South American blastomycosis) caused by *Paracoccidioides brasiliensis*.

IV amphotericin B is the drug of choice for initial treatment of severe paracoccidioidomycosis. Oral itraconazole is the drug of choice for the treatment of less severe or localized paracoccidioidomycosis and for follow-up in more severe infections after initial treatment with IV amphotericin B.

■ **Penicilliosis** Oral itraconazole is used in the treatment of penicilliosis† caused by *Penicillium marneffei*.

For the treatment of severe or disseminated *P. marneffei* infections, including in HIV-infected adults and adolescents, an initial regimen of IV amphotericin B followed by oral itraconazole is recommended. Oral itraconazole may be used alone for initial treatment of mild penicilliosis.

Chronic suppressive or maintenance therapy (secondary prophylaxis)† with oral itraconazole is recommended to prevent relapse of penicilliosis in HIV-infected adults and adolescents who respond to an initial treatment regimen of IV amphoteric B and/or oral itraconazole. Limited data indicate that secondary prophylaxis with oral itraconazole can be discontinued in those who are receiving antiretroviral therapy and have CD4⁺ T-cell counts that have remained greater than 100/mm³ for 6 months or longer. However, secondary prophylaxis should be reinitiated if the CD4⁺ T-cell count decreases to less than 100/mm³ or if penicilliosis recurs.

■ **Sporotrichosis** Itraconazole is used in the treatment of sporotrichosis† caused by *Sporothrix schenckii*.

IV amphotericin B is the drug of choice for initial treatment of severe, life-threatening sporotrichosis and sporotrichosis that is disseminated or has CNS involvement. Oral itraconazole is the drug of choice for the treatment of cutaneous, lymphocutaneous, or mild pulmonary or osteoarticular sporotrichosis and for follow-up treatment in more severe infections after a response has been obtained with IV amphotericin B.

■ **Zygomycosis** Itraconazole has been used in a limited number of patients for the treatment of basidiobolomycosis†, a zygomycosis caused by *Basidiobolus ranarum*. Itraconazole has been effective in a few patients for the treatment of subcutaneous basidiobolomycosis or the treatment of GI basidiobolomycosis.

B. ranarum has been isolated worldwide from decaying vegetation and soil and from the GI tracts of reptiles, amphibians, fish, and insectivorous bats (including in the US). Basidiobolomycosis most commonly occurs in tropical and subtropical regions such as eastern and western Africa and infection usually manifests as painless, subcutaneous nodules of the limbs, trunk, or buttocks secondary to traumatic inoculation. GI infections are extremely rare and possibly the result of ingestion of contaminated soil (especially near rivers or lakes) or fruits or vegetables contaminated with soil or feces from infected reptiles or amphibians.

From April 1994 through May 1999, 7 cases of GI basidiobolomycosis were identified in Arizona. Most cases of GI basidiobolomycosis have been successfully treated with oral itraconazole (400 mg daily given for 3–19 months) after partial surgical resection of the GI tract; however, it is unclear whether a clinical response would have been obtained if itraconazole had been used alone without surgical intervention. Although ketoconazole also has been reported to be effective in at least one patient, amphotericin B has been ineffective for the treatment of GI basidiobolomycosis in several patients.

■ **Empiric Therapy in Febrile Neutropenic Patients** Itraconazole (given IV initially followed by itraconazole oral solution; IV preparation no longer commercially available in the US) has been used for empiric therapy of presumed fungal infections in febrile neutropenic patients.

Clinical Experience Safety and efficacy of itraconazole for this indication has been evaluated in an open, randomized study in febrile neutropenic adults with hematologic malignancies; patients received either itraconazole (200 mg IV twice daily for 2 days, then 200 mg IV once daily from days 3–14 followed by itraconazole oral solution 200 mg twice daily to complete up to 28 days of therapy) or conventional IV amphotericin B (0.7–1 mg/kg daily for up to 28 days). The therapeutic success rate (defined as patient survival with resolution of fever and neutropenia within 28 days of therapy, absence of emergent fungal infections, use of study drug without premature discontinuance because of toxicity or lack of efficacy, and therapy for 3 or more days) was 47% for itraconazole and 38% for amphotericin B (intent-to-treat analysis). Although the overall response rate was higher in those receiving itraconazole, more patients receiving itraconazole discontinued the drug because of persistent fever or changed antifungal therapy because of fever and more patients receiving amphotericin B discontinued the drug because of intolerance.

Dosage and Administration

■ Reconstitution and Administration Itraconazole is administered orally.

Itraconazole also has been administered by IV infusion; however, an IV preparation of the drug is no longer commercially available in the US.

Oral Administration Bioavailability of oral itraconazole varies depending on whether the drug is administered as capsules or as an oral solution, and the manufacturer states that these preparations should not be used interchangeably.

The possibility that GI absorption of the drug may be decreased when gastric acid production is decreased (e.g., in patients with hypochlorhydria, including some individuals with human immunodeficiency virus [HIV] infection) should be considered. (See Pharmacokinetics: Absorption.)

Capsules. Itraconazole capsules should be administered *with* a full meal to ensure maximal absorption of the drug.

The capsules should not be used for the treatment of oropharyngeal or esophageal candidiasis; efficacy has not been established and this formulation may be less effective than the oral solution for these infections.

If itraconazole capsules are given in a dosage exceeding 200 mg daily, the daily dosage should be divided into 2 doses.

Oral Solution. Itraconazole oral solution should be administered *without* food to ensure maximal absorption of the drug.

For the treatment of oropharyngeal or esophageal candidiasis, the recommended dosage of itraconazole oral solution should be vigorously swished in the mouth (10 mL at a time) for several seconds and then swallowed.

The manufacturer states that data are limited to date regarding the safety of long-term use of itraconazole oral solution (i.e., longer than 6 months).

■ Dosage Because of differences in oral bioavailability, itraconazole capsules and oral solution should *not* be used interchangeably.

Itraconazole appears to undergo saturable metabolism in the liver; therefore, increases in dosage can result in more than proportional increases in plasma concentrations.

Dosage of itraconazole capsules should be based on the type and severity of infection, identity of the causative organism, and patient's response to therapy.

To ensure adequate plasma concentrations of itraconazole (especially in patients with life-threatening fungal infections), the Infectious Diseases Society of America (IDSA) and other experts recommend that itraconazole plasma concentrations be determined, usually after 2 weeks of therapy.

General Adult Dosage for Treatment of Serious, Life-threatening Systemic Fungal Infections For the treatment of life-threatening systemic fungal infections, the manufacturer states that oral itraconazole capsules should be initiated using a loading dosage. Although clinical studies evaluating the safety and efficacy of oral itraconazole capsules did not include a loading dosage, the manufacturer states that, based on pharmacokinetic considerations, oral itraconazole capsules should be initiated in life-threatening infections in adults using an initial loading dosage of 200 mg 3 times daily (600 mg daily) for the first 3 days of therapy. Subsequent therapy then can be continued at the usual oral dosage of 200–400 mg daily.

The manufacturer states that itraconazole therapy should be continued for at least 3 months and until clinical parameters and laboratory tests indicate that the active fungal infection has subsided. An inadequate period of treatment can result in recurrence of active infection.

Aspergillosis **Treatment of Aspergillosis in Adults.** For the treatment of pulmonary or extrapulmonary aspergillosis in adults who do not respond to or cannot tolerate IV amphotericin B, the recommended dosage of itraconazole capsules is 200–400 mg daily. For the treatment of invasive aspergillosis, the IDSA and other clinicians recommend a dosage of 200 mg 3 times daily for 3 days, then 200 mg twice daily.

For empiric or preemptive therapy of presumed aspergillosis, the IDSA recommends that itraconazole be given in a dosage of 200 mg twice daily.

Primary Prophylaxis to Prevent Aspergillosis in Adults. If itraconazole is used as an alternative for primary prophylaxis of aspergillosis† in immunocompromised individuals at high risk of invasive aspergillosis (i.e., neutropenic patients with acute myelogenous leukemia [AML] or myelodysplastic syndrome [MDS], hematopoietic stem cell transplant [HSCT] recipients with graft-versus-host disease [GVHD]), the IDSA recommends a dosage of 200 mg twice daily.

Blastomycosis **Treatment of Blastomycosis in Adults.** For the treatment of pulmonary or extrapulmonary blastomycosis in adults, the manufacturer recommends that itraconazole capsules be administered in an initial dosage of 200 mg once daily. If there is no apparent improvement or there is evidence of progression of the fungal infection at this dosage, the manufacturer recommends increasing the dosage in 100-mg increments daily up to a maximum dosage of 400 mg daily. Oral itraconazole dosages exceeding 200 mg daily should be divided into 2 doses daily.

For the treatment of mild to moderate pulmonary or mild to moderate disseminated blastomycosis (without CNS involvement) in adults, the IDSA recommends that itraconazole be given in a dosage of 200 mg 3 times daily for 3 days, then 200 mg once or twice daily for 6–12 months.

For the treatment of moderately severe to severe pulmonary or moderately severe to severe disseminated blastomycosis (without CNS involvement) in adults, the IDSA recommends an initial regimen of IV amphotericin B given for 1–2 weeks or until a response is obtained, followed by itraconazole given in a dosage of 200 mg 3 times daily for 3 days, then 200 mg twice daily. The total treatment duration should be 6–12 months for pulmonary blastomycosis or at least 12 months for disseminated extrapulmonary blastomycosis or for immunocompromised individuals.

For the treatment of CNS blastomycosis in adults, the IDSA recommends an initial regimen of IV amphotericin B given for 4–6 weeks, followed by itraconazole given in a dosage of 200 mg 2 or 3 times daily for at least 12 months and until CSF abnormalities resolve.

Prevention of Recurrence (Secondary Prophylaxis) of Blastomycosis in Adults. When itraconazole is used for prevention of recurrence (secondary prophylaxis) of blastomycosis† in immunosuppressed adults at risk, the IDSA recommends a dosage of 200 mg daily.

Life-long secondary prophylaxis may be necessary if immunosuppression cannot be reversed. In HIV-infected adults, the IDSA states that discontinuance of secondary prophylaxis against blastomycosis can be considered after at least 12 months if the patient is receiving antiretroviral therapy and $CD4^+$ T-cell counts have remained greater than 150/mm^3 for at least 6 months.

Treatment of Blastomycosis in Children. For the treatment of mild to moderate blastomycosis in children†, the IDSA recommends that itraconazole be given in a dosage of 10 mg/kg daily (up to 400 mg daily) for 6–12 months.

For the treatment of moderately severe to severe blastomycosis in children†, the IDSA recommends an initial regimen of IV amphotericin B given for 1–2 weeks, followed by itraconazole given in a dosage of 10 mg/kg daily (up to 400 mg daily) for a total treatment duration of 12 months.

Candida Infections **Treatment of Oropharyngeal Candidiasis in Adults and Adolescents.** For the treatment of oropharyngeal candidiasis in adults, the manufacturer recommends that itraconazole oral solution be given in a dosage of 200 mg (20 mL) daily for 1–2 weeks. Clinical signs and symptoms generally resolve within several days. When itraconazole oral solution is used for retreatment of oropharyngeal candidiasis in adults who have not responded to or are refractory to oral fluconazole therapy, the manufacturer recommends a dosage of 100 mg (10 mL) twice daily. A response to itraconazole in these patients generally is evident within 2–4 weeks; however, relapse may be expected shortly after the drug is discontinued. The manufacturer states that data are limited to date regarding the safety of long-term use of itraconazole oral solution (i.e., longer than 6 months).

For the treatment of oropharyngeal candidiasis, including fluconazole-refractory infections, in HIV-infected adults and adolescents†, the US Centers for Disease Control and Prevention (CDC), National Institutes of Health (NIH), and IDSA recommend that itraconazole oral solution be given in a dosage of 200 mg daily for 7–14 days.

Prevention of Recurrence (Secondary Prophylaxis) of Oropharyngeal Candidiasis in Adults and Adolescents. If long-term suppressive or maintenance therapy (secondary prophylaxis)† with itraconazole oral solution is used in HIV-infected adults or adolescents† with frequent or severe recurrences of oropharyngeal candidiasis, the CDC, NIH, and IDSA recommend a dosage of 200 mg daily.

Although only limited data are available regarding the safety of discontinuing secondary prophylaxis against oropharyngeal candidiasis in HIV-infected individuals, consideration can be given to discontinuing such prophylaxis if the $CD4^+$ T-cell count increases to 200/mm^3 in response to antiretroviral therapy.

Treatment of Oropharyngeal Candidiasis in Children. If itraconazole oral solution is used for the treatment of oropharyngeal candidiasis in HIV-infected infants and children†, the CDC, NIH, and IDSA recommend a dosage of 2.5 mg/kg twice daily (up to 200 mg daily) for 7–14 days.

If itraconazole oral solution is used for the treatment of fluconazole-refractory oropharyngeal candidiasis in HIV-infected infants and children†, the CDC, NIH, and IDSA recommend a dosage of 2.5 mg/kg twice daily (up to 200–400 mg daily) for 7–14 days.

Treatment of Esophageal Candidiasis in Adults and Adolescents. For the treatment of esophageal candidiasis in adults, the manufacturer recommends that itraconazole oral solution be given in a dosage of 100 mg (10 mL) daily; however, depending on the patient's response to the drug, a dosage up to 200 mg (20 mL) daily may be given. The manufacturer states that oral itraconazole therapy should be administered for a minimum of 3 weeks in patients with esophageal candidiasis, and should be continued for 2 weeks after symptoms resolve.

For the treatment of esophageal candidiasis, including fluconazole-refractory infections, in HIV-infected adults and adolescents† and other individuals, the CDC, NIH, and IDSA recommend that itraconazole oral solution be given in a dosage of 200 mg daily for 14–21 days.

Treatment of Esophageal Candidiasis in Children. If itraconazole oral solution is used for the treatment of esophageal candidiasis in HIV-infected infants and children†, the CDC, NIH, and IDSA recommend a dosage of 2.5 mg/kg twice daily or 5 mg/kg once daily for 14–21 days.

Treatment of Vulvovaginal Candidiasis in Adults and Adolescents. If itraconazole is used as an alternative for the treatment of vulvovaginal candidiasis†, some clinicians recommend a dosage of 200 mg twice daily for 1 day.

For the treatment of vulvovaginal candidiasis in HIV-infected adults and adolescents†, the CDC, NIH, and IDSA recommend that the oral solution be given in a dosage of 200 mg daily for 3–7 days.

Empiric Treatment of Suspected Candidiasis in Neutropenic Patients. If itraconazole is used as an alternative for initial empiric treatment of suspected candidiasis in neutropenic patients†, the IDSA recommends a dosage of 200 mg twice daily. The drug should not be used for empiric treatment in patients who previously received prophylaxis with an azole antifungal.

Coccidioidomycosis **Treatment of Coccidioidomycosis in Adults and Adolescents.** For the treatment of coccidioidomycosis†, the IDSA and others recommend that adults receive itraconazole in a dosage of 200 mg 2 or 3 times daily. Uncomplicated coccidioidal pneumonia generally is treated for 3–6 months; diffuse pneumonia and chronic progressive fibrocavitary pneumonia generally are treated for at least 1 year.

For the treatment of mild (nonmeningeal) coccidioidomycosis (e.g., focal pneumonia or positive coccidioidal serologic test alone) in HIV-infected adults and adolescents†, the CDC, NIH, and IDSA recommend that itraconazole be given in a dosage of 200 mg 3 times daily for 3 days, then 200 mg twice daily.

If itraconazole is used as an alternative to fluconazole for the treatment of meningeal coccidioidomycosis in HIV-infected adults and adolescents†, the CDC, NIH, and IDSA recommend a dosage of 200 mg 3 times daily for 3 days, then 200 mg twice daily. Consultation with an expert who has experience in treating coccidioidal meningitis is recommended.

Primary Prophylaxis to Prevent First Episode of Coccidioidomycosis in Adults and Adolescents. If itraconazole is used for primary prophylaxis against coccidioidomycosis† in HIV-infected adults and adolescents† who live in areas where the disease is endemic, have positive IgM or IgG serologic tests indicating an increased risk for development of active infection, and have CD4+ T-cell counts less than 250/mm³, the CDC, NIH, and IDSA recommend a dosage of 200 mg twice daily.

Consideration can be given to discontinuing primary prophylaxis against coccidioidomycosis if CD4+ T-cell counts remain greater than 250/mm³ for 6 months. Primary prophylaxis should be reinitiated if CD4+ T-cell counts decrease to less than 250/mm³.

Prevention of Recurrence (Secondary Prophylaxis) of Coccidioidomycosis in Adults and Adolescents. For long-term suppressive or maintenance therapy (secondary prophylaxis†) to prevent recurrence or relapse of coccidioidomycosis† in HIV-infected adults and adolescents† who have been adequately treated for the disease, the CDC, NIH, and IDSA recommend that itraconazole be given in a dosage of 200 mg twice daily.

In HIV-infected adults and adolescents with a history of adequately treated focal coccidioidal pneumonia, discontinuance of secondary prophylaxis against coccidioidomycosis can be considered after 12 months if they are receiving antiretroviral therapy and have CD4+ T-cell counts greater than 250/mm³.

In HIV-infected adults and adolescents with a history of adequately treated diffuse pulmonary or disseminated coccidioidomycosis (including meningeal infections), secondary prophylaxis against coccidioidomycosis should be continued lifelong, regardless of antiretroviral therapy or immune reconstitution.

Treatment of Coccidioidomycosis in Children. For the treatment of mild coccidioidomycosis (nonmeningeal) (e.g., focal pneumonia) in HIV-infected infants and children†, the CDC, NIH, and IDSA recommend that itraconazole be given in a dosage of 5–10 mg/kg twice daily for 3 days, then 2–5 mg/kg twice daily.

For the treatment of diffuse pulmonary or disseminated coccidioidomycosis (nonmeningeal) in HIV-infected infants and children†, the CDC, NIH, and IDSA recommend an initial regimen of IV amphotericin B given until a response is obtained, followed by itraconazole given in a dosage of 5–10 mg/kg twice daily for 3 days, then 2–5 mg/kg twice daily (up to 400 mg daily).

Uncomplicated coccidioidal pneumonia is generally treated for 3–6 months; diffuse pneumonia and chronic progressive fibrocavitary pneumonia generally are treated for at least 1 year.

Prevention of Recurrence (Secondary Prophylaxis) of Coccidioidomycosis in Children. For long-term suppressive or maintenance therapy (secondary prophylaxis) to prevent recurrence or relapse of coccidioidomycosis in HIV-infected infants and children† who have been adequately treated for the disease, the CDC, NIH, and IDSA recommend that itraconazole be given in a dosage of 2–5 mg/kg (up to 200 mg) twice daily.

Secondary prophylaxis against coccidioidomycosis should be continued lifelong in HIV-infected infants and children, regardless of antiretroviral therapy or immune reconstitution.

Cryptococcosis **Treatment of Cryptococcosis in Adults and Adolescents.** For the treatment of mild to moderate pulmonary cryptococcosis (nonmeningeal) in immunocompetent adults†, the IDSA states that itraconazole can be given in a dosage of 200 mg twice daily for 6–12 months.

As an alternative regimen for the treatment of cryptococcal meningitis in HIV-infected adults and adolescents†, the CDC, NIH, and IDSA recommend an initial (induction) regimen of IV amphotericin B given for at least 2 weeks, then a follow-up (consolidation) regimen of itraconazole 200 mg twice daily for 8 weeks or until CD4+ T-cell count remains at 200/mm³ or greater for at least 6 months as the result of antiretroviral therapy.

For the treatment of cryptococcal meningoencephalitis in HIV-infected adults†, the IDSA states that itraconazole given in a dosage of 200 mg twice daily for 10–12 weeks can be considered as an alternative regimen, although use of this regimen is discouraged and should be used only when all other alternative regimens have failed or are not available.

Some clinicians suggest that the oral solution may be preferred (instead of capsules) if itraconazole is used for the treatment of cryptococcosis.

Prevention of Recurrence (Secondary Prophylaxis) of Cryptococcosis in Adults and Adolescents. If itraconazole is used for long-term suppressive or maintenance therapy (secondary prophylaxis) to prevent recurrence or relapse of cryptococcosis in HIV-infected adults and adolescents† who have been adequately treated for the disease, the CDC, NIH, and IDSA recommend a dosage of 200 mg once or twice daily. There is some evidence that the twice-daily regimen is more effective for secondary prophylaxis than the once-daily regimen.

The IDSA states that consideration can be given to discontinuing secondary prophylaxis against cryptococcosis in HIV-infected adults who have received at least 1 year of antifungal treatment, are receiving antiretroviral therapy, have had undetectable or low plasma HIV RNA levels for at least 3 months, and have CD4+ T-cell counts of 100/mm³. If secondary prophylaxis against cryptococcosis is discontinued, the patient should be followed closely and serial cryptococcal serum antigen tests performed. Secondary prophylaxis against cryptococcosis should be reinitiated if CD4+ T-cell counts decrease to less than 100/mm³ and/or the serum cryptococcal antigen titer increases.

Other experts state that HIV-infected adults and adolescents with a history of cryptococcosis generally should receive life-long suppressive therapy to prevent recurrence unless immune reconstitution occurs in response to antiretroviral therapy. These experts state that consideration can be given to discontinuing secondary prophylaxis against cryptococcosis in HIV-infected adults and adolescents who are asymptomatic for cryptococcosis, are receiving antiretroviral therapy, and have had CD4+ T-cell counts of 200/mm³ or greater for more than 6 months. Secondary prophylaxis against cryptococcosis should be reinitiated if CD4+ T-cell counts decrease to less than 200/mm³.

Treatment of Cryptococcosis in Children. If itraconazole is used as an alternative regimen for the treatment of CNS cryptococcosis in HIV-infected infants and children†, the CDC, NIH, and IDSA recommend an initial (induction) regimen of IV amphotericin B given for at least 2 weeks, then a follow-up (consolidation) regimen of itraconazole given in a dosage of 200 mg 3 times daily for 3 days, then 5–10 mg/kg (maximum 200 mg) once or twice daily for at least 8 weeks.

Prevention of Recurrence (Secondary Prophylaxis) of Cryptococcosis in Children. If itraconazole is used for long-term suppressive or maintenance therapy (secondary prophylaxis) to prevent recurrence or relapse of cryptococcosis in HIV-infected infants or children† who have been adequately treated for the disease, the CDC, NIH, and IDSA recommend a dosage of 5 mg/kg (up to 200 mg) daily.

HIV-infected infants and children with a history of cryptococcosis usually should receive life-long secondary prophylaxis to prevent recurrence. Consideration can be given to discontinuing secondary prophylaxis in HIV-infected children 6 years of age or older who are asymptomatic for cryptococcosis and have received secondary prophylaxis for at least 6 months, have been receiving antiretroviral therapy for at least 6 months, and have had CD4+ T-cell counts of 200/mm³ or greater for at least 6 months. Secondary prophylaxis against cryptococcosis should be reinitiated if CD4+ T-cell count decreases to less than 200/mm³.

Histoplasmosis **Treatment of Histoplasmosis in Adults and Adolescents.** For the treatment of chronic cavitary pulmonary histoplasmosis or disseminated, nonmeningeal histoplasmosis, the manufacturer recommends that adults receive itraconazole capsules in a dosage of 200 mg once daily. If there is evidence of progression or no apparent improvement, dosage may be increased in 100-mg increments daily up to a maximum dosage of 400 mg daily. The usual duration of treatment is at least 12 months.

For the treatment of mild to moderate acute pulmonary histoplasmosis when treatment is considered necessary (i.e., symptomatic for at least 1 month), the IDSA recommends that itraconazole be given in a dosage of 200 mg 3 times daily for 3 days, then 200 mg once or twice daily for 6–12 weeks.

For the treatment of moderately severe to severe acute pulmonary histoplasmosis, the IDSA recommends an initial regimen of IV amphotericin B given for 1–2 weeks, followed by itraconazole given in a dosage of 200 mg 3 times daily for 3 days, then 200 mg twice daily for a total treatment duration of 12 weeks.

For the treatment of chronic cavitary pulmonary histoplasmosis, the IDSA recommends that itraconazole be given in a dosage of 200 mg 3 times daily for 3 days, then 200 mg once or twice daily for at least 1 year. Because of the risk of relapse, some clinicians prefer a duration of 18–24 months.

For the treatment of mild to moderate disseminated histoplasmosis, the IDSA recommends that itraconazole be given in a dosage of 200 mg 3 times daily for 3 days, then 200 mg twice daily for at least 1 year.

For the treatment of moderately severe to severe progressive disseminated histoplasmosis, the IDSA recommends an initial regimen of IV amphotericin B given for 1–2 weeks, followed by itraconazole given in a dosage of 200 mg 3 times daily for 3 days, then 200 mg twice daily for a total treatment duration of at least 12 months.

For the treatment of histoplasmosis with symptomatic mediastinal granuloma or with complications (pericarditis, rheumatologic syndromes, symptomatic mediastinal lymphadenitis) that require treatment with corticosteroids, the IDSA recommends that itraconazole be given in a dosage of 200 mg 3 times daily for 3 days, then 200 mg once or twice daily for 6–12 weeks.

For the treatment of less severe disseminated histoplasmosis in HIV-infected adults and adolescents†, the CDC, NIH, and IDSA recommend that itraconazole be given in a dosage of 200 mg 3 times daily for 3 days, then 200 mg twice daily for at least 12 months.

For the treatment of moderately severe to severe disseminated histoplasmosis in HIV-infected adults and adolescents†, the CDC, NIH, and IDSA recommend an initial regimen of IV amphotericin B given for at least 2 weeks or until a response is obtained, followed by itraconazole 200 mg 3 times daily for 3 days, then 200 mg twice daily for a total duration of at least 12 months and until histoplasmal antigen is undetectable.

For the treatment of CNS histoplasmosis† in HIV-infected adults and adolescents† or other adults, the CDC, NIH, and IDSA recommend an initial regimen of IV amphotericin B given for 4–6 weeks or until a response is obtained, followed by itraconazole 200 mg 2 or 3 times daily for at least 12 months and until CSF abnormalities resolve and histoplasmal antigen is undetectable.

Some clinicians suggest the oral solution may be preferred (instead of capsules) if itraconazole is used for the treatment of histoplasmosis.

Primary Prophylaxis to Prevent First Episode of Histoplasmosis in Adults and Adolescents. For primary prophylaxis to prevent histoplasmosis† in immunosuppressed adults, the IDSA recommends that itraconazole be given in a dosage of 200 mg daily.

If itraconazole is used for primary prophylaxis to prevent histoplasmosis† in HIV-infected adults and adolescents† with $CD4^+$ T-cell counts of 150/mm^3 or lower who are at high risk (occupational exposure, reside in a community hyperendemic for histoplasmosis), the CDC, NIH, and IDSA recommend a dosage of 200 mg daily.

Discontinuance of primary prophylaxis against histoplasmosis can be considered in HIV-infected adults and adolescents receiving antiretroviral therapy if $CD4^+$ T-cell counts exceed 150/mm^3 for 6 months. Primary prophylaxis against histoplasmosis should be reinitiated if $CD4^+$ T-cell count decreases to 150/mm^3 or lower.

Prevention of Recurrence (Secondary Prophylaxis) of Histoplasmosis in Adults and Adolescents. For long-term suppressive or maintenance therapy (secondary prophylaxis) to prevent recurrence or relapse of histoplasmosis in HIV-infected adults and adolescents†and other immunosuppressed adults who have been adequately treated for the disease, the CDC, NIH, and IDSA recommend that itraconazole be given in a dosage of 200 mg daily.

HIV-infected adults and adolescents with a history of histoplasmosis should receive life-long suppressive therapy to prevent recurrence. Consideration can be given to discontinuing secondary prophylaxis in HIV-infected adults and adolescents who have negative *Histoplasma* blood cultures, have serum *Histoplasma* antigen levels less than 2 ng/mL, have received itraconazole for at least 12 months, have been receiving antiretroviral therapy for at least 6 months, and have $CD4^+$ T-cell counts of 150/mm^3 or greater. Secondary prophylaxis against histoplasmosis should be reinitiated if $CD4^+$ T-cell count decreases to less than 150/mm^3.

Treatment of Histoplasmosis in Children. For the treatment of acute pulmonary histoplasmosis in children†, the IDSA recommends that itraconazole be given in a dosage of 5–10 mg/kg daily (up to 400 mg daily) in 2 divided doses.

For the treatment of progressive disseminated histoplasmosis in children†, the IDSA recommends an initial regimen of IV amphotericin B given for 2–4 weeks, followed by itraconazole given in a dosage of 5–10 mg/kg daily (up to 400 mg daily) in 2 divided doses for a total duration of 3 months. A longer duration may be necessary in children with severe disease or with immunosuppression or primary immunodeficiency syndromes.

For the treatment of mild disseminated histoplasmosis in HIV-infected infants and children†, the CDC, NIH, and IDSA recommend that itraconazole (oral solution) be given in a dosage of 2–5 mg/kg (up to 200 mg) 3 times daily for 3 days, then 2–5 mg/kg (up to 200 mg) twice daily for 12 months.

For the treatment of moderately severe to severe disseminated histoplasmosis in HIV-infected infants and children†, the CDC, NIH, and IDSA recommend an initial regimen of IV amphotericin B given for at least 1–2 weeks, followed by itraconazole (oral solution) given in a dosage of 2–5 mg/kg (up to 200 mg) 3 times daily for 3 days, then 2–5 mg/kg (up to 200 mg) twice daily for 12 months.

For the treatment of CNS histoplasmosis in HIV-infected infants and children†, the CDC, NIH, and IDSA recommend an initial regimen of IV amphotericin B given for 4–6 weeks, followed by itraconazole (oral solution) given in a dosage of 2–5 mg/kg (up to 200 mg) 3 times daily for 3 days, then 2–5 mg/kg (up to 200 mg) twice daily for at least 12 months and until CSF abnormalities resolve and histoplasmal antigen is undetectable.

Prevention of Recurrence (Secondary Prophylaxis) of Histoplasmosis in Children. For long-term suppressive or maintenance therapy (secondary prophylaxis) to prevent recurrence or relapse of histoplasmosis in HIV-infected infants or children† and other immunosuppressed children who have been adequately treated for the disease, the CDC, NIH, and IDSA recommend that itraconazole (oral solution) be given in a dosage of 5 mg/kg (up to 200 mg) twice daily.

HIV-infected infants and children with a history of histoplasmosis usually should receive life-long suppressive therapy to prevent recurrence. Consideration can be given to discontinuing secondary prophylaxis in HIV-infected children 6 years of age or older who have negative *Histoplasma* blood cultures, have serum *Histoplasma* antigen levels less than 2 ng/mL, have received itraconazole for at least 12 months, have been receiving antiretroviral therapy for at least 6 months, and have $CD4^+$ T-cell counts of 150/mm^3 or greater. Secondary prophylaxis against histoplasmosis should be reinitiated if $CD4^+$ T-cell counts decrease to less than 150/mm^3.

Microsporidiosis For the treatment of keratoconjunctivitis and sinusitis caused by *Encephalitozoon*†, itraconazole has been given in a dosage of 200 mg daily for 8 weeks.

For the treatment of disseminated microsporidiosis† caused by *Trachipleistophora* or *Anncaliia*, some clinicians recommend that itraconazole be given in a dosage of 400 mg daily in conjunction with oral albendazole.

Onychomycosis For the treatment of onychomycosis of the fingernails (without toenail involvement), itraconazole capsules are given in a pulse-dosing regimen that involves administering 200 mg of the drug twice daily during the first week, no itraconazole during weeks 2–4, and 200 mg of itraconazole twice daily during the fifth week.

For the treatment of onychomycosis of the toenails (with or without fingernail involvement), the recommended oral dosage of itraconazole capsules is 200 mg once daily for 12 consecutive weeks. A pulse-dosing regimen that involves administering itraconazole capsules in a dosage of 400 mg once daily for one week each month for 3 months† also has been effective for the treatment of onychomycosis of the toenails (tinea unguium).

Penicilliosis **Treatment of Penicilliosis.** For the treatment of severe penicilliosis†, an initial regimen of IV amphotericin B is given for 2 weeks, followed by oral itraconazole given in a dosage of 400 mg daily for 10 weeks. For the treatment of mild infections when an initial oral regimen in adequate, oral itraconazole in a dosage of 400 mg daily for 8 weeks is recommended.

Prevention of Recurrence (Secondary Prophylaxis) of Penicilliosis. For long-term suppressive or maintenance therapy (secondary prophylaxis) to prevent recurrence or relapse of penicilliosis† in HIV-infected adults and adolescents† who have been adequately treated, oral itraconazole should be given in a dosage of 200 mg daily. Secondary prophylaxis can be discontinued in those who are receiving antiretroviral therapy and have $CD4^+$ T-cell counts that have remained greater than 100/mm^3 for 6 months or longer. Secondary prophylaxis should be reinitiated if the $CD4^+$ T-cell count decreases to less than 100/mm^3.

Sporotrichosis **Treatment of Sporotrichosis in Adults.** For the treatment of cutaneous or lymphocutaneous sporotrichosis†, the IDSA and others recommend that adults receive itraconazole in a dosage of 200 mg once daily. If a response is not obtained, dosage may be increased to 200 mg twice daily. Treatment should be continued for 2–4 weeks after all lesions have resolved; the usual duration of treatment is 3–6 months.

For the treatment of osteoarticular sporotrichosis†, the IDSA states that adults should receive itraconazole in a dosage of 200 mg twice daily for at least 12 months. If used as follow-up after a response has been obtained with an initial regimen of IV amphotericin B, itraconazole should be continued for a total treatment duration of at least 12 months.

For the treatment of mild pulmonary sporotrichosis†, the IDSA recommends that adults receive itraconazole in a dosage of 200 mg twice daily for at least 12 months.

For the treatment of severe or life-threatening pulmonary or disseminated sporotrichosis†, the IDSA recommends that adults receive an initial regimen of IV amphotericin B given until a response is obtained, followed by itraconazole 200 mg twice daily continued for a total treatment duration of at least 12 months.

For the treatment of meningeal sporotrichosis†, the IDSA recommends that adults receive an initial regimen of IV amphotericin B given for at least 4–6 weeks and until a response is obtained, followed by itraconazole 200 mg twice daily continued for a total treatment duration of at least 12 months.

Some clinicians suggest that the oral solution may be preferred (instead of capsules) if itraconazole is used for the treatment of sporotrichosis.

Treatment of Sporotrichosis in Children. For the treatment of cutaneous or lymphocutaneous sporotrichosis in children†, the IDSA recommends that itraconazole be given in a dosage of 6–10 mg/kg daily (up to 400 mg daily). Treatment should be continued for 2–4 weeks after all lesions have resolved; the usual duration of treatment is 3–6 months.

For the treatment of disseminated sporotrichosis in children†, the IDSA recommends an initial regimen of IV amphotericin B given until a response is obtained, followed by itraconazole given in a dosage of 6–10 mg/kg daily (up to 400 mg daily) for a total duration of at least 12 months.

Empiric Therapy in Febrile Neutropenic Patients For empiric therapy of presumed fungal infections in febrile neutropenic patients, an initial IV regimen of itraconazole has been used (200 mg IV twice daily for 4 doses, then 200 mg IV once daily for up to 14 days; IV preparation no longer commercially available in the US). Treatment is then switched to itraconazole oral solution given in a dosage of 200 mg (20 mL) twice daily until clinically important neutropenia has resolved. Safety and efficacy of itraconazole administered for longer than 28 days for this indication are not known.

For empiric therapy of presumed fungal infections in patients with chemotherapy-induced neutropenia, the IDSA recommends that oral itraconazole be given in a dosage of 200 mg twice daily.

■ **Dosage in Renal and Hepatic Impairment** Only limited data are available on the use of itraconazole in patients with renal impairment, and the drug should be used with caution in such patients. (See Other Precautions and Contraindications under Cautions: Precautions and Contraindications.)

Only limited data are available on the use of itraconazole in patients with hepatic impairment, and the drug should be used with caution in such patients. (See Precautions Related to Hepatic Effects under Cautions: Precautions and Contraindications.)

Cautions

Itraconazole generally is well tolerated. However, serious potentially life-threatening adverse effects, including congestive heart failure (CHF), pulmonary edema, and hepatotoxicity, have occurred rarely in patients receiving itraconazole. In clinical studies evaluating itraconazole for the treatment of systemic fungal infections, adverse effects requiring discontinuance of the drug occurred in up to 11% of patients; the median duration of therapy before discontinuance was 81 days (range: 2–776 days). In patients receiving oral itraconazole capsules for the treatment of onychomycosis of the toenails or fingernails, adverse effects requiring temporary or permanent discontinuance of the drug occurred in 1–4% of patients. The most frequent adverse effects of itraconazole involve the GI tract, and the frequency of adverse effects may be increased during prolonged therapy.

■ **GI Effects** Adverse GI effects have been reported in about 1–11% of patients receiving itraconazole for the treatment of systemic fungal infections or oropharyngeal or esophageal candidiasis or for empiric anti-fungal therapy. These adverse GI effects usually are transient and respond to symptomatic treatment without alteration of itraconazole therapy; however, reduction of dosage or discontinuance of the drug occasionally may be required.

Nausea is the most frequently reported adverse effect of itraconazole, occurring in 9–11% of patients receiving the drug for the treatment of systemic fungal infections, oropharyngeal or esophageal candidiasis, or for empiric antifungal therapy. However, this effect occasionally has been reported to occur more frequently. Vomiting has occurred in about 5–7%, diarrhea in about 3–10%, and abdominal pain or anorexia in about 1–3% of patients being treated for systemic fungal infections, oropharyngeal or esophageal candidiasis, or for empiric antifungal prophylaxis. Constipation, dyspepsia, dysphagia, flatulence, gastritis, taste perversion, and ulcerative stomatitis also have been reported.

In patients receiving oral itraconazole capsules for the treatment of onychomycosis of the fingernails (a pulse-dosing regimen consisting of two 1-week treatment periods given 3 weeks apart), abdominal pain, constipation, dyspepsia, nausea, gingivitis, and ulcerative stomatitis were reported in 3–5%. In those receiving itraconazole capsules for the treatment of onychomycosis of the toenails (a continuous dosing regimen for 12 consecutive weeks), abdominal pain, diarrhea, dyspepsia, and flatulence were reported in 7% and constipation, gastritis, gastroenteritis, increased appetite, and nausea were reported in 3–4% of patients. Adverse GI effects requiring temporary or permanent discontinuance of itraconazole capsules occurred in 4% of those receiving the drug for the treatment of toenail infections.

■ **Dermatologic and Sensitivity Reactions** Rash has occurred in 3–9% of patients receiving itraconazole for the treatment of systemic fungal infections, oropharyngeal or esophageal candidiasis, or for empiric anti-fungal therapy. Rash tends to occur more frequently in immunocompromised patients who are receiving immunosuppressive therapy. Pruritus has occurred in up to 3% of patients with systemic fungal infections or oropharyngeal or esophageal candidiasis receiving itraconazole. Urticaria, angioedema, alopecia, and toxic epidermal necrolysis also have been reported in patients receiving itraconazole. In addition, anaphylaxis and Stevens-Johnson syndrome occurred rarely in patients receiving the drug.

In patients receiving oral itraconazole capsules for the treatment of onychomycosis of the fingernails or toenails, pruritus and rash were reported in 5–8% of patients; these adverse effects required temporary or permanent discontinuance of itraconazole capsules in 3%.

■ **Nervous System Effects** Headache and dizziness have been reported in 2–4% of patients receiving itraconazole for the treatment of systemic fungal infections, oropharyngeal or esophageal candidiasis, or for empiric anti-fungal prophylaxis. Somnolence, decreased libido, insomnia, depression, and tremor have occurred in up to 1% of patients. Although a causal relationship to itraconazole has not been established, neuropathy (including peripheral neuropathy) has occurred rarely in patients receiving the drug.

In patients receiving oral itraconazole capsules for the treatment of onychomycosis of the fingernails (a pulse-dosing regimen consisting of two 1-week treatment periods given 3 weeks apart), headache was reported in 8% and anxiety, depression, fatigue, and malaise were reported in 3%. In those receiving itraconazole capsules for the treatment of onychomycosis of the toenails (a continuous dosing regimen for 12 consecutive weeks), headache was reported in 10% and asthenia, dizziness, and tremor were reported in 2–4% of patients. Adverse nervous system effects (headache, malaise, vertigo) requiring temporary or permanent discontinuance of itraconazole capsules occurred in 1% of those receiving the drug for the treatment of toenail infections.

■ **Cardiovascular Effects** CHF, peripheral edema, and pulmonary edema have been reported rarely in patients receiving itraconazole for the treatment of systemic fungal infections and/or onychomycosis. Results from animal studies indicate that IV administration of itraconazole is associated with a dose-related negative inotropic effect. In addition, IV administration of itraconazole in healthy individuals (IV preparation no longer commercially available in the US) has resulted in transient, asymptomatic decreases in left ventricular ejection fraction (observed using gated SPECT imaging) which resolved before the next infusion, 12 hours later.

Heart failure has been reported most frequently in those receiving itraconazole in a dosage of 400 mg daily, but also has been reported in those receiving lower dosage.

The manufacturer states that itraconazole oral capsules should be discontinued in patients who develop CHF while receiving the drug. If CHF occurs during therapy with itraconazole oral solution, the manufacturer states that the patient should be carefully monitored and therapeutic options (including possible discontinuance of the drug) should be evaluated. (See Precautions Related to Cardiovascular Effects under Cautions: Precautions and Contraindications.)

Hypertension has been reported in up to 3% of patients receiving itraconazole for the treatment of systemic fungal infections and has been reported in less than 1% of patients receiving itraconazole for other uses.

Ventricular fibrillation secondary to itraconazole-induced hypokalemia has been reported in a patient with HIV infection and blastomycosis receiving high dosage of the drug (e.g., 400 mg twice daily). (See Cautions: Electrolyte and Metabolic Effects.) Serious adverse cardiovascular effects, including death, cardiac arrest, QT interval prolongation, ventricular tachycardia, and atypical ventricular tachycardia (torsades de pointes), have occurred rarely in patients receiving itraconazole concomitantly with certain drugs. (See Precautions related to Cardiovascular Effects under Cautions: Precautions and Contraindications.)

■ **Hepatic Effects** Hepatic function abnormalities, manifested principally as mild transient increases in serum liver enzyme concentrations, have occurred in about 3% of patients receiving itraconazole. However, serious hepatotoxicity, including liver failure and death, has occurred rarely and has been reported in patients with or without preexisting liver disease or a serious underlying medical condition. Hepatitis has been reported during postmarketing surveillance.

In patients receiving oral itraconazole capsules for the treatment of onychomycosis of the toenails (a continuous dosing regimen for 12 consecutive weeks), increased serum hepatic enzymes (greater than twice the upper limit of normal) that required temporary or permanent discontinuance of the drug have occurred in 4% of patients.

Itraconazole should be discontinued immediately and the risks and benefits of continuing therapy with the drug should be reassessed if signs and symptoms consistent with liver disease develop during therapy with the drug. (See Precautions Related to Hepatic Effects under Cautions: Precautions and Contraindications.)

■ **Electrolyte and Metabolic Effects** Hypokalemia has been reported in 2–9% of patients receiving itraconazole for the treatment of systemic fungal infections or oropharyngeal or esophageal candidiasis or for empiric antifungal prophylaxis. Itraconazole-induced hypokalemia may be mild to severe, may require potassium replacement and/or discontinuance of the drug, and has occurred principally at dosages of 400 mg daily or higher. (See Cautions: Precautions and Contraindications.) Edema (e.g., pedal) has occurred in up to 4% of patients with systemic fungal infections receiving itraconazole.

Adrenal insufficiency, gynecomastia, and male breast pain have occurred patients receiving the drug. Itraconazole generally does not appear to inhibit testicular or adrenal steroidogenesis substantially at usual dosages. However, at relatively high dosages (e.g., 600 mg daily or more) and/or with accumulation of the drug, adrenal suppression, which appears to be distinct from that associated with ketoconazole, may occur. Although a causal relationship to itraconazole has not been established, hypertriglyceridemia or hyperglycemia has been reported in patients receiving itraconazole.

■ **Genitourinary Effects** Albuminuria and impotence have occurred in about 1% of patients with systemic fungal infections receiving itraconazole. Urinary tract infection, cystitis, renal function abnormality, and menstrual disorder also have occurred in patients receiving itraconazole.

■ **Otic Effects** Transient or permanent hearing loss has been reported in patients receiving itraconazole. (See Cautions: Geriatric Precautions.) In some reported cases, the patient was also receiving quinidine, a drug that is contraindicated during itraconazole therapy. (See Drug Interactions: Antiarrhythmic Agents.)

If hearing loss occurs during itraconazole therapy, the drug should be discontinued. Although hearing loss usually resolves when itraconazole is discontinued, it can persist in some patients.

■ **Other Adverse Effects** Fatigue, fever, bursitis, myalgia, pain, herpes zoster infection, and injury have occurred in up to 7% of patients receiving itraconazole. Rhinitis, upper respiratory tract infection, sinusitis, and pharyngitis have been reported in up to 9% of itraconazole-treated patients. Neutropenia also has occurred in patients receiving the drug.

■ **Precautions and Contraindications** ***Precautions Related to Cardiovascular Effects*** CHF, peripheral edema, and pulmonary edema have been reported in immunocompromised or immunocompetent patients receiving itraconazole for the treatment of systemic fungal infections and also have been reported in immunocompetent patients receiving oral itraconazole capsules for the treatment of onychomycosis.

The manufacturer states that itraconazole capsules should *not* be used for the treatment of onychomycosis in patients with evidence of ventricular dysfunction, such as CHF or history of CHF, and should *not* be used for other indications in patients with evidence of ventricular dysfunction, unless benefits clearly outweigh risks. Itraconazole oral capsules should be discontinued in patients who develop CHF while receiving the drug.

The manufacturer states that itraconazole oral solution should not be used in patients with evidence of ventricular dysfunction, such as CHF or history of CHF, except for the treatment of life-threatening or other serious infections when benefits clearly outweigh risks. If CHF occurs in patients receiving the oral solution, the patient should be carefully monitored and therapeutic options (including possible discontinuance of the drug) should be evaluated.

Clinicians should carefully review the risks and benefits of itraconazole therapy in patients with risk factors for CHF (e.g., those with cardiac disease such as ischemic and valvular disease, clinically important pulmonary disease such as chronic obstructive pulmonary disease, or renal failure and other edematous disorders). If itraconazole is considered necessary in patients with risk factors for CHF, they should be informed of the signs and symptoms of CHF and carefully monitored during therapy.

Because itraconazole and its major metabolite, hydroxyitraconazole, are potent inhibitors of the cytochrome P-450 (CYP) 3A4 isoenzyme system, concomitant use of the antifungal with drugs metabolized by these enzymes can increase plasma concentrations of these drugs resulting in potential increases in their therapeutic and adverse effects. Serious adverse cardiovascular effects (QT prolongation, torsades de pointes, ventricular tachycardia, cardiac arrest, and/or sudden death) have been reported in patients receiving itraconazole concomitantly with certain drugs metabolized by CYP3A4 enzymes (e.g., cisapride [no longer available in the US only under a limited-access protocol], dofetilide, pimozide, quinidine, levomethadyl [no longer commercially available in the US]), and concomitant use with these drugs is contraindicated. (See Drug Interactions.)

Precautions Related to Hepatic Effects Because rare cases of serious hepatotoxicity have been reported with itraconazole, including some cases within the first week of therapy (see Cautions: Hepatic Effects), use of itraconazole is strongly discouraged in patients with increased serum hepatic enzymes, active liver disease, or a history of liver toxicity with other drugs, unless the potential benefits exceed the risks.

Itraconazole should be used with caution in patients with hepatic impairment since only limited data are available regarding use of the drug in such patients. The prolonged itraconazole elimination half-life reported in cirrhotic patients (see Pharmacokinetics) should be considered when deciding to initiate concomitant therapy with drugs that are metabolized by CYP3A4. (See Drug Interactions.)

Serum hepatic enzyme concentrations should be monitored in any patient with preexisting hepatic function abnormalities and in those who have experienced liver toxicity with other drugs. In addition, serum hepatic enzyme monitoring should be considered for all patients receiving itraconazole, especially those who receive itraconazole therapy continuously for longer than 1 month.

Itraconazole should be discontinued immediately and liver function testing performed if signs and symptoms consistent with liver disease develop during therapy. The risks and benefits of itraconazole should be reassessed in these patients.

Patients should be instructed to stop itraconazole immediately and contact their clinician if any signs or symptoms of liver dysfunction occur, including unusual fatigue, dark urine, pale stool, anorexia, nausea, vomiting, or jaundice, so that appropriate laboratory testing can be performed.

Other Precautions and Contraindications Itraconazole is contraindicated in patients with known hypersensitivity to the drug or any ingredient in the formulation. Although information concerning cross-sensitivity between itraconazole and other triazole or imidazole antifungals is not available, the manufacturer states that itraconazole should be used with caution in individuals hypersensitive to other azoles.

If neuropathy occurs that may be attributable to itraconazole, the drug should be discontinued.

Because itraconazole may cause hypokalemia, some clinicians recommended that serum potassium concentrations be monitored in patients receiving relatively high dosages and/or prolonged therapy with the drug. (See Cautions: Electrolyte and Metabolic Effects.)

Patients receiving itraconazole should be informed that hearing loss can occur and should be advised about the importance of discontinuing itraconazole and contacting a clinician if any symptoms of hearing loss occur. (See Cautions: Otic Effects.)

The manufacturer states that itraconazole oral solution has not been evaluated for the treatment of oropharyngeal and/or esophageal candidiasis in *severely* neutropenic patients. The oral solution is not recommended for initial treatment in patients at immediate risk of systemic candidiasis.

Variable itraconazole concentrations have been reported in cystic fibrosis patients receiving the oral solution. If itraconazole oral solution is used in cystic fibrosis patients and an adequate response is not obtained, consideration should be given to using alternative therapy. (See Cautions: Pediatric Precautions.)

Oral itraconazole should be used with caution in patients with renal impairment. Only limited data are available on the use of oral itraconazole in such patients. Wide interindividual variations in the area under the concentration-time curve (AUC) have been reported in patients with renal impairment. (See Pharmacokinetics.)

■ **Pediatric Precautions** The safety and efficacy of itraconazole in children younger than 18 years of age have not been established.

Itraconazole has been recommended by the Infectious Diseases Society of America (IDSA) and other experts for the treatment of some fungal infections (e.g., blastomycosis, oropharyngeal candidiasis, coccidioidomycosis†, histoplasmosis, sporotrichosis†) in children†, including HIV-infected infants, children, and adolescents†.

The manufacturer states that a limited number of patients 3–16 years of age with systemic nonmeningeal fungal infections have received itraconazole capsules in a dosage of 100 mg daily without unusual adverse effect. In addition, a limited number of pediatric patients 6 months to 12 years of age requiring systemic antifungal treatment have received itraconazole oral solution in a dosage of 5 mg/kg once daily for 2 weeks without any unusual adverse effects.

Data from a pharmacokinetic study evaluating itraconazole oral solution in patients with cystic fibrosis indicate that plasma itraconazole concentrations are variable in such patients and trough itraconazole concentrations attained in children younger than 16 years of age are lower than those in patients 16–28 years of age. If itraconazole oral solution is used in cystic fibrosis patients and an adequate response is not obtained, consideration should be given to initiating alternative therapy.

The long-term effects of itraconazole therapy on bone growth in children are not known. Data from animal studies have shown that itraconazole induces bone defects in rats receiving dosages as low as 20 mg/kg daily (2.5 times the maximum recommended human dosage). The defects included decreased bone plate activity, thinning of the zona compacta of large bones, and increased bone fragility. At a dosage of 80 mg/kg daily (10 times the maximum recommended human dosage) for longer than 1 year or 160 mg/kg daily (20 times the maximum recommended human dosage), the drug induced small tooth pulp with hypocellular appearance in some rats. Bone toxicity observed in animals has not been reported to date in adults receiving the drug.

■ **Geriatric Precautions** Itraconazole should be used with caution in geriatric patients.

Transient or permanent hearing loss has been reported in some geriatric patients receiving itraconazole. In some reported cases, the patient was also receiving quinidine, a drug that is contraindicated during itraconazole therapy. (See Drug Interactions: Antiarrhythmic Agents.)

■ **Mutagenicity and Carcinogenicity** There was no evidence of mutagenicity when itraconazole was assayed in appropriate bacterial, mammalian, and nonmammalian test systems.

There was no evidence of carcinogenicity in mice receiving oral itraconazole for 23 months at dosages up to 80 mg/kg daily (about 10 times the maximum recommended human dosage). There was a slight increase in the incidence of soft tissue sarcoma in male rats receiving 25 mg/kg daily (3.1 times the maximum recommended human dosage). These sarcomas may have been a consequence of hypercholesterolemia, a response to chronic itraconazole administration observed in rats but not in dogs or humans. An increase in the incidence of squamous cell carcinoma of the lung was observed in female rats receiving 50 mg/kg of itraconazole daily (6.25 times the maximum recommended human dosage). Although the occurrence of squamous cell carcinoma in the lung is extremely uncommon in untreated rats, the increased incidence in this study was not statistically significant.

Commercially available itraconazole oral solution and itraconazole injection contain hydroxypropyl-β-cyclodextrin (HP-β-CD) as an excipient. HP-β-CD has produced pancreatic adenocarcinomas in rat carcinogenicity studies but similar effects were not observed in a mouse carcinogenicity study. The clinical relevance of this finding is not known. It has been estimated that, based on body surface area comparisons, patients receiving the usual dosage of commercially available itraconazole oral solution would be exposed to concentrations of HP-β-CD that are equivalent to 1.7 times that the exposure of the lowest dose used in the rat study.

■ **Pregnancy, Fertility, and Lactation** ***Pregnancy*** Itraconazole has been shown to be teratogenic and embryotoxic in mice and rats. In addition, although a causal relationship with itraconazole has not been established, congenital abnormalities (skeletal, genitourinary tract, cardiovascular, ophthalmic) and chromosomal and multiple malformations have been reported during postmarketing experience when the drug was used in pregnant women.

There are no adequate and controlled studies evaluating itraconazole in pregnant women, and the drug should be used during pregnancy only when the potential benefits justify the possible risks to the fetus.

For the treatment of onychomycosis, use of itraconazole is contraindicated in pregnant women and also is contraindicated in women contemplating pregnancy. If itraconazole therapy for the treatment of onychomycosis is initiated in a woman of childbearing potential, the first dose of the drug should be given on the second or third day of the next normal menstrual period and measures should be taken to ensure that effective contraception is continued throughout itraconazole therapy and for 2 additional months following discontinuance of the drug.

In reproduction studies, itraconazole caused a dose-related increase in maternal toxicity, embryotoxicity, and teratogenicity in rats at dosages of approximately 40–160 mg/kg daily (5–20 times the maximum recommended human dosage) and in mice at dosages of approximately 80 mg/kg daily (10 times the maximum recommended human dosage). Teratogenicity consisted of major skeletal defects in rats and encephaloceles and/or macroglossia in mice.

Fertility Although parental toxicity was observed, reproduction studies in male and female rats receiving oral itraconazole dosages up to 40 mg/kg daily (5 times the maximum recommended human dosage) did not reveal evidence of impaired fertility. More severe parental toxicity, including death, occurred at a dosage of 160 mg/kg daily (20 times the maximum recommended human dosage).

Lactation Itraconazole is distributed into human milk and the expected benefits of itraconazole for the nursing woman should be weighed against the potential risk to the infant from exposure to the drug. Because of the potential for transmission of HIV to an uninfected child, the US Centers for Disease Control and Prevention (CDC) currently recommends that HIV-infected women *not* breastfeed infants.

Drug Interactions

■ **Antiarrhythmic Agents** Concomitant use of quinidine or dofetilide (antiarrhythmics that increase the QT interval) and itraconazole is contraindicated. Administration of itraconazole with quinidine or dofetilide would be expected to increase plasma concentrations of the antiarrhythmic agent which could result in serious adverse cardiovascular effects. Life-threatening cardiac dysrhythmias and/or sudden death have occurred in patients receiving quinidine concomitantly with itraconazole and/or other drugs that inhibit the cytochrome P-450 (CYP) 3A4 isoenzyme.

Concomitant use of disopyramide and itraconazole may result in increased plasma concentrations of the antiarrhythmic agent. Disopyramide and itraconazole should be used concomitantly with caution.

Concomitant use of digoxin and itraconazole may result in increased plasma concentrations of the antiarrhythmic agent, possibly as a result of inhibition of P-glycoprotein.

■ **Antilipemic Agents** Concomitant use of hydroxymethylglutaryl-CoA (HMG-CoA) reductase inhibitors (e.g., atorvastatin, cerivastatin, lovastatin, simvastatin) and itraconazole may increase plasma concentrations of these antilipemic agents resulting in increased effects and increased risk of toxicity (e.g., myopathy including rhabdomyolysis). Concomitant use of itraconazole and these antilipemic agents is contraindicated.

■ **Antiretroviral Agents** ***HIV Entry Inhibitors*** Concomitant use of maraviroc and itraconazole may result in increased concentrations of maraviroc. If maraviroc is used concomitantly with itraconazole, consideration should be given to reducing the maraviroc dosage to 150 mg twice daily.

HIV Protease Inhibitors (PIs) Pharmacokinetic interactions are likely if itraconazole is used in patients receiving HIV protease inhibitors (PIs) (e.g., atazanavir, darunavir, fosamprenavir, indinavir, lopinavir, nelfinavir, ritonavir, saquinavir, tipranavir), especially if *ritonavir-boosted* PI regimens are used. Concomitant use may result in altered serum concentrations of the PIs and/or the antifungal.

Atazanavir. If atazanavir (with or without low-dose ritonavir) is used in patients receiving itraconazole, increased concentrations of both itraconazole and atazanavir are possible and clinicians should consider monitoring itraconazole plasma concentrations to guide dosage adjustments of the antifungal. High itraconazole dosage (greater than 200 mg daily) is not recommended in patients receiving *ritonavir-boosted* atazanavir, unless plasma concentrations of the antifungal are used to guide dosage.

Darunavir. If *ritonavir-boosted* darunavir is used in patients receiving itraconazole, increased concentrations of both itraconazole and darunavir are possible and clinicians should consider monitoring itraconazole plasma concentrations to guide dosage adjustments of the antifungal. High itraconazole dosage (greater than 200 mg daily) is not recommended in patients receiving *ritonavir-boosted* darunavir, unless plasma concentrations of the antifungal are used to guide dosage.

Fosamprenavir. If fosamprenavir (with or without low-dose ritonavir) is used in patients receiving itraconazole, increased concentrations of both itraconazole and fosamprenavir are possible and clinicians should consider monitoring itraconazole plasma concentrations to guide dosage adjustments of the antifungal. High itraconazole dosage (greater than 200 mg daily) is not recommended in patients receiving *ritonavir-boosted* fosamprenavir, unless plasma concentrations of the antifungal are used to guide dosage.

Indinavir. If indinavir (with or without low-dose ritonavir) is used in patients receiving itraconazole, increased concentrations of both itraconazole and indinavir are possible and clinicians should consider monitoring itraconazole plasma concentrations to guide dosage adjustments of the antifungal.

If itraconazole is used concomitantly with indinavir (without low-dose ritonavir), some experts recommend that indinavir be given in a dosage of 600 mg every 8 hours and that itraconazole dosage should not exceed 200 mg twice daily. Appropriate dosage of *ritonavir-boosted* indinavir has not been established for patients receiving concomitant itraconazole; high itraconazole dosage (greater than 200 mg daily) is not recommended, unless plasma concentrations of the antifungal are used to guide dosage.

Lopinavir. If itraconazole is used with the fixed combination of lopinavir and ritonavir (lopinavir/ritonavir), some experts recommend that clinicians should consider not exceeding an itraconazole dosage of 200 mg daily or should consider monitoring itraconazole plasma concentrations.

Nelfinavir. If nelfinavir is used in patients receiving itraconazole, increased concentrations of both itraconazole and nelfinavir are possible and clinicians should consider monitoring itraconazole plasma concentrations to guide dosage adjustments of the antifungal.

Saquinavir. If *ritonavir-boosted* saquinavir is used in patients receiving itraconazole, altered plasma concentrations of both itraconazole and saquinavir are possible and clinicians should consider monitoring itraconazole plasma concentrations. Appropriate dosage for concomitant use has not been established, but decreased itraconazole dosage may be warranted.

Tipranavir. If *ritonavir-boosted* tipranavir is used in patients receiving itraconazole, increased concentrations of both itraconazole and tipranavir are possible and clinicians should consider monitoring itraconazole plasma concentrations to guide dosage adjustments of the antifungal.

Nonnucleoside Reverse Transcriptase Inhibitors (NNRTIs)

Efavirenz. Concomitant use of efavirenz and itraconazole results in decreased plasma concentrations and area under the concentration-time curve (AUC) of itraconazole and its major metabolite, hydroxyitraconazole, but does not affect efavirenz concentrations.

The manufacturer of efavirenz states that an alternative antifungal should be considered instead of itraconazole in patients receiving efavirenz. Some experts state that itraconazole plasma concentrations should be monitored in patients receiving efavirenz and dosage of the antifungal may need to be adjusted.

Etravirine. Concomitant use of etravirine and itraconazole may result in decreased itraconazole concentrations and increased etravirine concentrations. Dosage adjustment of itraconazole may be needed depending on other concomitantly administered drugs.

Nevirapine. Concomitant use of nevirapine and itraconazole may result in decreased plasma concentrations of itraconazole and increased nevirapine concentrations.

Itraconazole and nevirapine should not be used concomitantly. Some experts state that if itraconazole and nevirapine are used concomitantly, consideration should be given to monitoring plasma concentrations of both drugs.

Nucleoside Reverse Transcriptase Inhibitors (NRTIs)

Zidovudine. Concomitant use of zidovudine and itraconazole does not affect the pharmacokinetics of zidovudine.

■ **Astemizole and Terfenadine** Concomitant use of itraconazole and astemizole or terfenadine (drugs no longer commercially available in the US) is contraindicated. Rare cases of serious adverse cardiovascular effects, including death, ventricular tachycardia, and atypical ventricular tachycardia (torsades de pointes), have occurred in patients receiving itraconazole and terfenadine concomitantly. Similar effects have been reported when ketoconazole, a structurally similar antifungal, was used concomitantly with terfenadine. The antifungals appear to inhibit the metabolism of astemizole or terfenadine, probably via inhibition of the CYP isoenzyme system, resulting in increased plasma concentrations of unchanged drug (to measurable levels) and reduced clearance of the active desmethyl or carboxylic acid metabolite, respectively. Such alterations in the pharmacokinetics of these antihistamines may have been associated with prolongation of the QT and QT_c intervals.

■ **Benzodiazepines** Concomitant use of itraconazole and benzodiazepines (e.g., alprazolam, diazepam, oral midazolam, triazolam) may result in increased plasma concentrations of these benzodiazepines that could potentiate and prolong the sedative and hypnotic effects of the drugs. Concomitant use of itraconazole and oral midazolam or triazolam is contraindicated; if midazolam is administered parenterally in patients receiving itraconazole, special precaution and patient monitoring is required since the sedative effect of the benzodiazepine may be prolonged.

■ **Calcium-channel Blocking Agents** Itraconazole may inhibit metabolism of calcium-channel blocking agents (e.g., nifedipine, felodipine, verapamil). In addition, calcium-channel blocking agents can have negative inotropic effects, which may be additive to those of itraconazole. Edema has been reported in patients receiving itraconazole and a dihydropyridine calcium-channel blocker concomitantly.

Because of an increased risk of congestive heart failure (CHF), itraconazole should be used with caution in patients receiving a calcium-channel blocker and appropriate dosage adjustments may be necessary.

Concomitant use of itraconazole and nisoldipine is contraindicated because concomitant use of these drugs results in a clinically important increase in nisoldipine plasma concentrations that cannot be managed by dosage reduction.

■ **Carbamazepine** Concomitant use of carbamazepine and itraconazole may result in increased carbamazepine concentrations and decreased itraconazole concentrations.

■ **Cilostazol** Because cilostazol is metabolized by CYP3A4, concomitant use with itraconazole may result in increased cilostazol plasma concentrations.

■ **Cisapride** Concomitant use of itraconazole and cisapride (currently commercially available in the US only under a limited-access protocol) is contraindicated since itraconazole inhibits metabolism of cisapride and such use can result in increased plasma cisapride concentrations and increase the potential for serious adverse cardiovascular effects.

■ **Corticosteroids** Concomitant use of corticosteroids (e.g., budesonide, dexamethasone, fluticasone, methylprednisolone) and itraconazole may result in increased plasma concentrations of the corticosteroid.

■ **Eletriptan** Because eletriptan is metabolized by CYP3A4, concomitant use with itraconazole may result in increased eletriptan plasma concentrations.

■ **Ergot Alkaloids** Concomitant use of ergot alkaloids (dihydroergotamine, ergonovine, ergotamine, methylergonovine) and itraconazole may result in increased concentrations of the ergot alkaloid and may cause ergotism (i.e., risk for venospasm potentially leading to cerebral ischemia and/or ischemia of the extremities). Concomitant use of ergot alkaloids and itraconazole is contraindicated.

■ **Fentanyl** Concomitant use of fentanyl and itraconazole may result in increased plasma fentanyl concentrations and increased potential for fatal respiratory depression.

■ **Halofantrine** Concomitant use of halofantrine (not commercially available in the US) and itraconazole may result in increased plasma halofantrine concentrations increased risk of prolonged QT interval.Halofantrine and itraconazole should be used concomitantly with caution.

■ **Pimozide** Concomitant use of pimozide and itraconazole is contraindicated. Life-threatening cardiac dysrhythmias and/or sudden death have occurred in patients receiving pimozide concomitantly with itraconazole and/or other drugs that inhibit the CYP3A4 enzyme.

■ **Phosphodiesterase Type 5 Inhibitors** Itraconazole is a potent inhibitor of CYP3A4, and concomitant use in patients receiving a phosphodiesterase type 5 (PDE5) inhibitor (sildenafil, tadalafil, vardenafil) can substantially increase plasma concentrations of the PDE5 inhibitor and may increase the risk of adverse effects (e.g., hypotension, visual changes, priapism) associated with these agents.

Sildenafil The manufacturer of sildenafil recommends that a starting dose of 25 mg of sildenafil be considered in patients receiving itraconazole.

Tadalafil Although specific studies evaluating concomitant use of tadalafil and itraconazole are not available, the manufacturer of tadalafil recommends that patients receiving potent CYP3A4 inhibitors receive no more than 10 mg of tadalafil once every 72 hours. If a once-daily tadalafil regimen is used in patients receiving itraconazole, no more than 2.5 mg of tadalafil should be given once daily.

Vardenafil The manufacturer of vardenafil recommends that patients receiving itraconazole in a dosage of 400 mg daily should receive no more than a single 2.5-mg dose of vardenafil in a 24-hour period and those receiving itraconazole in a dosage of 200 mg daily should receive no more than a single 5-mg dose of vardenafil in a 24-hour period.

Spectrum

Itraconazole and its principal metabolite hydroxyitraconazole are active against many fungi, including yeasts and dermatophytes. The antifungal spectrum of activity of the drug is similar to that of fluconazole and ketoconazole, although differences in specific in vitro and in vivo activity on weight and pharmacodynamic bases exist. In addition, itraconazole more consistently exhibits clinically important activity against *Aspergillus*.

■ **Fungi** In vitro, the MIC_{90} of itraconazole for *C. guilliermondii, C. krusei, C. parapsilosis,* and *C. tropicalis* is 0.12–1 mcg/mL and the MIC_{90} of the drug for *C. albicans* and *C. glabrata* (formerly *Torulopsis glabrata*) is 0.12–4 mcg/mL. In a study evaluating in vitro susceptibility of clinical isolates of *C. dubliniensis* obtained from patients with or without human immunodeficiency virus (HIV) infection, these strains were inhibited by itraconazole concentrations of 0.03–0.5 mcg/mL. Some strains of *C. lusitaniae* are inhibited in vitro by itraconazole concentrations of 0.06–0.5 mcg/mL.

Aspergillus, including *A. fumigatus, A. flavus, A. niger*, and *A. terreus*, have been inhibited in vitro by itraconazole concentrations of 0.25–2 mcg/mL.

The MIC_{90} of itraconazole reported for *C. neoformans* is 0.5–1 mcg/mL. Some strains of *C. gattii* are inhibited in vitro by itraconazole concentrations of 0.12–2 mcg/mL.

Blastomyces dermatitidis generally is inhibited in vitro by itraconazole concentrations of 0.07 mcg/mL or less.

The MIC of itraconazole reported for clinical isolates of *Sporothrix schenckii* has ranged from 0.03–8 mcg/mL.

Several clinical isolates of *Basidiobolus ranarum* had itraconazole MICs of 1–8 mcg/mL.

Penicillium marneffei has been inhibited in vitro by itraconazole concentrations of 0.012–0.32 mcg/mL.

Some zygomycetes, including some strains of *Rhizopus, Mucor, Absidia, Rhizomucor, Cunninghamella*, and *Apophysomyces elegans*, are inhibited in vitro by itraconazole. There is some evidence that itraconazole is active in vitro against some strains of *Basidiobolus*, including *B. ranarum*.

Itraconazole is not active against *Fusarium, Scedosporium*, or *Scopulariopsis*, including *S. acremonium* and *S. brevicaulis*.

Resistance

Strains of fungi resistant to itraconazole have been isolated in vitro and from patients who received prolonged therapy with the drug. Itraconazole-resistant fungi, including *Candida*, may be cross-resistant to other azole antifungals (e.g., fluconazole, ketoconazole).

Pharmacokinetics

■ **Absorption** Following oral administration of itraconazole, bioavailability varies depending on whether the drug is administered as capsules or the oral solution; these preparations are not bioequivalent.

When administered under optimum conditions for GI absorption (oral solution under fasting conditions or oral capsules with food), itraconazole oral solution is more bioavailable than itraconazole capsules.

When a single 200-mg dose is given as capsules (with a meal), peak plasma concentrations are usually attained within 5 hours and average 302 ng/mL. When a single 200-mg dose of itraconazole is given as the oral solution (without food), peak plasma concentrations usually are attained within 2.2 hours and average 544 ng/mL.

When itraconazole capsules are used, bioavailability is maximal when administered with food. Food decreases the rate of absorption, but increases peak plasma concentrations and area under the concentration-time curve (AUC) of the oral capsules.

When itraconazole oral solution is used, bioavailability is maximal when administered under fasting conditions. Food decreases the rate and extent of absorption of the oral solution.

Oral absorption of itraconazole is impaired when gastric acid production is decreased. In fasting individuals with relative or absolute achlorhydria, such as individuals with human immunodeficiency virus (HIV) infection or those receiving a histamine H_2-receptor antagonist, peak plasma concentrations and AUC are increased when itraconazole oral capsules are administered with a cola beverage compared with administration with water.

In cirrhotic patients who received a single 100-mg itraconazole capsule, mean peak plasma concentrations were 47% lower, but overall exposure (based on AUC) was similar to that in healthy individuals. Data are not available regarding long-tem use in such patients.

Data from a single-dose study in uremic patients (mean creatinine clearance 13 mL/minute per 1.73 m^2) indicate that the AUC of itraconazole in these patients is slightly decreased compared with healthy individuals. Wide interindividual variations in AUC were reported in uremic patients and in patients undergoing hemodialysis or continuous ambulatory peritoneal dialysis (CAPD).

Data from a pharmacokinetic study evaluating itraconazole oral solution (2.5 mg/kg twice daily for 14 days) in patients with cystic fibrosis indicate that itraconazole concentrations are variable in such patients and trough concentrations attained in children younger than 16 years of age are lower than those in patients 16–28 years of age.

■ **Distribution** Itraconazole is 99.8% and hydroxyitraconazole is 99.5% bound to plasma proteins.

Itraconazole is highly lipophilic and is distributed into the nail matrix, bed, and plate following oral administration, persisting in these tissues for several months after discontinuance of the drug.

Itraconazole is distributed into human milk.

■ **Elimination** Itraconazole is metabolized principally in the liver by cytochrome P-450 (CYP) isoenzyme 3A4 (CYP3A4) to several metabolites. Hydroxyitraconazole, the major metabolite, has antifungal activity.

Saturable metabolism may occur with multiple dosing.

Approximately 40% of an itraconazole dose is eliminated in urine as inactive metabolites, less than 0.03% is eliminated in urine as unchanged drug, and 3–18% is eliminated in feces as unchanged drug.

In adults receiving itraconazole oral capsules (200 mg twice daily with a meal), the half-life of itraconazole is 64 hours and the half-life of hydroxyitraconazole is 56 hours at steady state.

In adults receiving itraconazole oral solution (200 mg daily without food), the half-life of itraconazole is 39.7 hours and the half-life of hydroxyitraconazole is 27.3 hours at steady state.

In children 6 months to 12 years of age receiving itraconazole oral solution (5 mg/kg once daily), the half-life of itraconazole is 35.8 hours and the half-life of hydroxyitraconazole is 17.7 hours at steady state.

In cirrhotic patients who received a single 100-mg itraconazole dose as capsules, the elimination half-life was 37 hours (compared with 16 hours following a single dose in healthy individuals). Data are not available regarding long-tem use of itraconazole in such patients.

Itraconazole is not appreciably removed by hemodialysis or peritoneal dialysis.

Chemistry and Stability

■ **Chemistry** Itraconazole, a synthetic triazole derivative, is an azole antifungal agent. The drug is structurally related to imidazole-derivative azole antifungal agents (e.g., butoconazole, clotrimazole, econazole, ketoconazole, oxiconazole); however, imidazoles have 2 nitrogens in the azole ring (imidazole ring) while itraconazole and other triazoles (e.g., fluconazole, terconazole) have 3 nitrogens in the ring (triazole ring). For additional information on the chemistry of triazoles, including structure-activity relationships, see Chemistry and Stability: Chemistry in Fluconazole 8:14.08.

Itraconazole is a 1:1:1:1 racemic mixture of 4 diastereomers (2 enantiomeric pairs), each possessing 3 chiral centers. The drug occurs as a white to slightly yellowish powder and is insoluble in water and very slightly soluble in alcohol.

Each mL of itraconazole oral solution contains 10 mg of itraconazole solubilized by 400 mg of hydroxypropyl-β-cyclodextrin as a molecular inclusion complex. The oral solution is clear and yellowish in color with a target pH of 2; the solution also contains hydrochloric acid, propylene glycol, sodium hydroxide, sodium saccharin, and sorbitol.

■ **Stability** Itraconazole capsules should be stored at a controlled room temperature of 15–25°C and protected from light and moisture. Itraconazole oral solution should be stored at 25°C or lower and should not be frozen.

Preparations

Excipients in commercially available drug preparations may have clinically important effects in some individuals; consult specific product labeling for details.

Itraconazole

Oral		
Capsules	100 mg*	**Itraconazole Capsules**
		Sporanox®, Ortho-McNeil-Janssen
Solution	10 mg/mL	**Sporanox®**, Centocor Ortho Biotech

*available from one or more manufacturer, distributor, and/or repackager by generic (nonproprietary) name

†Use is not currently included in the labeling approved by the US Food and Drug Administration

Posaconazole

■ Posaconazole, a synthetic triazole derivative, is an azole antifungal agent.

Uses

■ Prevention of Invasive Aspergillus and Candida Infections in Immunocompromised Individuals Oral posaconazole (delayed-release tablets, oral suspension) is used for prophylaxis of invasive *Aspergillus* and *Candida* infections in severely immunocompromised adults and adolescents 13 years of age and older at high risk of developing these infections, including hematopoietic stem cell transplant (HSCT) recipients with graft-versus-host disease (GVHD) or patients with hematologic malignancies and prolonged chemotherapy-associated neutropenia. Alternatively, IV posaconazole is used for such prophylaxis in adults 18 years of age or older.

For primary prophylaxis to prevent invasive aspergillosis in immunocompromised individuals at high risk for such infections (i.e., neutropenic patients with acute myelogenous leukemia [AML] or myelodysplastic syndrome [MDS], HSCT recipients with GVHD), the Infectious Diseases Society of America (IDSA) recommends posaconazole as the drug of choice; itraconazole and micafungin are recommended as alternatives.

IDSA recommends primary prophylaxis against *Candida* infections in neutropenic patients when the risk of invasive candida infection is substantial (e.g., allogeneic HSCT recipients, patients with acute leukemia undergoing intensive remission-induction or salvage-induction chemotherapy) and states that an azole antifungal (fluconazole, itraconazole, posaconazole, voriconazole) or IV echinocandin (caspofungin or micafungin) can be used. These experts state that antifungal prophylaxis is not recommended if the anticipated duration of neutropenia is less than 7 days. If primary prophylaxis is used to prevent invasive candidiasis in high-risk adults in intensive care settings, IDSA recommends fluconazole as the drug of choice and IV echinocandins (anidulafungin, caspofungin, micafungin) as alternatives.

Posaconazole is used for secondary prophylaxis to prevent relapse or recurrence of esophageal candidiasis† in HIV-infected adults and adolescents who have been adequately treated. (See Esophageal Candidiasis under Uses: Candida Infections.)

For additional information on prevention of fungal infections in immunocompromised patients, the current clinical practice guidelines from IDSA available at http://www.idsociety.org should be consulted.

Clinical Experience Safety and efficacy of posaconazole oral suspension for prophylaxis of invasive *Aspergillus* and *Candida* infections in adults and adolescents 13 years of age or older have been evaluated in a randomized, double-blind comparative study in HSCT recipients with GVHD and in a randomized, open-label comparative study in neutropenic patients receiving cytotoxic chemotherapy for acute myelogenous leukemia or myelodysplastic syndrome.

In the study in HSCT recipients 13 years of age or older with GVHD, patients were randomized to receive posaconazole oral suspension (200 mg 3 times daily) or fluconazole capsules (400 mg once daily) for up to 112 days. The mean duration of prophylaxis with posaconazole or fluconazole was 80 or 77 days, respectively. Results indicate that posaconazole and fluconazole prophylaxis produced similar rates of clinical failure (based on a composite endpoint of proven or probable invasive fungal infections, death, and/or treatment with systemic antifungals) at 16 weeks (33 versus 37%). Breakthrough infections caused by *Aspergillus* were reported in 2% of patients receiving posaconazole compared with 7% of patients receiving fluconazole during the fixed treatment period; the rate of breakthrough infections caused by *Candida* was similar with both drugs.

In the study in neutropenic patients receiving cytotoxic chemotherapy for acute myelogenous leukemia or myelodysplastic syndrome (study NCT00044486), patients were randomized to receive posaconazole oral suspension (200 mg 3 times daily) or either fluconazole oral suspension (400 mg once daily) or itraconazole oral solution (200 mg twice daily); the mean duration of prophylaxis was 29 days with posaconazole and 25 days with fluconazole or itraconazole. Clinical failure assessed up to 1 week after prophylaxis ended was lower in those receiving posaconazole (27%) than in those receiving fluconazole or itraconazole (42%); at 100 days after randomization, the clinical failure rate was 52 or 64%, respectively. Fewer breakthrough infections caused by *Aspergillus* were reported in patients receiving posaconazole than in those receiving fluconazole or itraconazole; the rates of breakthrough infections caused by *Candida* were similar.

Use of posaconazole delayed-release tablets for prophylaxis of invasive *Aspergillus* and *Candida* infections in adults and adolescents 13 years of age or older is supported by a phase 1/3b safety, tolerability, and pharmacokinetic study evaluating the delayed-release tablets in patients with hematologic malignancies at risk for these infections.

■ Candida Infections ***Oropharyngeal Candidiasis*** Oral posaconazole (oral suspension) is used for the treatment of oropharyngeal candidiasis in adults, including oropharyngeal candidiasis refractory to fluconazole and/or itraconazole.

For the treatment of mild oropharyngeal candidiasis, IDSA recommends topical treatment with clotrimazole lozenges or miconazole buccal tablets; nystatin (oral suspension or tablets) is the recommended alternative. For moderate to severe disease, IDSA recommends oral fluconazole. For fluconazole-refractory oropharyngeal candidiasis, IDSA recommends itraconazole oral solution or posaconazole oral suspension; oral voriconazole or amphotericin B oral suspension (not commercially available in US) are recommended as alternatives. Other alternatives for refractory oropharyngeal candidiasis are IV echinocandins (anidulafungin, caspofungin, micafungin) or IV amphotericin B.

For the treatment of oropharyngeal candidiasis in adults and adolescents with human immunodeficiency virus (HIV) infection, the US Centers for Disease Control and Prevention (CDC), National Institutes of Health (NIH), and IDSA recommend oral fluconazole as the preferred drug of choice for initial episodes. If topical therapy is used for the treatment of mild to moderate episodes, these experts recommend clotrimazole lozenges or miconazole buccal tablets. Alternatives for systemic treatment of oropharyngeal candidiasis in HIV-infected adults and adolescents are itraconazole oral solution or posaconazole oral suspension; nystatin oral suspension is an alternative if topical treatment is used. For fluconazole-refractory oropharyngeal infections in HIV-infected adults and adolescents, posaconazole oral suspension is preferred; itraconazole oral solution is an alternative.

Routine long-term suppressive or maintenance therapy (secondary prophylaxis) to prevent relapse or recurrence is not usually recommended in patients adequately treated for oropharyngeal candidiasis (including HIV-infected individuals) unless the patient has frequent or severe recurrences of oropharyngeal candidiasis. If secondary prophylaxis of oropharyngeal candidiasis is indicated, oral fluconazole is recommended; however, the potential for development of azole resistance should be considered.

For additional information on prophylaxis and treatment of oropharyngeal candidiasis, the current clinical practice guidelines from IDSA available at http://www.idsociety.org and current clinical practice guidelines from CDC, NIH, and IDSA on the prevention and treatment of opportunistic infections in HIV-infected individuals available at http://www.aidsinfo.nih.gov should be consulted.

Clinical Experience. In a randomized, evaluator-blinded study of posaconazole for the treatment of oropharyngeal candidiasis, HIV-infected adults 18 years of age or older with oropharyngeal candidiasis were randomized to receive posaconazole oral suspension (100 mg twice daily for 1 day, followed by 100 mg once daily for 13 days) or fluconazole oral suspension (100 mg twice daily for 1 day, followed by 100 mg once daily for 13 days). Patients evaluated for efficacy included those who received at least one dose of posaconazole or fluconazole and had a baseline oral swish culture positive for *Candida* (*C. albicans* was isolated from most patients). The clinical and mycologic cure rates after 14 days of antifungal therapy and clinical and mycologic relapse rates at 4 weeks posttreatment were similar for posaconazole and fluconazole. Clinical cure (defined as complete or partial resolution of all ulcers and/or plaques and symptoms) at day 14 was attained in 92 or 93% of those receiving posaconazole or fluconazole, respectively. The mycologic cure rate (defined as the absence of colony-forming units in quantitative culture at the end of the 14-day regimen) was 52 or 50% in those receiving posaconazole or fluconazole, respectively. At 4 weeks posttreatment, the rate of clinical relapse (defined as recurrence of signs or symptoms after initial cure or improvement) was 29 or 35% and the rate of mycologic relapse was 56 or 64% in patients receiving posaconazole or fluconazole, respectively.

Efficacy of posaconazole oral suspension for the treatment of oropharyngeal candidiasis refractory to fluconazole or itraconazole was evaluated in a phase 3, open-label, noncomparative study in HIV-infected adults 18 years of age or older. Oropharyngeal candidiasis was considered refractory to fluconazole or itraconazole if the infection failed to improve or worsened after the usual regimen of oral fluconazole (at least 100 mg daily for at least 10 consecutive days) or oral itraconazole (200 mg daily for at least 10 consecutive days) and treatment with these drugs had not been discontinued for more than 14 days prior to initiation of posaconazole. Of 199 adults enrolled in the study, 89 met these criteria for refractory oropharyngeal candidiasis. Forty-five adults with refractory oropharyngeal candidiasis received posaconazole oral suspension (400 mg twice daily for 3 days, followed by 400 mg once daily for 25 days); patients also received optional suppressive or maintenance therapy with the drug (400 mg twice daily 3 times weekly) for 3 additional months. As the result of a protocol amendment to simplify the regimen, the remaining 44 adults with refractory oropharyngeal candidiasis received oral posaconazole (400 mg twice daily for 28 days). Clinical cure or improvement was attained in 74% of patients overall; similar rates of clinical cure or improvement were attained in patients receiving the initial and increased dosage regimens (73 and 75%, respectively).

Esophageal Candidiasis Although safety and efficacy have not been established, oral posaconazole (oral suspension) has been effective for the treatment of esophageal candidiasis† refractory to oral fluconazole and/or itraconazole in HIV-infected adults and has been recommended as an alternative for the treatment of esophageal candidiasis.

Esophageal candidiasis requires treatment with a systemic antifungal (not a topical antifungal).

IDSA recommends oral fluconazole as the preferred drug of choice for the treatment of esophageal candidiasis; if oral therapy is not tolerated, IV fluconazole or an IV echinocandin (anidulafungin, caspofungin, micafungin) usually is recommended and IV amphotericin B is another alternative. For fluconazole-refractory esophageal candidiasis, IDSA recommends itraconazole oral solution or oral or IV voriconazole; alternatives for fluconazole-refractory disease are IV echinocandins (anidulafungin, caspofungin, micafungin) or IV amphotericin B. IDSA states that oral posaconazole (oral suspension or delayed-release tablets) could be considered as another alternative for the treatment of fluconazole-refractory esophageal candidiasis.

For the treatment of esophageal candidiasis in HIV-infected adults and adolescents, CDC, NIH, and IDSA recommend oral or IV fluconazole or itraconazole oral solution. Alternatives include oral or IV voriconazole, an IV echinocandin (caspofungin, micafungin, anidulafungin), or IV amphotericin B. For refractory esophageal candidiasis in HIV-infected adults and adolescents, including fluconazole-refractory infections, these experts recommend posaconazole oral suspension or itraconazole oral solution; alternatives include an IV echinocandin (anidulafungin, caspofungin, micafungin), oral or IV voriconazole, or IV amphotericin B.

Routine long-term suppressive or maintenance therapy (secondary prophylaxis) to prevent relapse or recurrence is not usually recommended in patients adequately treated for esophageal candidiasis (including HIV-infected individuals) unless the patient has frequent or severe recurrences of esophageal candidiasis. If secondary prophylaxis of esophageal candidiasis is indicated, oral fluconazole is recommended and posaconazole oral suspension is a possible alternative; however, the potential for development of azole resistance should be considered.

For additional information on prophylaxis and treatment of esophageal candidiasis, the current clinical practice guidelines from IDSA available at http://www.idsociety.org and current clinical practice guidelines from CDC, NIH, and IDSA on the prevention and treatment of opportunistic infections in HIV-infected individuals available at http://www.aidsinfo.nih.gov should be consulted.

■ **Aspergillosis** Although safety and efficacy have not been established, posaconazole has been effective in some patients when used as salvage therapy for the treatment of invasive aspergillosis† when other antifungals (e.g., voriconazole, amphotericin B, itraconazole) were ineffective or could not be used. In a limited study evaluating posaconazole salvage therapy, the overall success rate was 42% (median duration of treatment was 56 days); 39% of those with pulmonary aspergillosis and 53% of those with extrapulmonary aspergillosis responded to the posaconazole salvage regimen.

IDSA considers IV or oral voriconazole the drug of choice for primary treatment of invasive aspergillosis in most patients and IV amphotericin B the preferred alternative. For salvage therapy in patients refractory to or intolerant of primary antifungal therapy, IDSA recommends IV amphotericin B, an echinocandin (caspofungin or micafungin), posaconazole, or itraconazole. For empiric or preemptive therapy of presumed aspergillosis, IDSA recommends amphotericin B, caspofungin, itraconazole, or voriconazole.

For the treatment of invasive aspergillosis in HIV-infected adults and adolescents, CDC, NIH, and IDSA recommend voriconazole as the drug of choice; alternatives are IV amphotericin B, an IV echinocandin (anidulafungin, caspofungin, micafungin), and oral posaconazole.

Posaconazole is used for primary prophylaxis against invasive aspergillosis in immunocompromised individuals at high risk. (See Uses: Prevention of Invasive Aspergillus and Candida Infections in Immunocompromised Individuals.)

For additional information on prophylaxis and treatment of aspergillosis, the current clinical practice guidelines from IDSA available at http://www.idsociety.org and current clinical practice guidelines from CDC, NIH, and IDSA on the prevention and treatment of opportunistic infections in HIV-infected individuals available at http://www.aidsinfo.nih.gov should be consulted.

■ **Coccidioidomycosis** Although safety and efficacy have not been established, posaconazole has been used in some adults for the treatment of coccidioidomycosis† caused by *Coccidioides immitis*, and is recommended as an alternative for the treatment or prevention of these infections in HIV-infected individuals.

Antifungal treatment may not be necessary in patients with mild, uncomplicated coccidioidal pneumonia since such infections often are self-limited and may resolve spontaneously. However, antifungal treatment is recommended for patients with more severe or rapidly progressing coccidioidal infections, those with chronic pulmonary or disseminated infections, and immunocompromised or debilitated individuals (e.g., HIV-infected individuals, organ transplant recipients, those receiving immunosuppressive therapy, those with diabetes mellitus or cardiopulmonary disease).

IDSA and others state that an oral azole (fluconazole or itraconazole) usually is recommended for initial treatment of symptomatic pulmonary coccidioidomycosis and chronic fibrocavitary or disseminated (extrapulmonary) coccidioidomycosis. However, IV amphotericin B is recommended as an alternative and is preferred for initial treatment of severely ill patients who have hypoxia or rapidly progressing disease, for immunocompromised individuals, or when azole antifungals have been ineffective or cannot be used (e.g., pregnant women).

For the treatment of clinically mild coccidioidomycosis (e.g., focal pneumonia) in HIV-infected adults and adolescents, CDC, NIH, and IDSA recommend initial therapy with oral fluconazole or oral itraconazole. These experts state that, although clinical data are limited, oral voriconazole or posaconazole oral suspension may be used as an alternative for the treatment of clinically mild coccidioidomycosis† that has not responded to fluconazole or itraconazole.

HIV-infected individuals who have been adequately treated for coccidioidomycosis should receive long-term (usually life-long) secondary prophylaxis to prevent recurrence or relapse. Although oral fluconazole or oral itraconazole are the drugs of choice recommended by CDC, NIH, and IDSA for secondary prophylaxis to prevent recurrence or relapse of coccidioidomycosis in HIV-infected adults and adolescents, these experts state that oral voriconazole or posaconazole oral suspension can be used as an alternative for secondary prophylaxis of coccidioidomycosis† in patients who did not initially respond to fluconazole or itraconazole treatment.

For additional information on prophylaxis and treatment of coccidioidomycosis, the current clinical practice guidelines from IDSA available at http://www.idsociety.org and current clinical practice guidelines from CDC, NIH, and IDSA on the prevention and treatment of opportunistic infections in HIV-infected individuals available at http://www.aidsinfo.nih.gov should be consulted.

■ **Fusarium Infections** Although safety and efficacy have not been established, posaconazole has been effective in some patients for the treatment of infections caused by *Fusarium*†, including salvage therapy when other antifungals were ineffective or could not be used.

Amphotericin B and/or voriconazole has been recommended for the treatment of *Fusarium* infections in immunocompromised individuals; amphotericin B may be preferred for infections caused by *F. solani* or *F. verticillioides*. Some clinicians suggest that posaconazole may be an alternative for treatment of fusariosis in patients who fail to respond to or cannot tolerate other antifungals.

In an open-label, retrospective analysis of 21 patients with invasive fusariosis who received salvage therapy with posaconazole oral suspension, the overall response rate (complete or partial) was 48%; the response rate was 57–75% in those with localized infections (e.g., pulmonary infections), but was only 29–33% in those with disseminated infections (with or without pulmonary involvement). Most patients (95%) had received initial therapy with IV amphotericin B given for a median duration of 8 days (range: 2–38 days) and 81% met a criteria for refractory infection with or without intolerance to standard antifungal therapy.

■ **Histoplasmosis** Although safety and efficacy have not been established, posaconazole has been used in some patients for the treatment of histoplasmosis† caused by *Histoplasma capsulatum*, including salvage therapy, and is recommended as an alternative for the treatment of these infections.

The drugs of choice for the treatment of histoplasmosis are IV amphotericin B or oral itraconazole. IV amphotericin B is preferred for initial treatment of severe, life-threatening histoplasmosis, especially in immunocompromised patients such as those with HIV infection. Oral itraconazole generally is used for initial treatment of less severe disease (e.g., mild to moderate acute pulmonary histoplasmosis, chronic cavitary pulmonary histoplasmosis) and as follow-up therapy in the treatment of severe infections after a response has been obtained with IV amphotericin B. Other azole antifungals (fluconazole, ketoconazole, posaconazole, voriconazole) are considered second-line alternatives to itraconazole.

For the treatment of less severe disseminated histoplasmosis† in HIV-infected adults and adolescents, CDC, NIH, and IDSA recommend initial treatment with oral itraconazole. These experts state that, although clinical data are limited, oral voriconazole, oral posaconazole, or oral fluconazole may be used as an alternative for the treatment of less severe disseminated histoplasmosis in patients intolerant of itraconazole who are only moderately ill.

HIV-infected individuals who have been adequately treated for histoplasmosis should receive long-term suppressive or maintenance therapy (secondary prophylaxis) to prevent recurrence or relapse if they had severe disseminated or CNS infections or had to be retreated for a relapse after appropriate initial treatment. Oral itraconazole is the drug of choice for secondary prophylaxis of histoplasmosis in HIV-infected adults and adolescents. The role of posaconazole for secondary prophylaxis of histoplasmosis in HIV-infected patients has not been evaluated to date.

For additional information on prophylaxis and treatment of histoplasmosis, the current clinical practice guidelines from IDSA available at http://www.idsociety.org and current clinical practice guidelines from CDC, NIH, and IDSA on the prevention and treatment of opportunistic infections in HIV-infected individuals available at http://www.aidsinfo.nih.gov should be consulted.

■ **Mucormycosis** Although safety and efficacy have not been established, posaconazole has been effective in some patients when used as salvage therapy for the treatment of mucormycosis†, including infections caused by *Mucor* or *Rhizopus*, when other antifungals were ineffective or could not be used.

In a retrospective analysis of 91 patients with proven or probable zygomycosis who received salvage therapy with posaconazole, the overall response rate (complete or partial) was 60%. In another open-label analysis of 24 patients with zygomycosis, the overall response rate to posaconazole therapy was 79% (11 patients had a complete response, 8 patients had a partial response, 5 patients failed to respond).

IV amphotericin B usually is recommended as the drug of first choice for the treatment of mucormycosis (with or without surgical intervention). Some clinicians suggest that posaconazole is a possible alternative for the treatment of mucormycosis (e.g., when IV amphotericin B is ineffective or cannot be used) and may be useful for oral follow-up therapy in patients who have an initial response to IV amphotericin B and can tolerate an oral regimen.

Dosage and Administration

■ **Administration** Posaconazole is administered orally or by slow IV infusion.

Oral Administration Posaconazole is administered orally as an oral suspension or delayed-release tablets.

Posaconazole oral suspension and delayed-release tablets are not interchangeable because they require different dosages and frequencies of administration. The oral suspension and delayed-release tablets cannot be substituted for each other without a change in dosage. (See Dispensing and Dosage and Administration Precautions under Administration: Oral Administration, in Dosage and Administration.)

Posaconazole delayed-release tablets are labeled by FDA *only* for prophylaxis of invasive *Aspergillus* and *Candida* infections. Because the delayed-release tablets generally provide higher posaconazole exposures than the oral suspension under both fed and fasting conditions, the manufacturer states that the delayed-release tablets are the preferred preparation when oral posaconazole is used for such prophylaxis.

Patients with severe diarrhea or vomiting receiving posaconazole oral suspension or delayed-release tablets should be monitored closely for breakthrough fungal infections since plasma concentrations of the drug may be affected.

Dispensing and Dosage and Administration Precautions. FDA alerted healthcare professionals about the risk of medication errors with oral preparations of posaconazole. Because of differences in oral bioavailability, posaconazole oral suspension and posaconazole delayed-release tablets *cannot* be substituted for each other without a change in dosage and frequency of administration. There have been reports of errors occurring when the wrong oral preparation was prescribed and/or dispensed to patients without consideration for the different dosage and frequency of administration required for the other preparation. At least 1 fatality occurred in a patient who received incorrect dosage (underdosage) of posaconazole as the result of being provided with posaconazole oral suspension (instead of posaconazole delayed-release tablets) without consideration for the dosage and frequency of administration required for the oral suspension. In other cases, clinicians switched patients from posaconazole oral suspension to the delayed-release tablets and the delayed-release tablets were prescribed and/or dispensed without adjusting the dosage to that required for the delayed-release tablets. Adverse effects (e.g., nausea, vomiting, low serum potassium concentrations) were reported in some of these patients, possibly as the result of the incorrect dosage and higher posaconazole exposures.

To avoid medication errors, healthcare professionals should be aware that dosage recommendations for posaconazole oral suspension and posaconazole delayed-release tablets are *not* the same and that dosage recommendations for the specific oral preparation must be followed. (See Dosage and Administration: Dosage.) Prescribers should write posaconazole prescriptions that specify the dosage form, strength, and frequency of administration and pharmacists should request clarification from prescribers when the dosage form, strength, or frequency is not specified. In addition, patients should talk to their healthcare provider before they switch from one oral preparation to the other.

Oral Suspension. Posaconazole oral suspension should be administered during or immediately (i.e., within 20 minutes) following a full meal to enhance oral absorption and optimize plasma concentrations of the drug. Alternatively, if the patient cannot eat a full meal and if posaconazole delayed-release tablets and IV posaconazole are not options, each dose of posaconazole oral suspension should be administered with a liquid nutritional supplement or an acidic carbonated beverage (e.g., ginger ale).

If oral posaconazole is indicated for prophylaxis of invasive *Aspergillus* and *Candida* infections and the patient cannot eat a full meal, posaconazole delayed-release tablets should be used.

If the patient cannot eat a full meal and cannot tolerate an oral nutritional supplement or acidic carbonated beverage (e.g., ginger ale) and if posaconazole delayed-release tablets and IV posaconazole are not options, alternative antifungal therapy should be considered or the patient should be monitored closely for breakthrough fungal infections.

Posaconazole oral suspension should be shaken well prior to each dose. The oral suspension contains 40 mg of posaconazole per mL. Posaconazole oral suspension should be administered using the calibrated measuring spoon provided by the manufacturer that is designed to measure 2.5- and 5-mL doses. The calibrated spoon should be rinsed with water after each dose and before storage.

Although posaconazole oral suspension has been administered via nasogastric tube† with a liquid nutritional supplement, patients receiving the drug via a nasogastric tube should be monitored closely for breakthrough fungal infections since this route is associated with lower posaconazole concentrations than the oral route and may be associated with an increased risk of treatment failure.

Delayed-release Tablets. Posaconazole delayed-release tablets must be swallowed whole and should not be divided, crushed, or chewed.

The delayed-release tablets should be administered with food to enhance oral absorption and optimize posaconazole plasma concentrations.

Posaconazole delayed-release tablets are labeled by FDA *only* for prophylaxis of invasive *Aspergillus* and *Candida* infections in adults and adolescents 13 years of age or older.

IV Infusion IV posaconazole is administered by slow IV infusion; the drug should *not* be administered by rapid IV infusion or injection.

Posaconazole injection concentrate *must* be diluted in a compatible diluent prior to IV infusion.

Diluted posaconazole IV solutions *must* be administered through a 0.22-µm polyethersulfone (PES) or polyvinylidene difluoride (PVDF) filter.

Diluted posaconazole IV solutions should be administered by slow IV infusion into a central venous line (e.g., central venous catheter or peripherally inserted central catheter [PICC]). If a central venous line is not available (i.e., prior to placement of a central venous line, to bridge the period during which a central venous line is replaced, when the central venous line is in use for other treatment), a *single* dose of diluted posaconazole IV solution may be administered through a peripheral venous catheter.

Dilution. A single-dose vial of posaconazole injection concentrate containing 300 mg of the drug should be removed from the refrigerator and allowed to reach room temperature. Using proper aseptic technique, the contents of the 300-mg vial (16.7 mL) should be transferred to an IV bag or bottle containing a compatible diluent (i.e., 0.45 or 0.9% sodium chloride, 5% dextrose, 5% dextrose and 0.45 or 0.9% sodium chloride, potassium chloride 20 mEq in 5% dextrose). The resultant IV solution should contain a final posaconazole concentration of 1–2 mg/mL. Posaconazole should *not* be diluted using any other diluents since particulate formation may occur.

Posaconazole IV solutions should be used immediately after dilution; however, if not used immediately, diluted IV solutions may be refrigerated at 2–8° C for up to 24 hours.

Posaconazole IV solutions should be visually inspected for particulate matter prior to administration whenever solution and container permit. The IV solution should appear colorless to yellow; variations of color within this range do not affect the quality of the drug.

Any unused portion of the diluted IV solution should be discarded.

Rate of Administration. IV infusions of posaconazole should be given over 90 minutes into a central venous line (e.g., central venous catheter or PICC).

If a peripheral venous catheter must be used because a central venous catheter is not available (i.e., prior to placement of a central venous line, to bridge the period during which a central venous line is being replaced, when the central venous line is in use for other treatment), a *single* posaconazole dose may be given by slow IV infusion over 30 minutes through a peripheral venous catheter.

■ **Dosage** Posaconazole oral suspension and delayed-release tablets are *not* interchangeable and cannot be substituted for each other without a change in dosage and frequency of administration. (See Dispensing and Dosage and Administration Precautions under Administration: Oral Administration, in Dosage and Administration.)

Dosage recommendations for the specific posaconazole preparation must be followed.

Prevention of Invasive Aspergillus and Candida Infections in Immunocompromised Individuals The recommended dosage of posaconazole oral suspension for prevention of invasive *Aspergillus* or *Candida* infections in adults and children 13 years of age or older is 200 mg (5 mL of oral suspension containing 40 mg/mL) 3 times daily.

The recommended dosage of posaconazole delayed-release tablets for prevention of invasive *Aspergillus* or *Candida* infections in adults and children 13 years of age or older is 300 mg (three 100-mg delayed-release tablets) twice daily on day 1 (loading dosage), followed by 300 mg (three 100-mg delayed-release tablets) once daily thereafter (maintenance dosage).

If IV posaconazole is used for prevention of invasive *Aspergillus* or *Candida* infections in adults 18 years of age or older, the recommended dosage is 300 mg IV twice daily on day 1 (loading dosage), followed by 300 mg IV once daily thereafter (maintenance dosage).

The duration of antifungal prophylaxis is based on the patient's recovery from immunosuppression or neutropenia. Posaconazole prophylaxis has been continued for up to 12–16 weeks in clinical studies.

Candida Infections **Treatment of Oropharyngeal Candidiasis.** The recommended dosage of posaconazole oral suspension for the treatment of oropharyngeal candidiasis in adults is 100 mg (2.5 mL of oral suspension containing 40 mg/mL) twice daily on day 1 (loading dosage), followed by 100 mg (2.5 mL of oral suspension containing 40 mg/mL) once daily for 13 days (maintenance dosage).

If posaconazole oral suspension is used for the treatment of oropharyngeal candidiasis refractory to fluconazole and/or itraconazole, the manufacturer recommends that adults receive 400 mg (10 mL of oral suspension containing 40 mg/mL) twice daily and states that the duration of treatment should be based on clinical response and the severity of underlying disease. For the treatment of fluconazole-refractory oropharyngeal candidiasis, the Infectious Diseases Society of America (IDSA) recommends that posaconazole oral suspension be given in a dosage of 400 mg twice daily for 3 days, followed by 400 mg once daily for up to 28 days.

If posaconazole oral suspension is used as an alternative for the treatment of oropharyngeal candidiasis in adults and adolescents with human immunodeficiency virus (HIV) infection, the US Centers for Disease Control and Prevention (CDC), National Institutes of Health (NIH), and IDSA recommend a dosage of 400 mg twice daily on day 1, followed by 400 mg once daily for 7–14 days. For the treatment of fluconazole-refractory oropharyngeal candidiasis in HIV-infected adults and adolescents, these experts state that posaconazole oral suspension given in a dosage of 400 mg twice daily for 28 days has been effective in some patients. CDC, NIH, IDSA, and the American Academy of Pediatrics (AAP) state that data are insufficient to recommend use of posaconazole for the treatment of oropharyngeal candidiasis in HIV-infected children.

Treatment of Esophageal Candidiasis. If posaconazole oral suspension is used for the treatment of fluconazole-refractory esophageal candidiasis†, IDSA recommends a dosage of 400 mg twice daily. Alternatively, if posaconazole delayed-release tablets are used for the treatment of fluconazole-refractory esophageal candidiasis†, IDSA recommends a dosage of 300 mg once daily.

For the treatment of fluconazole-refractory esophageal candidiasis† in HIV-infected adults and adolescents, CDC, NIH, and IDSA state that posaconazole oral suspension given in a dosage of 400 mg twice daily for 28 days has been effective in some patients. CDC, NIH, IDSA, and AAP state that data are insufficient to recommend use of posaconazole for the treatment of esophageal candidiasis in HIV-infected children.

Prevention of Recurrence (Secondary Prophylaxis) of Esophageal Candidiasis. If long-term suppressive or maintenance therapy (secondary prophylaxis)† with oral posaconazole is used in HIV-infected adults and adolescents with frequent or severe recurrences of esophageal candidiasis, CDC, NIH, and IDSA recommend that posaconazole oral suspension be given in a dosage of 400 mg twice daily.

Although only limited data are available regarding the safety of discontinuing secondary prophylaxis against esophageal candidiasis in HIV-infected individuals, consideration can be given to discontinuing such prophylaxis when $CD4^+$ T-cell counts increase to greater than 200/mm^3 in response to antiretroviral therapy.

Aspergillosis If posaconazole oral suspension is used in adults for salvage therapy for the treatment of invasive aspergillosis† when other antifungals are ineffective or cannot be used, IDSA recommends an initial dosage of 200 mg 4 times daily until the disease stabilizes, followed by 400 mg twice daily thereafter. For salvage therapy in a clinical trial, posaconazole oral suspension has been given in a dosage of 400 mg twice daily or 200 mg 4 times daily for up to approximately 12 months.

If posaconazole oral suspension is used as an alternative for the treatment of invasive aspergillosis† in HIV-infected adults and adolescents, CDC, NIH, and IDSA recommend a dosage of 200 mg 4 times daily; after improvement occurs, dosage can be changed to 400 mg twice daily. The optimal duration of therapy in these patients has not been established, but antifungal therapy should be continued at least until the $CD4^+$ T-cell count increases to greater than 200/mm^3 as a result of potent antiretroviral therapy and there is evidence that the infection has resolved.

Coccidioidomycosis If posaconazole oral suspension is used as an alternative for the treatment of clinically mild coccidioidomycosis† (e.g., focal pneumonia) in HIV-infected adults and adolescents, a dosage of 200–400 mg twice daily is recommended by CDC, NIH, and IDSA.

If posaconazole oral suspension is used as an alternative for long-term suppressive or maintenance therapy (secondary prophylaxis)† to prevent relapse or recurrence of coccidioidomycosis in HIV-infected adults and adolescents who have completed initial treatment of the disease, a dosage of 200 mg twice daily is recommended by CDC, NIH, and IDSA. In HIV-infected patients who were treated for focal coccidioidal pneumonia and are receiving effective antiretroviral therapy, consideration can be given to discontinuing secondary prophylaxis against coccidioidomycosis after 12 months if $CD4^+$ T-cell counts are 250/mm^3 or higher, provided the patient is monitored for recurrence (e.g., serial chest radiographs, coccidioidal serology). HIV-infected patients who were treated for diffuse pulmonary, disseminated, or meningeal coccidioidomycosis usually require life-long secondary prophylaxis.

Fusarium Infections For salvage therapy in adults for the treatment of infections caused by *Fusarium*† when other antifungals were ineffective or could not be used, posaconazole oral suspension has been given in a dosage of 400 mg twice daily or 200 mg 4 times daily for up to 12 months or longer.

Histoplasmosis If posaconazole oral suspension is used as an alternative for the treatment of less severe disseminated histoplasmosis† in HIV-infected adults and adolescents who are only moderately ill, CDC, NIH, and IDSA recommend a dosage of 400 mg twice daily.

Mucormycosis For salvage therapy in adults for the treatment of mucormycosis† when other antifungals were ineffective or could not be used, posaconazole oral suspension has been given in a dosage of 400 mg twice daily or 200 mg 4 times daily.

In the treatment of mucormycosis† after a response has been obtained with an initial regimen of IV amphotericin B, some clinicians suggest that posaconazole oral suspension can be given for follow-up therapy in a dosage of 200 mg 3 or 4 times daily.

■ **Special Populations** ***Hepatic Impairment*** Dosage adjustments are not necessary if posaconazole oral suspension is used in patients with hepatic impairment (Child-Pugh class A, B, or C). However, discontinuance of the drug must be considered if clinical signs and symptoms consistent with liver disease develop that may be attributable to posaconazole. (See Hepatic Effects under Cautions: Warnings/Precautions.)

Dosage adjustments are not necessary if posaconazole delayed-release tablets or IV posaconazole is used in patients with hepatic impairment. However, specific studies have not been conducted to evaluate these posaconazole preparations in patients with hepatic impairment.

Renal Impairment Dosage adjustments are not necessary if posaconazole oral suspension or posaconazole delayed-release tablets are used in patients with mild, moderate, or severe renal impairment. However, because the area under the plasma concentration-time curve (AUC) is highly variable in patients with severe renal impairment receiving posaconazole oral suspension or delayed-release tablets, such patients should be monitored closely for breakthrough fungal infections. (See Renal Impairment under Warnings/Precautions: Specific Populations, in Cautions.)

IV posaconazole should be avoided in patients with moderate or severe renal impairment (estimated glomerular filtration rate [eGFR] less than 50 mL/minute) unless benefits of the IV preparation outweigh risks in such patients. The IV vehicle (betadex sulfobutyl ether sodium [SBECD]) contained in the posaconazole IV preparation is expected to accumulate in patients with moderate or severe renal impairment. If IV posaconazole is used in such patients, serum creatinine concentrations should be closely monitored and consideration given to switching to oral posaconazole if serum creatinine concentrations increase. (See Renal Impairment under Warnings/Precautions: Specific Populations, in Cautions.)

Because posaconazole is not dialyzable, the drug may be administered without regard to the timing of hemodialysis.

Geriatric Patients Dosage adjustments are not necessary when oral or IV posaconazole is used in geriatric adults 65 years of age or older.

Obese Patients Because pharmacokinetic modeling suggests that patients weighing more than 120 kg may have lower posaconazole exposures, such patients should be closely monitored for breakthrough fungal infections.

Other Special Populations Dosage adjustments are not necessary based on gender or race.

Cautions

■ **Contraindications** Posaconazole is contraindicated in patients with known hypersensitivity to posaconazole or other azole antifungals.

Concomitant use with sirolimus is contraindicated. (See Drug Interactions: Immunosuppressive Agents.)

Concomitant use with ergot alkaloids (e.g., ergotamine, dihydroergotamine) is contraindicated. (See Drug Interactions: Ergot Alkaloids.)

Concomitant use with drugs that are substrates for cytochrome P-450 (CYP) 3A4 and for which elevated plasma concentrations may be associated with prolonged QT interval corrected for rate (QT_c) and rare occurrences of torsades de pointes (e.g., pimozide, quinidine) is contraindicated. (See Drug Interactions: Drugs that Prolong the QT Interval.)

Concomitant use with HMG-CoA reductase inhibitors (statins) principally metabolized by CYP3A4 (e.g., atorvastatin, lovastatin, simvastatin) is contraindicated. (See Drug Interactions: HMG-CoA Reductase Inhibitors.)

■ **Warnings/Precautions** ***Sensitivity Reactions*** Allergic and/or hypersensitivity reactions, including rash and pruritus, have been reported in patients receiving posaconazole.

Data regarding cross-sensitivity among azole antifungals (e.g., fluconazole, isavuconazole [active metabolite of isavuconazonium], itraconazole, posaconazole, voriconazole) are not available. Posaconazole is contraindicated in patients hypersensitive to other azole antifungals.

Cardiovascular Effects Similar to some other azole antifungals (e.g., fluconazole, voriconazole), posaconazole has been associated with prolongation of the QT interval. Torsades de pointes has been reported during posaconazole therapy in some patients; one case occurred in a patient who was seriously ill and had multiple confounding risk factors (e.g., prior cardiotoxic chemotherapy, hypokalemia, concomitant drugs) that may have been contributory.

In a multiple time-matched ECG analysis in 173 healthy adults 18–85 years of age, administration of posaconazole oral suspension (400 mg twice daily with a high-fat meal) did not increase mean QT_c intervals. Multiple, time-matched ECGs were collected over a 12-hour period at baseline and at steady state. In a pooled analysis, the mean QT_c interval change from baseline was −5 msec following administration of the recommended posaconazole dose. Decreased QT_c interval (−3 msec) also was observed in a small number of individuals receiving placebo. The placebo-adjusted mean maximum QT_c interval change from baseline was −8 msec. No healthy individuals receiving posaconazole had a QT_c interval of 500 msec or higher or had an increase of 60 msec or more in their QT_c interval from baseline.

Posaconazole should be used with caution in patients with potentially proarrhythmic conditions and should not be used concomitantly with drugs that are metabolized by CYP3A4 and known to prolong the QT_c interval. (See Drug Interactions: Drugs that Prolong the QT Interval.)

Rigorous attempts should be made to correct electrolyte imbalances (i.e., potassium, magnesium, calcium) before initiating posaconazole therapy.

Hepatic Effects Serious hepatic effects, including cholestasis or hepatic failure (sometimes fatal), have been reported rarely during posaconazole therapy in patients with serious underlying medical conditions (e.g., hematologic malignancy). These severe hepatic effects generally have occurred in patients receiving posaconazole oral suspension in a dosage of 800 mg daily (400 mg twice daily or 200 mg 4 times daily) in clinical trials.

Less severe hepatic effects, including mild to moderate elevations in ALT, AST, alkaline phosphatase, total bilirubin, and/or clinical hepatitis, have been reported infrequently in clinical trials. Liver function test elevations generally were reversible following discontinuance of posaconazole and did not appear to be associated with increased plasma posaconazole concentrations; in some cases, test results returned to normal levels without interrupting posaconazole therapy and only rarely required discontinuance of the drug.

Liver function should be monitored (liver function tests, bilirubin) prior to and during posaconazole therapy. If abnormal liver function test results occur during posaconazole therapy, the patient should be monitored for the development of more severe hepatic injury using appropriate laboratory tests. Discontinuance of posaconazole must be considered if signs and symptoms consistent with liver disease develop that may be attributable to the drug.

Interactions Concomitant use of posaconazole and certain drugs may result in serious and/or life-threatening adverse effects as the result of higher exposures of the concomitant drug. Concomitant use of posaconazole and some drugs is contraindicated (e.g., sirolimus, drugs that are CYP3A4 substrates and are known to prolong the QT interval, HMG-CoA reductase inhibitors metabolized by CYP3A4, ergot alkaloids) or requires particular caution (e.g., cyclosporine, tacrolimus, midazolam). (See Cautions: Contraindications and see Drug Interactions.)

Specific Populations **Pregnancy.** There are no adequate and well-controlled studies in pregnant women. Posaconazole should be used during pregnancy only when potential benefits outweigh possible risks to the fetus.

The Infectious Diseases Society of America (IDSA) states that use of posaconazole should be avoided during pregnancy, especially during the first trimester.

Posaconazole has been shown to cause skeletal malformations (cranial malformations and missing ribs) when given to rats at dosages at least 1.4 times greater than a human dosage of the oral suspension of 400 mg twice daily (based on steady-state plasma concentrations). No malformations were seen in rabbits given a posaconazole dosage of 80 mg/kg (exposure levels 5.2 times higher than human exposures achieved with a dosage of the oral suspension of 400 mg twice daily); however, this dosage was associated with an increase in resorptions, reduction in body weight gain of females, and reduction in litter size.

Lactation. Posaconazole is distributed into milk in rats; it is not known whether the drug is distributed into milk in humans.

Because of the potential for serious adverse reactions in nursing infants, a decision should be made whether to discontinue nursing or posaconazole, taking into account the importance of the drug to the woman.

Pediatric Use. Safety and efficacy of posaconazole oral suspension and delayed-release tablets have not been established in children younger than 13 years of age.

Safety and efficacy of IV posaconazole have not been established in patients younger than 18 years of age.

The manufacturer states that use of posaconazole oral suspension or delayed-release tablets in pediatric patients 13–17 years of age is supported by evidence from adequate and well-controlled studies in adults.

Data from a limited number of pediatric patients 13–17 years of age who received posaconazole oral suspension (200 mg 3 times daily) for prophylaxis of invasive fungal infections indicate that the safety profile and mean steady-state plasma posaconazole concentrations in this age group are similar to those reported in adults 18 years of age or older.

Comparison of pharmacokinetic data from a limited number of pediatric patients 8–17 years of age who received posaconazole oral suspension (400 mg 2 times or 200 mg 4 times daily) for the treatment of invasive fungal infections† with pharmacokinetic data from adults 18 years of age or older indicates that mean steady-state plasma posaconazole concentrations in pediatric patients and adults are similar.

Posaconazole oral suspension has been used in a limited number of children 7 years of age† or older without unusual adverse effects.

The US Centers for Disease Control and Prevention (CDC), National Institutes of Health (NIH), IDSA, and American Academy of Pediatrics (AAP) state that data are insufficient to date to make recommendations regarding use of posaconazole in HIV-infected infants and children.

Geriatric Use. Although no overall differences in safety and pharmacokinetics were observed between geriatric and younger adults in clinical studies evaluating posaconazole oral suspension, posaconazole delayed-release tablets, or IV posaconazole, the possibility that some older patients may exhibit increased sensitivity to the drug cannot be ruled out.

Hepatic Impairment. Patients who develop evidence of hepatic impairment during posaconazole therapy (i.e., abnormal liver function test results) should be carefully monitored for the development of more severe hepatic injury. (See Hepatic Effects under Cautions: Warnings/Precautions.)

Although there are some differences in posaconazole pharmacokinetics in individuals with hepatic impairment compared with those with normal hepatic function, the manufacturer states that dosage adjustments are not considered necessary in patients with mild, moderate, or severe hepatic impairment. (See Hepatic Impairment under Dosage and Administration: Special Populations.)

Renal Impairment. Patients with severe renal impairment receiving posaconazole oral suspension or delayed-release tablets should be closely monitored for breakthrough fungal infections since the area under the plasma concentration-time curve (AUC) of posaconazole is highly variable in these patients.

IV posaconazole should not be used in patients with moderate or severe renal impairment (estimated glomerular filtration rate [eGFR] less than 50 mL/minute) unless potential benefits of the IV route justify the risks in such patients. Accumulation of the IV vehicle (SBECD) contained in the posaconazole IV preparation is expected in patients with moderate or severe renal impairment. If IV posaconazole is used in such patients, serum creatinine concentrations should be closely monitored. If serum creatinine concentrations increase, consideration should be given to switching to oral posaconazole.

■ **Common Adverse Effects** Adverse effects reported in 5% or more of patients receiving posaconazole include GI effects (nausea, vomiting, diarrhea, abdominal pain, anorexia, constipation, dry mouth, dyspepsia, flatulence, decreased appetite), fever, headache, increased sweating, rigors, chills, mucosal inflammation, dizziness, fatigue, edema (legs), asthenia, weakness, decreased weight, dehydration, hypertension, and hypotension. Vaginal hemorrhage, tachycardia, bacteremia, pneumonia, herpes simplex infection, cytomegalovirus infection, oral candidiasis, pharyngitis, musculoskeletal pain, arthralgia, back pain, petechiae, insomnia, coughing, dyspnea, epistaxis, rash, and pruritus also were reported in 5% or more of patients. Anemia, neutropenia, thrombocytopenia, hypocalcemia, hypokalemia, hypomagnesemia, hyperglycemia, increased AST, increased ALT, increased γ-glutamyltransferase (GGT, γ-glutamyl transpeptidase, GGPT), increased alkaline phosphatase, and bilirubinemia were reported in 2% or more of patients. Serious adverse effects, including fever and neutropenia, were reported more frequently when the drug was used in patients with refractory oropharyngeal candidiasis (especially in those severely immunocompromised by advanced HIV infection) than when used for prophylaxis.

Drug Interactions

■ **Drugs Metabolized by Hepatic Microsomal Enzymes** Posaconazole inhibits the metabolic activity of cytochrome P-450 (CYP) isoenzyme 3A4 (CYP3A4) and may increase plasma concentrations of other drugs metabolized by this hepatic enzyme.

Posaconazole does not appear to inhibit CYP isoenzymes 1A2, 2C8/9, 2D6, or 2E1.

■ **Drugs that Prolong the QT Interval** Potential pharmacokinetic interactions with drugs that are CYP3A4 substrates and prolong the QT interval corrected for rate (QT_c) (e.g., pimozide, quinidine). Potential increased plasma concentrations of the concomitantly used CYP3A4 substrate, which can result in QT interval prolongation and, rarely, torsades de pointes. Concomitant use of posaconazole and these drugs that prolong the QT_c interval is contraindicated.

■ **Drugs Affecting P-glycoprotein Transport** Because posaconazole is a substrate of P-glycoprotein (P-gp), inhibitors or inducers of the P-gp transport system may increase or decrease plasma posaconazole concentrations, respectively.

■ **Drugs Affecting Uridine Diphosphate-glucuronosyltransferase** Because posaconazole is principally metabolized via uridine diphosphate (UDP)-glucuronosyltransferase glucuronidation (UGT; phase 2 enzymes), inhibitors or inducers of UGT may increase or decrease posaconazole plasma concentrations, respectively.

■ **Antifungal Agents** ***Amphotericin B*** Although the clinical importance is unclear, the antifungal effects of posaconazole and amphotericin B usually have been synergistic in vitro against *Aspergillus* hyphae, but indifferent against *Aspergillus* conidia.

In vitro, the antifungal effects of posaconazole and amphotericin B were indifferent against *Rhizopus oryzae*; there was no evidence of synergism or antagonism.

■ **Antimycobacterial Agents** ***Rifabutin*** Concomitant use of rifabutin (300 mg once daily for 17 days) and posaconazole (200 mg once daily for 10 days) results in decreased peak plasma concentration and area under the plasma concentration-time curve (AUC) of posaconazole and increased peak plasma concentration and AUC of rifabutin; possible increased risk of rifabutin-associated adverse effects.

Concomitant use of rifabutin and posaconazole should be avoided unless benefits outweigh risks. If concomitant use is considered necessary, the patient should be closely monitored for breakthrough fungal infections. In addition, the patient should be monitored for adverse effects associated with increased rifabutin concentrations (e.g., uveitis, leukopenia) and complete blood counts should be assessed frequently.

■ **Antiretroviral Agents** ***HIV Integrase Inhibitors*** **Elvitegravir.** Possible pharmacokinetic interactions if posaconazole is used concomitantly with elvitegravir and a *ritonavir-boosted* HIV protease inhibitor (increased elvitegravir concentrations).

Possible pharmacokinetic interaction if posaconazole is used concomitantly with the fixed combination of elvitegravir, cobicistat, emtricitabine, and tenofovir disoproxil fumarate (EVG/c/FTC/TDF) (increased posaconazole, elvitegravir, and cobicistat concentrations). If posaconazole is used concomitantly with EVG/c/FTC/TDF, some experts state that posaconazole concentrations should be monitored.

HIV Nonnucleoside Reverse Transcriptase Inhibitors (NNRTIs) **Efavirenz.** Pharmacokinetic interaction (decreased posaconazole peak plasma concentrations and AUC) with efavirenz.

Concomitant use of efavirenz and posaconazole should be avoided unless benefits outweigh risks; if concomitant use is necessary, posaconazole plasma concentrations should be monitored and dosage adjusted accordingly.

Etravirine. Possible pharmacokinetic interaction if posaconazole is used concomitantly with etravirine (increased etravirine plasma concentrations, no change in posaconazole concentrations).

Some experts state that dosage adjustments are not needed when etravirine is used concomitantly with posaconazole; the manufacturer of etravirine states that dosage adjustment of posaconazole may be needed depending on other concomitantly administered drugs.

Rilpivirine. Possible pharmacokinetic interaction if posaconazole is used concomitantly with rilpivirine (increased rilpivirine concentrations).

Some experts state that dosage adjustments are not needed if rilpivirine is used concomitantly with posaconazole; however, because rilpivirine reduces ketoconazole exposure and effects of rilpivirine on posaconazole exposure have not been established, the patient should be monitored for breakthrough fungal infections.

HIV Nucleoside Reverse Transcriptase Inhibitors (NRTIs)

Lamivudine. No clinically important pharmacokinetic interactions when posaconazole is used concomitantly with lamivudine; dosage adjustments are not needed if lamivudine is used with posaconazole 200 mg daily.

Zidovudine. No clinically important pharmacokinetic interactions when posaconazole is used concomitantly with zidovudine; dosage adjustments are not needed if zidovudine is used with posaconazole 200 mg daily.

HIV Protease Inhibitors (PIs) **Atazanavir.** Pharmacokinetic interactions if posaconazole is used concomitantly with *ritonavir-boosted* or unboosted atazanavir (increased plasma concentrations and AUC of atazanavir); possible pharmacokinetic interactions if used concomitantly with *cobicistat-boosted* atazanavir (increased atazanavir concentrations).

If posaconazole is used concomitantly with *ritonavir-boosted*, *cobicistat-boosted*, or unboosted atazanavir, the patient should be frequently monitored for atazanavir-associated adverse effects and toxicity.

Darunavir. Possible pharmacokinetic interactions if posaconazole is used concomitantly with *ritonavir-boosted* or *cobicistat-boosted* darunavir (increased posaconazole, darunavir, and ritonavir or cobicistat concentrations).

If posaconazole and *ritonavir-boosted* or *cobicistat-boosted* darunavir are used concomitantly, patients should be monitored for increased posaconazole-, darunavir-, and ritonavir- or cobicistat-associated adverse effects and posaconazole plasma concentration monitoring should be considered.

Fosamprenavir. Pharmacokinetic interactions when posaconazole is used concomitantly with fosamprenavir (decreased posaconazole concentrations). Possible pharmacokinetic interactions if used concomitantly with *ritonavir-boosted* fosamprenavir (increased amprenavir [active metabolite of fosamprenavir] and posaconazole concentrations).

If posaconazole is used concomitantly with unboosted fosamprenavir, the patient should be closely monitored for breakthrough fungal infections; some experts state that posaconazole concentrations should be monitored.

If posaconazole is used concomitantly with *ritonavir-boosted* fosamprenavir, some experts state that posaconazole concentration monitoring should be considered and the patient should be monitored for amprenavir adverse effects.

Indinavir. No clinically important pharmacokinetic interactions when posaconazole is used concomitantly with indinavir; dosage adjustments are not needed if indinavir is used with posaconazole 200 mg daily.

Lopinavir. Possible pharmacokinetic interaction if posaconazole is used concomitantly with the fixed combination of lopinavir and ritonavir (lopinavir/ritonavir) (increased lopinavir and posaconazole concentrations). If posaconazole is used concomitantly with lopinavir/ritonavir, some experts state that posaconazole concentration monitoring should be considered and the patient should be monitored for lopinavir adverse effects.

Ritonavir. Pharmacokinetic interaction (increased ritonavir peak plasma concentrations and AUC) when used with low-dose ritonavir (100 mg once daily).

If ritonavir is used concomitantly with posaconazole, the patient should be frequently monitored for ritonavir adverse effects and toxicity.

Saquinavir. Possible pharmacokinetic interaction if posaconazole is used concomitantly with *ritonavir-boosted* saquinavir (increased saquinavir and posaconazole concentrations). If posaconazole is used concomitantly with *ritonavir-boosted* saquinavir, some experts state that posaconazole concentration monitoring should be considered and the patient should be monitored for saquinavir adverse effects.

Tipranavir. Possible pharmacokinetic interaction if posaconazole is used concomitantly with *ritonavir-boosted* tipranavir (increased tipranavir and posaconazole concentrations). If posaconazole is used concomitantly with *ritonavir-boosted* tipranavir, some experts state that posaconazole concentration monitoring should be considered and the patient should be monitored for tipranavir adverse effects.

■ **Benzodiazepines** Pharmacokinetic interaction if posaconazole is used concomitantly with midazolam (substantially increased peak plasma concentrations, AUC, and mean terminal half-life of midazolam), which may potentiate and prolong hypnotic and sedative effects of midazolam. Potential pharmacokinetic interaction (increased benzodiazepine plasma concentrations) with other benzodiazepines that are metabolized by CYP3A4 isoenzyme (e.g., alprazolam, triazolam).

If posaconazole is used in patients receiving midazolam or other benzodiazepines metabolized by CYP3A4 (e.g., alprazolam, triazolam), the patient must be closely monitored for adverse effects associated with high benzodiazepine concentrations and a benzodiazepine receptor antagonist must be available to reverse possible adverse effects.

■ **Caffeine** No clinically important pharmacokinetic interactions when posaconazole is used concomitantly with caffeine; dosage adjustments are not needed if caffeine is used concomitantly with posaconazole 200 mg daily.

■ **Calcium-channel Blocking Agents** Potential pharmacokinetic interaction (increased plasma concentrations of the calcium-channel blocker) if posaconazole is used concomitantly with calcium-channel blocking agents that are metabolized by CYP3A4 (e.g., diltiazem, felodipine, nicardipine, nifedipine, verapamil).

If posaconazole is used concomitantly with calcium-channel blocking agents metabolized by CYP3A4, the patient should be frequently monitored for adverse effects and toxicity associated with calcium-channel blockers; reduction of the calcium-channel blocker dosage may be needed.

■ **Digoxin** Pharmacokinetic interaction if posaconazole is used concomitantly with digoxin (increased digoxin plasma concentrations).

If digoxin is used concomitantly with posaconazole, digoxin plasma concentrations should be monitored.

■ **Ergot Alkaloids** Potential pharmacokinetic interactions if posaconazole is used concomitantly with ergot alkaloids (increased plasma concentrations of ergot alkaloids resulting in ergotism).

Concomitant use of ergot alkaloids (e.g., ergotamine, dihydroergotamine) and posaconazole is contraindicated.

■ **GI Drugs** *Antacids* No clinically important pharmacokinetic interactions have been reported when antacids were used concomitantly with posaconazole oral suspension or delayed-release tablets.

Dosage adjustments are not needed if posaconazole oral suspension or delayed-release tablets are used concomitantly with antacids.

Antidiarrhea Agents **Loperamide.** No clinically important pharmacokinetic interactions have been reported when loperamide was used concomitantly with posaconazole oral suspension; dosage adjustments are not needed when loperamide and posaconazole are used concomitantly.

Histamine H_2-receptor Antagonists Concomitant use of cimetidine and posaconazole oral suspension results in decreased peak plasma concentrations and AUC of posaconazole. Concomitant use of cimetidine and posaconazole oral suspension should be avoided unless benefits outweigh risks; if concomitant use is necessary, the patient should be closely monitored for breakthrough fungal infections.

No clinically important pharmacokinetic interactions have been reported when posaconazole oral suspension or delayed-release tablets were used concomitantly with other histamine H_2-receptor antagonists (e.g., ranitidine); dosage adjustments are not needed if posaconazole oral suspension or delayed-release tablets are used concomitantly with these drugs.

Metoclopramide Concomitant use of metoclopramide and posaconazole oral suspension results in decreased posaconazole mean peak plasma concentrations and AUC. If metoclopramide is used concomitantly with posaconazole oral suspension, the patient should be closely monitored for breakthrough fungal infections.

No clinically important pharmacokinetic interactions occurred when metoclopramide was used concomitantly with posaconazole delayed-release tablets. Dosage adjustments are not needed if metoclopramide is used concomitantly with posaconazole delayed-release tablets.

Proton-pump Inhibitors **Esomeprazole.** Concomitant use of esomeprazole and posaconazole oral suspension results in decreased posaconazole mean peak plasma concentrations and AUC. Concomitant use of esomeprazole and posaconazole oral suspension should be avoided unless benefits outweigh risks; if esomeprazole is used concomitantly with posaconazole oral suspension, the patient should be monitored closely for breakthrough fungal infections.

No clinically important pharmacokinetic interactions occurred when esomeprazole and posaconazole delayed-release tablets were used concomitantly; dosage adjustments are not necessary if posaconazole delayed-release tablets are used concomitantly with proton-pump inhibitors.

Omeprazole. Concomitant use of omeprazole and posaconazole oral suspension results in decreased posaconazole trough concentrations. If omeprazole is used concomitantly with posaconazole oral suspension, plasma posaconazole concentrations should be monitored or consideration given to switching to an alternative antifungal.

■ **Glipizide** Concomitant use of posaconazole and glipizide does not result in clinically important pharmacokinetic interactions; however, decreased blood glucose concentrations have been reported in healthy adults following concomitant use of glipizide and posaconazole.

Dosage adjustments are not needed if posaconazole and glipizide are used concomitantly, but blood glucose concentrations should be monitored.

■ **HCV Antivirals** *HCV Replication Complex Inhibitors*

Daclatasvir. Possible pharmacokinetic interaction if posaconazole is used concomitantly with daclatasvir (increased daclatasvir concentrations).

If daclatasvir and posaconazole are used concomitantly, a daclatasvir dosage of 30 mg once daily should be used.

HCV Protease Inhibitors **Simeprevir.** Possible pharmacokinetic interaction if posaconazole is used concomitantly with simeprevir (substantially increased simeprevir concentrations).

Concomitant use of simeprevir and posaconazole is not recommended.

■ **HMG-CoA Reductase Inhibitors** Concomitant use of posaconazole oral suspension (100 or 200 mg once daily for 13 days) and simvastatin (single 40-mg dose) results in substantially increased simvastatin concentrations and AUC. Similar pharmacokinetic interactions are likely if posaconazole is used concomitantly with other HMG-CoA reductase inhibitors (statins) metabolized by CYP3A4.

Because increased plasma concentrations of HMG-CoA reductase inhibitors can lead to rhabdomyolysis, concomitant use of posaconazole and HMG-CoA reductase inhibitors metabolized by CYP3A4 (e.g., atorvastatin, lovastatin, simvastatin) is contraindicated.

■ **Immunosuppressive Agents** ***Cyclosporine*** Pharmacokinetic interaction if cyclosporine is used concomitantly with posaconazole (increased cyclosporine concentrations, no change in posaconazole concentrations); elevated cyclosporine concentrations have been associated with serious adverse effects (e.g., nephrotoxicity, leukoencephalopathy, death).

If posaconazole is initiated in a patient receiving cyclosporine, the cyclosporine dosage should be reduced by approximately 25%. Trough cyclosporine concentrations should be monitored frequently during and following discontinuance of posaconazole therapy and cyclosporine dosage should be adjusted as required.

Sirolimus Pharmacokinetic interaction if sirolimus and posaconazole are used concomitantly (substantially increased sirolimus peak concentrations and AUC); possible sirolimus toxicity.

Concomitant use of sirolimus and posaconazole is contraindicated.

Tacrolimus Pharmacokinetic interaction if tacrolimus and posaconazole are used concomitantly (increased tacrolimus peak concentrations and AUC).

If posaconazole is initiated in a patient receiving tacrolimus, the tacrolimus dosage should be reduced by approximately 66%. Trough tacrolimus concentrations should be monitored frequently during and following discontinuance of posaconazole therapy and tacrolimus dosage should be adjusted as required.

■ **Phenytoin** Concomitant use of phenytoin (200 mg once daily for 10 days) and posaconazole (200 mg once daily for 10 days) results in decreased peak plasma concentrations and AUC of posaconazole and increased peak plasma concentrations and AUC of phenytoin.

Concomitant use of phenytoin and posaconazole should be avoided unless benefits outweigh risks. If concomitant use is necessary, the patient should be closely monitored for breakthrough fungal infections. In addition, plasma phenytoin concentrations should be assessed frequently and reduced phenytoin dosage considered.

■ **Pimozide** Possible pharmacokinetic interaction and potential for serious or life-threatening reactions (e.g., prolonged QT interval, torsades de pointes) if pimozide and posaconazole are used concomitantly.

Concomitant use of pimozide and posaconazole is contraindicated.

■ **Quinidine** Possible pharmacokinetic interaction and potential for serious or life-threatening reactions (e.g., prolonged QT interval, torsades de pointes) if quinidine and posaconazole are used concomitantly.

Concomitant use of quinidine and posaconazole is contraindicated.

■ **Vinca Alkaloids** Potential pharmacokinetic interaction if vinca alkaloids (e.g., vincristine, vinblastine) are used concomitantly with posaconazole (increased plasma concentrations of vinca alkaloids); possible increased risk of neurotoxicity.

If vinca alkaloids and posaconazole are used concomitantly, the patient should be monitored for manifestations of vinca alkaloid toxicity (i.e., neurotoxicity) and adjustment of the vinca alkaloid dosage should be considered.

Pharmacokinetics

■ **Absorption** When posaconazole oral suspension is administered over a dosage range of 50 mg twice daily to 400 mg twice daily, posaconazole exhibits dose-proportional increases in the area under the plasma concentration-time curve (AUC). In febrile neutropenic patients or those with refractory invasive fungal infections, no further increases in posaconazole exposure occur if dosage is increased from 400 mg twice daily to 600 mg twice daily. Following administration of posaconazole oral suspension, the median time to peak plasma concentrations of posaconazole is approximately 3–8 hours. Steady-state posaconazole concentrations are achieved at 7–10 days in patients receiving the oral suspension.

Posaconazole delayed-release tablets contain posaconazole mixed with a pH-sensitive polymer (hypromellose acetate succinate) that enhances oral bioavailability of the drug. The pH-sensitive polymer contained in the tablets limits release of posaconazole in the acidic pH of the stomach, allowing release of the drug in the elevated pH environment of the intestines. The polymer may also inhibit recrystallization of posaconazole in intestinal fluid, resulting in a greater portion of the drug being available for absorption. Several studies in solid organ transplant recipients or patients with hematologic malignancies indicate that posaconazole delayed-release tablets (300 mg once daily or 300 mg twice daily on day 1 followed by 300 mg once daily) result in consistently higher posaconazole plasma concentrations than posaconazole oral suspension (400 mg twice daily or 200 mg 3 or 4 times daily).

When posaconazole delayed-release tablets are administered in single or multiple doses up to 300 mg, posaconazole exhibits dose-proportional pharmacokinetics. Following administration of posaconazole delayed-release tablets, the median time to peak plasma concentrations is 4–5 hours. When posaconazole delayed-release tablets are given in a dosage of 300 mg twice daily on day 1 (loading dosage) followed by 300 mg once daily thereafter (maintenance dosage), steady-state posaconazole concentrations are achieved by day 6. The absolute bioavailability of posaconazole delayed-release tablets is approximately 54% under fasting conditions.

When IV posaconazole is given in single doses of 200–300 mg, posaconazole exhibits dose-proportional pharmacokinetics. The median time to peak plasma concentrations following IV administration of posaconazole is 1.5 hours.

In a crossover study in healthy adults who received a single 400-mg dose of posaconazole oral suspension orally or via a nasogastric tube† after a liquid nutritional supplement (Boost® Plus), the mean time to peak plasma concentrations of posaconazole was similar (4 hours) but mean peak plasma concentrations and AUC were 19 and 23% lower, respectively, when the dose was administered using a nasogastric tube. In some patients, posaconazole peak plasma concentrations and AUC were reduced substantially (up to approximately 50%) when the drug was administered via a nasogastric tube compared to when it was administered orally.

Data from a limited number of pediatric patients 13–17 years of age receiving posaconazole oral suspension (200 mg 3 times daily) for prophylaxis of invasive fungal infections indicate that mean steady-state posaconazole plasma concentrations in this age group are similar to those reported in adults.

Comparison of data from a limited number of pediatric patients 8–17 years of age who received posaconazole oral suspension (400 mg twice daily or 200 mg 4 times daily) for treatment of invasive fungal infections with data from adults indicates that mean steady-state posaconazole plasma concentrations in pediatric patients and adults are similar.

In individuals with mild, moderate, or severe hepatic impairment, the mean AUC of posaconazole following a single 400-mg dose of posaconazole oral suspension given after a high-fat meal was 43, 27, or 21% higher, respectively, and the mean peak plasma concentration was 1% higher, 40% higher, or 34% lower, respectively, compared with individuals with normal hepatic function.

Specific studies have not been performed to date to evaluate posaconazole pharmacokinetics following administration of the delayed-release tablets in individuals with hepatic impairment.

In individuals with mild or moderate renal impairment (estimated glomerular filtration rate [eGFR] 20–80 mL/minute per 1.73 m^2), posaconazole pharmacokinetics following a single dose of the oral suspension is similar to that reported in individuals with normal renal function. In individuals with severe renal insufficiency (eGFR less than 20 mL/minute per 1.73 m^2), the mean AUC of posaconazole following a single dose of posaconazole oral suspension is similar to that reported in individuals with normal renal function; however, the range of AUC estimates is highly variable compared with that in individuals with mild or moderate renal impairment.

The manufacturer states that renal impairment does not have a clinically important effect on the pharmacokinetics of posaconazole delayed-release tablets. However, although specific studies have not been performed to date using the delayed-release tablets, posaconazole exposures in patients with severe renal impairment receiving the tablets are expected to be highly variable.

Pharmacokinetic modeling suggests that posaconazole plasma concentrations may be lower in patients weighing more than 120 kg than in other patients. (See Other Special Populations under Dosage and Administration: Specific Populations.)

Food Food or a liquid nutritional supplement increases posaconazole plasma concentrations and AUC.

Following oral administration of a single 200-mg dose of posaconazole oral suspension with a nonfat or high-fat meal (approximately 50 g of fat), both the mean peak plasma concentration and AUC of the drug were approximately threefold or fourfold higher, respectively, compared with those observed following administration in the fasted state.

In a crossover study in healthy adults who received a single 400-mg dose of posaconazole oral suspension during or 20 minutes following a high-fat meal, mean peak plasma posaconazole concentrations and AUC were approximately threefold or fourfold higher, respectively, compared with those observed following administration in the fasted state. When the dose was administered 5 minutes prior to the high-fat meal, mean peak plasma posaconazole concentrations and AUC were similar to those observed when the drug is administered in the fasted state.

Following oral administration of a single 400-mg dose of posaconazole oral suspension with 240 mL of liquid nutritional supplement (Boost® Plus; 360 calories, 14 g fat), both the mean peak plasma concentration and AUC were approximately threefold higher than following administration in the fasted state. Bioavailability of posaconazole is lower if the posaconazole dose is administered with less than 240 mL of the liquid nutritional supplement; posaconazole bioavailability is about 20% lower if only 120 mL of the liquid nutritional supplement is used instead of 240 mL.

Following oral administration of a single 400-mg dose of posaconazole oral suspension with an acidic beverage (i.e., ginger ale) in healthy adults in the fasted state, mean peak plasma concentrations and AUC were increased by 92 and 70%, respectively, compared with those reported following administration of posaconazole alone in the fasted state.

Following oral administration of a single 300-mg dose of posaconazole as delayed-release tablets given with a high-fat meal, peak plasma concentrations and AUC were increased by 16 and 51%, respectively, compared with administration in the fasted state.

■ **Distribution** The mean volume of distribution of posaconazole is 261 L following IV administration.

Following oral administration of posaconazole oral suspension, the drug has been detected in skin and in pulmonary epithelial lining fluid and alveolar cell tissue.

Posaconazole is distributed into milk in rats; it is not known whether the drug is distributed into milk in humans.

Posaconazole is more than 98% bound to plasma proteins (primarily albumin).

■ **Elimination** Posaconazole is principally metabolized via uridine diphosphate (UDP)-glucuronosyltransferase UDP glucuronidation (UGT; phase 2 enzymes). Posaconazole circulates in plasma principally as the parent drug; the majority of circulating metabolites are glucuronide conjugates formed via UDP glucuronidation.

No major circulating posaconazole metabolites are formed via cytochrome P-450 (CYP) isoenzymes.

Following administration of posaconazole oral suspension, 71% of a posaconazole dose is recovered in feces (66% as the parent drug) over 120 hours; 13% of a dose is recovered in urine over 120 hours (less than 0.2% as the parent drug). Metabolites recovered in urine and feces represent approximately 17% of a dose.

The mean elimination half-life of posaconazole is 35 hours (range: 20–66 hours) following administration of the oral suspension and 26–31 hours following administration of the delayed-release tablets. Following IV infusion, the mean terminal elimination half-life of posaconazole is 27 hours.

In individuals with mild, moderate, or severe hepatic impairment, the mean apparent oral clearance following a single 400-mg dose of posaconazole oral suspension is decreased 18, 36, or 28%, respectively, compared with individuals with normal hepatic function. The elimination half-life of the drug is 39, 27, or 43 hours in those with mild, moderate, or severe hepatic impairment, respectively.

In patients with moderate or severe renal impairment (eGFR less than 50 mL/minute) receiving IV posaconazole, accumulation of the IV vehicle contained in the preparation (betadex sulfobutyl ether sodium [SBECD]) is expected to occur. (See Renal Impairment under Warnings/Precautions: Specific Populations, in Cautions.)

Description

Posaconazole, a triazole antifungal agent, is structurally similar to itraconazole. The drug inhibits the cytochrome P-450 (CYP)-dependent enzyme lanosterol 14-α-demethylase, thus inhibiting an essential step in fungal ergosterol biosynthesis and weakening the structure and function of the fungal cell membrane. Posaconazole may be fungicidal or fungistatic in action.

Posaconazole is commercially available for oral administration as an oral suspension or delayed-release tablets; a parenteral preparation also is available for IV administration. The oral suspension and delayed-release tablets are *not* interchangeable and cannot be directly substituted for each other since they have different pharmacokinetics and require different dosages and frequencies of administration. (See Dispensing and Dosage and Administration Precautions under Administration: Oral Administration, in Dosage and Administration.) The delayed-release tablets contain posaconazole mixed with a pH-sensitive polymer (hypromellose acetate succinate) that enhances oral bioavailability and results in higher plasma concentrations of the drug compared with the oral suspension. The pH-sensitive polymer in the tablets limits release of posaconazole in the acidic pH of the stomach, allowing release of the drug in the elevated pH environment of the intestines. The polymer may also inhibit recrystallization of posaconazole in intestinal fluid, resulting in a greater portion of the drug being available for absorption. (See Pharmacokinetics.)

Posaconazole is principally metabolized via uridine diphosphate (UDP)-glucuronosyltransferase-glucuronidation (UGT; phase 2 enzymes) and is a substrate for the P-glycoprotein transport system. Therefore, inhibitors or inducers of these metabolic pathways (e.g., rifabutin, phenytoin) may affect posaconazole plasma concentrations. Posaconazole is an inhibitor of CYP3A4; therefore, plasma concentrations of drugs predominantly metabolized by this isoenzyme (e.g., cyclosporine, tacrolimus, rifabutin, midazolam, phenytoin) may be increased by posaconazole. (See Drug Interactions.)

■ **Spectrum** Posaconazole is active in vitro against *Candida*, including *C. albicans*, *C. dubliniensis*, *C. fumata*, *C. glabrata*, *C. guilliermondii*, *C. kefyr*, *C. krusei*, *C. lipolytica*, *C. lusitaniae*, *C. metapsilosis*, *C. orthopsilosis*, *C. parapsilosis*, *C. pelliculosa*, *C. rugosa*, and *C. tropicalis*. Posaconazole is active in vitro against some fluconazole-resistant *Candida*, and has been active in vitro against some *C. albicans* isolates obtained from patients with infections refractory to fluconazole and/or itraconazole therapy.

Posaconazole has in vitro activity against *Aspergillus*, including *A. fumigatus*, *A. flavus*, *A. niger*, and *A. terreus*.

Posaconazole also has in vitro activity against *Blastomyces*, *Coccidioides immitis*, *C. posadasii*, *Cryptococcus neoformans*, *C. gattii*, *Histoplasma capsulatum*, and some strains of *Fusarium oxysporum* and *F. moniliforme*. The drug is active in vitro against some fungi in the order Mucorales, including *Rhizopus* (*R. arrhizus*, *R. microsporus*, *R. oryzae*), *Mucor* (*M. circinelloides*), *Lichtheimia* (formerly *Absidia*), *Cunninghamella* (*C. bertholletiae*), *Rhizomucor pusillus*, *Saksenaea*, *Syncephalastrum racemosum*, and *Apophysomyces* (*A. elegans*).

■ **Resistance** *C. albicans* and *C. glabrata* with decreased in vitro susceptibility to posaconazole have been reported. Such strains reportedly have developed in some patients receiving the drug for prophylaxis of fungal infections.

Posaconazole-resistant fungi may be cross-resistant to other azole antifungals (e.g., fluconazole, itraconazole).

Advice to Patients

Advise patients of the importance of taking posaconazole as directed by their healthcare provider and importance of reading the patient information provided by the manufacturer.

Advise patients that posaconazole oral suspension and posaconazole delayed-release tablets are *not* interchangeable and cannot be directly substituted for each other since they require different dosages and frequencies of administration. Importance of consulting their healthcare provider before switching from delayed-release tablets to oral suspension or vice versa.

If using posaconazole oral suspension, importance of taking each dose during or immediately (i.e., within 20 minutes) following a full meal or liquid nutritional supplement to ensure adequate GI absorption of the drug. Alternatively, the oral suspension may be taken with an acidic carbonated beverage (e.g., ginger ale). Advise patients to inform clinicians if they are unable to eat full meals or drink nutritional supplements.

If using posaconazole oral suspension, advise patients that if they miss a dose it should be taken as soon as it is remembered and the next dose should be taken at the usual time. If a missed dose is remembered near the time of the next dose, advise patients to skip the missed dose. The dose should not be doubled to replace a missed dose.

If using posaconazole delayed-release tablets, importance of taking each dose with food. Advise patients that the delayed-release tablets must be swallowed whole and should not be divided, crushed, or chewed.

If using posaconazole delayed-release tablets, advise patients that if they miss a dose and it is remembered within 12 hours after the scheduled time, the missed dose should be taken with food and the next dose should be taken at the usual time. If a missed dose is remembered more than 12 hours after the scheduled time, advise patients to skip the missed dose and resume the usual schedule. The dose should not be doubled to replace a missed dose.

Importance of informing clinicians of a history of allergic reactions to other antifungals (e.g., fluconazole, itraconazole, ketoconazole, voriconazole).

Importance of informing clinicians if currently taking drugs known to prolong QT interval corrected for rate (QT_c) that are metabolized by cytochrome P-450 (CYP) 3A4 (e.g., pimozide, quinidine).

Importance of informing clinicians if currently taking cyclosporine or tacrolimus.

Importance of immediately informing clinicians if a change in heart rate or heart rhythm occurs and informing clinicians of existing heart conditions or circulatory diseases. Posaconazole can be used with caution in patients with potentially proarrhythmic conditions.

Importance of immediately informing clinicians if itching, nausea or vomiting, yellowing of skin or eyes, extreme fatigue or flu-like symptoms, swelling in an arm or leg, or shortness of breath occurs.

Importance of informing clinicians of existing or contemplated concomitant therapy, including prescription and OTC drugs, and any concomitant illnesses (e.g., liver, kidney, or heart disease).

Importance of women informing clinicians if they are or plan to become pregnant or plan to breast-feed.

Importance of informing patients of other important precautionary information. (See Cautions.)

Overview® (see Users Guide). For additional information on this drug until a more detailed monograph is developed and published, the manufacturer's labeling should be consulted. It is *essential* that the manufacturer's labeling be consulted for more detailed information on usual cautions, precautions, contraindications, potential drug interactions, laboratory test interferences, and acute toxicity.

Preparations

Excipients in commercially available drug preparations may have clinically important effects in some individuals; consult specific product labeling for details.

Posaconazole

Oral		
Suspension	40 mg/mL	**Noxafil®**, Merck
Tablets, delayed-release	100 mg	**Noxafil®**, Merck
Parenteral		
Injection, for IV infusion only	18 mg/mL (300 mg)	**Noxafil®**, Merck

†Use is not currently included in the labeling approved by the US Food and Drug Administration

Voriconazole

■ Voriconazole, a triazole antifungal agent, is a synthetic derivative of fluconazole.

Uses

■ **Aspergillosis** Voriconazole is used for the treatment of invasive aspergillosis. Voriconazole has been evaluated in clinical studies for primary and salvage therapy of invasive aspergillosis, including treatment of invasive aspergillosis in patients intolerant of, or whose disease was refractory to, other antifungals. In these studies, the majority of isolates were *Aspergillus fumigatus.*

The Infectious Diseases Society of America (IDSA) considers voriconazole the drug of choice for primary treatment of invasive aspergillosis in most patients and IV amphotericin B the preferred alternative. For salvage therapy in patients refractory to or intolerant of primary antifungal therapy, IDSA recommends amphotericin B, caspofungin, micafungin, posaconazole, or itraconazole. For empiric or preemptive therapy of presumed aspergillosis, IDSA recommends amphotericin B, caspofungin, itraconazole, or voriconazole.

For the treatment of invasive aspergillosis in adults and adolescents with human immunodeficiency virus (HIV) infection, the US Centers for Disease Control and Prevention (CDC), National Institutes of Health (NIH), and IDSA recommend voriconazole as the drug of choice; IV amphotericin B, IV echinocandins (caspofungin, micafungin, anidulafungin), and oral posaconazole are recommended as alternatives. Voriconazole also is considered the drug of choice for treatment of invasive aspergillosis in HIV-infected children†; IV amphotericin B and IV caspofungin are alternatives.

Clinical Experience Efficacy of voriconazole as primary or salvage therapy for invasive aspergillosis was evaluated in an open-label, noncomparative study in 116 patients 18–79 years of age with definite or probable invasive aspergillosis. A complete or partial response was achieved in 48% of patients in this study, but lower response rates observed in patients with definite disease (38%) than in those with probable disease (58%).

In a randomized, nonblinded study of voriconazole as primary therapy for invasive aspergillosis, 277 patients 12–79 years of age with definite or probable invasive aspergillosis received voriconazole (6 mg/kg IV twice daily for 2 doses and then 4 mg/kg IV twice daily for at least 7 days followed by oral voriconazole 200 mg twice daily) or amphotericin B (1–1.5 mg/kg IV once daily) for up to 12 weeks. At the end of the study, a complete or partial response was achieved in 53% of patients randomized to receive voriconazole compared with 32% of those randomized to receive amphotericin B and the survival rate at the end of the study was 71 or 58%, respectively. Pooled analysis of data from this study and an additional study in patients intolerant of, or whose disease was refractory to, other antifungals indicate a response rate of 44 or 40% in patients with invasive infections caused by *A. fumigatus* or other *Aspergillus* species, respectively.

■ **Candidemia and Disseminated Candida Infections** Voriconazole is used for the treatment of candidemia in nonneutropenic patients and for the treatment of disseminated *Candida* infections involving the skin, abdomen, kidney, bladder wall, or wounds. The drug has been effective in *Candida albicans, C. tropicalis, C. parapsilosis, C. glabrata,* and *C. krusei* infections.

For the treatment of candidemia in *nonneutropenic* patients or for empiric treatment of suspected invasive candidiasis in such patients, the IDSA recommends fluconazole or an echinocandin (caspofungin, micafungin, anidulafungin) for initial therapy; amphotericin B is the preferred alternative. These experts state that voriconazole offers little advantage over fluconazole and generally has been reserved for step-down oral therapy for treatment of *C. krusei* candidiasis or for treatment of fluconazole-resistant, voriconazole-susceptible *C. glabrata* infections. Although an echinocandin is preferred for initial treatment of *C. glabrata* infections, if the patient initially received fluconazole or voriconazole, continuation of the azole antifungal until treatment completion is reasonable if the patient is clinically improved and follow-up culture results are negative.

For the treatment of candidemia in *neutropenic*† patients, the IDSA recommends an echinocandin (caspofungin, micafungin, anidulafungin) or amphotericin B for initial therapy; fluconazole is a reasonable alternative in those who are less critically ill or have not recently received an azole; voriconazole can be used as an alternative when broader antifungal coverage is required. An echinocandin is preferred for *C. glabrata* infections; fluconazole or amphotericin B is preferred for *C. parapsilosis* infections; an echinocandin, amphotericin B, or voriconazole is recommended for *C. krusei* infections. Although an echinocandin is preferred for initial treatment of *C. glabrata* infections, if the patient initially received fluconazole or voriconazole, continuation of the azole antifungal until treatment completion is reasonable if the patient is clinically improved and follow-up culture results are negative. For initial empiric treatment of suspected invasive candidiasis in *neutropenic*† patients, amphotericin B, caspofungin, or voriconazole is recommended; alternatives are fluconazole or itraconazole.

Voriconazole has been used prophylactically to reduce the incidence of candidiasis in patients at risk, including hematopoietic stem cell transplant recipients†.

Clinical Experience Efficacy of voriconazole for the treatment of candidemia and other disseminated or invasive infections caused by *Candida* was evaluated in an open-label comparative study in nonneutropenic patients with candidemia associated with clinical signs of infection. Patients were randomized to receive IV voriconazole (followed by oral voriconazole) or IV amphotericin B (followed by oral fluconazole); antifungal therapy was continued for a median of 15 days. In patients evaluated for efficacy, most infections were caused by *C. albicans* (46%), followed by *C. tropicalis* (19%), *C. parapsilosis* (17%), *C. glabrata* (15%), and *C. krusei* (1%). Analysis at 12 weeks after the end of therapy indicates that voriconazole is as effective as IV amphotericin B followed by oral fluconazole. A successful response (defined as resolution or improvement in all clinical signs and symptoms of infection, blood cultures negative for *Candida*, or infected deep tissue sites negative for *Candida* or resolution of all local signs of infection, and no systemic antifungal therapy other than study drugs) was observed in 41% of patients in each group.

Voriconazole has resulted in a favorable response in patients with invasive fungal infections (intra-abdominal infection, kidney and bladder wall infection, deep tissue abscess or wound infection, pneumonia/pleural space infection, skin lesions, suppurative phlebitis, hepatosplenic infection) caused by *Candida* whose disease was refractory to, or who were intolerant of, other antifungals.

■ **Oropharyngeal Candidiasis** Voriconazole has been used for the treatment of oropharyngeal candidiasis† refractory to other antifungals.

For the treatment of mild oropharyngeal candidiasis, the IDSA recommends topical treatment with clotrimazole lozenges or nystatin oral suspension; oral fluconazole is recommended for moderate to severe disease. For refractory oropharyngeal candidiasis, including fluconazole-refractory infections, itraconazole oral solution, oral posaconazole, or oral voriconazole is recommended. An IV echinocandin (caspofungin, micafungin, anidulafungin) or IV amphotericin B also are recommended as alternatives for refractory infections.

For the treatment of oropharyngeal candidiasis in HIV-infected adults and adolescents, the CDC, NIH, and IDSA recommend oral fluconazole as the drug of choice for initial episodes; if topical therapy is used for the treatment of mild to moderate episodes, the drugs of choice are miconazole buccal tablets or clotrimazole lozenges. Alternatives for systemic treatment of oropharyngeal candidiasis in HIV-infected adults and adolescents are itraconazole oral solution or oral posaconazole; nystatin oral suspension is an alternative if topical treatment is used. For fluconazole-refractory oropharyngeal infections in HIV-infected adults and adolescents, oral posaconazole is preferred; itraconazole oral solution is an alternative.

Although routine long-term suppressive or maintenance therapy (secondary prophylaxis) to prevent relapse or recurrence is not usually recommended in patients adequately treated for oropharyngeal candidiasis, patients with frequent or severe recurrences (including HIV-infected adults, adolescents, and children) may benefit from secondary prophylaxis with oral fluconazole or itraconazole oral solution; however, the potential for azole resistance should be considered.

■ **Esophageal Candidiasis** Voriconazole is used for the treatment of esophageal candidiasis. The drug has been effective in immunocompromised patients with esophageal candidiasis caused by *C. albicans, C. glabrata,* or *C. krusei.*

Esophageal candidiasis requires treatment with a systemic antifungal (not a topical antifungal).

The IDSA recommends oral fluconazole as the preferred drug of choice for the treatment of esophageal candidiasis; if oral therapy is not tolerated, IV fluconazole, IV amphotericin B, or an IV echinocandin (caspofungin, micafungin, anidulafungin) is recommended. For fluconazole-refractory infections, preferred alternatives are itraconazole oral solution, oral posaconazole, or oral or IV voriconazole; other alternatives are an IV echinocandin or IV amphotericin B.

For the treatment of esophageal candidiasis in HIV-infected adults and adolescents, the CDC, NIH, and IDSA recommend oral or IV fluconazole as the drug of choice and itraconazole oral solution as the preferred alternative. Other alternatives include oral or IV voriconazole, oral posaconazole, IV echinocandins (caspofungin, micafungin, anidulafungin), or IV amphotericin B. For refractory esophageal candidiasis, including fluconazole-refractory infections, in HIV-infected adults and adolescents, oral posaconazole is preferred; alternatives include itraconazole oral solution, IV amphotericin B, IV echinocandins (caspofungin, micafungin, anidulafungin), or oral or IV voriconazole.

Although routine long-term suppressive or maintenance therapy (secondary prophylaxis) to prevent relapse or recurrence is not usually recommended in patients adequately treated for esophageal candidiasis, patients with frequent or severe recurrences (including HIV-infected adults, adolescents, and children) may benefit from secondary prophylaxis with oral fluconazole or oral posaconazole; however, the potential for azole resistance should be considered.

Clinical Experience Efficacy of voriconazole has been evaluated in a comparative study in immunocompromised patients with esophageal candidiasis documented by endoscopy. Patients were randomized to receive oral voriconazole (200 mg twice daily) or oral fluconazole (200 mg once daily); antifungals were given for a median of 15 days. A successful response (defined as normal endoscopy at end of treatment or at least a 1 grade improvement over baseline endoscopic score) occurred in 98% of those who received voriconazole and in 95% of those who received fluconazole. In voriconazole-treated patients, mycologic eradication was achieved in 84% of those with *C. albicans* infection, in 57% of those with *C. glabrata* infection, and in the single patient with *C. krusei* infection.

■ **Coccidioidomycosis** Voriconazole has been used for the treatment of coccidioidomycosis† caused by *Coccidioides immitis* or *C. posadasii*, and is recommended as an alternative for the treatment or prevention of these infections.

Antifungal treatment may not be necessary in patients with mild, uncomplicated coccidioidal pneumonia since such infections often are self-limited and may resolve spontaneously. However, antifungal treatment is recommended for patients with more severe or rapidly progressing coccidioidal infections, those with chronic pulmonary or disseminated infections, and immunocompromised or debilitated individuals (e.g., HIV-infected individuals, organ transplant recipients, those receiving immunosuppressive therapy, those with diabetes or cardiopulmonary disease).

The IDSA and others state that an oral azole (fluconazole or itraconazole) usually is recommended for initial treatment of symptomatic pulmonary coccidioidomycosis and chronic fibrocavitary or disseminated (extrapulmonary) coccidioidomycosis. However, IV amphotericin B is recommended as an alternative and is preferred for initial treatment of severely ill patients who have hypoxia or rapidly progressing disease, for immunocompromised individuals, or when azole antifungals have been ineffective or cannot be used (e.g., pregnant women).

For the treatment of clinically mild coccidioidomycosis (e.g., focal pneumonia) in HIV-infected adults and adolescents, the CDC, NIH, and IDSA recommend initial therapy with oral fluconazole or oral itraconazole. These experts state that, although clinical data are limited, oral voriconazole or oral posaconazole may be used as an alternative for the treatment of clinically mild coccidioidomycosis† that has not responded to fluconazole or itraconazole.

HIV-infected individuals who have been adequately treated for coccidioidomycosis should receive long-term (usually life-long) secondary prophylaxis to prevent recurrence or relapse. Although oral fluconazole or oral itraconazole are the drugs of choice recommended by the CDC, NIH, and IDSA for secondary prophylaxis to prevent recurrence or relapse of coccidioidomycosis in HIV-infected adults and adolescents, these experts state that oral voriconazole or oral posaconazole can be used as an alternative for secondary prophylaxis of coccidioidomycosis† if the patient did not initially respond to fluconazole or itraconazole.

■ Exserohilum Infections

Amphotericin B has been used for the treatment of infections known or suspected to be caused by *Exserohilum rostratum*†.

Exserohilum is a common mold found in soil and on plants, especially grasses, and thrives in warm and humid climates. *E. rostratum* is considered an opportunistic human pathogen and rarely has been involved in human infections, including cutaneous and subcutaneous infections or keratitis, typically as the result of skin or eye trauma. More invasive infections (e.g., infections involving the sinuses, heart, lungs, or bones) and life-threatening infections also have been reported rarely, usually in immunocompromised individuals. In addition, *E. rostratum* was identified as the predominant pathogen in the 2012–2013 multistate outbreak of fungal meningitis and other fungal infections that occurred in the US in patients who received contaminated preservative-free methylprednisolone acetate injections prepared by a compounding pharmacy. *Exserohilum* infections cannot be transmitted person-to-person.

Although data are limited and the clinical relevance of in vitro testing remains uncertain, in vitro studies indicate that *Exserohilum* is inhibited by some triazole antifungals (e.g., voriconazole, itraconazole, posaconazole) and amphotericin B. Echinocandins (e.g., caspofungin, micafungin) have variable in vitro activity and fluconazole has poor in vitro activity against the fungus.

Exserohilum Infections Related to Contaminated Injections In September 2012, the CDC and US Food and Drug Administration (FDA) initiated investigations in response to fungal CNS infections (including some fatalities) reported in patients who received epidural injections of contaminated extemporaneously prepared methylprednisolone acetate injections from the New England Compounding Center (NECC). Subsequently, there were reports of joint infections and osteomyelitis in some patients who received intra-articular injections of methylprednisolone acetate from NECC, as well as infections possibly related to other NECC products.

Out of an abundance of caution at that time, the FDA recommended that health-care professionals and consumers not use any product that was produced by NECC, and the company recalled all products that were compounded at and distributed from its facility in Framingham, Massachusetts. Recall information is available at http://www.neccrx.com.

The predominant pathogen identified in samples taken from patients who received contaminated products from NECC has been *E. rostratum*; *Aspergillus* also was identified in an index patient and *Cladosporium cladosporioides* was recovered from several other patients. The presence of *E. rostratum* was confirmed in recalled lots of the contaminated products. Other organisms identified in unopened vials from these recalled lots were *C. cladosporioides*, *Bacillus subtilis*, *B. pumilus*, *Paecilomyces formosus*, *Rhodotorula laryngis*, and *Rhizopus stolonifer*; *Rhodotorula* and *Rhizopus* are not known to cause human disease and do not grow at human body temperature.

CDC data indicate that, as of September 6, 2013, there were a total of 750 cases of fungal infections (including 64 deaths) reported in 20 states that have been linked to 3 specific lots of contaminated methylprednisolone acetate injections. Although the majority of initial cases involved fungal meningitis (some with stroke), subsequent reports involved localized spinal or paraspinal infections (e.g., epidural abscess). More than 6 months after the outbreak related to contaminated products was first identified, the CDC continued to receive reports of patients presenting with localized spinal and paraspinal infections (e.g., epidural abscess, phlegmon, discitis, vertebral osteomyelitis, arachnoiditis, or other complications at or near the site of injection). These localized infections have occurred in patients with or without a diagnosis of fungal meningitis. In some patients being treated for fungal meningitis who had no previous evidence of localized infections, such infections were found at the site of injection using magnetic resonance imaging (MRI) studies. Some cases have occurred in patients without any previous evidence of infection or in those with persistent, worsening, or new symptoms.

Patients with meningitis generally presented 1–4 weeks or longer after receiving contaminated methylprednisolone acetate injections; the greatest risk for development of fungal meningitis appeared to be during the first 6 weeks after an epidural or paraspinal injection. Data from one group of patients indicate that the median time from the last injection with contaminated product to the date of the first MRI finding indicative of infection was 50 days (range 12–121 days) for all patients with a spinal or paraspinal infection, and the median time from the first positive lumbar puncture finding to the first positive MRI finding was 21 days for those with meningitis and spinal or paraspinal infections.

Clinicians treating fungal infections in patients who received contaminated methylprednisolone acetate injections from NECC should consult an infectious disease expert to assist with diagnosis, management, and follow-up, which may be complex and prolonged. A clinical consultant network for clinicians can be reached by calling CDC at 800-232-4636. Because of evidence of latent disease, the CDC cautions clinicians to maintain a high index of suspicion and remain vigilant for fungal infections in patients who received the contaminated methylprednisolone acetate injections, especially in those who have mild or baseline symptoms, and to consider MRI evaluation if clinically warranted.

In October 2012, the CDC released interim treatment guidance documents containing recommendations for empiric antifungal treatment of CNS and parameningeal infections and osteoarticular infections associated with the contaminated methylprednisolone acetate products. As additional information became available, these treatment guidance documents were updated and revised several times. Although the following information regarding the CDC recommendations for treatment of these fungal infections was current at the time the voriconazole monograph was finalized for publication, these recommendations may change and the most recent CDC guidance documents at http://www.cdc.gov/hai/outbreaks/meningitis.html should be consulted for the most current recommendations for selection of antifungal agents and the appropriate dosages and duration of treatment.

For the treatment of CNS infections (including meningitis, stroke, and arachnoiditis) and/or parameningeal infections (epidural or paraspinal abscess, discitis or osteomyelitis, and sacroiliac infection) in adults who received the contaminated methylprednisolone acetate injections, the CDC recommends voriconazole. In most patients with these CNS or parameningeal infections, voriconazole should be given IV initially and a transition to oral voriconazole considered only after the patient is clinically stable or improving. Initial treatment with oral voriconazole should be considered only in patients with mild disease who can be monitored closely. Use of IV amphotericin B liposomal *in addition* to IV voriconazole should be strongly considered in patients who present with severe disease and in patients who do not improve or experience clinical deterioration or manifest new sites of disease activity while receiving voriconazole monotherapy. IV amphotericin B liposomal also is an alternative in patients who are unable to tolerate voriconazole. IV amphotericin B liposomal is preferred over other lipid formulations of amphotericin B because of better CNS penetration. Because of limited data and associated toxicities, routine use of intrathecal amphotericin B is not recommended. Although posaconazole or itraconazole has been used in some patients who could not tolerate voriconazole or amphotericin B, efficacy of these drugs for the treatment of infections associated with the contaminated methylprednisolone acetate injections has not been established. Expert consultation is advised when making decisions regarding alternative regimens.

For the treatment of osteoarticular infections (discitis, vertebral osteomyelitis, and epidural abscess or osteoarticular infections not involving the spine) in adults who received intra-articular injections of contaminated methylprednisolone acetate, the CDC recommends voriconazole. Voriconazole should be given IV initially in those with more severe osteoarticular infections, clinical instability, discitis, vertebral osteomyelitis, or epidural abscess; a transition to oral voriconazole should be considered only after the patient is clinically stable or improving. Initial treatment with oral voriconazole should be considered only in patients with mild osteoarticular infections not involving the spine who can be monitored closely. Use of a lipid formulation of IV amphotericin B *in addition* to IV voriconazole should be considered in patients with severe osteoarticular infection and/or clinical instability. A lipid formulation of IV amphotericin B, posaconazole, or itraconazole are alternatives in patients who cannot tolerate voriconazole. Expert consultation is advised when making decisions regarding alternative regimens.

Adequate duration of antifungal treatment for *Exserohilum* infections associated with contaminated methylprednisolone acetate injections is unknown, but prolonged therapy is required. (See Exserohilum Infections under Dosage and Administration: Dosage.) In addition, close follow-up monitoring after completion of treatment is essential in all patients to detect potential relapse.

The CDC website at http://www.cdc.gov/hai/outbreaks/meningitis.html and FDA website at http://www.fda.gov/Drugs/DrugSafety/ucm322734.htm should be consulted for the most recent information regarding the contaminated NECC products and associated infections. The CDC website includes specific information regarding case definitions and diagnostic testing as well as management and treatment of these infections.

■ Fusarium and Scedosporium Infections

Voriconazole is used for the treatment of serious fungal infections caused by *Fusarium* (including *F. solani*) or *Scedosporium apiospermum* (asexual form of *Pseudallescheria boydii*) in patients intolerant of, or whose disease is refractory to, other antifungals.

For the treatment of fusariosis, the most appropriate antifungal should be selected based on in vitro susceptibility testing. Amphotericin B may be preferred for infections caused by *F. solani* or *F. verticillioides*; either voriconazole or amphotericin B are recommended for infections caused by other *Fusarium.*

For the treatment of scedosporiosis, some clinicians consider voriconazole the drug of choice and posaconazole the preferred alternative.

■ **Histoplasmosis** Voriconazole has been used for the treatment of histoplasmosis† caused by *Histoplasma capsulatum.*

The drugs of choice for the treatment of histoplasmosis are IV amphotericin B or oral itraconazole. IV amphotericin B is preferred for initial treatment of severe, life-threatening histoplasmosis, especially in immunocompromised patients such as those with HIV infection. Oral itraconazole generally is used for initial treatment of less severe disease (e.g., mild to moderate acute pulmonary histoplasmosis, chronic cavitary pulmonary histoplasmosis) and as follow-up therapy in the treatment of severe infections after a response has been obtained with IV amphotericin B. Other azole antifungals (fluconazole, ketoconazole, posaconazole, voriconazole) are considered second-line alternatives to oral itraconazole.

For the treatment of less severe disseminated histoplasmosis† in HIV-infected adults and adolescents, the CDC, NIH, and IDSA recommend initial treatment with oral itraconazole. These experts state that, although clinical data are limited, oral voriconazole or oral posaconazole may be used as an alternative for the treatment of less severe disseminated histoplasmosis in patients intolerant of itraconazole who are only moderately ill.

HIV-infected individuals who have been adequately treated for histoplasmosis should receive long-term suppressive or maintenance therapy (secondary prophylaxis) to prevent recurrence or relapse. Oral itraconazole is the drug of choice for secondary prophylaxis of histoplasmosis in HIV-infected adults and adolescents. The role of voriconazole for secondary prophylaxis of histoplasmosis in HIV-infected patients has not been evaluated to date.

■ **Penicilliosis** Voriconazole is used for treatment of penicilliosis† caused by *Penicillium marneffei.*

For the treatment of severe acute penicilliosis in HIV-infected adults and adolescents, the CDC, NIH, and IDSA recommend an initial regimen of IV amphotericin B liposomal followed by oral itraconazole. These experts state that a voriconazole regimen (IV initially, then oral) can be used as an alternative in patients with severe penicilliosis, including those who fail to respond to a regimen of amphotericin B followed by itraconazole.

For the treatment of mild penicilliosis† in HIV-infected adults and adolescents, the CDC, NIH, and IDSA recommend oral itraconazole as the drug of choice and oral voriconazole as an alternative.

HIV-infected patients who have been treated for penicilliosis should receive long-term suppressive or maintenance therapy (secondary prophylaxis) with oral itraconazole to prevent recurrence or relapse. (See Uses: Penicilliosis, in Itraconazole 8:14.08.) An optimal voriconazole regimen for secondary prophylaxis of penicilliosis has not been identified to date.

■ **Empiric Therapy in Febrile Neutropenic Patients** Voriconazole also has been used for empiric therapy of presumed fungal infections in febrile neutropenic patients†.

Clinical Experience Efficacy of voriconazole for empiric therapy in febrile neutropenic patients has been evaluated in an open-label, randomized, multicenter study in patients 12–82 years of age who were neutropenic following chemotherapy or stem cell transplantation. In this study, patients received voriconazole or amphotericin B liposomal for up to 3 days following neutrophil recovery, or for a maximum of 12 weeks. A response (based on a composite assessment including no breakthrough infections within 7 days of the completion of therapy, survival for 7 days following completion of therapy, discontinuance of the drug because of toxicity or lack of efficacy prior to recovery from neutropenia, resolution of fever during neutropenia, and complete or partial response in patients with baseline fungal infections by the completion of therapy) was obtained in 26 or 31% of patients receiving voriconazole or amphotericin B liposomal, respectively. The composite results failed to meet protocol-defined statistical criteria for concluding that voriconazole was not inferior to amphotericin B liposomal. Exploratory analyses of the individual elements of the composite measure suggested that breakthrough infections occurred in a smaller proportion of patients receiving voriconazole (1.9%) compared with amphotericin B liposomal (5%); exploratory analyses of the other individual elements of the composite measure failed to identify other substantial differences between the 2 regimens.

Dosage and Administration

■ **Administration** Voriconazole is administered orally or by slow IV infusion.

The IV route usually is used for initial treatment of systemic fungal infections, but may be switched to oral treatment when clinically indicated.

Electrolyte disturbances (e.g., hypokalemia, hypomagnesemia, hypocalcemia) should be corrected prior to initiation of voriconazole. (See IV Infusion under Dosage and Administration: Administration and see Cardiovascular Effects under Warnings/Precautions: General Precautions, in Cautions.)

Oral Administration Voriconazole film-coated tablets or oral suspension should be given at least 1 hour before or 1 hour after meals.

Reconstituted voriconazole oral suspension should be administered using the oral dispenser provided by the manufacturer and should not be mixed with other drugs or flavoring agents. Prior to withdrawal of each dose, the reconstituted oral suspension should be shaken for 10 seconds.

If a dose is missed, the missed dose should be taken as soon as possible; however, if it has been more than 6 hours since the missed dose, the next scheduled dose should be taken at the appropriate time. A double dose should not be taken.

Reconstitution. Voriconazole powder for oral suspension is reconstituted by adding 46 mL of water to the bottle containing 45 g of voriconazole to provide a suspension containing 40 mg/mL. The bottle should be shaken vigorously for about 1 minute.

The oral suspension should not be mixed with other drugs or additional flavoring agents. The reconstituted oral suspension should *not* be further diluted with water or any other vehicle and is stable for 14 days at 15–30°C.

IV Infusion Voriconazole IV solutions should *not* be administered concomitantly with short-term infusions of *concentrated* electrolytes, even if the 2 infusions are running in separate IV lines or cannulas. Voriconazole IV solutions may be administered at the same time as other IV solutions containing *nonconcentrated* electrolytes; however, the drug must be infused through a separate line.

Voriconazole IV solutions should *not* be administered concomitantly with any blood product, even if the 2 infusions are running in separate IV lines or cannulas.

Voriconazole IV solutions may be administered at the same time as total parenteral nutrition (TPN); however, the drug must be infused through a separate IV line. If infused through a multiple-lumen catheter, TPN must be administered using a different port from the one used for voriconazole.

Reconstitution and Dilution. For IV infusion, the contents of a single-use vial labeled as containing 200 mg of voriconazole should be reconstituted with exactly 19 mL of sterile water for injection to prepare a solution containing 10 mg/mL of the drug. The vial should be shaken until all the powder is dissolved. Reconstituted voriconazole solutions must be further diluted in a compatible IV infusion solution prior to administration. The reconstituted solutions should be used immediately since they contain no preservative; if not used immediately, reconstituted solutions should be stored for no longer than 24 hours at 2–8°C before being diluted and used.

To dilute reconstituted voriconazole solutions, calculate the volume of reconstituted solution required to administer the appropriate weight-based dose and then withdraw and discard a volume of diluent from the final infusion container that equals or exceeds that volume. The volume of diluent remaining in the container should be such that a final concentration of at least 0.5 mg/mL but not greater than 5 mg/mL will be achieved following addition of the reconstituted solution. The appropriate dose should then be withdrawn from the required number of reconstituted vials and added to the infusion container. Any unused portion of reconstituted solution should be discarded.

Rate of Administration. IV infusions of voriconazole should be given over 1–2 hours at a maximum rate of 3 mg/kg per hour. The drug should not be administered by rapid IV infusion.

■ **Dosage** In adults, the voriconazole 200-mg tablet and 40-mg/mL oral suspension are bioequivalent when administered using a loading dose regimen (400 mg every 12 hours) followed by maintenance dosage (200 mg every 12 hours).

In adults, an oral voriconazole dosage of 200 mg every 12 hours results in an area under the plasma-concentration time curve (AUC) similar to that achieved with an IV dosage of 3 mg/kg every 12 hours; an oral dosage of 300 mg every 12 hours results in an AUC similar to that reported with an IV dosage of 4 mg/kg every 12 hours.

Aspergillosis **Adult Dosage.** For the treatment of invasive aspergillosis, adults should receive an initial loading dose regimen of 6 mg/kg of voriconazole by IV infusion every 12 hours for 2 doses, followed by a maintenance dosage of 4 mg/kg by IV infusion every 12 hours for at least 7 days until the patient is clinically improved and can be switched to oral voriconazole. If this IV maintenance dosage cannot be tolerated, the maintenance dosage can be decreased to 3 mg/kg IV every 12 hours.

After an initial IV regimen, the recommended oral maintenance dosage of voriconazole in patients with invasive aspergillosis is 200 mg every 12 hours in patients weighing 40 kg or more or 100 mg every 12 hours in adults weighing less than 40 kg; if the therapeutic response is not adequate, the dosage may be increased to 300 mg every 12 hours in patients weighing 40 kg or more or 150 mg every 12 hours in those weighing less than 40 kg. If this dosage cannot be tolerated, the dosage may be decreased by increments of 50 mg to a minimum of 200 mg every 12 hours in those weighing 40 kg or more or 100 mg every 12 hours in adults weighing less than 40 kg.

The total duration of IV and oral therapy should be based on the severity of the patient's underlying disease, recovery from immunosuppression, and response to the drug. The optimal duration of therapy for aspergillosis is uncertain. In a clinical study in patients with invasive aspergillosis, the median duration of initial IV therapy was 10 days (range 2–90 days) and the median duration of maintenance oral therapy was 76 days (range 2–232 days). The Infectious Diseases Society of America (IDSA) recommends that treatment of invasive pulmonary aspergillosis be continued for at least 6–12 weeks and continued throughout the period of immunosuppression.

For the treatment of invasive aspergillosis in adults with human immunodeficiency virus (HIV) infection, the US Centers for Disease Control and Prevention (CDC), National Institutes of Health (NIH), and IDSA recommend an initial loading dose regimen of 6 mg/kg by IV infusion every 12 hours on day 1, followed by a maintenance dosage of 4 mg/kg by IV infusion every 12 hours. After clinical improvement, an oral dosage of 200 mg every 12 hours is recommended. The optimal duration of therapy in these patients has not been established, but antifungal therapy should be continued at least until the $CD4^+$ T-cell count increases to 200/mm^3 as a result of potent antiretroviral therapy and there is evidence that aspergillosis has resolved.

Pediatric Dosage. In children 12 years of age or older, an IV regimen of voriconazole that consists of a loading dose regimen of 6 mg/kg every 12 hours for 2 doses, followed by an IV maintenance regimen of 4 mg/kg every 12 hours has been recommended; the IV maintenance dosage should be decreased to 3 mg/kg every 12 hours if higher dosage is not tolerated.

In children 12 years of age or older weighing less than 40 kg, an oral regimen of voriconazole that consists of a loading dose regimen of 200 mg every 12 hours for 2 doses, followed by a maintenance dosage of 100 mg every 12 hours has been recommended; if the response is inadequate, the dosage may be increased to 150 mg every 12 hours. In children 12 years of age or older weighing 40 kg or more, an oral regimen of 400 mg every 12 hours for 2 doses, followed by a maintenance dosage of 200 mg every 12 hours has been recommended; if the response is inadequate, the dosage may be increased to 300 mg every 12 hours.

The IDSA recommends that pediatric patients receive 5–7 mg/kg IV every 12 hours for the treatment of invasive aspergillosis.

For the treatment of invasive aspergillosis in HIV-infected adolescents, some clinicians recommend an initial loading dose regimen of 6 mg/kg by IV infusion twice daily on day 1, followed by a maintenance dosage of 4 mg/kg by IV infusion twice daily. After clinical improvement, an oral dosage of 200 mg twice daily is recommended. The optimal duration of therapy in these patients has not been established, but antifungal therapy should be continued at least until the $CD4^+$ T-cell count increases to 200/mm^3 as a result of potent antiretroviral therapy and there is evidence of clinical response.

For the treatment of invasive aspergillosis in HIV-infected children†, some clinicians recommend an initial loading dose regimen of 8 mg/kg (maximum 400 mg) orally twice daily on day 1, followed by a maintenance dosage of 7 mg/kg (maximum 200 mg) orally twice daily. Alternatively, an initial loading dose regimen of 6–8 mg/kg given by IV infusion twice daily on day 1, followed by a maintenance dosage of 7 mg/kg (maximum 200 mg) given by IV infusion twice daily has been recommended. Treatment should be continued for at least 12 weeks; however, treatment duration should be individualized according to clinical response.

Candidemia and Disseminated Candida Infections **Adult Dosage.** The usual initial dosage of voriconazole for the treatment of candidemia and disseminated *Candida* infections in *nonneutropenic* adults is 6 mg/kg by IV infusion every 12 hours for 2 doses, followed by a maintenance dosage of 3–4 mg/kg by IV infusion every 12 hours until the patient can be switched to oral voriconazole. In clinical studies, patients with candidemia received 3 mg/kg every 12 hours and those with deep tissue infections received 4 mg/kg every 12 hours as salvage therapy. Dosage generally should be based on the nature and severity of the infection. If the patient cannot tolerate a dosage of 4 mg/kg, the dosage can be decreased to 3 mg/kg every 12 hours.

After an initial IV regimen, the usual oral dosage of voriconazole in *nonneutropenic* adults with candidemia and disseminated *Candida* infections is 200 mg every 12 hours in patients weighing 40 kg or more or 100 mg every 12 hours in those weighing less than 40 kg; if the therapeutic response is not adequate, the dosage may be increased to 300 mg every 12 hours in patients weighing 40 kg or more or 150 mg every 12 hours in adults weighing less than 40 kg. If this dosage is not tolerated, the dosage may be decreased by increments of 50 mg to a minimum of 200 mg every 12 hours in patients weighing 40 kg or more or 100 mg every 12 hours in adults weighing less than 40 kg.

If voriconazole is used for the treatment of candidemia in *neutropenic*† adults, the IDSA recommends an initial dosage of 6 mg/kg by IV infusion every 12 hours for 2 doses, followed by a maintenance dosage of 3 mg/kg by IV infusion every 12 hours.

The manufacturer recommends that treatment of candidemia be continued for at least 14 days after symptoms have resolved or the last positive culture, whichever is longer. The IDSA and others recommend that antifungal treatment for candidemia (without persistent fungemia or metastatic complications) be continued for 14 days after the first negative blood culture and resolution of signs and symptoms of candidemia.

Pediatric Dosage. In children 12 years of age or older, an IV regimen that consists of a loading dose regimen of 6 mg/kg every 12 hours for 2 doses, followed by an IV maintenance regimen of 4 mg/kg every 12 hours has been recommended; the IV maintenance dosage should be decreased to 3 mg/kg every 12 hours if higher dosage is not tolerated.

In children 12 years of age or older weighing less than 40 kg, an oral regimen of 200 mg every 12 hours for 2 doses, followed by a maintenance dosage of 100 mg every 12 hours has been recommended; if the response is inadequate, the dosage may be increased to 150 mg every 12 hours. In children 12 years of age or older weighing 40 kg or more, an oral regimen of 400 mg every 12 hours for 2 doses, followed by a maintenance dosage of 200 mg every 12 hours has been recommended; if the response is inadequate, the dosage may be increased to 300 mg every 12 hours.

The manufacturer recommends that treatment of candidemia be continued for at least 14 days after symptoms have resolved or the last positive culture, whichever is longer. The IDSA and others recommend that antifungal treatment for candidemia (without persistent fungemia or metastatic complications) be continued for 14 days after the first negative blood culture and resolution of signs and symptoms of candidemia.

Oropharyngeal Candidiasis **Adult Dosage.** For the treatment of oropharyngeal candidiasis† refractory to other antifungals, the IDSA and others recommend an oral voriconazole dosage of 200 mg twice daily.

The IDSA and others recommend that antifungal treatment for oropharyngeal candidiasis be continued for 7–14 days.

Esophageal Candidiasis **Adult Dosage.** The usual adult oral dosage of voriconazole for the treatment of esophageal candidiasis is 200 mg every 12 hours in patients weighing 40 kg or more or 100 mg every 12 hours in adults weighing less than 40 kg; if the therapeutic response is not adequate, the dosage may be increased to 300 mg every 12 hours in patients weighing 40 kg or more or 150 mg every 12 hours in adults weighing less than 40 kg. If this dosage is not tolerated, the dosage may be decreased by increments of 50 mg to a minimum of 200 mg every 12 hours in patients weighing 40 kg or more or 100 mg every 12 hours in adults weighing less than 40 kg.

For the treatment of esophageal candidiasis in HIV-infected adults, some clinicians recommend a voriconazole dosage of 200 mg twice daily given orally or by IV infusion.

The manufacturer recommends that treatment of esophageal candidiasis be continued for at least 14 days and for at least 7 days after symptoms resolve. The IDSA and others recommend that antifungal treatment of esophageal candidiasis be continued for 14–21 days after clinical improvement.

Pediatric Dosage. For the treatment of esophageal candidiasis in children 12 years of age or older weighing less than 40 kg, an oral regimen of 100 mg every 12 hours has been recommended. For children 12 years of age or older weighing 40 kg or more, an oral regimen of 200 mg every 12 hours has been recommended.

For the treatment of esophageal candidiasis in HIV-infected adolescents, some clinicians recommend a voriconazole dosage of 200 mg twice daily given orally or by IV infusion.

The manufacturer recommends that treatment of esophageal candidiasis be continued for at least 14 days and for at least 7 days after symptoms resolve. The IDSA and others recommend that antifungal treatment of esophageal candidiasis be continued for 14–21 days after clinical improvement.

Coccidioidomycosis If oral voriconazole is used as an alternative for the treatment of clinically mild coccidioidomycosis† (e.g., focal pneumonia) in HIV-infected adults and adolescents, a dosage of 200 mg twice daily is recommended by the CDC, NIH, and IDSA.

If oral voriconazole is used as an alternative for long-term suppressive or maintenance therapy (secondary prophylaxis)† to prevent relapse or recurrence of coccidioidomycosis in HIV-infected adults and adolescents who have completed initial treatment of the disease, a dosage of 200 mg twice daily is recommended by the CDC, NIH, and IDSA. In HIV-infected patients who were treated for focal coccidioidal pneumonia and are receiving effective antiretroviral therapy, consideration can be given to discontinuing secondary prophylaxis against coccidioidomycosis after 12 months if $CD4^+$ T-cell counts are 250/mm^3 or higher, provided the patient is monitored for recurrence (e.g., serial chest radiographs, coccidioidal serology). HIV-infected patients who were treated for diffuse pulmonary, disseminated, or meningeal coccidioidomycosis usually require life-long secondary prophylaxis.

Exserohilum Infections **Adult Dosage.** For the treatment of CNS and/or parameningeal infections known or suspected to be caused by *Exserohilum rostratum*† in adults who received injections of contaminated methylprednisolone acetate (see Uses: Exserohilum Infections), the CDC recommends that voriconazole be given in a dosage of 6 mg/kg every 12 hours. In most patients with these CNS or parameningeal infections, voriconazole should be given IV initially and a transition to oral voriconazole should be considered only after the patient is clinically stable or improving. Initial treatment with oral voriconazole should be considered only in those with mild disease who can be monitored closely.

For the treatment of osteoarticular infections known or suspected to be caused by *E. rostratum*† in adults who received intra-articular injections of contaminated methylprednisolone acetate (see Uses: Exserohilum Infections), the CDC recommends that voriconazole be given in a dosage of 6 mg/kg every 12 hours. For osteoarticular infections that do not involve the spine, voriconazole can be given in a dosage of 6 mg/kg every 12 hours for 2 doses, followed by 4 mg/kg every 12 hours. In most patients with osteoarticular infections, voriconazole should be given IV initially and a transition to oral voriconazole should be considered only after the patient is clinically stable or improving. Initial treatment with oral voriconazole should be considered only in those with mild infections who can be monitored closely.

Serum voriconazole concentrations should be measured in all patients on treatment day 5 and dosage adjusted if needed, aiming for trough concentrations of 2–5 mcg/mL. Serum concentrations should be monitored once weekly during the initial 4–6 weeks of treatment and whenever dosage changes are made, maintaining trough voriconazole concentrations of 2–5 mcg/mL. Voriconazole serum concentrations greater than 5 mcg/mL should be avoided because of the risk of neurotoxicity and other adverse effects.

Adequate duration of antifungal treatment for these *E. rostratum* infections is unknown, but prolonged treatment is required and should be based on disease severity and clinical response. A treatment duration of 6–12 months is probably necessary in patients who have severe CNS disease with complications (arachnoiditis, stroke), persistent CSF abnormalities, or underlying immunosuppression. In those with parameningeal infection, a minimum treatment duration of 3–6 months should be considered, and at least 6 months or longer probably is required for more severe disease (e.g., discitis, osteomyelitis) and in those with underlying immunosuppression or complications not amenable to surgical treatment. In those with osteoarticular infections, a minimum treatment duration of 3 months should be considered, and longer than 3 months is probably necessary in those with severe disease, bone infections, or underlying immunosuppression. After completion of treatment, close follow-up monitoring is essential in all patients to detect potential relapse.

An infectious disease expert and the most recent guidelines from the CDC should be consulted for information regarding the management of fungal infections in patients who received injections of potentially contaminated products. Clinicians should consult the CDC website at http://www.cdc.gov/hai/outbreaks/meningitis.html for the most recent recommendations regarding the drugs of choice, dosage, and duration of treatment of these infections.

Fusarium and Scedosporium Infections **Adult Dosage.** The recommended initial adult IV dosage of voriconazole for the treatment of infections caused by *Fusarium* or *Scedosporium apiospermum* is 6 mg/kg by IV infusion every 12 hours for 2 doses, followed by a maintenance dosage of 4 mg/kg by IV infusion every 12 hours until the patient can be switched to oral voriconazole. If this dosage is not tolerated, the IV maintenance dosage can be decreased to 3 mg/kg every 12 hours.

After an initial IV regimen, the usual oral dosage of voriconazole in patients with infections caused by *Fusarium* or *Scedosporium apiospermum* is 200 mg every 12 hours in those weighing 40 kg or more or 100 mg every 12 hours in adults weighing less than 40 kg; if the therapeutic response is not adequate, the dosage may be increased to 300 mg every 12 hours in those weighing 40 kg or more or 150 mg every 12 hours in adults weighing less than 40 kg. If this dosage cannot be tolerated, the dosage may be decreased by increments of 50 mg to a minimum of 200 mg every 12 hours in those weighing 40 kg or more or 100 mg every 12 hours in adults weighing less than 40 kg.

Total duration of therapy should be based on the severity of the patient's underlying disease, recovery from immunosuppression, and response to the drug.

Pediatric Dosage. In children 12 years of age of older, an IV regimen of voriconazole that consists of a loading dose regimen of 6 mg/kg every 12 hours for 2 doses, followed by an IV maintenance regimen of 4 mg/kg every 12 hours has been recommended the IV maintenance dosage should be decreased to 3 mg/kg every 12 hours if higher dosage is not tolerated.

In children 12 years of age or older weighing less than 40 kg, an oral regimen of voriconazole that consists of a loading dose regimen of 200 mg every 12 hours for 2 doses, followed by a maintenance dosage of 100 mg every 12 hours has been recommended; if the response is inadequate, the dosage may be increased to 150 mg every 12 hours. In children 12 years of age or older weighing 40 kg or more, an oral regimen of 400 mg every 12 hours for 2 doses, followed by a maintenance dosage of 200 mg every 12 hours has been recommended; if the response is inadequate, the dosage may be increased to 300 mg every 12 hours.

Total duration of therapy should be based on the severity of the patient's underlying disease, recovery from immunosuppression, and response to the drug.

Histoplasmosis If oral voriconazole is used as an alternative for the treatment of less severe disseminated histoplasmosis† in HIV-infected adults and adolescents who are only moderately ill (see Uses: Histoplasmosis), the CDC, NIH, and IDSA recommend a dosage of 400 mg twice daily for 2 doses followed by 200 mg twice daily.

Penicilliosis If voriconazole is used as an alternative for the treatment of severe acute penicilliosis in HIV-infected adults and adolescents, the CDC, NIH, and IDSA recommend an initial IV regimen of 6 mg/kg every 12 hours for 2 doses, followed by 4 mg/kg IV every 12 hours for at least 3 days, then an oral regimen of 200 mg twice daily for a maximum of 12 weeks.

If oral voriconazole is used as an alternative for the treatment of mild penicilliosis in HIV-infected adults and adolescents, the CDC, NIH, and IDSA recommend a dosage of 400 mg twice daily for 2 doses, followed by 200 mg twice daily for a maximum of 12 weeks.

■ **Special Populations** ***Hepatic Impairment*** In adults with mild-to-moderate hepatic cirrhosis (Child-Pugh class A or B), usual IV or oral loading dosages of voriconazole should be used, but IV or oral maintenance dosages should be decreased by 50%.

Voriconazole should be used in patients with severe hepatic impairment only if benefits outweigh risks; the drug has not been studied in patients with severe hepatic cirrhosis (Child-Pugh class C) or with chronic hepatitis B virus (HBV) or hepatitis C virus (HCV) infection. (See Hepatic Effects under Cautions: Warnings/Precautions.)

Renal Impairment Adjustment of oral voriconazole dosage is not necessary in patients with mild to severe renal impairment.

Because of potential accumulation of the IV vehicle (sulfobutyl ether β-cyclodextrin sodium [SBECD]), IV voriconazole should be avoided in patients with moderate or severe renal impairment (creatinine clearance less than 50 mL/minute); voriconazole should be administered orally in these patients unless potential benefits of the IV route outweigh risks. If IV voriconazole is used in patients with creatinine clearance less than 50 mL/minute, serum creatinine should be monitored closely; if increases occur, switching to oral voriconazole should be considered.

Geriatric Patients Dosage adjustment based on age is not necessary in geriatric adults.

Cautions

■ **Contraindications** Known hypersensitivity to voriconazole or any ingredient in the formulation.

Concomitant use with astemizole or terfenadine (drugs no longer commercially available in the US), carbamazepine, cisapride (currently commercially available in the US only under a limited-access protocol), ergot alkaloids (e.g., ergotamine, dihydroergotamine), pimozide, quinidine, rifabutin, rifampin, sirolimus, St. John's wort *(Hypericum perforatum)*, or long-acting barbiturates (e.g., phenobarbital, mephobarbital). (See Drug Interactions.)

Concomitant use with ritonavir (400 mg every 12 hours) is contraindicated. Concomitant use with low-dose ritonavir (100 mg every 12 hours) should be avoided, unless potential benefits outweigh risks. (See HIV Protease Inhibitors under Drug Interactions: Antiretroviral Agents.)

■ **Warnings/Precautions** ***Sensitivity Reactions*** Anaphylactoid reactions (e.g., flushing, fever, sweating, tachycardia, chest tightness, dyspnea, faintness, nausea, pruritus, rash) occurring immediately after initiation of voriconazole IV infusions have been reported rarely. Clinician should consider stopping the infusion if these reactions occur.

Serious cutaneous reactions (e.g., Stevens-Johnson syndrome, erythema multiforme, toxic epidermal necrolysis) and photosensitivity reactions have been reported rarely in patients receiving voriconazole. (See Dermatologic Effects under Warnings/Precautions: General Precautions, in Cautions.)

Data regarding cross-sensitivity with other azole antifungals are not available. Voriconazole should be used with caution in patients hypersensitive to other azoles.

Hepatic Effects Serious hepatic effects, including hepatitis, cholestasis, and fulminant hepatic failure, have been reported rarely in clinical trials. Hepatic effects (including hepatitis and jaundice) have occurred in patients with no identifiable risk factors.

Hepatic effects usually are reversible when voriconazole is discontinued; however, fatalities have occurred.

If abnormal liver function test results occur during voriconazole therapy, the patient should be monitored for the development of more severe hepatic injury using appropriate laboratory evaluations (particularly liver function tests and bilirubin). Discontinuance of voriconazole must be considered if signs and symptoms consistent with liver disease develop.

Ocular Effects Visual disturbances (e.g., abnormal vision, blurred vision, color vision change, photophobia) have been reported and may be related to high dosage and high plasma voriconazole concentrations.

There have been postmarketing reports of prolonged visual disturbances, including optic neuritis and papilledema, in patients receiving voriconazole.

Effect of voriconazole on visual function is unknown if duration of therapy exceeds 28 days. Monitor visual function (visual acuity, visual field, and color perception) if duration of therapy exceeds 28 days.

Fetal/Neonatal Morbidity and Mortality Voriconazole can cause fetal harm. Teratogenicity, embryotoxicity, and embryomortality have been demonstrated in animals.

If voriconazole is used during pregnancy or if the patient becomes pregnant while receiving voriconazole, clinicians should advise the patient of the potential hazard to the fetus. (See Pregnancy under Warnings/Precautions: Specific Populations, in Cautions.)

Pregnancy should be avoided. Women of childbearing potential should use effective contraception during voriconazole treatment. (See Drug Interactions: Estrogens and Progestins.)

Fructose or Galactose Intolerance Patients with a history of galactose intolerance, Lapp lactase deficiency, or glucose-galactose malabsorption should not be given voriconazole tablets since lactose is used in the manufacture of the tablets.

Patients with fructose intolerance, sucrase-isomaltase deficiency, or glucose-galactose malabsorption should not be given voriconazole oral suspension since the suspension contains sucrose.

Cardiovascular Effects Similar to other azole antifungals, voriconazole has been associated with prolongation of the QT interval. Arrhythmias (e.g., torsades de pointes), cardiac arrest, and sudden death have occurred rarely in patients receiving voriconazole. Most reported cases involved patients with multiple confounding risk factors (e.g., prior cardiotoxic chemotherapy, cardiomyopathy, hypokalemia, concomitant drugs) that may have been contributory.

Voriconazole should be used with caution in patients with potentially proarrhythmic conditions. Rigorous attempts should be made to correct electrolyte imbalances (i.e., potassium, magnesium, calcium) before initiating voriconazole therapy.

Laboratory Monitoring Hepatic function (liver function tests and bilirubin) should be evaluated prior to and during voriconazole therapy.

Serum electrolytes (i.e., potassium, magnesium, calcium) should be evaluated and any electrolyte abnormalities corrected prior to initiation of voriconazole therapy.

Renal function (e.g., serum creatinine concentrations) should be monitored in patients receiving voriconazole.

Patients with risk factors for acute pancreatitis (e.g., recent chemotherapy, hematopoietic stem cell transplantation [HSCT]) should be monitored for the development of pancreatitis during voriconazole therapy.

Dermatologic Effects Serious exfoliative cutaneous reactions (e.g., Stevens-Johnson syndrome, erythema multiforme, toxic epidermal necrolysis) have occurred rarely in patients receiving voriconazole. If an exfoliative cutaneous reaction occurs, voriconazole should be discontinued.

Photosensitivity skin reactions have been reported in patients receiving voriconazole. Patients receiving the drug should avoid intense or prolonged exposure to direct sunlight.

Squamous cell carcinoma of the skin and melanoma have been reported during long-term voriconazole therapy in patients with photosensitivity reactions. If a skin lesion consistent with squamous cell carcinoma or melanoma develops, voriconazole should be discontinued.

Renal Effects Acute renal failure has been reported in severely ill patients with other factors predisposing to impaired renal function (e.g., underlying conditions, concomitant nephrotoxic drugs).

Skeletal Effects Fluorosis and periostitis have been reported during long-term voriconazole therapy. If a patient develops skeletal pain and radiologic findings compatible with fluorosis or periostitis, voriconazole should be discontinued.

Specific Populations **Pregnancy.** Category D. (See Users Guide.)

Because voriconazole can cause fetal harm, it should not be used during pregnancy except when benefits for the mother clearly outweigh potential risks for the fetus.

In rats, voriconazole was teratogenic (cleft palates, hydronephrosis/hydroureter) at a dosage of 10 mg/kg (0.3 times the recommended human maintenance dosage [RMD] based on mg/m^2). Other effects in rats included reduced ossification of sacral and caudal vertebrae, skull, and pubic and hyoid bone; supernumerary ribs; anomalies of sternebrae; and dilatation of the ureter/renal pelvis. Reduced plasma estradiol concentrations in pregnant rats, increased gestational length, and dystocia (associated with increased perinatal pup mortality at a dosage of 10 mg/kg) also were reported. In rabbits, voriconazole was embryotoxic at a dosage of 100 mg/kg (6 times the RMD); increased embryomortality, reduced fetal weight, and increased incidence of skeletal variations, cervical ribs, and extrasternebral ossification sites also were reported.

Lactation. It is not known whether voriconazole is distributed into milk. Because many drugs are distributed into human milk and because of the potential for serious adverse reactions to voriconazole in nursing infants, a decision should be made whether to discontinue nursing or the drug, taking into account the importance of the drug to the mother.

Pediatric Use. Safety and efficacy of voriconazole have not been established in children younger than 12 years of age.

Voriconazole has been recommended for the treatment of fungal infections in children. Some clinicians consider voriconazole the drug of choice for the treatment of invasive aspergillosis in HIV-infected children†, but state that data are insufficient to recommend use of the drug for the treatment of candidemia or esophageal candidiasis in these children.

In one study, a limited number of pediatric patients 9 months to 15 years of age whose disease was refractory to, or who were intolerant of, other antifungals have received voriconazole for the treatment of aspergillosis, candidiasis, infections caused by *Scedosporium*, or other invasive fungal infections. At the completion of therapy, 45% of pediatric patients receiving voriconazole had a complete or partial response. Adverse effects in children receiving voriconazole were similar to those reported in adults.

There have been postmarketing reports of pancreatitis in pediatric patients receiving voriconazole. Children with risk factors for acute pancreatitis (e.g., recent chemotherapy, HSCT) should be monitored for the development of pancreatitis during voriconazole therapy.

In a population pharmacokinetic analysis of voriconazole concentrations in children 2 through 12 years of age who received various dosage regimens, systemic exposures of the drug (areas under the concentration-time curve [AUCs]) achieved with an IV dosage of 7 mg/kg twice daily or an oral dosage of 200 mg twice daily (oral suspension) were comparable to values observed in adults receiving usual dosages of the drug. Data from this study also indicated that loading doses do not appear to reduce the length of time required to reach steady-state in children 2 through 11 years of age and appear to offer little benefit in this age group. Based on a comparison of pharmacokinetic data from pediatric patients (2 years to less than 12 years of age) with data from adults, the manufacturer states that the predicted steady-state plasma voriconazole concentrations were similar in pediatric patients or adults (median concentration of 1.19 or 1.16 mcg/mL, respectively) at a maintenance IV dosage of 4 mg/kg every 12 hours in children or 3 mg/kg every 12 hours in adults.

Geriatric Use. Clinical experience with voriconazole in geriatric patients is limited. Plasma voriconazole concentrations are increased, but overall safety profile is similar to that in younger adults.

Hepatic Impairment. Patients with hepatic impairment should be monitored carefully for voriconazole toxicity, including hepatic effects. (See Hepatic Effects under Warnings/Precautions: Warnings, in Cautions.)

Voriconazole has not been evaluated in patients with severe hepatic cirrhosis (Child-Pugh class C) or with chronic hepatitis B virus (HBV) or hepatitis C virus (HCV) infection.

Voriconazole should be used in patients with severe hepatic impairment only if benefits outweigh risks. (See Dosage and Administration: Special Populations.)

Renal Impairment. IV voriconazole contains sulfobutyl ether β-cyclodextrin sodium (SBECD) which may accumulate in patients with moderate or severe renal impairment (creatinine clearance less than 50 mL/minute).

IV voriconazole should not be used in patients with creatinine clearance less than 50 mL/minute unless potential benefits outweigh risks. If IV voriconazole is used in these patients, serum creatinine concentrations should be monitored closely; if increases occur, consideration should be given to switching to oral voriconazole. (See Dosage and Administration: Special Populations.)

■ **Common Adverse Effects** Common adverse effects include visual disturbances (e.g., abnormal vision, blurred vision, color vision change, photophobia), GI effects (nausea, vomiting, diarrhea, abdominal pain), fever, rash, chills, headache, abnormalities in liver function test results, tachycardia, and hallucinations. The most commonly reported adverse effects resulting in discontinuance of voriconazole therapy include elevated liver function test results, rash, and visual disturbances.

Drug Interactions

■ **Drugs Affecting or Metabolized by Hepatic Microsomal Enzymes** Inhibitors or inducers of cytochrome P-450 (CYP) isoenzymes 2C9, 2C19, or 3A4 may increase or decrease plasma voriconazole concentrations, respectively. Voriconazole and its major metabolite inhibit the metabolic activity of CYP2C9, 2C19, and 3A4 and may increase plasma concentrations of other drugs metabolized by these hepatic enzymes. Voriconazole appears to be a less potent inhibitor of CYP3A4 than some other azoles (e.g., itraconazole, ketoconazole).

Because carbamazepine, long-acting barbiturates (e.g., phenobarbital, mephobarbital), ergot alkaloids, rifabutin, rifampin, ritonavir (400 mg every 12 hours), sirolimus, and St. John's wort *(Hypericum perforatum)* are inducers, inhibitors, and/or substrates of CYP isoenzymes, concomitant use with voriconazole is contraindicated.

■ **Drugs that Prolong the QT Interval** Potential pharmacokinetic interaction with CYP3A4 substrates that prolong the QT interval (e.g., cisapride [currently commercially available in the US only under a limited-access protocol], pimozide, quinidine, terfenadine [no longer commercially available in the US], astemizole [no longer commercially available in the US]). Potential increased plasma concentrations of the concomitantly administered CYP3A4 substrate, which can result in QT interval prolongation and rarely, torsades de pointes. Concomitant use of these drugs that prolong the QT interval and voriconazole is contraindicated.

■ **Alfentanil** Pharmacokinetic interaction (6- and 4-fold increase in mean area under the plasma concentration-time curve [AUC] and elimination half-life, respectively, of alfentanil) when voriconazole was administered concomitantly with alfentanil (patients also received and naloxone). Concomitant administration also resulted in an increased incidence of delayed and persistent alfentanil-induced nausea and vomiting.

If voriconazole is administered concomitantly with alfentanil or other opiate agonists metabolized by CYP3A4 (e.g., sufentanil), decreased dosage of the opiate agonist and extended close monitoring for opiate-related adverse events (e.g., respiratory depression) may be necessary.

■ **Antifungal Agents** ***Fluconazole*** Pharmacokinetic interaction with fluconazole (substantially increased plasma concentrations and AUC of voriconazole).

Concomitant use of fluconazole and voriconazole should be avoided. Patients should be monitored for voriconazole-related adverse effects if the drug is initiated within 24 hours after the last dose of fluconazole.

■ **Antiretroviral Agents** ***HIV Entry Inhibitors*** Possible pharmacokinetic interaction with maraviroc (increased maraviroc plasma concentrations). If used concomitantly, consider reducing the maraviroc dosage to 150 mg twice daily.

HIV Integrase Inhibitor **Elvitegravir.** Potential pharmacokinetic interaction with the fixed combination of elvitegravir, cobicistat, emtricitabine, and tenofovir disoproxil fumarate (increased concentrations of voriconazole, elvitegravir, and/or cobicistat).

Voriconazole and the fixed combination of elvitegravir, cobicistat, emtricitabine, and tenofovir disoproxil fumarate should not be used concomitantly unless potential benefits outweigh risks. If used concomitantly, consideration should be given to monitoring voriconazole concentrations and adjusting voriconazole dosage accordingly.

Raltegravir. Pharmacokinetic interaction with raltegravir unlikely; dosage adjustments not needed.

HIV Protease Inhibitors Pharmacokinetic interactions are likely if voriconazole is used in patients receiving HIV protease inhibitors (PIs) (e.g., atazanavir, darunavir, fosamprenavir, indinavir, lopinavir, nelfinavir, ritonavir, saquinavir, tipranavir), especially if *ritonavir-boosted* PI regimens are used. Concomitant use may result in altered serum concentrations of the PIs and/or the antifungal.

Atazanavir. Possible pharmacokinetic interaction with atazanavir (increased plasma concentrations of voriconazole and atazanavir); possible pharmacokinetic interaction with *ritonavir-boosted* atazanavir (decreased voriconazole concentrations).

If voriconazole is used concomitantly with atazanavir (without low-dose ritonavir), monitor for toxicities. Concomitant use with *ritonavir-boosted* atazanavir should be avoided unless benefits outweigh risks; if used concomitantly, consideration should be given to monitoring voriconazole concentrations and adjusting voriconazole dosage accordingly.

Darunavir. Possible pharmacokinetic interaction with *ritonavir-boosted* darunavir (decreased voriconazole concentrations).

Concomitant use with *ritonavir-boosted* darunavir should be avoided unless benefits outweigh risks; if used concomitantly, consideration should be given to monitoring voriconazole concentrations and adjusting voriconazole dosage accordingly.

Fosamprenavir. Possible pharmacokinetics interaction with fosamprenavir (increased fosamprenavir concentrations and/or increased voriconazole concentrations); possible pharmacokinetic interaction with *ritonavir-boosted* fosamprenavir (decreased voriconazole concentrations).

If voriconazole is used concomitantly with fosamprenavir (without low-dose ritonavir), monitor for toxicities. Concomitant use with *ritonavir-boosted* fosamprenavir should be avoided unless benefits outweigh risks; if used concomitantly, consideration should be given to monitoring voriconazole concentrations and adjusting voriconazole dosage accordingly.

Indinavir. Concomitant use of multiple doses of indinavir and voriconazole does not affect pharmacokinetics of either drug; dosage adjustments are not needed for either drug.

Possible pharmacokinetic interactions with *ritonavir-boosted* indinavir (decreased voriconazole concentrations). Concomitant use with *ritonavir-boosted* indinavir should be avoided unless benefits outweigh risks; if used concomitantly, consideration should be given to monitoring voriconazole concentrations and adjusting voriconazole dosage accordingly.

Lopinavir. Possible pharmacokinetic interaction with lopinavir/ritonavir (decreased voriconazole concentrations). Concomitant use should be avoided unless benefits outweigh risks; if used concomitantly, consideration should be given to monitoring voriconazole concentrations and adjusting voriconazole dosage accordingly.

Nelfinavir. Possible pharmacokinetic interaction with nelfinavir (increased nelfinavir concentrations and/or increased voriconazole concentrations) (without low-dose ritonavir); possible pharmacokinetic interactions with *ritonavir-boosted* nelfinavir (decreased voriconazole concentrations).

If voriconazole is used concomitantly with nelfinavir (without low-dose ritonavir), monitor for toxicities. Concomitant use with *ritonavir-boosted* nelfinavir should be avoided unless benefits outweigh risks; if used concomitantly, consideration should be given to monitoring voriconazole concentrations and adjusting voriconazole dosage accordingly.

Ritonavir. Pharmacokinetic interaction with full-dose ritonavir (400 mg every 12 hours) (mean 66% decrease in steady-state peak plasma voriconazole concentrations and mean 82% decrease in voriconazole AUC; no clinically important effect on ritonavir pharmacokinetics). Concomitant use of voriconazole and full-dose ritonavir (400 mg every 12 hours) is contraindicated.

Pharmacokinetic interaction with low-dose ritonavir (100 mg every 12 hours) (mean 24% decrease in steady-state peak plasma voriconazole concentrations and mean 39% decrease in voriconazole AUC; 24% decrease in steady-state peak ritonavir concentrations and 14% decrease in ritonavir AUC) . Concomitant use of voriconazole and low-dose ritonavir (100 mg every 12 hours) should be avoided unless benefits of such therapy outweigh risks; if used concomitantly, consideration should be given to monitoring voriconazole concentrations and adjusting voriconazole dosage accordingly.

Saquinavir. Possible pharmacokinetic interactions with saquinavir (increased saquinavir concentrations and/or increased voriconazole concentrations); possible pharmacokinetic interaction with *ritonavir-boosted* saquinavir (decreased voriconazole concentrations).

If voriconazole is used concomitantly with saquinavir (without low-dose ritonavir), monitor for toxicities. Concomitant use with *ritonavir-boosted* saquinavir should be avoided unless benefits outweigh risks; if used concomitantly, consideration should be given to monitoring voriconazole concentrations and adjusting voriconazole dosage accordingly.

Tipranavir. Possible pharmacokinetic interaction with *ritonavir-boosted* tipranavir (decreased voriconazole concentrations). Concomitant use with *ritonavir-boosted* tipranavir should be avoided unless benefits outweigh risks; if used concomitantly, consideration should be given to monitoring voriconazole concentrations and adjusting voriconazole dosage accordingly.

Nonnucleoside Reverse Transcriptase Inhibitors **Delavirdine.** Potential pharmacokinetic interaction with delavirdine (increased voriconazole concentrations). Monitor patients for voriconazole toxicities and clinical response.

Efavirenz. Concomitant use of voriconazole (400 mg every 12 hours for 1 day, then 200 mg every 12 hours for 8 days) and usual dosage of efavirenz (400 mg once daily for 9 days) reduced voriconazole peak plasma concentrations and AUC by 61 and 77%, respectively, and increased efavirenz peak plasma concentrations and AUC by 38 and 44%, respectively. When a lower dosage of voriconazole (400 mg once daily) was used concomitantly with a lower dosage of efavirenz (300 mg once daily), voriconazole peak plasma concentration was increased 23%, voriconazole AUC was decreased 7%, and efavirenz AUC was increased by 17%.

If concomitant use of efavirenz and voriconazole is necessary, voriconazole maintenance dosage should be increased to 400 mg every 12 hours and efavirenz dosage decreased to 300 mg once daily. After voriconazole therapy is discontinued, the initial dosage of efavirenz should be restored.

Etravirine. Possible pharmacokinetic interaction with etravirine (substantially increased etravirine plasma concentrations, increased voriconazole plasma concentrations). Because of limited data regarding the safety of increased etravirine concentrations, the manufacturer of etravirine states that caution is advised when the drug is administered concomitantly with voriconazole.

Although dosage adjustment is not needed for either drug, some experts state that consideration should be given to monitoring plasma concentrations of voriconazole.

Nevirapine. Potential pharmacokinetic interaction with nevirapine (decreased voriconazole concentrations, increased nevirapine concentrations). Monitor patients for nevirapine toxicity and monitor clinical response to voriconazole and/or voriconazole plasma concentrations.

Rilpivirine. Potential pharmacokinetic interaction (increased rilpivirine concentrations, unknown effect on voriconazole concentrations). Rilpivirine dosage adjustments are not needed; however, patients should be monitored for breakthrough fungal infections.

■ **Barbiturates** Potential pharmacokinetic interaction (decreased plasma voriconazole concentrations) with long-acting barbiturates (e.g., phenobarbital, mephobarbital) and risk of prolonged sedative effects. Concomitant use of long-acting barbiturates and voriconazole is contraindicated.

■ **Benzodiazepines** Potential pharmacokinetic interaction (increased plasma benzodiazepine concentrations and AUC) with benzodiazepines that are metabolized by CYP3A4 isoenzyme (e.g., diazepam, midazolam, triazolam, alprazolam). Monitor patient for manifestations of benzodiazepine toxicity and adjust benzodiazepine dosage as necessary.

■ **Calcium-channel Blocking Agents** Potential pharmacokinetic interaction (increased plasma concentrations of calcium-channel blocker) with calcium-channel blocking agents that are metabolized by CYP3A4 isoenzyme (e.g., felodipine). Monitor patient for manifestations of calcium-channel blocker toxicity and adjust dosage of the calcium-channel blocker as necessary.

■ **Carbamazepine** Potential pharmacokinetic interaction (decreased plasma voriconazole concentrations) with carbamazepine. Concomitant use of carbamazepine and voriconazole is contraindicated.

■ **Cimetidine** Pharmacokinetic interaction (increased voriconazole concentrations and AUC) with cimetidine; not considered clinically important and dosage adjustments not needed.

■ **Clopidogrel** Possible pharmacokinetic interaction (decreased plasma concentrations of the active metabolite of clopidogrel) and reduced antiplatelet effects of clopidogrel.

Concomitant use of clopidogrel and CYP2C19 inhibitors should be avoided since clopidogrel is metabolized to its active metabolite by CYP2C19; in vitro studies indicate voriconazole inhibits CYP2C19.

■ **Coumarin Anticoagulants** Pharmacokinetic interaction (increased prothrombin time) with coumarin anticoagulant. Monitor prothrombin time or other appropriate tests closely if a coumarin anticoagulant (e.g., warfarin) is used concomitantly with voriconazole; reduction of anticoagulant dosage may be necessary.

■ **Digoxin** No clinically important pharmacokinetic interaction; no dosage adjustments needed.

■ **Ergot Alkaloids** Potential pharmacokinetic interaction (increased plasma concentrations of ergot alkaloid). Concomitant use of ergot alkaloids (e.g., ergotamine, dihydroergotamine) and voriconazole is contraindicated.

■ **Estrogens and Progestins** Pharmacokinetic interaction with oral contraceptives containing ethinyl estradiol and norethindrone (increased peak plasma concentrations and AUC of ethinyl estradiol and norethindrone; increased peak plasma concentrations and AUC of voriconazole).

The manufacturer of voriconazole states that this pharmacokinetic interaction is unlikely to affect efficacy of the oral contraceptive. If concomitant therapy is necessary, monitor for oral contraceptive-related and voriconazole-related adverse events.

■ **Fentanyl** Pharmacokinetic interaction with IV fentanyl (decreased mean plasma fentanyl clearance and increased fentanyl AUC). If voriconazole is used concomitantly with IV, oral, or transdermal fentanyl, extended and frequent monitoring for respiratory depression and other fentanyl-associated adverse effects is recommended and fentanyl dosage should be reduced if warranted.

■ **HCV Protease Inhibitors** ***Boceprevir*** Potential pharmacokinetic interaction with boceprevir (increased voriconazole plasma concentrations).

Telaprevir Potential pharmacokinetic interaction with telaprevir (altered voriconazole plasma concentrations, increased telaprevir plasma concentrations). Although clinically important changes in the QT interval corrected for rate (QT_c) have not been reported with telaprevir, QT interval prolongation and torsades de pointes have been reported with voriconazole.

Voriconazole should be used in patients receiving telaprevir only if potential benefits outweigh risks. If the drugs are used concomitantly, caution is warranted and patients should be monitored clinically.

■ **HMG-CoA Reductase Inhibitors** Potential pharmacokinetic interaction (increased plasma concentrations of antilipemic agent) with HMG-CoA reductase inhibitors (i.e., statins) that are metabolized by CYP3A4 isoenzyme (e.g., lovastatin). Monitor patient for toxicities associated with HMG-CoA reductase inhibitors and adjust dosage of the antilipemic agent as necessary.

■ **Immunosuppressive Agents** ***Cyclosporine*** Pharmacokinetic interaction (increased plasma concentrations and AUC of cyclosporine).

When initiating voriconazole therapy in patients currently receiving cyclosporine, dosage of cyclosporine should be reduced by 50%. When voriconazole is discontinued, plasma concentrations of cyclosporine should be monitored frequently and dosage of the immunosuppressive agent adjusted as necessary.

Sirolimus Pharmacokinetic interaction (increased plasma concentrations and AUC of sirolimus).

Concomitant use of sirolimus and voriconazole is contraindicated.

Tacrolimus Pharmacokinetic interaction (increased plasma concentrations of tacrolimus).

When initiating voriconazole therapy in patients currently receiving tacrolimus, dosage of tacrolimus should be reduced to 33% of the original dose; plasma concentrations of tacrolimus should be monitored frequently. When voriconazole is discontinued, plasma concentrations of tacrolimus should be monitored frequently and dosage of the immunosuppressive agent adjusted as necessary.

■ **Macrolides** Concomitant use of voriconazole and azithromycin or erythromycin does not have a clinically important effect on voriconazole pharmacokinetics; effects on macrolide pharmacokinetics are not known. Dosage adjustments not needed.

■ **Methadone** Pharmacokinetic interaction (increased AUC and peak plasma concentrations of pharmacologically active *R*-methadone) and risk of toxicity (e.g., QT prolongation). Monitor patient for manifestation of methadone toxicity; adjust methadone dosage if necessary.

■ **Mycophenolic Acid** No clinically important effect on pharmacokinetics of mycophenolic acid or its major metabolite (mycophenolic acid glucuronide); dosage adjustments not needed.

■ **Nonsteroidal Anti-inflammatory Agents** If voriconazole is used concomitantly with a nonsteroidal anti-inflammatory agent (NSAIA) that is metabolized by CYP2C9 (e.g., celecoxib, diclofenac, ibuprofen, naproxen, lornoxicam [not commercially available in the US], meloxicam), increased plasma concentrations of the NSAIA are possible. Patients receiving voriconazole concomitantly with an NSAIA should be monitored closely for NSAIA-related adverse effects and toxicity and dosage of the NSAIA reduced if warranted.

Diclofenac Pharmacokinetic interaction with diclofenac (114% increase in peak plasma diclofenac concentrations and 78% increase in diclofenac AUC). If voriconazole is used concomitantly, reduced dosage of diclofenac may be necessary; patients should be monitored closely for NSAIA-related adverse effects and toxicity.

Ibuprofen Pharmacokinetic interaction (20% increase in peak plasma concentrations and 100% increase in AUC of the pharmacologically active isomer of ibuprofen). If voriconazole is used concomitantly, reduced dosage of ibuprofen may be necessary; patients should be monitored closely for NSAIA-related adverse effects and toxicity.

■ **Oxycodone** Pharmacokinetic interaction (increased peak plasma concentration, AUC, and elimination half-life of oxycodone); increased oxycodone-associated adverse visual effects (heterophoria, miosis). If voriconazole is used concomitantly with oxycodone, extended and frequent monitoring for oxycodone-associated adverse effects is recommended and reduced oxycodone dosage may be necessary to avoid opiate-related adverse effects.

■ **Phenytoin** Pharmacokinetic interaction (substantially decreased plasma voriconazole concentrations) with voriconazole 200 mg every 12 hours. Increasing the voriconazole dosage to 400 mg every 12 hours in patients receiving concomitant phenytoin results in plasma voriconazole concentrations that are essentially the same as those in patients receiving usual dosages of voriconazole (200 mg every 12 hours) without phenytoin. Pharmacokinetic interaction (increased plasma phenytoin concentrations) with voriconazole 400 mg every 12 hours.

When phenytoin and voriconazole are used concomitantly, increase IV maintenance dosage of voriconazole to 5 mg/kg every 12 hours and increase oral maintenance dosage of the drug to 400 mg every 12 hours in patients weighing 40 kg or more or 200 mg every 12 hours in those weighing less than 40 kg. Plasma phenytoin concentrations should be monitored frequently and the patient observed for potential phenytoin adverse effects.

■ **Pimozide** Possible pharmacokinetic interaction and potential for serious or life-threatening reactions (e.g., cardiac arrhythmias). Concomitant use of pimozide and voriconazole is contraindicated.

■ **Prednisolone** Pharmacokinetic interaction (increased concentration and AUC of prednisolone); no dosage adjustments needed.

■ **Proton-pump Inhibitors** Pharmacokinetic interaction (substantially increased plasma omeprazole concentrations and AUC, clinically unimportant increases in plasma voriconazole concentrations, GI absorption of voriconazole not affected) with omeprazole. In patients currently receiving omeprazole in dosages of 40 mg or more daily, reduce omeprazole dosage by one-half when voriconazole therapy is initiated. Adjustment of voriconazole dosage not needed.

Potential increased plasma concentrations of other proton-pump inhibitors that are metabolized by CYP2C19 isoenzyme.

■ **Quinidine** Possible pharmacokinetic interaction and potential for serious or life-threatening reactions (e.g., cardiac arrhythmias). Concomitant use of quinidine and voriconazole is contraindicated.

■ **Ranitidine** No pharmacokinetic interaction with ranitidine; dosage adjustments not needed.

■ **Rifampin and Rifabutin** Pharmacokinetic interaction with rifampin (substantially decreased plasma voriconazole concentrations and AUC). Pharmacokinetic interaction with rifabutin (clinically important decreased plasma voriconazole concentrations and decreased AUC of voriconazole, substantially increased plasma rifabutin concentrations and AUC).

Concomitant use of rifampin or rifabutin and voriconazole is contraindicated.

■ **St. John's Wort** Pharmacokinetic interaction (59% decrease in mean voriconazole AUC) following multiple doses of St. John's wort (Hypericum perforatum); no clinically important effect on voriconazole AUC when a single dose of St. John's wort and a single dose of voriconazole are used concomitantly. Because long-term use of St. John's wort could result in decreased voriconazole exposure, concomitant use of voriconazole and St. John's wort is contraindicated.

■ **Sulfonylurea Antidiabetic Agents** Potential pharmacokinetic interaction (increased plasma concentrations of antidiabetic agent) with sulfonylurea antidiabetic agents (e.g., tolbutamide, glipizide, glyburide). Monitor blood glucose concentrations and monitor patient for signs and symptoms of hypoglycemia; adjust dosage of antidiabetic agent as necessary.

■ **Venlafaxine** Pharmacokinetic interaction (increased venlafaxine AUC); if used concomitantly, monitor for venlafaxine-associated toxicity.

■ **Vinca Alkaloids** Potential pharmacokinetic interaction (increased plasma concentrations of vinca alkaloid). Monitor patient for manifestations of vinca alkaloid toxicity (i.e., neurotoxicity) and adjust dosage as necessary.

■ **Zolpidem** Pharmacokinetic interaction (increased peak plasma concentration and AUC of zolpidem and prolonged zolpidem half-life); monitor for zolpidem-associated toxicity and adjust dosage as necessary.

Description

Voriconazole, a triazole antifungal agent, is a synthetic derivative of fluconazole. Like other azole antifungals, voriconazole presumably exerts its antifungal activity by altering cellular membranes, resulting in increased permeability, secondary metabolic effects, and growth inhibition. Although the exact mechanism of action of voriconazole has not been fully determined, the drug inhibits cytochrome P-450-dependent sterol 14-α-demethylase in susceptible fungi, which leads to accumulation of C-14-methylated sterols (e.g., lanosterol) and decreased concentrations of ergosterol.

Voriconazole is active in vitro against *Aspergillus*, including *A. fumigatus*, *A. flavus*, *A. niger*, and *A. terreus*, and *Candida*, including *C. albicans*, *C. dubliniensis*, *C. fumata*, *C. glabrata*, *C. guilliermondii*, *C. kefyr*, *C. krusei*, *C. lipolytica*, *C. lusitaniae*, *C. metapsilosis*, *C. orthopsilosis*, *C. parapsilosis*, *C. pelliculosa*, *C. rugosa*, and *C. tropicalis*. Voriconazole is active in vitro against *Exserohilum rostratum*. The drug has variable activity in vitro against *Fusarium* (including *F. solani*) and *Scedosporium apiospermum*. Voriconazole is active in vitro against *Cryptococcus neoformans* and *C. gattii*. Fungi with reduced susceptibility to other azoles (e.g., fluconazole, itraconazole) may also have reduced susceptibility to voriconazole.

The pharmacokinetics of voriconazole are similar following IV or oral administration. Absorption of the drug is rapid and almost complete (oral bioavailability of 96%) when given in the fasting state. Peak plasma voriconazole concentrations are achieved 1–2 hours following a dose. In adults, steady-state concentrations are achieved within 24 hours if a loading dose is administered or after 5–7 days if a loading dose is not administered. Loading doses do not appear to reduce the length of time required to reach steady-state in children 2 through 11 years of age† and appear to offer little benefit in this age group. (See Pediatric Use under Warnings/Precautions: Specific Populations, in Cautions.) Voriconazole exhibits nonlinear, dose-dependent pharmacokinetics, apparently because of saturable first-pass metabolism or systemic clearance. In vitro studies indicate that voriconazole is extensively metabolized in the liver by cytochrome P-450 (CYP) isoenzymes 2C9, 2C19, and 3A4. (See Drug Interactions: Drugs Affecting or Metabolized by Hepatic Microsomal Enzymes.) The drug is primarily eliminated by hepatic metabolism with less than 2% of a dose eliminated as unchanged drug in the urine.

Advice to Patients

Importance of taking oral voriconazole at least 1 hour before or 1 hour after meals.

Advise patients that tablets contain lactose and should not be used in patients with galactose intolerance, Lapp lactase deficiency, or glucose-galactose malabsorption and that the oral suspension contains sucrose and is not recommended for those with fructose intolerance, sucrase-isomaltase deficiency, or glucose-galactose malabsorption.

Possibility of visual changes, including blurred vision and photophobia. Avoid driving, operating machinery, or performing hazardous tasks if visual changes occur; importance of not driving at night while taking voriconazole.

Possibility of photosensitivity reactions; importance of avoiding exposure to strong, direct sunlight during voriconazole therapy.

Importance of informing clinicians if any of the following symptoms develop during voriconazole therapy: changes in heart rate or rhythm, chest tightness, itching, yellowing of skin or eyes, extreme fatigue or flu-like symptoms, nausea or vomiting, visual changes, loss of appetite, changes in thinking, difficulty breathing, or seizures.

Importance of informing clinicians and discontinuing voriconazole if serious skin reactions (e.g., rash, hives, mouth sores, blisters, peeling skin) occur.

Importance of informing clinicians of existing or contemplated concomitant therapy, including prescription and OTC drugs, and any concomitant illnesses (e.g., liver disease, heart disease).

Importance of women informing clinicians if they are or plan to become pregnant or to breast-feed. Importance of contraceptive measures during voriconazole therapy.

Importance of advising patients of other important precautionary information. (See Cautions.)

Overview® (see Users Guide). For additional information on this drug until a more detailed monograph is developed and published, the manufacturer's labeling should be consulted. It is *essential* that the manufacturer's labeling be consulted for more detailed information on usual cautions, precautions, contraindications, potential drug interactions, laboratory test interferences, and acute toxicity.

Preparations

Excipients in commercially available drug preparations may have clinically important effects in some individuals; consult specific product labeling for details.

Voriconazole

Oral		
For suspension	200 mg/5 mL*	**Vfend®**, Pfizer **Voriconazole for Suspension**
Tablets, film-coated	50 mg*	**Vfend®**, Pfizer **Voriconazole Tablets**
	200 mg*	**Vfend®**, Pfizer **Voriconazole Tablets**
Parenteral		
For injection, for IV infusion only	200 mg*	**Vfend®**, Pfizer **Voriconazole for Injection**

*available from one or more manufacturer, distributor, and/or repackager by generic (nonproprietary) name

†Use is not currently included in the labeling approved by the US Food and Drug Administration

ECHINOCANDINS 8:14.16

Anidulafungin

■ Anidulafungin is a semisynthetic, echinocandin antifungal agent.

Uses

■ **Candida Infections** ***Candidemia and Other Invasive Candida Infections*** Anidulafungin is used for the treatment of candidemia and certain other invasive *Candida* infections (intra-abdominal abscess, peritonitis). The manufacturer states that safety and efficacy of anidulafungin have not been established for the treatment of endocarditis, osteomyelitis, or meningitis caused by *Candida*. In addition, the manufacturer states that data are insufficient to date to evaluate efficacy of anidulafungin for the treatment of candidemia or other invasive *Candida* infections in neutropenic patients.

For the treatment of candidemia in *nonneutropenic* patients or for empiric treatment of suspected invasive candidiasis in *nonneutropenic* patients in intensive care units (ICUs), the Infectious Diseases Society of America (IDSA) recommends an IV echinocandin (anidulafungin, caspofungin, micafungin) for *initial* therapy. IDSA states that fluconazole (IV or oral) is an acceptable alternative for *initial* therapy in selected patients, including those who are not critically ill and are unlikely to have infections caused by fluconazole-resistant *Candida*. If echinocandin- and azole-resistant *Candida* are suspected, IV amphotericin B is recommended; IV amphotericin B also is a reasonable alternative when echinocandins and fluconazole cannot be used because of intolerance, limited availability, or resistance. IDSA states that transition from the echinocandin (or amphotericin B) to fluconazole can be considered (usually within 5–7 days) in patients who are clinically stable, have isolates susceptible to fluconazole (e.g., *C. albicans*), and have negative repeat blood cultures after initial antifungal treatment. Although fluconazole has been considered the drug of choice for the treatment of infections caused by *C. parapsilosis* in nonneutropenic patients (based in part on concerns related to decreased in vitro susceptibility and resistance to echinocandins), IDSA states that there are no clinical studies to date indicating superiority of fluconazole over echinocandins for the treatment of *C. parapsilosis* infections.

For the treatment of candidemia in *neutropenic* patients†, IDSA recommends an IV echinocandin (anidulafungin, caspofungin, micafungin) or, alternatively, IV amphotericin B for *initial* therapy. Fluconazole is an alternative for *initial* therapy in those who are not critically ill and have had no prior exposure to azole antifungals and also can be used for step-down therapy during neutropenia in clinically stable patients who have fluconazole-susceptible isolates and documented bloodstream clearance. Voriconazole can be used as an alternative for *initial* therapy when broader antifungal coverage is required and also can be used as step-down therapy during neutropenia in clinically stable patients who have voriconazole-susceptible isolates and documented bloodstream clearance. For infections known to be caused by *C. krusei*, an echinocandin, amphotericin B, or voriconazole is recommended.

For the treatment of osteoarticular infections† (e.g., osteomyelitis, septic arthritis) caused by *Candida*, IDSA recommends *initial* treatment with fluconazole or an IV echinocandin (anidulafungin, caspofungin, micafungin) and follow-up treatment with fluconazole. If septic arthritis involves a prosthetic device that cannot be removed, long-term suppressive or maintenance therapy (secondary prophylaxis) with fluconazole is recommended if the isolate is susceptible.

For the treatment of endocarditis† (native or prosthetic valve) or implantable cardiac device infections† caused by *Candida*, IDSA recommends *initial* treatment with IV amphotericin B (with or without oral flucytosine) or an IV echinocandin (anidulafungin, caspofungin, micafungin) and follow-up treatment with fluconazole. If the isolate is susceptible, long-term suppressive or maintenance therapy (secondary prophylaxis) with fluconazole is recommended to prevent recurrence in those with native valve endocarditis who cannot undergo valve replacement and in those with prosthetic valve endocarditis.

For additional information on management of candidemia and disseminated candidiasis, the current clinical practice guidelines from IDSA available at http://www.idsociety.org should be consulted.

Clinical Experience. Safety and efficacy of anidulafungin for the treatment of candidemia or other forms of invasive candidiasis were evaluated in a phase 3, randomized, double-blind study in adults (97% were nonneutropenic, 61.6% had *C. albicans* infections). Patients were randomized to receive initial therapy with either IV anidulafungin (200-mg loading dose followed by 100 mg once daily) or IV fluconazole (800-mg loading dose followed by 400 mg once daily). After a minimum of 10 days of IV therapy, patients in both treatment groups were permitted to switch to oral fluconazole if they were afebrile for at least 24 hours, had blood cultures negative for *Candida*, and were able to tolerate oral therapy. The total duration of antifungal treatment was at least 14 days (maximum 42 days); 26% of those receiving IV anidulafungin and 28% of those receiving IV fluconazole switched to oral fluconazole. When data analysis was done using the modified intent-to-treat population, a successful global response consisting of clinical cure or improvement (defined as substantial but incomplete resolution of signs and symptoms of *Candida* infection without additional antifungal treatment) with documented or presumed microbiological eradication was observed in 74% of those in the anidulafungin group (median duration of 14 days of IV anidulafungin and 7 days of oral fluconazole) and in 56.8% of those in the fluconazole group (median duration of 11 days of IV fluconazole and 5 days of oral fluconazole). At 2 or 6 weeks posttreatment, a successful global response was maintained in 64.6 or 55.9%, respectively, of patients randomized to anidulafungin and 49.2 or 44.1%, respectively, of patients randomized to fluconazole.

Esophageal Candidiasis Anidulafungin is used for the treatment of esophageal candidiasis.

Esophageal candidiasis requires treatment with a systemic antifungal (not a topical antifungal).

IDSA recommends oral fluconazole as the preferred drug of choice for the treatment of esophageal candidiasis; if oral therapy is not tolerated, IV fluconazole or an IV echinocandin (anidulafungin, caspofungin, micafungin) usually is recommended and IV amphotericin B is another alternative. For fluconazole-refractory esophageal candidiasis, IDSA recommends itraconazole oral solution or oral or IV voriconazole; alternatives for fluconazole-refractory disease are IV echinocandins (anidulafungin, caspofungin, micafungin) or IV amphotericin B. IDSA states that oral posaconazole (oral suspension or delayed-release tablets) could be considered another alternative for the treatment of fluconazole-refractory esophageal candidiasis.

For the treatment of esophageal candidiasis in adults and adolescents with human immunodeficiency virus (HIV) infection, the Centers for Disease Control and Prevention (CDC), National Institutes of Health (NIH), and IDSA recommend IV or oral fluconazole or itraconazole oral solution. Alternatives include oral or IV voriconazole, an IV echinocandin (anidulafungin, caspofungin, micafungin), or IV amphotericin B. For refractory esophageal candidiasis in HIV-infected adults and adolescents, including fluconazole-refractory infections, these experts recommend posaconazole oral suspension or itraconazole oral solution; alternatives include an IV echinocandin (anidulafungin, caspofungin, micafungin), oral or IV voriconazole, or IV amphotericin B. Although data are limited, some experts state that an IV echinocandin (anidulafungin, caspofungin, micafungin) can be considered an alternative for the treatment of azole-refractory esophageal candidiasis in HIV-infected children†.

Routine long-term suppressive or maintenance therapy (secondary prophylaxis) to prevent relapse or recurrence is not usually recommended in patients adequately treated for esophageal candidiasis (including HIV-infected individuals) unless the patient has frequent or severe recurrences of esophageal candidiasis. If secondary prophylaxis of esophageal candidiasis is indicated, oral fluconazole or posaconazole oral suspension is recommended; however, the potential for development of azole resistance should be considered.

For additional information on management of esophageal candidiasis, the current clinical practice guidelines from IDSA available at http://www.idsociety.org and the current clinical practice guidelines from CDC, NIH, and IDSA on the prevention and treatment of opportunistic infections in HIV-infected individuals available at http://www.aidsinfo.nih.gov should be consulted.

Clinical Experience. There is some evidence that IV anidulafungin may be at least as effective as oral fluconazole for the treatment of esophageal candidiasis, but further study is needed since there also is some evidence that the relapse rate may be higher with anidulafungin.

In a phase 3, randomized, double-blind study designed to establish noninferiority of anidulafungin for the treatment of endoscopically and microbiologically confirmed esophageal candidiasis, adults received either IV anidulafungin (100-mg loading dose followed by 50 mg once daily) or oral fluconazole (200-mg loading dose followed by 100 mg once daily). Most patients who were tested for HIV were HIV-positive (85%) and most patients with culture-confirmed esophageal candidiasis had *C. albicans* infections (91%). Treatment groups were similar in demographic and other baseline characteristics. In the group of anidulafungin-treated patients, the age range was 16–69 years, the gender distribution was 42% male and 58% female, and the race distribution was 15% white, 49% black/African American, 15% Asian, 0.3% Hispanic, and 21% other races. Antifungal treatment was continued for 7 days after resolution of clinical symptoms (minimum duration of 14 days, maximum duration of 21 days). Efficacy was assessed by endoscopic examination at the end of treatment, and endoscopic success (cure or improvement) was similar following treatment with IV anidulafungin (97.4%) or oral fluconazole (98.7%); however, at 2 weeks posttreatment, the relapse rate based on recurrence of endoscopic lesions was higher with IV anidulafungin (53.3%) than with oral fluconazole (19.3%).

Oropharyngeal Candidiasis Anidulafungin is used as an alternative for the treatment of oropharyngeal candidiasis†.

For the treatment of mild oropharyngeal candidiasis, IDSA recommends topical treatment with clotrimazole lozenges or miconazole buccal tablets; nystatin (oral suspension or tablets) is the recommended alternative. For moderate to severe disease, IDSA recommends oral fluconazole. For fluconazole-refractory oropharyngeal candidiasis, IDSA recommends itraconazole oral solution or posaconazole oral suspension; oral voriconazole or amphotericin B oral suspension (not commercially available in the US) are recommended as alternatives. Other alternatives for refractory oropharyngeal candidiasis are an IV echinocandin (anidulafungin, caspofungin, micafungin) or IV amphotericin B.

For the treatment of oropharyngeal candidiasis in HIV-infected adults and adolescents, CDC, NIH, and IDSA recommend oral fluconazole as the preferred drug of choice for initial episodes. If topical therapy is used for the treatment of oropharyngeal candidiasis (e.g., mild to moderate episodes), these experts recommend clotrimazole lozenges or miconazole buccal tablets. Alternatives for systemic treatment of oropharyngeal candidiasis in HIV-infected adults and adolescents are itraconazole oral solution or posaconazole oral suspension; nystatin oral suspension is an alternative if topical treatment is used. For fluconazole-refractory oropharyngeal infections in HIV-infected adults and adolescents, posaconazole oral suspension is preferred; itraconazole oral solution is an alternative.

Routine long-term suppressive or maintenance therapy (secondary prophylaxis) to prevent relapse or recurrence is not usually recommended in patients adequately treated for oropharyngeal candidiasis (including HIV-infected individuals) unless the patient has frequent or severe recurrences of oropharyngeal candidiasis. If secondary prophylaxis of oropharyngeal candidiasis is indicated, oral fluconazole is recommended; however, the potential for development of azole resistance should be considered.

For additional information on management of oropharyngeal candidiasis, the current clinical practice guidelines from IDSA available at http://www.idsociety.org and the current clinical practice guidelines from CDC, NIH, and IDSA on the prevention and treatment of opportunistic infections in HIV-infected individuals available at http://www.aidsinfo.nih.gov should be consulted.

Clinical Experience. Efficacy of anidulafungin in the treatment of oropharyngeal candidiasis† was evaluated in a limited open-label, noncomparative study in 19 adults with confirmed azole-refractory oropharyngeal and/or esophageal candidiasis who received IV anidulafungin (100-mg loading dose on day 1 followed by 50 mg once daily) alone for 13–21 days. A total of 18 patients completed the study and were included in the modified intention to treat analysis. An overall clinical response was achieved in 94% of patients with oropharyngeal candidiasis; 61% (11/18) were considered cured and 33% (6/18) demonstrated improvement. At the follow-up visit 10–14 days after study completion, clinical success was maintained in 44% (8/18) of patients treated for oropharyngeal candidiasis. In one HIV-infected patient who had multiple prior episodes of oropharyngeal candidiasis and 2 prior episodes of esophageal candidiasis, treatment was considered a clinical and endoscopic failure.

Candida auris Infections Anidulafungin is used for the treatment of infections caused by *C. auris*, an emerging pathogen that has been associated with potentially fatal candidemia or other invasive infections.

C. auris, first identified in 2009, has now been reported as the cause of serious invasive infections (including fatalities) in multiple countries worldwide (e.g., Japan, South Korea, India, Kuwait, South Africa, Pakistan, United Kingdom, Venezuela, Colombia, US). As of May 2017, a total of 77 clinical cases of *C. auris* had been reported to CDC from 7 different states in the US. *C. auris* may be difficult to identify using standard in vitro methods and has been misidentified as *C. haemulonii*, *C. famata*, or *Rhodotorula glutinis*. A large percentage of *C. auris* clinical isolates are resistant to fluconazole and multidrug-resistant isolates with reduced susceptibility or resistance to all 3 major classes of antifungal agents (azoles, polyenes, echinocandins) have been reported.

Pending further accumulation of data, CDC has issued interim recommendations regarding laboratory diagnosis, treatment, and infection control measures for suspected or known *C. auris* infections. Based on limited data available to date, CDC recommends that an IV echinocandin (anidulafungin, caspofungin, micafungin) be used for initial treatment of invasive *C. auris* infections (e.g., bloodstream or intra-abdominal infections) in adults. CDC states that a switch to IV amphotericin B (lipid formulation) could be considered if the patient is clinically unresponsive to the echinocandin or fungemia persists longer than 5 days. Consultation with an infectious disease specialist is highly recommended.

Unless there is evidence of infection, CDC does not currently recommend antifungal treatment when *C. auris* is isolated only from noninvasive body sites (e.g., urine, external ear, wounds, respiratory secretions). Some individuals are colonized with *C. auris* in the axilla, groin, nose, external ear canal, oropharynx, urine, wounds, rectum, and stool; however, data are limited and the duration of *C. auris* colonization is unclear. Therefore, CDC recommends that infection control measures be observed for all patients with cultures yielding *C. auris*, including those with positive cultures only from noninvasive body sites.

Whenever *C. auris* infection is suspected, clinicians should immediately contact state or local public health authorities and the CDC (candidaauris@cdc.gov) for guidance. For additional information on diagnosis and management of *C. auris* infections, the interim recommendations and most recent information from CDC available at https://www.cdc.gov/fungal/diseases/candidiasis/candida-auris.html should be consulted.

■ **Aspergillosis** Safety and efficacy of anidulafungin for the treatment of invasive aspergillosis† have not been established, and only limited data are available regarding use of the drug for the treatment of such infections.

IDSA and other clinicians consider IV voriconazole the drug of choice for primary treatment of invasive aspergillosis in adult and pediatric patients, including those with HIV infection; IV amphotericin B or isavuconazonium sulfate (prodrug of isavuconazole) is usually recommended as an alternative for primary treatment. For salvage therapy in patients refractory to or intolerant of primary antifungal therapy, IDSA recommends IV amphotericin B, an IV echinocandin (caspofungin, micafungin), oral or IV posaconazole, or itraconazole oral suspension. IDSA states that echinocandins (either alone or in conjunction with other antifungals) may be effective for salvage therapy of invasive aspergillosis; however, routine use of echinocandin monotherapy is not recommended for primary treatment of invasive aspergillosis.

For additional information on management of aspergillosis, the current clinical practice guidelines from IDSA available at http://www.idsociety.org and the current clinical practice guidelines from CDC, NIH, and IDSA on the prevention and treatment of opportunistic infections in HIV-infected individuals available at http://www.aidsinfo.nih.gov should be consulted.

Dosage and Administration

■ **Administration** Anidulafungin is administered by slow IV infusion. The drug should *not* be given by rapid IV injection.

IV Infusion Anidulafungin should not be admixed or infused concomitantly with other drugs.

Strict aseptic technique should be observed when preparing anidulafungin solutions, since the drug contains no preservatives. Anidulafungin solutions should be inspected visually for particulate matter and discoloration and should not be used if discolored or if particulates are present.

Reconstitution and Dilution. Commercially available anidulafungin lyophilized powder for injection must be reconstituted and then further diluted prior to IV infusion.

Based on the indicated anidulafungin dosage, the appropriate number of vials labeled as containing 50 or 100 mg of anidulafungin should be reconstituted with 15 or 30 mL, respectively, of sterile water for injection to provide a solution containing 3.33 mg/mL.

The contents of the appropriate number of reconstituted vials should then be diluted in 50, 100, or 200 mL of 5% dextrose injection or 0.9% sodium chloride injection to provide an IV infusion solution containing 0.77 mg/mL. (See Table 1.)

Table 1. Instructions for Diluting Reconstituted Vials of Anidulafungin

Anidulafungin Dose Indicated	Number of Reconstituted Vials Required	Required Volume of Diluent (5% Dextrose Injection or 0.9% Sodium Chloride Injection)	Total Infusion Volume of 0.77-mg/mL Solution	Minimum Duration of Infusion (minutes)
50 mg	One 50-mg vial	50 mL	65 mL	45
100 mg	Two 50-mg vials or one 100-mg vial	100 mL	130 mL	90
200 mg	Four 50-mg vials or two 100-mg vials	200 mL	260 mL	180

Vials of lyophilized anidulafungin should be stored at 2–8°C, but may be exposed to temperatures up to 25°C for 96 hours and then returned to 2–8°C; the vials should not be frozen. Following reconstitution, anidulafungin solutions may be stored at temperatures up to 25°C for up to 24 hours. Reconstituted anidulafungin solutions that have been further diluted in 5% dextrose injection or 0.9% sodium chloride injection to a concentration of 0.77 mg/mL may be stored at temperatures up to 25°C for up to 48 hours or, alternatively, may be stored frozen for at least 72 hours.

Rate of Administration. IV infusions of anidulafungin should be given at a rate not exceeding 1.1 mg/minute (1.4 mL/minute). More rapid infusion may increase the risk of a histamine-mediated reaction. (See Sensitivity Reactions under Cautions: Warnings/Precautions.)

■ Dosage

Adult Dosage

Candidemia and Other Invasive Candida Infections. The recommended dosage of anidulafungin for the treatment of candidemia and certain other invasive *Candida* infections (intra-abdominal abscess, peritonitis) in *nonneutropenic* adults or *neutropenic*† adults is a single 200-mg loading dose on day 1, followed by 100 mg once daily.

When anidulafungin is used for initial treatment of candidemia or other invasive *Candida* infections, the Infectious Diseases Society of America (IDSA) states that a transition from the echinocandin to fluconazole can be considered (usually within 5–7 days) in patients who are clinically stable, have isolates susceptible to fluconazole (e.g., *C. albicans*), and have negative repeat blood cultures after initial antifungal treatment.

The duration of treatment should be based on the clinical response of the patient. The manufacturer recommends that anidulafungin therapy in patients with candidemia or other invasive *Candida* infections should be continued for at least 14 days after the last positive culture. IDSA recommends that antifungal treatment for candidemia (without persistent fungemia or metastatic complications) be continued for 2 weeks after documented clearance of *Candida* from the bloodstream, resolution of candidemia symptoms, and resolution of neutropenia.

If anidulafungin is used for *initial* treatment of osteoarticular infections† (e.g., osteomyelitis, septic arthritis) caused by *Candida*, IDSA recommends a dosage of 100 mg once daily in adults. After at least 2 weeks, treatment can be switched to fluconazole.

If anidulafungin is used for *initial* treatment of endocarditis† (native or prosthetic valve) or implantable cardiac device infections† caused by *Candida*, IDSA recommends a dosage of 200 mg once daily in adults. If the infection is caused by fluconazole-susceptible *Candida*, treatment can be switched to fluconazole after the patient is stabilized and *Candida* has been cleared from the bloodstream.

Esophageal Candidiasis. For the treatment of esophageal candidiasis in adults, the manufacturer recommends that a single 100-mg loading dose of anidulafungin be given on day 1, followed by 50 mg once daily.

If anidulafungin is used for the treatment of esophageal candidiasis, including fluconazole-refractory disease (see Esophageal Candidiasis under Uses: Candida Infections), IDSA recommends that adults receive anidulafungin in a dosage of 200 mg once daily.

If anidulafungin is used for the treatment of esophageal candidiasis in adults with human immunodeficiency virus (HIV) infection, the US Centers for Disease Control and Prevention (CDC), National Institutes of Health (NIH), and IDSA recommend a single 100-mg loading dose of anidulafungin on day 1, followed by 50 mg once daily.

The duration of treatment should be based on the clinical response of the patient. The manufacturer states that anidulafungin therapy in patients with esophageal candidiasis should be continued for at least 14 days and for at least 7 days following resolution of symptoms. CDC, NIH, and IDSA recommend that antifungal treatment of esophageal candidiasis be continued for 14–21 days.

Oropharyngeal Candidiasis. If anidulafungin is used for the treatment of oropharyngeal candidiasis†, IDSA recommends that adults receive a single 200-mg loading dose on day 1, followed by 100 mg once daily for 7–14 days.

Candida auris Infections. If anidulafungin is used for initial treatment of invasive *C. auris* infections (e.g., bloodstream or intra-abdominal infections), CDC recommends that adults receive a single 200-mg loading dose, followed by 100 mg once daily.

Aspergillosis. If anidulafungin is used for the treatment of invasive aspergillosis†, some experts recommend that adults receive a single 200-mg loading dose, followed by 100 mg daily.

The duration of treatment is based on the degree and duration of immunosuppression, disease site, and clinical response. IDSA recommends that antifungal treatment of invasive pulmonary aspergillosis be continued for at least 6–12 weeks.

Pediatric Dosage

General Dosing for Pediatric Patients. If anidulafungin is used in children†, the American Academy of Pediatrics (AAP) recommends a loading dose of 1.5–3 mg/kg, followed by 0.75–1.5 mg/kg once daily.

Candidemia and Other Invasive Candida Infections. If anidulafungin is used as for the treatment of invasive candidiasis in HIV-infected children 2 years of age or older†, some experts recommend an initial loading dose of 3 mg/kg on day 1, followed by 1.5 mg/kg once daily.

IDSA recommends that antifungal treatment for candidemia (without persistent fungemia or metastatic complications) be continued for 2 weeks after documented clearance of *Candida* from the bloodstream, resolution of candidemia symptoms, and resolution of neutropenia.

Esophageal Candidiasis. If anidulafungin is used as an alternative for the treatment of esophageal candidiasis in HIV-infected children 2 years of age or older†, some experts recommend an initial loading dose of 3 mg/kg on day 1, followed by 1.5 mg/kg (up to 100 mg) once daily.

For the treatment of esophageal candidiasis in HIV-infected adolescents†, CDC, NIH, and IDSA recommend a single 100-mg loading dose of anidulafungin on day 1, followed by 50 mg once daily.

CDC, NIH, and IDSA recommend that antifungal treatment of esophageal candidiasis be continued for 14–21 days.

■ Special Populations

Hepatic Impairment

Dosage adjustments are not necessary in patients with hepatic impairment (Child-Pugh class A, B, or C).

Renal Impairment

Dosage adjustments are not necessary in patients with renal impairment (including those receiving hemodialysis).

Because anidulafungin is not dialyzable, the drug may be administered without regard to the timing of hemodialysis.

Geriatric Patients

Dosage adjustments are not necessary in patients 65 years of age or older.

Cautions

■ Contraindications

Anidulafungin is contraindicated in patients with known hypersensitivity to the drug, other echinocandin antifungals (e.g., caspofungin, micafungin), or any ingredient in the formulation.

■ Warnings/Precautions

Sensitivity Reactions

Hypersensitivity Reactions. Anaphylactic reactions, including anaphylactic shock, have been reported in patients receiving anidulafungin. If such reactions occur, the drug should be discontinued and appropriate treatment administered.

Possible histamine-mediated symptoms (e.g., rash, urticaria, flushing, pruritus, dyspnea, hypotension) have occurred in patients receiving anidulafungin. These symptoms are infrequent when the infusion rate does not exceed 1.1 mg/minute.

Infusion-related adverse reactions (e.g., rash, urticaria, flushing, pruritus, bronchospasm, dyspnea, hypotension) have occurred in patients receiving anidulafungin and possibly may be histamine-mediated reactions. To reduce the occurrence of infusion-related adverse reactions, the infusion rate should not exceed 1.1 mg/minute.

Hepatic Effects

Abnormal liver function test results have been reported in healthy individuals and patients receiving anidulafungin. Hepatic abnormalities, including hepatic dysfunction, hepatitis, or worsening hepatic failure, have been reported in patients with serious underlying conditions receiving anidulafungin and multiple other drugs. A causal relationship to anidulafungin has not been established to date.

If abnormal liver function test results occur during anidulafungin therapy, the patient should be monitored for evidence of worsening hepatic function and the risks of continued anidulafungin therapy should be weighed against potential benefits.

Selection and Use of Antifungals

Prior to initiation of anidulafungin therapy, appropriate specimens for fungal cultures and other relevant laboratory studies (e.g., histopathology) should be obtained to isolate and identify causative organisms. The drug may be started pending availability of results, but antifungal therapy should be adjusted as needed when results become available.

Specific Populations

Pregnancy. Category B. (See Users Guide.)

There are no adequate and well-controlled studies of anidulafungin in pregnant women, and the manufacturer states that the drug should be used during pregnancy only if clearly needed.

In rats, anidulafungin crosses the placenta, is detected in fetal plasma, and has been associated with incomplete ossification of several bones.

Lactation. Anidulafungin is distributed into milk in rats; it is not known whether the drug is distributed into milk in humans.

Anidulafungin should be used with caution in nursing women.

Pediatric Use. Safety and efficacy of anidulafungin have not been established in pediatric patients 16 years of age or younger.

Anidulafungin has been used in a limited number of neutropenic children 2–17 years of age† without unusual adverse effects.

Although data are limited, some experts state that anidulafungin can be considered for first-line treatment of invasive candidiasis or for alternative treatment of esophageal candidiasis in children 2–17 years of age† with human immunodeficiency virus (HIV) infection.

Geriatric Use. Of the total number of patients treated with anidulafungin in clinical trials, 35% were 65 years of age or older and 18% were 75 years of age and older. Although no overall differences in safety and efficacy were observed between geriatric adults 65 years of age or older and younger adults in clinical trials and other clinical experience has not revealed any evidence of age-related differences, the possibility that some older patients may have increased sensitivity to the drug cannot be ruled out.

Dosage adjustments are not necessary when anidulafungin is used in geriatric patients.

Hepatic Impairment. Anidulafungin pharmacokinetics are not altered in adults with mild, moderate, or severe hepatic impairment (Child-Pugh class A, B, or C). Although the area under the concentration-time curve (AUC) of anidulafungin may be slightly decreased in those with Child-Pugh class C hepatic impairment, this is not considered clinically important.

Dosage adjustments are not necessary if anidulafungin is used in adults with mild, moderate, or severe hepatic impairment.

Renal Impairment. Anidulafungin pharmacokinetics are not altered in adults with mild, moderate, or severe renal impairment.

Dosage adjustments are not necessary if anidulafungin is used in adults with mild, moderate, or severe renal impairment.

■ **Common Adverse Effects** Adverse effects reported in 5% or more of patients receiving anidulafungin include GI effects (nausea, diarrhea, vomiting, dyspepsia), phlebitis/thrombophlebitis, hypokalemia, increased ALT, increased alkaline phosphatase, increased γ-glutamyltransferase (GGT, γ-glutamyl transpeptidase, GGPT), pyrexia, headache, rash, insomnia, anemia, and neutropenia.

Drug Interactions

■ **Drugs Affecting or Metabolized by Hepatic Microsomal Enzymes** Pharmacokinetic interactions unlikely. In vitro studies indicate that anidulafungin does not inhibit cytochrome P-450 (CYP) isoenzymes 1A2, 2B6, 2C8, 2C9, 2C19, 2D6, or 3A at clinically relevant concentrations. Anidulafungin is not a clinically important substrate, inducer, or inhibitor of CYP isoenzymes.

■ **Drugs Affecting or Affected by P-glycoprotein Transport** Anidulafungin is not an inhibitor or substrate of the P-glycoprotein transport system; pharmacokinetic interactions unlikely.

■ **Antifungal Agents** ***Amphotericin B*** No clinically important pharmacokinetic interactions if IV amphotericin B liposomal (AmBisome®) is used concomitantly with IV anidulafungin. Dosage of anidulafungin does not need to be adjusted if the drug is used concomitantly with IV amphotericin B liposomal.

In vitro, the antifungal effects of anidulafungin and amphotericin B usually have been additive against *Candida*, including *C. albicans*, *C. glabrata*, *C. krusei*, *C. parapsilosis*, and *C. tropicalis*. Although the combination usually has been indifferent against *Aspergillus* or *Fusarium*, antagonism occurred against some strains of *A. flavus* and *A. terreus* and synergism occurred against some strains of *A. fumigatus*. Clinical importance of these in vitro studies is unclear.

Fluconazole In vitro, the antifungal effects of anidulafungin and fluconazole have been additive or indifferent against *C. albicans* and *C. glabrata* and indifferent against *C. krusei*, *C. parapsilosis*, and *C. tropicalis*. Clinical importance of these in vitro studies is unclear.

Flucytosine In vitro, the antifungal effects of anidulafungin and flucytosine have been additive or indifferent against *C. albicans*, *C. glabrata*, *C. krusei*, *C. parapsilosis*, and *C. tropicalis*. Clinical importance of these in vitro studies is unclear.

Itraconazole In vitro, the antifungal effects of anidulafungin and itraconazole have been additive or indifferent against *Candida*, including *C. albicans*, *C. glabrata*, *C. krusei*, *C. parapsilosis*, and *C. tropicalis*. Although the antifungal effects of anidulafungin and itraconazole usually have been synergistic or indifferent against *Aspergillus*, the combination has been indifferent against *Fusarium*. Clinical importance of these in vitro studies is unclear.

Ketoconazole In vitro, the antifungal effects of anidulafungin and ketoconazole have been additive or indifferent against *C. albicans*, *C. glabrata*, *C. krusei*, and *C. parapsilosis*, but have been antagonistic against *C. tropicalis*. Clinical importance of these in vitro studies is unclear.

Voriconazole No clinically important pharmacokinetic interactions were reported when oral voriconazole was used concomitantly with IV anidulafungin in healthy adults.

If voriconazole and anidulafungin are used concomitantly, dosage adjustment not necessary for either drug.

■ **Immunosuppressive Agents** ***Cyclosporine*** Pharmacokinetic interaction with cyclosporine (22% increase in steady-state area under the concentration-time curve [AUC] of anidulafungin; no clinically important effect on steady-state peak anidulafungin plasma concentrations). Results of an in vitro study indicate that anidulafungin has no effect on cyclosporine metabolism.

If cyclosporine and anidulafungin are used concomitantly, dosage adjustments are not necessary for either drug.

Tacrolimus No clinically important pharmacokinetic interactions were reported when oral tacrolimus was used concomitantly with IV anidulafungin in healthy adults.

If tacrolimus and anidulafungin are used concomitantly, dosage adjustments are not necessary for either drug.

■ **Rifampin** No clinically important pharmacokinetic interactions when rifampin is used concomitantly with IV anidulafungin.

Dosage of anidulafungin does not need to be adjusted if the drug is used concomitantly with rifampin.

Description

Anidulafungin, a semisynthetic lipopeptide synthesized from a fermentation product of *Aspergillus nidulans*, is an echinocandin antifungal agent. Echinocandins (e.g., anidulafungin, caspofungin, micafungin) are glucan synthesis inhibitors and differ structurally and pharmacologically from other currently available antifungal agents.

Like other echinocandins, anidulafungin inhibits the synthesis of β(1,3)-D-glucan, an integral component of the fungal cell wall that is not present in mammalian cells. The drug may be fungistatic and fungicidal in action.

Anidulafungin undergoes slow chemical degradation at physiologic temperature and pH to a ring-opened peptide that lacks antifungal activity. The drug does not appear to undergo hepatic metabolism. Anidulafungin is not a clinically important substrate for and does not inhibit or induce cytochrome P-450 (CYP) isoenzymes and does not appear to have clinically important effects on the metabolism of drugs metabolized by these hepatic isoenzymes. The drug is more than 99% bound to plasma proteins. The elimination half-life of anidulafungin at steady state is approximately 27–52 hours. Steady-state concentrations are achieved within 24 hours of administration of the initial loading dose (twice the daily maintenance dosage); the estimated plasma accumulation factor during steady state is approximately 2. Anidulafungin is eliminated principally in feces via the biliary tract, mostly as degradation products of the drug. In healthy individuals, about 30% of a single IV dose of radiolabeled anidulafungin was recovered in feces over 9 days (less than 10% was unchanged drug); less than 1% of the dose is eliminated in urine.

■ **Spectrum** Anidulafungin is active in vitro against many *Candida*, including *C. albicans*, *C. dubliniensis*, *C. glabrata*, *C. guilliermondii*, *C. keyfri*, *C. krusei*, *C. lusitaniae*, *C. metapsilosis*, *C. orthopsilosis*, *C. parapsilosis*, and *C. tropicalis*. The drug has been active against some fluconazole-resistant strains of *C. albicans*, *C. glabrata*, and *C. krusei*.

Clinical isolates of *C. auris* (often misidentified as *C. haemulonii*, *C. famata*, or *Rhodotorula glutinis*) generally have been inhibited in vitro by anidulafungin concentrations of 0.125–1 mcg/mL.

Anidulafungin has in vitro activity against *Aspergillus*, including *A. flavus*, *A. fumigatus*, *A. niger*, and *A. terreus*.

Like other echinocandins, anidulafungin is not active against *Cryptococcus neoformans*, *Trichosporon*, *Fusarium*, or zygomycetes.

■ **Resistance** Although the clinical importance is unclear, *Candida* (e.g., *C. glabrata*) with reduced susceptibility to echinocandins have been reported. Some clinical isolates of *C. auris* have reduced susceptibility or resistance to anidulafungin in vitro (i.e., MICs 4 mcg/mL or greater).

Resistance to echinocandins usually is due to point mutations within the genes (FKS1 and FKS2) encoding for subunits in the glucan synthase enzyme complex.

The potential for development of resistance to anidulafungin or for cross-resistance with other echinocandins (caspofungin, micafungin) is not known. Anidulafungin has been active against some strains of *C. glabrata* resistant to caspofungin and *C. parapsilosis* resistant to caspofungin and micafungin.

Advice to Patients

Inform patients about the risk of developing abnormal liver function tests and/or hepatic dysfunction. Advise patients that liver function tests may be monitored during anidulafungin treatment.

Inform patients that anaphylactic reactions, including shock, have been reported in patients receiving anidulafungin. Advise patients that the drug may be discontinued and appropriate treatment administered if such reactions occur.

Inform patients that infusion-related adverse reactions, possibly histamine mediated, may occur and advise them of the importance of reporting symptoms (e.g., rash, urticaria, flushing, pruritus, dyspnea, hypotension) to their clinician.

Importance of informing clinicians of existing or contemplated concomitant therapy, including prescription and OTC drugs, and any concomitant illnesses.

Importance of women informing clinicians if they are or plan to become pregnant or plan to breast-feed.

Importance of informing patients of other important precautionary information. (See Cautions.)

Overview® (see Users Guide). For additional information on this drug until a more detailed monograph is developed and published, the manufacturer's labeling should be consulted. It is *essential* that the manufacturer's labeling be consulted for more detailed information on usual cautions, precautions, contraindications, potential drug interactions, laboratory test interferences, and acute toxicity.

Preparations

Excipients in commercially available drug preparations may have clinically important effects in some individuals; consult specific product labeling for details.

Anidulafungin

Parenteral		
For injection, for IV infusion	50 mg	Eraxis®, Pfizer
	100 mg	Eraxis®, Pfizer

†Use is not currently included in the labeling approved by the US Food and Drug Administration

Caspofungin Acetate

■ Caspofungin acetate is a semisynthetic, echinocandin antifungal agent.

Uses

■ **Aspergillosis** Caspofungin acetate is used for the treatment of invasive aspergillosis in adults, adolescents, and children 3 months of age and older whose disease is refractory to, or who are intolerant of, other antifungal agents. The drug has not been evaluated for initial therapy of invasive aspergillosis.

The Infectious Diseases Society of America (IDSA) and other clinicians consider IV voriconazole the drug of choice for primary treatment of invasive aspergillosis in adult and pediatric patients, including those with human immunodeficiency virus (HIV) infection; IV amphotericin B or isavuconazonium sulfate (prodrug of isavuconazole) is usually recommended as an alternative for primary treatment. For salvage therapy in patients refractory to or intolerant of primary antifungal therapy, IDSA recommends IV amphotericin B, an IV echinocandin (caspofungin, micafungin), oral or IV posaconazole, or itraconazole oral suspension. IDSA states that echinocandins (either alone or in conjunction with other antifungals) may be effective for salvage therapy of invasive aspergillosis; however, routine use of echinocandin monotherapy is not recommended for primary treatment of invasive aspergillosis.

For additional information on management of aspergillosis, the current clinical practice guidelines from IDSA available at http://www.idsociety.org and the current clinical practice guidelines from the Centers for Disease Control and Prevention (CDC), National Institutes of Health (NIH), and IDSA on the prevention and treatment of opportunistic infections in HIV-infected individuals available at http://www.aidsinfo.nih.gov should be consulted.

Clinical Experience Safety and efficacy of caspofungin for the treatment of invasive aspergillosis in adults whose disease is refractory to, or who are intolerant of, other antifungal agents (i.e., conventional amphotericin B, lipid-based amphotericin B, itraconazole) have been evaluated in an open-label, noncomparative study in 69 adults 18–80 years of age with definite or probable invasive aspergillosis who received a 70-mg loading dose followed by 50 mg once daily for a mean duration of 33.7 days (range: 1–162 days). Study patients consisted of those with infections categorized as refractory (i.e., disease progression or no improvement despite at least 7 days of therapy with amphotericin B [conventional or lipid-based formulation], itraconazole, or an investigational azole antifungal with activity against *Aspergillus*) or those who were intolerant of other antifungals (i.e., previous therapy associated with doubling of serum creatinine concentration or serum creatinine 2.5 mg/dL or greater, infusion-related toxicities, other acute reactions). A favorable response (defined as complete resolution or clinically meaningful improvement of all signs and symptoms of the infection and related radiographic findings) was observed in 41% of patients after at least 1 dose of caspofungin and in 50% of patients who received more than 7 days of treatment with the drug. Caspofungin therapy was associated with a favorable response rate in 36% of patients refractory to prior antifungal therapy and 70% of patients intolerant of prior antifungal therapy.

■ **Candida Infections** ***Candidemia and Other Invasive Candida Infections*** Caspofungin acetate is used for the treatment of candidemia and certain other invasive *Candida* infections (intra-abdominal abscess, peritonitis, pleural space infections) in adults, adolescents, and children 3 months of age and older. The drug has been effective in *C. albicans*, *C. glabrata*, *C. krusei*, *C. parapsilosis*, and *C. tropicalis* infections, principally in nonneutropenic patients. The manufacturer states that safety and efficacy of caspofungin have not been established for the treatment of endocarditis, osteomyelitis, or meningitis caused by *Candida*.

For the treatment of candidemia in *nonneutropenic* patients or for empiric treatment of suspected invasive candidiasis in *nonneutropenic* patients in intensive care units (ICUs), IDSA recommends an IV echinocandin (anidulafungin, caspofungin, micafungin) for *initial* therapy. IDSA states that fluconazole (IV or oral) is an acceptable alternative for *initial* therapy in selected patients, including those who are not critically ill and are unlikely to have infections caused by fluconazole-resistant *Candida*. If echinocandin- and azole-resistant *Candida* are suspected, IV amphotericin B is recommended; IV amphotericin B also is a reasonable alternative when echinocandins and fluconazole cannot be used because of intolerance, limited availability, or resistance. IDSA states that transition from the echinocandin (or amphotericin B) to fluconazole can be considered (usually within 5–7 days) in patients who are clinically stable, have isolates susceptible to fluconazole (e.g., *C. albicans*), and have negative repeat blood cultures after initial antifungal treatment. Although fluconazole has been considered the drug of choice for the treatment of infections caused by *C. parapsilosis* in nonneutropenic patients (based in part on concerns related to decreased in vitro susceptibility and resistance to echinocandins), IDSA states that there are no clinical studies to date indicating superiority of fluconazole over echinocandins for the treatment of *C. parapsilosis* infections.

For the treatment of candidemia in *neutropenic* patients, IDSA recommends an IV echinocandin (anidulafungin, caspofungin, micafungin) or, alternatively, IV amphotericin B for *initial* therapy. Fluconazole is an alternative in *initial* therapy in those who are not critically ill or have had no prior exposure to azole antifungals and also can be used for step-down therapy during neutropenia in clinically stable patients who have fluconazole-susceptible isolates and documented bloodstream clearance. Voriconazole can be used as an alternative for *initial* therapy when broader antifungal coverage is required and also can be used as step-down therapy during neutropenia in clinically stable patients who have voriconazole-susceptible isolates and documented bloodstream clearance. For infections known to be caused by *C. krusei*, an echinocandin, amphotericin B, or voriconazole is recommended.

For the treatment of osteoarticular infections† (e.g., osteomyelitis, septic arthritis) caused by *Candida*, IDSA recommends *initial* treatment with fluconazole or an IV echinocandin (anidulafungin, caspofungin, micafungin) and follow-up treatment with fluconazole. If septic arthritis involves a prosthetic device that cannot be removed, long-term suppressive or maintenance therapy (secondary prophylaxis) with fluconazole is recommended if the isolate is susceptible.

For the treatment of endocarditis† (native or prosthetic valve) or implantable cardiac device infections† caused by *Candida*, IDSA recommends *initial* treatment with IV amphotericin B (with or without oral flucytosine) or an IV echinocandin (anidulafungin, caspofungin, micafungin) and follow-up treatment with fluconazole. If the isolate is susceptible, long-term suppressive or maintenance therapy (secondary prophylaxis) with fluconazole is recommended to prevent recurrence in those with native valve endocarditis who cannot undergo valve replacement and in those with prosthetic valve endocarditis.

For additional information on management of candidemia and disseminated candidiasis, the current clinical practice guidelines from IDSA available at http://www.idsociety.org should be consulted.

Clinical Experience. Safety and efficacy of caspofungin for the treatment of candidemia or other invasive *Candida* infections were evaluated in a randomized, double-blind study in adults (87% were nonneutropenic). Patients were randomized to receive initial therapy with either IV caspofungin (70-mg loading dose on day 1 followed by 50 mg once daily) or IV amphotericin B deoxycholate (0.6–0.7 mg/kg daily for nonneutropenic patients; 0.7–1 mg/kg daily for neutropenic patients) for 14 days following the most recent positive *Candida* culture. After a minimum of 10 days of IV therapy, patients in both treatment groups were permitted to switch to oral fluconazole (400 mg daily) if they had a baseline *Candida* isolate susceptible to fluconazole and were nonneutropenic, were clinically improved, and had blood cultures negative for *Candida* for 48 hours; those with *C. krusei* or *C. glabrata* infections were not switched to oral fluconazole. A greater proportion of patients receiving amphotericin B deoxycholate compared with those receiving caspofungin switched to oral fluconazole (34.8 versus 24.8%, respectively). When data analysis was done using the modified intent-to-treat population, a favorable response (defined as complete resolution of signs and symptoms of *Candida* infection with documented or presumed microbiological eradication) was observed in 73.4% of those in the caspofungin group (mean duration of 12.1 days of IV caspofungin) and in 61.7% of those in the amphotericin B deoxycholate group (mean duration of 11.7 days of IV amphotericin B deoxycholate). The efficacy of caspofungin was comparable to that of amphotericin B deoxycholate at all time points evaluated (i.e., day 10 of IV therapy, completion of antifungal treatment, 2 weeks and 6–8 weeks after treatment) and at all sites of infection included in the study.

Results of a randomized, double-blind study in adults with invasive candidiasis that was designed to compare the safety and efficacy of a high dosage regimen of caspofungin (150 mg daily) and a dosage regimen that included a 70-mg loading dose on day 1 followed by 50 mg daily indicate that the higher dosage did not result in significant improvement in efficacy.

Esophageal Candidiasis Caspofungin acetate is used for the treatment of esophageal candidiasis in adults, adolescents, and children 3 months of age and older.

Esophageal candidiasis requires treatment with a systemic antifungal (not a topical antifungal).

IDSA recommends oral fluconazole as the preferred drug of choice for the treatment of esophageal candidiasis; if oral therapy is not tolerated, IV fluconazole or an IV echinocandin (anidulafungin, caspofungin, micafungin) usually is recommended and IV amphotericin B is another alternative. For fluconazole-refractory esophageal candidiasis, IDSA recommends itraconazole oral solution or IV or oral voriconazole; alternatives for fluconazole-refractory disease are an IV echinocandin (anidulafungin, caspofungin, micafungin) or IV amphotericin B. IDSA states that oral posaconazole (oral suspension or delayed-release tablets) could be considered another alternative for the treatment of fluconazole-refractory esophageal candidiasis.

For the treatment of esophageal candidiasis in HIV-infected adults and adolescents, CDC, NIH, and IDSA recommend IV or oral fluconazole or itraconazole oral solution. Alternatives include oral or IV voriconazole, an IV echinocandin (anidulafungin, caspofungin, micafungin), or IV amphotericin B. For refractory esophageal candidiasis in HIV-infected adults and adolescents, including fluconazole-refractory infections, these experts recommend posaconazole oral suspension or itraconazole oral solution; alternatives include an IV echinocandin (anidulafungin, caspofungin, micafungin), oral or IV voriconazole, or IV amphotericin B. Although data are limited, some experts state that an IV echinocandin (anidulafungin, caspofungin, micafungin) can be considered an alternative for treatment of azole-refractory esophageal candidiasis in HIV-infected children.

Routine long-term suppressive or maintenance therapy (secondary prophylaxis) to prevent relapse or recurrence is not usually recommended in patients adequately treated for esophageal candidiasis (including HIV-infected individuals) unless the patient has frequent or severe recurrences of esophageal candidiasis. If secondary prophylaxis of esophageal candidiasis is indicated, oral fluconazole or posaconazole oral suspension is recommended; however, the potential for development of azole resistance should be considered.

For additional information on management of esophageal candidiasis, the current clinical practice guidelines from IDSA available at http://www.idsociety.org and the current clinical practice guidelines from CDC, NIH, and IDSA on the prevention and treatment of opportunistic infections in HIV-infected individuals available at http://www.aidsinfo.nih.gov should be consulted.

Clinical Experience. Safety and efficacy of caspofungin for the treatment of esophageal candidiasis have been evaluated in a multicenter, noninferiority clinical study and in 2 smaller dose-ranging studies in adults with symptoms and microbiological documentation of esophageal candidiasis. The majority of patients in all 3 studies had advanced HIV infection ($CD4^+$ T-cell counts less than 50/mm^3). Patients in the multicenter, double-blind, noninferiority clinical study were randomized to receive either IV caspofungin (50 mg once daily) or IV fluconazole (200 mg once daily) for 7–21 days. Most patients in this study had both esophageal and oropharyngeal candidiasis at baseline. A favorable overall response (defined as complete resolution of clinical symptoms, with either total clearing of esophageal lesions [mucosal grade of 0] or a reduction in endoscopy score by at least 2 grade levels) at 5–7 days after completion of treatment was attained in 81.5 and 85.1% of patients in the caspofungin and fluconazole groups, respectively. The median time to symptom resolution in both groups was 4–5 days. The rate of relapse (defined as recurrence of clinical symptoms within 1 month after completion of treatment) at 2 and 4 weeks posttreatment was similar in those who received caspofungin (10.6 and 28.1%, respectively) or fluconazole (7.9 and 16.7%, respectively). The results from the 2 smaller dose-ranging studies corroborate the efficacy of caspofungin demonstrated in this study.

Oropharyngeal Candidiasis Although safety and efficacy of caspofungin for the treatment of oropharyngeal candidiasis have not been established, the drug has been recommended as an alternative for the treatment of oropharyngeal candidiasis†.

For the treatment of mild oropharyngeal candidiasis, IDSA recommends topical treatment with clotrimazole lozenges or miconazole buccal tablets; nystatin (oral suspension or tablets) is the recommended alternative. For moderate to severe disease, IDSA recommends oral fluconazole. For fluconazole-refractory oropharyngeal candidiasis, IDSA recommends itraconazole oral solution or posaconazole oral suspension; oral voriconazole or amphotericin B oral suspension (not commercially available in the US) are recommended as alternatives. Other alternatives for refractory oropharyngeal candidiasis are an IV echinocandin (anidulafungin, caspofungin, micafungin) or IV amphotericin B.

For the treatment of oropharyngeal candidiasis in HIV-infected adults and adolescents, CDC, NIH, and IDSA recommend oral fluconazole as the preferred drug of choice for initial episodes. If topical therapy is used for the treatment of oropharyngeal candidiasis (e.g., mild to moderate episodes), these experts recommend clotrimazole lozenges or miconazole buccal tablets. Alternatives for systemic treatment of oropharyngeal candidiasis in HIV-infected adults and adolescents are itraconazole oral solution or posaconazole oral suspension; nystatin oral suspension is an alternative if topical treatment is used. For fluconazole-refractory oropharyngeal infections in HIV-infected adults and adolescents, posaconazole oral suspension is preferred; itraconazole oral solution is an alternative.

Routine long-term suppressive or maintenance therapy (secondary prophylaxis) to prevent relapse or recurrence is not usually recommended in patients adequately treated for oropharyngeal candidiasis (including HIV-infected individuals) unless the patient has frequent or severe recurrences of oropharyngeal candidiasis. If secondary prophylaxis of oropharyngeal candidiasis is indicated, oral fluconazole is recommended; however, the potential for development of azole resistance should be considered.

For additional information on management of oropharyngeal candidiasis, the current clinical practice guidelines from IDSA available at http://www.idsociety.org and the current clinical practice guidelines from CDC, NIH, and IDSA on the prevention and treatment of opportunistic infections in HIV-infected individuals available at http://www.aidsinfo.nih.gov should be consulted.

Clinical Experience. In a randomized, double-blind study evaluating caspofungin for the treatment of endoscopically and microbiologically confirmed esophageal candidiasis, the majority of patients also had oropharyngeal candidiasis† in addition to esophageal candidiasis. Patients were randomized to receive either IV caspofungin (50 mg once daily) or IV fluconazole (200 mg once daily) for 7–21 days. Data for those with oropharyngeal infections indicate that a favorable response (based on resolution of symptoms and oropharyngeal lesions) 5–7 days after completion of treatment was achieved in 71.4% of those who received caspofungin and 83.3% of those who received fluconazole. However, the rate of relapse of oropharyngeal candidiasis (defined as recurrence of symptoms within 1 month of completion of treatment) was higher at 2 and 4 weeks posttreatment in those who received caspofungin (42.5 and 59%, respectively) than in those who received fluconazole (13.2 and 35.3%, respectively).

Safety and efficacy of caspofungin for the treatment of oropharyngeal candidiasis† and/or esophageal candidiasis in adults also have been evaluated in a phase 2 randomized, double-blind, dose-ranging study (98% had HIV infection, 79% had *C. albicans* infection). Patients were randomized to receive IV caspofungin (35, 50, or 70 mg once daily) or IV amphotericin B (0.5 mg/kg once daily) for 7–14 days. When data analysis was done using the modified intent-to-treat population, a favorable response (defined as complete resolution of symptoms and quantifiable improvement of mucosal lesions 3–4 days after completion of treatment) was achieved in a greater proportion of patients with oropharyngeal candidiasis who received caspofungin (84–93%) than in those who received amphotericin B (67%).

Candida auris Infections Caspofungin is used for the treatment of infections caused by *C. auris*, an emerging pathogen that has been associated with potentially fatal candidemia or other invasive infections.

C. auris, first identified in 2009, has now been reported as the cause of serious invasive infections (including fatalities) in multiple countries worldwide (e.g., Japan, South Korea, India, Kuwait, South Africa, Pakistan, United Kingdom, Venezuela, Colombia, US). As of May 2017, a total of 77 clinical cases of *C. auris* had been reported to CDC from 7 different states in the US. *C. auris* may be difficult to identify using standard in vitro methods and has been misidentified as *C. haemulonii*, *C. famata*, or *Rhodotorula glutinis*. A large percentage of *C. auris* clinical isolates are resistant to fluconazole and multidrug-resistant isolates with reduced susceptibility or resistance to all 3 major classes of antifungal agents (azoles, polyenes, echinocandins) have been reported.

Pending further accumulation of data, CDC has issued interim recommendations regarding laboratory diagnosis, treatment, and infection control measures for suspected or known *C. auris* infections. Based on limited data available to date, CDC recommends that an IV echinocandin (anidulafungin, caspofungin, micafungin) be used for initial treatment of invasive *C. auris* infections (e.g., bloodstream or intra-abdominal infections) in adults. CDC states that a switch to IV amphotericin B (lipid formulation) could be considered if the patient is clinically unresponsive to the echinocandin or fungemia persists longer than 5 days. Consultation with an infectious disease specialist is highly recommended.

Unless there is evidence of infection, CDC does not currently recommend antifungal treatment when *C. auris* is isolated only from noninvasive body sites (e.g., urine, external ear, wounds, respiratory secretions). Some individuals are colonized with *C. auris* in the axilla, groin, nose, external ear canal, oropharynx, urine, wounds, rectum, and stool; however, data are limited and the duration of *C. auris* colonization is unclear. Therefore, CDC recommends that infection control measures be observed for all patients with cultures yielding *C. auris*, including those with positive cultures only from noninvasive body sites.

Whenever *C. auris* infection is suspected, clinicians should immediately contact state or local public health authorities and the CDC (candidaauris@cdc.gov) for guidance. For additional information on diagnosis and management of *C. auris* infections, the interim recommendations and most recent information from CDC available at https://www.cdc.gov/fungal/diseases/candidiasis/candida-auris.html should be consulted.

■ **Empiric Therapy in Febrile Neutropenic Patients** Caspofungin acetate is used for empiric treatment of presumed fungal infections in febrile, neutropenic adults, adolescents, and children 3 months of age and older.

Clinical Experience Safety and efficacy of caspofungin for empiric therapy of presumed fungal infections in febrile neutropenic patients have been evaluated in a randomized, double-blind, noninferiority study in patients 16 years of age and older. In this study, patients received IV caspofungin (70-mg loading dose on day 1 followed by 50 mg once daily) or IV amphotericin B liposomal (3 mg/kg daily) until resolution of neutropenia or up to a maximum of 28 days (unless a fungal infection was documented). After 5 days of IV therapy, patients who remained febrile and clinically deteriorated could receive caspofungin 70 mg daily or amphotericin B liposomal 5 mg/kg daily. When data analysis was done using the modified intent-to-treat population, an overall favorable response (defined as resolution of fever during the neutropenic period, successful treatment of any baseline fungal infections, absence of emergent fungal infections up to 7 days after completion of study drug, patient survival for 7 days after empiric therapy, and use of study drug without premature discontinuance because of toxicity or lack of efficacy) was attained in 33.9 or 33.7% of those receiving caspofungin or amphotericin B liposomal, respectively.

Safety and efficacy of caspofungin for empiric treatment of presumed fungal infections in pediatric patients have been evaluated in a randomized, double-blind study comparing IV caspofungin (70-mg/m^2 loading dose on day 1 [up to 70 mg daily] followed by 50 mg/m^2 once daily) with IV amphotericin B liposomal (3 mg/kg daily) in patients 2–17 years of age with persistent fever and neutropenia. An overall favorable response was attained in 46.4 or 32% of those receiving caspofungin or amphotericin B liposomal, respectively.

Dosage and Administration

■ Administration

Caspofungin acetate is administered by slow IV infusion. The drug should *not* be given by rapid IV injection.

Caspofungin acetate should not be admixed or infused concomitantly with other drugs. Dextrose-containing diluents (e.g., 5% dextrose injection) should *not* be used.

IV Infusion

Reconstitution and Dilution. Commercially available caspofungin acetate lyophilized powder for injection must be reconstituted and then further diluted prior to IV infusion.

Vials of lyophilized caspofungin acetate should be stored at 2–8 °C and should be allowed to reach room temperature prior to reconstitution.

The 50- or 70-mg vial of caspofungin acetate should be reconstituted by adding 10.8 mL of 0.9% sodium chloride injection, sterile water for injection, bacteriostatic water for injection (with methylparaben and propylparaben), or bacteriostatic water for injection (with 0.9% benzyl alcohol) to provide a solution containing 5 or 7 mg/mL, respectively. The vial should be mixed gently until the drug is dissolved completely and a clear solution is obtained. The 50- and 70-mg vials are formulated to provide a slight overfill when reconstituted as directed, yielding 54.6 and 75.6 mg of caspofungin, respectively.

The reconstituted solution should be inspected for evidence of particulate matter or discoloration and should not be used if cloudy or if a precipitate has formed. After reconstitution and before dilution, the vial may be stored at a temperature of 25°C or less for up to 1 hour. After the reconstituted solution is diluted for IV administration, it may be stored at a temperature of 25°C or less for 24 hours or at a temperature of 2–8°C for 48 hours. Caspofungin vials are for single-use only, partially used vials of reconstituted solution should be discarded.

The appropriate volume of reconstituted solution (mL equivalent to the indicated loading or maintenance dose) should be withdrawn from the vial and added to 250 mL of 0.225%, 0.45%, or 0.9% sodium chloride injection or lactated Ringer's injection. Alternatively, the appropriate volume of reconstituted drug may be added to a reduced volume of 0.225%, 0.45%, or 0.9% sodium chloride injection or lactated Ringer's injection, provided the final concentration does not exceed 0.5 mg/mL.

For pediatric patients 3 months to 17 years of age, caspofungin vials should be reconstituted the same as for adults. After reconstitution, the appropriate volume of reconstituted solution equivalent to the calculated loading or maintenance dose based on a concentration of 5 mg/mL (if using the 50 mg vial) or 7 mg/mL (if using the 70 mg vial) should be withdrawn from the vial and added to 0.225%, 0.45%, or 0.9% sodium chloride injection or lactated Ringer's injection. The manufacturer recommends that the 50-mg vial (concentration of 5 mg/mL) be used for pediatric doses less than 50 mg and that the 70-mg vial (concentration of 7 mg/mL) be used for pediatric doses greater than 50 mg.

Rate of Administration. IV infusions of caspofungin acetate should be given over approximately 1 hour.

■ Dosage

Dosage of caspofungin acetate is expressed in terms of the salt.

Adult Dosage

Aspergillosis. The recommended dosage of caspofungin acetate for the treatment of invasive aspergillosis in adults whose disease is refractory to, or who are intolerant of, other antifungal therapy is a single loading dose of 70 mg on day 1, followed by 50 mg once daily thereafter.

The duration of treatment is based on the severity of the patient's underlying disease, recovery from immunosuppression, and clinical response. The Infectious Diseases Society of America (IDSA) recommends that antifungal treatment of invasive pulmonary aspergillosis be continued for at least 6–12 weeks.

Candidemia and Other Invasive Candida Infections. The recommended dosage of caspofungin acetate for the treatment of candidemia or certain other invasive *Candida* infections (intra-abdominal abscess, peritonitis, pleural space infections) in *nonneutropenic* or *neutropenic* adults is a single loading dose of 70 mg given on day 1, followed by 50 mg once daily thereafter.

When caspofungin acetate is used for initial treatment of candidemia or other invasive *Candida* infections, IDSA states that a transition from the echinocandin to fluconazole can be considered (usually within 5–7 days) in patients who are clinically stable, have isolates susceptible to fluconazole (e.g., *C. albicans*), and have negative repeat blood cultures after initial antifungal treatment.

The duration of treatment should be based on clinical and microbiological response. The manufacturer recommends that treatment be continued for at least 14 days after the last positive culture and states that those who remain persistently neutropenic may require a longer course of therapy pending resolution of neutropenia. IDSA recommends that antifungal treatment for candidemia (without persistent fungemia or metastatic complications) be continued for 2 weeks after documented clearance of *Candida* from the bloodstream, resolution of candidemia symptoms, and resolution of neutropenia.

If caspofungin acetate is used for *initial* treatment of osteoarticular infections† (e.g., osteomyelitis, septic arthritis) caused by *Candida*, IDSA recommends a dosage of 50–70 mg once daily in adults. After at least 2 weeks, treatment can be switched to fluconazole.

If caspofungin acetate is used for *initial* treatment of endocarditis† (native or prosthetic valve) or implantable cardiac device infections† caused by *Candida*, IDSA recommends a dosage of 150 mg once daily in adults. If the infection is caused by fluconazole-susceptible *Candida*, treatment can be switched to fluconazole after the patient is stabilized and *Candida* has been cleared from the bloodstream.

Esophageal Candidiasis. The manufacturer recommends that caspofungin acetate be given in a dosage of 50 mg once daily for the treatment of esophageal candidiasis in adults.

Although the manufacturer states that use of a 70-mg loading dose has not been evaluated for the treatment of esophageal candidiasis, IDSA recommends a single 70-mg loading dose on day 1, followed by 50 mg once daily for the treatment of esophageal candidiasis in adults.

For the treatment of esophageal candidiasis in adults with human immunodeficiency virus (HIV) infection, some experts recommend that caspofungin acetate be given in a dosage of 50 mg once daily.

The manufacturer recommends that treatment of esophageal candidiasis be continued for 7–14 days after resolution of symptoms. The Centers for Disease Control and Prevention (CDC), National Institutes of Health (NIH), and IDSA recommend that antifungal treatment of esophageal candidiasis be continued for 14–21 days.

Oropharyngeal Candidiasis. If caspofungin acetate is used for the treatment of oropharyngeal candidiasis†, IDSA recommends that adults receive a single 70-mg loading dose on day 1, followed by 50 mg once daily for 7–14 days.

Candida auris Infections. If caspofungin acetate is used for initial treatment of invasive *C. auris* infections (e.g., bloodstream or intra-abdominal infections), CDC recommends that adults receive a single 70-mg loading dose on day 1, followed by 50 mg once daily.

Empiric Therapy in Febrile Neutropenic Patients. The recommended dosage of caspofungin acetate for empiric therapy of presumed fungal infections in febrile neutropenic adults is a single loading dose of 70 mg given on day 1, followed by 50 mg once daily thereafter. If 50 mg once daily is well tolerated but does not provide an adequate clinical response, the manufacturer states that the dosage may be increased to 70 mg once daily.

The duration of empiric treatment should be based on clinical response and should be continued until neutropenia resolves. If a fungal infection is identified, the drug should be continued for at least 14 days after the last positive culture and for at least 7 days after both neutropenia and clinical symptoms resolve.

Pediatric Dosage

General Dosing for Pediatric Patients. Caspofungin acetate dosage for pediatric patients 3 months to 17 years of age is based on body surface area (BSA) calculated using the Mosteller Formula. The loading dose (in mg) should be calculated as BSA (m^2) x 70 mg/m^2 and the maintenance dose (in mg) should be calculated as BSA (m^2) x 50 mg/m^2.

Regardless of the patient's calculated dose, the maximum loading dose and maximum daily maintenance dosage in pediatric patients should not exceed 70 mg.

Aspergillosis. The recommended dosage of caspofungin acetate for pediatric patients 3 months to 17 years of age with invasive aspergillosis whose disease is refractory to, or who are intolerant of, other antifungal therapy is a single loading dose of 70 mg/m^2 given on day 1, followed by 50 mg/m^2 once daily thereafter. If 50 mg/m^2 once daily is well tolerated but does not provide an adequate clinical response, dosage may be increased to 70 mg/m^2 once daily.

The duration of treatment is based on the severity of the patient's underlying disease, recovery from immunosuppression, and clinical response. IDSA recommends that antifungal treatment of invasive pulmonary aspergillosis be continued for at least 6–12 weeks.

Candidemia and Other Invasive Candida Infections. The recommended dosage of caspofungin acetate for the treatment of candidemia or certain other invasive *Candida* infections (intra-abdominal abscess, peritonitis, pleural space infections) in pediatric patients 3 months to 17 years of age is a single loading dose of 70 mg/m^2 given on day 1, followed by 50 mg/m^2 once daily thereafter. If 50 mg/m^2 once daily is well tolerated but does not provide an adequate clinical response, dosage may be increased to 70 mg/m^2 once daily.

The duration of treatment should be based on clinical and microbiological response. The manufacturer recommends that treatment be continued for at least 14 days after the last positive culture and states that those who remain persistently neutropenic may require a longer course of therapy pending resolution of neutropenia. IDSA recommends that antifungal treatment for candidemia (without persistent fungemia or metastatic complications) be continued for 2 weeks after documented clearance of *Candida* from the bloodstream, resolution of candidemia symptoms, and resolution of neutropenia.

Esophageal Candidiasis. The recommended dosage of caspofungin acetate for the treatment of esophageal candidiasis in pediatric patients 3 months to 17 years of age is a single loading dose of 70 mg/m^2 given on day 1, followed by 50 mg/m^2 once daily thereafter. If 50 mg/m^2 once daily is well tolerated but does not provide an adequate clinical response, dosage may be increased to 70 mg/m^2 once daily.

For the treatment of esophageal candidiasis in HIV-infected adolescents, some experts recommend that caspofungin acetate be given in a dosage of 50 mg once daily.

The manufacturer recommends that treatment of esophageal candidiasis be continued for 7–14 days after resolution of symptoms. CDC, NIH, and IDSA recommend that antifungal treatment of esophageal candidiasis be continued for 14–21 days.

Empiric Therapy in Febrile Neutropenic Patients. The recommended dosage of caspofungin acetate for empiric treatment of presumed fungal infections in febrile neutropenic pediatric patients 3 months to 17 years of age is a single loading dose of 70 mg/m^2 given on day 1, followed by 50 mg/m^2 once daily thereafter. If 50 mg/m^2 once daily is well tolerated but does not provide an adequate clinical response, dosage may be increased to 70 mg/m^2 once daily.

The duration of empiric treatment should be based on clinical response and should be continued until neutropenia resolves. If a fungal infection is identified, the drug should be continued for at least 14 days after the last positive culture and for at least 7 days after neutropenia and clinical symptoms resolve.

■ **Special Populations** ***Hepatic Impairment*** Dosage adjustments are not necessary in adults with mild hepatic impairment (Child-Pugh score 5–6). When caspofungin acetate is used in adults with moderate hepatic impairment (Child-Pugh score 7–9), a dosage of 35 mg once daily following the initial 70-mg loading dose (if usually indicated) is recommended.

Data are not available regarding use of caspofungin acetate in adults with severe hepatic impairment (Child-Pugh score exceeding 9) or in pediatric patients with any degree of hepatic impairment.

Renal Impairment Dosage adjustments are not necessary in patients with renal impairment.

Because caspofungin is not dialyzable, supplementary doses are not required following hemodialysis.

Geriatric Patients Dosage adjustments are not necessary in patients 65 years of age or older.

Cautions

■ **Contraindications** Caspofungin acetate is contraindicated in patients with known hypersensitivity (e.g., anaphylaxis) to the drug or any ingredient in the formulation.

■ **Warnings/Precautions** ***Sensitivity Reactions*** **Hypersensitivity Reactions.** Anaphylaxis has been reported in patients receiving caspofungin. If such reactions occur, the drug should be discontinued and appropriate treatment administered.

Possible histamine-mediated symptoms (e.g., rash, facial swelling, pruritus, sensation of warmth, bronchospasm) have been reported in patients receiving caspofungin and may require discontinuance of the drug and/or administration of appropriate treatment.

There have been postmarketing reports of Stevens-Johnson syndrome (SJS) and toxic epidermal necrolysis (TEN) in patients receiving caspofungin. The drug should be used with caution in patients with a history of allergic skin reactions.

Hepatic Effects Abnormal liver function test results have been reported in healthy individuals and adult and pediatric patients receiving caspofungin. Hepatic abnormalities, including hepatic dysfunction, hepatitis, and hepatic failure, have been reported in some adult and pediatric patients with serious underlying conditions receiving caspofungin and multiple other drugs. A causal relationship to caspofungin has not been established to date.

Transient elevations in liver enzymes have been reported in patients receiving caspofungin and cyclosporine concomitantly. (See Cyclosporine under Drug Interactions: Immunosuppressive Agents.)

If abnormal liver function test results occur during caspofungin therapy, the patient should be monitored for evidence of worsening hepatic function and the risks of continued caspofungin therapy should be weighed against potential benefits.

Specific Populations **Pregnancy.** Category C. (See Users Guide.)

There are no adequate and well-controlled studies of caspofungin acetate in pregnant women, and the manufacturer states that the drug should be used during pregnancy only if potential benefits justify potential risks to the fetus.

In animals, embryofetal toxicity (increased resorptions, increased peri-implantation loss, incomplete ossification at multiple fetal sites) has been reported with caspofungin dosages about 2 times the recommended human dosage (based on body surface area comparisons).

Lactation. Caspofungin is distributed into milk in rats; it is not known whether the drug is distributed into milk in humans.

Caspofungin should be used with caution in nursing women.

Pediatric Use. Safety and efficacy of caspofungin have not been established in neonates and infants younger than 3 months of age. Although limited pharmacokinetic data are available for this age group, the manufacturer states that data are insufficient to date to establish a safe and effective dosage for treatment of neonatal candidiasis. In addition, invasive candidiasis in neonates has a higher rate of CNS and multi-organ involvement than do such infections in older patients, and data are insufficient to date regarding distribution of caspofungin into the CNS or regarding efficacy in the treatment of meningitis and endocarditis.

Caspofungin has not been evaluated in pediatric patients for the treatment of endocarditis, osteomyelitis, or meningitis caused by *Candida* or for initial therapy of invasive aspergillosis. The drug also has not been evaluated for use in pediatric patients with hepatic impairment.

Safety and efficacy of caspofungin for use in infants and children 3 months to 17 years of age for treatment of invasive aspergillosis in those refractory to or intolerant of other antifungals; for treatment of candidemia and certain other invasive *Candida* infections (intra-abdominal abscesses, peritonitis, pleural space infections) or esophageal candidiasis; and for empiric treatment of presumed fungal infections in febrile neutropenic patients is based on adequate and well-controlled studies in adults, pharmacokinetic data in pediatric patients, and additional data from prospective studies in this age group.

The manufacturer states that the overall safety profile of caspofungin in pediatric patients is comparable to that in adults. Adverse effects reported in 7% or more of pediatric patients receiving caspofungin include pyrexia, rash, decreased potassium, increased AST, diarrhea, increased ALT, chills, hypotension, vomiting, tachycardia, mucosal inflammation, hypertension, headache, erythema, central line infection, cough, respiratory distress, hypokalemia, abdominal pain, and pruritus.

Although data are limited, some experts state that caspofungin can be considered for first-line treatment of invasive candidiasis or for alternative treatment of esophageal candidiasis in children with human immunodeficiency virus (HIV) infection.

Geriatric Use. Clinical studies of caspofungin did not include a sufficient number of patients 65 years of age or older to determine whether they respond differently than younger individuals. Although no overall differences in efficacy or safety were observed between geriatric and younger adults, the possibility that some older patients may have increased sensitivity to the drug cannot be ruled out.

Although caspofungin plasma concentrations are increased slightly in men and women 65 years of age and older compared with young healthy males, dosage adjustments are not necessary in geriatric patients.

Hepatic Impairment. Although the area under the concentration-time curve (AUC) of caspofungin is increased slightly in adults with mild hepatic impairment (Child-Pugh score 5–6) compared with healthy adults, dosage adjustments are not necessary. A greater increase in AUC occurs in adults with moderate hepatic impairment (Child-Pugh score 7–9), and a dosage reduction is recommended in these patients. (See Hepatic Impairment under Dosage and Administration: Special Populations.)

Data are not available regarding use of caspofungin in adults with severe hepatic impairment or in pediatric patients with any degree of hepatic impairment.

Renal Impairment. Renal impairment does not have a clinically important effect on the pharmacokinetics of caspofungin. Dosage adjustments are not necessary in patients with renal impairment.

■ **Common Adverse Effects** Adverse effects reported in 5% or more of patients receiving caspofungin include pyrexia, diarrhea, chills, decreased potassium, increased alkaline phosphatase, decreased hemoglobin, hypotension, respiratory failure, increased ALT, fever, decreased hematocrit, phlebitis, vomiting, rash, increased AST, nausea, headache, increased bilirubin, septic shock, decreased leukocyte count, peripheral edema, cough, pneumonia, increased creatinine, anemia, abdominal pain, dyspnea, increased blood urea, pleural effusion, increased conjugated bilirubin, tachycardia, decreased albumin, decreased magnesium, rales, and sepsis.

Drug Interactions

■ **Drugs Affecting Or Metabolized by Hepatic Microsomal Enzymes** In vitro studies indicate that caspofungin does not inhibit and is a poor substrate for cytochrome P-450 (CYP) isoenzymes. The drug does not induce CYP3A4.

Concomitant use of caspofungin and drugs that induce CYP isoenzymes may result in clinically important decreases in plasma concentrations of caspofungin. It is not known which mechanism involved in caspofungin clearance may be inducible.

■ **Drugs Affecting or Affected by P-glycoprotein Transport** Caspofungin is not a substrate of the P-glycoprotein transport system; pharmacokinetic interactions unlikely.

■ **Antifungal Agents** ***Amphotericin B*** No evidence of pharmacokinetic interactions if caspofungin is used concomitantly with amphotericin B.

In vitro, the antifungal effects of caspofungin and amphotericin B have been synergistic or additive against some *Aspergillus*, including *A. fumigatus*, and some *Fusarium* species. In vitro, caspofungin and amphotericin B have shown indifferent or additive antifungal effects against *Candida glabrata*. Although the clinical importance is not known, the combination of caspofungin and amphotericin B has not demonstrated antagonistic antifungal effects against *A. fumigatus*, *C. albicans* (including azole-resistant strains), or other *Candida*.

Fluconazole In vitro, the antifungal effects of caspofungin and fluconazole have been synergistic against *C. glabrata*. No in vitro evidence of antagonistic antifungal effects against *C. albicans* (including azole-resistant strains) or against various other *Candida*.

Itraconazole No evidence of pharmacokinetic interactions if caspofungin is used concomitantly with itraconazole.

In vitro, the antifungal effects of caspofungin and itraconazole usually have been synergistic or additive against *Aspergillus*, including *A. fumigatus*.

Posaconazole In vitro, the antifungal effects of caspofungin and posaconazole usually have been synergistic against *Aspergillus* and *C. glabrata*.

Voriconazole In vitro, the antifungal effects of caspofungin and voriconazole have been additive against *C. glabrata*. In vitro, the antifungal effects of caspofungin and voriconazole have been indifferent, additive, or synergistic against some *Aspergillus*, including *A. fumigatus*. There was no in vitro evidence of antagonistic antifungal effects against *Aspergillus*.

■ **Antiretroviral Agents** ***Efavirenz*** Possible pharmacokinetic interaction (decreased caspofungin concentrations).

If caspofungin is used concomitantly with efavirenz, caspofungin dosage should be 70 mg once daily in adults and a dosage of 70 mg/m^2 (maximum 70 mg) once daily should be considered in pediatric patients.

Nelfinavir Pharmacokinetics of caspofungin are not affected by concomitant nelfinavir.

Nevirapine Possible pharmacokinetic interaction (decreased caspofungin concentrations).

If caspofungin is used concomitantly with nevirapine, caspofungin dosage should be 70 mg once daily in adults and a dosage of 70 mg/m^2 (maximum 70 mg) once daily should be considered in pediatric patients.

■ **Carbamazepine** Possible pharmacokinetic interaction (decreased caspofungin concentrations).

If caspofungin is used concomitantly with carbamazepine, caspofungin dosage should be 70 mg once daily in adults and a dosage of 70 mg/m^2 (maximum 70 mg) once daily should be considered in pediatric patients.

■ **Dexamethasone** Possible pharmacokinetic interaction (decreased caspofungin concentrations).

If caspofungin is used concomitantly with dexamethasone, caspofungin dosage should be 70 mg once daily in adults and a dosage of 70 mg/m^2 (maximum 70 mg) once daily should be considered in pediatric patients.

■ **Immunosuppressive Agents** ***Cyclosporine*** Concomitant use of caspofungin and cyclosporine increases the area under the concentration-time curve (AUC) of caspofungin by about 35%, but does not affect plasma concentrations of cyclosporine.

Transient elevations in ALT (SGPT) and AST (SGOT) have been reported when caspofungin and cyclosporine were used concomitantly in healthy adults and immunocompromised patients.

Caspofungin and cyclosporine should be used concomitantly with caution and only when potential benefits outweigh risks. If the drugs are used concomitantly, the patient should be monitored closely. If abnormal liver function test results occur, the risks and benefits of continuing concomitant therapy should be evaluated.

Mycophenolate No evidence of pharmacokinetic interactions if caspofungin is used concomitantly with mycophenolate.

Tacrolimus Concomitant use of caspofungin and tacrolimus reduces peak plasma concentrations and AUC of tacrolimus by 16 and 20%, respectively, but does not affect the pharmacokinetics of caspofungin.

Tacrolimus concentrations should be monitored in patients receiving concomitant caspofungin; tacrolimus dosage should be adjusted if appropriate.

■ **Phenytoin** Possible pharmacokinetic interaction (decreased caspofungin concentrations).

If caspofungin is used concomitantly with phenytoin, caspofungin dosage should be 70 mg once daily in adults and a dosage of 70 mg/m^2 (maximum 70 mg) once daily should be considered in pediatric patients.

■ **Rifampin** Concomitant use of caspofungin and rifampin results in a 30% decrease in trough plasma concentrations of caspofungin.

If caspofungin is used concomitantly with rifampin, caspofungin dosage should be 70 mg once daily in adults or 70 mg/m^2 (maximum 70 mg) once daily in pediatric patients.

Description

Caspofungin acetate, a semisynthetic lipopeptide synthesized from a fermentation product of *Glarea lozoyensis*, is an echinocandin antifungal agent. Echinocandins (e.g., anidulafungin, caspofungin, micafungin) are glucan synthesis inhibitors and differ structurally and pharmacologically from other currently available antifungal agents.

Like other echinocandins, caspofungin inhibits the synthesis of β(1,3)-D-glucan, an integral component of the fungal cell wall that is not present in mammalian cells. Depending on the concentration, the drug may be fungicidal against *Candida*, but usually is fungistatic against *Aspergillus*.

Following IV infusion of caspofungin acetate over 1 hour, plasma concentrations of caspofungin decline in a polyphasic manner. The drug is extensively (about 97%) protein bound (to albumin), with distribution (rather than excretion or biotransformation) being the predominant mechanism influencing plasma clearance. Caspofungin acetate is slowly metabolized in the liver via hydrolysis and *N*-acetylation. Following a single IV dose, 35 and 41% of the dose is eliminated in feces and urine, respectively, as the parent drug and metabolites.

■ **Spectrum** Caspofungin is active in vitro against *C. albicans*, *C. glabrata*, *C. guilliermondii*, *C. krusei*, *C. parapsilosis*, and *C. tropicalis*. The drug also is active in vitro against *C. dubliniensis*, *C. kefyr*, *C. lusitaniae*, *C. metapsilosis*, *C. orthopsilosis*, and *C. pseudotropicalis*. Caspofungin has been active against some *Candida*, including *C. glabrata* and *C. krusei*, resistant to fluconazole.

Clinical isolates of *C. auris* (often misidentified as *C. haemulonii*, *C. famata*, or *Rhodotorula glutinis*) generally have been inhibited in vitro by caspofungin concentrations of 0.06–1 mcg/mL.

Caspofungin is active in vitro against *Aspergillus*, including *A. fumigatus*, *A. flavus*, and *A. terreus*. The drug also is active in vitro against *A. niger*, *A. strictum*, and *A. versicolor*.

Like other echinocandins, caspofungin is not active against *Cryptococcus neoformans*, *Fusarium*, *Trichosporon*, or zygomycetes.

■ **Resistance** Strains of *Candida*, including *C. albicans*, *C. glabrata*, *C. krusei*, and *C. parapsilosis*, with reduced susceptibility or resistance to caspofungin have emerged in some patients who received the drug for treatment and, in some cases, were associated with clinical failures. Some clinical isolates of *C. auris* have reduced susceptibility or resistance to caspofungin in vitro (i.e., MICs 2 mcg/mL or greater).

Resistance to caspofungin has been associated with specific mutations in the FKS subunits of the glucan synthase enzyme. These mutations are associated with higher MICs and breakthrough infection. *Candida* with reduced susceptibility to caspofungin as a result of an increase in the chitin content of the fungal cell wall have also been identified, although the clinical importance of this phenomenon is unknown.

Some strains of *C. albicans* with reduced susceptibility to caspofungin may also have reduced susceptibility to micafungin.

Advice to Patients

Inform patients that anaphylactic reactions have been reported in patients receiving caspofungin acetate. Advise patients the drug can cause hypersensitivity reactions (e.g., rash, facial swelling, angioedema, pruritus, sensation of warmth, bronchospasm) and of the importance of contacting clinicians if any of these signs or symptoms occur.

Advise patients about isolated reports of serious hepatic effects (e.g., hepatitis, hepatic failure) associated with caspofungin and the importance of clinicians assessing the benefits versus risks of caspofungin therapy if abnormal liver function tests occur.

Importance of informing clinicians of existing or contemplated concomitant therapy, including prescription and OTC drugs, and any concomitant illnesses.

Importance of women informing clinicians if they are or plan to become pregnant or plan to breast-feed.

Importance of informing patients of other important precautionary information. (See Cautions.)

Preparations

Excipients in commercially available drug preparations may have clinically important effects in some individuals; consult specific product labeling for details.

Caspofungin Acetate

Parenteral

For injection, for IV infusion	50 mg*	Cancidas®, Merck
		Caspofungin Acetate for Injection
	70 mg*	Cancidas®, Merck
		Caspofungin Acetate for Injection

*available from one or more manufacturer, distributor, and/or repackager by generic (nonproprietary) name

†Use is not currently included in the labeling approved by the US Food and Drug Administration

Micafungin Sodium

■ Micafungin sodium is a semisynthetic, echinocandin antifungal agent.

Uses

■ **Candida Infections** ***Candidemia and Other Invasive Candida Infections*** Micafungin sodium is used for the treatment of candidemia, acute disseminated candidiasis, and certain other invasive *Candida* infections (peritonitis, abscesses). The manufacturer states that safety and efficacy of micafungin have not been established for the treatment of endocarditis, osteomyelitis, or meningitis caused by *Candida*.

For the treatment of candidemia in *nonneutropenic* patients or for empiric treatment of suspected invasive candidiasis in *nonneutropenic* patients in intensive care units (ICUs), the Infectious Diseases Society of America (IDSA) recommends an IV echinocandin (anidulafungin, caspofungin, micafungin) for *initial* therapy. IDSA states that fluconazole (IV or oral) is an acceptable alternative for *initial* therapy in selected patients, including those who are not critically ill and are unlikely to have infections caused by fluconazole-resistant *Candida*. If echinocandin- and azole-resistant *Candida* are suspected, IV amphotericin B is recommended; IV amphotericin B also is a reasonable alternative when echinocandins and fluconazole cannot be used because of intolerance, limited availability, or resistance. IDSA states that transition from the echinocandin (or amphotericin B) to fluconazole can be considered (usually within 5–7 days) in patients who are clinically stable, have isolates susceptible to fluconazole (e.g., *C. albicans*), and have negative repeat blood cultures after initial antifungal treatment. Although fluconazole has been considered the drug of choice for the treatment of infections caused by *C. parapsilosis* in nonneutropenic patients (based in part on concerns related to decreased in vitro susceptibility and resistance to echinocandins), IDSA states that there are no clinical studies to date indicating superiority of fluconazole over echinocandins for the treatment of *C. parapsilosis* infections.

For the treatment of candidemia in *neutropenic* patients, IDSA recommends an IV echinocandin (anidulafungin, caspofungin, micafungin) or, alternatively, IV amphotericin B for *initial* therapy. Fluconazole is an alternative for *initial* therapy in those who are not critically ill or have had no prior exposure to azole antifungals and also can be used for step-down therapy during neutropenia in clinically stable patients who have fluconazole-susceptible isolates and documented bloodstream clearance. Voriconazole can be used as an alternative for *initial* therapy when broader antifungal coverage is required and also can be used as step-down therapy during neutropenia in clinically stable patients who have voriconazole-susceptible isolates and documented bloodstream clearance. For infections known to be caused by *C. krusei*, an echinocandin, amphotericin B, or voriconazole is recommended.

For the treatment of osteoarticular infections† (e.g., osteomyelitis, septic arthritis) caused by *Candida*, IDSA recommends *initial* treatment with fluconazole or an IV echinocandin (anidulafungin, caspofungin, micafungin) and follow-up treatment with fluconazole. If septic arthritis involves a prosthetic device that cannot be removed, long-term suppressive or maintenance therapy (secondary prophylaxis) with fluconazole is recommended if the isolate is susceptible.

For the treatment of endocarditis† (native or prosthetic valve) or implantable cardiac device infections† caused by *Candida*, IDSA recommends *initial* treatment with IV amphotericin B (with or without oral flucytosine) or an IV echinocandin (anidulafungin, caspofungin, micafungin) and follow-up treatment with fluconazole. If the isolate is susceptible, long-term suppressive or maintenance therapy (secondary prophylaxis) with fluconazole is recommended to prevent recurrence in those with native valve endocarditis who cannot undergo valve replacement and in those with prosthetic valve endocarditis.

For additional information on management of candidemia and disseminated candidiasis, the current clinical practice guidelines from IDSA available at http://www.idsociety.org should be consulted.

Clinical Experience. Safety and efficacy of micafungin for the treatment of candidemia or other forms of invasive candidiasis were evaluated in a phase 3, randomized, double-blind, noninferiority study in 578 adults (8.7% were neutropenic, 48% had *C. albicans* infections). Patients were randomized to receive initial therapy with either IV micafungin (100 or 150 mg once daily) or IV caspofungin acetate (70-mg loading dose followed by 50 mg once daily). After a minimum of 10 days of IV therapy, patients were permitted to switch to oral fluconazole if the *Candida* isolate at baseline was susceptible to fluconazole and was not *C. krusei* or *C. glabrata* and if the patient was nonneutropenic, had improvement or resolution of clinical signs and symptoms, and had 2 blood cultures drawn at least 24 hours apart that were now negative for *Candida*. Patients with proven or suspected endocarditis, osteomyelitis, or meningitis due to *Candida* were excluded from the study. The median total duration of antifungal treatment (including switch to oral fluconazole) was 14 days (maximum 61 days); 20.9% of those receiving IV micafungin (100-mg regimen) and 21.2% of those receiving IV caspofungin acetate switched to oral fluconazole. At study completion, IV micafungin (100- and 150-mg regimens) was found to be noninferior to IV caspofungin acetate (50 mg daily), and the 100-mg micafungin regimen was as effective as the 150-mg micafungin regimen. Overall treatment success based on clinical response (defined as complete resolution or improvement in signs and symptoms and radiographic abnormalities of *Candida* infection without additional antifungal treatment) and mycologic response (documented or presumed microbiological eradication) at the end of the IV regimen was observed in 76.4% of those in the micafungin 100-mg group, 71.4% of those in the micafungin 150-mg group, and 72.3% of those in the caspofungin acetate 50-mg group. At 6 weeks posttreatment, the overall relapse rate was 36.3% in those who received micafungin (100-mg regimen) and 37% in those who received caspofungin.

In a multicenter, randomized, double-blind trial in 106 pediatric patients under 16 years of age with candidemia or other invasive candidiasis who received micafungin (2–4 mg/kg daily for those weighing up to 40 kg; 100–200 mg daily for those weighing over 40 kg) for a median duration of 15 days (range: 3–42 days), the overall treatment response rate (both clinical and mycologic response) was 73% and was similar to the 76% response rate in children who received amphotericin B liposomal (3–5 mg/kg daily); treatment success was independent of neutropenic status.

Esophageal Candidiasis Micafungin sodium is used for the treatment of esophageal candidiasis.

Esophageal candidiasis requires treatment with a systemic antifungal (not a topical antifungal).

IDSA recommends oral fluconazole as the preferred drug of choice for the treatment of esophageal candidiasis; if oral therapy is not tolerated, IV fluconazole or an IV echinocandin (anidulafungin, caspofungin, micafungin) usually is recommended and IV amphotericin B is another alternative. For fluconazole-refractory esophageal candidiasis, IDSA recommends itraconazole oral solution or oral or IV voriconazole; alternatives for fluconazole-refractory disease are an IV echinocandin (anidulafungin, caspofungin, micafungin) or IV amphotericin B. IDSA states that oral posaconazole (oral suspension or delayed-release tablets) could be considered another alternative for the treatment of fluconazole-refractory esophageal candidiasis.

For the treatment of esophageal candidiasis in adults and adolescents with human immunodeficiency virus (HIV) infection, the Centers for Disease Control and Prevention (CDC), National Institutes of Health (NIH), and IDSA recommend IV or oral fluconazole or itraconazole oral solution. Alternatives include oral or IV voriconazole, an IV echinocandin (anidulafungin, caspofungin, micafungin), or IV amphotericin B. For refractory esophageal candidiasis in HIV-infected adults and adolescents, including fluconazole-refractory infections, these experts recommend posaconazole oral suspension or itraconazole oral solution; alternatives include an IV echinocandin (anidulafungin, caspofungin, micafungin), oral or IV voriconazole, or IV amphotericin B. Although data are limited, some experts state that an IV echinocandin (anidulafungin, caspofungin, micafungin) can be considered an alternative for treatment of azole-refractory esophageal candidiasis in HIV-infected children†.

Routine long-term suppressive or maintenance therapy (secondary prophylaxis) to prevent relapse or recurrence is not usually recommended in patients adequately treated for esophageal candidiasis (including HIV-infected individuals) unless the patient has frequent or severe recurrences of esophageal candidiasis. If secondary prophylaxis of esophageal candidiasis is indicated, oral fluconazole or posaconazole oral suspension is recommended; however, the potential for development of azole resistance should be considered.

For additional information on management of esophageal candidiasis, the current clinical practice guidelines from IDSA available at http://www.idsociety.org and the current clinical practice guidelines from CDC, NIH, and IDSA on the prevention and treatment of opportunistic infections in HIV-infected individuals available at http://www.aidsinfo.nih.gov should be consulted.

Clinical Experience. In a randomized, double-blind study of micafungin sodium for the treatment of endoscopically confirmed esophageal candidiasis, adults received either micafungin (150 mg IV once daily) or fluconazole (200 mg IV once daily) for a median duration of 14 days (range: 1–33 days). Most patients in this study had both esophageal and oropharyngeal candidiasis at baseline (*C. albicans* was isolated from 96% of patients) and most patients had HIV infection ($CD4^+$ T-cell counts less than 100/mm^3). An endoscopic cure (defined as normal endoscopy [mucosal grade of 0] at end of treatment) was attained in 87.7% of those who received micafungin and 88% of those who received fluconazole. Clinical cure (defined as complete resolution of clinical symptoms including dysphagia, odynophagia, and retrosternal pain) was attained in 91.9% of patients in each group. The mycologic eradication rate (determined by culture and histologic or cytologic evaluation of esophageal biopsy/brushings obtained endoscopically at the end of treatment) was 74.6% in those who received micafungin and 77.6% in those who received fluconazole. The rate of relapse (defined as recurrence of clinical symptoms or endoscopic lesions) at 2 and 4 weeks posttreatment was similar in those who received micafungin (17.9 and 32.7%, respectively) or fluconazole (13.6 and 28.2%, respectively).

Oropharyngeal Candidiasis Although safety and efficacy of micafungin for the treatment of oropharyngeal candidiasis† have not been established, the drug has been recommended as an alternative for the treatment of oropharyngeal candidiasis.

For the treatment of mild oropharyngeal candidiasis, IDSA recommends topical treatment with clotrimazole lozenges or miconazole buccal tablets; nystatin (oral suspension or tablets) is the recommended alternative. For moderate to severe disease, IDSA recommends oral fluconazole. For fluconazole-refractory oropharyngeal candidiasis, IDSA recommends itraconazole oral solution or posaconazole oral suspension; oral voriconazole or amphotericin B oral suspension (not commercially available in the US) are recommended as alternatives. Other alternatives for refractory oropharyngeal candidiasis are an IV echinocandin (anidulafungin, caspofungin, micafungin) or IV amphotericin B.

For the treatment of oropharyngeal candidiasis in HIV-infected adults and adolescents, CDC, NIH, and IDSA recommend oral fluconazole as the preferred drug of choice for initial episodes. If topical therapy is used for the treatment of oropharyngeal candidiasis (e.g., mild to moderate episodes), these experts recommend clotrimazole lozenges or miconazole buccal tablets. Alternatives for systemic treatment of oropharyngeal candidiasis in HIV-infected adults and adolescents are itraconazole oral solution or posaconazole oral suspension; nystatin oral suspension is an alternative if topical treatment is used. For fluconazole-refractory oropharyngeal infections in HIV-infected adults and adolescents, posaconazole oral suspension is preferred; itraconazole oral solution is an alternative.

Routine long-term suppressive or maintenance therapy (secondary prophylaxis) to prevent relapse or recurrence is not usually recommended in patients adequately treated for oropharyngeal candidiasis (including HIV-infected individuals) unless the patient has frequent or severe recurrences of oropharyngeal candidiasis. If secondary prophylaxis of oropharyngeal candidiasis is indicated, oral fluconazole is recommended; however, the potential for development of azole resistance should be considered.

For additional information on management of oropharyngeal candidiasis, the current clinical practice guidelines from IDSA available at http://www.idsociety.org and the current clinical practice guidelines from CDC, NIH, and IDSA on the prevention and treatment of opportunistic infections in HIV-infected individuals available at http://www.aidsinfo.nih.gov should be consulted.

Clinical Experience. In a randomized, double-blind study in adults with endoscopically confirmed esophageal candidiasis who also had oropharyngeal candidiasis† and were treated with micafungin (150 mg IV once daily) or fluconazole (200 mg IV once daily), the clinical response rates for the oropharyngeal infections (based on resolution of signs and symptoms) were 83.5% in those treated with micafungin and 82.1% in those treated with fluconazole. However, the rate of relapse (defined as recurrence of symptoms and/or requirement of posttreatment systemic antifungal therapy) was higher at 2 and 4 weeks posttreatment in those who received micafungin (32.3 and 52.1%, respectively) than in those who received fluconazole (18.1 and 39.4%, respectively).

Candida auris Infections Micafungin is used for the treatment of infections caused by *C. auris*, an emerging pathogen that has been associated with potentially fatal candidemia or other invasive infections.

C. auris, first identified in 2009, has now been reported as the cause of serious invasive infections (including fatalities) in multiple countries worldwide (e.g., Japan, South Korea, India, Kuwait, South Africa, Pakistan, United Kingdom, Venezuela, Colombia, US). As of May 2017, a total of 77 clinical cases of *C. auris* had been reported to CDC from 7 different states in the US. *C. auris* may be difficult to identify using standard in vitro methods and has been misidentified as *C. haemulonii*, *C. famata*, or *Rhodotorula glutinis*. A large percentage of *C. auris* clinical isolates are resistant to fluconazole and multidrug-resistant isolates with reduced susceptibility or resistance to all 3 major classes of antifungal agents (azoles, polyenes, echinocandins) have been reported.

Pending further accumulation of data, CDC has issued interim recommendations regarding laboratory diagnosis, treatment, and infection control measures for suspected or known *C. auris* infections. Based on limited data available to date, CDC recommends that an IV echinocandin (anidulafungin, caspofungin, micafungin) be used for initial treatment of invasive *C. auris* infections (e.g., bloodstream or intra-abdominal infections) in adults. CDC states that a switch to IV amphotericin B (lipid formulation) could be considered if the patient is clinically unresponsive to the echinocandin or fungemia persists longer than 5 days. Consultation with an infectious disease specialist is highly recommended.

Unless there is evidence of infection, CDC does not currently recommend antifungal treatment when *C. auris* is isolated only from noninvasive body sites (e.g., urine, external ear, wounds, respiratory secretions). Some individuals are colonized with *C. auris* in the axilla, groin, nose, external ear canal, oropharynx, urine, wounds, rectum, and stool; however, data are limited and the duration of *C. auris* colonization is unclear. Therefore, CDC recommends that infection control measures be observed for all patients with cultures yielding *C. auris*, including those with positive cultures only from noninvasive body sites.

Whenever *C. auris* infection is suspected, clinicians should immediately contact state or local public health authorities and the CDC (candidaauris@cdc.gov) for guidance. For additional information on diagnosis and management of *C. auris* infections, the interim recommendations and most recent information from CDC available at https://www.cdc.gov/fungal/diseases/candidiasis/candida-auris.html should be consulted.

Prevention of Candida Infections in Hematopoietic Stem Cell Transplant Recipients Micafungin sodium is used for prophylaxis of *Candida* infections in hematopoietic stem cell transplant (HSCT) recipients.

Clinical Experience. Safety and efficacy of micafungin sodium compared with fluconazole for prophylaxis of *Candida* infections in HSCT recipients were evaluated in a randomized, double-blind study in adults and pediatric patients† undergoing autologous or syngeneic (46%) or allogeneic (54%) stem cell transplant. The autologous and syngeneic transplant recipients had underlying diseases that included multiple myeloma, non-Hodgkin's lymphoma, and Hodgkin's disease; the allogeneic transplant recipients had underlying diseases that included chronic myelogenous leukemia, acute myelogenous leukemia, acute lymphocytic leukemia, and non-Hodgkin's lymphoma. During the study, 22.4% of patients had proven graft-versus-host disease (GVHD) and 53.9% received immunosuppressive medications for treatment or prophylaxis of GVHD.

Patients were randomized to receive micafungin (50 mg IV once daily) or fluconazole (400 mg IV once daily) until neutrophil recovery (defined as an absolute neutrophil count [ANC] of 500/mm^3 or greater) up to a maximum of 42 days after transplant. The average duration of antifungal prophylaxis was 18 days (range: 1–51 days). Successful antifungal prophylaxis (defined as the absence of a proven, probable, or suspected systemic fungal infection during the period of prophylactic therapy and the absence of a proven or probable systemic fungal infection during the 4-week posttherapy period) was achieved in 80.7 or 73.7% of patients receiving micafungin or fluconazole, respectively. Systemic antifungal treatment was required after prophylaxis in 42% of those who received micafungin or fluconazole.

■ **Aspergillosis** Micafungin sodium, alone or in conjunction with other antifungals, has been used with some success as primary or salvage therapy for the treatment of invasive aspergillosis†.

IDSA and other clinicians consider IV voriconazole the drug of choice for primary treatment of invasive aspergillosis in adult and pediatric patients, including those with HIV infection; IV amphotericin B or isavuconazonium sulfate (prodrug of isavuconazole) is usually recommended as an alternative for primary treatment. For salvage therapy in patients refractory to or intolerant of primary antifungal therapy, IDSA recommends IV amphotericin B, an IV echinocandin (caspofungin, micafungin), oral or IV posaconazole, or itraconazole oral suspension. IDSA states that echinocandins (either alone or in conjunction with other antifungals) may be effective for salvage therapy of invasive aspergillosis; however, routine use of echinocandin monotherapy is not recommended for primary treatment of invasive aspergillosis.

For additional information on management of aspergillosis, the current clinical practice guidelines from IDSA available at http://www.idsociety.org and the current clinical practice guidelines from CDC, NIH, and IDSA on the prevention and treatment of opportunistic infections in HIV-infected individuals available at http://www.aidsinfo.nih.gov should be consulted.

Clinical Experience Efficacy of micafungin sodium in the treatment of invasive aspergillosis† was evaluated in an open-label, noncomparative study in 70 adults with confirmed or presumed invasive fungal infections who received IV micafungin (12.5–150 mg daily; dosage escalation permitted after 4–7 days at the same dosage) alone for 7–56 days. An overall clinical response was achieved in 60% (6/10) of patients with invasive pulmonary aspergillosis, 67% (6/9) of those with chronic necrotizing pulmonary aspergillosis, 55% (12/22) of those with pulmonary aspergilloma, 100% (6/6) of those with candidemia, and 71% (5/7) of those with esophageal candidiasis. The overall clinical response was lower in those with invasive aspergillosis (57%) than in those with candidiasis (79%).

Dosage and Administration

■ **Administration** Micafungin sodium is administered by slow IV infusion. The drug should *not* be given by rapid IV injection.

IV Infusion Micafungin should not be admixed or infused concomitantly with other drugs.

Strict aseptic technique must be observed when preparing micafungin solutions because the drug contains no preservatives.

If micafungin is administered via an existing IV line, the line should be flushed with 0.9% sodium chloride injection before the drug is infused.

To minimize the risk of infusion reactions, micafungin solutions with a concentration greater than 1.5 mg/mL should be administered IV via a central catheter.

Reconstitution and Dilution. Commercially available micafungin sodium lyophilized powder for injection must be reconstituted and then further diluted prior to administration.

Based on the indicated micafungin dosage, the appropriate number of vials labeled as containing 50 or 100 mg of micafungin should be reconstituted with 5 mL of 0.9% sodium chloride injection or 5% dextrose injection to provide a solution containing approximately 10 or 20 mg/mL, respectively. After the diluent has been added to the powder, the vial should be gently swirled; to minimize excessive foaming, the vial should not be shaken vigorously.

The appropriate volume of reconstituted micafungin solution should then be withdrawn from the vials and added to 100 mL of 0.9% sodium chloride injection or 5% dextrose injection.

The final solution for IV infusion should have a concentration of 0.5–4 mg/mL.

Vials of lyophilized micafungin must be stored at 25°C, but may be exposed to temperatures ranging from 15–30°C. Following reconstitution, micafungin solutions may be stored in the original vial at 25°C for up to 24 hours. Reconstituted micafungin solutions that have been further diluted in 0.9% sodium chloride injection or 5% dextrose injection may be stored at 25°C for up to 24 hours and should be protected from light; covering the infusion drip chamber or the IV tubing is not necessary during IV infusion of the drug.

Rate of Administration. IV infusions of micafungin should be given over 1 hour. More rapid infusion may increase the risk of a histamine-mediated reaction. (See Sensitivity Reactions under Cautions: Warnings/Precautions.)

■ **Dosage** Dosage of micafungin sodium is expressed in terms of micafungin.

A loading dose of micafungin is not required.

Adult Dosage **Candidemia and Other Invasive Candida Infections.** The recommended dosage of micafungin for the treatment of candidemia, acute disseminated candidiasis, and certain other invasive *Candida* infections (peritonitis, abscesses) in *nonneutropenic* or *neutropenic* adults is 100 mg once daily.

When micafungin is used for initial treatment of candidemia or other invasive *Candida* infections, the Infectious Diseases Society of America (IDSA) states that a transition from the echinocandin to fluconazole can be considered (usually within 5–7 days) in patients who are clinically stable, have isolates susceptible to fluconazole (e.g., *C. albicans*), and have negative repeat blood cultures after initial antifungal treatment.

IDSA recommends that antifungal treatment for candidemia (without persistent fungemia or metastatic complications) be continued for 2 weeks after documented clearance of *Candida* from the bloodstream, resolution of candidemia symptoms, and resolution of neutropenia. The mean duration of micafungin therapy in patients treated successfully in clinical trials was 15 days (range: 10–47 days).

If micafungin is used for *initial* treatment of osteoarticular infections† (e.g., osteomyelitis, septic arthritis) caused by *Candida*, IDSA recommends a dosage of 100 mg once daily in adults. After at least 2 weeks, treatment can be switched to fluconazole.

If micafungin is used for *initial* treatment of endocarditis† (native or prosthetic valve) or implantable cardiac device infections† caused by *Candida*, IDSA recommends a dosage of 150 mg once daily in adults. If the infection is caused by fluconazole-susceptible *Candida*, treatment can be switched to fluconazole after the patient is stabilized and *Candida* has been cleared from the bloodstream.

Esophageal Candidiasis. The recommended dosage of micafungin for the treatment of esophageal candidiasis in adults is 150 mg once daily.

If micafungin is used for the treatment of esophageal candidiasis in adults with human immunodeficiency virus (HIV) infection, the US Centers for Disease Control and Prevention (CDC), National Institutes of Health (NIH), and IDSA recommend a dosage of 150 mg daily.

CDC, NIH, and IDSA recommend that antifungal treatment of esophageal candidiasis be continued for 14–21 days. The mean duration of micafungin therapy in patients treated successfully in clinical trials was 15 days (range: 10–30 days).

Oropharyngeal Candidiasis. If micafungin is used for the treatment of oropharyngeal candidiasis†, IDSA recommends that adults receive 100 mg once daily for 7–14 days.

Candida auris Infections. If micafungin is used for initial treatment of invasive *C. auris* infections (e.g., bloodstream or intra-abdominal infections), CDC recommends that adults receive 100 mg once daily.

Prevention of Candida Infections in Hematopoietic Stem Cell Transplant Recipients. The recommended dosage of micafungin for the prevention of *Candida* infections in adult hematopoietic stem cell transplant (HSCT) recipients is 50 mg once daily.

The mean duration of micafungin therapy in patients who experienced successful antifungal prophylaxis in clinical trials was 19 days (range: 6–51 days).

Aspergillosis. If micafungin is used alone or in conjunction with other antifungals for salvage treatment of invasive aspergillosis†, IDSA and others recommend a dosage of 100–150 mg once daily in adults.

The duration of treatment is based on the degree and duration of immunosuppression, disease site, and clinical response. IDSA recommends that antifungal treatment of invasive pulmonary aspergillosis be continued for at least 6–12 weeks.

Pediatric Dosage

General Dosing for Pediatric Patients. If micafungin is used in children, the American Academy of Pediatrics (AAP) recommends a dosage of 2–10 mg/kg (up to 200 mg) once daily.

Candidemia and Other Invasive Candida Infections. For the treatment of candidemia, acute disseminated candidiasis and certain other invasive *Candida* infections (peritonitis, abscesses) in pediatric patients 4 months of age or older, the manufacturer recommends that micafungin be given in a dosage of 2 mg/kg (up to 100 mg) once daily.

If micafungin is used for the treatment of invasive candidiasis in HIV-infected children, some experts recommend a dosage of 5–7 mg/kg daily in infants weighing less than 15 kg and a dosage of 3–4 mg/kg daily in children 2–8 years of age weighing 40 kg or less. These experts recommend that children 9–17 years of age weighing 40 kg or less receive a dosage of 2–3 mg/kg daily and those weighing more than 40 kg receive 100 mg daily.

IDSA recommends that antifungal treatment for candidemia (without persistent fungemia or metastatic complications) be continued for 2 weeks after documented clearance of *Candida* from the bloodstream, resolution of candidemia symptoms, and resolution of neutropenia.

Esophageal Candidiasis. For the treatment of esophageal candidiasis in pediatric patients 4 months of age or older, the manufacturer recommends that micafungin be given in a dosage of 3 mg/kg once daily in those weighing 30 kg or less and 2.5 mg/kg (up to 150 mg) once daily in those weighing more than 30 kg.

If micafungin is used for the treatment of esophageal candidiasis in HIV-infected children, some experts recommend a dosage of 5–7 mg/kg daily in infants weighing less than 15 kg and a dosage of 3–4 mg/kg daily in children 2–8 years of age weighing 40 kg or less. These experts recommend that children 9–17 years of age weighing 40 kg or less receive a dosage of 2–3 mg/kg daily and those weighing more than 40 kg receive 100 mg daily.

If micafungin is used for the treatment of esophageal candidiasis in HIV-infected adolescents, CDC, NIH, and IDSA recommend a dosage of 150 mg daily.

CDC, NIH, and IDSA recommend that antifungal treatment of esophageal candidiasis be continued for 14–21 days.

Prevention of Candida Infections in Hematopoietic Stem Cell Transplant Recipients. If micafungin is used for the prevention of *Candida* infections in pediatric patients 4 months of age or older who are HSCT recipients, the recommended dosage is 1 mg/kg (up to 50 mg) once daily.

The mean duration of micafungin therapy in patients who experienced successful antifungal prophylaxis in clinical trials was 19 days (range: 6–51 days).

■ Special Populations

Hepatic Impairment

Dosage adjustments are not necessary in patients with mild, moderate, or severe hepatic impairment (Child-Pugh score 7–12).

Renal Impairment

Dosage adjustments are not necessary in patients with renal impairment.

Because micafungin is not dialyzable, supplemental doses are not required following hemodialysis.

Geriatric Patients

Dosage adjustments are not necessary in patients 65 years of age or older.

Cautions

■ Contraindications

Micafungin is contraindicated in patients with known hypersensitivity to the drug, other echinocandin antifungals (e.g., anidulafungin, caspofungin), or any ingredient in the formulation.

■ Warnings/Precautions

Sensitivity Reactions

Hypersensitivity Reactions. Serious hypersensitivity reactions (e.g., anaphylaxis and anaphylactoid reactions, including shock) have occurred in patients receiving micafungin.

Possible histamine-mediated symptoms (e.g., rash, pruritus, facial swelling, vasodilation) have occurred in patients receiving micafungin. Rapid IV infusion may increase the risk of histamine-mediated reactions. (See Rate of Administration under Dosage and Administration: Administration.)

If serious hypersensitivity reactions occur, the micafungin infusion should be discontinued and appropriate therapy initiated.

Hematologic Effects

Clinically important hemolysis and hemolytic anemia have been reported rarely in patients receiving micafungin. Transient acute intravascular hemolysis and hemoglobinuria (without clinically important anemia) was reported in a healthy individual receiving a 200-mg micafungin infusion in conjunction with oral prednisolone (20 mg daily).

If clinical or laboratory evidence of hemolysis or hemolytic anemia occur during micafungin therapy, the patient should be closely monitored for evidence of worsening hemolysis or hemolytic anemia and the risks of continued micafungin therapy should be weighed against potential benefits of the drug.

Hepatic Effects

Abnormal liver function test results have been reported in healthy individuals and patients receiving micafungin. Hepatic abnormalities, including clinically important hepatic dysfunction, hepatitis, and hepatic failure, have been reported in patients with serious underlying conditions receiving micafungin and multiple other drugs concomitantly.

If abnormal liver function test results occur during micafungin therapy, the patient should be monitored for the development of worsening hepatic function and the risks of continued micafungin therapy should be weighed against potential benefits of the drug.

Renal Effects

Increased BUN and serum creatinine concentrations have been reported in patients receiving micafungin. Clinically important renal dysfunction or acute renal failure have been reported rarely.

If abnormal renal function test results occur during micafungin therapy, the patient should be monitored for the development of worsening renal function.

Infusion Reactions

Possible histamine-mediated symptoms have been reported in patients receiving micafungin. (See Hypersensitivity Reactions under Warnings/Precautions: Sensitivity Reactions, in Cautions.)

Injection site reactions, including phlebitis and thrombophlebitis, have been reported in patients receiving micafungin dosages of 50–150 mg daily. These reactions tend to occur more often when IV infusions of the drug are given using a peripheral vein. To minimize the risk of infusion reactions, micafungin solutions with a concentration greater than 1.5 mg/mL should be administered IV via a central catheter. (See Dosage and Administration.)

Selection and Use of Antifungals

The manufacturer states that efficacy of micafungin has not been established for treatment of infections caused by fungi other than *Candida*.

Specific Populations

Pregnancy. Category C. (See Users Guide.)

There are no adequate and well-controlled studies of micafungin in pregnant women, and the manufacturer states that the drug should be used during pregnancy only if potential benefits outweigh potential risks to the fetus.

In rabbits, administration of micafungin in a dosage about 4 times the recommended human dosage (based on body surface area comparisons) resulted in increased abortions and visceral abnormalities (abnormal lobation of the lung, levocardia, retrocaval ureter, anomalous right subclavian artery, dilatation of the ureter).

Lactation. Micafungin is distributed into milk in rats; it is not known whether the drug is distributed into milk in humans.

Micafungin should be used with caution in nursing women.

Pediatric Use. Safety and efficacy of micafungin have not been established in pediatric patients younger than 4 months of age.

Safety and efficacy of micafungin in pediatric patients 4 months of age and older have been demonstrated based on evidence from adequate and well-controlled studies in adults and pediatric patients and additional pediatric pharmacokinetic and safety data.

Although data are limited, some experts state that micafungin can be considered for first-line treatment of invasive candidiasis or for alternative treatment of esophageal candidiasis in children with human immunodeficiency virus (HIV) infection.

Geriatric Use. Although no overall differences in safety and efficacy were observed between geriatric adults 65 years of age or older and younger adults in clinical trials and other clinical experience has not revealed any evidence of age-related differences, the possibility that some older patients may have increased sensitivity to the drug cannot be ruled out.

There are no clinically important differences in the pharmacokinetics of micafungin in healthy adults 66–78 years of age compared with those 20–24 years of age. Dosage adjustments are not necessary when micafungin is used in geriatric patients.

Hepatic Impairment. Peak plasma concentrations and area under the concentration-time curve (AUC) of micafungin are decreased by approximately

22% in adults with moderate hepatic impairment (Child-Pugh score 7–9) and by approximately 30% in adults with severe hepatic impairment (Child-Pugh score 10–12) compared with adults with normal hepatic function.

Dosage adjustments are not necessary if micafungin is used in patients with mild, moderate, or severe hepatic impairment.

Renal Impairment. In adults with severe renal impairment (creatinine clearance less than 30 mL/minute), peak plasma concentrations and AUC of micafungin are not altered compared with adults with normal renal function.

Dosage adjustments are not necessary if micafungin is used in patients with mild, moderate, or severe renal impairment.

■ **Common Adverse Effects** Adverse effects reported in 5% or more of patients receiving micafungin include GI effects (diarrhea, nausea, vomiting, abdominal pain, abdominal distention), pyrexia, infusion-related reactions, hypoglycemia, hypomagnesemia, hypernatremia, hyperkalemia, epistaxis, hematologic effects (thrombocytopenia, neutropenia, anemia), febrile neutropenia, increased AST, increased ALT, increased alkaline phosphatase, rash, pruritus, urticaria, headache, insomnia, anxiety, decreased urine output, hematuria, atrial fibrillation, and tachycardia. Injection site reactions (inflammation, phlebitis, thrombophlebitis) have been reported.

Drug Interactions

■ **Drugs Metabolized by Hepatic Microsomal Enzymes** Pharmacokinetic interactions unlikely with drugs metabolized by cytochrome P-450 (CYP) isoenzymes 1A2, 2C9, 2C19, 2D6, 2E1, and 3A4.

Although in vitro studies indicate that micafungin is a substrate for and a weak inhibitor of CYP3A, in vivo studies indicate that hydroxylation by CYP3A plays only a minor role in micafungin metabolism.

■ **Drugs Affecting or Affected by P-glycoprotein Transport** Micafungin is not an inhibitor or substrate of the P-glycoprotein transport system; pharmacokinetic interactions unlikely.

■ **Antifungal Agents** ***Amphotericin B*** Pharmacokinetics of micafungin are not affected by concomitant amphotericin B; micafungin dosage adjustments are not required.

In vitro, the antifungal effects of micafungin and amphotericin B have been additive or synergistic against *Aspergillus*; no in vitro evidence of antagonism.

Fluconazole No evidence of pharmacokinetic interactions when micafungin was used with oral or IV fluconazole; micafungin dosage adjustments are not required.

Itraconazole Pharmacokinetic interaction with itraconazole (increase in the peak plasma concentration and area under the concentration-time curve [AUC] of itraconazole; no effect on micafungin pharmacokinetics). Micafungin dosage adjustments are not required. Monitor for itraconazole toxicity and reduce itraconazole dosage if necessary.

Voriconazole No evidence of pharmacokinetic interactions when micafungin was used with voriconazole; micafungin dosage adjustments are not required.

In vitro evidence of additive antifungal effects against *Aspergillus*. In vitro, the antifungal effects of micafungin and voriconazole have usually been indifferent against *Candida*.

■ **Immunosuppressive Agents** ***Cyclosporine*** Possible pharmacokinetic interaction (decreased oral clearance and increased half-life of cyclosporine; no effect on micafungin pharmacokinetics). Although pharmacokinetic interactions between micafungin and cyclosporine probably are not clinically important in most patients, results of a study evaluating concomitant use of the drugs (a single cyclosporine dose and single or multiple micafungin doses) in healthy adults indicate that there is considerable interindividual variation, and a clinically important increase in cyclosporine half-life may occur in some patients. Micafungin dosage adjustments are not required if the drug is used concomitantly with cyclosporine. However, if micafungin is initiated or discontinued in patients receiving cyclosporine, some clinicians recommend that cyclosporine concentrations be monitored carefully and dosage of the immunosuppressive agent adjusted as needed.

Mycophenolate No evidence of pharmacokinetic interactions when micafungin was used with mycophenolate; micafungin dosage adjustments are not required.

Sirolimus Pharmacokinetic interaction (increased AUC of sirolimus; no change in peak sirolimus plasma concentrations; no effect on micafungin pharmacokinetics). Micafungin dosage adjustments are not required. Monitor for sirolimus toxicity and reduce sirolimus dosage if necessary.

Tacrolimus No evidence of pharmacokinetic interactions when micafungin was used with tacrolimus; micafungin dosage adjustments are not required.

■ **Nifedipine** Pharmacokinetic interaction with nifedipine (increase in the peak plasma concentration and AUC of nifedipine; no effect on micafungin pharmacokinetics). Micafungin dosage adjustments are not required. Monitor for nifedipine toxicity and reduce nifedipine dosage if necessary.

■ **Prednisolone** No evidence of pharmacokinetic interactions when micafungin was used with prednisolone; micafungin dosage adjustments are not required.

■ **Rifampin** Pharmacokinetics of micafungin were not affected by concomitant rifampin; micafungin dosage adjustments are not required.

■ **Ritonavir** Pharmacokinetics of micafungin were not affected by concomitant ritonavir; micafungin dosage adjustments are not required.

Description

Micafungin sodium, a semisynthetic lipopeptide synthesized from a fermentation product of *Coleophoma empetri* F-11899, is an echinocandin antifungal agent. Echinocandins (e.g., anidulafungin, caspofungin, micafungin) are glucan synthesis inhibitors and differ structurally and pharmacologically from other currently available antifungal agents.

Like other echinocandins, micafungin inhibits the synthesis of β(1,3)-D-glucan, an essential component of the fungal cell wall that is not present in mammalian cells. The drug may be fungistatic or fungicidal in action. Depending on concentration, micafungin may be fungicidal against some *Candida*, but usually is fungistatic against *Aspergillus*.

Micafungin appears to be metabolized slowly in the liver, principally via arylsulfatase with further metabolism by catechol-*O*-methyltransferase. Hydroxylation of micafungin by the cytochrome P-450 (CYP) 3A isoenzyme appears to be only a minor metabolic pathway. The drug is about 99% protein bound (primarily albumin and to a lesser extent α_1-acid glycoprotein). The elimination half-life of micafungin at steady state is approximately 13.4–17.2 hours in adults. Typically, 85% of the steady-state concentration is achieved after 3 days of once-daily IV micafungin. Micafungin is eliminated principally in feces. In healthy individuals, about 71% of a single IV dose of radiolabeled micafungin sodium was recovered in feces over 28 days.

■ **Spectrum** Micafungin is active in vitro against *Candida*, including *C. albicans*, *C. dubliniensis*, *C. glabrata*, *C. guilliermondii*, *C. krusei*, *C. lusitaniae*, *C. metapsilosis*, *C. orthopsilosis*, *C. parapsilosis*, and *C. tropicalis*.

Clinical isolates of *C. auris* (often misidentified as *C. haemulonii*, *C. famata*, or *Rhodotorula glutinis*) generally have been inhibited in vitro by micafungin concentrations of 0.03–2 mcg/mL.

Micafungin is active in vitro against *Aspergillus*, including *A. fumigatus*, *A. flavus*, *A. niger*, and *A. terreus*.

Like other echinocandins, micafungin is not active against *Cryptococcus neoformans*, *Trichosporon*, or zygomycetes.

■ **Resistance** Resistance to micafungin has been reported. *C. albicans* with reduced susceptibility or resistance to micafungin have been reported after long-term treatment with the drug. Resistance also has developed in *C. parapsilosis*. Some clinical isolates of *C. auris* have reduced susceptibility or resistance to micafungin in vitro (i.e., MICs 4 mcg/mL or greater).

Resistance to micafungin may be related to specific mutations in the FKS protein component of the glucan synthase enzyme.

Some *C. albicans* with reduced susceptibility to micafungin also have reduced susceptibility to caspofungin.

Advice to Patients

Inform patients about the possible benefits and risks associated with micafungin.

Inform patients about potential adverse effects associated with micafungin, including hypersensitivity reactions (anaphylaxis and anaphylactoid reactions including shock), hematologic effects (acute intravascular hemolysis, hemolytic anemia, hemoglobinuria), hepatic effects (abnormal liver function tests, hepatic impairment, hepatitis or worsening hepatic failure), and renal effects (elevated BUN and creatinine concentrations, renal impairment or acute renal failure). (See Cautions: Warnings/Precautions.)

Importance of informing clinicians if any unusual symptoms develop or if any known symptoms persist or worsen.

Importance of informing clinicians of existing or contemplated concomitant therapy, including prescription and OTC drugs, and any concomitant illnesses.

Importance of women informing clinicians if they are or plan to become pregnant or plan to breast-feed.

Importance of informing patients of other important precautionary information. (See Cautions.)

Overview® (see Users Guide). For additional information on this drug until a more detailed monograph is developed and published, the manufacturer's labeling should be consulted. It is *essential* that the manufacturer's labeling be consulted for more detailed information on usual cautions, precautions, contraindications, potential drug interactions, laboratory test interferences, and acute toxicity.

Preparations

Excipients in commercially available drug preparations may have clinically important effects in some individuals; consult specific product labeling for details.

Micafungin Sodium

Parenteral

For injection, for IV infusion	50 mg (of micafungin)	**Mycamine®**, Astellas
	100 mg (of micafungin)	**Mycamine®**, Astellas

†Use is not currently included in the labeling approved by the US Food and Drug Administration

POLYENES 8:14.28

Amphotericin B AmB, AmB-d, D-AMB, ABLC, L-AmB

■ Amphotericin B, a macrocyclic polyene, is an antifungal agent.

Uses

Conventional IV amphotericin B (formulated with sodium desoxycholate) is used for the treatment of potentially life-threatening fungal infections including aspergillosis, blastomycosis, systemic candidiasis, coccidioidomycosis, cryptococcosis, histoplasmosis, paracoccidioidomycosis†, sporotrichosis, and zygomycosis. The drug also has been used IV for empiric antifungal therapy in febrile neutropenic patients† or for prevention of fungal infections in other immunocompromised individuals† (e.g., cancer patients, bone marrow or solid organ transplant recipients). In addition, conventional IV amphotericin B is used for the treatment of certain protozoal infections, including leishmaniasis and primary amebic meningoencephalitis caused by *Naegleria fowleri*†.

Conventional IV amphotericin B should be used principally in patients with progressive, potentially life-threatening fungal infections and should not be used to treat noninvasive fungal infections (e.g., oral thrush, vaginal candidiasis, esophageal candidiasis) in immunocompetent patients with normal neutrophil counts. When necessary, conventional amphotericin B has been administered intrathecally† or intraventricularly† (either alone or in conjunction with systemic antifungal therapy) for the treatment of CNS infections caused by susceptible fungi. Conventional amphotericin B also has been administered by bladder irrigation† for the treatment of *Candida* cystitis, administered intraperitoneally† for the treatment of fungal peritonitis, and given intrabronchially† or by nebulization† for the treatment or prophylaxis of pulmonary fungal infections.

Amphotericin B lipid complex (Abelcet®) is labeled for the treatment of invasive fungal infections in patients who are refractory to or intolerant of conventional IV amphotericin B.

Amphotericin B liposomal (AmBisome®) is labeled for the treatment of infections caused by *Aspergillus*, *Candida*, or *Cryptococcus* that are refractory to conventional IV amphotericin B and for the treatment of these infections in patients who cannot receive conventional amphotericin B because of renal impairment or unacceptable toxicity. Amphotericin B liposomal also is labeled for the treatment of cryptococcal meningitis in patients with human immunodeficiency virus (HIV) infection, for empiric therapy of presumed fungal infections in febrile, neutropenic patients, and for the treatment of visceral leishmaniasis.

IV amphotericin B is considered a drug of choice for the treatment of many systemic infections caused by susceptible fungi, especially for initial treatment in patients with severe infections. Although clinical experience with lipid formulations of amphotericin B (amphotericin B lipid complex, amphotericin B liposomal) has been obtained principally from small, open-label studies and case reports, the lipid formulations of amphotericin B generally appear to be better tolerated (e.g., lower incidence of acute infusion reactions and adverse hematologic and renal effects) and may be preferred for some infections. Additional study is needed to determine the relative efficacy of these lipid formulations of amphotericin B compared with conventional IV amphotericin B for the treatment of severe, potentially life-threatening fungal infections.

■ **Aspergillosis** Conventional IV amphotericin B, amphotericin B lipid complex, and amphotericin B liposomal are used for the treatment of invasive aspergillosis caused by *Aspergillosis*.

The Infectious Diseases Society of America (IDSA) and other clinicians consider voriconazole the drug of choice for primary treatment of invasive aspergillosis in most patients, including HIV-infected patients. These experts state that IV amphotericin B liposomal or isavuconazonium sulfate (prodrug of isavuconazole) are the preferred alternatives for primary treatment of aspergillosis; IV amphotericin B lipid complex is another alternative. For salvage therapy in patients refractory to or intolerant of primary antifungal therapy, IV amphotericin B (a lipid formulation), an IV echinocandin (caspofungin, micafungin), oral or IV posaconazole, or itraconazole oral suspension are recommended. IDSA states that conventional IV amphotericin B and lipid formulations of amphotericin B are appropriate options for initial and salvage treatment of invasive aspergillosis when voriconazole cannot be used; however, conventional IV amphotericin B should be reserved for use in resource-limited settings when no alternative agents are available.

For the treatment of invasive aspergillosis in HIV-infected adults and adolescents, the US Centers for Disease Control and Prevention (CDC), National Institutes of Health (NIH), and IDSA recommend voriconazole as the drug of choice; IV amphotericin B (conventional or lipid formulation), IV echinocandins (anidulafungin, caspofungin, micafungin), and oral posaconazole are recommended as alternatives.

Clinical Experience Invasive aspergillosis (especially in immunocompromised patients) is difficult to diagnose and treat, and the overall response rate of invasive aspergillosis to conventional IV amphotericin B has been highly variable ranging from 14–83%. In a controlled study in immunocompromised adults and adolescents 12 years of age or older with invasive aspergillosis, patients were randomized to receive voriconazole (6 mg/kg IV twice daily on day 1, then 4 mg/kg IV twice daily for at least 7 days, followed by oral voriconazole 200 mg twice daily) or conventional amphotericin B (1–1.5 mg/kg IV once daily). A successful outcome (complete and partial responses) at week 12 in the modified intention-to-treat population (ITT) was achieved in 53% of those treated with voriconazole compared with 32% of those treated with amphotericin B. In addition, the survival rate at 12 weeks was 71% in the voriconazole group compared with 58% in the amphotericin B group.

In several studies involving patients with invasive aspergillosis, the response rates to amphotericin B lipid complex or amphotericin B liposomal have ranged from 32–69%.

Although conventional IV amphotericin B has been used in conjunction with other antifungals (e.g., flucytosine) for salvage therapy in some patients with invasive aspergillosis (e.g., CNS, endocarditis) that did not respond to conventional IV amphotericin B alone, it is unclear whether these combination regimens offer any benefit over use of IV amphotericin B alone and there are concerns related to possible drug interactions between amphotericin B and flucytosine. (See Flucytosine under Drug Interactions: Anti-infective Agents.)

For additional information on management of aspergillosis, the current clinical practice guidelines from IDSA available at http://www.idsociety.org and the current clinical practice guidelines from CDC, NIH, and IDSA on the prevention and treatment of opportunistic infections in HIV-infected individuals available at http://www.aidsinfo.nih.gov should be consulted.

■ **Blastomycosis** IV amphotericin B is used for the treatment of pulmonary and extrapulmonary blastomycosis caused by *Blastomyces dermatitidis*.

While both oral itraconazole and IV amphotericin B are considered drugs of choice for the treatment of blastomycosis, IV amphotericin B is preferred for initial treatment of severe blastomycosis, especially infections involving the CNS, and for initial treatment of presumptive blastomycosis in immunocompromised patients, including HIV-infected individuals. Oral itraconazole is the drug of choice for the treatment of nonmeningeal, non-life-threatening blastomycosis, including mild to moderate pulmonary blastomycosis or mild to moderate disseminated blastomycosis (without CNS involvement) and also is recommended for follow-up therapy in patients with more severe infections after an initial response has been obtained with IV amphotericin B.

When amphotericin B is used for the treatment of blastomycosis, conventional IV amphotericin B or a lipid formulation of amphotericin B can be used. However, IDSA and others state that a lipid formulation of amphotericin B (e.g., amphotericin B liposomal) may be preferred for the treatment of CNS blastomycosis since higher CSF concentrations may be obtained.

For additional information on management of blastomycosis, the current clinical practice guidelines from IDSA available at http://www.idsociety.org should be consulted.

■ **Candida Infections** IV amphotericin B is used for the treatment of disseminated or invasive infections caused by *Candida*, including candidemia, cardiovascular infections (endocarditis, pericarditis, myocarditis), and meningitis, and for the treatment of other serious infections caused by *Candida*, including osteoarticular infections (osteomyelitis, septic arthritis), peritonitis, intra-abdominal abscesses, urinary tract infections (symptomatic cystitis, pyelonephritis, urinary fungus balls), and endophthalmitis. The drug also is used for the treatment of certain severe or refractory mucocutaneous *Candida* infections (e.g., esophageal candidiasis†, oropharyngeal candidiasis†).

Amphotericin B generally is effective against infections caused by *C. albicans*, *C. glabrata*, *C. krusei*, *C. parapsilosis*, or *C. tropicalis*, and is a drug of choice for many infections caused by fluconazole-resistant *Candida*. Fluconazole-resistant *C. albicans* are being isolated with increasing frequency from patients who have received prior fluconazole therapy (especially in HIV-infected patients) and some *Candida* infections (e.g., candidemia) are increasingly caused by strains that are intrinsically resistant to fluconazole (e.g., *C. krusei*) or likely to have resistance or reduced susceptibility to fluconazole (e.g., *C. glabrata*).

For the treatment of candidemia in *nonneutropenic* patients or for empiric treatment of suspected invasive candidiasis† in *nonneutropenic* patients in intensive care units (ICUs), IDSA recommends an IV echinocandin (anidulafungin, caspofungin, micafungin) for *initial* therapy. IDSA states that fluconazole (IV or oral) is an acceptable alternative for *initial* therapy in selected patients, including those who are not critically ill and are unlikely to have infections caused by fluconazole-resistant *Candida*. If echinocandin- and azole-resistant *Candida* are suspected, IV amphotericin B (a lipid formulation) is recommended; IV amphotericin B (a lipid formulation) also is a reasonable alternative when echinocandins and fluconazole cannot be used because of intolerance, limited availability, or resistance. IDSA states that transition from the echinocandin (or amphotericin B) to fluconazole can be considered (usually within 5–7 days) in patients who are clinically stable, have isolates susceptible to fluconazole (e.g., *C. albicans*), and have negative repeat blood cultures after initial antifungal treatment.

For the treatment of candidemia in *neutropenic* patients, IDSA recommends an IV echinocandin (anidulafungin, caspofungin, micafungin) or, alternatively, IV amphotericin B (a lipid formulation) for *initial* therapy. Fluconazole is an alternative for *initial* therapy in those who are not critically ill or have had no prior exposure to azole antifungals and also can be used for step-down therapy during neutropenia in clinically stable patients who have fluconazole-susceptible isolates and documented bloodstream clearance. Voriconazole can be used as an alternative for *initial* therapy when broader antifungal coverage is required and also can be used as step-down therapy during neutropenia in clinically stable patients who have voriconazole-susceptible isolates and documented bloodstream clearance. For infections known to be caused by *C. krusei*, an echinocandin, amphotericin B (a lipid formulation), or voriconazole is recommended.

For the treatment of chronic disseminated (hepatosplenic) candidiasis, IDSA recommends initial treatment with IV amphotericin B (a lipid formulation) or an IV echinocandin (anidulafungin, caspofungin, micafungin) followed by oral fluconazole therapy.

For the treatment of CNS candidiasis, IDSA recommends initial treatment with IV amphotericin B liposomal (with or without oral flucytosine) and step-down treatment with fluconazole. Infected CNS devices (e.g., ventriculostomy drains, shunts, stimulators, prosthetic reconstructive devices, biopolymer wafers that deliver chemotherapy) should be removed if possible. If a ventricular device cannot be removed, IDSA states that conventional amphotericin B can be administered through the device. Conventional amphotericin B has been administered intrathecally† as an adjunct to systemic antifungal treatment in patients with *Candida* meningitis.

For the treatment of neonatal candidiasis, including CNS infections, conventional IV amphotericin B usually is the drug of choice for *initial* treatment. Although not routinely recommended in neonates, concomitant use of flucytosine can be considered as salvage therapy if CNS infections do not respond to initial therapy with IV amphotericin B alone. The IDSA and American Academy of Pediatrics (AAP) state that fluconazole can be considered for step-down treatment after an initial response has been obtained with IV amphotericin B. Fluconazole also is a reasonable alternative for initial treatment of neonatal candidiasis (without CNS involvement), provided the patient had not been receiving fluconazole prophylaxis and the causative agent is susceptible. Although lipid formulations of IV amphotericin B can be considered as alternatives for the treatment of neonatal candidiasis, these formulations should be used with caution in this age group, particularly in the presence of urinary tract involvement.

For the treatment of endocarditis (native or prosthetic valve) or implantable cardiac device infections caused by *Candida*, IDSA recommends *initial* treatment with a lipid formulation of IV amphotericin B (with or without oral flucytosine) or an IV echinocandin (anidulafungin, caspofungin, micafungin) and step-down treatment with fluconazole. If the isolate is susceptible, long-term suppressive or maintenance therapy (secondary prophylaxis) with fluconazole is recommended to prevent recurrence in those with native valve endocarditis who cannot undergo valve replacement and in those with prosthetic valve endocarditis.

Mucocutaneous or noninvasive *Candida* infections, such as esophageal, oropharyngeal, or vaginal candidiasis, usually can be adequately treated with an appropriate oral or topical antifungal; however, severe or refractory mucocutaneous infections (e.g., esophageal candidiasis†, oropharyngeal candidiasis†) caused by azole-resistant *Candida* or infections that fail to respond to such therapy may require IV amphotericin B therapy. In addition, IV amphotericin B has been recommended as an alternative for the treatment of esophageal candidiasis† in patients who cannot tolerate oral therapy.

Amphotericin B has been used for the treatment of urinary tract infections caused by *Candida*. IDSA states that antifungal treatment is not usually indicated in patients with asymptomatic cystitis, unless there is a high risk of disseminated candidiasis (e.g., neutropenic patients, low birthweight infants [less than 1.5 kg], patients undergoing urologic manipulations). For the treatment of symptomatic cystitis, pyelonephritis, or fungus balls likely to be caused by fluconazole-susceptible *Candida*, fluconazole is the drug of choice. If symptomatic cystitis is caused by fluconazole-resistant *Candida*, IDSA recommends conventional IV amphotericin B or oral flucytosine for infections caused by *C. glabrata* and conventional IV amphotericin B for infections caused by *C. krusei*. If pyelonephritis is caused by fluconazole-resistant *Candida*, conventional IV amphotericin B (with or without oral flucytosine) is recommended for *C. glabrata* and conventional IV amphotericin B is recommended for *C. krusei*. Although conventional amphotericin B has been administered by bladder irrigation† for the treatment of candiduria (funguria), such therapy has been controversial since candiduria may be self-limited in some patients (e.g., after changing or removing indwelling catheters) and the risks and benefits of bladder irrigation versus systemic antifungal treatment have not been clearly identified. IDSA states that bladder irrigation† with conventional amphotericin B is not generally recommended, but may be useful for patients with refractory, symptomatic cystitis caused by fluconazole-resistant *Candida* (e.g., *C. glabrata*, *C. krusei*) or as an adjunct to systemic antifungal therapy for the treatment of urinary fungus balls.

IDSA states that IV amphotericin B liposomal (with or without oral flucytosine) is the regimen of choice for the treatment of endophthalmitis caused by fluconazole- and voriconazole-resistant *Candida*. In patients with macular involvement, intravitreal† administration of conventional amphotericin B also is recommended to ensure prompt high levels of antifungal activity. Decisions regarding antifungal treatment and surgical intervention should be made jointly by an ophthalmologist and an infectious disease clinician.

Amphotericin B lipid complex has been effective when used in pediatric cancer patients with chronic disseminated candidiasis or other *Candida* infections. Liposomal amphotericin B has been used effectively for the treatment of disseminated *Candida* infections, and the overall response rate in patients with candidiasis who received the lipid formulation has been reported to be 56–70%.

***Candida auris* Infections** IV amphotericin B has been used for the treatment of infections caused by *C. auris*, an emerging pathogen that has been associated with potentially fatal candidemia or other invasive infections.

C. auris, first identified in 2009, has now been reported as the cause of serious invasive infections (including fatalities) in multiple countries worldwide (e.g., Japan, South Korea, India, Kuwait, South Africa, Pakistan, United Kingdom, Venezuela, Columbia, US). As of May 2017, a total of 77 clinical cases of *C. auris* had been reported to CDC from 7 different states in the US. *C. auris* may be difficult to identify using standard in vitro methods and has been misidentified as *C. haemulonii*, *C. famata*, or *Rhodotorula glutinis*. A large percentage of *C. auris* clinical isolates are resistant to fluconazole and multidrug-resistant isolates with reduced susceptibility or resistance to all 3 major classes of antifungal agents (azoles, polyenes, echinocandins) have been reported.

Pending further accumulation of data, CDC has issued interim recommendations regarding laboratory diagnosis, treatment, and infection control measures for suspected or known *C. auris* infections. Based on limited data available to date, CDC recommends that an IV echinocandin (anidulafungin, caspofungin, micafungin) be used for initial treatment of invasive *C. auris* infections (e.g., bloodstream or intra-abdominal infections) in adults. CDC states that a switch to IV amphotericin B (a lipid formulation) could be considered if the patient is clinically unresponsive to the echinocandin or fungemia persists longer than 5 days. Consultation with an infectious disease specialist is highly recommended.

Unless there is evidence of infection, CDC does not currently recommend antifungal treatment when *C. auris* is isolated only from noninvasive body sites (e.g., urine, external ear, wounds, respiratory secretions). Some individuals are colonized with *C. auris* in the axilla, groin, nose, external ear canal, oropharynx, urine, wounds, rectum, and stool; however, data are limited and the duration of *C. auris* colonization is unclear. Therefore, CDC recommends that infection control measures be observed for all patients with cultures yielding *C. auris*, including those with positive cultures only from noninvasive body sites.

Whenever *C. auris* infection is suspected, clinicians should immediately contact state or local public health authorities and the CDC (candidaauris@cdc.gov) for guidance. For additional information on diagnosis and management of *C. auris* infections, the interim recommendations and most recent information from CDC available at https://www.cdc.gov/fungal/diseases/candidiasis/candida-auris.html should be consulted.

■ **Coccidioidomycosis** IV amphotericin B is used for the treatment of coccidioidomycosis caused by *Coccidioides immitis* or *C. posadasii*.

IDSA states that antifungal treatment is not considered necessary in patients with newly diagnosed, uncomplicated coccidioidal pneumonia who have mild or nondebilitating symptoms, including those with an asymptomatic pulmonary nodule or cavity due to coccidioidomycosis and no overt immunocompromising conditions. However, antifungal treatment is recommended for patients with symptomatic chronic cavitary coccidioidal pneumonia, ruptured coccidioidal cavities, extrapulmonary soft tissue coccidioidomycosis, bone and joint coccidioidomycosis, or coccidioidal meningitis. Antifungal treatment of coccidioidomycosis also is usually recommended for patients who are immunocompromised or debilitated (e.g., HIV-infected individuals, organ transplant recipients, those receiving immunosuppressive therapy, those with diabetes or cardiopulmonary disease).

IDSA and others state that an oral azole (fluconazole or itraconazole) usually is recommended for initial treatment of symptomatic pulmonary coccidioidomycosis and chronic fibrocavitary or disseminated (extrapulmonary) coccidioidomycosis. However, IV amphotericin B is recommended as an alternative and is preferred for initial treatment of severely ill patients who have rapidly progressing or extrathoracic disseminated disease, for immunocompromised individuals, or when azole antifungals cannot be used (e.g., pregnant women).

For the treatment of clinically mild coccidioidomycosis (e.g., focal pneumonia) in HIV-infected adults, adolescents, or children, CDC, NIH, and IDSA recommend initial therapy with oral fluconazole or oral itraconazole. Although clinical data are limited, oral voriconazole or oral posaconazole may be used as alternatives in HIV-infected adults or adolescents for the treatment of clinically mild coccidioidomycosis† that has not responded to fluconazole or itraconazole.

For the treatment of severe (nonmeningeal) coccidioidomycosis (e.g., diffuse pulmonary or extrathoracic disseminated infections) in HIV-infected adults, adolescents, or children, CDC, NIH, and IDSA recommend initial therapy with IV amphotericin B (conventional or lipid formulation) followed by oral azole therapy. Alternatively, some experts recommend initial therapy with IV amphotericin B used in conjunction with an oral azole (fluconazole or itraconazole) followed by the oral azole alone.

For the treatment of coccidioidal meningitis, the regimen of choice in HIV-infected adults, adolescents, or children or other individuals is IV or oral fluconazole (with or without intrathecal† conventional amphotericin B). Other oral azoles (itraconazole, posaconazole, voriconazole) are considered alternatives for the treatment of coccidioidal meningitis in adults and adolescents. Patients who do not respond to fluconazole or itraconazole alone may be candidates for intrathecal† conventional amphotericin B (with or without continued azole therapy) or IV amphotericin B used in conjunction with intrathecal† conventional amphotericin B. Consultation with an expert who has experience in treating coccidioidal meningitis is recommended.

HIV-infected adults, adolescents, or children who have been adequately treated for coccidioidomycosis should receive long-term (usually life-long) secondary prophylaxis to prevent recurrence or relapse. Although oral fluconazole or oral itraconazole are the drugs of choice recommended by CDC, NIH, and IDSA for secondary prophylaxis to prevent recurrence or relapse of coccidioidomycosis in HIV-infected adults, adolescents, or children, these experts state that oral posaconazole or oral voriconazole can be used as an alternative for secondary prophylaxis of coccidioidomycosis in HIV-infected adults or adolescents who did not initially respond to fluconazole or itraconazole.

While data regarding use of lipid formulations of amphotericin B in the treatment of coccidioidomycosis are limited to date, amphotericin B lipid complex has been used with some success in a limited number of patients for the treatment of this infection. Some experts state that there is no evidence that lipid formulations of IV amphotericin B are more effective than conventional IV amphotericin B for the treatment of coccidioidomycosis.

For additional information on management of coccidioidomycosis, the current clinical practice guidelines from IDSA available at http://www.idsociety.org and the current clinical practice guidelines from CDC, NIH, and IDSA on the prevention and treatment of opportunistic infections in HIV-infected individuals available at http://www.aidsinfo.nih.gov should be consulted.

■ **Cryptococcosis** ***Treatment of Cryptococcosis*** IV amphotericin B is used for the treatment of infections caused by *Cryptococcus neoformans*, and generally is considered a drug of choice, especially for the treatment of cryptococcal meningitis. Because of reported in vitro and in vivo synergism, IDSA and other clinicians recommend concomitant use of amphotericin B and flucytosine for initial treatment of cryptococcal infections, especially in HIV-infected patients. Addition of flucytosine to the regimen appears to reduce the time required for sterilization of the CSF in those with CNS involvement and may decrease the risk of subsequent relapse and improve survival.

Conventional IV amphotericin had been the preferred amphotericin B formulation for the treatment of cryptococcosis, but IV amphotericin B liposomal may now be preferred, especially in patients who have or are predisposed to renal dysfunction. Conventional IV amphotericin B can be used if cost is an issue and the risk of renal dysfunction is low. Although data are limited, IV amphotericin B lipid complex is considered an alternative to IV amphotericin B liposomal or conventional IV amphotericin B for the treatment of cryptococcosis.

For the treatment of cryptococcal meningitis in HIV-infected adults, adolescents, and children, CDC, NIH, IDSA, and other clinicians state that the preferred regimen is initial (induction) therapy with IV amphotericin B (liposomal or conventional formulation) given in conjunction with flucytosine for at least 2 weeks until there is evidence of clinical improvement and negative CSF culture after repeat lumbar puncture, then follow-up (consolidation) therapy with oral fluconazole given for at least 8 weeks, followed by long-term suppressive or maintenance therapy (secondary prophylaxis) with oral fluconazole to complete at least 1 year of azole therapy.

For the initial (induction) phase of treatment of cryptococcal meningitis in HIV-infected adults and adolescents, IV amphotericin B (liposomal or conventional formulation) in conjunction with oral flucytosine is the preferred regimen. Alternative regimens for initial (induction) treatment of cryptococcal meningitis in HIV-infected adults and adolescents who cannot receive the preferred regimen are IV amphotericin B lipid complex given in conjunction with oral flucytosine; IV amphotericin B (liposomal or conventional formulation) given in conjunction with oral or IV fluconazole; IV amphotericin B (liposomal or conventional formulation) alone; oral or IV fluconazole given in conjunction with oral flucytosine; or oral or IV fluconazole alone. Alternative regimens may be less effective and are recommended only in patients who cannot tolerate or have not responded to the preferred regimen. IDSA states that use of intrathecal† or intraventricular† conventional amphotericin B in the treatment of cryptococcal meningitis generally is discouraged and is rarely necessary.

For the treatment of cryptococcal CNS infections in organ transplant recipients, IDSA recommends initial (induction) therapy with IV amphotericin B liposomal or IV amphotericin B lipid complex given in conjunction with oral flucytosine for at least 2 weeks, then follow-up (consolidation) therapy with oral fluconazole given for 8 weeks. If the induction regimen does not include flucytosine, it should be continued for at least 4–6 weeks. Conventional IV amphotericin B is not usually recommended for first-line treatment of cryptococcosis in transplant recipients because of the risk of nephrotoxicity. For organ transplant recipients with mild to moderate pulmonary cryptococcosis (without diffuse pulmonary infiltrates) or other mild to moderate cryptococcal infections not involving the CNS, IDSA recommends fluconazole given for 6–12 months.

In adults and children who do not have HIV infection and are not transplant recipients, IDSA states that the preferred regimen for the treatment of cryptococcal meningitis is initial (induction) therapy with conventional IV amphotericin B given in conjunction with oral flucytosine for at least 4 weeks (a 2-week period of induction therapy can be considered in those who are immunocompetent, are without uncontrolled underlying disease, and are at low risk for therapeutic failure), then follow-up (consolidation) therapy with oral fluconazole administered for an additional 8 weeks or longer.

For the treatment of mild to moderate pulmonary cryptococcosis (nonmeningeal) in immunocompetent or immunosuppressed adults or children, IDSA states that the regimen of choice is oral fluconazole given for 6–12 months. However, severe pulmonary cryptococcosis, cryptococcemia, and disseminated cryptococcal infections in immunocompetent or immunosuppressed adults, adolescents, or children should be treated using regimens recommended for cryptococcal meningitis.

Clinical Experience. In a randomized, multicenter study comparing conventional IV amphotericin B (mean dose of 0.4–0.5 mg/kg daily for 10 weeks with or without concomitant flucytosine) with oral fluconazole (400 mg on day 1 followed by 200–400 mg daily for 10 weeks) in HIV-infected patients with cryptococcal meningitis, therapy was effective in 40% of patients receiving amphotericin B and in 34% of those receiving fluconazole. Although overall mortality between patients receiving conventional amphotericin B and patients receiving fluconazole was similar (14% in patients receiving amphotericin B versus 18% in patients receiving fluconazole), mortality was higher during the first 2 weeks of therapy in patients receiving fluconazole (15% versus 8% in those receiving amphotericin B). CSF cultures were positive for an average of about 42 or 64 days in patients receiving conventional amphotericin B or fluconazole, respectively. In a double-blind multicenter trial in patients with AIDS-associated cryptococcal meningitis, the relative efficacy of initial therapy with conventional IV amphotericin B (0.7 mg/kg daily) given with flucytosine (100 mg/kg daily) or placebo for 2 weeks followed by oral fluconazole (800 mg daily for 2 days, then 400 mg daily for 8 weeks) or oral itraconazole (600 mg daily for 3 days, then 400 mg daily for 8 weeks) was evaluated. At 2 weeks, CSF cultures were negative in 60% of those who received amphotericin B with concomitant flucytosine compared with 51% of those who received amphotericin B alone. The clinical response to oral fluconazole or oral itraconazole for follow-up therapy was similar, but the rate of CSF sterilization at 10 weeks was higher in those who received fluconazole (72%) compared with those who received itraconazole (60%).

In a study evaluating safety and efficacy of IV amphotericin B lipid complex for the treatment of cryptococcal meningitis in HIV- infected patients, the lipid formulation was at least as effective as conventional IV amphotericin B for initial therapy in these patients and was associated with less hematologic and renal toxicity than the conventional formulation. An initial clinical response was obtained in 86% of patients who received amphotericin B lipid complex (5 mg/kg once daily during weeks 1 and 2, and 3 times weekly during weeks 3–6) and in 65% of those who received conventional IV amphotericin (0.7 mg/kg during weeks 1 and 2, and 1.2 mg/kg 3 times weekly during weeks 3–6); all patients received follow-up therapy with oral fluconazole for an additional 12 weeks). The overall response rate (resolution of all signs and symptoms and conversion of CNS, blood, and urine cultures to negative) was 38% in those who received amphotericin B lipid complex and 41% in those who received conventional IV amphotericin B.

Amphotericin B liposomal was compared with conventional amphotericin B for empiric treatment of cryptococcal meningitis in HIV-infected patients in a randomized, double-blind study in 267 patients (study 94-0-013). Patients were randomized to receive 11–21 days of IV amphotericin B liposomal (3 or 6 mg/kg daily) or conventional IV amphotericin B (0.7 mg/kg daily); this induction regimen was followed by oral fluconazole (400 mg daily for adults and 200 mg daily in a pediatric patient younger than 13 years of age) given to complete 10 weeks of protocol-directed therapy. At 2 weeks, the success rate (defined as CSF culture conversion) for mycologically evaluable patients (defined as all randomized patients who received at least 1 dose of study drug, had positive baseline CSF culture, and at least 1 follow-up culture) was 47.5% in those who received conventional amphotericin B and 58.3 or 48% in those who received amphotericin B liposomal in a dosage of 3 or 6 mg/kg daily, respectively. At 10 weeks, the success rate (defined as clinical success at week 10 plus CSF culture conversion at or prior to week 10) in those with documented cryptococcal meningitis at baseline was 53% in those who received conventional amphotericin B and 49% in those who received amphotericin B liposomal in a dosage of 6 mg/kg daily; the success rate was only 37% in those who received the lower dosage of amphotericin B liposomal. The survival rate at 10 weeks was similar in those receiving conventional amphotericin B (89%) or the higher dosage of amphotericin B liposomal (90%); the incidence of adverse effects (infusion reactions or adverse cardiovascular or renal effects) was lower in those receiving amphotericin B liposomal than in those receiving conventional amphotericin B. In another randomized study in HIV-infected patients with cryptococcal meningitis who received a 3-week course of liposomal amphotericin B (4 mg/kg daily) or a 3-week course of conventional IV amphotericin B (0.7 mg/kg daily) followed by a 7-week course of oral fluconazole (400 mg daily), the median time to negative CSF cultures was 7–14 days in those receiving amphotericin B liposomal compared with more than 21 days in those receiving conventional IV amphotericin B.

Prevention of Recurrence (Secondary Prophylaxis) of Cryptococcosis HIV-infected adults, adolescents, or children who have been adequately treated for cryptococcosis should receive long-term suppressive or maintenance therapy (secondary prophylaxis) to prevent recurrence. Oral fluconazole is the drug of choice for secondary prophylaxis of cryptococcosis in HIV-infected patients and other individuals who have had documented, adequately treated cryptococcal meningitis; some experts suggest that oral itraconazole is an alternative in those who cannot tolerate fluconazole, but the drug may be less effective than fluconazole in preventing relapse of cryptococcosis.

Although conventional IV amphotericin B has been used or recommended as an alternative for secondary prophylaxis to prevent relapse of cryptococcal meningitis† (e.g., in patients who could not receive azole antifungals), it is less effective and is associated with IV catheter-related infections. Results of a multicenter study comparing safety and efficacy of conventional IV amphotericin B (1 mg/kg once weekly) or oral fluconazole (200 mg once daily) for prevention of relapse of the disease in HIV-infected patients with negative cryptococcal cultures after initial adequate amphotericin B therapy indicate that the fluconazole regimen is more effective (in terms of preventing relapse of culture-positive meningitis) and better tolerated than the amphotericin B regimen for maintenance therapy in these patients.

***Cryptococcus gattii* Infections** Although data are limited, CDC, NIH, and IDSA state that recommendations for the treatment of CNS, pulmonary, or disseminated infections caused by *Cryptococcus gattii* and recommendations for long-term suppressive or maintenance therapy (secondary prophylaxis) of *C. gattii* infections are the same as the recommendations for *C. neoformans* infections. IDSA states that single, small cryptococcoma may be treated with oral fluconazole; however, induction therapy with a regimen of conventional IV amphotericin B and flucytosine given for 4–6 weeks, followed by consolidation therapy with fluconazole given for 6–18 months should be considered for very large or multiple cryptococcomas caused by *C. gattii*. Regimens that include amphotericin B (conventional or liposomal formulations), flucytosine, and fluconazole have been effective in a few patients with CNS infections known to be caused by *C. gattii*.

For additional information on management of cryptococcosis, the current clinical practice guidelines from IDSA available at http://www.idsociety.org and the current clinical practice guidelines from CDC, NIH, and IDSA on the prevention and treatment of opportunistic infections in HIV-infected individuals available at http://www.aidsinfo.nih.gov should be consulted.

■ **Histoplasmosis** IV amphotericin B is used for the treatment of histoplasmosis caused by *Histoplasma capsulatum*.

The drugs of choice for the treatment of histoplasmosis, including histoplasmosis in HIV-infected individuals, are IV amphotericin B and oral itraconazole. IV amphotericin B is preferred for initial treatment of severe, life-threatening histoplasmosis, especially in immunocompromised patients such as those with HIV infection. Oral itraconazole generally is used for initial treatment of less severe disease (e.g., mild to moderate acute pulmonary histoplasmosis, chronic cavitary pulmonary histoplasmosis) and as follow-up therapy in the treatment of severe infections after a response has been obtained with IV amphotericin B. Other azole antifungals (fluconazole, posaconazole, voriconazole) are considered second-line alternatives to itraconazole, but can be considered in patients who have less severe disease and cannot tolerate itraconazole.

For the treatment of moderately severe to severe acute pulmonary histoplasmosis in HIV-infected adults and adolescents, CDC, NIH, and IDSA recommend initial (induction) treatment with IV amphotericin B liposomal and follow-up treatment with oral itraconazole. Alternatively, if necessary because of cost or tolerability, IV amphotericin B lipid complex can be used.

For the treatment of progressive disseminated histoplasmosis in children, IDSA states that conventional IV amphotericin B or an initial regimen of conventional IV amphotericin B and follow-up treatment with oral itraconazole can be used. IDSA states that conventional amphotericin B usually is well tolerated in children, but a lipid formulation may be substituted if necessary.

For the treatment of moderately severe to severe disseminated histoplasmosis in HIV-infected infants and children, CDC, NIH, and IDSA recommend initial treatment with IV amphotericin B liposomal and follow-up treatment with oral itraconazole; conventional IV amphotericin B can be used as an alternative to the lipid formulation for initial treatment in these children. Although oral itraconazole may be used alone for the treatment of mild to moderate progressive disseminated histoplasmosis in children, including HIV-infected infants and children, this regimen is not recommended for more severe infections.

For the treatment of meningitis caused by *H. capsulatum* in HIV-infected adults, adolescents, or children and other individuals, CDC, NIH, and IDSA recommend initial (induction) treatment with IV amphotericin B liposomal and follow-up treatment with oral itraconazole. The liposomal formulation of amphotericin B generally is preferred for the treatment of CNS histoplasmosis since CSF concentrations may be higher with the liposomal formulation than with some other formulations. Conventional IV amphotericin B has been administered alone or in conjunction with intrathecal† administration of the drug for the treatment of meningitis caused by *H. capsulatum*.

HIV-infected adults, adolescents, or children who have been adequately treated for histoplasmosis should receive long-term suppressive or maintenance therapy (secondary prophylaxis) to prevent recurrence or relapse of histoplasmosis. Oral itraconazole is the drug of choice for secondary prophylaxis of histoplasmosis in HIV-infected patients.

For additional information on management of histoplasmosis, the current clinical practice guidelines from IDSA available at http://www.idsociety.org and the current clinical practice guidelines from CDC, NIH, and IDSA on the prevention and treatment of opportunistic infections in HIV-infected individuals available at http://www.aidsinfo.nih.gov should be consulted.

■ **Paracoccidioidomycosis** IV amphotericin B is used for the treatment of paracoccidioidomycosis† (South American blastomycosis) caused by *Paracoccidioides brasiliensis*.

IV amphotericin B is the drug of choice for initial treatment of severe paracoccidioidomycosis. Oral itraconazole is the drug of choice for the treatment of less severe or localized paracoccidioidomycosis and for follow-up therapy in more severe infections after initial treatment with IV amphotericin B.

■ **Penicilliosis** IV amphotericin B is used in the treatment of penicilliosis† caused by *Penicillium marneffei*.

Although oral itraconazole can be used alone for the treatment of mild penicilliosis, an initial regimen of IV amphotericin B is recommended for the treatment of severe or disseminated *P. marneffei* infections†.

For the treatment of severe, acute penicilliosis† in HIV-infected adults and adolescents, CDC, NIH, and IDSA recommend an initial regimen of IV amphotericin B liposomal followed by oral itraconazole. These experts state that a voriconazole regimen (IV initially, then oral) can be used as an alternative in patients with severe penicilliosis, including those who fail to respond to a regimen of IV amphotericin B followed by itraconazole.

HIV-infected patients who have been treated for penicilliosis should receive long-term suppressive or maintenance therapy (secondary prophylaxis) with oral itraconazole to prevent recurrence or relapse.

For additional information on management of penicilliosis, the current clinical practice guidelines from CDC, NIH, and IDSA on the prevention and treatment of opportunistic infections in HIV-infected individuals available at http://www.aidsinfo.nih.gov should be consulted.

■ **Sporotrichosis** IV amphotericin B is used in the treatment of disseminated, pulmonary, osteoarticular, and meningeal sporotrichosis caused by *Sporothrix schenckii*.

IV amphotericin B is the drug of choice for initial treatment of severe, life-threatening sporotrichosis and whenever sporotrichosis is disseminated or has CNS involvement. Oral itraconazole is the drug of choice for the treatment of cutaneous, lymphocutaneous, or mild pulmonary or osteoarticular sporotrichosis and for follow-up treatment of severe infections after a response has been obtained with IV amphotericin B.

Since sporotrichosis in immunocompromised patients (e.g., HIV-infected individuals) is particularly aggressive and difficult to treat, IV amphotericin B usually is the drug of choice for initial therapy in these patients; however, treatment failures occur. IDSA and other clinicians state that a lipid formulation of amphotericin B is preferred for the treatment of sporotrichosis since the lipid formulations generally are associated with fewer adverse effects.

For additional information on management of sporotrichosis, the current clinical practice guidelines from IDSA available at http://www.idsociety.org should be consulted.

■ **Exserohilum Infections** Amphotericin B has been used for the treatment of infections known or suspected to be caused by *Exserohilum rostratum*†.

Exserohilum is a common mold found in soil and on plants, especially grasses, and thrives in warm and humid climates. *E. rostratum* is considered an opportunistic human pathogen and rarely has been involved in human infections, including cutaneous and subcutaneous infections or keratitis, typically as the result of skin or eye trauma. More invasive infections (e.g., infections involving the sinuses, heart, lungs, or bones) and life-threatening infections also have been reported rarely, usually in immunocompromised individuals. In addition, *E. rostratum* was identified as the predominant pathogen in the 2012–2013 multistate outbreak of fungal meningitis and other fungal infections that occurred in the US in patients who received contaminated preservative-free methylprednisolone acetate injections prepared by a compounding pharmacy. *Exserohilum* infections cannot be transmitted person-to-person.

Although data are limited and the clinical relevance of in vitro testing remains uncertain, in vitro studies indicate that *Exserohilum* is inhibited by some triazole antifungals (e.g., voriconazole, itraconazole, posaconazole) and amphotericin B. Echinocandins (e.g., caspofungin, micafungin) have variable in vitro activity and fluconazole has poor in vitro activity against the fungus.

***Exserohilum* Infections Related to Contaminated Injections** In September 2012, the CDC and US Food and Drug Administration (FDA) initiated investigations in response to fungal CNS infections (including some fatalities) reported in patients who received epidural injections of contaminated extemporaneously prepared methylprednisolone acetate injections from the New England Compounding Center (NECC). Subsequently, there were reports of joint infections and osteomyelitis in some patients who received intra-articular injections of methylprednisolone acetate from NECC, as well as infections possibly related to other NECC products.

Out of an abundance of caution at that time, the FDA recommended that health-care professionals and consumers not use any product that was produced by NECC, and the company recalled all products that were compounded at and distributed from its facility in Framingham, Massachusetts.

E. rostratum was one of the predominant pathogen identified in samples taken from patients who received contaminated products from NECC; *Aspergillus* also was identified in an index patient and *Cladosporium cladosporioides* was recovered from several other patients. The presence of *E. rostratum* was confirmed in recalled lots of the contaminated products. Other organisms identified in unopened vials from recalled lots of corticosteroid products were *A. fumigatus*, *A. tubingensis*, various *Bacillus* species (including *Bacillus subtilis*), *Cladosporium*, *Paenibacillus*, and *Penicillium*.

CDC data indicate that, as of October 30, 2015, there were a total of 753 cases of fungal infections (including 64 deaths) reported in 20 states that have been linked to specific lots of contaminated methylprednisolone acetate injections. Although the majority of initial cases involved fungal meningitis (some with stroke), subsequent reports involved localized spinal or paraspinal infections (e.g., epidural abscess). More than 6 months after the outbreak related to contaminated products was first identified, CDC continued to receive reports of patients presenting with localized spinal and paraspinal infections (e.g., epidural abscess, phlegmon, discitis, vertebral osteomyelitis, arachnoiditis, or other complications at or near the site of injection). These localized infections occurred in patients with or without a diagnosis of fungal meningitis. In some patients being treated for fungal meningitis who had no previous evidence of localized infections, such infections were found at the site of injection using magnetic resonance imaging (MRI) studies. Some cases occurred in patients without any previous evidence of infection or in those with persistent, worsening, or new symptoms.

Patients with meningitis generally presented 1–4 weeks or longer after receiving contaminated methylprednisolone acetate injections; the greatest risk for development of fungal meningitis appeared to be during the first 6 weeks after an epidural or paraspinal injection. Data from one group of patients indicated that the median time from the last injection with contaminated product to the date of the first MRI finding indicative of infection was 50 days (range 12–121 days) for all patients with a spinal or paraspinal infection, and the median time from the first positive lumbar puncture finding to the first positive MRI finding was 21 days for those with meningitis and spinal or paraspinal infections.

Clinicians treating fungal infections in patients who received contaminated methylprednisolone acetate injections from NECC should consult an infectious disease expert to assist with diagnosis, management, and follow-up, which may be complex and prolonged. A clinical consultant network for clinicians can be reached by calling CDC at 800-232-4636.

Because of evidence of latent disease, CDC cautions clinicians to continue to remain vigilant for the possibility of infections in patients who received injections of NECC products and to consider such infections in the differential diagnosis when evaluating symptomatic patients who received such products. CDC recommends routine laboratory and microbiologic tests, including bacterial and fungal cultures, as necessary; MRI evaluations should be considered if clinically warranted.

CDC released interim treatment guidance documents containing recommendations for empiric antifungal treatment of CNS and parameningeal infections and osteoarticular infections associated with the contaminated methylprednisolone acetate products. These recommendations were based on evidence that *E. rostratum* was the predominant pathogen in the outbreak and consultation with experts.

For the treatment of CNS infections (including meningitis, stroke, and arachnoiditis) and/or parameningeal infections (epidural or paraspinal abscess, discitis or osteomyelitis, and sacroiliac infection) in adults who received contaminated corticosteroid injections, CDC recommends voriconazole. Use of IV amphotericin B liposomal *in addition* to voriconazole should be strongly considered in patients who present with severe disease and in patients who do not improve or experience clinical deterioration or manifest new sites of disease activity while receiving voriconazole monotherapy. IV amphotericin B liposomal also is recommended as an alternative in patients who unable to tolerate voriconazole. IV amphotericin B liposomal is preferred over other lipid formulations of amphotericin B because of better CNS penetration. Because of limited data and associated toxicities, routine use of intrathecal conventional amphotericin B is not recommended in these patients.

For the treatment of osteoarticular infections (discitis, vertebral osteomyelitis, and epidural abscess or osteoarticular infections not involving the spine) in adults who received intra-articular injections of contaminated corticosteroid products, CDC recommends voriconazole. Use of a lipid formulation of IV amphotericin B *in addition* to IV voriconazole should be considered in patients with severe osteoarticular infection and/or clinical instability. A lipid formulation of IV amphotericin B, posaconazole, or itraconazole are recommended as alternatives in patients who cannot tolerate voriconazole. Expert consultation is advised when making decisions regarding alternative regimens.

Adequate duration of antifungal treatment for infections associated with the contaminated corticosteroid injections is unknown, but prolonged therapy is required. (See Exserohilum Infections under Dosage: Amphotericin B Liposomal (AmBisome®), in Dosage and Administration.) In addition, close follow-up monitoring after completion of treatment is essential in all patients to detect potential relapse.

The CDC website at https://www.cdc.gov/hai/outbreaks/meningitis.html should be consulted for the most recent information regarding the contaminated NECC products and associated infections, including specific information regarding diagnosis and treatment of these infections.

■ **Fusarium Infections** Amphotericin B has been used for the treatment of serious fungal infections caused by *Fusarium*, and a lipid formulation of amphotericin B is recommended as a drug of choice for the treatment of these fungal infections.

For the treatment of fusariosis, the most appropriate antifungal should be selected based on in vitro susceptibility testing. Amphotericin B may be preferred for infections caused by *F. solani* or *F. verticillioides*; either voriconazole or amphotericin B are recommended for infections caused by other *Fusarium*. Some clinicians suggest that concomitant use of amphotericin B and voriconazole should be considered in patients with severe infections or immunosuppression.

■ **Zygomycosis** IV amphotericin B is used for the treatment of zygomycosis, including mucormycosis, caused by susceptible species of *Lichtheimia* (formerly *Absidia*), *Mucor*, or *Rhizopus* and for the treatment of infections caused by susceptible species of *Conidiobolus* or *Basidiobolus*. IV amphotericin B generally has been considered the drug of choice for these infections. However, in several cases of GI basidiobolomycosis caused by *Basidiobolus ranarum*, the response to amphotericin B (e.g., amphotericin B liposomal) was poor. Most cases of GI basidiobolomycosis reported to date have been successfully treated with oral itraconazole after partial surgical resection of the GI tract.

While most experience to date in treating zygomycosis has involved use of conventional IV amphotericin B, lipid formulations (amphotericin B lipid complex, amphotericin B liposomal) also have been used to treat these infections, including rhinocerebral and pulmonary mucormycosis in some patients who did not respond to conventional amphotericin B or had to discontinue conventional amphotericin B because of adverse renal effects.

■ **Empiric Therapy in Febrile Neutropenic Patients** Conventional IV amphotericin B†, amphotericin B lipid complex†, and amphotericin B liposomal are used for empiric therapy of presumed fungal infections in febrile, neutropenic patients who have not responded to empiric treatment with broad-spectrum antibacterial agents.

Because systemic fungal infections (e.g., *Candida*, *Aspergillus*) are present in up to one-third of neutropenic patients who remain febrile after a 7-day course of empiric broad-spectrum anti-infective therapy, IDSA and other clinicians recommend that consideration be given to administering empiric antifungal therapy (with or without a change in the antibacterial regimen) to neutropenic patients who have persistent or recurrent fever after 4–7 days of antibacterial therapy. Conventional IV amphotericin B historically has been considered the drug of choice for empiric antifungal treatment in such patients; however, lipid formulations of amphotericin B or other antifungals (e.g., caspofungin, voriconazole) also have been used.

Empiric therapy with conventional IV amphotericin B has been used in patients undergoing bone marrow transplantation (BMT) who have persistent fever despite 3–7 days of broad-spectrum antibacterial therapy, and such therapy was included in the Eastern Cooperative Oncology Group (ECOG) guidelines for the management of autologous and allogeneic BMT patients. If conventional IV amphotericin B is used for empiric antifungal therapy in febrile, neutropenic allogeneic BMT patients who are receiving cyclosporine, the potential for additive nephrotoxic effects should be considered before initiating such therapy. (See Drug Interactions: Nephrotoxic Drugs.)

Published protocols for the treatment of infections in febrile neutropenic patients should be consulted for specific recommendations regarding selection of the initial empiric anti-infective regimen, when to change the initial regimen, possible subsequent regimens, and duration of therapy in these patients. In addition, consultation with an infectious disease expert knowledgeable about infections in immunocompromised patients is advised.

Clinical Experience The relative efficacy of conventional IV amphotericin B and amphotericin B liposomal for empiric therapy in febrile, neutropenic patients has been evaluated in a randomized, double-blind, multicenter study that involved 687 adult and pediatric cancer patients 2–80 years of age who were febrile despite having received at least 5 days of empiric therapy with broad spectrum anti-infectives. The overall therapeutic success rate (defined as resolution of fever during the neutropenic period, successful treatment of any baseline fungal infections, absence of emergent fungal infections during therapy or within 7 days after completion of study drug, patient survival for at least 7 days after empiric therapy, and use of study drug without premature discontinuance because of toxicity or lack of efficacy) was 50.1% for amphotericin B liposomal and 49.4% for conventional amphotericin B. Emergent fungal infections were mycologically confirmed in 3.2% of those receiving amphotericin B liposomal and in 7.8% of those receiving conventional amphotericin B. While the overall success rate was similar in both groups, the group receiving amphotericin B liposomal had a lower incidence of documented emergent fungal infections and also had a lower incidence of acute infusion reactions and adverse renal effects than those receiving conventional amphotericin B. Amphotericin B liposomal also appeared to be as effective as conventional IV amphotericin B for empiric therapy of presumed fungal infections in several randomized, open label, multicenter studies that involved febrile neutropenic adults and pediatric patients undergoing chemotherapy for hematologic malignancy or as part of bone marrow transplantation.

■ **Prevention of Fungal Infections in Transplant Recipients, Cancer Patients, or Other Patients at High Risk** Conventional IV amphotericin B† and amphotericin B liposomal† have been used prophylactically in an attempt to reduce the incidence of fungal infections (e.g., aspergillosis, candidiasis) in neutropenic cancer patients† or patients undergoing BMT† or solid organ transplantation†. IV amphotericin B also has been used to prevent *Candida* infections in patients undergoing urologic procedures†.

Use of primary antifungal prophylaxis in cancer patients undergoing myelosuppressive therapy or patients undergoing BMT or solid organ transplantation has been controversial, particularly since such prophylaxis may predispose the patient to colonization with resistant fungi and/or result in the emergence of highly resistant organisms. Some clinicians discourage primary prophylaxis with antifungals except in certain carefully selected high-risk patients in whom potential benefits are expected to justify possible risks (e.g., patients in institutions that have a high incidence of fungal infections or circumstances where the frequency of systemic *Candida* infections is high). When primary antifungal prophylaxis is warranted in cancer patients or BMT or solid organ transplant recipients, IDSA and other clinicians generally prefer use of an oral azole antifungal.

For postoperative antifungal prophylaxis in recipients of solid organ transplants† at high risk for invasive candidiasis (i.e., liver, pancreas, or small bowel transplant recipients), IDSA recommends fluconazole or IV amphotericin B liposomal. IDSA states that the risk of invasive candidiasis in recipients of other solid organ transplants (e.g., kidney, heart) appears to be too low to warrant routine antifungal prophylaxis.

For high-risk patients undergoing urologic procedures†, IDSA states that fluconazole or conventional IV amphotericin B can be used for several days before and after the procedure to prevent *Candida* infections.

Conventional amphotericin B, amphotericin B lipid complex, and amphotericin B liposomal have been administered by nasal instillation† or nebulization† in an attempt to prevent aspergillosis in immunocompromised patients, including solid organ transplant recipients† (e.g., lung transplant recipients) and neutropenic chemotherapy patients†.

For additional information on prevention of fungal infections in neutropenic patients, the current clinical practice guidelines from IDSA available at http://www.idsociety.org should be consulted.

Clinical Experience When used for antifungal prophylaxis in cancer patients or patients undergoing BMT, conventional amphotericin B has been administered in usual IV dosages or, more frequently, as low-dose IV therapy (i.e., 0.1–0.25 mg/kg daily). Safety and efficacy of low-dose conventional IV amphotericin B for prophylaxis in neutropenic patients undergoing BMT have been evaluated in a prospective, randomized, placebo-controlled study. Patients undergoing autologous BMT were randomized to receive low-dose conventional IV amphotericin B (0.1 mg/kg daily) or placebo; any patient with persistent neutropenia and fever despite prophylaxis with low-dose amphotericin B and broad-spectrum antibacterial agent therapy was withdrawn from the study and given empiric therapy with a higher dosage of conventional IV amphotericin B (0.6 mg/kg daily). During the study, 8.8% of those receiving low-dose amphotericin B and 14.3% of those receiving placebo had mycologically confirmed fungal infections (*Candida*, *Aspergillus*); 6-week mortality was higher in those receiving placebo (11 deaths in those receiving placebo compared with 3 deaths in those receiving amphotericin B), but this difference did not appear to be related to fungal infections. Because there is some evidence that administration of low-dose conventional IV amphotericin B therapy to BMT patients can decrease the incidence posttransplant fungal infections, some clinicians suggest that secondary prophylaxis with low-dose conventional IV amphotericin B be considered for all transplant patients with a history of documented invasive aspergillosis since these patients are at risk for reactivation of the disease. However, there is evidence that prophylaxis with low-dose conventional IV amphotericin B may be ineffective in preventing posttransplant fungal infections in liver transplant patients since candidemia and invasive aspergillosis have been reported in liver transplant recipients receiving prophylaxis with conventional IV amphotericin B (0.5 mg/kg daily).

Data are accumulating regarding use of amphotericin B liposomal for antifungal prophylaxis in neutropenic cancer patients or BMT or transplant patients. Safety and efficacy of amphotericin B liposomal (2 mg/kg 3 times weekly) for antifungal prophylaxis in patients undergoing chemotherapy or BMT have been evaluated in a double-blind, placebo-controlled study. Systemic or superficial fungal infections were suspected in 42 or 46% of those receiving amphotericin B liposomal or placebo, respectively; however, while there were mycologically confirmed fungal infections in 3.4% of those receiving placebo, there were none in those receiving amphotericin B liposomal prophylaxis. There was fungal colonization of at least one site (fungal pathogen isolated but not associated with clinical or other evidence of disease) in 20 or 40% of those receiving amphotericin B liposomal or placebo, respectively. The mortality rate was similar in both groups (14–15%). In a limited placebo-controlled study in liver transplant recipients, there was no evidence of posttransplant fungal infections in those who received 5 days of amphotericin B liposomal prophylaxis (1 mg/kg daily initiated at the time of transplantation); 16% of patients who received placebo developed *C. albicans* infections posttransplant. However, in another study in liver transplant recipients who received amphotericin B liposomal for antifungal prophylaxis (1 mg/kg daily initiated after transplant and continued for 7 days), the regimen appeared to effectively prevent *Candida* infections but several patients developed posttransplant *Aspergillus* infections that were fatal.

■ Protozoal Infections

Leishmaniasis Conventional IV amphotericin B, amphotericin B lipid complex†, and amphotericin B liposomal have been used for the treatment of leishmaniasis.

Leishmaniasis is caused by more than 15–20 different species of *Leishmania* that are transmitted to humans by the bite of infected sand flies. *Leishmania* also can be transmitted via blood (e.g., blood transfusions, needles shared by IV drug abusers) and transmitted perinatally from mother to infant. In the Eastern Hemisphere, leishmaniasis is found most frequently in parts of Asia, the Middle East, Africa, and southern Europe; in the Western Hemisphere, the disease is found most frequently in Mexico and Central and South America and has been reported occasionally in Texas and Oklahoma. Leishmaniasis has been reported in short-term travelers to endemic areas and in immigrants and expatriates from such areas, and also has been reported in US military personnel and contract workers serving or working in endemic areas (e.g., Iraq, Afghanistan).

Leishmania infection in humans may cause uncomplicated cutaneous leishmaniasis, diffuse cutaneous leishmaniasis, mucosal leishmaniasis, visceral leishmaniasis, or post-kala-azar leishmaniasis and may be termed Old World (Eastern Hemisphere) or New World (Western Hemisphere). The specific form of leishmaniasis and disease severity depend on the *Leishmania* species involved, geographic area of origin, location of sand fly bite, and patient factors (e.g., nutritional and immune status). Treatment of leishmaniasis (e.g., drug, dosage, duration of treatment) must be individualized based on the region where the disease was acquired, likely infecting species, drug susceptibilities reported in the area of origin, form of the disease, and patient factors (e.g., age, pregnancy, immune status). No single treatment approach is appropriate for all possible clinical presentations. Consultation with clinicians experienced in management of leishmaniasis is recommended.

For assistance with diagnosis or treatment of leishmaniasis in the US, clinicians can contact CDC Parasitic Diseases Hotline at 404-718-4745 from 8:00 a.m. to 4:00 p.m. Eastern Standard Time or CDC Emergency Operation Center at 770-488-7100 after business hours and on weekends and holidays. CDC Drug Service should be contacted at 404-639-3670 for information on how to obtain antiparasitic drugs not commercially available in the US.

Cutaneous and Mucocutaneous Leishmaniasis. Conventional IV amphotericin B is used for the treatment of American cutaneous leishmaniasis, including infections caused by *Leishmania braziliensis* or *L. mexicana*, and for mucocutaneous leishmaniasis, including infections caused by *L. braziliensis*.

Although some cases of cutaneous leishmaniasis (usually Old World) may subside or resolve spontaneously over months or years, treatment of cutaneous leishmaniasis is recommended if there are multiple or large lesions, lesions are disabling or disfiguring or fail to heal within 6 months, the patient is immunocompromised, or dissemination to mucosal leishmaniasis is likely (e.g., New World disease caused by *L. braziliensis* or *L. panamensis*). Local treatment (e.g., topical paromomycin [not commercially available in the US], thermotherapy, intralesional pentavalent antimonials [not commercially available in the US], cryotherapy) may be appropriate in selected cases. For systemic treatment of cutaneous leishmaniasis, pentavalent antimonials (i.e., sodium stibogluconate or meglumine antimonate [drugs not commercially available in the US, but may be available from CDC]) usually are used. Other treatment options for cutaneous leishmaniasis include amphotericin B, miltefosine, pentamidine, and ketoconazole, especially when antimonials cannot be used because of tolerance or resistance.

Data are limited regarding use of lipid formulations of amphotericin B in the treatment of cutaneous leishmaniasis, but amphotericin B lipid complex† and amphotericin B liposomal† have been used in a limited number of patients for the treatment of cutaneous leishmaniasis. At least one patient with cutaneous leishmaniasis unresponsive to meglumine antimonate therapy was successfully treated with a 2-week regimen of IV amphotericin B liposomal (1.5 mg/kg daily) followed by a 4-week regimen of conventional IV amphotericin B (3 mg/kg once weekly).

Visceral Leishmaniasis. IV amphotericin B liposomal is used in the treatment of visceral leishmaniasis (also known as kala-azar) and is recommended by some clinicians as a drug of choice, especially for immunocompromised patients. Conventional IV amphotericin B† and amphotericin B lipid complex† also have been used for the treatment of visceral leishmaniasis.

Pentavalent antimonials (i.e., sodium stibogluconate or meglumine antimonate [drugs not commercially available in the US, but may available from CDC]) have historically been considered the drugs of first choice for initial treatment of visceral leishmaniasis; however, drug resistance and treatment failures have become a major concern in some areas (e.g., India, Nepal). Other treatment options for visceral leishmaniasis include amphotericin B, miltefosine, or paromomycin. Relapse of visceral leishmaniasis is common in immunocompromised patients (e.g., HIV-infected patients), regardless of the treatment regimen.

In a group of patients with visceral leishmaniasis who were infected in the Mediterranean basin with documented or presumed *L. infantum*, amphotericin B liposomal was associated with an overall success rate (clearance with no relapse during a follow-up period of 6 months or longer) of 96.5% in immunocompetent patients. In patients who were immunocompromised, amphotericin B liposomal therapy was able to initially clear the infection in 94.7% of patients; however, the overall success rate was only 11.8% and there was a high rate of relapse in these patients. The manufacturer states that data are inconclusive regarding efficacy of IV amphotericin B liposomal for the treatment of infections caused by *L. donovani* or *L. chagasi*.

Leishmaniasis in HIV-infected Individuals. Based on data from individuals who are not infected with HIV, CDC, NIH, and IDSA state that the drugs of choice for the treatment of cutaneous leishmaniasis in HIV-infected adults or adolescents are amphotericin B liposomal† or sodium stibogluconate (not commercially available in the US, but may be available from CDC). Possible alternatives are miltefosine, topical paromomycin (not commercially available in the US), intralesional pentavalent antimony (not commercially available in the US), or local heat therapy.

For the treatment of visceral leishmaniasis in HIV-infected adults and adolescents, CDC, NIH, and IDSA recommend amphotericin B liposomal as the drug of choice since the drug appears to have similar efficacy but is better tolerated in these patients than conventional amphotericin B or pentavalent antimony compounds. Alternatives for the treatment of visceral leishmaniasis in HIV-infected adults and adolescents include amphotericin B lipid complex†, conventional amphotericin B†, sodium stibogluconate (not commercially available in the US, but may be available from CDC), or miltefosine.

CDC, NIH, and IDSA recommend long-term suppressive or maintenance therapy (secondary prophylaxis)† to decrease the risk of relapse in HIV-infected adults and adolescents who have been treated for visceral leishmaniasis and have CD4+ T-cell counts less than 200/mm³. Although data are limited, these experts state that long-term suppressive or maintenance therapy (secondary prophylaxis) also should be offered to those who have been adequately treated for cutaneous leishmaniasis but are immunocompromised and have had multiple relapses. If secondary prophylaxis against leishmaniasis is indicated in HIV-infected adults and adolescents, CDC, NIH, and IDSA recommend use of amphotericin B liposomal† or amphotericin B lipid complex†; the alternative is sodium stibogluconate (not commercially available in the US, but may be available from CDC). The manufacturer of amphotericin B liposomal states that, while the drug may have a role for long-term suppressive therapy to prevent relapse of visceral leishmaniasis in HIV-infected individuals, the efficacy and safety of repeated courses of amphotericin B liposomal or maintenance therapy with the drug in immunocompromised individuals have not been evaluated to date.

If secondary prophylaxis against leishmaniasis is initiated in HIV-infected adults and adolescents, some experts state that consideration can be given to discontinuing such prophylaxis if CD4+ T-cell counts remain greater than 200–350/mm³ for at least 3–6 months in response to antiretroviral therapy. However, others suggest that such prophylaxis should be continued indefinitely.

Primary Amebic Meningoencephalitis Conventional IV amphotericin B has been used for the treatment of primary amebic meningoencephalitis caused by *Naegleria fowleri*†, a free-living ameba.

CNS infections caused by free-living ameba have a high mortality rate, and only a very limited number of cases have been successfully treated. Early diagnosis and aggressive treatment of these infections may increase the chance of survival. Although data are limited, most reported cases of *N. fowleri* have been treated empirically with multiple-drug regimens. Treatment regimens used or recommended for the treatment of *N. fowleri* infections include several anti-infectives (e.g., amphotericin B, azole antifungals [fluconazole], flucytosine, macrolides [azithromycin, clarithromycin], miltefosine, rifampin) and other therapies (e.g., dexamethasone, phenytoin, therapeutic hypothermia).

Based on multiple-drug regimens used to date in documented survivors, CDC recommends an anti-infective regimen that includes conventional amphotericin B (administered IV and intrathecally†), azithromycin, fluconazole, miltefosine, and rifampin for treatment of primary amebic meningoencephalitis caused by *N. fowleri*. Because there is some evidence that amphotericin B liposomal may be less effective than conventional amphotericin B in mice for the treatment of primary amebic meningoencephalitis caused by *N. fowleri*, the conventional formulation is preferred if amphotericin B is used for the treatment of primary amebic meningoencephalitis.

For assistance with diagnosis or treatment of patients with suspected free-living ameba infections, clinicians should contact the CDC Emergency Operation Center at 770-488-7100.

Dosage and Administration

■ **Reconstitution and Administration** ***Conventional Amphotericin B*** Conventional amphotericin B is administered by IV infusion. The drug also has been given intra-articularly†, intrapleurally†, intrathecally†, by nasal instillation† or nebulization†, and by bladder irrigation†.

Commercially available conventional amphotericin B for IV infusion must be reconstituted and diluted prior to administration. *The drug must not be prepared with any diluents other than those specified below since precipitation may occur. Strict aseptic technique must be observed.*

Conventional amphotericin B should be reconstituted to a concentration of 5 mg/mL by rapidly adding 10 mL of sterile water for injection *without bacteriostatic agent* to a vial labeled as containing 50 mg of drug. The sterile water diluent should be added to the vial using a sterile syringe (minimum needle size of 20 gauge) and the vial should be immediately shaken until the colloidal dispersion is clear. For IV infusion, the colloidal dispersion is further diluted, usually to a concentration of 0.1 mg/mL, with 500 mL of 5% dextrose injection (the dextrose injection must have a pH exceeding 4.2). Although the pH of commercially available 5% dextrose injection usually exceeds 4.2, the pH of each container of 5% dextrose injection should be determined and, if the pH is low, it may be adjusted with 1 or 2 mL of sterile buffer solution in accordance with the instructions provided by the manufacturers of conventional amphotericin B.

Reconstituted conventional amphotericin B or dilutions of the drug must not be used if precipitation or foreign matter is evident. An inline membrane filter may be used during IV administration of conventional amphotericin B; however, the mean pore diameter of the filter should *not* be less than 1 μm to ensure passage of the amphotericin B colloidal dispersion. IV infusions of conventional amphotericin B containing a drug concentration of 0.1 mg/mL or less should be used promptly after preparation.

Rate of Administration. IV infusions of conventional amphotericin B are given *slowly* over a period of approximately 2–6 hours, depending on the dose being administered.

Although IV infusions of conventional amphotericin B have been well tolerated in some patients when given over 1–2 hours, the manufacturers and many clinicians state that rapid IV infusions of conventional amphotericin B should be avoided since potentially serious adverse effects (e.g., hypotension, hypokalemia, arrhythmias, shock) may occur.

Amphotericin B Lipid Complex (Abelcet®) Amphotericin B lipid complex is administered by IV infusion. The drug also has been administered by nasal inhalation† or nebulization†.

Commercially available amphotericin B lipid complex injectable suspension concentrate must be diluted prior to IV infusion. The injectable suspension concentrate must be diluted in 5% dextrose injection to a concentration of 1 mg/mL; a concentration of 2 mg/mL may be appropriate for pediatric patients and patients with cardiovascular disease. Solutions containing sodium chloride or bacteriostatic agents should *not* be used to dilute amphotericin B lipid complex, and the drug should *not* be mixed with other drugs or with electrolytes.

To prepare IV infusions of amphotericin B lipid complex, vials labeled as containing 5 mg/mL should be shaken gently until there is no evidence of yellow sediment on the bottom of the vial. The appropriate dose should be withdrawn from the required number of vials into one or more sterile 20-mL syringes using an 18-gauge needle. The needle should be removed from the filled syringe and replaced with the 5-μm filter needle provided by the manufacturer; each filter needle may be used to filter the contents of up to four 100-mg vials of the drug. The filter needle should then be inserted into an IV container of 5% dextrose injection and the contents of the syringe injected into the container.

Prior to initiation of the infusion, the IV container of diluted drug should be shaken until the contents are thoroughly mixed; the infusion container should then be shaken every 2 hours if the infusion time exceeds 2 hours. Amphotericin B lipid complex diluted in 5% dextrose injection should not be used if there is any evidence of foreign matter in the solution.

The drug should be administered using a separate infusion line; if an existing IV line is used, it should be flushed with 5% dextrose injection before amphotericin B lipid complex is infused. An inline membrane filter should *not* be used during administration of amphotericin B lipid complex.

Rate of Administration. IV infusions of diluted amphotericin B lipid complex should be infused at a rate of 2.5 mg/kg per hour.

Amphotericin B Liposomal (AmBisome®) Amphotericin B liposomal is administered by IV infusion. The drug also has been administered by nasal inhalation† or nebulization†.

Amphotericin B liposomal must be reconstituted by adding 12 mL of sterile water for injection to a vial labeled as containing 50 mg of amphotericin B to provide a solution containing 4 mg/mL. Other diluents (e.g., diluents containing sodium chloride or a bacteriostatic agent) should *not* be used to reconstitute amphotericin B liposomal, and reconstituted solutions should *not* be admixed with other drugs. The appropriate amount of reconstituted amphotericin B liposomal should be withdrawn into a sterile syringe. The 5-μm sterile, disposable filter provided by the manufacturer should then be attached to the syringe and the syringe contents injected through the filter into the appropriate volume of 5% dextrose injection to provide a final concentration of 1–2 mg/mL. Lower concentrations (0.2–0.5 mg/mL) may be appropriate for infants and small children.

Amphotericin B liposomal may be infused through an in-line membrane filter provided the mean pore diameter of the filter is not less than 1 μm. The drug may be administered through an existing IV line; however, the line must be flushed with 5% dextrose injection prior to infusion of the antifungal. If this is not feasible, amphotericin B liposomal must be administered through a separate line.

Rate of Administration. IV infusions of amphotericin B liposomal should be given over a period of approximately 2 hours using a controlled infusion device. If the infusion is well tolerated, infusion time may be reduced to approximately 1 hour; however, the duration of infusion should be increased in patients who experience discomfort during infusion.

■ **Dosage** *Dosage of amphotericin B varies depending on whether the drug is administered as conventional amphotericin B (formulated with sodium desoxycholate), amphotericin B lipid complex, or amphotericin B liposomal. Dosage recommendations for the specific formulation being administered should be followed.*

Conventional Amphotericin B Dosage of conventional amphotericin B must be individualized and adjusted according to the patient's tolerance and clinical status (e.g., site and severity of infection, etiologic agent, cardiopulmonary and renal function status).

The manufacturers caution that under no circumstances should the total daily dose of conventional amphotericin B exceed 1.5 mg/kg. Overdosage can result in potentially fatal cardiac or cardiopulmonary arrest. (See Acute Toxicity.)

Prior to initiation of conventional IV amphotericin B therapy, a single test dose of the drug (1 mg in 20 mL of 5% dextrose injection) should be administered IV over 20–30 minutes and the patient carefully monitored (i.e., pulse and respiration rate, temperature, blood pressure) every 30 minutes for 2–4 hours. In patients with good cardiorenal function who tolerate the test dose, the manufacturers recommend that therapy be initiated with a daily dosage of 0.25 mg/kg (0.3 mg/kg in those with severe or rapidly progressing fungal infections) given as a single daily dose. In patients with impaired cardiorenal function and in patients who have severe reactions to the test dose, the manufacturers recommend that therapy be initiated with a smaller daily dosage (i.e., 5–10 mg). Depending on the patient's cardiorenal status, dosage may gradually be increased by 5–10 mg daily to a final daily dosage of 0.5–0.7 mg/kg.

The manufacturers state that the optimal dosage of conventional amphotericin B is unknown and data are insufficient to define total dosage and duration of treatment for eradication of specific fungal infections. Dosage up to 1 mg/kg daily or up to 1.5 mg/kg when given on alternate days is recommended by the manufacturers. When converting a daily IV dosage schedule to alternate-day therapy, dosage must be increased gradually every other day until it is twice the previous daily dosage.

If conventional amphotericin B therapy is discontinued for longer than 1 week, the manufacturers recommend that administration of the drug be resumed at the usual initial dosage of 0.25 mg/kg daily, and dosage should again be gradually increased.

Aspergillosis. For the treatment of invasive aspergillosis, conventional IV amphotericin B has been administered in a dosage of 0.5–1.5 mg/kg daily. The duration of treatment is based on the degree and duration of immunosuppression, disease site, and clinical response. The Infectious Diseases Society of America (IDSA) recommends that antifungal treatment of invasive pulmonary aspergillosis be continued for at least 6–12 weeks.

If conventional IV amphotericin B is used as an alternative for the treatment of invasive aspergillosis in HIV-infected adults or adolescents, the US Centers for Disease Control and Prevention (CDC), National Institutes of Health (NIH), and IDSA recommend a dosage of 1 mg/kg daily. The optimal duration of therapy in these patients has not been established, but antifungal therapy should be continued at least until CD4$^+$ T-cell counts exceed 200/mm^3 and there is evidence of resolution of aspergillosis.

Blastomycosis. For the treatment of blastomycosis, the usual dosage of conventional IV amphotericin B is 0.7–1 mg/kg once daily.

For the treatment of moderately severe to severe pulmonary or disseminated extrapulmonary blastomycosis (without CNS involvement), IDSA recommends that adults (including immunocompromised individuals) receive initial therapy with conventional IV amphotericin B in a dosage of 0.7–1 mg/kg once daily for 1–2 weeks or until improvement occurs, followed by oral itraconazole therapy. The total treatment duration should be 6–12 months for pulmonary blastomycosis or at least 12 months for disseminated extrapulmonary blastomycosis or for immunocompromised individuals.

For the treatment of severe blastomycosis in children, IDSA recommends initial therapy with conventional IV amphotericin B in a dosage of 0.7–1 mg/kg once daily, followed by oral itraconazole therapy for a total treatment duration of 12 months.

Candida Infections. For the treatment of disseminated or invasive *Candida* infections, the usual dosage of conventional IV amphotericin B in adults or pediatric patients is 0.5–1 mg/kg daily. The recommended duration of antifungal treatment for candidemia (without persistent fungemia or metastatic complications) is 2 weeks after documented clearance of *Candida* from the bloodstream, resolution of candidemia symptoms, and resolution of neutropenia.

For the treatment of neonatal candidiasis, including CNS infections, IDSA recommends that conventional IV amphotericin B be given in a dosage of 1 mg/kg daily. The recommended duration of antifungal treatment for uncomplicated neonatal candidiasis is 2 weeks after documented clearance of *Candida* from the bloodstream and resolution of candidemia symptoms. If neonatal candidiasis involves the CNS, antifungal treatment should be continued until resolution of all signs, symptoms, and CSF and radiologic abnormalities (if present).

If conventional IV amphotericin B is used as an alternative for the treatment of esophageal candidiasis† in adults who cannot tolerate oral therapy or have fluconazole-refractory infections, IDSA recommends a dosage of 0.3–0.7 mg/kg daily for 21 days. If conventional IV amphotericin B is used as an alternative for the treatment of esophageal candidiasis†, including fluconazole-refractory infections, in HIV-infected adults and adolescents, CDC, NIH, and IDSA recommend a dosage of 0.6 mg/kg daily for 14–21 days. If used as an alternative for the treatment of esophageal candidiasis† in HIV-infected infants and children, CDC, NIH, and IDSA recommend that conventional IV amphotericin B be given in a dosage of 0.3–0.7 mg/kg once daily for at least 3 weeks and for at least 2 weeks after resolution of symptoms.

If conventional IV amphotericin B is used as an alternative for the treatment of severe or refractory oropharyngeal candidiasis† (e.g., caused by fluconazole-resistant strains), IDSA recommends a dosage of 0.3 mg/kg daily.

For the treatment of symptomatic cystitis caused by fluconazole-resistant *Candida* (e.g., *C. glabrata*, *C. krusei*), IDSA recommends that conventional IV amphotericin B be given in a dosage of 0.3–0.6 mg/kg daily for 1–7 days. For the treatment of pyelonephritis caused by fluconazole-resistant *Candida*, conventional IV amphotericin B should be given in a dosage of 0.3–0.6 mg/kg daily (with or without oral flucytosine) for 1–7 days. The same regimen can be used for the treatment of urinary tract infections associated with fungus balls.

For the treatment of candiduria, conventional amphotericin B has been administered by bladder irrigation†. The optimal concentration of conventional amphotericin B for bladder irrigation†, method of irrigation (continuous or intermittent), and duration of therapy have not been established. For use as a continuous bladder irrigant†, conventional amphotericin B for injection has been reconstituted with sterile water for injection to a concentration of 50 mg/L and administered at a rate of 42 mL/hour for up to 15 days. Some clinicians suggest that lower concentrations (5–10 mg/L) may be acceptable based on usual susceptibilities of *Candida* and potential toxicity. IDSA states that a 5-day regimen of conventional amphotericin B administered by bladder irrigation† as a 50-mg/L solution in sterile water may be useful for treatment of symptomatic cystitis caused by fluconazole-resistant *Candida* (e.g., *C. glabrata*, *C. krusei*). For treatment of *Candida* urinary tract infections associated with fungus balls, IDSA states that 25–50 mg of conventional amphotericin B in 200–500 mL of sterile water administered by irrigation† through nephrostomy tubes (if present) is recommended.

Coccidioidomycosis. For the treatment of coccidioidomycosis, the usual dosage of conventional IV amphotericin B is 0.5–1.5 mg/kg daily. For the treatment of severe and/or rapidly progressive acute pulmonary or disseminated coccidioidomycosis (nonmeningeal), IV amphotericin B usually is used initially with follow-up therapy with oral fluconazole or oral itraconazole. The total duration of treatment usually is at least 1 year.

For the treatment of diffuse pulmonary or extrathoracic disseminated coccidioidomycosis (nonmeningeal) in HIV-infected adults and adolescents, CDC, NIH, and IDSA recommend initial therapy with conventional IV amphotericin B given in a dosage of 0.7–1 mg/kg daily until improvement occurs, then follow-up treatment with oral fluconazole or oral itraconazole.

For the treatment of diffuse pulmonary or disseminated coccidioidomycosis (nonmeningeal) in HIV-infected infants and children, CDC, NIH, and IDSA recommend initial therapy with conventional IV amphotericin B given in a dosage of 0.5–1 mg/kg once daily until improvement occurs, then follow-up treatment with oral fluconazole or oral itraconazole. The total duration of treatment should be 1 year.

HIV-infected adults, adolescents, or children who have been adequately treated for coccidioidomycosis should receive long-term suppressive or maintenance therapy (secondary prophylaxis) with oral fluconazole or oral itraconazole to prevent recurrence or relapse.

Cryptococcosis. If conventional IV amphotericin B is used for initial (induction) therapy in HIV-infected adults or adolescents with cryptococcal meningitis, CDC, NIH, and IDSA recommend a dosage of 0.7–1 mg/kg daily in conjunction with oral flucytosine (25 mg/kg 4 times daily) given for at least 2 weeks and until there is evidence of clinical improvement and negative CSF culture after repeat lumbar puncture, then follow-up (consolidation) therapy with oral or IV fluconazole alone given for at least 8 weeks.

If conventional IV amphotericin B is used for the treatment of cryptococcal meningitis in HIV-infected adults and adolescents who cannot receive flucytosine, CDC, NIH, and IDSA recommend initial (induction) therapy with a dosage of 0.7–1 mg/kg daily in conjunction with oral or IV fluconazole (800 mg daily) given for at least 2 weeks and until there is evidence of clinical improvement and negative CSF culture after repeat lumbar puncture, then follow-up (consolidation) therapy with oral or IV fluconazole alone given for at least 8 weeks. Alternatively, if necessary, IDSA states that conventional IV amphotericin B can be given alone in a dosage of 0.7–1 mg/kg daily for 4–6 weeks for initial (induction) therapy followed by the usual consolidation therapy.

For the treatment of cryptococcal meningitis in immunocompetent adults without HIV infection who are not transplant recipients, IDSA recommends a regimen than includes induction therapy with conventional IV amphotericin B in a dosage of 0.7–1 mg/kg daily and oral flucytosine (25 mg/kg 4 times daily) given for at least 4 weeks (6 weeks in those with neurologic complications), then consolidation therapy with oral fluconazole alone given for 8 weeks. If the patient is immunocompetent without uncontrolled, underlying disease and is at low risk for therapeutic failure, IDSA states that the induction regimen can be given for only 2 weeks, followed by consolidation therapy with oral fluconazole alone for 8 weeks. In those who cannot receive flucytosine, induction therapy with IV amphotericin B can be given in a dosage of 0.7–1 mg/kg daily alone for at least 6 weeks, then consolidation therapy with oral fluconazole alone given for 8 weeks.

For the treatment of CNS and disseminated cryptococcal infections in children, IDSA recommends a regimen that includes induction therapy with conventional IV amphotericin B in a dosage of 1 mg/kg daily and oral flucytosine (25 mg/kg daily 4 divided doses) given for 2 weeks, then consolidation therapy with oral fluconazole alone given for at least 8 weeks. In children without HIV infection who are not transplant recipients, the induction phase should be continued for at least 4 weeks (6 weeks in those with neurologic complications) before initiating the consolidation regimen.

For the treatment of cryptococcal meningitis in HIV-infected infants and children, CDC, NIH, and IDSA recommend a regimen that includes induction therapy with conventional IV amphotericin B in a dosage of 1 mg/kg once daily in conjunction with oral flucytosine (25 mg/kg 4 times daily) given for at least 2 weeks until there is evidence of clinical improvement and negative CSF culture after repeat lumbar puncture, then consolidation therapy with IV or oral fluconazole given alone for at least 8 weeks. In HIV-infected infants and children who cannot receive flucytosine, CDC, NIH, and IDSA recommend induction therapy with conventional IV amphotericin B in a dosage of 1–1.5 mg/kg once daily alone or in conjunction with fluconazole for at least 2 weeks until there is evidence of clinical improvement and negative CSF culture after repeat lumbar puncture, then consolidation therapy with IV or oral fluconazole alone for at least 8 weeks.

For the treatment of severe pulmonary or disseminated cryptococcosis (nonmeningeal) in HIV-infected infants and children, CDC, NIH, and IDSA recommend that conventional IV amphotericin B be given in a dosage of 0.7–1 mg/kg daily (with or without oral flucytosine). The same dosage can be used without flucytosine for localized disease (e.g., isolated pulmonary disease). The treatment duration depends on the patient's response and the site and severity of infection.

Severe pulmonary cryptococcosis, cryptococcemia, or disseminated cryptococcosis in immunocompetent or immunocompromised adults, adolescents, or children should be treated using a regimen recommended for cryptococcal meningitis.

HIV-infected adults, adolescents, or children who have been adequately treated for cryptococcosis should receive long-term suppressive or maintenance therapy (secondary prophylaxis) with oral fluconazole to prevent recurrence or relapse.

If conventional IV amphotericin B is used as an alternative to oral fluconazole for long-term suppressive or maintenance therapy (secondary prophylaxis)† to prevent recurrence or relapse of cryptococcosis in HIV-infected adults and adolescents or other adults and adolescents who were adequately treated for cryptococcal meningitis, IDSA recommends a dosage of 1 mg/kg once weekly.

Histoplasmosis. If conventional IV amphotericin B is used for the treatment of moderately severe to severe acute pulmonary histoplasmosis or progressive disseminated histoplasmosis, IDSA recommends that adults receive an initial regimen of 0.7–1 mg/kg daily for 1–2 weeks, followed by oral itraconazole. The total duration of treatment should be 12 weeks in those with acute pulmonary disease or at least 12 months in those with progressive disseminated disease.

For the treatment of progressive disseminated histoplasmosis in children, IDSA states that conventional IV amphotericin B can be given in a dosage of 1 mg/kg daily for 4–6 weeks or, alternatively, an initial regimen of 1 mg/kg daily can be given for 2–4 weeks followed by oral itraconazole for a total treatment duration of 3 months.

If conventional IV amphotericin B is used as an alternative for the treatment of moderately severe to severe disseminated histoplasmosis in HIV-infected infants or children, CDC, NIH, and IDSA recommend an initial regimen of 0.7–1 mg/kg once daily for at least 2 weeks or until a response is obtained, then follow-up treatment with oral itraconazole for 12 months.

HIV-infected adults, adolescents, or children and other immunosuppressed individuals who have been adequately treated for histoplasmosis should receive long-term suppressive or maintenance therapy (secondary prophylaxis) with oral itraconazole to prevent recurrence or relapse.

Paracoccidioidomycosis. For the treatment of paracoccidioidomycosis†, conventional IV amphotericin B has been given in a dosage of 0.4–0.5 mg/kg daily, although higher dosages (i.e., 1 mg/kg daily or, rarely, 1.5 mg/kg daily) have been used for the treatment of rapidly progressing, potentially fatal infections. Prolonged therapy usually is required. In severely ill patients, some clinicians recommend that conventional IV amphotericin B be given in a dosage of 0.7–1 mg/kg daily for initial treatment followed by oral itraconazole therapy.

Sporotrichosis. For the treatment of sporotrichosis, the manufacturers state that conventional IV amphotericin B has been given for up to 9 months with a total dose of up to 2.5 g.

For the treatment of osteoarticular sporotrichosis, severe or life-threatening pulmonary sporotrichosis, or disseminated sporotrichosis, IDSA recommends that adults receive conventional IV amphotericin B in a dosage of 0.7–1 mg/kg daily until a response is obtained, followed by oral itraconazole (200 mg twice daily) given for a total treatment duration of at least 12 months. IDSA and other clinicians state that a lipid formulation of amphotericin B may be preferred for the treatment of disseminated sporotrichosis.

For the treatment of meningeal sporotrichosis, IDSA recommends that adults receive conventional IV amphotericin B in a dosage of 0.7–1 mg/kg daily for at least 4–6 weeks, followed by oral itraconazole (200 mg twice daily) for a total treatment duration of at least 12 months. IDSA and other clinicians state that a lipid formulation of amphotericin B may be preferred (rather than conventional amphotericin B) for the treatment of meningeal sporotrichosis.

For the treatment of disseminated sporotrichosis in children, IDSA recommends that conventional IV amphotericin B be given in a dosage of 0.7 mg/kg daily until a response is obtained, followed by oral itraconazole for a total treatment duration of at least 12 months.

Zygomycosis. For the treatment of zygomycosis, including mucormycosis, the usual dosage of conventional IV amphotericin B is 1–1.5 mg/kg daily for 2–3 months. For the treatment of rhinocerebral phycomycosis, the manufacturer recommends a total treatment dose of at least 3 g. Although a total treatment dose of 3–4 g can cause lasting renal impairment, the manufacturer states that this is a reasonable minimum dosage if there is clinical evidence of invasion of deep tissue since such infections usually are rapidly fatal and an aggressive therapeutic approach is necessary.

Adjunctive Therapy in CNS Fungal Infections. For the treatment of CNS fungal infections (e.g., candidal, coccidioidal, or cryptococcal meningitis), intracisternal†, intraventricular†, or intrathecal† injection of conventional amphotericin B has been used in conjunction with IV administration. For intrathecal† administration, amphotericin B has been reconstituted with sterile water for injection to a concentration of 0.25 mg/mL. The usual initial dose is 0.025 mg (0.1 mL of the reconstituted injection diluted with 10–20 mL of CSF and administered by barbotage) 2 or 3 times per week. The dose is gradually increased until the maximum dose is reached that can be given without causing severe discomfort. This dose usually is 0.5–1 mg, although 0.2–0.3 mg may be effective in some infections and others (e.g., coccidioidal meningitis) may require up 1.5 mg; corticosteroids (10–15 mg of hydrocortisone in adults) usually are added to relieve headache. (See Drug Interactions: Corticosteroids.)

Empiric Therapy in Febrile Neutropenic Patients. For the empiric treatment of presumed fungal infections in febrile neutropenic patients†, conventional IV amphotericin B has been given in a dosage of 0.5–1 mg/kg daily.

Empiric antifungal therapy should be discontinued when neutropenia resolves. In those with prolonged neutropenia, IDSA suggests that such therapy may be discontinued after 2 weeks if the patient is clinically well and no discernible lesions are found by clinical evaluation, chest radiographs, or CT scans of abdominal organs. If the patient appears ill or is at high risk, consideration can be given to continuing empiric antifungal treatment throughout the neutropenic episode.

Prevention of Fungal Infections in Transplant Recipients, Cancer Patients, or Other Individuals at High Risk. For prophylaxis of fungal infections in neutropenic cancer patients† or patients undergoing bone marrow transplantation† (BMT), conventional IV amphotericin B has been administered in a dosage of 0.1 mg/kg daily.

For high-risk patients undergoing urologic procedures†, IDSA states that conventional IV amphotericin B can be given in a dosage of 0.3–0.6 mg/kg daily for several days before and after the procedure.

Leishmaniasis. For the treatment of American cutaneous leishmaniasis caused by *Leishmania braziliensis* or *L. mexicana* or the treatment of mucocutaneous leishmaniasis caused by *L. braziliensis*, conventional IV amphotericin B has been given in a dosage of 0.25–0.5 mg/kg daily, with dosage gradually increased until 0.5–1 mg/kg daily was reached, at which time the drug was given on alternate days. Duration of therapy depends on the severity of disease and response to the drug, but is generally 3–12 weeks and the total dose generally ranges from 1–3 g.

For the treatment of mucosal disease, some clinicians recommend that conventional IV amphotericin B be given in a dosage 0.5–1 mg/kg daily or every other day for 4–8 weeks.

Visceral leishmaniasis (also known as kala-azar) in adults and children has been treated with 0.5–1 mg/kg of conventional IV amphotericin B† administered on alternate days for 14–20 doses. Some clinicians recommend that adults and children with visceral leishmaniasis receive a total treatment dosage of 15–20 mg/kg of conventional IV amphotericin B† given as 1 mg/kg daily for 15–20 days or 1 mg/kg every second day for 4–8 weeks.

If conventional IV amphotericin B† is used as an alternative to amphotericin B liposomal in HIV-infected adults and adolescents with visceral leishmaniasis, CDC, NIH, and IDSA recommend a dosage of 0.5–1 mg/kg daily for a total treatment dosage of 1.5–2 g. Long-term suppressive or maintenance therapy (secondary prophylaxis) with amphotericin B liposomal may be indicated. (See Leishmaniasis under Dosage: Amphotericin B Liposomal [Ambisome®], in Dosage and Administration.)

Primary Amebic Meningoencephalitis. If conventional IV amphotericin B is used for the treatment of primary amebic meningoencephalitis caused by *Naegleria fowleri*†, a dosage of 1.5 mg/kg daily in 2 divided doses for 3 consecutive days, then 1 mg/kg IV once daily for 11 consecutive days, has been recommended. If conventional amphotericin B is administered intrathecally† for the treatment of primary amebic meningoencephalitis, a dosage of 1.5 mg once daily for 2 days, then 1 mg every other day for 8 days, has been recommended. If conventional amphotericin B is administered by both routes in the same patient, some clinicians state that the maximum total dosage in adults and children is 1.5 mg/kg daily. Amphotericin B should be used in conjunction with other anti-infectives. Consultation with a specialist at CDC is recommended. (See Primary Amebic Meningoencephalitis under Uses: Protozoal Infections.)

Amphotericin B Lipid Complex (Abelcet®) For the treatment of invasive fungal infections in adults and children, the manufacturer of amphotericin B lipid complex recommends a dosage of 5 mg/kg IV once daily.

Aspergillosis. If IV amphotericin B lipid complex is used as an alternative for the treatment of invasive aspergillosis, IDSA recommends a dosage of 5 mg/kg daily. The duration of treatment is based on the degree and duration of immunosuppression, disease site, and clinical response. IDSA recommends that antifungal treatment of invasive pulmonary aspergillosis be continued for at least 6–12 weeks.

If a lipid formulation of amphotericin B is used as an alternative for the treatment of invasive aspergillosis in HIV-infected adults and adolescents, CDC, NIH, and IDSA recommend a dosage of 5 mg/kg IV once daily. The optimal duration of therapy in these patients has not been established, but antifungal therapy should be continued at least until CD4+ T-cell counts exceed 200/mm^3 and there is evidence of resolution of aspergillosis.

Blastomycosis. If a lipid formulation of IV amphotericin B is used for the treatment of moderate to severe pulmonary or disseminated extrapulmonary blastomycosis (without CNS involvement), IDSA recommends that adults (including immunocompromised individuals) receive initial therapy with a dosage of 3–5 mg/kg once daily for 1–2 weeks or until improvement occurs, followed by oral itraconazole therapy. Total treatment duration should be 6–12 months for pulmonary blastomycosis or at least 12 months for disseminated extrapulmonary blastomycosis or for immunocompromised individuals.

If a lipid formulation of IV amphotericin B is used for the treatment of severe blastomycosis in children, IDSA recommends initial therapy with a dosage of 3–5 mg/kg daily, followed by oral itraconazole therapy for a total treatment duration of 12 months.

For the treatment of CNS blastomycosis, IDSA recommends that adults receive initial therapy with a lipid formulation of IV amphotericin B given in a dosage of 5 mg/kg daily for 4–6 weeks, followed by an oral azole (fluconazole, itraconazole, voriconazole) given for at least 12 months and until resolution of CSF abnormalities.

Candida Infections. If a lipid formulation of amphotericin B is used for initial treatment of candidemia or other invasive *Candida* infections in nonneutropenic or neutropenic adults, IDSA recommends a dosage of 3–5 mg/kg daily. These experts state that a transition to fluconazole can be considered (usually within 5–7 days) in nonneutropenic patients who are clinically stable, have isolates susceptible to fluconazole (e.g., *C. albicans*), and have negative repeat blood cultures after initial antifungal treatment. IDSA recommends that antifungal treatment for candidemia (without persistent fungemia or metastatic complications) be continued for 2 weeks after documented clearance of *Candida* from the bloodstream, resolution of candidemia symptoms, and resolution of neutropenia.

If a lipid formulation of amphotericin B is used for the treatment of chronic disseminated (hepatosplenic) candidiasis, IDSA recommends initial treatment with a dosage of 3–5 mg/kg daily for several weeks followed by oral fluconazole. Antifungal treatment should be continued until lesions resolve on repeat imaging (usually several months).

If a lipid formulation of amphotericin B is used for initial treatment of endocarditis (native or prosthetic valve) or implantable cardiac device infections caused by *Candida*, IDSA recommends a dosage of 3–5 mg/kg daily given with or without oral flucytosine. If the infection is caused by fluconazole-susceptible *Candida*, treatment can be transitioned to fluconazole after the patient is stabilized and *Candida* has been cleared from the bloodstream.

If a lipid formulation of amphotericin B is used as an alternative for the treatment of esophageal candidiasis†, including fluconazole-refractory infections, in HIV-infected adults and adolescents, CDC, NIH, and IDSA recommend a dosage of 3–4 mg/kg IV once daily for 14–21 days.

If a lipid formulation of amphotericin B is used for the treatment of invasive *C. auris* infections (e.g., bloodstream or intra-abdominal infections) in adults (see Candida auris Infections under Uses: Candida Infections), CDC recommends a dosage of 3–5 mg/kg IV daily.

Coccidioidomycosis. If a lipid formulation of IV amphotericin B is used for the treatment of diffuse pulmonary or extrathoracic disseminated coccidioidomycosis (nonmeningeal) in HIV-infected adults of adolescents, CDC, NIH, and IDSA recommend a dosage of 4–6 mg/kg daily until improvement occurs, then follow-up treatment with oral fluconazole or oral itraconazole.

If a lipid formulation of IV amphotericin B is used for the treatment of diffuse pulmonary or disseminated coccidioidomycosis (nonmeningeal) in HIV-infected infants and children, CDC, NIH, and IDSA recommend a dosage of 5 mg/kg once daily until improvement occurs, then follow-up treatment with oral fluconazole or oral itraconazole. The total duration of treatment should be 1 year.

HIV-infected adults, adolescents, or children who have been adequately treated for coccidioidomycosis should receive long-term suppressive or maintenance therapy (secondary prophylaxis) with oral fluconazole or oral itraconazole to prevent recurrence or relapse.

Cryptococcosis. If amphotericin B lipid complex is used for initial (induction) therapy in HIV-infected adults and adolescents with cryptococcal meningitis, CDC, NIH, and IDSA recommend a dosage of 5 mg/kg daily in conjunction with oral flucytosine (25 mg/kg 4 times daily) given for at least 2 weeks and until there is evidence of clinical improvement and negative CSF culture after repeat lumbar puncture, then follow-up (consolidation) therapy with oral or IV fluconazole given for at least 8 weeks. Alternatively, if necessary, IDSA states that IV amphotericin B lipid complex can be given alone in a dosage of 5 mg/kg daily for 4–6 weeks for initial (induction) therapy followed by the usual consolidation therapy.

For the treatment of CNS cryptococcosis in adult organ transplant recipients, IDSA recommends induction therapy with IV amphotericin B lipid complex in a dosage of 5 mg/kg daily and oral flucytosine (100 mg/kg daily in 4 divided doses) given for at least 2 weeks, then consolidation therapy with oral fluconazole given for 8 weeks followed by a maintenance regimen of oral fluconazole given for 6–12 months. If flucytosine cannot be used in the induction regimen, consideration should be given to continuing induction therapy with IV amphotericin B lipid complex for at least 4–6 weeks before initiating consolidation therapy with oral fluconazole.

For the treatment of cryptococcal meningitis in immunocompetent adults without HIV infection who are not transplant recipients and when conventional IV amphotericin B cannot be used (e.g., patients who have or are predisposed to renal dysfunction), IDSA recommends a regimen than includes induction therapy with IV amphotericin B lipid complex in a dosage of 5 mg/kg daily given with oral flucytosine (100 mg/kg daily in 4 divided doses) for at least 4 weeks (6 weeks in those with neurologic complications), then consolidation therapy with oral fluconazole given for 8 weeks. If the patient is immunocompetent without uncontrolled, underlying disease and is at low risk for therapeutic failure, IDSA states that the induction regimen can be given for only 2 weeks, followed by consolidation therapy with oral fluconazole for 8 weeks. In those who cannot receive flucytosine, induction therapy with IV amphotericin B lipid complex can be given in a dosage of 5 mg/kg daily alone for at least 6 weeks, then consolidation therapy with oral fluconazole given for 8 weeks.

If amphotericin B lipid complex is used for the treatment of cryptococcal meningitis in HIV-infected infants and children, CDC, NIH, and IDSA recommend induction therapy with 5 mg/kg once daily given with oral flucytosine for at least 2 weeks until there is evidence of clinical improvement and negative CSF culture after repeat lumbar puncture, then consolidation therapy with oral or IV fluconazole alone for at least 8 weeks.

For the treatment of CNS and disseminated cryptococcal infections in children who cannot receive conventional IV amphotericin B, IDSA recommends a regimen that includes induction therapy with IV amphotericin B lipid complex in a dosage of 5 mg/kg daily given with oral flucytosine (100 mg/kg daily in 4 divided doses) for 2 weeks, then consolidation therapy with oral fluconazole given for at least 8 weeks. In children without HIV infection who are not transplant recipients, the induction phase should be continued for at least 4 weeks (6 weeks in those with neurologic complications) before initiating the consolidation regimen.

If amphotericin B lipid complex is used in HIV-infected infants and children with severe pulmonary or disseminated cryptococcosis (nonmeningeal), CDC, NIH, and IDSA recommend a dosage of 5 mg/kg once daily (with or without oral flucytosine). The same dosage can be used without flucytosine for localized disease (e.g., isolated pulmonary disease). The treatment duration depends on the patient's response and site and severity of infection.

HIV-infected adults, adolescents, or children who have been adequately treated for cryptococcosis should receive long-term suppressive or maintenance therapy (secondary prophylaxis) with oral fluconazole to prevent recurrence or relapse.

Histoplasmosis. If IV amphotericin B lipid complex is used for the treatment of moderately severe to severe disseminated histoplasmosis in HIV-infected adults and adolescents, CDC, NIH, and IDSA recommend an initial (induction) regimen of 3 mg/kg daily given for at least 2 weeks or until a response is obtained, then follow-up treatment with oral itraconazole for at least 12 months.

HIV-infected adults, adolescents, or children and other immunosuppressed individuals who have been adequately treated for histoplasmosis should receive long-term suppressive or maintenance therapy (secondary prophylaxis) with oral itraconazole to prevent recurrence or relapse.

Empiric Therapy in Febrile Neutropenic Patients. For the empiric treatment of presumed fungal infections in febrile neutropenic patients†, amphotericin B lipid complex has been given in a dosage of 3–5 mg/kg daily.

Empiric antifungal therapy should be discontinued when neutropenia resolves. In those with prolonged neutropenia, IDSA suggests that such therapy may be discontinued after 2 weeks if the patient is clinically well and no discernible lesions are found by clinical evaluation, chest radiographs, or CT scans of abdominal organs. If the patient appears ill or is at high risk, consideration can be given to continuing empiric antifungal treatment throughout the neutropenic episode.

Leishmaniasis. For the treatment of visceral leishmaniasis† (kala-azar), amphotericin B lipid complex has been given in a dosage of 1–3 mg/kg once daily for 5–10 days.

If amphotericin B lipid complex is used for the treatment of cutaneous leishmaniasis† in HIV-infected adults and adolescents, CDC, NIH, and IDSA recommend a dosage of 2–4 mg/kg daily for a total treatment dosage of 20–60 mg/kg. Alternatively, a dosage of 4 mg/kg daily on days 1–5, 10, 17, 24, 31, and 38 for a total treatment dosage of 20–60 mg/kg can be used.

If amphotericin B lipid complex is used for long-term suppressive or maintenance therapy (secondary prophylaxis)† in HIV-infected adults and adolescents who have been adequately treated for visceral leishmaniasis, CDC, NIH, and IDSA recommend a dosage of 3 mg/kg once every 21 days. Some experts state that consideration can be given to discontinuing secondary prophylaxis against leishmaniasis in HIV-infected individuals who have $CD4^+$ T-cell counts that have remained greater than 200–350/mm^3 for 3–6 months or longer. Other clinicians suggest that secondary prophylaxis against leishmaniasis should be continued indefinitely in HIV-infected individuals.

Amphotericin B Liposomal (AmBisome®) For the treatment of systemic fungal infections, the usual dosage of IV amphotericin B liposomal for adults or children 1 month of age or older is 3–5 mg/kg once daily.

Aspergillosis. For the treatment of aspergillosis, the usual dosage of IV amphotericin B liposomal for adults or children 1 month of age or older is 3–5 mg/kg once daily. In the treatment of invasive aspergillosis, use of higher dosage (10 mg/kg daily) does not result in improved efficacy and is associated with an increased incidence of adverse effects (e.g., nephrotoxicity).

The duration of treatment is based on the degree and duration of immunosuppression, disease site, and clinical response. IDSA recommends that antifungal treatment of invasive pulmonary aspergillosis be continued for at least 6–12 weeks. In published studies, the median duration of amphotericin B liposomal therapy for the effective treatment of aspergillosis has ranged from 15–29 days.

If a lipid formulation of IV amphotericin B is used as an alternative for the treatment of invasive aspergillosis in HIV-infected adults, CDC, NIH, and IDSA recommend 5 mg/kg IV once daily. The optimal duration of therapy in these patients has not been established, but antifungal therapy should be continued at least until $CD4^+$ T-cell counts exceed 200/mm^3 and there is evidence of resolution of aspergillosis.

Blastomycosis. If a lipid formulation of IV amphotericin B is used for the treatment of moderate to severe pulmonary or disseminated extrapulmonary blastomycosis (without CNS involvement), IDSA recommends that adults (including immunocompromised individuals) receive initial therapy with a dosage of 3–5 mg/kg once daily for 1–2 weeks or until improvement occurs, followed by oral itraconazole therapy. The total treatment duration should be 6–12 months for pulmonary blastomycosis or at least 12 months for disseminated extrapulmonary blastomycosis or for immunocompromised individuals.

If a lipid formulation of IV amphotericin B is used for the treatment of severe blastomycosis in children, IDSA recommends initial therapy with a dosage of 3–5 mg/kg once daily, followed by oral itraconazole therapy for a total treatment duration of 12 months.

For the treatment of CNS blastomycosis, IDSA recommends that adults receive initial therapy with a lipid formulation of IV amphotericin B given in a dosage of 5 mg/kg once daily for 4–6 weeks, followed by oral azole therapy (fluconazole, itraconazole, voriconazole). The total duration of treatment should be at least 12 months and until CSF abnormalities resolve.

Candida Infections. For the treatment of systemic *Candida* infections, the usual dosage of IV amphotericin B liposomal for adults and children 1 month of age or older is 3–5 mg/kg once daily. In published studies, the median duration of amphotericin B liposomal therapy for the effective treatment of candidiasis has ranged from 15–29 days, although some *Candida* infections were effectively treated with a median duration of therapy of 5–7 days.

If a lipid formulation of IV amphotericin B is used for initial treatment of candidemia or other invasive *Candida* infections in nonneutropenic or neutropenic adults, IDSA recommends a dosage of 3–5 mg/kg daily. These experts state that a transition to fluconazole can be considered (usually within 5–7 days) in nonneutropenic patients who are clinically stable, have isolates susceptible to fluconazole (e.g., *C. albicans*), and have negative repeat blood cultures after initial antifungal treatment. IDSA recommends that antifungal treatment for candidemia (without persistent fungemia or metastatic complications) be continued for 2 weeks after documented clearance of *Candida* from the bloodstream, resolution of candidemia symptoms, and resolution of neutropenia.

If a lipid formulation of amphotericin B is used for the treatment of chronic disseminated (hepatosplenic) candidiasis, IDSA recommends initial treatment with a dosage of 3–5 mg/kg daily for several weeks followed by oral fluconazole. Antifungal treatment should be continued until lesions resolve on repeat imaging (usually several months).

If IV amphotericin B liposomal is used for treatment of CNS candidiasis, IDSA recommends a dosage of 5 mg/kg daily (with or without oral flucytosine). After a response is attained, transition to fluconazole can be considered. Antifungal treatment should be continued until signs and symptoms, CSF abnormalities, and radiologic abnormalities have resolved.

If a lipid formulation of IV amphotericin B is used for initial treatment of endocarditis (native or prosthetic valve) or implantable cardiac device infections caused by *Candida*, IDSA recommends a dosage of 3–5 mg/kg daily given with or without oral flucytosine. If the infection is caused by fluconazole-susceptible *Candida*, treatment can be transitioned to fluconazole after the patient is stabilized and *Candida* has been cleared from the bloodstream.

If a lipid formulation of IV amphotericin B is used as an alternative for the treatment of esophageal candidiasis†, including fluconazole-refractory infections, in HIV-infected adults and adolescents, CDC, NIH, and IDSA recommend a dosage of 3–4 mg/kg IV once daily for 14–21 days.

If IV amphotericin B liposomal is used for treatment of endophthalmitis caused by fluconazole- and voriconazole-resistant *Candida*, IDSA recommends a dosage of 3–5 mg/kg daily (with or without oral flucytosine). In patients with macular involvement, intravitreal administration of *conventional* IV amphotericin B† also is recommended to ensure prompt high levels of antifungal activity.

If a lipid formulation of IV amphotericin B is used for the treatment of invasive *C. auris* infections (e.g., bloodstream or intra-abdominal infections) in adults (see Candida auris Infections under Uses: Candida Infections), CDC recommends a dosage of 3–5 mg/kg IV daily.

Coccidioidomycosis. If a lipid formulation of IV amphotericin B is used for the treatment of diffuse pulmonary or extrathoracic disseminated coccidioidomycosis (nonmeningeal) in HIV-infected adults of adolescents, CDC, NIH, and IDSA recommend a dosage of 4–6 mg/kg daily until improvement occurs, then follow-up treatment with oral fluconazole or oral itraconazole.

If a lipid formulation of IV amphotericin B is used for the treatment of diffuse pulmonary or disseminated coccidioidomycosis (nonmeningeal) in HIV-infected infants and children, CDC, NIH, and IDSA recommend a dosage of 5 mg/kg daily until improvement occurs, then follow-up treatment with oral fluconazole or oral itraconazole. The total duration of treatment should be 1 year.

HIV-infected adults, adolescents, or children who have been adequately treated for coccidioidomycosis should receive long-term suppressive or maintenance therapy (secondary prophylaxis) with oral fluconazole or oral itraconazole to prevent recurrence or relapse.

Cryptococcosis. For empiric treatment of cryptococcosis in adults and children 1 month of age or older, the manufacturer recommends that IV amphotericin B liposomal be given in a dosage of 3–5 mg/kg daily. For the treatment of cryptococcal meningitis in HIV-infected adults and children 1 month of age or older, the manufacturer recommends that IV amphotericin B liposomal be given in a dosage of 6 mg/kg daily.

For the treatment of cryptococcal meningitis in HIV-infected adults and adolescents, CDC, NIH, and IDSA recommend a regimen than includes initial (induction) therapy with IV amphotericin B liposomal in a dosage of 3–4 mg/kg daily in conjunction with oral flucytosine (25 mg/kg 4 times daily) given for at least 2 weeks and until there is evidence of clinical improvement and negative CSF culture after repeat lumbar puncture, then follow-up (consolidation) therapy with oral or IV fluconazole given for at least 8 weeks.

For the treatment of cryptococcal meningitis in HIV-infected adults and adolescents who cannot receive flucytosine, CDC, NIH, and IDSA recommend initial (induction) therapy with IV amphotericin B liposomal given in a dosage of 3–4 mg/kg once daily in conjunction with oral or IV fluconazole (800 mg daily) for at least 2 weeks and until there is evidence of clinical improvement and negative CSF culture after repeat lumbar puncture, then follow-up (consolidation) therapy with oral or IV fluconazole alone given for at least 8 weeks. Alternatively, if necessary, a regimen of IV amphotericin B liposomal alone given in a dosage of 3–4 mg/kg once daily can be used for initial (induction) therapy followed by the usual consolidation therapy.

For the treatment of CNS cryptococcosis in adult organ transplant recipients, IDSA recommends induction therapy with IV amphotericin B liposomal in a dosage of 3–4 mg/kg daily and oral flucytosine (100 mg/kg daily in 4 divided doses) given for at least 2 weeks, then consolidation therapy with oral fluconazole given for 8 weeks followed by a maintenance regimen of oral fluconazole given for 6–12 months. Alternatively, if flucytosine cannot be used in the induction regimen, consideration should be given to using a regimen of IV amphotericin B liposomal in a dosage of 6 mg/kg daily given for at least 4–6 weeks followed by the usual consolidation therapy with oral fluconazole.

For the treatment of cryptococcal meningitis in immunocompetent adults without HIV infection who are not transplant recipients and when conventional IV amphotericin B cannot be used (e.g., patients who have or are predisposed to renal dysfunction), IDSA recommends a regimen than includes induction therapy with IV amphotericin B liposomal in a dosage of 3–4 mg/kg daily with oral flucytosine (100 mg/kg daily in 4 divided doses) given for at least 4 weeks (6 weeks in those with neurologic complications), then consolidation therapy with oral fluconazole given for 8 weeks. If the patient is immunocompetent without uncontrolled, underlying disease and is at low risk for therapeutic failure, IDSA states that the induction regimen can be given for only 2 weeks, followed by consolidation therapy with oral fluconazole for 8 weeks. In those who cannot receive flucytosine, induction therapy with IV amphotericin B liposomal alone given in a dosage of 3–4 mg/kg daily for at least 6 weeks can be used, followed by consolidation therapy with oral fluconazole given for 8 weeks.

For the treatment of CNS and disseminated cryptococcal infections in children who cannot receive conventional IV amphotericin B, IDSA recommends a regimen that includes induction therapy with IV amphotericin B liposomal in a dosage of 5 mg/kg daily with oral flucytosine (100 mg/kg daily in 4 divided doses) given for 2 weeks, then consolidation therapy with oral fluconazole given for at least 8 weeks. In children without HIV infection who are not transplant recipients, the induction phase should be continued for at least 4 weeks (6 weeks in those with neurologic complications) before initiating the consolidation regimen.

For the treatment of cryptococcal meningitis in HIV-infected infants and children, CDC, NIH, and IDSA recommend a regimen that includes induction therapy with IV amphotericin B liposomal in a dosage of 6 mg/kg once daily in conjunction with oral flucytosine (25 mg/kg 4 times daily) given for at least 2 weeks until there is evidence of clinical improvement and negative CSF culture after repeat lumbar puncture, then consolidation therapy with IV or oral fluconazole given alone for at least 8 weeks. In HIV-infected infants and children who cannot receive flucytosine, CDC, NIH, and IDSA recommend induction therapy with IV amphotericin B liposomal in a dosage of 6 mg/kg once daily alone or in conjunction with IV fluconazole for at least 2 weeks until there is evidence of clinical improvement and negative CSF culture after repeat lumbar puncture, then consolidation therapy with IV or oral fluconazole alone for at least 8 weeks.

If amphotericin B liposomal is used in HIV-infected infants and children with severe pulmonary or disseminated cryptococcosis (nonmeningeal), CDC, NIH, and IDSA recommend a dosage of 3–5 mg/kg once daily (with or without oral flucytosine). The same dosage can be used without flucytosine for localized disease (e.g., isolated pulmonary disease). The treatment duration depends on the patient's response and site and severity of infection.

HIV-infected adults, adolescents, or children who have been adequately treated for cryptococcosis should receive long-term suppressive or maintenance therapy (secondary prophylaxis) with oral fluconazole to prevent recurrence or relapse.

Histoplasmosis. For the treatment of moderately severe to severe acute pulmonary histoplasmosis, IDSA recommends that adults receive an initial regimen of IV amphotericin B liposomal given in a dosage of 3–5 mg/kg daily for 1–2 weeks, followed by oral itraconazole for a total treatment duration of 12 weeks. For the treatment of moderately severe to severe progressive disseminated histoplasmosis, IDSA recommends that adults receive an initial regimen of IV amphotericin B liposomal given in a dosage of 3 mg/kg daily for 1–2 weeks, followed by oral itraconazole for a total treatment duration of at least 12 months.

For the treatment of moderately severe to severe disseminated histoplasmosis in HIV-infected adults or adolescents, CDC, NIH, and IDSA recommend an initial (induction) regimen of IV amphotericin B liposomal in a dosage of 3 mg/kg once daily given for at least 2 weeks or until a response is obtained, then follow-up treatment with oral itraconazole for at least 12 months. In HIV-infected infants or children, CDC, NIH, and IDSA recommend an initial (induction) regimen of IV amphotericin B liposomal in a dosage of 3–5 mg/kg once daily given for at least 2 weeks or until a response is obtained, then follow-up treatment with oral itraconazole for 12 months.

For the treatment of CNS histoplasmosis in HIV-infected adults, adolescents, or children or other adults, CDC, NIH, and IDSA recommend an initial regimen of IV amphotericin B liposomal given in a dosage of 5 mg/kg once daily for 4–6 weeks and follow-up treatment with oral itraconazole given for a total treatment duration of at least 12 months and until abnormal CSF findings resolve and histoplasmal antigen is undetectable.

HIV-infected adults, adolescents, or children and other immunosuppressed individuals who have been adequately treated for histoplasmosis should receive long-term suppressive or maintenance therapy (secondary prophylaxis) with oral itraconazole to prevent recurrence or relapse.

Exserohilum Infections. If IV amphotericin B liposomal is used for the treatment of CNS and/or parameningeal infections known or suspected to be caused by *Exserohilum rostratum*† in adults who received injections of a contaminated corticosteroid product (see Uses: Exserohilum Infections), CDC recommends a dosage of 5–6 mg/kg daily. Higher dosage (7.5 mg/kg daily) may be considered in patients who are not improving, but the increased risk of nephrotoxicity should be considered. Administration of 1 L of 0.9% sodium chloride injection prior to IV infusion of amphotericin B liposomal may be considered to minimize risk of nephrotoxicity.

If IV amphotericin B liposomal is used for the treatment of osteoarticular infections known or suspected to be caused by *E. rostratum*† in adults who received intra-articular injections of a contaminated corticosteroid product (see Uses: Exserohilum Infections), CDC recommends a dosage of 5 mg/kg daily.

Adequate duration of antifungal treatment for infections related to contaminated corticosteroid products is unknown, but prolonged treatment is required and should be based on disease severity and clinical response. A treatment duration of 6–12 months is probably necessary in patients who have severe CNS disease with complications (arachnoiditis, stroke), persistent CSF abnormalities, or underlying immunosuppression. In those with parameningeal infection, a minimum treatment duration of 3–6 months should be considered, and at least 6 months or longer probably is required for more severe disease (e.g., discitis, osteomyelitis) and in those with underlying immunosuppression or complications not amenable to surgical treatment. In those with osteoarticular infections, a minimum treatment duration of 3 months should be considered, and longer than 3 months is probably necessary in those with severe disease, bone infections, or underlying immunosuppression. After completion of treatment, close follow-up monitoring is essential in all patients to detect potential relapse.

An infectious disease expert and the most recent guidelines from CDC should be consulted for information regarding the management of infections in patients who received injections of potentially contaminated products. Clinicians should consult the CDC website at https://www.cdc.gov/hai/outbreaks/meningitis.html for the most recent recommendations regarding the drugs of choice, dosage, and duration of treatment of these infections.

Penicilliosis. For the treatment of severe, acute penicilliosis† in HIV-infected adults and adolescents, CDC, NIH, and IDSA recommend that IV amphotericin B liposomal be given in a dosage of 3–5 mg/kg daily for 2 weeks, followed by oral itraconazole (200 mg twice daily) for 10 weeks.

After the patient has been adequately treated, long-term suppressive or maintenance therapy (secondary prophylaxis) with oral itraconazole is recommended to prevent recurrence or relapse.

Empiric Therapy in Febrile Neutropenic Patients. For the empiric treatment of presumed fungal infections in febrile neutropenic patients 1 month of age or older, the usual dosage of amphotericin B liposomal is 3 mg/kg once daily. In one limited study, the median duration of empiric therapy was 10.8 days.

Empiric antifungal therapy should be discontinued when neutropenia resolves. In those with prolonged neutropenia, IDSA suggests that such therapy may be discontinued after 2 weeks if the patient is clinically well and no discernible lesions are found by clinical evaluation, chest radiographs, or CT scans of abdominal organs. If the patient appears ill or is at high risk, consideration can be given to continuing empiric antifungal treatment throughout the neutropenic episode.

Prevention of Fungal Infections in Transplant Recipients, Cancer Patients, or Other Individuals at High Risk. For postoperative prophylaxis in liver, pancreas, or small bowel transplant recipients† at high risk of candidiasis, IDSA states that IV amphotericin B liposomal can be given in a dosage of 1–2 mg/kg daily for at least 7–14 days.

Leishmaniasis. For the treatment of visceral leishmaniasis (also known as kala-azar) in immunocompetent adults and children 1 month of age or older, the manufacturer recommends that amphotericin B liposomal be given in a dosage of 3 mg/kg once daily on days 1–5, then 3 mg/kg should be given once daily on days 14 and 21; a second course of the drug may be useful if the parasitic infection is not completely cleared with a single course. For the treatment of visceral leishmaniasis in immunocompromised adults and children 1 month of age or older, the manufacturer recommends that amphotericin B liposomal be given in a dosage of 4 mg/kg once daily on days 1–5, then 4 mg/kg once daily on days 10, 17, 24, 31, and 38; however, if the parasitic infection is not completely cleared after the first course or if relapses occur, an expert should be consulted regarding further treatment. Various other dosage regimens have been used, including 5–7.5 mg/kg or 10 mg/kg once daily for 2 consecutive days.

If amphotericin B liposomal is used for the treatment of cutaneous leishmaniasis† in HIV-infected adults and adolescents, CDC, NIH, and IDSA recommend a dosage of 2–4 mg/kg daily for a total treatment dosage of 20–60 mg/kg. Alternatively, a dosage of 4 mg/kg daily on days 1–5, 10, 17, 24, 31, and 38 for a total treatment dosage of 20–60 mg/kg can be used.

If amphotericin B liposomal is used for the treatment of visceral leishmaniasis in HIV-infected adults and adolescents, CDC, NIH, and IDSA recommend a dosage of 2–4 mg/kg daily for a total treatment dosage of 20–60 mg/kg. Alternatively, a dosage of 4 mg/kg daily on days 1–5, 10, 17, 24, 31, and 38 for a total treatment dosage of 20–60 mg/kg can be used.

If amphotericin B liposomal is used for long-term suppressive or maintenance therapy (secondary prophylaxis)† in HIV-infected adults and adolescents who have been adequately treated for visceral leishmaniasis and have CD4$^+$ T-cell counts less than 200/mm^3, CDC, NIH, and IDSA recommend a dosage of 4 mg/kg once every 2–4 weeks. Some experts state that consideration can be given to discontinuing secondary prophylaxis against leishmaniasis in HIV-infected adults and adolescents who have CD4$^+$ T-cell counts that have remained greater than 200–350/mm^3 for 3–6 months or longer. Other clinicians suggest that secondary prophylaxis against leishmaniasis should be continued indefinitely in HIV-infected individuals.

Cautions

Conventional IV amphotericin B is associated with a high incidence of adverse effects, and most patients who receive the drug experience potentially severe adverse effects at some time during the course of therapy. Acute infusion reactions (e.g., fever, shaking chills, hypotension, headache, anorexia, nausea, vomiting, tachypnea) and nephrotoxicity are common adverse reactions to conventional IV amphotericin B.

Although clinical experience with amphotericin B lipid complex (Abelcet®) and amphotericin B liposomal (AmBisome®) is limited to date, these drugs appear to be better tolerated than conventional IV amphotericin B. As with conventional IV amphotericin B, the most frequent adverse reactions to amphotericin B lipid complex or amphotericin B liposomal are acute infusion reactions; however, data accumulated to date indicate that lipid formulations of amphotericin B may be associated with a lower overall incidence of adverse effects and a lower incidence of hematologic and renal toxicity than the conventional formulation of the drug.

■ Acute Infusion Reactions

Acute infusion reactions consisting of fever, shaking chills, hypotension, anorexia, nausea, vomiting, headache, dyspnea, and tachypnea may occur 1–3 hours after initiation of IV infusions of conventional amphotericin B, amphotericin B lipid complex, or amphotericin B liposomal. These reactions are most severe and occur most frequently with initial doses and usually lessen with subsequent doses. Fever (with or without shaking chills) usually occurs within 15–20 minutes after IV infusions of conventional amphotericin B are started. The majority of patients receiving conventional IV amphotericin B (50–90%) exhibit some degree of intolerance to initial doses of the drug, even when therapy is initiated with low doses.

In a study designed to evaluate the incidence of infusion reactions occurring in patients receiving conventional IV amphotericin B, 71% of patients had at least one infusion-related reaction during the first 7 days of therapy; fever and chills occurred in 28–51% and nausea and headache occurred in 9–18% of patients. In patients receiving amphotericin B lipid complex, chills and fever have been reported in 14–18% of patients and nausea, vomiting, and hypotension have been reported in 8–9% of patients. In a large, double-blind study in adults and pediatric febrile neutropenic patients, infusion reactions (i.e., fever, chills/rigors, nausea, vomiting) occurred in 4–20% of those receiving the first dose of amphotericin B liposomal and 7–56% of those receiving the first dose of conventional IV amphotericin B. In a randomized study in HIV-infected patients with cryptococcal meningitis, infusion reactions (i.e., fever, chills/rigors, nausea, vomiting) occurred in 6–16% of those receiving amphotericin B liposomal (3 or 6 mg/kg daily) and 18–48% of those receiving conventional amphotericin B. There have been reports of flushing, back pain (with or without chest tightness), and chest pain occurring within a few minutes after initiation of IV infusions of amphotericin B liposomal; these reactions occasionally were severe but disappeared when the infusion was stopped. These symptoms do not occur with every dose and usually do not recur with subsequent doses given at a slower IV infusion rate.

Although the precise mechanism for these infusion reactions is not known, limited evidence indicates that amphotericin-induced increases in prostaglandin (e.g., PGE_2) synthesis may be involved. Aspirin, antipyretics (e.g., acetaminophen), antiemetics, meperidine, antihistamines (e.g., diphenhydramine), or corticosteroids have been used for the treatment or prevention of acute infusion reactions in patients receiving conventional IV amphotericin or other formulations of the drug. It has been suggested that meperidine (25–50 mg IV) may decrease the duration of shaking chills and fever occurring in association with IV infusion of amphotericin B. There is some evidence that IV administration of small doses of corticosteroids just prior to or during IV infusion of conventional amphotericin B may help decrease the severity of febrile and other systemic reactions; however, corticosteroids should be used only when necessary using minimal dosage for as short a period as possible. (See Drug Interactions: Corticosteroids.) Use of a premedication regimen (e.g., acetaminophen and diphenhydramine; acetaminophen, corticosteroid, and diphenhydramine) is not routinely recommended prior to the initial dose of any amphotericin B formulation, but can be administered promptly to treat a reaction if it occurs and then as pretreatment prior to subsequent doses.

Rapid IV infusion of conventional IV amphotericin B has been associated with a more severe reaction consisting of hypotension, hypokalemia, arrhythmias, and shock. Some of these adverse effects also have been reported rarely with amphotericin B lipid complex or amphotericin B liposomal. It may be difficult to determine whether these severe reactions indicate intolerance or hypersensitivity to the drug.

■ **Renal and Electrolyte Effects** Nephrotoxicity is the major dose-limiting toxicity reported with conventional IV amphotericin B, and nephrotoxicity occurs to some degree in the majority of patients receiving the drug. Adverse renal effects in patients receiving conventional IV amphotericin B include decreased renal function and renal function abnormalities such as azotemia, hypokalemia, hyposthenuria, renal tubular acidosis, and nephrocalcinosis. Increased BUN and serum creatinine concentrations have been reported. Hypokalemia and hypomagnesemia develop in a large proportion of patients, and hypocalcemia has been reported. Uric acid excretion is increased and nephrocalcinosis can occur. Renal tubular acidosis may be present without concurrent systemic acidosis. It has been suggested that hydration and sodium repletion prior to administration of IV amphotericin B may decrease the risk of nephrotoxicity, and supplemental alkali therapy may decrease complications related to renal tubular acidosis. Nephrotoxicity associated with conventional IV amphotericin B appears to involve several mechanisms, including a direct vasoconstrictive effect on renal arterioles that reduces glomerular and renal tubular blood flow and a lytic action on cholesterol-rich lysosomal membranes of renal tubular cells. On biopsy, juxtamedullary glomerulitis and intratubular and interstitial calcium deposits in the distal nephron are found. Although renal function usually improves within a few months after discontinuance of conventional amphotericin B therapy, some degree of permanent impairment may remain in some patients, especially in patients who received a large cumulative dose of the drug (exceeding 5 g) or concomitant therapy with other nephrotoxic drugs. Patients with higher serum low-density lipoprotein (LDL) concentrations appear to be more susceptible to amphotericin B-induced renal toxicity than those with lower concentrations.

Increased BUN and/or serum creatinine, hypokalemia, hypomagnesemia, and hypocalcemia also have been reported in patients receiving amphotericin B lipid complex or amphotericin B liposomal. While these formulations appear to be associated with a lower risk of nephrotoxicity than conventional IV amphotericin B and have been used in patients with preexisting renal impairment (in most cases resulting from prior therapy with conventional IV amphotericin B), additional experience with the drugs is necessary to more accurately determine the extent of nephrotoxicity that occurs with these formulations. In several studies when amphotericin B lipid complex was substituted for conventional IV amphotericin B in patients who developed nephrotoxicity while receiving the conventional formulation and had baseline serum creatinine concentrations of 2 mg/dL or greater, serum creatinine concentrations generally declined during therapy with the lipid formulations. In a randomized, double-blind study comparing safety and efficacy of amphotericin B liposomal or conventional IV amphotericin B for antifungal prophylaxis in febrile, neutropenic patients, nephrotoxicity occurred in about 19 or 34% of patients, respectively. In a randomized study in HIV-infected patients with cryptococcal meningitis, serum creatinine concentrations twofold higher than baseline concentrations were reported in 14–21% of those receiving amphotericin B liposomal (3 or 6 mg/kg daily) and in 33% of those receiving conventional amphotericin B.

Other adverse renal effects that have been reported in patients receiving conventional IV amphotericin B, amphotericin B lipid complex, or amphotericin B liposomal include anuria, oliguria, dysuria, decreased renal function, hematuria, urinary incontinence, renal tubular acidosis, and acute renal failure. Nephrogenic diabetes insipidus has been reported in patients receiving conventional IV amphotericin B.

■ **Hematologic Effects** Patients receiving conventional IV amphotericin B may develop normocytic, normochromic anemia. The anemia develops gradually and may not occur until after 10 weeks of therapy; it may be related either to a direct inhibition of erythrocytes or erythropoietin production or may be secondary to renal toxicity. The hematocrit rarely decreases below 20–25% and generally returns to baseline within several months following discontinuance of the drug. Anemia also has been reported rarely in patients receiving amphotericin B lipid complex or amphotericin B liposomal.

Other hematologic effects, including agranulocytosis, coagulation disorders, decreased or increased prothrombin, thrombocytopenia, leukopenia, eosinophilia, or leukocytosis, have been reported rarely in patients receiving conventional IV amphotericin B, amphotericin B lipid complex, or amphotericin B liposomal.

■ **Cardiopulmonary and Sensitivity Reactions** Various adverse cardiopulmonary effects, including hypotension, tachypnea, cardiac failure, cardiac arrest, cardiomyopathy, shock, pulmonary edema, hypersensitivity pneumonitis, arrhythmias (including ventricular fibrillation), dyspnea, and hypertension, have been reported in individuals receiving conventional IV amphotericin B.

Bronchospasm, wheezing, angioedema, and anaphylaxis or anaphylactoid reactions have been reported in patients receiving conventional IV amphotericin B or the lipid formulations of amphotericin B. If severe respiratory distress, anaphylaxis, or an anaphylactoid reaction occurs in a patient receiving amphotericin B, the drug should be discontinued immediately and the patient given appropriate therapy (e.g., epinephrine, corticosteroids, maintenance of an adequate airway, oxygen) as indicated. The manufacturer of amphotericin B lipid complex states that the drug is contraindicated in patients who have experienced severe respiratory distress after receiving a prior dose of the drug.

Cardiac enlargement with congestive heart failure occurred in a few patients receiving conventional IV amphotericin B with 20–40 mg of hydrocortisone sodium succinate added to each infusion. Congestive heart failure was considered to be due to amphotericin B-induced hypokalemic cardiopathy and corticosteroid-induced salt and fluid retention. (See Drug Interactions: Corticosteroids.) Following discontinuance of hydrocortisone and administration of oral potassium supplements, cardiac status returned to normal although conventional amphotericin B therapy was continued.

■ **GI Effects** In addition to the nausea and vomiting reported as part of acute infusion reactions to the drugs, other adverse GI effects have been reported in patients receiving conventional IV amphotericin B, amphotericin B lipid complex, or amphotericin B liposomal. These adverse effects include anorexia and weight loss, diarrhea, dyspepsia, cramping, epigastric pain, hemorrhagic gastroenteritis, GI hemorrhage, and melena. Alternate-day therapy may decrease the incidence of anorexia.

■ **Local Reactions** IV administration of conventional amphotericin B, amphotericin B lipid complex, or amphotericin B liposomal may cause erythema, pain, or inflammation at the injection site. Phlebitis or thrombophlebitis has been reported with conventional IV amphotericin B. The manufacturers of conventional IV amphotericin B and some clinicians suggest that the addition of 500–1000 units of heparin to the amphotericin B infusion, the use of a pediatric scalp-vein needle, or alternate-day therapy may decrease the incidence of thrombophlebitis. Extravasation of the drug causes local irritation.

■ **Nervous System Effects** Adverse neurologic effects that have been reported in patients receiving conventional IV amphotericin B, amphotericin B lipid complex, or amphotericin B liposomal include malaise, depression, confusion, dizziness, insomnia, somnolence, coma, anxiety,agitation, nervousness, abnormal thinking, hallucinations, tremor, seizures, myasthenia, hearing loss, tinnitus, transient vertigo, visual impairment, diplopia, peripheral neuropathy, encephalopathy, cerebrovascular accident, and extrapyramidal syndrome. Leukoencephalopathy has been reported following use of amphotericin B; literature reports suggest that total body irradiation may be a predisposition.

■ **Other Adverse Effects** Adverse musculoskeletal effects, including generalized pain, dystonia, and muscle, bone, or joint pain, have been reported in patients receiving conventional IV amphotericin B, amphotericin B lipid complex, or amphotericin B liposomal.

Rash (including maculopapular or vesiculobullous rash), purpura, pruritus, urticaria, sweating, exfoliative dermatitis, erythema multiforme, toxic epidermal necrolysis, Stevens-Johnson syndrome, alopecia, dry skin, skin discoloration, and ulcer have been reported in patients receiving amphotericin B.

Increased serum concentrations of AST (SGOT), ALT (SGPT), alkaline phosphatase, bilirubin, γ-glutamyltransferase (GGT, γ-glutamyltranspeptidase, GGTP), and LDH have been reported in patients receiving conventional IV amphotericin B, amphotericin B lipid complex, or amphotericin B liposomal. Acute liver failure, hepatotoxicity, hepatitis, jaundice, hyperglycemia, and hypoglycemia have been reported rarely.

Intrathecal† administration of conventional amphotericin B has produced headache, nausea and vomiting, urinary retention, pain along lumbar nerves, paresthesia, vision changes, and arachnoiditis.

■ **Precautions and Contraindications** Initial doses of conventional IV amphotericin B, amphotericin B lipid complex, or amphotericin B liposomal should be administered under close clinical observation by medically trained personnel. The fact that acute infusion reactions (e.g., fever, chills, hypotension, nausea, vomiting, headache, dyspnea, and tachypnea) often occur 1–3 hours after initiation of amphotericin B IV infusions (especially after the first few doses) and that severe reactions including anaphylaxis have been reported rarely should be considered. Conventional IV amphotericin B is associated with a high incidence of adverse effects and should be reserved principally for the treatment of progressive, potentially life-threatening fungal infections caused by susceptible organisms when the potential benefits of the drug outweigh its untoward and dangerous side effects.

Renal, hepatic, and hematologic function should be monitored in patients receiving conventional IV amphotericin B, amphotericin B lipid complex, or amphotericin B liposomal. Some clinicians suggest that renal function be monitored at least 2–3 times weekly during initial amphotericin B therapy and that hepatic and hematologic function be monitored 1–2 times weekly. Serum electrolytes (especially potassium and magnesium) and complete blood cell counts (CBCs) also should be monitored in patients receiving any of these drugs. Because of the drug's nephrotoxic potential, conventional IV amphotericin B should be used with caution in patients with reduced renal function and patients receiving any amphotericin B formulation concomitantly with a nephrotoxic drug should be closely monitored. (See Drug Interactions: Nephrotoxic Drugs.)

Conventional amphotericin B, amphotericin B lipid complex, and amphotericin B liposomal are contraindicated in patients who are hypersensitive to amphotericin B or any other component in the respective formulation. The manufacturers of conventional amphotericin B and amphotericin B liposomal suggest that use of these drugs can be considered in patients with hypersensitivity if the clinician determines that the benefits of such therapy outweigh the risks; however, they are contraindicated in patients who have had severe respiratory distress or a severe anaphylactic reaction while receiving the drugs.

■ **Pediatric Precautions** Although safety and efficacy of conventional IV amphotericin B in pediatric patients have not been established through adequate and well-controlled studies, the drug has been used effectively to treat systemic fungal infections in pediatric patients without unusual adverse effects. The manufacturers state that the lowest effective dosage of the drug should be employed whenever conventional IV amphotericin B is used in pediatric patients.

IV amphotericin B lipid complex generally is well tolerated in pediatric patients, and has been used for the treatment of invasive fungal infections in children 3 weeks to 16 years of age without unusual adverse effects. Acute infusion reactions (fever, chills, rigors) and anaphylaxis have been reported in pediatric patients receiving amphotericin B lipid complex and have necessitated discontinuance of the drug in these patients.

IV amphotericin B liposomal has been administered to pediatric patients 1 month to 16 years of age without any unusual adverse effects. Although safety and efficacy of the drug in neonates younger than 1 month of age have not been established to date, amphotericin B liposomal has been used in a limited number of neonates† for the treatment of severe fungal infections without any unusual adverse effects. Transient hypokalemia that responded to potassium supplementation was the only adverse effect reported in a group of neonates who received amphotericin B liposomal in a dosage of 1–5 mg/kg given by IV infusion over 0.5–1 hours. In a large, double-blind study comparing the safety and efficacy of amphotericin B liposomal and conventional IV amphotericin B, the incidence of chills, vomiting, hypokalemia, or hypertension in patients 16 years of age or younger ranged from 10–37% in those receiving amphotericin B liposomal and from 21–68% in those receiving the conventional formulation of the drug.

■ **Geriatric Precautions** While safety and efficacy of conventional IV amphotericin B, amphotericin B lipid complex, and amphotericin B liposomal have not been studied specifically in geriatric patients, no unusual age-related adverse effects have been reported when the drugs were used in patients 65 years of age or older.

Although clinical experience to date indicates that dosage modification is unnecessary when amphotericin B liposomal is used in geriatric patients, the manufacturer recommends that these patients be carefully monitored while receiving the drug.

■ **Mutagenicity and Carcinogenicity** There have been no long-term studies to date to evaluate the carcinogenic potential of conventional amphotericin B, amphotericin B lipid complex, or amphotericin B liposomal.

The mutagenic potential of conventional amphotericin B or amphotericin B liposomal has not been evaluated to date. There was no evidence of mutagenicity when amphotericin B lipid complex was evaluated using in vitro studies (e.g., bacterial reverse mutation assay, mouse lymphoma forward mutation assay, CHO chromosomal aberration assay) or in vivo studies (e.g., mouse bone marrow micronucleus assay) with or without metabolic activation.

■ **Pregnancy, Fertility, and Lactation** Safe use of amphotericin B during pregnancy has not been established. Conventional IV amphotericin B has been used to treat systemic fungal infections or visceral leishmaniasis in a limited number of pregnant women without obvious adverse effects to the fetus. While reproduction studies in rats and rabbits using conventional amphotericin B, amphotericin B lipid complex, or amphotericin B liposomal have not revealed evidence of harm to the fetus, rabbits receiving amphotericin B liposomal dosages equivalent to 0.5–2 times the usual human dosage experienced a higher rate of spontaneous abortions than the control group. However, animal reproduction studies are not always predictive of human response. There are no adequate or controlled studies to date using any amphotericin B formulation in pregnant women, and these drugs should be used during pregnancy only when clearly needed.

There have been no studies to date to determine whether conventional amphotericin B affects fertility. Studies in male and female rats using amphotericin B lipid complex at doses up to 0.32 times the usual human dose (based on body surface area) indicate that the drug does not affect fertility. When liposomal amphotericin was administered to rats in 10- or 15-mg/kg doses (equivalent to human doses of 1.6 or 2.4 mg/kg based on body surface area), there was evidence of an abnormal estrous cycle (prolonged diestrus) and decreased number of corpora lutea in female rats receiving the higher dosage but no effect on fertility or days to copulation; there were no effects on male reproductive function.

It is not known whether amphotericin B is distributed into human milk. Because many drugs are distributed into human milk and because of the potential for serious adverse reactions to amphotericin B in nursing infants if it were distributed, a decision should be made whether to discontinue nursing or the drug, taking into account the importance of the drug to the woman.

Drug Interactions

Systematic drug interaction studies have not been performed to date using amphotericin B lipid complex or amphotericin B liposomal. The fact that drug interactions reported with conventional IV amphotericin B could also occur with these lipid formulations of the drug should be considered.

■ **Nephrotoxic Drugs** Since nephrotoxic effects may be additive, the concurrent or sequential use of IV amphotericin B and other drugs with similar toxic potentials (e.g., aminoglycosides, cyclosporine, pentamidine) should be avoided, if possible. Great caution and intensive monitoring of renal function is recommended if any amphotericin B formulation is used concomitantly with a nephrotoxic agent.

Cyclosporine There is evidence from a prospective study in patients undergoing bone marrow transplantation (BMT) that concurrent initiation of cyclosporine and amphotericin B lipid complex therapy may be associated with increased nephrotoxicity. In a renal transplant recipient who was receiving cyclosporine and had stable whole blood cyclosporine concentrations, blood cyclosporine concentrations in the days after initiation of amphotericin B lipid complex therapy were more than twice those reported prior to initiation of antifungal therapy; however, this increase was transient and did not necessitate adjustment of cyclosporine dosage.

Pentamidine Acute, reversible renal failure occurred in at least 4 patients with human immunodeficiency virus (HIV) infection who received IV amphotericin B concomitantly with IV or IM pentamidine; there was no evidence of adverse renal effects in patients who received IV amphotericin B concomitantly with pentamidine administered by oral inhalation.

■ **Drugs Affected by Potassium Depletion** Because amphotericin B may induce hypokalemia, the drug may predispose patients receiving cardiac glycosides to glycoside-induced cardiotoxicity and may enhance the effects of skeletal muscle relaxants (e.g., tubocurarine). Serum potassium concentrations should be monitored closely in patients receiving any amphotericin B formulation concomitantly with a cardiac glycoside or skeletal muscle relaxant.

■ **Anti-infective Agents** ***Flucytosine*** In some in vitro studies, the combination of flucytosine and amphotericin B resulted in synergistic inhibition of strains of *Cryptococcus neoformans*, *Candida albicans*, and *C. tropicalis*. The suggested mechanism of the synergism is that the binding of amphotericin B to sterols in cell membranes increases the permeability of the cytoplasmic membrane, thus allowing greater penetration of flucytosine into the fungal cell. However, in a study evaluating the antifungal effects of the drugs in the presence of serum, the combination of amphotericin B and flucytosine was not additive or synergistic against *C. albicans*.

There is some evidence that concomitant use of amphotericin B and flucytosine may increase the toxicity of flucytosine, possibly by increasing cellular uptake and/or by decreasing renal excretion of the drug. Flucytosine and amphotericin B should be used concomitantly with caution. If flucytosine is used in conjunction with amphotericin B, especially in HIV-infected patients, serum flucytosine concentrations and blood cell counts should be monitored carefully. In addition, it has been suggested that flucytosine be initiated at a low dosage (i.e., 75–100 mg/kg daily) and subsequent dosage adjusted based on serum flucytosine concentrations.

Imidazole and Triazole Antifungal Agents Although the clinical importance is unclear, results of in vitro studies evaluating the antifungal effects of amphotericin B used concomitantly with imidazole- or triazole-derivative antifungals (e.g., clotrimazole, fluconazole, itraconazole, ketoconazole) against *C. albicans*, *C. pseudotropicalis*, *C. glabrata*, or *Aspergillus fumigatus* indicate that antagonism can occur with these combinations. Since amphotericin B exerts its antifungal activity by binding to sterols in the fungal cell membrane and imidazoles and triazoles act by altering the cell membrane, antagonism is theoretically possible; however, it is unclear whether such antagonism actually would occur in vivo. Results of studies evaluating combined use of amphotericin B and fluconazole, ketoconazole, or itraconazole in animal models of aspergillosis, candidiasis, or cryptococcosis have been conflicting. While antagonism occurred in some models (*A. fumigatus* infection in mice, rabbits, or rats treated with amphotericin B and fluconazole or itraconazole), these combinations resulted in additive or indifferent effects in other models (e.g., *C. albicans* or *C. neoformans* infection in mice or rabbits treated with amphotericin B and fluconazole). In a few studies evaluating the drugs in murine cryptococcosis or candidiasis, sequential use of an initial large dose of amphotericin B followed by an azole antifungal (e.g., fluconazole) was uniformly effective in prolonging survival and decreasing fungal burden. Because further study is needed regarding the interaction between amphotericin B and imidazole- or triazole-derivative antifungals (e.g., fluconazole, itraconazole, or ketoconazole), such combination therapy should be used with caution, particularly in immunocompromised patients.

Results of an in vitro study indicate that the combination of amphotericin B and fluconazole or itraconazole may be synergistic, additive, or indifferent against *Pseudallescheria boydii*; there was no evidence of antagonism.

Quinolones Norfloxacin may enhance the antifungal activity of some antifungals (e.g., amphotericin B, flucytosine, ketoconazole, nystatin). There are conflicting reports on this interaction, however, and in at least one in vitro study norfloxacin had no effect on the antifungal activity of amphotericin B. Further study is needed to evaluate the antifungal effect when norfloxacin is used in conjunction with an antifungal.

Rifabutin Results of an in vitro study indicate that the combination of rifabutin and amphotericin B may be additive or synergistic against *Aspergillus fumigatus*, *A. flavus*, *Fusarium solani*, *F. moniliforme*, *F. pallidoroseum* (formerly *F. semitectum*), and *F. proliferatum*; there was no evidence of antagonism with this combination. While rifabutin has no in vitro antifungal activity against *Aspergillus* or *Fusarium* when used alone, an antifungal effect was evident when the drug was used in combination with amphotericin B.

Zidovudine Results of a study in dogs indicate that concomitant administration of zidovudine and conventional amphotericin B (at 0.5 times the recommended human dosage) or amphotericin B lipid complex (at 0.16 or 0.5 times the recommended human dosage) for 30 days was associated with increased myelotoxicity and nephrotoxicity. Although the clinical importance of this animal study is unclear, renal and hematologic function should be closely monitored in patients receiving zidovudine concomitantly with amphotericin B.

■ **Antineoplastic Agents** The manufacturers state that antineoplastic agents (e.g., mechlorethamine) may enhance the potential for renal toxicity, bronchospasm, and hypotension in patients receiving amphotericin B and such concomitant therapy should be used only with great caution.

■ **Corticosteroids** Corticosteroids reportedly may enhance the potassium depletion caused by conventional amphotericin B. The manufacturers state that concomitant use of corticosteroids should be avoided, unless necessary to control adverse effects of conventional amphotericin B. In such cases, the corticosteroid should be administered using minimal dosage for as short a duration as possible.

If corticosteroids are used concomitantly with any amphotericin B formulation, serum electrolytes and cardiac function should be monitored closely.

■ **Leukocyte Transfusions** IV infusion of conventional amphotericin B during or shortly after leukocyte transfusions has rarely been associated with acute pulmonary reactions characterized by acute dyspnea, tachypnea, hypoxemia, hemoptysis, and diffuse interstitial infiltrates. The most severe pulmonary reactions have been reported when amphotericin B was administered within the first 4 hours after a leukocyte transfusion; respiratory deterioration appeared to contribute to death in at least 5 patients with such reactions.

It has been recommended that amphotericin B be used with caution in patients receiving leukocyte transfusions, especially in those with gram-negative septicemia. The manufacturer of amphotericin B lipid complex states that the drug should not be used concurrently with leukocyte transfusions. The manufacturers of conventional amphotericin B recommend that doses of the drug be separated in time as much as possible from leukocyte transfusions and that pulmonary function be monitored in patients receiving both therapies.

Acute Toxicity

■ **Manifestations** Acute overdosage of conventional amphotericin B may result in potentially fatal cardiac or cardiorespiratory arrest. Adverse cardiovascular effects, including hypotension, bradycardia, and cardiac arrest, have been reported in several pediatric patients who inadvertently received overdosage of conventional amphotericin B. One child who received conventional amphotericin B in a dosage of 4.6 mg/kg given by IV infusion over 2 hours experienced vomiting, followed by seizures, and cardiac arrest immediately after the infusion.

In patients who received 1 or more amphotericin B lipid complex doses of 7–13 mg/kg., serious acute reactions did not occur.

Information on acute toxicity of amphotericin B liposomal is not available. There was no reported dose-related toxicity following repeated daily doses up to 15 mg/kg in adult patients or up to 10 mg/kg in pediatric patients.

■ **Treatment** In the event of overdosage with any amphotericin B formulation, therapy with the drug should be discontinued and the patient's clinical status (e.g., cardiorespiratory, renal, and liver function, hematologic status, serum electrolytes) monitored. Supportive therapy should be administered as required. Amphotericin B is not removed by hemodialysis. The manufacturers of conventional amphoteric B state that the patient's condition should be stabilized, including correction of electrolyte abnormalities, prior to reinstituting the drug.

Mechanism of Action

Amphotericin B usually is fungistatic in action at concentrations obtained clinically, but may be fungicidal in high concentrations or against very susceptible organisms. Amphotericin B exerts its antifungal activity principally by binding to sterols (e.g., ergosterol) in the fungal cell membrane. As a result of this binding, the cell membrane is no longer able to function as a selective barrier and leakage of intracellular contents occurs. Cell death occurs in part as a result of permeability changes, but other mechanisms also may contribute to the in vivo antifungal effects of amphotericin B against some fungi. Amphotericin B is not active in vitro against organisms that do not contain sterols in their cell membranes (e.g., bacteria).

Binding to sterols in mammalian cells (such as certain kidney cells and erythrocytes) may account for some of the toxicities reported with conventional amphotericin B therapy. At usual therapeutic concentrations of amphotericin B, the drug does not appear to hemolyze mature erythrocytes, and the anemia seen with conventional IV amphotericin B therapy may result from the action of the drug on actively metabolizing and dividing erythropoietic cells.

Spectrum

Amphotericin B is active against most pathogenic fungi, including yeasts, and also is active against some protozoa. Amphotericin B is inactive against bacteria, rickettsiae, or viruses.

■ **Fungi** In vitro, amphotericin B concentrations of 0.03–1.0 mcg/mL usually inhibit *Aspergillus fumigatus*, *A. flavus*, *Coccidioides immitis*, *C. posadasii*, *Cryptococcus neoformans*, *C. gattii*, *Exophiala castellanii*, *E. spinifera*, *Histoplasma capsulatum*, *Rhodotorula*, and *Sporothrix schenckii*. *Blastomyces dermatitidis* may require slightly higher drug concentrations for inhibition.

Amphotericin B is active in vitro against most strains of *Candida*. In vitro, *C. albicans*, *C. dubliniensis*, *C. glabrata* (formerly *Torulopsis glabrata*), *C. krusei*, *C. parapsilosis*, and *C. tropicalis* usually are inhibited by amphotericin B concentrations of 0.03–1 mcg/mL. In a study evaluating in vitro susceptibility of clinical isolates of *C. dubliniensis* obtained from patients with or without human immunodeficiency virus (HIV) infection, these strains were inhibited by amphotericin B concentrations of 0.03–0.125 mcg/mL. While some strains of *C. lusitaniae* are inhibited in vitro by amphotericin B concentrations of 0.06–0.5 mcg/mL, other strains appear to be resistant to the drug. Clinical isolates of *C. auris* (often misidentified as *C. haemulonii*, *C. famata*, or *Rhodotorula glutinis*) generally have been inhibited in vitro by amphotericin B concentrations of 0.5–1 mcg/mL.

Some *Penicillium marneffei* isolates have been inhibited in vitro by amphotericin B concentrations of 0.002–4 mcg/mL, but other strains required concentrations as high as 32 mcg/mL for in vitro inhibition.

Many zygomycetes, including *Lichtheimia* (formerly *Absidia*), *Mucor*, *Rhizopus*, *Rhizomucor*, *Apophysomyces elegans*, and *Cunninghamella*, are inhibited in vitro by amphotericin B concentrations of 0.003–2 mcg/mL. Some clinical isolates of *Basidiobolus*, including *B. ranarum*, have amphotericin B MICs of 0.5–4 mcg/mL; however, other isolates are resistant to the drug. *Conidiobolus coronatus* has been inhibited in vitro by amphotericin B concentrations of 0.5–4 mcg/mL.

While some strains of *Pseudallescheria boydii* are inhibited in vitro by amphotericin B concentrations of 0.5 mcg/mL or less, most strains are resistant to the drug. Amphotericin B concentrations of 1–16 mcg/mL were necessary for in vitro inhibition of clinical isolates of *Scedosporium apiospermum* or *S. prolificans*, and these filamentous fungi probably are resistant to the drug.

Amphotericin B is active against *Exserohilum*, and *E. rostratum* has been inhibited in vitro by amphotericin B concentrations of 0.03–0.5 mcg/mL. In vitro studies of *E. rostratum* obtained from patients with infections related to injections of contaminated methylprednisolone acetate preparations (see Uses: Exserohilum Infections) indicate that the MIC of amphotericin B was 0.032–2 mcg/mL for these strains. However, the clinical relevance of MIC testing for *E. rostratum* remains uncertain, and MIC values indicating susceptibility have not been identified.

While many strains of *Fusarium* are resistant to amphotericin B, some strains of *F. solani*, *F. oxysporum*, and *F. verticillioides* have been inhibited in vitro by amphotericin B concentrations of 2–8 mcg/mL. Some strains of *Scopulariopsis*, including some strains of *S. acremonium* and *S. brevicaulis*, are inhibited in vitro by amphotericin B concentrations of 1–4 mcg/mL; other strains are resistant to the drug.

In one in vitro study, MICs of conventional amphotericin B reported for *B. dermatitidis*, *C. immitis*, *H. capsulatum*, *P. brasiliensis*, *C. albicans*, *C. tropicalis*, *C. parapsilosis*, and *C. neoformans* ranged from 0.125–2 mcg/mL. *C. glabrata* or *A. fumigatus* were inhibited in vitro by conventional amphotericin B concentrations of 1–2 mcg/mL; *A. flavus* was inhibited in vitro by conventional amphotericin B concentrations of 4 mcg/mL. In a study that evaluated the in vitro susceptibility of *C. albicans*, *C. parapsilosis*, *C. tropicalis*, and *C. glabrata* to several different amphotericin B formulations, MICs reported for conventional amphotericin B, amphotericin B lipid complex, or amphotericin B liposomal were 0.1–0.78, 0.2–0.78, or 0.2–6.25 mcg/mL, respectively. When *C. krusei* was tested, the MICs of conventional amphotericin B or amphotericin B lipid complex were 0.78–1.56 or 3.13–6.25 mcg/mL, respectively; however, MICs of amphotericin B liposomal reported for this organism were greater than 50 mcg/mL.

■ **Protozoa** Amphotericin B is active in vitro and in vivo against *Leishmania braziliensis*. The drug also is active in vitro and in vivo against *L. mexicana* and *L. donovani*, including antimony-resistant strains of the organisms. In vitro, amphotericin B concentrations of 1 mcg/mL result in complete elimination of *L. donovani* amastigotes in human monocyte-derived macrophages and *L. donovani* promastigotes in cell-free media. The drug also is active in vitro against *L. tropica*.

Amphotericin B is active in vitro and apparently in vivo against *Naegleria* spp., particularly *N. fowleri*. The drug has variable and limited activity in vitro against *Acanthamoeba castellanii* and *A. polyphaga*.

Resistance

Resistance to amphotericin B has been produced in vitro by serial passage of fungi in the presence of increasing concentrations of the drug, and resistant strains of some fungi (e.g., *Candida*) have been isolated from patients who received long-term therapy with conventional amphotericin B. Amphotericin B-resistant *Candida* are reported relatively infrequently; however, primary resistance to the drug occurs in some strains of *C. lusitaniae* and also occurs in *C. guilliermondii*. Some clinical isolates of *C. auris* have reduced susceptibility or resistance to amphotericin B in vitro (i.e., MIC 2 mcg/mL or greater).

While the clinical importance is unclear, fluconazole-resistant strains of *C. albicans* that were cross-resistant to amphotericin B have been isolated from a few immunocompromised individuals, including leukemia patients and patients with human immunodeficiency virus (HIV) infection. In addition, a few isolates of *Cryptococcus neoformans* resistant to fluconazole also have been resistant to amphotericin B.

Fungi resistant to conventional amphotericin B also may be resistant to amphotericin B lipid complex and amphotericin B liposomal.

Pharmacokinetics

The pharmacokinetics of amphotericin B vary substantially depending on whether the drug is administered as conventional amphotericin B (formulated with sodium desoxycholate), amphotericin B lipid complex, or amphotericin B liposomal, and pharmacokinetic parameters reported for one amphotericin B formulation should not be used to predict the pharmacokinetics of any other amphotericin B formulation.

In general, usual dosages of amphotericin B lipid complex result in lower serum concentrations of amphotericin B and greater volumes of distribution than those reported for the conventional formulation of the drug. Plasma drug concentrations attained after administration of amphotericin B liposomal generally are higher and the volume of distribution is lower than those reported for similar doses of conventional amphotericin B. The clinical importance of differences in pharmacokinetics of the various amphotericin B formulations has not been elucidated, and interpretation of serum or tissue concentrations of amphotericin B reported in published studies is complicated by the fact that many assays used to measure the drug do not differentiate between free amphotericin B and amphotericin B that is lipid-complexed, liposome-encapsulated, or protein-bound. It has been suggested that differences in the distribution and clearance of amphotericin B following administration of lipid-complexed or liposomal-encapsulated formulations relative to those reported following administration of conventional amphotericin B (i.e., increased uptake by the liver and spleen and decreased kidney concentrations) are one of several factors that may contribute to the improved toxicity profiles reported for these formulations; however, how these pharmacokinetic differences affect the therapeutic efficacy of the various formulations is unclear. The manufacturers' literature and specialized references should be consulted for information regarding the absorption, distribution, or elimination of amphotericin B administered as amphotericin B lipid complex or amphotericin B liposomal.

■ **Absorption** After an initial IV infusion of 1–5 mg of amphotericin B daily, with dosage gradually increased to 0.4–0.6 mg/kg daily, plasma concentrations ranging from approximately 0.5–2 mcg/mL were reported. Following a rapid initial decrease, plasma concentrations plateau at about 0.5 mcg/mL.

In one study, immediately after completion of IV infusion of 30 mg of amphotericin B (administered as conventional amphotericin B over a period of several hours), average peak serum concentrations were about 1 mcg/mL; when the dose was 50 mg, average peak serum concentrations were approximately 2 mcg/mL. Immediately after infusion, no more than 10% of the amphotericin B dose can be accounted for in serum. Average minimum serum concentrations (recorded just prior to the next drug infusion) of approximately 0.4 mcg/mL have been reported when 30-mg doses of conventional amphotericin B were given once daily or 60-mg doses were given every other day.

■ **Distribution** Information on the distribution of amphotericin B is limited.

The volume of distribution of the drug following administration of conventional amphotericin B has been reported to be 4 L/kg.

Amphotericin B concentrations attained in inflamed pleura, peritoneum, synovium, and aqueous humor following IV administration of conventional amphotericin B reportedly are about 60% of concurrent plasma concentrations. Penetration into vitreous humor is low.

Following IV administration of conventional amphotericin B, CSF concentrations of the drug rarely exceed 2.5% of concurrent serum concentrations. To achieve fungistatic CSF concentrations, the drug must usually be administered intrathecally†. In patients with meningitis, intrathecal† administration of 0.2–0.3 mg of conventional amphotericin B via a subcutaneous reservoir has produced peak CSF concentrations of 0.5–0.8 mcg/mL; 24 hours after the dose, CSF concentrations were 0.11–0.29 mcg/mL. Amphotericin B is removed from the CSF by arachnoid villi and appears to be stored in the extracellular compartment of the brain, which may act as a reservoir for the drug.

Low concentrations of amphotericin B are attained in amniotic fluid.

It is not known whether amphotericin B is distributed into milk.

Amphotericin B is more than 90% bound to plasma proteins.

■ **Elimination** The metabolic fate of amphotericin B in humans has not been fully elucidated.

Following IV administration of conventional amphotericin B in patients whose renal function is normal prior to therapy, the initial plasma half-life is approximately 24 hours. After the first 24 hours, the rate at which amphotericin B is eliminated decreases and an elimination half-life of approximately 15 days has been reported.

Conventional amphotericin B is eliminated very slowly (over weeks to months) by the kidneys; slow release of the drug from the peripheral compartment may account for the long elimination half-life. Over a 7-day period, the cumulative urinary excretion of a single dose of conventional amphotericin B is about 40% of the administered drug. It has been estimated that only about 2–5% of a total dose of amphotericin B is excreted in urine unchanged. When conventional IV amphotericin B therapy is discontinued, the drug can be detected in blood for up to 4 weeks and in urine for up to 4–8 weeks.

Amphotericin B is not hemodialyzable.

Chemistry and Stability

■ **Chemistry** Amphotericin B is an antifungal antibiotic produced by *Streptomyces nodosus*. The drug is an amphoteric polyene macrolide which occurs as a yellow to orange, odorless or practically odorless powder and is insoluble in water and in anhydrous alcohol. Each mg of amphotericin B contains not less than 750 mcg of anhydrous drug, and amphotericin A (a contaminant of amphotericin B) may be present in a concentration of not more than 5%. Because amphotericin B is amphoteric, it can form salts in acidic or basic media. Although the salts are more water soluble, they have less antifungal activity.

Various amphotericin B preparations are commercially available for parenteral administration. Amphotericin B formulated with sodium desoxycholate (conventional amphotericin B) was the first parenteral amphotericin B preparation to become commercially available. Because conventional amphotericin B is associated with certain dose-limiting toxicities (principally nephrotoxicity), various other formulations have been investigated with the goal of increasing the tolerability of amphotericin B without compromising the antifungal effects of the drug. As a result, amphotericin B now also is commercially available as amphotericin B lipid complex and amphotericin B liposomal. These formulations contain novel lipid-based drug delivery systems that may affect the pharmacokinetics and functional properties of amphotericin B and improve the toxicity profile of the drug.

Conventional Amphotericin B Conventional amphotericin B for injection contains amphotericin B and sodium desoxycholate. Amphotericin B is insoluble in water; presence of sodium desoxycholate in the formulation solubilizes amphotericin B during reconstitution with sterile water providing a colloidal dispersion of the drug. Commercially available conventional amphotericin B occurs as a sterile, yellow to orange lyophilized cake which may partially reduce to powder following manufacture. Each vial labeled as containing 50 mg of amphotericin B contains 41 mg of sodium desoxycholate and is buffered with 20.2 mg of sodium phosphates; at the time of manufacture, air in the vial is replaced with nitrogen.

Extemporaneous lipid emulsions of conventional IV amphotericin B have been prepared by diluting the drug in 20% fat emulsion (Intralipid®) in an attempt to provide a vehicle for amphotericin B that would decrease the nephrotoxicity of the drug; however, because of limited information on the safety and efficacy of these admixtures, lack of standardization, and the commercial availability of lipid formulations of amphotericin B, these extemporaneous lipid emulsions are not recommended.

Amphotericin B Lipid Complex Amphotericin B lipid complex (ABLC; Abelcet®) consists of a 1:1 molar ratio of amphotericin B complexed to a phospholipid vehicle composed of a 7:3 molar ratio of L-α-dimyristoylphosphatidylcholine (DMPC) to L-α-dimyristoylphosphatidylglycerol (DMPG). The amphotericin B-phospholipid complex has a microscopic, ribbon-like structure with a diameter of about 2–11 μm. Each mL of commercially available amphotericin B lipid complex suspension contains 5 mg of amphotericin B, 3.4 mg of DMPC, 1.5 mg of DMPG, and 9 mg of sodium chloride. The suspension occurs as a yellow, opaque liquid with a pH of 5–7.

Amphotericin B Liposomal Commercially available amphotericin B liposomal (L-AmB; AmBisome®) is a lyophilized powder containing amphotericin B intercalated into a unilamellar bilayer liposomal membrane. Liposomes are microscopic vesicles composed of a phospholipid bilayer capable of encapsulating drugs; the lipid bilayer separates the internal aqueous core from the external environment. The liposomal membranes used in commercially available amphotericin B liposomal have a diameter of less than 100 nm and consist of hydrogenated soy phosphatidylcholine (HSPC), cholesterol, distearoylphosphatidylglycerol, and alpha tocopherol. Commercially available amphotericin B liposomal also contains sucrose for isotonicity and disodium succinate hexahydrate as a buffer. Because of the amphophilic substances used in the membrane and the lipophilic nature of amphotericin B, the drug is an integral part of the overall structure of the liposomes. Reconstitution of commercially available amphotericin B liposomal with sterile water for injection results in a yellow, translucent suspension with a pH of 5–6.

■ **Stability** ***Conventional Amphotericin B*** Conventional amphotericin B powder for injection should be stored at 2–8°C and protected from light.

Following reconstitution with sterile water for injection, colloidal solutions of conventional amphotericin B containing 5 mg/mL should be protected from light and are stable for 24 hours at room temperature or 1 week when refrigerated.

Reconstituted colloidal solutions of conventional amphotericin B must be diluted *only* with 5% dextrose in water having a pH greater than 4.2 since the colloidal particles of the drug tend to coagulate quickly at pH less than 5. (See Reconstitution and Administration: Conventional Amphotericin B, in Dosage and Administration.) IV solutions of the drug containing 0.1 mg/mL or less should be used promptly after dilution. Although the manufacturers state that IV infusions of amphotericin B should be protected from light during administration, potency is unaffected if reconstituted dispersions or IV infusions of the drug are exposed to light for less than 8–24 hours.

Dilutions of amphotericin B apparently are compatible with limited amounts of heparin sodium and hydrocortisone sodium succinate or methylprednisolone sodium succinate. Specialized references should be consulted for specific compatibility information.

Amphotericin B Lipid Complex Commercially available amphotericin B lipid complex (Abelcet®) suspension for IV infusion should be refrigerated at 2–8°C and protected from light. Following dilution in 5% dextrose injection, amphotericin B lipid complex is stable for up to 48 hours at 2–8°C and for an additional 6 hours at room temperature. Amphotericin B lipid complex suspension and dilutions of the drug should not be frozen; any unused solutions of the drug should be discarded.

Amphotericin B Liposomal Commercially available lyophilized amphotericin B liposomal (AmBisome®) should be stored at 25°C or lower. Following reconstitution with sterile water for injection, liposomal amphotericin B solutions containing 4 mg/mL may be stored for up to 24 hours at 2–8°C and should not be frozen. IV infusions of amphotericin B liposomal should be initiated within 6 hours after dilution in 5% dextrose injection. Any partially used vials of the drug should be discarded.

Preparations

Excipients in commercially available drug preparations may have clinically important effects in some individuals; consult specific product labeling for details.

Amphotericin B

Parenteral

For injection, for IV infusion	50 mg*	**Amphotericin B for Injection**

*available from one or more manufacturer, distributor, and/or repackager by generic (nonproprietary) name

Amphotericin B Lipid Complex

Parenteral

Injectable suspension concentrate, for IV infusion	5 mg (of amphotericin B) per mL (100 mg)	**Abelcet®**, Sigma Tau

Amphotericin B Liposomal

Parenteral

For injection, for IV infusion	50 mg (of amphotericin B)	**AmBisome®**, Astellas (also promoted by Gilead Sciences)

†Use is not currently included in the labeling approved by the US Food and Drug Administration

Selected Revisions October 2017,

PYRIMIDINES 8:14.32

Flucytosine

5-Fluorocytosine

■ Flucytosine, a fluorinated pyrimidine analog, is a synthetic antifungal agent.

Uses

Flucytosine is used for the treatment of serious infections caused by susceptible *Candida* or *Cryptococcus neoformans*.

Flucytosine usually is used as an adjunct to IV amphotericin B, and should *not* be used alone in the treatment of systemic candidiasis and cryptococcosis. Use of flucytosine alone may be ineffective and may result in emergence of flucytosine resistance. Although concomitant use of flucytosine and amphotericin B is based on reported in vitro and in vivo synergistic effects, there is some evidence that combined use of the drugs may be associated with an increased risk of serious adverse effects, especially in immunocompromised patients such as those with human immunodeficiency virus (HIV) infection.

To optimize efficacy and reduce the risk of toxicity when flucytosine is used concomitantly with another antifungal, flucytosine dosage should be carefully adjusted based on serum concentrations of the drug and patients receiving such therapy should be monitored closely for adverse effects. (See Dosage and Administration: Dosage.) In addition, because of concerns related to intrinsic resistance or emergence of resistance to flucytosine, it has been recommended that in vitro susceptibility tests be performed prior to and during flucytosine therapy, whenever available.

■ **Candida Infections** Oral flucytosine is used in conjunction with IV amphotericin B for the treatment of serious *Candida* infections, including urinary tract or pulmonary infections, candidemia, endocarditis, meningitis, and endophthalmitis.

For the treatment of CNS candidiasis in adults, the Infectious Diseases Society of America (IDSA) recommends initial treatment with IV amphotericin B (with or without oral flucytosine) followed by step-down treatment with fluconazole.

For initial treatment of CNS candidiasis in neonates, IDSA and the American Academy of Pediatrics (AAP) recommend monotherapy with IV amphotericin B. Although oral flucytosine has been used in conjunction with IV amphotericin B for the treatment of severe invasive candidiasis, including CNS candidiasis, in pediatric patients†, this combination regimen is not usually recommended for the treatment of candidiasis in children, including HIV-infected children. AAP and other clinicians state that routine use of flucytosine for the treatment of meningitis in neonates† is not recommended because of concerns regarding toxicity. IDSA states that salvage therapy with a regimen of flucytosine and amphotericin B should be considered in neonates† *only* if there is no response to amphotericin B alone.

For the treatment of endocarditis (native or prosthetic valve) or implantable cardiac device infections caused by *Candida*, IDSA recommends initial treatment with a lipid formulation of IV amphotericin B (with or without oral flucytosine) or an IV echinocandin (anidulafungin, caspofungin, micafungin) followed by step-down treatment with fluconazole.

Oral flucytosine is used alone or in conjunction with IV amphotericin B for the treatment of certain urinary tract infections caused by *Candida*, especially fluconazole-resistant strains. IDSA states that antifungal treatment is not usually indicated in patients with asymptomatic cystitis, unless there is a high risk of disseminated candidiasis (e.g., neutropenic patients, low-birthweight infants [less than 1.5 kg], patients undergoing urologic manipulations). Fluconazole is the drug of choice for the treatment of symptomatic cystitis, pyelonephritis, or fungus balls likely to be caused by fluconazole-susceptible *Candida*. When fluconazole-resistant *C. glabrata* are likely, IV amphotericin B or oral flucytosine is recommended for symptomatic cystitis and IV amphotericin B (with or without oral flucytosine) or oral flucytosine alone is recommended for pyelonephritis.

For the treatment of endophthalmitis caused by fluconazole- and voriconazole-resistant *Candida*, IDSA states that IV amphotericin B liposomal (with or without oral flucytosine) is the regimen of choice. In patients with macular involvement, intravitreal administration of conventional amphotericin B also is recommended to ensure prompt high intraocular levels of antifungal activity. Decisions regarding antifungal treatment and surgical intervention should be made jointly by an ophthalmologist and an infectious disease clinician.

■ **Cryptococcosis** Oral flucytosine usually is used in conjunction with IV amphotericin B for the treatment of serious cryptococcal infections, including pulmonary infections, septicemia, and meningitis caused by *C. neoformans*. Concomitant use of amphotericin B and flucytosine for initial treatment of cryptococcosis appears to reduce the time required for sterilization of CSF in those with CNS involvement and may decrease the risk of subsequent relapse and improve survival. Oral flucytosine also has been used in conjunction with fluconazole for the treatment of cryptococcal meningitis in HIV-infected individuals. Flucytosine should *not* be used alone for the treatment of cryptococcosis.

For the treatment of cryptococcal meningitis in HIV-infected adults, adolescents, and children, the US Centers for Disease Control and Prevention (CDC), National Institutes of Health (NIH), IDSA, and other clinicians state that the preferred regimen is initial (induction) therapy with IV amphotericin B (liposomal or conventional formulation) given in conjunction with oral flucytosine for at least 2 weeks until there is evidence of clinical improvement and negative CSF cultures after repeat lumbar puncture, then follow-up (consolidation) therapy with oral or IV fluconazole given for at least 8 weeks, followed by long-term suppressive or maintenance therapy (secondary prophylaxis) with oral fluconazole to complete at least 1 year of azole therapy.

One alternative regimen for initial (induction) treatment of cryptococcal meningitis in HIV-infected adults, adolescents, and children who cannot receive the preferred regimen is oral or IV fluconazole used in conjunction with oral flucytosine. Alternative regimens may be less effective and are recommended only in patients who cannot tolerate or have not responded to the preferred regimen.

Although data are limited, CDC, NIH, and IDSA state that recommendations for the treatment of CNS, pulmonary, or disseminated infections caused by *C. gattii* and recommendations for long-term suppressive or maintenance therapy (secondary prophylaxis) of *C. gattii* infections are the same as the recommendations for *C. neoformans* infections. IDSA states that single, small cryptococcoma may be treated with oral fluconazole, but induction therapy with a regimen of IV amphotericin B and oral flucytosine given for 4–6 weeks, followed by consolidation therapy with fluconazole given for 6–18 months should be considered for very large or multiple cryptococcomas caused by *C. gattii*. Regimens that include IV amphotericin B (conventional or liposomal formulations), flucytosine, and fluconazole have been effective in a few patients with CNS infections known to be caused by *C. gattii*.

■ **Chromoblastomycosis** Oral flucytosine has been used alone or in conjunction with other antifungals for the treatment of chromoblastomycosis† (chromomycosis) caused by various dematiaceous fungi (e.g., *Cladosporium, Exophiala, Phialophora*). Optimum treatment of chromoblastomycosis has not been identified. Azole antifungals (usually itraconazole) or terbinafine have been effective and may be the preferred antifungals for the treatment of chromoblastomycosis; surgery and/or adjunctive use of other therapies (e.g., heat therapy, laser therapy, photodynamic therapy) may be indicated.

A regimen of itraconazole and flucytosine has been effective for the treatment of chromoblastomycosis in some patients and a regimen of posaconazole and flucytosine has been suggested as a possible alternative in refractory cases. Although amphotericin B has been used in conjunction with flucytosine for the treatment of chromoblastomycosis, this regimen is no longer recommended for such infections.

■ **Aspergillosis** Oral flucytosine has been used concomitantly with IV amphotericin B for the treatment of invasive aspergillosis† or other infections caused by *Aspergillus* (e.g., osteomyelitis and joint infections); however, it is unclear whether concomitant use of amphotericin B and flucytosine offers any benefit over use of amphotericin B alone for the treatment of invasive aspergillosis and there are concerns related to a possible increased incidence of adverse effects with concomitant therapy.

Voriconazole is considered the drug of choice for initial treatment of invasive aspergillosis in most patients and IV amphotericin B (a lipid formulation) is the preferred alternative.

■ **Free-living Ameba Infections** Flucytosine has been used in conjunction with other anti-infectives in a few patients for the treatment of free-living ameba infections†, including granulomatous amebic encephalitis or other infections caused by *Acanthamoeba*† or *Balamuthia mandrillaris*†.

CNS infections caused by free-living ameba have a high mortality rate, and only a very limited number of cases have been successfully treated. Early diagnosis and treatment with a multiple-drug regimen may increase the chance of survival. Although data are limited, most reported cases of *Acanthamoeba* and *B. mandrillaris* infection have been treated empirically with regimens that included a variety of anti-infectives (e.g., albendazole, amphotericin B, azole antifungals [fluconazole, itraconazole, ketoconazole], flucytosine, macrolides [azithromycin or clarithromycin], miltefosine, rifampin, pentamidine, sulfonamides [co-trimoxazole or sulfadiazine]).

For assistance with diagnosis or treatment of suspected free-living ameba infections, clinicians can contact the CDC Emergency Operations Center at 770-488-7100.

Dosage and Administration

■ Administration Flucytosine is administered orally. The manufacturer suggests that nausea and vomiting associated with oral flucytosine may be reduced or avoided if each dose is administered by ingesting the capsules a few at a time over a 15-minute period.

Flucytosine has been administered IV; however, a parenteral dosage form of the drug is not commercially available in the US. Flucytosine also has been administered topically as a cream, but topical preparations of the drug are not commercially available in the US.

For patients unable to swallow capsules, flucytosine oral suspensions containing 10 or 50 mg/mL have been prepared extemporaneously using the commercially available capsules of the drug.

■ Dosage Because prolonged serum flucytosine concentrations exceeding 100 mcg/mL may be associated with an increased risk of toxicity (e.g., adverse hematologic, GI, and hepatic effects), flucytosine dosage usually should be adjusted to ensure that peak serum concentrations of the drug remain below 100 mcg/mL. However, optimal target serum concentrations have not been identified, and a variety of target ranges have been recommended. The American Academy of Pediatrics (AAP), US Centers for Disease Control and Prevention (CDC), National Institutes of Health (NIH), Infectious Diseases Society of America (IDSA), and others generally recommend target serum flucytosine concentrations of 30–80 mcg/mL.

Some clinicians suggest that serum flucytosine concentrations should be measured beginning 3–5 days after initiation of the drug (or beginning after 3–5 doses) and then once or twice weekly during treatment and whenever there is evidence of toxicity or a change in renal function. Peak serum concentrations usually are measured using blood samples taken 2 hours after an oral dose.

Adult Dosage **General Adult Dosage.** The usual adult dosage of oral flucytosine recommended by the manufacturer is 50–150 mg/kg daily given in divided doses at 6-hour intervals. The manufacturer recommends that the lower dosage be used initially in patients with elevated BUN or serum creatinine concentrations.

To reduce the risk of toxicity in patients receiving flucytosine concomitantly with IV amphotericin B, some clinicians suggest that flucytosine therapy be initiated using a low dosage (i.e., 75 mg/kg daily given in 4 divided doses). Dosage can then be adjusted based on serum concentrations of flucytosine and the presence or absence of amphotericin B-associated renal toxicity.

Candida Infections. When used alone or in conjunction with IV amphotericin B for the treatment of *Candida* infections, IDSA recommends that oral flucytosine be given in a dosage of 25 mg/kg 4 times daily.

For the treatment of CNS candidiasis, IDSA recommends that flucytosine be given in a dosage of 25 mg/kg 4 times daily in conjunction with IV amphotericin B. After several weeks of concomitant therapy and when a response is attained, treatment can be transitioned to fluconazole step-down therapy. Antifungal treatment should be continued until all signs and symptoms, CSF abnormalities, and radiologic abnormalities resolve.

For the treatment of endocarditis (native or prosthetic valve) or implantable cardiac device infections caused by *Candida*, IDSA recommends that flucytosine be given in a dosage of 25 mg/kg 4 times daily in conjunction with IV amphotericin B. If the infection is caused by fluconazole-susceptible strains, treatment can be transitioned to fluconazole step-down therapy after the patient is clinically stable and *Candida* have been cleared from the bloodstream.

If flucytosine is used as an alternative for the treatment of symptomatic cystitis caused by fluconazole-resistant *C. glabrata*, IDSA recommends that the drug be given in a dosage of 25 mg/kg 4 times daily for 7–10 days.

For the treatment of pyelonephritis caused by fluconazole-resistant *C. glabrata*, IDSA recommends that flucytosine be given in a dosage of 25 mg/kg 4 times daily in conjunction with IV amphotericin B for up to 7 days. Alternatively, if flucytosine monotherapy is used, a dosage of 25 mg/kg 4 times daily for 2 weeks is recommended. These same regimens can be used for the treatment of *Candida* urinary tract infections associated with fungus balls.

For the treatment of *Candida* endophthalmitis caused by fluconazole- and voriconazole-resistant *Candida*, flucytosine should be given in a dosage of 25 mg/kg 4 times daily in conjunction with IV amphotericin B liposomal. The duration of treatment should be at least 4–6 weeks as determined by repeated examinations to verify resolution.

Cryptococcosis. When flucytosine is used in conjunction with another antifungal (e.g., IV amphotericin B, fluconazole) for the treatment of severe cryptococcal infections, a dosage of 100–150 mg/kg daily is recommended.

For the treatment of cryptococcal meningitis in HIV-infected adults and adolescents, CDC, NIH, and IDSA recommend a regimen than includes initial (induction) therapy with oral flucytosine in a dosage of 25 mg/kg 4 times daily in conjunction with IV amphotericin B (liposomal or conventional formulation) given for at least 2 weeks until there is evidence of clinical improvement and negative CSF cultures after repeat lumbar puncture, then follow-up (consolidation) therapy with oral or IV fluconazole alone.

As an alternative for the treatment of cryptococcal meningitis in HIV-infected adults and adolescents who cannot receive amphotericin B, CDC, NIH, and IDSA recommend initial (induction) therapy with oral flucytosine in a dosage of 25 mg/kg 4 times daily in conjunction with oral or IV fluconazole.

Free-living Ameba Infections. If flucytosine is used in conjunction with other anti-infectives for the treatment of free-living ameba infections†, including granulomatous amebic encephalitis or other infections caused by *Acanthamoeba*† or *Balamuthia mandrillaris*† (see Uses: Free-living Ameba Infections), some clinicians recommend a dosage of 37.5 mg/kg every 6 hours (up to 150 mg/kg daily). Higher dosage has been used in some patients.

Pediatric Dosage **General Pediatric Dosage.** If flucytosine is used in pediatric patients†, AAP recommends a dosage of 100 mg/kg daily given in divided doses every 6 hours.

Candidiasis. For salvage therapy of CNS candidiasis in neonates† who have not responded to initial treatment with IV amphotericin B alone, IDSA states that oral flucytosine can be given in a dosage of 25 mg/kg 4 times daily in conjunction with IV amphotericin B. After several weeks and when a response is attained, transition to fluconazole step-down therapy is recommended. Antifungal treatment should be continued until all signs, symptoms, CSF abnormalities, and radiologic abnormalities (if present) have resolved.

Cryptococcosis. For the treatment of CNS or disseminated cryptococcosis in children†, IDSA recommends an initial (induction) regimen of oral flucytosine given in a dosage of 100 mg/kg daily in 4 divided doses in conjunction with IV amphotericin B given for at least 2 weeks, then follow-up (consolidation) therapy with oral fluconazole alone for at least 8 weeks.

For the treatment of cryptococcal meningitis in HIV-infected infants and children†, CDC, NIH, IDSA, and other clinicians recommend a regimen than includes initial (induction) therapy with oral flucytosine in a dosage of 25 mg/kg 4 times daily in conjunction with IV amphotericin B given for at least 2 weeks until there is evidence of clinical improvement and negative CSF cultures after repeat lumbar puncture, then follow-up (consolidation) therapy with oral or IV fluconazole alone.

For the treatment of cryptococcal meningitis in HIV-infected infants and children† who cannot receive amphotericin B, CDC, NIH, IDSA, and other clinicians recommend initial (induction) therapy with oral flucytosine in a dosage of 25 mg/kg 4 times daily in conjunction with oral or IV fluconazole.

For the treatment of severe pulmonary or disseminated (non-CNS) cryptococcosis in HIV-infected infants and children†, CDC, NIH, IDSA, and other clinicians recommend that flucytosine be given in a dosage of 25 mg/kg 4 times daily in conjunction with IV amphotericin B. Treatment duration depends on the response and site and severity of infection.

■ Dosage in Renal Impairment In patients with impaired renal function, doses and/or frequency of administration of flucytosine must be modified in response to the degree of impairment and serum concentrations of the drug. Several methods of calculating flucytosine dosage for patients with impaired renal function have been proposed; however, for greater accuracy, dosage in these patients should be based on actual serum concentrations of the drug. Precise dosing is limited, since flucytosine is commercially available only as 250- and 500-mg capsules.

Some clinicians recommend that adults with creatinine clearances of 20–40 mL/minute receive 25 mg/kg of flucytosine every 12 hours and that those with creatinine clearances of 10–20 mL/minute receive 25 mg/kg once daily. In those with creatinine clearances less than 10 mL/minute, these clinicians recommend a flucytosine dosage of 25 mg/kg once every 48 hours.

Other clinicians recommend that the usual individual dose of flucytosine (12.5–37.5 mg/kg) be administered every 12 hours in patients with creatinine clearances of 20–40 mL/minute, every 24 hours in those with creatinine clearances of 10–20 mL/minute, and every 24–48 hours or longer (as determined by serum drug concentrations) in those with creatinine clearances less than 10 mL/minute. Alternatively, other clinicians have recommended that flucytosine doses of 12–35 mg/kg be administered at intervals equal to twice the half-life of the drug.

In patients undergoing hemodialysis, some clinicians recommend that flucytosine doses of 20–50 mg/kg be given once every 48–72 hours and that the doses be administered after dialysis.

Cautions

■ Hematologic Effects The most frequent adverse effects of flucytosine therapy appear to be related to the drug's effect on rapidly proliferating tissues, particularly the bone marrow. Anemia, leukopenia, pancytopenia, thrombocytopenia, eosinophilia, agranulocytosis, and aplastic anemia have been reported in patients receiving flucytosine.

Fatal bone marrow aplasia has been reported in some patients receiving flucytosine. Bone marrow toxicity can be irreversible and may lead to death in immunosuppressed patients.

The risk of bone marrow toxicity appears to be increased in patients who have hematologic disease and in those who are receiving or previously received radiation or drug therapy that depresses the bone marrow. The risk of adverse hematologic effects also may be increased in patients who have prolonged, high serum flucytosine concentrations (i.e., greater than 100 mcg/mL), particularly in those with renal dysfunction or during concomitant therapy with amphotericin B.

■ **GI Effects** Adverse GI effects, which are sometimes severe, have been reported in patients receiving flucytosine and have included anorexia, abdominal bloating, abdominal pain, diarrhea, dry mouth, duodenal ulcer, GI hemorrhage, nausea, vomiting, ulcerative colitis, and enterocolitis.

■ **Hepatic Effects** Increased hepatic enzyme concentrations (serum alkaline phosphatase, AST [SGOT], ALT [SGPT]) and increased serum bilirubin concentrations have been reported in patients receiving flucytosine. Hepatic dysfunction and jaundice have been reported.

Increased serum hepatic enzyme concentrations generally appear to be dose related and reversible. However, acute hepatic injury with possible fatal outcome has been reported in debilitated patients receiving flucytosine. In one patient, abnormal lactic dehydrogenase concentrations and sulfobromophthalein retention were attributed to hepatic necrosis, possibly resulting from flucytosine therapy.

■ **Renal Effects** Increased concentrations of BUN and serum creatinine have been reported in patients receiving flucytosine. Azotemia, crystalluria, and renal failure also have been reported.

■ **Nervous System Effects** Adverse nervous system effects that have been reported with flucytosine include ataxia, hearing loss, headache, paresthesia, parkinsonism, seizures, peripheral neuropathy, vertigo, and sedation. Confusion, hallucinations, and psychosis also have been reported.

An acute cerebellar syndrome with dysmetria and ataxia occurred in a patient receiving flucytosine concomitantly with amphotericin B. The syndrome resolved over the next 4 weeks following discontinuance of flucytosine, although mild dysmetria persisted.

■ **Dermatologic and Sensitivity Reactions** Rash, pruritus, urticaria, and photosensitivity have been reported with flucytosine. Allergic reactions and toxic epidermal necrolysis (Lyell syndrome) also have been reported.

Anaphylaxis, manifested as diffuse erythema, pruritus, conjunctival injection, fever, abdominal pain, edema, tachycardia, and hypotension, has been reported in at least one patient with acquired immunodeficiency syndrome (AIDS) receiving flucytosine therapy. Anaphylaxis recurred following rechallenge with the drug.

■ **Other Adverse Effects** Other adverse effects that have been reported with flucytosine include fatigue, pyrexia, hypoglycemia, hypokalemia, weakness, cardiac arrest, myocardial toxicity, ventricular dysfunction, chest pain, dyspnea, and respiratory arrest.

■ **Precautions and Contraindications** Flucytosine is contraindicated in patients hypersensitive to the drug.

Flucytosine should be used with extreme caution in patients with bone marrow depression and in patients with impaired renal function. Flucytosine is eliminated mainly by the kidneys and renal impairment may lead to accumulation of the drug and increase the risk of toxicity. Dosage of the drug should be adjusted in patients with renal impairment to prevent accumulation of the drug. (See Dosage and Administration: Dosage in Renal Impairment.)

Hematologic, renal, and hepatic status must be monitored closely during flucytosine therapy. Hematologic status (leucocyte and thrombocyte counts), renal function, hepatic function (serum alkaline phosphatase, AST, ALT), and electrolytes should be evaluated prior to initiation of flucytosine and at frequent intervals during therapy with the drug.

Because serum flucytosine concentrations exceeding 100 mcg/mL may be associated with an increased incidence of toxicity, especially GI effects (diarrhea, nausea, vomiting), hematologic effects (leukopenia, thrombocytopenia), and hepatic effects (hepatitis), flucytosine serum concentrations should be monitored and dosage adjusted to ensure that serum concentrations of the drug remain below 100 mcg/mL. (See Dosage and Administration: Dosage.)

■ **Pediatric Precautions** Safety and efficacy of flucytosine have not been systematically studied in children.

If flucytosine is used in neonates and infants†, serum concentrations of the drug should be closely monitored. Limited data regarding the pharmacokinetics of flucytosine in neonates indicate considerable interindividual variation in plasma concentrations attained, which does not correlate with gestational age. High plasma concentrations of the drug may accumulate in very low-birth-weight infants because of immature renal function.

Some clinicians state that flucytosine should be avoided in children† with severe renal impairment.

The manufacturer states that no unexpected adverse effects were reported when flucytosine was given to some neonates† in a dosage of 25–200 mg/kg daily (with or without concomitant amphotericin B). Hypokalemia and acidemia occurred in one neonate receiving flucytosine and amphotericin B concomitantly, and anemia was reported in another who received flucytosine monotherapy. Transient thrombocytopenia also has been reported in pediatric patients receiving flucytosine (with or without amphotericin B).

■ **Geriatric Precautions** Flucytosine dosage adjustment may be required in geriatric patients based on renal function. (See Dosage and Administration: Dosage in Renal Impairment.)

■ **Mutagenicity and Carcinogenicity** Flucytosine was not mutagenic in various in vitro studies using microbial (e.g., *Salmonella typhimurium*) test systems in the presence or absence of activating enzymes. In addition, there was no evidence of mutagenicity in repair assay systems.

The carcinogenic potential of flucytosine has not been adequately studied to date.

■ **Pregnancy, Fertility, and Lactation** ***Pregnancy*** Flucytosine was shown to be teratogenic in rats. When flucytosine was given to rats in a dosage of 40 mg/kg daily (0.051 times the human dosage) on days 7–13 of gestation, vertebral fusions occurred; at a dosage of 700 mg/kg daily (0.89 times the human dosage) on days 9–12 of gestation, cleft lip and palate and micrognathia were reported. In mice, flucytosine dosage of 400 mg/kg daily (0.236 times the human dosage) on days 7–13 of gestation was associated with a low incidence of cleft palate that was not statistically significant. Flucytosine was not teratogenic in rabbits when given in dosages up to 100 mg/kg daily (0.243 times the human dosage) on days 6–18 of gestation.

There are no adequate or controlled studies to date using flucytosine in pregnant women, and the drug should be used during pregnancy only when potential benefits justify possible risks to the fetus.

Fertility The effects of flucytosine on fertility or reproductive performance have not been adequately studied in animals.

Lactation It is not known whether flucytosine is distributed into human milk.

Because many drugs are distributed into human milk and because of the potential for serious adverse effects in nursing infants, a decision should be made whether to discontinue nursing or the drug, taking into account the importance of the drug to the mother.

Drug Interactions

■ **Drugs that Affect Renal Function** Because flucytosine is principally excreted by glomerular filtration, concomitant use of drugs that impair glomerular filtration may prolong the elimination half-life of flucytosine and increase the risk of toxicity. Flucytosine serum concentrations should be closely monitored if drugs that reduce glomerular filtration are used concomitantly.

■ **Myelosuppressive Agents** The risk of bone marrow toxicity may be increased if flucytosine is used concomitantly with other agents that depress the bone marrow. Because of potential additive effects on bone marrow, caution is advised if flucytosine is used concomitantly with other myelosuppressive drugs (e.g., zidovudine).

■ **Antifungal Agents** ***Amphotericin B*** In some in vitro studies, the combination of flucytosine and amphotericin B resulted in synergistic inhibition of *Cryptococcus neoformans*, *Candida albicans*, and *C. tropicalis*. The suggested mechanism of this synergism is that the binding of amphotericin B to sterols in cell membranes increases the permeability of the cytoplasmic membrane, thus allowing greater penetration of flucytosine into the fungal cell. However, in a study evaluating the antifungal effects of the drugs in the presence of serum, the combination of amphotericin B and flucytosine was not additive or synergistic against *C. albicans*.

There is some evidence that concomitant use of amphotericin B and flucytosine may increase the toxicity of flucytosine, possibly by increasing cellular uptake and/or by decreasing renal excretion of the drug.

If flucytosine is used in conjunction with amphotericin B, especially in patients with human immunodeficiency virus (HIV) infection, some clinicians suggest using a low initial dosage of flucytosine. In addition, serum flucytosine concentrations and blood cell counts should be carefully monitored and flucytosine dosage adjusted if needed. (See Dosage and Administration: Dosage.)

Azole Antifungal Agents The combination of flucytosine and fluconazole or itraconazole was synergistic, additive, or indifferent in vitro against *C. neoformans*; there was no evidence of antagonism. The combination of fluconazole and flucytosine generally did not exert a synergistic effect against *C. neoformans* isolates that had fluconazole MICs of 8 mcg/mL or greater. Synergism also has been demonstrated when the combination of fluconazole and flucytosine was evaluated in vivo in a murine model of cryptococcal meningitis. It has been suggested that synergism between the drugs may occur because fluconazole damages the fungal cell membrane allowing greater intracellular penetration of flucytosine.

■ **Cytarabine** Cytarabine (cytosine arabinoside) reportedly antagonizes the antifungal activity of flucytosine, possibly by competitive inhibition. Concomitant use of cytarabine and flucytosine is not recommended.

Laboratory Test Interferences

■ **Tests for Creatinine** There have been reports that flucytosine can cause markedly false elevations in serum creatinine values when certain test methods are used. Because flucytosine does not affect serum creatinine values when the Jaffé reaction or other alkaline picrate methods are used, such methods should be used to evaluate serum creatinine concentrations in patients receiving flucytosine.

Acute Toxicity

Limited information is available on the acute toxicity of flucytosine. Although there have been no reports to date of intentional overdosage of flucytosine, overdosage would be expected to produce pronounced manifestations of the known adverse effects of the drug. Prolonged serum flucytosine concentrations greater than 100 mcg/mL may be associated with an increased incidence of toxicity, especially GI effects (diarrhea, nausea, vomiting), hematologic effects (leukopenia, thrombocytopenia), and hepatic effects (hepatitis).

In the event of flucytosine overdosage, the manufacturer recommends prompt use of gastric lavage or an emetic. Because flucytosine is eliminated essentially unchanged in urine, adequate fluid intake should be maintained and IV fluids given if necessary. Hematologic parameters should be assessed frequently and liver and kidney function carefully monitored. Appropriate symptomatic therapy should be instituted if indicated. The manufacturer suggests that consideration be given to the use of hemodialysis in the management of flucytosine overdosage since the procedure readily removes the drug in anuric patients.

Mechanism of Action

Flucytosine may be fungistatic or fungicidal in action depending on the concentration of the drug. Two possible mechanisms of action have been identified for flucytosine. Flucytosine appears to enter fungal cells via the action of fungal-specific cytosine permease. Inside the cell, flucytosine is converted to fluorouracil (5-FU) by cytosine deaminase and then after several intermediate steps is converted to 5-fluorouridine triphosphate (FUTP). FUTP is incorporated into fungal RNA and interferes with protein synthesis. Flucytosine also appears to be converted to 5-fluorodeoxyuridine monophosphate, which noncompetitively inhibits thymidylate synthetase and interferes with DNA synthesis. Flucytosine does not appear to have antineoplastic activity.

Spectrum

Flucytosine is active in vitro and in clinical infections against *Candida albicans* and *Cryptococcus neoformans*.

Flucytosine is inactive against *Blastomyces dermatitidis, Coccidioides immitis, Histoplasma capsulatum, Paracoccidioides brasiliensis, Madurella*, dermatophytes (*Microsporum, Trichophyton, Epidermophyton*), and bacteria.

■ **Fungi** Flucytosine is active in vitro against most strains of *C. albicans, C. glabrata, C. guilliermondii, C. parapsilosis*, and *C. tropicalis*. In vitro, susceptible strains of *Candida* generally are inhibited by flucytosine concentrations of 4 mcg/mL or less.

Although some strains of *C. krusei* and *C. lusitaniae* may be susceptible to flucytosine in vitro, other strains are inhibited only by high concentrations of the drug and are considered resistant. Some clinical isolates of *C. auris* (often misidentified as *C. haemulonii, C. famata*, or *Rhodotorula glutinis*) have been susceptible to flucytosine in vitro; however, a wide range of minimum inhibitory concentrations (MICs) has been reported and reduced susceptibility or resistance to flucytosine occurs. *C. kefyr* usually is resistant to flucytosine.

Susceptible strains of *C. neoformans* generally are inhibited in vitro by flucytosine concentrations of 0.03–8 mcg/mL. Flucytosine concentrations of 0.25–2 mcg/mL inhibit some strains of *C. gattii*. However, some strains of *C. neoformans* and *C. gattii* are resistant to flucytosine.

There is some in vitro evidence that flucytosine has activity against some of the causative agents of chromoblastomycosis and phaeohyphomycosis, including some strains of *Cladophialophora, Phialophora verrucosa, Exophiala* (*E. castellanii, E. dermatitidis, E. spinifera*), and *Cladosporium*. Although some strains of *Fonsecaea* have been susceptible to flucytosine in vitro, the drug reportedly has limited or no activity against the organism.

Although *Sporothrix schenckii* usually is resistant to flucytosine, some strains may be inhibited in vitro by flucytosine concentrations of 0.6–2 mcg/mL. Some strains of *Penicillium marneffei* are inhibited in vitro by flucytosine concentrations of 0.002–0.25 mcg/mL.

Aspergillus generally are resistant to flucytosine, but rare strains may be inhibited in vitro by flucytosine concentrations of 4 mcg/mL or less.

Resistance

Resistance to flucytosine can be readily induced in vitro in *Candida* and *Cryptococcus neoformans*. Strains of *Candida* or *Cryptococcus* resistant to flucytosine have been isolated from patients who have never received the drug, and resistant strains of *Candida* and *C. neoformans* have emerged in patients receiving oral flucytosine alone or in conjunction with IV amphotericin B. Resistance to flucytosine can develop during monotherapy with the drug.

Resistance to flucytosine may be related to mutations that affect the production of fungal enzymes (e.g., uridine monophosphate pyrophosphorylase, cytosine permease, cytosine deaminase) important to the mechanism of action of the drug. Resistance also may result from mutations that result in increased production of pyrimidines.

Cross-resistance does not occur between flucytosine and amphotericin B.

Pharmacokinetics

■ **Absorption** Flucytosine is rapidly and almost completed absorbed from the GI tract. Bioavailability is 78–90% following oral administration. Food decreases the rate, but not the extent, of absorption.

In patients with normal renal function, peak serum flucytosine concentrations of 30–40 mcg/mL are reached within 2 hours following a single 2-g oral dose. In other studies in patients with normal renal function receiving a 6-week regimen of oral flucytosine (150 mg/kg daily given in divided doses every 6 hours) and concomitant IV amphotericin B, mean serum concentrations of flucytosine 1–2 hours after a dose were approximately 70–80 mcg/mL.

In a limited number of neonates† receiving oral flucytosine in a dosage of 25, 50, or 100 mg/kg daily for the treatment of systemic candidiasis, median peak serum concentrations after 5 days of treatment were 19.6, 27.7, and 83.9 mcg/mL, respectively, and the mean time to peak concentrations was 2.5 hours. There was considerable interindividual variation in serum concentrations, which did not correlate with gestational age, and some neonates had serum flucytosine concentrations greater than 100 mcg/mL.

Peak serum concentrations of flucytosine are higher, more prolonged, and reached more slowly in patients with impaired renal function. In anephric patients, peak serum concentrations may be 50% higher than those in patients with normal renal function. It has been recommended that steady-state serum flucytosine concentrations should not exceed 100 mcg/mL to avoid toxic effects.

■ **Distribution** Flucytosine is widely distributed into body tissues and fluids including liver, kidney, spleen, heart, bronchial secretions, joints, peritoneal fluid, brain, bile, bone, and aqueous humor.

Flucytosine is distributed into CSF following oral administration, and CSF concentrations may range from 60–100% of serum concentrations of the drug. In an infant† who received a 25-mg oral dose of flucytosine, CSF concentrations of the drug were 43 mcg/mL 3 hours after the dose. In a neonate† receiving oral flucytosine in a dosage of 120–150 mg/kg daily, CSF concentrations ranged from 20–67 mcg/mL.

Studies in pregnant rats indicate that flucytosine administered intraperitoneally crosses the placenta.

It is not known if flucytosine is distributed into milk.

The apparent volume of distribution of flucytosine is about 0.68 L/kg in healthy adults and has ranged from 0.4–0.7 L/kg in patients with renal failure.

In vitro studies indicate that flucytosine is approximately 2.9–4% bound to serum proteins over the range of therapeutic concentrations found in blood.

■ **Elimination** Only minimal amounts of flucytosine are metabolized in humans. The drug is deaminated (probably by gut bacteria) to fluorouracil. The area under the concentration-time curve (AUC) ratio of fluorouracil to flucytosine is 4%.

The elimination half-life of flucytosine in patients with normal renal function has been reported to range from 2.4–4.8. Half-life of the drug is prolonged in patients with renal impairment and has been reported to be 6–14 hours in those with creatinine clearances of 40 mL/minute, 12–15 hours in those with creatinine clearances of 20 mL/minute, 21–27 hours in those with creatinine clearances of 10 mL/minute, and 30–250 hours in those with creatinine clearances less than 10 mL/minute. Half-lives up to 1160 hours have been reported in a few patients with creatinine clearances less than 2 mL/minute. Some clinicians have suggested that the half-life of flucytosine in hours is approximately 5 or 6 times the serum creatinine concentration in mg/dL.

In a limited number of neonates and infants†, the median half-life of flucytosine was 7.4 hours.

Flucytosine is eliminated by the kidneys, principally by glomerular filtration without substantial tubular reabsorption. More than 90% of an oral dose of flucytosine is excreted unchanged in the urine. Urinary concentrations of flucytosine are generally 10–100 times greater than serum concentrations, although urinary drug concentrations are much lower in patients with impaired renal function. In one study, patients with flucytosine serum half-lives of 40–83 hours achieved urinary flucytosine concentrations of 42–500 mcg/mL within 24 hours after a single 2-g oral dose. Unabsorbed flucytosine is excreted unchanged in the feces.

Hepatic impairment does not affect the pharmacokinetics of flucytosine.

Flucytosine is readily removed by peritoneal dialysis and hemodialysis.

Chemistry and Stability

■ **Chemistry** Flucytosine, a synthetic antifungal agent, is a fluorinated pyrimidine analog structurally related to fluorouracil and floxuridine. Flucytosine occurs as a white to off-white, crystalline powder that is odorless or has a slight odor; the drug is sparingly soluble in water and slightly soluble in alcohol. The drug has pK_as of 2.9 and 10.71.

■ **Stability** Flucytosine capsules should be stored at 25°C, but may be exposed to temperatures ranging from 15–30°C.

Preparations

Excipients in commercially available drug preparations may have clinically important effects in some individuals; consult specific product labeling for details.

Flucytosine

Oral		
Capsules	250 mg*	**Ancobon®**, Valeant
		Flucytosine Capsules
	500 mg*	**Ancobon®**, Valeant
		Flucytosine Capsules

*available from one or more manufacturer, distributor, and/or repackager by generic (nonproprietary) name

†Use is not currently included in the labeling approved by the US Food and Drug Administration

ANTIMYCOBACTERIALS 8:16

ANTITUBERCULOSIS AGENTS 8:16.04

Bedaquiline Fumarate

TMC207, R207910

■ Bedaquiline, a diarylquinoline antimycobacterial, is an antituberculosis agent.

Uses

■ **Tuberculosis** ***Active Tuberculosis*** Bedaquiline fumarate is used in conjunction with other antituberculosis agents for the treatment of pulmonary multidrug-resistant tuberculosis (i.e., caused by *Mycobacterium tuberculosis* resistant to isoniazid and rifampin). The drug is designated an orphan drug by the US Food and Drug Administration (FDA) for use in the treatment of active tuberculosis.

The manufacturer states that bedaquiline must be used in conjunction with at least 3 other drugs selected based on results of in vitro susceptibility tests indicating that the patient's *M. tuberculosis* isolate is susceptible. If in vitro susceptibility test results are unavailable, treatment may be initiated using bedaquiline in conjunction with at least 4 other drugs to which the isolate is likely to be susceptible.

The manufacturer and some experts state that bedaquiline should be used *only* when an effective regimen for treatment of multidrug-resistant tuberculosis cannot otherwise be provided. The World Health Organization (WHO) interim guidance for use of bedaquiline suggests that the drug can be added to a WHO-recommended regimen for the treatment of multidrug-resistant tuberculosis in adults when an effective regimen containing 4 second-line drugs in addition to pyrazinamide cannot be designed or when there is documented evidence that the multidrug-resistant strain also is resistant to a fluoroquinolone. These experts state that bedaquiline should not be added alone as a single new drug to a failing regimen.

Safety and efficacy of bedaquiline for the treatment of drug-susceptible tuberculosis, extrapulmonary (e.g., CNS) tuberculosis, or latent tuberculosis infection have not been established. In addition, safety and efficacy for the treatment of infections caused by nontuberculous mycobacteria (NTM) have not been established. Use of bedaquiline in any of these settings is not recommended.

Patients with multidrug-resistant tuberculosis are at high risk for treatment failure and acquisition of further drug resistance. The American Thoracic Society (ATS), US Centers for Disease Control and Prevention (CDC), and Infectious Diseases Society of America (IDSA) recommend that such patients be referred to or that consultation be obtained from a specialized treatment center as identified by local or state health departments or the CDC.

For information on general principles used in the treatment of tuberculosis, see the Antituberculosis Agents General Statement 8:16.04.

Clinical Experience. Safety and efficacy of bedaquiline were evaluated in a double-blind, placebo-controlled phase 2 trial in 133 newly diagnosed adults with multidrug-resistant pulmonary tuberculosis. Patients were randomized to receive either bedaquiline (400 mg once daily for 2 weeks, followed by 200 mg 3 times weekly for 22 weeks) or placebo; patients in both treatment groups also received a background antituberculosis regimen (i.e., ethionamide, kanamycin, pyrazinamide, ofloxacin, and cycloserine/terizidone [not commercially available in the US] or available alternative). After 24 weeks, patients continued to receive the background antituberculosis treatment regimen for a total treatment duration of 18–24 months or for at least 12 months after the first confirmed negative culture. Time to sputum culture conversion (defined as the interval between the first dose of study drug and the date of the first of 2 consecutive negative sputum cultures collected at least 25 days apart) was shorter in patients receiving bedaquiline compared with patients receiving placebo (83 versus 125 days, respectively). The treatment success rate (sputum conversion without treatment discontinuance or death) at 24 weeks was 77.6% in patients receiving bedaquiline compared with 57.6% in patients receiving placebo; at 72 weeks, the treatment success rate was 70.1 and 56.1%, respectively.

In a smaller phase 2 trial, 44 adults with newly diagnosed, confirmed multidrug-resistant pulmonary tuberculosis were randomized to receive either bedaquiline (400 mg once daily for 2 weeks, followed by 200 mg 3 times weekly for weeks 3 through 8) or 8 weeks of placebo; all patients also received a 5-drug background antituberculosis regimen (i.e., ethionamide, kanamycin, pyrazinamide, ofloxacin, and cycloserine or terizidone [not commercially available in the US]). The primary efficacy end point was the time to conversion of sputum cultures from positive to negative. Patients who received bedaquiline had a decreased time to culture conversion and also had a 38.9 and 15.7% higher culture conversion rate at weeks 8 and 24, respectively, compared with patients who received placebo.

Data are limited to date regarding the use of bedaquiline for the treatment of multidrug-resistant tuberculosis in patients with human immunodeficiency virus (HIV) infection. (See HIV-infected Individuals under Warnings/Precautions: Other Warnings/Precautions, in Cautions.)

Dosage and Administration

■ **Administration** Bedaquiline is administered orally with food. The tablets should be swallowed whole with water.

Bedaquiline should be administered using directly observed (supervised) therapy (DOT).

■ **Dosage** Bedaquiline is commercially available as the fumarate salt; dosage is expressed in terms of bedaquiline.

Active Tuberculosis The recommended adult dosage of bedaquiline for the treatment of pulmonary multidrug-resistant tuberculosis is 400 mg once daily for 2 weeks, followed by 200 mg 3 times weekly (with at least 48 hours between doses) for 22 weeks (total of 24 weeks).

Bedaquiline must be used in conjunction with other antituberculosis agents. (See Active Tuberculosis under Uses: Tuberculosis.)

■ **Special Populations** ***Renal Impairment*** Bedaquiline dosage does not need to be adjusted in patients with mild or moderate renal impairment. The drug should be used with caution in patients with severe renal impairment or end-stage renal disease requiring hemodialysis or peritoneal dialysis. (See Renal Impairment under Warnings/Precautions: Specific Populations, in Cautions.)

Hepatic Impairment Bedaquiline dosage does not need to be adjusted in patients with mild or moderate hepatic impairment. The drug should be used with caution in patients with severe hepatic impairment and only when the benefits outweigh the risks. (See Hepatic Impairment under Warnings/Precautions: Specific Populations, in Cautions.)

Cautions

■ **Contraindications** The manufacturer states that there are no known contraindications to the use of bedaquiline.

■ **Warnings/Precautions** ***Warnings*** **Increased Mortality.** An increased risk of death was observed in patients receiving bedaquiline in a placebo-controlled clinical trial (11.4 versus 2.5%, based on data through week 120). In this study, there were 9 deaths in bedaquiline-treated patients; one death occurred during the 24 weeks of bedaquiline therapy and the median time to death for the other 8 patients was 329 days after the last dose of bedaquiline. Five of the 9 deaths in bedaquiline-treated patients and both deaths in placebo-treated patients were related to tuberculosis. The explanation for the imbalance in deaths in this study is not known; no correlation was demonstrated between death and sputum culture conversion, relapse, susceptibility to other antituberculosis drugs, HIV status, or disease severity.

Bedaquiline should be used *only* when an effective treatment regimen for multidrug-resistant tuberculosis cannot otherwise be provided.

Prolongation of QT Interval. Prolongation of the QT interval has occurred in patients receiving bedaquiline. Concomitant use of bedaquiline with other drugs associated with QT interval prolongation may result in additive or synergistic effects on the QT interval. (See Drug Interactions.) Documented cases of torsades de pointes have not been reported to date in patients receiving bedaquiline.

In a placebo-controlled clinical trial, mean increases in QT interval corrected for rate (QT_c, Fridericia method) after 1 week of treatment were greater in patients receiving bedaquiline compared with patients receiving placebo (9.9 versus 3.5 msec). The largest mean increase in QT_c during the 24 weeks of treatment occurred at 18 weeks (15.7 or 6.2 msec in patients receiving bedaquiline or placebo, respectively). Increases from baseline in QT interval persisted after bedaquiline was discontinued. There was no clear correlation between antecedent clinically important QT interval prolongation or clinically important dysrhythmia in any of the study patients who died.

In another trial, patients with no other treatment options received other QT interval-prolonging drugs, including clofazimine, concomitantly with bedaquiline. Additive QT interval prolongation, proportional to the number of additional QT interval-prolonging drugs, was observed. A mean increase in QT_c compared with baseline of 23.7 msec was observed in patients receiving bedaquiline without other QT interval-prolonging drugs compared with a mean increase of 30.7 msec in those receiving bedaquiline and at least 2 other QT interval-prolonging drugs. Although a QT_c segment duration exceeding 480 msec was not observed in any patient receiving bedaquiline without other QT interval-prolonging drugs, a QT_c segment duration exceeding 500 msec was observed in one patient receiving multiple QT interval-prolonging drugs.

ECGs should be performed before initiation of bedaquiline and at least at 2, 12, and 24 weeks after starting treatment. Serum concentrations of potassium, calcium, and magnesium should be measured at baseline and corrected if necessary. If QT interval prolongation is detected, electrolyte concentrations should be monitored.

The risk of QT interval prolongation may be increased in patients receiving other drugs that prolong the QT interval (e.g., clofazimine, fluoroquinolones, macrolides); patients with hypocalcemia, hypokalemia, or hypomagnesemia; or patients with a history of torsades de pointes, congenital long QT syndrome, hypothyroidism and bradyarrhythmias, or uncompensated heart failure. ECGs should be closely monitored in such patients.

Bedaquiline and all other drugs that may prolong the QT interval should be discontinued in patients who develop a clinically important ventricular arrhythmia or a QT_c greater than 500 msec (confirmed by repeat ECG). ECGs should be monitored frequently to confirm that the QT_c returns to baseline. If syncope occurs, an ECG should be performed to detect prolongation of the QT interval.

Bedaquiline has not been evaluated to date in patients with ventricular arrhythmias or recent myocardial infarction.

Concentrations of the major metabolite of bedaquiline (an *N*-monodesmethyl metabolite [M2]) appear to correlate with QT interval prolongation.

Other Warnings/Precautions **Hepatic Effects.** A higher incidence of adverse hepatic effects has been reported in patients receiving antituberculosis regimens containing bedaquiline compared with patients receiving regimens that did not contain the drug. Based on data from 2 clinical trials, reversible increases in serum aminotransferase concentrations to at least 3 times the upper limit of normal (ULN) were reported in 10.8 or 5.7% of patients receiving bedaquiline or placebo, respectively.

Liver function tests (AST, ALT, alkaline phosphatase, bilirubin) should be monitored at baseline, monthly during treatment, and as needed. Patients also should be monitored for symptoms of hepatic dysfunction.

If signs or symptoms of new or worsening liver dysfunction (e.g., clinically important elevation in serum aminotransferases and/or bilirubin, fatigue, anorexia, nausea, jaundice, dark urine, liver tenderness, hepatomegaly) develop, the patient should be promptly evaluated.

If AST or ALT increase to greater than 3 times the ULN, liver function tests should be repeated within 48 hours. In addition, patients should be tested for viral hepatitis and other hepatotoxic drugs should be discontinued.

Bedaquiline should be discontinued if elevated serum aminotransferase concentrations are accompanied by total bilirubin concentrations exceeding 2 times the ULN, serum aminotransferase concentrations exceed 8 times the ULN, or elevated aminotransferase concentrations persist for more than 2 weeks.

Alcohol and other hepatotoxic drugs or herbal products should be avoided in patients receiving bedaquiline, especially in those with diminished hepatic reserve.

HIV-infected Individuals. Data are limited to date regarding the use of bedaquiline in patients with human immunodeficiency virus (HIV) infection, including use in those receiving antiretroviral therapy. (See Drug Interactions: Antiretroviral Agents.) Some experts state that bedaquiline should be used with caution in HIV-infected individuals.

Selection and Use of Antimycobacterials. Specimens for microscopic examination and mycobacterial cultures and in vitro susceptibility testing should be obtained prior to initiation of antituberculosis therapy and periodically during treatment to monitor therapeutic response. The antituberculosis regimen should be modified as needed.

Bedaquiline must be used in conjunction with at least 3 other drugs to which the patient's multidrug-resistant *M. tuberculosis* isolate has been shown to be susceptible in vitro. If results of in vitro testing are not available, bedaquiline should be used in conjunction with at least 4 other drugs to which the patient's multidrug-resistant *M. tuberculosis* isolate is likely to be susceptible.

If the patient does not have sputum conversion or if relapse occurs following treatment, in vitro susceptibility testing should be performed to determine the bedaquiline MIC of the patient's isolate.

Compliance with the full course of antituberculosis therapy and all drugs included in the multiple-drug regimen is critical. Missed doses increase the risk of treatment failure and increase the likelihood that the patient's *M. tuberculosis* will develop resistance and will not be treatable.

To ensure compliance, the treatment regimen should be administered using directly observed (supervised) therapy (DOT).

Specific Populations **Pregnancy.** Category B. (See Users Guide.)

Lactation. Bedaquiline is distributed into milk in rats; it is not known whether the drug is distributed into human milk.

A decision should be made whether to discontinue nursing or bedaquiline, taking into account the importance of the drug to the woman.

Pediatric Use. Safety and efficacy of bedaquiline have not been established in patients younger than 18 years of age.

Geriatric Use. Clinical studies of bedaquiline did not include sufficient numbers of patients 65 years of age and older to determine whether geriatric patients respond differently than younger adults.

Hepatic Impairment. Bedaquiline has not been studied in patients with severe hepatic impairment. The drug should be used with caution in patients with severe hepatic impairment and only when the benefits outweigh the risks; such patients should be monitored for adverse effects.

Renal Impairment. Bedaquiline should be used with caution and with increased monitoring for adverse effects in patients with severe renal impairment or end-stage renal disease requiring hemodialysis or peritoneal dialysis.

■ **Common Adverse Effects** Adverse effects reported in 10% or more of patients receiving bedaquiline and more commonly than in patients receiving placebo include nausea, arthralgia, headache, hemoptysis, and chest pain.

Drug Interactions

■ **Drugs Affecting Hepatic Microsomal Enzymes** Bedaquiline is metabolized primarily by cytochrome P-450 (CYP) isoenzyme 3A4.

Concomitant use of bedaquiline with potent inhibitors of CYP3A4 (e.g., ketoconazole) may increase the area under the concentration-time curve (AUC) of bedaquiline and increase the risk of adverse effects associated with the drug. Concomitant use of bedaquiline and systemic drugs that are potent inhibitors of CYP3A4 for a duration longer than 14 consecutive days should be avoided, unless the benefits of concomitant use outweigh the risks. Patients receiving such concomitant therapy should be monitored for bedaquiline-related adverse effects.

Concomitant use of bedaquiline with potent inducers of CYP3A4, including rifamycins (e.g., rifampin, rifapentine, rifabutin), may reduce the AUC of bedaquiline and decrease the therapeutic effects of the drug. Concomitant use of bedaquiline with rifamycins or other potent inducers of CYP3A4 should be avoided.

■ **Drugs Metabolized by Hepatic Microsomal Enzymes** In vitro studies indicate that bedaquiline does not inhibit CYP isoenzymes 1A2, 2A6, 2C8/9/10, 2C19, 2D6, 2E1, 3A4, 3A4/5, or 4A to any clinically important extent and does not induce CYP isoenzymes 1A2, 2C9, 2C19, or 3A4. Therefore, bedaquiline is not expected to alter metabolism of CYP substrates.

■ **Drugs that Prolong the QT Interval** Pharmacologic interaction (increased risk of QT interval prolongation). Concomitant use with other drugs that prolong the QT interval (e.g., clofazimine, fluoroquinolones, macrolides) may result in additive or synergistic effects on the QT interval.

■ **Hepatotoxic Drugs** Pharmacologic interaction (increased risk of hepatotoxicity). Concomitant use with other hepatotoxic drugs or herbal products should be avoided, especially in patients with diminished hepatic reserve.

■ **Alcohol** Because of possible increased risk of hepatotoxicity, alcohol should be avoided in patients receiving bedaquiline, especially in those with diminished hepatic reserve.

■ **Antifungal Agents** ***Ketoconazole*** Concomitant use of bedaquiline (400 mg once daily for 14 days) and ketoconazole (400 mg once daily for 4 days) in healthy individuals increased bedaquiline AUC, peak plasma concentrations, and trough plasma concentrations by 22, 9, and 33%, respectively.

A greater effect on the QT interval corrected for rate (QT_c) was observed when multiple doses of bedaquiline and ketoconazole were administered concomitantly compared with multiple dosing of the individual drugs.

Concomitant use of bedaquiline and ketoconazole for a duration longer than 14 consecutive days should be avoided, unless the benefits of concomitant use outweigh the risks. Patients receiving such concomitant therapy should be monitored for bedaquiline-related adverse effects.

■ **Antimycobacterial Agents** ***Clofazimine*** Larger mean increases in QT_c compared with baseline were observed at week 24 in patients receiving clofazimine and bedaquiline concomitantly compared with patients receiving bedaquiline without clofazimine (31.9 versus 12.3 msec).

Because concomitant use of bedaquiline and clofazimine may increase the risk of QT interval prolongation, ECGs should be monitored closely during concomitant therapy.

Cycloserine In a placebo-controlled clinical trial in patients with multidrug-resistant tuberculosis, concomitant use of bedaquiline and cycloserine did not have a clinically important effect on the pharmacokinetics of cycloserine.

Ethambutol In a placebo-controlled clinical trial in patients with multidrug-resistant tuberculosis, concomitant use of bedaquiline and ethambutol did not have a clinically important effect on the pharmacokinetics of ethambutol.

Isoniazid Concomitant use of bedaquiline (400 mg once daily for 14 days), isoniazid (300 mg once daily for 5 days), and pyrazinamide (1 or 2 g once daily for 5 days) in healthy individuals did not result in clinically important changes in the AUC of any of the drugs.

Dosage adjustments are not needed for either bedaquiline or isoniazid if the drugs are used concomitantly.

Kanamycin In a placebo-controlled clinical trial in patients with multidrug-resistant tuberculosis, concomitant use of bedaquiline and kanamycin did not have a clinically important effect on the pharmacokinetics of kanamycin.

Pyrazinamide Concomitant use of bedaquiline (400 mg once daily for 14 days), isoniazid (300 mg once daily for 5 days), and pyrazinamide (1 or 2 g once daily for 5 days) in healthy individuals did not result in clinically important changes in the AUC of any of the drugs. In a placebo-controlled clinical trial in patients with multidrug-resistant tuberculosis, concomitant use of bedaquiline and pyrazinamide did not have a clinically important effect on the pharmacokinetics of pyrazinamide.

Dosage adjustments are not needed for either bedaquiline or pyrazinamide if the drugs are used concomitantly.

Rifamycins Concomitant use of bedaquiline (300 mg once daily) and rifampin (600 mg once daily for 21 days) in healthy individuals decreased the AUC of bedaquiline by 52%. Concomitant use of bedaquiline and other rifamycins (e.g., rifabutin, rifapentine) may also result in decreased bedaquiline concentrations and decreased therapeutic effects.

Concomitant use of bedaquiline and rifamycins (e.g., rifampin, rifabutin, rifapentine) should be avoided.

■ **Antiretroviral Agents** ***Efavirenz*** Concomitant use of bedaquiline (single 400-mg dose) with efavirenz (600 mg once daily) in healthy adults decreased the AUC of bedaquiline by 20% and increased peak plasma concentrations of the major metabolite of bedaquiline (an *N*-monodesmethyl metabolite [M2]), but did not affect the AUC of the M2 metabolite or the pharmacokinetics of efavirenz. This pharmacokinetic interaction does not appear to be clinically important.

Lopinavir/Ritonavir Concomitant use of bedaquiline (single 400-mg dose) with the fixed combination of lopinavir and ritonavir (lopinavir 400 mg/ritonavir 100 mg twice daily for 24 days) in healthy individuals increased the AUC of bedaquiline by 22%; mean peak plasma concentrations of bedaquiline were not substantially affected.

Bedaquiline and lopinavir/ritonavir should be used concomitantly with caution and only if benefits outweigh risks.

Nevirapine Concomitant use of bedaquiline (single 400-mg dose) with nevirapine (200 mg twice daily for 4 weeks) in patients with HIV infection did not have a clinically important effect on the AUC of bedaquiline. Dosage adjustment of bedaquiline is not necessary if the drug is used concomitantly with nevirapine.

■ **Macrolides** Because concomitant use of bedaquiline and macrolides may increase the risk of QT interval prolongation, ECGs should be monitored closely during concomitant therapy.

■ **Quinolones** Because concomitant use of bedaquiline and fluoroquinolones may increase the risk of QT interval prolongation, ECGs should be monitored closely during concomitant therapy.

Ofloxacin In a placebo-controlled clinical trial in patients with multidrug-resistant tuberculosis, concomitant use of bedaquiline and ofloxacin did not have a clinically important effect on the pharmacokinetics of ofloxacin.

Description

Bedaquiline, a diarylquinoline antimycobacterial, is an antituberculosis agent. Bedaquiline inhibits mycobacterial adenosine 5′-triphosphate (ATP) synthase, an enzyme that is essential for the generation of energy in *Mycobacterium tuberculosis*.

Bedaquiline is active in vitro against *M. tuberculosis*, including drug-susceptible *M. tuberculosis* and multidrug-resistant strains resistant to isoniazid, rifampin, ethambutol, ethionamide, pyrazinamide, streptomycin, and/or ofloxacin. The MIC of bedaquiline reported for clinical isolates of multidrug-resistant *M. tuberculosis* generally has ranged from 0.003–0.25 mcg/mL. Bedaquiline also is active in vitro against some other mycobacteria, including *M. avium*, *M. intracellulare*, *M. abscessus*, and *M. ulcerans*.

M. tuberculosis with reduced susceptibility or resistance to bedaquiline (4- to 133-fold increase in MIC) have been produced in vitro and strains with reduced susceptibility have emerged during treatment with the drug. Mutations in the *atpE* target gene have been identified as a mechanism of mycobacterial resistance to bedaquiline; other mechanisms of resistance also exist. Mycobacteria with natural resistance to bedaquiline include *M. xenopi*, *M. novocastrense*, and *M. shimoidei*.

Relative oral bioavailability of bedaquiline is increased twofold when the drug is administered with a standard meal (22 g fat, 558 calories) compared with administration under fasting conditions. Bedaquiline is metabolized primarily by cytochrome P-450 (CYP) isoenzyme 3A4. The major metabolite, an *N*-monodesmethyl metabolite (M2), has 4–6 times less antimycobacterial activity compared with the parent drug. Bedaquiline is eliminated mainly in feces; renal clearance of unchanged drug is negligible. The mean terminal elimination half-lives of bedaquiline and the M2 metabolite are similar and are approximately 5.5 months; the long half-life probably reflects slow release of the drug and metabolite from peripheral tissues.

Advice to Patients

Importance of providing patient a copy of the manufacturer's patient information (medication guide). Importance of the patient reading the medication guide prior to initiation of therapy and each time the prescription is refilled.

Importance of taking bedaquiline exactly as prescribed and completing the full course of therapy with bedaquiline and other antituberculosis drugs.

Advise patients that missed doses may decrease treatment effectiveness and increase the risk of developing resistance to bedaquiline and other antituberculosis drugs. If a dose of bedaquiline is missed during the first 2 weeks of therapy, the missed dose should be skipped and the usual dosing schedule continued. If a dose is missed after the first 2 weeks, the missed dose should be taken as soon as possible and the usual 3-times-weekly regimen resumed.

Importance of taking bedaquiline with food.

Importance of storing bedaquiline tablets in the original container and protecting the drug from light.

Advise patients that bedaquiline may be associated with serious adverse effects, including increased risk of death, heart rhythm abnormalities, and/or hepatitis.

Importance of informing clinicians of personal or family history of congenital QT interval prolongation or heart failure.

Importance of informing clinicians if symptoms suggestive of hepatotoxicity (e.g., nausea, vomiting, abdominal pain, fever, weakness, pruritus, fatigue, anorexia, jaundice, dark urine, light-colored stools) occur.

Potential for bedaquiline to cause nausea, arthralgia, headache, increased serum amylase concentrations, hemoptysis, chest pain, anorexia, or rash.

Importance of informing clinicians of existing or contemplated concomitant therapy, including prescription and OTC drugs and dietary or herbal products. Advise patients to abstain from alcohol and other hepatotoxic drugs or herbal products.

Importance of women informing clinicians if they are or plan to become pregnant or plan to breast-feed.

Importance of informing patients of other important precautionary information. (See Cautions.)

Overview® (see Users Guide). For additional information on this drug until a more detailed monograph is developed and published, the manufacturer's labeling should be consulted. It is *essential* that the manufacturer's labeling be consulted for more detailed information on usual cautions, precautions, contraindications, potential drug interactions, laboratory test interferences, and acute toxicity.

Preparations

Excipients in commercially available drug preparations may have clinically important effects in some individuals; consult specific product labeling for details.

Bedaquiline Fumarate

Oral

Tablets	100 mg (of bedaquiline)	**Sirturo®**, Janssen

Ethambutol Hydrochloride

■ Ethambutol hydrochloride is a synthetic antituberculosis agent.

Uses

■ **Tuberculosis** ***Active Tuberculosis*** Ethambutol is used in conjunction with other antituberculosis agents in the treatment of clinical tuberculosis.

The American Thoracic Society (ATS), US Centers for Disease Control and Prevention (CDC), and Infectious Diseases Society of America (IDSA) currently recommend several possible multiple-drug regimens for the treatment of culture-positive pulmonary tuberculosis. These regimens have a minimum duration of 6 months (26 weeks), and consist of an initial intensive phase (2 months) and a continuation phase (usually either 4 or 7 months). Ethambutol is considered a first-line antituberculosis agent for use in the initial phase of these regimens. In patients with previously untreated pulmonary tuberculosis, ethambutol usually is included in the initial phase of treatment in conjunction with isoniazid and rifampin (with or without pyrazinamide). In patients receiving a daily treatment regimen for the initial phase, the ATS, CDC, and IDSA state that ethambutol usually can be discontinued when in vitro susceptibility tests indicate that the strain of *Mycobacterium tuberculosis* is susceptible to isoniazid and rifampin. Ethambutol also is considered a first-line agent for use in multiple-drug regimens for the management of patients with drug-resistant pulmonary tuberculosis. For information on general principles used in the treatment of tuberculosis, see the Antituberculosis Agents General Statement 8:16.04.

■ **Myobacterium avium Complex (MAC) Infections** ***Treatment of MAC Infections*** Ethambutol is used in conjunction with other antituberculosis agents in the treatment of *Mycobacterium avium* complex (MAC) infections.† The ATS currently recommends that therapy for MAC pulmonary infections in HIV-negative patients consist of at least 3 drugs, including clarithromycin (500 mg twice daily) or azithromycin (250 mg daily or 500 mg 3 times weekly), rifabutin (300 mg daily) or rifampin (600 mg daily), and ethambutol (25 mg/kg daily for 2 months, then 15 mg/kg daily). In addition, the ATS recommends therapy that includes either clarithromycin or azithromycin combined with ethambutol and rifabutin for the treatment of disseminated MAC infection in HIV-infected patients. The choice of the drug regimen should be made in consultation with an expert. For further information on the treatment of MAC infections, see Management of Other Mycobacterial Infections: Mycobacterium avium Complex (MAC) Infections, in the Antituberculosis Agents General Statement 8:16.04.

Prevention of Recurrence To prevent recurrence of MAC infections, maintenance therapy (*secondary prophylaxis*) is recommended for all HIV-infected adults, adolescents, and children who have previously been treated for disseminated MAC infection. Unless there is clinical or laboratory evidence of macrolide resistance, the Prevention of Opportunistic Infections Working Group of the US Public Health Service and Infectious Diseases Society of America (USPHS/IDSA) recommends a regimen of clarithromycin (or azithromycin) in conjunction with ethambutol with or without rifabutin for secondary MAC prophylaxis†.

Secondary MAC prophylaxis after disseminated MAC infection in HIV-infected adults and adolescents generally is recommended for life, unless there is immune recovery in response to highly active antiretroviral therapy (HAART). There is some evidence that the risk for recurrence of MAC is low in adults and adolescents who have completed at least 12 months of MAC therapy, have remained asymptomatic with respect to MAC signs and symptoms, and have a sustained (e.g., for 6 months or longer) increase in $CD4^+$ T-cell counts to greater than 100/mm³ as the result of potent antiretroviral therapy. Based on these data and more extensive cumulative data regarding the safety of discontinuing secondary prophylaxis for other opportunistic infections, the USPHS/IDSA states that it is reasonable to consider discontinuance of secondary MAC prophylaxis in adults and adolescents meeting these criteria. To substantiate that the disease is no longer active, some experts would obtain a blood culture for MAC (even in asymptomatic patients) prior to discontinuing secondary MAC prophylaxis. The USPHS/IDSA recommends that secondary MAC prophylaxis be reinitiated if $CD4^+$ T-cell counts subsequently decrease to less than 100/mm³.

The safety of discontinuing secondary MAC prophylaxis in HIV-infected children whose $CD4^+$ T-cell count has increased in response to HAART has not been studied. Therefore, the USPHS/IDSA recommends that HIV-infected children with a history of disseminated MAC infection receive lifelong secondary MAC prophylaxis.

For additional information on prevention of recurrence of disseminated MAC infection, see Treatment and Prevention of Recurrence of Disseminated MAC Infection, under Management of Other Mycobacterial Diseases: Mycobacterium avium Complex (MAC) Infections, in the Antituberculosis Agents General Statement 8:16.04.

Dosage and Administration

■ Administration Ethambutol hydrochloride is administered orally.

■ Dosage ***Active Tuberculosis*** In the treatment of clinical tuberculosis, ethambutol should not be given alone. The drug is considered a first-line agent for use in patients with tuberculosis. Therapy for tuberculosis should be continued long enough to prevent relapse. The minimum duration of treatment currently recommended for patients with culture-positive pulmonary tuberculosis is 6 months (26 weeks), and recommended regimens consist of an initial intensive phase (2 months) and a continuation phase (usually either 4 or 7 months). However, completion of treatment is determined more accurately by the total number of doses and is not based solely on the duration of therapy. For information on general principles of antituberculosis therapy and recommendations regarding specific multiple-drug regimens and duration of therapy, see the Antituberculosis Agents General Statement 8:16.04.

Adult Dosage. The manufacturer states that the usual adult dosage of ethambutol hydrochloride for use in conjunction with other antituberculosis agents in previously untreated patients is 15 mg/kg once daily. In adults who have received previous antituberculosis therapy, the usual dosage recommended by the manufacturer for use in conjunction with other antituberculosis agents is 25 mg/kg daily for 60 days or until bacteriologic smears and cultures become negative, followed by 15 mg/kg daily.

The American Thoracic Society (ATS), US Centers for Disease Control and Prevention (CDC), and Infectious Diseases Society of America (IDSA) recommend that when ethambutol hydrochloride is used in an initial regimen that involves daily administration of antituberculosis agents, adults and children 15 years of age or older weighing 40–55 kg should receive a dosage of 800 mg, those weighing 56–75 kg should receive 1.2 g, and those weighing 76–90 kg should receive 1.6 g. The maximum daily dosage recommended is 1.6 g regardless of weight.

If ethambutol hydrochloride is used in an intermittent regimen that involves twice-weekly administration of antituberculosis agents, the ATS, CDC, and IDSA recommend that adults and children 15 years of age or older weighing 40–55 kg should receive a dosage of 2 g, those weighing 56–75 kg should receive 2.8 g, and those weighing 76–90 kg should receive 4 g. If a 3-times weekly regimen is used, adults weighing 40–55 kg should receive a dosage of 1.2 g, those weighing 56–75 kg should receive 2 g, and those weighing 76–90 kg should receive 2.4 g.

Pediatric Dosage. The manufacturer states that ethambutol hydrochloride is not recommended for use in children younger than 13 years of age. The ATS, CDC, and IDSA state that ethambutol should be used with caution in children in whom it may be difficult to monitor visual acuity (e.g., those younger than 5 years of age). If ethambutol hydrochloride is used in pediatric patients, the ATS, CDC, and IDSA recommend a dosage of 15–20 mg/kg daily (up to 1 g) or a dosage of 50 mg/kg twice weekly (up to 2.5 g). The American Academy of Pediatrics recommends a pediatric dosage of 15–25 mg/kg daily or 50 mg/kg twice weekly (up to 2.5 g).

Mycobacterium avium Complex (MAC) Infections **Adult Dosage.** When ethambutol hydrochloride is used in conjunction with other antituberculosis agents for the treatment of pulmonary *Mycobacterium avium* complex (MAC) infections† in adults *not* infected with the human immunodeficiency virus (HIV), a dosage of 25 mg/kg daily for 2 months, followed by 15 mg/kg daily thereafter, has been recommended by ATS. Therapy should continue until the patient has been culture negative for 1 year. When ethambutol hydrochloride is used in conjunction with other antituberculosis agents for the treatment of disseminated MAC infection†, a dosage of 15 mg/kg daily has been recommended by ATS.

For maintenance therapy to prevent recurrence of disseminated MAC infection (secondary prophylaxis)†, the Prevention of Opportunistic Infections Working Group of the US Public Health Service and the Infectious Diseases Society of America (USPHS/IDSA) recommends that adults or adolescents receive clarithromycin (500 mg twice daily) or azithromycin (500 mg once daily) in conjunction with ethambutol hydrochloride (15 mg/kg once daily), with or without rifabutin (300 mg once daily).

Pediatric Dosage. For maintenance therapy to prevent recurrence of disseminated MAC infection (secondary prophylaxis)†, the USPHS/IDSA recommends that infants and children receive clarithromycin (7.5 mg/kg [maximum 500 mg] daily) or azithromycin (5 mg/kg [maximum 250 mg] once daily) in conjunction with ethambutol hydrochloride (15 mg/kg [maximum 900 mg] once daily), with or without rifabutin (5 mg/kg [maximum 300 mg] once daily).

■ Dosage in Renal Impairment In patients with impaired renal function, doses and/or frequency of administration of ethambutol hydrochloride should be modified in response to the degree of renal impairment. Some clinicians suggest that if the creatinine clearance is 70–100 mL/minute, dosage of ethambutol hydrochloride should not exceed 15 mg/kg daily, and if the creatinine clearance is less than 70 mL/minute, dosage should be further reduced. Other clinicians have suggested that the usual dose be administered every 24–36 hours in patients with creatinine clearances of 10–50 mL/minute and every 48 hours in patients with creatinine clearances less than 10 mL/minute.

Cautions

■ Ocular Effects The most important adverse effect of ethambutol is optic neuritis with decreases in visual acuity, constriction of visual fields, central and peripheral scotomas, and loss of red-green color discrimination. The extent of ocular toxicity appears to be related to the dose and duration of ethambutol therapy. However, such toxicity also has been reported rarely after only a few days of therapy with the drug, and may represent an idiosyncratic reaction. Tests for visual acuity should be performed using a Snellen eye chart prior to and periodically during ethambutol therapy. Changes in visual acuity may be unilateral or bilateral; therefore, each eye must be tested separately and both eyes tested together. During 1–2 years of ethambutol therapy, some patients may develop a refractive error which must be corrected in order to obtain accurate test results; testing visual acuity through a pinhole eliminates the refractive error.

When ocular toxicity is detected early and ethambutol is discontinued promptly, the visual effects are generally reversible over a period of weeks or months. Patients have then received ethambutol again without recurrence of loss of visual acuity. Rarely, depending on the degree of impairment, recovery may be delayed for up to 1 year or more, or the effect may be irreversible. Care should be taken to be certain that variations in vision are not caused by underlying pathologic conditions (e.g., optic neuritis from other causes, cataracts, recurrent ocular inflammatory conditions, diabetic retinopathy).

■ Other Adverse Effects Other adverse effects of ethambutol include dermatitis, pruritus, headache, malaise, dizziness, fever, mental confusion, disorientation, possible hallucinations, joint pain, and rarely anaphylactoid reactions. GI upset, abdominal pain, nausea, vomiting, and anorexia have also occurred occasionally with ethambutol. Peripheral neuritis, with numbness and tingling of the extremities, has been reported infrequently. Increased serum uric acid concentrations and precipitation of acute gout have occurred occasionally in patients receiving ethambutol and are probably the result of decreased renal clearance of urate. Transient impairment of liver function, as indicated by abnormal liver function test results, has also occurred. Cholestatic jaundice, which appeared to be caused by ethambutol, has been reported in at least one patient who received the drug both alone and in conjunction with streptomycin.

■ Precautions and Contraindications Visual testing should be performed prior to initiating ethambutol therapy and then periodically during therapy with the drug. Testing should be done monthly in patients receiving more than 15 mg/kg daily. Examinations should include ophthalmoscopy, finger perimetry, and testing of color discrimination. Patients developing adverse ocular effects during ethambutol therapy may show subjective visual symptoms either before or simultaneously with decreases in visual acuity. All patients receiving the drug should be questioned periodically about blurred vision and other subjective visual symptoms and should be instructed to report to their physicians any such changes as soon as they are noticed. If substantial changes in visual acuity occur, ethambutol should be discontinued immediately. (See Cautions: Ocular Effects.)

Renal, hepatic, and hematopoietic tests should be performed periodically during long-term ethambutol therapy.

Ethambutol should be used with caution and in reduced dosage in patients with impaired renal function. The drug should also be used with caution in patients with ocular defects (e.g., cataracts, recurrent ocular inflammatory conditions, diabetic retinopathy) that make visual changes difficult to detect or evaluate; consideration should be given to whether the benefits of ethambutol therapy justify the possible ocular effects in these patients. Ethambutol is contraindicated in patients with optic neuritis unless clinical judgment deems it necessary that the drug be used. Ethambutol is also contraindicated in patients with known hypersensitivity to the drug.

■ Pediatric Precautions The manufacturer states that ethambutol should not be used in children younger than 13 years of age. The American Thoracic Society (ATS), US Centers for Disease Control and Prevention (CDC), and Infectious Diseases Society of America (IDSA) state that ethambutol should be used with caution in children in whom it may be difficult to monitor visual acuity (e.g., those younger than 5 years of age). These experts state that ethambutol usually is recommended for use in such children only when the strain of *Mycobacterium tuberculosis* involved is known or suspected to be resistant to isoniazid or rifampin or when the child has adult-type (upper lobe infiltration, cavity formation) tuberculosis.

■ Pregnancy Ethambutol has caused teratogenic effects in animals when used in high doses. Although safe use of the drugs during pregnancy has not been definitely established, ethambutol (combined with isoniazid or with isoniazid and rifampin) has been used to treat clinical tuberculosis in pregnant women and has not been reported to date to cause adverse effects on the fetus The manufacturer states that ethambutol should be used during pregnancy only when the potential benefits justify the possible risks to the fetus. The ATS, CDC, and IDSA state that ethambutol is considered safe for use in pregnant women.

Mechanism of Action

Ethambutol is bacteriostatic in action. Although the exact mechanism of action has not been fully elucidated, the drug appears to inhibit the synthesis of one or more metabolites in susceptible bacteria resulting in impairment of cellular metabolism, arrest of multiplication, and cell death. Ethambutol is active against susceptible bacteria only when they are undergoing cell division.

Spectrum

Ethambutol is a highly specific agent and is active only against organisms of the genus *Mycobacterium*. The drug is active in vitro and in vivo against *M. tuberculosis*, *M. bovis*, *M. marinum*, and some strains of *M. kansasii*, *M. avium*, *M. fortuitum*, and *M. intracellulare*. In vitro, the minimum inhibitory concentration (MIC) of ethambutol for most susceptible mycobacteria is 1–8 mcg/mL, depending on the culture media used.

Resistance

Natural and acquired resistance to ethambutol have been demonstrated in vitro and in vivo in strains of *M. tuberculosis*. In vitro, resistance to ethambutol appears to occur in a stepwise manner. Resistant strains of initially susceptible *M. tuberculosis* develop rapidly if ethambutol is used alone in the treatment of clinical tuberculosis. When ethambutol is combined with other antituberculosis agents in the treatment of the disease, emergence of resistant strains may be delayed or prevented. There is no evidence of cross-resistance between ethambutol and other antituberculosis agents currently available in the US.

Pharmacokinetics

■ **Absorption** Approximately 75–80% of an oral dose of ethambutol hydrochloride is rapidly absorbed from the GI tract. Absorption is not substantially affected when the drug is administered with food. Following a single oral ethambutol hydrochloride dose of 25 mg/kg, peak serum ethambutol concentrations of 2–5 mcg/mL are attained within 2–4 hours; serum concentrations of the drug are undetectable 24 hours after the dose. There is no evidence that accumulation of the drug occurs when ethambutol doses of 25 mg/kg are given once daily in patients with normal renal function. Serum concentrations of the drug are higher and accumulation may occur when ethambutol is used in patients with impaired renal function.

An agar-diffusion microbiologic assay may be used to determine serum and urine concentrations of ethambutol. Although the technique of this assay has not been published, it is based on inhibition of *M. smegmatis* (ATCC 607) and specific information can be obtained from the manufacturer (Lederle).

■ **Distribution** Ethambutol is widely distributed into most body tissues and fluids. Highest concentrations of the drug are found in erythrocytes, kidneys, lungs, and saliva; lower drug concentrations are found in ascitic fluid, pleural fluid, brain, and CSF. Peak intracellular concentrations of ethambutol in erythrocytes are about twice peak plasma concentrations and maintain this ratio for at least 24 hours after a single oral dose. In patients with meningitis, administration of an oral ethambutol hydrochloride dose of 25 mg/kg has produced peak CSF concentrations of the drug ranging from 0.15–2.0 mcg/mL.

Ethambutol crosses the placenta and is distributed into cord blood and amniotic fluid. Ethambutol is distributed into milk in concentrations approximately equal to plasma concentrations of the drug.

At a concentration of a 4.8 mcg/mL, ethambutol is approximately 8% bound to plasma proteins; at a concentration of 1.3 mcg/mL, the drug is approximately 22% bound to plasma proteins.

■ **Elimination** The plasma half-life of ethambutol is approximately 3.3 hours in patients with normal renal function. The half-life is prolonged in patients with impaired renal or hepatic function. In patients with renal failure, the half-life may be 7 hours or longer.

Ethambutol is partially inactivated in the liver by oxidation to an aldehyde intermediate, 2,2′-(ethylenediimino)-di-butyraldehyde, which is converted to the decarboxylic acid derivative, 2,2′-(ethylenediimino)-di-butyric acid. Within 24 hours, approximately 50% of an oral dose of ethambutol hydrochloride is excreted in urine as unchanged drug, and 8–15% is excreted as inactive metabolites. Unabsorbed ethambutol is excreted in feces as unchanged drug. Approximately 20–22% of an oral dose of the drug is excreted in feces as unchanged drug. Ethambutol is removed by peritoneal dialysis and to a lesser extent by hemodialysis.

Chemistry and Stability

■ **Chemistry** Ethambutol hydrochloride is a synthetic antituberculosis agent. The drug occurs as a white, crystalline powder and is freely soluble in water and soluble in alcohol. The drug has pK_as of 6.1 and 9.2.

■ **Stability** Ethambutol hydrochloride tablets should be protected from light, moisture, and excessive heat and should be stored in well-closed containers at 15–30°C.

Preparations

Excipients in commercially available drug preparations may have clinically important effects in some individuals; consult specific product labeling for details.

Ethambutol Hydrochloride

Oral		
Tablets, film-coated	100 mg*	Ethambutol Tablets Myambutol®, X-Gen
	400 mg*	Ethambutol Tablets Myambutol® (scored), X-Gen

*available from one or more manufacturer, distributor, and/or repackager by generic (nonproprietary) name

†Use is not currently included in the labeling approved by the US Food and Drug Administration

Isoniazid

Isonicotinic Acid Hydrazide, Isonicotinylhydrazide, INH

■ Isoniazid is a synthetic, isonicotinic acid-derivative antituberculosis agent.

Uses

■ **Tuberculosis** ***Active Tuberculosis*** Isoniazid is used in conjunction with other antituberculosis agents in the treatment of clinical tuberculosis.

The American Thoracic Society (ATS), US Centers for Disease Control and Prevention (CDC), and Infectious Diseases Society of America (IDSA) currently recommend several possible multiple-drug regimens for the treatment of culture-positive pulmonary tuberculosis. These regimens have a minimum duration of 6 months (26 weeks), and consist of an initial intensive phase (2 months) and a continuation phase (usually either 4 or 7 months). Isoniazid is considered a first-line antituberculosis agent for the treatment of all forms of tuberculosis caused by *Mycobacterium tuberculosis* known or presumed to be susceptible to the drug. For information on general principles used in the treatment of tuberculosis, see the Antituberculosis Agents General Statement 8:16.04.

Isoniazid is commercially available in the US alone or in fixed combination with rifampin (Rifamate®) or in fixed combination with rifampin and pyrazinamide (Rifater®). The fixed-combination preparation containing rifampin, isoniazid, and pyrazinamide (Rifater®) is designated an orphan drug by the US Food and Drug Administration (FDA) for use in the treatment of tuberculosis. Although oral isoniazid is preferred for the treatment of tuberculosis, the drug may be given IM for initial or retreatment of the disease when the drug cannot be given orally.

Latent Tuberculosis Infection Isoniazid usually is used alone for the treatment of latent tuberculosis infection to prevent the development of clinical tuberculosis. Previously, "preventive therapy" or "chemoprophylaxis" was used to describe a simple drug regimen (e.g., isoniazid monotherapy) used to prevent the development of active tuberculosis disease in individuals known or likely to be infected with *M. tuberculosis*. However, since use of such a regimen rarely results in true primary prevention (i.e., prevention of *infection* in individuals exposed to infectious tuberculosis), the ATS and CDC currently state that "treatment of latent tuberculosis infection" rather than "preventive therapy" more accurately describes the intended intervention and potentially will result in greater understanding and more widespread implementation of this tuberculosis control strategy.

Individuals at risk for developing tuberculosis include those who have been recently infected with *M. tuberculosis* and those who have clinical conditions that increase the risk of latent tuberculosis infection progressing to active disease. The likelihood that a positive tuberculin test represents a true infection with *M. tuberculosis* is influenced by the prevalence of infection in the population being tested. The ATS and CDC state that since the general population of the US has an estimated *M. tuberculosis* infection rate of 5–10% and the annual incidence of new tuberculosis infection without known exposure is estimated to be 0.01–0.1%, the tuberculin skin test has a low positive predictive value in individuals without a known or likely exposure to *M. tuberculosis*. To prioritize the use of resources for identifying those at risk for developing tuberculosis and minimize the incidence of false-positive tuberculin test results, the ATS and CDC currently recommend that tuberculin testing be targeted toward groups at high risk and discouraged in those at low risk. The ATS and CDC currently define positive (i.e., significant) tuberculin reactions (i.e., reactions highly likely to indicate true infection with *M. tuberculosis*) in terms of 3 cut-off points (i.e., levels of induration) based on the sensitivity, specificity, and prevalence of tuberculosis in different groups: 5 mm or more of induration for individuals at highest risk for developing clinical tuberculosis, 10 mm or more of induration for those with an increased probability of infection or with clinical conditions predisposing to enhanced progression of infection to active tuberculosis, and 15 mm or more of induration for individuals at low risk in whom tuberculin testing generally is not indicated. (See Tuberculosis under Interpretation: Mantoux Test, in Tuberculin 36:84.)

The following individuals or groups with clinical risk factors should be targeted for tuberculin testing and, if appropriate, treated for latent tuberculosis infection following exclusion of active tuberculosis disease:

- **Individuals with known or suspected human immunodeficiency virus (HIV) infection.** In several randomized, controlled trials, isoniazid therapy for 6–12 months substantially reduced the incidence of clinical tuberculosis in patients with HIV infection who had induration reactions to tuberculin skin tests of 5 mm or greater. HIV infection contributes most to an increased risk of progression of latent tuberculosis infection to the active disease, and patients of any age with HIV infection who have an induration reaction of 5 mm or greater to the Mantoux tuberculin skin test should receive therapy for latent tuberculosis infection after excluding the presence of clinically active tuberculosis, unless such therapy is medically contraindicated. In addition, falsely insignificant tuberculin reactions may occur in patients with human immunodeficiency virus (HIV) infection because of immunosuppression associated with this infection, and the ATS, CDC, and some clinicians recommend that patients with HIV infection and known exposure to active tuberculosis be given preventive therapy even in the presence of a negative (< 5 mm induration) tuberculin skin test reaction. Patients with HIV infection, whether symptomatic or asymptomatic, may be anergic, and it had previously been recommended that *all* individuals who were HIV seropositive be evaluated for cell-mediated immunity (delayed-type hypersensitivity) using at least two other antigens (i.e., mumps skin test antigen, candida, tetanus toxoid) at the time tuberculin skin testing was performed. However, the ATS and CDC no longer recommend anergy testing for use in identifying tuberculosis infection, including in HIV-infected individuals because the usefulness of such testing in identifying tuberculin-negative, HIV-infected individuals who might benefit from treatment of latent tuberculosis infection has not been demonstrated. Instead, the ATS, CDC, and some experts state that there may be selected situations in which evaluation of anergy may assist in guiding individual decisions about therapy for latent tuberculosis infection (e.g., in individuals with insignificant reactions to tuberculin from populations at high risk for *Mycobacterium tuberculosis* infection). (See Tuberculosis: Anergic Individuals at Risk of Tuberculosis, in Uses in Tuberculin 36:84.) Although therapy for latent tuberculosis infection in tuberculin-negative HIV-infected patients has not proven effective, therapy with isoniazid may be beneficial for tuberculin-negative children who are born to HIV-infected women and who are close contacts of an individual who has infectious tuberculosis, as well as in HIV-infected adults who reside or work in institutions (e.g., prisons, jails, homeless shelters) and are continually and unavoidably exposed to patients who have infectious tuberculosis. Some experts recommend continuing isoniazid therapy for latent tuberculosis infection indefinitely in HIV-infected individuals who have an ongoing high risk for exposure to *M. tuberculosis* (e.g., inmates of prisons in which the prevalence of tuberculosis is high). Since HIV-infected individuals are at risk for peripheral neuropathy, those receiving isoniazid should also be given pyridoxine. (See Cautions: Nervous System Effects.) Because the risk of tuberculosis appears to be increased in patients with HIV infection, and the association between tuberculosis and AIDS is most evident in IV drug abusers, attempts should be made to identify IV drug abusers who have a significant reaction to the Mantoux tuberculin skin test and to initiate isoniazid treatment of latent tuberculosis infection in such individuals regardless of their age.

The CDC states that HIV-infected patients with a history of prior untreated or inadequately treated tuberculosis that healed who have no history of adequate treatment for tuberculosis should receive therapy for latent tuberculosis infection regardless of their age or the results of tuberculin skin tests.

- **Close contacts of individuals with recently diagnosed clinical tuberculosis.** Contacts of individuals with infectious pulmonary tuberculosis who have a standard Mantoux tuberculin skin test induration reaction of 5 mm or more (significant reaction) and do not have a history of significant reactions in the past should be considered as recently infected and should, regardless of age, receive therapy for latent tuberculosis infection. The AAP states that regardless of the results of tuberculin skin testing, therapy for latent tuberculosis infection should be given to individuals exposed within the previous 3 months to a potentially contagious case of tuberculosis, especially contacts of immunologically impaired (e.g., HIV-infected) individuals and all household contacts younger than 4 years of age who are exposed to any adult with active tuberculosis, once clinical disease has been ruled out. The ATS and CDC state that children younger than 5 years of age should be treated for latent tuberculosis infection regardless of their tuberculin skin test results because of their susceptibility to severe disease. Recent contacts and household contacts of any age, particularly if they are from a population with a high prevalence of tuberculosis, also should receive treatment for latent tuberculosis infection even in the absence of a significant tuberculin test result. These contacts should be tested again 8–12 weeks after the last exposure to the infectious source and if they still have an insignificant reaction and exposure has ended, therapy may be discontinued.

The ATS, CDC, and AAP state that management of a neonate whose mother or other household contact has tuberculosis should be individualized. In an infant whose mother or other household contact has a significant reaction to the Mantoux tuberculin skin test and no evidence of current tuberculosis, the ATS and CDC state that a Mantoux tuberculin test (5 TU/0.1 mL) should be administered at 4–6 weeks of age and again at 3–4 months of age. The AAP states that management of a neonate whose mother (or household contact) has latent or active tuberculosis is based on categorization of the infection. If the mother (or household contact) has a normal chest radiograph and is asymptomatic, the mother or contact usually is a candidate for treatment of latent tuberculosis infection; the infant needs no special evaluation or therapy and need not be separated from the mother. However, if the mother (or household contact) has an abnormal chest radiograph, the AAP advises that the mother or contact and infant be separated until the mother or contact has been evaluated for clinical tuberculosis and, if active tuberculosis is found, is receiving appropriate antituberculosis therapy. (See Tuberculosis During Pregnancy under General Principles in Antituberculosis Therapy: Initial Treatment of Tuberculosis, in Uses in the Antituberculosis Agents General Statement 8:16.04.) Evaluation of other members of the household or extended family to whom the infant may later be exposed also is indicated. When the family cannot be tested promptly, the ATS and CDC state that administration of isoniazid 10 mg/kg daily to the infant should be considered until skin testing of the family has excluded contact with a case of active tuberculosis; isoniazid treatment in the mother also should be considered.

In a neonate whose mother has current tuberculosis, the AAP recommends that the infant be evaluated for congenital tuberculosis and tested for HIV infection. A chest roentgenogram and Mantoux tuberculin test should be performed at 4–6 weeks of age; if the results of these tests are negative, the infant should be tested again at 3–4 months and at 6 months of age. The ATS, CDC, and AAP state that the infant should receive isoniazid even if the tuberculin skin test and chest roentgenogram do not suggest tuberculosis since cell-mediated immunity of a degree sufficient to mount a significant reaction to tuberculin skin testing may not develop until as late as 6 months of age in an infant infected at birth. Isoniazid can be discontinued if the results of a Mantoux skin test are negative at 6 months of age (or at 3–4 months of age according to the AAP) and active tuberculosis is not present in family members or if active disease is being treated and family members are no longer contagious. The infant should be examined at monthly intervals during treatment. If nonadherence to the antituberculosis regimen by the mother is documented, the mother has sputum cultures or smears positive for acid-fast bacilli, and supervision is impossible, the ATS, CDC, and AAP state that administration of BCG vaccine to the infant may be considered. (See Uses: Tuberculosis, in BCG Vaccine 80:12.) However, the ATS, CDC, and AAP state that response to the vaccine in infants may be delayed and inadequate to prevent tuberculosis disease.

In a neonate whose mother has hematogenous spread of tuberculosis (e.g., meningitis, miliary disease, bone involvement), congenital tuberculosis in the infant is possible. If the infant is suspected of having congenital tuberculosis, the AAP recommends that a Mantoux tuberculin skin test, chest radiograph, lumber puncture, and appropriate cultures should be performed promptly, and regardless of the skin test results, treatment of the infant should be initiated promptly. (See Neonates under Treatment of Active Tuberculosis: Active Tuberculosis in Pediatric Patients in the Antituberculosis Agents General Statement 8:16.04.) If clinical and roentgenographic findings do not support the diagnosis of congenital tuberculosis, the infant should be separated from the mother until she is judged to be noninfectious. If the diagnosis of congenital tuberculosis is excluded, the AAP states that isoniazid should be given until the infant is 3–4 months old; the skin test should be repeated following isoniazid therapy. If the skin test is positive, isoniazid should be continued for a total of at least 9 months in HIV-negative children or for 9–12 months in HIV-infected children.

- Individuals receiving organ (e.g., renal, cardiac) transplants or prolonged corticosteroid or other immunosuppressive therapy. Although the exact risk is unknown, individuals receiving prednisone in daily dosages of 15 mg or more (or its equivalent) for at least 1 month are at increased risk for reactivation of tuberculosis; risk increases with increasing dosage and duration of corticosteroid therapy. Such individuals should receive treatment for latent tuberculosis infection if they have tuberculin skin test reactions of 5 mm or greater. The ATS and CDC further state that immunosuppressed individuals, including those with HIV infection, who are contacts of those with active tuberculosis should receive treatment for latent tuberculosis infection even in the absence of a significant tuberculin skin test upon repeated testing.
- Individuals with pulmonary fibrotic changes on chest radiographs that are consistent with prior, healed tuberculosis. Such individuals reportedly have a risk for progression to active tuberculosis of 2–13.6 cases per 1000 patient-years of observation and should receive treatment for latent tuberculosis infection when they have tuberculin induration reactions of 5 mm or more.
- Individuals with an induration reaction of 10 mm or more to the standard Mantoux tuberculin skin test who have other clinical conditions associated with an increased risk of tuberculosis, including those with silicosis, hematologic and reticuloendothelial diseases such as leukemias or lymphomas (e.g., Hodgkin's disease), individuals who have diabetes mellitus or chronic renal failure, and individuals known to be seronegative for HIV who inject illicit drugs. Individuals with clinical situations associated with substantial, rapid weight loss (10% or more of body weight) or chronic undernutrition, including intestinal (jejunoileal) bypass surgery for obesity, gastrectomy, or carcinomas of the head or neck and lung, should also receive isoniazid preventive therapy if they have an induration reaction of 10 mm or more to the standard Mantoux tuberculin skin test.

In addition, individuals in the following high-incidence groups who have induration reactions of 10 mm or greater to the Mantoux tuberculin skin test should be considered candidates for treatment of latent tuberculosis infection even if they have none of the risk factors listed above:

- Recent immigrants (within the past 5 years) from countries with a high prevalence of tuberculosis (e.g., Latin America, Asia, Africa).
- Residents of facilities for long-term care (e.g., correctional institutions, nursing homes, mental institutions), hospitals and other health-care facilities, residential facilities for patients with acquired immunodeficiency syn-

drome [AIDS], homeless shelters). Staff of facilities (e.g., correctional institutions, nursing homes, mental institutions, other health-care facilities, schools, child-care facilities) in which an individual with current tuberculosis would pose a risk to large numbers of susceptible individuals and mycobacteriology laboratory personnel, also may be considered for therapy of latent tuberculosis infection.

- Children younger than 4 years of age or infants, children, and adolescents exposed to adults in high-risk categories. Some evidence suggests that untreated infants with latent tuberculosis infection have up to a 40% risk of developing tuberculosis; the risk for progression of infection to active disease gradually decreases throughout childhood. Isoniazid therapy for latent tuberculosis infection is more effective in reducing the risk of clinical tuberculosis in children than in adults, with reported risk reductions of 70–90% in clinical trials. Therefore, such therapy is recommended in children and adolescents who have tuberculin skin test reactions of 10 mm of induration or greater following exposure to adults at high risk for tuberculosis infection or disease.

The ATS and CDC state that routine tuberculin skin testing is not recommended for populations at low-risk for latent tuberculosis infection. However, if tuberculin testing is conducted in such individuals (e.g., at a work site in which risk of exposure to tuberculosis is anticipated and an ongoing testing program is in place), treatment for latent tuberculosis infection may be considered in those who have a tuberculin reaction (induration of 15 mm or greater) based on an individual assessment of risks and benefits.

Prior to initiation of isoniazid therapy for latent tuberculosis infection, patients should be screened to exclude from therapy those with clinical tuberculosis, those who have previously received adequate therapy or for latent or active tuberculosis, those with acute or unstable liver disease of any etiology, and those with a history of severe adverse reactions to isoniazid or other conditions that may necessitate special precautions or contraindicate use of the drug. (See Cautions and also see Drug Interactions.) Because of the risk of inducing isoniazid resistance if the drug is used alone in an individual with current tuberculosis, one of the recommended regimens for treatment of tuberculosis should be used until the diagnosis is clarified. (See General Principles of Antituberculosis Therapy in the Antituberculosis Agents General Statement 8:16.04.) If the evaluation confirms that the patient has latent (not active) tuberculosis, multiple-drug therapy may be discontinued after 4 months in adults or 6 months in children.

Isoniazid Monotherapy. The ATS and CDC currently recommend a 9-month daily isoniazid regimen or, alternatively, a 9-month twice-weekly isoniazid regimen for both HIV-infected and HIV-negative adults. A 9-month daily or twice-weekly isoniazid regimen also is recommended for treatment of latent tuberculosis in most infants and children; some experts recommend that isoniazid be given for 9–12 months in HIV-infected children with latent tuberculosis infection.

Although a 9-month regimen is preferred, the ATS and CDC state that a 6-month daily isoniazid regimen or, alternatively, a 6-month twice-weekly isoniazid regimen can be used in HIV-negative adults. The 6-month regimens provide substantial protection and may offer a more cost-effective outcome than the 9-month regimen based on individual decisions by health departments or other providers. However, 6-month regimens are not recommended for children, HIV-infected individuals, or individuals with radiographic evidence of prior tuberculosis.

Isoniazid treatment for latent tuberculosis infection has been given for 6–12 months. Regimens shorter than 6 months may not be effective. A large (about 28,000 individuals), controlled, 5-year follow-up study conducted by the Committee on Prophylaxis of the International Union against Tuberculosis (IUAT) showed that administration of isoniazid for 3 months to individuals with a positive tuberculin skin test reaction and with previously untreated, fibrotic, pulmonary lesions was no more effective than placebo in preventing tuberculosis during the 5-year follow-up period, whereas a 6-month regimen was more effective than placebo. Studies comparing various lengths of isoniazid therapy (e.g., 3–12 months) for treatment of latent tuberculosis infection in patients not known to be infected with HIV indicate that the optimal duration appears to be 9 months and that therapy for longer than 12 months does not provide additional benefit. Although the benefit of a 12-month regimen was better than placebo, overall it was not substantially better than the 6-month regimen, principally because of patient noncompliance during the last 6 months of therapy. Among individuals with good compliance during the entire 12 months, the 12-month regimen was substantially more effective in preventing tuberculosis among patients with small pulmonary lesions than the 6-month regimen. Similar levels of protection against tuberculosis disease have been observed with isoniazid therapy for latent infection regardless of the patient's HIV serostatus or whether the drug was given intermittently twice weekly rather than daily (for 6 months). Therefore, although the recommended duration of therapy for latent tuberculosis infection is 9 months, the ATS and CDC suggest that every effort should be made to ensure compliance with isoniazid preventive therapy for at least 6 months.

The ATS and CDC state that completion of therapy for latent tuberculosis infection is based on the total number of administered drug doses, not the duration of therapy alone. Interruptions in antituberculosis preventive therapy because of drug toxicity or other reasons should be considered when calculating the point at which such therapy is to be discontinued. Regimens in which isoniazid is given daily should consist of at least 270 doses administered within 12 months (allowing for interruptions in the usual 9-month regimen). The 6-month isoniazid regimen should consist of at least 180 doses given within 9 months. Isoniazid regimens in which the drug is given twice weekly should consist of at least 76 doses administered within 12 months (for the 9-month regimen) or at least 52 doses within 9 months (or the 6-month regimen). Reinstitution of therapy in patients whose treatment has been interrupted might require a continuation of the regimen originally prescribed (as long as needed to complete the recommended duration of the particular regimen) or a complete renewal of the regimen. In either situation, when therapy is resumed after an interruption of 2 months or longer, a medical examination is indicated to rule out tuberculosis disease.

All patients receiving an intermittent (twice-weekly) isoniazid regimen for the treatment of latent tuberculosis infection should receive directly observed therapy (DOT); the ATS and CDC state that when feasible, DOT also should be used in some special settings (e.g., some institutional settings, community outreach programs, household contacts of patients with tuberculosis who are receiving home-based DOT). AAP states that when the patient cannot be relied on to adhere to daily isoniazid therapy, the drug may be given twice weekly by directly observed therapy (DOT), preferably after 1 month of daily therapy.

Alternative Regimens. While isoniazid monotherapy generally is the regimen of choice for the treatment of latent tuberculosis infection, a 4-month regimen of daily rifampin monotherapy can be used as an alternative regimen in both HIV-positive and HIV-negative patients, especially when isoniazid cannot be used because of resistance or intolerance. (See Latent Tuberculosis Infection under Uses: Tuberculosis, in Rifampin 8:16.04.)

Limited data suggest that a short-course (e.g., 2-month) regimen consisting of rifampin and pyrazinamide given daily is effective in treating latent tuberculosis infection in HIV-infected patients, and the ATS and CDC state that the efficacy of this regimen is not expected to differ in HIV-negative patients. However, hepatotoxicity (including some fatalities) has been reported in patients receiving rifampin and pyrazinamide regimens for the treatment of *latent* tuberculosis and, although multiple-drug regimens containing rifampin and pyrazinamide are still recommended for the treatment of *active* tuberculosis, the ATS, CDC, and IDSA now state that regimens containing both rifampin and pyrazinamide generally should not be offered for the treatment of *latent* tuberculosis in either HIV-infected or HIV-negative individuals. (See Cautions: Hepatic Effects, in Rifampin 8:16.04.)

HIV-infected Individuals. Factors to consider in selecting the appropriate regimen for treatment of latent tuberculosis infection in HIV-infected individuals include the likelihood that the infecting organism is susceptible to isoniazid (isoniazid is the preferred agent for isoniazid-susceptible *M. tuberculosis*), the potential for drug interactions with rifampin in patients receiving HIV protease inhibitors or NNRTIs, and the possibility of severe liver injury with pyrazinamide-containing regimens. Choice of therapy requires consultation with public health authorities if the infecting organism is resistant to isoniazid and rifampin.

Recommendations for treatment of latent tuberculosis infection in HIV-infected adults generally are similar to those for HIV-negative adults; however, the 6-month isoniazid monotherapy regimen usually is not recommended and use of rifabutin monotherapy may be necessary instead of rifampin monotherapy if there are concerns about drug interactions with antiretroviral agents the patient may be receiving. The ATS and CDC recommend that HIV-infected adults and adolescents with latent *M. tuberculosis* infection receive a 9-month regimen of isoniazid given daily or twice weekly; a 4-month regimen of rifampin or rifabutin given daily; or a 2 to 3-month regimen of rifampin and pyrazinamide given daily (this regimen no longer recommended in most patients).

For HIV-infected infants and children, recommended regimens for the treatment of latent tuberculosis infection are a 9- to 12-month regimen of isoniazid given daily or twice weekly or a 4- to 6-month regimen of rifampin given daily.

Pregnant Women. For pregnant women who are at risk for progression of latent tuberculosis infection to active disease, particularly those who have HIV infection or have been infected recently, the ATS and CDC state that the initiation or discontinuance of therapy for latent tuberculosis infection should not be delayed on the basis of pregnancy alone, even during the first trimester. For women whose risk of active disease is lower, some experts recommend delaying treatment until after delivery. Patients with HIV infection or radiographic evidence of prior tuberculosis should receive 9 rather than 6 months of isoniazid therapy. The ATS and CDC state that some experts would use rifampin and pyrazinamide as an alternative regimen for treatment of latent tuberculosis infection in HIV-infected pregnant women, although pyrazinamide should be avoided during the first trimester. The ATS and CDC state that a regimen of isoniazid administered daily or twice weekly for 9 or 6 months is recommended in these pregnant women who do not have HIV infection.

Drug-Resistant Latent Tuberculosis Infection. In individuals likely to be infected with *M. tuberculosis* organisms that are resistant to both isoniazid and rifampin and are at high risk for developing tuberculosis, the ATS and CDC recommend regimens consisting of pyrazinamide and ethambutol or pyrazinamide and a quinolone anti-infective (e.g., levofloxacin or ofloxacin) for 6–12 months if the organisms from the index case are known to be susceptible to these drugs. Immunocompetent contacts may be managed by observation alone or be treated with such regimens for 6 months; immunosuppressed individuals, including those with HIV infection, should be treated for 12 months. Clinicians should review the drug-susceptibility pattern of the *M. tuberculosis* strain isolated from the infecting source-patient before selecting a regimen for treating potentially multidrug-resistant tuberculosis infections. In individuals likely to have been infected with *M. tuberculosis* organisms that are resistant to both isoniazid and rifampin, the choice of drugs used for treatment of latent infection requires expert consultation. Prior to initiation of therapy for latent tuberculosis infection in patients with suspected multidrug-resistant tuberculosis, careful assessment to rule out active disease is necessary.

The AAP states that, until susceptibility test results are available, both rifampin and isoniazid should be given to contacts who are likely to have been infected by an index case with isoniazid-resistant tuberculosis. If the index case is proven to be excreting organisms that are completely resistant to isoniazid, isoniazid should be discontinued and rifampin given for a total of at least 6 months. The AAP recommends consultation with an expert in making decisions about therapy for latent tuberculosis infection in children with isoniazid and/or rifampin-resistant *M. tuberculosis*.

Dosage and Administration

■ **Administration** Isoniazid usually is administered orally. The drug may be given by IM injection when oral therapy is not possible.

The fixed-combination preparation containing isoniazid and rifampin (Rifamate®) and the fixed-combination preparation containing isoniazid, rifampin, and pyrazinamide (Rifater®) should be given either 1 hour before or 2 hours after a meal; the manufacturer states that Rifater® should be given with a full glass of water.

■ **Dosage** Oral and IM dosages of isoniazid are identical.

Active Tuberculosis In the treatment of clinical tuberculosis, isoniazid should not be given alone. The drug is considered a first-line agent for the treatment of all forms of tuberculosis. Therapy for tuberculosis should be continued long enough to prevent relapse. The minimum duration of treatment currently recommended for patients with culture-positive pulmonary tuberculosis is 6 months (26 weeks), and recommended regimens consist of an initial intensive phase (2 months) and a continuation phase (usually either 4 or 7 months). However, the American Thoracic Society (ATS), US Centers for Disease Control and Prevention (CDC), and the Infectious Diseases Society of America (IDSA) state that completion of treatment is determined more accurately by the total number of doses and should not be based solely on the duration of therapy. For information on general principles of antituberculosis therapy and recommendations regarding specific multiple-drug regimens and duration of therapy, see the Antituberculosis Agents General Statement 8:16.04.

Adult Dosage. The ATS, CDC, and IDSA recommend that when isoniazid is used in conjunction with other antituberculosis agents in a daily regimen, adults and children 15 years of age or older should receive an isoniazid dosage of 5 mg/kg (up to 300 mg) once daily.

When an intermittent multiple-drug regimen is used for the treatment of tuberculosis, the ATS, CDC, and IDSA recommend that adults and children 15 years of age or older receive isoniazid in a dosage 15 mg/kg (up to 900 mg) once, twice, or 3 times weekly.

Pediatric Dosage. Infants and children tolerate larger doses of isoniazid than do adults and may be given isoniazid in a dosage up to 10–20 mg/kg once daily, depending on the severity of the disease. The maximum dosage of isoniazid recommended by the manufacturers for children is 300–500 mg daily.

The ATS, CDC, IDSA, and American Academy of Pediatrics (AAP) recommend that when isoniazid is used in daily multiple-drug regimens in pediatric patients, an isoniazid dosage of 10–15 mg/kg (up to 300 mg) daily should be used. The AAP cautions that use of an isoniazid dosage exceeding 10 mg/kg daily in conjunction with rifampin may increase the incidence of hepatotoxicity.

When an intermittent multiple-drug regimen is used for the treatment of tuberculosis in pediatric patients, the ATS, CDC, IDSA, and AAP recommend an isoniazid dosage of 20–30 mg/kg (up to 900 mg) twice weekly.

Fixed-Combination Preparations. When isoniazid is administered as the fixed combination containing isoniazid and rifampin (Rifamate®) as part of a multiple-drug regimen for the treatment of pulmonary tuberculosis, the usual adult dosage of Rifamate® is 2 capsules (600 mg of rifampin and 300 mg of isoniazid) once daily. Although the fixed-combination preparation was formulated for daily regimens, the ATS, CDC, and IDSA state that Rifamate® can be used in twice-weekly regimens† provided additional isoniazid is administered concomitantly. When used in an intermittent multiple-drug regimen, these experts state that 2 capsules of Rifamate® (600 mg of rifampin and 300 mg of isoniazid) and an additional 600 mg of isoniazid (i.e., 900 mg of isoniazid total) may be given twice weekly using directly observed therapy (DOT). The manufacturer states that Rifamate® should *not* be used for the initial treatment of tuberculosis and should only be used after efficacy of the rifampin and isoniazid dosages contained in the fixed-combination preparation has been established by titrating the individual components in the patient.

When isoniazid is administered as the fixed combination containing isoniazid, rifampin, and pyrazinamide (Rifater®) in the initial phase (e.g., initial 2 months) of multiple-drug therapy for pulmonary tuberculosis, the manufacturer states that the adult dosage of Rifater® given as a single daily dose is 4 tablets (480 mg of rifampin, 200 mg of isoniazid, 1.2 g of pyrazinamide) in patients weighing 44 kg or less, 5 tablets (600 mg of rifampin, 250 mg of isoniazid, and 1.5 g of pyrazinamide) in those weighing 45–54 kg, and 6 tablets (720 mg of rifampin, 300 mg of isoniazid, 1.8 g of pyrazinamide) in patients weighing 55 kg or more. In individuals weighing more than 90 kg, additional pyrazinamide may need to be given in conjunction with the fixed-combination preparation to obtain an adequate dosage of this drug. The ratio of rifampin, isoniazid, and pyrazinamide in Rifater® may not be appropriate in children or adolescents under the age of 15 because of the higher mg/kg doses of isoniazid usually given in children compared with those given in adults.

Latent Tuberculosis Infection For treatment of latent tuberculosis infection, isoniazid usually is given as the sole antituberculosis drug for a minimum of 6 months. Every effort should be made to assure compliance for at least 6 months, since preventive therapy of shorter duration appears to provide little benefit. If drug administration cannot be directly observed, the use of spot testing of urine for isoniazid metabolites has been recommended for assessing compliance. The ATS and CDC currently recommend a 9-month daily isoniazid regimen or, alternatively, a 9-month twice-weekly isoniazid regimen for adults regardless of HIV infection status. Continuing isoniazid therapy for latent tuberculosis infection for longer than 12 months provides no additional benefit. It also is recommended that isoniazid therapy for latent tuberculosis infection be continued for 9–12 months in HIV-infected infants and children. The ATS and CDC state that completion of therapy for latent tuberculosis infection is determined more accurately by the total number of doses and should not be based solely on the duration of therapy. The 9-month daily isoniazid regimen should consist of at least 270 doses administered within 12 months (allowing for interruptions in the usual 9-month regimen) and the 6-month daily isoniazid regimen should consist of at least 180 doses given within 9 months. Isoniazid regimens in which the drug is given twice weekly should consist of at least 76 doses administered within 12 months (for the 9-month regimen) or at least 52 doses within 9 months (for the 6-month regimen). (See Latent Tuberculosis Infection under Uses: Tuberculosis.)

Adult Dosage. The usual adult dosage of isoniazid for treatment of latent tuberculosis infection is 5 mg/kg (up to 300 mg) once daily. If daily supervision is not possible in high-risk individuals who are likely to be noncompliant (e.g., the homeless, inmates of correctional facilities), the ATS and CDC recommend that a twice-weekly isoniazid regimen with direct supervision be used as an alternative to the preferred daily regimen; if this twice-weekly regimen is used, isoniazid is given in a dosage of 15 mg/kg (up to 900 mg) twice weekly.

Pediatric Dosage. For treatment of latent tuberculosis infection in infants and children, the ATS and CDC recommend an isoniazid dosage of 10–20 mg/kg (up to 300 mg) daily. The AAP and others recommend a pediatric isoniazid dosage of 10–15 mg/kg (up to 300 mg) daily. When compliance with the daily regimen cannot be assured, the ATS and CDC suggest that children may receive 20–40 mg/kg (up to 900 mg) twice weekly. The AAP and others suggest that, when an intermittent regimen is used, children should receive 20–30 mg/kg (up to 900 mg) of isoniazid twice weekly (under supervised administration) for 9 months, preferably after completion of 1 month of daily isoniazid therapy.

Cautions

■ **Nervous System Effects** Peripheral neuritis, usually preceded by paresthesia of the feet and hands, is the most common adverse effect of isoniazid and occurs most frequently in malnourished patients and those predisposed to neuritis (e.g., alcoholics, diabetics). Rarely, other adverse nervous system effects have also occurred including seizures, toxic encephalopathy, muscle twitching, ataxia, stupor, tinnitus, euphoria, memory impairment, separation of ideas and reality, loss of self-control, dizziness, and toxic psychosis. Neurotoxic effects may be prevented or relieved by the administration of 10–50 mg of pyridoxine hydrochloride daily during isoniazid therapy, and pyridoxine should be administered in malnourished patients, pregnant women, and those predisposed to neuritis (e.g., HIV-infected individuals). In addition, optic neuritis and atrophy have been reported with isoniazid.

■ **Hepatic Effects** Mild hepatic dysfunction, as evidenced by mild and transient increases in serum AST (SGOT), ALT (SGPT), and bilirubin concentrations, has occurred in approximately 10–20% of patients receiving isoniazid, usually during the first 4–6 months of therapy. In most cases, enzyme concentrations return to pretreatment values despite continuation of isoniazid, but progressive liver dysfunction, bilirubinuria, jaundice, and severe and sometimes fatal hepatitis have occurred rarely. The incidence of isoniazid-associated hepatitis is lowest in patients younger than 20 years of age and greatest in daily users of alcohol and patients 35 years of age or older. The American Academy of Pediatrics (AAP) states that the incidence of hepatitis during isoniazid therapy in otherwise healthy infants, children, and adolescents is rare and that routine determination of serum aminotransferase concentrations are not recommended. (See Cautions: Precautions and Contraindications.) The manufacturers state that progressive liver damage may occur in up to 2.3% of patients older than 50 years of age who receive isoniazid. However, data from one study suggest that hepatitis occurs in approximately 4.5% of patients older than 65 years of age who receive the drug. If symptoms of hepatitis or signs suggestive of hepatic damage occur during isoniazid therapy, the drug should be discontinued promptly. (See Cautions: Precautions and Contraindications.)

■ **Sensitivity Reactions** Hypersensitivity reactions, including fever, skin eruptions (morbilliform, maculopapular, purpuric, or exfoliative), lymphadenopathy, vasculitis, and, rarely, hypotension, have occurred rarely with isoniazid, usually 3–7 weeks following initiation of therapy. At the first sign of a hypersensitivity reaction, all drugs should be discontinued. If isoniazid is reinstituted, the drug should be restarted in small and gradually increasing doses only after symptoms have cleared. If there is any indication of recurrence of hypersensitivity, isoniazid should be discontinued immediately.

■ **Hematologic Effects** Adverse hematologic effects, including agranulocytosis, eosinophilia, thrombocytopenia, methemoglobinemia, and hemolytic, sideroblastic, or aplastic anemia, have occurred in patients receiving isoniazid.

■ **Other Adverse Effects** Other reported adverse effects of isoniazid include nausea, vomiting, epigastric distress, dryness of the mouth, pyridoxine deficiency, pellagra, hyperglycemia, metabolic acidosis, and urinary retention and gynecomastia in males. A systemic lupus erythematosus-like syndrome and a rheumatic syndrome with arthralgia have also occurred. IM administration of isoniazid has caused irritation at the site of injection.

■ **Precautions and Contraindications** Liver function tests should be performed periodically in patients receiving isoniazid. In addition, patients should be questioned monthly for signs and symptoms of liver disease and should be instructed to report to their physician any of the prodromal symptoms of hepatitis (e.g., persistent fatigue, weakness or fever exceeding 3 days, malaise, nausea, vomiting, unexplained anorexia). If these symptoms appear or if signs suggestive of hepatic damage occur, isoniazid should be discontinued promptly, since continued use of the drug in these patients has been reported to cause a more severe form of liver damage. Some clinicians recommend discontinuing isoniazid therapy if serum aminotransferase concentrations are more than 3–5 times higher than the upper limit of the normal range or if patients develop manifestations of hepatitis. Patients who have had signs or symptoms of hepatic damage during isoniazid therapy generally should receive alternative antituberculosis agents, but if isoniazid must be reinstituted, the drug should be restarted only after hepatic symptoms and laboratory abnormalities have cleared. Isoniazid should be restarted in very small and gradually increasing dosages and should be discontinued immediately if there is any indication of recurrent liver involvement.

The AAP states that the incidence of hepatitis during isoniazid therapy in children is rare and that routine determination of serum aminotransferase concentrations is not recommended. However, liver function tests should be monitored approximately monthly during the first several months of treatment in children with severe tuberculosis, especially meningitis and disseminated disease. The AAP states that monitoring of liver function tests should also be performed in patients with concurrent or recent liver disease, those receiving a high daily dose of isoniazid (more than 10 mg/kg daily) in combination with rifampin and/or pyrazinamide, those who are pregnant or within 6 weeks postpartum, those with clinical evidence of hepatotoxicity, and those with hepatobiliary tract disease from other causes, and those receiving other hepatotoxic drugs concomitantly (especially anticonvulsants). In most other patients, monthly clinical evaluations for 3 months, followed by evaluation every 1–3 months to observe for manifestations of hepatitis or other adverse effects of drug therapy, is appropriate.

Isoniazid should be used with caution in daily users of alcohol, individuals who inject illicit drugs, patients with chronic liver disease or severe renal impairment, and those with a history of prior therapy in whom isoniazid was discontinued because of adverse effects (e.g., headache, dizziness, nausea) possibly, but not definitely, related to the drug. Minor dosage adjustments may be necessary in patients with severe renal impairment. Limited data based on a retrospective analysis of isoniazid-associated hepatitis deaths suggest that the risk of fatal hepatitis associated with the drug may be increased in women, particularly black and Hispanic women, and during the postpartum period.

Periodic ophthalmologic examinations should be performed in patients who develop visual symptoms while receiving the drug. The manufacturers recommend that ophthalmologic examinations (including ophthalmoscopy) be performed prior to initiation of isoniazid therapy and periodically during therapy with the drug, even without the occurrence of visual symptoms; however, some clinicians question the necessity of this precaution.

Isoniazid should be used with caution in patients who are malnourished or predisposed to neuropathy (e.g., diabetics, alcoholics), and pyridoxine generally should be administered concomitantly. (See Cautions: Nervous System Effects.) The American Academy of Pediatrics (AAP) recommends concomitant pyridoxine therapy in children and adolescents who have an abnormally low milk and meat intake, in those with nutritional deficiencies (including all symptomatic HIV-infected children), in breast-feeding infants and their mothers, and pregnant women.

Isoniazid is contraindicated in patients with acute liver disease or a history of previous isoniazid-associated hepatic injury. Isoniazid preventive therapy should be deferred in patients with acute liver disease; however, the ATS and CDC state that seropositivity for hepatitis B surface antigen is not in itself a contraindication for such therapy. Isoniazid is also contraindicated in patients with a history of severe adverse reactions to the drug, including severe hypersensitivity reactions or drug fever, chills, and arthritis.

■ **Carcinogenicity** Isoniazid has been reported to induce pulmonary tumors in animals; however, there is no evidence to date to support carcinogenic effects in humans.

■ **Pregnancy and Lactation** No isoniazid-related congenital abnormalities have been observed in mammalian reproductive studies; however, it has been reported that isoniazid may exert an embryocidal effect when the drug is administered orally in pregnant rats and rabbits. Although safe use of the drugs during pregnancy has not been definitely established, isoniazid (combined with rifampin and/or ethambutol) has been used to treat clinical tuberculosis in pregnant women. The American Thoracic Society (ATS), US Centers for Disease Control and Prevention (CDC), and Infectious Diseases Society of America (IDSA) state that isoniazid is considered safe for use in pregnant women, but the risk of hepatitis may be increased in the peripartum period. The manufacturers state that the potential benefits of isoniazid therapy for latent tuberculosis infection during pregnancy should be weighed against the possible risks to the fetus. Use of antituberculosis agents for the treatment of latent tuberculosis infection in pregnant women is controversial. Some experts prefer to delay treatment until after delivery because pregnancy itself does not increase the risk for progression to disease and 2 studies suggest that there may be an increased risk of hepatotoxicity during pregnancy and the early postpartum period. However, the American Academy of Pediatrics (AAP) and other experts state that pregnant women who have positive tuberculin skin tests without evidence of clinical tuberculosis should receive therapy with isoniazid for latent tuberculosis infection if they are likely to have been infected recently or have high-risk medical conditions, especially human immunodeficiency virus (HIV) infection. The AAP recommends that such therapy begin after the first trimester.

If isoniazid is administered during pregnancy, concomitant administration of pyridoxine (25 mg daily) is recommended.

Because isoniazid crosses the placenta and is distributed into milk, neonates and breast-fed infants of isoniazid-treated mothers should be carefully observed for evidence of adverse effects.

Drug Interactions

■ **Antituberculosis Agents** There is some evidence that adverse nervous system effects of isoniazid, cycloserine, and ethionamide may be additive; therefore, isoniazid should be used with caution in patients receiving cycloserine or ethionamide.

Aminosalicylic acid appears to reduce the rate of acetylation of isoniazid; the effect is usually not clinically important.

Isoniazid inhibits multiplication of BCG; therefore BCG vaccine may not be effective if administered during therapy with the drug.

■ **Carbamazepine** Initiation of isoniazid therapy (200 or 300 mg daily) in patients receiving carbamazepine has resulted in increased serum concentrations of the anticonvulsant and symptoms of carbamazepine toxicity, including ataxia, headache, vomiting, blurred vision, drowsiness, and confusion. These symptoms of carbamazepine toxicity subsided either when carbamazepine dosage was decreased or when the antituberculosis agent was discontinued. This interaction presumably occurs because isoniazid inhibits hepatic metabolism of carbamazepine. In at least one patient, concomitant use of carbamazepine and isoniazid also appeared to increase the risk of isoniazid-induced hepatotoxicity, apparently because the anticonvulsant promoted the metabolism of isoniazid to its hepatotoxic metabolites. If carbamazepine and isoniazid are administered concomitantly, serum concentrations of the anticonvulsant should be closely monitored and the patient observed for evidence of carbamazepine toxicity; carbamazepine dosage should be decreased if necessary.

■ **Phenytoin** Isoniazid inhibits hepatic metabolism of phenytoin, resulting in increased plasma phenytoin concentrations and toxicity in some patients. Phenytoin toxicity occurs mainly in slow isoniazid inactivators and in patients receiving both isoniazid and aminosalicylic acid. Patients receiving isoniazid and phenytoin concurrently should be observed for evidence of phenytoin intoxication, and the dosage of the anticonvulsant should be reduced accordingly.

■ **Serotonergic Agents** Isoniazid appears to have some MAO-inhibiting activity. In addition, iproniazid, another antituberculosis agent structurally related to isoniazid that also possesses MAO-inhibiting activity, reportedly has resulted in serotonin syndrome in at least 2 patients when given in combination with meperidine. Pending further experience, clinicians should be aware of the potential for serotonin syndrome when isoniazid is given in combination with selective serotonin-reuptake inhibitor therapy or other serotonergic agents.

■ **Other Drugs** Aluminum hydroxide gel decreases GI absorption of isoniazid; isoniazid should be administered at least 1 hour before the antacid.

Coordination difficulties and psychotic episodes have occurred in patients receiving isoniazid and disulfiram concurrently, probably as a result of alterations in dopamine metabolism; concurrent administration of the drugs should be avoided.

Laboratory Test Interferences

■ **Tests for Urinary Glucose** Isoniazid reportedly causes false-positive results with cupric sulfate solution (Benedict's reagent and Clinitest®) for urine glucose determinations.

Acute Toxicity

■ **Manifestations** Overdosage of isoniazid has produced nausea, vomiting, dizziness, slurred speech, blurred vision, and visual hallucinations (including bright colors and strange designs). Symptoms of overdosage usually occur within 30 minutes to 3 hours following ingestion of the drug. After marked overdosage, respiratory distress and CNS depression, progressing rapidly from stupor to coma, severe intractable seizures, metabolic acidosis, acetonuria, and hyperglycemia have occurred. If untreated or treated inadequately, isoniazid overdosage may be fatal. Isoniazid-induced seizures are thought to be associated with decreased γ-aminobutyric acid (GABA) concentrations in the CNS, possibly resulting from inhibition by isoniazid of brain pyridoxal-5-phosphate activity.

■ **Treatment** In the management of isoniazid overdosage, an airway should be secured and adequate respiratory exchange established immediately. Seizures may be controlled with IV administration of diazepam or short-acting barbiturates and a dosage of pyridoxine hydrochloride equal to the amount of isoniazid ingested. Generally, 1–4 g of pyridoxine hydrochloride is given IV followed by 1 g IM every 30 minutes until the entire dose has been given. If seizures are controlled and overdosage is recent (within 2–3 hours), the stomach should be emptied by gastric lavage. Blood gases, serum electrolytes, glucose, and BUN determinations should be performed. Blood should be typed and cross-matched in case hemodialysis is required. IV sodium bicarbonate should be administered to control metabolic acidosis and repeated as needed; dosage should be adjusted on the basis of laboratory test results. Pyridoxine has also had a beneficial effect in correcting acidosis in some patients, possibly by controlling seizures and resulting lactic acidosis. Pyridoxine has been effective in treating isoniazid-induced seizures as well as other mental status changes associated with isoniazid overdosage. In several patients who remained comatose following initial treatment of seizures with diazepam and pyridoxine, administration of an additional 3- to 5-g dose of pyridoxine hydrochloride after 36–42 hours of coma resulted in complete awakening within 30 minutes. The fact that administration of high doses of pyridoxine can result in adverse neurologic effects should be considered whenever the drug is used in the treatment of isoniazid-induced seizures and/or coma.

Forced osmotic diuresis should be initiated as soon as possible following isoniazid overdosage to increase renal clearance of the drug and should be continued several hours after clinical improvement to ensure complete clearance of the drug and prevent relapse. Fluid intake and output should be monitored. In severe cases, hemodialysis or, if hemodialysis is not available, peritoneal dialysis should be used in conjunction with forced diuresis. In addition, measures should be taken to protect against hypoxia, hypotension, and aspiration pneumonitis.

Mechanism of Action

Isoniazid may be bacteriostatic or bactericidal in action, depending on the concentration of the drug attained at the site of infection and the susceptibility of the infecting organism. The exact mechanism of action of isoniazid has not been fully elucidated, but several mechanisms including interference with metabolism of bacterial proteins, nucleic acids, carbohydrates, and lipids have been proposed. One of the principal actions of the drug appears to be inhibition of mycolic acid synthesis in susceptible bacteria which results in loss of acid-fastness and disruption of the bacterial cell wall. Isoniazid is active against susceptible bacteria only when they are undergoing cell division. Susceptible bacteria may undergo 1 or 2 divisions before multiplication is arrested.

Spectrum

Isoniazid is a highly specific agent and is active only against organisms of the genus *Mycobacterium*. Isoniazid is active in vitro and in vivo against *M. tuberculosis*, *M. bovis*, and some strains of *M. kansasii*. In vitro, the minimum inhibitory concentration (MIC) for most susceptible mycobacteria is 0.02–0.2 mcg/mL in Lowenstein-Jensen media.

Resistance

Natural and acquired resistance to isoniazid have been demonstrated in vitro and in vivo in strains of *M. tuberculosis*. In vitro, resistance to isoniazid develops in a stepwise manner. The mechanism of resistance may be related to failure of the drug to penetrate or be taken up by the resistant bacteria. Resistant strains of initially susceptible bacteria develop rapidly if isoniazid is used alone in the treatment of clinical tuberculosis; however, development of resistance does not appear to be a major problem when the drug is used alone in preventive therapy. When isoniazid is combined with other antituberculosis agents in the treatment of clinical tuberculosis, emergence of resistant strains may be delayed or prevented.

Pharmacokinetics

■ **Absorption** Isoniazid is readily absorbed from the GI tract and from IM injection sites. When administered orally with food, the extent of absorption and peak plasma concentrations of the drug may be reduced. Following oral administration, peak plasma concentrations of the drug are attained within 1–2 hours. In general, plasma concentrations of the drug in rapid isoniazid inactivators are 20–50% of those in slow isoniazid inactivators. In one study in healthy fasting adults, plasma concentrations of isoniazid 6 hours after a single oral dose of 9 mg/kg averaged 4.5 mcg/mL in slow inactivators and 1 mcg/mL in rapid inactivators.

In a single-dose study in healthy fasting males, the extent of absorption (as measured by area under the plasma concentration-time curve) of isoniazid, rifampin, or pyrazinamide in dosages of 250 mg, 600 mg, or 1500 mg, respectively, was similar whether the drugs were administered individually as capsules (rifampin) and tablets (isoniazid and pyrazinamide) or as a fixed combination containing isoniazid 50 mg, rifampin 120 mg, and pyrazinamide 300 mg per tablet.

■ **Distribution** Isoniazid is distributed into all body tissues and fluids. CSF concentrations of the drug are reported to be 90–100% of concurrent plasma concentrations. Isoniazid is not substantially bound to plasma proteins. Isoniazid readily crosses the placenta. Isoniazid is distributed into milk in concentrations approximately equal to maternal plasma concentrations.

■ **Elimination** The plasma half-life of isoniazid in patients with normal renal and hepatic function ranges from 1–4 hours, depending on the rate of metabolism. The plasma half-life may be prolonged in patients with impaired hepatic function or severe renal impairment.

Isoniazid is inactivated in the liver, mainly by acetylation and dehydrazination. Metabolites of the drug include acetylisoniazid, isonicotinic acid, monoacetylhydrazine, diacetylhydrazine, and isonicotinyl glycine. The rate of acetylation is genetically determined and is subject to individual variation; however, it is usually constant for each person. Slow inactivation is an autosomal recessive trait and results from a relative deficiency of the hepatic enzyme *N*-acetyltransferase. Approximately 50% of whites and blacks are slow inactivators of isoniazid; the majority of native Alaskans, Japanese, and Chinese are rapid inactivators. Although more than 80% of native Alaskans, Japanese, and Chinese are rapid inactivators, some 30–50% overall would be homozygous rapid inactivators and the remaining would be heterozygous intermediate rapid inactivators.

The rate of isoniazid acetylation does not appear to alter efficacy when the drug is administered daily or 2 or 3 times weekly; however, a relationship between rapid inactivation and poor therapeutic response has been noted in once-weekly intermittent regimens.

Acetylation of acetylisoniazid results in the formation of monoacetylhydrazine which has been shown to be a potent hepatotoxin in animals. Microsomal metabolism of monoacetylhydrazine in animals results in production of a reactive acylating species capable of covalently binding with tissue macromolecules (i.e., liver protein) and subsequently causing hepatic necrosis. Although attempts have been made to correlate acetylator phenotype with risk of isoniazid-induced hepatotoxicity, published reports are equivocal, with some showing an association with slow inactivators and others showing an association with rapid inactivators. It has been suggested that acetylator phenotype is probably not a major determinant of isoniazid-induced hepatotoxicity, since the rate of acetylation of toxic monoacetylhydrazine to nontoxic diacetylhydrazine is also determined by acetylator phenotype. Thus, although rapid inactivators form more monoacetylhydrazine, they also inactivate it more rapidly.

In adults with normal renal function, approximately 75–96% of a 5-mg/kg oral dose of isoniazid is excreted in urine within 24 hours as unchanged drug and metabolites. Small amounts of the drug are also excreted in saliva, sputum, and feces. Isoniazid is removed by hemodialysis or peritoneal dialysis.

Chemistry and Stability

■ **Chemistry** Isoniazid is a synthetic, isonicotinic acid-derivative antituberculosis agent. The drug occurs as colorless or white crystals or as a white, crystalline powder and has solubilities of approximately 125 mg/mL in water and 20 mg/mL in alcohol at 25°C. Isoniazid injection is a clear, colorless to faintly greenish-yellow liquid; sodium hydroxide and/or hydrochloric acid may have been added during manufacture to adjust the pH to 6–7.

Oral isoniazid is commercially available alone, in fixed combination with rifampin, and in fixed combination with rifampin and pyrazinamide.

■ **Stability** Isoniazid preparations should be protected from light, air, and excessive heat. Isoniazid tablets should be stored in well-closed, light-resistant containers at a temperature less than 40°C, preferably between 15–30°C. Tablets containing the fixed combination of rifampin, isoniazid, and pyrazinamide (Rifater®) should be protected from excessive humidity and stored at 15–30°C.

Isoniazid injection should be protected from light and stored at a temperature less than 40°C, preferably between 15–30°C; freezing should be avoided. At low temperatures, isoniazid in solution tends to crystallize, and the injection should be warmed to room temperature to redissolve the crystals prior to use.

Preparations

Excipients in commercially available drug preparations may have clinically important effects in some individuals; consult specific product labeling for details.

Isoniazid

Powder*		
Oral		
Solution	50 mg/5 mL*	**Isoniazid Syrup**
Tablets	100 mg*	**Isoniazid Tablets**
	300 mg*	**Isoniazid Tablets**
Parenteral		
Injection	100 mg/mL*	**Isoniazid Injection**
		Nydrazid®, Sandoz

*available from one or more manufacturer, distributor, and/or repackager by generic (nonproprietary) name

Isoniazid Combinations

Oral		
Capsules	150 mg with Rifampin 300 mg*	**Isoniazid and Rifampin Capsules**
		Rifamate®, Sanofi-Aventis
Tablets	50 mg with Pyrazinamide 300 mg and Rifampin 120 mg	**Rifater®**, Sanofi-Aventis

*available from one or more manufacturer, distributor, and/or repackager by generic (nonproprietary) name

†Use is not currently included in the labeling approved by the US Food and Drug Administration

Selected Revisions January 2009,

Rifabutin

■ Rifabutin, a semisynthetic spiropiperidyl derivative of rifamycin S, is an ansamycin antibiotic that is an antimycobacterial agent.

Uses

■ **Mycobacterium avium Complex (MAC) Infections** ***Primary Prevention of Disseminated MAC Infection*** Rifabutin is used alone or in conjunction with azithromycin to prevent or delay the development of *Mycobacterium avium* complex (MAC) bacteremia and disseminated infections (*primary prophylaxis*) in patients with advanced human immunodeficiency virus (HIV) infection; rifabutin is designated an orphan drug by the US Food and Drug Administration (FDA) for this use. Prevention of disseminated MAC disease is an important goal in the management of patients with HIV infection and low helper/inducer ($CD4^+$, $T4^+$) T-cell counts because of the frequency with which the disease occurs in such patients and its associated morbidity. Current evidence indicates that MAC causes disseminated disease in a substantial proportion of HIV-infected patients and that prophylaxis with rifabutin, alone or combined with azithromycin, can reduce substantially the frequency of *M. avium* complex bacteremia and ameliorate clinical manifestations of the disease in patients with AIDS. Azithromycin or clarithromycin also is used alone to prevent disseminated MAC infection in HIV-infected patients. (See the sections on Primary Prevention of Disseminated MAC Infection, under Mycobacterium avium Complex (MAC) Infections, in Uses in Azithromycin 8:12.12.92 and Clarithromycin 8:12.12.92.) Prophylaxis with rifabutin or clarithromycin has been shown to improve survival in patients with advanced HIV infection. (See Primary Prevention of Disseminated MAC Infection, under Management of Other Mycobacterial Diseases: Mycobacterium avium Complex (MAC) Infections, in the Antituberculosis Agents General Statement 8:16.04.)

In controlled studies, patients with AIDS who received primary prophylaxis with rifabutin were one-half to one-third as likely to develop MAC bacteremia and its clinical manifestations as those receiving placebo. In 2 placebo-controlled studies in patients with AIDS whose $CD4^+$ T-cell counts were 200/mm^3 or less, MAC bacteremia occurred in 9–13% of patients receiving rifabutin prophylaxis compared with 22–28% of those receiving placebo. In addition, patients given the drug demonstrated fewer manifestations of disseminated MAC infection, including fever, night sweats, weight loss, fatigue, abdominal pain, anemia, and hepatic abnormalities. Most cases of therapeutic failure (e.g., development of MAC bacteremia despite rifabutin prophylaxis) occurred in patients whose $CD4^+$ T-cell count was 100/mm^3 or less on enrollment into the study. Although mortality rates in the individual studies were not significantly reduced with rifabutin prophylaxis, an analysis of the combined double-blind and open follow-up periods of these studies indicated that prophylaxis with the drug was associated with improved survival over a period of approximately 700 days of follow-up.

Rifabutin also has been used in conjunction with azithromycin for the prevention of disseminated infection caused by MAC in patients with advanced HIV infection. In a randomized, comparative study in patients with advanced HIV infection ($CD4^+$ T-cell counts less than 100/mm^3), prophylaxis with rifabutin (300 mg daily), azithromycin (1.2 g once weekly), or both drugs concomitantly was associated with a cumulative incidence of MAC infection at 1 year of 15.3, 7.6, or 2.8%, respectively. The risk of MAC infection (after adjustment for baseline $CD4^+$ counts) in patients receiving azithromycin prophylaxis was 47% lower than that with rifabutin prophylaxis, while prophylaxis with both drugs reduced the risk by 72% compared with rifabutin alone; survival among the 3 groups was similar. Although the overall incidence of adverse effects was similar among the 3 groups (i.e., 76, 86, or 90% of patients receiving rifabutin, azithromycin, or combined rifabutin-azithromycin prophylaxis, respectively), dose-limiting adverse effects (principally GI effects) occurred more frequently with combined azithromycin-rifabutin prophylaxis than with rifabutin or azithromycin alone. (See Primary Prevention of Disseminated Mycobacterium avium Complex (MAC) infection, in Uses in Azithromycin 8:12.12.92.)

Current evidence suggests that primary prophylaxis against disseminated MAC infection is superior to efforts aimed at early detection and treatment of the disease in terms of survival benefit. The Prevention of Opportunistic Infections Working Group of the US Public Health Service and the Infectious Diseases Society of America (USPHS/IDSA) currently recommends that primary prophylaxis against MAC disease be given to HIV-infected adults and adolescents (13 years of age or older) whose $CD4^+$ counts are less than 50/mm^3. Severely immunocompromised HIV-infected children younger than 13 years of age also should receive primary prophylaxis against MAC disease according to the following age-specific $CD4^+$ T-cell counts: children 6–13 years of age, less than 50/mm^3; children 2–6 years of age, less than 75/mm^3; children 1–2 years of age, less than 500/mm^3; and children younger than 1 year of age, less than 750/mm^3. The USPHS/IDSA currently states that clarithromycin or azithromycin alone is the preferred regimen for primary prophylaxis; alternatively, if these drugs cannot be tolerated, rifabutin may be used alone. In selecting a prophylactic regimen, consideration should be given to the potential for clinically important interactions between rifabutin, macrolide antibiotics (e.g., azithromycin, clarithromycin), and other drugs commonly used in HIV-infected patients, including HIV protease inhibitors (e.g., amprenavir, indinavir, lopinavir, nelfinavir, ritonavir, saquinavir) and nonnucleoside reverse transcriptase inhibitors (e.g., delavirdine, efavirenz, nevirapine). (See Drug Interactions: Antiretroviral Agents, and also see Patients Receiving Concurrent Antiretroviral Therapy, under Initial Treatment of Active Tuberculosis: Tuberculosis in HIV-infected Patients, in the Antituberculosis Agents General Statement 8:16.04.) Although the combination of azithromycin and rifabutin is more effective than azithromycin alone, the USPHS/IDSA currently does not recommend routine prophylaxis with the combination because of additional cost, increased incidence of adverse effects, potential for drug interactions, and absence of a difference in survival in patients receiving the combination compared with azithromycin alone. In addition, the USPHS/IDSA states that the combination of clarithromycin and rifabutin should not be used for primary MAC prophylaxis since such combined therapy is no more effective than clarithromycin alone and is associated with a higher incidence of adverse effects.

Before MAC prophylaxis is initiated, patients should be assessed to ensure that they do not have active infection with MAC, *M. tuberculosis*, or other mycobacterial diseases. If such active disease is present, appropriate anti-infective *treatment* should be initiated. Preventive therapy with rifabutin should not be initiated in patients with active *M. tuberculosis* since administration of the drug as *sole* antimycobacterial therapy in such patients would likely lead to development of tuberculosis that is resistant to both rifabutin and rifampin. Patients who develop symptoms compatible with active tuberculosis while receiving rifabutin prophylaxis should be evaluated immediately and appropriate therapy instituted with an effective combination of antituberculosis agents.

Current evidence indicates that primary MAC prophylaxis can be discontinued with minimal risk of developing disseminated MAC disease in HIV-infected adults and adolescents who have responded to highly active antiretroviral therapy (HAART) with an increase in $CD4^+$ T-cell counts to greater than 100/mm^3 that has been sustained for at least 3 months. The USPHS/IDSA states that discontinuance of primary prophylaxis is recommended in adults and adolescents meeting these criteria because prophylaxis appears to add little benefit in terms of disease prevention for MAC or bacterial infections, and discontinuance reduces the medication burden, the potential for toxicity, drug interactions, selection of drug-resistant pathogens, and cost. However, the USPHS/IDSA states that primary MAC prophylaxis should be restarted in adults and adolescents if $CD4^+$ T-cell counts decrease to less than 50–100/mm^3. (See Primary Prevention of Disseminated MAC Infection, under Management of Other Mycobacterial Diseases: Mycobacterium avium Complex (MAC) Infections, in the Antituberculosis Agents General Statement 8:16.04.)

Treatment and Secondary Prevention of Disseminated MAC Infection Rifabutin is designated an orphan drug by FDA for use in the treatment or prevention of recurrence of disseminated MAC infections†. For information on the use of rifabutin as a component of multiple-drug regimens for the *treatment or secondary prevention* of disseminated MAC infections, see Treatment or Secondary Prevention of Disseminated MAC Infection, under Management of Other Mycobacterial Diseases: Mycobacterium avium Complex (MAC) Infections, in the Antituberculosis Agents General Statement 8:16.04.

■ **Tuberculosis** ***Active Tuberculosis*** Rifabutin is used as an alternative to rifampin in multiple-drug regimens for the treatment of pulmonary tuberculosis†.

The American Thoracic Society (ATS), US Centers for Disease Control and Prevention (CDC), and Infectious Diseases Society of America (IDSA) currently recommend several possible multiple-drug regimens for the treatment of culture-positive pulmonary tuberculosis. These regimens have a minimum duration of 6 months (26 weeks), and consist of an initial intensive phase (2 months) and a continuation phase (usually either 4 or 7 months). Rifabutin is used as an alternative to rifampin and is considered a first-line antituberculosis agent for use in these regimens. The ATS, CDC, and IDSA state that use of rifabutin in the treatment of tuberculosis generally should be reserved for use in patients who cannot receive rifampin because of intolerance or because they are receiving other drugs (especially antiretroviral agents) that have a clinically important interaction with rifampin. For information on general principles used in the treatment of tuberculosis, see the Antituberculosis Agents General Statement 8:16.04.

Limited data in patients with previously untreated tuberculosis suggest that the efficacy of rifabutin in short-course (6–9-month) antituberculosis regimens compares favorably with that of rifampin in terms of bacteriologic conversion of sputum cultures and clinical improvement. Results of uncontrolled studies in a limited number of patients also suggest that rifabutin may provide some benefit in patients with multidrug-resistant pulmonary tuberculosis†, including those whose disease is resistant to rifampin and/or isoniazid. Additional well-controlled clinical trials are needed to confirm the efficacy of rifabutin for infections in patients with rifampin-resistant strains of *M. tuberculosis*.

HIV-infected Individuals. Data from a limited number of studies in patients with HIV infection and pulmonary tuberculosis also suggest similar efficacy and safety of short-course (6-month) antituberculosis regimens containing either rifampin or rifabutin in conjunction with isoniazid, ethambutol, and pyrazinamide. However, there is evidence that use of antituberculosis regimens that include once- or twice-weekly administration of rifamycins (e.g., rifabutin, rifampin, rifapentine) in HIV-infected patients with CD4+ T-cell counts less than 100/mm^3 is associated with an increased risk of acquired rifamycin resistance. Therefore, until additional data are available regarding this issue, the CDC recommends that HIV-infected individuals with CD4+ T-cell counts less than 100/mm^3 not receive rifamycin regimens for the treatment of active tuberculosis that involve once- or twice-weekly administration. These individuals should receive daily therapy during the initial phase, and daily or 3-times weekly regimens during the second phase; directly observed therapy also is recommended for both the daily and 3-times weekly regimens.

The fact that concomitant use of rifamycins and certain antiretroviral agents (e.g., HIV protease inhibitors, nonnucleoside reverse transcriptase inhibitors [NNRTIs]) can affect plasma concentrations of the antituberculosis agent and/or the antiretroviral agents must be considered when antituberculosis therapy is indicated for the treatment tuberculosis in HIV-infected patients. Because of the pharmacokinetic interactions between rifamycins and HIV protease inhibitors or NNRTIs and because rifabutin is a less potent inducer of cytochrome P-450 (CYP) isoenzymes than rifampin, the CDC and other experts previously stated that use of rifampin was contraindicated in patients receiving HIV protease inhibitors or NNRTIs and that use of rifabutin-containing regimens was the preferred alternative for the treatment of active tuberculosis in HIV-infected patients receiving these antiretroviral agents. However, the CDC and some experts now suggest that there are specific circumstances when HIV-infected patients with active tuberculosis can receive rifampin concomitantly with certain HIV protease inhibitors or certain NNRTIs. Rifampin can be used in patients receiving the following antiretroviral regimens (with appropriate dosage adjustments): efavirenz and 2 nucleoside reverse transcriptase inhibitors; ritonavir and 1 or 2 nucleoside reverse transcriptase inhibitors; or an antiretroviral regimen that includes both ritonavir and saquinavir. Rifabutin-containing regimens (with appropriate dosage adjustments) offer an alternative for HIV-infected patients receiving these and other antiretroviral regimens. Some advantages of rifabutin-containing antituberculosis regimens in HIV-infected patients include (1) less potential for drug interactions with drugs commonly prescribed in such patients (e.g., protease inhibitors, nonnucleoside reverse transcriptase inhibitors [NNRTIs], azole antifungal drugs, anticonvulsants, methadone), (2) potentially more reliable absorption in patients with advanced HIV disease, and (3) more tolerability in patients with rifampin-induced hepatotoxicity. (See Patients Receiving Concurrent Antiretroviral Therapy under Initial Treatment of Active Tuberculosis: Tuberculosis in HIV-Infected Patients, in the Antituberculosis Agents General Statement 8:16.04.)

Latent Tuberculosis Infection Rifabutin (with appropriate dosage adjustments) is used alone in a 4-month regimen or in conjunction with pyrazinamide in a 2- to 3-month regimen to *prevent* the development of clinical tuberculosis† in HIV-infected adults and adolescents. Previously, "preventive therapy" or "chemoprophylaxis" was used to describe a simple drug regimen (e.g., isoniazid monotherapy) used to prevent the development of active tuberculosis disease in individuals known or likely to be infected with *M. tuberculosis*. However, since use of such a regimen rarely results in true primary prevention (i.e., prevention of *infection* in individuals exposed to infectious tuberculosis), the ATS and CDC currently state that "treatment of latent tuberculosis infection" rather than "preventive therapy" more accurately describes the intended intervention and potentially will result in greater understanding and more widespread implementation of this tuberculosis control strategy. (See Uses: Treatment of Latent Tuberculosis Infection, in Isoniazid 8:16.04.)

While therapy with rifabutin in tuberculin-positive patients with HIV infection has not been evaluated in clinical trials, the ATS and CDC state that the use of rifabutin in these short-course, multiple-drug regimens for treatment of latent tuberculosis infection is valid for the same scientific principles that support its use in the treatment of active tuberculosis. When use of rifabutin is being considered for the treatment of latent tuberculosis infection in HIV-infected patients, the possibility that drug regimens or dosages may have to be altered because of clinically important pharmacokinetic interactions between rifabutin and certain antiretroviral agents (e.g., HIV protease inhibitors, NNRTIs) should be considered. (See Drug Interactions: Antiretroviral Agents.)

Dosage and Administration

■ **Administration** Rifabutin is administered orally. Administration of rifabutin with a high-fat meal decreases the rate but not the extent of absorption. Therefore, the drug generally can be given orally without regard to meals.

■ **Dosage** ***Mycobacterium avium Complex (MAC) Infection*** The usual dosage of rifabutin for primary prevention of *M. avium* complex (MAC) infection in adults and adolescents with advanced HIV infection is 300 mg once daily. Rifabutin in this dosage may be administered alone or concomitantly with the recommended dosage of azithromycin (1200 mg once weekly) for MAC prophylaxis. In patients who have a propensity to develop nausea, vomiting, or other GI upset, rifabutin may be administered with food and the dosage given as 150 mg twice daily.

When indicated for the prevention of recurrence of disseminated MAC infection (secondary prophylaxis or maintenance therapy)†, the Prevention of Opportunistic Infections Working Group of the US Public health Service and the Infectious Diseases Society of America (USPHS/IDSA) states that HIV-infected adults and adolescents can receive rifabutin in a dosage of 300 mg once daily in conjunction with azithromycin (500 mg once daily) or clarithromycin (500 mg twice daily) and ethambutol (15 mg/kg once daily).

Steady-state pharmacokinetics of rifabutin are more variable in geriatric patients older than 70 years of age and in symptomatic HIV-infected patients than in younger or healthy individuals. However, the manufacturer makes no specific recommendations for dosage adjustment in such patients. Steady-state pharmacokinetics of the drug during early stages of symptomatic HIV infection reportedly are similar to those in healthy individuals.

The manufacturer states that safety and efficacy of rifabutin for MAC prophylaxis in children have not been established; however, rifabutin has been used in a limited number of children (concomitantly with other antimycobacterial agents) for the treatment of MAC infection without unusual adverse effect. Although rifabutin dosages averaging 18.5 mg/kg (up to 25 mg/kg) or 8.6 mg/kg (up to 18.6 mg/kg) daily have been used for active treatment in infants 1 year of age or children 2–10 years of age, respectively, the manufacturer states that there is no evidence that dosages exceeding 5 mg/kg daily are required for MAC infection. The USPHS/IDSA states that HIV-infected children 6 years of age or older may receive rifabutin in a dosage of 300 mg once daily for primary MAC prophylaxis† as an alternative to the regimen of choice (azithromycin or clarithromycin monotherapy). If rifabutin is used in conjunction with clarithromycin (or azithromycin) and ethambutol for secondary MAC prophylaxis† in children, the USPHS/IDSA recommends a rifabutin dosage of 5 mg/kg (maximum 300 mg) once daily in conjunction with azithromycin 5 mg/kg (maximum 250 mg) once daily and ethambutol 15 mg/kg (maximum 900 mg) once daily.

Active Tuberculosis In the treatment of clinical tuberculosis†, rifabutin should not be given alone. The drug is considered a first-line agent for use in multiple-drug regimens in patients with pulmonary tuberculosis who cannot receive rifampin because of intolerance or because they are receiving other drugs (especially antiretroviral agents) that have a clinically important interaction with rifampin. Therapy for tuberculosis should be continued long enough to prevent relapse. The minimum duration of treatment currently recommended for patients with culture-positive pulmonary tuberculosis is 6 months (26 weeks), and recommended regimens consist of an initial intensive phase (2 months) and a continuation phase (usually either 4 or 7 months). However, completion of treatment is determined more accurately by the total number of doses and is not based solely on the duration of therapy. For information on general principles of antituberculosis therapy and recommendations regarding specific multiple-drug regimens and duration of therapy, see the Antituberculosis Agents General Statement 8:16.04.

Adult Dosage. When rifabutin is used in conjunction with other antituberculosis agents for the treatment of tuberculosis, the American Thoracic Society (ATS), US Centers for Disease Control and Prevention (CDC), Infectious Diseases Society of America (IDSA), and others recommend that adults and children 15 years of age or older receive a dosage of 5 mg/kg (up to 300 mg) given once daily or 5 mg/kg (up to 300 mg) given 2 or 3 times weekly.

The fact that rifabutin dosage may need to be altered if the drug is used for the treatment of tuberculosis in HIV-infected individuals receiving certain antiretroviral agents (e.g., HIV protease inhibitors, nonnucleoside reverse transcriptase inhibitors) should be considered. (See Drug Interactions: Antiretroviral Agents.) In addition, because of concerns that there may be an increased risk of acquired rifamycin resistance in HIV-infected individuals with CD4+ T-cell counts less than 100/mm^3 who receive intermittent rifamycin regimens, the ATS, CDC, and IDSA recommend that rifabutin be administered once daily or 3-times weekly and that rifabutin regimens that involve once- or twice-weekly administration be avoided in these HIV-infected individuals pending further accumulation of data. The CDC also recommends directly observed therapy (DOT) for both the daily and 3-times weekly regimens. (See Initial Treatment of Tuberculosis: Tuberculosis in HIV-Infected Patients, under General Principles in Antituberculosis Therapy in the Antituberculosis Agents General Statement 8:16.04.)

Pediatric Dosage. The ATS, CDC, and IDSA state that the appropriate dosage of rifabutin for use in conjunction with other antituberculosis agents for the treatment of tuberculosis in children has not been identified. However, the CDC has stated that a rifabutin dosage of 10–20 mg/kg (up to 300 mg) can be given daily or twice weekly in conjunction with other antituberculosis agents for the treatment of tuberculosis in children with HIV infection†.

Latent Tuberculosis Infection If rifabutin is used as monotherapy for the treatment of latent tuberculosis infection† in HIV-infected adults and adolescents, the recommended rifabutin dosage is 300 mg once daily for 4 months; some experts recommend that rifabutin monotherapy be continued for 4–6 months in HIV-infected individuals. When rifabutin is used in conjunction with pyrazinamide for the treatment of latent tuberculosis infection in HIV-infected adults and adolescents, the usual dosage of rifabutin is 300 mg once daily for 2–3 months.

■ **Dosage in Renal Impairment** Rifabutin concentrations reportedly are decreased in patients with impaired renal function as a result of decreased distribution and more rapid elimination of the drug. However, the clinical importance, if any, of this finding has not been determined, and the manufacturer currently makes no specific recommendations for modification of dosage in such patients.

Cautions

Rifabutin generally was well tolerated in controlled clinical trials. The most common adverse effects, including those that most frequently result in discontinuance of the drug, are rash, GI intolerance, and neutropenia. In controlled clinical trials in patients with severe HIV infection, adverse effects severe enough to require discontinuance occurred in 16% of patients receiving rifabutin and 8% of those receiving placebo. There is some evidence that adverse effects of rifabutin may be dose related. Because most HIV-infected patients receiving rifabutin to date have had serious underlying disease with multiple baseline symptomatology and clinical abnormalities and because many adverse effects that occurred in rifabutin-treated patients also occurred in patients receiving placebo, many reported effects may not be directly attributable to rifabutin. Adverse effects were reported in 51% of patients receiving rifabutin and 50% of those receiving placebo in controlled clinical trials.

■ **Hematologic Effects** The most common adverse effect of rifabutin is neutropenia (absolute neutrophil count [ANC] less than 750/mm^3), which occurred in 25% of patients with severe HIV infection receiving the drug in controlled clinical trials. Neutropenia occurred substantially more frequently in patients receiving rifabutin than in those receiving placebo. Neutropenia resulted in discontinuance of rifabutin therapy in 2% of patients receiving the drug in controlled clinical trials. Leukopenia (white blood cell [WBC] count less than 1500/mm^3) was reported in 17% of patients, anemia (hemoglobin concentration less than 8 g/dL) in 6%, and thrombocytopenia (platelet count less than 50,000/mm^3) in 5% of patients receiving rifabutin in controlled clinical trials. Although the frequency of thrombocytopenia in rifabutin-treated patients was not substantially greater than in patients receiving placebo, rifabutin has been clearly associated with thrombocytopenia in rare cases. Eosinophilia occurred in 1% of patients receiving rifabutin in controlled clinical trials. Hemolysis was reported in less than 1% of patients. Thrombotic thrombocytopenic purpura, which was attributed to rifabutin, was reported in a patient receiving the drug in a controlled clinical trial.

■ **Dermatologic and Hypersensitivity Reactions** The most frequent adverse dermatologic effect of rifabutin is rash, which occurred in 11% of patients with severe HIV infection receiving the drug in controlled clinical trials. Rash resulted in discontinuance of the drug in 4% of patients in controlled clinical trials. Skin discoloration and a flu-like syndrome each occurred in less than 1% of patients receiving rifabutin in controlled clinical trials. Rifabutin-induced skin discoloration may be orange or yellow in appearance, similar to that occurring with jaundice (pseudojaundice), but buccal or scleral mucosa is not affected. The discoloration generally is not associated with pruritus or other symptoms and subsides slowly after discontinuance of the drug.

■ **GI Effects** Nausea occurred in 6%, nausea and vomiting in 3%, and vomiting in 1% of patients with severe HIV infection receiving rifabutin in controlled clinical trials. Abdominal pain occurred in 4% of patients and taste perversion, diarrhea, dyspepsia, and eructation each occurred in 3% of patients receiving the drug in controlled clinical trials. Ageusia, which subsided with discontinuance of therapy, has been reported rarely. Anorexia and flatulence each occurred in 2% of patients receiving rifabutin in controlled clinical trials. GI intolerance to rifabutin resulted in discontinuance of the drug in 3% of patients in controlled clinical trials. In patients who have a propensity to develop nausea, vomiting, or other GI upset, rifabutin may be administered with food and the total daily dosage may be given as two divided doses.

Rifabutin-associated diarrhea and pseudomembranous colitis, caused by overgrowth of toxin-producing clostridia (e.g., *C. difficile*), have been reported rarely. Aphthous stomatitis also has been reported rarely in patients receiving high dosages of the drug.

■ **Nervous System Effects** Headache occurred in 3% of patients with severe HIV infection receiving rifabutin in controlled clinical trials. Fever occurred in 2% of patients and asthenia, insomnia, and nonspecific complaints of pain each occurred in 1% of patients receiving the drug. Although a causal relationship to rifabutin has not been established, seizures, paresthesia, aphasia, and confusion have been reported in patients receiving the drug.

■ **Musculoskeletal Effects** Myalgia occurred in 2% of patients with severe HIV infection receiving rifabutin in controlled clinical trials. Arthralgia and myositis each occurred in less than 1% of patients receiving the drug. The risk of rifabutin-induced arthralgia appears to be greatest in patients receiving a dosage of 1050 mg daily or higher. The arthralgia commonly involves the small joints of the hand and usually involves many joints; in some patients, periarticular swelling or joint tenderness may be present. The arthralgia was reversible following discontinuance of the drug.

■ **Ocular Effects** Uveitis, which may be unilateral or bilateral and is characterized by pain, redness, and possible temporary or permanent loss of vision, may occur occasionally in patients receiving rifabutin 300–900 mg daily in combination with other agents, particularly clarithromycin and/or fluconazole. (See Cautions: Precautions and Contraindications.) Uveitis also has occurred in association with arthralgia in a few patients receiving high dosages of the drug. In a patient receiving 2400 mg of rifabutin daily, severe uveitis manifested as unilateral panophthalmitis and reversible blindness responded slowly (over 6 weeks) to systemic corticosteroids and permanent discontinuance of rifabutin.

Rifabutin-induced uveitis occurs rarely when the drug is used as sole antimycobacterial therapy at the usual prophylactic dosage (i.e., 300 mg daily) for the prevention of *M. avium* complex (MAC) infections in patients with advanced HIV infection, even in combination with macrolide antibiotics or fluconazole. The risk of uveitis appears to be greatest in patients receiving higher dosages of rifabutin in combination with macrolide antibiotics (e.g., clarithromycin) or fluconazole, probably in part because of inhibition of rifabutin metabolism by these drugs and resulting increased plasma rifabutin concentrations. (See Drug Interactions: Rifabutin and Rifampin, in Clarithromycin 8:12.12.92 and in Fluconazole 8:14.08.) Mild to severe symptoms associated with the uveitis usually have resolved following discontinuance of rifabutin and treatment with topical corticosteroids and/or mydriatics; in severe cases, resolution of manifestations may require more aggressive therapy and be delayed for several weeks. If uveitis occurs in patients receiving rifabutin, the drug should be discontinued temporarily and the patient should have an ophthalmologic evaluation. In most mild cases, rifabutin therapy subsequently may be reinstituted; however, if signs or symptoms recur, the drug should be discontinued immediately.

Brown-orange discoloration of tears may occur during rifabutin therapy. In addition, permanent discoloration of soft contact lenses may occur.

■ **Hepatic Effects** Increased serum concentrations of ALT (SGPT) and AST (SGOT) (exceeding 150 U/L) occurred in 9 and 7% of patients with severe HIV infection, respectively, receiving rifabutin in controlled clinical trials. Increased serum alkaline phosphatase concentrations (exceeding 450 U/L) occurred in less than 1% of rifabutin-treated patients in controlled clinical trials. Hepatitis was reported in less than 1% of patients receiving the drug.

■ **Other Adverse Effects** Brown-orange discoloration of urine is common during rifabutin therapy. In controlled trials, such discoloration of urine was observed in 30% of patients, and should be anticipated. (See Cautions: Precautions and Contraindications.)

Chest pain occurred in 1% of patients with severe HIV infection receiving rifabutin in controlled clinical trials. Chest pressure or pain with dyspnea was reported in less than 1% of patients receiving the drug. Although a causal relationship to rifabutin has not been established, nonspecific T-wave changes on ECG have been reported in patients receiving the drug.

■ **Precautions and Contraindications** Because rifabutin may cause neutropenia or other adverse hematologic effects (e.g., thrombocytopenia), hematologic status should be monitored periodically during therapy with the drug.

Patients receiving rifabutin should be advised regarding manifestations of MAC infection and those of tuberculosis and to contact a physician if either develops or worsens during therapy with the drug.

The manufacturer states that preventive therapy with rifabutin should not be initiated in patients with active *M. tuberculosis* since administration of the drug as *sole* antimycobacterial therapy in such patients would likely lead to development of tuberculosis that is resistant to both rifabutin and rifampin. Patients who develop symptoms compatible with active tuberculosis while receiving rifabutin prophylaxis should be evaluated immediately and appropriate therapy instituted with an effective combination of antituberculosis agents.

Because uveitis may occur in patients receiving rifabutin, patients should be instructed to report to their physician manifestations such as eye pain, redness, or loss of vision which may be indicative of the inflammatory ocular condition. If uveitis occurs in patients receiving rifabutin, the drug should be discontinued temporarily and the patient should have an ophthalmologic evaluation. Appropriate treatment should be initiated as necessary. In most mild cases, rifabutin therapy subsequently may be reinstituted; however, if signs or symptoms recur, the drug should be discontinued immediately. Permanent discontinuance of the drug may be necessary if uveitis is severe.

A drug-induced lupus syndrome manifested principally by malaise, myalgias, arthritis, and peripheral edema has been reported in a few patients receiving rifabutin or rifampin concomitantly with ciprofloxacin and/or clarithromycin, known inhibitors of the hepatic P-450 enzyme system. (See Drug Interactions: Hepatic Microsomal Enzyme Induction, in Rifampin 8:16.04.) Careful surveillance for drug-induced lupus syndrome is advised when ciprofloxacin and/or clarithromycin are used concomitantly with a rifamycin. When rifabutin is administered to patients receiving oral contraceptives, consideration should be given to changing to a nonhormonal contraceptive method. Unlike rifampin, rifabutin does not appear to affect the acetylation of isoniazid.

Pharmacokinetic interactions between rifamycin derivatives (e.g., rifabutin, rifampin) and HIV protease inhibitors (e.g., amprenavir, indinavir, lopinavir, nelfinavir, ritonavir, saquinavir) or nonnucleoside reverse transcriptase inhibitors (e.g., delavirdine, efavirenz, nevirapine) have been reported or are expected to occur, which may complicate drug therapy for mycobacterial infections in HIV-infected patients. (See Drug Interactions: Antiretroviral Agents) and also see Treatment in Patients Receiving Concurrent Antiretroviral Therapy, under Initial Treatment of Active Tuberculosis: Tuberculosis in HIV-infected Patients, in the Antituberculosis Agents General Statement 8:16.04.)

Patients should be instructed to report to their physician manifestations such as joint stiffness, swelling, or tenderness or paresthesia which may be indicative of arthralgias or myositis.

Patients receiving rifabutin should be advised that the drug and its metabolites may impart a brown-orange color to urine, feces, saliva, sputum, perspiration, tears, and skin and that soft contact lenses worn during such therapy may be stained permanently.

Rifabutin is contraindicated in patients who have had clinically important hypersensitivity to the drug or to any other rifamycin (e.g., rifampin).

■ **Pediatric Precautions** The manufacturer states that safety and efficacy of rifabutin for prophylaxis against MAC infection in children have not been established. However, rifabutin reportedly has been used in a limited number of children (concomitantly with other antimycobacterial agents) for the treatment of MAC infection. Adverse effects reported were similar to those observed in adults and included leukopenia, neutropenia, and rash. In addition, rifabutin (5 mg/kg daily) was administered to a 3-month-old infant in combination with ethambutol as prophylaxis against MAC infection for 64 days without adverse effects.

■ **Geriatric Precautions** Although steady-state pharmacokinetics of rifabutin are more variable in geriatric individuals older than 70 years of age, the manufacturer makes no specific recommendations for dosage adjustment or monitoring precautions in such patients.

■ **Mutagenicity and Carcinogenicity** There was no evidence of mutagenicity when rifabutin was tested in vitro with the bacterial mutation assay (Ames test) using rifabutin-susceptible and -resistant strains. In addition, rifabutin was not mutagenic when tested in vitro using *Schizosaccharomyces pombe* P_1 and was not genotoxic in V-79 Chinese hamster cells, human lymphocytes in vitro, or mouse bone marrow cells in vivo.

Long-term studies in mice using rifabutin dosages up to 180 mg/kg daily (36 times the recommended human daily dosage) and in rats using rifabutin dosages up to 60 mg/kg daily (12 times the recommended human daily dosage) have not revealed evidence of carcinogenicity.

■ **Pregnancy, Fertility, and Lactation** Reproduction studies in rats and rabbits using rifabutin dosages up to 200 mg/kg daily (40 times the recommended human daily dosage) did not reveal evidence of teratogenicity. In rats receiving 200 mg/kg daily, decreased fetal viability occurred. An increase in fetal skeletal variants was observed in rats receiving rifabutin dosages of 40 mg/kg daily (8 times the recommended human daily dosage). In rabbits receiving rifabutin dosages of 80 mg/kg daily (16 times the recommended human daily dosage), maternotoxicity and an increase in fetal skeletal anomalies occurred. There are no adequate and controlled studies to date using rifabutin in pregnant women, and the drug should be used during pregnancy only when the potential benefits justify the possible risks to the fetus. The American Thoracic Society (ATS), US Centers for Disease Control and Prevention (CDC), and Infectious Diseases Society of America (IDSA) state that data are insufficient to date to recommend use of rifabutin in pregnant women.

Reproduction studies in male rats using rifabutin dosages of 160 mg/kg daily (32 times the recommended human daily dosage) revealed evidence of impaired fertility.

It is not known whether rifabutin is distributed into human milk. Because of the potential for serious adverse reactions to rifabutin in nursing infants, a decision should be made whether to discontinue nursing or the drug, taking into account the importance of the drug to the woman.

Drug Interactions

Rifabutin, like other rifamycins (e.g., rifampin) can induce hepatic microsomal enzymes which may result in drug interactions. Because of the structural similarity between rifampin and rifabutin and because rifampin is known to interact with numerous other drugs, rifabutin may be anticipated to have some effects on drugs known to be affected by rifampin (e.g., ketoconazole, cyclosporine, oral contraceptives). (See Drug Interactions in Rifampin 8:16.04.) In healthy individuals, rifabutin appears to induce hepatic microsomal enzymes to a lesser extent than rifampin, although the clinical relevance of this finding for drug interactions is not known.

■ **Antiretroviral Agents** Limited data suggest that rifamycin derivatives (e.g., rifabutin, rifampin) accelerate the metabolism of certain antiretroviral agents (i.e., HIV protease inhibitors, nonnucleoside reverse transcriptase inhibitors [NNRTIs]) by induction of hepatic cytochrome P-450 (CYP) oxidases, which may result in subtherapeutic plasma concentrations of some of these HIV protease inhibitors and NNRTIs. In addition, some HIV protease inhibitors and some NNRTIs (e.g., delavirdine) can reduce the metabolism of rifamycins, leading to increased plasma concentrations of rifamycins and an increased risk of toxicity and some other NNRTIs (e.g., efavirenz) can decrease plasma concentrations of rifabutin. The potential for alterations in the plasma concentrations of the antimycobacterial agents and/or HIV protease inhibitors or NNRTIs must be considered when antimycobacterial agents are indicated for the management of latent or active tuberculosis or the prophylaxis or treatment of *Mycobacterium avium* complex (MAC) infections in HIV-infected patients who are receiving or are being considered for antiretroviral therapy. Because the management of these patients is complex and must be individualized, experts in the management of mycobacterial infections in HIV-infected patients should be consulted.

HIV Protease Inhibitors Concomitant use of amprenavir and rifabutin can affect the pharmacokinetics of both drugs, resulting in a decrease in the area under the plasma concentration-time curve (AUC) of the protease inhibitor and a substantial increase in plasma concentrations and AUC of rifabutin. Because of this pharmacokinetic interaction, the manufacturer of amprenavir states that rifabutin dosage should be reduced to at least 50% of the usual dosage when concomitant use with amprenavir is necessary, and complete blood cell counts (CBCs) should be performed weekly and as clinically indicated to monitor for neutropenia. Although there is no published clinical experience, some experts state that usual dosage of amprenavir can be used concomitantly with a reduced dosage of rifabutin (150 mg once daily or 300 mg 2 or 3 times weekly) is a possibility.

Concomitant use of atazanavir sulfate and rifabutin results in increased serum concentrations of rifabutin and its metabolite. The manufacturer of atazanavir recommends that the rifabutin dosage be reduced up to 75% (e.g., 150 mg every other day or 3 times weekly) in patients receiving atazanavir.

Concomitant use of indinavir and rifabutin results in a decrease in the AUC of indinavir and a substantial increase in the AUC of rifabutin. Because of this pharmacokinetic interaction, the manufacturer of indinavir and some experts recommend that the dosage of indinavir be increased to 1000 mg every 8 hours and that the dosage of rifabutin be reduced by 50% (e.g., 150 mg once daily or 300 mg 2–3 times weekly) in patients receiving the drugs concomitantly. Some experts state that there is limited, but favorable, clinical experience with this dosage regimen.

Concomitant use of lopinavir and rifabutin results in increased concentrations of rifabutin and its metabolite. The manufacturer of the fixed combination containing lopinavir and ritonavir and some clinicians recommend that the rifabutin dosage be reduced by at least 75% to a maximum of 150 mg every other day or 3 times weekly in patients receiving lopinavir and ritonavir. Increased monitoring for adverse effect is warranted in patients receiving the fixed combination and rifabutin concomitantly, and further reductions in rifabutin dosage may be necessary.

Concomitant use of nelfinavir and rifabutin can result in alterations in the pharmacokinetics of both drugs. Because of the pharmacokinetic interaction between rifabutin and nelfinavir, the manufacturer of nelfinavir recommends that rifabutin dosage be decreased to 50% of the usual dosage in patients receiving nelfinavir and that a twice-daily regimen of nelfinavir (1250 mg twice daily) is the preferred regimen for patients receiving concomitant rifabutin. Some experts recommend increasing nelfinavir dosage to 1000 mg 3 times daily and decreasing rifabutin dosage to 150 mg once daily or 300 mg 3 times weekly. Others state that there is limited, but favorable, clinical experience with concomitant use of nelfinavir with a rifabutin dosage of 150 mg once daily or 300 mg 2 or 3 times weekly for the treatment of tuberculosis.

If ritonavir is used concomitantly with rifabutin, the manufacturer of ritonavir and some experts recommend that rifabutin dosage be decreased by at least 75% (e.g., reduced to 150 mg every other day or 3 times weekly); further dosage reduction may be needed. For the treatment of tuberculosis, some experts state that the need to use substantially reduced rifabutin dosage (150 mg 2 or 3 times weekly) is certain in tuberculosis patients receiving ritonavir concomitantly with another HIV protease inhibitor (e.g., saquinavir).

The manufacturer of saquinavir and some experts state that use of alternatives to rifabutin should be considered in patients receiving saquinavir hard gelatin capsules or liquid-filled (soft gelatin) capsules. Although pharmacokinetic data and clinical experience are limited, some experts state that concomitant use of saquinavir hard gelatin capsules and rifabutin is a possibility, provided the antiretroviral regimen also includes ritonavir and the rifabutin dosage is decreased to 150 mg 2 or 3 times weekly. Although pharmacokinetic data and clinical experience is limited, these experts state that saquinavir liquid-filled capsules probably may be given concomitantly with a rifabutin dosage of 300 mg daily or 300 mg 2 or 3 times weekly for the treatment of tuberculosis; however, rifabutin dosage should be decreased to 150 mg 2 or 3 times weekly if the antiretroviral regimen also contains ritonavir.

For specific information on the pharmacokinetic interactions between HIV protease inhibitors and rifabutin, see Antimycobacterial Agents under Drug Interactions: Anti-infective Agents, in the individual monographs in 8:18.08.08.

Nonnucleoside Reverse Transcriptase Inhibitors Concomitant use of rifabutin and delavirdine is not recommended.

The manufacturer of efavirenz states that the daily dosage of rifabutin should be increased by 50% in patients receiving efavirenz and that consideration should be given to doubling the rifabutin dose used in 2- or 3-times weekly regimens if efavirenz is used concomitantly. Some experts state that concomitant use of efavirenz with a rifabutin dosage of 450–600 mg daily or 600 mg 2 or 3 times weekly is a possibility, provided that the antiretroviral regimen does not include an HIV protease inhibitor.

The manufacturer of nevirapine states that concomitant use with rifabutin results in moderate increases in serum concentrations of the antimycobacterial agent and its metabolite; however, because of high interindividual variability, some patients may experience large increases in rifabutin concentrations and may be at higher risk of rifabutin toxicity. Therefore, caution is advised if nevirapine is used concomitantly with rifabutin. Although there is no published clinical experience regarding concomitant use of rifabutin and nevirapine, some experts suggest that, based on pharmacokinetic data, concomitant use of nevirapine with a rifabutin dosage of 300 mg daily or 2 or 3 times weekly is a possibility. Other experts state that no dosage adjustments are needed if nevirapine is used concomitantly with rifabutin, provided the antiretroviral regimen does not include an HIV protease inhibitor.

For specific information on the pharmacokinetic interactions between non-nucleoside reverse transcriptase inhibitors and rifabutin, see Antimycobacterial Agents under Drug Interactions: Anti-infective Agents, in the individual monographs in 8:18.08.16.

Nucleoside Reverse Transcriptase Inhibitors In HIV-infected patients receiving rifabutin (300 mg daily) and zidovudine (200 mg every 8 hours) concomitantly for 14 days, the mean elimination half-life of zidovudine decreased by 28% (from 1.5 to 1.1 hours); however, concomitant use of the drugs for 7 or 14 days did not substantially alter AUC, peak plasma drug concentration, or other pharmacokinetic parameters of zidovudine (i.e., less than 25% change in these parameters), and zidovudine dosage requirements are not expected to be altered by such concomitant therapy. In another study in HIV-infected patients designed to evaluate the effect of zidovudine on rifabutin pharmacokinetics, concomitant use of zidovudine (100 or 200 mg every 4 hours) and rifabutin (300 or 450 mg once daily) did not alter the pharmacokinetics of the antimycobacterial agent or its principal metabolite, and such use was not associated with any unusual adverse effects. In vitro studies indicate that rifabutin does not affect the inhibition of HIV by zidovudine.

Following addition of rifabutin to therapy with didanosine (167–375 mg daily given in 2 divided doses) in HIV-infected patients, no clinically important changes in the pharmacokinetics of either drug were observed.

Description

Rifabutin, a semisynthetic spiropiperidyl derivative of rifamycin S, is an ansamycin antibiotic. The drug is active in vitro and in vivo against *Mycobacterium avium* complex (MAC), including isolates obtained from patients with acquired immunodeficiency syndrome (AIDS). The MIC_{90} of rifabutin for susceptible MAC isolates is approximately 1 mcg/mL. The drug also is active against most other mycobacteria, including *M. leprae* and *M. tuberculosis*; some rifampin-resistant strains of *M. tuberculosis* are susceptible to rifabutin. Rifabutin has a spectrum of in vitro activity similar to that of rifampin against gram-positive and gram-negative organisms.

SumMon® (see Users Guide). For additional information on this drug until a more detailed monograph is developed and published, the manufacturer's labeling should be consulted. It is *essential* that the labeling be consulted for detailed information on the usual cautions, precautions, and contraindications concerning potential drug interactions and/or laboratory test interferences and for information on acute toxicity.

Preparations

Excipients in commercially available drug preparations may have clinically important effects in some individuals; consult specific product labeling for details.

Rifabutin

Oral

Capsules	150 mg	**Mycobutin®**, Pfizer

†Use is not currently included in the labeling approved by the US Food and Drug Administration

rifAMPin

Rifampicin

■ Rifampin is a rifamycin B-derivative antibiotic active against mycobacteria and some gram-positive and -negative bacteria.

Uses

■ **Tuberculosis** ***Active Tuberculosis*** Rifampin is used in conjunction with other antituberculosis agents for the treatment of clinical tuberculosis. For information on the general principles used in the treatment of tuberculosis, see the Antituberculosis Agents General Statement 8:16.04.

The American Thoracic Society (ATS), US Centers for Disease Control and Prevention (CDC), and Infectious Diseases Society of America (IDSA) currently recommend several possible multiple-drug regimens for the treatment of culture-positive pulmonary tuberculosis. These regimens have a minimum duration of 6 months (26 weeks), and consist of an initial intensive phase (2 months) and a continuation phase (usually either 4 or 7 months). Rifampin is considered a first-line antituberculosis agent for the treatment of all forms of tuberculosis caused by *Mycobacterium tuberculosis* known or presumed to be susceptible to the drug, and is an essential component of all short-course regimens. For information on general principles used in the treatment of tuberculosis, see the Antituberculosis Agents General Statement 8:16.04.

Rifampin is commercially available in the US alone or in fixed combination with isoniazid or in fixed combination with isoniazid and pyrazinamide (Rifater®). The fixed-combination preparation containing rifampin, isoniazid, and pyrazinamide (Rifater®) is designated an orphan drug by the US Food and Drug Administration (FDA) for use in this condition.

Oral rifampin is preferred for the treatment of tuberculosis, but the drug may be given IV for initial or retreatment of the disease when the drug cannot be given orally. IV rifampin is designated an orphan drug by the FDA for use in this condition.

HIV-infected Individuals. When use of rifampin in conjunction with other antituberculosis agents is being considered for the treatment of tuberculosis or other mycobacterial infections (e.g., *Mycobacterium avium* complex [MAC] infections) in patients with human immunodeficiency virus (HIV) infection, the possibility that concomitant use of certain drugs might be contraindicated or that dosages may have to be altered because of clinically important pharmacokinetic interactions between rifampin and certain antiretroviral agents (e.g., HIV protease inhibitors [PIs], nonnucleoside reverse transcriptase inhibitors [NNRTIs]) should be considered. The CDC and other experts state that concomitant use of rifampin and most PIs or NNRTIs usually is not recommended and that use of alternatives (e.g., rifabutin) may be preferred for the treatment of active tuberculosis in HIV-infected patients receiving PIs or NNRTIs. (See Drug Interactions: Antiretroviral Agents.)

There is evidence that use of antituberculosis regimens that include once- or twice-weekly administration of rifamycins (e.g., rifampin, rifabutin, rifapentine) in HIV-infected patients with CD4+ T-cell counts less than 100/mm³ is associated with an increased risk for acquired rifamycin resistance. Therefore, until additional data are available regarding this issue, the CDC recommends that HIV-infected individuals with CD4+ T-cell counts less than 100/mm³ not receive rifamycin regimens for the treatment of active tuberculosis that involve once- or twice-weekly administration. These individuals should receive daily therapy during the initial phase, and daily or 3-times weekly regimens during the second phase; directly observed therapy also is recommended for both the daily and 3-times weekly regimens.

Latent Tuberculosis Infection Rifampin is used alone or in conjunction with other antituberculosis agents for the treatment of latent tuberculosis infection to prevent the development of clinical tuberculosis, especially in individuals exposed to isoniazid-resistant *M. tuberculosis*. Previously, "preventive therapy" or "chemoprophylaxis" was used to describe a simple drug regimen (e.g., isoniazid monotherapy) used to prevent the development of active tuberculosis disease in individuals known or likely to be infected with *M. tuberculosis*. However, since use of such a regimen rarely results in true primary prevention (i.e., prevention of *infection* in individuals exposed to infectious tuberculosis), the ATS and CDC currently state that "treatment of latent tuberculosis infection" rather than "preventive therapy" more accurately describes the intended intervention and potentially will result in greater understanding and more widespread implementation of this tuberculosis control strategy.

Although a 9-month regimen of isoniazid monotherapy (once-daily or, alternatively, twice weekly) generally is considered the regimen of choice for the treatment of latent tuberculosis infection in most adult and pediatric patients and a 6-month regimen of isoniazid monotherapy (once-daily or, alternatively, 2 or 3 times weekly) is considered an acceptable alternative in some cases, a 4-month regimen (4–6 months in pediatric patients) of daily rifampin monotherapy also has been studied and can be considered as an alternative for the treatment of latent tuberculosis infection in selected individuals. Although a 2-month daily regimen of rifampin and pyrazinamide and a 2- to 3-month regimen of twice-weekly rifampin and pyrazinamide were previously recommended, these regimens have been associated with an increased risk of hepatotoxicity and generally should *not* be offered for the treatment of *latent* tuberculosis infection unless the potential benefits outweigh the risk of liver injury and death. (See Rifampin and Pyrazinamide Regimens under Tuberculosis: Treatment of Latent Tuberculosis, in Uses.)

Rifampin Monotherapy. A 4-month regimen of daily rifampin monotherapy is considered by the ATS and CDC to be an alternative regimen that can be used for the treatment of latent tuberculosis infection in both HIV-infected and HIV-seronegative adults. This rifampin regimen may be useful for those in whom isoniazid cannot be used because of drug resistance or intolerance.

In infants, children, and adolescents, a 6-month regimen of daily rifampin monotherapy is recommended by the CDC and AAP as an alternative to isoniazid monotherapy for the treatment of latent tuberculosis infection if the source case has isoniazid-resistant and rifampin-susceptible *M. tuberculosis* or if isoniazid is not tolerated despite careful education and efforts to alleviate mild isoniazid adverse effects. The AAP states that optimal regimens for treatment of latent tuberculosis infection in pediatric patients with strains resistant to both isoniazid and rifampin are unknown; however, a multiple-drug regimen and consultation with a tuberculosis specialist is indicated.

Rifampin and Pyrazinamide Regimens. Limited data suggest that a 2-month regimen consisting of rifampin and pyrazinamide given daily is effective in treating latent tuberculosis infection in HIV-infected patients, and the ATS and CDC state that the efficacy of this regimen is not expected to differ in HIV-negative patients. In a randomized, comparative study in HIV-infected adults, the efficacy and safety of a rifampin-pyrazinamide regimen given daily for 2 months was comparable to that of a 12-month regimen of isoniazid monotherapy for treatment of latent tuberculosis infection. An intermittent rifampin and pyrazinamide regimen that involves twice-weekly administration of the drugs for 2–3 months also may be effective for the treatment of latent tuberculosis infection when other regimens cannot be used.

Based on results in HIV-infected adults, the ATS and CDC previously recommended use of the 2-month daily rifampin and pyrazinamide regimen for HIV-infected or HIV-seronegative adults who were known contacts of patients with isoniazid-resistant, rifampin-susceptible tuberculosis. However, hepatotoxicity (including some fatalities) has been reported in patients receiving rifampin and pyrazinamide regimens for the treatment of latent tuberculosis and, although multiple-drug regimens containing rifampin and pyrazinamide are still recommended for the treatment of *active*tuberculosis, the ATS, CDC, and IDSA now state that regimens containing both rifampin and pyrazinamide generally should *not* be offered for the treatment of *latent*tuberculosis in either HIV-infected or HIV-negative individuals. The American Academy of Pediatrics (AAP) also states that the 2-month rifampin and pyrazinamide regimen is not recommended for children.

Based on a recent analysis of potential cofactors in patients with latent tuberculosis who developed hepatotoxicity while receiving a regimen of rifampin and pyrazinamide, this regimen should *never* be offered to patients who are currently taking other drugs associated with liver injury, patients who drink excessive amounts of alcohol (even if alcohol is discontinued during treatment), or patients with underlying liver disease or a history of isoniazid-associated liver injury. However, the ATS, CDC, and IDSA state that a rifampin and pyrazinamide regimen *might be considered* for the treatment of latent tuberculosis in carefully selected patients if the potential benefits of the regimen outweigh the risk for severe liver injury and death, but only when the preferred or alternative regimens (i.e., 9-month isoniazid regimens, 6-month isoniazid regimens, 4-month daily rifampin regimen) are judged unlikely to be completed and oversight can be provided by a clinician with expertise in the treatment of latent tuberculosis. An expert in the treatment of latent tuberculosis should be consulted before a regimen of rifampin and pyrazinamide is offered. If a rifampin and pyrazinamide regimen is used, patients should be informed of the potential for hepatotoxicity and certain precautions should be taken to ensure that the patient is closely monitored for adherence, tolerance, and adverse effects throughout the entire course of therapy. (See Precautions Related to Hepatotoxicity under Cautions: Precautions and Contraindications.)

HIV-infected Individuals. When use of rifampin is being considered for the treatment of latent tuberculosis infection in HIV-infected patients, the possibility that certain combinations of drugs might be contraindicated or drug dosages may have to be altered because of clinically important pharmacokinetic interactions between rifampin and certain antiretroviral agents (e.g., PIs, NNRTIs) should be considered. (See Drug Interactions: Antiretroviral Agents.) The ATS and CDC state that while therapy for latent tuberculosis infection with rifabutin in tuberculin-positive patients with HIV infection has not been evaluated in clinical trials, the use of rifabutin instead of rifampin in such regimens for treatment of latent *M. tuberculosis* infection is valid for the same scientific principles that support the use of rifabutin for the treatment of active tuberculosis. (See Uses: Tuberculosis, in Rifabutin 8:16.04.) However, the ATS and CDC state that substitution of rifapentine, a long-acting rifamycin, for rifampin in treatment regimens for latent tuberculosis infection currently is not recommended because the safety and efficacy of rifapentine in HIV-infected patients have not been established and drug interactions between rifapentine and PIs have not been adequately evaluated.

For HIV-infected adults who are receiving concomitant antiretroviral therapy that includes PIs or NNRTIs, recommended regimens for treatment of latent *M. tuberculosis* infection are a 9-month regimen of isoniazid given daily or twice weekly; a 4-month regimen of rifabutin given daily; or a 2-month regimen of rifabutin and pyrazinamide given daily. (See Rifabutin 8:16.04.)

For HIV-infected adults who are *not* receiving concomitant PIs or NNRTIs, recommended regimens for treatment of latent *M. tuberculosis* infection are the same as those for adults without HIV infection (i.e., usually a 9-month regimen of isoniazid given daily or twice weekly or a 4-month regimen of rifampin given daily).

Pregnant Women. The ATS and CDC state that treatment of latent tuberculosis infection in pregnant women who are at high risk for progression to active disease, particularly those who were infected recently or have HIV infection, should not be delayed on the basis of pregnancy alone, even during the first trimester. For women whose risk of active disease is lower, some experts recommend delaying treatment until after delivery

The preferred regimen for treatment of latent tuberculosis infection in pregnant women is a 6- or 9-month regimen of isoniazid monotherapy; those with HIV infection or radiographic evidence of prior tuberculosis should receive 9 rather than 6 months of isoniazid therapy. The ATS and CDC state that rifampin has been used to treat active tuberculosis in pregnant women† but there are no efficacy data to date to support use of the drug for treatment of latent tuberculosis infection in pregnant women. In addition, the ATS and CDC state that use of pyrazinamide can be considered in HIV-infected pregnant women after the first trimester of pregnancy but should be avoided in other pregnant women.

Drug-Resistant Latent Tuberculosis Infection. In individuals likely to be infected with *M. tuberculosis* that are resistant to both isoniazid and rifampin and who are at high risk for developing tuberculosis, the ATS and CDC recommend regimens consisting of pyrazinamide and ethambutol or pyrazinamide and a quinolone anti-infective (e.g., levofloxacin or ofloxacin) for 6–12 months if the organisms from the index case are known to be susceptible to these drugs. Immunocompetent contacts may be managed by observation alone or be treated with such regimens for 6 months; immunosuppressed individuals, including those with HIV infection, should be treated for 12 months. Clinicians should review the drug-susceptibility pattern of *M. tuberculosis* isolated from the infecting source-patient before selecting a regimen for treating potentially multiple-drug resistant tuberculosis infections. In individuals likely to have been infected with *M. tuberculosis* that are resistant to both isoniazid and rifampin, the choice of drugs used for treatment of latent infection requires expert consultation. Prior to initiation of therapy for latent tuberculosis infection in patients with suspected multidrug-resistant tuberculosis, careful assessment to rule out active disease is necessary.

The AAP states that, until susceptibility test results are available, both rifampin and isoniazid should be given to contacts who are likely to have been infected by an index case with isoniazid-resistant tuberculosis. If the index case is proven to be excreting organisms that are completely resistant to isoniazid, isoniazid should be discontinued and rifampin given for a total of at least 6 months. The AAP recommends consultation with an expert in making decisions about therapy for latent tuberculosis infection in children with isoniazid and/or rifampin-resistant *M. tuberculosis*.

Hematopoietic Stem Cell Transplant Recipients. Individuals who undergo hematopoietic stem cell transplant (HSCT) are at increased risk for progression from latent tuberculosis infection to active disease because of immunosuppression. The CDC, IDSA, and the American Society of Blood and Marrow Transplantation (ASBMT) have established guidelines for preventing opportunistic infections in HSCT recipients. These guidelines include recommendations regarding treatment of latent tuberculosis in HSCT candidates and recipients. All HSCT candidates should be screened for active and latent tuberculosis infection; although a tuberculin skin test can be administered, this test may not be reliable in patients who are immunocompromised. Therefore, clinicians should not rely solely on the test to determine whether latent tuberculosis infection is present and whether preventive therapy should be administered.

The CDC, IDSA, and ASBMT state that a regimen for the treatment of latent tuberculosis infection should be administered to all immunocompromised HSCT recipients or candidates (adults, adolescents, and children) who have been substantially exposed to someone with active, infectious (i.e., sputum-smear positive) pulmonary or laryngeal tuberculosis, regardless of tuberculin skin test results, and also should be administered to all HSCT recipients or candidates who have a positive skin test result and have not previously been treated and have no evidence of active tuberculosis.

A 9-month regimen of daily isoniazid monotherapy is the regimen of choice when treatment of latent tuberculosis infection is indicated in HSCT candidates or recipients. The 2-month regimen of daily rifampin and pyrazinamide is not recommended for HSCT candidates or recipients because of limited safety and efficacy data in these individuals, risk of hepatotoxicity, and substantial drug interactions that have been reported between rifampin and several drugs used in HSCT patients (e.g., cyclosporine, tacrolimus, corticosteroids, fluconazole). (See Precautions Related to Hepatotoxicity and see Drug Interactions.) The guidelines for preventing opportunistic infections in HSCT recipients should be consulted for additional information on preventing opportunistic infections in these patients and for information on hospital infection control, strategies for safe living after transplantation, and hematopoietic stem cell safety.

Completion of Treatment and Supervised Administration. The ATS and CDC state that completion of therapy for latent tuberculosis infection is based on the total number of administered doses of the antituberculosis agents, not the duration of therapy alone. If rifampin monotherapy regimen is used, at least 120 doses should be administered within 6 months. If a regimen in which a rifamycin (rifampin or rifabutin) and pyrazinamide is given daily, at least 60 doses should be administered within 3 months. Ideally, patients should receive the treatment regimens on a regular dosing schedule until completion of the indicated course; in practice, some doses may be missed requiring the course to be lengthened. Reinstitution of therapy in patients whose treatment has been interrupted might require a continuation of the regimen originally prescribed (as long as needed to complete the recommended duration of the particular regimen) or a complete renewal of the regimen if interruptions were frequent or prolonged enough to preclude completion of treatment as recommended. In either situation, when therapy is resumed after an interruption of 2 months or longer, a medical examination is indicated to rule out tuberculosis disease.

All patients receiving an intermittent (e.g., twice-weekly) dosing regimen for the treatment of latent tuberculosis infection should receive directly observed therapy (DOT). In addition, the ATS and CDC state that, when feasible, DOT also should be used in patients receiving 2-month regimens and in some special settings (e.g., some institutional settings, community outreach programs, household contacts of patients with tuberculosis who are receiving home-based DOT).

■ Mycobacterium avium Complex (MAC) Infections

Rifampin is used as an alternative to rifabutin in multiple-drug regimens for the treatment of *Mycobacterium avium* complex (MAC) pulmonary infections†. The ATS currently recommends that therapy for MAC pulmonary infections in HIV-negative adults consist of at least 3 drugs, including clarithromycin (500 mg twice daily) or azithromycin (250 mg daily or 500 mg 3 times weekly), rifabutin (300 mg daily) or rifampin (600 mg daily), and ethambutol (25 mg/kg daily for 2 months, then 15 mg/kg daily). The ATS states that the addition of streptomycin given intermittently (2 or 3 times weekly for at least 2 months) may be considered for patients with extensive disease. (See Treatment of Pulmonary and Localized Extrapulmonary Infections, under Management of Other Mycobacterial Diseases: Mycobacterium avium Complex [MAC] Infections, in the Antituberculosis Agents General Statement 8:16.04.)

When use of rifampin is being considered for the treatment of MAC infection in HIV-infected patients, the possibility that drug regimens or dosages may have to be altered because of clinically important pharmacokinetic interactions between rifampin and certain antiretroviral agents (e.g., PIs, NNRTIs) should be considered. (See Drug Interactions: Antiretroviral Agents.)

■ **Neisseria meningitidis Infections** Rifampin is used to eliminate meningococci from the nasopharynx of asymptomatic *Neisseria meningitidis* carriers. The drug also is used for chemoprophylaxis in close contacts of individuals with invasive meningococcal disease† when the risk of infection is high. Rifampin is *not* indicated for the *treatment* of *N. meningitidis* infections since rapid emergence of resistant strains of the organism may occur during long-term therapy with the drug. IV penicillin G generally is considered the drug of choice for the *treatment* of invasive disease caused by *N. meningitidis* and ceftriaxone or cefotaxime are alternative agents.

Patients with invasive meningococcal disease who have been treated with penicillin G or any anti-infective agent other than ceftriaxone or another third-generation cephalosporin may still be carriers of *N. meningitidis* and should receive an anti-infective regimen to eradicate nasopharyngeal carriage of the organism prior to hospital discharge. Rifampin, ceftriaxone, or ciprofloxacin can be used to eradicate nasopharyngeal carriage of *N. meningitidis*

Rifampin should not be used indiscriminately to eliminate meningococci from the nasopharynx of asymptomatic *N. meningitidis* carriers and should be used only when the risk of meningococcal meningitis is high. To avoid indiscriminate use of the drug, diagnostic laboratory procedures, including serotyping and susceptibility testing, should be performed to determine whether the carrier state exists and the appropriate drug therapy. Rifampin generally has been considered the drug of choice and is 72–90% effective in eradicating nasopharyngeal carriage of *N. meningitidis*. Alternatively, a single IM dose of ceftriaxone reportedly is 97–100% and a single oral dose of ciprofloxacin is 90–95% effective in eradicating nasopharyngeal carriage of the organism.

Chemoprophylaxis in Household and Other Close Contacts of Individuals with Invasive Meningococcal Disease When sporadic or cluster cases of meningococcal disease occur in the US, chemoprophylaxis is the principal means of preventing secondary cases in household and other close contacts of individuals with invasive disease. Recommended regimens for chemoprophylaxis against meningococcal disease include 2 days of oral rifampin therapy (not recommended in pregnant women), a single IM dose of ceftriaxone, or a single oral dose of ciprofloxacin (not recommended in individuals younger than 18 years of age unless no other regimen can be used and not recommended for pregnant or lactating women). Although the AAP and other clinicians suggest that rifampin is the drug of choice for chemoprophylaxis in pediatric patients in most instances, the CDC states that rifampin, ciprofloxacin, and ceftriaxone are all 90–95% effective and are all acceptable regimens for chemoprophylaxis. Sulfisoxazole is no longer included in CDC or AAP guidelines for chemoprophylaxis of meningococcal disease.

The attack rate for household contacts who do not receive chemoprophylaxis has been estimated to be 4 cases per 1000 individuals exposed, which is 500–800 times greater than that for the general population. A decision to administer chemoprophylaxis to close contacts of an individual with invasive meningococcal disease is based on the degree of risk. Throat and nasopharyngeal cultures are not useful in determining the need for chemoprophylaxis and may unnecessarily delay administration of the regimen. The CDC and AAP currently recommend that chemoprophylaxis be administered to contacts of individuals with invasive meningococcal disease only when the contacts are considered at high risk of infection. These high-risk individuals include household contacts (especially young children) and any individual who has slept or eaten frequently in the same dwelling with the index case; child care and nursery school contacts who were exposed during the 7 days before the onset of disease in the index case; individuals exposed directly to oropharyngeal secretions of the index case (e.g., through kissing or sharing toothbrushes, eating utensils, or drinking containers) during the 7 days before the onset of disease in the index case; and medical personnel who had intimate exposure (e.g., through mouth-to-mouth resuscitation, unprotected contact during endotracheal intubation or suctioning) to the index case during the 7 days before the onset of disease. Chemoprophylaxis is*not* routinely recommended for contacts considered at low risk of infection. Individuals considered in most circumstances as being at low risk include casual contacts with no history of direct exposure to the index case's oral secretions (e.g., school or work contacts); individuals who had only indirect contact with the index case (only contact was with a high-risk contact of the index case); and medical personnel who had no direct exposure to the index case's oral secretions.

When chemoprophylaxis is indicated in high risk contacts, it must be administered promptly (ideally within 24 hours after identification of the index case) since the attack rate of secondary disease is greatest in the few days following disease onset in the index case. All high-risk contacts should be informed that even if chemoprophylaxis is taken or started, the development of any suspicious clinical manifestation warrants early, rapid medical attention. Chemoprophylaxis probably is of limited or no value if administered more than 2 weeks after contact with the index case. If high-risk exposure to a new index case occurs more than 2 weeks after initial chemoprophylaxis, additional treatment is indicated.

Outbreak Control When an outbreak of meningococcal disease occurs in the US and the outbreak is caused by a vaccine-preventable meningococcal strain (i.e., serogroups A, C, Y, or W-135), large-scale vaccination programs with meningococcal polysaccharide vaccine in the appropriate target group is the principal control measure. (See Uses: Outbreak Control in Meningococcal Polysaccharide Vaccine 80:12.) Mass chemoprophylaxis programs (e.g., with rifampin, ceftriaxone, ciprofloxacin) in large population groups is not effective in most settings in which organization- or community-based outbreaks have occurred and disadvantages of such programs (e.g., costs, difficulty in ensuring simultaneous administration of the drugs to large populations, adverse effects of the drugs, emergence of resistant organisms) probably outweigh any possible benefit in disease prevention. However, when outbreaks involve small populations (e.g., a small organization such as a single school), administration of chemoprophylaxis to all individuals in the population may be considered. The CDC states that other measures, such as restricting travel to areas with a suspected meningococcal outbreak, closing schools or universities, or canceling sporting or social events, are *not* recommended to control meningococcal outbreaks in the US. In one reported outbreak of serogroup B meningococcal disease (a strain that cannot be prevented with currently available meningococcal polysaccharide vaccine) in a middle school, mass chemoprophylaxis with rifampin was 85% effective in eradicating carriage of meningococci and appeared to decrease transmission of the disease; however, rifampin-resistant isolates of *N. meningitidis* were recovered from some individuals who were carrying rifampin-susceptible strains prior to chemoprophylaxis. In an outbreak setting, some clinicians suggest that surveillance for rifampin resistance may be indicated and use of ciprofloxacin or ceftriaxone should be considered.

While the vast majority of cases of meningococcal disease in the US are sporadic, the frequency of outbreaks of group C meningococcal disease has increased in the US and Canada since 1991 and there also have been small outbreaks as well as statewide epidemics caused by serogroup B. As a result, the CDC has published guidelines for the evaluation and management of suspected meningococcal outbreaks that can be used by US public health professionals (e.g., epidemiologists in state and local health departments), and these guidelines can be consulted for further information. In addition, the Childhood and Respiratory Diseases Branch, Division of Bacteria and Mycotic Diseases, National Center for Infectious Diseases, CDC can be consulted on these and other issues regarding meningococcal disease (404-639-2215 or 404-639-3311).

■ **Prevention of Haemophilus influenzae Type b Infection** Rifampin is used for chemoprophylaxis in contacts of patients with *Haemophilus influenzae* type b (Hib) infection†. Rifampin is effective for eradicating oropharyngeal carriage of *H. influenzae* type b and is considered the most effective antimicrobial agent for eradicating carriage of the organism.

Unvaccinated household contacts of an individual with Hib infection are at increased risk of infection if they are younger than 4 years of age. In addition, asymptomatic colonization with Hib occurs more frequently in household contacts of all ages than in the general population. Rifampin is approximately 95% effective in eradicating Hib from the pharynx of carriers, and limited data indicate that rifampin prophylaxis also decreases the risk of secondary invasive illness in exposed household contacts. Although child-care and nursery school contacts of an individual with Hib infection also may be at increased risk of secondary disease, experts disagree about the magnitude of the risk. The risk of secondary disease in children attending child-care centers seems to be lower than that observed for age-susceptible household contacts, and secondary disease in child-care contacts is rare when all contacts are older than 2 years of age. Efficacy of rifampin in preventing disease in child-care groups is not established.

The AAP and US Public Health Service Advisory Committee on Immunization Practices (ACIP) state that rifampin is the drug of choice for chemoprophylaxis in contacts of patients with Hib infection. The AAP suggests the following guidelines for prophylaxis in household and child-care or nursery school contacts of patients with Hib infection:

■ ***Household Contacts***

- Rifampin prophylaxis is recommended for all household contacts (regardless of age) in households with at least 1 contact who is younger than 48 months of age and unimmunized or incompletely immunized against Hib.
- Rifampin prophylaxis is indicated for all members of the household when there is a child residing in the house who is immunocompromised (even if the child is older than 48 months of age).
- Rifampin prophylaxis is indicated for all household members in households with a child younger than 12 months of age who is unimmunized or incompletely immunized against Hib.
- Rifampin prophylaxis is *not* recommended for those households who do not have children younger than 48 months of age (other than the index case) or when all household contacts 12–48 months of age are immunocompetent and have been fully immunized against Hib.
- Household contacts are individuals residing with the infected (index) patient or nonresidents who spent 4 or more hours with the index patient for at least 5 of the 7 days preceding hospital admission of the index patient.
- Prophylaxis should be initiated as soon as possible, since the majority of secondary cases in households occur in the first week after hospitalization of the index patient. Because some secondary cases occur later, initiation of prophylaxis 7 days or longer after hospitalization of the index patient may still be of some benefit.

■ ***Child-care and Nursery School Contacts***

- Rifampin prophylaxis should be considered for all child-care and nursery school contacts (regardless of age) when 2 or more cases of Hib invasive disease have occurred within 60 days and unimmunized or incompletely immunized children attend the facility.

- When a single case has occurred, the advisability of rifampin prophylaxis in exposed child-care groups with unimmunized or incompletely immunized children is controversial, but many experts recommend no prophylaxis.

■ ***Index Patient***

- The index patient should receive rifampin prophylaxis if they are younger than 2 years of age or a member of a household with a susceptible contact and were treated with a regimen other than cefotaxime or ceftriaxone (e.g., ampicillin, chloramphenicol). Chemoprophylaxis usually is provided to the index patient just before discharge.

■ **Leprosy** Rifampin is used in conjunction with other anti-infective agents in multiple-drug regimens for the treatment of multibacillary leprosy†, paucibacillary leprosy†, and single-lesion paucibacillary leprosy†. Although single-drug regimens (e.g., dapsone monotherapy) were used in the past for the treatment of leprosy, the World Health Organization (WHO) and most clinicians currently recommend that rifampin-based multiple-drug regimens be used for the treatment of all forms of leprosy. These rifampin-based multiple-drug regimens generally are effective, well tolerated, and relatively inexpensive. They may reduce infectiousness of the patient more rapidly than single-drug regimens and may delay or prevent the emergence of resistant organisms. Rifampin-based multiple-drug regimens are necessary because of the increasing incidence of dapsone-resistant *Mycobacterium leprae*, and these regimens are designed to be effective against all strains of *M. leprae*, regardless of their susceptibility to dapsone.

Because rifampin is bactericidal against *M. leprae*, once-monthly administration of rifampin is the principal component of currently recommended multiple-drug regimens; dapsone and clofazimine are included in the regimens to prevent the emergence of rifampin-resistant *M. leprae*. Rifampin reportedly has greater bactericidal efficacy against *M. leprae* than any other single drug or combination of drugs that does not include rifampin, and once-monthly administration of rifampin is almost as effective against *M. leprae* as once-daily administration of the drug. The WHO states that elimination of *M. leprae* in patients receiving multiple-drug therapy principally is due to the bactericidal effect of the first several monthly doses of rifampin.

The relapse rate in leprosy patients treated with rifampin-based multiple-drug regimens appears to be low. The WHO states that retreatment with currently recommended multiple-drug regimens generally has been effective in reported cases of relapse, and rifampin-resistant strains of *M. leprae* have not been detected in relapsing patients. However, the susceptibility of *M. leprae* to rifampin has not been determined routinely in such patients and the true incidence of rifampin-resistant strains is unknown. Although rifampin-resistant *M. leprae* has been reported in a limited number of patients, these principally have been from areas where rifampin was administered either alone or with dapsone to patients with dapsone-resistant *M. leprae*. Therefore, the WHO states that rifampin-resistant strains of *M. leprae* currently is not a serious concern, but selective noncompliance with the recommended dapsone and/or clofazimine components of the multiple-drug regimens may facilitate emergence of such strains. Further, the WHO states that use of monotherapy with any one antileprosy agent uniformly results in development of resistance to that drug.

Because there is no specific vaccine available for the prevention of leprosy, early detection and effective treatment of all forms of the disease are the most effective measures available to prevent the spread of leprosy. However, while early detection and effective treatment may interrupt disease amplification within, and transmission by, human hosts and may prevent deformity in the individual with leprosy, it may not eliminate the disease. Leprosy (particularly multibacillary leprosy) patients are considered to be the principal source of new infection, and initiation of effective rifampin-based multiple-drug treatment rapidly stops shedding of *M. leprae* in nasal and upper respiratory secretions of leprosy patients, making them noninfectious. However, the epidemiologic effect of multiplication of *M. leprae* in humans is unknown; transmission continues to occur in areas where nonlepromatous patients predominate, and it is unclear whether asymptomatic infected individuals transmit infection. The exact modes of transmission and entry into susceptible individuals also are unknown, and the effects of socioeconomic and environmental factors on maintaining a leprosy epidemic are unclear. In addition, reservoirs of infection have been identified in species other than humans, and *M. leprae* may persist in soil or vegetation.

Duration of Therapy and Supervised Administration Until recently, the WHO and other clinicians recommended that multiple-drug therapy for the treatment of multibacillary leprosy be administered for 24 months. Because there is evidence that rifampin-based multiple-drug therapy is effective for the treatment of multibacillary leprosy even when the drugs are taken irregularly or for a substantially shorter duration, the WHO has revised their recommendations and currently states that a 12-month regimen of rifampin-based multiple-drug therapy can be used in most patients with multibacillary leprosy. A 6-month rifampin-based multiple-drug regimen is recommended for the treatment of paucibacillary leprosy, and a single-dose, rifampin-based multiple-drug regimen may be used in selected groups of patients with single-lesion paucibacillary leprosy.

Effective treatment of leprosy depends on compliance with the recommended multiple-drug regimens, and the WHO recommends supervised administration of some drug doses included in the regimens (e.g., once-monthly doses). However, the level of health-care services is inadequate in some countries where leprosy is endemic, and early supervision guidelines (i.e., monthly attendance on fixed days at leprosy clinics) proved to be unnecessarily rigid since it is not always possible for a health-care worker to supervise monthly drug administration. Although logistic problems associated with prolonged courses of administration remain, an alternative is to identify a family or community member who can supervise monthly drug administration when it is not possible for a health-care worker to do so. The WHO states that it may be assumed that individuals who show up for diagnosis and treatment may be considered to be sufficiently motivated to take full responsibility for their own care, provided they are appropriately educated regarding the importance of taking the daily and monthly components of multiple-drug therapy and the necessary duration of treatment. In such cases, more than a one-month supply of WHO-recommended drugs in blister packs may be provided to the patient.

The WHO states that multibacillary leprosy patients who have received 12 months of the recommended multiple-drug regimen or paucibacillary leprosy patients who have received 6 months of the recommended multiple-drug regimen usually can be considered cured. In patients who have been noncompliant, the multiple-drug regimens can be reinitiated and continued to complete the total number of recommended months of therapy (i.e., 12 or 6 months); however, patients who have been noncompliant for 12 consecutive months should be treated with an entirely new course of the recommended 12- or 6-month multiple-drug regimens.

Multibacillary Leprosy For the treatment of multibacillary leprosy (i.e., more than 5 lesions or skin smear positive for acid-fast bacteria), the WHO currently recommends a 12-month multiple-drug regimen of rifampin, clofazimine, and dapsone. Although the WHO and some clinicians state that 12 months of the recommended rifampin-based multiple-drug regimen is adequate for most multibacillary patients, there is concern that a 12-month regimen may not be of sufficient duration to be effective in patients with a high bacterial index. Therefore, the WHO currently recommends that after completing 12 months of treatment, a patient with a high bacterial index demonstrating no improvement and with evidence of deterioration should receive an additional 12 months of the multiple-drug regimen.

If a patient with multibacillary leprosy receiving the recommended rifampin-based multiple-drug regimen experiences severe adverse effects related to dapsone, the WHO states that dapsone may be discontinued and therapy continued with rifampin and clofazimine given in their usually recommended dosages. Ofloxacin and minocycline are bactericidal against *M. leprae* and are considered alternative agents that can be used in multibacillary leprosy patients who will not accept or cannot tolerate clofazimine or cannot receive rifampin because of a contraindication (e.g., hypersensitivity) or intolerance, intercurrent disease (e.g., chronic hepatitis), or infection with rifampin-resistant *M. leprae*. Clarithromycin has substantial bactericidal activity against *M. leprae* and has been used in the treatment of leprosy; however, clarithromycin has not been well tolerated in many patients, which limits its potential as an alternative drug. Although ethionamide was previously recommended as an alternative agent for use in multiple-drug regimens, it is associated with severe hepatotoxicity and the WHO no longer recommends use of the drug as an alternative to clofazimine in multiple-drug regimens.

Paucibacillary Leprosy For the treatment of paucibacillary leprosy† (i.e., 2–5 lesions), the WHO recommends a 6-month regimen of rifampin and dapsone. If a patient experiences severe adverse effects related to dapsone, dapsone may be discontinued and clofazimine substituted; the WHO recommends that clofazimine be administered for a duration of 6 months at the same dosage used in the treatment of multibacillary leprosy.

Single-lesion Paucibacillary Leprosy Patients with single-lesion paucibacillary leprosy (i.e., a single skin lesion with definite loss of sensation but without nerve trunk involvement) have been effectively treated with a single-dose rifampin-based multiple-drug regimen (ROM) that includes a single dose of rifampin, a single dose of ofloxacin, and single dose of minocycline. The single-dose ROM regimen was evaluated in a double-blind controlled study. Patients received the 6-month rifampin and dapsone regimen usually recommended for paucibacillary leprosy with single doses of placebo or received single doses of rifampin, ofloxacin, and minocycline and a 6-month regimen of placebo; patients were followed for an additional 12 months to determine response to treatment. Results at 18-month follow-up indicated that 51.8% of patients receiving the single-dose ROM regimen had marked improvement compared with 57.3% of those receiving the 6-month regimen. A complete cure (disappearance of the lesion and associated signs) was attained in 469 or 54.7% of those receiving the single-dose ROM or 6-month regimen, respectively. Treatment failure (i.e., no change or an increase in symptoms) occurred in 0.9% of patients in both treatment groups, and the incidence of adverse effects and leprosy reactions did not differ substantially between the groups.

Because the single-dose ROM regimen was almost as effective as the standard 6-month regimen in this study, and due to the considerable logistic advantage of a single-dose regimen compared with the 6-month regimen, the WHO states that the single-dose ROM regimen is an acceptable and cost-effective alternative regimen for the treatment of single-lesion paucibacillary leprosy in antileprosy programs that have detected a large number of patients (e.g., more than 1000 annually) with single-lesion paucibacillary leprosy. Use of the single-dose ROM regimen is considered to be especially advantageous in countries such as India, where over 50% of newly diagnosed leprosy patients are classified as having single-lesion leprosy. However, the WHO states that the single-dose ROM regimen should not be used in antileprosy programs that have detected few single-lesion paucibacillary patients since it involves additional logistic and information reporting problems for these programs. Because results of the controlled study indicated that the 6-month multiple-drug regimen may be more effective, some clinicians suggest that the 6-month regimen may be preferred unless operational issues of an antileprosy program make the single-dose ROM regimen more feasible.

In the US, the Gillis W. Long Hansen's Disease Center at 800-642-2477 should be contacted for further information on the treatment of leprosy.

■ **Anthrax** Strains of *Bacillus anthracis* that were associated with cases of inhalational or cutaneous anthrax that occurred in the US (Florida, New York, District of Columbia) during September and October 2001 in the context of an intentional release of anthrax spores (biologic warfare, bioterrorism) were susceptible to rifampin in vitro. Although limited clinical data are available regarding use of rifampin in the treatment of anthrax, rifampin was included in several multiple-drug regimens used in the treatment of patients who developed inhalational anthrax† following these bioterrorism-related anthrax exposures. These multiple-drug regimens include ciprofloxacin, rifampin, and clindamycin; ciprofloxacin, rifampin, and vancomycin; and ciprofloxacin, rifampin, and penicillin G. At least 2 patients who survived received a parenteral regimen of ciprofloxacin (400 mg every 8 hours), rifampin (300 mg every 12 hours), and clindamycin (900 mg every 8 hours) for treatment. Because of the rapid course of symptomatic inhalational anthrax and high mortality rate, prompt recognition of symptoms and early initiation of anti-infective therapy is essential. The CDC and other experts (e.g., US Working Group on Civilian Biodefense) recommend that treatment of inhalational anthrax that occurs as the result of exposure to anthrax spores in the context of bioterrorism should be initiated with a multiple-drug parenteral regimen that includes ciprofloxacin or doxycycline and 1 or 2 other anti-infectives predicted to be effective. Based on in vitro data, drugs that have been suggested as possibilities to augment ciprofloxacin or doxycycline in such multiple-drug regimens include rifampin, chloramphenicol, clindamycin, vancomycin, clarithromycin, imipenem, penicillin, or ampicillin. If meningitis is established or suspected, some clinicians suggest a multiple-drug regimen that includes ciprofloxacin (rather than doxycycline) and chloramphenicol, rifampin, or penicillin. Multiple-drug parenteral regimens also are recommended for the treatment of cutaneous anthrax if there are signs of systemic involvement, extensive edema, or lesions on the head and neck. For information on treatment of anthrax and recommendations for prophylaxis following exposure to anthrax spores, see Uses: Anthrax, in Ciprofloxacin 8:12.18.

■ **Bartonella Infections** Rifampin has been used in the treatment of infections caused by *Bartonella henselae*† (e.g., cat scratch disease, bacillary angiomatosis, peliosis hepatitis). Cat scratch disease generally is a self-limited illness in immunocompetent individuals and may resolve spontaneously in 2–4 months; however, some clinicians suggest that anti-infective therapy be considered for acutely or severely ill patients with systemic manifestations, particularly those with hepatosplenomegaly or painful lymphadenopathy, and such therapy probably is indicated in immunocompromised patients. Anti-infectives also may be indicated in patients with *B. henselae* infections who develop bacillary angiomatosis, neuroretinitis, or Parinaud's oculoglandular syndrome. While the optimum anti-infective regimen for the treatment of cat scratch disease or other *B. henselae* infections has not been identified, some clinicians recommend use of azithromycin, ciprofloxacin, erythromycin, co-trimoxazole, doxycycline, gentamicin, or rifampin. A regimen of erythromycin or doxycycline with or without rifampin has been used successfully in the treatment of *B. henselae* ocular infections.

■ **Brucellosis** Rifampin is used as an adjunct to other anti-infective agents for the treatment of brucellosis†. Tetracyclines generally are considered the drugs of choice for the treatment of brucellosis; however, concomitant use of another anti-infective (e.g., streptomycin or gentamicin and/or rifampin) may reduce the likelihood of disease relapse and usually is recommended in serious infections or when there are complications such as meningitis, endocarditis, or osteomyelitis.

Although many clinicians consider doxycycline and streptomycin (or gentamicin) the regimen of choice for the treatment of brucellosis, other experts recommend a regimen of a tetracycline (doxycycline) and rifampin. There is some evidence that the doxycycline-rifampin regimen may be less effective than the doxycycline-streptomycin regimen in some patients, possibly because of a pharmacokinetic interaction between rifampin and doxycycline that results in decreased plasma concentrations of the tetracycline. Although data are limited, alternative regimens that have been suggested for the treatment of brucellosis include co-trimoxazole with or without gentamicin or rifampin (recommended for use in children when tetracyclines are contraindicated); ciprofloxacin (or ofloxacin) and rifampin; and chloramphenicol with or without streptomycin.

For the treatment of acute, complicated brucellosis (e.g., skeletal disease, meningoencephalitis, endocarditis), some experts recommend a 3-drug regimen that includes doxycycline, an aminoglycoside (streptomycin or gentamicin), and rifampin; co-trimoxazole can be used instead of doxycycline in children younger than 8 years of age. Rifampin should not be used alone in the treatment of brucellosis.

Postexposure prophylaxis with anti-infectives is not generally recommended after possible exposure to endemic brucellosis; however, use of an anti-infective regimen recommended for the treatment of brucellosis (e.g., doxycycline and rifampin) should be considered following a high-risk exposure to *Brucella*. These high-risk exposures include percutaneous or mucous membrane exposure or aerosolization of infectious material in the laboratory or livestock husbandry setting or exposure in the context of biologic warfare or bioterrorism.

■ **Ehrlichia Infections** Although doxycycline is considered the drug of choice for infections caused by *Ehrlichia*, rifampin is an alternative for the treatment of infections caused by *E. phagocytophilia*†.

■ **Legionella Infections** In the treatment of infections caused by *Legionella pneumophila*† (Legionnaires' disease), rifampin is used as an adjunct to a macrolide (e.g., azithromycin, erythromycin), a fluoroquinolone (e.g., ciprofloxacin, ofloxacin, levofloxacin), or a tetracycline (e.g., doxycycline). Many clinicians consider azithromycin or a fluoroquinolone to be the preferred drugs for the treatment of Legionnaires' disease; some clinicians also consider erythromycin a drug of choice for this infection. A parenteral regimen usually is necessary for the initial treatment of severe disease, and rifampin may be added to the initial regimen in severely ill and/or immunocompromised patients. If *L. pneumophila* is identified in patients with community-acquired pneumonia, the Infectious Diseases Society of America (IDSA) recommends use of a macrolide (with or without rifampin) or a fluoroquinolone or, alternatively, a regimen of doxycycline (with or without rifampin).

■ **Rhodococcus Infections** Rifampin is used in conjunction with vancomycin for the treatment of infections caused by *Rhodococcus equi*†. *R. equi* has been identified as a cause of pulmonary infections (e.g., lung abscess) in immunocompromised individuals such as solid organ transplant recipients or patients with HIV infection. While optimum regimens for the treatment of these infections have not been identified, combination regimens usually are recommended. Some clinicians suggest that *R. equi* infections be treated with a regimen of vancomycin given with a fluoroquinolone, rifampin, a carbapenem (e.g., imipenem, meropenem), or amikacin.

■ **Staphylococcal and Streptococcal Infections** Rifampin is used as an adjunct to other anti-infective agents (e.g., third generation cephalosporins, vancomycin) for the treatment of serious infections such as bacteremia, pneumonia, and meningitis caused by penicillin-resistant *Streptococcus pneumoniae*† or oxacillin-resistant *Staphylococcus aureus* or *S. epidermidis*† (previously known as methicillin-resistant *S. aureus* or *S. epidermidis*). Rifampin should not be used alone in the treatment of these infections. (See Uses: Meningitis and Other CNS Infections in the Cephalosporins General Statement 8:12.06 and see Uses: Staphylococcal Infections and Uses: Streptococcal Infections in Vancomycin Hydrochloride 8:12.28.16.)

Dosage and Administration

■ **Reconstitution and Administration** Rifampin usually is administered orally. When oral therapy is not feasible, the drug may be given by IV infusion. Rifampin should *not* be administered IM or subcutaneously since local irritation and inflammation can occur.

Oral Administration Rifampin should be given orally either 1 hour before or 2 hours after a meal with a full glass of water to ensure maximum absorption. The fixed-combination preparation containing rifampin and isoniazid and the fixed-combination preparation containing isoniazid, rifampin, and pyrazinamide also should be given either 1 hour before or 2 hours after a meal with a full glass of water.

For patients who are unable to swallow the commercially available rifampin capsules, the contents of the capsules may be mixed with applesauce or jelly. Alternatively, a 1% rifampin suspension can be prepared by emptying the contents of four 300-mg or eight 150-mg capsules and mixing the contents vigorously with 20 mL of Syrup NF (simple syrup), and then further diluting with 100 mL of Syrup NF. Syrpalta® syrup (Emerson Laboratories), or Raspberry syrup (HumCo Laboratories) may also be used to prepare the suspension. The resulting suspensions contain 10 mg of rifampin per mL and are stable for 4 weeks when stored in a light-resistant (amber) glass or clear plastic bottle at room temperature (22–28°C) or refrigerated at 2–8°C. The extemporaneously prepared suspension must be shaken well prior to administration. The suspension is also suitable for use in children when lower doses are needed.

IV Infusion For IV infusion, rifampin powder for injection should be reconstituted by adding 10 mL of sterile water for injection to the vial labeled as containing 600 mg of rifampin to provide a solution containing 60 mg/mL. The vial should be swirled gently to facilitate dissolution of the drug. Immediately prior to administration, the appropriate dose of reconstituted solution may be added to 500 mL of 5% dextrose injection and infused at a rate that allows complete infusion within 3 hours. Alternatively, the appropriate dose of reconstituted solution may be added to 100 mL of 5% dextrose injection and infused at a rate that allows complete infusion within 30 minutes. The manufacturer states that the 500- and 100-mL IV infusion solutions containing rifampin should be prepared and administered within a total of 4 hours; precipitation of rifampin from the infusion solution may occur beyond this time period.

Extravasation during IV infusion of rifampin should be avoided. If local irritation or inflammation occurs at the site of infusion, the infusion should be discontinued and restarted at another site.

■ Dosage

Dosage of rifampin is identical for oral and IV administration.

Active Tuberculosis In the treatment of clinical tuberculosis, rifampin should not be given alone. The drug is considered a first-line agent for the treatment of all forms of tuberculosis and is an essential component of all short-course regimens. Therapy for tuberculosis should be continued long enough to prevent relapse. The minimum duration of treatment currently recommended for patients with culture-positive pulmonary tuberculosis is 6 months (26 weeks), and recommended regimens consist of an initial intensive phase (2 months) and a continuation phase (usually either 4 or 7 months). However, the American Thoracic Society (ATS), US Centers for Disease Control and Prevention (CDC), and the Infectious Diseases Society of America (IDSA) state that completion of treatment is determined more accurately by the total number of doses and should not be based solely on the duration of therapy. For information on general principles of antituberculosis therapy and recommendations regarding specific multiple-drug regimens and duration of therapy, see the Antituberculosis Agents General Statement 8:16.04.

Because of concerns that there may be an increased risk of acquired rifamycin resistance in HIV-infected individuals with $CD4^+$ T-cell counts less than 100/mm^3 who receive intermittent rifamycin regimens, the CDC recommends that rifampin be administered once daily or 3-times weekly and that rifampin regimens that involve once- or twice-weekly administration be avoided in these HIV-infected individuals pending further accumulation of data. The CDC also recommends directly observed therapy for both the daily and 3-times weekly regimens.

Adult Dosage. The manufacturer states that the usual dosage of rifampin for the treatment of active tuberculosis in adults is 10 mg/kg (up to 600 mg) once daily.

The ATS, CDC, and IDSA recommend that when rifampin is used in conjunction with other antituberculosis agents in a daily regimen, adults and children 15 years of age or older should receive a rifampin dosage of 10 mg/kg (up to 600 mg) once daily.

When an intermittent multiple-drug regimen is used, adults and children 15 years of age or older should receive a rifampin dosage of 10 mg/kg (up to 600 mg) 2 or 3 times weekly.

Pediatric Dosage. The manufacturer states that the usual dosage of rifampin for the treatment of active tuberculosis in children is 10–20 mg/kg (up to 600 mg) daily.

The ATS, CDC, IDSA, and American Academy of Pediatrics (AAP) recommend that when rifampin is used in daily multiple-drug regimens in pediatric patients, a dosage of 10–20 mg/kg (up to 600 mg) daily should be used.

If an intermittent multiple-drug regimen is used in pediatric patients, the ATS, CDC, IDSA, and AAP recommend a rifampin dosage of 10–20 mg/kg (up to 600 mg) twice weekly.

Fixed-Combination Preparations. When rifampin is administered as the fixed combination containing rifampin and isoniazid as part of a multiple-drug regimen for the treatment of pulmonary tuberculosis, the usual adult dosage is 2 capsules (600 mg of rifampin and 300 mg of isoniazid) once daily. Although the fixed-combination preparation was formulated for daily regimens, the ATS, CDC, and IDSA state that the fixed-combination preparation can be used in twice-weekly regimens† provided additional isoniazid is administered concomitantly. When used in an intermittent multiple-drug regimen, these experts state that 2 capsules of (600 mg of rifampin and 300 mg of isoniazid) and an additional 600 mg of isoniazid (i.e., 900 mg of isoniazid total) may be given twice weekly using directly observed therapy (DOT). The manufacturer states that the fixed combination containing rifampin and isoniazid should *not* be used for the initial treatment of tuberculosis and should only be used after efficacy of the rifampin and isoniazid dosages contained in the fixed-combination preparation has been established by titrating the individual components in the patient.

When rifampin is administered as the fixed combination containing isoniazid, rifampin, and pyrazinamide (Rifater®) in the initial phase (e.g., initial 2 months) of multiple-drug therapy for pulmonary tuberculosis, the manufacturer states that the adult dosage of Rifater® given as a single daily dose is 4 tablets (480 mg of rifampin, 200 mg of isoniazid, 1.2 g of pyrazinamide) in patients weighing 44 kg or less, 5 tablets (600 mg of rifampin, 250 mg of isoniazid, 1.5 g of pyrazinamide) in those weighing 45–54 kg, and 6 tablets (720 mg of rifampin, 300 mg of isoniazid, and 1.8 g of pyrazinamide) in those weighing 55 kg or more. This fixed-combination preparation provides a higher rifampin dosage than is usually used in the US because rifampin is less bioavailable in this formulation. In individuals weighing more than 90 kg, additional pyrazinamide should be given in conjunction with the fixed-combination preparation to obtain an adequate dosage of this drug. The ratio of rifampin, isoniazid, and pyrazinamide in Rifater® may not be appropriate in children or adolescents younger than 15 years of age because of the higher mg/kg doses of isoniazid usually given in children compared with those given in adults.

Treatment of Latent Tuberculosis Infection **Rifampin Monotherapy.** When daily rifampin monotherapy is used as an alternative regimen for the treatment of latent tuberculosis infection, the ATS and CDC recommend that adults receive a rifampin dosage of 10 mg/kg (up to 600 mg) daily for 4 months. The ATS, CDC, and AAP recommend that infants, children, and adolescents receive 10–20 mg/kg (up to 600 mg) daily for 4–6 months.

The ATS and CDC state that completion of treatment is determined more accurately by the total number of doses and should not be based solely on the duration of therapy. In adults, the rifampin monotherapy regimen should consist of at least 120 doses administered within 6 months (allowing for minor interruptions in the 4-month regimen).

Rifampin and Pyrazinamide Regimens. Because of the risk of hepatotoxicity, rifampin and pyrazinamide regimens should be used with caution and only in selected individuals with close clinical and laboratory monitoring throughout the course of treatment. To facilitate clinical assessment and laboratory monitoring of serum concentrations of AST (SGOT) and bilirubin at baseline and at 2, 4, 6, and 8 weeks, no more than a 2-week supply of rifampin and pyrazinamide should be dispensed at a time. (See Precautions Related to Hepatotoxicity under Cautions: Precautions and Contraindications.)

When a 2-month daily regimen of rifampin and pyrazinamide is used for the treatment of latent tuberculosis infection† when the potential benefits of the regimen outweigh the risk of severe liver injury and death (see Rifampin and Pyrazinamide Regimens under Tuberculosis: Latent Tuberculosis Infection, in Uses), the ATS and CDC recommend that adults receive a rifampin dosage of 10 mg/kg (up to 600 mg) daily in conjunction with pyrazinamide. This daily regimen should consist of at least 60 doses administered within 3 months (allowing for minor interruptions in the 2-month regimen).

If an intermittent (twice-weekly) regimen of rifampin and pyrazinamide is used for the treatment of latent tuberculosis infection when the potential benefits outweigh the risk of severe liver injury and death, the ATS and CDC recommend that adults receive a rifampin dosage of 10 mg/kg (up to 600 mg) given twice weekly for 2–3 months in conjunction with pyrazinamide given twice weekly. If this intermittent regimen is used, it should be given using DOT.

Neisseria meningitidis Infection **Elimination of Pharyngeal Carrier State.** When rifampin is used to eliminate meningococci from the nasopharynx of asymptomatic *Neisseria meningitidis* carriers, the recommended dosage in adults is 600 mg twice daily for 2 days. Children 1 month of age or older may receive rifampin in a dosage of 10 mg/kg twice daily for 2 days and children younger than 1 month of age may receive 5 mg/kg twice daily for 2 days.

Prophylaxis in Household or Other Close Contacts. When rifampin is used for chemoprophylaxis in close contacts of individuals with invasive meningococcal disease† when the risk of infection is high, adults should receive 600 mg every 12 hours for 2 days. The usual dosage of rifampin for chemoprophylaxis of meningococcal disease in children older than 1 month of age is 10 mg/kg (maximum dose 600 mg) every 12 hours for 2 days. Neonates 1 month of age or younger should receive 5 mg/kg every 12 hours for 2 days for chemoprophylaxis of meningococcal disease. When chemoprophylaxis is indicated in high-risk contacts, it must be administered promptly (ideally within 24 hours after identification of the index case) since the attack rate of secondary disease is greatest in the few days following disease onset in the index case. Chemoprophylaxis probably is of limited or no value if administered more than 2 weeks after contact with the index case.

Prevention of Haemophilus influenzae Type b Infection When indicated for prophylaxis of *Haemophilus influenzae* type b infection† in adults and children, the recommended dosage of rifampin is 20 mg/kg (maximum dose 600 mg) once daily for 4 consecutive days. Dosage for very young infants has not been established, but some clinicians recommend a dosage of 10 mg/kg once daily for 4 consecutive days in neonates younger than 1 month of age.

Leprosy **Multibacillary Leprosy.** For the treatment of multibacillary leprosy†, the World Health Organization (WHO) recommends that adults receive rifampin in a dosage of 600 mg once monthly in conjunction with clofazimine (50 mg once daily and 300 mg once monthly), and dapsone (100 mg daily) given for 12 months. Children 10–14 years of age with multibacillary leprosy should receive rifampin in a dosage of 450 mg once monthly in conjunction with clofazimine (50 mg every second day and 150 mg once monthly), and dapsone (50 mg daily) given for 12 months, and children younger than 10 years of age should receive an appropriately adjusted dosage (e.g., rifampin [300 mg monthly], clofazimine [50 mg twice weekly and 100 mg once monthly], and dapsone [25 mg daily]) given for 12 months. The WHO recommends supervised administration of some drug doses included in the regimen (e.g., once-monthly doses). While the 12-month regimen is adequate for most patients with multibacillary leprosy, the WHO recommends that multibacillary leprosy patients with a high bacteriologic index who demonstrate no improvement (with evidence of worsening) of leprosy following completion of the initial 12 months of treatment should receive an additional 12 months of therapy.

If a patient with multibacillary leprosy experiences severe adverse effects related to dapsone, dapsone may be discontinued from the regimen and therapy continued with rifampin and clofazimine given in the usually recommended dosages.

If a patient with multibacillary leprosy will not accept or cannot tolerate clofazimine, the WHO recommends supervised administration of a once-monthly rifampin-based multiple-drug regimen (ROM) that includes rifampin (600 mg once monthly), ofloxacin (400 mg once monthly), and minocycline (100 mg once monthly) given for 24 months.

For the treatment of multibacillary leprosy in adults who cannot receive rifampin because of a contraindication (e.g., hypersensitivity) or intolerance, intercurrent disease, or infection with rifampin-resistant *Mycobacterium leprae*, the WHO recommends supervised administration of a regimen of clofazimine (50 mg daily), ofloxacin (400 mg daily), and minocycline (100 mg daily) given for 6 months, followed by a regimen of clofazimine (50 mg daily) and ofloxacin

(400 mg daily) *or* minocycline (100 mg daily) given for at least an additional 18 months.

Paucibacillary Leprosy. For the treatment of paucibacillary leprosy†, the WHO recommends that adults receive rifampin in a dosage of 600 mg once monthly in conjunction with dapsone (100 mg daily) given for 6 months.

Children 10–14 years of age with paucibacillary leprosy should receive rifampin in a dosage of 450 mg once monthly in conjunction with dapsone (50 mg daily) given for 6 months, and children younger than 10 years of age should receive an appropriately adjusted dosage (e.g., rifampin [300 mg once monthly] in conjunction with dapsone [25 mg daily]) given for 6 months.

The WHO recommends supervised administration of some drug doses included in the regimen (e.g., once monthly doses).

If a patient with paucibacillary leprosy experiences severe adverse effects related to dapsone, dapsone may be discontinued from the regimen and clofazimine substituted (given in the dosage recommended for the treatment of multibacillary leprosy) for a period of 6 months.

Single-lesion Paucibacillary Leprosy. For the treatment of single-lesion paucibacillary leprosy† in certain patient groups (see Single-lesion Paucibacillary Leprosy under Uses: Leprosy), the WHO states that adults may receive a single-dose rifampin-based multiple-drug regimen (ROM) that includes a single 600-mg dose of rifampin, a single 400-mg dose of ofloxacin, and a single 100-mg dose of minocycline.

For the treatment of single-lesion paucibacillary leprosy, children 5–14 years of age may receive a single 300-mg dose of rifampin, a single 200-mg dose of ofloxacin, and a single 50-mg dose of minocycline, and children younger than 5 years of age should receive an appropriately adjusted dose of each drug.

Anthrax Although the optimum regimen for the treatment of inhalational anthrax remains to be established, limited experience indicates that early treatment with a multiple-drug parenteral regimen that includes a fluoroquinolone and at least one other active anti-infective may improve survival. Several patients with inhalational anthrax† have been treated successfully with a multiple-drug regimen that included IV rifampin 300 mg every 12 hours, IV ciprofloxacin 400 mg every 8 hours, and IV clindamycin 900 mg every 8 hours. Some clinicians suggest that rifampin be given in a dosage of 20 mg/kg IV daily if the drug is included in a multiple-drug regimen for the treatment of anthrax meningitis.

Brucellosis If rifampin is used in conjunction with a tetracycline (doxycycline), co-trimoxazole, or a fluoroquinolone (ciprofloxacin or ofloxacin) for the *treatment* of brucellosis†, a rifampin dosage of 15–20 mg/kg (up to 600–900 mg) daily usually is recommended in adults or pediatric patients. Some clinicians recommend a rifampin dosage of 0.6–1.2 g daily in conjunction with other anti-infectives. An oral regimen usually is effective for the treatment of brucellosis. The anti-infective regimen should be continued for 4–6 weeks to prevent relapse; however, more prolonged therapy may be necessary in serious infections or when there are complications (e.g., meningoencephalitis or endocarditis). Some clinicians state that 6–8 weeks of treatment may be necessary in patients with skeletal disease and at least 3 months (and possibly more than 6 months) of treatment may be necessary in those with meningoencephalitis or endocarditis.

If use of an anti-infective regimen is considered necessary for *prophylaxis* following a high-risk exposure to *Brucella*†, some experts recommend that the same regimen recommended for the treatment of brucellosis be given for 3–6 weeks.

Cautions

■ **GI Effects** The most frequent adverse effects of rifampin are GI disturbances, which include heartburn, epigastric distress, nausea, vomiting, anorexia, abdominal cramps, flatulence, and diarrhea. Rarely, adverse GI effects may be severe enough to require discontinuance of the drug. Although rifampin usually should be administered 1 hour before or 2 hours after food to ensure maximum absorption, adverse GI effects may be minimized by administering the drug during or immediately after a meal.

Although rifampin has some in vitro activity against *Clostridium difficile*, *C. difficile*-associated diarrhea and colitis (also known as antibiotic-associated pseudomembranous colitis) has been reported rarely in association with rifampin therapy and should be considered in the differential diagnosis of patients who develop diarrhea during or following therapy with the drug.

■ **Nervous System Effects** Headache, drowsiness, fatigue, ataxia, dizziness, inability to concentrate, mental confusion, behavioral changes, psychosis, visual disturbances, muscular weakness, myopathy, fever, generalized numbness, and pains in muscles, joints, and extremities have occurred, especially during the first few weeks of rifampin therapy.

■ **Hepatic Effects** Rifampin has caused transient increases in serum concentrations of AST (SGOT), ALT (SGPT), bilirubin, and alkaline phosphatase. Asymptomatic jaundice which subsided without discontinuance of the drug has occurred occasionally. However, hepatitis and fatalities associated with jaundice have been reported in patients with preexisting liver disease or in those who received other hepatotoxic agents concomitantly with rifampin. Rarely, hepatitis or a shocklike syndrome with hepatic involvement and abnormal liver function test results (thought to be allergic in nature) have been reported.

Hepatotoxicity with Combined Rifampin and Pyrazinamide Severe hepatic injuries, including some fatalities, have been reported in patients receiving regimens that contain both rifampin and pyrazinamide for the treatment of latent tuberculosis infection. Between October 2000 and June 2003, the US Centers for Disease Control and Prevention (CDC) received a total of 48 reports of severe hepatic injury (i.e., hospitalization or death) in patients with latent tuberculosis infection receiving a rifampin and pyrazinamide regimen; there were 11 fatalities. In many fatal cases, onset of hepatic injury occurred during the second month of the 2-month regimen. Some patients who died were receiving the rifampin and pyrazinamide regimen because they previously experienced isoniazid-associated hepatitis and some had risk factors for chronic liver disease (e.g., serologic evidence of previous hepatitis A or B infection, idiopathic nonalcoholic steatotic hepatitis, alcohol or parenteral drug abuse, concomitant use of other drugs associated with idiosyncratic hepatic injury). Although data are limited, there is no evidence to date that HIV-infected individuals receiving this regimen are at any increased risk for severe hepatitis. There is evidence that the rate of severe liver injury and death related to the use of rifampin and pyrazinamide are higher than the rates reported for isoniazid-associated liver injury in the treatment of latent tuberculosis infection. Based on these reports, rifampin and pyrazinamide regimens should be used for the treatment of *latent* tuberculosis only when the potential benefits outweigh the risk of liver injury and death. (See Cautions: Precautions and Contraindications.)

■ **Local, Sensitivity, and Dermatologic Reactions** Extravasation during IV infusion of rifampin has caused local irritation and inflammation. Extravasation should be avoided; if it occurs, the infusion should be discontinued and restarted at another site.

Hypersensitivity reactions characterized by a flu-like syndrome with episodes of fever, chills, and sometimes with headache, dizziness, and bone pain have occurred with rifampin. Edema of the face and extremities, decrease in blood pressure, and shock also have been reported. Dyspnea, sometimes accompanied by wheezing, may also occur. Occasionally, pruritus, urticaria, acneiform eruptions, rash, pemphigoid reactions, erythema multiforme including Stevens-Johnson syndrome, toxic epidermal necrolysis, vasculitis, eosinophilia, sore mouth, sore tongue, anaphylaxis, exfoliative dermatitis, and exudative conjunctivitis have also occurred. Anaphylaxis has been reported rarely. Some cutaneous reactions, including flushing and pruritus (with or without rash), are mild and self-limiting and do not appear to be hypersensitivity reactions to rifampin. More serious cutaneous reactions occur less frequently and do appear to be hypersensitivity reactions to the drug.

Hypersensitivity reactions, especially the flu-like syndrome, are usually associated with high-dose intermittent rifampin therapy (900–1200 mg twice weekly) or treatment that has been resumed after a lapse of days or weeks. These hypersensitivity reactions reportedly occur in about 1% of patients who receive 600 mg of rifampin twice weekly.

■ **Hematologic Effects** Thrombocytopenia, leukopenia, purpura, hemolytic anemia, hemolysis, hemoglobinuria, and decreased hemoglobin concentrations have occurred with rifampin. Acute hemolytic anemia has generally occurred only with intermittent rifampin therapy. Thrombocytopenia has been reported principally with high-dose intermittent rifampin therapy, but also has been reported rarely after rifampin therapy was discontinued and then resumed; thrombocytopenia occurs only rarely during daily rifampin therapy. Thrombocytopenia generally is reversible if rifampin is discontinued as soon as purpura occurs; cerebral hemorrhage and fatalities have been reported when rifampin therapy was continued or resumed after the appearance of purpura. In addition, disseminated intravascular coagulation has been reported rarely in patients receiving rifampin.

■ **Renal, Endocrine, and Metabolic Effects** Increased BUN and serum uric acid concentrations, light chain proteinuria, hematuria, renal insufficiency, interstitial nephritis, acute tubular necrosis, and acute renal failure have occurred infrequently with rifampin. Rifampin has also been associated with precipitation of adrenocortical insufficiency in a few patients with compromised adrenal function, possibly resulting from increased cortisol metabolism secondary to hepatic microsomal enzyme induction. Menstrual disturbances have also been reported.

Rifampin has been shown to decrease plasma concentrations of 25-hydroxy vitamin D (the major circulating metabolite of vitamin D) and/or 1α,25-dihydroxy vitamin D; isoniazid has similar effects and concomitant use of rifampin and isoniazid has been reported to alter vitamin D metabolism. In some cases, decreased plasma concentrations of vitamin D metabolites have been accompanied by decreased plasma calcium and phosphate concentrations and increased parathyroid hormone concentrations.

■ **Lupus-like Syndrome** A drug-induced lupus-like syndrome consisting principally of malaise, myalgias, arthritis, and peripheral edema and accompanied by positive antinuclear antibody (ANA) test results has been reported in a few patients receiving rifampin (450–600 mg daily) or rifabutin (300 mg daily). Manifestations of the syndrome disappeared within 1–10 weeks following discontinuance of rifamycin therapy despite continuation of other antimycobacterial therapy; one patient who was rechallenged with rifabutin had a relapse of symptoms. All patients were receiving concomitant therapy with clarithromycin and/or ciprofloxacin, known inhibitors of the cytochrome P-450 enzyme system, and it has been suggested that this syndrome may have been associated with elevated serum concentrations of the rifamycin (elevated serum rifampin concentration was documented in one patient) caused by inhibition of rifamycin metabolism. (See Drug Interactions: Drugs Undergoing Hepatic Metabolism.)

■ Precautions and Contraindications

Rifampin is contraindicated in patients with a history of hypersensitivity to the drug or any of the rifamycins.

Because rifampin used alone or in conjunction with other drugs has been associated with adverse hepatic effects (e.g., severe liver injury) and adverse hematologic effects (see Cautions: Hepatic Effects and see Cautions: Hematologic Effects), liver function (hepatic enzymes, bilirubin) and hematologic status (complete blood cell and platelet counts) should be assessed prior to initiation of rifampin therapy. Serum creatinine concentrations also should be assessed at baseline. Adult patients receiving rifampin generally should be seen at least monthly and questioned concerning adverse reactions; those reporting abnormalities should have follow-up, including laboratory monitoring, as necessary. Patients should be advised to contact their clinician immediately if they develop fever, loss of appetite, malaise, nausea and vomiting, darkened urine, yellowish discoloration of the skin and eyes, and/or pain or swelling of the joints during rifampin therapy Routine laboratory monitoring for drug-induced toxicity in patients with normal baseline tests generally is not necessary.

Although one manufacturer states that rifampin is not recommended for intermittent therapy, the American Thoracic Society (ATS), US Centers for Disease Control and Prevention (CDC), and Infectious Diseases Society of America (IDSA) currently recommend intermittent rifampin regimens that involve administration 2 or 3 times weekly for the treatment of uncomplicated pulmonary and most cases of extrapulmonary tuberculosis. (See General Principles in the Antituberculosis Agents General Statement 8:16.04.) and a once-monthly rifampin regimen is used in multiple-drug regimens for the treatment of leprosy†.

Precautions Related to Hepatotoxicity Rifampin should be used in patients with impaired liver function only when clearly necessary and only under strict medical supervision. If the drug is used in patients with impaired hepatic function, liver function tests should be performed every 2–4 weeks. The drug should be discontinued if signs of hepatocellular damage occur. In some cases, hyperbilirubinemia (resulting from competition between rifampin and bilirubin for excretory pathways in the liver) can occur shortly after initiation of rifampin therapy. An isolated report of a moderate increase in bilirubin and/or transaminase concentrations, therefore, is not in itself an indication to discontinue rifampin therapy; the decision to discontinue therapy should be made after repeating the tests, noting trends in the concentrations, and considering the test results in conjunction with the patient's clinical condition.

Because of reports of liver injury (including fatalities) when regimens containing rifampin and pyrazinamide were used in patients with *latent*tuberculosis infection, these regimens generally should *not* be offered to HIV-infected or HIV-negative patients. Regimens containing rifampin and pyrazinamide should be considered for the treatment of latent tuberculosis infection only when the potential benefits outweigh the risk of liver injury and death; when the preferred or alternative regimens (i.e., 9-month isoniazid regimens, 6-month isoniazid regimens, 4-month daily rifampin regimen) are judged unlikely to be completed; and when oversight can be provided by a clinician with expertise in the treatment of latent tuberculosis. A rifampin-pyrazinamide regimen should never be offered to patients who are currently taking other drugs associated with liver injury, patients who drink excessive amounts of alcohol (even if alcohol is discontinued during treatment), or patients with underlying liver disease or a history of isoniazid-associated liver injury. An expert in the treatment of latent tuberculosis should be consulted before a regimen of rifampin and pyrazinamide is offered. Individuals being considered for a 2-month rifampin-pyrazinamide regimen should be informed of potential hepatotoxicity, questioned regarding prior liver disease or history of adverse effects during treatment with isoniazid or other drugs, and cautioned against the concurrent use of potentially hepatotoxic drugs (including OTC drugs such as acetaminophen).

If a decision is made to use a rifampin-pyrazinamide regimen, serum AST and bilirubin concentrations should be measured at baseline and at 2, 4, 6, and 8 weeks and patients should be reassessed in person by a health-care provider at 2, 4, 6 and 8 weeks for adherence, tolerance, and adverse effects. To facilitate these periodic assessments, no more than a 2-week supply of the drugs should be dispensed at a time. Patients should be instructed to discontinue the rifampin-pyrazinamide regimen immediately and seek clinical consultation if abdominal pain, emesis, jaundice, or other manifestations of hepatitis develop. The drugs should be discontinued and not reinitiated in asymptomatic patients who have an AST concentration exceeding 5 times the upper limit of normal, in patients with symptoms of hepatitis who have an AST concentration exceeding the upper limit of normal, and in patients who have serum bilirubin concentrations exceeding the upper limit of normal (regardless of the presence or absence of symptoms).

Precautions in Leprosy Patients Effective therapy of leprosy with antileprosy agents (e.g., dapsone, clofazimine, rifampin) generally results in abrupt changes in the clinical state of the patient. These changes have been termed leprosy reactional states and can be classified into 2 types: reversal reactions (type 1) and erythema nodosum leprosum (ENL) or lepromatous lepra reactions (type 2). (See Cautions: Leprosy Reactional States, in Dapsone 8:16.92, and see Leprosy Reactional States under Uses: Leprosy, in Clofazimine 8:16.92). In the US, the Gillis W. Long Hansen's Disease Center at 800-642-2477 should be contacted for further information on the management of leprosy reactional states.

Although one manufacturer states that rifampin is not recommended for intermittent therapy, the World Health Organization (WHO) and many clinicians recommend that rifampin be given once monthly when used in recommended multiple-drug regimens for the treatment of leprosy†. Rifampin appears to be well tolerated in leprosy patients when administered once monthly as part of multiple-drug regimens. Most adverse effects reported in leprosy patients receiving the recommended rifampin regimens with one or more other drugs are mild. However, more severe adverse effects have been reported occasionally when rifampin was administered in leprosy patients, including renal failure, thrombocytopenia, flu-like syndrome, and hepatitis. Patients receiving intermittent therapy should be closely monitored for compliance and cautioned against intentional or accidental interruption of the dosage regimen.

Other Precautions and Contraindications Commercially available rifampin sterile powder for injection contains sodium formaldehyde sulfoxylate, a sulfite that may cause serious allergic-type reactions in certain susceptible individuals. The overall incidence of sulfite sensitivity in the general population is probably low, but in susceptible individuals, exposure to sulfites can result in acute bronchospasm or, less frequently, life-threatening anaphylaxis. Rifampin sterile powder for injection containing sodium formaldehyde sulfoxylate should be used with caution in atopic, nonasthmatic individuals.

Rifampin and its metabolites may impart a red-orange color to urine, feces, sputum, sweat, and tears; patients should be informed of this possibility. Soft contact lenses worn during rifampin therapy may become permanently stained.

To reduce development of drug-resistant bacteria and maintain effectiveness of rifampin and other antibacterials, the drug should be used only for the treatment or prevention of infections proven or strongly suspected to be caused by susceptible bacteria. When selecting or modifying anti-infective therapy, results of culture and in vitro susceptibility testing should be used. In the absence of such data, local epidemiology and susceptibility patterns should be considered when selecting anti-infectives for empiric therapy. Patients should be advised that antibacterials (including rifampin) should only be used to treat bacterial infections and not used to treat viral infections (e.g., the common cold). Patients also should be advised about the importance of completing the full course of therapy, even if feeling better after a few days, and that skipping doses or not completing therapy may decrease effectiveness and increase the likelihood that bacteria will develop resistance and will not be treatable with rifampin or other antibacterials in the future.

■ Pediatric Precautions

Rifampin is used in pediatric patients for the treatment of active tuberculosis and treatment of latent tuberculosis infection, to eliminate nasopharyngeal carriage of *Neisseria meningitidis*, for chemoprophylaxis against meningococcal disease† or *Haemophilus influenzae* type b (Hib) infection†, and for the treatment of leprosy.

Safety and efficacy of the fixed-combination preparation containing rifampin, isoniazid, and pyrazinamide (Rifater®) have not been established in children younger than 15 years of age; the ratio of rifampin and isoniazid contained in this preparation may not be appropriate in this age group since higher doses of isoniazid usually are used in pediatric patients.

■ Mutagenicity and Carcinogenicity

There was no evidence of mutagenicity when rifampin was tested in vitro and in vivo using bacteria, *Drosophila melanogaster*, or mice. However, in vitro studies indicate an increase in chromatid breaks in whole blood cell cultures exposed to rifampin and an increased frequency of chromosomal aberrations in lymphocytes obtained from patients treated with drug regimens that included rifampin, isoniazid, and pyrazinamide (with or without streptomycin).

In one strain of mice known to be particularly susceptible to the spontaneous development of hepatomas, there was an increase in hepatomas in the female mice after a year of rifampin at a dosage 2–10 times the maximum human dosage. There was no evidence of carcinogenicity in the male mice of this strain, in male or female mice of another strain, or in rats under similar experimental conditions. Although a causal relationship has not been definitely established, a few cases of accelerated growth of lung carcinoma has been reported in patients receiving rifampin.

■ Pregnancy, Fertility, and Lactation

An increased incidence of congenital malformations (principally spina bifida and cleft palate) has been reported in the offspring of mice and rats given rifampin in a dosage of 150–250 mg/kg daily during pregnancy. The incidence of these anomalies was dose dependent. In addition, imperfect osteogenesis and embryotoxicity occurred when rifampin doses up to 20 times the usual daily human dose were used in pregnant rabbits. The manufacturer states that isolated cases of fetal malformations have been reported. Although safe use of the drugs during pregnancy has not been definitely established, rifampin (combined with isoniazid and/or ethambutol) has been used to treat clinical tuberculosis in pregnant women. There are no adequate and controlled studies to date using rifampin in pregnant women, and the drug should be used during pregnancy only when the potential benefits justify the possible risks to the fetus. The American Thoracic Society (ATS), US Centers for Disease Control and Prevention (CDC), and Infectious Diseases Society of America (IDSA) state that rifampin is considered safe for use in pregnant women. The manufacturer states that neonates of rifampin-treated mothers should be carefully observed for evidence of adverse reactions.

Studies have not been performed to date to determine whether rifampin has an effect on fertility.

Since rifampin is distributed into milk and because animal studies indicate that the drug has a potential for tumorigenic effects, a decision should be made whether to discontinue nursing or the drug, taking into account the importance of the drug to the woman.

Drug Interactions

■ **Antiretroviral Agents** Rifamycin derivatives (e.g., rifampin, rifabutin) can accelerate the metabolism of certain antiretroviral agents (i.e., HIV protease inhibitors [PIs], nonnucleoside reverse transcriptase inhibitors [NNRTIs]) by induction of cytochrome P-450 (CYP) oxidases, which may result in subtherapeutic plasma concentrations of some of these PIs and NNRTIs. Rifampin also can affect the pharmacokinetics of some nucleoside reverse transcriptase inhibitors (e.g., zidovudine). In addition, PIs and some NNRTIs (e.g., delavirdine) reduce the metabolism of rifamycins, leading to increased plasma concentrations of rifamycins and an increased risk of toxicity. The potential for alterations in the plasma concentrations of antimycobacterial agent(s) and/or antiretroviral agent(s) must be considered when antimycobacterial agents are indicated for the management of latent or active tuberculosis or the prophylaxis or treatment of *Mycobacterium avium* complex (MAC) infections in HIV-infected patients who are receiving or are being considered for antiretroviral therapy. Because the management of these patients is complex and must be individualized, experts in the management of mycobacterial infections in HIV-infected patients should be consulted.

HIV Fusion Inhibitors Concomitant use of enfuvirtide and rifampin does not appear to have a clinically important effect on the pharmacokinetics of the HIV fusion inhibitor.

HIV Protease Inhibitors Because rifampin is a potent inducer of the CYP3A4 isoenzyme and can markedly reduce plasma concentrations of amprenavir, atazanavir, fosamprenavir, indinavir, lopinavir, nelfinavir, or saquinavir, concomitant use of rifampin and these PIs is contraindicated.

Concomitant use of rifampin and *ritonavir-boosted* indinavir is contraindicated. Concomitant use of rifampin (600 mg once daily) and *ritonavir-boosted* saquinavir (1 g of saquinavir and 100 mg of ritonavir twice daily) has resulted in drug-induced hepatotoxicity and marked increases in serum transaminase concentrations; therefore, concomitant use of rifampin with *ritonavir-boosted* saquinavir is contraindicated.

Because concomitant use of rifampin and ritonavir results in decreased ritonavir concentrations, the manufacturer of ritonavir and some clinicians state that other antimycobacterial agents (e.g., rifabutin) should be used instead of rifampin in patients receiving ritonavir.

For specific information on the pharmacokinetic interactions between PIs and rifampin, see Antimycobacterial Agents under Drug Interactions: Anti-infective Agents, in the individual monographs in 8:18.08.08.

Nonnucleoside Reverse Transcriptase Inhibitors Concomitant use of rifampin and delavirdine results in a substantial decrease in concentrations of the nonnucleoside reverse transcriptase inhibitor. Because of this pharmacokinetic interaction, concomitant use of rifampin and delavirdine is contraindicated.

Concomitant use of efavirenz and rifampin can result in decreased plasma concentrations and area under the plasma concentration-time curve (AUC) of the nonnucleoside reverse transcriptase inhibitor. The manufacturer of efavirenz states that the clinical importance of this pharmacokinetic interaction is unknown. Some experts recommend that consideration be given to increasing efavirenz dosage to 800 mg once daily when the drug is used in patients receiving rifampin.

Concomitant use of nevirapine and rifampin results in a substantial decrease in peak plasma concentrations and AUC of nevirapine, and the manufacturer of the nonnucleoside reverse transcriptase inhibitor states that the drugs should not be used concomitantly. Some experts state that because the virologic consequences are uncertain and because the potential for additive hepatotoxicity exists, concomitant use of rifampin and nevirapine is not recommended; however, if the drugs are used concomitantly, the patient should be closely monitored.

For specific information on the pharmacokinetic interactions between nonnucleoside reverse transcriptase inhibitors and rifampin, see Antimycobacterial Agents under Drug Interactions: Anti-infective Agents, in the individual monographs in 8:18.08.16.

Nucleoside and Nucleotide Reverse Transcriptase Inhibitors Concomitant use of rifampin and tenofovir disoproxil fumarate does not have a clinically important effect on the pharmacokinetics of either drug. Dosage adjustments are not necessary when the drugs are used concomitantly.

In a multiple-dose study in HIV-infected patients, concomitant use of zidovudine (200 mg every 8 hours) and rifampin (600 mg once daily) given for 14 days resulted in a 43% decrease in peak plasma concentrations of zidovudine, a 47% decrease in the AUC, and a 13% decrease in the plasma half-life of the antiretroviral agent.

■ **Drugs Undergoing Hepatic Metabolism** Rifampin induces certain cytochrome P-450 liver enzymes responsible for the metabolism of a number of drugs. Concurrent administration of rifampin and any of the following drugs may result in decreased plasma concentrations of the drugs; dosage adjustments may be required and, in some cases, concomitant use is contraindicated.

■ **Drugs with Induced Metabolism**

- β-Adrenergic agents
- Antiarrhythmic agents (disopyramide, mexiletine, quinidine)
- Anticonvulsants (phenytoin)
- Antifungal agents (fluconazole, itraconazole, ketoconazole)
- Antipsychotic agents (clozapine, haloperidol)
- Antiretroviral agents (see Drug Interactions: Antiretroviral Agents)
- Barbiturates
- Benzodiazepines (diazepam, midazolam, triazolam)
- Calcium-channel blocking agents (diltiazem, nifedipine, verapamil)
- Cardiac glycosides
- Chloramphenicol
- Clarithromycin
- Corticosteroids
- Dapsone
- Doxycycline
- Estrogens
- Fluoroquinolones (ciprofloxacin)
- Immunosuppressive agents (cyclosporine, tacrolimus)
- Narcotic analgesics (methadone)
- Oral anticoagulants
- Oral antidiabetic agents (sulfonylureas)
- Oral or other systemic hormonal contraceptives
- Progestins
- Quinine
- Theophyllines
- Tricyclic antidepressants (amitriptyline, nortriptyline)

Anticoagulants In patients receiving rifampin and oral anticoagulants concurrently, prothrombin times should be performed daily or as frequently as necessary to establish and maintain the required anticoagulant dosage.

Antifungal Agents Concomitant use of rifampin and fluconazole may result in decreased fluconazole AUCs and possible decreased efficacy of the antifungal. Depending on clinical circumstances, an increase in fluconazole dosage can be considered when the drugs are used concomitantly.

Concomitant use of rifampin and itraconazole may lead to decreased serum concentrations of itraconazole and possible decreased efficacy of the antifungal. In at least one patient receiving both rifampin and itraconazole, serum concentrations of the antifungal agent were undetectable. Concomitant use of rifampin and itraconazole is not recommended.

Concomitant use of rifampin and ketoconazole has resulted in decreased serum concentrations of ketoconazole, and the manufacturer of ketoconazole recommends that the drugs not be used concomitantly. In one patient receiving ketoconazole concomitantly with rifampin and isoniazid, serum concentrations of both rifampin and ketoconazole were decreased. Although administration of ketoconazole 12 hours after the rifampin dose resulted in therapeutic serum concentrations of rifampin, serum concentrations of ketoconazole were subtherapeutic regardless of when the doses were given. In addition, isoniazid and rifampin appeared to have an additive effect in reducing serum ketoconazole concentrations.

Immunosuppressive Agents Concomitant use of rifampin in transplant recipients (e.g., kidney, heart) who were receiving an immunosuppressive regimen that included cyclosporine has resulted in decreased serum concentrations of cyclosporine. If rifampin is used in transplant recipients or other individuals receiving cyclosporine, serum concentrations of the immunosuppressant should be monitored closely and appropriate dosage modifications made. Some clinicians suggest that rifampin should not be used in patients receiving cyclosporine.

Concomitant use of rifampin in a renal transplant recipient receiving tacrolimus has resulted in substantially decreased tacrolimus concentrations.

Oral Contraceptives When administered concurrently with oral contraceptives containing estrogen, rifampin has decreased the effectiveness of the contraceptives and has caused a high incidence of menstrual disorders (e.g., spotting, breakthrough bleeding); patients should be advised that the reliability of oral contraceptives may be affected by rifampin and an alternative form of contraception should be considered in patients receiving the drug.

Verapamil Marked (e.g., greater than 90%) reductions in bioavailability and peak serum concentrations of verapamil, accompanied by diminution or elimination of the drug's electrocardiographic and therapeutic effects, have occurred after concurrent administration of rifampin and oral but not IV verapamil; alternatives to rifampin should be considered in patients in whom oral verapamil therapy is deemed essential.

■ **Aminosalicylic Acid** Certain aminosalicylic acid preparations may impair GI absorption of rifampin, resulting in decreased serum concentrations of the drug. This effect appears to result from bentonite, an excipient used in preparations of aminosalicylic acid granules (not commercially available in the US).

■ **Antacids** Results of a pharmacokinetic study in healthy, fasting adults indicate that 20 mL of an aluminum and magnesium hydroxide antacid (Mylanta®) does not affect peak plasma concentrations or area under the concentration-time curve (AUC) of rifampin. However, the manufacturer of rifampin states that concomitant administration of rifampin and an antacid may reduce the absorption of rifampin and recommends that daily doses of rifampin be given at least 1 hour before ingestion of an antacid.

■ **Atovaquone** Concomitant use of rifampin and atovaquone is not recommended. Concomitant use of the drugs has resulted in decreased atovaquone concentrations and increased rifampin concentrations.

■ **Ciprofloxacin and Clarithromycin** A drug-induced lupus-like syndrome manifested principally by malaise, myalgias, arthritis, and peripheral edema has been reported in a few patients receiving rifampin or rifabutin concomitantly with ciprofloxacin and/or clarithromycin. (See Cautions: Lupus-like

Syndrome.) Serum rifampin concentrations available in one patient during such concomitant therapy were elevated compared with expected levels, presumably as a result of inhibition of rifampin metabolism by ciprofloxacin and/or clarithromycin, and careful surveillance for drug-induced lupus syndrome is advised when these drugs are used concomitantly with a rifamycin

■ **Clofazimine** Concomitant use of clofazimine in leprosy patients receiving rifampin alone or in conjunction with dapsone reportedly may decrease the rate of absorption of rifampin, delay the time to reach peak plasma rifampin concentrations, and result in a slight decrease in the area under the plasma concentration-time curve (AUC) of the drug. However, in a study in lepromatous leprosy patients receiving dapsone (100 mg daily) and rifampin (600 mg daily), concomitant use of clofazimine (100 mg daily) did not affect plasma rifampin concentrations or the AUC, plasma half-life, or urinary elimination of rifampin.

■ **Enalapril** Concomitant use of rifampin and enalapril has resulted in decreased concentrations of enalaprilat, the active metabolite of enalapril; dosage adjustments should be required.

■ **Halothane** Because of an increased risk of hepatotoxicity, concomitant use of rifampin and halothane should be avoided.

■ **Isoniazid** Because of an increased risk of hepatotoxicity, patients receiving rifampin and isoniazid concomitantly should be closely monitored for signs and symptoms of hepatotoxicity.

■ **Probenecid** There is some evidence that probenecid may compete with rifampin for hepatic uptake resulting in higher blood concentrations of the antituberculosis agent. However, this effect is not predictable, and the use of probenecid to increase the therapeutic efficacy of rifampin is not justified.

■ **Pyrazinamide** Severe liver injuries, including some fatalities, have been reported in patients receiving a 2-month daily regimen of rifampin and pyrazinamide for the treatment of latent tuberculosis infection. The 2-month daily rifampin and pyrazinamide regimen should be used with caution in selected individuals only and with close clinical and laboratory monitoring. (See Cautions: Precautions and Contraindications.)

■ **Sulfapyridine** Plasma concentrations of sulfapyridine may decrease if rifampin is used concomitantly, possibly due to alterations in the colonic bacteria responsible for the reduction of sulfasalazine to sulfapyridine and mesalamine.

Laboratory Test Interferences

Rifampin may cause cross-reactivity and false-positive results in urine screening tests for opiates that use Kinetic Interaction of Microparticles in Solution (KIMS) methods (e.g., Abuscreen OnLine opiates assay; Roche Diagnostic Systems). If opiate abuse is suspected, the finding should be confirmed by other diagnostic tests (e.g., gas chromatography/mass spectrometry).

Rifampin interferes with microbiologic assays for serum folate and vitamin B_{12}. Alternative test methods should be considered for patients receiving rifampin.

Rifampin reduces hepatic uptake of sulfobromophthalein sodium. To avoid false-positive sulfobromophthalein test results, the test should be completed prior to administration of the daily dose of rifampin.

In vitro studies indicate that serum rifampin concentrations greater than 100 mcg/mL, which might occur in acute overdosage, may cause false elevations in total serum bilirubin concentration determined by the modified Malloy method utilizing diazotized sulfanilic acid as a reagent.

Acute Toxicity

The LD_{50} of rifampin in mice, rats, and rabbits is 0.885, 1.72, and 2.12 g/kg, respectively. In humans, acute overdosage with rifampin doses up to 9–12 g in adults and one or two 100-mg/kg doses in children 1–4 years of age have not been fatal; however, fatalities in adults have been reported following ingestion of 14- to 60-g doses of the drug. Alcohol or a history of alcohol abuse was involved in some of these cases of fatal and nonfatal overdosage.

■ **Manifestations** Overdosage of rifampin produces symptoms that are principally extensions of common adverse reactions. These include nausea, vomiting, abdominal pain, pruritus, headache, lethargy, and brownish-red or orange discoloration of skin, urine, sweat, saliva, tears, and feces in proportion to the amount of drug ingested. Transient elevations in hepatic enzymes and/or bilirubin may occur. Following massive overdosage of rifampin, hepatic involvement can develop within a few hours and is manifested by liver enlargement (possibly with tenderness), jaundice, rapid increases in total and direct serum bilirubin and liver enzymes, and loss of consciousness. Hepatotoxicity may be more marked in patients with prior hepatic impairment. In addition, hypotension, sinus tachycardia, ventricular arrhythmias, seizures, and cardiac arrest have been reported in some cases of fatalities resulting from rifampin overdosages However, an effect upon the hematopoietic system, electrolyte concentrations, or acid-base balance is unlikely.

In one patient who ingested 12 g of rifampin, vomiting occurred 4 times within 1 hour of ingestion, and gastric lavage with 20 L of water was initiated 5 hours after ingestion. Plasma concentrations of rifampin in this patient were 400, 64, and 0.1 mcg/mL at 12, 24, and 72 hours, respectively, after the dose; urinary concentrations of the drug were 313, 625, and 78 mcg/mL at 30, 36, and 40 hours, respectively, after the dose. Results of liver function tests were only transiently increased for about 5 days after the overdosage and the patient's recovery was uneventful. Inadvertent administration of 1 or 2 rifampin doses of 100 mg/kg for chemoprophylaxis of *Haemophilus influenzae* type b infection (5 times the usual daily dose) in a group of children 1–4 years of age resulted in a glowing red discoloration of the skin, periorbital or facial edema, pruritus of the head, vomiting, headache, and diarrhea. Signs and symptoms of overdosage occurred within 0.5–4 hours after administration of the first or second excessive dose and lasted an average of 28 hours (range: 1–72 hours).

■ **Treatment** Treatment of rifampin overdosage consists of intensive supportive and symptomatic therapy. In acute rifampin overdosage, the stomach should be emptied by gastric lavage. Activated charcoal slurry then may be instilled into the stomach to adsorb any drug remaining in the GI tract. An antiemetic may be required to control severe nausea and vomiting. Active diuresis, with measured intake and output, may promote excretion of the drug. If serious hepatic impairment occurs which lasts more than 24–48 hours, bile drainage or hemodialysis may be indicated. Reversal of liver enlargement and improvement of impaired hepatic function usually occur within 72 hours in patients with previously adequate hepatic function.

Mechanism of Action

Rifampin may be bacteriostatic or bactericidal in action, depending on the concentration of the drug attained at the site of infection and the susceptibility of the infecting organism. Rifampin usually is rapidly bactericidal against *Mycobacterium leprae* in vivo.

Rifampin suppresses initiation of chain formation for RNA synthesis in susceptible bacteria by inhibiting DNA-dependent RNA polymerase. The β subunit of the enzyme appears to be the site of action. Rifampin is most active against susceptible bacteria when they are undergoing cell division; however, the drug also has some effect when bacteria are in the metabolic resting state. Although rifampin is reported to have an immunosuppressive effect in some animal experiments, this effect is probably not clinically important in humans.

Spectrum

Rifampin is active in vitro and in vivo against *Mycobacterium tuberculosis*, *M. bovis*, *M. marinum*, *M. kansasii*, and some strains of *M. fortuitum*, *M. avium* complex (MAC) , and *M. intracellulare*. Rifampin also is active against both dapsone-susceptible and dapsone-resistant *M. leprae* in experimental leprosy in mice.

Rifampin also is active in vitro against some gram-positive bacteria, including *Staphylococcus aureus* and *Bacillus anthracis*, and some gram-negative bacteria, including *Neisseria meningitidis*, *Haemophilus influenzae*, *Brucella melitensis*, and *Legionella pneumophila*. At very high concentrations, rifampin is active in vitro against *Chlamydia trachomatis*, poxviruses, and adenoviruses.

In vitro, most strains of *N. meningitidis* are inhibited by rifampin concentrations of 0.1–1 mcg/mL.

Clinical isolates of *Ehrlichia phagocytophila* have been inhibited in vitro by rifampin concentrations of 0.125 mcg/mL or less.

Results of in vitro susceptibility testing of 11 *B. anthracis* isolates that were associated with cases of inhalational or cutaneous anthrax that occurred in the US (Florida, New York, District of Columbia) during September and October 2001 in the context of an intentional release of anthrax spores (biologic warfare, bioterrorism) indicate that these strains had rifampin MICs of 0.5 mcg/mL or less. Based on interpretive criteria established for staphylococci, these strains are considered susceptible to rifampin.

■ **In Vitro Susceptibility Testing** The National Committee for Clinical Laboratory Standards (NCCLS) states that, if results of in vitro susceptibility testing indicate that a clinical isolate is *susceptible* to rifampin, then an infection caused by this strain may be appropriately treated with the dosage of the drug recommended for that type of infection and infecting species, unless otherwise contraindicated. If results indicate that a clinical isolate has *intermediate susceptibility* to rifampin, then the strain has a minimum inhibitory concentration (MIC) that approaches usually attainable blood and tissue concentrations and response rates may be lower than for strains identified as susceptible. Therefore, the intermediate category implies clinical applicability in body sites where the drug is physiologically concentrated or when a high dosage of the drug can be used. This intermediate category also includes a buffer zone which should prevent small, uncontrolled technical factors from causing major discrepancies in interpretation, especially for drugs with narrow pharmacotoxicity margins. If results of in vitro susceptibility testing indicate that a clinical isolate is *resistant* to rifampin, the strain is not inhibited by systemic concentrations of the drug achievable with usual dosage schedules and/or MICs fall in the range where specific microbial resistance mechanisms are likely and efficacy has not been reliable in clinical studies.

In vitro susceptibility testing of certain fastidious bacteria (e.g., *Haemophilus*, *Streptococcus*) requires use of specialized culture media, testing procedures, and interpretive criteria not required for most other bacteria.

Although results of susceptibility testing may indicate that strains of *Staphylococcus*, *Enterococcus*, or *S. pneumoniae* may be susceptible to rifampin, the drug should not be used alone in the treatment of infections caused by these organisms. (See Uses: Streptococcal and Staphylococcal Infections.)

Disk Susceptibility Tests When the disk-diffusion procedure is used to test susceptibility to rifampin, a disk containing 5 mcg of rifampin is used.

When the disk-diffusion procedure is performed according to NCCLS standardized procedures using NCCLS interpretive criteria, *Staphylococcus* or *Enterococcus* with growth inhibition zones of 20 mm or greater are susceptible to rifampin, those with zones of 17–19 mm have intermediate susceptibility, and those with zones of 16 mm or less are resistant to the drug.

When disk-diffusion susceptibility testing is performed according to NCCLS standardized procedures using *Haemophilus* test medium (HTM), *Haemophilus* with growth inhibition zones of 20 mm or greater are susceptible to rifampin, those with zones of 17–19 mm have intermediate susceptibility, and those with zones of 16 mm or less are resistant to the drug.

When the NCCLS standardized disk-diffusion procedure using Mueller-Hinton agar (supplemented with 5% sheep blood) is used to determine susceptibility of *S. pneumoniae*, *S. pneumoniae* with growth inhibition zones of 19 mm or greater are susceptible to rifampin, those with zones of 17–18 mm are have intermediate susceptibility, and those with zones of 16 mm or less are resistant to the drug.

NCCLS states that disk-diffusion susceptibility tests are unreliable for determining susceptibility of *Neisseria meningitidis* to rifampin; dilution susceptibility tests should be used to determine susceptibility of this organism.

Dilution Susceptibility Tests When dilution susceptibility testing is performed according to NCCLS standardized procedures using NCCLS interpretive criteria, *Staphylococcus* or *Enterococcus* with MICs of 1 mcg/mL or less are susceptible to rifampin, those with MICs of 2 mcg/mL have intermediate susceptibility, and those with MICs of 4 mcg/mL or greater are resistant to the drug. These same interpretive criteria apply when the appropriate NCCLS standardized procedures are used to test susceptibility of *Haemophilus* or *S. pneumoniae* to rifampin.

When dilution susceptibility testing is used, *N. meningitidis* with MICs of 1 mcg/mL or less are susceptible to rifampin, those with MICs of 2 mcg/mL have intermediate susceptibility, and those with MICs of 4 mcg/mL or greater are resistant to the drug. Rifampin is not likely to eradicate *N. meningitidis* from the nasopharynx of asymptomatic carriers when the organism is reported to be resistant using in vitro susceptibility procedures.

The in vitro susceptibility of mycobacteria to rifampin depends on the culture media used. Rifampin susceptibility powders are available for both direct and indirect methods of determining susceptibility of strains of mycobacteria. When determined in Middlebrook and Cohn 7H10 agar (7H10 agar) or other non-egg-containing media (e.g., Dubos), the minimum inhibitory concentration (MIC) of rifampin for most susceptible mycobacteria is 0.1–2 mcg/mL. When egg-containing media (e.g., Lowenstein-Jensen) are used, the MIC for most susceptible mycobacteria is 4–32 mcg/mL.

Resistance

Natural and acquired resistance to rifampin have been observed in vitro and in vivo in strains of *M. tuberculosis*, *M. kansasii*, *Neisseria meningitidis*, and most bacteria which are usually susceptible to the drug. In vitro, resistance to rifampin develops in a one-step process, probably as the result of modification of the β subunit of RNA polymerase. Resistant strains of initially susceptible organisms develop rapidly if rifampin is used alone in the treatment of clinical tuberculosis. When rifampin is combined with other antituberculosis agents in the treatment of the disease, emergence of resistant strains may be delayed or prevented. In patients with tuberculosis or the meningococcal carrier state, the small number of resistant strains of *M. tuberculosis* or *N. meningitidis* present within large populations of susceptible strains can rapidly become predominant.

Strains of *Staphylococcus aureus* and *Streptococcus pyogenes* (group A β-hemolytic streptococci) with rifampin resistance have been isolated from at least one patient who received rifampin monotherapy.

Strains of *M. leprae* resistant to rifampin have been reported rarely. Resistant strains of initially susceptible *M. leprae* have developed within 3–5 years in patients receiving rifampin alone for the treatment of leprosy.

Cross-resistance has been demonstrated only between rifampin and other rifamycin derivatives.

Pharmacokinetics

■ **Absorption** Rifampin is well absorbed from the GI tract. If rifampin is administered with food, peak plasma concentrations of the drug may be slightly reduced (by about 30%) and delayed. Following a single 600-mg oral dose of rifampin in healthy fasting adults in one study, peak plasma concentrations of the drug averaged 7 mcg/mL and were attained within 2–4 hours. However, there is considerable interpatient variation, and peak plasma concentrations of the drug may range from 4–32 mcg/mL.

In a single-dose study in healthy fasting males, the extent of absorption (as measured by area under the plasma concentration-time curve) of isoniazid, rifampin, or pyrazinamide in dosages of 250 mg, 600 mg, or 1500 mg, respectively, was similar whether the drugs were administered individually as capsules (rifampin) and tablets (isoniazid and pyrazinamide) or as a fixed combination (Rifater®) containing isoniazid 50 mg, rifampin 120 mg, and pyrazinamide 300 mg per tablet. The effect of food on the pharmacokinetics of Rifater® has not been determined to date.

Following IV infusion over 30 minutes of a single 300- or 600-mg dose of rifampin in healthy adult men, peak plasma concentrations of the drug average 9 or 17.5 mcg/mL, respectively, and plasma concentrations remain detectable for 8 or 12 hours, respectively. Plasma concentrations of the drug attained with the 600-mg dose are disproportionately higher (up to 50% higher) than expected based on those attained with the 300-mg dose. When 600-mg doses of rifampin are given once daily by IV infusion over 3 hours for 7 days, plasma concentrations of the drug average 5.8 mcg/mL 8 hours after completion of the infusion on the first day of therapy and 2.6 mcg/mL 8 hours after completion of the infusion on the 7th day of therapy.

In several studies in children receiving rifampin orally in a dosage of 10 mg/kg, peak serum rifampin concentrations ranged from 3.5–15 mcg/mL. In one study in fasting children 6–58 months of age who received 10 mg/kg of rifampin given orally (as an extemporaneously prepared oral suspension in simple syrup or as a dry powder mixed in applesauce), peak serum concentrations were attained 1 hour after the dose and averaged 10.7 or 11.5 mcg/mL, respectively. When a rifampin dose of approximately 300 mg/m^2 was given by IV infusion over 30 minutes to children 3 months to 12.8 years of age, peak serum rifampin concentrations at the end of the infusion averaged 26 mcg/mL. Following multiple doses in these children, peak concentrations of the drug ranged from 11.7–41.5 mcg/mL 1–4 days after initiation of therapy and 13.6–37.4 mcg/mL 5–14 days after initiation of therapy.

Plasma concentrations of rifampin are higher and more prolonged in patients with impaired hepatic function, especially in the presence of obstructive jaundice. There is no cumulative effect in patients with impaired renal function.

■ **Distribution** Rifampin is widely distributed into most body tissues and fluids including the liver, lungs, bile, pleural fluid, prostate, seminal fluid, ascitic fluid, CSF, saliva, tears, and bone. CSF concentrations of rifampin in patients with inflamed meninges are reported to be 10–20% of concurrent plasma concentrations of the drug. At a concentration of 10 mcg/mL, rifampin is 84–91% bound to plasma proteins. Rifampin crosses the placenta. Rifampin is distributed into milk.

■ **Elimination** The plasma half-life of rifampin following a single 600- or 900-mg oral dose in healthy adults is approximately 3.4–3.6 hours. During the first several weeks of continued daily administration of 600-mg oral doses of rifampin, there is a progressive decrease in plasma concentrations and half-life of the drug due to increased biliary excretion. In one study in adults with tuberculosis, the plasma half-life of rifampin was 1.7 hours after 3 months of daily 600-mg oral doses of the drug. The plasma half-life of the drug is increased in patients with renal impairment. In one study in individuals who received a single 900-mg oral dose of rifampin, the mean plasma half-life of the drug was 3.6 hours in healthy individuals, 5 hours in those with glomerular filtration rates of 30–50 mL/minute, 7.3 hours in those with rates less than 30 mL/minute, and 11 hours in anuric patients.

The plasma half-life of rifampin in children 6–58 months of age averages 2.9 hours following oral administration of a single 10-mg/kg dose of the drug. Plasma half-life of the drug in children 3 months to 12.8 years of age following IV doses of the drug was 1.04–3.81 hours during the first few days of therapy and decreased to 1.17–3.19 hours after 5–14 days of therapy.

Rifampin is metabolized in the liver to a deacetylated derivative which also possesses antibacterial activity. The drug and its deacetylated metabolite are excreted mainly via bile. Rifampin undergoes enterohepatic circulation and is largely reabsorbed, but the metabolite is not. Within 24 hours, 3–30% of a single 600-mg oral dose of rifampin is excreted in urine as unchanged drug and active metabolite. Approximately 60% of the oral dose is excreted in feces via biliary elimination. Plasma concentrations of rifampin are not appreciably affected by hemodialysis or peritoneal dialysis.

Chemistry and Stability

■ **Chemistry** Rifampin is a semisynthetic derivative of rifamycin B, an antibiotic derived from *Streptomyces mediterranei*. Rifampin occurs as a red-brown, crystalline powder and is very slightly soluble in water and slightly soluble in alcohol. The drug has a pK_a of 7.9.

Commercially available rifampin sterile powder for injection contains sodium formaldehyde sulfoxylate; sodium hydroxide may have been added to adjust pH.

Oral rifampin is commercially available alone, in fixed combination with isoniazid, and in fixed combination with isoniazid and pyrazinamide.

■ **Stability** Rifampin capsules should be stored in tight, light-resistant containers at a temperature of 30°C or less, preferably between 15–30°C. The capsules should not be exposed to excessive heat. Tablets containing the fixed combination of rifampin, isoniazid, and pyrazinamide (Rifater®) should be protected from excessive humidity and stored at 15–30°C.

Commercially available rifampin powder for injection should be protected from light and excessive heat (i.e., temperatures greater than 40°C). Following reconstitution with sterile water for injection, rifampin solutions containing 60 mg/mL are stable for 24 hours at room temperature. The manufacturer states that reconstituted solutions of rifampin that have been further diluted in 100 or 500 mL of 5% dextrose injection should be used within 4 hours of preparation. (See Reconstitution and Administration: IV Infusion, in Dosage and Administration.) A precipitate indicating incompatibility has been observed during simulated Y-site administration of rifampin (6 mg/mL in 0.9% sodium chloride) and diltiazem that is undiluted (5 mg/mL) or diluted (1 mg/mL in 0.9% sodium chloride).

Preparations

Excipients in commercially available drug preparations may have clinically important effects in some individuals; consult specific product labeling for details.

rifAMPin

Oral		
Capsules	150 mg*	**Rifadin**®, Sanofi-Aventis
		rifAMPin Capsules
	300 mg*	**Rifadin**®, Sanofi-Aventis
		rifAMPin Capsules
		Rimactane®, Amide Pharm
Parenteral		
For injection	600 mg*	**Rifadin**® **IV**, Sanofi-Aventis
		rifAMPin for Injection

*available from one or more manufacturer, distributor, and/or repackager by generic (nonproprietary) name

rifAMPin Combinations

Oral		
Capsules	300 mg with Isoniazid 150 mg*	**Rifamate**®, Sanofi-Aventis
		rifAMPin and Isoniazid Capsules
Tablets	120 mg with Isoniazid 50 mg and Pyrazinamide 300 mg	**Rifater**®, Sanofi-Aventis

*available from one or more manufacturer, distributor, and/or repackager by generic (nonproprietary) name

†Use is not currently included in the labeling approved by the US Food and Drug Administration

Rifapentine

■ Rifapentine, a long-acting semisynthetic cyclopentylpiperazinyl derivative of rifamycin SV, is an ansamycin antituberculosis antibiotic.

Uses

■ **Tuberculosis** ***Active Tuberculosis*** Rifapentine is used in conjunction with other antituberculosis agents in the treatment of clinical tuberculosis.

The American Thoracic Society (ATS), US Centers for Disease Control and Prevention (CDC), and Infectious Diseases Society of America (IDSA) currently recommend several possible multiple-drug regimens for the treatment of culture-positive pulmonary tuberculosis. These regimens have a minimum duration of 6 months (26 weeks), and consist of an initial intensive phase (2 months) and a continuation phase (usually either 4 or 7 months). Rifapentine is considered a first-line antituberculosis agent for use in intermittent regimens in patients with pulmonary tuberculosis. Although the manufacturer states that rifapentine can be used in both the initial and continuation phases of tuberculosis treatment, the ATS, CDC, and IDSA suggest that rifapentine not be used in the initial phase of treatment but can be used in certain patients for the continuation phase in a once-weekly regimen in conjunction with isoniazid. The ATS, CDC, and IDSA state that rifapentine can be used in patients with noncavitary pulmonary tuberculosis caused by susceptible *Mycobacterium tuberculosis* if sputum smears are negative at completion of the initial treatment phase, but the drug should not be used for the treatment of tuberculosis in individuals with human immunodeficiency virus (HIV) infection and, because of limited experience, should not be used in those with extrapulmonary tuberculosis. For information on general principles used in the treatment of tuberculosis, see the Antituberculosis Agents General Statement 8:16.04.

Clinical Experience. Safety and efficacy of rifapentine is based on a large, controlled international trial comparing the drug with rifampin in patients with pulmonary tuberculosis who received either drug concomitantly with at least one other antituberculosis agent in a regimen that consisted of an intensive phase for 2 months and a continuation phase for 4 subsequent months; all patients received pyridoxine (vitamin B_6) throughout the 6-month trial. The intensive phase of therapy included either rifapentine (600 mg twice weekly) or rifampin (450 or 600 mg daily depending on body weight) given in conjunction with isoniazid (300 mg daily), pyrazinamide (1.5 or 2 g daily depending on body weight), and ethambutol (800 mg or 1.2 g daily depending on body weight). The continuation phase of therapy (subsequent 4 months) evaluated a drug regimen consisting of rifapentine (600 mg once weekly) and isoniazid (600 or 900 mg once weekly depending on body weight) or a regimen of rifampin (450 or 600 mg twice weekly depending on body weight) and isoniazid (600 or 900 mg once weekly depending on body weight); pyrazinamide and ethambutol were discontinued. Sputum converted to negative in 87% of patients with tuberculosis receiving rifapentine-containing drug regimens and in 81% of patients receiving rifampin-containing regimens by the end of 6 months of therapy. Although rifapentine also has been studied in China and Hong Kong, the results of these studies were less than optimal since the oral formulation used produced low and variable bioavailability. Because rifapentine has a long half-life and can be administered intermittently (once weekly for the continuation phase or twice weekly for the intensive phase), some clinicians suggest that the drug may be particularly useful when patient compliance is a concern. In addition, intermittent rifapentine therapy may have operational advantages in implementing directly observed therapy. However, additional study and experience are needed to elucidate further the role of rifapentine vs. rifampin in multiple-drug regimens for the treatment of tuberculosis, particularly because of concerns about relapse.

The rate of relapse (reactivation of clinical tuberculosis) was higher in patients receiving rifapentine versus rifampin combination therapy, principally as a result of a higher rate of patient noncompliance with daily concomitant therapies during the intensive phase in rifapentine-treated patients. Failure for sputum to convert to negative during the intensive phase of short-course therapy also was associated with a greater risk of relapse for either treatment regimen as was male gender. Relapse or treatment failure at 6 months of follow-up occurred in 10% of patients receiving the rifapentine-containing regimens and in 5% of those receiving the rifampin-containing regimens. A small proportion of patients relapsing had in vitro evidence of rifampin- and rifapentine-resistant (genetic differences from baseline strains based on restriction fragment length polymorphism) or multidrug-resistant strains of tuberculosis. However, relapses in patients receiving rifapentine were *not* associated with mono-resistance to rifampin.

HIV-infected Individuals. Experience with rifapentine in patients with HIV infection and tuberculosis is limited, and the ATS, CDC, and IDSA state that use of the drug in antituberculosis regimens in such patients currently is not recommended. In an ongoing small clinical trial in patients with HIV infection and tuberculosis who were randomized to receive once-weekly rifapentine and daily isoniazid during the continuation phase (months 3–6) of therapy, the relapse rate was about twice that observed in HIV-negative patients with tuberculosis. Almost all (4 out of 5) cases of relapse in these HIV-infected patients who received rifapentine were associated with rifampin-resistant tuberculosis; relapse also was associated with late stages of HIV infection (e.g., lower CD4$^+$ T-cell counts compared with those whose disease did not relapse), extrapulmonary tuberculosis, and concomitant therapy with an azole-derivative antifungal. As with other antituberculosis agents used in HIV-infected patients, if rifapentine is used, a more aggressive (i.e., more frequent dosing) rifapentine-containing regimen should be employed during the continuation phase of short-course therapy. Based on these limited findings, once-weekly rifapentine dosing during the continuation phase of therapy should *not* be employed in HIV-infected patients. In addition, the possibility that drug regimens may have to be altered because of clinically important pharmacokinetic interactions between rifapentine and other drugs commonly used in these patients (e.g., HIV protease inhibitors such as indinavir, nelfinavir, ritonavir, saquinavir; azole antifungals; reverse transcriptase inhibitors) should be considered. The manufacturer recommends that rifapentine be used with extreme caution, if at all, in patients who are receiving an HIV protease inhibitor. (See Drug Interactions: Antimycobacterial Agents, in Indinavir, Nelfinavir, Ritonavir, and Saquinavir 8:18.08.08.) Because the management of these patients is complex and must be individualized, experts in the management of mycobacterial infections in HIV-infected patients should be consulted.

If tuberculosis is diagnosed in an HIV-infected patient in whom use of an HIV protease inhibitor is being considered but has not yet been initiated, a management strategy suggested by CDC is to complete the treatment of tuberculosis according to current ATS and CDC guidelines before adding the HIV protease inhibitor to the patient's antiretroviral regimen. In HIV-infected patients who already are receiving an HIV protease inhibitor when tuberculosis is diagnosed, the CDC has suggested several options for consideration. However, because the risks and benefits of these options are unknown, management decisions must be individualized on a case-by-case basis to provide optimal patient care. (See Initial Treatment of Tuberculosis: Active Tuberculosis in HIV-Infected Individuals, in the Antituberculosis Agents General Statement.)

Dosage and Administration

■ **Administration** Rifapentine is administered orally. Since the incidence of some adverse effects (e.g., vomiting, nausea, or GI upset) may be increased during fasting conditions, administration of rifapentine with food may be useful in patients with a history of such disorders. GI absorption of rifapentine is reduced (e.g., by 20–32% in the fasted state) in HIV-infected patients compared with healthy adults, but concomitant administration with food can increase the extent of GI absorption of the drug.

Rifapentine usually is given once or twice weekly, and the manufacturer recommends an interval of not less than 3 days (72 hours) between doses.

■ **Dosage** ***Active Tuberculosis*** In the treatment of clinical tuberculosis, rifapentine should not be given alone. The drug is considered a first-line agent for use in intermittent regimens in patients with pulmonary tuberculosis. Therapy for tuberculosis should be continued long enough to prevent relapse. The minimum duration of treatment currently recommended for patients with culture-positive pulmonary tuberculosis is 6 months (26 weeks), and recommended regimens consist of an initial intensive phase (2 months) and a continuation phase (usually either 4 or 7 months). However, completion of treatment is determined more accurately by the total number of doses and is not based solely on the duration of therapy. For information on general principles of antituberculosis therapy and recommendations regarding specific multiple-drug regimens and duration of therapy, see the Antituberculosis Agents General Statement 8:16.04.

The manufacturer states that the usual dosage of rifapentine for the treatment of pulmonary tuberculosis is an initial intensive phase of 600 mg of rifapentine twice weekly for 2 months in conjunction with other appropriated antituberculosis agents (e.g., isoniazid, pyrazinamide, ethambutol, streptomycin) followed by once-weekly administration of rifapentine (600 mg) and isoniazid for 4 additional months. The manufacturer also recommends concomitant administration of pyridoxine (vitamin B_6) in those who are malnourished, predisposed to neuropathy (e.g., alcoholics, diabetics), and in adolescents.

The American Thoracic Society (ATS), US Centers for Disease Control and Prevention (CDC), and Infectious Diseases Society of America (IDSA) currently do not recommend use of rifapentine during the initial intensive phase of tuberculosis treatment. However, these experts suggest that patients with pulmonary tuberculosis who have negative sputum smears at completion of an initial phase of treatment may receive rifapentine in conjunction with isoniazid for the continuation phase. When this regimen is used, the ATS, CDC, and IDSA recommend that adults and children 15 years of age or older receive rifapentine in a dosage of 10 mg/kg (600 mg) once weekly in conjunction with isoniazid (15 mg/kg [900 mg] once weekly) for 4 months (18 weeks).

■ **Dosage in Renal and Hepatic Impairment** While the half-life of rifapentine is prolonged in patients with mild to severe hepatic impairment, accumulation of the drug in patients receiving intermittent dosing (recommended once or twice weekly dosing) is unlikely. Results of a pharmacokinetic study in patients with hepatic dysfunction indicate that no dosage adjustments appear to be necessary in these patients, and the manufacturer makes no specific recommendations.

The effects of renal impairment on the elimination of rifapentine have not been evaluated. Studies using radiolabeled rifapentine indicate that 17% of a dose of the drug is excreted in urine, suggesting that renal impairment may not substantially affect elimination of the drug. The manufacturer makes no specific recommendations regarding dosage adjustments in patients with impaired renal function.

Cautions

■ **Contraindications** Known hypersensitivity to rifapentine, other rifamycins (e.g., rifampin and rifabutin), or any ingredient in the formulation.

■ **Warnings/Precautions** ***Warnings*** **Hepatic and Hematologic Effects.** Because multiple-drug antituberculosis regimens, including those that employ a rifamycin, can cause adverse hepatic and hematologic effects, liver function (hepatic enzymes, bilirubin) and hematologic status (complete blood cell and platelet counts) should be monitored at initiation of rifapentine therapy. Patients should be seen at least monthly during continued rifapentine therapy and questioned concerning adverse reactions; those reporting abnormalities should have follow-up, including laboratory monitoring, as necessary. Patients should be advised to contact their clinician immediately if they develop fever, loss of appetite, malaise, nausea and vomiting, darkened urine, yellowish discoloration of the skin and eyes, and/or pain or swelling of the joints during rifapentine therapy. Routine laboratory monitoring for drug-induced toxicity in patients with normal baseline tests generally is not necessary. However, if rifapentine is considered for use in patients with preexisting liver function abnormalities and/or liver disease, the drug should be used only if clinically necessary and with caution and close medical supervision; in addition to baseline tests, careful monitoring of liver function (particularly aminotransferases) should be repeated every 2–4 weeks during continued therapy. If signs or symptoms of liver disease develop or worsen, rifapentine should be discontinued. Hepatotoxicity of other antituberculosis agents that may be used in conjunction with rifapentine (e.g., isoniazid, pyrazinamide) should be considered.

Diarrhea and Colitis. *Clostridium difficile*-associated diarrhea and colitis (also known as antibiotic-associated pseudomembranous colitis) has been reported rarely during or following discontinuance of therapy with other rifamycins, including rifampin, and should be considered in the differential diagnosis of patients who develop diarrhea (particularly if severe or persistent) in association with rifapentine. If *C. difficile*-associated diarrhea and colitis is suspected, rifapentine should be discontinued and the patient should be treated with supportive and specific treatment as indicated.Mild cases may respond to discontinuance of the drug alone, but diagnosis and management of moderate to severe cases should include appropriate bacteriologic and other (e.g., identification of clostridial toxins) studies, and treatment with fluid, electrolyte, and protein supplementation as indicated; sigmoidoscopy (or other appropriate endoscopic examination) usually is reserved for special situations. If colitis is moderate to severe or is not relieved by discontinuance of rifapentine, appropriate anti-infective therapy (e.g., oral metronidazole or vancomycin) should be administered. Isolation of the patient also may be advisable. Agents inhibiting peristalsis are contraindicated in these patients.

Other Effects. The possibility that rifapentine may share the toxic profile of rifampin also should be considered. (See Cautions in Rifampin 8:16.04.)

General Precautions Patients should be advised that rifapentine, like other rifamycins, may impart a red-orange color to urine, feces, sputum, sweat, saliva, CSF, tears, breast milk, and tongue; patients should be informed of this possibility. Contact lenses or dentures worn during rifapentine therapy may become permanently stained.

Because of the ability of rifampin and possibly other rifamycins to induce various hepatic enzyme systems, including delta aminolevulinic acid synthetase, use of these drugs may be associated with an exacerbation of porphyria. Therefore, the manufacturer states that rifapentine should *not* be used in patients with porphyria.

Specific Populations **Pregnancy.** Category C. (See Users' Guide.)

Lactation. Not known whether rifapentine is distributed in milk; possibility of red-orange discoloration of breast milk exists because of known discoloration of other body fluids. (See Cautions: General Precautions.) Caution is advised if the drug is administered in nursing women.

Pediatric Use. The safety and efficacy of rifapentine in pediatric patients younger than 12 years of age have not been established.

Geriatric Use. Experience in those 65 years of age and older insufficient to determine whether they respond differently from younger adults. Careful titration of dosage is recommended because of the greater frequency of decreased hepatic, renal, and/or cardiac function and or concomitant disease and drug therapy in geriatric individuals.

Drug Interactions

■ **Drugs Affecting Hepatic Microsomal Enzymes** Rifapentine induces microsomal enzymes (i.e., cytochrome P-450 [CYP] 3A4 and 2C8/9 isoenzymes) responsible for the inactivation of a number of drugs including certain calcium-channel blocking agents (e.g., verapamil, diltiazem, nifedipine), certain antifungals (fluconazole, itraconazole, ketoconazole), opiate analgesics (e.g., methadone), oral antidiabetic agents (e.g., sulfonylureas), corticosteroids, cardiac glycosides, certain antiarrhythmic agents (e.g., disopyramide, mexiletine, quinidine, tocainide), certain anti-infectives (e.g., quinine, dapsone, chloramphenicol, clarithromycin, doxycycline, fluoroquinolones), certain reverse transcriptase inhibitors (e.g., delavirdine, zidovudine), certain immunosuppressants (e.g., cyclosporine, tacrolimus), and oral anticoagulants (e.g., warfarin). Concomitant use of rifapentine and any of these drugs may result in decreased plasma concentrations of the drugs, and dosage adjustments may be required. Concomitant use of rifapentine also may diminish the effects of barbiturates, anticonvulsants (e.g., phenytoin), benzodiazepines (e.g., diazepam), clofibrate [no longer commercially available in the US], theophylline, β-adrenergic blocking agents, haloperidol, levothyroxine, sildenafil, and tricyclic antidepressants (e.g., amitriptyline, nortriptyline); dosage adjustments of these agents also may be required.

Induction of cytochrome P-450 hepatic microsomal enzymes by rifapentine generally occurs within 4 days after the first dose and returns to baseline levels 14 days after discontinuing the drug. The magnitude of hepatic microsomal enzyme induction by rifapentine is dose- and dosing frequency-dependent; less enzyme induction occurs when 600 mg of rifapentine is given once every 72 hours versus daily administration. In vitro and in vivo enzyme induction studies have suggested that rifapentine induction potential may be less than that of rifampin but greater than that of rifabutin.

■ **Antiretroviral Agents** Because rifapentine has been shown to increase metabolism of HIV protease inhibitors, which may result in subtherapeutic plasma concentrations of these antiretroviral agents, rifapentine should be used with extreme caution, if at all, in HIV-infected patients taking these drugs. (See Uses.)

■ **Oral Contraceptives** Patients should be advised that the reliability of oral or other systemic hormonal contraceptives may be affected by concomitant rifapentine therapy, and consideration should be given to using alternative contraceptive measures.

■ **Antacids** In a large, international controlled trial, patients were advised to take the drug at least 1 hour before or 2 hours after ingestion of antacids. However, since no specific drug interaction studies have been performed, it is unknown whether an interaction between rifapentine and antacids exists.

Description

Rifapentine, a long-acting semisynthetic cyclopentylpiperazinyl derivative of rifamycin SV, is an ansamycin antibiotic. Rifapentine is a lipophilic compound that is similar structurally and pharmacologically to rifampin and rifabutin.

Rifapentine has an antibacterial spectrum of activity similar to that of rifampin; however, on a molar basis, rifapentine and its active 25-desacetyl metabolite generally are more active than rifampin against *Mycobacterium tuberculosis* and more active than rifampin but less active than rifabutin against *M. avium* complex (MAC). The clinical relevance of activity of rifapentine against other mycobacterial species has not been established.

Against nonmycobacterial organisms, rifapentine is active in vitro against some gram-negative bacteria such as *Brucella* species, *Legionella* species, *Neisseria* species, *Haemophilus influenza*, *Bordetella pertussis*, and *Bordetella parapertussis*. The drug also has inhibitory activity against some gram-positive bacteria including streptococci, staphylococci, *Corynebacterium pseudodiphtheriticum*, *Arcanobacterium haemolyticum* (formerly *Corynebacterium haemolyticum*), *A. pyogenes*, *Listeria* species, *Turicella otitidis*, *Brevibacterium* species, and *Oerskovia* species. Rifapentine generally was as active as or less active than rifampin against these bacteria. Like rifampin, rifapentine also is active in vitro against *Chlamydia* species but not against mycoplasma.

Natural and acquired resistance to rifapentine have been observed in vitro and in vivo in strains of *M. tuberculosis*. A high level of cross-resistance has been demonstrated between rifampin and other rifamycin derivatives such as rifapentine. Cross resistance has not been demonstrated between rifapentine and non-rifamycin antimycobacterial agents such as isoniazid or streptomycin.

Overview (see Users Guide). For additional information until a more detailed monograph is developed and published, the manufacturer's labeling should be consulted. It is *essential* that the manufacturer's labeling be consulted for more detailed information on usual cautions, precautions, contraindications, potential drug interactions, laboratory test interferences, and acute toxicity.

Preparations

Excipients in commercially available drug preparations may have clinically important effects in some individuals; consult specific product labeling for details.

Rifapentine

Oral		
Tablets, film-coated	150 mg	**Priftin**®, Sanofi-Aventis

Selected Revisions January 2009, © Copyright, January 2001, American Society of Health-System Pharmacists, Inc.

MISCELLANEOUS ANTIMYCOBACTERIALS 8:16.92

Dapsone

DDS

■ Dapsone, a synthetic sulfone, is an antimycobacterial and antiprotozoal agent.

Uses

■ **Leprosy** Dapsone is used in conjunction with other anti-infectives in multidrug therapy (MDT) for treatment of multibacillary and paucibacillary leprosy (Hansen's disease).

Dapsone was used alone for treatment of leprosy until the early 1980s; however, because the drug is slow acting and only weakly bactericidal against *Mycobacterium leprae*, prolonged or life-long dapsone monotherapy was necessary and led to poor patient compliance and emergence of dapsone-resistant strains. The World Health Organization (WHO) and US National Hansen's Disease Program (NHDP) recommend that MDT regimens that also include rifampin be used for the treatment of all forms of leprosy. MDT can rapidly kill *M. leprae*, render patients noninfectious after only a few days of treatment, delay or prevent emergence of resistant *M. leprae*, and reduce the risk of relapse after treatment is discontinued. MDT does not enhance the rate of clearance of dead *M. leprae* from the body; such clearance may take years and depends largely on the individual's immune response, which may be defective in leprosy patients. Reactive episodes reported in leprosy patients receiving treatment appear to be due to destruction of the bacilli and immune responses to released bacterial antigens. (See Cautions: Leprosy Reactional States.) MDT regimens recommended by NHDP for US patients differ from those recommended by WHO.

For treatment of multibacillary leprosy (i.e., 6 or more lesions or skin smear positive) in adults, WHO recommends a 12-month MDT regimen of dapsone (once daily), rifampin (once monthly), and clofazimine (once daily and once monthly). For treatment of paucibacillary leprosy (i.e., 1–5 lesions) in adults, WHO recommends a 6-month MDT regimen of dapsone (once daily) and rifampin (once monthly). Because of reports of relapse of leprosy in patients who were treated with dapsone monotherapy ("burnt-out cases"), WHO states that patients who previously received only dapsone should be retreated with a currently recommended MDT regimen, even if the disease appears bacteriologically and clinically inactive. Since 1995, WHO has provided MDT regimens at no cost for treatment of leprosy. Although there are some countries where leprosy is still highly endemic, most countries where leprosy was previously highly endemic have achieved elimination of the disease at the national level and are intensifying efforts at regional and district levels.

For US patients, NHDP recommends more prolonged treatment. NHDP recommends that adults with multibacillary leprosy (i.e., those who are skin smear positive and/or have a biopsy indicating more advanced disease) receive a 24-month MDT regimen of dapsone (once daily), rifampin (once daily), and clofazimine (once daily), and that adults with paucibacillary leprosy (i.e., those who are skin smear negative without evidence of more advanced disease on biopsy) receive a 12-month MDT regimen of dapsone (once daily) and rifampin (once daily). Clofazimine is no longer commercially available in the US, but may be obtained from NHDP under an investigational new drug (IND) protocol for treatment of leprosy. (See Clofazimine 8:16.92.) NHDP can provide MDT regimens at no cost for treatment of US leprosy patients. Data indicate that leprosy is rare in the US (total of approximately 6500 living patients, about 3300 requiring active medical management), although about 150–200 new cases are reported each year.

Treatment of leprosy is complicated and should be undertaken in consultation with a specialist familiar with the disease. In the US, clinicians should contact NHDP at 800-642-2477 on weekdays from 9:00 a.m. to 5:30 p.m. Eastern Standard Time or via email at nhdped@hrsa.gov for assistance with diagnosis or treatment of leprosy or assistance obtaining clofazimine for treatment of leprosy.

■ **Dermatitis Herpetiformis** Dapsone is used for treatment of dermatitis herpetiformis. A gluten-free diet is recommended for all patients with dermatitis herpetiformis, and strict adherence to such a diet can result in slow resolution of skin lesions (may take months to years) and improvement in GI symptoms. Dapsone is used as an adjunct to a gluten-free diet; in responsive patients, initiation of the drug usually results in a prompt decrease in pruritus and resolution of dermatitis herpetiformis skin lesions. Dapsone alone has no effect on the GI component of dermatitis herpetiformis. After several months when skin manifestations have responded to dapsone, some patients who adhere to a strict gluten-free diet may be able to decrease dosage or discontinue the drug; dapsone may then be reinitiated for brief periods as needed to control flares.

■ **Pneumocystis jirovecii Pneumonia** Dapsone is used as an alternative for treatment of *Pneumocystis jirovecii* (formerly *Pneumocystis carinii*) pneumonia† (PCP) and prevention of *P. jirovecii* infections†. Dapsone is designated an orphan drug by the US Food and Drug Administration (FDA) for treatment and prevention of PCP.

Treatment of Pneumocystis jirovecii Pneumonia Dapsone is used in conjunction with trimethoprim as an alternative for treatment of mild to moderate PCP†, including mild to moderate PCP in adults, adolescents, and children with human immunodeficiency virus (HIV) infection.

Co-trimoxazole is the drug of choice for treatment of mild, moderate, or severe PCP, including PCP in HIV-infected adults, adolescents, and children.

The US Centers for Disease Control and Prevention (CDC), National Institutes of Health (NIH), and Infectious Diseases Society of America (IDSA) state that alternative regimens for treatment of mild to moderate PCP in HIV-infected adults and adolescents are dapsone in conjunction with trimethoprim, primaquine in conjunction with clindamycin, or atovaquone alone. These experts state that dapsone in conjunction with trimethoprim may be as effective as co-trimoxazole for treatment of mild to moderate PCP and has fewer adverse effects, but is less convenient because of higher pill burden. Although efficacy and safety data are limited regarding use of dapsone in conjunction with trimethoprim for treatment of PCP in children, some clinicians also recommend the regimen as an alternative for treatment of mild to moderate PCP in children when co-trimoxazole cannot be used. The dapsone and trimethoprim regimen is not included in CDC, NIH, IDSA, and AAP recommendations for treatment of severe PCP.

There is evidence that a combination regimen of dapsone (100 mg once daily) and trimethoprim (20 mg/kg daily in 4 divided doses) given for 21 days is effective for treatment of initial episodes of mild to moderate PCP in patients with acquired immunodeficiency syndrome (AIDS), achieving a clinical response in 93% of patients in one study. Most patients exhibited clinical improvement within 6 days, and the regimen generally was well tolerated. Dapsone alone appears to be less effective than co-trimoxazole or the combination regimen of dapsone and trimethoprim for treatment of initial episodes of PCP in patients with AIDS.

Prevention of Pneumocystis jirovecii Infections Dapsone is used alone or in conjunction with pyrimethamine (and leucovorin) as an alternative for prevention of *P. jirovecii* infections† in HIV-infected adults, adolescents, and children who cannot tolerate co-trimoxazole.

Prevention of Initial Episode (Primary Prophylaxis). CDC, NIH, and IDSA recommend that primary prophylaxis to prevent initial episodes of PCP be initiated in HIV-infected adults and adolescents with $CD4^+$ T-cell counts less than 200/mm^3 or a history of oropharyngeal candidiasis. These experts state that primary PCP prophylaxis should be considered in HIV-infected adults and adolescents with $CD4^+$ T-cell percentages less than 14% or a history of an AIDS-defining illness who would not otherwise qualify for prophylaxis and also should be considered in those with $CD4^+$ T-cell counts greater than 200 but less than 250/mm^3 if frequent monitoring of $CD4^+$ T-cell counts (e.g., every 3 months) is not possible.

CDC, NIH, and IDSA state that primary PCP prophylaxis should be discontinued in HIV-infected adults and adolescents who have responded to antiretroviral therapy and have $CD4^+$ T-cell counts that have remained greater than 200/mm^3 for longer than 3 months. Discontinuance of primary PCP prophylaxis is recommended in these individuals since it appears to add little benefit in terms of disease prevention (PCP, toxoplasmosis, bacterial infections) and discontinuance reduces the medication burden, cost, and potential for drug toxicity, drug interactions, and selection of drug-resistant pathogens. Primary PCP prophylaxis should be reinitiated if $CD4^+$ T-cell counts decrease to less than 200/mm^3.

Co-trimoxazole is the drug of choice for primary PCP prophylaxis in HIV-infected adults and adolescents. CDC, NIH, and IDSA recommend that co-trimoxazole prophylaxis be continued, if clinically feasible, in individuals who experience adverse reactions to the drug that are not life-threatening; however, co-trimoxazole prophylaxis should be permanently discontinued and an alternative used in those with life-threatening adverse reactions to the drug.

Alternative regimens recommended by CDC, NIH, and IDSA for primary PCP prophylaxis in HIV-infected adults and adolescents who cannot tolerate co-trimoxazole are dapsone alone, dapsone in conjunction with pyrimethamine (and leucovorin), aerosolized pentamidine, atovaquone alone, or atovaquone in conjunction with pyrimethamine (and leucovorin). In HIV-infected adults or adolescents who cannot tolerate co-trimoxazole and are seropositive for *Toxoplasma gondii*, dapsone with pyrimethamine (and leucovorin), atovaquone alone, or atovaquone with pyrimethamine (and leucovorin) would provide prophylaxis against both PCP and toxoplasmosis.

Prevention of Recurrence (Secondary Prophylaxis). CDC, NIH, and IDSA recommend that HIV-infected adults and adolescents who have a history of PCP receive long-term suppressive or chronic maintenance therapy (secondary prophylaxis) to prevent recurrence.

Secondary PCP prophylaxis generally is administered for life, unless immune recovery occurs as a result of antiretroviral therapy. CDC, NIH, and IDSA state that secondary PCP prophylaxis generally can be discontinued in HIV-infected adults and adolescents who have responded to antiretroviral therapy and have CD4$^+$ T-cell counts that have remained greater than 200/mm^3 for longer than 3 months, but should be reinitiated if CD4$^+$ T-cell counts decrease to less than 200/mm^3. In addition, these experts state that it may be prudent to continue secondary PCP prophylaxis for life (regardless of CD4$^+$ T-cell count) if PCP occurred or recurred when CD4$^+$ T-cell counts were greater than 200/mm^3.

Co-trimoxazole is the drug of choice for secondary PCP prophylaxis in HIV-infected adults and adolescents. CDC, NIH, and IDSA recommend that co-trimoxazole prophylaxis be continued, if clinically feasible, in individuals who experience adverse reactions to the drug that are not life-threatening; however, co-trimoxazole prophylaxis should be permanently discontinued and an alternative used in those with life-threatening adverse reactions to the drug.

Alternative regimens recommended by CDC, NIH, and IDSA for secondary PCP prophylaxis in HIV-infected adults and adolescents who cannot tolerate co-trimoxazole are the same as those recommended for primary prophylaxis and include dapsone alone, dapsone in conjunction with pyrimethamine (and leucovorin), aerosolized pentamidine, atovaquone alone, or atovaquone in conjunction with pyrimethamine (and leucovorin). In HIV-infected adults or adolescents who cannot tolerate co-trimoxazole and are seropositive for *T. gondii*, dapsone with pyrimethamine (and leucovorin), atovaquone alone, or atovaquone with pyrimethamine (and leucovorin) would provide prophylaxis against both PCP and toxoplasmosis.

Primary and Secondary Prophylaxis in Children. CDC, NIH, IDSA, and American Academy of Pediatrics (AAP) recommend that primary prophylaxis to prevent initial episodes of PCP be initiated in HIV-infected children 1 to less than 6 years of age with CD4$^+$ T-cell counts less than 500/mm^3 or CD4$^+$ T-cell percentages less than 15% and in HIV-infected children 6–12 years of age with CD4$^+$ T-cell counts less than 200/mm^3 or CD4$^+$ T-cell percentages less than 15%. These experts recommend that all HIV-infected infants younger than 1 year of age (regardless of CD4$^+$ T-cell count or percentage) receive primary PCP prophylaxis. In addition, infants born to HIV-infected mothers should be considered for primary PCP prophylaxis beginning at 4–6 weeks of age and those with indeterminate HIV status should continue to receive prophylaxis until they are determined to be non-HIV-infected or presumptively non-HIV-infected. Those found to be HIV-infected should receive primary PCP prophylaxis throughout the first year of life; at 1 year of age, the need for continued PCP prophylaxis should be reassessed based on age-specific CD4$^+$ T-cell thresholds.

HIV-infected children who have a history of PCP should receive long-term suppressive or chronic maintenance therapy (secondary prophylaxis) to prevent recurrence.

CDC, NIH, IDSA, and AAP state that, in HIV-infected children who have received at least 6 months of antiretroviral therapy, discontinuance of primary or secondary PCP prophylaxis should be considered in those 1 to less than 6 years of age if CD4$^+$ T-cell counts have remained at 500/mm^3 or greater or CD4$^+$ T-cell percentages have remained at 15% or greater for more than 3 consecutive months and in those 6–12 years of age if CD4$^+$ T-cell counts have remained at 200/mm^3 or greater or CD4$^+$ T-cell percentages have remained at 15% or greater for more than 3 consecutive months. If primary or secondary PCP prophylaxis is discontinued in HIV-infected children, CD4$^+$ T-cell counts and CD4$^+$ T-cell percentages should be assessed every 3 months and PCP prophylaxis reinitiated if indicated based on age-specific CD4$^+$ T-cell thresholds.

Co-trimoxazole is the drug of choice for primary and secondary PCP prophylaxis in HIV-infected infants and children. CDC, NIH, IDSA, and AAP recommend that co-trimoxazole be continued, if clinically feasible, in individuals who experience adverse reactions to the drug that are not life-threatening; however, co-trimoxazole should be permanently discontinued and an alternative used in those with life-threatening adverse reactions to the drug.

Alternative regimens recommended by CDC, NIH, IDSA, and AAP for primary and secondary PCP prophylaxis in HIV-infected infants and children who cannot tolerate co-trimoxazole are dapsone (1 month of age or older), atovaquone (1 month of age or older), or aerosolized pentamidine (5 years of age or older).

■ **Toxoplasmosis** Dapsone is used in conjunction with pyrimethamine (and leucovorin) as an alternative for primary prophylaxis to prevent initial episodes of toxoplasmosis caused by *Toxoplasma gondii*† in HIV-infected adults, adolescents, and children. Dapsone is designated an orphan drug by FDA for toxoplasmosis prophylaxis in severely immunocompromised individuals with CD4$^+$ T-cell counts less than 100/ mm^3.

Dapsone is not included in CDC, NIH, IDSA, and AAP recommendations for treatment of toxoplasmosis in HIV-infected individuals or for chronic maintenance therapy to prevent relapse of toxoplasmosis (secondary prophylaxis) in HIV-infected individuals.

Prevention of Toxoplasmosis **Prevention of Initial Episode (Primary Prophylaxis).** CDC, NIH, and IDSA recommend primary prophylaxis against *T. gondii* encephalitis in HIV-infected adults and adolescents who are seropositive for *Toxoplasma* IgG antibody and have CD4$^+$ T-cell counts less than 100/mm^3.

CDC, NIH, and IDSA state that primary toxoplasmosis prophylaxis should be discontinued in HIV-infected adults and adolescents who have responded to antiretroviral therapy and have CD4$^+$ T-cell counts that have remained greater than 200/mm^3 for longer than 3 months. Discontinuance of primary toxoplasmosis prophylaxis is recommended in these individuals since it appears to add little benefit in terms of toxoplasmosis disease prevention and discontinuance reduces the medication burden, cost, and potential for toxicity, drug interactions, and selection of drug-resistant pathogens. Primary toxoplasmosis prophylaxis should be reinitiated in HIV-infected adults and adolescents if CD4$^+$ T-cell counts decrease to less than 100–200/mm^3.

Co-trimoxazole is the drug of choice for primary toxoplasmosis prophylaxis in HIV-infected adults and adolescents. Dapsone in conjunction with pyrimethamine (and leucovorin) is the preferred alternative for such prophylaxis in HIV-infected adults and adolescents who cannot tolerate co-trimoxazole. CDC, NIH, and IDSA state that other alternatives for primary toxoplasmosis prophylaxis in those who cannot tolerate co-trimoxazole are atovaquone alone or atovaquone in conjunction with pyrimethamine (and leucovorin).

Primary Prophylaxis in Children. Although specific levels of immunosuppression that increase the risk for *T. gondii* encephalitis in HIV-infected children are less well defined than those for HIV-infected adults and adolescents, CDC, NIH, IDSA, and AAP recommend primary prophylaxis against *T. gondii* encephalitis in toxoplasma-seropositive HIV-infected children younger than 6 years of age who have CD4$^+$ T-cell percentages less than 15% and in toxoplasma-seropositive HIV-infected children 6 years of age or older who have CD4$^+$ T-cell counts less than 100/mm^3.

The safety of discontinuing primary toxoplasmosis prophylaxis in HIV-infected children whose immunologic status improves in response to antiretroviral therapy has not been extensively studied. CDC, NIH, IDSA, and AAP state that primary toxoplasmosis prophylaxis should not be discontinued in HIV-infected children younger than 1 year of age. However, based on data from adults, these experts state that discontinuance of primary toxoplasmosis prophylaxis can be considered in HIV-infected children 1 to less than 6 years of age who have received at least 6 months of antiretroviral therapy and have CD4$^+$ T-cell percentages that have remained at 15% or greater for longer than 3 months. In HIV-infected children 6 years of age or older who have received at least 6 months of antiretroviral therapy, primary toxoplasmosis prophylaxis can be discontinued if CD4$^+$ T-cell counts have remained greater than 200/mm^3 for longer than 3 months. Primary toxoplasmosis prophylaxis should be reinitiated if CD4$^+$ T-cell percentages decrease to less than 15% in HIV-infected children younger than 6 years of age or if CD4$^+$ T-cell counts decrease to less than 100–200/mm^3 in HIV-infected children 6 years of age or older.

For primary toxoplasmosis prophylaxis in HIV-infected infants and children, the drug of choice is co-trimoxazole. Dapsone in conjunction with pyrimethamine (and leucovorin) is the preferred alternative for such prophylaxis in those 1 month of age or older who cannot tolerate co-trimoxazole. CDC, NIH, IDSA, and AAP state that atovaquone alone is another alternative for primary toxoplasmosis prophylaxis in HIV-infected children and adolescents 1 month of age or older; those 4–24 months of age can receive atovaquone alone or in conjunction with pyrimethamine (and leucovorin).

Dosage and Administration

■ **Administration** Dapsone is administered orally.

For administration to children, commercially available tablets of dapsone have been crushed and dissolved in strawberry syrup; however, studies evaluating bioavailability of the drug following administration of this preparation have not been published to date.

■ **Dosage** ***Leprosy*** **Treatment of Multibacillary Leprosy.** For treatment of multibacillary leprosy, the World Health Organization (WHO) recommends that adults receive dapsone in a dosage of 100 mg once daily in conjunction with rifampin (600 mg once monthly) and clofazimine (50 mg once daily and 300 mg once monthly) given for 12 months. WHO recommends that children 10–14 years of age with multibacillary leprosy receive dapsone in a dosage of 50 mg once daily in conjunction with rifampin (450 mg once monthly) and clofazimine (50 mg once every other day and 150 mg once monthly) given for 12 months. Children younger than 10 years of age should receive a 12-month regimen using appropriately adjusted dosage based on weight (e.g., dapsone 2 mg/kg once daily in conjunction with rifampin [10 mg/kg once monthly] and clofazimine [1 mg/kg once every other day]).

For US patients, the National Hansen's Disease Program (NHDP) recommends that adults with multibacillary leprosy receive dapsone in a dosage of 100 mg once daily in conjunction with rifampin (600 mg once daily) and clofazimine (50 mg once daily) given for 24 months. These experts recommend that children with multibacillary leprosy receive dapsone in a dosage of 1 mg/kg once daily in conjunction with rifampin (10–20 mg/kg [up to 600 mg] once daily) and clofazimine (1 mg/kg once daily or 2 mg/kg once every other day) given for 24 months.

Treatment of Paucibacillary Leprosy. For treatment of paucibacillary leprosy, WHO recommends that adults receive dapsone in a dosage of 100 mg once daily in conjunction with rifampin (600 mg once monthly) given for 6 months. WHO recommends that children 10–14 years of age with paucibacillary leprosy receive dapsone in a dosage of 50 mg once daily in conjunction with rifampin (450 mg once monthly) given for 6 months. Children younger than 10 years of age should receive a 6-month regimen using appropriately adjusted dosage based on weight (e.g., dapsone 2 mg/kg once daily in conjunction with rifampin [10 mg/kg once monthly]).

For US patients, NHDP recommends that adults with paucibacillary leprosy receive dapsone in a dosage of 100 mg once daily in conjunction with rifampin (600 mg once daily) given for 12 months. These experts recommend that children with paucibacillary leprosy receive dapsone in a dosage of 1 mg/kg once daily in conjunction with rifampin (10–20 mg/kg [up to 600 mg] once daily) given for 12 months.

Dermatitis Herpetiformis For treatment of dermatitis herpetiformis, dapsone dosage should be individually titrated to find the daily dosage that most effectively controls pruritus and lesions; daily dosage should then be reduced to a minimum maintenance dosage as soon as possible.

The manufacturer recommends that adults receive an initial dapsone dosage of 50 mg daily for treatment of dermatitis herpetiformis and, if full control is not achieved within the range of 50–300 mg daily, higher dosage may be tried. For treatment of dermatitis herpetiformis in children, the manufacturer recommends correspondingly smaller doses of dapsone.

Some clinicians state that dapsone dosages of 25–100 mg daily usually control symptoms of dermatitis herpetiformis.

Occasional new lesions (3 or 4 per week) may occur during dapsone maintenance therapy and are not generally an indication to alter maintenance dosage of the drug. Maintenance dosage of dapsone often can be reduced or the drug discontinued after several months in patients who adhere to a gluten-free diet. The manufacturer states that the average time for dapsone dosage reduction is 8 months (range 4 months to 2.5 years) and the average time before discontinuance of the drug is 29 months (range 6 months to 9 years).

Pneumocystis jirovecii Pneumonia **Treatment of Pneumocystis jirovecii Pneumonia.** When used as an alternative for treatment of mild to moderate *Pneumocystis jirovecii* (formerly *Pneumocystis carinii*) pneumonia† (PCP) in adults and adolescents 13 years of age or older, including those with human immunodeficiency virus (HIV) infection, dapsone is given in a dosage of 100 mg once daily for 21 days in conjunction with oral trimethoprim (5 mg/kg 3 times daily for 21 days).

Although efficacy and safety data are limited in children, some clinicians state that dapsone may be given in a dosage of 2 mg/kg (up to 100 mg) once daily for 21 days in conjunction with oral trimethoprim (5 mg/kg 3 times daily for 21 days) as an alternative for treatment of mild to moderate PCP in children younger than 13 years of age†.

Prevention of Initial Episode (Primary Prophylaxis). When dapsone monotherapy is used as an alternative for prevention of initial episodes (primary prophylaxis) of PCP† in adults and adolescents 13 years of age or older, including HIV-infected individuals, the usual dosage is 100 mg once daily or 50 mg twice daily. Alternatively, dapsone can be given in a dosage of 50 mg once daily in conjunction with oral pyrimethamine (50 mg once weekly) and oral leucovorin (25 mg once weekly) or, alternatively, in a dosage of 200 mg once weekly in conjunction with oral pyrimethamine (75 mg once weekly) and oral leucovorin (25 mg once weekly). The US Centers for Disease Control and Prevention (CDC), National Institutes of Health (NIH), and Infectious Diseases Society of America (IDSA) state that primary PCP prophylaxis should be discontinued in HIV-infected adults and adolescents if CD4$^+$ T-cell counts have remained greater than 200/mm^3 for longer than 3 months in response to antiretroviral therapy, but should be reinitiated if CD4$^+$ T-cell counts decrease to less than 200/mm^3. (See Prevention of Initial Episode [Primary Prophylaxis] under Pneumocystis jirovecii Pneumonia: Prevention of Pneumocystis jirovecii Infections, in Uses.)

When dapsone monotherapy is used as an alternative for primary PCP prophylaxis in HIV-infected children and infants 1 month of age or older†, CDC, NIH, IDSA, American Academy of Pediatrics (AAP), and others recommend a dosage of 2 mg/kg (up to 100 mg) once daily or 4 mg/kg (up to 200 mg) once weekly. In HIV-infected children 1 year of age or older who have received at least 6 months of antiretroviral therapy, CDC, NIH, IDSA, and AAP state that discontinuance of primary PCP prophylaxis should be considered based on age-related CD4$^+$ T-cell counts or CD4$^+$ T-cell percentages, but should be reinitiated if these parameters decrease below the age-related thresholds. (See Primary and Secondary Prophylaxis in Children under Pneumocystis jirovecii Pneumonia: Prevention of Pneumocystis jirovecii Infections, in Uses.)

Prevention of Recurrence (Secondary Prophylaxis). When dapsone monotherapy is used as an alternative for prevention of recurrence (secondary prophylaxis) of PCP† in adults and adolescents 13 years of age or older, including HIV-infected individuals, the usual dosage is 100 mg once daily or 50 mg twice daily. Alternatively, dapsone can be given in a dosage of 50 mg once daily in conjunction with oral pyrimethamine (50 mg once weekly) and oral leucovorin (25 mg once weekly) or, alternatively, in a dosage of 200 mg once weekly in conjunction with oral pyrimethamine (75 mg once weekly) and oral leucovorin (25 mg once weekly). CDC, NIH, and IDSA state that secondary PCP prophylaxis generally can be discontinued in HIV-infected adults and adolescents if CD4$^+$ T-cell counts have remained greater than 200/mm^3 for longer than 3 months in response to antiretroviral therapy, but should be reinitiated if CD4$^+$ T-cell counts decrease to less than 200/mm^3. However, secondary prophylaxis probably should be continued for life (regardless of CD4$^+$ T-cell count) if PCP occurred or recurred when CD4$^+$ T-cell counts were greater than 200/mm^3. (See Prevention of Recurrence [Secondary Prophylaxis] under Pneumocystis jirovecii Pneumonia: Prevention of Pneumocystis jirovecii Infections, in Uses.)

When dapsone monotherapy is used as an alternative for secondary prophylaxis of PCP in HIV-infected children and infants 1 month of age or older†, CDC, NIH, IDSA, AAP, and others recommend a dosage of 2 mg/kg (up to 100 mg) once daily or 4 mg/kg (up to 200 mg) once weekly. In HIV-infected children 1 year of age or older who have received at least 6 months of antiretroviral therapy, CDC, NIH, IDSA, and AAP state that discontinuance of secondary PCP prophylaxis should be considered based on age-related CD4$^+$ T-cell counts or CD4$^+$ T-cell percentages, but should be reinitiated if these parameters decrease below the age-related thresholds. (See Primary and Secondary Prophylaxis in Children under Pneumocystis jirovecii Pneumonia: Prevention of Pneumocystis jirovecii Infections, in Uses.)

Toxoplasmosis **Prevention of Initial Episode (Primary Prophylaxis).** When used as an alternative for primary prophylaxis of toxoplasmosis† in HIV-infected adults and adolescents, CDC, NIH, and IDSA recommend that dapsone be given in a dosage of 50 mg once daily in conjunction with pyrimethamine (50 mg once weekly) and oral leucovorin (25 mg once weekly). Alternatively, HIV-infected adults and adolescents can receive a dapsone dosage of 200 mg once weekly in conjunction with pyrimethamine (75 mg once weekly) and oral leucovorin (25 mg once weekly).

When used as an alternative for primary prophylaxis of toxoplasmosis† in HIV-infected children and infants 1 month of age or older, CDC, NIH, IDSA, and AAP recommend a dapsone dosage of 2 mg/kg or 15 mg/m^2 (up to 25 mg) once daily in conjunction with pyrimethamine (1 mg/kg [up to 25 mg] once daily) and oral leucovorin (5 mg once every 3 days).

CDC, NIH, and IDSA state that primary prophylaxis against toxoplasmosis should be discontinued in HIV-infected adults and adolescents who have CD4$^+$ T-cell counts that have remained greater than 200/mm^3 for longer than 3 months in response to antiretroviral therapy, but should be reinitiated if CD4$^+$ T-cell counts decrease to less than 100–200/mm^3. The safety of discontinuing primary prophylaxis against toxoplasmosis in HIV-infected children whose immunologic status improves in response to antiretroviral therapy has not been extensively studied. (See Prevention of Toxoplasmosis under Uses: Toxoplasmosis.)

Cautions

■ Hematologic Effects The most frequent adverse effects of dapsone are dose-related hemolytic anemia and methemoglobinemia. Hemolysis occurs in most patients receiving 200 mg or more of dapsone daily; however, symptomatic anemia occurs only occasionally. The manufacturer states that the hemoglobin level is generally decreased by 1–2 g/dL, the reticulocyte count is increased 2–12%, erythrocyte life span is shortened, and methemoglobinemia occurs in most patients receiving dapsone. Heinz body formation also occurs frequently. Unless severe, hemolysis or methemoglobinemia does not generally require discontinuance of dapsone therapy. These adverse hematologic effects occur in patients with or without glucose-6-phosphate dehydrogenase (G-6-PD) deficiency, but are most severe in patients with G-6-PD deficiency. Hemolysis and Heinz body formation may be exaggerated in patients with G-6-PD deficiency, methemoglobin reductase deficiency, or hemoglobin M. Hemolysis and methemoglobinemia may be poorly tolerated by patients with severe cardiopulmonary disease. In addition, dapsone-induced adverse hematologic effects may be poorly tolerated by some patients with acquired immunodeficiency syndrome (AIDS) receiving the drug for treatment of *Pneumocystis jirovecii* (formerly *Pneumocystis carinii*) pneumonia, since such patients may have preexisting anemia and/or hypoxemia. Generally, however, dapsone is well tolerated in AIDS patients, although asymptomatic methemoglobinemia has been reported in two-thirds of such patients receiving 100 mg of dapsone daily concomitantly with trimethoprim 20 mg/kg daily. (See Drug Interactions: Trimethoprim.) Methemoglobinemia has been reported substantially less frequently in AIDS patients receiving dapsone alone.

Cyanosis, which is usually associated with mild methemoglobinemia, may occur during dapsone therapy. Acute methemoglobinemia occurs rarely, but may result in anemia, vascular collapse, and death. Unless the patient has G-6-PD deficiency, acute methemoglobinemia should be treated with IV methylene blue. (See Acute Toxicity: Treatment.) Prophylactic administration of ascorbic acid, folate, and iron reportedly may prevent some of the adverse hematologic effects of dapsone.

Leukopenia has been reported occasionally during therapy with dapsone, and potentially fatal agranulocytosis and aplastic anemia have been reported rarely.

■ Leprosy Reactional States Effective treatment of leprosy with dapsone or other antileprosy agents generally results in abrupt changes in the clinical and immune status of the patient and many patients have reactive episodes (reactions) that may be mild to severe. Leprosy reactive episodes can occur before, during, or after treatment is completed and apparently result from destruction of *Mycobacterium leprae* and immune responses to released bacterial antigens. Reactive episodes are classified into 2 main types: reversal reactions (type 1) and erythema nodosum leprosum (ENL) reactions (type 2). Other reactions (e.g., neuritis or silent neuropathies, iridocyclitis, orchitis) also can occur independently of reactive episodes.

Reversal reactions (type 1) occur mainly in borderline tuberculoid, mid-borderline, and borderline lepromatous leprosy patients. Reversal reactions are usually evidenced by edema and erythema of pre-existing lesions. These reactions presumably occur because the patient is able to mount an enhanced delayed hypersensitivity response to the residual infection and this leads to swelling (reversal) of existing skin and nerve lesions. Existing lesions become erythematous and edematous and may ulcerate; fever and an increased leukocyte count frequently occur, and acute neuritis and loss of nerve function may develop.

ENL reactions (type 2) are recurrent immunologically mediated reactions that occur principally in patients with multibacillary leprosy (borderline lepromatous and lepromatous leprosy). While ENL reactions have been reported to occur in 10–50% of lepromatous leprosy patients and 25–30% of borderline lepromatous patients, these reactions have been reported less frequently in patients receiving currently recommended multidrug therapy (MDT) regimens that include clofazimine than in patients who received dapsone monotherapy. ENL reactions usually manifest with fever and painful erythematous nodules, but peripheral neuritis, orchitis, lymphadenitis, iridocyclitis, nephritis, periostitis, arthralgia, malaise, albuminuria, epistaxis, or depression may also occur. These reactions are considered to be a manifestation of the disease rather than an adverse reaction to antileprosy regimens.

Treatment of leprosy reactional states depends on the severity of manifestations; severe reactions may require hospitalization. In general, the usual antileprosy regimen is continued despite the occurrence of a leprosy reactional state and, if nerve injury or skin ulceration is threatened, corticosteroids are administered.

Reversal reactions that include neuritis or ulceration always require treatment with corticosteroids (e.g., prednisone 1 mg/kg daily); although only a short course of corticosteroid treatment may be needed if the patient has only minimally active disease and no neuritis, prolonged treatment (4–6 months) may be required in those with neuritis. Mild ENL reactions may require no treatment or only symptomatic measures (e.g., analgesics); treatment with corticosteroids generally is effective and is always indicated in those with acute neuritis since this may prevent permanent nerve injury. Thalidomide and clofazimine also are effective for treatment of ENL reactions. For additional information on treatment on ENL, see Uses: Erythema Nodosum Leprosum, in Thalidomide 92:20 and see Leprosy Reactional States under Uses: Leprosy, in Clofazimine 8:16.92.

Early diagnosis and treatment of leprosy reactional states is important since these reactions are associated with considerable morbidity, especially if chronic, recurrent ENL occurs.

Therapy for leprosy and leprosy reactional states should be undertaken in consultation with an expert in the treatment of leprosy. In the US, clinicians should contact the National Hansen's Disease Program (NHDP) at 800-642-2477 on weekdays from 9:00 a.m. to 5:30 p.m. Eastern Standard Time or via email at nhdped@hrsa.gov for information on management of leprosy reactional states.

■ **Dermatologic Reactions** Adverse cutaneous effects, which usually result from sensitization to dapsone, occur rarely during therapy with the drug. Cutaneous reactions include exfoliative dermatitis, toxic erythema, erythema multiforme, toxic epidermal necrolysis, morbilliform and scarlatiniform eruptions, urticaria, and erythema nodosum. If a new or toxic dermatologic reaction occurs during therapy with dapsone, the drug should be discontinued and appropriate therapy initiated. Rash reportedly occurs in about 30–40% of AIDS patients receiving dapsone concomitantly with trimethoprim, but less frequently in those receiving dapsone alone.

■ **Nervous System Effects** Peripheral neuropathy with motor loss has been reported rarely in patients receiving high dosage of dapsone (200–500 mg daily). If muscle weakness occurs during therapy with dapsone, the drug should be discontinued; complete recovery may occur if the drug is withdrawn, but may take many months to several years. The mechanism of recovery is reportedly by axonal regeneration, and some recovered patients have tolerated retreatment with dapsone using a lower dosage of the drug. Although peripheral neuropathy has not been reported to date in patients with leprosy receiving dapsone, presumably because lower dosage is used, this adverse effect may be difficult to distinguish from a leprosy reactional state.

Insomnia, headache, nervousness, vertigo, and psychosis have also been reported with dapsone.

■ **GI Effects** Adverse GI effects including anorexia, abdominal pain, nausea, and vomiting have occurred in patients receiving dapsone.

■ **Hepatic Effects** Toxic hepatitis and cholestatic jaundice have been reported with dapsone. Cholestatic jaundice may be a hypersensitivity reaction, and generally appears to be reversible following discontinuance of the drug. Adverse hepatic effects have occurred shortly after initiation of dapsone therapy and may be manifested by increased serum concentrations of alkaline phosphatase, AST, bilirubin, and LDH. Liver function test abnormalities reportedly occur more frequently during combined dapsone and trimethoprim therapy than during dapsone alone. Hyperbilirubinemia has also occurred during dapsone therapy and may occur more often in patients with G-6-PD deficiency.

■ **Renal and Electrolyte Effects** Albuminuria, nephrotic syndrome, and renal papillary necrosis have occurred rarely during dapsone therapy. Mild, generally asymptomatic hyperkalemia has been reported frequently in patients receiving combined dapsone and trimethoprim therapy, but serum potassium concentrations generally returned to normal during continued therapy.

■ **Other Adverse Effects** Blurred vision, tinnitus, fever, phototoxicity, hyperpigmented macules, hypoalbuminemia without proteinuria, drug-induced lupus erythematosus, and an infectious mononucleosis-like syndrome have been reported with dapsone. Tachycardia has also occurred with dapsone, particularly with excessive dosage of the drug.

■ **Precautions and Contraindications** Dapsone is contraindicated in patients who are hypersensitive to the drug or dapsone derivatives.

Dapsone should not be administered to patients with severe anemia; the anemia should be treated prior to initiation of dapsone therapy. Dapsone should be used with caution in patients with G-6-PD deficiency, methemoglobin reductase deficiency, or hemoglobin M. Dapsone should also be used with caution in patients who are exposed to other drugs or agents that are capable of inducing hemolysis (see Drug Interactions) and in patients with conditions associated with hemolysis (e.g., certain infections, diabetic ketosis). Some clinicians recommend that screening for G-6-PD deficiency be performed prior to initiating dapsone therapy in human immunodeficiency virus (HIV)-infected patients, and that hemoglobin and methemoglobin concentrations and hematocrit be monitored periodically in such patients, particularly those receiving the drug concomitantly with trimethoprim. (See Drug Interactions: Trimethoprim.)

Complete blood cell counts (CBCs) should be performed frequently during dapsone therapy. Some clinicians recommend that CBCs be performed weekly during the first month of therapy, monthly for the next 6 months, and every 6 months thereafter. If a substantial reduction in leukocytes, platelets, or hematopoiesis is evident, dapsone should be discontinued and the patient closely monitored.

Because toxic hepatitis and cholestatic jaundice have been reported with dapsone, liver function should be monitored, when feasible, before and during therapy with the drug. If any abnormality in liver function is evident, the drug should be discontinued until the source of the abnormality is established. Patients should be instructed to report to their clinician the presence of sore throat, fever, pallor, purpura, or jaundice during dapsone therapy.

Leprosy patients should be informed about the signs and symptoms of neuritis and cautioned about the importance of immediately reporting such signs and symptoms to a clinician. (See Cautions: Leprosy Reactional States.)

■ **Pediatric Precautions** Dapsone is labeled for treatment of leprosy and for treatment of dermatitis herpetiformis in children. The drug is generally considered to have no effect on growth, development, and functional development of children.

Although data are limited regarding efficacy and safety in children, some experts recommend a regimen of dapsone in conjunction with trimethoprim as an alternative for treatment of mild to moderate *Pneumocystis jirovecii* (formerly *Pneumocystis carinii*) pneumonia (PCP) in children† and recommend dapsone monotherapy as an alternative for primary and secondary prophylaxis of PCP in HIV-infected children 1 month of age or older† (see Uses: Pneumocystis jirovecii Pneumonia). In addition, dapsone in conjunction with pyrimethamine (and leucovorin) is recommended as an alternative for primary prophylaxis of toxoplasmosis in HIV-infected children 1 month of age or older† (see Uses: Toxoplasmosis).

■ **Mutagenicity and Carcinogenicity** Dapsone was not mutagenic in microbial tests using *Salmonella typhimurium*, with or without microsomal activation.

Dapsone has been found to be carcinogenic in animal studies. The drug has caused mesenchymal tumors in the spleen and peritoneum of male rats and female mice and thyroid carcinoma in female rats.

■ **Pregnancy, Fertility, and Lactation** Animal reproduction studies have not been performed with dapsone. Although dapsone has been used in pregnant women without evidence of fetal abnormalities, the drug should be used during pregnancy only when clearly needed.

In patients with leprosy, some clinicians recommend maintaining dapsone treatment during pregnancy. In addition, dapsone has been important for the management of dermatitis herpetiformis in some pregnant women.

Infertility has been reported in males receiving dapsone; in 2 patients, fertility was restored following discontinuance of the drug.

Because dapsone is distributed into milk and because of the tumorigenic potential demonstrated in animal studies, a decision should be made to discontinue nursing or the drug, taking into account the importance of the drug to the woman.

Drug Interactions

■ **Drugs Associated with Adverse Hematologic Effects** Because the drugs have similar adverse hematologic effects, concurrent use of a folic acid antagonist (e.g., pyrimethamine) and dapsone may result in an increased risk of these adverse effects. Agranulocytosis has developed during the second and third months of therapy in patients receiving concomitant treatment with weekly pyrimethamine and dapsone. If pyrimethamine is used concomitantly with dapsone, the patient should be monitored more frequently than usual for adverse hematologic effects.

Because effects may be additive, dapsone should be used with caution in patients with G-6-PD deficiency receiving or exposed to other drugs or agents which are capable of inducing hemolysis in these individuals (e.g., nitrite, aniline, phenylhydrazine, naphthalene, niridazole, nitrofurantoin, primaquine).

■ **Clofazimine** Results of several studies indicate that concomitant clofazimine does not affect the pharmacokinetics of dapsone, although a transient increase in urinary excretion of dapsone reportedly occurred in a few patients receiving concomitant therapy with the drugs. In a study in lepromatous leprosy patients receiving dapsone (100 mg daily) and rifampin (600 mg daily), concomitant administration of clofazimine (100 mg daily) did not affect plasma dapsone concentrations or the plasma half-life or urinary elimination of dapsone.

There is some evidence that dapsone may decrease or nullify some of the anti-inflammatory effects of clofazimine. In vitro, clofazimine and dapsone have opposing effects on neutrophil motility and lymphocyte transformation. Some clinicians suggest that this theoretically could adversely affect the efficacy of clofazimine in patients with erythema nodosum leprosum (ENL) reactions. Several borderline leprosy and lepromatous leprosy patients with severe, recurrent ENL reactions reportedly required higher clofazimine dosage to control these reactions when dapsone therapy was given concomitantly than when clofazimine was given alone. The manufacturer of clofazimine, however, suggests that further study is needed to confirm this interaction and states that it is advisable to continue treatment with both clofazimine and dapsone in patients who develop leprosy-associated inflammatory reactions, including ENL, during concomitant therapy with the drugs. There is no evidence to date that dapsone and clofazimine interfere with the antimycobacterial activity of each other.

■ **Didanosine** Failure of dapsone to prevent *Pneumocystis jirovecii* (formerly *Pneumocystis carinii*) pneumonia (PCP) was reported in about 40% of patients with human immunodeficiency virus (HIV) infection who were receiving didanosine concomitantly. This failure rate was substantially higher than that reported in other studies in which dapsone was *not* administered with didanosine or that were observed when didanosine was used in patients receiving co-trimoxazole or aerosolized pentamidine for prevention of PCP. Although the possibility of a pharmacokinetic interaction was not evaluated in these patients, it was suggested that the buffers present in the didanosine preparation, which provides a pH of 7–8 to facilitate GI absorption of the antiretroviral agent, may interfere with GI absorption of dapsone. Dapsone is insoluble at neutral pH, while solubility is facilitated at acidic pH. However, in a study in 6 healthy adults and 6 HIV-infected adults, the pharmacokinetics of dapsone was *not* affected when 100 mg of the drug was administered 5 minutes after a 200-mg dose of didanosine given as chewable/dispersible, buffered tablets (no longer commercially available in the US) in the patients, or 5 minutes after administration of placebo tablets containing the aluminum and magnesium buffer without didanosine, in the healthy individuals. It has been suggested that dapsone be administered at least 2 hours before didanosine, although some clinicians have observed prophylactic failure of dapsone despite such separation of dosing and therefore recommend that the drugs not be used concomitantly.

Concomitant use of dapsone (single 100-mg dose) and buffered didanosine (200 mg every 12 hours for 14 days) did not have a clinically important effect on peak plasma concentrations or area under the plasma concentration-time curve (AUC) of dapsone.

■ **Rifamycins** Concomitant use of rifabutin (300 mg daily) and dapsone (50 mg daily) in HIV-infected individuals decreased the AUC of dapsone by about 27–40%.

Rifampin may accelerate metabolism of dapsone; decreased serum dapsone concentrations (7–10 times lower) and increased urinary excretion of dapsone have been reported. Dosage adjustments may be necessary when rifampin and dapsone are used concomitantly; however, dosage adjustments are *not* required when rifampin and dapsone are used concomitantly for treatment of leprosy.

Rifapentine may accelerate metabolism of dapsone; dosage adjustments may be necessary if rifapentine and dapsone are used concomitantly.

■ **Trimethoprim** Concomitant use of dapsone and trimethoprim may increase serum dapsone concentrations and potentially increase the risk of adverse effects associated with dapsone. In a study in adults with acquired immunodeficiency syndrome (AIDS) who received oral dapsone (100 mg once daily) alone or in conjunction with oral trimethoprim (20 mg/kg daily) for treatment of PCP, plasma dapsone concentrations were 40% higher with the combined regimen than with dapsone alone and methemoglobinemia occurred more frequently with the combined regimen (67%) than with dapsone alone (11%). There also is some evidence that dapsone may increase plasma trimethoprim concentrations, but an increased risk of trimethoprim-associated adverse effects was not identified in this study.

Periodic monitoring for potential toxicity (e.g., methemoglobinemia) is recommended in patients receiving dapsone in conjunction with trimethoprim.

Acute Toxicity

■ **Manifestations** Overdosage of dapsone generally results in nausea, vomiting, and hyperexcitability within a few minutes to up to 24 hours later. Methemoglobin-induced depression, seizures, and severe cyanosis may occur and require prompt treatment. Hemolysis may occur 7–14 days after an acute ingestion.

■ **Treatment** In patients who do not have G-6-PD deficiency, dapsone-induced methemoglobinemia should be treated with methylene blue (1–2 mg/kg given by slow IV injection). The effect usually is complete within 30 minutes, but methylene blue may need to be readministered if methemoglobin reaccumulates. Alternatively, in nonemergency situations, methylene blue may be given orally in a dosage of 3–5 mg/kg every 4–6 hours. Methylene blue should not be administered to patients with G-6-PD deficiency, since methylene blue reduction depends on G-6-PD. Orally administered activated charcoal (20 g 4 times daily) has been shown to substantially enhance the elimination of dapsone and its monoacetyl derivative in several cases of acute dapsone overdosage, and some clinicians recommend it as a treatment of choice in the management of acute dapsone intoxication. Hemodialysis also enhances the elimination of dapsone and its monoacetyl derivative.

Mechanism of Action

Dapsone is bacteriostatic or weakly bactericidal in action against *Mycobacterium leprae*. The mechanism of action of dapsone has not been fully elucidated. Because the antibacterial activity of dapsone is inhibited by *p*-aminobenzoic acid (PABA), the drug probably has a mechanism of action similar to that of sulfonamides which involves inhibition of folic acid synthesis in susceptible organisms.

Some studies indicate that dapsone may inhibit the alternate pathway of complement activation and interfere with the myeloperoxidase-H_2O_2-halide-mediated cytotoxic system within neutrophils. In vitro studies indicate that dapsone stimulates neutrophil motility. The drug also appears to inhibit spontaneous and induced synthesis of prostaglandin E_2 by polymorphonuclear leukocytes obtained from healthy individuals or patients with leprosy.

The mechanism of action of dapsone in the treatment of dermatitis herpetiformis is unknown; dapsone only suppresses the disease, and cutaneous IgA and complement deposition are not affected by the drug. It has been suggested that dapsone may act as an immunomodulator when used in the treatment of dermatitis herpetiformis and other dermatologic diseases.

Spectrum

Dapsone is active in vivo against *Mycobacterium leprae*. Although *M. leprae* cannot be cultured in vitro, in vivo mouse footpad studies using *M. leprae* recovered from untreated patients with leprosy indicate that dapsone concentrations of 1–10 ng/mL generally inhibit susceptible strains of the organism. Dapsone is also active against *M. tuberculosis* and several other species of mycobacteria. In vitro, most susceptible strains of *M. tuberculosis* are inhibited by dapsone concentrations of 10 mcg/mL.

Dapsone also has some activity against *Pneumocystis jirovecii* (formerly *Pneumocystis carinii*) and *Plasmodium*.

Resistance

Resistant strains of initially susceptible *M. leprae* may develop during therapy with dapsone; resistance to the drug appears to develop in a slow, stepwise manner. It has been estimated that resistance to dapsone develops in 2–10% of patients with lepromatous leprosy who have received dapsone alone for many years. Resistance has been reported to occur as long as 5–24 years after initiation of dapsone therapy; resistance has been reported most frequently when the drug was given in low dosage or intermittently.

Although primary resistance to dapsone used to be reported only rarely, resistance to the drug has been reported with increasing frequency in *M. leprae* recovered from newly diagnosed cases of leprosy in patients who have not previously received therapy with a sulfone.

M. leprae resistant to both dapsone and clofazimine, but susceptible to rifampin, has been reported rarely.

Pharmacokinetics

■ **Absorption** Following oral administration, dapsone is rapidly and almost completely absorbed from the GI tract and peak serum concentrations of the drug are attained within 4–8 hours. When a dosage of 200 mg daily is used, steady-state serum concentrations of the drug range from 0.1–7 mcg/mL and average 2.3 mcg/mL after 8 days of therapy. Following oral administration of a single 100-mg oral dose of dapsone, serum concentrations of the drug range from 0.4–1.2 mcg/mL 24 hours after the dose. Trace amounts of dapsone may be found in serum for 8–12 days after oral administration of a single 200-mg dose of the drug or for as long as 35 days after discontinuance of repeated doses of the drug. Dapsone and its monoacetyl metabolite (MADDS) appear to undergo enterohepatic circulation.

■ **Distribution** The volume of distribution of dapsone is reportedly 1.5–2.5 L/kg in adults.

Dapsone is distributed into most body tissues. Dapsone is reportedly retained in skin, muscle, kidneys, and liver; trace concentrations of the drug may be present in these tissues up to 3 weeks after discontinuance of dapsone therapy. Dapsone is also distributed into sweat, saliva, sputum, and tears. The drug is also distributed into bile.

Although in one study using radiolabeled dapsone in patients with leprosy, higher concentrations of radioactivity were attained in diseased than in presumably healthy skin, other studies indicate little or no difference in sulfone content of healthy and diseased skin in patients with leprosy. Dapsone may not penetrate ocular tissue well, since eye lesions may develop or progress during therapy of leprosy even though the disease may be controlled or eliminated in other tissues.

Dapsone crosses the placenta. Dapsone is distributed into milk. In a woman receiving dapsone in a dosage of 50 mg daily, dapsone concentrations in milk were 1.1 mcg/mL; concurrent maternal serum concentrations of the drug were 1.6 mcg/mL.

Dapsone is 50–90% bound to plasma proteins. The major metabolite of dapsone, monoacetyldapsone, is almost completely bound to plasma proteins.

■ **Elimination** There are large interindividual variations in the plasma half-life of dapsone. The plasma half-life of dapsone may range from 10–83 hours and averages 20–30 hours.

Dapsone is acetylated in the liver to monoacetyl and diacetyl derivatives. The major metabolite of dapsone is monoacetyldapsone (MADDS). The rate of acetylation of dapsone is genetically determined and is subject to interindividual variation, although the rate is usually constant for each individual. The drug also is hydroxylated in the liver to hydroxylamine dapsone (NOH-DDS). NOH-DDS appears to be responsible for methemoglobinemia and hemolysis induced by the drug.

Approximately 20% of each dose of dapsone is excreted in urine as unchanged drug, 70–85% is excreted in urine as water-soluble metabolites, and a small amount is excreted in feces. Dapsone is excreted in urine as acid-labile mono-*N*-glucuronide and mono-*N*-sulfamate derivatives in addition to some unidentified metabolites.

Orally administered activated charcoal has been shown to substantially enhance the elimination of dapsone and its monoacetyl derivative in healthy adults and in several cases of acute dapsone overdosage. Hemodialysis also reportedly enhances the elimination of dapsone and its monoacetyl derivative.

Chemistry and Stability

■ **Chemistry** Dapsone is a synthetic sulfone anti-infective. Dapsone occurs as a white or creamy white, crystalline powder that has a slightly bitter taste. The drug is very slightly soluble in water and freely soluble in alcohol.

■ **Stability** Dapsone tablets should be stored at 20–25°C and protected from light. Dapsone may discolor following exposure to light.

Preparations

Excipients in commercially available drug preparations may have clinically important effects in some individuals; consult specific product labeling for details.

Dapsone

Oral		
Tablets	25 mg*	**Dapsone Tablets** (scored)
	100 mg*	**Dapsone Tablets** (scored)

*available from one or more manufacturer, distributor, and/or repackager by generic (nonproprietary) name

†Use is not currently included in the labeling approved by the US Food and Drug Administration

ANTIVIRALS 8:18

ANTIRETROVIRALS 8:18.08

Antiretroviral Agents General Statement

Classification of Antiretroviral Agents

Antiretroviral agents are synthetic antiviral agents that have antiviral activity against human immunodeficiency virus (HIV) and are used in the management of HIV infection. There are 6 different classes of antiretroviral agents commercially available in the US: HIV nucleoside reverse transcriptase inhibitors (NRTIs), HIV protease inhibitors (PIs), HIV nonnucleoside reverse transcriptase inhibitors (NNRTIs), HIV nucleotide reverse transcriptase inhibitors, HIV integrase inhibitors , and HIV entry and fusion inhibitors.

HIV NUCLEOSIDE REVERSE TRANSCRIPTASE INHIBITORS (NRTIs)

abacavir sulfate (ABC)	lamivudine (3TC)
didanosine (ddI)	stavudine (d4T)
emtricitabine (FTC)	zidovudine (ZDV, AZT)

HIV NRTIs are synthetic analogs of naturally occurring nucleosides. There currently are 6 HIV NRTIs commercially available in the US; others are under investigation. Zalcitabine was discontinued in late 2006 and is no longer commercially available in the US.

NRTIs are commercially available in the US as single-entity preparations. Several NRTIs also are commercially available in the US in fixed combinations that contain *only* NRTIs (dual NRTIs, triple NRTIs), including a fixed combination containing abacavir sulfate and lamivudine (abacavir/lamivudine), a fixed combination containing lamivudine and zidovudine (lamivudine/zidovudine), and a fixed combination containing abacavir sulfate, lamivudine, and zidovudine (abacavir/lamivudine/zidovudine). Abacavir also is commercially available in the US in fixed combination with lamivudine and dolutegravir (abacavir/dolutegravir/lamivudine). Emtricitabine also is commercially available in the US in various fixed combinations with a tenofovir prodrug (either tenofovir alafenamide fumarate [TAF] or tenofovir disoproxil fumarate [tenofovir DF; TDF]), including a fixed combination containing only emtricitabine and tenofovir alafenamide (emtricitabine/tenofovir alafenamide), a fixed combination containing only emtricitabine and tenofovir DF (emtricitabine/tenofovir DF), a fixed combination containing emtricitabine, rilpivirine, and tenofovir alafenamide (emtricitabine/rilpivirine/tenofovir alafenamide), a fixed combination containing emtricitabine, rilpivirine, and tenofovir DF (emtricitabine/rilpivirine/tenofovir DF), a fixed combination containing emtricitabine, tenofovir DF, and efavirenz (efavirenz/emtricitabine/tenofovir DF), a fixed combination containing bictegravir, emtricitabine, and tenofovir alafenamide (BIC/FTC/TAF), a fixed combination containing elvitegravir, cobicistat (a pharmacokinetic enhancer), emtricitabine, and tenofovir alafenamide (EVG/c/FTC/TAF), and a fixed combination containing elvitegravir, cobicistat (a pharmacokinetic enhancer), emtricitabine, and tenofovir DF (EVG/c/FTC/TDF).

NRTIs have a wider spectrum of antiviral activity than other currently available antiretrovirals. NRTIs are active in vitro against human retroviruses, including HIV type 1 (HIV-1) and HIV type 2 (HIV-2). Lamivudine and emtricitabine also are active against hepatitis B virus (HBV); abacavir, didanosine, and zidovudine have only limited activity against HBV. Abacavir, didanosine, and zidovudine are active against many animal retroviruses, including feline leukemia virus, Friend leukemia virus, Harvey murine sarcoma virus, murine leukemia virus, and simian T lymphotropic virus. HIV NRTIs generally have been inactive against other human or animal viruses tested, including herpes simplex virus (HSV) types 1 and 2, influenza virus, adenovirus, cytomegalovirus (CMV), respiratory syncytial virus (RSV), varicella zoster virus (VZV), and vaccinia virus.

NRTIs are prodrugs that are inactive until phosphorylated by cellular enzymes and converted into active triphosphate metabolites. The pharmacologically active triphosphate metabolites then compete with naturally occurring deoxynucleoside triphosphates for the active binding site on viral reverse transcriptase, an enzyme essential for viral replication. Once the triphosphate metabolites become incorporated into viral DNA, synthesis of the viral DNA chain is terminated since the metabolites lack a functional 3′-hydroxyl group preventing further 5′ to 3′ phosphodiester linkages.

HIV PROTEASE INHIBITORS (PIs)

atazanavir sulfate (ATV)	nelfinavir mesylate (NFV)
darunavir (DRV)	ritonavir (RTV)
fosamprenavir calcium (FPV)	saquinavir mesylate (SQV)
indinavir sulfate (IDV)	tipranavir (TPV)
lopinavir and ritonavir (LPV/r)	

HIV PIs are synthetic antiviral agents that were specifically designed based on the structure of HIV protease, an enzyme that plays an essential role in the HIV replication cycle. Using computer models of the enzyme and binding sites on the enzyme, a wide variety of compounds have been identified as potential inhibitors of HIV protease activity. There currently are 9 HIV PIs commercially available in the US. Amprenavir was discontinued in late 2007 and is no longer commercially available in the US; commercially available fosamprenavir is a prodrug that is hydrolyzed in vivo to amprenavir.

Lopinavir is commercially available in the US *only* in fixed combination with low-dose ritonavir (lopinavir/ritonavir). Atazanavir and darunavir are commercially available in the US as single-entity preparations or in fixed combination with the pharmacokinetic enhancer, cobicistat (atazanavir/cobicistat, darunavir/cobicistat). Other HIV PIs (fosamprenavir, indinavir, nelfinavir, ritonavir, saquinavir, tipranavir) are commercially available in the US *only* as single-entity preparations. HIV PIs usually are used in conjunction with a pharmacokinetic enhancer (i.e., low-dose ritonavir or cobicistat). (See Drug Interactions: Pharmacokinetic Enhancers.)

PIs have a very limited spectrum of antiviral activity. These drugs are active against HIV-1, but have variable activity against HIV-2. Darunavir, lopinavir, and saquinavir may be more active against HIV-2 than other currently available PIs. While indinavir and saquinavir have some activity against simian immunodeficiency virus, HIV PIs generally have been inactive against other human and animal viruses tested. On a molar basis, the PIs appear to be more active than either NRTIs or NNRTIs against susceptible HIV-1.

Currently available HIV PIs have similar mechanisms of action. These drugs inhibit replication of HIV-1 and HIV-2 by directly interfering with HIV protease activity. This prevents the formation of mature virions. Most of the drugs function as selective, competitive, reversible inhibitors of the enzyme. Although fosamprenavir calcium is a prodrug and has little or no antiviral activity until hydrolyzed in vivo to amprenavir, the antiretroviral activity of other HIV PIs does not depend on intracellular conversion to an active metabolite.

HIV NONNUCLEOSIDE REVERSE TRANSCRIPTASE INHIBITORS (NNRTIs)

delavirdine mesylate (DLV)
efavirenz (EFV)
etravirine (ETV)
nevirapine (NVP)
rilpivirine (RPV)

HIV NNRTIs are a group of structurally diverse synthetic antiretrovirals that have a similar mechanism of action. There currently are 5 HIV NNRTIs commercially available in the US.

NNRTIs are commercially available in the US as single-entity preparations. In addition, efavirenz is commercially available in the US in fixed combination with emtricitabine and tenofovir DF (efavirenz/emtricitabine/tenofovir DF) and rilpivirine is commercially available in the US in fixed combination with dolutegravir (dolutegravir/rilpivirine), in fixed combination with emtricitabine and tenofovir alafenamide (emtricitabine/rilpivirine/tenofovir alafenamide), or in fixed combination with emtricitabine and tenofovir DF (emtricitabine/rilpivirine/tenofovir DF).

NNRTIs have a very specific spectrum of antiviral activity. Currently available NNRTIs are active against HIV-1, but HIV-2 are intrinsically resistant to the drugs. NNRTIs also have been inactive against other human or animal viruses tested to date.

NNRTIs inhibit replication of HIV-1 by interfering with viral RNA- and DNA-directed polymerase activities of reverse transcriptase. The mechanism of action of NNRTIs differs from that of NRTIs. While NRTIs interfere with reverse transcriptase activity by becoming incorporated into the growing viral DNA chain, NNRTIs interfere with the function of reverse transcriptase by binding directly to the enzyme in a noncompetitive fashion. Unlike the NRTIs, the antiretroviral activity of NNRTIs does not depend on intracellular conversion to an active metabolite.

HIV NUCLEOTIDE REVERSE TRANSCRIPTASE INHIBITORS

tenofovir alafenamide fumarate (TAF)
tenofovir disoproxil fumarate (tenofovir DF; TDF)

HIV nucleotide reverse transcriptase inhibitors are a group of synthetic acyclic nucleoside phosphonates that have a similar mechanism of action. Tenofovir is the only nucleotide reverse transcriptase inhibitor commercially available in the US and, for purposes of therapeutic decisions, is grouped with the NRTI class of antiretrovirals. Tenofovir is commercially available as tenofovir alafenamide fumarate and tenofovir disoproxil fumarate (tenofovir DF; TDF).

For the treatment of HIV infection, tenofovir alafenamide is commercially available in the US *only* in fixed combination with emtricitabine (emtricitabine/tenofovir alafenamide), in fixed combination with emtricitabine and rilpivirine (emtricitabine/rilpivirine/tenofovir alafenamide), in fixed combination with bictegravir and emtricitabine (BIC/FTC/TAF), or in fixed combination with elvitegravir, cobicistat (a pharmacokinetic enhancer), and emtricitabine (EVG/c/FTC/TAF).

Tenofovir DF is commercially available in the US as single-entity preparations, and also is commercially available in fixed combination with emtricitabine (emtricitabine/tenofovir DF), in fixed combination with emtricitabine and efavirenz (efavirenz/emtricitabine/tenofovir DF), in fixed combination with emtricitabine and rilpivirine (emtricitabine/rilpivirine/tenofovir DF), and in fixed combination with elvitegravir, cobicistat (a pharmacokinetic enhancer), and emtricitabine (EVG/c/FTC/TDF).

Tenofovir alafenamide and tenofovir DF are both tenofovir prodrugs that are inactive until hydrolyzed in plasma to tenofovir and then converted intracellularly to the active metabolite tenofovir diphosphate. Tenofovir diphosphate competes with naturally occurring deoxyadenosine triphosphate and, after incorporation into viral DNA, synthesis of the viral DNA chain is terminated. Tenofovir alafenamide is more stable in blood and plasma and more efficiently converted intracellularly to tenofovir diphosphate than tenofovir DF, resulting in lower circulating levels of tenofovir and higher concentrations of the active metabolite within HIV target cells than those reported with tenofovir DF.

Tenofovir alafenamide and tenofovir DF are active against HIV-1, have some activity against HIV-2, and also have activity against HBV.

HIV INTEGRASE INHIBITORS

bictegravir (BIC)
dolutegravir (DTG)
elvitegravir (EVG)
raltegravir potassium (RAL)

HIV integrase inhibitors inhibit an HIV enzyme that integrates viral DNA into the infected cell's DNA.

Bictegravir, dolutegravir, elvitegravir, and raltegravir are all HIV integrase strand transfer inhibitors (INSTIs). The drugs inhibit the activity of HIV-1 integrase, an enzyme that integrates HIV DNA into the host cell genome. Integration is required for maintenance of the viral genome and for efficient viral gene expression and replication. Inhibition of integration prevents propagation of viral infection. Bictegravir, dolutegravir, elvitegravir, and raltegravir also appear to have some activity against HIV-2.

Bictegravir is commercially available in the US *only* in fixed combination with emtricitabine and tenofovir alafenamide fumarate (BIC/FTC/TAF). Dolutegravir is commercially available in the US as a single-entity preparation, in fixed combination with rilpivirine (dolutegravir/rilpivirine), and in fixed combination with abacavir sulfate and lamivudine (abacavir/dolutegravir/lamivudine). Elvitegravir is commercially available in the US *only* in fixed combination with cobicistat (a pharmacokinetic enhancer), emtricitabine, and either tenofovir alafenamide fumarate (EVG/c/FTC/TAF) or tenofovir DF (EVG/c/FTC/TDF). Raltegravir is commercially available in the US *only* as a single-entity preparation.

HIV ENTRY AND FUSION INHIBITORS

enfuvirtide (T-20)
ibalizumab-uiyk (IBA)
maraviroc (MVC)

HIV entry and fusion inhibitors are a group of antiretrovirals that have mechanisms of action that involve blocking HIV from entering human cells.

HIV entry inhibitors bind to receptors on immune cells used by HIV to enter cells. Maraviroc and ibalizumab-uiyk are both HIV entry inhibitors, but have different mechanisms of action.

Maraviroc is a CC chemokine receptor 5 (CCR5) antagonist. The drug is active against HIV-1; activity of CCR5 antagonists against HIV-2 needs further study. HIV can enter host cells by attaching to the $CD4^+$ T-cell receptor using 1 of 2 chemokine co-receptors, CCR5 or CXCR4. Maraviroc selectively binds to CCR5 on the cell membrane and prevents the interaction of HIV-1 glycoprotein 120 and CCR5 necessary for CCR5-tropic HIV-1 to enter cells. Maraviroc is commercially available in the US *only* as a single-entity preparation.

Ibalizumab-uiyk is a CD4-directed post-attachment HIV-1 inhibitor. The drug is a recombinant humanized monoclonal antibody that blocks HIV-1 from infecting $CD4^+$ T-cells by binding to domain 2 of CD4, thereby interfering with post-attachment steps required for the entry of HIV-1 into host cells and preventing viral transmission that occurs via cell-cell fusion. The binding of ibalizumab-uiyk to domain 2 of CD4 is specific and blocks HIV-1 entry into host cells without causing immunosuppression. The drug is active in vitro against CCR5- and CXCR4-tropic HIV-1 strains. Ibalizumab-uiyk is commercially available in the US *only* as a single-entity preparation.

HIV fusion inhibitors interfere with the fusion of HIV-1 to its target cell. Enfuvirtide is the only HIV fusion inhibitor commercially available in the US and is available *only* as a single-entity preparation. HIV fusion inhibitors have a very specific spectrum of antiviral activity. HIV fusion inhibitors are active against HIV-1, but are inactive against HIV-2. HIV fusion inhibitors interfere with entry of HIV-1 into target cells by blocking conformational changes in the HIV-1 glycoprotein that are required for fusion of the virus to the membrane of the host $CD4^+$ T-cell.

Guidelines for Use of Antiretroviral Agents

Therapeutic options for the treatment and prevention of HIV infection have increased, and recommendations concerning the use of antiretrovirals have evolved as the result of expanded knowledge concerning the immunopathogenesis of HIV, availability of several different classes of antiretrovirals (HIV nucleoside reverse transcriptase inhibitors [NRTIs], HIV protease inhibitors (PIs), HIV nonnucleoside reverse transcriptase inhibitors [NNRTIs], HIV nucleotide reverse transcriptase inhibitors, HIV integrase inhibitors [INSTIs], HIV entry and fusion inhibitors), and improvements in laboratory methods used to evaluate the rate of disease progression and response to antiretroviral therapy. Effective management of HIV infection must be based on up-to-date information about the biology and pathogenesis of HIV infection and currently available antiretrovirals.

Because pools of latently infected $CD4^+$ T-cells are established during the earliest stages of acute HIV infection and persist even in patients who have received potent multiple-drug antiretroviral regimens that suppress viral load to undetectable levels for prolonged periods, eradication of HIV infection cannot be achieved with currently available antiretroviral regimens and is not a realistic goal. The primary goals of antiretroviral therapy in the management of HIV infection are maximal and durable suppression of HIV viral load (as measured by plasma HIV-1 RNA levels), restoration and/or preservation of immunologic function, prevention or reduction of HIV-related morbidity and mortality, improvements in the duration and quality of life, and prevention of secondary transmission of HIV. These goals can best be met by the use of potent multiple-drug antiretroviral regimens that suppress HIV replication to undetectable levels, limit the potential for selection of resistant HIV strains, delay disease progression, and minimize drug-related toxicities and drug interactions. In addition, strategies that facilitate decisions regarding modification of antiretroviral regimens (e.g., clinical and laboratory monitoring), address comorbidities that can complicate antiretroviral therapy (e.g., coinfection with hepatitis B virus [HBV], hepatitis C virus [HCV], mycobacterial infections), maximize patient adherence to antiretroviral therapy, and minimize the risk of HIV transmission (e.g., through perinatal transmission, blood exposures, high-risk sexual and drug abuse behaviors) also are integral parts of management of HIV infection.

Antiretroviral regimens that were considered treatments of choice for the initial management of HIV infection in the past (e.g., monotherapy or 2-drug regimens that include only NRTIs) are suboptimal since clinical benefits associated with such therapy (i.e., delay in disease progression, decrease in incidence of opportunistic infections, improved survival) are not sustained over the long term. Potent antiretroviral regimens that include a minimum of 3 antiretroviral agents currently are recommended for the management of HIV infection in most adults, adolescents, and children. These treatment regimens usually are referred to as antiretroviral therapy (ART), combination antiretroviral therapy (combination ART or cART), or multiple-drug antiretroviral therapy, and also have been referred to as highly active antiretroviral therapy (HAART) to differentiate them from the less potent regimens previously used for management of HIV infection.

Most individuals who receive an appropriate multiple-drug antiretroviral regimen for initial antiretroviral therapy will achieve viral suppression in 8–24 weeks if they are adherent and do not harbor HIV with resistance mutations to the drugs included in the regimen. However, experience with various antiretroviral regimens has shown that the duration of clinical benefit from any one regimen may be limited and that optimal antiretroviral therapy involves continuous evaluation of the patient's response to the current regimen and appropriate modification of the regimen whenever the need for a change is indicated by increases in viral load (plasma HIV-1 RNA levels), disease progression, or drug toxicity or intolerance. While potent multiple-drug antiretroviral regimens may effectively decrease plasma HIV-1 RNA to undetectable levels for prolonged periods and provide substantial benefits in terms of immunologic, virologic, and clinical responses, no antiretroviral regimen evaluated to date can suppress HIV replication completely or eliminate the virus from the body. HIV apparently continues to persist in various tissues (e.g., lymphoid tissue, latently infected resting $CD4^+$ T-cells, CNS), and infectious HIV has been isolated from $CD4^+$ T-cells obtained from infected individuals whose plasma HIV-1 RNA levels had been suppressed below the limits of detection for 2 years or more. There also is evidence that discontinuing or briefly interrupting antiretroviral therapy in patients with viremia may be associated with rapid increases in plasma HIV-1 RNA levels, decreased $CD4^+$ T-cell counts, and increased risk of clinical progression.

Since information on, and experience with, available multiple-drug regimens are changing rapidly, experts in the management of patients with HIV infection should be consulted regarding the potential advantages and limitations of available therapeutic options. The choice of antiretrovirals to include in *initial* treatment regimens used in HIV-infected individuals who are antiretroviral naive (have not previously received antiretroviral therapy) and the most appropriate agents to use in subsequent regimens in antiretroviral-experienced (previously treated) individuals must be individualized based on the advantages and disadvantages of the drugs and on virologic, immunologic, and clinical characteristics of the individual patient. Some factors to be considered when selecting antiretrovirals to include in multiple-drug regimens are the antiretroviral potency of the agents, availability and cost of the agents, potential rate of development of resistance, potential pharmacokinetic interactions among the drugs and with other drugs that the patient may be receiving, dosing convenience, adverse effect profile, patient's pretreatment $CD4^+$ T-cell count, gender, pregnancy potential, results of drug-resistance testing, and the patient's ability to adhere to the dosage regimens involved.

While the most appropriate antiretroviral regimen cannot be defined for each clinical scenario, the US Department of Health and Human Services (HHS) Panel on Antiretroviral Guidelines for Adults and Adolescents, HHS Panel on Antiretroviral Therapy and Medical Management of Children Living with HIV, and HHS Panel on Treatment of Pregnant Women with HIV Infection and Prevention of Perinatal Transmission have developed comprehensive guidelines that provide information on selection and use of antiretrovirals for treatment or prophylaxis of HIV infection. These guidelines are based on current knowledge regarding the pathogenesis of HIV, results of clinical studies, and expert opinion and are available at http://www.aidsinfo.nih.gov. Guidelines on the use of antiretrovirals for the management of HIV infection also are available from the British HIV Association (BHIVA) and the International AIDS Society—USA Panel. For information on results of controlled clinical studies evaluating the safety and efficacy of currently available antiretrovirals and experience to date regarding various antiretroviral regimens, see the Uses sections in the individual drug monographs in 8:18.08.

■ Laboratory Monitoring

Diagnostic HIV Testing Early detection of HIV infection facilitates early initiation of antiretroviral treatment and can lead to improved health outcomes, including slower clinical progression and reduced mortality. Beginning in 2006, the US Centers for Disease Control and Prevention (CDC) began recommending routine HIV testing and screening for *all* adults and adolescents 13–64 years of age in *all* health-care settings, unless the patient declines (opt-out HIV screening). This strategy of providing routine HIV testing and screening, regardless of the perceived risk of infection, is considered essential for optimal management of the disease. In addition, HIV testing and screening is recommended as a standard of care for *all* pregnant women and for neonates born to women whose HIV status is unknown. (See HIV Testing During Pregnancy under Guidelines for Use of Antiretroviral Agents: Antiretroviral Therapy During Pregnancy.)

Plasma HIV-1 RNA Levels and $CD4^+$ T-cell Counts Decisions regarding initiation and modification of antiretroviral therapy are guided by plasma HIV-1 RNA levels (viral load), $CD4^+$ T-cell counts, and the clinical condition of the patient. Various other surrogate markers and laboratory parameters were used in the past to assess the risk of progression of HIV infection and evaluate efficacy of antiretrovirals (e.g., peripheral blood mononuclear cell [PBMC] HIV-1 titers, plasma concentrations or levels of HIV p24 core antigen [p24 *gag* protein], β_2-microglobulin, neopterin), but considerable experience showed that the most important surrogate markers are plasma HIV-1 RNA levels and $CD4^+$ T-cell counts and these have now been used for several decades to manage and monitor HIV infection. Monitoring of lymphocyte subsets other than $CD4^+$ T-cells (e.g., CD8, CD19) has not proven clinically useful, adds to costs, and is not routinely recommended.

Although plasma HIV-1 RNA levels are the most important indicator of response to antiretroviral therapy and are useful in predicting clinical progression, $CD4^+$ T-cell counts are the major laboratory indicator of immune function in HIV-infected patients and the strongest predictor of subsequent disease progression and survival. Measurement of $CD4^+$ T-cell count is particularly useful before initiating antiretroviral therapy; plasma HIV-1 RNA levels are particularly useful for monitoring effectiveness of antiretroviral therapy after it has been initiated.

Updated CDC surveillance case definitions for HIV infection now include information regarding age-specific $CD4^+$ T-cell counts; therefore, absolute $CD4^+$ T-cell counts are recommended for monitoring immune status in children of all ages, with $CD4^+$ T-cell percentages used as an alternative.

Recommended Frequency of Plasma HIV-1 RNA Level and $CD4^+$ T-cell Count Testing. Baseline $CD4^+$ T-cell counts and plasma HIV-1 RNA levels should be measured in *all* newly diagnosed HIV-infected patients to provide information on the virologic and immunologic status of the patient and the risk of disease progression. If a decision is made not to initiate antiretroviral therapy in HIV-infected adults or adolescents (see Guidelines for Use of Antiretroviral Agents: Initial Antiretroviral Therapy in Antiretroviral-naive Adults and Adolescents), $CD4^+$ T-cell counts should be measured every 3–6 months. If a decision is made not to initiate combination antiretroviral therapy in HIV-infected children (see Antiretroviral Therapy in Pediatric Patients: Initial Antiretroviral Therapy in Antiretroviral-naive Pediatric Patients), $CD4^+$ T-cell counts/$CD4^+$ T-cell percentages and plasma HIV-1 RNA levels should be measured every 3–4 months. Plasma HIV-1 RNA level monitoring is optional if the patient is not receiving antiretroviral therapy, but should be measured prior to initiation of antiretroviral therapy since some antiretrovirals or regimens are associated with poorer responses in patients with high baseline viral load.

The HHS Panel on Antiretroviral Guidelines for Adults and Adolescents recommends that plasma HIV-1 RNA levels be measured at the time antiretroviral therapy is initiated and within 2–4 weeks (but not later than 8 weeks) after initiation of treatment. If plasma HIV-1 RNA is still detectable 2–8 weeks after initiation of therapy, levels should be measured every 4–8 weeks until they decline to less than 200 copies/mL and then every 3–6 months thereafter. For patients receiving stable, suppressive antiretroviral therapy, plasma HIV-1 RNA levels are typically measured every 3–4 months; however, in adherent patients with consistent viral suppression who have had stable immunologic status for longer than 2 years, the interval for plasma HIV-1 RNA testing can be extended to every 6 months. Whenever a modification is made to the antiretroviral regimen (e.g., for regimen simplification or because of drug toxicity or intolerance), plasma HIV-1 RNA levels should be measured at the time the change is made and 2–8 weeks after the modification to confirm potency of the new regimen.

The HHS panel recommends that $CD4^+$ T-cell counts be measured at the time antiretroviral therapy is initiated or modified and every 3–6 months during the first 2 years of antiretroviral therapy, if viremia (plasma HIV-1 RNA levels consistently greater than 200 copies/mL) develops while the patient is receiving antiretroviral therapy, or if $CD4^+$ T-cell counts are less than 300 cells/mm^3. After the patient has received 2 years of antiretroviral therapy and has consistent viral suppression, $CD4^+$ T-cell counts can be measured every 12 months in those with counts of 300–500 cells/mm^3, and $CD4^+$ T-cell monitoring is considered optional in those with counts exceeding 500 cells/mm^3. If antiretroviral therapy is not initiated for any reason in an HIV-infected individual, the panel recommends that $CD4^+$ T-cell counts be measured every 3–6 months to assess the urgency for initiation of treatment and assess the need for prophylaxis against opportunistic infections reported in HIV-infected individuals.

Interpretation of Plasma HIV-1 RNA Levels and $CD4^+$ T-cell Counts. When evaluating response to an antiretroviral regimen, a threefold (0.5 $\log_{10}$) decrease or increase in plasma HIV-1 RNA levels generally is accepted as the minimally significant change in viral load. Optimal viral suppression generally is defined as a viral load persistently below the level of detection (plasma HIV-1 RNA level less than 20 to 75 copies/mL, depending on the assay used). Transient increases ("blips") in viral load (i.e., detectable low viral loads typically less than 400 copies/mL that return to undetectable) may occur in successfully treated patients and may not represent viral replication or virologic failure. Individuals who adhere to their antiretroviral regimen and do not have HIV resistant to the drugs in the treatment regimen generally achieve viral suppression 8–24 weeks after initiation of antiretroviral therapy. Although data on the association between persistently low level but quantifiable viremia (plasma HIV-1 RNA level less than 200 copies/mL) and virologic failure is conflicting, viral load persistently 200 copies/mL or greater should be considered virologic failure. (See Virologic Failure under Antiretroviral Therapy in Antiretroviral-experienced Adults and Adolescents: Definitions and Management of Treatment Regimen Failure.)

An adequate $CD4^+$ T-cell response for most patients on antiretroviral therapy is defined as an increase in $CD4^+$ T-cell count that averages 50–150 cells/mm^3 per year, generally with an accelerated response in the first 3 months. Subsequent increases with good virologic control show an average increase of approximately 50–100 cells/mm^3 per year for the subsequent few years until a plateau level is reached. A blunted increase in $CD4^+$ T-cell counts may occur despite virologic suppression if antiretroviral therapy was initiated in patients with low baseline $CD4^+$ T-cell counts or advanced age. A poor or suboptimal $CD4^+$ T-cell response in a patient with viral suspension is not necessarily an indication to modify a virologically suppressive antiretroviral regimen. (See Suboptimal Immunologic Response under Antiretroviral Therapy in Antiretroviral-experienced Adults and Adolescents: Definitions and Management of Treatment Regimen Failure.)

In Vitro Resistance Testing Drug resistance testing is performed using genotypic assays (detect drug resistance mutations present in the viral genes) or phenotypic assays (measure the virus's ability to replicate in the presence of different concentrations of antiretrovirals). Most genotypic assays involve sequencing the reverse transcriptase, protease, and integrase genes to detect mutations known to confer resistance to NRTIs, NNRTIs, PIs, and INSTIs; assays to detect mutations on the gp41 (envelope) gene also are available to provide information on resistance to HIV fusion inhibitors. Phenotypic assays can be used to detect resistance to NRTIs, NNRTIs, PIs, and INSTIs. Viral coreceptor (tropism) assay, a type of phenotypic assay, also is available to detect the presence of HIV with tropism that will not respond to CCR5 antagonists (see Coreceptor Tropism Assay under Guidelines for Use of Antiretroviral Agents: Laboratory Monitoring).

Genotypic assays can be performed rapidly, and results may be available within 1–2 weeks of collection of the sample. Phenotypic assays are more expensive to perform than genotypic assays, and results may be available within 2–3 weeks. Interpretation of results of genotypic assays requires knowledge of the mutations that the various antiretrovirals select for and knowledge regarding cross-resistance that may be conferred by certain mutations. Interpretation of results of phenotypic assays is complicated since data regarding the specific resistance level that is associated with drug failure may not be available. Although some resources are available to provide guidance regarding interpretation of genotypic drug-resistance testing (e.g., http://www.iasusa.org/content/essential-management-hiv-infection, http://hivdb.stanford.edu/), consultation with a specialist in HIV drug resistance is recommended to facilitate interpretation of genotypic and/or phenotypic assay results.

Although genotypic or phenotypic evidence of in vitro resistance to an antiretroviral suggests that the drug may not be effective in suppressing viral replication in vivo, such testing should not be used as the sole indicator that modifications need to be made to an antiretroviral regimen since factors other than viral resistance (e.g., poor adherence, pharmacokinetic interactions, drug potency) also affect virologic response to therapy and/or may contribute to disease progression. Some antiretroviral regimens can provide sustained viral suppression in vivo despite the presence of HIV-1 strains resistant to one of the components of the regimen. In addition, the absence of genotypic or phenotypic evidence of resistance does not necessarily predict a good response to a drug since minor variants may not be detected by current assays or resistance may be evolving at the time the assay is performed.

Recommendations Regarding In Vitro Resistance Testing. Baseline HIV drug-resistance testing is recommended for *all* newly diagnosed (antiretroviral-naive) HIV-infected adults, adolescents, or children. If antiretroviral therapy is deferred (see Guidelines for Use of Antiretroviral Agents: Initial Antiretroviral Therapy in Antiretroviral-naive Adults and Adolescents), drug-resistance testing should be repeated at the time initiation of therapy is being considered. Drug-resistance testing also is recommended whenever decisions are being made regarding modification of an antiretroviral regimen.

The HHS Panel on Antiretroviral Guidelines for Adults and Adolescents states that genotypic resistance testing is the preferred assay to guide selection of initial antiretroviral regimens in antiretroviral-naive patients and also may be the preferred assay to guide regimen modification in patients who have suboptimal virologic responses or virologic failure. Although definitive prospective data are not available to support use of genotypic over phenotypic assays in different clinical situations, genotypic testing usually is preferred because of faster turnaround time, lower cost, and enhanced sensitivity for detecting mixtures of wild-type and resistant virus. However, for patients with a complex treatment history and known or suspected complex drug resistance mutations (especially to PIs), results of both genotypic and phenotypic assays might provide critical and complementary information to guide selection of the most appropriate antiretroviral regimens.

Standard genotypic drug-resistance testing in antiretroviral-naive patients involves testing for mutations in the reverse transcriptase (RT) and protease (PR) genes. If transmitted INSTI resistance is a concern, additional testing with an INSTI genotype test may be indicated.

Drug-resistance testing should be performed to guide drug selection when modifications are being made in patients with virologic failure and plasma HIV-1 RNA levels exceeding 1000 copies/mL. In individuals with virologic failure who have plasma HIV-1 RNA levels greater than 500 but less than 1000 copies/mL, drug-resistance testing should be considered, but may be unsuccessful. Drug-resistance testing in the setting of virologic failure should be performed while the patient is receiving the failing regimen or, if not possible, within 4 weeks of discontinuance of the failing regimen. If it has been longer than 4 weeks since antiretrovirals were discontinued, drug-resistance testing may still provide useful information to guide therapy, although previously selected resistance mutations may be missed.

In vitro drug-resistance testing (i.e., genotypic resistance testing) is recommended for *all* pregnant women prior to initiation of antiretroviral therapy and for antiretroviral-experienced women entering pregnancy with detectable plasma HIV-1 RNA levels. Initiation of antiretroviral therapy before results of resistance testing are available may be necessary for optimal prevention of perinatal HIV transmission. (See Guidelines for Use of Antiretroviral Agents: Antiretrovirals for Prevention of Perinatal HIV Transmission.)

Drug-resistance testing is not usually recommended in patients with plasma HIV-1 RNA levels less than 500 copies/mL because the assays cannot be consistently performed with low HIV-1 RNA levels.

Coreceptor Tropism Assay A coreceptor tropism assay should be performed whenever use of a CC chemokine receptor 5 (CCR5) antagonist (e.g., maraviroc) is being considered. Some experts also recommend that this test be considered in patients who exhibit virologic failure while receiving a CCR5 antagonist.

Human Leukocyte Antigen (HLA)-B*5701 Screening Prior to initiation of abacavir or a fixed-combination preparation containing abacavir (abacavir/lamivudine; Epzicom®: abacavir/lamivudine/zidovudine; Trizivir®: abacavir/dolutegravir/lamivudine; Triumeq®), screening for the HLA-B*5701 allele is recommended. Screening also is recommended prior to reinitiating an abacavir-containing preparation in patients who previously tolerated the drug and whose HLA-B*5701 status is unknown. Individuals who carry this allele are at high risk for abacavir hypersensitivity reactions. Abacavir or abacavir-containing preparations should *not* be used in individuals who test positive for HLA-B*5701. If HLA-B*5701 screening is not readily available, some experts suggest that it is reasonable to initiate abacavir with appropriate clinical counseling and monitoring for signs of hypersensitivity reactions. (See Cautions: Hypersensitivity Reactions, in Abacavir Sulfate 8:18.08.20.)

Therapeutic Drug Monitoring Therapeutic drug monitoring of antiretrovirals is not recommended *routinely* in the management of HIV infection. However, information on plasma concentrations of antiretrovirals may be useful for patient management in certain situations, including when pharmacokinetic drug-drug or drug-food interactions are suspected, the patient has pathophysiologic states that result in impaired GI, hepatic, or renal function and altered drug pharmacokinetics, there are concerns regarding concentration-dependent toxicities, or expected virologic responses have not been attained in adherent patients. Consultation with a clinical pharmacist or pharmacologist with HIV expertise is recommended in such cases.

■ Adverse Effects

Although most patients receiving antiretroviral therapy do not experience treatment-limiting adverse effects, modification of the antiretroviral regimen may be necessary in some patients because of serious and/or potentially life-threatening adverse effects. Non-life-threatening toxicities usually can be handled by substituting another antiretroviral for the presumed causative drug without interrupting antiretroviral therapy. Acute, life-threatening toxicities (e.g., acute hypersensitivity reaction, lactic acidosis, liver and/or severe cutaneous toxicities) usually require immediate discontinuance of all antiretrovirals and reinitiation of an alternative regimen that is not associated with the same toxicities. A switch from an effective antiretroviral regimen to a new regimen must be done carefully and only when potential benefits of the change outweigh the potential complications of altering treatment. When a change in the regimen is indicated, the management strategy must be individualized to ensure that viral suppression is maintained. Expert consultation may be necessary.

Some adverse effects appear to be common to specific drug classes of commercially available antiretrovirals (e.g., NRTIs, PIs, NNRTIs, INSTIs). These adverse effects should be considered when selecting alternative agents. In some cases, adverse effects were initially reported to be strongly associated with one class of antiretroviral agents and then found to occur in patients receiving various antiretroviral regimens that may or may not have included these agents (e.g., adipogenic effects).

For specific information on adverse effects reported with the individual antiretroviral agents and precautions and contraindications associated with the drugs, see the Cautions sections in the individual monographs in 8:18.08.

HIV Nucleoside Reverse Transcriptase Inhibitors (NRTIs) **Hepatic Effects and Lactic Acidosis.** Lactic acidosis and severe hepatomegaly with steatosis, including fatalities, have been reported in patients receiving NRTIs (abacavir, didanosine, emtricitabine, lamivudine, stavudine, zidovudine). Most reported cases have involved women; obesity and long-term therapy with NRTIs also may be risk factors. Fatal and nonfatal lactic acidosis has been reported in pregnant women who received antiretroviral regimens that included both didanosine and stavudine, and these drugs should *not* be used concomitantly in pregnant women. (See Guidelines for Use of Antiretroviral Agents: Antiretroviral Therapy During Pregnancy.)

NRTIs should be used with caution in patients with hepatomegaly, hepatitis, or other known risk factors for liver disease; however, lactic acidosis and severe hepatomegaly with steatosis have been reported in patients with no known risk factors. NRTI therapy should be discontinued in any patient who develops clinical or laboratory findings suggestive of lactic acidosis or pronounced hepatotoxicity (which may include hepatomegaly and steatosis even in the absence of marked transaminase elevations).

The mechanism for the development of lactic acidosis and severe hepatomegaly with steatosis in patients receiving NRTIs has not been fully elucidated, but may occur as the result of inhibition of DNA γ-polymerase, an enzyme involved in mitochondrial DNA synthesis and mitochondrial replication. Results of in vitro tests indicate that all commercially available NRTIs inhibit mitochondrial DNA γ-polymerase; zalcitabine (no longer commercially available in the US) is the most potent inhibitor of mitochondrial DNA γ-polymerase followed by didanosine, stavudine, zidovudine, lamivudine, abacavir, and tenofovir. Inhibition of this enzyme and possibly other mitochondrial enzymes theoretically could lead to mitochondrial dysfunction and cellular toxicity. It also has been suggested that mitochondrial dysfunction may be a factor in the development of several other adverse effects reported in patients receiving NRTIs (e.g., cardiomyopathy, peripheral neuropathy, pancreatitis, bone marrow suppression, lipodystrophy).

The clinical prodrome of the lactic acidosis syndrome in patients receiving NRTIs may initially include nonspecific GI symptoms, weight loss, and fatigue and may be rapidly progressive with tachycardia, tachypnea, jaundice, muscular weakness, mental status changes, respiratory distress, pancreatitis, and organ failure. Mortality rates up to 50% have been reported, especially in patients with serum lactate concentrations exceeding 10 mmol/L. Laboratory evaluation may reveal hyperlactatemia (often exceeding 5 mmol/L); an increased anion gap; elevated aminotransferases, prothrombin time, bilirubin, lipase, and amylase; and decreased arterial pH, serum bicarbonate, and serum albumin.

Lipodystrophy. Lipoatrophy (loss of subcutaneous fat) has been reported in patients receiving zidovudine or other NRTIs; the incidence and severity of this effect are related to cumulative exposure. Fat loss, which is most evident in the face, limbs, and buttocks, may be only partially reversible and improvement may take months to years after switching to an alternative antiretroviral regimen.

HIV Protease Inhibitors (PIs) Several different adverse effects reported in patients receiving PIs (atazanavir, darunavir, fosamprenavir, indinavir, lopinavir, nelfinavir, ritonavir, saquinavir, tipranavir) appear to be common to this drug class, including hyperglycemic and diabetogenic effects, adipogenic effects, hyperlipidemia and hypercholesterolemia, and spontaneous bleeding episodes. Although a causal relationship has not been established in all cases, the possibility of these adverse effects should be considered whenever a PI is included in an antiretroviral regimen.

Hyperglycemic and Diabetogenic Effects. Hyperglycemia, new-onset diabetes mellitus, or exacerbation of preexisting diabetes mellitus has been reported during postmarketing surveillance in patients receiving PIs. Some patients required either initiation or dose adjustments of insulin or oral hypoglycemic agents; in some cases, diabetic ketoacidosis has occurred. The hyperglycemic or diabetic episodes generally resolve following discontinuance of PI therapy; however, hyperglycemia persisted in some patients, including a few without a known history of diabetes at baseline. HIV-infected patients with preexisting diabetes mellitus should be closely monitored during PI therapy, and the risk of new-onset diabetes mellitus should be considered in those without a history of the disease.

Patients receiving a PI should be advised about the warning signs of hyperglycemia and diabetes (e.g., increase thirst and hunger, unexplained weight loss, increased urination, fatigue, dry or itchy skin) and advised of the need to maintain ideal body weight. Some clinicians recommend that fasting blood glucose or glycosylated hemoglobin (hemoglobin A_{1c}; HbA_{1c}) be determined before antiretroviral therapy is initiated or modified and every 3–6 months if the previous results were abnormal.

Studies in HIV-negative patients given short courses of a PI suggest a direct causal effect of lopinavir/ritonavir and indinavir on insulin resistance; however, traditional risk factors (e.g., obesity, family history of diabetes) may be stronger risk factors for insulin resistance than use of any PIs. Although results of switch studies have been inconsistent, some experts suggest that patients experiencing insulin resistance while receiving lopinavir/ritonavir or *ritonavir-boosted* fosamprenavir may be switched to an NNRTI (nevirapine or rilpivirine), an INSTI, or atazanavir (without low-dose ritonavir).

Lipodystrophy. Lipohypertrophy (accumulation of fat under the skin) has been reported in patients receiving PI-based antiretroviral regimens; a causal relationship has not been established.

Redistribution or accumulation of body fat, including central obesity, dorsocervical fat enlargement (buffalo hump), peripheral wasting, breast enlargement, and general cushingoid appearance, has been reported in patients receiving PIs. These adipogenic effects have been reported most frequently with PIs; however, similar adipogenic effects also have been reported in patients receiving NRTIs without a PI. Adipogenic effects generally have been clinically apparent within 1–14 months after starting PI therapy. The incidence of lipodystrophy in patients receiving PI therapy is unclear, but has been variously reported to range from about 5–80% of patients.

The etiology of lipodystrophy reported in HIV patients receiving antiretrovirals may be multifactorial. Several different mechanisms have been suggested, including inhibition of several proteins involved in lipid and carbohydrate metabolism resulting in interference with adipocyte differentiation and apoptosis. Long-term consequences of adipogenic effects that occur during antiretroviral therapy are unknown, and data are insufficient to date to guide management of patients who develop these effects. Discontinuance of PIs has resulted in partial or complete resolution of symptoms in some patients. Some clinicians state that it may not be necessary to discontinue PI therapy on the basis of adipogenic effects alone. There is no clinical evidence that switching to any other currently recommended regimen will reverse weight or visceral fat gain.

Hyperlipidemia. Hypertriglyceridemia and hypercholesterolemia have been reported in patients receiving PIs. Patients receiving antiretroviral regimens that include PIs may have increases in fasting cholesterol, triglycerides, low-density lipoprotein (LDL)-cholesterol, and very-low-density lipoprotein (VLDL)-cholesterol levels with either no change or decreases in high-density lipoprotein (HDL)-cholesterol. Most commercially available PIs (including all *ritonavir-boosted* PIs) have been associated with increases in serum cholesterol and/or triglyceride concentrations. Increased triglyceride and LDL-cholesterol concentrations are reported more frequently with lopinavir/ritonavir and *ritonavir-boosted* fosamprenavir than with other *ritonavir-boosted* PIs. Hypertriglyceridemia and hypercholesterolemia have been reported with or without adipogenic effects and/or hyperglycemia, and the relationship between alterations in body fat and lipid levels is unclear. Although further study is needed, there is some concern that lipid abnormalities in patients receiving PI therapy possibly may increase the risk of coronary artery disease and pancreatitis.

Indications for monitoring and treatment of dyslipidemias in HIV-infected patients are the same as those for other individuals. Replacing the PI in the regimen with an antiretroviral with less propensity for causing hyperlipidemia may be indicated. There is some evidence that triglyceride and LDL-cholesterol concentrations improve after a switch from lopinavir/ritonavir to atazanavir (with or without low-dose ritonavir). Some experts suggest that patients experiencing dyslipidemia while receiving a *ritonavir-boosted* PI may be switched to an INSTI (dolutegravir, raltegravir), NNRTI (nevirapine, rilpivirine), or atazanavir (without low-dose ritonavir).

The fact that pharmacokinetic interactions between certain HMG-CoA reductase inhibitors and PIs can increase plasma concentrations of the HMG-CoA reductase inhibitor and increase the risk of statin-associated adverse effects should be considered. (See Drug Interactions: HMG-CoA Reductase Inhibitors.)

Cardiovascular Effects. Prolongation of the PR interval has been reported with some PIs, including atazanavir (with or without low-dose ritonavir), lopinavir/ritonavir, and *ritonavir-boosted* saquinavir. Prolongation of the QT interval and torsades de pointes have been reported in patients receiving lopinavir/ritonavir or *ritonavir-boosted* saquinavir.

Spontaneous Bleeding Episodes. Although a causal relationship has not been established, spontaneous bleeding episodes and hematuria have been reported in patients with hemophilia A or hemophilia B receiving PIs. Intracranial hemorrhage has been reported in patients receiving *ritonavir-boosted* tipranavir, including some fatalities; many of these patients had other medical conditions (e.g., CNS lesions, history of head trauma, recent neurosurgery, coagulation disorders, hypertension, alcohol abuse) or were receiving concomitant therapy (e.g., anticoagulants, antiplatelet agents) that may have caused or contributed to these events.

HIV Nonnucleoside Reverse Transcriptase Inhibitors (NNRTIs)

Dermatologic and Sensitivity Reactions. Rash is a common adverse effect reported with NNRTIs (e.g., delavirdine, efavirenz, etravirine, nevirapine), and potentially life-threatening hypersensitivity reactions have been reported. Although most cases of rash are mild to moderate and occur during the first few weeks of therapy, severe reactions, including Stevens-Johnson syndrome, toxic epidermal necrolysis, and hypersensitivity reactions characterized by rash, constitutional findings, and organ dysfunction (e.g., hepatic failure), have been reported in patients receiving the drugs. Fatalities have been reported.

Rash and hypersensitivity reactions occur more frequently with nevirapine than with other currently available NNRTIs. Nevirapine therapy is initiated using a low dosage during the first 14 days of therapy since this appears to reduce the frequency of rash.

NNRTIs should be immediately discontinued in any patient with signs or symptoms of severe skin reactions or hypersensitivity, including (but not limited to) rash or rash accompanied by fever, generalized malaise, fatigue, muscle or joint aches, blisters, oral lesions, conjunctivitis, facial edema, hepatitis, eosinophilia, angioedema, or GI symptoms such as nausea, vomiting, diarrhea, or abdominal pain. Patients who experience a serious rash or hypersensitivity reaction while receiving an NNRTI should be switched to an antiretroviral regimen without an NNRTI.

Hepatic Effects. Hepatotoxicity has been reported in patients receiving NNRTI-based regimens. Fulminant hepatitis progressing to fatal hepatic failure or requiring transplantation has been reported with efavirenz.

Among the NNRTIs, nevirapine has the greatest potential to cause hepatotoxicity, including serious and sometimes fatal hepatic necrosis. Female gender (including pregnant women) and higher $CD4^+$ T-cell count (exceeding 250 cells/mm^3 in women or exceeding 400 cells/mm^3 in men) are risk factors. The risk also is greatest during the first few months of nevirapine treatment. Because of the risk of hepatic events, nevirapine should *not* be initiated in women with $CD4^+$ T-cell counts exceeding 250 cells/mm^3 or in men with counts exceeding 400 cells/mm^3, unless the benefits outweigh the risks.

CNS Effects and Depressive Disorders. Some NNRTIs (efavirenz, rilpivirine) have been associated with CNS effects. Dizziness, abnormal dreams, abnormal thinking, agitation, amnesia, confusion, depersonalization, dizziness, euphoria, hallucinations, impaired concentration, insomnia, somnolence, and stupor have been reported with efavirenz. Serious adverse psychiatric symptoms, including severe depression, suicidal ideation, nonfatal suicide attempts, aggressive behavior, paranoid reactions, or manic reactions have been reported rarely. Depressive disorders, including depressed mood, depression, dysphoria, major depression, altered mood, negative thoughts, suicide attempt, and suicidal ideation, also have been reported with rilpivirine.

An association between efavirenz and suicidal ideation, suicide, and attempted suicide (especially among younger patients and those with a history of mental illness or substance abuse) was found in a retrospective analysis of several comparative trials. Patients receiving efavirenz should be informed that adverse CNS effects (e.g., dizziness, insomnia, impaired concentration, somnolence, abnormal dreams) may occur during the first few weeks of therapy and that the drug may impair their ability to perform hazardous activities requiring mental alertness or physical coordination such as operating machinery or driving a motor vehicle.

Patients receiving efavirenz or rilpivirine should be advised to seek immediate medical evaluation if they experience severe psychiatric or depressive symptoms so that a determination can be made regarding the likelihood that the symptoms are related to the drug and to determine if the benefits of continued therapy outweigh the risks.

Although adverse CNS effects generally improve with continued efavirenz treatment and usually resolve after the first 2–4 weeks of therapy, the patient should be switched from efavirenz to an alternative antiretroviral agent if symptoms persist or are intolerable. Some experts suggest a switch from efavirenz to an alternative NNRTI (etravirine, nevirapine, rilpivirine), a PI, or an INSTI.

Lipodystrophy. Lipohypertrophy has been reported in patients receiving efavirenz-containing antiretroviral regimens; a causal relationship has not been established.

HIV Nucleotide Reverse Transcriptase Inhibitors **Bone Effects.** Tenofovir DF has been associated with loss of bone mineral density (BMD) and increases in biochemical markers of bone metabolism in adults, suggesting increased bone turnover, and has been associated with decreased rate of BMD gain in pediatric patients. Osteomalacia associated with proximal renal tubulopathy, which may contribute to fractures, also has been reported in patients receiving tenofovir DF.

Loss of BMD reported with tenofovir DF is greater than that reported with NRTIs (e.g., abacavir, zidovudine, stavudine). In patients experiencing BMD effects while receiving tenofovir DF, a switch to an alternative antiretroviral agent has been shown to increase bone density, but the clinical importance of this increase remains uncertain. There is some evidence that tenofovir alafenamide is associated with smaller declines in BMD than tenofovir DF and increases in BMD have been reported in some patients who were switched from tenofovir DF to tenofovir alafenamide; however, the long-term impact of tenofovir alafenamide in patients with osteopenia or osteoporosis is unknown and close clinical monitoring is recommended in this setting. Some experts suggest that a switch to abacavir can be considered in patients who experience loss of BMD while receiving tenofovir DF, provided the patient is negative for HLA-B*5701.

Renal Effects. Renal impairment, including cases of acute renal failure and Fanconi syndrome (renal tubular injury with severe hypophosphatemia), have been reported in patients receiving tenofovir DF or fixed combinations containing tenofovir DF. The risk of adverse renal effects appears to be greater if tenofovir DF is used in antiretroviral regimens that include a pharmacokinetic enhancer (i.e., low-dose ritonavir or cobicistat), possibly as the result of increased tenofovir concentrations.

There is some evidence that tenofovir alafenamide has less impact on renal function, including renal biomarkers and proteinuria, than tenofovir DF. Improvements in renal biomarkers and proteinuria have been reported in some patients switched from tenofovir DF to tenofovir alafenamide and some experts suggest that this switch can be considered in those with creatinine clearances greater than 30 mL/minute; however, the long-term impact of tenofovir alafenamide in patients with preexisting renal disease (including overt proximal tubulopathy) is unknown, and close clinical monitoring is recommended in this setting. Some experts suggest that patients experiencing adverse renal effects while receiving tenofovir DF may be switched to abacavir, provided the patient is negative for HLA-B*5701.

Estimated creatinine clearance, urine glucose, and urine protein concentrations should be determined prior to initiating therapy and routinely monitored during therapy in all patients receiving tenofovir alafenamide or tenofovir DF; in addition, serum phosphorus should be monitored in those with chronic kidney diseases or at risk for renal impairment.

Dyslipidemia. Hypertriglyceridemia and increased LDL and HDL cholesterol (without a change in total cholesterol or HDL ratio) have been reported in patients receiving tenofovir alafenamide or tenofovir DF. There is some evidence that patients receiving the fixed combination EVG/c/FTC/TAF have experienced greater increases in serum triglycerides and serum LDL and HDL than patients receiving the fixed combination EVG/c/FTC/TDF.

HIV Integrase Inhibitors (INSTIs) **CNS Effects and Depressive Disorders.** Neuropsychiatric adverse events (sleep disturbances, depression, anxiety, suicidal ideation) have been reported with some INSTIs (e.g., dolutegravir, raltegravir), principally in patients with a history of psychiatric illnesses.

Hepatic Effects. Adverse hepatic effects have been reported in patients receiving dolutegravir-containing regimens.

In some patients receiving a dolutegravir-containing regimen, serum aminotransferase elevations were consistent with immune reconstitution syndrome or HBV reactivation, particularly in the setting where HBV therapy had been discontinued. Cases of hepatic toxicity, including elevated serum liver biochemistries, hepatitis, and acute liver failure, also have been reported in patients receiving a dolutegravir-containing regimen who had no preexisting hepatic disease or other identifiable risk factors. Drug-induced liver injury leading to liver transplant has been reported with abacavir/dolutegravir/lamivudine.

Musculoskeletal Effects. Raltegravir has been associated with increased serum creatine kinase (CK, creatine phosphokinase, CPK) concentrations, and muscle weakness, myopathy, and rhabdomyolysis have been reported rarely. A causal relationship to the drug has not been established.

Raltegravir should be used with caution in patients at increased risk of myopathy or rhabdomyolysis, including those receiving concomitant therapy with a drug associated with myopathy or rhabdomyolysis.

Lipodystrophy. Lipohypertrophy has been reported in patients receiving raltegravir-containing antiretroviral regimens; a causal relationship has not been established.

HIV Entry and Fusion Inhibitors Cough, pyrexia, upper respiratory tract infection, rash, musculoskeletal symptoms, abdominal pain, and dizziness have been reported in patients receiving maraviroc. Hepatotoxicity, sometimes preceded by signs of a systemic allergic reaction (e.g., pruritic rash, eosinophilia or elevated IgE concentrations), also has been reported in maraviroc-treated patients.

Diarrhea, dizziness, nausea, and rash have been reported in patients receiving IV ibalizumab-uiyk.

Local injection site reactions (pain, erythema, induration, nodules, cysts, pruritus, ecchymosis) occur in almost 100% of patients receiving enfuvirtide. In addition, hypersensitivity reactions that may include rash, fever, nausea, vomiting, chills, rigors, hypotension, and elevated serum transaminase concentrations have been reported in enfuvirtide-treated patients; these reactions may recur on rechallenge.

■ Drug Interactions

Drug Interactions Among the Antiretroviral Agents Considerable data are available regarding pharmacokinetic interactions among the various antiretrovirals, especially those involving PIs and NNRTIs. Some pharmacokinetic interactions between antiretrovirals can be used for therapeutic advantage, such as use of low-dose ritonavir to *boost* plasma concentrations of some other PIs (see Drug Interactions: Pharmacokinetic Enhancers). Other pharmacokinetic interactions among antiretrovirals result in decreased or suboptimal antiretroviral concentrations and reduced therapeutic effects or increased antiretroviral concentrations and increased toxicity. In some cases, dosage adjustment of one or more of the antiretrovirals is indicated because of a pharmacokinetic interaction; however, in other cases, concomitant use is contraindicated or should be avoided. Potential drug interactions among the antiretrovirals must be considered whenever selecting or changing drugs used in multiple-drug regimens. For information on drug interactions involving the antiretrovirals and recommendations regarding these interactions, see the Drug Interactions sections in the individual monographs in 8:18.08.

Pharmacokinetic Enhancers Concomitant use of a pharmacokinetic enhancer (pharmacokinetic booster) is necessary to improve the pharmacokinetic profile of most HIV PIs. HIV PIs usually are used in conjunction with low-dose ritonavir (*ritonavir-boosted* PI) or in conjunction with cobicistat (*cobicistat-boosted* PI). Ritonavir and cobicistat are both potent inhibitors of cytochrome P-450 (CYP) 3A4 and increase plasma concentrations of concomitantly administered drugs that are metabolized by this pathway. Unboosted HIV PIs (i.e., without low-dose ritonavir or cobicistat) are *not* recommended for *initial* antiretroviral therapy and unboosted darunavir, saquinavir, or tipranavir are *not* recommended at any time.

Low-dose ritonavir (100–400 mg daily) inhibits metabolism of HIV PIs and increases plasma concentrations and prolongs the plasma half-lives of the drugs. The antiretroviral activity of these regimens is due to the other PI since the dosage of ritonavir used (100–400 mg daily) is not considered a therapeutic dosage. A fixed-combination preparation of lopinavir and low-dose ritonavir is commercially available (lopinavir/ritonavir). Other *ritonavir-boosted* regimens involve administration of specified low doses of single-entity ritonavir at the same time as a single-entity preparation of the PI (e.g., atazanavir, darunavir, fosamprenavir, saquinavir, tipranavir).

Atazanavir and darunavir can be used with low-dose ritonavir (*ritonavir-boosted*) or with cobicistat (*cobicistat-boosted*). Although concomitant use of low-dose ritonavir or cobicistat increases peak plasma concentrations and area under the plasma concentration-time curve (AUC) of these HIV PIs, these pharmacokinetic enhancers are not interchangeable in antiretroviral regimens since low-dose ritonavir and cobicistat have different dosage and administration requirements and are associated with different adverse effects, precautions, contraindications, and drug interactions. When *cobicistat-boosted* atazanavir or *cobicistat-boosted* darunavir is included in an antiretroviral regimen, fixed-combination preparations containing the HIV PI and cobicistat (atazanavir/cobicistat, darunavir/cobicistat) are commercially available or, alternatively, single-entity atazanavir or single-entity darunavir can be administered at the same time as single-entity cobicistat.

Elvitegravir (an INSTI) also must be used in conjunction with a pharmacokinetic enhancer; the drug is administered in conjunction with cobicistat in the fixed combination EVG/c/FTC/TAF or the fixed combination EVG/c/FTC/TDF.

HCV Antivirals Although concurrent treatment of HIV and HCV in coinfected patients is feasible, such treatment can by complicated because of high pill burden, toxicities, and drug interactions.

If a decision is made to treat HCV infection in an HIV-infected patient receiving antiretroviral therapy, the antiretroviral regimen may need to be modified before HCV treatment is initiated. The possibility of overlapping toxicities and drug interactions between antiretrovirals and HCV direct-acting antivirals (DAAs), including HCV NS3/4A protease inhibitors (e.g., glecaprevir, paritaprevir, voxilaprevir), HCV NS5B polymerase inhibitors (e.g., dasabuvir, grazoprevir, sofosbuvir), and HCV NS5A replication complex inhibitors (e.g., daclatasvir, elbasvir, ledipasvir, ombitasvir, pibrentasvir, velpatasvir), should be considered. In addition, possible drug interactions between antiretrovirals and ribavirin and/or peginterferon also should be considered.

Concomitant use of some HCV DAAs and some HIV NRTIs (e.g., tenofovir DF), HIV NNRTIs (e.g., efavirenz, etravirine, nevirapine), HIV PIs (e.g., atazanavir, darunavir, fosamprenavir, lopinavir, ritonavir, saquinavir, tipranavir), or HIV INSTIs (e.g., dolutegravir, EVG/c/FTC/TDF, EVG/c/FTC/TAF) can affect plasma concentrations of one or both drugs. Therefore, concomitant use of certain HCV DAAs and certain antiretrovirals is not recommended or requires close monitoring for HIV and HCV treatment responses; in some cases, dosage adjustments may be needed. Concomitant use of ribavirin and certain NRTIs (didanosine, zidovudine) may increase the risk of NRTI-associated adverse effects (e.g., hepatotoxicity, pancreatitis, anemia) and is contraindicated or not recommended.

For information on drug interactions between antiretroviral agents and HCV DAAs and recommendations regarding these interactions, see the Drug Interactions sections in the individual antiretroviral monographs in 8:18.08 and the individual HCV antiviral monographs in 8:18.40.

Antimycobacterial Agents The fact that pharmacokinetic interactions between some antimycobacterial agents (e.g., rifabutin, rifampin) and some antiretrovirals (e.g., PIs, NNRTIs) have been reported or are expected to occur must be considered when antimycobacterial therapy is indicated for the treatment of active tuberculosis or latent tuberculosis infection or for the prophylaxis or treatment of *Mycobacterium avium* complex (MAC) infections in HIV-infected patients who are receiving or are being considered for antiretroviral therapy. Because the management of these patients is complex and must be individualized, experts in the management of mycobacterial infections in HIV-infected patients should be consulted.

HMG-CoA Reductase Inhibitors Concomitant use of certain HMG-CoA reductase inhibitors (statins) metabolized by CYP3A (e.g., atorvastatin, fluvastatin, lovastatin, pitavastatin, pravastatin, rosuvastatin, simvastatin) and certain PIs (atazanavir [with or without low-dose ritonavir or cobicistat], darunavir [with low-dose ritonavir or cobicistat], fosamprenavir [with or without low-dose ritonavir], indinavir, lopinavir/ritonavir, nelfinavir, *ritonavir-boosted* saquinavir, *ritonavir-boosted* tipranavir) or NNRTIs (e.g., delavirdine, efavirenz, etravirine, nevirapine) may increase plasma concentrations and AUC of the antilipemic agent and increase the risk of statin-associated adverse effects, including myopathy and rhabdomyolysis. Concomitant use of these drugs may be contraindicated or necessitate dosage adjustments.

For information on drug interactions between antiretroviral and statins and recommendations regarding these interactions, see the Drug Interactions sections in the individual monographs in 8:18.08.

Illicit Drugs Because PIs and NNRTIs affect a wide range of CYP enzymes, the potential exists for interactions with many classes of recreational (illicit) drugs that are metabolized by these enzymes. Life-threatening reactions and at least one fatality have been reported secondary to interactions between methylenedioxymethamphetamine (MDMA, ecstasy) or γ-hydroxybutyrate (GHB, liquid ecstasy) and PIs. (See Drug Interactions: CNS Agents, in Ritonavir 8:18.08.08.) MDMA undergoes demethylenation principally by CYP2D6 but also is metabolized by CYP1A2, CYP2B6, and CYP3A4; concomitant use with inhibitors of these enzymes (e.g., PIs, efavirenz) can result in substantial increases in MDMA exposure. Other amphetamines (e.g., methamphetamine; crystal meth, speed) also are metabolized by CYP2D6. In addition, metabolism of ketamine (special K) appears to be mediated principally by CYP2B6 and to a lesser extent by CYP3A4 and CYP2C9 and metabolism of PCP (angel dust, rocket fuel, killer weed) appears to be mediated by CYP3A4 and possibly by CYP2C11. Although metabolism of GHB has not been characterized, the drug may undergo first-pass metabolism mediated by the CYP isoenzyme system.

CYP3A4 appears to play only a small role in metabolism of cocaine and interactions between antiretrovirals and cocaine have not been described. However, further study is needed to more fully evaluate possible interactions between cocaine and antiretrovirals. Limited data suggest that CYP3A and CYP2C9 isoenzymes are involved in microsomal oxidation of tetrahydrocannabinol (THC), but the effects of THC are unlikely to be substantially attenuated by drugs that inhibit these enzymes. There is evidence that THC can decrease plasma concentrations of indinavir and concentrations of the active metabolite of nelfinavir (M8), but these effects are not likely to have a clinically important effect on efficacy of the antiretrovirals.

Because the margin of safety for many illicit drugs is narrow or poorly defined and the known or potential interactions between some of these drugs and antiretrovirals is complex and potentially life-threatening, patients should be advised of the risk of serious consequences if they use these drugs while receiving antiretroviral therapy. In addition, in HIV-infected patients being treated for opioid addiction with buprenorphine or methadone, the possibility of pharmacokinetic interactions between these drugs and PIs (e.g., atazanavir, fosamprenavir, lopinavir/ritonavir, nelfinavir, ritonavir, tipranavir), NRTIs (e.g., abacavir), and NNRTIs (e.g., efavirenz, etravirine, nevirapine) should be considered since dosage modifications or use of alternative antiretrovirals may be necessary.

■ Patient Adherence and Issues Related to Dosage and Administration

Adherence Patient adherence to recommended antiretroviral regimens (even when asymptomatic) is essential to the potential benefits of antiretroviral therapy. Adherence to antiretroviral regimens has been strongly correlated with HIV viral suppression, reduced development of HIV resistance, increased survival, and improved quality of life. Strict adherence to antiretroviral therapy also decreases the risk of HIV transmission. Early detection of nonadherence and initiation of appropriate strategies to improve adherence may prevent development of viral resistance and decrease the likelihood of virologic failure.

A variety of factors may affect patient adherence to recommended antiretroviral regimens and/or compromise effectiveness of the regimens, and these factors should be discussed with all patients. Factors that can affect adherence include the complexity of the regimen (e.g., frequency of dosing, pill burden), dietary restrictions, palatability of the drugs, intercurrent illnesses that may affect GI absorption or require additional therapies (e.g., wasting, anorexia), adverse effects associated with the antiretrovirals or other drugs the patient is receiving, drug interactions among the antiretrovirals and/or with other drugs the patient is receiving (e.g., antimycobacterial agents), psychosocial issues (e.g., depression or emotional crisis, homelessness, inadequate social support, dementia, psychosis), and active substance abuse.

Patients should receive and understand information about HIV disease and should be advised that the *initial* treatment regimen usually is the best chance for a simple regimen with long-term treatment success and prevention of drug resistance. At the time antiretroviral therapy is initiated, patients and patient caregivers should receive information about the specific antiretroviral regimen being prescribed and should be advised about the importance of adhering to the regimen. The likelihood of patient adherence to a complex drug regimen should be discussed and determined by the individual patient and clinician before therapy is initiated. Intensive follow-up is necessary to assess adherence to the regimen and to continue patient counseling.

Administration Instructions The fact that some antiretrovirals can be administered without regard to meals (abacavir, delavirdine, dolutegravir, emtricitabine, fosamprenavir, lamivudine, maraviroc, nevirapine, raltegravir, stavudine, tenofovir, tipranavir with low-dose ritonavir, zidovudine) while others should be given with a meal (atazanavir, darunavir, etravirine, lopinavir/ritonavir, nelfinavir, rilpivirine, ritonavir, saquinavir) or in the fasting state (didanosine, efavirenz, indinavir) to maximize bioavailability should be considered when selecting an antiretroviral regimen.

All drugs in the antiretroviral regimen should be started simultaneously (ideally within 1 or 2 days of each other). While a dose escalation regimen (lead-in period) is recommended when initiating nevirapine therapy, all other drugs should be initiated using usually recommended dosages.

Patients receiving antiretroviral therapy must be evaluated continuously for toxicity and disease progression. Short-term interruption (days to weeks) of antiretroviral therapy may be indicated because of drug toxicity, intercurrent illnesses that preclude oral therapy (e.g., gastroenteritis, pancreatitis), surgical procedures, or unavailability of a particular drug. When a short-term interruption (2 days or less) is required because of scheduled medical or surgical procedures or when an unanticipated short-term interruption is needed (e.g., severe or life-threatening toxicity, unexpected inability to take oral medications), all antiretrovirals in the regimen should be stopped simultaneously. However, if interruption of therapy for longer than 2–3 days is anticipated, the pharmacokinetic properties of the specific drugs should be considered. If all drugs in the regimen have similar half-lives, they should all be stopped simultaneously and then restarted simultaneously, taking into consideration food requirements. If the drugs in the regimen have differing half-lives, discontinuing all drugs simultaneously may result in functional monotherapy with the drug with the longest half-life. This is most likely to occur when an NNRTI (efavirenz, etravirine, nevirapine) is a component of the regimen, since detectable concentrations of these NNRTIs may persist for less than 1 week to more than 3 weeks after discontinuance and increase the risk of selection of NNRTI-resistant mutants. Although some experts recommend stopping the NNRTI and continuing the other antiretrovirals for a period of time to avoid functional monotherapy, the optimal time sequence for staggered discontinuance has not been determined. Alternatively, it has been suggested that the NNRTI can be replaced with a *ritonavir-boosted* or *cobicistat-boosted* PI for 4 weeks before all drugs in the regimen are discontinued simultaneously. The optimal time sequence for staggered discontinuance of regimen components or replacement of an NNRTI with a PI-based regimen has not been determined.

Severe acute exacerbations of hepatitis B virus (HBV) infection have been reported in HIV-infected patients discontinuing emtricitabine, lamivudine, or tenofovir DF. If any of these agents is discontinued in a patient coinfected with HBV, the patient should be closely monitored for hepatitis or hepatic flare.

Regimen Simplification Regimen simplification (i.e., modification of an effective regimen to reduce pill burden and/or dosing frequency, enhance tolerability, decrease dietary and fluid requirements) has been used in patients receiving a suppressive antiretroviral regimen to improve the patient's quality of life, maintain long-term adherence, avoid toxicities that may develop with prolonged antiretroviral therapy, and reduce the risk of virologic failure. To the extent possible, antiretroviral regimens should be simplified by reducing the number of daily doses and by minimizing drug interactions and adverse effects. Patients who can be considered for regimen simplification include those receiving regimens no longer recommended as preferred or alternative choices for initial therapy, those receiving regimens selected in the setting of treatment failure at a time when only limited data were available regarding resistance or drug interactions, and those receiving regimens selected prior to the availability of newer drugs or formulations that are more tolerable or have easier dosage regimens (e.g., once-daily dosing, fixed-combination preparations).

■ Initial Antiretroviral Therapy in Antiretroviral-naive Adults and Adolescents

The US Department of Health and Human Services (HHS) Panel on Antiretroviral Guidelines for Adults and Adolescents recommends that antiretroviral therapy be initiated in *all* HIV-infected adults and adolescents, regardless of the patient's $CD4^+$ T-cell count. Without antiretroviral therapy, most individuals with HIV infection will eventually develop progressive immunodeficiency marked by $CD4^+$ T-cell depletion and AIDS-defining illnesses and premature death.

Results of recent studies that addressed the optimal time to initiate antiretroviral therapy demonstrated a 50% reduction in morbidity and mortality among HIV-infected adults with $CD4^+$ T-cell counts exceeding 500/mm^3 who were randomized to receive immediate antiretroviral therapy compared with those randomized to receive deferred initiation of antiretroviral therapy. The magnitude of CD4+ T-cell count recovery appears to be directly correlated with counts at the time of initiation of antiretroviral therapy and many individuals who begin treatment when CD4+ T-cell counts are less than 350/mm³ never achieve counts greater than 500/mm³ despite long-term antiretroviral therapy. In addition, there is evidence that early initiation of effective antiretroviral therapy can reduce secondary transmission of HIV to sexual partners. Therefore, the HHS panel recommends prompt initiation of antiretroviral therapy in *all* patients diagnosed with HIV infection, including pregnant women not currently receiving antiretroviral therapy. (See Guidelines for Use of Antiretroviral Agents: Antiretroviral Therapy During Pregnancy.)

The decision to initiate antiretroviral therapy should always include consideration of a patient's comorbid conditions and their willingness and readiness to initiate treatment. On a case-by-case basis, there may be some situations when antiretroviral therapy is deferred because of clinical and/or psychosocial factors; however, the HHS panel recommends that antiretroviral therapy be initiated as soon as possible.

Recommended Regimens for Initial Antiretroviral Therapy in Adults and Adolescents Antiretroviral therapy in HIV-infected adults and adolescents who are antiretroviral naive (have not previously received antiretroviral therapy) should be initiated with a potent multiple-drug regimen. Treatment should be aggressive with the goal of maximal suppression of viral load to undetectable levels.

Based on clinical data and expert opinion, the HHS Panel on Antiretroviral Guidelines for Adults and Adolescents recommends that antiretroviral therapy in most antiretroviral-naive adults and adolescents be initiated with one of several recommended INSTI-based regimens that include an INSTI with 2 NRTIs (dual NRTIs). In certain clinical situations, these experts recommend that antiretroviral therapy be initiated with one of several recommended INSTI-, NNRTI-, or PI-based regimens that include an INSTI, NNRTI, or PI (and a pharmacokinetic enhancer) with dual NRTIs. Selection of a specific regimen should be individualized based on virologic efficacy, potential adverse effects, pill burden, dosing frequency, potential for drug interactions, results of resistance testing, comorbid conditions, and access to and cost of the drugs.

Table 1 provides the recommended INSTI-based antiretroviral regimens for *initial* treatment in most antiretroviral-naive adults and adolescents (i.e., regimens with demonstrated durable virologic efficacy, favorable tolerability and toxicity profiles, and ease of use).

Table 1. Recommended Antiretroviral Regimens for Initial Therapy in Most Antiretroviral-naive Adults and Adolescents

INSTI-based Regimens	**Dolutegravir** *with* abacavir[a] and lamivudine[b] (fixed combination abacavir/dolutegravir/lamivudine)
	or
	Dolutegravir *with* emtricitabine and tenofovir alafenamide[c] (single-entity dolutegravir and fixed combination FTC/TAF)
	or
	Dolutegravir *with* emtricitabine[b] and tenofovir DF[c] (single-entity dolutegravir and fixed combination FTC/TDF)
	or
	Elvitegravir, cobicistat, emtricitabine, and tenofovir alafenamide[c] (fixed combination EVG/c/FTC/TAF)
	or
	Elvitegravir, cobicistat, emtricitabine, and tenofovir DF[c] (fixed combination EVG/c/FTC/TDF)
	or
	Raltegravir *with* emtricitabine and tenofovir alafenamide[c] (single-entity raltegravir and fixed combination FTC/TAF)
	or
	Raltegravir *with* emtricitabine[b] and tenofovir DF[c] (single-entity raltegravir and fixed combination FTC/TDF)
	or
	Bictegravir, emtricitabine, and tenofovir alafenamide (fixed combination BIC/FTC/TAF)

[a] Use regimen containing abacavir *only* in those who are HLA-B*5701 negative.

[b] If use of the individual components is desirable (instead of a fixed combination), either lamivudine or emtricitabine can be used.

[c] TAF and tenofovir DF (TDF) are both tenofovir prodrugs. When choosing between TAF and TDF, consider adverse effects and access to and cost of the drugs. Adverse bone and renal effects reported less frequently with TAF than with TDF; dyslipidemia reported less frequently with TDF than with TAF.

Adapted from Guidelines for the Use of Antiretroviral Agents in Adults and Adolescents Living with HIV (May 30, 2018). Updates may be available at the US Department of Health and Human Services (HHS) AIDS Information (AIDSinfo) website (http://www.aidsinfo.nih.gov).

Table 2 provides the recommended PI-, NNRTI-, or INSTI-based antiretroviral regimens for *initial* treatment in antiretroviral-naive adults and adolescents in certain clinical circumstances (i.e., regimens that are effective and tolerable, but have some disadvantages compared with regimens recommended for most individuals, including less supporting data from randomized clinical trials). In certain clinical situations, one of these regimens may be the preferred regimen based on individual patient characteristics.

Table 2. Recommended Antiretroviral Regimens for Initial Therapy in Antiretroviral-naive Adults and Adolescents in Certain Clinical Situations

PI-based Regimens	*Cobicistat-boosted* or *ritonavir-boosted* **darunavir** *with* emtricitabine and tenofovir alafenamide[a]
	or
	Cobicistat-boosted or *ritonavir-boosted* **darunavir** *with* emtricitabine[b] and tenofovir DF[a]
	or
	Cobicistat-boosted or *ritonavir-boosted* **atazanavir** *with* emtricitabine and tenofovir alafenamide[a]
	or
	Cobicistat-boosted or *ritonavir-boosted* **atazanavir** *with* emtricitabine[b] and tenofovir DF[a]
	or
	Cobicistat-boosted or *ritonavir-boosted* **darunavir** *with* abacavir[c] and lamivudine[b]
	or
	Cobicistat-boosted or *ritonavir-boosted* **atazanavir**[d] *with* abacavir[c] and lamivudine[b]
NNRTI-based Regimens	**Efavirenz** *with* emtricitabine and tenofovir alafenamide[a]
	or
	Efavirenz *with* emtricitabine[b] and tenofovir DF[a]
	or
	Rilpivirine[e] *with* emtricitabine and tenofovir alafenamide[a]
	or
	Rilpivirine[e] *with* emtricitabine[b] and tenofovir DF[a]
INSTI-based Regimens	**Raltegravir**[d] *with* abacavir[c] and lamivudine[b]
Other Regimens to Consider when Abacavir, Tenofovir Alafenamide, and Tenofovir DF Cannot be Used	*Ritonavir-boosted* **darunavir** *with* **raltegravir** (twice daily)[c]
	or
	Lopinavir/ritonavir (twice daily) *with* lamivudine (or emtricitabine)

[a] TAF and tenofovir DF (TDF) are both tenofovir prodrugs. When choosing between TAF and TDF, consider adverse effects and access to and cost of the drugs. Adverse bone and renal effects reported less frequently with TAF than with TDF; dyslipidemia reported less frequently with TDF than with TAF.

[b] If use of the individual components is desirable (instead of a fixed combination), either lamivudine or emtricitabine can be used.

[c] Use regimens containing abacavir *only* in those who are HLA-B*5701 negative.

[d] Use regimen *only* in those with pretreatment viral load less than 100,000 copies/mL.

[e] Use regimen *only* in those with pretreatment viral load less than 100,000 copies/mL *and* CD4+ T-cell count greater than 200 cells/mm³.

Adapted from Guidelines for the Use of Antiretroviral Agents in Adults and Adolescents Living with HIV (May 30, 2018). Updates may be available at the US Department of Health and Human Services (HHS) AIDS Information (AIDSinfo) website (http://www.aidsinfo.nih.gov).

Recommended Dual NRTI Options. INSTI-, NNRTI-, and PI-based regimens usually recommended for *initial* treatment of antiretroviral-naive adults and adolescents include 2 NRTIs (dual NRTIs). These dual NRTI options are commonly referred to as the "backbone" of antiretroviral regimens. There are 6 commercially available NRTIs; in addition, tenofovir alafenamide and tenofovir DF (nucleotide reverse transcriptase inhibitors) are grouped with the NRTIs for purposes of therapeutic decisions. The choice of the specific dual NRTI option is based on virologic potency and durability, short- and long-term toxicity, and dosing convenience.

Tenofovir alafenamide and emtricitabine, tenofovir DF and emtricitabine (or lamivudine), or abacavir and lamivudine (or emtricitabine) are the dual NRTI options included in regimens recommended by the HHS Panel on Antiretroviral Guidelines for Adults and Adolescents for *initial* treatment in most antiretroviral-naive HIV-infected adults and adolescents and in most regimens recommended by these experts for *initial* treatment in antiretroviral-naive HIV-infected adults and adolescents in certain clinical situations. (See Table 1 and Table 2.)

Advantages of the dual NRTI option of tenofovir alafenamide and emtricitabine include less potential for adverse bone and kidney effects compared with the dual option of tenofovir DF and emtricitabine, substantially higher intracellular concentrations of the active tenofovir metabolite than those reported with tenofovir DF, activity against HBV, and availability of fixed-combination preparations. A fixed-combination preparation containing tenofovir alafenamide and emtricitabine (emtricitabine/tenofovir alafenamide; Descovy®) is commercially available for use in adults and pediatric patients weighing 35 kg or more and may be preferred to decrease pill burden and improve adherence when this dual NRTI option is used. In addition, the dual NRTI option of tenofovir alafenamide and emtricitabine is commercially available in fixed combination with either rilpivirine or *cobicistat-boosted* elvitegravir and both of these fixed-combination preparations provide a complete single-tablet regimen. Disadvantages of the dual option of tenofovir alafenamide and emtricitabine include greater increases in triglycerides and cholesterol than those reported with tenofovir DF, the need to monitor renal function, urine glucose, and urine protein in all patients, and the precaution that tenofovir alafenamide should not be used in patients with creatinine clearances less than 30 mL/minute. (See HIV Nucleotide Reverse Transcriptase Inhibitors under Guidelines for Use of Antiretroviral Agents: Adverse Effects.)

Advantages of the dual NRTI option of tenofovir DF and emtricitabine include a better virologic response than that reported with the dual NRTI option of abacavir and lamivudine when used in conjunction with *ritonavir-boosted* atazanavir or efavirenz in patients with baseline viral load of 100,000 copies/mL or greater, activity against HBV, a once-daily dosing regimen that can be administered without regard to meals, and availability of fixed-combination preparations. A fixed-combination preparation containing tenofovir DF and emtricitabine (emtricitabine/tenofovir DF; Truvada®) is commercially available for use in adults and pediatric patients weighing at least 17 kg and may be preferred to decrease pill burden and improve adherence when this dual NRTI option is used. In addition, the dual NRTI option of tenofovir DF and emtricitabine is commercially available in fixed combination with efavirenz or rilpivirine or *cobicistat-boosted* elvitegravir and each of these 3 fixed-combination preparations provides a complete single-tablet regimen. Disadvantages of the dual NRTI option of tenofovir DF and emtricitabine include potential adverse effects reported with tenofovir DF (e.g., bone effects, nephrotoxicity), the need to monitor renal function, urine glucose, and urine protein in all patients, and the precaution that tenofovir DF should be used with caution or avoided in patients with renal disease and osteoporosis. (See HIV Nucleotide Reverse Transcriptase Inhibitors under Guidelines for Use of Antiretroviral Agents: Adverse Effects.)

The dual NRTI option of abacavir and lamivudine (or emtricitabine) should be used *only* in those who are negative for HLA-B*5701. Advantages of the dual NRTI option of abacavir and lamivudine include a once-daily dosing regimen that can be administered without regard to meals, no reported nephrotoxicity, and availability of fixed-combination preparations. A fixed-combination preparation containing abacavir and lamivudine (abacavir/lamivudine; Epzicom®) is commercially available for use in adults and pediatric patients weighing 25 kg or more and may be preferred to decrease pill burden and improve adherence when this dual NRTI option is used. In addition, the dual NRTI option of abacavir and lamivudine is commercially available in fixed combination with dolutegravir and can be used in adults and pediatric patients weighing 40 kg or more to provide a complete single-tablet regimen (abacavir/dolutegravir/lamivudine; Triumeq®). Disadvantages include the need to test for the HLA B*5701 allele before initiation of abacavir (see Human Leukocyte Antigen (HLA)-B*5701 Screening under Guidelines for Use of Antiretroviral Agents: Laboratory Monitoring), inferior virologic response compared with that reported with the dual NRTI option of tenofovir DF and emtricitabine when used in conjunction with *ritonavir-boosted* atazanavir or efavirenz in patients with baseline viral load of 100,000 copies/mL or greater (difference in efficacy not evident in those with baseline viral load less than 100,000 copies/mL and no difference in efficacy when abacavir and lamivudine was used with dolutegravir), and potential adverse effects reported with abacavir, such as hypersensitivity reactions and adverse cardiovascular effects.

The dual option of zidovudine and lamivudine is no longer recommended for *initial* treatment regimens in nonpregnant antiretroviral-naive adults and adolescents because of greater toxicities (e.g., bone marrow suppression, GI effects, skeletal muscle myopathy, cardiomyopathy, mitochondrial toxicities such as lipoatrophy, lactic acidosis, and hepatic steatosis) than those reported with the recommended dual NRTI options. However, the dual NRTI option of zidovudine and lamivudine is recommended as an alternative dual NRTI option for *initial* treatment regimens in antiretroviral-naive pregnant women (see Safety and Choice of Antiretrovirals During Pregnancy under Guidelines for Use of Antiretroviral Agents: Antiretroviral Therapy During Pregnancy). In addition, the dual NRTI option of zidovudine and lamivudine (or emtricitabine) is a preferred option for *initial* treatment regimens in pediatric patients from birth to less than 6 years of age and an alternative option in pediatric patients 6 years of age or older (see Initial Antiretroviral Therapy in Antiretroviral-naive Pediatric Patients under Guidelines for Use of Antiretroviral Agents: Antiretroviral Therapy in Pediatric Patients). A fixed-combination preparation containing zidovudine and lamivudine (lamivudine/zidovudine; Combivir®) is commercially available for use in adults and pediatric patients weighing 30 kg or more and may be preferred to decrease pill burden and improve adherence when this dual NRTI option is used.

For HIV-infected adults and adolescents coinfected with HBV, the dual NRTI options of tenofovir alafenamide and emtricitabine or tenofovir DF and emtricitabine (or lamivudine) are preferred since these antiretrovirals all have some activity against HBV.

NRTI Pairings *Not* Recommended for Initial Therapy. A dual option of zidovudine and lamivudine is not usually recommended for *initial* treatment regimens in antiretroviral-naive adults and adolescents because of greater toxicities than the dual NRTI options of tenofovir alafenamide and emtricitabine, tenofovir DF and emtricitabine, or abacavir and lamivudine. (See Recommended Dual NRTI Options under Guidelines for Use of Antiretroviral Agents: Initial Antiretroviral Therapy in Antiretroviral-naive Adults and Adolescents.)

A dual NRTI option of didanosine and emtricitabine (or lamivudine) is *not* recommended for *initial* treatment regimens in antiretroviral-naive HIV-infected adults and adolescents because of inferior virologic efficacy, limited clinical trial experience in antiretroviral-naive patients, and didanosine toxicities (e.g., pancreatitis, peripheral neuropathy).

A dual NRTI option of stavudine and lamivudine is *not* recommended for *initial* treatment regimens in antiretroviral-naive adults and adolescents because of reported toxicities (e.g., lipoatrophy, peripheral neuropathy, hyperlactatemia including symptomatic and life-threatening lactic acidosis, hepatic steatosis, pancreatitis).

NRTI Pairings *Not* Recommended at Any Time. Concomitant use of lamivudine and emtricitabine is *not* recommended at any time because the drugs have similar resistance profiles and concomitant use provides no additional benefit.

A dual NRTI option of didanosine and stavudine is *not* recommended at any time. Concomitant use of didanosine and stavudine is associated with a high incidence of toxicities (e.g., peripheral neuropathy, pancreatitis, hyperlactatemia). Serious, sometimes fatal, lactic acidosis with hepatic steatosis with or without pancreatitis has been reported in HIV-infected pregnant women receiving these drugs concomitantly.

A dual NRTI option of didanosine and tenofovir DF is *not* recommended at any time because of increased didanosine concentrations and serious didanosine toxicities, potential for immunologic nonresponse and/or decline in $CD4^+$ T-cell counts, high rate of early virologic failure, and rapid selection of resistance mutations.

Concomitant use of stavudine and zidovudine is *not* recommended at any time because of antagonistic antiretroviral effects.

All-NRTI Regimens. All-NRTI regimens that include 3 or 4 NRTIs (without any drugs from another class) have been used but are not recommended for *initial* treatment in antiretroviral-naive adults and adolescents because such regimens have inferior virologic efficacy or have not been adequately studied.

A triple NRTI regimen that includes abacavir, lamivudine, and zidovudine has been used, and a fixed combination containing these 3 NRTIs is commercially available (abacavir/lamivudine/zidovudine; Trizivir®). Abacavir/lamivudine/zidovudine is intended only for regimens that require all 3 drugs, and clinicians should consider that data are limited regarding use of this fixed-combination preparation in patients with baseline viral loads exceeding 100,000 copies/mL. The HHS panel states that a triple NRTI regimen of abacavir, lamivudine, and zidovudine is *not* usually recommended since it has inferior virologic efficacy and should be used only when INSTI-, NNRTI-, or PI-based regimens cannot be used.

A triple NRTI regimen of lamivudine, tenofovir DF, and zidovudine has been used and has been shown to have antiretroviral activity; however, this regimen is *not* usually recommended and should be used only when other regimens are not desirable.

A quadruple NRTI regimen of abacavir, lamivudine, tenofovir DF, and zidovudine is *not* recommended for initial therapy in antiretroviral-naive HIV-infected adults and adolescents because of inferior virologic efficacy. In an open-label, pilot study, a quadruple NRTI regimen was compared with an NNRTI-based regimen of efavirenz with lamivudine and zidovudine and both regimens had similar efficacy and tolerability. However, a larger, open-label study comparing a similar quadruple NRTI regimen (abacavir, emtricitabine, tenofovir DF, zidovudine) with a standard NNRTI- or PI-based regimen found that substantially fewer patients receiving the quadruple NRTI regimen achieved plasma HIV-1 RNA levels below 200 copies/mL.

Antiretrovirals *Not* Recommended for Initial Therapy. Delavirdine is *not* recommended for use in NNRTI-based regimens for *initial* antiretroviral therapy in antiretroviral-naive adults and adolescents because of inferior antiretroviral activity compared with other NNRTIs (e.g., efavirenz, nevirapine) and has an inconvenient dosing schedule (i.e., 3-times daily dosing).

Etravirine is *not* recommended for use in NNRTI-based regimens for *initial* antiretroviral therapy since safety and efficacy have not been established in such patients.

Nevirapine is *not* recommended for *initial* treatment regimens in antiretroviral-naive adults and adolescents because it has been associated with serious and potentially fatal toxicity (hepatic events, severe rash, Stevens-Johnson syndrome, toxic epidermal necrolysis) and did not meet noninferiority criteria when compared to efavirenz.

Unboosted atazanavir (i.e., without low-dose ritonavir or cobicistat) is *not* recommended for *initial* treatment because it is less potent than *ritonavir-boosted* or *cobicistat-boosted* atazanavir.

Unboosted darunavir (i.e., without low-dose ritonavir or cobicistat) is *not* recommended for *initial* treatment because of inadequate bioavailability and because it has not been studied.

Fosamprenavir (with or without low-dose ritonavir) is *not* recommended for *initial* treatment regimens in antiretroviral-naive adults and adolescents. Regimens that include unboosted fosamprenavir may be associated with virologic failure and result in emergence of resistance, and clinical trial data regarding use of *ritonavir-boosted* fosamprenavir are more limited compared with clinical trial data available for other *ritonavir-boosted* PIs.

Indinavir (with or without low-dose ritonavir) is *not* recommended for *initial* therapy. Use of indinavir without low-dose ritonavir is not recommended because of potential for nephrolithiasis and crystalluria, an inconvenient dosage regimen (3-times daily dosing and the need to take it on an empty stomach or with a light meal), and fluid requirements. Use of *ritonavir-boosted* indinavir is *not* recommended because of a high incidence of nephrolithiasis and crystalluria and fluid requirements.

Lopinavir/ritonavir is *not* recommended for *initial* treatment regimens because of GI intolerance and because of higher ritonavir dose and higher pill burden than other *ritonavir-boosted* PIs.

Nelfinavir is *not* recommended for *initial* treatment regimens because of inferior virologic efficacy compared with some other PIs and high incidence of diarrhea.

Ritonavir as the sole PI is *not* recommended for *initial* therapy because of high pill burden, GI intolerance, and metabolic toxicity. However, low-dose ritonavir is used concomitantly with certain other PIs for therapeutic advantage (*ritonavir-boosted* PIs), and some recommended and alternative PI-based regimens for *initial* therapy include low-dose ritonavir.

Saquinavir without low-dose ritonavir is *not* recommended for *initial* therapy because of inadequate bioavailability and inferior virologic efficacy. *Ritonavir-boosted* saquinavir is *not* recommended for *initial* treatment regimens because of high pill burden and potential for adverse cardiovascular effects, including QT and PR prolongation.

Ritonavir-boosted tipranavir is *not* recommended for *initial* therapy because of inferior virologic efficacy and because of higher ritonavir dose and higher rate of adverse effects than other *ritonavir-boosted* PIs.

Enfuvirtide has *not* been evaluated for use in antiretroviral-naive patients.

Maraviroc is *not* recommended for *initial* treatment regimens because a coreceptor tropism assay (see Coreceptor Tropism Assay under Guidelines for Use of Antiretroviral Agents: Laboratory Monitoring) should be performed before the drug is initiated, there is no virologic benefit compared with other recommended regimens, and a twice-daily dosing regimen is required.

Antiretrovirals and Regimens *Not* Recommended at Any Time. The HHS Panel on Antiretroviral Guidelines for Adults and Adolescents states that delavirdine, didanosine, indinavir, nelfinavir, and stavudine are no longer recommended for treatment of HIV infection in adults and adolescents because of suboptimal antiviral potency, unacceptable toxicities, high pill burden, or pharmacologic concerns.

Monotherapy is *not* recommended for the treatment of HIV infection. Monotherapy with an NRTI is not recommended because it is inferior to dual NRTIs. Monotherapy with a PI is inferior to combination antiretroviral therapy. Monotherapy with an INSTI has resulted in virologic rebound and INSTI resistance.

Regimens that include 2 NRTIs alone (without a third antiretroviral) are considered suboptimal regimens and are *not* recommended at any time. Although 2-drug regimens that included 2 NRTIs were used in the past for initial antiretroviral therapy in antiretroviral-naive individuals, these regimens may be associated with initial declines in plasma HIV-1 RNA levels, are associated with rapid development of resistance, and are less effective in providing durable suppression of HIV replication than regimens that include 3 or more drugs and include at least 1 antiretroviral from another class.

Certain dual NRTI pairings are *not* recommended at any time because of inferior virologic efficacy, antagonistic antiretroviral effects, increased risk of toxicity, or insufficient data. (See NRTI Pairings Not Recommended at Any Time under Guidelines for Use of Antiretroviral Agents: Initial Antiretroviral Therapy in Antiretroviral-naive Adults and Adolescents.)

Certain triple NRTI regimens are *not* recommended at any time in antiretroviral-naive patients or antiretroviral-experienced patients because of a high rate of early virologic failure in clinical trials. (See All-NRTI Regimens under Guidelines for Use of Antiretroviral Agents: Initial Antiretroviral Therapy in Antiretroviral-naive Adults and Adolescents.)

Tenofovir alafenamide and tenofovir DF should *not* be administered concomitantly. Care should be taken to avoid inadvertent concomitant administration of these tenofovir prodrugs, especially during transition from one formulation to another. Data are not available regarding potential additive toxicity if tenofovir alafenamide and tenofovir DF are inadvertently used concomitantly.

Certain unboosted PIs (i.e., darunavir, saquinavir, tipranavir) should *not* be used at any time because of inadequate bioavailability.

Atazanavir and indinavir should *not* be used concomitantly since both of these PIs can cause hyperbilirubinemia and jaundice and the possibility exists that concomitant use may result in additive adverse effects.

Cobicistat and ritonavir should *not* be administered concomitantly. Inadvertent concomitant administration of both of these pharmacologic enhancers may result in additive CYP3A4 inhibition and further increases in concentrations of the antiretrovirals or other drugs that the patient is receiving. (See Drug Interactions: Pharmacokinetic Enhancers.)

Concomitant use of 2 NNRTIs is *not* recommended at any time because regimens that include 2 NNRTIs have been associated with a high incidence of adverse effects.

Etravirine should *not* be used concomitantly with *ritonavir-boosted* atazanavir, *ritonavir-boosted* fosamprenavir, or an *unboosted* PI at any time since etravirine may alter plasma concentrations of the PI and appropriate dosages for such regimens have not been established. In addition, etravirine should *not* be used concomitantly with *ritonavir-boosted* tipranavir at any time because of substantially decreased etravirine concentrations.

Because of the risk of hepatic events, nevirapine should *not* be initiated in antiretroviral-naive women with $CD4^+$ T-cell counts exceeding 250 cells/mm^3 or in men with counts exceeding 400 cells/mm^3, unless no other antiretroviral options are available and the patient is closely monitored.

■ Antiretroviral Therapy in Antiretroviral-experienced Adults and Adolescents

Optimal antiretroviral therapy involves continuous evaluation of the patient's tolerance and virologic and immunologic response to their current regimen. Regimen modification is indicated in individuals experiencing toxicity or intolerance to their current regimen and whenever there is evidence of treatment failure. In addition, consideration can be given to modifying an effective antiretroviral regimen in patients who are virologically suppressed if the change results in regimen simplification, promotes long-term adherence, enhances tolerability and decreases short- or long-term toxicity, prevents or mitigates drug interactions, eliminates food or fluid requirements, reduces the risk of virologic failure, or reduces costs.

Whenever a change in antiretroviral therapy is considered in antiretroviral-experienced patients, a review of the agents that the patient already has received is essential. Viral mutants will emerge in all HIV-infected patients over time; however, use of potent regimens that provide durable suppression of HIV replication are less likely to result in rapid emergence of resistant strains. The new regimen should include antiretrovirals that are predicted to provide maximal suppression of HIV replication while avoiding use of those that might be ineffective.

Management of Treatment Regimen Failure

Failure of an antiretroviral treatment regimen may be the result of poor patient adherence, poor tolerability, pharmacokinetic issues (including drug-food or drug-drug interactions), suboptimal virologic potency, and resistance factors. Failure of a regimen can be associated with virologic failure or suboptimal immunologic response.

Virologic Failure. Virologic suppression is defined as a confirmed plasma HIV-1 RNA level below the limits of detection. Virologic failure is defined as the inability of an antiretroviral regimen to achieve or maintain suppression of viral replication to plasma HIV-1 RNA levels less than 200 copies/mL. An incomplete virologic response is defined as 2 consecutive plasma HIV-1 RNA levels of 200 copies/mL or greater after 24 weeks of an antiretroviral regimen. Virologic rebound refers to confirmed plasma HIV-1 RNA levels of 200 copies/mL or greater after prior suppression of viremia. After virologic suppression, transient increases ("blips") in viral load may occasionally occur and may not represent virologic failure. Baseline plasma HIV-1 RNA levels may affect the time course of response and some regimens may take longer than others to suppress viremia.

Virologic failure can occur as the result of viral resistance or suboptimal adherence to the treatment regimen (e.g., because of intolerance/toxicity or complex dosage regimens). Other factors include suboptimal pharmacokinetics of the drugs, drug or food interactions, higher pretreatment or baseline plasma HIV-1 RNA levels, lower pretreatment or nadir $CD4^+$ T-cell counts, prior AIDS diagnosis, or prior treatment failure. Although it is not always possible to identify the cause of virologic failure, identifying the cause is beneficial since it can provide valuable information to use when modifying the treatment regimen.

Evaluation of virologic failure should include assessment of HIV disease severity, antiretroviral treatment history, plasma HIV-1 RNA and $CD4^+$ T-cell count trends over time, results of prior drug-resistance testing, concomitant therapy (including prescription and nonprescription drugs and dietary or herbal supplements), comorbidities (including substance abuse), and the patient's adherence to the treatment regimen (including dose, dosing frequency, and administration with or without food). When currently recommended antiretroviral regimens are used for *initial* treatment, HIV-infected patients have a high likelihood of achieving and maintaining plasma HIV-1 RNA levels below the lower limits of detection. If this does not occur or if virologic rebound occurs, resistance mutations to one or more components of the regimen may have developed. However, many patients with detectable viral loads are nonadherent to treatment; some of these patients may have minimal or no drug resistance while others may have extensive resistance. Management of patients with extensive resistance is complex and usually requires consultation with an HIV expert.

In patients experiencing virologic failure who have plasma HIV-1 RNA levels greater than 1000 copies/mL and with identified drug resistance, the antiretroviral regimen should be modified with the goal of maximal suppression of plasma HIV-1 RNA levels (i.e., below the lower limits of detection) and prevention of further selection of resistance mutations. This usually involves a change to a new regimen with at least 2 (preferably 3) fully active antiretrovirals.

In those with plasma HIV-1 RNA levels greater than 1000 copies/mL without identified drug resistance, virologic failure is almost always related to nonadherence and management usually involves a thorough assessment to determine the level of adherence and identify any food or drug interactions.

Because there is evidence that emergence of drug-resistance mutations often occurs when plasma HIV-1 RNA levels are 200 copies/mL or higher, especially when levels exceed 500 copies/mL, patients with plasma HIV-1 RNA levels persistently in the range of 200–1000 copies/mL should be considered as virologic failures, resistance testing should be performed in those with levels greater than 500 copies/mL, and regimen modification considered if there are sufficient therapeutic options.

The clinical implications of plasma HIV-1 RNA levels above the lower limits of detection but less than 200 copies/mL are controversial; there is no consensus on how to manage such patients, but the risk of emerging resistance is believed to be relatively low. Therefore, such patients may continue their current regimen and plasma HIV-1 RNA levels should be measured at least every 3 months to assess the need for a regimen change in the future.

Suboptimal Immunologic Response. Suboptimal immunologic response refers to failure to achieve and maintain an adequate $CD4^+$ T-cell response despite virologic suppression.

In antiretroviral-naive patients, the increase in $CD4^+$ T-cell counts in response to initial antiretroviral therapy usually is about 150 cells/mm^3 over the first year of treatment. After 4–6 years on a suppressive regimen, the $CD4^+$ T-cell count may plateau. Although there is no clear definition of suboptimal immunologic response, some studies describe it as a failure to increase $CD4^+$ T-cell count above a certain threshold (e.g., greater than 350 or 500 cells/mm^3) over a specified time period (e.g., 4–7 years). Alternatively, others have focused on an inability to increase $CD4^+$ T-cell counts by a certain threshold (e.g., greater than 50 or 100 cells/mm^3) over a given time period.

Factors associated with poor $CD4^+$ T-cell response include baseline $CD4^+$ T-cell counts less than 200/mm^3, older age, coinfection (e.g., HCV, HIV-2, human T-cell leukemia virus type 1 or 2 [HTLV-1, HTLV-2]), certain antiretrovirals, persistent immune activation, loss of regenerative potential of the immune system, comorbidities).

In the setting of virologic suppression, there is no consensus regarding how to manage suboptimal immunologic response. Although there is some evidence that persistently low $CD4^+$ T-cell counts in individuals receiving a suppressive antiretroviral regimen are associated with a small, but appreciable, risk of AIDS-related or non-AIDS-related morbidity and mortality, it is not clear whether suboptimal immunologic response in the setting of virologic suppression should prompt a modification of the antiretroviral regimen.

Considerations When Modifying an Antiretroviral Regimen If a change in the antiretroviral regimen is being made because of problems with adherence, use of commercially available fixed-combination preparations should be considered to reduce pill burden and simplify the regimen. Other conditions that may reduce adherence (e.g., depression, substance abuse) should be addressed.

If a change is being made because of pharmacokinetic issues, food/fasting requirements should be reviewed, the possibility of malabsorption assessed, and concomitant drugs and dietary supplements reviewed for possible drug-drug interactions and changes in the antiretroviral regimen and/or concomitant therapy should be made if possible.

Evaluation and management of antiretroviral-experienced patients experiencing virologic failure, especially those with extensive resistance, is complex, and consultation with an expert is recommended and considered critical.

Drug-resistance testing should be performed while the patient is taking the failing antiretroviral regimen or, if not possible, within 4 weeks of discontinuance of the failing regimen. If it has been longer than 4 weeks since antiretrovirals were discontinued, drug-resistance testing may still provide useful information to guide therapy, although previously selected resistance mutations may not be detected.

If a change is being made because of virologic failure, the goal of therapy is to reestablish virologic suppression (e.g., plasma HIV-1 RNA levels below the lower limits of detection). However, in some highly antiretroviral-experienced patients, maximal virologic suppression is not possible. In these cases, antiretroviral therapy should be continued with regimens designed to minimize toxicity, preserve $CD4^+$ T-cell counts, and delay clinical progression.

To design a new regimen for patients with virologic failure, the patient's treatment history and past and current resistance testing should be used to identify at least 2 (preferably 3) fully active drugs (i.e., drugs likely to have antiretroviral activity based on treatment history, drug-resistance testing, and/or a novel mechanism of action) that can be used in conjunction with an optimized background antiretroviral regimen.

In general, adding a single, fully active antiretroviral is *not* recommended because of the risk of rapid development of resistance to all drugs in the regimen. However, in select cases, adding a fully active *ritonavir-boosted* PI to a single active drug may result in a regimen that is as effective as a regimen that includes more antiretrovirals.

When no viable suppressive regimen can be constructed for a patient with extensive drug resistance, consideration can be given to enrolling the patient in a clinical trial of investigational antiretrovirals or contacting pharmaceutical sponsors that may have investigational agents available.

Discontinuing or briefly interrupting antiretroviral therapy is *not* recommended since such a strategy in patients with viremia may result in rapid increases in plasma HIV-1 RNA, decreased $CD4^+$ T-cell counts, and increased risk of clinical progression. Planned long-term interruptions of antiretroviral therapy are not recommended outside of controlled clinical trials.

Regimen Modification in the Setting of Virologic Suppression With currently available antiretroviral therapy, most patients living with HIV can achieve and maintain HIV viral suppression. In some virologically suppressed patients, it may be desirable to switch to a simplified or better tolerated regimen, provided the change maintains viral suppression without jeopardizing future treatment options. Regimen modification in the setting of viral suppression may be considered to reduce pill burden and dosing frequency, enhance tolerability and decrease short- or long-term toxicity, prevent or mitigate drug interactions, eliminate food or fluid requirements, or reduce costs.

Although 3-drug antiretroviral regimens are generally recommended when modifying an existing regimen in antiretroviral-experienced adults and adolescents who are virologically suppressed, there is some evidence that *certain* 2-drug regimens can maintain virologic suppression.

If a 2-drug antiretroviral regimen is being considered in antiretroviral-experienced patients who are virologically suppressed, the HHS Panel on Antiretroviral Guidelines for Adults and Adolescents states that a ritonavir-boosted PI (i.e., *ritonavir-boosted* atazanavir, *ritonavir-boosted* darunavir, lopinavir/ritonavir) in conjunction with lamivudine may be a reasonable option when use of tenofovir alafenamide, tenofovir DF, or abacavir is contraindicated or not desirable.

The HHS panel also states that a regimen of dolutegravir and rilpivirine can be a reasonable option when use of NRTIs is not desirable and when resistance to dolutegravir or rilpivirine is not expected. A fixed-combination preparation containing dolutegravir and rilpivirine (dolutegravir/rilpivirine) is commercially available and is labeled by FDA for use in antiretroviral-experienced adults to replace the current antiretroviral regimen in those who are virologically suppressed (i.e., plasma HIV-1 RNA levels less than 50 copies/mL) on a stable antiretroviral regimen for at least 6 months, have no known history of treatment failure, and are infected with HIV-1 with no known substitutions associated with resistance to dolutegravir or rilpivirine.

Strategies Not Recommended in the Setting of Virologic Suppression. Monotherapy is *not* recommended as a switching strategy in the setting of virologic suppression. Based on results of preliminary studies indicating that low-level viremia is more common in antiretroviral-experienced patients receiving monotherapy with a *ritonavir-boosted* HIV PI than in those receiving regimens that include a *ritonavir-boosted* HIV PI with HIV NRTIs, the HHS panel states that such monotherapy regimens generally should be avoided. These experts also state that dolutegravir monotherapy cannot be recommended in the setting of virologic suppression based on results of uncontrolled trials and cohorts indicating an unacceptable risk of virologic failure and subsequent development of resistance.

The HHS panel states that a 2-drug regimen of *ritonavir-boosted* atazanavir and raltegravir cannot be recommended because results of a randomized study in virologically suppressed patients indicated that a switch to such a regimen was associated with higher rates of virologic failure and treatment discontinuance than switching to a regimen of *ritonavir-boosted* atazanavir in conjunction with emtricitabine and tenofovir DF.

The HHS panel states that a 2-drug regimen of maraviroc and an HIV PI (with a pharmacologic enhancer) is not recommended based on results of a randomized, controlled trial in virologically suppressed patients. These experts also state that a 2-drug regimen of maraviroc and raltegravir is not recommended because of the rate of virologic relapse reported in a nonrandomized pilot study in virologically suppressed patients who were switched to such a regimen.

■ Antiretroviral Therapy in Pediatric Patients

The pathogenesis of HIV infection and the general virologic and immunologic principles of antiretroviral therapy that apply to HIV-infected adults also apply to HIV-infected pediatric patients; however, the treatment of HIV-infected neonates, children, and adolescents involves some unique pharmacologic, virologic, and immunologic considerations. In 1993, when the first set of guidelines regarding the use of antiretrovirals in the treatment of HIV-infected children were issued, monotherapy with zidovudine or didanosine was considered an appropriate regimen for initial therapy. However, based on subsequent studies evaluating multiple-drug antiretroviral regimens in pediatric patients and accumulation of data regarding the benefits of multiple-drug antiretroviral regimens in HIV-infected adults, treatment of HIV-infected pediatric patients should be initiated with a multiple-drug antiretroviral regimen that contains at least 3 drugs. Because recommendations for the management of HIV infection in neonates, children, and adolescents are rapidly evolving and increasingly complex, management of HIV-infected pediatric patients should be directed by a clinician with expertise in the treatment of pediatric and adolescent HIV infection, whenever possible, or such a specialist should be consulted regularly throughout the course of treatment to obtain the most up-to-date information.

The goals of combination antiretroviral therapy in treatment-naive pediatric patients are to prevent or reduce HIV-related mortality and morbidity, restore and/or preserve immune function as reflected by $CD4^+$ T-cell count, maximally suppress viral replication for as long as possible, prevent emergence of viral drug-resistance mutations, minimize drug toxicity, maintain normal physical growth and neurocognitive development, and improve quality of life.

Considerable information is available regarding use of NRTIs in pediatric patients. Zidovudine is labeled by FDA for treatment of HIV-1 infection in pediatric patients 4 weeks of age or older and for use in neonates for prevention of perinatal HIV transmission. (See Guidelines for Use of Antiretroviral Agents: Antiretrovirals for Prevention of Perinatal HIV Transmission.) Didanosine is labeled by FDA for treatment of HIV-1 infection in pediatric patients 2 weeks of age or older. Safety and efficacy of emtricitabine have been established in pediatric patients 3 months of age or older; FDA-approved labeling also includes emtricitabine dosage recommendations for infants 0–3 months of age. Abacavir and lamivudine are labeled for treatment of HIV-1 infection in pediatric patients 3 months of age or older. Stavudine is labeled for treatment of HIV-1 infection in pediatric patients, including neonates. Although single-entity tenofovir DF is labeled for use in pediatric patients 2 years of age or older, the fixed combination containing emtricitabine and tenofovir DF (emtricitabine/tenofovir DF) is labeled for treatment of HIV-1 infection in pediatric patients weighing at least 17 kg. Other fixed combinations containing tenofovir DF (efavirenz/emtricitabine/tenofovir DF, emtricitabine/rilpivirine/tenofovir

DF, EVG/c/FTC/TDF) are labeled for use in pediatric patients 12 years of age or older. The fixed combination EVG/c/FTC/TAF is labeled by FDA for treatment of HIV-1 infection in pediatric patients weighing 25 kg or more, the fixed combination emtricitabine/tenofovir alafenamide is labeled for use in pediatric patients weighing 35 kg or more, and the fixed combination emtricitabine/rilpivirine/tenofovir alafenamide is labeled for use in pediatric patients 12 years of age or older weighing 35 kg or more.

Data are available regarding the safety and efficacy of most PIs in pediatric patients. Lopinavir/ritonavir is labeled for treatment of HIV-1 infection in children 14 days of age or older *and* postmenstrual age at least 42 weeks (i.e., time elapsed since first day of the mother's last menstrual period to birth plus time elapsed after birth); ritonavir is labeled for use in children 1 month of age or older; and fosamprenavir is labeled for use in those 4 weeks of age or older. Atazanavir is labeled for use in children 3 months of age or older weighing 5 kg or more; because of the risk of kernicterus, atazanavir should *not* be used in neonates and infants younger than 3 months of age. Nelfinavir and *ritonavir-boosted* tipranavir are labeled for use in antiretroviral-experienced children 2 years of age or older. *Ritonavir-boosted* darunavir is labeled for use in children 3 years of age or older; because of toxicity and mortality observed in animal studies, darunavir should *not* be used in pediatric patients younger than 3 years of age. Only limited information is available regarding use of indinavir in pediatric patients and optimal dosage has *not* been identified. Safety and efficacy of saquinavir have *not* been established in pediatric patients younger than 16 years of age. Safety and efficacy of the fixed combinations containing atazanavir or darunavir with cobicistat (atazanavir/cobicistat, darunavir/cobicistat) have not been established in patients younger than 18 years of age.

Regarding use of NNRTIs in pediatric patients, nevirapine is labeled for use in pediatric patients 15 days of age or older and efavirenz is labeled for use in children 3 months of age or older weighing 3.5 kg or more. Etravirine is labeled for use in pediatric patients 6 years of age or older. Rilpivirine is labeled for use in pediatric patients 12 years of age or older weighing at least 35 kg. Safety and efficacy of delavirdine have *not* been established in pediatric patients younger than 16 years of age. The fixed combination efavirenz/emtricitabine/tenofovir DF and the fixed combination emtricitabine/rilpivirine/tenofovir DF are labeled for use in pediatric patients 12 years of age or older.

Regarding use of INSTIs in pediatric patients, single-entity raltegravir is labeled for use in pediatric patients 4 weeks of age or older and single-entity dolutegravir is labeled for use in pediatric patients weighing at least 30 kg. Although the fixed combination abacavir/dolutegravir/lamivudine is labeled for use in pediatric patients weighing 40 kg or more, safety and efficacy of the fixed combination dolutegravir/rilpivirine have not been established in pediatric patients. The fixed combination EVG/c/FTC/TAF is labeled for use in pediatric patients weighing 25 kg or more and the fixed combination EVG/c/FTC/TDF is labeled for use in pediatric patients 12 years of age or older weighing 35 kg or more. Safety and efficacy of the fixed combination BIC/FTC/TAF have not been established in pediatric patients younger than 18 years of age.

Only limited information is available regarding use of HIV entry and fusion inhibitors in pediatric patients. Enfuvirtide is labeled for treatment of HIV-1 infection in children 6 years of age or older. Maraviroc is labeled for use in pediatric patients 2 years of age or older weighing at least 10 kg. Safety and efficacy of ibalizumab-uiyk have not been established in pediatric patients.

Initial Antiretroviral Therapy in Antiretroviral-naive Pediatric Patients For *initial* treatment of HIV-infected pediatric patients, the HHS Panel on Antiviral Therapy and Medical Management of Children Living with HIV recommends antiretroviral therapy with a 3-drug regimen that includes a PI (*ritonavir-boosted*), NNRTI, or INSTI with 2 NRTIs (dual NRTIs). The choice of antiretroviral regimen should be individualized based on patient characteristics (especially age), efficacy, potential adverse effects, results of viral drug resistance testing, family preferences, and advantages and disadvantages of the specific regimen.

Based on data from clinical studies (preferably in children) demonstrating durable viral suppression with immunologic and clinical improvement, extent of pediatric experience, information regarding incidence and types of short- and long-term toxicity, availability and acceptability of pediatric drug formulations (including palatability, ease of preparation, volume of liquid dose required, pill size, and pill burden), dosing frequency, food and fluid requirements, and potential for drug interactions, the HHS Panel on Antiretroviral Therapy and Medical Management of Children Living with HIV recommends that antiretroviral therapy in antiretroviral-naive children be initiated with certain preferred or alternative PI-, NNRTI-, or INSTI-based regimens. Table 3 includes these preferred and alternative antiretroviral regimens for *initial* treatment in antiretroviral-naive pediatric patients.

Table 3. Preferred and Alternative Antiretroviral Regimens for Initial Therapy in Antiretroviral-naive Pediatric Patients.

Age	PI, NNRTI, or INSTI *with* Dual NRTIs[a]
Preferred Regimens:	
Neonates younger than 14 days of age[b]	NNRTI-based regimen: Nevirapine *with* 2 NRTIs **or** INSTI-based regimen: Raltegravir *with* 2 NRTIs
Children 14 days of age to less than 3 years of age	PI-based regimen: Lopinavir/ritonavir[c] *with* 2 NRTIs **or** INSTI-based regimen: Raltegravir *with* 2 NRTIs
Children 3 years to less than 6 years of age	PI-based regimen: *Ritonavir-boosted* atazanavir *with* 2 NRTIs **or** PI-based regimen: *Ritonavir-boosted* darunavir[d] (twice daily) *with* 2 NRTIs **or** INSTI-based regimen: Raltegravir *with* 2 NRTIs
Children 6 years to less than 12 years of age	PI-based regimen: *Ritonavir-boosted* atazanavir *with* 2 NRTIs **or** INSTI-based regimen: Dolutegravir[e] *with* 2 NRTIs
Adolescents 12 years of age or older and not sexually mature (SMR 1–3)	PI-based regimen: *Ritonavir-boosted* atazanavir *with* 2 NRTIs **or** INSTI-based regimen: Dolutegravir[e] *with* 2 NRTIs **or** PI-based regimen: *Ritonavir-boosted* darunavir[d] (once daily) *with* 2 NRTIs **or** INSTI-based regimen: EVG/c/FTC/TAF
Adolescents 12 years of age or older and sexually mature (SMR 4 or 5)	(See Table 1 and Table 2.)
Alternative Regimens:	
Children older than 14 days to less than 3 years of age	NNRTI-based regimen: Nevirapine *with* 2 NRTIs
Children 3 months to less than 3 years of age weighing at least 10 kg	PI-based regimen: *Ritonavir-boosted* atazanavir *with* 2 NRTIs
Children 3 years to less than 6 years of age	NNRTI-based regimen: Efavirenz *with* 2 NRTIs **or** PI-based regimen: Lopinavir/ritonavir *with* 2 NRTIs
Children 6 years to less than 12 years of age	PI-based regimen: *Ritonavir-boosted* darunavir[d] (twice daily) *with* 2 NRTIs **or** NNRTI-based regimen: Efavirenz *with* 2 NRTIs **or** INSTI-based regimen: EVG/c/FTC/TAF **or** PI-based regimen: Lopinavir/ritonavir *with* 2 NRTIs **or** INSTI-based regimen: Raltegravir *with* 2 NRTIs
Adolescents 12 years of age or older and not sexually mature (SMR 1–3)	NNRTI-based regimen: Efavirenz *with* 2 NRTIs **or** INSTI-based regimen: Raltegravir *with* 2 NRTIs **or** NNRTI-based regimen: Rilpivirine[f] *with* 2 NRTIs

[a] See Table 4 for information on dual NRTI options for use in pediatric patients.

[b] If treatment is initiated before 14 days of age, nevirapine or raltegravir are preferred agents because dosage information is available for this age group. Consultation with an expert in pediatric HIV infection is recommended since clinical trial data are not available suggesting that initiation of antiretroviral treatment within the first 14 days of life improves outcome compared with initiation after 14 days of age. Consider changing from nevirapine to lopinavir/ritonavir when the infant reaches 14 days of age with postmenstrual age 42 weeks or more.

[c] Lopinavir/ritonavir should *not* be used in neonates unless they are at least 14 days of age with postmenstrual age 42 weeks or more.

[d] Darunavir (once daily) should *not* be used in children younger than 12 years of age or weighing less than 40 kg or in patients who have HIV-1 with substitutions associated with darunavir resistance (V11I, V32I, L33F, I47V, I50V, I54L, I54M, T74P, L76V, I84V, L89V).

[e] Dolutegravir is recommended *only* in children and adolescents weighing at least 30 kg.

[f] Rilpivirine should *only* be used in adolescents 12 years of age or older weighing at least 35 kg who have pretreatment viral load 100,000 copies/mL or less.

Adapted from Guidelines for the Use of Antiretroviral Agents in Pediatric HIV Infection (May 22, 2018). Updates may be available at the US Department of Health and Human Services HIV/AIDS Information Services (AIDSinfo) website (http://www.aidsinfo.nih.gov).

Recommended Dual NRTI Options in Children. Use of 2 NRTIs (dual NRTIs) is recommended in all preferred and alternative PI-, NNRTI-, and INSTI-based regimens in pediatric patients. There are 6 commercially available NRTIs; in addition, tenofovir alafenamide and tenofovir DF (nucleotide reverse transcriptase inhibitors) are grouped with the NRTIs for purposes of therapeutic decisions. Table 4 includes recommendations of the HHS Panel on Antiretroviral Therapy and Medical Management of Children Living with HIV regarding preferred and alternative dual NRTIs for use in *initial* treatment regimens in pediatric patients.

Table 4. Dual NRTI Options for Use in Initial PI-, NNRTI-, or INSTI-based Regimens in Pediatric Patients

Age	Dual NRTI Option
Preferred Dual NRTI Options:	
Infants and children from birth to less than 3 months of age	zidovudine and lamivudine (or emtricitabine)
Children 3 months to less than 6 years of age	abacavir and lamivudine (or emtricitabine) or zidovudine and lamivudine (or emtricitabine)
Children and adolescents 6 years of age or older and not sexually mature (SMR 1–3)	abacavir and lamivudine (or emtricitabine) or tenofovir alafenamide and emtricitabine
Adolescents 12 years of age or older and sexually mature (SMR 4 or 5)	(See Table 1 and Table 2.)
Alternative Dual NRTI Options:	
Children 3 months of age or older	abacavir and zidovudine
Children 2–12 years of age	tenofovir DF and lamivudine (or emtricitabine)
Children and adolescents 6 years of age or older and not sexually mature (SMR 1–3)	zidovudine and lamivudine (or emtricitabine)
Dual NRTIs Not Recommended at Any Age:	lamivudine and emtricitabine (similar resistance profile, no additive benefit) abacavir and tenofovir DF (insufficient data) stavudine and zidovudine (antagonistic antiretroviral effects)

Adapted from Guidelines for the Use of Antiretroviral Agents in Pediatric HIV Infection (May 22, 2018). Updates may be available at the US Department of Health and Human Services HIV/AIDS Information Services (AIDSinfo) website (http://www.aidsinfo.nih.gov).

Antiretrovirals and Regimens *Not* Recommended in Children. Based on results of clinical trials in children and adults, monotherapy with any antiretroviral agent alone is considered a suboptimal regimen for treatment of HIV-infected children and is *not* recommended. Use of zidovudine monotherapy is appropriate only in HIV-exposed infants younger than 6 weeks of age when the drug is being used for prevention of perinatal transmission of HIV. (See Guidelines for Use of Antiretroviral Agents: Antiretrovirals for Prevention of Perinatal HIV Transmission.) If HIV infection is confirmed, the infant should be switched to a recommended multiple-drug antiretroviral regimen.

Dual NRTI regimens alone (2 NRTIs without any other antiretroviral) are considered suboptimal regimens for treatment of HIV-infected children and are *not* recommended. Use of 2 NRTIs alone is unlikely to result in sustained viral suppression and leads to the development of viral resistance. For children previously initiated on a dual NRTI regimen who have achieved viral suppression, some clinicians may opt to continue the regimen.

All-NRTI regimens, including triple NRTI regimens that include 3 NRTIs (without any drugs from another class), have been used but are not recommended for *initial* treatment in antiretroviral-naive children because of inferior virologic potency. In addition, a triple NRTI regimen of abacavir, tenofovir DF, and lamivudine (or emtricitabine) or triple NRTI regimen of didanosine, tenofovir DF, and lamivudine (or emtricitabine) are *not* recommended at any time in children because a high rate of early virologic failure was reported when these regimens were used in adults.

Regimens containing agents from 3 different drug classes (e.g., NRTI, NNRTI, and PI or INSTI, NRTI, and PI or NNRTI) are *not* recommended in children because of insufficient data.

Regimens that include didanosine or stavudine are *not* recommended at any time in children and concomitant use of didanosine and stavudine is contraindicated.

Regimens containing 2 PIs given in full dose are *not* recommended for *initial* treatment in children because of insufficient data and potential for added toxicities.

PI-based regimens that include unboosted atazanavir, darunavir, or tipranavir are *not* recommended at any time in pediatric patients because of poor oral bioavailability and inferior virologic activity compared with other PI-based regimens.

PI-based regimens that include once-daily *ritonavir-boosted* darunavir are *not* recommended for *initial* treatment in children younger than 12 years of age because of insufficient data.

PI-based regimens that include fosamprenavir (*ritonavir-boosted* or unboosted), indinavir (*ritonavir-boosted* or unboosted), lopinavir/ritonavir (once-daily dosing), nelfinavir (*ritonavir-boosted* or unboosted), saquinavir (*ritonavir-boosted* or unboosted), or full-dose ritonavir or ritonavir as the only PI are *not* recommended for *initial* treatment in children because of insufficient data or concerns related to toxicity, potency, or inconvenient dosing.

PI-based regimens that include *ritonavir-boosted* tipranavir are *not* recommended at any time in children because of rare reports of intracranial hemorrhage and because of higher ritonavir dose than other *ritonavir-boosted* PIs. Atazanavir and indinavir should *not* be used concomitantly at any time because of potential additional hyperbilirubinemia.

NNRTI-based regimens that include etravirine are *not* recommended for *initial* treatment in pediatric patients because of insufficient data . Nevirapine should *not* be used in NNRTI-based regimens for *initial* treatment in postpubertal girls with $CD4^+$ T-cell counts exceeding 250 /mm^3 or adolescent boys with $CD4^+$ T-cell counts exceeding 400/mm^3. In addition, efavirenz is *not* recommended at any time for children younger than 3 years of age or for sexually active female adolescents when reliable contraception cannot be assured.

Regimens containing an NNRTI and 3 NRTIs are not recommended for *initial* treatment in children because the added cost and complexity outweigh any benefits. In addition, regimens containing 2 NNRTIs are *not* recommended at any time in children because of increased toxicity.

The fixed combination of EVG/c/FTC/TAF is *not* recommended for treatment in children younger than 12 years of age because of insufficient data. The fixed combination of EVG/c/FTC/TDF is *not* recommended in children younger than 12 years of age or in adolescents 12 years of age or older at SMR 1–3.

Because of potential bone toxicity, regimens that include tenofovir DF are *not* recommended for *initial* treatment in children younger than 2 years of age.

Regimens that contain enfuvirtide or maraviroc are *not* recommended for *initial* treatment in children because of insufficient data.

Neonates and Infants Younger than 12 Months of Age. Antiretroviral therapy should be initiated in *all* HIV-infected infants younger than 12 months of age as soon as infection is confirmed, regardless of clinical status, immune status ($CD4^+$ T-cell count or percentage), or viral load. The risk of disease progression is greatest during the first year of life. At any given viral load or level of $CD4^+$ T-cell percentage, there is evidence that the 1-year risk of AIDS or death is substantially higher in younger than in older children, particularly in those younger than 12 months of age. The HHS Panel on Antiretroviral Therapy and Medical Management of Children Living with HIV recommends "urgent" initiation of combination antiretroviral therapy (i.e., within 1–2 weeks) in *all* HIV-infected children younger than 12 months of age.

The majority of pediatric HIV infections are acquired perinatally, and early identification of HIV-exposed neonates is important in providing effective treatment of these infants. Universal HIV counseling and HIV testing of all pregnant women is an important tool for identifying neonates at risk for HIV infection and is recommended as a standard of care for *all* pregnant women in the US. HIV screening should be a routine component of *preconception* care, since this allows women to know their HIV status before conception, and also should be included in the routine panel of *prenatal* screening tests for all pregnant women since this provides an opportunity for appropriate and timely interventions to decrease the risk of maternal-fetal transmission of the virus. (See HIV Testing During Pregnancy under Guidelines for Use of Antiretroviral Agents: Antiretroviral Therapy During Pregnancy.)

If maternal HIV serostatus was not determined during the prenatal or immediate postpartum period, diagnostic testing of the neonate is recommended as soon as possible after birth. Virologic diagnostic testing should be considered at birth for infants at high risk of HIV infection. Specific references should be consulted for information on diagnosis of HIV infection in pediatric patients, including infants with perinatal HIV exposure.

Beginning as soon as possible after delivery (preferably within 6–12 hours), *all* neonates born to HIV-infected woman should receive antiretroviral prophylaxis to reduce the risk of perinatal HIV transmission. (See Guidelines for Use of Antiretroviral Agents: Antiretrovirals for Prevention of Perinatal HIV Transmission.) If subsequent diagnostic testing indicates that a neonate receiving prophylaxis is HIV infected, the prophylaxis regimen should be discontinued and a multiple-drug regimen for treatment of pediatric HIV infection initiated.

Children 1 Year through 5 Years of Age. Although disease progression is less rapid in children 1 year of age or older than in younger children, children who have CDC stage 3-defining opportunistic infections are at high risk of disease progression and death.

The HHS Panel on Antiretroviral Therapy and Medical Management of Children Living with HIV recommends *urgent* initiation of combination antiretroviral therapy (i.e., within 1–2 weeks) in *all* HIV-infected children 1 year through 5 years of age who have CDC stage 3-defining opportunistic illnesses (regardless of immunologic or virologic status) or have CDC stage 3 immunodeficiency based on age-specific $CD4^+$ T-cell count or percentage (i.e., CD4 T-cell count less than 500/mm^3 or percentage less than 22% for children 1 year through 5 years of age).

Initiation of combination antiretroviral therapy is recommended in HIV-infected children 1 year through 5 years of age who have moderate HIV-related symptoms (as designated by CDC), plasma HIV-1 RNA levels exceeding 100,000 copies/mL, or CDC stage 2 immunodeficiency based on age-specific $CD4^+$ T-cell count or percentage (i.e., CD4 T-cell count 500–999/mm^3 or percentage 22–29% for children 1 year through 5 years of age).

Initiation of combination antiretroviral therapy also is recommended in HIV-infected children 1 through 5 years of age who are asymptomatic or have mild HIV-related symptoms (as designated by CDC) *and* have CDC stage 1 immunodeficiency based on age-specific $CD4^+$ T-cell count or percentage (i.e., CD4 T-cell count 1000/mm^3 or greater or percentage 30% or greater for children 1 year through 5 years of age). The relative benefits of initiating antiretroviral therapy in asymptomatic children with low viral burdens and high CD4+ T-cell counts generally outweigh potential risks.

The HHS Panel on Antiretroviral Therapy and Medical Management of Children Living with HIV recommends that, when *urgent* initiation of combination antiretroviral treatment is indicated in children 1 year through 5 years of age because of stage 3-defining opportunistic infections or CDC stage 3 immunodeficiency, discussions with parents/caregivers regarding adherence be expedited and intensive follow-up be provided during the first few weeks of treatment. In children 1 year through 5 years of age who have mild to moderate clinical symptoms or are asymptomatic, additional time can be taken prior to initiation of antiretroviral treatment so that issues regarding adherence can be fully assessed and addressed with the child and parents/caregivers; parents/caregivers of these children may choose to postpone therapy and, on a case-by-case basis, clinicians may elect to defer antiretroviral treatment based on clinical and/or psychosocial factors. If treatment is deferred, clinicians should closely monitor the child's virologic, immunologic, and clinical status every 3–4 months.

Children 6 Years of Age or Older. The HHS Panel on Antiretroviral Therapy and Medical Management of Children Living with HIV recommends *urgent* initiation of combination antiretroviral therapy (i.e., within 1–2 weeks) in *all* HIV-infected children 6 years of age or older who have CDC stage 3-defining opportunistic illnesses (regardless of immunologic or virologic status) or have CDC stage 3 immunodeficiency based on age-specific CD4+ T-cell count or percentage (i.e., CD4 T-cell count less than 200/mm^3 or percentage less than 14% for children 6 years of age or older).

Initiation of combination antiretroviral therapy is recommended in HIV-infected children 6 years of age or older who have moderate HIV-related symptoms (as designated by CDC), plasma HIV-1 RNA levels exceeding 100,000 copies/mL, or CDC stage 2 immunodeficiency based on age-specific CD4+ T-cell count or percentage (i.e., CD4 T-cell count 200–499/mm^3 or percentage 14–25% for children 6 years of age or older).

Initiation of combination antiretroviral therapy also is recommended in HIV-infected children 6 years of age or older who are asymptomatic or have mild HIV-related symptoms (as designated by CDC) and have CDC stage 1 immunodeficiency based on age-specific CD4+ T-cell count or percentage (i.e., CD4 T-cell count 500/mm^3 or greater or percentage 26% or greater for children 6 years of age or older). The relative benefits of initiating antiretroviral therapy in asymptomatic children with low viral burdens and high CD4+ T-cell counts generally outweigh potential risks.

The HHS Panel on Antiretroviral Therapy and Medical Management of Children Living with HIV recommends that, when *urgent* initiation of combination antiretroviral therapy is indicated in children 6 years of age or older because of stage 3-defining opportunistic infections or CDC stage 3 immunodeficiency, discussions with parents/caregivers regarding adherence be expedited and intensive follow-up be provided during the first few weeks of treatment. In children 6 years of age or older who have mild to moderate clinical symptoms or are asymptomatic, additional time can be taken prior to initiation of antiretroviral therapy so that issues regarding adherence can be fully assessed and addressed with the child and parents/caregivers; parents/caregivers of these children may choose to postpone therapy and, on a case-by-case basis, clinicians may elect to defer antiretroviral treatment based on clinical and/or psychosocial factors. If treatment is deferred, clinicians should closely monitor the child's virologic, immunologic, and clinical status every 3–4 months.

Adolescents. Antiretroviral therapy regimens in adolescents must be individualized since HIV-infected adolescents are a heterogeneous group in terms of mode of HIV infection. Many were infected with HIV through sexual exposure or IV drug use during adolescence and generally experience a clinical course that is similar to that of adults; such adolescents are treated most appropriately using the guidelines recommended for adults. (See Guidelines for Use of Antiretroviral Agents: Initial Antiretroviral Therapy in Antiretroviral-naive Adults and Adolescents.) There are, however, increasing numbers of adolescents who were either infected perinatally or in infancy through HIV-infected blood products and such adolescents have an extensive history of antiretroviral treatment and may have a unique clinical course that differs from that of adolescents infected later in life.

Dosage of antiretrovirals in adolescents generally is based on the stage of puberty, rather than strictly on the basis of age. Using the adolescent sexual maturity rating (SMR), adolescents in early puberty (SMR 1–3) are most appropriately treated using pediatric guidelines and dosages and those in late puberty (SMR 4 or 5) are most appropriately treated using adult guidelines and dosages. However, SMR and age are not necessarily directly predictive of the pharmacokinetics of some drugs and there may be some discrepancies between puberty stage-based dosing and age-based dosing since puberty may be delayed in children who acquired HIV perinatally.

Antiretroviral Therapy in Previously Treated Pediatric Patients

Consideration should be given to altering the initial antiretroviral regimen in HIV-infected pediatric patients if there is clinical, immunologic, or virologic evidence of disease progression or if there are signs of toxicity or intolerance or problems with adherence.

Consultation with a specialist who has extensive experience in the care of HIV-infected children is strongly advised when a change in antiretroviral therapy is being considered.

■ Antiretroviral Therapy During Pregnancy

Recommendations for use of antiretrovirals for treatment of HIV infection in pregnant HIV-infected women generally are the same as those for nonpregnant HIV-infected adults; therefore, women should receive optimal antiretroviral therapy regardless of pregnancy status. In the US, multiple-drug antiretroviral therapy with at least 3 drugs is considered the standard of care for the treatment of HIV infection in pregnant women and for prevention of perinatal HIV transmission, and multiple-drug therapy should be discussed with and offered to *all* HIV-infected pregnant women.

Decisions regarding the most appropriate drugs to include in antiretroviral regimens during pregnancy should be made on an individual basis and should involve collaboration between the pregnant woman, her obstetrician, and an HIV specialist. The clinical, virologic, and immunologic status of the woman, results of drug-resistance testing, presence of comorbidities, and the potential for teratogenicity and known and unknown benefits and risks of the drugs to the woman and her fetus should be considered. The HHS Panel on Treatment of Pregnant Women with HIV Infection and Prevention of Perinatal Transmission states that antiretrovirals with known benefit to the HIV-infected woman should not be withheld during pregnancy, unless there are known adverse effects to the mother, fetus, or infant and these adverse effects outweigh the benefits to the woman. (See Safety and Choice of Antiretrovirals During Pregnancy under Guidelines for Use of Antiretroviral Agents: Antiretroviral Therapy During Pregnancy.)

In most cases, HIV-infected women who become pregnant while receiving a multiple-drug antiretroviral regimen that is fully suppressive and well tolerated should continue that regimen during the intrapartum and postpartum period. Discontinuance or interruption of antiretroviral therapy during pregnancy can lead to an increase in viral load, decline in immune status, and disease progression and may increase the risk of perinatal HIV transmission. Women who are currently receiving an antiretroviral regimen that is *not* fully suppressive should be carefully evaluated for adherence and genotypic resistance and every effort should be made to achieve full virologic suppression through adherence interventions or changes in the regimen. Clinicians should consider that there are certain antiretrovirals that should not be continued in pregnant women because of toxicity risks (e.g., didanosine, stavudine, full-dose ritonavir) or that may be associated with low drug exposures during pregnancy and the potential for virologic failure (i.e., cobicistat-boosted elvitegravir) and that modification of the antiretroviral regimen may be indicated. HIV-infected women receiving antiretroviral therapy who present for antenatal care during the first trimester of pregnancy should be advised about the benefits and risks of antiretroviral drugs during this period and that continuation of antiretroviral therapy is recommended.

If an HIV-infected pregnant woman is treatment-naive or treatment-experienced but *not* currently receiving antiretroviral therapy, the HHS panel states that a multiple-drug antiretroviral regimen should be initiated as early in the pregnancy as possible (regardless of plasma HIV-1 RNA levels or CD4+ T-cell counts) and should be continued to maintain viral load below the limits of detection throughout the pregnancy (antepartum and intrapartum) and after delivery. Earlier initiation of antiretroviral treatment may be more effective in reducing perinatal HIV transmission, but the benefits of first trimester antiretroviral therapy should be weighed against first trimester fetal exposure and potential fetal effects of certain antiretroviral agents.

If an HIV-infected pregnant women has plasma HIV-1 RNA levels exceeding 1000 copies/mL (or unknown plasma HIV-1 RNA levels) near the time of delivery, she should receive an intrapartum IV zidovudine prophylaxis regimen initiated at the onset of labor (or 3 hours before scheduled cesarean delivery) and continued until delivery (unless contraindicated because of hypersensitivity) since this may further decrease the risk of perinatal HIV transmission. In addition, *all* neonates born to HIV-infected women (HIV-exposed neonates) should receive an antiretroviral regimen (either prophylaxis or empiric HIV therapy) initiated as soon as possible after birth (preferably within 6–12 hours) and continued for 4–6 weeks. (See Guidelines for Use of Antiretrovirals Agents: Antiretrovirals for Prevention of Perinatal HIV Transmission.)

To monitor maternal-fetal outcomes of pregnant women who receive antiretroviral agents during their pregnancy, an antiretroviral pregnancy registry has been established, and physicians are strongly encouraged to contact the registry at 800-258-4263 or http://www.APRegistry.com to enroll such women. Long-term follow-up of all infants born to women who received antiretroviral therapy during pregnancy is recommended to determine whether there are any late effects of such exposure.

HIV Testing During Pregnancy Since 1995, the USPHS, the American Academy of Pediatrics (AAP), and the American Congress of Obstetricians and Gynecologists (ACOG) have recommended universal HIV counseling and HIV testing (with consent) as a standard of care for *all* pregnant women in the US. This recommendation was made to facilitate optimal antiretroviral treatment of HIV-infected pregnant women, provide an opportunity for appropriate and timely interventions to decrease the risk of maternal-fetal transmission of the virus (antiretroviral therapy, scheduled cesarean delivery, avoidance of breast-feeding), and facilitate early identification and optimal treatment of perinatally infected children.

HIV testing should be a routine component of *preconception* care, since this allows women to know their HIV status before conception, and also should be included in the routine panel of *prenatal* screening tests for all pregnant women. Patients should be informed that HIV screening is recommended for all pregnant women and that the test will be performed unless they decline (opt-out screening).

To promote informed and timely therapeutic decisions, women should be tested for HIV as early as possible during *each* pregnancy. Women who decline the test early in prenatal care should be encouraged to be tested at a subsequent visit.

Repeat HIV testing is recommended during the third trimester of pregnancy in women who had initial negative tests if they are known to be at risk of acquiring HIV, are receiving care in facilities that have an HIV incidence in pregnant women of at least 1 per 1000 per year, are incarcerated, or reside in jurisdictions with elevated HIV incidence.

Expedited HIV testing (i.e., results available within 1 hour) should be performed at the time of labor or delivery in any woman with undocumented HIV status. Appropriate intrapartum and neonatal antiretroviral regimens for prevention of perinatal HIV transmission (see Guidelines for Use of Antiretroviral Agents: Antiretrovirals for Prevention of Perinatal HIV Transmission) should be initiated immediately based on results of the expedited test without waiting for confirmatory tests.

Women who were not tested for HIV before or during labor should undergo expedited HIV testing during the immediate postpartum period (or their infants should undergo expedited HIV testing). If results in the mother or infant are positive, an appropriate neonatal antiretroviral regimen should be initiated immediately.

Safety and Choice of Antiretrovirals During Pregnancy Data from human and/or animal studies indicate that abacavir, atazanavir, darunavir, didanosine, dolutegravir, efavirenz, elvitegravir, emtricitabine, enfuvirtide, etravirine, fosamprenavir, indinavir, lamivudine, lopinavir/ritonavir, maraviroc, nelfinavir, nevirapine, raltegravir, rilpivirine, ritonavir, saquinavir, stavudine, tenofovir, tipranavir, and zidovudine cross the placenta. Because ibalizumab-uiyk is a monoclonal antibody, the drug has the potential to cross the human placenta. Data are not available to date regarding whether bictegravir crosses the human placenta.

The HHS Panel on Treatment of Pregnant Women with HIV Infection and Prevention of Perinatal Transmission states that data from the antiretroviral pregnancy registry regarding first-trimester exposures are sufficient to detect at least a twofold increase in the risk of overall birth defects for darunavir, didanosine, efavirenz, indinavir, raltegravir, rilpivirine, and stavudine; however, no such increases have been detected to date. For abacavir, atazanavir, emtricitabine, lamivudine, lopinavir, nelfinavir, nevirapine, ritonavir, tenofovir DF, and zidovudine, sufficient numbers of first-trimester exposures have been monitored to detect at least a 1.5-fold increase in risk of overall birth defects and a twofold increase in risk of birth defects in the more common classes (cardiovascular and genitourinary systems); however, no such increases have been detected to date. These experts state that data for elvitegravir, etravirine, fosamprenavir, maraviroc, saquinavir, tenofovir alafenamide, and tipranavir are insufficient to date to assess the risk of teratogenicity in humans, but there was no evidence of teratogenicity in animals.

Although animal studies evaluating dolutegravir did not reveal evidence of teratogenicity or adverse fetal or developmental outcomes, neural tube defects have been reported rarely in infants born to women who received dolutegravir.

CNS or other malformations have been reported in cynomolgus monkeys receiving efavirenz during the first trimester and there have been at least 6 retrospective case reports and 1 prospective case report of CNS defects and 1 prospective case report of anophthalmia with facial clefts in humans. The HHS panel states that human data regarding first-trimester efavirenz exposures is sufficient to date to rule out a twofold increase in low-incidence birth defects such as neural tube defects.

Data regarding didanosine and nelfinavir in the Antiretroviral Pregnancy Registry indicate an increased rate of overall birth defects with these drugs compared with the US population-based Metropolitan Atlanta Congenital Defects Program (MACDP) surveillance data, but not when results were compared to the Texas Birth Defect Registry. No particular pattern of defects was detected with either didanosine or nelfinavir and the clinical relevance of this statistical finding is uncertain.

Data are not available regarding teratogenicity of enfuvirtide in humans.

HIV Nucleoside Reverse Transcriptase Inhibitors (NRTIs). Safety and efficacy of zidovudine in pregnant women have been established, and extensive information is available regarding use of the drug in pregnant women. In addition, there has been no evidence of human teratogenicity with abacavir, emtricitabine, lamivudine, stavudine, or tenofovir DF. Although the clinical importance is uncertain and there was no specific pattern of defects, data from the Antiretroviral Pregnancy Registry indicate that didanosine exposures in pregnant women are associated with an increased rate of birth defects compared to the general population.

The HHS Panel on Treatment of Pregnant Women with HIV Infection and Prevention of Perinatal Transmission states that the preferred dual NRTI options for use in multiple-drug antiretroviral treatment regimens in HIV-infected pregnant women are abacavir and lamivudine (should be used only in those negative for HLA-B*5701, may be administered as the fixed combination abacavir/lamivudine; Epzicom®) and tenofovir DF and either emtricitabine or lamivudine (should be used with caution in patients with renal insufficiency).

The dual NRTI option of zidovudine and lamivudine (may be administered as the fixed combination zidovudine/lamivudine; Combivir®) is considered an alternative option. Although zidovudine and lamivudine was previously considered a preferred dual NRTI option, it requires twice-daily dosing and is associated with higher rates of mild to moderate adverse effects (e.g., nausea, headache, reversible maternal and neonatal anemia and neutropenia) than the preferred options.

Didanosine and stavudine are *not* recommended for use in pregnant women because of reported toxicity. The dual NRTI option of didanosine and stavudine should *not* be used at any time, including during pregnancy. Pregnant women receiving these drugs should be switched to a preferred or alternative dual NRTI option.

Safety and pharmacokinetic data regarding use of tenofovir alafenamide during pregnancy are insufficient to date to recommend the drug for use in pregnant women.

HIV Protease Inhibitors (PIs). The HHS Panel on Treatment of Pregnant Women with HIV Infection and Prevention of Perinatal Transmission states that *ritonavir-boosted* atazanavir in conjunction with 2 NRTIs and *ritonavir-boosted* darunavir in conjunction with 2 NRTIs are the preferred PI-based regimens for *initial* treatment in antiretroviral-naive pregnant women. Because of insufficient pharmacokinetic and safety data, the HHS panel states that *cobicistat-boosted* atazanavir and *cobicistat-boosted* darunavir are *not* recommended during pregnancy.

When *ritonavir-boosted* atazanavir is used in pregnant women, some experts suggest that an increased dosage of atazanavir should be used during the second and third trimester. Atazanavir without low-dose ritonavir (unboosted atazanavir) should *not* be used in pregnant women.

When *ritonavir-boosted* darunavir is used in pregnant women, a twice-daily regimen should be used; once-daily regimens of *ritonavir-boosted* darunavir are *not* recommended during pregnancy.

Lopinavir/ritonavir is the alternative PI recommended by the HHS panel for use in conjunction with 2 NRTIs for *initial* treatment in antiretroviral-naive pregnant women. When lopinavir/ritonavir is used in pregnant women, a twice-daily regimen should be used; once-daily lopinavir/ritonavir regimens are *not* recommended during pregnancy. Some experts suggest that an increased dosage of twice-daily lopinavir/ritonavir should be used during the second and third trimesters of pregnancy (especially in antiretroviral-experienced pregnant women and women who start treatment during pregnancy with baseline plasma HIV-1 RNA levels exceeding 50 copies/mL) and state that, if the usual twice-daily lopinavir/ritonavir dosage is used, virologic response and lopinavir plasma concentrations should be monitored.

Ritonavir-boosted saquinavir is not recommended for *initial* treatment regimens in antiretroviral-naive pregnant women because of limited data regarding use in pregnant women, potential toxicities (e.g., risk of PR and QT prolongation, need for baseline ECGs), higher pill burden, and requirement for twice-daily dosing.

Data are insufficient to recommend routine use of *ritonavir-boosted* fosamprenavir for *initial* treatment regimens in antiretroviral-naive pregnant women. If fosamprenavir is used in pregnant women, the drug must be used with low-dose ritonavir (*ritonavir-boosted* fosamprenavir).

Ritonavir-boosted tipranavir is *not* recommended for *initial* treatment regimens in antiretroviral-naive pregnant women.

Because indinavir has a higher pill burden than many other PIs and may be associated with kidney stones, it is *not* recommended for *initial* treatment regimens in antiretroviral-naive pregnant women. If indinavir is used, it should be administered as *ritonavir-boosted* indinavir. Although hyperbilirubinemia has been reported in individuals receiving indinavir, it is not known whether use of indinavir in pregnant women exacerbates physiologic hyperbilirubinemia in their neonates.

Studies in nonpregnant adults indicate that the virologic response to nelfinavir may be lower than that reported with some other antiretrovirals (e.g., lopinavir/ritonavir, efavirenz). Therefore, the HHS panel states that nelfinavir is *not* recommended for *initial* treatment regimens in pregnant women.

Ritonavir should *not* be used alone as the sole PI in antiretroviral regimens in pregnant women.

The fact that hyperglycemia, new-onset diabetes mellitus, exacerbation of preexisting diabetes mellitus, and diabetic ketoacidosis have occurred in HIV-infected individuals receiving PIs should be considered when these drugs are used during pregnancy. In addition, pregnancy is itself a risk factor for hyperglycemia. Most data to date have not shown an increased risk of glucose intolerance in pregnant women receiving a PI-based antiretroviral regimen. HIV-infected women receiving antiretroviral therapy during pregnancy should undergo standard glucose screening at 24 to 28 weeks of gestation. Some experts would perform glucose screening before week 24 in women who were receiving a PI-based antiretroviral regimen prior to pregnancy, especially in those at increased risk for glucose intolerance.

Concomitant use of ergot alkaloids and PIs has been associated with exaggerated vasoconstrictive responses, and concomitant use is contraindicated. Therefore, some experts recommend that women receiving PIs who develop postpartum hemorrhage due to uterine atony should be treated for their postpartum hemorrhage with agents other than methylergonovine (e.g., carboprost, misoprostol, oxytocin, dinoprostone). These experts state that if the need for treatment outweighs the risk and alternative antiretrovirals are not available, methylergonovine can be used in the lowest dosage and shortest duration possible.

HIV Nonnucleoside Reverse Transcriptase Inhibitors (NNRTIs). The HHS Panel on Treatment of Pregnant Women with HIV Infection and Prevention of Perinatal Transmission states that there are no preferred NNRTI-based regimens for *initial* treatment in pregnant women.

Efavirenz in conjunction with 2 NRTIs is considered an alternative NNRTI-based regimen for *initial* treatment in antiretroviral-naive pregnant women. Although efavirenz is associated with adverse CNS and psychiatric symptoms (e.g., dizziness, fatigue, vivid dreams and/or nightmares, increased suicidality risk), it may be suitable if the drug is tolerated and the convenience of a fixed-combination preparation with a once-daily regimen is desired. Because of the potential risk of neural tube defects, the manufacturer states that efavirenz should not be used during the first trimester of pregnancy. The HHS panel states that antiretroviral regimens that do *not* include efavirenz should be strongly considered in women who are planning to become pregnant or are sexually active and not using effective contraception. However, if a woman becomes pregnant while receiving an efavirenz-based regimen and presents for antenatal care during the first trimester of pregnancy, the HHS panel suggests that the regimen can be continued if it is well tolerated and providing adequate virologic suppression. This strategy recognizes that the risk of neural tube defects is restricted to the first 5–6 weeks of pregnancy and that pregnancy is rarely recognized until after 4–6 weeks, and that unnecessary changes in antiretroviral regimens during pregnancy may be associated with loss of virologic control and an increased risk of perinatal HIV transmission.

Rilpivirine is another alternative NNRTI recommended by the HHS panel for use in conjunction with 2 NRTIs for *initial* treatment in antiretroviral-naive pregnant women. However, regimens containing rilpivirine should *only* be used in patients with pretreatment viral load less than 100,000 copies/mL *and* $CD4^+$ T-cell count greater than 200 cells/mm^3. Although some experts state that routine dosage adjustments are not necessary when rilpivirine is used in pregnant women, pharmacokinetics of the drug are highly variable during pregnancy and individual patients should be closely monitored.

Nevirapine in conjunction with 2 NRTIs is *not* recommended for *initial* treatment in antiretroviral-naive pregnant women because of the potential for adverse effects (e.g., hypersensitivity reactions, hepatotoxicity), a complex lead-in dosage regimen, and a low barrier for resistance. The HHS panel states that nevirapine should be used in pregnant women with pretreatment $CD4^+$ T-cell counts of 250/mm^3 or greater *only* if benefits clearly outweigh risks. The HHS panel states that nevirapine may be continued in women who become pregnant while receiving a suppressive nevirapine-based regimen, regardless of their $CD4^+$ T-cell count, as long as the drug is tolerated.

Etravirine is not recommended for *initial* treatment in antiretroviral-naive patients, including pregnant women.

Concomitant use of ergot alkaloids and certain NNRTIs (e.g., efavirenz, delavirdine) is contraindicated because of the risk for acute ergot toxicity. Concomitant use with other NNRTIs (e.g., nevirapine) is not recommended since decreased concentrations of the ergot alkaloids may occur. If methylergonovine is used for the management of postpartum hemorrhage and uterine atony in a woman receiving an NNRTI that is a CYP3A4 inducer (e.g., efavirenz, etravirine, nevirapine), additional uterotonic agents may be needed since the NNRTI could decrease concentrations of the ergot alkaloid resulting in an inadequate treatment effect.

HIV Integrase Inhibitors (INSTIs). The HHS Panel on Treatment of Pregnant Women with HIV Infection and Prevention of Perinatal Transmission states that raltegravir in conjunction with 2 NRTIs is the preferred INSTI-based regimen for *initial* treatment in antiretroviral-naive pregnant women. Data are available regarding the pharmacokinetics of raltegravir during pregnancy and dosage adjustments are not necessary; in addition, experience regarding use of the drug during pregnancy is accumulating. One disadvantage is that a twice-daily regimen of raltegravir is recommended in pregnant women.

Although dolutegravir in conjunction with 2 NRTIs has been considered an alternative INSTI-based regimen for *initial* treatment in antiretroviral-naive pregnant women, neural tube defects involving the brain, spine, and spinal cord have been reported in infants born to women who received dolutegravir. Preliminary results from an ongoing observational study in Botswana indicate a higher risk of neural tube defects in infants born to women who were receiving a dolutegravir-containing regimen at the time of conception or early in the first trimester of pregnancy. Pending further accumulation of data, the HHS Panel on Treatment of Pregnant Women with HIV Infection and Prevention of Perinatal Transmission and the other HHS antiretroviral panels recommend that dolutegravir *not* be initiated in pregnant women who are within 8 weeks from their last menstrual period. If a pregnant woman is already receiving a dolutegravir-containing regimen and it is within 8 weeks from her last menstrual period, the HHS panels recommend that the healthcare provider counsel the woman about the risks and benefits of the current regimen and, if other options are available, a switch to a regimen that does not contain dolutegravir is recommended. If a women is pregnant and it is at least 8 weeks from her last menstrual period, the HHS panels state that consideration can be given to initiating or continuing a dolutegravir-containing regimen *or* initiating or switching to a regimen that does not contain dolutegravir after weighing the risks and benefits. Clinicians can consult the National Perinatal HIV Hotline at 888-448-8765 for additional guidance.

The HHS Panel on Treatment of Pregnant Women with HIV Infection and Prevention of Perinatal Transmission states that safety and pharmacokinetic data are insufficient to recommend use of EVG/c/FTC/TAF or EVG/c/FTC/TDF for *initial* treatment in antiretroviral-naive pregnant women. For women already receiving EVG/c/FTC/TAF or EVG/c/FTC/TDF at the time of pregnancy, the HHS panel suggests switching to a recommended regimen. If the fixed-combination is continued during pregnancy, viral load should be monitored frequently and therapeutic drug monitoring (if available) may be useful.

Data are not available regarding use of the fixed combination BIC/FTC/TAF during pregnancy.

HIV Entry and Fusion Inhibitors. Enfuvirtide and maraviroc are *not* recommended for *initial* treatment in antiretroviral-naive pregnant women because safety and pharmacokinetic data are insufficient regarding use of these drugs during pregnancy. Data are not available regarding use of ibalizumab-uiyk during pregnancy.

■ Antiretrovirals for Prevention of Perinatal HIV Transmission

In the US, multiple-drug antiretroviral regimens are considered the standard of care for treatment of HIV-1 infection in pregnant women and for prevention of perinatal HIV transmission. The HHS Panel on Treatment of Pregnant Women with HIV Infection and Prevention of Perinatal Transmission states that *all* pregnant HIV-infected women in the US should receive multiple-drug antiretroviral therapy, regardless of the woman's plasma HIV-1 RNA level or $CD4^+$ T-cell count.

In addition, to further decrease the risk of perinatal HIV transmission, the HHS panel states that *all* pregnant HIV-infected women with plasma HIV-1 RNA levels exceeding 1000 copies/mL (or unknown plasma HIV-1 RNA levels) near the time of delivery should receive an intrapartum IV zidovudine prophylaxis regimen initiated at the onset of labor (or 3 hours before scheduled cesarean delivery) and continued until delivery (unless contraindicated because of hypersensitivity), regardless of their antepartum antiretroviral regimen and *all* neonates born to HIV-infected women (HIV-exposed neonates) should receive an antiretroviral regimen (either prophylaxis or empiric HIV therapy) initiated as soon as possible after birth (preferably within 6–12 hours) and continued for 4–6 weeks. This strategy of combined antepartum, intrapartum, and neonatal antiretrovirals reduces perinatal HIV transmission by several mechanisms, including lowering maternal antepartum viral load and providing pre- and postexposure prophylaxis in the infant. Ideally, decisions regarding management of HIV infection and prevention of perinatal HIV infection during pregnancy should involve collaboration between an HIV specialist, the pregnant woman, and her obstetrician.

Maternal and neonatal regimens recommended for prevention of perinatal HIV transmission in the US may differ from those used in other countries. A variety of simple or short-course antiretroviral regimens (e.g., single-dose intrapartum and neonatal nevirapine alone or in conjunction with short-course zidovudine with or without lamivudine, intrapartum zidovudine and lamivudine with neonatal zidovudine, intrapartum/neonatal zidovudine alone, neonatal zidovudine alone) have been used for prevention of perinatal HIV transmission in other countries or resource-limited settings (e.g., sub-Saharan Africa).

The current guidelines published by the HHS panel available at http://www.aidsinfo.nih.gov should be consulted for more specific information regarding prevention of perinatal transmission of HIV. In addition, clinicians can consult the National Perinatal HIV Hotline at 888-448-8765 for information regarding antiretroviral treatment of pregnant HIV-infected women and their infants and prevention of perinatal HIV transmission.

Risk of Perinatal HIV Transmission The rate of transmission of HIV infection from infected mothers (who have not received antiretroviral therapy) to their fetuses has been estimated to range from 7–65%, and appears to depend on a variety of factors, including the health status of the mother. With the implementation of universal prenatal HIV counseling and testing, antiretroviral prophylaxis, scheduled cesarean delivery, and avoidance of breast-feeding, the rate of perinatal HIV transmission has decreased to 2% or lower in the US.

Maternal-fetal transmission of HIV can occur in utero, intrapartum, or postpartum via breast-feeding. HIV has been detected in fetal tissue as early as 8–15 weeks of gestation. Based on presence or absence of HIV in cord blood or peripheral blood lymphocytes at birth, it has been estimated that HIV infection is acquired late in gestation or around the time of delivery in 50–70% of cases and earlier in the pregnancy in 30–50% of cases. HIV is distributed in milk, and postpartum transmission of HIV infection to infants can occur through breast-feeding, which is thought to be an important route of transmission in certain patient populations (e.g., in Africa, Haiti). Results of several studies in Africa indicate that the risk of HIV transmission through milk is continuous throughout the period of postpartum breast-feeding, but is greatest during the first 6 months postpartum.

A variety of clinical or biologic factors in the mother appear to influence the risk of maternal-fetal HIV transmission during pregnancy or delivery. The risk of perinatal HIV transmission in untreated women is greater in those with advanced symptomatic disease, high viral load, or low $CD4^+$ T-cell counts than in those with less advanced disease. In pregnant women receiving antiretroviral therapy, viral load and $CD4^+$ T-cell counts may affect the risk of HIV transmission. In one study of pregnant women, plasma HIV-1 RNA levels were significantly higher in those who transmitted the infection to their infants than in those who did not, and the risk of transmission generally increased with increasing maternal viral load. Results of another study indicated that maternal plasma HIV-1 RNA levels at the time of delivery were the strongest predictor of the risk of maternal-fetal transmission of the virus. However, a threshold for viral load below which there is no risk of HIV transmission has not been identified. The risk for perinatal HIV transmission appears to be low in women with plasma HIV-1 RNA levels that are undetectable or less than 1000 copies/mL; however, there have been reports of perinatal transmission of the virus in women with all levels of plasma HIV-1 RNA, including those with levels below the limits of detection. Therefore, use of antiretrovirals during pregnancy for prevention of perinatal HIV transmission is recommended in *all* HIV-infected pregnant women, regardless of plasma HIV-1 RNA levels.

Certain conditions that expose the neonate to large amounts of HIV-infected maternal blood and/or cervicovaginal secretions during labor and delivery (e.g., premature membrane rupture, abruptio placentae, invasive monitoring procedures) may increase the risk of transmission of the virus, even in women with low viral load. There is some evidence that mode of delivery (elective cesarean section, vaginal delivery) may affect the rate of perinatal HIV transmission. A scheduled cesarean delivery is recommended for prevention of perinatal transmission of HIV in women with plasma HIV RNA levels exceeding 1000 copies/mL near the time of delivery and for HIV-infected women with unknown plasma HIV RNA levels. The current guidelines published by the HHS Panel on Treatment of Pregnant Women with HIV Infection and Prevention of Perinatal Transmission available at http://www.aidsinfo.nih.gov should be consulted for specific information on maternal risks and current recommendations regarding when a scheduled cesarean section should be considered in HIV-infected women.

Intrapartum Zidovudine for Prevention of Perinatal HIV Transmission In addition to their current antiretroviral treatment regimen, the HHS Panel on Treatment of Pregnant Women with HIV Infection and Prevention of Perinatal Transmission states that *all* HIV-infected pregnant women with plasma HIV-1 RNA levels exceeding 1000 copies/mL (or unknown HIV-1 RNA levels) near the time of delivery should receive an intrapartum IV zidovudine prophylaxis regimen initiated at the onset of labor (or 3 hours before scheduled cesarean delivery) and continued until delivery (unless contraindicated because of hypersensitivity). These experts state that the intrapartum IV zidovudine prophylaxis regimen also may be considered in pregnant HIV-infected women with plasma HIV-1 RNA levels of 50–999 copies/mL near the time of delivery. Although data are inadequate to determine whether the intrapartum IV zidovudine prophylaxis regimen provides any additional protection against perinatal transmission of HIV in women with plasma HIV-1 RNA levels between 50 and 999 copies/mL, some experts would administer the IV zidovudine prophylaxis regimen to such women since the risk of HIV transmission is slightly higher (approximately 1–2% higher) when viral loads are 50–999 copies/mL compared to when viral loads are less than 50 copies/mL. The intrapartum IV zidovudine prophylaxis regimen is not necessary in HIV-infected women receiving an antiretroviral treatment regimen if they have plasma HIV-1 RNA levels of 50 copies/mL or less during late pregnancy and near delivery, provided there are no concerns related to maternal adherence to the treatment regimen.

If the intrapartum IV zidovudine prophylaxis regimen is indicated and the woman's current antiretroviral regimen includes oral zidovudine, IV zidovudine should be substituted for oral zidovudine until after delivery; other antiretrovirals included in the woman's treatment regimen can be continued orally during labor.

If zidovudine was not included in the antenatal antiretroviral treatment regimen because of known or suspected zidovudine resistance, the HHS panel states that the intrapartum IV zidovudine prophylaxis regimen is still recommended in women with plasma HIV-1 RNA levels exceeding 1000 copies/mL (or unknown HIV-1 RNA levels) near the time of delivery, unless the woman has a documented history of zidovudine hypersensitivity.

Antiretrovirals in HIV-exposed Neonates The HHS Panel on Treatment of Pregnant Women with HIV Infection and Prevention of Perinatal Transmission recommends that *all* neonates born to HIV-infected women (HIV-exposed neonates) receive an antiretroviral regimen (either prophylaxis or empiric HIV therapy) initiated as soon as possible after birth (preferably within 6–12 hours) and continued for 4–6 weeks. The choice of a neonatal antiretroviral prophylaxis regimen *or* a neonatal empiric HIV therapy regimen should be based on an assessment of the likelihood of perinatal HIV transmission.

In HIV-exposed neonates at low risk of perinatal HIV transmission (i.e., infants born to women who were receiving a recommended multiple-drug antiretroviral regimen during pregnancy with sustained viral suppression near delivery and no concerns related to maternal adherence to the treatment regimen), the HHS panel states that a 4-week zidovudine prophylaxis regimen can be used alone. These experts state that HIV-exposed neonates at higher risk of HIV acquisition (e.g., those born to HIV-infected women who did not receive antepartum or intrapartum antiretrovirals, received only intrapartum antiretrovirals, or received antepartum and intrapartum antiretrovirals with suboptimal viral suppression near delivery) should receive a 2-drug prophylaxis regimen that includes a 6-week zidovudine prophylaxis regimen *and* a 3-dose nevirapine prophylaxis regimen. Alternatively, the HHS panel states that neonates at highest risk can receive empiric HIV therapy with a 3-drug regimen of zidovudine, lamivudine, and nevirapine. The 3-drug empiric HIV therapy regimen serves as antiretroviral prophylaxis to prevent acquisition of HIV and also serves as early treatment for neonates who are later confirmed to have acquired HIV. The optimal duration of empiric HIV therapy in neonates at highest risk of HIV acquisition is unknown. Many experts recommend that the 3-drug regimen be continued for 6 weeks; others discontinue nevirapine and/or lamivudine if results of the neonate's HIV nucleic acid amplification test (NAAT) are negative, but recommend continuing zidovudine for 6 weeks.

Because safety and dosage data are not available, the HHS panel states that use of antiretrovirals other than zidovudine, lamivudine, and nevirapine cannot be recommended for premature HIV-exposed neonates (gestational age less than 37 weeks).

■ Antiretrovirals for Preexposure Prophylaxis for Prevention of HIV-1 Infection (PrEP) The fixed combination containing emtricitabine and tenofovir DF (emtricitabine/tenofovir DF; Truvada®) is used for preexposure prophylaxis (PrEP) in conjunction with safer sex practices to reduce the risk of sexually acquired HIV-1 in non-HIV-infected individuals at high risk. Other antiretroviral regimens also have been used or are being investigated for PrEP in high-risk individuals in an attempt to prevent acquisition of the virus, including oral tenofovir DF alone and/or topical antiretrovirals or microbicides (e.g., intravaginal tenofovir gel [not commercially available in the US]).

The principal interventions used for HIV prevention are screening, education, and counseling regarding high-risk behaviors (e.g., condom use, number of sex partners, risky sexual practices, substance abuse, sexually transmitted diseases), HIV testing and linkage to care, and early initiation of antiretroviral treatment in HIV-infected individuals. There is evidence that early initiation of effective multiple-drug antiretroviral regimens in HIV-infected individuals can play an important role in decreasing the risk of secondary HIV transmission through sexual contact. Effective antiretroviral regimens that decrease HIV concentrations in blood and genital secretions and strict adherence to such regimens in conjunction with risk-reduction measures may decrease, but cannot absolutely eliminate, the risk of secondary transmission of HIV to others. Although antiretroviral treatment that suppresses HIV replication and decreases plasma HIV-1 RNA to undetectable levels are associated with decreased HIV concentrations in genital secretions, HIV-1 RNA levels in plasma and genital secretions do not necessarily correlate in all patients. Data from discordant heterosexual couples and men who have sex with men (MSM) indicate that the risk of HIV transmission to an uninfected sexual partner may be substantially decreased when the HIV-infected individual has sustained plasma HIV-1 RNA levels below the limits of detection; however, the risk is not completely eliminated and can be affected by factors such as persistence of HIV in genital secretions, nonadherence to antiretroviral treatment regimens, presence of other sexually transmitted diseases, or increased high-risk behaviors (i.e., risk compensation). HIV transmission to a monogamous uninfected sexual partner from an HIV-infected individual with suppressed plasma viral load has been reported.

Data are accumulating regarding the safety and efficacy of emtricitabine/tenofovir DF PrEP in non-HIV-infected individuals, and it has been suggested that such PrEP may be an important strategy for HIV prevention in high-risk individuals in conjunction with adherence counseling and risk-reduction measures. However, use of PrEP has been controversial since it requires certain important considerations and precautions in the non-HIV-infected individual (e.g., selection criteria, strict adherence to the PrEP regimen, use of PrEP in conjunction with other prevention strategies, close clinical and laboratory monitoring). In addition, further study is needed to more fully evaluate efficacy in specific populations at risk (US populations, low resource settings, MSM, discordant heterosexual couples, injection drug abusers) and to evaluate adverse effects associated with long-term use of antiretrovirals in non-HIV-infected individuals. There also are cost considerations and concerns that use of PrEP may increase the incidence of HIV resistance (especially in nonadherent individuals) and complicate future treatment of HIV infection and that the benefits of PrEP may be offset by increases in high-risk behaviors (i.e., risk compensation).

Emtricitabine/Tenofovir DF Preexposure Prophylaxis for Prevention of HIV-1 Infection (PrEP) The fixed combination emtricitabine/tenofovir DF is labeled by FDA for PrEP in conjunction with safer sex practices to reduce the risk of sexually acquired HIV-1 infection in at-risk HIV-1-negative adults and adolescents weighing 35 kg or more. The manufacturer states that individuals at high risk for HIV-1 infection may include those with partner(s) known to be infected with HIV-1 or those engaging in sexual activity within a high prevalence area or social network and with 1 or more of the following factors: inconsistent or no condom use, diagnosis of sexually transmitted infections, exchange of sex for commodities (e.g., money, food, shelter, drugs), use of illicit drugs, alcohol dependence, incarceration, or partner(s) of unknown HIV-1 status with any of these risk factors.

Efficacy and safety of a once-daily regimen of emtricitabine/tenofovir DF for HIV-1 PrEP were evaluated in a multinational, randomized, double-blind, placebo-controlled, phase 3 trial (Preexposure Prophylaxis Initiative [iPrEx trial]; NCT00458393) that included 2499 HIV-seronegative men or transgender women (male at birth) who have sex with men and have evidence of high-risk behavior for HIV-1 infection. Study participants were randomized to receive emtricitabine/tenofovir DF (single tablet containing 200 mg of emtricitabine and 300 mg of tenofovir DF once daily) or placebo in conjunction with usual prevention strategies (i.e., monthly HIV-1 testing, risk-reduction counseling, condoms, diagnosis and management of sexually transmitted infections) and were followed for 4237 person-years. The primary outcome measure was the incidence of documented HIV seroconversion. There was a 42% reduction in the risk of HIV-1 seroconversion in the group receiving emtricitabine/tenofovir DF (48 individuals receiving emtricitabine/tenofovir DF and 83 individuals receiving placebo seroconverted). Results of a post-hoc case-control study of plasma and intracellular drug concentrations in about 10% of study participants indicated that efficacy of emtricitabine/tenofovir DF PrEP is strongly correlated with adherence since risk reduction appeared to be greatest in those with detectable intracellular tenofovir.

Efficacy and safety of a once-daily regimen of emtricitabine/tenofovir DF for HIV-1 PrEP in HIV-1-seronegative partners of serodiscordant heterosexual couples were evaluated in a randomized, double-blind, placebo-controlled, 3-arm trial (Partners Preexposure Prophylaxis [PrEP] trial; NCT00557245) that included 4758 serodiscordant couples in Kenya and Uganda. The uninfected partners were randomized to receive emtricitabine/tenofovir DF (single tablet containing 200 mg of emtricitabine and 300 mg of tenofovir DF once daily), tenofovir DF (300 mg of tenofovir DF once daily), or placebo (once daily). Study participants received monthly HIV-1 testing, adherence evaluations, sexual behavior assessments, and safety evaluations. Women received monthly pregnancy tests; if pregnancy occurred, the study drug was interrupted during pregnancy and breast-feeding. After 7827 person-years of follow-up, there were a total of 82 emergent HIV-1 seroconversions (overall observed seroincidence rate of 1.05 per 100 person-years). The risk reduction for the emtricitabine/tenofovir DF group relative to the placebo group was 75%. There were 13 seroconversions in partners randomized to emtricitabine/tenofovir DF and 52 seroconversions in partners randomized to placebo (2 and 3 seroconversions, respectively, occurred during interruption of PrEP for pregnancy). Results of a post-hoc case-control study of plasma and drug concentrations in about 10% of study participants indicated that efficacy of emtricitabine/tenofovir DF PrEP is strongly correlated with adherence since risk reduction appeared to be greatest in those with detectable plasma tenofovir.

CDC Recommendations for Preexposure Prophylaxis for Prevention of HIV-1 Infection (PrEP) CDC first issued comprehensive guidelines for clinicians in the US regarding the use of PrEP for prevention of HIV-1 infection in heterosexually active adults and MSM at substantial risk for sexual acquisition of the virus in 2014 and updated these guidelines in 2017. These CDC guidelines provide information on the safety and efficacy of PrEP and include recommendations regarding eligibility prescreening and testing, risk behavior assessment, counseling prior to and during PrEP, and clinical and laboratory follow-up during and after discontinuance of PrEP.

CDC states that PrEP is recommended as one prevention option for sexually active adult MSM in the US at substantial risk for acquiring HIV infection (i.e., those with an HIV-infected sexual partner, recent sexually transmitted bacterial infection, high number of sex partners, history of inconsistent or no condom use, commercial sex work). CDC also states that PrEP is recommended as one prevention option for adult heterosexually active men or women in the US who are at substantial risk for sexual acquisition of HIV infection (i.e., those with an HIV-infected sexual partner, recent sexually transmitted bacterial infection, high number of sex partners, history of inconsistent or no condom use, commercial sex work, in high-prevalence area or network). In addition, CDC states that PrEP is recommended as one prevention option for adult injection drug users in the US at substantial risk of HIV acquisition (i.e., those with an HIV-infected injecting partner and those sharing injection equipment or who recently received drug treatment but are currently injecting). CDC states that the risks and benefits of PrEP for adolescents should be weighed carefully in the context of local laws and regulations about autonomy in health-care decision-making by minors.

If PrEP is used, the recommended regimen for MSM, heterosexually active men and women, and injection drug users in the US is oral emtricitabine/tenofovir DF once daily (a fixed-combination tablet containing 200 mg of emtricitabine and 300 mg of tenofovir DF once daily). Because there is some evidence that use of oral tenofovir DF alone may be effective in heterosexually active men and women and in injection drug users, the CDC states that tenofovir DF monotherapy (300 mg once daily) can be considered an alternative regimen for PrEP only in these specific populations; tenofovir DF alone is *not* recommended for PrEP in MSM.

CDC states that other antiretrovirals (e.g., emtricitabine, tenofovir alafenamide) should *not* be used alone for PrEP and should *not* be used in addition to the recommended emtricitabine/tenofovir DF or tenofovir DF regimens. CDC also states that other dosage regimens of emtricitabine/tenofovir DF or tenofovir DF (e.g., intermittent, episodic) should *not* be used for PrEP.

Acute and chronic HIV infection must be excluded by symptom history and HIV testing immediately before PrEP is initiated. In addition, individuals receiving PrEP must be screened for HIV-1 infection at least once every 3 months. The emtricitabine/tenofovir DF PrEP regimen is inadequate for treatment of HIV-1 infection.

The CDC guidelines and other information regarding PrEP are available at https://www.cdc.gov/hiv/guidelines/preventing.html and should be consulted for more specific information.

■ **Antiretrovirals for Postexposure Prophylaxis following Occupational Exposure to HIV (PEP)** Antiretrovirals are used for postexposure prophylaxis of HIV infection following occupational exposure† (PEP) in health-care personnel and other individuals exposed via percutaneous injury (e.g., needlestick, cut with sharp object) or mucous membrane or nonintact skin (e.g., chapped, abraded, dermatitis) contact with blood, tissue, or other body fluids that might contain HIV.

The principal means of preventing occupationally acquired HIV infection is avoidance of blood and body fluid exposures through the use of safety and isolation practices and strategies outlined in guidelines from the Health Care Infection Control Practices Advisory Committee (HICPAC) and CDC regarding standard precautions for prevention of transmission of infectious agents in health-care settings. While adherence to these and other precautions decreases the incidence of occupational exposure to HIV, accidental exposures that put health-care personnel and others at risk of infection can still occur. There is direct and indirect evidence from animal and human studies that antiretroviral PEP can reduce the risk of HIV transmission and infection. Therefore, use of antiretroviral PEP is important in the management of occupational exposures to HIV.

In 2013, the US Public Health Service (USPHS) issued updated guidelines for management of occupational exposures to HIV and use of PEP following occupational exposures. Although the prior PEP guidelines required an assessment of the level of risk of HIV transmission and infection for each individual exposure incident and recommended either a 2- or 3-drug regimen based on the assessment of risk, the current PEP guidelines no longer require that the level of risk of the exposure be assessed to determine the appropriate number of drugs to include in the PEP regimen. The 2013 USPHS guidelines state that a PEP regimen that includes 3 (or more) antiretrovirals should be used for *all* occupational exposures associated with a risk of HIV transmission. These guidelines also include recommendations regarding preferred and alternative PEP regimens selected based on optimal tolerability and a convenient dosing schedule that encourages completion of the PEP regimen.

Occupational Exposures Associated with Risk of HIV Infection The risk of acquiring HIV following occupational exposure varies depending on the type and severity of exposure.

Types of exposures that place health-care personnel at risk for HIV infection include percutaneous injuries (e.g., needlestick, cut with a sharp object) or contact of mucous membrane or nonintact skin (e.g., when the exposed skin is chapped, abraded, or afflicted with dermatitis) with blood, tissue, or other potentially infectious body fluids from an HIV-infected individual. In addition to blood and body fluids contaminated with visible blood, potentially infectious body fluids include semen and vaginal secretions (these fluids have been implicated in sexual transmission of HIV infection, but have not been implicated in occupational transmission) and CSF and synovial, pleural, peritoneal, pericardial, or amniotic fluids (the risk of transmission of HIV from these fluids has not yet been determined). Other body fluids (e.g., urine, saliva, sputum, nasal secretions, feces, vomitus, sweat, tears) are not considered potentially infectious unless they are visibly bloody. There has been at least one case of documented HIV seroconversion in an individual unintentionally bitten by a patient with advanced HIV infection who, at the time of the bite, was having a tonic-clonic (grand mal) seizure and had saliva contaminated with visible blood. Although transmission of HIV by this route is rare, clinical evaluation must include the possibility that both the person bitten and the person who inflicted the bite were potentially exposed to HIV. Any direct contact (i.e., without barrier protection) to concentrated HIV in a research laboratory or production facility is considered an exposure that requires clinical evaluation and consideration of the need for PEP.

While the true incidence of HIV transmission following occupational exposure to HIV-positive material is unknown, the risk of transmission of the virus is greater following percutaneous exposures than following mucous membrane or skin exposures. The risk of transmission of HIV after occupational exposure to body fluids or tissues other than HIV-infected blood is unknown, but probably is considerably lower than for blood exposures.

Although the risk of HIV transmission associated with an occupational exposure from an HIV-positive individual with plasma HIV-1 RNA levels that are undetectable is thought to be very low, the possibility of transmission cannot be ruled out since HIV transmission has been reported from source individuals with undetectable viral load following sexual exposure and via perinatal transmission.

Percutaneous Exposure. The risk of HIV transmission following a percutaneous injury that results in exposure to HIV-positive blood has been estimated to be approximately 0.3%. The risk appears to be greatest for percutaneous exposures involving a large blood volume (indicated by a needle or other device visibly contaminated with the patient's blood, a procedure that involved a needle being placed directly in a vein or artery, or a deep injury) and/or a source patient with advanced HIV infection. There is evidence that more blood is transferred by deeper injuries and hollow-bore needles.

Mucous-membrane Exposure. The risk of HIV transmission for each episode of mucous membrane exposure to HIV-positive blood is probably too low to measure accurately, but has been estimated to be about 0.09%. In documented cases of HIV transmission following mucous membrane exposure, factors that appeared to contribute to transmission of the virus included a large volume of blood and prolonged duration of contact.

Skin Exposure. The risk of transmission following nonintact skin exposures to HIV-positive blood has not been precisely quantified, but is estimated to be less than that following mucous membrane exposures. There have been documented episodes of HIV transmission from nonintact skin exposures. Compared with exposures that involve intact skin, the risk of HIV transmission presumably would be increased for skin exposures involving an area where skin integrity is visibly compromised.

Choice of Antiretroviral Agents for Postexposure Prophylaxis following Occupational Exposure to HIV (PEP) Although recommendations for PEP initially involved zidovudine monotherapy and subsequently involved selection of a 2- or 3-drug regimen based on the level of risk, multiple-drug antiretroviral regimens that include 3 (or more) antiretroviral agents are now recommended for *all* occupational exposures associated with a risk of HIV transmission. Although the optimal number of antiretrovirals necessary for PEP remains unknown, the recommendation for use of 3 (or more) drugs is based on evidence that regimens that include 3 or more antiretrovirals agents are more effective than monotherapy and 2-drug regimens for the *treatment* of HIV infection and the fact that it is highly likely that occupational exposures to HIV-positive materials will involve resistant strains of HIV.

The USPHS states that the preferred regimen for PEP following an occupational exposure associated with a risk of HIV transmission is raltegravir in conjunction with emtricitabine and tenofovir DF (may be administered as the fixed combination emtricitabine/tenofovir DF; Truvada®). This regimen has a convenient dosing schedule and is potent, tolerable, and associated with minimal potential for drug interactions. These experts also recommend various alternative PEP regimens containing antiretrovirals selected based on known adverse effects and tolerability of the drugs, potential for drug interactions with other antiretrovirals in the regimen or other drugs the exposed individual may be taking, and convenient dosing schedules.

Because strains of HIV resistant to each of the currently available antiretrovirals have been reported and horizontal or vertical transmission of resistant strains can occur, consideration can be given to whether the HIV source is known or suspected to be infected with resistant HIV. If the source person's virus is known or suspected to be resistant to 1 or more antiretrovirals, drugs that the source person's virus is unlikely to be resistant to should be selected for the PEP regimen. Initiation of PEP should *not* be delayed while waiting results of resistance testing of the source person's virus; the regimen can be modified, if necessary, if results become available.

Although the USPHS has made the following recommendations regarding the choice of antiretrovirals to include in PEP regimens, consultation with an expert is recommended whenever possible. Initiation of PEP should *not* be delayed while waiting for expert consultation. (See Initiation and Duration of PEP under Antiretrovirals for Postexposure Prophylaxis following Occupational Exposure to HIV (PEP): Management of Occupational Exposures to HIV, in Guidelines for Use of Antiretroviral Agents.)

HIV Nucleoside Reverse Transcriptase Inhibitors (NRTIs) for PEP Regimens. The USPHS states that the preferred dual NRTI option for use in conjunction with an INSTI, NNRTI, or PI in PEP regimens is emtricitabine and tenofovir DF (may be administered as the fixed combination emtricitabine/tenofovir DF). Alternative dual NRTIs recommended by these experts for use in PEP regimens are tenofovir DF and lamivudine, zidovudine and lamivudine (may be administered as the fixed combination lamivudine/zidovudine; Combivir®), or zidovudine and emtricitabine.

Abacavir is considered an alternative NRTI for PEP regimens, but should be used for PEP *only* with expert consultation since HLA-B*5701 testing is required (see Human Leukocyte Antigen (HLA)-B*5701 Screening under Guidelines for Use of Antiretroviral Agents: Laboratory Monitoring) and such testing may not be available or practical prior to initiating PEP.

Stavudine is considered an alternative NRTI for PEP regimens, but should be used *only* with expert consultation. In addition, stavudine should *not* be used in conjunction with didanosine because of increased risk of toxicity.

Didanosine generally is *not* recommended for use in PEP regimens because of a higher risk for potentially serious or life-threatening adverse effects.

HIV Integrase Inhibitors (INSTIs) for PEP Regimens. The USPHS states that raltegravir in conjunction with emtricitabine and tenofovir DF is the preferred regimen for PEP following an occupational exposure to the virus. Raltegravir also can be used with the recommended alternative dual NRTIs.

These experts state that the fixed combination of elvitegravir, cobicistat, tenofovir DF, and emtricitabine (EVG/c/FTC/TDF) used alone is one of several alternative regimens recommended for PEP.

HIV Protease Inhibitors (PIs) for PEP Regimens. The USPHS states that PI-based regimens of *ritonavir-boosted* darunavir, *ritonavir-boosted* atazanavir, or the fixed combination of lopinavir/ritonavir in conjunction with 2 NRTIs are alternative regimens for PEP.

These experts state that PI-based regimens of fosamprenavir (with or without low-dose ritonavir) or *ritonavir-boosted* saquinavir in conjunction with 2 NRTIs can be considered alternative regimens for PEP, but should be used *only* with expert consultation.

Tipranavir generally is *not* recommended for use in PEP regimens because of a higher risk for potentially serious or life-threatening adverse effects.

Nelfinavir generally is *not* recommended for use in PEP regimens.

HIV Nonnucleoside Reverse Transcriptase Inhibitors (NNRTIs) for PEP Regimens. The USPHS states that NNRTI-based regimens of etravirine or rilpivirine in conjunction with 2 NRTIs are alternative regimens for PEP.

These experts state that efavirenz in conjunction with 2 NRTIs is an alternative regimen, but should be used for PEP *only* with expert consultation.

Because serious adverse effects were reported in individuals who received multiple-drug PEP regimens that included nevirapine, the drug is contraindicated for and should *not* be used in PEP regimens.

HIV Entry and Fusion Inhibitors for PEP Regimens. The USPHS states that enfuvirtide is an alternative antiretroviral for use in PEP regimens, but should be used *only* with expert consultation. Enfuvirtide is *not* usually recommended for PEP regimens since it is administered subcutaneously and is associated with significant adverse effects. In addition, patients receiving the drug may develop anti-enfuvirtide antibodies that could cause false-positive antibody tests in uninfected individuals.

These experts state that maraviroc is an alternative antiretroviral for use in PEP regimens, but should be used *only* with expert consultation. Maraviroc is *not* usually recommended for PEP regimens because of the potential for serious or life-threatening drug interactions and because a coreceptor tropism assay (see Coreceptor Tropism Assay under Guidelines for Use of Antiretroviral Agents: Laboratory Monitoring) should be performed using the source virus to ensure efficacy and such testing may not be available or practical prior to initiating PEP.

Safety and Efficacy of HIV Postexposure Prophylaxis (PEP)

Efficacy of PEP has been difficult to determine because of the low incidence of occupational exposures to HIV and the low seroconversion rate following such exposure. Results of a retrospective case-control study suggest that the risk for HIV infection in health-care personnel who received zidovudine monotherapy for PEP following percutaneous exposure to HIV-positive blood was reduced by approximately 81%. This study included data reported to national surveillance systems in the US, France, and United Kingdom on health-care personnel who had documented occupational percutaneous exposure to HIV-infected blood (i.e., needlestick injury or cut with a sharp object such as a scalpel or lancet) and no other concurrent exposure to HIV.

Prophylaxis Failures. There have been documented cases where PEP with zidovudine monotherapy failed to prevent transmission of HIV in health-care personnel or others exposed to the virus. Although zidovudine prophylaxis was initiated within 0.5–12 hours in most of these individuals, most experienced an acute retroviral illness 13–75 days (median: 22 days) after exposure and seroconverted within 6 months.

There has been at least one report of prophylaxis failure in a health-care personnel who received a 6-week multiple-drug PEP regimen (zidovudine, lamivudine, indinavir, and didanosine) initiated within 40 minutes following a needle-stick injury that occurred while drawing blood from a parenteral drug abuser who was infected with HIV and hepatitis C virus (HCV). The health-care worker became HIV-positive and HCV-positive about 6 weeks after PEP was finished; HIV isolated from the health-care worker had a mutation associated with low-level zidovudine resistance and HIV isolated from the source patient had a mutation associated with lamivudine resistance but not the one associated with low-level zidovudine resistance. There have been 2 other reports of health-care workers allegedly seroconverting despite PEP with a multiple-drug regimen after occupational exposure to HIV; however, epidemiologic investigations and viral sequence comparisons indicated that HIV transmission in these 2 cases did not occur as a result of the reported occupational exposure.

Adverse Effects of PEP Regimens. A substantial proportion of health-care personnel receiving previously recommended PEP regimens after occupational exposures to HIV experienced adverse effects and many were unable to complete a full 4-week prophylaxis regimen because of inability to tolerate the drugs.

Although there is no evidence to date that any unusual adverse effects occur when antiretrovirals are used in healthy individuals for PEP, multiple-drug PEP regimens can be associated with adverse effects and these effects may impact adherence to and/or completion of the regimen. Serious adverse effects (e.g., nephrolithiasis, hepatitis, pancytopenia) have been reported rarely in health-care personnel receiving antiretroviral regimens for PEP.

Information regarding tolerability of multiple-drug regimens previously used for PEP in health-care workers following occupational exposure to HIV is available from the Human Immunodeficiency Virus Postexposure Prophylaxis (HIV PEP) Registry, a prospective surveillance project that collected data from October 17, 1996 through March 31, 1999 and was sponsored by the CDC and 2 antiretroviral agent manufacturers. The registry (now closed) included data on 492 US health-care workers (71% female, median age: 37 years) who received PEP following an occupational exposure to HIV (63% received a regimen containing 3 or more antiretroviral agents). Overall, 76% of health-care workers for whom 4- to 6-week follow-up was available reported some symptom or adverse effect. The most frequent adverse effects were nausea (57%), fatigue/malaise (38%), headache (18%), vomiting (16%), and diarrhea (14%) and these effects generally were evident within 3–4 days after initiation of the PEP regimen. Of those who discontinued all drugs before completion of the PEP regimen, 50% did so because of adverse effects. A variety of PEP regimens were used (e.g., zidovudine monotherapy; zidovudine and lamivudine with or without indinavir; zidovudine, lamivudine, and saquinavir), and it was not possible to correlate toxicity with any particular drug. Although there were no reports of unusual adverse effects, serious adverse effects requiring dosage reduction or discontinuance of the PEP regimen (high fever and rash; adverse renal effects such as renal calculi, flank pain, and hematuria; adverse GI effects such as intractable vomiting or nausea; involuntary muscle movements or adverse ophthalmic effects) were reported in 6 health-care workers. All reported adverse effects resolved following completion or discontinuance of PEP.

Additional information regarding adverse effects reported in health-care workers who received multiple-drug regimens for PEP is available from individual case reports or small prospective and retrospective studies in individual health-care facilities. In one facility, 68 health-care workers received PEP (zidovudine and lamivudine with or without indinavir) and 75% reported at least one adverse effect; adverse effects were more frequent in those receiving the 3-drug regimen and many failed to complete the 28-day regimen because of adverse effects. In a small retrospective study, most individuals who discontinued or modified their PEP regimens did so because of intolerable adverse effects that appeared to be related to indinavir (e.g., uncontrollable vomiting, nausea, or reflux; urticaria; galactorrhea with hyperprolactinemia). In a prospective study in France that evaluated adverse effects reported with a PEP regimen of zidovudine, lamivudine, and nelfinavir, 85% experienced at least one adverse effect (diarrhea, nausea, and vomiting were reported most frequently) and 25% discontinued nelfinavir from the regimen because of adverse effects.

Because serious adverse effects, including hepatotoxicity (e.g., end-stage liver failure requiring transplantation, clinical hepatitis, and elevated serum

ALT and AST concentrations without clinical hepatitis), skin reaction, and/or rhabdomyolysis, were reported in individuals who received multiple-drug PEP regimens that included nevirapine, nevirapine is contraindicated for and should *not* be used for PEP.

Health-care personnel receiving PEP following an occupational exposure to HIV should be advised of the potential adverse effects and drug interactions associated with the regimen. Careful counseling about such effects may be necessary to improve adherence. In some cases, preemptive prescribing of antiemetic and antispasmodic agents may be useful to ameliorate adverse effects and may improve adherence to the PEP regimen.

Health-care personnel receiving PEP should be monitored for toxicity by testing at baseline and 2 weeks after initiation of the regimen. The scope of testing should be based on medical conditions in the exposed individual and the known and anticipated toxicities of the drugs included in the regimen. At a minimum, complete blood counts (CBCs) and renal and hepatic function should be monitored. Depending on the clinical situation, further diagnostic studies may be indicated (e.g., monitoring for hyperglycemia in a diabetic if the PEP regimen includes a PI).

If toxicity occurs, modification of the PEP regimen should be considered with expert consultation.

Management of Occupational Exposures to HIV Each health-care facility should develop institutional policies and protocols for management of occupational exposures that put health-care personnel and others at risk of HIV infection. These policies should include appropriate procedures for documenting and reporting such exposures, determining the HIV status of the source person, acquiring expert consultation from in-house infectious disease experts or outside experts, and appropriate immediate and follow-up postexposure testing, care, and counseling for the exposed individual.

Since the great majority of occupational exposures to HIV do not result in transmission of the virus, the potential benefits and risks of PEP (including the potential for severe toxicity and/or drug interactions) must be considered carefully and, whenever possible, decisions regarding PEP should be made in consultation with experts.

Assessment of the Type of Occupational Exposure and Associated Risk. An assessment of the likelihood of HIV transmission from the exposure should be made, taking into consideration information about the HIV source and the type of exposure. The exposure should be evaluated for potential to transmit HIV based on the type of body substance involved and the route and severity of the exposure.

Exposure to blood, tissue, other body fluid containing visible blood, or other potentially infectious fluid (e.g., semen, vaginal secretions, CSF, and synovial, pleural, peritoneal, pericardial, amniotic fluids) or tissue resulting from a percutaneous injury (i.e., needlestick or cut with a sharp object) or through contact of mucous membrane or nonintact skin (e.g., exposed skin that is chapped, abraded, or affected by dermatitis) are situations that pose a risk for HIV transmission and require further evaluation. Feces, nasal secretions, saliva, sputum, sweat, tears, urine, and vomitus are not considered potentially infectious unless they are visibly bloody.

Any direct contact (i.e., contact without barrier protection) with concentrated HIV in a research laboratory or production facility is considered an exposure that requires clinical evaluation to assess the need for PEP.

For human bites, the clinical evaluation must consider possible exposure of both the bite recipient and the person who inflicted the bite. While HIV transmission only rarely has been reported by this route, postexposure follow-up (including consideration of PEP) may be indicated if a bite results in blood exposure to either person involved.

Evaluation and Testing of the Source. The individual whose blood or body fluids are the source of an occupational exposure should be immediately evaluated for HIV infection and HIV antibody testing performed if indicated.

If the source individual is known to be HIV seropositive, information regarding their viral load, current and previous antiretroviral therapy, and genotypic or phenotypic viral resistance testing should be collected and may be considered when selecting the PEP regimen for the exposed individual. Initiation of PEP should *not* be delayed while acquiring this information.

If the exposure involved an HIV-infected source, information regarding whether or not the individual harbors drug-resistant HIV may or may not be available. Resistance testing of the source at the time of exposure will *not* provide results soon enough to influence selection of the PEP regimen. If the exposure involved an HIV-infected source known or suspected to harbor drug-resistant HIV, expert consultation is recommended regarding selection of an optimal PEP regimen. However, initiation of PEP should *not* be delayed while waiting for expert consultation. If drug resistance information about the source becomes available later in the course of PEP, additional expert consultation is recommended regarding possible modification of the PEP regimen.

If the exposure involved an HIV-infected source who had undetectable plasma HIV-1 RNA at the time of the exposure, this does *not* eliminate the possibility of HIV transmission and does *not* eliminate the need for PEP and follow-up testing in the exposed individual.

If the exposure involved a source individual who is HIV seronegative and has no clinical evidence of AIDS or symptoms of HIV infection, no further testing of the source is indicated. The likelihood of the source individual being in the window period of HIV infection before seroconversion (i.e., period between initial HIV infection and development of detectable HIV antibodies) is extremely small.

If the HIV status of the source individual is unknown, availability of rapid HIV testing facilitates timely decisions regarding the need for PEP in the exposed individual. Results of some HIV tests may be available within 30–60 minutes; however, initiation of PEP should *not* be delayed while waiting for test results. If the source individual is determined to be HIV negative, PEP should be discontinued and testing of the exposed individual is not necessary.

If the exposure source is unknown or cannot be tested (e.g., needle in disposal container or laundry), decisions regarding PEP should be made on an individual basis with expert consultation. Important considerations in these cases are the severity of the exposure and the epidemiologic likelihood of HIV exposure.

HIV testing of needles or other sharp instruments involved in an exposure (regardless of whether the source is known) is not recommended.

Initial Evaluation and Testing of Exposed Health-care Personnel. Following an occupational exposure, the exposed individual should be evaluated immediately and should be tested to establish HIV serostatus at the time of exposure. The exposed individual should be questioned regarding other drugs they may currently be taking and any current or underlying medical conditions or circumstances (e.g., pregnancy, breast-feeding, renal or hepatic disease) that may influence choice of antiretrovirals for a PEP regimen. A pregnancy test should be offered to all nonpregnant women of childbearing age whose pregnancy status is unknown.

If the source individual is found to be HIV seronegative, baseline HIV testing and further follow-up testing of the exposed individual normally is not necessary.

Regardless of whether PEP is initiated, follow-up reevaluation and counseling of the exposed individual is strongly recommended within 72 hours after the exposure to reassess the risks and benefits of PEP.

Initiation and Duration of PEP. If PEP is appropriate for the exposure and the exposed health-care worker elects to receive PEP, it should be initiated as soon as possible (preferably within hours) following the exposure. To ensure timely access to PEP, an occupational exposure should be regarded as an urgent medical concern. When the most appropriate regimen to administer is unclear, it probably is preferable to immediately initiate a PEP regimen while waiting for expert consultation.

Although there is some evidence from animal studies suggesting that prophylaxis is likely to be less effective when initiated more than 72 hours after exposure, the interval after which there is no benefit from PEP has not been defined in humans. If initiation of PEP is delayed, there is an increased likelihood that benefits might not outweigh risks. However, initiating PEP after a longer interval (e.g., 1 week) might still be considered for exposures associated with an extremely high risk of transmission.

The optimal duration of PEP is unknown. In animal models, the duration of PEP has been shown to influence success. Based on evidence that 4 weeks of PEP appeared protective in vitro and in animal and occupational studies, PEP should be administered for 4 weeks, if tolerated.

Follow-up and Counseling of Exposed Health-care Personnel. Health-care personnel with occupational exposure to HIV should receive postexposure testing, medical evaluation, and counseling regardless of whether they receive PEP.

Follow-up HIV testing should be performed at baseline and at 6 weeks, 12 weeks, and 6 months after the exposure to determine whether transmission of HIV occurred. Extended follow-up (e.g., for 12 months) is recommended for health-care personnel who become infected with HCV following exposure to a source coinfected with both HIV and HCV; however, it is unclear whether extended follow-up is necessary in other circumstances. Although rare cases of delayed HIV seroconversion have been reported, this probably does not warrant increasing the exposed individual's anxiety by routinely extending the duration of postexposure follow-up. However, this does not preclude a decision to extend follow-up in an individual situation based on the clinical judgment of the health-care provider. HIV testing should be performed in any health-care worker who has an illness that is compatible with an acute retroviral syndrome, regardless of the interval since exposure.

Exposed health-care workers should be advised to use measures to prevent secondary transmission of HIV during the follow-up period, especially during the first 6–12 weeks following the exposure. These individuals should be counseled to avoid donating blood or tissue, to use barrier contraception and avoid pregnancy, and to avoid breast-feeding if possible.

Exposed individuals should be advised of the potential adverse effects of the PEP regimen and that evaluation of certain symptoms should not be delayed (e.g., rash, fever, back or abdominal pain, pain on urination, blood in the urine, dark urine, yellowing of skin or whites of the eyes, symptoms of hyperglycemia such as increased thirst or frequent urination).

Individuals receiving PEP should be advised of the importance of adhering to and completing the recommended regimen.

Situations for Which Expert Consultation Regarding PEP Is Advised. Because evaluation and management of occupational exposures to HIV can be complex, clinicians should consult local experts and/or the National Clinicians' Postexposure Prophylaxis Hotline (PEPline) at 888-448-4911 or http://www.nccc.ucsf.edu/about_nccc/pepline/ whenever possible. At a minimum, the USPHS recommends expert consultation in the following situations:

- **Occupational exposure report is delayed (i.e., more than 72 hours after the exposure):** The interval after which there is no benefit from PEP is undefined.
- **Source is unknown (e.g., needle in sharps disposal container or laundry):** The use of PEP is decided on a case-by-case basis, taking into con-

sideration the severity of the exposure and epidemiologic likelihood of HIV exposure. Needles or other sharp instruments should *not* be tested for HIV.

- **Exposed individual is known or suspected to be pregnant or is breast-feeding:** Initiation of PEP should *not* be delayed while waiting for expert consultation.
- **Source virus is known or likely to be resistant to antiretroviral agents:** If the source individual's virus is known or suspected to be resistant to at least 1 of the drugs being considered for the PEP regimen, a regimen should be selected that includes antiretrovirals to which the source individual's virus is unlikely to be resistant. Initiation of PEP should *not* be delayed while waiting for results of resistance testing of the source individual's virus.
- **Toxicity occurs with the initial PEP regimen:** Symptoms (e.g., GI and others) often can be managed by prescribing antimotility and/or antiemetic agents without changing the PEP regimen. Counseling and support for management of adverse effects is important since symptoms are often exacerbated by anxiety.
- **Exposed individual has serious medical illness:** The risk of drug toxicity and drug interactions may be increased if the exposed individual has significant underlying illness (e.g., renal disease) or is already taking multiple medications.

USPHS Recommendations for HIV Postexposure Prophylaxis following Occupational Exposure (PEP) Current USPHS guidelines for management of occupational exposures to HIV and use of PEP include the following recommendations.

- **A PEP regimen containing 3 (or more) antiretroviral agents is recommended for all occupational exposures associated with risk of HIV infection.** These exposures include percutaneous injury or contact of mucous membrane or nonintact skin with blood, tissue, or other body fluids from a source person known or suspected to be infected with HIV.
- **The preferred PEP regimen is raltegravir in conjunction with emtricitabine and tenofovir DF (may be administered as the fixed combination emtricitabine/tenofovir DF).** This regimen has a convenient dosing schedule and is potent, tolerable, and associated with minimal drug interactions.
- **Alternative PEP regimens include certain PIs (ritonavir-boosted darunavir, ritonavir-boosted atazanavir, lopinavir/ritonavir) or certain NNRTIs (etravirine, rilpivirine) in conjunction with 2 NRTIs (dual NRTIs). The fixed combination containing elvitegravir (EVG/c/FTC/TDF) used alone is another recommended alternative PEP regimen.** Although alternative regimens that contain certain other antiretrovirals (i.e., efavirenz, enfuvirtide, fosamprenavir, maraviroc, saquinavir) in conjunction with 2 NRTIs can be used for PEP, these regimens should be used *only* with expert consultation.
- **The preferred dual NRTI option for use in PEP regimens is emtricitabine and tenofovir DF (may be administered as the fixed combination emtricitabine/tenofovir DF); alternative dual NRTI options are tenofovir DF and lamivudine, zidovudine and lamivudine (may be administered as the fixed combination lamivudine/zidovudine; Combivir®), or zidovudine and emtricitabine.**
- **PEP should be initiated as soon as possible (preferably within hours) following an occupational exposure associated with risk of HIV infection.** To ensure timely access to PEP, an occupational exposure should be regarded as an urgent medical concern and treated immediately.
- **PEP should be administered for 4 weeks, if tolerated.** Although optimal duration of PEP is unknown, 4 weeks has been protective in vitro and in animal and occupational studies.
- **Whenever possible, the HIV status of the source person should be determined to guide appropriate use of PEP.** Depending on the type of test used, results may be available within 30–60 minutes; however, initiation of PEP should *not* be delayed while waiting for HIV test results. If the source person is found to be HIV negative, PEP should be discontinued and follow-up HIV testing is not necessary in the exposed individual.
- **If the source person is known to harbor drug-resistant HIV, expert consultation is recommended to identify an optimal PEP regimen.** Initiation of PEP should *not* be delayed while waiting for expert consultation.
- **When PEP is prescribed, the exposed individual should be advised of the importance of adhering to and completing the regimen and advised about possible drug toxicities and drug interactions associated with the regimen.** To monitor for adverse effects, CBCs and renal and hepatic function tests should be performed at baseline and 2 weeks after initiation of PEP; additional testing may be indicated if abnormalities are detected or adverse effects occur.
- **Regardless of whether PEP is prescribed, the exposed individual should be reevaluated within 72 hours after the exposure.** This provides an opportunity to reassess the risks and benefits of PEP, helps ensure adherence and follow-up, and is especially important if additional information becomes available about the exposure incident or source individual.
- **Health-care personnel with occupational exposure to HIV should receive counseling at the time of exposure and at follow-up appointments.** These individuals should be advised to use precautions to prevent possible secondary transmission (e.g., avoidance of blood or tissue donations, use of barrier contraception and avoidance of pregnancy and breast-feeding), especially during the first 6–12 weeks after the exposure.
- **HIV testing should be used to monitor for seroconversion after occupational exposure to HIV.** HIV testing should be performed at baseline and at 6 weeks, 12 weeks, and 6 months after the exposure. Use of a fourth-generation combination HIV p24 antigen-HIV antibody test allows earlier detection of HIV infection; if a fourth generation test is used, HIV testing could be performed at baseline and at 6 weeks and 4 months after the exposure.
- **If HIV infection is identified in the exposed individual, the person should be referred to a specialist with expertise in HIV treatment.**
- **Clinicians seeking information and guidance regarding the management of an occupational exposure to HIV and additional information on PEP can consult the National Clinicians' Postexposure Prophylaxis Hotline (PEPline) at 888-448-4911 or http://nccc.ucsf.edu/clinician-consultation/pep-post-exposure-prophylaxis/.**
- **Any unusual or severe toxicity associated with PEP should be reported to the manufacturer and/or the FDA MedWatch program at 800-332-1088 or http://www.fda.gov/Safety/MedWatch/default.htm.**
- **Cases of occupationally acquired HIV or failures of PEP should be reported to the CDC at 404-639-2050.**

Adapted from Updated US Public Health Service Guidelines for the Management of Occupational Exposures to Human Immunodeficiency Virus and Recommendations for Postexposure Prophylaxis. Infect Control Hosp Epidemiol. 2013; 34: 875-92 (may be available at http://www.jstor.org/stable/10.1086/672271).

■ Antiretrovirals for Postexposure Prophylaxis following Sexual, Injection Drug Use, or other Nonoccupational Exposures to HIV (nPEP)

Antiretrovirals are used for postexposure prophylaxis of HIV infection following nonoccupational exposure† (nPEP) in individuals exposed to blood, genital secretions, or other potentially infectious body fluids that might contain HIV when that exposure represents a substantial risk for HIV transmission.

The most effective means for preventing HIV infection are methods that protect against exposure. Antiretroviral agents given after HIV exposure cannot replace behaviors that help avoid such exposure (e.g., sexual abstinence, sex in a mutually monogamous relationship with a noninfected partner, consistent and correct condom use, abstinence from injection drug use, consistent use of sterile equipment by those unable to cease injection drug use). However, data from animal transmission models, clinical studies evaluating antiretroviral prophylaxis for prevention of perinatal HIV transmission, observational studies evaluating use of PEP in health-care personnel following occupational exposures, and observational and case studies of antiretroviral prophylaxis following sexual exposures (e.g., sexual assault, inadvertent artificial insemination from an HIV-positive donor) or other nonoccupational exposures (e.g., needlestick injection, piercing, cutting with a sharp object) indicate that nPEP can reduce the risk of HIV infection following nonoccupational exposures.

In 2016, CDC issued updated guidelines for management of nonoccupational exposures to HIV and recommendations regarding use of nPEP following nonoccupational exposures. These guidelines include new evidence on efficacy and safety of nPEP, updated information on laboratory evaluation of the source and exposed individuals, recommendations regarding preferred and alternative 3-drug nPEP regimens, information on follow-up evaluations, and suggestions for transitioning between nPEP and PrEP when appropriate for certain individuals at risk for frequent, recurring HIV exposures.

Nonoccupational Exposures Associated with Risk of HIV Infection Nonoccupational exposures that place an individual at risk for HIV infection include direct mucosal (vagina, rectum, eye, mouth, other mucosal membranes), nonintact skin, percutaneous, or IV contact with potentially infectious body fluids that occur outside of health-care settings and do not involve perinatal exposures. Potentially infectious body fluids from HIV-infected individuals that are considered to be associated with a substantial risk for HIV transmission include blood, semen, vaginal secretions, rectal secretions, breast milk, or any body fluid visibly contaminated with blood. Regardless of the known or suspected HIV status of the source individual, other body fluids (e.g., urine, saliva, nasal secretions, sweat, tears) are considered negligible risks for HIV transmission following nonoccupational exposures unless they are visibly contaminated with blood.

Individuals who have had nonoccupational exposure to potentially infectious fluids of an HIV-infected individual are at highest risk for HIV infection, especially if the HIV-infected individual is not receiving antiretroviral therapy. Individuals who have had nonoccupational exposure to potentially infectious fluids of a person of unknown HIV status are at unknown risk for acquiring HIV infection. If the source is known to be from a group with a high prevalence of HIV infection (e.g., MSM, needle-sharing injection drug user), the risk for unrecognized HIV infection in the source is increased. If the source individual recently acquired HIV infection, the risk for HIV transmission may be particularly high since the viral burden in the blood and semen of such individuals may be particularly high.

Nonoccupational exposures to potentially infectious body fluids from an HIV-infected individual are associated with different levels of risk for HIV transmission depending on the route. The highest levels of risk are associated with blood transfusions, needle-sharing injection drug use, receptive anal intercourse, and percutaneous needle stick. Other types of sexual exposures are associated with a lower level of risk; biting, spitting, and thrown body fluids (e.g., semen, saliva) are associated with a negligible level of risk.

Management of Nonoccupational Exposure to HIV The decision to initiate nPEP should be individualized based on the HIV status of the potentially exposed individual, HIV status of the source of the body fluids, timing regarding when the most recent sexual, injection drug use, or other nonoccupational exposure occurred, frequency of HIV exposures, and the transmission risk associated with the exposure (i.e., whether the potentially infected body fluids and exposure routes are associated with a substantial risk of HIV transmission). The likelihood of exposure to and need for prophylaxis or treatment of other transmissible infections (e.g., gonorrhea, chlamydial infection, trichomoniasis, HBV, HCV) or other health consequences of the exposure event (i.e., pregnancy) also should be considered.

Following a nonoccupational exposure to HIV, initiation of nPEP usually is recommended when the exposed individual is HIV-negative, the source of the potentially infected body fluids is HIV-positive, the most recent exposure occurred within the last 72 hours, and the reported exposure represents a substantial risk for HIV transmission.

Because exposed individuals might not know whether they are already infected with HIV, baseline HIV testing should be performed on all individuals seeking evaluation for potential nonoccupational HIV exposure, preferably using rapid antigen/antibody (Ag/Ab) combination HIV tests. If the HIV status of the source individual is unknown and the reported exposure would represent a substantial risk for HIV transmission if the source was HIV-positive, the decision to administer nPEP should be determined on a case-by-case basis. If the source individual is available and consents, the individual should be evaluated clinically and undergo HIV testing, preferably using rapid Ag/Ab combination HIV tests. If the risk for HIV transmission associated with the exposure is high, nPEP can be initiated in the exposed individual and then continued or discontinued if the HIV status of the source individual can be determined.

Available data indicate that nPEP is most effective when initiated as soon as possible after exposure and is unlikely to be effective if initiated more than 72 hours after exposure. Therefore, nPEP is *not* recommended if an individual seeks care more than 72 hours after a potential nonoccupational exposure to HIV.

If the reported exposure represents no substantial risk of HIV transmission, nPEP is *not* recommended. In addition, nPEP should be used only for infrequent exposures. Individuals who engage in behaviors that result in frequent, recurrent exposures (e.g., HIV discordant sex partners who inconsistently use condoms, injection drug users who often share injection equipment) should *not* receive frequent, repeated courses of nPEP. Such individuals need risk-reduction interventions and, in some cases, consideration can be given to transitioning the patient to PrEP after completion of nPEP. (See Guidelines for Use of Antiretroviral Agents: Antiretrovirals for Preexposure Prophylaxis for Prevention of HIV-1 Infection (PrEP).)

CDC Recommendations for HIV Postexposure Prophylaxis following Nonoccupational Exposure (nPEP) Current CDC guidelines for management of nonoccupational exposures to HIV and use of nPEP include the following recommendations.

- **When an individual seeks care within 72 hours after a sexual, injection drug use, or other nonoccupational exposure to HIV, the HIV status of the exposed individual should be determined, the HIV status of the source individual should be determined (if possible), and the type of exposure (i.e., type of potentially infectious body fluids, exposure route) should be evaluated to determine whether the exposure represents with a substantial risk of HIV transmission.** HIV status should be determined using rapid Ag/Ab combined HIV tests whenever possible. If rapid HIV tests are unavailable, nPEP should be initiated in the exposed individual without delay if the source is known to have HIV infection and the reported exposure represents a substantial risk for HIV transmission; if the exposed individual is later determined to already be infected with HIV, nPEP can be changed to an appropriate antiretroviral treatment regimen.
- **nPEP is not indicated if the exposed individual is HIV-positive, if the source individual is HIV-negative, if it has been more than 72 hours since the most recent nonoccupational exposure to HIV, or if the exposure is determined to be associated with a negligible risk for HIV transmission.**
- **When indicated, nPEP should be initiated as soon as possible (within 72 hours) following nonoccupational exposure associated with a substantial risk of HIV transmission and should be continued for 28 days.**
- **An nPEP regimen containing 3 antiretroviral agents is recommended for all nonoccupational exposures associated with a substantial risk of HIV transmission.** Baseline serum creatinine and estimated creatinine clearance should be determined to aid in selection of the most appropriate nPEP regimen.
- **For adults and adolescents 13 years of age or older with normal renal function (creatinine clearance of 60 mL/minute or greater), the preferred nPEP regimen is raltegravir (or dolutegravir) in conjunction with emtricitabine and tenofovir DF (administered as the fixed combination emtricitabine/tenofovir DF).** The alternative nPEP regimen recommended for such individuals is *ritonavir-boosted* darunavir in conjunction with the fixed combination emtricitabine/tenofovir DF.
- **For adults and adolescents 13 years of age or older with renal impairment (creatinine clearance of 59 mL/minute or lower), the preferred nPEP regimen is raltegravir (or dolutegravir) in conjunction with zidovudine and lamivudine (dosage adjusted based on the degree of renal impairment).** The alternative nPEP regimen recommended for such individuals is *ritonavir-boosted* darunavir in conjunction with zidovudine and lamivudine (dosage adjusted based on the degree of renal impairment).
- **For children 2–12 years of age, the preferred nPEP regimen is raltegravir in conjunction with emtricitabine and tenofovir DF.** Alternative nPEP regimens recommended for such children are raltegravir (or lopinavir/ritonavir) in conjunction with zidovudine and lamivudine or lopinavir/ritonavir in conjunction with emtricitabine and tenofovir DF. A regimen of *ritonavir-boosted* darunavir in conjunction with emtricitabine and tenofovir DF is another alternative in children 3–12 years of age.
- **For infants 4 weeks to less than 2 years of age, the preferred nPEP regimen is raltegravir (or lopinavir/ritonavir) in conjunction with zidovudine and lamivudine.** The alternative nPEP regimen recommended for such infants is raltegravir (or lopinavir/ritonavir) in conjunction with zidovudine and emtricitabine.
- **When nPEP is prescribed, the exposed individual should be advised of the importance of adhering to and completing the regimen and advised about possible drug toxicities and drug interactions associated with the regimen.** Hematologic parameters and renal and hepatic function should be monitored as needed based on the antiretrovirals included in the nPEP regimen.
- **HIV testing should be used to monitor for seroconversion after nonoccupational exposure to HIV.** HIV testing should be repeated 4–6 weeks and 3 months after the exposure. Because HIV seroconversion may be delayed in individuals who acquire HIV and HCV simultaneously, exposed individuals who tested negative for HCV at baseline and positive for HCV at 4–6 weeks should be retested for HIV again 6 months after the exposure.
- **If HIV infection is identified in the exposed individual at baseline during initial evaluation or if there is laboratory evidence of HIV infection after initiation of nPEP, the individual should be referred to a specialist with expertise in HIV treatment.** If the individual is taking a 3-drug antiretroviral regimen for nPEP at the time of HIV infection diagnosis, the 3-drug regimen should be continued until the patient has been evaluated by an HIV specialist and an HIV treatment plan is initiated.
- **Expert consultation is advised when nPEP is indicated in certain exposed individuals (e.g., those with medical conditions such as renal impairment, pregnant women, children), when an antiretroviral regimen not included in the CDC guidelines is being considered, when the source virus is known or likely to be resistant to antiretroviral agents, or the healthcare provider is inexperienced in prescribing antiretrovirals.** Initiation of nPEP should *not* be delayed while waiting for expert consultation.
- **Clinicians seeking information and guidance regarding the management of a nonoccupational exposure to HIV and additional information on nPEP can consult the National Clinicians' Postexposure Prophylaxis Hotline (PEPline) at 888-448-4911 or http://nccc.ucsf.edu/clinician-consultation/pep-post-exposure-prophylaxis/.**
- **Any unusual or severe toxicity associated with nPEP should be reported to the manufacturer and/or the FDA MedWatch program at 800-332-1088 or http://www.fda.gov/Safety/MedWatch/default.htm.**

Adapted from US Centers from Disease Control and Prevention, US Department of Health and Human Services. Updated Guidelines for Antiretroviral Postexposure Prophylaxis after Sexual, Injection Drug Use, or Other Nonoccupational Exposure to HIV–United States, 2016 (may be available at http://www.cdc.gov/hiv/pdf/programresources/cdc-hiv-npep-guidelines.pdf).

For complete information on chemistry and stability, mechanism of action, spectrum, resistance, pharmacokinetics, efficacy, cautions, drug interactions, and dosage and administration of the antiretroviral agents, see the individual monographs in 8:18.08.

†Use is not currently included in the labeling approved by the US Food and Drug Administration

HIV PROTEASE INHIBITORS 8:18.08.08

Atazanavir Sulfate

ATV, ATV/rCobicistat-boosted Atazanavir, ATV/c, atazanavir/cobicistat

■ Atazanavir sulfate, an antiretroviral agent, is a human immunodeficiency virus (HIV) protease inhibitor (PI).

Uses

■ **Treatment of HIV Infection** Atazanavir with low-dose ritonavir (*ritonavir-boosted* atazanavir) is used in conjunction with other antiretroviral agents for the treatment of human immunodeficiency virus type 1 (HIV-1) infection in antiretroviral-naive (have not previously received antiretroviral therapy) or antiretroviral-experienced (previously treated) adults, adolescents, and children 3 months of age or older. The manufacturer advises that use of *ritonavir-boosted* atazanavir in antiretroviral-experienced patients should be guided by the number of baseline primary HIV protease inhibitor (PI) resistance substitutions.

Atazanavir with cobicistat (*cobicistat-boosted* atazanavir) is used in conjunction with other antiretroviral agents for the treatment of HIV-1 infection in treatment-naive or treatment-experienced adults. When *cobicistat-boosted* atazanavir is included in an antiretroviral regimen, the fixed-combination preparation containing both drugs (atazanavir/cobicistat) can be used or, alternatively, single-entity atazanavir and single-entity cobicistat can be administered at the same time. The manufacturer of atazanavir/cobicistat states that use of the fixed combination in antiretroviral-experienced patients should be guided by the number of baseline primary HIV PI resistance substitutions. Estimated creatinine clearance should be assessed in all patients prior to initiation of *cobicistat-boosted* atazanavir (administered as fixed combination atazanavir/cobicistat or, alternatively, as single-entity atazanavir and single-entity cobicistat). (See Renal Effects under Cautions: Warnings/Precautions.)

Although unboosted atazanavir (i.e., *without* low-dose ritonavir or cobicistat) has been used in conjunction with other antiretroviral agents for the treatment of HIV-1 infection in treatment-naive adults and adolescents 13 years of age or older who cannot tolerate ritonavir, unboosted atazanavir is *not* included in preferred or alternative regimens recommended for *initial* treatment in antiretroviral-naive patients because it is less potent than boosted atazanavir. In addition, unboosted atazanavir should *not* be used in antiretroviral-experienced patients with prior virologic failure.

Atazanavir usually is used with a pharmacokinetic enhancer (i.e., low-dose ritonavir or cobicistat). A pharmacokinetic enhancer (pharmacokinetic booster) is necessary to improve the pharmacokinetic profile of atazanavir. Although concomitant use of low-dose ritonavir or cobicistat with atazanavir increases peak plasma concentrations and area under the plasma concentration-time curve (AUC) of the HIV PI, these pharmacokinetic enhancers are not interchangeable in antiretroviral regimens since low-dose ritonavir and cobicistat have different dosage and administration requirements and are associated with different adverse effects, precautions, contraindications, and drug interactions. In addition, although *ritonavir-boosted* atazanavir may be used in adults, adolescents, and children 3 months of age or older, efficacy and safety of *cobicistat-boosted* atazanavir (administered as fixed-combination atazanavir/cobicistat or, alternatively, as single-entity atazanavir and single-entity cobicistat) have been established only in adults.

Ritonavir-boosted atazanavir, *cobicistat-boosted* atazanavir, or unboosted atazanavir should always be used in conjunction with one or more antiretroviral agents and should not be used alone for treatment of HIV-1 infection. *Ritonavir-boosted* atazanavir, *cobicistat-boosted* atazanavir, or unboosted atazanavir usually is used in an HIV PI-based regimen that includes 2 nucleoside reverse transcriptase inhibitors (NRTIs).

The most appropriate antiretroviral regimen cannot be defined for each clinical scenario and selection of specific antiretroviral agents for use in multiple-drug regimens should be individualized based on information regarding antiretroviral potency, potential rate of development of resistance, known toxicities, and potential for pharmacokinetic interactions as well as virologic, immunologic, and clinical characteristics of the patient. For information on the general principles and guidelines for use of antiretroviral therapy, including specific recommendations for initial therapy in antiretroviral-naive patients and recommendations for changing antiretroviral regimens, see the Antiretroviral Agents General Statement 8:18.08.

Antiretroviral-naive Adults and Adolescents For *initial* treatment in HIV-infected adults and adolescents who are antiretroviral-naive, the US Department of Health and Human Services (HHS) Panel on Antiretroviral Guidelines for Adults and Adolescents states that *ritonavir-boosted* atazanavir in conjunction with tenofovir alafenamide fumarate (TAF) and emtricitabine or *ritonavir-boosted* atazanavir in conjunction with tenofovir disoproxil fumarate (tenofovir DF) and emtricitabine (or lamivudine) are considered alternative PI-based regimens. These experts state that *cobicistat-boosted* atazanavir in conjunction with TAF and emtricitabine or *cobicistat-boosted* atazanavir in conjunction with tenofovir DF and emtricitabine (or lamivudine) are alternative PI-based regimens for *initial* treatment in antiretroviral-naive adults and adolescents†. In addition, these experts also state that *ritonavir-boosted* atazanavir or *cobicistat-boosted* atazanavir in conjunction with abacavir and lamivudine are other regimen options for *initial* treatment in antiretroviral-naive patients when recommended or alternative regimens cannot be used, but should be used *only* in patients with baseline plasma HIV RNA levels less than 100,000 copies/mL who are human leukocyte antigen (HLA)-B*5701 negative.

The HHS panel states that unboosted atazanavir (i.e., atazanavir *without* low-dose ritonavir or cobicistat) is *not* recommended for *initial* treatment because it is less potent than boosted atazanavir.

Clinical Experience. In an open-label, noninferiority study in antiretroviral-naive adults (study AI424-138; CASTLE study), a regimen of *ritonavir-boosted* atazanavir given once daily in conjunction with tenofovir DF and emtricitabine demonstrated antiviral efficacy similar to that of a regimen of the fixed combination of lopinavir and ritonavir (lopinavir/ritonavir) given twice daily in conjunction with tenofovir DF and emtricitabine. At week 48, 78 or 76% of adults receiving the regimen that included *ritonavir-boosted* atazanavir or the regimen that included lopinavir/ritonavir had plasma HIV-1 RNA levels less than 50 copies/mL, respectively. At week 96, 75 or 68% of adults receiving the regimen that included *ritonavir-boosted* atazanavir or the regimen that included lopinavir/ritonavir respectively, had plasma HIV-1 RNA levels less than 50 copies/mL.

Safety and efficacy of *cobicistat-boosted* atazanavir have been evaluated in a randomized, double-blind, active-controlled study in 692 treatment-naive HIV-infected adults (mean age 37 years, 83% male, 60% white, mean baseline plasma HIV-1 RNA level 4.8 $\log_{10}$ copies/mL, mean baseline $CD4^+$ T-cell count 352 cells/mm^3). All patients had a baseline estimated creatinine clearance greater than 70 mL/minute and were randomized in a 1:1 ratio to receive *cobicistat-boosted* atazanavir (single-entity atazanavir 300 mg once daily administered with single-entity cobicistat 150 mg once daily) or *ritonavir-boosted* atazanavir (single-entity atazanavir 300 mg once daily administered with single-entity ritonavir 100 mg once daily). All patients also received concomitant treatment with tenofovir DF and emtricitabine (administered as fixed-combination tablets containing tenofovir DF 300 mg and emtricitabine 200 mg once daily). At week 48, 85% of patients receiving the regimen that included *cobicistat-boosted* atazanavir and 87% of those receiving the regimen that included *ritonavir-boosted* atazanavir had plasma HIV-1 RNA levels less than 50 copies/mL. In addition, the mean increase from baseline in $CD4^+$ T-cell counts at week 48 was 213 cells/mm^3 in those receiving *cobicistat-boosted* atazanavir and 219 cells/mm^3 in those receiving *ritonavir-boosted* atazanavir.

Safety and efficacy of unboosted atazanavir used in conjunction with other antiretroviral agents have been evaluated in 2 randomized multicenter studies in antiretroviral-naive adults (study AI424-034 and AI424-008). In study AI424-034, 810 HIV-infected adults (mean age: 34 years; 65% male; 33% white; 36% Hispanic; mean baseline plasma HIV-1 RNA level: 4.8 $\log_{10}$ copies/mL; mean baseline $CD4^+$ T-cell count: 321 cells/mm^3) were randomized to receive atazanavir (400 mg once daily) or efavirenz (600 mg once daily) in conjunction with a fixed-combination preparation containing lamivudine and zidovudine (150 mg of lamivudine and 300 mg of zidovudine twice daily). Results of this study indicated that an initial regimen that includes atazanavir in conjunction with lamivudine and zidovudine is as effective as an initial regimen of efavirenz in conjunction with lamivudine and zidovudine. At week 48, 67 and 32% of adults receiving the regimen that included atazanavir and 62 and 37% of those receiving the regimen that included efavirenz had plasma HIV-1 RNA levels less than 400 or 50 copies/mL, respectively. In patients with high viral titers at baseline (i.e., 100,000 copies/mL or greater), the proportion of patients responding at week 48 to the regimen that included atazanavir was similar to the proportion responding to the regimen that included efavirenz. At week 48, increases in $CD4^+$ T-cell counts were greater in patients receiving the regimen that included atazanavir (increase of 176 cells/mm^3) than in those receiving the regimen that included efavirenz (increase of 160 cells/mm^3).

In study AI424-008, 467 HIV-infected adults (mean age: 35 years; 63% male; 55% white; mean baseline plasma HIV-1 RNA level: 4.7 $\log_{10}$ copies/mL; mean baseline $CD4^+$ T-cell count: 295 cells/mm^3) were randomized to receive unboosted atazanavir (600 or 400 mg once daily) or nelfinavir (1250 mg twice daily) in conjunction with lamivudine (150 mg twice daily) and stavudine (40 mg twice daily). In this study, an initial regimen of atazanavir, lamivudine, and stavudine was as effective as an initial regimen of nelfinavir, lamivudine, and stavudine. At week 48, 67 and 33% of adults receiving the regimen that included atazanavir (400 mg once daily) and 59 and 38% of those receiving the regimen that included nelfinavir had plasma HIV-1 RNA levels less than 400 or 50 copies/mL, respectively. At week 48, patients receiving the regimen that included atazanavir 400 mg once daily had greater increases in $CD4^+$ T-cell counts than those receiving the regimen that included nelfinavir (mean increase of 234 and 211 cells/mm^3, respectively). In an open-label extension study (study AI424-044), virologic response was maintained at a median of 108 weeks in patients receiving atazanavir, lamivudine, and stavudine.

Antiretroviral-experienced Adults and Adolescents If atazanavir is used in antiretroviral-experienced (previously treated) patients with prior virologic failure, *ritonavir-boosted* atazanavir or *cobicistat-boosted* atazanavir is used. Use of these regimens in antiretroviral-experienced patients should be guided by the number of baseline primary PI resistance substitutions. Unboosted atazanavir (i.e., *without* low-dose ritonavir or cobicistat) is *not* recommended in antiretroviral-experienced patients with prior virologic failure.

Clinical Experience. *Ritonavir-boosted* atazanavir has been evaluated in a randomized, open-label, multicenter study (study AI424-045) in 347 previously treated adults who experienced virologic failure with antiretroviral regimens that included HIV nonnucleoside reverse transcriptase inhibitors (NNRTIs), NRTIs, and/or PIs. Patients were randomized to receive *ritonavir-boosted* atazanavir (300 mg of atazanavir with 100 mg of ritonavir once daily), lopinavir/ritonavir (400 mg of lopinavir/100 mg of ritonavir twice daily) or atazanavir (400 mg once daily) with saquinavir (1.2 g once daily as soft gelatin capsules no longer commercially available in the US), each in conjunction with tenofovir DF 300 mg once daily and an additional NRTI. At 48 weeks, 55 or 38% of adults receiving the regimen that included *ritonavir-boosted* atazanavir and 57 or 45% of those receiving the regimen that included lopinavir/ritonavir had plasma HIV-1 RNA levels less than 400 or 50 copies/mL, respectively. Administration of *ritonavir-boosted* atazanavir in conjunction with tenofovir DF and an additional NRTI resulted in a mean decrease in plasma HIV-1 RNA levels of 1.58 $\log_{10}$ copies/mL at 48 weeks. Similarly, administration of lopinavir/ritonavir in conjunction with tenofovir DF and an additional NRTI resulted in a mean decrease in plasma HIV-1 RNA levels of 1.7 $\log_{10}$ copies/mL. The regimen of atazanavir, saquinavir, tenofovir DF, and one NRTI was less effective than the regimens of *ritonavir-boosted* atazanavir or lopinavir/ritonavir with tenofovir DF and an additional NRTI in this group of patients. (See Saquinavir under Antiretroviral Agents: HIV Protease Inhibitors, in Drug Interactions.) At 96 weeks, 44 or 33% of patients continuing a regimen containing *ritonavir-boosted* atazanavir maintained plasma HIV-1 RNA levels below 400 or 50 copies/mL, respectively. This was similar to 46 or 36%, respectively, of patient receiving a regimen containing lopinavir/ritonavir.

Although no longer recommended for antiretroviral-experienced patients, unboosted atazanavir was evaluated in a randomized, open-label, multicenter study (study AI424-043) in 300 previously treated adults who experienced virologic failure to one (but not more than one) antiretroviral regimen that included a PI. Patients were randomized to receive unboosted atazanavir (400 mg once daily) in conjunction with 2 NRTIs or lopinavir/ritonavir (400 mg of lopinavir/100 mg of ritonavir twice daily) in conjunction with 2 NRTIs. At week 48, 49 and 35% of adults receiving the regimen that included atazanavir and 69 and 53% of those receiving the regimen that included lopinavir/ritonavir had plasma HIV-1 RNA levels less than 400 or 50 copies/mL, respectively. Administration of atazanavir in conjunction with 2 NRTIs resulted in a mean decrease in viral load of 1.59 $\log_{10}$ copies/mL at 48 weeks; administration of lopinavir/ritonavir in conjunction with 2 NRTIs resulted in a mean decrease in viral load of 2.02 $\log_{10}$ copies/mL. Based on results of this study, a regimen that includes atazanavir without low-dose ritonavir is not recommended in adults who previously received a PI and experienced virologic failure.

Pediatric Patients *Ritonavir-boosted* atazanavir is used in conjunction with other antiretroviral agents for the treatment of HIV-1 infection in children 3 months of age or older weighing 5 kg or more.

For *initial* treatment in HIV-infected pediatric patients, the HHS Panel on Antiretroviral Therapy and Medical Management of HIV-infected Children recommends a regimen that includes a *ritonavir-boosted* PI, NNRTI, or integrase strand transfer inhibitor (INSTI) in conjunction with 2 NRTIs (dual NRTIs). These experts state that *ritonavir-boosted* atazanavir in conjunction with 2 NRTIs is a preferred regimen for *initial* treatment in children 3 years of age or older and an alternative regimen for *initial* treatment in children 3 months to less than 3 years of age weighing 5–25 kg. The panel states that unboosted atazanavir (i.e., *without* low-dose ritonavir) is *not* recommended for *initial* treatment in pediatric patients.

Efficacy and safety of *cobicistat-boosted* atazanavir (administered as atazanavir/cobicistat or, alternatively, as single-entity atazanavir and single-entity cobicistat) have not been established in patients younger than 18 years of age.

For further information on treatment of HIV infection in pediatric patients, see Guidelines for Use of Antiretroviral Agents: Antiretroviral Therapy in Pediatric Patients, in the Antiretroviral Agents General Statement 8:18.08.

Clinical Experience. Efficacy and safety of atazanavir capsules (with or without low-dose ritonavir) were evaluated in an open-label trial in 105 HIV-infected children 6 years to less than 18 years of age (PACTG 1020A). At week 96, 51 or 47% of antiretroviral-naive children and 34 or 24% of antiretroviral-experienced children had plasma HIV-1 RNA levels less than 400 or 50 copies/mL, respectively. At week 96, the median increase in absolute $CD4^+$ T-cell count from baseline was 335 cells/mm^3 in antiretroviral-naive children and 220 cells/mm^3 in antiretroviral-experienced children.

Efficacy and safety of *ritonavir-boosted* atazanavir oral powder were evaluated in 2 open-label, multicenter trials that included 134 pediatric patients 3 months to less than 11 years of age weighing 5 kg to less than 35 kg (PRINCE I and PRINCE II). Patients weighing 5 kg to less than 10 kg received either 150 or 200 mg of atazanavir (oral powder) and 80 mg of ritonavir (oral solution); those weighing 10 kg to less than 15 kg received 200 mg of atazanavir (oral powder) and 80 mg of ritonavir (oral solution); those weighing 15 kg to less than 25 kg received 250 mg of atazanavir (oral powder) and 80 mg of ritonavir (oral solution); and those weighing 25 kg to less than 35 kg received 300 mg of atazanavir (oral powder) and 100 of ritonavir. At 48 weeks, 79 or 54% of antiretroviral-naive children and 62 or 50% of antiretroviral-experienced children had achieved plasma HIV-1 RNA levels less than 400 or 50 copies/mL, respectively. The median increase in absolute $CD4^+$ T-cell count from baseline was 215 cells/mm^3 in antiretroviral-naive children and 133 cells/mm^3 in antiretroviral-experienced children; the median increase in T-cell percentage from baseline was 6 and 4%, respectively.

■ **Postexposure Prophylaxis following Occupational Exposure to HIV** *Ritonavir-boosted* atazanavir is used in conjunction with 2 NRTIs for postexposure prophylaxis of HIV infection following occupational exposure† (PEP) in health-care personnel and other individuals exposed via percutaneous injury (e.g., needlestick, cut with sharp object) or mucous membrane or nonintact skin (e.g., chapped, abraded, dermatitis) contact with blood, tissue, or other body fluids that might contain HIV.

The US Public Health Service (USPHS) states that the preferred regimen for PEP following an occupational exposure to HIV is a 3-drug regimen of raltegravir used in conjunction with emtricitabine and tenofovir DF (may be administered as the fixed combination emtricitabine/tenofovir DF; Truvada®). *Ritonavir-boosted* atazanavir and 2 NRTIs is one of several alternative regimens recommended when the preferred regimen cannot be used. The preferred dual NRTI option for use in PEP regimens is emtricitabine and tenofovir DF (may be administered as emtricitabine/tenofovir DF; Truvada®); alternative dual NRTIs are tenofovir DF and lamivudine, zidovudine and lamivudine (may be administered as the fixed combination lamivudine/zidovudine; Combivir®), or zidovudine and emtricitabine.

Because management of occupational exposures to HIV is complex and evolving, consultation with an infectious disease specialist, clinician with expertise in administration of antiretroviral agents, and/or the National Clinicians' Postexposure Prophylaxis Hotline (PEPline at 888-448-4911) is recommended whenever possible. However, initiation of PEP should not be delayed while waiting for expert consultation.

For information on types of occupational exposure to HIV and associated risk of infection, management of occupational exposure to HIV, efficacy and safety of postexposure prophylaxis, and recommendations regarding PEP, see Guidelines for Use of Antiretroviral Agents: Antiretrovirals for Postexposure Prophylaxis following Occupational Exposure to HIV (PEP), in the Antiretroviral Agents General Statement 8:18.08.

■ **Postexposure Prophylaxis following Nonoccupational Exposure to HIV** *Ritonavir-boosted* atazanavir is used in conjunction with other antiretrovirals for postexposure prophylaxis of HIV infection following nonoccupational exposure† (nPEP) in individuals who have had exposure to blood, genital secretions, or other potentially infectious body fluids that might contain HIV when the exposure represents a substantial risk for HIV transmission.

When nPEP is indicated following a nonoccupational exposure to HIV, the US Centers for Disease Control and Prevention (CDC) states that the preferred regimen in adults and adolescents 13 years of age or older with normal renal function is either raltegravir or dolutegravir used in conjunction with emtricitabine and tenofovir DF (administered as emtricitabine/tenofovir DF; Truvada®); the recommended alternative nPEP regimen in these patients is *ritonavir-boosted* darunavir used in conjunction with emtricitabine/tenofovir DF.

CDC states that *ritonavir-boosted* atazanavir is an alternative antiretroviral that can be used in nPEP regimens.

Consultation with an infectious disease specialist, clinician with expertise in administration of antiretroviral agents, and/or the National Clinicians' Postexposure Prophylaxis Hotline (PEPline at 888-448-4911) is recommended if nPEP is indicated in certain exposed individuals (e.g., pregnant women, children, those with medical conditions such as renal impairment) or if an antiretroviral regimen not included in the CDC guidelines is being considered, the source virus is known or likely to be resistant to antiretrovirals, or the healthcare provider is inexperienced in prescribing antiretrovirals. However, initiation of nPEP should not be delayed while waiting for expert consultation.

For additional information on nonoccupational exposure to HIV and recommendations regarding postexposure prophylaxis, see Guidelines for Use of Antiretroviral Agents: Antiretrovirals for Postexposure Prophylaxis following Sexual, Injection Drug Use, or other Nonoccupational Exposures to HIV (nPEP), in the Antiretroviral Agents General Statement 8:18.08.

Dosage and Administration

■ **Administration** Atazanavir is administered orally in conjunction with low-dose ritonavir (*ritonavir-boosted* atazanavir) once daily with food.

Alternatively, atazanavir is administered orally in conjunction with oral cobicistat (*cobicistat-boosted* atazanavir) once daily with food.

Atazanavir also has been administered orally unboosted (i.e., *without* low-dose ritonavir or cobicistat) once daily with food.

If atazanavir is used concomitantly with certain drugs (e.g., antacids, didanosine, histamine H_2-receptor antagonists, proton-pump inhibitors), dosage adjustments may be needed and/or doses of atazanavir and the other drug may need to be given at separate times. (See Drug Interactions.)

Ritonavir-boostedAtazanavir or Unboosted Atazanavir When *ritonavir-boosted* atazanavir is used, single-entity atazanavir is administered as capsules or oral powder with single-entity ritonavir capsules, tablets, or oral solution.

Capsules. Atazanavir capsules should be swallowed whole and should not be opened.

Capsules are used in adults, adolescents, and pediatric patients 6 years of age or older.

Atazanavir capsules usually are administered with low-dose ritonavir (*ritonavir-boosted* atazanavir), but may be used without low-dose ritonavir in adults and adolescents 13 years of age or older weighing 40 kg or more who are unable to tolerate ritonavir.

Atazanavir capsules should be stored at 25°C, but may be exposed to 15–30°C.

Oral Powder. Atazanavir oral powder is provided in single-use packets containing 50 mg of atazanavir; the oral powder *must* be mixed with food or beverage prior to administration.

The oral powder can be used in pediatric patients 3 months of age or older weighing 5 kg or more.

Atazanavir oral powder *must* be administered with low-dose ritonavir (*ritonavir-boosted* atazanavir). The dose of low-dose ritonavir should be administered immediately following the atazanavir dose.

The oral powder should be stored in the original packet at less than 30°C and should not be opened until ready to use. The oral powder preferably should be mixed with food (e.g., applesauce, yogurt), but may be mixed with a beverage (e.g., milk, infant formula, water) for infants who are able to drink from a cup. For infants younger than 6 months of age who cannot eat solid food or drink from a cup, the oral powder may be mixed with infant formula and administered using an oral dosing syringe. Administration using an infant bottle is not recommended because the full atazanavir dose may not be delivered.

The entire dose should be administered within 1 hour after the powder has been mixed with food or beverage; the mixture may be left at room temperature for up to 1 hour after preparation.

If mixing with food, packets containing atazanavir oral powder should be tapped to settle the powder and a clean pair of scissors used to cut along the dotted line. Using a spoon, the contents of the recommended number of packets should be mixed with at least 1 tablespoon of food (e.g., applesauce, yogurt) in a small container (e.g., cup, bowl). The mixture should be fed to the patient. Then, an additional 1 tablespoon of food should be added to the small container and mixed; the residual mixture should be fed to the patient.

If mixing with a beverage, packets containing atazanavir oral powder should be tapped to settle the powder and a clean pair of scissors used to cut along the dotted line. Using a spoon, the contents of the recommended number of packets should be mixed in a drinking cup with at least 30 mL of beverage. The patient should drink the mixture. Then, an additional 15 mL of beverage should be added to the drinking cup and mixed; the patient should drink the residual mixture. If water is used as the beverage, the patient also should eat food at the time of administration.

If mixing with liquid infant formula, packets containing atazanavir oral powder should be tapped to the settle powder and a clean pair of scissors used to cut along the dotted line. Using a spoon, the contents of the recommended number of packets should be mixed in a small medicine cup with 10 mL of prepared liquid infant formula. The entire mixture should be drawn into an oral dosing syringe and administered into the infant's right or left inner cheek. Then, an additional 10 mL of infant formula should be poured into the medicine cup to rinse off any remaining atazanavir oral powder. The residual mixture should be drawn into the oral dosing syringe and administered into the infant's right or left inner cheek.

Cobicistat-boosted Atazanavir When *cobicistat-boosted* atazanavir is used, fixed-combination tablets containing both drugs are commercially available (atazanavir/cobicistat). Alternatively, single-entity atazanavir is administered as capsules at the same time as single-entity cobicistat tablets.

■ Dosage

Single-entity atazanavir is commercially available as capsules or oral powder containing atazanavir sulfate; dosage is expressed in terms of atazanavir.

Atazanavir/cobicistat is commercially available as fixed-combination tablets containing atazanavir sulfate (300 mg of atazanavir) and cobicistat (150 mg).

Adult Dosage **Treatment of HIV Infection in Antiretroviral-naive Adults.** The recommended dosage of *ritonavir-boosted* atazanavir for the treatment of human immunodeficiency virus type 1 (HIV-1) infection in antiretroviral-naive adults is 300 mg of single-entity atazanavir once daily given in conjunction with single-entity ritonavir 100 mg once daily.

The recommended dosage of *cobicistat-boosted* atazanavir for the treatment of HIV-1 infection in antiretroviral-naive adults is 300 mg of atazanavir once daily with 150 mg of cobicistat once daily. When fixed-combination atazanavir/cobicistat is used, adults should receive 1 tablet (300 mg of atazanavir and 150 mg of cobicistat) once daily. Alternatively, adults can receive 300 mg of single-entity atazanavir (one 300-mg capsule) once daily given in conjunction with single-entity cobicistat 150 mg once daily.

If unboosted atazanavir (i.e., *without* low-dose ritonavir or cobicistat) is used for the treatment of HIV-1 infection in antiretroviral-naive adults unable to tolerate ritonavir, the recommended dosage is 400 mg of single-entity atazanavir once daily.

Treatment of HIV Infection in Antiretroviral-experienced Adults. The recommended dosage of *ritonavir-boosted* atazanavir for the treatment of HIV-1 infection in antiretroviral-experienced adults is 300 mg of single-entity atazanavir once daily given in conjunction with single-entity ritonavir 100 mg once daily.

The recommended dosage of *cobicistat-boosted* atazanavir for the treatment of HIV-1 infection in antiretroviral-experienced adults is 300 mg of atazanavir once daily with 150 mg of cobicistat once daily. When fixed-combination atazanavir/cobicistat is used, adults should receive 1 tablet (300 mg of atazanavir and 150 mg of cobicistat) once daily. Alternatively, adults can receive 300 mg of single-entity atazanavir (one 300-mg capsule) once daily given in conjunction with single-entity cobicistat 150 mg once daily.

Postexposure Prophylaxis following Occupational Exposure to HIV. For postexposure prophylaxis of HIV infection following occupational exposure† (PEP) in health-care personnel or other individuals, the preferred dosage of *ritonavir-boosted* atazanavir is 300 mg of atazanavir once daily with ritonavir 100 mg once daily. *Ritonavir-boosted* atazanavir is used in conjunction with 2 HIV nucleoside reverse transcriptase inhibitors (NRTIs). (See Uses: Postexposure Prophylaxis following Occupational Exposure to HIV.)

The PEP regimen should be initiated as soon as possible following occupational exposure (preferably within hours) and continued for 4 weeks, if tolerated.

Pediatric Dosage **Treatment of HIV Infection.** Dosage of atazanavir oral powder for the treatment of HIV-1 infection in pediatric patients 3 months of age or older weighing 5 kg or more is based on weight. (See Table 1.) Atazanavir oral powder *must* be used with low-dose ritonavir (*ritonavir-boosted* atazanavir).

Table 1: Dosage of *Ritonavir-boosted* Atazanavir for Pediatric Patients 3 Months of Age or Older Weighing 5 kg or More

Body Weight	Atazanavir Dosage (Oral Powder)	Ritonavir Dosage (Oral Solution)
5 to less than 15 kg	200 mg (4 packets) once daily[a]	80 mg once daily
15 to less than 25 kg	250 mg (5 packets) once daily	80 mg once daily
25 kg or more *and* not able to swallow capsules	300 mg (6 packets) once daily	100 mg once daily

[a] In patients weighing 5 to less than 10 kg who do not tolerate 200 mg (4 packets) of atazanavir oral powder *and* have not previously received an HIV protease inhibitor (PI), atazanavir oral powder in a dosage of 150 mg (3 packets) once daily may be used with close HIV viral load monitoring.

Dosage of atazanavir capsules for the treatment of HIV-1 infection in pediatric patients 6 years to less than 18 years of age is based on weight. (See Table 2.) Atazanavir capsules usually are used with low-dose ritonavir (*ritonavir-boosted* atazanavir).

Table 2: Dosage of *Ritonavir-boosted* Atazanavir for Pediatric Patients 6 Years to Less than 18 Years of Age

Body Weight	Atazanavir Dosage (Capsules)	Ritonavir Dosage
Less than 15 kg	Capsules not recommended	
15 to less than 20 kg	150 mg once daily	100 mg once daily
20 to less than 40 kg	200 mg once daily	100 mg once daily
40 kg or more	300 mg once daily	100 mg once daily

If unboosted atazanavir (i.e., *without* low-dose ritonavir or cobicistat) is used for the treatment of HIV-1 infection in antiretroviral-naive adolescents 13 years of age or older who weigh at least 40 kg and are unable to tolerate ritonavir, the recommended dosage is 400 mg of single-entity atazanavir once daily. Unboosted atazanavir should not be used in antiretroviral-experienced adolescents.

■ Special Populations

Hepatic Impairment If unboosted atazanavir (i.e., *without* low-dose ritonavir or cobicistat) is used in treatment-naive patients with hepatic impairment, a dosage of 400 mg once daily should be used in those with mild hepatic impairment (Child-Pugh class A) and a dosage of 300 mg once daily should be used in those with moderate hepatic impairment (Child-Pugh class B). Unboosted atazanavir should not be used in patients with severe hepatic impairment (Child-Pugh class C). (See Hepatic Impairment under Warnings/Precautions: Specific Populations, in Cautions.)

Ritonavir-boosted atazanavir and *cobicistat-boosted* atazanavir should not be used in patients with any degree of hepatic impairment.

Renal Impairment Dosage of *ritonavir-boosted* atazanavir or unboosted atazanavir does not need to be adjusted in patients with renal impairment who are *not* undergoing hemodialysis.

If *ritonavir-boosted* atazanavir is used in antiretroviral-naive patients with end-stage renal disease undergoing hemodialysis, the recommended dosage is 300 mg of single-entity atazanavir once daily given in conjunction with single-entity ritonavir 100 mg once daily.

Prior to initiation of *cobicistat-boosted* atazanavir (administered as fixed-combination atazanavir/cobicistat or, alternatively, as single-entity atazanavir and single-entity cobicistat), estimated creatinine clearance should be assessed. Some experts state that dosage adjustments are not necessary when *cobicistat-boosted* atazanavir is used in patients with renal impairment who do not require hemodialysis. However, these experts and the manufacturer state that *cobicistat-boosted* atazanavir should *not* be used in conjunction with tenofovir DF in patients with estimated creatinine clearances less than 70 mL/minute. (See Renal Impairment under Warnings/Precautions: Specific Populations, in Cautions.)

Ritonavir-boosted atazanavir, *cobicistat-boosted* atazanavir, or unboosted atazanavir should *not* be used in antiretroviral-experienced patients with end-stage renal disease undergoing hemodialysis.

Pregnant and Postpartum Women If atazanavir is used during pregnancy or the postpartum period, it should be administered as *ritonavir-*

boosted atazanavir. (See Pregnancy under Warnings/Precautions: Specific Populations, in Cautions.)

For the treatment of HIV-1 infection in pregnant or postpartum women, the manufacturer states that the usually recommended adult dosage of *ritonavir-boosted* atazanavir should be used during pregnancy or the postpartum period unless certain drugs are used concomitantly.

Some experts recommend that an increased dosage of *ritonavir-boosted* atazanavir (i.e., 400 mg of single-entity atazanavir once daily with single-entity ritonavir 100 mg once daily) should be used for treatment of HIV-1 infection in pregnant women during the second and third trimesters.

If *ritonavir-boosted* atazanavir is used during the second or third trimester in antiretroviral-experienced pregnant women who are also receiving either a histamine H_2-receptor antagonist *or* tenofovir DF, the manufacturer recommends a dosage of 400 mg of single-entity atazanavir once daily with single-entity ritonavir 100 mg once daily. *Ritonavir-boosted* atazanavir is not recommended in antiretroviral-experienced pregnant women receiving both a histamine H_2-receptor antagonist *and* tenofovir DF.

Cobicistat-boosted atazanavir should *not* be used in treatment-experienced pregnant women receiving a histamine H_2-receptor antagonist and/or tenofovir DF during the second or third trimester.

Cautions

■ **Contraindications** History of clinically important hypersensitivity reaction (e.g., Stevens-Johnson syndrome, erythema multiforme, toxic skin eruptions) to atazanavir sulfate or any ingredient in the formulation.

Concomitant use of *ritonavir-boosted* atazanavir, *cobicistat-boosted* atazanavir (administered as fixed-combination atazanavir/cobicistat or, alternatively, as single-entity atazanavir and single-entity cobicistat), or unboosted atazanavir (i.e., *without* low-dose ritonavir or cobicistat) with drugs highly dependent on cytochrome P-450 (CYP) isoenzyme 3A (CYP3A) or uridine diphosphate-glucuronosyltransferase (UGT) 1A1 for clearance and for which elevated plasma concentrations are associated with serious and/or life-threatening events (e.g., alfuzosin, cisapride, ergot alkaloids, indinavir, irinotecan, lovastatin, lurasidone, oral midazolam, pimozide, sildenafil used for treatment of pulmonary arterial hypertension [PAH], simvastatin, triazolam). In addition, concomitant use of *cobicistat-boosted* atazanavir and colchicine, dronedarone, lurasidone, or ranolazine is contraindicated. (See Drug Interactions.)

Concomitant use of *ritonavir-boosted* atazanavir, *cobicistat-boosted* atazanavir, or unboosted atazanavir with drugs that are strong inducers of CYP3A when such use may lead to decreased atazanavir exposures resulting in possible loss of virologic response (e.g., nevirapine, rifampin, St. John's wort [*Hypericum perforatum*]). (See Drug Interactions.)

■ **Warnings/Precautions** ***Sensitivity Reactions*** **Dermatologic Reactions.** Rash (generally mild to moderate maculopapular eruptions) occurred in 20% of patients receiving atazanavir in clinical studies. The median time to onset of rash was 7.3 weeks following initiation of atazanavir therapy and the median duration of rash was 1.4 weeks. Atazanavir generally was continued without interruption in these patients. If severe rash develops, atazanavir should to discontinued.

Stevens-Johnson syndrome, erythema multiforme, and toxic skin eruptions, including drug rash with eosinophilia and systemic symptoms (DRESS) syndrome, have been reported in patients receiving atazanavir.

Cardiovascular Effects Abnormalities in atrioventricular (AV) conduction, including prolongation of the PR interval, have occurred in individuals receiving atazanavir. Cardiac conduction abnormalities generally are limited to first-degree AV block; prolongation of the corrected QT (QT_c) interval observed in HIV-infected patients receiving atazanavir has not been directly attributed to the drug. Asymptomatic first-degree AV block was observed in 5.9 or 3–10.4% of patients in clinical trials receiving regimens that included atazanavir or comparator antiretrovirals (fixed combination of lopinavir and ritonavir [lopinavir/ritonavir], nelfinavir, efavirenz), respectively; second- or third-degree block was not observed.

Because of limited clinical experience in patients with preexisting cardiac conduction abnormalities (e.g., marked first-degree AV block, second- or third-degree AV block), ECG monitoring should be considered in such patients.

Caution is advised if atazanavir is used with other drugs that prolong the PR interval (e.g., some β-adrenergic blocking agents, some calcium-channel blocking agents, digoxin, verapamil, lopinavir/ritonavir). (See Drug Interactions.)

Renal Effects Because cobicistat decreases estimated creatinine clearance by inhibiting tubular secretion of creatinine without affecting actual renal glomerular function, this effect should be considered when interpreting changes in estimated creatinine clearance in patients receiving *cobicistat-boosted* atazanavir. This is particularly important in those needing creatinine clearance monitoring because of a medical condition or other concomitant drugs.

Estimated creatinine clearance should be assessed prior to initiating *cobicistat-boosted* atazanavir. Although cobicistat may cause only modest increases in serum creatinine and modest declines in estimated creatinine clearance without affecting renal glomerular function, the patient should be closely monitored for renal safety if there is an increase in serum creatinine of more than 0.4 mg/dL from baseline during *cobicistat-boosted* atazanavir therapy.

The manufacturer states that dosage recommendations are not available for drugs that require dosage adjustments in patients with renal impairment who are receiving *cobicistat-boosted* atazanavir. Therefore, alternative drugs that do not require dosage adjustments based on renal impairment should be considered in patients receiving *cobicistat-boosted* atazanavir.

New-onset or worsening renal impairment, including acute renal failure and Fanconi syndrome, has been reported in patients receiving cobicistat in an antiretroviral regimen that also included tenofovir disoproxil fumarate (tenofovir DF). In clinical trials, 1.5% of patients receiving *cobicistat-boosted* atazanavir concomitantly with tenofovir DF discontinued the drug because of adverse renal effects. None of these patients had renal impairment at baseline; laboratory findings showed evidence of proximal tubulopathy which improved following discontinuance of the drugs, but did not completely resolve in all patients.

Concomitant use of *cobicistat-boosted* atazanavir and tenofovir DF is not recommended in patients with estimated creatinine clearances less than 70 mL/minute. Whenever *cobicistat-boosted* atazanavir and tenofovir DF are used concomitantly, urine glucose and urine protein should be documented at baseline and estimated creatinine clearance, urine glucose, and urine protein should be routinely monitored throughout concomitant therapy. In addition, serum phosphorus should be monitored in those with or at risk for renal impairment. Concomitant use of a nephrotoxic agent is not recommended in patients receiving an antiretroviral regimen that includes *cobicistat-boosted* atazanavir and tenofovir DF.

Hyperbilirubinemia Because atazanavir is a competitive inhibitor of uridine diphosphate-glucuronosyltransferase (UGT) 1A1 (an enzyme that catalyzes the glucuronidation of bilirubin), reversible asymptomatic elevations in indirect (unconjugated) bilirubin occur in most patients receiving the drug. Total bilirubin concentrations at least 2.6 times the upper limit of normal (ULN) have been reported in 35–49% of patients receiving the drug in clinical trials; long-term safety data are not available for patients experiencing persistent elevations in total bilirubin exceeding 5 times the ULN. Increases in serum AST (SGOT) and/or ALT (SGPT) concentrations that occur with hyperbilirubinemia should be evaluated for etiologies other than hyperbilirubinemia.

If jaundice or scleral icterus that results from bilirubin elevations cause cosmetic concerns, alternative antiretroviral therapy can be considered; reduction of atazanavir dosage is not recommended (efficacy data not available for reduced dosages).

Hyperbilirubinemia has been observed in pregnant women receiving atazanavir, and neonates exposed to the drug in utero also are at risk of hyperbilirubinemia. (See Pregnancy under Warnings/Precautions: Specific Populations, in Cautions.)

Phenylketonuria Individuals with phenylketonuria (i.e., homozygous genetic deficiency of phenylalanine hydroxylase) and other individuals who must restrict their intake of phenylalanine should be advised that atazanavir oral powder contains aspartame (NutraSweet®), which is metabolized in the GI tract to phenylalanine.

Each packet of atazanavir oral powder (50 mg of atazanavir) contains 35 mg of phenylalanine. Atazanavir capsules do not contain phenylalanine.

Hepatic Effects HIV-infected patients with hepatitis B virus (HBV) or hepatitis C virus (HCV) coinfection or elevated serum transaminase concentrations prior to initiating atazanavir may be at increased risk for further transaminase elevations or hepatic decompensation.

If atazanavir is used in patients with underlying hepatic disease (e.g., HBV or HCV coinfection), appropriate laboratory tests should be performed to evaluate hepatic function prior to and during atazanavir treatment. (See Hepatic Impairment under Warnings/Precautions: Specific Populations, in Cautions.)

Nephrolithiasis and Cholelithiasis There have been postmarketing reports of nephrolithiasis and cholelithiasis in patients receiving atazanavir. Some patients required hospitalization for additional management or experienced complications.

If signs or symptoms of nephrolithiasis or cholelithiasis occur, temporary interruption or discontinuance of atazanavir therapy may be considered.

Interactions Atazanavir usually is used in conjunction with a pharmacokinetic enhancer (i.e., low-dose ritonavir or cobicistat) to improve the pharmacokinetic profile of atazanavir. When *ritonavir-boosted* atazanavir or *cobicistat-boosted* atazanavir is used, the cautions, precautions, contraindications, and drug interactions associated with atazanavir and the pharmacokinetic enhancer (i.e., low-dose ritonavir or cobicistat) should be considered.

Concomitant use of *ritonavir-boosted* atazanavir or *cobicistat-boosted* atazanavir with certain drugs is contraindicated or requires particular caution. Concomitant use with some drugs may result in clinically important adverse effects due to higher exposures of the concomitant drug or higher exposures of atazanavir and/or the pharmacokinetic enhancer (i.e., ritonavir or cobicistat). Concomitant use with other drugs may result in drug interactions leading to loss of therapeutic effect of *ritonavir-boosted* atazanavir or *cobicistat-boosted* atazanavir and possible development of resistance. Because ritonavir and cobicistat are inhibitors of CYP3A4, interactions with drugs affecting or metabolized by CYP3A4 are of particular concern. However, concomitant use of *cobicistat-boosted* atazanavir with other drugs may result in different drug interactions than those observed or expected with *ritonavir-boosted* atazanavir because of complex or unknown mechanisms of drug interactions.

Concomitant use of *ritonavir-boosted* atazanavir or *cobicistat-boosted* atazanavir with other drugs that are administered in conjunction with a pharmacokinetic enhancer (e.g., *ritonavir-boosted* HIV protease inhibitors [PIs], *ri-*

tonavir-boosted paritaprevir, elvitegravir) is not recommended. Dosage recommendations for such regimens have not been established and concomitant use of more than one pharmacokinetic enhancer may result in complex drug interactions, including decreased plasma concentrations of the antiretroviral agents leading to loss of therapeutic effect and development of resistance.

Potential drug interactions should be considered prior to and during use of *ritonavir-boosted* atazanavir or *cobicistat-boosted* atazanavir. Patients should be monitored for adverse reactions associated with other drugs used concomitantly with *ritonavir-boosted* atazanavir or *cobicistat-boosted* atazanavir. (See Drug Interactions.)

Hyperglycemic and Diabetogenic Effects Hyperglycemia (potentially persistent), new-onset diabetes mellitus, or exacerbation of preexisting diabetes mellitus has been reported in patients receiving HIV protease inhibitors (PIs); diabetic ketoacidosis can occur. Initiation of antidiabetic therapy (e.g., insulin, oral antidiabetic agents) or dosage adjustment of existing antidiabetic therapy may be required.

Immune Reconstitution Syndrome Patients receiving potent antiretroviral therapy may experience an immune reconstitution syndrome during the initial phase of therapy. Patients whose immune system responds to antiretroviral therapy may develop an inflammatory response to indolent or residual opportunistic infections (e.g., *Mycobacterium avium* complex [MAC], *M. tuberculosis*, cytomegalovirus [CMV], *Pneumocystis jirovecii* [formerly *P. carinii*]); this may necessitate further evaluation and treatment.

Autoimmune disorders (e.g., Graves' disease, polymyositis, Guillain-Barré syndrome) have also been reported to occur in the setting of immune reconstitution; however, the time to onset is variable and can occur many months after initiation of antiretroviral therapy.

Adipogenic Effects Redistribution or accumulation of body fat, including central obesity, dorsocervical fat enlargement ("buffalo hump"), peripheral wasting, facial wasting, breast enlargement, and general cushingoid appearance noted in patients receiving antiretroviral therapy.

The mechanism and long-term consequences of fat redistribution are unknown; a causal relationship has not been established.

Hemophilia A and B Increased bleeding, including spontaneous skin hematomas and hemarthrosis, has been reported in hemophilia A or B patients receiving HIV PIs; a causal relationship has not been established.

Increased hemostatic (e.g., antihemophilic factor) therapy may be needed.

HIV Resistance HIV-1 strains resistant to atazanavir may occur. Varying degrees of cross-resistance occur among the various HIV PIs. Resistance to atazanavir may not necessarily preclude subsequent use of other HIV PIs.

Specific Populations **Pregnancy.** Atazanavir has been evaluated in a limited number of women during pregnancy and the postpartum period. Available human and animal data suggest that atazanavir does not increase the risk of major birth defects overall compared to the background rate. No treatment-related malformations were observed in rats and rabbits using dosages that resulted in atazanavir exposures 0.7–1.2 times those reported with the usual human dosage of *ritonavir-boosted* atazanavir (300 mg of atazanavir once daily with ritonavir 100 mg once daily).

The US Department of Health and Human Services (HHS) Panel on Treatment of HIV-infected Pregnant Women and Prevention of Perinatal Transmission states that *ritonavir-boosted* atazanavir in conjunction with 2 HIV nucleoside reverse transcriptase inhibitors (NRTIs) is a preferred PI-based regimen for *initial* treatment in antiretroviral-naive pregnant women. Dosage adjustments may be necessary in certain pregnant women. (See Pregnant and Postpartum Women under Dosage and Administration: Special Populations.)

The manufacturer states that *cobicistat-boosted* atazanavir should be used during pregnancy only if potential benefits to the woman justify potential risks to the fetus. *Cobicistat-boosted* atazanavir should *not* be used in treatment-experienced pregnant women receiving a histamine H_2-receptor antagonist and/or tenofovir DF. The HHS panel states that data are insufficient to date to recommend *routine* use of *cobicistat-boosted* atazanavir for *initial* treatment in antiretroviral-naive pregnant women.

Unboosted atazanavir (i.e., *without* low-dose ritonavir or cobicistat) should *not* be used in pregnant or postpartum women.

Lactic acidosis, sometimes fatal, and symptomatic hyperlactatemia have occurred in pregnant women receiving atazanavir in conjunction with NRTIs.

Hyperbilirubinemia has occurred in pregnant women receiving atazanavir. In a clinical trial evaluating *ritonavir-boosted* atazanavir in conjunction with 2 NRTIs, 30–62% of pregnant women in the study developed hyperbilirubinemia (total bilirubin at least 2.6 times higher than the ULN). Although severe hyperbilirubinemia (bilirubin concentrations exceeding 20 mg/dL) was not observed in neonates born to women in the study, elevated bilirubin concentrations (4 mg/dL or greater) occurred in 28% of neonates within the first 24 hours of life. All neonates exposed to atazanavir in utero should be monitored for development of severe hyperbilirubinemia during the first few days of life.

Postpartum women should be monitored closely for adverse effects during the first 2 months after delivery since atazanavir concentrations and areas under the concentration-time curve (AUC) may be increased approximately 28–43% during the postpartum period.

Antiretroviral Pregnancy Registry at 800-258-4263 or http://www.apregistry.com.

Based on prospective reports from the Antiretroviral Pregnancy Registry of approximately 1600 live births following exposure to atazanavir-containing antiretroviral regimens during pregnancy (including 1037 first-trimester exposures), there was no difference in the rate of overall birth defects in those exposed to atazanavir-containing regimens compared with the estimated background risk of major birth defects (2–4% in the US population).

Lactation. Atazanavir is distributed into milk in low concentrations. It is not known whether ritonavir or cobicistat is distributed into human milk; cobicistat is distributed into milk in rats.

Because of the risk of adverse effects in the infant and the risk of HIV transmission, HIV-infected women should not breast-feed infants.

Pediatric Use. Because of the risk of kernicterus, atazanavir should not be used in neonates and infants younger than 3 months of age. In addition, any infant exposed to the drug in utero should be monitored closely. (See Pregnancy under Warnings/Precautions: Specific Populations, in Cautions.) Safety, efficacy, and pharmacokinetic profile of atazanavir have not been established in infants younger than 3 months of age.

Safety, efficacy, and pharmacokinetic profile of *ritonavir-boosted* atazanavir and unboosted atazanavir have been evaluated in pediatric patients 3 months of age or older weighing 5 kg or more. Adverse effects reported in pediatric patients 6 years to less than 18 years of age receiving atazanavir capsules were generally similar to those reported in adults. Adverse effects reported in pediatric patients weighing 5 kg or more receiving atazanavir oral powder were generally similar to those reported in pediatric patients receiving the capsules.

Safety and efficacy of *cobicistat-boosted* atazanavir (administered as atazanavir/cobicistat or, alternatively, as single-entity atazanavir and single-entity cobicistat) have not been established in patients younger than 18 years of age.

Geriatric Use. Experience in those 65 years of age or older is insufficient to determine whether they respond differently to *ritonavir-boosted* atazanavir, *cobicistat-boosted* atazanavir, or unboosted atazanavir than younger adults. Caution should be exercised in administration and monitoring because of age-related decreases in hepatic, renal, and/or cardiac function and concomitant disease or drug therapy in geriatric patients.

Hepatic Impairment. Atazanavir is principally metabolized and eliminated by the liver and increased plasma concentrations of atazanavir are expected in patients with moderate to severe hepatic impairment. Dosage adjustments are recommended when unboosted atazanavir (i.e., *without* low-dose ritonavir or cobicistat) is used in patients with mild or moderate hepatic impairment (Child-Pugh class A or B). (See Hepatic Impairment under Dosage and Administration: Special Populations.) Unboosted atazanavir should *not* be used in patients with severe hepatic impairment (Child-Pugh class C).

Ritonavir-boosted atazanavir and *cobicistat-boosted* atazanavir are *not* recommended in patients with any degree of hepatic impairment.

HIV-infected patients with chronic hepatitis B virus (HBV) or hepatitis C virus (HCV) coinfection and those with markedly increased AST (SGOT) or ALT (SGPT) concentrations prior to atazanavir therapy may be at increased risk for further elevations in hepatic enzyme concentrations or hepatic decompensation. Liver function should be evaluated prior to and periodically during atazanavir therapy in such patients.

Renal Impairment. Plasma concentrations of atazanavir are not markedly altered in individuals with severe renal impairment who are not undergoing hemodialysis. Although atazanavir is not appreciably removed by hemodialysis, plasma concentrations of the drug are lower in individuals undergoing dialysis.

Ritonavir-boosted atazanavir can be used in antiretroviral-naive patients with end-stage renal disease who are undergoing hemodialysis. (See Renal Impairment under Dosage and Administration: Special Populations.)

Ritonavir-boosted atazanavir, *cobicistat-boosted* atazanavir, and unboosted atazanavir should *not* be used in antiretroviral-experienced patients with end-stage renal disease who are undergoing hemodialysis.

Cobicistat has been shown to decrease estimated creatinine clearance without affecting renal glomerular function. Prior to initiation of *cobicistat-boosted* atazanavir (administered as fixed-combination atazanavir/cobicistat or, alternatively, as single-entity atazanavir and single-entity cobicistat), estimated creatinine clearance should be assessed. *Cobicistat-boosted* atazanavir should *not* be used in conjunction with tenofovir DF in patients with estimated creatinine clearances less than 70 mL/minute. (See Renal Effects under Cautions: Warnings/Precautions.)

■ Common Adverse Effects

The most common adverse effects in adults receiving *ritonavir-boosted* atazanavir or unboosted atazanavir in conjunction with other antiretrovirals are headache, nausea, jaundice/scleral icterus, abdominal pain, rash, vomiting, diarrhea, insomnia, peripheral neurologic symptoms, dizziness, myalgia, depression, and fever.

The most common adverse effects in adults receiving *cobicistat-boosted* atazanavir are jaundice, ocular icterus, and nausea.

The most common adverse effects in pediatric patients 6 years to less than 18 years of age receiving *ritonavir-boosted* atazanavir or unboosted atazanavir are elevated total bilirubin, cough, fever, jaundice/scleral icterus, rash, vomiting, diarrhea, neutropenia, headache, peripheral edema, extremity pain, nasal congestion, oropharyngeal pain, wheezing, rhinorrhea, and hypoglycemia.

The most common adverse effects in pediatric patients 3 months to 10 years of age receiving *ritonavir-boosted* atazanavir are neutropenia and elevated amylase, ALT, total bilirubin, and lipase concentrations.

Drug Interactions

When atazanavir is used with a pharmacokinetic enhancer (i.e., low-dose ritonavir or cobicistat), drug interactions associated with both atazanavir and the pharmacokinetic enhancer should be considered. Because low-dose ritonavir and cobicistat are associated with different drug interactions, interactions reported or expected with *ritonavir-boosted* atazanavir may differ from those reported or expected with *cobicistat-boosted* atazanavir.

The following drug interactions are based on studies using *ritonavir-boosted* atazanavir or unboosted atazanavir or studies using cobicistat alone. Drug interaction studies are not available to date using *cobicistat-boosted* atazanavir administered either as the fixed combination containing atazanavir and cobicistat (atazanavir/cobicistat) or as single-entity atazanavir given with single-entity cobicistat.

■ **Drugs Affecting or Metabolized by Hepatic Microsomal Enzymes** Atazanavir, ritonavir, and cobicistat are metabolized by cytochrome P-450 (CYP) isoenzyme 3A4. Atazanavir inhibits CYP3A and 2C8. Ritonavir and cobicistat inhibit CYP3A and 2D6.

Pharmacokinetic interactions are likely if *ritonavir-boosted, cobicistat-boosted*, or unboosted atazanavir is used concomitantly with drugs that are inducers or substrates of CYP3A with possible alteration in metabolism and concentrations of atazanavir and/or the other drug. Concomitant use of *ritonavir-boosted* atazanavir or *cobicistat-boosted* atazanavir with such drugs may lead to severe, life-threatening, or fatal events due to increased exposures of certain drugs, adverse effects due to increased exposures to *ritonavir-boosted* atazanavir or *cobicistat-boosted* atazanavir, or loss of therapeutic effect and possible development of resistance to atazanavir.

Concomitant use of *cobicistat-boosted* atazanavir with drugs primarily metabolized by CYP2D6 may result in increased plasma concentration of such drugs, increase or prolong therapeutic effects and adverse reactions of such drugs, and may require dosage adjustments or additional monitoring. Use of *cobicistat-boosted* atazanavir with drugs that are highly dependent on CYP2C8 for clearance and have narrow therapeutic ranges (e.g., paclitaxel, repaglinide) is not recommended.

Pharmacokinetic interactions also are possible when unboosted atazanavir is used with CYP2C8 substrates. Atazanavir is not expected to interact with CYP2C19, 2C9, 2D6, 2B6, 2A6, 1A2, or 2E1 substrates.

Cobicistat is metabolized by CYP2D6 to a minor extent. Based on in vitro data, cobicistat is not expected to induce CYP1A2 or 2B6; based on in vivo data, cobicistat is not expected to induce CYP3A to a clinically important extent. It is not known whether cobicistat induces CYP2C9 or 2C19, but any effect is expected to be minimal based on in vitro CYP3A induction data.

■ **Drugs Metabolized by Uridine diphosphate-glucuronosyltransferase 1A1** Atazanavir inhibits uridine diphosphate-glucuronosyltransferase (UGT) 1A1; pharmacokinetic interactions are possible with drugs that are UGT 1A1 substrates (altered metabolism of the other drug). It is not known whether cobicistat induces UGT 1A1, but any effect is expected to be minimal based on CYP3A induction data.

■ **Drugs Affected by P-glycoprotein Transport** Cobicistat is a P-gp inhibitor. Potential pharmacokinetic interactions if *cobicistat-boosted* atazanavir is used with drugs transported by P-gp (increased plasma concentrations of such drugs, which could increase or prolong their therapeutic effects and may be associated with adverse effects).

■ **Drugs Affecting or Affected by Other Membrane Transporters** Cobicistat inhibits breast cancer resistance protein (BCRP) and organic anion transporting polypeptide (OATP) 1B1 and 1B3. Potential pharmacokinetic interactions if *cobicistat-boosted* atazanavir is used concomitantly with drugs that are substrates of BCRP, OATP1B1, or OATP1B3 (increased plasma concentrations of such drugs, which could increase or prolong their therapeutic effects and may be associated with adverse effects).

Based on in vitro data, cobicistat is not expected to induce multidrug-resistance gene (MDR) 1 to a clinically important extent.

■ **Drugs Affecting Gastric pH** Atazanavir solubility decreases as pH increases; reduced plasma concentrations of atazanavir are expected if drugs that affect gastric pH (e.g., antacids, buffered medications, histamine H_2-receptor antagonists, proton-pump inhibitors) are used concomitantly. (See Drug Interactions: GI Drugs.)

■ **Acetaminophen** Pharmacokinetic interactions between acetaminophen and atazanavir are unlikely.

■ **Alfuzosin** Potential pharmacokinetic interactions with alfuzosin (increased alfuzosin plasma concentrations).

Concomitant use of alfuzosin and *ritonavir-boosted, cobicistat-boosted*, or unboosted atazanavir is contraindicated because increased alfuzosin concentrations may result in hypotension.

■ **Antiarrhythmic Agents** Possible pharmacokinetic interactions if certain antiarrhythmic agents (e.g., amiodarone, dofetilide, dronedarone, flecainide, systemic lidocaine, propafenone, quinidine) are used concomitantly with *ritonavir-boosted, cobicistat-boosted*, or unboosted atazanavir (increased plasma concentrations of the antiarrhythmic, which may increase the potential for serious and/or life-threatening adverse effects). In addition, possible pharmacokinetic interactions if disopyramide or mexiletine is used concomitantly with *cobicistat-boosted* atazanavir (increased concentrations of the antiarrhythmic).

Ritonavir-boosted, cobicistat-boosted, or unboosted atazanavir and antiarrhythmic agents should be used concomitantly with caution; plasma concentration monitoring of the antiarrhythmic agents, if available, should be considered.

Amiodarone Some experts state that if amiodarone is used concomitantly with *ritonavir-boosted* or *cobicistat-boosted* atazanavir, the patient should be monitored for amiodarone toxicity and consideration given to ECG and amiodarone plasma concentration monitoring.

Dronedarone Concomitant use of dronedarone and *cobicistat-boosted* atazanavir is contraindicated.

Some experts state that concomitant use of dronedarone and *ritonavir-boosted* or unboosted atazanavir also is contraindicated.

■ **Anticoagulants** ***Apixaban*** Possible pharmacokinetic interactions if apixaban is used concomitantly with *ritonavir-boosted, cobicistat-boosted*, or unboosted atazanavir (increased apixaban concentrations).

Concomitant use of *ritonavir-boosted, cobicistat-boosted*, or unboosted atazanavir with apixaban is not recommended.

Dabigatran Possible pharmacokinetic interactions if dabigatran is used concomitantly with *ritonavir-boosted* or *cobicistat-boosted* atazanavir (increased dabigatran concentrations).

Concomitant use of *ritonavir-boosted* or *cobicistat-boosted* atazanavir with dabigatran is not recommended in certain patients with renal impairment. Some experts state that concomitant use should be avoided in those with creatinine clearances less than 50 mL/minute.

Edoxaban Possible pharmacokinetic interactions if edoxaban is used concomitantly with *ritonavir-boosted, cobicistat-boosted*, or unboosted atazanavir (increased edoxaban concentrations).

Concomitant use of *ritonavir-boosted, cobicistat-boosted*, or unboosted atazanavir and edoxaban should be avoided.

Rivaroxaban Possible pharmacokinetic interactions if rivaroxaban is used concomitantly with *ritonavir-boosted, cobicistat-boosted*, or unboosted atazanavir (increased concentrations of rivaroxaban) and increased risk of bleeding.

Concomitant use of *ritonavir-boosted, cobicistat-boosted*, or unboosted atazanavir should be avoided.

Warfarin Potential pharmacokinetic interactions if warfarin is used concomitantly with *ritonavir-boosted* or unboosted atazanavir (increased or decreased plasma concentrations of warfarin) and potential for serious and/or life-threatening bleeding. The effect of *cobicistat-boosted* atazanavir on warfarin concentrations is not known.

If warfarin is used concomitantly with *ritonavir-boosted, cobicistat-boosted*, or unboosted atazanavir, the international normalized ratio (INR) should be monitored, especially when initiating or discontinuing atazanavir; warfarin dosage should be adjusted as needed.

Some experts state that if *ritonavir-boosted* atazanavir is switched to *cobicistat-boosted* atazanavir, the effect of cobicistat on warfarin concentrations is not expected to be equivalent to the effect of ritonavir on warfarin concentrations.

■ **Anticonvulsants** ***Carbamazepine*** Concomitant use of unboosted atazanavir and carbamazepine may decrease plasma concentrations of atazanavir and is not recommended.

Concomitant use of *ritonavir-boosted* atazanavir and carbamazepine may decrease plasma concentrations of atazanavir and increase plasma concentrations of the anticonvulsant. If *ritonavir-boosted* atazanavir is initiated in a patient already receiving a stable carbamazepine dosage, reduction of the anticonvulsant dosage may be needed. Some experts recommend that alternatives to carbamazepine should be considered in patients receiving *ritonavir-boosted* atazanavir or plasma concentrations of both drugs should be monitored and antiretroviral response assessed.

Concomitant use of *cobicistat-boosted* atazanavir and carbamazepine may decrease plasma concentrations of atazanavir and cobicistat and may result in loss of therapeutic effect and development of resistance. Concomitant use of *cobicistat-boosted* atazanavir and carbamazepine is contraindicated.

Eslicarbazepine Concomitant use of *cobicistat-boosted* atazanavir and eslicarbazepine may decrease atazanavir and cobicistat plasma concentrations. An alternative anticonvulsant or alternative antiretroviral therapy should be considered; if concomitant use of eslicarbazepine and *cobicistat-boosted* atazanavir is necessary, the patient should be monitored for lack or loss of virologic response.

Ethosuximide Possible pharmacokinetic interactions if ethosuximide is used concomitantly with *ritonavir-boosted, cobicistat-boosted*, or unboosted atazanavir (increased ethosuximide concentrations). If ethosuximide is used concomitantly with *ritonavir-boosted, cobicistat-boosted*, or unboosted atazanavir, the patient should be clinically monitored for ethosuximide toxicities.

Lamotrigine Concomitant use of unboosted atazanavir and lamotrigine is not expected to affect lamotrigine concentrations; dosage adjustments are not needed if lamotrigine is used concomitantly with unboosted atazanavir.

Concomitant use of *ritonavir-boosted* atazanavir and lamotrigine decreases lamotrigine plasma concentrations and decreases the area under the plasma concentration-time curve (AUC) by 32%. An alternative anticonvulsant should be considered in patients receiving *ritonavir-boosted* atazanavir. If lamotrigine is used concomitantly with *ritonavir-boosted* atazanavir, increased lamotrigine dosage may be needed and lamotrigine plasma concentration monitoring should be considered.

Data are not available regarding concomitant use of *cobicistat-boosted* atazanavir and lamotrigine. In patients receiving *cobicistat-boosted* atazanavir, an alternative anticonvulsant should be considered or lamotrigine plasma concentrations should be monitored.

Oxcarbazepine Concomitant use of *cobicistat-boosted* atazanavir and oxcarbazepine may decrease atazanavir and cobicistat plasma concentrations. An alternative anticonvulsant or alternative antiretroviral should be considered; if concomitant use of oxcarbazepine and *cobicistat-boosted* atazanavir is necessary, the patient should be monitored for lack or loss of antiretroviral response.

Phenobarbital and Phenytoin Concomitant use of unboosted atazanavir and phenobarbital or phenytoin may decrease plasma concentrations of atazanavir and is not recommended.

Concomitant use of *ritonavir-boosted* atazanavir and phenobarbital or phenytoin may decrease plasma concentrations or atazanavir and the anticonvulsant. If *ritonavir-boosted* atazanavir is used concomitantly with phenobarbital or phenytoin, adjustment of the anticonvulsant dosage may be needed. Some experts recommend that alternatives to phenobarbital and phenytoin should be considered in patients receiving *ritonavir-boosted* atazanavir or plasma concentrations of both drugs should be monitored and antiretroviral response assessed.

Concomitant use of *cobicistat-boosted* atazanavir and phenobarbital or phenytoin may decrease plasma concentrations of atazanavir and cobicistat and may result in loss of therapeutic effect and development of resistance. Concomitant use of *cobicistat-boosted* atazanavir and phenobarbital or phenytoin is contraindicated.

■ **Antifungal Agents** ***Fluconazole*** Pharmacokinetic interactions unlikely if *ritonavir-boosted* or *cobicistat-boosted* atazanavir is used with fluconazole (no clinically important changes in plasma concentrations of atazanavir or fluconazole).

Dosage adjustments are not necessary if *ritonavir-boosted* or *cobicistat-boosted* atazanavir is used with fluconazole.

Isavuconazonium Concomitant use of isavuconazonium sulfate (prodrug of isavuconazole) and *ritonavir-boosted, cobicistat-boosted*, or unboosted atazanavir may result in increased isavuconazole concentrations and altered atazanavir concentrations.

If isavuconazonium sulfate and *ritonavir-boosted, cobicistat-boosted*, or unboosted atazanavir are used concomitantly, the patient should be monitored for atazanavir-associated adverse effects and virologic efficacy and isavuconazole concentration monitoring should be considered.

Itraconazole Possible pharmacokinetic interactions if *ritonavir-boosted, cobicistat-boosted*, or unboosted atazanavir is used with itraconazole (increased plasma concentrations of itraconazole, atazanavir, and cobicistat).

If itraconazole is used with *ritonavir-boosted, cobicistat-boosted*, or unboosted atazanavir, consideration should be given to monitoring itraconazole plasma concentrations and adjusting itraconazole dosage accordingly. Caution is advised if high itraconazole dosage (more than 200 mg daily) is used in patients receiving *ritonavir-boosted* atazanavir. Specific dosage recommendations are not available for concomitant use of *cobicistat-boosted* atazanavir and itraconazole. Some experts state that itraconazole dosages exceeding 200 mg daily are not recommended in patients receiving *ritonavir-boosted* or *cobicistat-boosted* atazanavir, unless plasma itraconazole concentrations are used to guide dosage of the antifungal.

Ketoconazole Pharmacokinetic interactions unlikely if unboosted atazanavir is used with ketoconazole (no clinically important changes in atazanavir plasma concentrations).

Possible pharmacokinetic interactions if ketoconazole is used with *ritonavir-boosted* or *cobicistat-boosted* atazanavir (increased plasma concentrations of ketoconazole, atazanavir, and cobicistat). Caution is advised if high ketoconazole dosage (more than 200 mg daily) is used in patients receiving *ritonavir-boosted* atazanavir. Specific dosage recommendations are not available for concomitant use of *cobicistat-boosted* atazanavir and ketoconazole.

Posaconazole Pharmacokinetic interactions if posaconazole is used with *ritonavir-boosted* or unboosted atazanavir (increased plasma concentration and AUC of atazanavir); possible pharmacokinetic interactions if used concomitantly with *cobicistat-boosted* atazanavir (increased atazanavir concentrations).

If posaconazole is used with *ritonavir-boosted, cobicistat-boosted*, or unboosted atazanavir, the patient should be monitored for atazanavir-associated adverse effects.

Voriconazole Pharmacokinetic interactions if voriconazole is used with *ritonavir-boosted* atazanavir (decreased atazanavir and voriconazole plasma concentrations in patients with a functional CYP2C19 allele; decreased atazanavir concentrations and increased voriconazole concentrations in patients without a functional CYP2C19 allele). Possible pharmacokinetic interactions if voriconazole is used with unboosted atazanavir (altered voriconazole and atazanavir plasma concentrations). Data are not available regarding concomitant use of voriconazole and *cobicistat-boosted* atazanavir.

Concomitant use of voriconazole and *ritonavir-boosted* or *cobicistat-boosted* atazanavir is not recommended unless potential benefits outweigh risks. If voriconazole is used concomitantly with *ritonavir-boosted* or *cobicistat-boosted* atazanavir, patients should be monitored for voriconazole-associated adverse effects and loss of voriconazole or atazanavir efficacy; consideration should be given to monitoring voriconazole concentrations and adjusting voriconazole dosage accordingly.

If voriconazole is used concomitantly with unboosted atazanavir, the patient should be monitored for toxicities.

■ **Antimalarial Agents** ***Atovaquone and Proguanil*** Pharmacokinetic interactions if the fixed combination of atovaquone and proguanil (atovaquone/proguanil) is used concomitantly with *ritonavir-boosted* atazanavir (decreased atovaquone and proguanil plasma concentrations). Some experts state that an alternative antimalarial should be considered, if possible, in patients receiving *ritonavir-boosted* atazanavir.

■ **Antimycobacterial Agents** ***Bedaquiline*** Possible pharmacokinetic interactions if bedaquiline is used concomitantly with *ritonavir-boosted* or *cobicistat-boosted* atazanavir (increased bedaquiline concentrations); clinical importance is unknown.

Some experts state that bedaquiline may be used concomitantly with *ritonavir-boosted* or *cobicistat-boosted* atazanavir if potential benefits outweigh risks, but caution is advised and patients should be monitored for corrected QT (QT_c) interval prolongation and liver dysfunction.

Rifabutin Pharmacokinetic interactions if rifabutin is used concomitantly with *ritonavir-boosted* or unboosted atazanavir (increased peak plasma concentration and AUC of rifabutin and its metabolite). Possible pharmacokinetic interactions if rifabutin is used concomitantly with *cobicistat-boosted* atazanavir (increased rifabutin concentrations expected; effects on atazanavir and cobicistat concentrations unknown).

If rifabutin is used concomitantly with *ritonavir-boosted, cobicistat-boosted*, or unboosted atazanavir, dosage of the antimycobacterial agent should be reduced (e.g., 150 mg once every other day or 3 times weekly) and increased monitoring for rifabutin-associated adverse effects (e.g., neutropenia, uveitis) is warranted. Some experts recommend a rifabutin dosage of 150 mg once daily or 300 mg 3 times weekly and state that patients should be monitored for antimycobacterial response and therapeutic drug concentration monitoring should be considered.

Rifampin Pharmacokinetic interactions if rifampin is used concomitantly with *ritonavir-boosted, cobicistat-boosted*, or unboosted atazanavir (substantially decreased plasma concentrations of atazanavir) with possible loss of therapeutic effect of the antiretroviral agent and development of resistance.

Concomitant use of rifampin and *ritonavir-boosted, cobicistat-boosted*, or unboosted atazanavir is contraindicated. If a rifamycin is indicated in a patient receiving *ritonavir-boosted, cobicistat-boosted*, or unboosted atazanavir, some experts state that rifabutin should be considered as an alternative to rifampin.

Rifapentine Possible pharmacokinetic interactions if rifapentine is used concomitantly with *ritonavir-boosted, cobicistat-boosted*, or unboosted atazanavir (decreased atazanavir plasma concentrations). Concomitant use of *ritonavir-boosted, cobicistat-boosted*, or unboosted atazanavir and rifapentine is not recommended. HIV-infected tuberculosis patients treated with rifapentine have a higher rate of tuberculosis relapse than those treated with other rifamycin-based tuberculosis regimens; an alternative antimycobacterial agent is recommended in HIV-infected patients.

■ **Antineoplastic Agents** ***Dasatinib or Nilotinib*** Possible pharmacokinetic interactions if dasatinib or nilotinib is used concomitantly with *cobicistat-boosted* atazanavir (increased antineoplastic agent concentrations).

If dasatinib or nilotinib is used concomitantly with *cobicistat-boosted* atazanavir, decreased dosage of the antineoplastic agent may be necessary.

Irinotecan Pharmacokinetic interactions if irinotecan is used concomitantly with *ritonavir-boosted, cobicistat-boosted*, or unboosted atazanavir. Atazanavir inhibits UGT 1A1 and may interfere with the metabolism of irinotecan leading to an increase in irinotecan toxicity.

Concomitant use of irinotecan with *ritonavir-boosted, cobicistat-boosted*, or unboosted atazanavir is contraindicated.

Paclitaxel Possible pharmacokinetic interactions if paclitaxel is used concomitantly with unboosted atazanavir (increased plasma concentrations of paclitaxel); caution is advised.

Clinically important interactions are not expected if paclitaxel is used concomitantly with *ritonavir-boosted* atazanavir.

Concomitant use of paclitaxel and *cobicistat-boosted* atazanavir is *not* recommended.

Vinblastine or Vincristine Possible pharmacokinetic interactions if vinblastine or vincristine is used concomitantly with *cobicistat-boosted* atazanavir (increased antineoplastic agent concentrations).

If vincristine or vinblastine is used concomitantly with *cobicistat-boosted* atazanavir, the patient should be monitored for adverse hematologic or GI effects.

■ **Antipsychotic Agents** ***Lurasidone*** Possible pharmacokinetic interactions if lurasidone is used concomitantly with *ritonavir-boosted* or unboosted atazanavir (increased lurasidone concentrations). Potential for serious and/or life-threatening adverse effects if lurasidone is used concomitantly with *ritonavir-boosted* or *cobicistat-boosted* atazanavir.

Concomitant use of *ritonavir-boosted* or *cobicistat-boosted* atazanavir and lurasidone is contraindicated.

The manufacturer of atazanavir states that if concomitant use of unboosted atazanavir and lurasidone is necessary, lurasidone dosage should be reduced. Some experts state that unboosted atazanavir should not be used concomitantly with lurasidone.

Perphenazine, Risperidone, Thioridazine Possible pharmacokinetic interactions if *ritonavir-boosted* or *cobicistat-boosted* atazanavir is used concomitantly with perphenazine, risperidone, or thioridazine (increased plasma concentrations of the antipsychotic agent).

If perphenazine, risperidone, or thioridazine is used concomitantly with *ritonavir-boosted* or *cobicistat-boosted* atazanavir, a reduced dosage of the antipsychotic may be needed. Some experts state that the antipsychotic should be initiated using the lowest dosage, maintenance dosage should be adjusted as needed, and the patient should be monitored for toxicities associated with the antipsychotic.

Pimozide Concomitant use of pimozide and *ritonavir-boosted, cobicistat-boosted*, or unboosted atazanavir is contraindicated because of the potential for serious and/or life-threatening adverse effects (e.g., cardiac arrhythmias).

Quetiapine Pharmacokinetic interactions expected if quetiapine is used concomitantly with *ritonavir-boosted, cobicistat-boosted*, or unboosted atazanavir (increased quetiapine concentrations).

Alternative antiretroviral therapy should be considered. If *ritonavir-boosted, cobicistat-boosted*, or unboosted atazanavir is necessary in a patient receiving a stable dosage of quetiapine, the quetiapine dosage should be reduced to one-sixth of the original dosage and the patient should be monitored for quetiapine efficacy and adverse effects. If quetiapine is necessary in a patient receiving *ritonavir-boosted, cobicistat-boosted*, or unboosted atazanavir, some experts recommend that quetiapine should be initiated using the lowest dosage and titrated as needed.

■ Antiretroviral Agents *HIV Entry and Fusion Inhibitors*

Enfuvirtide. No in vitro evidence of antagonistic antiretroviral effects between atazanavir and enfuvirtide.

Maraviroc. Concomitant use of maraviroc and *ritonavir-boosted, cobicistat-boosted*, or unboosted atazanavir results in increased maraviroc plasma concentrations and AUC. If maraviroc is used concomitantly with *ritonavir-boosted, cobicistat-boosted*, or unboosted atazanavir, the recommended maraviroc dosage is 150 mg twice daily.

No in vitro evidence of antagonistic antiretroviral effects between atazanavir and maraviroc.

HIV Integrase Inhibitors (INSTIs) **Dolutegravir.** Concomitant use of dolutegravir and *ritonavir-boosted* or unboosted atazanavir results in increased dolutegravir AUC. Data are not available regarding concomitant use of dolutegravir and *cobicistat-boosted* atazanavir.

Some experts state that dosage adjustments are not necessary if dolutegravir is used concomitantly with *ritonavir-boosted, cobicistat-boosted*, or unboosted atazanavir.

Elvitegravir. Concomitant use of single-entity elvitegravir and *ritonavir-boosted* atazanavir results in increased trough plasma concentrations of elvitegravir but the AUC of elvitegravir and AUC of atazanavir are unaffected. If *ritonavir-boosted* atazanavir and single-entity elvitegravir are used concomitantly, some experts recommend that single-entity atazanavir 300 mg, single-entity ritonavir 100 mg, and single-entity elvitegravir 85 mg be given once daily. Data are not available regarding concomitant use of single-entity elvitegravir and *cobicistat-boosted* atazanavir and some experts state that *cobicistat-boosted* atazanavir should *not* be used concomitantly with single-entity elvitegravir.

Possible pharmacokinetic interactions if the fixed combination of elvitegravir, cobicistat, emtricitabine, and tenofovir disoproxil fumarate (EVG/c/FTC/TDF) is used concomitantly with *ritonavir-boosted* or unboosted atazanavir (altered concentrations of elvitegravir, cobicistat, and/or atazanavir). EVG/c/FTC/TDF should not be used concomitantly with *ritonavir-boosted, cobicistat-boosted*, or unboosted atazanavir.

Raltegravir. Concomitant use of raltegravir and *ritonavir-boosted* or unboosted atazanavir results in increased raltegravir plasma concentrations and AUC. Data are not available regarding concomitant use of raltegravir and *cobicistat-boosted* atazanavir.

Dosage adjustments are not necessary if raltegravir is used concomitantly with *ritonavir-boosted, cobicistat-boosted*, or unboosted atazanavir.

The antiretroviral effects of raltegravir and atazanavir are additive to synergistic against HIV-1 in vitro.

HIV Nonnucleoside Reverse Transcriptase Inhibitors (NNRTIs) There is no in vitro evidence of antagonistic antiretroviral effects between atazanavir and HIV nonnucleoside reverse transcriptase inhibitors (NNRTIs) (delavirdine, efavirenz, etravirine, nevirapine, rilpivirine). The antiretroviral effects of atazanavir and nevirapine may be additive to synergistic against HIV-1 in vitro.

Efavirenz. Concomitant use of efavirenz and unboosted atazanavir results in substantially decreased plasma concentrations and AUC of atazanavir, but no clinically important effects on efavirenz plasma concentrations. Depending on the specific regimen used, concomitant use of *ritonavir-boosted* atazanavir and efavirenz may increase atazanavir plasma concentrations and AUC. Concomitant use of efavirenz with *cobicistat-boosted* atazanavir may result in decreased plasma concentrations of atazanavir and cobicistat, but no change in efavirenz concentrations.

Unboosted atazanavir should not be used concomitantly with efavirenz in antiretroviral-naive or antiretroviral-experienced patients.

If *ritonavir-boosted* atazanavir is used concomitantly with efavirenz in antiretroviral-naive adults, a regimen of atazanavir 400 mg and ritonavir 100 mg once daily (with food) and efavirenz 600 mg once daily (without food, preferably at bedtime) is recommended. *Ritonavir-boosted* atazanavir should not be used concomitantly with efavirenz in antiretroviral-experienced patients.

If *cobicistat-boosted* atazanavir is used concomitantly with efavirenz in antiretroviral-naive adults, a regimen of single-entity atazanavir 400 mg and single-entity cobicistat 150 mg once daily (with food) and efavirenz 600 mg once daily (without food, preferably at bedtime) is recommended. *Cobicistat-boosted* atazanavir should not be used concomitantly with efavirenz in antiretroviral-experienced patients.

Etravirine. Pharmacokinetic interactions if etravirine is used concomitantly with *ritonavir-boosted* or unboosted atazanavir (increased etravirine plasma concentrations and AUC; decreased atazanavir plasma concentrations and AUC) with possible decreased antiretroviral efficacy. Pharmacokinetic interactions if etravirine is used concomitantly with *cobicistat-boosted* atazanavir (decreased atazanavir and cobicistat concentrations).

Concomitant use of etravirine and *ritonavir-boosted, cobicistat-boosted*, or unboosted atazanavir is not recommended.

If *ritonavir-boosted* atazanavir is used concomitantly with etravirine, some experts recommend a regimen of atazanavir 300 mg once daily and ritonavir 100 mg once daily in conjunction with usual etravirine dosage.

Nevirapine. Pharmacokinetic interactions if nevirapine is used concomitantly with *ritonavir-boosted* or unboosted atazanavir (substantially decreased atazanavir plasma concentrations and AUC with possible loss of therapeutic effect and development of resistance; increased nevirapine plasma concentrations and AUC and increased risk of nevirapine-associated adverse effects). Pharmacokinetic interactions if nevirapine is used concomitantly with *cobicistat-boosted* atazanavir (decreased cobicistat concentrations).

Concomitant use of nevirapine and *ritonavir-boosted, cobicistat-boosted*, or unboosted atazanavir is contraindicated.

Rilpivirine. Concomitant use of rilpivirine and *ritonavir-boosted, cobicistat-boosted*, or unboosted atazanavir may result in increased rilpivirine plasma concentrations, but is not expected to affect atazanavir plasma concentrations.

Some experts state that dosage adjustments are not needed if rilpivirine and *ritonavir-boosted, cobicistat-boosted*, or unboosted atazanavir are used concomitantly.

HIV Nucleoside and Nucleotide Reverse Transcriptase Inhibitors (NRTIs) In vitro studies indicate that antagonism does not occur between atazanavir and HIV-nucleoside reverse transcriptase inhibitors (NRTIs) (abacavir, didanosine, emtricitabine, lamivudine, stavudine, tenofovir, zidovudine).

Didanosine. Administration of buffered didanosine and atazanavir at the same time results in substantially decreased plasma concentrations and AUC of atazanavir and decreased plasma concentrations and AUC of didanosine. Administration of didanosine delayed-release capsules and atazanavir at the same time and with food results in decreased plasma concentrations and AUC of didanosine, but does not affect atazanavir plasma concentrations.

Ritonavir-boosted, cobicistat-boosted, or unboosted atazanavir should be administered (with food) at least 2 hours before or 1 hour after buffered or delayed-release didanosine preparations (without food).

Lamivudine and Zidovudine. No clinically important pharmacokinetic interactions reported when unboosted atazanavir (400 mg once daily) is used concomitantly with lamivudine (150 mg twice daily) and zidovudine (300 mg twice daily).

Tenofovir Alafenamide Fumarate. Concomitant use of *ritonavir-boosted* atazanavir and tenofovir alafenamide fumarate results in a 91% increase in the AUC of tenofovir.

Some experts state that dosage adjustments for tenofovir alafenamide are not necessary if the drug is used concomitantly with *ritonavir-boosted, cobicistat-boosted*, or unboosted atazanavir.

Tenofovir Disoproxil Fumarate. Pharmacokinetic interactions between tenofovir disoproxil fumarate (tenofovir DF) and *ritonavir-boosted, cobicistat-boosted*, or unboosted atazanavir (decreased atazanavir plasma concentrations and AUC; increased tenofovir plasma concentrations and AUC and possible increased risk of tenofovir-associated adverse effects, including renal disorders).

Unboosted atazanavir should not be used concomitantly with tenofovir DF.

If tenofovir DF and *ritonavir-boosted* atazanavir are used concomitantly, a regimen of atazanavir 300 mg, ritonavir 100 mg, and tenofovir DF 300 mg once daily with food is recommended. Patients should be monitored for tenofovir toxicity; tenofovir should be discontinued if tenofovir-associated adverse effects occur.

If tenofovir DF and *cobicistat-boosted* atazanavir are used concomitantly, a regimen of atazanavir 300 mg, cobicistat 150 mg, and tenofovir DF 300 mg once daily with food is recommended. Baseline estimated creatinine clearance, urine glucose, and urine protein should be assessed and patients should be monitored for tenofovir toxicity. Serum phosphorus concentrations should be monitored in patients with or at risk for renal impairment. Concomitant use of *cobicistat-boosted* atazanavir and tenofovir DF is not recommended in patients with estimated creatinine clearances less than 70 mL/minute.

If *ritonavir-boosted* atazanavir is used concomitantly with tenofovir DF *and* a histamine H_2-receptor antagonist in antiretroviral-experienced adults, the recommended dosage is atazanavir 400 mg, ritonavir 100 mg, and tenofovir DF 300 mg given once daily with food. Patients should be monitored for tenofovir toxicity.

If *cobicistat-boosted* atazanavir is used concomitantly with tenofovir DF *and* a histamine H_2-receptor antagonist in antiretroviral-experienced adults, some experts recommend single-entity atazanavir 400 mg and single-entity cobicistat 150 mg once daily with food. Patients should be monitored for tenofovir toxicity.

If an antiretroviral-experienced pregnant woman in the second or third trimester is receiving *ritonavir-boosted* atazanavir *and* either a histamine H_2-receptor antagonist *or* tenofovir DF, the recommended dosage is atazanavir 400 mg and ritonavir 100 mg once daily with food. Dosage recommendations are not available for pregnant women receiving both a histamine H_2-receptor antagonist *and* tenofovir in conjunction with *ritonavir-boosted* atazanavir.

HIV Protease Inhibitors (PIs) In vitro studies indicate that the antiretroviral effects of atazanavir and amprenavir (active metabolite of fosamprenavir) or saquinavir are synergistic, the antiretroviral effects of atazanavir and lopinavir are additive to synergistic, and the antiretroviral effects of atazanavir and tipranavir are additive to antagonistic. There is no in vitro evidence of antagonism between atazanavir and other HIV PIs (amprenavir, darunavir, indinavir, lopinavir, nelfinavir, ritonavir, saquinavir).

Darunavir. Concomitant use of atazanavir 300 mg once daily with *ritonavir-boosted* darunavir (darunavir 400 mg and ritonavir 100 mg twice daily [dosage differs from usually recommended dosage]) results in plasma concentrations of atazanavir that are similar to those attained with *ritonavir-boosted* atazanavir (atazanavir 300 mg and ritonavir 100 mg once daily) and plasma concentrations of darunavir similar to those attained without atazanavir.

The manufacturer of darunavir states that concomitant use of darunavir and *ritonavir-boosted* atazanavir is not recommended.

Fosamprenavir. Pharmacokinetic interactions between atazanavir and *ritonavir-boosted* fosamprenavir (decreased plasma concentrations and AUC of atazanavir; no change in plasma concentrations or AUC of amprenavir [active metabolite of fosamprenavir]); data not available regarding concomitant use of fosamprenavir (without low-dose ritonavir) and atazanavir.

Appropriate dosages for concomitant use of atazanavir and fosamprenavir (with or without low-dose ritonavir) with respect to safety and efficacy have not been established.

Indinavir. Both indinavir and atazanavir are associated with hyperbilirubinemia and additive adverse effects are possible.

Concomitant use of *ritonavir-boosted*, *cobicistat-boosted*, or unboosted atazanavir and indinavir is contraindicated.

Lopinavir. Because prolonged PR interval has been reported with both lopinavir and atazanavir, the fixed combination of lopinavir and ritonavir (lopinavir/ritonavir) and atazanavir should be used concomitantly with caution and clinical monitoring.

Ritonavir. Pharmacokinetic interactions if ritonavir is used concomitantly with atazanavir (increased plasma concentration and AUC of atazanavir). Low-dose ritonavir (100 mg once daily) is a pharmacokinetic enhancer (pharmacokinetic booster), and is used in conjunction with atazanavir for therapeutic advantage (*ritonavir-boosted* atazanavir). Additional pharmacokinetic interactions are possible if *ritonavir-boosted* atazanavir is used concomitantly with other HIV PIs and such use is not recommended.

Safety and efficacy of concomitant use of atazanavir and ritonavir dosages exceeding 100 mg once daily have not been established and such concomitant use is not recommended.

Concomitant use of *cobicistat-boosted* atazanavir with ritonavir or ritonavir-containing preparations is not recommended since cobicistat and ritonavir have similar effects on CYP3A.

Saquinavir. Concomitant use of atazanavir (300 mg once daily) and saquinavir (1.6 g once daily as Invirase®) and ritonavir (100 mg once daily) results in increased plasma concentrations and AUC of saquinavir (42 and 60%, respectively) and no change in plasma atazanavir concentrations. In a clinical study, a regimen of atazanavir, saquinavir, tenofovir, and a NRTI did not provide adequate efficacy. (See Clinical Experience under Treatment of HIV Infection: Antiretroviral-Experienced Adults and Adolescents, in Uses.)

Prolonged PR interval has been reported with both saquinavir and atazanavir and additive effects on the PR interval could occur.

Appropriate dosages for concomitant use of atazanavir and saquinavir (with or without low-dose ritonavir) with respect to safety and efficacy have not been established. Atazanavir and *ritonavir-boosted* saquinavir should be used concomitantly with caution and clinical monitoring.

Tipranavir. Pharmacokinetic interactions between *ritonavir-boosted* atazanavir and *ritonavir-boosted* tipranavir (decreased atazanavir plasma concentrations and AUC and increased tipranavir plasma concentrations and AUC).

Concomitant use of atazanavir (with or without low-dose ritonavir) and tipranavir is not recommended.

■ **Atovaquone** Concomitant use of *ritonavir-boosted* atazanavir and atovaquone does not affect atovaquone concentrations. Dosage adjustments are not needed if *ritonavir-boosted* atazanavir and atovaquone are used concomitantly.

■ **Benzodiazepines** ***Alprazolam*** Potential pharmacokinetic interactions if alprazolam is used concomitantly with *ritonavir-boosted*, *cobicistat-boosted*, or unboosted atazanavir (increased benzodiazepine plasma concentrations).

Although pharmacokinetic studies evaluating concomitant use are lacking, some experts state that other benzodiazepines not metabolized by CYP isoenzymes (e.g., lorazepam, oxazepam, temazepam) should be considered instead of alprazolam in patients receiving *ritonavir-boosted*, *cobicistat-boosted*, or unboosted atazanavir.

Clonazepam Potential pharmacokinetic interactions if clonazepam is used concomitantly with *ritonavir-boosted*, *cobicistat-boosted*, or unboosted atazanavir (increased clonazepam concentrations).

If clonazepam is used concomitantly with *cobicistat-boosted* atazanavir, clinical monitoring is recommended. Although pharmacokinetic studies evaluating concomitant use are lacking, some experts state that other benzodiazepines not metabolized by CYP isoenzymes (e.g., lorazepam, oxazepam, temazepam) should be considered instead of clonazepam in patients receiving *ritonavir-boosted*, *cobicistat-boosted*, or unboosted atazanavir.

Diazepam If diazepam is used concomitantly with *cobicistat-boosted* atazanavir, reduction of the diazepam dosage may be needed and the patient should be monitored for adverse effects. Some experts state that other benzodiazepines not metabolized by CYP isoenzymes (e.g., lorazepam, oxazepam, temazepam) should be considered instead of diazepam in patients receiving *ritonavir-boosted* or *cobicistat-boosted* atazanavir.

Midazolam or Triazolam Pharmacokinetic interactions if midazolam or triazolam is used concomitantly with *ritonavir-boosted*, *cobicistat-boosted*, or unboosted atazanavir (increased benzodiazepine plasma concentrations) and potential for serious and/or life-threatening adverse effects (e.g., prolonged or increased sedation or respiratory depression).

Concomitant use of oral midazolam or triazolam and *ritonavir-boosted*, *cobicistat-boosted*, or unboosted atazanavir is contraindicated.

Concomitant use of parenteral midazolam and *ritonavir-boosted*, *cobicistat-boosted*, or unboosted atazanavir should be undertaken with caution and in a monitored setting where respiratory depression and/or prolonged sedation can be managed. In addition, a reduced dosage of midazolam should be considered, especially if more than a single dose of midazolam is given. Some experts state that parenteral midazolam can be given in a single dose with caution in a monitored situation for procedural sedation in patients receiving *ritonavir-boosted*, *cobicistat-boosted*, or unboosted atazanavir.

■ ***β*-Adrenergic Blocking Agents** Possible pharmacokinetic interactions if certain *β*-adrenergic blocking agents metabolized by CYP2D6 (e.g., carvedilol, metoprolol, timolol) are used concomitantly with *ritonavir-boosted*, *cobicistat-boosted*, or unboosted atazanavir (increased concentrations of the *β*-adrenergic blocking agent).

If carvedilol, metoprolol, or timolol is used concomitantly with *ritonavir-boosted*, *cobicistat-boosted*, or unboosted atazanavir, clinical monitoring of the patient is recommended and reduction of the dosage of the *β*-adrenergic blocking agent may be needed. Alternatively, some experts state that use of *β*-adrenergic blocking agents that are not metabolized by CYP enzymes (e.g., atenolol, labetalol, nadolol, sotalol) should be considered.

In a pharmacokinetic study evaluating concomitant use of atazanavir 400 mg once daily with atenolol 50 mg once daily, no clinically important pharmacokinetic interactions were observed. Pharmacokinetic interactions are not expected if *cobicistat-boosted* atazanavir and atenolol are used concomitantly.

■ **Bosentan** Possible pharmacokinetic interactions if bosentan is used concomitantly with *ritonavir-boosted*, *cobicistat-boosted*, or unboosted atazanavir (increased bosentan plasma concentrations, decreased atazanavir and cobicistat plasma concentrations).

Unboosted atazanavir should not be used concomitantly with bosentan.

In patients who have been receiving *ritonavir-boosted* or *cobicistat-boosted* atazanavir for at least 10 days, bosentan should be initiated using a dosage of 62.5 mg once daily or every other day based on individual tolerability.

In patients who have been receiving bosentan, bosentan should be discontinued for at least 36 hours prior to initiating *ritonavir-boosted* or *cobicistat-boosted* atazanavir; after at least 10 days of *ritonavir-boosted* or *cobicistat-boosted* atazanavir therapy, bosentan can be resumed using a dosage of 62.5 mg once daily or every other day based on individual tolerability.

In patients switching from *ritonavir-boosted* atazanavir to *cobicistat-boosted* atazanavir, the current bosentan dosage should be maintained.

■ **Buspirone** Possible pharmacokinetic interactions if buspirone is used concomitantly with *ritonavir-boosted*, *cobicistat-boosted*, or unboosted atazanavir (increased buspirone concentrations).

If buspirone is used concomitantly with *ritonavir-boosted*, *cobicistat-boosted*, or unboosted atazanavir, buspirone dosage should be titrated, a lower buspirone dosage should be considered, and the patient should be monitored for prolonged or adverse effects.

■ **Calcium-channel Blocking Agents** Possible pharmacokinetic interactions if certain calcium-channel blocking agents (e.g., amlodipine, felodipine, nicardipine, nifedipine, verapamil) are used concomitantly with *ritonavir-boosted*, *cobicistat-boosted*, or unboosted atazanavir (increased concentrations of the calcium-channel blocking agent). These calcium-channel blocking agents should be used concomitantly with *ritonavir-boosted*, *cobicis-*

tat-boosted, or unboosted atazanavir with caution; dosage titration and clinical and ECG monitoring are recommended.

Pharmacokinetic interactions if diltiazem is used concomitantly with unboosted atazanavir (increased diltiazem plasma concentrations and AUC). Concomitant use of diltiazem with *ritonavir-boosted* or *cobicistat-boosted* atazanavir is expected to result in greater increases in diltiazem concentrations. Diltiazem and atazanavir should be used concomitantly with caution. If diltiazem is used concomitantly with *ritonavir-boosted, cobicistat-boosted*, or unboosted atazanavir, a 50% reduction in diltiazem dosage should be considered and ECG monitoring is recommended.

■ **Cobicistat** Pharmacokinetic interactions if cobicistat is used concomitantly with atazanavir (increased plasma concentrations and AUC of atazanavir). Cobicistat is a pharmacokinetic enhancer (pharmacokinetic booster) and is used in conjunction with atazanavir for therapeutic advantage (*cobicistat-boosted* atazanavir).

■ **Colchicine** Potential pharmacokinetic interactions if colchicine is used concomitantly with *ritonavir-boosted, cobicistat-boosted*, or unboosted atazanavir (increased colchicine plasma concentrations).

Concomitant use of colchicine and *ritonavir-boosted* or unboosted atazanavir is not recommended in patients with renal or hepatic impairment. Concomitant use of colchicine and *cobicistat-boosted* atazanavir is contraindicated in patients with renal or hepatic impairment.

When colchicine is used for *treatment* of gout flares in patients receiving *ritonavir-boosted, cobicistat-boosted*, or unboosted atazanavir, an initial colchicine dose of 0.6 mg should be given followed by 0.3 mg 1 hour later; the colchicine dose should be repeated no earlier than 3 days later.

When colchicine is used for *prophylaxis* of gout flares in patients receiving *ritonavir-boosted, cobicistat-boosted*, or unboosted atazanavir, colchicine dosage should be reduced to 0.3 mg once daily in those originally receiving 0.6 mg twice daily or decreased to 0.3 mg once every other day in those originally receiving 0.6 mg once daily.

When colchicine is used for treatment of familial Mediterranean fever (FMF) in patients receiving *ritonavir-boosted, cobicistat-boosted*, or unboosted atazanavir, a maximum colchicine dosage of 0.6 mg daily (may be given as 0.3 mg twice daily) should be used.

■ **Corticosteroids** ***Orally Inhaled or Intranasal Corticosteroids*** Possible pharmacokinetic interactions if fluticasone (orally inhaled or intranasal) is used concomitantly with unboosted atazanavir (increased fluticasone concentrations). Concomitant use of budesonide (orally inhaled or intranasal), fluticasone (orally inhaled or intranasal), or mometasone (orally inhaled or intranasal) with *ritonavir-boosted* or *cobicistat-boosted* atazanavir may result in increased concentrations of the corticosteroid and may result in adrenal insufficiency or Cushing's syndrome.

Fluticasone (orally inhaled or intranasal) and unboosted atazanavir should be used concomitantly with caution. Budesonide (orally inhaled or intranasal), fluticasone (orally inhaled or intranasal), and mometasone (orally inhaled or intranasal) should not be used concomitantly with *ritonavir-boosted* or *cobicistat-boosted* atazanavir unless potential benefits of the inhaled corticosteroid outweigh risks of systemic corticosteroid adverse effects. An alternative corticosteroid (e.g., beclomethasone) should be considered, especially when long-term use of the corticosteroid is anticipated.

Local Injections of Corticosteroids Concomitant use of intra-articular or other local injections of methylprednisolone, prednisolone, or triamcinolone with *ritonavir-boosted* or *cobicistat-boosted* atazanavir may result in increased concentrations of the corticosteroid and may result in adrenal insufficiency or Cushing's syndrome.

Ritonavir-boosted or *cobicistat-boosted* atazanavir should not be used concomitantly with local injections of methylprednisolone, prednisolone, or triamcinolone; other nonsteroidal therapies should be considered. If intra-articular corticosteroid therapy is required, an alternative antiretroviral that does not alter CYP3A4 activity should be considered (e.g., dolutegravir, raltegravir).

Systemic Corticosteroids Concomitant use of systemic budesonide or prednisone and *ritonavir-boosted, cobicistat-boosted*, or unboosted atazanavir may result in increased corticosteroid concentrations and may result in adrenal insufficiency or Cushing's syndrome. Systemic budesonide or prednisone should not be used concomitantly with *ritonavir-boosted, cobicistat-boosted*, or unboosted atazanavir unless potential benefits outweigh the risks of systemic corticosteroid adverse effects.

Concomitant use of systemic dexamethasone and *ritonavir-boosted, cobicistat-boosted*, or unboosted atazanavir may result in decreased atazanavir concentrations and possible decreased antiretroviral efficacy and development of atazanavir resistance. Systemic dexamethasone and *ritonavir-boosted, cobicistat-boosted*, or unboosted atazanavir should be used concomitantly with caution; alternative corticosteroids should be considered for long-term use.

■ **Co-trimoxazole** Clinically important interactions between co-trimoxazole and *ritonavir-boosted, cobicistat-boosted*, or unboosted atazanavir are unlikely.

■ **Dapsone** Clinically important interactions between dapsone and *ritonavir-boosted, cobicistat-boosted*, or unboosted atazanavir are unlikely.

■ **Digoxin** Pharmacokinetic interactions if digoxin is used concomitantly with *ritonavir-boosted* or *cobicistat-boosted* atazanavir (increased digoxin concentrations). Digoxin and *ritonavir-boosted* or *cobicistat-boosted* atazanavir should be used concomitantly with caution; the digoxin dosage should be titrated and digoxin plasma concentrations monitored.

■ **Eplerenone** Concomitant use of eplerenone and *ritonavir-boosted, cobicistat-boosted*, or unboosted atazanavir is expected to result in increased eplerenone concentrations.

Some experts state that concomitant use of eplerenone and *ritonavir-boosted, cobicistat-boosted*, or unboosted atazanavir is contraindicated.

■ **Ergot Alkaloids** Concomitant use of ergot alkaloids (e.g., dihydroergotamine, ergotamine, methylergonovine) and *ritonavir-boosted, cobicistat-boosted*, or unboosted atazanavir is contraindicated because of possible increased concentrations of the ergot alkaloids and potential for serious adverse effects (e.g., peripheral vasospasm, ischemia of the extremities and other tissues).

If a woman receiving atazanavir or any other PI as part of an antiretroviral regimen experiences uterine atony and excessive postpartum bleeding, methylergonovine maleate (Methergine®) should be used for treatment of the hemorrhage *only* if alternative treatments (e.g., carboprost, misoprostol, oxytocin, dinoprostone) cannot be used and the potential benefits of the ergot alkaloid outweigh the risks. In this situation, methylergonovine maleate should be used in the lowest dosage and shortest duration possible.

■ **Estrogens and Progestins** Pharmacokinetic interactions if oral contraceptives containing ethinyl estradiol and norgestimate or norethindrone are used concomitantly with *ritonavir-boosted* or unboosted atazanavir (increased or decreased plasma concentrations of ethinyl estradiol; increased plasma concentrations of the progestin). Data are not available regarding concomitant use of oral contraceptives and *cobicistat-boosted* atazanavir and possible effects on estrogen and progestin concentrations.

If *ritonavir-boosted* atazanavir is used with an oral contraceptive, caution is advised and use of an oral contraceptive preparation containing at least 35 mcg of ethinyl estradiol is recommended. If unboosted atazanavir is used with an oral contraceptive, caution is advised and use of an oral contraceptive preparation containing no more than 30 mcg of ethinyl estradiol is recommended.

Additional or alternative nonhormonal forms of contraception should be considered in patients receiving *ritonavir-boosted, cobicistat-boosted*, or unboosted atazanavir.

Data are not available regarding use of etonogestrel-releasing subdermal implant contraceptives in patients receiving *ritonavir-boosted, cobicistat-boosted*, or unboosted atazanavir; some experts recommend use of alternative or additional methods of contraception or use of alternative antiretrovirals.

Data are not available regarding use of other hormonal contraceptives (e.g., transdermal contraceptive preparations, contraceptive vaginal ring, injectable contraceptive preparations, oral contraceptive preparations containing progestins other than norgestimate or norethindrone, or oral contraceptive preparations containing less than 25 mcg of ethinyl estradiol) in patients receiving *ritonavir-boosted* or unboosted atazanavir. Alternative methods of contraception are recommended.

■ **Flibanserin** Concomitant use of flibanserin and *ritonavir-boosted, cobicistat-boosted*, or unboosted atazanavir is expected to increase flibanserin concentrations.

Some experts state that concomitant use of flibanserin and *ritonavir-boosted, cobicistat-boosted*, or unboosted atazanavir is contraindicated.

■ **GI Drugs** ***Antacids*** Potential pharmacokinetic interactions if antacids or buffered medications are given concomitantly with atazanavir (decreased oral absorption of atazanavir). *Ritonavir-boosted, cobicistat-boosted*, or unboosted atazanavir should be administered at least 2 hours before or 1–2 hours after antacids or buffered medications.

Cisapride Concomitant use of cisapride and *ritonavir-boosted, cobicistat-boosted*, or unboosted atazanavir is contraindicated because of possible increased cisapride plasma concentrations and potential for serious and/or life-threatening adverse effects (e.g., cardiac arrhythmias).

Histamine H_2-receptor Antagonists Atazanavir 400 mg once daily administered simultaneously with famotidine 40 mg twice daily results in a substantial decrease in plasma concentrations of atazanavir and possible loss of the therapeutic effect of the antiretroviral agent and development of resistance. Concomitant use of *ritonavir-boosted, cobicistat-boosted*, or unboosted atazanavir with famotidine (20 or 40 mg) may result in changes in the pharmacokinetics of atazanavir.

If *ritonavir-boosted* atazanavir is used in adults receiving a histamine H_2-receptor antagonist, a regimen of 300 mg of single-entity atazanavir once daily with single-entity ritonavir 100 mg once daily with food is recommended. Atazanavir and ritonavir should be given simultaneously with and/or at least 10 hours after the histamine H_2-receptor antagonist. For antiretroviral-naive patients, dosage of the histamine H_2-receptor antagonist should not exceed famotidine 40 mg twice daily (or equivalent). In antiretroviral-experienced patients, dosage of the histamine H_2-receptor antagonist should not exceed famotidine 20 mg twice daily (or equivalent).

If *cobicistat-boosted* atazanavir is used in adults receiving a histamine H_2-receptor antagonist, a regimen of 300 mg of atazanavir once daily with cobicistat 150 mg once daily (administered as fixed-combination atazanavir/cobicistat or as single-entity atazanavir with single-entity cobicistat) with food is recommended. *Cobicistat-boosted* atazanavir should be given simultaneously with and/or at least 10 hours after the histamine H_2-receptor antagonist. In antiretroviral-naive patients, dosage of the histamine H_2-receptor antagonist should not exceed famotidine 40 mg twice daily (or equivalent). In antiretroviral-experienced patients, dosage of the histamine H_2-receptor antagonist should not exceed famotidine 20 mg twice daily (or equivalent).

If unboosted atazanavir (i.e., *without* low-dose ritonavir or cobicistat) is used in antiretroviral-naive adults receiving a histamine H_2-receptor antagonist, a regimen of 400 mg of atazanavir once daily with food should be used and the dose given at least 2 hours before and at least 10 hours after a dose of the histamine H_2-receptor antagonist. Dosage of the histamine H_2-receptor antagonist should not exceed famotidine 40 mg daily (or equivalent) and a single dose of the histamine H_2-receptor antagonist should not exceed famotidine 20 mg (or equivalent) in these patients.

If *ritonavir-boosted* atazanavir is used in an antiretroviral regimen that includes tenofovir DF and a histamine H_2-receptor antagonist is used concomitantly, the recommended dosage for antiretroviral-experienced adults is atazanavir 400 mg, ritonavir 100 mg, and tenofovir DF 300 mg once daily with food. Single-entity atazanavir and single-entity ritonavir should be given simultaneously with and/or at least 10 hours after the histamine H_2-receptor antagonist. Dosage of the histamine H_2-receptor antagonist should not exceed famotidine 20 mg twice daily (or equivalent) in these patients.

The manufacturer states that concomitant use of the fixed combination atazanavir/cobicistat with tenofovir DF and a histamine H_2-receptor antagonist is not recommended in antiretroviral-experienced patients. If *cobicistat-boosted* atazanavir is used in an antiretroviral regimen that includes tenofovir DF and a histamine H_2-receptor antagonist is used concomitantly, the recommended dosage for antiretroviral-experienced adults is atazanavir 400 mg and cobicistat 150 mg once daily. Fixed-combination atazanavir/cobicistat or, alternatively, single-entity atazanavir and single-entity cobicistat should be given simultaneously with and/or at least 10 hours after the histamine H_2-receptor antagonist. Dosage of the histamine H_2-receptor antagonist should not exceed famotidine 20 mg twice daily (or equivalent) in these patients. (See Drug Interactions: Drugs Affecting Gastric pH.)

If *ritonavir-boosted* atazanavir is used in an antiretroviral-experienced pregnant woman in the second or third trimester of pregnancy who is receiving a histamine H_2-receptor antagonist, dosage should be increased to 400 mg of atazanavir once daily with ritonavir 100 mg once daily. Dosage recommendations are not available for pregnant women receiving both a histamine H_2-receptor antagonist *and* tenofovir in conjunction with atazanavir.

Proton-pump Inhibitors Concomitant use of omeprazole 40 mg once daily and *ritonavir-boosted* or unboosted atazanavir results in substantially decreased plasma concentrations of atazanavir and may result in loss of the therapeutic effect of the antiretroviral agent and development of resistance.

Unboosted atazanavir is not recommended in patients receiving a proton-pump inhibitor. An alternative acid-reducing agent should be used or, alternatively, *ritonavir-boosted* or *cobicistat-boosted* atazanavir should be used.

If *ritonavir-boosted* atazanavir is used in antiretroviral-naive adults receiving a proton-pump inhibitor, a regimen of 300 mg of single-entity atazanavir once daily with single-entity ritonavir 100 mg once daily with food is recommended. The proton-pump inhibitor must be administered approximately 12 hours before *ritonavir-boosted* atazanavir and dosage should not exceed omeprazole 20 mg daily (or equivalent).

If *cobicistat-boosted* atazanavir is used in antiretroviral-naive adults receiving a proton-pump inhibitor, the usual dosage of *cobicistat-boosted* atazanavir should be given (300 mg of atazanavir once daily with 150 mg of cobicistat once daily). The proton-pump inhibitor must be administered approximately 12 hours before *cobicistat-boosted* atazanavir and dosage should not exceed omeprazole 20 mg daily (or equivalent).

Proton-pump inhibitors should not be used in antiretroviral-experienced patients receiving *ritonavir-boosted* or *cobicistat-boosted* atazanavir.

■ **HCV Antivirals** ***HCV Polymerase Inhibitors*** **Dasabuvir.** Concomitant use of *ritonavir-boosted* atazanavir and the fixed combination of ombitasvir, paritaprevir, and ritonavir (ombitasvir/paritaprevir/ritonavir) with dasabuvir results in increased paritaprevir plasma concentrations and AUC, but atazanavir, dasabuvir, and ombitasvir concentrations are not substantially affected. (See Paritaprevir under HCV Antivirals: HCV Protease Inhibitors, in Drug Interactions.)

Data are not available regarding pharmacokinetic interactions between *cobicistat-boosted* atazanavir and ombitasvir/paritaprevir/ritonavir with dasabuvir.

Sofosbuvir. In clinical trials of sofosbuvir, elevated total bilirubin concentrations were observed in 94% of patients with hepatitis C virus (HCV) infection coinfected with HIV who were receiving atazanavir as part of an antiretroviral regimen, but was observed in only 1.5% of such patients *not* receiving atazanavir.

Sofosbuvir and Velpatasvir. Concomitant use of the fixed combination of sofosbuvir and velpatasvir (sofosbuvir/velpatasvir) with *ritonavir-boosted* atazanavir does not result in clinically important pharmacokinetic interactions.

Concomitant use of sofosbuvir/velpatasvir and *ritonavir-boosted* atazanavir in conjunction with the fixed combination of emtricitabine and tenofovir (emtricitabine/tenofovir DF) results in increased velpatasvir and tenofovir plasma concentrations and AUC. Patients should be monitored for tenofovir-associated adverse effects if sofosbuvir/velpatasvir is used concomitantly with any HIV antiretroviral regimen containing tenofovir DF.

HCV Protease Inhibitors **Paritaprevir.** Concomitant use of the fixed combination of ombitasvir/paritaprevir/ritonavir with *ritonavir-boosted* or unboosted atazanavir results in increased paritaprevir plasma concentrations and AUC, but atazanavir and ombitasvir concentrations are not substantially affected. The manufacturer of ombitasvir/paritaprevir/ritonavir states that concomitant use of *ritonavir-boosted* or unboosted atazanavir with this HCV fixed-combination drug is not recommended.

Concomitant use of *ritonavir-boosted* atazanavir and the fixed combination ombitasvir/paritaprevir/ritonavir with dasabuvir sodium results in increased paritaprevir concentrations and AUC, but atazanavir, ombitasvir, and dasabuvir concentrations are not substantially affected. Data are not available regarding pharmacokinetic interactions between *cobicistat-boosted* atazanavir and ombitasvir/paritaprevir/ritonavir with dasabuvir. If unboosted atazanavir and ombitasvir/paritaprevir/ritonavir with dasabuvir are used concomitantly, atazanavir should be given in a dosage of 300 mg once daily in the morning at the same time as the morning dose of ombitasvir/paritaprevir/ritonavir with dasabuvir. Atazanavir should be used *without* low-dose ritonavir and *without* cobicistat during HCV treatment with ombitasvir/paritaprevir/ritonavir with dasabuvir; *ritonavir-boosted* or *cobicistat-boosted* atazanavir can be substituted for unboosted atazanavir *after* HCV treatment is completed.

Simeprevir. Concomitant use of simeprevir and *ritonavir-boosted, cobicistat-boosted*, or unboosted atazanavir may alter (increase or decrease) plasma concentrations of simeprevir due to CYP3A4 inhibition or induction by the HIV PIs.

Concomitant use of simeprevir and *ritonavir-boosted, cobicistat-boosted*, or unboosted atazanavir is not recommended.

HCV Replication Complex Inhibitors **Daclatasvir.** Concomitant use of daclatasvir (20 mg once daily) with *ritonavir-boosted* atazanavir (300 mg of atazanavir and 100 mg of ritonavir once daily) results in increased daclatasvir peak plasma concentrations and AUC. Concomitant use of daclatasvir and *cobicistat-boosted* atazanavir may result in increased daclatasvir exposures. Clinically important changes in daclatasvir exposures are not expected if the drug is used concomitantly with unboosted atazanavir.

If daclatasvir and *ritonavir-boosted* or *cobicistat-boosted* atazanavir are used concomitantly, daclatasvir should be given in a dosage of 30 mg once daily.

If daclatasvir and unboosted atazanavir are used concomitantly, adjustment of daclatasvir dosage is not needed.

Elbasvir and Grazoprevir. Concomitant use of *ritonavir-boosted* atazanavir (300 mg of atazanavir and 100 mg of ritonavir once daily) and elbasvir (50 mg once daily) results in increased elbasvir concentrations. Concomitant use of *ritonavir-boosted* atazanavir (300 mg of atazanavir and 100 mg of ritonavir once daily) and grazoprevir (200 mg once daily) results in substantially increased grazoprevir concentrations due to OATP1B1 and 1B3 inhibition by *ritonavir-boosted* atazanavir. Concomitant use of *cobicistat-boosted* or unboosted atazanavir is expected to increase grazoprevir concentrations. Increased grazoprevir concentrations may increase the risk of ALT elevations.

Concomitant use of elbasvir/grazoprevir and *ritonavir-boosted, cobicistat-boosted*, or unboosted atazanavir is contraindicated.

Ledipasvir and Sofosbuvir. Concomitant use of the fixed combination of ledipasvir and sofosbuvir (ledipasvir/sofosbuvir) with *ritonavir-boosted* increases the AUCs of atazanavir and ledipasvir, but this is not considered clinically important. Concomitant use of ledipasvir/sofosbuvir and *cobicistat-boosted* atazanavir is not expected to result in any clinically important pharmacokinetic interactions. Dosage adjustments are not necessary if ledipasvir/sofosbuvir is used concomitantly with *ritonavir-boosted* or *cobicistat-boosted* atazanavir.

Concomitant use of ledipasvir/sofosbuvir and an HIV antiretroviral regimen that includes *ritonavir-boosted* or *cobicistat-boosted* atazanavir with emtricitabine and tenofovir DF may result in increased tenofovir concentrations. Safety of increased tenofovir concentrations in patients receiving ledipasvir/sofosbuvir and these HIV treatment regimens has not been established. Alternative HCV treatment or an alternative antiretroviral regimen should be considered to avoid increased tenofovir exposure, especially in patients at risk for renal toxicity. If concomitant use is necessary, the patient should be monitored for tenofovir-associated adverse effects.

Atazanavir. Concomitant use of *ritonavir-boosted* atazanavir (atazanavir 300 mg and ritonavir 100 mg) and ledipasvir/sofosbuvir increases the AUCs of atazanavir and ledipasvir by 33 and 113%, respectively, but does not have a clinically important effect on the pharmacokinetics of sofosbuvir. Dosage adjustments are not necessary if *ritonavir-boosted* atazanavir and ledipasvir/sofosbuvir are used concomitantly.

Ombitasvir. Concomitant use of the fixed combination of ombitasvir/paritaprevir/ritonavir and *ritonavir-boosted* or unboosted atazanavir results in substantially increased paritaprevir plasma concentrations and AUC, but atazanavir and ombitasvir concentrations are not substantially affected. The manufacturer of ombitasvir/paritaprevir/ritonavir states that concomitant use of *ritonavir-boosted* or unboosted atazanavir with this HCV fixed-combination drug is not recommended.

Concomitant use of *ritonavir-boosted* atazanavir and the fixed combination of ombitasvir, paritaprevir, and ritonavir (ombitasvir/paritaprevir/ritonavir) with dasabuvir sodium results in increased paritaprevir concentrations, but atazanavir concentrations are not substantially affected. Data are not available regarding pharmacokinetic interactions between *cobicistat-boosted* atazanavir and ombitasvir/paritaprevir/ritonavir with dasabuvir. (See Paritaprevir under HCV Antivirals: HCV Protease Inhibitors, in Drug Interactions.)

■ **HMG-CoA Reductase Inhibitors** Pharmacokinetic interactions with HMG-CoA reductase inhibitors (statins) metabolized by CYP3A isoenzyme. Concomitant use of *ritonavir-boosted, cobicistat-boosted*, or unboosted atazanavir and certain statins (e.g., atorvastatin, lovastatin, pitavastatin, rosuvastatin, simvastatin) may increase plasma concentrations and AUCs of the antilipemic agents and increase the risk of statin-associated adverse effects, including myopathy and rhabdomyolysis.

Atorvastatin If atorvastatin is used concomitantly with *ritonavir-boosted, cobicistat-boosted*, or unboosted atazanavir, atorvastatin dosage should be titrated carefully and the lowest necessary dosage used.

Fluvastatin If fluvastatin is used concomitantly with *cobicistat-boosted* atazanavir, fluvastatin dosage should be titrated carefully and the lowest necessary dosage used.

Lovastatin Concomitant use of lovastatin with *ritonavir-boosted, cobicistat-boosted*, or unboosted atazanavir is contraindicated.

Pitavastatin Concomitant use of atazanavir and pitavastatin results in a 31% increase in the AUC and a 60% increase in the peak plasma concentration of pitavastatin, but does not have a clinically important effect on atazanavir plasma concentrations.

Dosage adjustments are not necessary if *ritonavir-boosted, cobicistat-boosted*, or unboosted atazanavir is used concomitantly with pitavastatin.

Rosuvastatin If rosuvastatin is used concomitantly with *ritonavir-boosted, cobicistat-boosted*, or unboosted atazanavir, rosuvastatin dosage should not exceed 10 mg daily. Rosuvastatin dosage should be titrated carefully and the lowest necessary dosage used.

Simvastatin Concomitant use of simvastatin with *ritonavir-boosted, cobicistat-boosted*, or unboosted atazanavir is contraindicated.

■ **Immunosuppressive Agents** Pharmacokinetic interactions with certain immunosuppressive agents (e.g., cyclosporine, everolimus, sirolimus, tacrolimus); increased plasma concentrations of the immunosuppressive agent expected.

If cyclosporine, everolimus, sirolimus, or tacrolimus is used concomitantly with *ritonavir-boosted, cobicistat-boosted*, or unboosted atazanavir, plasma concentrations of the immunosuppressive agent should be monitored.

■ **Ivabradine** Concomitant use of ivabradine and *ritonavir-boosted, cobicistat-boosted*, or unboosted atazanavir is expected to result in increased ivabradine concentrations.

Some experts state that concomitant use of ivabradine and *ritonavir-boosted, cobicistat-boosted*, or unboosted atazanavir is contraindicated.

■ **Macrolides** ***Azithromycin*** Clinically important interactions between azithromycin and *ritonavir-boosted, cobicistat-boosted*, or unboosted atazanavir are unlikely.

Clarithromycin Pharmacokinetic interactions if clarithromycin is used concomitantly with *ritonavir-boosted* or unboosted atazanavir (increased plasma concentrations of clarithromycin, decreased plasma concentrations of 14-hydroxyclarithromycin, increased plasma concentrations of atazanavir). Because increased clarithromycin concentrations may result in prolongation of the corrected QT (QT_c) interval, a 50% reduction in clarithromycin dosage should be considered in patients receiving *ritonavir-boosted* or unboosted atazanavir. Alternative anti-infective therapy (e.g., azithromycin) should be considered.

Pharmacokinetic interactions if clarithromycin is used concomitantly with *cobicistat-boosted* atazanavir (increased atazanavir, cobicistat, and clarithromycin concentrations). An alternative anti-infective (e.g., azithromycin) should be considered in patients receiving *cobicistat-boosted* atazanavir.

Erythromycin Pharmacokinetic interactions if erythromycin is used concomitantly with *cobicistat-boosted* atazanavir (increased atazanavir, cobicistat, and erythromycin concentrations). An alternative anti-infective should be considered in patients receiving *cobicistat-boosted* atazanavir.

Clinically important interactions between unboosted atazanavir and erythromycin are unlikely.

Telithromycin Pharmacokinetic interactions if telithromycin is used concomitantly with *cobicistat-boosted* atazanavir (increased atazanavir, cobicistat, and telithromycin concentrations). An alternative anti-infective should be considered in patients receiving *cobicistat-boosted* atazanavir.

■ **Opiate Agonists, Opiate Partial Agonists, and Opiate Antagonists** ***Buprenorphine*** Pharmacokinetic interactions if buprenorphine is used concomitantly with *ritonavir-boosted* or unboosted atazanavir (increased buprenorphine and norbuprenorphine concentrations and AUC, possible decreased atazanavir concentrations when used without low-dose ritonavir). It is not known whether *cobicistat-boosted* atazanavir affects the pharmacokinetics of buprenorphine or the fixed combination of buprenorphine and naloxone.

Because of the potential for decreased atazanavir plasma concentrations, buprenorphine should not be used concomitantly with *unboosted* atazanavir.

If buprenorphine is used concomitantly with *ritonavir-boosted* atazanavir, the patient should be monitored for sedation and adverse cognitive effects and a reduced dosage of buprenorphine should be considered. In patients with a buprenorphine subdermal implant, it may be necessary to remove the implant and switch to a different buprenorphine formulation that permits dosage adjustments.

In patients receiving *cobicistat-boosted* atazanavir, buprenorphine or the fixed combination of buprenorphine and naloxone should be initiated using the lowest possible dosage and carefully titrated to the desired therapeutic effect. If initiating *cobicistat-boosted* atazanavir in patients already receiving buprenorphine or the fixed combination of buprenorphine and naloxone, dosage adjustments of buprenorphine or the fixed combination of buprenorphine and naloxone may be needed and the patient should be clinically monitored. In patients with a buprenorphine subdermal implant, it may be necessary to remove the implant and switch to a different buprenorphine formulation that permits dosage adjustments.

Fentanyl Possible pharmacokinetic interactions if fentanyl is used concomitantly with *ritonavir-boosted, cobicistat-boosted*, or unboosted atazanavir (increased fentanyl concentrations).

If fentanyl is used concomitantly with *ritonavir-boosted, cobicistat-boosted*, or unboosted atazanavir, the patient should be carefully monitored for therapeutic and adverse effects of fentanyl, including potentially fatal respiratory depression.

Methadone Pharmacokinetic interactions between methadone and unboosted atazanavir are unlikely. Adjustment of methadone dosage is not necessary in patients receiving unboosted atazanavir.

Pharmacokinetic interactions if methadone is used concomitantly with *ritonavir-boosted* atazanavir (decreased concentrations of *R*-methadone [active isomer]). Although adjustment of methadone dosage is not usually needed, patients should be closely monitored for signs of opiate withdrawal and methadone dosage increased as clinically indicated.

It is not known whether *cobicistat-boosted* atazanavir affects methadone pharmacokinetics. In patients receiving *cobicistat-boosted* atazanavir, methadone should be initiated at the lowest possible dosage and carefully titrated to the desired therapeutic effect. In patients initiating *cobicistat-boosted* atazanavir who are already receiving methadone, dosage adjustments of methadone may be needed and the patient should be clinically monitored.

Tramadol Pharmacokinetic interactions if tramadol is used concomitantly with *cobicistat-boosted* atazanavir (increased tramadol concentrations). If tramadol is used concomitantly with *cobicistat-boosted* atazanavir, decreased tramadol dosage may be needed and the patient should be monitored for efficacy and tramadol-associated adverse effects.

■ **Phosphodiesterase Type 5 Inhibitors** Concomitant use of *ritonavir-boosted, cobicistat-boosted*, or unboosted atazanavir and selective phosphodiesterase type 5 (PDE5) inhibitors (e.g., avanafil, sildenafil, tadalafil, vardenafil) is expected to result in substantially increased plasma concentrations of the PDE5 inhibitor and increase the risk of adverse effects associated with these agents (e.g., hypotension, syncope, visual disturbances, priapism).

Avanafil Avanafil should not be used in patients receiving *ritonavir-boosted* or *cobicistat-boosted* atazanavir.

Although specific data are not available, some experts state that if avanafil is used in patients receiving unboosted atazanavir, dosage of avanafil should not exceed 50 mg once every 24 hours.

Sildenafil Concomitant use of sildenafil (Revatio®) for treatment of pulmonary arterial hypertension (PAH) is contraindicated in patients receiving *ritonavir-boosted, cobicistat-boosted*, or unboosted atazanavir. Safe and effective dosages for concomitant use have not been established.

If sildenafil is used for treatment of erectile dysfunction in patients receiving *ritonavir-boosted, cobicistat-boosted*, or unboosted atazanavir, a reduced sildenafil dosage of 25 mg once every 48 hours should be used and the patient should be closely monitored for sildenafil-related adverse effects.

Tadalafil If tadalafil is indicated for treatment of PAH in patients who have been receiving *ritonavir-boosted, cobicistat-boosted*, or unboosted atazanavir for at least 1 week, tadalafil should be initiated at a dosage of 20 mg once daily and, if tolerated, dosage may be increased to 40 mg once daily. *Ritonavir-boosted, cobicistat-boosted*, or unboosted atazanavir should not be initiated in patients receiving tadalafil for treatment of PAH; tadalafil should be discontinued for at least 24 hours prior to initiating atazanavir. After at least 1 week, tadalafil may be resumed at a dosage of 20 mg once daily, and if tolerated, dosage may be increased to 40 mg once daily. In patients switching from *ritonavir-boosted* atazanavir to *cobicistat-boosted* atazanavir, the current tadalafil dosage should be maintained.

If tadalafil is used for treatment of erectile dysfunction in patients receiving *ritonavir-boosted, cobicistat-boosted*, or unboosted atazanavir, tadalafil dosage should not exceed 10 mg once every 72 hours and the patient should be closely monitored for tadalafil-related adverse effects.

If tadalafil is used for treatment of benign prostatic hyperplasia in patients receiving *ritonavir-boosted, cobicistat-boosted*, or unboosted atazanavir, tadalafil dosage should not exceed 2.5 mg once daily.

Vardenafil If vardenafil is used for treatment of erectile dysfunction in patients receiving unboosted atazanavir, vardenafil dosage should not exceed 2.5 mg once every 24 hours. The drugs should be used concomitantly with caution and the patient should be monitored for vardenafil-related adverse effects.

If vardenafil is used for treatment of erectile dysfunction in patients receiving *ritonavir-boosted* or *cobicistat-boosted* atazanavir, vardenafil dosage should not exceed 2.5 mg once every 72 hours. The drugs should be used concomitantly with caution and the patient should be monitored for vardenafil-related adverse effects.

■ **Ranolazine** Potential for serious and/or life-threatening adverse effects if *cobicistat-boosted* atazanavir is used concomitantly with ranolazine. Concomitant use of *cobicistat-boosted* atazanavir and ranolazine is contraindicated.

Some experts state that concomitant use of ranolazine and *ritonavir-boosted* or unboosted atazanavir is contraindicated.

■ **Repaglinide** Possible pharmacokinetic interactions if repaglinide is used concomitantly with unboosted atazanavir (increased concentrations of repaglinide); caution is advised. Clinically important interactions are not expected if repaglinide is used with *ritonavir-boosted* atazanavir.

Concomitant use of repaglinide and *cobicistat-boosted* atazanavir is not recommended

■ **St. John's Wort** Potential pharmacokinetic interactions with St. John's wort (*Hypericum perforatum*) (decreased atazanavir plasma concentrations); potential loss of therapeutic effect and development of resistance. Concomitant use of St. John's wort and *ritonavir-boosted, cobicistat-boosted*, or unboosted atazanavir is contraindicated.

■ **Salmeterol** Possible pharmacokinetic interactions if salmeterol is used concomitantly with *ritonavir-boosted, cobicistat-boosted*, or unboosted atazanavir (increased salmeterol concentrations) and increased risk of salmeterol-associated adverse cardiovascular effects, including QT interval prolongation, palpitations, and sinus tachycardia.

Concomitant use of salmeterol and *ritonavir-boosted, cobicistat-boosted*, or unboosted atazanavir is not recommended.

■ **Selective Serotonin-reuptake Inhibitors** Data are not available regarding possible pharmacokinetic interactions if selective serotonin-reuptake inhibitors (SSRIs), such as citalopram, escitalopram, fluoxetine, paroxetine, or sertraline, are used concomitantly with *ritonavir-boosted* or *cobicistat-boosted* atazanavir. If *ritonavir-boosted* atazanavir is used concomitantly with an SSRI, dosage of the SSRI should be titrated based on clinical response. If *cobicistat-boosted* atazanavir is used concomitantly with an SSRI, dosage of the SSRI should be titrated based on clinical response using the lowest possible initial or maintenance dosage.

Some experts state that concomitant use of fluvoxamine with *ritonavir-boosted* or *cobicistat-boosted* atazanavir may alter (increase or decrease) atazanavir concentrations. These experts state that an alternative to fluvoxamine should be considered.

■ **Suvorexant** Pharmacokinetic interactions expected if suvorexant is used concomitantly with *ritonavir-boosted, cobicistat-boosted*, or unboosted atazanavir (increased suvorexant concentrations). Some experts state that concomitant use is not recommended.

■ **Ticagrelor** Possible pharmacokinetic interactions if ticagrelor is used concomitantly with *ritonavir-boosted, cobicistat-boosted*, or unboosted atazanavir (increased ticagrelor concentrations expected). Some experts state that concomitant use should be avoided.

■ **Trazodone** Possible pharmacokinetic interactions if trazodone is used concomitantly with *ritonavir-boosted, cobicistat-boosted*, or unboosted atazanavir (increased plasma concentrations of trazodone); nausea, dizziness, hypotension, and syncope have been reported when trazodone was used with ritonavir. Caution is advised; a lower dosage of trazodone should be considered in patients receiving concomitant atazanavir. The patient should be monitored for therapeutic response and trazodone adverse effects (e.g., CNS effects, cardiovascular effects).

■ **Tricyclic Antidepressants** Potential pharmacokinetic interactions if amitriptyline, desipramine, doxepin, imipramine, or nortriptyline is used concomitantly with *ritonavir-boosted, cobicistat-boosted*, or unboosted atazanavir (increased plasma concentration of the tricyclic antidepressant); potential for serious and/or life-threatening adverse effects. Plasma concentrations of the tricyclic antidepressants should be monitored if used concomitantly with atazanavir. Some experts recommend that the lowest possible dosage of the tricyclic antidepressant should be used and dosage titrated based on plasma antidepressant concentrations and/or clinical assessment.

■ **Vorapaxar** Possible pharmacokinetic interactions if vorapaxar is used concomitantly with *ritonavir-boosted, cobicistat-boosted*, or unboosted atazanavir (increased vorapaxar concentrations expected). Some experts state that concomitant use should be avoided.

■ **Zolpidem** Potential pharmacokinetic interactions if zolpidem is used concomitantly with *ritonavir-boosted* or *cobicistat-boosted* atazanavir (increased zolpidem concentrations).

If zolpidem is used concomitantly with *ritonavir-boosted* or *cobicistat-boosted* atazanavir, some experts state that zolpidem should be initiated using a low dosage and dosage reduction may be needed.

Description

Atazanavir, a synthetic azapeptide, inhibits replication of human immunodeficiency virus type 1 (HIV-1) by interfering with HIV protease. During HIV replication, HIV protease cleaves viral polypeptide products of the *gag* and *gag-pol* genes to form structural proteins of the virion core and essential viral enzymes. By interfering with the formation of these essential proteins and enzymes, atazanavir blocks maturation of the virus and causes formation of nonfunctional, immature noninfectious virions. Atazanavir has some activity in vitro against HIV-2.

HIV-1 strains with reduced susceptibility to atazanavir can be produced in vitro and strains with reduced susceptibility to atazanavir have emerged during therapy with the drug. Varying degrees of cross-resistance occur among HIV protease inhibitors (PIs). Some HIV-1 isolates resistant to atazanavir may be cross-resistant to other HIV PIs (e.g., amprenavir [active metabolite of fosamprenavir], indinavir, lopinavir, nelfinavir, ritonavir, saquinavir).

Atazanavir is extensively metabolized by the hepatic cytochrome P-450 (CYP) enzyme system, principally CYP3A, and usually is administered with a pharmacokinetic enhancer (pharmacokinetic booster) to improve the pharmacokinetic profile of the drug. Atazanavir may be administered with low-dose ritonavir (*ritonavir-boosted* atazanavir) or with cobicistat (*cobicistat-boosted* atazanavir). Because ritonavir and cobicistat are potent inhibitors of CYP3A, concomitant administration with atazanavir results in increased peak plasma concentrations and area under the plasma concentration-time curve (AUC) of the HIV PI. The antiretroviral activity of *ritonavir-boosted* atazanavir or *cobicistat-boosted* atazanavir is due to atazanavir.

Atazanavir steady-state pharmacokinetic parameters reported with a once-daily regimen of *ritonavir-boosted* atazanavir (atazanavir 300 mg and ritonavir 100 mg) are similar to those reported with a once-daily regimen of *cobicistat-boosted* atazanavir (fixed-combination tablet containing atazanavir 300 mg and cobicistat 150 mg; atazanavir/cobicistat). In addition, atazanavir exposures following a single dose of atazanavir/cobicistat (atazanavir 300 mg and cobicistat 150 mg) are comparable to those attained following a single 300-mg dose of single-entity atazanavir (capsule) given with a single 150-mg dose of single-entity cobicistat (tablet). *Ritonavir-boosted* atazanavir, *cobicistat-boosted* atazanavir, or unboosted atazanavir is given with food to enhance bioavailability and minimize pharmacokinetic variability. Compared with administration in the fasting state, administration of *ritonavir-boosted* atazanavir with a light meal increases peak concentrations and AUC of atazanavir by 40 and 33%, respectively. Administration of *cobicistat-boosted* atazanavir (given as atazanavir/cobicistat) with a light meal increases peak concentrations and AUC of atazanavir by 42 and 28%, respectively. Mean half-life of atazanavir at steady state is 8.6–18.1 hours when administered as *ritonavir-boosted* atazanavir, approximately 7.5 hours when administered as atazanavir/cobicistat, and 6.5–7.9 hours when administered as unboosted atazanavir. When unboosted atazanavir is administered, the drug is eliminated principally in feces (79%) and urine (13%).

Advice to Patients

Critical nature of compliance with HIV therapy and importance of remaining under the care of a clinician. Importance of taking as prescribed; do not alter or discontinue antiretroviral regimen without consulting clinician.

Importance of using *ritonavir-boosted* atazanavir, *cobicistat-boosted* atazanavir, or unboosted atazanavir in conjunction with other antiretrovirals—not for monotherapy.

Antiretroviral therapy is not a cure for HIV infection; opportunistic infections and other complications associated with HIV disease may still occur.

Advise patients that sustained decreases in plasma HIV RNA have been associated with reduced risk of progression to AIDS and death.

Advise patients that effective antiretroviral regimens can decrease HIV concentrations in blood and genital secretions and strict adherence to such regimens in conjunction with risk-reduction measures may decrease, but cannot absolutely eliminate, the risk of secondary transmission of HIV to others. Importance of continuing to practice safer sex (e.g., using latex or polyurethane condoms to minimize sexual contact with body fluids), never sharing personal items that can have blood or body fluids on them (e.g., toothbrushes, razor blades), and never reusing or sharing needles.

Importance of reading patient information provided by the manufacturer.

When using *ritonavir-boosted* atazanavir, importance of taking single-entity atazanavir with food at the same time as single-entity ritonavir.

When using *cobicistat-boosted* atazanavir, importance of taking the fixed-combination tablet containing both drugs (atazanavir/cobicistat) with food; alternatively, importance of taking single-entity atazanavir with food and at the same time as single-entity cobicistat.

When using unboosted atazanavir, importance of taking with food.

If a dose of atazanavir is missed, it should be taken as soon as it is remembered and the next dose taken at the regularly scheduled time; if a dose is skipped, the next dose should not be doubled.

If a dose of *cobicistat-boosted* atazanavir is missed by less than 12 hours, the dose should be taken as soon as it is remembered and the next dose taken at the regularly scheduled time. If a dose of *cobicistat-boosted* atazanavir is missed by more than 12 hours, the dose should be skipped and the next dose taken at the regularly scheduled time. A double dose should not be taken to make up for a missed dose.

If atazanavir oral powder is used, importance of caregivers carefully following mixing and administration instructions.

If atazanavir oral powder is used, advise caregivers of patients with phenylketonuria that atazanavir oral powder contains phenylalanine.

Advise patients that ECG changes (PR prolongation) have occurred; importance of consulting clinician if dizziness or lightheadedness occurs.

Possibility of asymptomatic increases in indirect bilirubin that may be accompanied by yellowing of the skin or whites of the eyes; alternative antiretroviral therapy can be considered if these cosmetic changes are a concern.

Redistribution/accumulation of body fat may occur with antiretroviral therapy, with as yet unknown long-term health effects.

Advise patients that mild rash and severe skin reactions, including Stevens-Johnson syndrome, erythema multiforme, and toxic skin eruptions, have occurred. Importance of immediately discontinuing *ritonavir-boosted*, *cobicistat-boosted*, or unboosted atazanavir and contacting clinician if manifestations of severe skin reactions or hypersensitivity occur (e.g., severe rash or rash accompanied by shortness of breath, fever, general malaise, muscle or joint aches, blisters, oral lesions, conjunctivitis, facial edema).

Advise patients that kidney stones and/or gallstones have been reported and some patients required hospitalization or experienced complications; discontinuance of the drug may be necessary.

Importance of informing clinicians of existing or contemplated concomitant therapy, including prescription and OTC drugs and dietary or herbal supplements (e.g., St. John's wort), and any concomitant illnesses.

Advise patients receiving a selective phosphodiesterase type 5 (PDE5) inhibitor (e.g., sildenafil, tadalafil, vardenafil) that they may be at increased risk of PDE5 inhibitor-associated adverse effects (e.g., hypotension, visual disturbances, priapism) and that any symptoms should be promptly reported to clinician. Should not be used in patients receiving avanafil for treatment of erectile dysfunction or sildenafil for treatment of pulmonary arterial hypertension (PAH).

Importance of women informing clinicians if they are or plan to become pregnant or plan to breast-feed. Advise HIV-infected women not to breast-feed.

Importance of advising patients of other important precautionary information. (See Cautions.)

Overview® (see Users Guide). For additional information on this drug until a more detailed monograph is developed and published, the manufacturer's labeling should be consulted. It is *essential* that the manufacturer's labeling be consulted for more detailed information on usual cautions, precautions, contraindications, potential drug interactions, laboratory test interferences, and acute toxicity.

Preparations

Excipients in commercially available drug preparations may have clinically important effects in some individuals; consult specific product labeling for details.

Atazanavir Sulfate

Oral		
Powder	50 mg (of atazanavir) per packet	Reyataz®, Bristol-Myers Squibb
Capsules	150 mg (of atazanavir)	Reyataz®, Bristol-Myers Squibb
	200 mg (of atazanavir)	Reyataz®, Bristol-Myers Squibb
	300 mg (of atazanavir)	Reyataz®, Bristol-Myers Squibb

Atazanavir Sulfate Combinations

Oral		
Tablets, film-coated	300 mg (of atazanavir) with Cobicistat 150 mg	Evotaz®, Bristol-Myers Squibb

†Use is not currently included in the labeling approved by the US Food and Drug Administration

Darunavir

DRVCobicistat-boosted Darunavir, darunavir/cobicistat, DRV/c

■ Darunavir, an antiretroviral agent, is a human immunodeficiency virus (HIV) protease inhibitor (PI).

Uses

■ **Treatment of HIV Infection** Darunavir with low-dose ritonavir (*ritonavir-boosted* darunavir) is used in conjunction with other antiretroviral agents for the treatment of human immunodeficiency virus type 1 (HIV-1) infection in antiretroviral-naive (have not previously received antiretroviral therapy) or antiretroviral-experienced (previously treated) adults, adolescents, and children 3 years of age or older. The manufacturer advises that use of *ritonavir-boosted* darunavir in antiretroviral-experienced patients should be guided by results of genotypic and/or phenotypic viral resistance testing and the individual's prior antiretroviral treatment. Hepatic function should be assessed prior to initiation of *ritonavir-boosted* darunavir. (See Hepatic Effects under Cautions: Warnings/Precautions.)

Darunavir with cobicistat (*cobicistat-boosted* darunavir) is used in conjunction with other antiretroviral agents for the treatment of HIV-1 infection in treatment-naive or treatment-experienced adults. When *cobicistat-boosted* darunavir is included in an antiretroviral regimen, the fixed-combination preparation containing both drugs (darunavir/cobicistat) can be used or, alternatively, single-entity darunavir and single-entity cobicistat can be administered at the same time. The manufacturer of darunavir/cobicistat states that the fixed combination should not be used in patients who have HIV-1 with substitutions associated with darunavir resistance (V11I, V32I, L33F, I47V, I50V, I54L, I54M, T74P, L76V, I84V, L89V). In addition, use of darunavir/cobicistat in treatment-experienced patients should be guided by results of genotypic viral resistance testing; if such testing is not available, the fixed combination may be used in HIV protease inhibitor-naive (PI-naive) patients, but is not recommended in HIV PI-experienced patients. Estimated creatinine clearance should be assessed in all patients prior to initiation of *cobicistat-boosted* darunavir (administered as fixed-combination darunavir/cobicistat or, alternatively, as single-entity darunavir and single-entity cobicistat). (See Renal Effects under Cautions: Warnings/Precautions.)

Darunavir should *not* be used without a pharmacokinetic enhancer (i.e., low-dose ritonavir or cobicistat). A pharmacokinetic enhancer (pharmacokinetic booster) is necessary to improve the pharmacokinetic profile of darunavir. Although concomitant use of low-dose ritonavir or cobicistat with darunavir increases peak plasma concentrations and area under the plasma concentration-time curve (AUC) of the HIV protease inhibitor, these pharmacokinetic enhancers are not interchangeable in antiretroviral regimens since low-dose ritonavir and cobicistat have different dosage and administration requirements and are associated with different adverse effects, precautions, contraindications, and drug interactions. In addition, although *ritonavir-boosted* darunavir may be used in adults, adolescents, and children 3 years of age or older, efficacy and safety of *cobicistat-boosted* darunavir (administered as fixed-combination darunavir/cobicistat or, alternatively, as single-entity darunavir and single-entity cobicistat) have been established only in adults.

Ritonavir-boosted darunavir or *cobicistat-boosted* darunavir should always be used in conjunction with one or more other antiretroviral agents and should not be used alone for the treatment of HIV infection. *Ritonavir-boosted* darunavir or *cobicistat-boosted* darunavir usually is used in an HIV PI-based regimen that includes 2 nucleoside reverse transcriptase inhibitors (NRTIs).

The most appropriate antiretroviral regimen cannot be defined for each clinical scenario, and selection of specific antiretroviral agents for use in multiple-drug regimens should be individualized based on information regarding antiretroviral potency, potential rate of development of resistance, known toxicities, and potential for pharmacokinetic interactions as well as virologic, immunologic, and clinical characteristics of the patient. For information on the general principles and guidelines for use of antiretroviral therapy, including specific recommendations for initial therapy in antiretroviral-naive patients and recommendations for changing antiretroviral regimens, see the Antiretroviral Agents General Statement 8:18.08.

Antiretroviral-naive Adults and Adolescents For *initial* treatment in HIV-infected adults and adolescents, the US Department of Health and Human Services (HHS) Panel on Antiretroviral Guidelines for Adults and Adolescents states that *ritonavir-boosted* darunavir in conjunction with tenofovir alafenamide fumarate (TAF) and emtricitabine or *ritonavir-boosted* darunavir in conjunction with tenofovir disoproxil fumarate (tenofovir DF) and emtricitabine (or lamivudine) are recommended PI-based regimens. These experts state that *cobicistat-boosted* darunavir in conjunction with TAF and emtricitabine or *cobicistat-boosted* darunavir in conjunction with tenofovir DF and emtricitabine (or lamivudine) are alternative PI-based regimens for *initial* treatment in antiretroviral-naive adults and adolescents†. *Ritonavir-boosted* darunavir or *cobicistat-boosted* darunavir in conjunction with abacavir and lamivudine (or emtricitabine) are considered additional alternative PI-based regimens for *initial* treatment in antiretroviral-naive patients, but should be used *only* in patients with baseline plasma HIV RNA levels less than 100,000 copies/mL who are human leukocyte antigen (HLA)-B*5701 negative. In addition, these experts state that *ritonavir-boosted* darunavir in conjunction with raltegravir (twice daily) is another regimen option for *initial* treatment in antiretroviral-naive adults and adolescents when TAF, TDF, or abacavir cannot be used, but should be used *only* in patients with baseline plasma HIV RNA levels less than 100,000 copies/mL *and* $CD4^+$ T-cell counts exceeding 200 cells/mm^3.

Clinical Experience. The comparative safety and efficacy of *ritonavir-boosted* darunavir and the fixed combination of lopinavir and ritonavir (lopinavir/ritonavir) were evaluated in a phase 3, randomized, open-label study in 689 treatment-naive HIV-infected adults 18 years of age or older (study TMC114-C211, ARTEMIS). All patients had baseline plasma HIV-1 RNA levels of 5000 copies/mL or greater and were randomized to receive *ritonavir-boosted* darunavir (darunavir 800 mg once daily with ritonavir 100 mg once daily) or lopinavir/ritonavir (lopinavir 400 mg/ritonavir 100 mg twice daily or lopinavir 800 mg/ritonavir 200 mg once daily) in conjunction with tenofovir DF (300 mg once daily) and emtricitabine (200 mg once daily). Results at 48 weeks indicated noninferiority of *ritonavir-boosted* darunavir compared with lopinavir/ritonavir. At 192 weeks, 70% of patients receiving *ritonavir-boosted* darunavir and 61% of those receiving lopinavir/ritonavir had plasma HIV-1 RNA levels less than 50 copies/mL, and the median increase in $CD4^+$ T-cell count from baseline was 258 and 263 cells/mm^3, respectively. In patients receiving *ritonavir-boosted* darunavir, 81% of those with a confirmed virologic response less than 50 copies/mL at week 48 had undetectable levels at week 192 versus 68% of those receiving lopinavir/ritonavir. In the 192-week analysis, the *ritonavir-boosted* regimen was statistically superior to the lopinavir/ritonavir regimen in the intent-to-treat population (ITT).

The manufacturer of darunavir/cobicistat states that efficacy of the fixed combination is based on efficacy demonstrated in clinical trials of *ritonavir-boosted* darunavir. In addition, pharmacokinetic data indicate that a once-daily regimen of darunavir (800 mg) given in conjunction with cobicistat (150 mg) results in darunavir pharmacokinetic parameters that are comparable to those attained with a once-daily regimen of darunavir (800 mg) given in conjunction with low-dose ritonavir (100 mg).

Antiretroviral-experienced Adults **Clinical Experience.** The comparative efficacy of once- and twice-daily regimens of *ritonavir-boosted* darunavir was evaluated in a randomized, open-label study (study TMC114-C229) in 590 antiretroviral-experienced adults 18 years of age or older with baseline plasma HIV-1 RNA levels greater than 1000 copies/mL and no mutations associated with darunavir resistance (i.e., V11I, V32I, L33F, I47V, I50V, I54L, I54M, T74P, L76V, I84V, L89V). All patients had been receiving highly active antiretroviral therapy (HAART) for at least 12 weeks and then received *ritonavir-boosted* darunavir as a once-daily regimen (darunavir 800 mg once daily with ritonavir 100 mg once daily) or twice-daily regimen (darunavir 600 mg twice daily with ritonavir 100 mg twice daily) in conjunction with an optimized background antiretroviral regimen (OBR) consisting of at least 2 NRTIs. At 48 weeks, 69% of patients in each group had plasma HIV-1 RNA levels less than 50 copies/mL and the mean increase in $CD4^+$ T-cell count from baseline was similar (108 and 112 cells/mm^3).

The comparative safety and efficacy of *ritonavir-boosted* darunavir and lopinavir/ritonavir were evaluated in a phase 3, randomized, controlled, open-label study (study TMC114-C214; TITAN study) in 595 antiretroviral-experienced HIV-infected adults 18 years of age or older with baseline plasma HIV-1 RNA levels greater than 1000 copies/mL who had been receiving HAART for at least 12 weeks. Patients were randomized to receive *ritonavir-boosted* darunavir (darunavir 600 mg twice daily with ritonavir 100 twice daily) or lopinavir/ritonavir (lopinavir 400 mg/ritonavir 100 mg twice daily) in conjunction with an OBR consisting of at least 2 antiretrovirals (NRTIs with or without nonnucleoside reverse transcriptase inhibitors [NNRTIs]). At 96 weeks, 58% of patients receiving *ritonavir-boosted* darunavir and 52% of patients receiving lopinavir/ritonavir had plasma HIV-1 RNA levels less than 50 copies/mL and the median change in $CD4^+$ T-cell count from baseline was 81 and 93 cells/mm^3, respectively.

Ritonavir-boosted darunavir also was evaluated in 2 randomized, controlled, phase 2b studies (studies TMC114-C213 and TMC114-C202) in adults with clinically advanced HIV infection (baseline plasma HIV-1 RNA levels greater than 1000 copies/mL) who had received prior therapy with an antiretroviral regimen that included a PI, NRTI, and NNRTI and were receiving a stable PI-containing regimen for at least 8 weeks at study entry. All patients had at least 1 mutation in the HIV protease gene (D30N, M46I/L, G48V, I50L/V, V82A/F/S/T, I84V, L90M) at baseline. These studies were conducted in 2 phases: an initial dose-finding phase and a long-term phase in which patients randomized to receive *ritonavir-boosted* darunavir received 600 mg of darunavir and 100 mg of ritonavir twice daily. Patients were randomized to receive *ritonavir-boosted* darunavir in conjunction with an OBR or a comparator *ritonavir-boosted* PI in conjunction with an OBR (36% received lopinavir, 34% amprenavir or fosamprenavir, 35% saquinavir, 17% atazanavir; 98% of control group received a *ritonavir-boosted* PI regimen and 23% of these were dual-boosted PIs). At 96 weeks, 57% of those receiving *ritonavir-boosted* darunavir (recommended regimen) and an OBR and 10% of those receiving a comparator *ritonavir-boosted* PI and an OBR were virologic responders (achieved and maintained a reduction in plasma HIV-1 RNA levels of at least 1 log_{10} copies/mL below baseline); 39% of those receiving *ritonavir-boosted* darunavir and an OBR and 9% of those receiving the comparator PI-containing regimen and an OBR had plasma HIV-1 RNA levels less than 50 copies/mL.

Pediatric Patients *Ritonavir-boosted* darunavir is used in conjunction with other antiretroviral agents for the treatment of HIV-1 infection in children 3 years of age or older. The indication for antiretroviral-experienced pediatric patients is based on analyses of plasma HIV-1 RNA levels and $CD4^+$ T-cell counts from 2 open-label phase 2 trials (24-week analysis of a trial in children 6 to less than 18 years of age and 48-week analysis of a trial in children 3 to less than 6 years of age). The indication for antiretroviral-naive or antiretroviral-experienced pediatric patients with no mutations associated with darunavir resistance is based on 48-week analysis of an open-label phase 2 trial in antiretroviral-naive patients 12 to less than 18 years of age and pharmacokinetic modeling and simulation for patients 3 to less than 12 years of age.

Efficacy and safety of *cobicistat-boosted* darunavir (administered as fixed-combination darunavir/cobicistat or, alternatively, as single-entity darunavir and single-entity cobicistat) have not been established in patients younger than 18 years of age.

For *initial* treatment of HIV-infected pediatric patients, the HHS Panel on Antiretroviral Therapy and Medical Management of HIV-infected Children recommends a regimen that includes a *ritonavir-boosted* PI, NNRTI, or integrase strand transfer inhibitor (INSTI) in conjunction with 2 NRTIs (dual NRTIs). These experts state that *ritonavir-boosted* darunavir (twice daily) in conjunction with 2 NRTIs is a preferred regimen in children 3 years to less than 12 years of age and that once-daily *ritonavir-boosted* regimens should *not* be used in this age group. The panel also states that *ritonavir-boosted* darunavir (once daily) in conjunction with 2 NRTIs is a preferred regimen in children 12 years of age or older, but once-daily *ritonavir-boosted* darunavir regimens should *not* be used if darunavir resistance-associated substitutions are present. For further information on treatment of HIV infection in pediatric patients, see Antiretroviral Therapy in Pediatric Patients, in Guidelines for Use of Antiretroviral Agents in the Antiretroviral Agents General Statement 8:18.08.

Clinical Experience. Safety and efficacy of *ritonavir-boosted* darunavir in conjunction with other antiretroviral agents have been evaluated in an open-label study in 80 antiretroviral-experienced HIV-infected children 6 to less than 18 years of age weighing at least 20 kg (study TMC114-C212). These children (median age 14 years, 71% male, 54% Caucasian, 30% black, mean baseline plasma HIV-1 RNA level 4.64 log_{10} copies/mL, median baseline $CD4^+$ T-cell count 330 cells/mm^3) were randomized to receive *ritonavir-boosted* darunavir plus a background regimen consisting of at least 2 non-PI antiretroviral agents; 79% had previously received at least 1 NNRTI and 96% had previously received at least 1 PI. At week 24, 64 and 50% of children had plasma HIV-1 RNA levels less than 400 and 50 copies/mL, respectively; the mean $CD4^+$ T-cell count increase from baseline was 117 cells/mm^3.

Safety and efficacy also were evaluated in an open-label study in 21 antiretroviral-experienced HIV-infected children 3 to less than 6 years of age weighing 10 kg to less than 20 kg (study TMC114-C228). These children (median age 4.4 years, 48% male, 57% black, 29% Caucasian, mean baseline plasma HIV-1 RNA level 4.34 log_{10} copies/mL, median baseline $CD4^+$ T-cell count 927 cells/mm^3, median baseline $CD4^+$ percentage 27.7%) received a *ritonavir-boosted* regimen of darunavir oral suspension and ritonavir oral solution in addition to a background regimen consisting of at least 2 active non-PI drugs; all patients previously received 2 or more NRTIs, 62% previously received at least 1 NNRTI, and 76% previously received at least 1 HIV PI. At week 48, 1 child had discontinued treatment and 71% of the remaining 20 children had plasma HIV-1 RNA levels less than 50 copies/mL. The mean change in $CD4^+$ T-cell count from baseline was 187 cells/mm^3 and the mean increase in $CD4^+$ percentage from baseline was 4%.

In study TMC114-C230, safety and efficacy of *ritonavir-boosted* darunavir were evaluated in 12 antiretroviral-naive pediatric patients 12 to less than 18 years of age weighing at least 40 kg. Enrolled patients (median age 14.4 years, 33.3% male, 58.3% Caucasian, 41.7% black, mean baseline plasma HIV-1 RNA level 4.72 log_{10} copies/mL, median baseline $CD4^+$ T-cell count 282 cells/mm^3) received the adult recommended dosage of *ritonavir-boosted* darunavir (darunavir 800 mg once daily with ritonavir 100 mg once daily) in addition to background therapy consisting of at least 2 non-PI antiretroviral agents. At 48 weeks, data from the 12 patients indicated that 91.7 and 83.3% had plasma HIV-1 RNA levels less than 400 and 50 copies/mL, respectively. The mean increase in $CD4^+$ T-cell count from baseline was 221 cells/mm^3.

■ **Postexposure Prophylaxis following Occupational Exposure to HIV** *Ritonavir-boosted* darunavir is used in conjunction with 2 NRTIs for postexposure prophylaxis of HIV infection following occupational exposure† (PEP) in health-care personnel and other individuals exposed via percutaneous injury (e.g., needlestick, cut with sharp object) or mucous membrane or nonintact skin (e.g., chapped, abraded, dermatitis) contact with blood, tissue, or other body fluids that might contain HIV.

The US Public Health Service (USPHS) states that the preferred regimen for PEP following an occupational exposure to HIV is a 3-drug regimen of raltegravir used in conjunction with emtricitabine and tenofovir DF (may be administered as the fixed combination emtricitabine/tenofovir DF; Truvada®). These experts state that *ritonavir-boosted* darunavir and 2 NRTIs is one of several alternative regimens recommended when the preferred regimen cannot be used. The preferred dual NRTI option for use with *ritonavir-boosted* darunavir for PEP is emtricitabine and tenofovir DF (may be administered as emtricitabine/tenofovir DF; Truvada®); alternative dual NRTIs are tenofovir DF and lamivudine, zidovudine and lamivudine (may be administered as the fixed combination lamivudine/zidovudine; Combivir®), or zidovudine and emtricitabine.

Because management of occupational exposures to HIV is complex and evolving, consultation with an infectious disease specialist, clinician with expertise in administration of antiretroviral agents, and/or the National Clinicians' Postexposure Prophylaxis Hotline (PEPline at 888-448-4911) is recommended whenever possible. However, initiation of PEP should not be delayed while waiting for expert consultation.

For information on types of occupational exposure to HIV and associated risk of infection, management of occupational exposure to HIV, efficacy and safety of postexposure prophylaxis, and recommendations regarding PEP, see Guidelines for Use of Antiretroviral Agents: Antiretrovirals for Postexposure Prophylaxis (PEP) following Occupational Exposure to HIV, in the Antiretroviral Agents General Statement 8:18.08.

■ **Postexposure Prophylaxis following Nonoccupational Exposure to HIV** *Ritonavir-boosted* darunavir is used in conjunction with other antiretrovirals for postexposure prophylaxis of HIV infection following nonoccupational exposure† (nPEP) in individuals who have had exposure to blood, genital secretions, or other potentially infectious body fluids that might contain HIV when the exposure represents a substantial risk for HIV transmission.

When nPEP is indicated following a nonoccupational exposure to HIV, the US Centers for Disease Control and Prevention (CDC) states that the preferred regimen in adults and adolescents 13 years of age or older with normal renal function is either raltegravir or dolutegravir used in conjunction with emtricitabine and tenofovir DF (administered as emtricitabine/tenofovir DF; Truvada®); the recommended alternative nPEP regimen in these patients is *ritonavir-boosted* darunavir used in conjunction with emtricitabine/tenofovir DF.

Consultation with an infectious disease specialist, clinician with expertise in administration of antiretroviral agents, and/or the National Clinicians' Postexposure Prophylaxis Hotline (PEPline at 888-448-4911) is recommended if nPEP is indicated in certain exposed individuals (e.g., pregnant women, children, those with medical conditions such as renal impairment) or if an antiretroviral regimen not included in the CDC guidelines is being considered, the source virus is known or likely to be resistant to antiretrovirals, or the healthcare provider is inexperienced in prescribing antiretrovirals. However, initiation of nPEP should not be delayed while waiting for expert consultation.

For additional information on nonoccupational exposure to HIV and recommendations regarding postexposure prophylaxis, see Guidelines for Use of Antiretroviral Agents: Antiretrovirals for Postexposure Prophylaxis following Sexual, Injection Drug Use, or other Nonoccupational Exposures to HIV (nPEP), in the Antiretroviral Agents General Statement 8:18.08.

Dosage and Administration

■ **Administration** Darunavir is administered orally in conjunction with low-dose ritonavir (*ritonavir-boosted* darunavir) once or twice daily with food.

Alternatively, darunavir is administered orally in conjunction with cobicistat (*cobicistat-boosted* darunavir) once daily with food.

Darunavir should *not* be administered without low-dose ritonavir or cobicistat. Low-dose ritonavir and cobicistat are pharmacokinetic enhancers that improve the pharmacokinetic profile of darunavir.

Ritonavir-boosted Darunavir When *ritonavir-boosted* darunavir is used, single-entity darunavir is administered as tablets or oral suspension at the same time as single-entity ritonavir capsules, tablets, or oral solution.

Oral Suspension. Darunavir oral suspension should be used in patients who have difficulty swallowing tablets.

The oral suspension should be administered using the oral dosing syringe supplied by the manufacturer. If an 800-mg dose of darunavir is indicated, the dose should be given as two 4-mL administrations of the suspension using the oral dosing syringe.

Darunavir oral suspension should be stored in the original container at 25°C, but may be exposed to 15–30°C; the suspension should not be refrigerated or frozen and should not be exposed to excessive heat.

The oral suspension is a white to off-white opaque suspension and should be shaken prior to each dose.

Tablets. Darunavir tablets should be swallowed whole with a drink (e.g., water, milk).

Children weighing 15 kg or more should be assessed for the ability to swallow the darunavir tablets; darunavir oral suspension should be considered in those unable to reliably swallow tablets.

Cobicistat-boosted Darunavir When *cobicistat-boosted* darunavir is used, fixed-combination tablets containing both drugs are commercially available (darunavir/cobicistat). Alternatively, single-entity darunavir is administered as tablets or oral suspension at the same time as single-entity cobicistat tablets.

■ **Dosage** Single-entity darunavir is commercially available as an oral suspension and tablets containing darunavir ethanolate; dosage is expressed in terms of darunavir.

Darunavir/cobicistat is commercially available as fixed-combination tablets containing darunavir ethanolate (800 mg of darunavir) and cobicistat (150 mg).

Adult Dosage **Treatment of HIV Infection in Antiretroviral-naive Adults.** The recommended dosage of *ritonavir-boosted* darunavir for the treatment of human immunodeficiency virus type 1 (HIV-1) infection in antiretroviral-naive adults is 800 mg of single-entity darunavir (one 800-mg tablet or 8 mL of the oral suspension containing 100 mg/mL) once daily given in conjunction with single-entity ritonavir 100 mg once daily.

The recommended dosage of *cobicistat-boosted* darunavir for the treatment of HIV-1 infection in antiretroviral-naive adults without any substitutions associated with darunavir resistance is 800 mg of darunavir once daily given in conjunction with 150 mg of cobicistat once daily. When fixed-combination darunavir/cobicistat is used, adults should receive 1 tablet (800 mg of darunavir and 150 mg of cobicistat) once daily. Alternatively, adults can receive 800 mg of single-entity darunavir (one 800-mg tablet or 8 mL of the oral suspension containing 100 mg/mL) once daily given in conjunction with single-entity cobicistat 150 mg once daily. A *cobicistat-boosted* darunavir regimen that contains a darunavir dosage of 600 mg twice daily is *not* recommended.

Treatment of HIV Infection in Antiretroviral-experienced Adults. When *ritonavir-boosted* darunavir or *cobicistat-boosted* darunavir is used in antiretroviral-experienced patients, genotypic testing is recommended to identify substitutions associated with darunavir resistance (V11I, V32I, L33F, I47V, I50V, I54L, I54M, T74P, L76V, I84V, L89V).

For the treatment of HIV-1 infection in antiretroviral-experienced adults without any substitutions associated with darunavir resistance, the recommended dosage of *ritonavir-boosted* darunavir is 800 mg of single-entity darunavir (one 800-mg tablet or 8 mL of the oral suspension containing 100 mg/mL) once daily given in conjunction with single-entity ritonavir 100 mg once daily.

For the treatment of HIV-1 infection in antiretroviral-experienced adults with at least 1 substitution associated with darunavir resistance, the recommended dosage of *ritonavir-boosted* darunavir is 600 mg of single-entity darunavir (one 600-mg tablet or 6 mL of the oral suspension containing 100 mg/mL) twice daily with single-entity ritonavir 100 mg twice daily.

If genotypic testing is not feasible, a *ritonavir-boosted* regimen of 600 mg of single-entity darunavir (one 600-mg tablet or 6 mL of the oral suspension containing 100 mg/mL) twice daily with single-entity ritonavir 100 mg twice daily is recommended.

For the treatment of HIV-1 infection in antiretroviral-experienced adults without any substitutions associated with darunavir resistance, the recommended dosage of *cobicistat-boosted* darunavir is 800 mg of darunavir once daily in conjunction with 150 mg of cobicistat once daily. When fixed combination darunavir/cobicistat is used, adults should receive 1 tablet (800 mg of darunavir and 150 mg of cobicistat) once daily. Alternatively, adults can receive 800 mg of single-entity darunavir (one 800-mg tablet or 8 mL of the oral suspension containing 100 mg/mL) once daily given in conjunction with single-entity cobicistat 150 mg once daily. A *cobicistat-boosted* darunavir regimen that contains a darunavir dosage of 600 mg twice daily is *not* recommended.

Postexposure Prophylaxis following Occupational Exposure to HIV. For postexposure prophylaxis of HIV infection following occupational exposure† (PEP) in health-care personnel or other individuals, the preferred dosage of *ritonavir-boosted* darunavir is 800 mg of darunavir once daily with ritonavir 100 mg once daily. Alternatively, a dosage of 600 mg of darunavir twice daily with ritonavir 100 mg twice daily may be used. *Ritonavir-boosted* darunavir usually is used in conjunction with emtricitabine and tenofovir disoproxil fumarate (tenofovir DF). (See Uses: Postexposure Prophylaxis following Occupational Exposure to HIV.)

PEP should be initiated as soon as possible following occupational exposure to HIV (preferably within hours) and continued for 4 weeks, if tolerated.

Postexposure Prophylaxis following Nonoccupational Exposure to HIV. For postexposure prophylaxis of HIV infection following nonoccupational exposure† (nPEP), the usual adult dosage of *ritonavir-boosted* darunavir is 800 mg of darunavir once daily with ritonavir 100 mg once daily. *Ritonavir-boosted* darunavir usually is used in conjunction with emtricitabine and tenofovir DF. (See Uses: Postexposure Prophylaxis following Nonoccupational Exposure to HIV.)

The nPEP regimen should be initiated as soon as possible (within 72 hours) following nonoccupational exposure to HIV and continued for 28 days. If the exposed individual seeks care more than 72 hours after the exposure, nPEP is not recommended.

Pediatric Dosage To avoid medication errors, extra care should be used in calculating the dose, transcribing the medication order, dispensing the prescription, and providing dosing instructions.

Dosage of *ritonavir-boosted* darunavir in children 3 years to less than 18 years of age weighing at least 10 kg is based on weight. Pediatric dosage should not exceed the recommended dosage for antiretroviral-experienced adults.

Treatment of HIV Infection in Antiretroviral-naive Pediatric Patients. For the treatment of HIV-1 infection in antiretroviral-naive pediatric patients 3 years to less than 18 years of age weighing at least 10 kg, the recommended dosage of *ritonavir-boosted* darunavir oral suspension is based on weight (approximately 35 mg/kg once daily with ritonavir 7 mg/kg once daily in those weighing less than 15 kg). (See Table 1 and Table 2.)

Table 1. Dosage of *Ritonavir-boosted* Darunavir in Antiretroviral-naive Pediatric Patients 3 Years to Less Than 18 Years of Age Weighing 10 to Less Than 15 kg

Body Weight	Darunavir Dosage (Oral Suspension Containing 100 mg/mL)	Ritonavir Dosage (Oral Solution Containing 80 mg/mL)
≥10 to <11 kg	350 mg (3.6 mL[a]) once daily	64 mg (0.8 mL) once daily
≥11 to <12 kg	385 mg (4 mL[a]) once daily	64 mg (0.8 mL) once daily
≥12 to <13 kg	420 mg (4.2 mL) once daily	80 mg (1 mL) once daily
≥13 to <14 kg	455 mg (4.6 mL[a]) once daily	80 mg (1 mL) once daily
≥14 to <15 kg	490 mg (5 mL[a]) once daily	96 mg (1.2 mL) once daily

[a] Dosage (in mL) rounded up for convenient measuring using oral dosing syringe provided by manufacturer.

Table 2. Dosage of *Ritonavir-boosted* Darunavir in Antiretroviral-naive Pediatric Patients 3 Years to Less Than 18 Years of Age Weighing at Least 15 kg

Body Weight	Darunavir Dosage (Oral Suspension Containing 100 mg/mL or Tablets)	Ritonavir Dosage (Oral Solution Containing 80 mg/mL or 100-mg Capsules or Tablets)
≥15 to <30 kg	600 mg (6 mL) once daily	100 mg (1.25 mL) once daily
≥30 to <40 kg	675 mg (6.8 mL[a]) once daily	100 mg (1.25 mL) once daily
≥40 kg	800 mg (8 mL) once daily	100 mg (1.25 mL) once daily

[a] Dosage (in mL) rounded up for convenient measuring using oral dosing syringe provided by manufacturer.

Treatment of HIV Infection in Antiretroviral-experienced Pediatric Patients. When *ritonavir-boosted* darunavir is used in antiretroviral-experienced pediatric patients, genotypic testing is recommended to identify mutations associated with darunavir resistance (V11I, V32I, L33F, I47V, I50V, I54L, I54M, T74P, L76V, I84V, L89V).

For the treatment of HIV-1 infection in antiretroviral-experienced pediatric patients 3 years to less than 18 years of age weighing at least 10 kg without any mutations associated with darunavir resistance, the recommended dosage of *ritonavir-boosted* darunavir oral suspension is based on weight (approximately 35 mg/kg once daily with ritonavir 7 mg/kg once daily in those weighing less than 15 kg). (See Table 3 and Table 4.)

Table 3. Dosage of *Ritonavir-boosted* Darunavir in Antiretroviral-experienced Pediatric Patients 3 Years to Less Than 18 Years of Age Weighing 10 to Less Than 15 kg without Any Mutations Associated with Darunavir Resistance

Body Weight	Darunavir Dosage (Oral Suspension Containing 100 mg/mL)	Ritonavir Dosage (Oral Solution Containing 80 mg/mL)
≥10 to <11 kg	350 mg (3.6 mL[a]) once daily	64 mg (0.8 mL) once daily
≥11 to <12 kg	385 mg (4 mL[a]) once daily	64 mg (0.8 mL) once daily
≥12 to <13 kg	420 mg (4.2 mL) once daily	80 mg (1 mL) once daily
≥13 to <14 kg	455 mg (4.6 mL[a]) once daily	80 mg (1 mL) once daily
≥14 to <15 kg	490 mg (5 mL[a]) once daily	96 mg (1.2 mL) once daily

[a] Dosage (in mL) rounded up for convenient measuring using oral dosing syringe provided by manufacturer.

Table 4. Dosage of *Ritonavir-boosted* Darunavir in Antiretroviral-naive Pediatric Patients 3 Years to Less Than 18 Years of Age Weighing at Least 15 kg without Any Mutations Associated with Darunavir Resistance

Body Weight	Darunavir Dosage (Oral Suspension Containing 100 mg/mL or Tablets)	Ritonavir Dosage (Oral Solution Containing 80 mg/mL or 100-mg Capsules or Tablets)
≥15 to <30 kg	600 mg (6 mL) once daily	100 mg (1.25 mL) once daily
≥30 to <40 kg	675 mg (6.8 mL[a]) once daily	100 mg (1.25 mL) once daily
≥40 kg	800 mg (8 mL) once daily	100 mg (1.25 mL) once daily

[a] Dosage (in mL) rounded up for convenient measuring using oral dosing syringe provided by manufacturer.

For the treatment of HIV-1 infection in antiretroviral-experienced pediatric patients 3 years to less than 18 years of age weighing at least 10 kg with at least 1 mutation associated with darunavir resistance, the recommended dosage of *ritonavir-boosted* darunavir oral suspension is based on weight (approximately 20 mg/kg twice daily with ritonavir 3 mg/kg twice daily in those weighing less than 15 kg). (See Table 5 and Table 6.)

Table 5. Dosage of *Ritonavir-boosted* Darunavir in Antiretroviral-experienced Pediatric Patients 3 Years to Less Than 18 Years of Age Weighing 10 to Less Than 15 kg with at Least One Mutation Associated with Darunavir Resistance

Body Weight	Darunavir Dosage (Oral Suspension Containing 100 mg/mL)	Ritonavir Dosage (Oral Solution Containing 80 mg/mL)
≥10 to <11 kg	200 mg (2 mL) twice daily	32 mg (0.4 mL) twice daily
≥11 to <12 kg	220 mg (2.2 mL) twice daily	32 mg (0.4 mL) twice daily
≥12 to <13 kg	240 mg (2.4 mL) twice daily	40 mg (0.5 mL) twice daily
≥13 to <14 kg	260 mg (2.6 mL) twice daily	40 mg (0.5 mL) twice daily
≥14 to <15 kg	280 mg (2.8 mL) twice daily	48 mg (0.6 mL) twice daily

Table 6. Dosage of *Ritonavir-boosted* Darunavir in Antiretroviral-experienced Pediatric Patients 3 Years to Less Than 18 Years of Age Weighing at Least 15 kg with at Least One Mutation Associated with Darunavir Resistance

Body Weight	Darunavir Dosage (Oral Suspension Containing 100 mg/mL or Tablets)	Ritonavir Dosage (Oral Solution Containing 80 mg/mL or 100-mg Capsules or Tablets)
≥15 to <30 kg	375 mg (3.8 mL[a]) twice daily	48 mg (0.6 mL) twice daily
≥30 to <40 kg	450 mg (4.6 mL[a]) twice daily	60 mg (0.75 mL) twice daily
≥40 kg	600 mg (6 mL) twice daily	100 mg (1.25 mL) twice daily

[a] Dosage (in mL) rounded up for convenient measuring using oral dosing syringe provided by manufacturer.

■ **Special Populations** ***Hepatic Impairment*** Dosage of *ritonavir-boosted* darunavir or *cobicistat-boosted* darunavir does not need to be adjusted in patients with mild to moderate hepatic impairment (Child-Pugh class A or B). (See Hepatic Impairment under Warnings/Precautions: Specific Populations, in Cautions.)

Ritonavir-boosted darunavir or *cobicistat-boosted* darunavir should not be used in patients with severe hepatic impairment (Child-Pugh class C). (See Hepatic Impairment under Warnings/Precautions: Specific Populations, in Cautions.)

Renal Impairment Some experts state that dosage of *ritonavir-boosted* darunavir does not need to be adjusted in patients with renal impairment. (See Renal Impairment under Warnings/Precautions: Specific Populations, in Cautions.)

Prior to initiation of *cobicistat-boosted* darunavir (administered as fixed-combination darunavir/cobicistat or, alternatively, as single-entity darunavir and single-entity cobicistat), estimated creatinine clearance should be assessed. Although some experts state that dosage adjustments are not necessary when *cobicistat-boosted* darunavir is used in patients with renal impairment, these experts and the manufacturer state that *cobicistat-boosted* darunavir should *not* be used in conjunction with tenofovir DF in patients with estimated creatinine clearances less than 70 mL/minute. (See Renal Impairment under Warnings/Precautions: Specific Populations, in Cautions.)

Pregnant Women If darunavir is used during pregnancy, it should be administered as *ritonavir-boosted* darunavir.

For the treatment of HIV-1 infection in pregnant women, the recommended dosage of *ritonavir-boosted* darunavir is 600 mg of single-entity darunavir twice daily (one 600-mg tablet or 6 mL of the oral suspension containing 100 mg/mL twice daily) with single-entity ritonavir 100 mg twice daily.

The manufacturer states that a once-daily regimen of 800 mg of single-entity darunavir (one 800-mg tablet or 8 mL of the oral suspension containing 100 mg/mL once daily) with single-entity ritonavir 100 mg once daily should be considered during pregnancy *only* in women already stabilized on this once-daily regimen prior to pregnancy who are virologically suppressed (i.e., plasma HIV-1 RNA levels less than 50 copies/mL) and in whom a change to a twice-daily regimen may compromise tolerability or compliance. However, some experts state that once-daily regimens of *ritonavir-boosted* darunavir are *not* recommended in pregnant women.

Cautions

■ **Contraindications** Concomitant use of *ritonavir-boosted* darunavir or *cobicistat-boosted* darunavir (administered as fixed-combination darunavir/cobicistat or, alternatively, as single-entity darunavir and single-entity cobicistat) with drugs highly dependent on cytochrome P-450 (CYP) isoenzyme CYP3A for metabolism and for which elevated plasma concentrations are associated with serious and/or life-threatening events (e.g., alfuzosin, cisapride, dronedarone, ergot alkaloids, lovastatin, lurasidone, simvastatin, oral midazolam, triazolam, ranolazine, pimozide, sildenafil [Revatio®] for treatment of pulmonary arterial hypertension) is contraindicated. (See Drug Interactions.)

Concomitant use of *ritonavir-boosted* darunavir or *cobicistat-boosted* darunavir with drugs that may decrease darunavir concentrations resulting in possible loss of virologic response (e.g., rifampin, St. John's wort [*Hypericum perforatum*]) is contraindicated. (See Drug Interactions.)

Concomitant use of *cobicistat-boosted* darunavir and carbamazepine, phenobarbital, phenytoin, and the fixed combination of elbasvir and grazoprevir (elbasvir/grazoprevir) is contraindicated. (See Drug Interactions.)

Concomitant use of *ritonavir-boosted* darunavir or *cobicistat-boosted* darunavir with colchicine is contraindicated in patients with renal and/or hepatic impairment. (See Drug Interactions: Colchicine.)

■ **Warnings/Precautions** ***Sensitivity Reactions*** **Dermatologic Reactions.** Severe skin reactions, sometimes accompanied by fever and/or increases in serum transaminase concentrations, have occurred in patients receiving *ritonavir-boosted* darunavir. Stevens-Johnson syndrome has been reported rarely; toxic epidermal necrolysis, drug rash with eosinophilia and systemic symptoms, and acute, generalized exanthematous pustulosis also have been reported.

Rash (usually of mild to moderate intensity) has occurred in 10.3% of patients receiving *ritonavir-boosted* darunavir; rash usually occurs during the first 4 weeks of therapy. *Ritonavir-boosted* darunavir was continued without interruption in most patients.

Although rash was reported more frequently in antiretroviral-experienced patients receiving *ritonavir-boosted* darunavir and raltegravir than in those receiving *ritonavir-boosted* darunavir without raltegravir or raltegravir without *ritonavir-boosted* darunavir, rash that was considered drug related occurred at similar rates in all 3 groups; rash generally was mild to moderate in severity and did not limit therapy or require discontinuance.

Ritonavir-boosted darunavir or *cobicistat-boosted* darunavir should be discontinued immediately if manifestations of severe skin reactions occur (e.g., severe rash, rash accompanied by fever, general malaise, fatigue, muscle or joint aches, blisters, oral lesions, conjunctivitis, hepatitis, and/or eosinophilia).

Sulfonamide Sensitivity. Darunavir contains a sulfonamide moiety, which may cause allergic-type reactions in certain susceptible individuals. In clinical studies evaluating *ritonavir-boosted* darunavir, the incidence of rash in patients with a history of sulfonamide sensitivity was similar to that in patients without a history of sulfonamide sensitivity.

Ritonavir-boosted darunavir and *cobicistat-boosted* darunavir should be used with caution in patients with known hypersensitivity to sulfonamide-containing drugs.

Hepatic Effects Drug-induced hepatitis (e.g., acute hepatitis, cytolytic hepatitis) has occurred in patients receiving *ritonavir-boosted* darunavir in clinical studies. Patients with preexisting liver dysfunction, including HIV-infected patients coinfected with hepatitis B virus (HBV) or hepatitis C virus (HCV), have an increased risk for liver function abnormalities. There have been postmarketing reports of liver injury (in some cases fatal) in patients receiving *ritonavir-boosted* darunavir; liver injury generally has occurred in patients with advanced HIV infection who were receiving multiple concomitant drugs, were coinfected with HBV or HCV, and/or were developing immune reconstitution syndrome.

Appropriate laboratory tests should be performed to evaluate hepatic function prior to and periodically during treatment with *ritonavir-boosted* darunavir or *cobicistat-boosted* darunavir. Increased AST/ALT monitoring should be considered, especially during the first several months of therapy, in patients with hepatitis, cirrhosis, or elevated transaminase values prior to therapy. (See Hepatic Impairment under Warnings/Precautions: Specific Populations, in Cautions.)

Renal Effects Cobicistat decreases estimated creatinine clearance by inhibiting tubular secretion of creatinine without affecting actual renal glomerular function; this effect should be considered when interpreting changes in estimated creatinine clearance in patients receiving *cobicistat-boosted* darunavir. This is particularly important in those needing creatinine clearance monitoring because of a medical condition or other concomitant drugs.

Estimated creatinine clearance should be assessed prior to initiating *cobicistat-boosted* darunavir. Although cobicistat may cause only modest increases in serum creatinine and modest declines in estimated creatinine clearance without affecting renal glomerular function, the patient should be closely monitored for renal safety if there is an increase in serum creatinine of more than 0.4 mg/dL from baseline during *cobicistat-boosted* darunavir therapy.

The manufacturer states that dosage recommendations are not available for drugs that require dosage adjustments in patients with renal impairment who are receiving *cobicistat-boosted* darunavir. Therefore, alternative drugs that do not require dosage adjustments based on renal impairment should be considered in patients receiving *cobicistat-boosted* darunavir.

New-onset or worsening renal impairment, including acute renal failure and Fanconi syndrome, has been reported in patients receiving cobicistat in an antiretroviral regimen that also included tenofovir disoproxil fumarate (tenofovir DF). Concomitant use of *cobicistat-boosted* darunavir and tenofovir DF is not recommended in patients with estimated creatinine clearances less than 70 mL/minute or in patients who are receiving (or recently received) a nephrotoxic agent. Whenever *cobicistat-boosted* darunavir and tenofovir DF are used concomitantly, urine glucose and urine protein should be documented at baseline and estimated creatinine clearance, urine glucose, and urine protein should be routinely monitored throughout concomitant therapy. In addition, serum phosphorus should be monitored in those with or at risk for renal impairment.

Interactions Darunavir must be used in conjunction with a pharmacokinetic enhancer (i.e., low-dose ritonavir or cobicistat). Failure to administer darunavir with the recommended dosage of ritonavir or cobicistat will result in subtherapeutic darunavir concentrations and inadequate antiretroviral response. When *ritonavir-boosted* darunavir or *cobicistat-boosted* darunavir is used, the cautions, precautions, contraindications, and drug interactions associated darunavir and the pharmacokinetic enhancer (i.e., low-dose ritonavir or cobicistat) should be considered.

Concomitant use of *ritonavir-boosted* darunavir or *cobicistat-boosted* darunavir with certain drugs is contraindicated or requires particular caution. Concomitant use with some drugs may result in clinically important adverse effects, including severe, life-threatening, or fatal events, due to higher exposures of the concomitant drug or higher exposures of darunavir and/or the pharmacokinetic enhancer (i.e., low-dose ritonavir or cobicistat). Concomitant use with other drugs may result in drug interactions leading to loss of therapeutic effect of *ritonavir-boosted* darunavir or *cobicistat-boosted* darunavir and possible development of resistance. Because ritonavir and cobicistat are inhibitors of CYP3A4, interactions with drugs affecting or metabolized by CYP3A4 are of particular concern. However, concomitant use of *cobicistat-boosted* darunavir with other drugs may result in different drug interactions than those observed or expected with *ritonavir-boosted* darunavir because of complex or unknown mechanisms of drug interactions.

Concomitant use of *ritonavir-boosted* darunavir or *cobicistat-boosted* darunavir with other drugs that are administered in conjunction with a pharmacokinetic enhancer (e.g., *ritonavir-boosted* HIV protease inhibitors [PIs], *ritonavir-boosted* paritaprevir, elvitegravir) is not recommended. Dosage recommendations for such regimens have not been established and concomitant use of more than one pharmacokinetic enhancer may result in complex drug interactions, including decreased plasma concentrations of the antiretroviral agents leading to loss of therapeutic effect and development of resistance.

Darunavir, ritonavir, and cobicistat are all available as single-entity preparations. In addition, fixed-combination darunavir/cobicistat is commercially available. Care should be taken to ensure that therapy is not duplicated; darunavir/cobicistat should not be used concomitantly with any other preparations containing darunavir, cobicistat, or ritonavir.

Potential drug interactions should be considered prior to and during use of *ritonavir-boosted* darunavir or *cobicistat-boosted* darunavir. Patients should be monitored for adverse effects associated with other drugs used concomitantly with *ritonavir-boosted* darunavir or *cobicistat-boosted* darunavir. (See Drug Interactions.)

Hyperglycemic and Diabetogenic Effects Hyperglycemia (potentially persistent), new-onset diabetes mellitus, or exacerbation of preexisting diabetes mellitus has been reported in patients receiving HIV PIs; diabetic ketoacidosis has occurred. It may be necessary to initiate or adjust dosage of antidiabetic therapy (e.g., insulin, oral hypoglycemic agents).

Immune Reconstitution Syndrome Patients receiving antiretroviral therapy may experience an immune reconstitution syndrome during the initial phase of therapy. Patients whose immune system responds to antiretroviral therapy may develop an inflammatory response to indolent or residual opportunistic infections (e.g., *Mycobacterium avium* complex [MAC], *M. tuberculosis*, cytomegalovirus [CMV], *Pneumocystis jirovecii* [formerly *P. carinii*]); this may necessitate further evaluation and treatment.

Autoimmune disorders (e.g., Graves' disease, polymyositis, Guillain-Barré syndrome) have also been reported to occur in the setting of immune reconstitution; however, the time to onset is more variable and can occur many months after initiation of antiretroviral therapy.

Adipogenic Effects Redistribution or accumulation of body fat, including central obesity, dorsocervical fat enlargement ("buffalo hump"), peripheral wasting, facial wasting, breast enlargement, and general cushingoid appearance have been reported in patients receiving antiretroviral therapy. The mechanisms and long-term consequences of fat redistribution are unknown; a causal relationship has not been established.

Hemophilia A and B Increased bleeding, including spontaneous skin hematomas and hemarthrosis, has been reported in patients with hemophilia A or B receiving HIV PIs. Increased hemostatic therapy (e.g., antihemophilic factor) may be needed.

HIV Resistance Potential for cross-resistance among PIs not evaluated in patients receiving *ritonavir-boosted* darunavir. The possible effect of *ritonavir-boosted* darunavir therapy on subsequent therapy with other PIs is unknown.

Specific Populations **Pregnancy.** Available human and animal data suggest that darunavir does not increase the risk of major birth defects overall compared to the background rate.

The US Department of Health and Human Services (HHS) Panel on Treatment of HIV-infected Pregnant Women and Prevention of Perinatal Transmission states that, although safety and pharmacokinetic data are limited in pregnant women, *ritonavir-boosted* darunavir (darunavir 600 mg twice daily with ritonavir 100 mg twice daily) and 2 nucleoside reverse transcriptase inhibitors (NRTIs) is a preferred PI-based regimen for *initial* treatment in pregnant women. These experts state that once-daily regimens of *ritonavir-boosted* darunavir are *not* recommended in pregnant women.

The manufacturer states that *cobicistat-boosted* darunavir should be used during pregnancy only if potential benefits to the woman justify potential risks to the fetus. The HHS panel states that data are insufficient to date to recommend *routine* use of *cobicistat-boosted* darunavir for *initial* treatment in antiretroviral-naive pregnant women.

Pharmacokinetic data evaluating *ritonavir-boosted* darunavir in pregnant women indicate that darunavir and ritonavir exposures following administration of darunavir 800 mg once daily with ritonavir 100 mg once daily or darunavir 600 mg twice daily with ritonavir 100 mg twice daily generally are lower during pregnancy than exposures reported in postpartum women. In addition, reductions in plasma concentrations of unbound darunavir and ritonavir reported in pregnant women receiving a once-daily regimen of *ritonavir-boosted* darunavir are greater than reductions reported in pregnant women receiving a twice-daily regimen. (See Pregnant Women under Dosage and Administration: Special Populations.)

Antiretroviral Pregnancy Registry at 800-258-4263 or http://www.apregistry.com.

Based on prospective reports from the Antiretroviral Pregnancy Registry of approximately 532 live births following exposure to darunavir-containing antiretroviral regimens during pregnancy (including 333 first-trimester exposures), there was no difference in the rate of overall birth defects in those exposed to darunavir-containing regimens compared with the background rate of major birth defects in the US reference population of the Metropolitan Atlanta Congenital Defects Program (2.7%).

Lactation. It is not known whether darunavir, ritonavir, or cobicistat is distributed into human milk; darunavir and cobicistat are distributed into milk in rats.

Because of the risk of adverse effects in the infant and the risk of HIV transmission, HIV-infected women should not breast-feed infants.

Pediatric Use. Darunavir is not recommended in pediatric patients younger than 3 years of age since toxicity and mortality have been observed in juvenile rats given darunavir.

Safety, pharmacokinetic profile, and efficacy of *ritonavir-boosted* darunavir have been evaluated in antiretroviral-naive and antiretroviral-experienced pediatric patients 3 years to less than 18 years of age weighing at least 10 kg. Adverse effects reported in pediatric patients were similar to those reported in adults.

Safety and efficacy of *cobicistat-boosted* darunavir (administered as darunavir/cobicistat or, alternatively, as single-entity darunavir and single-entity cobicistat) have not been established in patients younger than 18 years of age.

Geriatric Use. Experience in those 65 years of age and older is insufficient to determine whether they respond differently to *ritonavir-boosted* darunavir or *cobicistat-boosted* darunavir than younger adults. Appropriate caution should be exercised in administration and monitoring because of age-related decreases in hepatic function and potential for concomitant disease and drug therapy.

Pharmacokinetics of darunavir do not differ substantially over an age range of 18–75 years of age.

Hepatic Impairment. Pharmacokinetics of *ritonavir-boosted* darunavir are not altered in patients with mild to moderate hepatic impairment (Child-Pugh class A or B); dosage adjustments are not needed in such individuals. Because darunavir pharmacokinetics have not been evaluated in patients with severe hepatic impairment, *ritonavir-boosted* darunavir is not recommended in patients with severe hepatic impairment. (See Hepatic Impairment under Dosage and Administration: Special Populations.)

Pharmacokinetics of *cobicistat-boosted* darunavir have not been evaluated in patients with mild to moderate hepatic impairment (Child-Pugh class A or B); there were no clinically important pharmacokinetic changes when cobicistat was used alone in individuals with mild or moderate hepatic impairment. Based on recommendations for *ritonavir-boosted* darunavir, dosage adjustments of *cobicistat-boosted* darunavir are not needed in patients with mild to moderate hepatic impairment (Child-Pugh class A or B). Pharmacokinetics of *cobicistat-boosted* darunavir or cobicistat alone have not been evaluated in patients with severe hepatic impairment (Child-Pugh class C), and *cobicistat-boosted* darunavir is not recommended in such patients. (See Hepatic Impairment under Dosage and Administration: Special Populations.)

Limited data indicate that darunavir exposure is not altered in HIV-infected patients coinfected with HBV or HCV.

The risk of liver function abnormalities, including severe hepatic adverse effects, is increased in patients with preexisting hepatic impairment (e.g., HBV or HCV infection).

Liver function should be monitored during the first several months of treatment with *ritonavir-boosted* darunavir when the drug is used in patients with underlying chronic hepatitis or cirrhosis or in patients with pretreatment elevated liver enzymes.

If there is evidence of new or worsening liver disease (e.g., fatigue, anorexia, nausea, jaundice, dark urine, liver tenderness, hepatomegaly, clinically important increases in hepatic enzyme concentrations), interruption or discontinuance of *ritonavir-boosted* darunavir or *cobicistat-boosted* darunavir should be considered.

Renal Impairment. Pharmacokinetics of darunavir are not altered in patients with moderate renal impairment (creatinine clearance 30–60 mL/minute). Data are not available on darunavir pharmacokinetics in patients with severe renal impairment or end-stage renal disease. Because renal clearance of darunavir is limited, decreased clearance of the drug is not expected in patients with renal impairment.

Cobicistat-boosted darunavir has not been studied in individuals with renal impairment. Cobicistat has been shown to decrease estimated creatinine clearance without affecting renal glomerular function. Prior to initiation of *cobicistat-boosted* darunavir (administered as fixed-combination darunavir/cobicistat or, alternatively, as single-entity darunavir and single-entity cobicistat), estimated creatinine clearance should be assessed. *Cobicistat-boosted* darunavir should *not* be used in conjunction with tenofovir DF in patients with estimated creatinine clearances less than 70 mL/minute. (See Renal Effects under Cautions: Warnings/Precautions.)

Darunavir, ritonavir, and cobicistat are highly bound to plasma proteins, and the drugs are unlikely to be removed by hemodialysis or peritoneal dialysis.

■ **Common Adverse Effects** The most common adverse effects reported in patients receiving *ritonavir-boosted* darunavir in conjunction with other antiretrovirals are diarrhea, nausea, vomiting, abdominal pain, headache, and rash.

Drug Interactions

Darunavir must be used with a pharmacokinetic enhancer (i.e., low-dose ritonavir or cobicistat), and drug interactions associated with both darunavir and the pharmacokinetic enhancer should be considered. Because low-dose ritonavir and cobicistat are associated with different drug interactions, interactions reported or expected with *ritonavir-boosted* darunavir may differ from those reported or expected with *cobicistat-boosted* darunavir.

The following drug interactions are based on studies using *ritonavir-boosted* darunavir or studies using cobicistat alone. Drug interaction studies are not available to date using *cobicistat-boosted* darunavir administered either as the fixed combination containing darunavir and cobicistat (darunavir/cobicistat) or as single-entity darunavir given with single-entity cobicistat.

■ **Drugs Affecting or Metabolized by Hepatic Microsomal Enzymes** Darunavir, ritonavir, and cobicistat inhibit cytochrome P-450 (CYP) isoenzymes 3A4 and 2D6; potential pharmacokinetic interaction with drugs metabolized by CYP3A or CYP2D6 (altered metabolism of drug metabolized by CYP3A or CYP2D6). Darunavir, ritonavir, and cobicistat are metabolized by CYP3A. Potential pharmacokinetic interactions with drugs that induce CYP3A (increased clearance of darunavir, ritonavir, or cobicistat, which may lead to loss of antiretroviral efficacy and development of resistance); potential pharmacokinetic interactions with drugs that inhibit CYP3A (increased plasma concentrations of darunavir, ritonavir, or cobicistat).

Caution is advised if *ritonavir-boosted* or *cobicistat-boosted* darunavir is used concomitantly with substrates, inhibitors, or inducers of CYP3A4; such drug interactions may lead to severe, life-threatening, or fatal events due to increased exposures of certain drugs, adverse effects due to increased exposures to *ritonavir-boosted* or *cobicistat-boosted* darunavir, or loss of therapeutic effect and possible development of resistance to darunavir.

Cobicistat is metabolized by CYP2D6 to a minor extent. Based on in vitro data, cobicistat is not expected to induce CYP1A2 or 2B6; based on in vivo data, cobicistat is not expected to induce CYP3A to a clinically important extent. It is not known whether cobicistat induces CYP2C9 or 2C19, but any effect is expected to be minimal based on in vitro CYP3A induction data.

■ **Drugs Affected by P-glycoprotein Transport** *Ritonavir-boosted* darunavir is an inhibitor of the P-glycoprotein (P-gp) transport system; cobicistat also is a P-gp inhibitor. Potential pharmacokinetic interactions if *ritonavir-boosted* or *cobicistat-boosted* darunavir is used with drugs transported by P-gp (increased plasma concentrations of such drugs, which could increase or prolong their therapeutic effects and may be associated with adverse effects).

In vitro data suggests that darunavir may be a P-gp substrate; potential pharmacokinetic interaction if darunavir is used concomitantly with drugs that inhibit P-gp (decreased clearance of darunavir and ritonavir, leading to increased plasma concentrations).

■ **Drugs Affecting or Affected by Other Membrane Transporters** Cobicistat inhibits breast cancer resistance protein (BCRP) and organic anion transporting polypeptide (OATP) 1B1 and 1B3. Potential pharmacokinetic interactions if *cobicistat-boosted* darunavir is used concomitantly with drugs that are substrates of BCRP, OATP1B1, or OATP1B3 (increased plasma concentrations of such drugs, which could increase or prolong their therapeutic effects and may be associated with adverse effects).

Based on in vitro data, cobicistat is not expected to induce multidrug-resistance gene (MDR) 1 to a clinically important extent. It is not known whether cobicistat induces uridine diphosphate-glucuronosyl transferase (UGT) 1A1, but any effect is expected to be minimal based on in vitro CYP3A induction data.

■ **Alfuzosin** Concomitant use of alfuzosin and *ritonavir-boosted* or *cobicistat-boosted* darunavir is contraindicated because of the potential for serious and/or life-threatening reactions (e.g., hypotension).

■ **Antiarrhythmic Agents** Possible pharmacokinetic interactions if certain antiarrhythmic agents (e.g., amiodarone, bepridil [no longer commercially available in the US], disopyramide, dronedarone, flecainide, systemic lidocaine, mexiletine, propafenone, quinidine) are used concomitantly with *ritonavir-boosted* or *cobicistat-boosted* darunavir (increased plasma concentrations of the antiarrhythmic agent).

Ritonavir-boosted or *cobicistat-boosted* darunavir and antiarrhythmic agents should be used concomitantly with caution; plasma concentration monitoring of the antiarrhythmic agents, if available, is recommended.

Amiodarone Some experts state that if amiodarone is used concomitantly with *ritonavir-boosted* or *cobicistat-boosted* darunavir, the patient should be monitored for amiodarone toxicity and consideration given to ECG and amiodarone plasma concentration monitoring.

Dronedarone Concomitant use of dronedarone and *ritonavir-boosted* or *cobicistat-boosted* darunavir is contraindicated.

■ **Anticoagulants** ***Apixaban*** Pharmacokinetic interactions if apixaban is used concomitantly with *ritonavir-boosted* or *cobicistat-boosted* darunavir (increased apixaban concentrations).

Concomitant use of *ritonavir-boosted* or *cobicistat-boosted* darunavir with apixaban is not recommended.

Dabigatran Pharmacokinetic interactions if dabigatran is used concomitantly with *ritonavir-boosted* or *cobicistat-boosted* darunavir (increased dabigatran concentrations).

Concomitant use of *ritonavir-boosted* or *cobicistat-boosted* darunavir with dabigatran is not recommended in certain patients with renal impairment, depending on the indication. Some experts state that concomitant use of dabigatran and *ritonavir-boosted* or *cobicistat-boosted* darunavir should be avoided in those with creatinine clearances less than 50 mL/minute.

Edoxaban Possible pharmacokinetic interactions if edoxaban is used concomitantly with *ritonavir-boosted* or *cobicistat-boosted* darunavir (increased edoxaban concentrations).

Concomitant use of *ritonavir-boosted* or *cobicistat-boosted* darunavir and edoxaban should be avoided.

Rivaroxaban Possible pharmacokinetic interactions if rivaroxaban is used concomitantly with *ritonavir-boosted* or *cobicistat-boosted* darunavir (increased rivaroxaban concentrations and increased risk of bleeding).

Concomitant use of *ritonavir-boosted* or *cobicistat-boosted* darunavir and rivaroxaban is not recommended.

Warfarin Pharmacokinetic interactions if warfarin is used concomitantly with *ritonavir-boosted* darunavir (decreased warfarin concentrations; no change in darunavir concentrations). The effect of *cobicistat-boosted* darunavir on warfarin concentrations is not known.

If warfarin is used concomitantly with *ritonavir-boosted* or *cobicistat-boosted* darunavir, the international normalized ratio (INR) should be monitored, especially when darunavir is initiated or discontinued; warfarin dosage should be adjusted as needed.

Some experts state that if *ritonavir-boosted* darunavir is switched to *cobicistat-boosted* darunavir, the effect of cobicistat on warfarin concentrations is not expected to be equivalent to the effect of ritonavir on warfarin concentrations.

■ **Anticonvulsants** ***Carbamazepine*** Pharmacokinetic interactions if carbamazepine is used concomitantly with *ritonavir-boosted* darunavir (increased carbamazepine concentrations; no change in darunavir concentrations). Dosage adjustments are not needed when initiating concomitant therapy with *ritonavir-boosted* darunavir and carbamazepine. However, plasma concentrations of carbamazepine should be monitored and dosage of the anticonvulsant adjusted to achieve the desired clinical effect.

Pharmacokinetic interactions if carbamazepine is used concomitantly with *cobicistat-boosted* darunavir (increased carbamazepine concentrations; decreased cobicistat concentrations; effect on darunavir concentrations unknown, but substantially decreased darunavir concentrations and loss of therapeutic effect and development of resistance are possible). Concomitant use of *cobicistat-boosted* darunavir and carbamazepine is contraindicated.

Eslicarbazepine Concomitant use of *cobicistat-boosted* darunavir and eslicarbazepine may decrease cobicistat plasma concentrations, but effects on darunavir concentrations are unknown. An alternative anticonvulsant or alternative antiretroviral therapy should be considered; if concomitant use of eslicarbazepine and *cobicistat-boosted* darunavir is necessary, the patient should be monitored for lack or loss of antiretroviral response.

Ethosuximide Possible pharmacokinetic interactions if ethosuximide is used concomitantly with *ritonavir-boosted* or *cobicistat-boosted* darunavir (increased ethosuximide concentrations). If ethosuximide is used concomitantly with *ritonavir-boosted* or *cobicistat-boosted* darunavir, the patient should be clinically monitored for ethosuximide toxicities.

Lamotrigine Possible pharmacokinetic interactions if lamotrigine is used concomitantly with *ritonavir-boosted* darunavir (decreased lamotrigine concentrations). An alternative anticonvulsant should be considered in patients receiving *ritonavir-boosted* darunavir. If lamotrigine is used concomitantly with *ritonavir-boosted* darunavir, increased lamotrigine dosage may be needed and lamotrigine plasma concentration monitoring should be considered.

Data are not available regarding concomitant use of *cobicistat-boosted* darunavir and lamotrigine. In patients receiving *cobicistat-boosted* darunavir, an alternative anticonvulsant should be considered or lamotrigine plasma concentrations should be monitored.

Oxcarbazepine Pharmacokinetic interactions if oxcarbazepine is used concomitantly with *cobicistat-boosted* darunavir (decreased cobicistat concentrations; effect on darunavir concentrations unknown). An alternative anticonvulsant or alternative antiretroviral should be considered; if concomitant use of oxcarbazepine and *cobicistat-boosted* darunavir is necessary, the patient should be monitored for lack or loss of antiretroviral response.

Phenobarbital and Phenytoin Possible pharmacokinetic interactions if phenobarbital or phenytoin is used concomitantly with *ritonavir-boosted* darunavir (decreased concentrations of the anticonvulsant; no change in darunavir concentrations). If *ritonavir-boosted* darunavir is used concomitantly with phenobarbital or phenytoin, plasma concentrations of the anticonvulsant should be monitored. Some experts suggest that alternatives to phenobarbital and phenytoin should be considered in patients receiving *ritonavir-boosted* darunavir.

Possible pharmacokinetic interactions if phenobarbital or phenytoin is used concomitantly with *cobicistat-boosted* darunavir (decreased cobicistat and darunavir concentrations expected and may result in loss of therapeutic effect and development of resistance). Concomitant use of *cobicistat-boosted* darunavir and phenobarbital or phenytoin is contraindicated.

■ **Antifungal Agents** ***Isavuconazonium*** Concomitant use of isavuconazonium sulfate (prodrug of isavuconazole) and *ritonavir-boosted* or *cobicistat-boosted* darunavir may result in increased isavuconazole concentrations and altered darunavir concentrations.

If isavuconazonium sulfate and *ritonavir-boosted* or *cobicistat-boosted* darunavir are used concomitantly, the patient should be monitored for darunavir-associated adverse effects and virologic efficacy and isavuconazole concentration monitoring should be considered.

Itraconazole Possible pharmacokinetic interactions if itraconazole is used concomitantly with *ritonavir-boosted* or *cobicistat-boosted* darunavir (increased itraconazole, darunavir, and cobicistat concentrations).

If itraconazole and *ritonavir-boosted* or *cobicistat-boosted* darunavir are used concomitantly, patients should be monitored for itraconazole-, darunavir-, and ritonavir- or cobicistat-associated adverse effects and consideration given to monitoring itraconazole plasma concentrations. High itraconazole dosage (exceeding 200 mg daily) is not recommended in patients receiving *ritonavir-boosted* or *cobicistat-boosted* darunavir, unless plasma concentrations of the antifungal are used to guide dosage.

Ketoconazole Pharmacokinetic interactions if ketoconazole is used concomitantly with *ritonavir-boosted* or *cobicistat-boosted* darunavir (increased ketoconazole, darunavir, and cobicistat concentrations).

If ketoconazole and *ritonavir-boosted* or *cobicistat-boosted* darunavir are used concomitantly, patients should be monitored for increased ketoconazole-, darunavir-, and ritonavir- or cobicistat-associated adverse effects. Ketoconazole dosage should not exceed 200 mg daily in patients receiving *ritonavir-boosted* darunavir.

Posaconazole Possible pharmacokinetic interactions if posaconazole is used concomitantly with *ritonavir-boosted* or *cobicistat-boosted* darunavir (increased darunavir and cobicistat concentrations; posaconazole concentrations may be increased).

If posaconazole and *ritonavir-boosted* or *cobicistat-boosted* darunavir are used concomitantly, patients should be monitored for increased posaconazole-, darunavir-, and ritonavir- or cobicistat-associated adverse effects; monitoring of posaconazole plasma concentrations should be considered.

Voriconazole Possible pharmacokinetic interactions if voriconazole is used concomitantly with *ritonavir-boosted* darunavir (decreased voriconazole concentrations). Data are not available regarding concomitant use of voriconazole and *cobicistat-boosted* darunavir.

Concomitant use of voriconazole and *ritonavir-boosted* or *cobicistat-boosted* darunavir is not recommended unless potential benefits outweigh risks. If voriconazole and *ritonavir-boosted* or *cobicistat-boosted* darunavir are used concomitantly, experts state that consideration should be given to monitoring voriconazole concentrations and adjusting voriconazole dosage accordingly.

■ **Antimalarial Agents** ***Artemether and Lumefantrine*** Concomitant use of the fixed combination of artemether and lumefantrine (artemether/lumefantrine) and *ritonavir-boosted* darunavir decreases plasma concentrations and area under the concentration-time curve (AUC) of artemether and the active metabolite of artemether (dihydroartemisinin), increases plasma concentrations and AUC of lumefantrine, and has no clinically important effect on plasma concentrations or AUC of darunavir. Concomitant use of artemether/lumefantrine and *cobicistat-boosted* darunavir is expected to result in increased lumefantrine concentrations; the effect on artemether concentrations is not known.

If artemether/lumefantrine is used concomitantly with *ritonavir-boosted* or *cobicistat-boosted* darunavir, the patient should be monitored for antimalarial efficacy and lumefantrine toxicity (e.g., QT interval prolongation). Although dosage adjustments are not needed when artemether/lumefantrine is used concomitantly with *ritonavir-boosted* darunavir, the drugs should be used concomitantly with caution.

■ **Antimycobacterial Agents** ***Bedaquiline*** Possible pharmacokinetic interactions if bedaquiline is used concomitantly with *ritonavir-boosted* or *cobicistat-boosted* darunavir (increased bedaquiline concentrations); clinical importance is unknown.

Some experts state that bedaquiline may be used concomitantly with *ritonavir-boosted* or *cobicistat-boosted* darunavir if potential benefits outweigh risks, but caution is advised and patients should be monitored for corrected QT (QT_c) interval prolongation and liver dysfunction.

Rifabutin Pharmacokinetic interactions if rifabutin is used concomitantly with *ritonavir-boosted* darunavir (increased rifabutin concentrations; increased darunavir concentrations). Possible pharmacokinetic interactions if rifabutin is used concomitantly with *cobicistat-boosted* darunavir (increased rifabutin concentrations expected; effects on darunavir and cobicistat concentrations unknown).

If rifabutin is used concomitantly with *ritonavir-boosted* or *cobicistat-boosted* darunavir, dosage of the antimycobacterial agent should be reduced (e.g., 150 mg once every other day; further dosage reduction may be necessary) and increased monitoring for rifabutin-associated adverse effects (e.g., neutropenia, uveitis) is warranted. Some experts recommend a rifabutin dosage of 150 mg once daily or 300 mg 3 times weekly and state that patients should be monitored for antimycobacterial response and therapeutic drug concentration monitoring should be considered.

Rifampin Possible pharmacokinetic interactions if rifampin is used concomitantly with *ritonavir-boosted* or *cobicistat-boosted* darunavir (substantially decreased darunavir concentrations) with possible loss of antiretroviral effects.

Concomitant use of *ritonavir-boosted* or *cobicistat-boosted* darunavir and rifampin is contraindicated. If a rifamycin is indicated in a patient receiving *ritonavir-boosted* or *cobicistat-boosted* darunavir, some experts state that rifabutin should be considered as an alternative to rifampin.

Rifapentine Possible pharmacokinetic interactions if rifapentine is used concomitantly with *ritonavir-boosted* or *cobicistat-boosted* darunavir (decreased darunavir concentrations). Concomitant use of *ritonavir-boosted* or *cobicistat-boosted* darunavir and rifapentine is not recommended. HIV-infected tuberculosis patients treated with rifapentine have a higher rate of tuberculosis relapse than those treated with other rifamycin-based tuberculosis regimens; an alternative antimycobacterial agent is recommended in HIV patients.

■ **Antineoplastic Agents** Possible pharmacokinetic interactions if certain antineoplastic agents (e.g, dasatinib, nilotinib, vinblastine, vincristine) are used concomitantly with *ritonavir-boosted* or *cobicistat-boosted* darunavir (increased antineoplastic agent concentrations).

If dasatinib or nilotinib is used concomitantly with *ritonavir-boosted* or *cobicistat-boosted* darunavir, reduction of the dosage of the antineoplastic agent may be needed.

If vincristine or vinblastine is used concomitantly with *ritonavir-boosted* or *cobicistat-boosted* darunavir, consideration should be given to temporarily withholding the antiretroviral regimen in patients who develop clinically important hematologic or GI adverse effects. If the antiretroviral regimen must be withheld for a prolonged period, consideration should be given to changing to a different antiretroviral regimen that does not include a CYP3A or P-gp inhibitor.

■ **Antipsychotic Agents** ***Lurasidone*** Potential for serious and/or life-threatening adverse effects if lurasidone is used concomitantly with *ritonavir-boosted* or *cobicistat-boosted* darunavir.

Concomitant use of *ritonavir-boosted* or *cobicistat-boosted* darunavir and lurasidone is contraindicated.

Perphenazine, Risperidone, and Thioridazine Possible pharmacokinetic interactions if *ritonavir-boosted* or *cobicistat-boosted* darunavir is used concomitantly with perphenazine, risperidone, or thioridazine (increased plasma concentrations of the antipsychotic agent).

If perphenazine, risperidone, or thioridazine is used concomitantly with *ritonavir-boosted* or *cobicistat-boosted* darunavir, a reduced dosage of the antipsychotic may be needed. Some experts state that the antipsychotic should be initiated using the lowest dosage, maintenance dosage should be adjusted as needed, and the patient should be monitored for toxicities associated with the antipsychotic.

Pimozide Potential for serious and/or life-threatening adverse effects (e.g., cardiac arrhythmias) if pimozide is used concomitantly with *ritonavir-boosted* or *cobicistat-boosted* darunavir.

Concomitant use of *ritonavir-boosted* or *cobicistat-boosted* darunavir and pimozide is contraindicated.

Quetiapine Pharmacokinetic interactions expected if quetiapine is used concomitantly with *ritonavir-boosted* or *cobicistat-boosted* darunavir (increased quetiapine concentrations).

Alternative antiretroviral therapy should be considered. If *ritonavir-boosted* or *cobicistat-boosted* darunavir is necessary in a patient receiving a stable dosage of quetiapine, the quetiapine dosage should be reduced to one-sixth of the original dosage and the patient monitored for quetiapine efficacy and adverse effects. If quetiapine is necessary in a patient receiving *ritonavir-boosted* or *cobicistat-boosted* darunavir, some experts recommend that quetiapine should be initiated using the lowest dosage and titrated as needed.

■ **Antiretroviral Agents** ***HIV Entry and Fusion Inhibitors***

Enfuvirtide. No in vitro evidence of antagonistic antiretroviral effects between darunavir and enfuvirtide.

Maraviroc. Pharmacokinetic interactions if maraviroc is used concomitantly with *ritonavir-boosted* or *cobicistat-boosted* darunavir (increased maraviroc plasma concentrations and AUC). If maraviroc is used concomitantly with *ritonavir-boosted* or *cobicistat-boosted* darunavir, the recommended maraviroc dosage is 150 mg twice daily.

No in vitro evidence of antagonistic antiretroviral effects between darunavir and maraviroc.

HIV Integrase Inhibitors (INSTIs) **Dolutegravir.** Concomitant use of dolutegravir and *ritonavir-boosted* darunavir does not appear to have a clinically important effect on the pharmacokinetics of either drug. Clinically important drug interactions are not expected if *cobicistat-boosted* darunavir is used with dolutegravir.

Dosage adjustments are not needed for either drug if *ritonavir-boosted* or *cobicistat-boosted* darunavir is used concomitantly with dolutegravir.

Elvitegravir. Concomitant use of *ritonavir-boosted* darunavir (darunavir 600 mg twice daily and ritonavir 100 mg twice daily) and elvitegravir (125 mg once daily) does not result in clinically important changes in darunavir or elvitegravir AUC or trough plasma concentrations. If elvitegravir is used concomitantly with *ritonavir-boosted* darunavir, the recommended elvitegravir dosage is 150 mg once daily concomitantly with darunavir 600 mg twice daily and ritonavir 100 mg twice daily. Concomitant use of elvitegravir and *cobicistat-boosted* darunavir is not recommended.

Concomitant use of the fixed combination of elvitegravir, cobicistat, emtricitabine, and tenofovir disoproxil fumarate (EVG/c/FTC/TDF) and *ritonavir-boosted* darunavir results in altered concentrations of elvitegravir, cobicistat, and/or darunavir. Concomitant use of *cobicistat-boosted* elvitegravir and *cobicistat-boosted* darunavir may result in decreased elvitegravir concentrations. Concomitant use of EVG/c/FTC/TDF and *ritonavir-boosted* or *cobicistat-boosted* darunavir is not recommended.

Raltegravir. Pharmacokinetic interactions if raltegravir is used concomitantly with *ritonavir-boosted* darunavir (decreased raltegravir AUC; no clinically important effect on pharmacokinetics of *ritonavir-boosted* darunavir). Although data are not available, clinically important drug interactions are not expected if *cobicistat-boosted* darunavir is used with raltegravir.

Dosage adjustments are not necessary if raltegravir and *ritonavir-boosted* or *cobicistat-boosted* darunavir are used concomitantly.

HIV Nonnucleoside Reverse Transcriptase Inhibitors (NNRTIs) No in vitro evidence of antagonistic antiretroviral effects between darunavir and NNRTIs, including delavirdine, efavirenz, etravirine, nevirapine, and rilpivirine.

Efavirenz. Concomitant use of *ritonavir-boosted* darunavir (darunavir 300 mg and ritonavir 100 mg twice daily) and efavirenz (600 mg once daily) increased the AUC of efavirenz by 21% and decreased the AUC of darunavir by 13%. The clinical importance of this interaction remains to be established. Concomitant use of *cobicistat-boosted* darunavir and efavirenz may result in decreased darunavir and cobicistat concentrations.

If efavirenz is used concomitantly with *ritonavir-boosted* darunavir, dosage adjustments are not necessary. However, some experts state that the patient should be monitored closely and consideration given to monitoring plasma drug concentrations.

Concomitant use of efavirenz and *cobicistat-boosted* darunavir is not recommended because of possible loss of therapeutic effect and development of resistance to darunavir.

Etravirine. Pharmacokinetic interactions if etravirine is used concomitantly with *ritonavir-boosted* darunavir (decreased etravirine plasma concentrations and AUC; no clinically important effect on darunavir plasma concentrations and AUC). Safety and efficacy of concomitant use of etravirine and *ritonavir-boosted* darunavir was established in phase 3 clinical studies. Concomitant use of etravirine and *cobicistat-boosted* darunavir may result in decreased cobicistat concentrations; the effects on darunavir pharmacokinetics are not known.

If etravirine is used with *ritonavir-boosted* darunavir, dosage adjustments are not needed.

Concomitant use of etravirine and *cobicistat-boosted* darunavir is not recommended; possible loss of therapeutic effect and development of resistance to darunavir.

Nevirapine. Pharmacokinetic interactions if nevirapine is used concomitantly with *ritonavir-boosted* darunavir (increased plasma concentrations of nevirapine and darunavir). Concomitant use of nevirapine and *cobicistat-boosted* darunavir may result in decreased cobicistat concentrations; the effects on darunavir pharmacokinetics are not known.

If nevirapine and *ritonavir-boosted* darunavir are used concomitantly, dosage adjustments are not needed.

Concomitant use of nevirapine and *cobicistat-boosted* darunavir is not recommended; possible loss of therapeutic effect and development of resistance to darunavir.

Rilpivirine. Concomitant use of rilpivirine and *ritonavir-boosted* darunavir has resulted in increased rilpivirine plasma concentrations and AUC, but did not have a clinically important effect on darunavir concentrations or AUC. Concomitant use of rilpivirine and *cobicistat-boosted* darunavir may result in increased rilpivirine concentrations, but clinically important changes in darunavir concentrations are not expected.

If rilpivirine and *ritonavir-boosted* or *cobicistat-boosted* darunavir are used concomitantly, dosage adjustments are not needed.

HIV Nucleoside and Nucleotide Reverse Transcriptase Inhibitors (NRTIs) No in vitro evidence of antagonistic antiretroviral effects between darunavir and NRTIs, including abacavir, didanosine, emtricitabine, lamivudine, stavudine, tenofovir, and zidovudine.

Pharmacokinetic interactions are not expected if abacavir, emtricitabine, lamivudine, stavudine, or zidovudine is used concomitantly with *ritonavir-boosted* or *cobicistat-boosted* darunavir. Dosage adjustments are not needed if *ritonavir-boosted* darunavir is used concomitantly with abacavir, emtricitabine, lamivudine, stavudine, or zidovudine.

Didanosine. Concomitant use of didanosine delayed-release capsules and *ritonavir-boosted* or *cobicistat-boosted* darunavir does not affect the pharmacokinetics of didanosine or darunavir. Dosage adjustments are not necessary, but didanosine doses should be given (without food) 1 hour before or 2 hours after *ritonavir-boosted* darunavir (with food) or *cobicistat-boosted* darunavir (with food).

Tenofovir Alafenamide Fumarate. Concomitant use of *ritonavir-boosted* darunavir and tenofovir alafenamide fumarate (TAF) or *cobicistat-boosted* darunavir and TAF does not substantially affect the AUC of tenofovir.

Some experts state that dosage adjustments are not needed if *ritonavir-boosted* or *cobicistat-boosted* darunavir is used concomitantly with TAF.

Tenofovir Disoproxil Fumarate. Pharmacokinetic interactions if tenofovir disoproxil fumarate (tenofovir DF) is used concomitantly with *ritonavir-boosted* darunavir (increased tenofovir plasma concentrations and AUC; increased darunavir plasma concentrations and AUC). Possible pharmacokinetic interactions if tenofovir DF is used concomitantly with *cobicistat-boosted* darunavir.

The manufacturer of darunavir states that the usual dosage of *ritonavir-boosted* darunavir can be used concomitantly with the usual dosage of tenofovir DF. Some experts state that the clinical importance of increased tenofovir DF exposures is unknown, and patients receiving *ritonavir-boosted* darunavir concomitantly with tenofovir DF should be monitored for tenofovir toxicity.

If *cobicistat-boosted* darunavir is used concomitantly with tenofovir DF, baseline estimated creatinine clearance, urine glucose, and urine protein should be assessed and patients should be monitored for tenofovir toxicity. Concomitant use of *cobicistat-boosted* darunavir with tenofovir DF is *not* recommended in patients with estimated creatinine clearances less than 70 mL/minute. (See Renal Effects under Cautions: Warnings/Precautions.)

HIV Protease Inhibitors (PIs) Concomitant use of *ritonavir-boosted* darunavir with other HIV PIs (except atazanavir) has not been studied. The manufacturer of darunavir states that concomitant use with other HIV PIs is not recommended.

No in vitro evidence of antagonistic antiretroviral effects between darunavir and amprenavir (active metabolite of fosamprenavir), atazanavir, indinavir, lopinavir, nelfinavir, ritonavir, saquinavir, or tipranavir.

Atazanavir. Concomitant use of atazanavir 300 mg once daily with *ritonavir-boosted* darunavir (darunavir 400 mg and ritonavir 100 mg twice daily [dosage differs from usually recommended dosage]) results in plasma concentrations of atazanavir that are similar to those attained with *ritonavir-boosted* atazanavir (atazanavir 300 mg and ritonavir 100 mg once daily) and plasma concentrations of darunavir similar to those attained without atazanavir.

The manufacturer of darunavir states that concomitant use of darunavir and *ritonavir-boosted* atazanavir is not recommended.

Indinavir. Concomitant use of *ritonavir-boosted* darunavir and indinavir results in increased peak plasma concentrations and AUCs of darunavir and indinavir.

Appropriate dosages for concomitant use of *ritonavir-boosted* darunavir and indinavir are not established.

Lopinavir. Concomitant use of *ritonavir-boosted* darunavir and the fixed combination of lopinavir and ritonavir (lopinavir/ritonavir) results in substantially decreased concentrations of darunavir and no change in lopinavir concentrations.

Concomitant use of lopinavir/ritonavir and *ritonavir-boosted* darunavir is not recommended; appropriate dosages for concomitant use with respect to safety and efficacy have not been established.

Ritonavir. Pharmacokinetic interactions if ritonavir is used concomitant with darunavir (increased plasma concentration and AUC of darunavir). Low-dose ritonavir is a pharmacokinetic enhancer (pharmacokinetic booster), and is used in conjunction with darunavir for therapeutic advantage (*ritonavir-boosted* darunavir).

Saquinavir. Concomitant use of *ritonavir-boosted* darunavir (darunavir 400 mg and ritonavir 100 mg twice daily) and saquinavir 1 g twice daily results in substantially decreased darunavir concentrations and no change in saquinavir concentrations.

Concomitant use of saquinavir and *ritonavir-boosted* darunavir is not recommended.

■ **Benzodiazepines** Possible pharmacokinetic interactions if certain benzodiazepines (e.g., alprazolam, diazepam, estazolam, midazolam, triazolam) are used concomitantly with *ritonavir-boosted* or *cobicistat-boosted* darunavir (increased plasma concentrations of the benzodiazepine).

Alprazolam Some experts state that other benzodiazepines not metabolized by CYP isoenzymes (e.g., lorazepam, oxazepam, temazepam) should be considered instead of alprazolam in patients receiving *ritonavir-boosted* or *cobicistat-boosted* darunavir.

Clonazepam Pharmacokinetic interactions if clonazepam is used concomitantly with *ritonavir-boosted* or *cobicistat-boosted* darunavir (increased clonazepam concentrations).

If clonazepam is used concomitantly with *ritonavir-boosted* or *cobicistat-boosted* darunavir, clinical monitoring is recommended. Although pharmacokinetic studies evaluating concomitant use are lacking, some experts state that other benzodiazepines not metabolized by CYP isoenzymes (e.g., lorazepam, oxazepam, temazepam) should be considered instead of clonazepam in patients receiving *ritonavir-boosted* or *cobicistat-boosted* darunavir.

Diazepam If diazepam is used concomitantly with *ritonavir-boosted* or *cobicistat-boosted* darunavir, diazepam dosage should be titrated, a lower diazepam dosage should be considered, and the patient should be monitored for adverse effects. Some experts state that other benzodiazepines not metabolized by CYP isoenzymes (e.g., lorazepam, oxazepam, temazepam) should be considered instead of diazepam in patients receiving *ritonavir-boosted* or *cobicistat-boosted* darunavir.

Estazolam If estazolam is used concomitantly with *ritonavir-boosted* or *cobicistat-boosted* darunavir, estazolam dosage should be titrated, a lower estazolam dosage should be considered, and the patient should be monitored for adverse effects.

Midazolam and Triazolam Concomitant use of midazolam or triazolam with *ritonavir-boosted* or *cobicistat-boosted* darunavir potentially could result in serious and/or life-threatening adverse effects (e.g., prolonged or increased sedation or respiratory depression).

Concomitant use of oral midazolam or triazolam with *ritonavir-boosted* or *cobicistat-boosted* darunavir is contraindicated.

Concomitant use of parenteral midazolam and *ritonavir-boosted* or *cobicistat-boosted* darunavir should be undertaken with caution and in a monitored setting where respiratory depression and/or prolonged sedation can be managed. In addition, a reduced dosage of midazolam should be considered, especially if more than a single dose of midazolam is given. Some experts state that parenteral midazolam can be given in a single dose with caution in a monitored situation for procedural sedation in patients receiving *ritonavir-boosted* or *cobicistat-boosted* darunavir.

■ **β-Adrenergic Blocking Agents** Possible pharmacokinetic interactions if *ritonavir-boosted* or *cobicistat-boosted* darunavir is used concomitantly with carvedilol, metoprolol, or timolol (increased plasma concentrations of the β-adrenergic blocking agent).

If carvedilol, metoprolol, or timolol is used concomitantly with *ritonavir-boosted* or *cobicistat-boosted* darunavir, clinical monitoring of the patient is recommended and reduction of the dosage of the β-adrenergic blocking agent may be needed. Alternatively, some experts state that use of β-adrenergic blocking agents that are not metabolized by CYP enzymes (e.g., atenolol, labetalol, nadolol, sotalol) should be considered.

■ **Bosentan** Possible pharmacokinetic interactions if bosentan is used concomitantly with *ritonavir-boosted* darunavir (increased bosentan concentrations). Possible pharmacokinetic interactions if bosentan is used concomitantly with *cobicistat-boosted* darunavir (increased bosentan concentrations; decreased darunavir and cobicistat concentrations).

In patients who have been receiving *ritonavir-boosted* or *cobicistat-boosted* darunavir for at least 10 days, bosentan should be initiated using a dosage of 62.5 mg once daily or every other day based on individual tolerability.

In patients who have been receiving bosentan, bosentan should be discontinued for at least 36 hours prior to initiating *ritonavir-boosted* or *cobicistat-boosted* darunavir; after at least 10 days of *ritonavir-boosted* or *cobicistat-boosted* darunavir therapy, bosentan can be resumed using a dosage of 62.5 mg once daily or every other day based on individual tolerability.

In patients switching from *ritonavir-boosted* darunavir to *cobicistat-boosted* darunavir, the current bosentan dosage should be maintained.

■ **Buspirone** Possible pharmacokinetic interactions if buspirone is used concomitantly with *ritonavir-boosted* or *cobicistat-boosted* darunavir (increased buspirone concentrations).

If buspirone is used concomitantly with *ritonavir-boosted* or *cobicistat-boosted* darunavir, buspirone dosage should be titrated, a lower buspirone dosage should be considered, and the patient should be monitored for prolonged or adverse effects.

■ **Calcium-channel Blocking Agents** Possible pharmacokinetic interactions if certain calcium-channel blocking agents (e.g., amlodipine, felodipine, nicardipine, nifedipine, verapamil) are used concomitantly with *ritonavir-boosted* or *cobicistat-boosted* darunavir (increased concentrations of the calcium-channel blocking agent). These calcium-channel blocking agents should be used concomitantly with *ritonavir-boosted* or *cobicistat-boosted* darunavir with caution; clinical monitoring of the patient is recommended.

Possible pharmacokinetic interactions if diltiazem is used concomitantly with *ritonavir-boosted* or *cobicistat-boosted* darunavir (increased diltiazem concentrations). Diltiazem should be used concomitantly with *ritonavir-boosted* or *cobicistat-boosted* darunavir with caution; diltiazem dosage should be adjusted based on clinical response and toxicities.

■ **Cobicistat** Pharmacokinetic interactions if cobicistat is used concomitantly with darunavir (increased plasma concentrations and AUC of darunavir). Cobicistat is a pharmacokinetic enhancer (pharmacokinetic booster) and is used in conjunction with darunavir for therapeutic advantage (*cobicistat-boosted* darunavir).

■ **Colchicine** Potential pharmacokinetic interactions if colchicine is used concomitantly with *ritonavir-boosted* or *cobicistat-boosted* darunavir (increased colchicine concentrations).

Concomitant use of colchicine and *ritonavir-boosted* or *cobicistat-boosted* darunavir is contraindicated in patients with renal or hepatic impairment because of the potential for serious and/or life-threatening effects in such patients.

When colchicine is used for *treatment* of gout flares in patients receiving *ritonavir-boosted* or *cobicistat-boosted* darunavir, an initial colchicine dose of 0.6 mg should be given followed by 0.3 mg 1 hour later; the colchicine dose should be repeated no earlier than 3 days later.

When colchicine is used for *prophylaxis* of gout flares in patients receiving *ritonavir-boosted* or *cobicistat-boosted* darunavir, colchicine dosage should be reduced to 0.3 mg once daily in those originally receiving 0.6 mg twice daily or decreased to 0.3 mg once every other day in those originally receiving 0.6 mg once daily.

When colchicine is used for treatment of familial Mediterranean fever (FMF) in patients receiving *ritonavir-boosted* or *cobicistat-boosted* darunavir, a maximum colchicine dosage of 0.6 mg daily (may be given as 0.3 mg twice daily) should be used.

■ **Corticosteroids** ***Orally Inhaled or Intranasal Corticosteroids*** Concomitant use of budesonide (inhaled or intranasal), fluticasone propionate (inhaled or intranasal), or mometasone (inhaled or intranasal) with *ritonavir-boosted* or *cobicistat-boosted* darunavir may result in increased concentrations of the corticosteroid and may result in adrenal insufficiency or Cushing's syndrome.

Budesonide (inhaled or intranasal), fluticasone (inhaled or intranasal), and mometasone (inhaled or intranasal) should not be used concomitantly with *ritonavir-boosted* or *cobicistat-boosted* darunavir unless potential benefits of the corticosteroid outweigh risks of systemic corticosteroid adverse effects. An alternative (e.g., beclomethasone) should be considered, especially when long-term use of the corticosteroid is anticipated.

Some experts state that concomitant use of beclomethasone (inhaled) and *ritonavir-boosted* darunavir does not result in clinically important pharmacokinetic interactions and dosage adjustments are not necessary if the drugs are used concomitantly. These experts also state that concomitant use of beclomethasone (inhaled) and *cobicistat-boosted* darunavir is not expected to result in clinically important pharmacokinetic interactions.

Local Injections of Corticosteroids Concomitant use of intra-articular or other local injections of methylprednisolone, prednisolone, or triamcinolone with *ritonavir-boosted* darunavir may result in increased concentrations of the corticosteroid and may result in adrenal insufficiency or Cushing's syndrome.

Ritonavir-boosted or *cobicistat-boosted* darunavir should not be used concomitantly with local injections of methylprednisolone, prednisolone, or triamcinolone; other nonsteroidal therapies should be considered. If intra-articular corticosteroid therapy is required, an alternative antiretroviral that does not alter CYP3A4 activity should be considered (e.g., dolutegravir, raltegravir).

Systemic Corticosteroids Concomitant use of systemic budesonide with *ritonavir-boosted* or *cobicistat-boosted* darunavir may increase corticosteroid concentrations and may result in adrenal insufficiency or Cushing's syndrome; decreased darunavir concentrations may also occur. Systemic budesonide should not be used concomitantly with *ritonavir-boosted* or *cobicistat-boosted* darunavir, unless potential benefits outweigh the risks of systemic corticosteroid adverse effects.

Concomitant use of systemic prednisone with *ritonavir-boosted* or *cobicistat-boosted* darunavir may increase corticosteroid concentrations and may result in adrenal insufficiency or Cushing's syndrome. Systemic prednisone should not be used concomitantly with *ritonavir-boosted* or *cobicistat-boosted* darunavir, unless potential benefits outweigh the risks of systemic corticosteroid adverse effects.

Concomitant use of systemic dexamethasone and *ritonavir-boosted* or *cobicistat-boosted* darunavir may result in decreased darunavir, ritonavir, or cobicistat concentrations and possible decreased antiretroviral efficacy. Systemic dexamethasone and *ritonavir-boosted* or *cobicistat-boosted* darunavir should be used concomitantly with caution; alternative corticosteroids should be considered for long-term use.

■ **Dextromethorphan** Pharmacokinetic interactions if dextromethorphan is used concomitantly with *ritonavir-boosted* darunavir (increased plasma concentrations of dextromethorphan).

■ **Digoxin** Pharmacokinetic interactions if digoxin is used concomitantly with *ritonavir-boosted* or *cobicistat-boosted* darunavir (increased digoxin concentrations).

Ritonavir-boosted darunavir and digoxin should be used concomitantly with caution. The lowest possible dosage of digoxin should be used; digoxin plasma concentrations should be monitored and digoxin dosage adjusted to obtain the desired clinical effect.

Cobicistat-boosted darunavir and digoxin should be used concomitantly with caution. Digoxin dosage should be titrated and digoxin plasma concentrations monitored.

■ **Eplerenone** Concomitant use of *ritonavir-boosted* or *cobicistat-boosted* darunavir and eplerenone is expected to result in increased eplerenone concentrations.

Some experts state that use of eplerenone and *ritonavir-boosted* or *cobicistat-boosted* darunavir is contraindicated.

■ **Ergot Alkaloids** Potential for serious and/or life-threatening adverse effects (e.g., peripheral vasospasm, ischemia of the extremities and other tissues) if ergot alkaloids (dihydroergotamine, ergotamine, methylergonovine) are used concomitantly with *ritonavir-boosted* or *cobicistat-boosted* darunavir. Concomitant use of ergot alkaloids with *ritonavir-boosted* or *cobicistat-boosted* darunavir is contraindicated.

If a woman receiving darunavir or any other PI as part of an antiretroviral regimen experiences uterine atony and excessive postpartum bleeding, methylergonovine maleate (Methergine®) should be used for treatment of the hemorrhage *only* if alternative treatments cannot be used and the potential benefits of the ergot alkaloid outweigh the risks. In this situation, methylergonovine maleate should be used in the lowest dosage and shortest duration possible.

■ **Estrogens and Progestins** Pharmacokinetic interactions if oral contraceptives containing ethinyl estradiol and norethindrone are used concomitantly with *ritonavir-boosted* darunavir (decreased ethinyl estradiol and norethindrone concentrations). Concomitant use of darunavir may also reduce efficacy of contraceptives containing only progestins. Data are not available regarding concomitant use of oral contraceptives and *cobicistat-boosted* darunavir and possible effects on estrogen and progestin concentrations.

Additional or alternative nonhormonal methods of contraception should be used in patients receiving *ritonavir-boosted* or *cobicistat-boosted* darunavir.

Data are not available regarding use of transdermal contraceptive preparations containing ethinyl estradiol and norelgestromin or etonogestrel-releasing subdermal implant contraceptives in patients receiving *ritonavir-boosted* or *cobicistat-boosted* darunavir; some experts recommend use of alternative or additional methods of contraception or use of alternative antiretrovirals.

■ **Flibanserin** Concomitant use of flibanserin and *ritonavir-boosted* or *cobicistat-boosted* darunavir is expected to increase flibanserin concentrations.

Some experts state that concomitant use of flibanserin and *ritonavir-boosted* or *cobicistat-boosted* darunavir is contraindicated.

■ **GI Drugs** Potential for serious and/or life-threatening adverse effects if cisapride is used concomitantly with *ritonavir-boosted* or *cobicistat-boosted* darunavir (e.g., cardiac arrhythmias). Concomitant use of *ritonavir-boosted* or *cobicistat-boosted* darunavir and cisapride is contraindicated.

Antacids Concomitant use of drugs affecting gastric acidity is not expected to alter darunavir exposures.

Clinically important drug interactions are not expected if antacids are used concomitantly with *cobicistat-boosted* darunavir.

Histamine H_2-receptor Antagonists No clinically important drug interactions are expected if histamine H_2-receptor antagonists (e.g., ranitidine) are used concomitantly with *ritonavir-boosted* or *cobicistat-boosted* darunavir.

Dosage adjustments are not needed if ranitidine or other histamine H_2-receptor antagonists are used concomitantly with *ritonavir-boosted* or *cobicistat-boosted* darunavir.

Proton-pump Inhibitors Pharmacokinetic interactions if omeprazole is used concomitantly with *ritonavir-boosted* darunavir (decreased plasma concentrations of omeprazole; no change in plasma concentrations of darunavir). If *ritonavir-boosted* darunavir is used concomitantly with omeprazole, the patient should be monitored for decreased omeprazole efficacy; an increase in omeprazole dosage should be considered in patients whose symptoms are not well controlled, but omeprazole dosages exceeding 40 mg daily should be avoided.

No clinically important drug interactions are expected if proton pump inhibitors (PPIs) are used concomitantly with *cobicistat-boosted* darunavir; dosage adjustments are not needed.

■ **HCV Antivirals** ***HCV Polymerase Inhibitors*** **Dasabuvir.** Concomitant use of *ritonavir-boosted* darunavir and the fixed combination of ombitasvir, paritaprevir, and ritonavir (ombitasvir/paritaprevir/ritonavir) with dasabuvir sodium results in decreased darunavir trough plasma concentrations. Concomitant use of *ritonavir-boosted* darunavir and ombitasvir/paritaprevir/ritonavir with dasabuvir is not recommended.

Data are not available regarding pharmacokinetic interactions between *cobicistat-boosted* darunavir and ombitasvir/paritaprevir/ritonavir with dasabuvir. Therefore, concomitant use of the drugs is not recommended.

Sofosbuvir. Concomitant use of sofosbuvir and *ritonavir-boosted* darunavir does not have a clinically important effect on the pharmacokinetics of either drug. Dosage adjustments are not needed.

Sofosbuvir and Velpatasvir. Concomitant use of the fixed combination of sofosbuvir and velpatasvir (sofosbuvir/velpatasvir) with *ritonavir-boosted* darunavir does not result in clinically important pharmacokinetic interactions.

Concomitant use of sofosbuvir/velpatasvir and *ritonavir-boosted* darunavir in conjunction with the fixed combination of emtricitabine and tenofovir DF (emtricitabine/tenofovir DF) results in increased tenofovir plasma concentrations and AUC. Patients should be monitored for tenofovir-associated adverse effects if sofosbuvir/velpatasvir is used concomitantly with any HIV antiretroviral regimen containing tenofovir DF.

HCV Protease Inhibitors **Paritaprevir.** Concomitant use of *ritonavir-boosted* darunavir and the fixed combination of ombitasvir/paritaprevir/ritonavir results in decreased darunavir trough plasma concentrations. The manufacturer of ombitasvir/paritaprevir/ritonavir states that the fixed combination can be taken at the same time as darunavir (800 mg) *without* low-dose ritonavir.

Concomitant use of *ritonavir-boosted* darunavir and ombitasvir/paritaprevir/ritonavir with dasabuvir sodium results in decreased darunavir trough plasma concentrations. Concomitant use of *ritonavir-boosted* darunavir and ombitasvir/paritaprevir/ritonavir with dasabuvir is not recommended.

It is not known whether pharmacokinetic interactions occur between *cobicistat-boosted* darunavir and ombitasvir/paritaprevir/ritonavir with dasabuvir; concomitant use of the drugs is not recommended.

Simeprevir. Concomitant use of simeprevir and *ritonavir-boosted* darunavir increases simeprevir plasma concentrations and AUC and also increases darunavir plasma concentrations. Concomitant use of simeprevir and *cobicistat-boosted* darunavir results in increased simeprevir concentrations.

Concomitant use of simeprevir and *ritonavir-boosted* or *cobicistat-boosted* darunavir is not recommended.

HCV Replication Complex Inhibitors **Daclatasvir.** Concomitant use of daclatasvir with *ritonavir-boosted* darunavir does not have a clinically important effect on daclatasvir or darunavir exposures.

Dosage adjustments are not needed if daclatasvir is used concomitantly with *ritonavir-boosted* or *cobicistat-boosted* darunavir.

Elbasvir and Grazoprevir. Concomitant use of *ritonavir-boosted* darunavir (600 mg of darunavir and 100 mg of ritonavir once daily) and elbasvir (50 mg once daily) results in increased elbasvir concentrations and AUC. Concomitant use of *ritonavir-boosted* darunavir (600 mg of darunavir and 100 mg of ritonavir once daily) and grazoprevir (200 mg once daily) results in substantially increased grazoprevir concentrations due to OATP1B1 and 1B3 inhibition by *ritonavir-boosted* darunavir. Concomitant use of *cobicistat-boosted* darunavir is expected to increase grazoprevir concentrations. Increased grazoprevir concentrations may increase the risk of ALT elevations.

Concomitant use of elbasvir/grazoprevir and *ritonavir-boosted* or *cobicistat-boosted* darunavir is contraindicated.

Ledipasvir and Sofosbuvir. Concomitant use of a once-daily regimen of *ritonavir-boosted* darunavir (darunavir 800 mg and ritonavir 100 mg) and either ledipasvir (90 mg once daily) or sofosbuvir (single 400-mg dose) does not have a clinically important effect on the pharmacokinetics of darunavir, ritonavir, ledipasvir, or sofosbuvir. Clinically important pharmacokinetic interactions are not expected if the fixed combination of ledipasvir and sofosbuvir (ledipasvir/sofosbuvir) is used concomitantly with *ritonavir-boosted* or *cobicistat-boosted* darunavir.

Dosage adjustments are not needed if ledipasvir/sofosbuvir is used concomitantly with *ritonavir-boosted* or *cobicistat-boosted* darunavir.

Concomitant use of ledipasvir/sofosbuvir and an HIV treatment regimen of *ritonavir-boosted* darunavir, emtricitabine, and tenofovir DF increases tenofovir concentrations. Safety of increased tenofovir concentrations in patients receiving ledipasvir/sofosbuvir concomitantly with an antiretroviral regimen that includes *ritonavir-boosted* darunavir and tenofovir DF has not been established. An alternative HCV treatment regimen or alternative antiretroviral regimen should be considered to avoid increased tenofovir exposures, especially in patients at risk for renal toxicity. If concomitant use is necessary, the patient should be monitored for tenofovir-associated adverse effects.

Ombitasvir. Concomitant use of *ritonavir-boosted* darunavir and the fixed combination of ombitasvir/paritaprevir/ritonavir results in decreased darunavir trough plasma concentrations. The manufacturer of ombitasvir/paritaprevir/ritonavir states that the fixed combination can be taken at the same time as darunavir (800 mg) *without* low-dose ritonavir.

Concomitant use of *ritonavir-boosted* darunavir and ombitasvir/paritaprevir/ritonavir with dasabuvir sodium results in decreased darunavir trough plasma concentrations. Concomitant use of *ritonavir-boosted* darunavir and ombitasvir/paritaprevir/ritonavir with dasabuvir is not recommended.

It is not known whether pharmacokinetic interactions occur between *cobicistat-boosted* darunavir and ombitasvir/paritaprevir/ritonavir with dasabuvir; concomitant use of the drugs is not recommended.

■ **HMG-CoA Reductase Inhibitors** Pharmacokinetic interactions with HMG-CoA reductase inhibitors (statins) metabolized by CYP3A isoenzyme. Concomitant use of *ritonavir-boosted* or *cobicistat-boosted* darunavir and certain statins (e.g., atorvastatin, fluvastatin, lovastatin, pravastatin, rosuvastatin, simvastatin) may increase plasma concentrations and AUCs of the antilipemic agents and increase the risk of statin-associated adverse effects, including myopathy and rhabdomyolysis.

Atorvastatin If atorvastatin is used concomitantly with *ritonavir-boosted* darunavir, atorvastatin dosage should not exceed 20 mg daily. Dosage of atorvastatin should be titrated carefully; the lowest necessary dosage should be used and the patient monitored for adverse effects.

If atorvastatin is used concomitantly with *cobicistat-boosted* darunavir, atorvastatin should be initiated at the lowest dosage and titrated to the lowest necessary dosage; the patient should be monitored for safety.

Lovastatin Concomitant use of lovastatin with *ritonavir-boosted* or *cobicistat-boosted* darunavir is contraindicated.

Pitavastatin Concomitant use of *ritonavir-boosted* darunavir (darunavir 800 mg and ritonavir 100 mg once daily) and pitavastatin (4 mg once daily) results in a 26% decrease in the AUC of pitavastatin, but does not have a clinically important effect on darunavir concentrations. Dosage adjustments are not necessary if pitavastatin is used concomitantly with *ritonavir-boosted* darunavir.

The effect of *cobicistat-boosted* darunavir on pitavastatin pharmacokinetics is not known. If pitavastatin is used concomitantly with *cobicistat-boosted* darunavir, pitavastatin should be initiated at the lowest dosage and titrated; the patient should be monitored for safety. Some experts state that dosage adjustments are not necessary if pitavastatin is used concomitantly with *cobicistat-boosted* darunavir.

Pravastatin If pravastatin is used concomitantly with *ritonavir-boosted* or *cobicistat-boosted* darunavir, dosage of pravastatin should be titrated carefully and the lowest necessary dosage used with close monitoring for adverse effects.

Rosuvastatin If rosuvastatin is used concomitantly with *ritonavir-boosted* or *cobicistat-boosted* darunavir, dosage of rosuvastatin should be titrated carefully and the lowest necessary dosage used with close monitoring for adverse effects.

Simvastatin Concomitant use of simvastatin with *ritonavir-boosted* or *cobicistat-boosted* darunavir is contraindicated.

■ **Immunosuppressive Agents** Pharmacokinetic interactions with cyclosporine, everolimus, sirolimus, tacrolimus (increased concentrations of the immunosuppressive agent expected).

If cyclosporine, sirolimus, or tacrolimus is used concomitantly with *ritonavir-boosted* or *cobicistat-boosted* darunavir, plasma concentrations of the immunosuppressive agent should be monitored.

Concomitant use of everolimus and *ritonavir-boosted* or *cobicistat-boosted* darunavir is not recommended.

■ **Ivabradine** Concomitant use of ivabradine and *ritonavir-boosted* or *cobicistat-boosted* darunavir is expected to result in increased ivabradine concentrations.

Some experts state that concomitant use of ivabradine and *ritonavir-boosted* or *cobicistat-boosted* darunavir is contraindicated.

■ **Macrolides** ***Clarithromycin*** Pharmacokinetic interactions if clarithromycin is used concomitantly with *ritonavir-boosted* darunavir (increased clarithromycin concentrations). Modification of the usual dosage of clarithromycin is not necessary in those with normal renal function; however, clarithromycin dosage should be reduced by 50% in those with creatinine clearances of 30–60 mL/minute and reduced by 75% in those with creatinine clearances less than 30 mL/minute. Some experts state that patients should be monitored for clarithromycin-related toxicities or an alternative macrolide (e.g., azithromycin) should be considered.

Pharmacokinetic interactions if clarithromycin is used concomitantly with *cobicistat-boosted* darunavir (increased darunavir, cobicistat, and clarithromycin concentrations). An alternative anti-infective should be considered in patients receiving *cobicistat-boosted* darunavir.

Erythromycin Pharmacokinetic interactions if *cobicistat-boosted* darunavir is used concomitantly with erythromycin (increased darunavir, cobicistat, and erythromycin concentrations). An alternative anti-infective should be considered in patients receiving *cobicistat-boosted* darunavir.

Telithromycin Pharmacokinetic interactions if *cobicistat-boosted* darunavir is used concomitantly with telithromycin (increased darunavir, cobicistat, and telithromycin concentrations). An alternative anti-infective should be considered in patients receiving *cobicistat-boosted* darunavir.

■ **Opiate Agonists, Opiate Partial Agonists, and Opiate Antagonists** ***Buprenorphine*** Pharmacokinetic interactions if buprenorphine or fixed combination of buprenorphine and naloxone is used concomitantly with *ritonavir-boosted* darunavir (increased norbuprenorphine concentrations and AUC). It is not known whether *cobicistat-boosted* darunavir affects the pharmacokinetics of buprenorphine or the fixed combination of buprenorphine and naloxone.

If buprenorphine or the fixed combination of buprenorphine and naloxone is used concomitantly with *ritonavir-boosted* darunavir, dosage adjustments are not needed but patients should be monitored. In patients with a buprenorphine subdermal implant, it may be necessary to remove the implant and switch to a different buprenorphine formulation that permits dosage adjustments.

In patients receiving *cobicistat-boosted* darunavir, buprenorphine or the fixed combination of buprenorphine and naloxone should be initiated using the lowest possible dosage and carefully titrated to the desired therapeutic effect. If initiating *cobicistat-boosted* darunavir in patients already receiving buprenorphine or the fixed combination of buprenorphine and naloxone, dosage adjustments of buprenorphine or the fixed combination of buprenorphine and naloxone may be needed and the patient should be clinically monitored. In patients with a buprenorphine subdermal implant, it may be necessary to remove the implant and switch to a different buprenorphine formulation that permits dosage adjustments.

Fentanyl Possible pharmacokinetic interactions if fentanyl is used concomitantly with *ritonavir-boosted* or *cobicistat-boosted* darunavir (increased fentanyl concentrations).

If fentanyl is used concomitantly with *ritonavir-boosted* or *cobicistat-boosted* darunavir, the patient should be carefully monitored for therapeutic and adverse effects of fentanyl, including potentially fatal respiratory depression.

Methadone Pharmacokinetic interactions if methadone is used concomitantly with *ritonavir-boosted* darunavir (decreased methadone concentrations). Adjustment of methadone dosage is not needed when *ritonavir-boosted* darunavir is initiated; however, patients should be closely monitored for opioid withdrawal since maintenance dosage of methadone may need to be adjusted in some patients.

It is not known whether *cobicistat-boosted* darunavir affects methadone pharmacokinetics. In patients receiving *cobicistat-boosted* darunavir, methadone should be initiated using the lowest possible dosage and carefully titrated to the desired therapeutic effect. If *cobicistat-boosted* darunavir is initiated in a patient already receiving methadone, dosage adjustments of methadone may be needed and the patient should be clinically monitored.

Oxycodone Possible pharmacokinetic interactions if oxycodone is used concomitantly with *cobicistat-boosted* darunavir. If the drugs are used concomitantly, the patient should be carefully monitored for therapeutic and adverse effects of oxycodone, including potentially fatal respiratory depression.

Tramadol Pharmacokinetic interactions if tramadol is used concomitantly with *cobicistat-boosted* darunavir (increased tramadol concentrations). If tramadol is used concomitantly with *cobicistat-boosted* darunavir, decreased tramadol dosage may be needed and the patient should be monitored for efficacy and tramadol-associated adverse effects.

■ **Phosphodiesterase Type 5 Inhibitors** Concomitant use of *ritonavir-boosted* or *cobicistat-boosted* darunavir and selective phosphodiesterase type 5 (PDE5) inhibitors (e.g., avanafil, sildenafil, tadalafil, vardenafil) is expected to result in substantially increased plasma concentrations of the PDE5 inhibitor and increase the risk of adverse effects associated with these agents (e.g., hypotension, visual disturbances, priapism, syncope).

Avanafil Concomitant use of avanafil and *ritonavir-boosted* or *cobicistat-boosted* darunavir is not recommended.

Sildenafil Concomitant use of sildenafil (Revatio®) for the treatment of pulmonary arterial hypertension (PAH) is contraindicated in patients receiving *ritonavir-boosted* or *cobicistat-boosted* darunavir. Safe and effective dosages for concomitant use of the drugs have not been established.

If sildenafil is used for the treatment of erectile dysfunction in patients receiving *ritonavir-boosted* or *cobicistat-boosted* darunavir, sildenafil dosage should not exceed 25 mg once every 48 hours and the patient should be closely monitored for sildenafil-related adverse effects.

Tadalafil If tadalafil (Adcirca®) is indicated for the treatment of PAH in patients who have been receiving *ritonavir-boosted* or *cobicistat-boosted* darunavir for at least 1 week, tadalafil should be initiated at a dosage of 20 mg once daily and, if tolerated, dosage may be increased to 40 mg once daily. *Ritonavir-boosted* or *cobicistat-boosted* darunavir should not be initiated in patients receiving tadalafil for the treatment of PAH; tadalafil therapy should be discontinued at least 24 hours prior to initiating *ritonavir-boosted* or *cobicistat-boosted* darunavir. After at least 1 week, tadalafil may be resumed at a dosage of 20 mg once daily and, if tolerated, dosage may be increased to 40 mg once daily. In patients switching from *ritonavir-boosted* darunavir to *cobicistat-boosted* darunavir, the current tadalafil dosage should be maintained.

If tadalafil is used for the treatment of erectile dysfunction in patients receiving *ritonavir-boosted* or *cobicistat-boosted* darunavir, tadalafil dosage should not exceed 10 mg once every 72 hours and the patient should be closely monitored for tadalafil-related adverse effects.

If tadalafil is used for the treatment of benign prostatic hyperplasia in patients receiving *ritonavir-boosted* or *cobicistat-boosted* darunavir, tadalafil dosage should not exceed 2.5 mg once daily.

Vardenafil If vardenafil is used for the treatment of erectile dysfunction in patients receiving *ritonavir-boosted* or *cobicistat-boosted* darunavir, vardenafil dosage should not exceed 2.5 mg once every 72 hours and the patient should be closely monitored for vardenafil-associated adverse effects.

■ **Ranolazine** Potential for serious and/or life-threatening adverse effects if *ritonavir-boosted* or *cobicistat-boosted* darunavir is used concomitantly with ranolazine.

Concomitant use of *ritonavir-boosted* or *cobicistat-boosted* darunavir and ranolazine is contraindicated.

■ **St. John's Wort** Potential pharmacokinetic interactions with St. John's wort (*Hypericum perforatum*) (decreased darunavir concentrations); potential for loss of virologic response. Concomitant use of St. John's wort and *ritonavir-boosted* or *cobicistat-boosted* darunavir is contraindicated.

■ **Salmeterol** Possible pharmacokinetic interactions if salmeterol is used concomitantly with *ritonavir-boosted* or *cobicistat-boosted* darunavir (increased salmeterol concentrations) and increased risk of salmeterol-associated adverse cardiovascular effects, including QT interval prolongation, palpitations, and sinus tachycardia. Concomitant use of salmeterol and *ritonavir-boosted* or *cobicistat-boosted* darunavir is not recommended.

■ **Selective Serotonin-reuptake Inhibitors** Pharmacokinetic interactions if paroxetine or sertraline is used concomitantly with *ritonavir-boosted* darunavir (decreased concentrations and AUCs of the selective serotonin-reuptake inhibitor [SSRI]; no change in darunavir concentrations). Dosage of the SSRI should be titrated based on clinical response. If *ritonavir-boosted* darunavir is initiated in a patient receiving a stable dosage of paroxetine or sertraline, the patient should be monitored for clinical response.

Possible pharmacokinetic interactions if paroxetine or sertraline is used concomitantly with *cobicistat-boosted* darunavir (effect on SSRI concentrations not known). Dosage of the SSRI should be carefully titrated based on clinical response using the lowest possible initial or maintenance dosage. Clinical monitoring of antidepressant response is recommended.

Some experts state that concomitant use of fluvoxamine with *ritonavir-boosted* or *cobicistat-boosted* darunavir may alter (increase or decrease) darunavir concentrations. These experts state that an alternative to fluvoxamine should be considered.

■ **Suvorexant** Pharmacokinetic interactions expected if suvorexant is used concomitantly with *ritonavir-boosted* or *cobicistat-boosted* darunavir (increased suvorexant concentrations expected). Some experts state that concomitant use is not recommended.

■ **Ticagrelor** Possible pharmacokinetic interactions if ticagrelor is used concomitantly with *ritonavir-boosted* or *cobicistat-boosted* darunavir (increased ticagrelor concentrations expected). Some experts state that concomitant use should be avoided.

■ **Trazodone** Possible pharmacokinetic interactions if trazodone is used concomitantly with *ritonavir-boosted* or *cobicistat-boosted* darunavir (increased plasma concentrations of trazodone); nausea, dizziness, hypotension, and syncope may occur. Lowest effective dosage of trazodone should be used and patients monitored for adverse CNS and cardiovascular effects.

■ **Tricyclic Antidepressants** Potential pharmacokinetic interactions if amitriptyline, desipramine, doxepin, imipramine, or nortriptyline is used concomitantly with *ritonavir-boosted* or *cobicistat-boosted* darunavir (increased plasma concentrations of the tricyclic antidepressant); possible increased risk of adverse effects (e.g., nausea, dizziness, hypotension, syncope).

The lowest possible dosage of the tricyclic antidepressant (e.g., amitriptyline, desipramine, doxepin, imipramine, nortriptyline) should be used in patients receiving *ritonavir-boosted* or *cobicistat-boosted* darunavir and dosage of the antidepressant titrated based on clinical assessment and/or plasma antidepressant concentrations.

■ **Vorapaxar** Possible pharmacokinetic interactions if vorapaxar is used concomitantly with *ritonavir-boosted* or *cobicistat-boosted* darunavir (increased vorapaxar concentrations expected). Some experts state that concomitant use should be avoided.

■ **Zolpidem** Potential pharmacokinetic interactions if zolpidem is used concomitantly with *ritonavir-boosted* or *cobicistat-boosted* darunavir (increased zolpidem concentrations). If zolpidem is used concomitantly with *ritonavir-boosted* or *cobicistat-boosted* darunavir, some experts state that zolpidem should be initiated using a low dosage and dosage reduction may be needed.

Description

Darunavir, a nonpeptidic sulfonamide derivative, inhibits replication of human immunodeficiency virus type 1 (HIV-1) by interfering with HIV protease. During HIV replication, HIV protease cleaves viral polypeptide products of the *gag* and *gag-pol* genes to form structural proteins of the virion core and essential viral enzymes. By interfering with the formation of these essential proteins and enzymes, darunavir blocks maturation of the virus and causes formation of nonfunctional, immature, noninfectious virions. Darunavir also has some in vitro activity against HIV type 2 (HIV-2).

Darunavir-resistant HIV-1, including strains with decreased susceptibility to other HIV protease inhibitors (PIs), have been reported. Varying degrees of cross-resistance occurs among HIV protease inhibitors (PIs). Although some HIV-1 isolates resistant to atazanavir, indinavir, lopinavir, nelfinavir, ritonavir, saquinavir, and/or tipranavir have remained susceptible to darunavir, some clinical isolates with reduced susceptibility to darunavir have been resistant to atazanavir, fosamprenavir, indinavir, lopinavir, and nelfinavir. Only limited cross-resistance appears to occur between tipranavir and darunavir.

Darunavir is extensively metabolized by the hepatic cytochrome P-450 (CYP) enzyme system, principally CYP3A, and must be administered with a pharmacokinetic enhancer (pharmacokinetic booster) to improve the pharmacokinetic profile of the drug. Darunavir should be administered with low-dose ritonavir (*ritonavir-boosted* darunavir) or with cobicistat (*cobicistat-boosted* darunavir). Because ritonavir and cobicistat are potent inhibitors of CYP3A, concomitant administration with darunavir results in increased peak plasma concentrations and area under the plasma concentration-time curve (AUC) of the HIV PI. The antiretroviral activity of *ritonavir-boosted* darunavir or *cobicistat-boosted* darunavir is due to darunavir.

Darunavir pharmacokinetic parameters reported with a once-daily regimen of *ritonavir-boosted* darunavir (darunavir 800 mg and ritonavir 100 mg) are similar to those reported with a once-daily regimen of *cobicistat-boosted* darunavir (darunavir 800 mg and cobicistat 150 mg). Food increases oral bioavailability of darunavir. Compared with administration in the fasting state, administration of *ritonavir-boosted* darunavir (given as single-entity darunavir tablets and single-entity ritonavir) with food increases peak plasma concentrations and AUC of darunavir by approximately 40%. Administration of *cobicistat-boosted* darunavir (given as fixed-combination tablets containing both drugs [darunavir/cobicistat]) with a high-fat meal increases peak plasma concentrations and AUC of darunavir by 127 and 70%, respectively. Darunavir has a half-life of 15 hours after administration of *ritonavir-boosted* darunavir and a half-life of 7 hours after administration of *cobicistat-boosted* darunavir. The drug is eliminated principally in feces (80%) and urine (14%).

Advice to Patients

Critical nature of compliance with HIV therapy and importance of remaining under the care of a clinician. Importance of taking as prescribed; do not alter or discontinue antiretroviral regimen without consulting clinician.

Importance of using darunavir with low-dose ritonavir (*ritonavir-boosted* darunavir) or with cobicistat (*cobicistat-boosted* darunavir). Importance of using *ritonavir-boosted* or *cobicistat-boosted* darunavir in conjunction with other antiretrovirals.

Antiretroviral therapy is not a cure for HIV infection; opportunistic infections and other complications associated with HIV disease may still occur.

Advise patients that effective antiretroviral regimens can decrease HIV concentrations in blood and genital secretions and strict adherence to such regimens in conjunction with risk-reduction measures may decrease, but cannot absolutely eliminate, the risk of secondary transmission of HIV to others. Importance of continuing to practice safer sex (e.g., using latex or polyurethane condoms to minimize sexual contact with body fluids), never sharing personal items that can have blood or body fluids on them (e.g., toothbrushes, razor blades), and never reusing or sharing needles.

Importance of reading patient information provided by the manufacturer.

When using *ritonavir-boosted* darunavir, importance of taking single-entity darunavir with food and at the same time as single-entity ritonavir. Importance of swallowing darunavir tablets whole with a drink (e.g., water, milk).

In patients taking *ritonavir-boosted* darunavir once daily, if a dose of darunavir or ritonavir is missed by less than 12 hours, the dose should be taken as soon as it is remembered and the next dose taken at the regularly scheduled time. If a dose of darunavir or ritonavir is missed by more than 12 hours, the dose should be skipped and the next dose taken at the regularly scheduled time. A double dose should not be taken to make up for a missed dose.

In patients taking *ritonavir-boosted* darunavir twice daily, if a dose of darunavir or ritonavir is missed by less than 6 hours, the dose should be taken as soon as it is remembered and the next dose taken at the regularly scheduled time. If a dose of darunavir or ritonavir is missed by more than 6 hours, the dose should be skipped and the next dose taken at the regularly scheduled time. A double dose should not be taken to make up for a missed dose.

When using *cobicistat-boosted* darunavir, importance of taking the fixed-combination tablet containing both drugs (darunavir/cobicistat) with food; alternatively, importance of taking single-entity darunavir with food and at the same time as single-entity cobicistat.

If a dose of *cobicistat-boosted* darunavir is missed by less than 12 hours, the dose should be taken as soon as it is remembered and the next dose taken at the regularly scheduled time. If a dose of *cobicistat-boosted* darunavir is missed by more than 12 hours, the dose should be skipped and the next dose taken at the regularly scheduled time. A double dose should not be taken to make up for a missed dose.

Advise patients that drug-induced hepatitis has occurred. Importance of notifying clinician if manifestations of liver disease occur (e.g., jaundice of skin or eyes; dark tea-colored urine; pale stools; nausea; vomiting; loss of appetite; pain, aching, or sensitivity in right upper quadrant of abdomen).

Advise patients that mild to severe skin reactions, have occurred. Importance of immediately discontinuing *ritonavir-boosted* or *cobicistat-boosted* darunavir and contacting clinician if manifestations of severe skin reactions occur (e.g., severe rash or rash accompanied by fever, general malaise, fatigue, muscle or joint aches, blisters, oral lesions, conjunctivitis, hepatitis, and/or eosinophilia).

Redistribution/accumulation of body fat may occur with antiretroviral therapy, with as yet unknown long-term health effects.

Importance of informing clinicians of existing or contemplated concomitant therapy, including prescription and OTC drugs and herbal products (e.g., St. John's wort), and any concomitant illnesses.

Advise patients receiving selective phosphodiesterase type 5 (PDE5) inhibitors (e.g., avanafil, sildenafil, tadalafil, vardenafil) that they may be at increased risk of PDE5 inhibitor-associated adverse effects (e.g., hypotension, visual changes, priapism) and that any symptoms should be promptly reported to a clinician. Should not be used concomitantly with sildenafil used for treatment of pulmonary arterial hypertension (PAH).

Importance of women using a reliable nonhormonal (e.g., barrier) method of contraception because of potential interactions with hormonal contraceptives.

Importance of women informing clinicians if they are or plan to become pregnant or plan to breast-feed. Advise HIV-infected women not to breast-feed.

Importance of advising patients of other important precautionary information. (See Cautions.)

Overview® (see Users Guide). For additional information on this drug until a more detailed monograph is developed and published, the manufacturer's labeling should be consulted. It is *essential* that the manufacturer's labeling be consulted for more detailed information on usual cautions, precautions, contraindications, potential drug interactions, laboratory test interferences, and acute toxicity.

Preparations

Excipients in commercially available drug preparations may have clinically important effects in some individuals; consult specific product labeling for details.

Darunavir Ethanolate

Oral		
Suspension	100 mg (of darunavir) per mL	**Prezista®**, Janssen
Tablets, film-coated	75 mg (of darunavir)	**Prezista®**, Janssen
	150 mg (of darunavir)	**Prezista®**, Janssen
	600 mg (of darunavir)	**Prezista®**, Janssen
	800 mg (of darunavir)	**Prezista®**, Janssen

Darunavir Ethanolate Combinations

Oral		
Tablets, film-coated	800 mg (of darunavir) with Cobicistat 150 mg	**Prezcobix®**, Janssen

†Use is not currently included in the labeling approved by the US Food and Drug Administration

Lopinavir and Ritonavir

LPV/r

■ Lopinavir and ritonavir (lopinavir/ritonavir) is a fixed combination of 2 human immunodeficiency virus (HIV) protease inhibitors (PIs); ritonavir, a potent inhibitor of hepatic cytochrome P-450 (CYP) 3A isoenzyme, decreases metabolism and increases plasma concentrations of lopinavir.

Uses

■ Treatment of HIV Infection The fixed combination of lopinavir and ritonavir (lopinavir/ritonavir) is used in conjunction with other antiretroviral agents for the treatment of human immunodeficiency virus type 1 (HIV-1) infection in adults, adolescents, and pediatric patients 14 days of age and older. Lopinavir/ritonavir is used in patients who are antiretroviral naive (have not previously received antiretroviral therapy) or antiretroviral experienced (received prior antiretroviral therapy).

Lopinavir/ritonavir usually is used in HIV protease inhibitor-based (PI-based) regimens that include lopinavir/ritonavir and 2 HIV nucleoside reverse transcriptase inhibitors (dual NRTIs).

The manufacturer advises that the following factors be considered when initiating lopinavir/ritonavir. Administration of lopinavir/ritonavir in conjunction with other active antiretroviral agents is associated with a greater likelihood of treatment response. Use of lopinavir/ritonavir should be guided by results of genotypic or phenotypic viral resistance testing and/or the individual's prior antiretroviral treatment. The number of lopinavir resistance-associated mutations at baseline affects virologic response to lopinavir/ritonavir. Once- or twice-daily administration of lopinavir/ritonavir may be used in adults infected with HIV-1 strains with less than 3 mutations associated with lopinavir resistance; twice-daily administration *must* be used in those with 3 or more viral mutations associated with lopinavir resistance. Once-daily administration of lopinavir/ritonavir is *not* recommended in pediatric patients, pregnant women, or patients receiving concomitant therapy with certain drugs. (See Dosage and Administration: Administration.)

The most appropriate antiretroviral regimen cannot be defined for each clinical scenario and selection of specific antiretroviral agents for use in multiple-drug regimens should be individualized based on information regarding antiretroviral potency, potential rate of development of resistance, known toxicities, and potential for pharmacokinetic interactions as well as virologic, immunologic, and clinical characteristics of the patient. For information on the general principles and guidelines for use of antiretroviral therapy, including specific recommendations for initial therapy in antiretroviral-naive patients and recommendations for changing antiretroviral regimens, see the Antiretroviral Agents General Statement 8:18.08.

Antiretroviral-naive Adults and Adolescents The US Department of Health and Human Services (HHS) Panel on Antiretroviral Guidelines for Adults and Adolescents states that lopinavir/ritonavir in conjunction with 2 NRTIs is *not* recommended for *initial* treatment regimens in antiretroviral-naive adults and adolescents because of GI intolerance and because of higher ritonavir dose and higher pill burden than other PI-based regimens. These experts state that a twice-daily lopinavir/ritonavir regimen used in conjunction with lamivudine (or emtricitabine) is an option that can be considered for *initial* treatment in antiretroviral-naive adults and adolescents when recommended or alternative regimens cannot be used, but should be used *only* when tenofovir alafenamide, tenofovir disoproxil fumarate (tenofovir DF), or abacavir cannot be used. Although a twice-daily lopinavir/ritonavir regimen used in conjunction with 2 NRTIs is an alternative PI-based regimen for *initial* treatment in HIV-infected pregnant women, once-daily lopinavir/ritonavir regimens are *not* recommended during pregnancy.

Clinical Experience. Results of a study in treatment-naive adults indicate that a regimen of lopinavir/ritonavir administered once daily in conjunction with 2 NRTIs (tenofovir DF and emtricitabine) is at least as effective as a regimen of lopinavir/ritonavir administered twice daily in conjunction with 2 NRTIs (tenofovir DF and emtricitabine) for initial treatment. In this randomized, open-label, multicenter study (study 730), 664 antiretroviral-naive adults (mean age 39 years; 78% male; 75% white; mean baseline plasma HIV-1 RNA level 5 $\log_{10}$ copies/mL; median baseline $CD4^+$ T-cell count 216 cells/mm^3) were randomized to receive a once-daily regimen of lopinavir/ritonavir (lopinavir 800 mg/ritonavir 200 mg once daily) in conjunction with tenofovir DF (300 mg once daily) and emtricitabine (200 mg once daily) or a twice-daily regimen of lopinavir/ritonavir (lopinavir 400 mg/ritonavir 100 mg twice daily) in conjunction with tenofovir DF (300 mg once daily) and emtricitabine (200 mg once daily). Through 48 weeks, 78% of those receiving the once-daily lopinavir/ritonavir regimen and 77% of those receiving the twice-daily lopinavir/ritonavir regimen achieved and maintained plasma HIV-1 RNA levels less than 50 copies/mL. At 48 weeks, the mean increase in $CD4^+$ T-cell count from baseline was 186 cells/mm^3 in those receiving the once-daily regimen and 198 cells/mm^3 in those receiving the twice-daily regimen.

Antiretroviral-experienced Adults and Adolescents **Clinical Experience.** Lopinavir/ritonavir has been evaluated for use in HIV-infected adults who were antiretroviral experienced. In a randomized, open-label, multicenter study (study 888), 288 HIV-infected adults who had previously received a PI-containing regimen (mean age 40 years; 86% male; 68% white; mean baseline plasma HIV-1 RNA level 4.1 $\log_{10}$ copies/mL; mean baseline $CD4^+$ T-cell count 322 cells/mm^3) were randomized to receive either lopinavir/ritonavir (lopinavir 400 mg/ritonavir 100 mg twice daily) in conjunction with nevirapine and NRTIs or an investigator-selected PI in conjunction with nevirapine and NRTIs. Through 48 weeks, 57% of those receiving the twice-daily lopinavir/ritonavir regimen and 33% of those receiving the investigator-selected PI regimen had plasma HIV-1 RNA levels less than 400 copies/mL. In addition, the mean increase in $CD4^+$ T-cell count from baseline was 111 cells/mm^3 in those receiving the lopinavir/ritonavir regimen and 112 cells/mm^3 in those receiving the investigator-selected PI regimen.

A once-daily lopinavir/ritonavir regimen (lopinavir 800 mg and ritonavir 200 mg once daily) was compared with a twice-daily regimen (lopinavir 400 mg/ritonavir 100 mg twice daily) in a randomized, open-label study (study 802) that included 599 HIV-infected adults who had detectable virologic loads while receiving their current antiretroviral regimen (55% had not previously received a PI; mean age 41 years; 66% male; 51% white; mean baseline plasma HIV-1 RNA level 4.3 $\log_{10}$ copies/mL; mean baseline $CD4^+$ T-cell count 254 cells/mm^3). All patients received at least 2 NRTIs in conjunction with lopinavir/ritonavir. Through 48 weeks, the mean increase in $CD4^+$ T-cell count from baseline was 135 cells/mm^3 in patients receiving the once-daily lopinavir/ritonavir regimen and 122 cells/mm^3 in those receiving the twice-daily lopinavir/ritonavir regimen.

Pediatric Patients Lopinavir/ritonavir is used in conjunction with other antiretroviral agents for the treatment of HIV-1 infection in pediatric patients 14 days of age and older. (See Pediatric Use under Warnings/Precautions: Specific Populations, in Cautions.)

For *initial* treatment in antiretroviral-naive pediatric patients, the HHS Panel on Antiretroviral Therapy and Medical Management of HIV-infected Children recommends a regimen that includes a *ritonavir-boosted* PI, nonnucleoside reverse transcriptase inhibitor (NNRTI), or integrase strand transfer inhibitor (INSTI) with 2 NRTIs (dual NRTIs). These experts state that lopinavir/ritonavir in conjunction with 2 NRTIs is the preferred antiretroviral regimen for *initial* treatment in neonates 14 days of age or older *with* postmenstrual age at least 42 weeks (i.e., time elapsed since first day of the mother's last menstrual period to birth plus time elapsed after birth) and *initial* treatment in infants younger than 2 years of age. In addition, these experts state that lopinavir/ritonavir in conjunction with 2 NRTIs is a preferred regimen for *initial* treatment in children 2 to less than 3 years of age and one of several preferred PI-based regimens in children 3 to less than 12 years of age.

For further information on treatment of HIV infection in pediatric patients, see Antiretroviral Therapy in Pediatric Patients, in the Antiretroviral Agents General Statement 8:18.08.

■ Postexposure Prophylaxis following Occupational Exposure to HIV Lopinavir/ritonavir is used in conjunction with 2 NRTIs for postexposure prophylaxis of HIV infection following occupational exposure† (PEP)

in health-care personnel and other individuals exposed via percutaneous injury (e.g., needlestick, cut with sharp object) or mucous membrane or nonintact skin (e.g., chapped, abraded, dermatitis) contact with blood, tissue, or other body fluids that might contain HIV.

The US Public Health Service (USPHS) states that the preferred regimen for PEP following an occupational exposure to HIV is a 3-drug regimen of raltegravir used in conjunction with emtricitabine and tenofovir DF (may be administered as the fixed combination emtricitabine/tenofovir DF; Truvada®). Lopinavir/ritonavir and 2 NRTIs is one of several alternative regimens recommended when the preferred regimen cannot be used. The preferred dual NRTI option for use in PEP regimens is emtricitabine and tenofovir DF (may be administered as emtricitabine/tenofovir DF; Truvada®); alternative dual NRTIs are tenofovir DF and lamivudine, zidovudine and lamivudine (may be administered as the fixed combination lamivudine/zidovudine; Combivir®), or zidovudine and emtricitabine.

Because management of occupational exposures to HIV is complex and evolving, consultation with an infectious disease specialist, clinician with expertise in administration of antiretroviral agents, and/or the National Clinicians' Postexposure Prophylaxis Hotline (PEPline at 888-448-4911) is recommended whenever possible. However, initiation of PEP should not be delayed while waiting for expert consultation.

For information on types of occupational exposure to HIV and associated risk of infection, management of occupational exposure to HIV, efficacy and safety of postexposure prophylaxis, and recommendations regarding PEP, see Guidelines for Use of Antiretroviral Agents: Antiretrovirals for Postexposure Prophylaxis following Occupational Exposure to HIV (PEP), in the Antiretroviral Agents General Statement 8:18.08.

■ Postexposure Prophylaxis following Nonoccupational Exposure to HIV Lopinavir/ritonavir is used in conjunction with other antiretrovirals for postexposure prophylaxis of HIV infection following nonoccupational exposure† (nPEP) in individuals who have had exposure to blood, genital secretions, or other potentially infectious body fluids that might contain HIV when the exposure represents a substantial risk for HIV transmission.

When nPEP is indicated following a nonoccupational exposure to HIV, the US Centers for Disease Control and Prevention (CDC) states that the preferred regimen in adults and adolescents 13 years of age or older with normal renal function is either raltegravir or dolutegravir used in conjunction with emtricitabine and tenofovir DF (administered as emtricitabine/tenofovir DF; Truvada®); the recommended alternative nPEP regimen in these patients is *ritonavir-boosted* darunavir used in conjunction with emtricitabine/tenofovir DF.

CDC states that lopinavir/ritonavir is an option that can be considered for use in nPEP regimens in adults and adolescents and is a preferred or alternative option for use in nPEP regimens in certain pediatric patients 4 weeks of age or older; however, expert consultation is recommended.

Consultation with an infectious disease specialist, clinician with expertise in administration of antiretroviral agents, and/or the National Clinicians' Postexposure Prophylaxis Hotline (PEPline at 888-448-4911) is recommended if nPEP is indicated in certain exposed individuals (e.g., pregnant women, children, those with medical conditions such as renal impairment) or if an antiretroviral regimen not included in the CDC guidelines is being considered, the source virus is known or likely to be resistant to antiretrovirals, or the healthcare provider is inexperienced in prescribing antiretrovirals. However, initiation of nPEP should not be delayed while waiting for expert consultation.

For additional information on nonoccupational exposure to HIV and recommendations regarding postexposure prophylaxis, see Guidelines for Use of Antiretroviral Agents: Antiretrovirals for Postexposure Prophylaxis following Sexual, Injection Drug Use, or other Nonoccupational Exposures to HIV (nPEP), in the Antiretroviral Agents General Statement 8:18.08.

Dosage and Administration

■ Administration The fixed combination of lopinavir and ritonavir (lopinavir/ritonavir) is administered orally once or twice daily.

A once-daily regimen of lopinavir/ritonavir should *not* be used in adults infected with human immunodeficiency virus type 1 (HIV-1) strains with 3 or more of the following mutations associated with lopinavir resistance: L10F/I/R/V, K20M/N/R, L24I, L33F, M36I, I47V, G48V, I54L/T/V, V82A/C/F/S/T, or I84V. Such patients should receive a twice-daily regimen of lopinavir/ritonavir.

A once- or twice-daily regimen of lopinavir/ritonavir may be used in adults infected with HIV-1 strains with less than 3 mutations associated with lopinavir resistance.

A once-daily regimen of lopinavir/ritonavir should *not* be used in patients younger than 18 years of age.

A once-daily regimen of lopinavir/ritonavir should *not* be used in pregnant women.

A once-daily regimen of lopinavir/ritonavir should *not* be used in patients receiving concomitant therapy with efavirenz, nelfinavir, or nevirapine or in those receiving certain anticonvulsants (carbamazepine, phenobarbital, phenytoin).

Lopinavir/ritonavir must be used in conjunction with other antiretrovirals.

Film-coated Tablets Lopinavir/ritonavir film-coated tablets can be taken without regard to food.

The tablets should be swallowed whole and should *not* be chewed, broken, or crushed.

Children who can reliably swallow an intact tablet may receive lopinavir/ritonavir tablets.

Oral Solution Lopinavir/ritonavir oral solution should be taken with food.

The oral solution should be administered using a calibrated dosing syringe.

Lopinavir/ritonavir oral solution can be used in adults and pediatric patients unable to swallow tablets, including pediatric patients with a body surface area less than 0.6 m^2. However, the oral solution contains 42.4% (v/v) alcohol and 15.3% (w/v) propylene glycol and should *not* be used in neonates with a postnatal age less than 14 days or a postmenstrual age less than 42 weeks (i.e., time elapsed since first day of mother's last menstrual period to birth plus time elapsed after birth). (See Pediatric Use under Warnings/Precautions: Specific Populations, in Cautions.)

Lopinavir/ritonavir oral solution should be avoided in pregnant women since it contains alcohol and propylene glycol. (See Precautions Associated with Alcohol and Propylene Glycol in the Oral Solution under Cautions: Warnings/Precautions.)

Dispensing and Administration Precautions Because of similarity in spelling between Kaletra® (the trade name for the fixed combination of lopinavir and ritonavir) and Keppra® (the trade name for levetiracetam, an anticonvulsant), the potential exists for dispensing errors involving these drugs. Therefore, extra care should be exercised in ensuring the accuracy of both oral and written prescriptions for Kaletra® and Keppra®. The manufacturer of Keppra® recommends that clinicians consider including the intended use of the particular drug on the prescription, in addition to alerting patients to carefully check the drug they receive and promptly bring any question or concern to the attention of the dispensing pharmacist. Some experts also recommend that pharmacists assess various measures of avoiding dispensing errors and implement them as appropriate (e.g., by verifying all orders for these drugs by spelling both the trade and generic names to prescribers, using computerized name alerts, attaching reminders to drug containers and pharmacy shelves, separating the drugs on pharmacy shelves, employing independent checks in the dispensing process, counseling patients). (See Dispensing and Administration Precautions under Cautions: Warnings/Precautions.)

One death has occurred as a result of inadvertent overdosage of lopinavir/ritonavir oral solution in an infant. Clinicians should be aware that lopinavir/ritonavir oral solution is highly concentrated (contains 80 mg of lopinavir and 20 mg of ritonavir per mL). A child should receive 5 mL or less of the oral solution per dose unless the child also is receiving certain other antiretroviral agents. To avoid medication errors and overdosage, extra care should be used in calculating the dose, transcribing the medication order, and dispensing the prescription. In addition, complete dosing instructions should be provided. (See Dispensing and Administration Precautions under Cautions: Warnings/Precautions.)

■ Dosage Lopinavir/ritonavir is commercially available as film-coated tablets containing 100 mg of lopinavir and 25 mg of ritonavir (100 mg of lopinavir/25 mg of ritonavir) or film-coated tablets containing 200 mg of lopinavir and 50 mg of ritonavir (200 mg of lopinavir/50 mg of ritonavir).

Each 5 mL of lopinavir/ritonavir oral solution contains 400 mg of lopinavir and 100 mg of ritonavir (400 mg of lopinavir/100 mg of ritonavir per 5 mL).

Adult Dosage **Treatment of HIV Infection in Adults *Not* Receiving Efavirenz, Nelfinavir, or Nevirapine.** For the treatment of HIV-1 infection in adults who are *not* receiving concurrent therapy with efavirenz, nelfinavir, or nevirapine, the usual dosage of the fixed combination of lopinavir/ritonavir is lopinavir 800 mg/ritonavir 200 mg once daily (given as 4 tablets containing 200 mg of lopinavir/50 mg of ritonavir once daily) or lopinavir 400 mg/ritonavir 100 mg twice daily (given as 2 tablets containing 200 mg of lopinavir/50 mg of ritonavir twice daily). Alternatively, if the oral solution containing 400 mg of lopinavir/100 mg of ritonavir per 5 mL is used, adults should receive 10 mL once daily or 5 mL twice daily.

The twice-daily regimen (not the once-daily regimen) *must* be used in adults infected with HIV-1 strains with 3 or more specific mutations associated with lopinavir resistance (i.e., L10F/I/R/V, K20M/N/R, L24I, L33F, M36I, I47V, G48V, I54L/T/V, V82A/C/F/S/T, I84V).

Treatment of HIV Infection in Adults Receiving Efavirenz, Nelfinavir, or Nevirapine. For the treatment of HIV-1 infection in adults receiving concurrent therapy with efavirenz, nelfinavir, or nevirapine, the usual dosage of the fixed combination of lopinavir/ritonavir is lopinavir 500 mg/ritonavir 125 mg twice daily (given as 2 tablets containing 200 mg of lopinavir/50 mg of ritonavir and 1 tablet containing 100 mg of lopinavir/25 mg of ritonavir twice daily). Alternatively, if the oral solution containing 400 mg of lopinavir/100 mg of ritonavir per 5 mL is used, adults receiving concurrent therapy with efavirenz, nelfinavir, or nevirapine, should receive lopinavir 520 mg/ritonavir 130 mg twice daily (6.5 mL twice daily).

Postexposure Prophylaxis following Occupational Exposure to HIV. For postexposure prophylaxis of HIV infection following occupational exposure† (PEP) in health-care personnel or other individuals, the preferred dosage of the fixed combination of lopinavir/ritonavir is lopinavir 400 mg/ritonavir 100 mg twice daily (given as 2 tablets containing 200 mg of lopinavir/50 mg of ritonavir twice daily). Alternatively, lopinavir 800 mg/ritonavir 200 mg once daily (given as 4 tablets containing 200 mg of lopinavir/50 mg of ritonavir once daily) can be used. Lopinavir/ritonavir is used in conjunction with 2 HIV nucleoside reverse transcriptase inhibitors (NRTIs). (See Uses: Postexposure Prophylaxis following Occupational Exposure to HIV.)

The PEP regimen should be initiated as soon as possible following occupational exposure to HIV (preferably within hours) and continued for 4 weeks, if tolerated.

Pediatric Dosage **Treatment of HIV Infection.** Dosage of lopinavir/ritonavir in children 14 days of age and older is based on body surface area or body weight. Pediatric dosage should *not* exceed adult dosage.

A once-daily regimen of lopinavir/ritonavir should *not* be used in pediatric patients younger than 18 years of age. (See Pediatric Use under Warnings/Precautions: Specific Populations, in Cautions.)

In infants 14 days to 6 months of age, the recommended dosage of lopinavir/ritonavir *based on body surface area* is 300 mg/m^2 of lopinavir and 75 mg/m^2 of ritonavir twice daily (given as the oral solution). Alternatively, the recommended dosage *based on body weight* is 16 mg/kg of lopinavir and 4 mg/kg of ritonavir twice daily (given as the oral solution). Lopinavir/ritonavir should *not* be used in conjunction with efavirenz, nelfinavir, or nevirapine in children younger than 6 months of age.

In children 6 months to 18 years of age *not* receiving concurrent therapy with efavirenz, nelfinavir, or nevirapine, the recommended dosage of lopinavir/ritonavir *based on body surface area* is 230 mg/m^2 of lopinavir and 57.5 mg/m^2 of ritonavir twice daily (given as the oral solution). Alternatively, the recommended dosage *based on body weight* is 12 mg/kg of lopinavir and 3 mg/kg of ritonavir twice daily in children weighing less than 15 kg or 10 mg/kg of lopinavir and 2.5 mg/kg of ritonavir twice daily in children weighing 15–40 kg (given as the oral solution). For dosage recommendations when lopinavir/ritonavir is given as tablets in these children 6 months to 18 years of age, see Table 1.

Table 1. Dosage of Lopinavir/Ritonavir Tablets for Treatment of HIV Infection in Children 6 Months to 18 Years of Age *Not* Receiving Efavirenz, Nelfinavir, or Nevirapine

Weight (kg)	Body Surface Area (m^2)	Number of Lopinavir/Ritonavir Tablets Containing 100 mg of Lopinavir and 25 mg of Ritonavir
15 to 25	0.6 to less than 0.9	2 tablets twice daily
greater than 25 to 35	0.9 to less than 1.4	3 tablets twice daily
greater than 35	1.4 or greater	4 tablets twice daily[a]

[a] Two lopinavir/ritonavir tablets containing 200 mg of lopinavir and 50 mg of ritonavir twice daily can be used instead of 4 tablets containing 100 mg of lopinavir and 25 mg of ritonavir twice daily.

In children 6 months to 18 years of age receiving concurrent therapy with efavirenz, nelfinavir, or nevirapine, dosage *based on body surface area* should be increased to 300 mg/m^2 of lopinavir and 75 mg/m^2 of ritonavir twice daily (given as the oral solution). Alternatively, the recommended dosage of the oral solution *based on body weight* is 13 mg/kg of lopinavir and 3.25 mg/kg of ritonavir twice daily in children weighing less than 15 kg or 11 mg/kg of lopinavir and 2.75 mg/kg of ritonavir twice daily in children weighing 15–45 kg (given as the oral solution). For dosage recommendations when lopinavir/ritonavir is given as tablets in these children 6 months to 18 years of age, see Table 2.

Table 2. Dosage of Lopinavir/Ritonavir Tablets for Treatment of HIV Infection in Children 6 Months to 18 Years of Age Receiving Efavirenz, Nelfinavir, or Nevirapine

Weight (kg)	Body Surface Area (m^2)	Number of Lopinavir/Ritonavir Tablets Containing 100 mg of Lopinavir and 25 mg of Ritonavir
15 to 20	0.6 to less than 0.8	2 tablets twice daily
greater than 20 to 30	0.8 to less than 1.2	3 tablets twice daily
greater than 30 to 45	1.2 to less than 1.7	4 tablets once daily[a]
greater than 45	1.7 or greater	5 tablets twice daily

[a] Two lopinavir/ritonavir tablets containing 200 mg of lopinavir and 50 mg of ritonavir twice daily can be used instead of 4 tablets containing 100 mg of lopinavir and 25 mg of ritonavir twice daily.

■ **Special Populations** ***Renal Impairment*** Pharmacokinetics of lopinavir have not been studied in patients with renal impairment, but renal clearance of the drug is negligible and a decrease in total body clearance is not expected in patients with impaired renal function.

The manufacturer does not make dosage recommendations for patients with renal impairment. Some experts state that once-daily lopinavir/ritonavir regimens should be avoided in those undergoing hemodialysis.

Hepatic Impairment Limited pharmacokinetic data are available in patients with mild to moderate hepatic impairment; pharmacokinetics have not been studied in patients with severe hepatic impairment.

Dosage recommendations for patients with hepatic impairment are not available; lopinavir/ritonavir should be used with caution in patients with hepatic impairment.

Pregnant Women For the treatment of HIV-1 infection in pregnant women infected with HIV-1 strains without lopinavir-associated resistance mutations, a dosage of lopinavir 400 mg/ritonavir 100 mg twice daily is recommended. The manufacturer states that data are insufficient to make dosage recommendations for pregnant women infected with HIV-1 strains with lopinavir-associated resistance mutations. Dosage adjustments are not needed in postpartum women.

Because of evidence that lopinavir plasma concentrations may be decreased in some pregnant women receiving usual lopinavir/ritonavir dosage (see Pregnancy under Warnings/Precautions: Specific Populations, in Cautions), some experts recommend that dosage of lopinavir/ritonavir be increased to lopinavir 600 mg/ritonavir 150 mg twice daily during the second and third trimesters, especially in HIV protease inhibitor-experienced (PI-experienced) pregnant women and those with baseline plasma HIV-1 RNA levels exceeding 50 copies/mL at the time antiretroviral treatment is initiated. If usual dosage is used during the second and third trimesters, these experts state that virologic response and lopinavir plasma concentrations should be monitored.

Once-daily lopinavir/ritonavir regimens are *not* recommended during pregnancy.

Lopinavir/ritonavir oral solution should be avoided in pregnant women since it contains alcohol and propylene glycol.

Cautions

■ **Contraindications** The fixed combination of lopinavir and ritonavir (lopinavir/ritonavir) is contraindicated in patients with a history of clinically important hypersensitivity reaction (e.g., toxic epidermal necrolysis, Stevens-Johnson syndrome, erythema multiforme, urticaria, angioedema) to lopinavir, ritonavir, or any other ingredient in the formulation.

Concomitant use of lopinavir/ritonavir with drugs that are highly dependent on cytochrome P-450 (CYP) isoenzyme 3A for metabolism and for which elevated plasma concentrations are associated with serious and/or life-threatening events (e.g., alfuzosin, cisapride, ergot alkaloids, oral midazolam, pimozide, triazolam, lovastatin, simvastatin, sildenafil used for treatment of pulmonary arterial hypertension) is contraindicated. (See Drug Interactions.)

Concomitant use of lopinavir/ritonavir with drugs that are potent inducers of CYP3A (e.g., rifampin, St. John's wort [*Hypericum perforatum*]) is contraindicated because such use is expected to result in suboptimal antiretroviral concentrations and may be associated with loss of virologic response and development of resistance. (See Drug Interactions.)

■ **Warnings/Precautions** ***Interactions*** Serious and/or life-threatening adverse effects, clinically important drug interactions, or loss of virologic effect can occur if lopinavir/ritonavir is used concomitantly with some drugs. The potential for drug interactions must be considered prior to and during lopinavir/ritonavir therapy. Clinicians should review all drugs the patient is receiving and should monitor for adverse effects during lopinavir/ritonavir therapy. (See Contraindications and see Drug Interactions.)

Precautions Associated with Alcohol and Propylene Glycol in the Oral Solution Lopinavir/ritonavir oral solution contains 42.4% (v/v) alcohol and 15.3% (w/v) propylene glycol. When administered concomitantly with propylene glycol, ethanol competitively inhibits metabolism of propylene glycol, which may lead to elevated propylene glycol concentrations. Preterm neonates† may be at increased risk of propylene glycol-associated adverse effects due to diminished ability to metabolize propylene glycol, thereby leading to accumulation and potential adverse events.

Life-threatening cardiac toxicity (including complete atrioventricular [AV] block, bradycardia, cardiomyopathy), lactic acidosis, acute renal failure, CNS depression, and respiratory complications leading to death have been reported, predominantly in preterm neonates† receiving lopinavir/ritonavir oral solution. Neonates, especially those born prematurely, are at risk of lopinavir, ethanol, and/or propylene glycol toxicity if they receive lopinavir/ritonavir oral solution. (See Pediatric Use under Warnings/Precautions: Specific Populations, in Cautions.)

Pancreatitis Pancreatitis (with or without marked elevations in triglycerides) has occurred in patients receiving lopinavir/ritonavir and has been fatal in some patients. Although a causal relationship to lopinavir/ritonavir has not been established, marked triglyceride elevations are a risk factor for pancreatitis. (See Lipid Effects under Cautions: Warnings/Precautions.)

Patients with advanced HIV disease may be at increased risk of elevated triglycerides and pancreatitis, and patients with a history of pancreatitis may be at increased risk for recurrence during lopinavir/ritonavir therapy. The possibility of pancreatitis should be considered in a patient who develops abdominal pain, nausea and vomiting, or elevated biochemical markers (e.g., increased serum amylase or lipase concentration), and therapy with lopinavir/ritonavir, as well as other antiretroviral therapy, should be suspended if clinically appropriate.

Hepatic Effects Cases of hepatic dysfunction, including some fatalities, have been reported during postmarketing experience; a causal relationship to lopinavir/ritonavir has not been established. Hepatic dysfunction generally has occurred in patients with advanced HIV infection receiving multiple concomitant drugs in the setting of chronic hepatitis or cirrhosis.

Elevated transaminase concentrations, with or without elevated bilirubin concentrations, have been reported in HIV-1 monoinfected patients and uninfected individuals as early as 7 days after initiation of lopinavir/ritonavir therapy in conjunction with other antiretroviral agents.

HIV-infected patients with hepatitis B virus (HBV) or hepatitis C virus (HCV) coinfection or marked elevations in transaminase concentrations prior to lopinavir/ritonavir therapy may be at increased risk for new-onset or worsening transaminase elevations or hepatic decompensation.

Appropriate laboratory tests should be performed to evaluate hepatic function prior to initiating lopinavir/ritonavir and periodically during treatment.

Increased AST/ALT monitoring should be considered in patients with hepatitis or cirrhosis, especially during the first several months of lopinavir/ritonavir therapy.

Hyperglycemic and Diabetogenic Effects Hyperglycemia (potentially persistent), new-onset diabetes mellitus, or exacerbation of preexisting diabetes mellitus has been reported in patients receiving HIV protease inhibitors (PIs); diabetic ketoacidosis has occurred. It may be necessary to initiate or adjust dosage of antidiabetic therapy (e.g., insulin, oral hypoglycemic agents).

Cardiovascular Effects Prolongation of the PR interval has occurred in individuals receiving lopinavir/ritonavir; second- or third-degree AV block has been reported. Lopinavir/ritonavir should be used with caution in patients with structural heart disease, cardiac conduction abnormalities, ischemic heart disease, or cardiomyopathies; these individuals may be at increased risk for cardiac conduction abnormalities. Caution is advised if lopinavir/ritonavir is used with other drugs that prolong the PR interval (e.g., some β-adrenergic blocking agents, digoxin, calcium-channel blockers, atazanavir), especially drugs metabolized by the cytochrome P-450 isoenzyme CYP 3A4.

Prolongation of the QT interval and torsades de pointes have been reported in patients receiving lopinavir/ritonavir during postmarketing experience. It is unclear whether these events were related directly to the drug. Lopinavir/ritonavir should not be used in patients who have or may develop prolongation of the QT interval (e.g., hypokalemia, congenital long QT syndrome, use of drugs known to prolong QT interval).

Immune Reconstitution Syndrome Patients receiving antiretroviral therapy may experience an immune reconstitution syndrome during the initial phase of therapy. Patients whose immune system responds to antiretroviral therapy may develop an inflammatory response to indolent or residual opportunistic infections (e.g., *Mycobacterium avium* complex [MAC], *M. tuberculosis*, cytomegalovirus [CMV], *Pneumocystis jirovecii* [formerly *P. carinii*]); this may necessitate further evaluation and treatment.

Autoimmune disorders (e.g., Graves' disease, polymyositis, Guillain-Barré syndrome) have also been reported to occur in the setting of immune reconstitution; however, the time to onset is more variable and can occur many months after initiation of antiretroviral therapy.

Adipogenic Effects Redistribution or accumulation of body fat, including central obesity, dorsocervical fat enlargement ("buffalo hump"), peripheral wasting, facial wasting, breast enlargement, and general cushingoid appearance has been reported in patients receiving HIV PIs. The mechanism and long-term consequences of fat redistribution are unknown; a causal relationship has not been established.

Lipid Effects Substantial increases in total serum cholesterol and triglyceride concentrations have occurred. Serum triglyceride and cholesterol concentrations should be determined before initiating therapy with lopinavir/ritonavir and monitored periodically during therapy with the drug; lipid disorders should be managed as clinically appropriate. (See Drug Interactions: HMG-CoA Reductase Inhibitors.)

Hemophilia A and B Increased bleeding, including spontaneous hematomas and hemarthrosis, have been reported in hemophilia A or B patients receiving HIV PIs; a causal relationship has not been established.

Increased hemostatic (e.g., antihemophilic factor) therapy may be needed.

HIV Resistance The potential for cross-resistance among PIs has not been fully evaluated in patients receiving lopinavir/ritonavir. The possible effect of lopinavir/ritonavir therapy on subsequent therapy with other PIs is unknown.

Dispensing and Administration Precautions Because of similarity in spelling between Kaletra® (the trade name for the fixed combination of lopinavir and ritonavir) and Keppra® (the trade name for levetiracetam, an anticonvulsant), the potential exists for dispensing errors involving these drugs. These medication errors may be associated with serious adverse events (e.g., status epilepticus) due to lack of appropriate therapy for seizures or with the risk of developing adverse effects associated with the use of lopinavir/ritonavir or levetiracetam in patients for whom the drug was not prescribed. Therefore, extra care should be exercised in ensuring the accuracy of both oral and written prescriptions for these drugs. The manufacturer of Keppra® recommends that clinicians consider including the intended use of the particular drug on the prescription in addition to alerting patients to carefully check the drug they receive and promptly bring any question or concern to the attention of the dispensing pharmacist. Some experts also recommend that pharmacists assess various measures of avoiding dispensing errors and implement them as appropriate (e.g., by verifying all orders for these drugs by spelling both the trade and generic names to prescribers, using computerized name alerts, attaching reminders to drug containers and pharmacy shelves, separating the drugs on pharmacy shelves, employing independent checks in the dispensing process, counseling patients).

Dispensing errors involving Kaletra® and Keppra® should be reported to the manufacturers, the USP Medication Errors Reporting program by phone (800-233-7767), or directly to the FDA MedWatch program by phone (800-FDA-1088), by fax (800-FDA-0178), by the Internet (http://www.fda.gov/Safety/MedWatch/default.htm) or by mail (FDA Safety Information and Adverse Event Reporting Program, FDA, 5600 Fishers Lane, Rockville, MD 20852-9787).

One death has occurred as a result of inadvertent overdosage of lopinavir/ritonavir oral solution. This overdose occurred in a 44-day-old HIV-infected infant given approximately 6.5 mL of lopinavir/ritonavir oral solution (10 times the calculated dose). The infant died 9 days later of cardiogenic shock. To avoid medication errors and minimize the risk for overdosage when the oral solution is used, extra care should be taken to ensure the accuracy of the prescription. (See Dispensing and Administration Precautions under Dosage and Administration: Administration.)

Specific Populations **Pregnancy.** Antiretroviral Pregnancy Registry at 800-258-4263 or http://www.apregistry.com.

Based on prospective reports from the Antiretroviral Pregnancy Registry that included over 3000 exposures to lopinavir-containing regimens (including over 1000 first trimester exposures), there was no difference in the risk of overall major birth defects for lopinavir compared with the background rate for major birth defects.

When lopinavir/ritonavir was administered to pregnant rats or rabbits, no treatment-related malformations were observed; however, embryonic and fetal developmental toxicities occurred in rats administered maternally toxic doses.

The HHS Panel on Treatment of HIV-infected Pregnant Women and Prevention of Perinatal Transmission states that lopinavir/ritonavir (twice daily) with 2 NRTIs is an alternative PI-based regimen for *initial* treatment of HIV-1 infection in pregnant women.

Once-daily lopinavir/ritonavir regimens are *not* recommended during pregnancy. Lopinavir/ritonavir oral solution should be avoided in pregnant women since it contains alcohol and propylene glycol.

Some experts recommend that lopinavir/ritonavir dosage be increased during the second and third trimesters, especially in HIV PI-experienced pregnant women and those with baseline plasma HIV-1 RNA levels exceeding 50 copies/mL at the time antiretroviral treatment is initiated. (See Pregnant Women under Dosage and Administration: Special Populations.) There is some evidence that pregnant women receiving usual dosage of lopinavir/ritonavir may have decreased lopinavir plasma concentrations compared with nonpregnant adults. Other evidence suggests that, although trough plasma concentrations of lopinavir are decreased during the second and third trimesters compared with 8 weeks postpartum and total clearance of the drug is increased during pregnancy, plasma concentrations of unbound lopinavir in pregnant women are not substantially different from those observed at 8 weeks postpartum or in nonpregnant women. The manufacturer of lopinavir/ritonavir states that decreases in lopinavir trough plasma concentrations observed during the second and third trimesters are not considered clinically important when usual dosage of lopinavir/ritonavir is used for the treatment of HIV-1 infection in pregnant women infected with HIV-1 strains without lopinavir-associated resistance mutations.

Lactation. Lopinavir and ritonavir are distributed into milk in rats. Lopinavir concentrations in human milk are very low or undetectable. Because of the risk of adverse effects in the infant and the risk of HIV transmission, HIV-infected women should not breast-feed infants.

Pediatric Use. Safety, efficacy, and pharmacokinetic profile of lopinavir/ritonavir have not been established in neonates younger than 14 days of age.

Because of possible toxicities, lopinavir/ritonavir oral solution should *not* be used in neonates with a postnatal age less than 14 days or a postmenstrual age less than 42 weeks (i.e., time elapsed since first day of mother's last menstrual period to birth plus time elapsed after birth).

Lopinavir/ritonavir oral solution contains 42.4% (v/v) alcohol and 15.3% (w/v) propylene glycol. Inadvertent ingestion of the oral solution or overdosage in an infant or young child may result in significant toxicity and is potentially lethal. (See Precautions Associated with Alcohol and Propylene Glycol in the Oral Solution under Cautions: Warnings/Precautions.)

There have been postmarketing reports of life-threatening cases of cardiac toxicity (including complete AV block, bradycardia, cardiomyopathy), lactic acidosis, acute renal failure, CNS depression, and respiratory complications leading to death, predominantly in preterm neonates† receiving lopinavir/ritonavir oral solution.

A safe and effective dose of lopinavir/ritonavir oral solution has not been established in neonates younger than 14 days of age† (whether born prematurely or full term). If the benefits of the oral solution for treatment of HIV infection in an infant immediately after birth are judged to outweigh potential risks, the infant should be monitored closely for increases in serum osmolality and serum creatinine and other signs of toxicity related to the oral solution. These toxicities include hyperosmolality with or without lactic acidosis, renal toxicity, CNS depression (including stupor, coma, apnea), seizures, hypotonia, cardiac arrhythmias, ECG changes, and hemolysis.

If lopinavir/ritonavir oral solution is used in preterm neonates† or in pediatric patients 14 days to 6 months of age, total amounts of alcohol and propylene glycol from all drugs that the child is receiving should be taken into account to avoid toxicity associated with these excipients.

Once-daily lopinavir/ritonavir regimens are *not* recommended in patients younger than 18 years of age. In a randomized study in pediatric patients younger than 18 years of age, the rate of viral rebound in those receiving a once-daily regimen of lopinavir/ritonavir did not meet noninferiority criteria compared with a twice-daily regimen of the drug.

Geriatric Use. Experience in those 65 years of age and older is insufficient to determine whether they respond differently from younger adults.

Use with caution in geriatric individuals because of age-related decreases in hepatic, renal, and/or cardiac function and concomitant disease and drug therapy.

Hepatic Impairment. Use with caution since lopinavir plasma concentrations may be increased. Risk of further transaminase elevations in HIV-infected patients with HBV or HCV coinfection or preexisting HIV-elevations in transaminases prior to initiation of lopinavir/ritonavir. Carefully monitor liver function in these patients.

■ **Common Adverse Effects** Adverse effects occurring in 5% or more of patients include diarrhea, nausea, vomiting, abdominal pain, fatigue (including asthenia), headache (including migraine), hypercholesterolemia, hypertriglyceridemia, musculoskeletal pain, and upper or lower respiratory tract infection. A higher incidence of diarrhea has been reported with a once-daily regimen of lopinavir/ritonavir compared with a twice-daily regimen.

Drug Interactions

■ **Drugs Affecting or Metabolized by Hepatic Microsomal Enzymes** The fixed combination of lopinavir and ritonavir (lopinavir/ritonavir) inhibits the cytochrome P-450 (CYP) isoenzyme 3A; potential pharmacokinetic interactions with drugs metabolized by CYP3A (altered metabolism of the drug metabolized by CYP3A). Concomitant use with some drugs that are CYP3A substrates is contraindicated; concomitant use with other drugs that are CYP3A substrates may require dosage adjustment or additional monitoring. Lopinavir and ritonavir are metabolized by CYP3A; potential pharmacokinetic interactions with drugs that inhibit or induce CYP3A (altered metabolism of lopinavir).

Lopinavir/ritonavir does not inhibit CYP isoenzymes 2D6, 2C9, 2C19, 2E1, 2B6, or 1A2.

■ **Drugs Metabolized by Glucuronidation** Lopinavir/ritonavir induces glucuronidation and may decrease plasma concentrations of drugs metabolized by glucuronidation.

■ **Alfuzosin** Pharmacokinetic interaction (increased alfuzosin plasma concentrations) may result in hypotension. Concomitant use of lopinavir/ritonavir and alfuzosin is contraindicated.

■ **Antiarrhythmic Agents** Possible pharmacokinetic interaction with amiodarone, bepridil (no longer commercially available in the US), dofetilide, flecainide, lidocaine (systemic), propafenone, and quinidine (increased plasma concentrations of the antiarrhythmic agent). Lopinavir/ritonavir and antiarrhythmic agents should be used concomitantly with caution and plasma concentrations of the antiarrhythmic agents should be monitored.

Some experts state that concomitant use of dronedarone and lopinavir/ritonavir is contraindicated.

■ **Anticoagulants** ***Apixaban*** Pharmacokinetic interaction with apixaban expected (increased apixaban concentrations).

Concomitant use of lopinavir/ritonavir and apixaban should be avoided.

Dabigatran Possible pharmacokinetic interaction with dabigatran (increased dabigatran concentrations).

Dosage adjustments are not needed in patients with creatinine clearances exceeding 50 mL/minute. Concomitant use of lopinavir/ritonavir and dabigatran should be avoided in patients with creatinine clearances less than 50 mL/minute.

Edoxaban Pharmacokinetic interaction with edoxaban (increased edoxaban concentrations).

Concomitant use of lopinavir/ritonavir and edoxaban should be avoided.

Rivaroxaban Pharmacokinetic interaction with rivaroxaban (increased rivaroxaban concentrations); possible increased risk of bleeding.

Concomitant use of lopinavir/ritonavir and rivaroxaban should be avoided.

Warfarin Possible pharmacokinetic interaction with warfarin (altered warfarin plasma concentrations).

If warfarin is used concomitantly with lopinavir/ritonavir, the international normalized ratio (INR) should be monitored, especially when lopinavir/ritonavir is initiation or discontinued; warfarin dosage should be adjusted as needed.

■ **Anticonvulsants** ***Carbamazepine, Phenobarbital, Phenytoin*** Possible pharmacokinetic interaction with carbamazepine, phenobarbital, phenytoin (decreased lopinavir plasma concentrations, increased or decreased anticonvulsant plasma concentrations); possible decreased antiretroviral efficacy.

Caution is advised if lopinavir/ritonavir is used concomitantly with carbamazepine, phenobarbital, or phenytoin; an alternative anticonvulsant should be considered. Alternatively, plasma concentrations of the anticonvulsant and lopinavir should be monitored and virologic response assessed.

A once-daily lopinavir/ritonavir regimen should not be used in patients receiving carbamazepine, phenobarbital, or phenytoin.

Ethosuximide Possible pharmacokinetic interaction with ethosuximide (increased ethosuximide concentrations).

If lopinavir/ritonavir and ethosuximide are used concomitantly, the patient should be monitored for ethosuximide toxicity.

Lamotrigine Pharmacokinetic interaction with lamotrigine (substantially decreased lamotrigine plasma concentrations and AUC; no clinically important effect on lopinavir/ritonavir plasma concentrations).

If lamotrigine is used concomitantly with lopinavir/ritonavir, increased lamotrigine dosage may be needed and therapeutic concentration monitoring of the anticonvulsant may be indicated, especially during dosage adjustment. Alternatively, use of a different anticonvulsant should be considered.

Valproate Sodium and Valproic Acid Possible pharmacokinetic interaction with valproate sodium or valproic acid (substantially increased lopinavir plasma concentrations and AUC, decreased plasma valproic acid concentrations). Exacerbated mania possibly related to decreased plasma valproic acid concentrations has been reported in a patient receiving lopinavir/ritonavir and 2 NRTIs.

If lopinavir/ritonavir is used concomitantly with valproate sodium or valproic acid, increased dosage of the anticonvulsant may be needed and therapeutic concentration monitoring of the anticonvulsant may be indicated, especially during dosage adjustment. In addition, patients should be monitored for virologic response and lopinavir-related toxicities.

■ **Antifungal Agents** ***Fluconazole*** Clinically important interactions with fluconazole are not expected.

Isavuconazonium Concomitant use of isavuconazonium sulfate (prodrug of isavuconazole) and lopinavir/ritonavir results in increased isavuconazole AUC and decreased lopinavir AUC.

If lopinavir/ritonavir and isavuconazonium sulfate are used concomitantly, monitoring of isavuconazole concentrations and virologic response should be considered.

Itraconazole Pharmacokinetic interaction with itraconazole (increased plasma concentrations of the antifungal agent). If used concomitantly, high itraconazole dosage (exceeding 200 mg daily) is not recommended; consider monitoring itraconazole plasma concentrations.

Ketoconazole Pharmacokinetic interaction with ketoconazole (increased concentrations of the antifungal agent). If used concomitantly, high ketoconazole dosage (exceeding 200 mg daily) is not recommended.

Voriconazole Possible pharmacokinetic interaction with voriconazole (decreased plasma concentrations and AUC of voriconazole). Voriconazole and lopinavir/ritonavir should not be used concomitantly unless potential benefits outweigh risks. If used concomitantly, some experts recommend monitoring voriconazole plasma concentrations and adjusting voriconazole dosage accordingly.

■ **Antimalarial Agents** ***Artemether and Lumefantrine*** Pharmacokinetic interaction with the fixed combination of artemether and lumefantrine (artemether/lumefantrine) (decreased plasma concentrations and AUC of artemether and the active metabolite of artemether [DHA], increased plasma concentrations and AUC of lumefantrine); clinical importance unknown.

If artemether/lumefantrine and lopinavir/ritonavir are used concomitantly, the patient should be monitored for antimalarial efficacy and lumefantrine toxicity.

Artesunate and Mefloquine Pharmacokinetic interaction with the fixed combination of artesunate and mefloquine (artesunate/mefloquine; not commercially available in the US) (decreased AUC of dihydroartemisinin and mefloquine; lopinavir concentrations not affected). The clinical importance of this interaction is not known.

If lopinavir/ritonavir and artesunate/mefloquine are used concomitantly, the patient should be closely monitored for efficacy of the antimalarial agent.

Atovaquone and Proguanil Pharmacokinetic interaction with the fixed combination of atovaquone and proguanil (atovaquone/proguanil) (decreased plasma atovaquone and proguanil concentrations). Some experts state that an alternative antimalarial agent should be considered, if possible, in patients receiving lopinavir/ritonavir.

■ **Antimycobacterial Agents** ***Bedaquiline*** Pharmacokinetic interaction with bedaquiline (increased bedaquiline AUC, but no substantial change in plasma bedaquiline concentrations); clinical importance unknown.

Bedaquiline and lopinavir/ritonavir should be used concomitantly with caution and only if potential benefits outweigh risks; some experts recommend that patients be monitored for prolongation of the QT interval corrected for heart rate (QT_c) and liver dysfunction.

Rifabutin Pharmacokinetic interaction with rifabutin (increased rifabutin and rifabutin metabolite plasma concentrations and AUCs).

The manufacturer of lopinavir/ritonavir states that if rifabutin is used concomitantly with lopinavir/ritonavir, dosage of the antimycobacterial agent should be reduced by at least 75% (i.e., maximum 150 mg every other day or 3 times weekly); increased monitoring for adverse effects is warranted. However, because the pharmacokinetic interaction between lopinavir/ritonavir and rifabutin has been studied in healthy individuals and lower rifabutin exposure has been reported in HIV-infected patients, some experts recommend a rifabutin dosage of 150 mg once daily or 300 mg 3 times weekly in patients receiving lopinavir/ritonavir and also recommend that rifabutin plasma concentrations and antimycobacterial activity be monitored.

Rifampin Pharmacokinetic interaction with rifampin (substantially decreased lopinavir plasma concentrations); possible decreased antiretroviral efficacy and increased risk of resistance.

Concomitant use of lopinavir and rifampin is contraindicated.

Rifapentine Possible pharmacokinetic interaction with rifapentine (decreased lopinavir plasma concentrations).

Concomitant use of lopinavir/ritonavir and rifapentine is not recommended.

■ **Antineoplastic Agents** ***Dasatinib or Nilotinib*** Pharmacokinetic interaction (increased dasatinib or nilotinib plasma concentrations). Possible increased risk of dasatinib- or nilotinib-associated adverse effects. A decrease in dose or adjustment of the dosing interval of dasatinib or nilotinib may be required in patients receiving a potent CYP3A inhibitor, such as lopinavir/ritonavir, concomitantly.

Vinca Alkaloids Concomitant use of vincristine or vinblastine and lopinavir/ritonavir may result in increased plasma concentrations of the vinca alkaloid and possible increased vinca alkaloid-associated adverse effects. The manufacturer of lopinavir/ritonavir states that temporarily withholding ritonavir-containing antiretroviral regimens should be considered in patients who develop substantial hematologic or GI toxicity from the vinca alkaloid. Alternatively, if the antiretroviral regimen must be withheld for a prolonged period, an antiretroviral regimen that does not include agents that inhibit CYP3A or the P-glycoprotein transport system should be considered.

■ **Antiplatelet Agents** ***Ticagrelor*** Pharmacokinetic interaction with ticagrelor expected (increased ticagrelor concentrations).

Concomitant use of lopinavir/ritonavir and ticagrelor should be avoided.

Vorapaxar Pharmacokinetic interaction with vorapaxar expected (increased vorapaxar concentrations).

Concomitant use of lopinavir/ritonavir and vorapaxar should be avoided.

■ **Antipsychotic Agents** ***Lurasidone*** Potential for serious and/or life-threatening adverse effects.

Concomitant use of lopinavir/ritonavir and lurasidone is contraindicated.

Perphenazine, Risperidone, Thioridazine Possible pharmacokinetic interaction with perphenazine, risperidone, or thioridazine (increased concentrations of the antipsychotic).

If perphenazine, risperidone, or thioridazine is used concomitantly with lopinavir/ritonavir, the antipsychotic should be initiated at the lowest dosage, maintenance dosage should be adjusted, and the patient monitored for toxicities associated with the antipsychotic.

Pimozide Potential for serious and/or life-threatening adverse effects (e.g., cardiac arrhythmias) with pimozide.

Concomitant use of lopinavir/ritonavir and pimozide is contraindicated.

Quetiapine Pharmacokinetic interaction with quetiapine expected (increased quetiapine concentrations).

Alternative antiretroviral therapy should be considered in patients receiving quetiapine. If lopinavir/ritonavir is necessary in a patient receiving a stable dosage of quetiapine, the quetiapine dosage should be reduced to one-sixth of the original dosage. If quetiapine is necessary in a patient receiving lopinavir/ritonavir, some experts recommend that quetiapine be initiated using the lowest dosage and titrated as needed. Patients receiving quetiapine and lopinavir/ritonavir concomitantly should be monitored for efficacy and adverse effects of the antipsychotic.

■ **Antiretroviral Agents** ***HIV Entry and Fusion Inhibitors***

Maraviroc. Pharmacokinetic interaction with maraviroc (substantially increased maraviroc plasma concentrations and AUC). If maraviroc is used concomitantly with lopinavir/ritonavir, the recommended dosage of maraviroc is 150 mg twice daily.

There is no in vitro evidence of antagonistic antiretroviral effects between maraviroc and lopinavir.

HIV Integrase Inhibitors (INSTIs) There is no in vitro evidence of antagonistic antiretroviral effects between lopinavir and dolutegravir or elvitegravir. The antiretroviral effects of lopinavir and raltegravir are additive to synergistic against HIV-1 in vitro.

Dolutegravir. Concomitant use of lopinavir/ritonavir (lopinavir 400 mg/ritonavir 100 mg twice daily) and dolutegravir (30 mg once daily) does not have a clinically important effect on the pharmacokinetics of dolutegravir or lopinavir.

Dosage adjustments are not necessary if dolutegravir is used with a once- or twice-daily regimen of lopinavir/ritonavir.

Elvitegravir. Possible pharmacokinetic interaction with *cobicistat-boosted* elvitegravir (altered concentrations of elvitegravir, cobicistat, and/or lopinavir).

Lopinavir/ritonavir should not be used concomitantly with *cobicistat-boosted* elvitegravir, including the fixed combination of elvitegravir, cobicistat, emtricitabine, and tenofovir disoproxil fumarate (EVG/c/FTC/TDF).

Raltegravir. Pharmacokinetic interaction between raltegravir and lopinavir/ritonavir (decreased raltegravir plasma concentrations; no change in lopinavir/ritonavir plasma concentrations); not considered clinically important.

Some experts state that dosage adjustments are not necessary if raltegravir and lopinavir/ritonavir are used concomitantly.

HIV Nonnucleoside Reverse Transcriptase Inhibitors (NNRTIs) No in vitro evidence of antagonistic antiretroviral effects between lopinavir and etravirine or rilpivirine.

Delavirdine. Concomitant use of delavirdine and lopinavir/ritonavir may result in increased plasma concentrations of lopinavir. Appropriate dosages for concomitant use of lopinavir/ritonavir and delavirdine with respect to safety and efficacy have not been established.

Efavirenz. Pharmacokinetic interaction with efavirenz (decreased lopinavir plasma concentrations).

A once-daily regimen of lopinavir/ritonavir should not be used in patients receiving efavirenz.

If a twice-daily regimen of lopinavir/ritonavir is used with efavirenz, adults should receive lopinavir 500 mg/ritonavir 125 mg (as tablets) twice daily with the usual dosage of efavirenz. Alternatively, adults may receive lopinavir 520 mg/ritonavir 130 mg (as the oral solution) twice daily with the usual dosage of efavirenz.

For dosage recommendations in pediatric patients receiving lopinavir/ritonavir and efavirenz concomitantly, see Treatment of HIV Infection under Dosage: Pediatric Dosage, in Dosage and Administration.

Etravirine. Pharmacokinetic interaction with etravirine (decreased etravirine plasma concentrations and AUC; decreased lopinavir plasma concentrations and AUC). Because the decrease in etravirine systemic exposure reported with concomitant lopinavir/ritonavir is similar to that reported in patients receiving etravirine concomitantly with *ritonavir-boosted* darunavir (a combination that has been found to be safe and effective), the usual dosage of etravirine can be used with the usual dosage of lopinavir/ritonavir.

Nevirapine. Pharmacokinetic interaction with nevirapine (decreased lopinavir plasma concentrations and AUC).

A once-daily regimen of lopinavir/ritonavir should not be used in patients receiving nevirapine.

If a twice-daily regimen of lopinavir/ritonavir is used with nevirapine, adults should receive lopinavir 500 mg/ritonavir 125 mg (as tablets) twice daily with the usual dosage of nevirapine. Alternatively, adults may receive lopinavir 520 mg/ritonavir 130 mg (as the oral solution) twice daily with the usual dosage of nevirapine.

For dosage recommendations in pediatric patients receiving lopinavir/ritonavir and nevirapine concomitantly, see Treatment of HIV Infection under Dosage: Pediatric Dosage, in Dosage and Administration.

Rilpivirine. Pharmacokinetic interaction with rilpivirine (increased rilpivirine plasma concentrations and AUC; no clinically important effect on lopinavir plasma concentrations or AUC).

Dosage adjustments are not needed if lopinavir/ritonavir and rilpivirine are used concomitantly.

HIV Nucleoside and Nucleotide Reverse Transcriptase Inhibitors (NRTIs) There were no clinically important pharmacokinetic interactions when lopinavir/ritonavir was used concomitantly with lamivudine or stavudine.

Although the clinical importance is unclear, lopinavir induces glucuronidation and has the potential to reduce abacavir or zidovudine plasma concentrations.

Didanosine. Because of conflicting instructions regarding administration of didanosine and administration of lopinavir/ritonavir oral solution with meals, didanosine should be given 1 hour before or 2 hours after lopinavir/ritonavir oral solution (given with food). Lopinavir/ritonavir tablets can be taken at the same time as didanosine.

Tenofovir Alafenamide. Concomitant use of tenofovir alafenamide (10 mg once daily) and lopinavir/ritonavir (lopinavir 800 mg/ritonavir 200 mg once daily) results in increased tenofovir plasma concentrations and AUC, but does not affect lopinavir concentrations. Some experts state that dosage adjustments are not necessary if lopinavir/ritonavir is used concomitantly with tenofovir alafenamide.

Clinically important drug interactions are not expected if lopinavir/ritonavir and the fixed combination of emtricitabine and tenofovir alafenamide (emtricitabine/tenofovir alafenamide) are used concomitantly.

Tenofovir Disoproxil Fumarate. Pharmacokinetic interaction with tenofovir DF (increased tenofovir AUC; no change in lopinavir plasma concentrations and AUC). Clinical importance of this interaction is unknown.

Patients receiving lopinavir/ritonavir and tenofovir DF concomitantly should be monitored for tenofovir toxicity; tenofovir DF should be discontinued if such effects occur.

HIV Protease Inhibitors (PIs) There is in vitro evidence of additive to antagonistic antiretroviral effects with nelfinavir or tipranavir and additive to synergistic effects with amprenavir (active metabolite of fosamprenavir), atazanavir, indinavir, or saquinavir. No in vitro evidence of antagonistic antiretroviral effects between lopinavir and atazanavir or darunavir.

Atazanavir. Because prolonged PR interval has been reported with both lopinavir and atazanavir, lopinavir/ritonavir and atazanavir should be used concomitantly with caution and clinical monitoring.

Darunavir. Concomitant use of *ritonavir-boosted* darunavir and lopinavir/ritonavir results in substantially decreased plasma concentrations of darunavir and no change in lopinavir plasma concentrations.

Concomitant use of lopinavir/ritonavir and *ritonavir-boosted* darunavir is not recommended; appropriate dosages for concomitant use with respect to safety and efficacy have not been established.

Fosamprenavir. Concomitant use of fosamprenavir (without low-dose ritonavir) and lopinavir/ritonavir results in decreased amprenavir plasma concentrations and AUC and unchanged lopinavir plasma concentrations and AUC. Concomitant use of *ritonavir-boosted* fosamprenavir and lopinavir/ritonavir results in decreased amprenavir plasma concentrations and AUC and altered lopinavir plasma concentrations and AUC (decreased or increased). An increased incidence of adverse effects has been reported when the drugs were used concomitantly.

Fosamprenavir (with or without low-dose ritonavir) should not be used concomitantly with lopinavir/ritonavir; appropriate dosages for concomitant use with respect to safety and efficacy have not been established.

Indinavir. Pharmacokinetic interaction with indinavir (increased plasma concentrations of indinavir). The manufacturer of lopinavir/ritonavir states that if these drugs are used concomitantly, the recommended dosage of lopinavir/ritonavir is lopinavir 400 mg/ritonavir 100 mg twice daily and the recommended dosage of indinavir is 600 mg twice daily.

A once-daily regimen of lopinavir/ritonavir has not been studied in patients receiving indinavir.

Nelfinavir. Pharmacokinetic interaction with nelfinavir (decreased plasma concentrations of lopinavir and increased plasma concentrations of nelfinavir and nelfinavir's metabolite M8). If these drugs are used concomitantly, adults should receive lopinavir 500 mg/ritonavir 125 mg (as tablets) twice daily with nelfinavir. Alternatively, adults may receive lopinavir 520 mg/ritonavir 130 mg (as the oral solution) twice daily. A once-daily regimen of lopinavir/ritonavir should not be used in patients receiving nelfinavir.

For dosage recommendations in pediatric patients receiving lopinavir/ritonavir and nelfinavir concomitantly, see Treatment of HIV Infection under Dosage: Pediatric Dosage, in Dosage and Administration.

Ritonavir. Pharmacokinetic interaction with lopinavir (increased plasma concentrations and AUC of lopinavir); used to therapeutic advantage in commercially available fixed-combination lopinavir/ritonavir. In patients receiving lopinavir/ritonavir, appropriate dosages of *additional* ritonavir with respect to safety and efficacy have not been established.

Saquinavir. Pharmacokinetic interaction between lopinavir/ritonavir and saquinavir (increased saquinavir plasma concentrations).

The manufacturer of saquinavir states that saquinavir and lopinavir/ritonavir should be used concomitantly with caution because of the potential for additive effects on QT and/or PR interval prolongation.

If saquinavir is used concomitantly with lopinavir/ritonavir, saquinavir should be given in a dosage of 1 g twice daily with lopinavir 400 mg/ritonavir 100 mg twice daily. Data from clinical studies indicate that saquinavir concentrations achieved with this dosage regimen are similar to those achieved when *ritonavir-boosted* saquinavir is given in a dosage of 1 g of saquinavir and 100 mg of ritonavir twice daily. A once-daily regimen of lopinavir/ritonavir has not been studied in patients receiving saquinavir.

Tipranavir. Concomitant use of *ritonavir-boosted* tipranavir and lopinavir/ritonavir decreased lopinavir plasma concentrations and AUC. Concomitant use of lopinavir/ritonavir and *ritonavir-boosted* tipranavir is not recommended.

■ **Atovaquone** Pharmacokinetic interaction with atovaquone (decreased plasma atovaquone concentrations); clinical importance unknown. Increased atovaquone dosage may be needed in patients receiving lopinavir/ritonavir.

■ **β-Adrenergic Blocking Agents** Possible pharmacokinetic interaction with certain β-adrenergic blocking agents (e.g., metoprolol, timolol) (increased β-adrenergic blocking agent concentrations).

If lopinavir/ritonavir is used concomitantly with a β-adrenergic blocking agent, dosage of the β-adrenergic blocking agent may need to be decreased and should be adjusted based on the patient's clinical response. Use of certain β-adrenergic blocking agents not metabolized by CYP isoenzymes (e.g., atenolol, labetalol, nadolol, sotalol) should be considered.

■ **Benzodiazepines** ***Midazolam or Triazolam*** Pharmacokinetic interaction with midazolam and triazolam (increased plasma benzodiazepine concentrations); potential for serious and/or life-threatening adverse effects (e.g., prolonged or increased sedation or respiratory depression).

Concomitant use of oral midazolam or triazolam with lopinavir/ritonavir is contraindicated. Concomitant use with oral midazolam is expected to result in higher plasma concentrations of midazolam than concomitant use with parenteral midazolam.

Caution is advised if parenteral midazolam is used with lopinavir/ritonavir; concomitant use of parenteral midazolam and lopinavir/ritonavir should be undertaken in a monitored setting where respiratory depression and/or prolonged sedation can be managed. In addition, use of a reduced dose of midazolam should be considered. Some experts state that parenteral midazolam can be given in a single dose with caution in a monitored situation for procedural sedation in patients receiving lopinavir/ritonavir.

Other Benzodiazepines Potential pharmacokinetic interaction with alprazolam, clonazepam, and diazepam (increased benzodiazepine plasma concentrations).

Although pharmacokinetic studies evaluating concomitant use with lopinavir/ritonavir are lacking, some experts recommend that use of benzodiazepines not metabolized by CYP isoenzymes (e.g., lorazepam, oxazepam, temazepam) should be considered since these drugs have less potential for interaction with PIs.

■ **Bosentan** Pharmacokinetic interaction (increased bosentan plasma concentrations).

In patients who have already been receiving lopinavir/ritonavir for at least 10 days, bosentan should be initiated using a dosage of 62.5 mg once daily or every other day based on individual tolerability.

In patients who have already been receiving bosentan, bosentan should be discontinued for at least 36 hours prior to initiating lopinavir/ritonavir; after at least 10 days of lopinavir/ritonavir therapy, bosentan can be resumed using a dosage of 62.5 mg once daily or every other day based on individual tolerability.

■ **Bupropion** Pharmacokinetic interaction (decreased plasma concentrations of bupropion and hydroxybupropion [active metabolite]).

If bupropion and lopinavir/ritonavir are used concomitantly, patients should be monitored for clinical response to bupropion and dosage of the antidepressant titrated as needed.

■ **Buspirone** Pharmacokinetic interaction with buspirone expected (increased buspirone concentrations).

When used concomitantly with lopinavir/ritonavir, a low buspirone dosage should be used with caution and dosage should be titrated based on the patient's clinical response.

■ **Calcium-channel Blocking Agents** Pharmacokinetic interaction with dihydropyridine calcium-channel blocking agents (e.g., felodipine, nicardipine, nifedipine) (increased plasma concentrations of the calcium-channel blocking agent). Use concomitantly with caution; clinical monitoring of the patient recommended.

Potential pharmacokinetic interaction with diltiazem (increased diltiazem plasma concentrations). Diltiazem and lopinavir/ritonavir should be used concomitantly with caution; and diltiazem dosage adjusted based on clinical response and toxicity.

■ **Cobicistat** Lopinavir/ritonavir should not be used concomitantly with the pharmacokinetic enhancer cobicistat because of the similar effects of cobicistat and ritonavir on CYP3A.

■ **Colchicine** Pharmacokinetic interaction (increased colchicine plasma concentrations).

Colchicine and lopinavir/ritonavir should not be used concomitantly in patients with renal or hepatic impairment.

When colchicine is used for *treatment* of gout flares in patients receiving lopinavir/ritonavir, an initial colchicine dose of 0.6 mg should be given followed by 0.3 mg 1 hour later; the colchicine dose should be repeated no earlier than 3 days later.

When colchicine is used for *prophylaxis* of gout flares in patients receiving lopinavir/ritonavir, colchicine dosage should be reduced to 0.3 mg once daily in those originally receiving 0.6 mg twice daily or decreased to 0.3 mg once every other day in those originally receiving 0.6 mg once daily.

When colchicine is used for treatment of familial Mediterranean fever (FMF) in patients receiving lopinavir/ritonavir, a maximum colchicine dosage of 0.6 mg daily (may be given as 0.3 mg twice daily) should be used.

■ **Corticosteroids** ***Orally Inhaled or Intranasal Corticosteroids*** Concomitant use of budesonide (orally inhaled or intranasal) or fluticasone (orally inhaled or intranasal) with lopinavir/ritonavir may result in increased concentrations of the corticosteroid and reduced serum cortisol concentrations, which may result in adrenal insufficiency or Cushing's syndrome.

Budesonide (orally inhaled or intranasal) and fluticasone (orally inhaled or intranasal) should not be used concomitantly with lopinavir/ritonavir unless potential benefits of the inhaled corticosteroid outweigh risks of systemic corticosteroid adverse effects. An alternative corticosteroid (e.g., beclomethasone) should be considered.

Some experts state that concomitant use of beclomethasone (orally inhaled or intranasal) and *ritonavir-boosted* PIs is not expected to result in clinically important pharmacokinetic interactions.

Local Injections of Corticosteroids Concomitant use of intra-articular or other local injections of methylprednisolone, prednisolone, or triamcinolone with lopinavir/ritonavir may result in increased concentrations of the corticosteroid and may result in adrenal insufficiency or Cushing's syndrome.

Lopinavir/ritonavir should not be used concomitantly with local injections of methylprednisolone, prednisolone, or triamcinolone; other nonsteroidal therapies should be considered. If intra-articular corticosteroid therapy is required, an alternative antiretroviral that does not alter CYP3A4 activity should be considered (e.g., dolutegravir, raltegravir).

Systemic Corticosteroids Concomitant use of systemic prednisone with lopinavir/ritonavir increases the area under the concentration-time curve (AUC) of prednisolone and may decrease lopinavir concentrations; concomitant use of systemic budesonide or dexamethasone with lopinavir/ritonavir may result in increased concentrations of the corticosteroid and decreased lopinavir concentrations. Concomitant use of these systemic corticosteroids and lopinavir/ritonavir may result in adrenal insufficiency or Cushing's syndrome and may decrease antiretroviral efficacy.

Systemic budesonide, dexamethasone, or prednisone should be used concomitantly with lopinavir/ritonavir with caution and only when potential benefits outweigh risks of systemic corticosteroid adverse effects, particularly for long-term use of the corticosteroid. An alternative to dexamethasone should be considered for long-term corticosteroid use.

■ **Co-trimoxazole** Clinically important interactions between co-trimoxazole and lopinavir/ritonavir are unlikely.

■ **Dapsone** Clinically important interactions between dapsone and lopinavir/ritonavir are unlikely.

■ **Disulfiram or Metronidazole** Alcohol contained in lopinavir/ritonavir oral solution may result in disulfiram-like reactions if the oral solution is used concomitantly with disulfiram or other drugs that produce this reaction (e.g., metronidazole).

■ **Eplerenone** Pharmacokinetic interaction with eplerenone expected (increased eplerenone concentrations).

Some experts state that concomitant use of eplerenone and lopinavir/ritonavir is contraindicated.

■ **Ergot Alkaloids** Potential for serious adverse effects (e.g., peripheral vasospasm, ischemia of the extremities and other tissues) with ergot alkaloids (e.g., dihydroergotamine, ergotamine, methylergonovine). Concomitant use with lopinavir/ritonavir is contraindicated.

If a woman receiving lopinavir/ritonavir or any other HIV protease inhibitor (PI) as part of an antiretroviral regimen experiences uterine atony and excessive postpartum bleeding, methylergonovine maleate (Methergine®) should be used for treatment of the hemorrhage *only* if alternative treatments (e.g., carboprost, misoprostol, oxytocin, dinoprostone) cannot be used and the potential benefits of the ergot alkaloid outweigh the risks. In this situation, methylergonovine maleate should be used in the lowest dosage and shortest duration possible.

■ **Estrogens and Progestins** Pharmacokinetic interaction with oral contraceptives containing estrogens and progestins (decreased ethinyl estradiol and norethindrone plasma concentrations). Alternative nonhormonal or additional methods of contraception should be used.

Concomitant use of lopinavir/ritonavir and IM medroxyprogesterone acetate resulted in increased peak plasma concentrations and AUC of medroxyprogesterone acetate, but did not result in clinically important effects on trough plasma concentrations of the progestin. Dosage adjustments are not necessary if lopinavir/ritonavir and medroxyprogesterone are used concomitantly.

Concomitant use of lopinavir/ritonavir and subcutaneous implants containing etonogestrel results in increased etonogestrel trough plasma concentrations and AUC. Dosage adjustments are not necessary if lopinavir/ritonavir is used concomitantly with subcutaneous implants containing etonogestrel.

Concomitant use of lopinavir/ritonavir and transdermal systems containing ethinyl estradiol and norelgestromin results in decreased AUC of ethinyl estradiol and increased AUC of norelgestromin. Dosage adjustments are not necessary if lopinavir/ritonavir and transdermal systems containing ethinyl estradiol and norelgestromin are used concomitantly.

■ **Flibanserin** Pharmacokinetic interaction with flibanserin expected (increased flibanserin concentrations).

Some experts state that concomitant use of flibanserin and lopinavir/ritonavir is contraindicated.

■ **Fluvoxamine** Possible pharmacokinetic interaction with fluvoxamine (altered concentrations of lopinavir/ritonavir). Alternative therapy should be considered.

■ **GI Drugs** ***Cisapride*** Concomitant use with cisapride may result in cardiac arrhythmias. Concomitant use of lopinavir/ritonavir and cisapride is contraindicated.

Histamine H_2-receptor Antagonists Concomitant use of ranitidine did not have a clinically important effect on plasma concentrations or AUC of lopinavir/ritonavir.

Dosage adjustments are not necessary if lopinavir/ritonavir is used concomitantly with a histamine H_2-receptor antagonist.

Proton-pump Inhibitors Concomitant use of omeprazole did not have a clinically important effect on plasma concentrations or AUC of lopinavir/ritonavir.

Dosage adjustments are not necessary if lopinavir/ritonavir is used concomitantly with a proton-pump inhibitor.

■ **HCV Antivirals** ***HCV Polymerase Inhibitor*** **Sofosbuvir and Velpatasvir.** Concomitant use of the fixed combination of sofosbuvir and velpatasvir (sofosbuvir/velpatasvir) with lopinavir/ritonavir does not have a clinically important effect on the pharmacokinetics of lopinavir/ritonavir.

HCV Protease Inhibitors **Simeprevir.** Concomitant use of simeprevir and lopinavir/ritonavir may increase plasma concentrations of simeprevir.

Concomitant use of simeprevir and lopinavir/ritonavir is not recommended.

HCV Replication Complex Inhibitors **Daclatasvir.** Concomitant use of lopinavir/ritonavir and daclatasvir results in decreased daclatasvir plasma concentrations and AUC, but this is not considered clinically important.

Dosage adjustments are not necessary if lopinavir/ritonavir and daclatasvir are used concomitantly.

Elbasvir and Grazoprevir. Concomitant use of lopinavir/ritonavir and elbasvir (50 mg once daily) results in increased elbasvir concentrations. Concomitant use of lopinavir/ritonavir and grazoprevir (200 mg once daily) results in substantially increased grazoprevir concentrations; increased grazoprevir concentrations may increase the risk of ALT elevations.

Concomitant use of elbasvir/grazoprevir and lopinavir/ritonavir is contraindicated.

Ledipasvir and Sofosbuvir. Concomitant use of the fixed combination of ledipasvir and sofosbuvir (ledipasvir/sofosbuvir) with lopinavir/ritonavir is not expected to result in clinically important pharmacokinetic interactions. Dosage adjustments are not needed if ledipasvir/sofosbuvir is used concomitantly with lopinavir/ritonavir.

Concomitant use of ledipasvir/sofosbuvir and an HIV antiretroviral regimen that includes lopinavir/ritonavir and tenofovir DF may result in increased tenofovir concentrations. Safety of increased tenofovir concentrations in patients receiving ledipasvir/sofosbuvir and these HIV treatment regimens has not been established. Alternative HCV treatment or an alternative antiretroviral regimen should be considered to avoid increased tenofovir exposure. If concomitant use is necessary, the patient should be monitored for tenofovir-associated adverse effects.

Ombitasvir, Paritaprevir, and Ritonavir. Concomitant use of lopinavir/ritonavir and the fixed combination of ombitasvir, paritaprevir, and ritonavir (ombitasvir/paritaprevir/ritonavir) with or without dasabuvir results in increased concentrations of paritaprevir.

Concomitant use of lopinavir/ritonavir and ombitasvir/paritaprevir/ritonavir with or without dasabuvir is not recommended.

■ **HMG-CoA Reductase Inhibitors** Pharmacokinetic interactions with HMG-CoA reductase inhibitors (statins) metabolized by CYP3A isoenzyme. Concomitant use of lopinavir/ritonavir and certain statins (e.g., atorvastatin, lovastatin, rosuvastatin, simvastatin) may increase plasma concentrations and AUC of the antilipemic agent and increase the risk of statin-associated adverse effects, including myopathy and rhabdomyolysis.

Atorvastatin If atorvastatin is used concomitantly with lopinavir/ritonavir, caution is advised and the lowest necessary atorvastatin dosage should be used.

Lovastatin Concomitant use of lovastatin with lopinavir/ritonavir is contraindicated.

Pitavastatin Pharmacokinetic interaction with pitavastatin (decreased plasma concentrations and AUC of pitavastatin and lopinavir); not considered clinically important.

Dosage adjustments are not necessary if pitavastatin is used concomitantly with lopinavir/ritonavir.

Pravastatin Pharmacokinetic interaction (increased pravastatin plasma concentrations and AUC); not considered clinically important.

Dosage adjustments are not necessary if pravastatin and lopinavir/ritonavir are used concomitantly.

Rosuvastatin If rosuvastatin is used concomitantly with lopinavir/ritonavir, rosuvastatin dosage should not exceed 10 mg daily. Rosuvastatin dosage should be titrated carefully and the lowest necessary dosage used.

Simvastatin Concomitant use of simvastatin with lopinavir/ritonavir is contraindicated.

■ **Immunosuppressive Agents** Pharmacokinetic interaction with cyclosporine, everolimus, sirolimus, tacrolimus expected (increased plasma concentrations of the immunosuppressive agent).

If lopinavir/ritonavir is used concomitantly with cyclosporine, everolimus, sirolimus, or tacrolimus, plasma concentrations of the immunosuppressive agent should be monitored. Some experts state that the immunosuppressive agent should be initiated with an adjusted dosage to account for potential increased concentrations of the drug and the patient should be monitored for toxicities. A specialist should be consulted if necessary.

■ **Ivabradine** Pharmacokinetic interaction with ivabradine expected (increased ivabradine concentrations).

Some experts state that concomitant use of ivabradine and lopinavir/ritonavir is contraindicated.

■ **Macrolides** Clinically important interactions between lopinavir/ritonavir and azithromycin or erythromycin are not expected.

Clarithromycin Pharmacokinetic interaction with clarithromycin (increased plasma concentrations of clarithromycin). Modification of the usual dosage of clarithromycin is not necessary in those with normal renal function; however, the clarithromycin dosage should be reduced by 50% in those with creatinine clearances of 30–60 mL/minute and reduced by 75% in those with creatinine clearances less than 30 mL/minute.

■ **Opiates and Opiate Partial Agonists** ***Buprenorphine*** No clinically important pharmacokinetic interactions if lopinavir/ritonavir is used concomitantly with buprenorphine (sublingual, buccal, or subdermal implant).

Dosage adjustments are not necessary if buprenorphine and lopinavir/ritonavir are used concomitantly; however, clinical monitoring is recommended. If the route of buprenorphine administration is changed from transmucosal to subdermal implantation, the patient should be monitored to ensure that the effect of buprenorphine is adequate and not excessive.

Fentanyl Pharmacokinetic interaction with fentanyl (increased fentanyl plasma concentrations).

Careful monitoring for therapeutic and adverse effects (e.g., potentially fatal respiratory depression) is recommended if fentanyl and lopinavir/ritonavir are used concomitantly.

Methadone Pharmacokinetic interaction with methadone (decreased plasma concentrations and AUC of methadone); opiate withdrawal symptoms are unlikely, but may occur.

If methadone and lopinavir/ritonavir are used concomitantly, patients should be monitored closely for signs of opiate withdrawal; increased methadone dosage may be necessary.

Oxycodone Pharmacokinetic interaction with oxycodone (increased oxycodone AUC).

If oxycodone and lopinavir/ritonavir are used concomitantly, patients should be monitored for opioid-related adverse effects; reduced oxycodone dosage may be necessary.

■ **Phosphodiesterase Type 5 Inhibitors** Concomitant use of lopinavir/ritonavir and selective phosphodiesterase type 5 (PDE5) inhibitors (e.g., avanafil, sildenafil, tadalafil, vardenafil) is expected to result in substantially increased plasma concentrations of the PDE5 inhibitor and increase the risk of adverse effects (e.g., hypotension, syncope, visual disturbances, priapism) associated with these agents.

Avanafil Avanafil should not be used in patients receiving lopinavir/ritonavir; safe and effective dosages for concomitant use have not been established.

Sildenafil Concomitant use of sildenafil (Revatio®) for treatment of pulmonary arterial hypertension (PAH) is contraindicated in patients receiving lopinavir/ritonavir. Safe and effective dosages for concomitant use have not been established.

Sildenafil should be used with caution for treatment of erectile dysfunction in patients receiving lopinavir/ritonavir; sildenafil dosage should not exceed 25 mg once every 48 hours and the patient should be monitored for sildenafil-related adverse effects.

Tadalafil If tadalafil (Adcirca®) is indicated for treatment of PAH in patients who have been receiving lopinavir/ritonavir for at least 1 week, tadalafil should be initiated at a dosage of 20 mg once daily and, if tolerated, dosage may be increased to 40 mg once daily. Lopinavir/ritonavir should not be initiated in patients receiving tadalafil for treatment of PAH; tadalafil should be discontinued for at least 24 hours prior to initiating lopinavir/ritonavir. After at least 1 week, tadalafil may be resumed at a dosage of 20 mg once daily and, if tolerated, dosage may be increased to 40 mg once daily.

Tadalafil should be used with caution for treatment of erectile dysfunction in patients receiving lopinavir/ritonavir; tadalafil dosage should not exceed 10 mg once every 72 hours. The patient should be monitored for tadalafil-related adverse effects.

If tadalafil is used for treatment of benign prostatic hyperplasia in patients receiving lopinavir/ritonavir, tadalafil dosage should not exceed 2.5 mg once daily.

Vardenafil Vardenafil should be used with caution for treatment of erectile dysfunction in patients receiving lopinavir/ritonavir; vardenafil dosage should not exceed 2.5 mg once every 72 hours and the patient should be monitored for vardenafil-related adverse effects.

■ **Salmeterol** Pharmacokinetic interaction (increased salmeterol plasma concentrations) may result in increased risk of salmeterol-associated adverse cardiovascular effects, including QT interval prolongation, palpitations, and sinus tachycardia. The manufacturer of lopinavir/ritonavir and some experts state that concomitant use of lopinavir/ritonavir and salmeterol is not recommended.

■ **Suvorexant** Pharmacokinetic interaction with suvorexant expected (increased suvorexant concentrations).

Some experts state that concomitant use of suvorexant and lopinavir/ritonavir is not recommended.

■ **Trazodone** Possible pharmacokinetic interaction if trazodone is used concomitantly with lopinavir/ritonavir (increased plasma concentrations of trazodone); nausea, dizziness, hypotension, and syncope were observed when trazodone and ritonavir were used concomitantly.

Trazodone and lopinavir/ritonavir should be used concomitantly with caution; a lower trazodone dosage should be considered and the patient monitored for adverse CNS and cardiovascular effects.

■ **Tricyclic Antidepressants** Potential pharmacokinetic interaction with amitriptyline, desipramine, doxepin, imipramine, or nortriptyline (increased plasma concentrations of the tricyclic antidepressant).

If lopinavir/ritonavir is used concomitantly with a tricyclic antidepressant, some experts recommend that the lowest possible dosage of the antidepressant should be used and dosage titrated based on plasma antidepressant concentrations and/or clinical assessment.

The manufacturer of lopinavir/ritonavir states that a drug interaction study using a single 100-mg dose of desipramine did not result in clinically important drug interactions between desipramine and lopinavir/ritonavir.

■ **Zolpidem** Possible pharmacokinetic interaction with zolpidem (increased zolpidem concentrations).

If zolpidem is used concomitantly with lopinavir/ritonavir, some experts state that zolpidem should be initiated using a low dosage and dosage reduction may be needed.

■ **Dietary and Herbal Supplements** ***St. John's wort (Hypericum perforatum)*** Potential pharmacokinetic interaction with St. John's wort (*Hypericum perforatum*) (substantially decreased lopinavir plasma concentrations); potential for loss of virologic response and possible resistance to lopinavir or other PIs. Concomitant use contraindicated.

Description

Lopinavir and ritonavir (lopinavir/ritonavir) is a fixed combination of 2 human immunodeficiency virus (HIV) protease inhibitors (PIs). Lopinavir is extensively metabolized by the hepatic cytochrome P-450 (CYP) enzyme system, principally the 3A isoenzyme. Because ritonavir is a potent inhibitor of CYP3A, concomitant administration of ritonavir and lopinavir results in decreased metabolism and increased plasma concentrations of lopinavir. The concentration of ritonavir present in the fixed combination, although sufficient to inhibit CYP3A, is much lower than ritonavir dosages that are used therapeutically. Therefore, the antiretroviral activity of lopinavir/ritonavir is due to lopinavir.

Lopinavir inhibits replication of HIV type 1 (HIV-1) by interfering with HIV protease. During HIV replication, HIV protease cleaves viral polypeptide products of the *gag* and *gag-pol* genes to form structural proteins of the virion core and essential viral enzymes. By interfering with the formation of these essential proteins and enzymes, lopinavir blocks maturation of the virus and causes formation of nonfunctional, immature, noninfectious virions. Lopinavir also has some in vitro activity against HIV type 2 (HIV-2).

Strains of HIV-1 resistant to lopinavir can be produced in cell culture, and the presence of ritonavir does not appear to influence selection of lopinavir-resistant HIV-1 in cell culture. Strains of HIV-1 resistant to lopinavir have emerged during therapy with the fixed combination of lopinavir and ritonavir. Although varying degrees of HIV cross-resistance have been observed among PIs, the potential for cross-resistance in HIV-1 isolates from patients treated with lopinavir/ritonavir remains to be more fully elucidated.

Advice to Patients

Critical nature of compliance with HIV therapy and importance of remaining under the care of a clinician. Importance of taking as prescribed; do not alter or discontinue antiretroviral regimen without consulting clinician.

Importance of using in conjunction with other antiretrovirals—not for monotherapy.

Antiretroviral therapy is not a cure for HIV infection; opportunistic infections and other complications associated with HIV disease may still occur.

Advise patients that sustained decreases in plasma HIV RNA have been associated with reduced risk of progression to AIDS and death.

Advise patients that effective antiretroviral regimens can decrease HIV concentrations in blood and genital secretions and strict adherence to such regimens in conjunction with risk-reduction measures may decrease, but cannot absolutely eliminate, the risk of secondary transmission of HIV to others. Importance of continuing to practice safer sex (e.g., using latex or polyurethane condoms to minimize sexual contact with body fluids), never sharing personal items that can have blood or body fluids on them (e.g., toothbrushes, razor blades), and never reusing or sharing needles.

Importance of reading patient information provided by the manufacturer.

Provide patient or their caregiver with complete dosing instructions. Advise patient or their caregiver to pay special attention to dosing instructions to minimize risk of accidental overdosage or underdosage. Importance of informing clinician if child's weight changes.

Importance of taking lopinavir/ritonavir as directed and importance of not missing a dose. If a dose is missed, the dose should be taken as soon as it is remembered and the next dose taken at the regularly scheduled time; if a dose is skipped, do not double the next dose.

When lopinavir/ritonavir tablets are used, doses may be taken with or without food. If also taking didanosine, both drugs may be taken at the same time without food.

When lopinavir/ritonavir oral solution is used, importance of taking with food. If also taking didanosine, take didanosine 1 hour before or 2 hours after lopinavir/ritonavir oral solution.

Advise patients that mild to severe skin reactions have occurred. Importance of contacting clinician if rash occurs.

Advise patients that liver disease (including fatalities) have been reported. Importance of notifying clinician if manifestations of liver disease occur (e.g., jaundice of skin or eyes, dark tea-colored urine, pale stools, itchy skin, loss of appetite, or pain, aching, or sensitivity in right upper quadrant of abdomen).

Advise patients that severe pancreatitis (including fatalities) has been reported. Importance of notifying clinician if manifestations of pancreatitis occur (e.g., nausea, vomiting, stomach pain).

Importance of informing clinicians if signs or symptoms of diabetes (e.g., frequent urination, excessive thirst, extreme hunger, unusual weight loss, increased blood glucose), or cardiac effects (e.g., dizziness, lightheadedness, heart rhythm changes, loss of consciousness) occur.

Redistribution/accumulation of body fat may occur with antiretroviral therapy, with as yet unknown long-term health effects.

Importance of informing clinicians of existing or contemplated concomitant therapy, including prescription and OTC drugs and herbal products (e.g., St. John's wort), as well as any concomitant illnesses.

Advise patients receiving a selective phosphodiesterase type 5 (PDE5) inhibitor (e.g., avanafil, sildenafil, tadalafil, vardenafil) that they may be at increased risk of PDE5 inhibitor-associated adverse effects (e.g., hypotension, syncope, visual disturbances, priapism) and that any symptoms should be promptly reported to their clinician. Lopinavir/ritonavir should not be used in patients receiving sildenafil for treatment of pulmonary arterial hypertension (PAH or avanafil).

If lopinavir/ritonavir oral solution is used in young infants, advise caregiver that the oral solution contains alcohol and propylene glycol which can cause serious adverse effects in neonates younger than 14 days of age (whether premature or full-term). Importance of immediately informing clinician if infant appears too sleepy or if their breathing has changed.

Importance of women using a reliable nonhormonal (e.g., barrier) method of contraception because of the potential interaction with hormonal contraceptives.

Importance of women informing clinicians if they are or plan to become pregnant or plan to breast-feed. Advise HIV-infected women not to breast-feed.

Importance of informing patients of other precautionary information. (See Cautions.)

Preparations

Excipients in commercially available drug preparations may have clinically important effects in some individuals; consult specific product labeling for details.

Lopinavir and Ritonavir

Oral Solution	Lopinavir 400 mg/5 mL and Ritonavir 100 mg/5 mL	Kaletra®, AbbVie
Tablets, film-coated	Lopinavir 100 mg and Ritonavir 25 mg	Kaletra®, AbbVie
	Lopinavir 200 mg and Ritonavir 50 mg	Kaletra®, AbbVie

†Use is not currently included in the labeling approved by the US Food and Drug Administration

HIV Integrase Inhibitors 8:18.08.12

Bictegravir Sodium, Emtricitabine, and Tenofovir Alafenamide Fumarate

BIC/FTC/TAF, BIC/TAF/FTC, BIC, FTC, TAF Fumarate, TAF

■ Bictegravir sodium, emtricitabine, and tenofovir alafenamide fumarate (BIC/FTC/TAF) is a fixed-combination antiretroviral agent containing bictegravir (human immunodeficiency virus [HIV] integrase strand transfer inhibitor [INSTI]), emtricitabine (HIV nucleoside reverse transcriptase inhibitor [NRTI]), and tenofovir alafenamide (HIV nucleotide reverse transcriptase inhibitor).

Uses

■ **Treatment of HIV Infection** The fixed combination of bictegravir sodium, emtricitabine, and tenofovir alafenamide fumarate (BIC/FTC/TAF) is used for the treatment of human immunodeficiency virus type 1 (HIV-1) infection in antiretroviral-naive (have not previously received antiretroviral therapy) or antiretroviral-experienced (previously treated) adults.

BIC/FTC/TAF is used alone as a complete regimen for the treatment of HIV-1 infection; concomitant use with other antiretroviral agents is not recommended.

The most appropriate antiretroviral regimen cannot be defined for each clinical scenario, and selection of specific antiretroviral agents for use in multiple-drug regimens should be individualized based on information regarding antiretroviral potency, potential rate of development of resistance, known toxicities, and potential for pharmacokinetic interactions as well as virologic, immunologic, and clinical characteristics of the patient. For information on the general principles and guidelines for use of antiretroviral therapy, including specific recommendations for initial therapy in antiretroviral-naive patients and recommendations for changing antiretroviral regimens, see the Antiretroviral Agents General Statement 8:18.08.

Antiretroviral-naive Adults For *initial* treatment in HIV-infected adults, the US Department of Health and Human Services (HHS) Panel on Antiretroviral Guidelines for Adults and Adolescents states that BIC/FTC/TAF is a recommended HIV integrase strand transfer inhibitor-based (INSTI-based) regimen for most antiretroviral-naive adults.

Clinical Experience. Efficacy and safety of BIC/FTC/TAF in antiretroviral-naive HIV-infected adults were evaluated in 2 randomized, double blind, active-control, noninferiority phase 3 studies (study 1489; NCT02607930 and study 1490; NCT02607956).

In study 1489, 629 antiretroviral-naive adults (mean age 34 years, 90% male, 57% white, 36% black, 3% Asian, 22% Hispanic/Latino, mean baseline plasma HIV-1 RNA level 4.4 $\log_{10}$ copies/mL, mean baseline CD4$^+$ T-cell count 464 cells/mm^3) were randomized in a 1:1 ratio to receive BIC/FTC/TAF (bictegravir 50 mg, emtricitabine 200 mg, tenofovir alafenamide 25 mg) once daily or the fixed combination of abacavir 600 mg, dolutegravir 50 mg, and lamivudine 300 mg (ABC/DTG/3TC) once daily. The primary end point was virologic response (defined as plasma HIV-1 RNA levels less than 50 copies/mL) at 48 weeks. Results at 48 weeks indicated that BIC/FTC/TAF is noninferior to ABC/DTG/3TC in the proportion of patients achieving virologic response (92 and 93%, respectively). The mean increase in CD4$^+$ T-cell count from baseline was 233 cells/mm^3 in those receiving BIC/FTC/TAF compared with 229 cells/mm^3 in those receiving ABC/DTG/3TC. Treatment outcomes were similar across subgroups (i.e., age, gender, race, baseline viral load, and baseline CD4$^+$ T-cell count).

In study 1490, 645 antiretroviral-naive adults (mean age 37 years, 88% male, 59% white, 31% black, 3% Asian, 25% Hispanic/Latino, mean baseline plasma HIV-1 RNA level 4.4 $\log_{10}$ copies/mL, mean baseline CD4$^+$ T-cell count 456 cells/mm^3) were randomized to receive BIC/FTC/TAF (bictegravir 50 mg, emtricitabine 200 mg, tenofovir alafenamide 25 mg) once daily or a regimen of dolutegravir 50 mg in conjunction with the fixed combination of emtricitabine 200 mg and tenofovir alafenamide 25 mg (emtricitabine/tenofovir alafenamide) once daily. The primary end point was virologic response (defined as plasma HIV-1 RNA levels less than 50 copies/mL) at 48 weeks. Results at 48 weeks indicated that BIC/FTC/TAF is noninferior to a regimen of dolutegravir and emtricitabine/tenofovir alafenamide in the proportion of patients achieving virologic response (89% and 93%, respectively). The mean increase in CD4$^+$ T-cell count from baseline was 180 cells/mm^3 in those receiving BIC/FTC/TAF compared with 201 cells/mm^3 in those receiving the regimen of dolutegravir and emtricitabine/tenofovir alafenamide. Treatment outcomes were similar across subgroups (i.e., age, gender, race, baseline viral load, and baseline CD4$^+$ T-cell count).

Antiretroviral-experienced Adults For use in antiretroviral-experienced adults, the manufacturer states that BIC/FTC/TAF can be used to replace the current antiretroviral regimen in those who have had plasma HIV-1 RNA levels less than 50 copies/mL on a stable antiretroviral regimen for at least 3 months, have no history of treatment failure, and are infected with HIV-1 with no known substitutions associated with resistance to the antiretroviral components of the fixed combination (i.e., bictegravir, emtricitabine, tenofovir).

Clinical Experience. Efficacy and safety of BIC/FTC/TAF in antiretroviral-experienced adults were evaluated in a randomized, double-blind, active-control, noninferiority phase 3 study (trial 1844; NCT02603120) and a randomized, open-label, active-control, noninferiority phase 3 study (trial 1878; NCT02603107).

In trial 1844, 563 previously treated adults with baseline plasma HIV-1 RNA levels less than 50 copies/mL for at least 3 months and no history of treatment failure (mean age 45 years, 89% male, 73% white, 22% black, 17% Hispanic/Latino, mean baseline CD4$^+$ T-cell count 723 cells/mm^3) were randomized to either switch to BIC/FTC/TAF (bictegravir 50 mg, emtricitabine 200 mg, tenofovir alafenamide 25 mg) once daily or continue their baseline antiretroviral regimen of ABC/DTG/3TC. At 48 weeks, 94% of those receiving BIC/FTC/TAF had plasma HIV-1 RNA levels less than 50 copies/mL compared with 95% of those who continued to receive ABC/DTG/3TC. The mean change in CD4$^+$ T-cell count from baseline was -31 cells/mm^3 in those receiving BIC/FTC/TAF compared with 4 cells/mm^3 in those who continued to receive ABC/DTG/3TC.

Trial 1878 included 577 previously treated adults with baseline plasma HIV-1 RNA levels less than 50 copies/mL for at least 6 months, no previous treatment with an INSTI, and no history of treatment failure (mean age 46 years, 83% male, 66% white, 26% black, 19% Hispanic/Latino, mean baseline CD4$^+$ T-cell count 663 cells/mm^3) were randomized to either switch to BIC/FTC/TAF (bictegravir 50 mg, emtricitabine 200 mg, tenofovir alafenamide 25 mg) once daily or continue their baseline antiretroviral regimen (at baseline, 15% were receiving *cobicistat-* or *ritonavir-boosted* atazanavir or darunavir concomitantly with the fixed combination of abacavir and lamivudine [abacavir/lamivudine], 85% were receiving *cobicistat-* or *ritonavir-boosted* atazanavir or darunavir concomitantly with the fixed combination of emtricitabine and tenofovir disoproxil fumarate [emtricitabine/tenofovir DF]). At 48 weeks, 92% of those receiving BIC/FTC/TAF had plasma HIV-1 RNA levels less than 50 copies/mL compared with 89% of those who continued to receive their baseline regimen. The mean change in CD4$^+$ T-cell count from baseline was 25 cells/mm^3 in those receiving BIC/FTC/TAF compared with 0 cells/mm^3 in those who continued to receive their baseline regimen.

Treatment outcomes in trial 1844 and trial 1878 were similar across subgroups (i.e., age, gender, race, and region).

Dosage and Administration

■ **Administration** The fixed combination of bictegravir sodium, emtricitabine, and tenofovir alafenamide fumarate (BIC/FTC/TAF) is administered orally once daily without regard to food.

Serum creatinine, estimated creatinine clearance, urine glucose, and urine protein should be determined prior to initiation of BIC/FTC/TAF and routinely monitored during treatment in all patients as clinically appropriate. In patients with chronic kidney disease, serum phosphorus also should be determined. (See Renal Impairment under Warnings/Precautions: Specific Populations, in Cautions.)

Patients should be tested for hepatitis B virus (HBV) infection prior to initiation of BIC/FTC/TAF. (See HIV-infected Individuals Coinfected with Hepatitis B Virus under Warnings/Precautions: Warnings, in Cautions.)

■ **Dosage** Fixed combination tablets of BIC/FTC/TAF contain bictegravir sodium, emtricitabine, and tenofovir alafenamide fumarate; dosage of bictegravir sodium is expressed in terms of bictegravir and dosage of tenofovir alafenamide fumarate is expressed in terms of tenofovir alafenamide.

Each fixed-combination tablet of BIC/FTC/TAF contains bictegravir 50 mg, emtricitabine 200 mg, and tenofovir alafenamide 25 mg.

Adult Dosage **Treatment of HIV Infection.** For the treatment of human immunodeficiency virus type 1 (HIV-1) infection in adults, the usual dosage of BIC/FTC/TAF is 1 tablet (50 mg of bictegravir, 200 mg of emtricitabine, and 25 mg of tenofovir alafenamide) once daily.

■ **Special Populations** ***Hepatic Impairment*** Dosage adjustments are not necessary if BIC/FTC/TAF is used in patients with mild or moderate hepatic impairment (Child-Pugh class A or B).

BIC/FTC/TAF is not recommended in patients with severe hepatic impairment (Child-Pugh class C). (See Hepatic Impairment under Warnings/Precautions: Specific Populations, in Cautions.)

Renal Impairment Dosage adjustments are not necessary if BIC/FTC/TAF is used in patients with estimated creatinine clearance of 30 mL/minute or greater.

BIC/FTC/TAF is not recommended in patients with estimated creatinine clearance less than 30 mL/minute. (See Renal Impairment under Warnings/Precautions: Specific Populations, in Cautions.)

Cautions

■ **Contraindications** Concomitant use of the fixed combination of bictegravir sodium, emtricitabine, and tenofovir alafenamide fumarate (BIC/FTC/TAF) and dofetilide is contraindicated since concomitant use may result in serious and/or life-threatening adverse effects due to possible increased dofetilide plasma concentrations. (See Drug Interactions.)

Concomitant use of BIC/FTC/TAF and rifampin is contraindicated since substantially decreased plasma bictegravir concentrations may occur and may result in loss of virologic response and development of resistance. (See Drug Interactions.)

■ **Warnings/Precautions** *Warnings* **HIV-infected Individuals Coinfected with Hepatitis B Virus.** HIV-infected patients should be tested for hepatitis B virus (HBV) infection before antiretroviral therapy is initiated.

In HIV-infected patients with HBV coinfection, severe acute exacerbations of HBV infection, including liver decompensation and liver failure, have occurred following discontinuance of preparations containing emtricitabine and/or tenofovir disoproxil fumarate (tenofovir DF). Such reactions could occur following discontinuance of BIC/FTC/TAF.

Hepatic function should be closely monitored with clinical and laboratory follow-up for at least several months after BIC/FTC/TAF is discontinued in patients coinfected with HIV-1 and HBV. If appropriate, initiation of HBV treatment may be warranted, especially in patients with advanced liver disease or cirrhosis.

Other Warnings and Precautions **Interactions.** The potential for drug interactions should be considered prior to and during treatment with BIC/FTC/TAF and the patient should be monitored for adverse effects associated with concomitant drugs.

Concomitant use of BIC/FTC/TAF with certain drugs may result in substantial drug interactions, which may lead to loss of therapeutic effect of BIC/FTC/TAF and possible development of resistance or possible adverse effects from increased exposures of concomitant drugs. (See Drug Interactions.)

Renal Toxicity. Renal impairment, including cases of acute renal failure and Fanconi syndrome (renal tubular injury with severe hypophosphatemia), has been reported in patients receiving tenofovir prodrugs (e.g., tenofovir DF).

There were no cases of Fanconi syndrome or proximal renal tubulopathy (PRT) in clinical trials evaluating BIC/FTC/TAF. In treatment-naive patients with estimated glomerular filtration rates (eGFRs) exceeding 30 mL/minute and in virologically suppressed patients with eGFRs exceeding 50 mL/minute who were switched to BIC/FTC/TAF, serious adverse renal effects occurred in less than 1% of patients.

Serum creatinine, estimated creatinine clearance, urine glucose, and urine protein should be determined prior to initiating BIC/FTC/TAF and routinely monitored during treatment in all patients as clinically appropriate. In patients with chronic kidney disease, serum phosphorus also should be determined. (See Renal Impairment under Warnings/Precautions: Specific Populations, in Cautions.)

BIC/FTC/TAF is not recommended in patients with estimated creatinine clearance less than 30 mL/minute.

Patients receiving a tenofovir prodrug who have impaired renal function or are receiving a nephrotoxic agent (e.g., nonsteroidal anti-inflammatory agents [NSAIAs]) are at increased risk of developing adverse renal effects. (See Drug Interactions: Drugs Affecting Renal Function.)

BIC/FTC/TAF should be discontinued in patients who develop clinically important decreases in renal function or evidence of Fanconi syndrome.

Lactic Acidosis and Severe Hepatomegaly with Steatosis. Lactic acidosis and severe hepatomegaly with steatosis, including fatalities, have been reported in patients receiving HIV nucleoside reverse transcriptase inhibitors (NRTIs), including emtricitabine and the tenofovir prodrug tenofovir DF, alone or in conjunction with other antiretrovirals.

BIC/FTC/TAF treatment should be interrupted in any patient who develops clinical or laboratory findings suggestive of lactic acidosis or pronounced hepatotoxicity (signs of hepatotoxicity may include hepatomegaly and steatosis even in the absence of marked increases in serum aminotransferase concentrations).

Immune Reconstitution Syndrome. Immune reconstitution syndrome has been reported in HIV-infected patients receiving multiple-drug antiretroviral therapy. During the initial phase of treatment, HIV-infected patients whose immune systems respond to antiretroviral therapy may develop an inflammatory response to indolent or residual opportunistic infections (e.g., *Mycobacterium avium*, *M. tuberculosis*, cytomegalovirus [CMV], *Pneumocystis jirovecii* [formerly *P. carinii*]); such response may necessitate further evaluation and treatment.

Autoimmune disorders (e.g., Graves' disease, polymyositis, Guillain-Barré syndrome) also have been reported to occur in the setting of immune reconstitution; however, the time to onset is more variable and can occur many months after initiation of antiretroviral therapy.

Use of Fixed Combinations. The usual cautions, precautions, contraindications, and interactions associated with each component of BIC/FTC/TAF should be considered. Cautionary information applicable to specific populations (e.g., pregnant or nursing women, individuals with hepatic or renal impairment, geriatric patients) should be considered for each drug in the fixed combination. For cautionary information related to emtricitabine, see Cautions in Emtricitabine 8:18.08.20.

BIC/FTC/TAF is used alone as a complete regimen for the treatment of HIV-1 infection and use in conjunction with other antiretrovirals is not recommended.

Specific Populations **Pregnancy.** Antiretroviral Pregnancy Registry at 800-258-4263 or http://www.apregistry.com.

There are insufficient data on human use of BIC/FTC/TAF during pregnancy.

In animals, there was no evidence of adverse developmental outcomes when the individual components of BIC/FTC/TAF were administered in rabbits at exposures that were not maternally toxic or in rats and mice at exposures greater than those achieved in humans at the recommended human dosage.

Some experts state that BIC/FTC/TAF is not recommended during pregnancy.

Lactation. It is not known whether bictegravir or tenofovir alafenamide is distributed into human milk. Emtricitabine is distributed into human milk. Bictegravir was detected in the plasma of nursing rat pups, likely due to the presence of bictegravir in milk. Tenofovir is distributed into milk in rats and rhesus monkey following administration of tenofovir DF; it is not known whether tenofovir alafenamide is distributed into animal milk.

It is not known whether BIC/FTC/TAF affects human milk production or affects the breast-fed infant.

Because of the risk of adverse effects in the infant and the risk of HIV transmission, HIV-infected women should not breast-feed infants.

Pediatric Use. Safety and efficacy of BIC/FTC/TAF have not been established in pediatric patients younger than 18 years of age.

Geriatric Use. Clinical studies of BIC/FTC/TAF did not include a sufficient number of patients 65 years of age and older to determine if they respond differently than younger adults.

Population pharmacokinetic analysis of HIV-infected adults receiving BIC/FTC/TAF in phase 3 clinical trials indicates that age does not have a clinically important effect on bictegravir or tenofovir alafenamide exposures in adults up to 74 years of age.

Hepatic Impairment. Mild hepatic impairment (Child-Pugh class A) does not have a clinically important effect on the pharmacokinetics of tenofovir alafenamide. Moderate hepatic impairment (Child-Pugh class B) does not have a clinically important effect on the pharmacokinetics of bictegravir or tenofovir alafenamide. Hepatic impairment is not expected to affect the pharmacokinetics of emtricitabine.

BIC/FTC/TAF is *not* recommended in patients with severe hepatic impairment (Child-Pugh class C). Data are not available to date regarding the pharmacokinetics or safety of BIC/FTC/TAF in such patients.

Renal Impairment. Serum creatinine, estimated creatinine clearance, urine glucose, and urine protein should be determined prior to initiating BIC/FTC/TAF and routinely monitored during treatment in all patients as clinically appropriate. In patients with chronic kidney disease, serum phosphorus also should be determined.

There are no clinically important differences in the pharmacokinetics of bictegravir, tenofovir alafenamide, or tenofovir in individuals with severe renal impairment compared with healthy individuals.

BIC/FTC/TAF is *not* recommended in patients with estimated creatinine clearance less than 30 mL/minute. (See Renal Toxicity under Warnings/Precautions: Other Warnings and Precautions, in Cautions.)

■ **Common Adverse Effects** Adverse effects reported in 5% or more of patients receiving BIC/FTC/TAF include diarrhea, nausea, headache, upper respiratory tract infection, nasopharyngitis, fatigue, arthralgia, and lymphadenopathy.

Drug Interactions

The following drug interactions are based on studies that used bictegravir sodium, emtricitabine, or tenofovir alafenamide fumarate alone or the fixed combination of bictegravir, emtricitabine, and tenofovir alafenamide fumarate (BIC/FTC/TAF) or are predicted to occur.

Potential drug interactions associated with each drug in the fixed combination should be considered.

■ **Drugs Affecting or Metabolized by Hepatic Microsomal Enzymes** Bictegravir is a substrate of cytochrome P-450 (CYP) isoenzyme 3A. The drug does not inhibit CYP isoenzymes (including CYP3A) at clinically relevant concentrations.

Emtricitabine is not a substrate of CYP isoenzymes; emtricitabine does not inhibit CYP1A2, 2A6, 2B6, 2C9, 2C19, 2D6, or 3A4.

Tenofovir alafenamide does not inhibit CYP isoenzymes (including CYP3A) at clinically relevant concentrations.

Potential pharmacokinetic interactions if BIC/FTC/TAF is used concomitantly with drugs that are potent inducers of CYP3A *and* also are inducers of uridine diphosphate-glucuronosyltransferase (UGT) 1A1 enzyme (decreased plasma concentrations of bictegravir; possible decreased antiretroviral efficacy and development of resistance).

Potential pharmacokinetic interactions if BIC/FTC/TAF is used concomitantly with drugs that are potent inhibitors of CYP3A *and* also are inhibitors of UGT1A1 (increased plasma concentrations of bictegravir).

■ Drugs Affecting or Metabolized by Uridine Diphosphate-glucuronosyltransferase Bictegravir is a substrate of UGT1A1. Bictegravir and tenofovir alafenamide do not inhibit UGT1A1.

Potential pharmacokinetic interactions if BIC/FTC/TAF is used concomitantly with drugs that are potent inducers of CYP3A *and* also are inducers of UGT1A1 (decreased plasma concentrations of bictegravir; possible decreased antiretroviral efficacy and development of resistance).

Potential pharmacokinetic interactions if BIC/FTC/TAF is used concomitantly with drugs that are potent inhibitors of CYP3A *and* also are inhibitors of UGT1A1 (increased plasma concentrations of bictegravir).

■ Drugs Affecting or Affected by P-glycoprotein Transport Tenofovir alafenamide is a substrate of P-glycoprotein (P-gp) transport. The drug does not inhibit P-gp.

Potential pharmacokinetic interactions if BIC/FTC/TAF is used concomitantly with drugs that induce P-gp (decreased absorption and decreased plasma concentrations of tenofovir alafenamide; possible decreased antiretroviral efficacy and development of resistance).

Potential pharmacokinetic interactions if BIC/FTC/TAF is used concomitantly with drugs that inhibit P-gp *and* breast cancer resistance protein (BCRP) (increased absorption and increased plasma concentrations of tenofovir alafenamide).

■ Drugs Affecting or Affected by Breast Cancer Resistance Protein Tenofovir alafenamide is a substrate of BCRP. The drug does not inhibit BCRP.

Potential pharmacokinetic interactions if BIC/FTC/TAF is used concomitantly with drugs that inhibit P-gp *and* BCRP (increased absorption and increased plasma concentrations of tenofovir alafenamide).

■ Drugs Affecting or Affected by Multidrug and Toxin Extrusion Transporter Bictegravir inhibits multidrug and toxin extrusion transporter (MATE) 1. Therefore, bictegravir may increase plasma concentrations of drugs eliminated by MATE1 (e.g., dofetilide).

Tenofovir alafenamide does not inhibit MATE1.

■ Drugs Affecting or Affected by Renal Organic Anion Transporters Bictegravir and tenofovir alafenamide do not inhibit renal organic anion transporter (OAT) 1 or OAT3.

Bictegravir and tenofovir alafenamide do not inhibit hepatic organic anion transporter polypeptide (OATP) 1B1 or OATP1B3.

■ Drugs Affecting or Affected by Renal Organic Cation Transporters Bictegravir inhibits renal organic cation transporter (OCT) 2. Therefore, bictegravir may increase plasma concentrations of drugs eliminated by OCT2 (e.g., dofetilide).

Bictegravir and tenofovir alafenamide do not inhibit OCT1. Tenofovir alafenamide does not inhibit OCT2.

■ Drugs Affecting or Affected by Bile Salt Export Pump Bictegravir and tenofovir alafenamide do not inhibit bile salt export pump (BSEP).

■ Drugs Affecting Renal Function The emtricitabine and tenofovir components of BIC/FTC/TAF are principally excreted by the kidneys by a combination of glomerular filtration and active tubular secretion.

Potential pharmacokinetic interactions if BIC/FTC/TAF is used concomitantly with drugs that reduce renal function or compete for active tubular secretion (e.g., acyclovir, aminoglycosides [gentamicin], cidofovir, ganciclovir, valacyclovir, valganciclovir, high-dose or multiple nonsteroidal anti-inflammatory agents [NSAIAs]); may result in increased concentrations of emtricitabine, tenofovir, and/or the concomitant drug and may increase the risk of adverse effects. Concomitant use of BIC/FTC/TAF and nephrotoxic drugs should be avoided.

■ α_1-Adrenergic Blocking Agents Pharmacokinetic interactions are not expected between bictegravir and α_1-adrenergic blocking agents (e.g., alfuzosin, doxazosin, silodosin, tamsulosin, terazosin); dosage adjustments are not necessary if BIC/FTC/TAF is used concomitantly with any of these drugs.

■ Anticoagulants ***Apixaban, Betrixaban, Dabigatran, Edoxaban, and Rivaroxaban*** Pharmacokinetic interactions are not expected if bictegravir is used concomitantly with certain anticoagulants (e.g., apixaban, betrixaban, dabigatran, edoxaban, rivaroxaban); dosage adjustments are not necessary if BIC/FTC/TAF is used concomitantly with any of these anticoagulants.

Warfarin Pharmacokinetic interactions are not expected if bictegravir is used concomitantly with warfarin; dosage adjustments are not necessary if BIC/FTC/TAF is used concomitantly with warfarin.

■ Anticonvulsants ***Carbamazepine and Oxcarbazepine*** Concomitant use of carbamazepine (300 mg twice daily) and tenofovir alafenamide (single 25-mg dose) in fixed combination with emtricitabine decreases peak plasma concentrations and area under the plasma concentration-time curve (AUC) of tenofovir alafenamide.

Concomitant use of bictegravir and carbamazepine or oxcarbazepine is expected to decrease bictegravir exposures. An alternative anticonvulsant or an alternative to BIC/FTC/TAF should be considered.

Eslicarbazepine Possible pharmacokinetic interactions if eslicarbazepine is used concomitantly with bictegravir (decreased bictegravir concentrations). An alternative anticonvulsant or alternative to BIC/FTC/TAF should be considered.

Ethosuximide Pharmacokinetic interactions are not expected if bictegravir is used concomitantly with ethosuximide; dosage adjustments are not necessary if BIC/FTC/TAF is used concomitantly with ethosuximide.

Lamotrigine Pharmacokinetic interactions are not expected if bictegravir is used concomitantly with lamotrigine; dosage adjustments are not necessary if BIC/FTC/TAF is used concomitantly with lamotrigine.

Phenobarbital and Phenytoin Concomitant use of BIC/FTC/TAF and phenobarbital or phenytoin is expected to decrease plasma concentrations of bictegravir and tenofovir alafenamide.

Concomitant use of BIC/FTC/TAF and phenobarbital or phenytoin is not recommended; an alternative anticonvulsant should be considered.

Valproic Acid Data are not available regarding concomitant use of valproic acid and bictegravir; valproic acid concentrations and virologic response should be monitored if valproic acid is used concomitantly with BIC/FTC/TAF.

■ Antidiabetic Agents ***Dapagliflozin and Saxagliptin*** Pharmacokinetic interactions are not expected if bictegravir is used concomitantly with dapagliflozin and/or saxagliptin; dosage adjustments are not necessary if BIC/FTC/TAF is used concomitantly with these antidiabetic agents.

Metformin Concomitant use of metformin hydrochloride (500 mg twice daily), bictegravir (50 mg once daily), and tenofovir alafenamide (25 mg once daily) increases metformin peak plasma concentrations by 1.3-fold, trough plasma concentrations by 1.4-fold, and AUC by 1.4-fold.

If BIC/FTC/TAF and metformin are used concomitantly, the benefits and risks of concomitant use should be considered and patients should be monitored for metformin adverse effects.

■ Antifungal Agents ***Isavuconazonium, Itraconazole, and Posaconazole*** Pharmacokinetic interactions are expected or possible if bictegravir is used concomitantly with isavuconazonium, itraconazole, or posaconazole (increased bictegravir concentrations). Some experts state that dosage adjustments are not necessary if BIC/FTC/TAF is used concomitantly with any of these antifungals.

Voriconazole Concomitant use of voriconazole (300 mg twice daily) and bictegravir (single 75-mg dose) under fasting conditions increases bictegravir AUC, but does not affect peak plasma concentrations of the drug. Some experts state that dosage adjustments are not necessary if BIC/FTC/TAF is used concomitantly with voriconazole.

■ Antimycobacterial Agents ***Rifabutin*** Concomitant use of rifabutin (300 mg once daily) and bictegravir (75 mg once daily) under fasting conditions decreases bictegravir peak plasma concentrations by 20%, AUC by 38%, and trough plasma concentrations by 56%. Concomitant use of rifabutin with BIC/FTC/TAF may decrease plasma concentrations of tenofovir alafenamide.

Concomitant use of rifabutin and BIC/FTC/TAF is not recommended.

Rifampin Concomitant use of rifampin (600 mg once daily) and bictegravir (single 75-mg dose) under fed conditions decreases bictegravir peak plasma concentrations by 28% and AUC by 75%. Concomitant use of rifampin and BIC/FTC/TAF may decrease plasma concentrations of tenofovir alafenamide.

Concomitant use of rifampin and BIC/FTC/TAF is contraindicated.

Rifapentine Pharmacokinetic interactions with rifapentine are expected (decreased bictegravir and tenofovir alafenamide plasma concentrations).

Concomitant use of rifapentine and BIC/FTC/TAF is not recommended.

■ Antiplatelet Agents ***Ticagrelor and Vorapaxar*** Pharmacokinetic interactions are not expected if bictegravir is used concomitantly with ticagrelor or vorapaxar; dosage adjustments are not necessary if BIC/FTC/TAF is used concomitantly with these antiplatelet agents.

■ Antipsychotic Agents Pharmacokinetic interactions are not expected if bictegravir is used concomitantly with aripiprazole, brexpiprazole, cariprazine, lurasidone, pimavanserin, pimozide, or quetiapine; dosage adjustments are not necessary if BIC/FTC/TAF is used concomitantly with any of these antipsychotic agents.

■ Antiretroviral Agents Fixed-combination BIC/FTC/TAF should not be used in conjunction with any other antiretrovirals.

HIV Nucleoside and Nucleotide Reverse Transcriptase Inhibitors (NRTIs) **Emtricitabine.** There is in vitro evidence of synergistic antiretroviral effects when bictegravir is used with emtricitabine.

Tenofovir Alafenamide Fumarate. There is in vitro evidence of synergistic antiretroviral effects when bictegravir is used with tenofovir alafenamide.

■ Benzodiazepines Concomitant use of midazolam with bictegravir and tenofovir alafenamide does not have a clinically important effect on midazolam concentrations.

Pharmacokinetic interactions are not expected if bictegravir is used concomitantly with midazolam or other benzodiazepines (e.g., clonazepam, clorazepate, diazepam, estazolam, flurazepam, triazolam); dosage adjustments are not necessary if BIC/FTC/TAF is used concomitantly with any of these benzodiazepines.

■ **Bupropion** Pharmacokinetic interactions are not expected if bictegravir is used concomitantly with bupropion; dosage adjustments are not necessary if BIC/FTC/TAF is used concomitantly with bupropion.

■ **Buspirone** Pharmacokinetic interactions are not expected if bictegravir is used concomitantly with buspirone; dosage adjustments are not necessary if BIC/FTC/TAF is used concomitantly with buspirone.

■ **Calcifediol** Pharmacokinetic interactions are not expected if bictegravir is used concomitantly with calcifediol; dosage adjustments are not necessary if BIC/FTC/TAF is used concomitantly with calcifediol.

■ **Calcium, Iron, Multivitamins, and Other Preparations Containing Polyvalent Cations** Pharmacokinetic interactions reported when a single 1.2-g dose of calcium carbonate was administered simultaneously with a single 50-mg dose of bictegravir in the fasting state (decreased peak plasma concentrations and AUC of bictegravir). No clinically important pharmacokinetic interactions were observed when a single 1.2-g dose of calcium carbonate was administered simultaneously with a single 50-mg dose of bictegravir under fed conditions.

Pharmacokinetic interactions reported when a single 324-mg dose of ferrous fumarate was administered simultaneously with a single 50-mg dose of bictegravir in the fasting state (decreased peak plasma concentrations and AUC of bictegravir). No clinically important pharmacokinetic interactions were observed when a single 324-mg dose of ferrous fumarate was administered simultaneously with a single 50-mg dose of bictegravir under fed conditions.

Concomitant use of BIC/FTC/TAF with laxatives, buffered preparations, or other preparations containing polyvalent cations may decrease plasma concentrations of bictegravir.

BIC/FTC/TAF and supplements containing calcium or iron can be administered simultaneously with food.

Routine administration of BIC/FTC/TAF in the fasting state simultaneously with or 2 hours *after* supplements containing calcium or iron is *not* recommended.

■ **Cardiac Drugs** ***Antiarrhythmic Agents*** **Disopyramide.** Pharmacokinetic interactions are possible if disopyramide is used with bictegravir (increased disopyramide concentrations).

Some experts state that disopyramide and BIC/FTC/TAF should be used concomitantly with caution and clinical monitoring.

Dofetilide. Concomitant use of dofetilide and BIC/FTC/TAF may increase dofetilide plasma concentrations and increase the risk of serious and/or life-threatening adverse effects.

Concomitant use of dofetilide and BIC/FTC/TAF is contraindicated.

Other Antiarrhythmic Agents. Pharmacokinetic interactions are not expected if bictegravir is used concomitantly with amiodarone, digoxin, dronedarone, flecainide, systemic lidocaine, mexiletine, propafenone, or quinidine; dosage adjustments are not necessary if BIC/FTC/TAF is used concomitantly with any of these antiarrhythmic agents.

β-Adrenergic Blocking Agents Pharmacokinetic interactions are not expected if bictegravir is used concomitantly with β-adrenergic blocking agents (e.g., metoprolol, timolol); dosage adjustments are not necessary if BIC/FTC/TAF is used concomitantly with any of these drugs.

Bosentan Pharmacokinetic interactions are possible if bictegravir is used concomitantly with bosentan (decreased bictegravir concentrations); some experts state that dosage adjustments are not necessary if BIC/FTC/TAF is used concomitantly with bosentan.

Calcium-channel Blocking Agents Pharmacokinetic interactions are possible if bictegravir is used concomitantly with diltiazem (increased bictegravir concentrations). Pharmacokinetic interactions are not expected if bictegravir is used concomitantly with other calcium-channel blocking agents.

Some experts state that dosage adjustments are not necessary if BIC/FTC/TAF is used concomitantly with diltiazem or other calcium-channel blocking agents.

Eplerenone, Ivabradine, Ranolazine, and Spironolactone Pharmacokinetic interactions are not expected if bictegravir is used concomitantly with eplerenone, ivabradine, ranolazine, or spironolactone; dosage adjustments are not necessary if BIC/FTC/TAF is used concomitantly with any of these drugs.

■ **Cisapride** Pharmacokinetic interactions are not expected if bictegravir is used concomitantly with cisapride; dosage adjustments are not necessary if BIC/FTC/TAF is used concomitantly with cisapride.

■ **Colchicine** Pharmacokinetic interactions are not expected if bictegravir is used concomitantly with colchicine; dosage adjustments are not necessary if BIC/FTC/TAF is used concomitantly with colchicine.

■ **Corticosteroids** ***Systemic Corticosteroids*** **Dexamethasone.** Pharmacokinetic interactions are possible if bictegravir is used concomitantly with systemic dexamethasone (decreased bictegravir concentrations).

Some experts state that an alternative to long-term systemic dexamethasone therapy or an alternative antiretroviral should be used. If concomitant use of BIC/FTC/TAF and systemic dexamethasone is considered necessary, virologic response should be monitored.

Other Systemic Corticosteroids. Pharmacokinetic interactions are not expected if bictegravir is used concomitantly with systemic betamethasone, budesonide, prednisone, or prednisolone; dosage adjustments are not necessary if BIC/FTC/TAF is used concomitantly with any of these systemic corticosteroids.

Orally Inhaled or Intranasal Corticosteroids Pharmacokinetic interactions are not expected if bictegravir is used concomitantly with orally inhaled or intranasal budesonide, ciclesonide, fluticasone, or mometasone; dosage adjustments are not necessary if BIC/FTC/TAF is used concomitantly with any of these orally inhaled or intranasal corticosteroids.

Local Injections of Corticosteroids Pharmacokinetic interactions are not expected if bictegravir is used concomitantly with local injections (e.g., intra-articular, epidural, intraorbital) of betamethasone, methylprednisolone, prednisolone, or triamcinolone; dosage adjustments are not necessary if BIC/FTC/TAF is used concomitantly with local injections of any of these corticosteroids.

■ **Dronabinol** Pharmacokinetic interactions are not expected if bictegravir is used concomitantly with dronabinol; dosage adjustments are not necessary if BIC/FTC/TAF is used concomitantly with dronabinol.

■ **Eluxadoline** Pharmacokinetic interactions are not expected if bictegravir is used concomitantly with eluxadoline; dosage adjustments are not necessary if BIC/FTC/TAF is used concomitantly with eluxadoline.

■ **Enzalutamide** Pharmacokinetic interactions are expected if bictegravir is used concomitantly with enzalutamide (decreased bictegravir concentrations). Some experts state that concomitant use of BIC/FTC/TAF and enzalutamide is contraindicated.

■ **Ergot Alkaloids and Derivatives** Pharmacokinetic interactions are not expected if bictegravir is used concomitantly with ergot alkaloids (e.g., dihydroergotamine, ergotamine, methylergonovine); dosage adjustments are not necessary if BIC/FTC/TAF is used concomitantly with these drugs.

■ **Estrogens and Progestins** ***Drospirenone, Medroxyprogesterone, and Progesterone*** Concomitant use of bictegravir and drospirenone, medroxyprogesterone, or micronized progesterone is not expected to affect concentrations of the hormone; dosage adjustments are not necessary if BIC/FTC/TAF is used concomitantly with drospirenone, medroxyprogesterone, or micronized progesterone.

Estradiol, Estrogen, and Conjugated Estrogens Concomitant use of bictegravir and estradiol, estrogen, or conjugated estrogens (equine or synthetic) is not expected to affect estrogen concentrations; dosage adjustments are not necessary if BIC/FTC/TAF is used concomitantly with estradiol, estrogen, or conjugated estrogens.

Ethinyl Estradiol and Norgestimate Concomitant use of the fixed combination of norgestimate and ethinyl estradiol with bictegravir or tenofovir alafenamide does not have a clinically important effect on ethinyl estradiol, norelgestromin, or norgestrel concentrations.

Clinically important pharmacokinetic interactions are not expected if BIC/FTC/TAF is used concomitantly with oral contraceptives containing ethinyl estradiol or norgestimate.

Data are not available regarding concomitant use of bictegravir with other hormonal contraceptives (e.g., transdermal contraceptive systems, vaginal ring, injections).

■ **Finasteride** Concomitant use of bictegravir and finasteride is not expected to affect finasteride concentrations; dosage adjustments are not necessary if BIC/FTC/TAF is used concomitantly with finasteride.

■ **Flibanserin** Pharmacokinetic interactions are not expected if bictegravir is used concomitantly with flibanserin; dosage adjustments are not necessary if BIC/FTC/TAF is used concomitantly with flibanserin.

■ **GI Drugs** ***Antacids*** Pharmacokinetic interactions reported when a single dose of antacid containing aluminum, magnesium, and simethicone was administered simultaneously with a single 50-mg dose of bictegravir in the fasting or fed state (decrease peak plasma concentrations and AUC of bictegravir). Similarly, decreased peak plasma concentrations and AUC of bictegravir were observed when a single 50-mg dose of the drug was administered in the fasting state 2 hours *after* the antacid.

No clinically important pharmacokinetic interactions were observed when a single 50-mg dose of bictegravir was administered in the fasting state 2 hours *before* the antacid.

Other cation-containing antacids also may decrease bictegravir plasma concentrations if used concomitantly with BIC/FTC/TAF.

BIC/FTC/TAF should be administered in the fasting state at least 2 hours *before* antacids containing aluminum, calcium, or magnesium. Administration of BIC/FTC/TAF concomitantly with or 2 hours *after* an antacid containing aluminum, calcium, or magnesium is *not* recommended.

Histamine H_2-receptor Antagonists Bictegravir does not have a clinically important effect on histamine H_2-receptor antagonists; dosage adjustments are not necessary if BIC/FTC/TAF is used concomitantly with these drugs.

Proton-pump Inhibitors Clinically important pharmacokinetic effects do not occur if bictegravir is used with a proton-pump inhibitor; dosage adjustments are not necessary if BIC/FTC/TAF is used concomitantly with proton-pump inhibitors.

Sucralfate Concomitant use of sucralfate and BIC/FTC/TAF may decrease plasma concentrations of bictegravir.

■ **Goserelin** Pharmacokinetic interactions are not expected if bictegravir is used concomitantly with goserelin; dosage adjustments are not necessary if BIC/FTC/TAF is used concomitantly with goserelin.

■ **HCV Antivirals** ***HCV Polymerase Inhibitors*** **Dasabuvir, Ombitasvir, Paritaprevir, and Ritonavir.** Data are not available regarding concomitant use of bictegravir and the fixed combination of dasabuvir, ombitasvir, paritaprevir, and ritonavir (dasabuvir/ombitasvir/paritaprevir/ritonavir; not commercially available in the US); some experts state that dosage adjustments are not necessary if BIC/FTC/TAF is used concomitantly with dasabuvir/ombitasvir/paritaprevir/ritonavir.

Sofosbuvir. Clinically important pharmacokinetic interactions are not expected if BIC/FTC/TAF is used concomitantly with sofosbuvir; dosage adjustments are not necessary if BIC/FTC/TAF is used concomitantly with sofosbuvir.

Sofosbuvir and Velpatasvir. Clinically important pharmacokinetic interactions are not expected if BIC/FTC/TAF is used concomitantly with the fixed combination of sofosbuvir and velpatasvir (sofosbuvir/velpatasvir); dosage adjustments are not necessary if BIC/FTC/TAF is used concomitantly with sofosbuvir/velpatasvir.

Sofosbuvir, Velpatasvir, and Voxilaprevir. Concomitant use of the fixed combination of sofosbuvir, velpatasvir, and voxilaprevir (sofosbuvir/velpatasvir/voxilaprevir) with bictegravir or tenofovir alafenamide does not have a clinically important effect on sofosbuvir, velpatasvir, voxilaprevir, bictegravir, or tenofovir alafenamide concentrations.

Clinically important pharmacokinetic interactions are not expected if BIC/FTC/TAF is used concomitantly with sofosbuvir/velpatasvir/voxilaprevir; dosage adjustments are not necessary if BIC/FTC/TAF is used concomitantly with sofosbuvir/velpatasvir/voxilaprevir.

HCV Protease Inhibitors **Glecaprevir and Pibrentasvir.** Concomitant use of bictegravir and the fixed combination of glecaprevir and pibrentasvir (glecaprevir/pibrentasvir) is not expected to alter bictegravir concentrations; dosage adjustments are not necessary if BIC/FTC/TAF is used concomitantly with glecaprevir/pibrentasvir.

HCV Replication Complex Inhibitors **Daclatasvir.** Data are not available regarding concomitant use of bictegravir and daclatasvir; some experts state that dosage adjustments are not necessary if BIC/FTC/TAF is used concomitantly with daclatasvir.

Elbasvir and Grazoprevir. Concomitant use of bictegravir and the fixed combination of elbasvir and grazoprevir (elbasvir/grazoprevir) is not expected to alter bictegravir concentrations; dosage adjustments are not necessary if BIC/FTC/TAF is used concomitantly with elbasvir/grazoprevir.

Ledipasvir and Sofosbuvir. Concomitant use of the fixed combination of ledipasvir and sofosbuvir (ledipasvir/sofosbuvir) with bictegravir or with tenofovir alafenamide does not have a clinically important effect on ledipasvir, sofosbuvir, bictegravir, or tenofovir alafenamide concentrations.

Clinically important pharmacokinetic interactions are not expected if BIC/FTC/TAF is used concomitantly with ledipasvir/sofosbuvir; dosage adjustments are not necessary if BIC/FTC/TAF is used concomitantly with ledipasvir/sofosbuvir.

■ **HMG-CoA Reductase Inhibitors** Pharmacokinetic interactions are not expected if bictegravir is used concomitantly with hydroxymethylglutaryl-CoA (HMG-CoA) reductase inhibitors (statins) (e.g., atorvastatin, lovastatin, pitavastatin, pravastatin, rosuvastatin, simvastatin); dosage adjustments are not necessary if BIC/FTC/TAF is used concomitantly with any of these drugs.

■ **Immunosuppressive Agents** Pharmacokinetic interactions are not expected if bictegravir is used concomitantly with immunosuppressive agents (e.g., cyclosporine, everolimus, sirolimus, tacrolimus); dosage adjustments are not necessary if BIC/FTC/TAF is used concomitantly with any of these drugs.

■ **Leuprolide** Pharmacokinetic interactions are not expected if bictegravir is used concomitantly with leuprolide; dosage adjustments are not necessary if BIC/FTC/TAF is used concomitantly with leuprolide.

■ **Macrolides** ***Clarithromycin*** Pharmacokinetic interactions are not expected if bictegravir is used concomitantly with clarithromycin; dosage adjustments are not necessary if BIC/FTC/TAF is used concomitantly with clarithromycin.

■ **Mitotane** Pharmacokinetic interactions are expected if bictegravir is used concomitantly with mitotane (decreased bictegravir concentrations). Some experts state that concomitant use of BIC/FTC/TAF and mitotane is contraindicated.

■ **Opiate Agonists, Opiate Partial Agonists, and Opiate Antagonists** ***Buprenorphine*** Pharmacokinetic interactions are not expected if bictegravir is used concomitantly with buprenorphine; dosage adjustments are not necessary if BIC/FTC/TAF is used concomitantly with buprenorphine.

Methadone Concomitant use of bictegravir and methadone does not result in clinically important pharmacokinetic interactions; dosage adjustments are not necessary if BIC/FTC/TAF is used concomitantly with methadone.

■ **Phosphodiesterase Type 5 Inhibitors** Pharmacokinetic interactions are not expected if bictegravir is used concomitantly with selective phosphodiesterase type 5 (PDE5) inhibitors (e.g., avanafil, sildenafil, tadalafil, vardenafil); dosage adjustments are not necessary if BIC/FTC/TAF is used concomitantly with any of these drugs.

■ **Salmeterol** Pharmacokinetic interactions are not expected if bictegravir is used concomitantly with salmeterol; dosage adjustments are not necessary if BIC/FTC/TAF is used concomitantly with salmeterol.

■ **Selective Serotonin-reuptake Inhibitors** Concomitant use of sertraline with tenofovir alafenamide does not have a clinically important effect on sertraline concentrations.

Pharmacokinetic interactions are not expected if bictegravir is used concomitantly with selective serotonin-reuptake inhibitors (SSRIs) (e.g., citalopram, escitalopram, fluoxetine, fluvoxamine, paroxetine, sertraline). Dosage adjustments are not necessary if BIC/FTC/TAF is used concomitantly with any of these SSRIs.

■ **St. John's Wort** Pharmacokinetic interactions are possible if St. John's wort (*Hypericum perforatum*) is used concomitantly with BIC/FTC/TAF (decreased concentrations of bictegravir and tenofovir alafenamide).

Concomitant use of St. John's wort and BIC/FTC/TAF is not recommended.

■ **Suvorexant** Pharmacokinetic interactions are not expected if bictegravir is used concomitantly with suvorexant; dosage adjustments are not necessary if BIC/FTC/TAF is used concomitantly with suvorexant.

■ **Testosterone** Concomitant use of bictegravir and testosterone is not expected to affect testosterone concentrations; dosage adjustments are not necessary if BIC/FTC/TAF is used concomitantly with testosterone.

■ **Trazodone** Pharmacokinetic interactions are not expected if bictegravir is used concomitantly with trazodone; dosage adjustments are not necessary if BIC/FTC/TAF is used concomitantly with trazodone.

■ **Tricyclic Antidepressants** Pharmacokinetic interactions are not expected if bictegravir is used concomitantly with tricyclic antidepressants (e.g., amitriptyline, desipramine, doxepin, imipramine, nortriptyline); dosage adjustments are not necessary if BIC/FTC/TAF is used concomitantly with any of these antidepressants.

■ **Zolpidem** Pharmacokinetic interactions are not expected if bictegravir is used concomitantly with zolpidem; dosage adjustments are not necessary if BIC/FTC/TAF is used concomitantly with zolpidem.

Description

The fixed combination of bictegravir sodium, emtricitabine, and tenofovir alafenamide fumarate (BIC/FTC/TAF) contains a human immunodeficiency virus (HIV) integrase strand transfer inhibitor (INSTI) antiretroviral (bictegravir; BIC), an HIV nucleoside reverse transcriptase inhibitor (NRTI) antiretroviral (emtricitabine; FTC), and a nucleotide reverse transcriptase inhibitor antiretroviral classified as an HIV NRTI (tenofovir alafenamide; TAF).

Bictegravir inhibits the activity of HIV-1 integrase, an enzyme that integrates HIV DNA into the host cell genome. Integration is required for viral replication; therefore, inhibition of integration prevents propagation of viral infection. Bictegravir is active against HIV-1 and also has some in vitro activity against HIV type 2 (HIV-2).

Emtricitabine is inactive until converted intracellularly to an active 5′-triphosphate metabolite. After conversion to the pharmacologically active metabolite, the drug acts as a reverse transcriptase inhibitor antiretroviral. Emtricitabine is active against HIV-1 and also has some in vitro activity against HIV-2.

Tenofovir alafenamide is a tenofovir prodrug and is inactive until hydrolyzed intracellularly by cathepsin A to form tenofovir and subsequently metabolized by cellular kinases to the active metabolite (tenofovir diphosphate). After conversion to the pharmacologically active metabolite, the drug acts as a reverse transcriptase inhibitor antiretroviral. Tenofovir is active against HIV-1 and has some in vitro activity against HIV-2; the drug also is active against hepatitis B virus (HBV).

HIV-1 resistant to bictegravir, emtricitabine, or tenofovir have been produced in vitro. In clinical trials evaluating BIC/FTC/TAF, no specific bictegravir or NRTI resistance-associated substitutions emerged in patients receiving BIC/FTC/TAF who were considered to be virologic treatment failures. There is some evidence that bictegravir may possess a higher barrier to resistance development than some other HIV INSTIs (e.g., elvitegravir, raltegravir). Cross-resistance between bictegravir and other HIV INSTIs (e.g., dolutegravir, elvitegravir, raltegravir) has been reported. Cross-resistance also occurs among HIV NRTIs.

Following oral administration of the components of BIC/FTC/TAF, peak plasma concentrations of bictegravir, emtricitabine, and tenofovir occur at 2–4, 1.5–2, and 0.5–2 hours, respectively. Administration of BIC/FTC/TAF components with a high-fat meal (approximately 800 kcal, 50% fat) increases mean systemic exposures of bictegravir and tenofovir by 24 and 63%, respectively, compared with administration in the fasting state; mean systemic exposures of emtricitabine are comparable to those observed with administration in the fasting state. Bictegravir is over 99%, emtricitabine is less than 4%, and tenofovir alafenamide is approximately 80% bound to plasma proteins. Bictegravir is metabolized by cytochrome P-450 (CYP) isoenzyme 3A and uridine diphosphate-glucuronosyltransferase (UGT) 1A1. Emtricitabine is converted intracellularly to the active 5′-triphosphate metabolite, but is not substantially metabolized further. Tenofovir alafenamide is hydrolyzed intracellularly in peripheral blood mononuclear cells (PBMCs) and macrophages by cathepsin A to form tenofovir (the major metabolite) which is then phosphorylated to the active metabolite tenofovir diphosphate; in vitro studies indicate tenofovir alafenamide also is converted to tenofovir by carboxylesterase 1 (CES1) in hepatocytes. Following a single dose of bictegravir, 60% is excreted in feces and 35% in urine. Emtricitabine is principally excreted in urine (70% of a dose) and to a lesser extent in feces (14% of a dose). Following a single dose of tenofovir alafenamide, 32% is excreted in feces and less than 1% is eliminated in urine. The median terminal plasma half-lives of bictegravir, emtricitabine, and tenofovir alafenamide are 17.3, 10.4, and 0.5 hours, respectively. The half-life of tenofovir diphosphate, the active metabolite of tenofovir alafenamide, is 150–180 hours within PBMCs.

Advice to Patients

Critical nature of compliance with HIV therapy and importance of remaining under the care of a clinician. Importance of taking as prescribed; do not alter or discontinue antiretroviral regimen without consulting clinician.

Advise patients that the fixed combination of bictegravir sodium, emtricitabine, and tenofovir alafenamide (BIC/FTC/TAF) is a complete regimen for treatment of HIV-1 infection and should *not* be used in conjunction with other antiretrovirals.

Antiretroviral therapy is not a cure for HIV infection; opportunistic infections and other complications associated with HIV disease may still occur.

Advise patients that early initiation of antiretroviral therapy and sustained decreases in plasma HIV RNA have been associated with reduced risk of progression to acquired immunodeficiency syndrome (AIDS) and death.

Advise patients that effective antiretroviral regimens can decrease HIV concentrations in blood and genital secretions and strict adherence to such regimens in conjunction with risk-reduction measures may decrease, but cannot absolutely eliminate, the risk of secondary transmission of HIV to others. Importance of continuing to practice safer sex (e.g., using latex or polyurethane condoms to minimize sexual contact with body fluids) and reducing high-risk behaviors (e.g., reusing or sharing needles).

Importance of reading patient information provided by the manufacturer.

Inform patients that testing for hepatitis B virus (HBV) infection is recommended before antiretroviral therapy is initiated. Also advise patients that severe acute exacerbations of HBV infection have been reported following discontinuance of emtricitabine and/or tenofovir disoproxil fumarate (tenofovir DF) in HIV-infected patients coinfected with HBV and may occur with BIC/FTC/TAF.

Advise patients that renal impairment, including cases of acute renal failure or Fanconi syndrome, has occurred in patients receiving tenofovir prodrugs. Importance of not using BIC/FTC/TAF concomitantly with or shortly after nephrotoxic agents (e.g., high-dose or multiple nonsteroidal anti-inflammatory agents [NSAIAs]).

Advise patients that lactic acidosis and severe hepatomegaly with steatosis, including fatalities, have occurred in patients receiving HIV nucleoside reverse transcriptase inhibitors (NRTIs), including emtricitabine and/or tenofovir DF, in conjunction with other antiretrovirals. Importance of contacting clinician if symptoms suggestive of lactic acidosis or pronounced hepatotoxicity (e.g., unusual muscle pain, shortness of breath or fast breathing, cold or blue hands and feet, dizziness or lightheadedness, fast or abnormal heartbeat, nausea, vomiting, unusual/unexpected stomach discomfort, weakness or unusual tiredness) occur.

Advise patients that signs and symptoms of inflammation from previous infections may occur soon after initiation of antiretroviral therapy in some individuals with advanced HIV infection (AIDS). These symptoms may be due to an improvement in immune response, enabling the body to fight infections that may have been present with no obvious symptoms. Importance of immediately informing a healthcare provider if any symptoms of infection occur.

Importance of informing clinicians of existing or contemplated concomitant therapy, including prescription and OTC drugs and herbal supplements (e.g., St. John's wort), as well as any concomitant illnesses.

Importance of women informing clinicians if they are or plan to become pregnant or plan to breast-feed. Advise HIV-infected women not to breast-feed.

Importance of informing patients of other important precautionary information. (See Cautions.)

Overview® (see Users Guide). For additional information on this drug until a more detailed monograph is developed and published, the manufacturer's labeling should be consulted. It is *essential* that the manufacturer's labeling be consulted for more detailed information on usual cautions, precautions, contraindications, potential drug interactions, laboratory test interferences, and acute toxicity.

Preparations

Excipients in commercially available drug preparations may have clinically important effects in some individuals; consult specific product labeling for details.

Bictegravir Sodium, Emtricitabine, and Tenofovir Alafenamide Fumarate

Oral

Tablets, film-coated	Bictegravir Sodium 50 mg (of bictegravir), Emtricitabine 200 mg, and Tenofovir Alafenamide Fumarate 25 mg (of tenofovir alafenamide)	**Biktarvy®**, Gilead

Dolutegravir Sodium

DTG, abacavir/dolutegravir/lamivudine, ABC/DTG/3TC, DTG/RPV, dolutegravir/rilpivirine

■ Dolutegravir sodium, an antiretroviral agent, is a human immunodeficiency virus (HIV) integrase strand transfer inhibitor (INSTI).

Uses

■ Treatment of HIV Infection Dolutegravir sodium is used in conjunction with other antiretroviral agents for the treatment of human immunodeficiency virus type 1 (HIV-1) infection in antiretroviral-naive (have not previously received antiretroviral therapy) or antiretroviral-experienced (previously treated) adults, adolescents, and children weighing at least 30 kg.

If an HIV integrase strand transfer inhibitor-based (INSTI-based) regimen of dolutegravir, abacavir, and lamivudine is used for the treatment of HIV-1 infection in treatment-naive or previously treated patients, a fixed-combination preparation containing all 3 drugs (abacavir/dolutegravir/lamivudine; Triumeq®) is commercially available and can be used in adults, adolescents, and pediatric patients weighing 40 kg or more. Abacavir/dolutegravir/lamivudine can be used alone as a complete treatment regimen or in conjunction with other antiretrovirals; however, the fixed combination should not be used alone in patients who have HIV-1 with clinically suspected or confirmed INSTI-resistance substitutions since it contains a dolutegravir dosage that is insufficient in such patients.

If a 2-drug regimen of dolutegravir and rilpivirine is used for the treatment of HIV-1 infection in certain treatment-experienced adults (see Antiretroviral-experienced Adults and Adolescents under Uses: Treatment of HIV infection), a fixed-combination preparation containing both drugs (dolutegravir/rilpivirine; Juluca®) is commercially available and can be used as an alternative to concomitant use of single-entity dolutegravir and single-entity rilpivirine. (See Dolutegravir Sodium and Rilpivirine Hydrochloride 8:18.08.12.)

The most appropriate antiretroviral regimen cannot be defined for each clinical scenario, and selection of specific antiretroviral agents for use in multiple-drug regimens should be individualized based on information regarding antiretroviral potency, potential rate of development of resistance, known toxicities, and potential for pharmacokinetic interactions as well as virologic, immunologic, and clinical characteristics of the patient. For information on the general principles and guidelines for use of antiretroviral therapy, including specific recommendations for initial therapy in antiretroviral-naive patients and recommendations for changing antiretroviral regimens, see the Antiretroviral Agents General Statement 8:18.08.

Antiretroviral-naive Adults and Adolescents For *initial* treatment in antiretroviral-naive HIV-infected adults and adolescents, dolutegravir usually is used in INSTI-based regimens that include dolutegravir and 2 HIV nucleoside reverse transcriptase inhibitors (dual NRTIs).

The US Department of Health and Human Services (HHS) Panel on Antiretroviral Guidelines for Adults and Adolescents states that dolutegravir in conjunction with tenofovir alafenamide fumarate (TAF) and emtricitabine or dolutegravir in conjunction with tenofovir disoproxil fumarate (tenofovir DF) and emtricitabine (or lamivudine) are recommended INSTI-based regimens for *initial* treatment in HIV-infected adults and adolescents. These experts also state that dolutegravir in conjunction with abacavir and lamivudine (or emtricitabine) is another recommended INSTI-based regimen for *initial* treatment in adults and adolescents, but should be used *only* in patients who are negative for human leukocyte antigen (HLA)-B*5701.

Clinical Experience. Efficacy and safety of dolutegravir in antiretroviral-naive HIV-1-infected adults have been evaluated in phase 3 randomized studies (SPRING-2, SINGLE, FLAMINGO).

SPRING-2 is an ongoing phase 3, randomized, active-controlled, double-placebo, noninferiority study in antiretroviral-naive HIV-1-infected adults with baseline plasma HIV-1 RNA levels of 1000 copies/mL or higher. Patients were randomized to receive dolutegravir 50 mg once daily or raltegravir 400 mg twice daily in conjunction with an investigator-selected dual NRTI regimen of either the fixed-combination preparation containing emtricitabine and tenofovir DF (emtricitabine/tenofovir DF) or fixed-combination preparation containing abacavir and lamivudine (abacavir/lamivudine). Baseline characteristics of the 822 study patients were similar in both treatment groups (median age 36 years, 87% male, 15% non-white, 11% with hepatitis B virus [HBV] and/or hepatitis C virus [HCV] coinfection, 2% Centers for Disease Control and Prevention [CDC] Class C, median baseline plasma HIV-1 RNA level 4.52 or 4.58 $\log_{10}$ copies/mL, median baseline $CD4^+$ T-cell count 359 or 362 cells/mm^3). At 96 weeks, 82% of patients in the dolutegravir group and 78% of those in the raltegravir group had plasma HIV-1 RNA levels less than 50 copies/mL; the median increase in $CD4^+$ T-cell count was 276 cells/mm^3 in the dolutegravir group and 264 cells/mm^3 in the raltegravir group.

SINGLE is a 96-week randomized, double-blind, active-controlled study in antiretroviral-naive HIV-1-infected adults evaluating the efficacy and safety of dolutegravir 50 mg once daily in conjunction with abacavir/lamivudine compared with the fixed-combination preparation containing efavirenz, emtricitabine, and tenofovir DF (efavirenz/emtricitabine/tenofovir DF) followed by an open-label phase through week 144. Baseline characteristics of the 833 study patients were similar in both treatment groups (median age 35 years, 16% female, 32% non-white, 7% with HCV coinfection, 4% CDC Class C, median plasma HIV-1 RNA level 4.68 $\log_{10}$ copies/mL, median baseline $CD4^+$ T-cell count 338 cells/mm^3). At 144 weeks, 71% of patients receiving dolutegravir with abacavir/lamivudine and 63% of those receiving efavirenz/emtricitabine/tenofovir DF achieved plasma HIV-1 RNA levels less than 50 copies/mL. The adjusted mean increase in CD4$^+$ T-cell count was 378 cells/mm^3 in those receiving dolutegravir and abacavir/lamivudine compared with 332 cells/mm^3 in those receiving efavirenz/emtricitabine/tenofovir DF.

FLAMINGO is an open-label, randomized, noninferiority study in antiretroviral-naive HIV-1-infected adults that compared the efficacy and safety of dolutegravir 50 mg once daily with that of *ritonavir-boosted* darunavir when the drugs were given in conjunction with an investigator-selected dual NRTI regimen of abacavir/lamivudine or emtricitabine/tenofovir DF. At baseline, the 484 study patients had a median age of 34 years, 15% were female, 28% were non-white, 25% had plasma HIV-1 RNA levels greater than 100,000 copies/mL, and 35% had CD4$^+$ T-cell counts less than 350 cells/mm^3. At 96 weeks, 80% of patients in the dolutegravir group achieved plasma HIV-1 RNA levels less than 50 copies/mL compared with 68% in the *ritonavir-boosted* darunavir group.

Antiretroviral-experienced Adults and Adolescents For the treatment of HIV-1 infection in antiretroviral-experienced adults and adolescents, dolutegravir usually is used in INSTI-based regimens that include dolutegravir in conjunction with an optimized background antiretroviral regimen (OBR).

A 2-drug regimen of dolutegravir and rilpivirine can be used to replace the current regimen in antiretroviral-experienced adults who are virologically suppressed (i.e., plasma HIV-1 RNA levels less than 50 copies/mL) on a stable antiretroviral regimen for at least 6 months, have no known history of treatment failure, and are infected with HIV-1 with no known substitutions associated with resistance to dolutegravir or rilpivirine. If such patients are switched to a 2-drug regimen of dolutegravir and rilpivirine, single-entity dolutegravir and single-entity rilpivirine can be used concomitantly or the commercially available fixed-combination dolutegravir/rilpivirine can be used. (See Dolutegravir Sodium and Rilpivirine Hydrochloride 8:18.08.12.)

Clinical Experience. The comparative efficacy and safety of dolutegravir in 715 antiretroviral-experienced, INSTI-naive HIV-1-infected adults are being studied in an ongoing phase 3, randomized, double-blind, active-controlled, double-placebo study (SAILING). All enrolled patients had previously received antiretroviral therapy (average duration 77 months of prior therapy) and had infections resistant to at least 2 classes of antiretrovirals (49% had HIV-1 resistant to at least 3 classes of antiretrovirals). Patients were randomized to receive dolutegravir 50 mg once daily or raltegravir 400 mg twice daily, each in conjunction with an investigator-selected OBR consisting of at least 1 fully active antiretroviral. Baseline characteristics were similar in both treatment groups (median age 43 years, 32% female, 50% non-white, 16% with HBV and/or HCV coinfection, 46% CDC Class C, 20% with plasma HIV-1 RNA levels greater than 100,000 copies/mL, 72% with CD4$^+$ T-cell counts less than 350 cells/mm^3). At 48 weeks, 71% of patients in the dolutegravir group and 64% of those in the raltegravir group had plasma HIV-1 RNA levels less than 50 copies/mL; CD4$^+$ T-cell counts were increased from baseline in both groups (mean change 162 cells/mm^3 in the dolutegravir group and 153 cells/mm^3 in the raltegravir group).

An open-label, single-arm, phase 3 study (VIKING-3) evaluated use of dolutegravir and an OBR in 183 antiretroviral-experienced adults with current or prior virologic failure on another INSTI-containing regimen (elvitegravir, raltegravir) and current or historical evidence of resistance to these other INSTIs. At baseline, most patients had HIV-1 resistant to other antiretroviral classes (79% with resistance to 2 or more NRTIs, 75% with resistance to at least 1 HIV nonnucleoside reverse transcriptase inhibitor [NNRTI], 71% with resistance to 2 or more HIV protease inhibitors [PIs]). At baseline, the median age of study patients was 48 years, 23% were female, 29% were non-white, 20% had HBV and/or HCV coinfection, median plasma HIV-1 RNA level was 4.38 $\log_{10}$ copies/mL, median CD4$^+$ T-cell count was 140 cells/mm^3, and median duration of prior antiretroviral therapy was 13–14 years. Patients received dolutegravir 50 mg twice daily with their current failing background regimen for 7 days; on day 8, dolutegravir was continued and the background regimen was further optimized if possible. The mean reduction in plasma HIV-1 RNA level on day 8 (primary efficacy end point) was 1.4 $\log_{10}$ copies/mL. At 48 weeks after initiation of dolutegravir, 63% of study patients had plasma HIV-1 RNA levels less than 50 copies/mL and the median increase in CD4$^+$ T-cell count was 80 cells/mm^3. The presence of INSTI-resistance substitutions at baseline affected the 48-week response rate. The response rate to the dolutegravir regimen was 74% in those who had HIV-1 without the Q148 resistance substitution present at baseline, but was 61% if the Q148H/R and G140S/A/C substitutions were present at baseline and 29% if the Q148H/R substitution plus 2 additional INSTI-resistance substitutions (T66A, L74I/M, E138A/K/T, G140S/A/C, Y143R/C/H, E157Q, G163S/E/K/Q, or G193E/R) were present at baseline.

In a randomized, double-blind, placebo-controlled, phase 3 study (VIKING-4), antiretroviral-experienced, dolutegravir-naive adults receiving a failing INSTI-based regimen that included elvitegravir or raltegravir were randomized to receive dolutegravir (50 mg twice daily) or placebo with their previous failing antiretroviral regimen for 7 days, followed by a single-arm, open-label regimen of dolutegravir (50 mg twice daily) in conjunction with an optimized antiretroviral regimen containing at least 1 fully active antiretroviral selected based on baseline resistance data. At baseline, all patients had plasma HIV-1 RNA levels of 1000 copies/mL or greater and HIV-1 with INSTI genotypic resistance; in addition, most patients had HIV-1 resistant to other antiretroviral classes (63% with resistance to 3 or more NRTIs, 53% with resistance to 2 or more NNRTIs, 67% with resistance to 2 or more PIs). The mean reduction in plasma HIV-1 RNA level on day 8 (primary efficacy end point) in those initially randomized to dolutegravir was 1.06 $\log_{10}$ copies/mL. At 48 weeks, 40% of all study patients had plasma HIV-1 RNA levels less than 50 copies/mL and the median increase in CD4$^+$ T-cell count was 125 cells/mm^3. The response rate at 48 weeks was 57% in those with HIV-1 without the Q148 resistance substitution present at baseline, but was only 25% if the Q148 substitution plus 1 or more additional INSTI-resistance substitutions were present at baseline.

Pediatric Patients Dolutegravir is used in conjunction with other antiretrovirals for the treatment of HIV-1 infection in antiretroviral-naive or antiretroviral-experienced adolescents and children weighing 30 kg or more. Safety and efficacy of dolutegravir have not been established in antiretroviral-experienced, INSTI-experienced pediatric patients with documented or clinically suspected resistance to other HIV INSTIs (e.g., elvitegravir, raltegravir).

For *initial* treatment in antiretroviral-naive HIV-infected pediatric patients, the HHS Panel on Antiretroviral Therapy and Medical Management of Children Living with HIV recommends a regimen that includes a *ritonavir-boosted* PI, NNRTI, or INSTI in conjunction with 2 NRTIs (dual NRTIs). These experts state that an INSTI-based regimen of dolutegravir and 2 NRTIs is a preferred regimen for *initial* antiretroviral therapy in pediatric patients 6 years of age or older weighing 30 kg or more.

Abacavir/dolutegravir/lamivudine is used alone or in conjunction with other antiretrovirals for the treatment of HIV-1 infection in pediatric patients weighing 40 kg or more.

For further information on treatment of HIV infection in pediatric patients, see Antiretroviral Therapy in Pediatric Patients, in Guidelines for Use of Antiretroviral Agents in the Antiretroviral Agents General Statement 8:18.08.

Clinical Experience. The pharmacokinetic profile, safety, and efficacy of dolutegravir in HIV-1-infected pediatric patients have been evaluated in a phase 1/phase 2 open-label, noncomparative study (IMPAACT P1093). Patients were stratified by age into cohort 1 (12 to less than 18 years of age) and cohort 2A (6 to less than 12 years of age). Baseline characteristics of the 46 pediatric patients included mean age 12 years (range 6–17 years), 54% female, 52% black, mean plasma HIV-1 RNA level of 4.6 $\log_{10}$ copies/mL, median CD4$^+$ T-cell count of 639 cells/mm^3, and median CD4$^+$ T-cell percentage of 23% (range 1–44%); most had previously received at least 1 NNRTI (50%) or PI (70%). Patients weighing 30 to less than 40 kg received dolutegravir 35 mg once daily in conjunction with an OBR and patients weighing 40 kg or more received dolutegravir 50 mg once daily in conjunction with an OBR. At 24 weeks, 70% of patients in cohort 1 and 61% of patients in cohort 2A achieved plasma HIV-1 RNA levels less than 50 copies/mL. At 48 weeks, 61% of patients in cohort 1 achieved plasma HIV-1 RNA levels less than 50 copies/mL. At 48 weeks, the median increase in CD4$^+$ T-cell count in cohort 1 was 84 cells/mm^3; at 24 weeks, the median increase in CD4$^+$ T-cell count in cohort 2A was 209 cells/mm^3.

■ **Postexposure Prophylaxis following Nonoccupational Exposure to HIV** Dolutegravir is used in conjunction with other antiretrovirals for postexposure prophylaxis of HIV infection following nonoccupational exposure† (nPEP) in individuals exposed to blood, genital secretions, or other potentially infectious body fluids that might contain HIV when the exposure represents a substantial risk for HIV transmission.

When nPEP is indicated following a nonoccupational exposure to HIV, the US Centers for Disease Control and Prevention (CDC) states that the preferred regimen in adults and adolescents 13 years of age or older with normal renal function is either raltegravir or dolutegravir used in conjunction with emtricitabine and tenofovir DF (administered as emtricitabine/tenofovir DF; Truvada®); the recommended alternative nPEP regimen in these patients is *ritonavir-boosted* darunavir used in conjunction with emtricitabine/tenofovir DF.

Consultation with an infectious disease specialist, clinician with expertise in administration of antiretroviral agents, and/or the National Clinicians' Postexposure Prophylaxis Hotline (PEPline at 888-448-4911) is recommended if nPEP is indicated in certain exposed individuals (e.g., pregnant women, children, those with medical conditions such as renal impairment) or if an antiretroviral regimen not included in the CDC guidelines is being considered, the source virus is known or likely to be resistant to antiretrovirals, or the healthcare provider is inexperienced in prescribing antiretrovirals. However, initiation of nPEP should not be delayed while waiting for expert consultation.

For additional information on nonoccupational exposure to HIV and recommendations regarding postexposure prophylaxis, see Guidelines for Use of Antiretroviral Agents: Antiretrovirals for Postexposure Prophylaxis following Sexual, Injection Drug Use, or other Nonoccupational Exposures to HIV (nPEP), in the Antiretroviral Agents General Statement 8:18.08.

Dosage and Administration

■ **Administration** Dolutegravir sodium is administered orally once or twice daily without regard to food.

Although administration with food increases the extent and decreases the rate of absorption of dolutegravir, this effect is not considered clinically important.

Single-entity dolutegravir (Tivicay®) is commercially available as tablets. Dolutegravir also is commercially available in fixed-combination tablets containing abacavir, dolutegravir, and lamivudine (abacavir/dolutegravir/lamivudine; Triumeq®). (See Fixed Combinations Containing Dolutegravir under Dosage and Administration: Administration.) In addition, dolutegravir is commercially available in fixed-combination tablets containing dolutegravir and rilpivirine (dolutegravir/rilpivirine; Juluca®). (For information on dolutegravir/rilpivirine, see Dolutegravir Sodium and Rilpivirine Hydrochloride 8:18.08.12.)

Dolutegravir is used in conjunction with other antiretrovirals.

Fixed Combinations Containing Dolutegravir Abacavir/dolutegravir/lamivudine tablets are administered orally once daily without regard to food.

Abacavir/dolutegravir/lamivudine can be used alone as a complete treatment regimen or used in conjunction with other antiretrovirals.

Abacavir/dolutegravir/lamivudine should not be used concomitantly with single-entity dolutegravir, unless needed for adjustment of dolutegravir dosage (e.g., when the fixed combination is used concomitantly with efavirenz, *ritonavir-boosted* fosamprenavir, *ritonavir-boosted* tipranavir, carbamazepine, or rifampin). When abacavir/dolutegravir/lamivudine *and* single-entity dolutegravir are both indicated, the daily dose of the fixed combination and the daily dose of the single-entity dolutegravir preparation should be administered 12 hours apart.

Because the antiretrovirals contained in abacavir/dolutegravir/lamivudine may also be available in single-entity or other fixed-combination preparations, care should be taken to ensure that therapy is not duplicated if the fixed combination is used in conjunction with other antiretrovirals. (See Precautions Related to Use of Fixed Combinations under Cautions: Precautions and Contraindications.)

For information on dolutegravir/rilpivirine, see Dolutegravir Sodium and Rilpivirine Hydrochloride 8:18.08.12.

■ **Dosage** Single-entity dolutegravir (Tivicay®) tablets contain dolutegravir sodium; dosage is expressed in terms of dolutegravir.

Abacavir/dolutegravir/lamivudine (Triumeq®) tablets contain abacavir sulfate, dolutegravir sodium, and lamivudine; dosages of the abacavir and dolutegravir components are expressed in terms of the bases.

A fixed-combination tablet containing 600 mg of abacavir, 50 mg of dolutegravir, and 300 mg of lamivudine taken in the fasted state is bioequivalent to a 50-mg dolutegravir tablet taken simultaneously with a fixed-combination tablet containing 600 mg of abacavir and 300 mg of lamivudine (abacavir/lamivudine) in the fasted state.

Adult Dosage **Treatment of HIV Infection in Antiretroviral-naive Adults.** For initial treatment of human immunodeficiency virus type 1 (HIV-1) infection in antiretroviral-naive adults, the recommended dosage of dolutegravir is 50 mg once daily.

If dolutegravir is used in antiretroviral-naive adults receiving concomitant therapy with certain uridine diphosphate-glucuronosyltransferase (UGT) 1A or cytochrome P-450 (CYP) 3A inducers (i.e., efavirenz, *ritonavir-boosted* fosamprenavir, *ritonavir-boosted* tipranavir, carbamazepine, rifampin), the drug should be given in a dosage of 50 mg twice daily. (See Drug Interactions.)

When abacavir/dolutegravir/lamivudine is used for the treatment of HIV-1 infection in antiretroviral-naive adults, the recommended dosage is 1 tablet (600 mg of abacavir, 50 mg of dolutegravir, and 300 mg of lamivudine) once daily.

If abacavir/dolutegravir/lamivudine is used in antiretroviral-naive adults receiving concomitant therapy with efavirenz, *ritonavir-boosted* fosamprenavir, *ritonavir-boosted* tipranavir, carbamazepine, or rifampin, patients should receive 1 tablet of the fixed combination (600 mg of abacavir, 50 mg of dolutegravir, and 300 mg of lamivudine) once daily *and* a 50-mg tablet of single-entity dolutegravir given once daily 12 hours after the daily dose of the fixed combination.

Treatment of HIV Infection in Antiretroviral-experienced Adults. For the treatment of HIV-1 infection in antiretroviral-experienced adults who have not previously received an HIV integrase strand transfer inhibitor (INSTI-naive), the recommended dosage of dolutegravir is 50 mg once daily.

For the treatment of HIV-1 infection in antiretroviral-experienced, INSTI-experienced adults who have certain INSTI-associated resistance substitutions or clinically suspected INSTI resistance, the recommended dosage of dolutegravir is 50 mg twice daily.

If dolutegravir is used in antiretroviral-experienced adults receiving concomitant therapy with certain UGT1A or CYP3A inducers (i.e., efavirenz, *ritonavir-boosted* fosamprenavir, *ritonavir-boosted* tipranavir, carbamazepine, rifampin), the drug should be given in a dosage of 50 mg twice daily. Whenever possible, alternative regimens that do not contain these inducers should be considered when dolutegravir is used in INSTI-experienced patients who have certain INSTI-associated resistance substitutions or clinically suspected INSTI resistance. (See Drug Interactions.)

When abacavir/dolutegravir/lamivudine is used for the treatment of HIV-1 infection in antiretroviral-experienced adults, the usual dosage is 1 tablet (600 mg of abacavir, 50 mg of dolutegravir, and 300 mg of lamivudine) once daily. The fixed combination should not be used alone in patients who have HIV-1 with clinically suspected or confirmed INSTI-resistance substitutions.

If abacavir/dolutegravir/lamivudine is used in antiretroviral-experienced adults receiving efavirenz, *ritonavir-boosted* fosamprenavir, *ritonavir-boosted* tipranavir, carbamazepine, or rifampin, patients should receive 1 tablet of the fixed combination (600 mg of abacavir, 50 mg of dolutegravir, and 300 mg of lamivudine) once daily *and* a 50-mg tablet of single-entity dolutegravir given once daily 12 hours after the daily dose of the fixed combination.

If a 2-drug regimen of dolutegravir and rilpivirine is used in certain antiretroviral-experienced adults (see Antiretroviral-experienced Adults and Adolescents under Uses: Treatment of HIV Infection), single-entity dolutegravir is given in a dosage of 50 mg once daily *with* single-entity rilpivirine (25 mg once daily). Alternatively, the commercially available fixed-combination dolutegravir/rilpivirine can be used. (See Dolutegravir Sodium and Rilpivirine Hydrochloride 8:18.08.12.)

Postexposure Prophylaxis following Nonoccupational Exposure to HIV. For postexposure prophylaxis of HIV infection following nonoccupational exposure† (nPEP) when the exposure represents a substantial risk for HIV transmission, the usual adult dosage of dolutegravir is 50 mg once daily in conjunction with 2 HIV nucleoside reverse transcriptase inhibitors (NRTIs). (See Uses: Postexposure Prophylaxis following Nonoccupational Exposure to HIV.)

The nPEP regimen should be initiated as soon as possible (within 72 hours) following nonoccupational exposure to HIV and continued for 28 days. If the exposed individual seeks care more than 72 hours after the exposure, nPEP is not recommended.

Pediatric Dosage **Treatment of HIV Infection in Antiretroviral-naive Pediatric Patients.** For initial treatment of HIV-1 infection in antiretroviral-naive children and adolescents weighing 30 to less than 40 kg, the recommended dosage of dolutegravir is 35 mg once daily (one 25-mg tablet and one 10-mg tablet once daily).

If dolutegravir is used in antiretroviral-naive children and adolescents weighing 30 to less than 40 kg receiving concomitant therapy with certain UGT1A or CYP3A inducers (i.e., efavirenz, *ritonavir-boosted* fosamprenavir, *ritonavir-boosted* tipranavir, carbamazepine, rifampin), the drug should be given in a dosage of 35 mg twice daily (one 25-mg tablet and one 10-mg tablet twice daily). (See Drug Interactions.)

For initial treatment of HIV-1 infection in antiretroviral-naive children and adolescents weighing 40 kg or more, the recommended dosage of dolutegravir is 50 mg once daily.

If dolutegravir is used in antiretroviral-naive children and adolescents weighing 40 kg or more receiving concomitant therapy with certain UGT1A or CYP3A inducers (i.e., efavirenz, *ritonavir-boosted* fosamprenavir, *ritonavir-boosted* tipranavir, carbamazepine, rifampin), the drug should be given in a dosage of 50 mg twice daily. (See Drug Interactions.)

When abacavir/dolutegravir/lamivudine is used for the treatment of HIV-1 infection in antiretroviral-naive pediatric patients weighing 40 kg or more, the recommended dosage is 1 tablet (600 mg of abacavir, 50 mg of dolutegravir, and 300 mg of lamivudine) orally once daily. If abacavir/dolutegravir/lamivudine is used in those receiving concomitant therapy with efavirenz, *ritonavir-boosted* fosamprenavir, *ritonavir-boosted* tipranavir, carbamazepine, or rifampin, patients should receive 1 tablet of the fixed combination (600 mg of abacavir, 50 mg of dolutegravir, and 300 mg of lamivudine) once daily *and* a 50-mg tablet of single-entity dolutegravir given once daily 12 hours after the daily dose of the fixed combination.

Treatment of HIV Infection in Antiretroviral-experienced Pediatric Patients. For the treatment of HIV-1 infection in antiretroviral-experienced, INSTI-naive children and adolescents weighing 30 to less than 40 kg, the recommended dosage of dolutegravir is 35 mg once daily (one 25-mg tablet and one 10-mg tablet once daily).

If dolutegravir is used in antiretroviral-experienced, INSTI-naive children and adolescents weighing 30 to less than 40 kg receiving concomitant therapy with certain UGT1A or CYP3A inducers (i.e., efavirenz, *ritonavir-boosted* fosamprenavir, *ritonavir-boosted* tipranavir, carbamazepine, rifampin), the drug should be given in a dosage of 35 mg twice daily (one 25-mg tablet and one 10-mg tablet twice daily). (See Drug Interactions.)

For the treatment of HIV-1 infection in antiretroviral-experienced, INSTI-naive children and adolescents weighing 40 kg or more, the recommended dosage of dolutegravir is 50 mg once daily.

If dolutegravir is used in antiretroviral-experienced, INSTI-naive children and adolescents weighing 40 kg or more receiving concomitant therapy with certain UGT1A or CYP3A inducers (i.e., efavirenz, *ritonavir-boosted* fosamprenavir, *ritonavir-boosted* tipranavir, carbamazepine, rifampin), the drug should be given in a dosage of 50 mg twice daily. (See Drug Interactions.)

Safety and efficacy of dolutegravir have not been established in INSTI-experienced pediatric patients with documented or clinically suspected resistance to other INSTIs (e.g., elvitegravir, raltegravir).

When abacavir/dolutegravir/lamivudine is used for the treatment of HIV-1 infection in antiretroviral-experienced pediatric patients weighing 40 kg or more, the recommended dosage is 1 tablet (600 mg of abacavir, 50 mg of dolutegravir, and 300 mg of lamivudine) orally once daily. If abacavir/dolutegravir/lamivudine is used in those receiving concomitant therapy with efavirenz, *ritonavir-boosted* fosamprenavir, *ritonavir-boosted* tipranavir, carbamazepine, or rifampin, patients should receive 1 tablet of the fixed combination (600 mg of abacavir, 50 mg of dolutegravir, and 300 mg of lamivudine) once daily *and* a 50-mg tablet of single-entity dolutegravir given once daily 12 hours after the daily dose of the fixed combination.

■ **Special Populations** ***Hepatic Impairment*** Dosage adjustment of dolutegravir is not necessary in patients with mild or moderate hepatic impairment (Child-Pugh class A or B). Dolutegravir should not be used in those with severe hepatic impairment (Child-Pugh class C). (See Hepatic Impairment under Warnings/Precautions: Specific Populations, in Cautions.)

Abacavir/dolutegravir/lamivudine should not be used in patients with mild hepatic impairment (Child-Pugh class A) since reduction of abacavir dosage is needed in such patients. The fixed combination is contraindicated in those with moderate or severe hepatic impairment (Child-Pugh class B or C). (See Hepatic Impairment under Warnings/Precautions: Specific Populations, in Cautions.)

Renal Impairment Dosage adjustment of dolutegravir is not necessary in antiretroviral-naive or antiretroviral-experienced, INSTI-naive patients with mild, moderate, or severe renal impairment.

In INSTI-experienced patients, dosage adjustment of dolutegravir is not needed in those with mild or moderate renal impairment. However, dolutegravir should be used with caution in patients with severe renal impairment who are INSTI-experienced and have certain INSTI-associated resistance substitutions or clinically suspected INSTI resistance. (See Renal Impairment under Warnings/Precautions: Specific Populations, in Cautions.)

The manufacturer makes no specific dosage recommendations regarding use of dolutegravir in patients requiring dialysis; it is unlikely that any type of renal replacement therapy would have a clinically important effect on the pharmacokinetics of dolutegravir. (See Renal Impairment under Warnings/Precautions: Specific Populations, in Cautions.)

Abacavir/dolutegravir/lamivudine should not be used in patients with creatinine clearances less than 50 mL/minute since reduction in lamivudine dosage is needed in such patients. (See Renal Impairment under Warnings/Precautions: Specific Populations, in Cautions.)

Geriatric Patients The manufacturer makes no specific dosage recommendations for dolutegravir in geriatric patients, but recommends caution because of possible age-related decreases in hepatic, renal, and/or cardiac function and concomitant disease and drug therapy. (See Geriatric Use under Warnings/Precautions: Specific Populations, in Cautions.)

Cautions

■ **Contraindications** Dolutegravir (Tivicay®) is contraindicated in patients with a previous hypersensitivity reaction to dolutegravir. The drug also is contraindicated in patients receiving dofetilide. (See Dofetilide under Drug Interactions: Antiarrhythmic Agents.)

The fixed combination containing abacavir, dolutegravir, and lamivudine (abacavir/dolutegravir/lamivudine; Triumeq®) is contraindicated in patients who have the human leukocyte antigen (HLA)-B*5701 allele or have had a previous hypersensitivity reaction to abacavir (regardless of HLA-B*5701 status). Abacavir/dolutegravir/lamivudine also is contraindicated in patients with a previous hypersensitivity reaction to dolutegravir or lamivudine, patients receiving dofetilide (see Dofetilide under Drug Interactions: Antiarrhythmic Agents), and patients with moderate or severe hepatic impairment (see Hepatic Impairment under Warnings/Precautions: Specific Populations, in Cautions). When abacavir/dolutegravir/lamivudine is used, the contraindications associated with each drug in the fixed combination should be considered. (See Precautions Related to Use of Fixed Combinations under Cautions: Warnings/Precautions.)

■ **Warnings/Precautions** ***Sensitivity Reactions*** **Hypersensitivity Reactions.** Hypersensitivity reactions were reported in less than 1% of patients receiving dolutegravir in phase 3 clinical trials. Reactions were manifested by rash and constitutional findings and, occasionally, organ dysfunction including liver toxicity.

If signs or symptoms of hypersensitivity reactions occur, dolutegravir, abacavir/dolutegravir/lamivudine, and any other suspect agents should be discontinued immediately. These signs or symptoms include, but are not limited to, severe rash or rash accompanied by fever, general malaise, fatigue, muscle or joint aches, blisters or peeling skin, oral blisters or lesions, conjunctivitis, facial edema, hepatitis, eosinophilia, angioedema, or difficulty breathing. Clinical status, including liver aminotransferases, should be monitored and appropriate therapy initiated.

A life-threatening reaction could occur if there is a delay in discontinuing dolutegravir, abacavir/dolutegravir/lamivudine, and any other suspect agents after the onset of a hypersensitivity reaction.

Hepatic Effects Adverse hepatic effects have been reported in patients receiving dolutegravir-containing regimens.

Patients with human immunodeficiency virus (HIV) infection and with hepatitis B virus (HBV) or hepatitis C virus (HCV) coinfection may be at increased risk for development or worsening of aminotransferase elevations. In some patients receiving a dolutegravir-containing regimen, serum aminotransferase elevations were consistent with immune reconstitution syndrome or HBV reactivation, particularly in the setting where HBV therapy had been discontinued.

Cases of hepatic toxicity, including elevated serum liver biochemistries, hepatitis, and acute liver failure, also have been reported in patients receiving a dolutegravir-containing regimen who had no preexisting hepatic disease or other identifiable risk factors. Drug-induced liver injury leading to liver transplant has been reported with abacavir/dolutegravir/lamivudine.

Patients receiving dolutegravir-containing regimens should be monitored for hepatotoxicity.

Fetal/Neonatal Morbidity and Mortality Neural tube defects involving the brain, spine, and spinal cord have been reported rarely in infants born to women who received dolutegravir. Preliminary results from an ongoing observational study indicate a higher risk of neural tube defects in infants born to women who were receiving dolutegravir at the time of conception or early in the first trimester of pregnancy.

Pending further accumulation of data, FDA and other experts recommend that women of childbearing potential should undergo pregnancy testing before a dolutegravir-containing regimen is initiated and should take measures to avoid pregnancy during treatment with such regimens. (See Pregnancy under Warnings/Precautions: Specific Populations, in Cautions.)

Interactions The potential for drug interactions should be considered prior to and during treatment with dolutegravir or abacavir/dolutegravir/lamivudine and the patient should be monitored for adverse effects associated with concomitant drugs.

Concomitant use of dolutegravir with certain drugs may result in drug interactions, which may lead to possible loss of therapeutic effect of dolutegravir and possible development of resistance or possible adverse effects from increased exposures of concomitant drugs.

HIV-infected Individuals Coinfected with HBV or HCV HIV-infected patients with HBV or HCV coinfection may be at increased risk of development or worsening of serum aminotransferase elevations. (See Hepatic Effects under Cautions: Warnings/Precautions.)

If abacavir/dolutegravir/lamivudine is used in HIV-infected patients coinfected with HBV or HCV, clinicians should consider that additional precautions apply to these coinfected patients. (See Precautions Related to Use of Fixed Combinations under Cautions: Warnings/Precautions.)

Precautions Related to Use of Fixed Combinations When abacavir/dolutegravir/lamivudine is used, the cautions, precautions, contraindications, and drug interactions associated with each drug in the fixed combination must be considered. Cautionary information applicable to specific populations (e.g., pregnant or nursing women, individuals with hepatic or renal impairment, geriatric patients) should be considered for each drug. For cautionary information related to abacavir and lamivudine, see Cautions in Abacavir Sulfate 8:18.08.20 and in Lamivudine 8:18.08.20.

If abacavir/dolutegravir/lamivudine is used, clinicians should consider that abacavir has been associated with serious and sometimes fatal hypersensitivity reactions, including multiple organ failure and anaphylaxis. Prior to initiation or reinitiation of abacavir/dolutegravir/lamivudine, all patients should be screened for the HLA-B*5701 allele, unless there is documentation of a previous HLA-B*5701 allele assessment. The patient's medical history also should be reviewed for prior exposure to any abacavir-containing preparation. Abacavir/dolutegravir/lamivudine is contraindicated in individuals with the HLA-B*5701 allele and in patients who have had a previous hypersensitivity reaction to abacavir or abacavir-containing preparations. Although individuals with the HLA-B*5701 allele are at higher risk for abacavir hypersensitivity reactions, such reactions have occurred in those without the allele. Abacavir/dolutegravir/lamivudine should be discontinued immediately if a hypersensitivity reaction is suspected, regardless of the patient's HLA-B*5701 status and even if other diagnoses are possible. Abacavir-containing preparations, including abacavir/dolutegravir/lamivudine, should *never* be restarted in a patient who experienced a hypersensitivity reaction since more severe reactions can occur within hours and may include life-threatening hypotension and death. If hypersensitivity is ruled out, the manufacturer of abacavir/dolutegravir/lamivudine states that the drug may be reinitiated, but *only* if medical care is readily accessible. There have been rare reports of life-threatening reactions within hours after reinitiation of abacavir-containing preparations in patients who discontinued abacavir for reasons other than hypersensitivity. Since it is not possible to determine whether a hypersensitivity reaction in patients receiving abacavir/dolutegravir/lamivudine is caused by abacavir or dolutegravir, abacavir-containing and dolutegravir-containing preparations should never be reinitiated in patients who stopped therapy with abacavir/dolutegravir/lamivudine because of a hypersensitivity reaction. (See Cautions: Hypersensitivity Reactions in Abacavir Sulfate 8:18.08.20.)

If abacavir/dolutegravir/lamivudine is used, clinicians should consider that lactic acidosis and severe hepatomegaly with steatosis, including fatalities, have been reported in patients receiving HIV nucleoside reverse transcriptase inhibitors (NRTIs) alone or in conjunction with other antiretrovirals. Abacavir/dolutegravir/lamivudine should be discontinued in patients with clinical or laboratory findings suggestive of lactic acidosis or pronounced hepatotoxicity, which may include hepatomegaly and steatosis even in the absence of marked increases in serum aminotransferase concentrations.

If abacavir/dolutegravir/lamivudine is used in HIV-infected patients coinfected with HBV, clinicians should consider that severe, acute exacerbations of HBV infection have been reported following discontinuance of lamivudine in patients coinfected with HIV and HBV. Hepatic function should be closely monitored with clinical and laboratory follow-up for at least several months after abacavir/dolutegravir/lamivudine is discontinued in HIV-infected patients coinfected with HBV and, if appropriate, initiation of HBV treatment may be warranted. Safety and efficacy of abacavir/dolutegravir/lamivudine have not been established for treatment of chronic HBV infection.

For information on precautions related to the fixed combination of dolutegravir and rilpivirine (dolutegravir/rilpivirine), see Dolutegravir Sodium and Rilpivirine Hydrochloride 8:18.08.12.

Adipogenic Effects Redistribution or accumulation of body fat, including central obesity, dorsocervical fat enlargement ("buffalo hump"), peripheral wasting, facial wasting, breast enlargement, and general cushingoid appearance, has been reported in patients receiving antiretroviral therapy.

The mechanisms and long-term consequences of fat redistribution are unknown; a causal relationship has not been established.

Immune Reconstitution Syndrome Immune reconstitution syndrome has been reported in HIV-infected patients receiving multiple-drug antiretroviral therapy, including dolutegravir. During the initial phase of treatment, HIV-infected patients whose immune systems respond to antiretroviral therapy may develop an inflammatory response to indolent or residual opportunistic infections (e.g., *Mycobacterium avium*, *M. tuberculosis*, cytomegalovirus [CMV], *Pneumocystis jirovecii* [formerly *P. carinii*], varicella-zoster virus [VZV]); such responses may necessitate further evaluation and treatment.

Autoimmune disorders (e.g., Graves' disease, polymyositis, Guillain-Barré syndrome) have also been reported to occur in the setting of immune reconstitution; however, the time to onset is more variable and can occur many months after initiation of antiretroviral therapy.

Specific Populations **Pregnancy.** Antiretroviral Pregnancy Registry at 800-258-4263 or http://www.apregistry.com.

Dolutegravir crosses the placenta and results of an ex vivo perfusion model indicate a high fetal-to-maternal ratio for the drug (0.6).

Preliminary results from an ongoing observational study in Botswana indicate a higher risk of neural tube defects in infants born to women who were receiving a dolutegravir-containing regimen at the time of conception or early in the first trimester of pregnancy. To date, there have been no reported cases of infants born with neural tube defects to women who received dolutegravir initiated later in pregnancy. FDA is conducting a comprehensive review of these results and any other data that become available.

Pending further accumulation of data, FDA and the US Department of Health and Human Services (HHS) Antiretroviral Guideline Panels recommend that women of childbearing potential (including those already receiving a dolutegravir-containing regimen) should be advised about the potential risk of neural tube defects if dolutegravir is taken near the time of conception or early in the first trimester of pregnancy and should be instructed to use effective contraception to avoid pregnancy during treatment with such regimens. Neural tube defects can occur early in pregnancy within the first 4 weeks (28 days) after conception or 6 weeks from the last menstrual period.

FDA and the HHS panels recommend that a pregnancy test be performed in all women of childbearing potential prior to initiation of a dolutegravir-containing regimen. The HHS panels recommend that dolutegravir *not* be initiated in pregnant women within 8 weeks of their last menstrual period. If a woman already receiving a dolutegravir-containing regimen is pregnant and is within 8 weeks of her last menstrual period, the HHS panels recommend that the healthcare provider counsel the woman about the risks and benefits of the current regimen; if other options are available, a switch to a regimen that does not contain dolutegravir is recommended. If a woman is pregnant and 8 or more weeks past her last menstrual period, the HHS panels state that consideration can be given to initiating or continuing a dolutegravir-containing regimen *or* initiating or switching to a regimen that does not contain dolutegravir after weighing the risks and benefits. Clinicians can consult the National Perinatal HIV Hotline at 888-448-8765 for additional guidance.

The manufacturer states that data are insufficient to date to adequately assess the risk of birth defects and miscarriage if dolutegravir is used during pregnancy.

Lactation. The manufacturer states that it is not known whether dolutegravir is distributed into human milk, affects human milk production, or affects the breast-fed infant.

There are some reports that dolutegravir is distributed into human milk in low concentrations; the drug is distributed into milk in rats.

Because of the risk of adverse effects in the infant and the risk of HIV transmission, HIV-infected women should not breast-feed infants.

Pediatric Use. Safety and efficacy of dolutegravir have not been established in pediatric patients weighing less than 30 kg. In addition, safety and efficacy of the drug have not been established in pediatric patients who previously received another HIV integrase strand inhibitor (INSTI-experienced) and have HIV-1 with documented or suspected resistance to other HIV INSTIs (e.g., elvitegravir, raltegravir). The safety profile of dolutegravir in children and adolescents 6 to less than 18 years of age is similar to that in adults.

Abacavir/dolutegravir/lamivudine should not be used in pediatric patients weighing less than 40 kg since dosage adjustments cannot be made. Safety and efficacy of abacavir/dolutegravir/lamivudine in pediatric patients weighing 40 kg or more is derived from pediatric trials that used the individual components of the fixed combination.

Geriatric Use. Experience in patients 65 years of age and older is insufficient to determine whether they respond differently to dolutegravir or abacavir/dolutegravir/lamivudine than younger adults.

Dolutegravir and abacavir/dolutegravir/lamivudine should be used with caution in geriatric patients because of age-related decreases in hepatic, renal, and/or cardiac function and potential for concomitant disease and drug therapy.

Hepatic Impairment. Dolutegravir should not be used in patients with severe hepatic impairment (Child-Pugh class C); pharmacokinetics of the drug have not been evaluated in such patients.

Pharmacokinetics of dolutegravir in patients with moderate hepatic impairment are similar to those in healthy individuals, and dosage adjustments are not needed when the drug is used in those with mild or moderate hepatic insufficiency (Child-Pugh class A or B).

In phase 3 trials, the safety profile of dolutegravir in patients with HBV or HCV coinfection was similar to that in patients without HBV or HCV; however, rates of AST and ALT abnormalities were increased in this subset of patients.

Abacavir/dolutegravir/lamivudine should not be used in adults with mild hepatic impairment (Child-Pugh class A). Because decreased abacavir dosage is recommended in patients with mild hepatic impairment, abacavir/dolutegravir/lamivudine should be switched to the single-entity components to allow adjustment of abacavir dosage in such patients. Abacavir/dolutegravir/lamivudine is contraindicated in adults with moderate or severe hepatic impairment (Child-Pugh class B or C).

Renal Impairment. Dolutegravir should be used with caution in patients with severe renal impairment who are INSTI-experienced and have certain INSTI-associated resistance mutations or clinically suspected INSTI resistance. Plasma concentrations of dolutegravir are decreased in patients with severe renal impairment, which may result in loss of therapeutic effects and development of resistance to the drug or other antiretrovirals.

Mild or moderate renal impairment does not have a clinically important effect on the pharmacokinetics of dolutegravir. Therefore, dosage adjustments are not needed when dolutegravir is used in antiretroviral-naive or antiretroviral-experienced, INSTI-naive patients with mild, moderate, or severe renal impairment. Dosage adjustments also are not needed when the drug is used in INSTI-experienced patients with mild or moderate renal impairment.

Dolutegravir has not been evaluated in patients requiring dialysis. Although there are no specific dosage recommendations for use of dolutegravir in this subset of patients, it is unlikely that any type of renal replacement therapy would have a clinically important effect on the pharmacokinetics of dolutegravir since the drug is highly bound to plasma proteins.

Dolutegravir has been shown to increase serum creatinine concentrations; however, it does not cause a clinically important change in glomerular filtration rate or renal plasma flow. Dolutegravir inhibits tubular secretion of creatinine by inhibiting renal organic cation transporter (OCT) 2 and, possibly, multidrug and toxin extrusion transporter (MATE) 1. (See Drug Interactions.)

Abacavir/dolutegravir/lamivudine should not be used in adults with creatinine clearances less than 50 mL/minute. Because lamivudine is substantially eliminated by the kidneys and decreased lamivudine dosage is recommended in patients with creatinine clearances less than 50 mL/minute, abacavir/dolutegravir/lamivudine should be switched to the single-entity components to allow adjustment of lamivudine dosage in such patients.

■ **Common Adverse Effects** Adverse effects reported in 2% or more of patients receiving dolutegravir include insomnia, headache, fatigue, diarrhea, hyperglycemia, decreased neutrophil count, and increased serum concentrations of aminotransferases, total bilirubin, creatine kinase, lipase, and cholesterol.

Drug Interactions

The following drug interactions are based on studies using dolutegravir. Drug interaction studies have not been performed to date using the fixed combination containing abacavir, dolutegravir, and lamivudine (abacavir/dolutegravir/lamivudine; Triumeq®). When abacavir/dolutegravir/lamivudine is used, interactions associated with each drug in the fixed combination should be considered.

■ **Drugs Affecting or Metabolized by Hepatic Microsomal Enzymes** Cytochrome P-450 (CYP) isoenzyme 3A plays a minor role in the metabolism of dolutegravir. Concomitant use with drugs that induce CYP3A may decrease dolutegravir plasma concentrations and decrease therapeutic effects of the drug. Concomitant use with drugs that inhibit CYP3A may increase dolutegravir plasma concentrations.

In vitro studies indicate that dolutegravir does not inhibit CYP isoenzymes 1A2, 2A6, 2B6, 2C8, 2C9, 2C19, 2D6, or 3A. Dolutegravir does not induce CYP1A2, 2B6, or 3A4 in vitro.

■ **Drugs Affecting or Metabolized by Uridine Diphosphate-glucuronosyltransferases** Dolutegravir is metabolized by uridine diphosphate-glucuronosyltransferase (UGT) 1A1 and in vitro studies indicate the drug is a substrate for UGT1A3 and UGT1A9. Pharmacokinetic interactions are possible with inducers of these enzymes (decreased plasma concentrations of dolutegravir and decreased therapeutic effects of the drug) or inhibitors of these enzymes (increased plasma concentrations of dolutegravir).

Dolutegravir does not inhibit UGT1A1 or UGT2B7 in vitro; pharmacokinetic interactions with drugs that are UGT1A1 or UGT2B7 substrates are not expected.

■ **Drugs Affecting or Affected by P-glycoprotein Transport** Dolutegravir is a substrate of the P-glycoprotein (P-gp) transport system. Pharmacokinetic interactions are possible with inducers of P-gp (decreased plasma concentrations of dolutegravir and decreased therapeutic effects of the drug) or inhibitors of P-gp (increased plasma concentrations of dolutegravir).

Dolutegravir does not inhibit P-gp-mediated transport in vitro; pharmacokinetic interactions with drugs that are P-gp substrates are not expected.

■ **Drugs Affecting or Affected by Bile Salt Export Pump** Dolutegravir does not inhibit the bile salt export pump (BSEP) in vitro; pharmacokinetic interactions with drugs that are substrates of BSEP are not expected.

■ **Drugs Affecting or Affected by Breast Cancer Resistance Protein** Dolutegravir is a substrate of breast cancer resistance protein (BCRP) in vitro. Pharmacokinetic interactions are possible with inducers of BCRP (decreased plasma concentrations of dolutegravir and decreased therapeutic effects of the drug) or inhibitors of BCRP (increased plasma concentrations of dolutegravir).

Dolutegravir does not inhibit BCRP in vitro; pharmacokinetic interactions with drugs that are substrates for BCRP are not expected.

■ **Drugs Affecting or Affected by Multidrug and Toxin Extrusion Transporter** Dolutegravir inhibits multidrug and toxin extrusion transporter (MATE) 1 in vitro. Therefore, dolutegravir may increase plasma concentrations of drugs eliminated by MATE1 (e.g., dofetilide, metformin).

■ **Drugs Affecting or Affected by Multidrug Resistance Protein** Dolutegravir does not inhibit multidrug resistance protein (MRP) 2 or MRP4 in vitro; pharmacokinetic interactions with drugs that are substrates for these transporters are not expected.

■ **Drugs Affecting or Affected by Renal Organic Anion Transporters** In vitro, dolutegravir inhibits renal organic anion transporter (OAT) 1 and OAT3. In vivo, dolutegravir does not alter plasma concentrations of OAT1 or OAT3 substrates (e.g., tenofovir, aminohippurate).

Dolutegravir does not inhibit organic anion transporter polypeptide (OATP) 1B1 or OATP1B3 in vitro; pharmacokinetic interactions with drugs that are substrates for these transporters are not expected. Dolutegravir is not a substrate of OATP1B1 or 1B3 in vitro.

■ **Drugs Affecting or Affected by Renal Organic Cation Transporters** In vitro, dolutegravir inhibits renal organic cation transporter (OCT) 2. Therefore, dolutegravir may increase plasma concentrations of drugs eliminated by OCT2 (e.g., dofetilide, metformin).

Dolutegravir does not inhibit OCT1 in vitro; pharmacokinetic interactions with drugs that are substrates for this transporter are not expected.

■ **Drugs that Increase Gastric pH** ***Antacids*** Antacids containing aluminum, calcium, or magnesium decrease peak plasma concentrations and area under the plasma concentration-time curve (AUC) of dolutegravir.

Dolutegravir and abacavir/dolutegravir/lamivudine should be administered at least 2 hours before or 6 hours after antacids containing polyvalent cations (e.g., aluminum, calcium, magnesium).

Proton-pump Inhibitors **Omeprazole.** Omeprazole does not have a clinically important effect on the pharmacokinetics of dolutegravir.

Dosage adjustments are not needed if dolutegravir is used concomitantly with omeprazole or other proton-pump inhibitors.

Sucralfate Sucralfate may decrease plasma concentrations of dolutegravir.

Dolutegravir and abacavir/dolutegravir/lamivudine should be administered at least 2 hours before or 6 hours after sucralfate.

■ **Antiarrhythmic Agents** ***Dofetilide*** Concomitant use of dofetilide and dolutegravir or abacavir/dolutegravir/lamivudine may increase dofetilide plasma concentrations and increase the risk of serious and/or life-threatening adverse effects.

Concomitant use of dofetilide and dolutegravir or abacavir/dolutegravir/lamivudine is contraindicated.

■ **Anticonvulsants** ***Carbamazepine*** Concomitant use of carbamazepine (300 mg twice daily) and dolutegravir (50 mg once daily) decreases peak plasma concentrations and AUC of dolutegravir.

If carbamazepine is used concomitantly with dolutegravir in adults or pediatric patients weighing 40 kg or more who are antiretroviral-naive or antiretroviral-experienced but have not previously received an HIV integrase strand transfer inhibitor (INSTI-naive), dolutegravir should be given in a dosage of 50 mg twice daily. If carbamazepine is used concomitantly with dolutegravir in pediatric patients weighing 30 to less than 40 kg who are antiretroviral-naive or antiretroviral-experienced but INSTI-naive, dolutegravir should be given in a dosage of 35 mg twice daily. (See Dosage and Administration: Dosage.) An alternative anticonvulsant should be considered in patients receiving dolutegravir who are INSTI-experienced and have HIV-1 with documented or suspected INSTI resistance.

If abacavir/dolutegravir/lamivudine is used concomitantly with carbamazepine, adults should receive 1 tablet of the fixed combination (600 mg of abacavir, 50 mg of dolutegravir, and 300 mg of lamivudine) once daily *and* a 50-mg tablet of single-entity dolutegravir given once daily 12 hours after the daily dose of the fixed combination.

Oxcarbazepine, Phenobarbital, and Phenytoin Oxcarbazepine, phenobarbital, and phenytoin induce metabolism of dolutegravir and cause decreased plasma concentrations of dolutegravir.

Concomitant use of oxcarbazepine, phenobarbital, or phenytoin and dolutegravir or abacavir/dolutegravir/lamivudine should be avoided since data are insufficient to make dosage recommendations. An alternative anticonvulsant should be considered.

■ **Antidiabetic Agents** ***Metformin*** Concomitant use of metformin hydrochloride (500 mg twice daily) and dolutegravir (50 mg once or twice daily) increases peak plasma concentrations and AUC of metformin.

If dolutegravir or abacavir/dolutegravir/lamivudine is initiated or discontinued in patients receiving metformin, blood glucose concentrations should be monitored and metformin dosage adjustments may be required; metformin hydrochloride dosage should not exceed 1 g daily during concomitant therapy. Some experts state that, if metformin is initiated in a patient receiving dolutegravir, the lowest metformin dosage should be used initially and dosage of the antidiabetic agent titrated to achieve glycemic control and minimize adverse GI effects.

■ **Antimycobacterial Agents** ***Rifabutin*** Rifabutin does not have a clinically important effect on the pharmacokinetics of dolutegravir.

Dosage adjustments are not needed if rifabutin and dolutegravir are used concomitantly.

Rifampin Concomitant use of rifampin and dolutegravir decreases plasma concentrations and AUC of dolutegravir.

If rifampin is used concurrently with dolutegravir in adults or pediatric patients weighing 40 kg or more who are antiretroviral-naive or antiretroviral-experienced but INSTI-naive, dolutegravir should be given in a dosage of 50 mg twice daily. If rifampin is used concurrently with dolutegravir in pediatric patients weighing 30 to less than 40 kg who are antiretroviral-naive or antiretroviral-experienced but INSTI-naive, dolutegravir should be given in a dosage of 35 mg twice daily. An alternative to rifampin (e.g., rifabutin) should be considered in patients receiving dolutegravir who are INSTI-experienced and have HIV-1 with documented or suspected INSTI resistance.

If abacavir/dolutegravir/lamivudine is used concurrently with rifampin, adults should receive 1 tablet of the fixed combination (600 mg of abacavir, 50 mg of dolutegravir, and 300 mg of lamivudine) once daily *and* a 50-mg tablet of single-entity dolutegravir given once daily 12 hours after the daily dose of the fixed combination. (See Dosage and Administration: Dosage.)

Rifapentine Clinically important decreases in dolutegravir plasma concentrations are expected if rifapentine is used concomitantly. Some experts state that rifapentine and dolutegravir should not be used concomitantly.

■ **Antiretroviral Agents** ***HIV Entry and Fusion Inhibitors*** There is no in vitro evidence of antagonistic antiretroviral effects between dolutegravir and enfuvirtide or maraviroc.

HIV Integrase Inhibitors (INSTIs) There is no in vitro evidence of antagonistic antiretroviral effects between dolutegravir and raltegravir.

HIV Nonnucleoside Reverse Transcriptase Inhibitors (NNRTIs) There is no in vitro evidence of antagonistic antiretroviral effects between dolutegravir and efavirenz or nevirapine.

Efavirenz. Concomitant use of efavirenz and dolutegravir decreases plasma concentrations and AUC of dolutegravir.

If efavirenz is used concurrently with dolutegravir in adults or pediatric patients weighing 40 kg or more who are antiretroviral-naive or antiretroviral-experienced but INSTI-naive, dolutegravir should be given in a dosage of 50 mg twice daily. If efavirenz is used concurrently with dolutegravir in pediatric patients weighing 30 to less than 40 kg who are antiretroviral-naive or antiretroviral-experienced but INSTI-naive, dolutegravir should be given in a dosage of 35 mg twice daily. Whenever possible, an alternative to efavirenz that is not a metabolic inducer should be considered when dolutegravir is used in INSTI-experienced patients who have HIV-1 with documented or suspected INSTI resistance.

If abacavir/dolutegravir/lamivudine is used concurrently with efavirenz, adults should receive 1 tablet of the fixed combination (600 mg of abacavir, 50 mg of dolutegravir, and 300 mg of lamivudine) once daily *and* a 50-mg tablet of single-entity dolutegravir given once daily 12 hours after the daily dose of the fixed combination. (See Dosage and Administration: Dosage.)

Etravirine. Concomitant use of etravirine and dolutegravir results in substantially decreased plasma concentrations and AUC of dolutegravir. The effect on dolutegravir pharmacokinetics is mitigated if *ritonavir-boosted* darunavir or the fixed combination of lopinavir and ritonavir (lopinavir/ritonavir) is used concomitantly with etravirine and dolutegravir and is expected to be mitigated if *ritonavir-boosted* atazanavir is used concomitantly with etravirine and dolutegravir.

Etravirine should not be used concomitantly with dolutegravir or abacavir/dolutegravir/lamivudine unless *ritonavir-boosted* atazanavir, *ritonavir-boosted* darunavir, or lopinavir/ritonavir is included in the regimen. However, concomitant use of etravirine and *ritonavir-boosted* atazanavir is *not* usually recommended.

If etravirine is used concomitantly with dolutegravir in patients who are antiretroviral-naive or antiretroviral-experienced without INSTI resistance, some experts state that dolutegravir should be given in a dosage of 50 mg once daily and *ritonavir-boosted* atazanavir, *ritonavir-boosted* darunavir, or lopinavir/ritonavir should also be included in the regimen. (See Dosage and Administration: Dosage.)

Nevirapine. Concomitant use of nevirapine and dolutegravir may decrease dolutegravir plasma concentrations and AUC.

The manufacturer states that nevirapine should not be used concomitantly with dolutegravir or abacavir/dolutegravir/lamivudine; data are insufficient to make dosage recommendations. Some experts state that dosage adjustments are not needed if nevirapine and dolutegravir are used concomitantly.

Rilpivirine. Concomitant use of rilpivirine and dolutegravir does not have a clinically important effect on the pharmacokinetics of either drug.

Dosage adjustments are not needed if rilpivirine and dolutegravir are used concomitantly.

HIV Nucleoside and Nucleotide Reverse Transcriptase Inhibitors (NRTIs) There is no in vitro evidence of antagonistic antiretroviral effects between dolutegravir and abacavir or stavudine.

Tenofovir. Concomitant use of tenofovir alafenamide fumarate (TAF) or tenofovir disoproxil fumarate (tenofovir DF) and dolutegravir does not have a clinically important effect on the pharmacokinetics of the tenofovir prodrug or dolutegravir.

Dosage adjustments are not needed if TAF or tenofovir DF is used concomitantly with dolutegravir.

HIV Protease Inhibitors (PIs) There is no in vitro evidence of antagonistic antiretroviral effects between dolutegravir and amprenavir (active metabolite of fosamprenavir) or lopinavir.

Atazanavir. Concomitant use of dolutegravir and *ritonavir-boosted* or unboosted atazanavir results in increased dolutegravir plasma concentrations and AUC, but does not appear to affect the pharmacokinetics of atazanavir. Data are not available regarding concomitant use of dolutegravir and *cobicistat-boosted* atazanavir.

Dosage adjustments are not needed if dolutegravir is used concomitantly with *cobicistat-boosted*, *ritonavir-boosted*, or unboosted atazanavir.

Darunavir. Concomitant use of dolutegravir and *ritonavir-boosted* darunavir decreases peak plasma concentrations and AUC of dolutegravir, but does not appear to affect the pharmacokinetics of darunavir. Clinically important drug interactions are not expected if *cobicistat-boosted* darunavir is used concomitantly with dolutegravir.

Dosage adjustments are not needed if dolutegravir is used concomitantly with *cobicistat-boosted* or *ritonavir-boosted* darunavir.

Fosamprenavir. Concomitant use of *ritonavir-boosted* fosamprenavir and dolutegravir decreases plasma concentrations and AUC of dolutegravir, but does not appear to affect the pharmacokinetics of fosamprenavir or ritonavir.

If *ritonavir-boosted* fosamprenavir is used concomitantly with dolutegravir in adults or pediatric patients weighing 40 kg or more who are antiretroviral-naive or antiretroviral-experienced but INSTI-naive, dolutegravir should be given in a dosage of 50 mg twice daily. If *ritonavir-boosted* fosamprenavir is used concomitantly with dolutegravir in pediatric patients weighing 30 to less than 40 kg who are antiretroviral-naive or antiretroviral-experienced but INSTI-naive, dolutegravir should be given in a dosage of 35 mg twice daily. Whenever possible, an alternative to *ritonavir-boosted* fosamprenavir that is not a metabolic inducer should be considered when dolutegravir is used in INSTI-experienced patients who have HIV-1 with documented or suspected INSTI resistance.

If abacavir/dolutegravir/lamivudine is used concomitantly with *ritonavir-boosted* fosamprenavir, adults should receive 1 tablet of the fixed combination (600 mg of abacavir, 50 mg of dolutegravir, and 300 mg of lamivudine) once daily *and* a 50-mg tablet of single-entity dolutegravir given once daily 12 hours after the daily dose of the fixed combination. (See Dosage and Administration: Dosage.)

Lopinavir. Concomitant use of lopinavir/ritonavir (lopinavir 400 mg/ritonavir 100 mg twice daily) and dolutegravir (30 mg once daily) does not have a clinically important effect on the pharmacokinetics of dolutegravir.

Dosage adjustments are not needed if dolutegravir is used concomitantly with lopinavir/ritonavir.

Tipranavir. Concomitant use of *ritonavir-boosted* tipranavir and dolutegravir decreases peak plasma concentrations and AUC of dolutegravir.

If *ritonavir-boosted* tipranavir is used concomitantly with dolutegravir in adults or pediatric patients weighing 40 kg or more who are antiretroviral-naive or antiretroviral-experienced but INSTI-naive, dolutegravir should be given in a dosage of 50 mg twice daily. If *ritonavir-boosted* tipranavir is used concomitantly with dolutegravir in pediatric patients weighing 30 to less than 40 kg who are antiretroviral-naive or antiretroviral-experienced but INSTI-naive, dolutegravir should be given in a dosage of 35 mg twice daily. Whenever possible, an alternative to *ritonavir-boosted* tipranavir that is not a metabolic inducer should be considered when dolutegravir is used in INSTI-experienced patients who have HIV-1 with documented or suspected INSTI resistance.

If abacavir/dolutegravir/lamivudine is used concomitantly with *ritonavir-boosted* tipranavir, adults should receive 1 tablet of the fixed combination (600 mg of abacavir, 50 mg of dolutegravir, and 300 mg of lamivudine) once daily *and* a 50-mg tablet of single-entity dolutegravir given once daily 12 hours after the daily dose of the fixed combination. (See Dosage and Administration: Dosage.)

■ **Benzodiazepines** ***Midazolam*** Dolutegravir does not have a clinically important effect on the AUC of midazolam.

Dosage adjustments are not needed if midazolam is used concomitantly with dolutegravir.

■ **Calcium, Iron, Multivitamins, and Other Preparations Containing Polyvalent Cations** ***Calcium, Iron, and Multivitamins*** Oral calcium supplements, oral iron preparations, or other oral supplements containing calcium or iron (e.g., multivitamins), may decrease plasma concentrations of dolutegravir when used concomitantly in the fasted state.

Dolutegravir or abacavir/dolutegravir/lamivudine should be administered at least 2 hours before or 6 hours after oral supplements containing calcium or iron . Alternatively, if dolutegravir or abacavir/dolutegravir/lamivudine is administered with food, the drugs can be used concomitantly with oral supplements containing calcium or iron.

Preparations Containing Polyvalent Cations Concomitant use of dolutegravir and drugs containing polyvalent cations (e.g., magnesium, aluminum, laxatives, buffered preparations) may decrease plasma concentrations of dolutegravir when used concomitantly in the fasted state.

Dolutegravir or abacavir/dolutegravir/lamivudine should be administered at least 2 hours before or 6 hours after drugs or preparations containing polyvalent cations.

■ **Corticosteroids** ***Prednisone*** Prednisone does not have a clinically important effect on the pharmacokinetics of dolutegravir.

Dosage adjustments are not needed if prednisone is used in patients receiving dolutegravir.

■ **Estrogens and Progestins** ***Estradiol, Estrogen, and Conjugated Estrogens*** Concomitant use of dolutegravir and estradiol, estrogen, or conjugated estrogens (equine or synthetic) may have variable effects on estrogen concentrations.

Some experts state that dosage adjustments are not needed if dolutegravir is used concomitantly with estradiol, estrogen, or conjugated estrogens.

Ethinyl Estradiol and Norgestimate Dolutegravir does not have a clinically important effect on the pharmacokinetics of hormonal contraceptives containing ethinyl estradiol or norgestimate.

Dosage adjustments are not needed if oral contraceptives containing norgestimate and ethinyl estradiol are used in patients receiving dolutegravir.

Drospirenone, Medroxyprogesterone, and Progesterone Pharmacokinetic interactions are not expected if dolutegravir is used concomitantly with drospirenone, medroxyprogesterone, or micronized progesterone.

Some experts state that dosage adjustments are not needed if dolutegravir is used concomitantly with drospirenone, medroxyprogesterone, or micronized progesterone.

■ **Finasteride** Pharmacokinetic interactions are not expected if dolutegravir is used concomitantly with finasteride.

Some experts state that dosage adjustments are not needed if dolutegravir is used concomitantly with finasteride.

■ **Goserelin** Pharmacokinetic interactions are not expected if dolutegravir is used concomitantly with goserelin.

Some experts state that dosage adjustments are not needed if dolutegravir is used concomitantly with goserelin.

■ **HCV Antivirals** ***HCV Polymerase Inhibitors*** **Sofosbuvir.** Concomitant use of sofosbuvir and dolutegravir is not expected to have clinically important effects on dolutegravir or sofosbuvir pharmacokinetics.

Dosage adjustments are not needed if sofosbuvir and dolutegravir are used concomitantly.

Sofosbuvir and Velpatasvir. No clinically important pharmacokinetic interactions were observed when the fixed combination of sofosbuvir and velpatasvir (sofosbuvir/velpatasvir) was used concomitantly with dolutegravir.

Dosage adjustments are not needed if sofosbuvir/velpatasvir and dolutegravir are used concomitantly.

Sofosbuvir, Velpatasvir, and Voxilaprevir. No clinically important pharmacokinetic interactions are expected if the fixed combination of sofosbuvir, velpatasvir, and voxilaprevir (sofosbuvir/velpatasvir/voxilaprevir) is used concomitantly with dolutegravir.

Some experts state that dosage adjustments are not needed if dolutegravir is used concomitantly with sofosbuvir/velpatasvir/voxilaprevir.

HCV Protease Inhibitors **Glecaprevir and Pibrentasvir.** Concomitant use of dolutegravir and the fixed combination of glecaprevir and pibrentasvir (glecaprevir/pibrentasvir) does not result in clinically important interactions.

Dosage adjustments are not needed if dolutegravir is used concomitantly with glecaprevir/pibrentasvir.

Simeprevir. No clinically important interactions are expected if simeprevir is used concomitantly with dolutegravir.

Some experts state that dosage adjustments are not needed if simeprevir and dolutegravir are used concomitantly.

HCV Replication Complex Inhibitors **Daclatasvir.** Concomitant use of daclatasvir and dolutegravir does not have a clinically important effect on the pharmacokinetics of either drug.

Dosage adjustments are not needed if daclatasvir and dolutegravir are used concomitantly.

Elbasvir and Grazoprevir. Concomitant use of dolutegravir and the fixed combination of elbasvir and grazoprevir (elbasvir/grazoprevir) does not result in clinically important changes in the pharmacokinetics of elbasvir, grazoprevir, or dolutegravir.

Dosage adjustments are not needed if elbasvir/grazoprevir is used concomitantly with dolutegravir.

Ledipasvir and Sofosbuvir. Concomitant use of the fixed combination of ledipasvir and sofosbuvir (ledipasvir/sofosbuvir) and dolutegravir does not have a clinically important effect on the pharmacokinetics of dolutegravir, ledipasvir, or sofosbuvir.

Some experts state that dosage adjustments are not needed if ledipasvir/sofosbuvir and dolutegravir are used concomitantly.

■ **Leuprolide** Pharmacokinetic interactions are not expected if dolutegravir is used concomitantly with leuprolide.

Some experts state that dosage adjustments are not needed if dolutegravir is used concomitantly with leuprolide.

■ **Nucleoside and Nucleotide Antivirals** There is no in vitro evidence of antagonistic antiviral effects between dolutegravir and adefovir or ribavirin.

■ **Opiate Agonists and Partial Agonists** ***Methadone*** Dolutegravir does not have a clinically important effect on the pharmacokinetics of methadone.

Dosage adjustments are not needed if methadone and dolutegravir are used concomitantly.

■ **Selective Serotonin-reuptake Inhibitors** Concomitant use of dolutegravir and citalopram does not have a clinically important effect on the pharmacokinetics of either drug. Pharmacokinetic interactions are not expected if dolutegravir is used concomitantly with other selective serotonin-reuptake inhibitors (SSRIs) .

Dosage adjustments are not needed if dolutegravir is used concomitantly with citalopram or other SSRIs.

■ **Spironolactone** Pharmacokinetic interactions are not expected if dolutegravir is used concomitantly with spironolactone.

Some experts state that dosage adjustments are not needed if dolutegravir is used concomitantly with spironolactone.

■ **Testosterone** Pharmacokinetic interactions are not expected if dolutegravir is used concomitantly with testosterone.

Some experts state that dosage adjustments are not needed if dolutegravir is used concomitantly with testosterone.

■ **Dietary and Herbal Supplements** ***St. John's Wort*** St. John's wort (*Hypericum perforatum*) induces metabolism of dolutegravir and causes decreased plasma concentrations of dolutegravir.

Concomitant use of St. John's wort with dolutegravir or abacavir/dolutegravir/lamivudine should be avoided.

Description

Dolutegravir sodium, an antiretroviral agent, is a human immunodeficiency virus (HIV) integrase strand transfer inhibitor (INSTI). Dolutegravir binds to the active site of HIV integrase and blocks the strand transfer step of retroviral DNA integration, which is essential for HIV replication. The drug is active against HIV type 1 (HIV-1) and also has in vitro activity against HIV type 2 (HIV-2). Dolutegravir is not active against hepatitis C virus (HCV).

Dolutegravir-resistant HIV-1 has been produced in vitro and has emerged during dolutegravir therapy. In initial clinical studies in antiretroviral-naive patients, dolutegravir treatment was not associated with emergence of INSTI resistance. Treatment-emergent INSTI resistance has been reported when dolutegravir was used in clinical studies in antiretroviral-experienced patients who had not previously received an INSTI (INSTI-naive) or patients who had previously received an INSTI (INSTI-experienced), including some patients with historical genotypic evidence of INSTI-resistance substitutions or phenotypic evidence of resistance to other INSTIs (elvitegravir, raltegravir). In some studies, treatment-emergent INSTI resistance was reported less frequently in those who received dolutegravir than those who received raltegravir, and it has been suggested that dolutegravir may possess a higher barrier to resistance than elvitegravir and raltegravir.

Although there is some evidence that dolutegravir has a different resistance profile than other HIV INSTIs and has been active in vitro against some HIV-1 strains resistant to other INSTIs (e.g., elvitegravir, raltegravir), cross-resistance between dolutegravir and other INSTIs (e.g., elvitegravir and/or raltegravir) has been reported. Dolutegravir has been active against HIV-1 resistant to HIV nucleoside reverse transcriptase inhibitors (NRTIs), HIV nonnucleoside reverse transcriptase inhibitors (NNRTIs), or HIV protease inhibitors (PIs).

Dolutegravir is commercially available as single-entity tablets (Tivicay®). Dolutegravir also is commercially available in fixed-combination tablets containing abacavir and lamivudine (abacavir/dolutegravir/lamivudine; Triumeq®); abacavir and lamivudine are both HIV NRTIs. In addition, dolutegravir is commercially available in fixed combination with rilpivirine (dolutegravir/rilpivirine); rilpivirine is an HIV NNRTI. (See Dolutegravir Sodium and Rilpivirine Hydrochloride 8:18.08.12.)

Following oral administration of 50 mg of dolutegravir once or twice daily, peak plasma concentrations of the drug are attained 2–3 hours after a dose. Steady state is achieved within approximately 5 days when a once-daily regimen is used. Although food increases the extent and decreases the rate of oral absorption of dolutegravir, the drug may be taken with or without food. Following oral administration in the fasted state, a single tablet of abacavir/dolutegravir/lamivudine (600 mg of abacavir, 50 mg of dolutegravir, and 300 mg of lamivudine) is bioequivalent to a 50-mg dolutegravir tablet taken simultaneously with a fixed-combination tablet containing 600 mg of abacavir and 300 mg of lamivudine (abacavir/lamivudine) in the fasted state. Dolutegravir is metabolized primarily by uridine diphosphate-glucuronosyltransferase (UGT) 1A1; cytochrome P-450 (CYP) isoenzyme 3A plays only a minor role in metabolism of the drug. Following an oral dose, 53% of the dose is eliminated unchanged in feces, 31% is eliminated in urine as metabolites, and less than 1% is eliminated in urine unchanged. Dolutegravir has a terminal half-life of approximately 14 hours. Clearance of dolutegravir is 32% lower and the area under the plasma concentration-time curve (AUC) of the drug is 46% higher in individuals with UGT1A1 genotypes conferring poor dolutegravir metabolism compared with results obtained in those with UGT1A1 genotypes associated with normal UGT1A1 metabolism.

Advice to Patients

Critical nature of compliance with human immunodeficiency virus (HIV) therapy and importance of remaining under the care of a clinician. Importance of taking as prescribed; do not alter or discontinue antiretroviral regimen without consulting clinician.

Importance of using single-entity dolutegravir (Tivicay®) in conjunction with other antiretrovirals—not for monotherapy. Fixed combination containing abacavir, dolutegravir, and lamivudine (abacavir/dolutegravir/lamivudine; Triumeq®) is used alone as a complete regimen for treatment of HIV-1 infection or may be used in conjunction with other antiretrovirals.

Antiretroviral therapy is not a cure for HIV infection; opportunistic infections and other complications associated with HIV disease may still occur.

Advise patients that early initiation of antiretroviral therapy and sustained decreases in plasma HIV RNA have been associated with reduced risk of progression to acquired immunodeficiency syndrome (AIDS) and death.

Advise patients that effective antiretroviral regimens can decrease HIV levels in blood and genital secretions and strict adherence to such regimens in conjunction with risk-reduction measures may decrease, but cannot absolutely eliminate, the risk of secondary transmission of HIV to others. Importance of continuing to practice safer sex (e.g., using latex or polyurethane condoms to minimize sexual contact with body fluids) and reducing high-risk behaviors (e.g., reusing or sharing needles).

Importance of reading patient information provided by the manufacturer.

If a dose of dolutegravir or abacavir/dolutegravir/lamivudine is missed and remembered 4 hours or more before the next scheduled time, the dose should be taken as soon as it is remembered and the next dose taken at the regularly scheduled time. If a missed dose of dolutegravir or abacavir/dolutegravir/lamivudine is remembered within 4 hours before the next dose is due, the dose should be skipped and the next dose taken at the regularly scheduled time. A double dose should not be taken to make up for a missed dose.

Importance of immediately discontinuing dolutegravir, abacavir/dolutegravir/lamivudine, and other suspect agents and seeking medical attention if rash occurs and is associated with fever, generally ill feeling, extreme tiredness, muscle or joint aches, breathing difficulty, blisters or peeling skin, oral blisters or lesions, eye inflammation, swelling of the face, eyes, lips, or mouth, and/or signs and symptoms of liver problems (e.g., yellowing of skin or whites of the eyes, dark or tea-colored urine, pale stools/bowel movements, nausea, vomiting, loss of appetite, or pain, aching, or sensitivity on right side below ribs).

Advise patients that hepatotoxicity has been reported in patients receiving dolutegravir and that monitoring for hepatotoxicity is recommended.

Advise patients that signs and symptoms of inflammation from previous infections may occur soon after initiation of antiretroviral therapy in some individuals. Importance of immediately informing clinicians if any signs or symptoms of infection occur.

Inform patients that redistribution/accumulation of body fat may occur with antiretroviral therapy, with as yet unknown long-term health effects.

Importance of informing clinicians of existing or contemplated concomitant therapy, including prescription and OTC drugs and herbal products, and any concomitant illnesses.

Importance of women informing clinicians if they are or plan to become pregnant or plan to breast-feed. (See Pregnancy under Warnings/Precautions: Specific Populations, in Cautions.) Advise HIV-infected women not to breast-feed.

Importance of advising patients of other important precautionary information. (See Cautions.)

Overview® (see Users Guide). For additional information on this drug until a more detailed monograph is developed and published, the manufacturer's labeling should be consulted. It is *essential* that the manufacturer's labeling be consulted for more detailed information on usual cautions, precautions, contraindications, potential drug interactions, laboratory test interferences, and acute toxicity.

Preparations

Excipients in commercially available drug preparations may have clinically important effects in some individuals; consult specific product labeling for details.

Dolutegravir Sodium

Oral		
Tablets, film-coated	10 mg (of dolutegravir)	**Tivicay®**, ViiV
	25 mg (of dolutegravir)	**Tivicay®**, ViiV
	50 mg (of dolutegravir)	**Tivicay®**, ViiV

Dolutegravir Sodium Combinations

Oral		
Tablets, film-coated	50 mg (of dolutegravir) with Abacavir Sulfate 600 mg (of abacavir) and Lamivudine 300 mg	**Triumeq®**, ViiV
	50 mg (of dolutegravir) with Rilpivirine Hydrochloride 25 mg (of rilpivirine)	**Juluca®**, ViiV

†Use is not currently included in the labeling approved by the US Food and Drug Administration

Dolutegravir Sodium and Rilpivirine Hydrochloride

dolutegravir/rilpivirine, DTG/RPV, DTG, RPV

■ Dolutegravir sodium and rilpivirine hydrochloride (dolutegravir/rilpivirine) is a fixed-combination antiretroviral agent containing dolutegravir (human immunodeficiency virus [HIV] integrase strand transfer inhibitor [INSTI]) and rilpivirine (HIV nonnucleoside reverse transcriptase inhibitor [NNRTI]).

Uses

■ **Treatment of HIV Infection** The fixed combination of dolutegravir sodium and rilpivirine hydrochloride (dolutegravir/rilpivirine) is used for the treatment of human immunodeficiency virus type 1 (HIV-1) infection in antiretroviral-experienced (previously treated) adults to replace the current antiretroviral regimen in those who are virologically suppressed (i.e., plasma HIV-1 RNA levels less than 50 copies/mL) on a stable antiretroviral regimen for at least 6 months, have no known history of treatment failure, and are infected with HIV-1 with no known substitutions associated with resistance to dolutegravir or rilpivirine.

Dolutegravir/rilpivirine is used alone as a complete regimen for the treatment of HIV-1 infection in certain antiretroviral-experienced adults; the manufacturer states that concomitant use with other antiretrovirals is not recommended.

The most appropriate antiretroviral regimen cannot be defined for each clinical scenario, and selection of specific antiretroviral agents for use in multiple-drug regimens should be individualized based on information regarding antiretroviral potency, potential rate of development of resistance, known toxicities, and potential for pharmacokinetic interactions as well as virologic, immunologic, and clinical characteristics of the patient. For information on the general principles and guidelines for use of antiretroviral therapy, including specific recommendations for initial therapy in antiretroviral-naive patients and recommendations for changing antiretroviral regimens, see the Antiretroviral Agents General Statement 8:18.08.

Antiretroviral-experienced Adults In antiretroviral-experienced adults, dolutegravir/rilpivirine can be used to replace the current antiretroviral regimen *only* in those who are virologically suppressed (i.e., plasma HIV-1 RNA levels less than 50 copies/mL) on a stable antiretroviral regimen for at least 6 months, have no known history of treatment failure, and are infected with HIV-1 with no known substitutions associated with resistance to dolutegravir or rilpivirine.

When considering a change to a 2-drug antiretroviral regimen in antiretroviral-experienced adults who are virologically suppressed on an effective regimen, the HHS Panel on Antiretroviral Guidelines for Adults and Adolescents states that a regimen of dolutegravir and rilpivirine can be a reasonable option when use of HIV nucleoside reverse transcriptase inhibitors (NRTIs) is not desirable and when resistance to dolutegravir or rilpivirine is not expected.

Clinical Experience. Efficacy and safety of a 2-drug antiretroviral regimen of dolutegravir and rilpivirine in antiretroviral-experienced adults were evaluated in 2 identically designed randomized, open-label, active-control, phase 3 noninferiority studies (SWORD-1 and SWORD-2). Patients enrolled in these studies were adults with plasma HIV-1 RNA levels less than 50 copies/mL for at least 6 months (median age 43 years, 22% female, 20% non-white, 11% with baseline $CD4^+$ T-cell count less than 350 cells/mm^3). At initial screening, all patients were on a stable suppressive antiretroviral regimen (i.e., an HIV integrase strand transfer inhibitor [INSTI], HIV nonnucleoside reverse transcriptase inhibitor [NNRTI], or HIV protease inhibitor [PI] in conjunction with 2 HIV NRTIs) for at least 6 months and had no known history of resistance to dolutegravir or rilpivirine. Patients were randomized in a 1:1 ratio to either switch to the 2-drug regimen of dolutegravir and rilpivirine (dolutegravir 50 mg and rilpivirine 25 mg) once daily or stay on their current antiretroviral regimen. The primary end point was virologic response (defined as plasma HIV-1 RNA levels less than 50 copies/mL) at 48 weeks. Pooled virologic outcomes at 48 weeks indicated that 95% of patients in both treatment groups had plasma HIV-1 RNA levels less than 50 copies/mL.

Dosage and Administration

■ **Administration** The fixed combination of dolutegravir and rilpivirine (dolutegravir/rilpivirine) is administered orally once daily with a meal. The manufacturer states that a protein drink alone does not constitute a meal. (See Description.)

■ **Dosage** Dolutegravir/rilpivirine is commercially available as fixed-combination tablets containing dolutegravir sodium and rilpivirine hydrochloride; dosages are expressed in terms of dolutegravir and rilpivirine, respectively.

Each fixed-combination tablet of dolutegravir/rilpivirine contains 50 mg of dolutegravir and 25 mg of rilpivirine.

Adult Dosage **Treatment of HIV Infection in Antiretroviral-experienced Adults.** For the treatment of human immunodeficiency virus type 1 (HIV-1) infection in certain antiretroviral-experienced adults (see Uses: Treatment of HIV Infection), the usual dosage of dolutegravir/rilpivirine is 1 tablet (50 mg of dolutegravir and 25 mg of rilpivirine) once daily.

Treatment of HIV Infection in Antiretroviral-experienced Adults Receiving Rifabutin. If dolutegravir/rilpivirine is used for the treatment of HIV-1 infection in certain antiretroviral-experienced adults (see Uses: Treatment of HIV Infection) receiving rifabutin, patients should receive 1 tablet of the fixed combination (50 mg of dolutegravir and 25 mg of rilpivirine) *and* a 25-mg tablet of single-entity rilpivirine once daily to provide a total rilpivirine dosage of 50 mg daily. (See Rifabutin under Drug Interactions: Antimycobacterial Agents.)

■ **Special Populations** ***Hepatic Impairment*** Dosage adjustment of dolutegravir/rilpivirine is not necessary in adults with mild or moderate hepatic impairment (Child-Pugh class A or B).

The effect of severe hepatic impairment (Child-Pugh class C) on the pharmacokinetics of dolutegravir/rilpivirine is not known and the manufacturer makes no specific dosage recommendations for such patients. (See Hepatic Impairment under Warnings/Precautions: Specific Populations, in Cautions.)

Renal Impairment Dosage adjustment of dolutegravir/rilpivirine is not necessary in adults with mild or moderate renal impairment (creatinine clearance 30 mL/minute or greater).

The manufacturer makes no specific dosage recommendations for those with severe renal impairment (creatinine clearance less than 30 mL/minute) or end-stage renal disease; increased monitoring for adverse effects is recommended in such individuals. (See Renal Impairment under Warnings/Precautions: Specific Populations, in Cautions.)

Geriatric Patients The manufacturer makes no specific dosage recommendations for dolutegravir/rilpivirine in geriatric patients, but recommends caution because of possible age-related decreases in hepatic, renal, and/or cardiac function and concomitant disease and drug therapy. (See Geriatric Use under Warnings/Precautions: Specific Populations, in Cautions.)

Cautions

■ **Contraindications** The fixed combination of dolutegravir and rilpivirine (dolutegravir/rilpivirine) is contraindicated in patients with a previous hypersensitivity reaction to dolutegravir or rilpivirine.

Concomitant use of dolutegravir/rilpivirine and dofetilide is contraindicated since concomitant use may result in serious and/or life threatening adverse effects due to possible increased dofetilide plasma concentrations. (See Drug Interactions.)

Concomitant use of dolutegravir/rilpivirine with drugs that induce cytochrome P-450 isoenzyme 3A (CYP3A) or drugs that elevate gastric pH is contraindicated since substantially decreased plasma rilpivirine concentrations may occur and may result in loss of virologic response. This includes concomitant use with certain anticonvulsants (carbamazepine, oxcarbazepine, phenobarbital, phenytoin), certain antimycobacterials (rifampin, rifapentine), systemic dexamethasone (given in multiple doses), proton-pump inhibitors (e.g., esomeprazole, lansoprazole, omeprazole, pantoprazole, rabeprazole), or certain herbal supplements (St. John's wort [*Hypericum perforatum*]). (See Drug Interactions.)

■ **Warnings/Precautions** ***Sensitivity Reactions*** Hypersensitivity reactions (e.g., rash, constitutional findings, and sometimes organ dysfunction, including liver injury) have been reported in patients receiving dolutegravir. These adverse effects were reported in less than 1% of patients receiving dolutegravir in phase 3 clinical trials.

Severe skin and hypersensitivity reactions, including cases of drug reaction with eosinophilia and systemic symptoms (DRESS), have been reported during postmarketing experience with rilpivirine-containing regimens. Some skin reactions were accompanied by constitutional symptoms such as fever; other skin reactions were associated with organ dysfunction, including elevated hepatic enzyme concentrations. During phase 3 clinical trials evaluating rilpivirine, treatment-associated rash with at least grade 2 severity was reported in 3% of patients.

Dolutegravir/rilpivirine should be immediately discontinued if signs or symptoms of severe skin or hypersensitivity reactions occur (including, but not limited to, severe rash or rash accompanied by fever, general malaise, fatigue, muscle or joint aches, blisters or peeling of the skin, mucosal involvement [oral blisters or lesions], conjunctivitis, facial edema, hepatitis, eosinophilia, angioedema, difficulty breathing). The patient's clinical status, including laboratory parameters with liver aminotransferases, should be monitored and appropriate therapy initiated. Delay in stopping dolutegravir/rilpivirine treatment after onset of a hypersensitivity reaction may result in a life-threatening reaction.

Hepatic Effects Adverse hepatic effects have been reported in patients receiving dolutegravir- or rilpivirine-containing regimens.

Patients with human immunodeficiency virus (HIV) infection and with hepatitis B virus (HBV) or hepatitis C virus (HCV) coinfection or markedly elevated serum aminotransferase concentrations prior to initiation of dolutegravir/rilpivirine may be at increased risk for development or worsening of aminotransferase elevations. In some patients receiving a dolutegravir-containing regimen, serum aminotransferase elevations were consistent with immune reconstitution syndrome or HBV reactivation, particularly in the setting where HBV therapy had been discontinued.

Cases of hepatic toxicity, including elevated serum liver biochemistries and hepatitis, also have been reported in patients receiving dolutegravir- or rilpivirine-containing regimens who had no preexisting hepatic disease or other identifiable risk factors. Drug-induced liver injury leading to acute liver failure has been reported with dolutegravir-containing regimens; drug-induced liver injury leading to liver transplant has been reported with the fixed combination of abacavir, dolutegravir, and lamivudine (abacavir/dolutegravir/lamivudine).

Patients receiving dolutegravir/rilpivirine should be monitored for hepatotoxicity.

Depressive Disorders Depressive disorders (depressed mood, depression, dysphoria, major depression, altered mood, negative thoughts, suicide attempt, suicidal ideation) have been reported in patients receiving dolutegravir and/or rilpivirine.

Patients experiencing severe depressive symptoms should be promptly evaluated to determine the likelihood that symptoms are related to dolutegravir/rilpivirine and to determine if the benefits of continued dolutegravir/rilpivirine therapy outweigh the risks.

Fetal/Neonatal Morbidity and Mortality Neural tube defects involving the brain, spine, and spinal cord have been reported rarely in infants born to women who received dolutegravir. Preliminary results from an ongoing observational study indicate a higher risk of neural tube defects in infants born to women who were receiving dolutegravir at the time of conception or early in the first trimester of pregnancy.

Pending further accumulation of data, FDA and other experts recommend that women of childbearing potential should undergo pregnancy testing before a dolutegravir-containing regimen is initiated and should take measures to avoid pregnancy during treatment with such regimens. (See Pregnancy under Warnings/Precautions: Specific Populations, in Cautions.)

Interactions The potential for drug interactions should be considered prior to and during treatment with dolutegravir/rilpivirine and the patient should be monitored for adverse effects associated with concomitant drugs.

Concomitant use of dolutegravir/rilpivirine with certain drugs may result in drug interactions, which may lead to possible loss of therapeutic effect of dolutegravir/rilpivirine and possible development of resistance or possible adverse effects from increased exposures of concomitant drugs.

Because prolongation of the QT interval corrected for rate (QT_c) has been reported in healthy individuals receiving rilpivirine in a dosage of 75 or 300 mg once daily (3 or 12 times higher, respectively, than the rilpivirine dose in dolutegravir/rilpivirine), use of alternative antiretrovirals should be considered in patients receiving a drug with a known risk of torsades de pointes.

HIV-infected Individuals Coinfected with HBV or HCV HIV-infected patients with HBV or HCV coinfection may be at increased risk for elevated aminotransferase concentrations during dolutegravir/rilpivirine therapy. (See Hepatic Effects under Cautions: Warnings/Precautions.)

Population pharmacokinetic analyses have not shown any clinically important effects on dolutegravir or rilpivirine exposures in HIV-infected individuals with HCV coinfection. Individuals with HBV coinfection were excluded from clinical studies evaluating dolutegravir/rilpivirine.

Precautions Related to Use of Fixed Combinations When dolutegravir/rilpivirine is used, the cautions, precautions, contraindications, and drug interactions associated with both drugs in the fixed combination must be considered. Cautionary information applicable to specific populations (e.g., pregnant or nursing women, individuals with hepatic or renal impairment, geriatric patients) should be considered for each drug. For cautionary information related to dolutegravir and rilpivirine, see Dolutegravir Sodium 8:18.08.12 and see Rilpivirine Hydrochloride 8:18.08.16.

Specific Populations **Pregnancy.** Antiretroviral Pregnancy Registry at 800-258-4263 or http://www.apregistry.com.

Dolutegravir crosses the placenta and results of an ex vivo perfusion model indicate a high fetal-to-maternal ratio for the drug (0.6). Rilpivirine also crosses the placenta.

Preliminary results from an ongoing observational study in Botswana indicate a higher risk of neural tube defects in infants born to women who were receiving a dolutegravir-containing regimen at the time of conception or early in the first trimester of pregnancy. To date, there have been no reported cases of infants born with neural tube defects to women who received dolutegravir initiated later in pregnancy. FDA is conducting a comprehensive review of these results and any other data that become available.

Pending further accumulation of data, FDA and the US Department of Health and Human Services (HHS) Antiretroviral Guideline Panels recommend that women of childbearing potential (including those already receiving a dolutegravir-containing regimen) should be advised about the potential risk of neural tube defects if dolutegravir is taken near the time of conception or early in the first trimester of pregnancy and should be instructed to use effective contraception to avoid pregnancy during treatment with such regimens. Neural tube defects can occur early in pregnancy within the first 4 weeks (28 days) after conception or 6 weeks from the last menstrual period.

FDA and the HHS panels recommend that a pregnancy test be performed in all women of childbearing potential prior to initiation of a dolutegravir-containing regimen. The HHS panels recommend that dolutegravir *not* be initiated in pregnant women within 8 weeks of their last menstrual period. If a woman already receiving a dolutegravir-containing regimen is pregnant and is within 8 weeks of her last menstrual period, the HHS panels recommend that the healthcare provider counsel the woman about the risks and benefits of the current regimen; if other options are available, a switch to a regimen that does not contain dolutegravir is recommended. If a woman is pregnant and 8 or more weeks past her last menstrual period, the HHS panels state that consideration can be given to initiating or continuing a dolutegravir-containing regimen *or* initiating or switching to a regimen that does not contain dolutegravir after weighing the risks and benefits. Clinicians can consult the National Perinatal HIV Hotline at 888-448-8765 for additional guidance.

The manufacturer states that data are insufficient to date to adequately assess the risk of birth defects and miscarriage in pregnant women receiving dolutegravir/rilpivirine.

In animal reproduction studies, no evidence of adverse developmental outcomes was observed with the components of dolutegravir/rilpivirine. During organogenesis in rabbits and rats, systemic exposures to dolutegravir were less than and 38 times, respectively, exposures at the recommended human dose; exposures to rilpivirine were 70 and 15 times, respectively, exposures at the recommended human dose. In rat pre- and post-natal development studies, maternal systemic exposures to dolutegravir and rilpivirine were approximately 32 and 63 times, respectively, the exposures of each component in humans at the recommended human dose.

Lactation. It is not known whether the components of dolutegravir/rilpivirine are distributed into human milk, affect human milk production, or affect the breast-fed infant.

There are some reports that dolutegravir is distributed into human milk in low concentrations; the drug is distributed into milk in rats.

It is not known whether rilpivirine is distributed into human milk; the drug has been detected in the plasma of rat pups exposed to rilpivirine through the milk of lactating rats.

Because of the risk of adverse effects in the infant and the risk of HIV transmission, HIV-infected women should not breast-feed infants.

Pediatric Use. Safety and efficacy of dolutegravir/rilpivirine have not been established in pediatric patients. Pharmacokinetics of the drug have not been evaluated in pediatric patients.

Geriatric Use. Clinical studies of dolutegravir/rilpivirine did not include a sufficient number of patients 65 years of age or older to determine whether they respond differently compared with younger patients. Population pharmacokinetic analyses indicate that age has no clinically important effect on the pharmacokinetics of dolutegravir or rilpivirine.

Dolutegravir/rilpivirine should be used with caution in geriatric patients because of age-related decreases in hepatic, renal, and/or cardiac function and potential for concomitant disease and drug therapy.

Hepatic Impairment. Dosage adjustments are not necessary if dolutegravir/rilpivirine is used in patients with mild or moderate hepatic impairment (Child-Pugh class A or B).

Dolutegravir exposures in individuals with moderate hepatic impairment (Child-Pugh class B) were similar to those observed in healthy individuals. The effect of severe hepatic impairment (Child-Pugh class C) on dolutegravir exposures has not been evaluated.

Rilpivirine exposures were 47 or 5% higher in individuals with mild or moderate hepatic impairment (Child-Pugh class A or B), respectively, compared with healthy individuals. The effect of severe hepatic impairment (Child-Pugh class C) on rilpivirine exposures has not been evaluated.

Renal Impairment. Increased monitoring for adverse effects is recommended if dolutegravir/rilpivirine is used in patients with severe renal impairment (creatinine clearance less than 30 mL/minute) or end-stage renal disease. Dosage adjustments are not necessary if dolutegravir/rilpivirine is used in patients with mild or moderate renal impairment (creatinine clearance 30 mL/minute or greater).

Population pharmacokinetic analyses indicate that mild and moderate renal impairment do not have a clinically important effect on dolutegravir pharmacokinetics. In individuals with severe renal impairment, dolutegravir area under the plasma concentration-time curve (AUC), peak plasma concentrations, and plasma concentrations measured 24 hours after dosing were 40, 23, and 43% lower, respectively, compared with healthy individuals. The pharmacokinetics of dolutegravir have not been evaluated in individuals requiring dialysis.

Population pharmacokinetic analyses indicate that mild renal impairment does not have a clinically important effect on rilpivirine pharmacokinetics. The pharmacokinetics of rilpivirine have not been evaluated in individuals with moderate or severe renal impairment, end-stage renal disease, or renal disease requiring dialysis.

■ **Common Adverse Effects** Adverse effects reported in 2% or more of patients receiving dolutegravir/rilpivirine include diarrhea and headache.

Drug Interactions

The following drug interactions are based on studies using the individual components of the fixed combination of dolutegravir and rilpivirine (dolutegravir/rilpivirine) or are predicted to occur with the fixed combination. When dolutegravir/rilpivirine is used, interactions associated with both drugs in the fixed combination should be considered.

■ **Drugs Affecting or Metabolized by Hepatic Microsomal Enzymes** Cytochrome P-450 (CYP) isoenzyme 3A plays a minor role in the metabolism of dolutegravir; rilpivirine is primarily metabolized by CYP3A4. Concomitant use with drugs that induce CYP3A may decrease dolutegravir and rilpivirine plasma concentrations, decrease therapeutic effects of the drugs, and may lead to resistance to rilpivirine or other HIV nonnucleoside reverse transcriptase inhibitors (NNRTIs). Concomitant use with drugs that inhibit CYP3A may increase dolutegravir and rilpivirine plasma concentrations.

In vitro studies indicate that dolutegravir does not inhibit CYP isoenzymes 1A2, 2A6, 2B6, 2C8, 2C9, 2C19, 2D6, or 3A. Dolutegravir does not induce CYP1A2, 2B6, or 3A4 in vitro. Rilpivirine is not likely to have a clinically important effect on exposures of drugs metabolized by CYP isoenzymes.

■ **Drugs Affecting or Metabolized by Uridine Diphosphate-glucuronosyltransferases** Dolutegravir is metabolized by uridine diphosphate-glucuronosyltransferase (UGT) 1A1, and in vitro studies indicate the drug also is a substrate for UGT1A3 and UGT1A9. Pharmacokinetic interactions are possible with inducers of these enzymes (decreased plasma concentrations of dolutegravir and decreased therapeutic effects of the drug) or inhibitors of these enzymes (increased plasma concentrations of dolutegravir).

Dolutegravir does not inhibit UGT1A1 or UGT2B7 in vitro.

■ Drugs Affecting or Affected by P-glycoprotein Transport Dolutegravir is a substrate of the P-glycoprotein (P-gp) transport system in vitro. Pharmacokinetic interactions are possible with inducers of P-gp (decreased plasma concentrations of dolutegravir and decreased therapeutic effects of the drug) or inhibitors of P-gp (increased plasma concentrations of dolutegravir).

Dolutegravir does not inhibit P-gp-mediated transport in vitro.

■ Drugs Affecting or Affected by Bile Salt Export Pump Dolutegravir does not inhibit the bile salt export pump (BSEP) in vitro.

■ Drugs Affecting or Affected by Breast Cancer Resistance Protein Dolutegravir is a substrate of breast cancer resistance protein (BCRP) in vitro. Pharmacokinetic interactions are possible with inducers of BCRP (decreased plasma concentrations of dolutegravir and decreased therapeutic effects of the drug) or inhibitors of BCRP (increased plasma concentrations of dolutegravir).

Dolutegravir does not inhibit BCRP in vitro.

■ Drugs Affecting or Affected by Multidrug and Toxin Extrusion Transporter Dolutegravir inhibits multidrug and toxin extrusion transporter (MATE) 1 in vitro. Therefore, dolutegravir may increase plasma concentrations of drugs eliminated by MATE1 (e.g., dofetilide, metformin).

■ Drugs Affecting or Affected by Multidrug Resistance Protein Dolutegravir does not inhibit multidrug resistance protein (MRP) 2 or MRP4 in vitro.

■ Drugs Affecting or Affected by Renal Organic Anion Transporters In vitro, dolutegravir inhibits renal organic anion transporter (OAT) 1 and OAT3. In vivo, dolutegravir does not alter plasma concentrations of OAT1 or OAT3 substrates (e.g., tenofovir, aminohippurate).

Dolutegravir does not inhibit organic anion transporter polypeptide (OATP) 1B1 or OATP1B3 in vitro. Dolutegravir is not a substrate of OATP1B1 or 1B3 in vitro.

■ Drugs Affecting or Affected by Renal Organic Cation Transporters In vitro, dolutegravir inhibits renal organic cation transporter (OCT) 2. Therefore, dolutegravir may increase plasma concentrations of drugs eliminated by OCT2 (e.g., dofetilide, metformin).

Dolutegravir does not inhibit OCT1 in vitro.

■ Drugs that Increase Gastric pH ***Antacids*** Antacids containing aluminum, calcium, or magnesium are expected to decrease plasma concentrations of rilpivirine and may result in loss of therapeutic response and lead to resistance to rilpivirine or other HIV NNRTIs. Antacids also decrease plasma concentrations and area under the concentration-time curve (AUC) of dolutegravir.

Dolutegravir/rilpivirine should be administered at least 4 hours before or 6 hours after antacids containing aluminum, calcium, or magnesium.

Histamine H_2-receptor Antagonists Concomitant use of rilpivirine (single dose) and famotidine (single dose taken 2 hours before rilpivirine) results in decreased rilpivirine plasma concentrations and AUC. Concomitant use of other histamine H_2-receptor antagonists (e.g., cimetidine, nizatidine, ranitidine) also may result in decreased rilpivirine plasma concentrations and loss of therapeutic response and may lead to resistance to rilpivirine or other HIV NNRTIs. Concomitant use of histamine H_2-receptor antagonists and dolutegravir is not expected to affect dolutegravir exposures.

Dolutegravir/rilpivirine should be administered at least 4 hours before or 12 hours after a histamine H_2-receptor antagonist.

Proton-pump Inhibitors Concomitant use of omeprazole and rilpivirine results in decreased rilpivirine plasma concentrations and AUC. Concomitant use of other proton-pump inhibitors (e.g., esomeprazole, lansoprazole, pantoprazole, rabeprazole) also may result in decreased rilpivirine plasma concentrations and loss of therapeutic response and may lead to resistance to rilpivirine or other HIV NNRTIs. Concomitant use of omeprazole and dolutegravir does not have a clinically important effect on the pharmacokinetics of dolutegravir.

Concomitant use of dolutegravir/rilpivirine and proton-pump inhibitors (e.g., esomeprazole, lansoprazole, omeprazole, pantoprazole, rabeprazole) is contraindicated.

Sucralfate Dolutegravir/rilpivirine should be administered at least 4 hours before or 6 hours after sucralfate.

■ Drugs that Prolong the QT Interval Because rilpivirine can prolong the QT interval corrected for rate (QT_c), an alternative to dolutegravir/rilpivirine should be considered in patients receiving drugs with a known risk of torsades de pointes. (See Interactions under Cautions: Warnings/Precautions.)

■ Acetaminophen Concomitant use of rilpivirine and acetaminophen does not have a clinically important effect on the pharmacokinetics of either drug.

■ Antiarrhythmic Agents ***Dofetilide*** Concomitant use of dofetilide and dolutegravir/rilpivirine may increase dofetilide plasma concentrations and increase the risk of serious and/or life-threatening adverse effects.

Concomitant use of dofetilide and dolutegravir/rilpivirine is contraindicated.

■ Anticonvulsants ***Carbamazepine*** Concomitant use of carbamazepine (300 mg twice daily) and dolutegravir (50 mg once daily) decreases peak plasma concentrations and AUC of dolutegravir. Concomitant use of carbamazepine and rilpivirine is expected to substantially decrease rilpivirine exposures, which may lead to loss of virologic response.

Concomitant use of carbamazepine and dolutegravir/rilpivirine is contraindicated.

Oxcarbazepine, Phenobarbital, and Phenytoin Oxcarbazepine, phenobarbital, and phenytoin are expected to decrease dolutegravir and rilpivirine exposures, which may lead to loss of virologic response.

Concomitant use of oxcarbazepine, phenobarbital, or phenytoin and dolutegravir/rilpivirine is contraindicated.

■ Antidiabetic Agents ***Metformin*** Concomitant use of metformin hydrochloride (500 mg twice daily) and dolutegravir (50 mg once or twice daily) increases peak plasma concentrations and AUC of metformin.

If dolutegravir/rilpivirine is initiated or discontinued in patients receiving metformin, blood glucose concentrations should be monitored and metformin dosage adjustments may be required; metformin hydrochloride dosage should not exceed 1 g daily during concomitant therapy.

■ Antimycobacterial Agents ***Rifabutin*** Concomitant use of rifabutin and rilpivirine results in decreased rilpivirine plasma concentrations and AUC. Rifabutin does not have a clinically important effect on the pharmacokinetics of dolutegravir.

If dolutegravir/rilpivirine is used concomitantly with rifabutin, the manufacturer recommends that patients receive 1 tablet of the fixed combination (50 mg of dolutegravir and 25 mg of rilpivirine) *and* a 25-mg tablet of single-entity rilpivirine once daily with a meal to provide a total rilpivirine dosage of 50 mg daily.

Rifampin and Rifapentine Concomitant use of rifampin and dolutegravir decreases plasma concentrations and AUC of dolutegravir. Concomitant use of rifampin and rilpivirine decreases plasma concentrations and AUC of rilpivirine and may result in loss of virologic response.

Concomitant use of rifapentine and dolutegravir/rilpivirine is expected to result in clinically important decreases in rilpivirine plasma concentrations and may lead to loss of virologic response; dolutegravir plasma concentrations also may be decreased.

Concomitant use of rifampin or rifapentine with dolutegravir/rilpivirine is contraindicated.

■ Antiretroviral Agents Dolutegravir/rilpivirine is a complete regimen for the treatment of human immunodeficiency virus type 1 (HIV-1) infection in certain antiretroviral-experienced adults (see Uses: Treatment of HIV Infection), and the manufacturer states that concomitant use with other antiretroviral agents is not recommended.

■ Benzodiazepines ***Midazolam*** Dolutegravir does not have a clinically important effect on the AUC of midazolam.

■ Calcium, Iron, Multivitamins, and Other Preparations Containing Polyvalent Cations ***Calcium, Iron, and Multivitamins*** Oral calcium supplements, oral iron preparations, or other oral supplements containing calcium or iron (e.g., multivitamins) may decrease plasma concentrations of dolutegravir when used concomitantly with dolutegravir/rilpivirine in the fasted state.

Dolutegravir/rilpivirine should be administered at least 4 hours before or 6 hours after oral supplements containing calcium or iron. Alternatively, if dolutegravir/rilpivirine is administered with food, the drug can be used concomitantly with oral supplements containing calcium or iron.

Preparations Containing Polyvalent Cations Concomitant use of dolutegravir/rilpivirine and drugs containing polyvalent cations (e.g., magnesium, aluminum, laxatives, buffered medications, cation-containing products) may decrease absorption of dolutegravir resulting in decreased plasma concentrations of the drug.

Dolutegravir/rilpivirine should be administered at least 4 hours before or 6 hours after drugs or preparations containing polyvalent cations.

■ Chlorzoxazone Concomitant use of rilpivirine and chlorzoxazone does not have a clinically important effect on the pharmacokinetics of either drug.

■ Corticosteroids ***Dexamethasone*** Concomitant use of systemic dexamethasone (multiple doses) with dolutegravir/rilpivirine may result in decreased plasma concentrations of rilpivirine and may lead to loss of virologic response.

Concomitant use of more than a single dose of dexamethasone with dolutegravir/rilpivirine is contraindicated.

Prednisone Prednisone does not have a clinically important effect on the pharmacokinetics of dolutegravir.

■ Digoxin Rilpivirine does not have a clinically important effect on digoxin pharmacokinetics.

■ **Estrogens and Progestins** Dolutegravir does not have a clinically important effect on the pharmacokinetics of norelgestromin.

Concomitant use of rilpivirine with ethinyl estradiol and norethindrone does not have a clinically important effect on rilpivirine, ethinyl estradiol, or norethindrone pharmacokinetics.

■ **HCV Antivirals** ***HCV Polymerase Inhibitors*** **Sofosbuvir.** In cirrhotic patients with HIV and hepatitis C virus (HCV) coinfection receiving dolutegravir and rilpivirine (with or without HIV nucleoside reverse transcriptase inhibitors [NRTIs]) concomitantly with simeprevir and sofosbuvir (with or without ribavirin), no clinically important drug interactions were observed.

HCV Protease Inhibitors **Simeprevir.** Concomitant use of simeprevir and rilpivirine does not have a clinically important effect on the pharmacokinetics of either drug.

In cirrhotic patients with HIV and HCV coinfection receiving dolutegravir and rilpivirine (with or without HIV NRTIs) concomitantly with simeprevir and sofosbuvir (with or without ribavirin), no clinically important drug interactions were observed.

HCV Replication Complex Inhibitors **Daclatasvir.** Concomitant use of daclatasvir and dolutegravir does not have a clinically important effect on the pharmacokinetics of either drug.

■ **HMG-CoA Reductase Inhibitors** Concomitant use of rilpivirine and atorvastatin does not have a clinically important effect on the pharmacokinetics of either drug.

■ **Macrolides** Concomitant use of dolutegravir/rilpivirine and clarithromycin, erythromycin, or telithromycin may result in increased rilpivirine plasma concentrations, but is not expected to affect dolutegravir concentrations. An alternative to these macrolides (e.g., azithromycin) should be considered whenever possible in patients receiving dolutegravir/rilpivirine.

■ **Opiate Agonists and Partial Agonists** ***Methadone*** Dolutegravir does not have a clinically important effect on the pharmacokinetics of methadone. Concomitant use of methadone and rilpivirine results in decreased methadone concentrations, but does not have a clinically important effect on rilpivirine concentrations or AUC.

Although adjustment of initial methadone dosage is not needed when methadone and dolutegravir/rilpivirine are used concomitantly, close clinical monitoring is recommended and adjustment of methadone maintenance dosage may be required in some patients.

■ **Phosphodiesterase Type 5 Inhibitors** ***Sildenafil*** Concomitant use of rilpivirine and sildenafil does not have a clinically important effect on the pharmacokinetics of either drug.

■ **St. John's Wort** Concomitant use of St. John's wort (*Hypericum perforatum*) and dolutegravir/rilpivirine may result in clinically important decreases in rilpivirine plasma concentrations and may lead to loss of virologic response to the drug; dolutegravir plasma concentrations also may be decreased.

Concomitant use of St. John's wort and dolutegravir/rilpivirine is contraindicated.

Description

Dolutegravir sodium and rilpivirine hydrochloride (dolutegravir/rilpivirine) is a fixed combination containing 2 human immunodeficiency virus (HIV) antiretrovirals. Dolutegravir is an HIV integrase strand transfer inhibitor (INSTI) and rilpivirine is a diarylpyrimidine HIV nonnucleoside reverse transcriptase inhibitor (NNRTI). There is no in vitro evidence of antagonistic anti-HIV effects between dolutegravir and rilpivirine.

Dolutegravir binds to the active site of HIV integrase and blocks the strand transfer step of retroviral DNA integration, which is essential for HIV replication. Rilpivirine noncompetitively inhibits HIV type 1 (HIV-1) reverse transcriptase. Strains of HIV-1 resistant to dolutegravir or rilpivirine have been produced in vitro and have emerged during clinical use. In clinical studies evaluating a 2-drug regimen of dolutegravir and rilpivirine in antiretroviral-experienced adults, virologic failure during treatment with the regimen was reported in 2 patients with detectable resistance substitutions at rebound. One patient had a dolutegravir resistance-associated substitution (G193E) at baseline without decreased susceptibility to dolutegravir; the other patient had an HIV NNRTI resistance-associated substitution (K101K/E) without decreased susceptibility to rilpivirine and without HIV INSTI-resistance-associated substitutions. HIV-1 resistant to some other HIV INSTIs (e.g., elvitegravir, raltegravir) may have reduced susceptibility or resistance to dolutegravir. Cross-resistance occurs among HIV NNRTIs and cross-resistance to efavirenz, etravirine, and/or nevirapine is likely after virologic failure and development of resistance to rilpivirine.

Following oral administration of dolutegravir, peak plasma concentrations of the drug are attained 3 hours after a dose. Administration with a moderate- or high-fat meal increases the area under the concentration-time curve (AUC) of dolutegravir by 1.9-fold. Dolutegravir is metabolized primarily by uridine diphosphate-glucuronosyltransferase (UGT) 1A1; cytochrome P-450 (CYP) isoenzyme 3A plays only a minor role in metabolism of the drug. Following an oral dose, 64% of the dose is eliminated in feces (53% as unchanged drug) and 31% is eliminated in urine as metabolites (less than 1% as unchanged drug). Dolutegravir has a half-life of 14 hours. In vitro studies indicate that dolutegravir is approximately 99% bound to plasma proteins.

Following oral administration of rilpivirine, peak plasma concentrations of the drug are generally attained 4 hours after a dose. Administration with a moderate- or high-fat meal increases the AUC of rilpivirine by 1.6- or 1.7-fold, respectively. If taken with only a protein-rich nutritional drink, rilpivirine exposures are 50% lower than when taken with a meal. Rilpivirine is primarily metabolized by CYP3A. Following an oral dose, 85% of the dose is eliminated in feces (25% as unchanged drug) and 6.5% is eliminated in urine (less than 1% as unchanged drug). The half-life of rilpivirine is 50 hours. In vitro studies indicate that rilpivirine is approximately 99% bound to plasma proteins.

Advice to Patients

Critical nature of compliance with human immunodeficiency virus (HIV) therapy and importance of remaining under the care of a clinician. Importance of taking as prescribed; do not alter or discontinue antiretroviral regimen without consulting clinician.

Fixed combination dolutegravir and rilpivirine (dolutegravir/rilpivirine) is used alone as a complete regimen for treatment of HIV-1 infection in certain antiretroviral-experienced adults.

Antiretroviral therapy is not a cure for HIV infection; opportunistic infections and other complications associated with HIV disease may still occur.

Advise patients that early initiation of antiretroviral therapy and sustained decreases in plasma HIV RNA have been associated with reduced risk of progression to acquired immunodeficiency syndrome (AIDS) and death.

Advise patients that effective antiretroviral regimens can decrease HIV levels in blood and genital secretions and strict adherence to such regimens in conjunction with risk-reduction measures may decrease, but cannot absolutely eliminate, the risk of secondary transmission of HIV to others. Importance of continuing to practice safer sex (e.g., using latex or polyurethane condoms to minimize sexual contact with body fluids) and reducing high-risk behaviors (e.g., reusing or sharing needles).

Importance of reading patient information provided by the manufacturer.

Importance of taking once daily with a meal; a protein drink alone does not constitute a meal.

If a dose of dolutegravir/rilpivirine is missed, the dose should be taken with a meal as soon as it is remembered. A double dose should not be taken to make up for a missed dose.

Importance of immediately discontinuing dolutegravir/rilpivirine and seeking medical attention if rash occurs and is associated with fever, generally ill feeling, extreme tiredness, muscle or joint aches, breathing difficulty, blisters or peeling skin, oral blisters or lesions, eye inflammation, swelling of the face, eyes, lips, or mouth, and/or signs and symptoms of liver problems (e.g., yellowing of skin or whites of the eyes, dark or tea-colored urine, pale stools/bowel movements, nausea, vomiting, loss of appetite, or pain, aching, or sensitivity on right side below ribs). Advise patients that close monitoring and appropriate laboratory testing or treatment may be required if a hypersensitivity reaction occurs.

Advise patients that depressive disorders (depressed mood, depression, dysphoria, major depression, altered mood, negative thoughts, suicide attempt, suicidal ideation) have been reported in patients receiving the components of dolutegravir/rilpivirine. Importance of immediately contacting clinician if depressive symptoms (e.g., feeling sad, hopeless, anxious, or restless; hurting oneself; having thoughts of hurting oneself) occur.

Advise patients that hepatotoxicity has been reported in patients receiving the components of dolutegravir/rilpivirine and that monitoring for hepatotoxicity is recommended.

Importance of informing clinicians of existing or contemplated concomitant therapy, including prescription and OTC drugs and herbal products, and any concomitant illnesses.

Importance of women informing clinicians if they are or plan to become pregnant or plan to breast-feed. (See Pregnancy under Warnings/Precautions: Specific Populations, in Cautions.) Advise HIV-infected women not to breast-feed.

Importance of advising patients of other important precautionary information. (See Cautions.)

Overview® (see Users Guide). For additional information on this drug until a more detailed monograph is developed and published, the manufacturer's labeling should be consulted. It is *essential* that the manufacturer's labeling be consulted for more detailed information on usual cautions, precautions, contraindications, potential drug interactions, laboratory test interferences, and acute toxicity.

Preparations

Excipients in commercially available drug preparations may have clinically important effects in some individuals; consult specific product labeling for details.

Dolutegravir Sodium and Rilpivirine Hydrochloride

Oral		
Film-coated tablets	Dolutegravir Sodium 50 mg (of dolutegravir) and Rilpivirine Hydrochloride 25 mg (of rilpivirine)	**Juluca®**, ViiV

Elvitegravir, Cobicistat, Emtricitabine, and Tenofovir Alafenamide Fumarate

EVG/c/FTC/TAF, EVG/c/TAF/FTC, EVG/COBI/FTC/TAF, EVG/COBI/TAF/FTC, EVG, COBI, FTC, TAF Fumarate, TAF

■ Elvitegravir, cobicistat, emtricitabine, and tenofovir alafenamide (EVG/c/FTC/TAF) is a fixed-combination antiretroviral agent containing elvitegravir (human immunodeficiency virus [HIV] integrase strand transfer inhibitor [INSTI]), cobicistat (pharmacokinetic enhancer), emtricitabine (HIV nucleoside reverse transcriptase inhibitor [NRTI]), and tenofovir alafenamide (HIV nucleotide reverse transcriptase inhibitor). Cobicistat, a mechanism-based cytochrome P-450 (CYP) 3A inhibitor, is included in the fixed combination to increase plasma concentrations of elvitegravir (*cobicistat-boosted* elvitegravir) and is not active against HIV.

Uses

■ **Treatment of HIV Infection** The fixed combination of elvitegravir, cobicistat, emtricitabine, and tenofovir alafenamide (EVG/c/FTC/TAF) is used for the treatment of human immunodeficiency virus type 1 (HIV-1) infection in antiretroviral-naive (have not previously received antiretroviral therapy) or antiretroviral-experienced (previously treated) adults and pediatric patients 12 years of age or older.

EVG/c/FTC/TAF is used alone as a complete regimen for the treatment of HIV-1 infection; concomitant use with other antiretroviral agents is not recommended. (See Drug Interactions: Antiretroviral Agents.)

The most appropriate antiretroviral regimen cannot be defined for each clinical scenario, and selection of specific antiretroviral agents for use in multiple-drug regimens should be individualized based on information regarding antiretroviral potency, potential rate of development of resistance, known toxicities, and potential for pharmacokinetic interactions as well as virologic, immunologic, and clinical characteristics of the patient. For information on the general principles and guidelines for use of antiretroviral therapy, including specific recommendations for initial therapy in antiretroviral-naive patients and recommendations for changing antiretroviral regimens, see the Antiretroviral Agents General Statement 8:18.08.

Antiretroviral-naive Adults For *initial* treatment in HIV-infected adults, the US Department of Health and Human Services (HHS) Panel on Antiretroviral Guidelines for Adults and Adolescents states that EVG/c/FTC/TAF is a recommended HIV integrase strand transfer inhibitor-based (INSTI-based) regimen.

Clinical Experience. The comparative efficacy and safety of EVG/c/FTC/TAF (Genvoya®) and the fixed combination of elvitegravir, cobicistat, emtricitabine, and tenofovir disoproxil fumarate (tenofovir DF) (EVG/c/FTC/TDF; Stribild®) were evaluated in 2 identical randomized, double blind, active-control, phase 3 noninferiority studies in antiretroviral-naive HIV-infected adults (study 104; NCT01780506 and study 111; NCT01797445). Patients enrolled in these studies were adults (mean age 36 years, 85% male, 57% white, 25% black, 10% Asian, 19% Hispanic, mean baseline plasma HIV-1 RNA level 4.5 $\log_{10}$ copies/mL, mean baseline CD4$^+$ T-cell count 427 cells/mm^3). Patients were randomized in a 1:1 ratio to receive EVG/c/FTC/TAF (elvitegravir 150 mg, cobicistat 150 mg, emtricitabine 200 mg, tenofovir alafenamide 10 mg) or EVG/c/FTC/TDF (elvitegravir 150 mg, cobicistat 150 mg, emtricitabine 200 mg, tenofovir DF 300 mg) once daily. The primary end point was virologic response (defined as HIV-1 RNA levels less than 50 copies/mL). At 48 weeks, results from each study showed that virologic response in patients receiving EVG/c/FTC/TAF was noninferior to virologic response in those receiving EVG/c/FTC/TDF. Pooled data from both studies at 48 weeks indicate that 92% of those receiving EVG/c/FTC/TAF had plasma HIV-1 RNA levels less than 50 copies/mL compared with 90% of those receiving EVG/c/FTC/TDF. The mean increase in CD4$^+$ T-cell count from baseline was 230 cells/mm^3 in those receiving EVG/c/FTC/TAF compared with 211 cells/mm^3 in those receiving EVG/c/FTC/TDF. At 96 weeks, 87% of patients receiving EVG/c/FTC/TAF and 85% of those receiving EVG/c/FTC/TDF had plasma HIV-1 RNA levels less than 50 copies/mL. The mean increase in CD4$^+$ T-cell count from baseline was 280 cells/mm^3 in those receiving EVG/c/FTC/TAF compared with 266 cells/mm^3 in those receiving EVG/c/FTC/TDF. Treatment outcomes were similar across subgroups (i.e., age, gender, race, baseline viral load, and baseline CD4$^+$ T-cell count).

Antiretroviral-experienced Adults For use in antiretroviral-experienced adults, the manufacturer states that EVG/c/FTC/TAF can be used to replace the current antiretroviral regimen in those who have had plasma HIV-1 RNA levels less than 50 copies/mL on a stable antiretroviral regimen for at least 6 months, have no history of treatment failure, and are infected with HIV-1 with no known substitutions associated with resistance to the antiretroviral components of the fixed combination (i.e., elvitegravir, emtricitabine, tenofovir).

Clinical Experience. The efficacy and safety of EVG/c/FTC/TAF in antiretroviral-experienced adults were evaluated in a randomized, open-label, active-control, phase 3 noninferiority study (study 109; NCT01815736). Patients enrolled in the study were adults with baseline plasma HIV-1 RNA levels less than 50 copies/mL for at least 6 months (mean age 41 years, 90% male, 67% white, 21% black, mean baseline CD4$^+$ T-cell count 705 cells/mm^3). At initial screening, all patients were on a suppressive antiretroviral regimen (i.e., *ritonavir-boosted* or *cobicistat-boosted* atazanavir in conjunction with the fixed combination of emtricitabine and tenofovir DF [42%], EVG/c/FTC/TDF [32%], or fixed combination of efavirenz, emtricitabine, and tenofovir DF [26%]) for at least 6 months and had no known history of resistance to the antiretroviral components of EVG/c/FTC/TAF. Patients were randomized in a 2:1 ratio to either switch to EVG/c/FTC/TAF (elvitegravir 150 mg, cobicistat 150 mg, emtricitabine 200 mg, tenofovir alafenamide 10 mg) or stay on their baseline antiretroviral regimen. The primary end point was virologic response (defined as HIV-1 RNA levels less than 50 copies/mL). At 96 weeks, 93% of those receiving EVG/c/FTC/TAF had plasma HIV-1 RNA levels less than 50 copies/mL compared with 89% of those who continued to receive their baseline antiretroviral regimen. The mean increase in CD4$^+$ T-cell count from baseline was 60 cells/mm^3 in those receiving EVG/c/FTC/TAF compared with 42 cells/mm^3 in those who continued to receive their baseline antiretroviral regimen.

HIV-infected Individuals with Renal Impairment **Clinical Experience.** The efficacy and safety of EVG/c/FTC/TAF in adults with mild to moderate renal impairment (estimated glomerular filtration rate [eGFR] 30–69 mL/minute) were evaluated in a single-arm, open-label study (study 112; NCT01818596). The study included 242 previously treated patients (mean age 58 years [26% 65 years of age or older], 79% male, 18% black, median baseline CD4$^+$ T-cell count 632 cells/mm^3) who were virally suppressed (plasma HIV-1 RNA levels less than 50 copies/mL) for at least 6 months on their existing antiretroviral regimen (65% had been receiving a regimen that included tenofovir DF) and also included 6 treatment-naive patients. All patients then received EVG/c/FTC/TAF (elvitegravir 150 mg, cobicistat 150 mg, emtricitabine 200 mg, tenofovir alafenamide 10 mg) once daily with food. The primary end point was the change in eGFR from baseline to 24 weeks; a secondary end point was the proportion of patients maintaining virologic control. In the previously treated patients, eGFR (using the Cockcroft-Gault equation) was reduced by 0.4 mL/minute at 24 weeks after switching to EVG/c/FTC/TAF and there was no appreciable change in estimated creatinine clearance from baseline through 48 weeks. At 96 weeks after switching to EVG/c/FTC/TAF, 88% of previously treated patients had maintained plasma HIV-1 RNA levels less than 50 copies/mL; 5 patients experienced virologic failure.

Pediatric Patients For *initial* treatment in HIV-infected children and adolescents, the HHS Panel on Antiretroviral Therapy and Medical Management of HIV-infected Children states that EVG/c/FTC/TAF is a preferred HIV INSTI-based regimen in children and adolescents 12 years of age or older weighing 35 kg or more, including adolescents in early puberty (sexual maturity rating [SMR] 1–3).

Clinical Experience. The efficacy and safety of EVG/c/FTC/TAF in treatment-naive adolescents 12 to less than 18 years of age were evaluated in an open-label study (study 106; NCT01854775). The study included 23 patients (mean age 14 years, 52% male, 83% black, 17% Asian, median baseline CD4$^+$ T-cell count 456 cells/mm^3, median CD4$^+$ percentage 23%, mean baseline plasma HIV-1 RNA level 4.8 $\log_{10}$ copies/mL). All patients received EVG/c/FTC/TAF (elvitegravir 150 mg, cobicistat 150 mg, emtricitabine 200 mg, tenofovir alafenamide 10 mg) once daily. The virologic response rate to EVG/c/FTC/TAF in these treatment-naive adolescents was similar to response rates observed in treatment-naive adults. At 48 weeks, 92% had achieved plasma HIV-1 RNA levels less than 50 copies/mL; the mean increase in CD4$^+$ T-cell count from baseline was 224 cells/mm^3. Virologic failure was observed in 3 adolescents; there was no evidence of treatment-emergent resistance to EVG/c/FTC/TAF.

Dosage and Administration

■ **Administration** The fixed combination of elvitegravir, cobicistat, emtricitabine, and tenofovir alafenamide (EVG/c/FTC/TAF) is administered orally once daily with food.

Serum creatinine, estimated creatinine clearance, serum phosphorus, urine glucose, and urine protein should be determined prior to initiation of EVG/c/FTC/TAF and routinely monitored during treatment in all patients. (See Renal Impairment under Warnings/Precautions: Specific Populations, in Cautions.)

Patients should be tested for hepatitis B virus (HBV) infection prior to initiation of EVG/c/FTC/TAF. (See HIV-infected Individuals Coinfected with Hepatitis B Virus under Warnings/Precautions: Warnings, in Cautions.)

■ **Dosage** Each fixed-combination tablet of EVG/c/FTC/TAF contains elvitegravir 150 mg, cobicistat 150 mg, emtricitabine 200 mg, and tenofovir alafenamide 10 mg.

Although tenofovir alafenamide is provided in the fixed combination as tenofovir alafenamide fumarate, dosage of this tenofovir component is expressed in terms of tenofovir alafenamide.

Adult Dosage **Treatment of HIV Infection.** For the treatment of human immunodeficiency virus type 1 (HIV-1) infection in adults, the usual dosage of EVG/c/FTC/TAF is 1 tablet (150 mg of elvitegravir, 150 mg of cobicistat, 200 mg of emtricitabine, and 10 mg of tenofovir alafenamide) once daily.

Pediatric Dosage **Treatment of HIV Infection.** For the treatment of HIV-1 infection in children and adolescents 12 years of age or older weighing at least 35 kg, the usual dosage of EVG/c/FTC/TAF is 1 tablet (150 mg of elvitegravir, 150 mg of cobicistat, 200 mg of emtricitabine, and 10 mg of tenofovir alafenamide) once daily.

■ **Special Populations** ***Hepatic Impairment*** Dosage adjustments are not necessary if EVG/c/FTC/TAF is used in patients with mild or moderate hepatic impairment (Child-Pugh class A or B).

EVG/c/FTC/TAF is not recommended in patients with severe hepatic impairment (Child-Pugh class C). (See Hepatic Impairment under Warnings/Precautions: Specific Populations, in Cautions.)

Renal Impairment Dosage adjustments are not necessary if EVG/c/FTC/TAF is used in patients with estimated creatinine clearance of 30 mL/minute or greater.

EVG/c/FTC/TAF should *not* be used in patients with estimated creatinine clearance less than 30 mL/minute. (See Renal Impairment under Warnings/Precautions: Specific Populations, in Cautions.)

Cautions

■ **Contraindications** Concomitant use of the fixed combination of elvitegravir, cobicistat, emtricitabine, and tenofovir alafenamide (EVG/c/FTC/TAF) with drugs highly dependent on cytochrome P-450 isoenzyme 3A (CYP3A) for metabolism and for which elevated plasma concentrations are associated with serious and/or life-threatening events (e.g., alfuzosin, cisapride, ergot alkaloids, lovastatin, lurasidone, oral midazolam, pimozide, sildenafil used for treatment of pulmonary arterial hypertension [PAH], simvastatin, triazolam) is contraindicated. (See Drug Interactions.)

Concomitant use of EVG/c/FTC/TAF with drugs that are potent inducers of CYP3A (e.g., carbamazepine, phenobarbital, phenytoin, rifampin, St. John's wort [*Hypericum perforatum*]) is contraindicated, since these drugs may decrease elvitegravir, cobicistat, and/or tenofovir alafenamide concentrations resulting in possible decreased antiretroviral efficacy and development of resistance. (See Drug Interactions.)

■ **Warnings/Precautions** ***Warnings*** **HIV-infected Individuals Coinfected with Hepatitis B Virus.** HIV-infected patients should be tested for hepatitis B virus (HBV) before antiretroviral therapy is initiated.

EVG/c/FTC/TAF is not indicated for treatment of chronic HBV infection, and safety and efficacy of EVG/c/FTC/TAF have not been established in HIV-infected patients coinfected with HBV.

In HIV-infected patients with HBV coinfection, severe acute exacerbations of HBV infection have occurred following discontinuance of preparations containing emtricitabine and/or tenofovir disoproxil fumarate (tenofovir DF). In some patients receiving emtricitabine, exacerbations of HBV have been associated with hepatic decompensation and hepatic failure. Such reactions could occur with EVG/c/FTC/TAF.

Hepatic function should be closely monitored with clinical and laboratory follow-up for at least several months after EVG/c/FTC/TAF is discontinued in patients coinfected with HIV and HBV. If appropriate, initiation of HBV treatment may be warranted, especially in patients with advanced liver disease or cirrhosis.

Other Warnings/Precautions **Renal Toxicity.** Renal impairment, including cases of acute renal failure and Fanconi syndrome (renal tubular injury with severe hypophosphatemia), has been reported in patients receiving tenofovir prodrugs (e.g., tenofovir DF).

There were no cases of Fanconi syndrome or proximal renal tubulopathy (PRT) in clinical trials evaluating EVG/c/FTC/TAF. In treatment-naive patients and virally suppressed patients who were switched to EVG/c/FTC/TAF and had estimated glomerular filtration rates (eGFRs) exceeding 50 mL/minute, serious adverse renal effects or discontinuance of the drug because of adverse renal effects occurred in less than 1% of patients. In a study of virally suppressed individuals with baseline eGFRs between 30–69 mL/minute who received EVG/c/FTC/TAF for a median duration of 43 weeks, the drug was permanently discontinued because of worsening renal function in 3% of those with baseline eGFRs between 30–50 mL/minute.

Cobicistat (a component of EVG/c/FTC/TAF) may cause a modest increase in serum creatinine and modest decrease in estimated creatinine clearance because of inhibition of tubular secretion of creatinine; there is a corresponding decrease in serum creatinine-based eGFR, but renal glomerular function is not affected. Elevated serum creatinine concentrations typically occurred within 2 weeks after the drug was initiated and generally were reversible after the drug was discontinued.

Serum creatinine, estimated creatinine clearance, serum phosphorus, urine glucose, and urine protein should be determined prior to initiating EVG/c/FTC/TAF and routinely monitored during treatment in all patients. (See Renal Impairment under Warnings/Precautions: Specific Populations, in Cautions.)

EVG/c/FTC/TAF should *not* be used in patients with estimated creatinine clearances less than 30 mL/minute.

Patients with a confirmed increase in serum creatinine of greater than 0.4 mg/dL from baseline while receiving EVG/c/FTC/TAF should be closely monitored for renal toxicity. EVG/c/FTC/TAF should be discontinued in patients who develop clinically important decreases in renal function or evidence of Fanconi syndrome.

Patients receiving a tenofovir prodrug who have impaired renal function or are receiving a nephrotoxic agent (e.g., nonsteroidal anti-inflammatory agents [NSAIAs]) are at increased risk of developing adverse renal effects. (See Drug Interactions: Drugs Affecting Renal Function.)

Lactic Acidosis and Severe Hepatomegaly with Steatosis. Lactic acidosis and severe hepatomegaly with steatosis, including fatalities, have been reported in patients receiving HIV nucleoside reverse transcriptase inhibitors (NRTIs), including emtricitabine and the tenofovir prodrug tenofovir DF, in conjunction with other antiretroviral agents.

EVG/c/FTC/TAF treatment should be interrupted in any patient who develops clinical or laboratory findings suggestive of lactic acidosis or pronounced hepatotoxicity (signs of hepatotoxicity may include hepatomegaly and steatosis even in the absence of marked increases in serum aminotransferase concentrations).

Bone Effects. Tenofovir prodrugs (tenofovir alafenamide, tenofovir DF) have been associated with decreases in bone mineral density (BMD). Declines in BMD reported in adults receiving tenofovir alafenamide have been smaller than those reported in adults receiving tenofovir DF. In addition, BMD increases have been reported when some adults were switched from a regimen containing tenofovir DF to a regimen containing tenofovir alafenamide.

In a pooled analysis of data from 2 clinical studies comparing efficacy and safety of EVG/c/FTC/TAF and the fixed combination of elvitegravir, cobicistat, emtricitabine, and tenofovir DF (EVG/c/FTC/TDF) for the treatment of HIV infection in antiretroviral-naive adults, the mean change in BMD from baseline to week 96 was assessed by dual-energy X-ray absorptiometry (DXA). At the lumbar spine, the mean decrease in BMD was −0.96% in patients treated with EVG/c/FTC/TAF compared with −2.79% in those treated with EVG/c/FTC/TDF; 12% of those treated with EVG/c/FTC/TAF and 26% of those treated with EVG/c/FTC/TDF had lumbar spine BMD declines that were 5% or more. At the total hip, the mean decrease in BMD was −0.67% in those treated with EVG/c/FTC/TAF compared with −3.28% in those treated with EVG/c/FTC/TDF. At the femoral neck, 11% of patients treated with EVG/c/FTC/TAF and 26% of those treated with EVG/c/FTC/TDF had BMD declines that were 7% or more. In a clinical study in virologically suppressed adults who were receiving an antiretroviral regimen that included tenofovir DF, mean BMD increased (2.12% at the lumbar spine, 2.44% at the total hip) in those switched to EVG/c/FTC/TAF, but decreased slightly (−0.09% at the lumbar spine, −0.46% at the total hip) in those who continued their baseline regimen.

The long-term clinical importance of BMD changes reported with tenofovir prodrugs is unknown.

Use of Fixed Combinations. The usual cautions, precautions, contraindications, and interactions associated with each component of EVG/c/FTC/TAF should be considered. Cautionary information applicable to specific populations (e.g., pregnant or nursing women, individuals with hepatic or renal impairment, geriatric patients) should be considered for each drug in the fixed combination. For cautionary information related to emtricitabine, see Cautions in Emtricitabine 8:18.08.20.

EVG/c/FTC/TAF is used alone as a complete regimen for the treatment of HIV-1 infection and should not be used in conjunction with other antiretroviral agents. (See Drug Interactions: Antiretroviral Agents.)

EVG/c/FTC/TAF should not be used concomitantly with any preparation that contains any of its components (elvitegravir, cobicistat, emtricitabine, tenofovir alafenamide). In addition, EVG/c/FTC/TAF should not be used concomitantly with any preparation containing tenofovir DF, lamivudine, adefovir dipivoxil, or ritonavir.

Immune Reconstitution Syndrome. Immune reconstitution syndrome has been reported in HIV-infected patients receiving multiple-drug antiretroviral therapy, including emtricitabine (a component of EVG/c/FTC/TAF). During the initial phase of treatment, HIV-infected patients whose immune systems respond to antiretroviral therapy may develop an inflammatory response to indolent or residual opportunistic infections (e.g., *Mycobacterium avium*, *M. tuberculosis*, cytomegalovirus [CMV], *Pneumocystis jirovecii* [formerly *P. carinii*]); such response may necessitate further evaluation and treatment.

Autoimmune disorders (e.g., Graves' disease, polymyositis, Guillain-Barré syndrome) have also been reported to occur in the setting of immune reconstitution; however, the time to onset is more variable and can occur many months after initiation of antiretroviral therapy.

Specific Populations **Pregnancy.** Antiretroviral Pregnancy Registry at 800-258-4263 or http://www.apregistry.com.

Prospective pregnancy data from the Antiretroviral Pregnancy Registry are not sufficient to date to adequately assess the risk of birth defects or miscarriage if EVG/c/FTC/TAF is used in pregnant women. Data from the Antiretroviral Pregnancy Registry available through January 2016 show no birth defects reported for elvitegravir or cobicistat and no difference in the overall risk of major birth defects for emtricitabine compared with the background rate of major birth defects in the US.

In animal studies, there was no evidence of adverse developmental effects when the components of EVG/c/FTC/TAF were administered separately during the period of organogenesis at elvitegravir, cobicistat, emtricitabine, and tenofovir alafenamide exposures up to 23, 3.8, 108, and 53 times higher, respectively, than human exposures at the recommended daily dosage.

The US Department of Health and Human Services (HHS) Panel on Treatment of HIV-infected Pregnant Women and Prevention of Perinatal Transmission states that data are insufficient to recommend routine use of EVG/c/FTC/TAF for *initial* treatment in antiretroviral-naive pregnant women.

Lactation. Elvitegravir and cobicistat are distributed into milk in rats. Tenofovir is distributed into milk in rats and rhesus monkey following administration of tenofovir DF; it is not known whether tenofovir alafenamide is distributed into animal milk. It is not known whether elvitegravir, cobicistat, or tenofovir alafenamide are distributed into human milk. Emtricitabine is distributed into human milk.

It is not known whether EVG/c/FTC/TAF affects human milk production or affects the breast-fed infant.

Because of the risk of adverse effects in the infant and the risk of HIV transmission, HIV-infected women should not breast-feed infants.

Pediatric Use. Safety and efficacy of EVG/c/FTC/TAF have not been established in pediatric patients younger than 12 years of age or in those weighing less than 35 kg.

The HHS Panel on Antiretroviral Therapy and Medical Management of HIV-infected Children states that EVG/c/FTC/TAF is a preferred antiretroviral regimen in children and adolescents 12 years of age or older weighing 35 kg or more, including adolescents in early puberty (sexual maturity rating [SMR] 1–3).

Clinical trial data indicate that the safety of EVG/c/FTC/TAF in HIV-1-infected, treatment-naive pediatric patients 12 to less than 18 years of age is similar to that reported in adults.

Following oral administration of EVG/c/FTC/TAF, tenofovir alafenamide exposures in adolescents 12 to less than 18 years of age were 23% lower than those observed in treatment-naive adults; this difference is not considered clinically important based on exposure-response relationships. Elvitegravir, cobicistat, and emtricitabine exposures in adolescents 12 to less than 18 years of age were similar to those observed in treatment-naive adults.

Geriatric Use. No differences in safety or efficacy of EVG/c/FTC/TAF have been observed between individuals 65 years of age and older and individuals 12 to less than 65 years of age.

Pharmacokinetics of EVG/c/FTC/TAF have not been fully evaluated in adults 65 years of age and older. Population pharmacokinetic analysis of EVG/c/FTC/TAF in HIV-infected individuals showed that age does not have a clinically important effect on tenofovir alafenamide exposures in adults up to 75 years of age.

Hepatic Impairment. Mild hepatic impairment (Child-Pugh class A) does not have a clinically important effect on the pharmacokinetics of tenofovir alafenamide. Moderate hepatic impairment (Child-Pugh class B) does not have a clinically important effect on the pharmacokinetics of elvitegravir, cobicistat, or tenofovir alafenamide and is not expected to affect the pharmacokinetics of emtricitabine.

EVG/c/FTC/TAF is *not* recommended in patients with severe hepatic impairment (Child-Pugh class C). Data are not available to regarding the pharmacokinetics or safety of EVG/c/FTC/TAF in such patients.

Renal Impairment. Serum creatinine, estimated creatinine clearance, serum phosphorus, urine glucose, and urine protein should be determined prior to initiating EVG/c/FTC/TAF and routinely monitored during treatment in all patients.

EVG/c/FTC/TAF should *not* be used in patients with estimated creatinine clearances less than 30 mL/minute; safety of the drug has not been established in such patients.

■ **Common Adverse Effects** Adverse effects reported in 5% or more of patients receiving EVG/c/FTC/TAF include nausea (10%), diarrhea (7%), fatigue (5%), and headache (6%).

Drug Interactions

The following drug interactions are based on studies that used elvitegravir, elvitegravir administered with cobicistat (*cobicistat-boosted* elvitegravir), elvitegravir administered with low-dose ritonavir (*ritonavir-boosted* elvitegravir), cobicistat alone, or the fixed combination of elvitegravir, cobicistat, emtricitabine, and tenofovir alafenamide (EVG/c/FTC/TAF) or are predicted to occur.

Potential drug interactions associated with each drug in the fixed combination should be considered.

■ **Drugs Affecting or Metabolized by Hepatic Microsomal Enzymes** Elvitegravir is a substrate of cytochrome P-450 (CYP) 3A and a weak inducer and weak inhibitor of CYP3A; elvitegravir is an inducer of CYP2C9. The drug does not inhibit CYP1A, 2A6, 2C9, 2C19, 2D6, or 2E1 in vitro.

Cobicistat is a substrate of CYP3A and, to a minor extent, CYP2D6; cobicistat also is an inhibitor of CYP3A and 2D6.

Emtricitabine is not a substrate of CYP enzymes; emtricitabine does not inhibit CYP1A2, 2A6, 2B6, 2C9, 2C19, 2D6, or 3A4.

Tenofovir alafenamide is a weak inhibitor of CYP3A in vitro, but is not an inhibitor or inducer of CYP3A in vivo. Tenofovir alafenamide does not induce or inhibit other CYP enzymes, including CYP1A2, 2B6, 2C8, 2C9, 2C19, or 2D6.

Potential pharmacokinetic interactions if EVG/c/FTC/TAF is used concomitantly with drugs that are principally metabolized by CYP3A or 2D6 (increased plasma concentrations of the concomitant drug). Concomitant use of EVG/c/FTC/TAF with some drugs that are CYP3A substrates and for which elevated plasma concentrations are associated with serious and/or life-threatening events is contraindicated.

Potential pharmacokinetic interactions if EVG/c/FTC/TAF is used concomitantly with drugs that induce CYP3A (decreased plasma concentrations of elvitegravir, cobicistat, and tenofovir alafenamide; possible decreased antiretroviral efficacy and development of resistance). Concomitant use of EVG/c/FTC/TAF with some drugs that are potent inducers of CYP3A is contraindicated.

Potential pharmacokinetic interactions if EVG/c/FTC/TAF is used concomitantly with drugs that inhibit CYP3A (increased plasma concentrations of cobicistat).

■ **Drugs Affected by P-glycoprotein Transport** Cobicistat is an inhibitor of P-glycoprotein (P-gp) transport; tenofovir alafenamide is a substrate of P-gp.

Potential pharmacokinetic interactions if EVG/c/FTC/TAF is used concomitantly with drugs that are P-gp substrates (increased plasma concentrations of the concomitant drug).

Drugs that inhibit P-gp may increase absorption of tenofovir alafenamide. Cobicistat (a P-gp inhibitor) increases tenofovir alafenamide concentrations when the drugs are administered as the fixed combination EVG/c/FTC/TAF; further increases in tenofovir alafenamide concentrations are not expected if an additional P-gp inhibitor is used concomitantly with EVG/c/FTC/TAF.

Drugs that induce P-gp are expected to decrease absorption of tenofovir alafenamide, resulting in decreased plasma concentrations of tenofovir alafenamide.

■ **Drugs Affected by Breast Cancer Resistance Protein** Cobicistat is an inhibitor of breast cancer resistance protein (BCRP); tenofovir alafenamide is a substrate of BCRP.

Potential pharmacokinetic interactions if EVG/c/FTC/TAF is used concomitantly with drugs that are substrates for BCRP (increased plasma concentrations of the concomitant drug).

Drugs that inhibit BCRP may increase absorption of tenofovir alafenamide. Cobicistat (a BCRP inhibitor) increases tenofovir alafenamide concentrations when the drugs are administered as the fixed combination EVG/c/FTC/TAF; further increases in tenofovir alafenamide concentrations are not expected if an additional BCRP inhibitor is used concomitantly with EVG/c/FTC/TAF.

■ **Drugs Affected by Organic Anion Transport Polypeptides** Elvitegravir and cobicistat are inhibitors of organic anion transport polypeptides (OATP) 1B1 and 1B3; tenofovir alafenamide is a substrate of OATP1B1 and 1B3.

Potential pharmacokinetic interactions if EVG/c/FTC/TAF is used concomitantly with drugs that are substrates for OATP1B1 or 1B3 (increased plasma concentrations of the concomitant drug).

■ **Drugs Metabolized by Uridine Diphosphate-glucuronosyltransferase** Elvitegravir is partially metabolized by uridine diphosphate-glucuronosyltransferase (UGT) 1A1/3 enzymes. Tenofovir alafenamide does not inhibit UGT1A1.

■ **Drugs Affecting Renal Function** The emtricitabine and tenofovir components of EVG/c/FTC/TAF are principally excreted by the kidneys by a combination of glomerular filtration and active tubular secretion.

Potential pharmacokinetic interactions if EVG/c/FTC/TAF is used concomitantly with drugs that reduce renal function or compete for active tubular secretion (e.g., acyclovir, aminoglycosides [gentamicin], cidofovir, ganciclovir, valacyclovir, valganciclovir, high-dose or multiple nonsteroidal anti-inflammatory agents [NSAIAs]); may result in increased concentrations of emtricitabine, tenofovir, and/or the concomitant drug and may increase the risk of adverse effects.

■ **Alfuzosin** Potential pharmacokinetic interaction with alfuzosin (increased plasma concentrations of alfuzosin); may result in hypotension.

Concomitant use of alfuzosin and EVG/c/FTC/TAF is contraindicated.

■ **Anticoagulants** ***Apixaban, Edoxaban, Rivaroxaban*** Pharmacokinetic interactions are expected if apixaban, edoxaban, or rivaroxaban is used concomitantly with EVG/c/FTC/TAF (increased anticoagulant concentrations).

Concomitant use of EVG/c/FTC/TAF and apixaban, edoxaban, or rivaroxaban should be avoided.

Dabigatran Potential pharmacokinetic interactions if dabigatran is used concomitantly with EVG/c/FTC/TAF (increased dabigatran concentrations).

Some experts state that dosage adjustments are not necessary if dabigatran and EVG/c/FTC/TAF are used concomitantly in patients with creatinine clearances exceeding 50 mL/minute, but the drugs should not be used concomitantly in those with creatinine clearances less than 50 mL/minute.

Warfarin The effect of concomitant use of warfarin and EVG/c/FTC/TAF on the pharmacokinetics of warfarin is unknown, but warfarin concentrations may be affected.

If warfarin is used concomitantly with EVG/c/FTC/TAF, the international normalized ratio (INR) should be monitored.

■ **Anticonvulsants** ***Carbamazepine, Phenobarbital, Phenytoin*** Concomitant use of carbamazepine and *cobicistat-boosted* elvitegravir results in decreased elvitegravir plasma concentrations and area under the plasma concentration-time curve (AUC); increased carbamazepine plasma concentrations and AUC also occur. Potential pharmacokinetic interactions if carbamazepine, phenobarbital, or phenytoin is used concomitantly with EVG/c/FTC/TAF (decreased elvitegravir, cobicistat, and tenofovir alafenamide plasma concentrations with possible decreased antiretroviral efficacy and development of resistance).

Concomitant use of EVG/c/FTC/TAF and carbamazepine, phenobarbital, or phenytoin is contraindicated.

Ethosuximide Potential pharmacokinetic interaction if ethosuximide is used concomitantly with EVG/c/FTC/TAF (increased ethosuximide plasma concentrations and decreased elvitegravir, cobicistat, and tenofovir alafenamide plasma concentrations).

If ethosuximide and EVG/c/FTC/TAF are used concomitantly, the patient should be monitored clinically.

Oxcarbazepine Potential pharmacokinetic interaction if oxcarbazepine is used concomitantly with EVG/c/FTC/TAF (decreased elvitegravir, cobicistat, and tenofovir alafenamide plasma concentrations). An alternative anticonvulsant should be considered.

■ **Antifungal Agents** ***Isavuconazonium*** Concomitant use of isavuconazonium sulfate (prodrug of isavuconazole) and EVG/c/FTC/TAF may result in increased isavuconazole, elvitegravir, and cobicistat concentrations.

If isavuconazonium sulfate and EVG/c/FTC/TAF are used concomitantly, the patient should be monitored for virologic efficacy and isavuconazole concentration monitoring should be considered.

Itraconazole Potential pharmacokinetic interactions with itraconazole (increased plasma concentrations of itraconazole, elvitegravir, and cobicistat).

If itraconazole and EVG/c/FTC/TAF are used concomitantly, itraconazole dosage should not exceed 200 mg daily.

Ketoconazole Pharmacokinetic interactions with ketoconazole (increased plasma concentrations of ketoconazole, elvitegravir, and cobicistat).

If ketoconazole and EVG/c/FTC/TAF are used concomitantly, ketoconazole dosage should not exceed 200 mg daily.

Posaconazole Potential pharmacokinetic interactions with posaconazole (increased plasma concentrations of posaconazole, elvitegravir, and cobicistat).

If posaconazole and EVG/c/FTC/TAF are used concomitantly, posaconazole plasma concentrations should be monitored.

Voriconazole Potential pharmacokinetic interactions with voriconazole (increased plasma concentrations of voriconazole, elvitegravir, and cobicistat).

Voriconazole and EVG/c/FTC/TAF should not be used concomitantly unless potential benefits outweigh risks.

■ **Antimycobacterial Agents** ***Rifabutin*** Pharmacokinetic interactions when *cobicistat-boosted* elvitegravir (elvitegravir 150 mg and cobicistat 150 mg once daily) was used concomitantly with rifabutin 150 mg once every other day (decreased elvitegravir plasma concentrations and AUC, increased 25-*O*-desacetyl-rifabutin concentrations and AUC relative to those achieved with rifabutin 300 mg once daily without concomitant *cobicistat-boosted* elvitegravir). Concomitant use of EVG/c/FTC/TAF also may decrease plasma concentrations of tenofovir alafenamide. Possible decreased antiretroviral efficacy and development of resistance.

Concomitant use of rifabutin and EVG/c/FTC/TAF is not recommended.

Rifampin Potential pharmacokinetic interactions with rifampin (decreased elvitegravir, cobicistat, and tenofovir alafenamide plasma concentrations); possible decreased antiretroviral efficacy and development of resistance.

Concomitant use of rifampin and EVG/c/FTC/TAF is contraindicated.

Rifapentine Potential pharmacokinetic interactions with rifapentine (decreased elvitegravir, cobicistat, and tenofovir alafenamide plasma concentrations); possible decreased antiretroviral efficacy and development of resistance.

Concomitant use of rifapentine and EVG/c/FTC/TAF is not recommended.

■ **Antiplatelet Agents** ***Ticagrelor, Vorapaxar*** Pharmacokinetic interactions are expected if ticagrelor or vorapaxar is used concomitantly with EVG/c/FTC/TAF (increased antiplatelet agent concentrations).

Concomitant use of EVG/c/FTC/TAF and ticagrelor or vorapaxar should be avoided.

■ **Antipsychotic Agents** ***Lurasidone*** Concomitant use of lurasidone and EVG/c/FTC/TAF may result in serious and/or life-threatening reactions.

Concomitant use of lurasidone and EVG/c/FTC/TAF is contraindicated.

Perphenazine, Risperidone, Thioridazine Potential pharmacokinetic interactions with antipsychotics, including perphenazine, risperidone, and thioridazine (increased antipsychotic plasma concentrations).

If EVG/c/FTC/TAF is used concomitantly with certain antipsychotics (e.g., perphenazine, risperidone, thioridazine), decreased dosage of the antipsychotic may be necessary.

Pimozide Potential pharmacokinetic interaction with pimozide (increased pimozide plasma concentrations); potential for serious and/or life-threatening adverse effects (e.g., cardiac arrhythmias).

Concomitant use of pimozide and EVG/c/FTC/TAF is contraindicated.

Quetiapine Pharmacokinetic interaction with quetiapine (increased quetiapine plasma concentrations expected).

Alternative antiretroviral therapy should be considered. If EVG/c/FTC/TAF is necessary in a patient receiving quetiapine, the quetiapine dosage should be reduced to one-sixth of the original dosage and the patient monitored for quetiapine-associated adverse effects.

■ **Antiretroviral Agents** EVG/c/FTC/TAF should not be used in conjunction with any other antiretroviral agents.

HIV Integrase Inhibitors (INSTIs) EVG/c/FTC/TAF contains elvitegravir and should not be used concomitantly with any preparation containing elvitegravir.

HIV Nucleoside and Nucleotide Reverse Transcriptase Inhibitors (NRTIs) **Emtricitabine.** EVG/c/FTC/TAF contains emtricitabine and should not be used concomitantly with any preparation containing emtricitabine.

Lamivudine. EVG/c/FTC/TAF and lamivudine (or preparations containing lamivudine) should not be used concomitantly.

Tenofovir Disoproxil Fumarate. EVG/c/FTC/TAF and tenofovir disoproxil fumarate (tenofovir DF) (or preparations containing tenofovir DF) should not be used concomitantly.

HIV Protease Inhibitors (PIs) **Ritonavir.** EVG/c/FTC/TAF and ritonavir (or preparations containing ritonavir) should not be used concomitantly.

■ **β-Adrenergic Blocking Agents** Potential pharmacokinetic interactions with β-adrenergic blocking agents, including metoprolol and timolol (increased β-adrenergic blocking agent plasma concentrations).

If EVG/c/FTC/TAF is used concomitantly with a β-adrenergic blocking agent, patients should be monitored clinically and decreased dosage of the β-adrenergic blocking agent may be necessary.

■ **Benzodiazepines** ***Diazepam*** Potential pharmacokinetic interaction with diazepam (increased diazepam plasma concentrations).

Concomitant use of diazepam and EVG/c/FTC/TAF should be undertaken in a monitored setting where respiratory depression and/or prolonged sedation can be managed. Some experts state that alternatives to diazepam (e.g., lorazepam, oxazepam, temazepam) should be considered.

Lorazepam Because lorazepam is not metabolized by CYP isoenzymes, clinically important effects on lorazepam plasma concentrations are not expected if used concomitantly with EVG/c/FTC/TAF.

Midazolam or Triazolam Potential pharmacokinetic interaction with midazolam or triazolam (increased benzodiazepine plasma concentrations); potential for serious and/or life-threatening adverse effects (e.g., prolonged or increased sedation or respiratory depression).

Concomitant use of oral midazolam or triazolam with EVG/c/FTC/TAF is contraindicated.

Concomitant use of parenteral midazolam and EVG/c/FTC/TAF should be undertaken in a monitored setting where respiratory depression and/or prolonged sedation can be managed. In addition, use of a reduced midazolam dosage should be considered, especially if more than a single dose of the drug will be administered.

Other Benzodiazepines Potential pharmacokinetic interactions with clonazepam, clorazepate, estazolam, or flurazepam (increased benzodiazepine plasma concentrations).

If clonazepam, clorazepate, estazolam, or flurazepam is initiated in a patient receiving EVG/c/FTC/TAF, some experts recommend a low initial dosage with close monitoring.

■ **Bosentan** Potential pharmacokinetic interaction with bosentan (increased bosentan plasma concentrations).

In patients who have already been receiving EVG/c/FTC/TAF for at least 10 days, bosentan should be initiated using a dosage of 62.5 mg once daily or every other day based on individual tolerability.

In patients who have already been receiving bosentan, bosentan should be discontinued for at least 36 hours prior to initiating EVG/c/FTC/TAF; after at least 10 days of EVG/c/FTC/TAF therapy, bosentan can be resumed using a dosage of 62.5 mg once daily or every other day based on individual tolerability.

■ **Bupropion** Potential pharmacokinetic interaction with bupropion (increased bupropion plasma concentrations).

If bupropion is used concomitantly with EVG/c/FTC/TAF, dosage of the antidepressant should be titrated carefully while monitoring for antidepressant response.

■ **Buspirone** Potential pharmacokinetic interaction with buspirone (increased buspirone plasma concentrations).

If buspirone is used concomitantly with EVG/c/FTC/TAF, patients should be monitored clinically; reduced buspirone dosage may be necessary.

■ **Calcium-channel Blocking Agents** Potential pharmacokinetic interactions with calcium-channel blocking agents, including amlodipine, diltiazem, felodipine, nicardipine, nifedipine, and verapamil (increased plasma concentrations of the calcium-channel blocking agent).

Calcium-channel blocking agents and EVG/c/FTC/TAF should be used concomitantly with caution; the patient should be clinically monitored.

■ **Calcium, Iron, Multivitamins, and Other Preparations Containing Polyvalent Cations** Oral calcium supplements, oral iron preparations, other oral supplements containing calcium, iron, aluminum, magnesium, or zinc (e.g., multivitamins), and laxatives or other preparations containing polyvalent cations may decrease plasma concentrations of elvitegravir when used concomitantly.

EVG/c/FTC/TAF should be administered at least 2 hours before or at least 6 hours after oral supplements containing calcium, iron, aluminum, magnesium, or zinc or other preparations (e.g., laxatives) containing polyvalent cations and patients should be monitored for antiretroviral efficacy.

■ **Cardiac Drugs** ***Antiarrhythmic Agents*** Potential pharmacokinetic interactions if EVG/c/FTC/TAF is used with certain antiarrhythmic agents (e.g., amiodarone, bepridil [no longer commercially available in the US], disopyramide, dronedarone, flecainide, lidocaine [systemic], mexiletine, propafenone, quinidine) (increased plasma concentrations of the antiarrhythmic agent). Concomitant use of digoxin (single 0.5-mg dose) and cobicistat (150 mg once daily) has resulted in increased plasma concentrations of digoxin.

EVG/c/FTC/TAF and antiarrhythmic agents or digoxin should be used concomitantly with caution; plasma concentrations of the antiarrhythmic agents or cardiac glycoside should be monitored, if possible.

Eplerenone Concomitant use of eplerenone and EVG/c/FTC/TAF is expected to result in increased eplerenone concentrations.

Some experts state that concomitant use of eplerenone and EVG/c/FTC/TAF is contraindicated.

Ivabradine Concomitant use of ivabradine and EVG/c/FTC/TAF is expected to result in increased ivabradine concentrations.

Some experts state that concomitant use of ivabradine and EVG/c/FTC/TAF is contraindicated.

Ranolazine Some experts state that ranolazine and EVG/c/FTC/TAF should not be used concomitantly.

■ **Cisapride** Potential pharmacokinetic interaction with cisapride (increased cisapride plasma concentrations); potential for serious and/or life-threatening adverse effects (e.g., cardiac arrhythmias).

Concomitant use of cisapride and EVG/c/FTC/TAF is contraindicated.

■ **Cobicistat** Pharmacokinetic interaction with elvitegravir (increased plasma concentrations and AUC of elvitegravir); occurs because cobicistat inhibits CYP3A. Cobicistat acts as a pharmacokinetic enhancer when used concomitantly with elvitegravir (*cobicistat-boosted* elvitegravir) and is used to therapeutic advantage in the EVG/c/FTC/TAF fixed combination.

Pharmacokinetic interaction with tenofovir alafenamide (increased tenofovir alafenamide plasma concentrations and AUC); occurs because cobicistat inhibits P-gp, BCRP, and OATP1B1 and 1B3.

Cobicistat does not antagonize the antiretroviral effects of elvitegravir, emtricitabine, or tenofovir.

■ **Colchicine** Potential pharmacokinetic interaction with colchicine (increased colchicine plasma concentrations).

Colchicine and EVG/c/FTC/TAF should not be used concomitantly in patients with renal or hepatic impairment.

When colchicine is used for *treatment* of gout flares in patients receiving EVG/c/FTC/TAF, an initial colchicine dose of 0.6 mg should be given followed by 0.3 mg 1 hour later; the colchicine course should be repeated no earlier than 3 days later.

When colchicine is used for *prophylaxis* of gout flares in patients receiving EVG/c/FTC/TAF, colchicine dosage should be reduced to 0.3 mg once daily in those originally receiving 0.6 mg twice daily or decreased to 0.3 mg once every other day in those originally receiving 0.6 mg once daily.

When colchicine is used for treatment of familial Mediterranean fever (FMF) in patients receiving EVG/c/FTC/TAF, a maximum colchicine dosage of 0.6 mg daily (may be given as 0.3 mg twice daily) should be used.

■ **Corticosteroids** ***Orally Inhaled or Intranasal Corticosteroids*** **Fluticasone.** Concomitant use of EVG/c/FTC/TAF and fluticasone (orally inhaled or intranasal) may increase plasma concentrations of fluticasone. Alternative corticosteroids should be considered, particularly if long-term therapy is required.

Local Injections of Corticosteroids Concomitant use of EVG/c/FTC/TAF and local injections (e.g., intra-articular, epidural, intraorbital) of methylprednisolone, prednisolone, or triamcinolone is expected to increase plasma concentrations of the corticosteroid and may result in adrenal insufficiency or Cushing's syndrome.

EVG/c/FTC/TAF should not be used concomitantly with local injections of methylprednisolone, prednisolone, or triamcinolone.

Systemic Corticosteroids **Dexamethasone.** Concomitant use with systemic dexamethasone may decrease elvitegravir and cobicistat plasma concentrations.

An alternative corticosteroid should be considered in patients receiving EVG/c/FTC/TAF.

■ **Ergot Alkaloids** Potential for serious and/or life-threatening adverse effects (e.g., peripheral vasospasm, ischemia of the extremities and other tissues) if EVG/c/FTC/TAF is used concomitantly with ergot alkaloids (e.g., dihydroergotamine, ergotamine, methylergonovine).

Concomitant use of ergot alkaloids and EVG/c/FTC/TAF is contraindicated.

■ **Estrogens and Progestins** Pharmacokinetic interactions with oral contraceptives containing ethinyl estradiol and norgestimate (decreased ethinyl estradiol plasma concentrations and increased norgestimate plasma concentrations).

Effects of increased norgestimate plasma concentrations are not established, but may include increased risk of insulin resistance, dyslipidemia, acne, and venous thrombosis. The potential risks and benefits of concomitant use of EVG/c/FTC/TAF and oral contraceptives containing ethinyl estradiol and norgestimate should be considered, particularly in women with risk factors for these effects.

Concomitant use of EVG/c/FTC/TAF with oral contraceptives containing progestins other than norgestimate or with other hormonal contraceptives (e.g., transdermal contraceptive systems, vaginal ring, injections) have not been studied; alternative nonhormonal methods of contraception should be considered.

■ **Flibanserin** Concomitant use of flibanserin and EVG/c/FTC/TAF is expected to increase flibanserin concentrations.

Some experts state that concomitant use of flibanserin and EVG/c/FTC/TAF is contraindicated.

■ **GI Drugs** ***Antacids*** Antacids containing aluminum, calcium, and/or magnesium decrease plasma concentrations and AUC of elvitegravir.

EVG/c/FTC/TAF should be given at least 2 hours before or at least 2 hours after antacids containing aluminum, calcium, or magnesium.

Histamine H_2-receptor Antagonists Concomitant use of famotidine and *cobicistat-boosted* elvitegravir did not have a clinically important effect on elvitegravir plasma concentrations or AUC.

Concomitant use of EVG/c/FTC/TAF and histamine H_2-receptor antagonists is not expected to result in clinically important drug interactions.

Proton-pump Inhibitors Concomitant use of omeprazole and *cobicistat-boosted* elvitegravir did not result in clinically important alterations in elvitegravir pharmacokinetics.

Concomitant use of EVG/c/FTC/TAF and proton-pump inhibitors is not expected to result in clinically important drug interactions.

Sucralfate Sucralfate may decrease plasma concentrations of elvitegravir if used concomitantly with EVG/c/FTC/TAF.

EVG/c/FTC/TAF should be administered at least 2 hours before or at least 6 hours after sucralfate and patients should be monitored for antiretroviral efficacy.

■ **HCV Antivirals** ***HCV Polymerase Inhibitors*** **Sofosbuvir.** Clinically important pharmacokinetic interactions are not expected if EVG/c/FTC/TAF is used concomitantly with sofosbuvir.

Sofosbuvir and EVG/c/FTC/TAF can be used concomitantly without dosage adjustments.

Sofosbuvir and Velpatasvir. No clinically important pharmacokinetic interactions were observed when EVG/c/FTC/TAF was used concomitantly with sofosbuvir or velpatasvir.

Concomitant use of the fixed combination of sofosbuvir and velpatasvir (sofosbuvir/velpatasvir) with *cobicistat-boosted* elvitegravir or with tenofovir alafenamide did not have a clinically important effect on elvitegravir or tenofovir alafenamide concentrations.

HCV Protease Inhibitors **Simeprevir.** Concomitant use of simeprevir and EVG/c/FTC/TAF is expected to increase plasma concentrations of simeprevir.

Concomitant use of simeprevir and EVG/c/FTC/TAF is not recommended.

HCV Replication Complex Inhibitors **Daclatasvir.** Concomitant use of daclatasvir and EVG/c/FTC/TAF may result in increased plasma concentrations of daclatasvir.

If daclatasvir and EVG/c/FTC/TAF are used concomitantly, daclatasvir should be given in a dosage of 30 mg once daily.

Dasabuvir, Ombitasvir, Paritaprevir, and Ritonavir. Data are not available regarding concomitant use of EVG/c/FTC/TAF and the fixed combination of dasabuvir, ombitasvir, paritaprevir, and ritonavir (dasabuvir/ombitasvir/paritaprevir/ritonavir).

Concomitant use of dasabuvir/ombitasvir/paritaprevir/ritonavir and EVG/c/FTC/TAF is not recommended.

Elbasvir and Grazoprevir. Concomitant use of the fixed combination of elbasvir and grazoprevir (elbasvir/grazoprevir) and EVG/c/FTC/TAF may result in increased elbasvir and grazoprevir plasma concentrations.

Concomitant use of elbasvir/grazoprevir and EVG/c/FTC/TAF is not recommended.

Ledipasvir and Sofosbuvir. Concomitant use of the fixed combination of ledipasvir and sofosbuvir (ledipasvir/sofosbuvir) with *cobicistat-boosted* elvitegravir or with tenofovir alafenamide does not have a clinically important effect on elvitegravir or tenofovir alafenamide concentrations.

Clinically important pharmacokinetic interactions are not expected if EVG/c/FTC/TAF is used concomitantly with ledipasvir or sofosbuvir. Dosage adjustments are not necessary.

■ **HMG-CoA Reductase Inhibitors** Concomitant use of certain hydroxymethylglutaryl-CoA (HMG-CoA) reductase inhibitors (statins) metabolized by CYP3A (e.g., atorvastatin, lovastatin, simvastatin) and EVG/c/FTC/TAF may increase plasma concentrations of the HMG-CoA reductase inhibitor resulting in increased effects and increased risk of statin-associated adverse effects, including myopathy and rhabdomyolysis.

Atorvastatin If atorvastatin is used concomitantly with EVG/c/FTC/TAF, the statin should be initiated at the lowest dosage and titrated carefully while monitoring for atorvastatin-associated adverse effects.

Lovastatin Concomitant use of lovastatin and EVG/c/FTC/TAF is contraindicated.

Rosuvastatin Pharmacokinetic interaction when rosuvastatin is used concomitantly with *cobicistat-boosted* elvitegravir (increased rosuvastatin plasma concentrations and AUC; no clinically important effect on elvitegravir pharmacokinetics).

Simvastatin Concomitant use of simvastatin and EVG/c/FTC/TAF is contraindicated.

■ **Immunosuppressive Agents** ***Cyclosporine*** Potential pharmacokinetic interactions with cyclosporine (increased plasma concentrations of cyclosporine, elvitegravir, and cobicistat).

If EVG/c/FTC/TAF is used concomitantly with cyclosporine, plasma concentrations of the immunosuppressive agent should be monitored and the patient monitored for adverse effects associated with EVG/c/FTC/TAF. Some experts state that the immunosuppressive agent should be initiated with a decreased dosage to compensate for anticipated alterations in immunosuppressive concentrations and the patient should be monitored for toxicities; consultation with a specialist may be necessary.

Everolimus, Sirolimus, or Tacrolimus Potential pharmacokinetic interactions with everolimus, sirolimus, or tacrolimus (increased plasma concentrations of the immunosuppressant agent).

If EVG/c/FTC/TAF is used concomitantly with everolimus, sirolimus or tacrolimus, plasma concentrations of the immunosuppressive agent should be monitored.

■ **Macrolides** ***Clarithromycin*** Potential pharmacokinetic interactions if EVG/c/FTC/TAF is used concomitantly with clarithromycin (increased plasma concentrations of the macrolide and cobicistat).

Modification of the usual dosage of clarithromycin is not necessary in those with creatinine clearances of 60 mL/minute or greater; however, clarithromycin dosage should be reduced by 50% in those with creatinine clearances of 50–60 mL/minute.

■ **Nucleoside and Nucleotide Antivirals** Potential pharmacokinetic interactions if EVG/c/FTC/TAF is used concomitantly with drugs that compete for active tubular secretion, including acyclovir, cidofovir, ganciclovir, valacyclovir, and valganciclovir; increased plasma concentrations of certain components of EVG/c/FTC/TAF (i.e., emtricitabine, tenofovir) or the concomitant drug may occur and increase the risk of adverse effects.

Adefovir EVG/c/FTC/TAF should not be used concomitantly with adefovir dipivoxil.

Entecavir or Famciclovir Clinically important interactions are not expected if EVG/c/FTC/TAF is used concomitantly with entecavir or famciclovir.

Ribavirin Clinically important interactions are not expected if EVG/c/FTC/TAF is used concomitantly with ribavirin.

■ **Opiate Agonists, Opiate Partial Agonists, and Opiate Antagonists** ***Buprenorphine*** Concomitant use of the fixed combination of buprenorphine and naloxone (buprenorphine/naloxone) with *cobicistat-boosted* elvitegravir increased plasma concentrations and AUC of buprenorphine and norbuprenorphine and decreased peak plasma concentrations and AUC of naloxone.

If buprenorphine/naloxone is used concomitantly with EVG/c/FTC/TAF, dosage adjustments are not necessary; however, patients should be monitored closely for sedation and adverse cognitive effects.

Patients who are receiving EVG/c/FTC/TAF and are switching from transmucosal buprenorphine to the subdermal implant should be monitored to ensure that the buprenorphine effect is adequate and not excessive.

Methadone Concomitant use of methadone and *cobicistat-boosted* elvitegravir did not result in clinically important alterations in methadone pharmacokinetics.

Concomitant use of methadone and EVG/c/FTC/TAF is not expected to result in clinically important drug interactions.

■ **Phosphodiesterase Type 5 Inhibitors** Concomitant use of EVG/c/FTC/TAF and selective phosphodiesterase type 5 (PDE5) inhibitors (e.g., sildenafil, tadalafil, vardenafil) is expected to result in increased plasma concentrations of the PDE5 inhibitor and increase the risk of adverse effects (e.g., hypotension, syncope, visual disturbances, priapism) associated with these agents.

Avanafil Data are not available regarding concomitant use of avanafil and EVG/c/FTC/TAF; concomitant use is not recommended.

Sildenafil Concomitant use of EVG/c/FTC/TAF is contraindicated in patients receiving sildenafil for treatment of pulmonary arterial hypertension (PAH).

If sildenafil is used for treatment of erectile dysfunction in a patient receiving EVG/c/FTC/TAF, sildenafil dosage should not exceed 25 mg once every 48 hours and the patient should be monitored for sildenafil-related adverse effects.

Tadalafil If tadalafil is used for treatment of PAH in a patient who has been receiving EVG/c/FTC/TAF for at least 1 week, tadalafil should be initiated at a dosage of 20 mg once daily and, if tolerated, dosage may be increased to 40 mg once daily. EVG/c/FTC/TAF should not be initiated in patients receiving tadalafil for treatment of PAH; tadalafil should be discontinued for at least 24 hours prior to initiating EVG/c/FTC/TAF. After at least 1 week, tadalafil may be resumed at a dosage of 20 mg once daily and, if tolerated, dosage may be increased to 40 mg once daily.

If tadalafil is used for treatment of erectile dysfunction in a patient receiving EVG/c/FTC/TAF, tadalafil dosage should not exceed 10 mg once every 72 hours and the patient should be monitored for tadalafil-related adverse effects.

Vardenafil If vardenafil is used for treatment of erectile dysfunction in a patient receiving EVG/c/FTC/TAF, vardenafil dosage should not exceed 2.5 mg once every 72 hours and the patient should be monitored for vardenafil-related adverse effects.

■ **Salmeterol** Potential pharmacokinetic interaction with salmeterol (increased salmeterol plasma concentrations); may result in increased risk of salmeterol-associated adverse cardiovascular effects, including QT interval prolongation, palpitations, and sinus tachycardia.

Concomitant use of salmeterol and EVG/c/FTC/TAF is not recommended.

■ **Selective Serotonin-reuptake Inhibitors (SSRIs)** Potential pharmacokinetic interaction with SSRIs (increased SSRI plasma concentrations). However, clinically important interactions are not expected if EVG/c/FTC/TAF is used concomitantly with sertraline.

If an SSRI is used concomitantly with EVG/c/FTC/TAF, dosage of the SSRI should be carefully titrated and antidepressant response monitored.

■ **Suvorexant** Pharmacokinetic interaction with suvorexant expected (increased suvorexant plasma concentrations).

Some experts state that concomitant use of suvorexant and EVG/c/FTC/TAF is not recommended.

■ **Trazodone** Potential pharmacokinetic interaction with trazodone (increased trazodone plasma concentrations).

If trazodone is used concomitantly with EVG/c/FTC/TAF, dosage of trazodone should be carefully titrated and antidepressant response monitored.

■ **Tricyclic Antidepressants** Potential pharmacokinetic interactions if EVG/c/FTC/TAF is used concomitantly with tricyclic antidepressants, including amitriptyline, desipramine, doxepin, imipramine, and nortriptyline (increased tricyclic antidepressant plasma concentrations). Increased desipramine plasma concentrations and AUC reported when used concomitantly with *cobicistat-boosted* elvitegravir.

If a tricyclic antidepressant is used concomitantly with EVG/c/FTC/TAF, the lowest initial dosage of the tricyclic antidepressant should be used and dosage of the antidepressant should be carefully titrated according to clinical response.

■ **Zolpidem** Possible pharmacokinetic interaction with zolpidem (increased zolpidem plasma concentrations).

If zolpidem is used concomitantly with EVG/c/FTC/TAF, patients should be monitored clinically; reduced zolpidem dosage may be necessary.

■ **Dietary and Herbal Supplements** ***St. John's Wort*** Potential pharmacokinetic interactions with St. John's wort (*Hypericum perforatum*) (decreased elvitegravir, cobicistat, and tenofovir alafenamide plasma concentrations); possible decreased antiretroviral efficacy and development of resistance.

Concomitant use of St. John's wort and EVG/c/FTC/TAF is contraindicated.

Description

The fixed combination of elvitegravir, cobicistat, emtricitabine, and tenofovir alafenamide (EVG/c/FTC/TAF) contains a human immunodeficiency virus (HIV) integrase strand transfer inhibitor (INSTI) antiretroviral (elvitegravir; EVG), a pharmacokinetic enhancer (cobicistat), an HIV nucleoside reverse transcriptase inhibitor (NRTI) antiretroviral (emtricitabine; FTC), and a nucleotide reverse transcriptase inhibitor antiretroviral classified as an HIV NRTI (tenofovir alafenamide; TAF). Cobicistat, a potent cytochrome P-450 (CYP) 3A inhibitor, is included in the fixed combination to increase plasma concentrations of elvitegravir (*cobicistat-boosted* elvitegravir).

Elvitegravir inhibits the activity of HIV-1 integrase, an enzyme that integrates HIV DNA into the host cell genome. Integration is required for viral replication. Inhibition of integration prevents propagation of viral infection. Elvitegravir is active against HIV-1 and also has some in vitro activity against HIV type 2 (HIV-2); the drug does not have activity against hepatitis B virus (HBV) or hepatitis C virus (HCV).

Cobicistat is a mechanism-based inhibitor of CYP3A and decreases metabolism and increases plasma concentrations of CYP3A substrates; cobicistat also is a weak inhibitor of CYP2D6, but does not inhibit CYP1A2, 2C9, or 2C19. Cobicistat is included in EVG/c/FTC/TAF for therapeutic advantage and acts as a pharmacokinetic enhancer to decrease elvitegravir metabolism and increase plasma concentrations of the drug (*cobicistat-boosted* elvitegravir). Cobicistat does not have any antiretroviral or antiviral activity and is not active against HIV-1, HBV, or HCV; cobicistat does not antagonize the antiretroviral activity of elvitegravir, emtricitabine, or tenofovir.

Emtricitabine is inactive until converted intracellularly to an active 5′-triphosphate metabolite. After conversion to the pharmacologically active metabolite, the drug acts as a reverse transcriptase inhibitor antiretroviral. Emtricitabine is active against HIV-1 and also has some in vitro activity against HIV-2.

Tenofovir alafenamide is a tenofovir prodrug and is inactive until hydrolyzed intracellularly by cathepsin A to form tenofovir and subsequently metabolized by cellular kinases to the active metabolite (tenofovir diphosphate). After conversion to the pharmacologically active metabolite, the drug acts as a reverse transcriptase inhibitor antiretroviral. Tenofovir alafenamide is more stable in blood and plasma and more efficiently converted intracellularly to tenofovir diphosphate than the tenofovir prodrug tenofovir disoproxil fumarate (tenofovir DF; TDF), resulting in higher concentrations of the active metabolite within HIV target cells and lower circulating concentrations of tenofovir than those reported with tenofovir DF. Tenofovir is active against HIV-1 and also has some in vitro activity against HIV-2; the drug also is active against HBV.

HIV-1 resistant to elvitegravir, emtricitabine, or tenofovir have been produced in vitro and have emerged during EVG/c/FTC/TAF therapy. In clinical trials evaluating EVG/c/FTC/TAF in antiretroviral-naive patients, genotypic resistance to elvitegravir, emtricitabine, and/or tenofovir was identified in patients who received EVG/c/FTC/TAF and were considered to be virologic treatment failures. Cross-resistance between elvitegravir and other HIV INSTIs (e.g., dolutegravir, raltegravir) has been reported. Cross-resistance also occurs among the HIV NRTIs.

Following an oral dose of EVG/c/FTC/TAF, peak plasma concentrations of elvitegravir and cobicistat occur at 4 and 3 hours, respectively, and peak plasma concentrations of emtricitabine and tenofovir occur at 3 and 1 hours, respectively. Administration of EVG/c/FTC/TAF with a high-fat meal (approximately 800 kcal, 50% fat) increases mean systemic exposures of elvitegravir by 87% compared with administration in the fasting state; changes in mean systemic exposures of cobicistat, emtricitabine, and tenofovir alafenamide are not clinically important compared with administration in the fasting state. Elvitegravir and cobicistat are approximately 99 and 98% bound to plasma proteins, respectively; emtricitabine and tenofovir alafenamide are less than 4% and approximately 80% bound to plasma proteins, respectively. Elvitegravir is metabolized principally by CYP3A isoenzymes, but also undergoes glucuronidation via uridine diphosphate-glucuronsyltransferase (UGT) 1A1/3 enzymes. Cobicistat is metabolized by CYP3A and, to a minor extent, by CYP2D6. Emtricitabine is not substantially metabolized. Tenofovir alafenamide is hydrolyzed intracellularly in peripheral blood mononuclear cells and macrophages by cathepsin A to form tenofovir (the major metabolite); in vitro, tenofovir alafenamide also is converted to tenofovir by carboxylesterase 1 in hepatocytes. Tenofovir alafenamide is metabolized by CYP3A to a minor extent. Elvitegravir and cobicistat are principally excreted in feces (94.8 and 86.2% of a dose, respectively) and to a lesser extent in urine (6.7 and 8.2% of a dose, respectively). Emtricitabine is principally excreted in urine (70% of a dose) and to a lesser extent in feces (13.7% of a dose). Following a single dose of tenofovir alafenamide, 31.7% is excreted in feces and less than 1% is excreted in urine. The median terminal plasma half-lives of elvitegravir, cobicistat, emtricitabine, and tenofovir alafenamide are 12.9, 3.5, 10, and 0.51 hours, respectively. The half-life of tenofovir diphosphate, the active metabolite of tenofovir alafenamide, is 150–180 hours within peripheral blood mononuclear cells.

Advice to Patients

Critical nature of compliance with HIV therapy and importance of remaining under the care of a clinician. Importance of taking as prescribed; do not alter or discontinue antiretroviral regimen without consulting clinician.

Antiretroviral therapy is not a cure for HIV infection; opportunistic infections and other complications associated with HIV disease may still occur.

Advise patients that sustained decreases in plasma HIV RNA have been associated with reduced risk of progression to acquired immunodeficiency syndrome (AIDS) and death.

Advise patients that effective antiretroviral regimens can decrease HIV concentrations in blood and genital secretions and strict adherence to such regimens in conjunction with risk-reduction measures may decrease, but cannot absolutely eliminate, the risk of secondary transmission of HIV to others. Importance of continuing to practice safer sex (e.g., using latex or polyurethane condoms to minimize sexual contact with body fluids), never sharing personal items that can have blood or body fluids on them (e.g., toothbrushes, razor blades), and never reusing or sharing needles.

Importance of reading patient information provided by the manufacturer.

Advise patients that the fixed combination of elvitegravir, cobicistat, emtricitabine, and tenofovir alafenamide (EVG/c/FTC/TAF) is a complete regimen for treatment of HIV-1 infection and should *not* be used in conjunction with other antiretroviral agents.

Importance of taking EVG/c/FTC/TAF with food.

Inform patients that testing for hepatitis B virus (HBV) infection is recommended before antiretroviral therapy is initiated. Also advise patients that severe acute exacerbations of HBV infection have been reported following discontinuance of emtricitabine and/or tenofovir DF in HIV-infected patients coinfected with HBV and may occur with EVG/c/FTC/TAF.

Advise patients that renal impairment, including cases of acute renal failure or Fanconi syndrome, has occurred. Importance of not using EVG/c/FTC/TAF concomitantly with or shortly after nephrotoxic agents (e.g., high-dose or multiple nonsteroidal anti-inflammatory agents [NSAIAs]).

Advise patients that lactic acidosis and severe hepatomegaly with steatosis, including fatalities, have occurred in patients receiving HIV nucleoside reverse transcriptase inhibitors (NRTIs), including emtricitabine and/or tenofovir disoproxil fumarate (tenofovir DF), in conjunction with other antiretrovirals. Importance of contacting clinician if symptoms suggestive of lactic acidosis or pronounced hepatotoxicity (e.g., nausea, vomiting, unusual/unexpected stomach discomfort, weakness) occur.

Advise patients that signs and symptoms of inflammation from previous infections may occur soon after initiation of antiretroviral therapy in some individuals with advanced HIV infection (AIDS). These symptoms may be due to an improvement in immune response, enabling the body to fight infections that may have been present with no obvious symptoms. Importance of immediately informing a healthcare provider if any symptoms of infection occur.

Importance of informing clinicians of existing or contemplated concomitant therapy, including prescription and OTC drugs and herbal supplements (e.g., St. John's wort), as well as any concomitant illnesses.

Importance of women informing clinicians if they are or plan to become pregnant or plan to breast-feed. Advise HIV-infected women not to breast-feed.

Importance of informing patients of other important precautionary information. (See Cautions.)

Overview® (see Users Guide). For additional information on this drug until a more detailed monograph is developed and published, the manufacturer's labeling should be consulted. It is *essential* that the manufacturer's labeling be consulted for more detailed information on usual cautions, precautions, contraindications, potential drug interactions, laboratory test interferences, and acute toxicity.

Preparations

Excipients in commercially available drug preparations may have clinically important effects in some individuals; consult specific product labeling for details.

Elvitegravir, Cobicistat, Emtricitabine, and Tenofovir Alafenamide Fumarate

Oral

Tablets, film-coated	Elvitegravir 150 mg, Cobicistat 150 mg, Emtricitabine 200 mg, and Tenofovir Alafenamide Fumarate 10 mg (of tenofovir alafenamide)	**Genvoya®**, Gilead

Elvitegravir, Cobicistat, Emtricitabine, and Tenofovir Disoproxil Fumarate

EVG/c/FTC/TDF, EVG/c/TDF/FTC, EVG/COBI/FTC/TDF, EVG/COBI/TDF/FTC, EVG, COBI, FTC, Tenofovir DF, TDF

■ Elvitegravir, cobicistat, emtricitabine, and tenofovir disoproxil fumarate (EVG/c/FTC/TDF) is a fixed-combination antiretroviral agent containing elvitegravir (human immunodeficiency virus [HIV] integrase strand transfer inhibitor [INSTI]), cobicistat (pharmacokinetic enhancer), emtricitabine (HIV nucleoside reverse transcriptase inhibitor), and tenofovir disoproxil fumarate (HIV nucleotide reverse transcriptase inhibitor). Cobicistat, a mechanism-based cytochrome P-450 (CYP) 3A inhibitor, is included in the fixed combination to increase plasma concentrations of elvitegravir (*cobicistat-boosted* elvitegravir) and is not active against HIV.

Uses

■ **Treatment of HIV Infection** The fixed combination of elvitegravir, cobicistat, emtricitabine, and tenofovir disoproxil fumarate (tenofovir DF) (EVG/c/FTC/TDF) is used for the treatment of human immunodeficiency virus type 1 (HIV-1) infection in antiretroviral-naive (have not previously received antiretroviral therapy) or antiretroviral-experienced (previously treated) adults and pediatric patients 12 years of age or older.

EVG/c/FTC/TDF is used alone as a complete regimen for the treatment of HIV-1 infection; concomitant use with other antiretroviral agents is not recommended. (See Drug Interactions: Antiretroviral Agents.)

The most appropriate antiretroviral regimen cannot be defined for each clinical scenario, and selection of specific antiretroviral agents for use in multiple-drug regimens should be individualized based on information regarding antiretroviral potency, potential rate of development of resistance, known toxicities, and potential for pharmacokinetic interactions as well as virologic, immunologic, and clinical characteristics of the patient. For information on the general principles and guidelines for use of antiretroviral therapy, including specific recommendations for initial therapy in antiretroviral-naive patients and recommendations for changing antiretroviral regimens, see the Antiretroviral Agents General Statement 8:18.08.

Antiretroviral-naive Adults For *initial* treatment in HIV-infected adults, the US Department of Health and Human Services (HHS) Panel on Antiretroviral Guidelines for Adults and Adolescents states that EVG/c/FTC/TDF is a recommended HIV integrase strand transfer inhibitor-based (INSTI-based) regimen.

Clinical Experience. The comparative efficacy and safety of EVG/c/FTC/TDF and the fixed combination of efavirenz, emtricitabine, and tenofovir DF (EFV/FTC/TDF; Atripla®) were evaluated in a randomized, active-control, phase 3 study in antiretroviral-naive HIV-infected adults (study 102; NCT01095796). All patients had baseline HIV-1 RNA levels of 5000 copies/mL or more, baseline creatinine clearances of at least 70 mL/minute, and were randomized to receive EVG/c/FTC/TDF (elvitegravir 150 mg, cobicistat 150 mg, emtricitabine 200 mg, tenofovir DF 300 mg) once daily with food or EFV/FTC/TDF (efavirenz 600 mg, emtricitabine 200 mg, tenofovir DF 300 mg) once daily in the fasting state. Patients enrolled in this study were adults 18 years of age or older (mean age 38 years, 89% male, 63% white, 28% black, 2% Asian, 24% Hispanic, mean baseline plasma HIV-1 RNA level 4.8 $\log_{10}$ copies/mL, mean baseline $CD4^+$ T-cell count 386 cells/mm^3). At 144 weeks, 80% of those receiving EVG/c/FTC/TDF had plasma HIV-1 RNA levels less than 50 copies/mL compared with 75% of those receiving EFV/FTC/TDF. The mean increase in $CD4^+$ T-cell count from baseline was 298 cells/mm^3 in those receiving EVG/c/FTC/TDF compared with 272 cells/mm^3 in those receiving EFV/FTC/TDF.

In a similarly designed phase 3 study, the comparative efficacy and safety of EVG/c/FTC/TDF and a regimen of *ritonavir-boosted* atazanavir in conjunction with tenofovir DF and emtricitabine was evaluated in antiretroviral-naive HIV-infected adults (study 103; NCT01106586). All patients had baseline HIV-1 RNA levels of 5000 copies/mL or more, baseline creatinine clearances of at least 70 mL/minute, and were randomized to receive EVG/c/FTC/TDF (elvitegravir 150 mg, cobicistat 150 mg, emtricitabine 200 mg, tenofovir DF 300 mg) once daily with food or atazanavir 300 mg and ritonavir 100 mg in conjunction with the fixed combination of emtricitabine 200 mg and tenofovir DF 300 mg (FTC/TDF; Truvada®) once daily with food. Patients enrolled in this study were adults 18 years of age or older (mean age 38 years, 90% male, 74% white, 17% black, 5% Asian, 16% Hispanic, mean baseline plasma HIV-1 RNA level 4.8 $\log_{10}$ copies/mL, mean baseline $CD4^+$ T-cell count 370 cells/mm^3). At 144 weeks, 78% of those receiving EVG/c/FTC/TDF had plasma HIV-1 RNA levels less than 50 copies/mL compared with 75% of those receiving *ritonavir-boosted* atazanavir with FTC/TDF. The mean increase in $CD4^+$ T-cell count from baseline was 261 cells/mm^3 in those receiving EVG/c/FTC/TDF compared with 269 cells/mm^3 in those receiving *ritonavir-boosted* atazanavir with FTC/TDF.

Antiretroviral-experienced Adults For use in antiretroviral-experienced adults, the manufacturer states that EVG/c/FTC/TDF can be used to replace the current antiretroviral regimen in those with plasma HIV-1 RNA levels less than 50 copies/mL on a stable antiretroviral regimen for at least 6 months who have no history of treatment failure and are infected with HIV-1 with no known substitutions associated with resistance to the antiretroviral components of the fixed combination (i.e., elvitegravir, emtricitabine, tenofovir).

Clinical Experience. The comparative efficacy and safety of EVG/c/FTC/TDF and an HIV PI-based regimen in antiretroviral-experienced adults were evaluated in a randomized, open-label, phase 3b noninferiority study (study 115; STRATEGY-PI; NCT01475838). Patients enrolled in the study were adults 18 years of age or older with baseline plasma HIV-1 RNA levels less than 50 copies/mL (mean age 41 years, 86% male, 80% white, 15% black, mean baseline $CD4^+$ T-cell count 610 cells/mm^3). At initial screening, all patients were receiving either their first or second antiretroviral regimen with no history of virologic failure, had no current evidence or history of resistance to the antiretroviral components of EVG/c/FTC/TDF, and had been receiving a *ritonavir-boosted* HIV PI (40% atazanavir, 40% darunavir, 17% lopinavir, 3% fosamprenavir, less than 1% saquinavir) in conjunction with the fixed combination of emtricitabine 200 mg and tenofovir DF 300 mg (FTC/TDF; Truvada®) for at least 6 months. Patients were randomized in a 2:1 ratio to either switch to EVG/c/FTC/TDF (elvitegravir 150 mg, cobicistat 150 mg, emtricitabine 200 mg, tenofovir DF 300 mg) or continue receiving their baseline HIV PI-based antiretroviral regimen. At 48 weeks, 94% of those receiving EVG/c/FTC/TDF had plasma HIV-1 RNA levels less than 50 copies/mL compared with 87% of those receiving a *ritonavir-boosted* HIV PI with FTC/TDF.

In a similarly designed study, the comparative efficacy and safety of EVG/c/FTC/TDF and an HIV nonnucleoside reverse transcriptase inhibitor-based (NNRTI-based) regimen in antiretroviral-experienced adults were evaluated in a randomized, open-label, phase 3b noninferiority study (study 121; STRATEGY-NNRTI; NCT01495702). Patients enrolled in the study were adults 18 years of age or older with baseline plasma HIV-1 RNA levels less than 50 copies/mL (mean age 41 years, 93% male, 78% white, 17% black, mean baseline $CD4^+$ T-cell count 588 cells/mm^3). At initial screening, all patients were receiving either their first or second antiretroviral regimen with no history of virologic failure, had no current evidence or history of resistance to the antiretroviral components of EVG/c/FTC/TDF, and had been receiving an HIV NNRTI in conjunction with the fixed combination of emtricitabine 200 mg and tenofovir DF 300 mg (FTC/TDF; Truvada®) for at least 6 months. Patients were randomized in a 2:1 ratio to either switch to EVG/c/FTC/TDF (elvitegravir 150 mg, cobicistat 150 mg, emtricitabine 200 mg, tenofovir DF 300 mg) or continue receiving their baseline NNRTI-based antiretroviral regimen. Randomization was stratified by use of efavirenz in the NNRTI-based regimen (78% were receiving efavirenz [74% as EFV/FTC/TDF; Atripla®]); 17% were receiving nevirapine, 4% were receiving rilpivirine (as emtricitabine/rilpivirine/tenofovir DF; Complera®), and 1% were receiving etravirine. At 48 weeks, 93% of those receiving EVG/c/FTC/TDF had plasma HIV-1 RNA levels less than 50 copies/mL compared with 88% of those receiving an HIV NNRTI with FTC/TDF.

Pediatric Patients EVG/c/FTC/TDF is used for the treatment of HIV-1 infection in children and adolescents 12 years of age or older weighing at least 35 kg who are antiretroviral naive. The fixed combination also can be used to replace the current antiretroviral regimen in those with plasma HIV-1 RNA levels less than 50 copies/mL on a stable antiretroviral regimen for at least 6 months who have no history of treatment failure and are infected with HIV-1 with no known substitutions associated with resistance to the antiretroviral components of the fixed combination (i.e., elvitegravir, emtricitabine, tenofovir).

The HHS Panel on Antiretroviral Therapy and Medical Management of HIV-infected Children states that EVG/c/FTC/TDF is not a preferred or alternative regimen for *initial* treatment in pediatric patients and is recommended *only* for children and adolescents 12 years of age or older weighing 35 kg or more who are in late puberty (sexual maturity rating [SMR] 4 or 5). These experts state that the fixed combination of elvitegravir, cobicistat, emtricitabine, and tenofovir alafenamide (EVG/c/FTC/TAF) is a preferred regimen in children 12 years of age or older weighing 35 kg or more, including adolescents in early puberty (SMR 1–3). For further information on treatment of HIV infection in pediatric patients, see Antiretroviral Therapy in Pediatric Patients, in Guidelines for Use of Antiretroviral Agents in the Antiretroviral Agents General Statement 8:18.08.

Clinical Experience. The efficacy and safety of EVG/c/FTC/TDF in antiretroviral-naive HIV-infected children 12 to less than 18 years of age weighing at least 35 kg were evaluated in an uncontrolled, open-label study. The study included 50 patients (mean age 15 years, 70% male, 68% black, 28% Asian, mean baseline plasma HIV-1 RNA level 4.6 $\log_{10}$ copies/mL, mean baseline $CD4^+$ T-cell count 399 cells/mm^3, mean $CD4^+$ percentage 20.9%) and all patients received EVG/c/FTC/TDF. At 48 weeks, 88% had plasma HIV-1 RNA levels less than 50 copies/mL; the mean increase in $CD4^+$ T-cell count from baseline was 229 cells/mm^3.

■ **Postexposure Prophylaxis following Occupational Exposure to HIV** EVG/c/FTC/TDF is used alone for postexposure prophylaxis of HIV infection following occupational exposure† (PEP) in health-care personnel and other individuals exposed via percutaneous injury (e.g., needlestick, cut with sharp object) or mucous membrane or nonintact skin (e.g., chapped, abraded, dermatitis) contact with blood, tissue, or other body fluids that might contain HIV.

The US Public Health Service (USPHS) states that the preferred regimen for PEP following an occupational exposure to HIV is a 3-drug regimen of raltegravir used in conjunction with emtricitabine and tenofovir DF (may be administered as the fixed combination emtricitabine/tenofovir DF; Truvada®). EVG/c/FTC/TDF used alone is one of several alternative regimens recommended when the preferred regimen cannot be used.

Because management of occupational exposures to HIV is complex and evolving, consultation with an infectious disease specialist, clinician with expertise in administration of antiretroviral agents, and/or the National Clinicians' Postexposure Prophylaxis Hotline (PEPline at 888-448-4911) is recommended whenever possible. However, initiation of PEP should not be delayed while waiting for expert consultation.

For information on types of occupational exposure to HIV and associated risk of infection, management of occupational exposure to HIV, efficacy and safety of postexposure prophylaxis, and recommendations regarding PEP, see Guidelines for Use of Antiretroviral Agents: Antiretrovirals for Postexposure Prophylaxis following Occupational Exposure to HIV (PEP), in the Antiretroviral Agents General Statement 8:18.08.

Dosage and Administration

■ **Administration** The fixed combination of elvitegravir, cobicistat, emtricitabine, and tenofovir disoproxil fumarate (tenofovir DF) (EVG/c/FTC/TDF) is administered orally once daily with food.

Serum creatinine, estimated creatinine clearance, serum phosphorus, urine glucose, and urine protein should be determined prior to initiation of EVG/c/FTC/TDF and routinely monitored during treatment in all patients. (See Renal Impairment under Warnings/Precautions: Specific Populations, in Cautions.)

Patients should be tested for hepatitis B virus (HBV) infection prior to initiation of EVG/c/FTC/TDF. (See HIV-infected Individuals Coinfected with Hepatitis B Virus under Warnings/Precautions: Warnings, in Cautions.)

■ **Dosage** Each fixed-combination tablet of EVG/c/FTC/TDF contains elvitegravir 150 mg, cobicistat 150 mg, emtricitabine 200 mg, and tenofovir DF 300 mg.

Adult Dosage **Treatment of HIV Infection.** For the treatment of human immunodeficiency virus type 1 (HIV-1) infection in adults, the usual dosage of EVG/c/FTC/TDF is 1 tablet (150 mg of elvitegravir, 150 mg of cobicistat, 200 mg of emtricitabine, and 300 mg of tenofovir DF) once daily.

Postexposure Prophylaxis following Occupational Exposure to HIV. For postexposure prophylaxis of HIV infection following occupational exposure† (PEP) in health-care personnel or other individuals, the recommended dosage of EVG/c/FTC/TDF is 1 tablet (150 mg of elvitegravir, 150 mg of cobicistat, 200 mg of emtricitabine, and 300 mg of tenofovir DF) once daily.

PEP should be initiated as soon as possible following occupational exposure to HIV (preferably within hours) and continued for 4 weeks, if tolerated.

Pediatric Dosage **Treatment of HIV Infection.** For the treatment of HIV-1 infection in children and adolescents 12 years of age or older weighing at least 35 kg, the usual dosage of EVG/c/FTC/TDF is 1 tablet (150 mg of elvitegravir, 150 mg of cobicistat, 200 mg of emtricitabine, and 300 mg of tenofovir DF) once daily.

■ **Special Populations** ***Hepatic Impairment*** Dosage adjustments are not necessary if EVG/c/FTC/TDF is used in adults with mild or moderate hepatic impairment (Child-Pugh class A or B).

EVG/c/FTC/TDF should not be used in patients with severe hepatic impairment (Child-Pugh class C). (See Hepatic Impairment under Warnings/Precautions: Specific Populations, in Cautions.)

Renal Impairment EVG/c/FTC/TDF should *not* be initiated in adults with estimated creatinine clearance less than 70 mL/minute.

If estimated creatinine clearance decreases to less than 50 mL/minute during EVG/c/FTC/TDF treatment, the drug should be discontinued. (See Renal Impairment under Warnings/Precautions: Specific Populations, in Cautions.)

Data are insufficient to make dosage recommendations for pediatric patients with renal impairment.

Geriatric Patients EVG/c/FTC/TDF should be used with caution in geriatric adults. (See Geriatric Use under Warnings/Precautions: Specific Populations, in Cautions.)

Cautions

■ Contraindications

Concomitant use of the fixed combination of elvitegravir, cobicistat, emtricitabine, and tenofovir disoproxil fumarate (tenofovir DF) (EVG/c/FTC/TDF) with drugs highly dependent on cytochrome P-450 isoenzyme 3A (CYP3A) for metabolism and for which elevated plasma concentrations are associated with serious and/or life-threatening events (e.g., alfuzosin, cisapride, ergot alkaloids, lovastatin, lurasidone, oral midazolam, pimozide, sildenafil used for treatment of pulmonary arterial hypertension [PAH], simvastatin, triazolam) is contraindicated. (See Drug Interactions.)

Concomitant use of EVG/c/FTC/TDF with drugs that are potent inducers of CYP3A and which may decrease elvitegravir and/or cobicistat concentrations resulting in possible decreased antiretroviral efficacy and development of resistance (e.g., carbamazepine, phenobarbital, phenytoin, rifampin, St. John's wort [*Hypericum perforatum*]) is contraindicated. (See Drug Interactions.)

■ Warnings/Precautions

Warnings **HIV-infected Individuals Coinfected with Hepatitis B Virus.** HIV-infected patients should be tested for hepatitis B virus (HBV) before antiretroviral therapy is initiated.

EVG/c/FTC/TDF is not indicated for treatment of chronic HBV infection, and safety and efficacy of EVG/c/FTC/TDF have not been established in HIV-infected patients coinfected with HBV.

In HIV-infected patients with HBV coinfection, severe acute exacerbations of HBV infection have occurred following discontinuance of emtricitabine or tenofovir DF (components of EVG/c/FTC/TDF). In some patients receiving emtricitabine, exacerbations of HBV have been associated with hepatic decompensation and hepatic failure.

Hepatic function should be closely monitored with clinical and laboratory follow-up for at least several months after EVG/c/FTC/TDF is discontinued in patients coinfected with HIV and HBV. If appropriate, initiation of HBV treatment may be warranted.

Other Warnings/Precautions **Renal Toxicity.** Renal impairment, including cases of acute renal failure and Fanconi syndrome (renal tubular injury with severe hypophosphatemia), have been reported in patients receiving tenofovir DF (a component of EVG/c/FTC/TDF).

In clinical trials, 1.9% of patients receiving EVG/c/FTC/TDF and up to 2.3% of patients receiving an active comparator discontinued treatment by 144 weeks because of adverse renal effects. Laboratory findings consistent with proximal renal tubular dysfunction resulting in discontinuance of the drugs occurred in 4 (0.6%) of patients receiving EVG/c/FTC/TDF during the first 48 weeks of treatment; estimated creatinine clearances less than 70 mL/minute were reported at baseline in 2 of the patients receiving EVG/c/FTC/TDF. Laboratory findings improved after EVG/c/FTC/TDF was discontinued, but did not completely resolve in all patients; no patient required renal replacement therapy.

Cobicistat (a component of EVG/c/FTC/TDF) may cause a modest increase in serum creatinine and modest decrease in estimated creatinine clearance due to inhibition of tubular secretion of creatinine; there is a corresponding decrease in serum creatinine-based estimated glomerular filtration rate (eGFR), but renal glomerular function is not affected. Elevated serum creatinine concentrations generally were reversible when the drug was discontinued.

Serum creatinine, estimated creatinine clearance, serum phosphorus, urine glucose, and urine protein should be determined prior to initiation of EVG/c/FTC/TDF and routinely monitored during treatment in all patients.

EVG/c/FTC/TDF should *not* be initiated in patients with estimated creatinine clearances less than 70 mL/minute, and the drug should be discontinued if estimated creatinine clearance decreases to less than 50 mL/minute during treatment. (See Renal Impairment under Dosage and Administration: Special Populations.)

Patients who experience a confirmed increase in serum creatinine of greater than 0.4 mg/dL from baseline while receiving EVG/c/FTC/TDF should be closely monitored for renal toxicity.

Because persistent or worsening bone pain, pain in extremities, fractures, and/or muscular pain or weakness may be manifestations of proximal renal tubulopathy, renal function should be promptly evaluated in patients at risk for renal dysfunction who present with such symptoms. (See Bone Effects under Warnings/Precautions: Other Warnings/Precautions, in Cautions.)

EVG/c/FTC/TDF should be avoided in patients who are receiving or have recently received a nephrotoxic agent (e.g., high-dose or multiple nonsteroidal anti-inflammatory agents [NSAIAs]). Acute renal failure has been reported after initiation of high-dose or multiple NSAIA therapy in HIV-infected patients at risk for renal dysfunction who appeared stable while receiving tenofovir DF. Hospitalization and renal replacement therapy were required in some patients. Alternatives to NSAIAs should be considered if such therapy is needed in patients at risks for renal dysfunction. (See Drug Interactions: Drugs Affecting Renal Function.)

Lactic Acidosis and Severe Hepatomegaly with Steatosis. Lactic acidosis and severe hepatomegaly with steatosis, including fatalities, have been reported in patients receiving HIV nucleoside reverse transcriptase inhibitors (NRTIs), including emtricitabine and tenofovir DF, in conjunction with other antiretroviral agents.

EVG/c/FTC/TDF treatment should be interrupted in any patient who develops clinical or laboratory findings suggestive of lactic acidosis or pronounced hepatotoxicity (signs of hepatotoxicity may include hepatomegaly and steatosis even in the absence of marked increases in serum aminotransferase concentrations).

Bone Effects. Decreases in bone mineral density (BMD) from baseline at lumbar spine and hip, increases in several biochemical markers of bone metabolism, and increased serum parathyroid hormone levels and 1,25 vitamin D levels have been reported during clinical trials of tenofovir DF (a component of EVG/c/FTC/TDF). The effects of tenofovir-associated changes in BMD on long-term bone health and future fracture risk are unknown.

Osteomalacia associated with proximal renal tubulopathy, which manifested as bone pain or pain in extremities and may contribute to fractures, has been reported in patients receiving tenofovir DF. Arthralgia and muscle pain or weakness also have been reported in patients with proximal renal tubulopathy. Hypophosphatemia and osteomalacia secondary to proximal renal tubulopathy should be considered in patients at risk for renal dysfunction who present with persistent or worsening bone or muscle symptoms while receiving preparations containing tenofovir DF. (See Renal Toxicity under Warnings/Precautions: Other Warnings/Precautions, in Cautions.)

In a clinical study evaluating safety and efficacy of EVG/c/FTC/TDF (study 103), the mean percentage decrease in BMD from baseline to week 144 in patients receiving EVG/c/FTC/TDF was similar to that in patients receiving a regimen of *ritonavir-boosted* atazanavir and the fixed combination of emtricitabine and tenofovir DF (FTC/TDF). The mean change from baseline in BMD at the lumbar spine or hip was −1.4 or −2.8%, respectively, in those receiving EVG/c/FTC/TDF and −3.7 or −3.8%, respectively, in those receiving *ritonavir-boosted* atazanavir with FTC/TDF. Data from clinical studies 102 and 103 indicate that 3.9% of those receiving EVG/c/FTC/TDF experienced bone fractures compared with 2.3% of those receiving a fixed combination containing efavirenz, emtricitabine, tenofovir DF (EFV/FTC/TDF) and 5.4% of those receiving *ritonavir-boosted* atazanavir and FTC/TDF. In clinical studies evaluating tenofovir DF in pediatric and adolescent patients, bone effects were similar to those reported in adults. (See Pediatric Use under Warnings/Precautions: Specific Populations, in Cautions.)

BMD monitoring should be considered for adult and pediatric patients who have a history of pathologic bone fracture or other risk factors for osteoporosis or bone loss. Although the effect of calcium and vitamin D supplementation was not studied, such supplementation may be beneficial for all patients. If bone abnormalities are suspected, appropriate consultation should be obtained.

Interactions. Concomitant use of EVG/c/FTC/TDF with certain drugs may result in clinically important interactions, including some that may decrease plasma concentrations of the antiretroviral agents leading to loss of therapeutic effect and possible development of resistance and some that may increase plasma concentrations of the antiretroviral agents and/or concomitant drugs leading to clinically important adverse reactions. (See Cautions: Contraindications and see Drug Interactions.)

The potential for drug interactions should be considered prior to and during EVG/c/FTC/TDF therapy. Drugs used concomitantly should be reviewed during EVG/c/FTC/TDF therapy and the patient should be monitored for adverse reactions associated with the concomitant drugs. (See Drug Interactions.)

Use of Fixed Combinations. The usual cautions, precautions, contraindications, and interactions associated with each component of EVG/c/FTC/TDF should be considered. Cautionary information applicable to specific populations (e.g., pregnant or nursing women, individuals with hepatic or renal impairment, geriatric patients) should be considered for each drug in the fixed combination. For cautionary information related to emtricitabine or tenofovir disoproxil fumarate, see Cautions in Emtricitabine 8:18.08.20 and in Tenofovir Disoproxil Fumarate 8:18.08.20.

EVG/c/FTC/TDF is used alone as a complete regimen for the treatment of HIV-1 infection and should not be used in conjunction with other antiretroviral agents. (See Drug Interactions: Antiretroviral Agents.)

EVG/c/FTC/TDF should not be used concomitantly with any preparation that contains any of its components (elvitegravir, cobicistat, emtricitabine, tenofovir DF). In addition, EVG/c/FTC/TDF should not be used concomitantly with any preparation containing lamivudine, adefovir dipivoxil, or ritonavir.

Immune Reconstitution Syndrome. Immune reconstitution syndrome has been reported in HIV-infected patients receiving multiple-drug antiretroviral therapy, including EVG/c/FTC/TDF. During the initial phase of treatment, HIV-infected patients whose immune systems respond to antiretroviral therapy may develop an inflammatory response to indolent or residual opportunistic infections (e.g., *Mycobacterium avium*, *M. tuberculosis*, cytomegalovirus [CMV], *Pneumocystis jirovecii* [formerly *P. carinii*]); such response may necessitate further evaluation and treatment.

Autoimmune disorders (e.g., Graves' disease, polymyositis, Guillain-Barré syndrome) have also been reported to occur in the setting of immune reconstitution; however, the time to onset is more variable and can occur many months after initiation of antiretroviral therapy.

Specific Populations **Pregnancy.** Antiretroviral Pregnancy Registry at 800-258-4263 or http://www.apregistry.com.

Prospective pregnancy data from the Antiretroviral Pregnancy Registry are not sufficient to date to adequately assess the risk of birth defects or miscarriage if EVG/c/FTC/TDF is used in pregnant women. Data from the Antiretroviral Pregnancy Registry available through January 2016 show no birth defects reported for elvitegravir or cobicistat and no difference in the overall risk of major birth defects for emtricitabine or tenofovir DF compared with the background rate of major birth defects in the US.

In animal studies, there was no evidence of adverse developmental effects when the components of EVG/c/FTC/TDF were administered separately during the period of organogenesis at elvitegravir, cobicistat, emtricitabine, and tenofovir DF exposures up to 23, 4.3, 120, and 19 times higher, respectively, than human exposures at the recommended daily dosage.

The US Department of Health and Human Services (HHS) Panel on Treatment of HIV-infected Pregnant Women and Prevention of Perinatal Transmission states that data are insufficient to recommend routine use of EVG/c/FTC/TDF for *initial* treatment in antiretroviral-naive pregnant women.

Lactation. Elvitegravir and cobicistat are distributed into milk in rats; it is not known whether these drugs are distributed into human milk. The emtricitabine and tenofovir components of EVG/c/FTC/TDF are distributed into human milk.

It is not known whether EVG/c/FTC/TDF affects human milk production or affects the breast-fed infant.

Because of the risk of adverse effects in the infant and the risk of HIV transmission, HIV-infected women should not breast-feed infants.

Pediatric Use. Safety and efficacy of EVG/c/FTC/TDF have not been established in pediatric patients younger than 12 years of age or in those weighing less than 35 kg.

The HHS Panel on Antiretroviral Therapy and Medical Management of HIV-infected Children states that EVG/c/FTC/TDF should be considered for *initial* treatment only in antiretroviral-naive HIV-infected children and adolescents 12 years of age or older weighing 35 kg or more if they are in late puberty (sexual maturity rating [SMR] 4 or 5). These experts state that the fixed combination of elvitegravir, cobicistat, emtricitabine, and tenofovir alafenamide (EVG/c/FTC/TAF) is preferred in children and adolescents 12 years of age or older weighing 35 kg or more.

Clinical trial data indicate that the safety profile of EVG/c/FTC/TDF in HIV-1-infected, treatment-naive pediatric patients 12 to less than 18 years of age is similar to that reported in adults.

Bone effects reported when tenofovir DF is used in pediatric and adolescent patients are similar to those reported in adults. In clinical studies, total body BMD gain in tenofovir DF-treated pediatric patients was less than that reported in control groups; skeletal growth appeared to be unaffected. Effects of tenofovir DF-associated changes in BMD and biochemical markers on long-term bone health and future fracture risk are unknown.

Following oral administration of EVG/c/FTC/TDF, elvitegravir and tenofovir exposures in children and adolescents 12 to less than 18 years of age were 30 and 37% higher, respectively, than those reported in adults; this difference is not considered clinically important based on exposure-response relationships. Cobicistat and emtricitabine exposures in children and adolescents 12 to less than 18 years of age were similar to those reported in adults.

Geriatric Use. Experience in adults 65 years of age and older is insufficient to determine whether they respond differently than younger adults.

EVG/c/FTC/TDF should be used with caution in geriatric patients because of age-related decreases in hepatic, renal, and/or cardiac function and potential for concomitant disease and drug therapy.

Hepatic Impairment. Moderate hepatic impairment (Child-Pugh class B) does not have a clinically important effect on the pharmacokinetics of elvitegravir, cobicistat, or tenofovir DF and is not expected to affect the pharmacokinetics of emtricitabine.

EVG/c/FTC/TDF is *not* recommended in patients with severe hepatic impairment (Child-Pugh class C). Data are not available to date regarding the pharmacokinetics or safety of EVG/c/FTC/TDF in such patients.

Renal Impairment. Serum creatinine, estimated creatinine clearance, serum phosphorus, urine glucose, and urine protein should be determined prior to initiating EVG/c/FTC/TDF and routinely monitored during treatment in all patients.

EVG/c/FTC/TDF should *not* be initiated in adults with estimated creatinine clearances less than 70 mL/minute. If estimated creatinine clearance decreases to less than 50 mL/minute during EVG/c/FTC/TDF treatment, the fixed-combination drug should be discontinued.

Data are insufficient to make dosage recommendations for pediatric patients with renal impairment.

■ **Common Adverse Effects** Adverse effects reported in 5% or more of patients receiving EVG/c/FTC/TDF are nausea (16%), diarrhea (12%), abnormal dreams (9%), and headache (7%).

Drug Interactions

The following drug interactions are based on studies that used elvitegravir, elvitegravir administered with cobicistat (*cobicistat-boosted* elvitegravir), elvitegravir administered with low-dose ritonavir (*ritonavir-boosted* elvitegravir), cobicistat alone, or the fixed combination of elvitegravir, cobicistat, emtricitabine, and tenofovir disoproxil fumarate (tenofovir DF) (EVG/c/FTC/TDF) or are predicted to occur.

Potential drug interactions associated with each drug in the fixed combination should be considered.

■ **Drugs Affecting or Metabolized by Hepatic Microsomal Enzymes** Elvitegravir is a substrate of cytochrome P-450 (CYP) 3A and a weak inducer and weak inhibitor of CYP3A; elvitegravir is an inducer of CYP2C9. The drug does not inhibit CYP1A, 2A6, 2C9, 2C19, 2D6, or 2E1 in vitro.

Cobicistat is a substrate of CYP3A and, to a minor extent, CYP2D6; cobicistat also is an inhibitor of CYP3A and 2D6.

Emtricitabine is not a substrate of CYP enzymes and does not inhibit CYP1A2, 2A6, 2B6, 2C9, 2C19, 2D6, or 3A4.

Tenofovir DF and tenofovir are not substrates of CYP enzymes; tenofovir does not inhibit CYP3A4, 2D6, 2C9, or 2E1, but may have a slight inhibitory effect on CYP1A.

Potential pharmacokinetic interactions if EVG/c/FTC/TDF is used concomitantly with drugs that are principally metabolized by CYP3A or 2D6 (increased plasma concentrations of the concomitant drug). Concomitant use of EVG/c/FTC/TDF with some drugs that are CYP3A substrates and for which elevated plasma concentrations are associated with serious and/or life-threatening events is contraindicated.

Potential pharmacokinetic interactions if EVG/c/FTC/TDF is used concomitantly with drugs that induce CYP3A (decreased plasma concentrations of elvitegravir and cobicistat and possible decreased antiretroviral efficacy and development of resistance). Concomitant use of EVG/c/FTC/TDF with some drugs that are potent inducers of CYP3A is contraindicated.

Potential pharmacokinetic interactions if EVG/c/FTC/TDF is used concomitantly with drugs that inhibit CYP3A (increased plasma concentrations of cobicistat).

■ **Drugs Affected by P-glycoprotein Transport** Cobicistat is an inhibitor of P-glycoprotein (P-gp) transport.

Potential pharmacokinetic interactions if EVG/c/FTC/TDF is used concomitantly with drugs that are P-gp substrates (increased plasma concentrations of the concomitant drug).

■ **Drugs Affected by Breast Cancer Resistance Protein** Cobicistat is an inhibitor of breast cancer resistance protein (BCRP).

Potential pharmacokinetic interactions if EVG/c/FTC/TDF is used concomitantly with drugs that are substrates for BCRP (increased plasma concentrations of the concomitant drug).

■ **Drugs Affected by Organic Anion Transport Polypeptides** Elvitegravir and cobicistat are inhibitors of organic anion transport polypeptides (OATP) 1B1 and 1B3.

Potential pharmacokinetic interactions if EVG/c/FTC/TDF is used concomitantly with drugs that are substrates for OATP1B1 or 1B3 (increased plasma concentrations of the concomitant drug).

■ **Drugs Affecting Renal Function** The emtricitabine and tenofovir components of EVG/c/FTC/TDF are principally excreted by the kidneys by a combination of glomerular filtration and active tubular secretion.

Potential pharmacokinetic interactions if EVG/c/FTC/TDF is used concomitantly with drugs that reduce renal function or compete for active tubular secretion (e.g., acyclovir, aminoglycosides [gentamicin], cidofovir, ganciclovir, valacyclovir, valganciclovir, high-dose or multiple nonsteroidal anti-inflammatory agents [NSAIAs]); may result in increased concentrations of emtricitabine, tenofovir, and/or the concomitant drug and may increase the risk of adverse effects.

■ **Alfuzosin** Potential pharmacokinetic interaction with alfuzosin (increased plasma concentrations of alfuzosin) may result in hypotension.

Concomitant use of alfuzosin and EVG/c/FTC/TDF is contraindicated.

■ **Anticoagulants** ***Apixaban, Edoxaban, Rivaroxaban*** Pharmacokinetic interactions are expected if apixaban, edoxaban, or rivaroxaban is used concomitantly with EVG/c/FTC/TDF (increased anticoagulant concentrations).

Concomitant use of EVG/c/FTC/TDF and apixaban, edoxaban, or rivaroxaban should be avoided.

Dabigatran Potential pharmacokinetic interactions if dabigatran is used concomitantly with EVG/c/FTC/TDF (increased dabigatran concentrations).

Some experts state that dosage adjustments are not necessary if dabigatran and EVG/c/FTC/TDF are used concomitantly in patients with creatinine clearances exceeding 50 mL/minute, but the drugs should not be used concomitantly in those with creatinine clearances less than 50 mL/minute.

Warfarin Potential pharmacokinetic interaction if warfarin is used concomitantly with EVG/c/FTC/TDF (altered warfarin concentrations).

If warfarin is used concomitantly with EVG/c/FTC/TDF, the international normalized ratio (INR) should be monitored and warfarin dosage adjusted accordingly.

■ **Anticonvulsants** ***Carbamazepine, Phenobarbital, Phenytoin*** Concomitant use of carbamazepine and *cobicistat-boosted* elvitegravir results in decreased elvitegravir plasma concentrations and area under the plasma concentration-time curve (AUC) and may lead to loss of antiretroviral efficacy and development of resistance; increased carbamazepine plasma concentrations and AUC also occur. Potential pharmacokinetic interactions if phenobarbital or phenytoin is used concomitantly with EVG/c/FTC/TDF (decreased elvitegravir and cobicistat plasma concentrations with possible decreased antiretroviral efficacy and development of resistance).

Concomitant use of EVG/c/FTC/TDF and carbamazepine, phenobarbital, or phenytoin is contraindicated.

Ethosuximide Potential pharmacokinetic interaction if ethosuximide is used concomitantly with EVG/c/FTC/TDF (increased ethosuximide plasma concentrations).

If ethosuximide and EVG/c/FTC/TDF are used concomitantly, the patient should be monitored clinically for ethosuximide-related adverse effects.

Oxcarbazepine Potential pharmacokinetic interaction if oxcarbazepine is used concomitantly with EVG/c/FTC/TDF (decreased elvitegravir and cobicistat plasma concentrations). An alternative anticonvulsant should be considered.

■ **Antifungal Agents** ***Isavuconazonium*** Concomitant use of isavuconazonium sulfate (prodrug of isavuconazole) and EVG/c/FTC/TDF may result in increased isavuconazole, elvitegravir, and cobicistat concentrations.

If isavuconazonium sulfate and EVG/c/FTC/TDF are used concomitantly, the patient should be monitored for virologic efficacy and isavuconazole concentration monitoring should be considered.

Itraconazole Potential pharmacokinetic interactions with itraconazole (increased itraconazole plasma concentrations expected, increased elvitegravir and cobicistat plasma concentrations possible).

If itraconazole and EVG/c/FTC/TDF are used concomitantly, itraconazole dosage should not exceed 200 mg daily. Consideration should be given to monitoring itraconazole plasma concentrations during concomitant therapy; some experts state that itraconazole dosages exceeding 200 mg daily should be used in patients receiving EVG/c/FTC/TDF only if itraconazole plasma concentrations are used to guide dosage of the antifungal.

Ketoconazole Pharmacokinetic interactions with ketoconazole (increased plasma concentrations of ketoconazole, elvitegravir, and cobicistat).

If ketoconazole and EVG/c/FTC/TDF are used concomitantly, ketoconazole dosage should not exceed 200 mg daily.

Posaconazole Potential pharmacokinetic interactions with posaconazole (increased plasma concentrations of posaconazole, elvitegravir, and cobicistat).

If posaconazole and EVG/c/FTC/TDF are used concomitantly, posaconazole plasma concentrations should be monitored.

Voriconazole Potential pharmacokinetic interactions with voriconazole (increased voriconazole plasma concentrations expected, increased elvitegravir and cobicistat plasma concentrations possible).

Voriconazole and EVG/c/FTC/TDF should not be used concomitantly unless potential benefits outweigh risks. If voriconazole and EVG/c/FTC/TDF are used concomitantly, some experts state that consideration should be given to using voriconazole plasma concentrations to guide dosage of the antifungal.

■ **Antimycobacterial Agents** ***Rifabutin*** Pharmacokinetic interactions when *cobicistat-boosted* elvitegravir (elvitegravir 150 mg and cobicistat 150 mg once daily) was used concomitantly with rifabutin 150 mg once every other day (decreased elvitegravir plasma concentrations and AUC, increased 25-*O*-desacetyl-rifabutin concentrations and AUC relative to those achieved with rifabutin 300 mg once daily without concomitant *cobicistat-boosted* elvitegravir); possible decreased antiretroviral efficacy and development of resistance.

Concomitant use of rifabutin and EVG/c/FTC/TDF is not recommended.

Rifampin Potential pharmacokinetic interactions with rifampin (decreased elvitegravir and cobicistat plasma concentrations); possible decreased antiretroviral efficacy and development of resistance.

Concomitant use of rifampin and EVG/c/FTC/TDF is contraindicated.

Rifapentine Potential pharmacokinetic interactions with rifapentine (decreased elvitegravir and cobicistat plasma concentrations); possible decreased antiretroviral efficacy and development of resistance.

Concomitant use of rifapentine and EVG/c/FTC/TDF is not recommended.

■ **Antiplatelet Agents** ***Ticagrelor, Vorapaxar*** Pharmacokinetic interactions are expected if ticagrelor or vorapaxar is used concomitantly with EVG/c/FTC/TDF (increased antiplatelet agent concentrations).

Concomitant use of EVG/c/FTC/TDF and ticagrelor or vorapaxar should be avoided.

■ **Antipsychotic Agents** ***Lurasidone*** Concomitant use of lurasidone and EVG/c/FTC/TDF may result in serious and/or life-threatening adverse effects.

Concomitant use of lurasidone and EVG/c/FTC/TDF is contraindicated.

Perphenazine, Risperidone, Thioridazine Potential pharmacokinetic interactions with antipsychotics, including perphenazine, risperidone, and thioridazine (increased antipsychotic plasma concentrations).

If EVG/c/FTC/TDF is used concomitantly with perphenazine, risperidone, or thioridazine, decreased dosage of the antipsychotic may be necessary. If perphenazine, risperidone, or thioridazine is initiated in a patient receiving EVG/c/FTC/TDF, some experts recommend a low starting dosage.

Pimozide Potential pharmacokinetic interaction with pimozide (increased pimozide plasma concentrations); potential for serious and/or life-threatening adverse effects (e.g., cardiac arrhythmias).

Concomitant use of pimozide and EVG/c/FTC/TDF is contraindicated.

Quetiapine Pharmacokinetic interaction with quetiapine expected (increased quetiapine plasma concentrations).

Alternative antiretroviral therapy should be considered. If EVG/c/FTC/TDF is necessary in a patient receiving a stable dosage of quetiapine, the quetiapine dosage should be reduced to one-sixth of the original dosage. If quetiapine is necessary in a patient receiving EVG/c/FTC/TDF, some experts recommend that quetiapine should be initiated using the lowest dosage and titrated as needed. Patients receiving quetiapine and EVG/c/FTC/TDF concomitantly should be closely monitored for quetiapine efficacy and adverse effects.

■ **Antiretroviral Agents** EVG/c/FTC/TDF should not be used in conjunction with any other antiretroviral agents.

HIV Entry and Fusion Inhibitors **Maraviroc.** Pharmacokinetic interactions with *ritonavir-boosted* elvitegravir (increased maraviroc plasma concentrations and AUC; no effect on elvitegravir pharmacokinetics).

Maraviroc and EVG/c/FTC/TDF should not be used concomitantly.

HIV Integrase Inhibitors (INSTIs) **Raltegravir.** Raltegravir and EVG/c/FTC/TDF should not be used concomitantly.

HIV Nonnucleoside Reverse Transcriptase Inhibitors (NNRTIs) Potential drug interactions with efavirenz, etravirine, nevirapine, or rilpivirine (altered plasma concentrations of elvitegravir, cobicistat, and/or the NNRTI).

EVG/c/FTC/TDF should not be used concomitantly with HIV NNRTIs.

HIV Nucleoside and Nucleotide Reverse Transcriptase Inhibitors (NRTIs) EVG/c/FTC/TDF contains emtricitabine and tenofovir DF and should not be used concomitantly with any preparation containing these or any other NRTIs.

HIV Protease Inhibitors (PIs) Potential pharmacokinetic interactions with atazanavir, *ritonavir-boosted* or *cobicistat-boosted* atazanavir, *ritonavir-boosted* or *cobicistat-boosted* darunavir, fosamprenavir (with or without low-dose ritonavir), fixed combination of lopinavir and ritonavir (lopinavir/ritonavir), *ritonavir-boosted* saquinavir, or *ritonavir-boosted* tipranavir (altered plasma concentrations of elvitegravir, cobicistat, and/or the HIV PI).

EVG/c/FTC/TDF should not be used concomitantly with HIV PIs.

Ritonavir. Ritonavir and cobicistat have similar effects on CYP3A. EVG/c/FTC/TDF and ritonavir (or preparations containing ritonavir) should not be used concomitantly.

■ **β-Adrenergic Blocking Agents** Potential pharmacokinetic interactions with β-adrenergic blocking agents, including metoprolol and timolol (increased β-adrenergic blocking agent plasma concentrations).

If EVG/c/FTC/TDF is used concomitantly with a β-adrenergic blocking agent, patients should be monitored clinically and decreased dosage of the β-adrenergic blocking agent may be necessary. Some experts state that alternative β-adrenergic blocking agents that are not metabolized by CYP isoenzymes (e.g., atenolol, labetalol, nadolol, sotalol) should be considered.

■ **Benzodiazepines** ***Midazolam or Triazolam*** Pharmacokinetic interaction with midazolam or triazolam (increased benzodiazepine plasma concentrations); potential for serious and/or life-threatening adverse effects (e.g., prolonged or increased sedation or respiratory depression).

Concomitant use of oral midazolam or triazolam with EVG/c/FTC/TDF is contraindicated.

Concomitant use of parenteral midazolam and EVG/c/FTC/TDF should be undertaken in a monitored setting where respiratory depression and/or prolonged sedation can be managed. In addition, use of a reduced midazolam dosage should be considered, especially if more than a single dose of the drug will be administered.

Other Benzodiazepines Potential pharmacokinetic interactions with clonazepam, clorazepate, diazepam, estazolam, or flurazepam (increased benzodiazepine plasma concentrations).

If clonazepam, clorazepate, diazepam, estazolam, or flurazepam is used concomitantly with EVG/c/FTC/TDF, patients should be monitored clinically. If a benzodiazepine is initiated in a patient receiving EVG/c/FTC/TDF, some experts recommend a low initial dosage with close monitoring. Alternatives to diazepam (e.g., lorazepam, oxazepam, temazepam) should be considered.

■ **Bosentan** Potential pharmacokinetic interaction with bosentan (increased bosentan plasma concentrations).

In patients who have already been receiving EVG/c/FTC/TDF for at least 10 days, bosentan should be initiated using a dosage of 62.5 mg once daily or every other day based on individual tolerability.

In patients who have already been receiving bosentan, bosentan should be discontinued for at least 36 hours prior to initiating EVG/c/FTC/TDF; after at least 10 days of EVG/c/FTC/TDF therapy, bosentan can be resumed using a dosage of 62.5 mg once daily or every other day based on individual tolerability.

■ **Bupropion** Potential pharmacokinetic interaction with bupropion (increased or decreased bupropion plasma concentrations).

If bupropion is used concomitantly with EVG/c/FTC/TDF, dosage of the antidepressant should be titrated carefully based on clinical response.

■ **Buspirone** Potential pharmacokinetic interaction with buspirone (increased buspirone plasma concentrations).

If buspirone is used concomitantly with EVG/c/FTC/TDF, patients should be monitored clinically; reduced buspirone dosage may be necessary. If buspirone is initiated in a patient receiving EVG/c/FTC/TDF, some experts recommend a low initial buspirone dosage.

■ **Calcium-channel Blocking Agents** Potential pharmacokinetic interactions with calcium-channel blocking agents, including amlodipine, diltiazem, felodipine, nicardipine, nifedipine, and verapamil (increased plasma concentrations of the calcium-channel blocking agent).

Calcium-channel blocking agents and EVG/c/FTC/TDF should be used concomitantly with caution; dosage of the calcium-channel blocking agent should be titrated and the patient monitored for efficacy and adverse effects.

■ **Calcium, Iron, Multivitamins, and Other Preparations Containing Polyvalent Cations** Oral calcium supplements, oral iron preparations, other oral supplements containing calcium, iron, aluminum, magnesium, or zinc (e.g., multivitamins), and laxatives or other preparations containing polyvalent cations may decrease plasma concentrations of elvitegravir when used concomitantly.

EVG/c/FTC/TDF should be administered at least 2 hours before or at least 6 hours after oral supplements containing calcium, iron, aluminum, magnesium, or zinc or other preparations (e.g., laxatives) containing polyvalent cations and patients should be monitored for antiretroviral efficacy.

■ **Cardiac Drugs** ***Antiarrhythmic Agents*** Potential pharmacokinetic interactions if EVG/c/FTC/TDF is used with amiodarone, bepridil (no longer commercially available in the US), digoxin, disopyramide, dronedarone, flecainide, lidocaine (systemic), mexiletine, propafenone, or quinidine (increased plasma concentrations of the antiarrhythmic agent or cardiac glycoside). Concomitant use of digoxin (single 0.5-mg dose) and cobicistat (single 150-mg dose) has resulted in increased plasma concentrations of digoxin.

EVG/c/FTC/TDF and antiarrhythmic agents or digoxin should be used concomitantly with caution; plasma concentrations of the antiarrhythmic agents or cardiac glycoside should be monitored, if possible.

Eplerenone Concomitant use of eplerenone and EVG/c/FTC/TDF is expected to result in increased eplerenone concentrations.

Some experts state that concomitant use of eplerenone and EVG/c/FTC/TDF is contraindicated.

Ivabradine Concomitant use of ivabradine and EVG/c/FTC/TDF is expected to result in increased ivabradine concentrations.

Some experts state that concomitant use of ivabradine and EVG/c/FTC/TDF is contraindicated.

Ranolazine Some experts state that ranolazine and EVG/c/FTC/TDF should not be used concomitantly.

■ **Cisapride** Potential pharmacokinetic interaction with cisapride (increased cisapride plasma concentrations); potential for serious and/or life-threatening adverse effects (e.g., cardiac arrhythmias).

Concomitant use of cisapride and EVG/c/FTC/TDF is contraindicated.

■ **Cobicistat** Pharmacokinetic interaction with elvitegravir (increased plasma concentrations and AUC of elvitegravir); occurs because cobicistat inhibits CYP3A. Cobicistat acts as a pharmacokinetic enhancer when used concomitantly with elvitegravir (*cobicistat-boosted* elvitegravir) and this effect is used to therapeutic advantage in the EVG/c/FTC/TDF fixed combination.

Pharmacokinetic interaction with emtricitabine and tenofovir (slightly increased emtricitabine plasma concentrations and AUC; slightly increased tenofovir plasma concentrations); not considered clinically important.

Cobicistat does not antagonize the antiretroviral effects of elvitegravir, emtricitabine, or tenofovir.

■ **Colchicine** Potential pharmacokinetic interaction (increased colchicine plasma concentrations expected).

Colchicine and EVG/c/FTC/TDF should not be used concomitantly in patients with renal or hepatic impairment.

When colchicine is used for *treatment* of gout flares in patients receiving EVG/c/FTC/TDF, an initial colchicine dose of 0.6 mg should be given followed by 0.3 mg 1 hour later; the colchicine course should be repeated no earlier than 3 days later.

When colchicine is used for *prophylaxis* of gout flares in patients receiving EVG/c/FTC/TDF, colchicine dosage should be reduced to 0.3 mg once daily in those originally receiving 0.6 mg twice daily or decreased to 0.3 mg once every other day in those originally receiving 0.6 mg once daily.

When colchicine is used for treatment of familial Mediterranean fever (FMF) in patients receiving EVG/c/FTC/TDF, a maximum colchicine dosage of 0.6 mg daily (may be given as 0.3 mg twice daily) should be used.

■ **Corticosteroids** ***Orally Inhaled or Intranasal Corticosteroids*** Concomitant use of EVG/c/FTC/TDF and fluticasone (orally inhaled or intranasal) or other corticosteroids whose exposures are substantially affected by potent CYP3A inhibitors (e.g., ciclesonide, mometasone) may increase plasma concentrations of the corticosteroid, which may result in adrenal insufficiency or Cushing's syndrome. Alternative corticosteroids (e.g., beclomethasone) should be considered in patients receiving EVG/c/FTC/TDF, particularly if long-term corticosteroid therapy is required.

Local Injections of Corticosteroids Concomitant use of EVG/c/FTC/TDF and local injections (e.g., intra-articular, epidural, intraorbital) of methylprednisolone, prednisolone, or triamcinolone is expected to increase plasma concentrations of the corticosteroid and may result in adrenal insufficiency or Cushing's syndrome.

EVG/c/FTC/TDF should not be used concomitantly with local injections of methylprednisolone, prednisolone, or triamcinolone.

Systemic Corticosteroids **Dexamethasone.** Concomitant use of systemic dexamethasone may decrease elvitegravir and cobicistat plasma concentrations and may lead to decreased antiretroviral efficacy and development of resistance.

An alternative corticosteroid should be considered in patients receiving EVG/c/FTC/TDF. If dexamethasone and EVG/c/FTC/TDF are used concomitantly, caution is recommended and virologic response should be monitored.

Other Systemic Corticosteroids. Concomitant use of EVG/c/FTC/TDF and systemic corticosteroids whose exposures are substantially affected by potent CYP3A inhibitors (e.g., betamethasone, budesonide, prednisone) may increase plasma concentrations of the corticosteroid, which may result in adrenal insufficiency or Cushing's syndrome. Alternative corticosteroids (e.g., prednisolone) should be considered in patients receiving EVG/c/FTC/TDF, particularly if long-term corticosteroid therapy is required.

■ **Ergot Alkaloids** Potential for serious and/or life-threatening adverse effects (e.g., peripheral vasospasm, ischemia of the extremities and other tissues) if EVG/c/FTC/TDF is used concomitantly with ergot alkaloids (e.g., dihydroergotamine, ergotamine, methylergonovine).

Concomitant use of ergot alkaloids and EVG/c/FTC/TDF is contraindicated.

■ **Estrogens and Progestins** Pharmacokinetic interactions with oral contraceptives containing ethinyl estradiol and norgestimate (decreased ethinyl estradiol plasma concentrations and AUC and increased norgestimate plasma concentrations and AUC). In a pharmacokinetic study evaluating concomitant use of EVG/c/FTC/TDF and a triphasic oral contraceptive containing ethinyl estradiol and norgestimate, the AUC and trough plasma concentration of ethinyl estradiol were decreased 25 and 44%, respectively, while the mean peak plasma concentration, AUC, and trough plasma concentration of norgestimate were increased 108, 126, and 167%, respectively, compared with use of the oral contraceptive alone.

Possible effects of increased norgestimate plasma concentrations are not established, but may include increased risk of insulin resistance, dyslipidemia, acne, and venous thrombosis. The potential risks and benefits of concomitant use of EVG/c/FTC/TDF and oral contraceptives containing ethinyl estradiol and norgestimate should be considered, particularly in women with risk factors for these effects.

Concomitant use of EVG/c/FTC/TDF with oral contraceptives containing progestins other than norgestimate or with other hormonal contraceptives (e.g., patch, vaginal ring, injections) has not been studied; alternative nonhormonal methods of contraception should be considered.

■ **Flibanserin** Concomitant use of flibanserin and EVG/c/FTC/TDF is expected to increase flibanserin concentrations.

Some experts state that concomitant use of flibanserin and EVG/c/FTC/TDF is contraindicated.

■ **GI Drugs** ***Antacids*** Pharmacokinetic interaction with antacids containing aluminum, calcium, and/or magnesium hydroxide (decreased plasma concentrations and AUC of elvitegravir).

EVG/c/FTC/TDF should be given at least 2 hours before or at least 2 hours after antacids containing aluminum, calcium, or magnesium.

Histamine H_2-receptor Antagonists Concomitant use of famotidine and *cobicistat-boosted* elvitegravir did not have a clinically important effect on elvitegravir plasma concentrations or AUC.

Concomitant use of EVG/c/FTC/TDF and histamine H_2-receptor antagonists is not expected to result in clinically important drug interactions.

Dosage adjustments are not necessary if EVG/c/FTC/TDF is used concomitantly with a histamine H_2-receptor antagonist.

Proton-pump Inhibitors Concomitant use of omeprazole and *cobicistat-boosted* elvitegravir did not result in clinically important alterations in elvitegravir pharmacokinetics.

Concomitant use of EVG/c/FTC/TDF and proton-pump inhibitors is not expected to result in clinically important drug interactions.

Dosage adjustments are not necessary if EVG/c/FTC/TDF is used concomitantly with a proton-pump inhibitor.

Sucralfate Sucralfate may decrease plasma concentrations of elvitegravir if used concomitantly with EVG/c/FTC/TDF.

EVG/c/FTC/TDF should be administered at least 2 hours before or at least 6 hours after sucralfate and patients should be monitored for antiretroviral efficacy.

■ **HCV Antivirals** ***HCV Polymerase Inhibitors*** **Sofosbuvir.** Clinically important pharmacokinetic interactions are not expected if EVG/c/FTC/TDF is used concomitantly with sofosbuvir.

Sofosbuvir and EVG/c/FTC/TDF can be used concomitantly without dosage adjustments.

Sofosbuvir and Velpatasvir. Concomitant use of the fixed combination of sofosbuvir and velpatasvir (sofosbuvir/velpatasvir) with EVG/c/FTC/TDF results in increased tenofovir exposures.

If sofosbuvir/velpatasvir and EVG/c/FTC/TDF are used concomitantly, the patient should be monitored for tenofovir-associated adverse effects.

HCV Protease Inhibitors **Simeprevir.** Concomitant use of simeprevir and EVG/c/FTC/TDF is expected to increase plasma concentrations of simeprevir.

Concomitant use of simeprevir and EVG/c/FTC/TDF is not recommended.

HCV Replication Complex Inhibitors **Daclatasvir.** Concomitant use of daclatasvir and EVG/c/FTC/TDF may result in increased plasma concentrations of daclatasvir.

If daclatasvir and EVG/c/FTC/TDF are used concomitantly, daclatasvir should be given in a dosage of 30 mg once daily.

Dasabuvir, Ombitasvir, Paritaprevir, and Ritonavir. Data are not available regarding concomitant use of EVG/c/FTC/TDF and the fixed combination of dasabuvir, ombitasvir, paritaprevir, and ritonavir (dasabuvir/ombitasvir/paritaprevir/ritonavir).

Concomitant use of EVG/c/FTC/TDF and dasabuvir/ombitasvir/paritaprevir/ritonavir is not recommended.

Elbasvir and Grazoprevir. Concomitant use of the fixed combination of elbasvir and grazoprevir (elbasvir/grazoprevir) and EVG/c/FTC/TDF may result in increased elbasvir and grazoprevir plasma concentrations.

Concomitant use of elbasvir/grazoprevir and EVG/c/FTC/TDF is not recommended.

Ledipasvir and Sofosbuvir. Concomitant use of the fixed combination of ledipasvir and sofosbuvir (ledipasvir/sofosbuvir) and EVG/c/FTC/TDF results in increased ledipasvir plasma concentrations and is expected to result in increased tenofovir plasma concentrations. Safety of increased tenofovir plasma concentrations in patients receiving ledipasvir/sofosbuvir and EVG/c/FTC/TDF concomitantly has not been established.

Ledipasvir/sofosbuvir and EVG/c/FTC/TDF should not be used concomitantly.

■ **HMG-CoA Reductase Inhibitors** Concomitant use of certain hydroxymethylglutaryl-CoA (HMG-CoA) reductase inhibitors (statins) metabolized by CYP3A (e.g., atorvastatin, lovastatin, simvastatin) and EVG/c/FTC/TDF may increase plasma concentrations of the HMG-CoA reductase inhibitor resulting in increased effects and increased risk of statin-associated adverse effects, including myopathy and rhabdomyolysis.

Atorvastatin If atorvastatin is used concomitantly with EVG/c/FTC/TDF, the statin should be initiated at the lowest dosage and titrated carefully while monitoring for atorvastatin-associated adverse effects.

Lovastatin Concomitant use of lovastatin and EVG/c/FTC/TDF is contraindicated.

Pitavastatin and Pravastatin Data are not available regarding concomitant use of EVG/c/FTC/TDF and pitavastatin or pravastatin.

Rosuvastatin Pharmacokinetic interaction when rosuvastatin is used concomitantly with *cobicistat-boosted* elvitegravir (increased rosuvastatin plasma concentrations and AUC; no clinically important effect on elvitegravir pharmacokinetics).

If rosuvastatin is used concomitantly with EVG/c/FTC/TDF, some experts recommend slowly titrating rosuvastatin dosage and using the lowest possible dosage.

Simvastatin Concomitant use of simvastatin and EVG/c/FTC/TDF is contraindicated.

■ **Immunosuppressive Agents** Potential pharmacokinetic interactions with cyclosporine, everolimus, sirolimus, or tacrolimus (increased plasma concentrations of the immunosuppressive agent).

If EVG/c/FTC/TDF is used concomitantly with cyclosporine, sirolimus, or tacrolimus, plasma concentrations of the immunosuppressive agent should be monitored and the patient monitored for toxicities. Some experts recommend an initial adjustment of cyclosporine, everolimus, sirolimus, or tacrolimus dosage to compensate for anticipated alterations in immunosuppressant metabolism; consultation with a specialist may be necessary.

■ **Macrolides** ***Clarithromycin*** Potential pharmacokinetic interactions (increased plasma concentrations of clarithromycin and cobicistat).

Modification of the usual dosage of clarithromycin is not necessary in those with creatinine clearances of 60 mL/minute or greater; however, clarithromycin dosage should be reduced by 50% in those with creatinine clearances of 50–60 mL/minute. EVG/c/FTC/TDF should not be used in those with creatinine clearances less than 50 mL/minute.

■ **Nucleoside and Nucleotide Antivirals** Potential pharmacokinetic interactions if EVG/c/FTC/TDF is used concomitantly with drugs that compete for active tubular secretion, including acyclovir, cidofovir, ganciclovir, valacyclovir, and valganciclovir; increased plasma concentrations of some of the components of EVG/c/FTC/TDF (i.e., emtricitabine, tenofovir) or the concomitant drug may occur and increase the risk of adverse effects.

Adefovir EVG/c/FTC/TDF should not be used concomitantly with adefovir.

Entecavir or Famciclovir Clinically important interactions are not expected if EVG/c/FTC/TDF is used concomitantly with entecavir or famciclovir.

Ribavirin Clinically important interactions are not expected if EVG/c/FTC/TDF is used concomitantly with ribavirin.

■ **Opiates Agonists, Opiate Partial Agonists, and Opiate Antagonists** ***Buprenorphine*** Concomitant use of the fixed combination of buprenorphine and naloxone (buprenorphine/naloxone) with *cobicistat-boosted* elvitegravir increased plasma concentrations and AUC of buprenorphine and norbuprenorphine and decreased peak plasma concentrations and AUC of naloxone.

If buprenorphine/naloxone is used concomitantly with EVG/c/FTC/TDF, dosage adjustments are not necessary; however, patients should be monitored closely for sedation and adverse cognitive effects.

Patients who are receiving EVG/c/FTC/TDF and are switching from transmucosal buprenorphine to the subdermal implant should be monitored to ensure that the buprenorphine effect is adequate and not excessive.

Methadone Concomitant use of methadone and *cobicistat-boosted* elvitegravir did not result in clinically important alterations in methadone pharmacokinetics.

Concomitant use of methadone and EVG/c/FTC/TDF is not expected to result in clinically important drug interactions; dosage adjustments are not necessary.

■ **Phosphodiesterase Type 5 Inhibitors** Concomitant use of EVG/c/FTC/TDF and selective phosphodiesterase type 5 (PDE5) inhibitors (e.g., sildenafil, tadalafil, vardenafil) is expected to result in increased plasma concentrations of the PDE5 inhibitor and increase the risk of adverse effects (e.g., hypotension, syncope, visual disturbances, priapism) associated with these agents.

Avanafil Data are not available regarding concomitant use of avanafil and EVG/c/FTC/TDF; concomitant use is not recommended.

Sildenafil Concomitant use of EVG/c/FTC/TDF is contraindicated in patients receiving sildenafil for treatment of pulmonary arterial hypertension (PAH).

If sildenafil is used for treatment of erectile dysfunction in a patient receiving EVG/c/FTC/TDF, sildenafil dosage should not exceed 25 mg once every 48 hours and the patient should be monitored for sildenafil-related adverse effects.

Tadalafil If tadalafil is used for treatment of PAH in a patient who has been receiving EVG/c/FTC/TDF for at least 1 week, tadalafil should be initiated at a dosage of 20 mg once daily and, if tolerated, dosage may be increased to 40 mg once daily. EVG/c/FTC/TDF should not be initiated in patients receiving tadalafil for treatment of PAH; tadalafil should be discontinued for at least 24 hours prior to initiating EVG/c/FTC/TDF. After at least 1 week, tadalafil may be resumed at a dosage of 20 mg once daily and, if tolerated, dosage may be increased to 40 mg once daily.

If tadalafil is used for treatment of erectile dysfunction in a patient receiving EVG/c/FTC/TDF, tadalafil dosage should not exceed 10 mg once every 72 hours and the patient should be monitored for tadalafil-related adverse effects. Some experts recommend initiating tadalafil at a dose of 5 mg.

Vardenafil If vardenafil is used for treatment of erectile dysfunction in a patient receiving EVG/c/FTC/TDF, vardenafil dosage should not exceed 2.5 mg once every 72 hours and the patient should be monitored for vardenafil-related adverse effects.

■ **Salmeterol** Potential pharmacokinetic interaction with salmeterol (increased salmeterol plasma concentrations) may result in increased risk of salmeterol-associated adverse cardiovascular effects, including QT interval prolongation, palpitations, and sinus tachycardia.

Concomitant use of salmeterol and EVG/c/FTC/TDF is not recommended.

■ **Selective Serotonin-reuptake Inhibitors** Potential pharmacokinetic interactions with certain selective serotonin-reuptake inhibitors (SSRIs), including citalopram, escitalopram, fluoxetine, paroxetine, and sertraline (increased SSRI plasma concentrations).

If citalopram, escitalopram, fluoxetine, paroxetine, or sertraline is used concomitantly with EVG/c/FTC/TDF, the lowest initial dosage of the SSRI should be used and dosage carefully titrated based on clinical response.

Fluvoxamine Potential pharmacokinetic interactions if fluvoxamine is used concomitantly with EVG/c/FTC/TDF (increased or decreased elvitegravir concentrations).

Some experts state that an alternative to fluvoxamine or an alternative to EVG/c/FTC/TDF should be considered.

■ **Suvorexant** Pharmacokinetic interaction with suvorexant expected (increased suvorexant plasma concentrations).

Some experts state that concomitant use of suvorexant and EVG/c/FTC/TDF is not recommended.

■ **Trazodone** Potential pharmacokinetic interaction with trazodone (increased trazodone plasma concentrations).

If trazodone is initiated in a patient receiving EVG/c/FTC/TDF, the lowest initial dosage of the antidepressant should be used and dosage carefully titrated according to response.

■ **Tricyclic Antidepressants** Potential pharmacokinetic interactions with tricyclic antidepressants, including amitriptyline, desipramine, doxepin, imipramine, and nortriptyline (increased tricyclic antidepressant plasma concentrations and AUC). Increased desipramine plasma concentrations and AUC reported when used concomitantly with cobicistat or EVG/c/FTC/TDF.

If a tricyclic antidepressant is initiated in a patient receiving EVG/c/FTC/

TDF, the lowest initial dosage of the antidepressant should be used and dosage carefully titrated based on clinical response and/or plasma concentrations of the antidepressant.

■ **Zolpidem** Pharmacokinetic interaction with zolpidem expected (increased zolpidem plasma concentrations).

If zolpidem is used concomitantly with EVG/c/FTC/TDF, patients should be monitored clinically; reduced zolpidem dosage may be necessary. If zolpidem is initiated in a patient receiving EVG/c/FTC/TDF, some experts recommend a low initial dosage.

■ **Dietary and Herbal Supplements** *St. John's Wort* Potential pharmacokinetic interactions with St. John's wort (*Hypericum perforatum*) (decreased elvitegravir and/or cobicistat plasma concentrations); possible decreased antiretroviral efficacy and development of resistance.

Concomitant use of St. John's wort and EVG/c/FTC/TDF is contraindicated.

Description

The fixed combination of elvitegravir, cobicistat, emtricitabine, and tenofovir disoproxil fumarate (EVG/c/FTC/TDF) contains a human immunodeficiency virus (HIV) integrase strand transfer inhibitor (INSTI) antiretroviral (elvitegravir; EVG), a pharmacokinetic enhancer (cobicistat; c), an HIV nucleoside reverse transcriptase inhibitor (NRTI) antiretroviral (emtricitabine; FTC), and a nucleotide reverse transcriptase inhibitor antiretroviral classified as an HIV NRTI (tenofovir disoproxil fumarate; tenofovir DF; TDF). Cobicistat, a potent cytochrome P-450 (CYP) 3A inhibitor, is included in the fixed combination to increase plasma concentrations of elvitegravir (*cobicistat-boosted* elvitegravir).

Elvitegravir inhibits the activity of HIV-1 integrase, an enzyme that integrates HIV DNA into the host cell genome. Integration is required for maintenance of the viral genome and for efficient viral gene expression and replication. Inhibition of integration prevents propagation of viral infection. Elvitegravir is active against HIV-1 and also has some in vitro activity against HIV type 2 (HIV-2); the drug does not have activity against hepatitis B virus (HBV) or hepatitis C virus (HCV).

Cobicistat is a mechanism-based inhibitor of CYP3A and decreases metabolism and increases plasma concentrations of CYP3A substrates; cobicistat also is a weak inhibitor of CYP2D6, but does not inhibit CYP1A2, 2C9, or 2C19. Cobicistat is included in EVG/c/FTC/TDF for therapeutic advantage and acts as a pharmacokinetic enhancer to decrease elvitegravir metabolism and increase plasma concentrations of the drug, resulting in trough concentrations of elvitegravir sufficient to allow for once-daily dosing (*cobicistat-boosted* elvitegravir). Cobicistat does not have any antiretroviral or antiviral activity and is not active against HIV-1, HBV, or HCV; cobicistat does not antagonize the antiretroviral activity of elvitegravir, emtricitabine, or tenofovir.

Emtricitabine is a prodrug and is inactive until converted intracellularly to an active 5′-triphosphate metabolite. After conversion to the pharmacologically active metabolite, the drug acts as a reverse transcriptase inhibitor antiretroviral. Emtricitabine is active against HIV-1 and also has some in vitro activity against HIV-2.

Tenofovir DF is a tenofovir prodrug and is inactive until it undergoes diester hydrolysis in vivo to tenofovir and is subsequently metabolized to the active metabolite (tenofovir diphosphate). After conversion to the pharmacologically active metabolite, the drug act as a reverse transcriptase inhibitor antiretroviral. Tenofovir is active against HIV-1 and also has some in vitro activity against HIV-2; the drug also is active against HBV.

HIV-1 resistant to elvitegravir, emtricitabine, or tenofovir have been produced in vitro and have emerged during EVG/c/FTC/TDF therapy. In clinical trials evaluating EVG/c/FTC/TDF in antiretroviral-naive patients, 1 or more primary mutations associated with resistance to elvitegravir, emtricitabine, and/or tenofovir were identified in HIV-1 isolates from 51% of patients who received EVG/c/FTC/TDF and were considered to be virologic treatment failures. Cross-resistance between elvitegravir and other HIV INSTIs (e.g., dolutegravir, raltegravir) has been reported. Cross-resistance also occurs among the HIV NRTIs.

Following an oral dose of EVG/c/FTC/TDF given with food, peak plasma concentrations of elvitegravir and cobicistat occur at 4 and 3 hours, respectively, and peak plasma concentrations of emtricitabine and tenofovir occur at 3 and 2 hours, respectively. Administration of EVG/c/FTC/TDF with a high-fat meal (approximately 800 kcal, 50% fat) increases mean systemic exposures of elvitegravir and tenofovir by 87 and 23%, respectively, compared with administration in the fasting state; mean systemic exposures of cobicistat and emtricitabine are decreased by 17 and 4%, respectively, compared with administration in the fasting state. Elvitegravir is approximately 99% and cobicistat is approximately 98% bound to plasma proteins; emtricitabine is less than 4% and tenofovir is less than 1% bound to plasma proteins. Elvitegravir is metabolized principally by CYP3A isoenzymes, but also undergoes glucuronidation via uridine diphosphate-glucuronosyltransferase (UGT) 1A1/3 enzymes. Cobicistat is metabolized by CYP3A and to a minor extent by CYP2D6. Although the cobicistat component of EVG/c/FTC/TDF acts as a pharmacokinetic enhancer for elvitegravir, cobicistat does not have any clinically important effects on the pharmacokinetics of emtricitabine or tenofovir DF. Elvitegravir and cobicistat are principally excreted in feces (94.8 and 86.2% of a dose, respectively) and to a lesser extent in urine (6.7 and 8.2% of a dose, respectively). Emtricitabine is principally excreted in urine (70% of a dose) and to a lesser extent in feces (13.7% of a dose); approximately 70–80% of a dose of TDF is excreted in urine. The median terminal plasma half-lives of elvitegravir, cobicistat, emtricitabine, and tenofovir are 12.9, 3.5, 10, and 12–18 hours, respectively.

Advice to Patients

Critical nature of compliance with HIV therapy and importance of remaining under the care of a clinician. Importance of taking as prescribed; do not alter or discontinue antiretroviral regimen without consulting clinician.

Antiretroviral therapy is not a cure for HIV infection; opportunistic infections and other complications associated with HIV disease may still occur.

Advise patients that sustained decreases in plasma HIV RNA have been associated with reduced risk of progression to acquired immunodeficiency syndrome (AIDS) and death.

Advise patients that effective antiretroviral regimens can decrease HIV concentrations in blood and genital secretions and strict adherence to such regimens in conjunction with risk-reduction measures may decrease, but cannot absolutely eliminate, the risk of secondary transmission of HIV to others. Importance of continuing to practice safer sex (e.g., using latex or polyurethane condoms to minimize sexual contact with body fluids), never sharing personal items that can have blood or body fluids on them (e.g., toothbrushes, razor blades), and never reusing or sharing needles.

Importance of reading patient information provided by the manufacturer.

Advise patients that the fixed combination of elvitegravir, cobicistat, emtricitabine, and tenofovir disoproxil fumarate (tenofovir DF) (EVG/c/FTC/TDF) is a complete regimen for treatment of HIV-1 infection and should *not* be used in conjunction with other antiretroviral agents.

Importance of taking EVG/c/FTC/TDF with food.

If a dose is missed, the dose should be taken as soon as it is remembered and the next dose taken at the regularly scheduled time. If a dose is skipped, a double dose should not be taken to make up for the missed dose.

Inform patients that testing for hepatitis B virus (HBV) infection is recommended before antiretroviral therapy is initiated. Also advise patients that severe acute exacerbations of HBV infection have been reported following discontinuance of emtricitabine or tenofovir DF in HIV-infected patients coinfected with HBV.

Advise patients that renal impairment, including cases of acute renal failure or Fanconi syndrome, has occurred. Importance of not using EVG/c/FTC/TDF concomitantly with or shortly after nephrotoxic agents (e.g., high-dose or multiple nonsteroidal anti-inflammatory agents [NSAIAs]).

Advise patients that lactic acidosis and severe hepatomegaly with steatosis, including fatalities, have occurred with emtricitabine and tenofovir (components of EVG/c/FTC/TDF). Importance of contacting clinician if symptoms suggestive of lactic acidosis or hepatotoxicity (e.g., nausea, vomiting, unusual/unexpected stomach discomfort, weakness) occur.

Advise patients that decreased bone mineral density (BMD) has occurred and that assessment of BMD should be considered in those with a history of pathologic bone fracture or other risk factors for osteoporosis or bone loss.

Advise patients that signs and symptoms of inflammation from previous infections may occur soon after initiation of antiretroviral therapy in some individuals with advanced HIV infection (AIDS). These symptoms may be due to an improvement in immune response, enabling the body to fight infections that may have been present with no obvious symptoms. Importance of immediately informing a healthcare provider if any symptoms of infection occur.

Importance of informing clinicians of existing or contemplated concomitant therapy, including prescription and OTC drugs and herbal products (e.g., St. John's wort), as well as any concomitant illnesses.

Importance of women informing clinicians if they are or plan to become pregnant or plan to breast-feed. Advise HIV-infected women not to breast-feed.

Importance of informing patients of other important precautionary information. (See Cautions.)

Overview® (see Users Guide). For additional information on this drug until a more detailed monograph is developed and published, the manufacturer's labeling should be consulted. It is *essential* that the manufacturer's labeling be consulted for more detailed information on usual cautions, precautions, contraindications, potential drug interactions, laboratory test interferences, and acute toxicity.

Preparations

Excipients in commercially available drug preparations may have clinically important effects in some individuals; consult specific product labeling for details.

Elvitegravir, Cobicistat, Emtricitabine, and Tenofovir Disoproxil Fumarate

Oral		
Tablets, film-coated	Elvitegravir 150 mg, Cobicistat 150 mg, Emtricitabine 200 mg, and Tenofovir Disoproxil Fumarate 300 mg	**Stribild®**, Gilead

†Use is not currently included in the labeling approved by the US Food and Drug Administration

Raltegravir Potassium

RAL, lamivudine/raltegravir, 3TC/RAL

■ Raltegravir potassium, an antiretroviral agent, is a human immunodeficiency virus (HIV) integrase strand transfer inhibitor (INSTI).

Uses

■ **Treatment of HIV Infection** Raltegravir potassium is used in conjunction with other antiretroviral agents for the treatment of human immunodeficiency virus type 1 (HIV-1) infection in antiretroviral-naive (have not previously received antiretroviral therapy) or antiretroviral-experienced (previously treated) adults, adolescents, and children 4 weeks of age or older.

Raltegravir usually is used in HIV integrase strand transfer inhibitor-based (INSTI-based) regimens that include raltegravir and 2 HIV nucleoside reverse transcriptase inhibitors (dual NRTIs).

If an INSTI-based regimen containing raltegravir, lamivudine, and other antiretrovirals is used for the treatment of HIV-1 infection, a fixed-combination preparation containing lamivudine and raltegravir (lamivudine/raltegravir; Dutrebis®) is commercially available and can be used in adults, adolescents, and pediatric patients 6 years of age or older weighing at least 30 kg to decrease pill burden and improve adherence. Lamivudine/raltegravir must be used in conjunction with other antiretrovirals.

The most appropriate antiretroviral regimen cannot be defined for each clinical scenario, and selection of specific antiretroviral agents for use in multiple-drug regimens should be individualized based on information regarding antiretroviral potency, potential rate of development of resistance, known toxicities, and potential for pharmacokinetic interactions as well as virologic, immunologic, and clinical characteristics of the patient. For information on the general principles and guidelines for use of antiretroviral therapy, including specific recommendations for initial therapy in antiretroviral-naive patients and recommendations for changing antiretroviral regimens, see the Antiretroviral Agents General Statement 8:18.08.

Antiretroviral-naive Adults and Adolescents For *initial* treatment in HIV-infected adults and adolescents, the US Department of Health and Human Services (HHS) Panel on Antiretroviral Guidelines for Adults and Adolescents states that raltegravir in conjunction with tenofovir alafenamide and emtricitabine or raltegravir in conjunction with tenofovir disoproxil fumarate (tenofovir DF) and emtricitabine (or lamivudine) are recommended INSTI-based regimens. These experts also state that raltegravir in conjunction with abacavir and lamivudine (or emtricitabine) is an INSTI-based regimen option for *initial* treatment in antiretroviral-naive adults and adolescents when recommended or alternative regimens cannot be used, but should be used *only* in patients who are negative for human leukocyte antigen (HLA)-B*5701. Raltegravir (twice daily) in conjunction with *ritonavir-boosted* darunavir is another option that can be considered for *initial* treatment in antiretroviral-naive adults and adolescents when recommended or alternative regimens cannot be used, but should be used *only* when tenofovir alafenamide, tenofovir DF, or abacavir cannot be used.

Clinical Experience. The comparative safety and efficacy of raltegravir and efavirenz have been evaluated in a phase 3, randomized, active-control study in antiretroviral-naive HIV-infected adults (STARTMRK [protocol 021]). All patients had baseline HIV-1 RNA levels greater than 5000 copies/mL and were randomized to receive raltegravir 400 mg twice daily or efavirenz 600 mg once daily in conjunction with tenofovir DF and emtricitabine. Patients enrolled in this study were adults 18 years of age or older (mean age 37–38 years, 81–82% male, 41–44% white, 8–12% black, 11–13% Asian, 21–24% Hispanic, median baseline plasma HIV-1 RNA level 5 $\log_{10}$ copies/mL, median baseline $CD4^+$ T-cell count 204–212 cells/mm^3). At 240 weeks, 66% of those receiving raltegravir had plasma HIV-1 RNA levels less than 50 copies/mL compared with 60% of those receiving efavirenz. The mean change in $CD4^+$ T-cell count from baseline was 295 cells/mm^3 in those receiving raltegravir compared with 236 cells/mm^3 in those receiving efavirenz.

In a double-blind, randomized study in antiretroviral-naive adults, a regimen of raltegravir, tenofovir DF, and lamivudine was as effective as a regimen of efavirenz, tenofovir DF, and lamivudine (based on decrease in plasma HIV-1 RNA levels). At 96 weeks, 83% in the raltegravir group and 84% in the efavirenz group had plasma HIV-1 RNA concentrations less than 50 copies/mL and both groups had similar increases in $CD4^+$ T-cell count (221 and 232 cells/mm^3, respectively).

The manufacturer of lamivudine/raltegravir states that the fixed combination has not been evaluated in clinical trials; safety and efficacy of the fixed combination are based on clinical trials that evaluated single-entity lamivudine and single-entity raltegravir. In addition, pharmacokinetic data indicate that a single dose of the fixed combination (150 mg of lamivudine and 300 mg of raltegravir) results in lamivudine and raltegravir exposures comparable to those attained when single-entity lamivudine (150 mg) is administered concomitantly with single-entity raltegravir (400 mg).

Antiretroviral-experienced Adults **Clinical Experience.** Raltegravir has been evaluated in 2 phase 3, randomized, double-blind, placebo-controlled, multicenter studies (BENCHMRK 1 [protocol 018], BENCHMRK 2 [protocol 019]) in antiretroviral-experienced adults with documented resistance to at least one nucleoside reverse transcriptase inhibitor (NRTI), nonnucleoside reverse transcriptase inhibitor (NNRTI), and HIV protease inhibitor (PI). Patients enrolled in these studies were adults 16 years of age or older (mean age 45 years, 88–89% male, 65–73% white, 11–14% black, 3% Asian, 8–11% Hispanic, median baseline plasma HIV-1 RNA level 4.7–4.8 $\log_{10}$ copies/mL, median baseline $CD4^+$ T-cell count 119–123 cells/mm^3) who had previously received multiple antiretroviral drugs (median number of previous antiretrovirals was 12) for a median duration of 10 years. All patients received an optimized background antiretroviral regimen (OBR; selected on the basis of the individual's prior antiretroviral treatment and results of genotypic/phenotypic viral resistance testing; median number of drugs in the OBR was 4). A total of 699 patients were randomized to receive raltegravir 400 mg twice daily or placebo in conjunction with an OBR; random assignment was stratified by degree of resistance to PIs at study entry (i.e., resistant to one PI or more than one PI [95–97% were resistant to more than one PI]) and use of enfuvirtide in the OBR (38% received enfuvirtide). At 96 weeks, pooled analysis of these 699 patients indicated that 55% of those randomized to raltegravir in conjunction with an OBR had plasma HIV-1 RNA levels less than 50 copies/mL compared with 27% of those randomized to placebo and an OBR; the mean increase in $CD4^+$ T-cell count was 118 and 47 cells/mm^3, respectively. At 156 weeks (after completion of the double-blind treatment period), 251 patients from the raltegravir group and 47 patients from the placebo group received open-label treatment with raltegravir 400 mg twice daily in conjunction with an OBR. At 240 weeks (after 84 weeks of open-label treatment), 77% of patients originally enrolled in the raltegravir group had plasma HIV-1 RNA levels less than 50 copies/mL compared with 81% of patients originally enrolled in the placebo group; the mean increase in $CD4^+$ T-cell count from baseline was 293 and 267 cells/mm^3, respectively.

Two phase 3 studies designed to evaluate the use of raltegravir and 2 NRTIs in patients who had been receiving a suppressive regimen of the fixed combination of lopinavir and ritonavir (lopinavir/ritonavir) and 2 NRTIs were terminated early based on 24-week data that failed to demonstrate non-inferiority of switching to raltegravir versus continuing the lopinavir/ritonavir regimen (SWITCHMRK 1 and 2). In these studies, a total of 352 HIV-1-infected patients who had been receiving a regimen of lopinavir/ritonavir and at least 2 NRTIs for longer than 3 months and had plasma HIV-1 RNA levels less than 50 copies/mL were randomized to either continue the lopinavir/ritonavir regimen or be switched to raltegravir (400 mg twice daily) with the NRTIs. At 24 weeks, combined analysis of the studies indicated that plasma HIV-1 RNA levels less than 50 copies/mL were maintained in 90% of those who continued the lopinavir/ritonavir regimen compared with 82% of those who were switched to the raltegravir regimen.

Pediatric Patients Raltegravir is used in conjunction with other antiretrovirals for the treatment of HIV-1 infection in pediatric patients 4 weeks of age or older.

Lamivudine/raltegravir is used in conjunction with other antiretrovirals for the treatment of HIV-1 infection in pediatric patients 6 years of age or older weighing at least 30 kg.

For *initial* treatment in HIV-infected pediatric patients, the HHS Panel on Antiretroviral Therapy and Medical Management of HIV-infected Children usually recommends a regimen that includes a *ritonavir-boosted* PI, NNRTI, or INSTI in conjunction with 2 NRTIs (dual NRTIs). These experts state that an INSTI-based regimen of raltegravir and 2 NRTIs is a preferred regimen for *initial* therapy in antiretroviral-naive pediatric patients 2–12 years of age. Although data are limited, these experts also state that an INSTI-based regimen of raltegravir in conjunction with 2 NRTIs can be used as an alternative regimen for *initial* therapy in antiretroviral-naive infants and children 4 weeks to less than 2 years of age weighing at least 3 kg.

For further information on treatment of HIV infection in pediatric patients, see Antiretroviral Therapy in Pediatric Patients, in Guidelines for Use of Antiretroviral Agents in the Antiretroviral Agents General Statement 8:18.08.

Clinical Experience. Safety and efficacy of raltegravir in conjunction with other antiretrovirals in pediatric patients have been evaluated in a phase 1/phase 2 open-label study (IMPAACT P1066) that included 126 antiretroviral-experienced HIV-infected children and adolescents 2–18 years of age. These pediatric patients were enrolled into the following cohorts based on age and received raltegravir in conjunction with an OBR: cohort I (12 to less than 18 years of age; 400 mg film-coated tablets), cohort IIa (6 to less than 12 years of age; 400 mg film-coated tablets), cohort IIb (6 to less than 12 years old; chewable tablets), and cohort III (2 to less than 6 years of age; chewable tablets). In the initial dose-finding stage, raltegravir dosage was selected to achieve raltegravir plasma exposures and trough concentrations similar to those reported in adults and acceptable short-term safety. After dose selection, additional patients were enrolled for evaluation of long-term safety, tolerability, and efficacy. Of the initial 126 patients in cohorts I, IIa, IIb, and III, 96 received the recommended dosage of raltegravir (median age 13 years, 51% female, 34% Caucasian, 59% black, mean baseline plasma HIV-1 RNA level 4.3 $\log_{10}$ copies/mL, median baseline $CD4^+$ T-cell count 481 cells/mm^3, median CD4 percentage 23%). A total of 93 of these patients completed 24 weeks of treatment and 91 completed 48 weeks of treatment. At week 24, 66 and 54% had achieved plasma HIV-1 RNA levels less than 400 and 50 copies/mL, respectively; the mean increase in $CD4^+$ T-cell count from baseline was 119 cells/mm^3, and the mean increase in $CD4^+$ T-cell percentage from baseline was 3.8%. At week 48, 74 and 57% had achieved plasma HIV-1 RNA levels less than 400 and 50 copies/mL, respectively; the mean increase in $CD4^+$ T-cell count from baseline was 156 cells/mm^3, and the mean increase in $CD4^+$ T-cell percentage from baseline was 4.6%.

IMPAACT P1066 also evaluated the safety and efficacy of raltegravir oral suspension in conjunction with an OBR in infants 4 weeks to less than 2 years of age (cohorts IV and V). The 26 infants enrolled in cohorts IV and V (median age 28 weeks, 35% female, 8% Caucasian, 85% black, mean baseline plasma HIV-1 RNA level 5.7 $\log_{10}$ copies/mL, median baseline CD4+ T-cell count 1400 cells/mm^3, median CD4 percentage 18.6%) had previously received antiretroviral therapy as prophylaxis for prevention of perinatal HIV transmission and/or as combination antiretroviral therapy for treatment of HIV infection. Of the 26 infants, 23 were included in the 24-week and 48-week efficacy analyses. At week 24, 61 and 39% had achieved plasma HIV-1 RNA levels less than 400 and 50 copies/mL, respectively; the mean increase in CD4+ T-cell count from baseline was 500 cells/mm^3, and the mean increase in CD4+ T-cell percentage from baseline was 7.5%. At week 48, 61 and 44% had achieved plasma HIV-1 RNA levels less than 400 and 50 copies/mL, respectively; the mean increase in CD4+ T-cell count from baseline was 492 cells/mm^3, and the mean increase in CD4+ T-cell percentage from baseline was 7.8%.

■ **Postexposure Prophylaxis following Occupational Exposure to HIV** Raltegravir is used in conjunction with 2 NRTIs for postexposure prophylaxis of HIV infection following occupational exposure† (PEP) in health-care personnel and other individuals exposed via percutaneous injury (e.g., needlestick, cut with sharp object) or mucous membrane or nonintact skin (e.g., chapped, abraded, dermatitis) contact with blood, tissue, or other body fluids that might contain HIV.

The US Public Health Service (USPHS) states that the preferred regimen for PEP following an occupational exposure to HIV is a 3-drug regimen of raltegravir used in conjunction with emtricitabine and tenofovir DF (may be administered as the fixed combination emtricitabine/tenofovir DF; Truvada®). Alternative dual NRTIs recommended for use with raltegravir for PEP are tenofovir DF and lamivudine, zidovudine and lamivudine (may be administered as the fixed combination lamivudine/zidovudine; Combivir®), or zidovudine and emtricitabine.

Because management of occupational exposures to HIV is complex and evolving, consultation with an infectious disease specialist, clinician with expertise in administration of antiretrovirals, and/or the National Clinicians' Postexposure Prophylaxis Hotline (PEPline at 888-448-4911) is recommended whenever possible. However, initiation of PEP should not be delayed while waiting for expert consultation.

For information on types of occupational exposure to HIV and associated risk of infection, management of occupational exposure to HIV, efficacy and safety of postexposure prophylaxis, and recommendations regarding PEP, see Guidelines for Use of Antiretroviral Agents: Antiretrovirals for Postexposure Prophylaxis (PEP) following Occupational Exposure to HIV, in the Antiretroviral Agents General Statement 8:18.08.

■ **Postexposure Prophylaxis following Nonoccupational Exposure to HIV** Raltegravir is used in conjunction with other antiretrovirals for postexposure prophylaxis of HIV infection following nonoccupational exposure† (nPEP) in individuals exposed to blood, genital secretions, or other potentially infectious body fluids that might contain HIV when the exposure represents a substantial risk for HIV transmission.

When nPEP is indicated following a nonoccupational exposure to HIV, the US Centers for Disease Control and Prevention (CDC) states that the preferred regimen in adults and adolescents 13 years of age or older with normal renal function is either raltegravir or dolutegravir used in conjunction with emtricitabine and tenofovir DF (administered as emtricitabine/tenofovir DF; Truvada®); the recommended alternative nPEP regimen in these patients is *ritonavir-boosted* darunavir used in conjunction with emtricitabine/tenofovir DF (Truvada®).

Consultation with an infectious disease specialist, clinician with expertise in administration of antiretroviral agents, and/or the National Clinicians' Postexposure Prophylaxis Hotline (PEPline at 888-448-4911) is recommended if nPEP is indicated in certain exposed individuals (e.g., pregnant women, children, those with medical conditions such as renal impairment) or if an antiretroviral regimen not included in the CDC guidelines is being considered, the source virus is known or likely to be resistant to antiretrovirals, or the healthcare provider is inexperienced in prescribing antiretrovirals. However, initiation of nPEP should not be delayed while waiting for expert consultation.

For additional information on nonoccupational exposure to HIV and recommendations regarding postexposure prophylaxis, see Guidelines for Use of Antiretroviral Agents: Antiretrovirals for Postexposure Prophylaxis following Sexual, Injection Drug Use, or other Nonoccupational Exposures to HIV (nPEP), in the Antiretroviral Agents General Statement 8:18.08.

Dosage and Administration

■ **Administration** Raltegravir potassium is administered orally twice daily without regard to food.

Single-entity raltegravir (Isentress®) is commercially available as chewable tablets, film-coated tablets, and oral suspension. Raltegravir also is commercially available in fixed-combination, film-coated tablets containing lamivudine and raltegravir (lamivudine/raltegravir; Dutrebis®). (See Fixed Combinations Containing Raltegravir under Dosage and Administration: Administration.)

Raltegravir is used in conjunction with other antiretrovirals.

Chewable Tablets Raltegravir chewable tablets may be chewed or swallowed whole. If necessary, the 100-mg chewable tablet can be divided into equal halves.

The chewable tablets are used in pediatric patients weighing at least 11 kg to less than 25 kg. The chewable tablets also may be used as an alternative in pediatric patients weighing 25 kg or more who are not able to swallow the film-coated tablets. (See Table 2.)

When the chewable tablets are used, the maximum dosage is 300 mg twice daily.

Film-coated Tablets Raltegravir film-coated tablets must be swallowed whole. The film-coated tablets are used in adults and pediatric patients weighing at least 25 kg.

Oral Suspension Raltegravir powder for oral suspension is provided in single-use packets containing 100 mg of raltegravir. Immediately prior to use, the powder contained in a single-use packet must be suspended in 5 mL of water to provide a suspension containing 20 mg/mL. The appropriate dosage of the oral suspension should then be administered orally using the dosing syringe provided by the manufacturer.

To prepare the oral suspension, the dosing syringe provided by the manufacturer should be used to measure and add 5 mL of water to the mixing cup provided by the manufacturer. The entire contents of a single-use packet of raltegravir for oral suspension should then be poured into the mixing cup; the mixing cup should then be closed tightly and gently swirled for 30–60 seconds. The oral suspension will appear cloudy. The recommended dosage of the oral suspension should be drawn into the dosing syringe and administered orally. After each use, the dosing syringe and mixing cup should be handwashed with warm water and dish soap, rinsed with water, and air dried.

Raltegravir oral suspension is used in pediatric patients 4 weeks of age and older weighing at least 3 kg and less than 20 kg. When the oral suspension is used, the maximum dosage is 100 mg twice daily.

Single-use packets of raltegravir powder for oral suspension should be stored at 20–25°C. The foil packets should not be opened until ready to use. After the contents of the packet are suspended in water, the oral suspension should be used within 30 minutes and any unused portion should be discarded.

Fixed Combinations Containing Raltegravir Lamivudine/raltegravir film-coated tablets are administered orally twice daily without regard to food.

Lamivudine/raltegravir film-coated tablets are used in adults and pediatric patients 6 years of age or older weighing at least 30 kg.

Lamivudine/raltegravir must be used in conjunction with other antiretrovirals.

Because the antiretrovirals contained in lamivudine/raltegravir may also be available in single-entity or other fixed-combination preparations, care should be taken to ensure that lamivudine/raltegravir is not used concomitantly with other preparations containing lamivudine, raltegravir, or emtricitabine. (See Precautions Related to Use of Fixed Combinations under Cautions: Precautions and Contraindications.)

■ **Dosage** Single-entity raltegravir (Isentress®) chewable tablets, film-coated tablets, and powder for oral suspension contain raltegravir potassium; dosage is expressed in terms of raltegravir.

Lamivudine/raltegravir (Dutrebis®) film-coated tablets contain raltegravir potassium and lamivudine; dosage of the raltegravir component is expressed in terms of raltegravir.

Single-entity raltegravir chewable tablets and oral suspension are *not* bioequivalent to single-entity raltegravir film-coated tablets. The chewable tablets or oral suspension should *not* be substituted for the 400-mg film-coated tablets.

A film-coated tablet of lamivudine/raltegravir containing 150 mg of lamivudine and 300 mg of raltegravir provides lamivudine and raltegravir exposures comparable to those attained when a 150-mg lamivudine tablet is administered concomitantly with a 400-mg raltegravir tablet. Because bioavailability of the raltegravir formulation contained in lamivudine/raltegravir is higher than that of the raltegravir formulation contained in the single-entity preparation, the 300-mg raltegravir dose in lamivudine/raltegravir provides raltegravir exposures comparable to those provided by a 400-mg dose of single-entity raltegravir.

Adult Dosage **Treatment of HIV Infection.** For the treatment of human immunodeficiency virus type 1 (HIV-1) infection in adults, the usual dosage of raltegravir (Isentress®) film-coated tablets is 400 mg twice daily (one 400-mg film-coated tablet twice daily).

When lamivudine/raltegravir (Dutrebis®) is used for the treatment of HIV-1 infection in adults, the usual dosage is 1 tablet (150 mg of lamivudine and 300 mg of raltegravir) twice daily. The maximum dosage of the fixed combination is 1 tablet (150 mg of lamivudine and 300 mg of raltegravir) twice daily.

Postexposure Prophylaxis following Occupational Exposure to HIV. For postexposure prophylaxis of HIV infection following occupational exposure† (PEP) in health-care personnel or other individuals, the recommended dosage of raltegravir (Isentress®) is 400 mg twice daily. Raltegravir usually is used in conjunction with emtricitabine and tenofovir disoproxil fumarate (tenofovir DF). (See Uses: Postexposure Prophylaxis following Occupational Exposure to HIV.)

PEP should be initiated as soon as possible following occupational exposure to HIV (preferably within hours) and continued for 4 weeks, if tolerated.

Postexposure Prophylaxis following Nonoccupational Exposure to HIV. For postexposure prophylaxis of HIV infection following nonoccupational exposure† (nPEP) when the exposure represents a substantial risk for HIV transmission, the usual adult dosage of raltegravir is 400 mg twice daily in conjunction with 2 HIV nucleoside reverse transcriptase inhibitors (NRTIs). (See Uses: Postexposure Prophylaxis following Nonoccupational Exposure to HIV.)

The nPEP regimen should be initiated as soon as possible (within 72 hours) following nonoccupational exposure to HIV and continued for 28 days. If the exposed individual seeks care more than 72 hours after the exposure, nPEP is not recommended.

Pediatric Dosage **Treatment of HIV Infection.** For the treatment of HIV-1 infection, infants and children 4 weeks of age or older weighing at least 3 kg to less than 11 kg should receive raltegravir (Isentress®) oral suspension in a dosage based on weight. (See Table 1.)

Pediatric patients weighing at least 11 kg to less than 20 kg may receive raltegravir oral suspension or raltegravir chewable tablets in a dosage based on weight. Those weighing at least 20 kg to less than 25 kg should receiving the chewable tablets in a dosage based on weight. (See Table 1.)

Table 1. Dosage of Raltegravir (Isentress® Oral Suspension or Chewable Tablets) in Pediatric Patients 4 Weeks of Age or Older Weighing at Least 3 kg to Less Than 25 kg

Body Weight (kg)	Dosage of Oral Suspension Containing 20 mg/mL	Dosage of Chewable Tablets
3 to <4	20 mg (1 mL) twice daily	Do not use
4 to <6	30 mg (1.5 mL) twice daily	Do not use
6 to <8	40 mg (2 mL) twice daily	Do not use
8 to <11	60 mg (3 mL) twice daily	Do not use
11 to <14	80 mg (4 mL) twice daily	75 mg twice daily (three 25-mg tablets twice daily)
14 to <20	100 mg (5 mL) twice daily	100 mg twice daily (one 100-mg tablet twice daily)
20 to <25	Do not use	150 mg twice daily (one and one-half 100-mg tablets twice daily)

For the treatment of HIV-1 infection, children and adolescents weighing at least 25 kg should receive raltegravir film-coated tablets in a dosage of 400 mg twice daily (one 400-mg film-coated tablet twice daily). Alternatively, those weighing at least 25 kg who are unable to swallow the film-coated tablets may receive the chewable tablets in a dosage based on weight. (See Table 2.)

Table 2. Alternative Dosage of Raltegravir (Isentress® Chewable Tablets) in Pediatric Patients Weighing at Least 25 kg and Unable to Swallow Film-coated Tablets

Body Weight (kg)	Dosage	Number of Chewable Tablets
25 to <28	150 mg twice daily	One and one-half 100-mg tablets twice daily
28 to <40	200 mg twice daily	Two 100-mg tablets twice daily
≥40	300 mg twice daily	Three 100-mg tablets twice daily

Weight-based dosage recommendations for raltegravir oral suspension and chewable tablets are based on a dosage of approximately 6 mg/kg twice daily. The maximum dosage of the oral suspension is 100 mg twice daily; the maximum dosage of the chewable tablet is 300 mg twice daily.

When lamivudine/raltegravir (Dutrebis®) is used for the treatment of HIV-1 infection in children 6 years of age or older weighing at least 30 kg or adolescents 16 years of age or older, the usual dosage is 1 tablet (150 mg of lamivudine and 300 mg of raltegravir) twice daily. The maximum dosage of the fixed combination is 1 tablet (150 mg of lamivudine and 300 mg of raltegravir) twice daily.

■ **Special Populations** ***Hepatic Impairment*** Dosage adjustment of raltegravir (Isentress®) is not needed in patients with mild to moderate hepatic impairment. Pharmacokinetics of raltegravir have not been studied in those with severe hepatic impairment.

Dosage adjustment of lamivudine/raltegravir (Dutrebis®) is not needed in patients with mild to moderate hepatic impairment. Safety and efficacy of the fixed combination have not been established in those with decompensated liver disease.

Renal Impairment Dosage adjustment of raltegravir (Isentress®) is not needed in patients with renal impairment. Because it is not known whether raltegravir is dialyzable, administering the drug before a dialysis session should be avoided.

Lamivudine/raltegravir (Dutrebis®) has not been evaluated in patients with renal impairment. The fixed combination should not be used in patients with creatinine clearances less than 50 mL/minute since reduction in lamivudine dosage is needed in such patients. (See Renal Impairment under Warnings/Precautions: Specific Populations, in Cautions.)

Geriatric Patients The manufacturer makes no specific dosage recommendations for raltegravir in geriatric patients, but recommends careful dosage selection because of possible age-related decreases in hepatic, renal, and/or cardiac function and concomitant disease and drug therapy. (See Geriatric Use under Warnings/Precautions: Specific Populations, in Cautions.)

Cautions

■ **Contraindications** The manufacturer of raltegravir (Isentress®) states that there are no known contraindications to use of the drug.

The fixed combination containing lamivudine and raltegravir (lamivudine/raltegravir; Dutrebis®) is contraindicated in patients with hypersensitivity to lamivudine, raltegravir, or any component of the fixed combination. When lamivudine/raltegravir is used, the contraindications associated with both drugs in the fixed combination should be considered. (See Precautions Related to Use of Fixed Combinations under Cautions: Warnings/Precautions.)

■ **Warnings/Precautions** ***Sensitivity Reactions*** **Severe Skin and Hypersensitivity Reactions.** Severe, potentially life-threatening skin reactions have been reported, including some fatalities. Stevens-Johnson syndrome, toxic epidermal necrolysis, and hypersensitivity reactions characterized by rash, constitutional findings, and organ dysfunction (including hepatic failure) have occurred.

Raltegravir, lamivudine/raltegravir, and any other suspect agents should be discontinued immediately if signs or symptoms of severe skin or hypersensitivity reactions occur, including (but not limited to) severe rash or rash accompanied by fever, general malaise, fatigue, muscle or joint aches, blisters, oral lesions, conjunctivitis, facial edema, hepatitis, eosinophilia, or angioedema. Clinical status, including liver aminotransferases, should be monitored and appropriate therapy initiated.

A life-threatening reaction could occur if there is a delay in discontinuing raltegravir, lamivudine/raltegravir, and any other suspect agents after the onset of severe rash.

■ **Phenylketonuria** Individuals with phenylketonuria (i.e., homozygous genetic deficiency of phenylalanine hydroxylase) and other individuals who must restrict their intake of phenylalanine should be advised that raltegravir (Isentress®) chewable tablets contain aspartame (NutraSweet®), which is metabolized in the GI tract to phenylalanine.

Each 25- or 100-mg raltegravir (Isentress®) chewable tablet provides approximately 0.05 or 0.1 mg of phenylalanine, respectively.

■ **Interactions** Concomitant use of raltegravir or lamivudine/raltegravir with drugs that are potent inducers of uridine diphosphate-glucuronosyltransferase (UGT) 1A1 (e.g., rifampin) may result in decreased plasma concentrations of raltegravir. (See Rifampin under Drug Interactions: Antimycobacterial Agents.)

■ **Musculoskeletal Effects** Increased serum creatine kinase (CK, creatine phosphokinase, CPK) concentrations, myopathy, and rhabdomyolysis have been reported in patients receiving raltegravir.

Raltegravir and lamivudine/raltegravir should be used with caution in patients at increased risk of myopathy or rhabdomyolysis including those receiving concomitant therapy with drugs known to cause myopathy or rhabdomyolysis (e.g., hydroxymethylglutaryl-CoA [HMG-CoA] reductase inhibitors [statins], fenofibrate, gemfibrozil, zidovudine) and those with a history of rhabdomyolysis, myopathy, or increased serum CK concentrations. Such patients should be closely monitored.

■ **Individuals with Hepatitis B Virus or Hepatitis C Virus Infection** Although the safety profile of raltegravir in patients with human immunodeficiency virus (HIV) infection and with hepatitis B virus (HBV) or hepatitis C virus (HCV) coinfection is similar to that in HIV-infected patients without HBV or HCV coinfection, increased AST and ALT concentrations were reported more frequently in coinfected patients.

If lamivudine/raltegravir is used in HIV-infected patients coinfected with HBV or HCV, clinicians should consider that additional precautions apply to these coinfected patients. (See Precautions Related to Use of Fixed Combinations under Cautions: Warnings/Precautions.)

■ **Precautions Related to Use of Fixed Combinations** When lamivudine/raltegravir is used, the cautions, precautions, contraindications, and drug interactions associated with both drugs in the fixed combination must be considered. Cautionary information applicable to specific populations (e.g., pregnant or nursing women, individuals with hepatic or renal impairment, geriatric patients) should be considered for each drug. For cautionary information related to lamivudine, see Cautions in Lamivudine 8:18.08.20.

Because the antiretrovirals contained in lamivudine/raltegravir may also be available in single-entity or other fixed-combination preparations, care should be taken to ensure that therapy is not duplicated when the fixed combination is used in conjunction with other antiretrovirals.

Lamivudine/raltegravir should not be used concomitantly with any preparation containing lamivudine, raltegravir, or emtricitabine.

If lamivudine/raltegravir is used, clinicians should consider that lactic acidosis and severe hepatomegaly with steatosis, including fatalities, have been reported in patients receiving HIV nucleoside reverse transcriptase inhibitors (NRTIs) alone or in conjunction with other antiretrovirals. Lamivudine/raltegravir should be discontinued in patients with clinical or laboratory findings suggestive of lactic acidosis or pronounced hepatotoxicity, which may include hepatomegaly and steatosis even in the absence of marked increases in serum aminotransferase concentrations.

If lamivudine/raltegravir is used in HIV-infected patients coinfected with HBV, clinicians should consider that severe, acute exacerbations of HBV infection have been reported following discontinuance of lamivudine in patients coinfected with HIV and HBV. Hepatic function should be closely monitored with clinical and laboratory follow-up for at least several months after lamivudine/raltegravir is discontinued in HIV-infected patients coinfected with HBV and, if appropriate, initiation of HBV treatment may be warranted. Safety and efficacy of lamivudine/raltegravir have not been established for treatment of chronic HBV infection.

If lamivudine/raltegravir is used in HIV-infected patients coinfected with HCV, clinicians should consider that hepatic decompensation, sometimes fatal, has been reported in some patients receiving HIV NRTIs (e.g., lamivudine) concomitantly with peginterferon alfa (or interferon alfa) with or without ribavirin. Such patients should be closely monitored for toxicity, especially hepatic decompensation. Discontinuance of lamivudine/raltegravir should be considered as medically appropriate. Dosage reduction or discontinuance of peginterferon alfa (or interferon alfa) and/or ribavirin also should be considered if worsening clinical toxicities, including hepatic decompensation (e.g., Child-Pugh score greater than 6), occur.

■ **Adipogenic Effects** Redistribution or accumulation of body fat, including central obesity, dorsocervical fat enlargement ("buffalo hump"), peripheral wasting, facial wasting, breast enlargement, and general cushingoid appearance, has been reported in patients receiving antiretroviral therapy.

The mechanisms and long-term consequences of fat redistribution are unknown; a causal relationship has not been established.

■ **Immune Reconstitution Syndrome** Immune reconstitution syndrome has been reported in HIV-infected patients receiving multiple-drug antiretroviral therapy, including raltegravir. During the initial phase of treatment, HIV-infected patients whose immune systems respond to antiretroviral therapy may develop an inflammatory response to indolent or residual opportunistic infections (e.g., *Mycobacterium avium*, *M. tuberculosis*, cytomegalovirus [CMV], *Pneumocystis jirovecii* [formerly *P. carinii*], varicella zoster virus [VZV]); such responses may necessitate further evaluation and treatment.

Autoimmune disorders (e.g., Graves' disease, polymyositis, Guillain-Barré syndrome) have also been reported to occur in the setting of immune reconstitution; however, the time to onset is more variable and can occur many months after initiation of antiretroviral therapy.

Specific Populations **Pregnancy.** Raltegravir (Isentress®): Category C. (See Users Guide.)

Lamivudine/raltegravir (Dutrebis®): Category C.

Antiretroviral Pregnancy Registry at 800-258-4263 or http://www.apregistry.com.

The manufacturer states that there are no adequate and well-controlled studies of raltegravir or lamivudine/raltegravir in pregnant women, and the drugs should be used during pregnancy only if potential benefits to the woman justify potential risks to the fetus.

The US Department of Health and Human Services (HHS) Panel on Treatment of HIV-infected Pregnant Women and Prevention of Perinatal Transmission states that raltegravir is the preferred HIV integrase strand transfer inhibitor (INSTI) for use in antiretroviral-naive pregnant women and a regimen of raltegravir in conjunction with 2 NRTIs is a preferred regimen for *initial* treatment in antiretroviral-naive pregnant women.

Raltegravir crosses the human placenta.

Lactation. Raltegravir is distributed into milk in rats; it is not known whether the drug is distributed into human milk.

Because of the risk of adverse effects in the infant and the risk of HIV transmission, HIV-infected women should not breast-feed infants.

Pediatric Use. Safety and efficacy of raltegravir (Isentress®) have not been established in pediatric patients younger than 4 weeks of age. The safety profile of raltegravir in infants, children, and adolescents 4 weeks to 18 years of age is similar to that in adults.

Lamivudine/raltegravir (Dutrebis®) should not be used in pediatric patients younger than 6 years or age or in patients weighing less than 30 kg.

Lamivudine/raltegravir should be used with caution in pediatric patients with a history of prior therapy with HIV NRTIs, a history of pancreatitis, or other clinically important risk factors for development of pancreatitis. The fixed combination should be discontinued immediately if there are clinical signs, symptoms, or laboratory abnormalities suggestive of pancreatitis.

Geriatric Use. Experience in adults 65 years of age and older is insufficient to determine whether they respond differently to raltegravir (Isentress®) or lamivudine/raltegravir (Dutrebis®) than younger adults.

Dosage of raltegravir should be selected with caution because of age-related decreases in hepatic, renal, and/or cardiac function and potential for concomitant disease and drug therapy.

If lamivudine/raltegravir is used in geriatric patients, renal function should be monitored. A switch from the fixed combination to single-entity lamivudine and single-entity raltegravir may be necessary in patients with reduced renal function. (See Renal Impairment under Warnings/Precautions: Specific Populations, in Cautions.)

Hepatic Impairment. Pharmacokinetics of raltegravir are not altered in adults with moderate hepatic impairment. Pharmacokinetics of the drug have not been studied in patients with severe hepatic impairment.

Patients with chronic HBV or HCV infection may be at increased risk for further elevations in hepatic enzyme concentrations.

Pharmacokinetics of lamivudine/raltegravir have not been studied in patients with hepatic impairment. Safety and efficacy of the fixed combination have not been established in patients with decompensated liver disease.

Renal Impairment. Pharmacokinetics of raltegravir are not altered in adults with severe renal impairment. It is not known whether raltegravir is removed by dialysis; administration of the drug before a dialysis session should be avoided.

Pharmacokinetics of lamivudine/raltegravir have not been studied in patients with renal impairment, and the fixed combination should not be used in patients with creatinine clearances less than 50 mL/minute. If lamivudine/raltegravir is used in patients likely to have decreased renal function, renal function should be monitored. Because lamivudine is substantially eliminated by the kidneys and decreased lamivudine dosage is recommended in patients with creatinine clearances less than 50 mL/minute, lamivudine/raltegravir should be switched to single-entity lamivudine and single-entity raltegravir to allow adjustment of lamivudine dosage in such patients.

■ **Common Adverse Effects** Adverse effects reported in 2% or more of patients receiving raltegravir in conjunction with other antiretrovirals include insomnia, headache, dizziness, nausea, fatigue, hyperglycemia, decreased neutrophil count, and increased serum concentrations of aminotransferases, total bilirubin, lipase, pancreatic amylase, creatine kinase, and cholesterol.

Drug Interactions

The following drug interactions are based on studies using raltegravir and a study using the fixed combination containing lamivudine and raltegravir (lamivudine/raltegravir). When lamivudine/raltegravir is used, interactions associated with both drugs in the fixed combination should be considered.

■ **Drugs Affecting or Metabolized by Hepatic Microsomal Enzymes** In vitro studies indicate that raltegravir does not inhibit cytochrome P-450 (CYP) isoenzymes 1A2, 2B6, 2C8, 2C9, 2C19, 2D6, or 3A. Raltegravir does not induce CYP1A2, 2B6, or 3A4. Raltegravir is not a substrate for CYP isoenzymes. Pharmacokinetic interactions are unlikely with drugs that are substrates for these isoenzymes.

Lamivudine/raltegravir is not expected to have clinically important effects on the pharmacokinetics of drugs that are substrates for CYP isoenzymes.

■ **Drugs Affecting or Metabolized by Uridine Diphosphate-glucuronosyltransferases** Raltegravir is metabolized by uridine diphosphate-glucuronosyltransferase (UGT) 1A1; pharmacokinetic interactions are possible with drugs that are potent inducers of UGT1A1 (decreased plasma concentrations of raltegravir) or inhibitors of UGT1A1 (increased plasma concentrations of raltegravir).

In vitro studies indicate that raltegravir does not inhibit UGT1A1 or 2B7. Therefore, raltegravir is not expected to affect the pharmacokinetics of drugs that are substrates for these enzymes.

Lamivudine/raltegravir is not expected to have clinically important effects on the pharmacokinetics of drugs that are substrates for UGT1A1 or 2B7; pharmacokinetic interactions are possible with drugs that are potent inducers of UGT1A1 (decreased plasma concentrations of raltegravir) or inhibitors of UGT1A1 (increased plasma concentrations of raltegravir).

■ **Drugs Affected by P-Glycoprotein Transport** Raltegravir does not inhibit P-glycoprotein (P-gp); pharmacokinetic interaction are unlikely with drugs that are P-gp substrates.

Lamivudine/raltegravir is not expected to have clinically important effects on the pharmacokinetics of drugs that are P-gp substrates.

■ **Drugs that Increase Gastric pH** ***Antacids*** Antacids containing aluminum and/or magnesium administered concomitantly with or 2 hours before or after raltegravir decrease peak plasma concentrations and area under the concentration-time curve (AUC) of raltegravir. Aluminum- and/or magnesium-containing antacids should *not* be used in patients receiving raltegravir or lamivudine/raltegravir; an alternative acid-reducing agent should be used.

Although concomitant use of antacids containing calcium carbonate decrease peak plasma concentrations and AUC of raltegravir, this interaction is not considered clinically important. Dosage adjustments are not necessary if calcium carbonate-containing antacids are used concomitantly with raltegravir or lamivudine/raltegravir.

Proton-pump Inhibitors Pharmacokinetic interaction between omeprazole and raltegravir (substantially increased raltegravir peak plasma concentrations and AUC); not considered clinically important. Raltegravir and lamivudine/raltegravir are not expected to have clinically important effects on the pharmacokinetics of other proton-pump inhibitors.

Dosage adjustments are not necessary if raltegravir or lamivudine/raltegravir is used concomitantly with omeprazole or other proton-pump inhibitors.

■ **Anticonvulsants** Effect of phenytoin or phenobarbital on the pharmacokinetics of raltegravir is unknown. Concomitant use of phenytoin and/or phenobarbital was prohibited in the expanded-access program due to their potential to affect the UGT1A1 pathway.

■ **Antifungal Agents** Raltegravir and lamivudine/raltegravir are not expected to have clinically important effects on the pharmacokinetics of azole antifungal agents.

■ **Antimycobacterial Agents** ***Rifabutin*** Pharmacokinetic interaction between rifabutin and raltegravir (increased raltegravir AUC). Some experts state that dosage adjustments are not necessary if raltegravir is used with rifabutin.

Rifampin Pharmacokinetic interaction between rifampin and raltegravir (decreased raltegravir plasma concentrations and AUC); rifampin is a potent inducer of UGT1A1.

If raltegravir is used in adults receiving rifampin, dosage of raltegravir film-coated tablets should be increased to 800 mg twice daily and patients should be monitored closely for virologic response. Some experts recommend that use of rifabutin (instead of rifampin) should be considered in patients receiving raltegravir. Data are insufficient to make dosage recommendations for concomitant use of raltegravir and rifampin in patients younger than 18 years of age.

Lamivudine/raltegravir should not be used concomitantly with rifampin. If concomitant use with rifampin is necessary, the fixed combination should be switched to single-entity lamivudine and single-entity raltegravir to allow adjustment of raltegravir dosage.

Rifapentine Pharmacokinetic interaction between rifapentine and raltegravir (altered raltegravir plasma concentrations and AUC). Although decreased raltegravir plasma concentrations were reported when a once-daily rifapentine regimen (600 mg once daily) was used concomitantly with raltegravir, decreased raltegravir plasma concentrations but increased raltegravir AUC were reported when a once-weekly rifapentine regimen (900 mg once weekly) was used with raltegravir.

Experts state that usual dosages can be used if a once-weekly rifapentine regimen is used in patients receiving raltegravir. However, a once-daily rifapentine regimen should not be used concomitantly with raltegravir.

■ Antiretroviral Agents

HIV Entry and Fusion Inhibitors **Enfuvirtide.** There is in vitro evidence of additive to synergistic antiretroviral effects between raltegravir and enfuvirtide.

Maraviroc. Pharmacokinetic interaction between maraviroc and raltegravir (decreased raltegravir plasma concentrations and AUC; decreased maraviroc plasma concentrations and AUC); not considered clinically important.

When maraviroc is used in conjunction with raltegravir in a regimen that does *not* include a potent CYP3A inhibitor or inducer, the recommended maraviroc dosage is 300 mg twice daily.

HIV Integrase Inhibitors **Dolutegravir.** There is no in vitro evidence of antagonistic antiretroviral effects between raltegravir and dolutegravir.

Elvitegravir. There is no in vitro evidence of antagonistic antiretroviral effects between raltegravir and elvitegravir.

HIV Nonnucleoside Reverse Transcriptase Inhibitors (NNRTIs) There is in vitro evidence of additive to synergistic antiretroviral effects between raltegravir and NNRTIs (delavirdine, efavirenz, nevirapine). There is no in vitro evidence of antagonistic antiretroviral effects between raltegravir and etravirine or rilpivirine.

Lamivudine/raltegravir is not expected to have clinically important effects on the pharmacokinetics of NNRTIs.

Efavirenz. Pharmacokinetic interaction between efavirenz and raltegravir (decreased plasma concentrations and AUC of raltegravir); not considered clinically important.

Dosage adjustments are not necessary if raltegravir or lamivudine/raltegravir is used concomitantly with efavirenz.

Etravirine. Pharmacokinetic interaction between etravirine and raltegravir (decreased raltegravir plasma concentrations and AUC; no clinically important effect on etravirine pharmacokinetics); not considered clinically important. Dosage adjustments are not necessary if raltegravir is used concomitantly with etravirine.

Concomitant use of lamivudine/raltegravir and etravirine does not have a clinically important effect on raltegravir exposures. Dosage adjustments are not necessary if lamivudine/raltegravir is used concomitantly with etravirine.

Nevirapine. Some experts state that dosage adjustments are not necessary if raltegravir is used concomitantly with nevirapine.

Rilpivirine. Pharmacokinetic interaction between rilpivirine and raltegravir (increased raltegravir plasma concentrations); not considered clinically important. Dosage adjustments are not necessary if rilpivirine and raltegravir are used concomitantly.

HIV Nucleoside and Nucleotide Reverse Transcriptase Inhibitors (NRTIs) There is in vitro evidence of additive to synergistic antiretroviral effects between raltegravir and NRTIs (abacavir, didanosine, lamivudine, stavudine, tenofovir, zidovudine).

Lamivudine. Raltegravir does not have a clinically important effect on the pharmacokinetics of lamivudine. Dosage adjustments are not necessary if lamivudine and raltegravir are used concomitantly.

Tenofovir. Pharmacokinetic interaction with tenofovir disoproxil fumarate (tenofovir DF) (increased raltegravir plasma concentrations and AUC; no clinically important effect on tenofovir pharmacokinetics); not considered clinically important.

Dosage adjustments are not necessary if raltegravir or lamivudine/raltegravir is used concomitantly with tenofovir DF.

HIV Protease Inhibitors (PIs) There is in vitro evidence of additive to synergistic antiretroviral effects between raltegravir and HIV PIs (amprenavir [active metabolite of fosamprenavir], atazanavir, indinavir, lopinavir, nelfinavir, ritonavir, saquinavir).

Lamivudine/raltegravir is not expected to have clinically important effects on the pharmacokinetics of HIV PIs.

Atazanavir. Pharmacokinetic interaction between raltegravir and *ritonavir-boosted* atazanavir or unboosted atazanavir (increased raltegravir plasma concentrations and AUC); not considered clinically important.

Dosage adjustments are not necessary if raltegravir or lamivudine/raltegravir is used concomitantly with *ritonavir-boosted* atazanavir, *cobicistat-boosted* atazanavir, or unboosted atazanavir.

Darunavir. Pharmacokinetic interaction between raltegravir and *ritonavir-boosted* darunavir (decreased raltegravir AUC; no clinically important effect on pharmacokinetics of *ritonavir-boosted* darunavir); not considered clinically important. Clinically important drug interactions are not expected if *cobicistat-boosted* darunavir is used concomitantly with raltegravir.

Dosage adjustments are not necessary if raltegravir or lamivudine/raltegravir is used concomitantly with *ritonavir-boosted* darunavir or *cobicistat-boosted* darunavir.

Fosamprenavir. Pharmacokinetic interaction between raltegravir and fosamprenavir or *ritonavir-boosted* fosamprenavir (decreased plasma concentrations and AUCs of raltegravir and amprenavir [active metabolite of fosamprenavir]). Appropriate dosages for concomitant use of raltegravir and fosamprenavir (with or without low-dose ritonavir) with respect to safety and efficacy have not been established. Some experts state that dosage adjustments are not necessary.

Lopinavir. Pharmacokinetic interaction between raltegravir and the fixed combination of lopinavir and ritonavir (lopinavir/ritonavir) (decreased raltegravir plasma concentrations; no change in lopinavir/ritonavir plasma concentrations). Some experts state that dosage adjustments are not necessary if raltegravir is used concomitantly with lopinavir/ritonavir.

Ritonavir. Pharmacokinetic interaction between raltegravir and low-dose ritonavir (decreased raltegravir peak plasma concentrations and AUC). Dosage adjustments are not necessary if raltegravir is used concomitantly with low-dose ritonavir; however, when low-dose ritonavir is used to boost plasma concentrations of other PIs, the possibility of drug interactions between raltegravir and the other PIs in the regimen should be considered.

Saquinavir. Some experts state that dosage adjustments are not necessary if raltegravir is used concomitantly with *ritonavir-boosted* saquinavir.

Tipranavir. Pharmacokinetic interaction between raltegravir and *ritonavir-boosted* tipranavir (decreased raltegravir plasma concentrations and AUC); not considered clinically important.

Dosage adjustments are not necessary if raltegravir or lamivudine/raltegravir is used concomitantly with *ritonavir-boosted* tipranavir.

■ Benzodiazepines

Raltegravir does not have a clinically important effect on the pharmacokinetics of midazolam.

■ Estrogens and Progestins

Raltegravir does not have a clinically important effect on the pharmacokinetics of hormonal contraceptives.

Dosage adjustments are not necessary if raltegravir or lamivudine/raltegravir is used concomitantly with hormonal contraceptives.

■ HCV Antivirals

HCV Polymerase Inhibitors **Dasabuvir.** Concomitant use of raltegravir and the fixed combination of ombitasvir, paritaprevir, and ritonavir (ombitasvir/paritaprevir/ritonavir) copackaged with dasabuvir sodium does not result in clinically important interactions.

Dosage adjustments are not necessary if raltegravir is used concomitantly with an HCV regimen that includes dasabuvir and ombitasvir, paritaprevir, and ritonavir.

Sofosbuvir. Pharmacokinetic interaction between sofosbuvir and raltegravir (decreased raltegravir plasma concentrations and AUC; no effect on sofosbuvir pharmacokinetics); not considered clinically important. Dosage adjustments are not necessary if sofosbuvir and raltegravir are used concomitantly.

Sofosbuvir and Velpatasvir. No clinically important pharmacokinetic interactions were observed when the fixed combination of sofosbuvir and velpatasvir (sofosbuvir/velpatasvir) was used concomitantly with raltegravir.

HCV Protease Inhibitors **Paritaprevir.** Concomitant use of raltegravir and ombitasvir/paritaprevir/ritonavir with or without dasabuvir sodium does not result in clinically important interactions.

Dosage adjustments are not necessary if raltegravir is used concomitantly with ombitasvir/paritaprevir/ritonavir with or without dasabuvir.

Simeprevir. Concomitant use of simeprevir and raltegravir does not have a clinically important effect on the pharmacokinetics of either drug; dosage adjustments are not necessary if simeprevir and raltegravir are used concomitantly.

HCV Replication Complex Inhibitors **Daclatasvir.** Although data are not available to date regarding concomitant use of raltegravir and daclatasvir, some experts state that dosage adjustments are not necessary if the drugs are used concomitantly.

Elbasvir and Grazoprevir. Concomitant use of raltegravir (single 400-mg dose) and elbasvir (single 50-mg dose) does not have a clinically important effect on the pharmacokinetics of either drug. Concomitant use of raltegravir (400 mg twice daily) and grazoprevir (200 mg once daily) results in increased raltegravir plasma concentrations and AUC, but does not affect grazoprevir plasma concentrations.

Dosage adjustments are not necessary if raltegravir is used concomitantly with the fixed combination of elbasvir and grazoprevir (elbasvir/grazoprevir).

Ledipasvir and Sofosbuvir. Concomitant use of raltegravir (400 mg twice daily) and either ledipasvir (90 mg once daily) or sofosbuvir (single 400-mg dose) did not have a clinically important effect on the pharmacokinetics of raltegravir, ledipasvir, or sofosbuvir. Clinically important pharmacokinetic interactions are not expected if the fixed combination of ledipasvir and sofosbuvir (ledipasvir/sofosbuvir) is used concomitantly with raltegravir.

Dosage adjustments are not necessary if ledipasvir/sofosbuvir is used concomitantly with raltegravir.

Ombitasvir. Concomitant use of raltegravir and ombitasvir/paritaprevir/ritonavir with or without dasabuvir sodium does not result in clinically important interactions.

Dosage adjustments are not necessary if raltegravir is used concomitantly with ombitasvir/paritaprevir/ritonavir with or without dasabuvir.

■ **HMG-CoA Reductase Inhibitors** Raltegravir and lamivudine/raltegravir are not expected to have clinically important effects on the pharmacokinetics HMG-CoA reductase inhibitors (statins).

■ **Opiates and Opiate Partial Agonists** Raltegravir and lamivudine/raltegravir are not expected to have a clinically important effect on the pharmacokinetics of opiate analgesics.

Buprenorphine Raltegravir does not have a clinically important effect on the pharmacokinetics of sublingual buprenorphine; clinically important pharmacokinetic interactions are not expected if raltegravir is used concomitantly with a buprenorphine subdermal implant.

Dosage adjustments are not necessary if raltegravir and buprenorphine are used concomitantly.

Methadone Raltegravir does not have a clinically important effect on the pharmacokinetics of methadone.

Dosage adjustments are not necessary if raltegravir or lamivudine/raltegravir is used concomitantly with methadone.

■ **Phosphodiesterase Type 5 Inhibitors** Lamivudine/raltegravir is not expected to have clinically important effects on the pharmacokinetics of phosphodiesterase type 5 inhibitors.

■ **Selective Serotonin-reuptake Inhibitors** ***Citalopram*** No clinically important pharmacokinetic interactions were reported when raltegravir and citalopram were used concomitantly.

Dosage adjustments are not necessary if raltegravir is used concomitantly with citalopram.

Description

Raltegravir potassium, an antiretroviral agent, is a human immunodeficiency virus (HIV) integrase strand transfer inhibitor (INSTI). Raltegravir inhibits the activity of HIV integrase, an enzyme that integrates HIV DNA into the host cell genome. Integration is required for maintenance of the viral genome and for efficient viral gene expression and replication. Inhibition of integration prevents propagation of viral infection. Raltegravir is active against HIV type 1 (HIV-1) and also has some in vitro activity against HIV type 2 (HIV-2).

Raltegravir-resistant HIV-1 have been produced in vitro and have emerged during raltegravir therapy. Cross-resistance between raltegravir and other INSTIs (e.g., dolutegravir, elvitegravir) has been reported.

Raltegravir is commercially available as single-entity chewable tablets, film-coated tablets, and oral suspension (Isentress®). Raltegravir also is commercially available in fixed-combination, film-coated tablets with lamivudine (lamivudine/raltegravir; Dutrebis®); lamivudine is an HIV nucleoside reverse transcriptase inhibitor (NRTI).

Following oral administration of 400 mg of raltegravir as film-coated tablets in fasting adults, peak plasma concentrations of the drug are attained approximately 3 hours after dosing and steady state is achieved within approximately 2 days when a twice-daily regimen is used. Although absolute bioavailability of raltegravir has not been established, oral bioavailability is higher with raltegravir chewable tablets or oral suspension compared with the film-coated tablets. Considerable interindividual variation has been reported in the pharmacokinetics of raltegravir. Although studies using 400-mg film-coated tablets of raltegravir indicate that food increases pharmacokinetic variability relative to fasting, raltegravir film-coated tablets, chewable tablets, or oral suspension may be administered with or without food. Bioavailability of the raltegravir formulation contained in lamivudine/raltegravir is higher than that of the raltegravir formulation contained in the single-entity preparation. Following oral administration of lamivudine/raltegravir in the fasting state, bioavailability of raltegravir is approximately 60% and the pharmacokinetics of the lamivudine and raltegravir components are similar to the pharmacokinetics reported when the drugs are administered as single-entity preparations. Raltegravir is metabolized mainly by uridine diphosphate-glucuronosyltransferase (UGT) 1A1. Following an oral dose of raltegravir, approximately 51% of the dose is eliminated in feces (as raltegravir) and 32% is eliminated in urine (as raltegravir and raltegravir glucuronide). Raltegravir has an apparent terminal half-life of approximately 9 hours. Common UGT1A1 genotypes associated with reduced UGT1A1 activity do not appear to have a clinically important effect on the pharmacokinetics of raltegravir in adults compared with wild-type UGT1A1 genotype.

Advice to Patients

Critical nature of compliance with HIV therapy and importance of remaining under the care of a clinician. Importance of taking as prescribed; do not alter or discontinue antiretroviral regimen without consulting clinician.

Importance of using single-entity raltegravir (Isentress®) or the fixed combination containing lamivudine and raltegravir (lamivudine/raltegravir; Dutrebis®) in conjunction with other antiretrovirals—not for monotherapy.

Antiretroviral therapy is not a cure for HIV infection; opportunistic infections and other complications associated with HIV disease may still occur.

Advise patients that sustained decreases in plasma HIV RNA have been associated with reduced risk of progression to acquired immunodeficiency syndrome (AIDS) and death.

Advise patients that effective antiretroviral regimens can decrease HIV concentrations in blood and genital secretions and strict adherence to such regimens in conjunction with risk-reduction measures may decrease, but cannot absolutely eliminate, the risk of secondary transmission of HIV to others. Importance of continuing to practice safer sex (e.g., using latex or polyurethane condoms to minimize sexual contact with body fluids), never sharing personal items that can have blood or body fluids on them (e.g., toothbrushes, razor blades), and never reusing or sharing needles.

Importance of reading patient information provided by the manufacturer.

If using raltegravir film-coated tablets, importance of swallowing whole; raltegravir chewable tablets can be chewed or swallowed whole.

If using raltegravir for oral suspension, importance of parents and/or caregivers reading the manufacturer's instructions for use before preparing and administering the drug. Instruct parents and/or caregivers that the oral suspension should be administered within 30 minutes of mixing.

Advise patients not to take aluminum- and/or magnesium-containing antacids during raltegravir or lamivudine/raltegravir treatment.

If a dose of raltegravir or lamivudine/raltegravir is missed, the dose should be taken as soon as it is remembered and the next dose taken at the regularly scheduled time. If a dose is skipped, a double dose should not be taken to make up for the missed dose.

Importance of informing clinician if unusual symptoms develop or known symptoms persist or worsen.

Advise patients that severe and potentially life-threatening rash has been reported. Importance of immediately discontinuing raltegravir or lamivudine/raltegravir and other suspect agents and seeking medical attention if rash occurs and is associated with fever, generally ill feeling, extreme tiredness, muscle or joint aches, breathing difficulty, blisters, oral lesions, eye inflammation, swelling of the face, eyes, lips, or mouth, and/or signs and symptoms of liver problems (e.g., yellowing of skin or whites of the eyes, dark or tea-colored urine, pale stools/bowel movements, nausea, vomiting, loss of appetite, or pain, aching, or sensitivity on the right side below ribs).

Importance of informing clinician if patient has a history of rhabdomyolysis, myopathy, or increased serum creatine kinase concentrations or is receiving drugs known to cause these conditions (e.g., hydroxymethylglutaryl-CoA [HMG-CoA] reductase inhibitors [statins], fenofibrate, gemfibrozil, zidovudine). Importance of immediately informing clinician if unexplained muscle pain, tenderness, or weakness occurs while receiving raltegravir.

Importance of informing clinicians of existing or contemplated concomitant therapy, including prescription and OTC drugs and herbal products, and any concomitant illnesses.

Importance of women informing clinicians if they are or plan to become pregnant or plan to breast-feed. Advise HIV-infected women not to breast-feed.

Importance of advising patients of other important precautionary information. (See Cautions.)

Redistribution/accumulation of body fat may occur with antiretroviral therapy with as yet unknown long-term health effects.

Overview® (see Users Guide). For additional information on this drug until a more detailed monograph is developed and published, the manufacturer's labeling should be consulted. It is *essential* that the manufacturer's labeling be consulted for more detailed information on usual cautions, precautions, contraindications, potential drug interactions, laboratory test interferences, and acute toxicity.

Preparations

Excipients in commercially available drug preparations may have clinically important effects in some individuals; consult specific product labeling for details.

Raltegravir Potassium

Oral		
For suspension	100 mg (of raltegravir) per packet	**Isentress®**, Merck
Tablets, chewable	25 mg (of raltegravir)	**Isentress®**, Merck
	100 mg (of raltegravir)	**Isentress®**, Merck
Tablets, film-coated	400 mg (of raltegravir)	**Isentress®**, Merck

Raltegravir Potassium Combinations

Oral		
Tablets, film-coated	300 mg (of raltegravir) with Lamivudine 150 mg	**Dutrebis®**, Merck

†Use is not currently included in the labeling approved by the US Food and Drug Administration

HIV Nonnucleoside Reverse Transcriptase Inhibitors 8:18.08.16

Efavirenz EFV, efavirenz/emtricitabine/tenofovir DF, EFV/TDF/FTC

■ Efavirenz, an antiretroviral agent, is a human immunodeficiency virus (HIV) nonnucleoside reverse transcriptase inhibitor (NNRTI).

Uses

■ **Treatment of HIV Infection** Efavirenz is used in conjunction with other antiretroviral agents for treatment of human immunodeficiency virus type 1 (HIV-1) infection in adults, adolescents, and pediatric patients 3 months of age or older.

Efavirenz usually is used in HIV nonnucleoside reverse transcriptase inhibitor-based (NNRTI-based) regimens that include efavirenz and 2 HIV nucleoside reverse transcriptase inhibitors (NRTIs).

If an NNRTI-based regimen of efavirenz, emtricitabine, and tenofovir disoproxil fumarate (tenofovir DF) is used for treatment of HIV-1 infection, a fixed-combination preparation containing all 3 drugs (efavirenz/emtricitabine/tenofovir DF; Atripla®) is commercially available and can be used in adults and pediatric patients 12 years of age or older weighing at least 40 kg to decrease pill burden and improve adherence. Efavirenz/emtricitabine/tenofovir DF can be used alone as a complete treatment regimen or in conjunction with other antiretrovirals.

Because of potential risks to the fetus, the manufacturer states that efavirenz (single entity or fixed combination) should not be used during the first trimester of pregnancy and pregnancy should be avoided during and for 12 weeks after therapy with the drug is discontinued. (See Pregnancy under Cautions: Pregnancy, Fertility, and Lactation.)

The most appropriate antiretroviral regimen cannot be defined for each clinical scenario, and selection of specific antiretroviral agents for use in such regimens should be individualized based on current knowledge regarding antiretroviral potency, potential rate of development of resistance, known toxicities, and potential for pharmacokinetic interactions as well as virologic, immunologic, and clinical characteristics of the patient. For information on the general principles and guidelines for use of antiretroviral therapy, including specific recommendations for initial therapy in antiretroviral-naive patients and recommendations for changing antiretroviral regimens, see the Antiretroviral Agents General Statement 8:18.08.

Antiretroviral-naive Adults and Adolescents For *initial* treatment in HIV-infected adults and adolescents who are antiretroviral-naive, the HHS Panel on Antiretroviral Guidelines for Adults and Adolescents states that efavirenz in conjunction with tenofovir alafenamide and emtricitabine or efavirenz in conjunction with tenofovir DF and emtricitabine (or lamivudine) are considered alternative NNRTI-based regimens. These experts also state that efavirenz in conjunction with abacavir and lamivudine (or emtricitabine) is another NNRTI-based regimen option for *initial* treatment in antiretroviral-naive adults and adolescents when recommended or alternative regimens cannot be used, but should be used *only* in patients with baseline plasma HIV RNA levels less than 100,000 copies/mL who are human leukocyte antigen (HLA)-B*5701 negative.

Study 006. Efavirenz has been evaluated for use in conjunction with 2 NRTIs or in conjunction with an HIV protease inhibitor (PI) in a phase 2 or 3 randomized, open-label study (study 006) in 1266 HIV-infected adults (mean age 36.5 years [range: 18–81 years], 83% male, 60% white, mean baseline CD4+ T-cell count 320 cells/mm³, mean baseline plasma HIV-1 RNA level 4.8 $\log_{10}$ copies/mL). Although a small number of patients included in study 006 had previously received NRTIs, most were antiretroviral-naive (had not previously received antiretroviral therapy) and none had previously received PIs, NNRTIs, or lamivudine. Patients were randomized to receive a 2-drug regimen of efavirenz (600 mg once daily) and indinavir (1 g every 8 hours); a 3-drug regimen of efavirenz (600 mg once daily), zidovudine (300 mg every 12 hours), and lamivudine (150 mg every 12 hours); or a 3-drug regimen of indinavir (800 mg every 8 hours), zidovudine (300 mg every 12 hours), and lamivudine (150 mg every 12 hours).

At 48 or 168 weeks, plasma HIV-1 levels were below 400 copies/mL in 57 or 40%, respectively, of those receiving efavirenz and indinavir; 69 or 48% of those receiving efavirenz, zidovudine, and lamivudine; and 50 or 29% of those receiving indinavir, zidovudine, and lamivudine. When an assay with lower limits of detection (50 copies/mL) was used to measure plasma HIV-1 levels at 48 or 168 weeks, plasma HIV-1 levels were below 50 copies/mL in 50 or 31%, respectively, of those receiving efavirenz and indinavir; 65 or 43% of those receiving efavirenz, zidovudine, and lamivudine; and 45 or 23% of those receiving indinavir, zidovudine, and lamivudine. Evaluation of CSF HIV-1 RNA levels in a limited number of individuals at week 17–35 indicated that all patients receiving an efavirenz regimen had CSF HIV-1 RNA levels below 400 copies/mL.

Study 934. Safety and efficacy of a regimen of efavirenz, emtricitabine, and tenofovir DF are based on results of a randomized, open-label study designed to demonstrate noninferiority of this regimen compared with a regimen of efavirenz, zidovudine, and lamivudine (study 934). In this study, 511 antiretroviral-naive HIV-infected patients (mean age 38 years, 86% male, 59% white, 23% black, median baseline plasma HIV-1 RNA level 5.01 $\log_{10}$ copies/mL [range: 3.56–6.54 $\log_{10}$ copies/mL], mean baseline CD4+ T-cell count 245 cells/mm³) were randomized to receive a once-daily regimen of efavirenz, emtricitabine, and tenofovir DF or a regimen of efavirenz once daily with the fixed combination of lamivudine and zidovudine (lamivudine/zidovudine; Combivir®) twice daily. The primary measure used to assess noninferiority of the regimen of efavirenz, emtricitabine, and tenofovir DF to the regimen of efavirenz, zidovudine, and lamivudine was plasma HIV-1 RNA levels at week 48, specifically the number of patients with HIV-1 RNA levels less than 400 copies/mL. The 487 patients without baseline resistance to efavirenz who underwent randomization and received treatment were the predefined population used for the primary endpoint analysis.

Through week 48, the regimen of efavirenz, emtricitabine, and tenofovir DF met the criteria for noninferiority to the regimen of efavirenz, zidovudine, and lamivudine. At week 48, 84 or 80% of adults receiving the efavirenz, tenofovir DF, and emtricitabine regimen and 73 or 70% of adults receiving the efavirenz, zidovudine, and lamivudine regimen had plasma HIV-1 RNA levels less than 400 or 50 copies/mL, respectively. At week 48, increases in CD4+ T-cell counts were greater in patients receiving the efavirenz, emtricitabine, and tenofovir DF regimen (mean increase of 190 cells/mm³) than in those receiving the efavirenz, zidovudine, and lamivudine regimen (mean increase of 158 cells/mm³). Virologic failure (i.e., individuals who failed to achieve virologic suppression or experienced rebound after achieving virologic suppression) was reported in 2% of those receiving efavirenz, emtricitabine, and tenofovir DF and in 4% of those receiving efavirenz, zidovudine, and lamivudine at week 48.

At 144 weeks, 64% of adults receiving the efavirenz, emtricitabine, and tenofovir DF regimen and 56% of those receiving the efavirenz, zidovudine, and lamivudine regimen had plasma HIV-1 RNA levels less than 50 copies/mL. The mean increase in CD4+ T-cell count from baseline in these groups was 312 and 271 cells/mm³, respectively, at 144 weeks.

Antiretroviral-experienced Adults **Study ACTG 364.** Efavirenz has been evaluated for use in antiretroviral-experienced patients in a phase 2, randomized, double-blind, placebo-controlled study (study ACTG 364) in 196 HIV-infected adults (mean age 41 years [range: 18–76 years], 88% male, 74% white, mean baseline CD4+ T-cell count 389 cells/mm³, mean baseline plasma HIV-1 RNA level 8,130 copies/mL). In ACTG 364, patients with extensive prior therapy with NRTIs in ACTG trials (ACTG 175, ACTG 302/303) who had plasma HIV-1 RNA levels above 500 copies/mL (median baseline plasma HIV-1 levels of 5000–7000 copies/mL) were randomized to receive a 3-drug regimen of efavirenz (600 mg once daily) and 2 NRTIs; a 4-drug regimen of efavirenz (600 mg once daily), nelfinavir (750 mg 3 times daily), and 2 NRTIs; or a 3-drug regimen of nelfinavir (750 mg 3 times daily) and 2 NRTIs. At study entry, patients were assigned a new open-label NRTI regimen.

At 48 weeks, plasma HIV-1 levels were below 500 copies/mL (500 copies/mL is the lower limit of the assay used) in 63% of those receiving efavirenz and 2 NRTIs; 71% of those receiving efavirenz, nelfinavir, and 2 NRTIs; and 41% of those receiving nelfinavir and 2 NRTIs (without efavirenz).

Study 073. Efficacy of the fixed combination efavirenz/emtricitabine/tenofovir DF was evaluated in a randomized, open-label study (study 073) in antiretroviral-experienced patients who had been receiving a suppressive regimen consisting of at least 2 NRTIs and a PI or NNRTI (mean age 43 years [range 22–73 years]), 88% male, 68% white, 29% black, median CD4+ T-cell count 516 cells/mm³). Patients had plasma HIV-1 RNA levels less than 200 copies/mL for at least 12 weeks on their existing regimen (96% had plasma HIV-1 levels less than 50 copies/mL), no known HIV-1 substitutions conferring resistance to the components of the fixed combination, and no history of virologic failure; patients were randomized to either switch to efavirenz/emtricitabine/tenofovir DF or continue their existing (baseline) regimen. At 48 weeks, 89 and 87% of those switched to efavirenz/emtricitabine/tenofovir DF had plasma HIV-1 RNA levels less than 200 and 50 copies/mL, respectively, compared with 88 and 85% of those who remained on their baseline regimen. This difference was not statistically significant. There was no change in CD4+ T-cell count from baseline in either group.

Pediatric Patients Efavirenz is used in conjunction with other antiretroviral agents for the treatment of HIV-1 infection in children 3 months of age or older weighing at least 3.5 kg.

The fixed combination efavirenz/emtricitabine/tenofovir DF can be used alone as a complete regimen or in conjunction with other antiretrovirals for the treatment of HIV-1 infection in pediatric patients 12 years of age or older weighing at least 40 kg.

For *initial* treatment in HIV-infected pediatric patients, the HHS Panel on Antiretroviral Therapy and Medical Management of HIV-infected Children recommends a regimen that includes a *ritonavir-boosted* PI, NNRTI, or integrase strand transfer inhibitor (INSTI) in conjunction with 2 NRTIs (dual NRTIs). These experts state that efavirenz and 2 NRTIs is a preferred regimen for *initial* treatment in children 3 to less than 12 years of age and an alternative regimen for *initial* treatment in adolescents 12 years of age and older who are not sexually mature. Although efavirenz can be used in children as young as 3 months of age, these experts state the drug is not recommended for *initial* treatment regimens in those 3 months to less than 3 years of age.

For further information on treatment of HIV infection in pediatric patients, see Antiretroviral Therapy in Pediatric Patients, in Guidelines for Use of antiretroviral Agents, in the Antiretroviral Agents General Statement 8:18.08.

Study AI266922. Safety and efficacy of efavirenz in conjunction with didanosine and emtricitabine were evaluated in an open-label trial (study AI266922) that included 37 antiretroviral-naive or antiretroviral-experienced pediatric patients 3 months to 6 years of age (median age 0.7 years, median baseline plasma HIV-1 RNA level 5.88 $\log_{10}$ copies/mL, median baseline $CD4^+$ T-cell count 1144 cells/mm^3, median baseline $CD4^+$ T-cell percentage 25%). At 48 weeks, plasma HIV-1 RNA levels were less than 400 or 50 copies/mL in 57 or 46%, respectively, of patients (intent-to-treat analysis). The median increase in $CD4^+$ T-cell count was 196 cells/mm^3 and the median increase in $CD4^+$ T-cell percentage was 6%.

Study PACTG 1021. Safety and efficacy of efavirenz in conjunction with didanosine and emtricitabine also were evaluated in an open-label trial (study PACTG 1021) that included 43 antiretroviral-naive pediatric patients 3 months to 21 years of age (median age 9.6 years, median baseline plasma HIV-1 RNA level 4.8 $\log_{10}$ copies/mL, median baseline $CD4^+$ T-cell count 367 cells/mm^3, median baseline $CD4^+$ T-cell percentage 18%). At 48 weeks, plasma HIV-1 RNA levels were less than 400 or 50 copies/mL in 77 or 70%, respectively, of patients (intent-to-treat analysis). The median increase in $CD4^+$ T-cell count was 238 cells/mm^3 and the median increase in $CD4^+$ T-cell percentage was 13%.

Study PACTG 382. Safety and efficacy of efavirenz in pediatric patients were evaluated in an open-label study (study PACTG 382) that included 102 antiretroviral-naive or antiretroviral-experienced pediatric patients 3 months to 16 years of age (median age 5.7 years, 87% antiretroviral-experienced, median baseline plasma HIV-1 RNA level 4.57 $\log_{10}$ copies/mL, median baseline $CD4^+$ T-cell count 755 cells/mm^3, median baseline $CD4^+$ T-cell percentage 30%). Patients received efavirenz in conjunction with nelfinavir and an NRTI. At 48 weeks, plasma HIV-1 RNA levels were less than 400 or 50 copies/mL in 57 or 43%, respectively, of patients (intent-to-treat analysis). The median increase in $CD4^+$ T-cell count was 128 cells/mm^3 and the median increase in $CD4^+$ T-cell percentage was 5%.

■ Postexposure Prophylaxis following Occupational Exposure to HIV Efavirenz is used in conjunction with 2 NRTIs for postexposure prophylaxis of HIV infection following an occupational exposure† (PEP) in healthcare personnel and other individuals exposed via percutaneous injury (e.g., needlestick, cut with sharp object) or mucous membrane or nonintact skin (e.g., chapped, abraded, dermatitis) contact with blood, tissue, or other body fluids that might contain HIV.

The US Public Health Service (USPHS) states that the preferred regimen for PEP following an occupational exposure to HIV is a 3-drug regimen of raltegravir used in conjunction with emtricitabine and tenofovir DF (may be administered as the fixed combination emtricitabine/tenofovir DF; Truvada®). These experts state that efavirenz and 2 NRTIs can be considered an alternative regimen, but should be used for PEP *only* with expert consultation. The preferred dual NRTI option for use in PEP regimens is emtricitabine and tenofovir DF (may be administered as the fixed combination emtricitabine/tenofovir DF; Truvada®); alternative dual NRTIs are tenofovir DF and lamivudine, lamivudine and zidovudine (may be administered as the fixed combination lamivudine/zidovudine; Combivir®), or zidovudine and emtricitabine.

Because management of occupational exposures to HIV is complex and evolving, consultation with an infectious disease specialist, clinician with expertise in administration of antiretroviral agents, and/or the National Clinicians' Postexposure Prophylaxis Hotline (PEPline at 888-448-4911) is recommended whenever possible. However, initiation of PEP should not be delayed while waiting for expert consultation.

For information on types of occupational exposure to HIV and associated risk of infection, management of occupational exposure to HIV, efficacy and safety of postexposure prophylaxis, and recommendations regarding PEP, see Guidelines for Use of Antiretroviral Agents: Antiretrovirals for Postexposure Prophylaxis following Occupational Exposure to HIV (PEP), in the Antiretroviral Agents General Statement 8:18.08.

■ Postexposure Prophylaxis following Nonoccupational Exposure to HIV Efavirenz is used in conjunction with other antiretrovirals for postexposure prophylaxis of HIV infection following nonoccupational exposure† (nPEP) in individuals exposed to blood, genital secretions, or other potentially infectious body fluids that might contain HIV when the exposure represents a substantial risk for HIV transmission.

When nPEP is indicated following a nonoccupational exposure to HIV, the US Centers for Disease Control and Prevention (CDC) states that the preferred regimen in adults and adolescents 13 years of age or older with normal renal function is either raltegravir or dolutegravir used in conjunction with emtricitabine and tenofovir DF (administered as emtricitabine/tenofovir DF; Truvada®); the recommended alternative nPEP regimen in these patients is *ritonavir-boosted* darunavir used in conjunction with emtricitabine/tenofovir DF (Truvada®).

CDC states that efavirenz is an alternative antiretroviral that can be used in nPEP regimens, but should be used in such regimens *only* with expert consultation.

Consultation with an infectious disease specialist, clinician with expertise in administration of antiretroviral agents, and/or the National Clinicians' Postexposure Prophylaxis Hotline (PEPline at 888-448-4911) is recommended if nPEP is indicated in certain exposed individuals (e.g., pregnant women, children, those with medical conditions such as renal impairment) or if an antiretroviral regimen not included in the CDC guidelines is being considered, the source virus is known or likely to be resistant to antiretrovirals, or the healthcare provider is inexperienced in prescribing antiretrovirals. However, initiation of nPEP should not be delayed while waiting for expert consultation.

For additional information on nonoccupational exposure to HIV and recommendations regarding postexposure prophylaxis, see Guidelines for Use of Antiretroviral Agents: Antiretrovirals for Postexposure Prophylaxis following Sexual, Injection Drug Use, or other Nonoccupational Exposures to HIV (nPEP), in the Antiretroviral Agents General Statement 8:18.08.

Dosage and Administration

■ Administration Efavirenz is administered orally once daily on an empty stomach, preferably at bedtime.

Because administration with food increases plasma efavirenz concentrations (see Pharmacokinetics: Absorption) and may increase the incidence of adverse effects, the drug should be taken on an empty stomach. Administration of efavirenz at bedtime may make adverse CNS effects (e.g., dizziness, insomnia, impaired concentration, somnolence, abnormal dreams) more tolerable.

Single-entity efavirenz is commercially available as capsules or tablets. Efavirenz also is commercially available in fixed-combination tablets containing efavirenz, emtricitabine, and tenofovir disoproxil fumarate (efavirenz/emtricitabine/tenofovir DF; Atripla®). (See Fixed Combinations Containing Efavirenz under Dosage and Administration: Administration.)

Efavirenz is used in conjunction with other antiretrovirals. Single-entity efavirenz should not be used concomitantly with efavirenz/emtricitabine/tenofovir DF, unless needed for adjustment of efavirenz dosage (e.g., when the fixed combination is used concomitantly with rifampin).

Efavirenz Capsules Efavirenz capsules should be swallowed whole.

For adults and pediatric patients 3 months of age or older not able to swallow capsules or tablets, efavirenz capsules may be opened and the contents administered by mixing with a small amount (1–2 teaspoonfuls) of soft food (capsule sprinkle method). The use of infant formula for mixing should be considered only for infants who cannot consume solid foods. The efavirenz mixture should be administered within 30 minutes after preparation, and the patient should *not* consume any additional food or infant formula for 2 hours after the mixture.

To mix the contents of efavirenz capsules with food, 1–2 teaspoonfuls of age-appropriate soft food (e.g., applesauce, grape jelly, yogurt) should be added to a small container. The appropriate number of efavirenz capsules (see Table 1) should be held horizontally over the small container, twisted open, and emptied. The contents of the capsules should be gently mixed into the soft food with a spoon and the entire mixture fed to the patient. Then, an additional 2 teaspoonfuls of soft food should be added to the small container, stirred to disperse any remaining efavirenz residue, and fed to the patient.

To mix the contents of efavirenz capsules with infant formula for infants not able to consume solid food, 10 mL (2 teaspoonfuls) of reconstituted room temperature infant formula should be added to a 30-mL medicine cup. The appropriate number of efavirenz capsules (see Table 1) should be held horizontally over the medicine cup, twisted open, and emptied. The contents of the capsules should be gently mixed into the infant formula using a small spoon. The infant formula mixture should be drawn up into a 10-mL oral dosing syringe and administered into the infant's right or left inner cheek. Then, an additional 10 mL of infant formula should be added to the medicine cup, stirred to disperse any remaining efavirenz residue, drawn up into the oral dosing syringe, and administered to the infant.

Efavirenz Tablets Efavirenz tablets should be swallowed whole; the tablets should not be broken or crushed.

Fixed Combinations Containing Efavirenz Efavirenz/emtricitabine/tenofovir DF (Atripla®) tablets are administered orally once daily on an empty stomach, preferably at bedtime. Administration at bedtime may make efavirenz-associated adverse CNS effects more tolerable. A fixed-combination tablet containing 600 mg of efavirenz, 200 mg of emtricitabine, and 300 mg of tenofovir DF is bioequivalent to a 600-mg tablet of efavirenz, 200-mg capsule of emtricitabine, and 300-mg tablet of tenofovir DF when taken in the fasting state. The fixed combination can be used alone as a complete treatment regimen or in conjunction with other antiretrovirals.

Efavirenz/emtricitabine/tenofovir DF should not be used concomitantly with single-entity efavirenz, unless needed for adjustment of the efavirenz dosage (e.g., when the fixed combination is used concomitantly with rifampin).

Because the antiretroviral agents contained in efavirenz/emtricitabine/tenofovir DF also are available in single-entity or other fixed-combination preparations, care should be taken to ensure that therapy is not duplicated if the fixed combination is used in conjunction with other antiretrovirals. (See Precautions Related to Use of Fixed Combinations under Cautions: Precautions and Contraindications.)

■ Dosage ***Adult Dosage*** **Treatment of HIV Infection.** The usual dosage of efavirenz (Sustiva®) for treatment of human immunodeficiency virus type 1 (HIV-1) infection in adults and adolescents is 600 mg once daily.

When efavirenz/emtricitabine/tenofovir DF (Atripla®) is used for treatment of HIV-1 infection, adults should receive 1 tablet (600 mg of efavirenz, 200 mg of emtricitabine, and 300 mg of tenofovir DF) once daily.

Treatment of HIV Infection in Patients Receiving Rifampin. If efavirenz (Sustiva®) is used for treatment of HIV-1 infection in patients receiving rifampin, those weighing 50 kg or more should receive an increased efavirenz dosage of 800 mg daily. (See Rifampin under Drug Interactions: Antimycobacterial Agents.)

If efavirenz/emtricitabine/tenofovir DF (Atripla®) is used for treatment of HIV-1 infection in patients receiving rifampin, those weighing 50 kg or more should receive 1 tablet of the fixed combination (600 mg of efavirenz, 200 mg of emtricitabine, and 300 mg of tenofovir DF) once daily *and* 200 mg of single-entity efavirenz (Sustiva®) once daily to provide a total efavirenz dosage of 800 mg daily.

Postexposure Prophylaxis following Occupational Exposure to HIV. For postexposure prophylaxis of HIV infection following occupational exposure† (PEP) in health-care personnel or other individuals, efavirenz is administered in a dosage of 600 mg once daily in conjunction with 2 HIV nucleoside reverse transcriptase inhibitors (NRTIs). (See Uses: Postexposure Prophylaxis following Occupational Exposure to HIV.)

PEP should be initiated as soon as possible following occupational exposure to HIV (preferably within hours) and continued for 4 weeks, if tolerated.

Pediatric Dosage Dosage of efavirenz (Sustiva®) in children 3 months of age or older weighing 3.5 to less than 40 kg is based on weight. (See Table 1.) Adolescents and children who weigh 40 kg or more may receive the usual adult dosage of efavirenz.

Table 1. Efavirenz (Sustiva®) Dosage in Children 3 Months of Age or Older

Weight in kg	Efavirenz Dosage	Number of Capsules or Tablets
3.5 to less than 5	100 mg once daily	Two 50-mg capsules
5 to less than 7.5	150 mg once daily	Three 50-mg capsules
7.5 to less than 15	200 mg once daily	One 200-mg capsule
15 to less than 20	250 mg once daily	One 200-mg *and* one 50-mg capsule
20 to less than 25	300 mg once daily	One 200-mg *and* two 50-mg capsules
25 to less than 32.5	350 mg once daily	One 200-mg *and* three 50-mg capsules
32.5 to less than 40	400 mg once daily	Two 200-mg capsules
40 or more	600 mg once daily	One 600-mg tablet *or* three 200-mg capsules

When efavirenz/emtricitabine/tenofovir DF (Atripla®) is used for treatment of HIV-1 infection in pediatric patients 12 years of age or older weighing at least 40 kg, the recommended dosage is 1 tablet (600 mg of efavirenz, 200 mg of emtricitabine, and 300 mg of tenofovir DF) once daily.

■ Dosage in Renal and Hepatic Impairment

Renal Impairment While the pharmacokinetics of efavirenz have not been specifically studied in patients with renal failure, renal clearance of the drug is negligible and clinically important decreases in efavirenz clearance are not anticipated if efavirenz is administered to patients with renal impairment. Some experts state that the usual dosage of efavirenz (Sustiva®) can be used in patients with impaired renal function.

When efavirenz/emtricitabine/tenofovir DF (Atripla®) is used, usual dosage can be used in patients with creatinine clearances of 50 mL/minute or greater. The fixed combination should *not* be used in those with creatinine clearances less than 50 mL/minute.

Hepatic Impairment Efavirenz dosage adjustments are not necessary in patients with mild hepatic impairment. Because efavirenz is extensively metabolized in the liver and because of limited clinical experience, the drug is not recommended in patients with moderate or severe hepatic impairment. (See Precautions Related to Hepatic Impairment and Hepatic Effects under Cautions: Precautions and Contraindications.)

When efavirenz/emtricitabine/tenofovir DF (Atripla®) is used, usual dosage can be used in patients with mild hepatic impairment; however, caution is advised. (See Precautions Related to Hepatic Impairment and Hepatic Effects under Cautions: Precautions and Contraindications.) The fixed combination should *not* be used in those with moderate or severe hepatic impairment.

Cautions

Information on the safety and efficacy of efavirenz has been obtained principally from phase 2 and 3 open-label studies in adults with asymptomatic or advanced human immunodeficiency virus (HIV) infection who received the recommended dosage of the drug in conjunction with HIV nucleoside reverse transcriptase inhibitors (NRTIs) and/or an HIV protease inhibitor (PI). Information also has been obtained from a phase 1 or 2 open-label study in HIV-infected children who received efavirenz in conjunction with nelfinavir and nucleoside antiretroviral agents.

The principal adverse effects of efavirenz in clinical studies include nervous system effects, psychiatric symptoms, and dermatologic effects. About 2.1% of adults receiving efavirenz in clinical trials discontinued the drug because of CNS effects and about 1.7 or 8.8% of adults or children 3–16 years of age, respectively, discontinued the drug because of rash.

Because many patients with HIV infection have serious underlying disease with multiple baseline symptomatology and clinical abnormalities and because many adverse effects that have been reported in patients receiving efavirenz also occur in HIV-infected patients not receiving the drug, a causal relationship between efavirenz and some adverse effects has not been established.

When the fixed combination containing efavirenz, emtricitabine, and tenofovir disoproxil fumarate (efavirenz/emtricitabine/tenofovir DF; Atripla®) is used, the adverse effects, precautions, and contraindications associated with each of the individual components should be considered. (See Precautions Related to Use of Fixed Combinations under Cautions: Precautions and Contraindications.)

■ Nervous System Effects and Psychiatric Symptoms

About 53% of adults receiving efavirenz (600 mg once daily) in controlled clinical studies reported adverse CNS effects such as abnormal dreams, abnormal thinking, agitation, amnesia, confusion, depersonalization, dizziness, euphoria, hallucinations, impaired concentration, insomnia, somnolence, and stupor; these adverse effects were reported in 25% of adults in the control groups not receiving efavirenz. These effects were described as mild (do not interfere with daily activities) in 33.3%, moderate (may interfere with daily activities) in 17.4%, or severe (interrupt usual daily activities) in 2% of patients receiving efavirenz and required discontinuance of the drug in 2.1%. Dizziness was reported in 28.1% and insomnia was reported in 16.3% of patients receiving the drug. Impaired concentration, somnolence, or abnormal dreams were reported in 6.2–8.3% and hallucinations were reported in 1.2% of patients. Treatment-emergent adverse CNS effects of moderate or severe intensity reported in adults receiving efavirenz in studies ACTG 364 and 006 include dizziness in 2–9%, insomnia in up to 7%, headache in 2–8%, impaired concentration in up to 5%, somnolence in up to 2%, and abnormal dreams in up to 3%. These adverse effects generally begin during the first 1–2 days of efavirenz therapy, improve with continued therapy, and usually resolve after the first 2–4 weeks of therapy. After 4 weeks of efavirenz therapy, the incidence of moderate or severe adverse CNS effects ranges from 5–9% in adults receiving efavirenz and 3–5% in those in the control groups not receiving the drug. Adverse CNS effects may be more tolerable if the daily dose of efavirenz is administered at bedtime.

Serious adverse psychiatric symptoms have been reported rarely in adults receiving efavirenz. Severe depression (2.4%), suicidal ideation (0.7%), nonfatal suicide attempts (0.5%), aggressive behavior (0.4%), paranoid reactions (0.4%), or manic reactions (0.2%) have been reported in patients receiving efavirenz in controlled clinical studies; these psychiatric symptoms were reported in up to 0.9% of those in the control groups not receiving the drug. Analysis of data from clinical studies indicates that treatment with efavirenz is associated with an increased occurrence of these psychiatric symptoms. Other factors associated with an increased occurrence of these psychiatric symptoms were a history of drug use (injection), history of psychiatric disorders, and treatment with an antipsychotic drug at study entry. Other psychiatric symptoms reported in controlled clinical studies in adults receiving efavirenz include depression (19%), anxiety (13%), and nervousness (7%); these symptoms were reported in 16, 9, or 2%, respectively, of those in the control groups not receiving the drug. Although a causal relationship with efavirenz has not been established, there have been occasional postmarketing reports of delusions, psychosis-like behavior, catatonia, and death by suicide in patients receiving efavirenz. In addition, aggressive reactions, agitation, emotional lability, mania, neurosis, and paranoia have been reported during postmarketing surveillance.

Seizures have been reported in adults and pediatric patients receiving efavirenz; seizures generally have occurred in patients with a history of seizures. Fatigue has been reported in up to 8% of adults receiving efavirenz in clinical studies.

Adverse nervous system effects reported during postmarketing surveillance include abnormal coordination, ataxia, hypoesthesia, paresthesia, neuropathy, and tremor.

Adverse CNS effects occurred in 18% of children receiving efavirenz in clinical studies.

■ Dermatologic and Sensitivity Reactions

Rash has occurred in 26% of adults receiving efavirenz in clinical studies and in 17% of adults in control groups not receiving the drug. Although treatment-emergent rash generally manifests as mild to moderate maculopapular skin eruptions (NCI grade 1 and 2 reactions), rash associated with blistering, moist desquamation, or ulceration (NCI grade 3 reaction) has been reported in about 1% of adults receiving efavirenz in clinical studies. The incidence of grade 4 rash (e.g., erythema multiforme, Stevens-Johnson syndrome) in patients receiving efavirenz in clinical studies or in the expanded access program has been reported to be 0.1%.

Rash occurs more frequently in children than adults and has been reported in 32% of patients 3 months to 21 years of age receiving efavirenz in clinical studies. NCI grade 3 rash occurred in 1.1%, and grade 4 rash and erythema multiforme occurred in 2.2% of pediatric patients.

Treatment-emergent rash generally occurs within the first 2 weeks of efavirenz therapy; median time to onset of rash in clinical studies in adults or children was 11 or 28 days, respectively. In most patients who continued efavirenz treatment, the rash resolves within 1 month (median duration 16 days).

Pruritus has been reported in up to 9% of patients receiving efavirenz in clinical studies. Other adverse dermatologic and sensitivity reactions occurring in postmarketing reports include allergic reaction, erythema multiforme, photoallergic dermatitis, and Stevens-Johnson syndrome.

Efavirenz should be discontinued in patients with life-threatening cutaneous reactions (e.g., Stevens-Johnson syndrome) and alternative therapy considered.

Although the drug should be discontinued in patients who experience serious rash (i.e., rash associated with blistering, desquamation, mucosal involvement, or fever), mild to moderate rash resolves in most patients within 1 month with continued efavirenz therapy. The median duration of rash in adults is 16 days.

Antihistamines and/or corticosteroids may improve tolerability and hasten resolution of rash. Therapy with efavirenz can be reinitiated in patients who temporarily interrupted therapy with the drug because of development of a rash. Although prophylaxis with antihistamines prior to initiating efavirenz in children can be considered, the efficacy of such a strategy for prevention of rash has not been determined.

Limited information is available on use of efavirenz in patients who discontinued nevirapine because of rash. When efavirenz was initiated in 19 patients who previously discontinued nevirapine because of rash, mild to moderate rash occurred in 9 of these patients while receiving efavirenz. In at least 2 adults who had experienced severe hypersensitivity reactions while receiving nevirapine, initiation of efavirenz with concomitant corticosteroid therapy (an 11-day prednisone regimen involving decreasing dosage) resulted in a mild rash in one patient but allowed use of efavirenz without any severe hypersensitivity reactions.

■ **Hepatic Effects** Substantial increases in serum concentrations of AST (SGOT) or ALT (SGPT) (more than 5 times the upper limit of normal) occurred in 2–8% of evaluated adults receiving efavirenz in clinical studies; the frequency of increases in AST or ALT in patients receiving efavirenz was similar to that in patients receiving regimens that did not include efavirenz. In patients who were seropositive for hepatitis B virus (HBV) and/or hepatitis C virus (HCV), substantial increases in serum concentrations of AST or ALT (more than 5 times the upper limit of normal) occurred in 13 or 20%, respectively, of adults receiving efavirenz and in 7 or 7%, respectively, of adults receiving regimens that did not include efavirenz.

Increases in γ-glutamyltransferase (GGT, GGPT) (more than 5 times the upper limit of normal) occurred in 5–8% of patients receiving efavirenz in clinical studies; the frequency of increases in GGT in patients receiving efavirenz was similar to that in patients receiving regimens that did not include efavirenz.

There have been postmarketing reports of hepatic failure and hepatitis in patients receiving efavirenz. A few cases of hepatic failure, including some in patients with no preexisting hepatic disease or other identifiable risk factors, were characterized by a fulminant course and required transplantation or resulted in death.

■ **GI Effects** Moderate or severe GI effects have been reported in up to 14% of adults receiving efavirenz in clinical studies. Nausea or diarrhea occurred in 2–14%, vomiting in up to 7%, dyspepsia in up to 3%, abdominal pain in 1–3%, and anorexia in up to 2% of patients receiving the drug. In addition, constipation and malabsorption have been reported during postmarketing surveillance.

■ **Cardiovascular and Lipid Effects** Prolongation of the QT interval corrected for rate (QT_c) has been reported in patients receiving efavirenz.

While the clinical importance remains to be determined, total serum cholesterol concentrations have been increased 10–20% in healthy individuals receiving efavirenz. In patients receiving a 3-drug regimen of efavirenz, zidovudine, and lamivudine, serum concentrations of nonfasting total cholesterol or high-density lipoprotein (HDL) cholesterol were increased approximately 20 or 25%, respectively; in patients receiving a 2-drug regimen of efavirenz and indinavir, these serum concentrations were increased approximately 40 or 35%, respectively. The effects of efavirenz on triglycerides and low-density lipoprotein (LDL) were not well characterized since serum samples were obtained under nonfasting conditions.

Flushing and palpitations have been reported during postmarketing surveillance.

■ **Immune Reconstitution Syndrome** Patients receiving antiretroviral therapy may experience an immune reconstitution syndrome during the initial phase of therapy. Patients whose immune system responds to antiretroviral therapy may develop an inflammatory response to indolent or residual opportunistic infections (e.g., *Mycobacterium avium* complex [MAC], *M. tuberculosis*, cytomegalovirus [CMV], *Pneumocystis jirovecii* [formerly *P. carinii*]); this may necessitate further evaluation and treatment.

Autoimmune disorders (e.g., Graves' disease, polymyositis, Guillain-Barré syndrome) have also been reported to occur in the setting of immune reconstitution; the time to onset is more variable and can occur many months after initiation of antiretroviral therapy.

■ **Adipogenic Effects** Redistribution or accumulation of body fat, including central obesity, dorsocervical fat enlargement ("buffalo hump"), peripheral wasting, facial wasting, breast enlargement, and cushingoid appearance have been reported in patients receiving antiretroviral therapy. The mechanisms and long-term consequences of these adipogenic effects are unknown. A causal relationship has not been established.

■ **Other Adverse Effects** Although a causal relationship has not been established, pancreatitis has been reported in a few patients receiving efavirenz. In addition, asymptomatic increases in serum amylase concentrations to greater than 1.5 times the upper limit of normal have been reported in 10% of patients receiving efavirenz compared with 6% of patients in control groups not receiving the drug.

In a clinical study (study 006), lipodystrophy occurred in 2.3% of patients receiving efavirenz and indinavir, 0.7% of patients receiving efavirenz, zidovudine, and lamivudine, and 1% of patients receiving indinavir, zidovudine, and lamivudine without efavirenz.

Moderate or severe pain has been reported in 1–13% of patients receiving efavirenz in clinical studies. Other adverse effects reported in patients receiving efavirenz during postmarketing surveillance include abnormal vision, arthralgia, asthenia, dyspnea, gynecomastia, myalgia, myopathy, and tinnitus.

■ **Precautions and Contraindications** Efavirenz is contraindicated in patients who have had a clinically important hypersensitivity reaction (e.g., Stevens-Johnson syndrome, erythema multiforme, toxic skin eruption) to efavirenz or any other ingredient in the formulation.

Fetal/Neonatal Morbidity and Mortality Because efavirenz may cause fetal harm if administered during the first trimester of pregnancy, women of childbearing potential should undergo pregnancy testing before efavirenz or efavirenz/emtricitabine/tenofovir DF is initiated and measures should be taken to avoid pregnancy during and for 12 weeks after therapy with efavirenz is discontinued. (See Cautions: Pregnancy, Fertility, and Lactation.)

Interactions Plasma concentrations of efavirenz may be altered if used concomitantly with drugs that are substrates, inhibitors, or inducers of cytochrome P-450 (CYP) 3A. (See Drug Interactions.)

Efavirenz induces CYP3A and 2B6 and may alter plasma concentrations of drugs metabolized by these enzymes. (See Drug Interactions.)

Precautions Related to Nervous System Effects and Psychiatric Symptoms Patients should be informed that adverse CNS effects (e.g., dizziness, insomnia, impaired concentration, somnolence, abnormal dreams) may occur during the first few weeks of efavirenz therapy and that the drug may impair their ability to perform hazardous activities requiring mental alertness or physical coordination such as operating machinery or driving a motor vehicle. In addition, patients receiving efavirenz should be informed that there is a potential for additive CNS effects if they use efavirenz concomitantly with psychoactive drugs or alcohol.

Serious psychiatric symptoms (e.g., severe depression, suicidal ideation, nonfatal suicide attempts, aggressive behavior, delusions, paranoia, manic or psychosis-like reactions) have been reported rarely in patients receiving efavirenz. Patients should be asked about any history of mental illness or substance abuse prior to initiation of efavirenz and should be advised to immediately seek medical evaluation if they experience severe psychiatric symptoms while receiving the drug. If it appears that the psychiatric symptoms may possibly be related to use of efavirenz, a determination should be made whether the drug should be discontinued after weighing the risks and benefits of continued therapy.

Seizures have occurred in patients receiving efavirenz, generally in those with a history of seizures. Caution is advised if the drug is used in patients with a history of seizures. In patients receiving anticonvulsants that are metabolized principally by the liver (e.g., phenytoin, phenobarbital), anticonvulsant plasma concentrations should be monitored. (See Anticonvulsants under Drug Interactions: CNS Agents.)

Precautions Related to Hepatic Impairment and Hepatic Effects Because efavirenz is extensively metabolized in the liver and because of limited clinical experience in patients with hepatic impairment, the manufacturer states that the drug should be used with caution in such patients. Efavirenz can be used with caution in patients with mild hepatic impairment without any dosage adjustments; however, the drugs are not recommended in patients with moderate or severe hepatic impairment since data are insufficient to determine whether dosage adjustments are necessary.

Serum liver enzyme concentrations should be assessed prior to and during efavirenz treatment in patients with underlying hepatic disease (including those with HBV and/or HCV infection), patients with markedly increased serum transaminase concentrations, and patients receiving other drugs associated with liver toxicity. Monitoring serum liver enzyme concentrations also should be considered in patients without preexisting hepatic dysfunction or other risk factors.

In patients with serum hepatic enzyme concentrations more than 5 times the upper limit of normal, the benefits of continued efavirenz therapy versus the risks of hepatotoxicity should be considered.

Precautions Related to Cardiovascular Effects Because QT_c interval prolongation has been reported with efavirenz, an alternative antiretroviral should be considered in patients at higher risk of torsades de pointes and in patients receiving a drug known to increase the risk of torsades de pointes. (See Drug Interactions.)

Precautions Related to Use of Fixed Combinations When efavirenz/emtricitabine/tenofovir DF is used, the cautions, precautions, contraindications, and drug interactions associated with each drug in the fixed combination must be considered. Cautionary information applicable to specific populations (e.g., pregnant or nursing women, individuals with hepatic or renal impairment, geriatric patients) should be considered for each drug. For cautionary information related to emtricitabine and tenofovir DF, see Cautions in the individual drug monographs.

Efavirenz/emtricitabine/tenofovir DF should not be used concomitantly with single-entity efavirenz, unless needed for adjustment of efavirenz dosage (e.g., when the fixed combination is used concomitantly with rifampin). (See Rifampin under Drug Interactions: Antimycobacterial Agents.)

Because the antiretroviral agents contained in efavirenz/emtricitabine/tenofovir DF also are available in single-entity or other fixed-combination preparations, care should be taken to ensure that therapy is not duplicated if the fixed combination is used in conjunction with other antiretroviral agents.

Efavirenz/emtricitabine/tenofovir DF should not be used concomitantly with any preparation containing emtricitabine or tenofovir DF. In addition, because of similarities between emtricitabine and lamivudine, the fixed combination should not be used concomitantly with any preparation containing lamivudine or with adefovir dipivoxil.

If efavirenz/emtricitabine/tenofovir DF is used, clinicians should consider that lactic acidosis and severe hepatomegaly with steatosis, including fatalities, have been reported in patients receiving NRTIs in conjunction with other antiretrovirals.

If efavirenz/emtricitabine/tenofovir DF is used, clinicians should consider that severe, acute HBV infection has been reported following discontinuance of emtricitabine or tenofovir DF in HIV-infected patients coinfected with HBV. The fixed combination is not labeled by the US Food and Drug Administration for treatment of chronic HBV infection, and safety and efficacy have not been established in HIV-infected patients coinfected with HBV. Patients should be closely monitored with both clinical and laboratory follow-up for at least several months after the fixed combination is discontinued in coinfected patients. If appropriate, initiation of HBV treatment may be warranted.

Other Precautions Because increased serum concentrations of total cholesterol and triglycerides have been reported in patients receiving efavirenz, cholesterol and triglyceride testing should be performed prior to and at periodic intervals during efavirenz therapy.

Patients should be advised that rash is a common side effect of efavirenz and, although rash usually goes away without any treatment change, it may be serious. Therefore, patients should promptly contact a clinician is rash occurs.

Redistribution or accumulation of body fat, including central obesity, dorsocervical fat enlargement (buffalo hump), peripheral wasting, facial wasting, breast enlargement, and general cushingoid appearance, have been reported in patients receiving antiretroviral therapy. The mechanisms responsible for these adipogenic effects and the long-term consequences of these effects are unknown. A causal relationship has not been established. Patients receiving efavirenz should be informed that redistribution or accumulation of body fat may occur in patients receiving antiretroviral therapy and that the cause and long-term consequences of these adipogenic effects are not known.

Patients should be informed that efavirenz in conjunction with other antiretroviral agents is not a cure for HIV infection and that opportunistic infections and other complications associated with HIV disease may still occur. Patients receiving efavirenz should be under close clinical observation by clinicians experienced in treatment of diseases associated with HIV infection, and patients should be advised to seek medical care if any clinically important change in their health status occurs. Patients receiving antiretroviral therapy must be continuously evaluated and therapeutic modifications made as appropriate.

Patients should be advised that effective antiretroviral regimens can decrease HIV concentrations in blood and genital secretions and strict adherence to such regimens in conjunction with risk-reduction measures may decrease, but cannot absolutely eliminate, the risk of secondary transmission of HIV to others. Patients should continue to practice safer sex (e.g., use latex or polyurethane condoms to minimize sexual contact with body fluids), never share personal items that can have blood or body fluids on them (e.g., toothbrushes, razor blades), and never reuse or share needles.

■ **Pediatric Precautions** Safety and efficacy of single-entity efavirenz (Sustiva®) have not been established in neonates and infants younger than 3 months of age or in those weighing less than 3.5 kg, and the drug should not be used in these pediatric patients. Some experts state that efavirenz is *not* recommended for *initial* treatment in antiretroviral-naive pediatric patients 3 months to less than 3 years of age.

Efavirenz/emtricitabine/tenofovir DF (Atripla®) should *not* be used in pediatric patients younger than 12 years of age or in those weighing less than 40 kg.

Adverse effects reported in pediatric patients 3 months to 21 years of age receiving efavirenz are similar to those reported in adults receiving the drug and include rash and adverse CNS and GI effects. Rash has been reported more frequently in children than adults (32 versus 26%) and the incidence of moderate to severe rash (NCI grade 3 or 4) has been greater in children than adults. Because of the high incidence of dermatologic reactions in children, antihistamines may be considered for the prevention of rash when initiating efavirenz in children; however, the efficacy of such a strategy has not been determined.

Efavirenz is not recommended in sexually active adolescent females of childbearing potential who desire to become pregnant or when reliable contraception cannot be ensured. (See Pregnancy under Cautions: Pregnancy, Fertility, and Lactation.)

■ **Geriatric Precautions** Safety and efficacy of efavirenz have not been evaluated systematically in geriatric patients. Dosage for geriatric patients should be selected carefully because of limited experience in this age group and because these individuals frequently have decreased hepatic, renal, and/or cardiac function and concomitant disease and drug therapy.

■ **Mutagenicity and Carcinogenicity** Efavirenz was not mutagenic or genotoxic in several in vitro and in vivo genotoxicity assays, including *Salmonella typhimurium* and *Escherichia coli* bacterial mutation assays, mammalian mutation assays in Chinese hamster ovary cells, chromosomal aberration assays in human peripheral blood lymphocytes or Chinese hamster ovary cells, and a mouse bone marrow micronucleus assay.

The carcinogenic potential of efavirenz has been evaluated in long-term studies in mice and rats. The incidence of hepatocellular adenomas and carcinomas and pulmonary alveolar/bronchiolar adenomas was increased above background rates in female mice but not in male mice. In rats, no increase in tumor incidence above background was observed at efavirenz exposure that were 0.1 (males) or 0.2 (females) times the human exposure at recommended dosages of the drug.

■ **Pregnancy, Fertility, and Lactation** ***Pregnancy*** Efavirenz may cause fetal harm if administered during the first trimester of pregnancy; however, some experts state that the relative risk with first-trimester exposure is unclear. There are retrospective case reports of neural tube defects in infants born to mothers who were exposed to efavirenz during the first trimester of pregnancy, but prospective pregnancy data are not sufficient to adequately assess this risk.

Reproduction studies in cynomolgus monkeys using efavirenz dosages of 60 mg/kg daily throughout pregnancy (gestation days 20–150) resulted in maternal efavirenz systemic exposure levels 1.3 times those reported with the recommended human dosage and fetal umbilical venous concentrations approximately 0.7 times maternal concentrations and malformations (i.e., anencephaly and unilateral anophthalmia, microphthalmia, cleft palate) in 3 of 20 fetuses/offspring. In rats, an efavirenz dosage of 200 mg/kg daily was associated with an increased incidence of early resorptions and 100 mg/kg daily was associated with early neonatal mortality. Reproduction studies in rabbits have not revealed evidence of harm to the fetus. Efavirenz crosses the placenta in cynomolgus monkeys, rats, and rabbits, and produces fetal blood concentrations in these species that are similar to maternal blood concentrations.

To monitor maternal-fetal outcomes of pregnant women exposed to antiretroviral agents, including efavirenz, the Antiretroviral Pregnancy Registry was established. Clinicians are encouraged to contact the registry at 800-258-4263 or http://www.APRegistry.com to report cases of prenatal exposure to antiretroviral agents.

Based on prospective reports from the Antiretroviral Pregnancy Registry of approximately 1000 live births following exposure to efavirenz (including more than 800 live births following first-trimester exposures), there was no difference between overall birth defects with efavirenz compared with the background birth defect rate (2.7% in the US reference population of the Metropolitan Atlanta Congenital Defects Program). An interim report issued in December 2014 that used data from the registry indicated that the prevalence of birth defects was 2.3% following first-trimester exposures to efavirenz. Defects reported prospectively in first-trimester exposures included a case of myelomeningocele and a case of anophthalmia that included severe oblique facial clefts and amniotic banding. There also have been at least 6 retrospective reports of CNS defects, including myelomeningocele, and all involved exposures during the first trimester. Although a causal relationship between efavirenz and these defects has not been established, similar defects were observed in preclinical studies of the drug.

A meta-analysis of data from 23 studies that included 2026 reports of live births following first-trimester exposures to efavirenz found no increased risk of overall birth defects in infants born to women receiving efavirenz during the first trimester compared with those receiving other antiretrovirals. However, the number of reported first trimester exposures remains insufficient to rule out a significant increase in low-incidence birth defects (incidence of neural tube defects in the general US population is 0.02–0.2%).

Women of childbearing potential should be advised about the teratogenic potential of efavirenz and should not receive single-entity efavirenz or efavirenz/emtricitabine/tenofovir DF until pregnancy is excluded. Such women should undergo pregnancy testing before initiation of therapy and should be instructed to avoid pregnancy during and for 12 weeks after discontinuance of therapy with efavirenz or efavirenz/emtricitabine/tenofovir DF and to notify a clinician if they desire to become pregnant or become pregnant while receiving a regimen containing efavirenz. Women of childbearing potential should use a reliable method of barrier contraception in addition to or instead of a hormonal contraceptive (oral or other hormonal contraceptive) while receiving efavirenz and for 12 weeks after the drug is discontinued. Hormonal contraceptives containing progesterone may have decreased effectiveness when used concomitantly with efavirenz. (See Drug Interactions: Estrogens and Progestins.)

The manufacturer states that efavirenz should not be used during the first trimester of pregnancy.

The US Department of Health and Human Services (HHS) Panel on Treatment of HIV-infected Pregnant Women and Prevention of Perinatal Transmission states that efavirenz in conjunction with 2 NRTIs is an alternative NNRTI-based regimen for *initial* treatment in antiretroviral-naive pregnant women, but may be a preferred NNRTI-based regimen for *initial* treatment in pregnant women when drug interactions with PI-based regimens are a concern or when the convenience of a fixed-combination, single-tablet, once-daily regimen is advantageous. However, these experts state that efavirenz should be avoided during the first 8 weeks of pregnancy. These experts also state that antiretroviral regimens that do not include efavirenz should be strongly considered in women who are planning to become pregnant or are sexually active and not using effective contraception, provided such regimens are acceptable to the provider and not expected to compromise the health of the woman.

If a pregnant woman already receiving an efavirenz-based regimen presents for antenatal care during the first trimester of pregnancy, the HHS panel suggests that the regimen can be continued if it is well tolerated and providing adequate virologic suppression. This strategy recognizes that the risk of neural tube defects is restricted to the first 5–6 weeks of pregnancy and pregnancy is rarely recognized until after 4–6 weeks, and that unnecessary changes in antiretroviral regimens during pregnancy may be associated with loss of virologic control and an increased risk of perinatal HIV transmission.

If efavirenz or a fixed combination containing efavirenz is used during the first trimester, or if the patient becomes pregnant while taking the drug, she should be apprised of the potential harm to the fetus.

Fertility Reproductive studies in rats have not revealed evidence of impaired fertility or reproductive performance in males or females receiving efavirenz and the drug did not affect male sperm. The reproductive performance of offspring of female rats given efavirenz was not affected.

Lactation Efavirenz is distributed into human milk

Because of the risk of transmission of HIV to an uninfected infant through breast milk, the US Centers for Disease Control and Prevention (CDC) and other experts recommend that HIV-infected women *not* breast-feed infants, regardless of antiretroviral therapy. Therefore, because of the potential for HIV transmission and the potential for serious adverse effects from efavirenz in infants if the drug were distributed into milk, women should be instructed not to breast-feed while they are receiving efavirenz.

Drug Interactions

The following drug interactions are based on studies using efavirenz. Drug interaction studies have not been performed using the fixed combination containing efavirenz, emtricitabine, and tenofovir disoproxil fumarate (efavirenz/emtricitabine/tenofovir DF; Atripla®). When efavirenz/emtricitabine/tenofovir DF is used, interactions associated with each drug in the fixed combination should be considered.

■ **Drugs Affecting or Metabolized by Hepatic Microsomal Enzymes** Metabolism of efavirenz is mediated principally by cytochrome P-450 (CYP) isoenzymes 3A and 2B6, and drugs that induce these isoenzymes are expected to reduce efavirenz plasma concentrations. Efavirenz has been shown to induce CYP enzymes resulting in induction of its own metabolism. Efavirenz induces CYP3A and 2B6, and may alter plasma concentrations of drugs metabolized by these enzymes.

In vitro, efavirenz inhibits CYP isoenzymes 2C9 and 2C19 (K_i values 8.5–17 μM) at clinically important concentrations, and the possibility exists that efavirenz may alter the pharmacokinetics of drugs metabolized by these isoenzymes. In vitro studies indicate that efavirenz does not inhibit the CYP isoenzyme 2E1 and is a weak inhibitor of 2D6 and 1A2 (K_i values of 82–160 μM).

■ **Anticoagulants** Concomitant use of efavirenz and warfarin is predicted to alter plasma warfarin concentrations resulting in increased or decreased effects of the anticoagulant. The international normalized ratio (INR) should be monitored in patients receiving efavirenz and warfarin concomitantly and warfarin dosage adjusted accordingly.

■ **Antifungal Agents** ***Fluconazole*** Concomitant use of fluconazole (200 mg daily) and efavirenz (400 mg daily) for 7 days in healthy individuals did not result in clinically important changes in the pharmacokinetics of either drug, and dosage adjustments are not necessary in patients receiving the drugs concomitantly.

Isavuconazonium Concomitant use of isavuconazonium sulfate (prodrug of isavuconazole) and efavirenz may result in decreased isavuconazole concentrations.

If isavuconazonium sulfate and efavirenz are used concomitantly, isavuconazole concentration monitoring should be considered and the patient should be monitored for antifungal efficacy. Adjustment of isavuconazonium sulfate dosage may be necessary.

Itraconazole Concomitant use of itraconazole (200 mg every 12 hours for 28 days) and efavirenz (600 mg once daily for 14 days) reduced peak plasma concentrations of itraconazole by 37% and the area under the plasma concentration-time curve (AUC) by 39%; there was no change in the peak plasma concentration or AUC of efavirenz. Failure to achieve therapeutic itraconazole concentrations has been reported in patients receiving efavirenz.

The manufacturer of efavirenz states that dosage recommendations for concomitant use of efavirenz and itraconazole are not available, and an alternative antifungal should be considered. Some experts state that concomitant use of itraconazole and efavirenz should be avoided; if the drugs are used concomitantly, plasma concentrations of itraconazole should be monitored closely and dosage of the antifungal adjusted accordingly.

Ketoconazole Although specific drug interaction studies with efavirenz and ketoconazole have not been performed to date, the possibility exists that efavirenz may decrease plasma concentrations of this antifungal.

Posaconazole Concomitant use of posaconazole (400 mg twice daily) and efavirenz (400 mg once daily) reduces peak plasma concentrations and AUC of posaconazole by 45 and 50%, respectively, but does not affect efavirenz concentrations.

Concomitant use of posaconazole and efavirenz should be avoided unless potential benefits outweigh risks. If the drugs are used concomitantly, plasma concentrations of posaconazole should be monitored and dosage of the antifungal adjusted accordingly.

Voriconazole Concomitant use of voriconazole (400 mg every 12 hours for 1 day, then 200 mg every 12 hours for 8 days) and efavirenz (400 mg once daily for 9 days) reduced peak plasma concentrations and AUC of voriconazole by 61 and 77%, respectively, and increased peak plasma concentrations and AUC of efavirenz by 38 and 44%, respectively.

If efavirenz and voriconazole are used concomitantly, the maintenance dosage of voriconazole should be increased to 400 mg every 12 hours and the efavirenz dosage should be reduced to 300 mg once daily. The 300-mg dose of efavirenz should be administered using the capsule preparations; the 600-mg tablet should not be broken in half in order to provide a 300-mg dose. Usual dosage of voriconazole and usual dosage of efavirenz should not be used concomitantly.

Concomitant use of voriconazole and the fixed combination efavirenz/emtricitabine/tenofovir DF is contraindicated.

■ **Antihistamine Drugs** Administration of cetirizine (10 mg as a single dose) and efavirenz (600 mg daily for 10 days) decreased the peak plasma concentration of cetirizine by 24% but had no substantial effect on the area under the plasma concentration time curve (AUC) of efavirenz. The manufacturer of efavirenz states that dosage adjustments are not necessary in patients receiving concomitant cetirizine.

■ **Antimalarial Agents** ***Artemether and Lumefantrine*** Concomitant use of the fixed combination of artemether and lumefantrine (artemether/lumefantrine) and efavirenz decreases plasma concentrations and AUC of artemether and the active metabolite of artemether (dihydroartemisinin) and decreases the AUC of lumefantrine.

Because of the risk of QT interval prolongation, the manufacturer of efavirenz states that alternatives to artemether/lumefantrine should be considered in patients receiving efavirenz. Some experts state that if artemether/lumefantrine and efavirenz are used concomitantly, the patient should be closely monitored for antimalarial efficacy and malaria recurrence.

Atovaquone and Proguanil Concomitant use of efavirenz and the fixed combination of atovaquone and proguanil (atovaquone/proguanil) decreases the AUC of atovaquone and proguanil.

Concomitant use of atovaquone/proguanil and efavirenz is not recommended. Some experts state that dosage recommendations are not available for concomitant use of atovaquone/proguanil and that alternatives to that fixed combination should be considered for malaria prophylaxis, if possible.

■ **Antimycobacterial Agents** ***Bedaquiline*** Concomitant use of bedaquiline and efavirenz may result in decreased bedaquiline concentrations.

Concomitant use of bedaquiline and efavirenz is not recommended.

Rifabutin Concomitant use of efavirenz and rifabutin has resulted in decreased plasma concentration of rifabutin and 25-*O*-desacetylrifabutin (an active metabolite). In a limited number of healthy individuals, concomitant use of rifabutin (300 mg once daily) and efavirenz (600 mg once daily) for 10–14 days reduced the peak plasma rifabutin concentration by 32% and the AUC of the drug by 38%; there was no change in the peak plasma concentration or AUC of efavirenz.

Because of this pharmacokinetic interaction, the manufacturer of efavirenz recommends that rifabutin dosage be increased by 50% and that doubling of rifabutin daily dosage be considered when the antimycobacterial agent is given 2 or 3 times weekly. Some clinicians suggest that rifabutin dosage be increased to 450–600 mg once daily or 600 mg 3 times weekly in patients receiving efavirenz, provided an HIV protease inhibitor (PI) is not included in the regimen.

Rifampin Concomitant use of efavirenz and rifampin has resulted in decreased plasma efavirenz concentrations and AUC. In a limited number of healthy individuals, concomitant use of rifampin (600 mg daily) and efavirenz (600 mg daily) for 7 days reduced peak plasma efavirenz concentrations by 20% and the AUC of the drug by 26%; there was no change in the peak plasma concentration or AUC of rifampin. The clinical importance of these reduced plasma efavirenz concentrations remains to be determined.

If efavirenz is used in conjunction with rifampin in patients weighing 50 kg or more, the manufacturer of efavirenz recommends that efavirenz dosage be increased to 800 mg once daily. Some experts suggest that an efavirenz dosage of 600 mg once daily can be used in patients weighing less than 60 kg if virologic response is monitored and therapeutic drug monitoring considered; these experts state that efavirenz dosage should be increased to 800 mg once daily in those weighing more than 60 kg.

If the fixed combination efavirenz/emtricitabine/tenofovir DF is used in patients receiving rifampin, the manufacturer recommends that those weighing at least 50 kg receive 1 tablet of the fixed combination (600 mg of efavirenz, 200 mg of emtricitabine, and 300 mg of tenofovir DF) once daily *and* 200 mg of single-entity efavirenz once daily to provide a total efavirenz dosage of 800 mg daily.

Rifapentine Efavirenz and rifapentine should not be used concomitantly. HIV-infected tuberculosis patients treated with rifapentine have a higher rate of tuberculosis relapse than those treated with other rifamycin-based tuberculosis regimens; an alternative antimycobacterial agent is recommended in HIV patients.

■ **Antiretroviral Agents** ***HIV Entry and Fusion Inhibitors***

Enfuvirtide. There is in vitro evidence of additive to synergistic antiretroviral effects between enfuvirtide and efavirenz.

Maraviroc. Concomitant use of maraviroc and efavirenz results in clinically important decreases in plasma maraviroc concentrations and AUC. If maraviroc is used concomitantly with efavirenz, the recommended dosage of maraviroc is 600 mg twice daily, provided the regimen does *not* include a potent CYP3A inhibitor.

There is no in vitro evidence of antagonistic antiretroviral effects between maraviroc and efavirenz.

HIV Integrase Inhibitors (INSTIs) **Dolutegravir.** Concomitant use of dolutegravir and efavirenz decreases plasma concentrations and AUC of dolutegravir, but does not appear to affect the pharmacokinetics of efavirenz.

If efavirenz is used concurrently with dolutegravir in adults or pediatric patients weighing 40 kg or more who are antiretroviral-naive or antiretroviral-experienced but INSTI-naive, dolutegravir should be given in a dosage of 50 mg twice daily. If efavirenz is used concurrently with dolutegravir in pediatric patients weighing 30 kg to less than 40 kg who are antiretroviral-naive or antiretroviral-experienced but INSTI-naive, dolutegravir should be given in a dosage of 35 mg twice daily. Whenever possible, an alternative to efavirenz that is not a metabolic inducer should be considered when dolutegravir is used in INSTI-experienced patients who have HIV-1 with documented or suspected INSTI resistance.

There is no in vitro evidence of antagonistic antiretroviral effects between dolutegravir and efavirenz.

Elvitegravir. Concomitant use of *cobicistat-boosted* elvitegravir and efavirenz may result in altered concentrations of elvitegravir, cobicistat, and efavirenz.

Cobicistat-boosted elvitegravir and efavirenz should not be used concomitantly.

Raltegravir. Concomitant use of raltegravir and efavirenz results in decreased plasma concentrations and AUC of raltegravir; these effects are not considered clinically important. Dosage adjustments are not necessary if raltegravir is used concomitantly with efavirenz.

There is in vitro evidence of additive to synergistic antiretroviral effects between raltegravir and efavirenz.

HIV Nonnucleoside Reverse Transcriptase Inhibitors (NNRTIs) Concomitant use of efavirenz and other NNRTIs (delavirdine, etravirine, nevirapine, rilpivirine) is *not* recommended.

Concomitant use of efavirenz and etravirine may result in decreased etravirine concentrations and loss of therapeutic effect.

Concomitant use of efavirenz and nevirapine results in decreased efavirenz concentrations and AUC; nevirapine concentrations are not affected. An increased incidence of adverse effects and no improvement in efficacy has been reported when these NNRTIs were used concomitantly.

Concomitant use of efavirenz and rilpivirine may result in decreased plasma rilpivirine concentrations.

HIV Nucleoside and Nucleotide Reverse Transcriptase Inhibitors (NRTIs) Results of in vitro studies using some NRTIs (e.g., abacavir, didanosine, emtricitabine, lamivudine, stavudine, tenofovir, zidovudine) indicate that the antiretroviral effects of efavirenz and these drugs are additive to synergistic against HIV-1.

Concomitant use of efavirenz (600 mg once daily for 14 days) and zidovudine (300 mg every 12 hours for 14 days) or lamivudine (150 mg every 12 hours for 14 days) does not affect plasma concentrations or AUCs of the NRTIs. Concomitant use of tenofovir DF and efavirenz does not affect plasma concentrations or AUCs of either drug. Clinically important pharmacokinetic interactions between efavirenz and other NRTIs (abacavir, emtricitabine, stavudine, tenofovir DF) are not expected.

Dosage adjustments are not necessary if efavirenz is used concomitantly with abacavir, emtricitabine, lamivudine, stavudine, tenofovir DF, or zidovudine.

Concomitant use of didanosine and efavirenz/emtricitabine/tenofovir DF should be undertaken with caution and patients should be monitored closely for didanosine-associated adverse effects (e.g., pancreatitis, lactic acidosis, neuropathy).

HIV Protease Inhibitors (PIs) Clinically important pharmacokinetic interactions may occur when efavirenz is used with some PIs.

Results of in vitro studies indicate that the antiretroviral effects of efavirenz and some PIs (amprenavir [active metabolite of fosamprenavir], indinavir, lopinavir, nelfinavir, ritonavir, saquinavir, tipranavir) are additive to synergistic against HIV-1. There is no in vitro evidence of antagonistic antiretroviral effects between efavirenz and atazanavir or darunavir.

Atazanavir. Concomitant use of unboosted atazanavir (without low-dose ritonavir or cobicistat) and efavirenz results in substantially decreased plasma concentration and AUC of atazanavir, but no clinically important effect on efavirenz concentrations. Depending on the specific regimen used, concomitant use of *ritonavir-boosted* atazanavir and efavirenz may increase atazanavir plasma concentrations and AUC. Concomitant use of *cobicistat-boosted* atazanavir with efavirenz results in decreased plasma concentrations of atazanavir and cobicistat, but no change in efavirenz concentrations.

Unboosted atazanavir (without low-dose ritonavir or cobicistat) should not be used concomitantly with efavirenz in antiretroviral-naive or antiretroviral-experienced patients.

If *ritonavir-boosted* atazanavir is used concomitantly with efavirenz in antiretroviral-naive adults, a regimen of atazanavir 400 mg and ritonavir 100 mg once daily (with food) and efavirenz 600 mg once daily (without food, preferably at bedtime) is recommended. *Ritonavir-boosted* atazanavir should not be used concomitantly with efavirenz in antiretroviral-experienced patients.

If *cobicistat-boosted* atazanavir is used concomitantly with efavirenz in antiretroviral-naive adults, a regimen of single-entity atazanavir 400 mg and single-entity cobicistat 150 mg once daily (with food) and efavirenz 600 mg once daily (without food, preferably at bedtime) is recommended. *Cobicistat-boosted* atazanavir should not be used concomitantly with efavirenz in antiretroviral-experienced patients.

Concomitant use of atazanavir (with or without low-dose ritonavir) and the fixed combination efavirenz/emtricitabine/tenofovir DF is not recommended; data are insufficient to make dosage recommendations.

Darunavir. Concomitant use of *ritonavir-boosted* darunavir (darunavir 300 mg and ritonavir 100 mg twice daily) and efavirenz (600 mg once daily) increased the AUC of efavirenz by 21% and decreased the AUC of darunavir by 13%. The clinical importance of this interaction remains to be established. Concomitant use of *cobicistat-boosted* darunavir and efavirenz may result in decreased darunavir and cobicistat concentrations and may result in loss of therapeutic effect and development of darunavir resistance.

If *ritonavir-boosted* darunavir is used concomitantly with efavirenz, dosage adjustments are not necessary. However, some experts state that the patient should be monitored closely and consideration given to monitoring plasma concentrations of darunavir and efavirenz.

Cobicistat-boosted darunavir should not be used concomitantly with efavirenz because of possible loss of therapeutic effect and development of resistance to darunavir.

Fosamprenavir. Concomitant use of efavirenz and fosamprenavir (without low-dose ritonavir) results in substantially decreased concentrations of amprenavir (the active metabolite of fosamprenavir). Appropriate dosages for concomitant use of fosamprenavir (without low-dose ritonavir) and efavirenz or efavirenz/emtricitabine/tenofovir DF with respect to safety and efficacy have not been established.

Depending on the specific regimen of *ritonavir-boosted* fosamprenavir used, concomitant use with efavirenz may affect amprenavir concentrations. Concomitant use of efavirenz (600 mg once daily) with fosamprenavir 1.4 g once daily and ritonavir 200 mg once daily does not affect peak plasma amprenavir concentrations, but decreases the AUC and trough plasma concentrations of amprenavir. When additional ritonavir is added this regimen and efavirenz (600 mg once daily) is used concomitantly with fosamprenavir 1.4 g once daily and ritonavir 300 mg once daily, the AUC and peak plasma concentrations of amprenavir are increased slightly and trough plasma amprenavir concentrations are not affected. When a twice-daily regimen of *ritonavir-boosted* fosamprenavir is used, concomitant use of efavirenz (600 mg once daily) with fosamprenavir 700 mg twice daily and ritonavir 100 mg twice daily does not affect amprenavir AUC or peak plasma concentrations, but decreases trough plasma amprenavir concentrations.

If *ritonavir-boosted* fosamprenavir is used in patients receiving efavirenz, the usual efavirenz dosage should be used with fosamprenavir 1.4 g once daily and ritonavir 300 mg once daily or, alternatively, fosamprenavir 700 mg twice daily and ritonavir 100 mg twice daily.

If a once-daily regimen of *ritonavir-boosted* fosamprenavir is used in patients receiving efavirenz/emtricitabine/tenofovir DF, ritonavir dosage should be increased to 300 mg once daily; if a twice-daily regimen of *ritonavir-boosted* fosamprenavir is used in patients receiving efavirenz/emtricitabine/tenofovir DF, ritonavir dosage should not be adjusted.

Indinavir. Concomitant use of indinavir and efavirenz decreases the AUC of indinavir, but does not have a clinically important effect on plasma concentrations or AUC of efavirenz.

The optimum dosage of indinavir for use in conjunction with efavirenz has not been established; increasing indinavir dosage to 1 g every 8 hours does not compensate for the increased indinavir metabolism due to efavirenz.

Lopinavir. Concomitant use of efavirenz (600 mg once daily) and the fixed combination containing lopinavir and ritonavir (lopinavir/ritonavir; 400 mg of lopinavir and 100 mg of ritonavir administered as capsules [no longer commercially available in the US] twice daily) for 9 days results in decreased trough plasma concentrations and AUCs of both lopinavir and efavirenz. Concomitant use of efavirenz (600 mg once daily) and lopinavir/ritonavir (600 mg of lopinavir and 150 mg of ritonavir administered as tablets twice daily) for 9 days results in an increased lopinavir peak plasma concentrations and AUC.

A once-daily regimen of lopinavir/ritonavir should not be used in patients receiving efavirenz.

If a twice-daily regimen of lopinavir/ritonavir is used in adult or pediatric patients receiving efavirenz, an increased lopinavir/ritonavir dosage is recommended. Dosage depends on the lopinavir/ritonavir preparation used (tablets, oral solution) and clinical characteristics of the patient. (For specific dosage recommendations, see Dosage and Administration: Dosage, in Lopinavir and Ritonavir 8:18.08.08.)

Nelfinavir. Concomitant use of nelfinavir (750 mg every 8 hours) and efavirenz (600 mg daily) for 7 days increased the peak plasma concentration and AUC of nelfinavir by 21 and 20%, respectively, and decreased the peak plasma concentration and AUC of efavirenz by 12%.

Dosage adjustments are not necessary if nelfinavir is used concomitantly with efavirenz.

Ritonavir. Concomitant use of ritonavir (500 mg every 12 hours for 8 days) and efavirenz (600 mg daily for 10 days) increased the AUC of each drug by about 20%. If ritonavir is used concomitantly with efavirenz or efavirenz/emtricitabine/tenofovir DF, serum hepatic enzymes should be monitored and the patient should be monitored for adverse effects (e.g., dizziness, nausea, paresthesia).

Saquinavir. Concomitant use of saquinavir and efavirenz can substantially decrease the peak plasma concentration and AUC of saquinavir. In one study, administration of saquinavir (1.2 g every 8 hours as Fortovase® [no longer commercially available in US]) and efavirenz (600 mg once daily) for 10 days decreased the peak plasma concentration and AUC of saquinavir by 50 and 62%, respectively, and decreased the peak plasma concentration and AUC of efavirenz by 12–13%.

The manufacturer of saquinavir states that concomitant use of *ritonavir-boosted* saquinavir and efavirenz is not recommended. Appropriate dosages for concomitant use of *ritonavir-boosted* saquinavir and efavirenz with respect to safety and efficacy have not been established.

Some experts state that the usual dosage of *ritonavir-boosted* saquinavir (1 g of saquinavir and 100 mg of ritonavir twice daily) may be used in patients receiving efavirenz.

Tipranavir. Concomitant use of efavirenz (600 mg once daily) and *ritonavir-boosted* tipranavir (tipranavir 500 mg twice daily with ritonavir 100 mg twice daily) results in decreased plasma concentrations and AUC of tipranavir but does not affect the pharmacokinetics of efavirenz. Pharmacokinetics of the PI are not affected if efavirenz (600 mg once daily) is used concomitantly with a higher dosage of *ritonavir-boosted* tipranavir (tipranavir 750 mg twice daily with ritonavir 200 mg twice daily).

Some experts state that dosage adjustments are not necessary if efavirenz and *ritonavir-boosted* tipranavir are used concomitantly.

■ **Atovaquone** Concomitant use of efavirenz and atovaquone decreases atovaquone AUC. To avoid concomitant use, some experts state that an alternative to atovaquone should be considered for the treatment of *Pneumocystis jirovecii* pneumonia (PCP) or toxoplasmosis or an alternative to efavirenz should be considered. If efavirenz and atovaquone are used concomitantly, the patient should be monitored for therapeutic efficacy of atovaquone.

■ **Cardiovascular Agents** ***Antilipemic Agents*** Concomitant use of efavirenz and certain hydroxymethylglutaryl-CoA (HMG-CoA) reductase inhibitors (statins), including atorvastatin, pravastatin, and simvastatin, results in decreased plasma concentrations of the antilipemic agent, but does not have a clinically important effect on efavirenz concentrations.

Atorvastatin. If atorvastatin is used concomitantly with efavirenz, atorvastatin dosage should be titrated based on lipid response and should not exceed the maximum recommended dosage.

Lovastatin. If lovastatin is used concomitantly with efavirenz, lovastatin dosage should be titrated based on lipid response and should not exceed the maximum recommended dosage. Lovastatin should be avoided if efavirenz is used concomitantly with a *ritonavir-boosted* PI.

Pitavastatin. Concomitant use of pitavastatin and efavirenz results in decreased AUC and increased peak plasma concentrations of pitavastatin; dosage adjustments are not necessary.

Pravastatin. If pravastatin is used concomitantly with efavirenz, pravastatin dosage should be titrated based on lipid response and should not exceed the maximum recommended dosage.

Rosuvastatin. Data are not available regarding concomitant use of rosuvastatin and efavirenz; if the drugs are used concomitantly, rosuvastatin dosage should be titrated based on lipid response and should not exceed the maximum recommended dosage.

Simvastatin. If simvastatin is used concomitantly with efavirenz, simvastatin dosage should be titrated based on lipid response and should not exceed the maximum recommended dosage. Simvastatin should be avoided if efavirenz is used in a regimen that includes a *ritonavir-boosted* PI.

Calcium-channel Blocking Agents Concomitant use of diltiazem and efavirenz results in decreased concentrations of diltiazem and slightly increased concentrations of efavirenz. If diltiazem is used concomitantly with efavirenz or efavirenz/emtricitabine/tenofovir DF, dosage of the calcium-channel blocking agent should be titrated based on clinical response; dosage of efavirenz or efavirenz/emtricitabine/tenofovir DF does not need to be adjusted.

Concomitant use of other calcium-channel blocking agents (e.g., felodipine, nicardipine, nifedipine, verapamil) is predicted to result in decreased concentrations of the calcium-channel blocking agent. If efavirenz is used concomitantly with any of these drugs, dosage of the calcium-channel blocking agent should be titrated based on clinical response.

■ **CNS Agents** ***Opiates and Opiate Partial Agonists***

Buprenorphine. Concomitant use of buprenorphine (sublingual or buccal) and efavirenz may decrease the AUC of buprenorphine and norbuprenorphine. Some experts state that dosage adjustments are not recommended, but patients should be monitored for withdrawal symptoms.

Data are not available regarding concomitant use of buprenorphine (subdermal implant) and efavirenz. If efavirenz is initiated after insertion of the buprenorphine implant, clinical monitoring is recommended.

Methadone. Administration of methadone (35–100 mg daily) and efavirenz (600 mg daily for 14–21 days) in HIV-infected individuals with a history of drug dependence decreased the peak plasma concentration and AUC of methadone by 45 and 52%, respectively, and resulted in manifestations of opiate withdrawal. The maintenance dosage of methadone was increased by an average of 22% to alleviate withdrawal symptoms.

Individuals receiving concurrent efavirenz and methadone therapy should be informed of this potential interaction and closely monitored for signs of opiate withdrawal; an increase in the maintenance dosage of methadone may be necessary in such individuals.

Anticonvulsants Concomitant use of efavirenz and carbamazepine results in decreased plasma concentrations and AUCs of efavirenz and carbamazepine. Concomitant use of efavirenz and phenobarbital or phenytoin may result in decreased plasma concentrations of the anticonvulsant and/or efavirenz. The manufacturer of efavirenz states that data are insufficient to make dosage recommendations for concomitant use of efavirenz and carbamazepine. If carbamazepine, phenobarbital, or phenytoin is used concomitantly with efavirenz, plasma concentrations of the anticonvulsant and efavirenz should be monitored. If possible, use of another anticonvulsant should be considered.

Concomitant use of efavirenz and valproic acid in HIV-infected adults does not affect the pharmacokinetics of either drug.

The manufacturer of efavirenz/emtricitabine/tenofovir DF states that data are insufficient to make dosage recommendations for concomitant use of the fixed combination and carbamazepine; an alternative anticonvulsant should be used.

Psychotherapeutic Agents Administration of efavirenz in patients receiving psychoactive drugs may result in increased CNS effects.

Bupropion. Concomitant use of bupropion and efavirenz decreases peak plasma concentrations and AUC of bupropion and increases peak plasma concentrations of hydroxybupropion (an active metabolite).

In patients receiving efavirenz, bupropion dosage should be titrated based on clinical response, but should not exceed the maximum recommended bupropion dosage.

Selective Serotonin-reuptake Inhibitors. Concomitant use of paroxetine and efavirenz does not result in clinically important drug interactions; dosage adjustments are not needed.

Concomitant use of sertraline and efavirenz results in decreased plasma concentrations and AUC of sertraline. Sertraline dosage adjustments should be guided by clinical response.

Pimozide. Efavirenz and pimozide should not be used concomitantly.

Sedatives and Hypnotics Concomitant use of efavirenz and midazolam or triazolam is expected to substantially increase concentrations of the benzodiazepine. Efavirenz and oral midazolam or triazolam should not be used concomitantly. Some experts state that parenteral midazolam can be given in a single dose with caution in a monitored situation for procedural sedation in patients receiving efavirenz.

Data are not available regarding concomitant use of alprazolam and efavirenz; if the drugs are used concomitantly, some clinicians suggest that patients be monitored for therapeutic effectiveness of the benzodiazepine.

Administration of lorazepam (2 mg as a single dose) and efavirenz (600 mg daily for 10 days) increased the peak plasma concentration of lorazepam by 16%, but did not affect the AUC of the drug. Dosage adjustments are not necessary in patients receiving lorazepam and efavirenz concomitantly.

■ **Corticosteroids** Concomitant use of dexamethasone and efavirenz may result in decreased efavirenz concentrations. If dexamethasone and efavirenz are used concomitantly, virologic response should be monitored; alternative corticosteroids should be considered for long-term use.

■ **Ergot Alkaloids** Efavirenz and ergot alkaloids (e.g., dihydroergotamine, ergotamine, methylergonovine) should not be used concomitantly.

If methylergonovine maleate (Methergine®) is used to treat postpartum hemorrhage in a woman receiving efavirenz, additional uterotonic agents may be needed since efavirenz potentially could decrease methylergonovine concentrations resulting in an inadequate treatment effect.

■ **Estrogens and Progestins** Concomitant use of efavirenz (600 mg once daily for 14 days) and an oral contraceptive containing 0.035 mg of ethinyl estradiol and 0.25 mg of norgestimate did not affect peak plasma concentrations or AUC of ethinyl estradiol, but resulted in substantially decreased peak plasma concentrations and AUC of norelgestromin and levonorgestrel (metabolites of norgestimate). Efavirenz concentrations were not affected by the oral contraceptive.

Concomitant use of efavirenz and etonogestrel subcutaneous implant has not been studied, but decreased etonogestrel concentrations are expected. There have been postmarketing reports of subcutaneous implant contraceptive failure in women receiving efavirenz.

Concomitant use of levonorgestrel subcutaneous implant and efavirenz has resulted in a 47% decrease in plasma concentrations of levonorgestrel. In addition, unintended pregnancies have been reported in women with a levonorgestrel implant who were receiving efavirenz.

Studies evaluating concomitant use of efavirenz and orally administered levonorgestrel demonstrate a 64–83% decrease in levonorgestrel AUC. Efficacy of levonorgestrel as an emergency contraceptive is expected to be decreased in women receiving efavirenz. In a study in healthy women, concomitant use of efavirenz (600 mg once daily) and oral levonorgestrel (two 0.75-mg doses 12 hours apart) resulted in an estimated 56% decrease in the AUC of the progestin compared with use of levonorgestrel alone. It is not known whether efavirenz has a similar effect when oral levonorgestrel is given as a single 1.5-mg dose.

Women of childbearing potential should use a reliable method of barrier contraception in addition to or instead of a hormonal contraceptive (e.g., oral or other hormonal contraceptive) during and for 12 weeks after efavirenz is discontinued.

■ **GI Drugs** Efavirenz and cisapride should not be used concomitantly.

Concomitant use of drugs that alter gastric pH is not expected to affect absorption of efavirenz. Systemic availability of efavirenz is not affected by concomitant use with an antacid or a histamine H_2-receptor antagonist (e.g., famotidine). Concomitant use of efavirenz and an antacid preparation containing aluminum hydroxide 400 mg, magnesium hydroxide 400 mg, and simethicone 40 mg/30 mL dose in healthy individuals did not alter the absorption of efavirenz. Dosage adjustments are not needed if efavirenz is used concomitantly with famotidine or antacids.

■ **HCV Antivirals** ***HCV Polymerase Inhibitors*** **Sofosbuvir.** Concomitant use of sofosbuvir (single 400-mg dose) and efavirenz (600 mg once daily as the fixed combination efavirenz/emtricitabine/tenofovir DF) does not have a clinically important effect on the pharmacokinetics of sofosbuvir.

Dosage adjustments are not needed if sofosbuvir and efavirenz are used concomitantly.

Sofosbuvir and Velpatasvir. Concomitant use of the fixed combination of sofosbuvir and velpatasvir (sofosbuvir/velpatasvir) and the fixed combination efavirenz/emtricitabine/tenofovir DF does not have a clinically important effect on the pharmacokinetics of sofosbuvir, efavirenz, or emtricitabine, but results in decreased velpatasvir plasma concentrations and AUC and increased tenofovir plasma concentrations and AUC.

Concomitant use of sofosbuvir/velpatasvir and efavirenz is not recommended.

HCV Protease Inhibitors **Simeprevir.** Concomitant use of simeprevir (150 mg once daily for 14 days) and efavirenz (600 mg once daily for 14 days) substantially decreased plasma concentrations and AUC of simeprevir and may result in loss of simeprevir therapeutic effects. There was no clinically important effect on efavirenz concentrations or AUC.

Concomitant use of simeprevir and efavirenz is not recommended.

HCV Replication Complex Inhibitors **Daclatasvir.** Concomitant use of daclatasvir (120 mg once daily) and efavirenz (600 mg daily) results in decreased daclatasvir trough concentrations.

If daclatasvir and efavirenz are used concomitantly, daclatasvir should be given in a dosage of 90 mg once daily.

Elbasvir and Grazoprevir. Concomitant use of efavirenz (600 mg once daily) and elbasvir (50 mg once daily) or grazoprevir (200 mg once daily) results in substantially decreased elbasvir or grazoprevir concentrations due to potent CYP3A induction by efavirenz, which may lead to loss of virologic response to the HCV antiviral. Concomitant use does not have a clinically important effect on efavirenz exposures.

Concomitant use of the fixed combination of elbasvir and grazoprevir (elbasvir/grazoprevir) and efavirenz is contraindicated.

Ledipasvir and Sofosbuvir. If the fixed combination of ledipasvir and sofosbuvir (ledipasvir/sofosbuvir) is used concomitantly with efavirenz, clinically important pharmacokinetic interactions are not expected. Concomitant use of the fixed combination efavirenz/emtricitabine/tenofovir DF and ledipasvir or sofosbuvir results in decreased ledipasvir concentrations, but does not have a clinically important effect on sofosbuvir or efavirenz concentrations.

Dosage adjustments are not necessary if ledipasvir/sofosbuvir and efavirenz are used concomitantly. If ledipasvir/sofosbuvir and efavirenz/emtricitabine/tenofovir DF are used concomitantly, patients should be monitored for tenofovir-associated adverse effects.

Ombitasvir, Paritaprevir, and Ritonavir. Concomitant use of efavirenz and the fixed combination of ombitasvir, paritaprevir, and ritonavir (ombitasvir/paritaprevir/ritonavir) with or without dasabuvir is poorly tolerated and has resulted in elevated liver enzymes.

Concomitant use of efavirenz and ombitasvir/paritaprevir/ritonavir with or without dasabuvir is contraindicated.

■ **Immunosuppressive Agents** Concomitant use of efavirenz and immunosuppressive agents metabolized by CYP3A (e.g., cyclosporine, sirolimus, tacrolimus) may result in decreased concentrations of the immunosuppressive agents, but is not expected to affect efavirenz concentrations.

If efavirenz or efavirenz/emtricitabine/tenofovir DF is used concomitantly with an immunosuppressive agent metabolized by CYP3A (e.g., cyclosporine, sirolimus, tacrolimus), dosage of the immunosuppressive agent may need to be adjusted. When efavirenz or efavirenz/emtricitabine/tenofovir DF is initiated or discontinued, plasma concentrations of the immunosuppressive agent should be monitored for at least 2 weeks until stable concentrations are reached.

■ **Macrolide Antibiotics** Because of the risk of QT interval prolongation, the manufacturer of efavirenz states that alternatives to macrolide antibiotics should be considered in patients receiving efavirenz.

Administration of azithromycin (600 mg as a single dose) and efavirenz (400 mg daily for 7 days) in healthy individuals did not result in clinically important changes in the pharmacokinetics of either drug, and the manufacturer of efavirenz states that dosage adjustments are not necessary in patients receiving the drugs concurrently.

Administration of clarithromycin (500 mg every 12 hours) and efavirenz (400 mg daily) for 7 days in healthy individuals decreased the peak plasma concentration and AUC of clarithromycin by 26 and 39%, respectively, and increased the peak plasma concentration and AUC of 14-hydroxyclarithromycin by 49 and 34%, respectively. Some experts recommend that alternatives to clarithromycin (e.g., azithromycin) be considered in patients receiving efavirenz.

■ **Phosphodiesterase Type 5 Inhibitors** ***Avanafil*** Data are not available regarding concomitant use of avanafil and efavirenz; concomitant use is not recommended.

■ **Dietary and Herbal Supplements** ***St. John's Wort (Hypericum perforatum)*** St. John's wort (*Hypericum perforatum*) and efavirenz should not be used concomitantly since such use is expected to result in suboptimal antiretroviral concentrations and may be associated with loss of virologic response and development of resistance. St. John's wort is an extract of hypericum and contains at least 7 different components that may contribute to its pharmacologic effects, including hypericin, pseudohypericin, and hyperforin. There is evidence that hypericum extracts can induce several different CYP isoenzymes, including CYP3A4 and CYP1A2, and also may induce the P-glycoprotein transport system. Therefore, it has be recommended that concomitant use of St. John's wort and PIs or NNRTIs metabolized by CYP isoenzymes be avoided. For further information on drug interactions between St. John's wort and drugs metabolized by CYP isoenzymes, see Drug Interactions: Dietary and Herbal Supplements, in Indinavir 8:18.08.08.

Laboratory Test Interferences

■ **Cannabinoid Assays** False-positive urine cannabinoid test results have been reported in healthy and HIV-infected individuals receiving efavirenz. Positive screening tests for cannabinoids in patients receiving efavirenz should be confirmed using a more specific test. Efavirenz does not bind to cannabinoid receptors.

Acute Toxicity

■ **Manifestations** Limited information is available on acute toxicity of efavirenz. Increased adverse CNS effects, including involuntary muscle contractions, have been reported in some patients who inadvertently took efavirenz in a dosage of 600 mg twice daily instead of the usually recommended adult dosage of 600 mg once daily.

■ **Treatment** If acute overdosage of efavirenz occurs, supportive and symptomatic treatment should be initiated and the patient observed closely. Activated charcoal may be administered to prevent absorption of drug. There is no known antidote for efavirenz overdosage. Hemodialysis or peritoneal dialysis is unlikely to remove substantial amounts of efavirenz from the body, and these procedures should not be relied on to enhance elimination of the drug.

Mechanism of Action

■ **Antiviral Effects** Although the complete mechanism(s) of antiviral activity of efavirenz has not been fully elucidated, the drug inhibits human immunodeficiency virus type 1 (HIV-1) by interfering with viral RNA- and DNA-directed polymerase activities of reverse transcriptase. Efavirenz binds directly to HIV-1 reverse transcriptase and exerts a virustatic effect by acting as a specific, noncompetitive HIV-1 reverse transcriptase inhibitor.

The mechanism of action of efavirenz appears to be similar to that of other HIV nonnucleoside reverse transcriptase inhibitors (NNRTIs) (e.g., delavirdine, etravirine, nevirapine) but differs from that of HIV nucleoside reverse transcriptase inhibitors (NRTIs) (e.g., abacavir, didanosine, lamivudine, stavudine, zidovudine). NRTIs require intracellular conversion to triphosphate metabolites, which then compete with naturally occurring deoxynucleoside triphosphates for incorporation into viral DNA by reverse transcriptase and cause premature viral DNA chain termination by preventing further 5′ to 3′ phosphodiester linkages. Efavirenz and other NNRTIs, however, are noncompetitive with respect to primer-template or nucleoside triphosphate binding and are specific for HIV-1 reverse transcriptase. The drugs bind directly to heterodimeric HIV-1 reverse transcriptase and appear to inhibit viral RNA- and DNA-dependent DNA polymerase activities by disrupting the catalytic site of the enzyme.

The binding site for NNRTIs on HIV-1 reverse transcriptase is near, but not at, the proposed site of active polymerization, in a deep pocket lying between the β sheets of the "palm" and at the base of the "thumb" subdomains of the enzyme's p66 subunit. In the absence of a NNRTI, the binding of deoxynucleoside triphosphate to the reverse transcriptase-template complex results in a change in the conformation of reverse transcriptase. This conformational change is followed by a magnesium-dependent chemical reaction in which deoxynucleoside triphosphate is incorporated into the newly forming viral DNA; the conformational change appears to be the rate-limiting step of the reverse transcriptase catalysis of viral DNA formation. Efavirenz and other NNRTIs appear to have no appreciable effect on the rate of or equilibrium constant for the conformational change but may slow the chemical reaction, which then becomes the rate-limiting step in the catalytic sequence. When NNRTIs bind to the reverse transcriptase-template complex, changes may occur in the position of aspartic acid carboxyl groups in reverse transcriptase so that magnesium ions are not in proper alignment for the chemical reaction to occur efficiently, and the reaction is slowed. Therefore, although the drug-reverse transcriptase-template complex may continue to bind deoxynucleoside triphosphate and to catalyze its incorporation into the newly forming viral DNA, it appears to do so at a slower rate.

■ **Cytotoxic Effects** Efavirenz is a highly specific inhibitor of HIV-1 reverse transcriptase and does not appear to interfere with the activity of cellular DNA polymerases, including human α-, β-, γ-, or δ-polymerases.

Results of in vitro studies using HIV-infected primary cells and a T-cell line indicate that efavirenz exerts cytotoxic properties at concentrations substantially greater than those required for antiretroviral activity (25.3 mcg/mL versus 0.474–0.947 mcg/mL).

Spectrum

Efavirenz has a very limited spectrum of activity. The drug has in vitro virustatic activity against human immunodeficiency virus type 1 (HIV-1), but is inactive against HIV type 2 (HIV-2).

■ **Retroviruses** Efavirenz is active in vitro against HIV-1 and may be active against both zidovudine-susceptible and -resistant strains. Efavirenz is inactive against HIV-2.

The antiretroviral activity of efavirenz has been evaluated in vitro in various cell culture systems including lymphoblastoid cell lines, peripheral blood mononuclear cells, and macrophage/monocyte cultures. Depending on the cell culture system used, the IC_{90-95} of efavirenz (concentration of the drug required to inhibit 90–95% of detectable replication) for HIV-1 (wild-type laboratory adapted strains and clinical isolates) has ranged from 0.474–7.9 ng/mL. The precise relationship between in vitro susceptibility of HIV-1 to efavirenz and inhibition of in vivo replication of the virus or clinical response to therapy with the drug has not been determined.

Resistance

Strains of HIV-1 with reduced susceptibility to efavirenz (i.e., greater than 380-fold increase in IC_{90} from baseline) have been produced in vitro by serial passage of the retrovirus in the presence of increasing concentrations of the drug. In addition, strains of HIV-1 resistant to efavirenz emerge rapidly if the drug is administered alone and also have been reported in patients receiving the drug in conjunction with other antiretroviral agents.

Although the complete mechanism(s) of resistance or reduced susceptibility to efavirenz has not been fully determined to date, mutation of HIV reverse transcriptase appears to be the principal mechanism of resistance. Acquisition of a single mutation can result in resistance to efavirenz. Like some other HIV-nonnucleoside reverse transcriptase inhibitors (NNRTIs), (e.g., delavirdine, nevirapine), exposure to efavirenz selects for mutations that usually involve the regions of HIV reverse transcriptase that include amino acid positions 98–108 and 179–190; mutations at amino acid position 225 also have been reported following exposure to efavirenz.

Efavirenz-resistant variants produced in vitro in the presence of increasing concentrations of the drug have contained one or more mutations including L100I, K103N, V108I, V179D, Y181C, and Y188L. Efavirenz-resistant variants isolated from patients receiving efavirenz in conjunction other antiretrovirals (i.e., indinavir or zidovudine and lamivudine) in clinical trials have included K103N, V108I, Y188L, G190S, K103N/V108I, L100I/K103N, or K103N/G190S. Mutations at amino acid positions 98, 101, 106, and 225 also have been reported in patients who received efavirenz. The mutation at amino acid position 103 (i.e., K103N) is the most frequently observed change.

Genotypic and/or phenotypic changes in HIV isolates have been monitored in patients receiving efavirenz in conjunction with other antiretrovirals (i.e., indinavir or zidovudine and lamivudine) in clinical studies. Nucleic acid sequencing of plasma virus from patients whose viral load rebounded while receiving efavirenz-containing regimens revealed the emergence of K103N reverse transcriptase-mutant viruses around the time of viral load rebound. Most patients subsequently developed variants that contained K103N in combination with additional linked mutations (i.e., L100I, V108I, P225H). Viral isolates with K103N, V108I, and/or Y188L mutations have a 20-fold or greater increase in efavirenz IC_{50} compared with baseline.

■ **Cross-resistance** Strains of HIV-1 resistant to efavirenz may be cross-resistant to some other NNRTIs. The resistance profile of efavirenz overlaps that of some other NNRTIs (e.g., delavirdine, nevirapine). The K103N mutation has been observed with delavirdine, efavirenz, and nevirapine and can cause broad cross-resistance among the agents; high-level cross-resistance is seen when K103N is present in combination with certain other mutations.

The potential for cross-resistance between efavirenz and nucleoside reverse transcriptase inhibitors (abacavir, didanosine, lamivudine, stavudine, zidovudine) is considered low because the drugs bind at different sites on reverse transcriptase and have different mechanisms of action. Limited information indicates that zidovudine-resistant HIV-1 isolates retain susceptibility to efavirenz. Because efavirenz and HIV protease inhibitors (e.g., amprenavir, indinavir, lopinavir, nelfinavir, ritonavir, saquinavir) have different enzyme targets, cross-resistance between efavirenz and these drugs is unlikely.

Pharmacokinetics

The pharmacokinetics of efavirenz have been studied in healthy individuals, adults with human immunodeficiency virus (HIV) infection, and HIV-infected children 3–16 years of age. The pharmacokinetics of efavirenz capsules (or capsule contents mixed with soft food or infant formula) in pediatric patients were predicted using a population pharmacokinetic model.

Results to date indicate that pharmacokinetic parameters of the drug in healthy individuals are similar to those in HIV-infected individuals. Pharmacokinetic studies have not revealed gender- or race-related differences in the pharmacokinetics of efavirenz. Pharmacokinetics of efavirenz are not affected by mild hepatic impairment (Child-Pugh class A); data are insufficient to determine whether moderate or severe hepatic impairment (Child-Pugh class B or C) affects pharmacokinetics of the drug. The pharmacokinetics of efavirenz have not been specifically studied in patients with renal impairment, and only very limited data are available to date.

■ **Absorption** Following oral administration of a single 100- to 1600-mg dose of efavirenz in healthy adults, peak plasma drug concentrations of 0.51–2.9 mcg/mL were attained within 5 hours. While administration of single oral doses of up to 1600 mg of efavirenz was associated with dose-related increases in peak plasma concentration and AUC, the increases were less than proportional and suggest reduced absorption of the drug at higher doses. Following oral administration of efavirenz 200, 400, or 600 mg once daily in HIV-infected adults, mean peak plasma concentration, mean trough plasma concentration, and AUC of the drug at steady-state were dose proportional. In HIV-infected adults receiving efavirenz 200, 400, or 600 mg once daily, peak plasma concentrations of the drug generally occur in 3–5 hours and steady-state plasma concentrations are achieved in 6–10 days. Following continued administration of efavirenz, plasma concentrations are lower than expected from single-dose studies, presumably because of increased clearance of the drug. In one study in individuals receiving efavirenz 200–400 mg once daily for 10 days, plasma concentrations of the drug were 22–42% lower than those predicted from single-dose studies.

Following oral administration of efavirenz 600 mg once daily in HIV-infected adults, peak plasma concentration, trough plasma concentration, and AUC of the drug at steady-state averaged 4.1 mcg/mL, 1.8 mcg/mL, and 58.1 mcg•hour/mL, respectively. Predicted steady-state peak plasma concentrations of efavirenz following administration of efavirenz capsules (or capsule contents mixed with soft food or infant formula) in HIV-infected pediatric patients weighing 3.5–5 kg (100 mg once daily), 7.5–10 kg (200 mg once daily), 15–20 kg (250 mg once daily), 20–25 kg (300 mg once daily), or 32.5–40 kg (400 mg once daily) are 5.81, 7.75, 6.47, 7.04, or 6.96 mcg/mL, respectively.

Following oral administration of a single 400-mg oral dose of efavirenz in individuals with chronic liver disease or healthy individuals, peak plasma concentrations averaged 1.2 or 1.8 mcg/mL, respectively, and AUC averaged 94.4 or 96.3 mcg•hour/mL, respectively.

Oral bioavailability of efavirenz may be affected by administration with food. Administration of a single 600-mg dose of efavirenz as capsules with a high-fat, high-calorie meal (894 kcal, 54 g fat, 54% of calories from fat) or a reduced-fat, normal-calorie meal (440 kcal, 2 g fat, 4% of calories from fat) increases peak plasma concentrations of the drug by 39 or 51%, respectively, and AUC by 22 or 17%, respectively, compared with administration in the fasting state. Administration of a single 600-mg dose of efavirenz as tablets with a high-fat, high-calorie meal (approximately 1000 kcal, 500–600 kcal from fat) increases peak plasma concentrations and AUC of the drug by 79 and 28%, respectively, compared with administration in the fasting state. Therefore, the manufacturer states that efavirenz should be administered on an empty stomach. In healthy adults who received a 600-mg efavirenz dose administered by opening 200-mg capsules and mixing the contents of 3 capsules with 2 teaspoonfuls of soft food (e.g., applesauce, grape jelly, yogurt) or infant formula, the AUC of efavirenz met bioequivalency criteria compared with intact capsules administered in the fasted state. (See Dosage and Administration: Administration.)

■ **Distribution** Distribution of efavirenz into body tissues and fluids has not been fully characterized. In rats and rhesus monkeys, the volume of distribution of efavirenz following IV administration is 2.4–4.4 L/kg suggesting extensive tissue distribution.

Following oral administration of efavirenz 200–600 mg once daily for 1 month or longer in HIV-infected adults, CSF concentrations of efavirenz were 0.26–1.19% of corresponding plasma concentrations. Low concentrations of efavirenz are found in CSF; however, the proportion of drug in CSF is about threefold higher than the nonprotein-bound fraction in plasma. In a study in HIV-infected patients who received efavirenz 600 mg once daily for 5 weeks or longer mean CSF concentrations of efavirenz were 0.011 mcg/mL (range: 0.002–0.019 mcg/mL) and concurrent mean plasma concentrations were 1.97 mcg/mL (range: 0.792–2.95 mcg/mL).

Efavirenz is about 99.5–99.75% bound to plasma proteins, principally albumin.

Efavirenz crosses the placenta in animals (e.g., rats, rabbits, primates) and concentrations of the drug in fetal blood in these species are similar to those in maternal blood. Efavirenz is distributed into human milk.

■ **Elimination** Efavirenz appears to induce its own metabolism. The terminal elimination half-life of efavirenz reported in single-dose studies is longer than that reported in multiple-dose studies and has averaged 52–76 hours after a single oral dose and 40–55 hours following administration of 200–400 mg daily for 10 days. In addition, following continued administration of efavirenz, plasma concentrations are lower than expected from single-dose studies, presumably because of increased clearance.

The terminal elimination half-life of efavirenz is prolonged in patients with chronic liver disease. Following oral administration of a single 400-mg dose of efavirenz, an elimination half-life of 152 or 118 hours was reported in individuals with or without chronic liver disease, respectively.

In one HIV-infected adult with anuric end-stage renal failure who was receiving efavirenz in a dosage of 600 mg once daily, peak and trough plasma concentrations were 2.58 and 0.65 mcg/mL and the plasma half-life was decreased to 10 hours.

The metabolic fate of efavirenz has not been fully determined, but the drug is metabolized in the liver. Efavirenz is principally metabolized by the cytochrome P-450 (CYP) isoenzymes 3A and 2B6 to several hydroxylated metabolites, which undergo subsequent glucuronidation.

Efavirenz is excreted principally in the feces, both as unchanged drug and metabolites. Excretion of efavirenz has been evaluated in individuals receiving 400 mg daily for 1 month. Following oral administration of 400 mg of radiolabeled efavirenz on day 8, 14–34% of the dose was excreted in urine (less than 1% as unchanged drug), and 16–61% was excreted in feces (predominantly as unchanged drug).

Because efavirenz is highly protein bound and less than 1% of the drug is excreted unchanged in urine, it is unlikely that substantial amounts of the drug would be removed from the body by hemodialysis or peritoneal dialysis. The pharmacokinetics of efavirenz were evaluated in an HIV-infected adult with anuric end-stage renal failure undergoing hemodialysis and results confirm that hemodialysis does not affect the pharmacokinetics of the drug.

Chemistry and Stability

■ **Chemistry** Efavirenz, an antiretroviral agent, is a human immunodeficiency virus (HIV) nonnucleoside reverse transcriptase inhibitor (NNRTI). The drug is a benzoxazinone derivative NNRTI. Efavirenz differs structurally from other commercially available NNRTIs (e.g., delavirdine, etravirine, nevirapine, rilpivirine) and also differs structurally from other currently available antiretroviral agents.

Efavirenz occurs as a white to slightly pink crystalline powder. The drug is practically insoluble in water having an aqueous solubility less than 10 mcg/mL at pH 1–8; however, solubility increases markedly at pH exceeding 10. Efavirenz has an aqueous pK_a of 10.2.

Efavirenz is commercially available for oral administration as single-entity capsules or tablets (Sustiva®). Efavirenz also is commercially available for oral administration in fixed-combination tablets containing efavirenz, emtricitabine, and tenofovir disoproxil fumarate (efavirenz/emtricitabine/tenofovir DF; Atripla®).

■ **Stability** Efavirenz capsules and tablets (Sustiva®) and efavirenz/emtricitabine/tenofovir DF fixed-combination tablets (Atripla®) should be stored at a controlled room temperature of 25°C, but may be exposed to temperatures ranging from 15–30°C.

Preparations

Excipients in commercially available drug preparations may have clinically important effects in some individuals; consult specific product labeling for details.

Efavirenz

Oral		
Capsules	50 mg	Sustiva®, Bristol-Myers Squibb
	200 mg	Sustiva®, Bristol-Myers Squibb
Tablets, film-coated	600 mg	Sustiva®, Bristol-Myers Squibb

Efavirenz Combinations

Oral		
Tablets, film-coated	600 mg with Emtricitabine 200 mg and Tenofovir Disoproxil Fumarate 300 mg	Atripla®, Bristol-Myers Squibb and Gilead

†Use is not currently included in the labeling approved by the US Food and Drug Administration

Nevirapine

NVP

■ Nevirapine, an antiretroviral agent, is a human immunodeficiency virus (HIV) nonnucleoside reverse transcriptase inhibitor (NNRTI).

Uses

■ **Treatment of HIV Infection** Nevirapine is used in conjunction with other antiretroviral agents for the treatment of human immunodeficiency virus type 1 (HIV-1) infection in adults, adolescents, and pediatric patients.

Because adults with high pretreatment $CD4^+$ T-cell counts are at increased risk for serious and life-threatening hepatotoxicity associated with nevirapine, the drug should *not* be initiated in women with pretreatment $CD4^+$ T-cell counts exceeding 250 cells/mm^3 or in men with $CD4^+$ T-cell counts exceeding 400 cells/mm^3 unless potential benefits outweigh risks. (See Cautions: Hepatic Effects.)

Nevirapine generally has been used in HIV nonnucleoside reverse transcriptase inhibitor-based (NNRTI-based) regimens that include nevirapine and 2 HIV nucleoside reverse transcriptase inhibitors (NRTIs).

The most appropriate antiretroviral regimen cannot be defined for each clinical scenario and selection of specific antiretroviral agents for use in such regimens should be individualized based on information regarding antiretroviral potency, potential rate of development of resistance, known toxicities, and potential for pharmacokinetic interactions as well as virologic, immunologic, and clinical characteristics of the patient. For information on the general principles and guidelines for use of antiretroviral therapy, including specific recommendations for initial therapy in antiretroviral-naive patients and recommendations for changing antiretroviral regimens, see the Antiretroviral Agents General Statement 8:18.08.

Antiretroviral-naive Adults The US Department of Health and Human Services (HHS) Panel on Antiretroviral Guidelines for Adults and Adolescents states that nevirapine is *not* recommended for *initial* treatment regimens in antiretroviral-naive adults and adolescents because it has been associated with serious and potentially fatal toxicity (e.g., hepatic events and severe rash, including Stevens-Johnson syndrome and toxic epidermal necrolysis) and did not meet noninferiority criteria when compared to efavirenz in clinical trials.

Study BI 1046. Safety and efficacy of nevirapine (200 mg once daily for the initial 2 weeks, then 200 mg every 12 hours) have been evaluated in conjunction with zidovudine (200 mg 3 times daily) with or without didanosine (125 or 200 mg twice daily) for initial antiretroviral therapy in a randomized, double-blind study in treatment-naive (had not previously received antiretroviral therapy) adults (study BI 1046). Study BI 1046 included 151 adults (median age 36 years) with baseline $CD4^+$ T-cell counts of 200–600 cells/mm^3 (mean 376 cells/mm^3) and mean baseline plasma HIV-1 RNA levels of 4.41 $\log_{10}$ copies/mL (25,704 copies/mL). Patients were randomized to receive a 3-drug regimen of zidovudine, didanosine, and nevirapine or a 2-drug regimen of zidovudine and didanosine or zidovudine and nevirapine.

The primary endpoint was the proportion of patients with plasma HIV-1 RNA levels less than 400 copies/mL and not previously failed at 48 weeks. At 48 weeks, the virologic response rate was 45% in those receiving the 3-drug regimen (zidovudine, didanosine, and nevirapine), 19% for those receiving zidovudine and didanosine, and 0% in those receiving nevirapine and zidovudine. The mean increase in $CD4^+$ T-cell count above baseline was 139 cells/mm^3 in those receiving the 3-drug regimen compared with 87% in those receiving zidovudine and didanosine.

Study 1100.1486. Safety and efficacy of nevirapine extended-release tablets were evaluated in a randomized, double-blind, double-dummy, phase 3 trial in antiretroviral-naive adults (85% male, 75% white, 20% black, 29% from North America) who received a regimen of nevirapine immediate-release tablets (200 mg once daily) for 14 days with 2 NRTIs (tenofovir and emtricitabine) and were then randomized to continue therapy with nevirapine immediate-release tablets (200 mg twice daily) or switch to nevirapine extended-release tablets (400 mg once daily) with the same background regimen of 2 NRTIs (study 1100.1486; VERxVE). At baseline, the mean plasma HIV RNA level was 4.7 $\log_{10}$ copies/mL and the mean $CD4^+$ T-cell count was 228 cells/mm^3; approximately 66% of patients had baseline plasma HIV RNA levels of 100,000 copies/mL or lower. At 96 weeks, 67% of those receiving immediate-release nevirapine and 69% of those receiving extended-release nevirapine had plasma HIV RNA levels less than 50 copies/mL and the mean change from baseline in $CD4^+$ T-cell count, adjusted for baseline HIV viral load stratum, was 222 or 244 cells/mm^3, respectively.

Antiretroviral-experienced Adults **Study BI 1090.** Nevirapine has been evaluated for use in conjunction with other antiretroviral agents in adults with advanced HIV-1 infection (study BI 1090). This study was a placebo-controlled, double-blind, randomized study that included 2,249 adults (median age 36.5 years, 79% male, 70% white, median baseline $CD4^+$ T-cell count 96 cells/mm^3, median baseline plasma HIV-1 RNA level 4.58 $\log_{10}$ copies/mL [38,291 copies/mL]; 89% had previously received antiretroviral therapy). Patients were randomized to receive nevirapine (200 mg once daily for 2 weeks, then 200 mg twice daily) and lamivudine (150 mg twice daily) with a background antiretroviral regimen or lamivudine with a background regimen; the background regimen was one NRTI (58%), 2 or more NRTIs (34%), or HIV protease inhibitors (PIs) and NRTIs (8%). Prior to study entry, 45% of patients had previously experienced an AIDS-defining clinical event.

At 48 weeks, 18% of those receiving a regimen that included nevirapine had plasma HIV-1 RNA levels less than 50 copies/mL compared with 2% of those not receiving the NNRTI. At 1 year, the change from baseline $CD4^+$ T-cell count for the overall trial population was 64 cells/mm^3 in those receiving nevirapine compared with 22 cells/mm^3 in those not receiving the drug. At 2 years, 16% of those receiving nevirapine had experienced events classified as US Centers for Disease Control (CDC) class C events compared to 21% of those in the control arm.

Study 1100.1526. Safety and efficacy of switching from nevirapine immediate-release tablets to nevirapine extended-release tablets was evaluated in an ongoing open-label, phase 3 trial in antiretroviral-experienced adults with HIV-1 RNA levels less than 50 copies/mL (approximately 50% had been receiving immediate-release nevirapine for at least 3 years; approximately 50% were receiving a background regimen of tenofovir and emtricitabine and the remaining patients were receiving abacavir [or zidovudine]) and lamivudine. Patients were randomized (2:1 ratio) to switch to nevirapine extended-release tablets (400 mg once daily) or continue therapy with nevirapine immediate-release tablets (200 mg twice daily) with their current background regimen of 2 NRTIs (study 1100.1526; TRANxITION). At 48 weeks after randomization, 93% of those receiving extended-release tablets and 91% of those receiving immediate-release tablets continued to have plasma HIV-1 RNA levels less than 50 copies/mL.

Pediatric Patients Nevirapine is used in conjunction with other antiretroviral agents for the treatment of HIV-1 infection in children 15 days of age or older (oral suspension or immediate-release tablets). Alternatively, nevirapine extended-release tablets may be used in pediatric patients 6 years of age or older.

For *initial* treatment in HIV-infected pediatric patients, the HHS Panel on Antiretroviral Therapy and Medical Management of HIV-infected Children recommends a *ritonavir-boosted* PI, NNRTI, or integrase strand transfer inhibitor (INSTI) in conjunction with 2 NRTIs (dual NRTIs).

The HHS panel states that nevirapine in conjunction with 2 NRTIs is an alternative (not a preferred) regimen for *initial* treatment in pediatric patients older than 14 days and less than 3 years of age. The fixed combination of lopinavir and ritonavir (lopinavir/ritonavir) in conjunction with 2 NRTIs is the preferred regimen for antiretroviral treatment in pediatric patients 14 days to less than 2 years of age and also a preferred regimen in those 2 years of age to less than 3 years of age.

Although nevirapine is only labeled by FDA for use in neonates 15 days of age or older, the HHS panel states that nevirapine and 2 NRTIs is the preferred regimen for *initial* antiretroviral treatment in neonates younger than 14 days of age† if HIV infection has been confirmed and a decision is made to initiate treatment in this age group. However, consultation with an expert in pediatric HIV infection is recommended since clinical trial data are not available suggesting that initiation of antiretroviral treatment within the first 14 days of life improves outcome compared with initiation after 14 days of age. If a regimen of nevirapine and 2 NRTIs is initiated in a neonate younger than 14 days of age†, the HHS panel states that a change to lopinavir/ritonavir and 2 NRTIs should be considered when the infant is 14 days of age with postmenstrual age at least 42 weeks (i.e., time elapsed since first day of the mother's last menstrual period to birth plus time elapsed after birth).

Nevirapine should *not* be used in postpubertal or adolescent girls with $CD4^+$ T-cell counts exceeding 250 cells/mm^3 or adolescent boys with $CD4^+$ T-cell counts exceeding 400 cells/mm^3, unless benefits clearly outweigh risks. (See Cautions: Hepatic Effects.)

For further information on treatment of HIV infection in pediatric patients, see Antiretroviral Therapy in Pediatric Patients, in Guidelines for Use of Antiretroviral Agents in the Antiretroviral Agents General Statement 8:18.08.

Study BI 1100.1368. Safety and efficacy of nevirapine in HIV-infected pediatric patients have been evaluated in an open-label, randomized study in treatment-naive children 3 months to 16 years of age (49% male, 81% black, 19% white, median baseline plasma HIV-1 RNA level 5.45 $\log_{10}$ copies/mL, median baseline $CD4^+$ T-cell count 527 cells/mm^3, 4% previously received antiretroviral therapy). Children received nevirapine oral suspension (dose based on body surface area or body weight; maximum 400 mg daily) in conjunction with lamivudine and zidovudine. At 48 weeks, 47% of patients had plasma HIV-1 RNA levels less than 400 copies/mL.

Safety and efficacy of nevirapine also have been evaluated in an open-label, phase 1 or 2 study that included 8 HIV-infected children 2–16 months of age who were treatment-naive. These pediatric patients received a 3-drug regimen of oral zidovudine (180 mg/m^2 given every 8 hours), oral didanosine (120 mg/m^2 given every 12 hours), and nevirapine (120 mg/m^2 given once daily for 28 days, then 200 mg/m^2 given every 12 hours). Plasma HIV-1 RNA levels were reduced at least 96% (a decrease of 1.5 $\log_{10}$ copies/mL) in 7 of 8 patients within 2–4 weeks of initiating therapy and, at 6 months, were still below baseline levels in 5 of 6 infants whose treatment started when they were 4 months of age or younger; the regimen was well tolerated in all patients.

Study 1100.1518. Nevirapine extended-release tablets were evaluated in an open-label, nonrandomized, crossover trial in 85 HIV-infected pediatric patients 3 to less than 18 years of age who had received at least 18 weeks of immediate-release nevirapine and had plasma HIV-1 RNA levels less than 50 copies/mL (55% female, 93% black, approximately 84% from Africa, median baseline $CD4^+$ T-cell count 925 cells/mm^3 [range 207–2057 cells/mm^3]). Following a 10-day period of treatment with immediate-release nevirapine, patients were switched to extended-release nevirapine in conjunction with other antiretrovirals. After 10 days of treatment with the extended-release preparation, steady-state pharmacokinetics were determined and 40 of the initial study patients were enrolled in an optional extension phase of the trial to evaluate safety and antiretroviral activity of extended-release nevirapine. At 24 weeks, 39 of these patients continued to have plasma HIV-1 RNA levels less than 50 copies/mL and 1 patient had discontinued the drug because of an adverse reaction. When the 39 patients were stratified according to age, median $CD4^+$ T-cell counts in those 3 to less than 6 years, 6 to less than 12 years, and 12 to less than 18 years of age were 1113, 853, and 682 cells/mm^3, respectively. These $CD4^+$ T-cell counts were similar to those observed at baseline.

■ Prevention of Perinatal HIV Transmission Nevirapine is used in conjunction with other antiretroviral agents for prophylaxis† or empiric HIV therapy† in neonates for prevention of perinatal HIV transmission†.

Although various nevirapine regimens have been used alone or in conjunction with other antiretrovirals for prevention of perinatal HIV transmission in limited-resource areas (e.g., sub-Saharan Africa), including single-dose intrapartum/neonatal nevirapine regimens (e.g., a single nevirapine dose given to the mother at the onset of labor and a single nevirapine dose given to the neonate within 72 hours after birth) and 6-week neonatal nevirapine regimens, single-dose nevirapine regimens (either alone or in conjunction with intrapartum/neonatal zidovudine regimens) are *not* recommended in the US. Maternal and neonatal regimens recommended for prevention of perinatal HIV transmission in the US may differ from those used in other countries.

In the US, multiple-drug antiretroviral regimens are considered the standard of care for treatment of HIV-1 infection in pregnant women and for prevention of perinatal HIV transmission. The HHS Panel on Treatment of Pregnant Women with HIV Infection and Prevention of Perinatal Transmission states that *all* pregnant HIV-infected women in the US should receive multiple-drug antiretroviral therapy, regardless of the woman's plasma HIV RNA level or $CD4^+$ T-cell count. In addition, to further decrease the risk of perinatal HIV transmission, the HHS panel states that pregnant HIV-infected women with plasma HIV-1 RNA levels exceeding 1000 copies/mL (or with unknown HIV RNA levels) near the time of delivery should receive an intrapartum IV zidovudine prophylaxis regimen initiated at the onset of labor (or 3 hours before scheduled cesarean delivery) and continued until delivery (unless contraindicated) and *all* neonates born to HIV-infected women (HIV-exposed neonates) should receive an antiretroviral regimen (either prophylaxis or empiric HIV therapy) initiated as soon as possible after birth (preferably within 6–12 hours) and continued for 4–6 weeks. HIV-exposed neonates at low risk of perinatal HIV acquisition (e.g., those born to an HIV-infected mother who received standard multiple-drug antiretroviral treatment during pregnancy with sustained viral suppression near the time of delivery and with no concerns related to maternal adherence to the treatment regimen) can receive a neonatal prophylaxis regimen that includes only zidovudine. However, a combination antiretroviral regimen that includes zidovudine *and* 1 or 2 additional antiretrovirals should be used in neonates at higher risk of HIV acquisition, including those born to HIV-infected women who did not receive antepartum or intrapartum antiretrovirals, received only intrapartum antiretrovirals, received antepartum and intrapartum antiretrovirals with suboptimal viral suppression near delivery (i.e., detectable plasma HIV RNA levels), or had primary or acute HIV infection during pregnancy or during breast-feeding. This strategy of combined antepartum, intrapartum, and neonatal antiretrovirals reduces perinatal HIV transmission by several mechanisms, including lowering maternal antepartum viral load and providing pre- and postexposure prophylaxis in the infant.

Antiretrovirals in HIV-exposed Neonates The choice of a neonatal antiretroviral prophylaxis regimen *or* a neonatal empiric HIV therapy† regimen should be based on an assessment of the likelihood of perinatal HIV transmission.

Although the HHS panel states that a 4-week zidovudine prophylaxis regimen can be used alone in HIV-exposed neonates at low risk, those at higher risk of HIV acquisition (e.g., those born to HIV-infected women who did not receive antepartum or intrapartum antiretrovirals, received only intrapartum antiretrovirals, or received antepartum and intrapartum antiretrovirals with suboptimal viral suppression near delivery) should receive a 2-drug prophylaxis regimen that includes a 6-week zidovudine prophylaxis regimen *and* a 3-dose nevirapine prophylaxis regimen. Alternatively, the HHS panel states that neonates at highest risk can receive empiric HIV therapy† with a 3-drug regimen of zidovudine, lamivudine, and nevirapine. The 3-drug empiric HIV therapy regimen serves as antiretroviral prophylaxis to prevent acquisition of HIV and also serves as early treatment for neonates who are later confirmed to have acquired HIV. The optimal duration of empiric HIV therapy in neonates at highest risk of HIV acquisition is unknown. Many experts recommend that the 3-drug regimen be continued for 6 weeks; others discontinue nevirapine and/or lamivudine if results of the neonate's HIV nucleic acid amplification test (NAAT) are negative, but recommend continuing the zidovudine regimen for 6 weeks.

Because safety and dosage data are not available, the HHS panel states that use of antiretrovirals other than zidovudine, lamivudine, and nevirapine cannot be recommended for premature HIV-exposed neonates (gestational age less than 37 weeks).

For information on the risk of perinatal transmission of HIV and additional information regarding recommendations for use of antiretroviral agents for prevention of perinatal HIV transmission, see Guidelines for Use of Antiretroviral Agents: Antiretrovirals for Prevention of Perinatal HIV Transmission, in the Antiretroviral Agents General Statement 8:18.08.

Clinicians can consult the National Perinatal HIV Hotline at 888-448-8765 for information regarding antiretroviral treatment of pregnant HIV-infected women and their infants and prevention of perinatal HIV transmission.

Dosage and Administration

■ Administration Nevirapine is administered orally without regard to food.

Nevirapine conventional (immediate-release) tablets and oral suspension are used in adults, adolescents, and pediatric patients 15 days of age or older.

Nevirapine extended-release tablets are used in adults, adolescents, and pediatric patients 6 years of age or older.

Nevirapine therapy usually should be initiated using a low dosage of immediate-release nevirapine for the first 14 days since this appears to reduce the frequency of rash. Nevirapine extended-release tablets should *not* be used during the *initial* 14 days of nevirapine therapy. Patients not currently receiving nevirapine may receive the extended-release tablets *after* a lead-in period of 14 days of low dosage of immediate-release nevirapine. Patients already receiving usual dosage of immediate-release nevirapine may be switched to the extended-release tablets without the 14-day lead-in period.

If mild to moderate rash without constitutional symptoms occurs during the initial 14-day period of low dosage of immediate-release nevirapine, dosage should *not* be increased until the rash has resolved. The low dosage should *not* be continued for longer than 28 days; if the rash has not resolved by day 28, nevirapine should be discontinued and an alternative antiretroviral agent selected.

If nevirapine therapy has been interrupted for more than 7 days for any reason and reinitiation of the drug is not contraindicated, the manufacturer states that the drug should be restarted using the recommended low initial dosage of immediate-release nevirapine for the first 14 days.

If signs or symptoms of severe skin or hypersensitivity reactions, including (but not limited to) severe rash or rash accompanied by fever, general malaise, fatigue, muscle or joint aches, blisters, oral lesions, conjunctivitis, facial edema, and/or hepatitis, eosinophilia, granulocytopenia, lymphadenopathy, and renal dysfunction, occur at any time during nevirapine therapy, the drug should be discontinued and should *not* be reinitiated. If nevirapine therapy is discontinued because of hepatitis or aminotransferase (transaminase) elevations associated with rash or other systemic symptoms, the drug should be permanently discontinued and *not* reinitiated after recovery. (See Cautions: Precautions and Contraindications.)

Extended-release Tablets Nevirapine extended-release tablets should be swallowed whole; the tablets must not be chewed, crushed, or divided.

When considering use of nevirapine extended-release tablets in a child 6 years of age or older, the child should be assessed for their ability to swallow tablets.

Oral Suspension Nevirapine oral suspension should be shaken gently prior to administration of each dose. The entire measured dose of suspension should be administered using an oral dosing syringe or, alternatively, a dosing cup. The oral syringe is recommended, particularly for volumes of 5 mL or less; if a dosing cup is used, it should be thoroughly rinsed with water and the rinse should also be administered to the patient.

■ **Dosage** ***Adult Dosage*** **Treatment of HIV Infection.** The usual initial dosage of nevirapine immediate-release tablets for the treatment of human immunodeficiency virus type 1 (HIV-1) infection in adults is 200 mg once daily for the first 14 days of therapy (lead-in period of low dosage). Dosage should then be increased to 200 mg twice daily in patients who do not experience rash or liver function test abnormalities with the lower dosage.

The usual dosage of nevirapine extended-release tablets for the treatment of HIV-1 infection in adults is 400 mg once daily, initiated *after* immediate-release nevirapine. Patients not currently receiving nevirapine should receive a lead-in period of low dosage of immediate-release nevirapine (200 mg once daily for 14 days) before being switched to the once-daily regimen of extended-release tablets. Patients already receiving a twice-daily regimen of usual dosage of immediate-release nevirapine may be switched to the extended-release tablets without the 14-day lead-in period.

Pediatric Dosage Dosage of nevirapine in pediatric patients is usually based on body surface area (BSA) calculated using the Mosteller formula. Investigational dosage based on weight has been recommended in certain neonates.

Treatment of HIV Infection. For *initial* treatment of HIV-1 infection in neonates younger than 14 days of age† (see Pediatric Patients under Uses: Treatment of HIV Infection), the US Department of Health and Human Services (HHS) Panel on Antiretroviral Therapy and Medical Management of HIV-infected Children recommends that those with gestational age of 34 to less than 37 weeks receive a nevirapine dosage of 4 mg/kg twice daily from birth to 1 week of age followed by a dosage of 6 mg/kg twice daily beginning at 1 week of age. These experts recommend that neonates younger than 14 days of age† with gestational age of 37 weeks or more receive a nevirapine dosage of 6 mg/kg twice daily.

For the treatment of HIV-1 infection in neonates, infants, and children 15 days of age or older, the manufacturer recommends an initial dosage of nevirapine oral suspension or immediate-release tablets of 150 mg/m² once daily for the first 14 days of therapy (lead-in period of low dosage). Dosage should then be increased to 150 mg/m² twice daily in patients who do not experience rash or liver function test abnormalities with the lower dosage. Dosage should not exceed 400 mg daily.

When extended-release nevirapine tablets are used for the treatment of HIV-1 infection in children 6 years to less than 18 years of age, the manufacturer recommends that those not currently receiving immediate-release nevirapine should be given nevirapine oral suspension or immediate-release tablets in a dosage of 150 mg/m² once daily (up to 200 mg daily) for 14 days (lead-in period of low dosage) before being switched to the recommended dosage of nevirapine extended-release tablets. After the lead-in period, pediatric patients 6 years of age or older with BSA 0.58–0.83 m² should receive 200 mg once daily, those with BSA 0.84–1.16 m² should receive 300 mg once daily, and those with BSA 1.17 m² or greater should receive 400 mg once daily. Dosage should not exceed 400 mg daily.

Some experts suggest that a higher nevirapine dosage is required for the treatment of HIV-1 infection in infants and children 1 month to younger than 8 years of age than in those 8 years of age or older. When immediate-release nevirapine is used, these experts recommend that infants and children 1 month to younger than 8 years of age receive a dosage of 200 mg/m² once daily for 14 days (lead-in period of low dosage) followed by 200 mg/m² twice daily (up to 200 mg twice daily) and that children 8 years of age or older receive a dosage of 120–150 mg/m² once daily for 14 days (lead-in period of low dosage) followed by 120–150 mg/m² twice daily (up to 200 mg twice daily). If extended-release tablets are used in those 6 to less than 8 years of age, these experts recommend 400 mg/m² once daily (up to 400 mg once daily). Some experts suggest that nevirapine can be initiated in pediatric patients 2 years of age or younger without a lead-in period of low dosage.

Adolescents can receive the usual adult dosage of nevirapine. (See Adult Dosage under Dosage and Administration: Dosage.)

Prevention of Perinatal HIV Transmission. When a 2-drug antiretroviral regimen of zidovudine and nevirapine is used for prophylaxis for prevention of perinatal HIV transmission† in neonates at higher risk of HIV acquisition (see Uses: Prevention of Perinatal HIV Transmission), the HHS Panel on Treatment of Pregnant Women with HIV Infection and Prevention of Perinatal Transmission recommends that 3 doses of oral nevirapine be given during the first week of life (first dose given within 48 hours of birth, second dose given 48 hours after first dose, third dose given 96 hours after second dose) *in addition* to the usual 6-week neonatal zidovudine prophylaxis regimen. These experts recommend that neonates with birth weight of 1.5–2 kg receive 8 mg of nevirapine for each of the 3 doses and that neonates with birth weight greater than 2 kg receive 12 mg of nevirapine for each of the 3 doses.

When empiric HIV therapy† is used for prevention of perinatal HIV transmission† in neonates at highest risk of HIV acquisition (see Uses: Prevention of Perinatal HIV Transmission), a 3-drug antiretroviral regimen of zidovudine, nevirapine, and lamivudine is recommended and should be initiated as soon as possible after birth (within 6–12 hours). The HHS Panel recommends that neonates with gestational age of 34 to less than 37 weeks receive 4 mg/kg of nevirapine twice daily from birth to 1 week of age followed by 6 mg/kg twice daily beginning at 1 week of age. Neonates with gestational age of 37 weeks or more should receive 6 mg/kg of nevirapine twice daily. Optimal duration of empiric HIV therapy† in HIV-exposed neonates at highest risk of HIV acquisition is unknown. Many experts recommend that the 3-drug regimen be continued for 6 weeks; others discontinue nevirapine and/or lamivudine if results of the neonate's HIV nucleic acid amplification test (NAAT) are negative, but recommend continuing the zidovudine regimen for 6 weeks.

Clinicians can consult the National Perinatal HIV Hotline at 888-448-8765 for information regarding selection of antiretrovirals, including dosage considerations, for prevention of perinatal HIV transmission.

■ **Dosage in Renal and Hepatic Impairment** ***Renal Impairment*** Modification of the usual dosage of nevirapine is not necessary in patients with creatinine clearances of 20 mL/minute or greater not requiring dialysis. However, because nevirapine is removed by dialysis, an additional 200-mg dose of immediate-release nevirapine should be administered following each dialysis treatment. Although nevirapine metabolites may accumulate in patients receiving dialysis, the clinical importance of this accumulation is unknown. The pharmacokinetics of nevirapine have not been evaluated in those with creatinine clearances less than 20 mL/minute.

Nevirapine extended-release tablets have not been studied in patients with renal impairment.

Hepatic Impairment Data are insufficient to date to determine the appropriate dosage of immediate-release nevirapine in patients with mild hepatic impairment (Child-Pugh Class A); some experts state that dosage adjustments are not necessary in these patients. Immediate-release nevirapine is contraindicated in patients with moderate or severe hepatic impairment (Child-Pugh Class B or C). (See Cautions: Precautions and Contraindications.)

Nevirapine extended-release tablets have not been studied in patients with hepatic impairment. Extended-release tablets are contraindicated in patients with moderate or severe hepatic impairment (Child-Pugh class B or C).

Cautions

The most frequently reported adverse effects in patients receiving nevirapine are rash, nausea, headache, fatigue, and abnormal liver function test results. Serious adverse reactions reported in patients receiving nevirapine include hepatitis, hepatic failure, Stevens-Johnson syndrome, toxic epidermal necrolysis, and hypersensitivity reactions. Hepatitis/hepatic failure may be associated with signs of hypersensitivity, including severe rash or rash accompanied by fever, general malaise, fatigue, muscle or joint aches, blisters, oral lesions, conjunctivitis, facial edema, eosinophilia, granulocytopenia, lymphadenopathy, or renal impairment.

Adverse effects reported with nevirapine extended-release tablets are similar to those reported with conventional (immediate-release) nevirapine tablets.

■ **Hepatic Effects** Severe, life-threatening (and in some cases fatal) hepatotoxicity, including fulminant and cholestatic hepatitis (e.g., transaminase elevations with or without hyperbilirubinemia, prolonged partial thromboplastin time, or eosinophilia), hepatic necrosis, and hepatic failure, have been reported in patients receiving nevirapine. Although clinical presentation varied, frequently occurring features included nonspecific prodromal signs and symptoms of fatigue, malaise, anorexia, nausea, jaundice, liver tenderness, and/or hepatomegaly, with or without initially abnormal serum transaminase concentrations; rash was observed in 50% of patients with symptomatic hepatic events. A diagnosis of hepatotoxicity should be considered even if liver function tests are initially normal or alternative diagnoses are possible. Some events, especially those with rash and other symptoms, have progressed over several days to hepatic failure with transaminase elevation, with or without hyperbilirubinemia, hepatic encephalopathy, prolonged partial thromboplastin time, and/or eosinophilia. These events may occur at any time during treatment. While the risk of hepatic events is greatest during the first 6 weeks of therapy, substantial risk continues through the first 18 weeks of therapy.

Patients with signs and symptoms of hepatitis must seek immediate medical attention, have serum transaminase concentrations measured, and be advised to discontinue nevirapine as soon as possible. If nevirapine is discontinued because of hepatitis or transaminase elevations associated with rash or other systemic symptoms, the drug should be permanently discontinued and *not* reinitiated.

Asymptomatic increases in serum AST or ALT (more than 5 times the upper limit of normal) have occurred in 6% of patients receiving nevirapine and in 6% of those in control groups. In clinical studies, symptomatic hepatic events (regardless of severity) occurred in 4% of patients receiving regimens that included nevirapine and in 1% of those in the control group. Women, including pregnant women, appear to be at higher risk of nevirapine-associated hepatic events than men. Symptomatic hepatic events (usually associated with rash) have been observed in 6% of women and in 2% of men during the first 6 weeks of treatment with a nevirapine-containing regimen.

In a clinical study in antiretroviral-naive patients who received initial treatment with nevirapine immediate-release tablets for 14 days and were then randomized to continue treatment with immediate-release tablets or be switched to nevirapine extended-release tablets, the incidence of any hepatic event was 9% in the immediate-release group and 6% in the extended-release group; the incidence of symptomatic hepatic events (anorexia, jaundice, vomiting) was 3 and 2%, respectively. Overall the incidence of symptomatic events in study patients was similar among men and women.

While all patients with higher $CD4^+$ T-cell counts prior to initiation of therapy with nevirapine are at increased risk for symptomatic hepatic events, the patients at highest risk are women with high $CD4^+$ T-cell counts at baseline. Symptomatic hepatic events were observed in 11% of women with $CD4^+$ T-cell counts exceeding 250 cells/mm^3 at baseline and in 6% of men with $CD4^+$ T-cell counts exceeding 400 cells/mm^3 at baseline.

Increased serum concentrations of AST or ALT prior to initiation of antiretroviral therapy and/or coinfection with hepatitis B virus (HBV) or hepatitis C virus (HCV) are associated with a greater risk of later symptomatic hepatic adverse effects (i.e., events that occur 6 or more weeks after initiation of nevirapine therapy) and asymptomatic increases in serum transaminase concentrations.

Serious hepatotoxicity has been reported in individuals not infected with HIV who received multiple doses of nevirapine as part of a 2- or 3-drug regimen for postexposure prophylaxis following occupational or nonoccupational exposure to HIV. Adverse hepatic effects in these individuals have included end-stage liver failure requiring transplantation, clinical hepatitis (e.g., jaundice, fever, nausea, vomiting, abdominal pain, and/or hepatomegaly), and elevated serum ALT and AST concentrations without clinical hepatitis. Nevirapine is contraindicated for and should not be included in regimens used for such prophylaxis. (See Cautions: Precautions and Contraindications)

Asymptomatic elevations in serum γ-glutamyltransferase (GGT, γ-glutamyltranspeptidase, GGTP) have been reported frequently in patients receiving nevirapine. Nevirapine therapy may be continued in patients who have asymptomatic elevations of GGT without elevations in other liver enzymes.

■ Dermatologic and Sensitivity Reactions The most frequently reported adverse reaction in patients receiving nevirapine is rash. Rash reported in patients receiving nevirapine usually is mild to moderate, consists of maculopapular erythematous cutaneous eruptions (with or without pruritus), and is located on the trunk, face, and extremities. In controlled studies, 13 or 6% of patients receiving nevirapine or placebo, respectively, experienced a mild to moderate rash (grade 1 or 2) during the first 6 weeks of therapy and 2% or less than 1% of patients receiving nevirapine or placebo, respectively, experienced a serious rash (grade 3 or 4). Women appear to be at higher risk of nevirapine-associated rash than men.

Severe and life-threatening skin reactions, including Stevens-Johnson syndrome, toxic epidermal necrolysis, and hypersensitivity reactions characterized by rash, constitutional findings, and organ dysfunction including hepatic failure, also have occurred in patients receiving nevirapine. Fatalities have been reported. There have been postmarketing reports of anaphylaxis, drug reaction with eosinophilia and systemic symptoms (DRESS), angioedema, bullous eruptions, ulcerative stomatitis, and urticaria.

Most cases of rash (including severe, life-threatening skin reactions and fatalities) have occurred within the first 4–6 weeks of nevirapine therapy. Initiating nevirapine therapy using a low dosage during the first 14 days of therapy appears to reduce the frequency of rash and is recommended for all patients. (See Dosage and Administration.) Risk factors for developing serious cutaneous reactions include failure to follow the low dosage regimen during the first 14 days of therapy and delay in discontinuing nevirapine after the onset of initial symptoms.

In a clinical study in antiretroviral-naive patients who received initial treatment with nevirapine immediate-release tablets for 14 days and were then randomized to continue treatment with immediate-release tablets or be switched to nevirapine extended-release tablets, the incidence of severe or life-threatening rash considered to be related to nevirapine was 1% in patients during the lead-in phase and also was 1% in patients subsequently randomized to immediate-release or to extended-release tablets.

Concomitant use of prednisone during the first 14 days of therapy in an attempt to prevent nevirapine-associated rash is *not* recommended. In a clinical trial of nevirapine immediate-release tablets, concomitant use of prednisone (40 mg daily during the first 14 days of nevirapine administration) was associated with an increased incidence and severity of rash during the first 6 weeks of nevirapine therapy.

Management of patients who develop rash while receiving nevirapine should be based on the type and severity of symptoms. Serum transaminase concentrations should be immediately evaluated in any patient experiencing rash, especially during the first 18 weeks of therapy. If signs or symptoms of severe skin or hypersensitivity reactions, including (but not limited to) severe rash or rash accompanied by fever, general malaise, fatigue, muscle or joint aches, blisters, oral lesions, conjunctivitis, facial edema, and/or hepatitis, eosinophilia, granulocytopenia, lymphadenopathy, and renal dysfunction, occur during nevirapine therapy, the drug should be discontinued and should *not* be reinitiated. Delay in discontinuing nevirapine after onset of rash may result in a more severe reaction. If nevirapine is discontinued because of severe skin rash, skin rash combined with increased serum transaminase concentrations or other symptoms, or hypersensitivity reaction, the drug should be permanently discontinued and *not* reinitiated. While nevirapine therapy generally can be continued in patients with mild or moderate rash (e.g., erythema, pruritus, diffuse erythematous macular or maculopapular rash), dosage should *not* be increased until the rash has resolved. Mild to moderate rash resolves within 2 weeks in about 50% of patients and within 1 month in about 75% of patients; these patients may be treated symptomatically with antihistamines, antipyretics, and/or nonsteroidal anti-inflammatory agents.

■ GI Effects Adverse GI effects, including nausea, diarrhea, vomiting, abdominal pain, and ulcerative stomatitis, have been reported in patients who received nevirapine in conjunction with other antiretroviral agents.

■ Adipogenic Effects Redistribution or accumulation of body fat, including central obesity, dorsocervical fat enlargement ("buffalo hump"), peripheral wasting, facial wasting, breast enlargement, and general cushingoid appearance, has been reported in patients receiving antiretroviral agents. The mechanisms responsible for these adipogenic effects and the long-term consequences of these effects are unknown. A causal relationship has not been established.

■ Immune Reconstitution Syndrome An inflammatory response to indolent or residual opportunistic infections (e.g., *Mycobacterium avium* complex [MAC], *M. tuberculosis*, cytomegalovirus [CMV], *Pneumocystis jirovecii* [formerly *P. carinii*]) has occurred in patients who have responded to initial antiretroviral therapy.

Autoimmune disorders (e.g., Graves' disease, polymyositis, Guillain-Barré syndrome) also have been reported to occur in the setting of immune reconstitution; however, the time to onset is more variable and can occur many months after initiation of antiretroviral therapy.

■ Other Adverse Effects Other adverse effects reported in patients receiving nevirapine include headache, fatigue, somnolence, paresthesia, arthralgia, rhabdomyolysis associated with dermatologic and/or hepatic events, myalgia, neutropenia, thrombocytopenia, granulocytopenia, and decreased hemoglobin concentrations.

■ Precautions and Contraindications Nevirapine is contraindicated in patients with moderate or severe hepatic impairment (Child-Pugh class B or C).

Nevirapine is contraindicated for and should not be included in regimens used for postexposure prophylaxis following occupational exposure to HIV (PEP) or postexposure prophylaxis following nonoccupational exposure to HIV (nPEP). (See Cautions: Hepatic Effects.)

Hepatotoxicity and Skin Reactions Intensive clinical and laboratory monitoring, including liver enzyme tests, is essential at baseline and during the initial 18 weeks of nevirapine therapy to detect potentially life-threatening hepatotoxicity and skin reactions. Extra vigilance is required during the first 6 weeks of therapy since this is the period of greatest risk.

The optimum frequency of monitoring during initial nevirapine therapy has not been established, but some clinicians recommend clinical and laboratory monitoring more often than once monthly and, in particular, recommend liver function tests at baseline, prior to dosage escalation, and at 2 weeks after dosage escalation. Severe liver disease occurs most frequently during the first 6 weeks of therapy, but can occur after this period. Therefore, clinical and laboratory monitoring should continue at frequent intervals after the initial 18-week period and throughout nevirapine therapy. Serum transaminase concentrations should be determined immediately whenever a patient experiences rash or signs or symptoms suggestive of hepatitis and/or hypersensitivity reactions during nevirapine therapy.

Nevirapine is contraindicated in patients with moderate or severe hepatic impairment (Child-Pugh class B or C). Because severe, life-threatening, and in some cases fatal hepatotoxicity, including fulminant and cholestatic hepatitis, hepatic necrosis, and hepatic failure, has occurred in patients receiving nevirapine, clinicians and patients should be vigilant for the appearance of signs or symptoms of hepatitis (e.g., fatigue, malaise, anorexia, nausea, jaundice, bilirubinemia, acholic stools, liver tenderness, hepatomegaly). (See Cautions: Hepatic Effects.) Patients should be advised to seek immediate medical attention and have serum transaminase concentrations measured and to discontinue the drug as soon as possible if signs or symptoms of hepatitis develop. A diagnosis of hepatotoxicity should be considered in this setting, even if liver function test results are initially normal or alternative diagnoses are possible. If nevirapine is discontinued because of hepatitis or transaminase elevations associated with rash or other systemic symptoms, the drug should *not* be reinitiated. Patients also should be advised that increased liver function test results and/or a history of HBV or HCV infection and CD4$^+$ T-cell counts exceeding 250 cells/mm^3 in women or 400 cells/mm^3 in men prior to initiation of antiretroviral therapy are associated with an increased risk of hepatic events with nevirapine; women also may be at higher risk of these events.

Severe and life-threatening skin reactions (e.g., Stevens-Johnson syndrome; toxic epidermal necrolysis; hypersensitivity reactions characterized by rash, constitutional findings, and organ dysfunction including hepatic failure), including some fatalities, have occurred in patients receiving nevirapine, usually during the first 6 weeks of therapy. Nevirapine should be immediately discontinued and *not* reinitiated in any patient who develops signs or symptoms of severe skin reactions or hypersensitivity reactions, including (but not limited to) severe rash or rash accompanied by fever, general malaise, fatigue, muscle or joint aches, blisters, oral lesions, conjunctivitis, facial edema, and/or hepatitis, eosinophilia, granulocytopenia, lymphadenopathy, and renal dysfunction. Delay in discontinuing nevirapine after onset of rash may result in a more severe reaction.

Patients receiving nevirapine should be warned of the signs and symptoms of nevirapine skin reactions and directed to immediately discontinue the drug and seek medical evaluation if severe rash, rash accompanied by other symptoms, or hypersensitivity occurs. Patients also should be instructed that if any rash occurs during the first 14 days of nevirapine therapy, dosage of the drug should *not* be increased until the rash has resolved.

If nevirapine is discontinued because of severe skin rash, skin rash combined with increased serum transaminase concentrations or other symptoms, or hypersensitivity reaction, the drug should be permanently discontinued and *not* reinitiated.

Other Precautions Patients should be advised that redistribution or accumulation of body fat may occur in patients receiving antiretroviral therapy and that the cause and long-term health effects of these conditions are as yet unknown. (See Cautions: Adipogenic Effects.)

Concomitant use of nevirapine and some other drugs may result in drug interactions, and patients should be instructed to inform their clinician of their use of other drugs, including prescription and nonprescription drugs or dietary or herbal supplements such as St. John's wort. (See Drug Interactions.)

Patients should be advised to immediately contact a clinician if they have any signs or symptoms of infection since inflammation from previous infections may occur soon after antiretroviral therapy is initiated. (See Cautions: Immune Reconstitution Syndrome.)

Nevirapine in conjunction with other antiretroviral agents is not a cure for HIV infection, and opportunistic infections and other complications associated with HIV disease may still occur. Patients receiving nevirapine should be under close clinical observation by clinicians experienced in treatment of diseases associated with HIV infection, and patients should be advised to seek medical care if any clinically important change in their health status occurs.

Patients should be advised that effective antiretroviral regimens can decrease HIV concentrations in blood and genital secretions and strict adherence to such regimens in conjunction with risk-reduction measures may decrease, but cannot absolutely eliminate, the risk of secondary transmission of HIV to others. Patients should continue to practice safer sex (e.g., using latex or polyurethane condoms to minimize sexual contact with body fluids), never share personal items that can have blood or body fluids on them (e.g., toothbrushes, razor blades), and never reuse or share needles.

Nevirapine should always be administered in conjunction with other antiretroviral agents and should *not* be used alone for treatment of HIV infection. Although nevirapine used in conjunction with other antiretroviral agents appears to be well tolerated, patients should be monitored closely for adverse effects. The usual precautions and contraindications of the other antiretrovirals in the regimen should be considered.

To avoid overdosage, nevirapine immediate-release preparations (tablets or oral suspension) and nevirapine extended-release tablets should *not* be used concomitantly.

The effect of nevirapine therapy on subsequent therapy with certain other HIV nonnucleoside reverse transcriptase inhibitors (NNRTIs) remains to be determined. (See Resistance: Cross-resistance.)

■ Pediatric Precautions

Safety and pharmacokinetics of nevirapine oral suspension have been evaluated in pediatric patients 15 days to less than 3 months of age. Safety, pharmacokinetics, and efficacy of nevirapine immediate-release tablets and oral suspension have been evaluated in pediatric patients 3 months to 18 years of age.

Nevirapine extended-release tablets can be used for treatment of HIV-1 infection in children 6 years of age or older based on pharmacokinetic, safety, and antiretroviral activity data from an open-label trial evaluating the drug in pediatric patients 3 to less than 18 years of age and efficacy data from adults. The extended-release tablets are not recommended in pediatric patients 3 to less than 6 years of age because pharmacokinetic data are insufficient to support use in this age group; the tablets are not recommended in those less than 3 years of age because of inability to swallow tablets.

Although safety and efficacy have only been established in neonates 15 days of age or older, immediate-release nevirapine is recommended by some experts for *initial* treatment of confirmed HIV infection in neonates younger than 14 days of age† (see Pediatric Patients under Uses: Treatment of HIV Infection). Immediate-release nevirapine also is recommended by some experts for prophylaxis† or empiric HIV therapy† for prevention of perinatal HIV transmission† in certain neonates 14 days of age or younger (see Uses: Prevention of Perinatal HIV Transmission).

The most frequently reported adverse effects in children were similar to those observed in adults; however, granulocytopenia occurred more frequently in children than in adults. Stevens-Johnson syndrome or Stevens-Johnson/toxic epidermal necrolysis transition syndrome has occurred rarely in children receiving nevirapine. Rash, allergic reaction, including anaphylaxis, also have been reported. Anemia has been observed in children during postmarketing surveillance; whether anemia was due to nevirapine or concomitant drug therapy has not been determined. Nevirapine generally has been well tolerated when used in neonates.

■ Geriatric Precautions

Clinical studies of nevirapine to date have not included sufficient numbers of adults 65 years of age or older to determine whether geriatric individuals respond differently to the drug than younger adults. In general, dosage for geriatric patients should be selected carefully since these individuals frequently have decreased hepatic, renal, and/or cardiac function and concomitant disease and drug therapy.

■ Mutagenicity and Carcinogenicity

Nevirapine was not mutagenic or clastogenic in a variety of in vitro and in vivo assays, including microbial assays for gene mutation (Ames test in *Salmonella* and *Escherichia coli*), mammalian cell gene mutation assays (Chinese hamster ovary [CHO] cells/ HGPRT), cytogenetic assays using a CHO cell line, and a mouse bone marrow micronucleus assay.

Long-term carcinogenicity studies in mice using nevirapine dosages of 0, 50, 375, or 750 mg/kg daily for 2 years revealed an increased incidence of hepatocellular adenomas and carcinomas at all dosages in males and at the 2 highest dosages in females. In similar studies in rats using nevirapine dosages of 0, 3.5, 17.5, or 35 mg/kg daily for 2 years, there was an increase in hepatocellular adenomas at all dosages in males and at the highest dosage in females. The mechanism of the carcinogenic potential is unknown. Systemic exposure (based on AUC) in these rodents was lower than that measured in humans receiving a dosage of 200 mg twice daily. Given the lack of genotoxic activity of nevirapine, the relevance to humans of the hepatocellular neoplasms reported in nevirapine-treated mice and rats is unknown.

■ Pregnancy, Fertility, and Lactation

Pregnancy To monitor maternal-fetal outcomes of pregnant women exposed to antiretroviral agents, including nevirapine, the Antiretroviral Pregnancy Registry was established through the collaboration of antiretroviral manufacturers and an advisory committee of practitioners. Clinicians are encouraged to contact the registry at 800-258-4263 or http://www.APRegistry.com to report cases of prenatal exposure to antiretroviral agents.

Data from the Antiretroviral Pregnancy Registry show no difference in the risk of overall major birth defects for nevirapine compared with the US reference population of the Metropolitan Atlanta Congenital Defects Program (MACDP). Registry data include over 2600 reports of nevirapine exposures during pregnancy resulting in live births, including over 1100 first-trimester exposures to the drug. The prevalence of birth defects in live births was 2.8% following first-trimester exposures to nevirapine-containing regimens and 3.2% following second- or third-trimester exposures to nevirapine-containing regimens.

The HHS Panel on Treatment of Pregnant Women with HIV Infection and Prevention of Perinatal Transmission states that nevirapine in conjunction with 2 HIV nucleoside reverse transcriptase inhibitors (NRTIs) is *not* recommended for *initial* treatment in antiretroviral-naive pregnant women because of greater potential for adverse events, complex lead-in dosage regimen, and low barrier for HIV resistance.

Severe hepatic events, including fatalities, have been reported in HIV-infected pregnant women receiving long-term nevirapine therapy as part of multiple-drug antiretroviral treatment. Because women (including pregnant women) with baseline CD4$^+$ T-cell counts exceeding 250 cells/mm^3 appear to be at higher risk of nevirapine-associated symptomatic and potentially fatal rash and hepatic toxicity, the drug should be initiated in such women with caution and only when potential benefits outweigh risks. (See Cautions: Precautions and Contraindications.) Nevirapine may be continued in women who become pregnant while receiving a suppressive nevirapine-based regimen, regardless of their CD4$^+$ T-cell count, as long as the drug is tolerated.

Fertility In reproduction studies in female rats, there was evidence of impaired fertility at nevirapine doses providing systemic exposure approximately equivalent to that provided by the usually recommended human dosage based on AUC.

Human data are insufficient to determine the risk of infertility in patients receiving nevirapine.

Females with reproductive potential should be advised that, based on results from fertility studies in rats, nevirapine may impair fertility and it is not known whether effects on fertility are reversible.

Lactation Nevirapine is distributed into milk. Following administration of a single 100- or 200-mg dose of nevirapine to pregnant women several hours before delivery, postpartum concentrations of the drug in milk have been reported to be 25–122% of maternal serum concentrations. In some studies in women receiving immediate-release nevirapine, median breast milk concentrations of the drug ranged from about 4–7 mg/mL and the median breast milk to maternal plasma concentration ratio ranged from 0.59–0.88. Rash and hyperbilirubinemia have been reported in infants exposed to nevirapine through breast milk.

Because of the risk of transmission of HIV to an uninfected infant through breast milk, the CDC and other experts recommend that HIV-infected women *not* breast-feed infants, regardless of antiretroviral therapy. Therefore, because of the potential for HIV transmission and the potential for serious adverse effects from nevirapine if the drug were distributed into milk, women should be instructed not to breast-feed while they are receiving nevirapine.

Drug Interactions

The following drug interactions are based on studies using nevirapine conventional (immediate-release) tablets and are expected to also apply to nevirapine extended-release tablets.

■ **Drugs Affected or Metabolized by Hepatic Microsomal Enzymes** Metabolism of nevirapine is mediated in part by the cytochrome P-450 (CYP) 3A4 and 2B6 isoenzymes, and plasma nevirapine concentrations may be decreased by concomitant use of drugs that induce these isoenzymes (e.g., rifabutin, rifampin) or may be increased by concomitant use of drugs that inhibit these isoenzymes (e.g., cimetidine, macrolides). In addition, nevirapine is an inducer of CYP3A4 and CYP2B6 and may alter the pharmacokinetics of drugs metabolized by these isoenzymes (e.g., HIV protease inhibitors). While principally an inducer of CYP3A4 and CYP2B6, nevirapine may also inhibit these enzymes; however, the drug may have only a minimal inhibitory effect on other substrates of CYP3A4 at therapeutic concentrations.

Nevirapine does not appear to affect plasma concentrations of drugs that are substrates of other CYP isoenzymes (e.g., 1A2, 2D6, 2A6, 2E1, 2C9, 2C19).

■ **Anticoagulants** ***Apixaban and Rivaroxaban*** Concomitant use of nevirapine and apixaban or rivaroxaban may result in decreased concentrations of the anticoagulant. Some experts state that alternative therapy should be considered.

Betrixaban, Dabigatran, and Edoxaban Concomitant use of nevirapine is not expected to affect concentrations of betrixaban, dabigatran, or edoxaban.

Dosage adjustments are not necessary if nevirapine is used concomitantly with betrixaban, dabigatran, or edoxaban.

Warfarin Concomitant use of nevirapine and warfarin is predicted to alter warfarin plasma concentrations resulting in increased or decreased effects of the anticoagulant. The in vitro interaction between nevirapine and warfarin is complex.

The international normalized ration (INR) should be closely monitored in patients receiving nevirapine and warfarin concomitantly and warfarin dosage adjusted accordingly.

■ **Anticonvulsants** ***Carbamazepine, Clonazepam, Phenobarbital, Phenytoin*** Concomitant use of nevirapine and certain anticonvulsants (carbamazepine, clonazepam, phenobarbital, phenytoin) may result in decreased plasma concentrations of the anticonvulsant and nevirapine.

Nevirapine and certain anticonvulsants (carbamazepine, clonazepam, phenobarbital, phenytoin) should be used concomitantly with caution. Anticonvulsant and nevirapine concentrations and antiretroviral response should be monitored; alternatively, use of another anticonvulsant can be considered.

Eslicarbazepine Concomitant use of eslicarbazepine and nevirapine may result in decreased nevirapine concentrations.

If eslicarbazepine and nevirapine are used concomitantly, antiretroviral response should be monitored and nevirapine plasma concentration monitoring considered; alternatively, a different anticonvulsant or different antiretroviral should be considered.

Ethosuximide Concomitant use of ethosuximide and nevirapine may result in decreased plasma concentrations of the anticonvulsant and nevirapine.

Nevirapine and ethosuximide should be used concomitantly with caution. Ethosuximide concentrations and antiretroviral response should be monitored.

■ **Antidiabetic Agents** ***Canagliflozin, Dapagliflozin, Empagliflozin, and Sitagliptin*** Concomitant use of nevirapine and canagliflozin, dapagliflozin, empagliflozin, or sitagliptin is not expected to affect concentrations of the oral antidiabetic agent. Dosage adjustments are not necessary.

Linagliptin and Saxagliptin Concomitant use of nevirapine and linagliptin or saxagliptin may result in decreased concentrations of the oral antidiabetic agent.

If nevirapine is used concomitantly with linagliptin or saxagliptin, glycemic control should be monitored.

■ **Antifungal Agents** ***Fluconazole*** Concomitant use of fluconazole and nevirapine does not appear to affect plasma concentrations or area under the concentration-time curve (AUC) of the antifungal agent; however, based on comparison with historical data, concomitant use results in about a 100% increase in nevirapine exposure.

Nevirapine and fluconazole should be used concomitantly with caution and patients closely monitored for nevirapine-associated adverse effects. Because of a possible increased risk of hepatotoxicity, some experts suggest that an alternative antiretroviral agent be considered in patients receiving fluconazole.

Isavuconazonium Concomitant use of isavuconazonium sulfate (prodrug of isavuconazole) and nevirapine may result in decreased isavuconazole concentrations.

If isavuconazonium sulfate and nevirapine are used concomitantly, adjustment of the antifungal dosage may be required. Monitoring of isavuconazole concentrations and antifungal response should be considered.

Itraconazole Itraconazole and nevirapine should not be used concomitantly since plasma concentrations of the antifungal may be decreased and antifungal efficacy may be reduced and nevirapine concentrations may be increased.

If itraconazole and nevirapine are used concomitantly, plasma concentrations of itraconazole should be monitored and dosage of the antifungal adjusted accordingly.

Ketoconazole Ketoconazole and nevirapine should not be used concomitantly since plasma concentrations of the antifungal may be decreased and antifungal efficacy may be reduced.

Concomitant use of ketoconazole (400 mg once daily) and nevirapine (200 mg once daily for 2 weeks followed by 200 mg twice daily for 2 weeks) in HIV-infected patients decreased ketoconazole peak plasma concentrations and AUC by 44 and 72%, respectively.

Posaconazole Concomitant use of posaconazole and nevirapine may result in increased nevirapine concentrations.

If posaconazole and nevirapine are used concomitantly, the patient should be monitored for nevirapine-associated adverse effects.

Voriconazole Concomitant use of voriconazole and nevirapine may result in decreased voriconazole concentrations and increased nevirapine concentrations. If the drugs are used concomitantly, patients should be monitored for adverse effects or toxicity and clinical response to voriconazole and/or plasma concentrations of the antifungal should be monitored.

■ **Antimalarial Agents** Concomitant use of the fixed combination of artemether and lumefantrine (artemether/lumefantrine) and nevirapine decreases the AUC of artemether and the active metabolite of artemether (dihydroartemisinin) and may alter (increase or decrease) the AUC of lumefantrine. Although the clinical importance of this interaction is unknown, patients should be closely monitored for antimalarial efficacy and lumefantrine toxicity.

■ **Antimycobacterial Agents** ***Bedaquiline*** Concomitant use of bedaquiline and nevirapine does not affect the AUC of bedaquiline. Dosage adjustments are not necessary if bedaquiline and nevirapine are used concomitantly.

Rifabutin Concomitant use of rifabutin and nevirapine results in a 28% increase in peak plasma concentrations and 17% increase in the AUC of rifabutin and similar increases in plasma concentrations and AUC of its major metabolite. However, because of interindividual variability, some patients may experience large increases in rifabutin exposure and may be at higher risk of rifabutin toxicity.

Nevirapine and rifabutin should be used concomitantly with caution. Some experts state that dosage adjustments are unnecessary if the drugs are used concomitantly.

Rifampin Concomitant use of rifampin and nevirapine results a greater than 50% decrease in nevirapine peak plasma concentration and AUC; peak plasma concentrations of rifampin are unaffected bit the AUC of rifampin is increased 11%.

Concomitant use of rifampin and nevirapine is not recommended.

Rifapentine Concomitant use of rifapentine and nevirapine may result in decreased nevirapine concentrations.

Concomitant use of rifapentine and nevirapine is not recommended.

■ **Antineoplastic Agents** Concomitant use of nevirapine and cyclophosphamide is predicted to result in decreased plasma concentrations of the antineoplastic agent. Appropriate dosages for concomitant use of cyclophosphamide and nevirapine have not been established.

■ **Antiplatelet Agents** ***Clopidogrel*** Concomitant use of clopidogrel and nevirapine is not expected to affect clopidogrel concentrations. Dosage adjustments are not necessary if clopidogrel and nevirapine are used concomitantly.

Prasugrel Concomitant use of prasugrel and nevirapine is not expected to affect prasugrel concentrations. Dosage adjustments are not necessary if prasugrel and nevirapine are used concomitantly.

Ticagrelor Concomitant use of ticagrelor and nevirapine is expected to result in decreased ticagrelor concentrations. Some experts state that alternative therapy should be considered.

■ **Antipsychotic Agents** ***Lurasidone, Pimozide, Quetiapine, and Thioridazine*** Concomitant use of nevirapine and lurasidone, pimozide, quetiapine, or thioridazine may result in decreased concentrations of the antipsychotic agent.

If nevirapine is used concomitantly with lurasidone, pimozide, quetiapine, or thioridazine, the patient should be monitored for effects of the antipsychotic agent.

Olanzapine Concomitant use of olanzapine and nevirapine is not expected to affect olanzapine concentrations. Dosage adjustments are not necessary if the drugs are used concomitantly.

■ **Antiretroviral Agents** *HIV Entry and Fusion Inhibitors* **Maraviroc.** Concomitant use of maraviroc and nevirapine does not affect the AUC of maraviroc. If nevirapine is used with maraviroc in a regimen that does *not* include an HIV PI or other potent CYP3A inhibitor, the recommended maraviroc dosage is 300 mg twice daily. If nevirapine is used with maraviroc in a regimen that includes a PI (except *ritonavir-boosted* tipranavir), the recommended maraviroc dosage is 150 mg twice daily.

There is no in vitro evidence of antagonistic antiretroviral effects between maraviroc and nevirapine.

HIV Integrase Inhibitors (INSTIs) **Dolutegravir.** Concomitant use of nevirapine and dolutegravir may decrease dolutegravir plasma concentrations and AUC. Nevirapine and dolutegravir should not be used concomitantly; data are insufficient to make dosage recommendations.

There is no in vitro evidence of antagonistic antiretroviral effects between dolutegravir and nevirapine.

Elvitegravir and Cobicistat. Concomitant use of nevirapine and the fixed combination of elvitegravir, cobicistat, emtricitabine, and tenofovir alafenamide (EVG/c/FTC/TAF) or the fixed combination of elvitegravir, cobicistat, emtricitabine, and tenofovir disoproxil fumarate (EVG/c/FTC/TDF) may result in altered (increased or decreased) concentrations of elvitegravir, cobicistat, and/or nevirapine.

Nevirapine should not be used concomitantly with EVG/c/FTC/TAF or EVG/c/FTC/TDF.

Raltegravir. Some experts state that dosage adjustments are not necessary if raltegravir is used concomitantly with nevirapine.

There is no in vitro evidence of antagonistic antiretroviral effects between raltegravir and nevirapine.

HIV Nonnucleoside Reverse Transcriptase Inhibitors (NNRTIs) Nevirapine should not be used concomitantly with other NNRTIs (delavirdine, efavirenz, etravirine, rilpivirine).

Concomitant use of nevirapine and delavirdine, etravirine, or rilpivirine may result in altered plasma concentrations of the drugs.

Efavirenz. Concomitant use of efavirenz and nevirapine results in a 12% decrease in peak plasma concentrations and a 28% decrease in the AUC of efavirenz. An increased incidence of adverse effects and no improvement in efficacy have been reported when these NNRTIs were used concomitantly.

Appropriate dosages for concomitant use of efavirenz and nevirapine with respect to safety and efficacy have not been established.

HIV Nucleoside Reverse Transcriptase Inhibitors (NRTIs) There is no in vitro evidence of antagonistic antiretroviral effects between nevirapine and NRTIs (e.g., abacavir, didanosine, emtricitabine, lamivudine, stavudine, tenofovir, zidovudine).

Didanosine. Concomitant use of didanosine and nevirapine does not appear to affect the pharmacokinetics of either drug.

Stavudine. Concomitant use of stavudine (30–40 mg twice daily) and nevirapine (200 mg once daily for 14 days, then 200 mg twice daily for 14 days) does not have a clinically important effect on peak plasma concentrations or AUC of stavudine.

Zidovudine. Concomitant use of zidovudine and nevirapine results in a 28 and 30% decrease in zidovudine peak plasma concentrations and AUC, respectively.

HIV Protease Inhibitors (PIs) There is no in vitro evidence of antagonistic antiretroviral effects between nevirapine and HIV PIs (e.g., amprenavir, atazanavir, darunavir, indinavir, nelfinavir, saquinavir, tipranavir).

Atazanavir. Concomitant use of *ritonavir-boosted* atazanavir with nevirapine results in substantially decreased atazanavir plasma concentrations and AUC with possible loss of therapeutic effect and development of resistance and also results in increased nevirapine plasma concentrations and AUC and increases the risk of nevirapine-associated adverse effects.

Concomitant use of *cobicistat-boosted* atazanavir with nevirapine may result in decreased concentrations of atazanavir and cobicistat.

Concomitant use of unboosted atazanavir with nevirapine may result in decreased atazanavir concentrations.

Concomitant use of nevirapine and *ritonavir-boosted, cobicistat-boosted,* or unboosted atazanavir is contraindicated.

Darunavir. Concomitant use of *ritonavir-boosted* darunavir and nevirapine results in increased plasma concentrations and AUC of darunavir and nevirapine. *Ritonavir-boosted* darunavir and nevirapine can be used concomitantly without dosage adjustments.

Concomitant use of *cobicistat-boosted* darunavir and nevirapine may result in decreased concentrations of darunavir and cobicistat. Nevirapine should not be used concomitantly with *cobicistat-boosted* darunavir.

Fosamprenavir. Concomitant use of nevirapine and fosamprenavir (without low-dose ritonavir) results in a 33% decrease in the AUC of amprenavir (active metabolite of fosamprenavir) and a 29% increase in the AUC of nevirapine. Concomitant use of nevirapine with twice-daily regimen of *ritonavir-boosted* fosamprenavir results in an 11% decrease in amprenavir AUC and 14% increase in nevirapine AUC.

Usual nevirapine dosage can be used concomitantly with a twice-daily regimen of *ritonavir-boosted* fosamprenavir (fosamprenavir 700 mg twice daily and ritonavir 100 mg twice daily). Concomitant use of nevirapine with a once-daily regimen of *ritonavir-boosted* fosamprenavir has not been studied.

Concomitant use of fosamprenavir (without low-dose ritonavir) and nevirapine is not recommended.

Indinavir. Concomitant use of nevirapine (200 mg once daily for 14 days, then 200 mg every 12 hours for 14 days) and indinavir (800 mg every 8 hours) decreased peak plasma concentrations and AUC of indinavir by 15 and 31%, respectively.

Appropriate dosages for concomitant use of nevirapine and indinavir with respect to safety and efficacy have not been established.

Lopinavir. Concomitant use of nevirapine and the fixed combination containing lopinavir and ritonavir (lopinavir/ritonavir) results in decreased lopinavir plasma concentrations and AUC.

A once-daily regimen of lopinavir/ritonavir should not be used in patients receiving nevirapine.

If a twice-daily regimen of lopinavir/ritonavir is used in patients receiving nevirapine, an increased lopinavir/ritonavir dosage is recommended. Dosage depends on the lopinavir/ritonavir preparation used (tablets, oral solution) and clinical characteristics of the patient. (For specific dosage recommendations, see Dosage and Administration: Dosage in Lopinavir and Ritonavir 8:18.08.08.)

Nelfinavir. Appropriate dosages for concomitant use of nelfinavir and nevirapine with respect to safety and efficacy have not been established.

In one study, concomitant use of nevirapine (200 mg once daily for 14 days, followed by 200 mg twice daily for 14 days) and nelfinavir (750 mg 3 times daily for 36 days) did not affect nelfinavir peak plasma concentrations or AUC, but resulted in a 32% decrease in trough plasma concentrations of the drug and a 62–66% decrease in plasma concentrations and AUC of the major nelfinavir metabolite (M8).

Ritonavir. Concomitant use of ritonavir and nevirapine in a limited number of HIV-infected patients did not result in clinically important changes in ritonavir plasma concentrations or AUC.

Saquinavir. Concomitant use of *ritonavir-boosted* saquinavir and nevirapine has not been evaluated.

Appropriate dosages for concomitant use of *ritonavir-boosted* saquinavir and nevirapine with respect to safety and efficacy have not been established.

Tipranavir. Concomitant use of nevirapine and *ritonavir-boosted* tipranavir does not result in clinically important effects on nevirapine concentrations and is not expected to affect tipranavir concentrations.

Some experts state that dosage adjustments are not necessary if nevirapine and *ritonavir-boosted* tipranavir are used concomitantly.

■ **Benzodiazepines** Concomitant use of nevirapine and alprazolam or diazepam may result in decreased concentrations of the benzodiazepine.

If nevirapine is used concomitantly with alprazolam or diazepam, the patient should be monitored for therapeutic effectiveness of the benzodiazepine.

■ **Bupropion** Concomitant use of bupropion and nevirapine decreases the AUC of bupropion. In patients receiving nevirapine, bupropion dosage should be titrated based on clinical response.

■ **Cardiovascular Agents** *Antiarrhythmic Agents* Concomitant use of nevirapine and antiarrhythmic agents (e.g., amiodarone, disopyramide, lidocaine) may result in decreased plasma concentrations of the antiarrhythmic agent. Appropriate dosages for concomitant use of these antiarrhythmic agents and nevirapine have not been established.

Calcium-channel Blocking Agents Concomitant use of nevirapine and calcium-channel blocking agents (diltiazem, nifedipine, verapamil) may result in decreased plasma concentrations of these agents. Appropriate dosages for concomitant use of these calcium-channel blocking agents and nevirapine have not been established.

If nevirapine is used concomitantly with diltiazem or verapamil, dosage of the calcium-channel blocking agent should be titrated based on clinical response.

■ **Corticosteroids** Concomitant use of dexamethasone and nevirapine may result in decreased nevirapine concentrations. If dexamethasone and nevirapine are used concomitantly, antiretroviral response should be monitored; an alternative corticosteroid should be considered for long-term therapy.

Concomitant use of prednisone (40 mg daily) during the first 14 days of nevirapine therapy is not recommended since it has been associated with an increased incidence and severity of rash during the first 6 weeks of nevirapine therapy. (See Cautions: Dermatologic and Sensitivity Reactions.)

■ **Dutasteride** Concomitant use of dutasteride and nevirapine may result in decreased dutasteride concentrations. Patients should be monitored and dosage of dutasteride adjusted if necessary.

■ **Ergot Alkaloids and Derivatives** Concomitant use of nevirapine and ergot alkaloids (e.g., dihydroergotamine, ergotamine, methylergonovine) is predicted to result in decreased plasma concentrations of the ergot alkaloid.

Appropriate dosages for concomitant use of ergotamine and nevirapine have not been established.

If methylergonovine maleate (Methergine®) is used to treat postpartum hemorrhage in a woman receiving nevirapine, additional uterotonic agents may be needed since nevirapine potentially could decrease methylergonovine concentrations resulting in an inadequate treatment effect.

■ **Estrogens and Progestins** ***Drospirenone, Medroxyprogesterone, and Progesterone*** Concomitant use of nevirapine and drospirenone, medroxyprogesterone, or micronized progesterone may result in decreased concentrations of the progestin.

If nevirapine is used concomitantly with drospirenone, medroxyprogesterone, or micronized progesterone, some experts state that the patient should be monitored and the lowest effective progestin dosage to achieve clinical effects should be used.

Estradiol and Conjugated Estrogens Concomitant use of nevirapine and estradiol or conjugated estrogens (equine or synthetic) may result in decreased estrogen concentrations.

If nevirapine is used concomitantly with estradiol or conjugated estrogens, some experts state that the patient should be monitored and the lowest effective estrogen dosage to achieve clinical effects should be used.

Ethinyl Estradiol and Norethindrone Concomitant use of nevirapine and an oral contraceptive containing 0.035 mg of ethinyl estradiol and 1 mg of norethindrone decreased the AUC of both hormones by about 20%.

Although ethinyl estradiol and norethindrone exposures may be decreased, concomitant use of nevirapine and oral contraceptives containing ethinyl estradiol and norethindrone in HIV-infected women does not appear to have an effect on pregnancy rates. Therefore, dosage adjustments are not necessary if nevirapine is used in patients receiving such oral contraceptives.

Etonogestrel and Levonorgestrel Concomitant use of nevirapine in patients with implants containing etonogestrel or levonorgestrel does not affect concentrations of the progestin; some experts state that dosage adjustments are not necessary.

■ **Finasteride** Concomitant use of finasteride and nevirapine may result in decreased finasteride concentrations. Patients should be monitored and dosage of finasteride adjusted if necessary.

■ **GI Drugs** ***Antacids*** Results of a study in 24 healthy adults indicate that concomitant use of a single 200-mg dose of immediate-release nevirapine and 30 mL of an antacid (Maalox®) does not affect the extent of absorption (AUC) of the antiretroviral agent. Immediate-release nevirapine may be administered with antacids.

Cisapride Concomitant use of nevirapine and cisapride is predicted to result in decreased plasma concentrations of cisapride. Appropriate dosages for concomitant use of cisapride and nevirapine have not been established.

■ **Goserelin** Concomitant use of goserelin and nevirapine is not expected to affect goserelin concentrations.

■ **HCV Antivirals** ***HCV Polymerase Inhibitors*** **Dasabuvir, Ombitasvir, Paritaprevir, and Ritonavir.** Concomitant use of nevirapine and the fixed combination of dasabuvir sodium, ombitasvir, paritaprevir, and ritonavir (dasabuvir/ombitasvir/paritaprevir/ritonavir) or the fixed combination of ombitasvir, paritaprevir, and ritonavir (ombitasvir/paritaprevir/ritonavir) copackaged with dasabuvir sodium (ombitasvir/paritaprevir/ritonavir with dasabuvir) may result in decreased concentrations of the HCV antivirals.

Nevirapine should not be used concomitantly with dasabuvir/ombitasvir/paritaprevir/ritonavir (fixed combination) or ombitasvir/paritaprevir/ritonavir with dasabuvir (copackaged).

Sofosbuvir and Velpatasvir. Concomitant use of nevirapine and the fixed combination of sofosbuvir and velpatasvir (sofosbuvir/velpatasvir) is expected to result in decreased velpatasvir concentrations.

Nevirapine and sofosbuvir/velpatasvir should not be used concomitantly.

Sofosbuvir, Velpatasvir, and Voxilaprevir. Concomitant use of nevirapine and the fixed combination of sofosbuvir, velpatasvir, and voxilaprevir (sofosbuvir/velpatasvir/voxilaprevir) is expected to result in decreased velpatasvir and voxilaprevir concentrations.

Nevirapine and sofosbuvir/velpatasvir/voxilaprevir should not be used concomitantly.

HCV Protease Inhibitors **Glecaprevir and Pibrentasvir.** Concomitant use of nevirapine and the fixed combination of glecaprevir and pibrentasvir (glecaprevir/pibrentasvir) may result in decreased glecaprevir and pibrentasvir concentrations.

Nevirapine and glecaprevir/pibrentasvir should not be used concomitantly.

Simeprevir. Concomitant use of simeprevir and nevirapine is expected to decrease simeprevir concentrations.

Simeprevir and nevirapine should not be used concomitantly.

HCV Replication Complex Inhibitors **Daclatasvir.** Concomitant use of daclatasvir and nevirapine decreases daclatasvir concentrations.

If nevirapine and daclatasvir are used concomitantly, daclatasvir should be given in a dosage of 90 mg once daily.

Elbasvir and Grazoprevir. Concomitant use of nevirapine and the fixed combination of elbasvir and grazoprevir (elbasvir/grazoprevir) is expected to result in decreased elbasvir and grazoprevir concentrations.

Nevirapine and elbasvir/grazoprevir should not be used concomitantly.

Ledipasvir and Sofosbuvir. Concomitant use of nevirapine and the fixed combination of ledipasvir and sofosbuvir (ledipasvir/sofosbuvir) is not expected to result in clinically important interactions. Dosage adjustments are not necessary if the drugs are used concomitantly.

■ **HMG-CoA Reductase Inhibitors** ***Atorvastatin*** Concomitant use of atorvastatin and nevirapine may result in decreased atorvastatin concentrations. If the drugs are used concomitantly, atorvastatin dosage should be adjusted based on lipid response and should not exceed the maximum recommended dosage.

Lovastatin Concomitant use of lovastatin and nevirapine may result in decreased plasma concentrations of the statin.

If lovastatin is used concomitantly with nevirapine, lovastatin dosage should be adjusted based on lipid response and should not exceed the maximum recommended dosage. Lovastatin should be avoided if nevirapine is used in a regimen that includes a *ritonavir-boosted* PI.

Pitavastatin and Rosuvastatin Concomitant use of nevirapine and pitavastatin or rosuvastatin is not expected to affect concentrations of the antilipemic agent.

Dosage adjustments are not needed if nevirapine is used concomitantly with pitavastatin or rosuvastatin.

Simvastatin Concomitant use of simvastatin and nevirapine may result in decreased plasma concentrations of the statin.

If simvastatin is used concomitantly with nevirapine, simvastatin dosage should be adjusted based on lipid response and should not exceed the maximum recommended dosage. Simvastatin should be avoided if nevirapine is used in a regimen that includes a *ritonavir-boosted* PI.

■ **Immunosuppressive Agents** Concomitant use of nevirapine and immunosuppressive agents such as cyclosporine, everolimus, tacrolimus, or sirolimus is predicted to result in decreased plasma concentrations of these agents. Appropriate dosages for concomitant use of these immunosuppressive agents and nevirapine have not been established. If nevirapine is used concomitantly with one of these immunosuppressive agents, increased dosage of the immunosuppressive agent may be necessary. Therapeutic drug monitoring of the immunosuppressive agent is recommended; consultation with a specialist may be necessary.

■ **Leuprolide** Concomitant use of leuprolide and nevirapine is not expected to affect leuprolide concentrations.

■ **Macrolides** ***Clarithromycin*** Concomitant use of clarithromycin and nevirapine has resulted in decreased clarithromycin concentrations and AUC and increased concentrations and AUC of its major metabolite (14-hydroxyclarithromycin). Because the clarithromycin metabolite has reduced activity against *Mycobacterium avium* complex (MAC), overall activity of the drug against this organism may be altered. Concomitant use may also result in increased nevirapine AUC.

Patients receiving nevirapine and clarithromycin concomitantly should be monitored for efficacy of the macrolide or an alternative to clarithromycin (e.g., azithromycin) should be used for treatment or prophylaxis of MAC.

■ **Nefazodone** Concomitant use of nefazodone and nevirapine is expected to result in decreased nefazodone concentrations and may result in increased nevirapine concentrations.

If nefazodone and nevirapine are used concomitantly, patients should be monitored for nefazodone therapeutic effects and dosage of the antidepressant should be titrated as needed. Patients also should be monitored for nevirapine-associated adverse effects.

■ **Opiate Agonists and Opiate Partial Agonists** ***Buprenorphine*** Concomitant use of sublingual or buccal formulations of buprenorphine and nevirapine does not result in a clinically important pharmacokinetic interaction; dosage adjustments are not necessary if the drugs are used concomitantly.

Data are not available regarding concomitant use of buprenorphine subdermal implants and nevirapine. If nevirapine is initiated after insertion of buprenorphine implants, clinical monitoring is recommended.

Fentanyl Concomitant use of fentanyl and nevirapine may decrease plasma concentrations of the opiate agonist. Appropriate dosages for concomitant use of fentanyl and nevirapine have not been established.

Methadone There have been reports of opiate withdrawal and subtherapeutic or decreased serum methadone concentrations following initiation of nevirapine therapy in individuals who were receiving long-term methadone treatment for opiate addiction; nevirapine concentrations are not affected.

Individuals receiving concomitant nevirapine and methadone therapy should be informed of this potential interaction and closely monitored for signs of opiate withdrawal when nevirapine therapy is initiated; an increase in methadone maintenance dosage may be necessary. If methadone dosage is increased during nevirapine therapy, patients should be monitored for methadone overdosage when the antiretroviral agent is discontinued.

■ **Phosphodiesterase Type 5 Inhibitors** Concomitant use of nevirapine and avanafil, sildenafil, tadalafil, or vardenafil may result in decreased concentrations of the phosphodiesterase (PDE) type 5 inhibitor. If nevirapine is used concomitantly with one of these drugs, an increase in dosage of the PDE type 5 inhibitor may be needed based on clinical effects.

■ **Quinupristin and Dalfopristin** Although specific studies are not available, it is possible that concomitant use of nevirapine and quinupristin and dalfopristin may result in increased nevirapine plasma concentrations since quinupristin and dalfopristin is a potent inhibitor of CYP3A4.

■ **Selective Serotonin-reuptake Inhibitors** *Citalopram and Escitalopram* Concomitant use of nevirapine and citalopram or escitalopram may result in decreased concentrations of the antidepressant. Dosage of the antidepressant should be titrated based on clinical response.

Fluoxetine, Fluvoxamine, and Paroxetine Concomitant use of nevirapine and fluoxetine, fluvoxamine, or paroxetine is not expected to affect concentrations of the antidepressant. If fluoxetine, fluvoxamine, or paroxetine is used concomitantly with nevirapine, no adjustment of the antidepressant dosage is required.

■ **Spironolactone** Concomitant use of spironolactone and nevirapine is not expected to affect spironolactone concentrations.

■ **Testosterone** Concomitant use of testosterone and nevirapine may result in decreased testosterone concentrations.

If testosterone and nevirapine are used concomitantly, some experts state that patients should be monitored for testosterone effects and dosage adjusted if needed.

■ **Trazodone** Concomitant use of trazodone and nevirapine may result in decreased trazodone concentrations. If the drugs are used concomitantly, patients should be monitored for trazodone therapeutic effects and dosage of the antidepressant titrated as needed.

■ **Dietary and Herbal Supplements** *St. John's Wort (Hypericum perforatum)* Concomitant use of St. John's wort (*Hypericum perforatum*) and nevirapine is expected to result in suboptimal antiretroviral concentrations and may be associated with loss of virologic response and development of resistance. St. John's wort is an extract of hypericum and contains at least 7 different components that may contribute to its pharmacologic effects, including hypericin, pseudohypericin, and hyperforin. There is evidence that hypericum extracts can induce several different CYP isoenzymes, including CYP3A4 and CYP1A2, and also may induce the *p*-glycoprotein transport system.

Concomitant use of nevirapine and St. John's wort is contraindicated.

Acute Toxicity

Limited information is available on acute toxicity of nevirapine. Overdosage of nevirapine (800–1800 mg/daily for up to 15 days) has resulted in edema, erythema nodosum, fatigue, fever, headache, insomnia, nausea, pulmonary infiltrates, rash, vertigo, vomiting, and weight decrease; these effects subsided following discontinuance of the drug. There is no known antidote for nevirapine overdosage.

Mechanism of Action

■ **Antiviral Effects** While the complete mechanism of antiviral activity of nevirapine has not been fully elucidated, the drug inhibits replication of human immunodeficiency virus type 1 (HIV-1) by interfering with viral RNA- and DNA-directed polymerase activities of reverse transcriptase. Nevirapine binds directly to HIV-1 reverse transcriptase and exerts a virustatic effect by acting as a specific, noncompetitive HIV-1 reverse transcriptase inhibitor.

The mechanism of action of nevirapine differs from that of HIV nucleoside reverse transcriptase inhibitors (NRTIs) (e.g., abacavir, didanosine, lamivudine, stavudine, zidovudine). NRTIs require intracellular conversion to triphosphate metabolites, which then compete with naturally occurring deoxynucleoside triphosphates for incorporation into viral DNA by reverse transcriptase and cause premature viral DNA chain termination by preventing further 5′ to 3′ phosphodiester linkages. Nevirapine, however, is noncompetitive with respect to primer-template or nucleoside triphosphate binding and is specific for HIV-1 reverse transcriptase. The drug binds directly to heterodimeric HIV-1 reverse transcriptase and appears to inhibit viral RNA- and DNA-dependent DNA polymerase activities by disrupting the catalytic site of the enzyme.

The binding site for nevirapine on HIV-1 reverse transcriptase is near, but not at the proposed site of active polymerization, in a deep pocket lying between the β sheets of the "palm" and at the base of the "thumb" subdomains of the enzyme's p66 subunit. In the absence of nevirapine, the binding of deoxynucleoside triphosphate to the reverse transcriptase-template complex results in a change in the conformation of reverse transcriptase. This conformational change is followed by a magnesium-dependent chemical reaction in which deoxynucleoside triphosphate is incorporated into the newly forming viral DNA; the conformational change appears to be the rate-limiting step of the reverse transcriptase catalysis of viral DNA formation. Nevirapine appears to have no appreciable effect on the rate of or equilibrium constant for the conformational change but may slow the chemical reaction, which then becomes the rate-limiting step in the catalytic sequence. When nevirapine binds to the reverse transcriptase-template complex, changes may occur in the position of aspartic acid carboxyl groups in reverse transcriptase so that magnesium ions are not in proper alignment for the chemical reaction to occur efficiently, and the reaction is slowed. Therefore, although the nevirapine-reverse transcriptase-template complex may continue to bind deoxynucleoside triphosphate and to catalyze its incorporation into the newly forming viral DNA, it appears to do so at a slower rate.

■ **Cytotoxic Effects** Nevirapine is a highly specific inhibitor of HIV-1 reverse transcriptase, and results of in vitro studies indicate that nevirapine does not appear to inhibit cellular DNA polymerases, including human α-, β-, γ-, or δ-polymerases.

Spectrum

Nevirapine has a very limited spectrum of antiviral activity. The drug has in vitro virustatic activity against human immunodeficiency virus type 1 (HIV-1), but is inactive against HIV type 2 (HIV-2) and animal retrovirus (e.g., feline leukemia virus). Although nevirapine has been reported to have some inhibitory activity against certain strains of simian immunodeficiency virus (e.g., SIV [agm3]), the drug has been inactive against other SIV strains tested (e.g., SIV [mac251], SIV [mndGB1]). In addition, nevirapine is inactive against picornaviridae, including rhinovirus, poliovirus type 1, and coxsackievirus type A13.

■ **Retroviruses** The antiretroviral activity of nevirapine has been evaluated in vitro in various cell culture systems including lymphoblastoid cell lines, peripheral blood mononuclear cells, and monocyte-derived macrophages. In human cord blood lymphocytes and human embryonic kidney cells, the concentration of nevirapine required to inhibit HIV-1 replication by 50% (EC_{50}) was 14–302 nM. Nevirapine appears to be active in vitro against both zidovudine-susceptible and -resistant strains of HIV-1.

Results of in vitro studies indicate that the antiretroviral activities of nevirapine and some HIV nucleoside reverse transcriptase inhibitors (e.g., abacavir, didanosine, emtricitabine, lamivudine, stavudine, tenofovir, zidovudine) or HIV protease inhibitors (e.g., amprenavir, atazanavir, indinavir, lopinavir, nelfinavir, saquinavir, tipranavir) may be additive to synergistic against HIV-1. In addition, nevirapine used in a 2-drug regimen with zidovudine or a 3-drug regimen with zidovudine and didanosine has resulted in increased in vitro and in vivo activity against HIV-1.

Resistance

Strains of human immunodeficiency virus type 1 (HIV-1) with reduced susceptibility to nevirapine (i.e., susceptibility that is 100- to 250-fold lower than baseline) have been produced in vitro, and the time to emergence of in vitro resistance was not altered when nevirapine was used in conjunction with several other HIV nonnucleoside reverse transcriptase inhibitors (NNRTIs). Although the clinical importance is unclear, strains of HIV-1 with in vitro resistance to nevirapine have emerged during therapy with the drug. For information on genotypic assays used to detect specific HIV-1 genetic variants (mutations) and phenotypic assays used to measure HIV-1 drug resistance and recommendations regarding these assays, see In Vitro Resistance Testing under Guidelines for Use of Antiretroviral Agents: Laboratory Monitoring, in the Antiretroviral Agents General Statement 8:18.08.

The mechanism(s) of resistance or reduced susceptibility to nevirapine has not been fully determined, but mutation of HIV reverse transcriptase appears to be involved. A single mutation may be sufficient to result in high-level resistance to nevirapine.

In phase 1 or 2 studies evaluating nevirapine monotherapy or nevirapine used in conjunction with zidovudine, 100% of 24 patients receiving the drug alone had HIV-1 isolates with decreased in vitro susceptibility to nevirapine (susceptibility more than 100-fold lower than baseline) and, in a few patients, these strains were evident after only 1 week of monotherapy. Isolates with reduced susceptibility to nevirapine had one or more nevirapine-associated resistance mutations including K103N, V106A, V108I, Y181C, Y188C, and G190A; regardless of dose, 80% of patients had isolates the Y181C mutation. Primary infection with HIV-1 strains highly resistant to nevirapine has been documented and occurred as the result of horizontal transmission from an individual who had received a regimen of zidovudine and nevirapine and harbored resistant strains.

■ **Cross-resistance** HIV-1 resistant to nevirapine may be cross-resistant to some other HIV nonnucleoside reverse transcriptase inhibitors (NNRTIs) (e.g., delavirdine, efavirenz).

In a study evaluating HIV-1 strains isolated from a limited number of patients, zidovudine-resistant HIV-1 isolates retained susceptibility to nevirapine and nevirapine-resistant isolates were susceptible to zidovudine and didanosine.

Because nevirapine and HIV protease inhibitors (e.g., amprenavir, indinavir, lopinavir, nelfinavir, ritonavir, saquinavir) have different enzyme targets, cross-resistance between nevirapine and these drugs is unlikely.

Pharmacokinetics

The pharmacokinetics of nevirapine have been studied in healthy adults, adults with human immunodeficiency virus type 1 (HIV-1) infection, and pediatric patients 14 days of age and older with HIV-1 infection. Studies to date have not revealed clinically important race-related differences in the pharmacokinetics of nevirapine. Studies in adults 18–68 years of age have not revealed any age-related differences in the pharmacokinetics of nevirapine; however, pharmacokinetics of the drug have not been extensively studied to date in geriatric adults older than 55–65 years of age.

The pharmacokinetics of nevirapine immediate-release tablets in pregnant women generally are similar to that reported in nonpregnant adults; dosage adjustments are not recommended during pregnancy. Data are not available regarding the pharmacokinetics of nevirapine extended-release tablets in pregnant women.

Immediate-release tablets containing nevirapine and the oral suspension containing nevirapine hemihydrate are bioequivalent and can be used interchangeably at doses up to 200 mg.

Bioavailability of 400 mg of nevirapine administered as extended-release tablets relative to 400 mg administered as conventional (immediate-release) tablets is approximately 75%.

■ Absorption Following oral administration of nevirapine immediate-release tablets or oral suspension in healthy or HIV-infected adults, the drug is readily (more than 90%) absorbed. Absolute bioavailability of nevirapine in 12 healthy adults was 93% following administration of a single 50-mg immediate-release tablet or 91% following administration of an oral solution of the drug. Peak plasma nevirapine concentrations average 2 mcg/mL and are attained within 4 hour after a single 200-mg dose in adults. Following multiple doses, peak plasma nevirapine concentrations appear to increase linearly in the dosage range of 200–400 mg daily. Nevirapine dosage of 400 mg daily resulted in steady-state trough plasma concentrations of 4.5 mcg/mL.

Following oral administration of a single 400-mg dose of nevirapine as an extended-release tablet in healthy adults, mean peak plasma concentrations were 2.06 mcg/mL and were attained at a median of approximately 24 hours. In a multiple-dose study in adults with HIV-1 infection who were switched from nevirapine immediate-release tablets to nevirapine extended-release tablets given under fasting conditions, the mean area under the concentration-time curve (AUC) and trough plasma concentrations after 19 days of the extended-release preparation were 82 mcg•hr/mL and 2.92 mcg/mL, respectively.

Following oral administration of multiple doses of nevirapine 150 mg/m^2 twice daily as the immediate-release oral suspension in HIV-infected pediatric patients, trough plasma concentrations averaged 4–6 mcg/mL. In HIV-infected children 6 to less than 18 years of age who were switched to nevirapine extended-release tablets after at least 18 weeks of immediate-release nevirapine, overall mean systemic nevirapine exposure with the extended-release preparation was similar to that reported for the immediate-release preparation. At steady state, the observed geometric mean ratios of extended-release nevirapine to immediate-release nevirapine were approximately 97% for trough plasma concentrations and 94% for AUCs; the ratio for peak plasma concentrations was lower and consistent with the once-daily extended-release preparation.

In 8 neonates who had serum nevirapine concentrations of 141–768 ng/mL at birth as the result of distribution across the placenta from their HIV-infected mothers who had received single 200-mg doses of the drug 3–7 hours prior to delivery (see Pharmacokinetics: Distribution), administration of a single 2-mg/kg dose of nevirapine to the neonates 48–78 hours after birth resulted in peak neonatal serum concentrations of 1355 ng/mL (range: 644–1607 ng/mL) at 2–24 hours after the dose. Serum nevirapine concentrations in these neonates 7 days after birth were estimated to be 215 ng/mL (range: 112–275 ng/mL) based on extrapolation from the concentration-time plots and the elimination rate constant.

Food Results of a study in 24 healthy adults indicate that when 200 mg of nevirapine as immediate-release tablets is administered with a high-fat meal (857 kcal, 50 g fat, 53% of calories from fat), the extent of absorption (AUC) is comparable to that observed under fasting conditions.

When nevirapine extended-release tablets were administered under fed conditions, the mean nevirapine AUC and trough plasma concentrations at steady state were 96.7 mcg•hr/mL and 3.15 mcg/mL, respectively. The bioavailability of 400 mg of nevirapine as extended-release tablets relative to 400 mg of the drug given as immediate-release tablets under fasted and fed conditions was 80 and 94%, respectively. The difference in bioavailability of nevirapine extended-release tablets under fasted or fed conditions is not considered clinically important.

■ Distribution Distribution of nevirapine into body tissues and fluids has not been fully characterized; however, animal studies indicate that the drug is widely distributed into most tissues. Nevirapine is highly lipophilic and is essentially nonionized at physiologic pH.

Following IV administration in healthy adults, the apparent volume of distribution of nevirapine is 1.21 L/kg, suggesting that the drug is widely distributed in humans.

In a study in 12 HIV-infected men receiving nevirapine in conjunction with lamivudine or stavudine, nevirapine was distributed into semen in concentrations that were approximately 60% of concurrent plasma concentrations.

Results of a study in 6 individuals indicate that nevirapine is distributed into CSF in concentrations that are 45% of concurrent plasma concentrations; this ratio is approximately equal to the fraction of the drug not bound to plasma proteins.

At plasma concentrations of 1–10 mcg/mL, nevirapine is approximately 60% bound to plasma proteins.

Nevirapine readily crosses the placenta in humans. In a limited number of HIV-infected pregnant women who received a single 100- or 200-mg oral dose of nevirapine 0.9–10.5 hours prior to delivery, cord blood concentrations of nevirapine were 74–123% of maternal serum concentrations and peak serum concentrations of the drug in the neonates of these women averaged 862 ng/mL (range: 257–1031 ng/mL) or 925 ng/mL (range: 62–2030 ng/mL), respectively. In pregnant HIV-infected women who received a regimen of nevirapine (200 mg once daily for 2 weeks followed by 200 mg twice daily), zidovudine, and lamivudine during the second and third trimester, cord blood concentrations (at delivery) and neonatal serum concentrations (24 hours after birth) of nevirapine were 76 and 60%, respectively, of maternal serum concentrations (at delivery). These neonatal concentrations were lower than those reported in neonates whose mothers received a single nevirapine dose during labor, possibly as the result of hepatic enzyme induction in the neonate after placental transfer.

Nevirapine is distributed into human milk. Following administration of a single 100- or 200-mg dose of nevirapine to pregnant women several hours before delivery, postpartum, concentrations of the drug in milk were 25–122% of maternal serum concentrations.

■ Elimination Nevirapine is extensively converted in vivo to several hydroxylated metabolites via cytochrome P-450 (CYP) oxidative metabolism. In vitro studies using human liver microsomes indicate that metabolism of nevirapine is mediated principally by CYP3A4, but other isoenzymes may also play a role in metabolism of the drug.

There is evidence that nevirapine induces CYP3A4 and CYP2B6 enzymes resulting in autoinduction of its own metabolism. The pharmacokinetics of autoinduction are characterized by an approximately 1.5- to 2-fold increase in the apparent oral clearance of nevirapine as treatment continues from a single dose to 2–4 weeks of dosing at a dosage of 200–400 mg daily. Autoinduction also results in a corresponding decrease in the terminal phase half-life of nevirapine in plasma from approximately 45 hours with a single dose to approximately 25–30 hours following multiple dosing using a dosage of 200–400 mg daily in adults.

In a study in 8 healthy adults who received 200 mg once daily for 2 weeks followed by 200 mg twice daily for 2 weeks to reach steady state and then received a single 50-mg dose of radiolabeled nevirapine, approximately 81% of the radiolabeled dose was recovered in urine and approximately 10% was recovered in feces over a period of 10 days. More than 80% of the radioactivity in urine consisted of glucuronide conjugates of hydroxylated metabolites. Therefore, CYP metabolism, glucuronide conjugation, and urinary excretion of glucuronidated metabolites represent the principal route of biotransformation and elimination of nevirapine in humans. Less than 5% of the radioactivity in urine (representing less than 3% of the total dose) consisted of unchanged drug.

Results of a study in a limited number of HIV-negative adults with mild, moderate, or severe renal impairment indicate that there are no clinically important changes in the pharmacokinetics of a single dose of nevirapine as immediate-release tablets in adults with impaired renal function. However, adults undergoing dialysis have a 44% reduction in the AUC of nevirapine after 1 week of nevirapine therapy; treatment and accumulation of the hydroxy metabolites of the drug also may occur. In an HIV-infected adult with end-stage renal failure on continuous ambulatory peritoneal dialysis who was receiving a regimen of nevirapine immediate-release tablets (200 mg twice daily), nelfinavir (1250 mg twice daily), and zidovudine (250 mg twice daily), peak and trough plasma concentrations of nevirapine were 4.7 and 2.6 mcg/mL, respectively, and the AUC_{0-12} was 46.6 mcg•hr/mL. The drug was removed by peritoneal dialysis, and concentrations in peritoneal dialysis fluid were approximately 50% of plasma concentrations.

Disposition of nevirapine was not altered in HIV-infected adults with mild, moderate, or severe hepatic fibrosis who received multiple doses of nevirapine immediate-release tablets (nevirapine 200 mg twice daily for at least 6 weeks); however, approximately 15% of these individuals had nevirapine trough concentrations that were twofold higher than the usual mean trough concentrations.

In a limited study in HIV-negative adults with mild or moderate hepatic impairment who received a single 200-mg dose of nevirapine as immediate-release tablets, most patients had no clinically important change in the pharmacokinetics of the drug. However, in one patient with moderate hepatic impairment (Child-Pugh Class B) and ascites, there was an increase in the AUC of nevirapine. Because nevirapine induces its own metabolism with multiple doses, a single-dose study may not reflect the impact of hepatic impairment on multiple-dose pharmacokinetics.

Nevirapine extended-release tablets have not been studied in patients with renal or hepatic impairment.

In a population substudy, women had a 13.8% lower clearance of nevirapine than men. These results could not be explained by body weight or body mass index differences between men and women.

Chemistry and Stability

■ Chemistry Nevirapine, an antiretroviral agent, is a human immunodeficiency virus (HIV) nonnucleoside reverse transcriptase inhibitor (NNRTI). The drug is a dipyridodiazepine derivative NNRTI. Nevirapine differs structurally from other commercially available NNRTIs (e.g., delavirdine, efavirenz, etravirine, rilpivirine) and also differs structurally from other currently available antiretroviral agents.

Nevirapine occurs as a white to off-white crystalline powder. The drug is commercially available for oral administration as conventional (immediate-release) tablets or extended-release tablets containing nevirapine and as an oral suspension containing nevirapine hemihydrate. Nevirapine oral suspension is a white to off-white suspension containing 50 mg of nevirapine (as the hemihydrate) per 5 mL; the oral suspension also contains carbomer 934P, methylparaben, propylparaben, sorbitol, sucrose, polysorbate 80, sodium hydroxide, and water.

■ Stability Commercially available nevirapine immediate-release tablets, extended-release tablets, and oral suspension should be stored at 25°C, but may be exposed to temperatures ranging from 15–30°C.

Preparations

Excipients in commercially available drug preparations may have clinically important effects in some individuals; consult specific product labeling for details.

Nevirapine

Oral		
Tablets	200 mg*	**Nevirapine Tablets**
		Viramune® (scored), Boehringer Ingelheim
Tablets, extended-release	100 mg*	**Nevirapine Extended-release Tablets**
		Viramune® XR, Boehringer Ingelheim
	400 mg*	**Nevirapine Extended-release Tablets**
		Viramune® XR, Boehringer Ingelheim

*available from one or more manufacturer, distributor, and/or repackager by generic (nonproprietary) name

Nevirapine Hemihydrate

Oral		
Suspension	50 mg (of nevirapine) per 5 mL*	**Nevirapine Oral Suspension**
		Viramune®, Boehringer Ingelheim

*available from one or more manufacturer, distributor, and/or repackager by generic (nonproprietary) name

†Use is not currently included in the labeling approved by the US Food and Drug Administration

Rilpivirine Hydrochloride

RPV, emtricitabine/rilpivirine/tenofovir alafenamide, RPV/FTC/TAF, RPV/TAF/FTC, RPV/TDF/FTC, emtricitabine/rilpivirine/tenofovir DF, RPV/FTC/TDF

■ Rilpivirine, an antiretroviral agent, is a human immunodeficiency virus (HIV) nonnucleoside reverse transcriptase inhibitor (NNRTI).

Uses

■ **Treatment of HIV Infection** Rilpivirine is used in conjunction with other antiretroviral agents for the treatment of human immunodeficiency virus type 1 (HIV-1) infection in adults and adolescents 12 years of age or older.

Rilpivirine usually is used in HIV nonnucleoside reverse transcriptase inhibitor-based (NNRTI-based) regimens that include rilpivirine and 2 HIV nucleoside reverse transcriptase inhibitors (NRTIs).

Single-entity rilpivirine is labeled by FDA for use in conjunction with other antiretrovirals for the treatment of HIV-1 infection in antiretroviral-naive (have not previously received antiretroviral therapy) adults and adolescents 12 years of age or older with plasma HIV-1 RNA levels of 100,000 copies/mL or less. Rilpivirine also is commercially available in fixed-combination preparations that contain emtricitabine and a tenofovir prodrug (either tenofovir alafenamide or tenofovir disoproxil fumarate [tenofovir DF]). These fixed combinations can be used in specific patient groups to decrease pill burden and improve compliance.

If an HIV NNRTI-based regimen of rilpivirine, emtricitabine, and tenofovir alafenamide is used for the treatment of HIV-1 infection, a fixed-combination preparation containing all 3 drugs (emtricitabine/rilpivirine/tenofovir alafenamide; Odefsey®) is commercially available and can be used in antiretroviral-naive adults and adolescents 12 years of age or older weighing at least 35 kg with baseline plasma HIV-1 RNA levels of 100,000 copies/mL or less. Emtricitabine/rilpivirine/tenofovir alafenamide also can be used to replace a stable antiretroviral regimen in *certain* antiretroviral-experienced (previously treated) patients who are virologically suppressed (i.e., plasma HIV-1 RNA levels less than 50 copies/mL). Emtricitabine/rilpivirine/tenofovir alafenamide is used alone as a complete regimen for the treatment of HIV-1 infection.

If an HIV NNRTI-based regimen of rilpivirine, emtricitabine, and tenofovir DF is used for the treatment of HIV-1 infection, a fixed-combination preparation containing all 3 drugs (emtricitabine/rilpivirine/tenofovir DF; Complera®) is commercially available and can be used in antiretroviral-naive adults and adolescents 12 years of age or older weighing at least 35 kg with baseline plasma HIV-1 RNA levels of 100,000 copies/mL or less. Emtricitabine/rilpivirine/tenofovir DF also can be used to replace a stable antiretroviral regimen in *certain* antiretroviral-experienced patients who are virologically suppressed (i.e., plasma HIV-1 RNA levels less than 50 copies/mL). Emtricitabine/rilpivirine/tenofovir DF is used alone as a complete regimen for the treatment of HIV-1 infection.

The manufacturer states that the following factors should be considered when initiating rilpivirine or emtricitabine/rilpivirine/tenofovir DF in antiretroviral-naive patients. In clinical studies evaluating rilpivirine, patients with baseline plasma HIV-1 RNA levels exceeding 100,000 copies/mL had greater rates of virologic failure than those with lower baseline HIV-1 RNA levels and patients with baseline $CD4^+$ T-cell counts less than 200 cells/mm^3 (regardless of HIV-1 RNA levels) had greater rates of virologic failure than those with higher baseline $CD4^+$ T-cell counts. Patients experiencing virologic failure while receiving a rilpivirine regimen had higher rates of overall treatment-emergent resistance and NNRTI-class cross-resistance than those receiving an efavirenz regimen. In addition, resistance to the HIV nucleoside reverse transcriptase inhibitors (NRTIs) tenofovir, lamivudine, and emtricitabine developed more frequently in patients receiving a rilpivirine regimen than in those receiving an efavirenz regimen.

The most appropriate antiretroviral regimen cannot be defined for each clinical scenario, and selection of specific antiretroviral agents for use in multiple-drug regimens should be individualized based on information regarding antiretroviral potency, potential rate of development of resistance, known toxicities, and potential for pharmacokinetic interactions as well as virologic, immunologic, and clinical characteristics of the patient. For information on the general principles and guidelines for use of antiretroviral therapy, including specific recommendations for initial therapy in antiretroviral-naive patients and recommendations for changing antiretroviral regimens, see the Antiretroviral Agents General Statement 8:18.08.

Antiretroviral-naive Adults and Adolescents For *initial* treatment in HIV-infected adults and adolescents who are antiretroviral-naive, the US Department of Health and Human Services (HHS) Panel on Antiretroviral Guidelines for Adults and Adolescents states that rilpivirine in conjunction with tenofovir alafenamide and emtricitabine or rilpivirine in conjunction with tenofovir DF and emtricitabine (or lamivudine) are alternative NNRTI-based regimens, but should be used *only* in patients with baseline plasma HIV-1 RNA levels less than 100,000 copies/mL *and* baseline $CD4^+$ T-cell count greater than 200 cells/mm^3.

Clinical Experience. Rilpivirine has been evaluated in 2 phase 3, randomized, double-blind, multicenter, noninferiority studies (studies TMC278-C209 [ECHO], TMC278-C215 [THRIVE]) in antiretroviral-naive adults with baseline plasma HIV-1 RNA levels of at least 5000 copies/mL. Patients enrolled in these studies were screened to ensure they had HIV-1 that did not have specific NNRTI resistance-associated mutations and were susceptible to NRTIs. Over 1300 patients (median age 36 years [range 18–78], 76% male, 60–61% white, 23–24% black, 11-14% Asian, median baseline plasma HIV-1 RNA level 5.0 log_{10} copies/mL, median baseline $CD4^+$ T-cell count 249–260 cells/mm^3) were randomized to receive rilpivirine 25 mg once daily or efavirenz 600 mg once daily. All patients received a background regimen of 2 NRTIs (dual NRTIs); patients enrolled in the ECHO study received a fixed combination of emtricitabine and tenofovir DF (emtricitabine/tenofovir DF) and patients enrolled in the THRIVE study received an investigator-selected dual NRTI option of emtricitabine and tenofovir DF, zidovudine and lamivudine, or abacavir and lamivudine. At 48 weeks, rilpivirine was noninferior to efavirenz in both studies. Based on pooled results at 48 weeks, 84% of those receiving rilpivirine and 2 NRTIs and 82% of those receiving efavirenz and 2 NRTIs had plasma HIV-1 RNA levels below 50 copies/mL. In addition, the mean increase in $CD4^+$ T-cell count from baseline at week 48 was 192 cells/mm^3 in patients receiving a rilpivirine regimen and 176 cells/mm^3 in those receiving an efavirenz regimen. Pooled results at week 96 showed that 76% of those receiving rilpivirine and 2 NRTIs and 77% of those receiving efavirenz and 2 NRTIs had plasma HIV-1 RNA levels below 50 copies/mL. The mean increase in $CD4^+$ T-cell count from baseline at week 96 was 228 cells/mm^3 in patients receiving a rilpivirine regimen and 219 cells/mm^3 in those receiving an efavirenz regimen.

Pooled data from the ECHO and THRIVE studies indicated that the virologic failure rate at week 96 (plasma HIV-1 RNA levels 50 copies/mL or greater) was 16 or 10% in those randomized to rilpivirine or efavirenz, respectively, and 2 NRTIs; most virologic failures occurred in the first 48 weeks. When results were stratified by baseline plasma HIV-1 RNA levels among patients randomized to receive rilpivirine, virologic failure occurred in 9% of patients with baseline plasma HIV-1 RNA levels of 100,000 copies/mL or less and in 24% of those with baseline levels exceeding 100,000 copies/mL.

Rilpivirine also has been evaluated in a randomized, active-controlled, phase 2b, dose-comparison study (TMC278-C204) in 368 antiretroviral-naive HIV-infected adults (median age 35 years, 67% male, 45% white, 24% black, 18% Asian) with baseline plasma HIV-1 RNA levels of at least 5000 copies/mL. Patients enrolled in this study had previously received no more than 2 weeks of treatment with NRTIs or HIV protease inhibitors (PIs), had not previously received any NNRTIs, and were screened to ensure they had HIV-1 that did not have specific NNRTI resistance-associated mutations and were susceptible to NRTIs. Patients received an investigator-selected background regimen of 2 NRTIs (lamivudine and zidovudine *or* emtricitabine and tenofovir DF; administered as fixed-combination preparations whenever possible) and were randomized (1:1:1:1) to receive open-label efavirenz (600 mg once daily) or 1 of 3 blinded rilpivirine dosage regimens (25, 75, or 150 mg once daily) for 96 weeks. At 96 weeks, 76% of patients receiving a regimen of rilpivirine 25 mg and 2 NRTIs and 71% of patients receiving a regimen of efavirenz and 2 NRTIs had plasma HIV-1 RNA levels below 50 copies/mL. The mean increase in $CD4^+$ T-cell count from baseline was 146 cells/mm^3 in those receiving rilpivirine 25 mg and 160 cells/mm^3 in those receiving efavirenz. At 96 weeks, patients originally randomized to any dose of rilpivirine were switched to an open label rilpivirine regimen of 25 mg once daily and 2 NRTIs for long-term follow-up. At 240 weeks, virologic suppression (plasma HIV-1 RNA levels below 50 copies/mL) was achieved in 60% of patients originally randomized to rilpivirine 25 mg and 57% of those randomized to efavirenz.

Efficacy of the fixed combination emtricitabine/rilpivirine/tenofovir alafenamide for the treatment of HIV-1 infection in antiretroviral-naive HIV-infected adults is based on results of clinical trials evaluating a regimen of rilpivirine and emtricitabine/tenofovir DF and clinical trials evaluating a regimen of elvitegravir, cobicistat, emtricitabine, and tenofovir alafenamide.

Antiretroviral-experienced Adults and Adolescents **Emtricitabine, Rilpivirine, and Tenofovir Alafenamide.** The fixed combination emtricitabine/rilpivirine/tenofovir alafenamide can be used to replace a stable antiretroviral regimen for the treatment of HIV-1 infection in antiretroviral-experienced adults and adolescents 12 years of age or older weighing at least 35 kg who have been virologically suppressed (i.e., plasma HIV-1 RNA levels less than 50 copies/mL) on their current regimen for at least 6 months, have no history of treatment failure, and are infected with HIV-1 with no known substitutions associated with resistance to the antiretroviral components of the fixed combination (i.e., emtricitabine, rilpivirine, tenofovir).

Efficacy of emtricitabine/rilpivirine/tenofovir alafenamide for the treatment of HIV-1 infection in antiretroviral experienced adults is based on results of clinical trials evaluating a regimen of rilpivirine and emtricitabine/tenofovir DF and clinical trials evaluating a regimen of elvitegravir, cobicistat, emtricitabine, and tenofovir alafenamide.

Emtricitabine, Rilpivirine, and Tenofovir DF. The fixed combination emtricitabine/rilpivirine/tenofovir DF can be used to replace a stable antiretroviral regimen for treatment of HIV-1 infection in antiretroviral-experienced adults and adolescents 12 years of age or older weighing at least 35 kg who have been virologically suppressed (i.e., plasma HIV-1 RNA levels less than 50 copies/mL) on their current regimen for at least 6 months, are currently receiving only their first or second antiretroviral regimen, have no history of virologic failure, and have no current evidence or history of resistance to emtricitabine, rilpivirine, or tenofovir DF.

The efficacy and safety of emtricitabine/rilpivirine/tenofovir DF have been evaluated in a randomized, open-label study (study 106) in 476 virologically suppressed HIV-infected adults (mean age 42 years, 88% male, 77% white, 17% black, 17% Hispanic, mean baseline $CD4^+$ T-cell count 584 cells/mm^3). Patients were receiving their first or second antiretroviral regimen with no history of virologic failure; had no history of resistance to emtricitabine, rilpivirine, or tenofovir DF; and were virologically suppressed (plasma HIV-1 RNA levels less than 50 copies/mL) for at least 6 months. Patients were randomized in a 2:1 ratio to switch to emtricitabine/rilpivirine/tenofovir DF for 48 weeks or to continue receiving their baseline antiretroviral regimen containing a *ritonavir-boosted* HIV protease inhibitor (PI) for 24 weeks and then switch to emtricitabine/rilpivirine/tenofovir DF for an additional 24 weeks. In patients initially switched to emtricitabine/rilpivirine/tenofovir DF, 89% maintained plasma HIV-1 RNA levels less than 50 copies/mL at 48 weeks; 90% of those who continued to receive their baseline regimen maintained plasma HIV-1 RNA levels less than 50 copies/mL at 24 weeks.

Pediatric Patients Rilpivirine is used in conjunction with other antiretroviral agents for the treatment of HIV-1 infection in adolescents 12 years of age or older weighing at least 35 kg.

The fixed combination emtricitabine/rilpivirine/tenofovir alafenamide or the fixed combination emtricitabine/rilpivirine/tenofovir DF can be used alone as a complete regimen for the treatment of HIV-1 infection in adolescents 12 years of age or older weighing at least 35 kg.

For *initial* treatment in pediatric patients, the HHS Panel on Antiretroviral Therapy and Medical Management of HIV-infected Children states that rilpivirine and 2 NRTIs is an alternative HIV NNRTI-based regimen in antiretroviral-naive adolescents 12 years of age or older weighing 35 kg or more, but should be used *only* in those with baseline plasma HIV-1 RNA levels less than 100,000 copies/mL.

Clinical Experience. The efficacy and safety of rilpivirine in conjunction with 2 NRTIs were evaluated in a single-arm, open-label, phase 2 study (TMC278-C213) in 36 treatment-naive pediatric patients 12 to less than 18 years of age weighing at least 32 kg (median age 14.5 years, 56% female, 89% black, 11% Asian, median baseline plasma HIV-1 RNA level 49,550 copies/mL, median baseline $CD4^+$ T-cell count 438 cells/mm^3). Of the 36 patients, 24 received rilpivirine in conjunction with emtricitabine and tenofovir DF. At week 48, virologic response (plasma HIV-1 RNA levels less than 50 copies/mL) was achieved in 79% of patients with baseline plasma HIV-1 RNA levels of 100,000 copies/mL or less compared with 50% of those with baseline HIV-1 RNA levels greater than 100,000 copies/mL. The mean increase in $CD4^+$ T-cell count from baseline was 201 cells/mm^3. In a subgroup of patients receiving rilpivirine in conjunction with emtricitabine and tenofovir DF who had baseline plasma HIV-1 RNA levels of 100,000 copies/mL or less, virologic response (plasma HIV-1 RNA levels less than 50 copies/mL) was achieved by 80% at 48 weeks and the mean increase in $CD4^+$ T-cell count from baseline was 225 cells/mm^3 at 48 weeks.

■ **Postexposure Prophylaxis following Occupational Exposure to HIV** Rilpivirine is used in conjunction with 2 NRTIs for postexposure prophylaxis of HIV infection following occupational exposure† (PEP) in health-care personnel and other individuals exposed via percutaneous injury (e.g., needlestick, cut with sharp object) or mucous membrane or nonintact skin (e.g., chapped, abraded, dermatitis) contact with blood, tissue, or other body fluids that might contain HIV.

The US Public Health Service (USPHS) states that the preferred regimen for PEP following an occupational exposure to HIV is a 3-drug regimen of raltegravir used in conjunction with emtricitabine and tenofovir DF (may be administered as the fixed combination emtricitabine/tenofovir DF; Truvada®). Rilpivirine and 2 NRTIs is one of several alternative regimens recommended when the preferred regimen cannot be used. The preferred dual NRTI option for use in PEP regimens is emtricitabine and tenofovir DF (may be administered as emtricitabine/tenofovir DF; Truvada®); alternative dual NRTIs are tenofovir DF and lamivudine, zidovudine and lamivudine (may be administered as the fixed combination lamivudine/zidovudine; Combivir®), or zidovudine and emtricitabine.

Because management of occupational exposures to HIV is complex and evolving, consultation with an infectious disease specialist, clinician with expertise in administration of antiretroviral agents, and/or the National Clinicians' Postexposure Prophylaxis Hotline (PEPline at 888-448-4911) is recommended whenever possible. However, initiation of PEP should not be delayed while waiting for expert consultation.

For information on types of occupational exposure to HIV and associated risk of infection, management of occupational exposure to HIV, efficacy and safety of postexposure prophylaxis, and recommendations regarding PEP, see Guidelines for Use of Antiretroviral Agents: Antiretrovirals for Postexposure Prophylaxis following Occupational Exposure to HIV (PEP), in the Antiretroviral Agents General Statement 8:18.08.

■ **Postexposure Prophylaxis following Nonoccupational Exposure to HIV** Rilpivirine is used in conjunction with 2 NRTIs for postexposure prophylaxis of HIV infection following nonoccupational exposure† (nPEP) in individuals exposed to blood, genital secretions, or other potentially infectious body fluids that might contain HIV when that exposure represents a substantial risk for HIV transmission.

When nPEP is indicated following a nonoccupational exposure to HIV, the US Centers for Disease Control and Prevention (CDC) states that the preferred regimen in adults and adolescents 13 years of age or older with normal renal function is either raltegravir or dolutegravir used in conjunction with emtricitabine and tenofovir DF (administered as emtricitabine/tenofovir DF; Truvada®) and the alternative nPEP regimen recommended in these patients is *ritonavir-boosted* darunavir used in conjunction with emtricitabine/tenofovir DF (Truvada®). CDC states that a regimen of rilpivirine and 2 NRTIs (may be administered as the fixed combination emtricitabine/rilpivirine/tenofovir DF; Complera®) is one of several other alternative regimens for nPEP.

Consultation with an infectious disease specialist, clinician with expertise in administration of antiretroviral agents, and/or the National Clinicians' Postexposure Prophylaxis Hotline (PEPline at 888-448-4911) is recommended if nPEP is indicated in certain exposed individuals (e.g., pregnant women, children, those with medical conditions such as renal impairment) or if an antiretroviral regimen not included in the CDC guidelines is being considered, the source virus is known or likely to be resistant to antiretrovirals, or the healthcare provider is inexperienced in prescribing antiretrovirals. However, initiation of nPEP should not be delayed while waiting for expert consultation.

For additional information on nonoccupational exposure to HIV and recommendations regarding postexposure prophylaxis, see Guidelines for Use of Antiretroviral Agents: Antiretrovirals for Postexposure Prophylaxis after Sexual, Injection Drug Use, or other Nonoccupational Exposures to HIV (nPEP), in the Antiretroviral Agents General Statement 8:18.08.

Dosage and Administration

■ **Administration** Rilpivirine hydrochloride is administered orally once daily with a meal.

Food enhances rilpivirine bioavailability. Systemic exposure is 40 or 50% lower if rilpivirine is administered under fasting conditions or with only a protein-rich nutritional drink (300 kcal, 8 grams of fat), respectively, compared with following a standard meal (533 kcal, 21 grams of fat) or high-fat meal (928 kcal, 56 grams of fat).

Single-entity rilpivirine hydrochloride is commercially available as tablets. Rilpivirine hydrochloride also is commercially available in fixed-combination tablets containing emtricitabine, rilpivirine hydrochloride, and tenofovir alafenamide (emtricitabine/rilpivirine/tenofovir alafenamide; Odefsey®) and in fixed-combination tablets containing emtricitabine, rilpivirine hydrochloride, and tenofovir disoproxil fumarate (emtricitabine/rilpivirine/tenofovir DF; Complera®). (See Fixed Combinations Containing Rilpivirine under Dosage and Administration: Administration.)

Rilpivirine is used in conjunction with other antiretrovirals. Single-entity rilpivirine should not be used concomitantly with emtricitabine/rilpivirine/tenofovir alafenamide. Single-entity rilpivirine should not be used concomitantly with emtricitabine/rilpivirine/tenofovir DF, unless needed for adjustment of rilpivirine dosage (e.g., when the fixed combination is used concomitantly with rifabutin).

Fixed Combinations Containing Rilpivirine Emtricitabine/rilpivirine/tenofovir alafenamide (Odefsey®) tablets are administered orally once daily with a meal. Each fixed-combination tablet contains 200 mg of emtricitabine, 25 mg of rilpivirine, and 25 mg of tenofovir alafenamide. The fixed combination is used alone as a complete treatment regimen.

Emtricitabine/rilpivirine/tenofovir DF (Complera®) tablets are administered orally once daily with a meal. A fixed-combination tablet containing 200 mg of emtricitabine, 25 mg of rilpivirine, and 300 mg of tenofovir DF taken with a meal is bioequivalent to a 200-mg emtricitabine capsule, 25-mg rilpivirine tablet, and 300-mg tenofovir DF tablet taken simultaneously with a meal. The fixed combination is used alone as a complete treatment regimen. Emtricitabine/rilpivirine/tenofovir DF should not be used concomitantly with single-entity rilpivirine, unless needed for adjustment of the rilpivirine dosage (e.g., when the fixed combination is used concomitantly with rifabutin).

Estimated creatinine clearance, urine glucose, and urine protein should be determined prior to initiation of emtricitabine/rilpivirine/tenofovir alafenamide or emtricitabine/rilpivirine/tenofovir DF and routinely monitored during treatment in all patients. In addition, serum phosphorous should be monitored in those with chronic kidney disease or at risk for renal impairment. (See Renal Impairment under Warnings/Precautions: Specific Populations, in Cautions.)

Because the antiretrovirals contained in emtricitabine/rilpivirine/tenofovir alafenamide and emtricitabine/rilpivirine/tenofovir DF also may be available in single-entity or other fixed-combination preparations, care should be taken to ensure that therapy is not duplicated if a fixed combination is used in conjunction with other antiretrovirals. (See Precautions Related to Use of Fixed Combinations under Cautions: Warnings/Precautions.)

■ **Dosage** Rilpivirine is commercially available as rilpivirine hydrochloride; dosage is expressed in terms of rilpivirine.

Adult Dosage **Treatment of HIV Infection in Antiretroviral-naive Adults.** For the treatment of human immunodeficiency virus type 1 (HIV-1) infection in antiretroviral-naive adults, the usual dosage of rilpivirine (Edurant®) is 25 mg once daily.

When emtricitabine/rilpivirine/tenofovir alafenamide (Odefsey®) is used for the treatment of HIV-1 infection in antiretroviral-naive adults, the usual dosage is 1 tablet (200 mg of emtricitabine, 25 mg of rilpivirine, and 25 mg of tenofovir alafenamide) once daily.

When emtricitabine/rilpivirine/tenofovir DF (Complera®) is used for the treatment of HIV-1 infection in antiretroviral-naive adults, the usual dosage is 1 tablet (200 mg of emtricitabine, 25 mg of rilpivirine, and 300 mg of tenofovir DF) once daily.

Treatment of HIV Infection in Antiretroviral-experienced Adults. When emtricitabine/rilpivirine/tenofovir alafenamide (Odefsey®) is used for the treatment of HIV-1 infection in previously treated adults, the usual dosage is 1 tablet (200 mg of emtricitabine, 25 mg of rilpivirine, and 25 mg of tenofovir alafenamide) once daily.

When emtricitabine/rilpivirine/tenofovir DF (Complera®) is used for the treatment of HIV-1 infection in previously treated adults, the usual dosage is 1 tablet (200 mg of emtricitabine, 25 mg of rilpivirine, and 300 mg of tenofovir DF) once daily.

Treatment of HIV Infection in Adults Receiving Rifabutin. If single-entity rilpivirine is used in conjunction with other antiretrovirals for the treatment of HIV-1 infection in adults receiving rifabutin, an increased rilpivirine dosage of 50 mg daily should be used. (See Rifabutin under Drugs Interactions: Antimycobacterial Agents.)

Concomitant use of emtricitabine/rilpivirine/tenofovir alafenamide (Odefsey®) and rifabutin is not recommended.

If emtricitabine/rilpivirine/tenofovir DF (Complera®) is used for the treatment of HIV-1 infection in adults receiving rifabutin, patients should receive 1 tablet of the fixed combination (200 mg of emtricitabine, 25 mg of rilpivirine, and 300 mg of tenofovir DF) once daily *and* a 25-mg tablet of single-entity rilpivirine once daily to provide a total rilpivirine dosage of 50 mg daily.

Postexposure Prophylaxis following Occupational Exposure to HIV. For postexposure prophylaxis of HIV infection following occupational exposure† (PEP) in health-care personnel or other individuals, rilpivirine is administered in a dosage of 25 mg once daily in conjunction with 2 HIV nucleoside reverse transcriptase inhibitors (NRTIs). (See Uses: Postexposure Prophylaxis following Occupational Exposure to HIV.) Alternatively, if emtricitabine/rilpivirine/tenofovir DF (Complera®) is used for PEP, the recommended dosage is 1 tablet (200 mg of emtricitabine, 25 mg of rilpivirine, and 300 mg of tenofovir DF) once daily.

The PEP regimen should be initiated as soon as possible following occupational exposure to HIV (preferably within hours) and continued for 4 weeks, if tolerated.

Postexposure Prophylaxis following Nonoccupational Exposure to HIV. When emtricitabine/rilpivirine/tenofovir DF (Complera®) is used as a complete regimen for postexposure prophylaxis of HIV infection following nonoccupational exposure† (nPEP), adults should receive 1 tablet (200 mg of emtricitabine, 25 mg of rilpivirine, and 300 mg of tenofovir DF) once daily.

The nPEP regimen should be initiated as soon as possible (within 72 hours) following nonoccupational exposure to HIV and continued for 28 days. If the exposed individual seeks care more than 72 hours after the exposure, nPEP is not recommended.

Pediatric Dosage **Treatment of HIV Infection in Antiretroviral-naive Pediatric Patients.** For the treatment of HIV-1 infection in antiretroviral-naive adolescents 12 years of age or older weighing at least 35 kg, the usual dosage of rilpivirine (Edurant®) is 25 mg once daily.

When emtricitabine/rilpivirine/tenofovir alafenamide (Odefsey®) is used for the treatment of HIV-1 infection in antiretroviral-naive adolescents 12 years of age or older weighing at least 35 kg, the usual dosage is 1 tablet (200 mg of emtricitabine, 25 mg of rilpivirine, and 25 mg of tenofovir alafenamide) once daily.

When emtricitabine/rilpivirine/tenofovir DF (Complera®) is used for the treatment of HIV-1 infection in antiretroviral-naive adolescents 12 years of age or older weighing at least 35 kg, the usual dosage is 1 tablet (200 mg of emtricitabine, 25 mg of rilpivirine, and 300 mg of tenofovir DF) once daily.

Treatment of HIV Infection in Antiretroviral-experienced Pediatric Patients. When emtricitabine/rilpivirine/tenofovir alafenamide (Odefsey®) is used for the treatment of HIV-1 infection in previously treated adolescents 12 years of age or older weighing at least 35 kg, the usual dosage is 1 tablet (200 mg of emtricitabine, 25 mg of rilpivirine, and 25 mg of tenofovir alafenamide) once daily.

When emtricitabine/rilpivirine/tenofovir DF (Complera®) is used for the treatment of HIV-1 infection in previously treated adolescents 12 years of age or older weighing at least 35 kg, the usual dosage is 1 tablet (200 mg of emtricitabine, 25 mg of rilpivirine, and 300 mg of tenofovir DF) once daily.

Treatment of HIV Infection in Pediatric Patients Receiving Rifabutin. If single-entity rilpivirine is used in conjunction with other antiretrovirals for the treatment of HIV-1 infection in adolescents 12 years of age or older weighing at least 35 kg receiving rifabutin, an increased rilpivirine dosage of 50 mg daily should be used. (See Rifabutin under Drugs Interactions: Antimycobacterial Agents.)

Concomitant use of emtricitabine/rilpivirine/tenofovir alafenamide (Odefsey®) and rifabutin is not recommended.

If emtricitabine/rilpivirine/tenofovir DF (Complera®) is used for the treatment of HIV-1 infection in adolescents 12 years of age or older weighing at least 35 kg receiving rifabutin, patients should receive 1 tablet of the fixed combination (200 mg of emtricitabine, 25 mg of rilpivirine, and 300 mg of tenofovir DF) once daily *and* a 25-mg tablet of single-entity rilpivirine once daily to provide a total rilpivirine dosage of 50 mg daily.

■ **Special Populations** ***Hepatic Impairment*** Dosage adjustment of rilpivirine (Edurant®) is not necessary for the treatment of HIV-1 infection in patients with mild or moderate hepatic impairment (Child-Pugh class A or B). Rilpivirine has not been studied in those with severe hepatic impairment (Child-Pugh class C).

When emtricitabine/rilpivirine/tenofovir alafenamide (Odefsey®) is used for the treatment of HIV-1 infection in patients with mild or moderate hepatic impairment (Child-Pugh class A or B), usual dosage can be used; the fixed combination has not been studied in those with severe hepatic impairment (Child-Pugh class C).

When emtricitabine/rilpivirine/tenofovir DF (Complera®) is used for the treatment of HIV-1 infection in patients with mild or moderate hepatic impairment (Child-Pugh class A or B), usual dosage can be used; the fixed combination has not been studied in those with severe hepatic impairment (Child-Pugh class C).

Renal Impairment Dosage adjustment of rilpivirine (Edurant®) is not necessary for the treatment of HIV-1 infection in patients with mild or moderate renal impairment. The manufacturer makes no specific dosage recommendations for those with severe renal impairment or end-stage renal disease; rilpivirine should be used with caution in such individuals. (See Renal Impairment under Warnings/Precautions: Specific Populations, in Cautions.)

When emtricitabine/rilpivirine/tenofovir alafenamide (Odefsey®) is used for the treatment of HIV-1 infection, usual dosage can be used in patients with estimated creatinine clearance of 30 mL/minute or greater; the fixed combination is *not* recommended in those with severe renal impairment (estimated creatinine clearance less than 30 mL/minute).

Emtricitabine/rilpivirine/tenofovir DF (Complera®) should *not* be used in patients with renal impairment that is moderate, severe, or end-stage (estimated creatinine clearance less than 50 mL/minute) or requires dialysis.

Cautions

■ **Contraindications** Concomitant use of rilpivirine with drugs that induce cytochrome P-450 isoenzyme 3A (CYP3A) or drugs that elevate gastric pH is contraindicated since substantially decreased plasma rilpivirine concentrations may occur and may result in loss of virologic response and development of resistance to rilpivirine and/or class resistance to human immunodeficiency virus (HIV) nonnucleoside reverse transcriptase inhibitors (NNRTIs). Concomitant use with certain anticonvulsants (carbamazepine, oxcarbazepine, phenobarbital, phenytoin), certain antimycobacterials (rifampin, rifapentine), systemic dexamethasone (given in multiple doses), proton-pump inhibitors (dexlansoprazole, esomeprazole, lansoprazole, omeprazole, pantoprazole, rabeprazole), or certain herbal supplements (St. John's wort [*Hypericum perforatum*]) is contraindicated. (See Drug Interactions.)

When the fixed combination containing emtricitabine, rilpivirine, and tenofovir alafenamide (emtricitabine/rilpivirine/tenofovir alafenamide; Odefsey®) or the fixed combination containing emtricitabine, rilpivirine, and tenofovir disoproxil fumarate (emtricitabine/rilpivirine/tenofovir DF; Complera®) is used, the contraindications associated with each drug in the fixed combination should be considered. (See Precautions Related to Use of Fixed Combinations under Cautions: Warnings/Precautions.)

■ **Warnings/Precautions** ***Dermatologic and Sensitivity Reactions*** Severe skin and hypersensitivity reactions, including cases of drug reaction with eosinophilia and systemic symptoms (DRESS), have been reported during postmarketing experience in patients receiving rilpivirine-containing antiretroviral regimens. While some skin reactions were accompanied by constitutional symptoms such as fever, other skin reactions were associated with organ dysfunction, including elevated serum concentrations of hepatic enzymes. During phase 3 studies of rilpivirine-containing antiretroviral regimens, treatment-associated rash with at least grade 2 severity was reported in 1–3% of patients. Most rashes were grade 1 or 2 and occurred in the first 4–6 weeks of therapy.

Rilpivirine, emtricitabine/rilpivirine/tenofovir alafenamide, or emtricitabine/rilpivirine tenofovir DF should be discontinued immediately if signs or symptoms of severe skin or hypersensitivity reactions develop (e.g., severe rash or rash accompanied by fever, blisters, mucosal involvement, conjunctivitis, facial edema, angioedema, hepatitis, or eosinophilia). Clinical status, including laboratory parameters, should be monitored and appropriate therapy initiated.

Interactions Concomitant use with certain drugs (e.g., drugs that may reduce rilpivirine concentrations, drugs known to increase the risk of torsades de pointes) is contraindicated or requires particular caution. (See Cautions: Contraindications and see Drug Interactions.)

Depressive Disorders Depressive disorders (depressed mood, depression, dysphoria, major depression, altered mood, negative thoughts, suicide attempt, suicidal ideation) have been reported in patients receiving rilpivirine. During phase 3 studies (ECHO and THRIVE studies), 9% of adults receiving rilpivirine reported depressive disorders compared with 8% of patients receiving efavirenz. While most depressive events were reported to be mild or moderate in severity, 1% of adults in each treatment group reported a grade 3 or 4 depressive disorder and 1% in each treatment group discontinued therapy as a result of a depressive disorder. Suicidal ideation was reported in 4 adults in each treatment group and suicide attempt was reported in 2 adults receiving rilpivirine.

During a phase 2 study evaluating rilpivirine in pediatric patients 12 to less than 18 years of age, the incidence of depressive disorders was 19.4%. While most depressive events were reported to be mild or moderate in severity, 5.6% of pediatric patients reported a grade 3 or 4 depressive disorder. Suicidal ideation and suicide attempt were reported in a pediatric patient.

Patients experiencing severe depressive symptoms should seek immediate medical evaluation to determine the likelihood that symptoms are related to rilpivirine and to determine if the benefits of continued rilpivirine therapy outweigh the risks.

Hepatotoxicity Adverse hepatic effects have been reported in patients receiving rilpivirine in conjunction with other antiretrovirals. Hepatotoxicity has been reported in patients receiving rilpivirine who had no preexisting hepatic disease or other risk factors.

HIV-infected patients with hepatitis B virus (HBV) or hepatitis C virus (HCV) coinfection or markedly elevated serum aminotransferase concentrations prior to initiation of rilpivirine may be at increased risk for development or worsening of aminotransferase elevations.

If rilpivirine, emtricitabine/rilpivirine/tenofovir alafenamide, or emtricitabine/rilpivirine/tenofovir DF is used in patients with underlying hepatic disease (e.g., HBV or HCV infection, markedly elevated aminotransferase concentrations), laboratory tests should be performed to evaluate hepatic function prior to and during rilpivirine treatment. Liver enzyme monitoring also should be considered in patients without preexisting hepatic disease or other risk factors.

Precautions Related to Use of Fixed Combinations When emtricitabine/rilpivirine/tenofovir alafenamide or emtricitabine/rilpivirine/tenofovir DF is used, the cautions, precautions, contraindications, and drug interactions associated with each drug in the fixed combination must be considered. Cautionary information applicable to specific populations (e.g., pregnant or nursing women, individuals with hepatic or renal impairment, geriatric patients) should be considered for each drug. For cautionary information related to emtricitabine and tenofovir DF, see Cautions in the individual drug monographs.

Because the antiretrovirals contained in emtricitabine/rilpivirine/tenofovir alafenamide and emtricitabine/rilpivirine/tenofovir DF also may be available in single-entity or other fixed-combination preparations, care should be taken to ensure that therapy is not duplicated if one of these fixed combinations is used in conjunction with other antiretrovirals.

Emtricitabine/rilpivirine/tenofovir DF should not be used concomitantly with single-entity rilpivirine, unless needed for adjustment of rilpivirine dosage (e.g., when the fixed combination is used concomitantly with rifabutin). (See Drug Interactions: Antimycobacterial Agents.)

Because of similarities between emtricitabine and lamivudine, fixed combinations containing emtricitabine should not be used concomitantly with any preparation containing lamivudine. In addition, fixed combinations containing tenofovir DF should not be used concomitantly with adefovir dipivoxil.

If emtricitabine/rilpivirine/tenofovir alafenamide or emtricitabine/rilpivirine/tenofovir DF is used, clinicians should consider that lactic acidosis and severe hepatomegaly with steatosis, including fatalities, have been reported in patients receiving nucleoside reverse transcriptase inhibitors (NRTIs) in conjunction with other antiretrovirals.

If emtricitabine/rilpivirine/tenofovir alafenamide or emtricitabine/rilpivirine/tenofovir DF is used, clinicians should consider that severe, acute exacerbations of HBV infection have been reported following discontinuance of emtricitabine and/or tenofovir DF in HIV-infected patients coinfected with HBV. The fixed combinations are not labeled for treatment of chronic HBV infection, and safety and efficacy have not been established in HIV-infected patients coinfected with HBV. Hepatic function should be closely monitored with both clinical and laboratory follow-up for at least several months after the fixed combination is discontinued in coinfected patients. If appropriate, initiation of HBV treatment may be warranted.

Adipogenic Effects Redistribution or accumulation of body fat, including central obesity, dorsocervical fat enlargement ("buffalo hump"), peripheral wasting, facial wasting, breast enlargement, and general cushingoid appearance, has been reported in patients receiving antiretroviral therapy. The mechanisms and long-term consequences of adipogenic effects are unknown; a causal relationship has not been established.

Immune Reconstitution Syndrome During the initial phase of treatment, HIV-infected patients whose immune systems respond to antiretroviral therapy may develop an inflammatory response to indolent or residual opportunistic infections (e.g., *Mycobacterium avium*, *M. tuberculosis*, cytomegalovirus [CMV], *Pneumocystis jirovecii* [formerly *P. carinii*]); such responses may necessitate further evaluation and treatment.

Autoimmune disorders (e.g., Graves' disease, polymyositis, Guillain-Barré syndrome) have also been reported to occur in the setting of immune reconstitution; however, the time to onset is more variable and can occur many months after initiation of antiretroviral therapy.

Specific Populations **Pregnancy.** Rilpivirine (Edurant®): Category B. (See Users Guide.)

Emtricitabine/rilpivirine/tenofovir alafenamide (Odefsey®): Insufficient human data to assess the risk of birth defects and miscarriage if used during pregnancy.

Emtricitabine/rilpivirine/tenofovir DF (Complera®): Category B.

Antiretroviral Pregnancy Registry at 800-258-4263 or http://www.APRegistry.com.

For *initial* treatment in antiretroviral-naive pregnant women, the US Department of Health and Human Services (HHS) Panel on Treatment of HIV-infected Pregnant Women and Prevention of Perinatal Transmission states that rilpivirine in conjunction with tenofovir DF and emtricitabine (or rilpivirine in conjunction with a preferred 2-NRTI backbone) is an alternative NNRTI-based regimen, but should be used *only* in patients with baseline plasma HIV-1 RNA levels less than 100,000 copies/mL *and* baseline $CD4^+$ T-cell count greater than 200 cells/mm^3.

Lactation. It is not known whether rilpivirine is distributed into human milk; however, the drug is distributed into milk in rats.

Because of the risk of adverse effects in the infant and the risk of HIV transmission, HIV-infected women should not breast-feed infants.

Pediatric Use. Safety and efficacy of single-entity rilpivirine (Edurant®) have *not* been established in pediatric patients younger than 12 years of age.

Emtricitabine/rilpivirine/tenofovir alafenamide (Odefsey®): Safety and efficacy have *not* been established in pediatric patients younger than 12 years of age or weighing less than 35 kg.

Emtricitabine/rilpivirine/tenofovir DF (Complera®): Safety and efficacy have *not* been established in pediatric patients younger than 12 years of age or weighing less than 35 kg.

Depressive disorders have been reported in pediatric patients 12 to less than 18 years of age receiving rilpivirine-containing regimens. (See Depressive Disorders under Cautions: Warnings/Precautions.)

Geriatric Use. Experience in those 65 years of age and older is insufficient to determine whether they respond differently to rilpivirine than younger adults. Dosage should be selected with caution because of age-related decreases in hepatic, renal, and/or cardiac function and potential for concomitant disease and drug therapy.

Hepatic Impairment. Rilpivirine (Edurant®), emtricitabine/rilpivirine/tenofovir alafenamide (Odefsey®), and emtricitabine/rilpivirine/tenofovir DF (Complera®) have not been studied in patients with severe hepatic impairment (Child-Pugh class C).

During phase 3 clinical trials evaluating rilpivirine, HIV-infected patients coinfected with HBV and/or HCV had a higher incidence of increased serum aminotransferase concentrations compared with those without coinfection. (See Hepatotoxicity under Cautions: Warnings/Precautions.)

Renal Impairment. Rilpivirine (Edurant®) should be used with caution and with increased monitoring for adverse effects in patients with severe renal impairment or end-stage renal disease since concentrations of the drug may be increased due to alterations in absorption, distribution, or metabolism. (See Renal Impairment under Dosage and Administration: Special Populations.)

Emtricitabine/rilpivirine/tenofovir alafenamide (Odefsey®) is *not* recommended in patients with severe renal impairment (estimated creatinine clearance less than 30 mL/minute).

Emtricitabine/rilpivirine/tenofovir DF (Complera®) should *not* be used in patients with renal impairment that is moderate, severe, or end-stage (estimated creatinine clearance less than 50 mL/minute) or requires dialysis.

■ **Common Adverse Effects** Adverse effects of moderate or severe intensity and reported in 2% or more of patients receiving rilpivirine include depressive disorders (see Depressive Disorders under Cautions: Warnings/Precautions), insomnia, headache, and rash. Increased serum AST and/or ALT concentrations (more than 2.5 times the upper limit of normal [ULN] were reported in 4–5% of patients receiving rilpivirine.

Drug Interactions

Most rilpivirine drug interaction studies reported to date used rilpivirine dosages of 75 or 150 mg once daily; these dosages are considerably higher than the usually recommended rilpivirine dosage (25 mg once daily).

The following drug interactions are based on studies using rilpivirine, the fixed combination of emtricitabine, rilpivirine, and tenofovir alafenamide (emtricitabine/rilpivirine/tenofovir alafenamide), the fixed combination of emtricitabine, rilpivirine, and tenofovir DF (emtricitabine/rilpivirine/tenofovir DF), or the individual components of the fixed combinations, or are predicted to occur. When emtricitabine/rilpivirine/tenofovir alafenamide or emtricitabine/rilpivirine/tenofovir DF is used, interactions associated with each drug in the fixed combination should be considered.

■ **Drugs Affecting or Metabolized by Hepatic Microsomal Enzymes** Rilpivirine is metabolized by the cytochrome P-450 (CYP) isoenzyme 3A. Concomitant use with drugs that induce CYP3A may result in decreased plasma rilpivirine concentrations and may result in possible loss of virologic response and development of resistance to rilpivirine or the human immunodeficiency virus (HIV) nonnucleoside reverse transcriptase inhibitor (NNRTI) class. Concomitant use with drugs that inhibit CYP3A may result in increased plasma rilpivirine concentrations.

When the recommended rilpivirine dosage (25 mg once daily) is used, it is unlikely to have clinically important effects on the pharmacokinetics of drugs that are metabolized by CYP isoenzymes.

■ **Drugs Affected by P-glycoprotein Transport** Tenofovir alafenamide, a component of emtricitabine/rilpivirine/tenofovir alafenamide, is a substrate of P-glycoprotein (P-gp) transport.

Concomitant use of emtricitabine/rilpivirine/tenofovir alafenamide and P-gp inhibitors may result in increased absorption of tenofovir alafenamide and may result in increased plasma concentrations of tenofovir alafenamide and increased adverse effects.

Concomitant use of emtricitabine/rilpivirine/tenofovir alafenamide and P-gp inducers is expected to decrease absorption of tenofovir alafenamide and may result in decreased plasma concentrations of tenofovir alafenamide leading to loss of therapeutic effect and development of resistance.

■ **Drugs that Increase Gastric pH** Concomitant use of rilpivirine and drugs that increase gastric pH may result in decreased plasma rilpivirine concentrations and may result in loss of virologic response and development of resistance to rilpivirine or the NNRTI class.

Antacids Potential pharmacokinetic interaction if antacids such as aluminum hydroxide, calcium carbonate, or magnesium hydroxide are used concomitantly with rilpivirine (decreased plasma rilpivirine concentrations).

Antacids and rilpivirine should be used concomitantly with caution; antacids should be administered at least 2 hours before or at least 4 hours after rilpivirine, emtricitabine/rilpivirine/tenofovir alafenamide, or emtricitabine/rilpivirine/tenofovir DF.

Histamine H_2-receptor Antagonists Concomitant use of famotidine and rilpivirine has resulted in decreased rilpivirine plasma concentrations and area under the concentration-time curve (AUC). Concomitant use of other histamine H_2-receptor antagonists (e.g., cimetidine, nizatidine, ranitidine) also may result in decreased rilpivirine plasma concentrations.

Histamine H_2-receptor antagonists and rilpivirine should be used concomitantly with caution; histamine H_2-receptor antagonists should be administered at least 12 hours before or at least 4 hours after rilpivirine, emtricitabine/rilpivirine/tenofovir alafenamide, or emtricitabine/rilpivirine/tenofovir DF.

Proton-pump Inhibitors Concomitant use of omeprazole and rilpivirine has resulted in decreased rilpivirine plasma concentrations and AUC. Concomitant use of other proton-pump inhibitors (e.g., dexlansoprazole, esomeprazole, lansoprazole, pantoprazole, rabeprazole) also may result in decreased rilpivirine plasma concentrations.

Concomitant use of proton-pump inhibitors (e.g., dexlansoprazole, esomeprazole, lansoprazole, omeprazole, pantoprazole, rabeprazole) and rilpivirine, emtricitabine/rilpivirine/tenofovir alafenamide, or emtricitabine/rilpivirine/tenofovir DF is contraindicated.

■ **Drugs that Prolong the QT Interval** Only limited data are available to date regarding the potential for pharmacodynamic interactions if rilpivirine is used concomitantly with drugs known to prolong the QT interval and increase the risk of torsades de pointes. Data from healthy individuals indicate that the recommended rilpivirine dosage (25 mg once daily) can result in increases in the corrected QT (QT_c) interval that are not considered clinically important; however, higher rilpivirine dosage (75 or 300 mg once daily) results in clinically important prolongation of the QT_c interval.

Caution is advised if rilpivirine or emtricitabine/rilpivirine/tenofovir DF is used concomitantly with drugs known to increase the risk of torsades de pointes. An alternative to emtricitabine/rilpivirine/tenofovir alafenamide should be considered in patients receiving drugs known to increase the risk of torsades de pointes.

■ **Nephrotoxic Drugs or Drugs Eliminated by Renal Excretion** The emtricitabine and tenofovir components of emtricitabine/rilpivirine/tenofovir alafenamide and emtricitabine/rilpivirine/tenofovir DF are primarily excreted renally by a combination of glomerular filtration and active tubular secretion.

Potential pharmacokinetic interactions if emtricitabine/rilpivirine/tenofovir alafenamide or emtricitabine/rilpivirine/tenofovir DF is used concomitantly with drugs that reduce renal function or compete for active tubular secretion (e.g., acyclovir, aminoglycosides [gentamicin], cidofovir, ganciclovir, valacyclovir, valganciclovir, high-dose or multiple nonsteroidal anti-inflammatory agents [NSAIAs]); increased plasma concentrations of emtricitabine, tenofovir, and/or the concomitant drug may occur and increase the risk of adverse effects.

■ **Acetaminophen** Clinically important pharmacokinetic interactions between rilpivirine and acetaminophen have not been observed; dosage adjustments are not needed.

■ **Anticonvulsants** Potential pharmacokinetic interactions when rilpivirine is used concomitantly with carbamazepine, oxcarbazepine, phenobarbital, or phenytoin (decreased plasma rilpivirine concentrations).

Concomitant use of anticonvulsants (carbamazepine, oxcarbazepine, phenobarbital, phenytoin) and rilpivirine, emtricitabine/rilpivirine/tenofovir alafenamide, or emtricitabine/rilpivirine/tenofovir DF is contraindicated.

■ **Antifungal Agents** Concomitant use of ketoconazole and rilpivirine has resulted in increased rilpivirine plasma concentrations and AUC and decreased ketoconazole plasma concentrations and AUC. Concomitant use of other azole antifungals (e.g., fluconazole, isavuconazonium, itraconazole, posaconazole, voriconazole) and rilpivirine also may result in increased rilpivirine plasma concentrations and decreased antifungal plasma concentrations. Concomitant use of an azole antifungal with emtricitabine/rilpivirine/tenofovir alafenamide may also result in increased tenofovir alafenamide concentrations.

When rilpivirine, emtricitabine/rilpivirine/tenofovir alafenamide, or emtricitabine/rilpivirine/tenofovir DF is used concomitantly with an azole antifungal (e.g., fluconazole, isavuconazonium, itraconazole, ketoconazole, posaconazole, voriconazole), dosage adjustments are not needed; however, patients should be monitored for breakthrough fungal infections.

■ **Antimycobacterial Agents** ***Rifampin and Rifapentine*** Concomitant use of rilpivirine and rifampin or rifapentine results in decreased rilpivirine plasma concentrations and AUC.

Concomitant use of rifampin or rifapentine with rilpivirine, emtricitabine/rilpivirine/tenofovir alafenamide, or emtricitabine/rilpivirine/tenofovir DF is contraindicated.

Rifabutin Concomitant use of rifabutin and rilpivirine results in decreased rilpivirine plasma concentrations and AUC.

If single-entity rilpivirine is used concomitantly with rifabutin, rilpivirine dosage should be increased to 50 mg once daily; if rifabutin is discontinued, the usual dosage of single-entity rilpivirine (25 mg once daily) should be resumed.

Concomitant use of rifabutin and emtricitabine/rilpivirine/tenofovir alafenamide results in decreased rilpivirine concentrations and may also result in decreased tenofovir alafenamide concentrations. Concomitant use of emtricitabine/rilpivirine/tenofovir alafenamide and rifabutin is not recommended.

If emtricitabine/rilpivirine/tenofovir DF is used concomitantly with rifabutin, the manufacturer recommends that patients receive 1 tablet of the fixed combination (25 mg of rilpivirine, 200 mg of emtricitabine, and 300 mg of tenofovir DF) once daily *and* a 25-mg tablet of single-entity rilpivirine once daily to provide a total rilpivirine dosage of 50 mg daily. (See Dosage and Administration: Dosage.)

■ **Antiretroviral Agents** ***HIV Entry and Fusion Inhibitors*** **Enfuvirtide.** No in vitro evidence of antagonistic antiretroviral effects between rilpivirine and enfuvirtide.

Maraviroc. No in vitro evidence of antagonistic antiretroviral effects between rilpivirine and maraviroc.

Clinically important pharmacokinetic interactions are not expected.

HIV Integrase Inhibitors (INSTIs) **Dolutegravir.** Concomitant use of dolutegravir and rilpivirine does not have a clinically important effect on the pharmacokinetics of either drug. Dosage adjustments are not needed if rilpivirine and dolutegravir are used concomitantly.

Elvitegravir. Concomitant use of rilpivirine and *cobicistat-boosted* elvitegravir may result in altered concentrations of elvitegravir, cobicistat, and/or rilpivirine. Rilpivirine and *cobicistat-boosted* elvitegravir should not be used concomitantly.

Concomitant use of rilpivirine and elvitegravir used in conjunction with a *ritonavir-boosted* HIV protease inhibitor (PI) is expected to increase rilpivirine plasma concentrations. Dosage adjustments are not needed if rilpivirine is used concomitantly with elvitegravir used in conjunction with a *ritonavir-boosted* HIV PI; however, the recommended dosage of elvitegravir depends on which *ritonavir-boosted* HIV PI is used.

Raltegravir. No in vitro evidence of antagonistic antiretroviral effects between rilpivirine and raltegravir.

Concomitant use of raltegravir and rilpivirine does not have a clinically important effect on plasma concentrations or AUC of raltegravir or rilpivirine. Dosage adjustments are not needed for either drug.

HIV Nonnucleoside Reverse Transcriptase Inhibitors (NNRTIs) No in vitro evidence of antagonistic antiretroviral effects between rilpivirine and NNRTIs (efavirenz, etravirine, nevirapine).

Concomitant use of delavirdine and rilpivirine may result in increased rilpivirine plasma concentrations; concomitant use of efavirenz, etravirine, or nevirapine may result in decreased rilpivirine plasma concentrations.

Concomitant use of rilpivirine and other NNRTIs (delavirdine, efavirenz, etravirine, nevirapine) is not recommended.

HIV Nucleoside and Nucleotide Reverse Transcriptase Inhibitors (NRTIs) No in vitro evidence of antagonistic antiretroviral effects between rilpivirine and HIV nucleoside reverse transcriptase inhibitors (NRTIs) (abacavir, didanosine, emtricitabine, lamivudine, stavudine, tenofovir, zidovudine).

Although not specifically studied, clinically important pharmacokinetic interactions are not expected if rilpivirine is used concomitantly with abacavir, emtricitabine, lamivudine, stavudine, or zidovudine.

Didanosine. Pharmacokinetic interactions were not observed when didanosine delayed-release capsules were administered 2 hours before rilpivirine. Although dosage adjustments are not needed if rilpivirine and didanosine are used concomitantly, didanosine should be administered (without food) at least 2 hours before or 4 hours after rilpivirine (with food).

Tenofovir. Concomitant use of tenofovir DF and rilpivirine has resulted in increased tenofovir plasma concentrations and AUC, but did not have a clinically important effect on rilpivirine plasma concentrations or AUC.

Dosage adjustments are not needed if tenofovir DF and rilpivirine are used concomitantly.

HIV Protease Inhibitors (PIs) No in vitro evidence of antagonistic antiretroviral effects between rilpivirine and HIV PIs (amprenavir [commercially available as fosamprenavir], atazanavir, darunavir, indinavir, lopinavir, nelfinavir, ritonavir, saquinavir, tipranavir).

Atazanavir. Concomitant use of rilpivirine and *ritonavir-boosted* atazanavir, *cobicistat-boosted* atazanavir, or unboosted atazanavir may result in increased rilpivirine plasma concentrations, but is not expected to affect atazanavir concentrations.

Dosage adjustments are not needed if rilpivirine is used concomitantly with *ritonavir-boosted*, *cobicistat-boosted*, or unboosted atazanavir.

Darunavir. Concomitant use of rilpivirine and *ritonavir-boosted* darunavir resulted in increased rilpivirine plasma concentrations and AUC, but did not have a clinically important effect on darunavir concentrations or AUC. Concomitant use of *cobicistat-boosted* darunavir and rilpivirine may increase rilpivirine plasma concentrations, but is not expected to affect darunavir concentrations.

Dosage adjustments are not needed if rilpivirine is used concomitantly with *ritonavir-boosted* or *cobicistat-boosted* darunavir.

Fosamprenavir. Concomitant use of rilpivirine and fosamprenavir or *ritonavir-boosted* fosamprenavir may result in increased rilpivirine plasma concentrations, but is not expected to affect amprenavir concentrations (active metabolite of fosamprenavir).

Dosage adjustments are not needed if fosamprenavir (with or without low-dose ritonavir) and rilpivirine are used concomitantly.

Indinavir. Concomitant use of rilpivirine and indinavir may result in increased rilpivirine plasma concentrations, but is not expected to affect indinavir concentrations.

Lopinavir. Concomitant use of rilpivirine and the fixed combination of lopinavir and ritonavir (lopinavir/ritonavir) increased rilpivirine plasma concentrations and AUC, but did not have a clinically important effect on lopinavir plasma concentrations or AUC.

Dosage adjustments are not needed if lopinavir/ritonavir and rilpivirine are used concomitantly.

Nelfinavir. Concomitant use of nelfinavir may result in increased rilpivirine plasma concentrations, but is not expected to affect nelfinavir concentrations.

Saquinavir. Concomitant use of rilpivirine and *ritonavir-boosted* saquinavir may result in increased rilpivirine plasma concentrations, but is not expected to affect saquinavir concentrations.

Dosage adjustments are not needed if *ritonavir-boosted* saquinavir and rilpivirine are used concomitantly.

Tipranavir. Concomitant use of rilpivirine and *ritonavir-boosted* tipranavir may result in increased rilpivirine plasma concentrations, but is not expected to affect tipranavir concentrations.

Dosage adjustments are not needed if *ritonavir-boosted* tipranavir and rilpivirine are used concomitantly.

■ **Benzodiazepines** Data are not available regarding concomitant use of rilpivirine and alprazolam; if the drugs are used concomitantly, patients should be monitored for alprazolam therapeutic effects.

Clinically important pharmacokinetic interactions are not expected if emtricitabine/rilpivirine/tenofovir alafenamide is used concomitantly with lorazepam or midazolam.

■ **Chlorzoxazone** Clinically important pharmacokinetic interactions between rilpivirine and chlorzoxazone have not been observed; dosage adjustments are not needed.

■ **Corticosteroids** Potential pharmacokinetic interaction if multiple doses of systemic dexamethasone are used concomitantly with rilpivirine (decreased plasma rilpivirine concentrations). Concomitant use of more than a single dose of dexamethasone with rilpivirine, emtricitabine/rilpivirine/tenofovir alafenamide, or emtricitabine/rilpivirine/tenofovir DF is contraindicated.

■ **Digoxin** Rilpivirine does not have a clinically important effect on digoxin pharmacokinetics.

■ **Estrogens and Progestins** Clinically important pharmacokinetic interactions have not been observed when usual rilpivirine dosage was used concomitantly with hormonal contraceptives containing ethinyl estradiol and norethindrone; dosage adjustments are not needed.

Clinically important pharmacokinetic interactions are not expected if emtricitabine/rilpivirine/tenofovir alafenamide is used concomitantly with the fixed combination of ethinyl estradiol and norgestimate.

■ **HCV Antivirals** ***HCV Polymerase Inhibitors*** **Sofosbuvir.** Concomitant use of sofosbuvir and rilpivirine does not have a clinically important effect on sofosbuvir or rilpivirine pharmacokinetics. Dosage adjustments are not needed for either drug.

Sofosbuvir and Velpatasvir. Concomitant use of the fixed combination of sofosbuvir and velpatasvir (sofosbuvir/velpatasvir) and rilpivirine did not result in clinically important pharmacokinetic interactions.

HCV Protease Inhibitors **Simeprevir.** Concomitant use of simeprevir and rilpivirine does not have a clinically important effect on simeprevir or rilpivirine pharmacokinetics. Dosage adjustments are not needed for either drug.

Clinically important pharmacokinetic interactions are not expected if emtricitabine/rilpivirine/tenofovir alafenamide is used concomitantly with simeprevir.

HCV Replication Complex Inhibitors **Daclatasvir.** Concomitant use of daclatasvir and rilpivirine is not expected to result in clinically important pharmacokinetic interactions.

Dosage adjustments are not needed if daclatasvir is used concomitantly with rilpivirine.

Elbasvir and Grazoprevir. Concomitant use of the fixed combination of elbasvir and grazoprevir (elbasvir/grazoprevir) and rilpivirine does not have a clinically important effect on elbasvir, grazoprevir, or rilpivirine pharmacokinetics.

Dosage adjustments are not needed if elbasvir/grazoprevir is used concomitantly with rilpivirine.

Ledipasvir and Sofosbuvir. Concomitant use of rilpivirine and the fixed combination of ledipasvir and sofosbuvir (ledipasvir/sofosbuvir) does not have clinically important effects on the pharmacokinetics of rilpivirine, ledipasvir, or sofosbuvir. Dosage adjustments are not necessary if rilpivirine and ledipasvir/sofosbuvir are used concomitantly.

Clinically important pharmacokinetic interactions are not expected if emtricitabine/rilpivirine/tenofovir alafenamide is used concomitantly with ledipasvir or sofosbuvir.

Concomitant use of emtricitabine/rilpivirine/tenofovir DF and ledipasvir/sofosbuvir does not have clinically important effects on the pharmacokinetics of rilpivirine, ledipasvir, or sofosbuvir, but results in increased tenofovir plasma concentrations and AUC. If emtricitabine/rilpivirine/tenofovir DF is used concomitantly with ledipasvir/sofosbuvir, the patient should be monitored for tenofovir-associated adverse effects.

Ombitasvir, Paritaprevir, and Ritonavir. Concomitant use of rilpivirine and the fixed combination of ombitasvir, paritaprevir, and ritonavir (ombitasvir/paritaprevir/ritonavir) with or without dasabuvir results in substantially increased plasma concentrations and AUC of rilpivirine and may increase the potential for QT interval prolongation.

Concomitant use of rilpivirine and ombitasvir/paritaprevir/ritonavir with or without dasabuvir is not recommended.

■ **HMG-CoA Reductase Inhibitors** Clinically important pharmacokinetic interactions have not been observed when atorvastatin and rilpivirine were used concomitantly; dosage adjustments are not needed.

Data are not available regarding concomitant use of pitavastatin and rilpivirine, but clinically important interactions are not expected and dosage adjustments are not needed.

■ **Macrolides** Concomitant use of rilpivirine and clarithromycin, erythromycin, or telithromycin may result in increased rilpivirine plasma concentrations, but is not expected to affect plasma concentrations of the macrolide. An alternative to these macrolides (e.g., azithromycin) should be considered whenever possible in patients receiving rilpivirine, emtricitabine/rilpivirine/tenofovir alafenamide, or emtricitabine/rilpivirine/tenofovir DF.

■ **Metformin** Rilpivirine does not have a clinically important effect on metformin pharmacokinetics.

■ **Opiates, Opiate Partial Agonists, and Opiate Antagonists** Clinically important pharmacokinetic interactions are not expected if emtricitabine/rilpivirine/tenofovir alafenamide is used concomitantly with buprenorphine or naloxone.

Methadone Concomitant use of methadone and usual rilpivirine dosage resulted in decreased methadone concentrations, but did not have a clinically important effect on rilpivirine concentrations or AUC.

Although adjustment of initial methadone dosage is not needed when methadone and rilpivirine are used concomitantly, close monitoring is recommended and methadone maintenance dosage may need to be adjusted in some patients.

■ **Phosphodiesterase Type 5 Inhibitors** ***Avanafil*** Data are not available regarding concomitant use of avanafil and rilpivirine; concomitant use is not recommended.

Sildenafil Clinically important pharmacokinetic interactions have not been observed when sildenafil and rilpivirine were used concomitantly; dosage adjustments are not needed.

■ **Ribavirin** Clinically important pharmacokinetic interactions between rilpivirine and ribavirin are not expected.

■ **St. John's Wort** Potential pharmacokinetic interaction if St. John's wort (*Hypericum perforatum*) is used concomitantly with rilpivirine (decreased plasma rilpivirine concentrations); may result in loss of therapeutic effect and development of resistance. Concomitant use of St. John's wort and rilpivirine, emtricitabine/rilpivirine/tenofovir alafenamide, or emtricitabine/rilpivirine/tenofovir DF is contraindicated.

Description

Rilpivirine, a diarylpyrimidine human immunodeficiency virus (HIV) nonnucleoside reverse transcriptase inhibitor (NNRTI), inhibits replication of HIV type 1 (HIV-1) by interfering with viral RNA- and DNA-directed polymerase activities of reverse transcriptase. Diarylpyrimidine NNRTIs (e.g., rilpivirine, etravirine) are capable of adapting to mutations in HIV-1 reverse transcriptase because of structural flexibility that allows for binding to the allosteric NNRTI binding pocket in a variety of conformations. Unlike other currently available NNRTIs, rilpivirine contains a cyanovinyl group that contributes to potency and maintains the drug's binding ability, despite the emergence of some resistance mutations. In vitro, rilpivirine is highly active against wild-type HIV-1, but has limited activity against HIV type 2 (HIV-2). Rilpivirine has been active against some clinical HIV-1 isolates resistant to other commercially available NNRTIs (delavirdine, efavirenz, nevirapine). However rilpivirine-resistant strains have been selected in cell culture and have emerged during clinical use.

Cross-resistance can occur between rilpivirine and other commercially available NNRTIs, and is expected in patients who have virologic failure while receiving a regimen that contains rilpivirine. Considerable cross-resistance occurs between rilpivirine and etravirine; up to 90% of rilpivirine-resistant isolates that developed in patients receiving rilpivirine in phase 3 clinical studies also were resistant to etravirine. In addition, patients experiencing virologic failure while receiving a rilpivirine regimen in phase 3 clinical studies were more likely to have developed NNRTI-class resistance and treatment-emergent resistance to nucleoside and HIV nucleotide reverse transcriptase inhibitors (NRTIs) than patients experiencing virologic failure while receiving an efavirenz regimen.

After oral administration, peak rilpivirine plasma concentrations are generally attained within 4–5 hours. Rilpivirine is primarily metabolized in the liver by cytochrome P-450 (CYP) isoenzyme 3A. After a single oral dose, an average of 85% of the dose is eliminated in feces (75% as metabolites) and 6% is eliminated in urine (only trace amounts as unchanged rilpivirine). The terminal elimination half-life of rilpivirine is approximately 50 hours. In individuals with mild (Child-Pugh class A) or moderate (Child-Pugh class B) hepatic impairment receiving multiple doses of rilpivirine, exposure to the drug was 47 or 5% higher, respectively, compared to healthy individuals. (See Hepatic Impairment under Warnings/Precautions: Specific Populations, in Cautions.) Coinfection with HIV and hepatitis B virus (HBV) and/or hepatitis C virus (HCV) does not appear to have a clinically important effect on exposure to the drug. Mild renal impairment does not have a clinically important effect on rilpivirine pharmacokinetics. Only limited data are available regarding pharmacokinetics of the drug in patients with moderate or severe renal impairment or end-stage renal disease, but rilpivirine concentrations may be increased as a result of altered absorption, distribution, or elimination. (See Renal Impairment under Specific Populations: Warnings/Precautions, in Cautions.) In vitro studies indicate that rilpivirine is approximately 99.7% bound to plasma proteins, primarily albumin. Because rilpivirine is highly bound to plasma proteins, peritoneal dialysis and hemodialysis are unlikely to result in clinically important removal of the drug. Clinically relevant differences in pharmacokinetics between men and women have not been observed. Based on population pharmacokinetic analysis, race is not expected to have a clinically relevant effect on rilpivirine exposure. Pharmacokinetics in treatment-naive HIV-1-infected pediatric patients 12 to less than 18 years of age receiving rilpivirine 25 mg once daily are similar to those observed in treatment-naive adult patients. In clinical trials, body weight in pediatric patients (ranging from 33–93 kg) did not have a clinically important effect on rilpivirine pharmacokinetics.

Advice to Patients

Critical nature of compliance with human immunodeficiency virus (HIV) therapy and importance of remaining under the care of a clinician. Importance of taking as prescribed; do not alter or discontinue antiretroviral regimen without consulting clinician.

Importance of using single-entity rilpivirine in conjunction with other antiretrovirals—not for monotherapy.

Fixed combination containing emtricitabine, rilpivirine, and tenofovir alafenamide (emtricitabine/rilpivirine/tenofovir alafenamide; Odefsey®) and fixed combination containing emtricitabine, rilpivirine, and tenofovir disoproxil fumarate (emtricitabine/rilpivirine/tenofovir DF; Complera®) are used alone as a complete regimen for treatment of HIV-1 infection.

Antiretroviral therapy is not a cure for HIV infection; opportunistic infections and other complications associated with HIV disease may still occur.

Advise patients that sustained decreases in plasma HIV RNA have been associated with reduced risk of progression to acquired immunodeficiency syndrome (AIDS) and death.

Advise patients that effective antiretroviral regimens can decrease HIV concentrations in blood and genital secretions and strict adherence to such regimens in conjunction with risk-reduction measures may decrease, but cannot absolutely eliminate, the risk of secondary transmission of HIV to others. Importance of continuing to practice safer sex (e.g., using latex or polyurethane condoms to minimize sexual contact with body fluids), never sharing personal items that can have blood or body fluids on them (e.g., toothbrushes, razor blades), and never reusing or sharing needles.

Importance of reading patient information provided by the manufacturer.

Importance of taking once daily with a meal; a protein drink alone does not constitute a meal. Food enhances absorption of rilpivirine.

If a missed dose of single-entity rilpivirine or emtricitabine/rilpivirine/tenofovir DF is remembered within 12 hours, it should be taken with a meal as soon as possible and the next dose taken at the regularly scheduled time. If the missed dose is remembered more than 12 hours after the scheduled time, the dose should be omitted and the next dose taken at the regularly scheduled time. Advise patients that doses that are larger or smaller than the prescribed dosage should not be taken at any time.

Advise patients that skin reactions ranging from mild to severe, including drug reaction with eosinophilia and systemic symptoms (DRESS), have been reported with rilpivirine-containing antiretroviral regimens. Instruct patients to immediately stop taking rilpivirine (single-entity or fixed-combination preparations) and contact a clinician if rash develops and is also associated with fever, blisters, mucosal involvement, eye inflammation (conjunctivitis), swelling of the face, eyes, lips, mouth, tongue, or throat which may lead to difficulty swallowing or breathing, or any signs and symptoms of liver problems.

Advise patients that depressive disorders (depressed mood, depression, dysphoria, major depression, altered mood, negative thoughts, suicide attempt, suicidal ideation) have been reported. Importance of immediately contacting clinician if depressive symptoms (e.g., feeling sad, hopeless, anxious, or restless; hurting oneself; having thoughts of hurting oneself) occur.

Advise patients that hepatotoxicity has been reported in patients receiving rilpivirine.

Inform patients that redistribution or accumulation of body fat may occur in patients receiving antiretroviral therapy and that the cause and long-term health effects of these conditions are unknown.

Importance of informing clinicians of existing or contemplated concomitant therapy, including prescription and OTC drugs and herbal supplements (e.g., St. John's wort), and any concomitant illnesses. (See Cautions: Contraindications.)

Importance of women informing clinicians if they are or plan to become pregnant or plan to breast-feed. Advise HIV-infected women not to breast-feed.

Importance of advising patients of other important precautionary information. (See Cautions.)

Overview® (see Users Guide). For additional information on this drug until a more detailed monograph is developed and published, the manufacturer's labeling should be consulted. It is *essential* that the manufacturer's labeling be consulted for more detailed information on usual cautions, precautions, contraindications, potential drug interactions, laboratory test interferences, and acute toxicity.

Preparations

Excipients in commercially available drug preparations may have clinically important effects in some individuals; consult specific product labeling for details.

Rilpivirine Hydrochloride

Oral

Tablets, film-coated	25 mg (of rilpivirine)	**Edurant®**, Janssen

Rilpivirine Hydrochloride Combinations

Oral

Tablets, film-coated	25 mg (of rilpivirine) with Emtricitabine 200 mg and Tenofovir Alafenamide Fumarate 25 mg (of tenofovir alafenamide)	**Odefsey®**, Gilead
	25 mg (of rilpivirine) with Emtricitabine 200 mg and Tenofovir Disoproxil Fumarate 300 mg	**Complera®**, Gilead

†Use is not currently included in the labeling approved by the US Food and Drug Administration

HIV Nucleoside and Nucleotide Reverse Transcriptase Inhibitors 8:18.08.20

Abacavir Sulfate

ABC, abacavir/lamivudine, ABC/3TC, ABC/DTG/3TC, ABC/3TC/ZDV, abacavir/lamivudine/zidovudine

■ Abacavir, an antiretroviral agent, is a human immunodeficiency virus (HIV) nucleoside reverse transcriptase inhibitor (NRTI).

Uses

■ **Treatment of HIV Infection** Abacavir is used in conjunction with other antiretroviral agents for the treatment of human immunodeficiency virus type 1 (HIV-1) infection in adults, adolescents, and pediatric patients 3 months of age or older.

Abacavir usually is used in conjunction with another HIV nucleoside reverse transcriptase inhibitor (NRTI) (dual NRTIs) and an HIV integrase strand transfer inhibitor (INSTI), HIV nonnucleoside reverse transcriptase inhibitor (NNRTI), or HIV protease inhibitor (PI) in INSTI-, NNRTI-, or PI-based regimens.

The fixed-combination preparation containing abacavir and lamivudine (abacavir/lamivudine; Epzicom®) is used in conjunction with other antiretrovirals for the treatment of HIV-1 infection in adults and pediatric patients weighing 25 kg or more.

The fixed-combination preparation containing abacavir, dolutegravir, and lamivudine (abacavir/dolutegravir/lamivudine; Triumeq®) is used alone as a complete treatment regimen or in conjunction with other antiretrovirals for the treatment of HIV-1 infection in adults 18 years of age or older.

The fixed-combination preparation containing abacavir, lamivudine, and zidovudine (abacavir/lamivudine/zidovudine; Trizivir®) is used alone as a complete treatment regimen or in conjunction with other antiretrovirals for the treatment of HIV-1 infection in adults and adolescents weighing 40 kg or more.

Abacavir has been used in triple and quadruple NRTI regimens (i.e., single-class NRTI regimens) that include abacavir and 2 or 3 other NRTIs. However, there is evidence that triple or quadruple NRTI regimens have inferior virologic efficacy. (See All-NRTI Regimens under Treatment of HIV Infection: Antiretroviral-naive Adults and Adolescents, in Uses.)

Abacavir and fixed-combination preparations containing abacavir (abacavir/lamivudine, abacavir/dolutegravir/lamivudine, abacavir/lamivudine/zidovudine) should *not* be used in individuals who test positive for the human leukocyte antigen (HLA)-B*5701 allele. (See Precautions Related to Hypersensitivity Reactions under Cautions: Precautions and Contraindications.)

The most appropriate antiretroviral regimen cannot be defined for each clinical scenario and selection of specific antiretroviral agents for use in such regimens should be individualized based on information regarding antiretroviral potency, potential rate of development of resistance, known toxicities, and potential for pharmacokinetic interactions as well as virologic, immunologic, and clinical characteristics of the patient. For information on the general principles and guidelines for use of antiretroviral therapy, including specific recommendations for initial therapy in antiretroviral-naive patients and recommendations for changing antiretroviral regimens, see the Antiretroviral Agents General Statement 8:18.08.

Antiretroviral-naive Adults and Adolescents

Dual NRTI Options. For *initial* treatment in HIV-infected adults and adolescents, the US Department of Health and Human Services (HHS) Panel on Antiretroviral Guidelines for Adults and Adolescents states that the dual NRTI option of abacavir and lamivudine is a recommended dual NRTI option for use in most INSTI-, NNRTI-, and PI-based regimens, but should be used *only* in patients who are HLA-B*5701 negative. This recommendation is based on safety and efficacy data from clinical trials, clinical experience, and availability of fixed combinations containing abacavir and lamivudine.

If the dual NRTI option of abacavir and lamivudine is used, the fixed combination containing both drugs (abacavir/lamivudine; Epzicom®) can be used in adults and adolescents to decrease pill burden and increase adherence. Abacavir/lamivudine must be used in conjunction with other antiretrovirals for treatment of HIV-1 infection and should be used with a drug from another class (not another NRTI).

The HHS panel states that dolutegravir in conjunction with the dual NRTI option of abacavir and lamivudine (or emtricitabine) is a recommended INSTI-based regimen for *initial* treatment in antiretroviral-naive adults and adolescents, but should be used *only* in those who are HLA-B*5701 negative. These experts also state that *ritonavir-boosted* darunavir or *cobicistat-boosted* darunavir in conjunction with abacavir and lamivudine (or emtricitabine) are alternative PI-based regimens for *initial* treatment in antiretroviral-naive adults and adolescents, but should be used *only* in those who are HLA-B*5701 negative. Other regimen options involving the dual NRTI option of abacavir and lamivudine (or emtricitabine) that can be considered for *initial* treatment in antiretroviral-naive adults include *ritonavir-boosted* or *cobicistat-boosted* atazanavir, efavirenz, or raltegravir in conjunction with abacavir and lamivudine (or emtricitabine); however, these options should be used *only* in those who are HLA-B*5701 negative *and* have baseline plasma HIV RNA levels less than 100,000 copies/mL.

All-NRTI Regimens. Abacavir has been included in NRTI regimens that include 3 or 4 NRTIs (without any drugs from another class). However, triple and quadruple NRTI regimens are *not* recommended for *initial* treatment in HIV-infected adults or adolescents because such regimens have inferior virologic efficacy or have not been adequately studied. In addition, regimens that only include NRTIs are *not* usually recommended in antiretroviral-experienced patients. (See Antiretroviral-experienced Adults and Adolescents under Uses: Treatment of HIV Infections.)

Abacavir has been used in a triple NRTI regimen that includes abacavir, lamivudine, and zidovudine. The fixed-combination preparation containing these 3 NRTIs (abacavir/lamivudine/zidovudine; Trizivir®) can be used in adults and adolescents weighing 40 kg or more. Abacavir/lamivudine/zidovudine is intended only for regimens that require all 3 drugs, and clinicians should consider that data are limited regarding use of this fixed-combination preparation in patients with baseline viral loads exceeding 100,000 copies/mL. Although a triple NRTI regimen of abacavir, lamivudine, and zidovudine offers the advantages of fewer drug interactions, low pill burden, and ease of administration (because of the commercially available fixed-combination preparation), and spares patients from potential adverse effects associated with PIs and NNRTIs, there is a high rate of virologic non-response when the regimen is used in treatment-naive patients. Therefore, experts state that a triple NRTI regimen that includes abacavir, lamivudine, and zidovudine is *not* recommended for *initial* therapy in antiretroviral-naive adults and adolescents and should be used only when other regimens cannot be used.

Safety and efficacy of the triple NRTI regimen of abacavir, lamivudine, and zidovudine were evaluated in a randomized, double-blind study (study CNA3005) in 562 HIV-infected, treatment-naive adults (median baseline $CD4^+$ T-cell counts 359–360/mm^3, median baseline plasma HIV-1 RNA levels 4.8–4.9 $\log_{10}$ copies/mL). Patients were randomized to receive a 3-drug regimen of abacavir (300 mg twice daily) and the fixed-combination preparation containing lamivudine and zidovudine (lamivudine/zidovudine; Combivir®; 150 mg of lamivudine and 300 mg of zidovudine twice daily) or a 3-drug regimen of indinavir (800 mg every 8 hours), lamivudine (150 mg twice daily), and zidovudine (300 mg twice daily). At week 48, 51% of patients in both treatment groups had plasma HIV-1 RNA levels less than 400 copies/mL and 40% of those receiving abacavir, lamivudine, and zidovudine and 46% of those receiving indinavir, lamivudine, and zidovudine had plasma HIV-1 RNA levels of 50 copies/mL or less (intent-to-treat analysis). In patients with baseline HIV-1 RNA levels exceeding 100,000 copies/mL, a greater proportion of those who received the indinavir-containing regimen (45%) had plasma HIV-1 RNA levels less than 50 copies/mL than those who received the abacavir-containing regimen (31%). The median change in $CD4^+$ T-cell count at 48 weeks was similar in both treatment groups.

A triple NRTI regimen of abacavir, lamivudine, and tenofovir disoproxil fumarate (tenofovir DF) is *not* recommended at any time in antiretroviral-naive or antiretroviral-experienced adults and adolescents because of a high rate of virologic failure. Interim analysis of a randomized, open-label study evaluating efficacy of a once-daily regimen of abacavir, lamivudine, and tenofovir DF compared with an NNRTI-based once-daily regimen of efavirenz, abacavir, and lamivudine in treatment-naive patients (ESS30009) indicated a high rate of early virologic nonresponse in those receiving the triple NRTI regimen (almost 50%). Based on these results, the abacavir, lamivudine, and tenofovir DF arm of the study was terminated. A high rate of virologic nonresponse also was reported in a pilot study evaluating this triple NRTI regimen. Several possible reasons for the poor response to this regimen have been proposed, but the ESS30009 investigators suggest that the most likely cause is a low genetic barrier to resistance because of synergistic selection from all 3 NRTIs for 2 specific resistance mutations (M184V and K65R).

A quadruple NRTI regimen of abacavir, lamivudine, tenofovir DF, and zidovudine is *not* recommended for *initial* treatment in antiretroviral-naive HIV-infected adults and adolescents because of inferior virologic efficacy. In an open-label pilot study, a quadruple NRTI regimen was compared with an NNRTI-based regimen of efavirenz with lamivudine and zidovudine, and both regimens had similar efficacy and tolerability. However, a larger, open-label study comparing a similar quadruple NRTI regimen (abacavir, emtricitabine, tenofovir DF, zidovudine) with a standard NNRTI- or PI-based regimen found that substantially fewer patients receiving the quadruple NRTI regimen achieved HIV-1 RNA levels below 200 copies/mL.

Dolutegravir, Abacavir, and Lamivudine. Efficacy and safety of an INSTI-based regimen of dolutegravir and the dual NRTI option of abacavir and lamivudine have been evaluated in a phase 3 randomized, double-blind, active-controlled study (SINGLE) in antiretroviral-naive HIV-1-infected adults. Patients were randomized to receive dolutegravir 50 mg once daily in conjunction with abacavir/lamivudine or the fixed-combination preparation containing efavirenz, emtricitabine, and tenofovir DF (efavirenz/emtricitabine/tenofovir DF) for a 96-week double-blind phase followed by an open-label phase through week 144. Baseline characteristics of the 833 study patients were similar in both treatment groups (median age 35 years, 16% female, 32% non-white, 7% with HCV coinfection, 4% CDC Class C, median plasma HIV-1 RNA level 4.68 $\log_{10}$ copies/mL, median baseline $CD4^+$ T-cell count 338 cells/mm^3). At 144 weeks, 71% of patients receiving dolutegravir with abacavir/lamivudine and 63% of those receiving efavirenz/emtricitabine/tenofovir DF achieved plasma HIV-1 RNA levels less than 50 copies/mL. The adjusted mean increase in $CD4^+$ T-cell count was 378 cells/mm^3 in those receiving dolutegravir and abacavir/lamivudine compared with 332 cells/mm³ in those receiving efavirenz/emtricitabine/tenofovir DF.

Efavirenz, Abacavir, and Lamivudine. Efficacy and safety of an NNRTI-based regimen of efavirenz and the dual NRTI option of abacavir and lamivudine have been evaluated in a randomized, double-blind study (study CNA30024) in 649 HIV-infected, treatment-naive adults (median baseline CD4⁺ T-cell count 264/mm³, median baseline plasma HIV-1 RNA level 4.79 $\log_{10}$ copies/mL). Patients were randomized to receive a 3-drug regimen of abacavir (300 mg twice daily), lamivudine (150 mg twice daily), and efavirenz (600 mg once daily) or a 3-drug regimen of zidovudine (300 mg twice daily), lamivudine (150 mg twice daily), and efavirenz (600 mg once daily). At week 48 (intent-to-treat analysis), about 69% of patients in both treatment groups had plasma HIV-1 RNA levels of 50 copies/mL or less. At week 48, the mean increase from baseline CD4⁺ T-cell count was 209/mm³ in those receiving abacavir, lamivudine, and efavirenz and 155/mm³ in those receiving zidovudine, lamivudine, and efavirenz.

The comparative efficacy of a once- or twice-daily abacavir regimen used with lamivudine in an NNRTI-based regimen was evaluated in a randomized, double-blind study (study CNA30021) in 770 HIV-infected, treatment-naive adults (median baseline CD4⁺ T-cell count 262/mm³ and median baseline plasma HIV-1 RNA level 4.89 $\log_{10}$ copies/mL). Patients were randomized to receive a regimen of abacavir (600 mg once daily), lamivudine (300 mg once daily), and efavirenz (600 mg once daily) or abacavir (300 mg twice daily), lamivudine (300 mg once daily), and efavirenz (600 mg once daily). At week 48 (intent-to-treat analysis), 64 or 65% of patients receiving abacavir once or twice daily, respectively, had plasma HIV-1 RNA levels less than 50 copies/mL. At week 48, the mean increase from baseline CD4⁺ T-cell count was 188/mm³ in those receiving abacavir once daily and 200/mm³ in those receiving abacavir twice daily.

Efficacy and safety of the fixed combination of abacavir and lamivudine (abacavir/lamivudine) in conjunction with efavirenz were evaluated in a randomized, open-label study (ASSERT study) in 385 HIV-infected, HLA-B*5701-negative, antiretroviral-naive adults (median baseline CD4⁺ T-cell count 240/mm³, median baseline plasma HIV-1 RNA level 5.06 $\log_{10}$ copies/mL). Patients were randomized to receive a 96-week NNRTI-based regimen of efavirenz and either abacavir/lamivudine or the fixed combination of emtricitabine and tenofovir DF (emtricitabine/tenofovir DF). At week 48, 59 or 67% of patients receiving abacavir/lamivudine in conjunction with efavirenz had achieved HIV-1 RNA levels below 50 or 400 copies/mL, respectively, compared with 71 or 77%, respectively, of those receiving emtricitabine/tenofovir DF in conjunction with efavirenz. Despite HLA-B*5701 testing to ensure that patients in the study were HLA-B*5701-negative, there were 6 cases of clinically suspected hypersensitivity reactions to abacavir.

PI-based Regimens. PI-based regimens that include the fixed combination of abacavir/lamivudine have been evaluated in an open-label study (KLEAN study) in 887 antiretroviral-naive adults (median baseline HIV-1 RNA level 5.1 $\log_{10}$ copies/mL, median CD4⁺ count 192/mm³). Patients were randomized to receive either *ritonavir-boosted* fosamprenavir (700 mg fosamprenavir twice daily and 100 mg ritonavir twice daily) or lopinavir/ritonavir (400 mg lopinavir/100 mg ritonavir twice daily) each in conjunction with abacavir/lamivudine (600 mg abacavir/300 mg lamivudine once daily). The time to loss of virologic response (TLOVR) analysis of the intent-to-treat exposed population (ITT-E) indicated that the proportion of patients achieving HIV-1 RNA levels less than 50 copies/mL at 48 weeks was similar between the 2 groups: 66% in the group receiving abacavir/lamivudine with *ritonavir-boosted* fosamprenavir and 65% in the group receiving abacavir/lamivudine with lopinavir/ritonavir. At the time of the 48-week analysis, there had been 32 cases of suspected abacavir hypersensitivity in the group receiving abacavir/lamivudine with *ritonavir-boosted* fosamprenavir and 21 cases in the group receiving abacavir/lamivudine with lopinavir/ritonavir. A long-term extension of the KLEAN study included 199 patients from the initial study who had plasma HIV-1 RNA levels less than 400 copies/mL at 48 weeks and continued to receive the PI-based regimen (abacavir/lamivudine was replaced with another dual NRTI option in 14 patients, principally because of suspected abacavir hypersensitivity) for a total of 144 weeks. At week 144, TLOVR analysis of the ITT-E extension population indicated that 73% of those receiving *ritonavir-boosted* fosamprenavir and 60% of those receiving lopinavir/ritonavir had plasma HIV-1 RNA levels less than 50 copies/mL. Both PI-based regimens were well tolerated and had similar safety profiles when used in conjunction with the fixed combination of abacavir/lamivudine over 144 weeks.

The comparative safety and efficacy of PI-based regimens of lopinavir/ritonavir with either the fixed combination of abacavir/lamivudine or the fixed combination of emtricitabine/tenofovir DF were evaluated in a randomized, double-blind, placebo-matched study (HEAT study) in 688 antiretroviral-naive adults (median baseline HIV-1 RNA level 4.9 $\log_{10}$ copies/mL, median CD4⁺ count 202/mm³). Patients were randomized to receive lopinavir/ritonavir (800 mg lopinavir/200 mg ritonavir once daily) and the dual NRTI option of abacavir/lamivudine (600 mg abacavir/300 mg lamivudine once daily) with emtricitabine/tenofovir DF placebo or the dual NRTI option of emtricitabine/tenofovir DF (200 mg emtricitabine/300 mg tenofovir DF once daily) with abacavir/lamivudine placebo. At week 48, similar proportions of the ITT-E population receiving the PI with abacavir/lamivudine or emtricitabine/tenofovir DF achieved HIV-1 RNA levels less than 50 copies/mL (68 or 67%, respectively). At week 96, 60 or 58% of the ITT-E population receiving the PI with abacavir/lamivudine or emtricitabine/tenofovir DF, respectively, maintained HIV-1 RNA levels less than 50 copies/mL. The median increase from baseline CD4⁺ T-cell count at week 96 in both groups also was similar (250 or 247 cells/mm³, respectively). Both regimens were well tolerated and had similar rates of treatment discontinuance (6%).

Data regarding efficacy of a dual NRTI option of abacavir/lamivudine fixed combination compared with that of emtricitabine/tenofovir DF fixed combination were obtained from a randomized, double-blind study in antiretroviral-naive adults that involved a PI-based regimen including open-label *ritonavir-boosted* atazanavir or an NNRTI-based regimen including open-label efavirenz (ACTG study A5202). Patients were stratified by baseline HIV-1 RNA levels (less than 100,000 copies/mL or 100,000 copies/mL or greater). Results of an interim analysis after a median 60 weeks of therapy indicated that patients with baseline HIV-1 RNA levels 100,000 copies/mL or greater receiving the dual NRTI option of abacavir/lamivudine had substantially shorter times to virologic failure compared with those receiving tenofovir DF/emtricitabine.

Antiretroviral-experienced Adults and Adolescents **All-NRTI Regimens.** Abacavir has been used in triple NRTI regimens in antiretroviral-experienced HIV-infected adults and adolescents, but triple NRTI regimens usually are not recommended because of inferior virologic efficacy or lack of data.

A triple NRTI regimen that includes abacavir (300 mg twice daily) and the fixed-combination preparation containing lamivudine and zidovudine (lamivudine/zidovudine; Combivir®; 150 mg of lamivudine and 300 mg of zidovudine twice daily) has been evaluated in a 48-week, open-label study in HIV-infected patients who previously received antiretroviral regimens that included 1 or 2 NRTIs without any other antiretroviral agents. At the start of the study, 34% of patients had baseline plasma HIV-1 RNA levels less than 400 copies/mL and 11% had levels less than 50 copies/mL; the median CD4⁺ T-cell count was 506/mm³. At 48 weeks, 82% of patients had plasma HIV-1 RNA levels less than 400 copies/mL and 56% had levels less than 50 copies/mL (intent-to-treat analysis). Patients with baseline HIV-1 RNA levels less than 5000 copies/mL were more likely to achieve levels less than 400 copies/mL at week 48 than those with baseline levels exceeding 5000 copies/mL. At 48 weeks, the median change from baseline CD4⁺ T-cell count was 66 cells/mm³. While triple NRTI regimens generally are *not* recommended, some experts state that a regimen of the fixed combination of abacavir, lamivudine, and zidovudine (abacavir/lamivudine/zidovudine) may be considered in patients when other regimens cannot be used.

Based on interim analysis of a study evaluating a triple NRTI regimen of abacavir, lamivudine, and tenofovir DF that indicated a high rate of early virologic nonresponse in treatment-naive patients receiving this regimen, a triple NRTI regimen of abacavir, lamivudine, and tenofovir DF is *not* recommended at any time in either antiretroviral-naive or antiretroviral-experienced patients.

In a study in 460 patients receiving a PI and 2 NRTIs who had maintained plasma HIV-1 RNA levels less than 200 copies/mL for at least 6 months but wished to change to a regimen that did not include a PI, patients were randomized to switch from their existing PI to abacavir, efavirenz, or nevirapine while maintaining the existing NRTIs. At 12 months, 13, 6, or 10% of patients switched to abacavir, efavirenz, or nevirapine, respectively, had experienced death, progression to acquired immunodeficiency syndrome (AIDS), or an increase in plasma HIV-1 RNA levels to 200 copies/mL or more (intent-to-treat analysis).

Dolutegravir, Abacavir, and Lamivudine. The comparative efficacy and safety of dolutegravir in conjunction with an investigator-selected optimized background antiretroviral regimen (OBR), including an OBR of abacavir in fixed combination with lamivudine (abacavir/lamivudine) in a limited number of patients, are being studied in 715 antiretroviral-experienced, INSTI-naive HIV-1-infected adults in an ongoing phase 3, randomized, double-blind, active-controlled, double-placebo study (SAILING). All enrolled patients had previously received antiretroviral therapy (average duration 77 months of prior therapy) and had infections resistant to at least 2 classes of antiretrovirals (49% had HIV-1 resistant to at least 3 classes of antiretrovirals). Patients were randomized to receive dolutegravir 50 mg once daily or raltegravir 400 mg twice daily, each in conjunction with an OBR consisting of at least 1 fully active antiretroviral; of those in the dolutegravir group, 8 patients received an OBR of abacavir/lamivudine. Baseline characteristics were similar in both treatment groups (median age 43 years, 32% female, 50% non-white, 16% with HBV and/or HCV coinfection, 46% CDC Class C, 20% with plasma HIV-1 RNA levels greater than 100,000 copies/mL, 72% with CD4⁺ T-cell counts less than 350 cells/mm³). At 48 weeks, 71% of patients in the dolutegravir group and 64% of those in the raltegravir group had plasma HIV-1 RNA levels less than 50 copies/mL; CD4⁺ T-cell counts were increased from baseline in both groups (mean change 162 cells/mm³ in the dolutegravir group and 153 cells/mm³ in the raltegravir group).

Pediatric Patients Abacavir is used in conjunction with other antiretroviral agents for treatment of HIV-1 infection in pediatric patients 3 months of age or older.

Abacavir/lamivudine is used in conjunction with other antiretrovirals for the treatment of HIV-1 infection in pediatric patients weighing 25 kg or more.

Abacavir/lamivudine/zidovudine is used for the treatment of HIV-1 infection in pediatric patients weighing 40 kg or more.

For *initial* treatment of HIV-infected pediatric patients, the HHS Panel on Antiretroviral Therapy and Medical Management of HIV-infected Children recommends a regimen that includes a *ritonavir-boosted* PI, NNRTI, or INSTI in conjunction with 2 NRTIs (dual NRTIs). These experts state that abacavir and lamivudine (or emtricitabine) is a preferred dual NRTI option and abacavir and zidovudine is an alternative dual NRTI option for use in PI-, NNRTI-, or INSTI-based regimens for *initial* treatment in antiretroviral-naive children 3 months of age or older who are HLA-B*5701 negative.

The dual NRTI options of abacavir and didanosine or abacavir and tenofovir DF are *not* recommended for use in *initial* antiretroviral regimens in antiretroviral-naive pediatric patients because of insufficient data.

Antiretroviral regimens that contain only NRTIs are *not* recommended for *initial* treatment in antiretroviral-naive children because of inferior virologic efficacy.

A triple NRTI regimen that includes abacavir, tenofovir DF, and either lamivudine or emtricitabine should *not* be used at any time in pediatric patients because of the high rate of early virologic failure reported in antiretroviral-naive adults. (See All-NRTI Regimens under Treatment of HIV Infections: Pediatric Patients, in Uses.)

For further information on treatment of HIV infection in pediatric patients, see Antiretroviral Therapy in Pediatric Patients, in the Antiretroviral Agents General Statement 8:18.08.

All-NRTI Regimens. Efficacy of a triple NRTI regimen of abacavir, lamivudine, and zidovudine in pediatric patients has been evaluated in a phase 3, randomized, double-blind study (study CNA3006) that included 205 HIV-infected children 3 months to 13 years of age (median age: 5.4 years, 56% female, 17% white, 50% African American, 30% Hispanic, median baseline $CD4^+$ T-cell percentage 27%, median baseline plasma HIV-1 RNA levels 4.6 $\log_{10}$ copies/mL); more than 50% had previously received NRTI therapy for longer than 2 years. Children were randomized to receive a 3-drug regimen of abacavir (8 mg/kg twice daily), lamivudine (4 mg/kg twice daily), and zidovudine (180 mg/m^2 twice daily) or a 2-drug regimen of lamivudine (4 mg/kg twice daily) and zidovudine (180 mg/m^2 twice daily). At week 16, the median $CD4^+$ T-cell count increase from baseline was 69 or $9/mm^3$ in those receiving the 3- or 2-drug regimen, respectively. At week 48, 17 or 2% of those receiving the 3- or 2-drug regimen, respectively, had plasma HIV-1 RNA levels of 400 copies/mL or less (as-treated analysis). The median decrease from baseline in plasma HIV-1 RNA was twofold to threefold greater in those receiving the 3-drug regimen than in those receiving the 2-drug regimen.

There is evidence from a limited study in HIV-infected children that a triple NRTI regimen of abacavir, lamivudine, and zidovudine can reduce CSF viral load. HIV-infected children who previously had received antiretroviral agent therapy were randomized to a 3-drug regimen of abacavir, lamivudine, and zidovudine or a 2-drug regimen of lamivudine and zidovudine, and baseline CSF HIV-1 RNA levels were determined. At week 16, 69% of those receiving the 3-drug regimen and 70% of those receiving the 2-drug regimen had undetectable CSF HIV-1 RNA (less than 100 copies/mL).

PI-based Regimens. Initial evidence from limited studies in treatment-naive pediatric patients 3 months to 13 years of age indicated that a 3-drug regimen that included 2 NRTIs (abacavir, lamivudine, or zidovudine) and nelfinavir can decrease plasma HIV-1 RNA levels to less than 400 copies/mL and substantially increase $CD4^+$ T-cells in these patients.

The comparative efficacy of 3 different NRTI options was evaluated in 128 antiretroviral-naive HIV-infected pediatric patients 3 months to 16 years of age (median age 5.4 years, median baseline CD4 percentage 22%, mean baseline HIV-1 RNA 5.1 $\log_{10}$ copies/mL) who were randomized to receive open-label dual NRTI options of abacavir and lamivudine, abacavir and zidovudine, or zidovudine and lamivudine with or without nelfinavir (Penta 5 study). Asymptomatic patients (n=55) were randomized to receive nelfinavir or placebo, while patients with more advanced HIV disease received open-label nelfinavir. At 48 weeks, intent-to-treat analysis indicated that reductions in plasma HIV-1 RNA levels were greater in children receiving an abacavir-containing dual NRTI option (decrease of 2.19 $\log_{10}$ copies/mL with abacavir and zidovudine or 2.63 $\log_{10}$ copies/mL with abacavir and lamivudine) than in those receiving the option containing zidovudine and lamivudine (decrease of 1.71 $\log_{10}$ copies/mL). At 5 years (intent-to-treat analysis in patients randomized to receive nelfinavir), plasma HIV-1 RNA levels were less than 50 copies/mL in 69% of those randomized to receive abacavir and lamivudine compared with 26 or 33% of those randomized to receive abacavir and zidovudine or zidovudine and lamivudine, respectively.

Once-daily versus Twice-daily Regimens. Efficacy and safety of abacavir and lamivudine in conjunction with other antiretrovirals were evaluated in a randomized, open-label, parallel-group study in 1206 HIV-1-infected treatment-naive infants, children, and adolescents 3 months to 17 years of age (ARROW). After a minimum of 36 weeks of treatment with a first-line regimen containing the dual NRTI option of abacavir and lamivudine (administered twice daily) in conjunction with a *ritonavir-boosted* PI or NNRTI, the comparative efficacy of a once- or twice-daily regimen of abacavir and lamivudine in conjunction with other antiretrovirals was evaluated in 669 patients weighing at least 25 kg (median age 5.5 years, 52% female, median time on twice-daily abacavir and lamivudine regimen 1.8 years). Patients were randomized in a 1:1 ratio to receive a once- or twice-daily regimen of abacavir and lamivudine (given as single-entity preparations or as abacavir/lamivudine) in conjunction with other antiretrovirals. At the time of randomization, 71% of those in the once-daily group and 75% of those in the twice-daily group were virologically suppressed. At 96 weeks, 67% of those receiving a once-daily regimen and 70% of those receiving a twice-daily regimen of abacavir and lamivudine achieved HIV-1 RNA levels less than 80 copies/mL.

■ Postexposure Prophylaxis following Occupational Exposure to HIV Abacavir is used in conjunction with other antiretroviral agents for postexposure prophylaxis of HIV infection following occupational exposure† (PEP) in health-care personnel and other individuals exposed via percutaneous injury (e.g., needlestick, cut with sharp object) or mucous membrane or nonintact skin (e.g., chapped, abraded, dermatitis) contact with blood, tissue, or other body fluids that might contain HIV.

The US Public Health Service (USPHS) states that the preferred regimen for PEP following an occupational exposure to HIV is a 3-drug regimen of raltegravir used in conjunction with emtricitabine and tenofovir DF (may be administered as the fixed combination emtricitabine/tenofovir DF; Truvada®). These experts state that abacavir is one of several alternative agents that may be used in PEP regimens, but should be used for PEP *only* with expert consultation since HLA-B*5701 testing is required and such testing may not be available or practical prior to initiating PEP.

Because management of occupational exposures to HIV is complex and evolving, consultation with an infectious disease specialist, clinician with expertise in administration of antiretroviral agents, and/or the National Clinicians' Postexposure Prophylaxis Hotline (PEPline at 888-448-4911) is recommended whenever possible. However, initiation of PEP should not be delayed while waiting for expert consultation.

For information on types of occupational exposure to HIV and associated risk of infection, management of occupational exposure to HIV, efficacy and safety of postexposure prophylaxis, and recommendations regarding PEP, see Guidelines for Use of Antiretroviral Agents: Antiretrovirals for Postexposure Prophylaxis following Occupational Exposure to HIV (PEP), in the Antiretroviral Agents General Statement 8:18.08.

■ Postexposure Prophylaxis following Nonoccupational Exposure to HIV Antiretrovirals are used for postexposure prophylaxis of HIV infection following nonoccupational exposure (nPEP) in individuals exposed to blood, genital secretions, or other potentially infectious body fluids that might contain HIV when the exposure represents a substantial risk for HIV transmission.

When nPEP is indicated following a nonoccupational exposure to HIV, the US Centers for Disease Control and Prevention (CDC) states that the preferred regimen in adults and adolescents 13 years of age or older with normal renal function is either raltegravir or dolutegravir used in conjunction with emtricitabine and tenofovir DF (administered as emtricitabine/tenofovir DF; Truvada®); the recommended alternative nPEP regimen in these patients is *ritonavir-boosted* darunavir used in conjunction with emtricitabine/tenofovir DF.

CDC states that abacavir should *not* be used in any nPEP regimens since the need for prompt initiation of nPEP does not allow time for HLA-B*5701 screening.

Consultation with an infectious disease specialist, clinician with expertise in administration of antiretroviral agents, and/or the National Clinicians' Postexposure Prophylaxis Hotline (PEPline at 888-448-4911) is recommended if nPEP is indicated in certain exposed individuals (e.g., pregnant women, children, those with medical conditions such as renal impairment) or if an antiretroviral regimen not included in the CDC guidelines is being considered, the source virus is known or likely to be resistant to antiretrovirals, or the healthcare provider is inexperienced in prescribing antiretrovirals. However, initiation of nPEP should not be delayed while waiting for expert consultation.

For additional information on nonoccupational exposure to HIV and recommendations regarding postexposure prophylaxis, see Guidelines for Use of Antiretroviral Agents: Antiretrovirals for Postexposure Prophylaxis following Sexual, Injection Drug Use, or other Nonoccupational Exposures to HIV (nPEP), in the Antiretroviral Agents General Statement 8:18.08.

Dosage and Administration

■ Administration Abacavir sulfate is administered orally once or twice daily without regard to meals.

Single-entity abacavir sulfate also is commercially available as an oral solution or tablets. Abacavir sulfate also is commercially available in fixed combination with other antiretrovirals. (See Fixed Combinations Containing Abacavir under Dosage and Administration: Administration.)

Abacavir is used in conjunction with other antiretrovirals. Single-entity abacavir should not be used concomitantly with any other abacavir-containing preparation.

Abacavir oral solution is used in pediatric patients or when a solid oral dosage form is inappropriate.

The scored 300-mg abacavir tablets are used in adults and may be used in children weighing 14 kg or greater who have undergone assessment demonstrating ability to reliably swallow tablets.

All patients should be screened for the human leukocyte antigen (HLA)-B*5701 allele before abacavir or a fixed-combination preparation containing abacavir is initiated or reinitiated, unless there is documentation of previous HLA-B*5701 allele assessment. Abacavir and abacavir-containing preparations are contraindicated in HLA-B*5701-positive individuals. (See Cautions: Hypersensitivity Reactions.)

Fixed Combinations Containing Abacavir Abacavir sulfate is commercially available in fixed-combination tablets containing abacavir and lamivudine (abacavir/lamivudine; Epzicom®), in fixed-combination tablets containing abacavir, dolutegravir, and lamivudine (abacavir/dolutegravir/lamivudine; Triumeq®), and in fixed-combination tablets containing abacavir, lamivudine, and zidovudine (abacavir/lamivudine/zidovudine; Trizivir®).

Abacavir/lamivudine (Epzicom®) tablets are administered orally once daily without regard to meals. A fixed-combination tablet containing 600 mg of abacavir and 300 mg of lamivudine is bioequivalent to two 300-mg tablets of abacavir and two 150-mg tablets of lamivudine given simultaneously. For the treatment of human immunodeficiency virus type 1 (HIV-1) infection, abacavir/lamivudine is used in conjunction with other antiretrovirals.

Abacavir/dolutegravir/lamivudine (Triumeq®) film-coated tablets are administered orally once daily without regard to food. A fixed-combination tablet containing 600 mg of abacavir, 50 mg of dolutegravir, and 300 mg of lamivudine is bioequivalent to a 50-mg tablet of dolutegravir administered simultaneously with a fixed-combination tablet containing 600 mg of abacavir and 300 mg of lamivudine. For the treatment of HIV-1 infection, abacavir/dolutegravir/lamivudine is used alone as a complete treatment regimen or in conjunction with other antiretrovirals.

Abacavir/lamivudine/zidovudine (Trizivir®) tablets are administered orally twice daily without regard to meals. A fixed-combination tablet containing 300 mg of abacavir, 150 mg of lamivudine, and 300 mg of zidovudine is bioequivalent to a 300-mg tablet of abacavir, a 150-mg tablet of lamivudine, and a 300-mg tablet of zidovudine administered simultaneously. For the treatment of human HIV-1 infection, abacavir/lamivudine/zidovudine is used alone as a complete treatment regimen or in conjunction with other antiretrovirals.

Because the antiretroviral agents contained in abacavir/lamivudine, abacavir/dolutegravir/lamivudine, and abacavir/lamivudine/zidovudine also are commercially available in single-entity or other fixed-combination preparations, care should be taken to ensure that therapy is not duplicated when a fixed combination is used in conjunction with other antiretrovirals. (See Precautions Related to Use of Fixed Combinations under Cautions: Precautions and Contraindications.)

■ Dosage

Abacavir is commercially available as abacavir sulfate; dosage is expressed in terms of abacavir.

Adult Dosage

Treatment of HIV Infection. The usual dosage of abacavir (Ziagen®) for the treatment of HIV-1 infection in adults is 600 mg once daily or 300 mg twice daily.

When abacavir/lamivudine (Epzicom®) is used for the treatment of HIV-1 infection, adults should receive 1 tablet (600 mg of abacavir and 300 mg of lamivudine) once daily.

When abacavir/dolutegravir/lamivudine (Triumeq®) is used for the treatment of HIV-1 infection, adults should receive 1 tablet (600 mg of abacavir, 50 mg of dolutegravir, and 300 mg of lamivudine) once daily.

When abacavir/lamivudine/zidovudine (Trizivir®) is used for the treatment of HIV-1 infection, adults should receive 1 tablet (300 mg of abacavir, 150 mg of lamivudine, and 300 mg of zidovudine) twice daily.

Postexposure Prophylaxis following Occupational Exposure to HIV. For postexposure prophylaxis of HIV infection following occupational exposure† (PEP) in health-care personnel or other individuals, abacavir is administered in a dosage of 600 mg once daily in conjunction with other antiretrovirals. (See Uses: Postexposure Prophylaxis following Occupational Exposure to HIV.)

The PEP regimen should be initiated as soon as possible following occupational exposure to HIV (preferably within hours) and continued for 4 weeks, if tolerated.

Pediatric Dosage

Treatment of HIV Infection. The usual dosage of abacavir oral solution (Ziagen®) for the treatment of HIV-1 infection in children and adolescents 3 months of age and older is 8 mg/kg (up to 300 mg) twice daily or 16 mg/kg (up to 600 mg) once daily. When the abacavir oral suspension is used for *initial* antiretroviral therapy in pediatric patients, some experts recommend that a twice-daily regimen be used initially and, based on response, consideration can then be given to switching to a once-daily regimen after approximately 24 weeks of therapy.

In pediatric patients 3 months of age or older weighing 14 kg or more who can reliably swallow tablets, the usual dosage of abacavir tablets (Ziagen®) for the treatment of HIV-1 infection is based on weight. (See Table 1 and Table 2.) Although a once- or twice-daily regimen of abacavir tablets can be used in pediatric patients, some experts recommend that a once-daily regimen be used.

Table 1. Twice-daily Regimen in Children and Adolescents Weighing ≥14 kg Able to Swallow Tablets (Ziagen® 300-mg Tablets)

Weight (kg)	AM Dose	PM Dose
14 to <20	150 mg (half tablet)	150 mg (half tablet)
20 to <25	150 mg (half tablet)	300 mg
≥25	300 mg	300 mg

Table 2. Once-daily Regimen in Children and Adolescents Weighing ≥14 kg Able to Swallow Tablets (Ziagen® 300-mg Tablets)

Weight (kg)	Once-daily Dose
14 to <20	300 mg
20 to <25	450 mg (one and one-half tablets)
≥25	600 mg (2 tablets)

When abacavir/lamivudine (Epzicom®) is used for the treatment of HIV-1 infection, children and adolescents weighing at least 25 kg should receive 1 tablet (600 mg of abacavir and 300 mg of lamivudine) once daily.

When abacavir/lamivudine/zidovudine (Trizivir®) is used for the treatment of HIV-1 infection, pediatric patients weighing 40 kg or more should receive 1 tablet (300 mg of abacavir, 150 mg of lamivudine, and 300 mg of zidovudine) twice daily.

Safety and efficacy of abacavir/dolutegravir/lamivudine (Triumeq®) have not been established in pediatric patients.

■ Dosage in Renal and Hepatic Impairment

Renal Impairment

Only limited information is available on the pharmacokinetics of abacavir in patients with impaired renal function, and the manufacturer provides no guidance on abacavir dosage adjustment in such patients. Some experts state that the usual dosage of abacavir can be used in adults and adolescents with impaired renal function.

Abacavir/lamivudine, abacavir/dolutegravir/lamivudine, and abacavir/lamivudine/zidovudine are *not* recommended in patients with creatinine clearance less than 50 mL/minute.

Hepatic Impairment

If abacavir (Ziagen®) is used in adults with mild hepatic impairment (Child-Pugh score 5–6), the manufacturer recommends that dosage of the drug for treatment of HIV-1 infection be reduced to 200 mg twice daily. To facilitate this dosage adjustment in these patients, the commercially available oral solution should be used (i.e., 10 mL twice daily). Abacavir is contraindicated in patients with moderate or severe hepatic impairment since safety, efficacy, and pharmacokinetics have not been established in these patients.

Abacavir/lamivudine, abacavir/dolutegravir/lamivudine, and abacavir/lamivudine/zidovudine are *not* recommended in patients with mild hepatic impairment and are contraindicated in those with moderate or severe hepatic impairment.

Cautions

Information on safety and efficacy of abacavir has been obtained principally from initial clinical studies in adult and pediatric patients with human immunodeficiency virus (HIV) infection who received the recommended dosage of the drug in conjunction with other antiretrovirals (e.g., lamivudine, zidovudine, efavirenz).

Although abacavir generally is well tolerated, potentially life-threatening hypersensitivity reactions have been reported in patients receiving the drug. (See Cautions: Hypersensitivity Reactions.)

When the fixed combination containing abacavir and lamivudine (abacavir/lamivudine), fixed combination containing abacavir, dolutegravir, and lamivudine (abacavir/dolutegravir/lamivudine), or fixed combination containing abacavir, lamivudine, and zidovudine (abacavir/lamivudine/zidovudine) is used, the adverse effects, precautions, and contraindications associated with each drug in the fixed combination should be considered. (See Precautions Related to Use of Fixed Combinations under Cautions: Precautions and Contraindications.)

■ Hypersensitivity Reactions

Serious, sometimes fatal, hypersensitivity reactions have been reported with abacavir or fixed-combination preparations containing abacavir (abacavir/lamivudine, abacavir/lamivudine/zidovudine). In clinical studies, hypersensitivity reactions have been reported in approximately 8% of patients receiving abacavir in conjunction with other antiretrovirals. In one controlled study (CNA30021), the incidence of severe hypersensitivity reactions was greater in adults receiving abacavir once daily (5%) than in those receiving abacavir twice daily (2%).

There is evidence that abacavir hypersensitivity is an immunologic reaction influenced by certain genetic factors. An association between presence of the human leukocyte antigen (HLA)-B*5701 allele and abacavir hypersensitivity has been established. Individuals who carry the HLA-B*5701 allele are at higher risk for abacavir hypersensitivity reactions, although hypersensitivity reactions have occurred in patients who do not carry the HLA-B*5701 allele.

Manifestations of hypersensitivity usually are apparent within the first 6 weeks of abacavir therapy (median time to onset is 9 days), but may occur at any time during therapy. Severe hypersensitivity reactions can occur within hours following rechallenge in patients with a prior history of hypersensitivity to the drug, and these reactions may include life-threatening hypotension and death. The most severe hypersensitivity reactions reported to date have been in individuals who were rechallenged with abacavir after a previous hypersensitivity reaction to the drug. There also have been reports of severe or fatal hypersensitivity reactions occurring after abacavir was reintroduced in patients with no identified history of abacavir hypersensitivity or with unrecognized manifestations of hypersensitivity to the drug. Although these patients had discontinued abacavir for reasons unrelated to hypersensitivity (e.g., interruption in drug supply, discontinuance of abacavir during treatment for other medical conditions), some may have had symptoms present before discontinuance of the drug that were consistent with hypersensitivity but were attributed to other medical conditions (e.g., acute onset respiratory disease, gastroenteritis, adverse reactions to other drugs). Most of the hypersensitivity reactions reported following reintroduction of abacavir in these patients were indistinguishable from hypersensitivity reactions associated with abacavir rechallenge (i.e., short time to onset, increased severity of symptoms, poor outcome including death). Hypersensitivity reactions can occur within hours after abacavir is reintroduced; however, in some cases, these reactions occurred days to weeks following reintroduction of the drug.

Hypersensitivity reactions reported in patients receiving abacavir are characterized by the appearance of manifestations indicating involvement of multiple organ and body systems; these reactions have occurred in association with anaphylaxis, liver failure, renal failure, hypotension, and death. The most frequent manifestations of abacavir hypersensitivity include signs or symptoms from at least 2 of the following groups: fever, rash, GI symptoms (including nausea, vomiting, diarrhea, abdominal pain), constitutional symptoms (including generalized malaise, fatigue, achiness), and respiratory symptoms (including pharyngitis, dyspnea, cough). Other signs and symptoms include lethargy, myalgia, chills, myolysis, headache, arthralgia, edema, tachycardia, abnormal chest radiographs (predominantly infiltrates, which may be localized), paresthesia, lymphadenopathy, and mucous membrane lesions (e.g., conjunctivitis, mouth ulceration). Respiratory symptoms, including cough, dyspnea, and pharyngitis, have been reported in approximately 20% of patients with hypersensitivity reactions to abacavir. Adult respiratory distress syndrome and respiratory failure have occurred in association with hypersensitivity reactions. Some patients who experienced fatal hypersensitivity reactions were initially diagnosed as having an acute respiratory disease (pneumonia, bronchitis, flu-like illness). Hypersensitivity reactions can occur without rash; if rash occurs, it usually is maculopapular or urticarial, but may be variable in appearance. Erythema multiforme has been reported. Laboratory abnormalities reported in patients experiencing a hypersensitivity reaction to abacavir include lymphopenia and increases in serum concentrations of liver enzymes, creatine kinase (CK, creatine phosphokinase, CPK), or creatinine.

Abacavir or fixed-combination preparations containing abacavir should be discontinued immediately in any individual who develops signs or symptoms suggesting hypersensitivity, regardless of HLA-B*5701 status and even when other diagnoses are possible. Clinical status, including liver function tests, should be monitored and appropriate therapy should be initiated. At least one fatality occurred in a patient who continued abacavir therapy despite experiencing a severe hypersensitivity reaction. Symptoms and laboratory abnormalities associated with abacavir hypersensitivity generally resolve following discontinuance of the drug. Abacavir and abacavir-containing preparations should *never* be reinitiated in any patient who experienced a hypersensitivity reaction while receiving the drug, regardless of the patient's HLA-B*5701 status; more severe symptoms may occur within hours and may include life-threatening hypotension and death. Similar severe reactions have also occurred rarely following the reintroduction of abacavir or abacavir-containing preparations in patients who have no history of abacavir hypersensitivity. (See Precautions Related to Hypersensitivity Reactions under Cautions: Precautions and Contraindications.)

Stevens-Johnson syndrome and toxic epidermal necrolysis have been reported during postmarketing experience in patients receiving abacavir concomitantly with other drugs known to be associated with these severe adverse effects. In such cases, abacavir should be discontinued and should not be reinitiated because of the possibility that the patient may have multiple drug sensitivities and because the clinical signs and symptoms of Stevens-Johnson syndrome and toxic epidermal necrolysis are similar to those of abacavir hypersensitivity. Erythema multiforme has been reported with use of abacavir.

■ **Hepatic Effects and Lactic Acidosis** Lactic acidosis and severe hepatomegaly with steatosis, including some fatalities, have been reported rarely in patients receiving abacavir or fixed-combination preparations containing abacavir (abacavir/lamivudine, abacavir/dolutegravir/lamivudine, abacavir/lamivudine/zidovudine) and have also been reported in patients receiving other HIV nucleoside reverse transcriptase inhibitors (NRTIs). Most reported cases have involved women; obesity and long-term therapy with an NRTI also may be risk factors. Cases also have been reported in patients with no known risk factors. (See Cautions: Hepatic Effects and Lactic Acidosis in Zidovudine 8:18.08.20.)

■ **GI Effects** Adverse GI effects have been reported in patients receiving abacavir. In adults receiving abacavir in conjunction with the fixed-combination preparation of lamivudine and zidovudine (lamivudine/zidovudine; Combivir®) in study CNA3005, nausea occurred in 19%, nausea and vomiting occurred in 10%, and diarrhea occurred in 7% of patients. In adults receiving abacavir in conjunction with lamivudine and efavirenz in study CNA30024, nausea, diarrhea, abdominal pain, gastritis, or other GI symptoms occurred in 6–7% and vomiting occurred in 2% of patients.

In one controlled study (CNA30021) evaluating once- or twice-daily abacavir in conjunction with lamivudine and efavirenz, the incidence of severe diarrhea was greater in those receiving abacavir once daily (2%) than in those receiving abacavir twice daily (0%).

In study CNA3006 in HIV-infected children 3 months to 13 years of age, nausea and vomiting occurred in 9% of those receiving abacavir in conjunction with lamivudine and zidovudine and in 2% of those receiving lamivudine and zidovudine without abacavir.

■ **Cardiovascular Effects** Myocardial infarction (MI) has been reported in some patients receiving abacavir.

In July 2008, analysis of data from a large observational study (D:A:D) evaluating short-term and long-term antiretroviral adverse effects in more than 33,000 HIV-infected patients indicated a possible increased risk of MI in patients with current or recent (within the previous 6 months) abacavir therapy. Based on this information, the FDA initiated a safety review of abacavir to assess the possible risk of MI. Studies have reported conflicting results regarding the possible association between the drug and MI risk. Several observational studies and a randomized controlled trial identified increased risk, while other randomized controlled trials and the manufacturer's safety database have not identified such a risk. In response, FDA conducted a meta-analysis of 26 randomized clinical trials that evaluated use of abacavir in adults. This meta-analysis did not identify an increased risk of MI in patients receiving abacavir. While clinicians should be aware of the conflicting data, the FDA recommends that clinicians continue to prescribe abacavir according to approved labeling and that patients not discontinue abacavir without consulting their clinician.

Although the clinical importance has not been determined, myocardial degeneration was found in mice and rats following administration of abacavir for 2 years (systemic exposure equivalent to 7–24 times the expected systemic exposure in humans).

■ **Adipogenic Effects** Redistribution or accumulation of body fat, including central obesity, dorsocervical fat enlargement ("buffalo hump"), peripheral wasting, facial wasting, breast enlargement, and general cushingoid appearance, has been reported in patients receiving antiretroviral agents. The mechanisms responsible for these adipogenic effects and the long-term consequences of these effects are unknown. A causal relationship has not been established.

■ **Immune Reconstitution Syndrome** Immune reconstitution syndrome has been reported in HIV-infected patients receiving multiple-drug antiretroviral therapy, including abacavir. During the initial phase of treatment, HIV-infected patients whose immune systems respond to antiretroviral therapy may develop an inflammatory response to indolent or residual opportunistic infections (e.g., *Mycobacterium avium complex* [MAC], *M. tuberculosis*, cytomegalovirus [CMV], *Pneumocystis jirovecii* [formerly *P. carinii*]); such responses may necessitate further evaluation and treatment.

Autoimmune disorders (e.g., Graves' disease, polymyositis, Guillain-Barré syndrome) also have been reported to occur in the setting of immune reconstitution; however, the time to onset is more variable and can occur many months after initiation of antiretroviral therapy.

■ **Other Adverse Effects** Headache, malaise and/or fatigue, sleep disorder, or anxiety have occurred in up to 13, 12, 10, or 5% of adults receiving abacavir in conjunction with other antiretroviral agents in clinical studies. Depressive disorders, dizziness, and musculoskeletal pain each have occurred in 6% of adults receiving abacavir in these studies.

Upper respiratory tract infections have been reported in 5% and bronchitis has been reported in 4% of adults receiving abacavir in clinical studies. Fever and/or chills, upper respiratory tract infections, pneumonia, and headache occurred in 9, 5, 4, and 1% of pediatric patients receiving abacavir in clinical studies.

The incidence of laboratory abnormalities (e.g., anemia, neutropenia, liver function test abnormalities, increases in CPK) reported in studies CNA30024, CNA3005, and CNA3006 in adults and children receiving a regimen that includes abacavir was similar to that reported in adults and children receiving regimens without abacavir.

Pancreatitis has been reported rarely in patients receiving abacavir.

Other adverse effects reported during postmarketing experience in patients receiving fixed-combination preparations containing abacavir (abacavir/lamivudine, abacavir/lamivudine/zidovudine) include stomatitis, hyperglycemia, weakness, lymphadenopathy, splenomegaly, posttreatment exacerbation of hepatitis B virus (HBV) infection, muscle weakness, rhabdomyolysis, paresthesia, peripheral neuropathy, seizures, abnormal breath sounds, wheezing, and alopecia. Cardiomyopathy, gynecomastia, anorexia, oral mucosal pigmentation, vasculitis, thrombocytopenia, and increased bilirubin concentrations also have been reported in patients receiving abacavir/lamivudine/zidovudine.

■ **Precautions and Contraindications** Abacavir and fixed combinations containing abacavir (abacavir/lamivudine, abacavir/dolutegravir/lamivudine, abacavir/lamivudine/zidovudine) are contraindicated in patients who have the HLA-B*5701 allele and in patients who have had a previous hypersensitivity reaction to abacavir or any ingredient in the formulation. Abacavir and abacavir-containing preparations should *not* be reinitiated in any patient who experienced an abacavir hypersensitivity reaction, regardless of the patient's HLA-B*5701 status. (See Precautions Related to Hypersensitivity Reactions under Cautions: Precautions and Contraindications.)

Abacavir, abacavir/lamivudine, abacavir/dolutegravir/lamivudine, and abacavir/lamivudine/zidovudine are contraindicated in patients with moderate or severe hepatic impairment. (See Other Precautions under Cautions: Precautions and Contraindications.) In addition, abacavir/dolutegravir/lamivudine is contraindicated in patients receiving dofetilide.

Precautions Related to Hypersensitivity Reactions Serious and sometimes fatal hypersensitivity reactions, with multiorgan involvement, have occurred in patients receiving abacavir or fixed-combination preparations containing abacavir. (See Cautions: Hypersensitivity Reactions.)

Prior to initiation or reinitiation of abacavir or a fixed-combination preparation containing abacavir, all patients should be screened for the HLA-B*5701 allele, unless there is documentation of a previous HLA-B*5701 allele assessment. The patient's medical history also should be reviewed for prior exposure to any abacavir-containing preparation. Abacavir and abacavir-containing preparations are contraindicated in individuals who test positive for HLA-B*5701. Such individuals are at higher risk for a hypersensitivity reaction; however, hypersensitivity reactions have occurred in patients who do not carry the HLA-B*5701 allele.

Prospective screening for the HLA-B*5701 allele should *not* be considered a substitute for close clinical observation and prompt identification and management of abacavir hypersensitivity whenever such reactions occur. A negative test result for HLA-B*5701 does not absolutely rule out the possibility of some form of hypersensitivity reaction. Although abacavir skin patch testing is used as a research tool, such testing should not be used in the clinical diagnosis of abacavir hypersensitivity.

Abacavir and abacavir-containing preparations should be discontinued immediately if a hypersensitivity reaction is suspected, regardless of HLA-B*5701 status and even when other diagnoses are possible (e.g., acute-onset respiratory diseases such as pneumonia, bronchitis, pharyngitis, or influenza; gastroenteritis; reactions to other drugs). Signs or symptoms of hypersensitivity include fever; rash; constitutional symptoms such as malaise, fatigue, achiness; GI symptoms such as nausea, vomiting, diarrhea, or abdominal pain; and respiratory symptoms such as pharyngitis, dyspnea, or cough. Because fatalities have been reported in patients who developed hypersensitivity reactions in which the initial presentation included respiratory symptoms, the diagnosis of hypersensitivity reaction should be carefully considered in any patient receiving abacavir who presents with symptoms of acute-onset respiratory disease, even if alternative respiratory diagnoses (pneumonia, bronchitis, pharyngitis, flu-like illness) are possible.

Abacavir and fixed-combination preparations containing abacavir should *never* be reinitiated in any patient who experienced a hypersensitivity reaction to abacavir, regardless of the patient's HLA-B*5701 status, since more severe symptoms may recur within hours and may include life-threatening hypotension and death. To minimize the risk of life-threatening hypersensitivity reactions, abacavir should be permanently discontinued if abacavir hypersensitivity cannot be ruled out (regardless of HLA-B*5701 allele status), even when other diagnoses are possible (e.g., acute-onset respiratory diseases, gastroenteritis, adverse reactions to other drugs). If hypersensitivity is ruled out, the manufacturer states that abacavir or other abacavir-containing preparations may be reinitiated, but *only* if medical care is readily accessible. Rarely, patients who discontinued abacavir for reasons other than hypersensitivity symptoms have experienced life-threatening reactions within hours of reinitiating abacavir.

Patients receiving abacavir or a fixed combination containing abacavir must be fully informed of the signs and symptoms of abacavir hypersensitivity reactions and directed to immediately contact their clinician if any such reaction occurs. Patients who have interrupted abacavir therapy for reasons other than manifestations of hypersensitivity (e.g., interruption in drug supply) should be advised that severe or fatal hypersensitivity reactions can occur following reintroduction of abacavir, and that abacavir reintroduction should be undertaken *only* after consultation with their clinician and HLA-B*5701 screening and *only* with continued monitoring for manifestations of hypersensitivity and if medical care can be readily accessed by the patient or others. To ensure that patients are fully informed regarding these potentially fatal hypersensitivity reactions, a copy of the manufacturer's medication guide and warning card should be dispensed to patients each time they are given a new or refill prescription of abacavir or abacavir-containing preparation and patients should be instructed to read this information and to carry the warning card with them. The medication guide and warning card include information on the potentially life-threatening hypersensitivity reactions that have been reported with abacavir, including information on how to recognize such a reaction if it occurs.

Precautions Related to Use of Fixed Combinations When abacavir/lamivudine, abacavir/dolutegravir/lamivudine, or abacavir/lamivudine/zidovudine is used, the cautions, precautions, contraindications, and drug interactions associated with each drug in the fixed combination must be considered. Cautionary information applicable to specific populations (e.g., pregnant or nursing women, individuals with hepatic or renal impairment, geriatric patients) should be considered for each drug. For cautionary information related to dolutegravir, lamivudine, and zidovudine, see Cautions in the individual drug monographs.

Because the antiretrovirals contained in abacavir/lamivudine, abacavir/dolutegravir/lamivudine, and abacavir/lamivudine/zidovudine also are available in single-entity or other fixed-combination preparations, care should be taken to ensure that therapy is not duplicated when a fixed combination is used in conjunction with other antiretrovirals.

Multiple abacavir-containing preparations should not be used concomitantly.

Abacavir/lamivudine should not be used concomitantly with any preparation containing abacavir or lamivudine. In addition, the fixed combination should not be used concomitantly with any preparation containing emtricitabine.

Abacavir/dolutegravir/lamivudine should not be used concomitantly with any preparation containing abacavir or lamivudine. In addition, the fixed combination should not be used concomitantly with any preparation containing emtricitabine.

Abacavir/lamivudine/zidovudine should not be used concomitantly with any preparation containing abacavir, lamivudine, or zidovudine. In addition, the fixed combination should not be used concomitantly with any preparation containing emtricitabine.

If abacavir/lamivudine, abacavir/dolutegravir/lamivudine, or abacavir/lamivudine/zidovudine is used in HIV-infected patients coinfected with HBV, clinicians should consider that severe, acute exacerbations of HBV infection have been reported following discontinuance of lamivudine in patients coinfected with HIV and HBV. Hepatic function should be closely monitored with clinical and laboratory follow-up for at least several months after abacavir/lamivudine, abacavir/dolutegravir/lamivudine, or abacavir/lamivudine/zidovudine is discontinued in HIV-infected patients coinfected with HBV and, if appropriate, initiation of HBV treatment may be warranted. (See Lamivudine 8:18.08.20.)

If abacavir/lamivudine/zidovudine is used, clinicians should consider that zidovudine has been associated with hematologic toxicity (including neutropenia and severe anemia), particularly in those with advanced HIV-1 disease, and that prolonged zidovudine use has been associated with symptomatic myopathy. Abacavir/lamivudine/zidovudine should be used with caution in patients who have bone marrow compromise evidenced by a granulocyte count less than 1000 cells/mm^3 or a hemoglobin concentration less than 9.5 g/dL. (See Zidovudine 8:18.08.20.)

Other Precautions Use of abacavir or other NRTIs has been associated with potentially fatal lactic acidosis and severe hepatomegaly with steatosis. (See Cautions: Hepatic Effects and Lactic Acidosis.) Abacavir should be administered with particular caution in patients with known risk factors for liver disease; however, lactic acidosis and severe hepatomegaly with steatosis have been reported in patients with no known risk factors. Abacavir therapy should be interrupted in any patient with clinical or laboratory findings suggestive of lactic acidosis or pronounced hepatotoxicity (signs of hepatotoxicity include hepatomegaly and steatosis even in the absence of marked increases in serum aminotransferase concentrations).

Patients should be advised that redistribution or accumulation of body fat may occur in patients receiving antiretroviral therapy and that the cause and long-term health effects of these conditions are as yet unknown. (See Cautions: Adipogenic Effects.)

Although there have been conflicting data regarding whether abacavir is associated with an increased risk of MI, an FDA safety analysis did not find an association. (See Cautions: Cardiovascular Effects.) As a precaution in patients receiving antiretroviral therapy (including abacavir), the patient's underlying risk for coronary heart disease (CHD) should be considered and measures taken to address risk factors for CHD (e.g., hypertension, hyperlipidemia, diabetes mellitus, smoking).

A reduction in dosage is recommended if abacavir is used in patients with mild hepatic impairment (Child-Pugh score 5–6). (See Dosage: Dosage in Renal and Hepatic Impairment under Dosage and Administration.) Safety, efficacy, and pharmacokinetics of abacavir have not been established in patients with moderate or severe hepatic impairment and the drug is contraindicated in such patients. Abacavir/lamivudine, abacavir/dolutegravir/lamivudine, and abacavir/lamivudine/zidovudine are *not* recommended in patients with mild hepatic impairment and are contraindicated in patients with moderate or severe hepatic impairment.

Abacavir in conjunction with other antiretroviral agents is not a cure for HIV infection, and patients receiving the drugs may continue to develop opportunistic infections and other complications associated with HIV disease. Patients should be informed of the critical nature of compliance with HIV therapy and the importance of remaining under the care of a clinician. Patients should be advised to take their antiretroviral regimen exactly as prescribed and to not alter or discontinue the regimen without consulting a clinician.

Patients should be advised that effective antiretroviral regimens can decrease HIV concentrations in blood and genital secretions and strict adherence to such regimens in conjunction with risk-reduction measures may decrease, but cannot absolutely eliminate, the risk of secondary transmission of HIV to others. Patients should continue to practice safer sex (e.g., use latex or polyurethane condoms to minimize sexual contact with body fluids), never share personal items that can have blood or body fluids on them (e.g., toothbrushes, razor blades), and never reuse or share needles.

■ Pediatric Precautions Safety and efficacy of single-entity abacavir tablets or oral solution (Ziagen®) have not been established in neonates and infants younger than 3 months of age. Use of abacavir in children 3 months of age and older is supported by pharmacokinetic trials and evidence from adequate and well-controlled trials in adults and pediatric patients. Adverse effects reported in children receiving abacavir are similar to those reported in adults receiving the drug (e.g., hypersensitivity reactions, adverse GI effects).

Abacavir/lamivudine (Epzicom®) should *not* be used in pediatric patients weighing less than 25 kg since dosage of the drugs cannot be adjusted individually.

Abacavir/lamivudine/zidovudine (Trizivir®) should *not* be used in pediatric patients weighing less than 40 kg since dosages of the drugs cannot be adjusted individually.

Safety and efficacy of abacavir/dolutegravir/lamivudine (Triumeq®) have not been established in pediatric patients.

■ Geriatric Precautions While clinical experience to date has not revealed age-related differences in response to abacavir, clinical studies evaluating abacavir have not included sufficient numbers of adults 65 years of age or older to determine whether geriatric patients respond differently than younger adults. Dosage of abacavir for geriatric patients should be selected carefully because of limited experience with the drug in this age group and because these individuals frequently have decreased hepatic, renal, and/or cardiac function and concomitant disease and drug therapy.

Clinical trials of abacavir/lamivudine, abacavir/dolutegravir/lamivudine, and abacavir/lamivudine/zidovudine did not include sufficient numbers of adults 65 years of age or older to determine whether they respond differently than younger adults. The fixed combinations should be used with caution in geriatric patients because of age-related decreases in hepatic, renal, and/or cardiac function and potential for concomitant disease and drug therapy.

■ **Mutagenicity and Carcinogenicity** Abacavir was not mutagenic in bacterial mutagenicity assays (with or without metabolic activation). Abacavir was mutagenic in a L5178Y mouse lymphoma assay without metabolic activation; the drug was not mutagenic in this assay with metabolic activation. In an in vitro cytogenetic study in human lymphocytes, abacavir induced chromosomal aberrations (with or without metabolic activation). Abacavir was clastogenic in male mice, but not in female mice, in an in vivo bone marrow micronucleus assay.

Studies to determine the carcinogenic potential of abacavir were performed in male and female mice and rats using dosages approximately 6–32 times the estimated human exposure based on the recommended human dosage (300 mg twice daily) and resulted in an increase in neoplasms and benign tumors. In mice and rats, neoplasms occurred in the preputial gland in males and in the clitoral gland of females; neoplasms also occurred in the liver of female rats. Benign tumors occurred in the liver and thyroid gland of female rats. The clinical importance of these carcinogenic effects reported in rodents is not known.

■ **Pregnancy, Fertility, and Lactation** ***Pregnancy*** Abacavir crosses the placenta and is distributed into cord blood in concentrations similar to maternal serum concentrations. (See Pharmacokinetics: Distribution.)

Data from the Antiretroviral Pregnancy Registry show no difference in the risk of overall major birth defects for abacavir compared with the background rate for major birth defects in the US reference population of the Metropolitan Atlanta Congenital Defects Program (MACDP). Registry data includes over 2000 prospective reports of abacavir exposures during pregnancy resulting in live births, including over 900 first trimester exposures to the drug.

In reproduction studies in rats, developmental toxicity (i.e., depressed fetal body weight, reduced crown-rump length) and fetal malformations (i.e., fetal anasarca, skeletal malformations) occurred at abacavir dosages associated with exposures 35 times the usual the human exposure (based on AUC). Embryonic and fetal toxicity (i.e., increased resorptions, decreased fetal body weights) and an increased incidence of stillbirth and lower body weights occurred at abacavir dosages associated with exposures approximately 17 times the usual human exposure. In reproduction studies in rabbits, there was no evidence of developmental toxicity and no increase in fetal malformations at abacavir dosages associated with exposure 8.5 times the usual human exposure (based on AUC).

The HHS Panel on Treatment of HIV-infected Pregnant Women and Prevention of Perinatal Transmission states that abacavir in conjunction with lamivudine is a preferred dual NRTI option for *initial* antiretroviral regimens in antiretroviral-naive pregnant women, but should be used *only* in those who test negative for the HLA-B*5701 allele.

A triple NRTI regimen of abacavir, lamivudine, and zidovudine is *not* recommended for *initial* treatment in antiretroviral-naive pregnant women because of inferior virologic efficacy.

To monitor maternal-fetal outcomes of pregnant women exposed to antiretroviral agents, including abacavir, the Antiretroviral Pregnancy Registry was established. Clinicians are encouraged to contact the registry at 800-258-4263 or http://www.APRegistry.com to report cases of prenatal exposure to antiretroviral drugs.

Fertility There was no evidence that abacavir affected fertility or reproductive performance in male or female rats when the drug was given in a dosage associated with exposures approximately 8 times the usual human exposure (based on body surface area).

Lactation Abacavir is distributed into human milk and has been detected in the plasma of at least one breast-feeding child. (See Pharmacokinetics: Distribution.)

Because of the risk of transmission of HIV to an uninfected infant through breast milk, the US Centers for Disease Control and Prevention (CDC) and other experts recommend that HIV-infected women *not* breast-feed infants, regardless of antiretroviral therapy. Therefore, because of the potential for HIV transmission and the potential for serious adverse effects from abacavir if the drug were distributed into milk, women should be instructed not to breast-feed while they are receiving abacavir.

Drug Interactions

The following drug interactions are based on studies using abacavir sulfate. Drug interaction studies have not been performed to date using the fixed combination containing abacavir and lamivudine (abacavir/lamivudine), fixed combination containing abacavir, dolutegravir, and lamivudine (abacavir/dolutegravir/lamivudine), or fixed combination containing abacavir, lamivudine, and zidovudine (abacavir/lamivudine/zidovudine). When a fixed combination is used, interactions associated with each drug in the fixed combination should be considered.

■ **Drugs Affecting Hepatic Microsomal Enzymes** In vitro studies indicate that abacavir does not inhibit the cytochrome P-450 (CYP) isoenzymes 2C9, 2D6, or 3A4. Therefore, clinically important drug interactions between abacavir and drugs metabolized by these isoenzymes are not expected.

■ **Alcohol** Although alcohol and abacavir are both metabolized by alcohol dehydrogenase, clinically important drug interactions are not expected between abacavir and alcohol. Following oral administration of a single oral dose of abacavir 600 mg and alcohol 0.7 g/kg (about 5 alcoholic drinks) in HIV-infected men, the area under the plasma concentration-time curve (AUC) of abacavir was increased 41% and the elimination half-life of the drug was increased 26%. There was no change in the pharmacokinetic parameters of alcohol and no evidence of disulfiram-type reactions in any of the men. Concomitant use of abacavir and alcohol has not been investigated in women.

■ **Antiretroviral Agents** ***HIV Entry and Fusion Inhibitors*** There is no in vitro evidence of antagonistic antiretroviral effects between maraviroc and abacavir.

HIV Integrase Inhibitors (INSTIs) Raltegravir and abacavir are additive or synergistic against HIV-1 in vitro. There is no in vitro evidence of antagonistic antiretroviral effects between abacavir and dolutegravir or elvitegravir.

Elvitegravir. Concomitant use of abacavir and elvitegravir, *ritonavir-boosted* elvitegravir, or *cobicistat-boosted* elvitegravir did not result in clinically important drug interactions.

HIV Nonnucleoside Reverse Transcriptase Inhibitors (NNRTIs) The antiretroviral effects of abacavir and nonnucleoside reverse transcriptase inhibitors (NNRTIs), including efavirenz and nevirapine, are additive or synergistic against HIV-1 in vitro. There is no in vitro evidence of antagonistic antiretroviral effects between abacavir and etravirine, nevirapine, or rilpivirine.

Although specific studies have not been performed, clinically important pharmacokinetic interactions between abacavir and delavirdine, efavirenz, nevirapine, or rilpivirine are not expected.

HIV Nucleoside and Nucleotide Reverse Transcriptase Inhibitors (NRTIs) Results of in vitro studies using HIV-1 indicate that the antiretroviral effects of abacavir are not antagonized by other nucleoside reverse transcriptase inhibitors (NRTIs), including didanosine, emtricitabine, lamivudine, stavudine, tenofovir disoproxil fumarate (tenofovir DF), and zidovudine.

Lamivudine and Zidovudine. Clinically important pharmacokinetic interactions have not been observed when abacavir, lamivudine, and zidovudine were used concurrently. In a crossover study evaluating concomitant use of single doses of abacavir (600 mg), lamivudine (150 mg), and zidovudine (300 mg) in HIV-infected individuals, the pharmacokinetic parameters of abacavir were unchanged when administered with lamivudine and/or zidovudine. The AUC of lamivudine was decreased 15% and the AUC of zidovudine increased 10% when used concomitantly with abacavir.

Tenofovir. Concomitant use of tenofovir DF (300 mg once daily) and abacavir (single 300-mg dose) resulted in a 12% increase in peak plasma concentrations of abacavir, but did not affect the AUC of abacavir; peak plasma concentrations and AUC of tenofovir were not affected.

HIV Protease Inhibitors (PIs) Abacavir and some HIV protease inhibitors (PIs) (e.g., amprenavir [commercially available as fosamprenavir], nelfinavir, tipranavir) are additive or synergistic against HIV-1 in vitro. There is no in vitro evidence of antagonistic antiretroviral effects between abacavir and amprenavir, atazanavir, or darunavir.

Darunavir. Although specific data are not available, pharmacokinetic interactions between abacavir and darunavir are not expected.

Fosamprenavir. A pharmacokinetic interaction between abacavir and fosamprenavir is unlikely.

Lopinavir. Although the clinical importance is unclear, lopinavir may induce glucuronidation, and concomitant use of abacavir and the fixed combination of lopinavir and ritonavir (lopinavir/ritonavir) has the potential to reduce plasma abacavir concentrations.

Tipranavir. Concomitant use of abacavir and *ritonavir-boosted* tipranavir results in a 35–44% decrease in the AUC of abacavir. The clinical importance of this pharmacokinetic interaction is not known, and appropriate dosages for concomitant use with respect to safety and efficacy have not been established.

■ **HCV Antivirals** ***HCV Protease Inhibitors*** **Simeprevir.** Clinically important pharmacokinetic interactions are not expected if abacavir is used concomitantly with simeprevir.

HCV Replication Complex Inhibitors **Elbasvir and Grazoprevir.** Clinically important pharmacokinetic interactions are not expected if abacavir is used concomitantly with the fixed combination of elbasvir and grazoprevir (elbasvir/grazoprevir).

Ledipasvir and Sofosbuvir. Clinically important pharmacokinetic interactions are not expected if abacavir is used concomitantly with the fixed combination of ledipasvir and sofosbuvir (ledipasvir/sofosbuvir).

■ **Opiates and Opiate Partial Agonists** ***Methadone*** Concomitant use of methadone and abacavir may increase clearance of methadone, but does not affect the pharmacokinetics of abacavir. In a limited number of HIV-infected individuals receiving maintenance therapy with methadone (40 or 90 mg daily), concomitant use of abacavir 600 mg twice daily (twice the usual recommended adult dosage) resulted in a 22% increase in methadone clearance.

Some experts state that dosage adjustments are not necessary in patients receiving methadone and abacavir concomitantly. The manufacturer of abacavir states that, although an increase in methadone dosage may be required in a small number of patients because of a pharmacokinetic interaction, most patients will not need modification of methadone dosage.

■ **Ribavirin** In vitro, ribavirin had no effect on the antiretroviral activity of abacavir against HIV-1.

Acute Toxicity

■ Manifestations Limited information is available on acute toxicity of abacavir. The acute lethal dose of the drug in humans is not known.

■ Treatment If acute overdosage of abacavir occurs, supportive and symptomatic treatment should be initiated and the patient observed closely. There is no known antidote for abacavir overdosage. It is not known whether hemodialysis or peritoneal dialysis will remove abacavir from the body.

Mechanism of Action

■ Antiviral Effects Following conversion to a pharmacologically active metabolite, abacavir apparently inhibits replication of retroviruses, including human immunodeficiency virus type 1 (HIV-1) and type 2 (HIV-2), by interfering with viral RNA-directed DNA polymerase (reverse transcriptase). The drug, therefore, exerts a virustatic effect against retroviruses by acting as a reverse transcriptase inhibitor.

Like other HIV nucleoside reverse transcriptase inhibitors (NRTIs), including didanosine, emtricitabine, lamivudine, stavudine, and zidovudine, the antiviral activity of abacavir appears to depend on intracellular conversion of the drug to a 5′-triphosphate metabolite. Carbovir triphosphate (carbocyclic guanosine triphosphate) and not unchanged abacavir appears to be the pharmacologically active form of the drug. Substantial differences exist in the rates at which human cells phosphorylate various NRTIs and in the enzymatic pathways involved.

Enzymatic conversion of abacavir to carbovir triphosphate appears to be complex and involves certain steps and enzymes that differ from those involved in the enzymatic conversion of dideoxynucleoside reverse transcriptase inhibitors. Abacavir is phosphorylated by adenosine phosphotransferase to abacavir monophosphate, which is converted to carbovir monophosphate by a cytosolic enzyme. Subsequently, carbovir monophosphate is phosphorylated by cellular kinases to carbovir triphosphate. Abacavir is not a substrate for enzymes (i.e., thymidine kinase, deoxycytidine kinase, adenosine kinase, mitochondrial deoxyguanosine kinase) known to phosphorylate other nucleoside analogs. Because phosphorylation of abacavir depends on cellular rather than viral enzymes, conversion of the drug to the active triphosphate derivative occurs in both virus-infected and uninfected cells. Carbovir triphosphate is a structural analog of deoxyguanosine-5′-triphosphate (dGTP), the usual substrate for viral RNA-directed DNA polymerase. Although other mechanisms may be involved in the antiretroviral activity of the drug, carbovir triphosphate appears to compete with deoxyguanosine-5′-triphosphate for viral RNA-directed DNA polymerase and incorporation into viral DNA. Following incorporation of carbovir triphosphate into the viral DNA chain instead of deoxyguanosine-5′-triphosphate, DNA synthesis is prematurely terminated because the absence of the 3′-hydroxy group on the drug prevents further 5′ to 3′ phosphodiester linkages.

■ Cytotoxic Effects Results of in vitro studies indicate that carbovir triphosphate interferes with activity of cellular DNA polymerases, including human α, β, γ, or ε-polymerases at concentrations substantially higher (90- to 2900-fold) than those required for antiretroviral activity.

In vitro cell-growth assays have been used to assess the cytotoxicity of abacavir for various cell lines. Results of these studies have shown that the drug is essentially nontoxic in a variety of human leukemic cell lines of T, B, and monocyte lineage, and in hepatitis B virus-producing liver tumor cell lines. The IC_{50} (concentration of the drug required to inhibit cell growth by 50%) in human leukemic cell lines exceeded 100 μM for IM-9 and CEM cell lines, and was about 20 μM in Molt-4F cells. In human leukemic cell lines, abacavir was a more potent inhibitor of cell growth than didanosine; the inhibitory potency of abacavir in some cell lines was similar to that of zidovudine.

Results of in vitro studies indicate that abacavir has a low potential for inhibition of hematopoiesis. In these studies, the IC_{50} for abacavir for granulocyte-monocyte colony-forming units (CFU-GM) and erythroid burst-forming unit (BFU-E) progenitors averaged 110 μM and was substantially greater than concentrations required for antiretroviral activity. In addition, abacavir does not alter intracellular deoxynucleoside triphosphate pools or affect thymidine incorporation into DNA at concentrations associated with antiretroviral activity.

Spectrum

Abacavir has a limited spectrum of antiviral activity. Following intracellular conversion to a pharmacologically active 5′-triphosphate metabolite, abacavir is active in vitro against human and animal retroviruses, including human immunodeficiency viruses type 1 (HIV-1) and type 2 (HIV-2) and feline immunodeficiency virus (Petaluma strain). Abacavir has some in vitro activity against hepatitis B virus (HBV) and cytomegalovirus (CMV), but has been inactive against other human viruses tested, including herpes simplex virus types 1 and 2, varicella-zoster virus, and influenza virus type A.

The antiretroviral activity of abacavir has been evaluated in vitro in various cell culture systems, including lymphoblastoid cell lines, macrophage/monocyte cultures, and peripheral blood mononuclear cells.

A concentration of abacavir of 1 μM is equivalent to 0.28 mcg/mL.

■ Retroviruses Abacavir is active in vitro against HIV-1 and HIV-2. In a study evaluating the in vitro antiretroviral activity of abacavir, didanosine, and zidovudine using peripheral blood lymphocytes inoculated with clinical isolates of HIV-1 obtained from individuals who were treatment naive (had not previously received antiretroviral agent therapy), abacavir was more active than didanosine and as active as zidovudine on a weight basis.

When tested against HIV-1_{IIIb} or HIV-1_{BaL}, the concentration of abacavir required to inhibit viral replication by 50% (EC_{50}) ranged from 3.7–5.8 or 0.07–1.0 μM, respectively. When tested against clinical isolates, the EC_{50} of abacavir was 0.26 μM. The EC_{50} of the drug ranged from 0.0015–1.05 μM against different HIV-1 clades (A–G) and 0.024–0.49 μM against HIV-2 isolates.

■ Other Viruses Although the clinical importance is unclear, abacavir has some activity in vitro against HBV. In cell culture using 2.2.15 cells derived from a human hepatoblastoma cell line that continuously produces HBV genome (Hep G2), the IC_{50} of abacavir was 7 μM based on measurement of intracellular DNA forms and 4.7 μM based on measurement of extracellular Dane particle production.

While plaque inhibition assays indicate that abacavir has some in vitro activity against CMV, ganciclovir has been reported to be 50- to 100-fold more active than abacavir against clinical isolates of CMV.

Resistance

Strains of human immunodeficiency virus type 1 (HIV-1) with reduced susceptibility to abacavir have been produced in vitro in cell culture by serial passage of the retrovirus in the presence of increasing concentrations of the drug. In addition, strains of HIV-1 with in vitro resistance to abacavir have emerged during therapy with the drug. For information on genotypic assays used to detect specific HIV-1 genetic variants (mutations), phenotypic assays used to measure HIV-1 drug resistance and recommendations regarding these assays, see In Vitro Resistance Testing under Guidelines for Use of Antiretroviral Agents: Laboratory Monitoring, in the Antiretroviral Agents General Statement 8:18.08.

Although the complete mechanism(s) of resistance or reduced susceptibility to abacavir has not been fully determined to date, mutation of HIV reverse transcriptase appears to be the principal mechanism of resistance. Acquisition of a single mutation can result in decreased susceptibility to abacavir; acquisition of multiple mutations generally is necessary for high-level resistance to the drug.

Abacavir-resistant variants produced in vitro in the presence of increasing concentrations of the drug have contained one or more amino acid substitutions including K65R, L74V, Y115F, or M184V/I. These same substitutions have been identified in HIV-1 variants isolated from patients receiving abacavir in clinical studies; the substitution at amino acid position 184 is the most frequently observed change in clinical isolates. Substitutions at amino acid positions M184V or I result in an approximately twofold decrease in abacavir susceptibility; substitutions at K65R, L74M, or Y115F with M184V or I confer a sevenfold to eightfold decrease in abacavir susceptibility. Combinations of these substitutions result in a greater than eightfold decrease in susceptibility.

In vitro studies indicate that resistance to abacavir does not develop rapidly; further study is needed to determine how rapidly abacavir-resistant isolates develop in vivo. Because of rapid viral proliferation and the inherent error rate of HIV reverse transcriptase, administration of a single antiretroviral agent or antiretroviral regimens that only partially suppress viral replication allows more rapid selection of resistant variants.

The frequency of abacavir-resistant HIV isolates existing in patients who are antiretroviral naive (have not previously received antiretroviral agent therapy) or have previously received antiretroviral agents other than abacavir has not been fully determined. Although the clinical importance is unclear, HIV variants containing mutations known to contribute to resistance to abacavir (e.g., M184V/I) have been isolated from individuals who have not previously received the drug.

■ Cross-resistance Cross-resistance between abacavir and other HIV nucleoside reverse transcriptase inhibitors (NRTIs), including didanosine, emtricitabine, lamivudine, tenofovir disoproxil fumarate (tenofovir DF), and stavudine, has been reported; There is evidence that HIV isolates that are highly resistant to multiple NRTIs also have reduced susceptibility to abacavir. Strains with the Q151M mutation (a mutation that appears to be associated with resistance against multiple NRTIs) also have reduced susceptibility to abacavir; these strains become highly resistant to abacavir when additional mutations conferring resistance to other nucleosides (e.g., V60I, K65R, V118I, M184V, T215Y) are present.

Pharmacokinetics

The pharmacokinetics of abacavir have been studied in adults with human immunodeficiency virus (HIV) infection and in HIV-infected children 3 months to 13 years of age.

There is some evidence from a multiple-dose study that mean peak plasma concentrations and area under the concentration-time curve (AUC) of abacavir may be 30 and 54% higher, respectively, in women than in men. However, in a population pharmacokinetic analysis, there was no gender difference in abacavir AUC normalized for lean body weight. Further study is needed to more fully evaluate the pharmacokinetics of abacavir during pregnancy. In one study, the AUC of abacavir was similar in pregnant and nonpregnant women, but peak plasma concentrations of the drug were slightly decreased and there was greater variability in AUC and oral clearance during pregnancy. Abacavir pharmacokinetics are similar between blacks and Caucasians.

Pharmacokinetics of abacavir have not been specifically studied in geriatric adults older than 65 years of age. In addition, only limited information is available on the pharmacokinetics of abacavir in individuals with renal or hepatic impairment.

The manufacturer states that commercially available abacavir sulfate tablets and oral solution are bioequivalent. In pediatric patients, abacavir exposure is expected to be similar regardless of whether the scored tablet or oral solution is administered.

A fixed-combination tablet containing abacavir 600 mg and lamivudine 300 mg (Epzicom®) is bioequivalent to two 300-mg tablets of abacavir and two 150-mg tablets of lamivudine given simultaneously. Results of a crossover study in fasting, healthy adults indicate that a fixed-combination tablet containing 300 mg of abacavir, 150 mg of lamivudine, and 300 mg of zidovudine (Trizivir®) is bioequivalent to a 300-mg tablet of abacavir, a 150-mg tablet of lamivudine, and a 300-mg tablet of zidovudine administered simultaneously.

In some early studies evaluating the pharmacokinetics of abacavir, the drug was administered orally as the succinate salt (a formulation not commercially available in the US).

Dosages and concentrations of abacavir sulfate or abacavir succinate are expressed in terms of the base.

■ **Absorption** Abacavir is rapidly absorbed following oral administration as the succinate or sulfate salts. The geometric mean absolute oral bioavailability of abacavir sulfate tablets is 83%. Studies using oral abacavir succinate (not commercially available in the US) indicate that peak plasma concentrations of the drug generally are attained 0.5–1.7 hours after a dose.

In HIV-infected adults receiving abacavir in a dosage of 300 mg twice daily (given as abacavir succinate), peak plasma concentration and AUC (0–12 hours) of the drug at steady-state averaged 3 mcg/mL and 6.02 mcg•hour/mL, respectively. In studies in HIV-infected adults employing oral abacavir dosages of 300–1200 mg daily (given as abacavir succinate), the pharmacokinetics of the drug were independent of the dose; results of studies using abacavir succinate indicate that increases in mean peak plasma concentration and AUC are not precisely proportional to dosage increases.

In HIV-infected children 3 months to 13 years of age who received 8 mg/kg of abacavir every 12 hours (given as an oral solution containing abacavir sulfate), steady-state peak plasma concentration and AUC of the drug averaged 3.71 mcg/mL and 9.8 mcg•hour/mL, respectively. Steady-state AUC in those 3 months to 2 years of age, older than 2 to 6 years of age, or older than 6 to 13 years of age averaged 8.67, 9.38, or 10.71 mcg•hour/mL, respectively. Pediatric patients receiving abacavir oral solution at the recommended dosage achieved plasma concentrations similar to those observed in adults; pediatric patients receiving abacavir oral tablets achieved plasma concentrations higher than those observed in pediatric patients receiving abacavir oral solution. In HIV-1-infected pediatric patients 3 months to 12 years of age, the AUC of abacavir reported in those receiving the oral solution or tablets administered once daily was comparable to the AUC reported in those receiving the same total daily dosage of the oral solution or tablets administered twice daily. Mean peak plasma concentrations reported with a once-daily regimen were 1.6- to 2.3-fold higher than those reported with a twice-daily regimen.

The pharmacokinetics of abacavir in pregnant women is similar to that reported in nonpregnant women; the AUC of the drug in pregnant women is similar to that reported in women 6–12 weeks postpartum and in nonpregnant individuals.

The pharmacokinetics of abacavir have been evaluated in patients with mild hepatic impairment (Child-Pugh score 5–6) and results indicate a mean increase of 89% in the AUC of the drug following a single 600-mg dose. Although the AUCs of metabolites of the drug were not affected by mild hepatic impairment, there was a decrease in the rates of formation and elimination of these metabolites. The pharmacokinetics of abacavir have not been studied in patients with moderate or severe hepatic impairment.

Food Presence of food in the GI tract does not have a clinically important effect on bioavailability of abacavir.

In a study in HIV-infected individuals who received a single 300-mg dose of abacavir (given as tablets containing abacavir sulfate), administration with food decreased peak plasma concentration 35% but decreased the AUC of the drug by only 5% compared with administration in the fasting state.

In a single-dose bioavailability study, food did not affect the extent of absorption of abacavir or lamivudine when the drugs were given as the commercially available fixed-combination tablet containing 600 mg of abacavir and 300 mg of lamivudine. In a crossover study in healthy adults, food did not affect the extent of absorption of abacavir, lamivudine, or zidovudine when the drugs were given as the commercially available fixed-combination tablet containing 300 mg of abacavir, 150 mg of lamivudine, and 300 mg of zidovudine (abacavir/lamivudine/zidovudine).

In a study in healthy adults using abacavir/dolutegravir/lamivudine, administration of the fixed combination with a high-fat meal decreased abacavir peak plasma concentrations by 23% and increased peak plasma concentrations and AUC of dolutegravir by 37 and 48%, respectively, compared with administration in the fasting state; lamivudine exposures were not affected.

■ **Distribution** Following oral administration, abacavir is extensively distributed. The apparent volume of distribution of the drug following IV administration in HIV-infected adults is 0.86 L/kg, suggesting distribution into extravascular spaces.

Following systemic administration, abacavir distributes into erythrocytes and CD4+ CEM cells by nonfacilitated diffusion. Following administration of radiolabeled abacavir, total blood- and plasma-drug related radioactivity are identical; these results indicate abacavir readily distributes into erythrocytes.

Abacavir is distributed into CSF. In HIV-infected adults receiving an antiretroviral regimen that included abacavir (usually 300 mg of abacavir twice daily), median CSF or plasma concentrations of the drug were 0.128 mcg/mL or 0.139 mcg/mL, respectively, and the estimated CSF half-life was 2.5 hours.

Abacavir is about 50% bound to plasma proteins; binding of abacavir to plasma proteins is independent of drug concentration.

Abacavir crosses the placenta. In several HIV-infected pregnant women who were receiving abacavir as part of a multiple-drug regimen, concentrations of the drug in cord blood were 0.21–1.8 mcg/mL and maternal serum concentrations were 0.15–1.83 in samples obtained at the time of delivery.

Abacavir is distributed into human milk. In a study in 15 women receiving abacavir at 1 month postpartum, the drug was distributed into milk (milk-to-plasma ratio of 0.85) and also was detected in the plasma of at least one breast-feeding child.

■ **Elimination** The plasma elimination half-life of abacavir following a single oral dose (given as abacavir sulfate) is about 1.5 hours. In HIV-infected children 3 months to 13 years of age who received 8 mg/kg of abacavir every 12 hours (given as an oral solution containing abacavir sulfate), steady-state plasma elimination half-life averaged 1.3 hours and was essentially the same as that reported after a single dose. Following IV administration of abacavir in adults, total clearance reportedly is 0.8 L/hour per kg.

In patients with mild hepatic impairment (Child-Pugh score 5–6), there is an increase of 58% in the half-life of abacavir after a single 600-mg dose of the drug. Following oral administration of a single 300-mg dose of abacavir to an individual with renal failure (glomerular filtration rate less than 10 mL/minute) undergoing peritoneal dialysis, the plasma elimination half-life of the drug was 1.33 hours.

Intracellularly, abacavir is phosphorylated to abacavir monophosphate by adenosine phosphotransferase; abacavir monophosphate is then converted to carbovir monophosphate in a reaction catalyzed by cytosolic enzymes and then to carbovir triphosphate by cellular kinases. Intracellular (host cell) conversion of abacavir to carbovir triphosphate is necessary for the antiviral activity of the drug. The in vitro intracellular half-life of carbovir triphosphate in CD4+ CEM cells is 3.3 hours.

Abacavir is metabolized by alcohol dehydrogenase to form the 5′-carboxylic acid and by glucuronyltransferase to form the 5′-glucuronide; these metabolites do not appear to have any antiviral activity. Any involvement of cytochrome P-450 isoenzymes in the metabolism of abacavir is limited.

Following oral administration of a 600-mg dose of radiolabeled abacavir, 82.2% of the dose is excreted in urine and 16% of the dose is excreted in feces. The 5′-carboxylic acid metabolite, 5′-glucuronide metabolite, and unchanged abacavir accounted for 30, 36, and 1.2%, respectively, of recovered radioactivity in urine; unidentified minor metabolites accounted for 15% of recovered radioactivity in urine.

Chemistry and Stability

■ **Chemistry** Abacavir, an antiretroviral agent, is a human immunodeficiency virus (HIV) nucleoside reverse transcriptase inhibitor (NRTI). Although abacavir is pharmacologically related to HIV dideoxynucleoside reverse transcriptase inhibitors (e.g., didanosine, lamivudine, stavudine, zidovudine), abacavir differs structurally from these drugs and also differs structurally from other currently available antiretroviral agents. Abacavir is a carbocyclic NRTI and contains a cyclopentenyl sugar moiety rather than the ribose moiety contained in dideoxynucleoside reverse transcriptase inhibitors and also lacks the glycosidic linkage between the heterocycle and carbohydrate moiety. Abacavir is an analog of guanine, a naturally occurring purine. Abacavir differs structurally from guanine by the presence of a cyclopropylamino group at position 6 on the carbohydrate ring; this substitution results in a lipophilic compound with high aqueous solubility. Abacavir is a prodrug and is not pharmacologically active until converted to carbovir triphosphate. (See Mechanism of Action.)

Abacavir sulfate occurs as a white to off-white solid and has a solubility of 77 mg/mL in distilled water at 25°C. The octanol/water (pH 7.1–7.3) partition coefficient (log P) for abacavir sulfate is approximately 1.2 at 25°C; the octanol/water coefficient for abacavir is higher than that for zidovudine (log P 0.09). Abacavir has a pK_a of 5.01.

Abacavir sulfate is commercially available for oral administration as single-entity tablets and oral solution (Ziagen®); dosage and concentration are expressed in terms of the base. Commercially available abacavir oral solution is a clear to opalescent yellowish solution containing 20 mg of abacavir per mL in a strawberry-banana flavored aqueous vehicle; the oral solution contains methylparaben and propylparaben as preservatives.

Abacavir also is commercially available for oral administration in fixed-combination tablets containing abacavir sulfate and lamivudine (abacavir/lamivudine; Epzicom®), fixed-combination tablets containing abacavir sulfate, dolutegravir, and lamivudine (abacavir/dolutegravir/lamivudine; Triumeq®), and fixed-combination tablets containing abacavir sulfate, lamivudine, and zidovudine (abacavir/lamivudine/zidovudine; Trizivir®).

■ **Stability** Abacavir sulfate tablets and oral solution (Ziagen®) should be stored at a controlled room temperature of 20–25°C. The oral solution may be refrigerated, but should not be frozen.

Abacavir/lamivudine fixed-combination tablets (Epzicom®), abacavir/dolutegravir/lamivudine fixed-combination tablets (Triumeq®), and abacavir/lamivudine/zidovudine fixed-combination tablets (Trizivir®) should be stored at 25°C, but may be exposed to temperatures ranging from 15–30°C.

Preparations

Excipients in commercially available drug preparations may have clinically important effects in some individuals; consult specific product labeling for details.

Abacavir Sulfate

Oral		
Solution	20 mg (of abacavir) per mL*	**Abacavir Sulfate Oral Solution**
		Ziagen®, ViiV
Tablets, film-coated, scored	300 mg (of abacavir)*	**Abacavir SulfateTablets**
		Ziagen®, ViiV

*available from one or more manufacturer, distributor, and/or repackager by generic (nonproprietary) name

Abacavir Sulfate Combinations

Oral		
Tablets, film-coated	300 mg (of abacavir) with Lamivudine 150 mg and Zidovudine 300 mg*	**Abacavir Sulfate, Lamivudine, and Zidovudine Tablets**
		Trizivir®, ViiV
	600 mg (of abacavir) with Lamivudine 300 mg*	**Abacavir Sulfate and Lamivudine Tablets**
		Epzicom®, ViiV
	600 mg (of abacavir) with Dolutegravir 50 mg and Lamivudine 300 mg	**Triumeq®**, ViiV

*available from one or more manufacturer, distributor, and/or repackager by generic (nonproprietary) name

†Use is not currently included in the labeling approved by the US Food and Drug Administration

Selected Revisions May 2017,

Emtricitabine

FTC, efavirenz/emtricitabine/tenofovir disoproxil fumarate, efavirenz/emtricitabine/tenofovir DF, EFV/FTC/TDF, EFV/TDF/FTC, TAF/FTC, TDF/FTC, RPV/TAF/FTC, RPV/TDF/FTC

■ Emtricitabine, an antiretroviral agent, is a human immunodeficiency virus (HIV) nucleoside reverse transcriptase inhibitor (NRTI).

REMS

FDA approved a REMS for emtricitabine to ensure that the benefits outweigh the risks. The REMS may apply to one or more preparations of emtricitabine and consists of the following: elements to assure safe use. See the FDA REMS page (https://www.accessdata.fda.gov/scripts/cder/rems/index.cfm).

Uses

■ **Treatment of HIV Infection** Emtricitabine is used in conjunction with other antiretroviral agents for the treatment of human immunodeficiency virus type 1 (HIV-1) infection in adults, adolescents, and pediatric patients.

Emtricitabine usually is used in multiple-drug regimens that include another HIV nucleoside reverse transcriptase inhibitor (NRTI) (dual NRTIs) and an HIV integrase strand transfer inhibitor (INSTI), HIV nonnucleoside reverse transcriptase inhibitor (NNRTI), or HIV protease inhibitor (PI) in INSTI-, NNRTI-, or PI-based regimens. Single-entity emtricitabine is labeled by FDA for use in conjunction with other antiretrovirals in all age groups. Emtricitabine also is commercially available in various fixed-combination preparations that contain a tenofovir prodrug (either tenofovir alafenamide fumarate or tenofovir disoproxil fumarate [tenofovir DF]) with or without a third antiretroviral. These fixed combinations can be used in specific patient groups to decrease pill burden and improve compliance.

If the dual NRTI option of emtricitabine and tenofovir alafenamide is used in conjunction with other antiretrovirals for the treatment of HIV-1 infection, a fixed-combination preparation containing both drugs (emtricitabine/tenofovir alafenamide; Descovy®) is commercially available and can be used in adults and adolescents 12 years of age or older weighing at least 35 kg. Emtricitabine/tenofovir alafenamide must be used in conjunction with other antiretrovirals for treatment of HIV-1.

If the dual NRTI option of emtricitabine and tenofovir DF is used in conjunction with other antiretrovirals for the treatment of HIV-1 infection, a fixed-combination preparation containing both drugs (emtricitabine/tenofovir DF; Truvada®) is commercially available and can be used in adults, adolescents, and children weighing at least 17 kg. Emtricitabine/tenofovir DF must be used in conjunction with other antiretrovirals for treatment of HIV-1.

If an NNRTI-based regimen of efavirenz, emtricitabine, and tenofovir DF is used for the treatment of HIV-1 infection, a fixed-combination preparation containing all 3 drugs (efavirenz/emtricitabine/tenofovir DF; Atripla®) is commercially available and can be used in adults and adolescents 12 years of age or older weighing at least 40 kg. Efavirenz/emtricitabine/tenofovir DF can be used alone as a complete treatment regimen or in conjunction with other antiretrovirals.

If an HIV NNRTI-based regimen of rilpivirine, emtricitabine, and tenofovir alafenamide is used for the treatment of HIV-1 infection, a fixed-combination preparation containing all 3 drugs (emtricitabine/rilpivirine/tenofovir alafenamide; Odefsey®) is commercially available and can be used in antiretroviral-naive adults and adolescents 12 years of age or older weighing at least 35 kg with baseline plasma HIV-1 RNA levels of 100,000 copies/mL or less. Emtricitabine/rilpivirine/tenofovir alafenamide also can be used to replace a stable antiretroviral regimen in *certain* antiretroviral-experienced (previously treated) patients who are virologically suppressed (i.e., plasma HIV-1 RNA levels less than 50 copies/mL). Emtricitabine/rilpivirine/tenofovir alafenamide is used alone as a complete regimen for the treatment of HIV-1 infection.

If an HIV NNRTI-based regimen of rilpivirine, emtricitabine, and tenofovir DF is used for the treatment of HIV-1 infection, a fixed-combination preparation containing all 3 drugs (emtricitabine/rilpivirine/tenofovir DF; Complera®) is commercially available and can be used in antiretroviral-naive adults and adolescents 12 years of age or older weighing at least 35 kg with baseline plasma HIV-1 RNA levels of 100,000 copies/mL or less. Emtricitabine/rilpivirine/tenofovir DF also can be used to replace a stable antiretroviral regimen in *certain* antiretroviral-experienced patients who are virologically suppressed (i.e., plasma HIV-1 RNA levels less than 50 copies/mL). Emtricitabine/rilpivirine/tenofovir DF is used alone as a complete treatment regimen.

A fixed-combination preparation of elvitegravir, cobicistat, emtricitabine, and tenofovir alafenamide (EVG/c/FTC/TAF; Genvoya®) and a fixed-combination preparation containing elvitegravir, cobicistat, emtricitabine, and tenofovir DF (EVG/c/FTC/TDF; Stribild®) also are commercially available for use alone as complete regimens for the treatment of HIV-1 infection. For information on EVG/c/FTC/TAF, see Elvitegravir, Cobicistat, Emtricitabine, and Tenofovir Alafenamide in 8:18.08.12. For information on EVG/c/FTC/TDF, see Elvitegravir, Cobicistat, Emtricitabine, and Tenofovir Disoproxil Fumarate in 8:18.08.12.

The most appropriate antiretroviral regimen cannot be defined for each clinical scenario and selection of specific antiretrovirals for use in multiple-drug regimens should be individualized based on information regarding antiretroviral potency, potential rate of development of resistance, known toxicities, and potential for pharmacokinetic interactions as well as virologic, immunologic, and clinical characteristics of the patient. For information on the general principles and guidelines for use of antiretroviral therapy, including specific recommendations for initial therapy in antiretroviral-naive patients and recommendations for changing antiretroviral regimens, see the Antiretroviral Agents General Statement 8:18.08.

Antiretroviral-naive Adults and Adolescents **Dual NRTI Options.** For *initial* treatment in HIV-infected adults and adolescents, the US Department of Health and Human Services (HHS) Panel on Antiretroviral Guidelines for Adults and Adolescents states that emtricitabine and tenofovir DF is a recommended dual NRTI option for use in most INSTI-, NNRTI-, and PI-based regimens. This recommendation is based on safety and efficacy data from clinical trials, long term clinical experience, and availability of fixed-combination preparations containing emtricitabine and tenofovir DF.

The HHS panel states that emtricitabine and tenofovir alafenamide is another recommended dual NRTI option for use in most INSTI-, NNRTI-, and PI-based regimens used for *initial* treatment in antiretroviral-naive adults and adolescents. This recommendation is based on safety and efficacy data from clinical trials, supportive bioequivalence data, and availability of fixed-combination preparations containing emtricitabine and tenofovir alafenamide.

Because all 3 drugs have activity against both HIV *and* hepatitis B virus (HBV), emtricitabine and tenofovir alafenamide or emtricitabine and tenofovir DF are preferred dual NRTI options for antiretroviral regimens used in HIV-infected patients coinfected with HBV.

A dual NRTI option of emtricitabine and didanosine is *not* recommended for *initial* antiretroviral regimens because of inferior virologic efficacy, limited clinical trial experience in antiretroviral-naive patients, and didanosine toxicities (e.g., pancreatitis, peripheral neuropathy).

Emtricitabine and lamivudine should *not* be used concomitantly at any time since the drugs have similar resistance profiles and concomitant use provides no additional benefit.

Efavirenz, Emtricitabine, and Tenofovir DF. Safety and efficacy of a regimen of efavirenz, emtricitabine, and tenofovir DF are based on results of a randomized, open-label study designed to demonstrate noninferiority of this regimen compared with a regimen of efavirenz, zidovudine, and lamivudine (study 934). In this study, 511 antiretroviral-naive HIV-infected patients (mean age 38 years, 86% male, 59% white, 23% black, median baseline plasma HIV-1 RNA level 5.01 $\log_{10}$ copies/mL [range: 3.56–6.54 $\log_{10}$ copies/mL], mean baseline CD4$^+$ T-cell count 245 cells/mm^3) were randomized to receive a once-daily regimen of efavirenz, emtricitabine, and tenofovir DF or a regimen of efavirenz once daily with the fixed combination of lamivudine and zidovudine (lamivudine/zidovudine; Combivir®) twice daily. The primary measure used to assess noninferiority of the regimen of efavirenz, emtricitabine, and tenofovir DF to the regimen of efavirenz and lamivudine/zidovudine was plasma HIV-1 RNA levels at week 48, specifically, the number of patients with HIV-1 RNA levels less than 400 copies/mL. The 487 patients without baseline resistance to efavirenz who underwent randomization and received treatment were the predefined population used for the primary endpoint analysis.

Through week 48, the regimen of efavirenz, emtricitabine, and tenofovir DF met the criteria for noninferiority to the regimen of efavirenz and lamivudine/zidovudine. At week 48, 84 or 80% of adults receiving the efavirenz, tenofovir DF, and emtricitabine regimen and 73 or 70% of adults receiving the efavirenz and lamivudine/zidovudine regimen had plasma HIV-1 RNA levels less than 400 or 50 copies/mL, respectively. At week 48, increases in CD4$^+$ T-cell counts were greater in patients receiving the efavirenz, emtricitabine, and tenofovir DF regimen (mean increase of 190 cells/mm^3) than in those receiving the efavirenz and lamivudine/zidovudine regimen (mean increase of 158 cells/mm^3). Virologic failure (i.e., individuals who failed to achieve virologic suppression or experienced rebound after achieving virologic suppression) was reported in 2% of those receiving efavirenz, emtricitabine, and tenofovir DF and in 4% of those receiving efavirenz and lamivudine/zidovudine at week 48.

At 144 weeks, 64% of adults receiving the efavirenz, emtricitabine, and tenofovir DF regimen and 56% of those receiving the efavirenz and lamivudine/zidovudine regimen had plasma HIV-1 RNA levels less than 50 copies/mL. The mean increase in CD4$^+$ T-cell count from baseline in these groups was 312 and 271 cells/mm^3, respectively, at 144 weeks.

Emtricitabine, Rilpivirine, and Tenofovir Alafenamide. Efficacy of the fixed combination emtricitabine/rilpivirine/tenofovir alafenamide for the treatment of HIV-1 infection in antiretroviral-naive HIV-infected adults is based on results of clinical trials evaluating a regimen of rilpivirine and emtricitabine/tenofovir DF and clinical trials evaluating a regimen of elvitegravir, cobicistat, emtricitabine, and tenofovir alafenamide.

Antiretroviral-experienced Adults and Adolescents The manufacturer states that a decision to use emtricitabine in previously treated patients should be based on the likelihood that the strain of HIV-1 is susceptible to the drug as assessed by laboratory testing (e.g., genotype testing, phenotype testing) and treatment history.

Study 303. Emtricitabine has been evaluated in a randomized, open-label, multicenter study (study 303) in 440 previously treated adults (mean age: 42 years; 86% male; 64% white; 13% Hispanic; 21% African American; median baseline plasma HIV-1 RNA level: 1.7 $\log_{10}$ copies/mL; mean baseline CD4$^+$ T-cell count: 527 cells/mm^3) who had received a lamivudine-containing regimen that also included 2 other antiretrovirals (background regimen) for at least 12 weeks prior to study entry and had plasma HIV-1 levels of 400 copies/mL or less. Patients in this study were randomized to receive emtricitabine in conjunction with stavudine or zidovudine and a PI or NNRTI or to continue their lamivudine-containing background regimen (i.e., lamivudine in conjunction with stavudine or zidovudine and a PI or NNRTI).

At week 48, 77 and 67% of adults receiving the regimen that included emtricitabine and 82 and 72% of those receiving the regimen that included lamivudine had plasma HIV-1 RNA levels less than 400 or 50 copies/mL, respectively. Virologic failure (i.e., individuals who failed to achieve virologic suppression or experienced rebound after achieving virologic suppression) was reported in 7% of those receiving the emtricitabine-containing regimen and in 8% of those receiving the lamivudine-containing regimen at week 48. Administration of the emtricitabine-containing regimen resulted in a mean increase in CD4$^+$ T-cell counts of 29 cells/mm^3; administration of the lamivudine-containing regimen resulted in a mean increase in CD4$^+$ T-cell counts of 61 cells/mm^3.

Efavirenz, Emtricitabine, and Tenofovir DF. Efficacy of the fixed combination efavirenz/emtricitabine/tenofovir DF (Atripla®) was evaluated in a randomized, open-label study (study 073) in antiretroviral-experienced patients who had been receiving a suppressive regimen consisting of at least 2 NRTIs and a PI or NNRTI (mean age 43 years [range 22–73 years]), 88% male, 68% white, 29% black, median CD4$^+$ T-cell count 516 cells/mm^3). Patients had plasma HIV-1 RNA levels less than 200 copies/mL for at least 12 weeks on their existing regimen (96% had plasma HIV-1 levels less than 50 copies/mL), no known HIV-1 substitutions conferring resistance to the components of the fixed combination, and no history of virologic failure; patients were randomized to either switch to efavirenz/emtricitabine/tenofovir DF or continue their existing (baseline) regimen.

At 48 weeks, 89 and 87% of those switched to efavirenz/emtricitabine/tenofovir DF had plasma HIV-1 RNA levels less than 200 and 50 copies/mL, respectively, compared with 88 and 85% of those who remained on their baseline regimen. This difference was not statistically significant. There was no change in CD4$^+$ T-cell count from baseline in either group.

Emtricitabine, Rilpivirine, and Tenofovir Alafenamide. The fixed combination emtricitabine/rilpivirine/tenofovir alafenamide (Odefsey®) can be used to replace a stable antiretroviral regimen for the treatment of HIV-1 in antiretroviral-experienced adults and adolescents 12 years of age or older weighing at least 35 kg who have been virologically suppressed (i.e., plasma HIV-1 RNA levels less than 50 copies/mL) on their current regimen for at least 6 months, have no history of treatment failure, and are infected with HIV-1 with no known substitutions associated with resistance to the antiretroviral components of the fixed combination (i.e., emtricitabine, rilpivirine, tenofovir).

Efficacy of emtricitabine/rilpivirine/tenofovir alafenamide for the treatment of HIV-1 infection in antiretroviral experienced adults is based on results of clinical trials evaluating a regimen of rilpivirine and emtricitabine/tenofovir DF and clinical trials evaluating a regimen of elvitegravir, cobicistat, emtricitabine, and tenofovir alafenamide.

Emtricitabine, Rilpivirine, and Tenofovir DF. The fixed combination emtricitabine/rilpivirine/tenofovir DF (Complera®) can be used to replace a stable antiretroviral regimen for treatment of HIV-1 infection in antiretroviral-experienced adults and adolescents 12 years of age or older weighing at least 35 kg who have been virologically suppressed (i.e., plasma HIV-1 RNA levels less than 50 copies/mL) on their current regimen for at least 6 months, are currently receiving only their first or second antiretroviral regimen, have no history of virologic failure, and have no current evidence or history of resistance to emtricitabine, rilpivirine, or tenofovir DF.

The efficacy and safety of emtricitabine/rilpivirine/tenofovir DF have been evaluated in a randomized, open-label study (study 106) in 476 virologically suppressed HIV-infected adults (mean age 42 years, 88% male, 77% white, 17% black, 17% Hispanic, mean baseline CD4$^+$ T-cell count 584 cells/mm^3). Patients were receiving their first or second antiretroviral regimen with no history of virologic failure; had no history of resistance to emtricitabine, rilpivirine, or tenofovir DF; and were virologically suppressed (plasma HIV-1 RNA levels less than 50 copies/mL) for at least 6 months. Patients were randomized in a 2:1 ratio to switch to emtricitabine/rilpivirine/tenofovir DF for 48 weeks or to continue receiving their baseline antiretroviral regimen containing a *ritonavir-boosted* HIV PI for 24 weeks and then switch to emtricitabine/rilpivirine/tenofovir DF for an additional 24 weeks. In patients initially switched to emtricitabine/rilpivirine/tenofovir DF, 89% maintained plasma HIV-1 RNA levels less than 50 copies/mL at 48 weeks; 90% of those who continued to receive their baseline regimen maintained plasma HIV-1 RNA levels less than 50 copies/mL at 24 weeks.

Pediatric Patients Emtricitabine is used in conjunction with other antiretroviral agents for the treatment of HIV-1 infection in pediatric patients.

The fixed combination emtricitabine/rilpivirine/tenofovir alafenamide or the fixed combination emtricitabine/rilpivirine/tenofovir DF can be used alone as a complete regimen for the treatment of HIV-1 infection in adolescents 12 years of age or older weighing at least 35 kg.

For *initial* treatment of HIV-infected pediatric patients, the HHS Panel on Antiretroviral Therapy and Medical Management of HIV-infected Children recommends a PI-, NNRTI-, or INSTI-based regimen that includes 2 NRTIs (dual NRTIs).

For use in *initial* treatment regimens in pediatric patients, the HHS panel states that emtricitabine and zidovudine is a preferred dual NRTI option for antiretroviral-naive neonates, infants, and children younger than 12 years of age and is an alternative dual NRTI option for antiretroviral-naive adolescents 12 years of age or older in early puberty (sexual maturity rating [SMR] 3). These experts also state that emtricitabine and abacavir is a preferred dual NRTI option in children 3 months of age or older and adolescents 12 years of age or older in early puberty (SMR 1–3) who are negative for human leukocyte antigen (HLA)-B*5701.

The HHS panel states that emtricitabine and tenofovir alafenamide is a preferred dual NRTI option for *initial* treatment regimens in antiretroviral-naive adolescents 12 years of age or older in early puberty (SMR 1–3) with estimated creatinine clearance 30 mL/minute or greater. These experts state that emtricitabine and tenofovir DF is an alternative dual NRTI option for use in antiretroviral-naive children and adolescents 12 years of age or older at SMR 3; however, because decreased bone mineral density (BMD) has been reported in adults and children receiving tenofovir DF, the panel states that the dual option of emtricitabine and tenofovir DF should be used in children 2 years or age or older or adolescents at SMR 1 or 2 *only* in special circumstances after weighing the potential risk of decreased BMD versus the benefits of the dual NRTI option.

Emtricitabine and didanosine is an alternative (not a preferred) dual NRTI option for *initial* treatment regimens in children 2 weeks of age or older.

Emtricitabine and lamivudine should *not* be used concomitantly at any time since the drugs have similar resistance profiles and concomitant use provides no additional benefit.

Antiretroviral regimens containing only NRTIs are *not* recommended for *initial* treatment in antiretroviral-naive pediatric patients because of inferior virologic efficacy.

A triple NRTI regimen that includes abacavir, tenofovir DF, and emtricitabine or a triple NRTI regimen that includes tenofovir DF, didanosine, and emtricitabine should *not* be used at any time in pediatric patients because of the high rate of early virologic failure reported in antiretroviral-naive adults.

For further information on treatment of HIV infection in pediatric patients, see Antiretroviral Therapy in Pediatric Patients, in the Antiretroviral Agents General Statement 8:18.08.

Clinical Experience. Safety and efficacy of emtricitabine in conjunction with other antiretrovirals have been evaluated in 3 open-label, nonrandomized studies in children 3 months to 21 years of age (mean age: 7.9 years; 49% male; 15% white; 24% Hispanic; 61% black; median baseline plasma HIV-1 RNA level: 4.6 $\log_{10}$ copies/mL; mean baseline CD4$^+$ T-cell count: 745 cells/mm^3) who were treatment naive or treatment experienced (i.e., virologic suppression on a lamivudine-containing regimen; emtricitabine substituted for lamivudine). At week 48, 86 or 73% of children had plasma HIV-1 RNA levels less than 400 or 50 copies/mL, respectively. The mean increase in CD4$^+$ T-cell counts was 232 cells/mm^3.

The pharmacokinetics and safety of emtricitabine were evaluated in a dose-finding study in 20 neonates born to HIV-infected mothers. (See Pediatric Use under Warnings/Precautions: Specific Populations, in Cautions.)

■ **Preexposure Prophylaxis for Prevention of HIV-1 Infection** The fixed combination containing emtricitabine and tenofovir DF (emtricitabine/tenofovir DF; Truvada®) is used for preexposure prophylaxis (PrEP) in conjunction with safer sex practices to reduce the risk of sexually-acquired HIV-1 in HIV-1-negative adults at high risk. The manufacturer states that this indication is based on clinical trials in men who have sex with men (MSM) at high risk for HIV-1 infection and in heterosexual HIV-serodiscordant couples.

Adults at high risk for HIV-1 infection include those with partner(s) known to be infected with HIV-1 or those engaging in sexual activity within a high prevalence area or social network and with 1 or more of the following factors: inconsistent or no condom use, diagnosis of sexually transmitted infections, exchange of sex for commodities (e.g., money, food, shelter, drugs), use of illicit drugs, alcohol dependence, incarceration, or partner(s) of unknown HIV-1 status with any of these risk factors.

PrEP with emtricitabine/tenofovir DF (Truvada®) is *not* always effective in preventing acquisition of HIV-1 infection and *must* be used as part of a comprehensive prevention strategy that includes safer sex practices. (See Precautions Related to HIV-1 Preexposure Prophylaxis [PrEP] under Cautions: Warnings/Precautions.)

For additional information on PrEP, see Guidelines for Use of Antiretroviral Agents: Antiretrovirals for Preexposure Prophylaxis for Prevention of HIV-1 Infection (PrEP), in the Antiretroviral Agents General Statement 8:18.08.

Clinical Experience Efficacy and safety of a once-daily regimen of emtricitabine/tenofovir DF for HIV-1 PrEP were evaluated in a multinational, randomized, double-blind, placebo-controlled, phase 3 trial (Preexposure Prophylaxis Initiative [iPrEx trial]; NCT00458393) that included 2499 HIV-seronegative men or transgender women (male at birth) who have sex with men and have evidence of high-risk behavior for HIV-1 infection. Study participants (mean age 27 years [range 18–67 years], 5% Asian, 9% black, 18% white, 72% Hispanic/Latino) were randomized to receive emtricitabine/tenofovir DF (a fixed-combination tablet containing 200 mg of emtricitabine and 300 mg of tenofovir DF once daily) or placebo in conjunction with usual prevention strategies (i.e., monthly HIV-1 testing, risk-reduction counseling, condoms, diagnosis and management of sexually transmitted infections) and were followed for 4237 person-years. The primary outcome measure was the incidence of documented HIV seroconversion. There was a 42% reduction in the risk of HIV-1 seroconversion in the group receiving emtricitabine/tenofovir DF (48 individuals receiving emtricitabine/tenofovir DF and 83 individuals receiving placebo seroconverted). Results of a post-hoc case-control study of plasma and intracellular drug concentrations in about 10% of study participants indicated that efficacy of emtricitabine/tenofovir DF PrEP is strongly correlated with adherence since risk reduction appeared to be greatest in those with detectable intracellular tenofovir DF.

Efficacy and safety of emtricitabine/tenofovir DF for PrEP in HIV-1-seronegative partners of serodiscordant heterosexual couples were evaluated in a randomized, double-blind, placebo-controlled, 3-arm trial (Partners Preexposure Prophylaxis [PrEP] trial; NCT00557245) that included 4758 serodiscordant couples in Kenya and Uganda. The infected partners had median plasma HIV-1 RNA levels of 3.9 $\log_{10}$ copies/mL and median $CD4^+$ T-cell counts of 495 cells/mm^3 (80% had $CD4^+$ T-cell counts of 350 cells/mm^3 or higher). The uninfected partners (mean age 33–34 years, 61–64% male) were randomized to receive emtricitabine/tenofovir DF (a fixed-combination tablet containing 200 mg of emtricitabine and 300 mg of tenofovir DF once daily), tenofovir DF (300 mg of tenofovir DF once daily), or placebo (once daily). Study participants received monthly HIV-1 testing, adherence evaluations, sexual behavior assessments, and safety evaluations. Women received monthly pregnancy tests; if pregnancy occurred, the study drug was interrupted during pregnancy and breast-feeding. After 7827 person-years of follow-up, there were a total of 82 emergent HIV-1 seroconversions (overall observed seroincidence rate of 1.05 per 100 person-years). The risk reduction for the emtricitabine/tenofovir DF group relative to the placebo group was 75%. There were 13 seroconversions in partners randomized to emtricitabine/tenofovir DF and 52 seroconversions in partners randomized to placebo (2 and 3 seroconversions, respectively, occurred during interruption of PrEP for pregnancy). Results of a post-hoc case-control study of plasma and drug concentrations in about 10% of study participants indicated that efficacy of emtricitabine/tenofovir DF PrEP is strongly correlated with adherence since risk reduction appeared to be greatest in those with detectable plasma tenofovir.

■ **Postexposure Prophylaxis following Occupational Exposure to HIV** Emtricitabine is used in conjunction with other antiretrovirals for postexposure prophylaxis of HIV infection following occupational exposure† (PEP) in health-care personnel and other individuals exposed via percutaneous injury (e.g., needlestick, cut with sharp object) or mucous membrane or nonintact skin (e.g., chapped, abraded, dermatitis) contact with blood, tissue, or other body fluids that might contain HIV.

The US Public Health Service (USPHS) states that the preferred regimen for PEP following an occupational exposure to HIV is a 3-drug regimen of raltegravir used in conjunction with emtricitabine and tenofovir DF (may be administered as the fixed combination emtricitabine/tenofovir DF; Truvada®). These experts recommend several alternative regimens that include an INSTI, NNRTI, or PI and 2 NRTIs (dual NRTIs). The preferred dual NRTI option for use in PEP regimens is emtricitabine and tenofovir DF (may be administered as the fixed combination emtricitabine/tenofovir DF; Truvada®); alternative dual NRTIs are tenofovir DF and lamivudine, lamivudine and zidovudine (may be administered as the fixed combination lamivudine/zidovudine; Combivir®), or zidovudine and emtricitabine.

Because management of occupational exposures to HIV is complex and evolving, consultation with an infectious disease specialist, clinician with expertise in administration of antiretroviral agents, and/or the National Clinicians' Postexposure Prophylaxis Hotline (PEPline at 888-448-4911) is recommended whenever possible. However, initiation of PEP should not be delayed while waiting for expert consultation.

For information on types of occupational exposure to HIV and associated risk of infection, management of occupational exposure to HIV, efficacy and safety of postexposure prophylaxis, and recommendations regarding PEP, see Guidelines for Use of Antiretroviral Agents: Antiretrovirals for Postexposure Prophylaxis following Occupational Exposure to HIV (PEP), in the Antiretroviral Agents General Statement 8:18.08.

■ **Postexposure Prophylaxis following Nonoccupational Exposure to HIV** Emtricitabine is used in conjunction with other antiretrovirals for postexposure prophylaxis of HIV infection following nonoccupational exposure† (nPEP) in individuals exposed to blood, genital secretions, or other potentially infectious body fluids that might contain HIV when that exposure represents a substantial risk for HIV transmission.

When nPEP is indicated following a nonoccupational exposure to HIV, the US Centers for Disease Control and Prevention (CDC) states that the preferred regimen in adults and adolescents 13 years of age or older with normal renal function is either raltegravir or dolutegravir used in conjunction with emtricitabine and tenofovir DF (administered as the fixed combination emtricitabine/tenofovir DF; Truvada®). The alternative nPEP regimen recommended in these patients is *ritonavir-boosted* darunavir used in conjunction with emtricitabine/tenofovir DF (Truvada®).

Consultation with an infectious disease specialist, clinician with expertise in administration of antiretroviral agents, and/or the National Clinicians' Postexposure Prophylaxis Hotline (PEPline at 888-448-4911) is recommended if nPEP is indicated in certain exposed individuals (e.g., pregnant women, children, those with medical conditions such as renal impairment) or if an antiretroviral regimen not included in the CDC guidelines is being considered, the source virus is known or likely to be resistant to antiretrovirals, or the healthcare provider is inexperienced in prescribing antiretrovirals. However, initiation of nPEP should not be delayed while waiting for expert consultation.

For additional information on nonoccupational exposure to HIV and recommendations regarding postexposure prophylaxis, see Guidelines for Use of Antiretroviral Agents: Antiretrovirals for Postexposure Prophylaxis after Sexual, Injection Drug Use, or other Nonoccupational Exposures to HIV (nPEP), in the Antiretroviral Agents General Statement 8:18.08.

Dosage and Administration

■ **Administration** Emtricitabine is administered orally once daily without regard to meals.

Single-entity emtricitabine is commercially available as 200-mg capsules or an oral solution containing 10 mg/mL.

Emtricitabine is used in conjunction with other antiretrovirals. Single-entity emtricitabine should not be used concomitantly with any other emtricitabine-containing preparation or with any preparation containing lamivudine.

Fixed Combinations Containing Emtricitabine Emtricitabine is commercially available in fixed-combination tablets containing emtricitabine and tenofovir alafenamide fumarate (emtricitabine/tenofovir alafenamide; Descovy®), fixed-combination tablets containing emtricitabine and tenofovir disoproxil fumarate (emtricitabine/tenofovir DF; Truvada®), fixed-combination tablets containing efavirenz, emtricitabine, and tenofovir DF (efavirenz/emtricitabine/tenofovir DF; Atripla), fixed-combination tablets containing rilpivirine, emtricitabine, and tenofovir alafenamide fumarate (emtricitabine/rilpivirine/tenofovir alafenamide; Odefsey®), and fixed-combination tablets containing emtricitabine, rilpivirine, and tenofovir DF (emtricitabine/rilpivirine/tenofovir DF; Complera®). In addition, emtricitabine is commercially available in fixed-combination tablets containing elvitegravir, cobicistat, emtricitabine, and tenofovir alafenamide fumarate (EVG/c/FTC/TAF; Genvoya®) and fixed-combination tablets containing elvitegravir, cobicistat, emtricitabine, and tenofovir DF (EVG/c/FTC/TDF; Stribild®). For information on EVG/c/FTC/TAF, see Elvitegravir, Cobicistat, Emtricitabine, and Tenofovir Alafenamide in 8:18.08.12. For information on EVG/c/FTC/TDF, see Elvitegravir, Cobicistat, Emtricitabine, and Tenofovir Disoproxil Fumarate in 8:18.08.12.

Emtricitabine/tenofovir alafenamide (Descovy®) tablets are administered orally once daily without regard to meals. For the treatment of human immunodeficiency virus type 1 (HIV-1) infection, emtricitabine/tenofovir alafenamide is used in conjunction with other antiretrovirals.

Emtricitabine/tenofovir DF (Truvada®) tablets are administered orally once daily without regard to meals. A fixed-combination tablet containing 200 mg of emtricitabine and 300 mg of tenofovir DF is bioequivalent to a 200-mg capsule of emtricitabine and a 300-mg tablet of tenofovir DF given simultaneously. For the treatment of human immunodeficiency virus type 1 (HIV-1) infection, emtricitabine/tenofovir DF is used in conjunction with other antiretrovirals. For preexposure prophylaxis (PrEP) for prevention of HIV-1 infection, emtricitabine/tenofovir DF is used alone without any other antiretrovirals.

Efavirenz/emtricitabine/tenofovir DF (Atripla®) tablets are administered orally once daily on an empty stomach, preferably at bedtime. Administration at bedtime may make efavirenz-related adverse CNS effects more tolerable. A fixed-combination tablet containing 600 mg of efavirenz, 200 mg of emtricitabine, and 300 mg of tenofovir DF is bioequivalent to a 600-mg tablet of efavirenz, 200-mg capsule of emtricitabine, and 300-mg tablet of tenofovir DF when taken in the fasting state. The fixed combination can be used alone as a complete treatment regimen or in conjunction with other antiretrovirals.

Emtricitabine/rilpivirine/tenofovir alafenamide (Odefsey®) tablets are administered orally once daily with a meal. The fixed combination is used alone as a complete treatment regimen.

Emtricitabine/rilpivirine/tenofovir DF (Complera®) tablets are administered orally once daily with a meal. A fixed-combination tablet containing 200 mg of emtricitabine, 25 mg of rilpivirine, and 300 mg of tenofovir DF taken with a meal is bioequivalent to a 200-mg emtricitabine capsule, 25-mg rilpivirine tablet, and 300-mg tenofovir DF tablet taken simultaneously with a meal. The fixed combination is used alone as a complete treatment regimen.

Because the antiretroviral agents contained in the fixed-combination preparations also may be available in single-entity or other fixed-combination preparations, care should be taken to ensure that therapy is not duplicated if a fixed combination is used in conjunction with other antiretrovirals. (See Precautions Related to Use of Fixed Combinations under Warnings/Precautions: Other Warnings/Precautions, in Cautions.)

■ Dosage

Emtricitabine (Emtriva®) capsules and oral solution are not bioequivalent. Bioavailability of the oral solution is 80% relative to that of the capsule.

Adult Dosage

Treatment of HIV Infection. For the treatment of HIV-1 infection in adults 18 years of age or older, the usual dosage of emtricitabine (Emtriva®) is 200 mg (as the capsule) once daily. Alternatively, when the oral solution containing 10 mg/mL is used, the usual dosage of emtricitabine (Emtriva®) is 240 mg (24 mL) once daily.

When emtricitabine/tenofovir alafenamide (Descovy®) is used in conjunction with other antiretrovirals for the treatment of HIV-1 infection, adults should receive 1 tablet (200 mg of emtricitabine and 25 mg of tenofovir alafenamide) once daily.

When emtricitabine/tenofovir DF (Truvada®) is used in conjunction with other antiretrovirals for the treatment of HIV-1 infection, adults should receive 1 tablet (200 mg of emtricitabine and 300 mg of tenofovir DF) once daily.

When efavirenz/emtricitabine/tenofovir DF (Atripla®) is used for the treatment of HIV-1 infection, adults should receive 1 tablet (600 mg of efavirenz, 200 mg of emtricitabine, and 300 mg of tenofovir DF) once daily.

When emtricitabine/rilpivirine/tenofovir alafenamide (Odefsey®) is used for the treatment of HIV-1 infection, adults should receive 1 tablet (200 mg of emtricitabine, 25 mg of rilpivirine, and 25 mg of tenofovir alafenamide) once daily.

When emtricitabine/rilpivirine/tenofovir DF (Complera®) is used for the treatment of HIV-1 infection, adults should receive 1 tablet (200 mg of emtricitabine, 25 mg of rilpivirine, and 300 mg of tenofovir DF) once daily.

Preexposure Prophylaxis for Prevention of HIV-1 Infection. When emtricitabine/tenofovir DF (Truvada®) is used for preexposure prophylaxis (PrEP) for prevention of HIV-1 infection in HIV-1-negative adults at high risk, the recommended dosage is 1 tablet (200 mg of emtricitabine and 300 mg of tenofovir DF) once daily.

PrEP should *only* be used in high-risk adults (see Uses: Preexposure Prophylaxis for Prevention of HIV-1 Infection) with confirmed HIV-1-negative status. PrEP should *not* be initiated if signs or symptoms of acute HIV-1 infection are present and recent (within the past month) exposure to HIV-1 is suspected. (See Precautions Related to HIV-1 Preexposure Prophylaxis [PrEP] under Cautions: Warnings/Precautions.)

Postexposure Prophylaxis following Occupational Exposure to HIV. For postexposure prophylaxis of HIV infection following occupational exposure† (PEP) in health-care personnel or other individuals, the recommended dosage of emtricitabine is 200 mg (as the capsule) once daily. Emtricitabine usually is used with tenofovir DF or zidovudine in conjunction with a recommended HIV integrase strand transferase inhibitor (INSTI), nonnucleoside reverse transcriptase inhibitor (NNRTI), or HIV protease inhibitor (PI). (See Uses: Postexposure Prophylaxis following Occupational Exposure to HIV.)

When emtricitabine/tenofovir DF (Truvada®) is used as the dual NRTI option in PEP† regimens, adults should receive 1 tablet (200 mg of emtricitabine and 300 mg of tenofovir DF) once daily in conjunction with a recommended INSTI, NNRTI, or PI. (See Uses: Postexposure Prophylaxis following Occupational Exposure to HIV.)

When emtricitabine/rilpivirine/tenofovir DF (Complera®) is used as a complete regimen for PEP†, adults should receive 1 tablet (200 mg of emtricitabine, 25 mg of rilpivirine, and 300 mg of tenofovir DF) once daily.

The PEP regimen should be initiated as soon as possible following occupational exposure to HIV (preferably within hours) and continued for 4 weeks, if tolerated.

Postexposure Prophylaxis following Nonoccupational Exposure to HIV. For postexposure prophylaxis of HIV infection following nonoccupational exposure† (nPEP) when the exposure represents a substantial risk for HIV transmission, the usual adult dosage of emtricitabine is 200 mg once daily in conjunction with other antiretrovirals. Emtricitabine usually is used in conjunction with tenofovir DF and a recommended or alternative INSTI, PI, or NNRTI. (See Uses: Postexposure Prophylaxis following Nonoccupational Exposure to HIV.)

When emtricitabine/tenofovir DF (Truvada®) is used as the dual NRTI option in nPEP† regimens, adults should receive 1 tablet (200 mg of emtricitabine and 300 mg of tenofovir DF) once daily in conjunction with a preferred or alternative INSTI, PI, or NNRTI.

When emtricitabine/rilpivirine/tenofovir DF (Complera®) is used as a complete regimen for nPEP†, adults should receive 1 tablet (200 mg of emtricitabine, 25 mg of rilpivirine, and 300 mg of tenofovir DF) once daily.

The nPEP regimen should be initiated as soon as possible (within 72 hours) following nonoccupational exposure to HIV and continued for 28 days. If the exposed individual seeks care more than 72 hours after the exposure, nPEP is not recommended.

Pediatric Dosage

Treatment of HIV Infection. For the treatment of HIV-1 infection in pediatric patients 3 months to 17 years of age, the usual dosage of emtricitabine (Emtriva®) is 6 mg/kg (as the oral solution containing 10 mg/mL) once daily (maximum 240 mg daily). Alternatively, children weighing more than 33 kg who can swallow an intact capsule may receive one 200-mg capsule once daily.

The usual dosage of emtricitabine (Emtriva®) for the treatment of HIV-1 infection in infants 0–3 months of age is 3 mg/kg (as the oral solution containing 10 mg/mL) once daily.

When emtricitabine/tenofovir alafenamide (Descovy®) is used in conjunction with other antiretrovirals for the treatment of HIV-1 infection in adolescents 12 years of age or older weighing at least 35 kg, the recommended dosage is 1 tablet (200 mg of emtricitabine and 25 mg of tenofovir alafenamide) once daily.

When emtricitabine/tenofovir DF (Truvada®) is used in conjunction with other antiretrovirals for the treatment of HIV-1 infection in children weighing at least 35 kg, the recommended dosage is 1 tablet (200 mg of emtricitabine and 300 mg of tenofovir DF) once daily. When emtricitabine/tenofovir DF (Truvada®) is used in conjunction with other antiretrovirals for the treatment of HIV-1 infection in children weighing 17 to less than 35 kg who are able to swallow a tablet, the recommended dosage is based on weight; a low-strength fixed-combination tablet of the drug should be used. (See Table 1.)

Table 1. Emtricitabine/tenofovir DF (Truvada®) Dosage for Treatment of HIV-1 Infection in Children Weighing 17 kg or more

Weight (kg)	Dosage of Emtricitabine/tenofovir DF given Once Daily
17 to less than 22 kg	1 tablet (100 mg of emtricitabine and 150 mg of tenofovir DF)
22 to less than 28 kg	1 tablet (133 mg of emtricitabine and 200 mg of tenofovir DF)
28 to less than 35 kg	1 tablet (167 mg of emtricitabine and 250 mg of tenofovir DF)
35 kg or more	1 tablet (200 mg of emtricitabine and 300 mg of tenofovir DF)

When efavirenz/emtricitabine/tenofovir DF (Atripla®) is used for the treatment of HIV-1 infection in adolescents 12 years of age or older weighing at least 40 kg, the recommended dosage is 1 tablet (600 mg of efavirenz, 200 mg of emtricitabine, and 300 mg of tenofovir DF) once daily.

When emtricitabine/rilpivirine/tenofovir alafenamide (Odefsey®) is used for the treatment of HIV-1 infection in adolescents 12 years of age or older weighing at least 35 kg, the usual dosage is 1 tablet (200 mg of emtricitabine, 25 mg of rilpivirine, and 25 mg of tenofovir alafenamide) once daily.

When emtricitabine/rilpivirine/tenofovir DF (Complera®) is used for the treatment of HIV-1 infection in adolescents 12 years of age or older weighing at least 35 kg, the usual dosage is 1 tablet (200 mg of emtricitabine, 25 mg of rilpivirine, and 300 mg of tenofovir DF) once daily.

■ Special Populations

Hepatic Impairment

While the pharmacokinetics of emtricitabine have not been specifically studied in patients with hepatic impairment, the drug is not metabolized by liver enzymes and clinically important changes in emtricitabine metabolism are not expected if the drug is used in patients with hepatic impairment.

If emtricitabine/tenofovir alafenamide (Descovy®) is used for the treatment of HIV-1 infection in patients with mild or moderate hepatic impairment (Child-Pugh class A or B), usual dosage can be used; the fixed combination has not been studied in those with severe hepatic impairment (Child-Pugh class C).

Emtricitabine/tenofovir DF (Truvada®) has not been studied in patients with hepatic impairment.

When efavirenz/emtricitabine/tenofovir DF (Atripla®) is used for the treatment of HIV-1 infection, usual dosage can be used in patients with mild hepatic impairment; however, caution is advised. The fixed combination is *not* recommended in those with moderate or severe hepatic impairment.

When emtricitabine/rilpivirine/tenofovir alafenamide (Odefsey®) is used for the treatment of HIV-1 infection in patients with mild or moderate hepatic impairment (Child-Pugh class A or B), usual dosage can be used; the fixed combination has not been studied in those with severe hepatic impairment (Child-Pugh class C).

When emtricitabine/rilpivirine/tenofovir DF (Complera®) is used for the treatment of HIV-1 infection in patients with mild or moderate hepatic impairment (Child-Pugh class A or B), usual dosage can be used; the fixed combination has not been studied in those with severe hepatic impairment (Child-Pugh class C).

Renal Impairment When emtricitabine (Emtriva®) is used for the treatment of HIV-1 infection in adults, dosage should be adjusted in those with creatinine clearance less than 50 mL/minute (see Table 2). The manufacturer states that data are insufficient to make emtricitabine dosage recommendations for treatment of HIV-1 infection in pediatric patients with renal impairment; however, a reduction in the dose and/or increase in dosing interval similar to adjustments for adults should be considered.

Table 2. Emtricitabine (Emtriva®) Dosage for Treatment of HIV-1 Infection in Adults with Renal Impairment

Creatinine Clearance (mL/minute)	Dosage of Capsules	Dosage of Oral Solution
30–49	200 mg every 48 hours	120 mg every 24 hours
15–29	200 mg every 72 hours	80 mg every 24 hours
less than 15	200 mg every 96 hours	60 mg every 24 hours
Hemodialysis patients	200 mg every 96 hours; on day of dialysis, give dose after the procedure	60 mg every 24 hours; on day of dialysis, give dose after the procedure

When emtricitabine/tenofovir alafenamide (Descovy®) is used for the treatment of HIV-1 infection, usual dosage can be used in patients with estimated creatinine clearance of 30 mL/minute or greater; the fixed combination is *not* recommended in those with severe renal impairment (estimated creatinine clearance less than 30 mL/minute).

When emtricitabine/tenofovir DF (Truvada®) is used for the treatment of HIV-1 infection in adults, usual dosage can be used in those with mild renal impairment (creatinine clearance 50–80 mL/minute), but calculated creatinine clearance, serum phosphorus, urine glucose, and urine protein should be monitored. If the fixed combination is used in adults with creatinine clearance of 30–49 mL/minute, dosage should be reduced to 1 tablet (200 mg of emtricitabine and 300 mg of tenofovir DF) once every 48 hours; clinical response and renal function should be monitored since dosage has not been evaluated clinically. Emtricitabine/tenofovir DF should *not* be used for treatment of HIV-1 infection in adults with creatinine clearances less than 30 mL/minute (including hemodialysis patients). Data are insufficient to make dosage recommendations for the fixed combination for treatment of HIV-1 infection in pediatric patients with renal impairment.

When emtricitabine/tenofovir DF (Truvada®) is used for PrEP for prevention of HIV-1 infection in HIV-1-negative adults at high risk, usual dosage can be used in those with creatinine clearances of 60 mL/minute or greater, but calculated creatinine clearance, serum phosphorus, urine glucose, and urine protein should be monitored. If creatinine clearance decreases while emtricitabine/tenofovir DF is being used for PrEP, potential causes should be evaluated and potential risks and benefits of continued use should be reassessed. Emtricitabine/tenofovir DF should *not* be used for PrEP in adults with creatinine clearances less than 60 mL/minute.

When efavirenz/emtricitabine/tenofovir DF (Atripla®) is used for the treatment of HIV-1 infection, usual dosage can be used in patients with creatinine clearance of 50 mL/minute or greater. The fixed combination should *not* be used in those with moderate or severe renal impairment (estimated creatinine clearances less than 50 mL/minute).

When emtricitabine/rilpivirine/tenofovir alafenamide (Odefsey®) is used for the treatment of HIV-1 infection, usual dosage can be used in patients with estimated creatinine clearance of 30 mL/minute or greater; the fixed combination is *not* recommended in those with severe renal impairment (estimated creatinine clearance less than 30 mL/minute).

Emtricitabine/rilpivirine/tenofovir DF (Complera®) should *not* be used in patients with renal impairment that is moderate, severe, or end-stage (estimated creatinine clearance less than 50 mL/minute) or requires dialysis.

Cautions

■ Contraindications

Emtricitabine is contraindicated in patients with known hypersensitivity to the drug or any ingredient in the formulation.

The manufacturer states that there are no known contraindications for use of the fixed combination of emtricitabine and tenofovir alafenamide (emtricitabine/tenofovir alafenamide; Descovy®).

The fixed combination containing emtricitabine and tenofovir disoproxil fumarate (emtricitabine/tenofovir DF; Truvada®) should *not* be used alone for treatment of HIV-1 infection and should *not* be used for preexposure prophylaxis of HIV-1 infection in individuals with unknown or positive HIV-1 status. (See Precautions Related to HIV-1 Preexposure Prophylaxis under Warnings/Precautions: Warnings, in Cautions.)

The fixed combination containing efavirenz, emtricitabine, and tenofovir DF (efavirenz/emtricitabine/tenofovir DF; Atripla®) is contraindicated in patients who have had a clinically important hypersensitivity reaction (e.g., Stevens-Johnson syndrome, erythema multiforme, toxic skin eruption) to efavirenz; because of the efavirenz component, concomitant use of this fixed combination and voriconazole is contraindicated.

Concomitant use of the fixed combination containing emtricitabine, rilpivirine, and tenofovir alafenamide (emtricitabine/rilpivirine/tenofovir alafenamide; Odefsey®) or fixed combination containing emtricitabine, rilpivirine, and tenofovir disoproxil fumarate (emtricitabine/rilpivirine/tenofovir DF; Complera®) and certain drugs that induce cytochrome P-450 isoenzyme 3A (CYP3A) or drugs that elevate gastric pH is contraindicated because of the rilpivirine component; substantially decreased plasma concentrations of rilpivirine may occur and may result in loss of virologic response and development of resistance to rilpivirine and/or class resistance to human immunodeficiency virus (HIV) nonnucleoside reverse transcriptase inhibitors (NNRTIs).

When emtricitabine/tenofovir alafenamide, emtricitabine/tenofovir DF, efavirenz/emtricitabine/tenofovir DF, emtricitabine/rilpivirine/tenofovir alafenamide, or emtricitabine/rilpivirine/tenofovir DF are used, the contraindications associated with each drug in the fixed combination should be considered. (See Precautions Related to Use of Fixed Combinations under Warnings/Precautions: Other Warnings/Precautions, in Cautions.)

■ Warnings/Precautions

Warnings **Lactic Acidosis and Severe Hepatomegaly with Steatosis.** Lactic acidosis and severe hepatomegaly with steatosis, including fatalities, have been reported in patients receiving HIV nucleoside reverse transcriptase inhibitors (NRTIs), including emtricitabine with or without a tenofovir prodrug, in conjunction with other antiretroviral agents. Most reported cases have involved women; obesity and long-term therapy with NRTIs also may be risk factors.

Caution should be observed when NRTIs are used in patients with known risk factors for liver disease; however, lactic acidosis and severe hepatomegaly with steatosis have been reported in patients with no known risk factors. Emtricitabine (single-entity or fixed-combination preparations) should be discontinued in any patient with clinical or laboratory findings suggestive of lactic acidosis or pronounced hepatotoxicity (signs of hepatotoxicity include hepatomegaly and steatosis even in the absence of marked increases in serum aminotransferase concentrations).

Individuals with Hepatitis B Virus Infection. Prior to initiating emtricitabine (single-entity or fixed-combination preparations) for treatment of human immunodeficiency virus type 1 (HIV-1) infection, the patient should be tested for chronic hepatitis B virus (HBV).

Although emtricitabine has some activity against HBV, single-entity or fixed-combination preparations containing emtricitabine are *not* indicated for treatment of chronic HBV infection.

Safety and efficacy of emtricitabine (single-entity or fixed-combination preparations) have not been established in patients with HBV and HIV-1 coinfection. However, when selecting components of an antiretroviral regimen for HIV-infected patients coinfected with HBV, some experts state that emtricitabine and tenofovir alafenamide or emtricitabine and tenofovir DF are preferred dual NRTI options in such patients since these antiretrovirals have activity against both HIV *and* HBV.

Severe acute exacerbations of HBV infection have been reported in HIV-infected patients following discontinuance of emtricitabine with or without a tenofovir prodrug. In some of these patients, exacerbations of HBV have been associated with hepatic decompensation and hepatic failure. Hepatic function should be closely monitored with clinical and laboratory follow-up for at least several months after stopping emtricitabine therapy (single-entity or fixed-combination preparations) in HIV-infected patients coinfected with HBV. If appropriate, initiation of treatment for HBV infection may be warranted.

Precautions Related to HIV-1 Preexposure Prophylaxis. Only the fixed combination containing emtricitabine and tenofovir DF (emtricitabine/tenofovir DF; Truvada®) should be used for PrEP. Emtricitabine should *not* be used alone for HIV-1 PrEP.

Emtricitabine/tenofovir DF should be used for HIV-1 PrEP *only* in HIV-1-negative adults at high risk.

A negative HIV-1 test should be confirmed immediately prior to initiation of emtricitabine/tenofovir DF for HIV-1 PrEP and screening for HIV-1 infection should be performed at least once every 3 months during PrEP. Individuals also should be tested for HBV prior to initiation of emtricitabine/tenofovir DF PrEP. (See Individuals with Hepatitis B Virus (HBV) Infection under Cautions: Warnings/Precautions.)

Emtricitabine/tenofovir DF PrEP is *not* always effective in preventing acquisition of HIV-1 infection.

Emtricitabine/tenofovir DF PrEP *must* be used as part of a comprehensive HIV prevention strategy that includes other prevention measures (e.g., safer sex practices). (See REMS.) All uninfected individuals should be counseled about safer sex practices that include consistent and correct use of condoms, knowledge of their own HIV-1 status and that of their partner(s), and regular testing for other sexually transmitted infections that can facilitate HIV-1 transmission (e.g., syphilis, gonorrhea). All HIV-negative individuals should be informed about and supported in their efforts to reduce sexual risk behavior.

Because emtricitabine/tenofovir DF alone does not constitute a complete antiretroviral regimen for treatment of HIV-1 infection, HIV-1 resistance-associated mutations may emerge if PrEP is used in individuals with undetected HIV-1 infection. Drug-resistant HIV-1 variants have been identified when emtricitabine/tenofovir DF PrEP was used in such individuals.

Clinicians should consider that many HIV-1 tests (e.g., rapid tests) detect anti-HIV antibodies and may not identify HIV-1 during the acute stage of infection. Prior to initiating emtricitabine/tenofovir DF PrEP, clinicians should evaluate HIV-negative individuals for current or recent signs or symptoms consistent with acute viral infection (e.g., fever, fatigue, myalgia, rash) and ask about any potential exposure events that may have occurred within the last month (e.g., unprotected sex, condom broke during sex with HIV-infected partner).

If clinical symptoms consistent with acute viral infection are present and recent (within 1 month) exposures to HIV-1 are suspected, initiation of emtricitabine/tenofovir DF PrEP should be delayed for at least 1 month and HIV-1 status reconfirmed or a test approved by the US Food and Drug Administration (FDA) for use as an aid in the diagnosis of HIV-1 infection, including acute or primary HIV-1 infection, should be used.

During emtricitabine/tenofovir DF PrEP, if symptoms consistent with acute HIV-1 infection develop following a potential exposure event, the drugs should be discontinued until negative infection status is confirmed using a test approved by FDA as an aid in the diagnosis of HIV-1 infection, including acute or primary HIV-1 infection.

Uninfected individuals should be counseled to strictly adhere to the recommended emtricitabine/tenofovir DF dosage schedule (see Preexposure Prophylaxis for Prevention of HIV-1 Infection under Dosage: Adult Dosage, in Dosage and Administration). Effectiveness of the fixed combination in reducing the risk of acquiring HIV-1 is strongly correlated with adherence as demonstrated by measurable tenofovir concentrations in clinical trials.

Adverse effects reported in HIV-negative adults receiving emtricitabine/tenofovir DF PrEP are similar to those reported in HIV-infected patients receiving the drugs for treatment of HIV-1 infection.

Other Warnings/Precautions

Precautions Related to Use of Fixed Combinations. When emtricitabine/tenofovir alafenamide, emtricitabine/tenofovir DF, efavirenz/emtricitabine/tenofovir DF, emtricitabine/rilpivirine/tenofovir alafenamide, or emtricitabine/rilpivirine/tenofovir DF is used, the cautions, precautions, contraindications, and drug interactions associated with each drug in the fixed combination must be considered. Cautionary information applicable to specific populations (e.g., pregnant or nursing women, individuals with hepatic or renal impairment, geriatric patients) should be considered for each drug. For cautionary information related to efavirenz, rilpivirine, and tenofovir DF, see Cautions in the individual drug monographs.

Because the antiretrovirals contained in the fixed-combination preparations also may be available in single-entity or other fixed-combination preparations, care should be taken to ensure that therapy is not duplicated when a fixed combination is used in conjunction with other antiretrovirals.

Multiple emtricitabine-containing preparations should not be used concomitantly.

Because of similarities between emtricitabine and lamivudine, emtricitabine (single-entity or fixed-combination preparations) should not be used concomitantly with any preparation containing lamivudine. In addition, fixed combinations containing tenofovir DF should not be used concomitantly with adefovir dipivoxil.

Adipogenic Effects. Redistribution or accumulation of body fat, including central obesity, dorsocervical fat enlargement ("buffalo hump"), peripheral wasting, breast enlargement, and general cushingoid appearance, has been reported in patients receiving antiretroviral therapy. The mechanism and long-term consequences of fat redistribution are unknown; a causal relationship has not been established.

Immune Reconstitution Syndrome. Immune reconstitution syndrome has been reported in HIV-infected patients receiving multiple-drug antiretroviral therapy, including emtricitabine. During the initial phase of treatment, HIV-infected patients whose immune systems respond to antiretroviral therapy may develop an inflammatory response to indolent or residual opportunistic infections (e.g., *Mycobacterium avium* complex [MAC], *M. tuberculosis*, cytomegalovirus [CMV], *Pneumocystis jirovecii* [formerly *P. carinii*]); such response may necessitate further evaluation and treatment.

Autoimmune disorders (e.g., Graves' disease, polymyositis, Guillain-Barré syndrome) have also been reported to occur in the setting of immune reconstitution; however, the time to onset is more variable and can occur many months after initiation of antiretroviral therapy.

Specific Populations

Pregnancy. Emtricitabine (Emtriva®): Category B. (See Users Guide)

Emtricitabine/tenofovir alafenamide (Descovy®): Insufficient human data to assess the risk of birth defects and miscarriage if used in pregnant women.

Emtricitabine/tenofovir DF (Truvada®): Category B.

Efavirenz/emtricitabine/tenofovir DF (Atripla®): Category D. (See Pregnancy under Cautions: Pregnancy, Fertility, and Lactation, in Efavirenz 8:18.08.16.)

Emtricitabine/rilpivirine/tenofovir alafenamide (Odefsey®): Insufficient human data to assess the risk of birth defects and miscarriage if used in pregnant women.

Emtricitabine/rilpivirine/tenofovir DF (Complera®): Category B.

Antiretroviral Pregnancy Registry at 800-258-4263 or http://www.APRegistry.com.

The US Department of Health and Human Services (HHS) Panel on Treatment of HIV-infected Pregnant Women and Prevention of Perinatal Transmission states that emtricitabine and tenofovir DF is a preferred dual NRTI option for use in conjunction with an HIV integrase strand transfer inhibitor (INSTI), HIV nonnucleoside reverse transcriptase inhibitor (NNRTI), or HIV protease inhibitor (PI) for *initial* treatment of HIV-1 infection in antiretroviral-naive pregnant women, and is a preferred dual NRTI option in pregnant women coinfected with HBV.

Some experts state that the dual NRTI option of emtricitabine and tenofovir DF used in conjunction with the fixed combination of lopinavir and ritonavir (lopinavir/ritonavir) is a preferred regimen for treatment of HIV type 2 (HIV-2) infection† in pregnant women.

If an HIV-1-negative woman receiving emtricitabine/tenofovir DF (Truvada®) for HIV-1 PrEP becomes pregnant, careful consideration should be given to whether the PrEP regimen should be continued, taking into account the potential increased risk of HIV-1 infection during pregnancy.

Lactation. Emtricitabine is distributed into human milk in low concentrations.

Because of the risk of adverse effects in the infant and the risk of HIV transmission, HIV-infected women should not breast-feed infants.

Pediatric Use. Safety and efficacy of emtricitabine (Emtriva®) have been established for treatment of HIV-1 infection in children 3 months of age and older.

The pharmacokinetics and safety of emtricitabine were evaluated in a dose-finding study in 20 neonates born to HIV-infected mothers. These neonates received zidovudine prophylaxis for 6 weeks. In addition, these neonates received 2 short courses of emtricitabine (3 mg/kg daily for 4 days per course) during the first 12 weeks of life. This dose was well tolerated and was not associated with any safety issues. Systemic exposure (area under the plasma concentration-time curve [AUC]) in infants 0–3 months of age receiving emtricitabine 3 mg/kg daily was similar to that reported in children 3 months to 17 years of age receiving emtricitabine 6 mg/kg daily. All neonates were HIV-1 negative at the end of the study (6 months postpartum); efficacy of emtricitabine for the prevention or treatment of HIV was not determined.

Emtricitabine/tenofovir alafenamide (Descovy®) should *not* be used in pediatric patients younger than 12 years of age or weighing less than 35 kg.

Safety and efficacy of emtricitabine/tenofovir DF (Truvada®) for treatment of HIV-1 infection have *not* been established in pediatric patients weighing less than 17 kg; safety and efficacy of this fixed combination for HIV-1 PrEP have *not* been established in pediatric patients.

Efavirenz/emtricitabine/tenofovir DF (Atripla®): Should *not* be used in pediatric patients younger than 12 years of age or weighing less than 40 kg.

Emtricitabine/rilpivirine/tenofovir alafenamide (Odefsey®): Safety and efficacy have *not* been established in pediatric patients younger than 12 years of age or weighing less than 35 kg.

Emtricitabine/rilpivirine/tenofovir DF (Complera®): Safety and efficacy have *not* been established in pediatric patients younger than 12 years of age or weighing less than 35 kg.

Geriatric Use. Experience in those 65 years of age or older is insufficient to determine whether they respond differently to emtricitabine (single-entity or fixed-combination preparations) than younger adults. Dosage should be selected with caution because of age-related decreases in hepatic, renal, and/or cardiac function and potential for concomitant disease and drug therapy.

Hepatic Impairment. Emtricitabine has not been studied in patients with hepatic impairment; impact of hepatic impairment is expected to be minimal. (See Hepatic Impairment under Dosage and Administration: Special Populations.)

Emtricitabine/tenofovir alafenamide (Descovy®) has not been studied in patients with severe hepatic impairment (Child-Pugh class C).

Emtricitabine/tenofovir DF (Truvada®) has not been studied in patients with hepatic impairment. Hepatic impairment does not have a substantial effect on tenofovir DF pharmacokinetics and is expected to have a minimal impact on emtricitabine pharmacokinetics.

Efavirenz/emtricitabine/tenofovir DF (Atripla®) is *not* recommended in patients with moderate or severe hepatic impairment.

Emtricitabine/rilpivirine/tenofovir alafenamide (Odefsey®) has not been studied in patients with severe hepatic impairment (Child-Pugh class C).

Emtricitabine/rilpivirine/tenofovir DF (Complera®) has not been studied in patients with severe hepatic impairment (Child-Pugh class C).

Renal Impairment. Emtricitabine is principally eliminated by the kidney and the pharmacokinetics of the drug are altered in patients with renal impairment. If renal function is impaired, dosage of single-entity emtricitabine (Emtriva®) must be adjusted based on creatinine clearance. (See Renal Impairment under Dosage and Administration: Special Populations.)

Emtricitabine/tenofovir alafenamide (Descovy®) is *not* recommended in patients with severe renal impairment (estimated creatinine clearance less than 30 mL/minute).

Emtricitabine/tenofovir DF (Truvada®) should *not* be used for treatment of HIV-1 infection in patients with creatinine clearance less than 30 mL/minute or in those with end-stage renal disease requiring dialysis; dosage adjustments are necessary when the drug is used for treatment of HIV-1 infection in those with creatinine clearance 30–49 mL/minute. (See Renal Impairment under Dosage and Administration: Special Populations.) Emtricitabine/tenofovir DF should *not* be used for PrEP in HIV-1 uninfected adults with creatinine clearance less than 60 mL/minute. If creatinine clearance decreases while emtricitabine/tenofovir DF is being used for PrEP, potential causes should be evaluated and potential risks and benefits of continued use should be reassessed.

Efavirenz/emtricitabine/tenofovir DF (Atripla®) should *not* be used in patients with moderate or severe renal impairment (estimated creatinine clearance less than 50 mL/minute,).

Emtricitabine/rilpivirine/tenofovir alafenamide (Odefsey®) is *not* recommended in patients with severe renal impairment (estimated creatinine clearance less than 30 mL/minute).

Emtricitabine/rilpivirine/tenofovir DF (Complera®) should *not* be used in patients with renal impairment that is moderate, severe, or end-stage (estimated creatinine clearance less than 50 mL/minute) or requires dialysis.

■ **Common Adverse Effects** The most common adverse effects in adults receiving emtricitabine in conjunction with other antiretrovirals are mild to moderate headache, diarrhea, nausea, and rash. Adverse effects reported in children 3 months to 21 years of age receiving emtricitabine in clinical studies have been similar to those in adults, with the exception of a higher frequency of hyperpigmentation.

Drug Interactions

The following drug interactions are based on studies using emtricitabine.

Drug interaction studies have also been performed using the fixed combination containing emtricitabine and tenofovir alafenamide (emtricitabine/tenofovir alafenamide; Descovy®), fixed combination containing emtricitabine and tenofovir disoproxil fumarate (emtricitabine/tenofovir DF; Truvada®), fixed combination containing efavirenz, emtricitabine, and tenofovir DF (efavirenz/emtricitabine/tenofovir DF; Atripla), fixed combination containing emtricitabine, rilpivirine, and tenofovir alafenamide (emtricitabine/rilpivirine/tenofovir alafenamide; Odefsey®), or fixed combination containing emtricitabine, rilpivirine, and tenofovir DF (emtricitabine/rilpivirine/tenofovir DF; Complera®). When a fixed combinations is used, interactions associated with each drug in the fixed combination should be considered.

■ **Drugs Metabolized by Hepatic Microsomal Enzymes** Pharmacokinetic interactions between emtricitabine and drugs metabolized by hepatic microsomal enzymes are unlikely. In vitro studies indicate that emtricitabine does not inhibit cytochrome P-450 (CYP) isoenzymes 1A2, 2A6, 2B6, 2C9, 2C19, 2D6, or 3A4.

■ **Drugs Metabolized by Uridine Diphosphate-glucuronosyltransferase** Pharmacokinetic interactions between emtricitabine and drugs metabolized by uridine diphosphate-glucuronosyltransferase are unlikely. Emtricitabine does not inhibit glucuronosyltransferase (uridine diphosphoglucuronosyltransferase, UDP-glucuronate β-D-glucuronosyltransferase [acceptor-unspecific]), an enzyme responsible for glucuronidation.

■ **Antiretroviral Agents** ***HIV Entry and Fusion Inhibitors*** **Maraviroc.** No in vitro evidence of antagonistic antiretroviral effects between maraviroc and emtricitabine.

HIV Nonnucleoside Reverse Transcriptase Inhibitors (NNRTIs) Although not specifically studied, clinically important pharmacokinetic interactions between rilpivirine and emtricitabine are unlikely.

In vitro evidence of additive or synergistic antiretroviral effects between emtricitabine and NNRTIs (e.g., delavirdine, efavirenz, nevirapine). No in vitro evidence of antagonistic antiretroviral effects between emtricitabine and etravirine or rilpivirine.

HIV Nucleoside and Nucleotide Reverse Transcriptase Inhibitors (NRTIs) In vitro evidence of additive to synergistic antiretroviral effects between emtricitabine and nucleoside and HIV nucleotide reverse transcriptase inhibitors (NRTIs) (e.g., abacavir, stavudine, tenofovir DF, zidovudine).

Lamivudine. Emtricitabine and lamivudine should not be used concomitantly. Because emtricitabine is an analog of lamivudine, the drugs have similar resistance profiles and concomitant use provides no additional benefit.

Stavudine. No clinically important pharmacokinetic interactions between emtricitabine and stavudine.

Tenofovir. No clinically important pharmacokinetic interactions between emtricitabine and tenofovir DF.

Zidovudine. Although not considered clinically important, concomitant use of emtricitabine (200 mg once daily for 7 days) and zidovudine (300 mg twice daily for 7 days) increased zidovudine peak plasma concentrations and area under the concentration-time curve (AUC) by 17 and 13%, respectively, but did not affect emtricitabine peak plasma concentrations or AUC.

HIV Protease Inhibitors (PIs) Although not specifically studied, pharmacokinetic interactions between darunavir and emtricitabine are unlikely.

No clinically important pharmacokinetic interactions between emtricitabine and indinavir.

In vitro evidence of additive or synergistic antiretroviral effects between emtricitabine and HIV PIs (e.g., amprenavir, nelfinavir, ritonavir, saquinavir, tipranavir). No in vitro evidence of antagonistic antiretroviral effects between emtricitabine and atazanavir or darunavir.

■ **Famciclovir** No clinically important pharmacokinetic interactions between emtricitabine and famciclovir.

■ **HCV Antivirals** ***HCV Polymerase Inhibitors*** **Sofosbuvir.** Concomitant use of emtricitabine and sofosbuvir does not have a clinically important effect on the pharmacokinetics of either drug. Dosage adjustments are not needed for either drug.

HCV Protease Inhibitors **Simeprevir.** No clinically important interactions are expected if simeprevir is used concomitantly with emtricitabine.

HCV Replication Complex Inhibitors **Elbasvir and Grazoprevir.** Clinically important pharmacokinetic interactions are not expected if emtricitabine is used concomitantly with the fixed combination of elbasvir and grazoprevir (elbasvir/grazoprevir).

Ledipasvir and Sofosbuvir. Clinically important pharmacokinetic interactions are not expected if emtricitabine is used concomitantly with the fixed combination of ledipasvir and sofosbuvir (ledipasvir/sofosbuvir).

Description

Emtricitabine, a synthetic antiretroviral agent, is a human immunodeficiency virus (HIV) nucleoside reverse transcriptase inhibitor (NRTI). Emtricitabine is inactive until converted intracellularly to an active 5′-triphosphate metabolite. Following conversion to the pharmacologically active metabolite, the drug apparently inhibits replication of human retroviruses by interfering with viral RNA-directed DNA polymerase (reverse transcriptase).

Emtricitabine is active against HIV type 1 (HIV-1) and also has some in vitro activity against HIV type 2 (HIV-2). The drug also has some activity against hepatitis B virus (HBV).

HIV-1 strains with reduced susceptibility to emtricitabine can be produced in vitro and strains with reduced susceptibility to the drug have emerged during emtricitabine therapy. These strains have contained a M184V/I mutation. HIV-1 strains with the M184V/I mutation have been resistant to lamivudine but retained susceptibility to didanosine, stavudine, tenofovir, zidovudine, delavirdine, efavirenz, and nevirapine.

Advice to Patients

Critical nature of compliance with human immunodeficiency virus (HIV) therapy and importance of remaining under the care of a clinician. Importance of taking as prescribed; do not alter or discontinue antiretroviral regimen without consulting clinician.

Importance of using emtricitabine (Emtriva®), fixed combination containing emtricitabine and tenofovir alafenamide (emtricitabine/tenofovir alafenamide; Descovy®) or fixed combination containing emtricitabine and tenofovir disoproxil fumarate (emtricitabine/tenofovir DF; Truvada®) in conjunction with other antiretrovirals for treatment of HIV-1 infection—not for monotherapy.

Fixed combination containing efavirenz, emtricitabine, and tenofovir DF (efavirenz/emtricitabine/tenofovir DF; Atripla®), fixed combination containing emtricitabine, rilpivirine, and tenofovir alafenamide (emtricitabine/rilpivirine/tenofovir alafenamide; Odefsey®), or fixed combination containing emtricitabine, rilpivirine, and tenofovir DF (emtricitabine/rilpivirine/tenofovir DF; Complera®) can be used alone as a complete regimen for treatment of HIV-1 infection.

Antiretroviral therapy is not a cure for HIV infection; opportunistic infections and other complications associated with HIV disease may still occur.

Advise HIV-infected patients that effective antiretroviral treatment regimens can decrease HIV-1 concentrations in blood and genital secretions and strict adherence to such regimens in conjunction with risk-reduction measures may decrease, but cannot absolutely eliminate, the risk of secondary transmission of HIV to others. Importance of continuing to practice safer sex (e.g., using latex or polyurethane condoms to minimize sexual contact with body fluids), never sharing personal items that can have blood or body fluids on them (e.g., toothbrushes, razor blades), and never reusing or sharing needles.

Emtricitabine/tenofovir DF (Truvada®) medication guide must be provided to and reviewed with all HIV-1-negative individuals each time the drug is dispensed for preexposure prophylaxis (PrEP) of HIV-1 infection. (See REMS.) Advise such individuals of the importance of confirming that they are HIV-1-negative before starting PrEP, importance of regular HIV-1 testing (at least every 3 months) during PrEP, importance of strictly adhering to recommended dosage schedule and not missing any doses of the drug, and importance of using a complete prevention strategy that also includes other measures (e.g., consistent condom use, testing for other sexually transmitted infections such as syphilis and gonorrhea that may facilitate HIV-1 transmission, reducing sexual risk behavior). Advise uninfected individuals that emtricitabine/tenofovir DF PrEP does not protect all individuals from acquiring HIV-1 and to report any symptoms of acute HIV-1 infection (e.g., fever, headache, fatigue, arthralgia, vomiting, myalgia, diarrhea, pharyngitis, rash, night sweats, cervical and inguinal adenopathy) immediately to a clinician.

Importance of reading patient information provided by the manufacturer.

Advise patients that lactic acidosis and severe hepatomegaly with steatosis, including fatalities, have occurred in patients receiving HIV nucleoside reverse transcriptase inhibitors (NRTIs), including emtricitabine, in conjunction with other antiretrovirals. Importance of contacting clinician if symptoms suggestive of lactic acidosis or pronounced hepatotoxicity (e.g., nausea, vomiting, unusual/unexpected stomach discomfort, weakness) occur.

Inform patients that testing for hepatitis B virus (HBV) infection is recommended before antiretroviral therapy is initiated. Also advise patients that severe acute exacerbations of HBV infection have been reported following discontinuance of emtricitabine (single-entity or fixed-combination preparations) in HIV-infected patients coinfected with HBV.

Inform patients that redistribution or accumulation of body fat may occur in patients receiving antiretroviral therapy and that the cause and long-term health effects of these conditions are unknown.

Importance of informing clinicians of existing or contemplated concomitant therapy, including prescription and OTC drugs and dietary and herbal products, as well as concomitant medical problems such as renal impairment.

Importance of women informing clinicians if they are or plan to become pregnant or plan to breast-feed. Advise HIV-infected women not to breast-feed.

Importance of informing patients of other precautionary information. (See Cautions.)

Overview® (see Users Guide). For additional information on this drug until a more detailed monograph is developed and published, the manufacturer's labeling should be consulted. It is *essential* that the manufacturer's labeling be consulted for more detailed information on usual cautions, precautions, contraindications, potential drug interactions, laboratory test interferences, and acute toxicity.

Preparations

Excipients in commercially available drug preparations may have clinically important effects in some individuals; consult specific product labeling for details.

Emtricitabine

Oral		
Capsules	200 mg	**Emtriva®**, Gilead
Solution	10 mg/mL	**Emtriva®**, Gilead

Emtricitabine Combinations

Oral		
Tablets, film-coated	100 mg with Tenofovir Disoproxil Fumarate 150 mg	**Truvada®**, Gilead
	133 mg with Tenofovir Disoproxil Fumarate 200 mg	**Truvada®**, Gilead
	167 mg with Tenofovir Disoproxil Fumarate 250 mg	**Truvada®**, Gilead
	200 mg with Tenofovir Disoproxil Fumarate 300 mg	**Truvada®**, Gilead
	200 mg with Tenofovir Alafenamide Fumarate 25 mg (of tenofovir alafenamide)	**Descovy®**, Gilead
	200 mg with Tenofovir Alafenamide Fumarate 25 mg (of tenofovir alafenamide) and Rilpivirine Hydrochloride 25 mg (of rilpivirine)	**Odefsey®**, Gilead
	200 mg with Tenofovir Disoproxil Fumarate 300 mg and Efavirenz 600 mg	**Atripla®**, Bristol-Myers Squibb and Gilead
	200 mg with Tenofovir Disoproxil Fumarate 300 mg and Rilpivirine Hydrochloride 25 mg (of rilpivirine)	**Complera®**, Gilead
	200 mg with Tenofovir Alafenamide Fumarate 10 mg (of tenofovir alafenamide), Elvitegravir 150 mg, and Cobicistat 150 mg	**Genvoya®**, Gilead
	200 mg with Tenofovir Disoproxil Fumarate 300 mg, Elvitegravir 150 mg, and Cobicistat 150 mg	**Stribild®**, Gilead

†Use is not currently included in the labeling approved by the US Food and Drug Administration

lamiVUDine

3TC, abacavir/lamiVUDine, ABC/3TC, ABC/DTG/3TC, ABC/3TC/ZDV, 3TC/ZDV, lamiVUDine/zidovudine

■ Lamivudine, an antiretroviral agent, is a human immunodeficiency virus (HIV) nucleoside reverse transcriptase inhibitor (NRTI) that is active against human immunodeficiency virus (HIV) and hepatitis B virus (HBV).

Uses

■ **Treatment of HIV Infection** Lamivudine is used in conjunction with other antiretroviral agents for the treatment of human immunodeficiency virus type 1 (HIV-1) infection in adults, adolescents, and pediatric patients.

Lamivudine usually is used in multiple-drug regimens that include another HIV nucleoside reverse transcriptase inhibitor (NRTI) (dual NRTIs) and an HIV integrase strand transferase inhibitor (INSTI), HIV nonnucleoside reverse transcriptase inhibitor (NNRTI), or HIV protease inhibitor (PI) in INSTI-, NNRTI-, or PI-based regimens. (See Dual NRTI Options under Treatment of HIV Infection: Antiretroviral-naive Adults and Adolescents, in Uses.)

If the dual NRTI option of lamivudine and zidovudine is used in conjunction with other antiretrovirals for the treatment of HIV-1 infection, a fixed-combination preparation containing both drugs (lamivudine/zidovudine; Combivir®, generic) is commercially available and can be used in adults, adolescents, and pediatric patients weighing 30 kg or more.

If the dual NRTI option of lamivudine and abacavir is used in conjunction with other antiretrovirals for the treatment of HIV-1 infection, a fixed-combination preparation containing both drugs (abacavir/lamivudine; Epzicom®, generic) is commercially available and can be used in adults, adolescents, and pediatric patients weighing 25 kg or more.

Lamivudine has been used in triple NRTI regimens (i.e., single-class NRTI regimens) that include lamivudine and 2 other NRTIs. A fixed-combination preparation containing abacavir, lamivudine, and zidovudine (abacavir/lamivudine/zidovudine; Trizivir®, generic) is commercially available and can be used alone or in conjunction with other antiretrovirals in adults, adolescents, and pediatric patients weighing 40 kg or more. (See All-NRTI Regimens under Treatment of HIV Infection: Antiretroviral-naive Adults and Adolescents, in Uses.)

The fixed-combination preparation containing abacavir, dolutegravir, and lamivudine (abacavir/dolutegravir/lamivudine; Triumeq®) is used alone as a complete treatment regimen or in conjunction with other antiretrovirals for the treatment of HIV-1 infection in adults, adolescents, and pediatric patients weighing 40 kg or more.

The most appropriate antiretroviral regimen cannot be defined for each clinical scenario and selection of specific antiretroviral agents for use in such regimens should be individualized based on information regarding antiretroviral potency, potential rate of development of resistance, known toxicities, and potential for pharmacokinetic interactions as well as virologic, immunologic, and clinical characteristics of the individual patient. For information on the general principles and guidelines for use of antiretroviral therapy, including specific recommendations for initial therapy in antiretroviral-naive patients and recommendations for changing antiretroviral regimens, see the Antiretroviral Agents General Statement 8:18.08.

Antiretroviral-naive Adults and Adolescents **Dual NRTI Options.** The US Department of Health and Human Services (HHS) Panel on Antiretroviral Guidelines for Adults and Adolescents states that the preferred dual NRTI options for use in most INSTI-, NNRTI-, and PI-based regimens recommended for *initial* treatment of HIV infection in antiretroviral-naive adults and adolescents are a tenofovir prodrug (either tenofovir alafenamide or tenofovir disoproxil fumarate [tenofovir DF]) and emtricitabine (or lamivudine). These experts state that abacavir and lamivudine (or emtricitabine) also is a recommended dual NRTI option for use in some *initial* treatment regimens in antiretroviral-naive adults and adolescents, but should be used *only* in those who are negative for human leukocyte antigen (HLA)-B*5701. If the dual NRTI option of abacavir and lamivudine is used in conjunction with other antiretrovirals, the fixed combination containing both drugs (abacavir/lamivudine) can be used in adults and adolescents weighing 25 kg or more.

The HHS panel states that the dual NRTI option of zidovudine and lamivudine is no longer recommended for *initial* treatment regimens in nonpregnant antiretroviral-naive adults and adolescents because it has greater toxicity than currently recommended dual NRTI options. However, zidovudine and lamivudine is recommended as an alternative (not a preferred) dual NRTI option for *initial* treatment regimens in antiretroviral-naive pregnant women (see Pregnancy under Cautions: Pregnancy, Fertility, and Lactation) and is a preferred dual NRTI option for *initial* treatment regimens in certain pediatric patients (see Pediatric Patients under Uses: Treatment of HIV Infection). When the dual NRTI option of lamivudine and zidovudine is used in conjunction with other antiretrovirals, the fixed-combination preparation containing both drugs (lamivudine/zidovudine) can be used in adults and adolescents weighing 30 kg or more.

A dual NRTI option of didanosine and lamivudine is *not* recommended for *initial* antiretroviral regimens because of inferior virologic efficacy, limited clinical trial experience in antiretroviral-naive patients, and didanosine-associated toxicities (e.g., pancreatitis, peripheral neuropathy).

A dual NRTI option of stavudine and lamivudine is *not* recommended for *initial* antiretroviral regimens because of reported toxicities.

Lamivudine and emtricitabine should *not* be used concomitantly at any time since the drugs have similar resistance profiles and minimal additive antiretroviral activity.

A tenofovir prodrug (either tenofovir alafenamide or tenofovir DF) and emtricitabine (or lamivudine) is the preferred dual NRTI option for antiretroviral regimens used in HIV-infected patients coinfected with hepatitis B virus (HBV). All 3 of these NRTIs (tenofovir, emtricitabine, lamivudine) have activity against both HIV and HBV, and regimens that contain only 1 of these 3 antiretrovirals are not recommended in HIV-infected patients coinfected with HBV.

All-NRTI Regimens. Lamivudine has been included in NRTI regimens that include 3 or 4 NRTIs (without any drugs from another class). However, triple and quadruple NRTI regimens are *not* recommended for *initial* treatment of HIV infection in antiretroviral-naive adults or adolescents because such regimens have inferior virologic efficacy. In addition, regimens that only include NRTIs are *not* usually recommended in antiretroviral-experienced patients. (See Antiretroviral-experienced Adults and Adolescents under Uses: Treatment of HIV Infection.)

Lamivudine has been used in a triple NRTI regimen that includes abacavir, lamivudine, and zidovudine. However, this triple NRTI regimen is *not* recommended for *initial* therapy in antiretroviral-naive adults and adolescents because of inferior virologic efficacy. If a triple NRTI regimen of abacavir, lamivudine, and zidovudine is used, the fixed-combination preparation containing these 3 NRTIs (abacavir/lamivudine/zidovudine) can be used in adults and adolescents weighing 40 kg or more. Clinicians should consider that data are limited regarding use of abacavir/lamivudine/zidovudine in patients with baseline viral loads exceeding 100,000 copies/mL.

A triple NRTI regimen of abacavir, lamivudine, and tenofovir DF is *not* recommended at any time in antiretroviral-naive or antiretroviral-experienced patients because of a high rate of virologic failure. Interim analysis of a randomized, open-label study evaluating efficacy of a once-daily regimen of abacavir, lamivudine, and tenofovir DF compared with an NNRTI-based once-daily regimen of efavirenz, abacavir, and lamivudine in treatment-naive patients (ESS30009) indicated a high rate of early virologic nonresponse in those receiving the triple NRTI regimen (almost 50%). Based on these results, the abacavir, lamivudine, and tenofovir DF arm of the study was terminated. A high rate of virologic nonresponse also was reported in a pilot study evaluating this triple NRTI regimen. Several possible reasons for the poor response to this regimen have been proposed, but the ESS30009 investigators suggested that the most likely cause is a low genetic barrier to resistance because of synergistic selection from all 3 NRTIs for 2 specific resistance mutations (M184V and K65R).

A quadruple NRTI regimen of abacavir, lamivudine, tenofovir DF, and zidovudine is *not* recommended for *initial* therapy in antiretroviral-naive HIV-infected adults and adolescents because of inferior virologic efficacy. In an open-label pilot study, a quadruple NRTI regimen was compared with an NNRTI-based regimen of efavirenz with lamivudine and zidovudine, and both regimens had similar efficacy and tolerability. However, a larger, open-label study comparing a similar quadruple NRTI regimen (abacavir, emtricitabine, tenofovir DF, zidovudine) with a standard NNRTI- or PI-based regimen found that substantially fewer patients receiving the quadruple NRTI regimen achieved HIV-1 RNA levels below 200 copies/mL.

Once-daily Versus Twice-daily Lamivudine Regimen. The comparative efficacy of a once- or twice-daily lamivudine regimen used in conjunction with zidovudine in an NNRTI-based regimen was evaluated in a 48-week, double-blind, randomized study (EPV20001) in 554 antiretroviral-naive adults (79% male, 50% Caucasian, median age 35 years, baseline $CD4^+$ T-cell count 69–1089/mm^3 [median 362/mm^3], median baseline plasma HIV-1 RNA level 4.66 $\log_{10}$ copies/mL). Patients were randomized to receive efavirenz (600 mg once daily) with zidovudine (300 mg twice daily) and either lamivudine 300 mg once daily or lamivudine 150 mg twice daily. Plasma HIV-1 RNA levels were less than 50 copies/mL through week 48 in 61% of patients receiving the once-daily lamivudine regimen and in 63% of those receiving the twice-daily lamivudine regimen. At week 48, the median increase in $CD4^+$ T-cell count was 144 cells/mm^3 or 146 cells/mm^3 in those receiving the once- or twice-daily lamivudine regimen, respectively. The virologic failure rate was 8% in both groups.

Antiretroviral-experienced Adults and Adolescents Although monotherapy or 2-drug regimens that include only NRTIs are no longer recommended for treatment of HIV infection, early studies evaluating the safety and efficacy of lamivudine in antiretroviral-experienced (previously-treated) patients used such regimens. These studies showed that patients who received lamivudine (150 or 300 mg every 12 hours) in conjunction with zidovudine (200 mg 3 times daily) for 24 weeks experienced greater increases in $CD4^+$ T-cell counts than those who received zidovudine monotherapy (200 mg 3 times daily) or zidovudine (200 mg 3 times daily) in conjunction with zalcitabine (0.75 mg 3 times daily; no longer commercially available in the US).

Lamivudine has been evaluated in a randomized, double-blind study (study NUCB3007; CAESAR study) in 1816 HIV-infected patients (baseline $CD4^+$ T-cell count 25–250/mm^3 [median 122/mm^3], 84% nucleoside-experienced, 16% treatment-naive). Oral lamivudine (with or without an NNRTI) was added to the patient's existing regimen (i.e., monotherapy with zidovudine [62%], a 2-drug regimen of zidovudine and didanosine or zalcitabine [38%]) and efficacy was assessed by disease progression or death over the following 12 months. The 12-month cumulative incidence of disease progression or death was 8.9–9.6% in patients randomized to receive lamivudine (with or without an NNRTI) in conjunction with their existing regimen and 19.6% in patients randomized to receive placebo in conjunction with their existing regimen. The 12-month cumulative mortality was 2.6–3 or 5.9% in patients randomized to receive lamivudine (with or without an NNRTI) or placebo, respectively, in conjunction with their existing regimen.

All-NRTI Regimens. Based on interim analysis of a study evaluating a triple NRTI regimen of abacavir, lamivudine, and tenofovir DF that indicated a high rate of early virologic nonresponse in antiretroviral-naive patients receiving this regimen, a triple NRTI regimen of abacavir, lamivudine, and tenofovir DF is *not* recommended in either antiretroviral-naive or antiretroviral-experienced patients. (See All-NRTI Regimens under Treatment of HIV Infection: Antiretroviral-naive Adults and Adolescents, in Uses.)

Pediatric Patients Lamivudine is used in conjunction with other antiretrovirals for the treatment of HIV-1 infection in children 3 months of age or older. In addition, the drug is recommended for use in conjunction with other antiretrovirals for the treatment of HIV infection in neonates and infants younger than 3 months of age† and for empiric HIV therapy† for prevention of perinatal HIV transmission in neonates. (See Uses: Prevention of Perinatal HIV Transmission.)

Lamivudine/zidovudine is used in conjunction with other antiretrovirals for the treatment of HIV-1 infection in pediatric patients weighing 30 kg or more.

Abacavir/lamivudine is used in conjunction with other antiretrovirals for the treatment of HIV-1 infection in pediatric patients weighing 25 kg or more.

Abacavir/lamivudine/zidovudine is used alone or in conjunction with other antiretrovirals for the treatment of HIV-1 infection in pediatric patients weighing 40 kg or more.

Abacavir/dolutegravir/lamivudine is used alone or in conjunction with other antiretrovirals for the treatment of HIV-1 infection in pediatric patients weighing 40 kg or more.

For *initial* treatment in antiretroviral-naive HIV-infected pediatric patients, the HHS Panel on Antiretroviral Therapy and Medical Management of HIV-infected Children recommends a *ritonavir-boosted* PI, NNRTI, or INSTI in conjunction with 2 NRTIs (dual NRTIs).

The HHS panel states that zidovudine and lamivudine (or emtricitabine) is a preferred dual NRTI option for use in *initial* treatment regimens in neonates, infants, and children younger than 12 years of age and an alternative dual NRTI option for use in adolescents 12 years of age or older with sexual maturity rating (SMR) 3. When the dual NRTI option of lamivudine and zidovudine is used, the fixed-combination preparation containing both drugs (lamivudine/zidovudine) can be used in pediatric patients weighing 30 kg or more.

These experts state that abacavir and lamivudine (or emtricitabine) is a preferred dual NRTI option in pediatric patients 3 months of age or older, including adolescents 12 years of age or older with SMR 1–3, but should be used *only* in those who are negative for HLA-B*5701.

The HHS panel states that tenofovir DF and lamivudine (or emtricitabine) is an alternative dual NRTI option for use in *initial* treatment regimens in adolescents with SMR 3. These experts state that, in special circumstances, tenofovir DF and lamivudine (or emtricitabine) also can be used in conjunction with other antiretrovirals for *initial* treatment regimens in children 2 years of age or older and in adolescents with SMR 1 or 2.

The HHS panel states that, in special circumstances, the dual NRTI option of didanosine and lamivudine (or emtricitabine) can be considered for *initial* treatment regimens in children 2 years of age or older and in adolescents with SMR 1 or 2.

Emtricitabine and lamivudine should *not* be used concomitantly at any time since the drugs have similar resistance profiles and no additive benefit.

Antiretroviral regimens that contain only NRTIs should *not* be used at any time for treatment of HIV infection in pediatric patients because of inferior virologic efficacy.

A triple NRTI regimen that includes abacavir, tenofovir DF, and either lamivudine or emtricitabine or a triple NRTI regimen that includes tenofovir DF, didanosine, and either lamivudine or emtricitabine should *not* be used at any time in pediatric patients because of the high rate of early virologic failure reported in antiretroviral-naive adults.

For further information on treatment of HIV infection in pediatric patients, see Antiretroviral Therapy in Pediatric Patients, in the Antiretroviral Agents General Statement 8:18.08.

■ Prevention of Perinatal HIV Transmission

Lamivudine is used in conjunction with other antiretrovirals for empiric HIV therapy† in neonates for prevention of perinatal HIV transmission†.

Although lamivudine has been used in some antepartum, intrapartum, and neonatal antiretroviral prophylaxis regimens for prevention of perinatal HIV transmission (e.g., resource-limited countries), lamivudine is not a component of intrapartum or neonatal prophylaxis regimens recommended in the US for prevention of perinatal HIV transmission. Maternal and neonatal regimens recommended for prevention of perinatal HIV transmission in the US may differ from those used in other countries.

In the US, multiple-drug antiretroviral regimens are considered the standard of care for treatment of HIV infection in pregnant women and for prevention of perinatal HIV transmission. The HHS Panel on Treatment of Pregnant Women with HIV Infection and Prevention of Perinatal Transmission states that *all* pregnant HIV-infected women in the US should receive multiple-drug antiretroviral therapy, regardless of the woman's plasma HIV-1 RNA level or $CD4^+$ T-cell count. In addition, to further decrease the risk of perinatal HIV transmission, the HHS panel states that *all* pregnant HIV-infected women with plasma HIV-1 RNA levels exceeding 1000 copies/mL (or unknown HIV-1 RNA levels) near the time of delivery should receive an intrapartum IV zidovudine prophylaxis regimen initiated at the onset of labor (or 3 hours before scheduled cesarean delivery) and continued until delivery (unless contraindicated) and *all* neonates born to HIV-infected women (HIV-exposed neonates) should receive an antiretroviral regimen (either prophylaxis or empiric HIV therapy) initiated as soon as possible after birth (preferably within 6–12 hours) and continued for 4–6 weeks. HIV-exposed neonates at low risk of perinatal HIV acquisition (e.g., those born to an HIV-infected mother who received standard multiple-drug antiretroviral treatment during pregnancy with sustained viral suppression near the time of delivery and with no concerns related to maternal adherence to the treatment regimen) can receive a prophylaxis regimen that includes only zidovudine. However, a combination antiretroviral regimen that includes zidovudine *and* 1 or 2 additional antiretrovirals should be used in neonates at higher risk of HIV acquisition, including those born to HIV-infected women who did not receive antepartum or intrapartum antiretrovirals, received only intrapartum antiretrovirals, received antepartum and intrapartum antiretrovirals with suboptimal viral suppression near delivery (i.e., detectable plasma HIV RNA levels), or had primary or acute HIV infection during pregnancy or during breast-feeding. This strategy of combined antepartum, intrapartum, and neonatal antiretrovirals reduces perinatal HIV transmission by several mechanisms, including lowering maternal antepartum viral load and providing pre- and postexposure prophylaxis in the infant.

Antiretrovirals in HIV-exposed Neonates The choice of a neonatal antiretroviral prophylaxis regimen *or* a neonatal empiric HIV therapy† regimen should be based on an assessment of the likelihood of perinatal HIV transmission.

Although the HHS panel states that a 4-week zidovudine prophylaxis regimen can be used alone in HIV-exposed neonates at low risk, those at higher risk of HIV acquisition (e.g., those born to HIV-infected women who did not receive antepartum or intrapartum antiretrovirals, received only intrapartum antiretrovirals, or received antepartum and intrapartum antiretrovirals with suboptimal viral suppression near delivery) should receive a 2-drug prophylaxis regimen that includes a 6-week zidovudine prophylaxis regimen *and* a 3-dose nevirapine prophylaxis regimen. Alternatively, the HHS panel states that neonates at highest risk can receive empiric HIV therapy† with a 3-drug regimen of zidovudine, lamivudine, and nevirapine. The 3-drug empiric HIV therapy regimen serves as antiretroviral prophylaxis to prevent acquisition of HIV and also serves as early treatment for neonates who are later confirmed to have acquired HIV. The optimal duration of empiric HIV therapy in neonates at highest risk of HIV acquisition is unknown. Many experts recommend that the 3-drug regimen be continued for 6 weeks; others discontinue nevirapine and/or lamivudine if results of the neonate's HIV nucleic acid amplification test (NAAT) are negative, but recommend continuing zidovudine for 6 weeks.

Because safety and dosage data are not available, the HHS panel states that use of antiretrovirals other than zidovudine, lamivudine, and nevirapine cannot be recommended for premature HIV-exposed neonates (gestational age less than 37 weeks).

For information on the risk of perinatal transmission of HIV and additional information regarding recommendations for use of antiretroviral agents for prevention of perinatal HIV transmission, see Guidelines for Use of Antiretroviral Agents: Antiretrovirals for Prevention of Perinatal HIV Transmission, in the Antiretroviral Agents General Statement 8:18.08.

Clinicians can consult the National Perinatal HIV Hotline at 888-448-8765 for information regarding antiretroviral treatment of pregnant HIV-infected women and their infants and prevention of perinatal HIV transmission.

■ **Postexposure Prophylaxis following Occupational Exposure to HIV** Lamivudine is used in conjunction with other antiretrovirals for postexposure prophylaxis of HIV infection following occupational exposure† (PEP) in health-care workers and other individuals exposed via percutaneous injury (e.g., needlestick, cut with sharp object) or mucous membrane or nonintact skin (e.g., chapped, abraded, dermatitis) contact with blood, tissue, or other body fluids that might contain HIV.

The US Public Health Service (USPHS) states that the preferred regimen for PEP following an occupational exposure to HIV is a 3-drug regimen of raltegravir used in conjunction with emtricitabine and tenofovir DF (may be administered as the fixed combination emtricitabine/tenofovir DF). These experts recommend several alternative regimens that include an INSTI, NNRTI, or PI and 2 NRTIs (dual NRTIs). The preferred dual NRTI option for use in PEP regimens is emtricitabine and tenofovir DF (may be administered as emtricitabine/tenofovir DF); alternative dual NRTIs are tenofovir DF and lamivudine, zidovudine and lamivudine (may be administered as the fixed combination lamivudine/zidovudine; Combivir®), or zidovudine and emtricitabine.

Because management of occupational exposures to HIV is complex and evolving, consultation with an infectious disease specialist, clinician with expertise in administration of antiretroviral agents, and/or the National Clinicians' Postexposure Prophylaxis Hotline (PEPline at 888-448-4911) is recommended whenever possible. However, initiation of PEP should not be delayed while waiting for expert consultation.

For information on types of occupational exposure to HIV and associated risk of infection, management of occupational exposure to HIV, efficacy and safety of postexposure chemoprophylaxis, and recommendations regarding postexposure prophylaxis, see Guidelines for Use of Antiretroviral Agents: Antiretrovirals for Postexposure Prophylaxis following Occupational Exposure to HIV (PEP), in the Antiretroviral Agents General Statement 8:18.08.

■ **Postexposure Prophylaxis following Nonoccupational Exposure to HIV** Lamivudine is used in conjunction with other antiretrovirals for postexposure prophylaxis of HIV infection following nonoccupational exposure† (nPEP) in individuals exposed to blood, genital secretions, or other potentially infectious body fluids that might contain HIV when that exposure represents a substantial risk for HIV transmission.

When nPEP is indicated following a nonoccupational exposure to HIV, the US Centers for Disease Control and Prevention (CDC) states that the preferred regimen in adults and adolescents 13 years of age or older with normal renal function is either raltegravir or dolutegravir used in conjunction with emtricitabine and tenofovir DF (administered as the fixed combination emtricitabine/tenofovir DF). In adults and adolescents 13 years of age or older with impaired renal function (creatinine clearance 59 mL/minute or less), CDC recommends a regimen of either raltegravir or dolutegravir used in conjunction with zidovudine and lamivudine.

Consultation with an infectious disease specialist, clinician with expertise in administration of antiretroviral agents, and/or the National Clinicians' Postexposure Prophylaxis Hotline (PEPline at 888-448-4911) is recommended if nPEP is indicated in certain exposed individuals (e.g., pregnant women, children, those with medical conditions such as renal impairment) or if an antiretroviral regimen not included in the CDC guidelines is being considered, the source virus is known or likely to be resistant to antiretrovirals, or the healthcare provider is inexperienced in prescribing antiretrovirals. However, initiation of nPEP should not be delayed while waiting for expert consultation.

For additional information on nonoccupational exposure to HIV and recommendations regarding postexposure prophylaxis, see Guidelines for Use of Antiretroviral Agents: Antiretrovirals for Postexposure Prophylaxis following Sexual, Injection Drug Use, or other Nonoccupational Exposures to HIV (nPEP), in the Antiretroviral Agents General Statement 8:18.08.

■ **Chronic Hepatitis B Virus Infection** Lamivudine is used for the treatment of chronic hepatitis B virus (HBV) infection associated with evidence of HBV replication and active liver inflammation in adults, adolescents, and pediatric patients 2 years of age or older.

Experts state that lamivudine is not considered a preferred antiviral for treatment of chronic HBV infection because a high rate of lamivudine-resistant HBV has been reported. The manufacturer states that lamivudine should be considered for treatment of chronic HBV infection *only* when alternative antiviral agents associated with a higher genetic barrier to resistance are not available or appropriate.

Safety and efficacy of lamivudine for the treatment of chronic HBV infection have *not* been established in patients with decompensated liver disease, liver transplant recipients, HBV-infected patients coinfected with HIV (see HIV-infected Individuals under Uses: Chronic Hepatitis B Virus Infection), or HBV-infected patients coinfected with hepatitis C virus (HCV) or hepatitis D virus (HDV).

The goal of antiviral therapy in patients with chronic HBV infection is to decrease the morbidity and mortality related to the infection (e.g., cirrhosis, hepatic failure, hepatocellular carcinoma). Sustained suppression of HBV replication has been associated with normalization of serum ALT concentrations, loss of hepatitis B e antigen (HBeAg) with or without detection of antibody to HBeAg (anti-HBe), and improvement in liver histology. Currently available therapies for chronic HBV infection (e.g., adefovir, entecavir, lamivudine, telbivudine, tenofovir alafenamide, tenofovir DF, interferon alfa, peginterferon alfa) are used in an attempt to provide an immunologic cure (hepatitis B surface antigen [HBsAg] loss and sustained HBV DNA suppression), but cannot provide a virologic cure (eradication of HBV).

Treatment of chronic HBV infection is complex and evolving, and specialized references and experts should be consulted. Information from the American Association for the Study of Liver Diseases (AASLD) regarding management of HBV infection, including recommendations for initial treatment, is available at https://www.aasld.org.

Adults Safety and efficacy of lamivudine for treatment of HBV infection were evaluated in 3 controlled studies in adults 16 years of age or older with compensated chronic HBV infection (serum HBsAg positive for at least 6 months) accompanied by evidence of HBV replication (positive for serum HBeAg and positive for serum HBV DNA as measured by a research solution hybridization assay) and persistently elevated serum ALT concentrations and/or chronic inflammation on liver biopsy compatible with a diagnosis of chronic viral hepatitis. Lamivudine treatment in patients with chronic HBV infection has been associated with histologic improvement on liver biopsy, decreases in HBV DNA, normalization of serum ALT concentrations, and HBeAg seroconversion (loss of HBeAg and development of antibody to HBeAg).

In a controlled study in Chinese patients with chronic HBV infection who received lamivudine 100 mg once daily, lamivudine 25 mg once daily, or placebo for 12 months, hepatic necroinflammatory activity improved in 56, 49, or 25% and deteriorated in 7, 8, or 26% of patients, respectively. Therapy with lamivudine 100 mg daily was associated with a reduction in the progression of fibrosis compared with placebo. At 12 months, HBeAg seroconversion occurred in 16, 13, or 4%, respectively, of patients receiving lamivudine 100 mg daily, 25 mg daily, or placebo. Therapy with lamivudine 100 mg daily was associated with a rapid and sustained reduction in HBV DNA (97% reduction at week 2, 98% reduction at week 52 compared with baseline) and sustained serum ALT response in 72% of patients; therapy with lamivudine 25 mg daily or placebo was associated with a 93 or 54% reduction in HBV DNA at week 52 and sustained ALT response in 65 or 24% of patients, respectively. In this study, therapy with lamivudine 100 mg daily was more effective than lamivudine 25 mg daily or placebo.

While therapy with lamivudine is associated with histologic improvement in most patients and is well tolerated, the optimum duration of therapy, the durability of HBeAg seroconversions occurring during treatment, and the relationship between treatment response and long-term outcomes such as hepatocellular carcinoma or decompensated cirrhosis remain to be determined. There is some evidence that efficacy of lamivudine may not be sustained during continued therapy. Results from 52-week studies in adults indicate that HBV DNA levels decrease to below the limits of detection in the majority of lamivudine-treated patients early in the course of treatment; however, assay-detectable HBV DNA reappears during treatment in approximately one-third of those who had an initial response. Strains of HBV with resistance to lamivudine have emerged during therapy with the drug, especially during long-term treatment. (See Resistance: Resistance in HBV.) Development of lamivudine-resistant HBV during treatment with the drug has been associated with decreased treatment responses evidenced by lower rates of HBeAg seroconversion and HBeAg loss and more frequent increases in HBV DNA levels and serum ALT concentrations after an initial response. Progression of HBV infection, including death, has been reported in some patients with lamivudine-resistant HBV.

Pediatric Patients Lamivudine is used for treatment of chronic HBV infection in children 2 years of age or older. Safety and efficacy of lamivudine was evaluated in a double-blind clinical study in 286 children and adolescents 2–17 years of age with compensated chronic HBV infection accompanied by evidence of HBV replication (positive serum HBeAg and positive for serum HBV DNA as measured by a research branched DNA [bDNA] assay) and persistently elevated serum ALT concentrations. Loss of HBeAg and reduction of HBV DNA to below the limits of detection of the research assay (evaluated at week 52) occurred in 23% of children who received 52 weeks of lamivudine (3 mg/kg once daily; maximum 100 mg once daily) compared with 13% of those who received placebo. In addition, normalization of serum ALT concentrations was achieved and maintained to week 52 more frequently in patients treated with lamivudine (55%) compared with placebo (13%). As in the controlled studies in adults, most lamivudine-treated pediatric patients had decreases in serum HBV DNA concentrations below the limits of detection early in treatment, but about one-third of subjects with this initial response had reappearance of detectable HBV DNA during treatment. Adolescents (13–17 years of age) showed less evidence of this treatment effect than younger children.

HIV-infected Individuals Safety and efficacy of lamivudine for treatment of chronic HBV infection in patients coinfected with HIV† have not been established.

HIV-infected patients coinfected with HBV often have higher HBV viral loads and are more likely to have detectable HBeAg, lower rates of HBeAg seroconversion, and an increased risk for and more rapid progression to cirrhosis, end-stage liver disease, and/or hepatocellular carcinoma compared with individuals not infected with HIV. Decisions to initiate HBV treatment in patients coinfected with HIV and HBV and the most appropriate drugs for HBV treatment in such patients depend on various factors, including the possible effects on replication of both HIV *and* HBV and whether the patient is currently receiving antiretroviral therapy. Specialized references should be consulted for specific information regarding the evaluation and management of chronic HBV infection in HIV-infected patients.

Although lamivudine is active against both HBV and HIV, it should *not* be used for treatment of chronic HBV infection in HIV-infected individuals who are not currently receiving antiretroviral therapy since dosages used for treatment of HBV infection are lower than those recommended for treatment of HIV infection and use of suboptimal dosages in HIV-infected individuals may allow for the selection of lamivudine-resistant HIV. In addition, emergence of lamivudine-resistant HBV has been reported in HIV-infected individuals who were coinfected with HBV and receiving lamivudine-containing antiretroviral regimens. Although a high rate of emergence of lamivudine-resistant HBV has been reported with long-term lamivudine therapy in HBV-infected patients without HIV infection, there is some evidence that the rate of emergence of HBV resistance may be even higher in HIV-infected individuals who receive the drug. Reactivation of chronic HBV has been reported in HIV-infected patients who received long-term lamivudine therapy, and fulminant and fatal reactivation of chronic HBV infection as the result of emergence of lamivudine-resistant HBV has been reported. (See Precautions Related to Treatment of Chronic HBV Infection under Cautions: Precautions and Contraindications.)

Transplant Recipients Safety and efficacy of lamivudine have *not* been established for treatment of HBV infection in organ transplant recipients. There is some evidence that lamivudine appears to reduce the risk of HBV reinfection in orthotopic liver transplant recipients†. However, further study is needed to define the role of lamivudine and other therapies for prevention and control of HBV recurrence in transplant recipients.

Dosage and Administration

■ **Administration** Lamivudine is administered orally once or twice daily without regard to meals.

For the treatment of human immunodeficiency virus type 1 (HIV-1) infection, lamivudine is commercially available as an oral solution containing 10 mg/mL or tablets containing 150 or 300 mg of the drug (Epivir®, generic). The 150-mg scored tablets are the preferred preparation in pediatric patients who weigh 14 kg or more and can swallow tablets. (See Cautions: Pediatric Precautions.) The oral solution should be used in those unable to safely and reliably swallow tablets. Lamivudine is used in conjunction with other antiretrovirals for the treatment of HIV-1 infection.

For the treatment of chronic hepatitis B virus (HBV) infection, lamivudine is commercially available as an oral solution containing 5 mg/mL or film-coated tablets containing 100 mg of the drug (Epivir-HBV®, generic). The 5-mg/mL oral solution should be used in patients requiring a dosage less than 100 mg and in children unable to reliably swallow tablets.

Lamivudine preparations labeled by FDA for treatment of chronic HBV infection should *not* be used in HIV-infected patients because they contain a lower dosage of the drug than that required for treatment of HIV-1 infection. If such preparations are used for the management of chronic HBV infection in a patient with unrecognized or untreated HIV infection, rapid emergence of HIV resistance is likely to result because of the subtherapeutic dose and the inappropriateness of monotherapy for HIV-infected individuals. (See Chronic Hepatitis B Virus Infection under Dosage and Administration: Dosage.)

Fixed Combinations Containing Lamivudine For the treatment of HIV infection, lamivudine is commercially available in fixed-combination tablets containing lamivudine and zidovudine (lamivudine/zidovudine; Combivir®, generic), fixed-combination tablets containing abacavir and lamivudine (abacavir/lamivudine; Epzicom®, generic), fixed-combination tablets containing abacavir, lamivudine, and zidovudine (abacavir/lamivudine/zidovudine; Trizivir®, generic), and fixed-combination tablets containing abacavir, dolutegravir, and lamivudine (abacavir/dolutegravir/lamivudine; Triumeq®).

Lamivudine/zidovudine tablets are administered orally twice daily without regard to meals. A fixed-combination tablet containing 150 mg of lamivudine and 300 mg of zidovudine is bioequivalent to one 150-mg tablet of lamivudine and one 300-mg tablet of zidovudine given simultaneously. Lamivudine/zidovudine is used in conjunction with other antiretrovirals. The fixed combination should *not* be used in pediatric patients weighing less than 30 kg, patients with renal impairment (i.e., creatinine clearance less than 50 mL/minute), patients with hepatic impairment, or patients who experience dose-limiting adverse effects.

Abacavir/lamivudine tablets are administered orally once daily without regard to meals. A fixed-combination tablet containing 600 mg of abacavir and 300 mg of lamivudine is bioequivalent to two 300-mg tablets of abacavir and two 150-mg tablets of lamivudine given simultaneously. Abacavir/lamivudine is used in conjunction with other antiretrovirals. The fixed combination should *not* be used in pediatric patients weighing less than 25 kg, patients with renal impairment (i.e., creatinine clearance less than 50 mL/minute), or patients with hepatic impairment (contraindicated in those with moderate or severe hepatic impairment).

Abacavir/lamivudine/zidovudine tablets are administered orally twice daily without regard to meals. A fixed-combination tablet containing 300 mg of abacavir, 150 mg of lamivudine, and 300 mg of zidovudine is bioequivalent to one 300-mg abacavir tablet, one 150-mg lamivudine tablet, and one 300-mg zidovudine tablet given simultaneously. Abacavir/lamivudine/zidovudine can be used alone as a complete treatment regimen or can be used in conjunction with other antiretrovirals. The fixed combination should *not* be used in pediatric patients weighing less than 40 kg, patients with renal impairment (i.e., creatinine clearance less than 50 mL/minute), patients with hepatic impairment (contraindicated in those with moderate or severe hepatic impairment), or others requiring dosage adjustment.

Abacavir/dolutegravir/lamivudine tablets are administered orally once daily without regard to meals. A fixed-combination tablet containing 600 mg of abacavir, 50 mg of dolutegravir, and 300 mg of lamivudine is bioequivalent to one 50-mg tablet of dolutegravir administered simultaneously with one fixed-combination tablet containing 600 mg of abacavir and 300 mg of lamivudine. Abacavir/dolutegravir/lamivudine can be used alone as a complete treatment regimen or can be used in conjunction with other antiretrovirals. The fixed combination should *not* be used in pediatric patients weighing less than 40 kg, patients with renal impairment (i.e., creatinine clearance less than 50 mL/minute), or patients with hepatic impairment (contraindicated in those with moderate or severe hepatic impairment).

■ **Dosage** ***Treatment of HIV Infection*** **Adult Dosage.** The usual dosage of lamivudine for the treatment of HIV-1 infection in adults is 150 mg twice daily or 300 mg once daily.

When lamivudine/zidovudine is used for the treatment of HIV-1 infection in adults weighing 30 kg or more, the recommended dosage is 1 tablet (150 mg of lamivudine and 300 mg of zidovudine) twice daily.

When abacavir/lamivudine is used for the treatment of HIV-1 infection in adults, the recommended dosage is 1 tablet (600 mg of abacavir and 300 mg of lamivudine) once daily.

When abacavir/lamivudine/zidovudine is used for the treatment of HIV-1 infection in adults weighing 40 kg or more, the recommended dosage is 1 tablet (300 mg of abacavir, 150 mg of lamivudine, and 300 mg of zidovudine) twice daily.

When abacavir/dolutegravir/lamivudine is used for the treatment of HIV-1 infection in adults weighing 40 kg or more, the recommended dosage is 1 tablet (600 mg of abacavir, 50 mg of dolutegravir, and 300 mg of lamivudine) once daily. If abacavir/dolutegravir/lamivudine is used in those receiving concomitant therapy with efavirenz, *ritonavir-boosted* fosamprenavir, *ritonavir-boosted* tipranavir, carbamazepine, or rifampin, patients should receive 1 tablet of the fixed combination (600 mg of abacavir, 50 mg of dolutegravir, and 300 mg of lamivudine) once daily *and* a 50-mg tablet of single-entity dolutegravir given once daily 12 hours after the daily dose of the fixed combination.

Pediatric Dosage. When lamivudine oral solution containing 10 mg/mL is used for the treatment of HIV-1 infection in pediatric patients 3 months of age or older, the recommended dosage is 5 mg/kg twice daily or 10 mg/kg once daily (up to 300 mg daily).

When lamivudine 150-mg scored tablets are used in pediatric patients 3 months of age or older who weigh 14 kg or more and are able to swallow tablets, the recommended dosage is based on weight (see Table 1 and Table 2). Data regarding efficacy of the once-daily regimen of lamivudine given as 150-mg scored tablets in pediatric patients 3 months of age or older is limited to those who transitioned from a twice-daily regimen to a once-daily regimen after 36 weeks of treatment.

Table 1. Twice-daily Lamivudine for Treatment of HIV-1 Infection in Pediatric Patients Weighing at least 14 kg (150-mg Tablets)

Weight (kg)	AM Dose	PM Dose
14 to <20	75 mg (half of 150-mg tablet)	75 mg (half of 150-mg tablet)
20 to <25	75 mg (half of 150-mg tablet)	150 mg (one 150-mg tablet)
≥25	150 mg (one 150-mg tablet)	150 mg (one 150-mg tablet)

Table 2. Once-daily Lamivudine for Treatment of HIV-1 Infection in Pediatric Patients Weighing at least 14 kg (150-mg Tablets)

Weight (kg)	Once-daily Dose
14 to <20	150 mg (one 150-mg tablet)
20 to <25	225 mg (one and one-half 150-mg tablets)
≥25	300 mg (two 150-mg tablets or one 300-mg tablet)

Some experts state that adolescents weighing less than 25 kg should receive lamivudine in a dosage of 4 mg/kg (up to 150 mg) twice daily and those weighing 25 kg or more should receive 150 mg twice daily or 300 mg once daily.

Although safety and efficacy of lamivudine in infants younger than 3 months of age have not been established, some experts suggest that neonates younger than 4 weeks of age† can receive lamivudine in a dosage of 2 mg/kg twice daily and infants 4 weeks of age or older† can receive a dosage of 4 mg/kg (up to 150 mg) twice daily. These experts state that once-daily regimens of lamivudine oral solution are not generally recommended in infants and young children.

When lamivudine/zidovudine is used for the treatment of HIV-1 infection in pediatric patients weighing 30 kg or more, the recommended dosage is 1 tablet (150 mg of lamivudine and 300 mg of zidovudine) twice daily.

When abacavir/lamivudine/zidovudine is used for the treatment of HIV-1 infection in pediatric patients weighing 40 kg or more, the recommended dosage is 1 tablet (300 mg of abacavir, 150 mg of lamivudine, and 300 mg of zidovudine) orally twice daily.

When abacavir/lamivudine is used for the treatment of HIV-1 infection in pediatric patients weighing 25 kg or more, the recommended dosage is 1 tablet (600 mg of abacavir and 300 mg of lamivudine) once daily.

When abacavir/dolutegravir/lamivudine is used for the treatment of HIV-1 infection in pediatric patients weighing 40 kg or more, the recommended dosage is 1 tablet (600 mg of abacavir, 50 mg of dolutegravir, and 300 mg of lamivudine) orally once daily. If abacavir/dolutegravir/lamivudine is used in those receiving concomitant therapy with efavirenz, *ritonavir-boosted* fosamprenavir, *ritonavir-boosted* tipranavir, carbamazepine, or rifampin, patients should receive 1 tablet of the fixed combination (600 mg of abacavir, 50 mg of dolutegravir, and 300 mg of lamivudine) once daily *and* a 50-mg tablet of single-entity dolutegravir given once daily 12 hours after the daily dose of the fixed combination.

Prevention of Perinatal HIV Transmission **Pediatric Dosage.** When empiric HIV therapy† is used for prevention of perinatal HIV transmission† in neonates at highest risk of HIV acquisition (see Uses: Prevention of Perinatal HIV Transmission), a 3-drug antiretroviral regimen of zidovudine, lamivudine, and nevirapine is recommended and should be initiated as soon as possible after birth (within 6–12 hours).

For empiric HIV therapy† in HIV-exposed neonates, experts recommend that lamivudine be given in a dosage of 2 mg/kg twice daily from birth to 4 weeks of age followed by 4 mg/kg twice daily from 4–6 weeks of age.

Optimal duration of empiric HIV therapy† in HIV-exposed neonates at highest risk of HIV acquisition is unknown. Many experts recommend that the 3-drug regimen be continued for 6 weeks; others discontinue nevirapine and/or lamivudine if results of the neonate's HIV nucleic acid amplification test (NAAT) are negative, but recommend continuing zidovudine for 6 weeks.

Clinicians can consult the National Perinatal HIV Hotline at 888-448-8765 for information regarding selection of antiretrovirals, including dosage considerations, for prevention of perinatal HIV transmission.

Postexposure Prophylaxis following Occupational Exposure to HIV For postexposure prophylaxis of HIV infection following occupational exposure† (PEP) in health-care personnel or other individuals, the preferred dosage of lamivudine is 300 mg once daily. Alternatively, lamivudine can be given in a dosage of 150 mg twice daily. Lamivudine usually is used with tenofovir DF or zidovudine in conjunction with a recommended HIV integrase strand transferase inhibitor (INSTI), HIV nonnucleoside reverse transcriptase inhibitor (NNRTI), or HIV protease inhibitor (PI). (See Uses: Postexposure Prophylaxis following Occupational Exposure to HIV.)

When lamivudine/zidovudine is used as the dual NRTI option in PEP† regimens, adults should receive 1 tablet (150 mg of lamivudine and 300 mg of zidovudine) twice daily in conjunction with a recommended INSTI, NNRTI, or PI. (See Uses: Postexposure Prophylaxis following Occupational Exposure to HIV.)

PEP should be initiated as soon as possible following occupational exposure to HIV (preferably within hours) and continued for 4 weeks, if tolerated.

Postexposure Prophylaxis following Nonoccupational Exposure to HIV For postexposure prophylaxis of HIV infection following nonoccupational exposure† (nPEP) in individuals with impaired renal function (creatinine clearance 59 mL/minute or less), lamivudine usually is used in conjunction with zidovudine and either raltegravir or dolutegravir. (See Uses: Postexposure Prophylaxis following Nonoccupational Exposure to HIV.) Lamivudine dosage should be adjusted based on the degree of renal impairment.

The nPEP regimen should be initiated as soon as possible (within 72 hours) following nonoccupational exposure to HIV and continued for 28 days. If it has been more than 72 hours since the exposure, nPEP is not recommended.

Chronic Hepatitis B Virus Infection For the treatment of chronic hepatitis B virus (HBV) infection in adults, lamivudine should be administered as the oral solution containing 5 mg/mL or tablets containing 100 mg of the drug. Prior to and periodically during lamivudine therapy for treatment of chronic HBV infection, the HIV status of the patient should be determined since the dosage of the drug used for treatment of HBV infection is lower than the dosage used for treatment of HIV infection and use of suboptimal dosages in HIV-infected individuals may allow for the selection of lamivudine-resistant HIV isolates. (See Precautions Related to Treatment of Chronic HBV Infection under Cautions: Precautions and Contraindications.)

Adult Dosage. When lamivudine (100-mg tablets or oral solution containing 5 mg/mL) is used for the treatment of chronic HBV infection in adults, the recommended dosage is 100 mg once daily.

Pediatric Dosage. When lamivudine (100-mg tablets or oral solution containing 5 mg/mL) is used for the treatment of chronic HBV infection in children 2 years of age or older, the recommended dosage is 3 mg/kg (up to 100 mg) once daily.

Duration of Therapy and Clinical and Laboratory Monitoring. The optimum duration of lamivudine therapy for treatment of chronic HBV infection is not known.

Patients receiving lamivudine for treatment of chronic HBV infection should be monitored regularly by a clinician experienced in the management of chronic HBV infection. During lamivudine therapy, events that may be considered as potentially reflecting loss of therapeutic response include combinations of such events as return of persistently elevated serum ALT concentrations, increasing levels of HBV DNA over time after an initial decline below the limits of detection of the assay, progression of clinical signs or symptoms of hepatic disease, and/or worsening of hepatic necroinflammatory findings. Such events should be taken into consideration when determining the advisability of continuing lamivudine therapy.

Patients should be informed that deterioration of liver disease has been reported following discontinuance of lamivudine therapy, and that they should discuss any change in regimen with their clinician. Patients also should be informed that emergence of lamivudine-resistant HBV and worsening of disease can occur during treatment, and they should promptly report any new symptoms to their clinician. (See Cautions: Precautions and Contraindications.)

■ Dosage in Renal and Hepatic Impairment

Treatment of HIV Infection Because lamivudine pharmacokinetics are not affected by hepatic impairment, dosage adjustments are not necessary when lamivudine is used for the treatment of HIV infection in patients with hepatic impairment. However, safety and efficacy have not been established in those with decompensated liver disease.

Because elimination of lamivudine may be reduced in patients with renal impairment, dosage of the drug should be decreased in those with creatinine clearances less than 50 mL/minute. If lamivudine is used for the treatment of HIV infection in adults and adolescents weighing 25 kg or more with impaired renal function, dosage of the drug should be adjusted based on creatinine clearance. (See Table 3.) The manufacturer states that data are insufficient to make dosage recommendations for HIV-infected pediatric patients with renal impairment; however, a reduction in the dose and/or an increase in the dosing interval should be considered.

Table 3. Lamivudine Dosage for Treatment of HIV-1 Infection in Adults and Adolescents with Renal Impairment Weighing 25 kg or More.

Creatinine Clearance (mL/minute)	Dosage
30–49	150 mg once daily
15–29	150 mg first dose, then 100 mg once daily
5–14	150 mg first dose, then 50 mg once daily
<5	50 mg first dose, then 25 mg once daily
Hemodialysis patients	Supplemental doses unnecessary after routine (4-hour) hemodialysis
Peritoneal dialysis patients	Supplemental doses unnecessary after peritoneal dialysis

Lamivudine/zidovudine should *not* be used for the treatment of HIV infection in patients with renal impairment (creatinine clearance less than 50 mL/minute) or in patients with hepatic impairment.

Abacavir/lamivudine, abacavir/lamivudine/zidovudine, and abacavir/dolutegravir/lamivudine should *not* be used for the treatment of HIV infection in patients with renal impairment (creatinine clearance less than 50 mL/minute) or in patients with hepatic impairment. Abacavir/lamivudine, abacavir/lamivudine/zidovudine, and abacavir/dolutegravir/lamivudine are contraindicated in those with moderate or severe hepatic impairment.

Chronic Hepatitis B Virus Infection Dosage adjustments are not necessary when lamivudine is used for the treatment of chronic HBV infection in patients with hepatic impairment. However, safety and efficacy have not been established in those with decompensated liver disease.

If lamivudine is used for treatment of chronic HBV infection in adults with impaired renal function, dosage of the drug should be adjusted based on creatinine clearance. (See Table 4.) The manufacturer states that data are insufficient to make specific dosage recommendations for pediatric patients with renal impairment.

Table 4. Lamivudine Dosage for the Treatment of Chronic HBV Infection in Adults with Renal Impairment.

Creatinine Clearance (mL/minute)	Dosage
30–49	100 mg first dose, then 50 mg once daily
15–29	100 mg first dose, then 25 mg once daily
5–14	35 mg first dose, then 15 mg once daily
<5	35 mg first dose, then 10 mg once daily
Hemodialysis patients	Supplemental doses unnecessary after routine (4-hour) hemodialysis
Peritoneal dialysis patients	Supplemental doses unnecessary after peritoneal dialysis

Cautions

Information on adverse effects of lamivudine has been obtained from clinical studies in adults with human immunodeficiency virus (HIV) infection who received the drug in conjunction with other antiretroviral agents (e.g., studies NUCA3001, NUCA3002, NUCB3001, NUCB3002, NUCB3007, EPV20001, EPV40001). In addition, information on adverse effects of lamivudine in patients with compensated chronic hepatitis B virus (HBV) infection has been obtained from 3 placebo-controlled studies where the drug was used alone for up to 68 weeks.

The most common adverse effects reported in HIV-infected adults receiving lamivudine in conjunction with other antiretroviral agents are nausea, fatigue and/or malaise, headache, nasal symptoms, diarrhea, and cough. The manufacturer states that the types and frequencies of adverse effects in HIV-infected patients receiving lamivudine 300 mg once daily are similar to those reported in patients receiving 150 mg twice daily. The most common adverse effects reported in clinical trials evaluating lamivudine in adults with chronic HBV infection are increased ALT concentrations; infections of the ear, nose, or throat; diarrhea; sore throat; and increased serum lipase concentrations.

Although lamivudine generally is well tolerated, serious adverse effects such as peripheral neuropathy, pancreatitis, and lactic acidosis and severe hepatomegaly with steatosis have been reported.

When the fixed combination containing lamivudine and zidovudine (lamivudine/zidovudine; Combivir®, generic), fixed combination containing abacavir and lamivudine (abacavir/lamivudine; Epzicom®, generic), fixed combination containing abacavir, lamivudine, and zidovudine (abacavir/lamivudine/zidovudine; Trizivir®, generic), or fixed combination containing abacavir, dolutegravir, and lamivudine (abacavir/dolutegravir/lamivudine; Triumeq®) is used, the adverse effects, precautions, and contraindications associated with each of the individual components should be considered. (See Precautions Related to Use of Fixed Combinations under Cautions: Precautions and Contraindications.)

■ Nervous System Effects

Peripheral neuropathy has been reported in adults receiving lamivudine, but has rarely resulted in interruption or discontinuance of therapy. In clinical studies NUCA3001, NUCA3002, NUCB3001, and NUCB3002 in HIV-infected adults receiving lamivudine in conjunction with zidovudine, neuropathy was reported in 12% of the patients. Weakness has been reported in patients receiving lamivudine during postmarketing experience.

In HIV-infected adults receiving lamivudine in conjunction with zidovudine, headache, malaise, fatigue, insomnia and other sleep disorders, dizziness, and depressive disorders were reported in 35, 27, 27, 11, 10, and 9%, respectively.

There have been postmarketing reports of paresthesia and peripheral neuropathy in patients receiving lamivudine for treatment of chronic HBV infection.

■ Pancreatitis

Pancreatitis has been reported in less than 0.5% of patients receiving lamivudine for treatment of HIV infection in controlled clinical studies; pancreatitis has been reported during postmarketing experience. However, the incidence of pancreatitis was reported to be 14–18% in HIV-infected pediatric patients receiving lamivudine in open-label studies. (See Cautions: Pediatric Precautions) Increased serum amylase concentrations (greater than 2 times the upper limit of normal) were reported 4.2 % of adults receiving lamivudine in conjunction with zidovudine in clinical studies NUCA3001, NUCA3002, NUCB3001, NUCB3002 and in 2.2% of adults receiving lamivudine in conjunction with other antiretroviral agents in clinical study NUCB3007.

In clinical studies in adults who received lamivudine for treatment of chronic HBV infection, increased serum lipase concentrations (at least 2.5 times the upper limit of normal) were reported in 10% of patients. There also have been postmarketing reports of pancreatitis.

■ Hepatic Effects and Lactic Acidosis

Lactic acidosis and severe hepatomegaly with steatosis, including some fatalities, have been reported rarely in patients receiving lamivudine and also have been reported in patients receiving other HIV nucleoside reverse transcriptase inhibitors (NRTIs) and other antiretrovirals. Most reported cases have involved women; obesity and long-term therapy with NRTIs also may be risk factors. Lamivudine should be used with caution in patients with known risk factors for liver disease; however, lactic acidosis and severe hepatomegaly with steatosis have been reported in patients with no known risk factors. (See Cautions: Precautions and Contraindications).

Increased serum concentrations of AST (SGOT), ALT (SGPT), and bilirubin have been reported in patients receiving lamivudine in conjunction with other antiretroviral agents for treatment of HIV infection. In clinical studies NUCA3001, NUCA3002, NUCB3001, and NUCB3002, increased serum concentrations of ALT (greater than 5 times the upper limit of normal), AST (greater than 5 times the upper limit of normal), or bilirubin (greater than 2.5 times the upper limit of normal) were reported in 3.7, 1.7, and 0.8% of patients, respectively. In another study (NUCB3007) evaluating patients receiving lamivudine in conjunction with other antiretroviral agents, the overall incidence of increased serum concentrations of ALT or AST (greater than 5 times the upper limit of normal) was 3.8 or 4%, respectively. The occurrence of increased levels of hepatic enzymes and bilirubin in these patients appears to be transient and resolves without dosage modification or discontinuance of therapy.

In clinical studies in adults who received 52 weeks of lamivudine for treatment of chronic HBV infection, serum ALT concentrations at least 2 times greater than baseline were reported in 27% and serum ALT concentrations at least 3 times greater than baseline were reported in 21% of patients during 16 weeks of follow-up after the drug was discontinued. Increased serum concentrations of ALT (at least 2 times greater than baseline) and absolute serum ALT concentrations exceeding 500 IU/L were reported in 15% of patients evaluated for up to 16 weeks after discontinuance of the drug; increased serum concentrations of ALT (at least 2 times greater than baseline) and increased serum bilirubin concentrations (greater than 2 times the upper limit of normal and at least 2 times greater than baseline) were reported in 0.7% of patients.

Hepatic decompensation, sometimes fatal, has been reported in HIV-infected patients coinfected with hepatitis C virus (HCV) receiving antiretroviral therapy concomitantly with interferon alfa (or peginterferon alfa) with or without ribavirin. (See Precautions Related to Treatment of HIV Infection under Cautions: Precautions and Contraindications and see Drug Interactions.)

■ GI Effects

In clinical studies NUCA3001, NUCA3002, NUCB3001, and NUCB3002 in HIV-infected adults, nausea, diarrhea, vomiting, anorexia and/or decreased appetite, abdominal pain, abdominal cramps, and dyspepsia were reported in 33, 18, 13, 10, 9, 6, and 5% of patients, respectively.

In clinical studies in adults receiving lamivudine for treatment of chronic HBV infection, diarrhea was reported in 14% of patients. There also have been postmarketing reports of stomatitis.

■ Dermatologic and Sensitivity Reactions

In studies NUCA3001, NUCA3002, NUCB3001, and NUCB3002 in HIV-infected adults receiving lamivudine in conjunction with zidovudine, rash was reported in 9% of patients. Anaphylaxis, urticaria, alopecia, rash, pruritus, erythema multiforme, and Stevens-Johnson syndrome have been reported in patients who received lamivudine or the fixed combination of lamivudine and zidovudine during postmarketing experience.

There have been postmarketing reports of alopecia, pruritus, and rash in patients receiving lamivudine for treatment of chronic HBV infection.

■ Hematologic Effects

In studies NUCA3001, NUCA3002, NUCB3001, and NUCB3002 in HIV-infected adults, anemia (hemoglobin concentration less than 8.0 g/dL) was reported in 2.9% of patients who received lamivudine in conjunction with zidovudine. In addition, neutropenia (neutrophil count less than 750/mm^3) occurred in 7.2% and thrombocytopenia (thrombocytes less than 50,000/mm^3) occurred in 0.4% of patients. In study NUCB3007 in HIV-infected adults, anemia (hemoglobin less than 8.0 g/dL) was reported in 2.2%, neutropenia (neutrophil count less than 750/mm^3) occurred in 15%, and thrombocytopenia (thrombocytes less than 50,000/mm^3) occurred in 2.8% of patients. The occurrence of neutropenia in these patients appears to be transient and resolves without dosage modification or discontinuation of therapy.

Thrombocytopenia has been reported in patients receiving lamivudine for treatment of chronic HBV infection. In clinical trials, thrombocytopenia (platelets less than 50,000/mm^3) was reported in 4% of patients receiving the drug.

Aplastic anemia, anemia (including severe anemia progressing on therapy), lymphadenopathy, pure red cell aplasia, and splenomegaly have been reported in patients receiving lamivudine or lamivudine/zidovudine during postmarketing experience.

■ Musculoskeletal Effects

Adverse musculoskeletal effects, including pain, myalgia, and arthralgia have been reported in 12, 8, and 5%, respectively, of HIV-infected patients who received lamivudine in studies NUCA3001, NUCA3002, NUCB3001, and NUCB3002.

In clinical studies evaluating lamivudine for treatment of chronic HBV infection, increased concentrations of creatine kinase (CK, creatine phosphokinase, CPK) exceeding 7 times the baseline concentration were reported in 9% of patients. Myalgia and arthralgia also have been reported.

Muscle weakness, cramps, CK (CPK) elevation, and rhabdomyolysis have been reported in patients receiving lamivudine or lamivudine/zidovudine during postmarketing experience.

■ Adipogenic Effects

Redistribution or accumulation of body fat, including central obesity, dorsocervical fat enlargement ("buffalo hump"), peripheral wasting, facial wasting, breast enlargement, and general cushingoid appearance, has been reported in patients receiving antiretroviral agents, including lamivudine or the fixed combination of lamivudine and ritonavir. The mechanisms responsible for these adipogenic effects and the long-term consequences of these effects are unknown. A causal relationship has not been established.

■ **Immune Reconstitution Syndrome** Patients receiving potent antiretroviral therapy may experience an immune reconstitution syndrome during the initial phase of therapy. Patients whose immune system responds to antiretroviral therapy may develop an inflammatory response to indolent or residual opportunistic infections (e.g., *Mycobacterium avium* complex [MAC], *M. tuberculosis*, cytomegalovirus [CMV], *Pneumocystis jirovecii* [formerly *P. carinii*]); this may necessitate further evaluation and treatment.

Autoimmune disorders (e.g., Graves' disease, polymyositis, Guillain-Barré syndrome) also have been reported to occur in the setting of immune reconstitution; however, the time to onset is more variable and can occur many months after initiation of antiretroviral therapy.

■ **Other Adverse Effects** Nasal signs and symptoms, cough, and fever or chills have been reported in 20, 18, and 10%, respectively, of HIV-infected patients who received lamivudine in studies NUCA3001, NUCA3002, NUCB3001, and NUCB3002. In adults who received lamivudine for treatment of chronic HBV infection, ear, nose, and throat infection was reported in 25% and sore throat was reported in 13% of patients. There also have been postmarketing reports of abnormal breath sounds/wheezing in patients receiving lamivudine for treatment of chronic HBV infection.

Hyperglycemia, cardiomyopathy, vasculitis, weakness have been reported in patients receiving lamivudine or lamivudine/zidovudine during postmarketing experience.

■ **Precautions and Contraindications** Lamivudine is contraindicated in patients with a history of hypersensitivity to the drug.

Lamivudine/zidovudine is contraindicated in patients with a history of hypersensitivity to lamivudine or zidovudine.

Abacavir/lamivudine is contraindicated in patients who have the human leukocyte antigen (HLA)-B*5701 allele; patients with a history of hypersensitivity to abacavir or lamivudine; and patients with moderate or severe hepatic impairment.

Abacavir/lamivudine/zidovudine is contraindicated in patients who have the HLA-B*5701 allele; patients with a history of hypersensitivity to abacavir, lamivudine, or zidovudine; and patients with moderate or severe hepatic impairment.

Abacavir/dolutegravir/lamivudine is contraindicated in patients who have the HLA-B*5701 allele; patients with a history of hypersensitivity to abacavir, dolutegravir, or lamivudine; patients receiving dofetilide; and patients with moderate or severe hepatic impairment.

Because lactic acidosis and severe hepatomegaly with steatosis, including fatalities, have been reported in patients receiving nucleoside analogs and other antiretrovirals (see Cautions: Hepatic Effects and Lactic Acidosis), lamivudine and fixed combinations containing lamivudine should be discontinued in any patient who develops clinical or laboratory findings suggestive of lactic acidosis or pronounced hepatotoxicity (which may include hepatomegaly and steatosis even in the absence of marked increases in serum aminotransferase concentrations). Lamivudine should be used with caution in patients with known risk factors for liver disease; however, lactic acidosis and severe hepatomegaly with steatosis have been reported in patients with no known risk factors.

Patients should be advised to immediately contact a clinician if they have any signs or symptoms of infection since inflammation from previous infections may occur soon after antiretroviral therapy is initiated. (See Cautions: Immune Reconstitution Syndrome.)

Patients should be advised that redistribution or accumulation of body fat may occur in patients receiving antiretroviral therapy and that the cause and long-term health effects of these conditions are as yet unknown. (See Cautions: Adipogenic Effects.)

Patients with renal impairment (i.e., creatinine clearances less than 50 mL/minute) may be at increased risk of adverse effects during lamivudine therapy because of decreased clearance of the drug; decreased dosage is recommended in such patients. Lamivudine dosage adjustments are recommended based on the degree of renal impairment. (See Dosage: Dosage in Renal and Hepatic Impairment.)

Individuals with diabetes mellitus and/or their caregivers should be informed that lamivudine oral solutions contain 200 mg of sucrose per mL.

Because of similarity in spelling between lamivudine and lamotrigine (Lamictal®, an anticonvulsant agent), several dispensing errors have been reported to the manufacturer. These medication errors may be associated with serious adverse effects either due to lack of appropriate therapy for seizures (e.g., in patients not receiving the prescribed anticonvulsant, lamotrigine, which may lead to status epilepticus) or due to the risk of developing adverse effects associated with the use of lamotrigine (e.g., serious rash) in patients for whom the drug was not prescribed and consequently not properly titrated. Therefore, the manufacturer cautions that extra care should be exercised in ensuring the accuracy of both oral and written prescriptions for lamotrigine (Lamictal®) and lamivudine. The manufacturer also recommends that pharmacists assess the measures of avoiding dispensing errors and implement them as appropriate (e.g., placing drugs with similar names apart from one another in product storage areas, patient counseling).

Precautions Related to Treatment of HIV Infection Patients should be advised of the importance of adhering to the prescribed antiretroviral regimen and the importance of remaining under the care of a clinician.

Patients should be advised that effective antiretroviral regimens can decrease HIV concentrations in blood and genital secretions and strict adherence to such regimens in conjunction with risk-reduction measures may decrease, but cannot absolutely eliminate, the risk of secondary transmission of HIV to others. Patients should continue to practice safer sex (e.g., consistent use of condoms).

Patients receiving lamivudine with peginterferon alfa (or interferon alfa) with or without ribavirin should be closely monitored for toxicity, especially hepatic decompensation, neutropenia, and anemia. HIV-infected patients coinfected with HCV should be informed that hepatic decompensation (sometimes fatal) has been reported when antiretrovirals were used concomitantly with interferon alfa with or without ribavirin. (See Drug Interactions: Interferon Alfa and Peginterferon Alfa.)

Precautions Related to Treatment of Chronic HBV Infection

Prior to and periodically during lamivudine therapy for treatment of chronic HBV infection, all patients should be offered HIV counseling and testing. Lamivudine preparations labeled by FDA for treatment of chronic HBV infection should *not* be used in patients coinfected with HIV since they contain a lower dose of lamivudine than preparations labeled for treatment of HIV-1 infection. If lamivudine preparations labeled for treatment of chronic HBV infection are used in patients with unrecognized or untreated HIV infection, rapid emergence of lamivudine-resistant HIV may occur and limit antiretroviral treatment options. If a decision is made to use lamivudine in patients coinfected with HBV and HIV, the drug should be used in dosages recommended for treatment of HIV infection and in conjunction with other antiretrovirals.

Patients receiving lamivudine for treatment of chronic HBV infection should be monitored regularly by a clinician experienced in the management of chronic HBV infection.

Posttreatment exacerbations of HBV infection and emergence of resistant strains of HBV have been reported following discontinuance of lamivudine therapy in non-HIV-infected patients. Exacerbations of HBV infection also have been reported when lamivudine was discontinued from antiretroviral regimens in HIV-infected patients coinfected with HBV. Such exacerbations of HBV infection have been detected principally by increases in serum ALT concentrations in addition to re-emergence of serum HBV DNA. Although most events appear to have been self-limited and the causal relationship to lamivudine discontinuance is unknown, some fatalities have been reported. Patients should be closely monitored with both clinical and laboratory follow-up for at least several months after stopping lamivudine treatment. There is insufficient evidence to determine whether reinitiation of therapy alters the course of posttreatment exacerbations of hepatitis.

Patients should be advised that the long-term benefits of lamivudine therapy in patients with chronic HBV infection are unknown at this time and that the relationship between treatment response and outcomes such as hepatocellular carcinoma and decompensated cirrhosis is unknown.

Patients should also be advised that lamivudine therapy has not been shown to reduce the risk of transmission of HBV to others via sexual conduct or blood contamination and that practices designed to prevent transmission of HBV should be maintained during therapy.

Lamivudine should not be used concomitantly with any preparation containing lamivudine or emtricitabine.

Precautions Related to Use of Fixed Combinations When lamivudine/zidovudine, abacavir/lamivudine, abacavir/lamivudine/zidovudine, or abacavir/dolutegravir/lamivudine is used, the usual cautions, precautions, contraindications, and drug interactions associated with each drug in the fixed combination must be considered. Cautionary information applicable to specific populations (e.g., pregnant or nursing women, individuals with hepatic or renal impairment, pediatric patients, geriatric patients) should be considered for each drug. For cautionary information related to abacavir, dolutegravir, or zidovudine, see Cautions in the individual drug monographs.

Lamivudine and fixed combinations containing lamivudine should not be used concomitantly with any preparation containing emtricitabine.

If abacavir/lamivudine, abacavir/lamivudine/zidovudine, or abacavir/dolutegravir/lamivudine is used, clinicians should consider that serious and sometimes fatal hypersensitivity reactions, with multiple organ involvement, have been reported in patients receiving abacavir or fixed combinations containing abacavir. Prior to initiation or reinitiation of abacavir/lamivudine, abacavir/lamivudine/zidovudine, or abacavir/dolutegravir/lamivudine, all patients should be screened for the HLA-B*5701 allele, unless there is documentation of a previous HLA-B*5701 allele assessment. The patient's medical history also should be reviewed for prior exposure to any abacavir-containing preparation. Abacavir-containing preparations are contraindicated in individuals who test positive for HLA-B*5701. Such individuals are at higher risk for hypersensitivity reactions; however, hypersensitivity reactions have occurred in patients who do not carry the HLA-B*5701 allele. Abacavir/lamivudine, abacavir/lamivudine/zidovudine, or abacavir/dolutegravir/lamivudine should be discontinued immediately if a hypersensitivity reaction is suspected, regardless of HLA-B*5701 status and even if other diagnoses are possible. The fixed combinations containing abacavir should be permanently discontinued if hypersensitivity cannot be ruled out. (See Abacavir Sulfate 8:18.08.20.)

If lamivudine/zidovudine or abacavir/lamivudine/zidovudine is used, clinicians should consider that zidovudine has been associated with hematologic toxicity (including neutropenia and severe anemia), particularly in those with advanced HIV-1 disease, and that prolonged zidovudine use has been associated with symptomatic myopathy. These fixed combinations should be used with caution in patients who have bone marrow compromise evidenced by a granulocyte count less than 1000 cells/mm^3 or a hemoglobin concentration less than 9.5 g/dL. (See Zidovudine 8:18.08.20.)

■ **Pediatric Precautions** Safety and efficacy of lamivudine (150-mg scored tablets, 300-mg tablets, oral solution containing 10 mg/mL) in conjunction with other antiretroviral agents for treatment of HIV infection have been established in children 3 months of age or older. Because there is some evidence that use of lamivudine oral solution in pediatric patients is associated with lower rates of virologic suppression, lower plasma lamivudine exposures, and more frequent emergence of lamivudine-resistant HIV-1, the 150-mg scored tablets are the preferred preparation in pediatric patients who weigh 14 kg or more and can swallow tablets.

Safety and efficacy of lamivudine (100-mg tablets, oral solution containing 5 mg/mL) for treatment of chronic HBV infection have been established in children 2 years of age or older. Adverse effects reported in HBV-infected children in this age group were similar to those reported in adults with HBV infection. Elevated serum aminotransferase (transaminase) concentrations were reported in some children after discontinuance of the drug. Safety and efficacy of lamivudine for treatment of HBV infection have not been established in children younger than 2 years of age.

In clinical studies in HIV-infected pediatric patients who received lamivudine in conjunction with zidovudine, paresthesia and peripheral neuropathies have been reported in up to 15% of patients. Pancreatitis, including some fatalities, has occurred in 14–18% of HIV-infected pediatric patients receiving lamivudine alone or in conjunction with other nucleoside antiretroviral agents. Other adverse effects reported in pediatric patients receiving lamivudine in conjunction with zidovudine were similar to those reported in adults and include GI effects, hepatic effects, sensitivity reactions, and hematologic effects.

Lamivudine should be used with caution in pediatric patients with a history of prior therapy with NRTIs, a history of pancreatitis, or significant risk factors for development of pancreatitis. If clinical signs, symptoms, or laboratory abnormalities suggestive of pancreatitis occur, lamivudine should be discontinued immediately. Parents or guardians should be advised to monitor pediatric patients for signs and symptoms of pancreatitis.

Limited data are available regarding safety of lamivudine in neonates†. Adverse effects reported in neonates who received lamivudine alone or in conjunction with zidovudine during the first week of life as part of a regimen for prevention of perinatal HIV transmission in 2 small, uncontrolled studies in Africa include increased liver function test results, anemia, diarrhea, electrolyte disturbances, hypoglycemia, jaundice and hepatomegaly, rash, respiratory infections, sepsis, and syphilis; 3 neonates died (one from gastroenteritis with acidosis and seizures, one from traumatic injury, and one from unknown causes). There were 2 other nonfatal gastroenteritis or diarrhea cases, including one with seizures; transient renal insufficiency associated with dehydration was reported in one infant. Because there were no control groups in these studies, causality is difficult to establish. However, it should be assumed that perinatally exposed neonates may be at risk for adverse effects similar to those reported in pediatric and adult HIV-infected patients receiving multiple-drug regimens containing lamivudine. The long-term effects of in utero and infant exposure to lamivudine are unknown.

Lamivudine/zidovudine should *not* be used in pediatric patients weighing less than 30 kg.

Abacavir/lamivudine should *not* be used in pediatric patients weighing less than 25 kg.

Abacavir/lamivudine/zidovudine should *not* be used in pediatric patients weighing less than 40 kg.

Abacavir/dolutegravir/lamivudine should *not* be used in pediatric patients weighing less than 40 kg.

■ **Geriatric Precautions** Clinical studies of lamivudine did not include sufficient numbers of patients 65 years of age and older to determine whether geriatric patients respond differently than younger patients. Lamivudine and fixed combinations containing lamivudine should be used with caution in geriatric patients because these individuals frequently have decreased hepatic, renal, and/or cardiac function and concomitant disease and drug therapy. (See Dosage and Administration: Dosage in Renal and Hepatic Impairment.)

■ **Mutagenicity and Carcinogenicity** Lamivudine was mutagenic in an L5178Y mouse lymphoma assay and clastogenic in a cytogenetic assay using cultured human lymphocytes. Lamivudine was not mutagenic in a microbial mutagenicity assay, an in vitro cell transformation assay, a rat micronucleus test, a rat bone marrow cytogenetic assay, and an assay for unscheduled DNA synthesis in rat liver. Lamivudine showed no evidence of in vivo genotoxic activity in the rat at oral doses up to 2 g/kg that produced plasma concentrations 35–45 times higher than those attained in humans receiving dosages recommended for treatment of HIV infection.

The carcinogenic potential of lamivudine has been studied in mice and rats. No evidence of carcinogenicity was seen in long-term studies in mice or rats receiving oral lamivudine dosages at exposures approximately 34 or 200 times higher, respectively, than those reported in humans receiving the recommended dosage for HBV infection and at exposures approximately 10 or 58 times higher, respectively, in humans receiving the recommended dosage for HIV infection.

■ **Pregnancy, Fertility, and Lactation** ***Pregnancy*** Lamivudine crosses the placenta and is distributed into cord blood in concentrations similar to maternal serum concentrations.

To monitor maternal-fetal outcomes of pregnant women exposed to antiretroviral agents, including lamivudine, the Antiretroviral Pregnancy Registry was established. Clinicians are encouraged to contact the registry at 800-258-4263 or http://www.APRegistry.com to report cases of prenatal exposure to antiretroviral agents.

Data from the Antiretroviral Pregnancy Registry show no difference in the risk of overall major birth defects for lamivudine compared with the background rate for major birth defects in the US reference population of the Metropolitan Atlanta Congenital Defects Program (MACDP). Registry data include over 11,000 prospective reports of lamivudine exposures during pregnancy resulting in live births, including over 4300 first-trimester exposures to the drug.

Reproduction studies in rats or rabbits using oral lamivudine dosages that resulted in plasma concentrations up to approximately 35 times higher than plasma concentrations attained with the recommended human dosage used for the treatment of HIV infection in adults have not revealed evidence of teratogenicity. Although there was evidence of early embryolethality in rabbits at exposure levels similar to those observed in humans, this effect was not seen in rats at exposure levels up to 35 times higher than those in humans.

The US Department of Health and Human Services (HHS) Panel on Treatment of Pregnant Women with HIV Infection and Prevention of Perinatal Transmission states that the preferred dual NRTI options for *initial* regimens used for treatment of HIV-1 infection in antiretroviral-naive pregnant women are abacavir and lamivudine (should be used only in those negative for HLA-B*5701) or tenofovir DF and emtricitabine (or lamivudine). Tenofovir DF and emtricitabine (or lamivudine) is the preferred dual NRTI option for treatment of HIV-1 infection in pregnant women coinfected with HBV. These experts state that zidovudine and lamivudine is an alternative dual NRTI option for *initial* regimens used for treatment of HIV infection in antiretroviral-naive pregnant women.

The American Association for the Study of Liver Diseases (AASLD) and other experts state that recommendations regarding use of antiviral therapy for the management of HBV infection in pregnant women generally are the same as those for other adults. AASLD suggests that hepatitis B surface antigen (HBsAg)-positive pregnant women with HBV DNA levels exceeding 200,000 IU/mL receive antiviral therapy since this may reduce the risk of perinatal transmission of HBV; however, preferred antiviral agents, exact viral load threshold, and optimal gestational week during the third trimester to initiate such therapy have not been clearly identified. Routine screening for HBV infection is recommended for *all* pregnant women. For prevention of perinatal transmission of HBV, US Public Health Service Advisory Committee on Immunization Practices (ACIP), American Academy of Pediatrics (AAP), and other experts state that infants born to HBsAg-positive women should receive their first dose of hepatitis B vaccine *and* a dose of hepatitis B immune globulin (HBIG) within 12 hours of birth.

Fertility There was no evidence that lamivudine affected fertility in rats that received the drug in dosages up to 4 g/kg daily resulting in plasma concentrations 47–70 times higher than those seen in humans receiving the recommended dosage for treatment of HIV infection or 70–104 times higher than those reported in humans receiving the usually recommended dosage for treatment of chronic HBV infection.

Lactation Lamivudine is distributed into milk in humans. It is not known whether the drug affects human milk production or affects the breast-fed infant.

Because of the risk of transmission of HIV to an uninfected infant through breast milk, the HHS Panel and the US Centers for Disease Control and Prevention (CDC) recommend that HIV-infected women *not* breast-feed infants, regardless of antiretroviral therapy. Therefore, because of the potential for HIV transmission and the potential for serious adverse effects from lamivudine in nursing infants, women should be instructed not to breast-feed while they are receiving lamivudine, lamivudine/zidovudine, abacavir/lamivudine, abacavir/lamivudine/zidovudine, or abacavir/dolutegravir/lamivudine.

If lamivudine is being used for treatment of chronic HBV infection, the benefits of breast-feeding and the importance of lamivudine to the woman should be considered along with the potential adverse effects on the breast-fed infant from the drug or from the underlying maternal condition.

Drug Interactions

The following drug interactions are based on studies using lamivudine. When the fixed combination containing lamivudine and zidovudine (lamivudine/zidovudine), fixed combination containing abacavir and lamivudine (abacavir/lamivudine), fixed combination containing abacavir, lamivudine, and zidovudine (abacavir/lamivudine/zidovudine), or fixed combination containing abacavir, dolutegravir, and lamivudine (abacavir/dolutegravir/lamivudine) is used, interactions associated with each drug in the fixed combination should be considered.

■ **Drugs Affecting or Affected by Membrane Transporters** Based on in vitro studies, lamivudine at clinically important concentrations is not expected to affect the pharmacokinetics of drugs that are substrates of organic anion transporter polypeptide 1B1/3 (OATP1B1/3), breast cancer resistance protein (BCRP), P-glycoprotein (P-gp), multidrug and toxin extrusion protein (MATE) 1 or MATE2-K, organic cation transporter (OCT) 1, OCT2, or OCT3.

Lamivudine is a substrate of P-gp and BCRP; however, it is unlikely that these transporters play a clinically important role in absorption of lamivudine. Therefore, concomitant use of drugs that are inhibitors of these efflux transporters is unlikely to affect the disposition and elimination of lamivudine.

Lamivudine is a substrate of MATE1, MATE2-K, and OCT2 in vitro.

■ **Antiretroviral Agents** ***HIV Entry and Fusion Inhibitors*** **Enfuvirtide.** In vitro studies indicate that the antiretroviral effects of enfuvirtide and lamivudine are additive to synergistic against HIV-1.

Maraviroc. Maraviroc does not have a clinically important effect on the pharmacokinetics of lamivudine.

There is no in vitro evidence of antagonistic antiretroviral effects between maraviroc and lamivudine.

HIV Integrase Inhibitors (INSTIs) **Raltegravir.** Raltegravir does not have a clinically important effect on the pharmacokinetics of lamivudine.

There is no in vitro evidence of antagonistic antiretroviral effects between raltegravir and lamivudine.

HIV Nonnucleoside Reverse Transcriptase Inhibitors (NNRTIs) In vitro studies indicate that the antiretroviral effects of lamivudine and delavirdine or efavirenz may be additive or synergistic against HIV-1. There is no in vitro evidence of antagonistic antiretroviral effects between lamivudine and etravirine, nevirapine, or rilpivirine.

Efavirenz. In a multiple-dose pharmacokinetic study in HIV-infected patients, concomitant use of efavirenz and lamivudine did not affect lamivudine peak plasma concentrations or area under the serum concentration-time curve (AUC).

Dosage adjustments are not necessary if efavirenz is used concomitantly with lamivudine.

Rilpivirine. Clinically important pharmacokinetic interactions are not expected if rilpivirine is used concomitantly with lamivudine.

HIV Nucleoside and Nucleotide Reverse Transcriptase Inhibitors (NRTIs) Results of in vitro studies indicate that the antiretroviral effects of lamivudine and some other HIV nucleoside reverse transcriptase inhibitors (NRTIs) (e.g. emtricitabine, stavudine, tenofovir) are additive to synergistic against HIV-1. There is no in vitro evidence of antagonistic antiretroviral effects between lamivudine and abacavir.

There is no in vitro evidence of antagonistic antiviral effects between lamivudine and tenofovir against hepatitis B virus (HBV).

Abacavir. In a crossover study evaluating concomitant use of single doses of abacavir (600 mg) and lamivudine (150 mg) in HIV-infected individuals, the AUC of lamivudine was decreased 15% and the pharmacokinetics of abacavir were not affected. This pharmacokinetic interaction is not considered clinically important.

Emtricitabine. Emtricitabine and lamivudine should not be used concomitantly. Because emtricitabine is an analog of lamivudine, the drugs have similar resistance profiles and minimal additive antiretroviral effects.

Stavudine. In a pharmacokinetic study evaluating concomitant use of a single dose of stavudine (40 mg) and lamivudine (150 mg) in HIV-infected individuals, peak plasma concentrations of stavudine were increased 12%, but the AUC of stavudine and the peak plasma concentration and AUC of lamivudine were not affected. This pharmacokinetic interaction is not considered clinically important.

Tenofovir. In a pharmacokinetic study evaluating concomitant use of tenofovir disoproxil fumarate (300 mg once daily for 7 days) and lamivudine (150 mg twice daily for 7 days), peak plasma concentrations of lamivudine were decreased 24%, but the AUC of lamivudine and the peak plasma concentration and AUC of tenofovir were not affected.

Zidovudine. Results of a study in asymptomatic HIV-infected patients who received a single 200-mg dose of zidovudine in conjunction with multiple doses of lamivudine (300 mg every 12 hours) indicate that concomitant use of the drugs does not have a clinically important effect on the pharmacokinetics of either drug. The AUC of zidovudine was increased 13%, but lamivudine concentrations were not affected.

Dosage adjustments are not necessary if lamivudine is used concomitantly with zidovudine.

HIV Protease Inhibitors (PIs) Lamivudine and some HIV protease inhibitors (PIs) (e.g., amprenavir [commercially available as fosamprenavir], nelfinavir, ritonavir, saquinavir, tipranavir) are additive or synergistic against HIV-1 in vitro. There is no in vitro evidence of antagonistic antiretroviral effects between lamivudine and atazanavir or darunavir.

Atazanavir. Concomitant use of atazanavir and lamivudine does not result in clinically important interactions.

No clinically important pharmacokinetic interactions were reported when unboosted atazanavir (400 mg once daily) was used concomitantly with lamivudine (150 mg twice daily) and zidovudine (300 mg twice daily).

Darunavir. Concomitant use of *ritonavir-boosted* darunavir and lamivudine does not result in clinically important interactions.

Dosage adjustments are not needed if *ritonavir-boosted* darunavir is used concomitantly with lamivudine.

Fosamprenavir. Pharmacokinetic interactions did not occur when a single 600-mg dose of amprenavir (active metabolite of fosamprenavir) was used concomitantly with a single 150-mg dose of lamivudine.

Lopinavir. There was no evidence of clinically important pharmacokinetic interactions when the commercially available fixed combination of lopinavir and ritonavir (lopinavir/ritonavir) and lamivudine were used concomitantly.

Nelfinavir. Concomitant use of lamivudine (single 150-mg dose) and nelfinavir (750 mg every 8 hours for 7–10 days) increased the AUC and peak plasma concentration of lamivudine by 10 and 31%, respectively.

Tipranavir. In multiple-dose pharmacokinetic studies in HIV-infected individuals, concomitant use of *ritonavir-boosted* tipranavir and lamivudine did not have any clinically important effects on lamivudine pharmacokinetics.

■ **Co-trimoxazole** In a crossover pharmacokinetic study in HIV-infected individuals, concomitant use of co-trimoxazole (160 mg of trimethoprim and 800 mg of sulfamethoxazole once daily for 5 days) and lamivudine (single 300-mg dose) resulted in a 43% increase in the AUC of lamivudine, but did not affect the pharmacokinetics of trimethoprim or sulfamethoxazole. Data are not available regarding concomitant use of lamivudine and higher dosages of co-trimoxazole.

■ **HCV Antivirals** ***HCV Polymerase Inhibitors*** **Dasabuvir, Ombitasvir, Paritaprevir, and Ritonavir.** Concomitant use of lamivudine and the fixed combination of dasabuvir sodium, ombitasvir, paritaprevir, and ritonavir (dasabuvir/ombitasvir/paritaprevir/ritonavir) or fixed combination of ombitasvir, paritaprevir, and ritonavir (ombitasvir/paritaprevir/ritonavir) copackaged with dasabuvir sodium does not result in clinically important interactions.

Dosage adjustments are not needed if lamivudine is used concomitantly with dasabuvir/ombitasvir/paritaprevir/ritonavir (fixed combination) or ombitasvir/paritaprevir/ritonavir with dasabuvir (copackaged).

HCV Protease Inhibitors **Glecaprevir and Pibrentasvir.** Concomitant use of lamivudine and the fixed combination of glecaprevir and pibrentasvir (glecaprevir/pibrentasvir) does not result in clinically important interactions.

Dosage adjustments are not needed if lamivudine is used concomitantly with glecaprevir/pibrentasvir.

Simeprevir. Clinically important pharmacokinetic interactions are not expected if simeprevir is used concomitantly with lamivudine.

HCV Replication Complex Inhibitors **Elbasvir and Grazoprevir.** Clinically important interactions are not expected if lamivudine is used concomitantly with the fixed combination of elbasvir and grazoprevir (elbasvir/grazoprevir).

Ledipasvir and Sofosbuvir. Clinically important pharmacokinetic interactions are not expected if lamivudine is used concomitantly with the fixed combination of ledipasvir and sofosbuvir (ledipasvir/sofosbuvir).

■ **Interferon Alfa and Peginterferon Alfa** Concomitant use of interferon alfa and lamivudine does not result in clinically important pharmacokinetic interactions. In healthy adults who received multiple doses of lamivudine and a single dose of interferon, the AUC of lamivudine was decreased 10% (not considered clinically important) and there was no effect on the pharmacokinetics of interferon.

Potentially fatal hepatic decompensation has been reported in HIV-infected patients coinfected with hepatitis C virus (HCV) receiving antiretroviral therapy concomitantly with interferon alfa with or without ribavirin. Patients receiving lamivudine concomitantly with interferon alfa (or peginterferon alfa) with or without ribavirin should be monitored closely for toxicities, especially hepatic decompensation, and consideration should be given to discontinuing lamivudine if medically appropriate. If worsening toxicities (e.g., hepatic decompensation with Child-Pugh scores greater than 6) occur, consideration should be given to immediately discontinuing or reducing dosage of interferon alfa (or peginterferon alfa) and/or ribavirin.

■ **Opiates and Opiate Partial Agonists** ***Buprenorphine*** There are no clinically important pharmacokinetic interactions between buprenorphine and lamivudine; dosage adjustments are not necessary if the drugs are used concomitantly.

■ **Ribavirin** In vitro studies indicate that ribavirin can reduce the phosphorylation of pyrimidine nucleoside analogs, including lamivudine. Ribavirin has decreased the in vitro antiretroviral activity of lamivudine.

Although there was no evidence of pharmacokinetic or pharmacodynamic interactions (e.g., loss of virologic suppression of HIV-1 or HCV) in HIV-infected patients coinfected with HCV who were receiving both lamivudine and ribavirin, potentially fatal hepatic decompensation has been reported in patients coinfected with HIV and HCV receiving antiretroviral therapy and interferon alfa with or without ribavirin. (See Drug Interactions: Interferon Alfa and Peginterferon Alfa.)

■ **Sorbitol** Concomitant use of sorbitol and lamivudine results in a sorbitol dose-dependent decrease in lamivudine exposures. When healthy adults received a single 300-mg dose of lamivudine oral solution alone or in conjunction with a single 3.2-, 10.2-, or 13.4-g dose of sorbitol in solution, peak plasma concentrations of lamivudine were decreased 28, 52, or 55%, respectively, and the AUC of lamivudine was decreased 20, 39, or 44%, respectively.

Concomitant use of lamivudine and sorbitol-containing preparations should be avoided whenever possible. If chronic concomitant use of sorbitol cannot be avoided in patients receiving lamivudine for the treatment of chronic HBV infection, more frequent monitoring of HBV viral load should be considered.

■ **Trimethoprim** Trimethoprim has been shown to increase lamivudine plasma concentrations. However, this interaction is not considered clinically important and lamivudine dosage adjustments are not needed.

Acute Toxicity

If overdosage of lamivudine occurs, the patient should be monitored and usual supportive treatment initiated as indicated. There is no known specific treatment for lamivudine overdosage. Because a negligible amount of lamivudine is removed by hemodialysis (4-hour session), continuous ambulatory peritoneal dialysis, and automated peritoneal dialysis, it is not known whether continuous hemodialysis would provide any clinical benefit in the treatment of overdosage.

Mechanism of Action

Following conversion to a pharmacologically active metabolite, lamivudine apparently inhibits replication of human retroviruses by interfering with viral RNA-directed DNA polymerase (reverse transcriptase). Lamivudine, therefore, exerts a virustatic effect against retroviruses by acting as a reverse transcriptase inhibitor.

Like other human immunodeficiency virus (HIV) nucleoside reverse transcriptase agents (NRTIs) (e.g., abacavir, didanosine, stavudine, zidovudine) and other nucleoside antiviral agents (e.g., acyclovir, ganciclovir, ribavirin), the antiviral activity of lamivudine appears to depend on intracellular conversion of the drug to a 5′-triphosphate metabolite; thus, 2′,3′-dideoxy,3′-thiacytidine-5′-triphosphate (3TC-TP) and not unchanged lamivudine appears to be the pharmacologically active form of the drug. 3TC-TP is a structural analog of deoxycytidine triphosphate (dC-TP), the natural substrate for reverse transcriptase (viral RNA-directed DNA polymerase). Although other mechanisms may be involved in the antiretroviral activity of the drug, 3TC-TP appears to compete with naturally occurring dC-TP for incorporation into viral DNA by reverse transcriptase. Following incorporation of 3TC-TP into the viral DNA chain instead of dC-TP, viral DNA synthesis is terminated prematurely because the absence of a 3′-hydroxy group on the oxathiolane ring prevents further 5′ to 3′ phosphodiester linkages.

Spectrum

Lamivudine is an antiviral agent that possesses in vitro virustatic activity against human immunodeficiency virus type 1 (HIV-1) and type 2 (HIV-2). The drug also is active against human hepatitis B virus (HBV), but appears to be inactive against other common human viruses (e.g., cytomegalovirus, Epstein-Barr virus, influenza virus, herpes simplex virus types 1 and 2, respiratory syncytial virus, varicella-zoster virus).

Resistance

■ **Resistance in HIV** Resistance to lamivudine can be produced in vitro in cell culture by serial passage of human immunodeficiency virus type 1 (HIV-1) in the presence of increasing concentrations of the drug, and strains of HIV-1 with in vitro resistance to lamivudine have emerged during therapy with the drug. Primary infection with lamivudine-resistant HIV-1 has been reported rarely in adults who were antiretroviral-naive (had not previously received antiretroviral agents). For information on genotypic assays used to detect specific HIV-1 genetic variants (mutations), phenotypic assays used to measure HIV-1 drug resistance and recommendations regarding these assays, see In Vitro Resistance Testing under Guidelines for Use of Antiretroviral Agents: Laboratory Monitoring, in the Antiretroviral Agents General Statement 8:18.08.

Cross-resistance occurs among the HIV nucleoside reverse transcriptase inhibitors (NRTIs). HIV isolates resistant to didanosine, lamivudine, stavudine, and zidovudine have been isolated from patients who received zidovudine in conjunction with didanosine for up to 2 years. Mutations identified in these multidrug-resistant isolates were A62V, V75I, F77L, F116Y, and Q151M.

■ **Resistance in HBV** Evidence of diminished treatment response has been reported in adult and pediatric patients with hepatitis B virus (HBV) infection following 52 weeks of lamivudine therapy. Lamivudine-resistant HBV develop M204V/I substitutions in the YMDD motif of the catalytic domain of HBV reverse transcriptase. These substitutions are frequently accompanied by other substitutions (V173L, L180M) that enhance lamivudine resistance or act as compensatory mutations improving replication efficiency. L80I and A181T substitutions also have been detected in lamivudine-resistant HBV.

In controlled clinical trials, YMDD-mutant HBV were detected in 19% of pediatric patients and in 24% (range: 16–32%) of adults who received lamivudine for 52 weeks. In follow-up studies of patients who continued to receive lamivudine therapy, the prevalence of YMDD mutations in pediatric patients increased from 24% at 12 months to 59% at 24 months and 64% at 36 months of lamivudine treatment. Similarly, in a follow-up study in adults, the prevalence of YMDD mutations was 18% at 1 year and 41, 53, and 69% at 2, 3, and 4 years, respectively.

Some lamivudine-resistant HBV remain susceptible to adefovir dipivoxil but have reduced susceptibility to entecavir and telbivudine. Other lamivudine-resistant HBV have reduced susceptibility to telbivudine and/or tenofovir.

Pharmacokinetics

■ **Absorption** Lamivudine is rapidly absorbed from the GI tract in patients with human immunodeficiency virus (HIV) or hepatitis B virus (HBV) infection. In HIV-infected patients or healthy individuals, peak plasma concentrations are achieved within 0.5–2 hours after a single dose.

The absolute bioavailability of lamivudine 150-mg scored tablets and oral solution in adults is similar (86 and 87%, respectively). In a crossover study in healthy adults evaluating the steady-state pharmacokinetics of lamivudine administered in a once-daily regimen (300-mg tablet once daily) or twice-daily regimen (150-mg tablet twice daily), the area under the plasma concentration-time curve (AUC) was similar with both regimens; however, peak plasma concentrations were 66% higher and trough concentrations were 53% lower with the once-daily regimen compared with the twice-daily regimen.

The absolute bioavailability of lamivudine tablets and lamivudine oral solution is lower in children than in adults. In addition, the relative bioavailability of the oral solution is approximately 40% lower than that of the tablets in children, despite no difference between the preparations in adults. It has been suggested that lower lamivudine exposures reported in pediatric patients receiving lamivudine oral solution are likely due to an interaction between lamivudine and concomitant solutions containing sorbitol (e.g., abacavir oral solution). (See Drug Interactions: Sorbitol.) Data from pharmacokinetic studies evaluating once- and twice-daily lamivudine regimens in HIV-1-infected pediatric patients 3 months through 12 years of age indicate that AUCs attained with once-daily regimens were similar to those attained with twice-daily regimens when comparing the dosage regimens within the same formulation (i.e., either tablets or the oral solution). However, mean peak plasma concentrations were approximately 80–90% higher with once-daily lamivudine regimens compared with twice-daily lamivudine regimens.

Results of a single-dose study in healthy, fasting individuals indicate that the commercially available fixed-combination tablet containing 150 mg of lamivudine and 300 mg of zidovudine (lamivudine/zidovudine) is bioequivalent to one 150-mg lamivudine tablet and one 300-mg zidovudine tablet given simultaneously.

Results of a single-dose crossover study indicate that the commercially available tablet containing 600 mg of abacavir and 300 mg of lamivudine (abacavir/lamivudine) is bioequivalent to two 300-mg tablets of abacavir and two 150-mg tablets of lamivudine administered simultaneously.

Results of a cross-over study in fasting, healthy adults indicate that the commercially available fixed-combination tablet containing 300 mg of abacavir, 150 mg of lamivudine, and 300 mg of zidovudine (abacavir/lamivudine/zidovudine) is bioequivalent to one 300-mg tablet of abacavir, one 150-mg tablet of lamivudine, and one 300-mg tablet of zidovudine administered simultaneously.

Results of a study in healthy, fasting individuals indicate that the commercially available fixed-combination tablet containing 600 mg of abacavir, 50 mg of dolutegravir, and 300 mg of lamivudine (abacavir/dolutegravir/lamivudine) is bioequivalent to one 50-mg tablet of dolutegravir administered simultaneously with one fixed-combination tablet containing 600 mg of abacavir and 300 mg of lamivudine (abacavir/lamivudine).

Pharmacokinetics of lamivudine in pregnant women are similar to that reported in nonpregnant adults and postpartum women.

Food Food does not appear to affect the AUC of lamivudine.

In a small study in HIV-infected patients, peak plasma concentrations of lamivudine were decreased 40% and the rate of absorption was reduced when lamivudine was administered with food, but clinically important decreases in systemic availability of the drug (AUC) were not observed.

■ **Distribution** The apparent volume of distribution of lamivudine is 1.3 L/kg, suggesting that the drug distributes into extravascular spaces. The volume of distribution is independent of dose and does not correlate with body weight.

Lamivudine is distributed into CSF. In HIV-infected children who received oral lamivudine in a dosage of 8 mg/kg daily, CSF concentrations ranged from 0.04–0.3 mcg/mL and were 5.6–30.9% of concurrent serum concentrations.

Lamivudine crosses the placenta and is distributed into cord blood and amniotic fluid. Lamivudine concentrations in amniotic fluid are typically twofold higher than maternal serum concentrations and have ranged from 1.2–2.5 mcg/mL or 2.1–5.2 mcg/mL when lamivudine dosage in the mother was 150 or 300 mg twice daily, respectively.

Lamivudine is distributed into milk.

Lamivudine is less than 36% bound to plasma proteins.

■ **Elimination** Lamivudine is not substantially metabolized by cytochrome P-450 (CYP) isoenzymes. Metabolism is a minor route of elimination of lamivudine; the only known metabolite is the trans-sulfoxide metabolite. The majority of a lamivudine dose is eliminated unchanged in urine by active organic cationic secretion. Within 12 hours after an oral dose, approximately 5% is excreted in urine as the trans-sulfoxide metabolite.

Intracellularly, lamivudine is phosphorylated and converted by cellular enzymes to the active 5′-triphosphate metabolite.

In single-dose studies in healthy individuals or patients with HIV or HBV infection, the mean plasma half-life of lamivudine was 5–7 hours. The plasma half-life in HIV-infected children 4 months to 14 years of age is 2 hours.

The pharmacokinetics of lamivudine are not altered in patients with hepatic impairment.

In patients with impaired renal function, peak plasma concentrations, AUC, and plasma half-life of lamivudine are increased.

Hemodialysis increases lamivudine clearance; however, the length of time of hemodialysis (4 hours) is insufficient to substantially alter mean lamivudine exposure after a single dose of the drug. Continuous ambulatory peritoneal dialysis and automated peritoneal dialysis have negligible effects on lamivudine clearance.

Chemistry and Stability

■ **Chemistry** Lamivudine, an antiretroviral agent, is a human immunodeficiency virus (HIV) nucleoside reverse transcriptase inhibitor (NRTI). The drug is a dideoxynucleoside reverse transcriptase inhibitor. Lamivudine is the negative enantiomer of a dideoxy analog of cytidine, and is structurally similar to zalcitabine (2′,3′-dideoxycytidine, ddC; no longer commercially available in the US). Lamivudine differs structurally from zalcitabine in that the 3′-carbon of the ribose ring is replaced with sulfur, forming an oxathiolane ring. The absence of a free 3′-hydroxyl group on the oxathiolane ring results in the inability of lamivudine to form phosphodiester linkages at this position. Both the positive and negative enantiomers of 2′,3′-dideoxy,3′-thiacytidine exhibit antiviral activity in vitro, but lamivudine appears to exhibit greater antiviral activity and to be considerably less cytotoxic than the positive enantiomer.

Lamivudine occurs as white to off-white, crystalline solid. The drug has a solubility of 70 mg/mL in water at 20°C.

Lamivudine is commercially available for oral administration as film-coated tablets and oral solution (Epivir®, Epivir-HBV®, generic). The oral solution containing 5 or 10 mg of lamivudine per mL is colorless to pale yellow, and also contains anhydrous citric acid, methylparaben, propylene glycol, propylparaben, sodium citrate (dihydrate), and 200 mg/mL of sucrose.

Lamivudine also is commercially available for oral administration in fixed-combination tablets containing lamivudine and zidovudine (lamivudine/zidovudine), fixed-combination tablets containing abacavir and lamivudine (abacavir/lamivudine), fixed-combination tablets containing abacavir, lamivudine, and zidovudine (abacavir/lamivudine/zidovudine), and fixed-combination tablets containing abacavir, dolutegravir, and lamivudine (abacavir/dolutegravir/lamivudine).

■ **Stability** Lamivudine tablets should be stored at 25°C, but may be exposed to temperatures ranging from 15–30°C.

Lamivudine oral solution containing 10 mg/mL should be stored in tightly closed bottles at 25°C. Lamivudine oral solution containing 5 mg/mL should be stored in tightly closed bottles at 20–25°C.

Lamivudine/zidovudine fixed-combination tablets should be stored at 2–30°C.

Abacavir/lamivudine fixed-combination tablets, abacavir/lamivudine/zidovudine fixed-combination tablets, and abacavir/dolutegravir/lamivudine fixed-combination tablets should be stored at 25°C, but may be exposed to temperatures ranging from 15–30°C.

Preparations

Excipients in commercially available drug preparations may have clinically important effects in some individuals; consult specific product labeling for details.

lamiVUDine

Oral		
Solution	5 mg/mL	**Epivir-HBV®**, GlaxoSmithKline
	10 mg/mL*	**Epivir®**, ViiV
		Lamivudine Oral Solution
Tablets, film-coated	100 mg*	**Epivir-HBV®**, GlaxoSmithKline
		Lamivudine Tablets
	150 mg*	**Epivir®** (scored), ViiV
		Lamivudine Tablets (scored)
	300 mg*	**Epivir®**, ViiV
		Lamivudine Tablets

*available from one or more manufacturer, distributor, and/or repackager by generic (nonproprietary) name

lamiVUDine Combinations

Oral		
Tablets, film-coated	150 mg with Abacavir Sulfate 300 mg (of abacavir) and Zidovudine 300 mg*	**Abacavir Sulfate, Lamivudine, and Zidovudine Tablets**
		Trizivir®, ViiV
	150 mg with Zidovudine 300 mg*	**Combivir®**, ViiV
		Lamivudine and Zidovudine Tablets
	300 mg with Abacavir Sulfate 600 mg (of abacavir)*	**Abacavir and Lamivudine Tablets**
		Epzicom®, ViiV
	300 mg with Abacavir Sulfate 600 mg (of abacavir), and Dolutegravir Sodium 50 mg (of dolutegravir)	**Triumeq®**, ViiV

*available from one or more manufacturer, distributor, and/or repackager by generic (nonproprietary) name

†Use is not currently included in the labeling approved by the US Food and Drug Administration

Tenofovir Disoproxil Fumarate

Tenofovir DF, TDF, efavirenz/emtricitabine/tenofovir disoproxil fumarate, efavirenz/emtricitabine/tenofovir DF, EFV/TDF/FTC, TDF/FTC, RPV/TDF/FTC

■ Tenofovir disoproxil fumarate (tenofovir DF), an antiretroviral agent, is a human immunodeficiency virus (HIV) nucleotide reverse transcriptase inhibitor that is active against HIV and hepatitis B virus (HBV).

REMS

FDA approved a REMS for tenofovir disoproxil fumarate (tenofovir DF) to ensure that the benefits outweigh the risks. The REMS may apply to one or more preparations of tenofovir DF and consists of the following: elements to assure safe use. See the FDA REMS page (https://www.accessdata.fda.gov/scripts/cder/rems/index.cfm).

Uses

■ **Treatment of HIV Infection** Tenofovir disoproxil fumarate (tenofovir DF) is used in conjunction with other antiretroviral agents for the treatment of human immunodeficiency virus type 1 (HIV-1) infection in adults, adolescents, and pediatric patients 2 years of age or older.

For purposes of therapeutic decisions, tenofovir DF is grouped with HIV nucleoside reverse transcriptase inhibitor (NRTI) antiretroviral agents. Tenofovir DF usually is used in multiple-drug regimens that include another NRTI (dual NRTIs) and an HIV integrase strand transfer inhibitor (INSTI), HIV nonnucleoside reverse transcriptase inhibitor (NNRTI), or HIV protease inhibitor (PI) in INSTI-, NNRTI-, or PI-based regimens. Single-entity tenofovir DF is labeled by FDA for use in conjunction with other antiretrovirals in adults, adolescents, and children 2 years of age or older. Tenofovir DF also is commercially available in various fixed-combination preparations that contain emtricitabine with or without a third antiretroviral. These fixed combinations can be used in specific patient groups to decrease pill burden and improve compliance.

If the dual NRTI option of tenofovir DF and emtricitabine is used in conjunction with other antiretrovirals for the treatment of HIV-1 infection, a fixed-combination preparation containing both drugs (emtricitabine/tenofovir DF; Truvada®) is commercially available and can be used in adults, adolescents, and children weighing at least 17 kg. Emtricitabine/tenofovir DF must be used in conjunction with other antiretrovirals for treatment of HIV-1.

If an HIV NNRTI-based regimen of efavirenz, emtricitabine, and tenofovir DF is used for the treatment of HIV-1 infection, a fixed-combination preparation containing all 3 drugs (efavirenz/emtricitabine/tenofovir DF; Atripla®) is commercially available and can be used in adults and adolescents 12 years of age or older weighing at least 40 kg. Efavirenz/emtricitabine/tenofovir DF can be used alone as a complete treatment regimen or in conjunction with other antiretrovirals.

If an HIV NNRTI-based regimen of rilpivirine, emtricitabine, and tenofovir DF is used for the treatment of HIV-1 infection, a fixed-combination preparation containing all 3 drugs (emtricitabine/rilpivirine/tenofovir DF; Complera®) is commercially available and can be used in antiretroviral-naive adults and adolescents 12 years of age or older weighing at least 35 kg with baseline plasma HIV-1 RNA levels of 100,000 copies/mL or less. Emtricitabine/rilpivirine/tenofovir DF also can be used to replace a stable antiretroviral regimen in *certain* antiretroviral-experienced (previously treated) patients who are virologically suppressed (i.e., plasma HIV-1 RNA levels less than 50 copies/mL). Emtricitabine/rilpivirine/tenofovir DF is used alone as a complete treatment regimen.

A fixed-combination preparation containing elvitegravir, cobicistat, emtricitabine, and tenofovir DF (EVG/c/FTC/TDF; Stribild®) also is commercially available for use alone as a complete regimen for the treatment of HIV-1 in adults. For information on EVG/c/FTC/TDF, see Elvitegravir, Cobicistat, Emtricitabine, and Tenofovir Disoproxil Fumarate in 8:18.08.12.

Tenofovir DF has been used in triple NRTI regimens, and some experts state that a regimen of tenofovir DF, zidovudine, and lamivudine may be considered in certain situations. However, triple NRTI regimens containing tenofovir DF, abacavir, and lamivudine or tenofovir DF, didanosine, and lamivudine are *not* recommended because of a high rate of virologic failure. (See All-NRTI Regimens under Treatment of HIV Infection: Antiretroviral-naive Adults and Adolescents, in Uses.)

The most appropriate antiretroviral regimen cannot be defined for each clinical scenario and selection of specific antiretroviral agents for use in multiple-drug regimens should be individualized based on information regarding antiretroviral potency, potential rate of development of resistance, known toxicities, and potential for pharmacokinetic interactions as well as virologic, immunologic, and clinical characteristics of the patient. For information on the general principles and guidelines for use of antiretroviral therapy, including specific recommendations for initial therapy in antiretroviral-naive patients and recommendations for changing antiretroviral regimens, see the Antiretroviral Agents General Statement 8:18.08.

Antiretroviral-naive Adults and Adolescents **Dual NRTI Options.** For *initial* treatment in HIV-infected adults and adolescents, the US Department of Health and Human Services (HHS) Panel on Antiretroviral Guidelines for

Adults and Adolescents states that the dual tenofovir DF and emtricitabine (or lamivudine) is a recommended dual NRTI option for use in most INSTI-, NNRTI-, and PI-based regimens. This recommendation is based on safety and efficacy data from clinical trials, long-term clinical experience, and availability of fixed-combination preparations containing tenofovir DF and emtricitabine.

Because all 3 drugs have activity against both HIV *and* hepatitis B virus (HBV), tenofovir DF and emtricitabine or tenofovir DF and lamivudine are preferred dual NRTI options for antiretroviral regimens used in HIV-infected patients coinfected with HBV.

A dual NRTI option of didanosine and tenofovir DF should *not* be used at any time because such regimens are associated with early virologic failure, rapid selection of resistant mutants, potential for immunologic nonresponse or decline in CD4+ T-cell counts, and increased didanosine concentrations and toxicities. Clinicians caring for patients who are clinically stable on a regimen containing didanosine and tenofovir DF should consider altering the NRTIs.

All-NRTI Regimens. Tenofovir DF has been included in NRTI regimens that include 3 or 4 NRTIs (without any drugs from another class). However, triple and quadruple NRTI regimens generally are *not* recommended for *initial* treatment in HIV-infected adults or adolescents because such regimens have inferior virologic efficacy or have not been adequately studied.

A triple NRTI regimen of zidovudine, lamivudine, and tenofovir DF has been used and has been shown to have antiretroviral activity; however, this regimen is *not* routinely recommended because of limited data comparing it with other options.

A quadruple NRTI regimen of abacavir, lamivudine, tenofovir DF, and zidovudine is *not* recommended for initial therapy in antiretroviral-naive HIV-infected adults and adolescents because of inferior virologic efficacy.

Study 903. Safety and efficacy of tenofovir DF in an NNRTI-based regimen in treatment-naive adults was evaluated in a double-blind, active-controlled study (study 903) in 600 adults (mean age 36 years, 74% male, 64% white, 20% African American, mean baseline CD4+ T-cell count 279 cells/mm^3, median baseline plasma HIV-1 RNA 77,600 copies/mL). At 144 weeks, 68% of those receiving a regimen of efavirenz, tenofovir DF, and lamivudine had plasma HIV-1 RNA levels less than 400 copies/mL compared with 62% of those receiving a regimen of efavirenz, stavudine, and lamivudine. In addition, 62% of those receiving the tenofovir DF regimen had plasma HIV-1 RNA levels less than 50 copies/mL compared with 58% in the comparator group. The mean increase from baseline CD4+ T-cell count was 263 or 283 cells/mm^3, respectively.

Efavirenz, Emtricitabine, and Tenofovir DF. Safety and efficacy of an NNRTI-based regimen that included tenofovir DF (efavirenz, emtricitabine, and tenofovir DF) was evaluated in a randomized, open-label study designed to demonstrate noninferiority of this regimen compared with a regimen of efavirenz, zidovudine, and lamivudine (study 934). In this study, 511 treatment-naive HIV-infected patients (mean age 38 years, 86% male, 59% white, 23% black, median baseline plasma HIV-1 RNA level 5.01 $\log_{10}$ copies/mL [range: 3.56–6.54 $\log_{10}$ copies/mL], mean baseline CD4+ T-cell count 245 cells/mm^3) were randomized to receive a once-daily regimen of efavirenz, emtricitabine, and tenofovir DF or a regimen of efavirenz once daily with the fixed combination of lamivudine and zidovudine (lamivudine/zidovudine; Combivir®) twice daily. The primary measure used to assess noninferiority of the regimen of efavirenz, emtricitabine, and tenofovir DF to the regimen of efavirenz and lamivudine/zidovudine was plasma HIV-1 RNA levels at week 48, specifically, the number of patients with HIV-1 RNA levels less than 400 copies/mL. The 487 patients without baseline resistance to efavirenz who underwent randomization and received treatment were the predefined population used for the primary endpoint analysis.

Through week 48, the regimen of efavirenz, emtricitabine, and tenofovir DF met the criteria for noninferiority to the regimen of efavirenz and lamivudine/zidovudine. At week 48, 84 or 80% of adults receiving the efavirenz, emtricitabine, and tenofovir DF regimen and 73 or 70% of adults receiving the efavirenz and lamivudine/zidovudine regimen had plasma HIV-1 RNA levels less than 400 or 50 copies/mL, respectively. At week 48, increases in CD4+ T-cell counts were greater in patients receiving the efavirenz, emtricitabine, and tenofovir DF regimen (mean increase of 190 cells/mm^3) than in those receiving the efavirenz and lamivudine/zidovudine regimen (mean increase of 158 cells/mm^3). Virologic failure (i.e., individuals who failed to achieve virologic suppression or experienced rebound after achieving virologic suppression) was reported in 2% of those receiving efavirenz, emtricitabine, and tenofovir DF and in 4% of those receiving efavirenz and lamivudine/zidovudine at week 48.

At 144 weeks, 64% of adults receiving the efavirenz, emtricitabine, and tenofovir DF regimen and 56% of those receiving the efavirenz and lamivudine/zidovudine regimen had plasma HIV-1 RNA levels less than 50 copies/mL. The mean increase in CD4+ T-cell count from baseline in these groups at 144 weeks was 312 and 271 cells/mm^3, respectively.

Antiretroviral-experienced Adults and Adolescents **Study 907.** In study 907, a placebo-controlled, randomized study in 550 previously treated HIV-infected adults (mean age 42 years, 85% male, 69% white, 17% African American, 12% Hispanic, mean duration of prior treatment 5.4 years, mean baseline CD4+ T-cell count 427 cells/mm^3; median baseline plasma HIV-1 RNA level 2340 copies/mL), addition of tenofovir DF to the existing antiretroviral regimen resulted in decreases in plasma HIV-1 RNA levels and increases in CD4+ T-cell counts. At 24 weeks, plasma HIV-1 RNA levels were less than 400 copies/mL in 40% of those receiving tenofovir DF compared with 11% of those receiving placebo; in addition, 19% of those receiving tenofovir DF had levels less than 50 copies/mL compared with 1% of those receiving placebo. After 24 weeks of blinded study, all patients received open-label tenofovir DF for an additional 24 weeks. At week 48, 28% of those who received tenofovir DF for the entire duration had plasma HIV-1 RNA levels less than 400 copies/mL.

Efavirenz, Emtricitabine, and Tenofovir DF. Efficacy of the fixed combination efavirenz/emtricitabine/tenofovir DF (Atripla®) was evaluated in a randomized, open-label study (study 073) in antiretroviral-experienced patients who had been receiving a suppressive regimen consisting of at least 2 NRTIs and a PI or NNRTI (mean age 43 years [range 22–73 years]), 88% male, 68% white, 29% black, median CD4+ T-cell count 516 cells/mm^3). Patients had plasma HIV-1 RNA levels less than 200 copies/mL for at least 12 weeks on their existing regimen (96% had plasma HIV-1 RNA levels less than 50 copies/mL), no known HIV-1 substitutions conferring resistance to the components of the fixed combination, and no history of virologic failure; patients were randomized to either switch to the fixed combination of efavirenz/emtricitabine/tenofovir DF or continue their existing (baseline) regimen. At 48 weeks, 89 and 87% of those switched to efavirenz/emtricitabine/tenofovir DF had plasma HIV-1 RNA levels less than 200 and 50 copies/mL, respectively, compared with 88 and 85% of those who remained on their baseline regimen. This difference was not statistically significant. There was no change in CD4+ T-cell count from baseline in either group.

Emtricitabine, Rilpivirine, and Tenofovir DF. The fixed combination emtricitabine/rilpivirine/tenofovir DF can be used to replace a stable antiretroviral regimen for treatment of HIV-1 infection in antiretroviral-experienced adults and adolescents 12 years of age or older weighing at least 35 kg who have been virologically suppressed (i.e., plasma HIV-1 RNA levels less than 50 copies/mL) on their current regimen for at least 6 months, are currently receiving only their first or second antiretroviral regimen, have no history of virologic failure, and have no current evidence or history of resistance to emtricitabine, rilpivirine, or tenofovir DF.

The efficacy and safety of emtricitabine/rilpivirine/tenofovir DF (Complera®) have been evaluated in a randomized, open-label study (study 106) in 476 virologically suppressed HIV-infected adults (mean age 42 years, 88% male, 77% white, 17% black, 17% Hispanic, mean baseline CD4+ T-cell count 584 cells/mm^3). Patients were receiving their first or second antiretroviral regimen with no history of virologic failure; had no history of resistance to emtricitabine, rilpivirine, or tenofovir DF; and were virologically suppressed (plasma HIV-1 RNA levels less than 50 copies/mL) for at least 6 months. Patients were randomized in a 2:1 ratio to switch to emtricitabine/rilpivirine/tenofovir DF for 48 weeks or to continue receiving their baseline antiretroviral regimen containing a *ritonavir-boosted* HIV PI for 24 weeks and then switch to emtricitabine/rilpivirine/tenofovir DF for an additional 24 weeks. In patients initially switched to emtricitabine/rilpivirine/tenofovir DF, 89% maintained plasma HIV-1 RNA levels less than 50 copies/mL at 48 weeks; 90% of those who continued to receive their baseline regimen maintained plasma HIV-1 RNA levels less than 50 copies/mL at 24 weeks.

Pediatric Patients Tenofovir DF is used in conjunction with other antiretroviral agents for treatment of HIV-1 infection in pediatric patients 2 years of age or older. Tenofovir DF is *not* recommended in children younger than 2 years of age because decreased bone mineral density (BMD) has been reported in adults and children. (See Bone Effects under Warnings/Precautions: Other Warnings/Precautions, in Cautions.)

The fixed combination emtricitabine/rilpivirine/tenofovir DF can be used alone as a complete regimen for the treatment of HIV-1 infection in adolescents 12 years of age or older weighing at least 35 kg.

For *initial* treatment of HIV-infected pediatric patients, the HHS Panel on Antiretroviral Therapy and Medical Management of HIV-infected Children recommends a PI-, NNRTI-, or INSTI-based regimen that includes 2 NRTIs (dual NRTIs).

For use in *initial* treatment regimens, the HHS panel states that tenofovir DF and emtricitabine is an alternative dual NRTI option for antiretroviral-naive children and adolescents with sexual maturity rating (SMR) 3; however, because decreased BMD has been reported in adults and children receiving tenofovir DF, the panel states that the dual option of tenofovir DF and emtricitabine should be used in children 2 years or age or older or adolescents at SMR 1 or 2 *only* in special circumstances after weighing the potential risk of decreased BMD versus the benefits of the dual NRTI option.

The dual NRTI option of tenofovir DF and abacavir is *not* recommended for use in *initial* treatment regimens in antiretroviral-naive pediatric patients because of insufficient data.

The dual NRTI option of tenofovir DF and didanosine is *not* recommended for use in *initial* treatment regimens in antiretroviral-naive pediatric patients because of a high rate of virologic failure.

Antiretroviral regimens containing only NRTIs are *not* recommended for *initial* treatment in antiretroviral-naive pediatric patients because of inferior virologic efficacy.

A triple NRTI regimen that includes abacavir, tenofovir DF, and either lamivudine or emtricitabine or a triple NRTI regimen that includes tenofovir DF, didanosine, and either lamivudine or emtricitabine should *not* be used at any time in pediatric patients because of the high rate of early virologic failure reported in antiretroviral-naive adults.

For further information on treatment of HIV infection in pediatric patients, see Antiretroviral Therapy in Pediatric Patients, in Guidelines for Use of Antiretroviral Agents in the Antiretroviral Agents General Statement 8:18.08.

Clinical Experience. Efficacy and safety of tenofovir DF in pediatric patients have been evaluated in a randomized study in 92 HIV-1-infected antiretroviral-experienced children 2 to less than 12 years of age (study 352). Patients had been receiving a suppressive regimen containing stavudine or zidovudine and were randomized to receive tenofovir DF instead of stavudine or zidovudine or to continue their original regimen. At 48 weeks, 89% of patients randomized to receive tenofovir DF and 90% of those who continued their original regimen had plasma HIV-1 RNA levels less than 400 copies/mL.

In a study in 87 antiretroviral-experienced pediatric patients 12 to less than 18 years of age (study 321) with mean baseline plasma HIV-1 RNA level of 4.6 $\log_{10}$ copies/mL and mean baseline $CD4^+$ T-cell count of 374 cells/mm^3 (90% harbored HIV-1 with NRTI resistance-associated substitutions at baseline), patients received tenofovir DF or placebo with an optimized background regimen (OBR) for 48 weeks. Overall, there was no difference in virologic response between the groups; subgroup analysis suggested that the lack of difference in virologic response may be attributable to imbalances between the treatment arms in baseline virus susceptibility to tenofovir DF and the OBR.

■ **Preexposure Prophylaxis for Prevention of HIV-1 Infection** The fixed combination containing emtricitabine and tenofovir DF (emtricitabine/tenofovir DF; Truvada®) is used for preexposure prophylaxis (PrEP) in conjunction with safer sex practices to reduce the risk of sexually acquired HIV-1 infection in HIV-1-negative adults at high risk. The manufacturer states that this indication is based on clinical trials in men who have sex with men (MSM) at high risk for HIV-1 infection and in heterosexual HIV-serodiscordant couples.

Adults at high risk for HIV-1 infection include those with partner(s) known to be infected with HIV-1 or those engaging in sexual activity within a high prevalence area or social network and with 1 or more of the following factors: inconsistent or no condom use, diagnosis of sexually transmitted infections, exchange of sex for commodities (e.g., money, food, shelter, drugs), use of illicit drugs, alcohol dependence, incarceration, or partner(s) of unknown HIV-1 status with any of these risk factors.

PrEP with emtricitabine/tenofovir DF (Truvada®) is *not* always effective in preventing acquisition of HIV-1 infection and *must* be used as part of a comprehensive prevention strategy that includes safer sex practices. (See Precautions Related to HIV-1 Preexposure Prophylaxis [PrEP] under Cautions: Warnings/Precautions.)

For additional information on PrEP, see Guidelines for Use of Antiretroviral Agents: Antiretrovirals for Preexposure Prophylaxis for Prevention of HIV-1 Infection (PrEP), in the Antiretroviral Agents General Statement 8:18.08.

Clinical Experience Efficacy and safety of a once-daily regimen of emtricitabine/tenofovir DF for HIV-1 PrEP were evaluated in a multinational, randomized, double-blind, placebo-controlled, phase 3 trial (Preexposure Prophylaxis Initiative [iPrEx trial]; NCT00458393) that included 2499 HIV-seronegative men or transgender women (male at birth) who have sex with men and have evidence of high-risk behavior for HIV-1 infection. Study participants (mean age 27 years [range 18–67 years], 5% Asian, 9% black, 18% white, 72% Hispanic/Latino) were randomized to receive emtricitabine/tenofovir DF (single tablet containing 200 mg of emtricitabine and 300 mg of tenofovir DF once daily) or placebo in conjunction with usual prevention strategies (i.e., monthly HIV-1 testing, risk-reduction counseling, condoms, diagnosis and management of sexually transmitted infections) and were followed for 4237 person-years. The primary outcome measure was the incidence of documented HIV seroconversion. There was a 42% reduction in the risk of HIV-1 seroconversion in the group receiving emtricitabine/tenofovir DF (48 individuals receiving emtricitabine/tenofovir DF and 83 individuals receiving placebo seroconverted). Results of a post-hoc case-control study of plasma and intracellular drug concentrations in about 10% of study participants indicated that efficacy of emtricitabine/tenofovir DF PrEP is strongly correlated with adherence since risk reduction appeared to be greatest in those with detectable intracellular tenofovir.

Efficacy and safety of emtricitabine/tenofovir DF for PrEP in HIV-1-seronegative partners of serodiscordant heterosexual couples were evaluated in a randomized, double-blind, placebo-controlled, 3-arm trial (Partners Preexposure Prophylaxis [PrEP] trial; NCT00557245) that included 4758 serodiscordant couples in Kenya and Uganda. The infected partners had median plasma HIV-1 RNA levels of 3.9 $\log_{10}$ copies/mL and median $CD4^+$ T-cell counts of 495 cells/mm^3 (80% had $CD4^+$ T-cell counts of 350 cells/mm^3 or higher). The uninfected partners (mean age 33–34 years, 61–64% male) were randomized to receive emtricitabine/tenofovir DF (single tablet containing 200 mg of emtricitabine and 300 mg of tenofovir DF once daily), tenofovir DF (300 mg of tenofovir DF once daily), or placebo (once daily). Study participants received monthly HIV-1 testing, adherence evaluations, sexual behavior assessments, and safety evaluations. Women received monthly pregnancy tests; if pregnancy occurred, the study drug was interrupted during pregnancy and breast-feeding. After 7827 person-years of follow-up, there were a total of 82 emergent HIV-1 seroconversions (overall observed seroincidence rate of 1.05 per 100 person-years). The risk reduction for the emtricitabine/tenofovir DF group relative to the placebo group was 75%. There were 13 seroconversions in partners randomized to emtricitabine/tenofovir DF and 52 seroconversions in partners randomized to placebo (2 and 3 seroconversions, respectively, occurred during interruption of PrEP for pregnancy). Results of a post-hoc case-control study of plasma and drug concentrations in about 10% of study participants indicated that efficacy of emtricitabine/tenofovir DF PrEP is strongly correlated with adherence since risk reduction appeared to be greatest in those with detectable plasma tenofovir.

■ **Postexposure Prophylaxis following Occupational Exposure to HIV** Tenofovir DF is used in conjunction with other antiretrovirals for postexposure prophylaxis of HIV infection following occupational exposure† (PEP) in health-care personnel and other individuals exposed via percutaneous injury (e.g., needlestick, cut with sharp object) or mucous membrane or nonintact skin (e.g., chapped, abraded, dermatitis) contact with blood, tissue, or other body fluids that might contain HIV.

The US Public Health Service (USPHS) states that the preferred regimen for PEP following an occupational exposure to HIV is a 3-drug regimen of raltegravir used in conjunction with emtricitabine and tenofovir DF (may be administered as the fixed combination emtricitabine/tenofovir DF; Truvada®). These experts recommend several alternative regimens that include an INSTI, NNRTI, or PI and 2 NRTIs (dual NRTIs). The preferred dual NRTI option for use in PEP regimens is emtricitabine and tenofovir DF (may be administered as the fixed combination emtricitabine/tenofovir DF; Truvada®); alternative dual NRTIs are tenofovir DF and lamivudine, lamivudine and zidovudine (may be administered as the fixed combination lamivudine/zidovudine; Combivir®), or zidovudine and emtricitabine.

Because management of occupational exposures to HIV is complex and evolving, consultation with an infectious disease specialist, clinician with expertise in administration of antiretroviral agents, and/or the National Clinicians' Postexposure Prophylaxis Hotline (PEPline at 888-448-4911) is recommended whenever possible. However, initiation of PEP should not be delayed while waiting for expert consultation.

For information on types of occupational exposure to HIV and associated risk of infection, management of occupational exposure to HIV, efficacy and safety of postexposure prophylaxis, and recommendations regarding PEP, see Guidelines for Use of Antiretroviral Agents: Antiretrovirals for Postexposure Prophylaxis following Occupational Exposure to HIV (PEP), in the Antiretroviral Agents General Statement 8:18.08.

■ **Postexposure Prophylaxis following Nonoccupational Exposure to HIV** Tenofovir DF is used in conjunction with other antiretrovirals for postexposure prophylaxis of HIV infection following nonoccupational exposure† (nPEP) in individuals exposed to blood, genital secretions, or other potentially infectious body fluids that might contain HIV when that exposure represents a substantial risk for HIV transmission.

When nPEP is indicated following a nonoccupational exposure to HIV, the US Centers for Disease Control and Prevention (CDC) states that the preferred regimen in adults and adolescents 13 years of age or older with normal renal function is either raltegravir or dolutegravir used in conjunction with emtricitabine and tenofovir DF (administered as the fixed combination emtricitabine/tenofovir DF; Truvada®). The alternative nPEP regimen recommended in these patients is *ritonavir-boosted* darunavir used in conjunction with emtricitabine/tenofovir DF (Truvada®).

Consultation with an infectious disease specialist, clinician with expertise in administration of antiretroviral agents, and/or the National Clinicians' Postexposure Prophylaxis Hotline (PEPline at 888-448-4911) is recommended if nPEP is indicated in certain exposed individuals (e.g., pregnant women, children, those with medical conditions such as renal impairment) or if an antiretroviral regimen not included in the CDC guidelines is being considered, the source virus is known or likely to be resistant to antiretrovirals, or the healthcare provider is inexperienced in prescribing antiretrovirals. However, initiation of nPEP should not be delayed while waiting for expert consultation.

For additional information on nonoccupational exposure to HIV and recommendations regarding postexposure prophylaxis, see Guidelines for Use of Antiretroviral Agents: Antiretrovirals for Postexposure Prophylaxis following Sexual, Injection Drug Use, or other Nonoccupational Exposures to HIV (nPEP), in the Antiretroviral Agents General Statement 8:18.08.

■ **Chronic Hepatitis B Virus Infection** Tenofovir DF is used for the treatment of chronic HBV infection in adults and adolescents 12 years of age or older. This indication is based principally on data from adults with hepatitis B e antigen (HBeAg)-positive or -negative chronic HBV infection with compensated liver function who had not previously received a nucleoside antiviral (nucleoside-naive) or were treatment experienced with documented resistance to lamivudine.

Tenofovir DF has been evaluated in only a limited number of patients with chronic HBV infection and decompensated liver disease. Data are insufficient to evaluate efficacy of tenofovir DF in patients with adefovir resistance-associated substitutions at baseline.

The goal of antiviral therapy in patients with chronic HBV infection is to decrease the morbidity and mortality related to the infection (e.g., cirrhosis, hepatic failure, hepatocellular carcinoma). Sustained suppression of HBV replication has been associated with normalization of serum ALT concentrations, loss of hepatitis B e antigen (HBeAg) with or without detection of antibody to HBeAg (anti-HBe), and improvement in liver histology. Currently available therapies for chronic HBV infection (e.g., adefovir, entecavir, lamivudine, telbivudine, tenofovir DF, interferon alfa, peginterferon alfa) are used in an attempt to provide an immunologic cure (HBsAg loss and sustained HBV DNA suppression), but cannot provide a virologic cure (eradication of HBV).

Treatment of chronic HBV infection is complex and evolving, and specialized references should be consulted. Information from the American Association for the Study of Liver Diseases (AASLD) regarding management of chronic HBV infection is available at http://www.aasld.org.

HBeAg-Positive Adults **Study 0103.** Efficacy of tenofovir DF for treatment of HBeAg-positive chronic HBV infection was evaluated in a phase 3, randomized, double-blind, active-controlled study (study 0103) in mainly nucleoside-naive adults with compensated liver function (mean baseline serum HBV DNA level 8.7 $\log_{10}$ copies/mL, mean serum ALT 147 IU/mL, mean baseline total Knodell Histology Activity Index [HAI] score 8.4). Patients received tenofovir DF 300 mg once daily or adefovir dipivoxil 10 mg once daily. Sixty-nine percent of patients in the study were male, 36% were Asian and 52% were Caucasian, 16% had received prior treatment with interferon alfa, and less than 5% had received treatment with a nucleoside. After 48 weeks of treatment, all patients were eligible to receive open-label tenofovir DF with no interruption in treatment.

At 48 weeks, 67% of patients receiving tenofovir DF had serum HBV DNA levels less than 400 copies/mL and histologic improvement (defined as a reduction of at least 2 points in the Knodell necroinflammatory score with no concurrent worsening of the Knodell fibrosis score) compared with 12% of those receiving adefovir. HBeAg seroconversion occurred in about 20 or 16% of those receiving tenofovir DF or adefovir, respectively; loss of hepatitis B surface antigen (HBsAg) occurred in 3 or 0% of those who received tenofovir DF or adefovir, respectively.

Through 384 weeks, 49% of patients originally randomized to tenofovir DF who subsequently received open-label tenofovir DF had HBV DNA levels less than 400 copies/mL, 42% had ALT normalization, 20% had HBeAg loss, and 13% had HBeAg seroconversion. In patients originally randomized to adefovir who subsequently received open-label tenofovir DF, 56% had HBV DNA levels less than 400 copies/mL, 50% had ALT normalization, 28% had HBeAg loss, and 19% had HBeAg seroconversion through 384 weeks. Rates of HBsAg loss and seroconversion were 11 and 8%, respectively, at week 384 in those initially randomized to tenofovir DF and 12 and 10%, respectively, in those initially randomized to adefovir.

Liver biopsies were obtained at baseline, 48 weeks, and 240 weeks from 328 patients in studies 102 (HBeAg-negative adults) and 103 (HBeAg-positive adults) who received continuing open-label treatment with tenofovir DF. The observed histological response rates in these patients were 80 and 88% at week 48 and 240, respectively. In patients with cirrhosis at baseline, 97 and 99% had improvement or no change in fibrosis score at week 48 and 240, respectively; 29 and 72% experienced regression of cirrhosis by week 48 and 240, respectively.

HBeAg-Negative Adults **Study 0102.** Efficacy of tenofovir DF for treatment of HBeAg-negative chronic HBV infection was evaluated in a phase 3, randomized, double-blind, active-controlled study (study 0102) in adults with compensated liver function (mean baseline serum HBV DNA level 6.9 $\log_{10}$ copies/mL, mean serum ALT 140 IU/mL, mean baseline total Knodell Histology Activity Index [HAI] score 7.8). Patients received tenofovir DF 300 mg once daily or adefovir dipivoxil 10 mg once daily for 48 weeks. Seventy-seven percent of patients in the study were male, 25% were Asian and 65% were Caucasian, 17% had received prior treatment with interferon alfa, and 18% had received treatment with a nucleoside (16% had received lamivudine). After 48 weeks of treatment, all patients were eligible to receive open-label tenofovir DF with no interruption in treatment.

At 48 weeks, 71% of patients receiving tenofovir DF had serum HBV DNA levels less than 400 copies/mL and histologic improvement (defined as a reduction of at least 2 points in the Knodell necroinflammatory score with no concurrent worsening of the Knodell fibrosis score) compared with 49% of those receiving adefovir.

At 384 weeks, 73% of patients originally randomized to tenofovir DF who subsequently received open-label tenofovir DF had HBV DNA levels less than 400 copies/mL and 63% had ALT normalization. In patients originally randomized to adefovir who subsequently received open-label tenofovir DF, 80% had HBV DNA levels less than 400 copies/mL and 70% had ALT normalization at 384 weeks. HBsAg loss and seroconversion rates were approximately 1% in both treatment groups at week 384.

Lamivudine-resistant Chronic HBV **Study 121.** Efficacy and safety of tenofovir DF for treatment of chronic HBV infection in adults with persistent viremia and genotypic evidence of lamivudine resistance were evaluated in a randomized, double-blind, active-controlled trial. Of the 141 adults randomized to receive tenofovir DF, mean age was 47 years, 74% were male, 59% were Caucasian, 37% were Asian, and mean baseline plasma HBV DNA was 6.4 $\log_{10}$ copies/mL. At baseline, 54% were HBeAg-negative, 46% were HBeAg-positive, and 56% had abnormal ALT. At 96 weeks, 89% of patients receiving tenofovir DF had HBV DNA levels less than 400 copies/mL, which was similar to comparator groups; 62% of patients with abnormal ALT at baseline experienced normalization. Of the 65 patients who were HBeAg-positive at baseline, 15% experienced HbeAg loss and 11% developed antibodies to HBsAg (anti-HBs) through week 96.

Across the combined chronic HBV treatment trials, there were insufficient data to establish efficacy in patents with adefovir resistance-associated substitutions.

Decompensated Liver Disease **Study 0108.** Efficacy of tenofovir DF for treatment of chronic HBV infection in adults with decompensated liver disease was evaluated in a small, randomized, double-blind, active-controlled trial (study 0108). At baseline, 69% of patients were HBeAg-negative and 31% were HBeAg-positive and patients had a mean Child-Pugh score of 7, mean Model for End-stage Liver Disease (MELD) score of 12, mean HBV DNA level of 5.8 $\log_{10}$ copies/mL, and mean serum ALT concentration of 61 IU/mL.

At 48 weeks, 70% of patients receiving tenofovir DF had HBV DNA levels less than 400 copies/mL and 46% had ALT normalization. The study was not designed to evaluate treatment effect on clinical end points such as progression of liver disease, need for liver transplantation, or death.

HIV-infected Individuals Because of the risk of development of HIV-1 resistance, tenofovir DF should *not* be used for treatment of chronic HBV infection in HIV-infected individuals who are not currently receiving antiretroviral therapy.

HIV-infected patients coinfected with HBV often have higher HBV viral loads and are more likely to have detectable HBeAg, lower rates of HBeAg seroconversion, and an increased risk for and more rapid progression to cirrhosis, end-stage liver disease, and/or hepatocellular carcinoma compared with individuals not infected with HIV. Decisions to initiate HBV treatment in patients coinfected with HIV and HBV and the most appropriate drugs for HBV treatment in such patients depend on various factors, including the possible effects on replication of both HIV *and* HBV and whether the patient is currently receiving antiretroviral therapy. Specialized references should be consulted for specific information regarding the evaluation and management of chronic HBV infection in HIV-infected patients.

Dosage and Administration

■ **Administration** Tenofovir disoproxil fumarate (tenofovir DF) is administered orally once daily without regard to meals.

Single-entity tenofovir DF (Viread®) is commercially available as tablets or oral powder.

Tenofovir DF oral powder contains 40 mg of tenofovir DF per g. The appropriate dosage of the oral powder should be measured using *only* the scoop provided by the manufacturer. The required number of scoops of the powder should be mixed with 2–4 ounces of soft food that can be swallowed without chewing (e.g., applesauce, baby food, yogurt), and the entire mixture immediately ingested to avoid a bitter taste. The oral powder should not be administered in a liquid since the powder may float to the top, even after stirring.

Single-entity tenofovir DF should not be used concomitantly with any other tenofovir-containing preparation.

Fixed Combinations Containing Tenofovir Tenofovir DF is commercially available in fixed-combination tablets containing emtricitabine and tenofovir DF (emtricitabine/tenofovir DF; Truvada®), fixed-combination tablets containing efavirenz, emtricitabine, and tenofovir DF (efavirenz/emtricitabine/tenofovir DF; Atripla), and fixed-combination tablets containing emtricitabine, rilpivirine, and tenofovir DF (emtricitabine/rilpivirine/tenofovir DF; Complera®). In addition, tenofovir DF is commercially available in fixed-combination tablets containing elvitegravir, cobicistat, emtricitabine, and tenofovir DF (EVG/c/FTC/TDF; Stribild®). For information on EVG/c/FTC/TDF), see Elvitegravir, Cobicistat, Emtricitabine, and Tenofovir Disoproxil Fumarate in 8:18.08.12.

Emtricitabine/tenofovir DF (Truvada®) tablets are administered orally once daily without regard to meals. A fixed-combination tablet containing 200 mg of emtricitabine and 300 mg of tenofovir DF is bioequivalent to a 200-mg capsule of emtricitabine and a 300-mg tablet of tenofovir DF given simultaneously. For the treatment of human immunodeficiency virus type 1 (HIV-1) infection, emtricitabine/tenofovir DF is used in conjunction with other antiretrovirals. For preexposure prophylaxis (PrEP) for prevention of HIV-1 infection, emtricitabine/tenofovir DF is used alone without any other antiretroviral.

Efavirenz/emtricitabine/tenofovir DF (Atripla®) tablets are administered orally once daily on an empty stomach, preferably at bedtime. Administration at bedtime may make efavirenz-related adverse CNS effects more tolerable. A fixed-combination tablet containing 600 mg of efavirenz, 200 mg of emtricitabine, and 300 mg of tenofovir DF is bioequivalent to a 600-mg tablet of efavirenz, 200-mg capsule of emtricitabine, and 300-mg tablet of tenofovir DF when taken in the fasting state. The fixed combination can be used alone as a complete regimen or used in conjunction with other antiretrovirals.

Emtricitabine/rilpivirine/tenofovir DF (Complera®) tablets are administered orally once daily with a meal. A fixed-combination tablet containing 200 mg of emtricitabine, 25 mg of rilpivirine, and 300 mg of tenofovir DF taken with a meal is bioequivalent to a 200-mg emtricitabine capsule, 25-mg rilpivirine tablet, and 300-mg tenofovir DF tablet taken simultaneously with a meal. The fixed combination can be used alone as a complete treatment regimen.

Because the antiretroviral agents contained in the fixed combination preparations also may be available in single-entity or other fixed-combination preparations, care should be taken to ensure that therapy is not duplicated if a fixed combination is used in conjunction with other antiretrovirals. (See Precautions Related to Use of Fixed Combinations under Warnings/Precautions: Other Warnings/Precautions, in Cautions.)

■ **Dosage** Although tenofovir DF is a prodrug that requires metabolism for activation (see Description), dosage of the drug is expressed in terms of the prodrug diester (i.e., tenofovir DF).

Dosage of tenofovir DF (Viread®) oral powder containing 40 mg/g is expressed as the number of scoops of powder. The scoop provided by the manufacturer delivers 1 g of powder for each level scoop.

Adult Dosage **Treatment of HIV Infection.** For the treatment of HIV-1 infection in adults, the usual dosage of tenofovir DF (Viread®) is 300 mg (one 300-mg tablet) once daily. Adults unable to swallow tablets can receive 300 mg once daily as the oral powder containing 40 mg of tenofovir DF per g (7.5 scoops of the powder using the scoop supplied by the manufacturer).

When emtricitabine/tenofovir DF (Truvada®) is used in conjunction with other antiretrovirals for the treatment of HIV-1 infection, adults should receive 1 tablet (200 mg of emtricitabine and 300 mg of tenofovir DF) once daily.

When efavirenz/emtricitabine/tenofovir DF (Atripla®) is used for the treatment of HIV-1 infection, adults should receive 1 tablet (600 mg of efavirenz, 200 mg of emtricitabine, and 300 mg of tenofovir DF) once daily.

When emtricitabine/rilpivirine/tenofovir DF (Complera®) is used for the treatment of HIV-1 infection, adults should receive 1 tablet (200 mg of emtricitabine, 25 mg of rilpivirine, and 300 mg of tenofovir DF) once daily.

Preexposure Prophylaxis for Prevention of HIV-1 Infection. When emtricitabine/tenofovir DF (Truvada®) is used for preexposure prophylaxis (PrEP) for prevention of HIV-1 infection in HIV-1-negative adults at high risk, the recommended dosage is 1 tablet (200 mg of emtricitabine and 300 mg of tenofovir DF) once daily.

PrEP should *only* be used in high-risk adults (see Uses: Preexposure Prophylaxis for Prevention of HIV-1 Infection) with confirmed HIV-1-negative status. PrEP should *not* be initiated if signs or symptoms of acute HIV-1 infection are present and recent (within the past month) exposure to HIV-1 is suspected. (See Precautions Related to HIV-1 Preexposure Prophylaxis [PrEP] under Cautions: Warnings/Precautions.)

Postexposure Prophylaxis following Occupational Exposure to HIV. For postexposure prophylaxis of HIV infection following occupational exposure† (PEP) in health-care personnel or other individuals, the recommended dosage of tenofovir DF (Viread®) is 300 mg once daily. Tenofovir DF usually is used with emtricitabine or lamivudine in conjunction with a recommended HIV integrase strand transferase inhibitor (INSTI), HIV nonnucleoside reverse transcriptase inhibitor (NNRTI), or HIV protease inhibitor (PI). (See Uses: Postexposure Prophylaxis following Occupational Exposure to HIV.)

When emtricitabine/tenofovir DF (Truvada®) is used as the dual NRTI option in PEP† regimens, adults should receive 1 tablet (200 mg of emtricitabine and 300 mg of tenofovir DF) once daily in conjunction with a recommended INSTI, NNRTI, or PI. (See Uses: Postexposure Prophylaxis following Occupational Exposure to HIV.)

When emtricitabine/rilpivirine/tenofovir DF (Complera®) is used as a complete regimen for PEP†, adults should receive 1 tablet (200 mg of emtricitabine, 25 mg of rilpivirine, and 300 mg of tenofovir DF) once daily.

The PEP regimen should be initiated as soon as possible following occupational exposure to HIV (preferably within hours) and continued for 4 weeks, if tolerated.

Postexposure Prophylaxis following Nonoccupational Exposure to HIV. For postexposure prophylaxis of HIV infection following nonoccupational exposure† (nPEP) when the exposure represents a substantial risk for HIV transmission, the usual adult dosage of tenofovir DF (Viread®) is 300 mg once daily in conjunction with other antiretrovirals. Tenofovir DF usually is used in conjunction with emtricitabine and a recommended or alternative INSTI, PI, or NNRTI. (See Uses: Postexposure Prophylaxis following Nonoccupational Exposure to HIV.)

When emtricitabine/tenofovir DF (Truvada®) is used as the dual NRTI option in nPEP† regimens, adults should receive 1 tablet (200 mg of emtricitabine and 300 mg of tenofovir DF) once daily in conjunction with a preferred† or alternative INSTI, PI, or NNRTI.

When emtricitabine/rilpivirine/tenofovir DF (Complera®) is used as a complete regimen for nPEP†, adults should receive 1 tablet (200 mg of emtricitabine, 25 mg of rilpivirine, and 300 mg of tenofovir DF) once daily.

The nPEP regimen should be initiated as soon as possible (within 72 hours) following nonoccupational exposure to HIV and continued for 28 days. If the exposed individual seeks care more than 72 hours after the exposure, nPEP is not recommended.

Chronic Hepatitis B Virus Infection. For the treatment of chronic hepatitis B virus (HBV) infection in adults, the usual dosage of tenofovir DF is 300 mg once daily. The optimum duration of tenofovir DF therapy in patients with chronic HBV infection is not known.

Pediatric Dosage **Treatment of HIV Infection.** For the treatment of HIV-1 infection in pediatric patients 2 to less than 12 years of age, the usual dosage of tenofovir DF (Viread®) is 8 mg/kg (up to 300 mg) once daily as a tablet or oral powder. In pediatric patients 2 years of age or older weighing 17 kg or more who can reliably swallow tablets, a single tablet containing the appropriate dosage should be given once daily (see Table 1). When the oral powder is used, the required number of scoops of the powder should be administered once daily (see Table 2).

For the treatment of HIV-1 infection in adolescents 12 years of age or older weighing at least 35 kg, the usual dosage of tenofovir DF is 300 mg (one 300-mg tablet) once daily. Patients unable to swallow tablets can receive 300 mg once daily as the oral powder containing 40 mg of tenofovir DF per g (7.5 scoops of the powder using the scoop supplied by the manufacturer).

Table 1. Tenofovir DF Dosage (Viread® Tablets) for Treatment of HIV-1 Infection in Pediatric Patients 2 Years of Age or Older Weighing 17 kg or More

Weight (kg)	Dosage (as Tablets) Once Daily
17 to less than 22	150 mg
22 to less than 28	200 mg
28 to less than 35	250 mg
35 or more	300 mg

Table 2. Tenofovir DF Dosage (Viread® Oral Powder) for Treatment of HIV-1 Infection in Pediatric Patients 2 Years of Age or Older

Weight (kg)	Dosage (as Oral Powder) Once Daily (40 mg of Tenofovir DF per Scoop)
10 to less than 12	80 mg (2 scoops)
12 to less than 14	100 mg (2.5 scoops)
14 to less than 17	120 mg (3 scoops)
17 to less than 19	140 mg (3.5 scoops)
19 to less than 22	160 mg (4 scoops)
22 to less than 24	180 mg (4.5 scoops)
24 to less than 27	200 mg (5 scoops)
27 to less than 29	220 mg (5.5 scoops)
29 to less than 32	240 mg (6 scoops)
32 to less than 34	260 mg (6.5 scoops)
34 to less than 35	280 mg (7 scoops)
35 or more	300 mg (7.5 scoops)

When emtricitabine/tenofovir DF (Truvada®) is used in conjunction with other antiretrovirals for the treatment of HIV-1 infection in children weighing at least 35 kg, the recommended dosage is 1 tablet (200 mg of emtricitabine and 300 mg of tenofovir DF) once daily. When emtricitabine/tenofovir DF is used in conjunction with other antiretrovirals for the treatment of HIV-1 infection in children weighing 17 to less than 35 kg who are able to swallow a tablet, recommended dosage is based on weight and a low-strength fixed-combination tablet of the drug should be used. (See Table 3.)

Table 3. Emtricitabine/Tenofovir DF (Truvada®) Dosage for Treatment of HIV-1 Infection in Children Weighing 17 kg or More

Weight (kg)	Dosage of Emtricitabine/Tenofovir DF Given Once Daily
17 to less than 22 kg	1 tablet (100 mg of emtricitabine and 150 mg of tenofovir DF)
22 to less than 28 kg	1 tablet (133 mg of emtricitabine and 200 mg of tenofovir DF)
28 to less than 35 kg	1 tablet (167 mg of emtricitabine and 250 mg of tenofovir DF)
35 kg or more	1 tablet (200 mg of emtricitabine and 300 mg of tenofovir DF)

When efavirenz/emtricitabine/tenofovir DF (Atripla®) is used for the treatment of HIV-1 infection in adolescents 12 years of age or older weighing at least 40 kg, the recommended dosage is 1 tablet (600 mg of efavirenz, 200 mg of emtricitabine, and 300 mg of tenofovir DF) once daily.

When emtricitabine/rilpivirine/tenofovir DF (Complera®) is used for the treatment of HIV-1 infection in adolescents 12 years of age or older weighing at least 35 kg, the usual dosage is 1 tablet (200 mg of emtricitabine, 25 mg of rilpivirine, and 300 mg of tenofovir DF) once daily.

Chronic Hepatitis B Virus Infection. For the treatment of chronic hepatitis B virus (HBV) infection in adolescents 12 years of age or older weighing at least 35 kg, the usual dosage of tenofovir DF is 300 mg once daily. The optimum duration of tenofovir DF therapy in patients with chronic HBV infection is not known.

■ Special Populations

Hepatic Impairment Dosage adjustments are not necessary when tenofovir DF (Viread®) is used for the treatment of HIV-1 infection or treatment of chronic HBV infection in patients with hepatic impairment.

Emtricitabine/tenofovir DF (Truvada®) has not been studied in patients with hepatic impairment.

When efavirenz/emtricitabine/tenofovir DF (Atripla®) is used for the treatment of HIV-1 infection, usual dosage can be used in patients with mild hepatic impairment; however, caution is advised. The fixed combination is not recommended in those with moderate or severe hepatic impairment.

When emtricitabine/rilpivirine/tenofovir DF (Complera®) is used for the treatment of HIV-1 infection in patients with mild or moderate hepatic impairment (Child-Pugh class A or B), usual dosage can be used; the fixed combination has not been studied in patients with severe hepatic impairment (Child-Pugh class C).

Renal Impairment When tenofovir DF (Viread®) is used for the treatment of HIV-1 infection in adults, dosage adjustments are not necessary in those with mild renal impairment (creatinine clearance 50–80 mL/minute), but calculated creatinine clearance, serum phosphorus, urine glucose, and urine protein should be monitored. Dosage of the drug should be adjusted in adults with creatinine clearances less than 50 mL/minute (see Table 4). Because safety and efficacy of these dosages have not been evaluated in clinical studies, clinical response to treatment and renal function should be closely monitored. The manufacturer states that dosage recommendations cannot be made for adults with creatinine clearances less than 10 mL/minute who are not undergoing hemodialysis since the pharmacokinetics of the drug have not been studied in such patients. The manufacturer states that data are not available to make to dosage recommendations for pediatric patients with renal impairment.

Table 4. Tenofovir DF (Viread®) Dosage for Treatment of HIV-1 Infection in Adults with Renal Impairment

Creatinine Clearance (mL/minute)	Dosage
30–49	300 mg once every 48 hours
10–29	300 mg once every 72–96 hours
Hemodialysis patients	300 mg once every 7 days or after a total of approximately 12 hours of hemodialysis (assuming 3 hemodialysis sessions/week each lasting approximately 4 hours); give dose after hemodialysis

When emtricitabine/tenofovir DF (Truvada®) is used for the treatment of HIV-1 infection in adults, usual dosage can be used in those with mild renal impairment (creatinine clearance 50–80 mL/minute), but calculated creatinine clearance, serum phosphorus, urine glucose, and urine protein should be monitored. If the fixed combination is used in adults with creatinine clearance of 30–49 mL/minute, dosage should be reduced to 1 tablet (200 mg of emtricitabine and 300 mg of tenofovir DF) once every 48 hours; clinical response and renal function should be monitored since dosage has not been evaluated clinically. Emtricitabine/tenofovir DF should not be used in adults with creatinine clearances less than 30 mL/minute (including hemodialysis patients). Data are insufficient to make dosage recommendations for the fixed combination for treatment of HIV-1 infection in pediatric patients with renal impairment.

When emtricitabine/tenofovir DF is used for PrEP for prevention of HIV-1 infection in HIV-1-negative adults at high risk, usual dosage can be used in those with creatinine clearances of 60 mL/minute or greater, but calculated creatinine clearance, serum phosphorus, urine glucose, and urine protein should be monitored. If creatinine clearance decreases while emtricitabine/tenofovir DF is being used for PrEP, potential causes should be evaluated and potential risks and benefits of continued use should be reassessed. Emtricitabine/tenofovir DF should *not* be used for PrEP in adults with creatinine clearances less than 60 mL/minute.

When efavirenz/emtricitabine/tenofovir DF (Atripla®) is used for the treatment of HIV-1 infection, usual dosage can be used in patients with creatinine clearances of 50 mL/minute or greater. The fixed combination should *not* be used in those with moderate or severe renal impairment (estimated creatinine clearances less than 50 mL/minute).

Emtricitabine/rilpivirine/tenofovir DF (Complera®) should *not* be used in patients with renal impairment that is moderate, severe, or end-stage (estimated creatinine clearance less than 50 mL/minute) or requires dialysis.

Cautions

■ Contraindications

The manufacturer states that there are no known contraindications to the use of tenofovir disoproxil fumarate (tenofovir DF).

The fixed combination containing emtricitabine and tenofovir DF (emtricitabine/tenofovir DF; Truvada®) should not be used alone for treatment of human immunodeficiency virus type 1 (HIV-1) infection and should not be used for preexposure prophylaxis of HIV-1 infection in individuals with unknown or positive HIV-1 status. (See Precautions Related to HIV-1 Preexposure Prophylaxis under Warnings/Precautions: Warnings, in Cautions.)

The fixed combination containing efavirenz, emtricitabine, and tenofovir DF (efavirenz/emtricitabine/tenofovir DF; Atripla®) is contraindicated in patients who have had a clinically important hypersensitivity reaction (e.g., Stevens-Johnson syndrome, erythema multiforme, toxic skin eruption) to efavirenz; because of the efavirenz component, concomitant use of this fixed combination and voriconazole is contraindicated.

Concomitant use of the fixed combination containing emtricitabine, rilpivirine, and tenofovir DF (emtricitabine/rilpivirine/tenofovir DF; Complera®) and certain drugs that induce cytochrome P-450 isoenzyme 3A (CYP3A) or drugs that elevate gastric pH is contraindicated because of the rilpivirine component; substantially decreased plasma concentrations of rilpivirine may occur and may result in loss of virologic response and development of resistance to rilpivirine and/or class resistance to human immunodeficiency virus (HIV) nonnucleoside reverse transcriptase inhibitors (NNRTIs).

When emtricitabine/tenofovir DF, efavirenz/emtricitabine/tenofovir DF, or emtricitabine/rilpivirine/tenofovir DF is used, the contraindications associated with each of the individual components should be considered. (See Precautions Related to Use of Fixed Combinations under Warnings/Precautions: Other Warnings/Precautions, in Cautions.)

■ Warnings/Precautions

Warnings

Hepatic Effects and Lactic Acidosis. Lactic acidosis and severe hepatomegaly with steatosis, including fatalities, have been reported in patients receiving HIV nucleoside reverse transcriptase inhibitors (NRTIs), including tenofovir DF, in conjunction with other antiretroviral agents. Most reported cases have involved women; obesity and long-term therapy with an NRTI also may be risk factors.

Caution should be observed when NRTIs are used in patients with known risk factors for liver disease; however, lactic acidosis and severe hepatomegaly with steatosis have been reported in patients with no known risk factors. Tenofovir DF (single-entity or fixed-combination preparations) should be discontinued in any patient with clinical or laboratory findings suggestive of lactic acidosis or pronounced hepatotoxicity (signs of hepatotoxicity include hepatomegaly and steatosis even in the absence of marked increases in serum aminotransferase concentrations).

Individuals with Hepatitis B Virus Infection. Prior to initiating tenofovir DF (single-entity or fixed-combination preparations) for treatment of HIV-1 infection, the patient should be tested for chronic hepatitis B virus (HBV).

Prior to initiation of tenofovir DF for treatment of chronic hepatitis B virus (HBV) infection, all patients should be offered HIV-1 testing.

In HIV-infected patients coinfected with HBV, tenofovir DF should be used in conjunction with other highly active antiretroviral agents. When selecting components of an antiretroviral regimen for HIV-infected patients coinfected with HBV, some experts state that tenofovir DF and emtricitabine (or lamivudine) are preferred dual NRTI options in such patients since these antiretrovirals have activity against both HIV *and* HBV.

Severe acute exacerbations of hepatitis have occurred following discontinuance of HBV therapy, including tenofovir DF therapy, in patients with HBV infection.

Hepatic function should be closely monitored with clinical and laboratory follow-up for at least several months after tenofovir DF is discontinued. If appropriate, resumption of anti-HBV therapy may be warranted.

Precautions Related to HIV-1 Preexposure Prophylaxis. Emtricitabine/tenofovir DF (Truvada®) should be used for HIV-1 PrEP *only* in HIV-1-negative adults at high risk.

A negative HIV-1 test should be confirmed immediately prior to initiation of emtricitabine/tenofovir DF for HIV-1 PrEP and screening for HIV-1 infection should be performed at least once every 3 months during PrEP. Individuals also should be tested for HBV prior to initiation of emtricitabine/tenofovir DF PrEP. (See Individuals with Hepatitis B Virus Infection under Cautions: Warnings/Precautions.)

Emtricitabine/tenofovir DF PrEP is *not* always effective in preventing acquisition of HIV-1 infection.

Emtricitabine/tenofovir DF PrEP *must* be used as part of a comprehensive HIV prevention strategy that includes other prevention measures (e.g., safer sex practices). (See REMS.) All uninfected individuals should be counseled about safer sex practices that include consistent and correct use of condoms, knowledge of their own HIV-1 status and that of their partner(s), and regular testing for other sexually transmitted infections that can facilitate HIV-1 transmission (e.g., syphilis, gonorrhea). All HIV-negative individuals should be informed about and supported in their efforts to reduce sexual risk behavior.

Because emtricitabine/tenofovir DF alone does not constitute a complete antiretroviral regimen for treatment of HIV-1 infection, HIV-1 resistance-associated mutations may emerge if PrEP is used in individuals with undetected HIV-1 infection. Drug-resistant HIV-1 variants have been identified when emtricitabine/tenofovir DF PrEP was used in such individuals.

Clinicians should consider that many HIV-1 tests (e.g., rapid tests) detect anti-HIV antibodies and may not identify HIV-1 during the acute stage of infection. Prior to initiating PrEP, clinicians should evaluate HIV-negative individuals for current or recent signs or symptoms consistent with acute viral infection (e.g., fever, fatigue, myalgia, rash) and ask about any potential exposure events that may have occurred within the last month (e.g., unprotected sex, condom broke during sex with HIV-infected partner).

If clinical symptoms consistent with acute viral infection are present and recent (within 1 month) exposures to HIV-1 are suspected, initiation of PrEP should be delayed for at least 1 month and HIV-1 status reconfirmed or a test approved by the US Food and Drug Administration (FDA) for use as an aid in the diagnosis of HIV-1 infection, including acute or primary HIV-1 infection, should be used.

During emtricitabine/tenofovir DF PrEP, if symptoms consistent with acute HIV-1 infection develop following a potential exposure event, the drugs should be discontinued until negative infection status is confirmed using a test approved by FDA as an aid in the diagnosis of HIV-1 infection, including acute or primary HIV-1 infection.

Uninfected individuals should be counseled to strictly adhere to the recommended emtricitabine/tenofovir DF dosage schedule (see Preexposure Prophylaxis for Prevention of HIV-1 Infection under Dosage: Adult Dosage, in Dosage and Administration). Effectiveness of the fixed combination in reducing the risk of acquiring HIV-1 is strongly correlated with adherence as demonstrated by measurable drug concentrations in clinical trials.

Adverse effects reported in HIV-negative adults receiving emtricitabine/tenofovir DF PrEP are similar to those reported in HIV-infected patients receiving the drugs for treatment of HIV-1 infection.

Other Warnings/Precautions

Renal Toxicity. Renal impairment, including cases of acute renal failure and Fanconi syndrome (renal tubular injury with severe hypophosphatemia), has been reported in patients receiving tenofovir DF.

Creatinine clearance should be calculated in all patients prior to and as clinically indicated during tenofovir DF therapy. Calculated creatinine clearance and serum phosphorus, urine glucose, and urine protein concentrations should be monitored prior to and periodically during tenofovir DF therapy in patients at risk for renal dysfunction, including those who had adverse renal effects while receiving adefovir dipivoxil.

Use of tenofovir DF should be avoided in patients who are receiving or have recently received nephrotoxic drugs (e.g., high-dose or multiple nonsteroidal anti-inflammatory agents [NSAIAs]). Acute renal failure has been reported after initiation of high-dose or multiple NSAIAs in HIV-infected patients with risk factors for renal dysfunction who appeared stable while receiving tenofovir DF. Some cases required hospitalization and renal replacement therapy. Alternatives to NSAIAs should be considered in patients at risk for renal dysfunction. If manifestations of proximal renal tubulopathy are present in patients at risk for renal dysfunction (i.e., persistent or worsening bone pain, pain in extremities, fractures, and/or muscular pain or weakness), renal function should be promptly evaluated.

Evidence of renal toxicity was reported in animal studies (increases in serum creatinine or BUN, glycosuria, proteinuria, phosphaturia, calciuria, decreases in serum phosphate); the relationship of renal abnormalities, particularly phosphaturia, to bone toxicity in animals is unknown.

Precautions Related to Use of Fixed Combinations. When emtricitabine/tenofovir DF, efavirenz/emtricitabine/tenofovir DF, or emtricitabine/rilpivirine/tenofovir DF is used, the usual cautions, precautions, contraindications, and drug interactions associated with each drug in the fixed combination must be considered. Cautionary information applicable to specific populations (e.g., pregnant or nursing women, individuals with hepatic or renal impairment, geriatric patients) should be considered for each drug. For cautionary information related to efavirenz, emtricitabine, and rilpivirine, see Cautions in the individual drug monographs.

Because the antiretrovirals contained in the fixed-combination preparations also may be available in single-entity or other fixed-combination preparations, take care to ensure that therapy is not duplicated if a fixed combination is used in conjunction with other antiretrovirals.

Multiple tenofovir-containing preparations should not be used concomitantly.

Preparations containing tenofovir DF should not be used concomitantly with adefovir dipivoxil. In addition, because of similarities between emtricitabine and lamivudine, fixed combinations containing emtricitabine should not be used concomitantly with any preparation containing lamivudine.

Bone Effects. In one clinical study (study 903), decreases from baseline in bone mineral density (BMD) at the lumbar spine, increases in levels of 4 biochemical markers of bone metabolism, increased serum parathyroid hormone levels, and increased 1,25 vitamin D levels were reported in HIV-infected adults receiving tenofovir DF concomitantly with lamivudine and efavirenz; these effects also were reported to a lesser extent in patients who received a regimen of stavudine, lamivudine, and efavirenz. With the exception of bone-specific alkaline phosphatase concentrations, these changes generally remained within the normal range. There were 4 bone fractures reported in patients receiving the regimen that contained tenofovir DF and 6 reported in those receiving the regimen that did not include tenofovir DF.

In 2 clinical studies (study 321 and study 352) in HIV-1-infected pediatric patients, effects on bone were similar to those observed in adults, suggesting increased bone turnover. Similar trends were observed in HBV-infected pediatric patients 12 to less than 18 years of age. In all pediatric studies, skeletal growth appeared to be unaffected.

The clinical importance of tenofovir DF-associated changes in BMD and biochemical markers on long-term bone health and fracture risk are unknown. BMD monitoring should be considered for adult and pediatric patients who have a history of pathologic bone fracture or other risk factors for osteoporosis or bone loss. Although the effect of calcium and vitamin D supplementation was not studied, such supplementation may be beneficial for all patients. If bone abnormalities are suspected, appropriate consultation should be obtained.

Osteomalacia associated with proximal renal tubulopathy, which may contribute to fractures, has been reported in patients receiving tenofovir DF; arthralgias and muscle pain or weakness have also been reported in patients with proximal renal tubulopathy. Hypophosphatemia and osteomalacia secondary to proximal renal tubulopathy should be considered in patients at risk of renal dysfunction who present with persistent or worsening bone or muscle symptoms while receiving products containing tenofovir DF.

Osteomalacia and decreases in BMD have been reported in toxicology studies in juvenile animals given high doses of tenofovir.

Adipogenic Effects. Redistribution or accumulation of body fat, including central obesity, dorsocervical fat enlargement ("buffalo hump"), peripheral wasting, facial wasting, breast enlargement, and general cushingoid appearance, has been reported with antiretroviral therapy. The mechanisms responsible for these adipogenic effects and the long-term consequences of these effects are unknown. A causal relationship has not been established.

Immune Reconstitution Syndrome. During the initial phase of treatment, HIV-infected patients whose immune systems respond to antiretroviral therapy may develop an inflammatory response to indolent or residual opportunistic infections (e.g., *Mycobacterium avium* complex [MAC], *M. tuberculosis*, cytomegalovirus [CMV], *Pneumocystis jirovecii* [formerly *P. carinii*]); such response may necessitate further evaluation and treatment.

Autoimmune disorders (e.g., Graves' disease, polymyositis, Guillain-Barré syndrome) have also been reported to occur in the setting of immune reconstitution; however, the time to onset is more variable and can occur many months after initiation of antiretroviral therapy.

Early Virologic Failure in HIV Infection. Triple NRTI regimens have less potent virologic activity than comparator HIV nonnucleoside reverse transcriptase (NNRTI)-based or HIV protease inhibitor (PI)-based regimens. Triple NRTI regimens are associated with early virologic failure and high rates of resistance. These regimens should be used with caution. Patients should be carefully monitored and consideration given to modifying the regimen.

Specific Populations

Pregnancy. Tenofovir DF (Viread®): Category B. (See Users Guide.)

Emtricitabine/tenofovir DF (Truvada®): Category B.

Efavirenz/emtricitabine/tenofovir DF (Atripla®): Category D. (See Pregnancy under Cautions: Pregnancy, Fertility, and Lactation in Efavirenz 8:18.08.16.)

Emtricitabine/rilpivirine/tenofovir DF (Complera®): Category B.

Antiretroviral Pregnancy Registry at 800-258-4263 or http://www.APRegistry.com.

The US Department of Health and Human Services (HHS) Panel on Treatment of HIV-infected Pregnant Women and Prevention of Perinatal Transmission states that tenofovir DF and either emtricitabine or lamivudine is a preferred dual NRTI option for use in conjunction with an HIV integrase strand transferase inhibitor (INSTI), NNRTI, or PI for *initial* treatment of HIV-1 infection in antiretroviral-naive pregnant women, and is a preferred dual NRTI option in pregnant women coinfected with HBV.

Some experts state that the dual NRTI option of tenofovir DF and emtricitabine used in conjunction with the fixed combination of lopinavir and ritonavir (lopinavir/ritonavir) is a preferred regimen for treatment of HIV type 2 (HIV-2) infection† in pregnant women.

If an HIV-1-negative woman receiving emtricitabine/tenofovir DF (Truvada®) for HIV-1 PrEP becomes pregnant, careful consideration should be given to whether the PrEP regimen should be continued, taking into account the potential increased risk of HIV-1 infection during pregnancy.

Lactation. Tenofovir is distributed into human milk in low concentrations.

Because of the risk of adverse effects in the infant and the risk of HIV transmission, HIV-infected women should not breast-feed infants.

Pediatric Use. Safety and efficacy of tenofovir DF (Viread®) have not been established in HIV-1-infected children younger than 2 years of age. Safety and efficacy of tenofovir DF (Viread®) for treatment of chronic HBV infection have not been established in children younger than 12 years of age weighing less than 35 kg.

Safety and efficacy of emtricitabine/tenofovir DF (Truvada®) for treatment of HIV-1 infection have *not* been established in pediatric patients weighing less than 17 kg; safety and efficacy of this fixed combination for HIV-1 PrEP have *not* been established in pediatric patients.

Efavirenz/emtricitabine/tenofovir DF (Atripla®) should *not* be used in pediatric patients younger than 12 years of age or weighing less than 40 kg. Safety and efficacy of emtricitabine/rilpivirine/tenofovir DF (Complera®) have *not* been established in pediatric patients younger than 12 years of age or weighing less than 35 kg.

Geriatric Use. Experience in those 65 years of age or older is insufficient to determine whether they respond differently to tenofovir DF (single-entity or fixed-combination preparations) than younger adults. Dosage should be selected with caution because of the greater frequency of decreased hepatic, renal, and/or cardiac function and of concomitant disease or drug therapy observed in geriatric individuals.

Hepatic Impairment. Limited data indicate that the pharmacokinetics of tenofovir are not substantially altered in patients with moderate or severe hepatic impairment. (See Hepatic Impairment under Dosage and Administration: Special Populations.)

Emtricitabine/tenofovir DF (Truvada®) has not been studied in patients with hepatic impairment. Hepatic impairment does not have a substantial effect on tenofovir DF pharmacokinetics and is expected to have a minimal effect on emtricitabine pharmacokinetics.

Efavirenz/emtricitabine/tenofovir DF (Atripla®) is *not* recommended in patients with moderate or severe hepatic impairment.

Emtricitabine/rilpivirine/tenofovir DF (Complera®) has not been studied in patients with severe hepatic impairment (Child-Pugh class C).

Renal Impairment. Tenofovir is principally eliminated by the kidney and the pharmacokinetics of the drug are likely to be affected by renal impairment. Dosage adjustments are necessary if tenofovir DF is used in patients with moderate or severe renal impairment. (See Renal Impairment under Dosage and Administration: Special Populations.)

Emtricitabine/tenofovir DF (Truvada®) should *not* be used for treatment of HIV-1 infection in patients with creatinine clearance less than 30 mL/minute or in those with end-stage renal disease requiring dialysis; dosage adjustments are necessary when the drug is used for treatment of HIV-1 infection in those with creatinine clearance 30–49 mL/minute. Emtricitabine/tenofovir DF should *not* be used for PrEP in HIV-1 uninfected adults with creatinine clearances less than 60 mL/minute. If creatinine clearance decreases while emtricitabine/tenofovir DF is being used for PrEP, potential causes should be evaluated and potential risks and benefits of continued use should be reassessed.

Efavirenz/emtricitabine/tenofovir DF (Atripla®) should *not* be used in patients with moderate or severe renal impairment (estimated creatinine clearances less than 50 mL/minute).

Emtricitabine/rilpivirine/tenofovir DF (Complera®) should *not* be used in patients with renal impairment that is moderate, severe, or end-stage (estimated creatinine clearance less than 50 mL/minute) or requires dialysis.

■ **Common Adverse Effects** The most common adverse effects in HIV-infected patients receiving tenofovir DF are rash, diarrhea, headache, pain, depression, asthenia, and nausea.

The most common adverse effects in patients with chronic HBV infection receiving tenofovir DF are GI effects (abdominal pain, nausea, vomiting, diarrhea), headache, insomnia, dizziness, fatigue, rash, pruritus, nasopharyngitis, back pain, and fever.

Drug Interactions

The following drug interactions are based on studies using tenofovir disoproxil fumarate (tenofovir DF).

Drug interaction studies have also been performed using the fixed combination containing efavirenz, emtricitabine, and tenofovir DF (efavirenz/emtricitabine/tenofovir DF; Atripla) or the fixed combination containing emtricitabine, rilpivirine, and tenofovir DF (emtricitabine/rilpivirine/tenofovir DF; Complera®). When a fixed combination is used, interactions associated with each drug in the fixed combination should be considered.

■ **Drugs Affecting or Metabolized by Hepatic Microsomal Enzymes** Pharmacokinetic interactions between tenofovir and drugs that are inhibitors or substrates of hepatic microsomal enzymes are unlikely. Tenofovir and its prodrug (tenofovir DF) are not substrates of cytochrome P-450 (CYP) isoenzymes; in vitro studies indicate tenofovir does not inhibit CYP isoenzymes 3A4, 2D6, 2C9, or 2E1, but may have a slight inhibitory effect on CYP1A.

■ **Drugs Affecting P-glycoprotein Transport** Tenofovir DF is a substrate of the P-glycoprotein (P-gp) transport system. Pharmacokinetic interactions are possible with inhibitors of P-gp (increased absorption of tenofovir DF).

■ **Drugs Affecting Breast Cancer Resistance Protein** Tenofovir DF is a substrate of breast cancer resistance protein (BCRP). Pharmacokinetic interactions are possible with inhibitors of BCRP (increased absorption of tenofovir DF).

■ **Nephrotoxic Drugs or Drugs Eliminated by Renal Excretion** Potential pharmacokinetic interaction between tenofovir and drugs that reduce renal function or that may compete with tenofovir for active renal tubular secretion (i.e., acyclovir, aminoglycosides [e.g., gentamicin], cidofovir, ganciclovir, valacyclovir, valganciclovir, high-dose or multiple nonsteroidal anti-inflammatory agents [NSAIAs]); increased plasma concentrations of tenofovir and/or the concomitantly administered drug may occur.

■ **Adefovir Dipivoxil** Concomitant use of adefovir dipivoxil and tenofovir DF may result in increased plasma concentrations of tenofovir and/or adefovir.

Tenofovir DF and adefovir dipivoxil should not be used concomitantly.

■ **Antiretroviral Agents** ***HIV Entry and Fusion Inhibitors***

Maraviroc. No in vitro evidence of antagonistic antiretroviral effects between maraviroc and tenofovir DF.

Tenofovir DF does not affect the pharmacokinetics of maraviroc.

HIV Integrase Inhibitors (INSTIs) **Dolutegravir.** Concomitant use of tenofovir DF and dolutegravir does not have a clinically important effect on the pharmacokinetics of either drug.

Dosage adjustments are not needed if dolutegravir is used concomitantly with tenofovir DF.

Raltegravir. In vitro evidence of additive to synergistic antiretroviral effects between raltegravir and tenofovir DF.

Pharmacokinetic interaction with raltegravir (increased raltegravir plasma concentrations and area under the concentration-time curve [AUC]; no clinically important effect on tenofovir pharmacokinetics). This interaction is not considered clinically important. Dosage adjustments are not needed if raltegravir is used concomitantly with tenofovir DF.

HIV Nonnucleoside Reverse Transcriptase Inhibitors (NNRTIs) No in vitro evidence of antagonistic antiretroviral effects between tenofovir and NNRTIs (delavirdine, efavirenz, etravirine, nevirapine, rilpivirine).

Efavirenz. Concomitant use of tenofovir DF and efavirenz does not affect plasma concentrations or AUC of either drug.

Dosage adjustments are not needed if efavirenz and tenofovir DF are used concomitantly.

Etravirine. Pharmacokinetic interaction with etravirine (decreased etravirine plasma concentrations and AUC; no clinically important effect on tenofovir plasma concentrations and AUC).

Dosage adjustments are not needed for either drug if etravirine and tenofovir DF are used concomitantly.

Rilpivirine. Concomitant use of tenofovir DF and rilpivirine has resulted in increased tenofovir plasma concentrations and AUC, but did not have any clinically important effects on rilpivirine plasma concentrations or AUC.

Dosage adjustments are not needed if rilpivirine and tenofovir DF are used concomitantly.

HIV Nucleoside Reverse Transcriptase Inhibitors (NRTIs) In vitro evidence of additive to synergistic antiretroviral effects between tenofovir and emtricitabine. No in vitro evidence of antagonistic antiretroviral effects between tenofovir and NRTIs (abacavir, didanosine, lamivudine, stavudine, zidovudine).

Abacavir. Concomitant use of tenofovir DF and abacavir does not have a clinically important effect on the pharmacokinetics of abacavir.

Didanosine. Depending on the specific didanosine dosage used, concomitant use of buffered didanosine (Videx®) or delayed-release capsules containing enteric-coated pellets of didanosine (Videx® EC) and tenofovir DF results in substantially increased didanosine plasma concentrations and AUC, but does not affect tenofovir pharmacokinetics. The mechanism of this interaction is unknown. Concomitant use of the drugs potentially could lead to didanosine-associated adverse effects (e.g., pancreatitis, lactic acidosis, neuropathy); concomitant use also has been associated with early virologic failure, rapid selection of resistant mutations, and immunologic nonresponse or decline in $CD4^+$ T-cell count.

When didanosine 250 mg enteric-coated capsules were used concomitantly with tenofovir DF and a light meal (373 kcal, 8.2 g fat), peak plasma concentrations of didanosine were decreased 20% and didanosine AUC was similar to that reported when the 400-mg didanosine enteric-coated capsules are used alone in the fasted state.

Concomitant use of didanosine and tenofovir DF should be avoided, and some experts state that didanosine and tenofovir DF should not be used concomitantly at any time. (See Dual NRTI Options under Treatment of HIV Infection: Antiretroviral-naive Adults and Adolescents, in Uses.) If didanosine and tenofovir DF are used concomitantly, the manufacturers recommend that a reduced didanosine dosage be used with caution and close monitoring for didanosine-associated adverse effects; didanosine should be discontinued if didanosine-associated adverse effects occur.

If didanosine delayed-release capsules are used with tenofovir DF, didanosine dosage should be decreased to 250 mg once daily in those weighing 60 kg or more with creatinine clearances of 60 mL/minute or greater or 200 mg once daily in those weighing less than 60 kg with creatinine clearances of 60 mL/minute or greater. Didanosine delayed-release capsules and tenofovir DF should be taken at the same time with a light meal (no more than 400 kcal, no more than 20% fat) or in the fasted state. The appropriate didanosine dosage in patients with creatinine clearance less than 60 mL/minute receiving tenofovir DF has not been established.

Emtricitabine. No clinically important pharmacokinetic interactions between emtricitabine and tenofovir DF.

Lamivudine. Concomitant use of tenofovir DF and lamivudine does not have a clinically important effect on the pharmacokinetics of lamivudine.

HIV Protease Inhibitors (PIs) In vitro evidence of additive antiretroviral effects between tenofovir DF and tipranavir. No in vitro evidence of antagonistic antiretroviral effects between tenofovir DF and HIV PIs (amprenavir, atazanavir, darunavir, indinavir, nelfinavir, ritonavir, saquinavir).

Atazanavir. Pharmacokinetic interaction between tenofovir DF and *ritonavir-boosted*, *cobicistat-boosted*, or unboosted atazanavir (decreased atazanavir plasma concentrations and AUC; increased tenofovir plasma concentrations and AUC and possible increased risk of tenofovir-associated adverse effects, including renal disorders).

Tenofovir DF and unboosted atazanavir (without low-dose ritonavir or cobicistat) should not be used concomitantly.

If tenofovir DF and *ritonavir-boosted* atazanavir are used concomitantly, a regimen of atazanavir 300 mg, ritonavir 100 mg, and tenofovir DF 300 mg given once daily with food is recommended. Patients should be monitored for tenofovir toxicity; tenofovir DF should be discontinued if tenofovir-associated adverse effects occur.

If tenofovir DF and *cobicistat-boosted* atazanavir are used concomitantly, a regimen of atazanavir 300 mg, cobicistat 150 mg, and tenofovir DF 300 mg once daily with food is recommended. Patients should be monitored for tenofovir toxicity. Concomitant use of *cobicistat-boosted* atazanavir and tenofovir DF is not recommended in patients with estimated creatinine clearances less than 70 mL/minute.

If *ritonavir-boosted* atazanavir is used concomitantly with tenofovir DF *and* a histamine H_2-receptor antagonist in antiretroviral-experienced adults, the recommended dosage is atazanavir 400 mg, ritonavir 100 mg, and tenofovir DF 300 mg once daily with food. Patients should be monitored for tenofovir toxicity.

If *cobicistat-boosted* atazanavir is used concomitantly with tenofovir DF *and* a histamine H_2-receptor antagonist in antiretroviral-experienced adults, the recommended dosage is atazanavir 400 mg, cobicistat 150 mg, and tenofovir DF 300 mg once daily with food. Patients should be monitored for tenofovir toxicity.

Darunavir. Pharmacokinetic interactions with *ritonavir-boosted* darunavir (increased tenofovir plasma concentrations and AUC; increased darunavir plasma concentrations and AUC). Possible pharmacokinetic interactions with *cobicistat-boosted* darunavir (increased tenofovir plasma concentrations).

The manufacturer of darunavir states that the usual dosage of *ritonavir-boosted* darunavir can be used concomitantly with the usual dosage of tenofovir DF. Some experts state that the clinical importance of increased tenofovir DF exposures is unknown, and patients receiving *ritonavir-boosted* darunavir concomitantly with tenofovir DF should be monitored for tenofovir toxicity.

If tenofovir DF is used concomitantly with *cobicistat-boosted* darunavir, patients should be monitored for tenofovir toxicity. Concomitant use of *cobicistat-boosted* darunavir with tenofovir DF is *not* recommended in patients with estimated creatinine clearances less than 70 mL/minute.

Indinavir. Pharmacokinetic interaction with indinavir (14% increase in peak plasma concentration of tenofovir; 11% decrease in peak plasma concentration of indinavir; no change in AUC of either drug).

Lopinavir. Pharmacokinetic interaction with the fixed combination of lopinavir and ritonavir (lopinavir/ritonavir) (increased tenofovir AUC; no change in lopinavir plasma concentrations and AUC).

Patients receiving lopinavir/ritonavir and tenofovir DF concomitantly should be monitored for tenofovir toxicity, and tenofovir DF should be discontinued if such effects occur.

Nelfinavir. No clinically important pharmacokinetic interaction between nelfinavir and tenofovir DF.

Saquinavir. Pharmacokinetic interaction with *ritonavir-boosted* saquinavir is not clinically important. Dosage adjustments are not needed when tenofovir DF is used with *ritonavir-boosted* saquinavir.

Tipranavir. Pharmacokinetic interaction with *ritonavir-boosted* tipranavir (decreased tipranavir concentrations and AUC; decreased tenofovir concentrations and AUC).

Dosage adjustments are not needed if tipranavir and tenofovir DF are used concomitantly.

■ **Entecavir** No in vitro evidence of antagonistic antiviral effects between tenofovir DF and entecavir.

No clinically important pharmacokinetic interaction between entecavir and tenofovir DF.

■ **Estrogens and Progestins** No clinically important pharmacokinetic interaction between oral contraceptives and tenofovir DF.

■ **Ganciclovir and Valganciclovir** Concomitant use of tenofovir DF and ganciclovir or valganciclovir may result in increased plasma concentrations of tenofovir and/or ganciclovir.

If tenofovir DF is used concomitantly with ganciclovir or valganciclovir, patients should be monitored for dose-related toxicities.

■ **HCV Antivirals** ***HCV Polymerase Inhibitors*** **Sofosbuvir.** Concomitant use of tenofovir DF and sofosbuvir does not have a clinically important effect on the pharmacokinetics of either drug.

Dosage adjustments are not needed for either drug if sofosbuvir is used concomitantly with tenofovir DF.

Sofosbuvir and Velpatasvir. Concomitant use of tenofovir DF and the fixed combination of sofosbuvir and velpatasvir (sofosbuvir/velpatasvir) may result in increased plasma concentrations of tenofovir.

If an antiretroviral regimen containing tenofovir DF is used concomitantly with sofosbuvir/velpatasvir, the patient should be monitored for tenofovir-associated adverse effects.

HCV Protease Inhibitors **Simeprevir.** Concomitant use of tenofovir DF and simeprevir results in slightly decreased simeprevir plasma concentrations and AUC, but does not have a clinically important effect on the pharmacokinetics of tenofovir DF.

Dosage adjustments are not needed for either drug if simeprevir is used concomitantly with tenofovir DF.

HCV Replication Complex Inhibitors **Daclatasvir.** Concomitant use of daclatasvir and tenofovir DF does not result in clinically important changes in the pharmacokinetics of either drug.

Elbasvir and Grazoprevir. Concomitant use of the fixed combination of elbasvir and grazoprevir (elbasvir/grazoprevir) and tenofovir DF does not result in clinically important changes in the pharmacokinetics of elbasvir, grazoprevir, or tenofovir. Dosage adjustments are not needed.

Ledipasvir and Sofosbuvir. Concomitant use of the fixed combination of ledipasvir and sofosbuvir (ledipasvir/sofosbuvir) and tenofovir DF results in increased tenofovir exposure.

Concomitant use of ledipasvir/sofosbuvir and antiretroviral regimens that include tenofovir DF and certain other antiretrovirals may result in increased tenofovir concentrations (e.g., efavirenz/emtricitabine/tenofovir DF, emtricitabine/rilpivirine/tenofovir DF, dolutegravir in conjunction with emtricitabine/tenofovir DF, any regimen that includes tenofovir DF and a *ritonavir-boosted* PI or tenofovir DF and cobicistat). Safety of increased tenofovir concentrations in patients receiving ledipasvir/sofosbuvir has not been established.

An alternative HCV treatment regimen or alternative antiretroviral regimen should be considered if the patient is receiving ledipasvir/sofosbuvir concomitantly with an antiretroviral regimen that contains tenofovir DF and a *ritonavir-boosted* PI or tenofovir DF and cobicistat; if concomitant use of ledipasvir/sofosbuvir and these antiretroviral regimens is necessary, the patient should be monitored for tenofovir-associated adverse effects. Patients also should be monitored for tenofovir-associated adverse effects if ledipasvir/sofosbuvir is used concomitantly with an HIV antiretroviral regimen that contains tenofovir DF without a *ritonavir-boosted* HIV PI or without cobicistat.

Ombitasvir, Paritaprevir, and Ritonavir. Concomitant use of emtricitabine/tenofovir DF and the fixed combination of ombitasvir, paritaprevir, and ritonavir (ombitasvir/paritaprevir/ritonavir) with or without dasabuvir does not result in clinically important interactions.

Dosage adjustments are not needed if emtricitabine/tenofovir DF is used concomitantly with ombitasvir/paritaprevir/ritonavir with or without dasabuvir.

■ **Opiates and Opiate Partial Agonists** ***Buprenorphine*** No clinically important pharmacokinetic interaction between buprenorphine and tenofovir DF.

Dosage adjustments are not necessary if buprenorphine and tenofovir DF are used concomitantly.

Methadone No clinically important pharmacokinetic interaction between methadone and tenofovir DF.

Dosage adjustments are not necessary if methadone and tenofovir DF are used concomitantly.

■ **Ribavirin** No clinically important pharmacokinetic interaction between ribavirin and tenofovir DF.

■ **Tacrolimus** Pharmacokinetic interaction is unlikely.

■ **Telbivudine** No in vitro evidence of antagonistic antiviral effects between tenofovir DF and telbivudine.

Description

Tenofovir disoproxil fumarate (tenofovir DF), a synthetic antiretroviral agent, is a human immunodeficiency virus (HIV) nucleotide reverse transcriptase inhibitor. Tenofovir DF is a prodrug and is inactive until it undergoes diester hydrolysis in vivo to tenofovir and is subsequently metabolized to the active metabolite (tenofovir diphosphate). After conversion to the pharmacologically active metabolite, tenofovir apparently inhibits replication of retroviruses, including HIV type 1 (HIV-1), by interfering with viral RNA-directed DNA polymerase (reverse transcriptase). In vitro and in vivo studies indicate that tenofovir is active against HIV-1 and hepatitis B virus (HBV); the drug also has some activity against HIV-2.

Like HIV nucleoside reverse transcriptase inhibitors (NRTIs), the antiviral activity of tenofovir depends on intracellular conversion to an active metabolite; however, tenofovir is a nucleotide containing a phosphonate group and the steps and enzymes involved in enzymatic conversion to the active metabolite differ from those involved in the conversion of NRTIs. Tenofovir is phosphorylated by cellular nucleotide kinases to tenofovir diphosphate; tenofovir diphosphate is a structural analog of deoxyadenosine-5′-triphosphate, the usual substrate for viral RNA-directed DNA polymerase. Although other mechanisms may be involved in the antiretroviral activities of the drug, tenofovir diphosphate appears to compete with deoxyadenosine-5′-triphosphate for viral RNA-directed DNA polymerase and for incorporation into viral DNA. Following incorporation of tenofovir diphosphate into the viral DNA chain, DNA synthesis is prematurely terminated because the absence of the 3′-hydroxy group on the drug prevents further 5′ to 3′ phosphodiester linkages.

Tenofovir diphosphate is a weak inhibitor of mammalian DNA α- and β-polymerases and mitochondrial DNA γ-polymerase. In vitro studies using human hepatoblastoma cells, skeletal muscle cells, or renal proximal tubule epithelial cells indicate that tenofovir has only a low potential to induce mitochondrial toxicity.

HIV-1 strains with reduced susceptibility to tenofovir DF can be produced in vitro and strains with reduced susceptibility to tenofovir have emerged during therapy with the drug. Resistant strains have contained a K65R substitution in reverse transcriptase. HIV-1 with a K70E substitution that results in low-level reduced susceptibility to tenofovir also have been selected in vitro and identified in clinical isolates.

Cross-resistance occurs between tenofovir and some NRTIs. The K65R and K70E substitutions selected by tenofovir also are selected in some patients treated with abacavir or didanosine; isolates with such substitutions may show reduced susceptibility to emtricitabine and lamivudine. Therefore, presence of the K65R or K70E substitution may result in cross-resistance between tenofovir and NRTIs. In vitro studies indicate that HIV isolates with multiple substitutions associated with zidovudine resistance have reduced susceptibility to tenofovir. Cross-resistance between tenofovir and HIV protease inhibitors (PIs) or HIV nonnucleoside reverse transcriptase inhibitors (NNRTIs) is unlikely.

Tenofovir inhibits HBV replication through competitive inhibition of viral reverse transcriptase. Although treatment-emergent amino acid substitutions have been reported in patients with HBV infection who received at least 24 weeks of tenofovir DF monotherapy and remained viremic, no specific substitutions occurred at a sufficient frequency to be associated with tenofovir resistance (genotypic and phenotypic analysis). Tenofovir may be active against some HBV strains that are resistant to adefovir and/or lamivudine. However, cross-resistance occurs among the HBV nucleoside/nucleotide reverse transcriptase inhibitors and some adefovir-, entecavir-, lamivudine-, or telbivudine-resistant HBV may have reduced susceptibility to tenofovir.

When a 300-mg tenofovir DF tablet is administered with a high-fat meal, plasma tenofovir concentrations and area under the plasma concentration-time curve (AUC) are increased; pharmacokinetics are not appreciably affected by administration with a light meal.

Advice to Patients

Critical nature of compliance with human immunodeficiency virus (HIV) therapy and importance of remaining under the care of a clinician. Importance of taking as prescribed; do not alter or discontinue antiretroviral regimen without consulting clinician.

Importance of using single-entity tenofovir disoproxil fumarate (Viread®) or fixed combination containing tenofovir DF and emtricitabine (emtricitabine/tenofovir DF; Truvada®) in conjunction with other antiretrovirals for treatment of HIV-1 infection—not for monotherapy.

Fixed combination containing efavirenz, emtricitabine, and tenofovir DF (efavirenz/emtricitabine/tenofovir DF; Atripla®) or fixed combination containing rilpivirine, emtricitabine, and tenofovir DF (emtricitabine/rilpivirine/tenofovir DF; Complera®) can be used alone as a complete regimen for treatment of HIV-1 infection.

Antiretroviral therapy is not a cure for HIV infection; opportunistic infections and other complications of HIV disease may still occur.

Advise HIV-infected patients that effective antiretroviral treatment regimens can decrease HIV-1 concentrations in blood and genital secretions and strict adherence to such regimens in conjunction with risk-reduction measures may decrease, but cannot absolutely eliminate, the risk of secondary transmission of HIV to others. Importance of continuing to practice safer sex (e.g., using latex or polyurethane condoms to minimize sexual contact with body fluids), never sharing personal items that can have blood or body fluids on them (e.g., toothbrushes, razor blades), and never reusing or sharing needles.

Emtricitabine/tenofovir DF (Truvada®) medication guide must be provided to and reviewed with all HIV-1-negative individuals each time the drug is dispensed for preexposure prophylaxis (PrEP) of HIV-1 infection. Advise such individuals of the importance of confirming that they are HIV-1-negative before starting PrEP, importance of regular HIV-1 testing (at least every 3 months) during PrEP, importance of strictly adhering to recommended dosage schedule and not missing any doses of the drug, and importance of using a complete prevention strategy that also includes other measures (e.g., consistent condom use, testing for other sexually transmitted infections such as syphilis and gonorrhea that may facilitate HIV-1 transmission, reducing sexual risk behavior). Advise uninfected individuals that emtricitabine/tenofovir DF PrEP does not protect all individuals from acquiring HIV-1 and to report any symptoms of acute HIV-1 infection (e.g., fever, headache, fatigue, arthralgia, vomiting, myalgia, diarrhea, pharyngitis, rash, night sweats, cervical and inguinal adenopathy) immediately to a clinician.

Importance of reading patient information provided by the manufacturer.

Inform patients that redistribution or accumulation of body fat may occur in patients receiving antiretroviral therapy and that the cause and long-term health effects of these conditions are unknown.

Importance of informing clinicians of existing or contemplated concomitant therapy, including prescription and OTC drugs and dietary or herbal products, as well as concomitant medical problems such as renal or hepatic impairment.

Importance of women informing clinicians if they are or plan to become pregnant or plan to breast-feed. Advise HIV-infected women not to breast-feed.

Importance of informing patients of other important precautionary information. (See Cautions.)

Overview® (see Users Guide). For additional information on this drug until a more detailed monograph is developed and published, the manufacturer's labeling should be consulted. It is *essential* that the manufacturer's labeling be consulted for more detailed information on usual cautions, precautions, contraindications, potential drug interactions, laboratory test interferences, and acute toxicity.

Preparations

Excipients in commercially available drug preparations may have clinically important effects in some individuals; consult specific product labeling for details.

Tenofovir Disoproxil Fumarate

Oral		
Powder	40 mg per g	Viread®, Gilead
Tablets, film-coated	150 mg	Viread®, Gilead
	200 mg	Viread®, Gilead
	250 mg	Viread®, Gilead
	300 mg	Viread®, Gilead

Tenofovir Disoproxil Fumarate Combinations

Oral		
Tablets, film-coated	150 mg with Emtricitabine 100 mg	Truvada®, Gilead
	200 mg with Emtricitabine 133 mg	Truvada®, Gilead
	250 mg with Emtricitabine 167 mg	Truvada®, Gilead
	300 mg with Emtricitabine 200 mg	Truvada®, Gilead
	300 mg with Emtricitabine 200 mg and Efavirenz 600 mg	Atripla®, Bristol-Myers Squibb and Gilead
	300 mg with Emtricitabine 200 mg and Rilpivirine Hydrochloride 25 mg (of rilpivirine)	Complera®, Gilead
	300 mg with Emtricitabine 200 mg, Elvitegravir 150 mg, and Cobicistat 150 mg	Stribild®, Gilead

†Use is not currently included in the labeling approved by the US Food and Drug Administration

Zidovudine

AZT, ZDV, ABC/3TC/ZDV, 3TC/ZDV, lamivudine/zidovudine

■ Zidovudine, an antiretroviral agent, is a human immunodeficiency virus (HIV) nucleoside reverse transcriptase inhibitor (NRTI).

Uses

■ **Treatment of HIV Infection** Oral and IV zidovudine are used in conjunction with other antiretroviral agents for the treatment of human immunodeficiency virus type 1 (HIV-1) infection in adults, adolescents, and pediatric patients who are antiretroviral-naive (have not previously received antiretroviral therapy) or antiretroviral-experienced (previously treated).

Zidovudine is used in multiple-drug regimens that include another HIV nucleoside reverse transcriptase inhibitor (NRTI) (dual NRTIs) and an HIV integrase strand transfer inhibitor (INSTI), HIV nonnucleoside reverse transcriptase inhibitor (NNRTI), or HIV protease inhibitor (PI) in INSTI-, NNRTI-, or PI-based regimens. (See Dual NRTI Options under Treatment of HIV Infection: Antiretroviral-naive Adults and Adolescents, in Uses.)

If the dual NRTI option of zidovudine and lamivudine is used in conjunction with other antiretrovirals for the treatment of HIV-1 infection, a fixed-combination preparation containing both drugs (lamivudine/zidovudine; Combivir®, generic) is commercially available and can be used in adults, adolescents, and children weighing 30 kg or more.

Zidovudine has been used in triple NRTI regimens (i.e., single-class NRTI regimens) that include zidovudine and 2 other NRTIs. A fixed-combination preparation containing abacavir, lamivudine, and zidovudine (abacavir/lamivudine/zidovudine; Trizivir®, generic) is commercially available and can be used alone or in conjunction with other antiretrovirals in adults, adolescents, and children weighing 40 kg or more who are negative for the human leukocyte antigen (HLA)-B*5701 allele. (See All-NRTI Regimens under Treatment of HIV Infection: Antiretroviral-naive Adults and Adolescents, in Uses.)

The most appropriate antiretroviral regimen cannot be defined for each clinical scenario and selection of specific antiretroviral agents for use in such regimens should be individualized based on information regarding antiretroviral potency, potential rate of development of resistance, known toxicities, and potential for pharmacokinetic interactions as well as virologic, immunologic, and clinical characteristics of the patient. For information on the general principles and guidelines for use of antiretroviral therapy, including specific recommendations for initial therapy in antiretroviral-naive patients and recommendations for changing antiretroviral regimens, see the Antiretroviral Agents General Statement 8:18.08.

Antiretroviral-naive Adults and Adolescents Although monotherapy and 2-drug regimens that include only NRTIs are no longer recommended for the treatment of HIV infection, early studies evaluating safety and efficacy of zidovudine for initial antiretroviral therapy in antiretroviral-naive HIV-infected adults used zidovudine monotherapy or 2-drug regimens of zidovudine and didanosine, lamivudine, or zalcitabine (no longer commercially available in the US). While results of these early studies indicated that zidovudine monotherapy or 2-drug NRTI regimens in antiretroviral-naive patients may be associated with initial declines in plasma HIV-1 RNA levels, subsequent studies showed that such regimens were less effective in providing durable suppression of HIV replication than 3-drug regimens that also included an agent from another class (i.e., PI or NNRTI).

Dual NRTI Options. The US Department of Health and Human Services (HHS) Panel on Antiretroviral Guidelines for Adults and Adolescents states that the preferred dual NRTI options for use in most INSTI-, NNRTI-, and PI-based regimens for *initial* treatment in antiretroviral-naive adults and adolescents are a tenofovir prodrug (either tenofovir alafenamide or tenofovir disoproxil fumarate [tenofovir DF]) and emtricitabine (or lamivudine) or abacavir and lamivudine (or emtricitabine).

The HHS panel states that the dual NRTI option of zidovudine and lamivudine is no longer recommended for *initial* treatment regimens in nonpregnant antiretroviral-naive adults and adolescents because it has greater toxicity than currently recommended dual NRTI options. However, zidovudine and lamivudine is recommended as an alternative (not a preferred) dual NRTI option for *initial* treatment regimens in antiretroviral-naive pregnant women (see Pregnancy under Cautions: Pregnancy, Fertility, and Lactation) and is a preferred dual NRTI option for *initial* treatment regimens in certain pediatric patients (see Pediatric Patients under Uses: Treatment of HIV-1 Infection). When the dual NRTI option of lamivudine and zidovudine is used in conjunction with other antiretrovirals, the fixed-combination preparation containing both drugs (lamivudine/zidovudine) can be used in adults and adolescents weighing 30 kg or more.

A dual NRTI option of zidovudine and stavudine should *not* be used at any time because in vitro and in vivo antagonistic antiretroviral effects have been reported.

All-NRTI Regimens. Zidovudine has been included in NRTI regimens that include 3 or 4 NRTIs (without any drugs from another class). However, triple and quadruple NRTI regimens are *not* recommended for *initial* treatment of HIV infection in antiretroviral-naive adults or adolescents because such regimens have inferior virologic efficacy. In addition, regimens that only include NRTIs are *not* usually recommended in antiretroviral-experienced patients.

(See Antiretroviral-experienced Adults and Adolescents under Uses: Treatment of HIV Infection.)

Zidovudine has been used in a triple NRTI regimen that includes abacavir, lamivudine, and zidovudine. However, this triple NRTI regimen is *not* recommended for *initial* therapy in antiretroviral-naive adults and adolescents because of inferior virologic efficacy. If a triple NRTI regimen of abacavir, lamivudine, and zidovudine is used, the fixed-combination preparation containing these 3 NRTIs (abacavir/lamivudine/zidovudine) can be used in adults and adolescents weighing 40 kg or more. Clinicians should consider that data are limited regarding use of abacavir/lamivudine/zidovudine in patients with higher baseline viral loads (plasma HIV-1 RNA levels exceeding 100,000 copies/mL).

A quadruple NRTI regimen of abacavir, lamivudine, tenofovir DF, and zidovudine is *not* recommended for initial therapy in antiretroviral-naive adults and adolescents because of inferior virologic activity. In an open-label pilot study, a quadruple NRTI regimen was compared with an NNRTI-based regimen of efavirenz with lamivudine and zidovudine and both regimens had similar efficacy and tolerability. However, a larger, open-label study comparing a similar quadruple NRTI regimen (abacavir, emtricitabine, tenofovir DF, zidovudine) with a standard NNRTI- or PI-based regimen found that substantially fewer patients receiving the quadruple NRTI regimen achieved HIV-1 RNA levels below 200 copies/mL.

Antiretroviral-experienced Adults and Adolescents Although monotherapy or 2-drug regimens that include only NRTIs are no longer recommended for treatment of HIV infection, early studies evaluating the safety and efficacy of zidovudine in antiretroviral-experienced (previously treated) patients used such regimens. Subsequent studies indicated that regimens that include zidovudine, another NRTI (e.g., lamivudine, didanosine), and a PI (e.g., indinavir, ritonavir, saquinavir) or NNRTI (e.g., nevirapine) were more effective in increasing CD4+ T-cell counts and decreasing plasma HIV-1 RNA levels in previously treated patients than zidovudine monotherapy or 2-drug NRTI regimens.

All-NRTI Regimens. Zidovudine has been used in triple NRTI regimens in antiretroviral-experienced HIV-infected adults and adolescents, but triple NRTI regimens are not recommended in such patients because of inferior virologic efficacy.

A triple NRTI regimen that includes abacavir (300 mg twice daily) and a fixed-combination preparation containing lamivudine and zidovudine (150 mg of lamivudine and 300 mg of zidovudine twice daily) has been evaluated in a 48-week, open-label study in HIV-infected patients who previously received antiretroviral regimens that included 1 or 2 NRTIs without any other antiretrovirals. At the start of the study, 34% of patients had baseline plasma HIV-1 RNA levels less than 400 copies/mL and 11% had levels less than 50 copies/mL; the median CD4+ T-cell count was 506/mm^3. At 48 weeks, 82% of patients had plasma HIV-1 RNA levels less than 400 copies/mL and 56% had levels less than 50 copies/mL (intent-to-treat analysis). Patients with baseline HIV-1 RNA levels less than 5000 copies/mL were more likely to achieve levels less than 400 copies/mL at week 48 than those with baseline levels exceeding 5000 copies/mL. At 48 weeks, the median change from baseline CD4+ T-cell count was 66 cells/mm^3.

Pediatric Patients Zidovudine is used in conjunction with other antiretrovirals for the treatment of HIV-1 infection in pediatric patients 4 weeks of age or older. In addition, the drug is used in neonates for prevention of perinatal HIV transmission as part of a regimen that includes intrapartum IV zidovudine prophylaxis in the mother and antiretroviral prophylaxis or empiric HIV therapy† in the neonate. (See Uses: Prevention of Perinatal HIV Transmission.)

Lamivudine/zidovudine is used in conjunction with other antiretrovirals for the treatment of HIV-1 infection in pediatric patients weighing 30 kg or more.

Abacavir/lamivudine/zidovudine is used alone or in conjunction with other antiretrovirals for the treatment of HIV-1 infection in pediatric patients weighing 40 kg or more.

For *initial* treatment of antiretroviral-naive HIV-infected pediatric patients, the HHS Panel on Antiretroviral Therapy and Medical Management of HIV-infected Children recommends a *ritonavir-boosted* PI, NNRTI, or INSTI in conjunction with 2 NRTIs (dual NRTIs).

The HHS panel states that zidovudine and lamivudine (or emtricitabine) is a preferred dual NRTI option for use in neonates, infants, and children younger than 12 years of age and an alternative dual NRTI option for use in adolescents 12 years of age or older with sexual maturity rating (SMR) 3. When the dual NRTI option of lamivudine and zidovudine is used, the fixed-combination preparation containing both drugs (lamivudine/zidovudine) can be used in pediatric patients weighing 30 kg or more.

Zidovudine and didanosine is an alternative (not a preferred) dual NRTI option that can be used in *initial* treatment regimens in children 2 weeks of age or older.

Zidovudine and abacavir is an alternative (not a preferred) dual NRTI option that can be used in *initial* treatment regimens in children 3 months of age or older who are negative for the HLA-B*5701 allele.

A dual NRTI option of zidovudine and stavudine should *not* be used at any time because of in vitro and in vivo antagonistic antiretroviral effects have been reported.

Antiretroviral regimens that contain only NRTIs should *not* be used at any time for treatment of HIV infection in pediatric patients because of inferior virologic efficacy.

For further information on treatment of HIV infection in pediatric patients, see Antiretroviral Therapy in Pediatric Patients, in the Antiretroviral Agents General Statement 8:18.08.

■ Prevention of Perinatal HIV Transmission

Zidovudine is used for the treatment of HIV-1 infection in pregnant women and also is used in pregnant HIV-infected women and their neonates to prevent perinatal transmission of HIV.

In the US, multiple-drug antiretroviral regimens are considered the standard of care for treatment of HIV-1 infection in pregnant women and for prevention of perinatal HIV transmission. The HHS Panel on Treatment of Pregnant Women with HIV Infection and Prevention of Perinatal Transmission states that *all* pregnant HIV-infected women in the US should receive multiple-drug antiretroviral therapy, regardless of the woman's plasma HIV-1 RNA level or CD4+ T-cell count. In addition, to further decrease the risk of perinatal HIV transmission, the HHS panel states that *all* pregnant HIV-infected women with plasma HIV-1 RNA levels exceeding 1000 copies/mL (or unknown HIV-1 RNA levels) near the time of delivery should receive an intrapartum IV zidovudine prophylaxis regimen initiated at the onset of labor (or 3 hours before scheduled cesarean delivery) and continued until delivery (unless contraindicated) and *all* neonates born to HIV-infected women (HIV-exposed neonates) should receive an antiretroviral regimen (either prophylaxis or empiric HIV therapy) initiated as soon as possible after birth (preferably within 6–12 hours) and continued for 4–6 weeks. HIV-exposed neonates at low risk of perinatal HIV acquisition (e.g., those born to an HIV-infected mother who received standard multiple-drug antiretroviral treatment during pregnancy with sustained viral suppression near the time of delivery and with no concerns related to maternal adherence to the treatment regimen) can receive a neonatal prophylaxis regimen that includes only zidovudine. However, a combination antiretroviral regimen that includes zidovudine *and* 1 or 2 additional antiretrovirals should be used in neonates at higher risk of HIV acquisition, including those born to HIV-infected women who did not receive antepartum or intrapartum antiretrovirals, received only intrapartum antiretrovirals, received antepartum and intrapartum antiretrovirals with suboptimal viral suppression near delivery (i.e., detectable plasma HIV RNA levels), or had primary or acute HIV infection during pregnancy or during breast-feeding. This strategy of combined antepartum, intrapartum, and neonatal antiretrovirals reduces perinatal HIV transmission by several mechanisms, including lowering maternal antepartum viral load and providing pre- and postexposure prophylaxis in the infant.

Maternal and neonatal regimens recommended for prevention of perinatal HIV transmission in the US may differ from those used in other countries (e.g., resource-limited countries).

Antiretrovirals in Pregnant HIV-infected Women The HHS panel recommends that *all* pregnant HIV-infected women in the US receive a potent multiple-drug antiretroviral regimen. If the antiretroviral regimen is well tolerated and providing adequate virologic suppression, it should be continued on schedule as much as possible during labor and delivery.

In addition to their current antiretroviral treatment regimen, the HHS panel states that *all* HIV-infected women with plasma HIV-1 RNA levels exceeding 1000 copies/mL (or unknown HIV-1 RNA levels) near the time of delivery should receive an intrapartum IV zidovudine prophylaxis regimen initiated at the onset of labor (or 3 hours before scheduled cesarean delivery) and continued until delivery. These experts state that the intrapartum IV zidovudine prophylaxis regimen also may be considered in pregnant HIV-infected women with plasma HIV-1 RNA levels of 50–999 copies/mL near the time of delivery. Although data are inadequate to determine whether the intrapartum IV zidovudine prophylaxis regimen provides any additional protection against perinatal transmission of HIV in women with plasma HIV-1 RNA levels between 50 and 999 copies/mL, some experts would administer the IV zidovudine prophylaxis regimen to such women since the risk of HIV transmission is slightly higher (approximately 1–2% higher) when viral loads are 50–999 copies/mL compared to when viral loads are less than 50 copies/mL. The intrapartum IV zidovudine prophylaxis regimen is not necessary in HIV-infected women receiving an antiretroviral treatment regimen if they have plasma HIV-1 RNA levels of 50 copies/mL or less during late pregnancy and near delivery, provided there are no concerns related to maternal adherence to the treatment regimen.

If the intrapartum IV zidovudine prophylaxis regimen is indicated and the woman's current antiretroviral regimen includes oral zidovudine, IV zidovudine should be substituted for oral zidovudine until after delivery; other antiretrovirals included in the woman's treatment regimen can be continued orally during labor.

If zidovudine was not included in the antenatal antiretroviral treatment regimen because of known or suspected zidovudine resistance, the HHS panel states that the intrapartum IV zidovudine prophylaxis regimen is still recommended in women with plasma HIV-1 RNA levels exceeding 1000 copies/mL (or unknown HIV-1 RNA levels) near the time of delivery, unless the woman has a documented history of zidovudine hypersensitivity.

Antiretrovirals in HIV-exposed Neonates The choice of a neonatal antiretroviral prophylaxis regimen *or* a neonatal empiric HIV therapy† regimen should be based on an assessment of the likelihood of perinatal HIV transmission.

In HIV-exposed neonates at low risk of perinatal HIV transmission (i.e., infants born to mothers who were receiving a recommended multiple-drug antiretroviral regimen during pregnancy with sustained viral suppression near delivery and no concerns related to maternal adherence to the treatment regimen), the HHS panel states that a 4-week zidovudine prophylaxis regimen can be used alone. These experts state that HIV-exposed neonates at higher risk of HIV acquisition (e.g., those born to HIV-infected women who did not receive antepartum or intrapartum antiretrovirals, received only intrapartum antiretrovirals, or received antepartum and intrapartum antiretrovirals with suboptimal viral suppression near delivery) should receive a 2-drug prophylaxis regimen that includes a 6-week zidovudine prophylaxis regimen *and* a 3-dose nevirapine prophylaxis regimen. Alternatively, the HHS panel states that neonates at highest risk can receive empiric HIV therapy† with a 3-drug regimen of zidovudine, lamivudine, and nevirapine. The 3-drug empiric HIV therapy regimen serves as antiretroviral prophylaxis to prevent acquisition of HIV and also serves as early treatment for neonates who are later confirmed to have acquired HIV. The optimal duration of empiric HIV therapy in neonates at highest risk of HIV acquisition is unknown. Many experts recommend that the 3-drug regimen be continued for 6 weeks; others discontinue nevirapine and/or lamivudine if results of the neonate's HIV nucleic acid amplification test (NAAT) are negative, but recommend continuing zidovudine for 6 weeks.

Because safety and dosage data are not available, the HHS panel states that use of antiretrovirals other than zidovudine, lamivudine, and nevirapine cannot be recommended for premature HIV-exposed neonates (gestational age less than 37 weeks).

For information on the risk of perinatal transmission of HIV and additional information regarding recommendations for use of antiretroviral agents for prevention of perinatal HIV transmission, see Guidelines for Use of Antiretroviral Agents: Antiretrovirals for Prevention of Perinatal HIV Transmission, in the Antiretroviral Agents General Statement 8:18.08.

Clinicians can consult the National Perinatal HIV Hotline at 888-448-8765 for information regarding antiretroviral treatment of pregnant HIV-infected women and their infants and prevention of perinatal HIV transmission.

■ Postexposure Prophylaxis following Occupational Exposure to HIV Oral zidovudine is used in conjunction with other antiretrovirals for postexposure prophylaxis of HIV infection following occupational exposure† (PEP) in health-care personnel and other individuals exposed occupationally via percutaneous injury (e.g., needlestick, cut with sharp object) or mucous membrane or nonintact skin (e.g., chapped, abraded, dermatitis) contact with blood, tissue, or other body fluids that might contain HIV.

The US Public Health Service (USPHS) states that the preferred regimen for PEP following an occupational exposure to HIV is a 3-drug regimen of raltegravir used in conjunction with emtricitabine and tenofovir DF (may be administered as the fixed combination emtricitabine/tenofovir DF). These experts recommend several alternative regimens that include an INSTI, NNRTI, or PI and 2 NRTIs (dual NRTIs). The preferred dual NRTI option for use in PEP regimens is emtricitabine and tenofovir DF (may be administered as emtricitabine/tenofovir DF); alternative dual NRTIs are tenofovir DF and lamivudine, lamivudine and zidovudine (may be administered as the fixed combination lamivudine/zidovudine), or zidovudine and emtricitabine.

Because management of occupational exposures to HIV is complex and evolving, consultation with an infectious disease specialist, clinician with expertise in administration of antiretroviral agents, and/or the National Clinicians' Postexposure Prophylaxis Hotline (PEPline at 888-448-4911) is recommended whenever possible. However, initiation of PEP should not be delayed while waiting for expert consultation.

For information on types of occupational exposure to HIV and associated risk of infection, management of occupational exposure to HIV, efficacy and safety of postexposure chemoprophylaxis, and recommendations regarding postexposure prophylaxis, see Guidelines for Use of Antiretroviral Agents: Antiretroviral Agents for Postexposure Prophylaxis following Occupational Exposure to HIV (PEP), in the Antiretroviral Agents General Statement 8:18.08.

■ Postexposure Prophylaxis following Nonoccupational Exposure to HIV Zidovudine is used in conjunction with other antiretrovirals for postexposure prophylaxis of HIV infection following nonoccupational exposure† (nPEP) in individuals exposed to blood, genital secretions, or other potentially infectious body fluids that might contain HIV when that exposure represents a substantial risk for HIV transmission.

When nPEP is indicated following a nonoccupational exposure to HIV, the US Centers for Disease Control and Prevention (CDC) states that the preferred regimen in adults and adolescents 13 years of age or older with normal renal function is either raltegravir or dolutegravir used in conjunction with emtricitabine and tenofovir DF (administered as the fixed combination emtricitabine/tenofovir DF). In adults and adolescents 13 years of age or older with impaired renal function (creatinine clearance 59 mL/minute or less), CDC recommends a regimen of either raltegravir or dolutegravir used in conjunction with zidovudine and lamivudine.

Consultation with an infectious disease specialist, clinician with expertise in administration of antiretroviral agents, and/or the National Clinicians' Postexposure Prophylaxis Hotline (PEPline at 888-448-4911) is recommended if nPEP is indicated in certain exposed individuals (e.g., pregnant women, children, those with medical conditions such as renal impairment) or if an antiretroviral regimen not included in the CDC guidelines is being considered, the source virus is known or likely to be resistant to antiretrovirals, or the healthcare provider is inexperienced in prescribing antiretrovirals. However, initiation of nPEP should not be delayed while waiting for expert consultation.

For additional information on nonoccupational exposure to HIV and recommendations regarding postexposure prophylaxis, see Guidelines for Use of Antiretroviral Agents: Antiretrovirals for Postexposure Prophylaxis following Sexual, Injection Drug Use, or other Nonoccupational Exposures to HIV (nPEP), in the Antiretroviral Agents General Statement 8:18.08.

Dosage and Administration

■ Reconstitution and Administration Zidovudine is administered orally or by intermittent or continuous IV infusion. Zidovudine should *not* be administered by rapid IV infusion or injection and should *not* be given IM.

When used for the treatment of human immunodeficiency virus (HIV) infection, zidovudine should be administered by intermittent IV infusion only until oral therapy can be substituted.

Oral Administration Zidovudine capsules, tablets, or oral solution should be administered without regard to meals. Although food may decrease peak plasma concentrations of zidovudine, the area under the concentration-time curve (AUC) is not affected.

Children who cannot reliably swallow an intact capsule or tablet should receive zidovudine oral solution.

IV Administration Commercially available zidovudine concentrate for IV infusion containing 10 mg of the drug per mL *must* be diluted prior to administration. The appropriate dose of zidovudine should be withdrawn from the vial and diluted in 5% dextrose injection to provide a solution containing no more than 4 mg of the drug per mL.

Zidovudine solutions should be inspected visually for particulate matter and discoloration prior to administration whenever solution and container permit; if either is present, the solution should be discarded.

Rate of Administration. Intermittent IV infusions of zidovudine should be given over 60 minutes in adults.

In neonates, intermittent IV infusions of zidovudine should be given over 30 minutes.

When used for intrapartum IV prophylaxis in pregnant HIV-infected women, an initial zidovudine dose should be given by IV infusion over 60 minutes followed by continuous IV infusion given at a rate of 1 mg/kg per hour.

Fixed Combinations Containing Zidovudine For treatment of HIV infection, zidovudine is commercially available in fixed-combination tablets containing lamivudine and zidovudine (lamivudine/zidovudine; Combivir®, generic) and fixed-combination tablets containing abacavir, lamivudine, and zidovudine (abacavir/lamivudine/zidovudine; Trizivir®, generic).

Lamivudine/zidovudine tablets are administered orally twice daily without regard to meals. A fixed-combination tablet containing 150 mg of lamivudine and 300 mg of zidovudine is bioequivalent to one 150-mg tablet of lamivudine and one 300-mg tablet of zidovudine given simultaneously. Lamivudine/zidovudine is used in conjunction with other antiretrovirals. The fixed combination should *not* be used in pediatric patients weighing less than 30 kg, patients with renal impairment (i.e., creatinine clearance less than 50 mL/minute), patients with hepatic impairment, or patients who experience dose-limiting adverse effects.

Abacavir/lamivudine/zidovudine tablets are administered orally twice daily without regard to meals. A fixed-combination tablet containing 300 mg of abacavir, 150 mg of lamivudine, and 300 mg of zidovudine is bioequivalent to a 300-mg abacavir tablet, a 150-mg lamivudine tablet, and a 300-mg zidovudine tablet given simultaneously. Abacavir/lamivudine/zidovudine can be used alone as a complete treatment regimen or can be used in conjunction with other antiretrovirals. The fixed combination should *not* be used in pediatric patients weighing less than 40 kg, patients with renal impairment (i.e., creatinine clearance less than 50 mL/minute), patients with hepatic impairment (contraindicated in those with moderate or severe hepatic impairment), or others requiring dosage adjustment.

■ Dosage ***Adult Dosage*** **Treatment of HIV Infection.** The recommended oral dosage of zidovudine for the treatment of HIV-1 infection in adults 18 years of age or older is 300 mg twice daily. Experts state that the usual dosage of oral zidovudine in adults can be given as 300 mg twice daily or 200 mg 3 times daily.

The recommended IV dosage of zidovudine for the treatment of HIV-1 infection in adults is 1 mg/kg every 4 hours.

When lamivudine/zidovudine is used for the treatment of HIV-1 infection in adults weighing 30 kg or more, the recommended dosage is 1 tablet (300 mg of zidovudine and 150 mg of lamivudine) orally twice daily.

When abacavir/lamivudine/zidovudine is used for the treatment of HIV-1 infection in adults weighing 40 kg or more, the recommended dosage is 1 tablet (300 mg of abacavir, 150 mg of lamivudine, and 300 mg of zidovudine) orally twice daily.

Prevention of Perinatal HIV Transmission. When the intrapartum IV zidovudine prophylaxis regimen is indicated for prevention of perinatal HIV transmission in pregnant HIV-infected women based on plasma HIV-1 RNA levels near the time of delivery (see Antiretrovirals in Pregnant HIV-infected Women under Uses: Prevention of Perinatal HIV Transmission), the IV prophylaxis regimen should be initiated at the start of labor (or 3 hours before scheduled cesarean delivery), regardless of the woman's current antiretroviral treatment regimen.

If the intrapartum IV zidovudine prophylaxis regimen is indicated in pregnant HIV-infected women, an initial zidovudine dose of 2 mg/kg should be given by IV infusion over 60 minutes followed by 1 mg/kg per hour given by continuous IV infusion until delivery. In those already receiving oral zidovudine as part of a multiple-drug antiretroviral treatment regimen, IV zidovudine should be substituted for oral zidovudine until after delivery; other antiretrovirals included in the woman's treatment regimen should be continued on schedule as much as possible during labor.

Postexposure Prophylaxis following Occupational Exposure to HIV. For postexposure prophylaxis of HIV infection following occupational exposure† (PEP) in health-care personnel or other individuals, the recommended dosage of oral zidovudine is 300 mg twice daily. Zidovudine usually is used with lamivudine or emtricitabine in conjunction with a recommended HIV integrase strand transferase inhibitor (INSTI), HIV nonnucleoside reverse transcriptase inhibitor (NNRTI), or HIV protease inhibitor (PI). (See Uses: Postexposure Prophylaxis following Occupational Exposure to HIV.)

When lamivudine/zidovudine is used as the dual NRTI option in PEP† regimens, adults should receive 1 tablet (150 mg of lamivudine and 300 mg of zidovudine) twice daily in conjunction with a recommended INSTI, NNRTI, or PI. (See Uses: Postexposure Prophylaxis following Occupational Exposure to HIV.)

PEP should be initiated as soon as possible following occupational exposure to HIV (preferably within hours) and continued for 4 weeks, if tolerated.

Postexposure Prophylaxis following Nonoccupational Exposure to HIV. For postexposure prophylaxis of HIV infection following nonoccupational exposure† (nPEP) in individuals with impaired renal function (creatinine clearance 59 mL/minute or less), oral zidovudine usually is used in conjunction with lamivudine and either raltegravir or dolutegravir. (See Uses: Postexposure Prophylaxis following Nonoccupational Exposure to HIV.) Zidovudine dosage should be adjusted based on the degree of renal impairment.

The nPEP regimen should be initiated as soon as possible (within 72 hours) following nonoccupational exposure to HIV and continued for 28 days. If it has been more than 72 hours since the exposure, nPEP is not recommended.

Pediatric Dosage Dosage of zidovudine in pediatric patients usually is based on body weight or, alternatively, body surface area. To avoid medication errors, extra care should be used in calculating the dose, transcribing the medication order, dispensing the prescription, and providing dosage instructions. Zidovudine dosage in pediatric patients should not exceed adult dosage.

Treatment of HIV Infection in Neonates. For the treatment of HIV-1 infection in premature neonates† (gestational age less than 30 weeks), experts recommend an oral zidovudine dosage of 2 mg/kg twice daily from birth to 4 weeks of age, 3 mg/kg twice daily from 4 weeks to 8–10 weeks of age, and 12 mg/kg twice daily in those older than 8–10 weeks of age.

For the treatment of HIV-1 infection in premature neonates† (gestational age 30 to less than 35 weeks), experts recommend an oral zidovudine dosage of 2 mg/kg twice daily from birth to 2 weeks of age, 3 mg/kg twice daily from 2 weeks to 6–8 weeks of age, and 12 mg/kg twice daily in those older than 6–8 weeks of age.

If oral zidovudine is used for the treatment of HIV-1 infection in full-term neonates† (gestational age 35 weeks or more), experts recommend a dosage of 4 mg/kg twice daily from birth to 4 weeks of age and 12 mg/kg twice daily in those older than 4 weeks of age. Alternatively, when a simplified weight-based dosage of zidovudine oral solution containing 10 mg/mL is used in full-term neonates (gestational age 35 weeks or more), experts recommend that those weighing 2 to less than 3 kg receive 10 mg (1 mL) twice daily, those weighing 3 to less than 4 kg receive 15 mg (1.5 mL) twice daily, and those weighing 4 to less than 5 kg receive 20 mg (2 mL) twice daily.

If IV zidovudine is used for the treatment of HIV-1 infection in full-term neonates† (gestational age 35 weeks or more), experts recommend 3 mg/kg twice daily from birth until 4 weeks of age and 9 mg/kg twice daily in those older than 4 weeks of age. For treatment of HIV-1 infection in premature neonates† (gestational age 30 to less than 35 weeks age), experts recommend an IV zidovudine dosage of 1.5 mg/kg twice daily from birth to 2 weeks of age, 2.3 mg/kg twice daily from 2 weeks to 6–8 weeks of age, and 9 mg/kg twice daily beginning at greater than 6–8 weeks of age. An IV zidovudine dosage of 1.5 mg/kg twice daily from birth to 4 weeks of age, 2.3 mg/kg twice daily from 4 weeks to 8–10 weeks of age, and 9 mg/kg twice daily beginning at greater than 8–10 weeks of age is recommended for the treatment of HIV-1 infection in premature neonates† (gestational age less than 30 weeks).

Treatment of HIV Infection in Infants and Children. For recommended weight-based dosage of oral zidovudine for the treatment of HIV-1 infection in infants and children 4 weeks of age or older weighing at least 4 kg, see Table 1.

Table 1. Oral Zidovudine Dosage Recommended for Treatment of HIV-1 Infection in Pediatric Patients 4 Weeks of Age or Older Weighing 4 kg or More

Body Weight (kg)	Twice-daily Dosage Regimen	Three-times-daily Dosage Regimen
4 to less than 9	12 mg/kg twice daily	8 mg/kg 3 times daily
9 to less than 30	9 mg/kg twice daily	6 mg/kg 3 times daily
30 or more	300 mg twice daily	200 mg 3 times daily

Alternatively, if body surface area is used to calculate dosage of oral zidovudine for the treatment of HIV-1 infection in pediatric patients 4 weeks of age or older, the manufacturer recommends 240 mg/m² twice daily or 160 mg/m² 3 times daily. Some experts recommend an oral dosage of 180–240 mg/m² every 12 hours for the treatment of HIV-1 infection in these pediatric patients.

When lamivudine/zidovudine is used for the treatment of HIV-1 infection in pediatric patients weighing 30 kg or more, the recommended dosage is 1 tablet (150 mg of lamivudine and 300 mg of zidovudine) orally twice daily.

When abacavir/lamivudine/zidovudine is used for the treatment of HIV-1 infection in pediatric patients weighing 40 kg or more, the recommended dosage is 1 tablet (300 mg of abacavir, 150 mg of lamivudine, and 300 mg of zidovudine) orally twice daily.

Prevention of Perinatal HIV Transmission. For prevention of perinatal HIV transmission in HIV-exposed neonates, zidovudine can be used alone for prophylaxis in neonates at low risk of perinatal HIV acquisition, but is used in conjunction with other antiretrovirals for prophylaxis or empiric HIV therapy† in neonates at higher risk of perinatal HIV acquisition. (See Antiretrovirals in HIV-exposed Neonates under Uses: Prevention of Perinatal HIV Transmission.)

When used for prophylaxis for prevention of perinatal HIV transmission in premature neonates (gestational age less than 30 weeks), experts recommend an oral zidovudine dosage of 2 mg/kg twice daily or an IV dosage of 1.5 mg/kg twice daily initiated as soon as possible after birth (within 6–12 hours). At 4 weeks of age, dosage should be increased to 3 mg/kg orally twice daily or 2.3 mg/kg IV twice daily and continued until 4–6 weeks of age, depending on the degree of risk of perinatal HIV transmission.

When used for prophylaxis for prevention of perinatal HIV transmission in premature neonates (gestational age of 30 weeks to less than 35 weeks), experts recommend an oral zidovudine dosage of 2 mg/kg twice daily or an IV dosage of 1.5 mg/kg twice daily initiated as soon as possible after birth (within 6–12 hours). At 2 weeks of age, dosage should be increased to 3 mg/kg orally twice daily or 2.3 mg/kg IV twice daily and continued until 4–6 weeks of age, depending on the degree of risk of perinatal HIV transmission.

When used for prophylaxis for prevention of perinatal HIV transmission in full-term neonates (gestational age 35 weeks or more), experts recommend that oral zidovudine be given in a dosage of 4 mg/kg twice daily, initiated as soon as possible after birth (within 6–12 hours) and continued until 4–6 weeks of age, depending on the degree of risk. Alternatively, when a simplified weight-based dosage of zidovudine oral solution containing 10 mg/mL is used in full-term neonates (gestational age 35 weeks or more), experts recommend that those weighing 2 to less than 3 kg receive 10 mg (1 mL) twice daily, those weighing 3 to less than 4 kg receive 15 mg (1.5 mL) twice daily, and those weighing 4 to less than 5 kg receive 20 mg (2 mL) twice daily. Full-term neonates unable to receive oral therapy can receive IV zidovudine in a dosage of 3 mg/kg twice daily given by IV infusion.

Although a 4-week zidovudine prophylaxis regimen may be used alone in HIV-exposed neonates at low risk of HIV acquisition (i.e., infants born to mothers who were receiving a recommended multiple-drug antiretroviral regimen during pregnancy with sustained viral suppression near delivery and no concerns related to maternal adherence to the treatment regimen), a 6-week zidovudine prophylaxis regimen used in conjunction with a 3-dose nevirapine prophylaxis regimen (2-drug prophylaxis regimen) is recommended for those at higher risk.

The manufacturer recommends that HIV-exposed neonates receive oral zidovudine in a dosage of 2 mg/kg every 6 hours, initiated within 12 hours of birth and continued through 6 weeks of age for prevention of perinatal HIV transmission. The manufacturer states that neonates unable to receive oral therapy should receive IV zidovudine in a dosage of 1.5 mg/kg every 6 hours (given by IV infusion over 30 minutes) initiated within 12 hours of birth and continued through 6 weeks of age.

When empiric HIV therapy† is used for prevention of perinatal HIV transmission in neonates at highest risk of HIV acquisition (see Uses: Prevention of Perinatal HIV Transmission), a 3-drug regimen of zidovudine, lamivudine, and nevirapine is recommended and should be initiated as soon as possible after birth (within 6–12 hours). Zidovudine dosage recommended for empiric HIV therapy† in neonates for prevention of perinatal HIV transmission is identical to that recommended for prophylaxis. Optimal duration of empiric HIV therapy in HIV-exposed neonates at highest risk of HIV acquisition is unknown. Many experts recommend that the 3-drug regimen be continued for 6 weeks; others discontinue nevirapine and/or lamivudine if results of the neonate's HIV nucleic acid amplification test (NAAT) are negative, but recommend continuing zidovudine for 6 weeks.

Clinicians can consult the National Perinatal HIV Hotline at 888-448-8765 for information regarding selection of antiretrovirals, including dosage considerations, for prevention of perinatal HIV transmission.

■ Dosage in Renal and Hepatic Impairment

Zidovudine dosage should be reduced in patients with severe renal impairment (i.e., creatinine clearance less than 15 mL/minute). Adults maintained on hemodialysis or peritoneal dialysis or with creatinine clearance less than 15 mL/minute should receive an oral zidovudine dosage of 100 mg every 6–8 hours or an IV dosage of 1 mg/kg every 6–8 hours.

Data are insufficient to recommend zidovudine dosage adjustments for patients with impaired hepatic function or liver cirrhosis. However, because plasma concentrations of zidovudine appear to be increased in patients with hepatic impairment and may increase the risk of adverse hematologic effects, frequent monitoring for hematologic toxicities is advised.

Lamivudine/zidovudine should *not* be used for treatment of HIV infection in patients with renal impairment (i.e., creatinine clearance less than 50 mL/minute) or in patients with hepatic impairment.

Abacavir/lamivudine/zidovudine should *not* be used for treatment of HIV infection in patients with renal impairment (i.e., creatinine clearance less than 50 mL/minute) or in patients with hepatic impairment. Abacavir/lamivudine/zidovudine is contraindicated in those with moderate or severe hepatic impairment.

Cautions

The most common adverse effects of zidovudine in adults are headache, malaise, nausea, anorexia, and vomiting. Because HIV-infected patients receiving zidovudine generally have serious underlying disease with multiple baseline symptomatology and clinical abnormalities and because many adverse effects that occurred in zidovudine-treated patients also occurred in patients receiving placebo, many reported effects may not be directly attributable to zidovudine. The frequency and severity of adverse effects associated with use of zidovudine in adults are greater in patients with more advanced disease at the time of initiation of therapy. In one study in asymptomatic patients receiving 100 mg of the drug orally 5 times daily for an average of longer than 1 year (range: 4 months to 2 years), only nausea occurred more frequently in patients receiving zidovudine than in those receiving placebo.

Adverse systemic effects reported with IV zidovudine are similar to those reported with oral zidovudine. However, long-term IV zidovudine therapy (i.e., longer than 2–4 weeks) has not been evaluated in adults and may enhance adverse hematologic effects.

When the fixed combination containing lamivudine and zidovudine (lamivudine/zidovudine; Combivir®, generic) or the fixed combination containing abacavir, lamivudine, and zidovudine (abacavir/lamivudine/zidovudine; Trizivir®, generic) is used, the adverse effects, precautions, and contraindications associated with each of the individual components should be considered. (See Precautions Related to Use of Fixed Combinations under Cautions: Precautions and Contraindications.)

■ Hematologic Effects

The major adverse effect of oral or IV zidovudine in patients with advanced symptomatic HIV-1 infection is bone marrow toxicity resulting in severe anemia and/or neutropenia. These adverse hematologic effects have been severe enough to require blood transfusions and discontinuance of zidovudine or dosage modification in up to 41% of patients receiving the drug.

Hematologic toxicity is causally related to zidovudine therapy, being directly related to dosage and duration of therapy with the drug, and has been reported most frequently in patients with advanced symptomatic HIV infection or low pretreatment hemoglobin concentrations, neutrophil counts, and CD4+ T-cell counts. Patients with low serum folate or vitamin B_{12} concentrations may be at increased risk for developing bone marrow toxicity during zidovudine therapy. There also are limited data suggesting that bone marrow of patients with fulminant acquired immunodeficiency syndrome (AIDS) may be more sensitive to zidovudine-induced toxicity than that of patients with less advanced disease (e.g., AIDS-related complex [ARC]).

In patients with asymptomatic HIV infection who received zidovudine in a dosage of 500 mg daily, anemia (hemoglobin concentration less than 8 g/dL) occurred in 1% and neutropenia (neutrophil count less than 750/mm^3) occurred in 2% of patients.

Anemia, as evidenced by a decrease in hemoglobin concentration, may occur as early as 2–4 weeks after initiation of zidovudine therapy, but occurs most commonly after 4–6 weeks of therapy. Anemia and granulocytopenia usually resolve when zidovudine is discontinued or when dosage is decreased. Biosynthetic hematopoietic agents, including filgrastim, a recombinant human granulocyte colony-stimulating factor (G-CSF), and sargramostim, a recombinant human granulocyte-macrophage colony-stimulating factor (GM-CSF), have been used in an effort to correct or minimize zidovudine-induced neutropenia. (See Uses: Neutropenia Associated with HIV Infection and Antiretroviral Therapy, in Filgrastim, Filgrastim-sndz, Tbo-filgrastim 20:16 and Sargramostim 20:16.) Severe, potentially fatal, but generally reversible, agranulocytosis or pancytopenia has occurred in some patients. Multiple blood transfusions may be required for treatment of severe anemia; however, a paradoxical erythrocytosis requiring phlebotomy has been reported rarely. Epoetin alfa, a recombinant human erythropoietin preparation, is used to treat the anemia associated with zidovudine. There is evidence that addition of epoetin alfa to the zidovudine regimen can increase and/or maintain the erythrocyte count as manifested by the hemoglobin concentration and hematocrit and decrease the need for red blood cell (RBC) transfusions; however, anemic zidovudine-treated patients with endogenous serum erythropoietin concentrations exceeding 500 mU/mL are unlikely to respond to epoetin alfa. In addition, epoetin alfa is not indicated for treatment of anemia in HIV-infected patients related to other factors (e.g., iron or folate deficiencies, hemolysis, GI bleeding). (See Uses: Anemia in HIV-infected Patients, in Epoetin Alfa 20:16.)

Zidovudine-induced anemia appears to result from impaired erythrocyte maturation; an increase in the mean corpuscular volume (MCV), which reflects megaloblastic changes, is often an early indicator of hematologic toxicity induced by the drug. Zidovudine-induced anemia is generally macrocytic and megaloblastic; however, a normocytic anemia associated with erythroid hypoplasia or aplasia has also been reported.

Exacerbation of anemia has been reported in HIV-infected patients coinfected with hepatitis C virus (HCV) who received zidovudine concomitantly with ribavirin; such concomitant use should be avoided. Concomitant use of zidovudine and myelosuppressive or cytotoxic drugs may increase the risk of hematologic toxicity. (See Drug Interactions.)

An increase in platelet count has occurred in some patients during zidovudine therapy, including some patients with HIV-associated thrombocytopenia. If an increase in platelet count occurs, it usually is evident during the first 1–2 weeks of therapy and may be maintained for at least the first 4–7 weeks of therapy. It has been suggested that the hematologic effects of zidovudine may be platelet sparing; however, thrombocytopenia has been reported rarely in patients receiving the drug. In one study, platelet counts decreased more than 50% from baseline values in 12% of patients receiving zidovudine and 5% of patients receiving placebo.

Aplastic anemia, hemolytic anemia, leukopenia, pancytopenia with marrow hypoplasia, and pure red cell aplasia have been reported in patients receiving zidovudine.

Lymphadenopathy has been reported in patients receiving zidovudine. Non-Hodgkin's lymphoma has been reported in patients with symptomatic HIV infection who have received long-term therapy with zidovudine either alone or in conjunction with other drugs (e.g., acyclovir). In one study in patients with AIDS or severe ARC, the incidence of non-Hodgkin's lymphoma was 14.5% in those who had received 13–35 months of regimens containing zidovudine. In this study, the estimated probabilities of developing non-Hodgkin's lymphoma were about 10, 29, and 46% by 24, 30, and 36 months of therapy, respectively. However, in another study in patients with AIDS or ARC receiving zidovudine, the probabilities of developing non-Hodgkin's lymphoma with continued therapy were substantially lower; the reasons for these differences are not known but may involve differences in antiretroviral therapy and severity of immunodeficiency at the start of therapy. In this study, the risk of developing non-Hodgkin's lymphoma appeared to be increased in patients with a history of Kaposi's sarcoma, cytomegalovirus infection, oral hairy leukoplakia, and possible herpes simplex infection. There also is some evidence that the risk of developing non-Hodgkin's lymphoma is increased by the degree of immunodeficiency (e.g., being increased substantially at CD4+ T-cell counts less than 50/mm^3). Non-Hodgkin's lymphoma is a complication of HIV infection, and it has been suggested that prolonged survival secondary to antiretroviral and other therapy in the setting of profound immunodeficiency rather than a direct carcinogenic effect of zidovudine is more likely responsible for the increased incidence of developing non-Hodgkin's lymphoma observed to date in patients with HIV infection; however, the possibility that zidovudine may have a direct role in the development of these tumors cannot be excluded, and additional study is necessary.

■ Nervous System Effects

Headache, which may be severe, has been reported in up to 63% of patients receiving zidovudine, malaise has been reported in up to 53%, and asthenia has been reported in 9–69%. Agitation, dizziness, fatigue, insomnia, paresthesia, and somnolence have been reported in up to 8% of patients, most frequently in those who received high dosage of the drug. In a study in patients with asymptomatic HIV infection receiving oral zidovudine in a dosage of 500 mg daily, asthenia, headache, or malaise occurred in 9, 63, or 53% of patients, respectively; these same effects occurred in 6, 53, or 45%, respectively, of patients receiving placebo.

Seizures have been reported in patients receiving zidovudine, most frequently in patients with advanced HIV disease. Neuropathy also has been reported.

Although a definite causal relationship was not established, a manic syndrome consisting of irritability, depression, reduced cognition, hallucinations, euphoria, flight of ideas, and/or delusional states has been reported in several patients receiving zidovudine; lithium and/or other psychotherapeutic agents have reduced manifestations of this syndrome, even during continued zidovudine therapy. In several patients with AIDS or ARC receiving zidovudine therapy, acute, transient meningoencephalitis occurred when dosage of the drug was reduced; it has been suggested that the dosage reduction allowed an increase in HIV replication within the brain. In a patient with AIDS who received zidovudine in a dosage of 200 mg every 4 hours, a neurotoxic reaction consisting of headache, confusion, aphasia, twitching, and focal seizures occurred within 48 hours after initiation of the drug. Neurotoxicity resolved within 48 hours after discontinuance of zidovudine, recurred within 72 hours after reinitiation of therapy with the drug, and appeared to contribute to the patient's death 36 hours later. A fatal neurotoxic reaction with focal seizures has occurred in at least one other patient who received zidovudine in an oral dosage of 200 mg every 4 hours. Although a causal relationship was not clearly established, neurotoxic effects (e.g., tonic-clonic seizures) were temporally associated with zidovudine therapy in another patient with AIDS; autopsy findings revealed evidence of encephalopathy.

Anxiety, confusion, depression, syncope, loss of mental acuity, vertigo, tremor, and back pain have been reported in patients receiving zidovudine; however, a definite causal relationship to the drug has not been established. In several patients, confusion and tremor were associated with high plasma concentrations of the drug.

■ GI Effects

Nausea has been reported in up to 51% and anorexia, constipation, diarrhea, dyspepsia, abdominal cramping or pain, and vomiting have been reported in 5–25% of patients receiving zidovudine. Nausea occurs most frequently in patients with more advanced HIV disease and those receiving higher zidovudine dosage. In patients with symptomatic HIV infection or early HIV disease receiving oral zidovudine in a dosage of 1200 mg daily, nausea occurred in 61–68% of patients receiving zidovudine and in 41–46% of patients receiving placebo. In a study in patients with asymptomatic HIV infection receiving oral zidovudine in a dosage of 500 mg daily, nausea occurred in 51% of those receiving zidovudine and 30% of those receiving placebo. In other studies in asymptomatic HIV-infected patients receiving zidovudine in a dosage of 100 mg 5 times daily, nausea was reported in about 3%.

Dysphagia, flatulence, mouth ulcer, oral mucosa pigmentation, and taste perversion have been reported in patients receiving zidovudine.

Esophageal ulceration, which was local in origin, has been reported in a few patients who swallowed their nightly doses of zidovudine capsules while in a recumbent position. To reduce the risk of esophageal irritation and ulceration, patients should be advised to swallow zidovudine capsules while in an upright position and with adequate amounts of fluid (e.g., at least 120 mL of water).

■ Musculoskeletal Effects Myopathy and myositis with pathologic changes, similar to that produced by HIV infection, have been associated with prolonged use of zidovudine. Severe necrotizing myopathy, which generally affected the legs, and a polymyositis-like syndrome have been reported occasionally in patients receiving zidovudine. In most cases, the myopathy or polymyositis syndrome was apparent after 6.5–12 months of zidovudine therapy and was characterized by myalgias, muscle tenderness and weakness, weight loss, atrophy, and increased serum concentrations of muscle enzymes (e.g., creatine kinase, LDH). In many reported cases, myopathy resolved within 1–2 weeks when the drug was discontinued; in other cases, manifestations resolved over a 6–8 week period. Zidovudine-associated myopathy reportedly occurs in 6–18% of patients receiving the drug for more than 6 months. However, necrotizing, noninflammatory myopathy with microvesicular degeneration of muscle fibers, normal serum concentrations of muscle enzymes, and little pain also has been reported in patients with AIDS who were not receiving zidovudine and appears to be related to the HIV infection. Zidovudine-associated myopathy may not be clinically distinguishable from HIV-associated myopathy. Zidovudine appeared to be at least partially responsible for myopathy in many patients since symptoms resolved following discontinuance of the drug and repeat muscle biopsies showed improved arrangement of muscle-fiber cells and a decrease in inflammatory lesions. Histologic and electron microscopic evaluation of muscle biopsies from patients with myopathy indicate that inflammatory infiltrates may be present in either HIV-associated or zidovudine-associated myopathy. However, ragged-red fibers suggestive of abnormal mitochondria have been a consistent feature in muscle biopsies from patients with zidovudine-associated myopathy, whereas normal mitochondria generally were present in biopsies from patients with HIV-associated myopathy who had never received zidovudine. It has been suggested that zidovudine may inhibit γ-DNA polymerase and interfere with mitochondrial DNA replication causing the development of abnormal mitochondria and a resultant energy shortage within the muscle cell. It appears that zidovudine-associated myopathy in patients with HIV infection may be the result of both a direct effect of the drug on mitochondria as well as immune-mediated mechanisms.

Myalgia, musculoskeletal pain, arthralgia, back pain, generalized pain, muscle spasm, and tremor have been reported in patients receiving zidovudine.

■ Dermatologic and Sensitivity Reactions Hypersensitivity reactions have been reported rarely in patients receiving zidovudine. Anaphylaxis, angioedema, Stevens-Johnson syndrome, and toxic epidermal necrolysis have been reported. In most reported cases, hypersensitivity reactions consisted of fever, rash, and pruritus; nausea, vomiting, anorexia, weakness, confusion, and elevated serum hepatic enzymes occurred in some patients. Cutaneous leukocytoclastic vasculitis, characterized by distinctive dermal perivascular inflammation without visceral involvement, has been reported in at least 2 patients receiving zidovudine. The vasculitis was associated with fever and appeared to be a hypersensitivity reaction. In addition, severe reactions consisting of pruritic rash on the abdomen, back, and extremities with fever, nausea, headache, vomiting, lymphocytopenia, and elevated liver enzymes have been reported in at least 2 otherwise healthy adults receiving zidovudine in conjunction with zalcitabine (no longer commercially available in the US) for postexposure prophylaxis of HIV following occupational exposure to the virus.

Dyspnea, fever, and rash have been reported in patients receiving zidovudine, but a causal relationship was not definitely established. In several reported cases, a causal relationship between low-grade fever (39–40°C) and zidovudine appeared to be demonstrated since fever started 5–7 days after initiation of therapy with the drug, persisted up to 5 days after the drug was discontinued, and recurred with rechallenge.

Pigmentation of fingernails and toenails has been reported occasionally in patients receiving zidovudine. A dark, bluish discoloration at the base of the fingernails was evident 2–6 weeks after initiation of zidovudine therapy in black patients with HIV infection; similar discoloration of the toenails occurred after 4 more weeks of therapy with the drug. A similar, but brownish-gray pigmentation of fingernails and toenails has also been reported in other patients (including some whites) receiving zidovudine. In some reported cases, pigmentation involved the entire nail; in other cases, there were transverse or longitudinal bands of color. Zidovudine-associated nail discoloration has been reported more frequently in black patients than in white or Hispanic patients, reportedly occurring in 67–81% of black patients compared with 20–31% of white or Hispanic patients. The cause of this nail pigmentation is unknown but may result from injury to the nail bed, matrix, and/or plate; increased stimulation of matrix melanocytes by zidovudine may be involved. Diffuse hyperpigmented macular skin lesions and hyperpigmentation of the oral mucosa also have been reported in several patients who had pigmentation of the nails during zidovudine therapy. It has been suggested that such hyperpigmentation may be an early indication of zidovudine hypersensitivity; however, this observation was based on limited data. Patients should be informed that discoloration of nails may occur during zidovudine therapy.

Other adverse dermatologic effects, including changes in skin pigmentation, pruritus, and urticaria, have been reported in patients receiving zidovudine, but a causal relationship has not been established.

■ Hepatic Effects and Lactic Acidosis Lactic acidosis and severe hepatomegaly with steatosis, including some fatalities, have been reported in patients receiving nucleoside analogs, including zidovudine. Most reported cases have involved women; obesity also may be a risk factor. Although lactic acidosis and severe hepatomegaly appear to be related, they have been reported both separately and together. Manifestations of hepatotoxicity included fever, malaise, weakness, nausea, vomiting, diarrhea, epigastric pain, and rapidly increasing serum transaminase concentrations. In fatalities associated with enlarged fatty liver, massive hepatomegaly with severe, diffuse macrovesicular steatosis of the liver were present without associated necrosis; most fatalities were reported in women, many of whom were mildly to moderately obese. Manifestations of lactic acidosis generally developed rapidly and included tachypnea and dyspnea, without evidence of systemic hypoxemia or tissue hypoxia. In fatalities associated with lactic acidosis, some of the deaths resulted from cardiovascular collapse secondary to progressive lactic acidosis; in other cases, lactic acidosis persisted or improved although the patient died within the next 15 months of other complications.

In most reported cases of lactic acidosis or hepatomegaly with steatosis, patients had received at least 6 months of zidovudine therapy. Similar cases of lactic acidosis and severe hepatomegaly with steatosis have been reported rarely in patients receiving other HIV nucleoside reverse transcriptase inhibitors (NRTIs) (e.g., abacavir, didanosine, stavudine). However, it is unclear whether these adverse effects are a direct result of nucleoside antiviral therapy since adverse hepatic effects, including hepatomegaly and mild to moderate macrovesicular steatosis, have been described in some AIDS patients in the absence of antiretroviral therapy or any apparent underlying etiology. Because results of in vitro studies indicate that the active metabolites of zidovudine and other nucleoside antiviral agents can exert an inhibitory effect on γ-polymerase, an enzyme involved in mitochondrial DNA synthesis, it has been suggested that this effect may be a factor in the development of lactic acidosis, as well as other adverse effects, in patients receiving the drugs. (See Mechanism of Action: Cytotoxic Effects.)

There also have been rare reports of zidovudine-associated hepatitis, including cholestatic hepatitis that recurred on rechallenge, and fulminant hepatic failure in patients who received zidovudine. Increases in liver function test results, including serum ALT, AST, LDH, and alkaline phosphatase concentrations, have been reported in some patients receiving zidovudine. In some reported cases, serum concentrations of these enzymes increased within 2–3 weeks after initiating zidovudine therapy but returned to pretreatment values when therapy with the drug was withheld and did not increase when therapy was restarted. Mild drug-associated increases in total bilirubin concentrations have been reported rarely in asymptomatic HIV-infected patients receiving zidovudine.

Hepatic decompensation, sometimes fatal, has been reported in HIV-infected patients coinfected with HCV who received antiretroviral therapy concomitantly with interferon alfa with or without ribavirin. (See Drug Interactions: Interferon Alfa and Peginterferon Alfa.)

■ Lipodystrophy Zidovudine treatment has been associated with lipoatrophy (loss of subcutaneous fat); the incidence and severity of this effect are related to cumulative exposure to the drug. Fat loss, which is most evident in the face, limbs, and buttocks, may be only partially reversible and improvement may take months to years after switching to an antiretroviral regimen that does not contain zidovudine. Patients receiving zidovudine or fixed combinations containing zidovudine should be regularly assessed for signs of lipoatrophy. If fat loss is suspected, therapy should be switched to an alternative antiretroviral regimen if feasible.

Redistribution or accumulation of body fat, including central obesity, dorsocervical fat enlargement ("buffalo hump"), peripheral wasting, facial wasting, breast enlargement, and general cushingoid appearance, has been reported in patients receiving antiretroviral agents. The mechanisms responsible for adipogenic effects and the long-term consequences of these effects are unknown. A causal relationship to antiretroviral therapy has not been established.

■ Immune Reconstitution Syndrome During initial treatment, patients who respond to antiretroviral therapy may develop an inflammatory response to indolent or residual opportunistic infections (e.g., *Mycobacterium avium complex* [MAC], *M. tuberculosis*, cytomegalovirus [CMV], *Pneumocystis jirovecii* [formerly *P. carinii*]); this may necessitate further evaluation and treatment.

Autoimmune disorders (e.g., Graves' disease, polymyositis, Guillain-Barré syndrome) have also been reported to occur in the setting of immune reconstitution; however, the time to onset is more variable and can occur many months after initiation of antiretroviral therapy.

■ Other Adverse Effects Dyspnea, epistaxis, hoarseness, pharyngitis, rhinitis, and sinusitis have been reported in patients receiving zidovudine; however a causal relationship was not established.

Other adverse effects reported in patients receiving zidovudine include amblyopia, hearing loss, photophobia, chills, macular edema, pancreatitis, flu syndrome, cardiomyopathy, chest pain, and rhabdomyolysis. Breast enlargement has been reported rarely in female patients and bilateral gynecomastia has been reported rarely in male patients receiving zidovudine.

IV administration of zidovudine may cause local reactions including pain and slight irritation at the infusion site. Phlebitis also has been reported rarely with IV zidovudine.

■ Precautions and Contraindications

Zidovudine is contraindicated in patients who have had a potentially life-threatening hypersensitivity reaction (e.g., anaphylaxis, Stevens-Johnson syndrome) to the drug or any ingredient in the formulation.

Lamivudine/zidovudine is contraindicated in patients with a history of hypersensitivity to lamivudine or zidovudine.

Abacavir/lamivudine/zidovudine is contraindicated in patients who have the human leukocyte antigen (HLA)-B*5701 allele; patients with a history of hypersensitivity to abacavir, lamivudine, or zidovudine; and patients with moderate or severe hepatic impairment.

Precautions Related to Hematologic Effects Zidovudine should be used with caution in patients who have bone marrow compromise evidenced by granulocyte count less than 1000 cells/mm^3 or hemoglobin concentration less than 9.5 g/dL. Zidovudine therapy has been associated with hematologic toxicity, including neutropenia and/or severe anemia, especially in patients with advanced HIV disease. (See Cautions: Hematologic Effects.)

Blood cell counts (CBCs) and indices of anemia (e.g., hemoglobin, mean corpuscular volume) should be performed prior to initiation of zidovudine therapy to establish baseline values and should then be monitored frequently during therapy with the drug, especially in patients with advanced HIV disease. Some experts recommend that CBCs with differentials should be measured 2–8 weeks after initiation of zidovudine treatment and every 3–6 months thereafter.

If substantial anemia (hemoglobin less than 7.5 g/dL or reduction of more than 25% from baseline) and/or neutropenia (granulocyte count less than 750 cells/mm^3 or reduction of more than 50% from baseline) occurs, interruption of zidovudine therapy may be necessary until there is evidence of bone marrow recovery. In patients who develop significant anemia, dosage interruption does not necessarily eliminate the need for blood transfusions. If marrow recovery occurs following dosage interruption, reinitiation of zidovudine therapy may be appropriate using adjunctive measures (e.g., epoetin alfa), depending on hematologic indices such as serum erythropoetin level and patient tolerance.

Patients should be informed that the major adverse effects of zidovudine are anemia and/or neutropenia and that the frequency and severity of these toxicities are greater in patients with more advanced disease and in those who initiate therapy later in the course of their infection. Patients should be advised of the extreme importance of CBC monitoring during zidovudine therapy, especially in patients with advanced symptomatic HIV-1 disease. Patients also should be advised that if hematologic toxicity develops, they may require transfusions or discontinuance of the drug.

Because exacerbation of anemia has been reported in HIV-infected patients coinfected with HCV who received zidovudine concomitantly with ribavirin, concomitant use of these drugs should be avoided. Clinicians should consider that concomitant use of zidovudine and myelosuppressive or cytotoxic drugs (e.g., ganciclovir, interferon alfa, ribavirin) may increase the risk of hematologic toxicity. (See Drug Interactions.)

Precautions Related to Use of Fixed Combinations When lamivudine/zidovudine or abacavir/lamivudine/zidovudine is used, the usual cautions, precautions, contraindications, and drug interactions associated with each drug in the fixed combination must be considered. Cautionary information applicable to specific populations (e.g., pregnant or nursing women, individuals with hepatic or renal impairment, pediatric patients, geriatric patients) should be considered for each drug. For cautionary information related to lamivudine and abacavir, see Cautions in the individual drug monographs.

If abacavir/lamivudine/zidovudine is used, clinicians should consider that serious and sometimes fatal hypersensitivity reactions, with multiple organ involvement, have been reported in patients receiving abacavir or fixed combinations containing abacavir. Prior to initiation or reinitiation of abacavir/lamivudine/zidovudine, all patients should be screened for the HLA-B*5701 allele, unless there is documentation of a previous HLA-B*5701 allele assessment. The patient's medical history also should be reviewed for prior exposure to any abacavir-containing preparation. Abacavir-containing preparations are contraindicated in individuals who test positive for HLA-B*5701. Such individuals are at higher risk for a hypersensitivity reaction; however, hypersensitivity reactions have occurred in patients who do not carry the HLA-B*5701 allele. Abacavir/lamivudine/zidovudine should be discontinued immediately if a hypersensitivity reaction is suspected, regardless of HLA-B*5701 status and even if other diagnoses are possible. The fixed combination should be permanently discontinued if hypersensitivity cannot be ruled out. (See Abacavir Sulfate 8:18.08.20.)

Lamivudine/zidovudine and abacavir/lamivudine/zidovudine should be used with caution in patients who have bone marrow compromise evidenced by granulocyte count less than 1000 cells/mm^3 or hemoglobin less than 9.5 g/dL. (See Precautions Related to Hematologic Effects under Cautions: Precautions and Contraindications.)

If lamivudine/zidovudine or abacavir/lamivudine/zidovudine is used, clinicians should consider that severe, acute exacerbations of hepatitis B virus (HBV) infection have been reported when lamivudine was discontinued from antiretroviral regimens in HIV-infected patients coinfected with HBV. Although a causal relationship to lamivudine discontinuance has not been established, patients receiving lamivudine-containing preparations should be closely monitored with both clinical and laboratory follow-up for at least several months after stopping treatment with the drug. Emergence of lamivudine-resistant HBV also has been reported in HIV-infected patients coinfected with HBV who were receiving lamivudine-containing antiretroviral regimens for treatment of HIV. (See Lamivudine 8:18.08.20.)

Other Precautions Because potentially life-threatening hypersensitivity reactions (e.g., anaphylaxis, Stevens-Johnson syndrome) have been reported in patients receiving zidovudine (see Cautions: Dermatologic and Sensitivity Reactions), patients should be informed that such reactions can occur and should be advised to immediately contact a clinician if they develop rash since this may be a sign of a more serious reaction.

Because lactic acidosis and severe hepatomegaly with steatosis, including fatalities, have been reported in patients receiving nucleoside analogs and other antiretrovirals (see Cautions: Hepatic Effects and Lactic Acidosis), zidovudine or fixed combinations containing zidovudine should be discontinued in any patient who develops clinical or laboratory findings suggestive of lactic acidosis or pronounced hepatotoxicity, which may include hepatomegaly and steatosis even in the absence of marked aminotransferase elevations.

Patients receiving zidovudine with peginterferon alfa (or interferon alfa) with or without ribavirin should be closely monitored for toxicity, especially hepatic decompensation, neutropenia, and anemia. HIV-infected patients coinfected with HCV should be informed that hepatic decompensation (sometimes fatal) has been reported when antiretrovirals were used concomitantly with interferon alfa with or without ribavirin. (See Drug Interactions: Interferon Alfa and Peginterferon Alfa.)

Because myopathy or myositis with pathologic changes (similar to that produced by HIV disease) has been reported in individuals who received long-term zidovudine therapy (see Cautions: Musculoskeletal Effects), patients should be informed about these adverse effects and questioned during routine visits about symptoms such as myalgia, loss of muscle mass, weight loss, and proximal muscle weakness. Elevations in serum concentrations of muscle enzymes (e.g., creatine kinase, LDH) may occur weeks before symptoms of myopathy and some clinicians recommend that serum creatine kinase concentrations be determined every 3 months in patients who have received zidovudine for 6–12 months or longer. Depending on the severity of musculoskeletal manifestations, interruption of zidovudine therapy or, preferably, dosage reduction should be considered in patients who develop myopathy during therapy with the drug. If manifestations of myopathy persist following discontinuance of zidovudine therapy, the drug probably should be reinstated since the myopathy may be related to the HIV infection. In patients with mild manifestations of myopathy, use of a nonsteroidal anti-inflammatory agent may be beneficial; the risks and benefits of corticosteroids for treatment of myopathy in patients with HIV infection have not been evaluated to date.

Patients should be advised to immediately contact a clinician if they have any signs or symptoms of infection since inflammation from previous infections may occur soon after antiretroviral therapy is initiated. (See Cautions: Immune Reconstitution Syndrome.)

Patients should be advised that loss of subcutaneous fat may occur during zidovudine therapy and that they will be regularly assessed for this effect during treatment with the drug. Patients also should be advised that redistribution or accumulation of body fat may occur in patients receiving antiretroviral therapy and that the cause and long-term health effects of these conditions are as yet unknown. (See Cautions: Lipodystrophy.)

A packaging component of zidovudine concentrate for IV infusion (i.e., vial stoppers) contains dry natural rubber (a latex derivative) which may cause allergic reactions in latex-sensitive individuals.

Patients should be advised of the importance of adhering to the prescribed antiretroviral regimen. Effective antiretroviral regimens can decrease HIV concentrations in blood and genital secretions and strict adherence to such regimens in conjunction with risk-reduction measures may decrease, but cannot absolutely eliminate, the risk of secondary transmission of HIV to others. Patients should continue to practice safer sex (e.g., consistent use of condoms).

Zidovudine should always be administered in conjunction with other antiretroviral agents and should not be used alone for treatment of HIV infection. The usual precautions and contraindications of the other antiretrovirals in the regimen should be considered during concomitant therapy.

Patients should be advised that certain drugs may interact with zidovudine and that certain drugs (e.g., ganciclovir, interferon alfa, ribavirin) may exacerbate zidovudine toxicity. (See Drug Interactions.)

Because zidovudine is eliminated principally by renal excretion following metabolism in the liver, patients with impaired renal or hepatic function or decreased hepatic blood flow may be at increased risk of toxicity from the drug. A reduction in zidovudine dosage is recommended in patients maintained on hemodialysis or peritoneal dialysis or with severe renal impairment (i.e., creatinine clearance less than 15 mL/minute). Although data are insufficient to recommend dosage adjustments for patients with impaired hepatic function or liver cirrhosis, frequent monitoring for hematologic toxicities is recommended in such patients since hepatic impairment increases plasma concentrations of zidovudine and may increase the risk of adverse hematologic effects. (See Dosage: Dosage in Renal and Hepatic Impairment.)

■ **Pediatric Precautions** Zidovudine generally has been well tolerated when used in neonates and children. The major adverse effects reported in children are similar to those reported in adults and include bone marrow toxicity resulting in anemia and/or neutropenia.

In one randomized, double-blind, placebo-controlled trial evaluating use of zidovudine for prevention of maternal-fetal transmission of HIV, the most common adverse effects in neonates were anemia (hemoglobin less than 9 g/dL) and neutropenia (less than 1000/mm³). Anemia occurred in 22% of infants who received zidovudine (2 mg/kg orally every 6 hours for 6 weeks beginning within 12 hours of birth) and in 12% of infants who received placebo. Mean hemoglobin concentrations in infants receiving zidovudine were less than 1 g/dL lower than hemoglobin concentrations in infants receiving placebo. No infants with anemia required transfusion and all hemoglobin concentrations spontaneously returned to normal within 6 weeks after completion of zidovudine therapy. Neutropenia was reported in 21% of infants who received zidovudine and 27% of infants who received placebo. The long-term consequences of in utero and infant exposure to zidovudine are unknown. (See Cautions: Pregnancy, Fertility, and Lactation.)

Lamivudine/zidovudine should *not* be used in pediatric patients weighing less than 30 kg.

Abacavir/lamivudine/zidovudine should *not* be used in pediatric patients weighing less than 40 kg.

■ **Geriatric Precautions** While clinical experience to date has not revealed age-related differences in response to zidovudine, clinical studies evaluating zidovudine, lamivudine/zidovudine, and abacavir/lamivudine/zidovudine have not included sufficient numbers of adults 65 years of age or older to determine whether geriatric patients respond differently than younger adults. Zidovudine and fixed combinations containing zidovudine should be used with caution in geriatric patients because these individuals frequently have decreased hepatic, renal, and/or cardiac function and concomitant disease and drug therapy.

■ **Mutagenicity and Carcinogenicity** Zidovudine was mutagenic in a 5178Y/TK± mouse lymphoma assay, positive in an in vitro cell transformation assay, clastogenic in a cytogenetic assay using cultured human lymphocytes, and positive in mouse and rat micronucleus tests following repeated doses. Zidovudine was negative in a cytogenetic study in rats given a single dose.

In carcinogenicity studies in mice, late-appearing (after 19 months) vaginal neoplasms (nonmetastasizing squamous cell carcinomas, squamous cell papilloma, squamous polyps) occurred in some of those receiving the highest zidovudine dosage (120 mg/kg daily and then 40 mg/kg daily after 90 days). One mouse receiving an intermediate dosage (60 mg/kg daily and then 30 mg/kg daily) developed vaginal squamous cell papilloma late in the study, but no vaginal neoplasms were observed in mice receiving the lowest dosage studied. In a similar study in rats, late-appearing (after 20 months) nonmetastasizing vaginal squamous cell carcinoma occurred in some rats receiving the highest oral dosages (600 mg/kg daily initially, 450 mg/kg daily starting on day 91, and then 300 mg/kg daily starting on day 279); no vaginal neoplasms occurred in rats receiving low or intermediate dosages. There were no other drug-related neoplasms observed in either sex of either species studied. At dosages that produced tumors in mice or rats, the estimated drug exposure (as measured by AUC) were approximately 3 or 24 times, respectively, the estimated human exposure at a dosage of 100 mg every 4 hours.

Transplacental carcinogenicity studies have been conducted in rodents. In one study in mice, zidovudine 20 or 40 mg/kg daily (zidovudine exposure equivalent to about 3 times the estimated human exposure at recommended dosages) was administered to the mother from gestation day 10 through parturition and lactation and then administered postnatally to the offspring for 24 months. An increased incidence of vaginal tumors was observed after 24 months; however, there was no observable increase in the incidence of tumors of the lung, liver, or any other organ in either male or female mice. In another study in pregnant mice, zidovudine was administered at maximally tolerated dosages of 12.5 or 25 mg daily (approximately 1000 mg/kg nonpregnant body weight or approximately 450 mg/kg of term body weight) from days 12–18 of gestation. There was an increase in the number of tumors in the lung, liver, and female reproductive tracts in the offspring of mice who received the higher zidovudine dosage. The clinical importance of these carcinogenic effects in rodents is not known.

■ **Pregnancy, Fertility, and Lactation** ***Pregnancy*** Zidovudine and its glucuronide metabolite cross the human placenta and are distributed into amniotic fluid, cord blood, and fetal blood and fetal liver, muscle, and CNS tissue.

To monitor maternal-fetal outcomes of pregnant women exposed to antiretroviral agents, including zidovudine, the Antiretroviral Pregnancy Registry was established. Clinicians are encouraged to contact the registry at 800-258-4263 or http://www.APRegistry.com to enroll such women.

Data from the Antiretroviral Pregnancy Registry show no difference in the overall risk of birth defects for zidovudine compared with the background rate for birth defects in the US reference population of the Metropolitan Atlanta Congenital Defects Program (MACDP). Registry data include over 13,000 prospective reports of zidovudine exposures during pregnancy resulting in live births, including over 4000 first-trimester exposures to the drug.

In a randomized, double-blind, placebo-controlled trial conducted in HIV-1-infected pregnant women to evaluate use of zidovudine for prevention of maternal-fetal transmission of HIV-1, there were no differences in pregnancy-related adverse events between treatment groups. Of the 363 neonates that were evaluated, congenital abnormalities occurred with similar frequency between neonates born to mothers who received zidovudine and neonates born to mothers who received placebo. The observed abnormalities included problems in embryogenesis (prior to 14 weeks) or were recognized on ultrasound before or immediately after initiation of study drug.

The US Department of Health and Human Services (HHS) Panel on Treatment of Pregnant Women with HIV Infection and Prevention of Perinatal Transmission states that zidovudine and lamivudine is an alternative dual NRTI option for *initial* regimens used for treatment of HIV infection in antiretroviral-naive pregnant women.

Fertility There was no evidence that zidovudine affected fertility (conception rates) when the drug was given to male and female rats in dosages up to 7 times the usual adult dosage based on body surface area.

Lactation Zidovudine is distributed into human milk.

Because of the risk of transmission of HIV to an uninfected infant through breast milk, the HHS Panel and the US Centers for Disease Control and Prevention (CDC) recommend that HIV-infected women *not* breast-feed infants, regardless of antiretroviral therapy. Therefore, because of the potential for HIV transmission and the potential for serious adverse effects from zidovudine in nursing infants, women should be instructed not to breast-feed while they are receiving zidovudine, lamivudine/zidovudine, or abacavir/lamivudine/zidovudine.

Drug Interactions

The following drug interactions are based on studies using zidovudine. Drug interaction studies have not been performed using the fixed combination containing lamivudine and zidovudine (lamivudine/zidovudine) or the fixed combination containing abacavir, lamivudine, and zidovudine (abacavir/lamivudine/zidovudine). When a fixed combination is used, interactions associated with each drug in the fixed combination should be considered.

■ **Acetaminophen** Concomitant use of acetaminophen reportedly resulted in an increased risk of granulocytopenia in patients receiving zidovudine; this potentiation of hematologic toxicity appeared to correlate with the duration of acetaminophen use. The exact mechanism of this possible interaction was not determined, but it was suggested that acetaminophen may competitively inhibit glucuronidation of zidovudine. However, further analysis of these data by the manufacturer failed to support the findings of an interaction, and there were no apparent alterations in the pharmacokinetics of zidovudine in several subsequent studies that evaluated concomitant short-term (for up to 7 days) use of acetaminophen and the drug; one study actually demonstrated an increase in zidovudine clearance during concurrent acetaminophen administration.

■ **Acyclovir** Neurotoxicity (profound drowsiness and lethargy), which recurred on rechallenge, has been reported in at least one HIV-infected patient who received acyclovir and zidovudine concomitantly Neurotoxicity was evident within 30–60 days after initiation of IV acyclovir therapy, persisted with some improvement when acyclovir was administered orally, and resolved following discontinuance of acyclovir in this patient. Acyclovir and zidovudine have been used concomitantly in other HIV-infected patients without evidence of increased toxicity.

Although the clinical importance is unclear, there is some evidence that acyclovir may potentiate the antiretroviral effect of zidovudine in vitro; acyclovir alone has only minimal antiretroviral activity.

■ **Antifungal Agents** ***Fluconazole*** Concomitant use of fluconazole appears to interfere with the metabolism and clearance of zidovudine. In one study in HIV-infected men who received zidovudine (200 mg every 8 hours) alone or in conjunction with fluconazole (400 mg daily), the area under the concentration-time curve (AUC) of zidovudine was increased 74% (range: 28–173%), peak serum zidovudine concentrations were increased 84% (range: −1 to 227%), and the terminal elimination half-life of the drug was increased 128% (range: −4 to 189%) in patients receiving concomitant fluconazole.

The manufacturer of zidovudine states that routine zidovudine dosage adjustments are not warranted in patients receiving concomitant fluconazole. However, it has been suggested that patients receiving concomitant zidovudine and fluconazole therapy should be monitored closely for zidovudine-associated adverse effects.

■ **Antimycobacterial Agents** The fact that pharmacokinetic interactions between some antimycobacterial agents (e.g., rifabutin, rifampin) and some antiretroviral agents (especially HIV protease inhibitors [PIs] and HIV nonnucleoside reverse transcriptase inhibitors [NNRTIs]) have been reported or are expected to occur must be considered when antimycobacterial therapy is indicated for treatment of active tuberculosis or latent tuberculosis infection or for the prophylaxis or treatment of *Mycobacterium avium* complex infection in HIV-infected patients who are receiving or are being considered for antiretroviral therapy. Because the management of these patients is complex and must be individualized, experts in the management of mycobacterial infections in HIV-infected patients should be consulted.

Zidovudine has been used concomitantly with antituberculosis agent therapy without evidence of substantially increased toxicity in patients with pulmonary tuberculosis and symptomatic HIV infection (acquired immunodeficiency syndrome [AIDS] or advanced AIDS-related complex [ARC]). In one study in a limited number of patients who received zidovudine concomitantly with an antituberculosis regimen of isoniazid and rifampin (with or without ethambutol) or a regimen of isoniazid, ethambutol, and pyrazinamide for 12 weeks, mild to moderate decreases in leukocyte counts occurred more frequently in the group that received concomitant therapy than in a control group that received zidovudine alone; however, there was no statistical difference between the groups in other reported adverse effects. In another study in adults with HIV infection and tuberculosis, zidovudine therapy administered concomitantly with an antituberculosis regimen (isoniazid, rifampin, pyrazinamide, and ethambutol initially, followed by isoniazid and rifampin) was well tolerated for up to 8 months or longer.

Rifabutin In one study in HIV-infected adults, concomitant use of rifabutin (300 mg once daily) and oral zidovudine (200 mg every 8 hours) did not affect most pharmacokinetic parameters of zidovudine, including AUC, peak plasma concentration, and renal clearance; the plasma half-life of zidovudine was decreased from 1.5 to 1.1 hours. In another study in HIV-infected patients designed to evaluate the effect of zidovudine on rifabutin pharmacokinetics, concomitant use of zidovudine (100 or 200 mg every 4 hours) and rifabutin (300 or 450 mg once daily) did not alter the pharmacokinetics of the antimycobacterial agent or its principal metabolite, and such use was not associated with any unusual adverse effects.

Rifampin In a multiple-dose study in HIV-infected patients, concomitant use of zidovudine (200 mg every 8 hours) and rifampin (600 mg once daily) for 14 days resulted in a 47% decrease in zidovudine AUC.

The manufacturer of zidovudine states that routine dosage adjustments are not necessary if rifampin and zidovudine are used concomitantly.

■ **Antiretroviral Agents** ***HIV Entry and Fusion Inhibitors***

Enfuvirtide. There is in vitro evidence of additive to synergistic antiretroviral effects between enfuvirtide and zidovudine.

Maraviroc. There is no in vitro evidence of antagonistic antiretroviral effects between maraviroc and zidovudine.

Maraviroc has no clinically important effect on zidovudine pharmacokinetics.

HIV Integrase Inhibitors (INSTIs) **Raltegravir.** There is no in vitro evidence of antagonistic antiretroviral effects between raltegravir and zidovudine.

HIV Nonnucleoside Reverse Transcriptase Inhibitors (NNRTIs) Results of in vitro cell culture studies indicate that the antiretroviral effects of zidovudine and delavirdine or efavirenz are additive to synergistic against HIV-1. There is no in vitro evidence of antagonistic antiretroviral effects between zidovudine and etravirine, nevirapine, or rilpivirine.

Delavirdine. Concomitant use of delavirdine and zidovudine does not affect the pharmacokinetics of either drug.

Efavirenz. Concomitant use of efavirenz (600 mg once daily for 14 days) and zidovudine (300 mg every 12 hours for 14 days) does not affect zidovudine peak plasma concentrations or AUC.

Dosage adjustments are not necessary if zidovudine and efavirenz are used concomitantly.

Nevirapine. Concomitant use of zidovudine and nevirapine results in a 28% and 30% decrease in zidovudine peak plasma concentrations and AUC, respectively.

Rilpivirine. Clinically important pharmacokinetic interactions are not expected if rilpivirine is used concomitantly with zidovudine.

HIV Nucleoside Reverse Transcriptase Inhibitors (NRTIs) Results of in vitro studies indicate that the antiretroviral effects of zidovudine and some other HIV nucleoside reverse transcriptase inhibitors (NRTIs) (e.g., didanosine, emtricitabine, lamivudine, tenofovir) are additive to synergistic against HIV-1. There is no in vitro evidence of antagonistic effects between abacavir and zidovudine.

Antagonistic antiretroviral effects have been reported in vitro and in vivo between zidovudine and stavudine.

Abacavir. Clinically important pharmacokinetic interactions have not been observed when abacavir was used concomitantly with zidovudine or lamivudine/zidovudine.

Didanosine. Concomitant use of buffered didanosine (200 mg every 12 hours for 3 days) and oral zidovudine (200 mg every 8 hours for 3 days) in HIV-infected patients decreased the peak plasma concentration and AUC of zidovudine by 17 and 10%, respectively, but did not affect the peak plasma concentration or AUC of didanosine. Results of a study in HIV-infected pediatric patients 3 months of age or older indicate that concomitant use of oral zidovudine and oral didanosine does not affect the AUC of either drug.

Emtricitabine. Although not considered clinically important, concomitant use of emtricitabine (200 mg once daily for 7 days) and zidovudine (300 mg twice daily for 7 days) increased zidovudine peak plasma concentrations and AUC by 17 and 13%, respectively, but did not affect emtricitabine peak plasma concentrations or AUC.

Lamivudine. Results of a study in asymptomatic HIV-infected patients who received a single 200-mg dose of zidovudine in conjunction with multiple doses of lamivudine (300 mg every 12 hours) indicate that concomitant use of the drugs does not have a clinically important effect on the pharmacokinetics of either drug. The AUC of zidovudine was increased 13%, but lamivudine concentrations were not affected.

Dosage adjustments are not necessary in patients receiving lamivudine and zidovudine concomitantly.

Stavudine. Zidovudine and stavudine should *not* be used concomitantly at any time because of in vitro and in vivo evidence of antagonistic antiretroviral effects.

Antagonism may occur because zidovudine and stavudine compete for cellular thymidine kinase that is needed for monophosphorylation of both drugs.

HIV Protease Inhibitors (PIs) The antiretroviral effects of zidovudine and some HIV protease inhibitors (PIs) (e.g., amprenavir [commercially available as fosamprenavir], indinavir, nelfinavir, ritonavir, saquinavir, tipranavir) are additive or synergistic against HIV-1 in vitro in cell culture. There is no in vitro evidence of antagonistic antiretroviral effects between zidovudine and atazanavir or darunavir.

Atazanavir. Concomitant use of zidovudine and atazanavir may decrease trough plasma concentrations of zidovudine, but does not affect the AUC of zidovudine. The clinical importance of this pharmacokinetic interaction is unknown.

Darunavir. Concomitant use of zidovudine and *ritonavir-boosted* darunavir does not result in clinically important pharmacokinetic interactions.

Fosamprenavir. Concomitant use of fosamprenavir (single 600-mg dose) and zidovudine (single 300-mg dose) increased zidovudine peak plasma concentrations and AUC by 40 and 31%, respectively. When amprenavir (single 600-mg dose) and zidovudine (single 300-mg dose) were used concomitantly, there was a 13% increase in the AUC of amprenavir, but no effect on amprenavir peak plasma concentrations.

Indinavir. Concomitant use of indinavir (1 g every 8 hours) and zidovudine (200 mg every 8 hours) for 1 week resulted in slightly increased indinavir peak plasma concentrations and AUC, slightly increased zidovudine AUC, and decreased zidovudine peak plasma concentrations. In a study in HIV-infected patients who received a 3-drug regimen of indinavir (800 mg every 8 hours), zidovudine (200 mg every 8 hours), and lamivudine (150 mg every 12 hours) for 7 days, peak plasma concentrations and AUC of indinavir and zidovudine were increased, but peak plasma concentrations and AUC of lamivudine were decreased.

Lopinavir. Although the clinical importance is unclear, lopinavir induces glucuronidation and has the potential to reduce zidovudine plasma concentrations.

Nelfinavir. Concomitant use of zidovudine (single 200-mg dose) and nelfinavir (750 mg every 8 hours for 7–10 days) resulted in a 35% decrease in the AUC of zidovudine and a 31% decrease in peak plasma concentrations of zidovudine; AUC and peak plasma concentrations of nelfinavir were not affected by concomitant zidovudine.

Routine zidovudine dosage adjustments are not warranted in patients receiving zidovudine and nelfinavir concomitantly.

Ritonavir. Concomitant use of oral zidovudine (200 mg every 8 hours) and oral ritonavir (300 mg every 6 hours) for 4 days decreased the peak plasma concentration and AUC of zidovudine by 27 and 25%, respectively, but did not affect the pharmacokinetics of ritonavir.

Dosage adjustments are not necessary in patients receiving zidovudine and ritonavir concomitantly.

Tipranavir. Concomitant use of *ritonavir-boosted* tipranavir decreases the AUC of zidovudine by approximately 35% and may also decrease peak plasma concentrations and AUC of tipranavir.

Some experts state that appropriate dosages for concomitant use of zidovudine and *ritonavir-boosted* tipranavir have not been established.

■ **Atovaquone** Concomitant use of zidovudine (200 mg every 8 hours) and atovaquone (750 mg every 12 hours with food) in 14 HIV-infected adults increased the AUC of zidovudine by about 31–35% and decreased zidovudine clearance by about 24%, but did not affect peak plasma concentrations of zidovudine or half-life of the drug. It was suggested that atovaquone inhibited glucuronidation of zidovudine. The pharmacokinetics of atovaquone were not affected by concomitant zidovudine.

Routine zidovudine dosage adjustments are not warranted in patients receiving zidovudine concomitantly with atovaquone, but patients should be monitored for zidovudine-associated adverse effects.

■ **Cidofovir** Cidofovir does not affect the pharmacokinetics of zidovudine. Cidofovir, however, *must* be given concomitantly with probenecid, a drug that can reduce zidovudine clearance. Since recommended regimens of cidofovir and probenecid are usually administered once every 1 or 2 weeks, the manufacturer of cidofovir recommends that zidovudine be temporarily discontinued or dosage reduced by 50% on the days that cidofovir and probenecid are administered. (See Drug Interactions: Probenecid.)

■ **Co-trimoxazole** In one study in a limited number of HIV-infected patients, concomitant use of oral zidovudine (250 mg every 12 hours) and oral co-trimoxazole (160 mg of trimethoprim and 800 mg of sulfamethoxazole twice daily 3 times weekly) did not alter the pharmacokinetics of zidovudine or its glucuronide metabolite.

■ **Dipyridamole** Although the clinical importance is unclear, in vitro studies using human monocyte/macrophage cells and T cells indicate that the antiviral activity of zidovudine against HIV-1 is enhanced by the presence of dipyridamole. Dipyridamole alone has little antiretroviral activity. Results of one study indicate that dipyridamole inhibits conversion of thymidine to thymidine triphosphate but does not interfere with conversion of zidovudine to its active triphosphate derivative. It has been suggested that dipyridamole potentiates the antiviral activity of zidovudine by decreasing cellular concentrations of thymidine triphosphate, which competes with zidovudine triphosphate for viral RNA-directed DNA polymerase and incorporation into viral DNA.

■ **Doxorubicin** Because there is in vitro evidence that doxorubicin inhibits phosphorylation of zidovudine to the active triphosphate metabolite and therefore could antagonize the antiretroviral activity of the drug, concomitant use doxorubicin and zidovudine should be avoided.

■ **Foscarnet** Although the clinical importance is unclear, results of in vitro tests indicate that the antiviral effects of foscarnet and zidovudine are additive or synergistic against HIV. In addition, in one study in a limited number of adults with symptomatic HIV infection, use of IV foscarnet (30 mg/kg every 8 hours) in conjunction with oral zidovudine (200 mg every 4 hours) apparently resulted in a transient additive effect since serum p24 antigen levels decreased during concomitant therapy and increased when foscarnet therapy was discontinued.

■ **Ganciclovir and Valganciclovir** Although the clinical importance is unclear, results of an in vitro study using H9 cells inoculated with HIV (strain HTLV-IIIB) indicate that ganciclovir antagonizes the antiretroviral activity of zidovudine against HIV. In addition, results of in vitro studies indicate that concomitant use of ganciclovir and zidovudine results in synergistic cytotoxicity.

Both ganciclovir and zidovudine alone produce direct, dose-dependent inhibitory effects on myeloid and erythroid progenitor cells, and concomitant use of zidovudine and ganciclovir (or valganciclovir) may increase the risk of hematologic toxicity or result in additive or synergistic myelotoxic effects. In several studies in patients with AIDS and cytomegalovirus infections, profound, intolerable myelosuppression, evidenced principally as severe neutropenia, occurred in all patients receiving ganciclovir (5 mg/kg IV 1–4 times daily) concomitantly with zidovudine (200 mg orally every 4 hours); anemia also occurred in many of these patients. Severe hematologic toxicity, which required a reduction in zidovudine dosage, also occurred in more than 80% of patients receiving ganciclovir (5 mg/kg IV 1–2 times daily) concomitantly with zidovudine (100 mg orally every 4 hours). The increased risk of hematologic toxicity does not appear to be related to a pharmacokinetic interaction between zidovudine and ganciclovir since there is no evidence that concomitant use affects the pharmacokinetic parameters of either drug.

Because of the risk of hematologic toxicity, concomitant use of zidovudine and ganciclovir is not recommended unless potential benefits outweigh risks. If combined therapy is considered necessary, the drugs must be used with extreme caution and hematologic parameters (e.g., hemoglobin, hematocrit, leukocyte count with differential) should be monitored frequently. HIV-infected patients should be counseled that concomitant use of zidovudine and ganciclovir may not be tolerated by some patients and may result in severe granulocytopenia (neutropenia).

■ **HCV Antivirals** ***HCV Protease Inhibitors*** **Simeprevir.** Clinically important interactions are not expected if simeprevir is used concomitantly with zidovudine.

■ **Hematopoietic Agents** Although the clinical importance is unclear, results of in vitro studies indicate that biosynthetic granulocyte-macrophage colony-stimulating factors (GM-CSFs) may potentiate the antiretroviral activity of zidovudine against HIV. In one in vitro study using monocyte/macrophage cell cultures, the presence of GM-CSF markedly enhanced the antiretroviral effect of zidovudine against a monocytotropic strain of HIV type 1 and against HIV-1 (strain HTLV-IIIB). A synergistic effect between GM-CSF and zidovudine also was evident in vitro in monocytic U-937 cells inoculated with HIV-1 (strain HTLV-IIIB). The mechanism of this synergistic effect has not been determined but may result from enhanced entry of zidovudine into infected cells and/or enhanced conversion of zidovudine monophosphate into the metabolically active triphosphate derivative. The fact that conflicting results have been obtained from studies evaluating the in vitro effects of biosynthetic GM-CSFs on replication of HIV when used alone and the fact that GM-CSFs appear to stimulate replication of some strains of HIV in vitro in certain cell cultures should be considered if sargramostim or any other biosynthetic GM-CSF is used in conjunction with zidovudine in patients with HIV infection.

■ **Interferon Alfa and Peginterferon Alfa** In vitro studies indicate that the antiretroviral activity of zidovudine and interferon alfa may be synergistic against HIV. There also is limited in vivo evidence of enhanced antiretroviral activity with combined therapy. Interferon alfa has been used concomitantly with zidovudine in patients with AIDS-related Kaposi's sarcoma, and there is evidence of clinical response, including good tumor response in some patients. Although concomitant use of zidovudine and interferon alfa does not appear to result in any major alterations in the pharmacokinetics of either drug, there may be a trend for increased AUC and decreased clearance of zidovudine after 3 weeks of concomitant therapy.

Depending on the dosage used, concomitant use of interferon alfa and zidovudine can be relatively well tolerated; however, concomitant use of the drugs can increase the risk of hematologic (e.g., neutropenia, thrombocytopenia) and hepatic toxicity. Potentially fatal hepatic decompensation has been reported in HIV-infected patients coinfected with hepatitis C virus (HCV) who received antiretroviral therapy concomitantly with interferon alfa with or without ribavirin. Patients receiving zidovudine with interferon alfa (or peginterferon alfa) with or without ribavirin should be closely monitored for toxicities, especially hepatic decompensation, neutropenia, and anemia. Discontinuance of zidovudine should be considered as medically appropriate. If worsening toxicities (e.g., hepatic decompensation with Child-Pugh scores greater than 6) occur, consideration should be given to immediately discontinuing or reducing dosage of interferon alfa (or peginterferon alfa) and/or ribavirin.

■ **Macrolides** Concomitant use of clarithromycin (500 mg twice daily) and zidovudine (100 mg 4 times daily for 7 days) decreased the AUC of zidovudine by 12% (range: 34% decrease to 14% increase).

Routine zidovudine dosage adjustments are not warranted in patients receiving zidovudine and clarithromycin concomitantly.

■ **Megestrol Acetate** Results of a pharmacokinetic study in HIV-infected adults indicate that concomitant use of megestrol acetate (800 mg) and oral zidovudine (100 mg) for 13 days results in a 14% decrease in the peak plasma concentration and about a 5% decrease in the AUC_{0-12} of zidovudine at steady-state. These effects were not considered clinically important.

■ **Myelosuppressive Agents** Drugs that are cytotoxic or myelosuppressive (e.g., amphotericin B, dapsone, doxorubicin, flucytosine, ganciclovir, interferon, pentamidine, vinblastine, vincristine) may increase the risk of hematologic toxicity and should be used with caution during zidovudine therapy.

■ **Opiates and Opiate Partial Agonists** ***Buprenorphine*** There are no clinically important pharmacokinetic interactions between buprenorphine and zidovudine; dosage adjustments are not necessary if the drugs are used concomitantly.

Methadone In one study in IV drug abusers with HIV infection who were receiving long-term methadone treatment for opiate addiction (30–90 mg daily), initiation of zidovudine therapy (200 mg orally every 4 hours) did not appear to have any clinically important effects on the pharmacokinetics of methadone and did not result in any evidence of narcotic withdrawal. However, the AUC of zidovudine was increased about 43% in patients receiving concomitant methadone compared with those receiving zidovudine alone. In another study in HIV-infected individuals who had been receiving methadone treatment for approximately 2 months, concomitant use of oral or IV zidovudine increased the zidovudine AUC by 29 or 41%, respectively, and reduced the clearance of zidovudine by about 26%. Methadone maintenance therapy did not appear to affect zidovudine pharmacokinetics is 5 pregnant women.

While the mechanism of this interaction requires further study, limited data indicate that methadone inhibits zidovudine glucuronidation, and also reduces renal clearance of zidovudine. Based on the results of the pharmacokinetic studies, it appears that the maintenance dose of methadone probably does not need to be adjusted when zidovudine therapy is initiated in patients receiving long-term methadone treatment.

Routine zidovudine dosage adjustments are not warranted in patients receiving zidovudine and methadone concomitantly, but patients should be monitored for zidovudine toxicity. In addition, the fact that IV drug abusers receiving methadone treatment also may be illicitly using other drugs (e.g., cannabis, cocaine, benzodiazepines, other opiate agonists) that have the potential to affect the pharmacokinetics of zidovudine should be considered when therapy with the antiretroviral agent is initiated in these patients.

■ **Phenytoin** Decreased plasma phenytoin concentrations have been reported in some patients receiving concomitant zidovudine and, in at least one patient, an increased phenytoin concentration was reported. In one study in adults with HIV infection receiving oral zidovudine therapy (200 mg every 4 hours), administration of a single 300-mg dose of phenytoin resulted in a 30% decrease in clearance of the antiretroviral agent; pharmacokinetics of phenytoin apparently was not affected.

■ **Probenecid** Concomitant use of probenecid may produce substantially higher and prolonged serum concentrations of zidovudine. In one study, concomitant use of probenecid (500 mg every 6 hours for 2 days) and zidovudine (2 mg/kg every 8 hours for 3 days) increased the AUC of zidovudine by 106%. Although limited information suggests that probenecid may inhibit glucuronidation and/or reduce renal excretion of zidovudine, there is some evidence suggesting that probenecid may principally inhibit metabolism rather than renal excretion of zidovudine, although renal excretion of its glucuronide metabolite appears to be inhibited.

In a study in patients with HIV infection who were receiving zidovudine, initiation of concomitant probenecid therapy (500 mg orally 3 times daily) resulted in flu-like symptoms, including myalgia, malaise, and/or fever and rash with maculopapular erythematous eruptions. These adverse effects generally developed during the first or second week of concomitant therapy and were severe enough to require discontinuance of probenecid therapy in some patients. It is unclear whether these adverse effects were the result of a drug interaction between zidovudine and probenecid or whether they reflect an increased potential for hypersensitivity reactions to probenecid in patients with HIV infection. Although some clinicians have suggested that probenecid's effect on the pharmacokinetics of zidovudine could be used to therapeutic advantage to decrease the dose and/or frequency of administration of zidovudine, other clinicians state that probenecid should be used with caution in patients receiving zidovudine.

The manufacturer of zidovudine states that routine zidovudine dosage adjustments are not warranted if probenecid and zidovudine are used concomitantly.

■ **Pyrimethamine** Results of one study indicate that zidovudine can antagonize the toxoplasmacidal action of pyrimethamine against *Toxoplasma gondii* in vitro and in vivo in mice and can interfere with the in vitro synergism of pyrimethamine and sulfadiazine against the organism. Although the clinical importance of this effect is unclear, it has been suggested that patients with HIV infection being treated for toxoplasmic encephalitis who also are receiving zidovudine should be monitored carefully for evidence of poor response to pyrimethamine. In vitro, trimethoprim and zidovudine have exhibited synergistic antibacterial activity in vitro against some gram-negative bacteria (i.e., *Citrobacter, Enterobacter, Escherichia, Klebsiella, Proteus, Providencia, Salmonella, Shigella*).

■ **Ribavirin** The manufacturer of zidovudine and some experts state that concomitant use of zidovudine and ribavirin is not recommended and should be avoided. If zidovudine and ribavirin are used concomitantly, caution is advised and patients should be closely monitored for virologic response and toxicities, especially hepatic decompensation and anemia.

In vitro, ribavirin antagonizes the antiviral activity of zidovudine against HIV. This antagonism appears to result from inhibition of zidovudine phosphorylation by ribavirin and/or phosphorylated ribavirin, possibly secondary to a ribavirin-induced increase in deoxythymidine triphosphate (dTTP) concentrations and a subsequent feedback inhibition of thymidine kinase. Increased dTTP concentrations might also interfere with the interaction of zidovudine triphosphate with HIV RNA-directed DNA polymerase (reverse transcriptase). Despite this in vitro antagonism, zidovudine has been used concomitantly with ribavirin (with or without interferon alfa) in some HIV-infected patients coinfected with HCV without evidence of an increase in HIV viral load and without evidence of pharmacokinetic interactions.

It has been suggested that concomitant use of ribavirin and NRTIs may increase the risk of mitochondrial dysfunction and associated toxicities (e.g., pancreatitis, lactic acidosis) reported with this group of antiretroviral agents. There have been several reports of lactic acidosis or pancreatitis occurring in HIV-infected patients coinfected with HCV who received antiretroviral therapy concomitantly with ribavirin and interferon alfa. These patients had been receiving long-term therapy with multiple-drug antiretroviral regimens that included one or more NRTIs (abacavir, didanosine, stavudine, zidovudine) and were clinically stable until lactic acidosis or pancreatitis developed 4–6 months after a regimen of ribavirin and interferon alfa was initiated for treatment of chronic HCV infection. Because ribavirin also is a nucleoside analog, it has been suggested that concomitant use of ribavirin and NRTIs may result in an adverse additive effect on mitochondrial function; however, other clinicians suggest that ribavirin may have potentiated the effects of the NRTIs through some other mechanism or that the viral diseases themselves may have been partly responsible for mitochondrial dysfunction in these patients.

■ **Valproic Acid** Concomitant use of valproic acid (250 or 500 mg every 8 hours) and oral zidovudine (100 mg every 8 hours) for 4 days in a limited number of HIV-infected adults resulted in an 80% increase in the AUC of zidovudine. The effect of concomitant zidovudine on the pharmacokinetics of valproic acid was not evaluated. Severe anemia has been reported following initiation of valproic acid therapy (500 mg twice daily) in an HIV-infected adult who was receiving an antiretroviral regimen that contained zidovudine, lamivudine, and abacavir; the patient had stable hematologic status at the time valproic acid was started.

The manufacturer of zidovudine states that routine zidovudine dosage adjustments are not warranted in patients receiving zidovudine and valproic acid concomitantly.

Acute Toxicity

■ **Manifestations** The IV or oral LD_{50} of zidovudine is greater than 750 or 3000 mg/kg, respectively, in rats and mice.

Acute overdosage of zidovudine (up to 50 g) have been reported in both adults and pediatric patients. There were no fatalities as a result of these overdosages and all patients recovered without permanent sequelae. Adverse effects reported following acute zidovudine overdosage include vomiting and nonspecific CNS effects such as fatigue, headache, dizziness, drowsiness, lethargy, and confusion. Although adverse hematologic effects, including anemia and a decrease in hemoglobin, occurred in a few patients following zidovudine overdosage, these effects were mild and transient and there was no evidence of prolonged bone marrow toxicity attributable to acute zidovudine overdosage. In at least one patient, acute overdosage of zidovudine was associated with bone marrow hypoplasia. Acute overdosage of zidovudine (10–40 g) alone or in conjunction with overdosage of a benzodiazepine and/or barbiturate has resulted in mild ataxia, lethargy, and fatigue. A single tonic-clonic (grand mal) seizure occurred in an adult who ingested 36 g of zidovudine in a single dose; no other cause could be identified. In another adult who inadvertently received 2.5 g (33 mg/kg) of zidovudine daily for 16 days, there was an increase in serum concentrations of AST (SGOT) and ALT (SGPT), but no evidence of bone marrow toxicity.

■ **Treatment** If acute overdosage of zidovudine occurs, the patient should be monitored for evidence of toxicity and supportive and symptomatic treatment should be initiated as required. Some clinicians suggest that the stomach be emptied by inducing emesis and that activated charcoal administered to prevent further absorption of unrecovered drug. Hemodialysis and peritoneal dialysis appear to have a negligible effect on the removal of zidovudine, but may enhance elimination of its primary metabolite (GZDV).

Mechanism of Action

■ **Antiviral Effects** Following conversion to a pharmacologically active metabolite, zidovudine apparently inhibits replication of retroviruses, including human immunodeficiency virus (HIV), by interfering with viral RNA-directed DNA polymerase (reverse transcriptase). Zidovudine, therefore, exerts a virustatic effect against retroviruses by acting as a reverse transcriptase inhibitor.

Like other HIV nucleoside reverse transcriptase inhibitors (NRTIs), including abacavir, didanosine, lamivudine, and stavudine, the antiviral activity of zidovudine appears to depend on intracellular conversion of the drug to a triphosphate metabolite. Zidovudine triphosphate and not unchanged zidovudine appears to be the pharmacologically active form of the drug. Zidovudine is converted to zidovudine monophosphate by cellular thymidine kinase; the monophosphate is phosphorylated to zidovudine diphosphate via cellular dTMP kinase (thymidylate kinase) and then to the triphosphate via other cellular enzymes. Formation of zidovudine diphosphate appears to be the rate-limiting step in the formation of zidovudine triphosphate. Neither zidovudine nor zidovudine monophosphate has in vitro activity against retroviruses; further study is needed to determine whether zidovudine diphosphate has antiretroviral activity. Because phosphorylation of zidovudine depends on cellular rather than viral enzymes, conversion of the drug to the active triphosphate derivative occurs in both virus-infected and uninfected cells.

Zidovudine triphosphate is a structural analog of thymidine triphosphate, the usual substrate for viral RNA-directed DNA polymerase. Although other mechanisms may be involved in the antiretroviral activity of the drug, zidovudine triphosphate appears to compete with thymidine triphosphate for viral RNA-directed DNA polymerase and incorporation into viral DNA. Following incorporation of zidovudine triphosphate into the viral DNA chain instead of thymidine triphosphate, DNA synthesis is prematurely terminated because the 3′-azido group of zidovudine prevents further 5′ to 3′ phosphodiester linkages. In addition, zidovudine monophosphate competitively inhibits dTMP kinase, resulting in decreased formation of thymidine triphosphate; thus, the drug can decrease concentrations of this natural substrate for RNA-directed DNA polymerase and facilitate binding of zidovudine triphosphate to the enzyme. The drug also appears to decrease 2′-deoxycytidine triphosphate concentrations, but the mechanism of this effect is not known. The contribution of these reductions in intracellular deoxynucleoside triphosphate concentrations on the antiretroviral and cytotoxic effects of zidovudine has not been fully elucidated.

In vitro studies indicate that the major in vivo metabolite of zidovudine, 3′-azido-3′-deoxy-5′-*O*-*β*-d-glucopyranuronosylthymidine (GZDV; formerly GAZT), does not have antiviral activity. GZDV does not antagonize the in vitro antiretroviral activity of zidovudine and does not compete with zidovudine triphosphate for viral RNA-directed DNA polymerase.

■ **Antibacterial Effects** Zidovudine is bactericidal against some gram-negative bacteria, including Enterobacteriaceae. Like the drug's antiviral action, the antibacterial action of zidovudine appears to result from premature termination of bacterial DNA synthesis secondary to incorporation of phosphorylated zidovudine in the bacterial DNA chain. In vitro exposure of susceptible bacteria to the drug results in bacterial elongation and death secondary to cell lysis. Unlike the antiviral action, the antibacterial action appears to depend on conversion of zidovudine to the active phosphorylated form via bacterial enzymes rather than via host enzymes. Zidovudine monophosphate, diphosphate, and triphosphate exhibit antibacterial activity in vitro, with the triphosphate being most active and the monophosphate being least active. Susceptibility of bacteria to zidovudine appears to depend in large part on the presence of bacterial thymidine kinase, an enzyme involved in phosphorylation of the drug. Organisms lacking thymidine kinase (e.g., *Mycobacterium avium, Pseudomonas aeruginosa*) are resistant to zidovudine, while those with relatively high concentrations of the enzyme (e.g., *Salmonella typhimurium*) are highly susceptible to the drug; in addition, mutants resistant to the drug have had relatively low concentrations of the enzyme. The antibacterial activity of zidovudine also appears to depend in part on other factors such as permeability of the organism to the drug.

■ **Cytotoxic Effects** Zidovudine triphosphate can bind to and inhibit some mammalian cellular DNA polymerases, particularly β- and γ-polymerases, in vitro. Zidovudine triphosphate and other dideoxynucleoside triphosphates appear to have a much greater affinity for viral RNA-directed DNA polymerase than for mammalian DNA polymerases. This differential sensitivity of mammalian and viral DNA polymerases to dideoxynucleoside triphosphates may account, in part, for some of the antiviral selectivity of these drugs in cells that phosphorylate them. However, inhibition of β- and γ-polymerases by these drugs may account, to some extent, for toxic effects associated with zidovudine and other NRTIs.

In vitro cell growth assays have been used to assess the cytotoxicity of zidovudine for various cell lines. Human fibroblasts and lymphocytes generally showed little inhibition of growth except at very high concentrations of the drug. In a colony-forming unit assay designed to assess the toxicity of the drug for human bone marrow, zidovudine exhibited a direct, dose-dependent inhibitory effect on erythroid and myeloid function in vitro; the ID_{50} of the drug was estimated to be less than 1.25 mcg/mL Results of an in vitro study using a human lymphoblastoid cell line (CEM) indicate that zidovudine inhibits mitochondrial DNA synthesis and stimulates lactic acid production in the cells. Results of in vitro tests indicate that all commercially available NRTIs inhibit mitochondrial DNA γ-polymerase; zalcitabine (no longer commercially available in the US) is the most potent inhibitor followed by didanosine, stavudine, lamivudine, zidovudine, and abacavir. Inhibition of this enzyme and other mitochondrial enzymes could lead to mitochondrial dysfunction and cellular toxicity. It has been suggested that mitochondrial dysfunction may be a factor in the development of several adverse effects reported in patients receiving zidovudine (e.g., myopathy, lactic acidosis, severe hepatomegaly with steatosis, bone marrow suppression, lipodystrophy).

Although further study is needed, zidovudine appears to alter nucleoside metabolism within host cells, resulting in decreased levels of thymidine triphosphate, 2′-deoxycytidine triphosphate, and several other deoxynucleoside triphosphates. Zidovudine-induced depletion of normal pyrimidine pools may contribute to the bone marrow toxicity reported during therapy with the drug.

Spectrum

Zidovudine has a limited spectrum of antiviral activity. Following intracellular conversion to a pharmacologically active metabolite, the drug is active in vitro against many human and animal retroviruses, including human immunodeficiency virus (HIV). Zidovudine also has some in vitro activity against hepatitis B virus (HBV) and Epstein-Barr virus, but has been inactive against other human or animal viruses tested.

The antiretroviral activity of zidovudine has been evaluated in vitro in cell culture systems, including lymphoblastic and monocytic cell lines and peripheral blood lymphocytes. A variety of methods, including assays for cytopathic effect inhibition, plaque inhibition, viral RNA-directed DNA polymerase (reverse transcriptase) activity, or retroviral antigens such as p24 core antigen (p24 *gag* protein), have been used to test in vitro susceptibility of retroviruses to zidovudine.

A concentration of 1 nmol/L of zidovudine is approximately equivalent to 0.27 ng/mL.

■ **Retroviruses** Zidovudine is active in vitro against human retroviruses, including HIV type 1 (HIV-1), HIV type 2 (HIV-2), and HTLV-I. The drug is also active in vitro against many animal retroviruses, including feline leukemia virus, Friend leukemia virus, Harvey murine sarcoma virus, murine leukemia virus, and simian T lymphotropic virus. In vitro on a weight basis, zidovudine generally is more active than didanosine against susceptible HIV-1.

The concentration of zidovudine required to inhibit viral replication by 50% (EC_{50}) or 90% (EC_{90}) for HIV-1 is 0.01– 0.49 μM or 0.1–9 μM, respectively. The EC_{50} of the drug for HIV obtained from treatment-naive patients (these isolates had no resistance mutations) has ranged from 0.005–0.11 μM. The EC_{50} of zidovudine has been 0.02 μM or less against different HIV-1 clades (A–G) and 0.004 μM or less against HIV-2 isolates.

In in vitro studies that measured RNA-directed DNA polymerase (reverse transcriptase) activity in H9 cells, phytohemagglutinin (PHA)-stimulated peripheral blood lymphocytes, or unstimulated peripheral blood lymphocytes, the ID_{90} (concentration of drug required to inhibit 90% of detectable HIV replication) of zidovudine was 0.13 mcg/mL or less when the drug was added shortly after the cells were inoculated with HIV. The ID_{50} (concentration of the drug required to produce a 50% decrease in supernatant RNA-directed DNA polymerase) in H9 cells or peripheral blood lymphocytes was 0.013 mcg/mL. At concentrations of 0.13 mcg/mL, zidovudine provided more than 90% protection from a strain of HIV (HTLV-IIIB)-induced cytopathic effects in 2 tetanus-specific T4 cell lines; p24 core antigen expression was undetectable at this concentration in these cells.

In an in vitro study in MT-4 cells, zidovudine inhibited replication of HIV when the drug was added to the cell cultures before inoculation with HIV or up to 20 hours after inoculation; however, the drug did not inhibit HIV replication when zidovudine was added 30–50 hours after inoculation. Zidovudine does not appear to inhibit HIV replication in chronically infected cells (i.e., those presumed to carry integrated HIV DNA).

■ **Other Viruses** Although the clinical importance is unclear, zidovudine has some activity in vitro against HBV. In cell culture using 2.2.15 (PR) cells derived from a human hepatoblastoma (HEP G2) cell line that continuously produces HBV genome, zidovudine was less active against the virus than didanosine when activity was based on reduction in extrachromosomal HBV DNA. Zidovudine also appears to have some in vitro activity against Epstein-Barr virus, although the clinical importance of this in vitro activity has not been determined to date.

Zidovudine is inactive in vitro against other viruses tested to date, including herpes simplex virus types 1 and 2, influenza virus, adenovirus, cytomegalovirus, respiratory syncytial virus, varicella-zoster virus, and vaccinia virus.

■ **Other Organisms** Zidovudine has some activity in vitro against gram-negative bacteria. In vitro, zidovudine concentrations of 0.005–0.5 mcg/mL inhibit some strains of *Citrobacter*, *Enterobacter*, *Escherichia coli*, *Klebsiella*, *Proteus vulgaris*, *Salmonella*, and *Shigella*. The clinical importance of this in vitro activity has not been determined to date, however, and limited data suggest that resistance to zidovudine develops rapidly in gram-negative bacteria. The drug appears to be only moderately active against *Yersinia enterocolitica*, *Vibrio cholerae*, *Haemophilus influenzae*, and *Proteus mirabilis*, with MIC_{50}s (minimum inhibitory concentration of the drug at which 50% of strains tested are inhibited) ranging from 6.2–12.5 mcg/mL, and inactive against *Bordetella*, *Campylobacter*, *Neisseria*, *Pseudomonas aeruginosa*, and *Serratia*.

Zidovudine is inactive against gram-positive bacteria, anaerobic bacteria, and *Mycobacteria*. Although zidovudine appeared to have some in vitro activity against *Mycoplasma*, including *M. fermentans*, in one in vitro study, results of several other studies indicate that zidovudine has no clinically important activity in vitro against *M. pneumoniae*, *M. hominis*, or *Ureaplasma urealyticum*. The drug is inactive against fungi, including *Candida albicans* and *Cryptococcus neoformans*.

Zidovudine concentrations of 1.9 mcg/mL reportedly inhibit *Giardia lamblia* in vitro, but the importance of this in vitro effect has not been determined. The drug has been inactive against other protozoa tested, including *Pneumocystis carinii*, *Leishmania donovani*, and *Toxoplasma gondii*.

Resistance

■ **Resistance in Retroviruses** HIV type 1 (HIV-1) strains with reduced susceptibility or resistance to zidovudine have been selected in vitro in cell culture and also have emerged during therapy with the drug. Zidovudine-resistant strains of HIV type 2 (HIV-2) also have been reported in patients who received the drug.

Emergence of zidovudine resistance appears to be a function of the duration of therapy with the drug, the severity of HIV disease, and the overall potency of the regimen in which it is used. Resistance is most likely to develop in patients with advanced HIV infection, those with low initial absolute $CD4^+$T-cell counts, and those receiving prolonged zidovudine therapy. The likelihood of developing in vitro resistance to zidovudine in HIV isolates obtained from patients with symptomatic HIV infection (acquired immunodeficiency syndrome [AIDS] or advanced AIDS-related complex [ARC]) who are receiving therapy with the drug increases with the duration of therapy; early studies using zidovudine monotherapy indicate that such resistance typically develops only after 6–9 months of continuous zidovudine therapy and occasionally has developed more rapidly (e.g., within 2 months). In one study in patients with symptomatic infection, almost 50% of isolates from patients receiving 6–9 months of zidovudine monotherapy were resistant, and resistance had developed in almost all patients (93%) by 36 months of therapy. The ID_{50} of zidovudine for HIV isolates obtained from patients with symptomatic infection who have received at least 1 year of zidovudine monotherapy frequently is 10–100 times higher than the ID_{50} of the drug for isolates obtained from these patients prior to initiation of therapy. In a study in which HIV isolates were obtained by cocultivation of peripheral blood lymphocytes with MT-2 cells and zidovudine's in vitro antiviral activity was assessed using a plaque reduction assay in HT4-6C cells, the ID_{50} of zidovudine for isolates obtained prior to or during the first 5 months of zidovudine monotherapy ranged from 0.003–0.013 mcg/mL, and the ID_{50} of the drug ranged from 0.016–1.07 and 0.011–1.6 mcg/mL for isolates obtained from patients who had received 6–11 and 12–30 months of zidovudine monotherapy, respectively. Although it has been suggested that zidovudine resistance may develop at a slower rate in patients with asymptomatic HIV infection than in those with more advanced disease, high-level zidovudine resistance has emerged in patients with asymptomatic infection, especially in those who received up to 3 years of zidovudine monotherapy.

The clinical importance of in vitro resistance to zidovudine has not been fully determined, and the quantitative relationship between in vitro susceptibility to zidovudine and clinical response to therapy with the drug remains to be established. The specific relationship between decreased in vitro susceptibility to zidovudine and clinical response to the drug and/or progression of HIV disease has not been defined. Results of some studies indicate that there may be a correlation between decreased in vitro susceptibility to zidovudine and poor clinical outcome in patients receiving the drug; however, additional factors apparently also are involved since a temporal relationship between the development of partial resistance to zidovudine and progression of HIV disease has not been clearly established. There is some evidence that the clinical progression of HIV infection may be more closely related to the presence of syncytium-inducing (SI) phenotypes of HIV than to the presence of zidovudine-resistant HIV. In some patients, there is no evidence that presence of zidovudine-resistant HIV isolates correlates with increased serum concentrations of HIV p24 core antigen; although the relationship between the amount of circulating virus and serum concentrations of HIV p24 core antigen has not been definitely established, serum concentrations of HIV p24 core antigen have been used to evaluate the in vivo response to antiviral therapy. In one study in children with advanced HIV disease who had been receiving zidovudine monotherapy for 9 months or longer, a clinically important correlation between zidovudine resistance and poor clinical outcome was apparent.

Specific mutations of HIV RNA-directed DNA polymerase (reverse transcriptase) at critical codons on the *pol* gene fragment have been associated with zidovudine resistance. Genotypic analyses of isolates selected in cell culture and recovered from zidovudine-treated patients showed thymidine analog mutations (TAMs) in the HIV-1 reverse transcriptase that include M41L, D67N, K70R, L210W, T215Y or F, and K219E/R/H/Q/N/Q. Development of resistance to zidovudine in HIV occurs in a progressive, stepwise manner, and each stepwise reduction in susceptibility appears to be associated with the acquisition of an additional mutation in the reverse transcriptase gene of the organism. The degree of zidovudine resistance appears to depend on the number and combination of these mutations. Acquisition of at least 3 mutations generally has resulted in HIV variants that are highly resistant to the drug; fewer mutations may result in variants that are partially susceptible. However, a single mutation reportedly has resulted in high-level zidovudine resistance in some strains. Because zidovudine is phosphorylated via host cell rather than viral enzymes, resistance of HIV to zidovudine would *not* result from production of virus-coded phosphorylating enzymes with altered substrate specificity or from decreased concentrations of virus-coded phosphorylating enzymes.

The frequency of zidovudine-resistant isolates existing in the general population is unknown. Primary infection with zidovudine-resistant HIV type 1 has been reported in adults who were zidovudine-naive (had not previously received zidovudine) and in infants born to HIV-infected mothers. This apparently occurred as the result of horizontal and vertical transmission from individuals who had been receiving long-term zidovudine monotherapy and harbored a high percentage of resistant HIV-1 variants. HIV isolates show considerable genetic variability, and patients with HIV infection who have received antiretroviral therapy harbor many related variants of the virus that change over time. There is some evidence that zidovudine-resistant isolates can revert to zidovudine-susceptible, but the frequency and rate at which the susceptible isolates emerge following discontinuance of the drug remain to be elucidated. Analysis of HIV isolates obtained from patients who have received 1–2 years of zidovudine monotherapy indicate that the ratio of wild-type, susceptible HIV strains to mutant, resistant HIV strains changes considerably following discontinuance of the drug in some, but not all, patients. The change from a mutant or mixed virus population to a wild-type population may require at least 1 year in some patients and appears to be affected by the duration of zidovudine therapy. It has been suggested that this may occur because of reversion of mutations to the wild-type, susceptible strains and/or selective outgrowth of the wild-type strains. In addition, one particular mutation in HIV (Thr215 to Tyr) that confers resistance to zidovudine apparently can be reversed or nullified by subsequent exposure to didanosine or zalcitabine. In this case, didanosine or zalcitabine causes a specific mutation (Leu74 to Val) that results in resistance to didanosine and zalcitabine but suppresses zidovudine resistance that results from the codon 215 mutation. In some patients harboring zidovudine-resistant strains of HIV, concomitant therapy with zidovudine and lamivudine restored phenotypic susceptibility to zidovudine.

■ **Cross-resistance** Cross-resistance has been reported among the HIV nucleoside reverse transcriptase inhibitors (NRTIs). TAM substitutions in HIV-1 reverse transcriptase selected by zidovudine can confer cross-resistance to abacavir, didanosine, stavudine, and tenofovir.

HIV isolates resistant to didanosine, lamivudine, stavudine, and zidovudine have been isolated from patients who received zidovudine in conjunction with didanosine for up to 2 years. Although some zidovudine-resistant HIV strains may be susceptible to didanosine, lamivudine, and/or stavudine in vitro, other zidovudine-resistant strains are cross-resistant to didanosine, lamivudine, and/or stavudine. In vitro studies indicate that HIV isolates with multiple mutations associated with zidovudine resistance have reduced susceptibility to tenofovir. Some zidovudine-resistant strains of HIV remain susceptible to emtricitabine in vitro.

■ **Resistance in Other Organisms** Limited data suggest that resistance to zidovudine develops rapidly in vitro in gram-negative bacteria, including *E. coli*, *Klebsiella*, *Proteus vulgaris*, *Salmonella*, and *Shigella*. Because the antibacterial effect of zidovudine depends on bacterial phosphorylating enzymes, bacterial resistance to the drug could result from alterations in these enzymes; emergence of resistant bacterial mutants deficient in thymidine kinase has been reported. Other mechanisms of bacterial resistance may also be involved.

Pharmacokinetics

Pharmacokinetics of zidovudine have been studied in adults with human immunodeficiency virus (HIV) infection, HIV-infected neonates, infants, and children up to 12 years of age, pregnant women, and adults with renal impairment. Pharmacokinetics of the drug have not been specifically studied in geriatric adults older than 65 years of age.

Pharmacokinetics of zidovudine in pediatric patients older than 3 months of age are similar to that reported in adults. However, zidovudine pharmacokinetics in neonates younger than 2 weeks of age, particularly premature neonates, are substantially different than those in adults. Results of a limited single-dose study indicate that gender does not affect the pharmacokinetics of zidovudine.

Pharmacokinetics of zidovudine in pregnant women are similar to that reported in nonpregnant adults. Results of studies evaluating use of oral zidovudine in women during the second and third trimesters of pregnancy indicate that, although the volume of distribution and clearance of the drug may be increased slightly in some patients during pregnancy, peak plasma concentrations and half-life of the drug generally are the same as those reported for other adults.

A concentration of 1 nmol/L of zidovudine is approximately equivalent to 0.27 ng/mL.

■ **Absorption** Following oral administration, zidovudine is well absorbed, but absorption shows considerable interindividual variation (range: 42–95%) and the drug appears to undergo first-pass metabolism. In adults, children, and neonates, about 65% (range: 50–89%) of an oral dose reaches systemic circulation as unchanged drug.

Results of some studies indicate that the rate of absorption and peak plasma concentrations of zidovudine may be increased substantially if the drug is taken with a meal. However, the manufacturer states that the extent of absorption of zidovudine as determined by the AUC is not affected by food.

The fixed-combination tablet containing 150 mg of lamivudine and 300 mg of zidovudine (Combivir®) is bioequivalent to one 150-mg tablet of lamivudine and one 300-mg tablet of zidovudine given simultaneously.

The fixed-combination tablet containing 300 mg of abacavir, 150 mg of lamivudine, and 300 mg of zidovudine (Trizivir®) is bioequivalent to one 300-mg abacavir tablet, one 150-mg lamivudine tablet, and one 300-mg zidovudine tablet given simultaneously.

Adults Zidovudine is rapidly absorbed from the GI tract, with peak serum concentrations generally occurring within 0.5–1.5 hours after an oral dose of the drug. In fasting adults, mean oral bioavailability of zidovudine is 64%. The AUC of zidovudine following administration of zidovudine tablets or oral solution is equivalent to that following administration of the capsules.

Following IV infusion of zidovudine, dose-independent pharmacokinetics are observed over the dosage range of 1–5 mg/kg. Following IV infusion over 1 hour of a single 2.5- or 5-mg/kg dose of zidovudine in adults with HIV infection, peak plasma concentrations of the drug immediately following completion of the infusion ranged from 1.07–1.6 or 1.6–2.7 mcg/mL, respectively. Following IV administration of zidovudine in a dosage of 2.5 mg/kg every 4 hours, mean steady-state peak plasma concentrations are 1.1 mcg/mL and trough concentrations are 0.1 mcg/mL.

Children In children 3 months to 12 years of age, zidovudine appears to have dose-dependent increases in plasma concentrations after administration of an oral solution over the dosage range of 90–240 mg/m² every 6 hours.

In one limited study in neonates and infants younger than 3 months of age born to HIV-infected mothers, zidovudine was well absorbed when administered orally; however, bioavailability decreased after 14 days of age. Following oral doses of 2–4 mg/kg, bioavailability of the drug averaged 89% in those 14 days of age or younger and 61% in those older than 14 days of age. In neonates 14 days of age or younger who received single 2-mg/kg oral doses of the drug or infants older than 14 days of age who received single 3-mg/kg oral doses, plasma zidovudine concentrations were greater than 0.267 mcg/mL for 4.12 or 2.25 hours, respectively, after the dose.

In children 14 months to 12 years of age with symptomatic HIV infection who received a single 80-mg/m² dose of zidovudine given by IV infusion over 1 hour, peak plasma concentrations of the drug averaged 1.58 mcg/mL; plasma concentrations were less than 0.27 mcg/mL within an hour following completion of the infusion. When these children received continuous IV infusion of zidovudine in a dosage of 0.5, 0.9, 1.4, or 1.8 mg/kg per hour, steady-state plasma concentrations of the drug averaged 0.51, 0.75, 0.83, or 1.2 mcg/mL, respectively.

■ **Distribution** There is limited information on the distribution of zidovudine into body tissue or fluids, but the drug appears to be widely distributed. The apparent volume of distribution of the drug in adults with HIV infection is 1.4–1.6 L/kg. In children 1–13 years of age with symptomatic HIV infection, the volume of distribution of zidovudine at steady state ranges from 22–64 L/m².

Zidovudine is distributed into CSF following oral or IV administration. The ratio of CSF/plasma concentrations of zidovudine reported in various studies in adults or children with HIV infection who received oral or IV therapy with the drug has ranged from 0.15–2.1. In one study in HIV-infected adults who received a single IV dose of zidovudine of 2.5 mg/kg by IV infusion over 1 hour, peak CSF concentrations averaged 0.35 mcg/mL (range: 0.11–0.96 mcg/mL) 1 hour after completion of the infusion and the ratio of peak CSF/plasma concentration was 0.17. In an adult who received an oral zidovudine dosage of 2 mg/kg every 8 hours, the CSF concentration of the drug 1.8 hours after a dose was about 0.04 mcg/mL and the CSF/plasma ratio was 0.15. However, CSF concentrations may not be good indicators of distribution of the drug into brain parenchyma. Studies in rats indicate that, although zidovudine readily distributes into CSF, distribution of the drug into brain interstitial fluid may be minimal.

Zidovudine is distributed into semen following oral administration; however, there is no evidence to date that presence of the drug in semen reduces the risk of transmission of HIV. In a limited number of HIV-infected men receiving oral zidovudine (200 mg every 4–6 hours), the ratio of semen/serum concentrations of the drug ranged from 1.3–20.4 in samples obtained 0.75–4.5 hours after dosing. In another study in antiretroviral-naive, HIV-infected men who received oral zidovudine (300 mg twice daily or 200 mg 3 times daily) and oral lamivudine (150 mg twice daily), the median ratio of semen/plasma concentrations of zidovudine was 5.9.

Zidovudine is less than 38% bound to plasma proteins.

Zidovudine and its glucuronide metabolite cross the human placenta and are distributed into cord blood and amniotic fluid as well as fetal liver, muscle, and CNS tissue. Concentrations of the drug and its metabolite in cord blood, fetal plasma, amniotic fluid, and fetal muscle tissue are similar to or exceed those in maternal plasma; only very low concentrations are distributed into fetal CNS tissue. The ratio of the glucuronide metabolite to zidovudine is higher in maternal blood than in fetal blood.

Zidovudine is distributed into milk. In a study in HIV-infected women who received a single 200-mg dose of zidovudine, concentrations of the drug in milk were similar to concurrent serum concentrations.

■ **Elimination** The plasma half-life of zidovudine in adults averages approximately 0.5–3 hours following oral or IV administration. Following IV administration of zidovudine in adults or children, plasma concentrations of the drug appear to decline in a biphasic manner. Half-life in adults is less than 10 minutes in the initial phase and 1 hour in the terminal phase.

Following IV administration over 1 hour of a single 80-, 120-, or 160-mg/m² dose in children 1–13 years of age with symptomatic HIV infection, the $t_{1/}$

$_{2\alpha}$ of zidovudine averaged 0.16–0.25 hours and the $t_{1/2\beta}$ averaged 1–1.7 hours. Plasma half-life of zidovudine generally is longer in neonates than in older children and adults but decreases with neonatal maturity. In one limited study in neonates and infants younger than 3 months of age, plasma half-life of zidovudine averaged 3.1 hours in those 14 days of age or younger and 1.9 hours in those older than 14 days of age. In a study in premature neonates (26–32 weeks' gestation; birthweight 0.7–1.9 kg), the serum half-life of zidovudine averaged 7.3 hours at an average postnatal age of 6.3 days and averaged 4.4 hours at an average postnatal age of 17.7 days.

Zidovudine is rapidly metabolized via glucuronidation in the liver principally to 3′-azido-3′-deoxy-5′-*O*-β-d-glucopyranuronosylthymidine (GZDV; formerly GAZT); zidovudine is also metabolized to GZDV in renal microsomes. GZDV has an apparent elimination half-life of 1 hour (range: 0.6–1.7 hours) and does not appear to have antiviral activity against HIV. In addition, two other hepatic metabolites of zidovudine have been identified as 3′-amino-3′-deoxythymidine (AMT) and its glucuronide derivative (GAMT). Intracellularly, in both virus-infected and uninfected cells, zidovudine is converted to zidovudine monophosphate by cellular thymidine kinase; the monophosphate derivative is phosphorylated to zidovudine diphosphate via cellular dTMP kinase (thymidylate kinase) and then to zidovudine triphosphate via other cellular enzymes. Intracellular (host cell) conversion of zidovudine to the triphosphate derivative is necessary for the *antiviral* activity of the drug. Activation for antibacterial action, however, does not depend on phosphorylation within host cells but rather depends on conversion within bacterial cells. (See Mechanism of Action.)

Zidovudine and GZDV are eliminated principally in urine via both glomerular filtration and tubular secretion. Following oral or IV administration in adults with HIV infection, total body clearance of zidovudine averages 1.6 L/hr per kg (range: 0.8–2.7 L/hr per kg) and renal clearance of the drug averages 0.34 L/hr per kg. In children 3 months to 12 years of age, the total body clearance averaged 1.85 L/hr per kg. In one limited study in neonates and infants younger than 3 months of age, total body clearance of the drug averaged 0.65 L/hr per kg in those 14 days of age or younger and 1.14 L/hr per kg in those older than 14 days of age.

Following oral administration of zidovudine in patients with HIV infection, 63–95% of the dose is excreted in urine; approximately 14–18% of the dose is excreted as unchanged zidovudine and 72–74% is excreted as GZDV within 6 hours. Following IV administration of the drug in adults or children with HIV infection, approximately 18–29% of the dose is excreted in urine as unchanged drug and 45–60% is excreted as GZDV within 6 hours.

In patients with impaired renal function, plasma concentrations of zidovudine may be increased and the half-life prolonged. In one study in adults with impaired renal function (creatinine clearances ranging from 6–31 mL/minute) without HIV infection, $t_{1/2\beta}$ of zidovudine averaged 1.4 hours and was similar to that reported for adults with HIV infection who had normal renal function. However, the $t_{1/2\beta}$ of GZDV in these adults with impaired renal function averaged 8 hours and was considerably prolonged compared with that reported for adults with HIV infection who had normal renal function.

In one study in adults with hemophilia and HIV infection who had elevated serum concentrations of AST, ALT, alkaline phosphatase, and γ-glutamyltransferase (GGT, γ-glutamyl transpeptidase, GGTP), pharmacokinetics of zidovudine after a single 300-mg oral dose showed considerable interindividual variation In some of these patients, pharmacokinetics of the drug could be described by a biexponential equation and the $t_{1/2\beta}$ of the zidovudine and GZDV averaged 1.3 and 1.2 hours, respectively. In some of these patients, pharmacokinetics of the drug was best described by a triexponential equation and the $t_{1/2\beta}$s were prolonged, averaging 48 and 5.2 hours, respectively.

Zidovudine clearance is decreased and plasma concentrations are increased in patients with hepatic impairment. In a limited number of HIV-infected patients with or without liver disease who received a single 250-mg oral dose of zidovudine, peak zidovudine plasma concentrations were attained within about an hour in both groups but averaged 8.3 mcg/mL in those with liver disease compared with 1.5 mcg/mL in those without liver disease; mean plasma half-life was 1.8 hours in those with liver disease compared with 0.5 hours in those without liver disease. In addition, peak plasma concentrations of GZDV were attained later in those with liver disease. (See Dosage and Administration: Dosage in Renal and Hepatic Impairment.)

Hemodialysis and peritoneal dialysis appear to have a negligible effect on removal of zidovudine, but may enhance elimination of GZDV. In anuric patients undergoing hemodialysis, the relative amount of a zidovudine dose eliminated via dialysis as unchanged drug compared with that eliminated via metabolism and dialysis of the metabolite appears to be minimal. The amount of drug removed during hemodialysis depends on several factors (e.g., type of coil used, dialysis flow rate). In anuric adults without HIV infection undergoing 4-hour periods of hemodialysis, plasma half-life of GZDV averaged 1.7 hours during dialysis and 52 hours between dialysis sessions. The manufacturer and some clinicians recommend that zidovudine be administered in a reduced dosage in patients undergoing hemodialysis or peritoneal dialysis. (See Dosage and Administration: Dosage in Renal and Hepatic Impairment.)

Chemistry and Stability

■ **Chemistry** Zidovudine, an antiretroviral agent, is a human immunodeficiency virus (HIV) nucleoside reverse transcriptase inhibitor (NRTI). The drug is a dideoxynucleoside reverse transcriptase inhibitor. Zidovudine is a thymidine analog which differs structurally from thymidine in that zidovudine contains a 3′-azido group rather than a 3′-hydroxyl group. Replacement of the 3′-hydroxyl group in the nucleoside results in the inability of zidovudine to form phosphodiester linkages at this position.

Zidovudine occurs as an odorless, white to beige, crystalline solid. The drug has solubilities of 20 mg/mL in water and 71 mg/mL in alcohol at 25°C

Zidovudine is commercially available for oral administration as capsules, film-coated tablets, and an oral solution; for parenteral administration, zidovudine is commercially available as a concentrate for IV infusion. Zidovudine also is commercially available for oral administration in fixed-combination tablets containing lamivudine and zidovudine (lamivudine/zidovudine) and fixed-combination tablets containing abacavir sulfate, lamivudine, and zidovudine (abacavir/lamivudine/zidovudine).

The oral solution containing 10 mg of zidovudine per mL is colorless to pale yellow and has a pH of 3–4. The oral solution contains sodium benzoate as a preservative and may contain sodium hydroxide to adjust pH.

Zidovudine injection for IV infusion is a clear, nearly colorless, sterile solution containing 10 mg of the drug per mL of water for injection. The injection has a pH of approximately 5.5 and contains no preservatives; hydrochloric acid and/or sodium hydroxide may be added during manufacture to adjust the pH.

■ **Stability** Commercially available zidovudine capsules and oral solution should be stored at 15–25°C. Zidovudine may not be adversely affected by short-term exposure to heat and sunlight, but capsules of the drug may become discolored or brittle as a result of such exposure and should be protected from light, heat, and moisture.

Zidovudine film-coated tablets should be stored at 20–25°C.

Commercially available zidovudine for injection concentrate for IV infusion should be stored at 15–25°C and protected from light. Following dilution in 5% dextrose injection, solutions containing 4 mg or less of zidovudine per mL are physically and chemically stable for 24 hours at room temperature or 48 hours when refrigerated at 2–8°C. However, because zidovudine for injection concentrate for IV infusion contains no preservatives, the manufacturer recommends that diluted solutions of the concentrate be administered within 8 hours if stored at 25°C or within 24 hours if refrigerated at 2–8°C to minimize the potential administration of a microbiologically contaminated solution.

Lamivudine/zidovudine fixed-combination tablets should be stored at 2–30°C.

Abacavir/lamivudine/zidovudine fixed-combination tablets should be stored at 25°C, but may be exposed to temperatures ranging from 15–30°C.

Preparations

Excipients in commercially available drug preparations may have clinically important effects in some individuals; consult specific product labeling for details.

Zidovudine

Oral		
Capsules	100 mg*	**Retrovir®**, ViiV
		Zidovudine Capsules
Solution	10 mg/mL*	**Retrovir® Syrup**, ViiV
		Zidovudine Oral Solution
Tablets, film-coated	300 mg*	**Zidovudine Tablets**
Parenteral		
For injection concentrate, for IV infusion only	10 mg/mL*	**Retrovir® Injection**, ViiV
		Zidovudine for Injection Concentrate

*available from one or more manufacturer, distributor, and/or repackager by generic (nonproprietary) name

Zidovudine Combinations

Oral		
Tablets, film-coated	300 mg with Abacavir Sulfate 300 mg (of abacavir) and Lamivudine 150 mg*	**Abacavir Sulfate, Lamivudine, and Zidovudine Tablets**
		Trizivir®, ViiV
	300 mg with Lamivudine 150 mg*	**Combivir®**, ViiV
		Lamivudine and Zidovudine Tablets

*available from one or more manufacturer, distributor, and/or repackager by generic (nonproprietary) name

†Use is not currently included in the labeling approved by the US Food and Drug Administration

Interferons 8:18.20

Peginterferon Alfa

■ Peginterferon alfa contains interferon alfa (recombinant DNA origin) covalently bound to monomethoxy polyethylene glycol (PEG). Peginterferon alfa-2a and peginterferon alfa-2b are used as antiviral agents. Peginterferon alfa-2b also is available in higher concentrations for use as an antineoplastic agent (see Peginterferon Alfa 10:00). For information on nonconjugated interferon alfa, see Interferon Alfa 8:18.20. and Interferon Alfa 10:00.

Uses

■ **Chronic Hepatitis B Virus Infection** Peginterferon alfa-2a (Pegasys®) is used for treatment of chronic HBV infection in adults with hepatitis B e antigen (HBeAg)-positive or -negative chronic HBV infection with compensated liver disease and evidence of viral replication and liver inflammation.

The goal of antiviral therapy in patients with chronic HBV infection is to achieve sustained suppression of HBV replication and remission of liver disease. The long-term goal of therapy is to prevent cirrhosis, hepatic failure, and hepatocellular carcinoma. Currently available therapies for chronic HBV infection (e.g., interferon alfa, peginterferon alfa, adefovir, entecavir, lamivudine, telbivudine, tenofovir) do not eradicate HBV and may have only limited long-term efficacy. Decisions on the appropriate time to initiate therapy and which drug to use should take into consideration the patient's age, severity of liver disease, likelihood of response, safety and efficacy of the drug, potential for selection of resistant HBV strains, potential for adverse reactions, costs, patient's pregnancy potential, and patient and provider preferences.

The American Association for the Study of Liver Diseases (AASLD) states that, unless contraindicated or ineffective, the drugs of choice for initial treatment of chronic HBV infection in patients with compensated liver disease are peginterferon alfa, entecavir, or tenofovir. Although efficacy of nonconjugated interferon alfa and peginterferon alfa are considered similar for treatment of chronic HBV infection, the dosing schedule for peginterferon alfa may be more convenient and is generally preferred instead of interferon alfa.

The AASLD states that treatment of HBV infection is indicated if the risk of liver-related morbidity and mortality in the near future (5–10 years) and the likelihood of achieving sustained HBV suppression during continued treatment are high. Treatment also is indicated if the risk of liver-related morbidity and mortality in the foreseeable future (10–20 years) and the likelihood of achieving sustained HBV suppression after a defined course of therapy are high. These experts state that treatment is *not* indicated if both the risk of liver-related morbidity or mortality in the next 20 years and the likelihood of achieving sustained HBV suppression after a defined course of treatment are low.

The manufacturer states that safety and efficacy of peginterferon alfa-2a have not been established for treatment of chronic HBV infection in patients coinfected with hepatitis C virus (HCV) or human immunodeficiency virus (HIV). Some experts suggest that peginterferon alfa is an alternative for treatment of HBV infection in some adults with HIV coinfection.

Treatment of chronic HBV infection is complex and rapidly evolving. Specialized references should be consulted for specific information regarding the evaluation and management of individuals with chronic HBV infection, including information on the choice of treatment regimens.

Clinical Experience Safety and efficacy of peginterferon alfa-2a for treatment of chronic HBV infection were assessed in 2 controlled clinical trials in adults with compensated liver disease and evidence of HBV replication (study 8 and study 9). Patients were randomized to receive 48 weeks of treatment with peginterferon alfa-2a monotherapy (180 mcg once weekly), peginterferon alfa-2a (180 mcg once weekly) in conjunction with oral lamivudine (100 mg once daily), or lamivudine monotherapy (100 mg once daily). At study entry, all patients had serum ALT concentrations between 1–10 times the upper limit of normal (ULN) and liver biopsy findings compatible with chronic hepatitis. Patients in study 8 were HBeAg-positive and had serum HBV levels exceeding 500,000 copies/mL; patients in study 9 were HBeAg-negative and had serum HBV levels exceeding 100,000 copies/mL.

At 24 weeks after treatment was completed (week 72), data from study 8 indicated that HBeAg seroconversion occurred in 32% of patients treated with peginterferon alfa-2a monotherapy compared with 19% of patients treated with lamivudine monotherapy. An HBV DNA response (HBV levels less than 100,000 copies/mL for HBeAg-positive patients and less than 20,000 copies/mL for HBe-Ag-negative patients) and ALT normalization occurred in 32 and 41%, respectively, of patients treated with peginterferon alfa-2a compared with 22 and 28%, respectively, of those treated with lamivudine.

Data from study 9 indicated that an HBV DNA response and ALT normalization occurred in 43 and 59%, respectively, of patients treated with peginterferon alfa-2a compared with 29 and 44%, respectively, of patients treated with lamivudine.

In studies 8 and 9, histologic improvement was evident on liver biopsy in 41 and 48%, respectively, of patients treated with peginterferon alfa-2a and 40 and 41%, respectively, of patients treated with lamivudine. Conclusions regarding comparative efficacy based on results of these studies are limited by the different mechanisms of action of peginterferon alfa-2a and lamivudine; most treatment effects of lamivudine are unlikely to persist 24 weeks after therapy is withdrawn. Concomitant use of peginterferon alfa-2a and lamivudine did not result in any additional sustained response compared with peginterferon monotherapy.

■ **Chronic Hepatitis C Virus Infection** Peginterferon alfa-2a (Pegasys®) and peginterferon alfa-2b (PegIntron®) are used in conjunction with oral ribavirin for treatment of chronic HCV infection in adults and pediatric patients with compensated liver disease. Because peginterferon alfa in conjunction with oral ribavirin is associated with higher response rates than nonconjugated interferon alfa in conjunction with oral ribavirin, peginterferon alfa (not interferon alfa) is recommended when an interferon is used for treatment of chronic HCV infection.

Peginterferon alfa (alfa-2a, alfa-2b) has been used alone for treatment of chronic HCV infection in patients with compensated liver disease; however, peginterferon alfa in conjunction with oral ribavirin is associated with substantially better response rates than peginterferon alfa monotherapy. Although the manufacturers state that peginterferon alfa without ribavirin should be considered *only* for treatment of chronic HCV infection in previously untreated patients when there are contraindications to or clinically important intolerance to oral ribavirin, experts state that peginterferon alfa monotherapy is *not* recommend for treatment of chronic HCV infection at any time.

Safety and efficacy of peginterferon alfa alone or in conjunction with oral ribavirin have not been established for treatment of chronic HCV infection in patients with HBV coinfection or in liver or other organ transplant recipients.

Peginterferon alfa usually is used in conjunction with oral ribavirin in multiple-drug regimens that include an HCV direct-acting antiviral (DAA). The most appropriate multiple-drug regimen depends on the specific HCV genotype and patient population involved. For the treatment of chronic HCV genotype 1 infection, peginterferon alfa has been used in conjunction with oral ribavirin and either simeprevir (an HCV protease inhibitor) or sofosbuvir (an HCV polymerase inhibitor). For the treatment of chronic HCV infection caused by other genotypes (e.g., genotypes 3, 4, 5, or 6), peginterferon alfa has been used in conjunction with oral ribavirin and sofosbuvir.

The goal of antiviral therapy in patients with chronic HCV infection is to achieve sustained suppression of HCV replication and prevent HCV-related complications (e.g., necroinflammation, fibrosis, cirrhosis, hepatocellular carcinoma) and death. Because chronic HCV infection evolves slowly over several decades, it is difficult to demonstrate that treatment prevents complications of liver disease. Short-term treatment outcomes are measured biochemically (normalization of serum ALT levels), virologically (absence of serum HCV RNA), and histologically (greater than 2-point improvement in necroinflammatory score with no worsening in fibrosis score). The most important virologic response is sustained virologic response (SVR), defined as the absence of HCV RNA from serum by a sensitive PCR assay 24 weeks following discontinuance of treatment. This is generally regarded as a "virologic cure," although liver cancer has been identified years later, especially if cirrhosis existed at the time SVR was achieved. Decisions regarding treatment of chronic HCV infection should be individualized, taking into consideration the severity of liver disease, HCV genotype, treatment history, potential for serious adverse reactions, likelihood of treatment response, presence of coexisting conditions, and the patient's readiness for treatment.

Because treatment of chronic HCV is complex and rapidly evolving, it is recommended that treatment be directed by clinicians who are familiar with the disease and that a specialist be consulted to obtain the most up-to-date information. Information from the American Association for the Study of Liver Diseases (AASLD), Infectious Diseases Society of America (IDSA), and International Antiviral Society–USA (IAS–USA) regarding diagnosis and management of HCV infection, including recommendations for initial treatment, is available at http://www.hcvguidelines.org.

Individuals Coinfected with HCV and HIV Because HCV infection tends to progress more rapidly in patients coinfected with HIV, the AASLD, US Centers for Disease Control and Prevention (CDC), National Institutes of Health (NIH), HIV Medicine Association of the Infectious Diseases Society of America (IDSA), and other experts state that all HIV-infected patients should be periodically screened for HCV and those coinfected with HCV should be offered treatment, provided there are no contraindications to such therapy. Optimal timing of initiation of HCV treatment relative to antiretroviral therapy has not been established. There is some evidence that HIV-infected patients with $CD4^+$ T-cell counts less than 200 cells/mm^3 receiving an HCV treatment regimen of oral ribavirin used in conjunction with peginterferon alfa have lower HCV treatment response rates and increased rates of toxicity compared to HIV-infected patients with $CD4^+$ T-cell counts exceeding 350 cells/mm^3. Some experts recommend that HCV treatment in patients with HCV and HIV coinfection should not be initiated until after at least 6 months of antiretroviral therapy, and state that initiation of HCV treatment is not usually recommended in HIV-infected patients with $CD4^+$ T-cell counts less than 200 cells/mm^3. The US Department of Health and Human Services (HHS) Panel on Antiretroviral Guidelines for Adults and Adolescents states that antiretroviral therapy should be initiated in all patients with HCV and HIV coinfection, including those with high $CD4^+$ T-cell counts and cirrhosis. In patients with HCV and HIV coinfection who have low $CD4^+$ T-cell counts (e.g., less than 200 cells/mm^3), the HHS panel recommends *prompt* initiation of antiretroviral therapy and states that initiation of HCV treatment may be delayed until the patient is stable on the HIV treatment regimen.

Peginterferon alfa has been used in multiple-drug regimens for the treatment of chronic HCV infection in patients coinfected with HIV. Peginterferon alfa-2a (Pegasys®) is labeled by the US Food and Drug Administration (FDA) for use alone or in conjunction with oral ribavirin for treatment of chronic HCV infection in adults with compensated liver disease who are coinfected with HIV and have clinically stable HIV disease with CD4+ T-cell counts exceeding 100 cells/mm³. Although the manufacturer of peginterferon alfa-2b (PegIntron®) states that safety and efficacy alone or in conjunction with oral ribavirin have not been established in patients with HCV and HIV coinfection, experts state that either peginterferon alfa-2a or peginterferon alfa-2b can be used in coinfected patients. For treatment of chronic HCV infection in HIV-infected adults, adolescents, and children 3 years of age or older, experts recommend that peginterferon alfa be used in conjunction with oral ribavirin and state that peginterferon alfa monotherapy should be used only if ribavirin is contraindicated. There is evidence that HCV treatment regimens that only include ribavirin and peginterferon alfa are associated with poor SVR rates, especially in patients with HCV and HIV coinfection.

Multiple-drug regimens that include various combinations of peginterferon alfa, oral ribavirin, and an HCV DAA (e.g., simeprevir, sofosbuvir) have been used for treatment of chronic HCV infection in patients coinfected with HIV. The most appropriate regimen depends on the HCV genotype and whether the patient is treatment naive or has relapsed after prior HCV treatment. Some experts state that multiple-drug regimens recommended for treatment of chronic HCV infection in patients coinfected with HIV are the same as those recommended for individuals without HIV infection, provided that potential drug interactions and overlapping toxicities between drugs in the HCV treatment regimen and drugs in the antiretroviral regimen are taken into consideration.

If peginterferon alfa is included in the HCV treatment regimen, potential drug interactions with HIV nucleoside reverse transcriptase inhibitors (e.g., didanosine, lamivudine, stavudine, zidovudine) should be considered. (See HIV Nucleoside Reverse Transcriptase Inhibitors [NRTIs] under Drug Interactions: Antiretroviral Agents.)

Treatment of HCV in patients coinfected with HIV can be complicated because of high pill burden, overlapping toxicities, and drug interactions. Because treatment in patients coinfected with HCV and HIV is complex and rapidly evolving, current recommendations regarding management of HCV infection (http://www.hcvguidelines.org) and management of HIV infection (http://www.aidsinfo.nih.gov) should be considered and expert consultation is recommended.

■ **Acute Hepatitis C Virus Infection** Peginterferon alfa (alfa-2a, alfa-2b) has been used alone or in conjunction with oral ribavirin for the treatment of acute HCV infection† in an attempt to prevent progression to chronic HCV infection.

There is evidence that patients with acute HCV infection have higher treatment response rates than those with chronic HCV infection and that treatment of the acute infection can reduce the risk that the disease will evolve to chronic infection. SVR rates of 62–90% or higher have been reported when peginterferon alfa or nonconjugated interferon alfa monotherapy or peginterferon alfa in conjunction with oral ribavirin was used for treatment of acute HCV infection. However, approximately 10–50% of patients with acute HCV infection have self-limited disease and spontaneous clearance of the virus without treatment; the spontaneous resolution rate varies depending on whether the acute infection is asymptomatic or symptomatic, the route of HCV transmission, and age at which the infection was acquired.

The optimum regimen (including dosage and duration of therapy) and optimum time to initiate treatment in such patients have not been established. To allow for spontaneous resolution, some experts suggest that it might be reasonable to delay initiation of treatment of acute HCV infection (especially in symptomatic patients) for 8–12 weeks after acute onset of hepatitis, unless HCV RNA levels are high and not declining; others suggest monitoring for 8–20 weeks after initial exposure. Although some experts recommend that treatment be offered to all HIV-infected patients with acute HCV infection, others recommend observing HIV-infected patients for 3–6 months before initiating HCV treatment, especially patients more likely to have spontaneous clearance after acute HCV infection (e.g., those with C/C IL28B genotype). Consultation with a specialist is advised to obtain the most up-to-date information regarding treatment of acute HCV infection.

■ **Postexposure Prophylaxis following Exposure to Hepatitis C Virus** Although peginterferon alfa-2b has been used in an attempt to provide postexposure prophylaxis of HCV† following occupational exposures to an HCV-positive source, such postexposure prophylaxis is not recommended.

The risk of HCV transmission following a single percutaneous exposure to an HCV-positive source is low, and the average incidence of anti-HCV seroconversion after accidental percutaneous exposure to an HCV-positive source has been estimated to be 1.8% (range: 0–7%). Mucous membrane or nonintact skin exposures to HCV-positive blood rarely result in HCV transmission and, although the risk from exposure to tissues or fluids other than HCV-infected blood has not been quantified, it is expected to be substantially lower than blood exposures.

The CDC and other experts state that postexposure prophylaxis with antiviral agents (e.g., peginterferon alfa or interferon alfa with or without oral ribavirin), immune globulin, or immunomodulators is not recommended following occupational or other exposures known or likely to involve an HCV-positive source, including penetrating injuries or nonintact skin exposures in bombings or other mass casualty settings. Postexposure management in the exposed individual involves early identification of HCV infection and appropriate antiviral treatment if indicated. To identify whether HCV infection occurred, some experts suggest evaluating ALT concentrations and anti-HCV at the time of exposure (within 7–14 days) and 4–6 months later and testing for HCV RNA at 4–6 weeks or at 2-week intervals.

■ **Chronic Hepatitis D Virus Infection** Peginterferon alfa-2b has been used with some limited success for the treatment of chronic HDV infection† in adults coinfected with HBV. Peginterferon alfa has been used alone or in conjunction with ribavirin or other antivirals (e.g., adefovir dipivoxil, emtricitabine, tenofovir disoproxil fumarate) in patients with HDV and HBV coinfections.

HDV infection only occurs in individuals infected with HBV since HDV depends on HBV for production of envelope proteins. HDV infection can be acquired as a coinfection with HBV, resulting in a more severe acute hepatitis with a higher mortality rate than acute HBV infection alone. HDV infection also can occur as a superinfection in HBV carriers and manifests as severe acute hepatitis in previously asymptomatic HBV carriers or as an exacerbation of underlying chronic HBV infection. HDV superinfection in HBV carriers almost always results in chronic infection with both viruses and is associated with a high risk of cirrhosis, hepatic decompensation, and hepatocellular carcinoma.

■ **Hepatitis E Virus Infection** Peginterferon alfa (alfa-2a, alfa-2b) has been used alone or in conjunction with ribavirin for treatment of chronic hepatitis E virus (HEV) infection†.

Chronic HEV infection has been reported almost exclusively among immunocompromised individuals, including solid organ transplant recipients, patients receiving cancer chemotherapy, and HIV-infected patients. Although optimal treatment of chronic HEV infection has not been identified, there is evidence that peginterferon alfa therapy is associated with a sustained virologic response in some solid organ transplant patients.

■ **Coronavirus Infections** ***Middle East Respiratory Syndrome (MERS)*** Peginterferon alfa (alfa-2a) has been used in conjunction with oral ribavirin for the treatment of Middle East respiratory syndrome† (MERS) caused by the Middle East respiratory syndrome coronavirus (MERS-CoV).

No specific treatment for MERS-CoV infection has been identified. In a retrospective, cohort study that included 44 patients with laboratory-confirmed MERS, the 14-day survival rate from the date of diagnosis was 70% in patients who were treated with a regimen of oral ribavirin and peginterferon alfa-2a (initiated within a median of 3 days from time of diagnosis; range 0–8 days) in addition to usual supportive care compared with a 14-day survival rate of 29% in the comparator group that only received usual supportive care. However, the 28-day survival rate was only 30% in patients who received the ribavirin and peginterferon alfa-2a treatment regimen compared with 17% in the comparator group. For additional information on MERS and MERS-CoV, see Middle East Respiratory Syndrome (MERS) under Uses: Coronavirus Infections in Ribavirin 8:18.32.

Information regarding evaluation, diagnosis, and management of MERS-CoV infection and guidance for individuals traveling to areas where MERS has been reported (e.g., the Middle East) is available at the CDC website at http://www.cdc.gov/coronavirus/mers/.

Dosage and Administration

■ **General** Several peginterferon alfa subtypes (alfa-2a, alfa-2b), dosage forms, and strengths are commercially available, and care should be taken to ensure that the correct preparation is used.

Because there are differences in the recommended indications and in the potencies and dosages between the commercially available peginterferon alfa preparations, it is recommended that the peginterferon alfa preparation selected for the patient be used throughout the treatment regimen. Patients should be cautioned *not* to change brands of peginterferon alfa without consulting their clinician.

■ **Reconstitution and Administration** Peginterferon alfa-2a (Pegasys®) and peginterferon alfa-2b (PegIntron®) are administered by subcutaneous injection once weekly.

Subcutaneous injections of peginterferon alfa-2a should be made into the abdomen or thigh. Subcutaneous injections of peginterferon alfa-2b should be made into the abdomen, outer surface of the upper arm, or thigh. Areas of the navel and waistline should be avoided. Injection sites should be rotated.

Peginterferon alfa-2a and peginterferon alfa-2b may be *self-administered* if the clinician determines that the patient and/or their caregiver are competent to safely administer the drug after appropriate training and with medical follow-up as necessary. Patients and/or their caregivers who administer peginterferon alfa in a home setting should be carefully instructed in the proper administration of the drug, including aseptic techniques. They should be cautioned against reuse of syringes and needles and should be supplied with a puncture-resistant container for the proper, safe disposal of such equipment after use. In addition, they should be provided with instructions on the proper disposal of full disposal containers.

Peginterferon Alfa-2a (Pegasys®) Peginterferon alfa-2a is administered undiluted.

Vials, prefilled syringes, and autoinjectors containing peginterferon alfa-2a should be stored in a refrigerator at 2–8°C, protected from light, and should not be frozen or shaken. Peginterferon alfa-2a should be allowed to reach room temperature before administration, but should not be kept out of a refrigerator for more than 24 hours.

Peginterferon alfa-2a should be inspected visually for particulate matter and discoloration prior to administration. The solution should be clear and colorless to light yellow, and should not be used if discolored or cloudy or if particulates are present. Vials, prefilled syringes, and autoinjectors containing peginterferon alfa-2a are for single-use only and any unused portions should be discarded.

Peginterferon Alfa-2b (PegIntron®) Peginterferon alfa-2b lyophilized powder for injection must be reconstituted prior to administration using *only* sterile water for injection. Prior to reconstitution, peginterferon alfa-2b should appear as a white to off-white powder or a tablet-shaped solid that is whole or in pieces. Strict aseptic technique must be observed since the drug and diluent contain no preservative.

Commercially available single-dose prefilled dual-chamber injection pens containing lyophilized peginterferon alfa-2b and sterile water for injection should be stored at 2–8°C and should not be frozen or exposed to heat. Peginterferon alfa-2b in the injection pens should be reconstituted according to the manufacturer's directions. The injection pen may be gently inverted to mix the contents, but should not be shaken. The needle provided by the manufacturer should be attached and the appropriate dose calibrated according to the manufacturer's directions.

Commercially available single-dose vials containing lyophilized peginterferon alfa-2b should be stored at 25°C, but may be exposed to temperatures ranging from 15–30°C. The vials should not be frozen or exposed to heat. Vials labeled as containing 50, 80, 120, or 150 mcg of peginterferon alfa-2b per 0.5 mL contain 74, 118.4, 177.6, or 222 mcg of the drug, respectively. The single-dose vials should be reconstituted by slowly adding 0.7 mL of the sterile water diluent provided by the manufacturer and gently swirling the vial; the vial should not be shaken.

Reconstituted peginterferon alfa-2b solutions should be clear and colorless and should be inspected visually for particulate matter and discoloration prior to administration; solutions should not be used if discolored or cloudy or if particulates are present.

Because peginterferon alfa-2b solutions contain no preservatives, reconstituted solutions in single-dose injection pens or single-dose vials should be used immediately, but may be stored for up to 24 hours at 2–8°C. Once the reconstituted vial has been entered, any unused portions should be discarded and should not be pooled. The single-dose injection pens should not be reused; any unused portion should be discarded.

■ Dosage

Modification of peginterferon dosage may be necessary if adverse effects occur. (See Dosage and Administration: Dosage Modification for Toxicity.)

Adult Dosage **Chronic HBV Infection (Peginterferon Alfa-2a [Pegasys®] Monotherapy).** When peginterferon alfa-2a is used for treatment of chronic hepatitis B virus (HBV) infection in adults, the recommended dosage is 180 mcg once weekly by subcutaneous injection for 48 weeks.

Chronic HCV Infection (Concomitant Peginterferon Alfa-2a [Pegasys®] and Oral Ribavirin). When peginterferon alfa-2a is used in conjunction with oral ribavirin for initial treatment of chronic hepatitis C virus (HCV) infection in adults with HCV monoinfection (without human immunodeficiency virus [HIV] infection), the usual dosage is 180 mcg once weekly by subcutaneous injection. The recommended duration of concomitant peginterferon alfa-2a and oral ribavirin treatment depends on HCV genotype. (See Table 1.)

Table 1. Adult Dosage of Peginterferon Alfa-2a (Pegasys®) for Concomitant Use with Oral Ribavirin for Chronic HCV Monoinfection

HCV Genotype	Pegasys® Dosage	Duration
1 (when used without HCV NS3/4A protease inhibitor)	180 mcg once weekly	48 weeks
4	180 mcg once weekly	48 weeks
2,3	180 mcg once weekly	24 weeks
5,6	Data insufficient to make dosage recommendations	

When peginterferon alfa-2a is used in conjunction with oral ribavirin for initial treatment of chronic HCV infection in adults with HCV and HIV coinfection, the usual dosage of peginterferon alfa-2a is 180 mcg once weekly by subcutaneous injection for a duration of 48 weeks, regardless of HCV genotype.

Consideration can be given to discontinuing HCV treatment if HCV RNA levels have not decreased at least 2 $\log_{10}$ from baseline at week 12 or are still detectable after 24 weeks of treatment.

The manufacturer states that safety and efficacy of peginterferon alfa-2a beyond 48 weeks of therapy have not been established.

For information on ribavirin dosage for concomitant use with peginterferon alfa for treatment of chronic HCV infection, see Chronic Hepatitis C Virus Infection under Dosage and Administration: Dosage, in Ribavirin 8:18.32.

For information on dosage of HCV direct-acting antivirals (DAAs) used in conjunction with peginterferon alfa and ribavirin for treatment of chronic HCV infection, including simeprevir (an HCV protease inhibitor) or sofosbuvir (an HCV polymerase inhibitor), see the individual monographs in HCV Antivirals 8:18.40.

Chronic HCV Infection (Concomitant Peginterferon Alfa-2b [PegIntron®] and Oral Ribavirin). When peginterferon alfa-2b is used in conjunction with oral ribavirin for treatment of chronic HCV infection in adults, the usual dosage is 1.5 mcg/kg once weekly by subcutaneous injection.

The appropriate volume of reconstituted peginterferon alfa-2b to be administered in conjunction with oral ribavirin is based on the specific single-dose prefilled injection pen or vial strength used and the patient's weight. (See Table 2.)

Table 2. Adult Dosage of Peginterferon Alfa-2b (PegIntron®) for Concomitant Use with Oral Ribavirin for Chronic HCV Infection

Weight	Prefilled Injection Pen or Vial Strength (mcg per 0.5 mL)	Once-Weekly Dose (mcg)	Volume of Reconstituted PegIntron® to Administer (mL)
less than 40 kg	50	50	0.5
40–50 kg	80	64	0.4
51–60 kg	80	80	0.5
61–75 kg	120	96	0.4
76–85 kg	120	120	0.5
86–105 kg	150	150	0.5
greater than 105 kg	Varies	Calculate based on weight	Volume may require more than 1 vial

In previously untreated (treatment-naive) adults, the usual duration of peginterferon alfa-2b and oral ribavirin treatment is 24 weeks for HCV genotype 2 or 3 or 48 weeks for HCV genotype 1. Consideration should be given to discontinuing HCV treatment if HCV RNA has not decreased at least 2 $\log_{10}$ from baseline at week 12 or remains detectable after 24 weeks of treatment.

For retreatment in adults following failure of prior therapy, the usual duration of treatment is 48 weeks regardless of HCV genotype. Consideration should be given to discontinuing HCV treatment if HCV RNA levels are still detectable at week 12 or if HCV RNA remains detectable after 24 weeks of treatment.

For information on ribavirin dosage for concomitant use with peginterferon alfa for treatment of chronic HCV infection, see Chronic Hepatitis C Virus Infection under Dosage and Administration: Dosage, in Ribavirin 8:18.32.

For information on dosage of HCV DAAs used in conjunction with peginterferon alfa and ribavirin for treatment of chronic HCV infection, including simeprevir (an HCV protease inhibitor) or sofosbuvir (an HCV polymerase inhibitor), see the individual monographs in HCV Antivirals 8:18.40.

Chronic HCV Infection (Peginterferon Alfa-2a [Pegasys®] Monotherapy). If peginterferon alfa-2a monotherapy is used for treatment of chronic HCV infection in previously untreated (treatment-naive) adults who cannot receive concomitant oral ribavirin, the usual dosage is 180 mcg once weekly by subcutaneous injection for 48 weeks. This dosage is recommended for adults without HIV coinfection and for those with HIV coinfection who have clinically stable HIV disease with $CD4^+$ T-cell counts exceeding 100 cells/mm³.

The manufacturer states that safety and efficacy of peginterferon alfa-2a beyond 48 weeks of therapy have not been established.

Chronic HCV Infection (Peginterferon Alfa-2b [PegIntron®] Monotherapy). If peginterferon alfa-2b monotherapy is used for treatment of chronic HCV infection in previously untreated (treatment-naive) adults who cannot receive concomitant oral ribavirin, the usual dosage is 1 mcg/kg once weekly by subcutaneous injection for 1 year.

The appropriate volume of reconstituted peginterferon alfa-2b to be administered is based on the specific single-dose prefilled injection pen or vial strength used and the patient's weight. (See Table 3.)

Table 3. Adult Dosage of Peginterferon Alfa-2b (PegIntron®) Monotherapy for Chronic HCV Infection

Weight (kg)	Prefilled Injection Pen or Vial Strength (mcg per 0.5 mL)	Once-Weekly Dose (mcg)	Volume of Reconstituted PegIntron® to Administer (mL)
45 or less	50	40	0.4
46–56	50	50	0.5
57–72	80	64	0.4
73–88	80	80	0.5
89–106	120	96	0.4
107–136	120	120	0.5
137–160	150	150	0.5

Acute HCV Infection (Peginterferon Alfa-2a [Pegasys®]). If peginterferon alfa-2a is used for the treatment of acute HCV infection†, some experts recommend a dosage of 180 mcg by subcutaneous injection once weekly for 24 weeks.

The optimum time to initiate treatment of acute HCV infection and optimum regimen (e.g., with or without oral ribavirin, dosage, duration of treatment) have not been established. Depending on the HCV genotype, HCV RNA response, and coexisting conditions (e.g., HIV infection), the recommended duration of treatment has ranged from 12–48 weeks.

If treatment is initiated and a response is not obtained, some experts recommend that patients be retreated using the standard of care for chronic HCV infection.

Acute HCV Infection (Peginterferon Alfa-2b [PegIntron®]). If peginterferon alfa-2b is used for the treatment of acute HCV infection†, some experts recommend a dosage of 1.5 mcg/kg by subcutaneous injection once weekly for 24 weeks.

The optimum time to initiate treatment of acute HCV infection and optimum regimen (e.g., with or without oral ribavirin, dosage, duration of treatment) have not been established. Depending on the HCV genotype, HCV RNA response, and coexisting conditions (e.g., HIV infection), the recommended duration of treatment has ranged from 12–48 weeks. If treatment is initiated and a response is not obtained, some experts recommend that patients be retreated using the standard of care for chronic HCV infection.

Chronic HDV Infection (Peginterferon Alfa-2a [Pegasys®]). For the treatment of chronic hepatitis D virus (HDV) infection†, peginterferon alfa-2a has been given in a dosage of 180 mcg by subcutaneous injection once weekly for 48 weeks.

Chronic HDV Infection (Peginterferon Alfa-2b [PegIntron®]). For the treatment of chronic HDV infection†, peginterferon alfa-2b has been given in a dosage of 1.5 mcg/kg by subcutaneous injection once weekly for 48 or 52 weeks.

Pediatric Dosage **Chronic HCV Infection (Concomitant Peginterferon Alfa-2a [Pegasys®] and Oral Ribavirin).** When peginterferon alfa-2a is used in conjunction with oral ribavirin for treatment of chronic HCV infection in pediatric patients 5 years of age and older, the usual dosage is 180 mcg/1.73 m^2 × body surface area (BSA) once weekly (maximum 180 mcg) by subcutaneous injection.

The recommended duration of treatment is 24 weeks for HCV genotype 2 or 3 and 48 weeks for other HCV genotypes.

For information on ribavirin dosage for concomitant use with peginterferon alfa for treatment of chronic HCV infection, see Chronic Hepatitis C Virus Infection under Dosage and Administration: Dosage, in Ribavirin 8:18.32.

Chronic HCV Infection (Concomitant Peginterferon Alfa-2b [PegIntron®] and Oral Ribavirin). When peginterferon alfa-2b is used in conjunction with oral ribavirin for initial treatment of chronic HCV infection in pediatric patients 3–17 years of age, the usual dosage is 60 mcg/m^2 once weekly by subcutaneous injection. Patients who reach their 18th birthday during treatment should continue receiving the pediatric dosage regimen for the remaining duration of treatment.

The recommended duration of treatment is 24 weeks for HCV genotype 2 or 3 and 48 weeks for genotype 1. With the exception of HCV genotypes 2 and 3, consideration can be given to discontinuing HCV treatment if HCV RNA has not decreased at least 2 $\log_{10}$ from baseline at week 12 or remains detectable after 24 weeks of treatment.

For information on ribavirin dosage for concomitant use with peginterferon alfa, see Chronic Hepatitis C Virus Infection under Dosage and Administration: Dosage, in Ribavirin 8:18.32.

■ Dosage Modification for Toxicity

Dosage of peginterferon alfa (alfa-2a, alfa-2b) should be adjusted in patients who develop adverse neuropsychiatric (i.e., depression) or hematologic effects, or other serious adverse effects or laboratory abnormalities. If serious adverse effects or laboratory abnormalities occur during concomitant peginterferon alfa and oral ribavirin therapy, dosage of one or both drugs should be modified, if appropriate, until the adverse reactions abate. If intolerance persists after dosage adjustments, both peginterferon alfa and oral ribavirin should be discontinued.

When dosage modification of peginterferon alfa-2a (Pegasys®) is required in adults because of adverse reactions (clinical and/or laboratory), an initial dosage reduction to 135 mcg once weekly is recommended; a further reduction to 90 mcg once weekly may be needed if the adverse reaction persists or recurs. If the adverse reaction abates, re-escalation of dosage may be considered.

If dosage modification of peginterferon alfa-2a (Pegasys®) is required in pediatric patients because of moderate to severe adverse reactions (clinical and/or laboratory), an initial dosage reduction to 135 mcg/1.73 m^2 × BSA usually is adequate; further dosage reductions to 90 mcg/1.73 m^2 × BSA or 45 mcg/1.73 m^2 × BSA may be needed in some cases. Up to 3 dosage modifications for toxicity can be made in pediatric patients before discontinuance of peginterferon alfa-2a and oral ribavirin therapy is considered.

If dosage modification of peginterferon alfa-2b (PegIntron®) is required because of adverse reactions in adults receiving concomitant therapy with peginterferon alfa-2b and oral ribavirin, a 2-step decrease from the original dosage of 1.5 mcg/kg once weekly is recommended (i.e., dosage should be decreased to 1 mcg/kg once weekly and then, if needed, further decreased to 0.5 mcg/kg once weekly). If dosage modification is required in adults receiving peginterferon alfa-2b monotherapy, the original dosage of 1 mcg/kg once weekly should be reduced to 0.5 mcg/kg once weekly.

If dosage modification of peginterferon alfa-2b (PegIntron®) is required in pediatric patients because of adverse reactions, a 2-step decrease from the original dosage of 60 mcg/m^2 once weekly is recommended (i.e., dosage should be decreased to 40 mcg/m^2 once weekly and then, if needed, further decreased to 20 mcg/m^2 once weekly).

For information on ribavirin dosage modification, see Dosage and Administration: Dosage in Ribavirin 8:18.32.

Depression **Adults.** If mild depression occurs in an adult receiving peginterferon alfa, usual dosage of the drug can be continued, but the patient should be evaluated once weekly (by office visit and/or phone). If moderate depression develops, dosage of the drug should be reduced and the patient evaluated once weekly (office visit at least every other week). If symptoms improve with the reduced dosage and remain stable for 4 weeks, then the reduced dosage can be continued or dosage can be increased to the usual dosage.

If moderate depression develops in an adult receiving peginterferon alfa-2a (Pegasys®), dosage should be decreased to 135 mcg once weekly (a reduction to 90 mcg once weekly may be needed in some cases).

If moderate depression develops in an adult receiving peginterferon alfa-2b (PegIntron®) concomitantly with oral ribavirin, peginterferon alfa-2b dosage should be reduced to 1 mcg/kg once weekly and, if needed, to 0.5 mcg/kg once weekly. If moderate depression develops in an adult receiving peginterferon alfa-2b monotherapy, dosage should be decreased to 0.5 mcg/kg once weekly.

If severe depression develops, peginterferon alfa should be permanently discontinued and psychiatric consultation provided.

Pediatric Patients. If depression occurs in pediatric patients receiving peginterferon alfa, the patient should be evaluated using the same criteria recommended for adults.

If a pediatric patient develops moderate depression while receiving peginterferon alfa-2a (Pegasys®), dosage should be reduced to 135 mcg/1.73 m^2 × BSA; further dosage reductions to 90 mcg/1.73 m^2 × BSA or 45 mcg/1.73 m^2 × BSA may be needed in some cases.

If a pediatric patient develops moderate depression while receiving peginterferon alfa-2b (PegIntron®), dosage should be decreased to 40 mcg/m^2 once weekly and, if needed, to 20 mcg/m^2 once weekly.

If severe depression develops, peginterferon alfa should be permanently discontinued and psychiatric consultation provided.

Hematologic Effects **Adults.** Dosage of peginterferon alfa-2a (Pegasys®) should be decreased to 135 mcg once weekly in adults with an absolute neutrophil count (ANC) less than 750/mm^3. If ANC is less than 500 cells/mm^3, peginterferon alfa-2a should be discontinued until ANC exceeds 1000 cells/mm^3; the drug can then be resumed at a dosage of 90 mcg once weekly with monitoring of the ANC. Peginterferon alfa-2a dosage also should be decreased to 90 mcg once weekly in adults with platelet counts less than 50,000/mm^3, but should be discontinued in those with platelet counts less than 25,000/mm^3. The manufacturer's information should be consulted for more specific recommendations regarding dosage modification for hematologic effects.

Dosage of peginterferon alfa-2b (PegIntron®) should be decreased in adults with leukocyte counts of 1000 to less than 1500/mm^3, neutrophil counts of 500 to less than 750/mm^3, or platelet counts of 25,000 to less than 50,000/mm^3. Both peginterferon alfa-2b and ribavirin should be permanently discontinued in adults with hemoglobin concentrations less than 8.5 g/dL, leukocyte counts less than 1000/mm^3, neutrophil counts less than 500/mm^3, or platelet counts less than 25,000/mm^3. In adults receiving peginterferon alfa-2b concomitantly with oral ribavirin who have a history of stable cardiac disease, peginterferon alfa-2b dosage should be decreased by 50% if hemoglobin concentrations decrease by 2 g/dL or more during any 4-week period and treatment should be discontinued if hemoglobin concentrations are less than 8.5 g/dL (or less than 12 g/dL after 4 weeks of reduced dosage). The manufacturer's information should be consulted for more specific recommendations regarding dosage modification for hematologic effects.

Pediatric Patients. If a pediatric patient receiving peginterferon alfa-2a (Pegasys®) develops neutropenia (less than 1000/mm^3) or decreased platelet counts (less than 50,000/mm^3), dosage modification or discontinuance is recommended depending on the severity of the hematologic effect. The manufacturer's information should be consulted for more specific recommendations regarding dosage modification for hematologic effects.

If a pediatric patient receiving peginterferon alfa-2b (PegIntron®) develops leukocyte counts of 1000 to less than 1500/mm^3, neutrophil counts of 500 to less than 750/mm^3, or platelet counts of 50,000 to less than 70,000/mm^3, dosage of peginterferon alfa-2b should be decreased. Both peginterferon alfa-2b and ribavirin should be permanently discontinued in pediatric patients who have hemoglobin concentrations less than 8.5 g/dL, leukocyte counts less than 1000/mm^3, neutrophil counts less than 500/mm^3, or platelet counts less than 50,000/mm^3. Pediatric patients with preexisting cardiac conditions should be closely monitored with weekly hematology evaluations if hemoglobin concentration decreases by 2 g/dL or more during any 4-week period and treatment should be discontinued if hemoglobin concentration is less than 8.5 g/dL (or less than 12 g/dL after 4 weeks of reduced dosage). The manufacturer's information should be consulted for more specific recommendations regarding dosage modification for hematologic effects.

■ Special Populations

Hepatic Impairment When peginterferon alfa-2a (Pegasys®) is used for treatment of chronic HBV infection in adults with elevated plasma ALT concentrations (greater than 5 times the upper limit of normal [ULN]), hepatic function should be monitored more frequently and consideration given to either reducing dosage to 135 mcg once weekly or temporarily discontinuing treatment. Treatment can be resumed after ALT flares subside. If ALT increases are persistent or severe (greater than 10 times the ULN), discontinuance of treatment should be considered. If ALT increases are progressive despite dosage reduction or are accompanied by increased bilirubin concentrations or evidence of hepatic decompensation, peginterferon alfa-2a therapy should be discontinued immediately.

When peginterferon alfa-2a is used for treatment of chronic HCV infection in adults with progressive ALT increases above baseline values, dosage should be reduced to 135 mcg once weekly and hepatic function monitored more frequently. Treatment can be resumed after ALT flares subside. If ALT increases are progressive despite dosage reduction or are accompanied by increased bilirubin concentrations or evidence of hepatic decompensation, peginterferon alfa-2a therapy should be discontinued immediately.

Renal Impairment When peginterferon alfa-2a (Pegasys®) is used in adults, those with creatinine clearances of 30–50 mL/minute can receive the usual dosage of 180 mcg once weekly, but dosage should be reduced to 135 mcg once weekly in those with creatinine clearance less than 30 mL/minute, including those with end-stage renal disease requiring hemodialysis. Peginterferon alfa-2a dosage in adults should be reduced to 90 mcg if severe adverse reactions or laboratory abnormalities occur; if intolerance persists, the drug should be discontinued. Data are not available regarding use of peginterferon alfa-2a in pediatric patients with renal impairment.

When peginterferon alfa-2b (PegIntron®) monotherapy is used in adults, dosage of the drug should be reduced by 25% in those with moderate renal impairment (creatinine clearance 30–50 mL/minute) and reduced by 50% in those with severe renal impairment (creatinine clearance 10–29 mL/minute), including those on hemodialysis. Peginterferon alfa-2b should be discontinued if renal function decreases during treatment. In pediatric patients receiving peginterferon alfa-2b with ribavirin capsules or oral solution (Rebetol®), both drugs should be discontinued if serum creatinine concentrations exceed 2 mg/dL.

Cautions

■ Contraindications

Known hypersensitivity reactions (e.g., urticaria, angioedema, bronchoconstriction, anaphylaxis, Stevens-Johnson syndrome, toxic epidermal necrolysis) to peginterferon alfa (alfa-2a, alfa-2b) or any ingredient in the formulation.

Autoimmune hepatitis.

Cirrhotic patients with hepatic decompensation (Child-Pugh score exceeding 6, class B and C) prior to or during treatment.

Use of peginterferon alfa-2a in cirrhotic patients with chronic hepatitis C virus (HCV) infection who are coinfected with human immunodeficiency virus (HIV) and have hepatic decompensation (Child-Pugh score 6 or greater) prior to treatment.

Use of peginterferon alfa-2a in neonates and infants (this preparation contains benzyl alcohol). (See Pediatric Use under Warnings/Precautions: Specific Populations, in Cautions.)

Concomitant use of ribavirin is contraindicated in women who are or may become pregnant, men whose female partners are pregnant, patients with known hypersensitivity (e.g., urticaria, angioedema, bronchoconstriction, anaphylaxis) to ribavirin or any ingredient in the formulation, patients with hemoglobinopathies (e.g., thalassemia major, sickle cell anemia), and patients receiving concomitant didanosine therapy, and usually is contraindicated in patients with creatinine clearance less than 50 mL/minute.

■ Warnings/Precautions

Warnings **Serious Disorders.** Peginterferon alfa (alfa-2a, alfa-2b) may cause or aggravate fatal or life-threatening neuropsychiatric, autoimmune, ischemic, and infectious disorders. Patients should be monitored closely with periodic clinical and laboratory evaluations and the drug discontinued in those with persistently severe or worsening signs or symptoms of these disorders. In many, but not all cases, these disorders resolve after peginterferon alfa is discontinued. (See Other Warnings/Precautions under Cautions: Warnings/Precautions.)

Precautions Related to Combination HCV Treatment Regimens. When peginterferon alfa is used in conjunction with oral ribavirin, the cautions, precautions, and contraindications associated with both drugs should be considered. (See Cautions in Ribavirin 8:18.32.)

Ribavirin may cause birth defects and/or death of the fetus. If oral ribavirin is used in conjunction with peginterferon alfa, extreme care must be taken to avoid pregnancy in female patients and in female partners of male patients. (See Cautions: Pregnancy, Fertility, and Lactation, in Ribavirin 8:18.32.)

Ribavirin causes hemolytic anemia, which can result in worsening of cardiac disease.

When peginterferon alfa is used in conjunction with oral ribavirin *and* an HCV direct-acting antiviral (DAA), such as simeprevir (an HCV protease inhibitor) or sofosbuvir (an HCV polymerase inhibitor), the cautions, precautions, and contraindications associated with the HCV DAA also should be considered. (See Cautions in the individual monographs in HCV Antivirals 8:18.40.)

Sensitivity Reactions Serious acute hypersensitivity reactions (urticaria, angioedema, bronchoconstriction, anaphylaxis) and cutaneous eruptions (vesiculobullous eruptions, Stevens Johnson syndrome, toxic epidermal necrolysis, erythroderma) have been reported during interferon alfa therapy.

If a hypersensitivity reaction occurs, peginterferon alfa and oral ribavirin should be discontinued immediately and appropriate supportive and symptomatic care provided. Transient rash does not necessitate interruption of treatment, but the drug should be discontinued if signs or symptoms of severe skin reactions occur.

Other Warnings/Precautions **Neuropsychiatric Effects.** Life-threatening or fatal neuropsychiatric events (suicide, suicidal and homicidal ideation, depression, relapse of drug addiction/overdose, aggressive behavior) have occurred during and after peginterferon alfa therapy in patients with and without a previous psychiatric disorder. Psychoses, hallucinations, aggressive behavior, bipolar disorder, and mania have been reported in patients receiving nonconjugated interferon alfa.

Treatment with interferons may be associated with exacerbated symptoms of psychiatric disorders in patients with both psychiatric and substance use disorders. If interferon treatment is initiated in a patient with current or prior psychiatric conditions or a history of substance use disorders, the need for drug screening and periodic health evaluation, including psychiatric symptom monitoring, should be considered. Early intervention for re-emergence or development of neuropsychiatric symptoms and substance use is recommended.

Peginterferon alfa should be used with extreme caution in any patient with a history of depression or psychiatric disorder. All patients receiving the drug should be monitored for evidence of depression and other psychiatric symptoms. Patients should be advised to report any sign or symptom of depression or suicidal ideation to their clinician.

In patients who develop mild depression, usual dosage of peginterferon alfa may be continued if the patient is evaluated once weekly and depression remains stable or improves. If moderate depression develops, dosage should be reduced and the patient evaluated once weekly. (See Dosage and Administration: Dosage Modification for Toxicity.)

If severe depression occurs, if psychiatric symptoms persist or worsen, or if suicidal ideation or aggressive behavior toward others is identified, peginterferon alfa should be discontinued immediately and psychiatric intervention instituted as indicated. The drug should not be reinitiated in such patients.

Cardiovascular Effects. Cardiovascular events, including hypotension, hypertension, supraventricular arrhythmia, tachycardia, cardiomyopathy, angina pectoris, and myocardial infarction, have been reported in patients receiving peginterferon alfa.

Peginterferon alfa should be used with caution and close monitoring in patients with preexisting cardiovascular disease, including a history of myocardial infarction and cardiac arrhythmias. Such patients should receive ECGs before initiation of therapy.

Because cardiac disease may be worsened by ribavirin-associated anemia, patients with a history of clinically important or unstable cardiac disease should *not* receive oral ribavirin in conjunction with peginterferon alfa. (See Hematologic Effects under Cautions: Oral Administration, in Ribavirin 8:18.32.)

Myelosuppression. Peginterferon alfa suppresses bone marrow function and may cause severe cytopenias. Aplastic anemia has been reported rarely in patients receiving alfa interferons. Concomitant ribavirin may potentiate neutropenia and lymphopenia induced by alfa interferons, including peginterferon alfa.

Severe thrombocytopenia and neutropenia occur more frequently in patients coinfected with HCV and HIV than in those not coinfected with HIV; serious infections or bleeding may occur.

Peginterferon alfa and concomitant oral ribavirin should be used with caution in patients with baseline neutrophil counts less than 1500/mm^3, baseline platelet counts less than 90,000/mm^3, baseline hemoglobin less than 10 g/dL, or a baseline risk of severe anemia (e.g., spherocytosis, history of GI bleeding).

Complete blood counts (CBCs) should be performed prior to and routinely during peginterferon alfa therapy. Dosage should be adjusted or the drug discontinued if necessary. (See Dosage and Administration: Dosage Modification for Toxicity.)

Autoimmune Disease. Development or exacerbation of autoimmune disorders (e.g., thyroiditis, thrombotic or idiopathic thrombocytopenic purpura, rheumatoid arthritis, myositis, interstitial nephritis, hepatitis, systemic lupus erythematosus, psoriasis) has been reported in patients receiving peginterferon alfa.

Peginterferon alfa should be used with caution in patients with autoimmune disorders.

Endocrine and Metabolic Effects. Peginterferon alfa may cause or aggravate hypothyroidism or hyperthyroidism. Hyperglycemia, hypoglycemia, and diabetes mellitus have developed in patients receiving the drug.

Patients with hypothyroidism, hyperthyroidism, or diabetes mellitus whose disease cannot be effectively treated should not receive peginterferon alfa. If these conditions develop during peginterferon alfa therapy and cannot be controlled with pharmacologic therapy, peginterferon alfa should be discontinued.

Ocular Effects. Decrease or loss of vision, retinopathy including macular edema, retinal artery or vein thrombosis, retinal hemorrhages and cotton-wool spots, optic neuritis, papilledema, and serous retinal detachment are induced or aggravated by peginterferon alfa or other interferon alfa preparations.

Baseline ophthalmologic examination should be performed in all patients prior to initiation of peginterferon alfa therapy. Patients with preexisting ophthalmologic disorders (e.g., diabetic or hypertensive retinopathy) should receive ophthalmologic examinations periodically during therapy.

A prompt and complete eye examination should be performed in any patient who develops ocular symptoms.

Peginterferon alfa should be discontinued in patients who develop new or worsening ophthalmologic disorders.

Cerebrovascular Disorders. Ischemic and hemorrhagic cerebrovascular events have been reported in patients receiving alfa interferons, including peginterferon alfa. Such events have occurred in patients with few or no reported risk factors for stroke, including patients younger than 45 years of age. Because these have been spontaneous reports, estimates of frequency and a causal relationship between alfa interferons and these events have not been established.

Hepatic Failure and Hepatitis Exacerbations. Patients with chronic HCV infection and cirrhosis may be at risk of hepatic decompensation and death during interferon alfa (including peginterferon alfa) therapy. Cirrhotic patients with HCV infection who are coinfected with HIV and are receiving highly active antiretroviral therapy (HAART) in conjunction with interferon alfa therapy (with or without oral ribavirin) appear to be at increased risk for development of hepatic decompensation compared with patients not receiving HAART. In most reported cases, patients were receiving HAART that included HIV nucleoside reverse transcriptase inhibitors (abacavir, didanosine, lamivudine, stavudine, zidovudine). (See HIV Nucleoside Reverse Transcriptase Inhibitors [NRTIs] under Drug Interactions: Antiretroviral Agents.)

Clinical status and hepatic function should be closely monitored during peginterferon therapy. Peginterferon alfa should be immediately discontinued if decompensation (Child-Pugh score 6 or greater) occurs.

Patients with chronic hepatitis B virus (HBV) infection may experience HBV exacerbations (characterized by transient and potentially severe increases in serum ALT concentrations) during treatment. Transient increases in ALT concentrations 5–10 times the upper limit of normal (ULN) have been reported in 25–27% of HBV patients receiving peginterferon alfa-2a (Pegasys®). Transient acute exacerbations (flares) of HBV with ALT concentrations greater than 10 times the ULN have been reported in 12% of hepatitis B e antigen (HBeAg)-negative patients and 18% of HBeAg-positive patients during treatment and in 7 and 12%, respectively, after treatment. Marked transaminase flares during treatment have been accompanied by other liver test abnormalities. If ALT flares occur, liver function should be monitored more frequently and a reduction in peginterferon alfa-2a dosage should be considered. If ALT increases are progressive despite dosage reduction or are accompanied by increased bilirubin concentrations or evidence of hepatic decompensation, the drug should be immediately discontinued.

Pulmonary Effects. Potentially life-threatening dyspnea, pulmonary infiltrates, pneumonia, bronchiolitis obliterans, interstitial pneumonitis, pulmonary hypertension, and sarcoidosis may be induced or aggravated by peginterferon alfa.

Peginterferon alfa and oral ribavirin therapy should be discontinued in patients who develop pulmonary infiltrates or pulmonary function impairment. Recurrence of respiratory failure has occurred with interferon rechallenge, and patients should be closely monitored if peginterferon alfa therapy is resumed.

Because fever and other flu-like symptoms have been associated with peginterferon alfa therapy, the drug should be used with caution in patients with debilitating medical conditions, such as those with a history of pulmonary disease (e.g., chronic obstructive pulmonary disease).

Infectious Complications. Serious and severe infections (bacterial, viral, fungal), some of which have resulted in death, have been observed in patients treated with alfa interferons, including peginterferon alfa. While fever may be associated with the flu-like syndrome commonly reported during interferon therapy, other causes of high or persistent fever must be ruled out, particularly in patients with neutropenia.

Appropriate anti-infective therapy should be initiated and discontinuance of peginterferon alfa considered in patients who develop severe infections.

Colitis. Fatal and nonfatal ulcerative and hemorrhagic/ischemic colitis has been observed within 12 weeks of initiation of interferon alfa treatment.

Peginterferon alfa should be discontinued immediately in patients who develop signs and symptoms of colitis (e.g., abdominal pain, bloody diarrhea, fever). Colitis usually resolves within 1–3 weeks after the drug is discontinued.

Pancreatitis. Pancreatitis, sometimes fatal, has occurred in patients receiving interferon alfa.

Peginterferon alfa should be discontinued in patients with signs and symptoms suggestive of pancreatitis; the drug should be permanently discontinue if a diagnosis of pancreatitis is established.

Peripheral Neuropathy. Peripheral neuropathy has been reported in patients receiving telbivudine concomitantly with an interferon alfa. (See Drug Interactions: Telbivudine.)

Triglycerides. Increased triglyceride concentrations have been reported in patients receiving alfa interferons, including peginterferon alfa. Elevated triglycerides should be managed as clinically appropriate.

Consideration should be given to discontinuing peginterferon alfa in patients with persistently elevated triglycerides (e.g., triglycerides exceeding 1000 mg/dL) and symptoms of potential pancreatitis (e.g., abdominal pain, nausea, vomiting).

Dental and Periodontal Disorders. Dental and periodontal disorders have been reported in patients receiving peginterferon alfa concomitantly with oral ribavirin; dry mouth may contribute to damage of teeth and oral mucous membranes during long-term treatment.

Patients should be advised to have regular dental examinations during treatment, brush their teeth thoroughly twice daily, and rinse their mouth thoroughly after vomiting.

Antibody Formation. As with other interferon alfa therapies, neutralizing antibodies may develop in patients receiving peginterferon alfa.

In patients with chronic HBV infection receiving peginterferon alfa-2a, 29% developed binding antibodies (13% developed low-titer neutralizing antibodies).

When antibody formation was assessed in patients with chronic HCV infection receiving peginterferon alfa-2a (with or without oral ribavirin), 9% developed binding antibodies to peginterferon alfa-2a (3% developed low-titer neutralizing antibodies). In HCV patients receiving peginterferon alfa-2b (with or without oral ribavirin), 2% developed low-titer neutralizing antibodies.

The clinical and pathologic importance of development of serum neutralizing antibodies is unknown. No apparent correlation of antibody development to clinical response or adverse events was observed. The percentage of individuals whose test results are considered positive for antibodies is highly dependent on the sensitivity and specificity of assays used. In addition, the observed incidence of antibody positivity in these assays may be influenced by several factors, including sample timing and handling, concomitant drug therapy, and underlying disease. For these reasons, comparison of the incidence of antibodies to different interferon or peginterferon preparations may be misleading.

Organ Transplant Recipients. As with other alfa interferons, liver and renal graft rejections have been reported when peginterferon alfa (with or without oral ribavirin) was used in organ transplant recipients.

Safety and efficacy of peginterferon alfa have not been established in patients with liver or other transplants.

Laboratory Monitoring. Assess organ system functions, including renal, hepatic, and hematopoietic, prior to and during peginterferon alfa therapy (with or without concomitant oral ribavirin).

Periodically monitor triglyceride concentrations.

In clinical studies in adults, CBCs and chemistries (liver function tests, uric acid) were measured at 1, 2, 4, 6, and 8 weeks or 2, 4, 8, and 12 weeks after initiation of therapy and then every 4–6 weeks or more frequently if abnormalities were found. In addition, thyrotropin (thyroid-stimulating hormone, TSH) was measured every 12 weeks.

In a clinical study in pediatric patients, hematologic and chemistry assessments were performed at 1, 3, 5, and 8 weeks after initiation of peginterferon alfa and then every 4 weeks.

Pregnancy screening tests should be performed in all women of childbearing potential prior to initiation of treatment; in those receiving concomitant oral ribavirin, pregnancy tests should be repeated once monthly during and for 6 months after discontinuing therapy.

Specific Populations **Pregnancy.** Peginterferon alfa (alfa-2a, alfa-2b) monotherapy: Category C. (See Users Guide.)

Concomitant peginterferon alfa (alfa-2a, alfa-2b) and oral ribavirin: Category X. (See Users Guide.) (See Concomitant Oral Ribavirin, under Warnings/Precautions: Warnings, in Cautions.)

Lactation. It is not known whether peginterferon alfa is distributed into milk. A decision should be made whether to discontinue nursing or the drug, taking into account the importance of the drug to the woman and potential risks to the infant.

Pediatric Use. Safety and efficacy of peginterferon alfa-2a (Pegasys®) have not been established in children younger than 5 years of age.

Safety and efficacy of peginterferon alfa-2b (PegIntron®) have not been established in children younger than 3 years of age. Concomitant therapy with peginterferon alfa-2b and ribavirin capsules or oral solution (Rebetol®) should not be used in pediatric patients with serum creatinine concentrations greater than 2 mg/dL.

Adverse effects reported in pediatric patients receiving peginterferon alfa generally are similar to those reported in adults receiving the drug and include fever and influenza-like illness, hematologic effects (e.g., neutropenia, thrombocytopenia), upper respiratory tract infection, headache, GI effects (e.g., vomiting, anorexia), rash, pruritus, musculoskeletal pain, fatigue, irritability, insomnia, and injection site reactions.

Delays in weight and height increases compared with baseline have been reported in pediatric patients receiving peginterferon alfa and oral ribavirin therapy. Decreased weight and height for age z-scores as well as percentiles of the normative population have been reported. Data from pediatric patients receiving peginterferon alfa-2a and oral ribavirin indicate that at the end of treatment 43% of patients experienced a weight percentile decrease of 15 percentiles or more and 25% experienced a height percentile decrease of 15 percentiles or more on the normative growth curves. Most children had returned to baseline normative growth curve percentiles for weight and height at the end of 2-year follow-up after completion of treatment (mean weight for age percentile was 64% at baseline and 60% at 2 years posttreatment, mean height percentile was 54% at baseline and 56% at 2 years posttreatment).

Data from an open-label trial in pediatric patients 3 through 17 years of age receiving peginterferon alfa-2b and oral ribavirin indicated that weight and height gain generally lagged behind that predicted by normative population data for the entire length of treatment. Results show that 70% of pediatric patients experienced severely inhibited growth velocity while receiving treatment; 24% of pediatric patients treated for 24 weeks and 40% of pediatric patients treated for 48 weeks experienced a height-for-age percentile decrease of 15 percentiles or more at the end of the 5-year long-term follow-up. Although rebound growth and weight gain occurred in most pediatric patients following completion of treatment, long-term follow-up data in pediatric patients indicate that peginterferon alfa-2b and oral ribavirin treatment may induce a growth inhibition that results in reduced final adult height in some patients.

Peginterferon alfa-2a (Pegasys®) is contraindicated in neonates and infants; each mL contains 10 mg of benzyl alcohol as a preservative. Although a causal relationship has not been established, administration of injections preserved with benzyl alcohol has been associated with toxicity (e.g., neurologic) in neonates and infants, which are sometimes fatal. Toxicity appears to have resulted from administration of large amounts (i.e., 100–400 mg/kg daily) of benzyl alcohol in these neonates. Although use of drugs preserved with benzyl alcohol should be avoided in neonates whenever possible, the American Academy of Pediatrics (AAP) states that the presence of small amounts of the preservative in a commercially available injection should not proscribe its use when indicated in neonates.

Geriatric Use. Experience in those 65 years of age and older is insufficient to determine whether they respond differently than younger adults. One manufacturer states that younger patients generally have higher virologic response rates than older patients (e.g., patients older than 40 years of age).

Peginterferon alfa should be used with caution in geriatric patients. Adverse reactions related to alfa interferons, such as CNS, cardiac, and systemic (e.g., flu- like) effects may be more severe in geriatric patients than in younger adults.

Because geriatric patients may have decreased renal function and because patients with renal impairment may be at increased risk of drug-induced toxicity, patients in this age group should be monitored closely and dosage adjusted accordingly. (See Renal Impairment under Dosage and Administration: Special Populations.)

Renal Impairment. Peginterferon alfa should be used with caution and close clinical monitoring in patients with renal impairment.

Dosage adjustments are required in those with creatinine clearance less than 30 mL/minute (peginterferon alfa-2a [Pegasys®]) or 50 mL/minute or less (peginterferon alfa-2b [PegIntron®]). (See Renal Impairment under Dosage and Administration: Special Populations.)

Peginterferon alfa-2a and oral ribavirin tablets (Copegus®) should be used concomitantly with caution in those with creatinine clearance of 50 mL/minute or less. Other ribavirin preparations are contraindicated if creatinine clearance is less than 50 mL/minute.

Concomitant peginterferon alfa-2b and oral ribavirin therapy is contraindicated in those with creatinine clearance less than 50 mL/minute. (See Drug Interactions: Ribavirin.)

Hepatic Impairment. Patients with chronic HBV infection may be at risk for transient acute exacerbations (flares) of HBV infection during treatment. (See Hepatic Failure and Hepatitis Exacerbations under Warnings/Precautions: Other Warnings/Precautions, in Cautions.)

Patients with chronic HCV infection with cirrhosis may be at risk of hepatic decompensation and death. Clinical status and hepatic function should be closely monitored and peginterferon alfa should be immediately discontinued if decompensation (Child-Pugh score 6 or greater) occurs. (See Hepatic Failure and Hepatitis Exacerbations under Warnings/Precautions: Other Warnings/Precautions, in Cautions.)

If elevated plasma ALT concentrations occur, hepatic function should be monitored more frequently and dosage adjustments or discontinuance of peginterferon alfa may be necessary. (See Hepatic Impairment under Dosage and Administration: Special Populations.)

Race. For reasons as yet unknown, response rates have been lower in black and Hispanic patients and higher in Asian patients compared with white patients. Although black patients had a higher proportion of poor prognostic factors compared with white patients, experience with these patients was insufficient to allow meaningful conclusions about differences in response rates after adjusting for these prognostic factors.

■ Common Adverse Effects Almost all (more than 96%) of patients with chronic HCV infection receiving peginterferon alfa (alfa-2a, alfa-2b) experience adverse effects at some time during the course of treatment. The most common adverse effects of peginterferon alfa in patients with chronic HCV infection are flu-like symptoms (fatigue/asthenia, headache, myalgia, pyrexia, rigors), neuropsychiatric effects (insomnia, depression, anxiety/emotional lability/irritability), and hematologic effects (e.g., neutropenia, thrombocytopenia). Some common adverse effects (e.g., fever, headache) tend to diminish in intensity and frequency with continued therapy. In clinical studies in patients with chronic HCV infection receiving the drug alone or in conjunction with oral ribavirin, 10–16% of patients discontinued peginterferon alfa therapy and 16–42% required dosage modifications because of adverse effects.

Adverse effects reported in patients with chronic HBV infection receiving peginterferon alfa-2a are similar to those reported in patients with chronic HCV infection receiving the drug. In addition, exacerbations of hepatitis have been reported in those with HBV. In clinical studies in patients with chronic HBV infection, 5% discontinued peginterferon alfa-2a therapy and 40% required dosage modifications because of adverse effects.

The most common reasons for dosage modification in patients receiving peginterferon alfa in clinical studies were hematologic abnormalities (e.g., anemia, neutropenia, thrombocytopenia) and elevated ALT concentrations. Incidences of adverse hematologic effects appear to be greater in patients receiving concomitant therapy with peginterferon alfa and oral ribavirin than in those receiving peginterferon alfa monotherapy. (See Drug Interactions: Ribavirin.)

Drug Interactions

■ Drugs Metabolized by Hepatic Microsomal Enzymes Studies using peginterferon alfa-2a (Pegasys®) indicated potential pharmacokinetic interactions with drugs metabolized by cytochrome P-450 (CYP) isoenzyme 1A2 (e.g., theophylline), but did not identify pharmacokinetic interactions with representative drugs metabolized by CYP isoenzymes 2C9, 2C19, 2D6, or 3A4.

Studies using peginterferon alfa-2b (PegIntron®) and representative drugs metabolized by CYP1A2 (caffeine), CYP2C8/9 (tolbutamide), CYP2D6 (dextromethorphan), and CYP3A4 (midazolam) indicated variable effects on CYP2C8/9 and CYP2D6 activity (including possible increases) but no clinically important effects on CYP1A2 or CYP3A4. The effects on CYP2C19 activity were not assessed.

■ Azathioprine Severe pancytopenia (marked decreases in erythrocytes, neutrophils, and platelets) and bone marrow suppression have been reported in some patients receiving azathioprine concomitantly with peginterferon alfa and oral ribavirin. These effects generally occurred within 3–7 weeks after initiation of concomitant therapy, reversed within 4–6 weeks after all 3 drugs were discontinued, and did not recur when either azathioprine or the regimen of peginterferon alfa and oral ribavirin was reinitiated alone. These adverse effects may occur because ribavirin inhibits inosine monophosphate dehydrogenase which may result in accumulation of 6-methylthioinosine monophosphate, an azathioprine metabolite associated with myelotoxicity.

If azathioprine and peginterferon alfa and oral ribavirin are used concomitantly, complete blood counts (CBCs), including platelet counts, should be monitored weekly for the first month, twice monthly during the second and third months of treatment, and then monthly or more frequently if necessary. If pancytopenia develops, all 3 drugs (azathioprine, peginterferon alfa, ribavirin) should be discontinued and peginterferon alfa and oral ribavirin therapy should not be restarted with concomitant azathioprine.

■ Antiretroviral Agents ***HIV Nucleoside Reverse Transcriptase Inhibitors (NRTIs)*** Hepatic decompensation, including some fatalities, have been reported in cirrhotic patients with chronic hepatitis C virus (HCV) infection who were coinfected with human immunodeficiency virus (HIV) and receiving nucleoside reverse transcriptase inhibitor (NRTI) antiretroviral agents and peginterferon alfa and oral ribavirin concomitantly. Patients receiving peginterferon alfa and NRTIs concomitantly should be monitored closely for toxicities. If worsening toxicities are observed, consideration should be given to discontinuing or reducing the dosage of peginterferon alfa and/or ribavirin; if decompensation occurs (Child-Pugh score 6 or greater), HCV treatment should be discontinued immediately.

Since concomitant use of didanosine and ribavirin are contraindicated because of reports of fatal hepatic failure, peripheral neuropathy, pancreatitis, and symptomatic hyperlactatemia/lactic acidosis, didanosine should not be used in patients receiving concomitant peginterferon alfa and oral ribavirin therapy.

Severe neutropenia (absolute neutrophil count [ANC] less than 500/mm^3) and severe anemia (hemoglobin less than 8 g/dL) have been reported more frequently in HCV patients receiving peginterferon alfa and oral ribavirin therapy concomitantly with zidovudine compared with patients receiving the regimen without concomitant zidovudine. If the drugs are used concomitantly, discontinuance of zidovudine should be considered as medically appropriate. If worsening clinical toxicities, including hepatic decompensation, occur, dosage reduction or discontinuance of peginterferon alfa and oral ribavirin therapy should be considered.

■ HCV Antivirals ***HCV Polymerase Inhibitors*** **Sofosbuvir.** There was no in vitro evidence of antagonism of antiviral effects between sofosbuvir and interferon against HCV when tested using nonconjugated interferon alfa.

HCV Protease Inhibitors **Simeprevir.** Concomitant use of simeprevir with ribavirin and peginterferon alfa does not affect simeprevir concentrations or AUC compared with use of simeprevir alone.

There was no in vitro evidence of antagonism of antiviral effects between simeprevir and interferon against HCV when tested using nonconjugated interferon.

HCV Replication Complex Inhibitors **Daclatasvir.** Concomitant use of daclatasvir with peginterferon alfa is not expected to result in any clinically important interactions.

■ Methadone Concomitant use of methadone and peginterferon alfa may increase methadone concentrations. Although the clinical importance is unknown, patients receiving the drugs concomitantly should be monitored for signs and symptoms of methadone toxicity.

■ Ribavirin Concomitant use of ribavirin, peginterferon alfa, and NRTIs in cirrhotic patients with HCV and HIV coinfection has been associated with hepatic decompensation, including some fatalities. (See HIV Nucleoside Reverse Transcriptase Inhibitors [NRTIs] under Drug Interactions: Antiretroviral Agents.)

Ribavirin may potentiate the hematologic effects (anemia, neutropenia, lymphopenia) induced by peginterferon alfa. (See Myelosuppression under Warnings/Precautions: Other Warnings/Precautions, in Cautions.)

There is no evidence of a pharmacokinetic interaction between ribavirin and peginterferon alfa-2a.

Peginterferon alfa-2a (Pegasys®) and oral ribavirin tablets (Copegus®) should be used concomitantly with caution in patients with creatinine clearance of 50 mL/minute or less. When used concomitantly, ribavirin dosage should be reduced if creatinine clearance is 50 mL/minute or less and peginterferon alfa-2a dosage should be decreased if creatinine clearance is 30 mL/minute or less. Concomitant use of peginterferon alfa-2a and other ribavirin preparations is contraindicated in patients with creatinine clearance less than 50 mL/minute.

Concomitant use of peginterferon alfa-2b (PegIntron®) and oral ribavirin is contraindicated in patients with creatinine clearance less than 50 mL/minute.

■ **Telbivudine** Peripheral neuropathy has been reported when telbivudine was used concomitantly with an interferon alfa. In one study, increased risk and severity of peripheral neuropathy occurred in patients receiving peginterferon alfa-2a concomitantly with telbivudine compared with those receiving telbivudine alone.

Safety and efficacy of concomitant use of telbivudine with any interferon for treatment of chronic HBV infection have not been established.

■ **Theophylline** Concomitant use of theophylline and peginterferon alfa-2a (Pegasys®) increased the area under the plasma concentration-time curve (AUC) of theophylline by 25% because of inhibition of CYP1A2. Plasma theophylline concentrations should be routinely monitored and appropriate dosage adjustments considered.

Description

Peginterferon alfa (alfa-2a, alfa-2b) is an antiviral agent. Peginterferon alfa contains interferon alfa (recombinant DNA origin) covalently bound to polyethylene glycol (PEG) monomethoxy ether. As a result of conjugation with PEG, the apparent clearance of peginterferon alfa-2a is 100 times lower and the mean half-life is 16 times greater than that reported for nonconjugated interferon alfa-2a. The apparent clearance of peginterferon alfa-2b is 7 times lower and the mean half-life is 5 times greater than that reported for nonconjugated interferon alfa-2b. Consequently, peginterferon preparations can be administered once weekly.

Although the precise mechanisms of antiviral activity of peginterferon alfa have not been fully elucidated, interferons with antiviral activity appear to bind to specific membrane receptors on cell surfaces and initiate a complex sequence of intracellular events, including induction of certain enzymes, suppression of cell proliferation, various immunomodulating activities, and inhibition of viral replication in virus-infected cells.

Advice to Patients

Advise patients receiving peginterferon alfa about appropriate use of the drug and the expected benefits and risks. Importance of reading the manufacturer's patient information and medication guide.

Importance of taking the once-weekly dose of peginterferon alfa on the same day and approximately same time of day each week during treatment.

If a dose of peginterferon alfa-2a (Pegasys®) is missed and remembered within 2 days, take the missed dose as soon as it is remembered and take the next dose on the usually scheduled day. If a missed dose if remembered more than 2 days late, the patient should consult their clinician for instructions. Also advise patients to consult their clinician if the full dose is not received (e.g., leakage occurs around the injection site).

Importance of remaining well hydrated, especially during initial treatment.

Importance of not reusing or sharing syringes, needles, autoinjectors, or injection pens. Importance of proper disposal of vials, syringes, needles, autoinjectors, and injection pens.

Caution patients not to change brands of peginterferon alfa without consulting their clinician.

Advise patients with hepatitis B virus (HBV) infection that it is not known whether peginterferon alfa-2a treatment will prevent transmission of HBV infection to others or prevent HBV-associated complications (cirrhosis, liver failure, liver cancer).

Advise patients with hepatitis C virus (HCV) infection that it is not known whether peginterferon alfa alone or in conjunction with oral ribavirin) will prevent transmission of HCV infection to others or prevent long-term HCV-associated complications (cirrhosis, liver failure, liver cancer). Importance of taking precautions to prevent transmission of HCV during treatment or in the event of treatment failure. If taking concomitant oral ribavirin, importance of taking the drug with food.

Advise patients to avoid drinking alcohol to reduce the chance of further injury to the liver.

Advise patients that laboratory evaluations are required before starting and periodically during treatment.

Importance of reporting any sign or symptom of depression or suicidal ideation to clinician. Advise patients that the drug may need to be immediately discontinued and psychiatric intervention instituted in severe cases.

Importance of immediately reporting trouble breathing, chest pain, severe stomach or lower back pain, bloody diarrhea or bloody bowel movements, high fever, bruising, bleeding, or decreased vision.

Caution patients that dizziness, confusion, somnolence, and fatigue may occur and to avoid driving or operating machinery.

Advise patients to maintain good oral hygiene, including brushing their teeth twice daily and rinsing their mouth after vomiting.

Importance of informing clinicians of existing or contemplated concomitant therapy, including herbal supplements, prescription and OTC drugs, as well as concomitant illnesses.

Importance of women informing clinicians if they are or plan to become pregnant or plan to breast-feed.

If concomitant oral ribavirin is used, advise patients of the teratogenic/embryocidal risks associated with ribavirin and the necessity of females of childbearing potential and male patients with female partners of childbearing age practicing effective contraception during and for 6 months after ribavirin therapy.

Importance of advising patients of other important precautionary information. (See Cautions.)

Overview® (see Users Guide). For additional information on this drug until a more detailed monograph is developed and published, the manufacturer's labeling should be consulted. It is *essential* that the manufacturer's labeling be consulted for more detailed information on usual cautions, precautions, contraindications, potential drug interactions, laboratory test interferences, and acute toxicity.

Preparations

Excipients in commercially available drug preparations may have clinically important effects in some individuals; consult specific product labeling for details.

Peginterferon Alfa-2a

Parenteral		
Injection, for subcutaneous use	135 mcg/0.5 mL	**Pegasys®** (available as single-dose prefilled autoinjectors), Genentech
	180 mcg/0.5 mL	**Pegasys®** (available as single-dose prefilled autoinjectors or single-dose prefilled syringes), Genentech
	180 mcg/mL	**Pegasys®** (available as single-dose vials), Genentech

Peginterferon Alfa-2b

Parenteral		
For injection, for subcutaneous use	50 mcg/0.5 mL	**PegIntron®** (available as single-dose prefilled dual-chambered injection pens with sterile water for injection diluent or as single-dose vials with 1.25 mL vial sterile water for injection diluent, Safety-Lok® syringes with safety sleeve, and alcohol swabs), Schering
	80 mcg/0.5 mL	**PegIntron®** (available as single-dose prefilled dual-chambered injection pens with sterile water for injection diluent or as single-dose vials with 1.25 mL vial sterile water for injection diluent, Safety-Lok® syringes with safety sleeve, and alcohol swabs), Schering
	120 mcg/0.5 mL	**PegIntron®** (available as single-dose prefilled dual-chambered injection pens with sterile water for injection diluent or as single-dose vials with 1.25 mL vial sterile water for injection diluent, Safety-Lok® syringes with safety sleeve, and alcohol swabs), Schering
	150 mcg/0.5 mL	**PegIntron®** (available as single-dose prefilled dual-chambered injection pens with sterile water for injection diluent or single-dose vials with 1.25 mL vial sterile water for injection diluent, Safety-Lok® syringes with safety sleeve, and alcohol swabs), Schering

†Use is not currently included in the labeling approved by the US Food and Drug Administration

Selected Revisions October 2015, © Copyright, January 2002, American Society of Health-System Pharmacists, Inc.

MONOCLONAL ANTIBODIES 8:18.24

Palivizumab

■ Palivizumab, a biosynthetic humanized form of a murine monoclonal antibody to the F surface glycoprotein of respiratory syncytial virus (RSV), is a highly specific antiviral agent.

Uses

Palivizumab is a highly specific monoclonal antibody that is used to provide passive immunity to respiratory syncytial virus (RSV) for the prevention of serious RSV lower respiratory tract infections in infants at high risk for RSV disease. Palivizumab is not indicated and should not be used for the *treatment* of RSV infection.

Palivizumab prophylaxis is recommended for infants younger than 24 months of age who have chronic lung disease (CLD) (e.g., bronchopulmonary dysplasia BPD]), a history of premature birth (gestational age of 35 weeks or less), or hemodynamically significant congenital heart disease (CHD). Palivizumab administered once monthly during the RSV season has been shown to effectively reduce the severity of RSV lower respiratory tract infection and reduce the frequency and duration of RSV-related hospitalizations in these high-risk infants; however, current evidence does not suggest that palivizumab prophylaxis can reduce the severity of RSV illness in patients who ultimately require hospitalization. Thus, the principal benefit of palivizumab prophylaxis established to date has been in reducing the need for RSV hospitalization.

The need for and efficacy of palivizumab prophylaxis following institutional RSV outbreaks† (e.g., in neonatal intensive care units) has not been studied to date, and the major means of preventing RSV illness in such situations is strict observance of infection control practices.

Decisions to administer palivizumab prophylaxis during the RSV season to infants at high risk for RSV-associated morbidity and mortality should be individualized. In addition to chronologic age, gestational age, and presence of CLD (e.g., BPD, cystic fibrosis), other factors may be taken into consideration. These include conditions that predispose to respiratory complications (e.g., other cardiopulmonary conditions, neurologic disease in very low-birthweight infants, impaired immune function, anticipated cardiac surgery, exposure to cigarette smoke in the home); conditions that increase the risk of exposure to RSV (e.g., time of year a premature infant is discharged from a neonatal intensive care unit, multiple births [e.g., twins], number of young siblings, crowding in the home, attendance at a child-care facility); local epidemiologic data regarding RSV-related hospitalizations; and the cost-benefit, feasibility, and tolerability of monthly palivizumab injections. Consultation with neonatologists, intensive care specialists, infectious disease specialists, or pulmonologists may be necessary.

■ Risks of RSV Exposure and Infection RSV is an enveloped RNA virus that is classified as a member of the Paramyxovirus family. The virus is the most common cause of lower respiratory tract illness in infants, and at least 95% of all children have serologic evidence of previous RSV infection by 2 years of age. While most children and adults with RSV infection have limited infections and an uncomplicated recovery, infants are at increased risk for progression of the RSV infection and development of severe lower respiratory tract illness. Severe RSV-related illness requiring hospitalization occurs most frequently in those younger than 3 months of age, and the virus is the most common cause of serious lower respiratory tract infection and rehospitalization in premature infants with or without CLD (e.g., BPD). Severe RSV illness also can occur in adults, particularly the elderly and those with compromised immune function. While both humoral and cell-mediated immunity appear to be involved in the response to natural RSV infection, primary RSV infection does not provide long-term immunity against the virus and reinfection with RSV is common in infants, children, and adults.

Outbreaks of RSV infection occur every year in the US. The RSV season generally occurs from October to May, with RSV-related hospitalizations peaking in December or January; however, the RSV season varies regionally. RSV subgroups A and B appear to circulate concurrently, but subgroup A is more prevalent and is associated with more severe illness. The principal mode of transmission of RSV appears to be through direct contact (e.g., hand-to-nose and hand-to-eye). While fomite transmission may play a limited role in transmission of the virus, aerosolization is not generally involved. The incubation period for RSV averages 5 days (range: 2–8 days). RSV initially replicates in the nasopharynx, resulting in coryza and congestion with or without low-grade fever. Two to five days after initial infection, RSV may spread to the lower respiratory tract resulting in manifestations such as cough, dyspnea, and wheezing. Infected individuals generally shed the virus from 3–8 days after infection, but young infants may shed the virus for up to 4 weeks.

Infants at particular risk for severe RSV lower respiratory tract infection and RSV-related morbidity and mortality include those with a history of premature birth, those with cardiopulmonary conditions (e.g., BPD, cystic fibrosis, or other CLD; CHD), and those with immunodeficiency or compromised immune function. Low levels of passively acquired maternal RSV-neutralizing antibodies may contribute to the increased risk for severe RSV-related illness in premature infants. Premature infants born at 32 weeks of gestation or earlier have significantly lower levels of maternal anti-RSV antibodies at birth than those born after 32 weeks of gestation. Full-term infants tend to have less severe RSV-related illness during the first few weeks of life when titers of maternal RSV-neutralizing antibodies are highest, but may have severe RSV-related illness after these antibody levels have decreased.

Infants with RSV lower respiratory tract infection often present with bronchiolitis, and such infants generally have tachypnea, cough, retractions, wheezing, rales, clear coryza, nasal congestion (with or without flaring), and minimal or no fever. These infants may be hypoxic and thoracic radiographs often reveal pulmonary infiltrates and/or hyperinflation. Leukocyte counts and differentials generally are normal except for an occasional increase in immature cells. Infants infected during the first month of life may have atypical manifestations including low-grade fever, irritability, poor appetite, and infrequently apnea. Such infants often are hospitalized for suspected septicemia.

During the first year of life, 15–22% of RSV- infected children will experience lower respiratory tract involvement, and 0.5–2% of infected children will require hospitalization; the need for hospitalization increases in high-risk children. A review of admissions data at one institution during an RSV season revealed that the median duration of hospitalization for infants with lower respiratory tract infection related to RSV was 3 days; 11 or 8% of these infants required intensive care or intubation and ventilation, respectively. In a review of US hospital discharge summaries from 16 states, the average duration of hospitalization for such infants was 5.2 days overall but increased to 13.7 days for those who both had comorbidities (e.g., congenital anomalies of the heart or circulatory system, chronic pulmonary heart disease, disorders related to short gestation or low birthweight) and required mechanical ventilation; substantially higher average hospitalization durations (e.g., 24.3 days) were reported in some states for those with comorbidities who required ventilatory assistance. Fatalities related to RSV infection are rare in otherwise healthy infants. Mortality rates in infants who require hospitalization for RSV infection range from 0.5–3.5%; however, RSV-related mortality rates are higher in those with underlying pulmonary or heart disease and in those requiring ventilatory support.

■ Prevention of Serious RSV Lower Respiratory Tract Disease

Palivizumab is labeled for the prevention of serious lower respiratory tract disease caused by RSV in pediatric patients at high risk for RSV disease. Efficacy and safety of the drug were established in infants 24 months of age and younger with CLD (i.e., BPD), a history of prematurity (gestational age of 35 weeks or less and who were 6 months of age or younger at study entry), or hemodynamically significant CHD. The American Academy of Pediatrics (AAP) and other experts state that palivizumab is the drug of choice for most high-risk infants when RSV prophylaxis is indicated. Although respiratory syncytial virus immune globulin (RSV-IGIV) also has been used for prevention of serious RSV disease in high-risk infants, RSV-IGIV is no longer commercially available in the US.

The AAP and other experts currently recommend that palivizumab prophylaxis be considered for infants younger than 24 months of age with CLD who are receiving or have received medical therapy (e.g., oxygen, bronchodilator, diuretics, corticosteroids) within the 6 months before the upcoming RSV season. The AAP states that infants with more severe CLD may benefit clinically from palivizumab prophylaxis administered during 2 consecutive RSV seasons, especially those continuing to require medical therapy for respiratory or cardiac dysfunction. There currently are only limited data on the efficacy of palivizumab during the second RSV season, but children with CLD or CHD who require ongoing medical therapy may experience severe RSV infections.

Premature Infants Palivizumab is labeled for the prevention of serious RSV lower respiratory tract infection in premature infants born at 35 weeks of gestation or earlier who may or may not have BPD. However, current AAP and other recommendations for the use of RSV immunoprophylaxis in premature infants with or without BPD but without additional risk factors (see below) generally address those born at 32 weeks of gestation or earlier. In these infants, major risk factors to consider are gestational age and chronologic age at the start of the RSV season. The AAP and other experts state that RSV immunoprophylaxis may be beneficial in infants who have a gestational age of 28 weeks or less and a chronologic age of 12 months or less at the start of the RSV season and in those with a gestational age of 29–32 weeks and a chronologic age of 6 months or less at the start of the RSV season. AAP states that, once a child qualifies for initiation of prophylaxis at the start of the RSV season, prophylaxis be continued throughout the season and not be stopped when the child reaches 6 or 12 months of age.

Because of the large number of children born between 32–35 weeks' gestation and because of the cost of RSV immunoprophylaxis, the cost-benefit of administering prophylaxis to this large group must be considered carefully. Most experts recommend that prophylaxis in this population be reserved for those at greatest risk of severe infection who are younger than 6 months of age at the start of the RSV season. Epidemiologic data suggest that RSV infection is more likely to lead to hospitalization for these infants if the following additional risk factors are present: child-care attendance, school-aged siblings, exposure to environmental air pollutants, congenital airway abnormalities, or severe neuromuscular disease. However, since no single risk factor causes a very large increase in the rate of hospitalization and the risk is additive as the number of risk factors for an individual infant increases, AAP recommends that prophylaxis be considered for infants between 32–35 weeks' gestation only if 2 or more of these additional risk factors are present.

Important risk factors that can be addressed by the family of premature infants include eliminating exposure to tobacco smoke and avoiding crowds or other situations where exposure to infected individuals cannot be controlled. AAP states that high-risk infants should never be exposed to tobacco smoke; tobacco smoke control measures are far less costly than palivizumab prophylaxis. In addition, whenever feasible, participation in child care should be restricted for high-risk infants during the RSV season. Caregivers should be instructed on the importance of careful hand hygiene. In addition, all high-risk infants and their contacts who are 6 months of age or older should be vaccinated against influenza.

Infants and Children with Congenital Heart Disease Palivizumab is labeled for the prevention of serious RSV lower respiratory tract infection in pediatric patients with hemodynamically significant CHD. AAP states that infants younger than 24 months of age with cyanotic and acyanotic CHD will benefit from RSV prophylaxis.

AAP recommends that decisions regarding RSV prophylaxis in children with CHD be made based on the degree of physiologic cardiovascular compromise. These experts state that infants younger than 12 months of age with CHD most likely to benefit from such prophylaxis include those receiving medications to control congestive heart failure, those with moderate or severe pulmonary hypertension, and those with cyanotic heart disease. However, infants who are not at increased risk from RSV and who should not generally receive prophylaxis include those with hemodynamically insignificant heart disease (e.g., secundum atrial septal defect, small ventricular septal defect, pulmonic stenosis, uncomplicated aortic stenosis, mild coarctation of the aorta, patent ductus arteriosus); infants with lesions adequately corrected by surgery (unless they continue to require medication for congestive heart failure); and infants with mild cardiomyopathy who are not receiving medical therapy.

Infants and Children with Immunodeficiencies Palivizumab has not been evaluated in randomized trials in immunocompromised pediatric patients, and the AAP states that current data are insufficient to develop specific recommendations for use of RSV immunoprophylaxis in all immunocompromised patients. There is evidence that infants and children with severe immunodeficiency† (e.g., severe combined immunodeficiency, severe T-cell dysfunction, or severe acquired immunodeficiency syndrome [AIDS]) are at increased risk for severe RSV illness and prolonged shedding of RSV. The role, if any, of RSV immunoprophylaxis in immunocompromised infants and children receiving induction chemotherapy† during the RSV season and in those receiving allogeneic bone marrow transplants† (BMT), especially in communities experiencing RSV outbreaks prior to engraftment, remains to be established; however, studies (e.g., in BMT recipients) are under way. The role, if any, of RSV immunoprophylaxis in patients with cystic fibrosis†, children with neuromuscular disease† or abnormalities of the diaphragm†, and infants with gastroesophageal reflux† and chronic aspiration† also remains to be established.

Clinical Experience Safety and efficacy of palivizumab in the prevention of RSV have been evaluated in 2 multicenter, randomized, double-blind, placebo-controlled studies. In one study (IMpact-RSV-trial), palivizumab was evaluated in infants with BPD who were 24 months of age or younger and required ongoing medical treatment (e.g., supplemental oxygen, corticosteroids, bronchodilators, or diuretics within the past 6 months) and in infants with a history of prematurity (gestational age of 35 weeks or less) who were 6 months of age or younger at the time of study entry. In the second study, palivizumab was evaluated in children with hemodynamically significant CHD who were 24 months of age or younger. In these studies, 15-mg/kg doses of palivizumab or placebo was administered by IM injection once monthly for 5 doses during the RSV season, beginning in mid-November through mid-December. The patients were observed over 150 days for efficacy and safety. Participation in these studies was completed by 96–99% of the patients and 92–93% of patients received all 5 doses of palivizumab or placebo.

In the IMpact-RSV trial, the incidence of RSV hospitalization was 4.8 or 10.6% with palivizumab or placebo, respectively, representing a 55% reduction in RSV hospitalization in patients treated with the drug. In patients with BPD at enrollment, the incidence of RSV hospitalization was 7.9 or 12.8% with palivizumab or placebo, respectively, representing a 39% reduction in RSV hospitalization secondary to drug therapy. In patients with a history of prematurity but not BPD at enrollment, the incidence of RSV hospitalization was 1.8 or 8.1% with palivizumab or placebo, respectively, representing a 78% reduction in RSV hospitalization secondary to drug therapy. In the study in children with CHD, the incidence of RSV hospitalization was 5.3 or 9.7% with palivizumab or placebo, respectively, representing a 45% reduction in RSV hospitalization in patients treated with the drug. In children with cyanotic congenital heart lesions (e.g., pulmonary atresia with ventricular septal defect, pulmonary atresia with intact septum, tetralogy of Fallot), the incidence of RSV hospitalization was 5.6 or 7.9% with palivizumab or placebo, respectively, representing a 29% reduction in RSV hospitalization secondary to drug therapy. In children who did not have cyanotic congenital heart lesions, the incidence of RSV hospitalization was 5 or 11.8% with palivizumab or placebo, respectively, representing a 58% reduction in RSV hospitalization secondary to drug therapy.

The incidence of admission to the intensive care unit (ICU) during hospitalization for RSV infection was lower in patients treated with palivizumab. Overall, the clinical trial data do not suggest that RSV illness was less severe among palivizumab versus placebo recipients who required hospitalization because of RSV infection. In the IMpact-RSV trial, neither the incidence and mean duration of hospitalization for respiratory illness unrelated to RSV disease nor the incidence of otitis media was altered by palivizumab therapy; the need for assisted (mechanical) ventilation also was not altered by drug therapy. Whether prophylaxis with palivizumab has any effect on RSV sequelae (e.g., long-term pulmonary complications) or mortality is not known.

It remains to be established whether RSV immunoprophylaxis early in life will alter the incidence of hyperactive airways and asthma later in life.

Dosage and Administration

■ **Administration** Palivizumab is administered IM, preferably in the anterolateral aspect of the thigh. Aseptic technique should be followed. IM administration into the gluteal muscle should not be routine because of the risk of damage to the sciatic nerve. Although palivizumab also has been administered by IV infusion† over 3–5 minutes in a limited number of infants, the manufacturer states that the currently available formulation of the drug is intended for IM injection *only*.

Palivizumab should be administered undiluted immediately after withdrawal from the vial. The vial is for single-use only and any unused portion should be discarded.

Volumes of palivizumab exceeding 1 mL should be injected IM as a divided dose.

The first dose of palivizumab should be administered prior to the RSV season and additional doses given once monthly throughout the RSV season. In the northern hemisphere, the RSV season typically commences in November and lasts through April, but it may begin earlier or persist later in certain communities. AAP states that in most seasons and in most regions of the northern hemisphere, the first dose of palivizumab should be given at the beginning of November and the last dose given at the beginning of March and that these 5 doses usually are sufficient to provide protection during the entire season. However, decisions about the specific duration of prophylaxis should be individualized according to the duration of the local RSV season. AAP recommends that clinicians consult local health departments or diagnostic virology laboratories or the CDC to determine the epidemiology of RSV in their area.

Infants who become infected with RSV while receiving palivizumab should continue receiving the usual monthly doses of the monoclonal antibody for the duration of the RSV season.

■ **Dosage** The usual dosage of palivizumab for prevention of serious lower respiratory tract disease caused by RSV in pediatric patients at high risk for RSV disease is 15 mg/kg once monthly. The first dose of palivizumab should be given prior to the beginning of the RSV season and subsequent doses should be given once monthly until the end of the season.

Because serum concentrations of palivizumab decrease after cardiopulmonary bypass, patients undergoing cardiopulmonary bypass should receive a supplemental 15-mg/kg dose of palivizumab as soon as possible after the procedure (even if this is sooner than 1 month after the last dose). Thereafter, the usual doses should be given once monthly.

Cautions

Palivizumab generally is well tolerated following IM administration in infants, and the incidences of adverse effects overall and by body system in controlled studies were similar for patients receiving the drug compared with placebo. However, severe acute hypersensitivity reactions, including anaphylaxis, have been reported rarely during postmarketing surveillance.

Description of the safety of palivizumab was derived principally from the studies that established the efficacy of palivizumab for prophylaxis of respiratory syncytial virus (RSV) infection (IMpact-RSV trial and the study in children with congenital heart disease [CHD]).

In the studies that evaluated efficacy of palivizumab, adverse effects that occurred in greater than 1% of patients who received palivizumab and at an incidence that exceeded that of placebo by at least 1% included upper respiratory infection, otitis media, fever, rhinitis, hernia, and elevated serum AST (SGOT) concentration.

In the IMpact-RSV trial, the overall incidences of adverse effects judged by clinical investigators as being treatment related were 11 and 10% for palivizumab and placebo, respectively; palivizumab was discontinued because of adverse effects (i.e., vomiting, diarrhea, fever) in 0.3% of patients in this study. Death occurred in 4 of the 1002 patients (0.4%) treated with palivizumab and 5 of the 500 patients (1%) who received placebo in this study, but no death was considered directly attributable to the drug.

Data from postmarketing surveillance indicate that the character and frequency of adverse effects observed in pediatric patients receiving 6 or more monthly doses of palivizumab during a single RSV season are similar to those observed after the first 5 monthly doses.

■ **Dermatologic and Sensitivity Reactions** Rash occurs frequently in children receiving palivizumab. Rash judged by clinical investigators as being treatment related occurred in 0.9 or 0.2% of patients who received palivizumab or placebo, respectively, in the IMpact-RSV trial.

Injection-site reactions have been reported. Reactions at the IM injection site generally were mild and of short duration and included erythema, pain, induration/swelling, and bruising; no serious reaction at the site of injection was reported.

Severe acute hypersensitivity reactions have been reported rarely following initial or subsequent doses of palivizumab during postmarketing surveillance. Anaphylaxis has been reported rarely (fewer than 1 case per 100,000 patients) following reexposure to the drug. In the event of anaphylaxis or severe allergic reaction, appropriate therapy (e.g., epinephrine) and supportive care should be provided. Hypersensitivity reactions to palivizumab may include dyspnea, cyanosis, respiratory failure, urticaria, pruritus, angioedema, hypotonia, and unresponsiveness. Hypersensitivity reactions reported to date have not been fatal. Palivizumab prophylaxis should be discontinued in patients who experience a severe hypersensitivity reaction; the drug may be continued with caution in patients who have experienced a milder reaction.

In the IMpact-RSV trial, the incidence of anti-palivizumab antibody after the fourth dose of palivizumab was 0.7 or 1.1% in patients who received palivizumab or placebo, respectively; overall, the incidence of such antibody titers exceeding 1:40 were 1.2 or 2.8%, respectively. Antibodies were directed to the Fc rather than Fab fragment and therefore were not true anti-idiotypic antibodies. In addition, they generally were single elevations which were not sustained and not associated with adverse reactions. Of 56 pediatric patients who received palivizumab for a second RSV season, one patient had transient, low-titer reactivity that was not associated with adverse effects or alteration in serum concentrations of the drug. Immunogenicity was not assessed in the study in children with CHD. In other studies in which palivizumab was administered by IM or IV injection for up to 5 monthly doses, low-level anti-palivizumab antibody titers (1:10–1:40) were observed in some patients who received palivizumab or placebo, but the antibody reactivity was transient and not specific for the drug.

Data on the incidence of anti-palivizumab antibody are based on the percentage of patients with tests considered positive for palivizumab antibodies detected with ELISA; these results are highly dependent on the sensitivity and specificity of the ELISA assay. Other factors that may influence the observed incidence of positive results for antibody include the manner in which samples are handled, concomitant therapy with other drugs, and underlying disease. Therefore, comparing the incidence of antibodies to palivizumab versus that with other drugs may be misleading.

■ **Respiratory Effects** In controlled clinical studies, upper respiratory infection occurred in 50.6 or 47.4% of patients who received palivizumab or placebo, respectively. In the IMpact-RSV trial, this adverse event was judged by clinical investigators as being treatment related in only 0.5 or 0.4% of patients, respectively. In clinical studies, otitis media occurred in 36.4 or 34.6% of patients who received the drug or placebo, respectively, and rhinitis occurred in 26.8 or 24.6% of patients, respectively. Cough and wheezing have occurred in palivizumab-treated children.

■ **Other Adverse Effects** In controlled clinical studies, fever was reported in 27.1 or 25.2% of patients who received drug or placebo, respectively. Hernia occurred in 4.1 or 2.6% of patients, respectively, and serum AST concentrations increased in 3 or 1.7% of patients, respectively.

In children with CHD, cyanosis was reported more frequently in those receiving palivizumab (9.1%) than in those receiving placebo (6.9%). Cyanosis was considered a serious adverse event in 3.6 or 2.2% of patients receiving drug or placebo, respectively; most of these serious events occurred in children with cyanotic congenital heart lesions. In the 30 days following a serious cyanotic event, similar proportions of palivizumab-treated children and placebo-treated children had earlier than planned or urgent surgery (2.2 and 1.9%) or died (1 patient in each group). Arrhythmia occurred in 3.1 or 1.7% of children with CHD who received drug or placebo, respectively; events reported as arrhythmia were judged not related to the drug.

Diarrhea, vomiting, and gastroenteritis have occurred in palivizumab-treated patients.

■ **Precautions and Contraindications** Palivizumab currently is intended for IM use only. Caution should be observed with IM administration of any drug, including palivizumab, to patients with thrombocytopenia or any disorder of coagulation.

Safety and efficacy of palivizumab for the *treatment* of established RSV disease remain to be established; therefore, such use currently is *not* recommended.

Severe acute hypersensitivity reactions, including anaphylaxis, have occurred rarely in patients receiving palivizumab. Appropriate supportive care and therapy (e.g., epinephrine) should be initiated immediately if anaphylaxis or another severe allergic reaction occurs.

Palivizumab should not be administered to pediatric patients with a history of a severe reaction to the drug or any ingredient in the formulation (e.g., murine protein).

■ **Mutagenicity and Carcinogenicity** Studies to determine the mutagenic or carcinogenic potential of palivizumab have not been performed to date.

■ **Pregnancy, Fertility, and Lactation** Animal reproduction studies have not been performed with palivizumab, and it is also not known whether the drug can cause fetal harm when administered to pregnant women. However, use of palivizumab currently is intended only for pediatric patients who would not be of childbearing potential.

Studies have not been conducted to evaluate palivizumab for reproductive toxicity, and the potential for the drug to affect reproductive capacity is not known.

Because palivizumab currently is intended for use only in pediatric patients who would not be of lactating potential, the potential for the drug to distribute into breast milk has not been determined.

Drug Interactions

Formal studies have not been conducted to evaluate potential interactions between palivizumab and other drugs.

Palivizumab does not interfere with the immune response to vaccines. Similar proportions of patients who received palivizumab or placebo in the study that established the efficacy of palivizumab also received concomitantly vaccines that are administered routinely during childhood, influenza virus vaccine, bronchodilators, and/or corticosteroids without any evidence of an incremental increase in adverse effects.

Acute Toxicity

Data are not available from clinical studies to describe the acute toxicity of palivizumab.

Toxicity was not observed in rabbits given a single 50-mg/kg dose of palivizumab by IM or subcutaneous injection.

Mechanism of Action

Palivizumab is a highly selective antiviral agent that is active only against respiratory syncytial virus (RSV). The drug is a potent, RSV-neutralizing, monoclonal antibody that neutralizes and inhibits fusion of the virus, resulting in inhibition of viral replication. The neutralizing antibody characteristics of palivizumab are targeted against the F surface glycoprotein of the virus, which is one of 2 surface proteins (the other is G) principally responsible for viral recognition and entry into cells; the F glycoprotein promotes fusion of the viral envelope with the infected (host) cell membrane during the early stage of infection. The F glycoprotein also is expressed on the surface of infected cells and is responsible for subsequent fusion with other cells resulting in syncytia formation. Thus, by binding to the F surface glycoprotein of RSV, palivizumab may directly neutralize the virus and/or block entry of the virus into the cell and/or may prevent syncytia formation. Antibodies to the F surface glycoprotein of RSV exhibit a high degree of cross-reactivity between the 2 major strains of the virus (subgroups A and B), and palivizumab has been shown to effectively neutralize both strains in vitro.

Spectrum

Palivizumab exhibits a narrow spectrum of antiviral activity, being active only against respiratory syncytial virus (RSV). The drug is active against both subgroup A and B, the 2 major strains of RSV. Palivizumab neutralized all 57 clinical isolates of RSV (34 subgroup A and 23 subgroup B) tested in vitro in one study. In vivo in an animal model of RSV infection, pulmonary replication of RSV subgroup A and B was reduced by a mean of 99% (2-log, 100-fold) at serum palivizumab concentrations of approximately 25–30 mcg/mL, and viral replication was reduced in all animals by a minimum of 99% at serum concentrations of 40 mcg/mL or more. The in vivo neutralizing activity of the drug has been confirmed in a clinical trial in RSV-infected pediatric patients as evidenced by a lower recovery of RSV from lower respiratory tract secretions in palivizumab-treated patients compared with placebo recipients.

Evidence from animal studies indicates that palivizumab administration does not interfere with the development of a protective immune response to RSV.

Resistance

Strains of respiratory syncytial virus (RSV) resistant to palivizumab have been isolated in vitro under laboratory conditions in which the virus was manipulated to create a mutant strain. However, all contemporary clinical isolates of subgroup A and B of RSV tested to date have been susceptible to the drug. In addition, evidence from animal studies indicates that exposure of RSV to subinhibitory concentrations of palivizumab does not enhance viral replication or pathology nor does it promote emergence of resistant variants; in fact, treatment with palivizumab appeared to protect the animals against infection from subsequent RSV challenge despite systemic clearance of the drug. Because escape mutants (resistant viruses) have been associated with other monoclonal antibodies, the possibility that they could occur with palivizumab should be considered.

Pharmacokinetics

■ **Absorption** Palivizumab is well absorbed following IM injection in infants, reaching concentrations that exceed 40 mcg/mL within 2 days after a single 15-mg/kg dose and that peak within 5–7 days after a dose. Following IM injection of 15-mg/kg doses at monthly intervals in pediatric patients 24 months of age and younger without congenital heart disease (CHD), including patients 6 months of age and younger who were born prematurely at 35 weeks' gestation or less, serum concentrations of palivizumab measured 30 days after administration of a dose (i.e., trough concentrations) averaged 37–49, 57–69, 68–70, 70–72, and 73 mcg/mL after the first, second, third, fourth, and fifth doses, respectively. Following IM injection of 15-mg/kg doses at monthly intervals in pediatric patients with CHD, trough concentrations were 55.5 and 90.8 mcg/mL after the first and fourth doses, respectively.

Trough serum palivizumab concentrations following monthly IV infusions over 2–5 minutes of 15-mg/kg doses of the drug in pediatric patients averaged 61, 71, 89, and 97 mcg/mL after the first, second, third, and fourth doses, respectively. Trough serum concentrations exceeded 40 mcg/mL in 66, 86, 91, and 96% of these pediatric patients following IM injection of the first, second, third, and fourth dose, respectively, and in 71 and 76% of patients following IV infusion of the first and second dose, respectively. Based on animal models of inhibition of RSV replication (see Spectrum), the target trough serum palivizumab concentrations in these studies were 25–30 mcg/mL, but ideally 40 mcg/mL. Pediatric patients administered palivizumab IM for a second RSV season were observed to have average trough serum concentrations of the drug of 61 and 86 mcg/mL 30 days after the first and fourth doses, respectively.

A mean decrease in palivizumab serum concentrations of 58% has been reported following surgical procedures that involve cardiopulmonary bypass. In pediatric patients 24 months of age or younger with hemodynamically significant CHD receiving the recommended dosage of palivizumab, serum palivizumab concentrations before cardiopulmonary bypass averaged 98 mcg/mL and concentrations after bypass averaged 41.4 mcg/mL.

Based on data from IM and IV pharmacokinetic studies in pediatric patients, monthly dosing of palivizumab at 15 mg/kg should be adequate to maintain trough serum concentrations that exceed the ideal target throughout the dosing period (except in children undergoing cardiopulmonary bypass). Lower doses (i.e., 3 or 10 mg/kg IV, or 5 or 10 mg/kg IM) resulted in inadequate trough concentrations in dose-ranging studies.

■ **Distribution** Transient nonspecific anti-palivizumab binding has been observed in a small proportion of patients treated with the drug, but such binding was not associated with alterations in the pharmacokinetic profile of palivizumab.

■ **Elimination** The elimination half-life of palivizumab is similar to that of human IgG_1 antibody, averaging about 18 days in healthy adults and 19–27 days in pediatric patients 24 months of age and younger, including patients 6 months of age and younger who were born prematurely at 35 weeks' gestation or less.

Chemistry and Stability

■ **Chemistry** Palivizumab, a biosynthetic humanized form of a murine monoclonal antibody to the F surface glycoprotein of respiratory syncytial virus (RSV), is a highly specific antiviral agent. The drug is prepared from cultures of genetically altered mouse myeloma cells using recombinant DNA technology. These cells have been modified by addition of the V_H and V_L genes from a palivizumab-resistant variant of the Long (a subgroup A) strain of RSV to produce murine monoclonal antibody 1129 (MAb 1129), which is humanized (to minimize the risk of inducing a human antimurine antibody response, especially with repeated administration) using the human K102 germline V_L and the Cor and CE-1 V_H framework regions. The humanized 1129 monoclonal antibody ($IgG_{1\kappa}$), designated MEDI-493, is directed to an epitope in the A antigenic site of the F (i.e., fusion) glycoprotein of respiratory syncytial virus (RSV). Its composite sequences of amino acids are 95% human and 5% murine. The resultant humanized molecule is unlikely to elicit an antimurine immune response (anti-idiotypic antibody), yet the binding affinity and specificity for the RSV F glycoprotein of the original murine monoclonal antibody are retained.

Palivizumab is composed of amino acids sequenced in 2 heavy chains and 2 light chains and has a molecular weight of approximately 148,000 daltons. The humanized monoclonal antibody in the form of palivizumab is a genetically engineered chimeric molecule that results from grafting an antigen (i.e., RSV)-recognition site derived from a murine monoclonal antibody onto a human immunoglobulin backbone. The human heavy chain of palivizumab was derived from the constant domains of human IgG_1 and the variable framework regions of the V_H genes Cor and Cess. The human light chain was derived from the constant domain of Cκ and the variable framework regions of the V_L gene K104 with Jκ-4. The murine sequences of amino acids were derived from a murine monoclonal antibody (MAb 1129) through a process that involved grafting onto the human antibody framework the regions that determine murine complementarity.

Palivizumab injection is a sterile, preservative-free solution of the drug; the injection contains histidine and glycine as excipients. Palivizumab injection is clear or slightly opalescent and has a pH of 6.

■ **Stability** Commercially available palivizumab injection should be stored at 2–8°C in the original container and should *not* be frozen.

Preparations

Excipients in commercially available drug preparations may have clinically important effects in some individuals; consult specific product labeling for details.

Palivizumab

Parenteral

Injection, for IM use only	50 mg/0.5 mL	**Synagis®**, MedImmune (also marketed by Ross)
	100 mg/1 mL	**Synagis®**, MedImmune (also marketed by Ross)

†Use is not currently included in the labeling approved by the US Food and Drug Administration

Selected Revisions June 2006, © Copyright, January 1999, American Society of Health-System Pharmacists, Inc.

NEURAMINIDASE INHIBITORS 8:18.28

Oseltamivir Phosphate

■ Oseltamivir phosphate is a prodrug of oseltamivir carboxylate, a sialic acid analog and neuraminidase inhibitor antiviral agent that is pharmacologically related to zanamivir and active against influenza A and B viruses.

Uses

■ **Treatment of Seasonal Influenza A and B Virus Infections** Oseltamivir is used for the *treatment* of acute, uncomplicated illness caused by influenza A or B viruses in adults, adolescents, and pediatric patients 2 weeks of age or older. Although safety and efficacy have not been established in neonates younger than 2 weeks of age†, oseltamivir also is recommended when *treatment* of influenza is necessary in this age group.

The US Centers for Disease Control and Prevention (CDC), US Public Health Service Advisory Committee on Immunization Practices (ACIP), and American Academy of Pediatrics (AAP) recommend antiviral treatment of seasonal influenza illness as soon as possible in all individuals with suspected or confirmed influenza if they require hospitalization or have severe, complicated, or progressive illness (regardless of vaccination status or underlying illness). These experts also recommend early empiric antiviral treatment in individuals with suspected or confirmed influenza of any severity who are at high risk for influenza-related complications because of age or underlying medical conditions. Individuals at increased risk for influenza-related complications include children younger than 2 years of age; adults 65 years of age or older; individuals of any age with chronic pulmonary (including asthma), cardiovascular (except hypertension alone), renal, hepatic, hematologic (including sickle cell disease), or metabolic disorders (including diabetes mellitus); individuals with neurologic and neurodevelopmental conditions (including disorders of the brain, spinal cord, peripheral nerve, and muscle such as cerebral palsy, epilepsy [seizure disorders], stroke, intellectual disability [mental retardation], moderate to severe developmental delay, muscular dystrophy, or spinal cord injury); individuals with immunosuppression (including that caused by medications or human immunodeficiency virus [HIV] infection); women who are pregnant or up to 2 weeks postpartum; individuals younger than 19 years of age receiving long-term aspirin therapy; American Indians or Alaskan natives; morbidly obese individuals with a body mass index (BMI) of 40 or greater; and residents of any age in nursing homes or other long-term care facilities.

CDC, ACIP, and AAP also state that empiric antiviral treatment can be considered in previously healthy, symptomatic individuals with suspected or confirmed seasonal influenza who are not known to be at increased risk of developing severe or complicated illness if such treatment can be initiated within 48 hours of illness onset. Although these individuals typically do not require treatment, early empiric antiviral treatment might provide some benefit (e.g., shortened duration of illness). The use of antiviral treatment in such individuals should be based on clinical judgment and is not necessary in those who are already beginning to recover. In areas with limited availability of antiviral agents, local public health authorities might provide additional guidance about prioritizing use of antivirals within groups at higher risk for complications.

When treatment of seasonal influenza is indicated, an appropriate antiviral agent should be initiated as soon as possible after illness onset (ideally within 48 hours), and should *not* be delayed while waiting for laboratory confirmation. The manufacturer states that oseltamivir should be used for the treatment of influenza only in patients who have been symptomatic for no more than 48 hours. However, although clinical benefit is greatest when oseltamivir is initiated within 48 hours of onset of influenza symptoms, there is some evidence from observational studies of hospitalized patients that antiviral treatment may still be beneficial when initiated up to 4 or 5 days after illness onset. Therefore, CDC, ACIP, and AAP recommend that antiviral treatment be initiated in all patients with severe, complicated, or progressive illness attributable to influenza and all hospitalized patients and patients at increased risk of influenza complications (either hospitalized or outpatient) who have suspected or confirmed influenza, even if it has been more than 48 hours after illness onset. Decisions regarding use of empiric antiviral treatment in outpatients, especially high-risk patients, should be based on disease severity and progression, age, underlying medical conditions, likelihood of influenza, and time since onset of symptoms. If empiric antiviral treatment is considered warranted in previously healthy, symptomatic outpatients not considered at increased risk of influenza complications, such treatment should be initiated within 48 hours after illness onset, but some experts state treatment can be considered in such patients even if it has been more than 48 hours after illness onset.

An age-appropriate neuraminidase inhibitor antiviral agent (oral oseltamivir, IV peramivir, inhaled zanamivir) should be used when treatment of suspected or confirmed acute, uncomplicated influenza is indicated in outpatients. Oseltamivir usually is the preferred neuraminidase inhibitor in hospitalized patients and patients with severe or complicated influenza because of the lack of data regarding use of IV peramivir or inhaled zanamivir in such patients. Although controlled clinical trials evaluating oseltamivir for the treatment of influenza generally only included patients with acute, uncomplicated influenza illness, observational studies indicate that oseltamivir reduces severe clinical outcomes in patients hospitalized with influenza. Limited data suggest that oral oseltamivir usually is well absorbed in critically ill influenza patients, including patients in intensive care units and those requiring continuous renal replacement therapy and/or extracorporeal membrane oxygenation, but there have been rare reports of suspected decreased oral absorption of the drug in patients with decreased gastric motility or GI bleeding. For the treatment of hospitalized patients with severe influenza who cannot tolerate or absorb oral oseltamivir (e.g., because of suspected or known gastric stasis, malabsorption, or GI bleeding), CDC states that use of IV peramivir or investigational IV zanamivir may be considered. Use of investigational IV zanamivir also should be considered for treatment of severe influenza caused by oseltamivir-resistant strains. Oseltamivir is the preferred antiviral agent for treatment of suspected or confirmed influenza in pregnant women. (See Pregnancy under Cautions: Pregnancy, Fertility, and Lactation.)

Viral surveillance data available from local and state health departments and CDC should be considered when selecting an antiviral for treatment of seasonal influenza. Strains of circulating influenza viruses and the antiviral susceptibility of these strains constantly evolve, and the possibility that emergence of oseltamivir-resistant influenza virus may decrease effectiveness of the drug should be considered. Although influenza A and B viruses circulating in the US during the last few years generally have been susceptible to oseltamivir (see Resistance), clinicians should consult the most recent information.

CDC issues recommendations concerning the use of antiviral agents for the treatment of influenza, and these recommendations are updated as needed during each influenza season. Information regarding influenza surveillance and updated recommendations for treatment of seasonal influenza are available from CDC at http://www.cdc.gov/flu.

Clinical Experience **Adults and Adolescents.** Efficacy of oseltamivir for the treatment of seasonal influenza in adults 18 years of age or older has been established in randomized placebo-controlled studies in which the predominant influenza infection was influenza A; only a limited number of adults in studies to date have been infected with influenza B. When initiated within 40 hours of onset of symptoms in otherwise healthy adults 18–65 years of age with uncomplicated influenza, the drug has decreased the severity of influenza symptoms (i.e., nasal congestion, sore throat, cough, aches, fatigue, headache, chills/sweats) and shortened the average duration of these symptoms by about 1.3 days. When used in geriatric patients 65 years of age or older, oseltamivir has reduced the time to symptom improvement by 1 day.

Analysis of data from several studies indicated that adults who received oseltamivir for seasonal influenza had a lower incidence of respiratory complications requiring anti-infective therapy and hospitalization. Individuals who initiate therapy sooner (i.e., no later than 24 hours after symptom onset) exhibit greater benefit (e.g., a 2-day decrease in symptom duration). Oseltamivir therapy also has reduced the magnitude and duration of viral replication.

Efficacy and safety of oseltamivir for the treatment of seasonal influenza in adolescents 13–17 years of age are supported by data from adequate and well-controlled trials in adults, adolescents, and younger pediatric patients and safety data in adolescents.

Children 1–12 Years of Age. Efficacy and safety of oseltamivir for the treatment of seasonal influenza in children 1–12 years of age was established in a double-blind, placebo-controlled study in children infected with influenza A (67%) or influenza B (33%). When used in these children within 48 hours of symptom onset, the drug reduced influenza symptoms (i.e., cough, coryza, duration of fever) and shortened the average duration of illness by about 1.5 days. Data from this study also indicate that children who received oseltamivir had a lower incidence of newly diagnosed otitis media (a common secondary complication of influenza) than those who received placebo.

The manufacturer states that efficacy could not be established in pediatric patients with asthma. In a study in children 6–12 years of age with asthma who received oseltamivir or placebo for the treatment of acute influenza virus infection, use of oseltamivir improved pulmonary function and reduced the risk of influenza-induced asthma exacerbations. When initiated within 48 hours of symptom onset, oseltamivir shortened the duration of illness in these children by about 24 hours; however, if initiated within 24 hours of symptom onset, oseltamivir shortened the duration of illness by about 40 hours.

Infants Younger than 1 Year of Age. Efficacy and safety of oseltamivir for the treatment of seasonal influenza in infants 2 weeks to less than 1 year of age are supported by adequate and well-controlled studies in adults and older pediatric patients and 2 open-label studies in 136 pediatric patients 2 weeks to less than 1 year of age. In addition, data from these 2 studies indicate that plasma concentrations of oseltamivir in pediatric patient 2 weeks to less than 1 year of age are similar to or greater than plasma concentrations observed in older pediatric patients and adults.

Immunocompromised Individuals. Although the manufacturer states that efficacy of oseltamivir for the *treatment* of influenza in immunocompromised patients has not been established, oseltamivir has been used to treat seasonal influenza A or B virus infections in bone marrow transplant (BMT) recipients† in a prospective, uncontrolled study. This study provides some evidence that oseltamivir treatment (75 mg twice daily for 5 days) may prevent influenza complications and is not associated with any unusual adverse effects in these patients. Oseltamivir also has been used for the treatment of influenza infections in hematopoietic stem cell transplant (HSCT) recipients†. Treatment with oseltamivir prevented progression to pneumonia in influenza-infected HSCT recipients in a small study.

■ Prevention of Seasonal Influenza A and B Virus Infections

Oseltamivir is used for *prophylaxis* of influenza A or B virus infections in adults, adolescents, and children 1 year of age or older.

Annual vaccination with seasonal influenza virus vaccine, as recommended by ACIP, is the primary means of preventing seasonal influenza and its severe complications. Prophylaxis with an appropriate antiviral agent active against circulating influenza strains is considered an adjunct to vaccination for the control and prevention of influenza.

Decisions regarding use of antivirals for prophylaxis of influenza should be based on the exposed person's risk for influenza complications, vaccination status, the type and duration of contact, recommendations from local or public health authorities, and clinical judgment. In general, postexposure prophylaxis should be used only if it can be initiated within 48 hours of the most recent exposure. Indiscriminate use of antivirals for prophylaxis may promote resistance or reduce availability of antiviral agents for treatment. In areas with limited availability of antiviral agents, local public health authorities might provide additional guidance about prioritizing use of antiviral prophylaxis within groups at higher risk for influenza complications. In certain situations, CDC or local public health authorities might recommend that antiviral agents be reserved for treatment and that prophylaxis be used only in certain limited situations.

When seasonal influenza viruses are circulating in the community, postexposure prophylaxis with oseltamivir or zanamivir can be considered for certain individuals, including those at high risk of developing influenza complications for whom influenza vaccine is contraindicated, unavailable, or expected to have low efficacy (e.g., immunocompromised individuals). Other possible candidates for antiviral postexposure prophylaxis include unvaccinated health care personnel, public health workers, and first responders with unprotected, close-contact exposure to a patient with confirmed, probable, or suspected influenza during the time when the patient was infectious. Antiviral prophylaxis also can be considered for controlling influenza outbreaks in nursing and long-term care facilities or other closed or semi-closed settings with large numbers of individuals at high risk for influenza complications. In individuals at high risk of influenza complications who receive influenza virus vaccine inactivated, use of prophylaxis can be considered during the 2 weeks after vaccination to provide protection until an adequate immune response develops. (See Drug Interactions: Influenza Virus Vaccines.)

Viral surveillance data available from local and state health departments and CDC should be considered when selecting an antiviral for the prophylaxis of influenza. Strains of circulating influenza viruses and the antiviral susceptibility of these strains constantly evolve, and the possibility that emergence of oseltamivir-resistant influenza virus may decrease effectiveness of the drug should be considered. Although influenza A and B viruses circulating in the US during the last few years generally have been susceptible to oseltamivir (see Resistance), clinicians should consult the most recent information.

CDC issues recommendations concerning the use of antiviral agents for prophylaxis of influenza, and these recommendations are updated as needed during each influenza season. Information regarding influenza surveillance and updated recommendations for prevention of seasonal influenza are available from CDC at http://www.cdc.gov/flu.

Clinical Experience **Adults and Adolescents.** Results of community studies in healthy, unvaccinated adults indicate that oseltamivir is about 82% effective in preventing febrile, laboratory-confirmed influenza illness. Efficacy of oseltamivir in preventing naturally occurring influenza illness has been demonstrated in seasonal prophylaxis studies and in postexposure prophylaxis studies in household contacts. The efficacy end point for these studies was the incidence of laboratory-confirmed clinical influenza, which was defined as oral temperature exceeding 37.2°C with at least one respiratory symptom (cough, sore throat, nasal congestion) and at least one constitutional symptom (aches and pain, fatigue, headache, chills/sweats) all occurring within a single 24-hour period and either a positive virus isolation or a fourfold increase in virus antibody titer from baseline.

In 2 seasonal prophylaxis studies in healthy, unvaccinated adults 18–65 years of age who received oseltamivir (75 mg once daily) or placebo for 42 days during a community outbreak, pooled analysis indicates that the incidence of laboratory-confirmed clinical influenza was 1 or 5% in those receiving oseltamivir or placebo, respectively. In a seasonal prophylaxis study in geriatric residents of skilled nursing facilities (80% vaccinated, 14% with chronic airway obstructive disorders, 43% with cardiac disorders) who received oseltamivir (75 mg once daily) or placebo for 42 days, the incidence of laboratory-confirmed clinical influenza was less than 1 or 4% of those receiving oseltamivir or placebo, respectively.

In a postexposure prophylaxis study in household contacts (13 years of age or older) of influenza-infected index cases (not treated with antivirals) who received oseltamivir (75 mg once daily) or placebo for 7 days within 48 hours of onset of symptoms in the index case, the incidence of laboratory-confirmed clinical influenza was 1 or 12% of those receiving oseltamivir or placebo, respectively. In another postexposure prophylaxis study, there was evidence that oseltamivir prophylaxis effectively reduced the secondary spread of influenza within households when given to household contacts of index patients who were receiving the drug for treatment.

Children 1–12 Years of Age. Efficacy of oseltamivir in preventing naturally occurring influenza illness in children 1–12 years of age was evaluated in a randomized, open-label, postexposure prophylaxis study. In this study, oseltamivir prophylaxis was used during a documented community influenza outbreak and was given to adults and children 1 year of age or older residing in households that had an index patient with an influenza-like illness who was receiving oseltamivir for treatment. The efficacy parameter for this study was the incidence of laboratory-confirmed clinical influenza (defined as oral temperature 37.8°C or higher with cough and/or coryza occurring within a single 48-hour period and either a positive virus isolation or a fourfold or greater increase in virus antibody titer from baseline). In household contacts 1–12 years of age not shedding virus at baseline, the incidence of laboratory-confirmed clinical influenza was 3 or 17% in those receiving oseltamivir or placebo, respectively. The overall incidence of influenza illness in children who received oseltamivir prophylaxis was higher than that in adults and adolescents 13 years of age or older who received such prophylaxis.

Immunocompromised Individuals. Although the manufacturer states that efficacy of oseltamivir for prevention of influenza in immunocompromised patients has not been established, the drug has been used for prophylaxis of influenza in some immunocompromised individuals†, including cancer patients, BMT recipients, HSCT recipients, and solid organ transplant recipients.

In a prospective, uncontrolled study, oseltamivir was used for prophylaxis of influenza in cancer patients† 6.3–23.4 years of age who were immunocompromised because of current or recent chemotherapy or BMT. There were no laboratory-confirmed cases of influenza in the study participants; however, a few patients withdrew from the study because of adverse GI effects.

Safety and efficacy of oseltamivir for prevention of seasonal influenza in immunocompromised patients were evaluated in a double-blind, placebo-controlled study that included 475 immunocompromised adults, adolescents, and pediatric patients 1–12 years of age who had received solid organ transplants (liver, kidney, liver and kidney) or HSCT. The median time since solid organ transplant was 1105 days in those randomized to placebo and 1379 days in those randomized to oseltamivir prophylaxis; the median time since HSCT transplant was 424 days in those randomized to placebo and 367 days in those randomized to oseltamivir. Approximately 40% of patients had received influenza vaccine prior to study entry. The primary efficacy endpoint was the incidence of confirmed clinical influenza, defined as oral temperature exceeding 37.2°C plus cough and/or coryza (all recorded within 24 hours) plus either a positive virus culture or a fourfold increase in virus antibody titers from baseline. The incidence of confirmed clinical influenza was 3% in the placebo group and 2% in the oseltamivir group; this difference was not statistically significant. The safety profile of oseltamivir reported in these immunocompromised patients (up to 12 weeks of prophylaxis) was similar to that reported in other clinical trials evaluating oseltamivir prophylaxis.

■ **Avian Influenza A Virus Infections** Oseltamivir is used for the treatment or prevention of infections caused by susceptible avian influenza A viruses† (e.g., H5N1, H7N3, H7N7, H7N9).

Risk of Exposure and Infection Although avian influenza A viruses usually do not infect humans, infection with these viruses has been reported following exposure to infected poultry. It can be anticipated that human cases of avian influenza A will continue to be detected in countries where these viruses circulate in wild birds, outbreaks occur in poultry, and close human contact with poultry is common (e.g., backyard flocks, markets).

Since 2003, avian influenza A (H5N1) infection in poultry or wild birds has been reported in parts of Asia, Africa, the Pacific, Eastern Europe, and the Middle East. World Health Organization (WHO) data indicate that there were 668 confirmed human cases of highly pathogenic avian influenza A (H5N1) infection (including 393 fatalities) reported in 16 countries from 2003 to October 2014. These human cases occurred in Azerbaijan, Bangladesh, Cambodia, Canada, China, Djibouti, Egypt, Indonesia, Iraq, Laos, Myanmar, Nigeria, Pakistan, Thailand, Turkey, and Vietnam.

In March 2013, a novel avian influenza A (H7N9) virus causing human infection was identified in China. By June 2013, 132 human cases had been confirmed in mainland China and Taiwan. From February 2013 to February 2014, the WHO had received reports of 355 human cases of avian influenza A (H7N9) infection (including 112 fatalities). To date, no cases have been reported in animals or humans in the US. Most reported cases of avian influenza A (H7N9) infection have involved severe respiratory illness, including pneumonia and acute respiratory distress syndrome (ARDS), and approximately 27% of identified cases have been fatal. Many of the infected individuals had close contact with poultry (chickens or ducks) and the source of infection is assumed to be infected poultry or contaminated environments. Preliminary investigations of patients and close contacts have not revealed evidence of sustained human-to-human transmission of influenza A (H7N9), but limited nonsustained human-to-human transmission of the virus could not be excluded in a few family clusters.

In addition, confirmed human cases of H7N2, H7N3, H7N7, and H9N2 avian influenza A infection and illness have been reported, including a few cases in Australia, Canada, Italy, Mexico, the Netherlands, the United Kingdom, and the US. Most of these infections occurred in association with poultry outbreaks and mainly resulted in conjunctivitis and mild upper respiratory symptoms. There was a large outbreak of avian influenza A (H7N7) in commercial poultry farms in the Netherlands in 2003 that resulted in large numbers of human cases of H7N7 infection (principally conjunctivitis and influenza-like illnesses). Human infection with avian influenza A (H10N8) also has been reported rarely in China.

Experience to date indicates that human cases of avian influenza infection are rare and that these viruses do not transmit easily from poultry to humans. Most, but not all, human cases reported to date have been linked to direct contact with infected poultry, uncooked poultry products, or surfaces contaminated with infected poultry feces or respiratory secretions. Sustained person-to-person transmission of avian influenza viruses has not been reported to date, but clustering and limited person-to-person transmission of H5N1 and H7N9 viruses has been reported. Most clusters of human infection with avian influenza A (H5N1) reported to date have included documented exposure to birds. Person-to-person transmission of H7N7 has occurred among household contacts during the outbreak of that virus that occurred in the Netherlands.

In humans, avian influenza A viruses can cause typical influenza illness (fever, cough, sore throat, muscle aches), conjunctivitis, or respiratory disease; however, severe illness can occur, especially with highly pathogenic avian influenza (H5N1) and avian influenza A (H7N9). The fatality rate in patients hospitalized with H5N1 infection has been high (exceeding 50%). In one group of patients in Vietnam with severe H5N1 infections, the median time to death was 9 days (range 6–17 days) with or without treatment.

Avian influenza A virus strains isolated during the past several years (including H5N1 and H7N9 strains causing human illness) generally have been resistant to adamantanes (amantadine, rimantadine). Most avian influenza A virus strains (e.g., H5N1, H7N7, H7N9, H9N2) have been susceptible to oseltamivir and zanamivir in vitro. However, avian influenza A (H5N1) and avian influenza A (H7N9) isolates that have reduced susceptibility or are resistant to oseltamivir in vitro have been reported. (See Spectrum and see Resistance.)

The most recent information regarding avian influenza A infections is available at the WHO website at http://www.who.int/influenza/human_animal_interface/en/ and the CDC website at http://www.cdc.gov/flu/avianflu/.

Travelers. CDC does not currently recommend that the general public avoid travel to any of the countries that have had poultry outbreaks or human cases of highly pathogenic avian influenza A (H5N1) or avian influenza A (H7N9). However, CDC recommends that travelers to these areas take certain precautions to reduce the risks. CDC recommends that travelers to countries where highly pathogenic avian influenza A (H5N1) is endemic or countries with known poultry outbreaks of the virus avoid direct contact with all birds (poultry such as chickens and ducks, wild birds), especially contact with sick or dead poultry. Travelers also should avoid places such as poultry farms and markets where live poultry are raised, kept, or sold and avoid contact with surfaces that might be contaminated with poultry feces or secretions. Uncooked (raw) or undercooked poultry or poultry products should *not* be consumed, and care should be taken when preparing these foods. Because influenza viruses are destroyed by heat, all foods from poultry that comes from these areas (including eggs and poultry blood) should be thoroughly cooked; egg yolks should not be runny or liquid and poultry meat should be cooked to a temperature of 74°C.

Additional information for travelers can be obtained at the CDC website at http://wwwnc.cdc.gov/travel/content/avian-flu-asia.aspx.

Treatment and Prevention of Avian Influenza A Infections CDC and WHO state that oseltamivir is the drug of choice for the treatment or prophylaxis of infections caused by highly pathogenic avian influenza A (H5N1)†. Zanamivir is considered an alternative.

Oseltamivir also is considered the drug of choice for the treatment of infections known or presumed to be caused by avian influenza A (H7N9), especially in hospitalized patients and patients with severe or complicated illness. Because of limited data, zanamivir is not recommended for the treatment of severe avian influenza A (H7N9) infections, but may be considered in those with uncomplicated infections. Either oseltamivir or zanamivir can be used for prophylaxis in close contacts of patients with confirmed or probable avian influenza A (H7N9) infections.

Only limited data are available to date regarding treatment of human cases of avian influenza A virus infections. Data from observational studies indicate that early initiation of oseltamivir therapy is associated with a reduction in mortality in influenza A (H5N1)-infected patients. Some data indicate a survival rate of 83% when oseltamivir treatment is initiated within 2 days of symptom onset compared with a survival rate of 21% if initiated 3–8 days after symptom onset. Because this virus continues to replicate for prolonged periods of time, treatment with oseltamivir is warranted even in patients who present for care in the later stages of illness. The optimum dosage and duration of oseltamivir treatment for avian influenza A (H5N1) infections are unknown, but high doses and prolonged duration of therapy may be needed in some patients. Although some individuals with avian influenza A (H5N1) infections who were treated with oseltamivir died, it is unclear whether these deaths were related to a lack of efficacy, a delay in diagnosis and initiation of oseltamivir treatment, or the dosage regimen used.

■ **Variant Influenza Virus Infections** Oseltamivir is used for the treatment of infections cause by variant influenza viruses†.

Influenza viruses that circulate in swine are called swine influenza viruses when isolated from swine, but are called variant influenza viruses when isolated from humans. Human infection with influenza A (H1N1) variant (H1N1v), influenza A (H1N2) variant (H1N2v), and influenza A (H3N2) variant (H3N2v) have been detected in the US. Limited data to date indicate that variant influenza viruses are susceptible to neuraminidase inhibitor antivirals (oseltamivir, peramivir, zanamivir).

CDC states that management of infections caused by variant influenza viruses is similar to management of seasonal influenza virus infections. CDC recommends early initiation of oseltamivir for treatment of hospitalized patients, those with severe and progressive illness, and any high-risk patient with suspected or confirmed variant influenza virus infection. Antiviral treatment with a neuraminidase inhibitor also is recommended for outpatients with suspected influenza, including variant influenza virus infection, if the individual is considered at high risk for influenza complications. CDC states that antiviral treatment also can be considered for any previously healthy, symptomatic outpatient not at high risk who has confirmed or suspected variant virus infection on the basis of clinical judgment, if treatment can be initiated within 48 hours of illness onset.

CDC does not recommend antiviral prophylaxis before or after exposure to swine.

■ **Pandemic Influenza** Oseltamivir is used for the treatment or prevention of pandemic influenza† caused by susceptible strains of influenza virus.

Influenza viruses can cause seasonal epidemics and, occasionally, pandemics during which rates of illness and death from influenza-related complications can increase dramatically worldwide. The most recent influenza pandemic occurred during 2009 and was related to a novel influenza A (H1N1) strain, influenza A (H1N1)pdm09. Influenza A strains also were involved in prior influenza pandemics occurring in 1918 (H1N1), 1957 (H2N2; originated in China), and 1968 (H3N2; originated in Hong Kong).

On June 11, 2009, the WHO declared that the first global influenza pandemic in 41 years was occurring and issued a pandemic alert regarding influenza A (H1N1)pdm09, previously referred to as the novel 2009 influenza A (H1N1) virus or swine-origin influenza A (H1N1) virus. Influenza outbreaks caused by the influenza A (H1N1)pdm09 virus were reported in several countries, including the US, beginning in March and April 2009. The virus is a triple-reassortant swine influenza virus with genes from human, swine, and avian influenza A viruses and contains a unique combination of gene segments not previously reported among human or swine influenza A in the US or elsewhere. The influenza A (H1N1)pdm09 virus is antigenically distinct from previous human influenza A (H1N1) viruses that had been in circulation since 1977, and widespread transmission of the virus occurred since most individuals had no preexisting antibody to the strain. In the US, the 2009 influenza A (H1N1)pdm09 pandemic was characterized by a substantial increase in influenza activity that peaked in late October and early November 2009 and returned to seasonal baseline levels by January 2010. During the pandemic, more than 99% of influenza viruses circulating in the US were the influenza A (H1N1)pdm09 virus; more than 60 million Americans become ill with the virus and more than 270,000 hospitalizations and 12,500 deaths were reported. In August 2010, the WHO declared that the world was in a post-pandemic period. Since that time, influenza A (H1N1)pdm09 has become a seasonal influenza virus and continues to circulate with other seasonal influenza viruses.

The spread of the highly pathogenic H5N1 strain of avian influenza A in poultry in Asia and other countries that has been occurring since 2003 may represent a future pandemic threat. (See Uses: Avian Influenza A Virus Infections.)

For information on pandemic influenza preparation and response, including use of antiviral agents, the CDC pandemic influenza website (https://www.cdc.gov/flu/pandemic-resources/index.htm) should be consulted.

Dosage and Administration

■ Administration

Oseltamivir phosphate is administered orally without regard to meals, although administration with meals may improve GI tolerability.

Oseltamivir phosphate is commercially available as 30-, 45-, and 75-mg capsules and as a powder for oral suspension that is reconstituted to provide an oral suspension containing 6 mg of oseltamivir per mL.

Reconstituted oseltamivir phosphate oral suspension is preferred for patients who cannot swallow capsules. Alternatively, if the powder for oral suspension is not available from the manufacturer or wholesaler, the appropriate strength of commercially available oseltamivir capsules can be administered by opening the capsules and mixing the contents with a sweet liquid (e.g., regular or sugar-free chocolate syrup, corn syrup, caramel topping, light brown sugar dissolved in water).

During emergency situations if the powder for oral suspension is not available *and* the appropriate strength of oseltamivir capsules is not available to mix with sweetened liquids, an emergency supply of oseltamivir phosphate oral suspension can be prepared extemporaneously by a pharmacist using the commercially available 75-mg capsules of the drug. (See Extemporaneous Oral Suspensions under Dosage and Administration: Administration.)

Reconstitution

The commercially available oseltamivir phosphate powder for oral suspension should be reconstituted at the time of dispensing. The bottle should be tapped to thoroughly loosen the white powder and then the amount of water specified on the bottle should be added; the bottle should be shaken for 15 seconds.

The reconstituted oral suspension contains 6 mg/mL; each 12.5 mL of the suspension contains 75 mg of oseltamivir. An oral dosing device that can accurately measure the appropriate volume in mL should be provided with the reconstituted suspension. Patients and/or caregivers should be counseled on how to use the oral dosing dispenser to correctly measure and administer the appropriate dose.

The suspension should be shaken well prior to each dose.

Extemporaneous Oral Suspensions

If necessary for use during emergency situations, an oral suspension containing 6 mg/mL can be prepared extemporaneously by a pharmacist using 75-mg capsules and simple syrup, cherry syrup vehicle (Humco®), or Ora-Sweet® SF (Paddock).

Extemporaneous oral suspensions should be used *only* if the commercially available powder for oral suspension *and* appropriate strength of commercially available oseltamivir capsules are not available from the manufacturer or wholesalers. The manufacturer's information should be consulted for specific directions on how to prepare extemporaneous oral suspensions of the drug.

■ Dosage

Dosage of oseltamivir phosphate is expressed in terms of oseltamivir.

Treatment of Seasonal Influenza A and B Virus Infections

When indicated for the *treatment* of seasonal influenza, oseltamivir should be initiated as soon as possible (preferably within 48 hours of symptom onset). Although efficacy has only been established when oseltamivir treatment is initiated no more than 48 hours after onset of symptoms, there is some evidence from observational studies in hospitalized patients that antiviral treatment may still be beneficial when initiated up to 4 or 5 days after illness onset. (See Uses: Treatment of Seasonal Influenza A and B Virus Infections.)

Oseltamivir usually is given for 5 days for the *treatment* of seasonal influenza. However, hospitalized patients with severe infections (e.g., those with prolonged infection or those admitted into an intensive care unit) or individuals with immunosuppression may require longer than 5 days of treatment.

Adults and Adolescents 13 Years of Age or Older. For the *treatment* of influenza in adults (including geriatric adults) and adolescents 13 years of age and older, the recommended dosage of oseltamivir is 75 mg twice daily for 5 days. Each dose can be given as a single 75-mg capsule or 12.5 mL of oral suspension containing 6 mg/mL.

Children 1–12 Years of Age. Dosage of oseltamivir for the *treatment* of influenza in children 1–12 years of age is based on weight. (See Table 1.)

Table 1. Oseltamivir Dosage for Treatment of Seasonal Influenza A and B in Children 1–12 Years of Age

Weight (kg)	Daily Dosage (mg)	Daily Dosage (Volume of Reconstituted Oral Suspension Containing 6 mg/mL)	Daily Dosage (Capsules)
≤15	30 mg twice daily for 5 days	5 mL twice daily for 5 days	One 30-mg capsule twice daily for 5 days
15.1–23	45 mg twice daily for 5 days	7.5 mL twice daily for 5 days	One 45-mg capsule twice daily for 5 days
23.1–40	60 mg twice daily for 5 days	10 mL twice daily for 5 days	Two 30-mg capsules twice daily for 5 days
≥40.1	75 mg twice daily for 5 days	12.5 mL twice daily for 5 days	One 75-mg capsule twice daily for 5 days

Infants Younger than 1 Year of Age. For the *treatment* of influenza in infants 2 weeks to less than 1 year of age, the manufacturer recommends that oseltamivir be given in a dosage of 3 mg/kg twice daily for 5 days.

For the *treatment* of influenza in neonates and infants younger than 1 year of age, the American Academy of Pediatrics (AAP) recommends that oseltamivir be given in a dosage of 3.5 mg/kg twice daily for 5 days in infants 9 through 11 months of age and 3 mg/kg twice daily for 5 days in *full-term* neonates and infants through 8 months of age. Although safety and efficacy have not been established in neonates younger than 2 weeks of age† (see Cautions: Pediatric Precautions), AAP states that, because of the known safety profile of the drug, oseltamivir can be used for the *treatment* of influenza in neonates from birth† if indicated.

Weight-based oseltamivir dosage recommended for *full-term* infants may be excessive in *preterm* neonates since clearance of the drug is slower in those with immature renal function. Limited data suggest that, if oseltamivir is considered necessary for *treatment* of influenza in *preterm* neonates†, dosage should be based on postmenstrual age (i.e., gestational age plus chronological age). AAP and US Centers for Disease Control and Prevention (CDC) recommend an oseltamivir dosage of 1 mg/kg twice daily in *preterm* neonates with postmenstrual age less than 38 weeks, 1.5 mg/kg twice daily in those with postmenstrual age of 38 through 40 weeks, and 3 mg/kg twice daily in those with postmenstrual age exceeding 40 weeks. For *treatment* of influenza in extremely premature neonates (postmenstrual age less than 28 weeks), a pediatric infectious disease expert should be consulted.

Prevention of Seasonal Influenza A and B Virus Infections

When indicated for *prophylaxis* of seasonal influenza following close contact with an infected individual, oseltamivir should be initiated within 48 hours of exposure. Protection lasts as long as oseltamivir is continued.

CDC recommends that antiviral *prophylaxis* be continued for 10 days after a household exposure and 7 days after the most recent exposure in other situations. For *prophylaxis* of influenza when an outbreak is occurring in a long-term care facility (e.g., nursing home) or hospital, CDC recommends that antiviral *prophylaxis* be continued for a minimum of 2 weeks and up to 7 days after the last known case of influenza is identified.

The manufacturer states that oseltamivir *prophylaxis* may be continued for up to 6 weeks in immunocompetent individuals and for up to 12 weeks in immunocompromised individuals during community outbreaks.

Adults and Adolescents 13 Years of Age or Older. For *prophylaxis* of influenza in adults (including geriatric adults) and adolescents 13 years of age or older following close contact with an infected individual or during community outbreaks, the recommended dosage of oseltamivir is 75 mg once daily. The manufacturer states that oseltamivir *prophylaxis* should be continued for at least 10 days following close contact with an infected individual; during community outbreaks, prophylaxis may be continued for up to 6 weeks in immunocompetent individuals and for up to 12 weeks in immunocompromised individuals.

Children 1–12 Years of Age. Dosage of oseltamivir for *prophylaxis* of influenza in children 1–12 years of age following close contact with an infected individual or during community outbreaks is based on weight. (See Table 2.)

Table 2. Oseltamivir Dosage for Prevention of Seasonal Influenza A and B in Children 1–12 Years of Age

Weight (kg)	Daily Dosage (mg)	Daily Dosage (Volume of Reconstituted Oral Suspension Containing 6 mg/mL)[a]	Daily Dosage (Capsules)[a]
≤15	30 mg once daily for 10 days	5 mL once daily for 10 days	One 30-mg capsule once daily for 10 days
15.1–23	45 mg once daily for 10 days	7.5 mL once daily for 10 days	One 45-mg capsule once daily for 10 days
23.1–40	60 mg once daily for 10 days	10 mL once daily for 10 days	Two 30-mg capsules once daily for 10 days
≥40.1	75 mg once daily for 10 days	12.5 mL once daily for 10 days	One 75-mg capsule once daily for 10 days

[a] The manufacturer states that oseltamivir *prophylaxis* in pediatric patients should be continued for 10 days following close contact with an infected individual; during community outbreaks, *prophylaxis* may be continued for up to 6 weeks in immunocompetent individuals or for up to 12 weeks in immunocompromised individuals.

Infants Younger than 1 Year of Age. Although safety and efficacy have not been established for *prophylaxis* of influenza in infants younger than 1 year of age† (see Cautions: Pediatric Precautions), CDC and the US Public Health Service Advisory Committee on Immunization Practices (ACIP) state that infants 3 months to less than 1 year of age† can receive oseltamivir in a dosage of 3 mg/kg once daily for 10 days if considered necessary for prevention of influenza. For *prophylaxis* of influenza, AAP recommends a dosage of 3.5 mg/kg once daily for 10 days in infants 9 through 11 months of age† and 3 mg/kg once daily for 10 days in infants 3 through 8 months of age†.

Because of limited safety and efficacy data, CDC, ACIP, and AAP state that oseltamivir should *not* be used for *prophylaxis* of influenza in *full-term* or *preterm* infants younger than 3 months of age† unless the situation is judged critical.

Avian Influenza A Virus Infections **Treatment.** Only limited data are available to date regarding *treatment* of infections caused by avian influenza A (H1N1) or avian influenza A (H7N9)†, and the optimum dosage and duration of oseltamivir for treatment of these infections, especially severe or complicated infections, are unknown.

Some clinicians suggest that the twice-daily oseltamivir dosage usually recommended for the treatment of seasonal influenza A and B virus infection can be used for the *treatment* of avian influenza A virus infections† in adults and pediatric patients. (See Treatment of Seasonal Influenza A and B Virus Infections under Dosage and Administration: Dosage.) Although some experts have suggested that severely ill hospitalized patients or immunocompromised patients may benefit from treatment with a higher oseltamivir dosage (i.e., 150 mg twice daily in adults with normal renal function), oral oseltamivir is adequately absorbed in critically ill patients and limited data from those with severe influenza, including some with avian influenza A (H1N1) infection, suggest that higher dosage may not provide additional clinical benefit. Although 5 days of treatment may be adequate for uncomplicated illness, a longer duration of treatment (i.e., 7–10 days) should be considered in severely ill hospitalized patients and may be necessary in immunosuppressed individuals.

Treatment should be initiated as early as possible and may be most beneficial if initiated within 2 days of symptom onset. However, because the viruses continue to replicate for prolonged periods of time, treatment with oseltamivir is warranted even if initiated more than 48 hours after onset of illness or in patients who present for care in the later stages of illness.

Prevention. If oseltamivir is used for *prophylaxis* of highly pathogenic avian influenza A (H5N1) infection in close contacts†, CDC and WHO state that the once-daily oseltamivir dosage usually recommended for prophylaxis of seasonal influenza A and B virus infections can be used in adults and pediatric patients. (See Prevention of Seasonal Influenza A and B Virus Infections under Dosage and Administration: Dosage.) Prophylaxis should be continued for 7–10 days after the last known exposure.

If oseltamivir is used for *prophylaxis* of avian influenza virus A (H7N9) infection in close contacts†, CDC recommends that the twice-daily oseltamivir dosage usually recommended for *treatment* of seasonal influenza A and B virus infections be given for 5–10 days. (See Treatment of Seasonal Influenza A and B Virus Infections under Dosage and Administration: Dosage.)

Oseltamivir has been given in a dosage of 75 mg daily for prophylaxis in exposed individuals during an outbreak of avian influenza A (H7N7).

Pandemic Influenza Oseltamivir dosage usually recommended for the *treatment* or *prophylaxis* of seasonal influenza A or B infections is considered the *minimum* dosage required for the treatment or prophylaxis of influenza in a pandemic situation†. (See Treatment of Seasonal Influenza A and B Virus Infections and see Prevention of Seasonal Influenza A and B Virus Infections under Dosage and Administration: Dosage.)

■ **Dosage in Renal and Hepatic Impairment** ***Hepatic Impairment*** Dosage adjustments are not needed in patients with mild to moderate hepatic impairment (Child-Pugh score 9 or less). The safety and pharmacokinetics of the drug have not been evaluated in those with severe hepatic impairment.

Renal Impairment Dosage of oseltamivir for the treatment or prevention of influenza should be adjusted in adults with creatinine clearance of 10–60 mL/minute and in those with end-stage renal disease (ESRD; creatinine clearance 10 mL/minute or less) undergoing hemodialysis or continuous peritoneal dialysis. (See Table 3 and Table 4.)

Oseltamivir is *not* recommended in adults with ESRD who are *not* undergoing dialysis.

Although dosage recommendations are not available for pediatric patients with renal impairment, CDC states that oseltamivir dosage recommendations for adults with renal impairment may be useful for treatment or prevention of influenza in children with renal impairment who weigh more than 40 kg.

Table 3. Oseltamivir Dosage for Treatment of Influenza in Adults with Renal Impairment

Creatinine Clearance (mL/minute)	Dosage
>30 to 60	30 mg twice daily for 5 days
>10 to 30	30 mg once daily for 5 days
≤10 (ESRD receiving hemodialysis)	30 mg given immediately and then 30 mg after each hemodialysis cycle for maximum of 5 days[a]
≤10 (ESRD receiving continuous peritoneal dialysis)	Single 30-mg dose given immediately[b]
ESRD not receiving dialysis	Not recommended

[a] Dosage assumes 3 hemodialysis sessions in the 5-day period. If influenza symptoms developed during the 48 hours between hemodialysis sessions, give initial oseltamivir dose immediately and give the posthemodialysis dose regardless of when initial dose was given.
[b] Data derived from studies in patients undergoing continuous ambulatory peritoneal dialysis (CAPD).

Table 4. Oseltamivir Dosage for Prevention of Influenza in Adults with Renal Impairment[a]

Creatinine Clearance (mL/minute)	Dosage
>30 to 60	30 mg once daily for ≥10 days
>10 to 30	30 mg once every other day for ≥10 days
≤10 (ESRD receiving hemodialysis)	30 mg given immediately and then 30 mg after alternate hemodialysis cycles
≤10 (ESRD receiving continuous peritoneal dialysis)	30 mg given immediately and then 30 mg once weekly[b]
ESRD not receiving dialysis	Not recommended

[a] The manufacturer states that *prophylaxis* with oseltamivir during community outbreaks may be continued for up to 6 weeks in immunocompetent individuals or for up to 12 weeks in immunocompromised individuals.
[b] Data derived from studies in patients undergoing CAPD.

Geriatric Patients Dosage adjustments are not needed in geriatric patients. (See Cautions: Geriatric Precautions.)

Cautions

Oseltamivir generally is well tolerated. Adverse effects occurring in 1% or more of adults and at an incidence greater than that with placebo include GI effects (nausea, vomiting, diarrhea, abdominal pain), headache, bronchitis, insomnia, and vertigo. In one study in frail older individuals residing in residential homes or sheltered accommodations, the incidence of adverse effects reported in those receiving oseltamivir was similar to that reported in those receiving placebo.

Safety data from dose-ranging studies indicate that a 5-day course of oseltamivir 150 mg twice daily or a 6-week course of oseltamivir 75 mg twice daily are tolerated as well as the usual recommended dosage for treatment or prophylaxis of influenza.

Adverse effects occurring in 1% or more of children receiving oseltamivir for the treatment of influenza include vomiting, abdominal pain, epistaxis, otic disorder, and conjunctivitis. GI effects, especially vomiting, were the most frequently reported adverse effects in children receiving the drug for prophylaxis of influenza.

■ **Dermatologic and Hypersensitivity Reactions** Anaphylaxis and serious dermatologic reactions (toxic epidermal necrolysis, Stevens-Johnson syndrome, erythema multiforme) have been reported in patients receiving oseltamivir, including pediatric patients.

Rash, swelling of the face or tongue, allergy, dermatitis, eczema, or urticaria has been reported during postmarketing experience.

■ **Nervous System Effects** Headache has occurred in about 2% of adults receiving oseltamivir for treatment of influenza and in about 18% of adults receiving the drug for prophylaxis of influenza.

Neuropsychiatric Events Adverse neurologic and/or psychiatric effects have been reported in patients receiving oseltamivir (principally children in Japan). The contribution of oseltamivir to these events has not been established.

Adverse neuropsychiatric events (e.g., agitation, anxiety, self-injury, delirium, hallucinations, altered level of consciousness, confusion, nightmares, delusions, abnormal behavior, seizures), which occasionally were fatal, have been reported in patients receiving oseltamivir. Cases generally had an abrupt onset and rapid resolution.

Postmarketing reports of self-injury and delirium principally have involved children in Japan. The contribution of oseltamivir to these events has not been established. (See Cautions: Pediatric Precautions.)

Influenza itself can be associated with a variety of neurologic and behavioral symptoms (e.g., hallucinations, delirium, abnormal behavior) and fatalities can occur. Although such events may occur in the setting of encephalitis or encephalopathy, they can occur without obvious severe disease.

■ **GI Effects** Nausea, with or without vomiting, has been reported in up to 10% of adults and adolescents 13 years of age or older receiving oseltamivir. Nausea usually occurs after the initial dose and resolves within 1–2 days; administration of the drug with food improves GI tolerance. In pediatric patients in clinical studies, vomiting was reported in 16% of children 1–12 years of age and diarrhea or vomiting was reported in up to 7 or 9%, respectively, of pediatric patients 2 weeks to less than 1 year of age.

GI bleeding and hemorrhagic colitis have been reported during postmarketing experience.

■ **Other Adverse Effects** Hepatitis or abnormal liver function test values have been reported during postmarketing experience.

Arrhythmia, hypothermia, or metabolic events (e.g., deterioration in diabetes control) has been reported during postmarketing experience.

■ **Precautions and Contraindications** Oseltamivir is contraindicated in patients with known hypersensitivity to the drug or any ingredient in the formulation. If an allergic reaction occurs or is suspected, oseltamivir should be discontinued and appropriate treatment initiated. Patients and/or their caregivers should be advised of the risk of severe allergic reactions (including anaphylaxis) or serious skin reactions and should be instructed to discontinue oseltamivir and immediately contact a clinician if an allergic-like reaction occurs or is suspected.

Because there have been postmarketing reports of neuropsychiatric events (e.g., self-injury, delirium) in influenza patients receiving oseltamivir (see Neuropsychiatric Events under Cautions: Nervous System Effects), patients with influenza (especially children) should be closely monitored for signs of abnormal behavior during oseltamivir treatment. Patients and/or their caregivers should be instructed to contact a clinician if there are any signs of unusual behavior during oseltamivir treatment. If neuropsychiatric symptoms develop, the risks and benefits of continued therapy with oseltamivir should be evaluated.

Efficacy of oseltamivir has not been established in patients with chronic cardiac disease and/or pulmonary disease; however, no difference in incidence of complications between drug and placebo has been observed in these populations. Safety and efficacy have not been established in those with any medical condition severe or unstable enough to require inpatient care.

Although efficacy of oseltamivir for treatment or prevention of influenza in immunocompromised patients has not been established, safety of oseltamivir prophylaxis has been demonstrated for up to 12 weeks in immunocompromised patients. The drug has been used for treatment or prevention of influenza in some immunocompromised individuals†, including bone marrow transplant (BMT) recipients, hematopoietic stem cell transplant (HSCT) recipients, solid organ transplant recipients, and chemotherapy patients. (See Uses.)

There is no evidence that oseltamivir is effective for illness caused by any organisms other than influenza viruses. Serious bacterial infections may begin with influenza-like symptoms or may coexist with or occur as complications of influenza. There is no evidence that oseltamivir prevents such complications. Clinicians should consider the potential for secondary bacterial infections; if such infections occur, they should be treated appropriately.

Oseltamivir is not a substitute for annual vaccination with a seasonal influenza vaccine (influenza virus vaccine inactivated, influenza vaccine live intranasal, influenza vaccine recombinant). Although antiviral agents used for treatment or prevention of influenza, including oseltamivir, may be used concomitantly with or at any time before or after influenza virus vaccine inactivated, these antivirals may inhibit the vaccine virus contained in influenza vaccine live intranasal. (See Influenza Virus Vaccines under Drug Interactions.)

When the commercially available oral suspension containing 6 mg/mL is used, each 75-mg dose of oseltamivir contains 2 g of sorbitol. Patients with hereditary fructose intolerance should be informed that this amount of sorbitol exceeds the maximum daily limit of sorbitol for such individuals and may result in dyspepsia and diarrhea.

Safety and pharmacokinetics of oseltamivir have not been evaluated in patients with severe hepatic impairment.

Patients with renal impairment (i.e., creatinine clearance of 60 mL/minute or less) may be at increased risk of adverse effects during oseltamivir therapy because of decreased clearance of the drug; dosage adjustments are recommended when oseltamivir is used in adults with creatinine clearance of 10–60 mL/minute or adults with end-stage renal disease (ESRD; creatinine clearance 10 mL/minute or less) undergoing hemodialysis or continuous peritoneal dialysis. Oseltamivir is *not* recommended in adults with ESRD who are *not* undergoing dialysis. (See Renal Impairment under Dosage and Administration: Dosage in Renal and Hepatic Impairment.)

■ **Pediatric Precautions** Safety and efficacy of oseltamivir for the *treatment* of influenza have not been established in infants younger than 2 weeks of age.

Safety and efficacy of oseltamivir for *prophylaxis* of influenza have not been established in infants younger than 1 year of age.

When used for the *treatment* of influenza, the safety profile of oseltamivir observed in neonates and infants 2 weeks to less than 1 year of age has been consistent with the safety profile for the drug established in adults and pediatric patients older than 1 year of age. Data from open-label studies evaluating oseltamivir for *treatment* of influenza in infants 2 weeks to less than 1 year of age (including some premature infants with a postconceptional age of at least 36 weeks) indicated that the safety profile was similar across this young age range, and that vomiting, diarrhea, and diaper rash were the most frequently reported adverse effects. In addition, serum concentrations of oseltamivir in these infants were similar to or greater than those observed in older children and adults.

Young children, especially those younger than 2 years of age, are at increased risk of influenza infection, hospitalization, and complications. During the 2009 influenza A (H1N1)pdm09 pandemic, the US Food and Drug Administration (FDA) issued an Emergency Use Authorization (EUA) that temporarily allowed use of oseltamivir for emergency treatment or prevention of these infections in infants younger than 1 year of age†. Although the EUA expired in June 2010, the American Academy of Pediatrics (AAP) states that, because of the known safety profile of the drug, use of oseltamivir for the *treatment* of influenza in *full-term* or *preterm* neonates from birth† or for *prevention* of influenza in infants 3 months of age or older† is appropriate if indicated. However, because of limited safety and efficacy data, the US Public Health Service Advisory Committee on Immunization Practices (ACIP) and AAP state that oseltamivir is not recommended for *prevention* of influenza in infants younger than 3 months of age† unless the situation is judged critical. (See Dosage and Administration: Dosage.)

Unusual adverse neurologic and/or psychiatric effects, including self-injury, delirium, hallucinations, mental confusion, abnormal behavior, seizures, and encephalitis, have been reported in children 16 years of age and younger receiving oseltamivir. These effects have been reported principally in children in Japan. There also have been reports of deaths (12 as of November 2005) in Japanese children receiving oseltamivir. These deaths were attributed to sudden death (4), cardiorespiratory arrest (4), suicide (1), pneumonia (1), asphyxiation (1), and acute pancreatitis with cardiopulmonary arrest (1). In many cases, a relationship to oseltamivir was difficult to assess because of concomitantly used drugs, comorbid conditions, and/or lack of adequate detail in reports.

There is no evidence that Japanese patients have a pharmacodynamic predisposition for adverse effects since they do not metabolize oseltamivir differently or achieve higher drug concentrations compared with US patients. However, unusual neurologic manifestations of influenza (influenza-associated encephalitis or encephalopathy) have been documented in Japan, and Japanese pediatricians describe a syndrome of rapid onset of fever accompanied by seizures and altered consciousness that progresses to coma within a few days of flu symptom onset. This syndrome has frequently resulted in death or substantial neurologic sequelae. Currently available information suggests that increased reports of neuropsychiatric events in Japanese children receiving oseltamivir are most likely related to an increased awareness of influenza-associated encephalopathy, increased access to the drug in the Japanese population, and a coincident period of intensive monitoring for potential adverse effects. Therefore, based on available information, the FDA states that it is unable to conclude that a causal relationship exists between oseltamivir and reported pediatric deaths.

■ **Geriatric Precautions** Safety of oseltamivir for the treatment of influenza in geriatric individuals has been established in clinical studies. In addition, safety and efficacy were demonstrated in geriatric individuals (many with cardiac and/or respiratory disease) residing in nursing homes who received oseltamivir for up to 42 days for the prevention of influenza.

When the total number of patients studied in oseltamivir clinical trials is considered, 20% of those in studies evaluating the drug for the treatment of influenza were 65 years of age or older (7% were 75 years of age or older) and 23% of those in studies evaluating the drug for the prevention of influenza were 65 years or older (16% were 75 years of age or older). No overall differences in efficacy or safety were observed between geriatric and younger adults, and other clinical experience revealed no evidence of age-related differences.

Oseltamivir dosage adjustments based solely on age are not necessary for geriatric patients older than 65 years of age.

■ **Mutagenicity and Carcinogenicity** Oseltamivir was not mutagenic in the Ames microbial test, the human lymphocyte chromosome assay, or the mouse micronucleus test; oseltamivir was mutagenic in the Syrian hamster embryo cell transformation assay. Oseltamivir carboxylate was not mutagenic in the Ames microbial test, the L5178Y mouse lymphoma assay, or the Syrian hamster embryo cell transformation assay.

Oseltamivir was not carcinogenic in studies in rats or mice.

■ **Pregnancy, Fertility, and Lactation** ***Pregnancy*** There are no adequate and well-controlled studies using oseltamivir in pregnant women, and the drug should be used during pregnancy only when potential benefits outweigh possible risks to the fetus.

Pregnant women are at increased risk for severe complications from influenza, which may lead to adverse pregnancy and/or fetal outcomes including maternal death, still births, birth defects, preterm delivery, low birthweight, and small size for gestational age.

The US Centers for Disease Control and Prevention (CDC) and ACIP state that pregnancy is not considered a contraindication to use of oseltamivir for treatment or prevention of influenza and that oseltamivir regimens recommended for such infections in pregnant women are the same as those for other adults.

CDC and ACIP state that oseltamivir may be preferred when a neuraminidase inhibitor is indicated for the treatment of suspected or confirmed influenza in women who are pregnant or up to 2 weeks postpartum, but the drug of choice for prophylaxis of influenza is less clear. Zanamivir may be preferred by some clinicians for prophylaxis in pregnant women because of its limited systemic absorption; however, respiratory complications that may be associated with zanamivir because of its route of administration should be considered, especially in women at risk for respiratory problems.

Although data are insufficient to make a definitive assessment of the risk, prospective and retrospective observational studies that included approximately 1500 women exposed to oseltamivir during pregnancy (including approximately 400 women exposed during the first trimester) suggest that the observed rate of congenital malformations following oseltamivir exposures during any trimester was not greater than that reported in the general population. In animal studies, there was a dose-dependent increase in the incidence rates of a variety of minor skeletal abnormalities and variants in offspring of rats and rabbits exposed to maternally toxic dosages (approximately 100 and 50 times the human exposure, respectively), but the individual incidence rate of each skeletal abnormality or variant remained within the background rates of occurrence in the species studied.

Fertility No effects on fertility, mating performance, or early embryonic development were observed in rats given oseltamivir at doses up to 100 times the human systemic exposure of oseltamivir carboxylate.

Lactation Limited data indicate that oseltamivir and its active metabolite, oseltamivir carboxylate, are distributed into human milk in low concentrations that are considered unlikely to cause toxicity in nursing infants.

Oseltamivir should be used with caution in nursing women.

Drug Interactions

■ **Drugs Affected or Metabolized by Hepatic Microsomal Enzymes** Oseltamivir phosphate and its active metabolite, oseltamivir carboxylate, are not metabolized by and do not inhibit cytochrome P-450 (CYP) isoenzymes; interactions with drugs that are substrates for or inhibitors of these enzymes are unlikely.

■ **Acetaminophen** Concomitant use of acetaminophen and oseltamivir does not result in clinically important pharmacokinetic interactions; dosage adjustments are not needed.

■ **Amantadine and Rimantadine** Concomitant use of oseltamivir and amantadine or rimantadine does not result in clinically important pharmacokinetic interactions; dosage adjustments are not needed if oseltamivir is used concomitantly with amantadine or rimantadine.

■ **Amoxicillin** Concomitant use of amoxicillin and oseltamivir does not result in clinically important pharmacokinetic interactions; dosage adjustments are not needed.

■ **Antacids** Concomitant use of oseltamivir and antacids containing magnesium hydroxide, aluminum hydroxide, or calcium carbonate does not result in clinically important pharmacokinetic interactions; dosage adjustments are not needed.

■ **Anticoagulants** Concomitant use of oseltamivir and warfarin does not result in clinically important pharmacokinetic interactions; dosage adjustments are not needed.

■ **Aspirin** Concomitant use of aspirin and oseltamivir does not result in clinically important pharmacokinetic interactions; dosage adjustments are not needed.

■ **Cimetidine** Concomitant use of cimetidine and oseltamivir does not affect plasma concentrations of oseltamivir or oseltamivir carboxylate. Dosage adjustments are not needed.

■ **Influenza Virus Vaccines** Influenza virus vaccine inactivated (IIV) may be administered concomitantly with or at any time before or after oseltamivir. Although drug interaction studies have not been conducted to evaluate the immune response to IIV in patients receiving oseltamivir, oseltamivir therapy does not appear to impair normal humoral antibody response to infection in patients with naturally or experimentally acquired influenza.

Safety and efficacy of concomitant use of oseltamivir and influenza vaccine live intranasal (LAIV) have not been evaluated. Because influenza antiviral agents, including oseltamivir, reduce replication of influenza viruses, these antivirals potentially could decrease the immune response and decrease efficacy of the live intranasal vaccine. LAIV should not be administered until at least 48 hours after oseltamivir is discontinued and oseltamivir should not be administered until at least 2 weeks after administration of LAIV. If oseltamivir is administered concomitantly with LAIV, revaccination should be considered if appropriate. The US Public Health Service Advisory Committee on Immunization Practices (ACIP) states that individuals who received oseltamivir 2 days before to 14 days after LAIV may be revaccinated with either IIV or influenza vaccine recombinant (RIV).

■ **Peramivir** There was no evidence of drug interactions when IV peramivir was used concomitantly with oral oseltamivir.

■ **Probenecid** Concomitant use of oseltamivir with probenecid results in a twofold increase in systemic exposure to oseltamivir carboxylate because of decreased renal tubular secretion. However, this pharmacokinetic interaction is not expected to be clinically important and the usual oseltamivir dosage can be used in patients receiving probenecid.

Mechanism of Action

Oseltamivir phosphate is a prodrug and has little, if any, pharmacologic activity until hydrolyzed in vivo to oseltamivir carboxylate. Oseltamivir is pharmacologically related to zanamivir; oseltamivir, like zanamivir, differs pharmacologically from other currently available antiviral agents.

Oseltamivir carboxylate is a potent selective competitive inhibitor of the influenza virus neuraminidase, an enzyme essential for viral replication in vivo. Neuraminidase cleaves terminal sialic acid residues from glycoconjugates to enable the release of virus from infected cells, prevents the formation of viral aggregates after release from host cells, and possibly facilitates viral invasion of the upper airways.

Neuraminidase inhibitors interfere with the release of progeny influenza virus from infected host cells, thus preventing infection of new host cells and halting the spread of infection. Because replication of influenza virus in the respiratory tract reaches its peak between 24 and 72 hours after the onset of illness, neuraminidase inhibitors must be administered as early as possible.

Spectrum

Oseltamivir (as oseltamivir carboxylate, the active metabolite of oseltamivir phosphate) exhibits potent antiviral activity in vitro against both influenza A and B viruses. Oseltamivir appears to be a potent and selective inhibitor of all influenza A neuraminidase subtypes (i.e., N1–N9) tested to date.

Oseltamivir has been shown to be active in vitro and in vivo in animal studies against a recombinant influenza A virus containing the H1 and N1 genes of the 1918 pandemic human influenza virus.

Viral surveillance data indicate that the majority of seasonal influenza A (H3N2), influenza A (H1N1)pdm09, and influenza B viruses circulating during influenza seasons 2011–2012 through 2016–2017 have been susceptible to oseltamivir in vitro; resistance was reported rarely. (See Resistance.)

In vitro studies indicate that oseltamivir is active against avian influenza A viruses, including avian influenza A (H5N1) and some other avian influenza A viruses (e.g., H7N7, H7N9, H9N2, H10N8). However, avian influenza A (H5N1) and avian influenza A (H7N9) with reduced in vitro susceptibility or resistance to oseltamivir have been reported rarely. (See Resistance.)

Resistance

The major mechanisms of resistance to neuraminidase inhibitors (i.e., oseltamivir, zanamivir) that have been identified in vitro are viral neuraminidase mutations that affect the ability of the drugs to inhibit the enzyme and hemagglutinin mutations that reduce viral dependence on neuraminidase activity.

Influenza A and B viruses with decreased susceptibility to oseltamivir due to viral neuraminidase mutations have been produced in vitro and observed in clinical isolates.

Hemagglutinin substitutions selected in cell culture and associated with reduced susceptibility to oseltamivir include A11T, K173G, and R453M in influenza A (H3N2) and H99Q in influenza B (Yamagata lineage). In some cases, hemagglutinin substitutions were selected in conjunction with known neuraminidase resistance substitutions and may contribute to reduced susceptibility to oseltamivir; however, the impact of hemagglutinin substitutions on antiviral activity of oseltamivir in humans is unknown and likely depends on the influenza strain.

Influenza A virus variants with reduced susceptibility to oseltamivir include substitutions in neuraminidase N1 (i.e., I117V, E119V, R152K, Y155H, F174V, D199G/N, I223K/R/T/V, S247N, G249R+I267V, H275Y, N295S, Q313R+I427T, N325K, R368K) and in neuraminidase N2 (i.e., E41G, E119I/V, D151V, I222L/V, N294S, Q226H, R292K, SASG245–248 deletion, S247P). Influenza B virus variants with reduced susceptibility to oseltamivir recovered from patients receiving the drug or identified during viral surveillance include E117A, P139S, G140R, R150K, I221L/T/V, D197E/N/Y, A245D/S/T, H273Y, N294S, R374K, and G407S. The H275Y substitution in influenza A (H1N1) has been the major substitution associated with resistance to oseltamivir. In the event of an H5N1 pandemic, the N1 mutation at position 274 would be important because this is associated with a greater than 600-fold increase in inhibitory concentrations for oseltamivir in enzyme inhibition assays. Viruses that have neuraminidase mutations generally have reduced virulence. Although it has been suggested that these mutant viruses may have some degree of compromised infectivity and transmissibility compared with wild-type viruses, person-to-person transmission of oseltamivir-resistant variants of influenza A (H1N1) has been documented.

■ **Resistance in Influenza A and B Viruses** Strains of *seasonal* influenza with decreased in vitro susceptibility to oseltamivir have emerged in posttreatment isolates obtained from 1.3% of adults and adolescents and 8.6% of pediatric patients 1–12 years of age who received the drug in clinical studies of naturally acquired influenza infection. In pediatric treatment studies, the rate of treatment-emergent resistance to oseltamivir was 27–37% in children with influenza A (H1N1) and 3–18% in children with influenza A (H3N2). In one group of Japanese children who received oseltamivir for the treatment of seasonal influenza, oseltamivir-resistant mutants were detected in 18% of patients posttreatment. Resistant strains of influenza A and influenza B viruses have emerged in immunocompromised patients who received oseltamivir therapy.

In the US, almost all *seasonal* influenza A (H1N1) strains tested in 2008, 2009, and the beginning of 2010 were resistant to oseltamivir. During the 2010–2011 influenza season, the former *seasonal* influenza A (H1N1) was rarely detected and almost all circulating influenza A (H1N1) reported since that time have been the 2009 pandemic influenza A (H1N1)pdm09 virus. Oseltamivir-resistant strains of influenza A (H1N1)pdm09 have been reported rarely.

Viral surveillance data from the 2013–2014 influenza season indicated that 1.2% of influenza A (H1N1)pdm09 isolates were resistant to oseltamivir and 1.3% were resistant to peramivir; all isolates were susceptible to zanamivir. Resistance in influenza A (H1N1)pdm09 has emerged during oseltamivir treatment or prophylaxis, including in immunosuppressed individuals with prolonged viral replication during oseltamivir treatment and in individuals who developed influenza illness while receiving oseltamivir prophylaxis. Emergence of oseltamivir-resistant influenza A (H1N1)pdm09 has been reported to occur within 48 hours after initiation of oseltamivir treatment. Transmission of oseltamivir-resistant influenza A (H1N1)pdm09 is rare, but has been documented. To date, almost all influenza A (H1N1)pdm09 with the H275Y N1 amino acid substitution were resistant to oseltamivir and peramivir, but susceptible to zanamivir.

Data from the US Centers for Disease Control and Prevention (CDC) regarding influenza isolates collected in the US from October 2016 until May 2017 indicate that all influenza A (H3N2), influenza A (H1N1)pdm09, and influenza B isolates tested were susceptible to oseltamivir, zanamivir, and peramivir. Data from the World Health Organization (WHO) regarding influenza isolates collected from September 2016 until February 2017 indicate that all influenza A (H3N2) isolates tested were susceptible to oseltamivir, but several isolates of influenza A (H1N1)pdm09 and influenza B (Victoria lineage) had reduced susceptibility to the neuraminidase inhibitor antivirals.

■ Resistance in Avian Influenza A Virus Avian influenza A (H5N1) with reduced in vitro susceptibility or resistance to oseltamivir have been reported. In a patient with influenza A (H5N1) infection who received prophylaxis with oseltamivir (75 mg once daily for 3 days) immediately followed by oseltamivir treatment (75 mg twice daily for 7 days), isolates obtained on the third day of oseltamivir prophylaxis had mutations associated with oseltamivir resistance (these isolates remained susceptible to zanamivir). In 2 patients in Vietnam who received oseltamivir for treatment of avian influenza A (H5N1) infection, isolates had an amino acid substitution (H274Y) associated with high-level oseltamivir resistance; both patients subsequently died.

Avian influenza A (H7N9) isolates with reduced susceptibility or resistance to oseltamivir have been reported. In a few patients with avian influenza A (H7N9) infection who were receiving oseltamivir for treatment, oseltamivir resistance emerged and was associated with treatment failure and adverse clinical outcomes. Genetic analyses of isolates from an ongoing epidemic of avian influenza A (H7N9) that has been occurring in China since October 2016 indicate that approximately 7–9% of isolates tested (many may have been collected after antiviral treatment was started) have known or suspected markers for reduced susceptibility to one or more neuraminidase inhibitor antivirals.

■ Cross-resistance Cross-resistance between oseltamivir and other neuraminidase inhibitors (e.g., peramivir, zanamivir) has been reported in influenza A and B viruses. However, because oseltamivir, peramivir, and zanamivir bind to different sites on the neuraminidase enzyme or interact differently with the binding sites, cross-resistance among the drugs is variable.

Some strains may have reduced susceptibility to oseltamivir and/or peramivir, but are susceptible to zanamivir; other strains may have reduced susceptibility to zanamivir, but are susceptible to oseltamivir and/or peramivir. To date, influenza A (H1N1)pdm09 isolates with the H275Y mutation are cross-resistant to oseltamivir and peramivir, but susceptible to zanamivir. Avian influenza A (H5N1) with the H274Y mutation that are resistant to oseltamivir have been susceptible to zanamivir in vitro.

Reduced in vitro susceptibility to all 3 drugs (oseltamivir, peramivir, zanamivir) has been observed in influenza A with R292K or N294S resistance-associated neuraminidase substitutions and in influenza B virus with R371K resistance-associated neuraminidase substitution. Cross-resistance to both oseltamivir and zanamivir has been reported in vitro in influenza B with I222T, D198E/N, R371K, or G402S resistance-associated neuraminidase substitutions. The H275Y (N1 numbering) or N294S (N2 numbering) oseltamivir resistance-associated substitutions observed in the N1 neuraminidase subtype and the E119V or N294S oseltamivir resistance-associated substitutions observed in the N2 subtype (N2 numbering) are associated with reduced in vitro susceptibility to oseltamivir, but not zanamivir. The Q136K and K150T zanamivir resistance-associated substitutions observed in N1 neuraminidase or the S250G zanamivir resistance-associated substitutions observed in influenza B virus neuraminidase confer reduced in vitro susceptibility to zanamivir, but not oseltamivir. Influenza A (H1N1)pdm09 with the H275Y N1 amino acid substitution are cross-resistant to oseltamivir and peramivir, but susceptible to zanamivir in vitro. Avian influenza A (H5N1) isolates with the H274Y mutation that are resistant to oseltamivir have been susceptible to zanamivir in vitro.

An amino acid substitution that confers cross-resistance between neuraminidase inhibitors (oseltamivir, peramivir, zanamivir) and adamantane derivatives (M2 ion channel inhibitors; amantadine, rimantadine) has not been identified. However, influenza strains that have a neuraminidase substitution that confers resistance to neuraminidase inhibitors and also have an M2 substitution that confers resistance to M2 ion channel inhibitors may be resistant to both classes of influenza antivirals. The clinical relevance of phenotypic cross-resistance evaluations has not been established.

Pharmacokinetics

■ Absorption Oseltamivir phosphate is readily absorbed following oral administration and then extensively converted by hepatic esterases to the active metabolite, oseltamivir carboxylate. Following oral administration of oseltamivir 75 mg twice daily for multiple days in healthy adults, peak plasma concentrations of oseltamivir or oseltamivir carboxylate were 65 or 348 ng/mL, respectively. Following oral administration of oseltamivir phosphate, oseltamivir carboxylate is detectable in plasma within 30 minutes; peak concentrations of oseltamivir carboxylate are attained within 3–4 hours. The absolute bioavailability of oseltamivir carboxylate is 80% following oral administration of oseltamivir phosphate. Plasma concentrations of oseltamivir carboxylate are proportional to dosage up to an oseltamivir dosage of 500 mg twice daily.

Administration of oseltamivir phosphate with food has no effect on peak plasma concentrations or area under the plasma concentration-time curve (AUC) of oseltamivir carboxylate.

Pharmacokinetic data indicate that a dosage of 3 mg/kg twice daily in neonates and infants 2 weeks to less than 1 year of age result in oseltamivir concentrations similar to or higher than those reported in adults and children 1 year of age or older receiving usual dosage of the drug.

Following oral administration of oseltamivir phosphate in geriatric individuals (65–78 years of age), systemic exposure to oseltamivir carboxylate at steady-state is about 25–35% higher compared with younger adults receiving the same dosage.

In individuals with varying degrees of renal impairment receiving 100 mg of oseltamivir phosphate twice daily (about 1.3 times the maximum recommended dosage) for 5 days, oseltamivir carboxylate exposure increases with declining renal function. In patients undergoing continuous ambulatory peritoneal dialysis (CAPD), peak concentrations of oseltamivir carboxylate following a single 30-mg dose of oseltamivir or once-weekly oseltamivir was approximately threefold higher than peak concentrations in patients with normal renal function receiving 75 mg twice daily.

Limited data in patients with cirrhosis indicate that hepatic carboxylesterase activity in patients with moderate hepatic impairment is sufficient to metabolize oseltamivir phosphate to oseltamivir carboxylate. Systemic exposure to oseltamivir carboxylate in individuals with mild or moderate hepatic impairment is comparable to that in individuals without hepatic impairment.

■ Distribution Following oral administration of oseltamivir phosphate, oseltamivir carboxylate is distributed throughout the body, including into the upper and lower respiratory tract.

It is not known whether oseltamivir or oseltamivir carboxylate crosses the placenta in humans; placental transfer of oseltamivir carboxylate has been demonstrated in rats and rabbits.

Oseltamivir and oseltamivir carboxylate are distributed into milk.

Oseltamivir phosphate is 42% bound to plasma proteins; oseltamivir carboxylate is 3% bound to plasma proteins.

■ Elimination Oseltamivir phosphate is extensively (greater than 90%) converted to oseltamivir carboxylate (the active metabolite), principally by hepatic esterases. Oseltamivir carboxylate is not further metabolized.

Oseltamivir phosphate and oseltamivir carboxylate are not metabolized by cytochrome P-450 (CYP) enzymes.

Oseltamivir carboxylate is eliminated (greater than 99%) by renal excretion; less than 20% of an oral radiolabeled dose of oseltamivir phosphate is eliminated in feces.

The plasma half-life of oseltamivir phosphate is 1–3 hours; half-life of oseltamivir carboxylate is 6–10 hours. Half-lives observed in geriatric individuals are similar to those observed in younger adults.

Clearance of both oseltamivir phosphate and oseltamivir carboxylate is increased in younger pediatric patients compared with adults. Total clearance of oseltamivir carboxylate decreases linearly with increasing age (up to 12 years of age); pharmacokinetics in those 12 years of age or older is similar to that in adults.

Renal clearance of oseltamivir carboxylate decreases linearly with creatinine clearance.

Chemistry and Stability

■ Chemistry Oseltamivir phosphate is a carbocyclic transition state sialic acid analog. Oseltamivir differs structurally from zanamivir (another sialic acid analog) by the absence of glycerol and guanidino groups. These structural modifications in oseltamivir result in a compound with substantially improved oral bioavailability compared with that of zanamivir.

Oseltamivir phosphate occurs as a white, crystalline solid with a bitter taste. Oseltamivir phosphate has an aqueous solubility of 588 mg/mL at 25°C.

■ Stability Oseltamivir phosphate capsules should be stored at 25°C, but may be exposed to temperatures ranging from 15–30°C.

Oseltamivir phosphate powder for oral suspension should be stored at 25°C, but may be exposed to temperatures ranging from 15–30°C. The reconstituted oral suspension should be stored at 2–8°C for up to 17 days. Alternatively, the reconstituted suspension may be stored for up to 10 days at 25°C and may be exposed to temperatures ranging from 15–30°C during this time. The reconstituted oral suspension should not be frozen.

Extemporaneous oral suspensions of oseltamivir phosphate prepared according to the manufacturer's directions using commercially available 75-mg capsules of the drug are stable for 5 weeks when refrigerated at 2–8°C or for 5 days when stored at room temperature (25°C).

Preparations

Excipients in commercially available drug preparations may have clinically important effects in some individuals; consult specific product labeling for details.

Oseltamivir Phosphate

Oral		
Capsules	30 mg (of oseltamivir)	**Tamiflu®**, Genentech
	45 mg (of oseltamivir)	**Tamiflu®**, Genentech
	75 mg (of oseltamivir)	**Tamiflu®**, Genentech
For suspension	6 mg (of oseltamivir) per mL	**Tamiflu®**, Genentech

†Use is not currently included in the labeling approved by the US Food and Drug Administration

Selected Revisions November 2017,

Peramivir

■ Peramivir is a neuraminidase inhibitor antiviral active against influenza A and B viruses.

Uses

■ Treatment of Seasonal Influenza A and B Virus Infections

Peramivir is used for the *treatment* of acute, uncomplicated illness caused by influenza A or B viruses in adults, adolescents, and children 2 years of age or older who have been symptomatic for no longer than 2 days.

Although peramivir has been used for the treatment of serious influenza† in some patients, efficacy of the drug has not been established in patients with serious influenza requiring hospitalization.

The US Centers for Disease Control and Prevention (CDC), Advisory Committee on Immunization Practices (ACIP), Infectious Diseases Society of America (IDSA), and American Academy of Pediatrics (AAP) recommend that antiviral treatment be initiated as soon as possible in all individuals with suspected or confirmed influenza who require hospitalization or have severe, complicated, or progressive illness (regardless of vaccination status or underlying illness). These experts also recommend early empiric antiviral treatment in individuals with suspected or confirmed influenza of any severity if they are at high risk for influenza-related complications because of age or underlying medical conditions (regardless of vaccination status). Individuals at increased risk for influenza-related complications include children younger than 5 years of age (especially those younger than 2 years of age); adults 65 years of age or older; individuals of any age with certain chronic medical or immunosuppressive conditions; women who are pregnant or up to 2 weeks postpartum; individuals younger than 19 years of age receiving long-term aspirin therapy; American Indians or Alaskan natives; morbidly obese individuals with a body mass index (BMI) of 40 or greater; and residents of any age in nursing homes or other long-term care facilities.

CDC, ACIP, IDSA, and AAP also state that empiric antiviral treatment can be considered in previously healthy, symptomatic individuals with suspected or confirmed seasonal influenza who are not known to be at increased risk of developing severe or complicated illness (regardless of vaccination status), if such treatment can be initiated within 48 hours of illness onset. Although these individuals typically do not require treatment, early empiric antiviral treatment might provide some benefit (e.g., shortened duration of illness). The use of antiviral treatment in such individuals should be based on clinical judgment and is not necessary in those who are already beginning to recover.

If treatment of seasonal influenza is indicated, an appropriate antiviral should be initiated as soon as possible after illness onset (ideally within 48 hours), and should *not* be delayed while waiting for laboratory confirmation. Because there is some evidence from observational studies evaluating use of oseltamivir in hospitalized patients that antiviral treatment may still be beneficial in such patients when initiated as late as 4 or 5 days after illness onset, CDC, ACIP, and AAP recommend that appropriate antiviral treatment be initiated in all patients with severe, complicated, or progressive illness attributable to influenza and all hospitalized patients and patients at increased risk of influenza complications (either hospitalized or outpatient) who have suspected or confirmed influenza, even if it has been more than 48 hours since illness onset. Decisions regarding use of empiric antiviral treatment in outpatients, especially high-risk patients, should be based on disease severity and progression, age, underlying medical conditions, likelihood of influenza, and time since onset of symptoms.

For the treatment of suspected or confirmed severe, complicated influenza in hospitalized patients or outpatients, oseltamivir is the preferred influenza antiviral because of the lack of data regarding use of IV peramivir, inhaled zanamivir, and oral baloxavir marboxil in such patients. CDC states that data are insufficient regarding use of IV peramivir for the treatment of severe influenza in hospitalized patients or outpatients; however, use of the drug should be considered for the treatment of severe influenza† in patients who cannot tolerate or absorb oral or enterically administered oseltamivir (e.g., because of suspected or known gastric stasis, malabsorption, or GI bleeding).

If an antiviral is used for the treatment of suspected or confirmed acute, uncomplicated influenza in otherwise healthy outpatients, CDC, IDSA, and other experts state that any age-appropriate influenza antiviral (oseltamivir, peramivir, zanamivir, baloxavir marboxil) can be used if not contraindicated.

Viral surveillance data available from local and state health departments and CDC should be considered when selecting an antiviral for the treatment of seasonal influenza. Strains of circulating influenza viruses and the antiviral susceptibility of these strains constantly evolve, and the possibility that emergence of resistant strains may decrease effectiveness of influenza antivirals should be considered. Although influenza A and B viruses circulating in the US during the last few years generally have been susceptible to peramivir (see Description: Resistance), clinicians should consult the most recent information.

CDC issues recommendations concerning the use of antivirals for the treatment of influenza, and these recommendations are updated as needed during each influenza season. Information regarding influenza surveillance and updated recommendations for treatment of seasonal influenza are available from CDC at http://www.cdc.gov/flu.

Clinical Experience **Acute, Uncomplicated Influenza in Adults.** Efficacy and safety of peramivir for the treatment of acute, uncomplicated influenza in adults were evaluated in randomized, controlled studies in otherwise healthy adults with documented influenza infection (study 621). The majority of patients enrolled in these studies had infections caused by seasonal influenza A; only a limited number of patients had infections caused by seasonal influenza B. In a placebo-controlled study in adults 20–65 years of age with documented influenza infection, peramivir (single 600-mg IV dose) initiated in an outpatient setting within 48 hours of onset of symptoms decreased the median duration of influenza symptoms (i.e., nasal congestion, sore throat, cough, aches or pains in muscles or joints, fatigue, headache, feverishness) by approximately 21 hours and decreased the median time to recovery of normal temperature (oral temperature less than 37°C) by approximately 12 hours compared with placebo. In a phase 3, double-blind, randomized study in adults 20 years of age or older with documented influenza infection who received treatment in an outpatient setting within 48 hours of onset of symptoms, peramivir (single 600-mg IV dose) was noninferior to oseltamivir (75 mg orally twice daily for 5 days) based on median time to alleviation of influenza symptoms.

Acute, Uncomplicated Influenza in Pediatric Patients 2–17 years of Age. Efficacy and safety of peramivir for the treatment of acute, uncomplicated influenza in pediatric patients 2–17 years of age were evaluated in a randomized, multicenter, open-label, active-controlled trial (study 305). At study entry, patients had fever (oral temperature 37.8°C or greater) with at least one respiratory symptom (cough or rhinitis) or a positive influenza rapid antigen test and were randomized to receive a single dose of IV peramivir (12 mg/kg [up to 600 mg] in those 2–12 years of age or 600 mg in those 13–17 years of age) or a 5-day regimen of oral oseltamivir (twice daily). Antiviral treatment was initiated within 48 hours of onset of symptoms and adjunctive use of fever-reducing medications was allowed. The primary end point was the safety of peramivir compared to oseltamivir as measured by adverse events, laboratory analysis, vital signs, and physical examination. Secondary end points included efficacy outcomes such as time to resolution of influenza symptoms and time to resolution of fever; however, the trial was not powered to detect statistically significant differences in the secondary end points. A total of 69 pediatric patients received IV peramivir (median age 7.9 years, 55% male, 58% infected with influenza A virus, 36% infected with influenza B virus, 6% coinfected with both influenza A and B viruses). The median time to alleviation of combined influenza symptoms was 79 hours in those treated with peramivir and 107 hours in those treated with oseltamivir; the median time to recovery to normal temperature (less than 37°C) was 40 and 28 hours, respectively.

Serious Influenza Requiring Hospitalization. Efficacy and safety of peramivir for the treatment of influenza in patients requiring hospitalization† were evaluated in a phase 3, randomized, double-blind, placebo-controlled study that included adults and children 6 years of age or older. Patients who were hospitalized with influenza and had been symptomatic for less than 72 hours were randomized to receive the usual standard of care in conjunction with a 5-day regimen of peramivir (600 mg IV once daily in adults; 10 mg/kg IV once daily [up to 600 mg daily] in children and adolescents) or placebo. The primary end point was time to clinical resolution (defined as time from initiation of study treatment until at least 4 of 5 vital sign abnormalities, including body temperature and oxygen saturation, had been resolved for at least 24 hours). A preplanned interim analysis indicated that there was no clinically important difference in the median time to clinical resolution in those treated with peramivir (41.8 hours) or placebo (48.9 hours), although there was some evidence that peramivir provided some benefit in time to clinical resolution in those who had been symptomatic for less than 48 hours prior to treatment and in those who required treatment in an intensive care unit (ICU). The study was terminated after the interim analysis because of practical considerations regarding the ability to obtain a sample size adequate for further evaluation.

■ Avian Influenza A Virus Infections

Neuraminidase inhibitors (oseltamivir, peramivir, zanamivir) have been used for the treatment of infections caused by susceptible avian influenza A viruses†.

Experience to date indicates that avian influenza A viruses do not easily transmit from wild or domestic birds, water fowl, or poultry to humans, but human infections may rarely occur and have been linked to contact with live or dead infected birds or poultry, uncooked poultry products, or surfaces contaminated with infected poultry feces or respiratory secretions. Recent human cases generally have involved a highly pathogenic Asian strain of avian influenza A (H5N1) that has been circulating since 2003 in poultry in Asia, Africa, the Pacific, Eastern Europe, and the Middle East or a novel avian influenza A (H7N9) virus that was first identified in China in March 2013.

Worldwide, most avian influenza viruses isolated in wild birds, water fowl, or poultry have been designated as low pathogenic strains; however, highly pathogenic avian influenza (HPAI) strains are occasionally detected. Since December 2014, HPAI viruses (H5N1, H5N2, H5N8) have been reported in wild birds, water fowl, and/or domestic poultry (commercial or backyard flocks) in the US (e.g., Arkansas, California, Idaho, Iowa, Minnesota, Missouri, Nebraska, North Dakota, Oregon, South Dakota, Utah, Washington, Wisconsin). Although CDC states that the risk of human infection with these HPAI H5 viruses is considered low in the US, human infection is possible since other closely related HPAI H5 viruses in Asia and other countries have caused sporadic cases of human respiratory illness. The HPAI (H5N1) strain reported in poultry outbreaks in the US is a new reassortant virus that is genetically different from the highly pathogenic Asian strain of influenza A (H5N1) that has caused human infections in Asia and other countries and has been associated with a high mortality rate.

Appropriate use of a neuraminidase inhibitor antiviral (oral oseltamivir, IV peramivir, inhaled zanamivir) is an important component of response and control measures to treat avian influenza A virus infections and help reduce the risk of additional human infections. For the treatment of severe, complicated, or progressive avian influenza A infections in hospitalized patients or outpatients, including infections caused by avian influenza A (H7N9), avian influenza A (H5N1), or novel avian influenza A H5 viruses, CDC recommends oseltamivir as the antiviral of choice. For the treatment of hospitalized patients with severe influenza who cannot tolerate or absorb oral oseltamivir (e.g., because of suspected or known gastric stasis, malabsorption, or GI bleeding), CDC states that use of IV peramivir or investigational IV zanamivir may be considered. For the treatment of uncomplicated avian influenza A infections in outpatients, CDC states that oral oseltamivir, inhaled zanamivir, or IV peramivir may be used. When antiviral prophylaxis is indicated in close contacts of individuals with confirmed or probable infection with avian influenza A viruses associated with severe disease or with potential to cause severe disease, CDC recommends oral oseltamivir or inhaled zanamivir.

For additional information on avian influenza A virus infections, see Uses: Avian Influenza A Virus Infections in Oseltamivir 8:18.28.

The most recent information regarding treatment and prevention of avian influenza A infections is available from CDC at http://www.cdc.gov/flu/avianflu/ or WHO at https://www.who.int/influenza/human_animal_interface/en/.

■ **Pandemic Influenza** Peramivir is recommended as an alternative for the treatment of pandemic influenza† caused by susceptible strains of influenza virus.

Influenza viruses can cause seasonal epidemics and, occasionally, pandemics during which rates of illness and death from influenza-related complications can increase dramatically worldwide. The most recent influenza pandemic occurred during 2009 and was related to a novel influenza A (H1N1) strain, influenza A (H1N1)pdm09. During the 2009 influenza A (H1N1)pdm09 pandemic, FDA issued an Emergency Use Authorization (EUA) that temporarily allowed use of peramivir for the treatment of serious pandemic influenza virus infection in certain hospitalized adults and pediatric patients†.

On June 11, 2009, the WHO declared that the first global influenza pandemic in 41 years was occurring and issued a pandemic alert regarding influenza A (H1N1)pdm09, previously referred to as the novel 2009 influenza A (H1N1) virus or swine-origin influenza A (H1N1) virus. Influenza outbreaks caused by the influenza A (H1N1)pdm09 virus were reported in several countries, including the US, beginning in March and April 2009. The virus is a triple-reassortant swine influenza virus with genes from human, swine, and avian influenza A viruses and contains a unique combination of gene segments not previously reported among human or swine influenza A in the US or elsewhere. The influenza A (H1N1)pdm09 virus is antigenically distinct from previous human influenza A (H1N1) viruses that had been in circulation since 1977, and widespread transmission of the virus occurred since most individuals had no preexisting antibody to the strain. In the US, the 2009 influenza A (H1N1)pdm09 pandemic was characterized by a substantial increase in influenza activity that peaked in late October and early November 2009 and returned to seasonal baseline levels by January 2010. During the pandemic, more than 99% of influenza viruses circulating in the US were the influenza A (H1N1)pdm09 virus; more than 60 million Americans become ill with the virus and more than 270,000 hospitalizations and 12,500 deaths were reported. In August 2010, the WHO declared that the world was in a post-pandemic period. Influenza A (H1N1)pdm09 had become a seasonal influenza virus and still continues to circulate with other seasonal influenza viruses.

The spread of the highly pathogenic Asian strain of influenza A (H5N1) in poultry in Asia, Africa, the Pacific, Eastern Europe, and the Middle East that has been occurring since 2003 and has caused human infections (including fatalities) represents a potential future pandemic threat. In addition, the novel avian influenza A (H7N9) virus that was first identified in China in March 2013 and has been causing sporadic human infections has pandemic potential. (See Uses: Avian Influenza A Virus Infections, in Oseltamivir 8:18.28.)

Dosage and Administration

■ **Administration** Peramivir is administered by IV infusion.

IV Administration Peramivir injection concentrate for IV use containing 10 mg of the drug per mL must be diluted prior to IV infusion.

Peramivir is compatible with 0.9% or 0.45% sodium chloride, 5% dextrose, or lactated Ringer's injection. Solutions of the drug are compatible with materials commonly used for administration (e.g., polyvinyl chloride and polyvinyl chloride-free infusion bags, polypropylene syringes, polyethylene tubing).

Peramivir solutions should *not* be mixed with or administered simultaneously with other drugs.

Vials of peramivir injection concentrate for IV use contain no preservatives or bacteriostatic agents and are intended for single use only.

Dilution. The appropriate dose of peramivir injection concentrate for IV use containing 10 mg/mL should be withdrawn from the vial and diluted in 0.9% sodium chloride injection, 0.45% sodium chloride injection, 5% dextrose injection, or lactated Ringer's injection to achieve a maximum total volume of 100 mL.

Following dilution, peramivir solutions should be administered immediately. Alternatively, diluted peramivir solutions may be stored for up to 24 hours at 2–8°C. Refrigerated solutions should be allowed to reach room temperature and then administered immediately. Unused portions should be discarded 24 hours after dilution.

Peramivir solutions should appear clear and colorless and should be inspected visually for particulate matter and discoloration prior to administration.

Rate of Administration. Peramivir solutions should be administered by IV infusion over 15–30 minutes.

■ **Dosage** ***Adult Dosage*** **Treatment of Seasonal Influenza A and B Virus Infections.** For the *treatment* of acute, uncomplicated influenza in adults 18 years of age or older, the recommended dosage of peramivir is a single 600-mg dose given by IV infusion within 2 days of symptom onset.

Treatment of Avian Influenza A Virus Infections. If peramivir is used for the *treatment* of avian influenza virus infections†, including avian influenza A (H7N9), avian influenza A (H5N1), and novel avian influenza A H5 viruses, the US Centers for Disease Control and Prevention (CDC) recommends that adults receive a dosage of 600 mg given IV once daily for 5 days or longer. Only limited data are available regarding use of peramivir for the treatment of these infections.

Pediatric Dosage **Treatment of Seasonal Influenza A and B Virus Infections.** For the *treatment* of acute, uncomplicated influenza in children 2–12 years of age, the recommended dosage of peramivir is a single dose of 12 mg/kg (up to 600 mg) given by IV infusion within 2 days of symptom onset.

For the *treatment* of acute, uncomplicated influenza in adolescents 13 years of age or older, the recommended dosage of peramivir is a single 600-mg dose given by IV infusion within 2 days of symptom onset.

Treatment of Avian Influenza A Virus Infections. If peramivir is used for the *treatment* of avian influenza virus infections†, including avian influenza A (H7N9), avian influenza A (H5N1), and novel avian influenza A H5 viruses, CDC recommends that children receive a dosage of 10 mg/kg (up to 600 mg) given IV once daily for 5 days or longer. Only limited data are available regarding use of peramivir for the treatment of these infections.

■ **Special Populations** ***Hepatic Impairment*** Peramivir has not been studied in patients with hepatic impairment; clinically important alterations in peramivir pharmacokinetics are not expected in such patients.

Renal Impairment Dosage of peramivir should be decreased in patients with creatinine clearances less than 50 mL/minute.

For the *treatment* of acute, uncomplicated influenza in pediatric patients 2–12 years of age with renal impairment, a single dose of 4 mg/kg is recommended in those with creatinine clearances of 30–49 mL/minute and a single dose of 2 mg/kg is recommended in those with creatinine clearances of 10–29 mL/minute.

For the *treatment* of acute, uncomplicated influenza in adults and adolescents 13 years of age or older with renal impairment, a single 200-mg dose of peramivir is recommended in those with creatinine clearances of 30–49 mL/minute and a single 100-mg dose of the drug is recommended in those with creatinine clearances of 10–29 mL/minute.

If peramivir is used in patients with chronic renal impairment maintained on hemodialysis, dosage should be adjusted based on renal function and the drug should be administered after hemodialysis. (See Renal Impairment under Warnings/Precautions: Specific Populations, in Cautions.)

Geriatric Adults Dosage adjustments based solely on age are not necessary in geriatric patients.

Cautions

■ **Contraindications** Peramivir is contraindicated in patients with known serious hypersensitivity (e.g., anaphylaxis, erythema multiforme, Stevens-Johnson syndrome) to the drug or any ingredient in the formulation.

■ **Warnings/Precautions** ***Sensitivity Reactions*** **Hypersensitivity Reactions.** Serious dermatologic reactions (erythema multiforme, Stevens-Johnson syndrome) have been reported in patients receiving peramivir. Anaphylactic/anaphylactoid reactions, exfoliative dermatitis, and rash also have been reported during postmarketing experience.

If anaphylaxis or a serious skin reaction occurs or is suspected, peramivir should be discontinued and appropriate treatment initiated.

Neuropsychiatric and CNS Effects Delirium and abnormal behavior leading to injury have been reported during postmarketing experience in patients with influenza receiving neuraminidase inhibitors, including peramivir. Most cases involved pediatric patients and generally had an abrupt onset and rapid resolution. The role of peramivir in these events has not been established.

Influenza itself can be associated with a variety of neurologic and behavioral symptoms (e.g., hallucinations, delirium, abnormal behavior) that sometimes result in fatalities. Although such events may occur in the setting of encephalitis or encephalopathy, they can occur in patients with uncomplicated influenza.

Patients with influenza should be closely monitored for signs of abnormal behavior.

Differential Diagnosis When making treatment decisions in patients with suspected influenza, clinicians should consider the possibility of primary or concomitant bacterial infections for which peramivir would be ineffective.

Serious bacterial infections may begin with influenza-like symptoms or may coexist with or occur as complications of influenza. There is no evidence that peramivir prevents such complications.

There is no evidence that peramivir is effective for illness caused by any organisms other than influenza A or B.

Influenza Vaccination Influenza antivirals, including peramivir, are not a substitute for annual vaccination with a seasonal influenza vaccine (influenza virus vaccine inactivated, influenza vaccine live intranasal, influenza vaccine recombinant).

Although influenza antivirals, including peramivir, may be used concomitantly with or at any time before or after influenza virus vaccine inactivated or influenza vaccine recombinant, such antivirals may inhibit the vaccine virus contained in influenza vaccine live intranasal and decrease efficacy of this vaccine. (See Influenza Vaccines under Drug Interactions: Vaccines.)

Specific Populations **Pregnancy.** Data regarding use of peramivir in pregnant women are insufficient to determine whether the drug is associated with a risk of adverse developmental outcomes.

In animal reproduction studies, no adverse embryofetal effects were observed in pregnant rats when peramivir was administered by IV injection once daily at the maximum feasible dosage, resulting in systemic drug exposures approximately 8 times those in humans at the recommended dosage. However, when peramivir was administered to pregnant rats by continuous IV infusion, fetal abnormalities (reduced renal papilla, dilated ureters) were observed. In rabbits, peramivir administered by IV injection once daily during organogenesis at exposures 8 times those in humans at the recommended dosage resulted in developmental toxicity (abortion or premature delivery) at maternally toxic doses.

Pregnant women are at increased risk for severe complications from influenza, which may lead to adverse pregnancy and/or fetal outcomes including maternal death, stillbirths, birth defects, preterm delivery, low birthweight, and small size for gestational age.

The US Centers for Disease Control and Prevention (CDC) states that only limited data are available regarding use of peramivir for the treatment of influenza in pregnant women. These experts state that oseltamivir is the preferred antiviral for the treatment of suspected or confirmed influenza in women who are pregnant or up to 2 weeks postpartum.

Lactation. It is not known whether peramivir is distributed into human milk, affects milk production, or has any effects on breast-fed infants. Peramivir is distributed into milk in rats. (See Extent under Pharmacokinetics: Distribution.)

The benefits of breast-feeding and the importance of peramivir to the woman should be considered along with potential adverse effects on the breast-fed child from the drug or from the underlying maternal condition.

Pediatric Use. Safety and efficacy of peramivir have not been established in pediatric patients younger than 2 years of age.

Safety and efficacy of peramivir for the treatment of acute, uncomplicated influenza in pediatric patients 2–17 years of age have been established and are supported by evidence from adequate and well-controlled trials of the drug in adults and additional data from a randomized, open-label, active-controlled trial in pediatric patients in this age group. Data from the open-label pediatric study indicated that the safety profile of the drug in pediatric patients 2–17 years of age generally is similar to that reported in adults. Adverse effects reported in 2% or more of pediatric patients treated with peramivir and not reported in adults include vomiting, fever, and tympanic membrane erythema.

Geriatric Use. Clinical studies of peramivir did not include sufficient numbers of patients 65 years of age and older to determine whether geriatric patients respond differently than younger adults. Other reported clinical experience has not identified differences in responses between geriatric and younger adults.

Peramivir pharmacokinetics in geriatric adults are similar to the pharmacokinetics of the drug reported in younger adults; therefore, dosage adjustments based solely on age are not necessary in adults 65 years of age and older.

Hepatic Impairment. The pharmacokinetics of peramivir have not been studied in patients with hepatic impairment; however, hepatic function is not expected to substantially affect pharmacokinetics of peramivir since the drug does not undergo clinically important metabolism.

Renal Impairment. The mean area under the plasma concentration-time curve (AUC) of peramivir following IV administration of a single 2-mg/kg dose was increased by 28, 302, or 412% in adults with creatinine clearances of 50–79, 30–49, or 10–29 mL/minute, respectively, compared with AUCs reported in individuals with normal renal function. Pharmacokinetics of peramivir have not been evaluated in pediatric patients with renal impairment.

Dosage of peramivir should be adjusted in patients with creatinine clearances less than 50 mL/minute. (See Renal Impairment under Dosage and Administration: Special Populations.)

■ **Common Adverse Effects** Adverse effects occurring in 2% or more of adults receiving peramivir include diarrhea, constipation, insomnia, and hypertension.

Drug Interactions

■ **Drugs Affected or Metabolized by Hepatic Microsomal Enzymes** Peramivir is not metabolized by and does not induce or inhibit cytochrome P-450 (CYP) isoenzymes. Drug interactions with drugs that are substrates or inhibitors of these enzymes are unlikely.

■ **Drugs Affecting or Affected by P-glycoprotein Transport System** Peramivir is not a substrate for and is not an inhibitor of the P-glycoprotein (P-gp) transport system.

■ **Antivirals** ***Oseltamivir*** There was no evidence of pharmacokinetic interactions when oseltamivir (single 75-mg oral dose) was used concomitantly with peramivir (single 600-mg IV dose).

There was no in vitro evidence of antagonistic antiviral effects between oseltamivir and peramivir when the combination was evaluated in cell cultures infected with influenza A (H1N1).

Rimantadine There was no evidence of pharmacokinetic interactions when rimantadine (single 100-mg oral dose) was used concomitantly with peramivir (single 600-mg IV dose).

There was no in vitro evidence of antagonistic antiviral effects between rimantadine and peramivir when the combination was evaluated in cell cultures infected with influenza A (H1N1) or influenza A (H3N2).

Zanamivir Concomitant use of zanamivir and peramivir is not recommended.

■ **Estrogens and Progestins** There was no evidence of pharmacokinetic interactions when oral contraceptives containing ethinyl estradiol and levonorgestrel were used concomitantly with peramivir.

■ **Probenecid** There was no evidence of pharmacokinetic interactions when probenecid was used concomitantly with peramivir.

■ **Vaccines** ***Influenza Vaccines*** Although concomitant use of peramivir and influenza virus vaccine inactivated (IIV) or influenza vaccine recombinant (RIV) has not been evaluated, the Advisory Committee on Immunization Practices (ACIP) states that antivirals used for the treatment of influenza have no effect on the immune response to inactivated influenza vaccines and these vaccines may be administered simultaneously with or at any time before or after influenza antivirals.

Safety and efficacy of concomitant use of peramivir and influenza vaccine live intranasal (LAIV) have not been studied. However, because influenza antivirals, including peramivir, inhibit replication of influenza viruses, these antivirals potentially could decrease the immune response to LAIV and efficacy of the vaccine. LAIV should not be administered until at least 48 hours after peramivir is discontinued and, if feasible, influenza antivirals should be avoided until at least 14 days after administration of LAIV. If peramivir is administered within 2 weeks after LAIV, the LAIV dose should be repeated at least 48 hours after the last dose of influenza antiviral. Alternatively, ACIP states that individuals who received an influenza antiviral 2 days before to 14 days after LAIV may be revaccinated using age-appropriate IIV or RIV.

Pharmacokinetics

■ **Absorption** ***Bioavailability*** Following IV infusion over 30 minutes, peak serum concentrations of peramivir are attained at the end of the infusion. Accumulation of the drug is negligible following multiple doses for up to 10 days.

There is a linear relationship between the dose of peramivir and exposure parameters (peak plasma concentrations, area under the plasma concentration-time curve [AUC]) of the drug.

■ **Distribution** ***Extent*** Following IV administration, peramivir is well distributed within extracellular fluid spaces, including the nose and throat.

It is not known whether peramivir is distributed into human milk. Peramivir is distributed into milk in rats; peak milk concentrations are attained 0.75 hours after an IV dose in rats and the milk to plasma AUC ratio is approximately 0.5.

Plasma Protein Binding Peramivir is less than 30% bound to plasma proteins.

■ **Elimination** ***Metabolism*** Peramivir does not undergo clinically important metabolism.

The drug is not a substrate for and does not affect cytochrome P-450 (CYP) isoenzymes.

Elimination Route Following IV administration of peramivir, approximately 90% of the dose is eliminated unchanged in urine, principally by glomerular filtration.

Peramivir is removed by hemodialysis; systemic exposure is decreased 73–81% in patients undergoing hemodialysis.

Half-life The plasma half-life of peramivir following a single 600-mg IV dose in healthy adults is approximately 20 hours.

Special Populations In children 2–12 years of age, the pharmacokinetics of peramivir following a single 12-mg/kg IV dose of the drug are similar to the pharmacokinetics reported in adults following a single 600-mg IV dose of the drug. Peramivir pharmacokinetics following a single 600-mg IV dose in adolescents 13–17 years of age are similar to the pharmacokinetics reported in adults following a single 600-mg IV dose.

In adults with creatinine clearances of 50–79, 30–49, or less than 30 mL/minute, the AUC of peramivir was increased by 28, 302, or 412%, respectively, compared with those with normal renal function. Pharmacokinetics of peramivir have not been evaluated in pediatric patients with renal impairment.

Although the pharmacokinetics of peramivir have not been studied in patients with hepatic impairment, substantial alterations in peramivir pharmacokinetics are not expected in such patients since the drug does not undergo clinically important metabolism.

Peramivir pharmacokinetics in geriatric individuals are similar to the pharmacokinetics in younger adults.

Description

Peramivir is a neuraminidase inhibitor antiviral and is pharmacologically related to other neuraminidase inhibitors (e.g., oseltamivir, zanamivir).

Peramivir is a potent selective competitive inhibitor of the influenza virus neuraminidase, an enzyme essential for viral replication. Neuraminidase cleaves terminal sialic acid residues from glycoconjugates to enable the release of virus from infected cells, prevents the formation of viral aggregates after release from host cells, and possibly facilitates viral invasion of the upper airways.

■ **Spectrum** Peramivir exhibits potent antiviral activity in vitro against both influenza A and B viruses.

Viral surveillance data indicate that the majority of seasonal influenza A (H3N2), influenza A (H1N1)pdm09, and influenza B viruses circulating worldwide, including in the US, during recent influenza seasons have been susceptible to neuraminidase inhibitors (oseltamivir, peramivir, zanamivir) in vitro; resistance to peramivir has been reported only rarely.

Peramivir has been active in vitro in cell culture against some avian influenza A viruses, including some strains of avian influenza A (H5N1) and (H7N9).

■ **Resistance** The major mechanisms of resistance to neuraminidase inhibitors that have been identified in vitro are viral neuraminidase mutations that affect the ability of the drugs to inhibit the enzyme and hemagglutinin mutations that reduce viral dependence on neuraminidase activity. The clinical importance of decreased in vitro susceptibility to peramivir is not known.

Resistance to peramivir has been produced in vitro by serial passage of influenza virus in the presence of increasing concentrations of the drug. In addition, influenza A and B viruses with reduced susceptibility to peramivir due to mutations in viral neuraminidase or hemagglutinin have been observed rarely in clinical isolates.

Influenza A virus variants with reduced in vitro susceptibility to peramivir have included those with substitutions in neuraminidase N1 (i.e., N58D, I211T, I223R/V, G147R, S247N, H275Y) or neuraminidase N2 (i.e., E119V, Q136K, D151A/E/G/N/V, K249E, R292K, N294S, Q391K). Influenza B virus variants with reduced in vitro susceptibility to peramivir have included those with E105K, D197N, I221T/V, H134Y, P139S, D197E/N/Y, A200T, H273Y, H275Y, R374K, H431Y, or T146I substitutions.

Hemagglutinin mutations associated with reduced susceptibility to peramivir include D125S and R208K (influenza A H1N1); N63K, G78D, N145D, and K189E (influenza A H3N2); and T139N, G141E, R162M, D195N, T198N, and Y319H (influenza B).

Cross-resistance between peramivir and other neuraminidase inhibitors (e.g., oseltamivir, zanamivir) has been reported in influenza A and B viruses. However, because oseltamivir, peramivir, and zanamivir bind to different sites on the neuraminidase enzyme or interact differently with the binding sites, cross-resistance among the drugs is variable. Some influenza strains have reduced in vitro susceptibility to peramivir and/or oseltamivir, but are susceptible to zanamivir; other strains have reduced in vitro susceptibility to zanamivir, but are susceptible to oseltamivir and/or peramivir. Reduced in vitro susceptibility to all 3 drugs (oseltamivir, peramivir, zanamivir) has been observed in influenza A with R292K, N294S, or N142S resistance-associated neuraminidase substitutions and in influenza B virus with R371K resistance-associated neuraminidase substitution. To date, influenza A (H1N1)pdm09 isolates with the H275Y amino acid substitutions are cross-resistant to oseltamivir and peramivir, but susceptible to zanamivir in vitro.

Cross-resistance between peramivir and baloxavir, a polymerase acidic (PA) endonuclease inhibitor antiviral, is not expected since neuraminidase inhibitors and baloxavir have different mechanisms of action against influenza viruses. However, influenza viruses with substitutions that confer resistance to neuraminidase inhibitors may also have amino acid substitutions in the PA protein that confer resistance to baloxavir. The clinical relevance of phenotypic cross-resistance evaluations has not been established.

Amino acid substitutions that confer cross-resistance between neuraminidase inhibitors (oseltamivir, peramivir, zanamivir) and adamantane derivatives (M2 ion channel inhibitors; amantadine, rimantadine) have not been identified. However, influenza strains that have a neuraminidase substitution that confers resistance to neuraminidase inhibitors and also have an M2 substitution that confers resistance to M2 ion channel inhibitors may be resistant to both classes of influenza antivirals.

Advice to Patients

Advise patients of the risk of severe allergic reactions (including anaphylaxis) or serious skin reactions with peramivir and the importance of immediately seeking medical attention if an allergic-like reaction occurs or is suspected.

Advise patients of the risk of neuropsychiatric reactions in patients with influenza and the importance of immediately contacting a clinician if they experience signs of abnormal behavior after receiving peramivir.

Importance of informing clinicians of existing or contemplated concomitant therapy, including prescription and OTC drugs, as well as any concomitant illnesses.

Importance of women informing clinicians if they are or plan to become pregnant or plan to breast-feed.

Importance of informing patients of other important precautionary information. (See Cautions.)

Overview® (see Users Guide). For additional information on this drug until a more detailed monograph is developed and published, the manufacturer's labeling should be consulted. It is *essential* that the manufacturer's labeling be consulted for more detailed information on usual cautions, precautions, contraindications, potential drug interactions, laboratory test interferences, and acute toxicity.

Preparations

Excipients in commercially available drug preparations may have clinically important effects in some individuals; consult specific product labeling for details.

Peramivir

Parenteral		
Concentrate, for injection, for IV use	10 mg/mL	Rapivab®, Seqirus

†Use is not currently included in the labeling approved by the US Food and Drug Administration

Zanamivir

■ Zanamivir, a sialic acid derivative, is a neuraminidase inhibitor antiviral agent that is pharmacologically related to oseltamivir and active against influenza A and B viruses.

Uses

■ Treatment of Seasonal Influenza A and B Virus Infections

Zanamivir is used for the symptomatic *treatment* of uncomplicated acute illness caused by susceptible influenza A or B viruses in adults, adolescents, and children 7 years of age or older who have been symptomatic for no longer than 2 days.

Efficacy of zanamivir for the treatment of influenza is *not* established in patients with underlying airways disease (e.g., asthma, chronic obstructive pulmonary disease [COPD]). Zanamivir is *not* recommended in patients with underlying airways disease because of the risk of serious bronchospasm. (See Individuals with Asthma or COPD under Cautions.) Treatment with zanamivir has not been shown to reduce the risk of transmission of influenza to others.

The US Centers for Disease Control and Prevention (CDC), US Public Health Service Advisory Committee on Immunization Practices (ACIP), American Academy of Pediatrics (AAP), and others recommend antiviral treatment initiated as soon as possible in all individuals with suspected or confirmed influenza who require hospitalization or have severe, complicated, or progressive illness (regardless of vaccination status or underlying illness). These experts also recommend early empiric antiviral treatment in individuals with suspected or confirmed influenza of any severity if they are at high risk of developing influenza-related complications because of age or underlying medical conditions. Individuals at increased risk for influenza-related complications include children younger than 2 years of age; adults 65 years of age or older; individuals of any age with certain chronic medical or immunosuppressive conditions; women who are pregnant or up to 2 weeks postpartum; individuals younger than 19 years of age receiving long-term aspirin therapy; American Indians or Alaskan natives; morbidly obese individuals with a body mass index (BMI) of 40 or greater; and residents of any age in nursing homes or other long-term care facilities. (See Uses: Treatment of Seasonal Influenza A and B Virus Infections, in Oseltamivir Phosphate 8:18.28.)

The CDC, ACIP, and AAP also state that empiric antiviral treatment can be considered in previously healthy, symptomatic individuals with suspected or confirmed influenza who are not known to be at increased risk of developing severe or complicated illness if such treatment can be initiated within 48 hours of illness onset. Although these individuals typically do not require treatment, early empiric antiviral treatment might provide some benefit (e.g., shortened duration of illness). The use of antiviral treatment in such individuals should be based on clinical judgment and is not necessary in those who are already beginning to recover. In areas with limited availability of antiviral agents, local public health authorities might provide additional guidance about prioritizing use of antiviral treatment within groups at higher risk for influenza complications.

If treatment of seasonal influenza is indicated, an appropriate antiviral agent should be initiated as early as possible since benefit is greatest if started within 48 hours of symptom onset. However, because there is some evidence that antiviral treatment initiated up to 96 hours after illness onset might still be beneficial in reducing morbidity and mortality in hospitalized patients and in those with severe, complicated, or progressive illness, some experts state that antiviral treatment can be initiated more than 48 hours after illness onset in these patients. Decisions regarding initiation of antiviral treatment should not be delayed while waiting for laboratory confirmation.

When treatment of seasonal influenza is indicated, oseltamivir or zanamivir usually is recommended. Oseltamivir is preferred for hospitalized patients and patients with severe or complicated influenza because of the lack of data regarding use of inhaled zanamivir in such patients. However, the CDC states that use of investigational IV zanamivir† may be considered for hospitalized patients with severe influenza if they cannot tolerate or absorb oral oseltamivir (e.g., because of suspected or known gastric stasis, malabsorption, or GI bleeding) or have infections caused by oseltamivir-resistant strains. Although safety and efficacy of IV zanamivir have not been established, an investigational aqueous solution of zanamivir for IV administration may be available either by enrollment in an ongoing clinical trial or under an emergency investigational new drug (EIND) protocol. Requests to determine a patient's eligibility for an ongoing clinical trial of IV zanamivir or requests to use IV zanamivir under an EIND should be made by contacting the manufacturer's clinical support help desk by email (gskclinicalsupportHD@gsk.com) or by phone (877-626-8019 or 866-341-9160).

Viral surveillance data available from local and state health departments and the CDC should be considered when selecting an antiviral agent for the treatment of seasonal influenza. Strains of circulating influenza viruses and the antiviral susceptibility of these strains constantly evolve, and the possibility that emergence of zanamivir-resistant influenza virus may decrease effectiveness of the drug should be considered. Although influenza A and B viruses circulating in the US during the last few years generally have been susceptible to zanamivir, clinicians should consult the most recent information.

The CDC issues recommendations concerning the use of antiviral agents for the treatment of influenza, and these recommendations are updated as needed during each influenza season. Information regarding influenza surveillance and updated recommendations for the treatment of seasonal influenza are available from the CDC at http://www.cdc.gov/flu.

Clinical Experience Efficacy of zanamivir for the treatment of influenza has been established in randomized placebo-controlled studies in which the predominant influenza infection was seasonal influenza A; a smaller number of patients in these studies were infected with seasonal influenza B. When used within 2 days of onset of symptoms in otherwise healthy adults, adolescents, and children with uncomplicated influenza, the drug has decreased viral shedding in adults and adolescents and reduced the degree and duration of fever, headache, myalgia, cough, and sore throat in adults, adolescents, and children. Zanamivir therapy generally has been associated with a median 1- to 1.5-day decrease in the duration of symptoms, although those who initiate therapy sooner (i.e., no later than 30 hours after symptom onset) and those with more pronounced illness may exhibit greater benefit (e.g., a 3-day decrease in symptom duration).

The comparative efficacy of oseltamivir versus zanamivir in the treatment of influenza A or B virus infections caused by susceptible strains have not been evaluated.

■ Prevention of Seasonal Influenza A and B Virus Infections

Zanamivir is used for *prophylaxis* of influenza virus infection caused by susceptible influenza A or B viruses in adults, adolescents, and children 5 years of age and older.

Safety and efficacy of zanamivir have been established for prophylaxis of seasonal influenza in household settings and during community outbreaks; the manufacturer states that efficacy of the drug has *not* been established for prophylaxis of seasonal influenza in nursing home settings.

Annual vaccination with seasonal influenza virus vaccine, as recommended by the ACIP, is the primary means of preventing seasonal influenza and its severe complications. Prophylaxis with an appropriate antiviral agent active against circulating influenza strains is considered an adjunct to vaccination for the control and prevention of influenza in certain individuals.

Decisions regarding use of antivirals for prophylaxis of influenza should be based on the exposed person's risk for influenza complications, the type and duration of contact, recommendations from local or public health authorities, and clinical judgment. In general, postexposure prophylaxis should be used only if it can be initiated within 48 hours of the most recent exposure. Indiscriminate use of antivirals for prophylaxis may promote resistance or reduce availability of antiviral agents for treatment. In areas with limited availability of antiviral agents, local public health authorities might provide additional guidance about prioritizing use of antiviral prophylaxis within groups at higher risk for influenza complications. In certain situations, the CDC or local public health authorities might recommend that antiviral agents be reserved for treatment and that prophylaxis be used only in certain limited situations.

When seasonal influenza viruses are circulating in the community, postexposure prophylaxis with oseltamivir or zanamivir can be considered for certain individuals, including those at high risk of developing influenza complications for whom influenza vaccine is contraindicated, unavailable, or expected to have low efficacy (e.g., immunocompromised individuals). Other possible candidates for antiviral prophylaxis include unvaccinated health care personnel, public health workers, and first responders with unprotected, close-contact exposure to a patient with confirmed, probable, or suspected influenza during the time when the patient was infectious. Antiviral prophylaxis also can be considered for controlling influenza outbreaks in nursing and long-term care facilities or other closed or semi-closed settings with large numbers of individuals at high risk for influenza complications. In individuals at high risk of influenza complications who receive influenza virus vaccine inactivated, use of prophylaxis can be considered during the 2 weeks after vaccination to provide protection until an adequate immune response develops. (See Drug Interactions: Influenza Virus Vaccines.)

Viral surveillance data available from local and state health departments and the CDC should be considered when selecting an antiviral for prophylaxis of influenza. Strains of circulating influenza viruses and the antiviral susceptibility of these strains constantly evolve, and the possibility that emergence of zanamivir-resistant influenza virus may decrease effectiveness of the drug should be considered. Although influenza A and B viruses circulating in the US during the last few years generally have been susceptible to zanamivir, clinicians should consult the most recent information.

The CDC issues recommendations concerning the use of antiviral agents for prophylaxis of influenza, and these recommendations are updated as needed during each influenza season. Information regarding influenza surveillance and updated recommendations for prevention of seasonal influenza are available from the CDC at http://www.cdc.gov/flu.

Clinical Experience Efficacy of zanamivir for prevention of seasonal influenza was demonstrated in postexposure prophylaxis studies in households and seasonal prophylaxis studies during community outbreaks of influenza. The primary efficacy endpoint in these studies was the incidence of symptomatic, laboratory-confirmed influenza, which was defined as the presence of at least 2 symptoms (oral temperature 37.8°C or higher, feverishness, cough, headache, sore throat, myalgia) and laboratory confirmation by culture, polymerase chain reaction (PCR), or seroconversion.

In the placebo-controlled studies evaluating zanamivir for postexposure prophylaxis in household contacts of an index case, each household (including all household members 5 years of age or older) was randomized to receive zanamivir (10 mg once daily for 10 days) or placebo initiated within 1.5 days of symptom onset in the index cases. The proportion of households with at least 1 new case of symptomatic, laboratory-confirmed influenza was 4.1% in the groups that received zanamivir and 19% in the groups that received placebo.

In a placebo-controlled seasonal prophylaxis study in university students (86% were unvaccinated), the incidence of symptomatic, laboratory-confirmed influenza was 2% in those who received zanamivir (10 mg once daily for 28 days) and 6.1% in those who received placebo during a community outbreak. In another seasonal prophylaxis study in adults and children 12–94 years of age (33% were unvaccinated), the incidence of symptomatic, laboratory-confirmed influenza was 0.2% in those who received zanamivir and 1.4% in those who received placebo during a community outbreak.

■ Avian Influenza A Virus Infections

Zanamivir is used for the treatment or prevention of infections caused by susceptible avian influenza A viruses†.

The CDC and World Health Organization (WHO) state that oseltamivir is the drug of choice for the treatment or prophylaxis of infections caused by highly pathogenic avian influenza A (H5N1) and zanamivir is an alternative.

Oseltamivir also is considered the drug of choice for the treatment of infections caused by avian influenza A (H7N9), especially in hospitalized patients and patients with severe or complicated illness. Because of limited data, zanamivir is not recommended for the treatment of severe avian influenza A (H7N9) infections, but may be considered in those with uncomplicated infections. Either oseltamivir or zanamivir can be used for prophylaxis in close contacts of patients with confirmed or probable avian influenza A (H7N9) infection.

The CDC states that use of investigational IV zanamivir† may be considered for hospitalized patients with severe influenza A (H7N9) infection who cannot tolerate or absorb oral oseltamivir (e.g., because of suspected or known gastric stasis, malabsorption, or GI bleeding) or have infections caused by oseltamivir-resistant strains. In addition, if influenza A (H7N9) infection is confirmed in an individual who received more than 2 days of oseltamivir prophylaxis, oseltamivir should be discontinued as soon as possible and treatment with inhaled zanamivir initiated. If progressive lower respiratory symptoms subsequently develop, the patient should be hospitalized and treated with investigational IV zanamivir†. (See Dosage and Administration: Administration.)

For additional information on avian influenza A virus infections, see Uses: Avian Influenza A Virus Infections in Oseltamivir 8:18.28.

■ **Pandemic Influenza** Zanamivir is used for the treatment or prevention of pandemic influenza caused by susceptible strains of influenza virus.

Influenza viruses can cause seasonal epidemics and, occasionally, pandemics during which rates of illness and death from influenza-related complications can increase dramatically worldwide. The most recent influenza pandemic occurred during 2009 and was related to a novel influenza A (H1N1) strain, influenza A (H1N1)pdm09.

Influenza outbreaks caused by influenza A (H1N1)pdm09 virus, previously referred to as the novel 2009 influenza A (H1N1) virus or swine-origin influenza A (H1N1) virus, were reported in several countries, including the US, beginning in March and April 2009. The virus is a triple-reassortant swine influenza virus with genes from human, swine, and avian influenza A viruses and contains a unique combination of gene segments not previously reported in the US or elsewhere. The influenza A (H1N1)pdm09 virus is antigenically distinct from seasonal human influenza A (H1N1) viruses that had been in circulation since 1977, and widespread transmission of the virus occurred since most individuals had no preexisting antibody to the strain. In the US, the 2009 influenza A (H1N1)pdm09 pandemic was characterized by a substantial increase in influenza activity that peaked in late October and early November 2009 and returned to seasonal baseline levels by January 2010. During that time, more than 99% of influenza viruses circulating in the US were the influenza A (H1N1)pdm09 virus. In August 2010, the WHO declared that the world was in a post-pandemic period. Since that time, influenza A (H1N1)pdm09 has become a seasonal influenza virus and continues to circulate with other seasonal viruses.

The spread of the highly pathogenic H5N1 strain of avian influenza A in poultry in Asia and other countries that has been occurring since 2003 may represent a potential future pandemic threat. (See Uses: Avian Influenza A Virus Infections, in Oseltamivir 8:18.28.)

Dosage and Administration

■ **Administration** Zanamivir powder for inhalation is administered *only* by oral inhalation using the inhaler (Diskhaler®) provided by the manufacturer.

Zanamivir has been administered IV†, but a parenteral dosage form of the drug is not commercially available in the US. An investigational aqueous solution of zanamivir for IV administration may be available for use in hospitalized patients with severe or complicated influenza (see Uses: Treatment of Seasonal Influenza A and B Virus Infections) either by enrollment in an ongoing clinical trial or under an emergency investigational new drug (EIND) protocol. Requests to determine a patient's eligibility for an ongoing clinical trial of IV zanamivir or requests to use IV zanamivir under an EIND should be made by contacting the manufacturer's clinical support help desk by email (gskclinicalsupportHD@gsk.com) or by phone (877-626-8019 or 866-341-9160).

Zanamivir powder for inhalation must **not** *be used to prepare an extemporaneous solution and must* **not** *be administered using a nebulizer or mechanical ventilator*. (See Administration Precautions under Cautions: Warnings/Precautions.)

Oral Inhalation Zanamivir powder for inhalation is commercially available in a disk containing 4 foil blisters of the drug (Rotadisk®) and is provided with an inhaler (Diskhaler®) that is used to deliver the drug to the respiratory tract.

The commercially available powder for inhalation should *not* be removed from its foil blister packaging.

The manufacturer's instructions should be consulted for information on how to load the Rotadisk® onto the drug delivery system (Diskhaler®) and how to use the Diskhaler® to administer the drug.

Patients should be instructed in the safe and effective use of the Diskhaler®, and instructions should include a demonstration whenever possible.

Patients scheduled to use an inhaled bronchodilator at the same time as zanamivir should use the bronchodilator before zanamivir.

■ **Dosage** ***Treatment of Seasonal Influenza A and B Virus Infections*** For the *treatment* of influenza infection in adults, adolescents, and children 7 years of age or older, the usual dosage of zanamivir is 2 inhalations (one 5-mg blister per inhalation for a total dose of 10 mg) twice daily (about 12 hours apart) for 5 days. Two doses should be administered the first day provided there is an interval of at least 2 hours between doses. On subsequent days, zanamivir doses should be administered about 12 hours apart (e.g., morning and evening) at about the same time each day.

Zanamivir treatment should be initiated within 2 days after the onset of symptoms and usually is continued for 5 days. Although efficacy has not been established if treatment is initiated more than 2 days after onset of symptoms, there is some evidence that antiviral treatment initiated up to 96 hours after onset of symptoms may still be beneficial in reducing morbidity and mortality in hospitalized patients and in those with severe, complicated, or progressive influenza. In addition, patients hospitalized with severe infections (e.g., those with prolonged infection or admitted into an intensive care unit) or individuals with immunosuppression may require more than 5 days of antiviral treatment.

Prevention of Seasonal Influenza A and B Virus Infections

Household Setting. For *prophylaxis* of influenza in adults, adolescents, and children 5 years of age or older in household settings, the usual dosage of zanamivir is 2 inhalations (one 5-mg blister per inhalation for a total dose of 10 mg) once daily for 10 days. The daily dose should be administered at approximately the same time each day.

Efficacy of zanamivir for prophylaxis in household settings is not established if the drug is initiated more than 1.5 days after the onset of symptoms in the index case.

Community Outbreak. For *prophylaxis* of influenza in adults and adolescents in community settings, the usual dosage of zanamivir is 2 inhalations (one 5-mg blister per inhalation for a total dose of 10 mg) once daily for 28 days. The daily dose should be administered at approximately the same time each day.

Efficacy of zanamivir for prophylaxis in community outbreaks is not established if the drug is initiated more than 5 days after the outbreak is identified in the community. The safety and efficacy of zanamivir prophylaxis given for longer than 28 days have not been evaluated.

Outbreaks in Long-term Care Facilities or Hospitals. For *prophylaxis* of influenza when an outbreak is occurring among high-risk individuals in a long-term care facility (e.g., nursing home) or hospital, the usual adult dosage of zanamivir is 2 inhalations (one 5-mg blister per inhalation for a total dose of 10 mg) once daily. In such situations, the US Centers for Disease Control and Prevention (CDC) recommends that antiviral prophylaxis be continued for a minimum of 2 weeks and up to 7 days after the last known case of influenza is identified.

Avian Influenza A Virus Infections **Treatment.** If zanamivir is used for the *treatment* of uncomplicated infections caused by avian influenza A viruses†, some experts recommend that the twice-daily zanamivir dosage usually recommended for the treatment of seasonal influenza A and B virus infections be used in adults and pediatric patients. (See Treatment of Seasonal Influenza A and B Virus Infections under Dosage and Administration: Dosage.)

Zanamivir administered by oral inhalation is not recommended for the treatment of severe avian influenza virus A virus infections. (See Uses: Avian Influenza A Virus Infections.)

Prophylaxis. If zanamivir is used for *prophylaxis* of highly pathogenic avian influenza virus A (H5N1) infection† in close contacts, the CDC and WHO state that the once-daily zanamivir dosage usually recommended for prophylaxis of seasonal influenza A and B virus infections can be used in adults and pediatric patients. (See Prevention of Seasonal Influenza A and B Virus Infections under Dosage and Administration: Dosage.) Prophylaxis should be continued for 7–10 days after the last known exposure.

If zanamivir is used for *prophylaxis* of avian influenza virus A (H7N9) infection† in close contacts, the CDC recommends that the twice-daily zanamivir dosage usually recommended for *treatment* of seasonal influenza A and B virus infections be given for 5–10 days. (See Treatment of Seasonal Influenza A and B Virus Infections under Dosage and Administration: Dosage.)

■ **Special Populations** Dosage adjustment is not needed in patients with renal impairment, but the potential for drug accumulation should be considered. (See Renal Impairment under Warnings/Precautions: Specific Populations, in Cautions.)

Cautions

■ **Contraindications** Zanamivir is contraindicated in individuals with a history of a hypersensitivity reaction to zanamivir or any ingredient in the formulation (e.g., milk proteins contained in the lactose vehicle).

■ **Warnings/Precautions** ***Respiratory Effects*** Serious bronchospasm, including fatalities, have been reported in patients receiving zanamivir; some (but not all) of these patients had chronic underlying pulmonary disease (e.g., asthma, chronic obstructive pulmonary disease [COPD]). (See Individuals with Asthma or COPD under Cautions.) Many of these cases were reported during postmarketing surveillance and causality to the drug is difficult to assess.

Some patients without prior respiratory disease also may have respiratory abnormalities from acute respiratory infection that could resemble adverse drug reactions or increase vulnerability to adverse drug reactions.

Zanamivir should be discontinued in any patient who experiences bronchospasm or decline in respiratory function; immediate treatment and hospitalization may be required.

Individuals with Asthma or COPD Zanamivir is not recommended for the treatment or prophylaxis of influenza in individuals with underlying airways disease (e.g., asthma, COPD) because of the risk of serious bronchospasm.

Bronchospasm has occurred when zanamivir was used in patients with mild or moderate asthma (but without acute influenza-like illness). When used in patients with acute influenza-like illness superimposed on underlying asthma or COPD, a greater than 20% decline in the forced expiratory volume in 1 second (FEV_1) occurred in more patients receiving the drug than in those receiving placebo.

The benefits and risks should be considered carefully if use of zanamivir is considered for a patient with underlying respiratory disease. If a decision is made to use the drug in such patients, monitor respiratory function carefully and have appropriate supportive care available, including short-acting β-adrenergic bronchodilators.

Sensitivity Reactions **Hypersensitivity Reactions.** Allergic-like reactions (e.g., oropharyngeal edema, serious skin rash, anaphylaxis) have been reported in patients receiving zanamivir.

If an allergic reaction occurs or is suspected, zanamivir should be discontinued immediately and appropriate treatment initiated.

Neuropsychiatric and CNS Effects There have been postmarketing reports of delirium and abnormal behavior leading to self-injury, principally involving children in Japan. The contribution of zanamivir to these events has not been established.

Influenza itself can be associated with a variety of neurologic and behavioral symptoms (e.g., seizures, hallucinations, delirium, abnormal behavior) and fatalities can occur. Although such events may occur in the setting of encephalitis or encephalopathy, they can occur without obvious severe disease.

Patients should be closely monitored for signs of abnormal behavior. If neuropsychiatric symptoms develop, the risks and benefits of continued therapy with zanamivir should be evaluated.

There have been postmarketing reports of vasovagal-like episodes shortly after oral inhalation of zanamivir.

Concomitant Illness Safety and efficacy for treatment or prophylaxis of influenza have not established in patients with high-risk underlying medical conditions. (see Individuals with Asthma or COPD under Cautions)

No data are available regarding use of zanamivir in patients with severe or unstable medical conditions that may require inpatient care.

Differential Diagnosis When making treatment decisions in patients with suspected influenza, consider the possibility of primary or concomitant bacterial infection for which zanamivir would be ineffective.

Serious bacterial infections may begin with influenza-like symptoms or may coexist with or occur as complications of influenza. There is no evidence that zanamivir prevents such complications.

There is no evidence that zanamivir is effective for illness caused by any organisms other than influenza A or B.

Administration Precautions Zanamivir powder for inhalation *must* be administered using *only* the inhaler (Diskhaler®) provided by the manufacturer. The powder should *not* be removed from its foil blister packaging (Rotadisk®).

Zanamivir powder for inhalation must **not** *be made into an extemporaneous solution for administration by nebulization or mechanical ventilation.* **No** *attempt should be made to reconstitute or solubilize the powder in liquid;* **no** *attempt should be made to administer the drug in a nebulizer or mechanical ventilator.*

Safety and efficacy have *not* been established for administration by nebulization. Lactose in the formulation may obstruct or interfere with proper functioning of mechanical ventilator equipment. There have been reports of hospitalized patients with influenza who received extemporaneous solutions made with the powder and administered by nebulization or mechanical ventilation; at least 1 death occurred when lactose in the formulation apparently obstructed the proper functioning of the equipment.

Patients should be instructed in the safe and effective use of the drug delivery system (Diskhaler®) provided by the manufacturer. Instructions on use of the inhaler should include a demonstration whenever possible.

Some geriatric patients may need assistance with the inhaler.

Children should be under adult supervision with close attention to use of the inhaler. (See Cautions: Pediatric Use.)

Prior Use No data are available regarding safety and efficacy of repeated courses of zanamivir for treatment of influenza.

Influenza Vaccination Zanamivir is not a substitute for annual vaccination with a seasonal influenza vaccine (influenza virus vaccine inactivated, influenza vaccine live intranasal, influenza vaccine recombinant).

Although antiviral agents used for treatment or prevention of influenza, including zanamivir, may be used concomitantly with or at any time before or after influenza virus vaccine inactivated, these antiviral agents may inhibit the vaccine virus contained in influenza vaccine live intranasal. (See Influenza Virus Vaccines under Drug Interactions.)

Specific Populations **Pregnancy.** Category C. (See Users Guide.)

Pregnant women are at increased risk for severe complications and death from influenza. The US Centers for Disease Control and Prevention (CDC) and US Public Health Service Advisory Committee on Immunization Practices (ACIP) state that pregnancy is not considered a contraindication to use of zanamivir for the treatment or prevention of influenza and that zanamivir regimens recommended for such infections in pregnant women are the same as those for other adults.

The CDC and ACIP state that oseltamivir may be preferred when a neuraminidase inhibitor is indicated for the treatment of suspected or confirmed influenza in women who are pregnant or up to 2 weeks postpartum, but the drug of choice for prophylaxis of influenza is less clear. Zanamivir may be preferred by some clinicians for prophylaxis in pregnant women because of its limited systemic absorption; however, respiratory complications that may be associated with zanamivir because of its route of administration should be considered, especially in women at risk for respiratory problems.

Lactation. Zanamivir should be used with caution in nursing women.

Zanamivir is distributed into milk in rats; it is not known whether the drug is distributed into human milk.

Pediatric Use. Safety and efficacy for *treatment* of influenza have not been established in children younger than 7 years of age. Some clinical studies evaluating zanamivir have included children 5–6 years of age†; however, there is some evidence that the drug is not as effective in these children as in older children and adults.

Safety and efficacy for *prophylaxis* of influenza have not been established in children younger than 5 years of age. Safety and efficacy in adolescents and children 5 years of age or older for *prophylaxis* of influenza are similar to adults.

Some young children may have suboptimal inspiratory flow rates through the drug delivery system (Diskhaler®). When considering use of zanamivir in pediatric patients, clinicians should carefully evaluate the ability of the child to use the inhaler.

Children should receive zanamivir only under adult supervision and with close attention to proper use of the inhaler. The supervising adult should be instructed on proper use of the inhaler.

Geriatric Use. Safety and efficacy for *treatment* of influenza in geriatric adults 65 years of age or older is similar to that reported in younger adults.

Safety and efficacy for *prophylaxis* of influenza in geriatric adults 65 years of age or older in household or community settings are similar to that reported in younger adults. Efficacy has *not* been established for *prophylaxis* of influenza in geriatric individuals in nursing home settings.

The possibility exists of greater sensitivity to the drug in some older individuals.

Some geriatric patients may need assistance with the drug delivery system (Diskhaler®).

Hepatic Impairment. The pharmacokinetics of zanamivir have not been studied in patients with hepatic impairment.

Renal Impairment. Safety and efficacy of zanamivir have not been documented in patients with severe renal impairment. Although zanamivir systemic exposure is limited after oral inhalation, the potential for drug accumulation should be considered.

■ **Common Adverse Effects** Adverse effects occurring in 1–3% or more of adults and children 12 years of age or older include diarrhea; nausea; vomiting; nasal signs and symptoms; bronchitis; sinusitis; cough; ear, nose, and throat infections; headache; and dizziness. No adverse effect occurred at an incidence greater than 3%. Adverse effects occurring in up to 5% of children 5–12 years of age include ear, nose, and throat infections; vomiting; nausea; and diarrhea. Bronchospasm and allergic-like reactions, including oropharyngeal edema and serious rash, have been reported. Some adverse effects may be related to the lactose vehicle (contains milk proteins) used in the powder for oral inhalation formulation.

Drug Interactions

Zanamivir not metabolized by and does not affect cytochrome P-450 (CYP) enzymes, including CYP1A1, 1A2, 2A6, 2C9, 2C18, 2D6, 2E1, or 3A4. Drug interactions with drugs that are substrates or inhibitors of these enzymes unlikely.

■ **Influenza Virus Vaccines** Zanamivir does not interfere with the antibody response to influenza virus vaccine inactivated (IIV). Inactivated influenza vaccines may be administered concomitantly with or at any time before or after zanamivir.

Safety and efficacy of concomitant use of zanamivir and influenza vaccine live intranasal (LAIV) have not been studied. Because influenza antiviral agents, including zanamivir, reduce replication of influenza viruses and may inhibit the vaccine virus, LAIV should not be administered until at least 48 hours after zanamivir is discontinued and zanamivir should not be administered until at least 2 weeks after administration of LAIV, unless medically indicated. If zanamivir is administered within 2 weeks after LAIV, the US Public Health Service Advisory Committee on Immunization Practices (ACIP) recommends that the LAIV dose be repeated 48 hours or more after the last dose of the antiviral agent. Alternatively, individuals who received zanamivir 2 days before to 14 days after LAIV may be revaccinated with either IIV or influenza vaccine recombinant (RIV).

Pharmacokinetics

■ **Absorption** ***Bioavailability*** Following oral inhalation of zanamivir, approximately 4–17% of the inhaled dose is absorbed systemically.

Absolute bioavailability averages 2% following oral inhalation; peak serum concentrations are attained within 1–2 hours.

Special Populations In pediatric patients younger than 12 years of age with signs and symptoms of respiratory illness, zanamivir serum concentrations may be low or undetectable following oral inhalation because of inadequate or absent inspiratory flow rates. (See Pediatric Use under Cautions.)

■ **Distribution** ***Extent*** Zanamivir is delivered to the epithelial lining of the respiratory tract following oral inhalation. The amount of the drug in the respiratory tract depends on patient factors such as inspiratory flow rate; it may be present in sputum and nasal washings for at least 12 hours after a dose.

Zanamivir crosses the placenta in animals.

Zanamivir is distributed into milk in animals; it is not known whether the drug is distributed into human milk.

Plasma Protein Binding Zanamivir is less than 10% bound to plasma proteins.

■ **Elimination** ***Metabolism*** Zanamivir is not metabolized.

The drug is not a substrate for and does not affect cytochrome P-450 (CYP) isoenzymes.

Elimination Route Following oral inhalation, absorbed zanamivir is excreted unchanged in urine within 24 hours; unabsorbed drug is excreted in feces.

Half-life The serum half-life of zanamivir following oral inhalation is 2.5–5.1 hours.

Special Populations The half-life of zanamivir is prolonged in individuals with renal impairment; studies using IV zanamivir indicate that the half-life is 4.7 hours in those with mild to moderate renal impairment and 18.5 hours in those with severe renal impairment.

Description

Zanamivir, a sialic acid derivative, is a neuraminidase inhibitor antiviral agent. Zanamivir is pharmacologically related to oseltamivir and, like oseltamivir, is pharmacologically unrelated to other currently available antiviral agents.

Zanamivir is a potent selective competitive inhibitor of the influenza virus neuraminidase, an enzyme essential for viral replication. Neuraminidase cleaves terminal sialic acid residues from glycoconjugates to enable the release of virus from infected cells, prevent the formation of viral aggregates after release from host cells, and possibly decrease viral inactivation by respiratory mucus.

Zanamivir exhibits potent antiviral activity in vitro against both influenza A and B viruses and is active against amantadine- and rimantadine-resistant isolates. Viral surveillance data indicate that almost all seasonal influenza A (H3N2), influenza A (H1N1)pdm09, and influenza B viruses circulating during recent influenza seasons have been susceptible to zanamivir in vitro. In vitro studies indicate that zanamivir generally is active against some avian influenza A viruses, including avian influenza A H5N1, H6N1, H7N7, H7N9, and H9N2. Zanamivir is active against some influenza strains, including some influenza A (H1N1)pdm09 strains, resistant to oseltamivir in vitro.

Resistance to zanamivir has been produced in vitro by serial passage of influenza virus in the presence of increasing concentrations of the drug. Although the risk of emergence of zanamivir resistance in clinical isolates has not been quantified, resistant strains of influenza B have emerged in immunocompromised patients receiving the drug. In addition, seasonal influenza A (H3N2) and influenza A (H1N1)pdm09 with in vitro resistance to zanamivir have been reported rarely.

Influenza strains cross-resistant to oseltamivir and zanamivir have been generated in cell culture; only limited data are available regarding possible emergence of clinical isolates with cross-resistance to both drugs. Mutations at positions 152 or 292 can confer cross-resistance between oseltamivir and zanamivir. To date, influenza A (H1N1)pdm09 isolates with the H275Y mutation and avian influenza A (H5N1) with the H274Y mutation that are resistant to oseltamivir were susceptible to zanamivir.

Advice to Patients

Importance of understanding proper inhalation technique and use of the drug delivery system (Diskhaler®); importance of reading the patient instructions for use.

Importance of initiating zanamivir treatment as soon as possible after appearance of influenza symptoms (within 2 days after symptom onset); efficacy not established if treatment begins after 48 hours of symptoms.

Advise patients that zanamivir treatment does not reduce the risk of transmission of influenza virus to others.

Advise patients of the possible risk of bronchospasm, especially in those with chronic underlying respiratory disease (e.g., asthma, chronic obstructive pulmonary disease [COPD]); importance of patients with asthma or COPD having a short-acting inhaled β-adrenergic bronchodilator readily available.

Advise patients using an inhaled bronchodilators at the same time as zanamivir of the importance of using the bronchodilator first.

Importance of discontinuing zanamivir and promptly contacting a clinician if there is an increase in respiratory symptoms (e.g., wheezing, dyspnea, signs or symptoms of bronchospasm) or if symptoms of an allergic reaction occur.

Importance of immediately contacting a clinician if patient demonstrates signs of unusual behavior. Influenza patients, particularly children and adolescents, may be at increased risk of seizures, confusion, or abnormal behavior early in their illness and should be closely observed for signs of unusual behavior. Such events are uncommon, but may occur after starting zanamivir treatment or when influenza is not treated and can result in accidental injury to the patient.

Importance of informing clinicians of existing or contemplated concomitant therapy, including prescription and OTC drugs, as well as any concomitant illnesses.

Importance of women informing clinicians if they are or plan to become pregnant or plan to breast-feed.

Importance of informing patients of other important precautionary information. (See Cautions.)

Overview (see Users Guide). For additional information until a more detailed monograph is developed and published, the manufacturer's labeling should be consulted. It is *essential* that the manufacturer's labeling be consulted for more detailed information on usual cautions, precautions, contraindications, potential drug interactions, laboratory test interferences, and acute toxicity.

Preparations

Excipients in commercially available drug preparations may have clinically important effects in some individuals; consult specific product labeling for details.

Zanamivir

Oral Inhalation		
Powder for inhalation (contained in Rotadisk® foil pack)	5 mg per inhalation	**Relenza®** (with Diskhaler®), GlaxoSmithKline

†Use is not currently included in the labeling approved by the US Food and Drug Administration

Selected Revisions April 2014, © Copyright, September 1999, American Society of Health-System Pharmacists, Inc.

NUCLEOSIDES AND NUCLEOTIDES 8:18.32

Acyclovir
Acyclovir Sodium

Aciclovir, Acycloguanosine, ACV

■ Acyclovir is a synthetic purine nucleoside analog antiviral agent derived from guanine and is active against Herpesviridae.

Uses

IV acyclovir sodium is used for the treatment of initial and recurrent mucocutaneous herpes simplex virus (HSV-1 and HSV-2) infections and the treatment of varicella-zoster infections in immunocompromised adults and children; for the treatment of severe first episodes of genital herpes infections in immunocompetent individuals; and for the treatment of HSV encephalitis and neonatal HSV infections. Acyclovir is used orally for the treatment of initial and recurrent episodes of genital herpes; for the acute treatment of herpes zoster (shingles, zoster) in immunocompetent individuals; and for the treatment of varicella (chickenpox) in immunocompetent individuals.

For topical uses of acyclovir, see 84:04.06.

■ **Mucocutaneous, Ocular, and Systemic Herpes Simplex Virus (HSV) Infections** Acyclovir is considered the drug of choice for the treatment of mucocutaneous herpes simplex virus (HSV) infections in immunocompromised adults, adolescents, and children and also is considered the drug of choice for the treatment of severe HSV infections such as HSV encephalitis and neonatal HSV infections.

Controlled studies of initial and recurrent mucocutaneous HSV-1 and HSV-2 infections (e.g., orofacial, esophageal, genital, nasal, labial) in immunocompromised adults and children have shown that IV acyclovir therapy decreases the duration of viral shedding (time from onset of therapy until the last positive culture), the duration of pain and itching, the time required for crusting and healing of lesions, and the duration of positive cultures. In one study, the median duration of viral shedding was 3 days in acyclovir-treated patients compared with 17 days in placebo-treated patients; pain ceased within 10 days of initiating therapy in acyclovir-treated patients compared with 16 days in placebo-treated patients. The time required for crusting and healing of lesions was 7 and 14 days, respectively, in acyclovir-treated patients compared with 14 and 28 days, respectively, in placebo-treated patients. IV acyclovir was not effective in reducing the frequency or delaying the onset of subsequent recurrent infection with HSV-1, HSV-2, or other herpesviruses or in eliminating an established latent infection.

Acyclovir has been used for the treatment of orolabial HSV infections, including gingivostomatitis, in adults and children; the drug is not effective or is minimally effective for the prevention of recurrence of herpes labialis† in immunocompetent individuals.

Oral or IV acyclovir has been reported to be effective in the treatment of eczema herpeticum† caused by HSV in several patients with a history of atopic dermatitis; the drug decreased fever and/or the appearance of new lesions, and promoted crusting and healing of lesions.

HIV-Infected Individuals Acyclovir generally is considered the drug of choice for the treatment of primary or recurrent mucocutaneous HSV infections in individuals with human immunodeficiency virus (HIV) infection. Mucocutaneous HSV infections in HIV-infected individuals can involve severe lesions that persist longer than those in immunocompetent individuals. Infections often progress to visceral disease and CNS or disseminated HSV may occur. HSV oral lesions in HIV-infected individuals generally are erosive, painful ulcerations that persist for several weeks and can extend to the esophagus. While these lesions may heal spontaneously, initiation of oral acyclovir at the onset of symptoms is recommended since severe pain and local tissue destruction may occur; IV acyclovir may be necessary for severe cases.

In patients with advanced HIV infection, reactivation of HSV frequently occurs and can result in chronic, persistent mucocutaneous disease that may be severe. The Prevention of Opportunistic Infections Working Group of the US Public Health Service and the Infectious Diseases Society of America (USPHS/IDSA) has established guidelines for the prevention of opportunistic infections in HIV-infected individuals that include recommendations concerning prevention of exposure to opportunistic pathogens, prevention of first disease episodes, and prevention of disease recurrence. The USPHS/IDSA does *not* currently recommend primary prophylaxis against initial episodes of HSV infection in HIV-infected adults, adolescents, or children. In addition, the

USPHS/IDSA does not recommend routine chronic suppressive or maintenance therapy (secondary prophylaxis) against HSV disease in HIV-infected individuals since acute episodes generally can be treated successfully with acyclovir. However, long-term prophylaxis against recurrence of HSV can be considered for adults, adolescents, and children who have frequent or severe recurrences. If secondary prophylaxis of HSV disease is indicated in HIV-infected adults or adolescents, the USPHS/IDSA and other experts recommend use of oral acyclovir, oral famciclovir, or oral valacyclovir as the regimen of choice. If indicated in infants and children, the USPHS/IDSA and other experts recommend oral acyclovir.

HIV-infected patients receiving acyclovir may develop acyclovir-resistant strains of HSV; these infections have been reported most often in patients with advanced HIV infection or those who have received long-term acyclovir therapy. IV foscarnet or IV cidofovir can be used for the management of HSV infections in HIV-infected patients when the HSV infection is known or suspected of being caused by acyclovir-resistant strains. Additional study is needed to determine whether long-term suppression of HSV reduces or facilitates the emergence of drug-resistant strains of the virus and to determine optimal strategies for suppressive therapy of acyclovir-resistant HSV infections. It has been postulated that alternating the use of antiviral agents (e.g., acyclovir, foscarnet) may prevent emergence and subsequent predominance of drug-resistant isolates.

Ocular HSV Infections Oral acyclovir (400 mg 5 times daily) has been used for the treatment of HSV keratitis† in HIV-infected patients. Long-term antiviral therapy may be necessary to prevent recurrent ocular HSV disease in these patients. Oral acyclovir (400 mg twice daily for 12 months) has been used for the prevention of recurrent ocular HSV disease† in immunocompetent adults and children 12 years of age or older who had an episode of ocular HSV disease (blepharitis, conjunctivitis, epithelial keratitis, stromal keratitis, iritis) in one or both eyes within the preceding 12 months. Results of one study in adults indicate that long-term oral acyclovir (400 mg twice daily for up to 18 months) is effective in decreasing the number of HSV recurrences. Oral acyclovir (400 mg twice daily for 6 months) has been used to prevent HSV recurrences in patients undergoing penetrating keratoplasty for herpetic eye disease. The optimum duration of prophylaxis remains to be determined.

HSV Encephalitis Controlled studies in adults and children 6 months of age or older have shown that IV acyclovir is effective for the treatment of HSV encephalitis. Many clinicians consider acyclovir the drug of choice for the treatment of HSV encephalitis, and the American Academy of Pediatrics (AAP) and other experts also consider acyclovir the drug of choice for the treatment of neonatal HSV infections involving the CNS.

HSV encephalitis and neonatal HSV infections of the CNS are associated with substantial morbidity and mortality despite antiviral treatment. In one study in patients 6 months to 79 years of age with brain biopsy-proven HSV encephalitis randomized to receive 10 days of IV acyclovir (10 mg/kg every 8 hours) or IV vidarabine (15 mg/kg daily; no longer commercially available in the US), the overall mortality rate at 12 months was 25% in those who received acyclovir versus 59% in those who received vidarabine. Morbidity assessments at 12 months indicated that 32% of patients who received acyclovir were functioning normally or had only mild neurologic sequelae (e.g., decreased attention span); the remaining survivors had moderate (e.g., hemiparesis, speech impediment, seizures) or severe (continuous supportive care required) sequelae. Patients who were younger than 30 years of age and those with less severe neurologic involvement at the time of treatment had the best outcome. Initiation of acyclovir early in the course of the infection (prior to the development of semicoma or coma) may enhance its efficacy.

Neonatal HSV Infections The AAP, US Centers for Disease Control and Prevention (CDC), and other experts consider IV acyclovir the drug of choice for the treatment of mucosal, cutaneous, CNS, or disseminated HSV infections in neonates.

Neonatal HSV infection is associated with substantial morbidity and mortality, and approximately 25% of neonates with disseminated HSV disease die despite antiviral therapy. Because the risk of morbidity and mortality increases substantially with systemic (CNS or disseminated) infection compared with mucocutaneous infection, early recognition of neonates with HSV infection confined to the skin, eyes, and mouth and early initiation of antiviral therapy are important. The AAP recommends that IV acyclovir therapy be initiated in all neonates with HSV infection, irrespective of presenting clinical findings. In addition, the AAP states that infants with HSV disease that has ocular involvement should received a topical ophthalmic antiviral agent (e.g., trifluridine, vidarabine) in addition to parenteral therapy.

In one study in infants with neonatal HSV disease who were randomized to receive a 10-day regimen of IV acyclovir (10 mg/kg every 8 hours) or vidarabine (30 mg/kg daily; no longer commercially available in the US), mortality at 1 year in the acyclovir group was 0/54 in those with localized disease (limited to skin, eye, and/or mouth), 5/35 in those with CNS infections, and 11/18 in those with visceral organ involvement such as hepatitis or pneumonitis with or without CNS involvement.

Relapse of neonatal HSV disease involving the skin, eyes, mouth, or CNS can occur after acyclovir therapy is discontinued; however, optimal management of these recurrences has not been established. The safety and efficacy of long-term suppressive or intermittent acyclovir therapy for neonates with HSV disease of the skin, eyes, and mouth are being evaluated.

The care of infants exposed to HSV during delivery depends on the status of the mother's infection and mode of delivery; infants exposed to HSV during birth should be monitored carefully in consultation with a specialist. Most experts recommend that women with recurrent genital herpetic lesions at the onset of labor should deliver by cesarean section to prevent neonatal herpes. However, cesarean section does not completely eliminate the risk for HSV transmission to the infant. Women without symptoms or signs of genital herpes can deliver vaginally. The AAP states that all neonates born to women with active genital HSV lesions, regardless of whether the child was delivered by vaginal or cesarean delivery, should be observed carefully and viral cultures for HSV should be obtained 24–48 hours after birth. Because the infection rate in infants born by vaginal delivery to mothers with recurrent genital herpes infection is low, most experts recommend that these infants not be given empiric acyclovir therapy. These infants should be observed for signs of infection and undergo surveillance cultures. For neonates whose mothers have presumed or proven primary genital herpes infection, some experts recommend empiric acyclovir treatment at birth (despite the fact that data are not available to support the efficacy of such a strategy) because the risk of infection in these neonates may exceed 50%; other experts would only initiate acyclovir therapy if HSV cultures are positive. All infants with neonatal herpes should be evaluated and treated with acyclovir. Symptoms suggestive of neonatal HSV infection include skin or scalp rash (especially vesicular lesions) and unexplained clinical manifestations (such as respiratory distress, seizures, signs of sepsis). The fact that neonatal HSV infection can occur as late as 4–6 weeks after delivery should be considered.

Hematopoietic Stem Cell Transplant Recipients The CDC, the Infectious Diseases Society of America (IDSA), and the American Society of Blood and Marrow Transplantation (ASBMT) have established guidelines for preventing opportunistic infections in hematopoietic stem cell transplant (HSCT) recipients. These guidelines recommend that candidates for HSCT whose screening tests before HSCT are seropositive for HSV receive acyclovir to prevent HSV recurrence†. Acyclovir prophylaxis is initiated at the beginning of the conditioning regimen and continued until engraftment occurs or mucositis resolves (approximately 30 days after HSCT). Routine prophylaxis for longer than 30 days is not recommended. Prophylaxis is not indicated for HSCT recipients who are seronegative for HSV.

■ **Genital Herpes** ***Treatment of First Episode Infections*** Acyclovir is used in the treatment of initial episodes of genital herpes. First episode genital herpes infections occur in patients experiencing their first vesicular or ulcerative lesion of the genitalia and can be either a true primary infection or a non-primary infection. Primary infections frequently are asymptomatic, in which case the first symptomatic episode actually represents a reactivated recurrent infection. Individuals with true primary HSV infections lack antibody to HSV-1 and/or HSV-2 in their serum.

The severity of first episodes of genital herpes may vary from asymptomatic to disabling; however, untreated primary infections are generally characterized by severe and prolonged symptoms (average duration of 14 days) and a large number of lesions (average duration of 24 days). Symptoms of primary genital herpes usually appear 2–20 days (average: 6 days) following sexual contact with an individual who has a symptomatic or asymptomatic genital herpes infection. Untreated non-primary infections are generally less severe, of shorter duration, and involve fewer systemic complications; lesions of non-primary infections are present for an average of 14 days. Viral shedding occurs in both primary and non-primary infections, and usually lasts about 12 days in untreated primary infections and 7 days in untreated non-primary infections.

Because many patients with first episodes of genital herpes present with mild clinical symptoms but later develop severe or prolonged symptoms, the CDC states that most patients with initial genital herpes should receive antiviral therapy. The CDC and some clinicians recommend that first episodes of genital herpes in immunocompetent adults and adolescents should be treated with a regimen of oral acyclovir (400 mg 3 times daily or 200 mg 5 times daily for 7–10 days), oral famciclovir (250 mg 3 times daily for 7–10 days), or oral valacyclovir (1 g twice daily for 7–10 days). Oral acyclovir also can be used for the treatment of first episodes of genital herpes in pediatric patients. Topical antiviral agents are not recommended for the treatment of genital herpes since these agents offer only minimal clinical benefit.

Controlled studies have shown that oral acyclovir is effective for the treatment of first episodes of genital herpes in immunocompetent patients. Several studies have shown that oral acyclovir therapy decreases viral shedding and the time required for crusting and healing of lesions; in some patients, the formation of new lesions and the duration of pain, pruritus, or dysuria were decreased.

IV acyclovir should be used for the initial treatment of genital herpes when the infection is severe or when there are complications that necessitate hospitalization, including disseminated infection, pneumonitis, hepatitis, CNS involvement (e.g., meningitis, encephalitis). Controlled studies of severe first episodes of genital herpes in immunocompetent individuals have shown that IV acyclovir decreases viral shedding (time from onset of therapy until last positive culture) from genital and cervical lesions, the time necessary for crusting and healing of lesions, the duration of positive cultures, the formation of new lesions, the duration of dysuria and abnormal vaginal discharge, and the degree and duration of pain and pruritus. In one study, the duration of viral shedding was 2 days in acyclovir-treated patients compared with 8 days in placebo-treated patients; the time required for healing of lesions was 7 days in acyclovir-treated patients compared with 15 days in placebo-treated patients.

No substantial reduction in the duration of pain was noted in acyclovir-treated patients compared with placebo-treated patients.

Oral acyclovir has been used at higher dosages (400 mg 5 times daily) for the treatment of first episodes of herpes proctitis†.

Episodic Treatment of Recurrent Infections Oral acyclovir is used in the treatment of recurrent episodes of genital herpes in immunocompetent adults and adolescents. Antiviral therapy for recurrent genital herpes can be given episodically to ameliorate or shorten the duration of lesions or can be given continuously as suppressive therapy to reduce the frequency of recurrences. For episodic treatment of recurrent genital herpes in immunocompetent adults and adolescents, the CDC and some clinicians recommend oral acyclovir (400 mg 3 times daily for 5 days, 800 mg twice daily for 5 days, or 800 mg 3 times daily for 2 days), oral famciclovir (125 mg twice daily for 5 days or 1 g twice daily for 1 day), or oral valacyclovir (500 mg twice daily for 3 days or 1 g once daily for 5 days). Episodic antiviral therapy should be initiated within 1 day of lesion onset or during the prodrome that precedes some outbreaks.

Suppressive Therapy of Recurrent Infections Oral acyclovir is used for chronic suppressive therapy of recurrent genital herpes in immunocompetent adults and adolescents. Data are not available regarding use of acyclovir for suppressive therapy in children. The CDC states that suppressive antiviral therapy can reduce the frequency of genital herpes recurrences by 70–80% in patients who have frequent recurrences (i.e., 6 or more per year) and many patients report no symptomatic outbreaks during such therapy. Quality of life often is improved in patients who receive suppressive therapy rather than episodic treatment for recurrent genital herpes. For chronic suppressive therapy of recurrent genital herpes, the CDC and some clinicians recommend that immunocompetent adults and adolescents receive a regimen of oral acyclovir (400 mg twice daily), oral famciclovir (250 mg twice daily), or oral valacyclovir (500 mg or 1 g once daily). The CDC states that data suggest that famciclovir and valacyclovir are as effective as acyclovir in terms of clinical outcome, although the 500-mg once-daily valacyclovir regimen might be less effective than the acyclovir regimen or other valacyclovir regimens in patients who have very frequent recurrences (i.e., 10 or more episodes per year).

Controlled studies have shown that prophylactic administration of oral acyclovir for suppressive therapy may reduce the frequency and/or severity of subsequent recurrent genital herpes infections or delay the onset of subsequent episodes in immunocompetent patients and can prevent clinical recurrences of genital herpes infections in a substantial proportion of patients. The efficacy of prophylactic administration of oral acyclovir therapy in patients with recurrent herpes proctitis remains to be established. In a study in patients with frequent recurrences of genital herpes infections (6 or more per year) receiving chronic suppressive therapy (400 mg of oral acyclovir twice daily), 45, 52, and 63% of patients were free of recurrences during the first, second, and third years, respectively; serial analyses of 3-month recurrence rates revealed that 71–87% were recurrence free during each quarter, and the annual frequency of recurrences during the third year of therapy relative to the baseline frequency was reduced in 97% of patients. The proportion of these patients (i.e., those receiving chronic suppressive therapy) who remained recurrence free during the first year of the study was substantially higher than that of another group of patients who received intermittent (initiated within 48 hours of onset of a herpes episode) therapy instead; in addition, approximately 25% of patients who received chronic suppressive therapy for 3 years remained recurrence free during the entire period.

Safety and efficacy of oral acyclovir for suppressive therapy of recurrent genital herpes infections have been established in patients receiving daily therapy for up to 5–6 years. Because the frequency of recurrent episodes diminishes over time in many patients, the manufacturer and CDC recommend that suppressive antiviral therapy be discontinued periodically (e.g., once yearly) to assess the need for continued therapy.

HIV-Infected Individuals Immunocompromised individuals may have prolonged or severe episodes of genital, perianal, or oral herpes; HSV lesions are common in those with human immunodeficiency virus (HIV) infection and may be severe, painful, and atypical. (See Uses: Mucocutaneous Herpes Simplex Virus Infections.)

The CDC states that episodic treatment or suppressive therapy with oral antiviral agents often is beneficial in HIV-infected individuals with genital herpes. While the drugs of choice for episodic treatment or suppressive therapy of genital herpes in HIV-infected individuals are the same as those in immunocompetent individuals, higher dosages and/or more prolonged therapy may be necessary. For episodic treatment of recurrences of genital herpes in HIV-infected individuals, the CDC recommends a 5- to 10-day regimen of oral acyclovir (400 mg 3 times daily), oral famciclovir (500 mg twice daily), or oral valacyclovir (1 g twice daily). If chronic suppressive therapy of recurrent genital herpes is used in HIV-infected individuals, the CDC recommends oral acyclovir (400–800 mg 2–3 times daily), oral famciclovir (500 mg twice daily), or oral valacyclovir (500 mg twice daily).

Although rare, clinically important resistance to acyclovir is more likely to occur with prolonged or repeated therapy in severely immunocompromised patients with active lesions. Acyclovir-resistant HSV are resistant to valacyclovir and most strains also are resistant to famciclovir. The potential clinical benefits of acyclovir therapy in immunocompromised patients must be weighed against the potential for selecting resistant HSV strains. If presence of acyclovir-resistant HSV are suspected, specimens should be obtained for in vitro susceptibility testing. Patients whose therapy for the prevention or treatment of recurrence fails because of resistance should be managed in consultation with an expert. IV foscarnet can be used for the management of severe HSV infections known or suspected of being caused by acyclovir-resistant strains; IV foscarnet (40 mg/kg every 8 hours given until clinical resolution is attained) often is effective for the treatment of acyclovir-resistant genital herpes.

Pregnant Women Although safe use of acyclovir during pregnancy has not been established, the CDC states that oral acyclovir may be used to treat first episodes of genital herpes or severe recurrent genital herpes in pregnant women and that IV acyclovir may be used to treat severe HSV infection in pregnant women.

The risk for transmission of HSV to the neonate from an infected mother during vaginal delivery is high (30–50%) among women who acquire genital herpes near the time of delivery (primary infections) and low (0–5%) among women with histories of recurrent genital herpes at term or women who acquire genital herpes during the first half of pregnancy. Administration of acyclovir late in pregnancy in women who have recurrent genital herpes decreases the frequency of recurrences at term and reduces the frequency of cesarean sections; many clinicians recommend such treatment. There are no data to support administration of acyclovir to HSV-seropositive women who do not have a history of genital herpes. Because the risk of herpes is high in infants of women who acquire genital herpes in late pregnancy, such women should be managed in consultation with an HSV expert. Some experts recommend acyclovir therapy and/or routine cesarean section in these women to decrease the risk of transmission of HSV to the neonate. (See Pregnancy under Cautions: Pregnancy, Fertility, and Lactation.)

Patient Counseling and Management of Sexual Partners Counseling of infected individuals and their sex partners is critical to management of genital herpes. The goals of such counseling are to help patients understand and cope with the infection and to prevent sexual and perinatal transmission of the virus. Antiviral therapy offers clinical benefit to most symptomatic patients and is the mainstay of management; however, genital herpes is a recurrent, lifelong viral infection. Although antiviral therapy can be used to control the symptoms and signs of genital herpes episodes, it cannot eradicate latent HSV or affect the risk, frequency, or severity of recurrences of genital herpes following discontinuance of antiviral therapy.

The majority of genital herpes infections are transmitted by individuals unaware that they have the infection or by individuals who are asymptomatic when transmission occurs. Patients should be advised that acyclovir is not a cure for genital herpes, and there are no data evaluating whether acyclovir prevents transmission of HSV to others. Because genital herpes is a sexually transmitted disease, patients should be advised to avoid sexual contact with uninfected partners when lesions and/or prodromal symptoms are present. In addition, patients should be advised that sexual transmission of the virus can occur during asymptomatic periods and that suppressive antiviral therapy reduces, but does not eliminate, subclinical viral shedding.

Sex partners of individuals with genital herpes should be advised that they may be infected even if they have no symptoms. Asymptomatic partners of patients with genital herpes should be questioned regarding a history of genital lesions, educated to recognize symptoms of genital herpes, and offered type-specific serologic testing to determine whether risk for HSV acquisition exists. Antiviral therapy is not recommended for sex partners who do not have clinical manifestations of infection, but symptomatic sex partners of individuals with genital herpes should be evaluated and treated.

The risk for neonatal HSV infection should be discussed with all genital herpes patients, including men. Pregnant women and women of childbearing potential who have genital herpes should inform their providers who care for them during pregnancy as well as those who will care for their neonate.

Information to assist patients and clinicians in counseling regarding genital herpes is available at http://www.ashastd.org and http://www.ihmf.org.

■ **Varicella-Zoster Infections** ***Varicella (Chickenpox)*** Oral acyclovir is used in the treatment of varicella (chickenpox) in immunocompetent adults and children to reduce the severity and duration of the illness. Use of oral acyclovir therapy (initiated within 24 hours of the onset of rash) in otherwise healthy children, postpubertal adolescents, or adults with varicella can decrease the appearance of new lesions, accelerate vesicle healing (vesicles often progress directly from the maculopapular stage to the crusted or healed stage), reduce new vesicle formation by the second day of treatment, and reduce the frequency, duration, and/or severity of fever, pruritus, and constitutional symptoms (e.g., anorexia, lethargy, coryza). In one study in otherwise healthy children 2–12 years of age, nearly all patients receiving oral acyclovir therapy initiated within 24 hours of the onset of rash developed only mild illness of 3–4 days duration with manifestations characteristic of the infection, whereas untreated children generally developed more severe disease of longer duration and many had progressive cutaneous lesions that persisted for more than 6 days.

Some patients who received oral acyclovir therapy reportedly had decreased numbers of residual hypopigmented lesions 4 weeks after initial appearance of rash, and it has been suggested that this possibly indicates a reduction in cutaneous sequelae. However, the clinical relevance, if any, of this finding remains to be established. There currently is no evidence that acyclovir therapy for acute varicella in immunocompetent patients can affect the frequency and/or severity of early complications associated with the disease, in part because such complications generally are uncommon even in untreated individuals. In addition, there currently is no evidence that such therapy can affect the frequency and/or severity of subsequent herpes zoster (shingles, zoster) later in life. It remains to be established whether acyclovir can affect transmission of varicella within households. Current regimens, in which acyclovir is initiated within 24 hours of the appearance of rash, have not reduced such transmission, possibly because therapy was initiated after the period of greatest infectivity. Many clinicians suggest that amelioration, rather than prevention, of varicella in otherwise healthy household contacts should be the principal goal of therapy since prevention could result in the individual being at ongoing risk of primary infection at an older age when manifestations of the disease generally are more severe.

Oral acyclovir therapy in immunocompetent patients generally does not appear to affect antibody response to varicella-zoster infection when measured 1 month and 1 year following treatment with the drug, although somewhat reduced response occasionally has been observed 1 month following treatment with the drug. However, some theoretical concern persists since use of acyclovir in patients with primary herpes simplex infection may result in decreased humoral and cellular immune responses in some patients. Although these altered responses generally have not been associated with increased rates of recurrence or relapse of herpes simplex, the severity of the first subsequent episode of the disease may be increased. Some clinicians also have raised theoretical concerns that potential pathophysiologic and/or immunologic alterations induced by early treatment of varicella infection may predispose to subsequent development of, or more severe, herpes zoster infection, but such concerns have been questioned and remain to be substantiated. Acyclovir should *not* be used prophylactically in an attempt to prevent infection or illness in otherwise healthy children exposed to varicella.

Because of the usually benign course of varicella, the current lack of evidence of effect of acyclovir therapy on early and delayed complications of the disease, and the lack of established substantial cost-benefit of such therapy, the role of acyclovir in the treatment of varicella in otherwise healthy patients currently is controversial. Therefore, the AAP and other clinicians state that oral acyclovir *should not be used routinely* in otherwise healthy children with uncomplicated varicella since administration within 24 hours of rash results in only a modest decrease in symptoms. However, use of oral acyclovir may be considered in certain individual cases when family or clinical circumstances justify the drug's modest benefit and only when the drug can be initiated within the first 24 hours after the onset of rash. The AAP and other clinicians state that use of acyclovir can be considered for otherwise healthy individuals at increased risk of moderate to severe varicella, including those older than 12 years of age, those who contract the disease from siblings or other household contacts, those with chronic cutaneous or pulmonary disorders, those receiving long-term salicylate therapy, and those receiving short, intermittent, or aerosolized courses of corticosteroids. Although it is not known whether children receiving short, intermittent, or aerosolized courses of corticosteroid therapy are at increased risk of complicated or severe varicella, the AAP states that use of acyclovir to minimize the likelihood of severe disease should be considered for these children since no data currently exist to confirm their immunocompetence. Because these children are unlikely to have clinically important immunosuppression, oral acyclovir may used; however, children immunocompromised because of high-dose corticosteroid therapy should receive IV acyclovir therapy. If possible, corticosteroid therapy should be discontinued after known exposure to varicella.

The fact that it may be difficult to recognize varicella and initiate acyclovir therapy soon enough after onset of rash to be of appreciable benefit in many patients, particularly the index case, should be considered. Oral acyclovir provides maximum benefit when initiated as soon as possible after the first manifestation of varicella appears; little if any benefit is apparent if treatment is delayed (e.g., for 48 hours after onset of rash).

IV acyclovir is used for the treatment of varicella in immunocompromised adults and children and many clinicians currently consider IV acyclovir the drug of choice for the treatment of varicella in immunocompromised patients. In immunocompromised adults and children with varicella, IV acyclovir therapy may produce negative viral cultures, decrease the appearance of new lesions, and promote the crusting of lesions; the drug also appears to prevent disseminated, life-threatening infection in some patients. Although limited data suggest that oral acyclovir also may be beneficial in some immunocompromised children with varicella†, the AAP states that oral therapy generally is not recommended for these patients because of poor oral bioavailability. However, high dosage of oral acyclovir has been used in highly selected immunocompromised patients perceived to be at lower risk of developing severe varicella, such as HIV-infected patients with relatively normal $CD4^+$ T-cell counts and children with leukemia in whom careful follow-up is assured. Acyclovir has been used IV in immunocompetent adults for the treatment of complicated varicella (e.g., pneumonia, encephalitis). IV acyclovir therapy appeared to be effective in the treatment of varicella-zoster pneumonia in at least one immunocompetent adult; however, it could not be conclusively determined that the drug was responsible for resolution of infection. In addition, efficacy of the drug may be reduced substantially if initiation of acyclovir is delayed until the disease has advanced to pneumonitis, particularly in immunocompromised patients; therefore, early initiation of therapy is recommended.

Herpes Zoster (Shingles, Zoster) Controlled studies have shown that oral acyclovir is effective for the acute treatment of herpes zoster (shingles, zoster) in immunocompetent adults. Oral acyclovir may prevent the appearance of new lesions, decrease viral shedding, decrease the severity and/or duration of pain, promote healing and crusting of lesions, and reduce the prevalence of localized zoster-associated neurologic manifestations (paresthesia, dysesthesia, or hyperesthesia) in immunocompetent adults with localized herpes zoster, at least when given in high dosages within 2 days of the onset of rash. In these studies, acyclovir was particularly effective in adults 50 years of age or older. In immunocompetent adults, high-dose oral acyclovir therapy also may ameliorate cutaneous manifestations, if initiated within 72 hours of rash onset, and acute pain, and may reduce some anterior inflammatory ocular complications (pseudodendritic keratopathy, stromal keratitis, uveitis), if initiated within 7 days of rash onset, but not early cutaneous and external ocular complications (e.g., lid margin vesiculation, conjunctivitis, corneal hypoesthesia, episcleritis). Longer than usual courses of acyclovir (e.g., 21-day therapy) appear to be associated only with marginal additional benefits with regard to the incidence, duration, and severity of pain during the acute phase of the disease in immunocompetent patients when compared with those receiving a 7-day course of therapy. Therefore, because of cost considerations and insufficient evidence of clinical benefits to support such prolonged use, acyclovir therapies longer than 10 days' duration are not recommended for treatment of acute herpes zoster in immunocompetent individuals.

The effect of oral acyclovir on postherpetic neuralgia remains to be clearly determined. In most studies to date, the drug did not appear to prevent postherpetic neuralgia; however, there is some evidence that high-dose therapy may reduce the occurrence of pain in the second and third months after treatment and the associated local neurologic symptoms 3–6 months after treatment. In a limited number of patients with acute herpes zoster, addition of corticosteroids to acyclovir therapy did not appear to influence incidence or severity of postherpetic neuralgia. In one double-blind, placebo-controlled study in immunocompetent adults older than 50 years of age with localized herpes zoster, patients were randomized to received oral acyclovir (800 mg 5 times daily for 21 days) with oral prednisone (daily dosage of 60 mg for days 1–7, then 30 mg for days 8–14 and 15 mg for days 15–21), oral acyclovir with placebo, oral prednisone with placebo, or 2 placebos. Patients were evaluated for persistence of pain and quality of life (i.e., return to 100% usual activity, return to uninterrupted sleep, cessation of analgesic therapy); acute neuritis was assessed during the first month and chronic pain was assessed for up to 6 months. While patients who received prednisone had a shorter duration of acute pain and improved quality of life during the first month after disease onset compared with those who did not receive the drug, the incidence of pain at 3 or 6 months was similar in all 4 treatment groups.

IV acyclovir is used for the treatment of herpes zoster infections in immunocompromised patients, and some clinicians suggest that IV acyclovir is the preferred antiviral agent for the treatment of primary or disseminated herpes zoster in immunocompromised patients, including HIV-infected patients. IV acyclovir also has been used for the treatment of herpes zoster in immunocompetent patients† who have both localized and disseminated infections. In a placebo-controlled study in immunocompromised patients with herpes zoster, reductions in cutaneous and visceral dissemination were greater in those who received IV acyclovir (500 mg/m² every 8 hours for 7 days) compared with those who received placebo. In a limited number of immunocompetent adults and immunocompromised adults and children with localized and disseminated herpes zoster infections, IV acyclovir therapy appeared to decrease pain and fever, prevent the appearance of new lesions, produce negative cultures, and promote crusting and healing of lesions; however, the principal therapeutic effect of acyclovir in immunocompromised patients appears to be in preventing progression of disease as manifested by cutaneous or visceral dissemination. IV acyclovir therapy has also produced rapid clinical response in a limited number of immunocompetent and immunocompromised patients with herpes zoster-associated encephalitis. There is no evidence that IV acyclovir prevents postherpetic neuralgia.

Oral acyclovir has been used for the treatment of dermatomal herpes zoster in immunocompromised patients†, including transplant recipients and HIV-infected patients.

IV acyclovir (10 mg/kg 3 times daily for 7 days) followed by oral acyclovir (800 mg 3–5 times daily) as maintenance therapy has been used for the treatment of herpes zoster ophthalmicus† in HIV-infected patients.

Several cases of acyclovir-resistant varicella-zoster virus infections have been reported in adults and children with acquired immunodeficiency syndrome (AIDS) following chronic suppressive courses of therapy with the drug; because pretreatment isolates were not obtained, it is not known whether the original virus developed resistance or a resistant strain was selected during chronic therapy. Another case of therapeutic failure secondary to resistant varicella-zoster has been reported in an immunocompromised patient; however, limited data to date suggest that resistance of the virus to acyclovir occurs only rarely, but additional study and experience are necessary.

■ **Cytomegalovirus Infections** Acyclovir generally is ineffective in the treatment of cytomegalovirus (CMV) infections†. IV acyclovir therapy reportedly reduced fever, improved radiographic findings of pneumonia, and resulted in negative blood cultures in some immunocompromised patients with pneumonia caused by CMV. However, in one randomized study in HIV-infected patients, there was no evidence that oral acyclovir therapy suppressed CMV excretion in these patients. IV acyclovir therapy produced little clinical improvement in several infants with congenital CMV infection.

Oral acyclovir has been used for the prevention of CMV disease in organ transplant recipients† considered at risk for the disease. There are conflicting data concerning the effectiveness of the drug for this use, however, and further study is necessary. There is some evidence that IV acyclovir may be effective for suppression of CMV infections in some immunocompromised patients undergoing bone marrow transplantation. Results of a randomized, double-blind study in bone marrow allograft recipients at risk for developing CMV infection (i.e., CMV-seropositive or -seronegative recipients of bone marrow from a CMV-seropositive donor) indicate that in patients who received acyclovir (IV [given 500 mg/m^2 3 times daily beginning 5 days before bone marrow transplantation until 30 days after transplantation] followed by either placebo or oral acyclovir [800 mg 4 times daily for 6 months]) the probability of developing CMV infection and delaying its onset was reduced compared with those receiving oral acyclovir (200-400 mg 4 times daily beginning 5 days before bone marrow transplantation until 30 days after transplantation) followed by placebo. If acute CMV infection developed in patients receiving oral acyclovir followed by placebo, it occurred at a median time of 41 days after transplantation while if the infection developed in patients receiving IV acyclovir followed by placebo or oral acyclovir, it occurred at a median time of 54 or 57 days, respectively. In addition, survival rate appeared to be increased in patients receiving IV acyclovir followed by oral acyclovir therapy, compared with those receiving oral acyclovir followed by placebo. While IV acyclovir also has been used in an attempt toprevent CMV disease in patients undergoing autologous bone marrow transplantation†, the drug does not appear to be effective for this use. In one retrospective study in CMV-seropositive autologous bone marrow recipients, patients who received IV acyclovir (500 mg/m^2 every 8 hours beginning 5 days before transplantation and continued to day 30) did not have a lower incidence of CMV disease and CMV pneumonia during the first 200 days after transplantation than a control group of CMV-seropositive autograft recipients who did not receive the drug.

There is some evidence that high-dose, oral acyclovir therapy may decrease the incidence of CMV disease in certain renal transplant patients, and results of one study indicate that the drug may decrease the incidence of CMV infection in some liver transplant patients. Although some clinicians recommend use of high-dose, oral acyclovir in renal transplant patients, there is little evidence to date that use of oral acyclovir (with or without concomitant immune globulin IV) is associated with a clinically important effect on CMV infection or disease in patients undergoing heart, lung, liver, or kidney transplantation who are considered at risk. In one randomized study in patients undergoing liver transplantation, acyclovir (10 mg/kg IV every 8 hours from day 1 after transplantation until discharge, then 800 mg orally 4 times daily until day 100) was less effective than ganciclovir (6 mg/kg daily IV from day 1–30 after transplantation, then 6 mg/kg daily 5 days weekly until day 100) in preventing CMV disease in these patients. During the first 120 days after the procedure, CMV infections occurred in 38% of those receiving acyclovir and in only 5% of those receiving ganciclovir.

Acyclovir is not effective in preventing CMV disease in HIV-infected individuals, and the drug is not recommended for this use in such patients.

Acyclovir is not effective in preventing CMV disease in hematopoietic stem cell transplant (HSCT) recipients, and the drug is not recommended for this use in such patients. Ganciclovir is the drug of choice for this indication.

■ Epstein-Barr Virus Infections and Disorders

Because acyclovir exhibits in vitro activity against Epstein-Barr virus (EBV), the drug has been used in the treatment of uncomplicated or complicated infectious mononucleosis, chronic infectious mononucleosis, and various disorders (e.g., oral hairy leukoplakia) associated with EBV infections†. While the role of acyclovir in EBV infections remains to be more fully elucidated, current evidence suggests that efficacy of the drug is variable and probably depends on the linear or circular state of EBV DNA, clonality of EBV-infected cells, immune responsiveness of the host, and role of ongoing EBV replication in the pathophysiology of the infection.

Although high-dose oral acyclovir or IV acyclovir has transiently inhibited oropharyngeal shedding of EBV in patients with uncomplicated or complicated infectious mononucleosis, therapy with the drug generally has had little clinical benefit in immunocompetent patients with signs and symptoms of infectious mononucleosis† or in immunocompromised patients with EBV infections†. There are some reports that IV acyclovir may decrease fever and interstitial pneumonitis and improve lymphocyte CD4$^+$/CD8$^+$ ratio in patients with chronic infectious mononucleosis; however, these effects do not occur in all patients who receive the drug.

In a limited number of HIV-infected patients, oral acyclovir therapy was effective in producing clinical regression of oral hairy leukoplakia† (apparently caused by EBV), which recurred following discontinuance of the drug; leukoplakia in patients with acquired immunodeficiency syndrome (AIDS) appeared to be less responsive than in patients whose HIV infection had not progressed to this stage. Some clinicians suggest that, because oral hairy leukoplakia is benign and usually asymptomatic, it may not require treatment. If treatment is required, topical therapy (e.g., topical trichloracetic acid, glycolic acid, podophyllum resin) may be effective; oral acyclovir can be used in severe cases. However, all of these should be considered palliative since the condition recurs when treatment is discontinued. While there is some evidence that oral acyclovir may suppress oral hairy leukoplakia†, the benefit of prolonged suppressive therapy with acyclovir is questionable because such use could promote emergence of acyclovir-resistant HSV in HIV-infected patients.

Acyclovir appeared to produce a beneficial response in several patients with an atypical EBV-associated syndrome manifested as fever, interstitial pneumonitis, pancytopenia, and extremely high titers of antibody to replicative antigens of EBV. IV acyclovir has been reported to be effective in some renal allograft recipients for the treatment of the early stages of posttransplant EBV-associated polyclonal B-cell lymphoproliferative disorders†; however, the drug does not appear to be effective once the tumor progresses into monoclonal lymphoma.

Because Epstein-Barr virus (EBV) has been suggested as a cause of chronic fatigue syndrome (chronic Epstein-Barr virus syndrome), acyclovir has been used in a limited number of patients for the treatment of this condition. However, in a placebo-controlled study in adults with chronic (average duration of 6.8 years), debilitating fatigue, oral acyclovir therapy (3.2 g daily for 30 days) was no more effective than placebo in ameliorating symptoms of the syndrome and there was no correlation between clinical improvement and reduction in EBV antibody levels.

Dosage and Administration

■ Reconstitution and Administration

Acyclovir is administered orally and acyclovir sodium is administered by slow IV infusion at a constant rate over at least 1 hour. Acyclovir sodium should *not* be administered by rapid IV infusion (over less than 10 minutes) or rapid IV injection. (See Cautions: Renal Effects.) Acyclovir sodium also should *not* be administered orally or by IM or subcutaneous injection and should *not* be applied topically or to the eye.

Oral Administration Food does not appear to affect oral absorption of acyclovir, and the drug may be administered without regard to meals.

For oral administration, acyclovir is commercially available as capsules, tablets, or an oral suspension. The commercially available capsules and oral suspension are bioequivalent; in addition, one commercially available 800-mg tablet of acyclovir is bioequivalent to four 200-mg capsules of the drug.

IV Infusion Prior to IV infusion, commercially available acyclovir sodium powder for injection must be reconstituted and then diluted with a compatible IV solution or the commercially available acyclovir sodium concentrate for injection containing acyclovir 50 mg/mL must be diluted with a compatible IV solution. Infusion concentrations of 7 mg/mL or lower are recommended.

Acyclovir sodium powder for injection is reconstituted by adding 10 or 20 mL of sterile water for injection to a vial labeled as containing 500 mg or 1 g of acyclovir, respectively, to provide a solution containing 50 mg/mL. For use in most patients, the appropriate dose of reconstituted solution should then be withdrawn from the vial and diluted with 50–125 mL of a compatible IV infusion solution. (See Chemistry and Stability: Stability.) Before withdrawing the dose of acyclovir, the vial containing the reconstituted solution should be shaken well to ensure complete dissolution of the drug. For use in fluid-restricted patients, the appropriate dose of reconstituted solution can be diluted in a ratio of about 1 part reconstituted solution of acyclovir to 9 parts infusion solution; however, because of the risk of adverse effects (e.g., phlebitis), concentrations of the infusion generally should not exceed 7 mg/mL. In addition, higher concentrations (e.g., 10 mg/mL) may produce phlebitis or inflammation at the infusion site if inadvertent extravasation occurs. Reconstituted acyclovir sodium solutions should be used within 12 hours and reconstituted solutions that have been further diluted in a compatible infusion solution should be used within 24 hours. (See Chemistry and Stability: Stability.)

Rate of Administration. Acyclovir sodium solutions generally should be given by IV infusion at a constant rate over a 1-hour period. Because of the risk of adverse renal effects (see Cautions: Renal Effects), diluted solutions of acyclovir *should not be infused over a period less than 1 hour.*

■ Oral Dosage

Mucocutaneous, Ocular, and Systemic Herpes Simplex Virus Infections **Treatment of Mucocutaneous HSV Infections.** When oral acyclovir is used for the *treatment* of mucocutaneous HSV infections in immunocompromised adults†, including those infected with human immunodeficiency virus (HIV), some clinicians recommend a dosage of 400 mg every 4 hours while awake (5 times daily) for 7–14 days. For the treatment of these infections in immunocompromised children†, the American Academy of Pediatrics (AAP) recommends an oral dosage of 1 g daily given in 3–5 divided doses for 7–14 days.

For the treatment of orolabial HSV infections in HIV-infected adults, the US Centers for Disease Control and Prevention (CDC) recommends an oral acyclovir dosage of 400 mg 3 times daily for 7–14 days. For the treatment of mild symptomatic HSV gingivostomatitis† in HIV-infected children, CDC recommends a dosage of 20 mg/kg (up to 400 mg) 3 times daily for 7–14 days. A dosage of 15 mg/kg (up to 200 mg) 5 times daily for 7 days has been used for the treatment of HSV gingivostomatitis† in immunocompetent children 1–6 years of age.

Chronic Suppressive and Maintenance Prophylaxis of HSV. When oral acyclovir is used for chronic suppressive or maintenance *prophylaxis* (secondary prophylaxis) of HSV† in HIV-infected adults or adolescents who have frequent or severe recurrences of HSV disease, a dosage of 200 mg 3 times daily or 400 mg twice daily has been recommended by the Prevention of Opportunistic Infections Working Group of the US Public Health Service and the Infectious Diseases Society of America (USPHS/IDSA).

The USPHS/IDSA recommends that HIV-infected infants and children who have frequent or severe recurrences of HSV receive oral acyclovir in a dosage of 80 mg/kg daily given in 3 or 4 divided doses for suppressive therapy.

Ocular HSV Infections. For the treatment of HSV keratitis† in HIV-infected patients, oral acyclovir has been given in a dosage of 400 mg 5 times daily; long-term antiviral therapy may be necessary to prevent recurrent ocular HSV disease in these patients. For the prevention of recurrent ocular HSV disease† in immunocompetent adults and children 12 years of age or older, oral acyclovir has been given in a dosage of 400 mg twice daily for 12–18 months. For prevention of recurrent ocular HSV disease† following penetrating keratoplasty for herpetic eye disease, oral acyclovir has been given in a dosage of 400 mg twice daily for 6 months. Optimum duration of prophylaxis remains to be determined.

Hematopoietic Stem Cell Transplant Recipients. When oral acyclovir is used for the prevention of recurrent HSV disease† in HSV-seropositive adults and adolescents undergoing hematopoietic stem cell transplantation (HSCT), some clinicians recommend an acyclovir dosage of 200 mg 3 times daily. For HSV-seropositive children, clinicians recommend an oral acyclovir dosage of 0.6–1 g daily given in 3–5 divided doses.

Acyclovir therapy is initiated at the beginning of the conditioning regimen and continued until engraftment occurs or mucositis resolves (i.e., approximately 30 days after HSCT). Routine prophylaxis for longer than 30 days is not recommended.

Genital Herpes **Treatment of Initial Episodes in Immunocompetent Individuals.** For the treatment of initial episodes of genital herpes in immunocompetent individuals, the dosage of oral acyclovir recommended by the manufacturer is 200 mg every 4 hours while awake (5 times daily) for 10 days. The CDC and other clinicians state that the usual dosage of oral acyclovir for the treatment of initial genital herpes in immunocompetent adults or adolescents is 400 mg 3 times daily or 200 mg 5 times daily given for 7–10 days. The CDC states that the duration of therapy may be extended if healing is incomplete after 10 days.

For the treatment of initial episodes of genital herpes in immunocompetent children, the AAP recommends a dosage of 40–80 mg/kg daily (maximum 1 g daily) given in 3 or 4 divided doses for 5–10 days.

If acyclovir is used for the treatment of initial episodes of herpes proctitis† in adults, an oral acyclovir dosage of 400 mg 5 times daily for 10 days or until clinical resolution occurs has been used. Alternatively, some clinicians recommend an oral dosage of 800 mg every 8 hours for 7–10 days for the treatment of initial episodes of herpes proctitis.

Episodic Treatment of Recurrent Episodes. For the episodic treatment of recurrent genital herpes in immunocompetent adults, the manufacturer recommends a dosage of 200 mg every 4 hours while awake (5 times daily) for 5 days. The CDC states that the usual dosage of oral acyclovir for the episodic treatment of recurrent genital herpes in immunocompetent adults and adolescents is 400 mg 3 times daily for 5 days, 800 mg twice daily for 5 days, or 800 mg 3 times daily for 2 days.

In HIV-infected adults and children, the CDC recommends a dosage of 400 mg 3 times daily given for 5–10 days for episodic treatment of recurrent episodes; alternatively, acyclovir can be given for 7–14 days. Acyclovir should be initiated at the earliest prodromal sign or symptom of recurrence or within 1 day of the onset of lesions.

Chronic Suppressive Therapy of Recurrent Episodes. For chronic suppressive therapy of recurrent episodes of genital herpes in immunocompetent adults and adolescents, the usual dosage of oral acyclovir is 400 mg orally twice daily. Alternatively, the manufacturer states that dosages of 200 mg orally 3–5 times daily have been be used.

In HIV-infected adults and adolescents, the CDC recommends a dosage of 400–800 mg 2- or 3-times daily for chronic suppressive therapy of recurrent genital herpes. Oral acyclovir has been used for chronic suppressive therapy for up to 5–6 years; however, the manufacturer and CDC recommend that suppressive antiviral therapy be discontinued periodically (e.g., once yearly) to assess the need for continued therapy.

Varicella-Zoster Infections **Varicella (Chickenpox).** For the treatment of varicella (chickenpox) in immunocompetent adults and children 2 years of age and older, the recommended oral dosage of acyclovir is 20 mg/kg (maximum 800 mg per dose) 4 times daily for 5 days. The manufacturer recommends that adults and children who weigh more than 40 kg receive 800 mg orally 4 times daily for 5 days and that children 2 years of age and older weighing 40 kg or less receive 20 mg/kg 4 times daily (maximum daily dosage 80 mg/kg) for 5 days. While lower dosages of oral acyclovir also have been used in immunocompetent children with varicella, some evidence indicates that such dosages may be less effective than the currently recommended dosage. Although the manufacturer states that safety and efficacy of oral acyclovir have not been adequately studied for children younger than 2 years of age, the AAP states that certain children older than 12 months of age† may receive the currently recommended oral dosage of the drug but that data are insufficient to make a recommendation for children 12 months of age or younger. For HIV-infected children with mild immunosuppression and mild varicella, CDC recommends oral acyclovir 20 mg/kg (maximum 800 mg per dose) 4 times daily for 7 days or until no new lesions appear for 48 hours.

If oral acyclovir is used for the treatment of varicella, the drug must be initiated at the earliest sign or symptom of infection. Oral acyclovir offers maximum benefit when initiated as soon as possible after the first manifestation of chickenpox appears; little if any benefit is apparent if treatment is delayed (e.g., for 48 hours after onset of rash). AAP recommends that oral acyclovir therapy be initiated within the first 24 hours after the onset of rash.

Herpes Zoster (Shingles, Zoster). For the treatment of acute herpes zoster (shingles, zoster) in immunocompetent adults and children 12 years of age or older, the recommended oral dosage of acyclovir is 800 mg every 4 hours 5 times daily (4 g daily) for 5–10 days, preferably initiated within 48 hours of rash onset. Acyclovir also has been used for longer periods (e.g., for 21 days) in the management of acute herpes zoster in immunocompetent patients.

For HIV-infected children with mild immunosuppression and mild zoster, CDC recommends oral acyclovir 20 mg/kg (maximum 800 mg per dose) 4 times daily for 7–10 days.

For the treatment of acute herpes zoster ophthalmicus† in immunocompetent adults, an acyclovir oral dosage of 600 mg every 4 hours 5 times daily (3 g daily) for 10 days, preferably initiated within 72 hours but no later than 7 days of rash onset, has been used.

For the treatment of dermatomal herpes zoster in immunocompromised patients†, including transplant recipients or HIV-infected adults, acyclovir has been given in a dosage of 800 mg orally 5 times daily for 10 days.

■ **IV Dosage** Dosage of acyclovir sodium is expressed in terms of acyclovir. The manufacturer states that the maximum dosage of IV acyclovir is 20 mg/kg every 8 hours. The manufacturer recommends that obese patients receive IV acyclovir dosages based on ideal body weight.

Mucocutaneous and Systemic Herpes Simplex Virus Infections

Treatment of Mucocutaneous HSV Infections. For the treatment of mucocutaneous HSV infections in immunocompromised patients, including HIV-infected individuals, the usual IV dosage of acyclovir for adults and children 12 years of age or older with normal renal function (i.e., creatinine clearance greater than 50 mL/minute per 1.73 m^2) is 5 mg/kg every 8 hours (15 mg/kg daily) for 7–14 days; in children younger than 12 years of age, the recommended dosage is 10 mg/kg every 8 hours for 7–14 days.

For the treatment of moderate to severe symptomatic HSV gingivostomatitis† in HIV-infected children, CDC recommends an IV acyclovir dosage of 5–10 mg/kg 3 times daily for 7–14 days.

Treatment of HSV Encephalitis. For the treatment of HSV encephalitis, the recommended IV dosage of acyclovir for adults and children 12 years of age or older is 10–15 mg/kg every 8 hours. In children between 3 months and 12 years of age, the recommended IV dosage is 20 mg/kg every 8 hours. The manufacturer recommends 10 days of IV acyclovir therapy for the treatment of HSV encephalitis; however, because relapses have been reported after only 10 days' treatment, some clinicians recommend a longer duration of parenteral treatment (e.g., 14–21 days).

Treatment of Neonatal HSV Infection. For the treatment of neonatal HSV infection in infants from birth to 3 months of age, the manufacturer recommends an IV acyclovir dosage of 10 mg/kg every 8 hours for 10 days. The AAP and other clinicians recommend an IV acyclovir dosage of 20 mg/kg every 8 hours for 14–21 days; however, the manufacturer states that safety and efficacy of doses greater than 10 mg/kg for the treatment of neonatal HSV infection have not been established. The AAP states that IV acyclovir should be given for 14 days if disease is limited to the skin, eye, and mouth or for 21 days if disease is disseminated or involves the CNS.

Hematopoietic Stem Cell Transplant Recipients. For the prevention of recurrent HSV disease† in HSV-seropositive adults and adolescents undergoing hematopoietic stem cell transplantation (HSCT), some clinicians recommend an IV acyclovir dosage of 250 mg/m^2 every 12 hours. For HSV-seropositive children, some clinicians recommend an IV acyclovir dosage of 250 mg/m^2 every 8 hours or 125 mg/m^2 every 6 hours. Therapy can be switched to oral acyclovir when appropriate. Acyclovir therapy is initiated at the beginning of the conditioning regimen and continued until engraftment occurs or mucositis resolves (i.e., approximately 30 days after HSCT). Routine prophylaxis for longer than 30 days is not recommended.

Genital Herpes For the treatment of severe first episodes of genital herpes, the usual IV dosage of acyclovir for immunocompetent adults and children 12 years of age and older is 5–10 mg/kg every 8 hours. The manufacturer and some clinicians states that IV acyclovir should be given for 5–7 days; the CDC states that IV acyclovir should be given for 2–7 days or until clinical improvement occurs and then an oral antiviral agent should be substituted to complete at least 10 days of therapy.

Varicella-Zoster Infections For the treatment of varicella (chickenpox) or herpes zoster (shingles, zoster) in immunocompromised adults and children 12 years of age and older with normal renal function, the manufacturer recommends an IV dosage of acyclovir of 10 mg/kg every 8 hours for 7 days. In children younger than 12 years of age, the manufacturer recommends an IV acyclovir dosage of 20 mg/kg every 8 hours for 7 days.

For the treatment of varicella in HIV-infected adults, CDC recommends an IV dosage of 10 mg/kg every 8 hours for 7–10 days. Therapy can be switched to oral acyclovir (800 mg 4 times daily) after defervescence if there is no evidence of visceral involvement.

For the treatment of varicella in immunocompetent children 2 years of age or older, AAP recommends an IV acyclovir dosage of 30 mg/kg daily in divided doses or 500 mg/m^2 every 8 hours for 7–10 days. For the treatment of varicella in immunocompromised children younger than 1 year of age, AAP and others recommend an IV acyclovir dosage of 10 mg/kg every 8 hours for 7–10 days. For immunocompromised children 1 year of age and older, AAP recommends 500 mg/m^2 every 8 hours for 7–10 days; other experts recommend 30 mg/kg daily in divided doses.

For the treatment of herpes zoster in immunocompromised children younger than 12 years of age, AAP recommends an IV acyclovir dosage of 20 mg/kg every 8 hours for 7–10 days. For immunocompromised children 12 years of age or older, AAP recommends an IV acyclovir dosage of 10 mg/kg every

8 hours for 7 days. For the treatment of herpes zoster in immunocompetent children younger than 1 year of age, AAP recommends an IV acyclovir dosage of 10 mg/kg every 8 hours for 7–10 days. For immunocompetent children 1 year of age and older, AAP recommends 500 mg/m² every 8 hours for 7–10 days; other experts recommend 30 mg/kg daily in divided doses.

For the treatment of extensive multidermatomal zoster or zoster with trigeminal nerve involvement in HIV-infected children with severe immunosuppression, CDC recommends an IV acyclovir dosage of 10 mg/kg 3 times daily for 7–10 days.

■ **Dosage in Renal Impairment** In patients with impaired renal function, doses and/or frequency of administration of acyclovir must be modified in response to the degree of impairment. Generally, the decrease in total body clearance of acyclovir is directly related to the decrease in body-surface-area-corrected creatinine clearance; however, clearance of acyclovir is usually greater than predicted from creatinine clearance, since the drug undergoes some renal tubular secretion.

Oral Dosage Based on pharmacokinetic studies of IV acyclovir in patients with renal impairment, the manufacturer recommends the following oral dosage of acyclovir based on the usual dosage regimen and the patient's creatinine clearance (see Table 1):

Table 1: Oral Dosage Adjustment in Patients with Renal Impairment.

Usual Dosage Regimen	Creatinine Clearance (mL/min per 1.73 m²)	Adjusted Dosage Regimen
200 mg every 4 h 5 times daily	>10	No adjustment necessary
	0–10	200 mg every 12 h
400 mg every 12 h	>10	No adjustment necessary
	0–10	200 mg every 12 h
800 mg every 4 h 5 times daily	>25	No adjustment necessary
	10–25	800 mg every 8 h
	0–10	800 mg every 12 h

Because acyclovir is removed by hemodialysis, the manufacturer recommends that patients undergoing hemodialysis receive a supplemental oral dose of the drug immediately after each dialysis period. The manufacturer states that supplemental doses of oral acyclovir do not appear to be necessary following peritoneal dialysis.

For HIV-infected patients with impaired renal function, the following oral dosages of acyclovir have been suggested based on a usual dosage regimen of 200–800 mg every 4–6 hours and the patient's creatinine clearance (see Table 2):

Table 2: Oral Dosage Adjustment in HIV-Infected Patients with Impaired Renal Function.

Creatinine Clearance (mL/min per 1.73 m²)	Adjusted Dosage Regimen
>80	No adjustment necessary
50–80	200–800 mg every 6–8 h
25–50	200–800 mg every 8–12 h
10–25	200–800 mg every 12–24 h
<10	200–400 mg every 24 h
Hemodialysis	supplement usual dose after each hemodialysis

Parenteral Dosage The manufacturer recommends the following IV dosage of acyclovir based on the patient's creatinine clearance (see Table 3):

Table 3: IV Dosage Adjustment in Patients with Renal Impairment.

Creatinine Clearance (mL/min per 1.73 m²)	Percent of Recommended Dose	Dosing Interval (hours)
>50	100%	8
25–50	100%	12
10–25	100%	24
0–10	50%	24

The manufacturer states that patients undergoing hemodialysis may require a supplemental acyclovir dose after each dialysis period. The patient's dosing schedule should be adjusted so that an additional dose is administered after each dialysis. Alternatively in patients undergoing hemodialysis, some clinicians recommend that 2.5 mg/kg be administered every 24 hours and that an additional 2.5-mg/kg dose be administered after each dialysis period.

Other IV acyclovir dosage regimens have been suggested for patients with end-stage renal disease. In one regimen, an initial loading dose of 93–185 mg/m², a maintenance dosage of 35–70 mg/m² every 8 hours, and a dose of 56–185 mg/m² immediately after dialysis have been used. Alternatively, an initial loading dose of 250–500 mg/m², a maintenance dosage of 250–500 mg/m² every 48 hours, and a dose of 150–500 mg/m² immediately after dialysis have been suggested.

Because acyclovir is removed by continuous ambulatory peritoneal dialysis (CAPD) to a lesser extent than by hemodialysis, the manufacturer states that supplemental doses of acyclovir do not appear to be necessary following CAPD.

For HIV-infected patients with impaired renal function, the following IV dosages of acyclovir have been suggested based on a usual dosage regimen of 5 mg/kg every 8 hours and the patient's creatinine clearance:

Table 4: IV Dosage Adjustment in HIV-Infected Patients with Impaired Renal Function.

Creatinine Clearance (mL/min per 1.73 m²)	Adjusted Dosage Regimen
greater than 80	No adjustment necessary
50–80	No adjustment necessary
25–50	5 mg/kg every 12–24 hours
10–25	5 mg/kg every 12–24 hours
less than 10	2.5 mg/kg every 24 hours
Hemodialysis	administer usual dose after hemodialysis

Cautions

Adverse reactions generally have been minimal following oral or IV administration of acyclovir. However, potentially serious reactions (e.g., renal failure, thrombotic thrombocytopenic purpura/hemolytic uremic syndrome) can occur and fatalities have been reported.

■ **Local Effects** The most frequent adverse effects of IV acyclovir are local reactions at the injection site. Inflammation or phlebitis has been reported in approximately 9% of patients. Severe local inflammatory reactions, including tissue necrosis, have occurred following infusion of acyclovir into extravascular tissues.

■ **Renal Effects** Increased BUN and/or serum creatinine concentrations, anuria, and hematuria have been reported in patients receiving acyclovir. Abnormal urinalysis (characterized by an increase in formed elements in urine sediment) and pain or pressure on urination have been reported rarely with IV acyclovir.

Transient increases in BUN and/or serum creatinine concentrations and decreases in creatinine clearance occur in about 5–10% of patients receiving IV acyclovir, and have been reported most frequently when the drug was administered by rapid (over less than 10 minutes) IV infusion rather than over the recommended period for IV infusion (at least 1 hour).

Renal failure, resulting in death in some patients, has occurred in patients receiving acyclovir. The risk of adverse renal effects during IV acyclovir therapy depends on the patient's degree of hydration, urine output, concomitant therapy (i.e., other nephrotoxic drugs), preexisting renal disease, and the rate of administration of acyclovir. Precipitation of the drug in the renal tubules can occur when the solubility of free acyclovir in the collecting duct is exceeded or following rapid IV administration of the drug; ensuing renal tubular damage may result in acute renal failure. In some cases, alterations in renal function during IV acyclovir therapy progress to acute renal failure; however, in most cases, alterations in renal function are transient and resolve spontaneously or following improved hydration and electrolyte balance, dosage adjustment, or discontinuance of the drug.

■ **Nervous System Effects** Headache is one of the most common nervous system adverse effects of oral acyclovir, occurring in about 2% of patients receiving the drug as chronic suppressive therapy. Aggressive behavior, agitation, ataxia, coma, confusion, decreased consciousness, delirium, dizziness, encephalopathy, hallucinations, obtundation, paresthesia, psychosis, seizures, somnolence, and tremors have been reported during oral or IV acyclovir therapy and these effects may be marked, particularly in older adults or patients with renal impairment. In patients receiving oral acyclovir for the treatment of herpes zoster (shingles, zoster), malaise was reported in 11.5% of patients receiving the drug and 11.1% of those receiving placebo.

Encephalopathic effects including lethargy, obtundation, tremors, confusion, hallucinations, agitation, seizures, and coma have occurred in approximately 1% of patients receiving IV acyclovir. Agitation, delirium, diaphoresis, dizziness, headache, lightheadedness, somnolence, and psychosis have occurred rarely. Coarse tremor and clonus developed in at least one immunocompromised patient during IV acyclovir therapy. Cerebral edema, coma, and death, probably resulting from cerebral anoxia, occurred during IV acyclovir therapy in an immunocompromised bone marrow transplant patient with pneumonitis.

■ **GI Effects** Nausea, vomiting, and diarrhea are among the most common adverse effects of oral acyclovir. In a study in patients receiving oral acyclovir for treatment of recurrent genital herpes, nausea occurred in about 5% and diarrhea in about 2% of patients receiving the drug for chronic suppressive therapy and these adverse GI effects occurred in 2.4–2.7% of those receiving episodic treatment of recurrences. In patients receiving oral acyclovir for the treatment of initial episodes of genital herpes, nausea and/or vomiting occurred in 2.7%. Diarrhea was reported in 3.2% of patients receiving the drug for the treatment of varicella (chickenpox). GI distress also has been reported in patients receiving oral acyclovir.

Nausea and/or vomiting have been reported in about 7% of patients receiving IV acyclovir therapy (mainly occurring in nonhospitalized patients receiving acyclovir dosages of 10 mg/kg 3 times daily). Anorexia, diarrhea, and GI distress also have been reported with IV acyclovir.

■ **Hematologic Effects** Anemia, leukocytoclastic vasculitis, leukopenia, lymphadenopathy, and thrombocytopenia have been reported in patients receiving oral acyclovir.

Anemia, disseminated intravascular coagulation, hemoglobinemia, hemolysis, leukocytoclastic vasculitis, leukocytosis, leukopenia, lymphadenopathy, neutropenia, neutrophilia, thrombocytopenia, and thrombocytosis have been reported rarely in patients receiving IV acyclovir.

■ **Dermatologic and Sensitivity Reactions** Rash, pruritus, or urticaria occasionally occurs during oral or IV acyclovir therapy. Alopecia and angioedema have been reported. At least one case of erythematous rash and vasculitis has been reported following administration of IV acyclovir to an immunocompromised patient exposed to chickenpox; however, this reaction has not been directly attributed to the drug.

Anaphylaxis has been reported rarely in patients receiving oral or IV acyclovir. Stevens-Johnson syndrome, erythema multiforme, photosensitivity rash, and toxic epidermal necrolysis have occurred rarely in patients receiving acyclovir.

■ **Other Adverse Effects** Fever and pain have been reported in patients receiving oral or IV acyclovir. Elevated liver function test results, hepatitis, hyperbilirubinemia, jaundice, hypotension, myalgia, peripheral edema, thirst, and visual abnormalities have been reported rarely in patients receiving oral or IV acyclovir.

■ **Precautions and Contraindications** Oral and IV acyclovir are contraindicated in patients who develop hypersensitivity to acyclovir or valacyclovir.

Patients receiving acyclovir for the treatment of genital herpes should be advised that the drug is not a cure for genital herpes and that, because genital herpes is a sexually transmitted disease, they should avoid sexual contact while visible lesions are present since there is a risk of infecting their sexual partner. (See Patient Counseling and Management of Sexual Partners under Uses: Genital Herpes.) If acyclovir is used for chronic suppressive therapy of genital herpes, the drug should be discontinued after 1 year of therapy so that the frequency and severity of the patient's genital herpes infection can be reevaluated to determine the need for continuing acyclovir therapy. Oral acyclovir has been used for suppressive therapy of genital herpes in immunocompetent adults for up to 5–6 years without evidence of long-term adverse effects.

All patients receiving oral acyclovir should be instructed to consult their clinician if severe or troublesome adverse effects occur during acyclovir therapy. Female patients receiving the drug should be instructed to consult their physician if they become pregnant or intend to become pregnant or if they intend to breast-feed. (See Cautions: Pregnancy, Fertility, and Lactation.)

The manufacturer states that the recommended dosage and duration of acyclovir therapy should not be exceeded. The manufacturer also cautions that both the dose and dosage interval should be carefully adjusted in patients with renal failure or in patients undergoing hemodialysis to prevent drug accumulation, decrease the risk of toxicity, and maintain adequate plasma concentrations of acyclovir. The manufacturer states that when dosage adjustment is required, they should be based on estimated creatinine clearance. (See Dosage and Administration: Dosage in Renal Impairment.)

Acyclovir should be used with caution in patients receiving other nephrotoxic drugs concurrently since the risk of acyclovir-induced renal impairment and/or reversible CNS symptoms is increased in these patients. Adequate hydration should be maintained in patients receiving acyclovir; however, in patients with encephalitis, the recommended hydration should be balanced by the risk of cerebral edema. Because the risk of acyclovir-induced renal impairment is increased during rapid IV administration of the drug, acyclovir should be given only by slow IV infusion (over at least 1 hour).

Parenteral acyclovir therapy can cause signs and symptoms of encephalopathy. (See Cautions: Nervous System Effects.) The manufacturer states that acyclovir should be used with caution in patients with underlying neurologic abnormalities and in patients with serious renal, hepatic, or electrolyte abnormalities or substantial hypoxia. The drug also should be used with caution in patients who have manifested prior neurologic reactions to cytotoxic drugs or those receiving intrathecal methotrexate or interferon.

■ **Pediatric Precautions** The manufacturer states that safety and efficacy of *oral* acyclovir in children younger than 2 years of age have not been established.

■ **Geriatric Precautions** In a clinical study evaluating use of oral acyclovir for the treatment of herpes zoster (shingles, zoster) in immunocompetent adults 50 years of age or older, approximately 65% of patients were 65 years of age or older and more than 30% were 75 years of age or older. There was no overall difference in effectiveness for time to cessation of new lesion formation or time to healing between geriatric patients and younger adults. However, the duration of pain after healing was longer in those 65 years of age and older and nausea, vomiting, and dizziness were reported more frequently in geriatric patients. Clinical studies evaluating IV acyclovir have not included sufficient numbers of patients 65 years of age or older to determine whether they respond differently than younger patients.

Geriatric patients are more likely than younger adults to have adverse CNS effects (e.g., coma, confusion, hallucinations, somnolence) during acyclovir therapy. Geriatric patients also are more likely to have adverse renal effects during acyclovir therapy and to have reduced renal function requiring dosage adjustment. Acyclovir dosage should be carefully selected for this age group and it may be useful to monitor renal function.

■ **Mutagenicity and Carcinogenicity** Mutagenic changes and chromosomal damage have occurred in vitro in human lymphocytes and mouse lymphoma cells at acyclovir concentrations at least 25 times greater than plasma drug concentrations achievable with usual dosage in humans. In other in vitro microbial and mammalian cell assays, no evidence of mutagenicity or inconclusive results were observed. The manufacturer states that acyclovir was tested in 16 in vitro and in vivo genetic toxicity assays and was positive in 5 of these assays.

In lifetime bioassays in rats and mice receiving single daily dosages of up to 450 mg/kg administered by gastric lavage, there was no statistically significant difference in the incidence of tumors between treated and control animals and no evidence that acyclovir shortened the latency of tumors. Maximum plasma concentrations in the mouse or rat bioassay were 3–6 or 1–2 times, respectively, the usual human concentrations (based on steady-state plasma concentrations observed in humans receiving 200 or 800 mg of acyclovir orally 5 times daily).

Evidence of mutagenicity or carcinogenicity in humans has not been reported to date.

■ **Pregnancy, Fertility, and Lactation** ***Pregnancy*** There are no adequate and controlled studies to date using acyclovir in pregnant women, and the drug should be used during pregnancy only when the potential benefits justify the possible risks to the fetus.

Acyclovir administered during organogenesis was not teratogenic in the mouse (450 mg/kg daily orally), rabbit (50 mg/kg daily subcutaneously or IV), or rat (50 mg/kg daily subcutaneously). These dosages resulted in plasma concentrations that were 106, 11, and 22 times, respectively, the steady-state plasma concentrations observed in humans receiving 200 or 800 mg of acyclovir orally 5 times daily. However, in nonstandard tests in rats, fetal abnormalities (e.g., head and tail anomalies) and maternal toxicity were observed with subcutaneous acyclovir. Acyclovir crosses the placenta in humans and the clinical relevance of these animal findings currently is not known.

IV acyclovir has been used during the second or third trimester of pregnancy without apparent adverse effects to the fetus. The US Centers for Disease Control and Prevention (CDC) state that first clinical episodes of genital herpes occurring during pregnancy may be treated with oral acyclovir and that use of IV acyclovir therapy may be indicated for the treatment of severe maternal HSV infections. Preliminary data suggest that acyclovir treatment late in pregnancy might reduce the frequency of cesarean sections among women who have recurrent genital herpes by diminishing the frequency of recurrences at term. The risk for HSV is high in infants born to women who acquired genital herpes in late pregnancy, and such women should be managed in consultation with an HSV specialist. Some experts recommend acyclovir therapy in this circumstance, some recommend routine cesarean section to reduce the risk for neonatal HSV, and others recommend both. (See Pregnant Women under Uses: Genital Herpes.)

Many clinicians do not recommend use of oral acyclovir in pregnant adolescents or women with uncomplicated varicella because the risk or benefit to the fetus currently is not known. However, other clinicians recommend use of oral acyclovir for the treatment of varicella in pregnant women, especially during the second and third trimesters. In addition, use of IV acyclovir is recommended in pregnant women with serious complications of varicella such as extensive cutaneous disease, high fever, or systemic symptoms. It is not known whether acyclovir administered to the mother prevents congenital varicella syndrome (i.e., low birthweight, hypotrophic limbs, ocular abnormalities, brain damage, mental retardation) in the neonate.

To monitor fetal outcomes of pregnant women exposed either inadvertently or intentionally to systemic acyclovir, the manufacturer established a prospective registry of acyclovir use during pregnancy and collected data from 1984 to April 1999. A total of 749 pregnancies were followed over this time period involving 756 outcomes, and comparison of registry data with birth defect surveillance data revealed no evidence of an increased risk for birth defects in infants of mothers treated with acyclovir during the first trimester of pregnancy. However, the sample size of the registry is insufficient to evaluate the risk for less common defects or to permit reliable or definitive conclusions regarding the safety of acyclovir in pregnant women and their developing fetuses.

Fertility Reproduction studies using oral acyclovir dosages of 450 mg/kg daily in mice and subcutaneous dosages of 25 mg/kg daily in rats have not revealed evidence of impaired fertility. Following subcutaneous dosages of 50 mg/kg daily in rats and rabbits, a decrease in implantation efficiency was observed; decreases in the numbers of corpora lutea, implantation sites, and live fetuses were observed in rats. No effect on implantation efficiency was observed in rabbits following IV dosages of 50 mg/kg daily. Although no drug-related reproductive effects were observed in rabbits following IV dosages of 50 mg/kg daily, increases in fetal resorptions and corresponding decreases in litter size were observed following IV dosages of 100 mg/kg daily. Following intraperitoneal acyclovir dosages of 320 or 80 mg/kg daily in male rats for 1 or 6 months, respectively, testicular atrophy was observed; some evidence of recovery of sperm production was apparent 30 days after discontinuance of the drug. Aspermatogenesis was observed in dogs following IV dosages of 100 and 200 mg/kg daily for 31 days. No adverse testicular effects were observed in dogs given IV dosages of 50 mg/kg daily for one month or given 60 mg/kg daily for one year. In a controlled study in men receiving chronic oral acyclovir (400 mg or 1 g daily) therapy, there was no evidence of clinically important effects on sperm count, motility, or morphology during 6 months of therapy and 3 months of posttreatment follow-up.

Lactation Limited data indicate that acyclovir is distributed into milk, generally in concentrations greater than concurrent maternal plasma concentrations, and can be absorbed by nursing infants. Acyclovir should be administered to nursing women with caution and only when indicated.

Drug Interactions

■ **Antifungal Agents** Amphotericin B has been shown to potentiate the antiviral effect of acyclovir against pseudorabies virus in vitro when both drugs are added to the culture medium. Ketoconazole and acyclovir have shown dose-dependent, synergistic, antiviral activity against herpes simplex virus types 1 and 2 (HSV-1 and -2) in in vitro replication studies. The clinical importance of these interactions has not been established, and additional study is necessary to determine potential antiviral synergy between these antifungal agents and acyclovir.

■ **Probenecid** Concomitant administration of probenecid and acyclovir has reportedly increased the mean plasma half-life and area under the plasma concentration-time curve (AUC) and decreased urinary excretion and renal clearance of acyclovir. In one study following oral administration of a 1-g dose of probenecid 1 hour prior to a 1-hour IV infusion of acyclovir 5 mg/kg, the half-life and AUC for acyclovir increased by 18% and 40%, respectively, and urinary excretion and renal clearance of acyclovir decreased by 13% and 32%, respectively. This interaction may result from competitive inhibition of the renal secretion of acyclovir by probenecid.

■ **Interferon** The manufacturer states that IV acyclovir should be used with caution in patients receiving interferon. In vitro, when acyclovir and interferon are both added to cultures of herpes simplex virus type 1 (HSV-1), the drugs have an additive or synergistic antiviral effect; however, the clinical importance of this interaction is not known.

■ **Methotrexate** The manufacturer states that IV acyclovir should be used with caution in patients receiving intrathecal methotrexate.

■ **Zidovudine** Acyclovir has been used concomitantly with zidovudine in some patients with human immunodeficiency virus (HIV) infections without evidence of increased toxicity; however, neurotoxicity (profound drowsiness and lethargy), which recurred on rechallenge, has been reported in at least one patient with acquired immunodeficiency syndrome (AIDS) during concomitant therapy with the drugs. Neurotoxicity was evident within 30–60 days after initiation of IV acyclovir therapy, persisted with some improvement when acyclovir was administered orally, and resolved following discontinuance of acyclovir in this patient. Because use of acyclovir for the treatment and prevention of opportunistic infections may be necessary in patients receiving zidovudine, such patients should be monitored closely during combined therapy.

Acute Toxicity

Acyclovir overdosage involving ingestion of up to 20 g of the drug have been reported. Overdosage of IV acyclovir has been reported following administration of rapid IV injections or inappropriately high doses and in patients with fluid and electrolyte imbalance, resulting in elevations in BUN and serum creatinine concentration and subsequent renal failure. Other adverse effects reported with acyclovir overdosage include agitation, coma, lethargy, and seizures. At renal concentrations exceeding 2.5 mg/mL, acyclovir crystals may precipitate in the renal tubules, possibly causing renal dysfunction and eventual renal failure and anuria. (See Cautions: Renal Effects.)

If acute renal failure and anuria occur, use of hemodialysis should be considered until renal function is restored. A 6-hour period of hemodialysis may result in a 60% decrease in plasma acyclovir concentrations. Data are limited regarding peritoneal dialysis but this method does not appear to appreciably remove the drug.

Mechanism of Action

Acyclovir exerts its antiviral effect against herpes simplex viruses (HSV) and varicella-zoster virus by interfering with DNA synthesis and inhibiting viral replication. The exact mechanisms of action against other susceptible viruses have not been fully elucidated.

In cells infected with herpesvirus in vitro, the antiviral activity of acyclovir appears to depend principally on the intracellular conversion of the drug to acyclovir triphosphate. Acyclovir is converted to acyclovir monophosphate principally via virus-coded thymidine kinase (TK); the monophosphate is phosphorylated to the diphosphate via cellular guanylate kinase and then to the triphosphate via other cellular enzymes (e.g., phosphoglycerate kinase, pyruvate kinase, phosphoenolpyruvate carboxykinase). In uninfected cells in vitro, acyclovir is only minimally phosphorylated by cellular (host cell) enzymes. The formation of acyclovir monophosphate appears to be the rate-limiting step in the formation of acyclovir triphosphate. In vitro studies have shown that the extent of formation of acyclovir monophosphate, diphosphate, and triphosphate by both uninfected and virus-infected cells is directly related to the concentration of acyclovir in the culture medium. Acyclovir also is apparently converted to acyclovir triphosphate by other mechanisms since the drug has some activity against several viruses that apparently do not code for viral TK (e.g., Epstein-Barr virus, cytomegalovirus). In vitro studies indicate that acyclovir triphosphate is produced in low concentrations via unidentified cellular phosphorylating enzymes in cells infected with Epstein-Barr virus and cytomegalovirus.

In vitro studies with HSV indicate that acyclovir triphosphate is the pharmacologically active form of the drug; the triphosphate functions as both a substrate for and preferential inhibitor of viral DNA polymerase. In herpesviruses, acyclovir triphosphate inhibits DNA synthesis by competing with deoxyguanosine triphosphate for viral DNA polymerase and incorporation principally into viral DNA. In vitro in herpesviruses, acyclovir can be incorporated into growing chains of DNA via viral DNA polymerase and to a much lesser extent via cellular α-DNA polymerase. Viral DNA polymerase exhibits a 10- to 30-fold or greater affinity in vitro for acyclovir triphosphate than does cellular α-DNA polymerase. Following incorporation of acyclovir triphosphate into the DNA chain, DNA synthesis is terminated. In vitro studies have shown that acyclovir triphosphate also partially inhibits the synthesis of γ-polypeptides within cells that are infected with herpesvirus. Acyclovir has minimal pharmacologic effects in vitro in uninfected cells since uptake of the drug into these cells is poor, phosphorylation of acyclovir and intracellular formation of acyclovir triphosphate are minimal, and cellular α-DNA polymerase has a low affinity for acyclovir triphosphate.

Non-phosphorylated acyclovir, acyclovir monophosphate, and acyclovir diphosphate are thought to have minimal or no effect on viral or cellular α-DNA polymerase and therefore have no antiviral activity.

The antiviral activity of acyclovir against Epstein-Barr virus and cytomegalovirus (CMV) appears to differ from that against HSV. The antiviral activity against Epstein-Barr virus may result from increased sensitivity of its viral DNA polymerase to inhibition by low concentrations of acyclovir triphosphate (formed via cellular phosphorylating enzymes). The antiviral activity against human CMV may result from inhibition of virus-specific polypeptide synthesis; such inhibition requires high concentrations of acyclovir or its triphosphate in vitro. In vitro studies indicate that DNA polymerase of murine CMV is substantially more sensitive to inhibition by acyclovir triphosphate than that of human CMV; this difference in sensitivity appears to correlate with the difference in in vitro susceptibility of murine and human CMV to the drug. Further studies are needed to evaluate the antiviral activity of acyclovir against Epstein-Barr virus and CMV.

Spectrum

Following intracellular conversion to a pharmacologically active triphosphate metabolite, acyclovir is active in vitro against various Herpesviridae including herpes simplex virus types 1 and 2 (HSV-1 and HSV-2), varicella-zoster virus, Epstein-Barr virus, herpesvirus simiae (B virus), and cytomegalovirus (CMV).

■ **In Vitro Susceptibility Testing** Various methods (e.g., cytopathic effect inhibition, plaque inhibition, dye-uptake, disk-agar diffusion) have been used to test the in vitro susceptibility of viruses to acyclovir. The results and interpretations of these tests are method dependent. Although IDs (inhibitory doses) and EDs (effective doses) of acyclovir for various viruses have been reported, a standardized method for determining these values does not currently exist. In addition, the relationship between in vitro susceptibility of viruses to acyclovir and clinical response has not been determined. In viral susceptibility testing, 1 mcg of acyclovir per mL is approximately equivalent to 4.4 μmol/L.

■ **Herpesviridae** In several studies using a cytopathic effect inhibition assay (CPE-inhibition assay), the ID_{50} (concentration of drug required to produce 50% inhibition of viral cytopathic effect or plaque formation) of acyclovir reported for susceptible strains of HSV-1 ranged from 0.02–0.7 mcg/mL; in studies using a plaque inhibition assay, the ID_{50} of the drug reported for susceptible HSV-1 was 0.018–0.043 mcg/mL. In several studies using a CPE-inhibition assay, the ID_{50} of acyclovir reported for susceptible strains of HSV-2 ranged from 0.01–3.2 mcg/mL; in studies using a plaque inhibition assay, the ID_{50} of the drug reported for susceptible HSV-2 was 0.027–0.36 mcg/mL. In several studies using a plaque inhibition assay, the ID_{50} of acyclovir for susceptible strains of varicella-zoster ranged from 0.34–1.43 mcg/mL.

In several studies using a cytohybridization assay, the ID_{50} of acyclovir for susceptible strains of Epstein-Barr virus ranged from 1.4–1.6 mcg/mL. In several studies using a plaque inhibition assay, the ID_{50} of acyclovir for susceptible strains of herpes simiae ranged from 5–10 mcg/mL.

Acyclovir is much less active against CMV than against many other Herpesviridae. This may occur because CMV does not produce thymidine kinase (TK) and therefore is less able than other viruses to phosphorylate acyclovir to its pharmacologically active triphosphate derivative. In several studies using a plaque inhibition assay, the ID_{50} of acyclovir for susceptible strains of CMV ranged from 2 to greater than 50 mcg/mL.

Acyclovir is inactive against vaccinia virus, adenovirus type 5, and several RNA viruses. Preliminary data indicate that acyclovir may inhibit replication of hepatitis B virus; however, additional study of the susceptibility of this virus to acyclovir is needed.

Resistance

Resistance to acyclovir in Herpesviridae can result from qualitative and quantitative changes in viral thymidine kinase (TK) and/or DNA polymerase. Since the antiviral activity of acyclovir generally appears to depend on phosphorylation of the drug to acyclovir triphosphate (see Mechanism of Action), resistance to the drug may result from low concentrations or absence of virus-coded TK in infected cells or from alterations in substrate specificity of virus-coded TK. Other mechanisms of resistance to acyclovir may also exist.

Acyclovir resistance in HSV-1 and HSV-2 may result from production of a virus-coded TK with altered substrate specificity or from an impaired ability to produce active virus-coded TK; either of these mechanisms may result in minimal amounts or absence of phosphorylated drug. Resistance to acyclovir in varicella-zoster may result from production of a virus-coded TK or DNA polymerase with altered substrate specificity or from an impaired ability to produce active virus-coded TK or DNA polymerase. The relative resistance of Epstein-Barr virus and cytomegalovirus (CMV) compared with HSV-1 and HSV-2 is thought to result from the inability of Epstein-Barr virus and CMV to code for virus-specific TK. In addition, although cellular TK may be present, its low affinity for acyclovir may result in concentrations of acyclovir triphosphate that are insufficient to effectively inhibit the DNA polymerase of Epstein-Barr virus or CMV. Presence of virus-coded TK is not the only determinant of susceptibility to acyclovir. Cells infected with vaccinia virus produce virus-coded TK, but the enzyme does not phosphorylate acyclovir and the drug does not inhibit replication of the virus. In addition to qualitative or quantitative alterations in virus-coded TK, resistance of herpesviruses to acyclovir may result from production of an altered DNA polymerase capable of synthesizing DNA in the presence of acyclovir triphosphate.

Clinical isolates of HSV or varicella-zoster with reduced susceptibility to acyclovir have been obtained from immunocompromised individuals, especially those with advanced human immunodeficiency virus (HIV) infection. It has been suggested that repeated treatment of recurrent viral infections with acyclovir may favor the selection of preexisting, or development of drug-resistant strains. While most of the acyclovir-resistant mutants isolated from immunocompromised individuals have been found to be TK-deficient, other mutants involving the viral TK gene (TK partial and TK altered) and DNA polymerase have been isolated. TK-negative mutants may cause severe disease in infants and immunocompromised adults, and the possibility of acyclovir resistance should be considered in patients who show poor clinical response to the drug.

Although lack of virus-coded TK is apparently responsible for resistance in some strains of viruses, this lack has also been associated with a loss of or decrease in virulence in some strains. In addition, in one study, inoculation of mice with acyclovir-resistant HSV-1 mutants afforded protection against infection with virulent acyclovir-susceptible HSV-1 strains.

During the course of an acute or asymptomatic herpesvirus infection, the virus usually leaves the initial site of infection and invades other cells and tissues where it establishes a site of latent infection. HSV-1, HSV-2, and varicella-zoster are thought to establish latent infections principally within the ganglia. Animal studies indicate that colonization of sensory neurons by HSV-1 may occur as soon as 24–48 hours after initial infection and latency may develop within 2–3 weeks. Epstein-Barr virus and CMV are thought to establish latent infections within B cells and leukocytes, respectively. The exact nature of the virus during the latent state is not well understood; however, current evidence suggests that the virus is not actively replicating and, therefore, would not be susceptible to the antiviral action of drugs such as acyclovir. Despite the host's immunity, latency usually persists for life and the virus can be periodically reactivated by various stimuli (e.g., fever, stress, trauma, exposure to sunlight, menstruation, sexual intercourse, immunosuppression). Once reactivated, the virus usually reinfects the site(s) of initial infection. Acyclovir is apparently unable to eliminate an established latent infection. Acyclovir-resistant HSV mutants appear to be less capable of establishing latent infections than susceptible strains.

Pharmacokinetics

In the studies described in the Pharmacokinetics section involving IV administration of the drug, acyclovir was administered as the sodium salt; dosages and concentrations of the drug are expressed in terms of acyclovir. A concentration of 1 mcg of acyclovir per mL is approximately equivalent to 4.4 μmol/L.

The pharmacokinetics of acyclovir in children generally are similar to that reported in adults.

Acyclovir plasma concentrations are higher in geriatric patients than in younger adults, in part due to age-related changes in renal function.

■ **Absorption** ***Oral Administration*** Absorption of acyclovir from the GI tract is variable and incomplete. It is estimated that 10–30% of an oral dose of the drug is absorbed. Some data suggest that GI absorption of acyclovir may be saturable; in a crossover study in which acyclovir was administered orally to healthy adults as 200-mg capsules, 400-mg tablets, or 800-mg tablets 6 times daily, the extent of absorption decreased with increasing dose, resulting in bioavailabilities of 20, 15, or 10%, respectively. The manufacturer states that this decrease in bioavailability appears to be a function of increasing dose, not differences in dosage forms. In addition, steady-state peak and trough plasma acyclovir concentrations were not dose proportional over the oral dosing range of 200–800 mg 6 times daily, averaging 0.83 and 0.46, 1.21 and 0.63, or 1.61 and 0.83 mcg/mL for the 200-, 400-, or 800-mg dosing regimens, respectively.

Peak plasma concentrations of acyclovir usually occur within 1.5–2.5 hours after oral administration.

In immunocompromised individuals, steady-state peak and trough plasma acyclovir concentrations averaged 0.49–0.56 and 0.29–0.31 mcg/mL, respectively, following oral administration of 200 mg every 4 hours, 1.2 and 0.62 mcg/mL, respectively, following oral administration of 400 mg every 4 hours, and 2.8 and 1.8 mcg/mL, respectively, following oral administration of 800 mg (as capsules) every 4 hours. In another study in immunocompromised individuals, steady-state peak and trough plasma acyclovir concentrations averaged 1.4 and 0.55 mcg/mL, respectively, following oral administration of 800 mg (as capsules) every 6 hours.

Food does not appear to affect absorption of acyclovir.

The commercially available capsules and oral suspension are bioequivalent; in addition, one commercially available 800-mg tablet of acyclovir is bioequivalent to four 200-mg capsules of the drug.

IV Infusion Results of studies in adults with normal renal function receiving single acyclovir doses ranging from 0.5- to 15-mg/kg or multiple doses ranging from 2.5- to 15-mg/kg every 8 hours indicate that plasma concentrations of the drug are dose proportional.

In adults with normal renal function receiving 5 or 10 mg/kg of acyclovir IV over 1 hour every 8 hours, mean steady-state peak plasma concentrations were 9.8 or 22.9 mcg/mL, respectively, and trough plasma concentrations were 0.7 or 1.9 mcg/mL. In a multiple-dose study in adults with malignancies and normal renal and liver function, 1-hour IV infusions of 2.5, 5, 10, or 15 mg/kg of acyclovir every 8 hours resulted in mean steady-state peak serum concentrations of 5.1, 9.8, 20.7, and 23.6 mcg/mL, respectively, and mean steady-state trough serum concentrations of 0.5, 0.7, 2.3, and 2 mcg/mL, respectively.

In several studies in adults with malignancies and normal renal and hepatic function, IV infusion over 1 hour of a single acyclovir dose of 0.5, 1, 2.5, or 5 mg/kg resulted in serum concentrations of the drug that averaged 0.7–1.4, 1.4–2.5, 3.4–4.9, or 7.7 mcg/mL, respectively, at the end of the infusion and 0.14, 0.27, 0.34, or 0.93 mcg/mL, respectively, 6 hours after the end of the infusion.

Serum concentrations in children 3 months to 16 years of age receiving IV acyclovir 10 mg/kg or 20 mg/kg every 8 hours are similar to those achieved in adults receiving IV acyclovir 5 mg/kg or 10 mg/kg every 8 hours. In a multiple-dose study in neonates up to 3 months of age, IV infusion over 1 hour of 5, 10, or 15 mg/kg of acyclovir every 8 hours resulted in mean steady-state peak serum concentrations of 6.8, 13.9, or 19.6 mcg/mL, respectively, and mean steady-state trough serum concentrations of 1.2, 2.3, or 3.1 mcg/mL, respectively. In another multiple-dose study in pediatric patients, IV infusion over 1 hour of 250 or 500 mg/m^2 of acyclovir every 8 hours resulted in mean steady-state peak serum concentrations of 10.3 or 20.7 mcg/mL, respectively.

In a single-dose study in adults with end-stage renal disease, a 1-hour IV infusion of 2.5 mg/kg of acyclovir resulted in serum concentrations of the drug that averaged 8.5, 4, 2.3, 2, and 1.5 mcg/mL at 1, 2, 8, 12, and 24 hours after the start of infusion, respectively. When these patients underwent hemodialysis, predialysis (48 hours after the start of drug infusion) and postdialysis (54.5 hours after the start of drug infusion) plasma acyclovir concentrations were 0.6 and 0.3 mcg/mL, respectively.

■ **Distribution** Acyclovir is widely distributed into body tissues and fluids including the brain, kidney, saliva, lung, liver, muscle, spleen, uterus, vaginal mucosa and secretions, CSF, and herpetic vesicular fluid. The drug also is distributed into semen, achieving concentrations about 1.4 and 4 times those in plasma during chronic oral therapy at dosages of 400 mg and 1 g daily, respectively.

The apparent volume of distribution of acyclovir is reported to be 32.4–61.8 L/1.73 m^2 in adults and 28.8, 31.6, 42, or 51.2–53.6 L/1.73 m^2 in neonates up to 3 months of age, children 1–2 years, 2–7 years, or 7–12 years of age, respectively.

In vitro, acyclovir is approximately 9–33% bound to plasma proteins at plasma concentrations of 0.41–5.2 mcg/mL.

Following IV infusion, acyclovir generally diffuses well into CSF. In patients with uninflamed meninges, CSF concentrations of acyclovir are reported to be approximately 50% of concurrent serum acyclovir concentrations.

Acyclovir crosses the placenta. Limited data indicate that the drug is distributed into milk, generally in concentrations greater than concurrent maternal plasma concentrations, possibly via an active transport mechanism.

■ **Elimination** Plasma concentrations of acyclovir appear to decline in a biphasic manner. In adults with normal renal function, the half-life of acyclovir in the initial phase ($t_{1/2\alpha}$) averages 0.34 hours and the half-life in the terminal phase ($t_{1/2\beta}$) averages 2.1–3.5 hours. In adults with renal impairment, both $t_{1/2\alpha}$ and $t_{1/2\beta}$ may be prolonged, depending on the degree of renal impairment. In a study in adults with anuria, the $t_{1/2\alpha}$ of acyclovir averaged 0.71 hours. In several studies, the $t_{1/2\beta}$ of acyclovir averaged 3, 3.5, or 19.5 hours in adults with creatinine clearances of 50–80 or 15–50 mL/minute per 1.73 m^2 or with anuria, respectively. In patients undergoing hemodialysis, the $t_{1/2\beta}$ of acyclovir during hemodialysis averaged 5.4–5.7 hours.

In neonates, the half-life of acyclovir depends principally on the maturity of renal mechanisms for excretion as determined by gestational age, chronologic age, and weight. In children older than 1 year of age, the half-life of the drug appears to be similar to that of adults. The $t_{1/2\beta}$ averages 3.8–4.1, 1.9, 2.2–2.8, or 3.6 hours in neonates up to 3 months of age, children 1–2 years, 2–12 years, or 12–17 years of age, respectively.

Acyclovir is metabolized partially to 9-carboxymethoxymethylguanine (CMMG) and minimally to 8-hydroxy-9-(2-hydroxyethoxymethyl)guanine. In vitro, acyclovir also is metabolized to acyclovir monophosphate, diphosphate, and triphosphate in cells infected with herpesviruses, principally by intracellular phosphorylation of the drug by virus-coded thymidine kinase (TK) and several cellular enzymes. (See Mechanism of Action.)

Acyclovir is excreted principally in urine via glomerular filtration and tubular secretion. Most of a single IV dose of acyclovir is excreted in urine as unchanged drug within 24 hours after administration. In adults with normal renal function, approximately 30–90% of a single IV dose is excreted unchanged in urine within 72 hours; approximately 8–14% and less than 0.2%

are excreted in urine as CMMG and 8-hydroxy-9-(2-hydroxyethoxy-methyl)guanine, respectively, within 72 hours. In a study in neonates up to 2 months of age, 62–72% of a single dose was excreted in urine unchanged. Less than 2% of a single IV dose of acyclovir is recovered in feces and only trace amounts in expired CO_2; the drug apparently does not accumulate in tissues.

Total body clearance of acyclovir is reported to be 327, 248, 190, or 29 mL/minute per 1.73 m^2 in patients with creatinine clearances of greater than 80, 50–80, 15–50, or 0 mL/minute per 1.73 m^2, respectively.

Oral administration of 1 g of probenecid 1 hour before a single 1-hour IV infusion of 5 mg/kg of acyclovir increased the plasma half-life and the area under the plasma concentration-time curve, produced higher and more prolonged plasma concentrations, and decreases the renal clearance of acyclovir. The volume of distribution of acyclovir does not appear to be affected by concomitant administration of oral probenecid. (See Drug Interactions: Probenecid.)

Acyclovir is removed by hemodialysis. The amount of acyclovir removed during hemodialysis depends on several factors (e.g., type of coil used, dialysis flow-rate); a 6-hour period of hemodialysis in one study removed into the dialysate approximately 60% of a single 2.5-mg/kg dose of acyclovir when the dose was given by a 60-minute IV infusion 48 hours prior to dialysis. Data are limited, but peritoneal dialysis and blood exchange transfusions do not appear to appreciably remove the drug.

Chemistry and Stability

■ **Chemistry** Acyclovir is a synthetic purine nucleoside analog derived from guanine. The drug differs structurally from guanine by the presence of an acyclic side chain. Acyclovir is commercially available for parenteral use as the sodium salt and for oral use as the base. Potency of commercially available acyclovir sodium powder or concentrate for injection is expressed in terms of acyclovir.

Acyclovir occurs as a white, crystalline powder and has a maximum solubility of 2.5 mg/mL in water at 25°C. The drug has pK_as of 2.27 and 9.25. Commercially available acyclovir sodium powder for injection occurs as a white, crystalline, lyophilized powder. Acyclovir sodium has a maximum solubility of greater than 100 mg/mL in water at 25°C, but at physiologic pH and 37°C the drug is almost completely un-ionized and has a maximum solubility of 2.5 mg/mL. The sodium salt of acyclovir contains 4.2 mEq of sodium per gram of acyclovir. Following reconstitution with sterile water for injection, acyclovir sodium solutions containing 50 mg of acyclovir per mL have a pH of approximately 11 and are clear and colorless.

■ **Stability** Acyclovir capsules and tablets should be stored in tight, light-resistant containers at 15–25°C. Acyclovir suspension should be stored at 15–25°C.

Commercially available acyclovir sodium powder for injection should be stored at 15–25°C. Following reconstitution with sterile water for injection, acyclovir sodium solutions containing 50 mg of acyclovir per mL are stable for 12 hours. Refrigeration of the reconstituted solution may result in formation of a precipitate which will redissolve at room temperature; potency of the drug does not appear to be affected by precipitation and subsequent redissolution. Acyclovir sodium also is compatible with bacteriostatic water for injection containing *benzyl alcohol*, exhibiting the stability noted above for sterile water for injection; however, use of this diluent is not recommended because of the potential risk of benzyl alcohol exposure if such reconstituted drug were administered to a neonate. Bacteriostatic water for injection containing *parabens* should *not* be used to reconstitute acyclovir sodium powder for injection since this diluent is incompatible with the drug and may cause precipitation.

The manufacturer states that acyclovir sodium is physically and chemically compatible for 24 hours at 25°C when diluted with 50–100 mL of a standard, commercially available electrolyte and/or dextrose solution. Although yellowish discoloration may occur when acyclovir sodium is diluted with greater than 10% dextrose, potency of the drug is not affected. The manufacturer states that acyclovir sodium is incompatible with biologic and/or colloidal fluids (e.g., blood products, protein-containing solutions).

Preparations

Excipients in commercially available drug preparations may have clinically important effects in some individuals; consult specific product labeling for details.

Acyclovir

Oral		
Capsules	200 mg*	**Acyclovir Capsules®**
		Zovirax®, GlaxoSmithKline
Suspension	200 mg/5 mL*	**Acyclovir Suspension**
		Zovirax®, GlaxoSmithKline
Tablets	400 mg*	**Acyclovir Tablets®**
		Zovirax®, GlaxoSmithKline
	800 mg*	**Acyclovir Tablets®**
		Zovirax®, GlaxoSmithKline

*available from one or more manufacturer, distributor, and/or repackager by generic (nonproprietary) name

Acyclovir Sodium

Parenteral		
For injection, concentrate, for IV infusion only	50 mg (of acyclovir) per mL (500 mg, 1 g)*	**Acyclovir Sodium Injection**
For injection, for IV infusion only	500 mg (of acyclovir)*	**Acyclovir Sodium for Injection**
		Zovirax®, GlaxoSmithKline
	1 g (of acyclovir)*	**Acyclovir Sodium for Injection**
		Zovirax®, GlaxoSmithKline

*available from one or more manufacturer, distributor, and/or repackager by generic (nonproprietary) name

†Use is not currently included in the labeling approved by the US Food and Drug Administration

Selected Revisions January 2007,

Adefovir Dipivoxil ADV

■ Adefovir dipivoxil is a prodrug of adefovir, an acyclic nucleotide analog antiviral agent that is active against human hepatitis B virus (HBV) and certain other viruses.

Uses

■ **Chronic Hepatitis B Virus Infection** Adefovir dipivoxil is used for the treatment of chronic hepatitis B virus (HBV) infection in adults and adolescents 12 years of age and older with evidence of active HBV replication and either persistent elevations in serum aminotransferase (ALT or AST) concentrations or histologic evidence of active liver disease. This indication is based on histologic, virologic, biochemical, and serologic responses in adults with hepatitis B e antigen (HBeAg)-positive or HBeAg-negative chronic HBV infection with compensated liver function and with clinical evidence of lamivudine-resistant HBV with either compensated or decompensated liver function. For adolescents 12 years of age or older, this indication is based on virologic and biochemical responses in patients in this age group with HBeAg-positive chronic HBV infection with compensated liver function.

The goal of antiviral therapy in patients with chronic HBV infection is to decrease the morbidity and mortality related to the infection (e.g., cirrhosis, hepatic failure, hepatocellular carcinoma). Sustained suppression of HBV replication has been associated with normalization of serum ALT concentrations, loss of HBeAg with or without detection of antibody to HBeAg (anti-HBe), and improvement in liver histology. Currently available therapies for chronic HBV infection (e.g., adefovir, entecavir, lamivudine, telbivudine, tenofovir alafenamide, tenofovir disoproxil fumarate [tenofovir DF], interferon alfa, peginterferon alfa) are used in an attempt to provide an immunologic cure (HBsAg loss and sustained HBV DNA suppression), but cannot provide a virologic cure (eradication of HBV).

Treatment of chronic HBV infection is complex and evolving, and specialized references and experts should be consulted. Information from the American Association for the Study of Liver Diseases (AASLD) regarding management of HBV infection, including recommendations for initial treatment, is available at https://www.aasld.org.

HBeAg-Positive Adults Efficacy of adefovir dipivoxil for the management of HBeAg-positive chronic HBV infection was evaluated in a phase III, randomized, double-blind, placebo-controlled study (study 437) in adults with active HBV replication (median baseline serum HBV DNA levels of 8.36 log_{10} copies/mL), persistent elevations in serum ALT concentrations (median elevations 2.3 times the upper limit of normal), and histologic evidence of active liver disease (median baseline total Knodell Histology Activity Index [HAI] scores of 10). Seventy-four percent of patients in the study were male, 59% were Asian, 36% were Caucasian, and 24 or 2% had prior treatment with interferon alfa or lamivudine, respectively.

Data analysis at 48 weeks indicated that 53% of patients receiving adefovir dipivoxil in a dosage of 10 mg daily had histologic improvement (defined as a reduction of at least 2 points in the Knodell necroinflammatory score with no concurrent worsening of the Knodell fibrosis score) compared with 25% of those receiving placebo. Forty-eight percent of patients receiving adefovir dipivoxil (10 mg daily) had normal serum ALT concentrations (i.e., biochemical response) at week 48 compared with 16% of those receiving placebo. In addition, the mean decrease in serum HBV DNA levels from baseline was 3.57 log_{10} copies/mL at week 48 in those receiving adefovir dipivoxil compared with a decrease of 0.98 log_{10} copies/mL in those receiving placebo. Twenty-one percent of patients who received adefovir dipivoxil (10 mg daily) had undetectable levels of serum HBV DNA (defined as less than 400 copies/mL by a polymerase chain reaction [PCR] assay) at week 48 compared with 0% of those who received placebo. Loss of HBeAg and seroconversion to anti-HBe also occurred in 24 and 12% of patients, respectively, who received adefovir dipivoxil (10 mg daily) compared with 11 and 6%, respectively, of those who received placebo. Although this study initially included a treatment arm that involved administering adefovir dipivoxil in a dosage of 30 mg daily, this arm of the study was discontinued at 48 weeks based on data from a phase II study indicating that the higher dosage might be associated with mild, reversible nephrotoxicity. At 48 weeks, patients who were receiving adefovir dipivoxil in a dosage of 10 mg daily were re-randomized to receive either continued treatment with 10 mg daily or placebo and those who were receiving placebo were all given adefovir dipivoxil 10 mg daily for an additional 48 weeks. There was evidence that treatment with adefovir dipivoxil 10 mg daily for up to 72 weeks resulted in continued maintenance of mean reductions in serum HBV DNA levels observed at week 48 and an increase in the proportion of patients with ALT normalization and/or HBeAg seroconversion. In one study in patients who received adefovir dipivoxil for up to 240 weeks (4.6 years), the median change from baseline serum HBV DNA at study week 144, 192, and 240 was −3.69, −3.55, and −4.05 log_{10} copies/mL, respectively, and 48% of patients had confirmed HBeAg seroconversion at week 240. The effect of continued adefovir dipivoxil therapy on seroconversion is unknown.

HBeAg-Negative Adults Efficacy of adefovir dipivoxil for the management of HBeAg-negative, anti-HBe- and HBV-DNA-positive chronic HBV infection was evaluated in a phase III, randomized, double-blind, placebo-controlled study (study 438) in 184 adults with active HBV replication (median baseline serum HBV DNA levels of 7.08 log_{10} copies/mL by a PCR-based assay), persistent elevations in serum ALT concentrations (median elevations 2.3 times the upper limit of normal), and histologic evidence of active liver disease (median baseline total HAI scores of 10). Eighty-three percent of patients in the study were male, 66% were Caucasian, 30% were Asian, and 41 or 8% had prior treatment with interferon alfa or lamivudine, respectively.

Data analysis at 48 weeks indicated that 64% of patients who received adefovir dipivoxil (10 mg daily) had histologic improvement (defined as a reduction of at least 2 points in the Knodell necroinflammatory score with no concurrent worsening of the Knodell fibrosis score) compared with 33–35% of those who received placebo. Serum ALT concentrations also normalized at week 48 in 72% of patients who received adefovir dipivoxil compared with 29% of those who received placebo. In addition, the mean decrease in serum HBV DNA levels from baseline was 3.65 log_{10} copies/mL at week 48 in patients receiving adefovir dipivoxil 10 mg daily compared with a mean decrease of 1.32 log_{10} copies/mL in those receiving placebo. Fifty-one percent of patients who received adefovir dipivoxil had undetectable levels of serum HBV DNA (defined as less than 400 copies/mL by a PCR-based assay) at week 48 compared with 0% of those who received placebo. After 48 weeks, patients receiving adefovir dipivoxil were re-randomized to continue the drug or to receive placebo and those receiving placebo were all given adefovir dipivoxil for an additional 48 weeks. Data analysis of patients who received continuous adefovir dipivoxil therapy for 96 weeks indicates that 71% had serum HBV DNA levels less than 1000 copies/mL, 73% had normalization of serum ALT concentrations, and 74 or 89% of patients with available liver biopsy results at year 2 had improvements in necroinflammation or fibrosis, respectively. After 96 weeks, patients who were receiving adefovir dipivoxil were able to enroll in an open-label study that involved using the drug for an additional 144 weeks. Data analysis of patients who received continuous adefovir dipivoxil therapy for 192 weeks (placebo-adefovir group) indicates that 71–73% had serum HBV DNA levels less than 1000 copies/mL, 73–74% had normalization of serum ALT concentrations, and 86 or 73% of patients with available liver biopsy results had improvements in necroinflammation or fibrosis, respectively. Data analysis of patients who received continuous adefovir dipivoxil therapy for 240 weeks (adefovir-adefovir group) indicates that 67% had serum HBV DNA levels less than 1000 copies/mL, 66–69% had normalization of serum ALT concentrations, and 83 or 75% of patients with available liver biopsy results had improvement in necroinflammation or fibrosis, respectively.

Because patients with HBeAg-negative chronic HBV infections rarely have hepatitis B surface antigen (HBsAg) seroconversion, these patients are likely to require long-term antiviral therapy. While there is evidence that adefovir dipivoxil monotherapy continued for at least 96 weeks may provide some benefits, further study is needed to determine the effect of such therapy on clearance of HBsAg and the frequency of virologic and biochemical relapse after discontinuance of the drug. In addition, further study is needed to investigate the possibility of emergence of adefovir-resistant strains of HBV with long-term therapy with the drug. Although there was no evidence of emergence of HBV resistant to adefovir dipivoxil during 48-week clinical studies evaluating adefovir dipivoxil monotherapy in HBV- infected patients, there are concerns about the potential for such resistance with single-agent use of the drug for long-term treatment of chronic HBV infection. This concern is based in part on experience with use of monotherapy with lamivudine (a nucleoside antiviral agent) for the treatment of chronic HBV infection. (See Patients with Lamivudine-Resistant HBV under Uses: Chronic Hepatitis B Virus Infection.) Although the clinical importance is unclear, there is evidence that reduced susceptibility to adefovir dipivoxil develops in some patients during long-term use. (See Resistance in HBV under Description: Resistance.)

HBeAg-Positive Pediatric Patients Efficacy of adefovir dipivoxil for the management of HBeAg-positive chronic HBV infection in adolescents was evaluated in a phase III, randomized, double-blind, placebo-controlled study (study 518) that included adolescents 12–17 years of age with active HBV replication (median baseline serum HBV DNA levels of 8.69–8.85 log_{10} copies/mL) and elevated serum ALT concentrations at baseline (median elevations 2.3 times the upper limit of normal). Seventy-five percent of adolescents 12–17 years of age in the study were male, 22% were Asian, and 75% were Caucasian. Data analysis at 48 weeks indicated that 23% of adolescents receiving adefovir dipivoxil (10 mg daily) had HBV DNA levels less than 1000 copies/mL with normalization of serum ALT concentrations compared with none of those receiving placebo.

Although study 518 also evaluated efficacy and safety of adefovir dipivoxil for the treatment of chronic HBV infection in pediatric patients 2–11 years of age†, the drug was no more effective than placebo in patients younger than 12 years of age. Adefovir dipivoxil is not recommended for and should not be used in children younger than 12 years of age.

Pre- and Post-Liver Transplantation Patients Adefovir dipivoxil has been shown to be well tolerated and to achieve significant reduction in serum HBV DNA levels and improvement in biochemical indices (e.g., ALT, bilirubin, albumin, prothrombin time [PT]) and Child-Pugh scores in a clinical trial involving HBeAg-positive and HBeAg-negative, compensated and decompensated, pre- and post-liver transplant patients with clinical evidence of lamivudine resistance. In one open-label, uncontrolled study (study 435) in adults, a 48-week regimen of adefovir dipivoxil monotherapy resulted in a mean decrease from baseline serum HBV DNA levels of 3.5–3.7 or 4 log_{10} copies/mL in pre- or post-liver transplant patients, respectively; these reductions occurred regardless of baseline patterns of lamivudine-resistant HBV DNA polymerase mutations. In addition, normalization of serum ALT, bilirubin, or albumin concentrations occurred in 74–77 or 51%, 58–60 or 76%, and 76–80 or 81% of pre- or post-liver transplant patients, respectively, at 48 weeks. Normalization of PT occurred in 84–85 or 56% of pre- or post-liver transplant patients, respectively. Child-Pugh scores remained stable or improved in 96 or 93% of pre- or post-liver transplant patients, respectively. The clinical importance of these findings as they relate to clinical outcomes is as yet unknown.

Patients with Lamivudine-Resistant HBV Adefovir dipivoxil has been evaluated for the treatment of chronic HBV infection in patients with clinical evidence of lamivudine-resistant YMDD mutant strains of HBV. Lamivudine-resistant strains of HBV have been reported in up to 24–32% of patients after 1 year of lamivudine monotherapy and in up to 70% of patients after 4–5 years of such treatment; however, there is in vitro evidence that adefovir usually is active against these lamivudine-resistant HBV. Data from a randomized, double-blind, active-controlled study (study 461) in patients 16–65 years of age suggest that adefovir dipivoxil monotherapy is as effective as a regimen of adefovir dipivoxil and lamivudine and more effective than lamivudine monotherapy in decreasing serum HBV DNA in patients with clinical and virologic evidence of lamivudine-resistant HBV. Data analysis at 48 weeks indicates that time-weighted average serum HBV DNA levels decreased approximately 3–4 log_{10} copies/mL in patients who received adefovir dipivoxil alone or in conjunction with lamivudine compared with a time-weighted average decrease of 0 log_{10} copies/mL in those who received lamivudine monotherapy. An increase in the proportion of patients with ALT normalization, HBeAg loss, and/or HBeAg seroconversion also was observed at week 48 in patients receiving adefovir dipivoxil alone or in conjunction with lamivudine. The clinical importance of these findings as they relate to clinical outcomes are unknown.

Dosage and Administration

■ **Administration** Adefovir dipivoxil is administered orally without regard to food.

■ **Dosage** ***Adult Dosage*** **Chronic Hepatitis B Virus Infection.** For the treatment of chronic hepatitis B virus (HBV) infection in adults, the usual dosage of adefovir dipivoxil is 10 mg once daily.

The optimal duration of adefovir dipivoxil therapy in patients with chronic HBV infection is not known. The drug has been continued for up to 5 years in controlled clinical studies in adults.

Pediatric Dosage **Chronic Hepatitis B Virus Infection.** For the treatment of chronic HBV infection in adolescents 12 years of age or older, the usual dosage of adefovir dipivoxil is 10 mg once daily.

The optimal duration of adefovir dipivoxil therapy in patients with chronic HBV infection is not known. The drug has been continued for up to 5 years in controlled clinical studies in adults.

■ **Special Populations** ***Hepatic Impairment*** Dosage adjustments are not necessary in patients with hepatic impairment.

Renal Impairment The dosing interval of adefovir dipivoxil should be adjusted in adults with preexisting renal impairment (i.e., baseline creatinine clearances less than 50 mL/minute). (See Table 1.)

Table 1: Dosage of Adefovir Dipivoxil for Treatment of HBV Infection in Adults with Renal Impairment

Creatinine Clearance (mL/min)	Dosage
30–49	10 mg once every 48 hours
10–29	10 mg once every 72 hours
Less than 10 (not undergoing hemodialysis)	Dosage recommendations not available
Hemodialysis patients	10 mg once every 7 days following dialysis

The safety and efficacy of these dosage guidelines for adults with renal impairment have not been clinically evaluated. The manufacturers state these dosage guidelines were derived from data for patients with preexisting renal impairment and may not be appropriate for patients in whom renal impairment evolves during therapy with the drug. Therefore, clinical response and renal function should be monitored closely.

The safety and efficacy of adefovir dipivoxil have not been studied in adolescents 12 years of age or older with renal impairment. Data are insufficient to make dosage recommendations for adolescents 12 years of age or older with underlying renal impairment; the drug should be used with caution and renal function monitored closely in such adolescents.

Geriatric Patients Dosage of adefovir dipivoxil should be selected with caution in geriatric patients because of possible age-related decreases in renal function, and patients should be monitored closely. (See Geriatric Use under Warnings/Precautions: Specific Populations, in Cautions.)

Cautions

■ **Contraindications** Adefovir dipivoxil is contraindicated in patients with known hypersensitivity to the drug or any ingredient in the formulation.

■ **Warnings/Precautions** *Warnings* **Exacerbation of Hepatitis.** Severe acute exacerbations of hepatitis have been reported following discontinuance of hepatitis B virus (HBV) therapy, including adefovir dipivoxil therapy.

In clinical studies, exacerbations of hepatitis (ALT elevations at least 10 times the upper limit of normal) occurred in up to 25% of patients following discontinuance of adefovir dipivoxil, usually within 12 weeks after discontinuance. These exacerbations generally occurred in the absence of hepatitis B e antigen (HBeAg) seroconversion and presented as elevations in ALT and reemergence of viral replication.

Although these exacerbations appeared to be self-limited or resolved with reinitiation of therapy, severe exacerbations (including fatalities) have been reported.

In patients with compensated liver function, exacerbations of hepatitis generally have not been accompanied by hepatic decompensation. However, patients with advanced liver disease or cirrhosis may be at higher risk for hepatic decompensation than those with compensated liver function.

Hepatic function should be closely monitored with both clinical and laboratory follow-up for at least several months after adefovir dipivoxil is discontinued. If appropriate, resumption of HBV therapy may be warranted.

Nephrotoxicity. Nephrotoxicity, characterized by a delayed onset, is the principal dose-limiting toxicity of adefovir dipivoxil and also may occur in patients receiving chronic (long-term) therapy with the recommended dosage of the drug.

Delayed onset of gradual increases in serum creatinine and decreases in serum phosphorus were the treatment-limiting toxicities of adefovir dipivoxil therapy in clinical studies evaluating use of high dosages of the drug for the treatment of human immunodeficiency virus (HIV) infection† (60 or 120 mg daily) or use of high dosages for the treatment of chronic HBV infection (30 mg daily).

Long-term administration of adefovir dipivoxil in dosages recommended for the treatment of HBV infection (10 mg daily) also may result in delayed nephrotoxicity. By week 96 or week 240, 2 or 3% of patients who received adefovir dipivoxil had serum creatinine increases of 0.5 mg/dL or greater from baseline (by Kaplan Meier estimates), respectively.

In pre- or postliver transplant patients receiving the usually recommended dosage of the drug (10 mg daily), most of whom had some degree of baseline renal insufficiency, 37 or 32% had increases in serum creatinine concentrations of 0.3 mg/dL or greater from baseline by week 48, respectively, and 53 or 51% had serum creatinine increases of 0.3 mg/dL or greater from baseline by week 96, respectively.

Although the overall risk of nephrotoxicity is low in patients with adequate renal function, the possibility of nephrotoxicity should be considered in patients at risk of or having underlying renal dysfunction and in those receiving concomitant therapy with nephrotoxic agents. (See Drug Interactions: Nephrotoxic Drugs or Drugs Eliminated by Renal Excretion.)

Renal function should be monitored closely in all patients receiving adefovir dipivoxil, especially those with preexisting renal impairment or other risks for renal impairment. Dosage adjustments may be necessary. (See Renal Impairment under Dosage and Administration: Special Populations.)

HBV-infected Individuals Coinfected with HIV. Use of adefovir dipivoxil for the treatment of chronic HBV infection in patients with unrecognized or untreated HIV infection may result in emergence of HIV resistance. Although adefovir has some in vitro activity against HIV, dosage of the drug used for the treatment of HBV infection (10 mg daily) has not been shown to suppress HIV RNA levels in HIV-infected patients.

Some experts state that adefovir dipivoxil alone or in conjunction with other antivirals should *not* be used for the treatment of HBV infection in HIV-infected patients.

HIV antibody testing should be offered to all patients prior to initiating adefovir dipivoxil therapy.

Lactic Acidosis and Severe Hepatomegaly with Steatosis. Lactic acidosis and severe hepatomegaly with steatosis, including some fatalities, have been reported in patients receiving nucleoside analogs alone or in conjunction with antiretrovirals. Most reported cases have involved women; obesity and long-term therapy with nucleoside reverse transcriptase inhibitors also may be risk factors.

Nucleoside analogs should be used with particular caution in patients with known risk factors for liver disease; however, lactic acidosis and severe hepatomegaly with steatosis have been reported in patients with no known risk factors.

Adefovir dipivoxil therapy should be discontinued in any patient with clinical or laboratory findings suggestive of lactic acidosis or pronounced hepatotoxicity (which may include hepatomegaly and steatosis even in the absence of marked aminotransferase elevations).

HBV Resistance. Resistance to adefovir dipivoxil may result in hepatitis B viral load rebound, which may lead to exacerbation of HBV infection; if the patient has impaired hepatic function, this may lead to liver decompensation and death.

To reduce risk of clinical resistance in patients with lamivudine-resistant HBV, adefovir dipivoxil should be used in conjunction with lamivudine; adefovir dipivoxil should not be used as monotherapy.

Patients with serum HBV DNA levels greater than 1000 copies/mL after 48 weeks of adefovir dipivoxil treatment are at greater risk of developing clinical resistance. To reduce risk of clinical resistance in patients receiving monotherapy with adefovir dipivoxil, treatment modification should be considered if serum HBV DNA levels remain greater than 1000 copies/mL with continued treatment.

Concomitant Use with Other Drugs. Adefovir dipivoxil should not be used concomitantly with tenofovir disoproxil fumarate (tenofovir DF) or fixed-combination preparations containing tenofovir DF.

Specific Populations **Pregnancy.** Category C. (See Users Guide.)

To monitor maternal-fetal outcomes of pregnant women exposed to adefovir dipivoxil, clinicians are encouraged to contact the pregnancy registry at 800-258-4263 to enroll such women.

There are no adequate, well-controlled studies of adefovir dipivoxil in pregnant women. The drug should be used during pregnancy only if potential benefits justify potential risks to the fetus.

There was no evidence of embryotoxicity or teratogenicity in rats or rabbits at systemic exposures 23 or 40 times, respectively, exposures in humans at the therapeutic dosage. However, embryotoxicity and increased incidence of fetal malformations (anasarca, depressed eye bulge, umbilical hernia, kinked tail) occurred in rats at adefovir dipivoxil exposures 38 times human exposures at the therapeutic dosage.

The American Association for the Study of Liver Diseases (AASLD) and other experts state that recommendations regarding antiviral therapy for the management of HBV infection in pregnant women generally are the same as those for other adults. AASLD also suggests that hepatitis B surface antigen (HBsAg)-positive pregnant women with HBV DNA levels exceeding 200,000 IU/mL receive antiviral therapy since this may reduce the risk of perinatal transmission of HBV; however, preferred antiviral agents, exact viral load threshold, and optimal gestational week during the third trimester to initiate such therapy have not been clearly identified.

Data are not available regarding the effect of adefovir dipivoxil therapy during pregnancy on transmission of HBV to the infant. Routine screening for HBV infection is recommended for *all* pregnant women. For prevention of perinatal transmission of HBV, US Public Health Service Advisory Committee on Immunization Practices (ACIP), American Academy of Pediatrics (AAP), and other experts state that infants born to HBsAg-positive women should receive their first dose of hepatitis B vaccine *and* a dose of hepatitis B immune globulin (HBIG) within 12 hours of birth.

Lactation. It is not known whether adefovir dipivoxil is distributed into milk.

A decision should be made to discontinue nursing or adefovir dipivoxil, taking into account the importance of the drug to the woman.

Pediatric Use. Safety and efficacy of adefovir dipivoxil have not been established in children younger than 12 years of age. (See HBeAg-Positive Pediatric Patients under Uses: Chronic Hepatitis B Virus Infection.)

Geriatric Use. Experience in those 65 years of age or older is insufficient to determine whether geriatric adults respond differently than younger adults.

Adefovir dipivoxil should be used with caution in geriatric patients because of age-related decreases in hepatic, renal, and/or cardiac function and concomitant disease and drug therapy.

Renal Impairment. Dosage adjustments are recommended for adults with creatinine clearance less than 50 mL/minute. (See Renal Impairment under Dosage and Administration: Special Populations.)

Adefovir dipivoxil has not been evaluated in adolescents 12 years of age or older with renal impairment. The drug should be used with caution in such adolescents and renal function should be monitored closely.

■ **Common Adverse Effects** Adverse effects reported in 3% or more of patients with adequate renal function who received adefovir dipivoxil for 48 weeks in clinical studies include asthenia (13%), headache (9%), abdominal pain (9%), nausea (5%), flatulence (4%), diarrhea (3%) and dyspepsia (3%); these frequencies were similar to those observed in patients receiving placebo (2–14%).

Adverse effects reported in 2% or greater of pre- and post-liver transplantation patients who received adefovir dipivoxil in clinical studies include asthenia, abdominal pain, headache, nausea, vomiting, diarrhea, increases in ALT and AST, pruritus, rash, increases in creatinine, renal failure, and renal insufficiency. In addition, transient serum phosphorus concentrations less than 2 mg/dL were observed in approximately 2% of these patients; adefovir dipivoxil therapy was continued and the patients did not require phosphorus supplementation. Four percent (19 of 467) of pre- and post-liver transplantation patients discontinued adefovir dipivoxil therapy because of adverse renal effects. However, a causal relationship to changes in serum creatinine and serum phosphorus is difficult to assess because of the presence of multiple concomitant risk factors for renal dysfunction in these patients.

Drug Interactions

■ **Drugs Affecting or Metabolized by Hepatic Microsomal Enzymes** Adefovir dipivoxil is not an inhibitor or a substrate for any of the major cytochrome P-450 (CYP) isoenzymes, including CYP1A2, CYP2C9, CYP2C19, CYP2D6, or CYP3A4; pharmacokinetic interactions unlikely. However, the potential for adefovir dipivoxil to induce CYP isoenzymes is unknown.

■ **Nephrotoxic Drugs or Drugs Affecting Eliminated by Renal Excretion** Potential increased risk of nephrotoxicity in patients receiving other nephrotoxic drugs (e.g., aminoglycosides, cyclosporine, tacrolimus, vancomycin, certain nonsteroidal anti-inflammatory agents [NSAIAs]); patients should be monitored closely.

Potential pharmacokinetic interactions with drugs that compete for active tubular secretion (increased plasma concentration of adefovir dipivoxil and/or the other drug); patients should be monitored closely.

■ **Acetaminophen** No pharmacokinetic interactions with acetaminophen.

■ **Antiretroviral Agents** ***HIV Nucleoside and Nucleotide Reverse Transcriptase Inhibitors (NRTIs)*** **Didanosine.** No pharmacokinetic interactions with didanosine delayed-release capsules containing enteric-coated pellets.

Lamivudine. No pharmacokinetic interactions with lamivudine.

Additive antiviral effects against hepatitis B virus (HBV).

Tenofovir Disoproxil Fumarate. Tenofovir disoproxil fumarate (tenofovir DF) and adefovir dipivoxil should not be used concomitantly.

■ **Co-trimoxazole** No pharmacokinetic interactions with co-trimoxazole.

■ **Entecavir** No clinically important pharmacokinetic interactions with entecavir.

■ **Ibuprofen** Pharmacokinetic interaction (33% increase in peak plasma concentration and 23% increase in area under the plasma concentration-time curve [AUC] of adefovir dipivoxil; no effect on pharmacokinetics of ibuprofen). Clinical importance unknown. This pharmacokinetic interaction may occur because of increased oral bioavailability of adefovir.

■ **Immunosuppressive Agents** No pharmacokinetic interactions with tacrolimus.

Effect of adefovir dipivoxil on cyclosporine concentrations not known.

Concomitant use of adefovir dipivoxil and cyclosporine or tacrolimus may increase the risk of nephrotoxicity.

■ **Telbivudine** No pharmacokinetic interactions with telbivudine.

In vitro studies indicate additive antiviral effects between telbivudine and adefovir against HBV.

Description

Adefovir dipivoxil is a prodrug of adefovir, an acyclic nucleotide analog antiviral agent active against human hepatitis B virus (HBV). Following initial diester hydrolysis in vivo to form adefovir, the drug undergoes subsequent phosphorylation by cellular enzymes to form its active metabolite, adefovir diphosphate. Adefovir diphosphate inhibits HBV DNA polymerase (reverse transcriptase) by competing with the natural substrate deoxyadenosine triphosphate and by causing DNA chain termination after its incorporation into viral DNA. Adefovir diphosphate is a weak inhibitor of human DNA polymerases, including α- and γ-polymerases.

■ **Spectrum** Adefovir is active in vitro and in vivo against human HBV. The drug also has some in vitro activity against certain other human viruses, including herpes simplex virus types 1 and 2 (HSV-1 and HSV-2), human immunodeficiency virus types 1 and 2 (HIV-1 and HIV-2), human papillomavirus (HPV), Epstein-Barr virus, and varicella zoster virus, but has not been shown to be effective in clinical infections caused by these viruses.

Adefovir is active in vivo against some lamivudine-resistant HBV isolates and has demonstrated anti-HBV activity (median reduction in serum HBV DNA levels of 4.1 $\log_{10}$ copies/mL) against clinical isolates of HBV containing lamivudine-associated mutations. In vitro studies indicate that adefovir is active against HBV variants containing substitutions that confer resistance to lamivudine (rtL180M, rtM204I, rtM204V, rtL180M + rtM204V, rtV173L + rtL180M + rtM204V) or entecavir (rtT184G, rtS202I, rtM250V). (See Patients with Lamivudine-Resistant HBV under Uses: Chronic Hepatitis B Virus Infection.)

■ **Resistance** ***Resistance in HBV*** Although the clinical importance is unclear, there is evidence that HBV with reduced susceptibility to adefovir dipivoxil develop in some patients during long-term use of the drug.

There was no evidence of emergence of HBV resistant to adefovir dipivoxil during 48-week clinical studies evaluating adefovir dipivoxil monotherapy in HBV-infected patients; however, resistance or diminished virologic response was reported in some patients with HBV infection following at least 56 weeks of adefovir dipivoxil monotherapy.

Genotypic analysis of isolates obtained from patients who showed renewed evidence of HBV replication while receiving adefovir dipivoxil indicates that mutations at rtN236T and rtA181T/V are associated with resistance to adefovir. After 96 weeks of adefovir dipivoxil monotherapy, the N236T mutation was detected in 2 patients (1.6% of patients) and this mutation was associated with reduced in vitro susceptibility to the drug. In studies of patients who received adefovir dipivoxil for up to 5 years, mutations associated with adefovir resistance developed in 20–42% of patients.

Cross-resistance can occur among the nucleoside and nucleotide antivirals used for treatment of HBV. Some strains of HBV may be cross-resistant to both adefovir and lamivudine. Preliminary data suggest that the N236T mutation alone does not confer cross-resistance to lamivudine since isolates with the mutation remained susceptible to lamivudine in vitro and in vivo, but cross-resistance to adefovir and lamivudine can occur in isolates with the rtA181V mutation. In vitro studies indicate that some HBV with mutations associated with adefovir resistance may have decreased susceptibility to entecavir. Some adefovir-resistant HBV (e.g., those with adefovir resistance-associated substitution rtA181V, rtA181S, rt181T) have reduced susceptibility to telbivudine; other strains (e.g., those with rtN236T substitution) remain susceptible to telbivudine. HBV isolates with rtA181T, rtA181V, or rtN236T single adefovir resistance-associated substitutions also have less than twofold reduced susceptibility to tenofovir alafenamide. Isolates with double adefovir resistance-associated substitutions of rtA181V *and* rtN236T have 3.7-fold reduced susceptibility to tenofovir alafenamide.

Advice to Patients

Advise patient of the risks and benefits of adefovir dipivoxil and other alternatives for treatment of hepatitis B virus (HBV) infection and importance of reading the patient package insert for the drug before starting treatment.

Importance of remaining under the care of a clinician while taking adefovir dipivoxil and not discontinuing the drug without first informing a clinician.

Importance of following a regular dosage schedule and avoiding missed doses.

Risk of exacerbations of hepatitis when adefovir dipivoxil is discontinued and importance of close monitoring of liver function and HBV levels for several months or longer after the drug is stopped.

Risk of nephrotoxicity and importance of monitoring renal function during treatment, especially in those with preexisting renal impairment or other risks for renal impairment.

Importance of immediately reporting any signs or symptoms of lactic acidosis (e.g., weakness/fatigue, unusual muscle pain, trouble breathing, stomach pain with nausea and vomiting, cold intolerance especially in the arms and legs, dizziness or feeling light-headed, fast or irregular heart beat) or any signs or symptoms of hepatotoxicity (e.g., jaundice, dark urine, bowel movements light in color, anorexia, nausea, stomach pain). Importance of reporting any other unusual symptoms or any known symptom persists or worsens.

Risk of rapid emergence of human immunodeficiency virus (HIV) resistance in HBV-infected patients with unrecognized or untreated HIV infection; importance of HIV antibody testing prior to initiation of adefovir dipivoxil therapy and any time during therapy if possible exposure to HIV occurs.

Advise patients with lamivudine-resistant HBV that they should receive adefovir dipivoxil in conjunction with lamivudine and should not receive adefovir dipivoxil monotherapy.

Advise patients that the optimal duration of treatment and the relationship between treatment response and long-term outcomes of HBV infection (hepatocellular carcinoma, decompensated cirrhosis) are not known.

Importance of informing clinician of existing or contemplated concomitant therapy, including prescription and OTC drugs, and any concomitant illnesses.

Importance of women immediately informing clinician if they are or plan to become pregnant or plan to breast-feed.

Importance of advising patients of other important precautionary information. (See Cautions.)

Preparations

Excipients in commercially available drug preparations may have clinically important effects in some individuals; consult specific product labeling for details.

Adefovir Dipivoxil

Oral		
Tablets	10 mg*	Adefovir Dipivoxil Tablets
		Hepsera®, Gilead

*available from one or more manufacturer, distributor, and/or repackager by generic (nonproprietary) name

†Use is not currently included in the labeling approved by the US Food and Drug Administration

Cidofovir

Vistide, CDV

■ Cidofovir, an acyclic nucleotide analog (acyclic nucleoside phosphonate), is an antiviral agent active against herpesviruses and certain other viruses.

Uses

■ **Treatment of Cytomegalovirus Infection and Disease** ***Cytomegalovirus Retinitis*** Cidofovir is used for initial treatment (induction therapy) and maintenance therapy (secondary prophylaxis) of cytomegalovirus (CMV) retinitis in adults with human immunodeficiency virus (HIV) infection, including those with acquired immunodeficiency syndrome (AIDS). The drug also is used for the management of CMV retinitis in HIV-infected adolescents and children†. Safety and efficacy of cidofovir have not been established for the treatment of other CMV infections (e.g., pneumonitis, gastroenteritis), congenital or neonatal CMV disease, or CMV disease in individuals not infected with HIV.

Like other antivirals, cidofovir is not a cure for CMV retinitis. Although cidofovir can induce stabilization or improvement of ocular manifestations of CMV retinitis, the retinitis may relapse and/or progress during or after discontinuance of the drug.

Retinitis is the most common clinical manifestation of CMV end-organ disease in HIV-infected patients and ideally should be managed in consultation with an ophthalmologist familiar with the diagnosis and treatment of retinal diseases. Antiviral regimens for initial treatment of CMV retinitis in HIV-infected individuals should be selected based on the location and severity of CMV retinal lesions, severity of underlying immunosuppression, concomitant drug therapy, and the patient's ability to adhere to the treatment regimen. The antiviral regimen used for maintenance therapy of CMV retinitis in HIV-infected individuals should be selected with consideration for the location of the CMV retinal lesions, vision in the contralateral eye, the patient's immunologic and virologic status, and the patient's response to antiretroviral therapy.

For the management of immediate sight-threatening CMV retinal lesions (i.e., within 1.5 mm of the fovea) in HIV-infected adults and adolescents, the US Centers for Disease Control and Prevention (CDC), National Institutes of Health (NIH), and HIV Medicine Association of the Infectious Diseases Society of America (IDSA) state that the preferred regimen is initial treatment (induction therapy) with intravitreal ganciclovir or intravitreal foscarnet (1–4 doses given over a period of 7–10 days) in conjunction with oral valganciclovir (twice daily for 14–21 days) followed by maintenance therapy (secondary prophylaxis) with oral valganciclovir (once daily). One alternative regimen recommended by these experts for management of sight-threatening CMV retinitis in HIV-infected adults and adolescents is intravitreal ganciclovir or intravitreal foscarnet (1–4 doses given over a period of 7–10 days) in conjunction with IV cidofovir (once weekly for 2 weeks) followed by maintenance therapy (secondary prophylaxis) with IV cidofovir (once every other week). Use of systemic antivirals (without an intravitreal antiviral) usually is adequate for the management of CMV retinitis in patients who have only small peripheral lesions.

For the management of CMV retinitis in HIV-infected pediatric patients, CDC, NIH, IDSA, and others state that IV ganciclovir is the drug of choice for initial treatment (induction therapy) and is one of several options for maintenance therapy (secondary prophylaxis). These experts state that IV cidofovir has not been studied in children with CMV disease, but is a possible alternative for the management of CMV retinitis in HIV-infected children† when other options cannot be used.

Because of the risk of relapse, HIV-infected patients who have received adequate initial treatment of CMV retinitis should receive chronic maintenance therapy (secondary prophylaxis) until immune reconstitution occurs as a result of effective antiretroviral therapy. CDC, NIH, and IDSA state that consideration can be given to discontinuing maintenance therapy of CMV retinitis in HIV-infected adults and adolescents if CMV lesions have been treated for at least 3–6 months and are inactive and there has been a sustained (i.e., 3–6 months) increase in $CD4^+$ T-cell count to greater than 100/mm^3 in response to antiretroviral therapy. The safety of discontinuing maintenance therapy of CMV retinitis in HIV-infected pediatric patients has not been well studied; however, CDC, NIH, IDSA, and others state that consideration can be given to discontinuing such maintenance therapy in HIV-infected children who are receiving antiretroviral therapy and have a sustained (i.e., greater than 6 months) increase in $CD4^+$ T-cell percentage to greater than 15% (children younger than 6 years of age) or an increase in $CD4^+$ T-cell count to greater than 100/mm^3 (children 6 years of age or older). These experts state that a decision to discontinue maintenance therapy of CMV retinitis should be made in consultation with an ophthalmologist and, if maintenance therapy is discontinued, the patient should continue to receive regular ophthalmologic monitoring (optimally every 3–6 months) for early detection of CMV relapse or immune reconstitution uveitis. If $CD4^+$ T-cell count decreases to less than 100/mm^3 (adults, adolescents, children 6 years of age or older) or if $CD4^+$ T-cell percentage decreases to less than 15% (children younger than 6 years of age), maintenance therapy of CMV retinitis should be reinitiated.

For additional information on the management of CMV retinitis and other CMV infections in HIV-infected individuals, the current clinical practice guidelines from CDC, NIH, and IDSA on the prevention and treatment of opportunistic infections in HIV-infected individuals available at http://www.aidsinfo.nih.gov should be consulted.

Clinical Experience. Efficacy of cidofovir for the treatment of previously untreated CMV retinitis and the treatment of CMV retinitis that relapsed (progressed) despite prior therapy with other antivirals has been established in several phase 2/3 controlled trials in HIV-infected patients.

In one trial (study 106) in which previously untreated patients with peripheral CMV retinitis received either immediate or delayed (until progression) cidofovir therapy (induction with 5 mg/kg IV once weekly for 2 weeks, then maintenance therapy with 5 mg/kg IV once every other week), the median time to progression of CMV retinitis as evidenced by changes in retinal photographs was 120 or 22 days for the immediate or delayed groups, respectively. However, because of the limited number of patients in the immediate-treatment group who continued to receive cidofovir therapy over time (only 3 of 25 patients received the drug for 120 days or longer), estimates of the median time to progression are imprecise. For alternative indicators of retinal progression or drug discontinuance, the median times for the immediate- and delayed-treatment groups were 52 and 22 days, respectively. Estimates of clinical efficacy from this trial may not be directly comparable to estimates reported for other therapies.

In an open-label, dose-response trial (study 107) in which HIV-infected patients with relapsing CMV retinitis received cidofovir 5 mg/kg IV once weekly for 2 weeks (induction) followed by either 5 or 3 mg/kg IV once every other week (maintenance therapy), the median time to CMV retinitis progression as evidenced by changes in retinal photographs was 115 or 49 days, respectively. For alternative indicators of retinal progression or drug discontinuance, the median times for the 5- and 3-mg/kg maintenance therapy groups were 49 and 35 days, respectively. In this trial, patients had been diagnosed with CMV retinitis approximately 1 year prior to randomization and had undergone a median of 4 prior courses of systemic antiviral therapy (ganciclovir and/or foscarnet) and 20% had received intraocular antiviral therapy active against CMV.

■ **Mucocutaneous Herpes Simplex Virus Infections** IV cidofovir has been used for the management of mucocutaneous infections caused by acyclovir-resistant herpes simplex virus types 1 and 2† (HSV-1 and HSV-2) in immunocompromised patients, including HIV-infected individuals.

The drugs of choice for the management of orolabial lesions or initial or recurrent genital lesions caused by HSV are valacyclovir, famciclovir, and acyclovir. For the management of mucocutaneous lesions caused by acyclovir-resistant HSV in HIV-infected adults and adolescents†, CDC, NIH, and IDSA recommend IV foscarnet as the drug of choice and state that IV cidofovir is a potential alternative. These experts also recommend IV foscarnet as the drug of choice for the management of acyclovir-resistant HSV infections in HIV-infected children† and state that IV cidofovir is recommended for infections caused by HSV resistant to acyclovir and foscarnet.

Although a topical preparation of cidofovir is not commercially available in the US, the drug has been used topically† for the management of mucocutaneous HSV infections†, including genital herpes†, caused by acyclovir-resistant strains. CDC, NIH, and IDSA suggest that topical cidofovir (extemporaneously prepared) can be considered another option for the treatment of acyclovir-resistant genital herpes†.

■ **Adenovirus Infections** Although safety and efficacy have not been established and data are limited, cidofovir has been used with some success for the treatment of adenovirus infections† in some immunocompromised patients (e.g., allogeneic hematopoietic stem cell transplant recipients, solid organ transplant recipients).

■ **Varicella-Zoster Virus Infections** Cidofovir has been recommended as a possible alternative for the management of varicella-zoster virus (VZV) infections†.

The preferred antivirals for the management of acute, localized herpes zoster (shingles) in HIV-infected adults and adolescents are acyclovir, famciclovir, and valacyclovir. For the management of proven or suspected acyclovir-resistant VZV infections† in HIV-infected adults or adolescents, CDC, NIH, and IDSA recommend IV foscarnet and state that IV cidofovir is a possible alternative.

Although optimal regimens for the management of progressive outer retinal necrosis caused by VZV† in HIV-infected individuals have not been identified, CDC, NIH, and IDSA recommend treatment with at least one IV antiviral (acyclovir, ganciclovir, foscarnet, cidofovir) used in conjunction with at least one intravitreal antiviral (ganciclovir or foscarnet). The prognosis for visual preservation in patients with progressive outer retinal necrosis caused by VZV is poor and such infections should be managed in consultation with an ophthalmologist.

■ **Smallpox** ***Smallpox Vaccination Complications*** Cidofovir is recommended as an alternative for the treatment of certain serious complications of smallpox vaccination†, including eczema vaccinatum, progressive vaccinia, severe generalized vaccinia, and aberrant vaccinia infection caused by inadvertent autoinoculation (if severe because of large numbers of lesions, toxicity, or pain). While cidofovir has antiviral activity against vaccinia virus in vitro and in animal models, safety and efficacy of the drug for the treatment of complications of smallpox vaccination have not been determined and the possible benefits for this use are not known.

Vaccinia immune globulin IV (VIGIV) is considered first-line treatment for serious complications of smallpox vaccination.

If VIGIV alone is inadequate or if VIGIV is not readily available, certain antivirals (e.g., cidofovir, tecovirimat, brincidofovir) may be considered for the treatment of complications of smallpox vaccination after consultation with CDC.

For assistance with diagnosis and management of suspected complications of smallpox vaccination, clinicians should contact their state or local health department or the CDC Emergency Operations Center at 770-488-7100.

Treatment of Smallpox The role, if any, of cidofovir in the treatment of smallpox† remains to be determined. Cidofovir is active in vitro against poxviruses, including variola virus (the causative agent of smallpox), and has in vivo activity in mice against cowpox and vaccinia virus. Although limited in vitro and in vivo data suggest that cidofovir might prove useful in preventing smallpox infection if administered within 1–2 days after exposure, there is no evidence that the antiviral would be more effective than smallpox vaccination in this early period. Data are not available to date regarding the safety and efficacy of cidofovir for the treatment or prevention of smallpox in humans and it has been suggested that the potential usefulness of the drug for the treatment of smallpox may be limited because of the need for IV administration and potential renal toxicity. The US Working Group on Civilian Biodefense and US Army Medical Research Institute of Infectious Diseases, while acknowledging the potential activity of cidofovir against the virus, state that clinical efficacy in the treatment of smallpox has not been established for any antiviral agent to date.

■ **Monkeypox** Although no specific treatments are available for monkeypox infection, CDC states that human monkeypox outbreaks can be controlled through use of smallpox vaccine, VIGIV, and certain antivirals (e.g., cidofovir, tecovirimat, brincidofovir). Monkeypox virus is an orthopoxvirus closely related to the causative agent of smallpox.

Efficacy of cidofovir for the treatment of human monkeypox† remains to be established; however, the drug is active in vitro against monkeypox and has in vivo activity against the virus in animal models. While it is not known whether an individual with severe monkeypox infection would benefit from treatment with an antiviral (e.g., cidofovir, brincidofovir), CDC states that use of an antiviral may be considered in such patients.

If an outbreak of human monkeypox occurs in the US, CDC will establish updated guidelines regarding use of smallpox vaccine, VIGIV, or antivirals for treatment of monkeypox infection and/or postexposure prophylaxis of exposed individuals.

Dosage and Administration

■ **General** Renal function *must* be assessed prior to initiation of cidofovir and monitored during therapy with the drug.

Cidofovir *must* not be initiated in patients with serum creatinine concentration exceeding 1.5 mg/dL, calculated creatinine clearance of 55 mL/minute or less, or urine protein concentration of 100 mg/dL or greater (equivalent to 2+ or greater). (See Renal Impairment under Dosage and Administration: Special Populations.)

Patients *must* receive adequate hydration prior to each dose of cidofovir.

A regimen of oral probenecid *must* be administered concomitantly with each dose of cidofovir.

The recommended dosage of cidofovir and recommended frequency and rate of administration of the drug *must* not be exceeded.

Hydration To reduce the risk of cidofovir-induced nephrotoxicity, patients should receive at least 1 L of 0.9% sodium chloride infused IV over 1–2 hours immediately before each IV infusion of cidofovir.

For patients who can tolerate additional fluid, an additional 1 L of 0.9% sodium chloride should be administered; this second IV infusion of 0.9% sodium chloride should be initiated either concomitantly with or immediately after the cidofovir IV infusion and should be administered over 1–3 hours.

Volume repletion and maintenance are particularly important in patients with potential volume depletion secondary to conditions such as chronic diarrhea, poor fluid intake, or wasting related to human immunodeficiency virus (HIV) infection.

Concomitant Probenecid To reduce the risk of cidofovir-induced nephrotoxicity, a regimen of oral probenecid must be administered concomitantly with each dose of cidofovir. Cidofovir undergoes renal tubular secretion, suggesting that use of probenecid may reduce the risk of cidofovir renal toxicity by decreasing concentrations of the drug within proximal tubular cells.

For each dose of cidofovir, the recommended regimen of *oral probenecid* is 2 g given 3 hours prior to initiation of the cidofovir IV infusion, followed by 1-g doses given 2 and 8 hours after completion of the cidofovir IV infusion, for a total *probenecid* dose of 4 g.

To reduce the risk of nausea and/or vomiting associated with oral probenecid, food can be ingested prior to each probenecid dose and concomitant administration of an effective antiemetic can be considered. For patients who develop allergic or other hypersensitivity manifestations with probenecid, appropriate prophylactic or therapeutic use of antihistamines and/or acetaminophen can be considered. Because concomitant probenecid is required, cidofovir is contraindicated in patients with a history of severe hypersensitivity to probenecid or other sulfa-containing drugs since probenecid is contraindicated in such patients.

Because probenecid can affect the pharmacokinetics of many drugs, a careful assessment should be made of other drugs that the patient may be receiving. (See Drug Interactions: Probenecid.)

■ **Administration** Cidofovir is administered by slow IV infusion using a controlled-infusion device (e.g., pump).

Although cidofovir has been administered by intravitreal injection†, a preparation specifically for intravitreal administration is not commercially available in the US and the manufacturer states that *direct intraocular injection of the currently available IV preparation of cidofovir (even if diluted) is contraindicated since such administration has been associated with iritis, ocular hypotony, and permanent visual impairment.*

Cidofovir has been administered topically† as a gel or cream for the management of certain mucocutaneous viral infections (e.g., acyclovir-resistant herpes simplex virus [HSV] infections). Although topical preparations of cidofovir are not commercially available in the US, a topical gel containing 1% cidofovir has been prepared extemporaneously using the IV preparation of cidofovir.

IV Infusion Cidofovir *must* be administered using a controlled-infusion device (e.g., pump).

Cidofovir is commercially available as a concentrate for injection containing 75 mg of cidofovir per mL and *must* be diluted prior to IV infusion.

Cidofovir concentrate should appear clear and colorless and should not be used if it appears discolored or contains particles.

Caution should be exercised when preparing, administering, and discarding solutions of cidofovir according to guidelines for handling mutagenic substances. If cidofovir concentrate for injection or a diluted solution of the drug comes in contact with the skin or mucosa, the affected area should be washed immediately and thoroughly with soap and water. Partially used vials of cidofovir and diluted solutions of the drug should be discarded by high temperature incineration.

Dilution. For IV infusion, the appropriate dose of cidofovir concentrate for injection containing 75 mg/mL should be withdrawn from the vial and diluted in 100 mL of 0.9% sodium chloride injection in a compatible infusion container (e.g., PVC, glass, ethylene/propylene copolymer). The entire volume of diluted solution should then be administered by IV infusion.

Diluted solutions of cidofovir should be administered within 24 hours of preparation and should *not* be refrigerated or frozen to extend the storage period beyond this 24-hour limit. However, if a diluted solution will not be used immediately, it may be prepared in advance and refrigerated at 2–8°C for up to 24 hours; the refrigerated diluted solution should be allowed to reach room temperature before administration and should be administered within 24 hours of initial preparation.

Compatibility of cidofovir with Ringer's, lactated Ringer's, or bacteriostatic infusion fluids has not been evaluated.

Rate of Administration. IV infusions of cidofovir should be given at a constant rate over 1 hour using a controlled-infusion device (e.g., pump).

To minimize the risk of nephrotoxicity, the IV dose must *not* be infused over a shorter time period.

■ **Dosage** Cidofovir is commercially available as the dihydrate; dosage is expressed in terms of anhydrous drug.

Adult Dosage **Cytomegalovirus Retinitis.** For the treatment of cytomegalovirus (CMV) retinitis in HIV-infected adults with serum creatinine concentration of 1.5 mg/dL or less, a calculated creatinine clearance exceeding 55 mL/minute, and urine protein concentration less than 100 mg/dL (equivalent to less than 2+), the recommended dosage of IV cidofovir for initial treatment (induction therapy) is 5 mg/kg once weekly for 2 consecutive weeks. In patients with immediate sight-threatening CMV retinal lesions (i.e., within 1.5 mm of the fovea), the US Centers for Disease Control and Prevention (CDC), National Institutes of Health (NIH), and HIV Medicine Association of the Infectious Diseases Society of America (IDSA) recommend that initial treatment also include an appropriate intravitreal antiviral. (See Cytomegalovirus Retinitis under Uses: Treatment of Cytomegalovirus Infection and Disease.)

After completion of initial treatment, the recommended dosage of IV cidofovir for maintenance therapy (secondary prophylaxis) of CMV retinitis in HIV-infected adults is 5 mg/kg once every 2 weeks (i.e., every other week). If renal function declines during cidofovir therapy, maintenance dosage must be reduced or the drug discontinued depending on the degree of impairment. (See Renal Impairment under Dosage and Administration: Special Populations.)

Decisions regarding discontinuance of maintenance therapy of CMV retinitis in HIV-infected individuals who have been treated for at least 3–6 months, have inactive CMV retinal lesions, and have achieved immune reconstitution as the result of antiretroviral therapy should be made in consultation with an ophthalmologist. (See Cytomegalovirus Retinitis under Uses: Treatment of Cytomegalovirus Infection and Disease.)

Mucocutaneous Herpes Simplex Virus Infections. For the management of mucocutaneous herpes simplex virus type 1 and 2 (HSV-1 and HSV-2) infections† known or suspected to be caused by acyclovir-resistant strains in immunocompromised individuals, including HIV-infected adults, the recommended dosage of IV cidofovir is 5 mg/kg once weekly for a treatment duration of 2–4 weeks or longer until a response is obtained. CDC states that a cidofovir dosage of 5 mg/kg IV once weekly may be effective for the management of acyclovir-resistant genital herpes.

For the topical treatment of mucocutaneous HSV infections†, including genital herpes†, caused by acyclovir-resistant HSV, an extemporaneously prepared gel† containing cidofovir 1% has been applied topically once daily for 5 days. If an extemporaneously prepared gel containing cidofovir 1% is used for the topical treatment of acyclovir-resistant HSV lesions in HIV-infected individuals, a treatment duration of 3–4 weeks or longer is recommended depending on clinical response.

Pediatric Dosage **Cytomegalovirus Retinitis.** If cidofovir is used as an alternative for the management of CMV retinitis in HIV-infected adolescents†, CDC, NIH, IDSA, and others recommend initial treatment (induction therapy) with a dosage of 5 mg/kg IV once weekly for 2 consecutive weeks.

After completion of initial treatment, the recommended dosage of cidofovir for maintenance therapy (secondary prophylaxis) in HIV-infected adolescents† is 5 mg/kg IV once every 2 weeks (i.e., every other week). If renal function declines during cidofovir therapy, dosage must be reduced or the drug discontinued depending on the degree of impairment. (See Renal Impairment under Dosage and Administration: Special Populations.)

Decisions regarding discontinuance of maintenance therapy of CMV retinitis in HIV-infected individuals who have been treated for at least 3–6 months, have inactive CMV retinal lesions, and have achieved immune reconstitution as the result of antiretroviral therapy should be made in consultation with an ophthalmologist. (See Cytomegalovirus Retinitis under Uses: Treatment of Cytomegalovirus Infection and Disease.)

Mucocutaneous Herpes Simplex Virus Infections. For the management of mucocutaneous HSV-1 or HSV-2 infections† known or suspected to be caused by acyclovir-resistant strains in HIV-infected adolescents†, the recommended dosage of cidofovir is 5 mg/kg IV once weekly for a treatment duration of 2–4 weeks or longer until a response is obtained.

For the topical treatment of mucocutaneous HSV infections†, including genital herpes†, caused by acyclovir-resistant HSV, an extemporaneously prepared gel† containing cidofovir 1% has been applied topically once daily for 5 days. If an extemporaneously prepared gel containing cidofovir 1% is used for the topical treatment of acyclovir-resistant HSV lesions in HIV-infected individuals, a treatment duration of 3–4 weeks or longer is recommended depending on clinical response.

■ **Special Populations** ***Hepatic Impairment*** The manufacturer makes no specific dosage recommendation for use of cidofovir in patients with hepatic impairment; the effect of hepatic impairment on the pharmacokinetics of the drug has not been evaluated to date.

Renal Impairment Initiation of cidofovir is contraindicated in patients with serum creatinine concentration exceeding 1.5 mg/dL, calculated creatinine clearance of 55 mL/minute or less, or urine protein concentration of 100 mg/dL or greater (equivalent to proteinuria of 2+ or greater).

If serum creatinine concentration increases by 0.3–0.4 mg/dL above baseline during cidofovir therapy, the dose must be reduced to 3 mg/kg. If this occurs in HIV-infected adults or adolescents† receiving cidofovir for maintenance therapy (secondary prophylaxis) of CMV retinitis, dosage of the drug should be reduced to 3 mg/kg once every 2 weeks (i.e., every other week).

If serum creatinine concentration increases by 0.5 mg/dL or more above baseline or if proteinuria of 3+ or greater develops, cidofovir *must* be discontinued.

Patients who develop 2+ proteinuria in the face of a stable serum creatinine during cidofovir therapy should be observed carefully (including close monitoring of serum creatinine and urinary protein) to detect potential deterioration that would warrant dose reduction or discontinuance of the drug.

Geriatric Patients Dosage of cidofovir for geriatric patients should be selected with caution because of age-related decreases in renal function. (See Geriatric Use under Warnings/Precautions: Specific Populations, in Cautions.)

Cautions

■ **Contraindications** Initiation of cidofovir is contraindicated in patients with serum creatinine concentration exceeding 1.5 mg/dL, calculated creatinine clearance of 55 mL/minute or less, or urine protein concentration of 100 mg/dL or greater (equivalent to proteinuria of 2+ or greater).

Cidofovir is contraindicated in patients receiving other drugs with nephrotoxic potential. (See Drug Interactions: Nephrotoxic Drugs.)

Cidofovir is contraindicated in patients hypersensitive to the drug. Cidofovir also is contraindicated in patients with a history of clinically severe hypersensitivity to probenecid or other sulfa-containing drugs since an oral probenecid regimen *must* be given in conjunction with each cidofovir dose.

Direct intraocular injection of cidofovir is contraindicated; intraocular injection of the drug has been associated with iritis, ocular hypotony, and permanent vision impairment.

■ **Warnings/Precautions** ***Warnings*** **Renal Effects.** Dose-dependent nephrotoxicity is the major dose-limiting toxicity associated with cidofovir. In clinical trials in patients with cytomegalovirus (CMV) retinitis, renal toxicity (manifested by an increase in serum creatinine concentration of 0.4 mg/dL or greater, decrease in creatinine clearance to 55 mL/minute or less, or proteinuria of 2+ or greater) occurred in 59% of patients receiving cidofovir at the recommended maintenance dosage of 5 mg/kg IV every other week.

There have been reports of severe renal impairment in patients receiving the drug, including acute renal failure resulting in dialysis and/or contributing to death, in patients who received as few as 1 or 2 doses of cidofovir. In some patients, there were associated risk factors for nephrotoxicity, such as preexisting mild renal insufficiency or cidofovir administration proximal to completion of aminoglycoside therapy in a patient with preexisting normal serum creatinine concentrations. In some patients, renal function failed to return to baseline following discontinuance of cidofovir therapy.

Proteinuria may be an early sign of cidofovir-induced nephrotoxicity. In patients who develop proteinuria during cidofovir therapy, the manufacturer recommends that IV hydration be administered and the test repeated. If renal function deteriorates during cidofovir therapy, dosage reduction or discontinuance of the drug may be required. (See Renal Impairment under Dosage and Administration: Special Populations.) Continued administration of cidofovir may lead to additional proximal tubular cell injury, which may result in glycosuria; decreases in serum phosphate, uric acid, and bicarbonate concentrations; increases in serum creatinine concentrations; and/or acute renal failure which may require dialysis.

A diagnosis of Fanconi syndrome, manifested as multiple abnormalities of proximal renal tubular function, has been reported in 1% of patients receiving cidofovir. (See Metabolic Acidosis under Warnings/Precautions: Other Warnings and Precautions, in Cautions.)

To reduce the risk of nephrotoxicity, IV hydration with 0.9% sodium chloride injection is required prior to administration of each cidofovir dose and a regimen of oral probenecid is required with each cidofovir dose. (See Dosage and Administration: General.) In addition, concomitant use of cidofovir and potentially nephrotoxic drugs is contraindicated and at least 7 days should elapse between discontinuance of such drugs and administration of cidofovir. (See Drug Interactions: Nephrotoxic Drugs.)

Prior to initiation of cidofovir therapy, renal function *must* be assessed. The drug is contraindicated and should *not* be initiated in patients with serum creatinine concentration exceeding 1.5 mg/dL, calculated creatinine clearance of 55 mL/minute or less, or urine protein concentration of 100 mg/dL or greater (equivalent to proteinuria of 2+ or greater). Because serum creatinine concentrations may not provide an accurate assessment of renal function in patients with severe acquired immunodeficiency deficiency syndrome (AIDS) and CMV retinitis, Cockcroft-Gault calculations should be used *initially* to estimate creatinine clearance more precisely when determining the eligibility of such patients to receive cidofovir; for subsequent assessments, serum creatinine and *not* Cockcroft-Gault calculations of creatinine clearance should be used.

During cidofovir therapy, renal function (i.e., serum creatinine concentration and urine protein) *must* be determined within 48 hours prior to *each* dose of cidofovir, and the cidofovir dose should be adjusted or withheld as appropriate based on any changes in renal function. (See Renal Impairment under Dosage and Administration: Special Populations.)

Hematologic Effects. Neutropenia may occur during cidofovir therapy. In clinical trials in patients with CMV retinitis, neutropenia (500/mm^3 or less) occurred in 24% of patients receiving recommended maintenance dosages of cidofovir; 39% of these patients received treatment with filgrastim (G-CSF).

Neutrophil counts should be monitored during cidofovir therapy.

Carcinogenic and Mutagenic Potential. Cidofovir should be considered a potential carcinogen in humans. In animal studies, the drug was carcinogenic and mutagenic.

In rats receiving cidofovir by subscapular subcutaneous injection, mammary adenocarcinomas were observed in the females at dosages as low as 0.6 mg/kg once weekly (equivalent to 0.04 times the human systemic exposure achieved at recommended IV dosages); the first mass was detected after 6 doses of cidofovir. In another study in rats receiving IV cidofovir, mammary adenocarcinomas were observed in females and Zymbal gland carcinomas were observed in males and females at a dosage of 15 mg/kg once weekly (equivalent to 1.1 times the human systemic exposure achieved at recommended IV dosages).

In mutagenicity studies in mice, an increase in micronucleated polychromatic erythrocytes was seen at cidofovir dosages of 2 g/kg or greater (equivalent to approximately 65 times the maximum recommended human IV dose). Cidofovir has induced chromosomal aberrations in human peripheral blood lymphocytes in vitro without metabolic activation, but there was no evidence of mutagenicity in microbial mutagenicity assays involving *Salmonella typhimurium* (Ames) and *Escherichia coli* in the presence and absence of metabolic activation.

Effects on Fertility. Cidofovir has caused reduced testes weight and hypospermia in animals and it is possible that such effects could occur in humans and cause infertility.

Although cidofovir caused inhibition of spermatogenesis in rats and monkeys, no adverse effects on fertility or reproduction were observed in male rats receiving IV cidofovir at dosages up to 15 mg/kg once weekly (equivalent to 1.1 times the recommended human dosage) for 13 consecutive weeks.

In female rats receiving IV cidofovir at a dosage of 1.2 mg/kg once weekly (equivalent to 0.09 times the recommended human dosages) for up to 6 weeks prior to mating and for 2 weeks after mating, decreased litter size, decreased live births per litter, and increased early resorptions per litter were observed. In peri- and postnatal development studies in female rats receiving subcutaneous injections of cidofovir at dosages up to 1 mg/kg daily from day 7 of gestation through day 21 postpartum (approximately 5 weeks), there were no observed adverse effects on viability, growth, behavior, sexual maturation, or reproductive capacity in the offspring.

Women of childbearing potential and men should be advised to use an effective method of contraception during cidofovir therapy and for certain periods of time after the drug is discontinued. (See Pregnancy under Warnings/Precautions: Specific Populations, in Cautions.)

Selection and Use of Antivirals. Cidofovir is labeled by the FDA *only* for the treatment of CMV retinitis in patients with human immunodeficiency virus (HIV) infection, including those with AIDS.

Safety and efficacy of the drug have not been established for the treatment of other CMV infections or for the treatment of CMV disease in individuals not infected with HIV.

Other Warnings and Precautions **Administration Precautions.** Cidofovir should be administered *only* by IV infusion. The commercially available IV preparation of the drug must *not* be administered by intraocular injection because iritis, ocular hypotony, and permanent visual impairment have been reported when this route was used.

Patients *must* receive IV hydration prior to each cidofovir dose and *must* receive a regimen of oral probenecid concomitantly with each cidofovir dose. (See Dosage and Administration: General.)

Because of the potential for nephrotoxicity, the recommended cidofovir dosage, frequency, and rate of administration *must* not be exceeded. (See Dosage and Administration.)

Ophthalmologic Effects. Decreased intraocular pressure (IOP) may occur during cidofovir therapy. In some cases, decreased IOP has been associated with decreased visual acuity. Among patients in clinical trials who received IV cidofovir doses of 5 mg/kg for maintenance therapy of CMV retinitis and whose IOP was monitored, 24% experienced at least a 50% decrease in IOP from baseline and severe hypotony (i.e., IOP of 0–1 mm Hg) was reported in 3 patients. The risk of ocular hypotony may be increased in patients with preexisting diabetes mellitus.

Uveitis or iritis has been reported in patients in clinical trials receiving IV cidofovir for the treatment of CMV retinitis. Among those receiving IV cidofovir maintenance therapy of CMV retinitis, uveitis or iritis was reported in 11%.

Patients receiving cidofovir should receive periodic ophthalmic examinations to monitor IOP and visual acuity and to monitor for symptoms of uveitis or iritis.

If anterior uveitis or iritis develops, appropriate therapy (e.g., topical corticosteroids with or without cycloplegic therapy) should be considered as indicated.

Metabolic Acidosis. Decreased serum bicarbonate associated with proximal tubule injury and renal wasting syndrome (including Fanconi syndrome) has been reported in patients receiving cidofovir. Decreased serum bicarbonate concentration (16 mEq/L or less) has been reported in 16% of cidofovir-treated patients.

Fatal cases of metabolic acidosis in association with liver dysfunction and pancreatitis have been reported in patients receiving cidofovir.

Specific Populations **Pregnancy.** There are no adequate and well-controlled studies to date using cidofovir in pregnant women. Cidofovir should be used during pregnancy only if potential benefits justify potential risks to the fetus.

In animal studies, embryotoxicity (reduced fetal body weights) and maternal toxicity were observed in rats and rabbits receiving IV cidofovir at dosages of 1.5 and 1 mg/kg daily, respectively, during organogenesis. In rabbits receiving IV cidofovir in a dosage of 1 mg/kg daily, maternal toxicity and an increased incidence of fetal external, soft tissue, and skeletal anomalies (meningocele, short snout, and short maxillary bones) were observed.

Women of childbearing potential should be informed that cidofovir is embryotoxic in animals and should be advised to use an effective method of contraception during and for at least 1 month after cidofovir therapy.

Men should be advised to use a reliable method of barrier contraception during and for at least 3 months after cidofovir therapy.

Lactation. It is not known whether cidofovir is distributed into human milk.

Since there is a potential for adverse effects in nursing infants and because carcinogenicity has been shown in animal studies, cidofovir should not be used in breast-feeding women.

Because of the risk of adverse effects in the infant and the risk of HIV transmission, HIV-infected women should not breast-feed infants.

Pediatric Use. Safety and efficacy of cidofovir have not been established in pediatric patients younger than 18 years of age.

Because of the risks of potential long-term carcinogenic and reproductive toxicity, cidofovir should be used with extreme caution in children† with AIDS. The manufacturer states that the drug should be used in children *only* after careful evaluation and *only* when potential benefits outweigh risks.

Some experts state that cidofovir has not been studied in children with CMV disease, but can be considered for the management of CMV retinitis in HIV-infected children† if other options cannot be used.

Geriatric Use. Safety and efficacy of cidofovir have not been evaluated in geriatric patients older than 60 years of age.

Because geriatric patients frequently have reduced glomerular filtration, particular attention should be paid to monitoring renal function prior to and during cidofovir therapy in this age group, and dosage should be modified in response to changes in renal function. (See Renal Impairment under Dosage and Administration: Special Populations.)

Renal Impairment. Initiation of cidofovir is contraindicated in patients with serum creatinine concentration exceeding 1.5 mg/dL, calculated creatinine clearance of 55 mL/minute or less, or urine protein concentration of 100 mg/dL or greater (equivalent to proteinuria of 2+ or greater).

Pharmacokinetic data in individuals with renal impairment (creatinine clearance as low as 11 mL/minute) indicate that cidofovir clearance decreases proportionally with creatinine clearance.

High-flux hemodialysis reduces serum cidofovir concentrations by approximately 75%.

■ **Common Adverse Effects** Adverse effects reported in 15% or more of patients receiving cidofovir (with concomitant probenecid regimen) include nephrotoxicity (proteinuria, elevated serum creatinine), nausea and/or vomiting, fever, neutropenia, asthenia, headache, rash, infection, alopecia, diarrhea, pain, anemia, decreased IOP, anorexia, dyspnea, chills, increased cough, oral moniliasis, and decreased serum bicarbonate.

Drug Interactions

■ **Nephrotoxic Drugs** Concomitant use of cidofovir and nephrotoxic drugs (e.g., aminoglycosides [amikacin, gentamicin, tobramycin], amphotericin B, foscarnet, nonsteroidal anti-inflammatory agents, IV pentamidine, vancomycin) may increase the risk of nephrotoxicity and is contraindicated. Such drugs *must* be discontinued at least 7 days prior to initiating cidofovir therapy.

■ **Foscarnet** Concomitant use of foscarnet and cidofovir is contraindicated. Foscarnet must be discontinued at least 7 days prior to initiating cidofovir therapy. In addition, because the risk of cidofovir-associated nephrotoxicity is increased in patients who previously received foscarnet, such patients must be monitored closely after cidofovir is initiated.

■ **Probenecid** Concomitant use of probenecid and cidofovir decreases renal clearance of cidofovir to a level consistent with creatinine clearance, suggesting that probenecid blocks active renal tubular secretion of cidofovir. This pharmacokinetic interaction is used to therapeutic advantage to reduce the risk of cidofovir-associated nephrotoxicity.

Because a regimen of oral probenecid *must* be administered with each dose of cidofovir (see Concomitant Probenecid under Dosage and Administration: General), drug interactions reported for probenecid must also be considered in patients receiving cidofovir. Probenecid interacts with the metabolism or renal tubular excretion of many drugs (e.g., acetaminophen, acyclovir, angiotensin-converting enzyme inhibitors, aminosalicylic acid, barbiturates, benzodiazepines, bumetanide, famotidine, furosemide, methotrexate, nonsteroidal anti-inflammatory agents, theophylline, zidovudine).

■ **Zidovudine** Although concomitant use of cidofovir (without probenecid) and zidovudine does not affect zidovudine pharmacokinetics, probenecid reduces metabolic clearance of zidovudine.

Patients receiving zidovudine may continue taking the antiretroviral agent while receiving cidofovir therapy. However, on the days that the patient receives a dose of cidofovir, zidovudine should be temporarily discontinued or, alternatively, the zidovudine dosage should be reduced by 50% because the probenecid regimen used concomitantly with the cidofovir dose can increase zidovudine concentrations.

Description

Cidofovir, an acyclic nucleotide analog of cytosine (acyclic nucleoside phosphonate), is an antiviral agent.

Cidofovir is a prodrug and exhibits no antiviral activity until converted intracellularly to the active metabolite, cidofovir diphosphate. Unlike other nucleoside and nucleotide antivirals that require conversion within viral cells to an active metabolite (e.g., acyclovir, ganciclovir), the presence of the phosphonate group in cidofovir is believed to account for the drug's ability to become phosphorylated by cellular (host cell) enzymes to its active intracellular metabolite without initial virus-dependent phosphorylation by viral nucleoside kinases.

Cidofovir is converted intracellularly by pyrimidine nucleoside monophosphate kinase to cidofovir monophosphate, which is further converted to the diphosphate and cidofovir phosphate-choline via other cellular enzymes. Cidofovir diphosphate is a viral DNA polymerase inhibitor and exerts its antiviral effects by interfering with DNA synthesis and inhibiting viral replication. Cidofovir diphosphate stops replication of viral DNA by competitive inhibition of viral DNA polymerase (an enzyme encoded by CMV UL54 gene), incorporation and termination of the growing viral DNA chain, and inactivation of the viral DNA polymerase. The inhibitory activity of cidofovir diphosphate is highly selective because of its greater affinity for viral DNA polymerases than for human DNA polymerases.

The pharmacokinetics of IV cidofovir have been evaluated in patients with human immunodeficiency virus (HIV) infection when the drug was given with or without a regimen of oral probenecid. In patients with normal renal function, approximately 80–100% of a dose of IV cidofovir (without oral probenecid) was recovered unchanged in urine within 24 hours. Renal clearance of cidofovir (without oral probenecid) is greater than creatinine clearance, indicating that renal tubular secretion contributes to cidofovir elimination. Following IV administration of cidofovir (with oral probenecid regimen), approximately 70–85% of the dose was excreted unchanged in urine within 24 hours. Renal clearance of cidofovir (with oral probenecid regimen) is consistent with creatinine clearance, indicating that probenecid blocks renal tubular secretion of cidofovir. This effect of probenecid on the pharmacokinetics of cidofovir is used to therapeutic advantage, and a regimen of oral probenecid must be given with each dose of cidofovir. (See Concomitant Probenecid under Dosage and Administration: General.) In vitro studies indicate that cidofovir is less than 6% bound to plasma or serum proteins. In one patient who received a single cidofovir dose of 5 mg/kg by IV infusion over 1 hour (with IV prehydration and concomitant oral probenecid regimen), cidofovir serum concentrations were 8.7 mcg/mL at 15 minutes after completion of the infusion and the drug was undetectable in CSF.

■ **Spectrum** Following intracellular conversion of cidofovir to the pharmacologically active diphosphate metabolite, the drug has in vitro and in vivo inhibitory activity against human herpesviruses, including cytomegalovirus (CMV), herpes simplex virus types 1 and 2 (HSV-1 and HSV-2), varicella-zoster virus (VZV), and Epstein-Barr virus (EBV). The drug also has in vitro activity against adenovirus, human papillomavirus (HPV), and human polyomavirus.

Cidofovir has in vitro activity against poxviruses, including vaccinia virus (cowpox), monkeypox, and variola virus (the causative agent of smallpox). Studies in mice indicate that cidofovir has in vivo activity against vaccinia virus. In vivo activity against monkeypox has been demonstrated in animal models.

Because of the drug's ability to become phosphorylated to its active metabolite without dependence on virally encoded kinases, cidofovir has been shown to exert its antiviral effect on acyclovir-resistant strains of HSV and ganciclovir-resistant strains of CMV. Cidofovir has been shown to exhibit greater in vitro activity against CMV than ganciclovir. In vitro and in vivo studies indicate that cidofovir diphosphate has an extended intracellular half-life, which may result in the drug's ability to exert a prolonged antiviral effect, and activation to the diphosphate by cellular rather than virally encoded enzymes as well as the extended intracellular half-life offer protection against subsequent viral infection in uninfected cells.

■ **Resistance** CMV isolates with reduced susceptibility to cidofovir have been selected in vitro in the presence of high concentrations of the drug, and the possibility of cidofovir-resistant CMV should be considered in patients with CMV retinitis who fail to respond to cidofovir or experience recurrent CMV retinitis progression during therapy with the drug.

Some cidofovir-resistant CMV isolates selected in vitro following exposure to increasing concentrations of cidofovir have been cross-resistant to ganciclovir, but remained susceptible to foscarnet. Ganciclovir-resistant or ganciclovir- and foscarnet-resistant isolates that were cross-resistant to cidofovir have been obtained from drug-naive patients and patients who were treated with ganciclovir with or without foscarnet. Although CMV strains with ganciclovir-resistance caused by mutations in DNA polymerase (UL54) are likely to be cross-resistant to cidofovir, strains with ganciclovir resistance secondary only to mutations in CMV UL97 may remain susceptible to cidofovir. Clinical isolates exhibiting high-level resistance to ganciclovir due to mutations in both CMV UL54 and UL97 have been cross-resistant to cidofovir. Cidofovir is active in vitro against some, but not all, CMV isolates resistant to foscarnet.

Advice to Patients

Advise patients that cidofovir is not a cure for cytomegalovirus (CMV) retinitis; progression of retinitis may continue during or following treatment. Advise patients that regular ophthalmologic examinations are necessary. Other manifestations of CMV disease may also occur.

Advise patients with human immunodeficiency virus (HIV) infection who are receiving zidovudine to temporarily discontinue zidovudine or decrease the zidovudine dose by 50% on days cidofovir is administered because the probenecid regimen used with each cidofovir dose reduces metabolic clearance of zidovudine.

Inform patients that the major toxicity of cidofovir is renal impairment; dosage modifications, including reduction, interruption, and, possibly, discontinuance of the drug may be required. Importance of close monitoring of renal function (routine urinalysis, serum creatinine) during cidofovir therapy.

Importance of receiving IV hydration prior to each cidofovir dose and importance of taking the recommended regimen of oral probenecid with each cidofovir dose to minimize the risk of cidofovir-associated nephrotoxicity.

Inform patients of possible adverse effects associated with the probenecid regimen, including headache, nausea, vomiting, and hypersensitivity reactions (e.g., rash, fever, chills, anaphylaxis). Advise patients that taking probenecid after a meal or concomitant use of an antiemetic may decrease nausea; antihistamines and/or acetaminophen can be used to ameliorate hypersensitivity reactions.

Inform patients that cidofovir has caused tumors (principally mammary adenocarcinomas) in rats and that the drug should be considered a potential carcinogen in humans.

Inform patients that cidofovir has caused reduced testes weight and hypospermia in animals and such effects may occur in humans and cause infertility.

Importance of informing clinician of existing or contemplated concomitant therapy, including prescription and OTC drugs, as well as any concomitant illnesses.

Importance of women informing clinicians if they are or plan to become pregnant or plan to breast-feed. Inform women of childbearing potential that cidofovir is embryotoxic in animals and should not be used during pregnancy.

Advise women of childbearing potential to use effective contraception during and for 1 month after cidofovir therapy. Advise men to practice barrier contraceptive methods during and for 3 months after cidofovir treatment.

Importance of advising patients of other important precautionary information. (See Cautions.)

Overview® (see Users Guide). For additional information on this drug until a more detailed monograph is developed and published, the manufacturer's labeling should be consulted. It is *essential* that the manufacturer's labeling be consulted for more detailed information on usual cautions, precautions, contraindications, potential drug interactions, laboratory test interferences, and acute toxicity.

Preparations

For the treatment of serious complications of smallpox vaccination† or the treatment of human monkeypox†, cidofovir is stored in the US Strategic National Stockpile (SNS). The SNS ensures that certain drugs and medical supplies are readily available to prevent or treat specific diseases, including during public health emergencies, and is managed by the US Department of Health and Human Services (HHS) Office of the Assistant Secretary for Preparedness and Response (ASPR). To request a drug from the SNS, state health departments can contact the US Centers for Disease Control and Prevention (CDC) Emergency Operations Center at 770-488-7100 or the HHS Secretary's Operations Center at 202-619-7800.

Excipients in commercially available drug preparations may have clinically important effects in some individuals; consult specific product labeling for details.

Cidofovir

Parenteral		
Concentrate, for injection, for IV infusion only	75 mg (of anhydrous cidofovir) per mL*	**Cidofovir Injection**

*available from one or more manufacturer, distributor, and/or repackager by generic (nonproprietary) name

†Use is not currently included in the labeling approved by the US Food and Drug Administration

Entecavir

ETV

■ Entecavir, a synthetic purine nucleoside analog derived from guanine, is an antiviral agent that is active against human hepatitis B virus (HBV).

Uses

■ **Chronic Hepatitis B Virus Infection** Entecavir is used for the treatment of chronic hepatitis B virus (HBV) infection in adults and pediatric patients 2 years of age and older with evidence of active HBV replication and either persistent elevations in serum aminotransferase (ALT or AST) concentrations or histologic evidence of active liver disease.

The indication for use of entecavir in adults is based on clinical trial data in adults and adolescents 16 years of age or older with hepatitis B e antigen (HBeAg)-positive or HBeAg-negative chronic HBV infection with compensated liver disease who were nucleoside-naive (had not previously received treatment with nucleoside antivirals) or had lamivudine-refractory HBV; although most study patients had compensated liver disease, a limited number had decompensated liver disease. The indication for use of the drug in pediatric patients is based on clinical trial data in nucleoside-naive pediatric patients 2 years of age and older and in a limited number of lamivudine-experienced patients with HBeAg-positive chronic HBV infection and compensated liver disease.

Entecavir has not been evaluated for the treatment of chronic HBV infection in patients with human immunodeficiency virus (HIV) coinfection who were not receiving antiretroviral therapy; the drug should *not* be used for the treatment of HBV infection in such patients. (See HBV-infected Individuals Coinfected with HIV under Warning/Precautions: Warnings, in Cautions.)

Only limited data are available regarding the efficacy and safety of entecavir for the treatment of HBV infection in liver transplant recipients. (See Liver Transplant Recipients under Uses: Chronic Hepatitis B Infection and see Liver Transplant Recipients under Warnings/Precautions: Warnings, in Cautions.)

The goal of antiviral therapy in patients with chronic HBV infection is to decrease the morbidity and mortality related to the infection (e.g., cirrhosis, hepatic failure, hepatocellular carcinoma). Sustained suppression of HBV replication has been associated with normalization of serum ALT concentrations, loss of HBeAg with or without detection of antibody to HBeAg (anti-HBe), and improvement in liver histology. Currently available therapies for chronic HBV infection (e.g., adefovir, entecavir, lamivudine, telbivudine, tenofovir alafenamide, tenofovir disoproxil fumarate [tenofovir DF], interferon alfa, peginterferon alfa) are used in an attempt to provide an immunologic cure (HBsAg loss and sustained HBV DNA suppression), but cannot provide a virologic cure (eradication of HBV).

Treatment of chronic HBV infection is complex and evolving, and specialized references and experts should be consulted. Information from the American Association for the Study of Liver Diseases (AASLD) regarding management of chronic HBV infection, including recommendations for initial treatment, is available at https://www.aasld.org.

HBeAg-Positive Adults Efficacy of entecavir for the management of HBeAg-positive chronic HBV infection was evaluated in a phase III, randomized, double-blind, active-controlled study (AI463022) in nucleoside-naive adults with active HBV replication (median baseline serum HBV DNA levels 9.66 log_{10} copies/mL), persistent elevations in serum ALT concentrations (mean serum ALT of 143 IU/L), and histologic evidence of active liver disease (mean Knodell necroinflammatory score of 7.8). Seventy-five percent of patients in the study were male, 57% were Asian, 40% were Caucasian, and 13% had prior treatment with interferon alfa.

Data analysis at 48 weeks indicated that 72% of patients who received entecavir in a dosage of 0.5 mg daily had histologic improvement (defined as a reduction of at least 2 points in the Knodell necroinflammatory score with no concurrent worsening of the Knodell fibrosis score) compared with 62% of those who received lamivudine in a dosage of 100 mg daily. Sixty-eight percent of patients receiving entecavir (0.5 mg daily) had normal serum ALT concentrations (i.e., biochemical response) at week 48 compared with 60% of those receiving lamivudine (100 mg daily). In addition, the mean decrease in serum HBV DNA levels from baseline was 6.86 log_{10} copies/mL at week 48 in those receiving entecavir compared with a decrease of 5.39 log_{10} copies/mL in those receiving lamivudine. Sixty-seven percent of patients who received entecavir had undetectable levels of serum HBV DNA (defined as less than 300 copies/mL by a polymerase chain reaction [PCR] assay) at week 48 compared with 36% of those who received lamivudine. Seroconversion to anti-HBe also occurred in 21 or 18% of patients who received entecavir or lamivudine, respectively. The optimal duration of therapy with entecavir is not known. According to the study protocol, patients who met the response criteria (determined at 48 weeks based on HBV virologic suppression [less than 0.7 MEq/mL by bDNA assay] and loss of HBeAg [in HBeAg-positive patients] or ALT normalization [less than 1.25 times the upper limit of normal in HBeAg-negative patients]) discontinued therapy at week 52 while patients who did not meet the response criteria continued treatment through week 96 or until they met the response criteria. Twenty-one percent of patients treated with entecavir who met the response criteria discontinued entecavir at 52 weeks per protocol; 82% of these patients maintained such a response during an additional 24 weeks of posttreatment follow-up. Approximately 69% of patients treated with entecavir continued treatment for up to 96 weeks; 74% of these patients had undetectable levels of serum HBV DNA after the last dose of the drug and 79% had normal ALT concentrations. Seroconversion to anti-HBe occurred in 11% of patients receiving entecavir.

HBeAg-Negative Adults Efficacy of entecavir for the management of HBeAg-negative, anti-HBe- and HBV-DNA-positive chronic HBV infection was evaluated in a phase III, randomized, double-blind, active-controlled study (AI463027) in nucleoside-naive adults with active HBV replication (median baseline serum HBV DNA levels 7.58 log_{10} copies/mL by a PCR-based assay), persistent elevations in serum ALT concentrations (mean serum ALT of 142 IU/L), and histologic evidence of active liver disease (mean Knodell necroinflammatory score of 7.8). Seventy-six percent of patients in the study were male, 58% were Caucasian, 39% were Asian, and 13% had prior treatment with interferon alfa.

Data analysis at 48 weeks indicated that 70% of patients who received entecavir (0.5 mg daily) had histologic improvement (defined as a reduction of at least 2 points in the Knodell necroinflammatory score with no concurrent worsening of the Knodell fibrosis score) compared with 61% of those who received lamivudine (100 mg daily). Serum ALT concentrations also normalized at week 48 in 78% of patients who received entecavir compared with 71% of those who received lamivudine. In addition, the mean decrease in serum HBV DNA levels from baseline was 5.04 log_{10} copies/mL at week 48 in patients receiving entecavir compared with a mean decrease of 4.53 log_{10} copies/mL in those receiving lamivudine. Ninety percent of patients who received entecavir had undetectable levels of serum HBV DNA (defined as less than 300 copies/mL by PCR assay) at week 48 compared with 72% of those who received lamivudine. Eighty-five percent of patients treated with entecavir met the response criteria (determined at 48 weeks based on HBV virologic suppression [less than 0.7 MEq/mL by bDNA assay] and loss of HBeAg) and discontinued entecavir at 52 weeks per protocol; very few of these patients had undetectable levels of serum HBV DNA and 46% of patients maintained normal ALT concentrations during an additional 24 weeks of follow-up.

Adults with Lamivudine-refractory HBV Entecavir has been evaluated for the treatment of lamivudine-refractory chronic HBV infection in a phase III, randomized, double-blind, active-controlled study (AI463026) in adults with active HBV replication (median baseline serum HBV DNA levels 9.36 log_{10} copies/mL), persistent elevations in serum ALT concentrations (mean serum ALT of 128 IU/L), and histologic evidence of compensated liver disease (mean Knodell necroinflammatory score of 6.5). Seventy-six percent of patients in the study were male, 37% were Asian, 62% were Caucasian, and 52% had prior treatment with interferon alfa.

Patients in the study had previously received lamivudine therapy for a mean duration of 2.7 years and lamivudine-resistant mutations were identified at baseline in 85% of patients. Patients were randomized to switch (without a washout or an overlap period) from lamivudine to entecavir (1 mg daily) or to continue lamivudine (100 mg daily) for 52 weeks. Data analysis at 48 weeks indicated that 55% of patients switched to entecavir had histologic improvement (defined as a reduction of at least 2 points in the Knodell necroinflammatory score with no concurrent worsening of the Knodell fibrosis score) compared with 28% of those who continued to receive lamivudine. Sixty-one percent of patients receiving entecavir had normal serum ALT concentrations (i.e., biochemical response) at week 48 compared with 15% of those receiving lamivudine. In addition, the mean decrease in serum HBV DNA levels from baseline was 5.11 log_{10} copies/mL at week 48 in those receiving entecavir compared with a decrease of 0.48 log_{10} copies/mL in those receiving lamivudine. Nineteen percent of patients who received entecavir had undetectable levels of serum HBV DNA (defined as less than 300 copies/mL by PCR assay) at week 48 compared with 1% of those who received lamivudine. Seroconversion to anti-HBe occurred in 8 or 3% of patients who received entecavir or lamivudine, respectively. Approximately 55% of patients treated with entecavir continued treatment for up to 96 weeks; 40% of these patients had undetectable levels of serum HBV DNA, 81% had normal ALT concentrations, and 10% achieved seroconversion.

Adults with Decompensated Liver Disease Entecavir has been evaluated for the treatment of chronic HBV infection in patients with decompensated liver disease in a randomized, open-label study (AI463048). The study included 191 adults with HBeAg-positive or HBeAg-negative chronic HBV infection and evidence of hepatic decompensation (Child-Turcotte-Pugh score of 7 or higher) (mean age 52 years, 74% male, 54% Asian, 33% Caucasian, 5% black, baseline HBV DNA levels 7.83 log_{10} copies/mL, mean ALT concentration 100 U/L, 54% HBeAg-positive, 35% with evidence of lamivudine resistance, baseline mean Child-Turcotte-Pugh score 8.6). Patients were randomized to receive entecavir 1 mg once daily or adefovir dipivoxil 10 mg once daily. At 48 weeks, 57 or 20% of patients receiving entecavir or adefovir dipivoxil, respectively, achieved undetectable levels of HBV DNA (less than 300 copies/mL [the lower limit of quantification]) and 61 or 67% of patients, respectively, had stable or improved Child-Turcotte-Pugh scores.

HBeAg-Positive Pediatric Patients Efficacy, safety, and pharmacokinetics of entecavir in pediatric patients were initially evaluated in 53 pediatric patients 2 years to less than 18 years of age with chronic HBV infection (HBeAg-positive) with compensated liver disease and elevated ALT concentration (study AI463028); 24 patients were treatment-naive and 19 patients were previously treated with lamivudine (lamivudine-experienced). Nucleoside-naive (had not previously received treatment with nucleoside antivirals) patients received entecavir in a dosage of 0.015 mg/kg (up to 0.5 mg) once daily and lamivudine-experienced patients received 0.03 mg/kg (up to 1 mg) once daily. At 48 weeks, 58 or 47% of treatment-naive or lamivudine-experienced patients, respectively, achieved HBV DNA levels less than 50 IU/mL; ALT concentrations normalized in 83 or 95% of patients, respectively.

Efficacy and safety of entecavir in pediatric patients were confirmed in an ongoing randomized, placebo-controlled, double-blind study (AI463189) in 180 pediatric patients 2 years to less than 18 years of age who were nucleoside-naive with HBeAg-positive chronic HBV infection, compensated liver disease, and elevated ALT concentrations (mean HBV DNA levels 8.1 log_{10} IU/mL, mean ALT concentrations 103 U/L). Patients were randomized in a 2:1 ratio to receive entecavir in a dosage of 0.015 mg/kg (up to 0.5 mg) once daily or placebo. At 48 weeks, 24% of patients receiving entecavir met the composite primary efficacy end point of HBeAg seroconversion *and* serum HBV DNA levels less than 50 IU/mL. An HBV DNA level less than 50 IU/mL was achieved in 46 or 2% of patients receiving entecavir or placebo, respectively; ALT normalization and HBeAg seroconversion were attained in 67 or 24%, respectively, of patients receiving entecavir compared with 22 or 12%, respectively, of patients receiving placebo.

HBV-infected Individuals Coinfected with HIV Efficacy of entecavir for the treatment of chronic HBV infection in HIV-infected patients was evaluated in a phase III, randomized, double-blind, active-controlled study (AI463038) in patients receiving highly active antiretroviral therapy (HAART) that included lamivudine. These HIV-infected patients had recurrent HBV viremia (99% were HBeAg-positive), active HBV replication (median baseline serum HBV DNA levels 9.13 log_{10} copies/mL), and persistent elevations in serum ALT concentrations (mean serum ALT of 71.5 IU/L). Patients continued HAART (including lamivudine 300 mg daily) and were randomized to receive concurrent therapy with entecavir (1 mg daily) or placebo for 24 weeks followed by an additional 24-week open-label period during which all patients received entecavir (1 mg daily).

Analysis of limited data at 24 weeks indicated that 6% of patients who received entecavir in conjunction with lamivudine-containing HAART had undetectable levels of serum HBV DNA (defined as less than 300 copies/mL by PCR assay) compared with 0% of those who received placebo and lamivudine-containing HAART. Thirty-four percent of patients receiving the regimen that included entecavir had normal serum ALT concentrations (i.e., biochemical response) at week 24 compared with 8% of those who did not receive entecavir. In addition, the mean decrease in serum HBV DNA levels from baseline was 3.65 log_{10} copies/mL at week 24 in those receiving the regimen that included entecavir compared with an increase of 0.11 log_{10} copies/mL in those receiving a lamivudine-containing HAART regimen alone. Median serum HIV-1 RNA levels remained stable at approximately 2 log_{10}/mL during the 24-week blinded study period.

HBV-infected patients coinfected with HIV often have higher HBV viral loads, more rapid disease progression, and an increased risk of HBV-related liver complications and death than those not infected with HIV. Decisions regarding when to initiate treatment of HBV and which HBV treatment regimen to use in HIV-infected patients must be individualized and such patients should be treated in consultation with an expert.

Entecavir should *not* be used for the treatment of HBV infection in HIV-infected patients who are not receiving antiretroviral therapy. Although the drug has not been systematically evaluated in HIV-infected patients with HBV who were *not* receiving concomitant antiretroviral therapy, limited clinical experience suggests there is a potential for development of HIV resistance in such patients. (See HBV-infected Individuals Coinfected with HIV under Warning/Precautions: Warnings, in Cautions.)

Liver Transplant Recipients Efficacy and safety of entecavir in liver transplant recipients were evaluated in a single-arm, open-label trial that included 65 patients who received a liver transplant for complications of chronic HBV infection. Patients had HBV DNA levels less than 172 IU/mL and 89% had HBeAg-negative disease at the time of transplant; mean age was 49 years, 82% were male, 39% were white, and 37% were Asian. All patients received entecavir 1 mg once daily in addition to usual posttransplant management, including hepatitis B immune globulin (HBIG). Of the 53 patients who completed the trial and had HBV DNA levels tested at or after 72 weeks of posttransplant treatment, all achieved HBV DNA levels less than 50 IU/mL. Of the 61 evaluable patients, all lost HBsAg posttransplant and 2 patients experienced recurrence of measurable HBsAg without recurrence of HBV viremia.

Dosage and Administration

■ **Administration** Entecavir is administered orally.

Because presence of food in the GI tract may decrease the rate and extent of absorption, entecavir should be administered on an empty stomach at least 2 hours before or 2 hours after meals.

The oral solution should be administered using the oral dosing spoon according to the patient instructions provided by the manufacturer. The oral solution contains 0.05 mg of entecavir per mL and should *not* be diluted or mixed with water or any other liquid.

■ **Dosage** ***Adult Dosage*** **Chronic Hepatitis B Virus Infection.** For the treatment of chronic hepatitis B virus (HBV) infection in nucleoside-naive (have not previously received treatment with nucleoside antivirals) adults with compensated liver disease, the recommended dosage of entecavir is 0.5 mg once daily. Adults with compensated liver disease and a history of HBV viremia while receiving lamivudine or with HBV known to have lamivudine- or telbivudine-associated resistance mutations (rtM204I/V ± rtL180M, rtL80I/V, or rtV173L) should receive entecavir in a dosage of 1 mg once daily.

For the treatment of HBV infection in adults with decompensated liver disease, the recommended dosage of entecavir is 1 mg once daily.

The optimal duration of entecavir therapy in patients with chronic HBV infection is not known.

Pediatric Dosage **Chronic Hepatitis B Virus Infection.** Dosage of entecavir for the treatment of chronic HBV infection in pediatric patients 2 years of age and older weighing at least 10 kg is based on weight. (See Table 1.) For patients weighing 30 kg or less, entecavir oral solution should be used.

Table 1: Dosage of Entecavir for Treatment of HBV Infection in Pediatric Patients 2 Years of Age or Older Weighing 10 kg or More

Body Weight	Dosage of Oral Solution Containing 0.05 mg/mL in Treatment-naive Patients	Dosage of Oral Solution Containing 0.05 mg/mL in Lamivudine-experienced Patients
10–11 kg	0.15 mg (3 mL) once daily	0.3 mg (6 mL) once daily
>11 to 14 kg	0.2 mg (4 mL) once daily	0.4 mg (8 mL) once daily
>14 to 17 kg	0.25 mg (5 mL) once daily	0.5 mg (10 mL) once daily
>17 to 20 kg	0.3 mg (6 mL) once daily	0.6 mg (12 mL) once daily
>20 to 23 kg	0.35 mg (7 mL) once daily	0.7 mg (14 mL) once daily
>23 to 26 kg	0.4 mg (8 mL) once daily	0.8 mg (16 mL) once daily
>26 to 30 kg	0.45 mg (9 mL) once daily	0.9 mg (18 mL) once daily
>30 kg	0.5 mg (10 mL) once daily[a]	1 mg (20 mL) once daily[b]

[a] Treatment-naive pediatric patients weighing more than 30 kg may receive 0.5 mg (10 mL) of entecavir oral solution containing 0.05 mg/mL once daily *or* one 0.5-mg tablet of entecavir once daily.

[b] Lamivudine-experienced pediatric patients weighing more than 30 kg may receive 1 mg (20 mL) of entecavir oral solution containing 0.05 mg/mL once daily *or* one 1-mg tablet of entecavir once daily.

For the treatment of chronic HBV infection in nucleoside-naive (have not previously received treatment with nucleoside antivirals) adolescents 16 years of age and older, the recommended dosage of entecavir is 0.5 mg once daily. Adolescents 16 years of age and older with a history of HBV viremia while receiving lamivudine or with HBV known to have lamivudine- or telbivudine-associated resistance mutations (rtM204I/V ± rtL180M, rtL80I/V, or rtV173L) should receive entecavir in a dosage of 1 mg once daily.

The optimal duration of entecavir therapy in patients with chronic HBV infection is not known.

■ **Special Populations** ***Hepatic Impairment*** Dosage adjustments are not necessary in patients with hepatic impairment.

Renal Impairment Dosage of entecavir should be adjusted in adults with preexisting renal impairment (i.e., baseline creatinine clearances less than 50 mL/minute), including patients undergoing hemodialysis or continuous ambulatory peritoneal dialysis (CAPD). (See Table 2.) The manufacturer states that the once-daily regimens are preferred.

Table 2. Dosage of Entecavir for Treatment of HBV Infection in Adults with Renal Impairment

Creatinine Clearance (mL/min)	Nucleoside-naive Individuals	Lamivudine-refractory HBV or Decompensated Liver Disease
30 to <50	0.25 mg once daily[a] *or* 0.5 mg once every 48 hours	0.5 mg once daily *or* 1 mg once every 48 hours
10 to <30	0.15 mg once daily[a] *or* 0.5 mg once every 72 hours	0.3 mg once daily[a] *or* 1 mg once every 72 hours
<10, undergoing hemodialysis[b] or CAPD	0.05 mg once daily[a] *or* 0.5 mg once every 7 days	0.1 mg once daily[a] *or* 1 mg once every 7 days

[a] For doses less than 0.5 mg, entecavir oral solution should be used.

[b] When a dose is indicated on a hemodialysis day, the dose should be given after the hemodialysis session.

Although data are insufficient to recommend specific dosage adjustments in pediatric patients 2 years of age or older with renal impairment, the manufacturer states that dose reductions or increases in dosing interval similar to those recommended for adults with renal impairment should be considered.

Geriatric Patients Dosage of entecavir for geriatric patients should be selected with caution because of possible age-related decreases in renal function and patients should be monitored closely. (See Geriatric Use under Warnings/Precautions: Specific Populations, in Cautions.)

Cautions

■ **Contraindications** The manufacturers state there are no known contraindications to use of entecavir.

■ **Warnings/Precautions** ***Warnings*** **Exacerbations of Hepatitis.** Severe acute exacerbations of hepatitis have been reported following discontinuance of hepatitis B virus (HBV) therapy, including entecavir therapy.

In studies that evaluated safety of entecavir, exacerbations of hepatitis or ALT flare was defined as ALT elevations greater than 10 times the upper limit of normal (ULN) and greater than 2 times baseline serum concentrations. In clinical studies (AI463022, AI463027, AI463026), ALT flare occurred in 2, 8, or 12% of nucleoside-naive HBeAg-positive, nucleoside-naive HBeAg-negative, or lamivudine-refractory patients, respectively, following discontinuance of entecavir. The median time to exacerbations of hepatitis was 23 weeks. Rates of post-treatment ALT flare may be higher if entecavir therapy is discontinued without regard to previous response to therapy.

Exacerbations of hepatitis also have been reported during entecavir treatment of HBV, but generally resolved with continued therapy. In clinical studies, exacerbations of hepatitis (e.g., ALT elevations greater than 10 times the ULN and greater than 2 times baseline serum concentrations) occurring during therapy generally were associated with a reduction in viral load of at least of 2 $\log_{10}$ copies/mL that preceded or coincided with the ALT elevations.

Hepatic function should be closely monitored with both clinical and laboratory follow-up for at least several months after entecavir is discontinued. If appropriate, resumption of anti-HBV therapy may be warranted.

HBV-infected Individuals Coinfected with HIV. Use of entecavir for treatment of chronic HBV infection in patients with unrecognized or untreated human immunodeficiency virus (HIV) infection may result in emergence of HIV isolates with resistance to HIV nucleoside reverse transcriptase inhibitors (NRTIs).

Prior to initiation of entecavir therapy, all patients should be offered HIV testing.

Entecavir has not been systematically evaluated in HBV-infected patients coinfected with HIV who were not receiving concomitant antiretroviral therapy.

Because of the possible risk of emergence of NRTI-resistant HIV, entecavir should *not* be used for the treatment of HBV in HIV-infected patients who are not receiving antiretroviral therapy.

Entecavir has not been systematically evaluated for the treatment of HIV infection and such use is not recommended.

Lactic Acidosis and Severe Hepatomegaly with Steatosis. Lactic acidosis and severe hepatomegaly with steatosis, including some fatalities, have been reported in patients receiving nucleoside analogs alone or in conjunction with antiretrovirals. Most reported cases have involved women; obesity and long-term therapy with nucleoside reverse transcriptase inhibitors also may be risk factors.

Lactic acidosis in patients receiving entecavir often is reported in association with hepatic decompensation, other serious medical conditions, or drug exposures. Patients with decompensated liver disease may be at higher risk of lactic acidosis.

Nucleoside analogs should be used with particular caution in patients with known risk factors for liver disease; however, lactic acidosis and severe hepatomegaly with steatosis have been reported in patients with no known risk factors.

Entecavir therapy should be discontinued in any patient with clinical or laboratory findings suggestive of lactic acidosis or pronounced hepatotoxicity (which may include hepatomegaly and steatosis even in the absence of marked aminotransferase elevations).

Liver Transplant Recipients. Limited data are available regarding safety and efficacy of entecavir in liver transplant recipients. In an open-label, post-liver transplant trial, the frequency and nature of adverse events were consistent with those expected in patients who have received a liver transplant and the known safety profile of entecavir.

If entecavir is necessary in liver transplant recipients who have received or are receiving an immunosuppressive agent that may affect renal function (e.g., cyclosporine, tacrolimus), renal function should be carefully monitored prior to and during entecavir treatment. (See Drug Interactions: Immunosuppressive Agents.)

Specific Populations **Pregnancy.** Category C. (See Users Guide)

To monitor maternal-fetal outcomes of pregnant women exposed to entecavir, clinicians are encouraged to contact the pregnancy registry at 800-258-4263 to enroll such women.

There are no adequate, well-controlled studies of entecavir in pregnant women. The drug should be used during pregnancy only if potential benefits justify potential risks to the fetus.

There was no evidence of teratogenicity in rats or rabbits at entecavir exposures approximately 28 or 212 times, respectively, human exposures achieved at the highest recommended human dose of 1 mg daily.

The American Association for the Study of Liver Diseases (AASLD) and other experts state that recommendations regarding antiviral therapy for the management of HBV infection in pregnant women generally are the same as those for other adults. AASLD also suggests that hepatitis B surface antigen (HBsAg)-positive pregnant women with HBV DNA levels exceeding 200,000 IU/mL receive antiviral therapy since this may reduce the risk of perinatal transmission of HBV; however, preferred antiviral agents, exact viral load threshold, and optimal gestational week during the third trimester to initiate such therapy have not been clearly identified.

Data are not available regarding the effect of entecavir therapy during pregnancy on transmission of HBV to the infant. Routine screening for HBV infection is recommended for *all* pregnant women. For prevention of perinatal transmission of HBV, the US Public Health Service Advisory Committee on Immunization Practices (ACIP), American Academy of Pediatrics (AAP), and other experts state that infants born to HBsAg-positive women should receive their first dose of hepatitis B vaccine *and* a dose of hepatitis B immune globulin (HBIG) within 12 hours of birth.

Lactation. Entecavir is distributed into milk in rats; it is not known whether the drug is distributed into human milk.

A decision should be made to discontinue nursing or entecavir, taking into account the importance of the drug to the woman.

Pediatric Use. Safety and efficacy of entecavir have not been established in children younger than 2 years of age.

The manufacturer states that only limited data are available on use of entecavir in lamivudine-experienced pediatric patients and the drug should be used in such patients only if potential benefits justify potential risks to the child. Since some pediatric patients may require long-term or lifetime management of chronic active HBV infection, consideration should be given to the impact of entecavir use on future treatment options.

Geriatric Use. Experience in those 65 years of age and older is insufficient to determine whether they respond differently than younger adults.

Entecavir should be used with caution in geriatric patients. The drug is substantially excreted by the kidneys, and the risk of entecavir-induced toxicity may be increased in patients with impaired renal function. Because geriatric patients may have decreased renal function, select dosage based on degree of renal impairment; it also may be useful to monitor renal function in such patients. (See Dosage and Administration: Special Populations.)

Renal Impairment. Dosage adjustments are recommended for patients with creatinine clearance less than 50 mL/minute, including patients undergoing hemodialysis or continuous ambulatory peritoneal dialysis (CAPD). (See Renal Impairment under Dosage and Administration: Special Populations.)

Hispanic Patients. The manufacturers state that safety and efficacy of entecavir have not been established in the US Hispanic population because of low enrollment of such patients in clinical trials.

Race. There are no substantial race-related differences in entecavir pharmacokinetics.

■ **Common Adverse Effects** Adverse effects reported in 3% or more of patients with compensated liver disease who received entecavir in clinical trials include headache, fatigue, dizziness, and nausea. Diarrhea, dyspepsia, vomiting, somnolence, and insomnia also have been reported. The most common laboratory abnormalities reported in clinical trials of entecavir are ALT elevations (greater than 5 times the ULN), hematuria, lipase elevations (at least 2.1 times the ULN), glycosuria, hyperbilirubinemia (greater than 2 times the ULN), ALT elevations (greater than 10 times the ULN and greater than 2 times baseline serum concentrations), fasting hyperglycemia (greater than 250 mg/dL), and creatinine increases (at least 0.5 mg/dL).

Adverse effects reported in 10% or more of patients with decompensated liver disease who received entecavir in clinical trials include peripheral edema, ascites, pyrexia, hepatic encephalopathy, and upper respiratory infection.

Drug Interactions

■ **Drugs Affecting or Metabolized by Hepatic Microsomal Enzymes** Entecavir is not a substrate for and does not inhibit or induce cytochrome P-450 (CYP) isoenzymes. Entecavir does not inhibit CYP isoenzymes 1A2, 2C9, 2C19, 2D6, 3A4, 2B6, or 2E1. Entecavir does not induce CYP isoenzymes 1A2, 2C9, 2C19, 3A4, 3A5, or 2B6. Pharmacokinetic interactions with drugs metabolized by CYP isoenzymes are unlikely.

■ **Nephrotoxic Drugs or Drugs Eliminated by Renal Excretion** Potential pharmacokinetic interactions with drugs that reduce renal function or that may compete with entecavir for active renal tubular secretion; increased serum concentrations of entecavir or the concomitantly used drug may occur. Although the effect of concomitant use of such drugs with entecavir has not been specifically studied, patients receiving entecavir in conjunction with other drugs that may affect renal function or are excreted renally should be monitored closely for adverse effects.

■ **Adefovir Dipivoxil** No clinically important pharmacokinetic interactions with adefovir dipivoxil.

■ **Antiretroviral Agents** ***HIV Nucleoside and Nucleotide Reverse Transcriptase Inhibitors (NRTIs)*** No pharmacokinetic interactions between entecavir and lamivudine or tenofovir disoproxil fumarate (tenofovir DF).

In vitro evidence indicates that concurrent use of human immunodeficiency virus (HIV) nucleoside reverse transcriptase inhibitors (NRTIs) and entecavir is unlikely to reduce the antiretroviral activity of the HIV NRTIs (abacavir, didanosine, lamivudine, stavudine, tenofovir, zidovudine) against HIV.

In vitro, concurrent use of HIV NRTIs (abacavir, didanosine, lamivudine, stavudine, tenofovir, zidovudine) does not reduce or antagonize the antiviral activity of entecavir against HBV.

■ **Immunosuppressive Agents** Possible pharmacokinetic interactions with cyclosporine or tacrolimus (increased entecavir serum concentrations because of altered renal function).

In a small pilot study, entecavir exposures in HBV-infected liver transplant recipients receiving a stable dose of cyclosporine or tacrolimus were approximately twofold higher than those observed in healthy individuals with normal renal function. Altered renal function contributed to the increase in entecavir exposure in these patients. The potential for pharmacokinetic interactions between entecavir and cyclosporine or tacrolimus was not formally evaluated.

Renal function should be monitored prior to and during entecavir treatment in patients (e.g., transplant patients) receiving cyclosporine, tacrolimus, or other immunosuppressive agents that may affect renal function.

Pharmacokinetics

■ **Absorption** ***Bioavailability*** Entecavir is well absorbed following oral administration.

Peak plasma concentrations are attained within 0.5–1.5 hours after a dose. Steady-state concentrations are achieved after 6–10 days of once-daily administration with approximately 2-fold accumulation.

Commercially available entecavir tablets and oral solution are bioequivalent.

Food Food delays absorption, decreases peak plasma concentrations, and decreases the area under the plasma concentration-time curve (AUC) of entecavir.

■ **Distribution** ***Extent*** Entecavir is extensively distributed into tissues.

Entecavir is distributed into milk in rats; it is not known whether the drug is distributed into human milk.

Plasma Protein Binding Entecavir is approximately 13% bound to serum proteins in vitro.

■ **Elimination** ***Metabolism*** Following oral administration, entecavir undergoes phosphorylation by cellular enzymes to form the active metabolite, entecavir triphosphate.

Entecavir is partially metabolized to glucuronide and sulfate conjugates.

Elimination Route Entecavir is excreted principally in urine by both glomerular filtration and tubular secretion. Approximately 62–73% of an oral dose is eliminated unchanged in urine.

Hemodialysis removes approximately 13% of a dose in 4 hours; CAPD removes approximately 0.3% of a dose over 7 days.

Half-life The terminal elimination half-life of entecavir is approximately 128–149 hours.

Special Populations Adults with moderate or severe hepatic impairment (without hepatitis B virus [HBV] infection): Pharmacokinetics of entecavir are similar to those reported in adults without hepatic impairment.

Adults with impaired renal function (without HBV infection): Entecavir plasma concentrations and AUC are increased and clearance of the drug is decreased compared with adults without renal impairment..

Geriatric adults: AUC of entecavir is increased compared with younger adults, possibly as the result of age-related changes in renal function.

Pediatric patients 2 years to less than 18 years of age with compensated liver disease: Entecavir exposures in those who are nucleoside inhibitor-naive receiving the oral solution in a dosage of 0.015 mg/kg (up to 0.5 mg) once daily are similar to exposures observed in adults receiving a 0.5-mg tablet once daily. Exposures in those who are lamivudine-experienced receiving the oral solution in a dosage of 0.03 mg/kg (up to 1 mg) once daily are similar to exposures observed in adults receiving a 1-mg tablet once daily.

Description

Entecavir, a synthetic purine nucleoside analog derived from guanine, is an antiviral agent that is active against human hepatitis B virus (HBV). The drug undergoes phosphorylation by cellular enzymes to form its active metabolite, entecavir triphosphate. By competing with the natural substrate deoxyguanosine triphosphate, entecavir triphosphate inhibits activities of HBV DNA polymerase (reverse transcriptase) including base priming, reverse transcription of the negative strand from the pregenomic messenger RNA, and synthesis of the positive strand of HBV DNA.

Entecavir is excreted principally in urine via glomerular filtration and tubular secretion. Entecavir is not a substrate for and does not inhibit or induce cytochrome P-450 (CYP) isoenzymes.

■ **Spectrum** Entecavir is active in vitro and in vivo against human HBV, including some strains of lamivudine-resistant HBV. The drug also has limited in vitro activity against certain other human viruses, including herpes simplex virus types 1 and 2 (HSV-1 and HSV-2), varicella zoster virus, and cytomegalovirus, but has not been shown to be effective in clinical infections caused by these viruses.

■ **Resistance** ***Resistance in HBV*** There is some evidence that HBV with reduced susceptibility to entecavir can develop slowly in some patients during long-term therapy. In nucleoside-naive patients receiving entecavir for up to 96 weeks, viral rebound due to resistance occurred in less than 1% of patients. In lamivudine-refractory patients, viral rebound due to entecavir resistance occurred in 1% of patients after the first year of therapy and in 9% of patients during the second year of therapy.

Resistance to entecavir occurs in a 2-step process, with initial selection of M204V/I mutation followed by amino acid substitutions at rtI169, rtT184, stS202, or rtM250.

Cross-resistance can occur among the nucleoside and nucleotide antivirals used for treatment of HBV. Lamivudine- and telbivudine-resistant HBV with reduced in vitro susceptibility to entecavir have been reported. Adefovir-resistant HBV may have reduced susceptibility to entecavir in vitro. HBV isolates from lamivudine-refractory patients who failed entecavir therapy have retained in vitro susceptibility to adefovir.

Advice to Patients

Importance of providing a copy of the manufacturer's patient information.

Importance of taking entecavir exactly as prescribed and not discontinuing or interrupting therapy unless instructed by a clinician; importance of regular medical follow-up.

Patients should be advised that deterioration of liver disease has occurred when entecavir therapy is discontinued and that any change in treatment should be discussed with the clinician.

Importance of taking entecavir on an empty stomach at least 2 hours before or 2 hours after meals, preferably at the same time each day.

Importance of protecting oral solution from light. Importance of using the calibrated dosing spoon provided, holding the spoon in a vertical position and filling it gradually to the mark corresponding to the prescribed dose, and rinsing it well after each use.

Importance of liver function test monitoring and immediate reporting of potential exacerbations of hepatitis following discontinuance of entecavir therapy.

Importance of immediately reporting any signs or symptoms of lactic acidosis (e.g., weakness/fatigue, unusual muscle pain, trouble breathing, stomach pain with nausea and vomiting, feeling cold especially in arms and legs, dizziness or feeling light-headed, fast or irregular heart beat) or hepatotoxicity (e.g., jaundice, dark urine, bowel movements light in color, anorexia, nausea, stomach pain) or any other new symptoms.

Critical nature of HBV therapy compliance. Entecavir therapy is not a cure for HBV infection. HBV transmission via sexual contact, sharing needles, or blood contamination is not prevented by entecavir therapy.

Patients should be advised of available measures to prevent spread of HBV infection to close contacts.

Importance of testing for HIV prior to initiation of entecavir therapy. Advise patients that if they have HIV infection and are not receiving effective HIV treatment, entecavir may increase the risk of HIV resistance.

Importance of informing clinicians of existing or contemplated concomitant therapy, including prescription and OTC drugs and dietary or herbal supplements, and any concomitant illnesses (e.g., renal disease).

Importance of women informing clinicians if they are or plan to become pregnant or plan to breast-feed.

Importance of informing patients of other important precautionary information. (See Cautions.)

Overview® (see Users Guide). For additional information on this drug until a more detailed monograph is developed and published, the manufacturer's labeling should be consulted. It is *essential* that the manufacturer's labeling be consulted for more detailed information on usual cautions, precautions, contraindications, potential drug interactions, laboratory test interferences, and acute toxicity.

Preparations

Excipients in commercially available drug preparations may have clinically important effects in some individuals; consult specific product labeling for details.

Entecavir

Oral		
Solution	0.05 mg/mL	**Baraclude®**, Bristol-Myers Squibb
Oral		
Tablets, film-coated	0.5 mg*	**Baraclude®**, Bristol-Myers Squibb
		Entecavir Tablets
	1 mg*	**Baraclude®**, Bristol-Myers Squibb
		Entecavir Tablets

*available from one or more manufacturer, distributor, and/or repackager by generic (nonproprietary) name

Famciclovir

■ Famciclovir (FCV), a synthetic, acyclic purine nucleoside analog antiviral, is a prodrug of the antiviral penciclovir and is active against herpesviruses and hepatitis B virus.

Uses

Oral famciclovir is used for the treatment of acute, localized herpes zoster (shingles, zoster). Oral famciclovir also is used for the treatment of genital herpes infections and for the suppression of recurrent episodes of genital herpes in immunocompetent adults. The drug also is used for the treatment of recurrent mucocutaneous herpes simplex virus (HSV) infections in adults with human immunodeficiency virus (HIV) infection. In addition, oral famciclovir is used for the episodic treatment of herpes labialis (perioral herpes, cold sores, fever blisters) in immunocompetent adults.

■ **Genital Herpes** ***Treatment of First Episodes*** Although the manufacturer states that efficacy of famciclovir for the treatment of initial episodes of genital herpes simplex virus (HSV) infection† has not been established, famciclovir is considered a drug of choice for the treatment of initial episodes of genital herpes. Because many patients with first episodes of genital herpes present with mild clinical symptoms but later develop severe or prolonged symptoms, the US Centers for Disease Control and Prevention (CDC) states that most patients with initial genital herpes should receive antiviral therapy. The CDC and some clinicians recommend that first episodes of genital herpes be treated with a regimen of oral acyclovir (400 mg 3 times daily or 200 mg 5 times daily for 7–10 days), oral famciclovir (250 mg 3 times daily given for 7–10 days), or oral valacyclovir (1 g twice daily given for 7–10 days).

Studies have been initiated to compare the relative efficacy of oral famciclovir and oral acyclovir for the treatment of initial episodes of genital herpes in immunocompetent adults, and preliminary results indicate that oral famciclovir (125, 250, 500, or 750 mg 3 times daily) is as effective as oral acyclovir (200 mg 5 times daily) in terms of time to complete healing of lesions, resolution of symptoms, and time to cessation of viral shedding.

Episodic Treatment of Recurrent Episodes Oral famciclovir is used in the treatment of recurrent episodes of genital herpes in immunocompetent adults. Antiviral therapy for recurrent genital herpes can be given episodically to ameliorate or shorten the duration of lesions or can be given continuously as suppressive therapy to reduce the frequency of recurrences. For episodic treatment of recurrent genital herpes, the CDC and some clinicians recommend oral acyclovir (400 mg 3 times daily for 5 days, 800 mg twice daily for 5 days, or 800 mg 3 times daily for 2 days), oral famciclovir (125 mg twice daily for 5 days or 1 g twice daily for 1 day), or oral valacyclovir (500 mg twice daily for 3 days or 1 g once daily for 5 days). Episodic antiviral therapy should be initiated within 1 day of lesion onset or during the prodrome that precedes some outbreaks. The manufacturer states that patients should be advised to initiate oral famciclovir at the first sign or symptom of an episode and that there are no data on the effectiveness of the drug initiated more than 6 hours after the onset of signs and symptoms of a recurrent episode.

Efficacy of oral famciclovir for the episodic treatment of recurrent genital herpes has been evaluated in randomized double-blind, placebo-controlled studies. In one study involving 329 immunocompetent adults who self-initiated treatment within 6 hours of appearance of lesions or onset of symptoms of recurrence, the median time to lesion healing of nonaborted lesions and resolution of all symptoms was 4.3 and 3.3 days, respectively, in patients who received oral famciclovir (1 g twice daily for 1 day) compared with 6.1 and 5.4 days, respectively, in those who received placebo. The proportion of patients with aborted lesions (no development beyond erythema) was larger in the famciclovir group than in the placebo group (23 versus 13%).

Combined data from 2 studies involving 626 otherwise healthy adults who self-initiated treatment within 6 hours of appearance of lesions or onset of symptoms of recurrence indicate that the median time to lesion healing and cessation of viral shedding was 4 and 1.8 days, respectively, in patients who received oral famciclovir (125 mg twice daily for 5 days) compared with 5 and 3.4 days, respectively, in those who received placebo. The median time to resolution of all symptoms was 3.2 days in those who received famciclovir versus 3.8 days in placebo-treated patients. There is no evidence that higher dosages of famciclovir (i.e., 250 or 500 mg twice daily) provide additional benefit in terms of time to lesion healing or relief of symptoms in immunocompetent adults.

Suppressive Therapy of Recurrent Episodes Famciclovir is used for chronic suppressive therapy of recurrent genital herpes in immunocompetent adults. The CDC states that suppressive antiviral therapy can reduce the frequency of genital herpes recurrences by 70–80% in patients who have frequent recurrences (i.e., 6 or more per year) and many patients report no symptomatic outbreaks during such therapy. For chronic suppressive therapy of recurrent genital herpes, the CDC and some clinicians recommend a regimen of oral acyclovir (400 mg twice daily), oral famciclovir (250 mg twice daily), or oral valacyclovir (500 mg or 1 g once daily). The CDC states that data suggest that therapy with famciclovir or valacyclovir is as effective as acyclovir in terms of clinical outcome, although the 500 mg once-daily valacyclovir regimen might be less effective than acyclovir or other valacyclovir regimens in patients who have very frequent recurrences (i.e., 10 or more episodes per year).

In a study of patients with frequent recurrences of genital herpes infections (6 or more per year), 39 or 29% of those receiving famciclovir suppressive therapy (250 mg twice daily) were free of recurrences at 6 or 12 months, respectively, and 10 or 6% of those receiving placebo were free of recurrences at these time points. Safety and efficacy of oral famciclovir for suppressive therapy of recurrent genital herpes infections have been established in patients receiving daily therapy for up to 1 year.

HIV-Infected Individuals Immunocompromised individuals may have prolonged or severe episodes of genital, perianal, or oral herpes; HSV lesions are common in those with human immunodeficiency virus (HIV) infection and may be severe, painful, and atypical. (See Uses: Mucocutaneous Herpes Simplex Virus Infections.)

The CDC states that episodic treatment or suppressive therapy with oral antiviral agents often is beneficial in HIV-infected individuals with genital herpes. While the drugs of choice for episodic treatment or suppressive therapy of genital herpes in HIV-infected individuals are the same as those in immunocompetent adults, higher dosages and/or more prolonged therapy may be necessary. For episodic treatment of recurrences of genital herpes in HIV-infected individuals, the CDC recommends a 5- to 10-day regimen of oral acyclovir (400 mg 3 times daily), oral famciclovir (500 mg twice daily), or oral valacyclovir (1 g twice daily). For daily suppressive therapy of recurrent genital herpes in HIV-infected individuals, the CDC recommends oral acyclovir (400–800 mg 2–3 times daily), oral famciclovir (500 mg twice daily), or oral valacyclovir (500 mg twice daily).

Patient Counseling and Management of Sexual Partners Counseling of infected individuals and their sex partners is critical to management of genital herpes. The goals of such counseling are to help patients understand and cope with the infection and to prevent sexual and perinatal transmission of the virus. Antiviral therapy offers clinical benefit to most symptomatic patients and is the mainstay of management; however, genital herpes is a recurrent, life-long viral infection. Although antiviral therapy can be used to control the symptoms and signs of genital herpes episodes, it cannot eradicate latent HSV or affect the risk, frequency, or severity of recurrences of genital herpes when antiviral therapy is discontinued.

The majority of genital herpes infections are transmitted by individuals unaware that they have the infection or by individuals who are asymptomatic when transmission occurs. Patients should be advised that famciclovir is not a cure for genital herpes, and there are no data evaluating whether famciclovir prevents transmission of HSV to others. Because genital herpes is a sexually transmitted disease, patients should be advised to avoid sexual contact with uninfected partners when lesions and/or prodromal symptoms are present. In addition, patients should be advised that sexual transmission of the virus can occur during asymptomatic periods and that suppressive antiviral therapy reduces, but does not eliminate, subclinical viral shedding.

Sex partners of individuals with genital herpes should be advised that they may be infected even if they have no symptoms. Asymptomatic partners of patients with genital herpes should be questioned regarding a history of genital lesions, educated to recognize symptoms of genital herpes, and offered type-specific serologic testing to determine whether risk for HSV acquisition exists. Antiviral therapy is not recommended for sexual partners who do not have clinical manifestations of infection, but symptomatic sex partners of individuals with genital herpes should be evaluated and treated.

The risk for neonatal HSV infection should be discussed with all genital herpes patients, including men. Pregnant women and women of childbearing age who have genital herpes should inform their providers who care for them during pregnancy as well as those who will care for their neonates.

Information to assist patients and clinicians in counseling regarding genital herpes is available at http://www.ashastd.org and http://www.ihmf.org. For further information on treatment of initial or recurrent episodes of genital herpes or suppression of recurrent infections, see Uses: Genital Herpes in Acyclovir 8:18.32.

■ **Herpes Labialis** Famciclovir is used for the episodic treatment of herpes labialis (perioral herpes, cold sores, fever blisters) in immunocompetent adults.

Efficacy of a 1-day regimen of famciclovir was evaluated in healthy adults with a history of recurrent cold sores. Patients were randomized to famciclovir 1.5 g as a single dose, famciclovir 750 mg twice daily for 1 day, or placebo; patients self-initiated therapy within 1 hour of symptom onset. The median time to lesion healing of nonaborted lesions and resolution of symptoms (pain and tenderness) was 4.4 and 1.7 days, respectively, in patients who received the single-dose oral famciclovir regimen compared with 6.2 and 2.9 days, respectively, in those who received placebo. There was no difference between the famciclovir-treated and placebo-treated patients in aborted lesions (no development beyond the papular stage).

■ **Mucocutaneous Herpes Simplex Virus Infections** Oral famciclovir is used for the treatment of recurrent mucocutaneous HSV infections (HSV-1 and HSV-2) in HIV-infected adults. The CDC, National Institutes of Health (NIH), Infectious Diseases Society of America (IDSA), and other experts state that orolabial HSV infections in HIV-infected individuals may be treated with oral acyclovir, oral famciclovir, or oral valacyclovir. IV acyclovir usually is indicated for *initial* treatment of moderate to severe mucocutaneous HSV infections in HIV-infected individuals but may be switched to oral antiviral therapy (acyclovir, famciclovir, valacyclovir) after lesions begin to regress. If acyclovir-resistant HSV is suspected, IV foscarnet or IV cidofovir is recommended for treatment.

In a comparative study in HIV-infected patients (40% had $CD4^+$ T-cell counts below 200/mm^3) with recurrent mucocutaneous HSV infections (54% with anogenital lesions, 35% with orolabial lesions) who initiated therapy within 48 hours of the onset of lesions, oral famciclovir (500 mg twice daily for 7 days) was as effective as oral acyclovir (400 mg 5 times daily for 7 days) in reducing formation of new lesions and time to complete healing. (See HIV-infected Individuals under Uses: Genital Herpes.)

Famciclovir also has been recommended for chronic suppressive or maintenance therapy (secondary prophylaxis) against HSV disease† in HIV-infected adults or adolescents with frequent or severe recurrences. In patients with advanced HIV infection, reactivation of HSV frequently occurs and can result in chronic, persistent mucocutaneous disease that may be severe. The Prevention of Opportunistic Infections Working Group of the US Public Health Service and the Infectious Diseases Society of America (USPHS/IDSA) has established guidelines for the prevention of opportunistic infections in HIV-infected individuals that include recommendations concerning prevention of exposure to opportunistic pathogens, prevention of first disease episodes, and prevention of disease recurrence. The USPHS/IDSA does *not* recommend primary prophylaxis against initial episodes of HSV infection in HIV-infected adults, adolescents, or children. In addition, the USPHS/IDSA does not recommend routine chronic suppressive or maintenance therapy (secondary prophylaxis) against HSV disease in HIV-infected individuals since acute episodes of mucocutaneous disease generally can be treated successfully with acyclovir. However, these and other experts state that long-term prophylaxis against recurrence of HSV disease can be considered for HIV-infected adults, adolescents, and children who have frequent or severe recurrences. If secondary prophylaxis is indicated in HIV-infected adults or adolescents, the USPHS/IDSA, CDC, NIH, IDSA, and other experts recommend use of oral acyclovir, oral famciclovir, or oral valacyclovir. If indicated in infants and children, the USPHS/IDSA and other experts recommend use of oral acyclovir.

■ **Herpes Zoster (Shingles, Zoster)** Oral famciclovir is used for the treatment of acute, localized herpes zoster (shingles, zoster) in immunocompetent adults. Some clinicians suggest that the drugs of choice for the treatment of herpes zoster in immunocompetent adults are oral acyclovir, oral famciclovir, or oral valacyclovir.

Efficacy of famciclovir in the treatment of acute, localized herpes zoster has been evaluated in a randomized, double-blind, placebo-controlled trial in immunocompetent adults and in a dose-ranging, double-blind trial in immunocompetent adults who were randomized to receive oral famciclovir (250, 500, or 750 mg 3 times daily for 7 days) or oral acyclovir (800 mg every 4 hours 5 times daily for 7 days). Results of these studies indicate that famciclovir may prevent the appearance of new lesions, decrease the duration of viral shedding, decrease the duration of pain, and promote healing and crusting of lesions in immunocompetent adults with localized herpes zoster when given within 72 hours of the onset of rash, particularly if initiated within 48 hours of rash onset. Like acyclovir, famciclovir does not appear to *prevent* the development of postherpetic neuralgia; the drug significantly *decreases the median duration* of neuralgia, particularly in patients older than 50 years of age. In comparative studies, 7 days of oral therapy with famciclovir (250–750 mg 3 times daily) was comparably effective to 7 days of oral therapy with acyclovir (800 mg 5 times daily). There were no statistically significant differences in the duration of postherpetic neuralgia between famciclovir- and acyclovir-treated patients.

Oral famciclovir has been used in a limited number of patients for the treatment of ophthalmic herpes zoster† or disseminated herpes zoster† or for the treatment of herpes zoster in immunocompromised patients; however, the manufacturer states that efficacy of famciclovir for the treatment of these infections has not been established. The CDC and other experts state that oral famciclovir or oral valacyclovir is the treatment of choice for localized dermatomal herpes zoster in HIV-infected adults or adolescents.

■ **Hepatitis B Virus Infection** Famciclovir has been used for the management of chronic hepatitis B virus (HBV) infection† in a limited number of patients. The drug also has been evaluated for the control of HBV recurrence in organ or bone marrow transplant recipients†. While there is some evidence suggesting that famciclovir (250–500 mg 3 times daily) is effective for the management of HBV infection, further study is needed to establish safety and efficacy.

The CDC, NIH, IDSA, and other experts state that famciclovir is *not* recommended for the treatment of HBV infection in HIV-infected individuals since the drug is less active than lamivudine against HBV and is not active against lamivudine-resistant HBV.

Dosage and Administration

■ **Administration** Famciclovir is administered orally without regard to meals. Food does not affect the systemic bioavailability or elimination of famciclovir.

■ **Dosage** *Genital Herpes* **Treatment of First Episodes.** If oral famciclovir is used for the treatment of initial episodes of genital herpes simplex virus (HSV) infection† in immunocompetent adults or adolescents, the US Centers for Disease Control and Prevention (CDC) and other clinicians recommend that adults receive 250 mg 3 times daily for 7–10 days. The CDC states that the duration of treatment may be extended if healing is incomplete after 10 days of therapy.

In HIV-infected individuals, the CDC and other clinicians recommend a dosage of 500 mg twice daily for 7–14 days for the treatment of initial episodes of genital HSV infection.

Episodic Treatment of Recurrent Episodes. For the episodic treatment of recurrent genital herpes in immunocompetent adults, the dosage of oral famciclovir recommended by the manufacturer is 1 g twice daily for 1 day. The CDC and other clinicians recommend a dosage of 1 g twice daily for 1 day or 125 mg twice daily for 5 days.

In HIV-infected individuals, the CDC and other clinicians recommend a dosage of 500 mg twice daily for 5–10 days for the episodic treatment of recurrent genital herpes; alternatively, this dosage can be given for 7–14 days.

Patients should be advised to initiate famciclovir therapy at the first sign or symptom of an episode. Data are not available concerning efficacy of oral famciclovir initiated more than 6 hours after the onset of signs or symptoms of a recurrent episode of genital herpes.

Suppressive Therapy of Recurrent Episodes. For chronic suppressive therapy of recurrent episodes of genital herpes in immunocompetent adults, the recommended dosage of oral famciclovir is 250 mg every 12 hours.

In HIV-infected individuals, the CDC recommends a dosage of 500 mg twice daily for suppressive therapy of recurrent episodes of genital herpes. The manufacturer states that chronic suppressive therapy with oral famciclovir may be given for up to 1 year. Because the frequency of recurrent episodes diminishes over time in many patients, the CDC recommends that suppressive antiviral therapy be discontinued periodically (e.g., once yearly) to assess the need for continued therapy.

Herpes Labialis For the treatment of herpes labialis (perioral herpes, cold sores, fever blisters) in immunocompetent adults, the recommended dosage of oral famciclovir is 1.5 g given as a single dose.

Treatment should be initiated at the first prodromal symptom of a cold sore (e.g., tingling, itching, burning).

Mucocutaneous Herpes Simplex Virus Infections For the treatment of recurrent mucocutaneous HSV infections (i.e., orolabial or anogenital lesions) in adults with human immunodeficiency virus (HIV) infection, the usual dosage of oral famciclovir is 500 mg every 12 hours for 7 days. Some experts recommend a duration of 7–14 days.

If oral famciclovir is used for chronic suppressive or maintenance prophylaxis (secondary prophylaxis) of HSV† in HIV-infected adults and adolescents who have frequent or severe recurrences of HSV disease, a dosage of 250 mg twice daily has been recommended by the Prevention of Opportunistic Infections Working Group of the US Public Health Service and the Infectious Diseases Society of America (USPHS/IDSA).

Herpes Zoster For the treatment of acute, localized herpes zoster (shingles, zoster) in immunocompetent adults, the recommended dosage of oral famciclovir is 500 mg every 8 hours for 7 days.

For the treatment of local dermatomal herpes zoster in HIV-infected adults†, the CDC and other experts recommend 500 mg of famciclovir three times daily for 7–10 days.

Therapy should be initiated promptly after herpes zoster is diagnosed. Efficacy of famciclovir initiated more than 72 hours after rash onset has not been established.

■ **Dosage in Renal and Hepatic Impairment** *Dosage in Renal Impairment* Famciclovir is eliminated mainly by the kidneys via tubular secretion and glomerular filtration. In patients with moderately or severely impaired renal function, the frequency of administration of famciclovir should be decreased in response to the degree of impairment as indicated by creatinine clearance.

Because penciclovir (the active metabolite) is readily removed from plasma during hemodialysis, famciclovir should be administered after each hemodialysis session when the drug is used for the treatment of herpes zoster, treatment of recurrent mucocutaneous HSV infections in HIV-infected patients, or suppression of recurrent genital herpes. Famciclovir is administered once as a single dose after a hemodialysis session when the drug is used for the treatment of recurrent genital herpes or treatment of recurrent herpes labialis. The manufacturer recommends that a famciclovir dose (250 mg for patients with herpes zoster, 250 mg for HIV-infected patients with recurrent mucosal or cutaneous HSV infection, or 125 mg for patients receiving the drug for suppression of recurrent genital herpes) be administered following each hemodialysis session. The manufacturer recommends that a famciclovir dose (250 mg for patients with recurrent genital herpes, 250 mg for patients with recurrent herpes labialis) be administered once as a single dose after a hemodialysis session.

Genital Herpes. For episodic treatment of recurrent genital herpes in immunocompetent adults, the manufacturer states that patients with creatinine clearances of 60 mL/minute or greater may receive the usual oral famciclovir dosage of 1 g every 12 hours for 1 day. However, those with creatinine clearances of 40–59 mL/minute should receive 500 mg every 12 hours for 1 day, those with clearances of 20–39 mL/minute should receive 500 mg given as a single dose, and those with creatinine clearances less than 20 mL/minute should receive 250 mg given as a single dose.

For chronic suppressive therapy of recurrent genital herpes in immunocompetent adults with impaired renal function, the manufacturer states that patients with a creatinine clearance of 40 mL/minute or greater may receive the usual oral famciclovir dosage of 250 mg every 12 hours; those with creatinine clearances of 20–39 mL/minute or less than 20 mL/minute should receive 125 mg every 12 or 24 hours, respectively.

Herpes Labialis. For episodic treatment of recurrent herpes labialis in immunocompetent adults, the manufacturer states that patients with creatinine clearances of 60 mL/minute or greater may receive the usual oral famciclovir dosage of 1.5 g given as a single dose. However, those with creatinine clearances of 40–59 mL/minute should receive a single 750-mg dose, those with clearances of 20–39 mL/minute should receive a single 500-mg dose, and those with creatinine clearances less than 20 mL/minute should receive a single 250-mg dose.

Mucocutaneous Herpes Simplex Virus Infections. For the treatment of recurrent mucocutaneous HSV infections in HIV-infected adults with impaired renal function, the manufacturer states that patients with creatinine clearances of 40 mL/minute or greater may receive the usual oral famciclovir dosage of 500 mg every 12 hours; however those with creatinine clearances of 20–39 mL/minute should receive 500 mg once every 24 hours, and those with creatinine clearances less than 20 mL/minute should receive 250 mg once every 24 hours.

Herpes Zoster. For the treatment of localized herpes zoster in immunocompetent adults, the manufacturer states that patients with creatinine clearances of 60 mL/minute or greater may receive the usual oral famciclovir dosage of 500 mg every 8 hours. However, those with creatinine clearances of 40–59 mL/minute should receive 500 mg every 12 hours, those with creatinine clearances of 20–39 mL/minute should receive 500 mg once every 24 hours, and those with creatinine clearances less than 20 mL/minute should receive 250 mg once every 24 hours.

Dosage in Hepatic Impairment Famciclovir is metabolized mainly in the liver to the active drug penciclovir. In patients with well-compensated chronic liver disease such as chronic hepatitis, chronic alcohol abuse, or primary biliary cirrhosis, bioavailability of penciclovir was not affected. Therefore, modification of famciclovir dosage is not necessary in patients with well-compensated liver disease. The manufacturer does not make specific recommendations for patients with uncompensated hepatic impairment, since the pharmacokinetics of famciclovir has not been evaluated in these patients.

Cautions

Famciclovir is well tolerated in immunocompetent patients with herpes zoster, genital herpes, or herpes labialis with an adverse effect profile similar to that of placebo. The most common adverse effects of the drug in both types of patients are headache, nausea, and diarrhea, and adverse effects usually are mild or moderate in severity. In controlled clinical trials in immunocompetent patients with herpes zoster, less than 1% of patients discontinued famciclovir as a result of severe adverse effects.

Similar adverse effects have been reported when famciclovir was used in patients with human immunodeficiency virus (HIV) infection, and the most frequent adverse effects in these patients are headache, nausea, and diarrhea.

■ **Nervous System Effects** The most common adverse effect of famciclovir is headache, which occurred in approximately 23% of patients receiving the drug (versus in 18% of placebo recipients) in a large, controlled clinical trial for herpes zoster. Headache resulted in discontinuance of famciclovir in less than 1% of patients in clinical trials for herpes zoster or genital herpes. Fatigue was reported in 4.4% of patients receiving the drug (versus in 3.4% of placebo recipients) in a large, controlled clinical trial for herpes zoster. Dizziness, fever, paresthesia, and somnolence have occurred in patients receiving famciclovir in this clinical trial for herpes zoster.

Headache or fatigue occurred in 16 or 4%, respectively, of HIV-infected patients receiving famciclovir in clinical studies.

■ **GI Effects** The most frequent adverse GI effect of famciclovir is nausea which occurred in approximately 13% of patients receiving the drug (versus in 11.6% in placebo recipients) in a large, controlled clinical trial for herpes zoster. Nausea resulted in discontinuance of famciclovir in less than 1% of patients in clinical trials for herpes zoster or genital herpes. Diarrhea was reported in approximately 8% of patients (5% of placebo recipients) and vomiting in approximately 5% of patients (3.4% of placebo recipients) in a large, controlled clinical trial for herpes zoster. Vomiting only rarely resulted in discontinuance of famciclovir in clinical trials for herpes zoster or genital herpes. Constipation, anorexia, abdominal pain, flatulence, and dyspepsia have occurred in patients receiving famciclovir in clinical trials for herpes zoster. Acute necroticohemorrhagic pancreatitis resulting in death has been reported following famciclovir administration for severe hepatitis B virus infection in a kidney graft recipient who was receiving cyclosporine concomitantly; a causal relationship to famciclovir was not established.

Nausea, diarrhea, vomiting, or abdominal pain has been reported in 11, 7, 5, or 3%, respectively, of HIV-infected patients receiving famciclovir in clinical studies.

■ **Hepatic Effects** Increased serum concentrations of ALT (SGPT) occurred in 1.4–2.4% of patients receiving famciclovir in clinical trials for herpes zoster or genital herpes. Increased serum concentrations of alkaline phosphatase, total bilirubin, and albumin each occurred rarely in patients receiving the drug in clinical trials for herpes zoster or genital herpes.

■ **Other Adverse Effects** Pruritus occurred in approximately 4% of patients (versus in about 3% of placebo recipients) receiving famciclovir in a large, controlled clinical trial for herpes zoster. Worsening of herpes zoster manifestations or complications has been reported in patients receiving the drug. Pharyngitis, sinusitis, injury, generalized pain, rigors, back pain, and arthralgia have occurred in patients receiving famciclovir in this clinical trial for herpes zoster. Increased serum phosphate concentrations occurred in 1.6% of patients receiving famciclovir in a large, placebo-controlled clinical trial for herpes zoster, and increased serum sodium or potassium concentrations and abnormal leukocyte counts each occurred rarely in patients receiving the drug in clinical trials for herpes zoster or genital herpes. Purpura has been reported rarely.

Acute renal failure has been reported in patients with renal disease who received doses of famciclovir that were inappropriately high for their level of renal function.

■ **Precautions and Contraindications** Famciclovir is contraindicated in patients with known hypersensitivity to the drug.

The manufacturer recommends that the dosage interval of famciclovir be adjusted carefully in patients with impaired renal function to prevent drug accumulation while maintaining adequate plasma concentrations of penciclovir, the active metabolite of famciclovir. (See Dosage and Administration: Dosage in Renal and Hepatic Impairment.)

Concomitant administration of famciclovir and probenecid or other drugs that are excreted extensively by active renal tubular secretion may result in increased plasma concentrations of penciclovir.

Each 125-, 250-, or 500-mg tablet of famciclovir contains 26.9, 53.7, or 107.4 mg of lactose, respectively. Patients with a history of galactose intolerance, severe lactase deficiency, or glucose-galactose malabsorption should not be given famciclovir tablets.

■ **Pediatric Precautions** Safety and efficacy of famciclovir in children younger than 18 years of age have not been established.

■ **Geriatric Precautions** Safety and efficacy of famciclovir in geriatric patients have not been specifically studied to date; however, in clinical studies of famciclovir for the treatment of herpes zoster involving over 800 patients, approximately 56% of the patients were 50 years of age or older, 30% were 65 years of age or older, and 13% were 75 years of age and older. As in the overall population of patients, headache and nausea were the most frequently reported adverse effects among geriatric patients. Although no overall differences were observed between geriatric and younger patients in the type or frequency of adverse effects in clinical studies, the possibility that some older patients may exhibit increased sensitivity to the drug cannot be ruled out. Based on comparisons from different studies of the oral administration of famciclovir, the mean renal clearance of penciclovir (the active metabolite of famciclovir) was 22% lower and the area under the plasma concentration-time curve (AUC) for penciclovir was 40% higher in healthy geriatric individuals 65–79 years of age than in healthy younger individuals.

Clinical studies of famciclovir for the treatment of recurrent herpes simplex did not include a sufficient number of patients 65 years of age or older to determine whether geriatric patients respond differently than younger adults

Caution is advised when famciclovir is used in geriatric patients. The greater frequency of decreased hepatic, renal, and/or cardiac function and of concomitant disease and drug therapy observed in the elderly should be considered.

■ **Mutagenicity and Carcinogenicity** Famciclovir and penciclovir (the active metabolite of famciclovir) did not show evidence of genotoxicity in in vitro tests for gene mutations in bacteria (*Salmonella typhimurium* and *Escherichia coli*) or unscheduled DNA synthesis in mammalian HeLa 83 cells at doses up to 10,000 and 5000 mcg/plate, respectively. Famciclovir was not mutagenic in the L5178Y mouse lymphoma assay at a concentration of 5000 mcg/mL, in the in vivo mouse micronucleus test at a dose of 4.8 g/kg, or in the rat dominant lethal study at a dose of 5 g/kg. Famciclovir caused increases in polyploidy in human lymphocytes in vitro in the absence of chromosomal damage at a concentration of 1200 mcg/mL. Penciclovir was mutagenic in the L5178Y mouse lymphoma assay for gene mutation/chromosomal aberrations, with and without metabolic activation at a concentration of 1000 mcg/mL. In human lymphocytes, penciclovir caused chromosomal aberrations in the absence of metabolic activation at a concentration of 250 mcg/mL. Penciclovir caused an increased incidence of micronuclei in mouse bone marrow in vivo when administered IV at a dose highly toxic to bone marrow (500 mg/kg) but not when administered orally.

Two-year dietary carcinogenicity studies of famciclovir were performed in rats and mice. After 7–8 months of drug administration, dosage was decreased from 750 to 600 mg/kg daily in female rats and in male and female mice and from 300 to 240 mg/kg daily in male rats to ensure long-term survival. An increase in the incidence of mammary adenocarcinoma was seen in female rats receiving 600 mg/kg daily (1.5–9 times the human systemic exposure at the recommended oral dosage of 500 mg 3 times daily or 125 mg twice daily based on the 24-hour AUC for penciclovir). Marginal increases in the incidence of subcutaneous tissue fibrosarcomas or squamous cell carcinomas of the skin were seen in female rats and male mice, respectively, at a dosage of 600 mg/kg daily (0.4–2.4 times the human systemic exposure based on the 24-hour AUC for penciclovir). No increases in tumor incidence occurred in male rats receiving dosages up to 240 mg/kg daily (0.9–5.4 times the human systemic exposure) or in female mice receiving dosages up to 600 mg/kg daily (0.4–2.4 times the human systemic exposure).

There currently is no evidence of mutagenicity or carcinogenicity in humans.

■ **Pregnancy, Fertility, and Lactation** Reproduction studies using oral famciclovir dosages up to 1 g/kg daily in rats and rabbits (approximately 3.6–21.6 and 1.8–10.8 times the human systemic exposure to penciclovir, respectively, based on AUC comparisons) and IV dosages of 360 mg/kg daily in rats (2–12 times the human dose based on body surface area comparisons) or 120 mg/kg daily in rabbits (1.5–9 times the human dose based on body surface area comparisons) have not revealed evidence of adverse effects on embryofetal development. Similar studies using IV penciclovir dosages up to 80 mg/kg daily in rats (0.4–2.6 times the human dose based on body surface area comparisons) or 60 mg/kg daily in rabbits (0.7–4.2 times the human dose based on body surface area comparisons) also did not reveal evidence of adverse effects on embryofetal development. There are no adequate and well-controlled studies to date using famciclovir in pregnant women, and the drug should be used during pregnancy only when clearly needed.

To monitor maternal-fetal outcome of pregnant women exposed to famciclovir, the manufacturer maintains a Famciclovir Pregnancy Registry. The registry may be contacted by calling 888-669-6682.

Reproduction studies using famciclovir or penciclovir in rats, mice, and dogs revealed evidence of testicular toxicity following repeated oral administration of high dosages. Testicular changes, including atrophy of the seminiferous tubules, reduction in sperm count, and/or increased incidence of sperm with abnormal morphology or reduced motility, were observed. The degree of toxicity was related to dose and duration of exposure. In male rats, decreased fertility was observed following 10 weeks of dosing at 500 mg/kg daily (1.9–11.4 times the human AUC). Administration of famciclovir to male rats in dosages of 50 mg/kg daily (0.2–1.2 times the human systemic exposure based on AUC comparisons) for 26 weeks did not reveal evidence of sperm or testicular toxicity. Testicular toxicity was observed following administration of dosages of 600 mg/kg daily (0.4–2.4 times the human systemic exposure based on AUC comparisons) for 104 weeks in male mice and dosages of 150 mg/kg daily (1.7–10.2 times the human system exposure based on AUC comparisons) for 26 weeks in male dogs. No effect on spermatogenesis was observed in human males with genital herpes following oral famciclovir dosages of 250 mg twice daily for 18 weeks.

Reproduction studies using oral famciclovir dosages up to 1 g/kg daily (3.6–21.6 times the human systemic exposure based on AUC comparisons) in female rats have not revealed evidence of impaired fertility or reproductive performance.

It is not known whether famciclovir or penciclovir is distributed into milk in humans. Following oral administration of famciclovir to lactating rats, penciclovir was distributed into breast milk at concentrations higher than those observed in plasma. Data on safety of famciclovir in infants currently is not available.

Drug Interactions

Famciclovir not metabolized by CYP isoenzymes.

■ **Drugs Eliminated by Renal Excretion** Potential increased plasma penciclovir concentrations when used concomitantly with other drugs eliminated by active renal tubular secretion (e.g., probenecid).

■ **Drugs Metabolized by Aldehyde Oxidase** Potential pharmacokinetic interaction with other drugs metabolized by aldehyde oxidase.

Pharmacokinetics

■ **Absorption** ***Bioavailability*** Famciclovir, a prodrug of penciclovir, is rapidly and well absorbed following oral administration and metabolized to penciclovir. Little or no prodrug is present in plasma or urine.

Absolute bioavailability of penciclovir is 77% following oral administration of famciclovir; peak penciclovir plasma concentrations attained within 0.5–0.9 hours.

Pharmacokinetics in HIV-infected patients similar to healthy individuals.

Food Administration of famciclovir with food decreases peak penciclovir plasma concentrations and delays time to peak concentrations but does not affect penciclovir AUC.

■ **Distribution** ***Extent*** Not known whether penciclovir crosses the placenta or is distributed into human milk.

Plasma Protein Binding Penciclovir <20% bound to plasma proteins.

■ **Elimination** ***Metabolism*** Famciclovir is deacetylated and oxidized to penciclovir. Penciclovir is phosphorylated to penciclovir triphosphate (the active metabolite) in cells infected with HSV-1, HSV-2, or VZV. The inactive metabolite 6-deoxy penciclovir is converted to penciclovir by aldehyde oxidase.

Famciclovir not metabolized by CYP enzymes.

Elimination Route Famciclovir eliminated principally by the kidneys as penciclovir and other metabolites. 73% of an oral famciclovir dose eliminated in urine and 27% eliminated in feces within 72 hours.

Half-life Elimination half-life of penciclovir after oral administration of famciclovir 1.6–3 hours.

Intracellular half-life of penciclovir triphosphate in cells infected with HSV-1 or HSV-2 is 10 and 20 hours, respectively; intracellular half-life in VZV-infected cells is 7–14 hours.

Special Populations AUC of penciclovir not affected when oral famciclovir used in patients with well-compensated chronic liver disease (chronic hepatitis, chronic ethanol abuse, primary biliary cirrhosis). Pharmacokinetics not evaluated in severe uncompensated hepatic impairment.

Renal clearance decreased and terminal elimination half-life increased in patients with renal impairment; half-life 6.2 hours if Cl_{cr} 20–39 mL/minute and 13.4 hours if Cl_{cr} <20 mL/minute.

AUC may be greater and renal clearance decreased in geriatric patients ≥65 years of age, presumably because of decreased renal function.

Description

Famciclovir (FCV) is a synthetic, acyclic purine nucleoside analog derived from guanine. The drug is the diacetyl 6-deoxy ester of penciclovir (PCV); penciclovir is structurally related to ganciclovir but pharmacologically and microbiologically related to acyclovir. Famciclovir is a prodrug of penciclovir and exhibits no antiviral activity until hydrolyzed in vivo to penciclovir and its active metabolites (e.g., penciclovir triphosphate).

Following metabolism of famciclovir in the intestinal wall and liver to penciclovir and intracellular conversion to the active triphosphate, the drug is active against various Herpesviridae including herpes simplex virus types 1 and 2 (HSV-1 and HSV-2), varicella-zoster virus, and Epstein-Barr virus (EBV). The drug also is active against hepatitis B virus (HBV). The drug exhibits only limited activity in vitro against cytomegalovirus (CMV).

Preparations

Excipients in commercially available drug preparations may have clinically important effects in some individuals; consult specific product labeling for details.

Famciclovir

Oral		
Tablets, film-coated	125 mg	**Famvir®**, Novartis
	250 mg	**Famvir®**, Novartis
	500 mg	**Famvir®**, Novartis

†Use is not currently included in the labeling approved by the US Food and Drug Administration

Ganciclovir Sodium

Nordeoxyguanosine, DHPG, GCV

■ Ganciclovir, a synthetic nucleoside analog of guanine, is an antiviral agent active against herpesviruses.

Uses

■ **Treatment of Cytomegalovirus Infection and Disease** Ganciclovir is used for the management of cytomegalovirus (CMV) retinitis in immunocompromised patients, including individuals with human immunodeficiency virus (HIV) infection. Ganciclovir also has been used for the management of other CMV infections (e.g., GI infections†, pneumonitis†, CNS infections†) in immunocompromised patients, but experience with the drug in these extraocular infections is less extensive.

Like other herpesviruses, CMV usually establishes a site(s) of latent infection following primary infection with the virus. Latency usually persists for life and the virus can be reactivated by various stimuli (e.g., immunosuppression), especially during periods of impaired cell-mediated immunity. Reactivation of the virus may result in subclinical infections or active end-organ CMV disease (e.g., retinitis, GI infections, pneumonitis, encephalitis), including serious, potentially life-threatening CMV disease.

Cytomegalovirus Retinitis Ganciclovir is used for initial treatment (induction therapy) and maintenance therapy (secondary prophylaxis) of CMV retinitis in immunocompromised adults, including those with HIV infection and acquired immunodeficiency syndrome (AIDS), those with iatrogenic (e.g., chemotherapy-induced) immunosuppression, and transplant recipients. The drug also is used for the management of CMV retinitis in HIV-infected pediatric patients†.

Like other antivirals, ganciclovir is not a cure for CMV retinitis. Although ganciclovir can induce stabilization or improvement of ocular manifestations, the retinitis may relapse and/or progress during or after discontinuance of the drug.

Retinitis is the most common clinical manifestation of CMV end-organ disease in HIV-infected patients and ideally should be managed in consultation with an ophthalmologist familiar with the diagnosis and treatment of retinal diseases. Antiviral regimens for initial treatment of CMV retinitis in HIV-infected individuals should be selected based on the location and severity of CMV retinal lesions, severity of underlying immunosuppression, concomitant drug therapy, and the patient's ability to adhere to the treatment regimen. The antiviral regimen used for maintenance therapy of CMV retinitis in HIV-infected individuals should be selected with consideration for the location of the CMV retinal lesions, vision in the contralateral eye, the patient's immunologic and virologic status, and the patient's response to antiretroviral therapy.

For the management of immediate sight-threatening CMV retinal lesions (i.e., within 1.5 mm of the fovea) in HIV-infected adults and adolescents, the US Centers for Disease Control and Prevention (CDC), National Institutes of Health (NIH), and the HIV Medicine Association of the Infectious Diseases Society of America (IDSA) state that the preferred regimen is initial treatment (induction therapy) with intravitreal ganciclovir† or intravitreal foscarnet (1–4 doses given over a period of 7–10 days) in conjunction with oral valganciclovir (twice daily for 14–21 days) followed by maintenance therapy (secondary prophylaxis) with oral valganciclovir (once daily). One alternative regimen recommended by these experts for management of sight-threatening CMV retinitis in HIV-infected adults and adolescents is intravitreal ganciclovir† or intravitreal foscarnet (1–4 doses given over a period of 7–10 days) in conjunction with IV ganciclovir (twice daily for 14–21 days) followed by maintenance therapy (secondary prophylaxis) with oral valganciclovir (once daily). Use of systemic antivirals (without an intravitreal antiviral) usually is adequate for the management of CMV retinitis in patients who have only small peripheral lesions.

For the management of CMV retinitis in HIV-infected pediatric patients†, CDC, NIH, IDSA, and others state that IV ganciclovir is the drug of choice for initial treatment (induction therapy) and is one of several options for maintenance therapy (secondary prophylaxis). These experts state that oral valganciclovir is an option for the management of CMV retinitis in HIV-infected pediatric patients and can be considered for induction and/or maintenance therapy in adolescents and older children who can receive the recommended adult dosage of the drug and can also be considered in children who are able to transition from initial IV ganciclovir therapy to an oral regimen to complete treatment and/or for maintenance therapy. Data are limited regarding use of intravitreal antivirals in children, and intravitreal injections are impractical in most children.

Because of the risk of relapse, HIV-infected patients who have received adequate initial treatment of CMV retinitis should receive chronic maintenance therapy (secondary prophylaxis) until immune reconstitution occurs as a result of effective antiretroviral therapy. CDC, NIH, and IDSA state that consideration can be given to discontinuing maintenance therapy of CMV retinitis in HIV-infected adults and adolescents if CMV lesions have been treated for at least 3–6 months and are inactive and there has been a sustained (i.e., 3–6 months) increase in $CD4^+$ T-cell count to greater than 100/mm^3 in response to antiretroviral therapy. The safety of discontinuing maintenance therapy of CMV retinitis in HIV-infected pediatric patients has not been well studied; however, CDC, NIH, IDSA, and others state that consideration can be given to discontinuing such maintenance therapy in HIV-infected children who are receiving antiretroviral therapy and have a sustained (i.e., greater than 6 months) increase in $CD4^+$ T-cell percentage to greater than 15% (children younger than 6 years of age) or an increase in $CD4^+$ T-cell count to greater than 100/mm^3 (children 6 years of age or older). These experts state that a decision to discontinue maintenance therapy of CMV retinitis should be made in consultation with an ophthalmologist and, if maintenance therapy is discontinued, the patient should continue to receive regular ophthalmologic monitoring (optimally every 3–6 months) for early detection of CMV relapse or immune reconstitution uveitis. If $CD4^+$ T-cell count decreases to less than 100/mm^3 (adults, adolescents, children 6 years of age or older) or if $CD4^+$ T-cell percentage decreases to less than 15% (children younger than 6 years of age), maintenance therapy of CMV retinitis should be reinitiated.

For additional information on management of CMV retinitis and other CMV infections in HIV-infected individuals, the current clinical practice guidelines from CDC, NIH, and IDSA on the prevention and treatment of opportunistic infections in HIV-infected individuals available at http://www.aidsinfo.nih.gov should be consulted.

Clinical Experience. Efficacy of IV ganciclovir for the management of CMV retinitis has been established in uncontrolled and randomized controlled studies.

Initial ocular response (improvement or stabilization of vision and/or other ophthalmologic findings) reportedly occurs in 70–80% or more of immunocompromised patients receiving IV ganciclovir induction therapy. Stabilization of retinal lesions usually is apparent within 2 weeks of initiating ganciclovir therapy, although optimum clinical response to induction therapy may be delayed for several weeks to a month after initiating the drug. Ophthalmologic evidence of response to ganciclovir therapy may include decreased retinal opacification and inflammation, improvement in ocular hemorrhage and vasculitis (vascular sheathing) and in visual acuity, and development of atrophic changes in previously inflamed retinal areas, although reversal of resultant visual abnormalities may not occur. Stabilization or improvement in visual acuity reportedly occurs in 50% or more of patients receiving induction therapy with the drug and depends in part on the extent of macular (more specifically, foveal) and optic nerve involvement; however, such visual improvement rarely is dramatic, and rhegmatogenous retinal detachment can develop as a consequence of ganciclovir-induced resolution of retinitis, especially in patients with AIDS. (See Cautions: Ocular Effects.) In one study, visual acuity stabilized in 73%, improved (by more than 2 lines on the Snellen chart) in 15%, and deteriorated in 12% of ganciclovir-treated AIDS patients; there was no foveal involvement in those patients whose acuity improved. Extraocular (e.g., blood, urine) virologic response (negative cultures and/or decreased viral shedding) reportedly occurs in almost all ganciclovir-treated patients with CMV retinitis and usually is apparent within several days to 2 weeks after initiating therapy; however, a direct relationship between extraocular virologic response and clinical improvement of the retinitis has not been demonstrated.

In a retrospective, nonrandomized analysis of data from a study in 41 patients with AIDS and CMV retinitis who received IV ganciclovir induction therapy (5 mg/kg every 12 hours) for 14–21 days followed by IV ganciclovir maintenance therapy (5 mg/kg once daily every day or 6 mg/kg once daily 5 days each week), treatment with ganciclovir resulted in a delay in median time from diagnosis to initial retinitis progression compared with untreated patients (71 days versus 29 days).

In a randomized, prospective study in a limited number of patients with AIDS and peripheral CMV retinitis who received IV ganciclovir that was either initiated immediately or deferred, the median time to retinitis progression was 50 versus 13.5 days for those receiving immediate versus deferred ganciclovir treatment. This study indicates that all patients with HIV-related CMV retinitis, regardless of whether the lesions are peripheral or central, should be offered CMV treatment.

Extraocular Cytomegalovirus Infections

Although safety and efficacy of ganciclovir have not been established for the treatment of extraocular CMV infections, the drug has been used in immunocompromised patients for the management of CMV GI disease† and/or pneumonitis†, and, less frequently, for the management of CMV encephalitis†, hepatic†, cardiac†, and/or other CMV infections†.

GI Infections. Ganciclovir has been used for the management of CMV GI infections†, including colitis†, esophagitis†, gastritis†, and rectal disease†.

There is evidence that the clinical response rate of CMV GI infections† to ganciclovir is similar to or less than that of CMV retinitis. Approximately 70% or more of immunocompromised patients with CMV GI infections exhibit stabilization or improvement of the infection with ganciclovir induction therapy. Similarly, there is clearing of viremia and/or viruria and decreased viral shedding, with the frequency of virologic response usually exceeding clinical response. Response generally is apparent within 1–2 weeks of initiating therapy with the drug. In patients with colitis, response to ganciclovir therapy usually manifests as a reduction in stool frequency and diarrhea and in abdominal pain. In patients with esophagitis, response to the drug usually manifests as a reduction in dysphagia and odynophagia and in esophageal and epigastric pain. Improvement in rectal ulcers usually is observed in those with rectal disease, and weight gain also may be observed in response to ganciclovir therapy in patients with CMV GI infections.

Relapse, usually based on symptomatic recurrence or worsening but occasionally confirmed histologically, has occurred following ganciclovir induction therapy and discontinuance of the drug in immunosuppressed patients with CMV GI infections†. In some patients, particularly those with AIDS, long-term maintenance and/or intermittent induction therapy with the drug may be required.

CDC, NIH, and IDSA state that IV ganciclovir usually is the preferred antiviral for initial management of CMV GI disease† in HIV-infected adults and that a transition to oral valganciclovir may be considered when the patient can tolerate and absorb oral drugs. These experts state that IV foscarnet is a possible alternative to IV ganciclovir for the management of CMV esophagitis or colitis in those who cannot receive ganciclovir or have infections caused by ganciclovir-resistant CMV.

Pneumonitis. Ganciclovir has been used for the treatment of CMV pneumonitis† with variable results; in part, this variability in response appears to depend on the patient's underlying immunologic disorder. Clinical outcome in bone marrow transplant (BMT) recipients treated with ganciclovir alone has been particularly disappointing. Although CMV can be isolated from the respiratory tract of many AIDS patients, the virus rarely is the only pulmonary pathogen recovered, and its role as the principal pathogen in these patients has not been fully defined; in one study in AIDS patients with serious pulmonary disorders, CMV was isolated in 17% of patients but was the sole pathogen isolated in only 4%. Coexistent infections also may be present in organ (e.g., kidney) and BMT recipients, but presence of the virus as the principal pulmonary pathogen in these patients is better defined, especially in BMT recipients. Response to ganciclovir therapy appears to be better if the infection is treated early in its course; therefore, prompt recognition and diagnosis of the infection and initiation of ganciclovir therapy appear important.

There is some evidence that the clinical response rate of CMV pneumonitis† to ganciclovir therapy alone generally is less than that of CMV retinitis, especially in BMT recipients. In some studies, approximately 50–60% of immunocompromised patients with CMV pneumonitis exhibited clinical improvement with ganciclovir induction therapy alone. Up to about 80% of patients whose immunodeficiency resulted from AIDS or organ transplantation exhibited a clinical response to therapy with the drug alone, whereas response rates reportedly have ranged from 10–45% in BMT recipients receiving the drug alone. Response to ganciclovir therapy usually manifests as improvement in respiratory symptoms and function; radiographic evidence of response usually is somewhat delayed. Evidence of virologic response occurs in almost all ganciclovir-treated patients with CMV pneumonitis, even in those who do not respond clinically. CMV pneumonitis may be less likely to require maintenance therapy after initial treatment than CMV retinitis.

The reasons for the poor response to ganciclovir monotherapy in BMT recipients with CMV pneumonitis† have not been fully elucidated, but in part the poor response may depend on differences in immunologic responses to the infection. Untreated CMV pneumonitis may be fatal in 85% or more of BMT recipients. These patients are more prone than AIDS or organ transplant recipients to develop respiratory failure and die despite pulmonary and extrapulmonary (e.g., blood, urine) clearing of the virus during ganciclovir therapy. There is animal and human evidence to suggest that CMV pneumonitis in BMT recipients is a complex immunopathologic disease. While it is possible that poor response in these patients may result from progressive infection, it has been suggested that a pulmonary immunologic reaction to the infection (e.g., secondary to a T-cell-mediated cytotoxic effect against viral and/or HLA antigens expressed on infected pulmonary cells) and/or exacerbation of the infection by some underlying factor not related to CMV (e.g., graft-versus-host disease, radiation/chemotherapy-induced inflammation, pulmonary toxicity from high oxygen concentrations used during ventilatory support) may be responsible. An association between graft-versus-host disease and development of CMV pneumonitis has been observed in humans and animals. In addition, an association between presence of functional T cells and development of CMV pneumonitis has been observed in animals and is further supported by the more favorable clinical response of the pneumonitis observed in AIDS patients in whom cytotoxic cellular immune responses generally are poorer.

For the management of well-documented CMV pneumonitis† in HIV-infected adults, CDC, NIH, and IDSA state that either IV ganciclovir or IV foscarnet is a reasonable choice.

Neurologic Disease. Ganciclovir has been used with variable results in immunosuppressed patients with CMV encephalitis†. Neurologic and magnetic resonance imaging findings improved with induction and/or maintenance therapy with the drug in some of these patients, while other patients failed to respond. Many patients with CMV encephalitis also have other active CMV infections.

A combination regimen of IV ganciclovir and IV foscarnet has been used for the management of CMV neurologic disease† (e.g., CMV encephalitis or myelitis), and is recommended by CDC, NIH, IDSA, and others for such infections in HIV-infected individuals.

Congenital Cytomegalovirus Disease

Although safety and efficacy of ganciclovir have not been established in neonates or infants with congenital CMV infection, the drug has been used for the management of symptomatic congenital CMV disease† when an antiviral was indicated.

Transmission of CMV from infected mothers to their fetuses occurs as a result of maternal viremia and transplacental infection. Perinatal infection also can occur from exposure of the neonate to CMV shedding in the mother's genital tract. Approximately 10% of neonates with congenital CMV infection are symptomatic at birth; mortality in symptomatic infants is about 10% and approximately 50–90% of symptomatic surviving neonates experience substantial morbidity (e.g., mental retardation, sensorineural hearing loss, microcephaly, seizures). The risk of congenital CMV infection resulting from primary maternal CMV infection may be higher and the disease may be more severe than that resulting from reactivation of maternal CMV infection.

Because there is some evidence that antivirals (i.e., ganciclovir, valganciclovir) may help prevent hearing deterioration and/or improve developmental delay in neonates and infants with moderate to severe symptomatic congenital CMV disease, the American Academy of Pediatrics (AAP) and other clinicians state that use of an antiviral regimen should be considered in such neonates if it can be initiated within the first month of life. Antivirals are not usually recommended for neonates with asymptomatic congenital CMV infection or only mildly symptomatic infection without evidence of CNS involvement.

AAP and others recommend that a 6-month regimen of oral valganciclovir be considered in neonates with moderate to severe symptomatic congenital CMV disease (with or without CNS involvement). A 6-week regimen of IV ganciclovir either alone or followed by a regimen of oral valganciclovir (continued until up to 12 months of age) also has been used in neonates with symptomatic congenital CMV disease.

CDC, NIH, IDSA, and others state that IV ganciclovir can be considered for initial treatment of symptomatic congenital CMV disease with CNS involvement in HIV-exposed or HIV-infected infants†.

Decisions regarding antiviral treatment in neonates with congenital CMV disease should be made in consultation with a pediatric infectious diseases specialist. Because of the risk of serious sequelae (e.g., late-onset hearing loss), long-term ophthalmologic and audiologic monitoring is necessary in patients with congenital CMV infection, regardless of antiviral treatment.

■ Prevention of Cytomegalovirus Infection and Disease IV ganciclovir is used for prophylaxis to prevent CMV infection and disease in solid organ transplant recipients, BMT recipients, and hematopoietic stem cell transplant (HSCT) recipients considered at high risk for the disease. The drug also has been used for preemptive treatment of CMV infection and disease† in transplant recipients.

CMV infection in transplant recipients can occur either as a primary infection in CMV-seronegative recipients of organs and cells from CMV-positive donors or as reactivation of latent CMV infection in CMV-seropositive recipients. CMV infection in transplant recipients is associated with substantial morbidity and mortality. The risk for CMV infection or reactivation is greatest during the first 3 months after transplantation and depends on several factors, including the serologic status of the recipient and donor, CMV-specific T-cell immunity in the recipient, and immunosuppressive regimens used in the recipient. Certain antiviral strategies have been used to prevent severe, life-threatening CMV disease in transplant recipients, including antiviral prophylaxis (initiated posttransplantation and continued for at least 3 months) and/or preemptive antiviral treatment (i.e., initiated when CMV infection is detected, but before clinical progression to symptomatic CMV disease). These antiviral strategies each have certain advantages and disadvantages.

Specialized references should be consulted for specific information regarding prevention and management of CMV infections in BMT, HSCT, or solid organ transplant recipients.

Clinical Experience In a randomized, double-blind, placebo-controlled study in 149 cardiac allograft recipients at risk for developing CMV disease (i.e., CMV-seropositive or CMV-seronegative recipients of an organ from a CMV-seropositive donor), patients who received IV ganciclovir (5 mg/kg twice daily for 14 days beginning 1 day after cardiac allotransplantation, followed by 6 mg/kg once daily for 5 days per week for an additional 2 weeks) had a substantial decrease in the overall incidence of CMV disease compared with those receiving placebo. During the 120-day period following transplantation, 16% of patients who received ganciclovir developed acute CMV disease (GI infection, pneumonitis, myocarditis, CMV syndrome) compared with 43% of patients who received placebo. However, a clinically important decrease in the incidence of CMV disease was evident only in those cardiac allograft recipients who were CMV-seropositive before transplantation; patients who were at highest risk for serious disease (CMV-seronegative recipients of hearts from CMV-seropositive donors) did not have a clinically important decrease in the incidence of CMV disease. In patients who were CMV-seropositive prior to transplantation, 9% of those who received ganciclovir developed CMV disease compared with 46% who received placebo. In patients who were CMV-seronegative prior to transplantation and received hearts from CMV-positive donors, 35% of those who received ganciclovir developed CMV disease compared with 29% who received placebo. If acute CMV disease developed in patients receiving placebo, it occurred at an average of 45 or 56 days after transplantation in CMV-seropositive patients or CMV-seronegative recipients of CMV-seropositive hearts, respectively. If it developed in patients receiving ganciclovir, it occurred at an average of 71 days after transplantation.

In a randomized study in patients undergoing liver transplantation, IV ganciclovir (6 mg/kg daily from day 1–30 after transplantation, then 6 mg/kg daily 5 days weekly until day 100) was more effective than acyclovir (10 mg/kg IV every 8 hours from day 1 after transplantation until discharge, then 800 mg orally 4 times daily until day 100) in preventing CMV disease in these patients. During the first 120 days after the procedure, CMV infection occurred in only 5% of patients receiving ganciclovir but occurred in 38% of those receiving acyclovir. Symptomatic CMV disease developed in less than 1% of patients receiving ganciclovir and in 10% of those receiving acyclovir. Ganciclovir reduced the incidence of CMV disease in both CMV-seropositive and -seronegative individuals.

In several randomized, double-blind, placebo-controlled studies in bone marrow allograft recipients with asymptomatic CMV infection (CMV-positive culture of urine, throat, or blood) who were at risk for developing CMV disease, patients who received IV ganciclovir (5 mg/kg twice daily for 5–7 days, followed by 5 mg/kg once daily until 100 days after transplantation) had a substantial decrease in the incidence of CMV disease compared with those receiving placebo. During the 100-day period following transplantation, 0–3% of patients receiving ganciclovir and 29–43% of patients receiving placebo developed CMV disease. During the first 6-month period following transplantation, 9–16% of patients who had received ganciclovir and 32–43% of patients who had received placebo developed CMV disease. In one study, the overall survival rate 100 and 180 days after transplantation was higher in patients who had received ganciclovir. In another study, mortality at 100 and 180 days after transplantation was similar in both groups; it was suggested that this lack of difference in survival may have occurred because of a reduction in excess deaths in the placebo group since any patient who began to excrete the virus was removed from the study and given ganciclovir. The incidence of neutropenia was higher in patients receiving ganciclovir compared with those receiving placebo. In another study in bone marrow allograft recipients, patients were evaluated for presence of pulmonary CMV by bronchoscopy with bronchoalveolar lavage at days 35 and 49 after transplantation. Those patients with histologic, immunologic, or virologic evidence of asymptomatic pulmonary CMV infection were identified as at risk for developing interstitial pneumonia and randomly assigned to receive IV ganciclovir (5 mg/kg twice daily for 14 days followed by 5 mg/kg once daily 5 days per week until 120 days after transplantation) or no ganciclovir treatment. The incidence of subsequent interstitial pneumonia was lower in patients who received ganciclovir; interstitial pneumonia developed in 20% of those who received ganciclovir and 70% of those who received no antiviral therapy.

■ Varicella-Zoster Virus Infections Although optimal regimens for the management of progressive outer retinal necrosis caused by varicella-zoster virus† (VZV) in HIV-infected individuals have not been identified, CDC, NIH, and IDSA recommend treatment with at least one IV antiviral (acyclovir, ganciclovir, foscarnet, cidofovir) used in conjunction with at least one intravitreal antiviral (ganciclovir or foscarnet). Some experts recommend a regimen of IV ganciclovir and/or IV foscarnet used in conjunction with intravitreal† ganciclovir and/or intravitreal foscarnet. The prognosis for visual preservation in patients with progressive outer retinal necrosis caused by VZV is poor and such infections should be managed in consultation with an ophthalmologist.

Dosage and Administration

■ Reconstitution and Administration Ganciclovir is administered by IV infusion.

Ganciclovir should not be administered by rapid IV infusion or direct IV injection since potentially toxic plasma concentrations of the drug may result.

Ganciclovir should *not* be administered by IM or subcutaneous injection because reconstituted and diluted solutions of the drug are alkaline (pH of 11) and may cause severe tissue irritation.

Ganciclovir has been administered by intravitreal injection†; however, a preparation of the drug specifically for intravitreal administration is not commercially available in the US.

Ganciclovir has been administered orally, but oral preparations of the drug are no longer commercially available in the US.

Females of childbearing potential should be tested for pregnancy prior to initiation of ganciclovir. (See Cautions: Pregnancy, Fertility, and Lactation.)

Renal function should be assessed prior to initiation of ganciclovir and monitored during therapy with the drug; dosage should be adjusted as necessary.

Complete blood counts with differential and platelet counts should be performed frequently during ganciclovir therapy, especially in those who developed cytopenias during previous therapy with ganciclovir or other nucleoside analogs and in those with neutrophil counts less than 1000/mm^3 prior to initiation of ganciclovir. (See Cautions: Hematologic Effects.)

Patients receiving ganciclovir should be adequately hydrated.

The recommended dosage of ganciclovir and the recommended frequency and rate of administration of the drug should not be exceeded.

IV Infusion IV infusions of ganciclovir should be given via a large peripheral or central vein. To avoid phlebitis and pain at the IV infusion site, the drug preferably should be administered using a plastic cannula and infused into a vein that will provide adequate blood flow for rapid dilution and distribution of the drug.

For IV infusion, single-dose vials of lyophilized ganciclovir sodium labeled as containing 500 mg of ganciclovir are reconstituted by adding 10 mL of preservative-free sterile water for injection to provide a solution containing 50 mg/mL. The vial should be gently swirled until the drug is completely wetted and a clear reconstituted solution is obtained. Bacteriostatic water for injection containing parabens should *not* be used to reconstitute ganciclovir sodium. (See Chemistry and Stability: Stability.) The appropriate dose of reconstituted solution should then be withdrawn from the vial and diluted in a compatible IV infusion solution (usually 100 mL). Solutions containing ganciclovir concentrations exceeding 10 mg/mL are not recommended for IV infusion.

Alternatively, if the commercially available ganciclovir sodium concentrate for injection for IV use containing 500 mg of ganciclovir (50 mg/mL) is used, the single-dose vial of solution should be shaken and the appropriate dose withdrawn from the vial and diluted in a compatible IV infusion solution (usually 100 mL). Solutions containing ganciclovir concentrations exceeding 10 mg/mL are not recommended for IV infusion.

Alternatively, commercially available single-dose IV bags containing 500 mg of ganciclovir in 250 mL of 0.8% sodium chloride (2 mg/mL) can be used for IV infusion without further dilution. The premixed solution in the bag should appear clear. If any crystals have formed in the solution, the bag should be gently shaken to redissolve the crystals prior to use. Any unused portions of the premixed solution should be discarded.

Ganciclovir solutions should be inspected visually for discoloration and particulate matter prior to administration; if either is present, the solution should be discarded.

Ganciclovir lyophilized powder and solutions of the drug should be handled cautiously because of the high pH of some preparations and because of the mutagenic and/or carcinogenic potential of the drug (see Cautions: Mutagenicity and Carcinogenicity). The use of disposable gloves is recommended. If ganciclovir powder or solutions of the drug contact the skin or mucous membranes, the affected area should be washed immediately and thoroughly with soap and water. If the drug comes in contact with the eyes, the eyes should flushed thoroughly with water.

Since ganciclovir shares some of the properties of cytotoxic drugs (i.e., mutagenicity, carcinogenicity), the manufacturers state that consideration should be given to handling and disposing the drug according to guidelines issued for cytotoxic drugs. For further information on the handling of cytotoxic drugs, see the ASHP Guidelines on Handling Hazardous Drugs at http://ahfs-druginformation.com.

Rate of Administration. Ganciclovir solutions should be administered by IV infusion at a constant rate over 1 hour.

Dosage

Ganciclovir is commercially available as the base and as ganciclovir sodium; dosage is expressed in terms of ganciclovir.

Adult Dosage

Cytomegalovirus Retinitis. For the treatment of cytomegalovirus (CMV) retinitis in adults with normal renal function (creatinine clearance of 70 mL/minute or greater), including those with human immunodeficiency virus (HIV) infection, the recommended dosage of IV ganciclovir for initial treatment (induction therapy) is 5 mg/kg every 12 hours for 14–21 days. In patients with immediate sight-threatening CMV retinal lesions (i.e., within 1.5 mm of the fovea), the US Centers for Disease Control and Prevention (CDC), National Institutes of Health (NIH), and HIV Medicine Association of the Infectious Diseases Society of America (IDSA) recommend that initial treatment also include an appropriate intravitreal antiviral. (See Cytomegalovirus Retinitis under Uses: Treatment of Cytomegalovirus Infection and Disease.)

After completion of initial treatment, the usual dosage of IV ganciclovir for maintenance therapy (secondary prophylaxis) of CMV retinitis in adults with normal renal function is 5 mg/kg once daily. Alternatively, IV ganciclovir can be given in a dosage of 6 mg/kg once daily 5 days each week for maintenance therapy.

Decisions regarding discontinuance of maintenance therapy of CMV retinitis in HIV-infected individuals who have received CMV treatment for at least 3–6 months, have inactive CMV retinal lesions, and have achieved immune reconstitution as the result of antiretroviral therapy should be made in consultation with an ophthalmologist. (See Cytomegalovirus Retinitis under Uses: Treatment of Cytomegalovirus Infection and Disease.)

Cytomegalovirus Esophagitis or Colitis. For the treatment of CMV GI infections† in adults with normal renal function, a ganciclovir dosage of 5 mg/kg IV every 12 hours for 14–21 days has been used for initial treatment (induction); alternatively, a dosage of 2.5 mg/kg IV every 8 hours also has been used. If maintenance therapy is required, dosages comparable to those used for maintenance therapy of CMV retinitis have been used.

For the management of CMV esophagitis† or colitis† in HIV-infected adults, CDC, NIH, and IDSA recommend that IV ganciclovir be given in a dosage of 5 mg/kg every 12 hours and state that a switch to oral valganciclovir can be made after the patient can absorb and tolerate oral therapy. These experts recommend that antiviral therapy be continued for 21–42 days or until signs and symptoms of the infection have resolved. Maintenance therapy (secondary prophylaxis) usually is not necessary, but should be considered if relapse occurs.

Cytomegalovirus Pneumonitis. For the treatment of CMV pneumonitis† in adults with normal renal function, a ganciclovir dosage of 5 mg/kg IV every 12 hours for 14–21 days has been used for initial treatment (induction); alternatively, a dosage of 2.5 mg/kg IV every 8 hours also has been used. If maintenance therapy is required, dosages comparable to those used for maintenance therapy of CMV retinitis have been used.

If IV ganciclovir is used for the management of well-documented CMV pneumonitis† in HIV-infected adults, CDC, NIH, and IDSA state that the same dosage recommended for the management of CMV retinitis in HIV-infected adults should be used. The optimal duration of treatment in such patients has not been established.

Cytomegalovirus Neurologic Disease. If IV ganciclovir is used for the management of CMV neurologic disease† in HIV-infected adults, CDC, NIH, and IDSA state that the same dosage recommended for the management of CMV retinitis in HIV-infected adults should be used in conjunction with IV foscarnet. The optimal duration of treatment in such patients has not been established.

Prevention of Cytomegalovirus Infection and Disease in Transplant Recipients. For prophylaxis to prevent CMV infection and disease in transplant recipients with normal renal function, the manufacturers recommend that IV ganciclovir be given in a dosage of 5 mg/kg every 12 hours for 7–14 days followed by a maintenance dosage of 5 mg/kg once daily 7 days each week or 6 mg/kg once daily 5 days each week. Prophylaxis should be continued until 100–120 days posttransplantation.

Some experts recommend that IV ganciclovir be given in a dosage of 5 mg/kg once daily for prophylaxis of CMV infection and disease in transplant recipients with normal renal function. These experts recommend that antiviral prophylaxis be continued for 3 months in CMV-seropositive recipients of solid organs (kidney, pancreas, kidney/pancreas, liver, heart) and for 3–6 months in CMV-seronegative recipients of solid organs (kidney, pancreas, kidney/pancreas, liver, heart) from CMV-seropositive donors.

If IV ganciclovir is used for preemptive treatment of CMV infection in solid organ transplant recipients†, a dosage of 5 mg/kg twice daily is recommended in those with normal renal function.

Varicella-Zoster Virus Infections. For the management of progressive outer retinal necrosis caused by varicella-zoster virus† (VZV) in HIV-infected adults, CDC, NIH, and IDSA state that a regimen that includes IV ganciclovir in a dosage of 5 mg/kg every 12 hours (used with or without IV foscarnet) in conjunction with intravitreal ganciclovir† (used with or without intravitreal foscarnet) can be considered.

Pediatric Dosage

Cytomegalovirus Retinitis. For initial treatment (induction therapy) of CMV retinitis in pediatric patients†, including HIV-infected children†, CDC, NIH, IDSA, and others recommend that IV ganciclovir be given in a dosage of 5 mg/kg IV every 12 hours for 14–21 days (may be increased to 7.5 mg/kg every 12 hours if needed). After completion of initial treatment, these experts recommend that pediatric patients receive IV ganciclovir in a dosage of 5 mg/kg once daily for 5–7 days each week for maintenance therapy (secondary prophylaxis).

Decisions regarding discontinuance of maintenance therapy of CMV retinitis in HIV-infected individuals who have inactive CMV retinal lesions and have achieved immune reconstitution as the result of antiretroviral therapy should be made in consultation with an ophthalmologist. (See Cytomegalovirus Retinitis under Uses: Treatment of Cytomegalovirus Infection and Disease.)

CNS or Disseminated Cytomegalovirus Infections. For initial treatment (induction therapy) of CNS infections caused by CMV in HIV-infected children†, CDC, NIH, IDSA, and others recommend that IV ganciclovir be given in a dosage of 5 mg/kg every 12 hours in conjunction with IV foscarnet. Initial treatment should be continued until symptomatic improvement.

For initial treatment (induction therapy) of disseminated CMV infections in HIV-infected children†, CDC, NIH, IDSA, and others state that IV ganciclovir be given in a dosage of 5 mg/kg IV every 12 hours (may be increased to 7.5 mg/kg every 12 hours if needed). Initial treatment should be continued for 14–21 days.

After completion of initial treatment, the recommended dosage of IV ganciclovir for maintenance therapy (secondary prophylaxis) of CNS or disseminated CMV infections in HIV-infected children† is 5 mg/kg once daily for 5–7 days each week.

Congenital Cytomegalovirus Disease. If IV ganciclovir is used for the management of symptomatic congenital CMV disease† when an antiviral is indicated (see Congenital Cytomegalovirus Disease under Uses: Treatment of Cytomegalovirus Infection and Disease), the American Academy of Pediatrics (AAP) and other clinicians recommend a dosage of 6 mg/kg twice daily.

AAP and other clinicians recommend that, if an antiviral is indicated, it should be initiated within the first month of life and continued for a total of 6 months. If IV ganciclovir is used initially, treatment should be transitioned to oral valganciclovir when the infant is able to tolerate and absorb oral drugs.

Prevention of Cytomegalovirus Infection and Disease in Transplant Recipients. For prophylaxis to prevent CMV infection and disease in pediatric transplant recipients†, some clinicians recommend that IV ganciclovir be given in a dosage of 5 mg/kg every 12 hours for 5–7 days (or 7–14 days) followed by a maintenance regimen of 5 mg/kg once daily 7 days each week or 6 mg/kg once daily 5 days each week. Prophylaxis should be continued for 100–120 days posttransplantation.

Other clinicians recommend that IV ganciclovir be given in a dosage of 5 mg/kg once daily for prophylaxis in pediatric transplant recipients† and that antiviral prophylaxis be continued for 3 months or longer depending on the immune status of the recipient and type of transplant.

If IV ganciclovir is used for preemptive treatment of CMV infection in pediatric patients†, a dosage of 5 mg/kg twice daily for 7–14 days followed by 5 mg/kg once daily has been recommended.

Varicella-Zoster Virus Infections. For the management of progressive outer retinal necrosis caused by VZV in HIV-infected children†, CDC, NIH, IDSA, and others state that a regimen that includes IV ganciclovir given in a dosage of 5 mg/kg every 12 hours (used with IV foscarnet) in conjunction with intravitreal ganciclovir† (used with or without intravitreal foscarnet) can be considered.

Dosage in Renal Impairment

In patients with impaired renal function, doses and/or frequency of administration of ganciclovir must be modified in response to the degree of impairment.

Dosage should be based on the patient's measured or estimated creatinine clearance. The patient's creatinine clearance (Ccr) can be estimated by using the following formulas:

$$Ccr\ male = \frac{(140 - age) \times weight}{72 \times serum\ creatinine}$$

$$Ccr\ female = 0.85 \times Ccr\ male$$

where age is in years, weight is in kg, and serum creatinine is in mg/dL.

When IV ganciclovir is used for the management of CMV retinitis in adults with renal impairment, the manufacturers recommend the following dosage for initial treatment (induction therapy) and maintenance therapy (secondary prophylaxis) based on creatinine clearance. (See Table 1.)

Table 1. Dosage of IV Ganciclovir for Management of CMV Retinitis in Adults with Renal Impairment

Creatinine Clearance (mL/minute)	Initial Treatment (Induction) Dosage	Maintenance Dosage
50–69	2.5 mg/kg every 12 hours	2.5 mg/kg every 24 hours
25–49	2.5 mg/kg every 24 hours	1.25 mg/kg every 24 hours
10–24	1.25 mg/kg every 24 hours	0.625 mg/kg every 24 hours
Less than 10	1.25 mg/kg 3 times weekly	0.625 mg/kg 3 times weekly

In adults undergoing hemodialysis, dosage of IV ganciclovir for initial treatment (induction therapy) of CMV retinitis should not exceed 1.25 mg/kg 3 times weekly and dosage for maintenance therapy should not exceed 0.625 mg/kg 3 times weekly. Because hemodialysis may reduce ganciclovir plasma concentrations by approximately 50% (see Pharmacokinetics: Elimination), dosing of the drug should be timed so that doses administered on the days of dialysis are given shortly after completion of dialysis.

Cautions

Adverse reactions to ganciclovir occur frequently, but usually are reversible following discontinuance of therapy with the drug. Because most patients receiving ganciclovir have serious underlying disease with multiple baseline symptomatology and clinical abnormalities and are receiving multiple drugs concomitantly and because clinical studies generally did not include a placebo control, it is difficult to establish whether a causal relationship to ganciclovir exists for many reported adverse effects.

Adverse effects reported in 20% of more of patients receiving ganciclovir in clinical trials include hematologic effects (leukopenia, neutropenia, thrombocytopenia, anemia), pyrexia, GI effects (diarrhea, nausea, decreased appetite, abdominal pain), catheter-associated effects (sepsis), hyperhidrosis, asthenia, headache, cough, dyspnea, and increased creatinine concentrations. In clinical trials evaluating ganciclovir in patients with cytomegalovirus (CMV) retinitis, adverse reactions necessitated discontinuance of the drug in 9% of patients.

■ **Hematologic Effects** Hematologic toxicity, including granulocytopenia (neutropenia), anemia, thrombocytopenia, and pancytopenia, have been reported in patients receiving ganciclovir. Hematologic effects, which may be severe, are one of the most common adverse reactions to the drug.

Neutropenia (absolute neutrophil count less than 1000/mm^3), which is potentially fatal, has been reported in up to 25–60% of patients receiving ganciclovir and is the most common dose-limiting adverse effect of the drug. Absolute neutrophil count declines to less than 500/mm^3 in approximately 15–25% of patients receiving the drug for the treatment of CMV infection. Granulocytopenia (neutropenia) usually develops early in treatment (e.g., during the first or second week of induction therapy), but can occur at any time. In most cases, interruption of ganciclovir therapy or a decrease in dosage will result in increased neutrophil counts, which usually is evident within 3–7 days; however, prolonged or irreversible neutropenia has occurred, and bacterial or fungal sepsis and subsequent death have been reported occasionally in patients with ganciclovir-induced neutropenia. Neutropenia has recurred following reinitiation of ganciclovir therapy, occasionally even at reduced dosage. If severe neutropenia (absolute neutrophil count less than 500/mm^3) occurs, ganciclovir therapy is not recommended.

Patients with human immunodeficiency virus (HIV) infection and acquired immunodeficiency syndrome (AIDS) may be at greater risk of developing neutropenia compared with other immunosuppressed patients receiving the drug. There also is limited evidence to suggest that bone marrow transplant (BMT) recipients may be at greater risk than organ transplant recipients for developing ganciclovir-induced neutropenia, but the possibility exists that other factors (e.g., concurrently administered drugs) may have contributed to the observed differences. In controlled studies in patients who received IV ganciclovir for prevention of CMV disease following transplantation, the absolute neutrophil count decreased to 1000/mm^3 or less in 7% of cardiac allograft recipients (mean duration of IV ganciclovir 28 days) and in 41% of bone marrow allograft recipients (mean duration of IV ganciclovir 45 days); 11% of cardiac allograft recipients who received placebo and 23% of bone marrow allograft recipients who did not receive ganciclovir therapy also had neutrophil counts this low.

Thrombocytopenia occurs frequently in patients receiving ganciclovir, developing in approximately 20% of patients who receive the drug. Interruption of ganciclovir therapy or a decrease in dosage usually results in increased platelet counts. Patients with low baseline platelet counts (less than 100,000/mm^3) appear to be more prone to develop this reaction. In addition, patients who are iatrogenically immunosuppressed appear to be at greater risk than AIDS patients of developing thrombocytopenia, which occurred in 46 and 14% of such patients, respectively, in one study. In controlled studies in patients who received IV ganciclovir for prevention of CMV disease following transplantation, platelet counts decreased to less than 25,000/mm^3 in 3% of cardiac allograft recipients (mean duration of IV ganciclovir 28 days) and in 32% of bone marrow allograft recipients (mean duration of IV ganciclovir 45 days); 1% of cardiac allograft recipients who received placebo and 28% of bone marrow allograft recipients who did not receive ganciclovir therapy in these studies also had platelet counts this low. If the platelet count declines to less than 25,000/mm^3, ganciclovir therapy is not recommended.

Leukopenia has been reported in 41% and anemia has been reported in 25% of patients receiving ganciclovir for maintenance therapy of CMV retinitis. Anemia with hemoglobin concentrations less than 6.5 g/dL occurred in 5% of patients. If hemoglobin concentrations decline to less than 8 g/dL, ganciclovir therapy is not recommended.

Pancytopenia and bone marrow failure have been reported in clinical studies in patients receiving ganciclovir for the treatment of CMV retinitis or in transplant recipients receiving the drug for prophylaxis of CMV. Hemolytic anemia, agranulocytosis, and granulocytopenia have been reported during postmarketing experience in patients receiving ganciclovir.

Although experience is limited, intravitreal injection† of ganciclovir does not appear to be associated with appreciable systemic toxicity and this route has been suggested as an alternative to IV ganciclovir in patients with CMV retinitis in whom hematologic toxicity is not tolerated.

Ganciclovir-induced neutropenia and thrombocytopenia appear to result from a direct, dose-dependent myelotoxic effect of the drug. This effect probably results from nonspecific activation of the drug by cellular (host cell) enzymes and subsequent inhibition of cellular DNA synthesis, particularly in rapidly dividing cells (e.g., in bone marrow). In vitro, ganciclovir has been shown to exhibit dose-dependent inhibitory effects on both myeloid and erythroid human progenitor cells, with erythroid precursors being slightly less sensitive than myeloid precursors to the cytotoxic effects. In one in vitro study, ganciclovir exhibited substantial and acyclovir minimal cytotoxic effects as determined by inhibition of colony formation of human granulocyte-macrophage precursors, which could in part explain the apparent differences in in vivo hematologic toxicity of these drugs.

Careful monitoring for potential hematologic toxicity is necessary during ganciclovir therapy. (See Cautions: Precautions and Contraindications.)

■ **Ocular Effects** Rhegmatogenous retinal detachment has been reported in patients with CMV retinitis, both before and after initiation of ganciclovir therapy; however, the relationship between ganciclovir and retinal detachment is not known. Such detachment is thought to result from the hastening of the involutional stage of the disease in which the retina thins as necrotic tissue is mobilized and edema fluid resorbs; these changes predispose the retina to tears and detachment. Retinal detachment has been reported in 11–30% of ganciclovir-treated patients with CMV retinitis. This complication appears to occur more frequently in AIDS patients than in other immunosuppressed patients and may be related to the inability of AIDS patients to form firm scar tissue, secondary to impaired inflammatory responses, as the retina heals.

Intravitreal injection† of ganciclovir (0.05–0.1 mL of a solution containing 2–8 mg/mL) did not produce any apparent oculotoxic effects in animal studies or in a limited number of patients being treated for CMV retinitis. In one study in several patients with CMV retinitis, there was no evidence during 77–244 days of observation of oculotoxic effects (e.g., lens changes, anterior segment or vitreal inflammation, retinal detachment) associated with intravitreal injection of 9–30 (mean: 16.6) doses of the drug per eye. In a study in rabbits, intravitreal injection of single ganciclovir doses ranging from 10–400 mcg at concentrations of 1–20 mcg/mL produced no discernible ophthalmologic or histologic changes in the eye or in electroretinographic B waves.

Although intravitreal injection† of ganciclovir has been well tolerated, local reactions, such as foreign body sensation, small conjunctival or vitreal hemorrhage, and mattering, have been associated with such administration. In addition, conjunctival scarring and scleral induration have been observed occasionally in patients receiving multiple intravitreal injections of the drug. Staphylococcal endophthalmitis, which responded to intravitreal antibacterial therapy alone or combined with systemic therapy, has been reported in several patients receiving intravitreal ganciclovir. In addition, rhegmatogenous retinal detachment occurred in several patients during intravitreal injection; while this complication also has been associated with IV ganciclovir therapy, the possibility exists that local trauma associated with intravitreal injection may have contributed to its occurrence in these patients.

■ **Nervous System Effects** Adverse nervous system effects, including headache, insomnia, dizziness, paresthesia, hypoesthesia, seizures, somnolence, and tremor, have been reported in clinical studies in patients receiving ganciclovir for the treatment of CMV retinitis or in transplant recipients receiving the drug for prophylaxis of CMV. Peripheral neuropathy has been reported in 9% of patients receiving IV ganciclovir for maintenance therapy of CMV retinitis. Dysesthesia, dysphasia, extrapyramidal disorder, facial paralysis, amnesia, anosmia, myelopathy, cerebrovascular accident, third cranial nerve paralysis, aphasia, encephalopathy, and intracranial hypertension have been reported during postmarketing experience in patients receiving ganciclovir. In some cases, observed nervous system effects may have resulted from causes other than the drug itself, such as opportunistic infections (e.g., toxoplasmosis, cryptococcosis) or HIV encephalopathy, and this possibility should be considered in any ganciclovir-treated patient who develops such effects.

Psychiatric disorders, including depression, confused state, anxiety, agitation, psychotic disorder, abnormal thinking, and abnormal dreams, have been reported in clinical studies in patients receiving ganciclovir for the treatment of CMV retinitis or in transplant recipients receiving the drug for prophylaxis of CMV. Irritability and hallucinations have been reported during postmarketing experience in patients receiving ganciclovir.

■ **GI Effects** Diarrhea, decreased appetite, and vomiting have been reported in 44, 14, and 13% of patients, respectively, receiving IV ganciclovir for maintenance treatment of CMV retinitis. Other adverse GI effects that have been reported in clinical studies in patients receiving ganciclovir for the treatment of CMV retinitis or in transplant recipients receiving the drug for prophylaxis of CMV include nausea, GI perforation, abdominal pain, dyspepsia, flatulence, constipation, mouth ulceration, dysphagia, abdominal distention, pancreatitis, eructation, dysgeusia, and dry mouth. Intestinal ulcer has been reported during postmarketing experience in patients receiving ganciclovir.

■ **Renal and Genitourinary Effects** Increased serum creatinine concentrations have been reported when IV ganciclovir was used in geriatric patients or in transplant patients, including transplant patients receiving concomitant therapy with nephrotoxic drugs (e.g., cyclosporine, amphotericin B). In a placebo-controlled study in cardiac allograft recipients, increased serum creatinine concentrations (2.5 mg/dL or greater) occurred in 18% of those receiving IV ganciclovir and 4% of those receiving placebo. In a study in bone marrow allograft recipients, 20% of patients receiving ganciclovir had serum creatinine concentrations of 2.5 mg/dL or greater whereas no patients receiving placebo had these increased concentrations. In a study in bone marrow allograft recipients, increased serum creatinine concentrations were not reported in patients receiving ganciclovir.

Kidney failure, abnormal renal function, urinary frequency, and hematuria have been reported in clinical studies in patients receiving ganciclovir for the treatment of CMV retinitis or in transplant recipients receiving the drug for prophylaxis of CMV. Renal tubular disorder and hemolytic uremic syndrome have been reported during postmarketing experience in patients receiving ganciclovir.

■ **Local Effects** Inflammation, edema, phlebitis, and/or pain at the site of IV infusion have been reported in patients receiving ganciclovir and probably are related to the high pH of the infusion solution. (See Dosage and Administration: Reconstitution and Administration.) To minimize the risk of phlebitis, the use of a vein with adequate blood flow is recommended to allow for rapid dilution and distribution of the drug.

Infection at the IV catheter site and other catheter-associated events (e.g., sepsis) have been reported in patients receiving IV ganciclovir.

Intravitreal injection† of ganciclovir in a limited number of animals and humans did not appear to produce oculotoxic effects, although other local ocular effects occasionally were observed. (See Cautions: Ocular Effects.)

■ **Other Adverse Effects** Pyrexia has been reported in 48% of patients receiving IV ganciclovir for maintenance therapy of CMV retinitis. Other adverse effects reported in 5–13% of patients receiving IV ganciclovir include sepsis, infection, hyperhidrosis, chills, and pruritus.

Hypersensitivity, including anaphylactic or allergic reactions, have been reported in patients receiving ganciclovir.

■ **Precautions and Contraindications** Ganciclovir is contraindicated in patients who have had a clinically important hypersensitivity reaction (e.g., anaphylaxis) to ganciclovir, valganciclovir, or any component of the formulation.

Because ganciclovir therapy is associated with hematologic toxicity (e.g., neutropenia, anemia, and/or thrombocytopenia), complete blood counts with differential and platelet counts should be monitored frequently in all patients, especially in those with renal impairment, baseline neutrophil counts less than $1000/mm^3$, or a history of leukopenia during treatment with ganciclovir or other nucleoside analogs and in those receiving myelosuppressive drugs or radiation therapy. Ganciclovir is not recommended in patients with absolute neutrophil counts less than $500/mm^3$, platelet counts less than $25,000/mm^3$, or hemoglobin concentrations less than 8 g/dL. Patients should be informed about the potential hematologic toxicities of the drug and the importance of close monitoring of blood cell counts.

Because plasma concentrations and half-life of ganciclovir are increased in patients with renal impairment, the drug should be used with caution in such patients and dosage should be adjusted based on the degree of renal impairment. (See Dosage and Administration: Dosage in Renal Impairment.) Renal function monitoring is essential in all patients receiving ganciclovir therapy, especially in geriatric patients and in transplant recipients receiving concomitant nephrotoxic drugs (e.g., cyclosporine, amphotericin B). (See Drug Interactions.) Patients receiving ganciclovir should be adequately hydrated since the drug is almost entirely excreted renally and normal clearance depends on adequate renal function. Patients should be informed that ganciclovir has been associated with decreased renal function and that serum creatinine concentrations or creatinine clearance should be monitored during treatment with the drug and that dosage adjustments are necessary in patients with renal impairment.

Safety and efficacy of ganciclovir have not been evaluated in patients with hepatic impairment.

Frequent ophthalmologic examinations are necessary in patients being treated for CMV retinitis to monitor status of the CMV retinitis and assess for other retinal abnormalities. Patients should be informed that ganciclovir is not a cure for CMV retinitis and that they may continue to experience progression and/or recurrence of the retinitis during or following treatment with the drug. Patients also should be advised about the necessity of frequent ophthalmologic examinations and that some patients may require more frequent ophthalmologic follow-up.

Patients should be advised that ganciclovir may cause seizures, dizziness, and/or confusion, which may affect cognitive abilities (e.g., ability to drive or operate machinery).

Patients should be advised that animal data suggest that ganciclovir is a potential carcinogen. (See Cautions: Mutagenicity and Carcinogenicity.)

Patients should be advised that ganciclovir may cause temporary or permanent inhibition of spermatogenesis in males and suppression of fertility in females. (See Cautions: Pregnancy, Fertility, and Lactation.)

Because of the mutagenic potential of ganciclovir and the potential for fetal harm, women of reproductive potential should undergo pregnancy testing before initiation of ganciclovir. In addition, females of childbearing potential should use effective contraception during and for at least 30 days after ganciclovir therapy and male patients should use barrier contraceptive methods during and for at least 90 days after ganciclovir therapy. (See Cautions: Pregnancy, Fertility, and Lactation.)

■ **Pediatric Precautions** Safety and efficacy of ganciclovir have not been established in pediatric patients.

Granulocytopenia and thrombocytopenia were the most common adverse effects reported in pediatric patients† who received ganciclovir in clinical trials.

Although the pharmacokinetics of IV ganciclovir reported in pediatric patients are similar to those reported in adults (see Pharmacokinetics), safety and efficacy of such ganciclovir exposures in pediatric patients have not been established.

■ **Geriatric Precautions** Clinical studies of ganciclovir did not include sufficient numbers of patients 65 years of age or older to determine whether geriatric patients respond differently than younger adults. Dosage in geriatric patients generally should be selected carefully, taking into account the greater frequency of decreased hepatic, renal, and/or cardiac function and of concomitant disease and drug therapy in the elderly.

Because geriatric patients may have decreased renal function and because patients with renal impairment may be at increased risk of ganciclovir-induced toxicity, particular attention should be paid to evaluating renal function prior to and during ganciclovir therapy in this age group. If evidence of renal impairment exists or develops, appropriate dosage adjustments should be made. (See Dosage and Administration: Dosage in Renal Impairment.)

■ **Mutagenicity and Carcinogenicity** Based on animal data, ganciclovir should be considered a potential carcinogen in humans.

Ganciclovir increased mutations in mouse lymphoma cells and DNA damage in human lymphocytes in vitro at concentrations between 50–500 and 250–2000 mcg/mL, respectively. In the mouse micronucleus assay, ganciclovir was clastogenic at doses of 150 and 500 mg/kg (2.8–10 times exposures attained in humans with the recommended human dose), but such effects were not observed at doses comparable to the recommended human dose. Ganciclovir was not mutagenic in the Ames *Salmonella* assay at concentrations of 500–5000 mcg/mL.

Ganciclovir was carcinogenic in mice at mean drug exposures equal to those attained in humans with the recommended dose of 5 mg/kg. At exposures 1.4 times the human exposure at the recommended human dose, there was a significant increase in the incidence of tumors of the preputial gland in males, forestomach (nonglandular mucosa) in males and females, and reproductive tissues (ovaries, uterus, mammary gland, clitoral gland, vagina) and liver in females. At exposures 0.1 times the human exposure at the recommended human dose, there was a slightly increased incidence of tumors in the preputial and harderian glands in males, forestomach in males and females, and liver in females. Carcinogenic effects were not observed in mice at exposures estimated to be 0.01 times those attained in humans with the recommended human dose.

■ **Pregnancy, Fertility, and Lactation** ***Pregnancy*** Animal data indicate that ganciclovir has the potential to cause fetal toxicity, including birth defects, in humans. Data regarding use of ganciclovir in pregnant women are inadequate to establish whether the drug poses a risk to pregnancy outcomes. Ganciclovir appears to cross the placenta based on ex vivo experiments with human placenta and at least one case report in a pregnant woman.

In animal studies, ganciclovir caused maternal and fetal toxicity and embryofetal mortality in pregnant mice and rabbits and teratogenic effects in rabbits at systemic exposures that were approximately 2 times those attained in humans at the recommended human dose. IV ganciclovir administered to pregnant mice (108 mg/kg daily) and rabbits (60 mg/kg daily) and administered to female mice (90 mg/kg) prior to mating, during gestation, and during lactation resulted in fetal resorptions in at least 85% of the mice and rabbits. Fetal growth retardation, embryolethality, and teratogenic effects (cleft palate, anophthalmia/microphthalmia, hydrocephaly, brachygnathia, aplastic organs [kidney, pancreas]) were reported in the rabbits. In pre/postnatal development studies in mice, maternal/fetal toxicity and embryolethality were observed and included hypoplasia of the testes and seminal vesicles in male offspring, as well as pathologic changes in the nonglandular region of the stomach.

Although most maternal CMV infections are asymptomatic or may be associated with a self-limited mononucleosis-like syndrome, CMV infections in pregnant immunocompromised patients (e.g., HIV-infected patients with AIDS, transplant recipients) may be symptomatic and result in substantial maternal morbidity and mortality. Perinatal transmission of CMV from an infected mother to her fetus can occur resulting in congenital CMV infection and disease. (See Congenital Cytomegalovirus Disease under Uses: Treatment of Cytomegalovirus Infection and Disease.)

Females of childbearing potential should undergo pregnancy testing before initiation of ganciclovir.

Females of childbearing potential should use effective contraception during and for at least 30 days after ganciclovir therapy and male patients should use effective barrier contraceptive methods during and for at least 90 days after ganciclovir therapy.

Fertility Based on animal data and limited human data, ganciclovir at the usually recommended dosages may cause temporary or permanent inhibition of spermatogenesis in men and may cause suppression of fertility in women.

In female mice, ganciclovir caused decreased mating behavior, decreased fertility, and increased incidence of embryolethality at exposures approximately 1.7 times those attained in humans at the recommended human dose. Ganciclovir caused decreased fertility in male mice and hypospermatogenesis in male mice and dogs following oral or IV doses ranging from 0.2–10 mg/kg. Systemic exposures at the lowest dose associated with toxicity in each species ranged from 0.03–0.1 times the human exposures attained with the recommended human dose.

In a small, open-label, nonrandomized clinical study, adult male renal transplant patients receiving CMV prophylaxis with valganciclovir (prodrug of ganciclovir) for up to 200 days posttransplantation were followed for 6 months after the drug was discontinued and data compared with an untreated control group. Among 24 evaluable patients in the valganciclovir group, the mean sperm density at the end-of-treatment visit was *decreased* by 11 million/mL from baseline; whereas, among 14 evaluable patients in the control group, the mean sperm density at the end-of-treatment visit had *increased* by 33 million/mL. However, at the final follow-up visit, the mean sperm density among 20 evaluable patients in the valganciclovir group was comparable to that observed among 10 evaluable patients in the untreated control group (mean sperm density increased by 41 or 43 million/mL from baseline, respectively).

Patients receiving ganciclovir should be advised that the drug may be associated with infertility.

Lactation It is not known whether ganciclovir is distributed into human milk, affects the breast-fed infant, or affects milk production. The drug is distributed into milk in lactating rats; the milk-to-serum ratio at steady state is approximately 1.6 in rats.

Because of the potential for serious adverse reactions to ganciclovir in breast-fed infants, nursing women should be instructed not to breast-feed while they are receiving the drug. HIV-infected mothers should be instructed not to breast-feed their infants because of the risk of transmission of HIV.

Drug Interactions

Drug interaction studies with ganciclovir were performed in patients with normal renal function. In patients with renal impairment, concomitant use of ganciclovir and other drugs eliminated by renal excretion may result in increased concentrations of ganciclovir and the concomitant drug and such patients should be closely monitored for toxicity associated with ganciclovir and the concomitant drug.

■ **Antibacterial Agents** ***Imipenem and Cilastatin Sodium*** Generalized seizures have occurred in several patients who received concomitant therapy with the fixed combination of imipenem and cilastatin sodium (imipenem/cilastatin) and ganciclovir. While the mechanism of this potential interaction is not known, the seizures resolved in all but one patient when both imipenem/cilastatin and ganciclovir or just imipenem/cilastatin was discontinued. In the patient whose seizures failed to resolve following discontinuance of imipenem/cilastatin, continued seizures were attributed to encephalitis rather than the drugs.

Because of the risk of seizures, concomitant use of imipenem/cilastatin and ganciclovir is not recommended.

Trimethoprim Concomitant use of trimethoprim and oral ganciclovir (no longer commercially available in the US) did not affect the pharmacokinetics of either drug.

Because of possible increased toxicity, concomitant use of trimethoprim and ganciclovir should be considered only if potential benefits outweigh risks.

Other Antibacterials Because of possible increased toxicity if ganciclovir is used with certain anti-infectives (e.g., co-trimoxazole, dapsone, pentamidine, sulfamethoxazole), concomitant use of ganciclovir and such anti-infectives should be considered only if potential benefits outweigh risks.

■ **Antifungal Agents** ***Amphotericin B*** Concomitant use of amphotericin B and ganciclovir may result in increased serum creatinine concentrations.

Renal function should be monitored if amphotericin B and ganciclovir are used concomitantly.

Flucytosine Because of possible increased toxicity, concomitant use of flucytosine and ganciclovir should be considered only if potential benefits outweigh risks.

■ **Antiretroviral Agents** ***Didanosine*** Although the clinical importance is unclear, there is some in vitro evidence that ganciclovir may antagonize the antiretroviral activity of didanosine against human immunodeficiency virus (HIV).

Concomitant use of didanosine (200 mg every 12 hours) with IV ganciclovir (5 mg/kg twice daily) has resulted in a 70% increase in the area under the plasma concentration-time curve (AUC_{0-12}) and 49% increase in peak plasma concentrations of didanosine, but did not affect the pharmacokinetics of ganciclovir.

Patients receiving didanosine and ganciclovir concomitantly should be monitored closely for didanosine toxicity (e.g., pancreatitis).

Tenofovir Concomitant use of ganciclovir and tenofovir alafenamide or tenofovir disoproxil fumarate may result in increased serum concentrations of ganciclovir and/or tenofovir and patients should be monitored for dose-related tenofovir toxicities.

Zidovudine Although the clinical importance is unclear, there is some in vitro evidence that ganciclovir may antagonize the antiretroviral activity of zidovudine against HIV.

Concomitant use of zidovudine with ganciclovir can increase the risk of hematologic toxicity. Both zidovudine and ganciclovir alone produce direct, dose-dependent inhibitory effects on myeloid and erythroid progenitor cells, and combined use of the drugs may result in additive or synergistic myelotoxic effects. In several studies in patients with acquired immunodeficiency syndrome (AIDS) and cytomegalovirus (CMV) infection, profound, intolerable myelosuppression, evidenced principally as severe neutropenia, occurred in all patients receiving oral zidovudine (200 mg every 4 hours) concomitantly with IV ganciclovir (5 mg/kg 1–4 times daily); anemia also occurred in many of these patients. Severe hematologic toxicity, which required a reduction in zidovudine dosage, also occurred in more than 80% of patients receiving oral zidovudine (100 mg every 4 hours) concomitantly with IV ganciclovir (5 mg/kg 1–2 times daily). Several other patients with initially stable hematologic findings on ganciclovir alone, developed prolonged pancytopenia during concomitant therapy with oral zidovudine and IV ganciclovir. The increased risk of hematologic toxicity does not appear to be related to a pharmacokinetic interaction between ganciclovir and zidovudine.

Because of the risk of hematologic toxicity, concomitant use of zidovudine and ganciclovir should be considered only if potential benefits outweigh risks. If combined therapy is considered necessary, the drugs should be used with extreme caution and careful monitoring of hematologic function.

■ **Antiviral Agents** ***Foscarnet*** Concomitant use of ganciclovir and foscarnet does not affect the pharmacokinetics of either drug. However, ganciclovir and foscarnet are physically incompatible and must not be admixed.

Foscarnet has exhibited additive or synergistic antiviral activity with ganciclovir in vitro against CMV and herpes simplex virus type 2 (HSV-2). There was no in vitro evidence of antagonistic antiviral effects between ganciclovir and foscarnet.

In addition, combined therapy with the drugs may be effective in the treatment of CMV infection resistant to either drug alone. In several AIDS patients with CMV retinitis and/or GI infections that progressed during therapy with either ganciclovir or foscarnet alone, concomitant use of the drugs appeared to effectively reduce the symptoms and halt progression of the disease. Concomitant therapy was effective in some patients who previously had received monotherapy with both drugs. Although the incidence of anemia during concomitant therapy was higher than that reported during use of ganciclovir alone, adverse effects were not severe enough to require discontinuance of concomitant therapy.

Letermovir In vitro, there was no evidence of antagonistic anti-CMV effects between letermovir and ganciclovir.

■ **Immunosuppressive Agents** Patients receiving immunosuppressive agents (e.g., azathioprine, cyclosporine, corticosteroids) may require decreased dosages or temporary withdrawal of these drugs during ganciclovir therapy to prevent excessive suppression of bone marrow or the immune system.

Cyclosporine When oral cyclosporine at therapeutic doses was used concomitantly with IV ganciclovir (5 mg/kg every 12 hours) in liver allograft recipients, there was no evidence of any change in cyclosporine whole blood concentrations. However, concomitant use of these drugs may increase serum creatinine concentrations.

If ganciclovir is used concomitantly with cyclosporine, renal function should be monitored.

Mycophenolate Mofetil Concomitant use of mycophenolate mofetil and ganciclovir in patients with normal renal function does not affect the pharmacokinetics of either drug.

Because of possible increased risk, the patient should be monitored for hematologic and renal toxicity if mycophenolate mofetil and ganciclovir are used concomitantly.

Tacrolimus Because of possible increased toxicity, concomitant use of tacrolimus and ganciclovir should be considered only if potential benefits outweigh risks.

■ **Myelosuppressive Drugs** Concomitant use of ganciclovir and myelosuppressive drugs may have additive toxicity. Such drugs include dapsone, pentamidine, pyrimethamine, flucytosine, cytotoxic antineoplastic agents (e.g., vincristine, vinblastine, doxorubicin, hydroxyurea), amphotericin B, co-trimoxazole, or other nucleoside analogs. These drugs should be used concomitantly with ganciclovir only when the potential benefits of such therapy are thought to outweigh the possible risks. In addition, the possibility that AIDS patients may be at particular risk for potential toxicity during combined therapy should be considered, since such patients appear to be at increased risk of hematologic toxicity with some of these drugs alone (e.g., co-trimoxazole).

■ **Probenecid** Concomitant use of probenecid (500 mg every 6 hours) with oral ganciclovir (no longer commercially available in the US) has resulted in a 53% increase in the AUC of ganciclovir and a 22% decrease in renal clearance of ganciclovir.

If probenecid and ganciclovir are used concomitantly, reduced ganciclovir dosage may be required and the patient should be monitored for ganciclovir toxicity.

Acute Toxicity

The acute lethal dose of ganciclovir in humans is not known.

Overdosages of IV ganciclovir, including some fatalities, have been reported during clinical trials and postmarketing experience. In general, overdosage may be expected to produce toxicities that are extensions of the drug's pharmacologic and adverse effects. Ganciclovir overdosage has resulted in hematologic toxicity (pancytopenia, leukopenia, neutropenia, granulocytopenia, thrombocytopenia, bone marrow failure), hepatotoxicity (hepatitis, liver function disorder), renal toxicity (worsening of hematuria, acute kidney injury, elevated creatinine concentration), GI toxicity (abdominal pain, diarrhea, vomiting), and neurotoxicity (seizure).

Management of ganciclovir overdosage generally involves symptomatic and supportive care. Because the drug is removed by dialysis (see Pharmacokinetics: Elimination), hemodialysis or peritoneal dialysis might be useful in the management of overdosage. Adequate hydration should be maintained. Protective measures for neutropenia may be necessary until bone marrow function returns; use of hematopoietic growth factors should be considered in patients with cytopenias.

Mechanism of Action

Ganciclovir exerts its antiviral effect on human cytomegalovirus (CMV) and other human herpesviruses by interfering with DNA synthesis via competition with deoxyguanosine for incorporation into viral DNA and thereby inhibiting viral DNA polymerase as well as being incorporated into growing viral DNA chains.

Ganciclovir is a prodrug and exhibits no antiviral activity until converted intracellularly to the active metabolite, ganciclovir triphosphate. In CMV-infected cells, ganciclovir is initially phosphorylated to ganciclovir monophosphate by the viral protein kinase pUL97. Further phosphorylation occurs by cellular kinases to produce the pharmacologically active ganciclovir triphosphate. Ganciclovir triphosphate is a viral DNA polymerase inhibitor that competitively inhibits viral DNA polymerase pUL54. The drug also is incorporated into growing DNA chains as a false nucleotide, thus interfering with chain elongation (prematurely terminating DNA synthesis) and/or resulting in formation of a mutant DNA chain and thereby inhibiting viral replication.

Because conversion of ganciclovir to the pharmacologically active triphosphate is largely dependent on viral kinase, phosphorylation of the drug occurs preferentially in virus-infected cells. The formation of ganciclovir monophosphate appears to be the rate-limiting step in the formation of ganciclovir triphosphate. In vitro in herpesviruses, ganciclovir triphosphate functions both as substrate for, and a preferential inhibitor of, viral DNA polymerase and as a false nucleotide base. In cells infected with herpes simplex virus type 1 or 2 (HSV-1 or HSV-2) or varicella-zoster virus (VZV), ganciclovir is converted to ganciclovir monophosphate via virus-coded thymidine kinase. The pathway for conversion to the monophosphate in cells infected with CMV or Epstein-Barr virus (EBV) differs since these viruses do not code for thymidine kinase. A cellular deoxyguanosine kinase, found in the cytosol and in mitochondria, may be involved. In CMV-infected cells, increased concentrations of deoxyguanosine kinase (mitochondrial origin) have been detected, suggesting that the virus may induce production of the enzyme.

Ganciclovir is virustatic in action. Following removal of the drug from the culture medium in vitro, viral DNA synthesis (which previously was inhibited) resumes, resulting in restored viral replication. In addition, clinical evidence of reactivated disease suggests that ganciclovir acts principally to suppress virus activity and that eradication of the virus does not occur.

During the course of an acute or asymptomatic herpesvirus infection, the virus usually leaves the initial site of infection and invades other cells and tissues where it establishes a latent infection. HSV-1, HSV-2, and VZV are thought to establish latent infections principally within the ganglia. CMV and Epstein-Barr virus are thought to establish latent infections within leukocytes and B cells, respectively. CMV also may establish a site of latent infection in solid organ tissue (e.g., lung, kidney). The exact nature of the virus in the latent state is not well understood; however, evidence suggests that the virus is not actively replicating and, therefore, would not be susceptible to the action of antiviral agents such as ganciclovir. Despite the host's immunity, herpesvirus latency usually persists for life and the viruses can be reactivated periodically by various stimuli, including immunosuppression. Reactivation of latent CMV has been specifically linked to pregnancy and to decreases in host immunocompetence, either iatrogenic or via disease process (i.e., acquired immunodeficiency syndrome). Once reactivated, the virus usually reinfects the site of initial infection. Ganciclovir, like other antivirals, is unable to eliminate an established latent infection, as demonstrated in animal tests.

Spectrum

Following intracellular conversion of ganciclovir to the pharmacologically active ganciclovir triphosphate, the drug is active against human herpesviruses, including cytomegalovirus (CMV), herpes simplex virus types 1 and 2 (HSV-1 and HSV-2), and varicella-zoster virus (VZV). Although the clinical importance is unclear, ganciclovir has some in vitro activity against Epstein-Barr virus (EBV) and human herpesvirus type 6 and type 8. Ganciclovir is not active against human immunodeficiency virus (HIV).

Resistance

Cytomegalovirus (CMV) isolates resistant to ganciclovir have been selected in vitro in the presence of increasing concentrations of the drug. Ganciclovir-resistant CMV have been reported in ganciclovir-naive patients and may emerge in patients receiving prolonged treatment or prophylaxis with the drug. The possibility of ganciclovir-resistant CMV should be considered in patients who show poor clinical response or relapse or experience persistent viral shedding during ganciclovir therapy.

Several mechanisms of resistance to ganciclovir apparently exist. Since the antiviral activity of ganciclovir depends on phosphorylation of the drug to ganciclovir triphosphate (see Mechanism of Action), resistance to the drug may result from decreased phosphorylation. In some viruses, such as herpes simplex virus (HSV) and varicella-zoster virus (VZV), resistance to ganciclovir might result from low or absent concentrations of virus-coded thymidine kinase or from alterations in substrate specificity of the enzyme. However, other mechanisms also appear to be involved since some thymidine-kinase deficient or mutant strains of acyclovir-resistant HSV are susceptible to ganciclovir.

Ganciclovir resistance usually is the result of amino acid substitutions in the viral protein kinase pUL97 and/or the viral DNA polymerase pUL54. Certain pUL97 ganciclovir resistance-associated substitutions (e.g., M460V/I, H520Q, C529G, A594V, L595S, C603W) have been reported most frequently in clinical isolates. Numerous other pUL97 and pUL54 ganciclovir resistance-associated mutations also have been reported.

Cross-resistance can occur between ganciclovir and some other antivirals (e.g., acyclovir, cidofovir, foscarnet). Certain amino acid substitutions selected in vitro in cell culture following exposure of CMV to ganciclovir, cidofovir, or foscarnet have resulted in cross-resistance. Amino acid substitutions in pUL54 that confer cross-resistance between ganciclovir and cidofovir generally have involved the exonuclease domains and region V of the viral DNA polymerase. A variety of amino acid substitutions have conferred cross-resistance between ganciclovir and foscarnet, but concentrate at and between regions II and III of viral DNA polymerase.

Pharmacokinetics

Dosages and concentrations of ganciclovir sodium are expressed in terms of ganciclovir. A concentration of 1 mcg of ganciclovir per mL is approximately equivalent to 3.92 μmol/L.

■ **Absorption** Following IV administration of ganciclovir given in a dosage of 5 mg/kg every 12 hours by IV infusion over 1 hour, peak plasma concentrations of the drug ranged from 8.3–9 mcg/mL. In immunocompromised patients with cytomegalovirus (CMV) infection and normal renal function who received 2.5 mg/kg of ganciclovir every 8 hours by IV infusion over 1 hour, peak and trough plasma concentrations of the drug averaged 4.09–5.36 (range: 1.66–7.78 mcg/mL) and 0.33–1.07 mcg/mL (range: 0.2–1.66 mcg/mL), respectively. In a limited number of such patients receiving 5 mg/kg every 8 hours by IV infusion over 1 hour, peak and trough plasma concentrations averaged 6.53–11.41 and 1.13–2.23 mcg/mL, respectively. Following IV administration, ganciclovir exhibits linear pharmacokinetics over the dosage range of 1.6–5 mg/kg. Accumulation of the drug does not appear to occur in patients with normal renal function receiving IV dosages of 3–15 mg/kg daily in divided doses.

Studies have not been performed to specifically evaluate the pharmacokinetics of IV ganciclovir in geriatric adults 65 years of age and older.

In a limited number of neonates 2–49 days of age†, IV administration of a ganciclovir dose of 4 or 6 mg/kg resulted in peak plasma concentrations of 5.5 or 7 mcg/mL, respectively. In pediatric patients 9 months to 12 years of age† who received IV ganciclovir (single or multiple doses of 5 mg/kg every 12 hours), peak plasma concentrations of the drug were 7.9 mcg/mL.

Limited data regarding intravitreal injection† of ganciclovir suggest that minimal systemic absorption of the drug occurs, although adequate intravitreal ganciclovir concentrations appear to be achievable with this route. In a patient with CMV retinitis receiving five 200-mcg intravitreal doses of ganciclovir over 15 days, plasma concentrations of the drug were less than 0.1 mcg/mL. A vitreous humor concentration of 1.17 mcg/mL and an aqueous humor concentration of 0.66 mcg/mL were achieved 51.4 hours after the initial dose in this patient, and a vitreous humor concentration of 0.1 mcg/mL was achieved 97.3 hours after the fourth dose. Data from rabbits also indicate that antiviral intravitreal concentrations of the drug are achievable with small intravitreal but *not* subconjunctival doses of ganciclovir. Following intravitreal injection of a single 400-mcg dose in rabbits, vitreous humor ganciclovir concentrations averaged 543, 423, 57.7, 16, 2.02, and 1.2 mcg/mL at 2, 5, 12, 24, 48, and 60 hours after injection. Following subconjunctival injection of a single 1.25-mg dose in rabbits, ganciclovir concentrations at 1, 2, 3, and 8 hours after injection averaged 0.09, 0.31, 0.16, and 0.02 mcg/mL, respectively, in vitreous humor and 2.18, 3.27, 2.22, and 0.07 mcg/mL, respectively, in aqueous humor.

■ **Distribution** Following IV administration, ganciclovir is widely distributed. Autopsy findings in several patients who had been receiving IV ganciclovir suggest that the drug concentrates in the kidneys, with substantially lower concentrations occurring in lung, liver, brain, and testes. While efficacy of ganciclovir in CMV pneumonitis has been reported to be substantially less than in some other CMV infections (e.g., retinitis), lung ganciclovir concentrations that exceed the ID_{50} for CMV appear to be achievable with usual IV dosages of the drug. Concentrations attained in lung and liver were 99 and 92%, respectively, of those attained concurrently in heart/blood in several adults receiving the drug IV. Following IV administration in mice, ganciclovir was distributed widely, achieving highest concentrations in the kidney and lowest concentrations in the brain. Substantial distribution of ganciclovir into lung, liver, heart, spleen, stomach, intestines, muscle, and testes also occur, exceeding concurrent blood concentrations in these tissues; concentrations achieved in brain, eyes, and fat were lower than concurrent blood concentrations. Accumulation of the drug did not appear to occur, although measurable concentrations persisted for at least 30 hours in stomach, liver, and intestines in these animals. In addition, there was no evidence of testicular ganciclovir accumulation in several men receiving 15 mg/kg IV daily for 8–13 days.

The volume of distribution of ganciclovir at steady state following IV administration is 0.74 L/kg. The volume of distribution appears to be reduced in patients with renal impairment.

Data on intraocular concentrations of ganciclovir following IV administration are limited, but it appears that the drug has good ocular distribution following administration by this route. In one adult patient, subretinal ganciclovir concentrations were 0.87 and 2 times concurrent plasma concentrations at 5.5 and 8 hours after IV administration, respectively. In another adult patient, aqueous and vitreous humor ganciclovir concentrations were 0.4 and 0.6 times simultaneous plasma concentrations, respectively, at 2.5 hours after IV infusion of the drug; at 21 hours after IV infusion, plasma concentrations were undetectable, while the vitreous humor concentration was still 0.2 mcg/mL. Following intravitreal injection† of ganciclovir in an adult with CMV retinitis, the apparent volume of distribution in vitreous humor was 11.7 mL, suggesting that the drug may distribute into the retina.

Ganciclovir crosses the blood-brain barrier. Following IV administration in several adult patients, ganciclovir concentrations in CSF at 0.25–5.7 hours after a dose ranged from 0.31–0.68 mcg/mL and averaged 41% (range: 24–70%) of corresponding plasma concentration of the drug. Autopsy findings revealed similar evidence of CNS distribution of the drug in several other patients, with brain tissue concentrations of ganciclovir averaging 38% of corresponding blood concentrations.

Ganciclovir appears to cross the placenta based on ex vivo experiments with human placenta and at least one case report in a pregnant woman.

It is not known whether ganciclovir is distributed into milk in humans, but the drug is distributed into milk following IV administration in rats.

Ganciclovir is 1–2% bound to plasma proteins at drug concentrations of 0.5–51 mcg/mL.

■ **Elimination** Following IV administration in adults with normal renal function, the half-life of ganciclovir is 3.5 hours. Plasma concentrations of the drug may be higher and the elimination half-life prolonged in patients with impaired renal function. In a limited number of immunocompromised patients with renal impairment who received IV ganciclovir doses ranging from 1.25–5 mg/kg, mean plasma half-life of the drug was 4.4 hours in those with creatinine clearances of 25–59 mL/minute and 10.7 hours in those with creatinine clearances less than 25 mL/minute. In adults with moderate to severe renal impairment (creatinine clearances less than 50 mL/minute per 1.73 m^2), the terminal half-life ($t_{1/2\beta}$) of IV ganciclovir ranged from 4.4–30 hours, depending on the degree of impairment.

Although the pharmacokinetics of ganciclovir have not been specifically evaluated in geriatric patients, renal clearance decreases with age and decreased ganciclovir total body clearance and prolonged half-life of the drug are expected in adults 65 years of age and older.

In a limited number of neonates 2–49 days of age† who received IV ganciclovir, the plasma half-life of the drug was 2.4 hours. In pediatric patients 9 months to 12 years of age† who received IV ganciclovir, the plasma half-life of the drug also was approximately 2.4 hours.

Following intravitreal injection† of ganciclovir in a patient with CMV retinitis, the elimination half-life of the drug from the vitreous humor was estimated to be 13.3 hours. In this patient, intravitreal ganciclovir concentrations were estimated to exceed the ID_{50} (0.66 mcg/mL) of the virus for about 62 hours after a single 200-mcg intravitreal dose. In rabbits, the elimination half-life from vitreous humor after intravitreal injection of a single 400-mcg dose was 8.6 hours, and intravitreal ganciclovir concentrations exceeded the ID_{50} (range: 0.24–1.5 mcg/mL) of many strains of CMV for at least 60 hours.

With the exception of intracellular phosphorylation of the drug (see Mechanism of Action), ganciclovir does not appear to be metabolized appreciably in humans. The drug appears to undergo little, if any, extrarenal elimination, and approximately 90–99% of an IV dose is excreted unchanged in urine. Renal excretion of ganciclovir appears to occur principally via glomerular filtration and active tubular secretion.

Total body clearance of ganciclovir from plasma reportedly averages 170–203 mL/minute per 1.73 m^2 in adults with normal renal function. Total body clearance of the drug is decreased in adults with renal impairment and appears to correlate positively with creatinine clearance. In a limited number of patients, total body clearance from plasma averaged 128, 57, or 30 mL/minute in adults with creatinine clearances of 50–79, 25–49, or less than 25 mL/minute, respectively.

Ganciclovir is removed by hemodialysis. The amount of ganciclovir removed during hemodialysis depends on several factors (e.g., type of coil used, dialysis flow rate); however, in several patients, a 4-hour period of hemodialysis removed into the dialysate approximately 40–50% of a dose.

Chemistry and Stability

■ **Chemistry** Ganciclovir, a synthetic nucleoside analog of guanine, is an antiviral agent. Ganciclovir is structurally and pharmacologically related to acyclovir, differing from acyclovir only by the addition of a second terminal hydroxymethyl group at C-2 of the acyclic side chain on the ribose ring. Compared with acyclovir, this structural difference results in substantially increased antiviral activity against cytomegalovirus (CMV) and less selectivity for viral DNA.

Ganciclovir occurs as a white to off-white powder and has an aqueous solubility of 2.6 mg/mL at 25°C. Aqueous solubility of the drug is relatively constant over a pH range of 3.5–8.5, but increases substantially in strongly acidic or basic solutions. The drug has pK_as of 2.2 and 9.4.

Ganciclovir is commercially available for IV use as the monosodium salt, which is formed in situ by the addition of sodium hydroxide during the manufacturing process. At physiologic pH, ganciclovir sodium exists as the unionized form with a solubility of approximately 6 mg/mL at 37°C. Potency of ganciclovir sodium is expressed in terms of ganciclovir.

Commercially available ganciclovir sodium sterile powder for IV use provided in single-use vials containing 500 mg of ganciclovir occurs as a white to off-white lyophilized powder. The lyophilized powder has an aqueous solubility that is greater than 50 mg/mL at 25°C. Following reconstitution of the powder with preservative-free sterile water for injection, ganciclovir sodium solutions containing 50 mg of ganciclovir per mL are alkaline with a pH of 11 and are colorless.

Commercially available sterile ganciclovir sodium concentrate for IV use provided in single-use vials containing 500 mg of ganciclovir (50 mg/mL) should appear as a clear solution.

Commercially available premixed injection for IV use containing 500 mg of ganciclovir in 250 mL of 0.8% sodium chloride (2 mg/mL) is provided in single-use polymeric IV bags. The premixed solution has a pH of 7.5 and does not contain any preservatives.

■ **Stability** Ganciclovir sodium lyophilized powder for IV use provided in single-use vials should be stored at 25°C, but may be exposed to temperatures ranging from 15–30°C. Following reconstitution with sterile water for injection, ganciclovir sodium solutions containing 50 mg of ganciclovir per mL are stable for 12 hours at 25°C and should not be refrigerated or frozen. Bacteriostatic water for injection containing parabens should *not* be used for reconstitution of ganciclovir sodium since a precipitate may form. The manufacturer states that reconstituted ganciclovir sodium that has been further diluted in 0.9% sodium chloride or other compatible IV infusion solution should be stored under refrigeration at 2–8°C and used within 24 hours. The solution should not be frozen.

Ganciclovir sodium concentrate for IV use containing 500 mg of ganciclovir (50 mg/mL) provided in single-use vials should be stored at 25°C, but may be exposed to temperatures ranging from 15–30°C. Following dilution in 0.9% sodium chloride or other compatible IV infusion solution, the manufacturer states that the solution should be stored under refrigeration at 2–8°C and used within 24 hours. The solution should not be frozen.

The premixed injection for IV use containing 500 mg of ganciclovir in 250 mL of 0.8% sodium chloride (2 mg/mL) provided in single-use IV bags should be stored at 20–25°C, but may be exposed to temperatures ranging from 15–30°C. Crystals may form in the premixed solution if it is exposed during transportation or storage to temperatures lower than recommended; the crystals should redissolve if the bag is gently shaken.

At a concentration of 10 mg or less of ganciclovir per mL, ganciclovir sodium is physically and chemically stable in the following IV solutions: 0.9% sodium chloride, 5% dextrose, Ringer's, or lactated Ringer's. Solutions containing approximately 2.5 mg of ganciclovir per mL reportedly are physically and chemically stable for at least 5 days at 4–25°C in 0.9% sodium chloride injection or 5% dextrose injection. Although sterility of the solutions was not assessed, results of one study indicate that ganciclovir is stable for up to 35 days when diluted in 0.9% sodium chloride or 5% dextrose to a concentration of 1 or 5 mg/mL and stored in polyvinyl chloride (PVC) containers at 5°C or 25°C. In another study, ganciclovir was stable for up to 28 days when diluted in 0.9% sodium chloride or 5% dextrose to a concentration of 5 or 10 mg/mL and stored in PVC containers at 4°C or -20°C or stored in ADFuse syringes (Healthtek) at 4°C. Protection of diluted ganciclovir sodium solutions from usual room light is not necessary. The drug does not appear to adsorb appreciably to PVC containers.

Preparations

Excipients in commercially available drug preparations may have clinically important effects in some individuals; consult specific product labeling for details.

Ganciclovir

Parenteral

Injection, for IV infusion only	2 mg/mL (500 mg) in 0.8% Sodium Chloride*	**Ganciclovir Injection**

*available from one or more manufacturer, distributor, and/or repackager by generic (nonproprietary) name

Ganciclovir Sodium

Parenteral

Concentrate, for injection, for IV infusion only	50 mg (of ganciclovir) per mL (500 mg)*	**Ganciclovir Injection**
For injection, for IV infusion only	500 mg (of ganciclovir)*	**Cytovene®-IV**, Roche **Ganciclovir Sodium for Injection**

*available from one or more manufacturer, distributor, and/or repackager by generic (nonproprietary) name

†Use is not currently included in the labeling approved by the US Food and Drug Administration

Ribavirin

Tribavirin, RBV, RTCA

■ Ribavirin is a synthetic nucleoside antiviral agent that has a broad spectrum of antiviral activity against both RNA and DNA viruses.

Uses

■ **Hepatitis C Virus Infection** ***Chronic Hepatitis C Virus Infection*** For treatment of chronic HCV infection, oral ribavirin *must* be used as part of a multiple-drug regimen and should *not* be used alone.

Oral ribavirin has been used in conjunction with peginterferon alfa-2a (Pegasys®) or peginterferon alfa-2b (PegIntron®) for treatment of chronic hepatitis C virus (HCV) infection in adults and pediatric patients with compensated liver disease. Safety and efficacy of oral ribavirin in conjunction with peginterferon alfa or interferon alfa have *not* been established for treatment of chronic HCV infection in patients with decompensated liver disease, patients with hepatitis B virus (HBV) coinfection, or in liver or other organ transplant recipients. Although oral ribavirin was used in conjunction with nonconjugated interferon alfa-2b in the past for the treatment of chronic HCV infection, regimens that include nonconjugated interferon are associated with lower response rates than regimens that include peginterferon alfa and such regimens are no longer included in recommendations for the treatment of chronic HCV infection.

Oral ribavirin usually is used in multiple-drug regimens that include one or more HCV direct-acting antivirals (DAAs) with or without peginterferon alfa. Ribavirin has been used in regimens that include simeprevir (an HCV protease inhibitor), ribavirin, and peginterferon alfa; regimens that include sofosbuvir (an HCV polymerase inhibitor) and ribavirin with or without peginterferon alfa; regimens that include simeprevir (an HCV protease inhibitor), sofosbuvir (an HCV polymerase inhibitor), and ribavirin; regimens that include the fixed combination of ombitasvir (an HCV replication complex inhibitor), paritaprevir (an HCV protease inhibitor), and ritonavir (ombitasvir/paritaprevir/ritonavir) and ribavirin; or regimens that include the fixed combination ombitasvir/paritaprevir/ritonavir with dasabuvir and with ribavirin. The most appropriate multiple-drug regimen depends on the specific HCV genotype and patient population involved.

Because treatment of chronic HCV is complex and rapidly evolving, it is recommended that treatment be directed by clinicians who are familiar with the disease and that a specialist be consulted to obtain the most up-to-date information. Information from the American Association for the Study of Liver Diseases (AASLD), Infectious Diseases Society of America (IDSA), and International Antiviral Society–USA (IAS–USA) regarding diagnosis and management of HCV infection, including recommendations for initial treatment, is available at http://www.hcvguidelines.org.

Pediatric Patients. Oral ribavirin is designated an orphan drug by the US Food and Drug Administration (FDA) for treatment of chronic HCV infection in pediatric patients. Ribavirin oral capsules (Rebetol®, Ribasphere®) and oral solution (Rebetol®) are used in conjunction with peginterferon alfa-2b (PegIntron®) or nonconjugated interferon alfa-2b for treatment of chronic HCV infection in children 3 years of age or older with compensated liver disease. Oral ribavirin tablets (Copegus®) are used in conjunction with peginterferon alfa-2a (Pegasys®) for initial treatment of chronic HCV infection in children 5 years of age or older with compensated liver disease. Similar to data in adults, sustained virologic response (SVR) rates in those receiving a regimen or oral ribavirin and peginterferon alfa have been lower in children infected with HCV genotype 1 than in those infected with other genotypes.

In a multicenter study in 107 children 3–17 years of age with compensated chronic HCV infection who were previously untreated (52% female, 89% Caucasian, 67% infected with HCV genotype 1), a regimen of oral ribavirin (Rebetol® 15 mg/kg daily) and peginterferon alfa-2b (60 mcg/m^2 once weekly) was given for 24 weeks (genotype 2, genotype 3 with baseline HCV RNA level less than 600,000 IU/mL) or 48 weeks (HCV genotypes 1 and 4, genotype 3 with baseline HCV RNA level of 600,000 IU/mL or greater). The overall SVR (defined as undetectable plasma HCV RNA at 24 weeks after treatment) rate was 65%. In children who received a 24-week regimen, the SVR rate was 93% in those with genotype 2 infections and 100% in those with genotype 3 infections and baseline HCV RNA level less than 600,000 IU/mL. In children who received a 48-week regimen, the SVR rate was 53% in those with genotype 1 infections, 80% in those with genotype 4 infections, and 67% in those with genotype 3 infections and baseline HCV RNA level of 600,000 IU/mL or greater.

In a study in 114 children 5–17 years of age with chronic HCV infection, compensated liver disease, and detectable HCV RNA who were previously untreated, patients were randomized to receive a 48-week regimen of oral ribavirin (Copegus® 15 mg/kg daily) and peginterferon alfa-2a (180 mcg/1.73 $m^2 \times$ body surface area [BSA] once weekly) or monotherapy with peginterferon alfa-2a (180 mcg/1.73 $m^2 \times$ BSA once weekly). Overall, SVR (defined as undetectable plasma HCV RNA [less than 50 IU/mL] on or after week 68) was attained in 53% of those treated with peginterferon alfa-2a and oral ribavirin compared with 20% of those treated with peginterferon alfa-2a monotherapy. In those treated with the combination regimen, the SVR rate was 47% in those with genotype 1 infections and 80% in those with non-genotype-1 infections.

Individuals Coinfected with HCV and HIV. Because HCV infection tends to progress more rapidly in patients coinfected with human immunodeficiency virus (HIV), the AASLD, US Centers for Disease Control and Prevention (CDC), National Institutes of Health (NIH), HIV Medicine Association of the Infectious Diseases Society of America (IDSA), and other experts state that all HIV-infected patients should be periodically screened for HCV and those diagnosed with HCV should be offered HCV treatment, provided there are no contraindications to such therapy. Optimal timing of initiation of HCV treatment relative to antiretroviral therapy has not been established. There is some evidence that HIV-infected patients with $CD4^+$ T-cell counts less than 200 cells/mm^3 receiving an HCV treatment regimen of ribavirin used in conjunction with peginterferon alfa have lower HCV treatment response rates and increased rates of toxicity compared to HIV-infected patients with $CD4^+$ T-cell counts exceeding 350 cells/mm^3. Some experts recommend that HCV treatment in patients with HCV and HIV coinfection should not be initiated until after at least 6 months of antiretroviral therapy, and state that initiation of HCV treatment is not usually recommended in HIV-infected patients with $CD4^+$ T-cell counts less than 200 cells/mm^3. The US Department of Health and Human Services (HHS) Panel on Antiretroviral Guidelines for Adults and Adolescents states that antiretroviral therapy should be initiated in all patients coinfected with HCV and HIV, including those with high $CD4^+$ T-cell counts and cirrhosis. In patients with HCV and HIV coinfection who have low $CD4^+$ T-cell counts (e.g., less than 200 cells/mm^3), the HHS panel recommends *prompt* initiation of antiretroviral therapy and states that initiation of HCV treatment may be delayed until the patient is stable on the HIV treatment regimen.

Oral ribavirin has been used in conjunction with peginterferon alfa for treatment of chronic HCV infection in adults with compensated liver disease who are coinfected with HIV. Although some ribavirin manufacturers state that safety and efficacy of oral ribavirin used in conjunction with peginterferon alfa-2b (PegIntron®) or interferon alfa-2b (Intron® A) have not been established in patients with HCV and HIV coinfection, other ribavirin manufacturers state that initial studies evaluating safety and efficacy of oral ribavirin used in conjunction with peginterferon alfa-2a for treatment of chronic HCV infection included clinically stable HIV-infected adults with $CD4^+$ T-cell counts greater than 100 cells/mm^3. There is evidence that HCV treatment regimens that only include ribavirin and peginterferon alfa are associated with poor SVR rates, especially in patients with HCV and HIV coinfection.

Various multiple-drug regimens that include one or more HCV DAAs (e.g., sofosbuvir and ribavirin with or without peginterferon alfa; sofosbuvir and simeprevir with ribavirin) have been used for treatment of chronic HCV infection in patients coinfected with HIV. The most appropriate regimen depends on the HCV genotype and whether the patient is treatment naive or has relapsed after prior HCV treatment. Some experts state that multiple-drug regimens recommended for treatment of chronic HCV infection in patients coinfected with HIV are the same as those recommended for individuals without HIV infection, provided that potential drug interactions and overlapping toxicities between drugs in the HCV treatment regimen and drugs in the antiretroviral regimen are taken into consideration.

If ribavirin is included in the HCV multiple-drug treatment regimen in HIV-infected patients, potential drug interactions with HIV nucleoside reverse transcriptase inhibitors (e.g., didanosine, lamivudine, stavudine, zidovudine) should be considered. (See HIV Nucleoside Reverse Transcriptase Inhibitors under Drug Interactions: Antiretroviral Agents.)

Treatment of chronic HCV infection in patients coinfected with HIV can by complicated because of high pill burden, overlapping toxicities, and drug interactions. Because treatment in patients coinfected with HCV and HIV is complex and rapidly evolving, current recommendations regarding management of HCV infection (http://www.hcvguidelines.org) and management of HIV infection (http://www.aidsinfo.nih.gov) should be considered and expert consultation is recommended.

Acute Hepatitis C Virus Infection Oral ribavirin has been used in conjunction with peginterferon alfa (alfa-2a, alfa-2b) for treatment of acute HCV infection† in an attempt to prevent progression to chronic HCV infection.

There is evidence that patients with acute HCV infection have higher treatment response rates than those with chronic HCV infection and that treatment of the acute infection can reduce the risk that the disease will evolve to chronic infection. SVR rates of 62–90% or higher have been reported when peginterferon alfa or nonconjugated interferon alfa monotherapy or peginterferon alfa in conjunction with oral ribavirin was used for treatment of acute HCV infection. However, approximately 10–50% of patients with acute HCV infection have self-limited disease and spontaneous clearance of the virus without treatment; the spontaneous resolution rate varies depending on whether the acute infection is asymptomatic or symptomatic, the route of HCV transmission, and age at which the infection was acquired.

The optimum regimen (including dosage and duration of therapy) and optimum time to initiate treatment in patients with acute HCV infection have not been established. To allow for spontaneous resolution, some experts suggest that it might be reasonable to delay initiation of treatment of acute HCV infection (especially in symptomatic patients) for 8–12 weeks after acute onset of hepatitis, unless HCV RNA levels are high and not declining; others suggest monitoring for 8–20 weeks after initial exposure.

Although some experts recommend that treatment be offered to all HIV-infected patients with acute HCV infection, others recommend observing HIV-infected patients for 3–6 months before initiating HCV treatment, especially patients more likely to have spontaneous clearance after acute HCV infection (e.g., those with C/C IL28B genotype).

Consultation with a specialist is advised to obtain the most up-to-date information regarding treatment of acute HCV infection.

■ **Hepatitis E Virus Infection** Oral ribavirin has been used alone or in conjunction with peginterferon alfa for treatment of chronic hepatitis E virus (HEV) infection†.

Chronic HEV infection has been reported almost exclusively among immunocompromised individuals, including solid organ transplant recipients, patients receiving cancer chemotherapy, and HIV-infected patients. Although optimal treatment of chronic HEV infection has not been identified, there is evidence that ribavirin monotherapy is associated with a sustained virologic response in some solid organ transplant recipients.

■ **Respiratory Syncytial Virus Infection** Ribavirin is used via nasal and oral inhalation (Virazole®) for treatment of severe lower respiratory tract infections (i.e., bronchiolitis and/or pneumonia) caused by respiratory syncytial virus (RSV) in hospitalized infants and young children.

The manufacturer states that use of ribavirin nasal and oral inhalation therapy should be considered *only* for infants and small children with *severe* RSV lower respiratory tract infections and that use in mechanically ventilated patients should be undertaken *only* by clinicians and support staff familiar with the mode of administration and the specific ventilator being used. The American Academy of Pediatrics (AAP) states that ribavirin nasal and oral inhalation therapy may be considered for selected patients with documented, potentially life-threatening RSV infection, but *routine* use of the drug is *not* recommended.

Efficacy of ribavirin therapy in RSV infection depends on prompt initiation of the drug following the onset of signs and symptoms. Ribavirin inhalation therapy is *not* a substitute for usual supportive respiratory therapy and fluid management in patients with severe respiratory tract infection.

When indicated, ribavirin nasal and oral inhalation therapy may be started pending results of definitive diagnostic tests, particularly when the clinical diagnosis is compatible with RSV infection during the RSV season (usually November to April), but the drug generally should be discontinued if RSV lower respiratory tract infection is not documented. Appropriate specimens (i.e., respiratory tract secretions) for rapid identification of RSV should be obtained prior to initiating or during the first 24 hours of ribavirin therapy. Rapid diagnostic methods for identification of RSV include demonstration of RSV viral antigen in respiratory tract secretions using immunofluorescence or enzyme-linked immunosorbent assay (ELISA). The fact that false-positive or false-negative test results may occur with these rapid diagnostic methods should be considered. Test results from other diagnostic procedures that use culture techniques generally are not available for 1–5 days.

High-risk Infants and Children Ribavirin nasal and oral inhalation therapy is used for treatment of *severe* lower respiratory tract infections caused by RSV in hospitalized infants and young children.

Outbreaks of RSV infection usually occur annually during the winter and early spring. RSV is one of the most common diseases of early childhood. Most infants are infected during the first year of life, and essentially all children have been infected with RSV at least once by their second birthday. Most previously healthy infants and young children with RSV infection do not exhibit signs and/or symptoms of lower respiratory tract infection or only exhibit manifestations of mild, self-limited infection that does not require hospitalization or antiviral therapy (e.g., ribavirin). Mild RSV lower respiratory tract infections in previously healthy patients in this age group generally improve within a few days with supportive care and do not require treatment with ribavirin nasal and oral inhalation therapy; if hospitalization is required, it usually is of shorter duration than that required for a complete course of ribavirin inhalation therapy (i.e., 3–7 days).

The severity of RSV respiratory tract infection and its attendant risk to the patient may be increased in infants and young children with an underlying compromising condition (e.g., prematurity, cardiopulmonary disease, immunodeficiency). In infants with preexisting cardiac and respiratory disease (i.e., bronchopulmonary dysplasia and/or congenital heart disease), ribavirin inhalation therapy may increase the rate of improvement in clinical manifestations of the infection, especially during the first 24 hours after initiating therapy. The drug has also been effective in treatment of pneumonia associated with severe RSV and/or parainfluenza infections in immunocompromised infants (e.g., infants with severe combined immunodeficiency disease [SCID]), decreasing viral shedding in respiratory tract secretions and promoting improvement in clinical manifestations of pneumonia, including arterial blood gases, cough, fever, and respiratory rate. However, complete recovery occurred only after bone marrow transplantation in these immunocompromised infants, suggesting that a healthy, intact host immune system is necessary for complete recovery from RSV infection in immunocompromised patients, even following ribavirin inhalation therapy.

Clinical Experience. Results of some placebo-controlled studies have indicated that ribavirin inhalation therapy can improve clinical manifestations of RSV lower respiratory tract infection in hospitalized infants with severe infection, especially when therapy was initiated within the first 3 days following onset of infection. The effect of such therapy on short- and long-term morbidity and on mortality remains to be more fully elucidated.

In some studies, ribavirin-treated infants generally experienced a more rapid improvement in cough, respiratory rate, rales, chest recession, and/or heart rate compared with infants receiving the placebo, but the duration of wheezing did not appear to be substantially affected by the drug. Ribavirin inhalation therapy has also decreased the duration and amount of viral shedding in respiratory tract secretions, although reported effects on viral shedding have been inconsistent, in part because such effects generally do not seem to become apparent until several days after initiation of therapy (e.g., after 3 days). Clinical manifestations of RSV infection, including arterial oxygen saturation, lethargy, cough, and rales, have improved as early as 3 days following initiation of inhalation therapy with the drug in some infants. In addition, in a limited number of infants with severe pneumonia associated with RSV infection, prolonged inhalation therapy (e.g., 7–22 days) reportedly has been effective in promoting recovery in most children and has decreased viral shedding in respiratory tract secretions.

In some of the initial studies, the use of sterile water instead of saline for the placebo control has been criticized because of the potential for sterile water to cause bronchospasm and potentially affect outcomes. Subsequent randomized studies performed using a saline control have produced inconsistent results. Studies that assessed outcomes such as length of hospitalization, length of intensive care stay, and duration of illness have not generally revealed differences between patients receiving ribavirin and those receiving placebo. Studies that evaluated the effects of aerosolized ribavirin treatment on outcomes such as symptoms and clinical severity have also yielded inconsistent results. Some studies reported improved clinical scores on days 1–4 of ribavirin treatment, quicker improvement of some symptoms (e.g., cough and crepitation), reduced nasal viral shedding at end of treatment, and greater improvements in blood gas values. Other studies did not indicate a benefit from ribavirin treatment for such outcomes. In a study in children with mild RSV illness and underlying disease (bronchopulmonary dysplasia, congenital heart disease), early treatment with aerosolized ribavirin resulted in a greater rate of improvement of clinical scores, reduced oxygen requirements, and greater oxygen saturation.

Results of long-term follow-up studies have been inconsistent. One study indicated a decreased incidence of 2 or more wheezing episodes during the 6 years following ribavirin treatment for RSV infection versus placebo, but no differences in overall respiratory illness or symptoms during the same period. A 1-year follow-up study of patients who received aerosolized ribavirin in conjunction with usual treatment versus usual treatment alone for RSV infection indicated a decreased incidence of reactive airway disease and respiratory tract infections in those who received ribavirin. A follow-up study of 5 years' duration found no differences in annual rates, timing, or severity of lower respiratory tract illness, nor were there differences observed in pulmonary function.

Mechanically Ventilated Patients The manufacturer states that ribavirin inhalation therapy may be used in patients requiring mechanical ventilator assistance; however, such therapy should be undertaken only by clinicians and support staff familiar with this mode of administration and with the specific ventilator being used, and strict attention must be paid to procedures that have been shown to minimize accumulation of drug precipitate in the equipment. (See Nasal and Oral Inhalation under Cautions: Precautions and Contraindications and see Nasal and Oral Inhalation under Dosage and Administration: Reconstitution and Administration.)

Clinical Experience. In one randomized, double-blind, controlled study in infants (mean age 1.4 months) requiring mechanical ventilation for respiratory failure caused by RSV, ribavirin inhalation therapy at the recommended dosage resulted in decreases compared with placebo in the duration of mechanical ventilation required from 9.9 to 4.9 days and in the duration of required supplemental oxygen from 13.5 to 8.7 days; there were no technical difficulties with ribavirin inhalation therapy during the study. Intensive patient management and monitoring techniques were used during the study, including endotracheal tube suctioning every 1–2 hours, arterial blood gas monitoring every 2–6 hours, and recording of proximal airway pressure, ventilatory rate, and F_IO_2 every hour. In addition, certain procedures were performed to reduce the risk of precipitation of ribavirin and possible ventilator malfunction (e.g., heated wire tubing, 2 bacterial filters connected in series in the expiratory limb of the ventilator with filter changes every 4 hours, water column pressure release valves to monitor internal ventilator pressures installed when connecting ventilator circuits to the SPAG-2).

Adults Although the manufacturer states that ribavirin nasal and oral inhalation therapy is *not* indicated for use in adults, aerosolized ribavirin has been used alone or in conjunction with IV† ribavirin for the treatment of severe RSV infection in previously healthy adults†. Aerosolized ribavirin also has been used alone or in conjunction with immune globulin IV (IGIV) for treatment of RSV infection in immunocompromised adults†, including bone marrow or hematopoietic cell transplant recipients. In addition, IV† ribavirin has been used for treatment of RSV infection in a limited number of adult lung transplant recipients†.

■ **Viral Hemorrhagic Fevers** Ribavirin is used orally and/or IV† for treatment of certain viral hemorrhagic fevers†, including Lassa fever†, hemorrhagic fever with renal syndrome (HFRS) caused by Hantavirus infection†, some infections caused by New World arenaviruses†, and Crimean-Congo hemorrhagic fever†. Although parenteral ribavirin is not commercially available in the US, it is available for compassionate use protocols for treatment of viral hemorrhagic fevers. (See Parenteral Administration under Dosage and Administration: Administration.)

Viral hemorrhagic fevers are a diverse group of infections caused by RNA viruses from 5 viral families, including Arenaviridae (e.g., Lassa virus [Lassa fever], Junin virus [Argentine hemorrhagic fever], Lujo virus, Machupo virus

[Bolivian hemorrhagic fever], Guanarito virus [Venezuelan hemorrhagic fever], Sabia virus [Brazilian hemorrhagic fever]), Bunyaviridae (e.g., Hantavirus infections, Crimean-Congo hemorrhagic fever, Rift Valley fever), Filoviridae (e.g., Ebola hemorrhagic fever, Marburg hemorrhagic fever), Flaviviridae (e.g., dengue hemorrhagic fever, yellow fever, Kyasanur Forest disease, Omsk hemorrhagic fever, Alkhurma viruses), and Paramyxoviridae. Ribavirin has been used for the management of various viral hemorrhagic fevers; however, the drug provides benefit only in some (not all) of these infections. Ribavirin has some activity against Arenaviridae and Bunyaviridae, but is *inactive* against Filoviridae (including Ebola and Marburg viruses) and most Flaviviridae.

The principal clinical features of viral hemorrhagic fevers usually result from microvascular damage and changes in vascular permeability. Although certain types of hemorrhagic fever viruses can cause relatively mild illnesses, many of these viruses cause severe, life-threatening disease. Specific clinical manifestations vary by the type of viral hemorrhagic fever, but initially often include fever, fatigue, dizziness, myalgia, prostration, loss of strength, and exhaustion. Severe cases often exhibit signs of bleeding under the skin, in internal organs, and from body orifices (e.g., mouth, eyes, ears), but death rarely results from blood loss per se. Severely ill patients may exhibit shock and neurologic (e.g., nervous system abnormalities, coma, seizures, delirium), pulmonary, and hematopoietic involvement. Some viral hemorrhagic fevers may result in renal failure, which is proportional in many cases to the degree of cardiovascular compromise but integral to the disease process in hemorrhagic fever with renal syndrome.

Risks of Exposure and Infection The viruses that cause viral hemorrhagic fevers are principally zoonotic (i.e., they reside naturally in and depend on an animal reservoir host or arthropod vector for replication and survival) and are distributed worldwide. Because each virus is associated with one or more particular host species, the virus and associated disease usually occur only in areas where the host species lives and the risk of contracting naturally occurring viral hemorrhagic fevers usually is restricted geographically to these respective areas. However, humans occasionally become infected by a host that has been exported from its native habitat. Naturally occurring viral hemorrhagic fevers can be transmitted to humans when human activities overlap with activities of infected reservoir hosts or vectors. Transmission can occur through contact with the urine, feces, saliva, or other body excretions of rodent reservoirs or through the bites of arthropod vectors (e.g., mosquitoes, ticks). Transmission also can occur through the care and slaughter of infected livestock or consumption of raw meat from infected animals. Some of these viruses (e.g., those associated with Ebola, Marburg, Lassa fever, and Crimean-Congo hemorrhagic fevers) can be spread from person to person.

Person-to-person transmission of viral hemorrhagic fevers can occur directly via close contact with infected individuals or their body fluids or cadavers or indirectly via contact with objects contaminated with infected body fluids. In addition, some of the viruses (including Lassa fever virus, Crimean-Congo hemorrhagic fever virus and Ebola and Marburg viruses) are associated with aerosol nosocomial spread. Although humans are not a natural reservoir for the viruses, patients with viral hemorrhagic fever often harbor significant quantities of virus in blood and other body fluids and secretions. Therefore, nosocomial transmission and secondary infections in contacts and health-care personnel have been reported, especially if infection control procedures are inadequate.

The US Army Medical Research Institute of Infectious Diseases (USAMRIID) and US Working Group on Civilian Biodefense state that there is a risk that human infection with viruses that cause hemorrhagic fevers could occur as the result of biologic warfare or bioterrorism since most hemorrhagic fever viruses can be transmitted by aerosols. (See Viral Hemorrhagic Fevers in the Context of Biologic Warfare or Bioterrorism under Uses: Viral Hemorrhagic Fevers.)

Information on diagnosis and management of viral hemorrhagic fevers is available from the Viral Special Pathogens Branch of CDC at http://www.cdc.gov/ncezid/dhcpp/vspb/diseases.html or at 404-639-1115. Any suspected cases of viral hemorrhagic fever occurring in individuals residing in or requiring evacuation to the US should immediately be reported to local health authorities and the CDC Viral Special Pathogens Branch at 404-639-1115 or the CDC Emergency Operations Center at 770-488-7100.

Travelers. Although the risk for travelers is considered to be low, travelers to endemic areas are at increased risk of exposure to viral hemorrhagic fevers if they are engaging in animal research or are healthcare workers or others providing care for patients in the community, particularly when an outbreak of viral hemorrhagic fever is occurring. Healthcare workers should observe standard precautions, including contact and droplet precautions, when working with patients if viral hemorrhagic fever is suspected. In addition, direct contact with corpses of patients suspected of having died of Ebola, Marburg, or Old World arenavirus infection should be avoided.

Travelers should avoid contact with host or vector species (e.g., rodents, bats, livestock) and should not visit locations where an outbreak of viral hemorrhagic fever is occurring. Travelers to areas where Rift Valley fever or Crimean-Congo hemorrhagic fever is endemic are at increased risk and should avoid direct contact with livestock and should minimize their exposure to mosquito bites by using insecticide-treated bed nets and insect repellants. Contact with or consumption of primates, bats, and other bushmeat should be avoided. In addition, direct contact with corpses of patients suspected of having died of Ebola, Marburg, or Old World arenavirus infection should be avoided.

Lassa Fever Ribavirin has been effective when used orally and/or IV† for treatment of Lassa fever†, and is considered the drug of choice for treatment of the disease.

Lassa fever is a severe, often fatal, hemorrhagic fever caused by Lassa virus, an Arenavirus that can be transmitted to humans from asymptomatically infected rodents (multimammate rats). Transmission to humans can occur via inhalation of primary aerosols from rodent urine, by ingestion of contaminated food, or by direct contact of broken skin with rodent excreta. Rodent infestation and inappropriate food storage increase the risk of human infection. Person-to-person transmission of Lassa fever has been reported (including transmission to health-care workers) and usually occurs because of contact with blood, tissue, secretions, or excretions from an infected individual; transmission via aerosols also has been reported. Lassa fever is endemic in portions of West Africa (including areas in Sierra Leone, Guinea, Liberia, and Nigeria).

Ribavirin treatment has been associated with decreased morbidity and mortality in patients with Lassa fever, and appears to be more effective than Lassa immune plasma therapy (convalescent plasma obtained from survivors of the disease) or no therapy. Ribavirin is most effective when initiated early in the course of the infection (within 6–7 days of onset of symptoms). Patients need intensive supportive care, including maintenance of appropriate fluid and electrolyte balance, oxygenation, and blood pressure, as well as treatment of any complicating infections.

When treating patients with Lassa fever, strict barrier precautions (use of gloves, gowns, masks, goggles) should be used to minimize exposure to patient blood and other body fluids. Although use of oral ribavirin for postexposure prophylaxis of Lassa fever† in high-risk contacts of patients with Lassa fever (i.e., individuals who, within 3 weeks of diagnosis of Lassa fever in a patient, have mucous membrane contact [e.g., kissing, sexual intercourse] with the infected patient, or who have had a needle stick or other penetrating injury involving contact with the patient's secretions, excretions, blood, tissue, or other body fluids during this period) has been suggested, efficacy of the drug for such prophylaxis has never been studied in humans. Therefore, oral ribavirin prophylaxis is not usually recommended for exposed individuals. Instead, the CDC recommends that a treatment regimen of IV† ribavirin be used in contacts with clinical evidence of the infection during the incubation period.

Hantavirus Infections **Hemorrhagic Fever with Renal Syndrome (HFRS).** Ribavirin has been used IV† for treatment of hemorrhagic fever with renal syndrome† (HFRS), and has been designated an orphan drug by FDA for treatment of this condition. HFRS is caused by Hantaan virus (a Hantavirus) and related Bunyaviridae and is characterized by hemorrhagic fever associated with vascular instability, shock, and severe renal insufficiency resulting from acute interstitial nephritis; a subsequent diuretic phase is then observed

When administered IV† within 4–7 days after the onset of fever, ribavirin has been shown to be effective in decreasing the viremia, renal dysfunction, vascular instability, and mortality of HFRS. Patients also need intensive supportive care, including avoidance of transporting patients, supportive care for shock, prevention of overhydration (particularly with crystalloid solution), dialysis for complications of renal failure, control of hypertension during the oliguric phase, and early recognition of possible myocardial failure with appropriate therapy.

Hantavirus Pulmonary Syndrome (HPS). A Hantavirus infection named Hantavirus pulmonary syndrome (HPS) was recognized in the US, principally among residents of the Southwest. HPS is mainly produced by a strain of Hantavirus named Sin Nombre (Muerto Canyon) virus, most closely related to the Prospect Hill strain of Hantavirus. Available data strongly suggest that the deer mouse (*Peromyscus maniculatus*) is the principal reservoir of Sin Nombre virus. Although the overall incidence of HPS is unknown, the syndrome appears to be widespread geographically since HPS has been reported in areas outside of the Southwest. Humans are thought to be at risk for infection after exposure to rodent excreta or saliva, either through aerosols or direct inoculation. There currently is *no* evidence of arthropod vectors of hantavirus transmission. Manifestations of HPS, while sharing some clinical manifestations of other Hantavirus infections (e.g., HFRS), do not include the prominent renal involvement and hemorrhagic manifestations previously described with Hantavirus infections. Instead, HPS is characterized by abrupt onset of fever or hypothermia and myalgias, variably accompanied by headache, chills, cough, dyspnea, nausea, vomiting, diarrhea, hypotension, tachycardia, tachypnea, and abdominal distress, followed by a precipitous onset of rapidly progressive bilateral interstitial infiltrates resembling radiographic changes of adult respiratory distress syndrome (ARDS) and frequently by shock; most cases to date have been fatal.

Optimum therapy for treatment of HPS remains to be established, but is principally symptomatic and supportive. Prompt supportive management of pulmonary edema, severe hypoxemia, and hypotension during the first 24–48 hours, including avoidance of excessive fluid administration and early use of inotropic and vasopressor agents, appears particularly important. Based on in vitro antiviral activity and limited experience in treating other Hantavirus infections (e.g., HFRS) and various hemorrhagic fevers (e.g., Lassa fever), IV† ribavirin had been used for treatment of HPS†. From June 1993 through August 1994, IV ribavirin† (administered as a loading dose of 30 mg/kg followed by 15 mg/kg every 6 hours for 4 days and then 7.5 mg/kg every 8 hours for 6 days) was available under an open-label investigational new drug (IND) protocol from CDC for treatment of HPS. However, in July 1994, experts from outside CDC reviewed the results of this open-label IND protocol and concluded that, while ribavirin generally was well tolerated in patients with HPS, the drug had no clear positive influence on the outcome of such infection. Therefore, enrollment under the IND protocol was closed in September 1994. A total of 140 patients were enrolled in the study and 37 completed a 7- to 10-day regimen of ribavirin; reasons for early termination of treatment included death, alternate diagnosis, adverse effects, negative HPS testing, clinical improvement, and drug shortage. Placebo-controlled, randomized clinical studies have been initiated to evaluate ribavirin for treatment of HPS. Clinicians and public health officials should remain alert for individuals with unexplained bilateral interstitial infiltrates accompanied by fever; appropriate specimens should be collected for serologic and diagnostic tests from these individuals. Suspected cases of HPS should be reported to CDC through corresponding state health departments.

Crimean-Congo Hemorrhagic Fever Ribavirin has been used orally or IV† with some success in a limited number of patients for treatment of Crimean-Congo hemorrhagic fever† (CCHF). Although experience with ribavirin in the treatment and prevention of CCHF is substantially more limited than that with Lassa fever, CDC states that use of ribavirin to treat the disease and to prevent infection in high-risk contacts seems reasonable based on in vitro susceptibility data for this and other Bunyaviridae. CDC recommends that similar procedures for care, including isolation and body fluid precautions and therapy, recommended for Lassa fever be followed for patients with Crimean-Congo hemorrhagic fever and their contacts; however, additional study and experience are necessary.

Viral Hemorrhagic Fevers caused by Filoviridae and Flaviviridae Ribavirin is *inactive* in vitro against Filoviridae, including Ebola and Marburg viruses, and is *not* effective for treatment of Ebola hemorrhagic fever or Marburg hemorrhagic fever. Ribavirin also is *inactive* against most Flaviviridae.

Viral Hemorrhagic Fevers in the Context of Biologic Warfare or Bioterrorism Because of the potential risk that viruses that cause hemorrhagic fever might be used in the context of biologic warfare or bioterrorism, the Working Group on Civilian Biodefense and other experts (e.g., USAMRIID) have made recommendations for treatment of viral hemorrhagic fevers in such a setting. Ribavirin is recommended for the treatment of clinically evident viral hemorrhagic fever in the context of biologic warfare or bioterrorism† when the disease is caused by an Arenavirus (e.g., Lassa fever, New World hemorrhagic fever) or Bunyavirus (e.g., Rift Valley fever) or is of unknown etiology. Although safety and efficacy of oral or IV† ribavirin have not been established in children or in pregnant women, experts (i.e., the Working Group on Civilian Biodefense) recommend that children or pregnant women with clinically evident viral hemorrhagic fever caused by an Arenavirus or Bunyavirus or of unknown etiology should receive ribavirin since the benefits are likely to outweigh the risks of such therapy. In addition to use of ribavirin when indicated, treatment of patients with viral hemorrhagic virus infection requires intensive supportive care with careful maintenance of fluid and electrolyte balance, circulatory volume, and blood pressure.

Preemptive administration of ribavirin or postexposure prophylaxis with the drug in the absence of clinical signs of infection in individuals with known or presumed exposure to a hemorrhagic fever virus in the context of biologic warfare or bioterrorism is not currently recommended. Individuals with known or presumed exposure to a hemorrhagic fever virus and all known high-risk contacts (i.e., individuals who have mucous membrane contact with an infected patient) and close contacts (i.e., individuals who live with, shake hands or hug, process laboratory specimens, or care for an infected patient [prior to initiation of appropriate precautions]) should be placed under medical surveillance for 21 days after the potential exposure or last contact with the infected patient. Exposed individuals and contacts who develop a temperature of 38.3°C or higher should receive ribavirin for the presumptive treatment of viral hemorrhagic fever† unless there is an alternative diagnosis or the etiologic agent is a filovirus or flavivirus. Only high-risk or close contacts of patients with Rift Valley fever or Flavivirus infection who processed laboratory specimens from an infected patient prior to initiation of appropriate precautions require medical surveillance since these viruses are not transmitted from person to person.

■ **Adenovirus Infections** Ribavirin has been used IV† with some success for treatment of infections caused by adenovirus† in immunocompromised adults and children, including bone marrow or stem cell transplant recipients, solid organ transplant recipients (e.g., liver, kidney), and patients with leukemia or severe combined immunodeficiency. However, safety and efficacy of the drug for treatment of adenovirus infections have not been established. Experience is limited to date and further study is needed to determine the role of ribavirin in the treatment of adenovirus infections.

In most reported cases, ribavirin was used in critically ill patients with severe adenovirus infections (e.g., hemorrhagic cystitis, nephritis, respiratory tract infections, GI infections, disseminated disease); these patients received multiple treatment modalities and it is difficult to determine whether the drug contributed to a favorable outcome. In some patients, IV† ribavirin was used in conjunction with IV cidofovir. There is evidence that not all patients respond to ribavirin therapy and that the drug is unlikely to be of benefit if initiated late in the course of severe infections.

In addition to being used in patients with severe adenovirus infections, ribavirin has been used for preemptive therapy in several immunocompromised patients who were asymptomatic, but had clinical cultures positive for adenovirus. However, the possible benefits and risks of the drug in such patients have not been determined since asymptomatic adenovirus infections often resolve spontaneously.

■ **Coronavirus Infections** ***Severe Acute Respiratory Syndrome (SARS)*** IV† and/or oral ribavirin has been used empirically in some adults and a limited number of children with severe acute respiratory syndrome† (SARS), alone or in conjunction with systemic corticosteroids. SARS was first reported in Asia during early 2003 and then spread to many other areas of the world, including North America, South America, and Europe. By July 2003, more than 8000 SARS cases and 780 deaths were reported from 29 countries worldwide. A new human pathogen, a member of the coronavirus family, was identified as the causative agent and was named the SARS coronavirus (SARS-CoV). Although person-to-person transmission of SARS-CoV does not appear to be occurring anywhere in the world at the present time, it could recur and future outbreaks of SARS-CoV are possible.

Because SARS can be fatal (overall case-fatality rate 10%, which can increase to more than 50% in patients older than 60 years of age), various empiric therapies were attempted. SARS may be difficult to differentiate from influenza or bacterial pneumonia early in the course of the infection, and patients were treated with multiple anti-infective regimens aimed at presumptively treating known bacterial pathogens of atypical pneumonia. In addition, because some early evidence suggested that a paramyxovirus might be the causative pathogen, ribavirin therapy (with or without corticosteroids) was used for empiric therapy in some patients.

The clinical benefits of the various anti-infective regimens employed in the treatment of SARS, including ribavirin, were disappointing. Results from several in vitro studies using isolates obtained from infected patients indicated that ribavirin concentrations that inhibit ribavirin-susceptible viruses do *not* inhibit replication or cell-to-cell transmission of SARS-CoV. In a retrospective analysis of SARS patients in Toronto, ribavirin was used for empiric therapy in 88% of patients but was temporally associated with clinically important toxicity and was discontinued in 18%. Because the most efficacious therapeutic regimen, if any, remains to be established, suspected cases should be reported to local health departments and managed according to the most recent recommendations of the WHO (http://www.who.int/csr/sars/guidelines/en/) and US Centers for Disease Control and Prevention (CDC; http://www.cdc.gov/sars/index.html).

Middle East Respiratory Syndrome (MERS) Ribavirin has been used in conjunction with an interferon (e.g., peginterferon alfa-2a, interferon alfa-2b) for the treatment of Middle East respiratory syndrome† (MERS) caused by the Middle East respiratory syndrome coronavirus (MERS-CoV).

MERS was first reported in September 2012 in patients in Saudi Arabia. Most cases of MERS-CoV infection have involved severe respiratory illness requiring hospitalization, although some cases involved only mild or asymptomatic disease. The case-fatality rate for MERS has been reported to range from 36–50%. Human cases generally have been attributed to human-to-human transmission of MERS-CoV, but the virus does not appear to pass easily from person to person unless there is close contact (e.g., providing unprotected care to a MERS patient) and sustained human-to-human transmission has not been reported to date. Although MERS-CoV is a zoonotic virus that is transmitted to humans from contact with infected animals, the route of transmission from animals to humans has not been fully identified. Dromedary camels appear to be a major reservoir host for MERS-CoV and an animal source for human infections, but the exact role of camels in direct or indirect transmission of the virus to humans is unknown.

MERS-CoV appears to be circulating throughout the Arabian Peninsula, primarily in Saudi Arabia, and the majority of MERS cases reported since 2012 have occurred in Saudi Arabia. As of August 28 2015, there were 1,474 laboratory-confirmed cases of MERS reported to the World Health Organization (WHO), including 515 deaths. MERS cases have been reported in the Middle East (Iran, Jordan, Kuwait, Lebanon, Oman, Qatar, Saudi Arabia, United Arab Emirates, Yemen), Europe (Austria, France, Germany, Greece, Italy, Netherlands, Turkey, United Kingdom), Africa (Algeria, Egypt, Tunisia), Asia (China, Malaysia, Philippines, Republic of Korea, Thailand), and North America (US). The majority of MERS cases that have occurred outside the Middle East have been directly or indirectly linked through travel or residence to the Middle East. Although an outbreak of MERS was reported in the Republic of Korea (South Korea) beginning in May 2015 and has involved at least 185 cases and 36 deaths, these were related to a traveler from the Middle East and linked to healthcare facilities where MERS patients were treated. There were 2 confirmed cases reported in the US in 2014; both individuals had recently lived and worked in Saudi Arabia before arriving in the US.

No specific treatment for MERS-CoV infection has been identified. Because there is some evidence that ribavirin and interferon are active against the MERS-CoV virus in vitro and in animal studies and because of prior experience using ribavirin in patients with SARS, a regimen of oral ribavirin in conjunction with an interferon (e.g., peginterferon alfa-2a, interferon alfa-2b) has been used in some patients with MERS-CoV infection. In a retrospective, observational study of 5 patients who received oral ribavirin and interferon in conjunction with systemic corticosteroids, no patients survived; however, it is unclear whether this outcome was because the regimen was ineffective or because treatment was initiated late in the course of the disease (range 10–22 days after hospital admission). In a retrospective, cohort study that included 44 patients with laboratory-confirmed MERS, the 14-day survival rate from the date of diagnosis was 70% in patients who were treated with a regimen of oral ribavirin and peginterferon alfa-2a (initiated within a median of 3 days from time of diagnosis; range 0–8 days) in addition to usual supportive care compared with a 14-day survival rate of 29% in the comparator group that only received usual supportive care. However, the 28-day survival rate was only 30% in patients who received the ribavirin and peginterferon alfa-2a treatment regimen compared with 17% in the comparator group.

CDC states that MERS-CoV infection should be considered in the differential diagnosis of individuals who develop respiratory symptoms within 14 days after traveling from countries in or near the Arabian peninsula and all suspected cases should be reported to state or local health departments. Information regarding evaluation, diagnosis, and management of MERS-CoV infection and guidance for individuals traveling to areas where MERS has been reported (e.g., the Middle East) is available at the CDC website at http://www.cdc.gov/coronavirus/mers/.

Dosage and Administration

■ **Reconstitution and Administration** ***Oral Administration*** Ribavirin capsules, tablets, and oral solution are administered orally with food.

Ribavirin capsules should not be opened, crushed, or broken.

If use of Copegus® 200-mg tablets is considered in children 5 years of age or older, clinicians should ensure that the child can reliably swallow the tablets.

Ribavirin oral solution containing 40 mg of ribavirin per mL is recommended (instead of capsules) in children 3 years of age or older weighing less than 47 kg. The oral solution may be used in any patient 3 years of age or older, regardless of weight.

Patients should be well hydrated during oral ribavirin therapy, especially during initial treatment.

Nasal and Oral Inhalation Commercially available ribavirin sterile powder (Virazole®) is intended for administration *only* as a solution via nasal and oral inhalation using the Valeant small-particle aerosol generator (SPAG) Model SPAG-2 available from the manufacturer. The SPAG-2 aerosol generator is intended for administration of ribavirin inhalation *only* and should *not* be used for the administration of other drugs. Prior to administration of ribavirin inhalation, the operator's manual provided by the manufacturer should be reviewed to assure thorough familiarity with the use and operation of the SPAG-2 aerosol generator. *Ribavirin inhalation should not be administered using any other aerosol generator and should not be administered concomitantly with other drug solutions for nebulization.*

In patients not requiring mechanical ventilation, ribavirin solution for nebulization should be administered from the SPAG-2 aerosol generator via an oxygen hood. If an oxygen hood cannot be used, the solution may be administered from the SPAG-2 aerosol generator via a face mask or oxygen tent; however, the volume and condensation area of the solution for nebulization are larger in an oxygen tent, and this may alter delivery dynamics of the drug.

When ribavirin inhalation therapy is used in patients who require assisted ventilation, either a pressure or volume cycle ventilator may be used in conjunction with the SPAG-2. *Administration of ribavirin inhalation therapy in patients requiring mechanical ventilator assistance should be undertaken only by physicians and support staff who are familiar with this mode of administration of the drug and with the specific ventilator being used. In addition, strict attention must be paid to procedures that have been shown to minimize accumulation of ribavirin precipitate in the ventilator.* The endotracheal tubes of mechanically ventilated patients should be suctioned every 1–2 hours and pulmonary pressure should be monitored frequently (every 2–4 hours). In order to minimize the risk of ribavirin precipitation in either pressure or volume cycle ventilators, heated wire connective tubing should be used and bacterial filters should be placed in series in the expiratory limb of the system; the filters should be changed frequently (e.g., every 4 hours). In addition, to indicate presence of elevated ventilator pressures, water column pressure release valves should be used in the ventilator circuit for pressure cycle ventilators and also may be used in the ventilator circuit for volume cycle ventilators. Some clinicians have inserted a one-way valve in the inspiratory line of the ventilator (a pressure-limited, Healthdyne 102 infant ventilator) circuit proximal to the T-shaped connector to prevent the ribavirin solution from entering the humidifier or the ventilator, another one-way valve between the SPAG-2 aerosol generator and this T-shaped connector to prevent loss of volume from the SPAG-2 apparatus, and a disposable exhalation valve in the expiratory line to prevent the ribavirin from entering the ventilator. This entire system was inspected every 2 hours, temperature was maintained at 36–37°C to minimize drug precipitation, a high- and low-pressure alarm (in addition to the ventilator alarm) was connected to the inspiratory line of the circuit to warn of occlusion of the ventilator alarm tubing or any inadvertent circuit disruption, and the drying-chamber flow was reduced or stopped to avoid delivering excess pressure. In addition, the one-way valves and exhalation valve were changed every 4 hours regardless of the amount of precipitate present, the endotracheal tube was instilled with a 0.9% sodium chloride solution and cleared at least every 2 hours, the tubing was changed every 8 hours, and the patient was monitored continuously by pulse oximetry. Regardless of the method used, constant monitoring (e.g., in an intensive care setting) of the patient and the apparatus is necessary. The SPAG-2 manual should be consulted for detailed administration instructions.

Reconstitution and Dilution. Ribavirin sterile powder (Virazole®) is initially reconstituted by adding a minimum of 75 mL of sterile water for injection or inhalation (additive free) to a vial labeled as containing 6 g of ribavirin and shaking well. This initial solution should then be transferred to a sterile 500-mL reservoir for the SPAG-2 aerosol generator, and further diluted with sterile water for injection or inhalation (additive free) to a final volume of 300 mL to provide a solution containing 20 mg/mL.

Diluents containing any additive should *not* be used for reconstitution of ribavirin.

Ribavirin solutions should be inspected visually for particulate matter and discoloration prior to administration. After the solution has been placed in the SPAG-2 reservoir, any unused solution remaining in the reservoir should be discarded within 24 hours and prior to adding any newly reconstituted solution (e.g., when remaining amount of solution in reservoir is low).

Rate of Administration. When reconstituted and diluted ribavirin solution containing 20-mg/mL is delivered using the SPAG-2 aerosol generator according to the manufacturer's instructions, the average aerosol concentration for a 12-hour delivery period is 190 mcg/L.

The manufacturer recommends that the 20-mg/mL solution be administered via the SPAG-2 aerosol generator at a rate of about 15 L/minute when using an oxygen hood or tent or about 12 L/minute when using a face mask.

Parenteral Administration Ribavirin has been administered IV†.

A parenteral preparation of ribavirin is not commercially available in the US, but is available for compassionate use protocols for treatment of viral hemorrhagic fevers† such as Lassa fever†, Hantavirus infections†, and Crimean-Congo hemorrhagic fever†. To obtain IV† ribavirin for emergency use, clinicians should contact the US Food and Drug Administration (FDA) at 301-736-3400 for compassionate use authorization and also contact the manufacturer (Valeant Pharmaceuticals) at 800-548-5100.

■ **Dosage** ***Chronic Hepatitis C Virus Infection*** For treatment of chronic hepatitis C virus (HCV) infection, oral ribavirin *must* be used in conjunction with other drugs as part of a multiple-drug regimen.

Oral ribavirin may be used in conjunction with peginterferon alfa for the treatment of chronic HCV infection; although no longer recommended, ribavirin was used in the past in conjunction with nonconjugated interferon alfa.

For treatment of chronic HCV infection, oral ribavirin usually is used in multiple-drug regimens that include one or more HCV direct-acting antivirals (DAAs) with or without peginterferon alfa. Ribavirin has been used in regimens that include simeprevir (an HCV protease inhibitor), ribavirin, and peginterferon alfa; regimens that include sofosbuvir (an HCV polymerase inhibitor) and ribavirin with or without peginterferon alfa; regimens that include simeprevir (an HCV protease inhibitor), sofosbuvir (an HCV polymerase inhibitor), and ribavirin; regimens that include the fixed combination of ombitasvir (an HCV replication complex inhibitor), paritaprevir (an HCV protease inhibitor), and ritonavir (ombitasvir/paritaprevir/ritonavir) and ribavirin; or regimens that include the fixed combination ombitasvir/paritaprevir/ritonavir with dasabuvir and with ribavirin. The most appropriate multiple-drug regimen depends on the specific HCV genotype and patient population involved.

Dosage and duration of oral ribavirin treatment in patients with chronic HCV infection depend on body weight, HCV genotype, specific treatment regimen used, response to treatment, and tolerability of the regimen. Modification of ribavirin dosage may be necessary if adverse effects occur.

For information on dosage of peginterferon alfa or interferon alfa used in conjunction with oral ribavirin for treatment of chronic HCV infection, see Dosage and Administration: Dosage, in Peginterferon Alfa 8:18.20 and see Dosage and Administration: Dosage in Interferon Alfa 8:18.20.

For information on dosage of HCV DAAs used in conjunction with oral ribavirin (with or without peginterferon alfa) for treatment of chronic HCV infection, see the individual monographs in HCV Antivirals 8:18.40.

Adult Dosage. When oral ribavirin *capsules* (Rebetol®, Ribasphere®) are used in conjunction with peginterferon alfa-2b (PegIntron®) for treatment of chronic HCV infection, the usual adult dosage is 800–1400 mg daily based on body weight. (See Table 1.) The recommended duration of concomitant peginterferon alfa-2b and oral ribavirin treatment depends on HCV genotype, history of prior treatment, and response to treatment. (See Table 2.)

Table 1. Adult Dosage of Ribavirin Capsules (Rebetol®, Ribasphere®) for Concomitant Use with Peginterferon Alfa-2b (PegIntron® A).

Weight	Total Daily Dosage of Ribavirin (Capsules)	Recommended Ribavirin Dosage Regimen (Capsules)
65 kg or less	800 mg	400 mg in morning and 400 mg in evening
66–80 kg	1 g	400 mg in morning and 600 mg in evening
81–105 kg	1.2 g	600 mg in morning and 600 mg in evening
greater than 105 kg	1.4 g	600 mg in morning and 800 mg in evening

Table 2. Duration of Treatment with Ribavirin Capsules (Rebetol®, Ribasphere®) and Peginterferon Alfa-2b (PegIntron®) in Adults.

Patient Type and Response	HCV Genotype	Duration	Considerations
Treatment-naive	1	48 weeks	Consider discontinuing HCV treatment if HCV RNA has not decreased at least 2 $\log_{10}$ by week 12 or remains detectable after 24 weeks of treatment
Treatment-naive	2,3	24 weeks	
Prior failure	Any	48 weeks	Consider discontinuing HCV treatment if HCV RNA still detectable at week 12 or remains detectable after 24 weeks of treatment

When oral ribavirin *tablets* (Copegus®, generic) are used in conjunction with peginterferon alfa-2a (Pegasys®) for initial treatment of chronic HCV infection in adults with HCV monoinfection (without coexisting HIV infection), the usual dosage is 800–1200 mg daily. The recommended duration of concomitant peginterferon alfa-2a and oral ribavirin treatment depends on HCV genotype. (See Table 3.)

Table 3. Adult Dosage of Ribavirin Tablets (Copegus®, generic) for Concomitant Use with Peginterferon Alfa-2a (Pegasys®) for Chronic HCV Monoinfection

HCV Genotype	Ribavirin Dosage (Tablets)	Duration
1,4	1 g daily (500 mg twice daily) in those weighing less than 75 kg or 1.2 g daily (600 mg twice daily) in those weighing 75 kg or more	48 weeks
2,3	800 mg daily (400 mg twice daily)	24 weeks
5,6	Data insufficient to make dosage recommendations	

When oral ribavirin *tablets* (Copegus®, generic) are used in conjunction with peginterferon alfa-2a (Pegasys®) for initial treatment of chronic HCV infection in adults with HCV and HIV coinfection, the usual dosage is 800 mg daily in 2 divided doses for a duration of 48 weeks, regardless of HCV genotype. However, some experts suggest that HIV-infected adults with HCV genotypes 1, 4, 5, or 6 receive a weight-based ribavirin dosage of 1 g daily (i.e., 600 mg in morning and 400 mg in evening) if they weigh less than 75 kg or 1.2 g daily (i.e., 600 mg in morning and 600 mg in evening) if they weigh 75 kg or more.

If oral ribavirin *capsules* (Rebetol®, Ribasphere®) are used in conjunction with nonconjugated interferon alfa-2b (Intron A®) for treatment of chronic HCV infection, the manufacturers recommend a ribavirin dosage of 1 g daily (400 mg in morning and 600 mg in evening) for adults weighing 75 kg or less and 1.2 g daily (600 mg in morning and 600 mg in evening) for adults weighing more than 75 kg. The duration of treatment depends on prior treatment, HCV genotype, and treatment response. The manufacturers state that concomitant nonconjugated interferon alfa-2b and oral ribavirin therapy should be continued for 24–48 weeks in treatment-naive patients, but discontinuance of treatment should be considered in patients who have not achieved HCV RNA levels below the limit of detection at 24 weeks. If concomitant therapy is used in patients who relapsed after prior nonconjugated interferon monotherapy, the manufacturers recommend a treatment duration of 24 weeks.

Pediatric Dosage. When ribavirin *capsules* (Rebetol®, Ribasphere®) or *oral solution* (Rebetol®) is used in conjunction with peginterferon alfa-2b (PegIntron®) or nonconjugated interferon alfa-2b (Intron® A) for treatment of chronic HCV infection in children 3–17 years of age, the manufacturers recommend a ribavirin dosage of 15 mg/kg daily in 2 divided doses. (See Table 4.) The recommended duration of treatment is 24 weeks in those with HCV genotype 2 or 3 or 48 weeks in those with HCV genotype 1. Discontinuance of HCV treatment should be considered if HCV RNA has not decreased by at least 2 $\log_{10}$ from baseline at treatment week 12 or if HCV RNA is detectable at treatment week 24. Patients who reach their 18th birthday during treatment should continue receiving the pediatric dosage regimen for the remaining duration of treatment.

Table 4. Pediatric Dosage of Ribavirin Capsules (Rebetol®, Ribasphere®) or Oral Solution (Rebetol®) for Concomitant Use with Peginterferon Alfa-2b (PegIntron®) or Nonconjugated Interferon Alfa-2b (Intron® A)

Weight	Ribavirin Dosage (Capsules, Oral Solution)
Less than 47 kg	15 mg/kg daily, given as oral solution in 2 divided doses
47–59 kg	400 mg in morning and 400 mg in evening
60–73 kg	400 mg in morning and 600 mg in evening
greater than 73 kg	600 mg in morning and 600 mg in evening

When ribavirin *tablets* (Copegus®) are used in conjunction with peginterferon alfa-2a (Pegasys®) for treatment of chronic HCV infection in children 5 years of age or older capable of swallowing tablets, the manufacturers recommend a ribavirin dosage of approximately 15 mg/kg daily in divided doses. (See Table 5.) Patients who reach their 18th birthday during treatment should continue receiving the pediatric dosage regimen for the remaining duration of treatment. The recommended duration of treatment is 24 weeks for HCV genotype 2 or 3 and 48 weeks for other HCV genotypes.

Table 5. Pediatric Dosage of Ribavirin Tablets (Copegus®) for Concomitant Use with Peginterferon Alfa-2a (Pegasys®)

Weight	Copegus® Dosage (Tablets)
23–33 kg	200 mg in morning and 200 mg in evening
34–46 kg	200 mg in morning and 400 mg in evening
47–59 kg	400 mg in morning and 400 mg in evening
60–74 kg	400 mg in morning and 600 mg in evening
greater than 75 kg	600 mg in morning and 600 mg in evening

Dosage Modification for Toxicity (Adult Dosage). If serious adverse effects or laboratory changes occur when oral ribavirin is used in conjunction with peginterferon alfa or nonconjugated interferon alfa in adults with chronic HCV infection, dosage of one or both drugs should be modified, if appropriate, until the adverse reactions abate. If intolerance persists after dosage adjustments, both drugs should be discontinued.

When ribavirin *capsules* (Rebetol®, Ribasphere®) are used in adults, ribavirin dosage should be decreased by 200 mg daily (or by 400 mg daily in those originally receiving 1.4 g daily) if hemoglobin decreases to 8.5 to less than 10 g/dL; an additional dosage reduction of 200 mg daily may be used if needed. Both ribavirin and peginterferon alfa or nonconjugated interferon alfa should be permanently discontinued in adults with hemoglobin concentrations less than 8.5 g/dL, leukocyte counts less than 1000/mm^3, neutrophil counts less than 500/mm^3, or platelet counts less than 25,000/mm^3. In adults receiving ribavirin *capsules* concomitantly with peginterferon alfa or nonconjugated interferon alfa who have a history of stable cardiovascular disease, ribavirin dosage should be decreased by 200 mg daily if hemoglobin decreases by 2 g/dL or more during any 4-week period and treatment should be discontinued if hemoglobin concentrations are less than 8.5 g/dL (or less than 12 g/dL after 4 weeks of reduced dosage).

When ribavirin *tablets* (Copegus®, generic) are used in adults without cardiac disease, ribavirin dosage should be decreased to 600 mg daily (200 mg in morning and 400 mg in evening) if hemoglobin decreases to less that 10 g/dL; the drug should be discontinued if hemoglobin decreases to less than 8.5 g/dL. When ribavirin *tablets* are used in adults with a history of stable cardiac disease, ribavirin dosage should be decreased to 600 mg daily (200 mg in morning and 400 mg in evening) if hemoglobin decreases by 2 g/dL or more during any 4-week period; the drug should be discontinued if hemoglobin decreases to less than 12 g/dL after 4 weeks of reduced dosage. In patients who have had ribavirin *tablets* withheld, an attempt may be made to reinitiate the drug at a dosage of 600 mg daily after the toxicity has resolved or decreased in severity; dosage may then be increased to 800 mg daily if tolerated. The usual maximum recommended adult dosage of 1–1.2 g daily (see Table 3) should *not* be resumed.

The manufacturer's information should be consulted for more specific recommendations regarding dosage modification for hematologic or other adverse effects.

Dosage Modification for Toxicity (Pediatric Dosage). If serious adverse effects or laboratory changes occur when oral ribavirin is used in conjunction with peginterferon alfa or nonconjugated interferon alfa in pediatric patients with chronic HCV infection, dosage of one or both drugs should be modified, if appropriate, until the adverse reactions abate. If intolerance persists after dosage adjustments, both drugs should be discontinued.

When ribavirin *capsules* (Rebetol®, Ribasphere®) or *oral solution* (Rebetol®) is used in children 3–17 years of age, ribavirin dosage should be decreased from 15 mg/kg daily to 12 mg/kg daily and; if needed, to 8 mg/kg daily if hemoglobin decreases to less than 10 g/dL. Both ribavirin and peginterferon alfa or nonconjugated interferon alfa should be permanently discontinued in pediatric patients with hemoglobin concentrations less than 8.5 g/dL, leukocyte counts less than 1000/mm^3, neutrophil counts less than 500/mm^3, or platelet counts less than 50,000/mm^3. Pediatric patients with preexisting cardiac conditions receiving ribavirin *capsules* concomitantly with peginterferon alfa or nonconjugated interferon alfa should be closely monitored with weekly hematology evaluations if hemoglobin concentration decreases by 2 g/dL or more during any 4-week period and treatment should be discontinued if hemoglobin concentration is less than 8.5 g/dL (or less than 12 g/dL after 4 weeks of reduced dosage).

When ribavirin *tablets* (Copegus®) are used in children 5 years of age or older without cardiac disease, ribavirin dosage should be decreased if hemoglobin decreases to less than 10 g/dL and should be discontinued if hemoglobin decreases to less than 8.5 g/dL. When ribavirin *tablets* are used in children 5 years of age or older with a history of stable cardiac disease, ribavirin dosage should be decreased if hemoglobin decreases by 2 g/dL or more during any 4-week period and the drug should be discontinued if hemoglobin decreases to less than 12 g/dL after 4 weeks of reduced dosage. In children requiring dosage reduction, a decreased ribavirin dosage of 200 mg daily (200 mg in morning) should be used in those weighing 23–33 kg, 400 mg daily (200 mg in morning and 200 mg in evening) should be used in those weighing 34–59 kg, or 600 mg daily (200 mg in morning and 400 mg in evening) should be used in those weighing 60 kg or more.

The manufacturer's information should be consulted for more specific recommendations regarding dosage modification for hematologic or other adverse effects.

Respiratory Syncytial Virus Infection When ribavirin is used via nasal and oral inhalation (Virazole®) for treatment of severe lower respiratory tract infections caused by RSV in hospitalized infants and young children, the drug should be initiated as soon as possible following the onset of signs and symptoms of infection. Dose and administration schedule of ribavirin inhalation therapy for infants who require mechanical ventilation is the same as that for infants who do not require assisted ventilation.

For treatment of severe RSV infection, a SPAG-2 aerosol generator with an oxygen hood, face mask, or oxygen tent should be used to deliver the reconstituted and diluted ribavirin solution containing 20 mg/mL continuously for 12–18 hours daily for 3–7 days. The manufacturer recommends that the mist be delivered at a rate of about 15 L/minute when using an oxygen hood or tent or about 12 L/minute when using a face mask. The average aerosol concentration for a 12-hour delivery period is 190 mcg/L.

When administered as recommended, the dose of ribavirin delivered to the respiratory tract via the small-particle aerosol generator can be *estimated* using the following equation:

$$\text{dose delivered to respiratory tract} = \text{minute volume (liters)} \times \text{duration of inhalation (minutes)} \times \text{0.19 mg/L (nebulized ribavirin concentration)} \times \text{0.7 (fraction of inhaled dose deposited in respiratory tract)}$$

The manufacturer states that the duration of a course of ribavirin inhalation therapy for RSV infection should be a minimum of 3 days but should not exceed 7 days. Some clinicians indicate that more prolonged and/or repeated therapy with the drug may be necessary in infants with preexisting cardiac and/or respiratory disease or immunocompromised infants (e.g., infants with severe combined immunodeficiency disease [SCID]) with severe lower respiratory tract infection caused by RSV. Therapy with ribavirin inhalation is intended as an adjunct to usual supportive respiratory therapy and fluid management in patients with RSV infection. (See Nasal and Oral Inhalation under Cautions: Precautions and Contraindications.)

Viral Hemorrhagic Fevers **Lassa Fever.** For the treatment of Lassa fever†, the US Centers for Disease Control and Prevention (CDC), US Army Medical Research Institute of Infectious Diseases (USAMRIID), and other experts recommend IV† ribavirin given in a regimen consisting of an initial loading dose of 30 mg/kg (up to 2 g), followed by a dosage of 16 mg/kg (up to 1 g) every 6 hours for 4 days and then 8 mg/kg (up to 500 mg) every 8 hours for 6 days for a total treatment course of 10 days.

Hantavirus Infections. For treatment of hemorrhagic fever with renal syndrome† (HFRS) caused by Hantaan (a Hantavirus) and related Bunyaviridae, IV† ribavirin has been administered in a limited number of patients as an initial loading dose of 33 mg/kg followed by a dosage of 16 mg/kg every 6 hours for 4 days and then 8 mg/kg every 8 hours for 3 days for a total treatment course of 7 days

Crimean-Congo Hemorrhagic Fever. For treatment of Crimean-Congo hemorrhagic fever†, the CDC, USAMRIID, and other experts recommend an adult IV† ribavirin regimen consisting of an initial loading dose of 30 mg/kg (up to 2 g), followed by a dosage of 16 mg/kg (up to 1 g) every 6 hours for 4 days and then 8 mg/kg (up to 500 mg) every 8 hours for 6 days for a total treatment course of 10 days. Alternatively, a 10-day regimen of oral ribavirin consisting of an initial loading dose of 30 mg/kg, followed by 15 mg/kg every 6 hours for 4 days and then 7.5 mg/kg every 8 hours for 6 days has been effective for treatment of Crimean-Congo hemorrhagic fever† in some patients.

For the prevention of Crimean-Congo hemorrhagic fever† in high-risk contacts, the CDC has recommended an oral ribavirin dosage of 500–600 mg every 6 hours for 7–10 days for adults and children older than 9 years of age and an oral dosage of 400 mg every 6 hours for children 6–9 years of age. Dosage for children younger than 6 years of age has not been established. The prophylactic efficacy of various dosages of oral ribavirin remains to be established, and the CDC continues to periodically reassess its recommendations based on accumulating experience. Some clinicians suggest that, based on dose-response experience in the treatment of active disease with low degrees of viremia, oral dosages lower than those recommended by CDC may prove effective for prophylaxis and that pediatric dosages adjusted by body weight or surface area would be more appropriate, especially for prepubertal children. Because of the prolonged elimination half-life of the drug, consideration may be given to administering an initial IV† loading dose in high-risk contacts if the interval between exposure and initiation of prophylaxis is several days.

Viral Hemorrhagic Fevers in the Context of Biologic Warfare or Bioterrorism. For the treatment of clinically evident viral hemorrhagic fever in the context of biologic warfare or bioterrorism† when the disease is caused by an Arenavirus or Bunyavirus or is of unknown etiology, some experts (e.g., the US Working Group on Civilian Biodefense, USAMRIID) recommend that adults or children receive an IV† ribavirin regimen consisting of an initial loading dose of 30 mg/kg (maximum 2 g), followed by a dosage of 16 mg/kg (maximum 1 g) every 6 hours for 4 days and then 8 mg/kg (maximum 500 mg) every 8 hours for 6 days. The IV regimen is recommended for contained casualty settings.

Alternatively, a 10-day regimen of oral ribavirin should be used for treatment of these viral hemorrhagic fevers when the parenteral ribavirin preparation cannot be obtained or would be impractical (e.g., when large numbers of individuals require treatment in a mass casualty setting). When an oral ribavirin regimen is used, the US Working Group on Civilian Biodefense and USAMRIID recommend that adults receive an initial loading dose of 2000 mg followed by 1200 mg daily given in 2 divided doses for those weighing more than 75 kg or 1000 mg daily (400 mg in morning and 600 mg in evening) for those weighing 75 kg or less. If an oral ribavirin regimen is used in children, these experts recommend an initial loading dose of 30 mg/kg followed by 15 mg/kg daily given in 2 divided doses.

Preemptive administration of ribavirin or postexposure prophylaxis in the absence of clinical signs of infection in individuals with known or presumed exposure to a hemorrhagic fever virus in the context of biologic warfare or bioterrorism is not recommended. However, individuals with known or presumed exposure to a hemorrhagic fever virus and all known high-risk contacts (i.e., individuals who have mucous membrane contact with an infected patient) and close contacts (i.e., individuals who live with, shake hands or hug, process laboratory specimens, or care for an infected patient [prior to initiation of appropriate precautions]) should be placed under medical surveillance for 21 days after the potential exposure or last contact with the infected patient. Exposed individuals and contacts who develop a temperature of 38.3°C or higher should receive presumptive treatment of viral hemorrhagic fever† using the ribavirin regimens recommended for treatment of clinically evident viral hemorrhagic fever, unless there is an alternative diagnosis or the etiologic agent is found to be a filovirus or a flavivirus. Although medical surveillance is not necessary for close or high risk contacts of patients diagnosed with Rift Valley fever or a flavivirus since these specific viruses are not transmitted person to person, surveillance is recommended for individuals who processed laboratory specimens from these patients prior to initiation of appropriate precautions since these viruses can be transmitted in the laboratory setting.

Adenovirus Infections For treatment of severe infections caused by adenovirus† in immunocompromised adults, IV† ribavirin has been given in a regimen consisting of an initial loading dose of 33 mg/kg, followed by a dosage of 16 mg/kg every 6 hours for 4 days and then 8 mg/kg every 8 hours for another 3 days or longer until relevant cultures were negative for adenovirus.

For treatment of severe infections caused by adenovirus† in immunocompromised children, IV† ribavirin has been given in a dosage of 25 mg/kg daily in 3 divided doses on day 1, followed by 15 mg/kg daily given in 3 divided doses on days 2–10. Alternatively, a dosage of 15 mg/kg daily for 10 days has been used for treatment of adenovirus infections in children.

■ Dosage in Renal and Hepatic Impairment ***Renal Impairment*** The manufacturer states that dosage of ribavirin *tablets* (Copegus®) should be reduced in adults with creatinine clearance of 50 mL/minute or less. When Copegus® is used for treatment of chronic HCV infection, adults with creatinine clearance of 30–50 mL/minute should receive alternating doses of 200 mg and 400 mg every other day and adults with creatinine clearance less than 30 mL/minute or undergoing hemodialysis should receive 200 mg daily. Dosage should not be reduced any further; if severe adverse effects or laboratory abnormalities occur, the drug should be discontinued. Data are insufficient to make dosage recommendations for use of Copegus® in pediatric patients with renal impairment.

Ribavirin capsules (Rebetol®, Ribasphere®), tablets (Ribasphere®), and oral solution (Rebetol®) are contraindicated in patients with creatinine clearance less than 50 mL/minute. In pediatric patients receiving ribavirin capsules or oral solution (Rebetol®) with peginterferon alfa-2b or nonconjugated interferon alfa-2b, both drugs should be discontinued if serum creatinine concentrations exceed 2 mg/dL.

Hepatic Impairment Although the effect of hepatic impairment on the pharmacokinetics of oral ribavirin has not been fully evaluated, peak plasma concentrations are increased depending on the severity of hepatic impairment. (See Oral Administration under Pharmacokinetics: Absorption.)

Cautions

■ Oral Administration Oral ribavirin used in conjunction with peginterferon alfa or nonconjugated interferon alfa usually is well tolerated, but the combination can cause a variety of serious adverse reactions that may require dosage reduction or discontinuance. Important adverse effects reported with concomitant oral ribavirin and peginterferon alfa or interferon alfa therapy include severe depression and suicidal ideation, hemolytic anemia, suppression of bone marrow function, autoimmune and infectious disorders, ophthalmologic disorders, cerebrovascular disorders, pulmonary dysfunction, colitis, pancreatitis, and diabetes. In clinical studies, 6–19% of patients receiving combination therapy in clinical studies discontinued therapy because of adverse effects. The most common reasons for discontinuance were psychiatric symptoms, flu-like syndrome (lethargy, fatigue, headache), adverse dermatologic effects, adverse GI effects, and adverse hematologic effects (anemia, neutropenia, thrombocytopenia).

Adverse effects reported with oral ribavirin in conjunction with peginterferon alfa-2a in patients coinfected with hepatitis C virus (HCV) and human immunodeficiency virus (HIV) generally are similar to those reported in patients with HCV monoinfection (without HIV infection). However, adverse hematologic effects (anemia, neutropenia, thrombocytopenia), weight decrease, and mood alteration have been reported more frequently in those coinfected with HCV and HIV. In addition, there is an increased risk of hepatic decompensation in cirrhotic HCV patients coinfected with HIV receiving antiretroviral therapy and interferon alfa with or without oral ribavirin.

For information on the adverse effects associated with peginterferon alfa or interferon alfa, see Cautions in Peginterferon Alfa 8:18.20 and see Cautions in Interferon Alfa 8:18.20.

Hematologic Effects The primary toxicity or oral ribavirin is hemolytic anemia (hemoglobin less than 10 g/dL). Ribavirin appears to produce a dose- and time-dependent, reversible anemia, especially during oral or IV† use of the drug in dosages of 1.2 g or higher daily (about 15–17 mg/kg daily) for more than 10 days. (See Effects on Erythrocytes under Cautions: Nasal and Oral Inhalation.)

Anemia has been reported in 10–13% of patients receiving oral ribavirin in conjunction with peginterferon alfa or interferon alfa in clinical studies evaluating this regimen for treatment of HCV infection. Anemia also has been reported in patients receiving oral or IV† ribavirin for treatment or prevention of Lassa fever or Hantavirus infections;

Ribavirin-associated anemia generally occurs within 1–2 weeks following initiation of oral ribavirin therapy, and the maximum hemoglobin decrease usually occurs during the first 8 weeks of therapy. Anemia may be mild and reversible within 2–4 weeks after discontinuance of the drug, although severe anemia which may require transfusion can occur, and complete reversal occasionally may be delayed for several months after discontinuance of ribavirin.

Reversible increases in bilirubin and uric acid concentrations may occur as the result of hemolytic anemia. In clinical studies, these alterations occurred most frequently in patients previously diagnosed with Gilbert's syndrome and were generally moderate and reversed within 4 weeks of treatment discontinuance. An association with hepatic dysfunction or clinical morbidity has not been established.

Ribavirin-induced anemia may result in deterioration in cardiac function and/or exacerbation of the symptoms of coronary disease; fatal and nonfatal myocardial infarctions have been reported in patients with ribavirin-associated anemia.

Hepatic Effects Transient increases in serum bilirubin, AST (SGOT), and ALT (SGPT) concentrations have occurred during use of oral or IV† ribavirin.

Patients with chronic HCV infection and cirrhosis may be at risk of hepatic decompensation and death during peginterferon alfa or interferon alfa therapy. Such patients who are coinfected with HIV and receiving highly active antiretroviral therapy (HAART) in conjunction with interferon alfa-2a therapy (with or without ribavirin) appear to be at increased risk for development of hepatic decompensation compared with patients not receiving HAART.

Respiratory Effects Adverse pulmonary effects, including dyspnea, pulmonary infiltrates, pneumonitis, pulmonary hypertension, pneumonia (including some fatalities), coughing, pharyngitis, rhinitis, and sinusitis, have occurred in patients receiving oral ribavirin in clinical studies. In addition, sarcoidosis or exacerbation of sarcoidosis has been reported.

Nervous System Effects Psychiatric events including insomnia, irritability, and depression have occurred in 26–39, 23–32, and 23–25% of patients, respectively, receiving oral ribavirin in conjunction with interferon alfa-2b in clinical studies. Suicidal ideation or attempts has been reported in about 1% of adults receiving such therapy in clinical studies; these events were more common in adolescents than adults.

Other Adverse Effects Serious skin reactions, including vesiculobullous eruptions, reactions in the spectrum of Stevens-Johnson syndrome with varying degrees of skin and mucosal involvement, and erythroderma, have been reported in patients receiving peginterferon alfa-2a with or without ribavirin.

Dental and periodontal disorders have been reported in patients receiving ribavirin in conjunction with peginterferon alfa or interferon alfa. Dry mouth may result in damage to teeth and oral mucous membranes during long-term treatment.

Hearing disorder, vertigo, and pancreatitis have been reported in patients receiving oral ribavirin in conjunction with peginterferon alfa or interferon alfa.

■ **Nasal and Oral Inhalation** Information on adverse effects of ribavirin inhalation therapy has been obtained principally from clinical studies conducted prior to 1986, from a controlled study conducted in 1989–1990, and from postmarketing surveillance reports. The most common adverse effects associated with inhalation of the drug appear to include respiratory and cardiovascular effects; these effects generally occur infrequently.

Although a definite causal relationship to the drug has not been established, serious adverse effects have occasionally occurred during ribavirin inhalation therapy in severely ill infants with underlying life-threatening conditions, many of whom required assisted respiration. Death has occurred in 20 patients during or shortly after discontinuance of ribavirin inhalation therapy, but a causal relationship to the drug was not clearly established. The long-term toxic potential of the drug in children has not been fully elucidated.

Respiratory Effects Worsening of respiratory function has occurred, sometimes suddenly, during ribavirin inhalation therapy in infants with RSV infections or in adults† with chronic obstructive pulmonary disease (COPD) or asthma. In infants with underlying life-threatening conditions, inhalation of the drug has been associated with aggravation and worsening of respiratory function, apnea, and physical dependence on assisted respiration. In adults with COPD or asthma, therapy with the drug frequently has been associated with deterioration in pulmonary function, and dyspnea and chest soreness have occurred in several adults with asthma. Minor pulmonary function abnormalities have also been observed in healthy adults receiving ribavirin inhalation. Bronchospasm, pulmonary edema, hypoventilation, cyanosis, dyspnea, bacterial pneumonia, pneumothorax, apnea, atelectasis, and ventilator dependence also have been associated with ribavirin inhalation therapy. Several deaths that were characterized as possibly related to ribavirin inhalation therapy by the treating physician occurred in infants who experienced worsening respiratory status related to bronchospasm while receiving the drug.

Ribavirin inhalation therapy in patients who require assisted respiration has resulted in mechanical problems caused by precipitation of the drug in the respiratory apparatus, including the endotracheal tube and other tubing, and may result in inadequate assisted respiration and gas exchange in these patients. Increases in positive inspiratory and end-expiratory pressures have occurred in these patients as a result of drug precipitation and subsequent malfunction or obstruction of valves in the respiratory apparatus, and pneumothorax can result from such alterations in the pressures of the apparatus. Accumulation of fluid in tubing of the apparatus ("rain out") has also occurred. There have been several deaths reported in infants with RSV who were undergoing assisted respiration while receiving ribavirin inhalation therapy. In these cases, death was attributed to mechanical ventilator malfunction caused by precipitation of the drug within the ventilator apparatus that led to excessively high pulmonary pressures and diminished oxygenation. Whenever ribavirin inhalation therapy is used in a patient requiring mechanical ventilator assistance, strict attention must be paid to procedures that have been shown to minimize the accumulation of drug precipitate. (See Nasal and Oral Inhalation under Cautions: Precautions and Contraindications and see Nasal and Oral Inhalation under Dosage and Administration: Reconstitution and Administration.)

Additional study is needed to determine the safety of prolonged and multiple courses of ribavirin inhalation therapy. In a study in developing ferrets, inhalation of ribavirin dosages of 60 mg/kg for 10 or 30 days resulted in inflammatory and possible emphysematous changes in the lungs, and proliferative changes were observed following dosages of 131 mg/kg for 30 days; however, the relevance of these findings to humans is not known. The manufacturer states that prolonged courses of ribavirin inhalation therapy are not recommended; some clinicians caution that prolonged or multiple courses of ribavirin inhalation therapy could potentially affect respiratory tract physiology secondary to biochemical changes and that high concentrations of the drug could affect respiratory membranes.

Cardiovascular Effects Adverse cardiovascular effects, including cardiac arrest, hypotension, bradycardia, and cardiac glycoside intoxication, have been reported in patients receiving ribavirin inhalation therapy. In addition, bigeminy, bradycardia, and tachycardia have occurred with ribavirin inhalation in patients with underlying congenital heart disease. Cardiac lesions were observed in mice and rats receiving ribavirin inhalation dosages of 30 and 36 mg/kg daily, respectively, for 4 weeks, and in monkeys and rats receiving oral dosages of 120 and 154–200 mg/kg daily, respectively, for 1–6 months; however, the relevance of this finding to humans is not known.

Effects on Erythrocytes Although anemia was not reported with ribavirin inhalation therapy in several controlled clinical trials, most of these infants and young children who received the drug via inhalation were not evaluated 1–2 weeks following discontinuance of the drug, when evidence of ribavirin-induced anemia is most likely. Reversible anemia, reticulocytosis, and hemolytic anemia have been reported in postmarketing experience of patients receiving the drug via inhalation.

Studies in animals and humans have shown that ribavirin and/or its metabolites accumulate in erythrocytes and persist for prolonged periods (e.g., weeks or longer) following administration of the drug, possibly because of minimal phosphatase activity in these cells. (See Pharmacokinetics: Distribution and Elimination.)

Ribavirin appears to produce a dose- and time-dependent, reversible anemia, especially during oral or IV use of the drug in dosages of 1.2 g or higher daily (about 15–17 mg/kg daily) for more than 10 days. Ribavirin-induced anemia appears to result from hemolysis of erythrocytes and inhibition of late stages of erythrocyte maturation in bone marrow. The drug does not appear to affect erythrocyte stem cells. Ribavirin also does not appear to affect the maturation of leukocyte precursors or leukocytes and may increase the production of megakaryocytes and thrombocytes.

Other Adverse Effects Rash, erythema of the eyelids, and conjunctivitis have occurred in patients receiving ribavirin inhalation therapy. These effects usually resolve within hours after ribavirin therapy is discontinued.

Adverse hepatic effects, including increased transaminase concentrations, have not been observed during ribavirin inhalation therapy.

Environmental Exposure of Health-care Personnel and Visitors The potential risks, particularly for long-term and cumulative effects, associated with environmental exposure to aerosolized ribavirin by health-care personnel and visitors while in contact with patients undergoing inhalation therapy with the drug currently have not been elucidated but acute effects do not appear to be substantial. However, because of animal evidence of ribavirin's teratogenic potential and absence of data defining safe levels of aerosol exposure to the drug, some experts and clinicians state that such exposure of pregnant women and possibly those who may become pregnant may represent a risk to the fetus. Evidence from several studies in which health-care personnel were exposed to ribavirin while in contact with patients undergoing ribavirin inhalation therapy revealed minimal concentrations of the drug in urine or erythrocytes (in only a single sample) and undetectable concentrations in plasma or serum, and no adverse effects attributable to the drug in these personnel. However, only a limited number of personnel were studied. In one study, urinary concentrations of ribavirin were measurable in 65% of nurses caring for children receiving aerosolized ribavirin via a variety of administration methods and in 15% of respiratory therapists, with creatinine-corrected urinary concentrations of the drug averaging 4.25 (range: less than 0.25 up to 35) ng of ribavirin per mg of creatinine.

The most frequent adverse effects reported to date in health-care personnel exposed to aerosolized ribavirin include eye irritation (which may be more likely in contact lens wearers) and headache, which usually were mild and reversible following discontinuance of exposure. Nasal and/or throat irritation, pharyngitis, lacrimation, nausea, dizziness, fatigue, rash, bronchospasm, rhinitis, chest pain, and nasal congestion also have been reported in health-care personnel in contact with patients undergoing ribavirin inhalation therapy. A causal relationship between many of these adverse effects and ribavirin exposure has not been established. In most cases, these adverse effects resolved within minutes to hours of discontinuing close exposure to aerosolized ribavirin and few of the personnel exposed to aerosolized drug required medical attention. Ribavirin can precipitate on contact lenses of health-care personnel exposed to aerosolized drug, and such precipitation may be associated with conjunctivitis. Therefore, it has been suggested that contact lens wearers use eyeglasses rather than contact lenses or, alternatively, use protective goggles while potentially in contact with aerosolized ribavirin.

Evidence from several studies indicates that measurable exposure of health-care personnel to the drug can occur, the level of which depends on the method of drug administration to the patient and probably other factors including length of exposure, number of patients treated in a room simultaneously, room ventilation, administration schedule, integrity of the small-particle aerosol generator, and variations in work practices (e.g., turning off the small-particle aerosol generator before manipulating the delivery apparatus). In a few of these studies in which personal-breathing-zone area air samples from health-care personnel (nurses and respiratory therapists) and bedside area air samples were collected, the highest levels of exposure occurred during contact with patients receiving the drug via a tracheostomy tube, followed by those receiving the drug via an oxygen hood or tent, and the lowest level occurred during contact with those receiving the drug via a ventilator that included an in-line filter in the expiratory line. An exposure level intermediate to the tent/hood and the ventilator was observed during contact with a patient receiving the drug via a face mask, and exposure levels higher than those with a ventilator but lower than those with a face mask were observed with an aerosol delivery hood that included a vacuum exhaust filtration system (available from Valeant) or with a croup tent (croupette). Exposure levels observed with an aerosol delivery hood combined with a scavenging tent were lower than those with an aerosol delivery hood alone and similar to those with a ventilator. Ribavirin concentrations in personal area air samples reportedly averaged 579 mcg/m^3 (range: 390–828 mcg/m^3) for personnel in contact with patients receiving the drug via a tracheostomy tube, 485 mcg/m^3 (range: 26–1692 mcg/m^3) for those in contact with patients receiving the drug via an oxygen hood, 161 mcg/m^3 (range: 69–316 mcg/m^3) for those in contact with patients receiving the drug via an oxygen tent, 25–34 mcg/m^3 (range: 1–91 mcg/m^3) for those in contact with patients receiving the drug via an aerosol delivery hood with a vacuum exhaust filtration system, 23 mcg/m^3 (range: 12–28 mcg/m^3 for those in contact with patients receiving the drug via a croup tent, 6 mcg/m^3 (range: undetectable to 12 mcg/m^3) for those in contact with patients receiving the drug via an aerosol delivery hood combined with a scavenging tent, and 6 or less mcg/m^3 for those in contact with patients receiving the drug via a ventilator; concentrations in bedside area air samples generally substantially exceeded those in personal area air samples In a pilot study involving one patient receiving ribavirin via a double-tent system (consisting of an oxygen tent canopy over an oxygen hood), undetectable concentrations of ribavirin were found in personal-breathing-zone area air samples from health-care personnel and in bedside area samples. However, further studies are needed to evaluate the double-tent system. In addition, theoretical estimates based on exposure data from these studies indicate that the amount of ribavirin that potentially could be absorbed systemically by personnel receiving relatively high-level exposure (e.g., during contact with patients receiving the drug via an oxygen tent) could potentially represent a risk to the fetus.

Until potential risks of exposure are more clearly delineated, health-care personnel who provide direct care to patients receiving aerosolized ribavirin and are pregnant, lactating, or in relationships of likely reproductive potential should be counseled about risk-reduction strategies, including alternative job responsibilities. Visitors (including family members) of patients receiving aerosolized ribavirin also should be advised of the potential risks associated with exposure to the drug since they may spend considerable time in close proximity to the patient's bedside. Data currently available cannot be extrapolated reliably to assess possible risks to individuals working elsewhere in a room or ward where ribavirin is being administered via aerosolization. However, measurable concentrations of ribavirin have been detected in the air at nurses' stations located near the rooms of patients receiving ribavirin inhalation therapy via an oxygen hood, an aerosol delivery hood, a croup tent, or an aerosol delivery hood in combination with a scavenging tent. Such measurable exposure may have resulted from positive pressure or inadequate negative pressure in patient rooms.

Because of uncertainties about potential risk, procedures to minimize environmental exposure to aerosolized ribavirin generally should be developed. Whenever possible, patients receiving ribavirin inhalation therapy should be located in rooms where potential exposure of personnel and other patients is minimized (e.g., private rooms with adequate ventilation or, preferably, the National Institute for Occupational Safety and Health [NIOSH] recommends isolation rooms that are under negative pressure and have adequate air exchange and exhaust to the outside). Use of gowns, gloves, goggles, and masks, which already may be part of the usual procedures for minimizing nosocomial spread of RSV when in contact with infected patients, has been suggested, although the level of protection provided is not known. Some experts, including NIOSH, state that use of surgical masks by health-care personnel caring for ribavirin-treated patients probably is unlikely to provide an effective means for reducing environmental exposure to the drug, and therefore currently is not recommended by these experts as a primary protective measure. However, use of alternative, appropriately designed (e.g., for adequate particle-size filtration) and well-fitted face masks (e.g., 3M Company model 9970) or powered air-purifying respirators may provide protection. In deciding the method of administration of ribavirin inhalation therapy, current data on associated exposure levels should be considered, and, whenever possible, methods associated with the lowest levels of exposure employed. Except when immediate care is necessary, the small-particle aerosol generator should be turned off (using a remote switch) temporarily, but for at least 5–10 minutes before entering the room, when attending to the patient and when handling the respiratory apparatus. In addition, the air pressure of the ribavirin treatment room should be evaluated (e.g., using tissue paper at the ajar doorway) and ideally be negative relative to the hallway prior to initiation of a treatment session. An aerosol delivery hood intended for use in administering oxygen and aerosolized ribavirin and that includes a vacuum exhaust filtration system has recently become available from the manufacturer of ribavirin (Valeant) and reportedly can substantially reduce the risk of aerosol emission into the environment during ribavirin inhalation therapy. Other devices, procedures, and precautions to minimize environmental exposure to aerosolized ribavirin have been suggested, and occupational safety or other experts should be consulted for additional information. NIOSH currently is gathering additional information on potential risks associated with environmental exposure to aerosolized ribavirin by health-care personnel; results of these evaluations will be made available by NIOSH upon completion.

■ Precautions and Contraindications *Oral Administration*

Oral ribavirin is contraindicated in patients with known hypersensitivity to ribavirin or any component of the formulations. The drug should be discontinued immediately and appropriate therapy initiated if an acute hypersensitivity reaction (e.g., urticaria, angioedema, bronchoconstriction, anaphylaxis) occurs. The drug should also be discontinued in patients with manifestations of severe skin reactions (e.g., Stevens-Johnson syndrome, toxic epidermal necrolysis, erythema multiforme).

Oral ribavirin is contraindicated in women who are or may become pregnant and also is contraindicated in male partners of pregnant women. (See Pregnancy under Cautions: Pregnancy, Fertility, and Lactation.)

Oral ribavirin is contraindicated in patients with hemoglobinopathies (e.g., thalassemia, sickle cell anemia).

Concomitant use of oral ribavirin and didanosine is contraindicated. (See Increased Risk of Adverse Effects under Antiretroviral Agents: HIV Nucleoside Reverse Transcriptase Inhibitors, in Drug Interactions.)

Oral ribavirin capsules (Rebetol®, Ribasphere®), tablets (generic), and oral solution (Rebetol®) are contraindicated in patients with creatinine clearance less than 50 mL/minute.

Use of oral ribavirin and peginterferon alfa or interferon alfa is contraindicated in patients with autoimmune hepatitis.

Use of ribavirin *tablets* (Copegus®, generic) in conjunction with peginterferon alfa-2a is contraindicated in cirrhotic patients with chronic HCV monoinfection (without coexisting HIV infection) who have hepatic decompensation (Child-Pugh score greater than 6; class B and C) prior to or during treatment.

Use of ribavirin *tablets* (Copegus®, generic) in conjunction with peginterferon alfa-2a is contraindicated in cirrhotic patients with chronic HCV infection who are coinfected with HIV and have hepatic decompensation (Child-Pugh score 6 or greater) prior to or during treatment.

Hematologic and Cardiac Precautions. Patients receiving oral ribavirin should be monitored for the development of anemia. (See Hematologic Effects under Cautions: Oral Administration.) Since ribavirin-associated anemia usually occurs within 1–2 weeks after initiation of oral ribavirin therapy, hemoglobin or hematocrit should be determined before initiating therapy, at weeks 2 and 4 (or more frequently if needed), and then as clinically appropriate. Other standard hematologic tests, including complete and differential white blood cell counts and platelet counts, also should be performed prior to and periodically during oral ribavirin therapy. Ribavirin should be used with caution in patients with baseline risk of severe anemia (e.g., spherocytosis, history of GI bleeding).

The manufacturers state that the entry criteria used in clinical studies evaluating safety and efficacy of oral ribavirin (Copegus®) and peginterferon alfa-2a for treatment of chronic HCV infection can be considered a guideline for acceptable baseline values for initiation of therapy. These studies required that hemoglobin be at least 12 g/dL in women and at least 13 g/dL in men with HCV monoinfection (without concomitant HIV infection) or at least 11 g/dL in women and at least 12 g/dL in men coinfected with HCV and HIV. In addition, these studies required that platelet counts be at least 90,000/mm^3 (as low as 75,000/mm^3 in those with cirrhosis or 70,000/mm^3 in those coinfected with HCV and HIV) and that absolute neutrophil counts (ANCs) be at least 1500/mm^3.

If use of IV† ribavirin therapy is being considered, some clinicians recommend that baseline hemoglobin concentrations of 8 g/dL or less should be corrected prior to initiation of the drug and patients monitored closely throughout the course of treatment.

Because ribavirin-induced anemia may exacerbate preexisting cardiac disease and fatal and nonfatal myocardial infarctions have been reported in patients with ribavirin-associated anemia, patients should be assessed for underlying cardiac disease before initiation of ribavirin therapy. Those with preexisting cardiac disease should have ECGs before the drug is initiated and should be appropriately monitored during therapy. If there is any deterioration of cardiovascular status, oral ribavirin should be suspended or discontinued.

Oral ribavirin should not be used in patients with a history of substantial or unstable cardiac disease.

Precautions Related to Combination HCV Treatment Regimens. Oral ribavirin monotherapy is *not* effective and should *not* be used for treatment of chronic HCV infection.

When oral ribavirin is used in conjunction with peginterferon alfa or interferon alfa, the cautions, precautions, and contraindications associated with both oral ribavirin and peginterferon alfa or interferon alfa should be considered. (See Cautions in Peginterferon Alfa 8:18.20 and in Interferon Alfa 8:18.20.)

Safety and efficacy of oral ribavirin in conjunction with peginterferon alfa or interferon alfa have *not* been established in liver or other organ transplant recipients, patients coinfected with HCV and hepatitis B virus (HBV), or patients with HCV infection and decompensated liver disease.

Safety and efficacy of ribavirin *capsules* (Rebetol®, Ribasphere®) in conjunction with peginterferon alfa or nonconjugated interferon alfa-2b have not been established in chronic HCV patients coinfected with HIV.

Some manufacturers state that safety and efficacy of ribavirin *tablets* (Copegus®, generic) in conjunction with peginterferon alfa-2a have not been established in chronic HCV patients who have not responded to interferon therapy or are coinfected with HIV and have $CD4^+$ T-cell counts less than $100/mm^3$.

Safety and efficacy of oral ribavirin in conjunction with peginterferon alfa or interferon alfa for treatment of infections caused by HIV, adenovirus, RSV, parainfluenza, or influenza virus have not been established and this regimen should *not* be used for these indications.

Patients receiving oral ribavirin in conjunction with peginterferon alfa or interferon alfa for treatment of chronic HCV infection should be advised that the effect of such treatment on transmission of the virus is not known and that appropriate precautions should be taken to prevent transmission.

Patients who experience pulmonary infiltrates or a deterioration in pulmonary function while receiving oral ribavirin with peginterferon alfa or interferon alfa should be closely monitored and, if appropriate, the drugs should be discontinued.

Oral ribavirin in conjunction with peginterferon alfa or interferon alfa should be suspended in patients with manifestations of pancreatitis and discontinued in those with confirmed pancreatitis.

When oral ribavirin is used in a multiple-drug regimen that includes one or more HCV direct-acting antivirals (DAAs), including those classified as HCV protease inhibitors (e.g., paritaprevir, simeprevir), HCV polymerase inhibitors (e.g., dasabuvir, sofosbuvir), or HCV replication complex inhibitors (e.g., ombitasvir), the cautions, precautions, and contraindications associated with the HCV DAAs also should be considered. (See Cautions in the individual monographs in HCV Antivirals 8:18.40.)

Other Precautions. Thyroid function should be assessed prior to and periodically during oral ribavirin therapy. In clinical studies evaluating use of oral ribavirin (Copegus®) and peginterferon alfa-2a for treatment of chronic HCV infection, study entry criteria required thyrotropin (thyroid-stimulating hormone, TSH) and thyroxine (T_4) concentrations within normal limits or adequately controlled thyroid function.

Patients should be advised to have regular dental examinations during treatment, brush their teeth thoroughly twice daily, and rinse their mouth thoroughly after vomiting.

Nasal and Oral Inhalation Ribavirin inhalation therapy is contraindicated in patients with known hypersensitivity to the drug or any ingredient in the formulation and also is contraindicated in women who are or may become pregnant.

Ribavirin nasal and oral inhalation therapy is *not* a substitute for usual supportive respiratory therapy and fluid management in infants and young children with severe lower respiratory tract infection caused by respiratory syncytial virus (RSV), and careful monitoring of respiratory function and fluid balance in these patients is necessary. Although the manufacturer states that use of ribavirin inhalation currently is recommended only for pediatric patients with severe RSV lower respiratory tract infection, if the inhalation is used in other patients†, careful monitoring of respiratory function is necessary during inhalation therapy. Because initiation of ribavirin inhalation therapy in infants has been associated with sudden deterioration of respiratory function, the drug should be discontinued if sudden worsening of respiratory function occurs following initiation of therapy with the drug; ribavirin should be reintroduced only with extreme caution and continuous monitoring, and consideration should be given to concomitant administration of bronchodilators.

Use of ribavirin inhalation therapy in patients requiring mechanical ventilator assistance should be undertaken only by physicians and support staff familiar with this mode of administration and the specific ventilator being used. Because ribavirin may precipitate in the respiratory apparatus in patients requiring mechanical ventilation and can cause mechanical ventilator dysfunction and associated increased pulmonary pressures, strict attention should be given to procedures that have been shown to minimize the accumulation of ribavirin precipitates in the apparatus. These procedures include use of bacterial filters in series in the expiratory limb of the ventilator circuit with frequent changes (e.g., every 4 hours), water column pressure release valves to indicate elevated ventilator pressures, frequent monitoring of these devices and verification that ribavirin crystals have not accumulated within the ventilator circuitry, and frequent suctioning and monitoring of the patient. (See Nasal and Oral Inhalation under Dosage and Administration: Reconstitution and Administration.)

Patients receiving ribavirin inhalation therapy for longer than 1–2 weeks should be monitored for the development of anemia (see Effects on Erythrocytes under Cautions: Nasal and Oral Inhalation); monitoring for this adverse effect generally is not considered necessary in patients receiving the inhalation for 7 days or less. The risk of developing anemia and need for close monitoring are increased in patients receiving systemic (e.g., oral, IV) ribavirin therapy.

The manufacturer states that although ribavirin inhalation currently is not intended for use in adults, clinicians should be aware that the drug is teratogenic in animals and ribavirin therapy should *not* be initiated in women of childbearing potential. (See Pregnancy under Cautions: Pregnancy, Fertility, and Lactation.) Some experts state that potential risk of environmental exposure to aerosolized ribavirin by pregnant health-care personnel or visitors should be considered. (See Environmental Exposure of Health-care Personnel and Visitors under Cautions: Nasal and Oral Inhalation.)

■ Pediatric Precautions

Safety and efficacy of aerosolized ribavirin (ribavirin nasal and oral inhalation) have been established for treatment of RSV infection in infants and young children.

Safety and efficacy of ribavirin oral capsules (Rebetol®, Ribasphere®) or ribavirin oral solution (Rebetol®) in conjunction with peginterferon alfa-2b or nonconjugated interferon alfa-2b have not been established for treatment of chronic HCV infection in children younger than 3 years of age. When deciding whether to use such regimens in HCV-infected children, evidence of disease progression (hepatic inflammation, fibrosis), prognostic factors for response, HCV genotype, and viral load should be considered. The benefits of such treatment should be weighed against adverse effects reported in pediatric patients. Concomitant therapy with ribavirin capsules or oral solution (Rebetol®) and peginterferon alfa-2b or nonconjugated interferon alfa-2b should not be used in pediatric patients with serum creatinine concentrations greater than 2 mg/dL.

Safety and efficacy of ribavirin tablets (Copegus®) in conjunction with peginterferon alfa-2b have not been established for treatment of chronic HCV infection in children younger than 5 years of age. Some manufacturers state that safety and efficacy of ribavirin tablets have not been established in patients younger than 18 years of age.

Adverse effects reported with oral ribavirin in conjunction with peginterferon alfa or interferon alfa in pediatric patients generally are similar to those reported in adults. In clinical studies in children, 2–13% of patients discontinued oral ribavirin and interferon alfa therapy because of adverse effects; dosage modifications were required in 25–30%, usually because of anemia, neutropenia, or weight loss. Among patients receiving concomitant therapy with ribavirin capsules and interferon alfa-2b, injection site disorders, fever, anorexia, vomiting, and emotional lability were reported more frequently in pediatric patients than in adults; however, fatigue, dyspepsia, arthralgia, insomnia, irritability, impaired concentrations, dyspnea, and pruritus were reported less frequently in pediatric patients than in adults. Overall, suicidal ideation or attempts occurred more frequently in pediatric patients (2.4%) than in adults (1%) during or after therapy; most of these children were adolescents. Like adults, other adverse psychiatric effects (depression, emotional lability, somnolence), anemia, and neutropenia were also reported in pediatric patients.

Delays in weight and height gain compared with baseline have been reported in pediatric patients receiving peginterferon alfa and oral ribavirin therapy. Decreased weight and height for age z-scores as well as percentiles of the normative population have been reported. Data from pediatric patients receiving peginterferon alfa-2a and oral ribavirin indicate that at the end of treatment 43% experienced a weight percentile decrease of 15 percentiles or more and 25% experienced a height percentile decrease of 15 percentiles or more on the normative growth curves. Most children had returned to baseline normative growth curve percentiles for weight and height at the end of 2-year follow-up after completion of treatment (mean weight for age percentile was 64% at baseline and 60% at 2 years posttreatment, mean height percentile was 54% at baseline and 56% at 2 years posttreatment).

Data from an open-label trial in pediatric patients 3 through 17 years of age receiving peginterferon alfa-2b and oral ribavirin indicated that weight and height gain generally lagged behind that predicted by normative population data for the entire length of treatment. During a 48-week treatment course, there was a decrease in the rate of linear growth (mean percentile assignment decrease of 7%) and a decrease in the rate of weight gain (mean percentile assignment decrease of 9%). Although a general reversal of these trends was noted during the 24-week posttreatment period, long-term follow-up data in pediatric patients indicate that oral ribavirin and peginterferon alfa-2b treatment may induce a growth inhibition that results in reduced final adult height in some patients.

■ Geriatric Precautions

Clinical studies of oral ribavirin used in conjunction with peginterferon alfa or interferon alfa did not include sufficient numbers of patients 65 years of age and older to determine whether geriatric patients respond differently than younger patients. In clinical trials, geriatric patients had a higher frequency of anemia (67%) than did younger patients (28%).

Oral ribavirin should be used with caution in geriatric patients, usually initiating therapy at the lower end of the usual dosage range to reflect the greater frequency of decreased hepatic, renal, and/or cardiac function and of concomitant disease and drug therapy observed in this population. Because ribavirin is known to be substantially excreted by the kidney, and because patients with renal impairment are at increased risk of ribavirin-induced toxicity, renal function should be monitored closely and dosage adjusted accordingly. Oral ribavirin capsules (Rebetol®, Ribasphere®), tablets (generic), and oral solution (Rebetol®) should *not* be used in geriatric patients with creatinine clearance less than 50 mL/minute; dosage of ribavirin tablets (Copegus®) should be adjusted for patients with creatinine clearance less than 50 mL/minute. (See Renal Impairment under Dosage and Administration: Dosage in Renal and Hepatic Impairment.)

■ **Mutagenicity and Carcinogenicity** Ribavirin increased the incidence of cell transformations and mutations in mouse Balb/c 3T3 fibroblasts at concentrations of 0.015 mg/mL and in L5178Y lymphoma cells at concentrations of 0.03–5 mg/mL (without metabolic activation). In vitro, in L5178Y cells with the addition of a metabolic activation fraction, there were modest increases in mutation rates (3–4 times higher) at ribavirin concentrations of 3.75–10 mg/mL. In the mouse micronucleus assay, ribavirin was clastogenic at IV doses of 20–200 mg/kg (estimated human equivalent of 1.67–16.7 mg/kg based on body surface area adjustment for a 60-kg adult); however, the drug was not mutagenic in a dominant lethal assay in rats at intraperitoneal doses of 50–200 mg/kg administered for 5 days (estimated human equivalent of 7.14–28.6 mg/kg based on body surface area adjustment for the adult).

The carcinogenic potential of ribavirin has not been fully determined. Results of a chronic feeding study in rats receiving 16–100 mg/kg daily (estimated human equivalent of 2.3–14.3 mg/kg daily based on body surface area adjustment for the adult) suggest that ribavirin may induce benign mammary, pancreatic, pituitary, and adrenal tumors. Preliminary results of 2 oral gavage oncogenicity studies in mice and rats receiving 18–24 months of ribavirin are inconclusive as to the carcinogenic potential of the drug but demonstrate a relationship between chronic ribavirin exposure and increased incidences of vascular lesions (microscopic hemorrhages) in mice and retinal degeneration in rats. The mice and rats in these studies received 20–75 and 10–40 mg/kg, respectively, of ribavirin daily (estimated human equivalent of 1.67–6.25 and 1.43–5.71 mg/kg, respectively, daily based on body surface area adjustment for the adult).

■ **Pregnancy, Fertility, and Lactation** ***Pregnancy*** Ribavirin may cause fetal toxicity and/or death. The drug has been shown to be teratogenic and/or embryocidal in almost all animal species tested to date. Malformations of the skull, palate, eye, jaw, limbs, skeleton, and GI tract have been reported in animal studies. The incidence and severity of teratogenic effects increase with increasing dosage.

Oral ribavirin is contraindicated in women who are or may become pregnant and also is contraindicated in male partners of such women.

Extreme care should be exercised to avoid pregnancy in female patients receiving ribavirin and in female partners of male patients receiving ribavirin. In addition, based on a multiple-dose ribavirin half-life of 12 days, pregnancy also should be avoided in female patients and in female partners of male patients for 6 months after oral ribavirin is discontinued (e.g., 15 half-lives of clearance for ribavirin). Oral ribavirin should not be initiated until a report of a negative pregnancy test has been obtained; the pregnancy test should be performed immediately prior to initiating therapy. Women of childbearing potential and men with female partners of childbearing potential should be counseled about effective contraception and must use 2 reliable forms of contraception during and, because of the long half-life of the drug, for 6 months following completion of therapy. Pregnancy tests should be performed monthly during and for 6 months after the drug is discontinued. If ribavirin is inadvertently administered during pregnancy or if the patient becomes pregnant while receiving the drug or up to 6 months after discontinuance, the patient should be informed of the potential hazard to the fetus. If pregnancy occurs in a patient or in the partner of a patient receiving oral ribavirin or during the 6 months following completion of therapy, clinicians and patients are encouraged to report such cases to the ribavirin pregnancy registry at 800-593-2214.

Ribavirin nasal and oral inhalation is contraindicated in women who are or may become pregnant. In addition, because of animal evidence of the drug's teratogenic potential, some experts state that environmental exposure to aerosolized ribavirin by pregnant health-care personnel or visitors may represent a risk to the fetus. Whether a potential risk exists for women exposed to aerosolized ribavirin in the environment who may become pregnant remains controversial, but some experts and clinicians state that such women at least should be advised of the drug's teratogenic potential. (See Environmental Exposure of Health-care Personnel and Visitors under Cautions: Nasal and Oral Inhalation.)

Evidence of teratogenicity was observed following a single oral ribavirin dose of 2.5 mg/kg in hamsters and following oral dosages of 1 mg/kg daily in rats. Abnormalities of the skull, brain, skin, palate, eye, jaw, skeleton, and GI tract were observed in rats receiving oral ribavirin dosages of 10, 30, 60, or 90 mg/kg daily on days 6–15 of gestation and in hamsters receiving oral and/or parenteral dosages of 2.5–5 or 25 mg/kg on days 7–9 or 12–15 of gestation, respectively. Reproduction studies in rats using oral ribavirin dosages of 60 and 90 mg/kg daily have shown decreases in the number of live births and in fetal survival (first and second generation). Reproduction studies in hamsters using an IV ribavirin dose of 5 mg/kg on day 8 of gestation have shown an increased rate of resorption. Ribavirin has been shown to produce skeletal malformations in rabbits receiving oral dosages of 0.3 mg/kg daily and was embryocidal in rabbits receiving oral dosages of 1 mg/kg daily. When administered orally in dosages of 120 mg/kg daily in baboons, however, ribavirin showed no evidence of teratogenic or embryocidal effects.

Fertility The effect of ribavirin on fertility in male or female animals has not been fully investigated. In studies in mice, ribavirin dosages of 35–150 mg/kg daily (estimated human equivalent of 2.92–12.5 mg/kg daily based on body surface area adjustment for the adult) resulted in seminiferous tubule atrophy, decreased sperm concentrations, and increased numbers of sperm with abnormal morphology; partial recovery of sperm production was apparent 3–6 months after the drug was discontinued. Ribavirin has been shown to produce testicular lesions (e.g., tubular atrophy) in adult rats receiving oral dosages of 16 mg/kg daily (estimated human equivalent of 2.29 mg/kg daily based on body surface area adjustment for the adult); lower dosages were not tested. In addition, sperm abnormalities have occurred in mice following oral ribavirin doses of 15–150 mg/kg daily (estimated human equivalent of 1.25–12.5 mg/kg/day, based on body surface area adjustment for a 60-kg adult; 0.1–0.8 times the maximum human 24-hour dose of ribavirin) administered for 3 or 6 months. Essentially total recovery from ribavirin-induced testicular toxicity was apparent within 1 or 2 spermatogenesis cycles following discontinuance of the drug. However, ribavirin is known to accumulate in intracellular components of cells from which the drug is cleared very slowly, and it is not yet known whether ribavirin contained in sperm will exert a potential teratogenic effect upon fertilization of the ova.

Oral ribavirin should be used with caution in fertile men. Men receiving oral ribavirin are advised to take every precaution (i.e., effective contraception using 2 reliable forms) to avoid risk of pregnancy in their female partners during and for 6 months following completion of therapy.

Lactation Ribavirin has been shown to be toxic to lactating animals and their offspring. It is not known whether ribavirin is distributed into milk following nasal or oral inhalation or oral administration in humans.

Because of the potential for serious adverse reactions to oral ribavirin in nursing infants, a decision should be made whether to discontinue nursing or to delay or discontinue oral ribavirin therapy taking into account the importance of the drug to the woman.

Drug Interactions

The following drug interactions are based on studies using oral ribavirin. Studies have not been performed to evaluate potential drug interactions in infants receiving ribavirin nasal and oral inhalation concomitantly with other drugs (e.g., digoxin, diuretics, respiratory smooth muscle relaxants such as theophylline, anti-infectives, antimetabolites, other antiviral agents).

■ **Drugs Affecting or Metabolized by Hepatic Microsomal Enzymes** In vitro studies indicate that ribavirin does not inhibit and is not a substrate for cytochrome P-450 (CYP) enzymes. Therefore, there is little potential for drug interactions with drugs affecting or metabolized by CYP enzymes; no effect on the pharmacokinetics of representative drugs metabolized by CYP2C9, 2C19, 2D6, or 3A4 have been reported.

■ **Antacids** Although the clinical importance is unknown, concomitant administration of a single dose of oral ribavirin and a single dose of antacid containing magnesium, aluminum, and simethicone (Mylanta®) decreased the mean area under the plasma concentration-time curve (AUC) of ribavirin by 14%.

■ **Antiretroviral Agents** ***HIV Nucleoside Reverse Transcriptase Inhibitors*** There is evidence that concomitant use of ribavirin and human immunodeficiency virus (HIV) nucleoside reverse transcriptase inhibitors (NRTIs) may increase the risk of certain adverse effects associated with mitochondrial dysfunction (e.g., potentially fatal hepatic failure, peripheral neuropathy, pancreatitis, symptomatic hyperlactatemia/lactic acidosis).

Although there have been some reports that ribavirin may potentiate the antiretroviral activity of didanosine, there is evidence from in vitro studies that ribavirin may antagonize the antiretroviral activity of some other NRTIs (e.g., lamivudine, stavudine, zidovudine).

Concomitant use of oral ribavirin and lamivudine, stavudine, or zidovudine in patients coinfected with hepatitis C virus (HCV) and HIV did not result in pharmacokinetic (e.g., alterations in plasma concentrations of active metabolites) or pharmacodynamic (e.g., loss of HIV/HCV virologic suppression) interactions.

Increased Risk of Adverse Effects. Concomitant use of oral ribavirin and didanosine is contraindicated because there have been reports of fatal hepatic failure, peripheral neuropathy, pancreatitis, and symptomatic hyperlactatemia/lactic acidosis in patients receiving the drugs concomitantly.

Concomitant use of oral ribavirin and zidovudine is not recommended because of the potential for worsening anemia. If ribavirin and zidovudine are used concomitantly, caution is advised and patients should be closely monitored for virologic response and toxicities, particularly anemia, hepatic decompensation, and neutropenia. An increased incidence of severe neutropenia (absolute neutrophil count [ANC] less than 500/mm^3) and severe anemia (hemoglobin less than 8 g/dL) was reported in patients coinfected with HCV and HIV who were receiving zidovudine in conjunction with peginterferon alfa-2a and oral ribavirin compared with those not receiving zidovudine. In patients receiving zidovudine concomitantly with interferon alfa and ribavirin, consideration should be given to discontinuing zidovudine, as medically appropriate. In patients receiving established HIV and HCV treatment, consideration should be given to replacing zidovudine.

Oral ribavirin should be used concomitantly with stavudine with caution.

Patients receiving oral ribavirin and interferon alfa or peginterferon alfa concomitantly with NRTIs should be closely monitored for treatment-associated toxicities, particularly hepatic decompensation and anemia. Dosage reduction or discontinuance of peginterferon alfa (or interferon alfa) and/or oral ribavirin should be considered if worsening toxicities occur. The concomitant regimen should be discontinued if hepatic decompensation occurs. Prescribing information for the specific NRTI should be consulted for guidance regarding toxicity management.

Cirrhotic patients with chronic HCV infection who are coinfected with HIV and receiving antiretroviral therapy concomitantly with a regimen of interferon alfa or peginterferon alfa and oral ribavirin may be at increased risk of potentially fatal hepatic decompensation compared with those not receiving highly active antiretroviral therapy (HAART). There have been several reports of lactic acidosis or pancreatitis occurring in HIV-infected patients coinfected with HCV who received antiretroviral therapy concomitantly with ribavirin and interferon alfa therapy. These patients had been receiving long-term therapy with antiretroviral regimens that included one or more NRTIs (abacavir, didanosine, lamivudine, stavudine, zidovudine) and were clinically stable until lactic acidosis or pancreatitis developed 4–6 months after a regimen of ribavirin and interferon alfa was initiated for treatment of chronic HCV infection. In addition, hepatic decompensation (including some fatalities) were reported in a study evaluating a regimen of peginterferon alfa-2a and oral ribavirin in patients coinfected with HCV and HIV; all those who developed hepatic decompensation were cirrhotic at baseline and were receiving NRTIs (e.g., abacavir, didanosine, lamivudine, stavudine, zidovudine).

Because ribavirin also is a nucleoside analog, it has been suggested that concomitant use of ribavirin and NRTIs may result in an adverse additive effect on mitochondrial function; however, it also has been suggested that ribavirin may have potentiated the adverse effects of the NRTIs through some other mechanism or that the viral diseases themselves may have been partly responsible for mitochondrial dysfunction in these patients.

Synergism and/or Antagonism. Results of in vitro tests in various cell cultures and peripheral blood lymphocytes indicate that ribavirin may potentiate the antiretroviral effects of didanosine against HIV by promoting formation of didanosine-5′-triphosphate (ddA-TP), the metabolically active metabolite of didanosine. Conversely, there is some evidence from in vitro studies that ribavirin antagonizes the antiretroviral activity of some other NRTIs (e.g., stavudine, zidovudine). The mechanism by which ribavirin antagonizes the antiretroviral effects of these NRTIs has not been elucidated but it has been suggested that ribavirin may interfere with phosphorylation steps that convert the drugs to their active triphosphate metabolite, deoxythymidine triphosphate (dT-TP) or dideoxycytidine-5′-triphosphate (ddC-TP), respectively. Despite this in vitro antagonism, antiretroviral regimens that include zidovudine or stavudine have been used concomitantly with ribavirin (with or without interferon alfa or peginterferon alfa) in some HIV-infected patients coinfected with HCV without evidence of an increase in HIV viral load.

■ **Azathioprine** Severe pancytopenia (marked decreases in erythrocytes, neutrophils, and platelets) and bone marrow suppression have been reported in some patients receiving azathioprine concomitantly with peginterferon alfa and oral ribavirin. Such effects generally occurred within 3–7 weeks after initiation of concomitant therapy, reversed within 4–6 weeks after all 3 drugs were discontinued, and did not recur when either azathioprine or the regimen of peginterferon alfa and oral ribavirin was reinitiated alone. These adverse effects may occur because ribavirin inhibits inosine monophosphate dehydrogenase, which may result in accumulation of 6-methylthioinosine monophosphate, an azathioprine metabolite associated with myelotoxicity.

If azathioprine and a regimen of peginterferon alfa and oral ribavirin are used concomitantly, complete blood counts (CBCs), including platelet counts, should be monitored weekly for the first month, twice monthly during the second and third months of treatment, and then monthly or more frequently if necessary. If pancytopenia develops, all 3 drugs (azathioprine, ribavirin, peginterferon alfa) should be discontinued and peginterferon alfa and oral ribavirin therapy should not be restarted with concomitant azathioprine.

■ **HCV Antivirals** ***HCV Polymerase Inhibitors*** **Dasabuvir.** There is no in vitro evidence of antagonism between the fixed combination of ombitasvir, paritaprevir, and dasabuvir (ombitasvir/paritaprevir/dasabuvir) and ribavirin against HCV.

Sofosbuvir. There is no in vitro evidence of antagonism between sofosbuvir and ribavirin against HCV.

HCV Protease Inhibitors **Paritaprevir.** There is no in vitro evidence of antagonism between the fixed combination ombitasvir/paritaprevir/dasabuvir and ribavirin against HCV.

Simeprevir. Concomitant use of simeprevir with ribavirin and peginterferon alfa does not affect simeprevir concentrations or AUC compared with use of simeprevir alone.

In vitro, simeprevir and ribavirin have additive effects against HCV; there is no in vitro evidence of antagonism between simeprevir and ribavirin against HCV.

HCV Replication Complex Inhibitors **Daclatasvir.** Concomitant use of daclatasvir with ribavirin is not expected to result in any clinically important interactions.

Ombitasvir. There is no in vitro evidence of antagonism between the fixed combination ombitasvir/paritaprevir/dasabuvir and ribavirin against HCV.

■ **Interferons** Concomitant use of ribavirin, peginterferon alfa, and HIV NRTIs in cirrhotic patients with HCV and HIV coinfection has been associated with hepatic decompensation, including some fatalities. (See HIV Nucleoside Reverse Transcriptase Inhibitors under Drug Interactions: Antiretroviral Agents.)

Ribavirin may potentiate the hematologic effects (anemia, neutropenia, lymphopenia) induced by interferon alfas, including peginterferon alfa.

There is no evidence of a pharmacokinetic interaction between ribavirin and peginterferon alfa-2a.

Laboratory Test Interferences

The manufacturer states that the effect of ribavirin on laboratory tests has not been evaluated.

Acute Toxicity

■ **Pathogenesis** The oral LD_{50} of ribavirin has been reported to be 2 g (estimated human equivalent dose of 0.17 g/kg, based on body surface area) and 5.3 g/kg in mice and rats, respectively, and the intraperitoneal LD_{50} has been reported to be 0.9–1.3 and 2 g/kg, respectively.

Ribavirin accumulates in human erythrocytes and remains in the body for weeks or longer after administration of the drug.

■ **Manifestations** In animals, overdosage of ribavirin produces anorexia; lethargy; muscle weakness; prostration; GI effects, including hemorrhage, diarrhea, and vomiting; and death.

In humans, acute ingestion of up to 20 g of ribavirin as capsules (Rebetol®) has been reported and was associated with an increased incidence and severity of the usual adverse effects of the drug. The manufacturers state that overdosage of ribavirin inhalation solution or ribavirin tablets (Copegus®) has not been reported to date. However, hypocalcemia and hypomagnesemia have been observed when dosages up to and exceeding 4 times the recommended maximum dosage of oral ribavirin were administered IV†.

■ **Treatment** There is no specific antidote for ribavirin, and hemodialysis and peritoneal dialysis are not effective for treatment of ribavirin overdosage. While ribavirin is removed by hemodialysis with an extraction ratio of 50%, because of the large volume of distribution of the drug, plasma exposure is not expected to change with hemodialysis.

Mechanism of Action

■ **Antiviral Effect** The exact mechanism of action of the antiviral activity of ribavirin has not been fully elucidated, but the drug appears to exert its antiviral activity by interfering with RNA and DNA synthesis and subsequently inhibiting protein synthesis and viral replication. The antiviral activity of the drug results principally in an intracellular virustatic effect in cells infected with ribavirin-sensitive RNA or DNA viruses; however, specific mechanisms of action of the drug may vary depending on the virus. In virus-infected cells in vitro, ribavirin generally exhibits a greater affinity for inhibition of viral DNA and RNA synthesis than cellular (host cell) DNA and RNA synthesis. However, in vesicular stomatitis virus-infected cells in vitro, the drug appeared to exhibit a greater affinity for inhibition of cellular than viral RNA synthesis. Inhibition of cellular RNA synthesis usually occurs only at in vitro concentrations higher than those necessary for inhibition of cellular DNA synthesis. Ribavirin is reportedly cytotoxic in some viral-infected cells (e.g., cells infected with the polycythemia-inducing strain of Friend virus, herpes simplex type 1 virus, or enterovirus 72 [formerly hepatitis A virus]) and in uninfected cells, resulting in inhibition of cell division, DNA and RNA synthesis, and subsequent protein synthesis. The cytotoxic effect of the drug usually occurs only at concentrations 100–200 times those necessary to inhibit viral DNA synthesis or viral replication. The antiviral and cytotoxic activities of ribavirin appear to be reversible following removal of the drug.

The antiviral activity of ribavirin appears to depend principally on intracellular conversion of the drug to ribavirin-5′triphosphate and -monophosphate.Ribavirin-5′diphosphate exhibits minimal antiviral activity compared with the monophosphate or triphosphate. Ribavirin is readily absorbed across the cellular plasma membrane, probably via a nucleoside transport mechanism. The drug is then converted via cellular enzymes to deribosylated ribavirin (the 1,2,4-triazole-3-carboxamide) and phosphorylated to ribavirin-5′monophosphate, -diphosphate, and -triphosphate. Phosphorylation of ribavirin occurs principally in virus-infected cells, but also occurs in uninfected cells. Ribavirin is converted to ribavirin-5′monophosphate via adenosine kinase; the monophosphate is phosphorylated to the diphosphate and triphosphate via other cellular enzymes, including adenosine kinase. The enzyme deoxyadenosine kinase may also participate in the phosphorylation of ribavirin. Formation of ribavirin-5′monophosphate appears to be the rate-limiting step in the formation of ribavirin-5′triphosphate. The extent of phosphorylation of ribavirin by both uninfected and virus-infected cells in vitro is directly related to the extracellular (e.g., in the culture medium) concentration of the drug. Ribavirin-5′triphosphate is the principal intracellular form of the drug, with only approximately 4 and 12% of the phosphorylated metabolites present as ribavirin-5′diphosphate and -monophosphate, respectively. Transit of the drug out of cells appears to occur only after dephosphorylation via phosphatases.

Reversal of the antiviral activity of ribavirin by guanosine, adenosine, or xanthosine suggests that the pharmacologic activity of ribavirin, which is structurally similar to these cellular metabolites, involves guanosine nucleotides.

Guanosine nucleotides and phosphorylated ribavirin are substrates for many of the same enzyme systems, but guanosine and its nucleotides are not substrates for adenosine kinase.

In vitro studies with influenza virus indicate that ribavirin 5′triphosphate functions as a preferential inhibitor of viral RNA polymerase. Ribavirin-5′triphosphate competes with adenosine-5′triphosphate and guanosine-5′triphosphate for viral RNA polymerase. Inhibition of cellular (host cell) RNA polymerase reportedly is minimal and reversible. In vitro studies with influenza virus have shown that ribavirin-5′triphosphate also inhibits viral replication by inhibiting guanylyltransferase and methyltransferase, enzymes necessary for the addition of guanosine triphosphate to the 5′ terminus ("cap") of viral messenger RNA (mRNA), and by competing with guanosine for incorporation into the 5′ terminus of viral mRNA. Although the rate of synthesis of mRNA does not appear to be affected, the efficiency of translation of mRNA in viral replication is decreased by about 80%. Viruses in which the 5′ mRNA terminus is naturally absent (e.g., poliovirus) are generally not substantially inhibited by ribavirin.

Ribavirin-5′monophosphate appears to exhibit minimal antiviral activity relative to ribavirin-5′triphosphate; however, the monophosphate does function as a competitive inhibitor of IMP dehydrogenase (inosine monophosphate dehydrogenase), the enzyme necessary for synthesis of guanosine monophosphate. Compared with the monophosphate of the drug, the diphosphate only minimally inhibits this enzyme. Inhibition of IMP dehydrogenase results in depletion of intracellular nucleotide pools of guanosine triphosphate, but has only minimal effects on the rates of RNA and DNA synthesis. Further study is necessary to determine the importance of ribavirin-5′monophosphate and the inhibition of IMP dehydrogenase and subsequent depletion of intracellular nucleotide pools in the regulation of other cellular enzyme activity.

In vitro studies indicate that ribavirin inhibits phosphorylation of thymidine at drug concentrations of 2 μmol/L (0.5 mcg/mL) and that DNA synthesis is inhibited only at drug concentrations of 200 μmol/L (50 mcg/mL). Unlike acyclovir, ribavirin appears to be incorporated minimally, if at all, into growing chains of DNA and RNA. In vitro studies with vaccinia virus have shown that the virus DNA fails to coat in the presence of ribavirin, resulting in incomplete viral particles.

Ribavirin reportedly does not induce interferon production.

■ Effects on Host Immune Responses Ribavirin reportedly has only minimal inhibitory effects on host immune responses; however, evidence regarding specific effects of the drug on these responses is conflicting, and the effects appear to depend on cellular drug concentrations, with low and high ribavirin concentrations producing stimulation and inhibition of immune responses, respectively. The clinical importance of these effects is not known, however, and additional study is necessary. The manufacturer states that stimulation of cellular and/or humoral immune responses may not contribute to the virustatic activity of ribavirin in humans.

In animals, ribavirin has produced lymphoid atrophy of the thymus, spleen, and lymph nodes. The drug has also decreased cellular and humoral (e.g., antibody formation against some viruses) immune responses in animals at dosages approximately 10–20 times the usual human dosage. At lower dosages, stimulation of antibody formation against some viruses has been reported. The drug has been shown to stimulate T cells (T-lymphocytes) indirectly by inhibiting splenic suppressor cells and to produce a dose-dependent inhibition of antigen- and mitogen-induced proliferation of lymphocytes without affecting cell survival. In human infants, antibody formation against respiratory syncytial virus (RSV) has decreased during therapy with ribavirin, but the clinical importance of this finding is not known. The drug has been shown to have little, if any, effect on antibody formation against influenza A or B or measles virus in infected patients. Decreases in antibody formation during viral infections may result from decreases in antigenic stimulation secondary to ribavirin-induced inhibition of viral replication or from a direct inhibition of antibody formation by the drug. Ribavirin may indirectly inhibit RSV-specific immunoglobulin E and histamine, which are increased in infants who have wheezing in association with RSV infection, by decreasing RSV and attendant antigenic stimulation.

Ribavirin has also been reported to have some antitumor activity, which may in part depend on the drug's immunologic effects. The drug has inhibited tumor growth in animals infected with transplanted adenovirus tumors, possibly by simultaneously inhibiting humoral immune responses and stimulating cellular immune responses, thereby enhancing tumor cell rejection. The apparent antitumor activity of ribavirin may also result, in part, from interference with RNA synthesis in virus-infected cells or interference with cellular enzymes necessary for cell transformation rather than from direct antitumor activity.

Spectrum

Ribavirin has a spectrum of antiviral activity that is broader than that of other currently available antiviral agents. Ribavirin is active in vitro against many RNA viruses, including various Arenaviridae, Bunyaviridae, Orthomyxoviridae, Paramyxoviridae, Picornaviridae, Reoviridae, Retroviridae, and Togaviridae. The drug also is active in vitro against many DNA viruses, including various Adenoviridae, Herpesviridae, and Poxviridae. However, some viruses inhibited by ribavirin in vitro appear to be less susceptible to the drug in vivo.

■ In Vitro Susceptibility Testing Various methods (e.g., cytopathic effect inhibition, immunofluorescence, plaque inhibition, reverse transcriptase activity, solid phase radioimmunoassay, virus titer reduction, viral hemagglutinin inhibition) have been used to test in vitro susceptibility of viruses to ribavirin. Results and interpretations of these tests are method dependent and results may be substantially affected by the cell type used for the in vitro culture. In addition, the relationship between in vitro susceptibility of viruses to ribavirin and clinical response has not been determined. In viral susceptibility testing, 1 mcg of ribavirin per mL is approximately equivalent to 4 μmol/L.

■ RNA Viruses Ribavirin is active in vitro against many RNA viruses including respiratory syncytial virus (RSV); many strains of influenza A and B viruses; measles virus; subacute sclerosing panencephalitis virus; parainfluenza viruses; mumps virus; enterovirus 72 (formerly hepatitis A virus); human rhinoviruses; human reovirus 1, 2, and 3; human rotavirus; Colorado tick fever virus; human immunodeficiency virus (HIV); Crimean-Congo hemorrhagic fever virus; Junin virus (causes Argentine hemorrhagic fever); various hantaviruses (including those causing Korean hemorrhagic fever and hantavirus pulmonary syndrome); yellow fever virus; Lassa fever virus; and Machupo virus (causes Bolivian hemorrhagic fever). The drug also has antiviral activity in vivo against hantavirus, Lassa fever virus, and Rift Valley fever virus. Some viruses, including arboviruses, rhinoviruses, and rotaviruses, that are inhibited in vitro by ribavirin may not be inhibited in vivo.

In cell culture, ribavirin preferentially affects RSV-infected rather than uninfected cells. In studies using a plaque inhibition assay, plaques of susceptible strains of RSV were reduced by 50–98% by ribavirin concentrations of 3–30 mcg/mL, but plaque reduction appears to be method dependent, and the clinical importance of this in vitro effect is not known. The MIC of ribavirin reported for susceptible strains of influenza A has ranged from 0.01–3.2 mcg/mL using cytopathic effect (CPE) inhibition, virus titer reduction, or viral hemagglutinin inhibition. The IC_{50} (concentration of drug required to produce 50% inhibition of plaque formation) for H0N1, H1N1, H_{SW}1N1, H2N2, and H3N2 strains of influenza A has ranged from 2.8–8.5 mcg/mL.

The MIC of ribavirin for susceptible strains of influenza B has been reported to range from 0.01–3.2 mcg/mL using CPE inhibition, virus titer reduction, or viral hemagglutinin inhibition. The IC_{50} for susceptible strains of influenza B ranged from 2.6–6.3 mcg/mL using a plaque inhibition assay. The MIC for strains of subacute sclerosing panencephalitis virus has ranged from 10–50 mcg/mL using CPE inhibition, and the MIC reported for susceptible strains of measles virus has ranged from 0.003–10 mcg/mL using CPE or plaque inhibition or virus titer reduction.

The MIC of ribavirin reported for susceptible strains of parainfluenza virus (1, 2, or 3) has ranged from 3.2–32 mcg/mL using CPE or plaque inhibition, virus titer reduction, or viral hemagglutinin inhibition. The MIC for susceptible strains of mumps virus is 0.1–10 mcg/mL, and that for susceptible strains of human rhinoviruses has ranged from 10–32 mcg/mL, although some strains of human rhinoviruses have been reported to have MICs up to 100 mcg/mL. The MIC of ribavirin reported for susceptible strains of human reovirus has ranged from 0.32–10 mcg/mL, and has been reported to be 0.1–1 mcg/mL for susceptible strains of human rotavirus and 3.2 mcg/mL for susceptible strains of Colorado tick fever virus.

In studies using immunofluorescence or reverse transcriptase activity, human immunodeficiency virus (HIV) was inhibited by ribavirin concentrations of 10–100 mcg/mL; however, in a study using CPE inhibition, the cytopathic effect of HIV against ATH8 cells was not inhibited by concentrations up to 100 mcg/mL.

In a study using solid phase radioimmunoassay, enterovirus 72 (formerly hepatitis A virus) was partially inhibited by ribavirin concentrations of 25 mcg/mL and was substantially inhibited by concentrations of 62.5 or 125 mcg/mL; however, the latter concentrations were also cytotoxic to infected cells.

The ED_{50} (dose required to produce 50% inhibition of plaque formation) of ribavirin for Hantaan virus has been reported to be 15–16 mcg/mL.

Although the clinical importance is unclear, ribavirin has some activity against West Nile virus (WNV) in vitro. In one in vitro study in human neural cells, high doses of ribavirin inhibited replication and cytopathogenicity of WNV. In another study using a primate cell system infected with WNV, high doses of ribavirin were protective against the virus and a cytotoxic effect occurred with very high doses. Further study is needed to determine whether ribavirin has in vivo activity against WNV and to determine whether the drug might provide any benefits in the treatment of clinical infection caused by the virus. However, based on these preliminary in vitro studies, it has been suggested that very high IV dosages of ribavirin would be required to attain serum concentrations of the drug that might be potentially effective.

Results from several in vitro studies using isolates obtained from patients with severe acute respiratory syndrome (SARS) indicate that ribavirin concentrations that inhibit ribavirin-susceptible viruses do *not* inhibit replication or cell-to-cell transmission of the coronavirus that has been identified as the causative agent of SARS (SARS-CoV). There is some evidence that ribavirin is active in vitro against the coronavirus identified as the causative agent of Middle East respiratory syndrome (MERS-CoV).

Ribavirin generally is inactive against poliovirus, Ebola virus (causes Ebola hemorrhagic fever), Marburg virus (causes Marburg hemorrhagic fever), and coxsackieviruses. In one study, however, ribavirin was active against group B coxsackievirus 3 in vitro and in vivo in mice.

■ DNA Viruses Ribavirin has antiviral activity in vitro against many DNA viruses including herpes simplex types 1 (HSV-1) and 2 (HSV-2); human cytomegalovirus; and human adenovirus. However, cytomegalovirus may not be susceptible to the drug in vivo. In vitro, ribavirin has some activity against variola virus, vaccinia virus and other orthopoxviruses including camelpox, cowpox, and monkeypox. Although ribavirin was active against cowpox virus in a mouse model, the in vivo activity of the drug against poxvirus infections (including smallpox) in humans has not been evaluated to date.

Using CPE or plaque inhibition or virus titer reduction, the MIC of ribavirin reported for susceptible strains of HSV-1 or -2 has generally ranged from 0.32–3.2 mcg/mL; however, MICs up to 100 mcg/mL have been reported for some strains of these viruses. The MIC for susceptible strains of human cytomegalovirus has ranged from 10–32 mcg/mL using CPE inhibition or virus titer reduction, and that for susceptible strains of vaccinia virus has ranged from 0.1–3.2 mcg/mL using CPE or plaque inhibition or virus titer reduction. However, MICs up to 50 mcg/mL have been reported for some strains of vaccinia. The MIC for susceptible strains of human adenovirus has ranged from 10–32 mcg/mL, although the MIC has ranged up to 200 mcg/mL for some strains.

In cell culture using a plaque inhibition assay, plaques of simian varicella-zoster virus were reduced 50% by ribavirin concentrations of 50 mcg/mL; however, the drug appears to have little, if any, activity against human varicella-zoster virus. Ribavirin has been reported to produce a dose-related inhibition of hepatitis B surface antigen (HBsAg) production in vitro; however, the importance of this in vitro effect has not been determined and the drug has failed to alter production of hepatitis B antigens in several in vivo studies in animals and in humans.

■ Other Organisms Ribavirin is slightly active in vitro against some gram-negative aerobic bacteria and some fungi. *Brucella suis*, *Pseudomonas aeruginosa*, and *Phialophora verrucosa* are reportedly inhibited by ribavirin concentrations of 5.25–12.5 mcg/mL. Ribavirin concentrations of 500 mcg/mL or greater may be necessary to inhibit other bacteria and fungi.

Resistance

Development of in vitro or in vivo resistance to the antiviral activity of ribavirin has not been fully evaluated. Unlike some other currently available antiviral agents (e.g., acyclovir, amantadine), resistance to ribavirin does not appear to develop during repeated exposure of most susceptible viruses to the drug. The lack of development of resistance in susceptible viruses may result from ribavirin's multiple mechanisms of antiviral action. (See Mechanism of Action: Antiviral Effect.)

Pharmacokinetics

In the Pharmacokinetics section, 1 mcg of ribavirin per mL is approximately equivalent to 4 μmol/L.

■ Absorption ***Nasal and Oral Inhalation*** Ribavirin is absorbed systemically from the respiratory tract following nasal and oral inhalation. The bioavailability of ribavirin administered via nasal and oral inhalation has not been determined but may depend on the method of drug delivery during nebulization (i.e., oxygen hood, face mask, oxygen tent). At a constant flow rate, the amount of drug delivered to the respiratory tract theoretically is directly related to the concentration of nebulized drug solution and the duration of inhalation therapy. In addition, alterations in the method of aerosol delivery can affect the amount of drug reaching the respiratory tract. The fraction of an inhaled dose of ribavirin that is deposited in the respiratory tract during oral and nasal inhalation of a nebulized solution containing 190 mcg/L using a small-particle aerosol generator has been estimated to average about 70%, but the actual amount deposited depends on several factors including respiratory rate and tidal volume. The fraction of a nasally and orally inhaled dose of ribavirin that is swallowed and absorbed from the GI tract has not been determined.

Peak plasma ribavirin concentrations generally appear to occur at the end of the inhalation period when the drug is inhaled orally and nasally using a small-particle aerosol generator, and increase with increasing duration of the inhalation period. Following nasal and oral inhalation (via face mask) of 0.82 mg/kg per hour for 2.5 hours daily for 3 days in a limited number of pediatric patients, peak plasma ribavirin concentrations averaged 0.19 (range: 0.11–0.388) mcg/mL. Peak plasma ribavirin concentrations averaged 0.275 (range: 0.21–0.35) or 1.1 (range: 0.45–2.18) mcg/mL in a limited number of patients inhaling 0.82 mg/kg per hour for 5 or 8 hours daily, respectively, for 3 days, and averaged 1.7 (range: 0.38–3.58) mcg/mL in a limited number of pediatric patients inhaling 0.82 mg/kg per hour via face mask, mist tent, or respirator for 20 hours daily for 5 days. Highest plasma concentrations for a given dosage of ribavirin appear to be achieved in patients receiving the drug from the aerosol generator via an endotracheal tube. The manufacturer states that peak plasma ribavirin concentrations achieved with nasal and oral inhalation of usual dosages of the drug are less than concentrations that reportedly reduce respiratory syncytial virus (RSV) plaque formation by 85–98%. (See Spectrum: RNA Viruses.)

Concentrations of ribavirin achieved in respiratory tract secretions in patients inhaling the drug nasally and orally are likely to be substantially greater than those achieved in plasma. In a limited number of pediatric patients who received a nasally and orally inhaled ribavirin dose of 0.82 mg/kg per hour for 8 hours daily for 3 days, peak concentrations of the drug in respiratory tract secretions (from endotracheal tube) ranged from 250–1925 mcg/mL. In pediatric patients who received 0.82 mg/kg per hour via nasal and oral inhalation for 20 hours daily for 5 days, ribavirin concentrations in respiratory tract secretions (from endotracheal tube) ranged from 313–28,250 mcg/mL during therapy, with peak concentrations averaging 3075 (range: 313–7050) mcg/mL at the end of therapy. Concentrations of ribavirin achieved in respiratory tract secretions via nasal and oral inhalation are likely to be substantially greater than concentrations necessary to inhibit plaque formation of susceptible strains of RSV in vitro. However, RSV is found within virus-infected cells in the respiratory tract, and it is not known whether ribavirin concentrations in plasma or respiratory tract secretions better reflect the intracellular concentrations of the drug.

Oral Administration Ribavirin is rapidly absorbed following oral administration, with peak plasma concentrations of the drug occurring within 1–3 hours after multiple doses. However, the absolute bioavailability of ribavirin averages only 64% following oral administration because the drug undergoes first-pass metabolism.

Oral bioavailability of ribavirin appears to be increased when the drug is administered with a high-fat meal. Concomitant administration of oral ribavirin (as capsules or tablets) with a high-fat meal increases the peak ribavirin plasma concentration and area under the plasma concentration-time curve (AUC). Results of a single-dose study indicate that peak plasma concentration and AUC of ribavirin reportedly increase by 70% when ribavirin capsules are administered with a high-fat meal (31.6 g protein, 57.4 g carbohydrate, 53.8 g fat; 841 kcal). Peak plasma concentration and AUC of ribavirin reportedly increase by 66 and 42%, respectively, when ribavirin tablets are administered with a high-fat meal.

There is extensive accumulation of ribavirin following multiple (twice daily) doses of the drug, such that peak plasma ribavirin concentrations at steady state are fourfold higher than those following a single dose. Following oral administration of single or multiple 600-mg doses of ribavirin (as capsules), mean peak plasma concentrations in adults average 0.782 or 3.7 mcg/mL, respectively. In patients weighing more than 75 kg, ribavirin 1.2 g daily (as tablets) given with food for 12 weeks resulted in peak plasma ribavirin concentrations of 2.7 mcg/mL.

In children 5–16 years of age, mean peak plasma concentrations average 3.3 mcg/mL following ribavirin dosages of 15 mg/kg twice daily (as capsules).

Following oral administration of a single 400-mg dose of ribavirin (as capsules), the AUC was twofold or threefold greater in those with creatinine clearances of 30–60 or 10–30 mL/minute, respectively, compared with individuals with normal renal function.

In a small number of individuals with end-stage renal disease receiving hemodialysis, a ribavirin dosage (as tablets) of 200 mg daily provided plasma ribavirin exposures approximately 20% lower than those observed in individuals with normal renal function receiving recommended dosages.

Following oral administration of a single 600-mg dose of ribavirin (as capsules), the AUC of ribavirin was not altered in individuals with mild, moderate, or severe hepatic dysfunction compared to controls. However, mean peak plasma concentration was increased twofold in those with severe hepatic impairment (Child-Pugh class C) compared to controls.

■ Distribution Following nasal and oral inhalation, highest ribavirin concentrations are found in the respiratory tract and erythrocytes. Following parenteral administration of single doses in monkeys and baboons, ribavirin and/or its metabolites are distributed in highest concentrations into skeletal muscle; blood cells, principally erythrocytes; and liver.

Studies in animals and humans have shown that ribavirin and/or its metabolites accumulate in erythrocytes. The extent of accumulation of ribavirin and/or its metabolites in erythrocytes following inhalation of the drug has not been established, but, following oral administration of a single 3-mg/kg dose, erythrocyte concentrations of the drug have been reported to peak within approximately 4 days, exceeding concurrent plasma concentrations at 4 days by about 100-fold, and then declining with a half-life of about 40 days (the half-life of erythrocytes). During the initial 1–2 hours following oral administration of a single dose of the drug, erythrocyte concentrations increase at a rate similar to plasma concentrations; thereafter, erythrocyte concentrations continue to increase for about 4 days as plasma drug concentrations decline. Approximately 3% of a single ribavirin dose is present in erythrocytes 72 hours after oral administration.

Ribavirin appears to distribute slowly into CSF. Following chronic (4–7 weeks) oral administration of ribavirin in patients with acquired immunodeficiency syndrome (AIDS) or AIDS-related complex (ARC), CSF concentrations of the drug were approximately 70% of concurrent plasma concentrations. It is not known whether ribavirin crosses the placenta or distributes into milk in humans. The drug appears to be only minimally bound to plasma proteins.

■ Elimination Plasma concentrations of ribavirin appear to decline in a manner dependent on the route of drug administration. Following nasal and oral inhalation in a limited number of pediatric patients, the plasma half-life of ribavirin averaged about 9.5 (range: 6.5–11) hours. Following oral administration of a single dose of the drug in a limited number of healthy adults, plasma ribavirin concentrations declined in a multiphasic manner, with half-lives averaging 24 hours 10–80 hours after the dose and 48 hours or longer in the terminal phase. In adults with chronic hepatitis C infection, plasma half-life of ribavirin averages 43.6 hours after a single 600-mg oral dose and averages 298 hours at steady state (reached by approximately 4 weeks) in those receiving a dosage of 600 mg twice daily. The terminal half-life of ribavirin following a single oral 800-, 1000-, or 1200-mg dose of ribavirin capsules is about 120–170 hours.

Based on limited data, the half-life of ribavirin in respiratory tract secretions following nasal and oral inhalation for 3 days reportedly is approximately 1.4–2.5 hours. Elimination of the drug from the respiratory tract may result from distribution across respiratory membranes, clearance by macrophages in the respiratory tract, and/or upward ciliary activity.

Ribavirin is metabolized principally to deribosylated ribavirin (the 1,2,4-triazole-3-carboxamide), probably in the liver; the antiviral activity of 1,2,4-triazole-3-carboxamide against various RNA and DNA viruses is reportedly similar to ribavirin. The drug is also metabolized to 1,2,4-triazole-3-carboxylic acid. In vitro, ribavirin has been shown to be metabolized to ribavirin-5′monophosphate, -diphosphate, and -triphosphate, principally by intracellular phosphorylation of the drug via adenosine kinase and other cellular enzymes. It is likely that phosphorylation in vivo is necessary for the antiviral activity of the drug. (See Mechanism of Action: Antiviral Effect.) Ribavirin also undergoes phosphorylation in erythrocytes, principally to ribavirin-5′-triphosphate; approximately 81, 16, and 3% of drug metabolized in erythrocytes is present as ribavirin-5′triphosphate, -diphosphate, and -monophosphate, respectively. It has been suggested that prolonged distribution of the drug in erythrocytes may result from minimal phosphatase activity in these cells, with transit of the drug out of cells dependent on dephosphorylation via phosphatases.

Results of in vitro studies using both human and rat livers microsome preparations indicated little or no cytochrome P-450 (CYP) enzyme-mediated metabolism of ribavirin; ribavirin is not a substrate of CYP isoenzymes.

Ribavirin is excreted principally in urine. In healthy adults with normal renal function, approximately 53% of a single oral dose is excreted in urine within 72–80 hours, with about 33% excreted within the first 24 hours. Approximately 37, 30, and 30% of the fraction excreted in urine appears as unchanged drug, 1,2,4-triazole-3-carboxamide, and 1,2,4-triazole-3-carboxylic acid, respectively, within 1.5–2 hours, and approximately 17, 50, and 22%, respectively, within 24 hours. About 15% of a single oral dose is excreted in feces within 72 hours. Little, if any, ribavirin appears to be eliminated in expired CO_2.

The pharmacokinetics of ribavirin tablets (Copegus®) have been evaluated in patients with chronic HCV infection and varying degrees of renal impairment (moderate, severe, or requiring hemodialysis). Among those with creatinine clearances of 50 mL/minute or less, the apparent clearance of ribavirin was approximately 30% of values observed in patients with normal renal function. Based on these results, pharmacokinetic modeling has provided a basis for dosage adjustments of Copegus® in such patients. (See Renal Impairment under Dosage and Administration: Dosage in Renal and Hepatic Impairment.)

Chemistry and Stability

■ **Chemistry** Ribavirin is a synthetic nucleoside antiviral agent. Ribavirin is structurally similar to guanosine, xanthosine, and pyrazofurin (pyrazomycin). The drug differs structurally from guanosine in that the D-ribose of the nucleoside is attached to a 1,2,4-triazole-3-carboxamide moiety rather than a purine ring. The ribavirin structure is necessary to maintain the drug's antiviral activity; alterations in either the D-ribose moiety or the triazole or carboxamide moieties result in a substantial loss of antiviral activity. However, acetylation or phosphorylation of the ribosyl hydroxyl groups or conversion of the carboxamide group of the triazole carboxamide moiety to a carboxamidine moiety does not affect the drug's antiviral activity, since conversion of these compounds back to ribavirin occurs intracellularly.

Ribavirin occurs as a white, crystalline powder that is tasteless and odorless. At 25°C, the maximum aqueous solubility of ribavirin is 142 mg/mL and the drug is slightly soluble in alcohol.

Ribavirin is commercially available for nasal or oral inhalation as a powder for inhalation solution (Virazole®). For oral administration, ribavirin is commercially available as capsules (Rebetol®, Ribasphere®, generic), oral solution (Rebetol®), or tablets (Copegus®, generic).

Commercially available ribavirin powder for inhalation solution occurs as a white, sterile, lyophilized powder. When reconstituted and diluted in sterile water for injection or inhalation (additive free) as directed, ribavirin solutions containing 20 mg/mL are clear and colorless, have an osmolarity of 82 mOsm/L, and have a pH of 5–6.9. When these solutions are administered as directed using the Valeant small-particle aerosol generator (SPAG) Model SPAG-2, the SPAG-2 delivers a mist containing about 190 mcg of ribavirin per L as nebulized particles having a median mass diameter of 1.3 μm, with 95% of the particles having a mass diameter less than 5 μm.

■ **Stability** Commercially available ribavirin powder for inhalation solution should be stored in tight containers in a dry place at 25°C, but may be exposed to temperatures ranging from 15–30°C. Ribavirin inhalation solutions contain no preservatives and are stable for 24 hours when stored under sterile conditions at a room temperature of 20–30°C. Following addition of the reconstituted solution to the reservoir of the SPAG-2, any unused solution remaining in the reservoir should be discarded within 24 hours and prior to adding any newly reconstituted solution (e.g., when remaining amount of solution in reservoir is low).

Ribavirin capsules or tablets should be stored at 25°C, but may be exposed to temperatures ranging from 15–30°C.

Ribavirin oral solution should be stored at 2–8°C or at 25°C, but may be exposed to temperatures ranging from 15–30°C.

Preparations

Excipients in commercially available drug preparations may have clinically important effects in some individuals; consult specific product labeling for details.

Ribavirin

Nasal and Oral Inhalation		
For inhalation solution	6 g	**Virazole®**, Valeant
Oral		
Capsules	200 mg*	**Rebetol®**, Merck
		Ribasphere®, Kadmon
		Ribavirin Capsules
Solution	40 mg/mL	**Rebetol®**, Merck
Tablets, film-coated	200 mg*	**Copegus®**, Genentech
		Ribavirin Tablets
	400 mg*	**Ribavirin Tablets**
	500 mg*	**Ribavirin Tablets**
	600 mg*	**Ribavirin Tablets**

*available from one or more manufacturer, distributor, and/or repackager by generic (nonproprietary) name

†Use is not currently included in the labeling approved by the US Food and Drug Administration

Selected Revisions October 2015, © Copyright, November 1986, American Society of Health-System Pharmacists, Inc.

Tenofovir Alafenamide Fumarate

TAF, TAF Fumarate

■ Tenofovir alafenamide fumarate, an antiviral agent, is a nucleotide reverse transcriptase inhibitor that is active against hepatitis B virus (HBV) and human immunodeficiency virus (HIV).

Uses

Tenofovir alafenamide fumarate is used for the treatment of chronic hepatitis B virus (HBV) infection.

Tenofovir alafenamide fumarate also is used for the treatment of human immunodeficiency virus (HIV) infection. For information on use of the drug as an antiretroviral agent, see section 8:18.08.

■ **Chronic Hepatitis B Virus Infection** Tenofovir alafenamide fumarate is used for the treatment of HBV infection in adults with compensated liver disease. Safety and efficacy of tenofovir alafenamide fumarate have not been established in patients with decompensated cirrhosis (Child-Pugh class B or C), and the drug is not recommended for treatment of HBV infection in such patients.

The goal of antiviral therapy in patients with chronic HBV infection is to decrease the morbidity and mortality related to the infection (e.g., cirrhosis, hepatic failure, hepatocellular carcinoma). Sustained suppression of HBV replication has been associated with normalization of serum ALT concentrations, loss of hepatitis B e antigen (HBeAg) with or without detection of antibody to HBeAg (anti-HBe), and improvement in liver histology. Currently available therapies for chronic HBV infection (e.g., adefovir, entecavir, lamivudine, telbivudine, tenofovir alafenamide, tenofovir disoproxil fumarate [tenofovir DF], interferon alfa, peginterferon alfa) are used in an attempt to provide an immunologic cure (HBsAg loss and sustained HBV DNA suppression), but cannot provide a virologic cure (eradication of HBV).

Treatment of chronic HBV infection is complex and evolving, and specialized references and experts should be consulted. Information from the American Association for the Study of Liver Diseases (AASLD) regarding management of HBV infection, including recommendations for initial treatment, is available at https://www.aasld.org.

Clinical Experience Efficacy and safety of tenofovir alafenamide fumarate for the treatment of HBV infection were evaluated in 2 randomized, double-blind, active-controlled studies in treatment-naive (have not previously received nucleoside or nucleotide antivirals) and previously treated adults with compensated liver disease (study 108 and study 110). The primary efficacy end point in both studies was the proportion of patients with plasma HBV DNA levels less than 29 IU/mL at week 48.

In study 108, 425 adults with chronic HBV infection who were negative for serum HBeAg (mean age 46 years, 61% male; 72% Asian, 25% White, 2% Black; 24% HBV genotype B infection, 38% HBV genotype C infection, 31% HBV genotype D infection; 21% previously treated; mean baseline plasma HBV DNA level 5.8 $\log_{10}$ IU/mL; mean serum ALT concentration 94 units/L, 9% with history of cirrhosis) were randomized in a 2:1 ratio to receive tenofovir alafenamide fumarate (25 mg of tenofovir alafenamide once daily) or tenofovir DF (300 mg once daily) for 48 weeks. Concomitant use of other nucleoside or nucleotide antivirals or interferons was not permitted. At 48 weeks, 94 or 93% of patients receiving tenofovir alafenamide or tenofovir DF, respectively, had plasma HBV DNA levels less than 29 IU/mL. In patients with baseline serum ALT concentrations above the upper limit of normal (based on AASLD criteria), normalized ALT concentrations were achieved by 50% of those treated with tenofovir alafenamide and 32% of those treated with tenofovir DF.

In study 110, 873 adults with chronic HBV infection who were positive for serum HBeAg (mean age 38 years, 64% male; 82% Asian, 17% White, 1% Black or other races; 17% HBV genotype B infection, 52% HBV genotype C infection, 23% HBV genotype D infection; 26% previously treated; mean baseline plasma HBV DNA level 7.6 $\log_{10}$ IU/mL; mean serum ALT concentration 120 units/L, 7% with history of cirrhosis) were randomized in a 2:1 ratio to receive tenofovir alafenamide fumarate (25 mg of tenofovir alafenamide once daily) or tenofovir DF (300 mg once daily) for 48 weeks. Concomitant use of other nucleoside or nucleotide antivirals or interferons was not permitted. At 48 weeks, 64 or 67% of patients receiving tenofovir alafenamide or tenofovir DF, respectively, had plasma HBV DNA levels less than 29 IU/mL. In patients with baseline serum ALT concentrations above the upper limit of normal (based on AASLD criteria), normalized ALT concentrations were achieved by 45% of those treated with tenofovir alafenamide and 36% of those treated with tenofovir DF.

Dosage and Administration

General Prior to initiation of tenofovir alafenamide fumarate for the treatment of chronic hepatitis B virus (HBV) infection, patients should be tested for human immunodeficiency virus type 1 (HIV-1) infection. The drug should *not* be used alone in patients with HBV and HIV coinfection. (See Individuals with HBV and HIV Coinfection under Warnings/Precautions: Other Warnings/ Precautions, in Cautions.)

Serum creatinine, serum phosphorus, estimated creatinine clearance, urine glucose, and urine protein should be assessed prior to initiation of tenofovir alafenamide fumarate and monitored as clinically indicated during treatment with the drug. (See New Onset or Worsening Renal Impairment under Warnings/Precautions: Other Warnings/Precautions, in Cautions.)

Administration Tenofovir alafenamide fumarate is administered orally once daily with food.

Dosage Dosage of tenofovir alafenamide fumarate is expressed in terms of tenofovir alafenamide.

Adult Dosage **Treatment of Chronic HBV Infection.** For the treatment of chronic HBV infection in adults, the recommended dosage of tenofovir alafenamide is 25 mg once daily.

Special Populations ***Hepatic Impairment*** Dosage adjustments are not necessary if tenofovir alafenamide is used in patients with mild hepatic impairment (Child-Pugh class A).

Tenofovir alafenamide is *not* recommended in patients with decompensated hepatic impairment (Child-Pugh class B or C). (See Hepatic Impairment under Warnings/Precautions: Specific Populations, in Cautions.)

Renal Impairment Dosage adjustments are not necessary if tenofovir alafenamide is used in patients with mild, moderate, or severe renal impairment.

Tenofovir alafenamide is *not* recommended in patients with end-stage renal disease (creatinine clearance less than 15 mL/minute). (See Renal Impairment under Warnings/Precautions: Specific Populations, in Cautions.)

Geriatric Patients Limited data suggest that there are no clinically important differences in the pharmacokinetics of tenofovir alafenamide or tenofovir in geriatric patients compared with younger adults. (See Geriatric Use under Warnings/Precautions: Specific Populations, in Cautions.)

Cautions

Contraindications The manufacturer states that there are no contraindications to the use of tenofovir alafenamide fumarate.

Warnings/Precautions ***Warnings*** **Severe Acute Exacerbation of HBV Infection after Discontinuance of Treatment.** Severe acute exacerbations of hepatitis B virus (HBV) infection may occur following discontinuance of HBV treatment, including tenofovir alafenamide.

Hepatic function should be closely monitored with clinical and laboratory follow-up for at least several months after tenofovir alafenamide is discontinued. If appropriate, resumption of HBV treatment may be warranted.

Other Warnings/Precautions **Individuals with HBV and HIV Coinfection.** Safety and efficacy of tenofovir alafenamide have not been established in patients with HBV and human immunodeficiency virus type 1 (HIV-1) coinfection.

Tenofovir alafenamide is *not* used alone for the treatment of HIV-1 infection and should *not* be used alone for treatment of HBV infection in patients with HBV and HIV-1 coinfection because of the risk of development of HIV-1 resistance.

Prior to initiation of tenofovir alafenamide for the treatment of chronic HBV infection, all patients should be offered HIV antibody testing and, if positive, an appropriate antiretroviral regimen recommended for patients with HBV and HIV-1 coinfection should be used.

New Onset or Worsening Renal Impairment. Renal impairment, including cases of acute renal failure and Fanconi syndrome (renal tubular injury with severe hypophosphatemia), has been reported in HIV-infected patients receiving tenofovir prodrugs (e.g., tenofovir DF) and similar effects have been reported in animal toxicology studies.

No cases of Fanconi syndrome or proximal renal tubulopathy (PRT) were reported in clinical trials evaluating tenofovir alafenamide for treatment of chronic HBV infection.

In a pooled analysis of 2 clinical studies in adults with chronic HBV infection (studies 108 and 110), the median baseline estimated glomerular filtration rate (eGFR) was 106 or 105 mL/minute prior to treatment with tenofovir alafenamide or tenofovir DF, respectively. Mean serum creatinine concentrations increased by less than 0.1 mg/dL and median serum phosphorus concentrations decreased by 0.1 mg/dL in both treatment groups. The median change in eGFR from baseline was −1.2 mL/minute in patients treated with tenofovir alafenamide compared with −5.4 mL/minute in those treated with tenofovir DF. The long-term clinical importance of these renal laboratory changes on the incidence of adverse effects reported with these tenofovir prodrugs is not known.

Patients receiving a tenofovir prodrug who have impaired renal function or are receiving nephrotoxic agents (e.g., nonsteroidal anti-inflammatory agents [NSAIAs]) are at increased risk of developing adverse renal effects. (See Drug Interactions: Nephrotoxic Drugs or Drugs Eliminated by Renal Excretion.)

Serum creatinine, serum phosphorous, estimated creatinine clearance, urine glucose, and urine protein should be assessed in all patients prior to initiating tenofovir alafenamide and monitored as clinically appropriate during treatment with the drug.

Tenofovir alafenamide should be discontinued in patients who develop clinically important decreases in renal function or evidence of Fanconi syndrome.

Lactic Acidosis and Severe Hepatomegaly with Steatosis. Lactic acidosis and severe hepatomegaly with steatosis, including fatalities, have been reported in patients receiving nucleoside or nucleotide analogs (e.g., the tenofovir prodrug tenofovir disoproxil fumarate [tenofovir DF]) alone or in conjunction with other antiretroviral agents.

Tenofovir alafenamide should be suspended in any patient who develops clinical or laboratory findings suggestive of lactic acidosis or pronounced hepatotoxicity (signs of hepatotoxicity may include hepatomegaly and steatosis even in the absence of marked increases in serum aminotransferase concentrations).

Bone Effects. In animal studies and clinical trials, tenofovir prodrugs (tenofovir alafenamide, tenofovir DF) have been associated with decreases in bone mineral density (BMD) and increases in biochemical markers of bone metabolism, suggestive of increased bone turnover. The long-term clinical importance of these BMD changes is not known.

In a pooled analysis of 2 clinical studies in adults with chronic HBV infection (study 108 and study 110), the mean percentage change in BMD from baseline to week 48 was assessed by dual-energy X-ray absorptiometry (DXA). At the lumbar spine, the mean percentage change in BMD was −0.6% in patients treated with tenofovir alafenamide compared with −2.4% in those treated with tenofovir DF; 6% of those treated with tenofovir alafenamide and 20% of those treated with tenofovir DF had lumbar spine BMD declines that were 5% or more. At the total hip, the mean percentage change in BMD was −0.2% in patients treated with tenofovir alafenamide compared with −1.9% in those treated with tenofovir DF. At the femoral neck, 3% of patients treated with tenofovir alafenamide and 6% of those treated with tenofovir DF had BMD declines that were 7% or greater.

Specific Populations **Pregnancy.** Data are not available regarding use of tenofovir alafenamide in pregnant women.

In animal studies, there was no evidence of impaired fertility or harm to the fetus. Adverse developmental effects were not observed when tenofovir alafenamide was administered during organogenesis to rats or rabbits in dosages that resulted in exposures equal to or 51 times higher, respectively, than human exposures reported with the recommended daily dosage of tenofovir alafenamide.

If tenofovir alafenamide is used during pregnancy or the patient becomes pregnant while receiving the drug, the patient should be enrolled in the Antiretroviral Pregnancy Registry (APR) at 800-258-4263.

Lactation. It is not known whether tenofovir alafenamide and its metabolites are distributed into human milk, affect human milk production, or have effects on the breast-fed infant. Tenofovir is distributed into milk of lactating rats and rhesus monkeys receiving tenofovir DF.

The benefits of breast-feeding and the importance of tenofovir alafenamide to the woman should be considered along with the potential adverse effects on the breast-fed infant from the drug or from the underlying maternal condition.

Pediatric Use. Safety and efficacy of tenofovir alafenamide have not been established in pediatric patients younger than 18 years of age.

Geriatric Use. Clinical trials of tenofovir alafenamide did not include sufficient numbers of patients 65 years of age and older to determine if they respond differently than younger adults.

Hepatic Impairment. Safety and efficacy of tenofovir alafenamide have not been established in patients with decompensated cirrhosis (Child-Pugh class B or C), and the drug is not recommended in such patients.

Dosage adjustments are not necessary if tenofovir alafenamide is used in patients with mild hepatic impairment (Child-Pugh class A). In individuals with mild hepatic impairment, tenofovir alafenamide and tenofovir plasma exposures are 7.5 and 11% lower, respectively, compared with exposures reported in those with normal hepatic function.

Renal Impairment. Pharmacokinetics of tenofovir alafenamide have not been studied in patients with end-stage renal disease (estimated creatinine clearance less than 15 mL/minute), and the drug is not recommended in such patients.

Dosage adjustments are not necessary if tenofovir alafenamide is used in patients with mild, moderate, or severe renal impairment. In individuals with severe renal impairment, tenofovir alafenamide and tenofovir plasma exposures are 1.9- and 5.7-fold higher, respectively, compared with exposures reported in those with normal renal function.

■ **Common Adverse Effects** Adverse effects reported in 5% or more of patients with compensated liver disease receiving tenofovir alafenamide for the treatment of HBV infection include headache, abdominal pain, fatigue, cough, nausea, and back pain.

Drug Interactions

The following drug interactions are based on studies that used tenofovir alafenamide fumarate or are predicted to occur.

■ **Drugs Affecting or Metabolized by Hepatic Microsomal Enzymes** Tenofovir alafenamide is a weak inhibitor of cytochrome P-450 (CYP) isoenzyme 3A in vitro; tenofovir alafenamide does not induce or inhibit other CYP isoenzymes, including CYP1A2, 2B6, 2C8, 2C9, 2C19, or 2D6.

■ **Drugs Affecting or Affected by P-glycoprotein Transport System and Breast Cancer Resistance Protein** Tenofovir alafenamide is a substrate of the P-glycoprotein (P-gp) transport system and breast cancer resistance protein (BCRP). Drugs that strongly affect P-gp transport or BCRP activity may lead to changes in tenofovir alafenamide absorption.

Concomitant use of tenofovir alafenamide and P-gp inducers is expected to decrease absorption of tenofovir alafenamide and may result in decreased plasma concentrations and loss of therapeutic effect of tenofovir alafenamide.

Concomitant use of tenofovir alafenamide and inhibitors of P-gp or BCRP may increase absorption of tenofovir alafenamide resulting in increased plasma concentrations of the drug.

■ **Nephrotoxic Drugs or Drugs Eliminated by Renal Excretion** Tenofovir is principally excreted by a combination of glomerular filtration and active tubular secretion. Concomitant use of tenofovir alafenamide with drugs that reduce renal function or compete for active tubular secretion (e.g., acyclovir, cidofovir, ganciclovir, valacyclovir, valganciclovir, gentamicin, high-dose or multiple nonsteroidal anti-inflammatory agents [NSAIAs]) may increase concentrations of tenofovir and other drugs that are renally eliminated, which may increase the risk of adverse effects.

■ **Anticonvulsants** ***Carbamazepine*** Concomitant use of carbamazepine (300 mg twice daily) and the fixed combination of emtricitabine and tenofovir alafenamide (emtricitabine/tenofovir alafenamide) substantially decreases tenofovir alafenamide plasma concentrations and AUC.

If tenofovir alafenamide and carbamazepine are used concomitantly, dosage of tenofovir alafenamide should be increased to 50 mg once daily.

Oxcarbazepine, Phenobarbital, and Phenytoin Concomitant use of tenofovir alafenamide and oxcarbazepine, phenobarbital, or phenytoin is expected to decrease tenofovir alafenamide plasma concentrations.

Concomitant use of tenofovir alafenamide and oxcarbazepine, phenobarbital, or phenytoin is not recommended.

■ **Antifungal Agents** No clinically important pharmacokinetic interactions were reported when tenofovir alafenamide was used concomitantly with itraconazole or ketoconazole.

■ **Antimycobacterial Agents** Concomitant use of tenofovir alafenamide and rifabutin, rifampin, or rifapentine is expected to decrease plasma concentrations of tenofovir alafenamide.

Concomitant use of tenofovir alafenamide and rifabutin, rifampin, or rifapentine is not recommended.

■ **Cobicistat** Concomitant use of cobicistat (150 mg once daily) and tenofovir alafenamide (8 mg once daily) results in increased peak plasma concentrations and AUC of tenofovir alafenamide.

■ **Estrogens and Progestins** No clinically important pharmacokinetic interactions were reported when tenofovir alafenamide was used concomitantly with ethinyl estradiol or norgestimate.

■ **HBV Antivirals** There is no in vitro evidence of antagonistic anti-HBV effects between tenofovir and other HBV nucleoside or nucleotide reverse transcriptase inhibitor antivirals (e.g., entecavir, lamivudine, telbivudine).

■ **HCV Antivirals** ***HCV Polymerase Inhibitors*** **Sofosbuvir.** No clinically important pharmacokinetic interactions were reported when tenofovir alafenamide was used concomitantly with sofosbuvir.

HCV Replication Complex Inhibitors **Ledipasvir and Sofosbuvir.** No clinically important pharmacokinetic interactions were reported when tenofovir alafenamide was used concomitantly with the fixed combination of ledipasvir and sofosbuvir (ledipasvir/sofosbuvir).

■ **Midazolam** No clinically important pharmacokinetic interactions were reported when tenofovir alafenamide was used concomitantly with midazolam.

■ **Sertraline** No clinically important pharmacokinetic interactions were reported when tenofovir alafenamide was used concomitantly with sertraline.

■ **St. John's Wort** Concomitant use of St. John's wort (*Hypericum perforatum*) and tenofovir alafenamide is expected to decrease plasma concentrations of tenofovir alafenamide.

Concomitant use of tenofovir alafenamide and St. John's wort is not recommended.

Description

Tenofovir alafenamide fumarate is a nucleotide reverse transcriptase inhibitor antiviral agent.

Tenofovir alafenamide fumarate is a phosphonamidate prodrug of tenofovir (2'-deoxyadenosine monophosphate analog) and is inactive until converted intracellularly to the active metabolite (tenofovir diphosphate). Tenofovir alafenamide enters primary hepatocytes by passive diffusion and by the hepatic uptake transporters organic anion transport protein (OATP) 1B1 and 1B3. The prodrug is converted to tenofovir within hepatocytes by hydrolysis (principally by carboxylesterase 1 [CES1]) and is subsequently phosphorylated by cellular kinases to tenofovir diphosphate. Tenofovir diphosphate is active against hepatitis B virus (HBV) and human immunodeficiency virus type-1 (HIV-1) and has some in vitro activity against HIV-2.

Tenofovir diphosphate inhibits HBV replication through incorporation into viral DNA by HBV reverse transcriptase, which results in DNA chain termination. Tenofovir diphosphate is a weak inhibitor of mammalian DNA polymerases, including mitochondrial DNA polymerase γ, and there is no evidence of toxicity to mitochondria in cell culture.

The antiviral activity of tenofovir alafenamide was assessed in a transient transfection assay (HepG2 cells) against a panel of HBV clinical isolates representing genotypes A–H. The EC_{50} (50% effective concentration) for tenofovir alafenamide ranged from 34.7–134.4 nM, with an overall mean EC_{50} of 86.6 nM. The CC_{50} (50% cytotoxicity concentration) for the drug in HepG2 cells was greater than 44,400 nM.

In a pooled analysis of clinical studies evaluating tenofovir alafenamide fumarate for treatment of HBV infection in treatment-naive and previously treated patients, genotypic resistance analysis was performed on paired baseline and on-treatment HBV isolates from those who either experienced virologic breakthrough (2 consecutive visits with plasma HBV DNA levels greater than or equal to 69 IU/mL [400 copies/mL] after having been less than 69 IU/mL, or a 1-$\log_{10}$ or greater increase in HBV DNA from nadir) through week 48 or had plasma HBV DNA levels greater than or equal to 69 IU/mL at early discontinuation at or after week 24. Treatment-emergent amino acid substitutions in the HBV reverse transcriptase domain, all occurring at polymorphic positions, were observed in 25% (5/20) of HBV isolates evaluated; however, no specific substitutions occurred at a sufficient frequency to be associated with resistance to tenofovir alafenamide fumarate.

HBV isolates resistant to some other nucleoside or nucleotide antivirals used for the treatment of HBV infection (e.g., adefovir, entecavir, lamivudine) may also have reduced susceptibility to tenofovir. HBV isolates with lamivudine resistance-associated substitutions rtM204V/I and entecavir resistance-associated substitutions rtT184G, rtS202G, or rtM250V in the presence of rtL180M and rtM204V result in less than twofold reduced susceptibility to tenofovir alafenamide. HBV isolates with rtA181T, rtA181V, or rtN236T single adefovir resistance-associated substitutions also have less than twofold reduced susceptibility to tenofovir alafenamide. Isolates with double adefovir resistance-associated substitutions of rtA181V *and* rtN236T have 3.7-fold reduced susceptibility to tenofovir alafenamide. The clinical importance of these substitutions is not known.

Following oral administration of tenofovir alafenamide fumarate, peak plasma concentrations of tenofovir alafenamide occur at approximately 0.5 hours after the dose. Tenofovir alafenamide is hydrolyzed to tenofovir intracellularly within hepatocytes by CES1 to tenofovir; tenofovir alafenamide also is hydrolyzed to tenofovir intracellularly within peripheral blood mononuclear cells (PBMCs) and macrophages by cathepsin A. Tenofovir undergoes phosphorylation, resulting in the pharmacologically active metabolite (tenofovir diphosphate). Tenofovir alafenamide is metabolized by cytochrome P-450 (CYP) isoenzyme 3A to a minor extent. After administration of tenofovir alafenamide fumarate with a high-fat meal, the area under the plasma concentration-time curve increases by 1.65-fold relative to administration in the fasting state. Tenofovir alafenamide is approximately 80% bound to plasma proteins. Following a single oral dose of tenofovir alafenamide fumarate (25 mg of tenofovir alafenamide), 32% of the dose is excreted in feces and less than 1% is eliminated in urine. The median terminal plasma half-life of tenofovir alafenamide is 0.5 hours.

Advice to Patients

Importance of reading patient information provided by the manufacturer.

Importance of taking tenofovir alafenamide fumarate with food and importance of taking the drug on a regular dosing schedule and avoiding missed doses since this may result in development of resistance.

Importance of informing patients that severe acute exacerbations of hepatitis B virus (HBV) infection have been reported following discontinuance of HBV treatment, including tenofovir alafenamide. Advise patients not to discontinue tenofovir alafenamide without first informing a clinician.

Importance of informing patients that if they have or develop human immunodeficiency virus (HIV) infection and are not receiving effective HIV treatment, use of tenofovir alafenamide alone may increase the risk of development of resistance to HIV treatment.

Advise patients that renal impairment, including cases of acute renal failure or Fanconi syndrome, has been reported in patients receiving tenofovir products.

Advise patients that lactic acidosis and severe hepatomegaly with steatosis, including fatalities, have occurred in patients receiving drugs similar to tenofovir alafenamide. Importance of immediately contacting a clinician and discontinuing tenofovir alafenamide if clinical symptoms suggestive of lactic acidosis or pronounced hepatotoxicity occur.

Importance of informing clinicians of existing or contemplated concomitant therapy, including prescription and OTC drugs and dietary or herbal products, as well as any concomitant illnesses.

Importance of women informing clinicians if they are or plan to become pregnant or plan to breast-feed. Inform patients that there is a pregnancy registry to monitor fetal outcomes of pregnant women exposed to tenofovir alafenamide. (See Pregnancy under Warnings/Precautions: Specific Populations, in Cautions.)

Importance of informing patients of other important precautionary information. (See Cautions.)

Overview® (see Users Guide). For additional information on this drug until a more detailed monograph is developed and published, the manufacturer's labeling should be consulted. It is *essential* that the manufacturer's labeling be consulted for more detailed information on usual cautions, precautions, contraindications, potential drug interactions, laboratory test interferences, and acute toxicity.

Preparations

Excipients in commercially available drug preparations may have clinically important effects in some individuals; consult specific product labeling for details.

Tenofovir Alafenamide Fumarate

Oral		
Tablets, film-coated	25 mg (of tenofovir alafenamide)	**Vemlidy®**, Gilead

valACYclovir Hydrochloride

■ Valacyclovir, the L-valine ester of acyclovir, is an antiviral agent that is a prodrug of acyclovir and is active against herpes viruses.

Uses

Oral valacyclovir is used for the treatment of initial and recurrent episodes of genital herpes infections in immunocompetent adults and adolescents and for the suppression of recurrent episodes of genital herpes in immunocompetent adults and adolescents and individuals infected with human immunodeficiency virus (HIV). Valacyclovir also is used for the episodic treatment of herpes labialis (perioral herpes, cold sores, fever blisters) in adults and adolescents and for the treatment of acute, localized herpes zoster (shingles, zoster) in adults and adolescents.

The manufacturer states that safety and efficacy of valacyclovir in immunocompromised patients have not been established for any use other than suppression of genital herpes and safety and efficacy of the drug have not been established for any use in prepubertal pediatric patients.

■ **Genital Herpes** ***Treatment of First Episodes*** Oral valacyclovir is used in the treatment of initial episodes of genital herpes simplex virus (HSV-2) infection in immunocompetent adults and adolescents. Because many patients with first episodes of genital herpes present with mild clinical symptoms but later develop severe or prolonged symptoms, the US Centers for Disease Control and Prevention (CDC) states that most patients with initial genital herpes should receive antiviral therapy. The CDC and some clinicians recommend that first episodes of genital herpes be treated with a regimen of oral acyclovir (400 mg 3 times daily or 200 mg 5 times daily for 7–10 days), oral famciclovir (250 mg 3 times daily for 7–10 days), or oral valacyclovir (1 g twice daily for 7–10 days).

Oral valacyclovir appears to be as effective as oral acyclovir in the treatment of first episodes of genital herpes. Efficacy of oral valacyclovir (1 g twice daily for 10 days) was compared with that of oral acyclovir (200 mg 5 times daily for 10 days) in a randomized, double-blind trial in immunocompetent adults who presented for treatment within 72 hours of the onset of symptoms. Results of this study indicate that, for both drugs, the median time to lesion healing was 9 days, the median time to cessation of pain was 5 days, and the median time to cessation of viral shedding was 3 days.

Episodic Treatment of Recurrent Episodes Oral valacyclovir is used in the treatment of recurrent episodes of genital herpes in immunocompetent adults and adolescents. Antiviral therapy for recurrent genital herpes can be given episodically to ameliorate or shorten the duration of lesions or can be given continuously as suppressive therapy to reduce the frequency of recurrences. For episodic treatment of recurrent genital herpes, the CDC and some clinicians recommend oral acyclovir (400 mg 3 times daily for 5 days, 800 mg twice daily for 5 days, or 800 mg 3 times daily for 2 days), oral famciclovir (125 mg twice daily for 5 days or 1 g twice daily for 1 day), or oral valacyclovir (500 mg twice daily for 3 days or 1 g once daily for 5 days). Episodic antiviral therapy should be initiated within 1 day of lesion onset or during the prodrome that precedes some outbreaks. The manufacturer states that patients should be advised to initiate oral valacyclovir at the first sign or symptoms of an episode and that there are no data on the effectiveness of the drug initiated more than 24 hours after the onset of signs and symptoms of a recurrent episode.

Efficacy of oral valacyclovir in the treatment of recurrent episodes of genital herpes has been evaluated in 3 double-blind (2 of them placebo-controlled) studies in which immunocompetent adults self-initiated therapy within 24 hours of the first sign or symptom of a recurrent genital herpes episode. In one study, the median time to lesion healing and cessation of pain was 4 and 3 days, respectively, in those randomized to receive oral valacyclovir (500 mg twice daily for 5 days) compared with 6 and 4 days, respectively, in those randomized to receive placebo. The median time to cessation of viral shedding was 2 days in those who received valacyclovir versus 4 days in those who received placebo. Results of this study were duplicated in a second study.

There is evidence that a 3-day regimen of oral valacyclovir is as effective as a 5-day regimen of the drug for the episodic treatment of recurrent genital herpes. In a double-blind study, patients were randomized to receive valacyclovir 500 mg twice daily for 3 or 5 days (patients receiving the 3-day regimen received placebo on days 4 and 5). The median time to lesion healing was about 4.5 days and the median time to cessation of pain was about 3 days in both treatment groups.

Suppressive Therapy of Recurrent Episodes Valacyclovir is used for chronic suppressive therapy of recurrent genital herpes in immunocompetent and HIV-infected adults and adolescents. The CDC states that suppressive antiviral therapy can reduce the frequency of genital herpes recurrences by 70–80% in patients who have frequent recurrences (i.e., 6 or more per year) and many patients report no symptomatic outbreaks during such therapy. For chronic suppressive therapy of recurrent genital herpes, the CDC and some clinicians recommend a regimen of oral acyclovir (400 mg twice daily), oral famciclovir (250 mg twice daily), or oral valacyclovir (500 mg or 1 g once daily). The CDC states that data suggest that famciclovir and valacyclovir are as effective as acyclovir in terms of clinical outcome, although the 500 mg once-daily valacyclovir regimen might be less effective than the acyclovir regimen or other valacyclovir regimens in patients who have very frequent recurrences (i.e., 10 or more episodes per year).

Efficacy of oral valacyclovir for chronic suppressive therapy of recurrent genital herpes infections has been evaluated in a double-blind, placebo-controlled study in immunocompetent adults with a history of frequent recurrences (6 or more per year). Patients were randomized to receive oral valacyclovir (1 g once daily), oral acyclovir (400 mg twice daily), or placebo. At 6 months, 55% of those receiving valacyclovir and 54% of those receiving acyclovir were free of recurrences compared with only 7% of those receiving placebo; at 12 months, 34% of patients in both groups receiving antiviral therapy were still free of recurrences. When valacyclovir is used for suppressive therapy in immunocompetent individuals, the risk of heterosexual transmission to susceptible partners is reduced. (See Reduction of Transmission under Uses: Genital Herpes.)

Efficacy of oral valacyclovir for suppressive therapy of recurrent genital herpes has been evaluated in HIV-infected adults 18 years of age or older (median HIV-1 RNA level 2.6 $\log_{10}$ copies/mL and median CD4$^+$ T-cell count 336/mm^3 at study entry) with a history of frequent recurrences (4 or more per year). At 6 months, 65% of those receiving valacyclovir were free of recurrences compared with 26% of those receiving placebo. Safety and efficacy of valacyclovir for suppression of recurrent genital herpes in patients with advanced HIV disease (CD4$^+$ T-cell counts less than 100/mm^3) have not been established.

Safety and efficacy of oral valacyclovir for suppressive therapy of recurrent genital herpes infections have been established in immunocompetent patients receiving daily therapy for up to 1 year; safety and efficacy for this indication have been established in HIV-infected patients receiving daily therapy for up to 6 months.

Reduction of Transmission When valacyclovir is used for suppressive therapy of genital herpes in immunocompetent individuals, the risk of heterosexual transmission to susceptible partners is reduced. Transmission of genital herpes was assessed in a double-blind, placebo-controlled study in monogamous, heterosexual, immunocompetent couples discordant for HSV-2 infection; the infected partner received valacyclovir (500 mg once daily) or placebo for 8 months. Clinically symptomatic HSV-2 infection developed in 0.5% of susceptible individuals whose partner received valacyclovir and in 2.2% of those whose partner received placebo. Acquisition of HSV-2 was observed in 1.9% of susceptible individuals whose partner received valacyclovir and in 3.6% of those whose partner received placebo. Efficacy for reducing transmission of HSV-2 has not been established in individuals with multiple partners or in non-heterosexual couples.

HIV-infected Individuals Immunocompromised individuals may have prolonged or severe episodes of genital, perianal, or oral herpes; HSV-2 lesions are common in those with human immunodeficiency virus (HIV) infection and may be severe, painful, and atypical. (See Uses: Mucocutaneous Herpes Simplex Virus Infections.)

The CDC states that episodic treatment or suppressive therapy with oral antiviral agents often is beneficial in HIV-infected individuals with genital herpes. While the drugs of choice for episodic treatment or suppressive therapy of genital herpes in HIV-infected individuals are the same as those in immunocompetent individuals, higher dosages and/or more prolonged therapy may be necessary. Although safety and efficacy of valacyclovir for treatment of genital herpes have not been established in immunocompromised patients, CDC recommends valacyclovir for the treatment of genital herpes in HIV-infected individuals†. For episodic treatment of recurrences of genital herpes in HIV-infected individuals, the CDC recommends a 5- to 10-day regimen of oral acyclovir (400 mg 3 times daily), oral famciclovir (500 mg twice daily), or oral valacyclovir (1 g twice daily). Valacyclovir is used for suppression of recurrent genital herpes in HIV-infected individuals. For chronic suppressive therapy of recurrent genital herpes, CDC recommends oral acyclovir (400–800 mg 2–3 times daily), oral famciclovir (500 mg twice daily), or oral valacyclovir (500 mg twice daily).

Patient Counseling and Management of Sexual Partners Counseling of infected individuals and their sex partners is critical to management of genital herpes. The goals of such counseling are to help patients understand and cope with the infection and to prevent sexual and perinatal transmission of the virus. Antiviral therapy offers clinical benefit to most symptomatic patients and is the mainstay of management; however, genital herpes is a recurrent, life-long viral infection. Use of valacyclovir for suppressive therapy in immunocompetent individuals is associated with reduced risk of heterosexual transmission to susceptible partners. However, antiviral therapy does not eradicate latent HSV-2 or affect the risk, frequency, or severity of recurrences of genital herpes following discontinuance of therapy.

The majority of genital herpes infections are transmitted by individuals unaware that they have the infection or by individuals who are asymptomatic when transmission occurs. Patients should be advised that valacyclovir is not a cure for genital herpes. While use of valacyclovir for suppressive therapy is associated with a reduced risk of heterosexual transmission, safer sex practices should be used even in patients receiving suppressive therapy. Because genital herpes is a sexually transmitted disease, patients should be advised to avoid sexual contact with uninfected partners when lesions and/or prodromal symptoms are present. In addition, patients should be advised that sexual transmission of the virus can occur during asymptomatic periods and that suppressive antiviral therapy reduces, but does not eliminate, subclinical viral shedding.

Sex partners of individuals with genital herpes should be advised that they may be infected even if they have no symptoms. Asymptomatic partners of patients with genital herpes should be questioned regarding a history of genital lesions, educated to recognize symptoms of genital herpes, and offered type-specific serologic testing to determine whether risk for HSV-2 acquisition exists. Antiviral therapy is not recommended for sex partners who do not have clinical manifestations of infection, but symptomatic sex partners of individuals with genital herpes should be evaluated and treated.

The risk for neonatal HSV-2 infection should be discussed with all genital herpes patients, including men. Pregnant women and women of childbearing age who have genital herpes should inform their providers who care for them during pregnancy as well as those who will care for their neonate.

Information to assist patients and clinicians in counseling regarding genital herpes is available at http://www.ashastd.org and http://www.ihmf.org. For further information on treatment of initial or recurrent episodes of genital herpes or suppression of recurrent infections, see Uses: Genital Herpes in Acyclovir 8:18.32.

■ **Herpes Labialis** Valacyclovir is used for the episodic treatment of herpes labialis (perioral herpes, cold sores, fever blisters) in adults and adolescents.

Efficacy of a short-duration regimen of valacyclovir was evaluated in healthy adults and adolescents 12 years of age or older with a history of recurrent cold sores (at least 3 episodes in the past year). Patients were randomized to 1-day treatment (valacyclovir 2 g twice daily), 2-day treatment (valacyclovir 2 g twice daily on day 1 then valacyclovir 1 g twice daily on day 2), or placebo; patients self-initiated therapy at the earliest prodromal symptom and before clinical signs of a cold sore (most initiated treatment within 2 hours of symptom onset). The mean duration of the cold sore episode was reduced by about 1 day in patients receiving valacyclovir compared with those given placebo; the 2-day regimen was not more effective than the 1-day regimen. The proportion of valacyclovir-treated patients with prevented and/or blocked cold sore lesions (44–46%) was essentially the same as the proportion of patients given placebo (38%).

The manufacturer states that safety and efficacy of valacyclovir for the treatment of cold sores in immunocompromised patients have not been established.

■ **Mucocutaneous Herpes Simplex Virus Infections** Oral valacyclovir has been used for the treatment of recurrent mucocutaneous HSV-1 infections in HIV-infected adults† and for chronic suppressive or maintenance therapy (secondary prophylaxis) against HSV-1 disease in HIV-infected individuals†.

In patients with advanced HIV infection, reactivation of HSV-1 frequently occurs and can result in chronic, persistent mucocutaneous disease that may be severe. The Prevention of Opportunistic Infections Working Group of the US Public Health Service and the Infectious Diseases Society of America (USPHS/IDSA) has established guidelines for the prevention of opportunistic infections in HIV-infected individuals that include recommendations concerning prevention of exposure to opportunistic pathogens, prevention of first disease episodes, and prevention of disease recurrence. The USPHS/IDSA does not currently recommend primary prophylaxis against initial episodes of HSV-1 infection in HIV-infected adults, adolescents, or children. In addition, the USPHS/IDSA does not recommend routine chronic suppressive or maintenance therapy (secondary prophylaxis) against HSV-1 disease in HIV-infected individuals since acute episodes generally can be treated successfully with acyclovir. However, long-term prophylaxis against recurrence of HSV-1 can be considered for adults, adolescents, and children who have frequent or severe recurrences. If secondary prophylaxis of HSV-1 disease is indicated in HIV-infected adults or adolescents, the USPHS/IDSA recommends oral acyclovir or oral famciclovir as the drugs of choice and oral valacyclovir as an alternative. If indicated in infants and children, the USPHS/IDSA recommends oral acyclovir. If acyclovir-resistant HSV-1 is suspected, IV foscarnet or IV cidofovir can be used to treat the infection.

■ **Herpes Zoster** Oral valacyclovir is used for the treatment of acute, localized herpes zoster (shingles, zoster) in immunocompetent adults. Some clinicians suggest that the drugs of choice for the treatment of herpes zoster in immunocompetent adults are oral acyclovir, oral famciclovir, or oral valacyclovir.

Efficacy of oral valacyclovir in the treatment of acute, localized herpes zoster has been evaluated in a randomized, double-blind, placebo-controlled trial in immunocompetent adults younger than 50 years of age and in a double-blind trial in immunocompetent adults 50 years of age or older who were randomized to receive oral valacyclovir (1 g every 8 hours for 7 or 14 days) or oral acyclovir (800 mg 5 times daily for 7 days). Results of these studies indicate that valacyclovir may prevent the appearance of new lesions, decrease viral shedding, decrease the duration of pain, and promote healing and crusting of lesions in immunocompetent adults with localized herpes zoster, at least when given within 72 hours of onset of rash. In one study, there was no evidence of additional benefit on pain duration when valacyclovir was initiated within 48 hours versus between 48–72 hours of rash onset; however, the effect of time on other clinical endpoints (e.g., appearance of new lesions, viral shedding) was not determined, and antiviral therapy for herpes zoster generally is most effective when initiated within 48 hours of rash onset. Like acyclovir, valacyclovir does not appear to *prevent* the development of postherpetic neuralgia; the drug may *decrease the median duration* of neuralgia, particularly in patients older than 50 years of age. In comparative studies, 7 or 14 days of oral valacyclovir (1 g 3 times daily) was as effective as 7 days of oral acyclovir (800 mg 5 times daily) in reducing the duration of virus shedding and accelerating the resolution of herpes zoster-associated pain and cutaneous healing in patients 50 years of age or older, and the drugs exhibited comparable safety profiles. Although there was a trend toward a shorter median duration of postherpetic pain with the valacyclovir regimens compared with the acyclovir regimen in patients 50 years of age or older, the difference was not statistically significant. The principal potential benefits relative to acyclovir are valacyclovir's improved oral bioavailability and resultant more convenient dosing regimen. In these studies, there were no gender-related differences in safety or efficacy.

Valacyclovir has been used for the treatment of localized dermatomal herpes zoster in HIV-infected adults or adolescents†. If cutaneous lesions are extensive or there is clinical evidence of visceral involvement, IV acyclovir should be used for initial treatment.

The manufacturer states that the efficacy of valacyclovir in the treatment of disseminated herpes zoster or for the treatment of herpes zoster in immunocompromised patients has not been established.

■ **Prevention of Cytomegalovirus Disease** ***HIV-infected Individuals*** Although some evidence indicates that use of valacyclovir for prophylaxis of cytomegalovirus (CMV) disease in HIV-infected individuals† reduces the incidence of CMV disease in these patients, the USPHS/IDSA states that valacyclovir should not be used for primary prophylaxis against CMV in HIV-infected individuals because an unexplained trend toward increased mortality has been observed in HIV-infected patients receiving the drug for such prophylaxis.

Transplant Recipients Valacyclovir has been evaluated for the prevention of CMV disease in renal transplant recipients† considered at risk for the disease. Results of a randomized placebo-controlled study in renal transplant recipients at risk of developing CMV infection (i.e., CMV-seropositive or -seronegative recipients of a kidney from a CMV-seropositive donor) indicate that in patients who received valacyclovir (2 g four times daily, dosage reduced for those with a creatinine clearance less than 75 mL/minute) the probability of CMV disease was reduced compared with those receiving placebo.

Although valacyclovir is being investigated for prophylaxis of CMV disease in hematopoietic stem cell transplant (HSCT) recipients†, the CDC, IDSA, and American Society of Blood and Marrow Transplantation (ASBMT) state the valacyclovir currently is not recommended for this use since it is presumed to be less effective against CMV than ganciclovir.

Dosage and Administration

■ **Administration** Valacyclovir hydrochloride is administered orally without regard to meals. Food does not affect systemic bioavailability of the drug.

Patients should maintain adequate hydration during valacyclovir treatment.

■ **Dosage** Dosage of valacyclovir hydrochloride is expressed in terms of valacyclovir.

Valacyclovir dosage modification according to renal function may be necessary in geriatric patients, depending on the underlying renal status of the patient. (See Dosage and Administration: Dosage in Renal and Hepatic Impairment.)

Genital Herpes **Treatment of First Episodes.** For the treatment of initial episodes of genital herpes simplex virus (HSV-2) infection in immunocompetent adults and adolescents, the dosage of oral valacyclovir recommended by the manufacturer, the US Centers for Disease Control and Prevention (CDC), and other clinicians is 1 g twice daily for 7–10 days. The manufacturer recommends a duration of 10 days; the CDC states that the usual duration of treatment is 7–10 days but that this may be extended if healing is incomplete after 10 days.

In HIV-infected adults and adolescents†, the CDC and other experts recommend 1 g twice daily for 7–14 days for the treatment of initial episodes of genital herpes.

Valacyclovir has been most effective when administered within 48 hours of the onset of signs and symptoms of genital herpes; efficacy of the drug initiated more than 72 hours after the onset of signs and symptoms has not been established.

Episodic Treatment of Recurrent Episodes. For the episodic treatment of recurrent genital herpes in immunocompetent adults and adolescents, the manufacturer and some clinicians recommend that oral valacyclovir be given in a dosage of 500 mg twice daily for 3 days. The CDC states that oral valacyclovir can be given in a dosage of 500 mg twice daily for 3 days or 1 g once daily for 5 days for the episodic treatment of recurrent genital herpes in immunocompetent adults and adolescents.

In HIV-infected adults and adolescents†, the CDC recommends a dosage of 1 g twice daily for 5–10 days for the episodic treatment of recurrent genital herpes. Alternatively, treatment may be continued for 7–14 days in these patients.

Patients should be advised to initiate valacyclovir therapy at the first sign or symptom of an episode. Data are not available concerning efficacy of oral valacyclovir initiated more than 24 hours after the onset of signs or symptoms of a recurrent episode of genital herpes.

Suppressive Therapy of Recurrent Episodes. For chronic suppression of recurrent episodes of genital herpes in immunocompetent adults and adolescents, the usual dosage of oral valacyclovir is 1 g once daily; however, a dosage of 500 mg once daily may be used in patients with infrequent recurrences. The manufacturer states that those with a history of 9 or fewer recurrences per year may receive 500 mg once daily for chronic suppressive therapy; the CDC cautions that the 500 mg once daily regimen might be less effective in those who have very frequent recurrences (i.e., 10 or more per year).

In HIV-infected adults and adolescents, the usual dose of oral valacyclovir for chronic suppression of recurrent episodes of genital herpes is 500 mg twice daily.

Data are not available to date concerning efficacy and safety of oral valacyclovir administered for more than 1 year in immunocompetent patients or for more than 6 months in HIV-infected patients for chronic suppressive therapy of recurrent genital herpes infections.

Because the frequency of recurrent episodes diminishes over time in many patients, the CDC recommends that suppressive antiviral therapy be discontinued periodically (e.g., once yearly) to assess the need for continued therapy.

Reduction of Transmission. For reduction of transmission of genital herpes in patients with a history of 9 or fewer recurrences per year, the recommended dosage of oral valacyclovir for the infected partner is 500 mg once daily. Valacyclovir is used in conjunction with safer sex practices.

Efficacy for reducing transmission in discordant couples has not been established beyond 8 months.

Herpes Labialis For the treatment of herpes labialis (perioral herpes, cold sores, fever blisters) in immunocompetent adults and adolescents, the recommended dosage of oral valacyclovir is 2 g every 12 hours for 1 day; initiate at the first prodromal symptom of a cold sore (e.g., tingling, itching, burning). Efficacy has not been established if initiated after development of clinical signs of a cold sore (e.g., papule, vesicle, ulcer).

Mucocutaneous Herpes Simplex Virus Infections If oral valacyclovir is used for chronic suppressive or maintenance prophylaxis (secondary prophylaxis) of HSV† in HIV-infected adults and adolescents who have frequent or severe recurrences of HSV disease, a dosage of 500 mg twice daily has been recommended by the Prevention of Opportunistic Infections Working Group of the US Public Health Service and the Infectious Diseases Society of America (USPHS/IDSA).

Herpes Zoster (Shingles, Zoster) For the treatment of acute, localized herpes zoster (shingles, zoster) in immunocompetent adults and adolescents, the recommended dosage of oral valacyclovir is 1 g 3 times daily at 8-hour intervals for 7 days.

Therapy should be initiated at the earliest sign or symptom of herpes zoster, preferably within 48 hours of rash onset. Efficacy of oral valacyclovir initiated longer than 72 hours after rash onset has not been established. Limited evidence indicates that extending the valacyclovir regimen to 14 days in immunocompetent adults with acute, localized herpes zoster does not provide additional clinical benefit.

For the treatment of local dermatomal herpes zoster in HIV-infected adults or adolescents†, the CDC and others recommend 1 g of valacyclovir 3 times daily for 7–10 days.

■ **Dosage in Renal and Hepatic Impairment** The manufacturer states that valacyclovir should be used with caution in patients receiving potentially nephrotoxic agents because this may increase the risk of renal dysfunction and/or reversible CNS manifestations. In patients with impaired renal function, doses and/or frequency of administration of valacyclovir must be modified in response to the degree of impairment.

For the treatment of first episodes of genital herpes in immunocompetent adults with impaired renal function, the manufacturer states that patients with creatinine clearances of 30 mL/minute per 1.73 m^2 or greater may receive the usual oral valacyclovir dosage of 1 g every 12 hours; however, those with creatinine clearances of 10–29 or less than 10 mL/minute per 1.73 m^2 should receive 1 g or 500 mg, respectively, once every 24 hours. For the episodic treatment of recurrent genital herpes in immunocompetent adults with impaired renal function, patients with creatinine clearances of 30 mL/minute per 1.73 m^2 may receive the usual dosage of 500 mg every 12 hours, but those with clearances of 29 mL/minute per 1.73 m^2 or less should receive 500 mg once every 24 hours.

For chronic suppression of recurrent episodes of genital herpes in immunocompetent adults with renal impairment, those with creatinine clearances of 30 mL/minute per 1.73 m^2 or greater may receive the usually recommended dosage of oral valacyclovir. Patients with creatinine clearances less than 30 mL/minute per 1.73 m^2 should receive 500 mg once every 24 hours; alternatively, those with a history of 9 or fewer recurrences per year may receive 500 mg once every 48 hours.

For chronic suppression of recurrent episodes of genital herpes in HIV-infected adults with renal impairment, those with creatinine clearances of 30 mL/minute per 1.73 m^2 or greater may receive the usually recommended dosage of oral valacyclovir and those with creatinine clearances less than 30 mL/minute per 1.73 m^2 should receive 500 mg once every 24 hours.

For the treatment of herpes labialis (cold sores) in patients with renal impairment, patients with creatinine clearances of 50 mL/minute or greater per 1.73 m^2 may receive the usual oral valacyclovir dosage of 2 g every 12 hours for 1 day. Those with creatinine clearances of 30–49 mL/minute per 1.73 m^2 should receive 1 g every 12 hours for 1 day, those with creatinine clearances of 10–29mL/minute per 1.73 m^2 should receive 500 mg every 12 hours for 1 day, and those with creatinine clearances less than 10 mL/minute per 1.73 m^2 should receive a single 500-mg dose.

For the treatment of acute, localized herpes zoster in adults, the manufacturer states that patients with creatinine clearances of 50 mL/minute or greater per 1.73 m^2 may receive the usual oral valacyclovir dosage of 1 g every 8 hours. Those with creatinine clearances of 30–49 mL/minute per 1.73 m^2 should receive 1 g every 12 hours, and those with creatinine clearances of 10–29 or less than 10 mL/minute per 1.73 m^2 should receive 1 g or 500 mg, respectively, once every 24 hours.

Because acyclovir is removed by hemodialysis, the manufacturer states that patients undergoing hemodialysis may require a supplemental dose of valacyclovir after each dialysis period. However, if usual dosing coincides with a valacyclovir dose being administered soon after hemodialysis and subsequent dialysis takes place toward the end of the dosing interval, a supplemental dose would not be necessary.

Information regarding use of valacyclovir in patients undergoing peritoneal dialysis is not available. Based on experience with acyclovir, the manufacturer states that supplemental doses of valacyclovir do not appear to be necessary following peritoneal dialysis, either continuous ambulatory peritoneal dialysis (CAPD) or continuous arteriovenous hemofiltration/dialysis (CAVHD).

The rate but not the extent of conversion of valacyclovir to acyclovir may be reduced in patients with moderate (biopsy-proven cirrhosis) or severe (with and without ascites and biopsy-proven cirrhosis) hepatic impairment. Therefore, the manufacturer states that dosage modification is not necessary for patients with cirrhosis.

Cautions

■ **Contraindications** Known hypersensitivity or intolerance to valacyclovir, acyclovir, or any component of the formulation.

■ **Warnings/Precautions** ***Warnings*** **Hematologic Effects.** Thrombotic thrombocytopenic purpura/hemolytic uremic syndrome (sometimes fatal) reported in patients with advanced HIV infection and in allogeneic bone marrow or renal transplant recipients receiving high dosages (8 g daily).

General Precautions **Renal Effects.** Use of inappropriately high dosage for the level of renal function has resulted in acute renal failure in patients with underlying renal disease. Acyclovir may precipitate in renal tubules if solubility exceeds 2.5 mg/mL in intratubular fluid.

Adequate hydration should be maintained during therapy.

If acute renal failure and anuria occur, hemodialysis recommended until normal renal function returns.

CNS Effects. Use of inappropriately high dosage for the level of renal function has resulted in CNS symptoms in patients with underlying renal disease.

Genital Herpes. Valacyclovir is not a cure for genital herpes. Patients should avoid sexual contact while lesions and/or symptoms are present due to risk of infecting sexual partners. Infection can be transmitted in the absence of symptoms through asymptomatic viral shedding. Although use of valacyclovir for suppressive therapy in immunocompetent individuals with genital herpes decreases the risk for heterosexual transmission, safer sex practices also should be used. Efficacy for reducing transmission not established in individuals with multiple partners or in non-heterosexual couples. Type-specific serologic testing of asymptomatic partners of individuals with genital herpes can determine whether risk for HSV-2 acquisition exists. Valacyclovir has not been shown to reduce transmission of sexually transmitted infections other than HSV-2.

Although recommended by CDC and others for episodic treatment of genital herpes or chronic suppressive therapy of recurrent episodes in HIV-infected adults and adolescents, manufacturer says efficacy not established for treatment of genital herpes in HIV-infected individuals and safety and efficacy not established for chronic suppressive therapy in those with advanced HIV disease (CD4$^+$ T-cell count <100/mm^3).

Herpes Labialis. Valacyclovir is not a cure for cold sores. Treatment should not exceed a single day; therapy beyond 1 day does not provide additional clinical benefits. Because of high dosage, use caution when prescribing valacyclovir for treatment of cold sores in geriatric individuals or those with renal impairment.

Herpes Zoster. Safety and efficacy not established for treatment of disseminated herpes zoster or for treatment of herpes zoster in immunocompromised individuals.

Specific Populations

Pregnancy. Category B.

Lactation. Acyclovir distributed into human milk following oral administration of valacyclovir. Use valacyclovir with caution.

Pediatric Use. Safety and efficacy not established in prepubertal children.

Geriatric Use. Increased risk of adverse renal or CNS effects. CNS effects reported more frequently in geriatric adults than in younger adults include agitation, hallucinations, confusion, delirium, and encephalopathy. In herpes zoster, longer duration of pain after healing (post-herpetic neuralgia) than in younger adults. Consider age-related decreases in renal function when selecting dosage and adjust dosage if necessary. (See Renal Impairment under Dosage and Administration.)

Renal Impairment. Decreased clearance; increased risk of adverse renal and CNS effects in patients with underlying renal disease receiving high dosages. Adjust dosage as necessary. (See Renal Impairment under Dosage and Administration.)

■ **Common Adverse Effects** Headache, nausea, vomiting.

Drug Interactions

■ **Antacids** Concomitant use of valacyclovir and aluminum- or magnesium-containing antacids does not affect the pharmacokinetics of acyclovir; no dosage adjustments are necessary.

■ **Cimetidine** Concomitant use of valacyclovir and cimetidine may increase peak plasma concentrations and AUC of acyclovir. This pharmacokinetic interaction is not considered clinically important in patients with normal renal function; no dosage adjustments are necessary in these patients.

■ **Digoxin** Concomitant use of valacyclovir and digoxin does not affect the pharmacokinetics of acyclovir or digoxin; no dosage adjustments are necessary.

■ **Probenecid** Concomitant use of valacyclovir and probenecid may increase peak plasma concentrations and AUC of acyclovir. This pharmacokinetic interaction is not considered clinically important in patients with normal renal function and no dosage adjustments are necessary in these patients.

■ **Thiazide Diuretics** Concomitant use of valacyclovir and thiazide diuretics does not affect the pharmacokinetics of acyclovir; no dosage adjustments are necessary.

Description

Valacyclovir, the L-valine ester of acyclovir, is an antiviral agent. Valacyclovir is a prodrug and exhibits no antiviral activity until hydrolyzed in the intestinal wall and/or liver to acyclovir and subsequently to its active metabolite (acyclovir triphosphate). Valacyclovir is commercially available as the hydrochloride salt and differs structurally from acyclovir by the presence of the l-amino acid, valine, attached to the 5′-hydroxyl group of the nucleoside and by the presence of the monohydrochloride salt. These structural modifications result in substantially increased GI absorption of valacyclovir and resultant plasma acyclovir concentrations compared with those achieved orally with the parent drug acyclovir, which is poorly absorbed from the GI tract.

Valacyclovir is rapidly converted to acyclovir in vivo and subsequently to the pharmacologically active triphosphate metabolite, which has in vitro and in vivo inhibitory activity against herpes simplex virus types 1 (HSV-1) and 2 (HSV-2), varicella-zoster virus (VZV), and cytomegalovirus (CMV). Acyclovir triphosphate exerts its antiviral effect on HSV and VZV by interfering with DNA synthesis and inhibiting viral replication. The inhibitory activity of acyclovir triphosphate is highly selective because of its affinity for the enzyme thymidine kinase encoded by HSV and VZV; however, other mechanisms may be involved since the drug exhibits activity against viruses that apparently do not code for this enzyme. Virus-coded thymidine kinase converts acyclovir into acyclovir monophosphate, a nucleotide analog. The monophosphate is further converted to the diphosphate via cellular guanylate kinase and then to the triphosphate via other cellular enzymes. In vitro, acyclovir triphosphate stops replication of herpes viral DNA by competitive inhibition of viral DNA polymerase, incorporation and termination of the growing viral DNA chain, and inactivation of the viral DNA polymerase. For additional information, see Mechanism of Action in Acyclovir 8:18.32.

Overview® (see Users Guide). For additional information on this drug until a more detailed monograph is developed and published, the manufacturer's labeling should be consulted. It is *essential* that the manufacturer's labeling be consulted for more detailed information on usual cautions, precautions, contraindications, potential drug interactions, laboratory test interferences, and acute toxicity.

Preparations

Excipients in commercially available drug preparations may have clinically important effects in some individuals; consult specific product labeling for details.

valACYclovir Hydrochloride

Oral		
Tablets, film-coated	500 mg (of valacyclovir)	**Valtrex® Caplets,** GlaxoSmithKline
	1 g (of valacyclovir)	**Valtrex® Caplets,** GlaxoSmithKline

†Use is not currently included in the labeling approved by the US Food and Drug Administration

valGANciclovir Hydrochloride

ValcyteVGCV

■ Valganciclovir, a prodrug of ganciclovir, is an antiviral agent; after in vivo conversion to an active metabolite, the drug is active against herpes viruses.

Uses

■ **Treatment of Cytomegalovirus Infection and Disease** ***Cytomegalovirus Retinitis*** Valganciclovir hydrochloride is used for initial treatment (induction therapy) and maintenance therapy (secondary prophylaxis) of cytomegalovirus (CMV) retinitis in adults with human immunodeficiency virus (HIV) infection, including those with acquired immunodeficiency syndrome (AIDS). The drug also is used for the management of CMV retinitis in certain HIV-infected pediatric patients†.

Like others antivirals, valganciclovir is not a cure for CMV retinitis; the retinitis may relapse and/or progress during or after discontinuance of the drug.

Retinitis is the most common clinical manifestation of CMV end-organ disease in HIV-infected patients and ideally should be managed in consultation with an ophthalmologist familiar with the diagnosis and treatment of retinal diseases. Antiviral regimens for initial treatment of CMV retinitis in HIV-infected individuals should be selected based on the location and severity of the CMV retinal lesions, severity of underlying immunosuppression, concomitant drug therapy, and the patient's ability to adhere to the treatment regimen. The antiviral regimen used for maintenance therapy of CMV retinitis in HIV-infected individuals should be selected with consideration for the location of the CMV retinal lesions, vision in the contralateral eye, the patient's immunologic and virologic status, and the patient's response to antiretroviral therapy.

For the management of immediate sight-threatening CMV retinal lesions (i.e., within 1.5 mm of the fovea) in HIV-infected adults and adolescents, the US Centers for Disease Control and Prevention (CDC), National Institutes of Health (NIH), and HIV Medicine Association of the Infectious Diseases Society of America (IDSA) state that the preferred regimen is initial treatment (induction therapy) with intravitreal ganciclovir or intravitreal foscarnet (1–4 doses given over a period of 7–10 days) in conjunction with oral valganciclovir (twice daily for 14–21 days) followed by maintenance therapy (secondary prophylaxis) with oral valganciclovir (once daily). One alternative regimen recommended by these experts for management of sight-threatening CMV retinitis in HIV-infected adults and adolescents is intravitreal ganciclovir or intravitreal foscarnet (1–4 doses given over a period of 7–10 days) in conjunction with IV ganciclovir (twice daily for 14–21 days) followed by maintenance therapy (secondary prophylaxis) with oral valganciclovir (once daily). Use of systemic antivirals (without an intravitreal antiviral) usually is adequate for the management of CMV retinitis in patients who have only small peripheral lesions.

For the management of CMV retinitis in HIV-infected pediatric patients, CDC, NIH, IDSA, and others state that IV ganciclovir is the drug of choice for initial treatment (induction therapy) and is one of several options for maintenance therapy (secondary prophylaxis). These experts state that oral valganciclovir is an option for the management of CMV retinitis in HIV-infected pediatric patients† and can be considered for induction and/or maintenance therapy in adolescents and older children who can receive the recommended adult dosage of the drug and can also be considered in children who are able to transition from initial IV ganciclovir therapy to an oral regimen to complete treatment and/or for maintenance therapy.

Because of the risk of relapse, HIV-infected patients who have received adequate initial treatment of CMV retinitis should receive chronic maintenance therapy (secondary prophylaxis) until immune reconstitution occurs as a result of effective antiretroviral therapy. CDC, NIH, and IDSA state that consideration can be given to discontinuing maintenance therapy of CMV retinitis in HIV-infected adults and adolescents if CMV lesions have been treated for at least 3–6 months and are inactive and there has been a sustained (i.e., 3–6 months) increase in CD4$^+$ T-cell count to greater than 100/mm^3 in response to antiretroviral therapy. The safety of discontinuing maintenance therapy of CMV retinitis in HIV-infected pediatric patients has not been well studied; however, CDC, NIH, IDSA, and others state that consideration can be given to discontinuing such maintenance therapy in HIV-infected children who are receiving antiretroviral therapy and have a sustained (i.e., greater than 6 months) increase in CD4+ T-cell percentage to greater than 15% (children younger than 6 years of age) or increase in CD4+ T-cell count to greater than 100/mm^3 (children 6 years of age or older). These experts state that a decision to discontinue maintenance therapy of CMV retinitis should be made in consultation with an ophthalmologist and, if maintenance therapy is discontinued, the patient should continue to receive regular ophthalmologic monitoring (optimally every 3–6 months) for early detection of CMV relapse or immune reconstitution uveitis. If CD4+ T-cell count decreases to less than 100/mm^3 (adults, adolescents, children 6 years of age or older) or if CD4+ T-cell percentage decreases to less than 15% (children younger than 6 years of age), maintenance therapy of CMV retinitis should be reinitiated.

For additional information on the management of CMV retinitis and other CMV infections in HIV-infected individuals, the current clinical practice guidelines from CDC, NIH, and IDSA on the prevention and treatment of opportunistic infections in HIV-infected individuals available at http://www.aidsinfo.nih.gov should be consulted.

Clinical Experience. In a randomized, open-label, comparative study (study WV15376) in HIV-infected adults with AIDS (median age 39 years, baseline plasma HIV-1 RNA levels of 4.9 $\log_{10}$, median CD4+ T-cell count of 23/mm^3, 91% male, 53% white, 31% Hispanic, 11% black) with previously untreated CMV retinitis, oral valganciclovir (900 mg twice daily for 21 days followed by 900 mg once daily for 7 days) was as effective as IV ganciclovir (5 mg/kg twice daily for 21 days followed by 5 mg/kg once daily for 7 days) in delaying CMV retinitis progression based on a masked evaluation of retinal photographs at week 4 of the study (the primary outcome measure).

All patients enrolled in study WV15376 received maintenance therapy with open-label valganciclovir after week 4; the median time to photographically determined first CMV retinitis progression in patients who had received initial treatment (induction therapy) with oral valganciclovir or IV ganciclovir was 180 days (mean: 226) or 126 days (mean: 219), respectively.

Extraocular Cytomegalovirus Infections Safety and efficacy of valganciclovir have not been established for the management of extraocular CMV infections.

CDC, NIH, and IDSA state that IV ganciclovir usually is the preferred antiviral for initial management of CMV GI disease (e.g., colitis, esophagitis) in HIV-infected adults and that a transition to oral valganciclovir may be considered when the patient can tolerate and absorb oral drugs. These experts also state that oral valganciclovir can be considered for initial management of CMV esophagitis† or colitis† in patients with GI symptoms that do not interfere with oral absorption.

Congenital Cytomegalovirus Disease Although safety and efficacy of valganciclovir have not been established in neonates or infants with congenital CMV infection, the drug has been used for the management of symptomatic congenital CMV disease† when an antiviral was indicated.

Transmission of CMV from infected mothers to their fetuses occurs as a result of maternal viremia and transplacental infection. Perinatal infection also can occur from exposure of the neonate to CMV shedding in the mother's genital tract. Approximately 10% of children with congenital CMV infection are symptomatic at birth; mortality in symptomatic infants is about 10% and approximately 50–90% of symptomatic surviving neonates experience substantial morbidity (e.g., mental retardation, sensorineural hearing loss, microcephaly, seizures). The risk of congenital CMV infection resulting from primary maternal CMV infection may be higher and the disease may be more severe than that resulting from reactivation of maternal CMV infection.

Because there is some evidence that antivirals (i.e., ganciclovir, valganciclovir) may help prevent hearing deterioration and/or improve developmental delay in neonates and infants with moderate to severe symptomatic congenital CMV disease, the American Academy of Pediatrics (AAP) and other clinicians state that use of an antiviral regimen should be considered in such neonates if it can be initiated within the first month of life. Antivirals are not usually recommended for neonates with asymptomatic congenital CMV infection or only mildly symptomatic infection without evidence of CNS involvement.

A 6-month regimen of oral valganciclovir has been used in neonates with symptomatic congenital CMV disease (with or without CNS involvement), and there is some evidence that this regimen is associated with some improvement in audiologic and neurodevelopmental outcomes at 12 and 24 months compared with a 6-week regimen of oral valganciclovir. A 6-week regimen of IV ganciclovir either alone or followed by a regimen of oral valganciclovir (continued until up to 12 months of age) also has been used in neonates with symptomatic congenital CMV disease. CDC, NIH, IDSA, and others state that IV ganciclovir can be considered for initial treatment in HIV-exposed or HIV-infected infants with symptomatic congenital CMV disease with CNS involvement.

Decisions regarding antiviral treatment in neonates with congenital CMV disease should be made in consultation with a pediatric infectious diseases specialist. Because of the risk of serious sequelae (e.g., late-onset hearing loss), long-term ophthalmologic and audiologic monitoring is necessary in patients with congenital CMV infection, regardless of antiviral treatment.

■ **Prevention of Cytomegalovirus Infection and Disease** Valganciclovir hydrochloride is used for prophylaxis to prevent CMV infection and disease in certain adult and pediatric solid organ transplant recipients at high risk for the disease. The drug also has been used for prophylaxis or preemptive treatment of CMV infection and disease in hematopoietic stem cell transplant (HSCT) recipients† at risk for the disease.

CMV infection in transplant recipients can occur either as a primary infection in CMV-seronegative recipients of organs and cells from CMV-positive donors or as reactivation of latent CMV infection in CMV-seropositive recipients. CMV infection in transplant recipients is associated with substantial morbidity and mortality. The risk for CMV infection or reactivation is greatest during the first 3 months after transplantation and depends on several factors, including the serologic status of the recipient and donor, CMV-specific T-cell immunity in the recipient, and immunosuppressive regimens used in the recipient. Certain antiviral strategies have been used to prevent severe, life-threatening CMV disease in transplant recipients, including antiviral prophylaxis (initiated posttransplantation and continued for at least 3 months) and/or preemptive antiviral treatment (i.e., initiated when CMV infection is detected, but before clinical progression to symptomatic CMV disease). These antiviral strategies each have certain advantages and disadvantages.

Specialized references should be consulted for specific information regarding prevention and management of CMV infections in HSCT or solid organ transplant recipients.

Solid Organ Transplant Recipients Valganciclovir hydrochloride is used for prophylaxis to prevent CMV infection and disease in adult kidney, heart, and kidney-pancreas transplant recipients considered at high risk (CMV-seronegative recipient of an organ from a CMV-seropositive donor). The drug also is used for prophylaxis to prevent CMV infection and disease in pediatric kidney transplant recipients 4 months to 16 years of age and pediatric heart transplant recipients 1 month to 16 years of age considered at high risk (CMV-seronegative recipient of an organ from a CMV-seropositive donor).

Valganciclovir also has been used for preemptive treatment of CMV infection in solid organ transplant recipients† (e.g., kidney, heart, pancreas); however, safety and efficacy of the drug have not been established for preemptive treatment of CMV infections in transplant recipients.

Although safety and efficacy of valganciclovir have not been established in adult or pediatric liver transplant recipients and low efficacy was reported in one study in adult patients (see Clinical Experience under Prevention of Cytomegalovirus Infection and Disease: Solid Organ Transplant Recipients, in Uses), the drug has been used and is recommended by some clinicians for prophylaxis or preemptive treatment of CMV infection in liver transplant recipients†.

Clinical Experience. Safety and efficacy of valganciclovir for prevention of CMV disease in 372 solid organ transplant recipients were evaluated in a double-blind, double-dummy, active comparator study (study PV16000) in heart, liver, kidney, and kidney-pancreas transplant patients at high risk (CMV-seronegative recipient of an organ from a CMV-seropositive donor). Patients were randomized to receive oral valganciclovir (900 mg once daily) or oral ganciclovir (1 g 3 times daily; not commercially available in the US) initiated within 10 days of transplantation and continued until 100 days after transplantation. During the first 6 months following transplantation, 12% of those receiving valganciclovir and 15% of those receiving ganciclovir developed CMV disease (CMV syndrome and/or tissue-invasive disease). However, in liver transplant recipients, the incidence of CMV disease was greater in those receiving valganciclovir (19%) than in those receiving ganciclovir (12%); tissue-invasive CMV disease was reported most frequently. Mortality at 6 months was 3.7% in the oral valganciclovir group and 1.6% in the oral ganciclovir group.

Safety and efficacy of a longer duration (200 days) of valganciclovir prophylaxis against CMV disease in kidney transplant recipients were established in a double-blind, placebo-controlled trial that included 326 adult kidney transplant patients at high risk (CMV-seronegative recipient of an organ from a CMV-seropositive donor). Patients were randomized to receive valganciclovir prophylaxis (900 mg once daily) starting within 10 days of transplantation and continued for either 200 days posttransplantation or for 100 days posttransplantation followed by placebo for 100 days. At 1 year posttransplantation, the incidence of CMV disease was about 17% in those who received 200 days of valganciclovir prophylaxis compared with 37% in those who received only 100 days of such prophylaxis. There was no overall difference in the safety profile between the 2 groups.

Safety and pharmacokinetics of oral valganciclovir for prevention of CMV disease in pediatric patients were established in an open-label study of 63 solid organ transplant (i.e., kidney, liver, heart, kidney-liver) recipients 4 months to 16 years of age. These pediatric patients received once-daily valganciclovir (tablets or oral solution) given in a dose calculated based on body surface area (BSA) and estimated creatinine clearance (modified Schwartz formula) and limited to a maximum dosage of 900 mg daily. Valganciclovir treatment was initiated within 10 days posttransplantation and continued for a maximum of 100 days (median duration was approximately 92 days). Systemic ganciclovir exposures in these pediatric solid organ transplant patients were somewhat higher compared with exposures reported in adult solid organ transplant patients receiving the drug at a dosage of 900 mg once daily. Although CMV viremia was reported in 11% of patients in this study, CMV disease was not reported in any pediatric patient up to 26 weeks posttransplantation. Use of valganciclovir for the prevention of CMV disease in pediatric kidney or heart transplant recipients 4 months to 16 years of age at high risk for the disease is based on pharmacokinetic, safety, and efficacy data from this open-label study and efficacy extrapolated from a study in adults.

Valganciclovir in pediatric patients also was evaluated in an open-label tolerability study that included 57 renal transplant recipients 1 month to 16 years of age who were at risk for developing CMV disease. All patients received once-daily valganciclovir (tablets or oral solution) given in a dose calculated based on BSA and modified creatinine clearance. Valganciclovir treatment was initiated within 10 days posttransplantation and continued for a maximum of 200 days. No cases of CMV syndrome or tissue-invasive CMV disease were reported within the first 12 months posttransplantation.

Hematopoietic Stem Cell Transplant Recipients Valganciclovir has been used for prophylaxis or preemptive treatment of CMV infection and disease in HSCT recipients†.

Dosage and Administration

■ Administration Valganciclovir hydrochloride is administered orally as tablets or an oral solution and should be given with food.

Adults should receive valganciclovir tablets (not the oral solution). Valganciclovir tablets should not be broken or crushed.

Valganciclovir oral solution is the preferred dosage form for pediatric patients. Valganciclovir tablets should be used in pediatric patients *only* if the calculated dose is within 10% of the tablet strength (i.e., a single 450-mg tablet may be used if the calculated dose is 405–495 mg). (See Pediatric Dosage under Dosage and Administration: Dosage.)

Patients receiving valganciclovir should be adequately hydrated.

Females of childbearing potential should be tested for pregnancy prior to initiation of valganciclovir. (See Pregnancy under Warnings/Precautions: Specific Populations, in Cautions.)

Because of the mutagenic and/or carcinogenic potential of valganciclovir, the tablets, powder for oral solution, and reconstituted oral solutions of the drug should be handled carefully according to guidelines issued for cytotoxic drugs. (See Handling and Disposal under Warnings/Precautions: Other Warnings/Precautions, in Cautions.)

Oral Solution Valganciclovir hydrochloride powder for oral solution should be reconstituted at the time of dispensing by adding 91 mL of purified water to provide a solution containing 250 mg of valganciclovir per 5 mL. After tapping the bottle to loosen the powder, the water should be added in 2 approximately equal portions and the bottle should be shaken for about 1 minute after each addition. Following reconstitution, the solution is colorless to brownish yellow.

The reconstituted oral solution should be stored at 2–8°C for up to 49 days and should not be frozen.

Just prior to each dose, the oral solution should be shaken for about 5 seconds.

The appropriate dose of the reconstituted oral solution should be administered using the bottle adapter and dosing dispenser provided by the manufacturer.

■ Dosage Dosage of valganciclovir hydrochloride is expressed in terms of valganciclovir.

Adult Dosage **Cytomegalovirus Retinitis.** For initial treatment (induction therapy) of cytomegalovirus (CMV) retinitis in adults with normal renal function (creatinine clearance 60 mL/minute or greater), the recommended dosage of valganciclovir tablets is 900 mg orally twice daily for 21 days. The US Centers for Disease Control and Prevention (CDC), National Institutes of Health (NIH), and HIV Medicine Association of the Infectious Diseases Society of America (IDSA) recommend that initial treatment (induction therapy) be continued for 14–21 days in adults with human immunodeficiency virus (HIV) infection. In patients with immediate sight-threatening CMV retinal lesions (i.e., within 1.5 mm of the fovea), these experts recommend that initial treatment also include an appropriate intravitreal antiviral. (See Cytomegalovirus Retinitis under Uses: Treatment of Cytomegalovirus Infection and Disease.)

After completion of initial treatment or in patients with inactive CMV retinitis, the recommended dosage of valganciclovir tablets for maintenance therapy (secondary prophylaxis) in adults with normal renal function is 900 mg orally once daily.

Decisions regarding discontinuance of maintenance therapy of CMV retinitis in HIV-infected individuals who have received CMV treatment for at least 3–6 months, have inactive CMV retinal lesions, and have achieved immune reconstitution as the result of antiretroviral therapy should be made in consultation with an ophthalmologist. (See Cytomegalovirus Retinitis under Uses: Treatment of Cytomegalovirus Infection and Disease.)

Cytomegalovirus Esophagitis or Colitis. If oral valganciclovir is used for the management of CMV esophagitis† or colitis† in HIV-infected adults, CDC, NIH, and IDSA recommend a dosage of 900 mg every 12 hours for 21–42 days or until signs and symptoms of the infection have resolved. Maintenance therapy (secondary prophylaxis) usually is not necessary, but should be considered if relapse occurs.

Prevention of Cytomegalovirus Infection and Disease in Transplant Recipients. For prophylaxis to prevent CMV infection and disease in adult *heart* or *kidney-pancreas* transplant recipients, the usual dosage of valganciclovir tablets is 900 mg once daily initiated within 10 days of transplantation and continued until 100 days posttransplantation. Some experts recommend that antiviral prophylaxis be continued for 3–6 months in CMV-seronegative recipients of heart, liver†, or pancreas transplants from CMV-seropositive donors.

For prophylaxis to prevent CMV infection and disease in adult *kidney* transplant recipients, the usual dosage of valganciclovir tablets is 900 mg once daily initiated within 10 days of transplantation and continued until 200 days posttransplantation. Some experts recommend that antiviral prophylaxis be continued for 6 months in CMV-seronegative recipients of kidney transplants from CMV-seropositive donors.

If oral valganciclovir is used for preemptive treatment of CMV infection in solid organ transplant recipients†, a dosage of 900 mg twice daily is recommended in those with normal renal function.

Pediatric Dosage **Cytomegalovirus Retinitis.** If oral valganciclovir is used for initial treatment (induction therapy) of CMV retinitis in HIV-infected older children† and adolescents† who can receive adult dosage, CDC, NIH, IDSA, and others recommend a dosage of 900 mg twice daily for 14–21 days.

If oral valganciclovir is used for maintenance therapy (secondary prophylaxis) of CMV retinitis in HIV-infected older children† and adolescents† who can receive adult dosage, CDC, NIH, IDSA, and others recommend a dosage of 900 mg once daily.

Decisions regarding discontinuance of maintenance therapy of CMV retinitis in HIV-infected individuals who have been treated at least 3–6 months, have inactive CMV retinal lesions, and have achieved immune reconstitution as the result of antiretroviral therapy should be made in consultation with an ophthalmologist. (See Cytomegalovirus Retinitis under Uses: Treatment of Cytomegalovirus Infection and Disease.)

Congenital Cytomegalovirus Disease. If oral valganciclovir is used for the management of symptomatic congenital CMV disease† when an antiviral is indicated (see Congenital Cytomegalovirus Disease under Uses: Treatment of Cytomegalovirus Infection and Disease), the American Academy of Pediatrics (AAP) and other clinicians recommend a dosage of 16 mg/kg twice daily.

AAP and other clinicians recommend that, if an antiviral is indicated, it should be initiated within the first month of life and continued for a total of 6 months. If IV ganciclovir is used initially, treatment should be transitioned to oral valganciclovir when the infant is able to tolerate and absorb oral drugs.

Prevention of Cytomegalovirus Infection and Disease in Transplant Recipients. For prophylaxis to prevent CMV infection and disease in pediatric *heart* transplant patients 1 month to 16 years of age, oral valganciclovir should be given once daily initiated within 10 days of transplantation and continued until 100 days posttransplantation.

For prophylaxis to prevent CMV infection and disease in pediatric *kidney* transplant patients 4 months to 16 years of age, oral valganciclovir should be given once daily initiated within 10 days of transplantation and continued until 200 days posttransplantation.

The pediatric dose of oral valganciclovir for prevention of CMV infection and disease should be individualized based on body surface area (BSA) and estimated creatinine clearance (Cl_{cr}, modified Schwartz formula), and is calculated using the following pediatric dosage equation:

$$\text{Pediatric dose (in mg)} = 7 \times \text{BSA (in m}^2) \times Cl_{cr} \text{ (modified Schwartz formula)}$$

$$\text{Modified Schwartz formula for } Cl_{cr} \text{ (in mL/minute per 1.73 m}^2) = \frac{k \times \text{height (in cm)}}{\text{serum creatinine (in mg/dL)}}$$

Where k =
0.33 for infants less than 1 year of age with low birth weight for gestational age
0.45 for infants less than 1 year of age with birth weight appropriate for gestational age
0.45 for children 1 to less than 2 years of age
0.55 for girls 2 to less than 16 years of age
0.55 for boys 2 to less than 13 years of age
0.7 for boys 13–16 years of age

To prevent overdosage in pediatric patients, the estimated creatinine clearance used to calculate the pediatric dose should not exceed 150 mL/minute per 1.73 m², regardless of the value calculated using the modified Schwartz formula. If the estimated creatinine clearance exceeds 150 mL/minute per 1.73 m², the value of 150 mL/minute per 1.73 m² should be used to calculate the dose for that patient. The calculated dose should be rounded to the nearest 10-mg increment. The *maximum* dose in pediatric patients is 900 mg.

■ Special Populations ***Renal Impairment*** In patients with impaired renal function, dosage and/or frequency of administration of valganciclovir must be modified in response to the degree of impairment.

Dosage for adults with renal impairment should be based on the patient's creatinine clearance, which can be estimated using the following formula:

$$Ccr\ male = \frac{(140 - age) \times weight}{72 \times serum\ creatinine}$$

$$Ccr\ female = 0.85 \times Ccr\ male$$

where age is in years, weight is in kg, and serum creatinine is in mg/dL.

Dosage for pediatric patients with renal impairment can be calculated using the usually recommended pediatric dosage equation since this is based on both BSA and estimated creatinine clearance. (See Pediatric Dosage under Dosage and Administration: Dosage.)

Valganciclovir should not be used in adults undergoing hemodialysis (creatinine clearance less than 10 mL/minute). (See Renal Impairment under Warnings/Precautions: Specific Populations, in Cautions.)

Cytomegalovirus Retinitis. When valganciclovir is used for initial treatment (induction therapy) and maintenance therapy (secondary prophylaxis) of CMV retinitis in adults with renal impairment, dosage should be based on the patient's creatinine clearance. (See Table 1.)

Table 1. Dosage of Valganciclovir for Management of CMV Retinitis in Adults with Renal Impairment

Creatinine Clearance (mL/minute)	Initial Treatment (Induction) Dosage	Maintenance Dosage
40–59	450 mg twice daily	450 mg once daily
25–39	450 mg once daily	450 mg once every 2 days
10–24	450 mg once every 2 days	450 mg twice weekly
Less than 10 (hemodialysis patients)	Not recommended	Not recommended

Geriatric Patients Dosage of valganciclovir for geriatric patients should be selected with caution, usually starting at the low end of the dosage range, because of age-related decreases in hepatic, renal, and/or cardiac function. Renal function should be assessed before and during valganciclovir therapy and appropriate dosage adjustments made as necessary. (See Geriatric Use under Warnings/Precautions: Specific Populations, in Cautions.)

Cautions

■ Contraindications

Valganciclovir is contraindicated in patients who have had a clinically important hypersensitivity reaction (e.g., anaphylaxis) to valganciclovir, ganciclovir, or any ingredient in the formulation.

■ Warnings/Precautions

Warnings **Hematologic Effects.** Severe leukopenia, neutropenia, anemia, thrombocytopenia, pancytopenia, and bone marrow failure (including aplastic anemia) have been reported in patients receiving valganciclovir or ganciclovir. Cytopenia may occur at any time during valganciclovir therapy and the degree of cytopenia may increase with continued therapy with the drug. Cell counts usually begin to return to baseline within 3–7 days after valganciclovir is discontinued.

Complete blood cell counts (CBCs) with differential and platelet counts should be performed frequently, especially in infants and in patients with baseline neutrophil counts less than 1000/mm^3, in those who previously experienced leukopenia while receiving ganciclovir or other nucleoside analogs, and in those with renal impairment. Because oral valganciclovir results in comparatively increased plasma ganciclovir concentrations compared with oral ganciclovir (not commercially available in the US), more frequent monitoring for cytopenias may be warranted if therapy is changed from oral ganciclovir to valganciclovir.

Valganciclovir should be avoided in patients with absolute neutrophil counts less than 500/mm^3, platelet counts less than 25,000/mm^3, or hemoglobin concentrations less than 8 g/dL.

Valganciclovir should be used with caution in patients with preexisting cytopenias and in those who have received or are receiving concomitant myelosuppressive drugs or irradiation.

In patients experiencing severe leukopenia, neutropenia, anemia, and/or thrombocytopenia, treatment with hematopoietic growth factors may be considered.

Impairment of Fertility. Animal data from studies using ganciclovir and limited data from patients receiving valganciclovir indicate that valganciclovir may cause temporary or permanent inhibition of spermatogenesis in males and may cause suppression of fertility in females.

In a small, open-label, nonrandomized clinical study, adult male renal transplant patients receiving cytomegalovirus (CMV) prophylaxis with oral valganciclovir for up to 200 days posttransplantation were followed for 6 months after the drug was discontinued and data compared with an untreated control group. Among 24 evaluable patients in the valganciclovir group, the mean sperm density at the end-of-treatment visit was *decreased* by 11 million/mL from baseline; whereas, among 14 evaluable patients in the control group, the mean sperm density at the end-of-treatment visit had *increased* by 33 million/mL. However, at the final follow-up visit, the mean sperm density among 20 evaluable patients in the valganciclovir group was comparable to that observed among 10 evaluable patients in the untreated control group (mean sperm density increased by 41 or 43 million/mL from baseline, respectively).

Patients receiving valganciclovir should be advised that the drug may be associated with infertility.

Teratogenesis. Animal data from studies using ganciclovir indicate that valganciclovir may cause fetal toxicity and has the potential to cause birth defects if administered to pregnant women.

In studies in pregnant mice and rabbits receiving ganciclovir at dosages resulting in 2 times the human exposure, maternal toxicity and embryofetal toxicity (e.g., fetal resorptions, embryofetal mortality) was observed. In addition, teratogenic effects (cleft palate, anophthalmia/microphthalmia, hydrocephalus, brachygnathia, aplastic organs [kidney, pancreas]) were reported in rabbits.

Females of childbearing potential should undergo pregnancy testing before valganciclovir is initiated.

Females of childbearing potential should be advised to use an effective method of contraception during and for at least 30 days after valganciclovir is discontinued. Male patients should be advised to use a reliable method of barrier contraception during and for at least 90 days after valganciclovir is discontinued.

Mutagenicity and Carcinogenicity. Animal studies using ganciclovir indicate the drug is mutagenic and carcinogenic.

Valganciclovir should be considered a potential carcinogen in humans.

Other Warnings/Precautions **Renal Effects.** Acute renal failure may occur in geriatric patients (with or without renal impairment), patients receiving potentially nephrotoxic drugs, and inadequately hydrated patients.

Adequate hydration should be maintained in all patients.

Valganciclovir should be used with caution in geriatric patients and in patients receiving concomitant therapy with potentially nephrotoxic drugs.

Dosage adjustment of valganciclovir is recommended in patients with renal impairment. (See Renal Impairment under Dosage and Administration: Special Populations.)

Handling and Disposal. Because valganciclovir is considered a potential teratogen and carcinogen, caution should be exercised when handling the drug. Valganciclovir tablets should not be broken or crushed. Direct contact of broken or crushed tablets, powder for oral solution, or reconstituted oral solution with skin or mucous membranes should be avoided. If such contact occurs, skin should be washed thoroughly with soap and water; eyes should be rinsed thoroughly with water. For further information on handling of cytotoxic drugs, see the ASHP Guidelines on Handling Hazardous Drugs at http://ahfsdruginformation.com.

Specific Populations **Pregnancy.** In animal studies, ganciclovir caused maternal and fetal toxicity, embryofetal mortality, and teratogenicity. Valganciclovir is expected to have reproductive toxicity similar to ganciclovir. (See Teratogenesis under Warnings/Precautions: Warnings, in Cautions.)

Data are not available regarding use of valganciclovir in pregnant women to establish the presence or absence of drug-associated risk. An ex vivo placental model indicates that ganciclovir crosses the human placenta by passive diffusion and is not saturable over a concentration range of 1–10 mg/mL.

Although most maternal CMV infections are asymptomatic or may be associated with a self-limited mononucleosis-like syndrome, CMV infections in pregnant immunocompromised patients (e.g., those with human immunodeficiency virus [HIV] infection and acquired immunodeficiency syndrome [AIDS], transplant recipients) may be symptomatic and result in substantial maternal morbidity and mortality. Perinatal transmission of CMV from infected mothers to their neonates can occur resulting in congenital CMV infection and disease. (See Congenital Cytomegalovirus Disease under Uses: Treatment of Cytomegalovirus Infection and Disease.)

Females of childbearing potential should undergo pregnancy testing before initiation of valganciclovir. In addition, pregnancy should be avoided in female patients receiving valganciclovir and in females with male partners receiving valganciclovir.

Females of childbearing potential should be advised to use an effective method of contraception during and for at least 30 days after valganciclovir therapy and male patients should be advised to use a reliable method of barrier contraception during and for at least 90 days after valganciclovir therapy.

Lactation. It is not known whether valganciclovir or ganciclovir is distributed into human milk, affects the breast-fed infant, or affects milk production. Animal data from studies using ganciclovir indicate that the drug is distributed into milk of lactating rats.

Because of the potential for serious adverse effects in nursing infants, valganciclovir is not recommended in breast-feeding women. HIV-infected mothers should be instructed not to breast-feed their infants because of the risk of transmission of HIV.

Pediatric Use. Safety and efficacy of valganciclovir have not been established in pediatric patients younger than 1 month of age.

Use of valganciclovir for the prevention of CMV disease in pediatric *heart* transplant recipients 1 month to 16 years of age is based on safety and pharmacokinetic data from 2 studies in pediatric solid organ transplant recipients and is supported by efficacy data from studies in adult solid organ transplant recipients.

Use of valganciclovir for the prevention of CMV disease in pediatric *kidney* transplant recipients 4 months to 16 years of age is based on safety, tolerability, and pharmacokinetic data from 2 open-label studies in solid organ transplant recipients in this age group and is supported by efficacy data from studies in adult solid organ transplant recipients.

Safety and efficacy of valganciclovir have not been established for prevention of CMV disease in pediatric heart transplant recipients younger than 1 month of age, pediatric kidney transplant recipients younger than 4 months of age, or pediatric liver transplant recipients of any age.

The safety profile of valganciclovir in pediatric patients generally is similar to that observed in adults. However, upper respiratory tract infection, pyrexia, nasopharyngitis, anemia, abdominal pain, and neutropenia have been reported more frequently in pediatric patients than in adults.

Geriatric Use. Safety and efficacy of valganciclovir have not been specifically evaluated in geriatric patients 65 years of age or older and there were insufficient numbers of individuals in this age group in clinical studies to determine whether they respond differently than younger adults. Pharmacokinetics of the drug have been not studied in geriatric patients.

Because geriatric individuals frequently have decreased renal function and because valganciclovir is substantially excreted by the kidneys, particular attention should be paid to assessing renal function before and during valganciclovir therapy in this age group. If evidence of renal impairment exists or develops, appropriate dosage adjustments should be made. In general, dosage should be selected carefully, usually starting at the low end of the dosage range, taking into account the greater frequency of decreased hepatic, renal, and/or cardiac function and of concomitant disease and drug therapy observed in the elderly.

Hepatic Impairment. Safety and efficacy of valganciclovir have not been evaluated in patients with hepatic impairment.

Renal Impairment. The major route of elimination of valganciclovir is renal excretion as ganciclovir. If renal function is impaired, dosage of valganciclovir must be adjusted based on measured or estimated creatinine clearance. (See Renal Impairment under Dosage and Administration: Special Populations.)

Hemodialysis reduces plasma concentrations of ganciclovir by approximately 50%. Valganciclovir should not be used in adults undergoing hemodialysis (creatinine clearance less than 10 mL/minute) because the appropriate daily dose for such patients is lower than 450 mg (i.e., would require breaking a tablet); such patients should receive ganciclovir instead.

■ **Common Adverse Effects** Adverse effects occurring in 20% or more of adults receiving valganciclovir include diarrhea, pyrexia, fatigue, nausea, tremor, neutropenia, anemia, leukopenia, thrombocytopenia, headache, insomnia, urinary tract infection, and vomiting.

Adverse effects occurring in 20% or more of pediatric patients receiving valganciclovir include diarrhea, pyrexia, upper respiratory tract infection, urinary tract infection, vomiting, neutropenia, leukopenia, and headache.

Drug Interactions

No formal drug interaction studies have been performed using valganciclovir. However, valganciclovir is rapidly and extensively converted to ganciclovir and interactions reported with ganciclovir are expected to occur in patients receiving valganciclovir.

Drug interaction studies with ganciclovir were performed in patients with normal renal function. In patients with renal impairment, concomitant use of valganciclovir and other drugs eliminated by renal excretion may result in increased concentrations of ganciclovir and the concomitant drug and such patients should be closely monitored for toxicity associated with ganciclovir and the concomitant drug.

■ **Antibacterial Agents** ***Imipenem and Cilastatin Sodium*** Generalized seizures have been reported in patients who received ganciclovir concomitantly with the fixed combination of imipenem and cilastatin sodium (imipenem/cilastatin).

Concomitant use of valganciclovir and imipenem/cilastatin is not recommended.

Trimethoprim Concomitant use of ganciclovir and trimethoprim does not affect the pharmacokinetics of either drug.

Because of the potential for increased toxicity (e.g., nephrotoxicity), concomitant use of valganciclovir and trimethoprim should be considered only if potential benefits outweigh potential risks.

Other Antibacterials Because of the potential for increased toxicity (e.g., myelosuppression, nephrotoxicity) if valganciclovir is used with certain anti-infectives (e.g., co-trimoxazole, dapsone, pentamidine), concomitant use of valganciclovir and such anti-infectives should be considered only if potential benefits outweigh potential risks.

■ **Antifungal Agents** ***Amphotericin B*** If valganciclovir and amphotericin B are used concomitantly, renal function should be monitored since there is a potential for increased serum creatinine concentrations.

Flucytosine Because of the potential for increased toxicity (e.g., myelosuppression, nephrotoxicity), concomitant use of valganciclovir and flucytosine should be considered only if potential benefits outweigh potential risks.

■ **Antineoplastic Agents** Because of the potential for increased toxicity (e.g., myelosuppression, nephrotoxicity), concomitant use of valganciclovir and certain antineoplastic agents (e.g., doxorubicin, hydroxyurea, vinblastine, vincristine) should be considered only if potential benefits outweigh potential risks.

■ **Antiretroviral Agents** ***Didanosine*** Concomitant use of ganciclovir and didanosine increases peak plasma concentrations and area under the plasma concentration-time curve (AUC) of didanosine, but does not affect the pharmacokinetics of ganciclovir.

If valganciclovir and didanosine are used concomitantly, the patient should be closely monitored for didanosine toxicity (e.g., pancreatitis).

Tenofovir Concomitant use of valganciclovir and tenofovir alafenamide or tenofovir disoproxil fumarate may result in increased serum concentrations of ganciclovir and/or tenofovir; patients receiving such concomitant therapy should be monitored for dose-related toxicities.

Zidovudine Concomitant use of ganciclovir and zidovudine has resulted in additive or synergistic bone marrow toxicity.

If valganciclovir and zidovudine are used concomitantly, there is an increased risk of hematologic toxicity. Concomitant use of valganciclovir and zidovudine should be considered only if potential benefits outweigh potential risks.

■ **Immunosuppressive Agents** ***Cyclosporine*** Concomitant use of ganciclovir and cyclosporine does not appear to affect cyclosporine whole blood concentrations.

If valganciclovir and cyclosporine are used concomitantly, renal function should be monitored since there is potential for increased serum creatinine concentrations.

Mycophenolate Mofetil Concomitant use of ganciclovir and mycophenolate mofetil in patients with normal renal function does not affect the pharmacokinetics of either drug.

If valganciclovir and mycophenolate mofetil are used concomitantly, the patient should be monitored for hematologic and renal toxicity because of increased risk.

Tacrolimus Because of the potential for increased toxicity (e.g., nephrotoxicity) if valganciclovir is used with tacrolimus, concomitant use should be considered only if potential benefits outweigh potential risks.

■ **Probenecid** Concomitant use of ganciclovir and probenecid decreases renal clearance and increases the AUC of ganciclovir.

If valganciclovir and probenecid are used concomitantly, dosage of valganciclovir may need to be reduced and the patient should be monitored for evidence of ganciclovir toxicity.

Description

Valganciclovir, the L-valyl ester of ganciclovir, is an antiviral agent. Valganciclovir is a prodrug and exhibits no antiviral activity until converted by intestinal and hepatic esterases to ganciclovir and subsequently to the active form ganciclovir triphosphate.

Valganciclovir is commercially available as the hydrochloride salt and differs structurally from ganciclovir by the presence of the L-amino acid, valine, attached to the 2-hydroxyl group of the nucleoside and by the presence of the monohydrochloride salt. These structural modifications result in substantially increased GI absorption of valganciclovir relative to oral ganciclovir (no longer commercially available in the US), resulting in plasma ganciclovir concentrations comparable to those achieved with IV ganciclovir.

Valganciclovir is rapidly converted to ganciclovir in vivo and subsequently phosphorylated within cytomegalovirus (CMV)-infected cells to ganciclovir triphosphate. Since initial phosphorylation of ganciclovir depends largely on the presence of a viral kinase (pUL97), phosphorylation occurs preferentially in virus-infected cells. Ganciclovir triphosphate is a viral DNA polymerase inhibitor and exerts its antiviral activity on CMV by inhibiting the viral DNA polymerase. Other mechanisms also are involved. For additional information, see Mechanism of Action in Ganciclovir 8:18.32.

The absolute bioavailability of ganciclovir following oral administration of valganciclovir is about 60%. Results from pharmacokinetic studies in adults indicate that oral administration of valganciclovir 900 mg once daily with food provides a mean area under the plasma concentration-time curve$_{0\text{–}24\text{ hour}}$ (AUC$_{0\text{–}24\text{ hour}}$) for ganciclovir comparable to that following IV ganciclovir 5 mg/kg once daily. However, at these dosages, oral valganciclovir produces lower peak plasma ganciclovir concentrations than IV ganciclovir.

■ **Spectrum** Following conversion of valganciclovir to the pharmacologically active ganciclovir triphosphate, the drug is active against human herpes viruses, including CMV, herpes simplex virus types 1 and 2 (HSV-1 and HSV-2), and varicella-zoster virus (VZV). Although the clinical importance is unclear, ganciclovir has some in vitro activity against Epstein-Barr virus (EBV) and human herpes viruses types 6 and 8 (HHV-6 and HHV-8). Ganciclovir is not active against human immunodeficiency virus type 1 (HIV-1).

■ **Resistance** CMV isolates with reduced susceptibility or resistance to ganciclovir have been selected in vitro in the presence of the drug. CMV resistant to ganciclovir may emerge after prolonged treatment or prophylaxis with the drug, and the possibility of ganciclovir-resistant CMV should be considered in patients who show poor clinical response or relapse or experience persistent viral shedding during valganciclovir therapy.

Resistance can occur as the result of amino acid substitutions in the viral protein kinase pUL97 and/or the viral DNA polymerase pUL54. Certain pUL97 ganciclovir resistance-associated substitutions (e.g., M460V/I, H520Q, C529G, A594V, L595S, C603W) have been reported most frequently in clinical isolates. Numerous other pUL97 and pUL54 ganciclovir resistance-associated mutations also have been reported.

Cross-resistance can occur between ganciclovir and some other antivirals (e.g., acyclovir, cidofovir, foscarnet). Certain amino acid substitutions selected in vitro in cell culture following exposure of CMV to ganciclovir, cidofovir, or foscarnet have resulted in cross-resistance. Amino acid substitutions in pUL54 that confer cross-resistance between ganciclovir and cidofovir generally have involved the exonuclease domains and region V of the viral DNA polymerase. A variety of amino acid substitutions have conferred cross-resistance between ganciclovir and foscarnet, but concentrate at and between regions II and III of viral DNA polymerase.

Advice to Patients

Importance of reading the patient information and instructions for use provided by the manufacturer.

Importance of taking valganciclovir with food. Inform adults that they should receive valganciclovir tablets, not valganciclovir oral solution.

Inform patients that valganciclovir may cause granulocytopenia (neutropenia), anemia, thrombocytopenia, and elevated creatinine concentrations and that dosage modification or discontinuance of the drug may be required. Necessity of frequent monitoring of blood cell counts, platelet counts, and serum creatinine concentrations.

Advise patients that valganciclovir may cause seizures, dizziness, and/or confusion, which may affect tasks requiring alertness (e.g., ability to drive or operate machinery).

When valganciclovir is used for the management of cytomegalovirus (CMV) retinitis, advise patients that the drug is not a cure for CMV retinitis; progression of retinitis may occur during or after treatment with valganciclovir. Advise patients that regular ophthalmologic examinations during valganciclovir therapy (at least every 4–6 weeks) are necessary and some patients require more frequent follow-up.

Importance of informing clinicians of existing or contemplated concomitant therapy, including prescription and OTC drugs, as well as any concomitant illnesses.

Advise patients that valganciclovir is a potential carcinogen.

Advise patients that valganciclovir may cause temporary or permanent female and male infertility.

Advise females of reproductive potential that the drug causes birth defects in animals.

Importance of women informing clinicians if they are or plan to become pregnant or plan to breast-feed. Advise women to avoid pregnancy and to not breast-feed infants.

Importance of both women and men using effective contraception during valganciclovir therapy. Advise females of reproductive potential to use effective contraception during and for at least 30 days after valganciclovir therapy. Advise male patients to use effective barrier contraception during and for at least 90 days after valganciclovir therapy.

Importance of advising patients of other important precautionary information. (See Cautions.)

Overview® (see Users Guide). For additional information on this drug until a more detailed monograph is developed and published, the manufacturer's labeling should be consulted. It is *essential* that the manufacturer's labeling be consulted for more detailed information on usual cautions, precautions, contraindications, potential drug interactions, laboratory test interferences, and acute toxicity.

Preparations

Excipients in commercially available drug preparations may have clinically important effects in some individuals; consult specific product labeling for details.

valGANciclovir Hydrochloride

Oral		
For solution	250 mg (of valganciclovir) per 5 mL*	**Valcyte®**, Roche **Valganciclovir for Oral Solution**
Tablets, film-coated	450 mg (of valganciclovir)*	**Valcyte®**, Roche **Valganciclovir Tablets**

*available from one or more manufacturer, distributor, and/or repackager by generic (nonproprietary) name

†Use is not currently included in the labeling approved by the US Food and Drug Administration

HCV Antivirals 8:18.40

HCV Polymerase Inhibitors 8:18.40.16

Sofosbuvir SOF

■ Sofosbuvir, an antiviral, is a nucleotide analog hepatitis C virus (HCV) nonstructural 5B (NS5B) polymerase inhibitor.

Uses

■ **Chronic Hepatitis C Virus Infection** Sofosbuvir is used in conjunction with other antivirals for the treatment of chronic hepatitis C virus (HCV) genotype 1, 2, 3, or 4 infection in treatment-naive (previously untreated) or previously treated adults without cirrhosis or with compensated cirrhosis, including those with human immunodeficiency virus (HIV) coinfection and those with hepatocellular carcinoma awaiting liver transplantation. Although data are limited, sofosbuvir also has been used in conjunction with other antivirals for the treatment of chronic HCV infection caused by genotype 5† or genotype 6†.

Sofosbuvir is used in conjunction with other antivirals for the treatment of HCV genotype 2 or 3 in treatment-naive or previously treated pediatric patients 12 years of age and older without cirrhosis or with compensated cirrhosis.

Sofosbuvir *must* be used in conjunction with other antivirals as part of a multiple-drug regimen and should *not* be used alone for the treatment of chronic HCV infection. The drug is used in a multiple-drug regimen that includes sofosbuvir and ribavirin (with or without peginterferon alfa), a multiple-drug regimen that includes sofosbuvir and simeprevir, or a multiple-drug regimen that includes sofosbuvir and daclatasvir (with or without ribavirin). Sofosbuvir also is used in conjunction with ledipasvir, and a fixed combination containing ledipasvir and sofosbuvir (ledipasvir/sofosbuvir) is commercially available. For information on clinical studies evaluating efficacy and safety of the fixed combination ledipasvir/sofosbuvir for the treatment of chronic HCV infection, see Uses in Ledipasvir and Sofosbuvir 8:18.40.24. In addition, sofosbuvir is commercially available in fixed combination with velpatasvir (sofosbuvir/velpatasvir).

The specific multiple-drug regimen and duration of treatment with sofosbuvir and other antivirals depend on the HCV genotype and patient population. (See Dosage and Administration: Dosage.)

Because the treatment of chronic HCV infection is complex and rapidly evolving, it is recommended that treatment be directed by clinicians who are familiar with the disease and that a specialist be consulted to obtain the most up-to-date information. Information from the American Association for the Study of Liver Diseases (AASLD), Infectious Diseases Society of America (IDSA), and International Antiviral Society–USA (IAS–USA) regarding diagnosis and management of HCV infection, including recommendations for initial treatment, is available at http://www.hcvguidelines.org.

HCV Genotype 1 Infection **Sofosbuvir in Conjunction with Daclatasvir and Ribavirin.** Efficacy and safety of daclatasvir in conjunction with sofosbuvir *and* ribavirin for the treatment of chronic HCV genotype 1 infection were evaluated in a phase 3, open-label clinical trial (ALLY-1; NCT02032875) that included 113 treatment-naive or previously treated adults with cirrhosis or HCV recurrence after liver transplantation (median age 59 years, 67% male, 96% white, 4% black, 1% Asian, 59% treatment experienced, 71% with baseline HCV RNA levels 800,000 IU/mL or greater, 58% HCV genotype 1a, 19% HCV genotype 1b, 4% HCV genotype 2, 15% HCV genotype 3, 4% HCV genotype 4, 1% HCV genotype 6, 77% with IL28B rs12979860 non-CC genotype). Those previously treated with a regimen that included an HCV nonstructural 5A (NS5A) replication complex inhibitor (HCV NS5A inhibitor) were excluded. All patients in ALLY-1 received a 12-week regimen of daclatasvir (60 mg once daily) in conjunction with sofosbuvir (400 mg once daily) *and* ribavirin (daily dosage of 600 mg or less initially; titrated up to 1 g daily if tolerated) and were monitored for 24 weeks after treatment completion. The primary end point was SVR12 (defined as plasma HCV RNA level less than 25 IU/mL [the lower limit of quantification] at 12 weeks after the end of treatment). The overall SVR12 rates in the 86 patients with HCV genotype 1 infection were 82% in those with cirrhosis and 95% in transplant recipients. The SVR12 rates were similar in treatment-naive or previously treated patients and were comparable regardless of age, gender, IL28B allele status, or baseline HCV RNA level.

ALLY-1 included 60 patients with cirrhosis (20% Child-Pugh class A, 53% Child-Pugh class B, and 27% Child-Pugh class C); 35% had baseline Model for End-stage Liver Disease (MELD) scores of 15 or greater. Following a 12-week treatment regimen of daclatasvir in conjunction with sofosbuvir *and* ribavirin, the SVR12 rate was 76% in cirrhotic patients with HCV genotype 1a infection and 100% in cirrhotic patients with HCV genotype 1b infection. When results were subdivided based on Child-Pugh class, the SVR12 rate was 91, 92, or 50% in those with Child-Pugh class A, B, or C, respectively. There was evidence that efficacy of the daclatasvir regimen was lower in cirrhotic patients with HCV genotype 1a infection when NS5A resistance-associated polymorphisms at amino acid positions M28, Q30, L31, or Y93 were present at baseline.

Sofosbuvir in Conjunction with Peginterferon Alfa and Ribavirin. Efficacy and safety of sofosbuvir in conjunction with peginterferon alfa and ribavirin for the treatment of chronic HCV infection were evaluated in an open-label, single-arm, phase 3 study (NEUTRINO; NCT01641640) that included 327 treatment-naive (previously untreated) adults (median age 54 years, 64% male, 79% white, 17% black, 14% Hispanic or Latino, 17% with cirrhosis of the liver). Of these, 292 patients (89%) were infected with HCV genotype 1 and the remainder were infected with HCV genotype 4, 5, or 6. Patients with hepatitis B virus (HBV) or HIV coinfection were excluded. All patients received a 12-week regimen of sofosbuvir 400 mg once daily, ribavirin (1 g daily in those weighing less than 75 kg or 1.2 g daily in those weighing 75 kg or more; given orally in divided doses), and peginterferon alfa-2a (180 mcg subcutaneously once weekly). When all patients (regardless of genotype) were evaluated, substantially more patients (90%) achieved a sustained virologic response at 12 weeks after the end of treatment (SVR12; defined as plasma HCV RNA level less than 25 IU/mL [the lower limit of quantification] at 12 weeks after the end of treatment) compared with the predefined historical control SVR rate of 60%. When only the 292 patients infected with HCV genotype 1 were evaluated, the SVR12 rate was 89% (92% for HCV genotype 1a and 82–83% for HCV genotype 1b). Overall, there were no substantial differences in SVR12 rates according to HCV genotype, race, or ethnic group. However, patients with cirrhosis had lower SVR12 rates than those without cirrhosis (80 and 92%, respectively) and patients with non-CC IL28B genotypes had lower SVR12 rates than those with the CC IL29B genotype (87 and 98%, respectively).

Sofosbuvir in Conjunction with Simeprevir. Efficacy and safety of simeprevir in conjunction with sofosbuvir for the treatment of chronic HCV genotype 1 infection were evaluated in an open-label, randomized, phase 2 trial (COSMOS; NCT01466790) and 2 open-label, phase 3 trials (OPTIMIST-1; NCT02114177 and OPTIMIST-2; NCT02114151).

The COSMOS trial included previously treated adults with METAVIR fibrosis score F0-F2 (cohort 1) or treatment-naive or previously treated adults with METAVIR fibrosis score F3-F4 and compensated liver disease (cohort 2).

Cohort 1 included 80 patients *without* advanced hepatic fibrosis who were prior null responders to treatment with peginterferon alfa and ribavirin (median age 56 years, 61% male, 41% METAVIR fibrosis score F0 or F1, 59% METAVIR fibrosis score F2, 98% with baseline HCV RNA levels exceeding 800,000 IU/mL, 78% HCV genotype 1a [50% of these with NS3 Q80K polymorphism at baseline]). Cohort 2 included 87 patients *with* advanced hepatic fibrosis who were treatment-naive or prior null responders to peginterferon alfa and ribavirin (median age 58 years, 67% male, 53% METAVIR fibrosis score F3, 47% METAVIR fibrosis score F4 [cirrhosis], 84% with baseline HCV RNA levels exceeding 800,000 IU/mL, 78% HCV genotype 1a [40% of these with NS3 Q80K polymorphism at baseline], 54% prior null responders, 46% treatment-naive). Patients were randomized to receive 12 or 24 weeks of simeprevir (150 mg once daily) and sofosbuvir (400 mg once daily) with or without ribavirin. The primary end point was SVR12 (defined as plasma HCV RNA level less than 25 IU/mL [the lower limit of quantification] at 12 weeks after planned end of treatment). Pooled data from both cohorts showed that the overall SVR12 rate was 95% in patients with METAVIR fibrosis score of F0–F3 who received 12 weeks of treatment and 96% in patients with METAVIR fibrosis score of F4 who received 24 weeks of treatment. Results showed that the addition of ribavirin to the simeprevir and sofosbuvir regimen did not increase response rates compared with the 2-drug regimen *without* ribavirin.

OPTIMIST-1 included 310 treatment-naive or previously treated adults without cirrhosis (median age 56 years, 53–56% male, 78–81% white, 16–20% black, median baseline HCV RNA levels 683,000–685,000 IU/mL, 75% HCV genotype 1a [40–42% of these with NS3 Q80K polymorphism at baseline], 66–74% treatment-naive, 26–34% previously treated). Patients were randomized in a 1:1 ratio to receive an 8- or 12-week regimen of simeprevir (150 mg once daily) and sofosbuvir (400 mg once daily). Sustained virologic response (SVR12; defined as plasma HCV RNA level less than 25 IU/mL [the lower limit of quantification] at 12 weeks after planned end of treatment) was achieved in 97% of patients who received the 12-week regimen compared with 83% of patients who received the 8-week regimen. The SVR12 rate in those receiving the 12-week regimen was substantially higher than the historical control SVR rate of 87%; the SVR rate in those receiving the 8-week regimen was *not* substantially higher than the historical control SVR rate.

OPTIMIST-2 included 103 treatment-naive or previously treated adults with compensated cirrhosis (median age 58 years, 81% male, 81% white, 19% black, median baseline HCV RNA levels 680,000 IU/mL, 70% HCV genotype 1a [47% of these with NS3 Q80K polymorphism at baseline], 49% treatment-naive, 51% previously treated). All patients received a 12-week regimen of simeprevir (150 mg once daily) and sofosbuvir (400 mg once daily). Sustained virologic response (SVR12; defined as plasma HCV RNA level less than 25 IU/mL [the lower limit of quantification] at 12 weeks after planned end of treatment) was achieved in 83% of patients; this SVR12 rate was higher than a composite historical control SVR rate reported for cirrhotic patients with HCV genotype 1 infection (70%). However, a 24-week regimen is recommended if sofosbuvir is used in conjunction with simeprevir for the treatment of HCV genotype 1 infection in adults with compensated cirrhosis (Child-Pugh class A).

HCV Genotype 2 or 3 Infection **Sofosbuvir in Conjunction with Daclatasvir.** Although data are limited, a regimen of daclatasvir in conjunction with sofosbuvir has been used for the treatment of chronic HCV infection caused by genotype 2.

Efficacy and safety of daclatasvir in conjunction with sofosbuvir for the treatment of chronic HCV genotype 3 infection have been evaluated in a phase 3, open-label clinical trial (ALLY-3; NCT02032901) that included 152 treatment-naive or previously treated adults (median age 55 years, 59% male, 66% treatment-naive, 90% white, 5% Asian, 4% black, 76% with baseline HCV RNA levels 800,000 IU/mL or greater, 21% with compensated cirrhosis, 40% with IL28B rs12979860 CC genotype). Of the 51 patients in whom a previous treatment failed, most had received prior treatment with a regimen of peginterferon alfa and ribavirin, 7 patients had received prior treatment with a sofosbuvir-based regimen, and 2 patients had received prior treatment with an investigational HCV cyclophilin inhibitor. Those previously treated with a regimen that included an HCV NS5A inhibitor were excluded. All patients in ALLY-3 received a 12-week regimen of daclatasvir (60 mg once daily) in conjunction with sofosbuvir (400 mg once daily) and were monitored for 24 weeks after treatment completion. The primary end point was SVR12 (defined as plasma HCV RNA level less than 25 IU/mL [the lower limit of quantification] at 12 weeks after the end of treatment). The overall SVR12 rate in patients with HCV genotype 3 infection was 89% (90% in treatment-naive patients and 86% in previously treated patients). The SVR12 rate was lower in patients with cirrhosis (63%) than in those without cirrhosis (96%). There was evidence that efficacy of the daclatasvir regimen also was lower in patients with HCV genotype 3 infection who had NS5A polymorphisms present at baseline. The SVR12 rates were comparable regardless of HCV treatment history, age, gender, IL28B allele status, or baseline HCV RNA level.

Sofosbuvir in Conjunction with Ribavirin in Adults. Safety and efficacy of sofosbuvir in conjunction with ribavirin for the treatment of chronic HCV genotype 2 or 3 infection have been evaluated in four phase 3 clinical trials (FISSION, FUSION, VALANCE, POSITRON). In each trial, sofosbuvir was given in conjunction with ribavirin (1 g daily in those weighing less than 75 kg or 1.2 g daily in those weighing 75 kg or more; given orally in divided doses). The primary end point in each trial was SVR12 (defined as plasma HCV RNA level less than 25 IU/mL [the lower limit of quantification] at 12 weeks after the end of treatment).

FISSION (NCT01497366), a randomized, open-label, active-controlled phase 3 study, evaluated the safety and efficacy of sofosbuvir in conjunction with ribavirin in 499 treatment-naive adults with HCV genotype 2 or 3 infection (median age 50 years, 66% male, 87% white, 3% black, 14% Hispanic or Latino, 20% with cirrhosis of the liver, 28% HCV genotype 2 infection, 72% HCV genotype 3 infection). Patients with HBV or HIV coinfection were excluded. Patients were randomized to receive a 12-week regimen of sofosbuvir 400 mg once daily in conjunction with ribavirin (1 g daily in those weighing less than 75 kg or 1.2 g daily in those weighing 75 kg or more; given orally in divided doses) or a 24-week regimen of peginterferon alfa-2a (180 mcg subcutaneously once weekly) in conjunction with ribavirin (800 mg daily given orally in divided doses). In patients with HCV genotype 2 infection, SVR12 rates were 95 or 78% in the sofosbuvir group or active-control group, respectively. In patients with HCV genotype 3 infection, SVR12 rates were suboptimal (56 or 63% in the sofosbuvir group or active-control group, respectively). In those who received sofosbuvir, HCV genotype 3 infection and cirrhosis of the liver were associated with lower SVR12 rates.

FUSION (NCT01604850), a randomized, double-blind phase 3 study, evaluated the safety and efficacy of sofosbuvir in conjunction with ribavirin in 201 previously treated adults with HCV genotype 2 or 3 infection who did not achieve SVR with a previous interferon-based regimen (median age 56 years, 70% male, 87% white, 3% black, 9% Hispanic or Latino, 34% with cirrhosis of the liver, 63% HCV genotype 3 infection, 75% with previous relapse). Patients were randomized to receive a 16-week regimen of sofosbuvir 400 mg once daily in conjunction with ribavirin or a 12-week regimen of sofosbuvir 400 mg once daily in conjunction with ribavirin followed by 4 weeks of matching placebo. Demographic and baseline characteristics were balanced between groups. In patients with HCV genotype 2 infection, SVR12 rate was 82% in those treated with the 12-week regimen of sofosbuvir in conjunction with ribavirin; the SVR12 rate in patients with HCV genotype 2 infection treated with the 16-week regimen of sofosbuvir in conjunction with ribavirin was not substantially increased compared with the 12-week regimen. In patients with HCV genotype 3 infection, SVR12 rates were suboptimal regardless of whether the 12- or 16-week treatment regimen was used. In both groups, HCV genotype 3 and cirrhosis of the liver were associated with lower SVR12 rates.

VALENCE (NCT0168720), a randomized, placebo-controlled phase 3 trial, evaluated sofosbuvir in conjunction with ribavirin in 419 adults infected with HCV genotype 2 or 3 who were treatment-naive *or* previously treated and did not achieve SVR with an interferon-based regimen (median age 51 years, 60% male, 78% HCV genotype 3 infection, 58% previously treated). Patients were randomized to receive 12 weeks of sofosbuvir 400 mg once daily in conjunction with ribavirin or a placebo-only regimen. Based on emerging data, the trial was unblinded prior to completion and treatment regimens were modified for certain groups; patients infected with HCV genotype 2 received the originally planned 12-week regimen of sofosbuvir in conjunction with ribavirin; patients infected with HCV genotype 3 received sofosbuvir in conjunction with ribavirin for 24 weeks. Those who received placebo (85 patients) and those with HCV genotype 3 infection who received only 12 weeks of treatment (11 patients) were not included in the efficacy analysis. SVR12 was achieved by 93% of patients with HCV genotype 2 infection treated with the 12-week regimen of sofosbuvir in conjunction with ribavirin and 84–85% of patients with HCV genotype 3 infection treated with the 24-week regimen of sofosbuvir in conjunction with ribavirin. The SVR12 rate was 97 or 93% in treatment-naive patients with HCV genotype 2 or 3 infection, respectively, and 90 or 77% in previously treated patients with HCV genotype 2 or 3 infection, respectively.

POSITRON (NCT01542788), a randomized, double-bind, placebo-controlled phase 3 study, evaluated a regimen of sofosbuvir in conjunction with ribavirin in treatment-naive and previously treated adults with HCV genotype 2 or 3 infection who were intolerant, ineligible, or unwilling to receive treatment with an interferon-containing regimen. In this study, 278 patients (median age 54 years, 54% male, 91% white, 5% black, 11% Hispanic or Latino, 16% with cirrhosis of the liver, 49% HCV genotype 3 infection, 81% treatment-naive) were randomized to receive a 12-week treatment regimen of sofosbuvir 400 mg once daily in conjunction with ribavirin or a regimen of matching placebo only. Demographic and baseline characteristics were balanced between groups. In patients with HCV genotype 2 infection, the SVR12 rate was 93% in those treated with sofosbuvir in conjunction with ribavirin compared with 0% in those treated with placebo. In patients with HCV genotype 3 infection treated with sofosbuvir in conjunction with ribavirin, the SVR12 rate was suboptimal (61%).

Sofosbuvir in Conjunction with Ribavirin in Pediatric Patients. Safety and efficacy of sofosbuvir in conjunction with ribavirin for the treatment of chronic HCV genotype 2 or 3 infection in pediatric patients 12 years of age and older weighing at least 35 kg were evaluated in a phase 2, open-label study (Study 1112). In this study, 50 patients (median age 15 years, 42% female, 90% white, 4% black, 4% Hispanic/Latino, 2% Asian, 26% HCV genotype 2, 74% HCV genotype 3, 18% previously treated, 66% with baseline HCV RNA levels exceeding 800,000 IU/mL, 74% with non-CC IL28B alleles) received sofosbuvir in conjunction with ribavirin. The duration of treatment was 12 weeks in patients with HCV genotype 2 infection and 24 weeks in those with HCV genotype 3 infection. SVR12 was achieved in 97 or 100% of patients with HCV genotype 2 or 3 infection, respectively. No patient experienced on-treatment virologic failure or relapse.

HCV Genotype 4 Infection **Sofosbuvir in Conjunction with Peginterferon Alfa and Ribavirin.** Safety and efficacy of sofosbuvir in conjunction with peginterferon alfa and ribavirin for the treatment of chronic HCV infection were evaluated in an open-label, single-arm study (NEUTRINO) that included 327 treatment-naive adults (median age 54 years, 64% male, 79% white, 17%

black, 14% Hispanic or Latino, 17% with cirrhosis of the liver) infected with HCV genotype 1, 4, 5, or 6. Of these, 28 patients (9%) were infected with HCV genotype 4. Patients with HBV or HIV coinfection were excluded. All patients received a 12-week regimen of sofosbuvir 400 mg once daily in conjunction with oral ribavirin and subcutaneous peginterferon alfa-2a. Of the 28 patients with HCV genotype 4 infection, 27 patients (96%) achieved SVR12.

HCV Genotype 5 or 6 Infection **Sofosbuvir in Conjunction with Peginterferon Alfa and Ribavirin.** Safety and efficacy of sofosbuvir in conjunction with peginterferon alfa and ribavirin for the treatment of chronic HCV infection were studied in an open-label, single-arm study (NEUTRINO) that included 327 treatment-naive adults (median age 54 years, 64% male, 79% white, 17% black, 14% Hispanic or Latino, 17% with cirrhosis of the liver) infected with HCV genotype 1, 4, 5, or 6. Of these, 1 patient was infected with HCV genotype 5, and 6 patients were infected with HCV genotype 6. Patients with HBV or HIV coinfection were excluded. All patients received a 12-week regimen of sofosbuvir 400 mg once daily in conjunction with oral ribavirin and subcutaneous peginterferon alfa-2a. All 7 patients with HCV genotype 5 or 6 infection achieved SVR12.

HCV-infected Individuals Coinfected with HIV **Sofosbuvir in Conjunction with Daclatasvir.** In a phase 3, open-label trial (ALLY-2; NCT02032888), efficacy and safety of daclatasvir in conjunction with sofosbuvir were evaluated for the treatment of chronic HCV infection in 153 adults coinfected with HIV-1 (median age 53 years, 88% male, 63% white, 33% black, 68% with HCV genotype 1a, 15% with HCV genotype 1b, 8% with HCV genotype 2, 7% with HCV genotype 3, 2% with HCV genotype 4, 66% HCV treatment-naive, 80% with baseline HCV RNA levels 800,000 IU/mL or greater, 16% with compensated cirrhosis, 73% with IL28B rs12979860 non-CC genotype). Those previously treated with a regimen that included an HCV NS5A inhibitor were excluded. All patients who received a 12-week regimen of daclatasvir (60 mg once daily; dosage adjusted when necessary based on concomitant HIV antiretroviral agents) in conjunction with sofosbuvir (400 mg once daily) also received concomitant antiretroviral therapy, including HIV protease inhibitor-based regimens (*ritonavir-boosted* atazanavir, *ritonavir-boosted* darunavir, fixed combination of lopinavir and ritonavir [lopinavir/ritonavir]), HIV nonnucleoside reverse transcriptase inhibitor-based regimens (efavirenz, nevirapine, or rilpivirine), HIV integrase inhibitor-based regimens (raltegravir or dolutegravir), or a regimen that included only HIV nucleoside reverse transcriptase inhibitors (abacavir, emtricitabine, and zidovudine). The SVR12 rate was 97% in patients with HCV genotype 1 infection and HIV coinfection (91% in cirrhotic patients and 98% in noncirrhotic patients) and 100% in those with HCV genotype 3 infection and HIV coinfection. The SVR12 rates in these coinfected patients were comparable regardless of HCV treatment history, age, race, gender, IL28B allele status, HCV genotype 1 subtype, or baseline HCV RNA level. Treatment of HCV infection in these HIV-infected patients did not appear to interfere with maintenance of HIV virologic suppression. Data were insufficient to determine SVR12 and outcomes in those with HCV genotype 2, 4, 5, or 6 infection and HIV coinfection.

Sofosbuvir in Conjunction with Ribavirin. Efficacy and safety of sofosbuvir in conjunction with ribavirin for the treatment of chronic HCV infection in patients with HIV coinfection were studied in 2 open-label, nonrandomized, phase 3 studies (PHOTON-1, PHOTON-2).

In PHOTON-1, the safety and efficacy of sofosbuvir in conjunction with ribavirin were evaluated in 223 adults with HCV genotype 1, 2, or 3 infection who were coinfected with HIV type 1 (HIV-1). All patients with HCV genotype 1 infection were treatment-naive; patients with HCV genotype 2 or 3 were either treatment-naive or previously treated. Patients had $CD4^+$ T-cell counts greater than 500 cells/mm^3 and were not receiving antiretroviral therapy *or* were receiving antiretroviral therapy and had virologically suppressed HIV-1 (plasma HIV-1 levels less than 50 copies/mL) and $CD4^+$ T-cell counts greater than 200 cells/mm^3. Patients received sofosbuvir 400 mg once daily in conjunction with ribavirin (1 g daily in those weighing less than 75 kg or 1.2 g daily in those weighing 75 kg or more; given orally in divided doses) for 12 or 24 weeks depending on HCV genotype and prior treatment history. In treatment-naive patients with HCV genotype 1 infection who received a 24-week treatment regimen, the SVR12 rate was 76%. In treatment-naive patients with HCV genotype 2 or 3 infection who received a 12-week treatment regimen, the SVR12 rate was 88 or 67%, respectively. In previously treated patients with HCV genotype 2 or 3 infection who received a 24-week treatment regimen, the SVR12 rate was 92 or 94%, respectively. Overall, $CD4^+$ T-cell percentages did not change during HCV treatment. The median $CD4^+$ T-cell count decreased by 85 or 84 cells/mm^3 in patients receiving sofosbuvir in conjunction with ribavirin for 12 or 24 weeks, respectively.

In PHOTON-2, the safety and efficacy of sofosbuvir in conjunction with ribavirin were evaluated in 274 adults with HCV genotype 1, 2, 3, or 4 infection who were coinfected with HIV-1. All patients with HCV genotype 1 or 4 infection were treatment-naive; patients with HCV genotype 2 or 3 infection were either treatment-naive or previously treated. Patients had $CD4^+$ T-cell counts greater than 500 cells/mm^3 and were not receiving antiretroviral therapy *or* were receiving antiretroviral therapy and had virologically suppressed HIV-1 (plasma HIV-1 levels less than 50 copies/mL) and $CD4^+$ T-cell counts greater than 200 cells/mm^3. Patients received sofosbuvir 400 mg once daily in conjunction with ribavirin (1 g daily in those weighing less than 75 kg or 1.2 g daily in those weighing 75 kg or more) for 24 weeks, but treatment-naive patients with genotype 2 infection received this regimen for 12 weeks. In treatment-naive patients with HCV genotype 1, 3, or 4 infection who received a 24-week treatment regimen, the SVR12 rate was 85, 91, or 84%, respectively. In treatment-naive patients with HCV genotype 2 infection who received a 12-week treatment regimen, the SVR12 rate was 89%. In previously treated patients with HCV genotype 2 or 3 infection who received a 24-week treatment regimen, the SVR12 rate was 83 or 86%, respectively. Overall, $CD4^+$ T-cell percentages were largely unaffected during HCV treatment. The median decrease in $CD4^+$ T-cell count from baseline to end of HCV treatment was 39 or 91 cells/mm^3 in those who received sofosbuvir in conjunction with ribavirin for 12 or 24 weeks, respectively.

HCV-infected Individuals with Hepatocellular Carcinoma Awaiting Liver Transplantation **Sofosbuvir in Conjunction with Ribavirin.** In an open-label trial, the safety and efficacy of sofosbuvir in conjunction with ribavirin were evaluated in HCV-infected adults with hepatocellular carcinoma awaiting liver transplantation. All patients met Milan criteria (defined as the presence of a solitary tumor 5 cm or less in diameter or no more than 3 tumor nodules, each 3 cm or less in diameter, and no extrahepatic manifestations of the cancer or evidence of vascular invasion by tumor). A treatment regimen of sofosbuvir 400 mg once daily in conjunction with ribavirin (1–1.2 g daily based on weight) was given to patients prior to liver transplantation in order to prevent post-transplantation reinfection. The duration of treatment was 24–48 weeks or until the time of liver transplantation, whichever occurred first. An interim analysis showed that 61 patients had received sofosbuvir in conjunction with ribavirin (74% HCV genotype 1 infection, 72% baseline Child-Pugh-Turcotte [CPT] score less than 7, 100% with baseline unadjusted MELD score of 14 or less). Of these, 41 patients underwent liver transplantation. Interim results showed that the post-transplant virologic response rate (defined as HCV RNA level below the lower limit of quantification at 12 weeks after transplantation) was 64% in the 36 evaluable patients.

Dosage and Administration

■ **General** For the treatment of chronic hepatitis C virus (HCV) infection, sofosbuvir *must* be used in conjunction with other antivirals and should *not* be used alone.

The specific multiple-drug regimen and duration of treatment depend on the HCV genotype and patient population.

Prior to initiating sofosbuvir for treatment of HCV infection, all patients should be tested for evidence of current or prior hepatitis B virus (HBV) infection by measuring hepatitis B surface antigen (HBsAg), hepatitis B surface antibody (anti-HBs), and hepatitis B core antibody (anti-HBc). (See Risk of HBV Reactivation in Patients Coinfected with HCV and HBV under Warnings/Precautions: Warnings, in Cautions.)

Sofosbuvir dosage should *not* be reduced for any reason. If serious adverse reactions potentially related to other antivirals included in the multiple-drug regimen occur, dosage adjustment (dosage modification) or discontinuance of these drugs may be necessary according to the respective manufacturer's prescribing information. If other antivirals in the multiple-drug regimen are discontinued for any reason, sofosbuvir also should be discontinued.

For information on dosage and administration of the fixed combination containing ledipasvir and sofosbuvir (ledipasvir/sofosbuvir), see Dosage and Administration in Ledipasvir and Sofosbuvir 8:18.40.24.

For information on dosage and administration of the fixed combination containing sofosbuvir and velpatasvir (sofosbuvir/velpatasvir), see Dosage and Administration in Sofosbuvir and Velpatasvir 8:18.40.16.

■ **Administration** Sofosbuvir is administered orally once daily without regard to food.

If a dose of sofosbuvir is missed, it should be taken that day as soon as it is remembered and the regular dosing schedule should be resumed the next day. No more than a single 400-mg dose of sofosbuvir should be taken on any calendar day.

■ **Adult Dosage** ***HCV Genotype 1 Infection*** **Sofosbuvir in Conjunction with Daclatasvir.** If sofosbuvir is used in conjunction with daclatasvir for the treatment of chronic HCV genotype 1 infection in adults *without* cirrhosis, the recommended dosage of sofosbuvir is 400 mg once daily in conjunction with daclatasvir (60 mg once daily). Both drugs are continued for 12 weeks.

If sofosbuvir is used in conjunction with daclatasvir for the treatment of chronic HCV genotype 1 infection in adults with compensated cirrhosis (Child-Pugh class A), the recommended dosage of sofosbuvir is 400 mg once daily in conjunction with daclatasvir (60 mg once daily). The manufacturer of daclatasvir recommends that both drugs be continued for 12 weeks. Some experts recommend a treatment duration of 24 weeks in patients with compensated cirrhosis and state that consideration can be given to adding ribavirin to the sofosbuvir and daclatasvir regimen.

If sofosbuvir is used in conjunction with daclatasvir *and* ribavirin for the treatment of chronic HCV genotype 1 infection in adults with decompensated cirrhosis (Child-Pugh class B or C), the recommended dosage of sofosbuvir is 400 mg once daily in conjunction with daclatasvir (60 mg once daily) *and* ribavirin. The usual duration of treatment is 12 weeks, but the optimal duration of treatment in patients with HCV genotype 1 infection who have cirrhosis has not been established. If a regimen of sofosbuvir and daclatasvir (without ribavirin) is used for the treatment of HCV genotype 1 infection in patients with decompensated cirrhosis who cannot receive ribavirin, some experts recommend a treatment duration of 24 weeks. HCV-infected patients with decompensated cirrhosis should be referred to an expert for treatment (ideally at a liver transplant center).

Sofosbuvir in Conjunction with Peginterferon Alfa and Ribavirin. If sofosbuvir is used in conjunction with peginterferon alfa and ribavirin for the treatment of chronic HCV genotype 1 infection in treatment-naive adults *without* cirrhosis or with compensated cirrhosis (Child-Pugh class A), the recommended dosage of sofosbuvir is 400 mg once daily in conjunction with peginterferon alfa *and* ribavirin for a duration of 12 weeks.

Sofosbuvir in Conjunction with Ribavirin. If sofosbuvir is used in conjunction with ribavirin for the treatment of chronic HCV genotype 1 infection in adults unable to receive peginterferon alfa (interferon-ineligible patients), the recommended dosage of sofosbuvir is 400 mg once daily in conjunction with ribavirin for a duration of 24 weeks.

Sofosbuvir in Conjunction with Simeprevir. If sofosbuvir is used in conjunction with simeprevir for the treatment of chronic HCV genotype 1 infection in adults, the recommended dosage of sofosbuvir is 400 mg once daily in conjunction with simeprevir (150 mg once daily with food). Both drugs are continued for 12 or 24 weeks, depending on whether or not the patient has compensated cirrhosis (Child-Pugh class A). (See Table 1.) For the treatment of HCV genotype 1 infection in patients with compensated cirrhosis, some experts state that consideration can be given to adding ribavirin to the 24-week regimen of sofosbuvir and simeprevir.

Table 1. Recommended Treatment Duration of Sofosbuvir in Conjunction with Simeprevir in Adults with HCV Genotype 1 Infection.

Patient Type	Duration of Sofosbuvir in Conjunction with Simeprevir
Treatment-naive or previously treated[a] adults (*without* cirrhosis)	12 weeks
Treatment-naive or previously treated[a] adults (*with* compensated cirrhosis)	24 weeks

[a] Previously treated defined as patients with prior relapse, prior partial response, or prior null response who failed prior interferon-based treatment.

HCV Genotype 2 Infection **Sofosbuvir in Conjunction with Daclatasvir.** If sofosbuvir is used in conjunction with daclatasvir (without ribavirin) for the treatment of chronic HCV genotype 2 infection in adults *without* cirrhosis or with compensated cirrhosis, some experts recommended a sofosbuvir dosage of 400 mg once daily in conjunction with daclatasvir (60 mg once daily). These experts recommend a treatment duration of 12 weeks in those *without* cirrhosis and a treatment duration of 16–24 weeks in those with compensated cirrhosis.

If sofosbuvir is used in conjunction with daclatasvir *and* ribavirin for the treatment of chronic HCV genotype 2 infection in adults with decompensated cirrhosis (Child-Pugh class B or C), some experts recommend a sofosbuvir dosage of 400 mg once daily in conjunction with daclatasvir (60 mg once daily) *and* ribavirin for a treatment duration of 12 weeks. HCV-infected patients with decompensated cirrhosis should be referred to an expert for treatment (ideally at a liver transplant center).

Sofosbuvir in Conjunction with Ribavirin. For the treatment of chronic HCV genotype 2 infection in treatment-naive or previously treated (defined as patients who failed an interferon-based regimen with or without ribavirin) adults *without* cirrhosis or with compensated cirrhosis (Child-Pugh class A), the recommended dosage of sofosbuvir is 400 mg once daily in conjunction with ribavirin for a duration of 12 weeks.

HCV Genotype 3 Infection **Sofosbuvir in Conjunction with Daclatasvir.** If sofosbuvir is used in conjunction with daclatasvir for the treatment of chronic HCV genotype 3 infection in adults *without* cirrhosis, the recommended dosage of sofosbuvir is 400 mg once daily in conjunction with daclatasvir (60 mg once daily). Both drugs are continued for 12 weeks.

If sofosbuvir is used in conjunction with daclatasvir for the treatment of chronic HCV genotype 3 infection in adults with compensated cirrhosis (Child-Pugh class A), the recommended dosage of sofosbuvir is 400 mg once daily in conjunction with daclatasvir (60 mg once daily) *and* ribavirin. The usual duration of treatment is 12 weeks, but the optimal duration of treatment in patients with HCV genotype 3 infection who have cirrhosis has not been established. Some experts recommend a duration of 24 weeks for the treatment of HCV genotype 3 infection in patients with compensated cirrhosis and state that a regimen of sofosbuvir and daclatasvir *without* ribavirin may be considered.

If sofosbuvir is used in conjunction with daclatasvir for the treatment of chronic HCV genotype 3 infection in adults with decompensated cirrhosis (Child-Pugh class B or C), the recommended dosage of sofosbuvir is 400 mg once daily in conjunction with daclatasvir (60 mg once daily) *and* ribavirin. The usual duration of treatment is 12 weeks, but the optimal duration of treatment in patients with HCV genotype 3 infection who have cirrhosis has not been established. HCV-infected patients with decompensated cirrhosis should be referred to an expert for treatment (ideally at a liver transplant center).

Sofosbuvir in Conjunction with Ribavirin. For the treatment of chronic HCV genotype 3 infection in treatment-naive or previously treated (defined as patients who failed an interferon based regimen with or without ribavirin) adults without cirrhosis or with compensated cirrhosis (Child-Pugh class A), the recommended dosage of sofosbuvir is 400 mg once daily in conjunction with ribavirin for a duration of 24 weeks.

HCV Genotype 4 Infection **Sofosbuvir in Conjunction with Daclatasvir.** If sofosbuvir is used in conjunction with daclatasvir for the treatment of chronic HCV genotype 4 infection in adults with decompensated cirrhosis (Child-Pugh class B or C), the recommended dosage of sofosbuvir is 400 mg once daily in conjunction with daclatasvir (60 mg once daily) *and* ribavirin for a duration of 12 weeks. If a regimen of sofosbuvir and daclatasvir (without ribavirin) is used for the treatment of HCV genotype 4 infection in patients with decompensated cirrhosis who cannot receive ribavirin, some experts recommend a treatment duration of 24 weeks. HCV-infected patients with decompensated cirrhosis should be referred to an expert for treatment (ideally at a liver transplant center).

Sofosbuvir in Conjunction with Peginterferon Alfa and Ribavirin. For the treatment of chronic HCV genotype 4 infection in treatment-naive adults *without* cirrhosis or with compensated cirrhosis (Child-Pugh class A), the recommended dosage of sofosbuvir is 400 mg once daily in conjunction with peginterferon alfa *and* ribavirin for a duration of 12 weeks.

HCV Genotype 5 or Genotype 6 Infection **Sofosbuvir in Conjunction with Peginterferon Alfa and Ribavirin.** The manufacturer states that data are insufficient to make sofosbuvir dosage recommendations for treatment of chronic HCV infection caused by genotype 5† or 6†. Some experts state that adults with HCV genotype 5 or 6 infection can receive 400 mg of sofosbuvir once daily in conjunction with peginterferon alfa *and* ribavirin for a duration of 12 weeks.

HCV-infected Individuals Coinfected with HIV Sofosbuvir dosage and sofosbuvir multiple-drug treatment regimens and duration of therapy recommended for the treatment of chronic HCV genotype 1, 2, 3, or 4 infection in adults coinfected with human immunodeficiency virus (HIV) generally are the same as those recommended for adults without HIV coinfection.

HCV-infected Individuals with Hepatocellular Carcinoma Awaiting Liver Transplantation **Sofosbuvir in Conjunction with Ribavirin.** For the treatment of chronic HCV infection and prevention of post-transplantation reinfection, adults with hepatocellular carcinoma awaiting liver transplantation may receive sofosbuvir in a dosage of 400 mg once daily in conjunction with ribavirin for up to 48 weeks or until the time of liver transplantation, whichever occurs first.

■ **Pediatric Dosage** ***HCV Genotype 2 Infection*** **Sofosbuvir in Conjunction with Ribavirin.** For the treatment of chronic HCV genotype 2 infection in treatment-naive or previously treated (defined as patients who failed an interferon-based regimen with or without ribavirin) pediatric patients 12 years of age and older weighing at least 35 kg *without* cirrhosis or with compensated cirrhosis (Child-Pugh class A), the recommended dosage of sofosbuvir is 400 mg once daily in conjunction with ribavirin for a duration of 12 weeks.

HCV Genotype 3 Infection **Sofosbuvir in Conjunction with Ribavirin.** For the treatment of chronic HCV genotype 2 infection in treatment-naive or previously treated pediatric patients 12 years of age and older weighing at least 35 kg *without* cirrhosis or with compensated cirrhosis (Child-Pugh class A), the recommended dosage of sofosbuvir is 400 mg once daily in conjunction with ribavirin for a duration of 24 weeks.

■ **Special Populations** ***Hepatic Impairment*** Sofosbuvir dosage adjustments are not needed in patients with mild, moderate, or severe hepatic impairment (Child-Pugh class A, B, or C). (See Hepatic Impairment under Warnings/Precautions: Specific Populations, in Cautions.)

Renal Impairment Sofosbuvir dosage adjustments are not needed in patients with mild or moderate renal impairment.

The manufacturer states that dosage recommendations cannot be made for patients with severe renal impairment (estimated glomerular filtration rate [eGFR] less than 30 mL/minute per 1.73 m^2) or end-stage renal disease (ESRD); safety and efficacy of sofosbuvir have not been established in such patients. (See Renal Impairment under Warnings/Precautions: Specific Populations, in Cautions.)

Geriatric Patients Sofosbuvir dosage adjustments are not needed in geriatric patients.

Cautions

■ **Contraindications** Because sofosbuvir *must* be used in conjunction with other antivirals, the contraindications for all antivirals included in the multiple-drug regimen should be considered. (See Precautions Related to Multiple-drug Treatment Regimens under Cautions: Warnings/Precautions.)

Sofosbuvir used in conjunction with ribavirin or in conjunction with peginterferon alfa *and* ribavirin is contraindicated in women who are pregnant or may become pregnant and men whose female partners are pregnant. (See Precautions Related to Multiple-drug Treatment Regimens under Warnings/Precautions: Other Warnings/Precautions, in Cautions.)

■ **Warnings/Precautions** ***Warnings*** **Risk of HBV Reactivation in Patients Coinfected with HCV and HBV.** Reactivation of hepatitis B virus (HBV) infection has been reported during postmarketing experience when direct-acting antivirals (DAAs) were used for the treatment of chronic hepatitis C virus (HCV) infection in patients with HBV coinfection. In some cases, HBV reactivation resulted in fulminant hepatitis, hepatic failure, and death.

HBV reactivation (defined as an abrupt increase in HBV replication manifested as a rapid increase in serum HBV DNA levels or detection of hepatitis B surface antigen [HBsAg] in an individual who was previously HBsAg negative and hepatitis B core antibody [anti-HBc] positive) has been reported in patients with HCV and HBV coinfection who were receiving HCV treatment with a regimen that included HCV DAAs without interferon alfa. Reactivation also may be accompanied by hepatitis (i.e., increased aminotransferase concentrations) and, in severe cases, may lead to increased bilirubin concentrations, liver failure, or death. Data to date indicate that HBV reactivation usually occurs within 4–8 weeks after initiation of HCV treatment. Patients with HBV reactivation have been heterogeneous in terms of HCV genotype and in terms of baseline HBV disease. While some patients with HBV reactivation were HBsAg positive, others had serologic evidence of resolved HBV infection (i.e., HBsAg negative and anti-HBc positive). HBV reactivation also has been reported in patients receiving certain immunosuppressant or chemotherapeutic drugs; the risk of reactivation associated with HCV DAAs may be increased in such patients.

The mechanism for HBV reactivation in patients with HCV and HBV coinfection receiving HCV DAAs is unknown. Although HCV DAAs are not known to cause immunosuppression, HBV reactivation in coinfected patients may result from a complex interplay of host immunologic responses in the setting of infection with 2 hepatitis viruses.

Prior to initiating treatment with an HCV DAA, including sofosbuvir, all patients should be screened for evidence of current or prior HBV infection by measuring HBsAg, anti-HBs, and anti-HBc. If there is serologic evidence of HBV infection, baseline HBV DNA levels should be measured.

Patients with evidence of current or prior HBV infection should be monitored for clinical and laboratory signs (i.e., HBsAg, HBV DNA levels, serum aminotransferase concentrations, bilirubin concentrations) of hepatitis flare or HBV reactivation during and after treatment with HCV DAAs, including sofosbuvir. Appropriate management for HBV infection should be initiated as clinically indicated.

Patients with HCV and HBV coinfection receiving sofosbuvir should be advised to immediately contact a clinician if they develop any signs or symptoms of serious liver injury (e.g., fatigue, weakness, loss of appetite, nausea and vomiting, yellowing of the eyes or skin, light-colored bowel movements).

When making decisions regarding HBV monitoring or HBV treatment in coinfected patients, consultation with a clinician who has expertise in managing HBV infection is recommended.

Other Warnings/Precautions **Cardiovascular Effects.** Symptomatic bradycardia, sometimes requiring pacemaker intervention, has been reported during postmarketing experience in patients receiving amiodarone concomitantly with an HCV treatment regimen containing sofosbuvir in conjunction with another HCV DAA, including ledipasvir, simeprevir, or an investigational HCV NS5A replication complex inhibitor. Fatal cardiac arrest was reported in a patient receiving amiodarone concomitantly with the fixed combination of ledipasvir and sofosbuvir (ledipasvir/sofosbuvir). In most reported cases, bradycardia occurred within hours to days after HCV treatment was initiated in patients receiving amiodarone, but has been observed up to 2 weeks after initiation of HCV treatment. Bradycardia generally resolved after HCV treatment was discontinued. The mechanism for this adverse cardiovascular effect is unknown.

Patients who may be at increased risk for symptomatic bradycardia if amiodarone is used concomitantly with an HCV treatment regimen containing sofosbuvir with another DAA include those also receiving a β-adrenergic blocking agent, those with underlying cardiac comorbidities, and/or those with advanced liver disease.

Concomitant use of amiodarone with an HCV treatment regimen containing sofosbuvir with another DAA is *not* recommended. If there are no alternative HCV treatment options and sofosbuvir with another DAA must be used in a patient receiving amiodarone, the patient should be advised about the risk of serious symptomatic bradycardia before HCV treatment is initiated. Cardiac monitoring should be performed in an inpatient setting during the first 48 hours of concomitant use of amiodarone and a regimen containing sofosbuvir with another DAA; heart rate monitoring should then be performed daily (outpatient or self-monitoring) through at least the first 2 weeks of concomitant use. Similar cardiac monitoring is recommended in patients who discontinued amiodarone just prior to initiation of a regimen containing sofosbuvir with another DAA or if there are no other treatment options and amiodarone must be initiated in a patient already receiving sofosbuvir with another DAA.

Patients receiving amiodarone concomitantly with a regimen containing sofosbuvir with another DAA should be advised to immediately contact a clinician if they develop signs or symptoms of bradycardia (e.g., near-fainting or fainting, dizziness, lightheadedness, malaise, weakness, excessive tiredness, shortness of breath, chest pain, confusion, memory problems).

Hematologic Effects. Anemia has been reported in patients receiving sofosbuvir in conjunction with ribavirin or in conjunction with peginterferon alfa *and* ribavirin. In clinical trials, anemia was reported in 21% of patients who received 12 weeks of treatment with sofosbuvir, peginterferon alfa, and ribavirin compared with 12% of patients who received 24 weeks of treatment with peginterferon alfa and ribavirin without sofosbuvir. In addition, hemoglobin concentrations less than 10 g/dL were reported in 23% of patients who received 12 weeks of treatment with sofosbuvir, peginterferon alfa, and ribavirin compared with 14% of patients who received 24 weeks of treatment with peginterferon alfa and ribavirin without sofosbuvir.

Interactions. Concomitant use of sofosbuvir with drugs that are inducers of the P-glycoprotein (P-gp) transport system in the intestine (e.g., rifampin, St. John's wort) is not recommended since this may result in substantially decreased sofosbuvir plasma concentrations and could lead to reduced therapeutic effect of sofosbuvir. (See Drug Interactions.)

Precautions Related to Multiple-drug Treatment Regimens. Sofosbuvir *must* be used in conjunction with other antivirals. The cautions, precautions, contraindications, and drug interactions associated with each drug in the multiple-drug regimen should be considered. Cautionary information applicable to specific populations (e.g., pregnant or nursing women, individuals with hepatic or renal impairment, geriatric patients) also should be considered for each drug.

Sofosbuvir should *not* be used concomitantly with the fixed combination of ledipasvir and sofosbuvir (ledipasvir/sofosbuvir) or the fixed combination containing sofosbuvir and velpatasvir (sofosbuvir/velpatasvir).

When sofosbuvir is used in conjunction with another HCV DAA (simeprevir, daclatasvir), the cautions, precautions, and contraindications associated with the other DAA also should be considered. (See Cautions in Daclatasvir 8:18.40.24.)

When sofosbuvir is used in conjunction with ribavirin or in conjunction with peginterferon alfa *and* ribavirin, the cautions, precautions, and contraindications associated with ribavirin and/or peginterferon alfa also should be considered. (See Cautions in Ribavirin 8:18.32 and see Cautions in Peginterferon Alfa 8:18.20.) Clinicians should consider that ribavirin may cause fetal toxicity and/or death and extreme care *must* be taken to avoid pregnancy in female patients and in female partners of male patients receiving the ribavirin-containing regimen. Women of childbearing potential should have a negative pregnancy test immediately prior to initiating ribavirin therapy and pregnancy tests should be performed monthly during and for 6 months after ribavirin treatment is completed. Women of childbearing potential (and their male partners) and male patients (and their female partners) *must* use at least 2 forms of effective contraception during and for 6 months after ribavirin treatment is completed. (See Cautions: Pregnancy, Fertility, and Lactation, in Ribavirin 8:18.32.)

Specific Populations **Pregnancy.** There are no adequate and well-controlled studies using sofosbuvir in pregnant women. In animal studies, no adverse developmental outcomes were observed at sofosbuvir exposures greater than those attained in humans using the recommended dosage.

When sofosbuvir is used in conjunction *with* ribavirin, clinicians should consider that ribavirin may cause fetal toxicity and/or death and extreme care must be taken to avoid pregnancy in female patients and in female partners of male patients receiving the ribavirin-containing regimen. (See Cautions: Pregnancy, Fertility, and Lactation, in Ribavirin 8:18.32.)

Lactation. It is not known whether sofosbuvir or its metabolites are distributed into human milk.

The predominant metabolite of sofosbuvir (GS-331007) is distributed into milk in rats (milk concentrations approximately 10% of the maternal plasma concentrations 1 hour after a single 20-mg/kg dose). GS-331007 had no apparent effects on the nursing pups.

The benefits of breast-feeding and the importance of sofosbuvir to the woman should be considered along with the potential adverse effects on the breast-fed child from the drug or from the underlying maternal condition.

When sofosbuvir is used in conjunction *with* ribavirin, the potential for adverse reactions to ribavirin in nursing infants should be considered and a decision should be made whether to discontinue nursing or the ribavirin-containing regimen, taking into account the importance of the treatment regimen to the woman. (See Precautions Related to Multiple-drug Treatment Regimens under Warnings/Precautions: Other Warnings/Precautions, in Cautions .)

Pediatric Use. Safety and efficacy of sofosbuvir for the treatment of HCV genotype 2 or 3 have not been established in children younger than 12 years of age or weighing less than 35 kg.

Safety and efficacy of sofosbuvir for the treatment of HCV genotype 1 or 4 infection have not been established in pediatric patients of any age.

Adverse effects and pharmacokinetics of sofosbuvir in pediatric patients 12 years of age and older with HCV genotype 2 or 3 infection are similar to those observed in adults.

Geriatric Use. There are no clinically important differences in response rates to sofosbuvir in patients 65 years of age or older compared with younger adults.

Population pharmacokinetic analysis in HCV-infected adults 19–75 years of age indicates there are no clinically important age-related differences in sofosbuvir or GS-331007 exposure in this age group.

Hepatic Impairment. Safety and efficacy of sofosbuvir have not been established in patients with decompensated cirrhosis or in post-liver transplant patients.

The safety profile of sofosbuvir used in conjunction with ribavirin in HCV-infected adults with hepatocellular carcinoma awaiting liver transplantation is similar to that observed in HCV-infected adults in phase 3 clinical trials.

Renal Impairment. Safety and efficacy of sofosbuvir have not been established in patients with severe renal impairment (estimated glomerular filtration rate [eGFR] less than 30 mL/minute per 1.73 m^2) or patients with end-stage renal disease (ESRD) requiring hemodialysis.

In individuals without HCV infection with severe renal impairment or ESRD requiring hemodialysis, a single 400-mg dose of sofosbuvir results in sofosbuvir and GS-331007 plasma exposures that are substantially higher than those reported in individuals with normal renal function.

■ Common Adverse Effects

Sofosbuvir in conjunction with ribavirin: Adverse effects reported in more than 20% of patients include fatigue and headache.

Sofosbuvir in conjunction with peginterferon alfa *and* ribavirin: Adverse effects reported in more than 20% of patients include fatigue, headache, nausea, insomnia, and anemia.

Sofosbuvir in conjunction with simeprevir: Adverse effects reported in more than 10% of patients include fatigue, headache, nausea, dizziness, diarrhea, insomnia, pruritus, and rash.

Sofosbuvir in conjunction with daclatasvir: Adverse effects reported in 5% or more of patients include headache, fatigue, nausea, diarrhea, and insomnia.

Drug Interactions

■ Drugs Affecting or Affected by P-glycoprotein Transport System Sofosbuvir is a substrate of the P-glycoprotein (P-gp) transport system; GS-331007, the predominant metabolite, is not a P-gp substrate. Pharmacokinetic interactions are possible with drugs that are inducers of P-gp in the intestine (e.g., rifampin, St. John's wort), which may decrease sofosbuvir plasma concentrations leading to reduced therapeutic effect of the HCV antiviral. Concomitant use of sofosbuvir and P-gp inhibitors may cause increased plasma concentrations of sofosbuvir without increasing plasma concentrations of GS-331007.

Sofosbuvir and GS-331007 are not inhibitors of P-gp; pharmacokinetic interactions are unlikely with drugs that are P-gp substrates.

■ Drugs Affecting or Affected by Breast Cancer Resistance Protein Sofosbuvir is a substrate of breast cancer resistance protein (BCRP); GS-331007 is not a BCRP substrate. Inhibitors of BCRP may increase plasma concentrations of sofosbuvir without increasing plasma concentrations of GS-331007.

Sofosbuvir and GS-331007 are not BCRP inhibitors; pharmacokinetic interactions are unlikely with drugs that are BCRP substrates.

■ Antiarrhythmic Agents ***Amiodarone*** Concomitant use of amiodarone and a hepatitis C virus (HCV) treatment regimen containing sofosbuvir with another HCV direct-acting antiviral (DAA), including ledipasvir or simeprevir, may result in serious symptomatic bradycardia and is not recommended. If there are no alternative HCV treatment options and a regimen of sofosbuvir with another DAA must be used in a patient receiving amiodarone, the patient should be advised about the risk of serious symptomatic bradycardia and cardiac monitoring should be performed in an inpatient setting during the first 48 hours of concomitant use and then heart rate monitoring (outpatient or self-monitoring) should be performed daily through at least the first 2 weeks of concomitant use. Similar cardiac monitoring is recommended in patients who discontinued amiodarone just prior to initiation of a regimen of sofosbuvir with another DAA or if there are no other treatment options and amiodarone must be initiated in a patient already receiving such sofosbuvir regimens. (See Cardiovascular Effects under Cautions: Warnings/Precautions.)

The effect of concomitant use of amiodarone and sofosbuvir on plasma concentrations of amiodarone and sofosbuvir is unknown.

■ Anticonvulsants Concomitant use of sofosbuvir and certain anticonvulsants (i.e., carbamazepine, oxcarbazepine, phenobarbital, phenytoin) is expected to decrease plasma concentrations of sofosbuvir and GS-331007, which may lead to decreased therapeutic effect of sofosbuvir. Concomitant use of these anticonvulsants and sofosbuvir is not recommended.

■ Antimycobacterial Agents ***Rifabutin*** Rifabutin is expected to decrease plasma concentrations of sofosbuvir and GS-331007, which may lead to decreased therapeutic effect of sofosbuvir. Concomitant use of rifabutin and sofosbuvir is not recommended.

Rifampin Concomitant use of rifampin, an inducer of P-gp in the intestine, and sofosbuvir may decrease plasma concentrations of sofosbuvir and GS-331007 and may lead to decreased therapeutic effect of sofosbuvir. Concomitant use of rifampin and sofosbuvir is not recommended.

Rifapentine Rifapentine is expected to decrease plasma concentrations of sofosbuvir and GS-331007, which may lead to decreased therapeutic effect of sofosbuvir. Concomitant use of rifapentine and sofosbuvir is not recommended.

■ Antiretroviral Agents ***HIV Entry and Fusion Inhibitors*** **Maraviroc.** Concomitant use of maraviroc and sofosbuvir is not expected to affect maraviroc pharmacokinetics.

Some experts recommend a maraviroc dosage of 300 mg twice daily in patients receiving sofosbuvir.

HIV Integrase Inhibitors (INSTIs) **Dolutegravir.** Concomitant use of sofosbuvir and dolutegravir is not expected to result in clinically important pharmacokinetic interactions; dosage adjustments are not necessary if the drugs are used concomitantly.

Elvitegravir. Concomitant use of elvitegravir and sofosbuvir is not expected to result in clinically important pharmacokinetic interactions.

Clinically important interactions are not expected if sofosbuvir is used concomitantly with the fixed combination of elvitegravir, cobicistat, emtricitabine, and tenofovir alafenamide (EVG/c/FTC/TAF); dosage adjustments are not necessary if the drugs are used concomitantly.

Raltegravir. Concomitant use of raltegravir and sofosbuvir does not have a clinically important effect on the pharmacokinetics of either drug; dosage adjustments are not necessary if the drugs are used concomitantly.

HIV Nonnucleoside Reverse Transcriptase Inhibitors (NNRTIs) **Efavirenz.** Concomitant use of efavirenz and sofosbuvir does not have a clinically important effect on the pharmacokinetics of either drug. Dosage adjustments are not needed.

Rilpivirine. Concomitant use of rilpivirine and sofosbuvir does not have a clinically important effect on the pharmacokinetics of either drug. Dosage adjustments are not needed.

HIV Nucleoside and Nucleotide Reverse Transcriptase Inhibitors (NRTIs) **Emtricitabine.** Concomitant use of emtricitabine and sofosbuvir does not have a clinically important effect on the pharmacokinetics of either drug. Dosage adjustments are not needed.

Tenofovir Disoproxil Fumarate. Concomitant use of tenofovir disoproxil fumarate and sofosbuvir does not have a clinically important effect on the pharmacokinetics of either drug. Dosage adjustments are not needed.

HIV Protease Inhibitors (PIs) **Atazanavir.** In clinical trials of sofosbuvir, elevated total bilirubin concentration was observed in 94% of HCV-infected patients coinfected with human immunodeficiency virus (HIV) who were receiving atazanavir as part of an antiretroviral regimen, but was observed in only 1.5% of such patients *not* receiving atazanavir.

Darunavir. Concomitant use of *ritonavir-boosted* darunavir and sofosbuvir does not have a clinically important effect on the pharmacokinetics of either drug. Dosage adjustments are not needed.

Tipranavir. Concomitant use of *ritonavir-boosted* tipranavir and sofosbuvir is expected to decrease plasma concentrations of sofosbuvir and GS-331007, which may lead to decreased therapeutic effect of sofosbuvir.

Concomitant use of *ritonavir-boosted* tipranavir and sofosbuvir is not recommended.

■ Estrogens and Progestins When studied in healthy women, concomitant use of sofosbuvir and an oral contraceptive containing ethinyl estradiol and norgestimate did not have a clinically important effect on the pharmacokinetics of ethinyl estradiol or norgestimate and its active metabolites (norelgestromin, norgestrel). Concomitant use of sofosbuvir is not expected to affect efficacy of oral contraceptives containing ethinyl estradiol and norgestimate. Dosage adjustments are not needed for either drug when sofosbuvir is used concomitantly with oral contraceptives.

■ HCV Antivirals ***HCV Protease Inhibitors*** **Simeprevir.** Concomitant use of simeprevir (150 mg once daily) and sofosbuvir (400 mg once daily) resulted in slightly increased plasma concentrations and area under the plasma concentration-time curve (AUC) of sofosbuvir, but did not have a clinically important effect on simeprevir plasma concentrations. Dosage adjustments are not needed for either drug.

HCV Replication Complex Inhibitors **Daclatasvir.** Concomitant use of daclatasvir and sofosbuvir does not result in clinically important changes in the pharmacokinetics of daclatasvir.

Elbasvir and Grazoprevir. Concomitant use of sofosbuvir and the fixed combination of elbasvir and grazoprevir (elbasvir/grazoprevir) does not result in clinically important pharmacokinetic interactions. Dosage adjustments are not needed.

■ Immunosuppressive Agents ***Cyclosporine*** Concomitant use of cyclosporine and sofosbuvir results in increased sofosbuvir exposure. However, dosage adjustments are not needed.

Tacrolimus Concomitant use of tacrolimus and sofosbuvir does not have a clinically important effect on the pharmacokinetics of either drug. Dosage adjustments are not needed.

■ Interferons There is no in vitro evidence of antagonistic anti-HCV effects between interferon alfa and sofosbuvir.

■ Methadone Concomitant use of methadone and sofosbuvir does not have a clinically important effect on the pharmacokinetics of either drug. Dosage adjustments are not needed.

■ Ribavirin There is no in vitro evidence of antagonistic anti-HCV effects between ribavirin and sofosbuvir.

■ St. John's Wort Concomitant use of St. John's wort (*Hypericum perforatum*), an inducer of P-gp in the intestine, and sofosbuvir may cause decreased plasma concentrations of sofosbuvir and GS-331007. St. John's wort and sofosbuvir should not be used concomitantly.

■ Warfarin In patients receiving warfarin, subtherapeutic international normalized ratios (INRs) have been reported after initiation of sofosbuvir-containing HCV treatment regimens.

INR should be closely monitored when initiating or discontinuing sofosbuvir-containing regimens in patients receiving warfarin.

Description

Sofosbuvir is a nucleotide analog hepatitis C virus (HCV) nonstructural 5B (NS5B) polymerase inhibitor. The drug is a direct-acting antiviral (DAA) with activity against HCV. Sofosbuvir is a prodrug that is converted in the liver to a pharmacologically active uridine analog triphosphate (GS-461203), which can be incorporated into HCV RNA by NS5B polymerase and acts as an RNA chain terminator. GS-461203 does not inhibit human DNA and RNA polymerases and does not inhibit mitochondrial RNA polymerase. In vitro studies using biochemical and cell-based replicon assays indicate that the pharmacologically active metabolite of sofosbuvir has activity against HCV genotypes 1a, 1b, 2a, 2b, 3a, 4a, 5a, and 6a.

Certain amino acid substitutions in NS5B polymerase (e.g., S282T) of HCV genotype 1b, 2 a, 2b, 3a, 4a, 5a, or 6a have been selected in cell culture and have been associated with reduced susceptibility to sofosbuvir in vitro in replicon studies. In biochemical assays, recombinant NS5B polymerase from HCV genotypes 1b, 2a, 3a, and 4a expressing the S282T substitution showed reduced susceptibility to GS-461203. In phase 3 clinical trials, treatment-emergent amino acid substitutions (e.g., L159F, V321A) were detected in patients with HCV genotype 3a infection, but these substitutions did not appear to be associated with changes in phenotypic susceptibility to the drug. In a study in

HCV-infected patients with hepatocellular carcinoma awaiting liver transplantation, the L159F substitution emerged in several patients with genotype 1a or 1b infection who experienced virologic failure (breakthrough and relapse) and the presence of L159F and/or C316N at baseline in patients with genotype 1b infection was associated with breakthrough and relapse after transplantation. In replicon studies, the S282T substitution associated with reduced susceptibility to sofosbuvir did not affect susceptibility to ribavirin or HCV NS5A inhibitors. In addition, sofosbuvir was active against HCV replicons with the ribavirin-associated substitutions of T390I and F415Y or HCV replicons with variants associated with resistance to HCV NS3/4A protease inhibitors.

Following oral administration, peak plasma concentrations of sofosbuvir and the predominant metabolite (GS-331007) occur at approximately 0.5–2 and 2–4 hours, respectively, after the dose. Sofosbuvir undergoes intracellular metabolic activation in the liver involving hydrolysis by human cathepsin A (CatA) or carboxylesterase 1 (CES1) and phosphoramidate cleavage by histidine triad nucleotide-binding protein 1 (HINT1). Then, phosphorylation occurs by the pyrimidine nucleotide biosynthesis pathway, resulting in the pharmacologically active metabolite (GS-461203). Subsequently, desphosphorylation results in the formation of GS-331007, the predominant circulating metabolite, which does not have anti-HCV activity. After a single 400-mg oral dose of sofosbuvir, unchanged drug and GS-331007 account for approximately 4% and 90% of systemic exposure, respectively. Administration with a high-fat meal does not substantially affect sofosbuvir or GS-331007 peak plasma concentrations or area under the plasma concentration-time curve (AUC) relative to administration in the fasting state. Sofosbuvir is approximately 61–65% bound to plasma proteins. Following a single 400-mg oral dose of sofosbuvir, 80% of the dose is eliminated in urine (78% of this as GS-331007), 14% is excreted in feces, and 2.5% is eliminated in expired air. The median terminal half-lives of sofosbuvir and GS-331007 are 0.4 and 27 hours, respectively.

In HCV-infected patients with moderate or severe hepatic impairment (Child-Pugh class B or C) who received sofosbuvir 400 mg daily for 7 days, sofosbuvir AUC was 126 or 143% higher, respectively, and GS-331007 AUC was 18 or 9% higher, respectively, compared with patients with normal hepatic function. Population pharmacokinetic analysis in HCV-infected patients indicates that cirrhosis has no clinically important effect on sofosbuvir and GS-331007 exposure. Following a single 400-mg dose, patients with mild, moderate, or severe renal impairment had sofosbuvir AUCs that were 61, 107, or 171% higher, respectively, and GS-331007 AUCs that were 55, 88, or 451% higher, respectively, compared with patients with normal renal function. Population pharmacokinetic analysis indicates that age (range 19–75 years), race, and gender do not have clinically important effects on sofosbuvir pharmacokinetics.

Advice to Patients

Importance of using sofosbuvir in conjunction with other antivirals; sofosbuvir should *not* be used alone.

Advise patients not to reduce sofosbuvir dosage; if antivirals in the multiple-drug regimen are discontinued for any reason, sofosbuvir also should be discontinued.

Sofosbuvir may be taken with or without food.

Inform patients that reactivation of hepatitis B virus (HBV) infection has occurred in coinfected patients being treated for hepatitis C virus (HCV) infection. Importance of informing clinician of any history of HBV infection or other liver problems (e.g., cirrhosis). Importance of immediately contacting a clinician if any signs or symptoms of serious liver injury (e.g., fatigue, weakness, loss of appetite, nausea and vomiting, yellowing of the eyes or skin, light-colored bowel movements) occur. (See Risk of HBV Reactivation in Patients Coinfected with HCV and HBV under Warnings/Precautions: Warnings, in Cautions.)

If a regimen containing sofosbuvir with another hepatitis C virus (HCV) direct-acting antiviral (DAA) is used in a patient receiving amiodarone, advise the patient about the risk of serious symptomatic bradycardia and the importance of immediately contacting a clinician if signs or symptoms of bradycardia (e.g., near-fainting or fainting, dizziness, lightheadedness, malaise, weakness, excessive tiredness, shortness of breath, chest pain, confusion, memory problems) occur. (See Cardiovascular Effects under Warnings/Precautions: Other Warnings/Precautions, in Cautions.)

Inform patients that the effect of HCV treatment on transmission of HCV is unknown; patients should take appropriate precautions to prevent transmission of the virus during treatment or in the event of treatment failure.

Importance of informing clinicians of existing or contemplated concomitant therapy, including prescription and OTC drugs and dietary or herbal supplements, as well as any concomitant illnesses.

Importance of women informing clinicians if they are or plan to become pregnant or plan to breast-feed. If sofosbuvir is used in a multiple-drug regimen that includes ribavirin, advise men and women of the importance of using 2 forms of effective contraception during and for 6 months after ribavirin therapy. (See Precautions Related to Multiple-drug Treatment Regimens under Warnings/Precautions: Other Warnings/Precautions, in Cautions.)

Importance of informing patients of other important precautionary information. (See Cautions.)

Overview® (see Users Guide). For additional information on this drug until a more detailed monograph is developed and published, the manufacturer's labeling should be consulted. It is *essential* that the manufacturer's labeling be consulted for more detailed information on usual cautions, precautions, contraindications, potential drug interactions, laboratory test interferences, and acute toxicity.

Preparations

Excipients in commercially available drug preparations may have clinically important effects in some individuals; consult specific product labeling for details.

Sofosbuvir

Oral		
Tablets, film-coated	400 mg	**Sovaldi®**, Gilead

Sofosbuvir Combinations

Oral		
Tablets, film-coated	400 mg with Ledipasvir 90 mg	**Harvoni®**, Gilead
Tablets, film-coated	400 mg with Velpatasvir 100 mg	**Epclusa®**, Gilead

†Use is not currently included in the labeling approved by the US Food and Drug Administration

Sofosbuvir and Velpatasvir SOF

■ Sofosbuvir and velpatasvir (sofosbuvir/velpatasvir) is a fixed combination containing 2 hepatitis C virus (HCV) antivirals; sofosbuvir is a nucleotide analog HCV nonstructural 5B (NS5B) polymerase inhibitor and velpatasvir is an HCV nonstructural 5A (NS5A) replication complex inhibitor (NS5A inhibitor).

Uses

■ Chronic Hepatitis C Virus Infection The fixed combination of sofosbuvir and velpatasvir (sofosbuvir/velpatasvir) is used for the treatment of chronic hepatitis C virus (HCV) genotype 1, 2, 3, 4, 5, or 6 infection in treatment-naive (previously untreated) or previously treated adults, including those with cirrhosis (compensated or decompensated).

Sofosbuvir/velpatasvir is used alone or in conjunction with ribavirin, depending on certain patient factors (e.g., presence of decompensated cirrhosis).

Because the treatment of chronic HCV infection is complex and rapidly evolving, it is recommended that treatment be directed by clinicians who are familiar with the disease and that a specialist be consulted to obtain the most up-to-date information. Information from the American Association for the Study of Liver Diseases (AASLD), Infectious Diseases Society of America (IDSA), and International Antiviral Society–USA (IAS–USA) regarding diagnosis and management of HCV infection, including recommendations for initial treatment, is available at http://www.hcvguidelines.org.

HCV Genotype 1 Infection Efficacy and safety of sofosbuvir/velpatasvir for the treatment of chronic HCV genotype 1 infection in adults have been evaluated in 2 randomized, phase 3 trials (ASTRAL-1 [NCT02201940] and ASTRAL-4 [NCT02201901]). The primary end point in both studies was sustained virologic response at 12 weeks after the end of treatment (SVR12; defined as plasma HCV RNA level less than 15 IU/mL [the lower limit of quantification] at 12 weeks after end of treatment).

ASTRAL-1, a double-blind, placebo-controlled trial, included 740 treatment-naive or previously treated adults with chronic HCV genotype 1, 2, 4, 5, or 6 infection who were noncirrhotic or had compensated cirrhosis (median age 56 years, 60% male, 74% with baseline HCV RNA levels 800,000 IU/mL or greater, 69% with non-CC IL28B alleles [CT or TT], 32% previously treated, 19% with compensated cirrhosis). Patients who previously received treatment with an HCV nonstructural 5A (NS5A) replication complex inhibitor (NS5A inhibitor) or HCV nonstructural 5B (NS5B) polymerase inhibitor and patients with human immunodeficiency virus (HIV) or hepatitis B virus (HBV) coinfection were excluded. Those with HCV genotype 1, 2, 4, or 6 infection were randomized in a 5:1 ratio to receive a 12-week regimen of sofosbuvir/velpatasvir (a fixed-combination tablet containing 400 mg of sofosbuvir and 100 mg of velpatasvir) or placebo once daily. Of the 210 patients with HCV genotype 1a infection treated with sofosbuvir/velpatasvir, 98% achieved SVR12; of the 118 patients with HCV genotype 1b infection treated with sofosbuvir/velpatasvir, 99% achieved SVR12. No patients treated with placebo achieved SVR12. Among the 121 patients with compensated cirrhosis (regardless of HCV genotype), 99% achieved SVR12.

ASTRAL-4, an open-label trial, included 267 treatment-naive or previously treated adults with chronic HCV genotype 1, 2, 3, 4, or 6 infection with decompensated cirrhosis (Child-Pugh class B). Patients who previously received treatment with an HCV NS5A inhibitor or HCV NS5B polymerase inhibitor and patients with HIV or HBV coinfection were excluded. Patients were randomized in a 1:1:1 ratio to receive sofosbuvir/velpatasvir (a fixed-combination tablet containing 400 mg of sofosbuvir and 100 mg of velpatasvir) once daily with or without ribavirin for 12 weeks or sofosbuvir/velpatasvir once daily alone for 24 weeks. Baseline characteristics were balanced among treatment groups (median age 59 years, 70% male, 56% with baseline HCV RNA levels 800,000 IU/mL or greater, 76% with non-CC IL28B alleles [CT or TT], 55% previously treated, 95% had baseline Model for End-stage Liver Disease [MELD] scores of 15 or lower). Of the 68 patients with HCV genotype 1 infection treated with a regimen of sofosbuvir/velpatasvir in conjunction *with* ribavirin for 12 weeks, 96% achieved SVR12 (94 or 100% of those with HCV genotype 1a or 1b, respectively). SVR12 was achieved in 88 or 92% of patients with HCV genotype 1 infection treated with a regimen of sofosbuvir/velpatasvir alone for 12 or 24 weeks, respectively.

HCV Genotype 2 Infection Efficacy and safety of sofosbuvir/velpatasvir for the treatment of chronic HCV genotype 2 infection in adults have been evaluated in 3 randomized, phase 3 trials (ASTRAL-1 [NCT02201940], ASTRAL-2 [NCT02220998], and ASTRAL-4 [NCT02201901]). The primary end point in each study was sustained virologic response at 12 weeks after the end of treatment (SVR12; defined as plasma HCV RNA level less than 15 IU/mL [the lower limit of quantification] at 12 weeks after end of treatment).

ASTRAL-1, a double-blind, placebo-controlled trial, included 740 treatment-naive or previously treated adults with chronic HCV genotype 1, 2, 4, 5, or 6 infection who were noncirrhotic or had compensated cirrhosis (median age 56 years, 60% male, 74% with baseline HCV RNA levels 800,000 IU/mL or greater, 69% with non-CC IL28B alleles [CT or TT], 32% previously treated, 19% with compensated cirrhosis). Patients who previously received treatment with an HCV NS5A inhibitor or HCV NS5B polymerase inhibitor and patients with HIV or HBV coinfection were excluded. Those with HCV genotype 1, 2, 4, or 6 infection were randomized in a 5:1 ratio to receive sofosbuvir/velpatasvir (a fixed-combination tablet containing 400 mg of sofosbuvir and 100 mg of velpatasvir) once daily or placebo for 12 weeks. Of the 104 patients with HCV genotype 2 infection treated with sofosbuvir/velpatasvir, 100% achieved SVR12; no patients treated with placebo achieved SVR12. Among the 121 patients with compensated cirrhosis (regardless of HCV genotype), 99% achieved SVR12.

ASTRAL-2, an open-label trial, included 266 treatment-naive or previously treated adults with chronic HCV genotype 2 infection (median age 58 years, 59% male, 80% with baseline HCV RNA levels 800,000 IU/mL or greater, 62% with non-CC IL28B alleles [CT or TT], 15% previously treated, 14% with compensated cirrhosis). Those with clinical evidence of hepatic decompensation and those with HIV or HBV coinfection were excluded. Patients were randomized in a 1:1 ratio to receive a 12-week regimen of sofosbuvir/velpatasvir (a fixed-combination tablet containing 400 mg of sofosbuvir and 100 mg of velpatasvir) once daily or a regimen of sofosbuvir 400 mg once daily in conjunction with ribavirin. SVR12 was achieved by substantially more patients treated with sofosbuvir/velpatasvir compared with those treated with sofosbuvir in conjunction with ribavirin (99 and 94%, respectively).

ASTRAL-4, an open-label trial, included 267 treatment-naive or previously treated adults with chronic HCV genotype 1, 2, 3, 4, or 6 infection with decompensated cirrhosis (Child-Pugh class B). Patients who previously received treatment with an HCV NS5A inhibitor or HCV NS5B polymerase inhibitor and patients with HIV or HBV coinfection were excluded. Patients were randomized in a 1:1:1 ratio to receive sofosbuvir/velpatasvir (a fixed-combination tablet containing 400 mg of sofosbuvir and 100 mg of velpatasvir) once daily with or without ribavirin for 12 weeks or sofosbuvir/velpatasvir once daily alone for 24 weeks. Baseline characteristics were balanced among treatment groups (median age 59 years, 70% male, 56% with baseline HCV RNA levels 800,000 IU/mL or greater, 76% with non-CC IL28B alleles [CT or TT], 55% previously treated, 95% had baseline MELD scores of 15 or lower). Of the 4 patients with HCV genotype 2 infection treated with sofosbuvir/velpatasvir in conjunction *with* ribavirin for 12 weeks, 100% achieved SVR12; of the 8 patients with HCV genotype 2 infection treated with sofosbuvir/velpatasvir alone for 12 or 24 weeks, 88% achieved SVR12.

HCV Genotype 3 Infection Efficacy and safety of sofosbuvir/velpatasvir for the treatment of chronic HCV genotype 3 infection in adults have been evaluated in 2 randomized, phase 3 trials (ASTRAL-3 [NCT02201953] and ASTRAL-4 [NCT02201901]). The primary end point in both studies was sustained virologic response at 12 weeks after the end of treatment (SVR12; defined as plasma HCV RNA level less than 15 IU/mL [the lower limit of quantification] at 12 weeks after end of treatment).

ASTRAL-3, an open-label trial, included 552 treatment-naive or previously treated adults with chronic HCV genotype 3 infection (median age 52 years, 62% male, 70% with baseline HCV RNA levels 800,000 IU/mL or greater, 61% with non-CC IL28B alleles [CT or TT], 26% previously treated, 30% with compensated cirrhosis). Those with clinical evidence of hepatic decompensation and those with HIV or HBV coinfection were excluded. Patients were randomized in a 1:1 ratio to receive sofosbuvir/velpatasvir (a fixed-combination tablet containing 400 mg of sofosbuvir and 100 mg of velpatasvir) once daily for 12 weeks or a regimen of sofosbuvir 400 mg once daily in conjunction *with* ribavirin for 24 weeks. SVR12 was achieved by substantially more patients treated with a 12-week regimen of sofosbuvir/velpatasvir compared with those treated with a 24-week regimen of sofosbuvir in conjunction *with* ribavirin (95 and 80%, respectively). In patients with compensated cirrhosis, SVR12 was achieved in 91% of those treated with sofosbuvir/velpatasvir and in 66% of those treated with sofosbuvir in conjunction with ribavirin; similar SVR12 rates were observed in previously treated patients.

ASTRAL-4, an open-label trial, included 267 treatment-naive or previously treated adults with chronic HCV genotype 1, 2, 3, 4, or 6 infection with decompensated cirrhosis (Child-Pugh class B). Patients who previously received treatment with an HCV NS5A inhibitor or HCV NS5B polymerase inhibitor and patients with HIV or HBV coinfection were excluded. Patients were randomized in a 1:1:1 ratio to receive sofosbuvir/velpatasvir (a fixed-combination tablet containing 400 mg of sofosbuvir and 100 mg of velpatasvir) once daily with or without ribavirin for 12 weeks or sofosbuvir/velpatasvir once daily alone for 24 weeks. Baseline characteristics were balanced among treatment groups (median age 59 years, 70% male, 56% with baseline HCV RNA levels 800,000 IU/mL or greater, 76% with non-CC IL28B alleles [CT or TT], 55% previously treated, 95% had baseline MELD scores of 15 or lower). Of the 13 patients with HCV genotype 3 infection treated with sofosbuvir/velpatasvir in conjunction *with* ribavirin for 12 weeks, 85% achieved SVR12; of the 26 patients with HCV genotype 3 infection treated with sofosbuvir/velpatasvir alone for 12 or 24 weeks, 50% achieved SVR12.

HCV Genotype 4 Infection Efficacy and safety of sofosbuvir/velpatasvir for the treatment of chronic HCV genotype 4 infection in adults have been evaluated in 2 randomized, phase 3 trials (ASTRAL-1 [NCT02201940] and ASTRAL-4 [NCT02201901]). The primary end point in both studies was sustained virologic response at 12 weeks after the end of treatment (SVR12; defined as plasma HCV RNA level less than 15 IU/mL [the lower limit of quantification] at 12 weeks after end of treatment).

ASTRAL-1, a double-blind, placebo-controlled trial, included 740 treatment-naive or previously treated adults with chronic HCV genotype 1, 2, 4, 5, or 6 infection who were noncirrhotic or had compensated cirrhosis (median age 56 years, 60% male, 74% with baseline HCV RNA levels 800,000 IU/mL or greater, 69% with non-CC IL28B alleles [CT or TT], 32% previously treated, 19% with compensated cirrhosis). Patients who previously received treatment with an HCV NS5A inhibitor or HCV NS5B polymerase inhibitor and patients with HIV or HBV coinfection were excluded. Those with HCV genotype 1, 2, 4, or 6 infection were randomized in a 5:1 ratio to receive sofosbuvir/velpatasvir (a fixed-combination tablet containing 400 mg of sofosbuvir and 100 mg of velpatasvir) once daily or placebo for 12 weeks. Of the 116 patients with HCV genotype 4 infection treated with sofosbuvir/velpatasvir, 100% achieved SVR12; no patients treated with placebo achieved SVR12. Among the 121 patients with compensated cirrhosis (regardless of HCV genotype), 99% achieved SVR12.

ASTRAL-4, an open-label trial, included 267 treatment-naive or previously treated adults with chronic HCV genotype 1, 2, 3, 4, or 6 infection with decompensated cirrhosis (Child-Pugh class B). Patients who previously received treatment with an HCV NS5A inhibitor or HCV NS5B polymerase inhibitor and patients with HIV or HBV coinfection were excluded. Patients were randomized in a 1:1:1 ratio to receive sofosbuvir/velpatasvir (a fixed-combination tablet containing 400 mg of sofosbuvir and 100 mg of velpatasvir) once daily with or without ribavirin for 12 weeks or sofosbuvir/velpatasvir once daily alone for 24 weeks. Baseline characteristics were balanced among treatment groups (median age 59 years, 70% male, 56% with baseline HCV RNA levels 800,000 IU/mL or greater, 76% with non-CC IL28B alleles [CT or TT], 55% previously treated, 95% had baseline MELD scores of 15 or lower). Of the 2 patients with HCV genotype 4 infection treated with sofosbuvir/velpatasvir in conjunction *with* ribavirin for 12 weeks, both achieved SVR12; similarly, all 6 patients with HCV genotype 4 infection treated with sofosbuvir/velpatasvir alone for 12 or 24 weeks achieved SVR12.

HCV Genotype 5 Infection Efficacy and safety of sofosbuvir/velpatasvir for the treatment of HCV genotype 5 infection in treatment-naive or previously treated adults have been evaluated in a double-blind, placebo-controlled trial (ASTRAL-1 [NCT02201940]). The study included 740 treatment-naive or previously treated adults with chronic HCV genotype 1, 2, 4, 5, or 6 infection who were noncirrhotic or had compensated cirrhosis (median age 56 years, 60% male, 74% with baseline HCV RNA levels 800,000 IU/mL or greater, 69% with non-CC IL28B alleles [CT or TT], 32% previously treated, 19% with compensated cirrhosis). Patients who previously received treatment with an HCV NS5A inhibitor or HCV NS5B polymerase inhibitor and patients with HIV or HBV coinfection were excluded. All 35 patients with HCV genotype 5 infection received sofosbuvir/velpatasvir (a fixed-combination tablet containing 400 mg of sofosbuvir and 100 mg of velpatasvir) once daily for 12 weeks and were not randomized to other treatment groups due to the low prevalence of HCV genotype 5 infection in the regions where the study took place. SVR12 was achieved by 97% of patients with HCV genotype 5 infection. Among the 121 patients with compensated cirrhosis (regardless of HCV genotype), 99% achieved SVR12.

Although criteria for the ASTRAL-4 (NCT02201901) study allowed inclusion of patients with HCV genotype 5 infection, no patients with HCV genotype 5 infection were enrolled. Therefore, efficacy and safety of sofosbuvir/velpatasvir have not been evaluated to date in patients with HCV genotype 5 infection and decompensated cirrhosis.

HCV Genotype 6 Infection Efficacy and safety of sofosbuvir/velpatasvir for the treatment of chronic HCV genotype 6 infection in adults have been evaluated in 2 randomized, phase 3 trials (ASTRAL-1 [NCT02201940] and ASTRAL-4 [NCT02201901]). The primary end point in both studies was sustained virologic response at 12 weeks after the end of treatment (SVR12; defined as plasma HCV RNA level less than 15 IU/mL [the lower limit of quantification] at 12 weeks after end of treatment).

ASTRAL-1, a double-blind, placebo-controlled trial, included 740 treatment-naive or previously treated adults with chronic HCV genotype 1, 2, 4, 5, or 6 infection who were noncirrhotic or had compensated cirrhosis (median age 56 years, 60% male, 74% with baseline HCV RNA levels 800,000 IU/mL or greater, 69% with non-CC IL28B alleles [CT or TT], 32% previously treated, 19% with compensated cirrhosis). Patients who previously received treatment with an HCV NS5A inhibitor or HCV NS5B polymerase inhibitor and patients with HIV or HBV coinfection were excluded. Those with HCV genotype 1, 2, 4, or 6 infection were randomized in a 5:1 ratio to receive sofosbuvir/velpatasvir (a fixed-combination tablet containing 400 mg of sofosbuvir and 100 mg of velpatasvir) once daily or placebo for 12 weeks. Of the 41 patients with HCV genotype 6 infection treated with sofosbuvir/velpatasvir, 100% achieved SVR12. No patients treated with placebo achieved SVR12. Among the 121 patients with compensated cirrhosis (regardless of HCV genotype), 99% achieved SVR12.

ASTRAL-4, an open-label trial, included 267 treatment-naive or previously treated adults with chronic HCV genotype 1, 2, 3, 4, or 6 infection with decompensated cirrhosis (Child-Pugh class B). Patients who previously received treatment with an HCV NS5A inhibitor or HCV NS5B polymerase inhibitor and patients with HIV or HBV coinfection were excluded. Patients were randomized in a 1:1:1 ratio to receive sofosbuvir/velpatasvir (a fixed-combination tablet containing 400 mg of sofosbuvir and 100 mg of velpatasvir) once daily with or without ribavirin for 12 weeks or sofosbuvir/velpatasvir alone for 24 weeks. Baseline characteristics were balanced among treatment groups (median age 59 years, 70% male, 56% with baseline HCV RNA levels 800,000 IU/mL or greater, 76% with non-CC IL28B alleles [CT or TT], 55% previously treated, 95% had baseline MELD scores of 15 or lower). One patient with HCV genotype 6 infection was enrolled in the study and achieved SVR12 after receiving a regimen of sofosbuvir/velpatasvir alone for 24 weeks.

Dosage and Administration

■ General

For the treatment of chronic hepatitis C virus (HCV) infection, sofosbuvir and velpatasvir (sofosbuvir/velpatasvir) is used alone or in conjunction with ribavirin.

The specific regimen is based on certain patient factors (e.g., presence of decompensated cirrhosis).

Prior to initiating sofosbuvir/velpatasvir for treatment of HCV infection, all patients should be tested for evidence of current or prior hepatitis B virus (HBV) infection by measuring hepatitis B surface antigen (HBsAg), hepatitis B surface antibody (anti-HBs), and hepatitis B core antibody (anti-HBc). (See Risk of HBV Reactivation in Patients Coinfected with HCV and HBV under Warnings/Precautions: Warnings, in Cautions.)

■ Administration

Sofosbuvir/velpatasvir is administered orally once daily without regard to food.

■ Dosage

Sofosbuvir/velpatasvir is commercially available as fixed-combination tablets containing 400 mg of sofosbuvir and 100 mg of velpatasvir.

Chronic Hepatitis C Virus Infection **HCV Genotype 1, 2, 3, 4, 5, or 6 Infection.** For the treatment of chronic HCV genotype 1, 2, 3, 4, 5, or 6 infection in adults without cirrhosis or with compensated cirrhosis (Child-Pugh class A), the recommended dosage of sofosbuvir/velpatasvir is 1 tablet (400 mg of sofosbuvir and 100 mg of velpatasvir) once daily. A treatment duration of 12 weeks is recommended.

For the treatment of chronic HCV genotype 1, 2, 3, 4, 5, or 6 infection in adults with decompensated cirrhosis (Child-Pugh class B or C), the recommended dosage of sofosbuvir/velpatasvir is 1 tablet (400 mg of sofosbuvir and 100 mg of velpatasvir) once daily in conjunction *with* ribavirin. A treatment duration of 12 weeks is recommended. If sofosbuvir/velpatasvir (without ribavirin) is used for the treatment of HCV genotype 1, 4, 5, or 6 infection in patients with decompensated cirrhosis who cannot receive ribavirin, some experts recommend a treatment duration of 24 weeks. HCV-infected patients with decompensated cirrhosis should be referred to an expert for treatment (ideally at a liver transplant center).

■ Special Populations

Hepatic Impairment Sofosbuvir/velpatasvir dosage adjustments are not necessary in adults with mild, moderate, or severe hepatic impairment (Child-Pugh class A, B, or C). (See Hepatic Impairment under Warnings/Precautions: Specific Populations, in Cautions.)

Renal Impairment Sofosbuvir/velpatasvir dosage adjustments are not necessary in adults with mild or moderate renal impairment.

Dosage recommendations are not available for patients with severe renal impairment (estimated glomerular filtration rate [eGFR] less than 30 mL/minute per 1.73 m^2) or end-stage renal disease (ESRD); safety and efficacy have not been established in such patients. (See Renal Impairment under Warnings/Precautions: Specific Populations, in Cautions.)

Geriatric Patients Sofosbuvir/velpatasvir dosage adjustments are not necessary in geriatric patients.

Cautions

■ Contraindications

If the fixed combination containing sofosbuvir and velpatasvir (sofosbuvir/velpatasvir) is used in conjunction *with* ribavirin, the contraindications to ribavirin also apply. (See Precautions Related to Fixed Combinations and Multiple-drug Treatment Regimens under Warnings/Precautions: Other Warnings/Precautions, in Cautions.)

■ Warnings/Precautions

Warnings **Risk of HBV Reactivation in Patients Coinfected with HCV and HBV.** Reactivation of hepatitis B virus (HBV) infection has been reported during postmarketing experience when direct-acting antivirals (DAAs) were used for the treatment of chronic hepatitis C virus (HCV) infection in patients with HBV coinfection. In some cases, HBV reactivation resulted in fulminant hepatitis, hepatic failure, and death.

HBV reactivation (defined as an abrupt increase in HBV replication manifested as a rapid increase in serum HBV DNA levels or detection of hepatitis B surface antigen [HBsAg] in an individual who was previously HBsAg negative and hepatitis B core antibody [anti-HBc] positive) has been reported in patients with HCV and HBV coinfection who were receiving HCV treatment with a regimen that included HCV DAAs without interferon alfa. Reactivation also may be accompanied by hepatitis (i.e., increased aminotransferase concentrations) and, in severe cases, may lead to increased bilirubin concentrations, liver failure, or death.

Data to date indicate that HBV reactivation usually occurs within 4–8 weeks after initiation of HCV treatment. Patients with HBV reactivation have been heterogeneous in terms of HCV genotype and in terms of baseline HBV disease. While some patients with HBV reactivation were HBsAg positive, others had serologic evidence of resolved HBV infection (i.e., HBsAg negative and anti-HBc positive). HBV reactivation also has been reported in patients receiving certain immunosuppressant or chemotherapeutic drugs; the risk of reactivation associated with HCV DAAs may be increased in such patients.

The mechanism for HBV reactivation in patients with HCV and HBV coinfection receiving HCV DAAs is unknown. Although HCV DAAs are not known to cause immunosuppression, HBV reactivation in coinfected patients may result from a complex interplay of host immunologic responses in the setting of infection with 2 hepatitis viruses.

Prior to initiating treatment with an HCV DAA, including sofosbuvir/velpatasvir, all patients should be screened for evidence of current or prior HBV infection by measuring HBsAg, hepatitis B surface antibody (anti-HBs), and anti-HBc. If there is serologic evidence of HBV infection, baseline HBV DNA levels should be measured.

Patients with evidence of current or prior HBV infection should be monitored for clinical and laboratory signs (i.e., HBsAg, HBV DNA levels, serum aminotransferase concentrations, bilirubin concentrations) of hepatitis flare or HBV reactivation during and after treatment with HCV DAAs, including sofosbuvir/velpatasvir. Appropriate management for HBV infection should be initiated as clinically indicated.

Patients with HCV and HBV coinfection receiving sofosbuvir/velpatasvir should be advised to immediately contact a clinician if they develop any signs or symptoms of serious liver injury (e.g., fatigue, weakness, loss of appetite, nausea and vomiting, yellowing of the eyes or skin, light-colored bowel movements).

When making decisions regarding HBV monitoring or HBV treatment in coinfected patients, consultation with a clinician who has expertise in managing HBV infection is recommended.

Other Warnings/Precautions **Cardiovascular Effects.** Symptomatic bradycardia, sometimes requiring pacemaker intervention, has been reported during postmarketing experience in patients receiving amiodarone concomitantly with an HCV treatment regimen containing sofosbuvir in conjunction with daclatasvir or simeprevir. Symptomatic bradycardia, including a fatal cardiac arrest, has been reported in patients receiving amiodarone concomitantly with the fixed combination containing ledipasvir and sofosbuvir (ledipasvir/sofosbuvir).

In most reported cases, bradycardia occurred within hours to days after HCV treatment was initiated in patients receiving amiodarone, but has been observed up to 2 weeks after initiation of HCV treatment. Bradycardia generally resolved after HCV treatment was discontinued. The mechanism for this adverse cardiovascular effect is unknown.

Patients who may be at increased risk for symptomatic bradycardia if amiodarone is used concomitantly with an HCV treatment regimen containing sofosbuvir and another HCV DAA include those also receiving a β-adrenergic blocking agent, those with underlying cardiac comorbidities, and/or those with advanced liver disease.

Concomitant use of amiodarone with sofosbuvir/velpatasvir is *not* recommended. If there are no alternative HCV treatment options and sofosbuvir/velpatasvir must be used in a patient receiving amiodarone, the patient should be advised about the risk of serious symptomatic bradycardia before sofosbuvir/velpatasvir is initiated. Cardiac monitoring should be performed in an inpatient setting during the first 48 hours of concomitant use of amiodarone and sofosbuvir/velpatasvir; heart rate monitoring should then be performed daily (outpatient or self-monitoring) through at least the first 2 weeks of concomitant use. Similar cardiac monitoring is recommended in patients who discontinued amiodarone just prior to initiation of sofosbuvir/velpatasvir or if there are no other treatment options and amiodarone must be initiated in a patient already receiving sofosbuvir/velpatasvir.

Patients receiving amiodarone concomitantly with sofosbuvir/velpatasvir should be advised to immediately contact a clinician if they develop signs or symptoms of bradycardia (e.g., near-fainting or fainting, dizziness, lightheadedness, malaise, weakness, excessive tiredness, shortness of breath, chest pain, confusion, memory problems).

Interactions. Concomitant use of sofosbuvir/velpatasvir and inducers of the P-glycoprotein (P-gp) transport system and/or moderate or potent inducers of cytochrome P-450 (CYP) isoenzyme 2B6, 2C8, or 3A4 (e.g., carbamazepine and other anticonvulsants, rifampin, St. John's wort [*Hypericum perforatum*]) may result in substantially decreased plasma concentrations of sofosbuvir and/or velpatasvir and may lead to reduced therapeutic effect of sofosbuvir/velpatasvir. Concomitant use of such drugs with sofosbuvir/velpatasvir is not recommended. (See Drug Interactions.)

Precautions Related to Fixed Combinations and Multiple-drug Treatment Regimens. When sofosbuvir/velpatasvir is used, the cautions, precautions, contraindications, and drug interactions associated with both drugs in the fixed combination must be considered. Cautionary information applicable to specific populations (e.g., pregnant or nursing women, individuals with hepatic or renal impairment, geriatric patients) should be considered for each drug. (For cautionary information specific for sofosbuvir, see Cautions in Sofosbuvir 8:18.40.16.)

When sofosbuvir/velpatasvir is used in conjunction *with* ribavirin, the cautions, precautions, and contraindications associated with ribavirin also should be considered. (See Cautions in Ribavirin 8:18.32.) Ribavirin may cause fetal toxicity and/or death and extreme care *must* be taken to avoid pregnancy in female patients and in female partners of male patients receiving ribavirin-containing regimens. Women of childbearing potential should have a negative pregnancy test immediately prior to initiating ribavirin and pregnancy tests should be performed monthly during and for 6 months after ribavirin treatment is completed. Women of childbearing potential (and their male partners) and male patients (and their female partners) *must* use at least 2 forms of effective contraception during and for 6 months after ribavirin treatment is completed. (See Cautions: Pregnancy, Fertility, and Lactation, in Ribavirin 8:18.32.)

Specific Populations **Pregnancy.** Adequate data are not available regarding use of sofosbuvir/velpatasvir in pregnant women. In animal studies, there was no evidence that sofosbuvir or velpatasvir affected fetal development at the dosages tested.

When sofosbuvir/velpatasvir is used in conjunction *with* ribavirin, clinicians should consider that ribavirin may cause fetal toxicity and/or death and extreme care must be taken to avoid pregnancy in female patients and in female partners of male patients receiving the ribavirin-containing regimen. (See Cautions: Pregnancy, Fertility, and Lactation, in Ribavirin 8:18.32.)

Lactation. It is not known whether sofosbuvir/velpatasvir and metabolites are distributed into human milk.

The predominant metabolite of sofosbuvir (GS-331007) is distributed into milk in rats; velpatasvir is distributed into milk in rats and has been detected in plasma of suckling rat pups. GS-331007 and velpatasvir had no apparent effects on the nursing pups.

The benefits of breast-feeding and the importance of sofosbuvir/velpatasvir to the woman should be considered along with the potential adverse effects on the breast-fed child from the drug or from the underlying maternal condition.

When sofosbuvir/velpatasvir is used in conjunction *with* ribavirin, the potential for adverse reactions to ribavirin in nursing infants should be considered and a decision should be made whether to discontinue nursing or the ribavirin-containing regimen, taking into account the importance of the regimen to the woman. (See Precautions Related to Fixed Combinations and Multiple-drug Treatment Regimens under Warnings/Precautions: Other Warnings/Precautions, in Cautions.)

Pediatric Use. Safety and efficacy of sofosbuvir/velpatasvir have not been established in pediatric patients younger than 18 years of age.

Geriatric Use. No overall differences in safety and efficacy of sofosbuvir/velpatasvir have been observed between patients 65 years of age and older and younger adults. However, greater sensitivity in some older individuals cannot be ruled out.

Hepatic Impairment. In HCV-infected individuals with moderate or severe hepatic impairment (Child-Pugh class B or C), sofosbuvir (400 mg daily for 7 days) results in sofosbuvir and GS-331007 plasma exposures higher than those reported in individuals with normal hepatic function. In individuals with moderate or severe hepatic impairment (Child-Pugh class B or C) without HCV infection, a single 100-mg dose of velpatasvir results in plasma exposures similar to those reported when the same dose is given to individuals with normal hepatic function.

When velpatasvir/sofosbuvir is used in conjunction *with* ribavirin in patients with decompensated cirrhosis (Child-Pugh class B or C), clinical and hepatic laboratory monitoring is recommended as clinically indicated.

Renal Impairment. In individuals with mild, moderate, or severe renal impairment without HCV infection, a single 400-mg dose of sofosbuvir results in sofosbuvir and GS-331007 plasma exposures higher than those reported in individuals with normal renal function. In those with end-stage renal disease (ESRD), sofosbuvir and GS-331007 exposures were higher when the drug was administered 1 hour before or 1 hour after hemodialysis compared with exposures in those with normal renal function; a 4-hour hemodialysis session removed approximately 18% of the dose.

In individuals with severe renal impairment without HCV infection, velpatasvir pharmacokinetics following a single 100-mg dose of the drug are similar to pharmacokinetics reported in healthy individuals.

■ **Common Adverse Effects** Sofosbuvir/velpatasvir in patients without cirrhosis or with compensated cirrhosis: Adverse effects reported in 10% or more of patients include headache, fatigue, nasopharyngitis, nausea, and insomnia.

Sofosbuvir/velpatasvir in conjunction *with* ribavirin in patients with decompensated cirrhosis: Adverse effects reported in 10% or more of patients include fatigue, anemia, nausea, headache, insomnia, diarrhea, muscle spasm, dyspnea, and cough.

Drug Interactions

The following drug interactions are based on studies using the fixed combination containing sofosbuvir and velpatasvir (sofosbuvir/velpatasvir), sofosbuvir alone, or velpatasvir alone, or are predicted to occur. When sofosbuvir/velpatasvir is used, interactions associated with both drugs in the fixed combination should be considered.

■ **Drugs Affecting or Metabolized by Hepatic Microsomal Enzymes** In vitro studies indicate slow metabolic turnover of velpatasvir by cytochrome P-450 (CYP) isoenzymes 2B6, 2C8, and 3A4; velpatasvir does not inhibit CYP isoenzymes at clinically relevant concentrations.

Pharmacokinetic interactions are possible with moderate or potent inducers of CYP2B6, 2C8, or 3A4, which may decrease sofosbuvir and/or velpatasvir plasma concentrations leading to reduced therapeutic effect of sofosbuvir/velpatasvir. Concomitant use of sofosbuvir/velpatasvir with moderate or potent inducers of CYP2B6, 2C8, or 3A4 is not recommended.

Although inhibitors of CYP2B6, 2C8, or 3A4 may increase velpatasvir plasma concentrations, sofosbuvir/velpatasvir may be used concomitantly with inhibitors of CYP2B6, 2C8, or 3A4.

■ **Drugs Affecting or Affected by P-glycoprotein Transport System** Velpatasvir is an inhibitor of the P-glycoprotein (P-gp) transport system; sofosbuvir and the predominant sofosbuvir metabolite (GS-331007) are not inhibitors of P-gp. Concomitant use of sofosbuvir/velpatasvir and P-gp substrates may affect intestinal absorption of P-gp substrates and increase exposure of such drugs.

Sofosbuvir and velpatasvir are substrates of P-gp; GS-331007 is not a P-gp substrate. Pharmacokinetic interactions are possible with P-gp inducers, which may decrease sofosbuvir and/or velpatasvir plasma concentrations leading to reduced therapeutic effect of sofosbuvir/velpatasvir. Concomitant use of sofosbuvir/velpatasvir with P-gp inducers is not recommended.

Inhibitors of P-gp may increase plasma concentrations of sofosbuvir and/or velpatasvir without increasing plasma concentrations of GS-331007. Sofosbuvir/velpatasvir may be used concomitantly with P-gp inhibitors.

■ **Drugs Affecting or Affected by Breast Cancer Resistance Protein** Velpatasvir is an inhibitor of breast cancer resistance protein (BCRP); sofosbuvir and GS-331007 are not BCRP inhibitors. Concomitant use of sofosbuvir/velpatasvir and BCRP substrates may affect intestinal absorption of BCRP substrates and increase exposure of such drugs.

Sofosbuvir and velpatasvir are substrates of BCRP; GS-331007 is not a BCRP substrate. Inhibitors of BCRP may increase plasma concentrations of sofosbuvir and/or velpatasvir without increasing plasma concentrations of GS-331007. Sofosbuvir/velpatasvir may be used concomitantly with BCRP inhibitors.

■ **Drugs Affecting or Affected by Organic Anion Transporting Polypeptides** Velpatasvir is transported by organic anion transporting polypeptide (OATP) 1B1 and 1B3. Velpatasvir inhibits OATP1B1, 1B3, and 2B1, but does not inhibit OATP1A2 at clinically relevant concentrations.

Concomitant use of sofosbuvir/velpatasvir and OATP1B1, 1B3, or 2B1 substrates may affect intestinal absorption of OATP1B1, 1B3, or 2B1 substrates and increase exposure of such drugs.

■ **Drugs Affecting or Affected by Other Membrane Transporters** Velpatasvir does not inhibit organic anion transporter (OAT) 1, OAT3, organic cation transporter (OCT) 1, OCT2, multidrug and toxin extrusion protein (MATE) 1, or uridine diphosphate-glucuronosyl transferase (UGT) 1A1 at clinically relevant concentrations.

■ **Drugs Affecting Gastric pH** The solubility of velpatasvir decreases as pH increases. Therefore, drugs that increase gastric pH are expected to decrease velpatasvir plasma concentrations.

Antacids Administration of sofosbuvir/velpatasvir and antacids (e.g., aluminum and magnesium hydroxides) should be separated by 4 hours.

Histamine H_2-Receptor Antagonists H_2-receptor antagonists may be administered concurrently with or 12 hours apart from sofosbuvir/velpatasvir; dosage of the H_2-receptor antagonist should not exceed dosages comparable to famotidine 40 mg twice daily.

Proton-pump Inhibitors Concomitant use of sofosbuvir/velpatasvir and proton-pump inhibitors (e.g., omeprazole) is not recommended.

If concomitant use of sofosbuvir/velpatasvir and omeprazole is considered necessary, sofosbuvir/velpatasvir should be administered with food 4 hours before omeprazole 20 mg. Use of sofosbuvir/velpatasvir with other proton-pump inhibitors has not been studied.

■ **Antiarrhythmic Agents** ***Amiodarone*** Concomitant use of amiodarone and sofosbuvir/velpatasvir may result in serious symptomatic bradycardia and is not recommended. If there are no alternative hepatitis C virus (HCV) treatment options and a regimen of sofosbuvir/velpatasvir must be used in a patient receiving amiodarone, the patient should be advised about the risk of serious symptomatic bradycardia and cardiac monitoring should be performed in an inpatient setting during the first 48 hours of concomitant use and then heart rate monitoring (outpatient or self-monitoring) should be performed daily through at least the first 2 weeks of concomitant use. Similar cardiac monitoring is recommended in patients who discontinued amiodarone just prior to initiation of sofosbuvir/velpatasvir or if there are no other treatment options and amiodarone must be initiated in a patient already receiving sofosbuvir/velpatasvir. (See Cardiovascular Effects under Warnings/Precautions: Other Warnings/Precautions, in Cautions.)

The effect of concomitant use of amiodarone and sofosbuvir/velpatasvir on plasma concentrations of amiodarone, sofosbuvir, and velpatasvir is unknown.

■ **Anticonvulsants** Concomitant use of sofosbuvir/velpatasvir and certain anticonvulsants (i.e., carbamazepine, oxcarbazepine, phenobarbital, phenytoin) is expected to decrease sofosbuvir and velpatasvir plasma concentrations. Concomitant use of sofosbuvir/velpatasvir with such anticonvulsants is not recommended.

■ **Antifungal Agents** No clinically important pharmacokinetic interactions were observed when a single 100-mg dose of velpatasvir was used concomitantly with ketoconazole (200 mg twice daily).

■ **Antimycobacterial Agents** ***Rifabutin*** Rifabutin is expected to decrease plasma concentrations of sofosbuvir and velpatasvir.

Concomitant use of rifabutin and sofosbuvir/velpatasvir is not recommended.

Rifampin Concomitant use of rifampin (600 mg once daily) and velpatasvir (single 100-mg dose) or sofosbuvir (single 400-mg dose) results in decreased plasma concentrations and area under the plasma concentration-time curves (AUCs) of sofosbuvir and velpatasvir. Concomitant use of rifampin (single 600-mg dose) and velpatasvir (single 100-mg dose) results in increased velpatasvir plasma concentrations and AUC.

Concomitant use of rifampin and sofosbuvir/velpatasvir is not recommended.

Rifapentine Rifapentine is expected to decrease plasma concentrations of sofosbuvir and velpatasvir.

Concomitant use of rifapentine and sofosbuvir/velpatasvir is not recommended.

■ **Antiretroviral Agents** ***HIV Integrase Inhibitors (INSTIs)***

Dolutegravir. No clinically important pharmacokinetic interactions were observed when sofosbuvir/velpatasvir was used concomitantly with dolutegravir.

Elvitegravir. Concomitant use of sofosbuvir/velpatasvir and the fixed combination of elvitegravir, cobicistat, emtricitabine, and tenofovir disoproxil fumarate (tenofovir DF) (EVG/c/FTC/TDF) does not have a clinically important effect on the pharmacokinetics of sofosbuvir, velpatasvir, elvitegravir, cobicistat, or emtricitabine, but results in increased tenofovir plasma concentrations and AUC. Patients should be monitored for tenofovir-associated adverse effects if sofosbuvir/velpatasvir is used concomitantly with EVG/c/FTC/TDF.

No clinically important pharmacokinetic interactions were observed when the fixed combination of elvitegravir, cobicistat, emtricitabine, and tenofovir alafenamide (EVG/c/FTC/TAF) was used concomitantly with sofosbuvir or velpatasvir.

Raltegravir. Concomitant use of sofosbuvir/velpatasvir and an HIV antiretroviral regimen of raltegravir in conjunction with the fixed combination of emtricitabine and tenofovir DF (emtricitabine/tenofovir DF) does not have a clinically important effect on the pharmacokinetics of raltegravir or emtricitabine, but results in increased tenofovir plasma concentrations and AUC.

Patients should be monitored for tenofovir-associated adverse effects if sofosbuvir/velpatasvir is used concomitantly with any HIV antiretroviral regimen containing tenofovir DF.

HIV Nonnucleoside Reverse Transcriptase Inhibitors (NNRTIs)

Efavirenz. Concomitant use of the fixed combination of efavirenz, emtricitabine, and tenofovir DF (efavirenz/emtricitabine/tenofovir DF) and sofosbuvir/velpatasvir does not have a clinically important effect on the pharmacokinetics of sofosbuvir, but results in decreased velpatasvir plasma concentrations and AUC and increased tenofovir plasma concentrations and AUC.

Concomitant use of sofosbuvir/velpatasvir with HIV antiretroviral regimens containing efavirenz is not recommended.

Rilpivirine. Concomitant use of the fixed combination of emtricitabine, rilpivirine, and tenofovir DF (emtricitabine/rilpivirine/tenofovir DF) and sofosbuvir/velpatasvir does not have a clinically important effect on the pharmacokinetics of sofosbuvir, velpatasvir, emtricitabine, or rilpivirine, but results in increased tenofovir plasma concentrations and AUC.

Patients should be monitored for tenofovir-associated adverse effects if sofosbuvir/velpatasvir is used concomitantly with any HIV antiretroviral regimen containing tenofovir DF.

HIV Nucleoside and Nucleotide Reverse Transcriptase Inhibitors (NRTIs) **Emtricitabine.** No clinically important pharmacokinetic interactions were observed when sofosbuvir/velpatasvir was used concomitantly with emtricitabine.

Tenofovir. Concomitant use of sofosbuvir/velpatasvir and HIV antiretroviral regimens that include tenofovir DF and certain other antiretroviral agents may result in increased tenofovir plasma concentrations, including the fixed-combination preparations of EVG/c/FTC/TDF, emtricitabine/rilpivirine/tenofovir DF, raltegravir in conjunction with emtricitabine/tenofovir DF, *ritonavir-boosted* atazanavir in conjunction with emtricitabine/tenofovir DF, and *ritonavir-boosted* darunavir in conjunction with emtricitabine/tenofovir DF.

Patients should be monitored for tenofovir-associated adverse effects if sofosbuvir/velpatasvir is used concomitantly with any HIV antiretroviral regimen containing tenofovir DF.

HIV Protease Inhibitors (PIs) **Atazanavir.** Concomitant use of *ritonavir-boosted* atazanavir and sofosbuvir/velpatasvir does not result in clinically important pharmacokinetic interactions.

Concomitant use of *ritonavir-boosted* atazanavir in conjunction with emtricitabine/tenofovir DF and sofosbuvir/velpatasvir results in increased velpatasvir and tenofovir plasma concentrations and AUC. Patients should be monitored for tenofovir-associated adverse effects if sofosbuvir/velpatasvir is used concomitantly with any HIV antiretroviral regimen containing tenofovir DF.

Darunavir. Concomitant use of *ritonavir-boosted* darunavir and sofosbuvir/velpatasvir does not result in clinically important pharmacokinetic interactions.

Concomitant use of *ritonavir-boosted* darunavir in conjunction with emtricitabine/tenofovir DF and sofosbuvir/velpatasvir results in decreased sofosbuvir and velpatasvir plasma concentrations and AUC and increased tenofovir plasma concentrations and AUC. Patients should be monitored for tenofovir-associated adverse effects if sofosbuvir/velpatasvir is used concomitantly with any HIV antiretroviral regimen containing tenofovir DF.

Lopinavir. Concomitant use of the fixed combination of lopinavir and ritonavir (lopinavir/ritonavir) in conjunction with emtricitabine/tenofovir DF and sofosbuvir/velpatasvir does not have a clinically important effect on the pharmacokinetics of sofosbuvir or velpatasvir.

Tipranavir. Concomitant use of *ritonavir-boosted* tipranavir and sofosbuvir/velpatasvir is expected to decrease sofosbuvir and velpatasvir plasma concentrations.

Concomitant use of *ritonavir-boosted* tipranavir and sofosbuvir/velpatasvir is not recommended.

■ **Digoxin** Concomitant use of velpatasvir and a single 0.25-mg dose of digoxin results in increased digoxin plasma concentrations and AUC.

Therapeutic concentration monitoring of digoxin is recommended if the drug is used concomitantly with sofosbuvir/velpatasvir.

■ **Estrogens and Progestins** Concomitant use of sofosbuvir or velpatasvir and an oral contraceptive containing ethinyl estradiol and norgestimate did not have a clinically important effect on the pharmacokinetics of ethinyl estradiol or norgestimate and its active metabolites (norelgestromin, norgestrel).

■ **HCV Antivirals** ***HCV Polymerase Inhibitors*** In vitro in replicon studies, there was no evidence of antagonistic anti-HCV effects between velpatasvir and sofosbuvir or between velpatasvir and other HCV nonstructural 5B (NS5B) polymerase inhibitors tested.

HCV Protease Inhibitors In vitro in replicon studies, there was no evidence of antagonistic anti-HCV effects between velpatasvir and an HCV NS3/4A protease inhibitor.

HCV Replication Complex Inhibitors In vitro in replicon studies, there was no evidence of antagonistic anti-HCV effects between velpatasvir and ledipasvir, an HCV NS5A replication complex inhibitor (NS5A inhibitor).

■ **HMG-CoA Reductase Inhibitors** ***Atorvastatin*** Concomitant use of sofosbuvir/velpatasvir and atorvastatin is expected to increase plasma concentrations of atorvastatin, which is associated with increased risk of myopathy and rhabdomyolysis.

If sofosbuvir/velpatasvir and atorvastatin are used concomitantly, the patient should be closely monitored for HMG-CoA reductase inhibitor-associated adverse effects (e.g., myopathy, rhabdomyolysis).

Pravastatin No clinically important pharmacokinetic interactions were observed when velpatasvir (100 mg once daily) was used concomitantly with pravastatin (single 40-mg dose).

Rosuvastatin Concomitant use of velpatasvir (100 mg once daily) and rosuvastatin (single 10-mg dose) results in substantially increased rosuvastatin plasma concentrations and AUC, which is associated with increased risk of myopathy and rhabdomyolysis.

If sofosbuvir/velpatasvir and rosuvastatin are used concomitantly, rosuvastatin dosage should not exceed 10 mg daily.

■ **Immunosuppressive Agents** ***Cyclosporine*** No clinically important pharmacokinetic interactions were observed when cyclosporine (single 600-mg dose) was used concomitantly with sofosbuvir (single 400-mg dose) or velpatasvir (single 100-mg dose).

Tacrolimus No clinically important pharmacokinetic interactions were observed when tacrolimus (single 5-mg dose) was used concomitantly with sofosbuvir (single 400-mg dose).

■ **Interferons** In vitro in replicon studies, there was no evidence of antagonistic anti-HCV effects between sofosbuvir and interferon alfa or between velpatasvir and interferon alfa.

■ **Methadone** No clinically important pharmacokinetic interactions were observed when sofosbuvir (400 mg once daily) was used concomitantly with methadone hydrochloride (30–130 mg daily).

■ **Ribavirin** In vitro in replicon studies, there was no evidence of antagonistic anti-HCV effects between sofosbuvir and ribavirin or between velpatasvir and ribavirin.

■ **St. John's Wort** Concomitant use of St. John's wort (*Hypericum perforatum*) and sofosbuvir/velpatasvir may result in clinically important decreases in sofosbuvir and velpatasvir plasma concentrations.

Concomitant use of sofosbuvir/velpatasvir and St. John's wort is not recommended.

■ **Topotecan** Concomitant use of sofosbuvir/velpatasvir and topotecan is expected to increase topotecan plasma concentrations.

Concomitant use of sofosbuvir/velpatasvir and topotecan is not recommended.

■ **Warfarin** In patients receiving warfarin, subtherapeutic international normalized ratios (INRs) have been reported after initiation of sofosbuvir-containing HCV treatment regimens.

INR should be closely monitored when initiating or discontinuing sofosbuvir-containing regimens (e.g., sofosbuvir/velpatasvir) in patients receiving warfarin.

Description

Sofosbuvir and velpatasvir (sofosbuvir/velpatasvir) is a fixed combination containing 2 hepatitis C virus (HCV) antivirals. Sofosbuvir is a nucleotide analog HCV nonstructural 5B (NS5B) polymerase inhibitor. Velpatasvir is an HCV nonstructural 5A (NS5A) replication complex inhibitor (NS5A inhibitor). Both drugs are direct-acting antivirals (DAAs) with activity against HCV. There was no in vitro evidence of antagonistic anti-HCV effects between sofosbuvir and velpatasvir when the combination was evaluated in HCV replicon studies.

Sofosbuvir is a prodrug that is converted in the liver to a pharmacologically active uridine analog triphosphate (GS-461203), which can be incorporated into HCV RNA by NS5B polymerase and acts as an RNA chain terminator. In vitro studies using biochemical and cell-based replicon assays indicate that GS-461203 has activity against HCV genotypes 1b, 2a, 3a, and 4a. Sofosbuvir has shown in vitro activity against full-length or chimeric replicons of HCV genotypes 1a, 1b, 2a, 2b, 3a, 4a, 4d, 5a, and 6a (mean concentration of the drug required to inhibit viral replication by 50% [EC_{50}] has ranged from 14–110 nM).

Velpatasvir inhibits the HCV NS5A protein, which is required for viral replication. Velpatasvir has shown in vitro activity against full-length or chimeric replicons of HCV genotypes 1a, 1b, 2a, 2b, 3a, 4a, 4d, 5a, 6a, and 6e (mean EC_{50} has ranged from 0.002–0.13 nM).

Certain amino acid substitutions in NS5B polymerase of HCV genotypes 1b, 2a, 2b, 3a, 4a, 5a, and 6a have been selected in cell culture and have been associated with reduced susceptibility to sofosbuvir in vitro in replicon studies. In all replicon genotypes tested, the S282T substitution was associated with reduced susceptibility to sofosbuvir; in genotypes 2a, 5, and 6 replicons, an M289L substitution developed along with the S282T substitution. Treatment-emergent NS5B resistance-associated substitutions were detected in phase 3 clinical trials evaluating sofosbuvir/velpatasvir in patients with HCV genotype 3a infection (e.g., L314F, L314I, L314P) who experienced virologic failure.

Certain amino acid substitutions in NS5A of HCV genotype 1a (e.g., L31V, Y93H/N), genotype 1b (e.g., L31V, Y93H), genotype 2a (e.g., F28S, Y93H), genotype 3a (e.g., Y93H/S), genotype 4a (e.g., Y93H), and genotype 6 (e.g., L31V, P32A/L/Q/R) have been selected in cell culture and have been associated with reduced susceptibility to velpatasvir in vitro in replicon studies. Combinations of these NS5A substitutions often resulted in greater reductions in susceptibility to velpatasvir compared with a single NS5A substitution. Treatment-emergent NS5A resistance-associated substitutions were detected in phase 3 clinical trials evaluating sofosbuvir/velpatasvir in patients with HCV genotype 1a (e.g., Y93N, Q30R, H58D), genotype 1b (e.g., L31M/V, Y93H), genotype 1c/h (e.g., Y93H, K24M/T, L31I/V), or genotype 3a (e.g., Y93H, M28T/V, S38P/Y, P58L, A30V, H58T) infection who experienced virologic failure. Some of these patients also had baseline NS5A polymorphisms at resistance-associated amino acid positions.

Sofosbuvir and velpatasvir are active against HCV with substitutions associated with resistance to other HCV DAAs that have different mechanisms of action (e.g., HCV NS5B polymerase inhibitors, HCV NS3 protease inhibitors). Efficacy of sofosbuvir/velpatasvir has not been established in patients in whom previous treatment with a regimen that included an NS5A inhibitor failed.

Following oral administration of sofosbuvir/velpatasvir, peak plasma concentrations of sofosbuvir occur approximately 0.5–1 hour after the dose and peak plasma concentrations of velpatasvir occur 3 hours after the dose. Administration of sofosbuvir/velpatasvir with a moderate-fat (approximately 600 kcal, 30% fat) or high-fat (approximately 800 kcal, 50% fat) meal increased sofosbuvir exposures by 60 or 78%, respectively, and increased velpatasvir exposures by 34 or 21%, respectively.

Sofosbuvir is a prodrug that undergoes intracellular metabolic activation in the liver (hydrolysis by human cathepsin A [CatA] or carboxylesterase 1 [CES1], phosphoramidate cleavage by histidine triad nucleotide-binding protein 1 [HINT1], and phosphorylation by pyrimidine nucleotide biosynthesis pathway). This results in formation of the pharmacologically active metabolite, GS-461203; desphosphorylation subsequently occurs leading to formation of GS-331007 (the predominant circulating metabolite), which has no anti-HCV activity. Sofosbuvir is approximately 61–65% bound to plasma proteins. The major route of elimination is renal clearance (glomerular filtration and active tubular secretion). Following a single 400-mg oral dose of sofosbuvir, 80% is eliminated in urine (mainly as GS-331007), 14% is excreted in feces, and 2.5% is eliminated in expired air. The median terminal plasma half-lives of sofosbuvir and GS-331007 are 0.5 and 25 hours, respectively.

Velpatasvir is metabolized by cytochrome P-450 (CYP) isoenzymes 2B6, 2C8, and 3A4. The drug is greater than 99.5% bound to plasma proteins. The major route of elimination of velpatasvir is biliary excretion (approximately 77% excreted as the parent drug). Following a single 100-mg oral dose of velpatasvir, 94% is excreted in feces and 0.4% is eliminated in urine. The median terminal plasma half-life of velpatasvir is 15 hours.

Advice to Patients

Importance of reading patient information provided by the manufacturer.

Advise patients that the fixed-combination preparation of sofosbuvir and velpatasvir (sofosbuvir/velpatasvir) should be taken once daily (with or without food) on a regular dosing schedule.

Importance of taking the recommended dosage of sofosbuvir/velpatasvir for the recommended duration of treatment; importance of not missing doses.

Inform patients that reactivation of hepatitis B virus (HBV) infection has occurred in patients being treated for hepatitis C virus (HCV) infection who were coinfected with HBV. Importance of informing clinician of any history of HBV infection or other liver problems (e.g., cirrhosis). Importance of immediately contacting a clinician if any signs or symptoms of serious liver injury (e.g., fatigue, weakness, loss of appetite, nausea and vomiting, yellowing of the eyes or skin, light-colored bowel movements) occur. (See Risk of HBV Reactivation in Patients Coinfected with HCV and HBV under Warnings/Precautions: Warnings, in Cautions.)

If sofosbuvir/velpatasvir is used in a patient receiving amiodarone, advise the patient about the risk of serious symptomatic bradycardia and the importance of immediately contacting a clinician if signs or symptoms of bradycardia (e.g., near-fainting or fainting, dizziness, lightheadedness, malaise, weakness, excessive tiredness, shortness of breath, chest pain, confusion, memory problems) occur. (See Cardiovascular Effects under Warnings/Precautions: Other Warnings/Precautions, in Cautions.)

Importance of informing clinicians of existing or contemplated concomitant therapy, including prescription and OTC drugs and dietary or herbal supplements, as well as any concomitant illnesses.

Importance of women informing clinicians if they are or plan to become pregnant or plan to breast-feed. If used in conjunction with ribavirin, advise men and women of importance of using 2 forms of effective contraception during and for 6 months after ribavirin therapy. (See Precautions Related to Fixed Combinations and Multiple-drug Treatment Regimens under Warnings/Precautions: Other Warnings/Precautions, in Cautions.)

Importance of informing patients of other important precautionary information. (See Cautions.)

Overview® (see Users Guide). For additional information on this drug until a more detailed monograph is developed and published, the manufacturer's labeling should be consulted. It is *essential* that the manufacturer's labeling be consulted for more detailed information on usual cautions, precautions, contraindications, potential drug interactions, laboratory test interferences, and acute toxicity.

Preparations

Excipients in commercially available drug preparations may have clinically important effects in some individuals; consult specific product labeling for details.

Sofosbuvir and Velpatasvir

Oral

Tablets, film-coated	Sofosbuvir 400 mg and Velpatasvir 100 mg	**Epclusa®**, Gilead

Sofosbuvir, Velpatasvir, and Voxilaprevir SOF

■ Sofosbuvir, velpatasvir, and voxilaprevir (sofosbuvir/velpatasvir/voxilaprevir) is a fixed combination containing 3 hepatitis C virus (HCV) antivirals; sofosbuvir is a nucleotide analog HCV nonstructural 5B (NS5B) polymerase inhibitor, velpatasvir is an HCV nonstructural 5A (NS5A) replication complex inhibitor (NS5A inhibitor), and voxilaprevir is an HCV nonstructural 3/4A (NS3/4A) protease inhibitor.

Uses

■ **Chronic Hepatitis C Virus Infection** The fixed combination of sofosbuvir, velpatasvir, and voxilaprevir (sofosbuvir/velpatasvir/voxilaprevir) is used for the treatment of chronic hepatitis C virus (HCV) genotype 1, 2, 3, 4, 5, or 6 infection in adults previously treated with an HCV regimen containing an HCV nonstructural 5A (NS5A) replication complex inhibitor (NS5A inhibitor), including those with compensated cirrhosis.

Sofosbuvir/velpatasvir/voxilaprevir also is used for the treatment of HCV genotype 1a or 3 infection in adults previously treated with an HCV regimen containing sofosbuvir *without* an HCV NS5A inhibitor, including those with compensated cirrhosis. Clinical trial data to date indicate that sofosbuvir/velpatasvir/voxilaprevir does not provide any additional benefit over the fixed combination of sofosbuvir and velpatasvir (sofosbuvir/velpatasvir) for the treatment of HCV genotype 1b, 2, 4, 5, or 6 infection in adults previously treated with sofosbuvir *without* an HCV NS5A inhibitor.

Although sofosbuvir/velpatasvir/voxilaprevir has been used for treatment of chronic HCV infection caused by HCV genotypes 1, 2, 3, 4, 5, or 6 in some treatment-naive† (previously untreated) adults, the drug is not labeled by FDA for use in such patients.

Because the treatment of chronic HCV infection is complex and rapidly evolving, it is recommended that treatment be directed by clinicians who are familiar with the disease and that a specialist be consulted to obtain the most up-to-date information. Information from the American Association for the Study of Liver Diseases (AASLD) and Infectious Diseases Society of America (IDSA) regarding diagnosis and management of HCV infection, including recommendations for initial treatment, is available at http://www.hcvguidelines.org.

HCV Genotype 1 Infection Efficacy and safety of sofosbuvir/velpatasvir/voxilaprevir for the treatment of chronic HCV genotype 1 infection in adults have been evaluated in 3 randomized, phase 3 trials (POLARIS-1, PO-

LARIS-2, and POLARIS-4). The primary end point in each study was sustained virologic response at 12 weeks after the end of treatment (SVR12; defined as plasma HCV RNA level less than 15 IU/mL [the lower limit of quantification] at 12 weeks after end of treatment).

POLARIS-1, a double-blind, placebo-controlled trial, included 415 adults with chronic HCV genotype 1, 2, 3, 4, 5, or 6 infection who were noncirrhotic or had compensated cirrhosis and had previously failed treatment with an HCV regimen containing an HCV NS5A inhibitor (median age 59 years, 77% male, 74% with baseline HCV RNA levels 800,000 IU/mL or greater, 41% with compensated cirrhosis). Patients were previously treated with HCV treatment regimens containing ledipasvir (51%), daclatasvir (27%), ombitasvir (11%), velpatasvir (7%), or elbasvir (3%). Those with HCV genotype 1 infection were randomized in a 1:1 ratio to receive a 12-week regimen of sofosbuvir/velpatasvir/voxilaprevir (a fixed-combination tablet containing 400 mg of sofosbuvir, 100 mg of velpatasvir, and 100 mg of voxilaprevir) or placebo once daily. Of the 101 patients with HCV genotype 1a infection treated with sofosbuvir/velpatasvir/voxilaprevir, 96% achieved SVR12; of the 45 patients with HCV genotype 1b infection treated with sofosbuvir/velpatasvir/voxilaprevir, 100% achieved SVR12. No patients treated with placebo achieved SVR12.

POLARIS-4, a randomized, open-label trial, included 333 previously treated adults with chronic HCV genotype 1, 2, 3, or 4 infection who were noncirrhotic or had compensated cirrhosis and had previously failed treatment with an HCV regimen that included a direct acting antiviral (DAA), but did *not* include an HCV NS5A inhibitor (median age 58 years, 77% male, 75% with baseline HCV RNA levels 800,000 IU/mL or greater, 81% with non-CC IL28B alleles [CT or TT], 46% with compensated cirrhosis). Patients whose only DAA exposure was an HCV NS3/4A protease inhibitor were excluded. Those with HCV genotype 1 infection were randomized in a 1:1 ratio to receive sofosbuvir/velpatasvir/voxilaprevir (a fixed-combination tablet containing 400 mg of sofosbuvir, 100 mg of velpatasvir, and 100 mg of voxilaprevir) or sofosbuvir/velpatasvir (a fixed-combination tablet containing 400 mg of sofosbuvir and 100 mg of velpatasvir) once daily for 12 weeks. Of the 54 patients with HCV genotype 1 infection treated with a regimen of sofosbuvir/velpatasvir/voxilaprevir, 96% achieved SVR12 (97 or 94% of those with HCV genotype 1a or 1b, respectively). Of the 40 patients with HCV genotype 1 infection treated with a regimen of sofosbuvir/velpatasvir, 85% achieved SVR12 (82 or 92% of those with HCV genotype 1a or 1b, respectively).

POLARIS-2, a randomized, open-label trial, evaluated sofosbuvir/velpatasvir/voxilaprevir in adults with any genotype of HCV infection who were treatment naive or previously failed treatment with an HCV regimen that did not include a DAA. Enrolled patients were noncirrhotic or had compensated cirrhosis, although those with HCV genotype 3 infection were excluded if they had cirrhosis. Patients were randomized in a 1:1 ratio to receive sofosbuvir/velpatasvir/voxilaprevir (a fixed-combination tablet containing 400 mg of sofosbuvir, 100 mg of velpatasvir, and 100 mg of voxilaprevir) once daily for 8 weeks or sofosbuvir/velpatasvir (a fixed-combination tablet containing 400 mg of sofosbuvir and 100 mg of velpatasvir) once daily for 12 weeks. Results showed that the 8-week regimen of sofosbuvir/velpatasvir/voxilaprevir in these patients did *not* meet noninferiority criteria when compared with the 12-week regimen of sofosbuvir/velpatasvir (overall SVR12 achieved by 95 or 98% of patients, respectively).

HCV Genotype 2 Infection Efficacy and safety of sofosbuvir/velpatasvir/voxilaprevir for the treatment of chronic HCV genotype 2 infection in adults have been evaluated in 3 randomized, phase 3 trials (POLARIS-1, POLARIS-2, and POLARIS-4). The primary end point in each study was sustained virologic response at 12 weeks after the end of treatment (SVR12; defined as plasma HCV RNA level less than 15 IU/mL [the lower limit of quantification] at 12 weeks after end of treatment).

POLARIS-1, a double-blind, placebo-controlled trial, included 415 adults with chronic HCV genotype 1, 2, 3, 4, 5, or 6 infection who were noncirrhotic or had compensated cirrhosis and had previously failed treatment with an HCV regimen containing an HCV NS5A inhibitor (median age 59 years, 77% male, 74% with baseline HCV RNA levels 800,000 IU/mL or greater, 41% with compensated cirrhosis). Patients were previously treated with HCV treatment regimens containing ledipasvir (51%), daclatasvir (27%), ombitasvir (11%), velpatasvir (7%), or elbasvir (3%). All enrolled patients with HCV genotype 2 infection received a 12-week regimen of sofosbuvir/velpatasvir/voxilaprevir (a fixed-combination tablet containing 400 mg of sofosbuvir, 100 mg of velpatasvir, and 100 mg of voxilaprevir) once daily. Of the 5 patients with HCV genotype 2 infection treated with sofosbuvir/velpatasvir/voxilaprevir, 100% achieved SVR12.

POLARIS-4, a randomized, open-label trial, included 333 previously treated adults with chronic HCV genotype 1, 2, 3, or 4 infection who were noncirrhotic or had compensated cirrhosis and had previously failed treatment with an HCV regimen that included a DAA, but did *not* include an HCV NS5A inhibitor (median age 58 years, 77% male, 75% with baseline HCV RNA levels 800,000 IU/mL or greater, 81% with non-CC IL28B alleles [CT or TT], 46% with compensated cirrhosis). Patients whose only DAA exposure was an HCV NS3/4A protease inhibitor were excluded. Those with HCV genotype 2 infection were randomized in a 1:1 ratio to receive sofosbuvir/velpatasvir/voxilaprevir (a fixed-combination tablet containing 400 mg of sofosbuvir, 100 mg of velpatasvir, and 100 mg of voxilaprevir) or sofosbuvir/velpatasvir (a fixed-combination tablet containing 400 mg of sofosbuvir and 100 mg of velpatasvir) once daily for 12 weeks. Of the 31 patients with HCV genotype 2 infection treated with a regimen of sofosbuvir/velpatasvir/voxilaprevir, 100% achieved SVR12. Of the 33 patients with HCV genotype 2 infection treated with a regimen of sofosbuvir/velpatasvir, 97% achieved SVR12.

POLARIS-2, a randomized, open-label trial, evaluated sofosbuvir/velpatasvir/voxilaprevir in adults with any genotype of HCV infection who were treatment naive or previously failed treatment with an HCV regimen that did not include a DAA. Enrolled patients were noncirrhotic or had compensated cirrhosis, although those with HCV genotype 3 infection were excluded if they had cirrhosis. Patients were randomized in a 1:1 ratio to receive sofosbuvir/velpatasvir/voxilaprevir (a fixed-combination tablet containing 400 mg of sofosbuvir, 100 mg of velpatasvir, and 100 mg of voxilaprevir) once daily for 8 weeks or sofosbuvir/velpatasvir (a fixed-combination tablet containing 400 mg of sofosbuvir and 100 mg of velpatasvir) once daily for 12 weeks. Results showed that the 8-week regimen of sofosbuvir/velpatasvir/voxilaprevir did *not* meet noninferiority criteria in these patients when compared with the 12-week regimen of sofosbuvir/velpatasvir (overall SVR12 achieved by 95 or 98% of patients, respectively).

HCV Genotype 3 Infection Efficacy and safety of sofosbuvir/velpatasvir/voxilaprevir for the treatment of chronic HCV genotype 3 infection in adults have been evaluated in 4 randomized, phase 3 trials (POLARIS-1, POLARIS-2, POLARIS-3, and POLARIS-4). The primary end point in each study was sustained virologic response at 12 weeks after the end of treatment (SVR12; defined as plasma HCV RNA level less than 15 IU/mL [the lower limit of quantification] at 12 weeks after end of treatment).

POLARIS-1, a double-blind, placebo-controlled trial, included 415 adults with chronic HCV genotype 1, 2, 3, 4, 5, or 6 infection who were noncirrhotic or had compensated cirrhosis and had previously failed treatment with an HCV regimen containing an HCV NS5A inhibitor (median age 59 years, 77% male, 74% with baseline HCV RNA levels 800,000 IU/mL or greater, 41% with compensated cirrhosis). Patients were previously treated with HCV treatment regimens containing ledipasvir (51%), daclatasvir (27%), ombitasvir (11%), velpatasvir (7%), or elbasvir (3%). All patients with HCV genotype 3 infection received a 12-week regimen of sofosbuvir/velpatasvir/voxilaprevir (a fixed-combination tablet containing 400 mg of sofosbuvir, 100 mg of velpatasvir, and 100 mg of voxilaprevir) once daily. Of the 78 patients with HCV genotype 3 infection treated with sofosbuvir/velpatasvir/voxilaprevir, 95% achieved SVR12.

POLARIS-4, a randomized, open-label trial, included 333 previously treated adults with chronic HCV genotype 1, 2, 3, or 4 infection who were noncirrhotic or had compensated cirrhosis and had previously failed treatment with an HCV regimen that included a DAA, but did *not* include an HCV NS5A inhibitor (median age 58 years, 77% male, 75% with baseline HCV RNA levels 800,000 IU/mL or greater, 81% with non-CC IL28B alleles [CT or TT], 46% with compensated cirrhosis). Patients whose only DAA exposure was an HCV NS3/4A protease inhibitor were excluded. Those with HCV genotype 3 infection were randomized in a 1:1 ratio to receive sofosbuvir/velpatasvir/voxilaprevir (a fixed-combination tablet containing 400 mg of sofosbuvir, 100 mg of velpatasvir, and 100 mg of voxilaprevir) or sofosbuvir/velpatasvir (a fixed-combination tablet containing 400 mg of sofosbuvir and 100 mg of velpatasvir) once daily for 12 weeks. Of the 54 patients with HCV genotype 3 infection treated with a regimen of sofosbuvir/velpatasvir/voxilaprevir, 96% achieved SVR12. Of the 52 patients with HCV genotype 3 infection treated with a regimen of sofosbuvir/velpatasvir, 85% achieved SVR12.

POLARIS-2, a randomized, open-label trial, evaluated sofosbuvir/velpatasvir/voxilaprevir in adults with any genotype of HCV infection who were treatment naive or previously failed treatment with an HCV regimen that did not include a DAA. Enrolled patients were noncirrhotic or had compensated cirrhosis, although those with HCV genotype 3 infection were excluded if they had cirrhosis. Patients were randomized in a 1:1 ratio to receive sofosbuvir/velpatasvir/voxilaprevir (a fixed-combination tablet containing 400 mg of sofosbuvir, 100 mg of velpatasvir, and 100 mg of voxilaprevir) once daily for 8 weeks or sofosbuvir/velpatasvir (a fixed-combination tablet containing 400 mg of sofosbuvir and 100 mg of velpatasvir) once daily for 12 weeks. Results showed that the 8-week regimen of sofosbuvir/velpatasvir/voxilaprevir did *not* meet noninferiority criteria in these patients when compared with the 12-week regimen of sofosbuvir/velpatasvir (overall SVR12 achieved by 95 or 98% of patients, respectively).

POLARIS-3, a randomized, open-label trial, evaluated sofosbuvir/velpatasvir/voxilaprevir in treatment-naive patients with HCV genotype 3 infection who also had compensated cirrhosis. Patients were randomized in a 1:1 ratio to receive sofosbuvir/velpatasvir/voxilaprevir (a fixed-combination tablet containing 400 mg of sofosbuvir, 100 mg of velpatasvir, and 100 mg of voxilaprevir) once daily for 8 weeks or a fixed combination of sofosbuvir and velpatasvir (a fixed-combination tablet containing 400 mg of sofosbuvir and 100 mg of velpatasvir) once daily for 12 weeks. SVR12 was achieved by 96% of patients in each group. Both groups exceeded the performance goal of 83%, but the two groups were not statistically compared with each other.

HCV Genotype 4 Infection Efficacy and safety of sofosbuvir/velpatasvir/voxilaprevir for the treatment of chronic HCV genotype 4 infection in adults have been evaluated in 3 randomized, phase 3 trials (POLARIS-1, POLARIS-2, and POLARIS-4). The primary end point in each study was sustained virologic response at 12 weeks after the end of treatment (SVR12; defined as plasma HCV RNA level less than 15 IU/mL [the lower limit of quantification] at 12 weeks after end of treatment).

POLARIS-1, a double-blind, placebo-controlled trial, included 415 adults with chronic HCV genotype 1, 2, 3, 4, 5, or 6 infection who were noncirrhotic or had compensated cirrhosis and had previously failed treatment with an HCV regimen containing an HCV NS5A inhibitor (median age 59 years, 77% male, 74% with baseline HCV RNA levels 800,000 IU/mL or greater, 41% with compensated cirrhosis). Patients were previously treated with HCV treatment regimens containing ledipasvir (51%), daclatasvir (27%), ombitasvir (11%), velpatasvir (7%), or elbasvir (3%). All patients with HCV genotype 4 infection received a 12-week regimen of sofosbuvir/velpatasvir/voxilaprevir (a fixed-combination tablet containing 400 mg of sofosbuvir, 100 mg of velpatasvir, and 100 mg of voxilaprevir) once daily. Of the 22 patients with HCV genotype 4 infection treated with sofosbuvir/velpatasvir/voxilaprevir, 91% achieved SVR12.

POLARIS-4, a randomized, open-label trial, included 333 previously treated adults with chronic HCV genotype 1, 2, 3, or 4 infection who were noncirrhotic or had compensated cirrhosis and had previously failed treatment with an HCV regimen that included a DAA, but did *not* include an HCV NS5A inhibitor (median age 58 years, 77% male, 75% with baseline HCV RNA levels 800,000 IU/mL or greater, 81% with non-CC IL28B alleles [CT or TT], 46% with compensated cirrhosis). Patients whose only DAA exposure was an HCV NS3/4A protease inhibitor were excluded. All patients with HCV genotype 4 infection received sofosbuvir/velpatasvir/voxilaprevir (a fixed-combination tablet containing 400 mg of sofosbuvir, 100 mg of velpatasvir, and 100 mg of voxilaprevir) once daily for 12 weeks. Of the 18 patients with HCV genotype 4 infection treated with a regimen of sofosbuvir/velpatasvir/voxilaprevir, 100% achieved SVR12.

POLARIS-2, a randomized, open-label trial, evaluated sofosbuvir/velpatasvir/voxilaprevir in adults with any genotype of HCV infection who were treatment naive or previously failed treatment with an HCV regimen that did not include a DAA. Enrolled patients were noncirrhotic or had compensated cirrhosis, although those with HCV genotype 3 infection were excluded if they had cirrhosis. Patients were randomized in a 1:1 ratio to receive sofosbuvir/velpatasvir/voxilaprevir (a fixed-combination tablet containing 400 mg of sofosbuvir, 100 mg of velpatasvir, and 100 mg of voxilaprevir) once daily for 8 weeks or sofosbuvir/velpatasvir (a fixed-combination tablet containing 400 mg of sofosbuvir and 100 mg of velpatasvir) once daily for 12 weeks. Results showed that the 8-week regimen of sofosbuvir/velpatasvir/voxilaprevir did *not* meet noninferiority criteria in these patients when compared with the 12-week regimen of sofosbuvir/velpatasvir (overall SVR12 achieved by 95 or 98% of patients, respectively).

HCV Genotype 5 Infection Efficacy and safety of sofosbuvir/velpatasvir/voxilaprevir for the treatment of chronic HCV genotype 5 infection in adults have been evaluated in 2 randomized, phase 3 trials (POLARIS-1 and POLARIS-2). The primary end point in both studies was sustained virologic response at 12 weeks after the end of treatment (SVR12; defined as plasma HCV RNA level less than 15 IU/mL [the lower limit of quantification] at 12 weeks after end of treatment).

POLARIS-1, a double-blind, placebo-controlled trial, included 415 adults with chronic HCV genotype 1, 2, 3, 4, 5, or 6 infection who were noncirrhotic or had compensated cirrhosis and had previously failed treatment with an HCV regimen containing an HCV NS5A inhibitor (median age 59 years, 77% male, 74% with baseline HCV RNA levels 800,000 IU/mL or greater, 41% with compensated cirrhosis). Patients were previously treated with HCV treatment regimens containing ledipasvir (51%), daclatasvir (27%), ombitasvir (11%), velpatasvir (7%), or elbasvir (3%). The single patient with HCV genotype 5 infection enrolled in the study received a 12-week regimen of sofosbuvir/velpatasvir/voxilaprevir (a fixed-combination tablet containing 400 mg of sofosbuvir, 100 mg of velpatasvir, and 100 mg of voxilaprevir) once daily and achieved SVR12.

POLARIS-2, a randomized, open-label trial, evaluated sofosbuvir/velpatasvir/voxilaprevir in adults with any genotype of HCV infection who were treatment naive or previously failed treatment with an HCV regimen that did not include a DAA. Enrolled patients were noncirrhotic or had compensated cirrhosis, although those with HCV genotype 3 infection were excluded if they had cirrhosis. Patients were randomized in a 1:1 ratio to receive sofosbuvir/velpatasvir/voxilaprevir (a fixed-combination tablet containing 400 mg of sofosbuvir, 100 mg of velpatasvir, and 100 mg of voxilaprevir) once daily for 8 weeks or sofosbuvir/velpatasvir (a fixed-combination tablet containing 400 mg of sofosbuvir and 100 mg of velpatasvir) once daily for 12 weeks. Results showed that the 8-week regimen of sofosbuvir/velpatasvir/voxilaprevir did *not* meet noninferiority criteria in these patients when compared with the 12-week regimen of sofosbuvir/velpatasvir (overall SVR12 achieved by 95 or 98% of patients, respectively).

HCV Genotype 6 Infection Efficacy and safety of sofosbuvir/velpatasvir/voxilaprevir for the treatment of chronic HCV genotype 6 infection in adults have been evaluated in 2 randomized, phase 3 trials (POLARIS-1 and POLARIS-2). The primary end point in both studies was sustained virologic response at 12 weeks after the end of treatment (SVR12; defined as plasma HCV RNA level less than 15 IU/mL [the lower limit of quantification] at 12 weeks after end of treatment).

POLARIS-1, a double-blind, placebo-controlled trial, included 415 adults with chronic HCV genotype 1, 2, 3, 4, 5, or 6 infection who were noncirrhotic or had compensated cirrhosis and had previously failed treatment with an HCV regimen containing an HCV NS5A inhibitor (median age 59 years, 77% male, 74% with baseline HCV RNA levels 800,000 IU/mL or greater, 41% with compensated cirrhosis). Patients were previously treated with HCV treatment regimens containing ledipasvir (51%), daclatasvir (27%), ombitasvir (11%), velpatasvir (7%), or elbasvir (3%). All patients with HCV genotype 6 infection received a 12-week regimen of sofosbuvir/velpatasvir/voxilaprevir (a fixed-combination tablet containing 400 mg of sofosbuvir, 100 mg of velpatasvir, and 100 mg of voxilaprevir) once daily. Of the 6 patients with HCV genotype 6 infection treated with sofosbuvir/velpatasvir/voxilaprevir, 100% achieved SVR12.

POLARIS-2, a randomized, open-label trial, evaluated sofosbuvir/velpatasvir/voxilaprevir in adults with any genotype of HCV infection who were treatment naive or previously failed treatment with an HCV regimen that did not include a DAA. Enrolled patients were noncirrhotic or had compensated cirrhosis, although those with HCV genotype 3 infection were excluded if they had cirrhosis. Patients were randomized in a 1:1 ratio to receive sofosbuvir/velpatasvir/voxilaprevir (a fixed-combination tablet containing 400 mg of sofosbuvir, 100 mg of velpatasvir, and 100 mg of voxilaprevir) once daily for 8 weeks or sofosbuvir/velpatasvir (a fixed-combination tablet containing 400 mg of sofosbuvir and 100 mg of velpatasvir) once daily for 12 weeks. Results showed that the 8-week regimen of sofosbuvir/velpatasvir/voxilaprevir did *not* meet noninferiority criteria in these patients when compared with the 12-week regimen of sofosbuvir/velpatasvir (overall SVR12 achieved by 95 or 98% of patients, respectively).

Dosage and Administration

■ **General** Prior to initiating the fixed combination of sofosbuvir, velpatasvir, and voxilaprevir (sofosbuvir/velpatasvir/voxilaprevir) for treatment of chronic hepatitis C virus (HCV) infection, all patients should be tested for evidence of current or prior hepatitis B virus (HBV) infection by measuring hepatitis B surface antigen (HBsAg), hepatitis B surface antibody (anti-HBs), and hepatitis B core antibody (anti-HBc). (See Risk of HBV Reactivation in Patients Coinfected with HCV and HBV under Warnings/Precautions: Warnings, in Cautions.)

Prior to and during treatment, appropriate laboratory tests should be performed to evaluate liver function. (See Hepatic Impairment under Warnings/Precautions: Specific Populations, in Cautions.)

■ **Administration** Sofosbuvir/velpatasvir/voxilaprevir is administered orally once daily with food.

■ **Dosage** Sofosbuvir/velpatasvir/voxilaprevir is commercially available as fixed-combination tablets containing 400 mg of sofosbuvir, 100 mg of velpatasvir, and 100 mg of voxilaprevir.

Chronic Hepatitis C Virus Infection **HCV Genotype 1, 2, 3, 4, 5, or 6 Infection.** For the treatment of chronic HCV genotype 1, 2, 3, 4, 5, or 6 infection in adults who previously failed treatment with an HCV regimen containing an HCV NS5A replication complex inhibitor (NS5A inhibitor) and who are noncirrhotic or have compensated cirrhosis (Child-Pugh class A), the recommended dosage of sofosbuvir/velpatasvir/voxilaprevir is 1 tablet (400 mg of sofosbuvir, 100 mg of velpatasvir, and 100 mg of voxilaprevir) once daily. A treatment duration of 12 weeks is recommended.

HCV Genotype 1a or 3 Infection. For the treatment of chronic HCV genotype 1a or 3 infection in adults who previously failed treatment with an HCV regimen containing sofosbuvir *without* an HCV NS5A inhibitor and who are noncirrhotic or have compensated cirrhosis (Child-Pugh class A), the recommended dosage of sofosbuvir/velpatasvir/voxilaprevir is 1 tablet (400 mg of sofosbuvir, 100 mg of velpatasvir, and 100 mg of voxilaprevir) once daily. A treatment duration of 12 weeks is recommended.

■ **Special Populations** ***Hepatic Impairment*** Dosage adjustments are not necessary if sofosbuvir/velpatasvir/voxilaprevir is used in adults with mild hepatic impairment (Child-Pugh class A).

Sofosbuvir/velpatasvir/voxilaprevir is not recommended in adults with moderate or severe hepatic impairment (Child-Pugh class B or C). (See Hepatic Impairment under Warnings/Precautions: Specific Populations, in Cautions.)

Renal Impairment Dosage adjustments are not necessary if sofosbuvir/velpatasvir/voxilaprevir is used in adults with mild or moderate renal impairment.

Dosage recommendations are not available for patients with severe renal impairment (estimated glomerular filtration rate [eGFR] less than 30 mL/minute per 1.73 m^2) or end-stage renal disease (ESRD); safety and efficacy have not been established in such patients. (See Renal Impairment under Warnings/Precautions: Specific Populations, in Cautions.)

Geriatric Patients Dosage adjustments are not necessary if sofosbuvir/velpatasvir/voxilaprevir is used in geriatric patients. (See Geriatric Use under Warnings/Precautions: Specific Populations, in Cautions.)

Cautions

■ **Contraindications** Concomitant use of the fixed combination of sofosbuvir, velpatasvir, and voxilaprevir (sofosbuvir/velpatasvir/voxilaprevir) and rifampin is contraindicated.

■ **Warnings/Precautions** ***Warnings*** **Risk of HBV Reactivation in Patients Coinfected with HCV and HBV.** Reactivation of hepatitis B virus (HBV) infection has been reported during postmarketing experience when direct-acting antivirals (DAAs) were used for the treatment of chronic hepatitis C virus (HCV) infection in patients with HBV coinfection. In some cases, HBV reactivation resulted in fulminant hepatitis, hepatic failure, and death.

HBV reactivation (defined as an abrupt increase in HBV replication manifested as a rapid increase in serum HBV DNA levels or detection of hepatitis B surface antigen [HBsAg] in an individual who was previously HBsAg negative and hepatitis B core antibody [anti-HBc] positive) has been reported in patients with HCV and HBV coinfection who were receiving HCV treatment with a regimen that included HCV DAAs without interferon alfa. Reactivation also may be accompanied by hepatitis (i.e., increased aminotransferase concentrations) and, in severe cases, may lead to increased bilirubin concentrations, liver failure, or death.

Data to date indicate that HBV reactivation usually occurs within 4–8 weeks after initiation of HCV treatment. Patients with HBV reactivation have been heterogeneous in terms of HCV genotype and in terms of baseline HBV disease. While some patients with HBV reactivation were HBsAg positive, others had serologic evidence of resolved HBV infection (i.e., HBsAg negative and anti-HBc positive). HBV reactivation also has been reported in patients receiving certain immunosuppressant or chemotherapeutic drugs; the risk of reactivation associated with HCV DAAs may be increased in such patients.

The mechanism for HBV reactivation in patients with HCV and HBV coinfection receiving HCV DAAs is unknown. Although HCV DAAs are not known to cause immunosuppression, HBV reactivation in coinfected patients may result from a complex interplay of host immunologic responses in the setting of infection with 2 hepatitis viruses.

Prior to initiating treatment with an HCV DAA, including sofosbuvir/velpatasvir/voxilaprevir, all patients should be screened for evidence of current or prior HBV infection by measuring HBsAg, hepatitis B surface antibody (anti-HBs), and anti-HBc. If there is serologic evidence of HBV infection, baseline HBV DNA levels should be measured.

Patients with evidence of current or prior HBV infection should be monitored for clinical and laboratory signs (i.e., HBsAg, HBV DNA levels, serum aminotransferase concentrations, bilirubin concentrations) of hepatitis flare or HBV reactivation during and after treatment with HCV DAAs, including sofosbuvir/velpatasvir/voxilaprevir. Appropriate management for HBV infection should be initiated as clinically indicated.

Patients with HCV and HBV coinfection receiving sofosbuvir/velpatasvir/voxilaprevir should be advised to immediately contact a clinician if they develop any signs or symptoms of serious liver injury (e.g., fatigue, weakness, loss of appetite, nausea and vomiting, yellowing of the eyes or skin, light-colored bowel movements).

When making decisions regarding HBV monitoring or HBV treatment in coinfected patients, consultation with a clinician who has expertise in managing HBV infection is recommended.

Other Warnings/Precautions **Cardiovascular Effects.** Symptomatic bradycardia, sometimes requiring pacemaker intervention, has been reported during postmarketing experience in patients receiving amiodarone concomitantly with an HCV treatment regimen containing sofosbuvir in conjunction with daclatasvir or simeprevir. Symptomatic bradycardia, including a fatal cardiac arrest, has been reported in patients receiving amiodarone concomitantly with the fixed combination containing ledipasvir and sofosbuvir (ledipasvir/sofosbuvir).

In most reported cases, bradycardia occurred within hours to days after HCV treatment was initiated in patients receiving amiodarone, but has been observed up to 2 weeks after initiation of HCV treatment. Bradycardia generally resolved after HCV treatment was discontinued. The mechanism for this adverse cardiovascular effect is unknown.

Patients who may be at increased risk for symptomatic bradycardia if amiodarone is used concomitantly with an HCV treatment regimen containing sofosbuvir and another HCV DAA include those also receiving a β-adrenergic blocking agent, those with underlying cardiac comorbidities, and/or those with advanced liver disease.

Concomitant use of amiodarone with sofosbuvir/velpatasvir/voxilaprevir is *not* recommended. If there are no alternative HCV treatment options and sofosbuvir/velpatasvir/voxilaprevir must be used in a patient receiving amiodarone, the patient should be advised about the risk of serious symptomatic bradycardia before sofosbuvir/velpatasvir/voxilaprevir is initiated. Cardiac monitoring should be performed in an inpatient setting during the first 48 hours of concomitant use of amiodarone and sofosbuvir/velpatasvir/voxilaprevir; heart rate monitoring should then be performed daily (outpatient or self-monitoring) through at least the first 2 weeks of concomitant use. Similar cardiac monitoring is recommended in patients who discontinued amiodarone just prior to initiation of sofosbuvir/velpatasvir/voxilaprevir or if there are no other treatment options and amiodarone must be initiated in a patient already receiving sofosbuvir/velpatasvir/voxilaprevir.

Patients receiving amiodarone concomitantly with sofosbuvir/velpatasvir/voxilaprevir should be advised to immediately contact a clinician if they develop signs or symptoms of bradycardia (e.g., near-fainting or fainting, dizziness, lightheadedness, malaise, weakness, excessive tiredness, shortness of breath, chest pain, confusion, memory problems).

Interactions. Concomitant use of sofosbuvir/velpatasvir/voxilaprevir and inducers of the P-glycoprotein (P-gp) transport system and/or moderate or potent inducers of cytochrome P-450 (CYP) isoenzyme 2B6, 2C8, or 3A4 (e.g., carbamazepine and other anticonvulsants, St. John's wort [*Hypericum perforatum*]) may result in clinically important decreases in plasma concentrations of sofosbuvir, velpatasvir, and/or voxilaprevir and may lead to reduced therapeutic effect of sofosbuvir/velpatasvir/voxilaprevir. Concomitant use of such drugs with sofosbuvir/velpatasvir/voxilaprevir is not recommended. (See Drug Interactions.)

Precautions Related to Fixed Combinations. When sofosbuvir/velpatasvir/voxilaprevir is used, the cautions, precautions, contraindications, and drug interactions associated with each drug in the fixed combination must be considered. Cautionary information applicable to specific populations (e.g., pregnant or nursing women, individuals with hepatic or renal impairment, geriatric patients) should be considered for each drug.

Specific Populations **Pregnancy.** Adequate data are not available regarding use of sofosbuvir/velpatasvir/voxilaprevir in pregnant women. In animal studies, there was no evidence that sofosbuvir, velpatasvir, or voxilaprevir affected fetal development at exposures greater than those in humans receiving the recommended human dosage.

Lactation. It is not known whether sofosbuvir/velpatasvir/voxilaprevir or their metabolites are distributed into human milk, affect milk production, or have effects on the breast-fed infant.

The predominant metabolite of sofosbuvir (GS-331007) is distributed into milk in rats; velpatasvir is distributed into milk in rats and has been detected in plasma of suckling rat pups; and voxilaprevir has been detected in plasma of suckling rat pups. GS-331007, velpatasvir, and voxilaprevir had no apparent effects on nursing pups.

The benefits of breast-feeding and the importance of sofosbuvir/velpatasvir/voxilaprevir to the woman should be considered along with the potential adverse effects on the breast-fed child from the drug or from the underlying maternal condition.

Pediatric Use. Safety and efficacy of sofosbuvir/velpatasvir/voxilaprevir have not been established in pediatric patients younger than 18 years of age.

Geriatric Use. No overall differences in safety and efficacy of sofosbuvir/velpatasvir/voxilaprevir have been observed between patients 65 years of age and older and younger adults. However, greater sensitivity in some older individuals cannot be ruled out.

Population pharmacokinetic analysis in HCV-infected adults up to 85 years of age indicates that age does not have a clinically important effect on sofosbuvir, GS-331007, velpatasvir, or voxilaprevir exposures.

Hepatic Impairment. Safety and efficacy of sofosbuvir/velpatasvir/voxilaprevir have not been established in HCV-infected patients with moderate or severe hepatic impairment (Child-Pugh class B or C) and the drug is not recommended in such patients.

In August 2019, FDA reported that the use of glecaprevir/pibrentasvir, elbasvir/grazoprevir, or sofosbuvir/velpatasvir/voxilaprevir to treat chronic hepatitis C in patients with moderate to severe liver impairment has resulted in rare cases of worsening liver function or liver failure. FDA noted that all these medicines contain an HCV protease inhibitor and are not indicated for use in patients with moderate to severe liver impairment. In most patients, symptoms resolved or new onset worsening of liver function improved after stopping the medicine. Health care professionals should continue to prescribe these drugs as indicated in the prescribing information for patients without liver impairment or with mild liver impairment (Child-Pugh A). The severity of liver disease should be assessed at baseline and patients should be closely monitored for signs and symptoms of worsening liver function. Assessment of baseline liver disease and close monitoring are especially important in patients with preexisting significant liver problems or risk factors, such as hepatocellular carcinoma or alcohol abuse, which can also contribute to clinical worsening of liver function or liver failure during treatment. These medicines should be discontinued in patients who develop signs and symptoms of liver decompensation or as clinically indicated.

In HCV-infected individuals with moderate or severe hepatic impairment (Child-Pugh class B or C), sofosbuvir (400 mg daily for 7 days) results in sofosbuvir and GS-331007 plasma exposures higher than those reported in individuals with normal hepatic function.

In individuals with moderate or severe hepatic impairment (Child-Pugh class B or C) without HCV infection, a single 100-mg dose of velpatasvir results in plasma exposures similar to those reported when the same dose is given to individuals with normal hepatic function.

In individuals with moderate or severe hepatic impairment (Child-Pugh class B or C) without HCV infection, a single 100-mg dose of voxilaprevir results in plasma exposures substantially higher than those reported in individuals with normal hepatic function.

Renal Impairment. Safety and efficacy of sofosbuvir/velpatasvir/voxilaprevir have not been established in patients with severe renal impairment (estimated glomerular filtration rate [eGFR] less than 30 mL/minute per 1.73 m^2) or end-stage renal disease (ESRD) requiring hemodialysis, and dosage recommendations are not available for such patients.

In individuals with mild, moderate, or severe renal impairment without HCV infection, a single 400-mg dose of sofosbuvir results in sofosbuvir and GS-331007 plasma exposures higher than those reported in individuals with normal renal function. In those with ESRD, sofosbuvir and GS-331007 exposures were higher when the drug was administered 1 hour before or 1 hour after hemodialysis compared with exposures in those with normal renal function; a 4-hour hemodialysis session removed approximately 18% of the dose.

In individuals with severe renal impairment without HCV infection, velpatasvir pharmacokinetics following a single 100-mg dose of the drug are similar to pharmacokinetics reported in healthy individuals. Velpatasvir is not expected to be removed to any clinically important extent by hemodialysis.

In individuals with severe renal impairment without HCV infection, voxilaprevir pharmacokinetics following a single 100-mg dose of the drug are similar to pharmacokinetics reported in healthy individuals. Voxilaprevir is not expected to be removed to any clinically important extent by hemodialysis.

■ **Common Adverse Effects** Adverse effects reported in 5% or more of patients receiving sofosbuvir/velpatasvir/voxilaprevir include headache, fatigue, diarrhea, nausea, asthenia, and insomnia.

Drug Interactions

The following drug interactions are based on studies using the fixed combination containing sofosbuvir, velpatasvir, voxilaprevir (sofosbuvir/velpatasvir/voxilaprevir), the fixed combination of sofosbuvir and velpatasvir (sofosbuvir/velpatasvir), sofosbuvir alone, velpatasvir alone, or voxilaprevir alone, or are predicted to occur. When sofosbuvir/velpatasvir/voxilaprevir is used, interactions associated with each drug in the fixed combination should be considered.

■ **Drugs Affecting or Metabolized by Hepatic Microsomal Enzymes** In vitro studies indicate slow metabolic turnover of velpatasvir by cytochrome P-450 (CYP) isoenzymes 2B6, 2C8, and 3A4 and slow metabolic turnover of voxilaprevir by CYP3A4 and, to a lesser extent, 1A2 and 2C8. Sofosbuvir and the predominant metabolite of sofosbuvir (GS-331007) do not inhibit or induce CYP isoenzymes; velpatasvir and voxilaprevir do not inhibit CYP isoenzymes at clinically important concentrations.

Pharmacokinetic interactions are possible with moderate or potent inducers of CYP2B6, 2C8, or 3A4, which may decrease sofosbuvir, velpatasvir, and/or voxilaprevir plasma concentrations potentially leading to reduced therapeutic effect of sofosbuvir/velpatasvir/voxilaprevir. Concomitant use of sofosbuvir/velpatasvir/voxilaprevir with moderate or potent inducers of CYP2B6, 2C8, or 3A4 is not recommended.

Although inhibitors of CYP2B6, 2C8, or 3A4 may increase velpatasvir and/or voxilaprevir plasma concentrations, sofosbuvir/velpatasvir/voxilaprevir may be used concomitantly with inhibitors of CYP2B6, 2C8, or 3A4.

■ **Drugs Affecting or Affected by P-glycoprotein Transport System** Velpatasvir and voxilaprevir are inhibitors of the P-glycoprotein (P-gp) transport system; sofosbuvir and GS-331007 are not inhibitors of P-gp. Concomitant use of sofosbuvir/velpatasvir/voxilaprevir and P-gp substrates may alter the exposure of such drugs.

Sofosbuvir, velpatasvir, and voxilaprevir are substrates of P-gp; GS-331007 is not a P-gp substrate. Pharmacokinetic interactions are possible with P-gp inducers, which may decrease sofosbuvir, velpatasvir, and/or voxilaprevir plasma concentrations potentially leading to reduced therapeutic effect of sofosbuvir/velpatasvir/voxilaprevir. Concomitant use of sofosbuvir/velpatasvir/voxilaprevir with P-gp inducers is not recommended.

Inhibitors of P-gp may increase plasma concentrations of sofosbuvir, velpatasvir, and/or voxilaprevir without increasing plasma concentrations of GS-331007. Sofosbuvir/velpatasvir/voxilaprevir may be used concomitantly with P-gp inhibitors.

■ **Drugs Affecting or Affected by Breast Cancer Resistance Protein** Velpatasvir and voxilaprevir are inhibitors of breast cancer resistance protein (BCRP); sofosbuvir and GS-331007 are not BCRP inhibitors. Pharmacokinetic interactions are possible if sofosbuvir/velpatasvir/voxilaprevir and BCRP substrates are used concomitantly; altered exposure of such drugs may occur. Concomitant use of sofosbuvir/velpatasvir/voxilaprevir and BCRP substrates is not recommended.

Sofosbuvir, velpatasvir, and voxilaprevir are substrates of BCRP; GS-331007 is not a BCRP substrate. Inhibitors of BCRP may increase plasma concentrations of sofosbuvir, velpatasvir, and/or voxilaprevir without increasing plasma concentrations of GS-331007. Sofosbuvir/velpatasvir/voxilaprevir may be used concomitantly with BCRP inhibitors.

■ **Drugs Affecting or Affected by Organic Anion Transporting Polypeptides** Velpatasvir and voxilaprevir inhibit organic anion transporting polypeptide (OATP) 1B1 and 1B3; velpatasvir also inhibits OATP2B1, but does not inhibit OATP1A2 at clinically relevant concentrations. Sofosbuvir and GS-331007 do not inhibit OATP1B1 or 1B3. Concomitant use of sofosbuvir/velpatasvir/voxilaprevir and OATP1B1, 1B3, or 2B1 substrates may alter exposures of such drugs.

Voxilaprevir and, to a lesser extent, velpatasvir are substrates of OATP1B1 and 1B3. Inhibitors of OATP may substantially increase plasma concentrations of voxilaprevir. Therefore, concomitant use of sofosbuvir/velpatasvir/voxilaprevir and OATP inhibitors is not recommended.

■ **Drugs Affecting or Affected by Other Membrane Transporters** Sofosbuvir and GS-331007 do not inhibit organic cation transporter (OCT) 1; GS-331007 does not inhibit organic anion transporter (OAT) 1, OAT3, OCT2, or multidrug and toxin extrusion protein (MATE) 1. Sofosbuvir and GS-331007 do not inhibit or induce uridine diphosphate-glucuronosyl transferase (UGT) 1A1.

Velpatasvir and voxilaprevir do not inhibit OAT1, OAT3, OCT1, OCT2, MATE1, or UGT1A1 at clinically relevant concentrations.

■ **Drugs Affecting Gastric pH** The solubility of velpatasvir decreases as pH increases. Therefore, drugs that increase gastric pH are expected to decrease velpatasvir plasma concentrations.

Antacids Administration of sofosbuvir/velpatasvir/voxilaprevir and antacids (e.g., aluminum and magnesium hydroxide) should be separated by 4 hours.

Histamine H_2-Receptor Antagonists H_2-receptor antagonists may be administered concurrently with or staggered from sofosbuvir/velpatasvir/voxilaprevir; dosage of the H_2-receptor antagonist should not exceed dosages comparable to famotidine 40 mg twice daily.

Proton-pump Inhibitors Administration of omeprazole 20 mg 2 hours before or 4 hours after sofosbuvir/velpatasvir/voxilaprevir results in decreased velpatasvir plasma concentrations and AUC.

Sofosbuvir/velpatasvir/voxilaprevir may be administered with omeprazole 20 mg. Use of sofosbuvir/velpatasvir/voxilaprevir with other proton-pump inhibitors has not been studied.

■ **Antiarrhythmic Agents** ***Amiodarone*** Concomitant use of amiodarone and sofosbuvir/velpatasvir/voxilaprevir may result in serious symptomatic bradycardia and is not recommended. If there are no alternative hepatitis C virus (HCV) treatment options and a regimen of sofosbuvir/velpatasvir/voxilaprevir must be used in a patient receiving amiodarone, the patient should be advised about the risk of serious symptomatic bradycardia and cardiac monitoring should be performed in an inpatient setting during the first 48 hours of concomitant use and then heart rate monitoring (outpatient or self-monitoring) should be performed daily through at least the first 2 weeks of concomitant use. Similar cardiac monitoring is recommended in patients who discontinued amiodarone just prior to initiation of sofosbuvir/velpatasvir/voxilaprevir or if there are no other treatment options and amiodarone must be initiated in a patient already receiving sofosbuvir/velpatasvir/voxilaprevir. (See Cardiovascular Effects under Warnings/Precautions: Other Warnings/Precautions, in Cautions.)

The effect of concomitant use of amiodarone and sofosbuvir/velpatasvir/voxilaprevir on plasma concentrations of amiodarone, sofosbuvir, velpatasvir, and voxilaprevir is unknown.

■ **Anticoagulants** ***Dabigatran*** Concomitant use of sofosbuvir/velpatasvir/voxilaprevir once daily and a single 75-mg dose of dabigatran etexilate results in 2.9- and 2.6-fold increased dabigatran peak plasma concentrations and area under the plasma concentration-time curve (AUC), respectively.

If sofosbuvir/velpatasvir/voxilaprevir and dabigatran are used concomitantly, clinical effects of the anticoagulant should be monitored; recommendations from the manufacturer of dabigatran etexilate should be consulted regarding dosage modifications.

■ **Anticonvulsants** Concomitant use of sofosbuvir/velpatasvir/voxilaprevir and certain anticonvulsants (i.e., carbamazepine, oxcarbazepine, phenobarbital, phenytoin) is expected to decrease sofosbuvir, velpatasvir, and voxilaprevir plasma concentrations.

Concomitant use of sofosbuvir/velpatasvir/voxilaprevir and carbamazepine, oxcarbazepine, phenobarbital, or phenytoin is not recommended.

■ **Antifungal Agents** ***Ketoconazole*** No clinically important pharmacokinetic interactions were observed when sofosbuvir/velpatasvir was used concomitantly with ketoconazole.

No clinically important pharmacokinetic interactions were observed when a single 100-mg dose of velpatasvir was used concomitantly with ketoconazole (200 mg twice daily).

Voriconazole No clinically important pharmacokinetic interactions were observed when sofosbuvir/velpatasvir/voxilaprevir was used concomitantly with voriconazole.

No clinically important pharmacokinetic interactions were observed when a single 100-mg dose of voxilaprevir was used concomitantly with voriconazole (200 mg twice daily).

■ **Antimycobacterial Agents** ***Rifabutin*** Rifabutin is expected to decrease plasma concentrations of sofosbuvir, velpatasvir, and voxilaprevir.

Concomitant use of rifabutin and sofosbuvir/velpatasvir/voxilaprevir is not recommended.

Rifampin Concomitant use of rifampin (600 mg once daily) and sofosbuvir (single 400-mg dose), velpatasvir (single 100-mg dose), or voxilaprevir (single 100-mg dose) results in decreased plasma concentrations and AUCs of sofosbuvir, velpatasvir, and voxilaprevir. Concomitant use of rifampin (single 600-mg dose) and velpatasvir (single 100-mg dose) or voxilaprevir (single 100-mg dose) results in increased velpatasvir or voxilaprevir plasma concentrations and AUC.

Concomitant use of rifampin and sofosbuvir/velpatasvir/voxilaprevir is contraindicated.

Rifapentine Rifapentine is expected to decrease plasma concentrations of sofosbuvir, velpatasvir, and voxilaprevir.

Concomitant use of rifapentine and sofosbuvir/velpatasvir/voxilaprevir is not recommended.

■ **Antineoplastic Agents** Concomitant use of sofosbuvir/velpatasvir/voxilaprevir and imatinib, irinotecan, lapatinib, methotrexate, mitoxantrone, or topotecan is not recommended.

■ **Antiretroviral Agents** ***HIV Entry and Fusion Inhibitors*** **Maraviroc.** Concomitant use of maraviroc and sofosbuvir/velpatasvir/voxilaprevir is not expected to affect maraviroc pharmacokinetics.

Dosage adjustments are not necessary if maraviroc is used concomitantly with sofosbuvir/velpatasvir/voxilaprevir.

HIV Integrase Inhibitors (INSTIs) **Dolutegravir.** No clinically important pharmacokinetic interactions were observed when dolutegravir was used concomitantly with sofosbuvir/velpatasvir.

Dosage adjustments are not necessary if dolutegravir is used concomitantly with sofosbuvir/velpatasvir/voxilaprevir.

Elvitegravir. No clinically important pharmacokinetic interactions were observed when the fixed combination of elvitegravir, cobicistat, emtricitabine, and tenofovir alafenamide (EVG/c/FTC/TAF) was used concomitantly with sofosbuvir/velpatasvir/voxilaprevir. Dosage adjustments are not necessary if sofosbuvir/velpatasvir/voxilaprevir is used concomitantly with EVG/c/FTC/TAF; however, some experts state that consideration should be given to monitoring for hepatotoxicity.

If sofosbuvir/velpatasvir/voxilaprevir is used concomitantly with the fixed combination of elvitegravir, cobicistat, emtricitabine, and tenofovir disoproxil fumarate (EVG/c/FTC/TDF), increased tenofovir concentrations may occur. Patients should be monitored for tenofovir-associated adverse effects if sofosbuvir/velpatasvir/voxilaprevir is used concomitantly with EVG/c/FTC/TDF. In addition, some experts state that consideration should be given to monitoring for hepatotoxicity.

Raltegravir. No clinically important pharmacokinetic interactions were observed when raltegravir was used concomitantly with sofosbuvir/velpatasvir.

Concomitant use of sofosbuvir/velpatasvir and an HIV antiretroviral regimen of raltegravir in conjunction with the fixed combination of emtricitabine and tenofovir DF (emtricitabine/tenofovir DF) did not have a clinically important effect on the pharmacokinetics of raltegravir or emtricitabine, but tenofovir plasma concentrations and AUC were increased.

Dosage adjustments are not necessary if raltegravir is used concomitantly with sofosbuvir/velpatasvir/voxilaprevir.

If sofosbuvir/velpatasvir/voxilaprevir is used concomitantly with an HIV antiretroviral regimen that includes raltegravir and tenofovir DF, patients should be monitored for tenofovir-associated adverse effects.

HIV Nonnucleoside Reverse Transcriptase Inhibitors (NNRTIs) **Efavirenz.** Decreased velpatasvir and voxilaprevir concentrations are expected if efavirenz is used concomitantly with sofosbuvir/velpatasvir/voxilaprevir.

Concomitant use of the fixed combination of efavirenz, emtricitabine, and tenofovir DF (efavirenz/emtricitabine/tenofovir DF) and sofosbuvir/velpatasvir did not have a clinically important effect on the pharmacokinetics of sofosbuvir, but velpatasvir plasma concentrations and AUC were decreased and tenofovir plasma concentrations and AUC were increased.

Concomitant use of efavirenz and sofosbuvir/velpatasvir/voxilaprevir is not recommended.

Etravirine. Concomitant use of the etravirine and sofosbuvir/velpatasvir/voxilaprevir is expected to result in decreased velpatasvir and voxilaprevir plasma concentrations.

Concomitant use of etravirine and sofosbuvir/velpatasvir/voxilaprevir is not recommended.

Nevirapine. Concomitant use of nevirapine and sofosbuvir/velpatasvir/voxilaprevir is expected to result in decreased velpatasvir and voxilaprevir plasma concentrations.

Concomitant use of nevirapine and sofosbuvir/velpatasvir/voxilaprevir is not recommended.

Rilpivirine. No clinically important pharmacokinetic interactions are expected if rilpivirine is used concomitantly with sofosbuvir/velpatasvir/voxilaprevir.

Concomitant use of the fixed combination of emtricitabine, rilpivirine, and tenofovir alafenamide and sofosbuvir/velpatasvir/voxilaprevir did not have a clinically important effect on the pharmacokinetics of sofosbuvir, velpatasvir, or voxilaprevir.

Concomitant use of the fixed combination of emtricitabine, rilpivirine, and tenofovir DF (emtricitabine/rilpivirine/tenofovir DF) and sofosbuvir/velpatasvir/voxilaprevir did not have a clinically important effect on the pharmacokinetics of emtricitabine or rilpivirine, but tenofovir plasma concentrations and AUC were increased.

Dosage adjustments are not necessary if rilpivirine is used concomitantly with sofosbuvir/velpatasvir/voxilaprevir.

If sofosbuvir/velpatasvir/voxilaprevir is used concomitantly with an HIV antiretroviral regimen that contains rilpivirine and tenofovir DF, patients should be monitored for tenofovir-associated adverse effects.

HIV Nucleoside and Nucleotide Reverse Transcriptase Inhibitors (NRTIs) **Emtricitabine.** No clinically important pharmacokinetic interactions were observed when sofosbuvir/velpatasvir/voxilaprevir was used concomitantly with emtricitabine.

Tenofovir. No clinically important pharmacokinetic interactions were observed when sofosbuvir/velpatasvir/voxilaprevir was used concomitantly with tenofovir alafenamide.

Concomitant use of sofosbuvir/velpatasvir/voxilaprevir and HIV antiretroviral regimens that include tenofovir DF and certain other antiretroviral agents, including EVG/c/FTC/TDF, emtricitabine/rilpivirine/tenofovir DF, raltegravir in conjunction with emtricitabine/tenofovir DF, or *ritonavir-boosted* darunavir in conjunction with emtricitabine/tenofovir DF, may result in increased tenofovir DF concentrations.

Dosage adjustments are not necessary if tenofovir alafenamide or tenofovir DF is used concomitantly with sofosbuvir/velpatasvir/voxilaprevir. However, patients should be monitored for tenofovir-associated adverse effects if sofosbuvir/velpatasvir/voxilaprevir is used concomitantly with any HIV antiretroviral regimen containing tenofovir DF. In addition, some experts state that consideration should be given to monitoring for hepatotoxicity if sofosbuvir/velpatasvir/voxilaprevir is used concomitantly with EVG/c/FTC/TAF or EVG/c/FTC/TDF.

HIV Protease Inhibitors (PIs) **Atazanavir.** Concomitant use of *ritonavir-boosted* atazanavir and sofosbuvir/velpatasvir/voxilaprevir results in substantially increased voxilaprevir peak plasma concentrations and AUC.

Concomitant use of sofosbuvir/velpatasvir/voxilaprevir and *ritonavir-boosted*, *cobicistat-boosted*, or unboosted atazanavir is not recommended.

Darunavir. No clinically important pharmacokinetic interactions were observed when sofosbuvir/velpatasvir/voxilaprevir was used concomitantly with *ritonavir-boosted* darunavir in conjunction with emtricitabine/tenofovir DF, but tenofovir plasma concentrations and AUC were increased.

Dosage adjustments are not necessary if *ritonavir-boosted* or *cobicistat-boosted* darunavir is used concomitantly with sofosbuvir/velpatasvir/voxilaprevir.

Lopinavir. Pharmacokinetic interactions are expected if the fixed combination of lopinavir and ritonavir (lopinavir/ritonavir) is used concomitantly with sofosbuvir/velpatasvir/voxilaprevir (increased voxilaprevir concentrations).

Concomitant use of lopinavir/ritonavir and sofosbuvir/velpatasvir/voxilaprevir is not recommended.

Tipranavir. Pharmacokinetic interactions are expected if *ritonavir-boosted* tipranavir is used concomitantly with sofosbuvir/velpatasvir/voxilaprevir (decreased sofosbuvir and velpatasvir plasma concentrations); the effect of *ritonavir-boosted* tipranavir on voxilaprevir concentrations is not known.

Concomitant use of *ritonavir-boosted* tipranavir and sofosbuvir/velpatasvir/voxilaprevir is not recommended.

■ **Digoxin** Concomitant use of velpatasvir 100 mg once daily and a single 0.25-mg dose of digoxin results in increased digoxin concentrations and AUC.

If sofosbuvir/velpatasvir/voxilaprevir and digoxin are used concomitantly, therapeutic concentration monitoring of digoxin is recommended.

■ **Estrogens and Progestins** Concomitant use of sofosbuvir/velpatasvir/voxilaprevir and an oral contraceptive containing ethinyl estradiol and norgestimate does not have a clinically important effect on the pharmacokinetics of ethinyl estradiol or norgestimate.

■ **Gemfibrozil** Concomitant use of sofosbuvir/velpatasvir/voxilaprevir and gemfibrozil does not result in clinically important pharmacokinetic interactions.

■ **HCV Antivirals** In vitro in replicon studies, there was no evidence of antagonistic anti-HCV effects between sofosbuvir and velpatasvir or voxilaprevir.

In vitro in replicon studies, there was no evidence of antagonistic anti-HCV effects between velpatasvir and voxilaprevir.

■ **HMG-CoA Reductase Inhibitors** ***Atorvastatin*** Concomitant use of sofosbuvir/velpatasvir once daily and a single 40-mg dose of atorvastatin results in increased atorvastatin peak plasma concentrations and AUC, which is associated with increased risk of myopathy and rhabdomyolysis.

If sofosbuvir/velpatasvir/voxilaprevir and atorvastatin are used concomitantly, the lowest atorvastatin dosage should be used. If higher atorvastatin dosages are required, the lowest necessary dosage should be used taking into account the risks and benefits.

Fluvastatin, Lovastatin, and Simvastatin Concomitant use of sofosbuvir/velpatasvir/voxilaprevir with fluvastatin, lovastatin, or simvastatin may increase concentrations of the statin, which is associated with increased risk of myopathy and rhabdomyolysis.

If sofosbuvir/velpatasvir/voxilaprevir is used concomitantly with fluvastatin, lovastatin, or simvastatin, the lowest statin dosage should be used. If higher statin dosages are required, the lowest necessary dosage should be used taking into account the risks and benefits.

Pitavastatin Concomitant use of sofosbuvir/velpatasvir/voxilaprevir and pitavastatin may increase pitavastatin concentrations, which is associated with increased risk of myopathy and rhabdomyolysis.

Concomitant use of sofosbuvir/velpatasvir/voxilaprevir and pitavastatin is not recommended.

Pravastatin Concomitant use of sofosbuvir/velpatasvir/voxilaprevir once daily and a single 40-mg dose of pravastatin results in increased pravastatin peak plasma concentrations and AUC, which is associated with increased risk of myopathy and rhabdomyolysis.

If sofosbuvir/velpatasvir/voxilaprevir and pravastatin are used concomitantly, the pravastatin dose should not exceed 40 mg.

Rosuvastatin Concomitant use of sofosbuvir/velpatasvir/voxilaprevir and rosuvastatin (single 10-mg dose) results in substantially increased rosuvastatin plasma concentrations and AUC, which is associated with increased risk of myopathy and rhabdomyolysis.

Concomitant use of sofosbuvir/velpatasvir/voxilaprevir and rosuvastatin is not recommended.

■ **Immunosuppressive Agents** ***Cyclosporine*** Concomitant use of cyclosporine (single 600-mg dose) and voxilaprevir (single100-mg dose) results in substantially increased voxilaprevir peak plasma concentrations and AUC. Increased sofosbuvir or velpatasvir exposures are observed when cyclosporine (single 600-mg dose) is used concomitantly with sofosbuvir (single 400-mg dose) or velpatasvir (single 100-mg dose).

Concomitant use of sofosbuvir/velpatasvir/voxilaprevir and cyclosporine is not recommended.

Tacrolimus No clinically important pharmacokinetic interactions were observed when tacrolimus (single 5-mg dose) was used concomitantly with sofosbuvir (single 400-mg dose).

■ **Methadone** No clinically important pharmacokinetic interactions were observed when sofosbuvir (400 mg once daily) was used concomitantly with methadone hydrochloride (30–130 mg daily).

■ **St. John's Wort** Concomitant use of St. John's wort (*Hypericum perforatum*) and sofosbuvir/velpatasvir/voxilaprevir may result in clinically important decreases in sofosbuvir, velpatasvir, and voxilaprevir plasma concentrations.

Concomitant use of sofosbuvir/velpatasvir/voxilaprevir and St. John's wort is not recommended.

■ **Sulfasalazine** Concomitant use of sulfasalazine and sofosbuvir/velpatasvir/voxilaprevir is not recommended.

■ **Warfarin** In patients receiving warfarin, subtherapeutic international normalized ratios (INRs) have been reported after initiation of sofosbuvir-containing HCV treatment regimens. INR fluctuations have been reported in patients receiving warfarin and sofosbuvir/velpatasvir/voxilaprevir concomitantly.

If a sofosbuvir-containing regimen (e.g., sofosbuvir/velpatasvir/voxilaprevir) is used in patients receiving warfarin, INR should be frequently monitored at the time of initiation, during treatment, and after discontinuance of the sofosbuvir-containing regimen.

Description

Sofosbuvir, velpatasvir, and voxilaprevir (sofosbuvir/velpatasvir/voxilaprevir) is a fixed combination containing 3 hepatitis C virus (HCV) antivirals. Sofosbuvir is a nucleotide analog HCV nonstructural 5B (NS5B) polymerase inhibitor. Velpatasvir is an HCV nonstructural 5A (NS5A) replication complex inhibitor (NS5A inhibitor). Voxilaprevir is an HCV nonstructural 3/4A (NS3/4A) protease inhibitor. All three drugs are direct-acting antivirals (DAAs) with activity against HCV. There is no in vitro evidence of antagonistic anti-HCV effects between sofosbuvir and velpatasvir or voxilaprevir and no in vitro evidence of antagonistic anti-HCV effects between velpatasvir and voxilaprevir.

Sofosbuvir is a prodrug that is converted in the liver to a pharmacologically active uridine analog triphosphate (GS-461203), which can be incorporated into HCV RNA by NS5B polymerase and acts as an RNA chain terminator. In vitro studies using biochemical assays indicate that GS-461203 has activity against HCV genotypes 1b, 2a, 3a, and 4a. Sofosbuvir has shown in vitro activity against full-length or chimeric replicons of HCV genotypes 1a, 1b, 2a, 2b, 3a, 4a, 4d, 5a, and 6a (median concentration of the drug required to inhibit viral replication by 50% [EC_{50}] has ranged from 15–110 nM).

Velpatasvir inhibits the HCV NS5A protein, which is required for viral replication. Velpatasvir has shown in vitro activity against full-length or chimeric replicons of HCV genotypes 1a, 1b, 2a, 2b, 3a, 4a, 4d, 4r, 5a, 6a, and 6e (median EC_{50} has ranged from 0.002–0.13 nM).

Voxilaprevir reversibly binds to the active site of HCV NS3/4A protease, thereby blocking enzyme activity essential for viral replication (i.e., blocking cleavage of the HCV-encoded polyproteins into mature forms of NS3, NS4A, NS4B, NS5A, and NS5B). In vitro studies using biochemical assays indicate that voxilaprevir has activity against HCV genotypes 1b and 3a. Voxilaprevir has shown in vitro activity against full-length or chimeric replicons of HCV genotypes 1a, 1b, 2a, 2b, 3a, 4a, 4d, 4r, 5a, 6a, 6e, and 6n (median EC_{50} has ranged from 0.2–6.6 nM).

Certain amino acid substitutions in NS5B polymerase of HCV genotypes 1b, 2a, 2b, 3a, 4a, 5a, and 6a have been selected in cell culture and have been associated with reduced susceptibility to sofosbuvir in vitro in replicon studies. In all replicon genotypes tested, the S282T substitution was associated with reduced susceptibility to sofosbuvir; in genotypes 2a, 5, and 6 replicons, an M289L substitution developed along with the S282T substitution. Treatment-emergent NS5B resistance-associated substitutions were not detected in patients who experienced virologic failure or relapsed with sofosbuvir/velpatasvir/voxilaprevir in phase 3 clinical trials (POLARIS-1, POLARIS-4).

Certain amino acid substitutions in NS5A of HCV genotype 1a (e.g., L31V, Y93H/N), genotype 1b (e.g., L31V, Y93H), genotype 2a (e.g., F28S, Y93H), genotype 3a (e.g., Y93H/S), genotype 4a (e.g., Y93H), and genotype 6 (e.g., L31V, P32A/L/Q/R) have been selected in cell culture and have been associated with reduced susceptibility to velpatasvir in vitro in replicon studies. Combinations of these NS5A substitutions often resulted in greater reductions in susceptibility to velpatasvir compared with a single NS5A substitution. Treatment-emergent NS5A resistance-associated substitutions were detected in phase 3 clinical trials evaluating sofosbuvir/velpatasvir/voxilaprevir in patients with HCV genotype 1a (e.g., L31M, Y93H, K24R), genotype 3a (e.g., E92K), or genotype 4 (e.g., Y93H) infection who relapsed or experienced virologic failure. Some of these patients also had baseline NS5A polymorphisms at resistance-associated amino acid positions.

Certain amino acid substitutions in NS3/4A protease inhibitor resistance-associated positions of HCV genotypes 1a (e.g., A156 L/T), 1b (e.g., A156T/V), 2a (e.g., A156L/V), 3a (e.g., A156T/V), 4a (e.g., A156L/T/V), 5a, and 6a have been selected in cell culture and have been associated with reduced susceptibility to voxilaprevir in vitro in replicon studies. Combinations of these NS3 substitutions often resulted in greater reductions in susceptibility to voxilaprevir compared with a single NS3 substitution. Treatment-emergent NS3 resistance-associated substitutions were detected in phase 3 clinical trials evaluating sofosbuvir/velpatasvir/voxilaprevir in patients with HCV genotype 1a (e.g., V36A) or genotype 3a (e.g., Q41K, V55A, R155M) infection who relapsed.

Sofosbuvir, velpatasvir, and voxilaprevir are each active against HCV with substitutions associated with resistance to other HCV DAAs that have different mechanisms of action. Cross-resistance is possible among the HCV NS5A inhibitors and among the HCV NS3/4A protease inhibitors.

Following oral administration of sofosbuvir/velpatasvir/voxilaprevir, peak plasma concentrations of sofosbuvir occur 2 hours after the dose and peak plasma concentrations of velpatasvir and voxilaprevir both occur 4 hours after the dose. Administration of sofosbuvir/velpatasvir/voxilaprevir with food increases sofosbuvir exposures by 64–144%, increases velpatasvir exposures by 40–166%, and increases voxilaprevir exposures by 112–435%.

Sofosbuvir is a prodrug that undergoes intracellular metabolic activation in the liver (hydrolysis by human cathepsin A [CatA] or carboxylesterase 1 [CES1], phosphoramidate cleavage by histidine triad nucleotide-binding protein 1 [HINT1], and phosphorylation by pyrimidine nucleotide biosynthesis pathway). This results in formation of the pharmacologically active metabolite, GS-461203; desphosphorylation subsequently occurs leading to formation of GS-331007 (the predominant circulating metabolite), which has no anti-HCV activity. Sofosbuvir is approximately 61–65% bound to plasma proteins. The major route of elimination is renal clearance (glomerular filtration and active tubular secretion). Following a single oral dose of sofosbuvir, 80% is eliminated in urine (mainly as GS-331007) and 14% is excreted in feces. The median terminal plasma half-lives of sofosbuvir and GS-331007 are 0.5 and 29 hours, respectively.

Velpatasvir is metabolized by cytochrome P-450 (CYP) isoenzymes 2B6, 2C8, and 3A4. The drug is greater than 99% bound to plasma proteins. The major route of elimination of velpatasvir is biliary excretion (approximately 77% excreted as the parent drug). Following a single oral dose of velpatasvir, 94% is excreted in feces and 0.4% is eliminated in urine. The median terminal plasma half-life of velpatasvir is 17 hours.

Voxilaprevir is metabolized by CYP3A4. The drug is greater than 99% bound to plasma proteins. The major route of elimination of velpatasvir is biliary excretion (approximately 40% excreted as the parent drug). Following a single oral dose of voxilaprevir, 94% is excreted in feces and no drug is eliminated in urine. The median terminal plasma half-life of velpatasvir is 33 hours.

Advice to Patients

Importance of reading patient information provided by the manufacturer.

Advise patients that the fixed-combination preparation of sofosbuvir, velpatasvir, and voxilaprevir (sofosbuvir/velpatasvir/voxilaprevir) should be taken once daily with food on a regular dosing schedule.

Importance of taking the recommended dosage of sofosbuvir/velpatasvir/voxilaprevir for the recommended duration of treatment; importance of not missing doses.

Inform patients that reactivation of hepatitis B virus (HBV) infection has occurred in patients being treated for hepatitis C virus (HCV) infection who were coinfected with HBV. Importance of informing clinician of any history of HBV infection or other liver problems (e.g., cirrhosis). Importance of immediately contacting a clinician if any signs or symptoms of serious liver injury (e.g., fatigue, weakness, loss of appetite, nausea and vomiting, yellowing of the eyes or skin, light-colored bowel movements) occur. (See Risk of HBV Reactivation in Patients Coinfected with HCV and HBV under Warnings/Precautions: Warnings, in Cautions.)

If sofosbuvir/velpatasvir/voxilaprevir is used in a patient receiving amiodarone, advise the patient about the risk of serious symptomatic bradycardia and the importance of immediately contacting a clinician if signs or symptoms of bradycardia (e.g., near-fainting or fainting, dizziness, lightheadedness, malaise, weakness, excessive tiredness, shortness of breath, chest pain, confusion, memory problems) occur. (See Cardiovascular Effects under Warnings/Precautions: Other Warnings/Precautions, in Cautions.)

Importance of informing clinicians of existing or contemplated concomitant therapy, including prescription and OTC drugs and dietary or herbal supplements, as well as any concomitant illnesses.

Importance of women informing clinicians if they are or plan to become pregnant or plan to breast-feed.

Importance of informing patients of other important precautionary information. (See Cautions.)

Overview® (see Users Guide). For additional information on this drug until a more detailed monograph is developed and published, the manufacturer's labeling should be consulted. It is *essential* that the manufacturer's labeling be consulted for more detailed information on usual cautions, precautions, contraindications, potential drug interactions, laboratory test interferences, and acute toxicity.

Preparations

Excipients in commercially available drug preparations may have clinically important effects in some individuals; consult specific product labeling for details.

Sofosbuvir, Velpatasvir, and Voxilaprevir

Oral		
Tablets, film-coated	Sofosbuvir 400 mg, Velpatasvir 100 mg, and Voxilaprevir 100 mg	Vosevi®, Gilead

†Use is not currently included in the labeling approved by the US Food and Drug Administration

HCV PROTEASE INHIBITORS 8:18.40.20

Glecaprevir and Pibrentasvir

■ Glecaprevir and pibrentasvir (glecaprevir/pibrentasvir) is a fixed combination containing 2 hepatitis C virus (HCV) antivirals; glecaprevir is an HCV nonstructural 3/4A (NS3/4A) protease inhibitor and pibrentasvir is an HCV nonstructural 5A (NS5A) replication complex inhibitor (NS5A inhibitor).

Uses

■ **Chronic Hepatitis C Virus Infection** The fixed combination of glecaprevir and pibrentasvir (glecaprevir/pibrentasvir) is used for the treatment of chronic hepatitis C virus (HCV) genotype 1, 2, 3, 4, 5, or 6 infection in treatment-naive (previously untreated) or previously treated adults and pediatric patients 12 years of age and older without cirrhosis or with compensated cirrhosis, including liver or kidney transplant recipients and those with human immunodeficiency virus (HIV) coinfection.

Because the treatment of chronic HCV infection is complex and rapidly evolving, it is recommended that treatment be directed by clinicians who are familiar with the disease and that a specialist be consulted to obtain the most up-to-date information. Information from the American Association for the Study of Liver Diseases (AASLD) and Infectious Diseases Society of America (IDSA) regarding diagnosis and management of HCV infection, including recommendations for initial treatment, is available at http://www.hcvguidelines.org.

HCV Genotype 1 Infection Efficacy and safety of glecaprevir/pibrentasvir for the treatment of chronic HCV genotype 1 infection in adults have been evaluated in 4 clinical trials (ENDURANCE-1, EXPEDITION-1, EXPEDITION-4, and MAGELLAN-1). The primary end point in each study was sustained virologic response at 12 weeks after the end of treatment (SVR12; defined as plasma HCV RNA level less than 15 IU/mL [the lower limit of quantification] at 12 weeks after end of treatment).

ENDURANCE-1 (NCT02604017), an open-label, randomized, phase 3 trial, included 703 treatment-naive or previously treated adults with chronic HCV genotype 1 infection who were noncirrhotic, including patients with HIV type 1 (HIV-1) coinfection (median age 52–53 years, 49% male, 84% white, 4% black, 13% with baseline HCV RNA levels 6 million IU/mL or greater, 38% previously treated). Previously treated patients had treatment experience with regimens containing interferon, peginterferon, ribavirin, and/or sofosbuvir, but no prior treatment experience with an HCV NS3/4A protease inhibitor or HCV NS5A inhibitor. Patients were randomized in a 1:1 ratio to receive glecaprevir/pibrentasvir (300 mg of glecaprevir and 120 mg of pibrentasvir) once daily for 8 or 12 weeks. SVR12 was achieved in 99.1% of patients treated with the 8-week regimen and 99.7% of those treated with the 12-week regimen.

EXPEDITION-1 (NCT02642432), an open-label, single-arm, phase 3 trial, included 146 treatment-naive or previously treated adults with chronic HCV genotype 1, 2, 4, 5, or 6 infection with compensated cirrhosis (median age 60 years, 62% male, 82% white, 10% black, 12% with baseline HCV RNA levels 6 million IU/mL or greater, 25% previously treated). Previously treated patients had prior treatment experience with regimens containing interferon, peginterferon, ribavirin, and/or sofosbuvir, but no prior treatment experience with an HCV NS3/4A protease inhibitor or HCV NS5A inhibitor. All patients received glecaprevir/pibrentasvir (300 mg of glecaprevir and 120 mg of pibrentasvir) once daily for 12 weeks. Of the 90 patients with HCV genotype 1 infection, 99% achieved SVR12.

EXPEDITION-4 (NCT02651194), an open-label, single-arm, phase 3 trial, included 104 treatment-naive or previously treated adults with chronic HCV genotype 1, 2, 3, 4, 5, or 6 infection who were noncirrhotic or had compensated cirrhosis; all patients also had severe renal impairment (chronic kidney disease stages 4 and 5). Patients had a median age of 57 years, 76% were male, 62% were white, 24% were black, 82% were receiving hemodialysis, 19% had compensated cirrhosis, and 42% were previously treated; 53, 15, 11, 19, 1, and 1% had HCV genotype 1, 2, 3, 4, 5, or 6 infection, respectively. Previously treated patients had treatment experience with regimens containing interferon, peginterferon, ribavirin, and/or sofosbuvir, but no prior treatment experience with an HCV NS3/4A protease inhibitor or HCV NS5A inhibitor. All patients received glecaprevir/pibrentasvir (300 mg of glecaprevir and 120 mg of pibrentasvir) once daily for 12 weeks. Overall, 98% of patients achieved SVR12. The presence of renal impairment did not affect efficacy of glecaprevir/pibrentasvir; dosage adjustments were not required.

MAGELLAN-1 (NCT02446717), a multi-part, randomized, open-label, phase 2 trial, included previously treated adults with HCV genotype 1 or 4 infection who previously failed a treatment regimen containing an HCV NS5A inhibitor and/or HCV NS3/4A protease inhibitor. In part 1 of the trial, 50 patients with HCV genotype 1 infection were randomized to receive a 12-week regimen of glecaprevir/pibrentasvir (200 mg of glecaprevir and 80 mg of pibrentasvir) once daily (arm A), glecaprevir/pibrentasvir (300 mg of glecaprevir and 120 mg of pibrentasvir) once daily in conjunction with ribavirin (arm B), or glecaprevir/pibrentasvir (300 mg of glecaprevir and 120 mg of pibrentasvir) once daily (arm C). The protocol was later amended to halt enrollment for arm A (lower dosage) so that glecaprevir/pibrentasvir dosage was optimized. In part 2 of the trial, 91 patients with HCV genotype 1 or 4 infection who were noncirrhotic or had compensated cirrhosis were randomized in a 1:1 ratio to receive glecaprevir/pibrentasvir (300 mg of glecaprevir and 120 mg of pibrentasvir) once daily for 12 or 16 weeks (arms D and E, respectively). Patients (part 1 and part 2) had a median age of 56 years, 75% were male, 72% were white, 26% were black, 97% had HCV genotype 1 infection, 33% were previously treated with an HCV NS5A inhibitor *and* an HCV NS3/4A protease inhibitor, 30% were previously treated with an HCV NS5A inhibitor (HCV NS3/4A inhibitor-naive), 37% were previously treated with an HCV NS3/4A protease inhibitor (HCV NS5A inhibitor-naive), and 19% had compensated cirrhosis. In HCV NS5A inhibitor-experienced (HCV NS3/4A protease inhibitor-naive) patients, SVR12 was achieved in 90 or 94% of those who received the 12- or 16-week treatment regimen, respectively. In HCV NS3/4A protease inhibitor-experienced (HCV NS5A inhibitor-naive) patients, SVR12 was achieved in 92 or 100% of those who received the 12- or 16-week treatment regimen, respectively. Those who were previously treated with an HCV NS5A inhibitor *and* an HCV NS3/4A protease inhibitor and received either 12 or 16 weeks of treatment had SVR12 rates of 80% and these patients had higher rates of virologic failure and treatment-emergent drug resistance compared with the other patient groups. Because of higher rates of virologic failure and treatment-emergent drug resistance, data do not support use of glecaprevir/pibrentasvir for treatment of HCV genotype 1 infection in patients who failed previous treatment with a regimen containing both an HCV NS5A inhibitor *and* an HCV NS3/4A protease inhibitor.

HCV Genotype 2 Infection Efficacy and safety of glecaprevir/pibrentasvir for the treatment of chronic HCV genotype 2 infection in adults have been evaluated in 3 clinical trials (SURVEYOR-2, EXPEDITION-1, and EXPEDITION-4). The primary end point in each study was sustained virologic response at 12 weeks after the end of treatment (SVR12; defined as plasma HCV RNA level less than the lower limit of quantification [15 or 25 IU/mL depending on assay used] at 12 weeks after end of treatment).

SURVEYOR-2 (NCT02243293), a multi-arm, multi-part, open-label, phase 2 trial, evaluated glecaprevir/pibrentasvir with or without ribavirin in adults with HCV genotype 2, 3, 4, 5, or 6 infection who were treatment naive or previously treated, including those with compensated cirrhosis. Previously treated patients had treatment experience with regimens containing interferon, peginterferon, ribavirin, and/or sofosbuvir, but no prior treatment experience with an HCV NS3/4A protease inhibitor or HCV NS5A inhibitor. Part 2 of the study included 54 noncirrhotic patients with HCV genotype 2 infection and part 4 of the study included 143 noncirrhotic patients with genotype 2 infection (a total of 197 patients in part 2 and part 4 combined). All 197 of these patients received glecaprevir/pibrentasvir (300 mg of glecaprevir and 120 mg of pibrentasvir) for 8 weeks. SVR12 was achieved in 98% of patients with HCV genotype 2 infection (part 2 and part 4 combined).

EXPEDITION-1 (NCT02642432), an open-label, single-arm, phase 3 trial, included 146 treatment-naive or previously treated adults with chronic HCV genotype 1, 2, 4, 5, or 6 infection with compensated cirrhosis (median age 60 years, 62% male, 82% white, 10% black, 12% with baseline HCV RNA levels 6 million IU/mL or greater, 25% previously treated). Previously treated patients had prior treatment experience with regimens containing interferon, peginterferon, ribavirin, and/or sofosbuvir, but no prior treatment experience with an HCV NS3/4A protease inhibitor or HCV NS5A inhibitor. All patients received glecaprevir/pibrentasvir (300 mg of glecaprevir and 120 mg of pibrentasvir) once daily for 12 weeks. Of the 31 patients with HCV genotype 2 infection, 100% achieved SVR12.

EXPEDITION-4 (NCT02651194), an open-label, single-arm, phase 3 trial, included 104 treatment-naive or previously treated adults with chronic HCV genotype 1, 2, 3, 4, 5, or 6 infection who were noncirrhotic or had compensated cirrhosis; all patients also had severe renal impairment (chronic kidney disease stages 4 and 5). Patients had a median age of 57 years, 76% were male, 62% were white, 24% were black, 82% were receiving hemodialysis, 19% had compensated cirrhosis, and 42% were previously treated; 53, 15, 11, 19, 1, and 1% had HCV genotype 1, 2, 3, 4, 5, or 6 infection, respectively. Previously treated patients had treatment experience with regimens containing interferon, peginterferon, ribavirin, and/or sofosbuvir, but no prior treatment experience with an HCV NS3/4A protease inhibitor or HCV NS5A inhibitor. All patients received glecaprevir/pibrentasvir (300 mg of glecaprevir and 120 mg of pibrentasvir) once daily for 12 weeks. Overall, 98% of patients achieved SVR12. The presence of renal impairment did not affect the efficacy of glecaprevir/pibrentasvir and dosage adjustments were not required.

HCV Genotype 3 Infection Efficacy and safety of glecaprevir/pibrentasvir for the treatment of chronic HCV genotype 3 infection in adults have been evaluated in 3 clinical trials (ENDURANCE-3, SURVEYOR-2, and EXPEDITION-4). The primary end point in each study was sustained virologic response at 12 weeks after the end of treatment (SVR12; defined as plasma HCV RNA level less than the lower limit of quantification [15 or 25 IU/mL depending on assay used] at 12 weeks after end of treatment).

ENDURANCE-3 (NCT02640157), a partially randomized, open-label, active-controlled, phase 3 trial, evaluated the efficacy of glecaprevir/pibrentasvir in treatment-naive, noncirrhotic patients with HCV genotype 3 infection (median age 47–49 years, 52% male, 88% white, 2% black, 22% with baseline HCV RNA levels 6 million IU/mL or greater). Patients were randomized in a 2:1 ratio to receive glecaprevir/pibrentasvir (300 mg of glecaprevir and 120 mg of pibrentasvir) once daily for 12 weeks or a regimen of sofosbuvir in conjunction with daclatasvir for 12 weeks. The study subsequently included an additional nonrandomized study arm evaluating an 8-week regimen of glecaprevir/pibrentasvir (300 mg of glecaprevir and 120 mg of pibrentasvir) once daily. SVR12 was achieved in 95 or 97% of patients with HCV genotype 3 infection treated with glecaprevir/pibrentasvir or a regimen of sofosbuvir in conjunction with daclatasvir, respectively. SVR12 was achieved in 95% of those in the nonrandomized arm treated with an 8-week regimen of glecaprevir/pibrentasvir. These data indicated that 8- and 12-week regimens of glecaprevir/pibrentasvir have similar efficacy in noncirrhotic patients with HCV genotype 3 infection.

SURVEYOR-2 (NCT02243293), a multi-arm, multi-part, open-label, phase 2 trial, evaluated glecaprevir/pibrentasvir with or without ribavirin in adults with HCV genotype 2, 3, 4, 5, or 6 infection who were treatment-naive or previously treated, including those with compensated cirrhosis. Previously treated patients had treatment experience with regimens containing interferon, peginterferon, ribavirin, and/or sofosbuvir, but no prior treatment experience with an HCV NS3/4A protease inhibitor or HCV NS5A inhibitor. In part 3 of the study, previously treated, noncirrhotic patients with HCV genotype 3 infection were randomized to receive glecaprevir/pibrentasvir (300 mg of glecaprevir and 120 mg of pibrentasvir) once daily for 12 or 16 weeks. In addition, a 12- or 16- week regimen of glecaprevir/pibrentasvir (300 mg of glecaprevir and 120 mg of pibrentasvir) once daily was evaluated in patients with HCV genotype 3 infection who had compensated cirrhosis and were treatment naive or previously treated, respectively. SVR12 was achieved in 98% of patients with HCV genotype 3 infection who were treatment naive and had compensated cirrhosis. In a pooled analysis of all previously treated patients with HCV genotype 3 infection (with or without compensated cirrhosis), SVR12 was achieved in 96% of patients.

EXPEDITION-4 (NCT02651194), an open-label, single-arm, phase 3 trial, included 104 treatment-naive or previously treated adults with chronic HCV genotype 1, 2, 3, 4, 5, or 6 infection who were noncirrhotic or had compensated cirrhosis; all patients also had severe renal impairment (chronic kidney disease stages 4 and 5). Patients had a median age of 57 years, 76% were male, 62% were white, 24% were black, 82% were receiving hemodialysis, 19% had compensated cirrhosis, and 42% were previously treated; 53, 15, 11, 19, 1, and 1% had HCV genotype 1, 2, 3, 4, 5, or 6 infection, respectively. Previously treated patients had treatment experience with regimens containing interferon, peginterferon, ribavirin, and/or sofosbuvir, but no prior treatment experience with an HCV NS3/4A protease inhibitor or HCV NS5A inhibitor. All patients received glecaprevir/pibrentasvir (300 mg of glecaprevir and 120 mg of pibrentasvir) once daily for 12 weeks. Overall, 98% of patients achieved SVR12. The presence of renal impairment did not affect the efficacy of glecaprevir/pibrentasvir and dosage adjustments were not required.

HCV Genotype 4 Infection Efficacy and safety of glecaprevir/pibrentasvir for the treatment of chronic HCV genotype 4 infection in adults have been evaluated in 4 clinical trials (SURVEYOR-2, ENDURANCE-4, EXPEDITION-1, and EXPEDITION-4). The primary end point in each study was sustained virologic response at 12 weeks after the end of treatment (SVR12; defined as plasma HCV RNA level less than the lower limit of quantification [15 or 25 IU/mL depending on assay used] at 12 weeks after end of treatment).

SURVEYOR-2 (NCT02243293), a multi-arm, multi-part, open-label, phase 2 trial, evaluated glecaprevir/pibrentasvir with or without ribavirin in adults with HCV genotype 2, 3, 4, 5, or 6 infection who were treatment naive or previously treated, including those with compensated cirrhosis. Previously treated patients had treatment experience with regimens containing interferon, peginterferon, ribavirin, and/or sofosbuvir, but no prior treatment experience with an HCV NS3/4A protease inhibitor or HCV NS5A inhibitor. In one arm of the study, there were 46 patients with HCV genotype 4 infection; 39 were treatment naive and 7 were previously treated. All 46 patients received glecaprevir/pibrentasvir (300 mg of glecaprevir and 120 mg of pibrentasvir) once daily for 8 weeks. SVR12 was achieved in 93% of patients with HCV genotype 4 infection.

ENDURANCE-4 (NCT02636595), a single-arm, open-label, phase 3 trial, evaluated the efficacy and safety of glecaprevir/pibrentasvir in noncirrhotic treatment-naive and previously treated patients with HCV genotype 4, 5, or 6 infection. Previously treated patients had prior treatment experience with regimens containing interferon, peginterferon, ribavirin, and/or sofosbuvir, but no prior treatment experience with an HCV NS3/4A protease inhibitor or HCV NS5A inhibitor. There were 76 patients with HCV genotype 4 infection; 45 were treatment naive and 31 were previously treated. All 76 patients received glecaprevir/pibrentasvir (300 mg of glecaprevir and 120 mg of pibrentasvir) once daily for 12 weeks. SVR12 was achieved in 99% of patients with HCV genotype 4 infection.

EXPEDITION-1 (NCT02642432), an open-label, single-arm, phase 3 trial, included 146 treatment-naive or previously treated adults with chronic HCV genotype 1, 2, 4, 5, or 6 infection with compensated cirrhosis (median age 60 years, 62% male, 82% white, 10% black, 12% with baseline HCV RNA levels 6 million IU/mL or greater, 25% previously treated). Previously treated patients had prior treatment experience with regimens containing interferon, peginterferon, ribavirin, and/or sofosbuvir, but no prior treatment experience with an HCV NS3/4A protease inhibitor or HCV NS5A inhibitor. All patients received glecaprevir/pibrentasvir (300 mg of glecaprevir and 120 mg of pibrentasvir) once daily for 12 weeks. Of the 16 patients with HCV genotype 4 infection, 100% achieved SVR12.

EXPEDITION-4 (NCT02651194), an open-label, single-arm, phase 3 trial, included 104 treatment-naive or previously treated adults with chronic HCV genotype 1, 2, 3, 4, 5, or 6 infection who were noncirrhotic or had compensated cirrhosis; all patients also had severe renal impairment (chronic kidney disease stages 4 and 5). Patients had a median age of 57 years, 76% were male, 62% were white, 24% were black, 82% were receiving hemodialysis, 19% had compensated cirrhosis, and 42% were previously treated; 53, 15, 11, 19, 1, and 1% had HCV genotype 1, 2, 3, 4, 5, or 6 infection, respectively. Previously treated patients had treatment experience with regimens containing interferon, peginterferon, ribavirin, and/or sofosbuvir, but no prior treatment experience with an HCV NS3/4A protease inhibitor or HCV NS5A inhibitor. All patients received glecaprevir/pibrentasvir (300 mg of glecaprevir and 120 mg of pibrentasvir) once daily for 12 weeks. Overall, 98% of patients achieved SVR12. The presence of renal impairment did not affect the efficacy of glecaprevir/pibrentasvir and dosage adjustments were not required.

HCV Genotype 5 Infection Efficacy and safety of glecaprevir/pibrentasvir for the treatment of chronic HCV genotype 5 infection in adults have been evaluated in 6 clinical trials (SURVEYOR-2, ENDURANCE-4, SURVEYOR-1, EXPEDITION-1, EXPEDITION-4, and ENDURANCE-5, 6). The primary end point in each study was sustained virologic response at 12 weeks after the end of treatment (SVR12; defined as plasma HCV RNA level less than the lower limit of quantification [15 or 25 IU/mL depending on assay used] at 12 weeks after end of treatment).

SURVEYOR-2 (NCT02243293), a multi-arm, multi-part, open-label, phase 2 trial, evaluated glecaprevir/pibrentasvir with or without ribavirin in adults with HCV genotype 2, 3, 4, 5, or 6 infection who were treatment naive or previously treated, including those with compensated cirrhosis. Previously treated patients had treatment experience with regimens containing interferon, peginterferon, ribavirin, and/or sofosbuvir, but no prior treatment experience with an HCV NS3/4A protease inhibitor or HCV NS5A inhibitor. There were 2 patients with HCV genotype 5 infection who received glecaprevir/pibrentasvir (300 mg of glecaprevir and 120 mg of pibrentasvir) once daily for 8 weeks. SVR12 was achieved in both patients with HCV genotype 5 infection.

ENDURANCE-4 (NCT02636595), a single-arm, open-label, phase 3 trial, evaluated the efficacy and safety of glecaprevir/pibrentasvir in noncirrhotic treatment-naive and previously treated patients with HCV genotype 4, 5, or 6 infection. Previously treated patients had treatment experience with regimens containing interferon, peginterferon, ribavirin, and/or sofosbuvir, but no prior treatment experience with an HCV NS3/4A protease inhibitor or HCV NS5A inhibitor. There were 26 patients with HCV genotype 5 infection; 20 were treatment naive and 6 were previously treated. All 26 patients received glecaprevir/pibrentasvir (300 mg of glecaprevir and 120 mg of pibrentasvir) once daily for 12 weeks. SVR12 was achieved in 100% of patients with HCV genotype 5 infection.

EXPEDITION-1 (NCT02642432), an open-label, single-arm, phase 3 trial, included 146 treatment-naive or previously treated adults with chronic HCV genotype 1, 2, 4, 5, or 6 infection with compensated cirrhosis (median age 60 years, 62% male, 82% white, 10% black, 12% with baseline HCV RNA levels 6 million IU/mL or greater, 25% previously treated). Previously treated patients had prior treatment experience with regimens containing interferon, peginterferon, ribavirin, and/or sofosbuvir, but no prior treatment experience with an HCV NS3/4A protease inhibitor or HCV NS5A inhibitor. All patients received glecaprevir/pibrentasvir (300 mg of glecaprevir and 120 mg of pibrentasvir) once daily for 12 weeks. Of the 2 patients with HCV genotype 5 infection, both achieved SVR12.

EXPEDITION-4 (NCT02651194), an open-label, single-arm, phase 3 trial, included 104 treatment-naive or previously treated adults with chronic HCV genotype 1, 2, 3, 4, 5, or 6 infection who were noncirrhotic or had compensated cirrhosis; all patients also had severe renal impairment (chronic kidney disease stages 4 and 5). Patients had a median age of 57 years, 76% were male, 62% were white, 24% were black, 82% were receiving hemodialysis, 19% had compensated cirrhosis, and 42% were previously treated; 53, 15, 11, 19, 1, and 1% had HCV genotype 1, 2, 3, 4, 5, or 6 infection, respectively. Previously treated patients had prior treatment experience with regimens containing interferon, peginterferon, ribavirin, and/or sofosbuvir, but no prior treatment experience with an HCV NS3/4A protease inhibitor or HCV NS5A inhibitor. All patients received glecaprevir/pibrentasvir (300 mg of glecaprevir and 120 mg of pibrentasvir) once daily for 12 weeks. Overall, 98% of patients achieved SVR12. The presence of renal impairment did not affect the efficacy of glecaprevir/pibrentasvir and dosage adjustments were not required.

ENDURANCE-5,6 (NCT02966795), an open-label, single-arm, phase 3b trial, included 84 treatment-naive or previously treated adults with chronic

HCV genotype 5 or 6 infection who were noncirrhotic or had compensated cirrhosis. Of the 23 patients with HCV genotype 5 infection, median age was 68 years, 43% were male, 91% were white, 13% had compensated cirrhosis, and 17% were previously treated. Noncirrhotic patients received glecaprevir/pibrentasvir (300 mg of glecaprevir and 120 mg of pibrentasvir) once daily for 8 weeks and those with compensated cirrhosis received the same glecaprevir/pibrentasvir dosage for 12 weeks. Of the patients with HCV genotype 5 infection, 95.7% achieved SVR12.

HCV Genotype 6 Infection Efficacy and safety of glecaprevir/pibrentasvir for the treatment of chronic HCV genotype 6 infection in adults have been evaluated in 5 clinical trials (SURVEYOR-2, ENDURANCE-4, SURVEYOR-1, EXPEDITION-1, EXPEDITION-4, and ENDURANCE-5, 6). The primary end point in each study was sustained virologic response at 12 weeks after the end of treatment (SVR12; defined as plasma HCV RNA level less than the lower limit of quantification [15 or 25 IU/mL depending on assay used] at 12 weeks after end of treatment).

SURVEYOR-2 (NCT02243293), a multi-arm, multi-part, open-label, phase 2 trial, evaluated glecaprevir/pibrentasvir with or without ribavirin in adults with HCV genotype 2, 3, 4, 5, or 6 infection who were treatment naive or previously treated, including those with compensated cirrhosis. Previously treated patients had treatment experience with regimens containing interferon, peginterferon, ribavirin, and/or sofosbuvir, but no prior treatment experience with an HCV NS3/4A protease inhibitor or HCV NS5A inhibitor. There were 10 patients with HCV genotype 6 infection; 8 were treatment naive and 2 were previously treated. All 10 patients received glecaprevir/pibrentasvir (300 mg of glecaprevir and 120 mg of pibrentasvir) once daily for 8 weeks. SVR12 was achieved in 88% of patients with HCV genotype 6 infection.

ENDURANCE-4 (NCT02636595), a single-arm, open-label, phase 3 trial, evaluated the efficacy and safety of glecaprevir/pibrentasvir in noncirrhotic treatment-naive and previously treated patients with HCV genotype 4, 5, or 6 infection. Previously treated patients had treatment experience with regimens containing interferon, peginterferon, ribavirin, and/or sofosbuvir, but no prior treatment experience with an HCV NS3/4A protease inhibitor or HCV NS5A inhibitor. There were 19 patients with HCV genotype 6 infection; 17 were treatment naive and 2 were previously treated. All 19 patients received glecaprevir/pibrentasvir (300 mg of glecaprevir and 120 mg of pibrentasvir) once daily for 12 weeks. SVR12 was achieved in 100% of patients with HCV genotype 6 infection. An additional 11 noncirrhotic patients with HCV genotype 6 infection were evaluated in another phase 2 study, SURVEYOR-1 (NCT002243280). These patients also received glecaprevir/pibrentasvir (300 mg of glecaprevir and 120 mg of pibrentasvir) for 12 weeks and SVR12 was achieved in 100% of this subset of patients.

EXPEDITION-1 (NCT02642432), an open-label, single-arm, phase 3 trial, included 146 treatment-naive or previously treated adults with chronic HCV genotype 1, 2, 4, 5, or 6 infection with compensated cirrhosis (median age 60 years, 62% male, 82% white, 10% black, 12% with baseline HCV RNA levels 6 million IU/mL or greater, 25% previously treated). Previously treated patients had prior treatment experience with regimens containing interferon, peginterferon, ribavirin, and/or sofosbuvir, but no prior treatment experience with an HCV NS3/4A protease inhibitor or HCV NS5A inhibitor. All patients received glecaprevir/pibrentasvir (300 mg of glecaprevir and 120 mg of pibrentasvir) once daily for 12 weeks. Of the 7 patients with HCV genotype 6 infection, 100% achieved SVR12.

EXPEDITION-4 (NCT02651194), an open-label, single-arm, phase 3 trial, included 104 treatment-naive or previously treated adults with chronic HCV genotype 1, 2, 3, 4, 5, or 6 infection who were noncirrhotic or had compensated cirrhosis; all patients also had severe renal impairment (chronic kidney disease stages 4 and 5). Patients had a median age of 57 years, 76% were male, 62% were white, 24% were black, 82% were receiving hemodialysis, 19% had compensated cirrhosis, and 42% were previously treated; 53, 15, 11, 19, 1, and 1% had HCV genotype 1, 2, 3, 4, 5, or 6 infection, respectively. Previously treated patients had treatment experience with regimens containing interferon, peginterferon, ribavirin, and/or sofosbuvir, but no prior treatment experience with an HCV NS3/4A protease inhibitor or HCV NS5A inhibitor. All patients received glecaprevir/pibrentasvir (300 mg of glecaprevir and 120 mg of pibrentasvir) once daily for 12 weeks. Overall, 98% of patients achieved SVR12. The presence of renal impairment did not affect the efficacy of glecaprevir/pibrentasvir and dosage adjustments were not required.

ENDURANCE-5,6 (NCT02966795), an open-label, single-arm, phase 3b trial, included 84 treatment-naive or previously treated adults with chronic HCV genotype 5 or 6 infection who were noncirrhotic or had compensated cirrhosis. Of the 61 patients with HCV genotype 6 infection, median age was 54 years, 48% were male, 7% were white, 92% were Asian, 10% had compensated cirrhosis, and 7% were previously treated. Noncirrhotic patients received glecaprevir/pibrentasvir (300 mg of glecaprevir and 120 mg of pibrentasvir) once daily for 8 weeks and those with compensated cirrhosis received the same glecaprevir/pibrentasvir dosage for 12 weeks. Of the patients with HCV genotype 6 infection, 98.4% achieved SVR12.

Transplant Recipients Efficacy and safety of glecaprevir/pibrentasvir for the treatment of chronic HCV genotype 1, 2, 3, 4, or 6 infection in treatment-naive or previously treated adults who were noncirrhotic and had received a kidney or liver transplant were evaluated in a single-arm, open-label, phase 3 clinical trial (MAGELLAN-2; NCT02692703). Of the 100 patients included in the study, 66% were treatment-naive and 34% were previously treated with interferon, peginterferon, ribavirin, and/or sofosbuvir; all patients with HCV genotype 3 infection were treatment-naive. Patients had a median age of 60 years, 75% were male, 8% were black, 80% had received liver transplants, 20% had received kidney transplants, and 11% had normal renal function at baseline; 57, 13, 24, 4, or 2% had HCV genotype 1, 2, 3, 4, or 6 infection, respectively. All patients received glecaprevir/pibrentasvir (300 mg of glecaprevir and 120 mg of pibrentasvir) once daily for 12 weeks. Concomitant use of immunosuppressive agents was allowed (e.g., cyclosporine [dosage less than 100 mg daily], tacrolimus, sirolimus, everolimus, azathioprine, mycophenolic acid, low-dose corticosteroids [prednisone or prednisolone dosage not exceeding 10 mg daily at baseline]). The primary end point was sustained virologic response at 12 weeks after end of treatment (SVR12; defined as plasma HCV RNA level less than 15 IU/mL [the lower limit of quantification] at 12 weeks after end of treatment). SVR12 was achieved in 98% of patients; one patient experienced relapse and no patients experienced on-treatment virologic failure.

HCV-infected Individuals Coinfected with HIV Efficacy and safety of glecaprevir/pibrentasvir for the treatment of chronic HCV infection in adults with HIV coinfection have been evaluated in 2 clinical trials (ENDURANCE-1, EXPEDITION-2). The primary end point in each study was sustained virologic response at 12 weeks after end of treatment (SVR12; defined as plasma HCV RNA level less than 15 IU/mL [the lower limit of quantification] at 12 weeks after end of treatment).

ENDURANCE-1 (NCT02604017), an open-label, randomized, phase 3 trial, included 703 treatment-naive or previously treated adults with chronic HCV genotype 1 infection who were noncirrhotic, including 33 patients with HIV-1 coinfection. Previously treated patients had treatment experience with regimens containing interferon, peginterferon, ribavirin, and/or sofosbuvir, but no prior treatment experience with an HCV NS3/4A protease inhibitor or HCV NS5A inhibitor. Patients were randomized in a 1:1 ratio to receive glecaprevir/pibrentasvir (300 mg of glecaprevir and 120 mg of pibrentasvir) once daily for 8 or 12 weeks. Overall, SVR12 was achieved in 99.1% of patients treated with the 8-week regimen and 99.7% of those treated with the 12-week regimen. In the subset of patients with HIV-1 coinfection, 100% achieved SVR12.

EXPEDITION-2 (NCT02738138), a nonrandomized, open-label, phase 3 trial, included 153 treatment-naive or previously treated adults with chronic HCV infection and HIV-1 coinfection. Previously treated patients had treatment experience with regimens containing interferon, peginterferon, ribavirin, and/or sofosbuvir. Patients had a median age of 45 years, 84% were male, 16% were black, and 11% had compensated cirrhosis; 63, 7, 17, 11, or 2% had HCV genotype 1, 2, 3, 4, or 6 infection, respectively. All patients with HCV genotype 3 infection were treatment-naive. Noncirrhotic patients or those with compensated cirrhosis received glecaprevir/pibrentasvir (300 mg of glecaprevir and 120 mg of pibrentasvir) once daily for 8 or 12 weeks, respectively. SVR12 was achieved in 98% of patients with HCV and HIV-1 coinfection (100% of noncirrhotic patients and 93% of patients with compensated cirrhosis).

Pediatric Patients Efficacy and safety of glecaprevir/pibrentasvir for the treatment of chronic HCV infection in treatment-naive or previously treated noncirrhotic pediatric patients 12 to less than 18 years of age were evaluated in a nonrandomized, open-label, phase 2/3 trial (DORA [Part 1]; NCT03067129). Patients received glecaprevir/pibrentasvir (300 mg of glecaprevir and 120 mg of pibrentasvir) once daily for 8 or 16 weeks; treatment duration was chosen to match adult durations based on HCV genotype and prior treatment experience. Of the 47 patients included in the study, median age was 14 years (range: 12–17 years), mean weight was 59 kg (range: 32–109 kg), 55% were female, 9% were black, 77% were treatment-naive, 23% were previously treated with interferon, and 4% had HIV-1 coinfection; 79, 6, 9, or 6% had HCV genotype 1, 2, 3, or 4 infection, respectively. The primary end point was sustained virologic response at 12 weeks after end of treatment (SVR12; defined as plasma HCV RNA level less than 15 IU/mL [the lower limit of quantification] at 12 weeks after end of treatment). The overall SVR12 rate in these pediatric patients was 100%.

Dosage and Administration

■ **General** Prior to initiating the fixed combination of glecaprevir and pibrentasvir (glecaprevir/pibrentasvir) for treatment of chronic hepatitis C virus (HCV) infection, all patients should be tested for evidence of current or prior hepatitis B virus (HBV) infection by measuring hepatitis B surface antigen (HBsAg), hepatitis B surface antibody (anti-HBs), and hepatitis B core antibody (anti-HBc). (See Risk of HBV Reactivation in Patients Coinfected with HCV and HBV under Warnings/Precautions: Warnings, in Cautions.)

Prior to and during treatment, appropriate laboratory tests should be performed to evaluate liver function. (See Hepatic Impairment under Warnings/Precautions: Specific Populations, in Cautions.)

■ **Administration** Glecaprevir/pibrentasvir is administered orally once daily with food.

■ **Dosage** Glecaprevir/pibrentasvir is commercially available as fixed-combination tablets containing 100 mg of glecaprevir and 40 mg of pibrentasvir.

Adult Dosage **HCV Genotype 1, 2, 3, 4, 5, or 6 Infection.** For the treatment of chronic HCV genotype 1, 2, 3, 4, 5, or 6 infection in treatment-naive (previously untreated) or previously treated adults, the recommended dosage of glecaprevir/pibrentasvir is 3 tablets (total of 300 mg of glecaprevir and 120 mg of pibrentasvir) once daily. The treatment duration depends on the HCV genotype, the patient's previous HCV treatment experience, and presence of cirrhosis. (See Tables 1 and 2.)

Table 1. Recommended Treatment Duration of Glecaprevir/Pibrentasvir in Treatment-naive Adults with HCV Genotype 1, 2, 3, 4, 5, or 6 Infection.

HCV Genotype	Hepatic Impairment	Duration of Glecaprevir/Pibrentasvir
HCV genotype 1, 2, 3, 4, 5, or 6 infection	Noncirrhotic	8 weeks
	Compensated cirrhosis (Child-Pugh class A)	12 weeks

Table 2. Recommended Treatment Duration of Glecaprevir/Pibrentasvir in Previously Treated Adults with HCV Genotype 1, 2, 3, 4, 5, or 6 Infection.

HCV Genotype	Treatment Experience	Hepatic Impairment	Duration of Glecaprevir/Pibrentasvir
HCV genotype 1 infection	Previously treated *without* HCV NS3/4A protease inhibitors or HCV NS5A inhibitors[a]	Noncirrhotic	8 weeks
		Compensated cirrhosis (Child-Pugh class A)	12 weeks
	Previously treated with an HCV NS5A inhibitor; no prior treatment with HCV NS3/4A protease inhibitors[b]	Noncirrhotic	16 weeks
		Compensated cirrhosis	16 weeks
	Previously treated with an HCV NS3/4A protease inhibitor; no prior treatment with HCV NS5A inhibitors[c]	Noncirrhotic	12 weeks
		Compensated cirrhosis	12 weeks
HCV genotype 2, 4, 5, or 6 infection	Previously treated *without* HCV NS3/4A protease inhibitors or HCV NS5A inhibitors[a]	Noncirrhotic	8 weeks
		Compensated cirrhosis	12 weeks
HCV genotype 3 infection	Previously treated *without* HCV NS3/4A protease inhibitors or HCV NS5A inhibitors[a]	Noncirrhotic	16 weeks
		Compensated cirrhosis	16 weeks

[a] Previously received HCV regimen containing interferon, peginterferon, ribavirin, and/or sofosbuvir; no previous treatment with HCV NS3/4A protease inhibitors or HCV NS5A inhibitors.

[b] In clinical trials, patients previously received HCV regimens containing the fixed combination of ledipasvir and sofosbuvir (ledipasvir/sofosbuvir) or daclatasvir in conjunction with peginterferon *and* ribavirin.

[c] In clinical trials, patients previously received HCV regimens containing simeprevir (no longer commercially available) in conjunction with sofosbuvir or simeprevir, boceprevir, or telaprevir (drugs no longer commercially available) in conjunction with peginterferon *and* ribavirin.

HCV-infected Individuals with HIV Coinfection. Glecaprevir/pibrentasvir dosage and duration of therapy recommended for the treatment of chronic HCV genotype 1, 2, 3, 4, 5, or 6 infection in adults coinfected with human immunodeficiency virus type 1 (HIV-1) generally are the same as those recommended for adults without HIV coinfection. (See Drug Interactions: Antiretroviral Agents.)

Liver or Kidney Transplant Recipients. For the treatment of chronic HCV genotype 1, 2, 3, 4, 5, or 6 infection in treatment-naive or previously treated adults who are liver or kidney transplant recipients, the recommended dosage of glecaprevir/pibrentasvir is 3 tablets (total of 300 mg of glecaprevir and 120 mg of pibrentasvir) once daily.

The manufacturer states that a treatment duration of 12 weeks usually is recommended in liver or kidney transplant recipients. However, the manufacturer states that a treatment duration of 16 weeks is recommended in those with HCV genotype 1 infection who were previously treated with an HCV NS5A inhibitor, but have not received an HCV NS3/4A protease inhibitor, and in those with HCV genotype 3 infection who were previously treated with regimens containing interferon, peginterferon, ribavirin, and/or sofosbuvir, but have not received an HCV NS3/4A protease inhibitor or HCV NS5A inhibitor.

Some experts state that adult liver transplant recipients who are treatment-naive or previously treated (with or without decompensated cirrhosis) can receive glecaprevir/pibrentasvir in a dosage of 3 tablets (total of 300 mg of glecaprevir and 120 mg of pibrentasvir) once daily for 12 weeks for the treatment of HCV genotype 1, 2, 3, 4, 5, or 6 infection.

For adult kidney transplant recipients with HCV genotype 1, 2, 3, 4, 5, or 6 infection who are treatment-naive or previously treated (with or without compensated cirrhosis), some experts state that glecaprevir/pibrentasvir (3 tablets [total of 300 mg of glecaprevir and 120 mg of pibrentasvir] once daily) for 12 weeks' duration is a recommended treatment option.

Pediatric Dosage **HCV Genotype 1, 2, 3, 4, 5, or 6 Infection.** For the treatment of chronic HCV genotype 1, 2, 3, 4, 5, or 6 infection in treatment-naive or previously treated pediatric patients 12 years of age or older weighing at least 45 kg, the recommended dosage of glecaprevir/pibrentasvir is 3 tablets (total of 300 mg of glecaprevir and 120 mg of pibrentasvir) once daily. The treatment duration depends on the HCV genotype, the patient's previous HCV treatment experience, and presence of cirrhosis. (See Tables 3 and 4.)

Table 3. Recommended Treatment Duration of Glecaprevir/Pibrentasvir in Treatment-naive Pediatric Patients 12 Years of Age or Older with HCV Genotype 1, 2, 3, 4, 5, or 6 Infection.

HCV Genotype	Hepatic Impairment	Duration of Glecaprevir/Pibrentasvir
HCV genotype 1, 2, 3, 4, 5, or 6 infection	Noncirrhotic	8 weeks
	Compensated cirrhosis (Child-Pugh class A)	12 weeks

Table 4. Recommended Treatment Duration of Glecaprevir/Pibrentasvir in Previously Treated Pediatric Patients 12 Years of Age or Older with HCV Genotype 1, 2, 3, 4, 5, or 6 Infection.

HCV Genotype	Treatment Experience	Hepatic Impairment	Duration of Glecaprevir/Pibrentasvir
HCV genotype 1 infection	Previously treated *without* HCV NS3/4A protease inhibitors or HCV NS5A inhibitors[a]	Noncirrhotic	8 weeks
		Compensated cirrhosis (Child-Pugh class A)	12 weeks
	Previously treated with an HCV NS5A inhibitor; no prior treatment with HCV NS3/4A protease inhibitors[b]	Noncirrhotic	16 weeks
		Compensated cirrhosis	16 weeks
	Previously treated with an HCV NS3/4A protease inhibitor; no prior treatment with HCV NS5A inhibitors[c]	Noncirrhotic	12 weeks
		Compensated cirrhosis	12 weeks
HCV genotype 2, 4, 5, or 6 infection	Previously treated *without* HCV NS3/4A protease inhibitors or HCV NS5A inhibitors[a]	Noncirrhotic	8 weeks
		Compensated cirrhosis	12 weeks
HCV genotype 3 infection	Previously treated *without* HCV NS3/4A protease inhibitors or HCV NS5A inhibitors[a]	Noncirrhotic	16 weeks
		Compensated cirrhosis	16 weeks

[a] Previously received HCV regimen containing interferon, peginterferon, ribavirin, and/or sofosbuvir; no previous treatment with HCV NS3/4A protease inhibitors or HCV NS5A inhibitors.

[b] In clinical trials, patients previously received HCV regimens containing the fixed combination of ledipasvir and sofosbuvir (ledipasvir/sofosbuvir) or daclatasvir in conjunction with peginterferon *and* ribavirin.

[c] In clinical trials, patients previously received HCV regimens containing simeprevir (no longer commercially available) in conjunction with sofosbuvir or simeprevir, boceprevir, or telaprevir (drugs no longer commercially available) in conjunction with peginterferon *and* ribavirin.

HCV-infected Individuals with HIV Coinfection. Glecaprevir/pibrentasvir dosage and duration of therapy recommended for the treatment of chronic HCV genotype 1, 2, 3, 4, 5, or 6 infection in pediatric patients 12 years of age or older weighing at least 45 kg who are coinfected with HIV-1 generally are the same as those recommended for pediatric patients without HIV coinfection. (See Drug Interactions: Antiretroviral Agents.)

Transplant Recipients. For the treatment of chronic HCV genotype 1, 2, 3, 4, 5, or 6 infection in treatment-naive or previously treated pediatric patients 12 years of age or older weighing at least 45 kg who are liver or kidney transplant recipients, the recommended dosage of glecaprevir/pibrentasvir is 3 tablets (total of 300 mg of glecaprevir and 120 mg of pibrentasvir) once daily.

The manufacturer states that a treatment duration of 12 weeks usually is recommended in liver or kidney transplant recipients. However, the manufacturer states that a treatment duration of 16 weeks is recommended in those with HCV genotype 1 infection who were previously treated with an HCV NS5A inhibitor, but have not received an HCV NS3/4A protease inhibitor, and in those with HCV genotype 3 infection who were previously treated with regimens containing interferon, peginterferon, ribavirin, and/or sofosbuvir, but have not received an HCV NS3/4A protease inhibitor or HCV NS5A inhibitor.

■ **Special Populations** ***Hepatic Impairment*** Dosage adjustments of glecaprevir/pibrentasvir are not necessary in patients with mild hepatic impairment (Child-Pugh class A).

Glecaprevir/pibrentasvir is not recommended in patients with moderate hepatic impairment (Child-Pugh class B) and is contraindicated in those with severe hepatic impairment (Child-Pugh class C). (See Hepatic Impairment under Warnings/Precautions: Specific Populations, in Cautions.)

Renal Impairment Dosage adjustments of glecaprevir/pibrentasvir are not necessary in patients with mild, moderate, or severe renal impairment, including those receiving hemodialysis. Glecaprevir and pibrentasvir are not removed by hemodialysis to any clinically important extent. (See Renal Impairment under Warnings/Precautions: Specific Populations, in Cautions.)

Geriatric Patients Dosage adjustments of glecaprevir/pibrentasvir are not necessary in geriatric patients. (See Geriatric Use under Warnings/Precautions: Specific Populations, in Cautions.)

Cautions

■ **Contraindications** The fixed combination of glecaprevir and pibrentasvir (glecaprevir/pibrentasvir) is contraindicated in patients with severe hepatic impairment (Child-Pugh class C).

Concomitant use of glecaprevir/pibrentasvir with atazanavir or rifampin is contraindicated. (See Drug Interactions.)

■ **Warnings/Precautions** ***Warnings*** **Risk of HBV Reactivation in Patients Coinfected with HCV and HBV.** Reactivation of hepatitis B virus (HBV) infection has been reported during postmarketing experience when direct-acting antivirals (DAAs) were used for the treatment of chronic hepatitis C virus (HCV) infection in patients with HBV coinfection. In some cases, HBV reactivation resulted in fulminant hepatitis, hepatic failure, and death.

HBV reactivation (defined as an abrupt increase in HBV replication manifested as a rapid increase in serum HBV DNA levels or detection of hepatitis B surface antigen [HBsAg] in an individual who was previously HBsAg negative and hepatitis B core antibody [anti-HBc] positive) has been reported in patients with HCV and HBV coinfection who were receiving HCV treatment with a regimen that included HCV DAAs without HBV antiviral therapy. Reactivation also may be accompanied by hepatitis (i.e., increased aminotransferase concentrations) and, in severe cases, may lead to increased bilirubin concentrations, liver failure, or death.

Data to date indicate that HBV reactivation usually occurs within 4–8 weeks after initiation of HCV treatment. Patients with HBV reactivation have been heterogeneous in terms of HCV genotype and in terms of baseline HBV disease. While some patients with HBV reactivation were HBsAg positive, others had serologic evidence of resolved HBV infection (i.e., HBsAg negative and anti-HBc positive). HBV reactivation also has been reported in patients receiving certain immunosuppressant or chemotherapeutic drugs; the risk of reactivation associated with HCV DAAs may be increased in such patients.

The mechanism for HBV reactivation in patients with HCV and HBV coinfection receiving HCV DAAs is unknown. Although HCV DAAs are not known to cause immunosuppression, HBV reactivation in coinfected patients may result from a complex interplay of host immunologic responses in the setting of infection with 2 hepatitis viruses.

Prior to initiating treatment with an HCV DAA, including glecaprevir/pibrentasvir, all patients should be screened for evidence of current or prior HBV infection by measuring HBsAg, hepatitis B surface antibody (anti-HBs), and anti-HBc. If there is serologic evidence of HBV infection, baseline HBV DNA levels should be measured.

Patients with evidence of current or prior HBV infection should be monitored for clinical and laboratory signs (i.e., HBsAg, HBV DNA levels, serum aminotransferase concentrations, bilirubin concentrations) of hepatitis flare or HBV reactivation during and after treatment with HCV DAAs, including glecaprevir/pibrentasvir. Appropriate management for HBV infection should be initiated as clinically indicated.

Patients with HCV and HBV coinfection receiving glecaprevir/pibrentasvir should be advised to immediately contact a clinician if they develop any signs or symptoms of serious liver injury (e.g., fatigue, weakness, loss of appetite, nausea and vomiting, yellowing of the eyes or skin, light-colored bowel movements).

When making decisions regarding HBV monitoring or HBV treatment in coinfected patients, consultation with a clinician who has expertise in managing HBV infection is recommended.

Other Warnings and Precautions **Interactions.** Concomitant use of glecaprevir/pibrentasvir with certain drugs (i.e., carbamazepine, efavirenz, St. John's wort) may result in clinically important decreases in glecaprevir and pibrentasvir plasma concentrations and may lead to reduced therapeutic effect of glecaprevir/pibrentasvir. Concomitant use with such drugs is not recommended. (See Drug Interactions.)

Precautions Related to Fixed Combinations. When glecaprevir/pibrentasvir is used, the cautions, precautions, contraindications, and drug interactions associated with each drug in the fixed combination must be considered. Cautionary information applicable to specific populations (e.g., pregnant or nursing women, individuals with hepatic or renal impairment, geriatric patients) should be considered for each drug.

Specific Populations **Pregnancy.** Adequate data are not available regarding use of glecaprevir/pibrentasvir in pregnant women. In animal studies, there was no evidence of adverse effects on fetal development at glecaprevir or pibrentasvir exposures 53 or 51 times greater, respectively, than human exposures at the recommended human dosage.

Lactation. It is not known whether glecaprevir and pibrentasvir are distributed into human milk, affect human milk production, or have effects on the breast-fed infant.

Glecaprevir and pibrentasvir are distributed into milk in rodents, but no apparent effects on growth and postnatal development were observed in nursing pups.

The benefits of breast-feeding and the importance of glecaprevir/pibrentasvir to the woman should be considered along with potential adverse effects on the breast-fed child from the drug or from the underlying maternal condition.

Pediatric Use. Safety, efficacy, and pharmacokinetics of glecaprevir/pibrentasvir have not been established in pediatric patients younger than 12 years of age.

Safety and efficacy of glecaprevir/pibrentasvir for the treatment of HCV genotype 1, 2, 3, or 4 infection in pediatric patients 12 years of age or older weighing at least 45 kg are based on safety, efficacy, and pharmacokinetic data from an open-label phase 2/3 trial in treatment-naive or previously treated noncirrhotic pediatric patients (DORA [Part 1]). Trial data indicated that safety and efficacy of glecaprevir/pibrentasvir in these pediatric patients are consistent with those observed in HCV-infected adults receiving the drug in clinical trials.

Safety and efficacy of glecaprevir/pibrentasvir for the treatment of HCV genotype 5 or 6 infection in pediatric patients 12 years of age or older weighing at least 45 kg and for treatment of HCV infection in pediatric patients 12 years of age or older who weigh at least 45 kg and are cirrhotic or have received a kidney and/or liver transplant are supported by data indicating that glecaprevir and pibrentasvir systemic exposures in pediatric patients in this age group are comparable to those reported in adults.

Geriatric Use. No overall differences in safety and efficacy of glecaprevir/pibrentasvir have been observed between patients 65 years of age and older and younger adults. Pooled analysis of data from 9 clinical trials (phase 2 or 3) that evaluated safety and efficacy of glecaprevir/pibrentasvir for the treatment of chronic HCV infection in adults indicated that, in the subset of patients with severe renal impairment, those 65 years of age and older had a higher incidence of adverse effects (79 or 68%, respectively) and treatment-related adverse effects (57 or 46%, respectively) compared with younger adults.

Hepatic Impairment. Safety and efficacy of glecaprevir/pibrentasvir have not been established in patients with moderate hepatic impairment (Child-Pugh class B) and the drug is not recommended in such patients. Glecaprevir/pibrentasvir is contraindicated in patients with severe hepatic impairment (Child-Pugh class C).

In August 2019, FDA reported that the use of glecaprevir/pibrentasvir, elbasvir/grazoprevir, or sofosbuvir/velpatasvir/voxilaprevir to treat chronic hepatitis C in patients with moderate to severe liver impairment has resulted in rare cases of worsening liver function or liver failure. FDA noted that all these medicines contain an HCV protease inhibitor and are not indicated for use in patients with moderate to severe liver impairment. In most patients, symptoms resolved or new onset worsening of liver function improved after stopping the medicine. Health care professionals should continue to prescribe these drugs as indicated in the prescribing information for patients without liver impairment or with mild liver impairment (Child-Pugh A). The severity of liver disease should be assessed at baseline and patients should be closely monitored for signs and symptoms of worsening liver function. Assessment of baseline liver disease and close monitoring are especially important in patients with pre-existing significant liver problems or risk factors, such as hepatocellular carcinoma or alcohol abuse, which can also contribute to clinical worsening of liver function or liver failure during treatment. These medicines should be discontinued in patients who develop signs and symptoms of liver decompensation or as clinically indicated.

In HCV-infected individuals with compensated cirrhosis (Child-Pugh class A), administration of glecaprevir/pibrentasvir results in glecaprevir exposures approximately twofold higher than those reported in HCV-infected individuals without cirrhosis; pibrentasvir exposures are similar to those observed in HCV-infected individuals without cirrhosis.

In individuals with moderate or severe hepatic impairment (Child-Pugh class B or C), administration of glecaprevir/pibrentasvir results in glecaprevir plasma exposures twofold and 11-fold higher, respectively, than those reported in individuals with normal hepatic function; pibrentasvir plasma exposures are 26 and 114% higher, respectively, than those reported in individuals with normal hepatic function.

Renal Impairment. In individuals with mild, moderate, severe, or end-stage renal impairment without HCV infection, glecaprevir and pibrentasvir exposures were up to 56 and 46% higher, respectively, than exposures reported in individuals with normal renal function. In dialysis-dependent individuals without HCV infection, pibrentasvir and glecaprevir exposures were similar with or without dialysis (up to 18% difference).

In HCV-infected individuals with end-stage renal disease (with or without dialysis), glecaprevir and pibrentasvir exposures were 86 and 54% higher, respectively, than exposures reported in individuals with normal renal function.

■ **Common Adverse Effects** Adverse effects reported in 5% or more of patients receiving glecaprevir/pibrentasvir include pruritus, headache, fatigue, nausea, diarrhea, asthenia, nasopharyngitis, and urinary tract infection.

Drug Interactions

■ **Drugs Affecting or Metabolized by Hepatic Microsomal Enzymes** Glecaprevir and pibrentasvir are weak inhibitors of cytochrome P-450 (CYP) isoenzymes 3A and 1A2. Clinically important pharmacokinetic interactions are not expected if the fixed combination of glecaprevir and pibrentasvir (glecaprevir/pibrentasvir) is used concomitantly with substrates of CYP3A, 1A2, 2C9, 2C19, or 2D6.

Pharmacokinetic interactions are possible with inducers of CYP3A4, which may decrease glecaprevir and pibrentasvir plasma concentrations.

■ **Drugs Affecting or Affected by P-glycoprotein Transport System** Glecaprevir and pibrentasvir are inhibitors of the P-glycoprotein (P-gp) transport system. Concomitant use of glecaprevir/pibrentasvir and P-gp substrates may increase exposure of such drugs.

Glecaprevir and pibrentasvir are substrates of P-gp. Pharmacokinetic interactions are possible with P-gp inducers, which may decrease glecaprevir and pibrentasvir plasma concentrations. Pharmacokinetic interactions are possible with P-gp inhibitors, which may increase glecaprevir and pibrentasvir plasma concentrations.

■ **Drugs Affecting or Affected by Breast Cancer Resistance Protein** Glecaprevir and pibrentasvir are inhibitors of breast cancer resistance protein (BCRP). Concomitant use of glecaprevir/pibrentasvir and BCRP substrates may increase exposure of such drugs.

Glecaprevir and pibrentasvir are substrates of BCRP. Pharmacokinetic interactions are possible with BCRP inducers, which may decrease glecaprevir and pibrentasvir plasma concentrations. Pharmacokinetic interactions are possible with BCRP inhibitors, which may increase glecaprevir and pibrentasvir plasma concentrations.

■ **Drugs Affecting or Affected by Organic Anion Transporting Polypeptides** Glecaprevir and pibrentasvir are inhibitors of organic anion transporting polypeptide (OATP) 1B1 and 1B3. Concomitant use of glecaprevir/pibrentasvir and OATP1B1 or 1B3 substrates may increase exposure of such drugs.

Glecaprevir is a substrate of OATP1B1 and 1B3. Pharmacokinetic interactions are possible with OATP1B1 and 1B3 inducers, which may decrease glecaprevir plasma concentrations. Pharmacokinetic interactions are possible with OATP1B1 and 1B3 inhibitors, which may increase glecaprevir plasma concentrations.

■ **Drugs Affecting or Affected by Other Membrane Transporters** Glecaprevir and pibrentasvir are weak inhibitors of uridine diphosphate-glucuronosyl transferase (UGT) 1A1. Clinically important pharmacokinetic interactions are not expected if glecaprevir/pibrentasvir is used concomitantly with substrates of UGT1A1 or 1A4.

■ **Angiotensin II Receptor Antagonists** No clinically important pharmacokinetic interactions were observed when losartan or valsartan was used concomitantly with glecaprevir/pibrentasvir.

Dosage adjustments are not necessary if losartan or valsartan is used concomitantly with glecaprevir/pibrentasvir.

■ **Anticoagulants** ***Dabigatran*** Concomitant use of dabigatran etexilate (single 150-mg dose) and glecaprevir/pibrentasvir (300 mg of glecaprevir and 120 mg of pibrentasvir once daily) results in increased dabigatran peak plasma concentrations and area under the concentration-time curve (AUC).

If dabigatran etexilate and glecaprevir/pibrentasvir are used concomitantly in patients with renal impairment, the recommendations from the manufacturer of dabigatran etexilate regarding dosage modifications for concomitant use with P-gp inhibitors should be followed.

Warfarin If warfarin is used in patients receiving treatment for hepatitis C virus (HCV) infection, including treatment with glecaprevir/pibrentasvir, fluctuations in the international normalized ratio (INR) may occur. INR should be closely monitored during HCV treatment and after treatment is completed.

■ **Anticonvulsants** ***Carbamazepine*** Concomitant use of carbamazepine (200 mg twice daily) and glecaprevir/pibrentasvir (300 mg of glecaprevir and 120 mg of pibrentasvir as a single dose) results in clinically important decreases in glecaprevir and pibrentasvir plasma concentrations and AUCs, which may lead to reduced therapeutic effect of glecaprevir/pibrentasvir.

Concomitant use of carbamazepine and glecaprevir/pibrentasvir is not recommended.

Lamotrigine No clinically important pharmacokinetic interactions were observed when lamotrigine was used concomitantly with glecaprevir/pibrentasvir.

Dosage adjustments are not necessary if lamotrigine is used concomitantly with glecaprevir/pibrentasvir.

Phenytoin Concomitant use of phenytoin and glecaprevir/pibrentasvir may result in decreased glecaprevir and pibrentasvir plasma concentrations and may lead to reduced therapeutic effect of glecaprevir/pibrentasvir.

Concomitant use of phenytoin and glecaprevir/pibrentasvir is not recommended.

■ **Antimycobacterial Agents** ***Rifampin*** Concomitant use of rifampin (600 mg once daily) and a single dose of glecaprevir/pibrentasvir (300 mg of glecaprevir and 120 mg of pibrentasvir) results in clinically important decreases in plasma concentrations and AUCs of glecaprevir and pibrentasvir and may lead to reduced therapeutic effect of glecaprevir/pibrentasvir. Concomitant use of rifampin (single 600-mg dose) and glecaprevir/pibrentasvir results in increased glecaprevir plasma concentrations and AUC.

Concomitant use of rifampin and glecaprevir/pibrentasvir is contraindicated.

■ **Antiretroviral Agents** ***HIV Entry and Fusion Inhibitors*** **Maraviroc.** Concomitant use of maraviroc and glecaprevir/pibrentasvir is not expected to affect maraviroc pharmacokinetics.

Dosage adjustments are not necessary if maraviroc is used concomitantly with glecaprevir/pibrentasvir.

HIV Integrase Inhibitors (INSTIs) **Bictegravir.** Concomitant use of bictegravir and glecaprevir/pibrentasvir is not expected to alter bictegravir concentrations.

Dosage adjustments are not necessary if bictegravir is used concomitantly with glecaprevir/pibrentasvir.

Dolutegravir. No clinically important pharmacokinetic interactions were observed when the fixed combination of abacavir, dolutegravir, and lamivudine (abacavir/dolutegravir/lamivudine) was used concomitantly with glecaprevir/pibrentasvir.

Dosage adjustments are not necessary if dolutegravir is used concomitantly with glecaprevir/pibrentasvir.

Elvitegravir. Concomitant use of the fixed combination of elvitegravir, cobicistat, emtricitabine, and tenofovir alafenamide (EVG/c/FTC/TAF) and glecaprevir/pibrentasvir results in increased plasma concentrations and AUCs of glecaprevir and pibrentasvir and increased AUC of elvitegravir.

Dosage adjustments are not necessary if *cobicistat-boosted* elvitegravir is used concomitantly with glecaprevir/pibrentasvir.

Raltegravir. Concomitant use of raltegravir and glecaprevir/pibrentasvir results in increased plasma concentrations and AUC of raltegravir.

Dosage adjustments are not necessary if raltegravir is used concomitantly with glecaprevir/pibrentasvir.

HIV Nonnucleoside Reverse Transcriptase Inhibitors (NNRTIs) **Doravirine.** Concomitant use of doravirine and glecaprevir/pibrentasvir is expected to result in increased plasma concentrations of doravirine.

Dosage adjustments are not necessary if doravirine is used concomitantly with glecaprevir/pibrentasvir.

Efavirenz. Concomitant use of efavirenz and glecaprevir/pibrentasvir may result in decreased glecaprevir and pibrentasvir plasma concentrations and may lead to reduced therapeutic effect of glecaprevir/pibrentasvir.

Concomitant use of efavirenz and glecaprevir/pibrentasvir is not recommended.

Etravirine. Concomitant use of etravirine and glecaprevir/pibrentasvir may result in decreased glecaprevir and pibrentasvir plasma concentrations.

Concomitant use of etravirine and glecaprevir/pibrentasvir is not recommended.

Nevirapine. Concomitant use of nevirapine and glecaprevir/pibrentasvir may result in decreased glecaprevir and pibrentasvir plasma concentrations.

Concomitant use of nevirapine and glecaprevir/pibrentasvir is not recommended.

Rilpivirine. Concomitant use of rilpivirine and glecaprevir/pibrentasvir results in increased plasma concentrations and AUC of rilpivirine; this is not considered clinically important. Concomitant use does not affect glecaprevir and pibrentasvir concentrations.

Dosage adjustments are not necessary if rilpivirine is used concomitantly with glecaprevir/pibrentasvir.

HIV Nucleoside and Nucleotide Reverse Transcriptase Inhibitors (NRTIs) **Abacavir.** No clinically important pharmacokinetic interactions were observed when abacavir/dolutegravir/lamivudine was used concomitantly with glecaprevir/pibrentasvir.

Dosage adjustments are not necessary if abacavir is used concomitantly with glecaprevir/pibrentasvir.

Emtricitabine. Concomitant use of the fixed combination of elvitegravir, cobicistat, emtricitabine, and tenofovir alafenamide (EVG/c/FTC/TAF) and glecaprevir/pibrentasvir results in increased plasma concentrations and AUCs of glecaprevir and pibrentasvir.

Dosage adjustments are not necessary if emtricitabine is used concomitantly with glecaprevir/pibrentasvir.

Lamivudine. No clinically important pharmacokinetic interactions were observed when abacavir/dolutegravir/lamivudine was used concomitantly with glecaprevir/pibrentasvir.

Dosage adjustments are not necessary if lamivudine is used concomitantly with glecaprevir/pibrentasvir.

Tenofovir. Concomitant use of EVG/c/FTC/TAF and glecaprevir/pibrentasvir results in increased plasma concentrations and AUCs of glecaprevir and pibrentasvir, but does not affect tenofovir concentrations or AUC. Concomitant use of the fixed combination of efavirenz, emtricitabine, and tenofovir disoproxil fumarate (tenofovir DF; TDF) and glecaprevir/pibrentasvir results in increased plasma concentrations and AUC of tenofovir.

Dosage adjustments are not necessary if tenofovir alafenamide or tenofovir DF is used concomitantly with glecaprevir/pibrentasvir.

HIV Protease Inhibitors (PIs) **Atazanavir.** Concomitant use of *ritonavir-boosted* atazanavir (300 mg of atazanavir and 100 mg of ritonavir once daily) and glecaprevir/pibrentasvir (300 mg of glecaprevir and 120 mg of pibrentasvir once daily) results in 4-, 14.3-, and 6.5-fold increases in glecaprevir peak plasma concentrations, trough plasma concentrations, and AUC, respectively, and 1.3-, 2.3-, and 1.6-fold increases in pibrentasvir peak plasma concentrations, trough plasma concentrations, and AUC, respectively. Concomitant use may result in increased ALT concentrations.

Concomitant use of glecaprevir/pibrentasvir and *ritonavir-boosted*, *cobicistat-boosted*, or unboosted atazanavir is contraindicated.

Darunavir. Concomitant use of *ritonavir-boosted* darunavir (800 mg of darunavir and 100 mg of ritonavir once daily) and glecaprevir/pibrentasvir (300 mg of glecaprevir and 120 mg of pibrentasvir once daily) results in 3.1-, 8.2-, and 5-fold increases in glecaprevir peak plasma concentrations, trough plasma concentrations, and AUC, respectively, and 1.7-fold increases in pibrentasvir trough plasma concentrations.

Concomitant use of glecaprevir/pibrentasvir and *ritonavir-boosted* or *cobicistat-boosted* darunavir is not recommended.

Lopinavir. Concomitant use of the fixed combination of lopinavir 400 mg and ritonavir 100 mg (lopinavir/ritonavir once daily) and glecaprevir/pibrentasvir (300 mg of glecaprevir and 120 mg of pibrentasvir once daily) results in 2.6-, 18.6-, and 4.4-fold increases in glecaprevir peak plasma concentrations, trough plasma concentrations, and AUC, respectively, and 1.4-, 5.2-, and 2.5-fold increases in pibrentasvir peak plasma concentrations, trough plasma concentrations, and AUC, respectively.

Concomitant use of lopinavir/ritonavir and glecaprevir/pibrentasvir is not recommended.

Ritonavir. Concomitant use of ritonavir and glecaprevir/pibrentasvir is expected to increase plasma concentrations of glecaprevir and pibrentasvir.

Concomitant use of ritonavir and glecaprevir/pibrentasvir is not recommended.

Tipranavir. Concomitant use of *ritonavir-boosted* tipranavir and glecaprevir/pibrentasvir is expected to increase plasma concentrations of glecaprevir and pibrentasvir.

Concomitant use of *ritonavir-boosted* tipranavir and glecaprevir/pibrentasvir is not recommended.

■ **Benzodiazepines** No clinically important pharmacokinetic interactions were observed when midazolam was used concomitantly with glecaprevir/pibrentasvir.

Dosage adjustments are not necessary if midazolam is used concomitantly with glecaprevir/pibrentasvir.

■ **Caffeine** No clinically important pharmacokinetic interactions were observed when caffeine was used concomitantly with glecaprevir/pibrentasvir.

Dosage adjustments are not necessary if caffeine is used concomitantly with glecaprevir/pibrentasvir.

■ **Calcium-channel Blocking Agents** ***Amlodipine and Felodipine*** No clinically important pharmacokinetic interactions were observed when amlodipine or felodipine was used concomitantly with glecaprevir/pibrentasvir.

Dosage adjustments are not necessary if amlodipine or felodipine is used concomitantly with glecaprevir/pibrentasvir.

■ **Dextromethorphan** No clinically important pharmacokinetic interactions were observed when dextromethorphan was used concomitantly with glecaprevir/pibrentasvir.

Dosage adjustments are not necessary if dextromethorphan is used concomitantly with glecaprevir/pibrentasvir.

■ **Digoxin** Concomitant use of digoxin and glecaprevir/pibrentasvir increases digoxin exposures.

Serum digoxin concentrations should be measured prior to and monitored during concomitant glecaprevir/pibrentasvir therapy. Digoxin serum concentrations should be reduced by decreasing the digoxin dosage by 50% or modifying the frequency of administration of the drug.

■ **Estrogens and Progestins** Concomitant use of glecaprevir/pibrentasvir and an oral contraceptive containing ethinyl estradiol and norgestimate or levonorgestrel results in increased plasma concentrations and AUC of ethinyl estradiol, norgestrel, and norgestromin, which may increase the risk of ALT elevations; concomitant use is not expected to affect glecaprevir or pibrentasvir concentrations.

Concomitant use of glecaprevir/pibrentasvir and ethinyl estradiol-containing preparations (e.g., combined oral contraceptives) is not recommended.

Dosage adjustments are not necessary if glecaprevir/pibrentasvir is used concomitantly with norethindrone or other progestin-only contraceptives.

■ **HCV Antivirals** ***HCV Polymerase Inhibitors*** **Sofosbuvir.** No clinically important pharmacokinetic interactions were observed when sofosbuvir was used concomitantly with glecaprevir/pibrentasvir.

Dosage adjustments are not necessary if sofosbuvir is used concomitantly with glecaprevir/pibrentasvir.

■ **HMG-CoA Reductase Inhibitors** ***Atorvastatin*** Concomitant use of atorvastatin (10 mg once daily) and glecaprevir/pibrentasvir (400 mg of glecaprevir and 120 mg of pibrentasvir once daily) results in 22- and 8.3-fold increases in atorvastatin peak plasma concentrations and AUC, respectively, which may increase the risk of myopathy and rhabdomyolysis.

Concomitant use of atorvastatin and glecaprevir/pibrentasvir is not recommended.

Fluvastatin Concomitant use of fluvastatin and glecaprevir/pibrentasvir may increase plasma concentrations of fluvastatin, which may increase the risk of myopathy and rhabdomyolysis.

If fluvastatin and glecaprevir/pibrentasvir are used concomitantly, the lowest dosage of fluvastatin should be used. If higher fluvastatin dosages are required, the lowest necessary dosage should be used taking into account the risks and benefits.

Lovastatin Concomitant use of lovastatin (10 mg once daily) and glecaprevir/pibrentasvir (300 mg of glecaprevir and 120 mg of pibrentasvir once daily) results in 5.7- and 4.1-fold increases in lovastatin peak plasma concentrations and AUC, respectively, which may increase the risk of myopathy and rhabdomyolysis.

Concomitant use of lovastatin and glecaprevir/pibrentasvir is not recommended.

Pitavastatin Concomitant use of pitavastatin and glecaprevir/pibrentasvir may increase plasma concentrations of pitavastatin, which may increase the risk of myopathy and rhabdomyolysis.

If pitavastatin and glecaprevir/pibrentasvir are used concomitantly, the lowest dosage of pitavastatin should be used. If higher pitavastatin dosages are required, use the lowest necessary dosage taking into account the risks and benefits.

Pravastatin Concomitant use of pravastatin (10 mg once daily) and glecaprevir/pibrentasvir (400 mg of glecaprevir and 120 mg of pibrentasvir once daily) results in 2.2- and 2.3-fold increases in pravastatin peak plasma concentrations and AUC, respectively, which may increase the risk of myopathy and rhabdomyolysis.

If pravastatin is used concomitantly with glecaprevir/pibrentasvir, the pravastatin dosage should be reduced by 50%.

Rosuvastatin Concomitant use of rosuvastatin (5 mg once daily) and glecaprevir/pibrentasvir (400 mg of glecaprevir and 120 mg of pibrentasvir once daily) results in 5.6- and 2.2-fold increases in rosuvastatin peak plasma concentrations and AUC, respectively, which may increase the risk of myopathy and rhabdomyolysis.

If rosuvastatin is used concomitantly with glecaprevir/pibrentasvir, the rosuvastatin dosage should not exceed 10 mg.

Simvastatin Concomitant use of simvastatin (5 mg once daily) and glecaprevir/pibrentasvir (300 mg of glecaprevir and 120 mg of pibrentasvir once daily) results in 10.7- and 4.5-fold increases in simvastatin peak plasma concentrations and AUC, respectively, which may increase the risk of myopathy and rhabdomyolysis.

Concomitant use of simvastatin and glecaprevir/pibrentasvir is not recommended.

■ **Immunosuppressive Agents** ***Cyclosporine*** Concomitant use of low-dose cyclosporine (single 100-mg dose) and glecaprevir/pibrentasvir (300 mg of glecaprevir and 120 mg of pibrentasvir once daily) results in 1.3-, 1.3-, and 1.4-fold increases in glecaprevir peak plasma concentrations, trough plasma concentrations, and AUC, respectively, and 1.3-fold increases in pibrentasvir trough plasma concentrations. Concomitant use of high-dose cyclosporine (single 400-mg dose) and glecaprevir/pibrentasvir (300 mg of glecaprevir and 120 mg of pibrentasvir once daily) results in 4.5- and 5-fold increases in glecaprevir peak plasma concentrations and AUC, respectively, and 1.9-fold increases in pibrentasvir AUC. Cyclosporine exposures following single 100- or 400-mg doses are not substantially affected by concomitant glecaprevir/pibrentasvir.

Concomitant use of cyclosporine and glecaprevir/pibrentasvir is not recommended in patients receiving stable cyclosporine dosages exceeding 100 mg daily.

Tacrolimus No clinically important pharmacokinetic interactions were observed when tacrolimus was used concomitantly with glecaprevir/pibrentasvir.

Dosage adjustments are not necessary if tacrolimus is used concomitantly with glecaprevir/pibrentasvir.

■ **Opiate Agonists, Opiate Partial Agonists, and Opiate Antagonists** No clinically important pharmacokinetic interactions were observed when methadone, buprenorphine, naloxone, or the fixed combination of buprenorphine and naloxone (buprenorphine/naloxone) was used concomitantly with glecaprevir/pibrentasvir.

Dosage adjustments are not necessary if methadone, buprenorphine, naloxone, or buprenorphine/naloxone is used concomitantly with glecaprevir/pibrentasvir.

■ **Proton-pump Inhibitors** No clinically important pharmacokinetic interactions were observed when omeprazole (20 mg once daily) was used concomitantly with glecaprevir/pibrentasvir (single dose of 300 mg of glecaprevir and 120 mg of pibrentasvir). Concomitant use of omeprazole (40 mg once daily) given 1 hour before glecaprevir/pibrentasvir (single dose of 300 mg of glecaprevir and 120 mg of pibrentasvir) decreased peak plasma concentrations and AUC of glecaprevir, but did not affect plasma concentrations or AUC of pibrentasvir. Concomitant use of glecaprevir/pibrentasvir and omeprazole given in a dose of 40 mg has been reported to decrease glecaprevir exposures by 51%.

In a clinical study evaluating glecaprevir/pibrentasvir for the treatment of chronic HCV genotype 1, 2, 4, 5, or 6 infection (EXPEDITION-1), 21% of patients reported concomitant use of a proton-pump inhibitor (PPI); PPI use did not appear to affect rates of sustained virologic response at 12 weeks after end of treatment (SVR12). In a pooled analysis of data from 9 clinical trials (phase 2 or 3) that evaluated efficacy and safety of glecaprevir/pibrentasvir for the treatment of chronic HCV infection in adults, 263 patients were identified who received a PPI during the trial; 59% received low PPI doses (omeprazole 20 mg daily [or equivalent]) and 41% received high PPI doses (at least 1 dose greater than omeprazole 20 mg daily [or equivalent]). SVR12 rates were 97.4% in those receiving low PPI doses and 96.3% in those receiving high PPI doses.

The manufacturer states that dosage adjustments are not necessary if omeprazole is used concomitantly with glecaprevir/pibrentasvir. Some clinicians recommend that long-term concomitant use of glecaprevir/pibrentasvir and omeprazole 40 mg once daily should be avoided.

■ **St. John's Wort** Concomitant use of St. John's wort (*Hypericum perforatum*) and glecaprevir/pibrentasvir may result in clinically important decreases in glecaprevir and pibrentasvir plasma concentrations and may lead to reduced therapeutic effect of glecaprevir/pibrentasvir.

Concomitant use of St. John's wort and glecaprevir/pibrentasvir is not recommended.

■ **Tolbutamide** No clinically important pharmacokinetic interactions were observed when tolbutamide was used concomitantly with glecaprevir/pibrentasvir.

Dosage adjustments are not necessary if tolbutamide is used concomitantly with glecaprevir/pibrentasvir.

Description

Glecaprevir and pibrentasvir (glecaprevir/pibrentasvir) is a fixed combination containing 2 hepatitis C virus (HCV) antivirals. Glecaprevir is an HCV nonstructural 3/4A (NS3/4A) protease inhibitor. Pibrentasvir is an HCV nonstructural 5A (NS5A) replication complex inhibitor (NS5A inhibitor). Both drugs are direct-acting antivirals (DAAs) with activity against HCV. There was no in vitro evidence of antagonistic anti-HCV effects between glecaprevir and pibrentasvir when the combination was evaluated in HCV genotype 1 replicon cell culture assays.

Glecaprevir binds to the active site of HCV NS3/4A protease, thereby blocking enzyme activity essential for viral replication (i.e., blocking cleavage of the HCV-encoded polyproteins into mature forms of NS3, NS4A, NS4B, NS5A, and NS5B). In vitro studies using biochemical assays indicate that glecaprevir has activity against clinical isolates of HCV genotypes 1a, 1b, 2a, 2b, 3a, 4a, 5a, and 6a. In HCV replicon assays, glecaprevir has shown in vitro activity against laboratory and clinical isolates of HCV genotypes 1a, 1b, 2a, 2b, 3a, 4a, 4d, 5a, and 6a (median EC_{50} ranging from 0.08–4.6 nM).

Pibrentasvir inhibits the HCV NS5A protein, which is required for viral replication and virion assembly. In HCV replicon assays, pibrentasvir has shown in vitro activity against laboratory and clinical isolates of HCV genotypes 1a, 1b, 2a, 2b, 3a, 4a, 4b, 4d, 5a, 6a, 6e, and 6p (median EC_{50} ranging from 0.5–4.3 nM).

Certain amino acid substitutions in NS3/4A protease inhibitor resistance-associated positions of HCV genotypes 1a (e.g., D168F/Y), 1b, 2a, 3a (e.g., Q168R), 4a, and 6a (e.g., D168A/G/H/V/Y) have been selected in cell culture and have been associated with reduced susceptibility to glecaprevir in vitro in replicon studies. Emergence of amino acid substitutions occurred most commonly at NS3 positions A156 or D/Q168. The combination of NS3 resistance-associated substitutions Y56H and D/Q168 resulted in greater reductions in glecaprevir susceptibility. Treatment-emergent NS3 resistance-associated substitutions were detected in clinical trials evaluating glecaprevir/pibrentasvir in patients with HCV genotype 1 (e.g., A156V, V36A/M, Y56H, R155K/T, A156G/T/V, D168A/T) or genotype 3 (e.g., Y56H/N, Q80K/R, A156G, Q168L/R) infection who experienced virologic failure.

Certain amino acid substitutions in NS5A of HCV genotype 1a (e.g., Q30D/deletion, Y93D/H/N, H58D *and* Y93H, M28G), genotype 1b (e.g., P32-deletion), genotype 2a (e.g., F28S *and* M31I, P29S *and* K30G), and genotype 3a (e.g., Y93H) have been selected in cell culture and have been associated with reduced susceptibility to pibrentasvir in vitro in replicon studies. Combinations of these NS5A substitutions often resulted in greater reductions in susceptibility to pibrentasvir compared with a single NS5A substitution. Treatment-emergent NS5A resistance-associated substitutions were detected in clinical trials evaluating glecaprevir/pibrentasvir in patients with HCV genotype 1 (e.g., Q30R, L31M, M28A/G, L28M, P29Q/R, Q30K/R, H58D, Y93H/N) or genotype 3a (e.g., S24F, M28G/K, A30G/K, L31F, P58T, Y93H) infection who experienced virologic failure. Some of these patients also had baseline NS5A polymorphisms at resistance-associated amino acid positions.

Cross-resistance is possible between glecaprevir and other HCV NS3/4A protease inhibitors and between pibrentasvir and other HCV NS5A inhibitors. Cross-resistance is not expected between glecaprevir/pibrentasvir and sofosbuvir, peginterferon, or ribavirin.

Following oral administration of glecaprevir/pibrentasvir in healthy individuals, peak plasma concentrations of glecaprevir and pibrentasvir occur 5 hours after the dose. Administration of glecaprevir/pibrentasvir with a moderate- to high-fat meal increased glecaprevir exposures by 83–163% and increased pibrentasvir exposures by 40–53% relative to administration in the fasting state.

Glecaprevir is metabolized to some extent by cytochrome P-450 (CYP) isoenzyme 3A. The drug is 97.5% bound to plasma proteins. The major route of elimination is biliary and fecal excretion. Following a single oral dose of glecaprevir, 92.1% of the dose is excreted in feces and 0.7% is eliminated in urine. The plasma half-life of glecaprevir is 6 hours.

Pibrentasvir is only minimally metabolized. The drug is more than 99.9% bound to plasma proteins. The major route of elimination is biliary and fecal excretion. Following a single oral dose of pibrentasvir, 96.6% of the dose is excreted in feces; no drug is eliminated in urine. The plasma half-life of pibrentasvir is 13 hours.

Advice to Patients

Importance of reading patient information provided by the manufacturer.

Advise patients that the fixed-combination preparation of glecaprevir and pibrentasvir (glecaprevir/pibrentasvir) should be taken once daily with food on a regular dosing schedule.

Importance of taking the recommended dosage of glecaprevir/pibrentasvir for the recommended duration of treatment; importance of not missing doses.

If a dose is missed and remembered less than 18 hours after the scheduled administration time, advise patient to take glecaprevir/pibrentasvir as soon as possible and then take the next dose at the usual time. If a dose is missed and remembered more than 18 hours after the schedule administration time, advise patient to skip the missed dose and take the next dose at the usual time.

Inform patients that reactivation of hepatitis B virus (HBV) infection has occurred in patients being treated for hepatitis C virus (HCV) infection who were coinfected with HBV. Importance of informing clinician of any history of HBV infection or other liver problems (e.g., cirrhosis). Importance of immediately contacting a clinician if any signs or symptoms of serious liver injury (e.g., fatigue, weakness, loss of appetite, nausea and vomiting, yellowing of the eyes or skin, light-colored bowel movements) occur. (See Risk of HBV Reactivation in Patients Coinfected with HCV and HBV under Warnings/Precautions: Warnings, in Cautions.)

Advise patients that glecaprevir/pibrentasvir may interact with some drugs. Importance of informing clinicians of existing or contemplated concomitant therapy, including prescription and OTC drugs and dietary or herbal supplements, as well as any concomitant illnesses.

Importance of women informing clinicians if they are or plan to become pregnant or plan to breast-feed.

Importance of informing patients of other important precautionary information. (See Cautions.)

Overview® (see Users Guide). For additional information on this drug until a more detailed monograph is developed and published, the manufacturer's labeling should be consulted. It is *essential* that the manufacturer's labeling be consulted for more detailed information on usual cautions, precautions, contraindications, potential drug interactions, laboratory test interferences, and acute toxicity.

Preparations

Excipients in commercially available drug preparations may have clinically important effects in some individuals; consult specific product labeling for details.

Glecaprevir and Pibrentasvir

Oral		
Tablets, film-coated	Glecaprevir 100 mg and Pibrentasvir 40 mg	**Mavyret®**, AbbVie

HCV Replication Complex Inhibitors 8:18.40.24

Elbasvir and Grazoprevir EBR, GZR

■ Elbasvir and grazoprevir (elbasvir/grazoprevir) is a fixed combination containing 2 hepatitis C virus (HCV) antivirals; elbasvir is an HCV nonstructural 5A (NS5A) replication complex inhibitor (NS5A inhibitor) and grazoprevir is an HCV nonstructural 3/4A (NS3/4A) protease inhibitor.

Uses

■ **Chronic Hepatitis C Virus Infection** The fixed combination of elbasvir and grazoprevir (elbasvir/grazoprevir) is used for the treatment of chronic hepatitis C virus (HCV) genotype 1 or genotype 4 infection in adults who are treatment-naive (previously untreated) or in whom prior treatment with peginterferon alfa and ribavirin (with or without an HCV protease inhibitor) failed, including those with compensated liver disease (with or without cirrhosis) and those with human immunodeficiency virus (HIV) coinfection.

Elbasvir/grazoprevir is used alone or in conjunction with ribavirin, depending on HCV genotype and certain patient factors (e.g., previous treatment experience, presence of baseline polymorphisms).

Because efficacy of a 12-week regimen of elbasvir/grazoprevir for the treatment of HCV genotype 1a infection is reduced when 1 or more NS5A resistance-associated polymorphisms at certain amino acid positions (28, 30, 31, 93) are present at baseline, screening for NS5A resistance-associated polymorphisms is recommended prior to initiation of treatment in patients with HCV genotype 1a infection. (See Dosage and Administration: General.)

Because the treatment of chronic HCV infection is complex and rapidly evolving, it is recommended that treatment be directed by clinicians who are familiar with the disease and that a specialist be consulted to obtain the most up-to-date information. Information from the American Association for the Study of Liver Diseases (AASLD), Infectious Diseases Society of America (IDSA), and International Antiviral Society–USA (IAS–USA) regarding diagnosis and management of HCV infection, including recommendations for initial treatment, is available at http://www.hcvguidelines.org.

HCV Genotype 1 Infection **Treatment-naive Adults.** Efficacy and safety of elbasvir/grazoprevir for the treatment of chronic HCV genotype 1 infection in treatment-naive adults have been evaluated in a randomized, double-blind, placebo-controlled, phase 3 trial (C-EDGE TN; NCT02105467). A total of 421 treatment-naive adults with chronic HCV genotype 1, 4, or 6 infection (noncirrhotic or with compensated cirrhosis) were randomized in a 3:1 ratio to receive elbasvir/grazoprevir (a fixed-combination tablet containing 50 mg of elbasvir and 100 mg of grazoprevir once daily) or placebo for 12 weeks. Those with decompensated liver disease and those with HIV coinfection were excluded. Patients who initially received placebo then received open-label elbasvir/grazoprevir for 12 weeks (deferred-treatment group). The primary end point was sustained virologic response at 12 weeks after the end of treatment (SVR12; defined as plasma HCV RNA level less than 15 IU/mL [the lower limit of quantification] at 12 weeks after end of treatment). The study included 382 patients with HCV genotype 1 infection (288 in the immediate-treatment group, 94 in the deferred-treatment group); among those in the immediate-treatment group, the median age was 55 years, 56% were male, 72% had baseline HCV RNA levels exceeding 800,000 IU/mL, 55% had HCV genotype 1a infection, 67% had non-CC IL28B alleles, and 24% had cirrhosis. SVR12 was achieved in 95% of patients with HCV genotype 1 infection in the immediate-treatment group (92 or 98% of those with HCV genotype 1a or 1b infection, respectively).

Previously Treated Adults. Efficacy and safety of elbasvir/grazoprevir for the treatment of chronic HCV genotype 1 infection in previously treated adults have been evaluated in a randomized, open-label, phase 3 trial (C-EDGE TE) and a single-arm, open-label, phase 2 trial (C-SALVAGE). The primary end point in both studies was SVR12 (defined as plasma HCV RNA level less than 15 IU/mL [the lower limit of quantification] at 12 weeks after end of treatment).

C-EDGE TE (NCT02105701) included 414 noncirrhotic or cirrhotic adults with chronic HCV genotype 1 or genotype 4 infection (with or without HIV coinfection) who previously failed a treatment regimen of peginterferon alfa and ribavirin. Patients were randomized in a 1:1:1:1 ratio to receive elbasvir/grazoprevir (a fixed-combination tablet containing 50 mg of elbasvir and 100 mg of grazoprevir once daily) for 12 or 16 weeks or elbasvir/grazoprevir once daily in conjunction *with* ribavirin for 12 or 16 weeks. C-EDGE TE included approximately 374 previously treated patients with HCV genotype 1 infection (median age 57 years, 64% male, 78% with baseline HCV RNA levels exceeding 800,000 IU/mL, 60% with HCV genotype 1a infection, 79% with non-CC IL28B alleles, 34% with cirrhosis). In those with HCV genotype 1 infection, SVR12 was achieved in 94% of patients treated with elbasvir/grazoprevir alone for 12 weeks and in 97% of those treated with elbasvir/grazoprevir *with* ribavirin for 16 weeks.

C-SALVAGE (NCT02105454) included 79 noncirrhotic or cirrhotic adults with HCV genotype 1 infection who previously failed a treatment regimen of peginterferon alfa, ribavirin, and an HCV protease inhibitor (e.g., boceprevir, simeprevir, telaprevir) (median age 55 years, 58% male, 63% with baseline HCV RNA levels exceeding 800,000 IU/mL, 38% with HCV genotype 1a infection, 97% with non-CC IL28B alleles, 43% with cirrhosis, 46% with baseline NS3 resistance-associated substitutions). All patients received elbasvir/grazoprevir (a fixed-combination tablet containing 50 mg of elbasvir and 100 mg of grazoprevir once daily) in conjunction *with* ribavirin for 12 weeks. SVR12 was achieved in 96% of patients overall; 4% of patients did not achieve SVR12 and experienced relapse after the end of treatment. The SVR12 rates were similar in those with HCV genotype 1a or 1b infection, cirrhotic or noncirrhotic patients, and those with varying response to previous HCV treatments. All patients who achieved SVR12 also achieved SVR24 (defined as plasma HCV RNA level less than 15 IU/mL [the lower limit of quantification] at 24 weeks after end of treatment).

HCV Genotype 4 Infection **Treatment-naive Adults.** Efficacy and safety of elbasvir/grazoprevir for the treatment of chronic HCV genotype 4 infection in treatment-naive adults have been evaluated in a randomized, open-label, phase 2 trial (C-SCAPE), a randomized, double-blind, placebo-controlled, phase 3 trial (C-EDGE TN), and an open-label, single-arm, phase 3 trial (C-EDGE COINFECTION).

In C-SCAPE (NCT01932762), 20 treatment-naive, noncirrhotic adults with HCV genotype 4 infection were randomized to receive elbasvir/grazoprevir (a fixed-combination tablet containing 50 mg of elbasvir and 100 mg of grazoprevir once daily) alone or in conjunction *with* ribavirin for 12 weeks. The primary end point was sustained virologic response at 12 weeks after the end of treatment (SVR12; defined as plasma HCV RNA level less than 25 IU/mL [the lower limit of quantification] at 12 weeks after end of treatment).

In C-EDGE TN (NCT02105467), treatment-naive adults with chronic HCV genotype 1, 4, or 6 infection (without cirrhosis or with compensated cirrhosis) were randomized in a 3:1 ratio to receive elbasvir/grazoprevir (a fixed-combination tablet containing 50 mg of elbasvir and 100 mg of grazoprevir once daily) or placebo for 12 weeks. Those who initially received placebo then received open-label elbasvir/grazoprevir for 12 weeks (deferred-treatment group). The primary end point was sustained virologic response at 12 weeks after the end of treatment (SVR12; defined as plasma HCV RNA level less than 15 IU/mL [the lower limit of quantification] at 12 weeks after end of treatment). The immediate-treatment group in C-EDGE TN included 18 treatment-naive patients with HCV genotype 4 infection.

In C-EDGE COINFECTION (NCT02105662), treatment-naive adults with HCV genotype 1, 4, or 6 infection coinfected with HIV received elbasvir/grazoprevir (a fixed-combination tablet containing 50 mg of elbasvir and 100 mg of grazoprevir once daily) for 12 weeks. The primary end point was sustained virologic response at 12 weeks after the end of treatment (SVR12; defined as plasma HCV RNA level less than 15 IU/mL [the lower limit of quantification] at 12 weeks after end of treatment). C-EDGE COINFECTION included 28 treatment-naive patients with HCV genotype 4 infection.

When data from these 3 studies were combined, a total of 66 treatment-naive adults with HCV genotype 4 infection received 12 weeks of treatment with elbasvir/grazoprevir and SVR12 was achieved in 97% of these patients.

Previously Treated Adults. Efficacy and safety of elbasvir/grazoprevir for the treatment of chronic HCV genotype 4 infection in previously treated adults have been evaluated in a randomized, open-label, phase 3 trial, C-EDGE TE (NCT02105701). This trial included cirrhotic or noncirrhotic adults with chronic HCV genotype 1, 4, or 6 (with or without HIV coinfection) who previously failed a treatment regimen of peginterferon alfa and ribavirin. Patients were randomized in a 1:1:1:1 ratio to receive elbasvir/grazoprevir (a fixed-combination tablet containing 50 mg of elbasvir and 100 mg of grazoprevir once daily) for 12 or 16 weeks or elbasvir/grazoprevir once daily in conjunction *with* ribavirin for 12 or 16 weeks. The primary end point was SVR12 (defined as plasma HCV RNA level less than 15 IU/mL [the lower limit of quantification] at 12 weeks after end of treatment). In C-EDGE TE, a total of 37 previously treated patients with HCV genotype 4 infection received a 12- or 16-week regimen of elbasvir/grazoprevir with or without ribavirin. Among the 8 patients who received a 16-week regimen of elbasvir/grazoprevir *with* ribavirin, the SVR12 rate was 100%.

HCV-infected Individuals Coinfected with HIV Efficacy and safety of elbasvir/grazoprevir for the treatment of HCV genotype 1, 4, or 6 infection in treatment-naive adults coinfected with HIV have been evaluated in an open-label, single-arm, phase 3 study (C-EDGE COINFECTION; NCT02105662). A total of 218 HCV-infected patients who were coinfected with HIV (mean age 49 years, 84% male, 58% with baseline HCV RNA levels exceeding 800,000 IU/mL, 66% with HCV genotype 1a infection, 20% with HCV genotype 1b infection, 13% with HCV genotype 4 infection, 1% with HCV genotype 6 infection, 65% with non-CC IL28B alleles, 16% with METAVIR F4 [cirrhosis], 97% receiving HIV antiretroviral therapy and with undetectable HIV RNA levels) received elbasvir/grazoprevir (a fixed-combination tablet containing 50 mg of elbasvir and 100 mg of grazoprevir once daily) for 12 weeks. The primary end point was SVR12 (defined as plasma HCV RNA level less than 15 IU/mL [the lower limit of quantification] at 12 weeks after end of treatment). SVR12 was achieved in 96% of patients overall (97, 96, or 96% of those with HCV genotype 1a, 1b, or 4 infection, respectively).

HCV-infected Individuals with Severe Renal Impairment Efficacy and safety of elbasvir/grazoprevir for the treatment of HCV genotype 1 infection in treatment-naive or previously treated adults with severe renal impairment were evaluated in a randomized, double-blind, placebo-controlled phase 3 study (C-SURFER; NCT02092350). A total of 235 patients with compensated liver disease (with or without cirrhosis) and with stage 4 or 5 chronic kidney disease (estimated glomerular filtration rate [eGFR] 15–29 mL/minute per 1.73 m^2 or less than 15 mL/minute per 1.73 m^2, respectively, including those undergoing hemodialysis) were randomized in a 1:1 ratio to receive elbasvir/grazoprevir (a fixed-combination tablet containing 50 mg of elbasvir and 100 mg of grazoprevir once daily) or placebo for 12 weeks. Patients who initially received placebo then received open-label elbasvir/grazoprevir for 12 weeks (deferred-treatment group). In addition, 11 patients in an intensive pharmacokinetic group received open-label treatment with elbasvir/grazoprevir once daily for 12 weeks. The primary end point was sustained virologic response at 12 weeks after the end of treatment (SVR12; defined as plasma HCV RNA level less than 15 IU/mL [the lower limit of quantification] at 12 weeks after end of treatment). A total of 122 patients were included in the immediate-treatment group and intensive pharmacokinetic group (median age 58 years, 75% male, 57% with baseline HCV RNA levels exceeding 800,000 IU/mL, 72% with non-CC IL28B alleles, 52% with HCV genotype 1a infection, 6% with cirrhosis). SVR12 was achieved in 94% of patients in the pooled immediate-treatment group and intensive pharmacokinetic group (97 or 92% of those with HCV genotype 1a or 1b infection, respectively). SVR12 was achieved in 95% of those without cirrhosis compared with 86% of those with cirrhosis and in 100% of those with stage 4 renal impairment compared with 93% of those with stage 5 renal impairment.

Dosage and Administration

■ **General** For the treatment of chronic hepatitis C virus (HCV) infection, elbasvir and grazoprevir (elbasvir/grazoprevir) is used alone or in conjunction with ribavirin.

The specific regimen and duration of treatment is based on HCV genotype and certain patient factors (e.g., previous treatment experience, presence of baseline polymorphisms). Relapse rates following treatment are affected by baseline patient and viral factors and differ between treatment regimens and treatment duration for certain subgroups.

Screening for the presence of HCV nonstructural 5A (NS5A) resistance-associated polymorphisms is recommended prior to initiation of elbasvir/grazoprevir in patients with HCV genotype 1a infection to determine the appropriate treatment regimen and treatment duration.

Prior to initiating elbasvir/grazoprevir for treatment of HCV infection, all patients should be tested for evidence of current or prior hepatitis B virus (HBV) infection by measuring hepatitis B surface antigen (HBsAg), hepatitis B surface antibody (anti-HBs), and hepatitis B core antibody (anti-HBc). (See Risk of HBV Reactivation in Patients Coinfected with HCV and HBV under Warnings/Precautions: Warnings, in Cautions.)

Prior to and during treatment, appropriate laboratory tests should be performed to evaluate liver function. (See Hepatic Effects under Warnings/Precautions: Other Warnings/Precautions, in Cautions.)

■ **Administration** Elbasvir/grazoprevir is administered orally once daily without regard to food.

■ **Dosage** Elbasvir/grazoprevir is commercially available as fixed-combination tablets containing 50 mg of elbasvir and 100 mg of grazoprevir.

Chronic Hepatitis C Virus Infection **HCV Genotype 1a Infection.** For the treatment of HCV genotype 1a infection in adults, the recommended dosage of elbasvir/grazoprevir is 1 tablet (50 mg of elbasvir and 100 mg of grazoprevir) once daily. Elbasvir/grazoprevir is used alone in patients *without* baseline NS5A polymorphisms who are treatment-naive or were previously treated with peginterferon alfa and ribavirin, but is used in conjunction with ribavirin in those *with* baseline NS5A polymorphisms or in those previously treated with peginterferon alfa, ribavirin, and an HCV protease inhibitor. (See Table 1.)

A treatment duration of 12 weeks is recommended for most patients, but a treatment duration of 16 weeks is recommended in those *with* baseline NS5A polymorphisms. (See Table 1.)

Table 1. Recommended Treatment Regimen and Duration of Elbasvir/Grazoprevir for HCV Genotype 1a Infection in Adults with or without Cirrhosis.

Patient Type	Multiple-drug Regimen	Duration of Treatment
Treatment-naive or previously treated[a] *without* baseline NS5A polymorphisms[b]	Elbasvir/grazoprevir	12 weeks
Treatment-naive or previously treated[a] *with* baseline NS5A polymorphisms[b]	Elbasvir/grazoprevir *with* ribavirin[c]	16 weeks
Previously treated with an HCV protease inhibitor[d,e]	Elbasvir/grazoprevir *with* ribavirin[c]	12 weeks

[a] Previously treated defined as patients who failed treatment with peginterferon alfa and ribavirin.

[b] NS5A resistance-associated polymorphisms at amino acid positions 28, 30, 31, or 93.

[c] Use weight-based ribavirin dosage in patients with creatinine clearance >50 mL/minute (800 mg daily in those <66 kg, 1 g daily in those 66–80 kg, 1.2 g daily in those 81–105 kg, 1.4 g daily in those >105 kg); give ribavirin daily dosage in 2 divided doses with food.

[d] Previously treated with an HCV protease inhibitor defined as patients who failed treatment with a regimen of peginterferon alfa, ribavirin, and an HCV NS3/4A protease inhibitor (e.g., boceprevir, simeprevir, telaprevir).

[e] The optimal elbasvir/grazoprevir-based regimen and duration of treatment not established for patients with HCV genotype 1a infection who previously failed treatment with peginterferon alfa, ribavirin, and an HCV protease inhibitor and have 1 or more baseline NS5A resistance-associated polymorphisms at positions 28, 30, 31, and 93.

HCV Genotype 1b Infection. For the treatment of HCV genotype 1b infection in adults, the recommended dosage of elbasvir/grazoprevir is 1 tablet (50 mg of elbasvir and 100 mg of grazoprevir) once daily. Elbasvir/grazoprevir is used alone in patients who are treatment-naive or were previously treated with peginterferon alfa and ribavirin, but is used in conjunction with ribavirin in those previously treated with peginterferon alfa, ribavirin, and an HCV protease inhibitor. (See Table 2.)

A treatment duration of 12 weeks is recommended. (See Table 2.)

Table 2. Recommended Treatment Regimen and Duration of Elbasvir/Grazoprevir for HCV Genotype 1b Infection in Adults with or without Cirrhosis.

Patient Type	Multiple-drug Regimen	Duration of Treatment
Treatment-naive or previously treated[a]	Elbasvir/grazoprevir	12 weeks
Previously treated with an HCV protease inhibitor[b]	Elbasvir/grazoprevir *with* ribavirin[c]	12 weeks

[a] Previously treated defined as patients who failed treatment with peginterferon alfa and ribavirin.

[b] Previously treated with an HCV protease inhibitor defined as patients who failed treatment with a regimen of peginterferon alfa, ribavirin, and an HCV NS3/4A protease inhibitor (e.g., boceprevir, simeprevir, telaprevir).

[c] Use weight-based ribavirin dosage in patients with creatinine clearance >50 mL/minute (800 mg daily in those <66 kg, 1 g daily in those 66–80 kg, 1.2 g daily in those 81–105 kg, 1.4 g daily in those >105 kg); give ribavirin daily dosage in 2 divided doses with food.

HCV Genotype 4 Infection. For the treatment of HCV genotype 4 infection in adults, the recommended dosage of elbasvir/grazoprevir is 1 tablet (50 mg of elbasvir and 100 mg of grazoprevir) once daily. Elbasvir/grazoprevir is used alone in patients who are treatment-naive, but is used in conjunction with ribavirin in those previously treated with peginterferon alfa and ribavirin. (See Table 3.)

A treatment duration of 12 weeks is recommended for treatment-naive patients, but a treatment duration of 16 weeks is recommended in patients previously treated with peginterferon alfa and ribavirin. (See Table 3.)

Table 3. Recommended Treatment Regimen and Duration of Elbasvir/Grazoprevir for HCV Genotype 4 Infection in Adults with or without Cirrhosis.

Patient Type	Multiple-drug Regimen	Duration of Treatment
Treatment-naive	Elbasvir/grazoprevir	12 weeks
Previously treated[a]	Elbasvir/grazoprevir *with* ribavirin[b]	16 weeks

[a] Previously treated defined as patients who failed treatment with peginterferon alfa and ribavirin.

[b] Use weight-based ribavirin dosage in patients with creatinine clearance >50 mL/minute (800 mg daily in those <66 kg, 1 g daily in those 66–80 kg, 1.2 g daily in those 81–105 kg, 1.4 g daily in those >105 kg); give ribavirin daily dosage in 2 divided doses with food.

HCV-infected Individuals Coinfected with HIV. For the treatment of chronic HCV genotype 1 or genotype 4 infection in adults with human immunodeficiency virus (HIV) coinfection, the same elbasvir/grazoprevir dosage and same HCV genotype-specific multiple-drug regimen and treatment duration recommended for HCV-infected patients without HIV coinfection should be used. (See Table 1, Table 2, and Table 3.)

■ **Special Populations** ***Hepatic Impairment*** Dosage adjustments of elbasvir/grazoprevir are not needed in patients with mild hepatic impairment (Child-Pugh class A).

Elbasvir/grazoprevir is contraindicated in those with moderate or severe hepatic impairment (Child-Pugh class B or C). (See Hepatic Impairment under Warnings/Precautions: Specific Populations, in Cautions.)

Renal Impairment Dosage adjustments of elbasvir/grazoprevir are not needed in patients with mild, moderate, or severe renal impairment, including those requiring hemodialysis. (See Renal Impairment under Warnings/Precautions: Specific Populations, in Cautions.)

Geriatric Patients Dosage adjustments of elbasvir/grazoprevir are not needed in geriatric patients. (See Geriatric Use under Warnings/Precautions: Specific Populations, in Cautions.)

Cautions

■ **Contraindications** The fixed combination of elbasvir and grazoprevir (elbasvir/grazoprevir) is contraindicated in patients with moderate or severe hepatic impairment (Child-Pugh class B or C). (See Hepatic Impairment under Warnings/Precautions: Specific Populations, in Cautions.)

Concomitant use of elbasvir/grazoprevir with certain drugs (e.g., inhibitors of organic anion transporting polypeptides [OATP] 1B1 and 1B3, potent inducers of cytochrome P-450 [CYP] 3A, efavirenz) is contraindicated. (See Drug Interactions.)

When elbasvir/grazoprevir is used in conjunction *with* ribavirin, the contraindications for ribavirin apply. (See Precautions Related to Fixed Combinations and Multiple-drug Treatment Regimens under Warnings/Precautions: Other Warnings/Precautions, in Cautions.)

■ **Warnings/Precautions** ***Warnings*** **Risk of HBV Reactivation in Patients Coinfected with HCV and HBV.** Reactivation of hepatitis B virus (HBV) infection has been reported during postmarketing experience when direct-acting antivirals (DAAs) were used for the treatment of chronic hepatitis C virus (HCV) infection in patients with HBV coinfection. In some cases, HBV reactivation resulted in fulminant hepatitis, hepatic failure, and death.

HBV reactivation (defined as an abrupt increase in HBV replication manifested as a rapid increase in serum HBV DNA levels or detection of hepatitis B surface antigen [HBsAg] in an individual who was previously HBsAg negative and hepatitis B core antibody [anti-HBc] positive) has been reported in patients with HCV and HBV coinfection who were receiving HCV treatment with a regimen that included HCV DAAs without interferon alfa. Reactivation also may be accompanied by hepatitis (i.e., increased aminotransferase concentrations) and, in severe cases, may lead to increased bilirubin concentrations, liver failure, or death. Data to date indicate that HBV reactivation usually occurs within 4–8 weeks after initiation of HCV treatment. Patients with HBV reactivation have been heterogeneous in terms of HCV genotype and in terms of baseline HBV disease. While some patients with HBV reactivation were HBsAg positive, others had serologic evidence of resolved HBV infection (i.e., HBsAg negative and anti-HBc positive). HBV reactivation also has been reported in patients receiving certain immunosuppressant or chemotherapeutic drugs; the risk of reactivation associated with HCV DAAs may be increased in such patients.

The mechanism for HBV reactivation in patients with HCV and HBV coinfection receiving HCV DAAs is unknown. Although HCV DAAs are not known to cause immunosuppression, HBV reactivation in coinfected patients may result from a complex interplay of host immunologic responses in the setting of infection with 2 hepatitis viruses.

Prior to initiating treatment with an HCV DAA, including elbasvir/grazoprevir, all patients should be screened for evidence of current or prior HBV infection by measuring HBsAg, anti-HBs, and anti-HBc. If there is serologic evidence of HBV infection, baseline HBV DNA levels should be measured.

Patients with evidence of current or prior HBV infection should be monitored for clinical and laboratory signs (i.e., HBsAg, HBV DNA levels, serum aminotransferase concentrations, bilirubin concentrations) of hepatitis flare or HBV reactivation during and after treatment with HCV DAAs, including elbasvir/grazoprevir. Appropriate management for HBV infection should be initiated as clinically indicated.

Patients with HCV and HBV coinfection receiving elbasvir/grazoprevir should be advised to immediately contact a clinician if they develop any signs or symptoms of serious liver injury (e.g., fatigue, weakness, loss of appetite, nausea and vomiting, yellowing of the eyes or skin, light-colored bowel movements).

When making decisions regarding HBV monitoring or HBV treatment in coinfected patients, consultation with a clinician who has expertise in managing HBV infection is recommended.

Other Warnings/Precautions

Hepatic Effects. In clinical trials evaluating elbasvir/grazoprevir with or without ribavirin, increased ALT concentrations (exceeding 5 times the upper limit of normal [ULN]) were reported in 1% of patients, usually at 8 weeks or longer after initiation of treatment (mean onset 10 weeks; range 6–12 weeks). ALT elevations usually were asymptomatic and resolved with ongoing treatment or completion of treatment. Increased rates of late-onset ALT elevations were reported in patients with increased grazoprevir plasma concentrations and in certain patient groups (e.g., 65 years of age or older, Asian descent, females). The incidence of late-onset ALT elevations did not appear to be affected by presence of cirrhosis or treatment duration.

In clinical trials, increased bilirubin concentrations (exceeding 2.5 times the ULN) were reported in 6% of patients receiving elbasvir/grazoprevir in conjunction *with* ribavirin compared with less than 1% of patients receiving elbasvir/grazoprevir alone. These bilirubin increases were predominately indirect bilirubin and typically were not associated with increased ALT concentrations.

Hepatic laboratory testing should be performed prior to initiation of elbasvir/grazoprevir, at treatment week 8, and as clinically indicated. (See Hepatic Impairment under Warnings/Precautions: Specific Populations, in Cautions.) For patients receiving 16 weeks of elbasvir/grazoprevir treatment, additional hepatic laboratory testing should be performed at treatment week 12.

If ALT concentrations remain persistently greater than 10 times the ULN, discontinuance of elbasvir/grazoprevir should be considered. If ALT elevations are accompanied by signs or symptoms of liver inflammation or increasing conjugated bilirubin, alkaline phosphatase, or international normalized ratio (INR), the drug should be discontinued. Patients should be advised to immediately contact a clinician if they have onset of fatigue, weakness, lack of appetite, nausea and vomiting, jaundice, or discolored feces.

Interactions. Concomitant use of elbasvir/grazoprevir and certain drugs is contraindicated or not recommended. Concomitant use with some drugs may result in drug interactions leading to loss of therapeutic effect and possible development of resistance to elbasvir/grazoprevir. Certain other drug interactions may result in clinically important adverse reactions due to increased exposures of the concomitant drugs or components of elbasvir/grazoprevir.

Potential drug interactions should be considered prior to and during elbasvir/grazoprevir treatment. Drugs used concomitantly with elbasvir/grazoprevir should be reviewed during the course of treatment and the patient should be monitored for adverse reactions associated with these drugs. (See Drug Interactions.)

Precautions Related to Fixed Combinations and Multiple-drug Treatment Regimens. When elbasvir/grazoprevir is used, the cautions, precautions, contraindications, and drug interactions associated with both drugs in the fixed combination must be considered. Cautionary information applicable to specific populations (e.g., pregnant or nursing women, individuals with hepatic or renal impairment, geriatric patients) should be considered for each drug.

When elbasvir/grazoprevir is used in conjunction *with* ribavirin, the cautions, precautions, and contraindications associated with ribavirin also should be considered. (See Cautions in Ribavirin 8:18.32.) Ribavirin may cause fetal toxicity and/or death and extreme care *must* be taken to avoid pregnancy in female patients and in female partners of male patients receiving ribavirin-containing regimens. Women of childbearing potential should have a negative pregnancy test immediately prior to initiating ribavirin and pregnancy tests should be performed monthly during and for 6 months after ribavirin treatment is completed. Women of childbearing potential (and their male partners) and male patients (and their female partners) *must* use at least 2 forms of effective contraception during and for 6 months after ribavirin treatment is completed. (See Cautions: Pregnancy, Fertility, and Lactation, in Ribavirin 8:18.32.)

Specific Populations

Pregnancy. Adequate data are not available regarding use of elbasvir/grazoprevir in pregnant women. Animal reproduction studies using elbasvir or grazoprevir have not revealed evidence of fetal harm at exposures greater than those attained with recommended human dosage.

When elbasvir/grazoprevir is used in conjunction *with* ribavirin, clinicians should consider that ribavirin may cause fetal toxicity and/or death and extreme care must be taken to avoid pregnancy in female patients and in female partners of male patients receiving the ribavirin-containing regimen. (See Cautions: Pregnancy, Fertility, and Lactation, in Ribavirin 8:18.32.)

Lactation. It is not known whether elbasvir/grazoprevir is distributed into human milk, affects human milk production, or affects the breast-fed infant. Both elbasvir and grazoprevir are distributed into milk in rats.

The benefits of breast-feeding and the importance of elbasvir/grazoprevir to the woman should be considered along with the potential adverse effects on the breast-fed child from the drug or from the underlying maternal condition.

When elbasvir/grazoprevir is used in conjunction *with* ribavirin, the potential for adverse reactions to ribavirin in nursing infants should be considered and a decision should be made whether to discontinue nursing or the ribavirin-containing regimen, taking into account the importance of the treatment regimen to the woman. (See Precautions Related to Fixed Combinations and Multiple-drug Treatment Regimens under Warnings/Precautions: Other Warnings/Precautions, in Cautions.)

Pediatric Use. Safety and efficacy of elbasvir/grazoprevir have not been established in pediatric patients younger than 18 years of age.

Pharmacokinetics of elbasvir/grazoprevir have not been evaluated in pediatric patients.

Geriatric Use. In clinical trials, a higher rate of late-onset ALT elevations was reported in individuals 65 years of age and older. (See Hepatic Effects under Warnings/Precautions: Other Warnings/Precautions, in Cautions.)

In population pharmacokinetic analyses, the areas under the plasma concentration-time curves (AUCs) of elbasvir and grazoprevir are estimated to be increased by 16 and 45%, respectively, in individuals 65 years of age and older compared with AUCs in younger adults.

Hepatic Impairment. Elbasvir/grazoprevir is contraindicated in patients with moderate or severe hepatic impairment (Child-Pugh class B or C) because increased grazoprevir plasma concentrations are expected and the risk of ALT elevations is increased in these patients. Data are insufficient regarding efficacy and safety of elbasvir/grazoprevir in HCV-infected patients with moderate hepatic impairment.

In August 2019, FDA reported that the use of glecaprevir/pibrentasvir, elbasvir/grazoprevir, or sofosbuvir/velpatasvir/voxilaprevir to treat chronic hepatitis C in patients with moderate to severe liver impairment has resulted in rare cases of worsening liver function or liver failure. FDA noted that all these medicines contain an HCV protease inhibitor and are not indicated for use in patients with moderate to severe liver impairment. In most patients, symptoms resolved or new onset worsening of liver function improved after stopping the medicine. Health care professionals should continue to prescribe these drugs as indicated in the prescribing information for patients without liver impairment or with mild liver impairment (Child-Pugh A). The severity of liver disease should be assessed at baseline and patients should be closely monitored for signs and symptoms of worsening liver function. Assessment of baseline liver disease and close monitoring are especially important in patients with preexisting significant liver problems or risk factors, such as hepatocellular carcinoma or alcohol abuse, which can also contribute to clinical worsening of liver function or liver failure during treatment. These medicines should be discontinued in patients who develop signs and symptoms of liver decompensation or as clinically indicated.

Efficacy and safety of elbasvir/grazoprevir have not been established in liver transplant recipients or pretransplant patients.

In population pharmacokinetic analyses of elbasvir and grazoprevir in adults with mild, moderate, or severe hepatic impairment (Child-Pugh class A, B, or C) without HCV infection, the AUC of grazoprevir is increased by 1.7-, 5-, and 12-fold, respectively, compared with AUCs reported in adults with normal hepatic function. There are no clinically important differences in the AUCs of elbasvir in adults with mild, moderate, or severe hepatic impairment compared with AUCs reported in adults with normal hepatic function.

Although elbasvir AUCs in HCV-infected adults with compensated cirrhosis are similar to those reported in HCV-infected adults without cirrhosis, grazoprevir AUCs in HCV-infected adults with compensated cirrhosis are 1.65-fold higher than those reported in HCV-infected adults without cirrhosis.

Renal Impairment. In population pharmacokinetic analyses of elbasvir and grazoprevir in adults with severe renal impairment (not dependent on dialysis) and adults requiring hemodialysis, the AUC of elbasvir was increased by 46 and 25%, respectively, and the AUC of grazoprevir was increased by 40 and 10%, respectively, compared with adults without severe renal impairment. These changes in elbasvir and grazoprevir exposures in HCV-infected adults with renal impairment (with or without hemodialysis) are not considered clinically important.

Elbasvir and grazoprevir are not removed by hemodialysis; the drugs are unlikely to be removed by peritoneal dialysis since they are highly bound to plasma proteins.

Race. In clinical trials, a higher rate of late-onset ALT elevations was observed in Asians. (See Hepatic Effects under Warnings/Precautions: Other Warnings/Precautions, in Cautions.) In population pharmacokinetic analyses, elbasvir and grazoprevir AUCs were estimated to be increased by 15 and 50%, respectively, in Asians compared with AUCs reported in Caucasians; dosage adjustments are not needed based on race.

Estimated elbasvir and grazoprevir exposures in Black or African American individuals are comparable to those reported in Caucasians.

Gender. In clinical trials, a higher rate of late-onset ALT elevations was observed in females. (See Hepatic Effects under Warnings/Precautions: Other Warnings/Precautions, in Cautions.)

In population pharmacokinetic analyses, elbasvir and grazoprevir AUCs were estimated to be increased by 50 and 30%, respectively, in females compared with AUCs reported in males; dosage adjustments are not needed based on gender.

■ **Common Adverse Effects** Elbasvir/grazoprevir: Adverse effects reported in 5% or more of patients include fatigue, headache, insomnia, dizziness, nausea, diarrhea, upper respiratory tract infection, and arthralgia.

Elbasvir/grazoprevir in conjunction *with* ribavirin: Adverse effects reported in 5% or more of patients include fatigue, headache, asthenia, nausea, vomiting, diarrhea, constipation, upper abdominal pain, insomnia, anemia, decreased hemoglobin concentrations, elevated total bilirubin concentrations, and elevated triacylglycerol lipase concentrations.

Drug Interactions

The following drug interactions are based on studies that used the fixed combination of elbasvir and grazoprevir (elbasvir/grazoprevir), elbasvir alone, or grazoprevir alone, or are predicted drug interactions that may occur with elbasvir/grazoprevir. When elbasvir/grazoprevir is used, interactions associated with both drugs in the fixed combination should be considered.

■ **Drugs Affecting or Metabolized by Hepatic Microsomal Enzymes** Elbasvir and grazoprevir are both substrates of cytochrome P-450 (CYP) isoenzyme 3A. Elbasvir does not inhibit CYP3A in vitro; grazoprevir is a weak inhibitor of CYP3A in vivo.

Pharmacokinetic interactions are possible if elbasvir/grazoprevir is used concomitantly with moderate or potent inducers of CYP3A (decreased elbasvir and grazoprevir concentrations and possible loss of therapeutic effect) or potent inhibitors of CYP3A (increased elbasvir and grazoprevir concentrations).

Concomitant use of elbasvir/grazoprevir and potent CYP3A inducers is contraindicated and concomitant use with moderate CYP3A inducers is not recommended. Concomitant use of elbasvir/grazoprevir and certain potent CYP3A inhibitors is not recommended.

In vitro, elbasvir and grazoprevir both inhibit CYP1A2, 2B6, 2C8, 2C9, 2C19, and 2D6. However, clinically important pharmacokinetic interactions are not expected if elbasvir/grazoprevir is used concomitantly with substrates of these CYP isoenzymes. Based on in vitro data, it is unlikely that administration of multiple doses of elbasvir or grazoprevir would induce metabolism of drugs metabolized by CYP1A2, 2B6, or 3A.

■ **Drugs Affecting or Affected by P-glycoprotein Transport** Elbasvir and grazoprevir are both substrates of P-glycoprotein (P-gp) transport; the role of intestinal P-gp in absorption of elbasvir and grazoprevir appears to be minimal.

In vitro, elbasvir inhibits P-gp; grazoprevir is not an inhibitor of P-gp.

■ **Drugs Affecting or Affected by Breast Cancer Resistance Protein** Elbasvir and grazoprevir are both inhibitors of intestinal breast cancer resistance protein (BCRP). Concomitant use of elbasvir/grazoprevir and drugs that are BCRP substrates may result in increased concentrations of such substrate drugs.

■ **Drugs Affecting or Affected by Organic Anion Transport Polypeptides** Grazoprevir is a substrate and inhibitor of organic anion transporting polypeptide (OATP) 1B1 and 1B3. Elbasvir is not a substrate of OATP1B.

Pharmacokinetic interactions are possible if elbasvir/grazoprevir is used concomitantly with OATP1B1 or 1B3 inhibitors (increased grazoprevir concentrations). Concomitant use of elbasvir/grazoprevir and OATP1B1 or 1B3 inhibitors that are known or expected to substantially increase grazoprevir plasma concentrations is contraindicated.

■ **Drugs Affecting or Affected by Other Enzymes** In vitro, elbasvir and grazoprevir do not inhibit carboxylesterase (CES) 1, CES2, cathepsin A (CatA), or uridine diphosphate-glucuronosyl transferase (UGT) 1A1. Clinically important pharmacokinetic interactions are not expected if elbasvir/grazoprevir is used concomitantly with CES1, CES2, CatA, or UGT1A1 substrates.

■ **Drugs Affecting Gastric pH** ***Antacids*** Dosage adjustments are not needed if antacids are used concomitantly with elbasvir/grazoprevir.

Histamine H_2-receptor Antagonists Concomitant use of famotidine and elbasvir/grazoprevir does not result in clinically important changes in the pharmacokinetics of elbasvir or grazoprevir.

Dosage adjustments are not needed if a histamine H_2-receptor antagonist is used concomitantly with elbasvir/grazoprevir.

Proton-pump Inhibitors Concomitant use of pantoprazole and elbasvir/grazoprevir does not result in clinically important changes in the pharmacokinetics of elbasvir or grazoprevir.

Dosage adjustments are not needed if a proton-pump inhibitor is used concomitantly with elbasvir/grazoprevir.

■ **Antibacterial Agents** ***Penicillins*** **Nafcillin.** Concomitant use of nafcillin and elbasvir/grazoprevir may result in decreased elbasvir and grazoprevir concentrations due to moderate CYP3A induction by nafcillin, which may lead to reduced therapeutic effect of the HCV antiviral.

Concomitant use of nafcillin and elbasvir/grazoprevir is not recommended.

■ **Anticonvulsants** ***Carbamazepine*** Concomitant use of carbamazepine and elbasvir/grazoprevir may result in substantially decreased elbasvir and grazoprevir concentrations due to potent CYP3A induction by carbamazepine, which may lead to loss of virologic response to the HCV antiviral.

Concomitant use of carbamazepine and elbasvir/grazoprevir is contraindicated.

Phenytoin Concomitant use of phenytoin and elbasvir/grazoprevir may result in substantially decreased elbasvir and grazoprevir concentrations due to potent CYP3A induction by phenytoin, which may lead to loss of virologic response to the HCV antiviral.

Concomitant use of phenytoin and elbasvir/grazoprevir is contraindicated.

■ **Antifungal Agents** ***Ketoconazole*** In healthy adults, concomitant use of ketoconazole (400 mg once daily) and elbasvir (single 50-mg dose) or grazoprevir (single 100-mg dose) results in increased plasma concentrations and areas under the plasma concentration-time curves (AUCs) of elbasvir and grazoprevir, which may increase the overall risk of hepatotoxicity.

Concomitant use of ketoconazole and elbasvir/grazoprevir is not recommended.

■ **Antimycobacterial Agents** ***Rifampin*** Concomitant use of rifampin (single 600-mg oral or IV dose) and elbasvir (single 50-mg dose) results in slightly increased elbasvir plasma concentrations and AUC. Although specific studies are not available, concomitant use of multiple doses of rifampin and elbasvir is expected to result in clinically important decreases in elbasvir plasma concentrations because of potent CYP3A induction and may lead to loss of virologic response to the HCV antiviral.

Concomitant use of rifampin (single 600-mg oral or IV dose) and grazoprevir (single 200-mg dose) results in substantially increased grazoprevir plasma concentrations and AUC, presumably due to OATP1B1 inhibition by rifampin. However, concomitant use of multiple doses of rifampin and grazoprevir results in clinically important decreases in grazoprevir concentrations, most likely because of the mixed effects of rifampin on OATP1B (inhibition) and CYP3A4 (induction) and may lead to loss of virologic response to the HCV antiviral.

Concomitant use of rifampin and elbasvir/grazoprevir is contraindicated.

■ **Antiretroviral Agents** ***HIV Entry and Fusion Inhibitors*** **Maraviroc.** Data are not available regarding concomitant use of maraviroc and elbasvir/grazoprevir.

HIV Integrase Inhibitors (INSTIs) **Dolutegravir.** Concomitant use of dolutegravir and elbasvir/grazoprevir does not result in clinically important changes in the pharmacokinetics of elbasvir, grazoprevir, or dolutegravir. Dosage adjustments are not needed.

Elvitegravir. Concomitant use of the fixed combination of elvitegravir, cobicistat, emtricitabine, and tenofovir disoproxil fumarate (EVG/c/FTC/TDF) and elbasvir/grazoprevir results in increased elbasvir and grazoprevir concentrations. Concomitant use of the fixed combination of elvitegravir, cobicistat, emtricitabine, and tenofovir alafenamide (EVG/c/FTC/TAF) and elbasvir/grazoprevir is expected to result in increased elbasvir and grazoprevir concentrations.

Concomitant use of elbasvir/grazoprevir and EVG/c/FTC/TAF or EVG/c/FTC/TDF is not recommended.

Raltegravir. Concomitant use of raltegravir and elbasvir/grazoprevir does not result in clinically important changes in the pharmacokinetics of elbasvir, grazoprevir, or raltegravir. Dosage adjustments are not needed.

HIV Nonnucleoside Reverse Transcriptase Inhibitors (NNRTIs) **Efavirenz.** Concomitant use of efavirenz (600 mg once daily) and elbasvir (50 mg once daily) or grazoprevir (200 mg once daily) results in substantially decreased elbasvir or grazoprevir concentrations due to potent CYP3A induction by efavirenz, which may lead to loss of virologic response to the HCV antiviral.

Concomitant use of efavirenz and elbasvir/grazoprevir is contraindicated.

Etravirine. Concomitant use of etravirine and elbasvir/grazoprevir may result in decreased elbasvir and grazoprevir concentrations due to moderate

CYP3A induction by etravirine, which may lead to reduced therapeutic effect of the HCV antiviral.

Concomitant use of etravirine and elbasvir/grazoprevir is not recommended.

Rilpivirine. Concomitant use of rilpivirine and elbasvir/grazoprevir does not result in clinically important changes in the pharmacokinetics of elbasvir, grazoprevir, or rilpivirine. Dosage adjustments are not needed.

HIV Nucleoside and Nucleotide Reverse Transcriptase Inhibitors (NRTIs) **Abacavir.** Clinically important pharmacokinetic interactions are not expected if abacavir is used concomitantly with elbasvir/grazoprevir.

Emtricitabine.. Clinically important pharmacokinetic interactions are not expected if emtricitabine is used concomitantly with elbasvir/grazoprevir.

Lamivudine. Clinically important pharmacokinetic interactions are not expected if lamivudine is used concomitantly with elbasvir/grazoprevir.

Tenofovir. Concomitant use of tenofovir disoproxil fumarate (tenofovir DF) and elbasvir or grazoprevir does not result in clinically important changes in the pharmacokinetics of elbasvir, grazoprevir, or tenofovir. Dosage adjustments are not needed.

HIV Protease Inhibitors (PIs) **Atazanavir.** Concomitant use of *ritonavir-boosted* atazanavir (300 mg of atazanavir and 100 mg of ritonavir once daily) and elbasvir (50 mg once daily) results in increased elbasvir concentrations. Concomitant use of *ritonavir-boosted* atazanavir (300 mg of atazanavir and 100 mg of ritonavir once daily) and grazoprevir (200 mg once daily) results in substantially increased grazoprevir concentrations due to OATP1B1 and 1B3 inhibition by *ritonavir-boosted* atazanavir. Increased grazoprevir concentrations may increase the risk of ALT elevations.

Concomitant use of elbasvir/grazoprevir and *ritonavir-boosted, cobicistat-boosted,* or unboosted atazanavir is contraindicated.

Darunavir. Concomitant use of *ritonavir-boosted* darunavir (600 mg of darunavir and 100 mg of ritonavir twice daily) and elbasvir (50 mg once daily) results in increased elbasvir concentrations. Concomitant use of *ritonavir-boosted* darunavir (600 mg of darunavir and 100 mg of ritonavir twice daily) and grazoprevir (200 mg once daily) results in substantially increased grazoprevir concentrations due to OATP1B1 and 1B3 inhibition by *ritonavir-boosted* darunavir. Increased grazoprevir concentrations may increase the risk of ALT elevations.

Concomitant use of elbasvir/grazoprevir and *ritonavir-boosted* or *cobicistat-boosted* darunavir is contraindicated.

Fosamprenavir. Data are not available regarding concomitant use of elbasvir/grazoprevir and fosamprenavir or *ritonavir-boosted* fosamprenavir.

Lopinavir. Concomitant use of the fixed combination of lopinavir and ritonavir (lopinavir/ritonavir) and elbasvir (50 mg once daily) results in increased elbasvir concentrations. Concomitant use of lopinavir/ritonavir and grazoprevir (200 mg once daily) results in substantially increased grazoprevir concentrations due to OATP1B1 and 1B3 inhibition by lopinavir/ritonavir. Increased grazoprevir concentrations may increase the risk of ALT elevations.

Concomitant use of lopinavir and elbasvir/grazoprevir is contraindicated.

Ritonavir. Concomitant use of ritonavir (100 mg twice daily) and grazoprevir (single 200-mg dose) results in increased grazoprevir concentrations.

Saquinavir. Pharmacokinetic interactions are expected if saquinavir and elbasvir/grazoprevir are used concomitantly (substantially increased grazoprevir concentrations due to potent OATP1B1 and 1B3 inhibition by saquinavir). Increased grazoprevir concentrations may increase the risk of ALT elevations.

Concomitant use of elbasvir/grazoprevir and saquinavir or *ritonavir-boosted* saquinavir is contraindicated.

Tipranavir. Pharmacokinetic interactions are expected if tipranavir and elbasvir/grazoprevir are used concomitantly (substantially increased grazoprevir concentrations due to potent OATP1B1 and 1B3 inhibition by tipranavir). Increased grazoprevir concentrations may increase the risk of ALT elevations.

Concomitant use of elbasvir/grazoprevir and *ritonavir-boosted* tipranavir is contraindicated.

■ **Benzodiazepines** ***Midazolam*** Concomitant use of midazolam (single 2-mg dose) and grazoprevir (200 mg once daily) results in a 34% increase in midazolam exposures due to weak CYP3A inhibition by grazoprevir.

■ **Bosentan** Possible pharmacokinetic interactions if bosentan and elbasvir/grazoprevir are used concomitantly (decreased elbasvir and grazoprevir concentrations due to moderate CYP3A induction by bosentan, which may lead to reduced therapeutic effect of the HCV antiviral).

Concomitant use of bosentan and elbasvir/grazoprevir is not recommended.

■ **Cardiac Agents** ***Digoxin*** Concomitant use of digoxin (single 0.25-mg dose) and elbasvir (50 mg once daily) does not result in clinically important changes in digoxin plasma concentrations or AUC.

Dosage adjustments are not needed if digoxin is used concomitantly with elbasvir/grazoprevir.

■ **Corticosteroids** ***Prednisone*** Concomitant use of prednisone and elbasvir/grazoprevir does not result in clinically important changes in the pharmacokinetics of elbasvir, grazoprevir, or prednisone. Dosage adjustments are not needed.

■ **Entecavir** Clinically important pharmacokinetic interactions are not expected if entecavir is used concomitantly with elbasvir/grazoprevir.

■ **Estrogens and Progestins** Concomitant use of elbasvir or grazoprevir with an oral contraceptive containing ethinyl estradiol and levonorgestrel does not result in clinically important changes in the pharmacokinetics of ethinyl estradiol or levonorgestrel. Dosage adjustments are not needed.

■ **HCV Antivirals** ***HCV Polymerase Inhibitors*** **Sofosbuvir.** Concomitant use of sofosbuvir and elbasvir/grazoprevir does not result in clinically important pharmacokinetic interactions. Dosage adjustments are not needed.

■ **HMG-CoA Reductase Inhibitors** ***Atorvastatin*** Concomitant use of atorvastatin (single 10-mg dose) and elbasvir (50 mg once daily) in conjunction with grazoprevir (200 mg once daily) results in increased atorvastatin plasma concentrations and AUC.

If atorvastatin is used concomitantly with elbasvir/grazoprevir, atorvastatin dosage should not exceed 20 mg once daily.

Fluvastatin Possible pharmacokinetic interaction if fluvastatin and elbasvir/grazoprevir are used concomitantly (increased fluvastatin concentrations).

If fluvastatin and elbasvir/grazoprevir are used concomitantly, the lowest necessary dosage of fluvastatin should be used and the patient should be closely monitored for statin-associated adverse effects (e.g., myopathy).

Lovastatin Possible pharmacokinetic interaction if lovastatin and elbasvir/grazoprevir are used concomitantly (increased lovastatin concentrations).

If lovastatin and elbasvir/grazoprevir are used concomitantly, the lowest necessary dosage of lovastatin should be used and the patient should be closely monitored for statin-associated adverse effects (e.g., myopathy).

Pitavastatin Concomitant use of pitavastatin (single 1-mg dose) and grazoprevir (200 mg once daily) does not have a clinically important effect on the pharmacokinetics of pitavastatin. Dosage adjustments are not needed.

Pravastatin Concomitant use of pravastatin (single 40-mg dose) and elbasvir (50 mg once daily) in conjunction with grazoprevir (200 mg once daily) does not have a clinically important effect on the pharmacokinetics of pravastatin. Dosage adjustments are not needed.

Rosuvastatin Concomitant use of rosuvastatin (single 10-mg dose) and elbasvir (50 mg once daily) in conjunction with grazoprevir (200 mg once daily) results in increased rosuvastatin plasma concentrations and AUC.

If rosuvastatin is used concomitantly with elbasvir/grazoprevir, rosuvastatin dosage should not exceed 10 mg once daily.

Simvastatin Possible pharmacokinetic interaction if simvastatin and elbasvir/grazoprevir are used concomitantly (increased simvastatin concentrations).

If simvastatin and elbasvir/grazoprevir are used concomitantly, the lowest necessary dosage of simvastatin should be used and the patient should be closely monitored for statin-associated adverse effects (e.g., myopathy).

■ **Immunosuppressive Agents** ***Cyclosporine*** Concomitant use of cyclosporine (single 400-mg dose) and elbasvir (50 mg once daily) in conjunction with grazoprevir (200 mg once daily) results in increased elbasvir plasma concentrations and AUC and substantially increased grazoprevir plasma concentrations and AUC. Substantially increased grazoprevir concentrations are caused by OATP1B1 and 1B3 inhibition by cyclosporine and may increase the risk of ALT elevations.

Concomitant use of cyclosporine and elbasvir/grazoprevir is contraindicated.

Tacrolimus Concomitant use of tacrolimus (single 2-mg dose) and elbasvir (50 mg once daily) in conjunction with grazoprevir (200 mg once daily) results in a 43% increase in tacrolimus exposures due to weak CYP3A inhibition by grazoprevir; elbasvir and grazoprevir concentrations are not affected.

If tacrolimus and elbasvir/grazoprevir are used concomitantly, tacrolimus whole blood concentrations, renal function, and tacrolimus-associated adverse effects should be monitored frequently.

■ **Modafinil** Possible pharmacokinetic interactions if modafinil and elbasvir/grazoprevir are used concomitantly (decreased elbasvir and grazoprevir concentrations due to moderate CYP3A induction by modafinil, which may lead to reduced therapeutic effect of the HCV antiviral).

Concomitant use of modafinil and elbasvir/grazoprevir is not recommended.

■ **Montelukast** Concomitant use of montelukast and grazoprevir does not result in clinically important changes in the pharmacokinetics of montelukast.

■ **Mycophenolate** Concomitant use of mycophenolate mofetil and elbasvir in conjunction with grazoprevir does not result in clinically important changes in elbasvir, grazoprevir, or mycophenolic acid plasma concentrations or AUC. Dosage adjustments are not needed.

■ **Opiate Agonists and Opiate Partial Agonists** ***Buprenorphine*** Concomitant use of the fixed combination of buprenorphine and naloxone (buprenorphine/naloxone) and elbasvir does not result in clinically important effects on plasma concentrations or AUCs of elbasvir or buprenorphine. Concomitant use of buprenorphine/naloxone and grazoprevir does not result in clinically important effects on plasma concentrations or AUC of buprenorphine. Dosage adjustments are not needed.

Methadone Concomitant use of methadone does not result in clinically important effects on plasma concentrations or AUCs of elbasvir or grazoprevir. Dosage adjustments are not needed.

■ **Phosphate Binders** Concomitant use of sevelamer carbonate or calcium acetate and elbasvir/grazoprevir does not result in clinically important changes in the pharmacokinetics of elbasvir or grazoprevir.

Dosage adjustments are not needed if elbasvir/grazoprevir is used concomitantly with phosphate binders.

■ **Ribavirin** Concomitant use of ribavirin and elbasvir/grazoprevir does not have clinically important effects on peak plasma concentrations or AUCs of elbasvir or grazoprevir compared with administration of elbasvir/grazoprevir alone. Dosage adjustments are not needed if elbasvir/grazoprevir is used in conjunction with ribavirin.

There was no in vitro evidence of antagonistic anti-HCV effects between ribavirin and elbasvir or ribavirin and grazoprevir when the combinations were evaluated in HCV replicon studies.

■ **St. John's Wort** Concomitant use of St. John's wort (*Hypericum perforatum*) and elbasvir/grazoprevir may result in substantially decreased elbasvir and grazoprevir concentrations due to potent CYP3A induction by St. John's wort, which may lead to loss of virologic response to the HCV antiviral.

Concomitant use of St. John's wort and elbasvir/grazoprevir is contraindicated.

Description

Elbasvir and grazoprevir (elbasvir/grazoprevir) is a fixed combination containing 2 hepatitis C virus (HCV) antivirals. Elbasvir is an HCV nonstructural 5A (NS5A) replication complex inhibitor (NS5A inhibitor). Grazoprevir is an HCV nonstructural 3/4A (NS3/4A) protease inhibitor. Both drugs are direct-acting antivirals (DAAs) with activity against HCV. There was no in vitro evidence of antagonistic anti-HCV effects between elbasvir and grazoprevir when the combination was evaluated in HCV replicon studies.

Elbasvir targets HCV NS5A protein, which is required for viral replication and virion assembly. In vitro studies using cell-based replicon assays indicate that elbasvir has activity against HCV genotypes 1a, 1b, and 4.

Grazoprevir inhibits HCV NS3/4A protease, which is required for viral replication. Inhibition of NS3/4A protease prevents proteolytic cleavage of the HCV-encoded polyprotein to form mature forms of NS3, NS4A, NS4B, NS5A, and NS5B. In vitro studies using cell-based replicon assays indicate that grazoprevir has activity against HCV genotypes 1a, 1b, and 4.

Certain amino acid substitutions in NS5A of HCV genotypes 1a, 1b, and 4 have been selected in cell culture and have been associated with reduced susceptibility to elbasvir in vitro in replicon studies. In HCV genotype 1a replicons, single M28A/G/T, Q30D/E/H/K/R, L31M/V, H28D, and Y93C/H/N substitutions in NS5A are associated with reduced susceptibility to elbasvir (up to 2000-fold lower); in HCV genotype 1b replicons, single L28M, L31F, and Y93H substitutions in NS5A are associated with reduced susceptibility to elbasvir (up to17-fold lower). In HCV genotype 4 replicons, single L30S, M31V, and Y93H substitutions in NS5A are associated with reduced susceptibility to elbasvir (up to 23-fold lower). In general, combinations of elbasvir resistance-associated substitutions further reduce elbasvir antiviral activity in HCV genotypes 1a, 1b, and 4 replicons. In phase 2 and 3 clinical trials, treatment-emergent amino acid substitutions in NS5A were detected in patients with HCV genotype 1a infection (M28A/G/T, Q30H/K/R/Y, L31F/M/V, H58D, Y93H/N/S), HCV genotype 1b infection (L28M, L31F/V, Y93H), or HCV genotype 4 infection (L28S/T, M31I/V, P58D, Y93H) experiencing virologic failure.

Certain amino acid substitutions in NS3 of HCV genotypes 1a, 1b, and 4 have been selected in cell culture and have been associated with reduced susceptibility to grazoprevir in vitro in replicon studies. In HCV genotype 1a replicons, single Y56H, R155K, A156G/T/V, and D168A/E/G/N/S/V/Y substitutions in NS3 are associated with reduced susceptibility to grazoprevir (up to 81-fold lower); in HCV genotype 1b replicons, single F43S, Y56F, V107I, A156S/T/V, and D168A/G/V substitutions in NS3 are associated with reduced susceptibility to grazoprevir (up to 375-fold lower). In HCV genotype 4 replicons, single D168A/V substitutions in NS3 are associated with reduced susceptibility to grazoprevir (up to 320-fold lower). In general, combinations of grazoprevir resistance-associated substitutions further reduce grazoprevir antiviral activity in HCV genotypes 1a, 1b, and 4 replicons. In phase 2 and 3 clinical trials, treatment-emergent amino acid substitutions in NS3 were detected in patients with HCV genotype 1a infection (V36L/M, Y56H, V107I, R155I/K, A156G/T/V, V158A, D168A/G/N/V/Y), HCV genotype 1b infection (Y56F, V107I, A156T), or HCV genotype 4 infection (A156M/T/V, D168A/G, V170I) experiencing virologic failure.

Cross-resistance among HCV NS5A inhibitors and among HCV NS3/4A protease inhibitors is possible. Efficacy of elbasvir/grazoprevir has not been established in patients in whom previous treatment with a regimen that included an HCV NS5A inhibitor failed. Only limited data are available regarding efficacy of elbasvir/grazoprevir in patients who previously failed treatment with a regimen of peginterferon alfa, ribavirin, and an HCV NS3/4A protease inhibitor (e.g., boceprevir, simeprevir, telaprevir) and have HCV NS3 resistance-associated substitutions at baseline prior to administration of elbasvir/grazoprevir. Elbasvir and grazoprevir are active against HCV with amino acid substitutions associated with resistance to HCV NS5B polymerase inhibitors.

Following oral administration of elbasvir/grazoprevir in HCV-infected adults, peak plasma concentrations of elbasvir and grazoprevir occur approximately 3 and 2 hours, respectively, after the dose. Although not considered clinically important, administration of elbasvir/grazoprevir with a high-fat meal (approximately 900 kcal, 500 kcal from fat) in healthy adults decreases the area under the plasma concentration-time curve (AUC) and peak plasma concentrations of elbasvir by approximately 11 and 15%, respectively, and increases the AUC and peak plasma concentrations of grazoprevir by approximately 1.5- and 2.8-fold, respectively, relative to administration in the fasting state. When a once-daily regimen of elbasvir/grazoprevir is used, steady-state concentrations of elbasvir and grazoprevir are attained within approximately 6 days. Concomitant use of elbasvir and grazoprevir does not have a clinically important effect on the pharmacokinetics of either drug compared with administration alone.

Elbasvir pharmacokinetics are similar in healthy and HCV-infected adults; elbasvir exposures increase in a dose-proportional manner over the dosage range of 5–200 mg once daily. Grazoprevir exposures are approximately two-fold higher in HCV-infected adults compared with healthy adults; studies using grazoprevir dosages of 10–800 mg once daily in HCV-infected adults indicate that peak plasma concentrations and AUC increase in a more-than-dose-proportional manner. Preclinical studies indicate that elbasvir is distributed into most tissues (including the liver) and grazoprevir is distributed principally into the liver, which is likely facilitated by active transport of the drug through organic anion transporting polypeptide (OATP) 1B1 and 1B3 liver uptake transporters. Elbasvir and grazoprevir are both partially eliminated by oxidative metabolism, principally by cytochrome P-450 (CYP) 3A; both drugs are extensively (99.9 and 98.8%, respectively) bound to plasma proteins (e.g., serum albumin, α_1-acid glycoprotein). Both elbasvir and grazoprevir are eliminated principally in feces. Over 90% of each dose is excreted in feces and less than 1% is excreted in urine. In HCV-infected adults, the geometric mean apparent terminal half-lives of elbasvir and grazoprevir are approximately 24 and 31 hours, respectively.

Advice to Patients

Advise patients that the fixed-combination preparation of elbasvir and grazoprevir (elbasvir/grazoprevir) should be taken once daily (with or without food) on a regular dosing schedule.

Inform patients that reactivation of hepatitis B virus (HBV) infection has occurred in coinfected patients being treated for hepatitis C virus (HCV) infection. Importance of informing clinician of any history of HBV infection or other liver problems (e.g., cirrhosis). Importance of immediately contacting a clinician if any signs or symptoms of serious liver injury (e.g., fatigue, weakness, loss of appetite, nausea and vomiting, yellowing of the eyes or skin, light-colored bowel movements) occur. (See Risk of HBV Reactivation in Patients Coinfected with HCV and HBV under Warnings/Precautions: Warnings, in Cautions.)

Advise patients that elbasvir/grazoprevir should be stored in the original container to protect the drug from moisture.

Importance of taking the recommended dosage of elbasvir/grazoprevir for the recommended duration of treatment; importance of not missing or skipping doses.

Advise patients to watch for early warning signs of liver inflammation (e.g., fatigue, weakness, lack of appetite, nausea and vomiting) as well as later signs (e.g., jaundice, discolored feces) and to immediately contact a clinician if such manifestations occur.

Importance of informing clinicians of existing or contemplated concomitant therapy, including prescription and OTC drugs and dietary or herbal supplements, as well as any concomitant illnesses.

Importance of women informing clinicians if they are or plan to become pregnant or plan to breast-feed. If used in conjunction with ribavirin, advise men and women of importance of using 2 forms of effective contraception during and for 6 months after ribavirin therapy. (See Precautions Related to Fixed Combinations and Multiple-drug Treatment Regimens under Warnings/Precautions: Other Warnings/Precautions, in Cautions.)

Importance of informing patients of other important precautionary information. (See Cautions.)

Overview® (see Users Guide). For additional information on this drug until a more detailed monograph is developed and published, the manufacturer's labeling should be consulted. It is *essential* that the manufacturer's labeling be consulted for more detailed information on usual cautions, precautions, contraindications, potential drug interactions, laboratory test interferences, and acute toxicity.

Preparations

Excipients in commercially available drug preparations may have clinically important effects in some individuals; consult specific product labeling for details.

Elbasvir and Grazoprevir

Oral

Tablets, film-coated	Elbasvir 50 mg and Grazoprevir 100 mg	**Zepatier®**, Merck

Ledipasvir and Sofosbuvir LDV, SOF

■ Ledipasvir and sofosbuvir (ledipasvir/sofosbuvir) is a fixed combination containing 2 hepatitis C virus (HCV) antivirals; ledipasvir is an HCV nonstructural 5A (NS5A) replication complex inhibitor (NS5A inhibitor) and sofosbuvir is a nucleotide analog HCV nonstructural 5B (NS5B) polymerase inhibitor.

Uses

■ **Chronic Hepatitis C Virus Infection** The fixed combination of ledipasvir and sofosbuvir (ledipasvir/sofosbuvir) is used for the treatment of chronic hepatitis C virus (HCV) genotype 1 infection in treatment-naive (previously untreated) or previously treated adults, including those with cirrhosis (compensated or decompensated), liver transplant recipients, and those with human immunodeficiency virus (HIV) coinfection.

Ledipasvir/sofosbuvir is used for the treatment of chronic HCV genotype 4 infection in treatment-naive or previously treated adults, including those with compensated cirrhosis, liver transplant recipients, and those with HIV coinfection.

Ledipasvir/sofosbuvir is used for the treatment of chronic HCV genotype 5 or 6 infection in treatment-naive or previously treated adults, including those with compensated cirrhosis or HIV coinfection.

Ledipasvir/sofosbuvir also is used for the treatment of chronic HCV genotype 1, 4, 5, or 6 infection in treatment-naive or previously treated pediatric patients 12 years of age and older, including those with compensated cirrhosis or HIV coinfection.

Ledipasvir/sofosbuvir is used alone or in conjunction with ribavirin, depending on HCV genotype and certain patient factors (e.g., presence of compensated or decompensated cirrhosis, liver transplantation).

Because the treatment of chronic HCV infection is complex and rapidly evolving, it is recommended that treatment be directed by clinicians who are familiar with the disease and that a specialist be consulted to obtain the most up-to-date information. Information from the American Association for the Study of Liver Diseases (AASLD), Infectious Diseases Society of America (IDSA), and International Antiviral Society–USA (IAS–USA) regarding diagnosis and management of HCV infection, including recommendations for initial treatment, is available at http://www.hcvguidelines.org.

HCV Genotype 1 Infection **Treatment-naive Adults.** Efficacy and safety of ledipasvir/sofosbuvir for the treatment of chronic HCV genotype 1 infection in treatment-naive adults have been evaluated in 2 randomized, open-label, phase 3 trials (ION-1 [NCT01701401] and ION-3 [NCT01851330]). The primary end point for both studies was sustained virologic response at 12 weeks after the end of treatment (SVR12; defined as plasma HCV RNA level less than 25 IU/mL [the lower limit of quantification] at 12 weeks after end of treatment).

In ION-1, 865 treatment-naive cirrhotic or noncirrhotic adults with chronic HCV genotype 1 infection (median age 54 years, 59% male, 79% with baseline HCV RNA levels 800,000 IU/mL or greater, 67% with HCV genotype 1a infection, 70% with non-CC IL28B alleles [CT or TT], 16% with cirrhosis) were randomized to receive ledipasvir/sofosbuvir (a fixed-combination tablet containing 90 mg of ledipasvir and 400 mg of sofosbuvir once daily) with or without ribavirin for 12 or 24 weeks. Of the 213 patients treated with ledipasvir/sofosbuvir *without* ribavirin for 12 weeks, 99% achieved SVR12. No additional benefit was observed with the addition of ribavirin or with the extended 24-week treatment duration. In patients who received the 12-week regimen of ledipasvir/sofosbuvir *without* ribavirin, the SVR12 rate was 98% in those with HCV genotype 1a infection and 100% in those with HCV genotype 1b infection. In a subgroup analysis of patients with or without cirrhosis who received the 12-week regimen of ledipasvir/sofosbuvir *without* ribavirin, 94% of those with cirrhosis and 99% of those without cirrhosis achieved SVR12.

ION-3 evaluated ledipasvir/sofosbuvir in 647 treatment-naive, noncirrhotic patients with chronic HCV genotype 1 infection. Patients were randomized to receive ledipasvir/sofosbuvir (a fixed-combination tablet containing 90 mg of ledipasvir and 400 mg of sofosbuvir once daily) with or without ribavirin for 8 weeks or ledipasvir/sofosbuvir (a fixed-combination tablet containing 90 mg of ledipasvir and 400 mg of sofosbuvir once daily) alone for 12 weeks. Baseline characteristics were balanced among treatment groups (median age 55 years, 58% male, 81% with baseline HCV RNA levels 800,000 IU/mL or greater, 80% with HCV genotype 1a infection, 73% with non-CC IL28B alleles [CT or TT]). SVR12 was achieved in 94 or 96% of patients treated with ledipasvir/sofosbuvir *without* ribavirin for 8 or 12 weeks, respectively. No additional benefit was observed with the addition of ribavirin to the 8-week treatment regimen. Among patients with baseline HCV RNA levels less than 6 million IU/mL, the SVR12 rate was 97 or 96% in patients treated with ledipasvir/sofosbuvir *without* ribavirin for 8 or 12 weeks, respectively; 2% of patients in both treatment groups experienced relapse. In patients who received the 12-week regimen of ledipasvir/sofosbuvir *without* ribavirin, the SVR12 rate was 96% in those with HCV genotype 1a infection and 98% in those with HCV genotype 1b infection.

Previously Treated Adults. Efficacy and safety of ledipasvir/sofosbuvir for the treatment of chronic HCV genotype 1 infection in previously treated adults have been evaluated in a randomized, open-label, phase 3 trial (ION-2; NCT01768286) and a randomized, double-blind, placebo-controlled, phase 2 trial (SIRIUS; NCT01965535). The primary end point for both studies was SVR12 (defined as plasma HCV RNA level less than 25 IU/mL [the lower limit of quantification] at 12 weeks after end of treatment).

ION-2 included 440 cirrhotic or noncirrhotic adults with chronic HCV genotype 1 infection who previously failed therapy with an interferon-based regimen, including regimens containing an HCV protease inhibitor. Patients were randomized to receive ledipasvir/sofosbuvir (a fixed-combination tablet containing 90 mg of ledipasvir and 400 mg of sofosbuvir once daily) with or without ribavirin for 12 or 24 weeks. Baseline characteristics were balanced among treatment groups (median age 57 years, 65% male, 89% with baseline HCV RNA levels 800,000 IU/mL or greater, 79% with HCV genotype 1a infection, 88% with non-CC IL28B alleles, 20% with cirrhosis, 47% failed prior therapy with peginterferon alfa and ribavirin, 53% failed prior therapy with peginterferon alfa, ribavirin, and an HCV protease inhibitor). SVR12 was achieved in 94 or 99% of patients treated with ledipasvir/sofosbuvir *without* ribavirin for 12 or 24 weeks, respectively. Use of ribavirin in conjunction with ledipasvir/sofosbuvir did not affect response rates, regardless of treatment duration. In patients who received a 12- or 24-week regimen of ledipasvir/sofosbuvir *without* ribavirin, the SVR rate was 95 or 99%, respectively, in those with HCV genotype 1a infection and 87 or 100%, respectively, in those with HCV genotype 1b infection. In a subgroup analysis of patients with or without cirrhosis, the SVR12 rate in those treated with ledipasvir/sofosbuvir *without* ribavirin was 86 or 100% with the 12- or 24-week regimen, respectively, in those with cirrhosis and 95 or 99% with the 12- or 24-week regimen, respectively, in those without cirrhosis.

SIRIUS included 155 adults with chronic HCV genotype 1 infection who had compensated cirrhosis and previously failed therapy with peginterferon alfa and ribavirin *and* failed subsequent therapy with peginterferon alfa, ribavirin, and an HCV protease inhibitor. Patients were randomized in a 1:1 ratio to receive ledipasvir/sofosbuvir (a fixed-combination tablet containing 90 mg of ledipasvir and 400 mg of sofosbuvir once daily) in conjunction with ribavirin for a duration of 12 weeks or ledipasvir/sofosbuvir *without* ribavirin for a duration of 24 weeks. Demographics and baseline characteristics were balanced among treatment groups (median age 56 years, 74% male, 97% white, 63% with HCV genotype 1a infection, 94% with non-CC IL28B alleles [CT or TT]). The SVR12 rate was 96% in patients treated with a 12-week regimen of ledipasvir/sofosbuvir *with* ribavirin and 97% in those treated with a 24-week regimen of ledipasvir/sofosbuvir alone.

HCV Genotype 4 Infection Efficacy and safety of ledipasvir/sofosbuvir for the treatment of chronic HCV genotype 4 infection in treatment-naive or previously treated adults with or without cirrhosis have been evaluated in an open-label, phase 2 trial (Study 1119; NCT02081079). The primary end point was sustained virologic response at 12 weeks after the end of treatment (SVR12; defined as plasma HCV RNA level less than 15 IU/mL [the lower limit of quantification] at 12 weeks after end of treatment). Study 1119 included 22 treatment-naive patients (mean age 52 years, 50% male, 5% with cirrhosis) and 22 previously treated patients (mean age 50 years, 77% male, 41% with cirrhosis) who received ledipasvir/sofosbuvir (a fixed-combination tablet containing 90 mg of ledipasvir and 400 mg of sofosbuvir once daily) for 12 weeks. The overall SVR12 rate was 93%; SVR12 rates were similar based on prior HCV treatment history and cirrhosis status.

HCV Genotype 5 Infection Efficacy and safety of ledipasvir/sofosbuvir for the treatment of chronic HCV genotype 5 infection in treatment-naive or previously treated adults with or without cirrhosis have been evaluated in an open-label, phase 2 trial (Study 1119; NCT02081079). The primary end point was sustained virologic response at 12 weeks after the end of treatment (SVR12; defined as plasma HCV RNA level less than 15 IU/mL [the lower limit of quantification] at 12 weeks after end of treatment). Study 1119 included 21 treatment-naive patients (mean age 61 years, 50% male, 100% white, 14% with cirrhosis) and 20 previously treated patients (mean age 64 years, 50% male, 100% white, 30% with cirrhosis) who received ledipasvir/sofosbuvir (a fixed-combination tablet containing 90 mg of ledipasvir and 400 mg of sofosbuvir once daily) for 12 weeks. The overall SVR12 rate was 93%; SVR12 rates were similar based on prior HCV treatment history and cirrhosis status.

HCV Genotype 6 Infection Efficacy and safety of ledipasvir/sofosbuvir for the treatment of chronic HCV genotype 6 infection in treatment-naive or previously treated adults have been evaluated in an open-label trial (ELECTRON-2). The primary end point was sustained virologic response at 12 weeks after the end of treatment (SVR12; defined as plasma HCV RNA level less than 15 IU/mL [the lower limit of quantification] at 12 weeks after end of treatment). A total of 25 patients with or without cirrhosis received ledipasvir/sofosbuvir (a fixed-combination tablet containing 90 mg of ledipasvir and 400 mg of sofosbuvir once daily) for 12 weeks. The overall SVR12 was 96%; SVR12 rates were similar based on prior HCV treatment history and cirrhosis status.

Transplant Recipients Efficacy and safety of ledipasvir/sofosbuvir in conjunction with ribavirin for the treatment of HCV genotype 1 or genotype 4 infection in 670 treatment-naive or previously treated adults who were liver transplant recipients and/or had decompensated liver disease were evaluated in 2 identical, open-label, phase 2 trials (SOLAR-1 and SOLAR-2). Study patients were enrolled in 1 of 7 groups based on liver transplantation status and severity of hepatic impairment; those with Child-Pugh scores greater than 12 were excluded. Within each group, patients were randomized in a 1:1 ratio to receive either a 12- or 24-week regimen of ledipasvir/sofosbuvir with ribavirin; patients with decompensated cirrhosis received an initial ribavirin dosage of 600 mg daily regardless of transplantation status and ribavirin dosage adjustments were performed according to ribavirin prescribing information. Demographics and baseline characteristics were balanced across the treatment groups (median age 59 years, 77% male, 91% white, 94% with HCV genotype 1 infection, 6% with HCV genotype 4 infection, 78% failed previous HCV therapy). The primary end point was SVR12 (defined as plasma HCV RNA level less than 15 IU/mL [the lower limit of quantification] at 12 weeks after end of treatment).

In patients with HCV genotype 1 infection enrolled in SOLAR-1 and SOLAR-2, the SVR12 rates observed with the 12- and 24-week regimens of ledipasvir/sofosbuvir in conjunction with ribavirin were similar. Pooled SVR12 rates for patients with HCV genotype 1 infection who were liver transplant recipients and received the 12-week regimen were 95% in those with METAVIR score F0–F3 and 98, 89, or 57% in those with Child-Pugh class A, B, or C, respectively. Pooled SVR12 rates in pretransplant patients with HCV genotype 1 infection were 87 or 88% in those with Child-Pugh class B or C, respectively. The relapse rate was 7% in those with HCV genotype 1 infection *with* baseline NS5A polymorphisms at baseline and 5% in those with HCV genotype 1 infection *without* NS5A polymorphisms at baseline. In patients with HCV genotype 4 infection who received the 12-week regimen of ledipasvir/sofosbuvir with ribavirin, SVR12 rates in transplant recipients without cirrhosis or with compensated cirrhosis were similar to SVR12 rates reported in those with HCV genotype 1 infection. Data were insufficient to determine the SVR rates in transplant recipients or pretransplant patients who had HCV genotype 4 infection and decompensated cirrhosis.

HCV-infected Individuals Coinfected with HIV Efficacy and safety of ledipasvir/sofosbuvir for the treatment of chronic HCV genotype 1 or genotype 4 infection in adults coinfected with HIV-1 have been evaluated in an open-label, phase 3 trial (ION-4; NCT02073656). Patients were HCV treatment-naive or had failed previous HCV treatment with a regimen of peginterferon alfa and ribavirin (with or without an HCV protease inhibitor) or a regimen of sofosbuvir and ribavirin. The primary end point was sustained virologic response at 12 weeks after the end of treatment (SVR12; defined as plasma HCV RNA level less than 25 IU/mL [the lower limit of quantification] at 12 weeks after end of treatment). A total of 335 adults (median age 52 years, 82% male, 61% white, 34% black, 75% with HCV genotype 1a infection, 23% with HCV genotype 1b infection, 2% with HCV genotype 4 infection, 76% with non-CC IL28B alleles [CT or TT], 20% with compensated cirrhosis, 55% previously treated) received ledipasvir/sofosbuvir (a fixed-combination tablet containing 90 mg of ledipasvir and 400 mg of sofosbuvir once daily) for 12 weeks. All patients also were receiving a stable HIV antiretroviral regimen (emtricitabine and tenofovir disoproxil fumarate [tenofovir DF] in conjunction with efavirenz, rilpivirine or raltegravir). The overall SVR12 rate was 96%; SVR12 rates were similar based on prior HCV treatment history and cirrhosis status. However, black patients had lower SVR12 rates compared with patients of other races (90 versus 99%, respectively) and the relapse rate was 9% in black patients (all patients who relapsed had non-CC IL28B alleles). HCV treatment did not appear to interfere with maintenance of HIV virologic suppression; the percentage of $CD4^+$ T-cells remained stable and there was no evidence of HIV-1 virologic rebound in any patient during the study.

Pediatric Patients Efficacy and safety of ledipasvir/sofosbuvir for the treatment of HCV genotype 1 infection in treatment-naive or previously treated pediatric patients 12 years of age and older (with or without compensated cirrhosis) were evaluated in a phase 2, open-label study (Study 1116). In this study, 100 pediatric patients (median age 15 years, 63% female, 90% white, 13% Hispanic/Latino, 7% black, 2% Asian, 20% previously treated, 55% with baseline HCV RNA levels 800,000 IU/mL or greater, 81% with HCV genotype 1a infection, 76% with non-CC IL28B alleles, 1% with known compensated cirrhosis) received ledipasvir/sofosbuvir once daily for 12 weeks. The majority of pediatric patients in this study had been infected with HCV through vertical transmission from their mothers. SVR12 was achieved by 98% of treatment-naive pediatric patients and 100% of previously treated pediatric patients. No patient experienced on-treatment virologic failure or relapse.

Efficacy and safety of ledipasvir/sofosbuvir for the treatment of HCV genotype 4, 5, or 6 infection in treatment-naive or previously treated pediatric patients 12 years of age and older (with or without compensated cirrhosis) is supported by data indicating comparable plasma exposures for ledipasvir, sofosbuvir, and G-331007 (predominant metabolite of sofosbuvir) in adults and adolescents with HCV genotype 1 infection and similar efficacy and plasma exposures across HCV genotypes 1, 4, 5, and 6 in adults.

Dosage and Administration

■ **General** For the treatment of chronic hepatitis C virus (HCV) infection, ledipasvir and sofosbuvir (ledipasvir/sofosbuvir) is used alone or in conjunction with ribavirin.

The specific regimen and duration of treatment is based on HCV genotype and certain patient factors (e.g., presence of compensated or decompensated cirrhosis, liver transplantation). Relapse rates following treatment are affected by baseline host and viral factors and differ between treatment durations for certain subgroups.

Prior to initiating ledipasvir/sofosbuvir for treatment of HCV infection, all patients should be tested for evidence of current or prior hepatitis B virus (HBV) infection by measuring hepatitis B surface antigen (HBsAg), hepatitis B surface antibody (anti-HBs), and hepatitis B core antibody (anti-HBc). (See Risk of HBV Reactivation in Patients Coinfected with HCV and HBV under Warnings/Precautions: Warnings, in Cautions.)

Prior to and during treatment, appropriate laboratory tests should be performed to evaluate liver function, especially in patients with decompensated cirrhosis receiving a regimen of ledipasvir/sofosbuvir in conjunction with ribavirin. (See Hepatic Impairment under Warnings/Precautions: Specific Populations, in Cautions.)

■ **Administration** Ledipasvir/sofosbuvir is administered orally once daily without regard to food.

■ **Dosage** Ledipasvir/sofosbuvir is commercially available as fixed-combination tablets containing 90 mg of ledipasvir and 400 mg of sofosbuvir.

Adult Dosage **HCV Genotype 1 Infection.** For the treatment of chronic hepatitis C virus (HCV) genotype 1 infection in adults, the recommended dosage of ledipasvir/sofosbuvir is 1 tablet (90 mg of ledipasvir and 400 mg of sofosbuvir) once daily. Ledipasvir/sofosbuvir is used alone for the treatment of HCV genotype 1 infection in patients without cirrhosis or with compensated cirrhosis (Child-Pugh class A), but is used in conjunction with ribavirin for the treatment of HCV genotype 1 infection in those with decompensated cirrhosis (Child-Pugh class B or C) and in liver transplant recipients. (See Table 1.)

A treatment duration of 12 weeks is recommended for most patients with HCV genotype 1 infection, but a treatment duration of 24 weeks is recommended for previously treated patients with compensated cirrhosis (Child-Pugh class A). (See Table 1.) If ledipasvir/sofosbuvir (without ribavirin) is used for the treatment of HCV genotype 1 infection in patients with decompensated cirrhosis who cannot receive ribavirin, some experts recommend a treatment duration of 24 weeks. HCV-infected patients with decompensated cirrhosis should be referred to an expert for treatment (ideally at a liver transplant center).

Table 1. Recommended Treatment Regimen and Duration of Ledipasvir/Sofosbuvir for HCV Genotype 1 Infection in Adults.

Patient Type	Treatment Regimen	Duration of Treatment
Treatment-naive *without* cirrhosis	Ledipasvir/sofosbuvir	12 weeks[a]
Treatment-naive *with* compensated cirrhosis	Ledipasvir/sofosbuvir	12 weeks
Previously treated[b] *without* cirrhosis	Ledipasvir/sofosbuvir	12 weeks
Previously treated[b] *with* compensated cirrhosis	Ledipasvir/sofosbuvir	24 weeks[c]
Treatment-naive or previously treated[b] *with* decompensated cirrhosis	Ledipasvir/sofosbuvir *and* ribavirin[d]	12 weeks
Treatment-naive or previously treated[b] liver transplant recipients *without* cirrhosis or *with* compensated cirrhosis	Ledipasvir/sofosbuvir *and* ribavirin[e]	12 weeks

[a] Manufacturer states treatment duration of 8 weeks can be considered in treatment-naive patients *without* cirrhosis who have pretreatment HCV RNA levels less than 6 million IU/mL. Some experts recommend treatment duration of 8 weeks for HCV genotype 1 infection in treatment-naive patients *without* cirrhosis who are nonblack, do *not* have HIV coinfection, and have pretreatment HCV RNA levels less than 6 million IU/mL.

[b] Previously treated defined as patients who failed treatment with peginterferon alfa and ribavirin with or without an HCV protease inhibitor.

[c] Alternatively, a regimen of ledipasvir/sofosbuvir *and* ribavirin for a duration of 12 weeks can be considered in previously treated patients with compensated cirrhosis who are eligible to receive ribavirin.

[d] In patients with decompensated cirrhosis, the starting ribavirin dosage is 600 mg daily and can be titrated up to weight-based ribavirin dosage (up to 1 g daily for patients <75 kg or up to 1.2 g daily for those ≥75 kg); give ribavirin daily dosage in 2 divided doses with food. If ribavirin starting dosage not well tolerated, reduce dosage as clinically indicated based on hemoglobin levels.

[e] Use weight-based ribavirin dosage (1 g daily for patients <75 kg or 1.2 g daily for those ≥75 kg); give ribavirin daily dosage in 2 divided doses with food.

HCV Genotype 4 Infection. For the treatment of chronic HCV genotype 4 infection in adults, the recommended dosage of ledipasvir/sofosbuvir is 1 tablet (90 mg of ledipasvir and 400 mg of sofosbuvir) once daily. Ledipasvir/sofosbuvir is used alone for the treatment of HCV genotype 4 infection in patients without cirrhosis or in those with compensated cirrhosis (Child-Pugh class A), but is used in conjunction with ribavirin for the treatment of HCV genotype 4 infection in liver transplant recipients. (See Table 2.)

For the treatment of HCV genotype 4 infection in adults with decompensated cirrhosis† (Child-Pugh class B or C), some experts recommend a 12-week regimen of ledipasvir/sofosbuvir given in a dosage of 1 tablet (90 mg of ledipasvir and 400 mg of sofosbuvir) once daily in conjunction *with* ribavirin. If ledipasvir/sofosbuvir (without ribavirin) is used for the treatment of HCV genotype 4 infection in patients with decompensated cirrhosis who cannot receive ribavirin, these experts recommend a treatment duration of 24 weeks. HCV-infected patients with decompensated cirrhosis should be referred to an expert for treatment (ideally at a liver transplant center).

Table 2. Recommended Treatment Regimen and Duration of Ledipasvir/Sofosbuvir for HCV Genotype 4 Infection in Adults.

Patient Type	Treatment Regimen	Duration of Treatment
Treatment-naive *without* cirrhosis or *with* compensated cirrhosis	Ledipasvir/sofosbuvir	12 weeks
Previously treated[a] *without* cirrhosis or *with* compensated cirrhosis	Ledipasvir/sofosbuvir	12 weeks
Treatment-naive or previously treated[a] liver transplant recipients *without* cirrhosis or *with* compensated cirrhosis	Ledipasvir/sofosbuvir *and* ribavirin[b]	12 weeks

[a] Previously treated defined as patients who failed treatment with peginterferon alfa and ribavirin with or without an HCV protease inhibitor.

[b] Use weight-based ribavirin dosage (1 g daily for patients <75 kg or 1.2 g daily for those ≥75 kg); give ribavirin daily dosage in 2 divided doses with food.

HCV Genotype 5 or 6 Infection. For the treatment of chronic HCV genotype 5 or 6 infection in adults, the recommended dosage of ledipasvir/sofosbuvir is 1 tablet (90 mg of ledipasvir and 400 mg of sofosbuvir) once daily for 12 weeks. (See Table 3.)

For the treatment of HCV genotype 5 or 6 infection in adults with decompensated cirrhosis† (Child-Pugh class B or C), some experts recommend a 12-week regimen of ledipasvir/sofosbuvir given in a dosage of 1 tablet (90 mg of ledipasvir and 400 mg of sofosbuvir) once daily in conjunction *with* ribavirin. If ledipasvir/sofosbuvir (without ribavirin) is used for the treatment of HCV genotype 5 or 6 infection in patients with decompensated cirrhosis who cannot receive ribavirin, these experts recommend a treatment duration of 24 weeks. HCV-infected patients with decompensated cirrhosis should be referred to an expert for treatment (ideally at a liver transplant center).

Table 3. Recommended Treatment Regimen and Duration of Ledipasvir/Sofosbuvir for HCV Genotype 5 or 6 Infection.

Patient Type	Treatment Regimen	Duration of Treatment
Treatment-naive *without* cirrhosis or *with* compensated cirrhosis	Ledipasvir/sofosbuvir	12 weeks
Previously treated[a] *without* cirrhosis or *with* compensated cirrhosis	Ledipasvir/sofosbuvir	12 weeks

[a] Previously treated defined as patients who failed treatment with peginterferon alfa and ribavirin with or without an HCV protease inhibitor.

HCV-infected Adults Coinfected with HIV. For the treatment of chronic HCV genotype 1, 4, 5, or 6 infection in adults with human immunodeficiency virus (HIV) coinfection, the same ledipasvir/sofosbuvir dosage and same HCV genotype-specific multiple-drug regimen and treatment duration recommended for HCV-infected patients without HIV coinfection should be used. (See Table 1, Table 2, and Table 3.)

Pediatric Dosage **HCV Genotype 1 Infection.** For the treatment of chronic HCV genotype 1 infection in pediatric patients 12 years of age and older weighing at least 35 kg, the recommended dosage of ledipasvir/sofosbuvir is 1 tablet (90 mg of ledipasvir and 400 mg of sofosbuvir) once daily. (See Table 4.)

A treatment duration of 12 weeks is recommended for most patients with HCV genotype 1 infection, but a treatment duration of 24 weeks is recommended for previously treated patients with compensated cirrhosis (Child-Pugh class A). (See Table 4.)

Table 4. Recommended Treatment Regimen and Duration of Ledipasvir/Sofosbuvir for HCV Genotype 1 Infection in Pediatric Patients 12 Years of Age and Older.

Patient Type	Treatment Regimen	Duration of Treatment
Treatment-naive *without* cirrhosis	Ledipasvir/sofosbuvir	12 weeks
Treatment-naive *with* compensated cirrhosis	Ledipasvir/sofosbuvir	12 weeks
Previously treated[a] *without* cirrhosis	Ledipasvir/sofosbuvir	12 weeks
Previously treated[a] *with* compensated cirrhosis	Ledipasvir/sofosbuvir	24 weeks

[a] Previously treated defined as patients who failed treatment with an interferon-based regimen with or without ribavirin.

HCV Genotype 4, 5, or 6 Infection. For the treatment of chronic HCV genotype 4, 5, or 6 infection in treatment-naive or previously treated pediatric patients 12 years of age and older weighing at least 35 kg, the recommended dosage of ledipasvir/sofosbuvir is 1 tablet (90 mg of ledipasvir and 400 mg of sofosbuvir) once daily for 12 weeks. (See Table 5.)

Table 5. Recommended Treatment Regimen and Duration of Ledipasvir/Sofosbuvir for HCV Genotype 4, 5, or 6 Infection in Pediatric Patients 12 Years of Age and Older.

Patient Type	Treatment Regimen	Duration of Treatment
Treatment-naive *without* cirrhosis or *with* compensated cirrhosis	Ledipasvir/sofosbuvir	12 weeks
Previously treated[a] *without* cirrhosis or *with* compensated cirrhosis	Ledipasvir/sofosbuvir	12 weeks

[a] Previously treated defined as patients who failed treatment with an interferon-based regimen with or without ribavirin.

HCV-infected Pediatric Patients Coinfected with HIV. For the treatment of chronic HCV genotype 1, 4, 5, or 6 infection in pediatric patients 12 years of age and older weighing at least 35 kg with HIV coinfection, the same ledipasvir/sofosbuvir dosage and same HCV genotype-specific multiple-drug regimen and treatment duration recommended for HCV-infected patients without HIV coinfection should be used. (See Table 4 and Table 5.)

■ **Special Populations** ***Hepatic Impairment*** Ledipasvir/sofosbuvir dosage adjustments are not necessary in adults with mild, moderate, or severe hepatic impairment (Child-Pugh class A, B, or C). (See Hepatic Impairment under Warnings/Precautions: Specific Populations, in Cautions.)

Renal Impairment Ledipasvir/sofosbuvir dosage adjustments are not necessary in adults with mild or moderate renal impairment.

Dosage recommendations are not available for patients with severe renal impairment (estimated glomerular filtration rate [eGFR] less than 30 mL/minute per 1.73 m^2) or end-stage renal disease (ESRD); safety and efficacy have not been established in such patients. (See Renal Impairment under Warnings/Precautions: Specific Populations, in Cautions.)

Geriatric Patients Ledipasvir/sofosbuvir dosage adjustments are not necessary in geriatric patients.

Cautions

■ **Contraindications** If the fixed combination containing ledipasvir and sofosbuvir (ledipasvir/sofosbuvir) is used in conjunction with ribavirin, the contraindications to ribavirin also apply. (See Precautions Related to Fixed Combinations and Multiple-drug Treatment Regimens under Warnings/Precautions: Other Warnings/Precautions, in Cautions.)

■ **Warnings/Precautions** ***Warnings*** **Risk of HBV Reactivation in Patients Coinfected with HCV and HBV.** Reactivation of hepatitis B virus (HBV) infection has been reported during postmarketing experience when direct-acting antivirals (DAAs) were used for the treatment of chronic hepatitis C virus (HCV) infection in patients with HBV coinfection. In some cases, HBV reactivation resulted in fulminant hepatitis, hepatic failure, and death.

HBV reactivation (defined as an abrupt increase in HBV replication manifested as a rapid increase in serum HBV DNA levels or detection of hepatitis B surface antigen [HBsAg] in an individual who was previously HBsAg negative and hepatitis B core antibody [anti-HBc] positive) has been reported in patients with HCV and HBV coinfection who were receiving HCV treatment with a regimen that included HCV DAAs without interferon alfa. Reactivation also may be accompanied by hepatitis (i.e., increased aminotransferase concentrations) and, in severe cases, may lead to increased bilirubin concentrations, liver failure, or death. Data to date indicate that HBV reactivation usually occurs within 4–8 weeks after initiation of HCV treatment. Patients with HBV reactivation have been heterogeneous in terms of HCV genotype and in terms of baseline HBV disease. While some patients with HBV reactivation were HBsAg positive, others had serologic evidence of resolved HBV infection (i.e., HBsAg negative and anti-HBc positive). HBV reactivation also has been reported in patients receiving certain immunosuppressant or chemotherapeutic drugs; the risk of reactivation associated with HCV DAAs may be increased in such patients.

The mechanism for HBV reactivation in patients with HCV and HBV coinfection receiving HCV DAAs is unknown. Although HCV DAAs are not known to cause immunosuppression, HBV reactivation in coinfected patients may result from a complex interplay of host immunologic responses in the setting of infection with 2 hepatitis viruses.

Prior to initiating treatment with an HCV DAA, including ledipasvir/sofosbuvir, all patients should be screened for evidence of current or prior HBV infection by measuring HBsAg, anti-HBs, and anti-HBc. If there is serologic evidence of HBV infection, baseline HBV DNA levels should be measured.

Patients with evidence of current or prior HBV infection should be monitored for clinical and laboratory signs (i.e., HBsAg, HBV DNA levels, serum aminotransferase concentrations, bilirubin concentrations) of hepatitis flare or HBV reactivation during and after treatment with HCV DAAs, including ledipasvir/sofosbuvir. Appropriate management for HBV infection should be initiated as clinically indicated.

Patients with HCV and HBV coinfection receiving ledipasvir/sofosbuvir should be advised to immediately contact a clinician if they develop any signs or symptoms of serious liver injury (e.g., fatigue, weakness, loss of appetite, nausea and vomiting, yellowing of the eyes or skin, light-colored bowel movements).

When making decisions regarding HBV monitoring or HBV treatment in coinfected patients, consultation with a clinician who has expertise in managing HBV infection is recommended.

Sensitivity Reactions Angioedema and rash, sometimes with blisters or angioedema-like swelling, has been reported during postmarketing experience.

Other Warnings/Precautions **Cardiovascular Effects.** Symptomatic bradycardia, sometimes requiring pacemaker intervention, has been reported during postmarketing experience in patients receiving amiodarone concomitantly with an HCV treatment regimen containing sofosbuvir in conjunction with another HCV DAA. Symptomatic bradycardia, including a fatal cardiac arrest, has been reported in patients receiving amiodarone concomitantly with the fixed combination containing ledipasvir and sofosbuvir (ledipasvir/sofosbuvir). In most reported cases, bradycardia occurred within hours to days after HCV treatment was initiated in patients receiving amiodarone, but has been observed up to 2 weeks after initiation of HCV treatment. Bradycardia generally resolved after HCV treatment was discontinued. The mechanism for this adverse cardiovascular effect is unknown.

Patients who may be at increased risk for symptomatic bradycardia if amiodarone is used concomitantly with an HCV treatment regimen containing sofosbuvir and another DAA include those also receiving a β-adrenergic blocking agent, those with underlying cardiac comorbidities, and/or those with advanced liver disease.

Concomitant use of amiodarone with ledipasvir/sofosbuvir is *not* recommended. If there are no alternative HCV treatment options and ledipasvir/sofosbuvir must be used in a patient receiving amiodarone, the patient should be advised about the risk of serious symptomatic bradycardia before ledipasvir/sofosbuvir is initiated. Cardiac monitoring should be performed in an inpatient setting during the first 48 hours of concomitant use of amiodarone and ledipasvir/sofosbuvir; heart rate monitoring should then be performed daily (outpatient or self-monitoring) through at least the first 2 weeks of concomitant use. Similar cardiac monitoring is recommended in patients who discontinued amiodarone just prior to initiation of ledipasvir/sofosbuvir or if there are no other treatment options and amiodarone must be initiated in a patient already receiving ledipasvir/sofosbuvir.

Patients receiving amiodarone concomitantly with ledipasvir/sofosbuvir should be advised to immediately contact a clinician if they develop signs or symptoms of bradycardia (e.g., near-fainting or fainting, dizziness, lightheadedness, malaise, weakness, excessive tiredness, shortness of breath, chest pain, confusion, memory problems).

Interactions. Concomitant use of ledipasvir/sofosbuvir and inducers of the P-glycoprotein (P-gp) transport system (e.g., rifampin, St. John's wort [*Hypericum perforatum*]) may decrease ledipasvir and sofosbuvir plasma concentrations and may lead to reduced therapeutic effect of ledipasvir/sofosbuvir. Concomitant use of ledipasvir/sofosbuvir and P-gp inducers is not recommended. (See Drug Interactions.)

Precautions Related to Fixed Combinations and Multiple-drug Treatment Regimens. When ledipasvir/sofosbuvir is used, the cautions, precautions, contraindications, and drug interactions associated with both drugs in the fixed combination must be considered. Cautionary information applicable to specific populations (e.g., pregnant or nursing women, individuals with hepatic or renal impairment, geriatric patients) should be considered for each drug. (For cautionary information specific for sofosbuvir, see Cautions in Sofosbuvir 8:18.40.16.)

Ledipasvir/sofosbuvir should not be used concomitantly with any other preparation containing sofosbuvir.

When ledipasvir/sofosbuvir is used in conjunction with ribavirin, the cautions, precautions, and contraindications associated with ribavirin also should be considered. (See Cautions in Ribavirin 8:18.32.) Ribavirin may cause fetal toxicity and/or death and extreme care *must* be taken to avoid pregnancy in female patients and in female partners of male patients receiving ribavirin-containing regimens. Women of childbearing potential should have a negative pregnancy test immediately prior to initiating ribavirin and pregnancy tests should be performed monthly during and for 6 months after ribavirin treatment is completed. Women of childbearing potential (and their male partners) and male patients (and their female partners) *must* use at least 2 forms of effective contraception during and for 6 months after ribavirin treatment is completed. (See Cautions: Pregnancy, Fertility, and Lactation, in Ribavirin 8:18.32.)

Specific Populations **Pregnancy.** Adequate data are not available regarding use of ledipasvir/sofosbuvir in pregnant women. In animal studies, neither ledipasvir nor sofosbuvir affected fetal development at the dosages tested.

When ledipasvir/sofosbuvir is used in conjunction *with* ribavirin, clinicians should consider that ribavirin may cause fetal toxicity and/or death and extreme care must be taken to avoid pregnancy in female patients and in female partners of male patients receiving the ribavirin-containing regimen. (See Cautions: Pregnancy, Fertility, and Lactation, in Ribavirin 8:18.32.)

Lactation. It is not known whether ledipasvir/sofosbuvir or their metabolites are distributed into human milk.

The predominant metabolite of sofosbuvir (GS-331007) is distributed into milk in rats, and ledipasvir has been detected in plasma of suckling rat pups. Ledipasvir and GS-331007 had no apparent effects on the nursing pups.

The benefits of breast-feeding and the importance of ledipasvir/sofosbuvir to the woman should be considered along with the potential adverse effects on the breast-fed child from the drug or from the underlying maternal condition.

When ledipasvir/sofosbuvir is used in conjunction *with* ribavirin, the potential for adverse reactions to ribavirin in nursing infants should be considered and a decision should be made whether to discontinue nursing or the ribavirin-containing regimen, taking into account the importance of the regimen to the woman. (See Precautions Related to Fixed Combinations and Multiple-drug Treatment Regimens under Warnings/Precautions: Other Warnings/Precautions, in Cautions.)

Pediatric Use. Safety and efficacy of ledipasvir/sofosbuvir have not been established in pediatric patients younger than 12 years of age or weighing less than 35 kg. Safety and efficacy also have not been established in pediatric patients with decompensated cirrhosis or in pediatric liver transplant recipients.

Pharmacokinetics of ledipasvir/sofosbuvir in pediatric patients 12 years of age and older weighing at least 35 kg with HCV genotype 1 infection are comparable to pharmacokinetics observed in adults.

Geriatric Use. No overall differences in safety and efficacy of ledipasvir/sofosbuvir have been observed between patients 65 years of age and older and younger adults. However, greater sensitivity in some older individuals cannot be ruled out.

Hepatic Impairment. In individuals with severe hepatic impairment (Child-Pugh class C) without HCV infection, a single 90-mg dose of ledipasvir results in plasma exposures similar to those reported when the same dose is given to individuals with normal hepatic function. In HCV-infected individuals with moderate or severe hepatic impairment (Child-Pugh class B or C), sofosbuvir (400 mg daily for 7 days) results in sofosbuvir and GS-331007 plasma exposures higher than those reported in individuals with normal hepatic function.

When ledipasvir/sofosbuvir is used in conjunction with ribavirin in patients with decompensated cirrhosis (Child-Pugh class B or C), clinical and hepatic laboratory monitoring is recommended as clinically indicated.

Renal Impairment. Safety and efficacy of ledipasvir/sofosbuvir have not been established in patients with severe renal impairment (estimated glomerular filtration rate [eGFR] less than 30 mL/minute per 1.73 m^2) or end-stage renal disease (ESRD) requiring hemodialysis.

In individuals with severe renal impairment without HCV infection, ledipasvir pharmacokinetics following a single 90-mg dose of the drug are similar to pharmacokinetics reported in healthy individuals. In individuals with severe renal impairment or ESRD requiring hemodialysis without HCV infection, a single 400-mg dose of sofosbuvir results in sofosbuvir and GS-331007 plasma exposures that are substantially higher than those reported in individuals with normal renal function.

Although hemodialysis removes the predominant metabolite of sofosbuvir (GS-331007), it is unlikely that ledipasvir will be substantially removed by dialysis since it is highly bound to plasma proteins.

HCV-infected Individuals Coinfected with HIV. The safety profile of ledipasvir/sofosbuvir in individuals with HCV genotype 1 or genotype 4 infection and HIV-1 coinfection generally has been comparable to that reported in HCV-infected individuals without HIV-1 coinfection.

■ **Common Adverse Effects** Ledipasvir/sofosbuvir: Adverse effects reported in 5% or more of patients receiving ledipasvir/sofosbuvir include fatigue, headache, nausea, diarrhea, abdominal pain, insomnia or sleep disorder, irritability, rash, pruritus, dry skin, arthralgia, myalgia, back pain, asthenia, cough, upper respiratory tract infection, and dizziness.

Ledipasvir/sofosbuvir in conjunction with ribavirin: Adverse effects reported in 5% or more of patients receiving ledipasvir/sofosbuvir in conjunction with ribavirin include fatigue, headache, nausea, diarrhea, insomnia, asthenia, cough, bronchitis, dyspnea, irritability, pruritus, dry skin, myalgia, and decreased hemoglobin.

Drug Interactions

The following drug interactions are based on studies using the fixed combination containing ledipasvir and sofosbuvir (ledipasvir/sofosbuvir), ledipasvir alone, or sofosbuvir alone. When ledipasvir/sofosbuvir is used, interactions associated with both drugs in the fixed combination should be considered.

■ **Drugs Affecting or Affected by P-glycoprotein Transport System** Ledipasvir is an inhibitor of the P-glycoprotein (P-gp) transport system; sofosbuvir and the predominant sofosbuvir metabolite (GS-331007) are not inhibitors of P-gp. Concomitant use of ledipasvir and P-gp substrates may increase intestinal absorption of such drugs.

Ledipasvir and sofosbuvir are substrates of P-gp; GS-331007 is not a P-gp substrate. Pharmacokinetic interactions are possible with P-gp inducers (e.g., rifampin, St. John's wort), which may decrease ledipasvir and sofosbuvir plasma concentrations leading to reduced therapeutic effect of ledipasvir/sofosbuvir. Concomitant use of ledipasvir/sofosbuvir with P-gp inducers is not recommended.

■ **Drugs Affecting or Affected by Breast Cancer Resistance Protein** Ledipasvir is an inhibitor of breast cancer resistance protein (BCRP); sofosbuvir and GS-331007 are not BCRP inhibitors. Concomitant use of ledipasvir and BCRP substrates may increase intestinal absorption of such drugs.

Ledipasvir and sofosbuvir are substrates of BCRP; GS-331007 is not a BCRP substrate. Inhibitors of BCRP may increase plasma concentrations of ledipasvir and sofosbuvir without increasing plasma concentrations of GS-331007.

■ **Drugs Affecting or Affected by Other Membrane Transporters** At concentrations exceeding those achieved in the clinical setting, ledipasvir inhibits organic anion transporting polypeptide (OATP) 1B1, OATP1B3, and the bile salt export pump (BSEP).

Ledipasvir does not inhibit organic anion transporter (OAT) 1, OAT3, organic cation transporter (OCT) 1, OCT2, multidrug and toxin extrusion protein (MATE) 1, multidrug resistance-associated protein (MRP) 2, or MRP4.

■ **Drugs Affecting Gastric pH** The solubility of ledipasvir decreases as pH increases. Therefore, drugs that increase gastric pH are expected to decrease ledipasvir plasma concentrations.

Antacids Administration of ledipasvir/sofosbuvir and antacids (e.g., aluminum and magnesium hydroxides) should be separated by 4 hours.

Histamine H_2-Receptor Antagonists H_2-receptor antagonists may be administered concomitantly with or 12 hours apart from ledipasvir/sofosbuvir; dosage of the H_2-receptor antagonist should not exceed dosages comparable to famotidine 40 mg twice daily.

Proton-pump Inhibitors Proton-pump inhibitors in dosages comparable to omeprazole 20 mg once daily or lower may be administered concomitantly with ledipasvir/sofosbuvir under fasting conditions.

■ **Antiarrhythmic Agents** ***Amiodarone*** Concomitant use of amiodarone and ledipasvir/sofosbuvir may result in serious symptomatic bradycardia and is not recommended. If there are no alternative hepatitis C virus (HCV) treatment options and a regimen of ledipasvir/sofosbuvir must be used in a patient receiving amiodarone, the patient should be advised about the risk of serious symptomatic bradycardia and cardiac monitoring should be performed in an inpatient setting during the first 48 hours of concomitant use and then heart rate monitoring (outpatient or self-monitoring) should be performed daily through at least the first 2 weeks of concomitant use. Similar cardiac monitoring is recommended in patients who discontinued amiodarone just prior to initiation of ledipasvir/sofosbuvir or if there are no other treatment options and amiodarone must be initiated in a patient already receiving ledipasvir/sofosbuvir. (See Cardiovascular Effects under Warnings/Precautions: Other Warnings/Precautions, in Cautions.)

The effect of concomitant use of amiodarone and ledipasvir/sofosbuvir on plasma concentrations of amiodarone, ledipasvir, and sofosbuvir is unknown.

■ **Anticonvulsants** Concomitant use of ledipasvir/sofosbuvir and certain anticonvulsants (i.e., carbamazepine, oxcarbazepine, phenobarbital, phenytoin) is expected to decrease ledipasvir and sofosbuvir plasma concentrations, leading to reduced therapeutic effect of ledipasvir/sofosbuvir. Concomitant use of ledipasvir/sofosbuvir with these anticonvulsants is not recommended.

■ **Antimycobacterial Agents** ***Rifabutin*** Rifabutin is expected to decrease plasma concentrations of ledipasvir and sofosbuvir, which may lead to decreased therapeutic effect of ledipasvir/sofosbuvir. Concomitant use of rifabutin and ledipasvir/sofosbuvir is not recommended.

Rifampin Concomitant use of rifampin (a P-gp inducer) and ledipasvir/sofosbuvir may result in a clinically important decrease in plasma concentrations of ledipasvir and sofosbuvir and may lead to decreased therapeutic effect of ledipasvir/sofosbuvir. Concomitant use of rifampin and ledipasvir/sofosbuvir is not recommended.

Rifapentine Rifapentine is expected to decrease plasma concentrations of ledipasvir and sofosbuvir, which may lead to decreased therapeutic effect of ledipasvir/sofosbuvir. Concomitant use of rifapentine and ledipasvir/sofosbuvir is not recommended.

■ **Antiretroviral Agents** ***HIV Entry and Fusion Inhibitors***

Maraviroc. Concomitant use of ledipasvir/sofosbuvir and maraviroc is not expected to affect the pharmacokinetics of maraviroc.

Some experts recommend a maraviroc dosage of 300 mg twice daily in patients receiving ledipasvir/sofosbuvir.

HIV Integrase Inhibitors (INSTIs) **Dolutegravir.** Concomitant use of ledipasvir/sofosbuvir and dolutegravir is not expected to result in clinically important pharmacokinetic interactions.

Concomitant use of ledipasvir/sofosbuvir and a human immunodeficiency virus (HIV) antiretroviral regimen of dolutegravir in conjunction with the fixed combination of emtricitabine and tenofovir disoproxil fumarate (emtricitabine/tenofovir DF) is expected to result in increased plasma concentrations and area under the plasma concentration-time curve (AUC) of tenofovir.

Elvitegravir. Concomitant use of ledipasvir/sofosbuvir and elvitegravir with cobicistat (*cobicistat-boosted* elvitegravir) increases peak plasma concentrations and area under the AUC of ledipasvir and cobicistat, but does not have clinically important effects on the pharmacokinetics of sofosbuvir or elvitegravir.

Concomitant use of ledipasvir/sofosbuvir and the fixed combination of elvitegravir, cobicistat, emtricitabine, and tenofovir disoproxil fumarate (EVG/c/FTC/TDF) is expected to result in increased tenofovir and ledipasvir concentrations. Safety of increased tenofovir concentrations in patients receiving ledipasvir/sofosbuvir and EVG/c/FTC/TDF concomitantly has not been established. Concomitant use of ledipasvir/sofosbuvir and EVG/c/FTC/TDF is not recommended.

Concomitant use of ledipasvir/sofosbuvir and the fixed combination of elvitegravir, cobicistat, emtricitabine, and tenofovir alafenamide (EVG/c/FTC/TAF) does not result in clinically important effects on the pharmacokinetics of any of the drugs.

Concomitant use of ledipasvir/sofosbuvir and single-entity elvitegravir used in conjunction with a *ritonavir-boosted* HIV protease inhibitor (PI) is not expected to have a clinically important effect on elvitegravir concentrations. If used concomitantly, dosage recommendations for the HIV PI should be followed.

Raltegravir. Concomitant use of raltegravir (400 mg twice daily) and either ledipasvir (90 mg once daily) or sofosbuvir (single 400-mg dose) did not have a clinically important effect on the pharmacokinetics of raltegravir, ledipasvir, or sofosbuvir.

HIV Nonnucleoside Reverse Transcriptase Inhibitors (NNRTIs)

Efavirenz. Concomitant use of efavirenz and ledipasvir/sofosbuvir may decrease ledipasvir plasma concentrations and AUC, but has no clinically important effect on sofosbuvir or efavirenz pharmacokinetics. Dosage adjustments are not necessary if efavirenz and ledipasvir/sofosbuvir are used concomitantly.

Concomitant use of the fixed combination of efavirenz, emtricitabine, and tenofovir DF (efavirenz/emtricitabine/tenofovir DF) and ledipasvir/sofosbuvir does not have a clinically important effect on the pharmacokinetics of efavirenz or sofosbuvir, but results in decreased ledipasvir plasma concentrations and AUC and increased tenofovir plasma concentrations and AUC. If ledipasvir/sofosbuvir is used concomitantly with an HIV antiretroviral regimen that includes efavirenz in conjunction with emtricitabine and tenofovir DF, the patient should be monitored for tenofovir-associated adverse effects.

Etravirine. Concomitant use of etravirine and ledipasvir/sofosbuvir is not expected to result in clinically important drug interactions. Dosage adjustments are not necessary if etravirine and ledipasvir/sofosbuvir are used concomitantly.

Nevirapine. Concomitant use of nevirapine and ledipasvir/sofosbuvir is not expected to result in clinically important drug interactions. Dosage adjustments are not necessary if nevirapine and ledipasvir/sofosbuvir are used concomitantly.

Rilpivirine. Concomitant use of rilpivirine and ledipasvir/sofosbuvir does not have clinically important effects on the pharmacokinetics of rilpivirine, ledipasvir, or sofosbuvir. Dosage adjustments are not necessary if rilpivirine and ledipasvir/sofosbuvir are used concomitantly.

Concomitant use of the fixed combination of emtricitabine, rilpivirine, and tenofovir DF (emtricitabine/rilpivirine/tenofovir DF) and ledipasvir/sofosbuvir does not have clinically important effects on the pharmacokinetics of rilpivirine, ledipasvir, or sofosbuvir, but results in increased tenofovir plasma concentrations and AUC. If ledipasvir/sofosbuvir is used concomitantly with an HIV antiretroviral regimen that includes emtricitabine/rilpivirine/tenofovir DF, the patient should be monitored for tenofovir-associated adverse effects.

HIV Nucleoside and Nucleotide Reverse Transcriptase Inhibitors (NRTIs) No clinically important pharmacokinetic interactions are expected if ledipasvir/sofosbuvir is used concomitantly with abacavir, emtricitabine, or lamivudine.

Abacavir and Lamivudine. Concomitant use of the fixed combination of abacavir and lamivudine (abacavir/lamivudine) and ledipasvir/sofosbuvir does not have a clinically important effect on the pharmacokinetics of abacavir, lamivudine, ledipasvir, or sofosbuvir.

Tenofovir. Concomitant use of ledipasvir/sofosbuvir and HIV antiretroviral regimens that include tenofovir DF and certain other antiretroviral agents may result in increased tenofovir concentrations, including the fixed-combination preparations of EVG/c/FTC/TDF, efavirenz/emtricitabine/tenofovir DF, emtricitabine/rilpivirine/tenofovir DF, dolutegravir in conjunction with emtricitabine/tenofovir DF, or any regimen that includes tenofovir DF and a *ritonavir-boosted* PI or tenofovir DF and the fixed combination of atazanavir and cobicistat (atazanavir/cobicistat) or fixed combination or darunavir and cobicistat (darunavir/cobicistat).

Safety of increased tenofovir concentrations in patients receiving ledipasvir/sofosbuvir and these antiretroviral regimens has not been established. Concomitant use of ledipasvir/sofosbuvir with EVG/c/FTC/TDF is not recommended. An alternative HCV treatment regimen or alternative antiretroviral regimen should be considered if the patient is receiving ledipasvir/sofosbuvir concomitantly with an antiretroviral regimen containing tenofovir DF and a *ritonavir-boosted* PI, atazanavir/cobicistat, or darunavir/cobicistat; if concomitant use of ledipasvir/sofosbuvir and these antiretroviral regimens is necessary, the patient should be monitored for tenofovir-associated adverse effects.

Patients also should be monitored for tenofovir-associated adverse effects if ledipasvir/sofosbuvir is used concomitantly with an HIV antiretroviral regimen that contains tenofovir DF without a *ritonavir-boosted* HIV PI or cobicistat.

HIV Protease Inhibitors (PIs) Concomitant use of ledipasvir/sofosbuvir and any HIV antiretroviral regimen that includes tenofovir DF and a *ritonavir-boosted* PI (e.g., *ritonavir-boosted* atazanavir, *ritonavir-boosted* darunavir, *ritonavir-boosted* fosamprenavir, fixed combination of lopinavir and ritonavir [lopinavir/ritonavir], *ritonavir-boosted* saquinavir) or tenofovir DF and atazanavir/cobicistat or darunavir/cobicistat may result in increased tenofovir concentrations. Safety of increased tenofovir concentrations in patients receiving ledipasvir/sofosbuvir and these HIV treatment regimens has not been established. Alternative HCV treatment or an alternative antiretroviral regimen should be considered to avoid increased tenofovir exposure, especially in patients at risk for renal toxicity. If concomitant use of ledipasvir/sofosbuvir and any of these HIV PI regimens is necessary, the patient should be monitored for tenofovir-associated adverse effects.

Atazanavir. Concomitant use of *ritonavir-boosted* atazanavir (atazanavir 300 mg and ritonavir 100 mg) and ledipasvir/sofosbuvir increases the AUCs of atazanavir and ledipasvir by 33 and 113%, respectively, but does not have a clinically important effect on the pharmacokinetics of sofosbuvir. Dosage adjustments are not necessary if *ritonavir-boosted* atazanavir and ledipasvir/sofosbuvir are used concomitantly.

Concomitant use of atazanavir/cobicistat and ledipasvir/sofosbuvir is not expected to result in clinically important pharmacokinetic interactions. Dosage adjustments are not necessary if atazanavir/cobicistat and ledipasvir/sofosbuvir are used concomitantly.

Darunavir. Concomitant use of *ritonavir-boosted* darunavir once daily (darunavir 800 mg and ritonavir 100 mg) and either ledipasvir (90 mg once daily) or sofosbuvir (single 400-mg dose) does not have a clinically important effect on the pharmacokinetics of darunavir, ritonavir, ledipasvir, or sofosbuvir.

Concomitant use of darunavir/cobicistat and ledipasvir/sofosbuvir is not expected to results in clinically important pharmacokinetic interactions. Dosage adjustments are not necessary if darunavir/cobicistat and ledipasvir/sofosbuvir are used concomitantly.

Tipranavir. Concomitant use of *ritonavir-boosted* tipranavir and ledipasvir/sofosbuvir is expected to decrease ledipasvir and sofosbuvir concentrations, leading to reduced therapeutic effect of ledipasvir/sofosbuvir.

Concomitant use of *ritonavir-boosted* tipranavir and ledipasvir/sofosbuvir is not recommended.

■ **Calcium-channel Blockers** Concomitant use of ledipasvir/sofosbuvir and verapamil is not expected to result in any clinically important drug interactions.

■ **Digoxin** Concomitant use of ledipasvir/sofosbuvir and digoxin may increase digoxin concentrations. Therapeutic concentration monitoring of digoxin is recommended if used concomitantly with ledipasvir/sofosbuvir.

■ **Estrogens and Progestins** When studied in healthy women, concomitant use of ledipasvir or sofosbuvir and an oral contraceptive containing ethinyl estradiol and norgestimate did not have a clinically important effect on the pharmacokinetics of ethinyl estradiol or norgestimate and its active metabolites (norelgestromin, norgestrel). Concomitant use of ledipasvir/sofosbuvir is not expected to affect efficacy of oral contraceptives containing ethinyl estradiol and norgestimate.

■ **HCV Antivirals** ***HCV Polymerase Inhibitors*** **Sofosbuvir.** Ledipasvir/sofosbuvir should not be used concomitantly with any other preparation containing sofosbuvir.

HCV Protease Inhibitors **Simeprevir.** When studied in healthy adults, concomitant use of ledipasvir (30 mg once daily) and simeprevir (150 mg once daily) resulted in increased ledipasvir and simeprevir concentrations.

Concomitant use of ledipasvir/sofosbuvir and simeprevir is not recommended.

■ **HMG-CoA Reductase Inhibitors** ***Pravastatin*** Concomitant use of ledipasvir/sofosbuvir and pravastatin is not expected to result in any clinically important drug interactions.

Rosuvastatin Concomitant use of a ledipasvir/sofosbuvir and rosuvastatin may result in increased rosuvastatin concentrations, which is associated with increased risk of myopathy and rhabdomyolysis. Concomitant use of ledipasvir/sofosbuvir and rosuvastatin is not recommended.

■ **Immunosuppressive Agents** ***Cyclosporine*** Cyclosporine pharmacokinetics are not affected by ledipasvir or sofosbuvir. Concomitant use of ledipasvir/sofosbuvir and cyclosporine is not expected to result in any clinically important drug interactions.

Tacrolimus Concomitant use of ledipasvir/sofosbuvir and tacrolimus is not expected to result in any clinically important drug interactions.

■ **Methadone** Methadone pharmacokinetics are not affected by ledipasvir or sofosbuvir. Concomitant use of ledipasvir/sofosbuvir and methadone is not expected to result in any clinically important drug interactions.

■ **St. John's Wort** Concomitant use of St. John's wort (*Hypericum perforatum*) and ledipasvir/sofosbuvir may result in a clinically important decrease in ledipasvir and sofosbuvir plasma concentrations because of P-gp induction by St. John's wort and may result in loss of therapeutic effect of ledipasvir/sofosbuvir. Concomitant use of ledipasvir/sofosbuvir and St. John's wort is not recommended.

■ **Warfarin** In patients receiving warfarin, subtherapeutic international normalized ratios (INRs) have been reported after initiation of sofosbuvir-containing regimens, including ledipasvir/sofosbuvir.

INR should be closely monitored when initiating or discontinuing ledipasvir/sofosbuvir in patients receiving warfarin.

Description

Ledipasvir and sofosbuvir is a fixed combination containing 2 hepatitis C virus (HCV) antivirals. Ledipasvir is an HCV nonstructural 5A (NS5A) replication complex inhibitor (NS5A inhibitor). Sofosbuvir is a nucleotide analog HCV nonstructural 5B (NS5B) polymerase inhibitor. Both drugs are direct-acting antivirals (DAAs) with activity against HCV. There was no in vitro evidence of antagonistic anti-HCV effects between ledipasvir and sofosbuvir when the combination was evaluated in HCV replicon studies.

Ledipasvir targets HCV NS5A protein, which is required for viral replication. In vitro studies using cell-based replicon assays indicate that ledipasvir has activity against HCV genotypes 1a and 1b. Ledipasvir also has some antiviral activity against HCV genotypes 4a, 5a, and 6a, but substantially lower activity against HCV genotype 6e.

Sofosbuvir is a prodrug that is converted in the liver to a pharmacologically active uridine analog triphosphate (GS-461203), which can be incorporated into HCV RNA by NS5B polymerase and acts as an RNA chain terminator. In vitro studies using biochemical and cell-based replicon assays indicate that GS-461203 has activity against HCV genotypes 1a, 1b, 4a, 5a, and 6a.

Certain amino acid substitutions in NS5A of HCV genotype 1a (e.g., Y93H, Q30E) and genotype 1b (e.g., Y93H) have been selected in cell culture and have been associated with reduced susceptibility to ledipasvir in vitro in replicon studies. In phase 2 and 3 clinical trials evaluating ledipasvir/sofosbuvir in patients with HCV genotype 1 infection, treatment-emergent NS5A resistance-associated substitutions (e.g., K24R, M28T/V, Q30R/H/K/L, L31M/V, H58D/P, and/or Y93H/N/C) were detected in patients with HCV genotype 1a infection who experienced virologic failure, and treatment-emergent resistance-associated substitutions (e.g., L31V/M/I, R30Q, and/or Y93H/N) were detected in patients with HCV genotype 1b infection who experienced virologic failure. Some of these patients also had baseline NS5A polymorphisms at resistance-associated amino acid positions. In clinical trials evaluating ledipasvir/sofosbuvir in patients with HCV genotype 4, 5, or 6 infection, patients with relapse who had NS5A sequencing data available had pretreatment NS5A resistance-associated polymorphisms (single polymorphism or combinations at positions 24, 28, 30, 31 and 58); NS5A resistance-associated substitutions Y93C or L28V emerged posttreatment in a few of the patients with HCV genotype 4 relapse who also had NS5A polymorphisms pretreatment.

Certain amino acid substitutions in NS5B polymerase of HCV genotypes 1b, 4a, 5a, and 6a have been selected in cell culture and have been associated with reduced susceptibility to sofosbuvir in vitro in replicon studies. In all replicon genotypes tested, the S282T substitution was associated with reduced susceptibility to sofosbuvir; in genotypes 5 and 6 replicons, an M289L substitution developed along with the S282T substitution. Although the clinical importance is unknown, treatment-emergent NS5B resistance-associated substitutions (e.g., L159, V321, D61G, A112T, E237G, S473T, S282T, L320V/I, V321I) were detected in phase 3 clinical trials evaluating ledipasvir/sofosbuvir in patients with HCV genotype 1 infection. Treatment-emergent sofosbuvir resistance-associated NS5B substitution S282T has been reported at the time of relapse in patients with HCV genotype 4, 5, or 6 infection who received ledipasvir/sofosbuvir in clinical trials; treatment-emergent nucleotide inhibitor substitution M289I also was reported in a patient with HCV genotype 5 relapse.

Cross-resistance between ledipasvir and other NS5A inhibitors is expected; efficacy of ledipasvir/sofosbuvir has not been established in patients in whom previous treatment with other regimens that included an NS5A inhibitor failed. Ledipasvir and sofosbuvir are both active against HCV with amino acid substitutions associated with resistance to other classes of HCV DAAs that have different mechanisms of action (e.g., HCV NS5B nonnucleoside inhibitors, HCV NS3 protease inhibitors).

Following oral administration of ledipasvir/sofosbuvir, peak plasma concentrations of ledipasvir occur approximately 4–4.5 hours after the dose and peak plasma concentrations of sofosbuvir and the predominant sofosbuvir metabolite (GS-331007; accounts for more than 90% of total systemic exposure) occur approximately 0.8–1 and 3.5–4 hours, respectively, after the dose. Administration with a moderate-fat (approximately 600 kcal, 25–30% fat) or high-fat (approximately 1000 kcal, 50% fat) meal does not substantially affect ledipasvir or GS-331007 exposures relative to administration in the fasting state; sofosbuvir peak plasma concentrations are not affected, but the AUC of the drug is increased approximately twofold.

Ledipasvir appears to undergo slow oxidative metabolism by an unknown mechanism; however, systemic exposure is almost exclusively the parent drug. The drug is greater than 99.8% bound to plasma proteins. The major route of elimination of ledipasvir is biliary excretion. Following a single 90-mg oral dose of ledipasvir, 86% is excreted in feces (70% as unchanged ledipasvir, 2.2% as the oxidative metabolite) and 1% is excreted in urine. Following oral administration of ledipasvir/sofosbuvir, the median terminal half-life of ledipasvir is 47 hours.

Sofosbuvir is a prodrug that undergoes intracellular metabolic activation in the liver (hydrolysis by human cathepsin A [CatA] or carboxylesterase 1 [CES1], phosphoramidate cleavage by histidine triad nucleotide-binding protein 1 [HINT1], and phosphorylation by pyrimidine nucleotide biosynthesis pathway). This results in formation of the pharmacologically active metabolite, GS-461203; desphosphorylation subsequently occurs leading to formation of GS-331007 (the predominant circulating metabolite), which has no anti-HCV activity. Sofosbuvir is approximately 61–65% bound and GS-331007 is minimally bound to plasma proteins. The major route of elimination is renal clearance. Following a single 400-mg oral dose of sofosbuvir, 80% is eliminated in urine (mainly as GS-331007), 14% is excreted in feces, and 2.5% is eliminated in expired air. Following oral administration of ledipasvir/sofosbuvir, the median terminal half-lives of sofosbuvir and GS-331007 are 0.5 and 27 hours, respectively.

In individuals with severe hepatic impairment (Child-Pugh class C) without HCV infection, AUC of ledipasvir after a single 90-mg dose is similar to that observed in individuals with normal hepatic function. In HCV-infected individuals with moderate or severe hepatic impairment (Child-Pugh class B or C), sofosbuvir AUC is 126 or 143% higher, respectively, compared with HCV-infected individuals with normal hepatic function; GS-331007 AUC is 18 or 9% higher, respectively. Population pharmacokinetic analysis in HCV-infected patients indicates that cirrhosis has no clinically important effect on ledipasvir, sofosbuvir, or GS-331007 exposure. Following a single 90-mg dose, there were no clinically important differences in ledipasvir pharmacokinetics between individuals with severe renal impairment without HCV infection and healthy individuals. In individuals with mild, moderate, or severe renal impairment without HCV infection, sofosbuvir AUC is 61, 107, or 171% higher, respectively, compared with individuals with normal renal function; GS-331007 AUC is 55, 88, or 451% higher, respectively. Although not considered clinically important, population pharmacokinetic analysis in HCV-infected individuals indicates that peak plasma concentrations and AUC of ledipasvir are 58 and 77% higher, respectively, in females than in males; gender does not affect sofosbuvir or GS-331007 exposure. Population pharmacokinetic analysis indicates that age (range 18–80 years) and race do not have clinically important effects on ledipasvir, sofosbuvir, or GS-331007 exposures.

Advice to Patients

Advise patients that the fixed-combination preparation of ledipasvir and sofosbuvir (ledipasvir/sofosbuvir) should be taken once daily (with or without food) on a regular dosing schedule.

Inform patients that reactivation of hepatitis B virus (HBV) infection has occurred in coinfected patients being treated for hepatitis C virus (HCV) infection. Importance of informing clinician of any history of HBV infection or other liver problems (e.g., cirrhosis). Importance of immediately contacting a clinician if any signs or symptoms of serious liver injury (e.g., fatigue, weakness, loss of appetite, nausea and vomiting, yellowing of the eyes or skin, light-colored bowel movements) occur. (See Risk of HBV Reactivation in Patients Coinfected with HCV and HBV under Warnings/Precautions: Warnings, in Cautions.)

Importance of taking the recommended dosage of ledipasvir/sofosbuvir for the recommended duration of treatment; importance of not missing or skipping doses.

If ledipasvir/sofosbuvir is used in a patient receiving amiodarone, advise the patient about the risk of serious symptomatic bradycardia and the importance of immediately contacting a clinician if signs or symptoms of bradycardia (e.g., near-fainting or fainting, dizziness, lightheadedness, malaise, weakness, excessive tiredness, shortness of breath, chest pain, confusion, memory problems) occur. (See Cardiovascular Effects under Warnings/Precautions: Other Warnings/Precautions, in Cautions.)

Importance of informing clinicians of existing or contemplated concomitant therapy, including prescription and OTC drugs and dietary or herbal supplements, as well as any concomitant illnesses.

Importance of women informing clinicians if they are or plan to become pregnant or plan to breast-feed. If used in conjunction with ribavirin, advise men and women of importance of using 2 forms of effective contraception during and for 6 months after ribavirin therapy. (See Precautions Related to Fixed Combinations and Multiple-drug Treatment Regimens under Warnings/Precautions: Other Warnings/Precautions, in Cautions.)

Importance of informing patients of other important precautionary information. (See Cautions.)

Overview® (see Users Guide). For additional information on this drug until a more detailed monograph is developed and published, the manufacturer's labeling should be consulted. It is *essential* that the manufacturer's labeling be consulted for more detailed information on usual cautions, precautions, contraindications, potential drug interactions, laboratory test interferences, and acute toxicity.

Preparations

Excipients in commercially available drug preparations may have clinically important effects in some individuals; consult specific product labeling for details.

Ledipasvir and Sofosbuvir

Oral		
Tablets, film-coated	Ledipasvir 90 mg and Sofosbuvir 400 mg	Harvoni®, Gilead

†Use is not currently included in the labeling approved by the US Food and Drug Administration

MISCELLANEOUS ANTIVIRALS 8:18.92

Baloxavir Marboxil BXM

■ Baloxavir marboxil is a prodrug of baloxavir, a polymerase acidic (PA) endonuclease inhibitor antiviral agent active against influenza A and B viruses.

Uses

■ Treatment of Seasonal Influenza A and B Virus Infections

Baloxavir marboxil is used for the *treatment* of acute, uncomplicated influenza caused by influenza A or B viruses in adults and adolescents 12 years of age or older who have been symptomatic for no longer than 48 hours. Efficacy of baloxavir marboxil administered more than 48 hours after onset of influenza symptoms has not been evaluated.

Data are not available to date regarding use of baloxavir marboxil for the *treatment* of severe or complicated influenza in either hospitalized patients or outpatients. Data also are not available to date regarding use of baloxavir marboxil for *prophylaxis* of influenza infections.

The US Centers for Disease Control and Prevention (CDC), Advisory Committee on Immunization Practices (ACIP), Infectious Diseases Society of America (IDSA), American Academy of Pediatrics (AAP), and others recommend that antiviral treatment be initiated as soon as possible in all individuals with suspected or confirmed influenza who require hospitalization or have severe, complicated, or progressive illness (regardless of vaccination status or underlying illness). These experts also recommend early empiric antiviral treatment in individuals with suspected or confirmed influenza of any severity if they are at high risk of developing influenza-related complications because of age or underlying medical conditions (regardless of vaccination status). Individuals at increased risk for influenza-related complications include children younger than 5 years of age (especially those younger than 2 years of age); adults 65 years of age or older; individuals of any age with certain chronic medical or immunosuppressive conditions; women who are pregnant or up to 2 weeks postpartum; individuals younger than 19 years of age receiving long-term aspirin therapy; American Indians or Alaskan natives; morbidly obese individuals with a body mass index (BMI) of 40 or greater; and residents of any age in nursing homes or other long-term care facilities.

CDC, ACIP, IDSA, and AAP also state that empiric antiviral treatment can be considered in previously healthy, symptomatic individuals with suspected or confirmed influenza who are not known to be at increased risk of developing severe or complicated illness (regardless of vaccination status), if such treatment can be initiated within 48 hours of illness onset. Although these individuals typically do not require treatment, early empiric antiviral treatment might provide some benefit (e.g., shortened duration of illness). The use of antivirals in such individuals should be based on clinical judgment and is not necessary in those who are already beginning to recover.

If treatment of influenza is indicated, an appropriate antiviral should be initiated as soon as possible after illness onset (ideally within 48 hours) and should not be delayed while waiting for laboratory confirmation. Because there is some evidence from observational studies evaluating use of oseltamivir in hospitalized patients that antiviral treatment may still be beneficial in such patients when initiated as late as 4 or 5 days after illness onset, CDC, ACIP, and AAP recommend that appropriate antiviral treatment be initiated in all patients with severe, complicated, or progressive illness attributable to influenza and all hospitalized patients and patients at increased risk of influenza complications (either hospitalized or outpatient) who have suspected or confirmed influenza, even if it has been more than 48 hours since illness onset. Decisions regarding use of empiric antiviral treatment in outpatients, especially high-risk patients, should be based on disease severity and progression, age, underlying medical conditions, likelihood of influenza, and time since onset of symptoms.

For the treatment of suspected or confirmed severe, complicated influenza in hospitalized patients or outpatients, oseltamivir is the preferred antiviral because of the lack of data regarding use of inhaled zanamivir, IV peramivir, and oral baloxavir marboxil in such patients. Oseltamivir also is the preferred antiviral for the treatment of suspected or confirmed influenza in women who are pregnant or up to 2 weeks postpartum.

If an antiviral is used for the treatment of suspected or confirmed acute, uncomplicated influenza in otherwise healthy outpatients, CDC, IDSA, and other experts state that any age-appropriate influenza antiviral (oseltamivir, zanamivir, peramivir, baloxavir marboxil) can be used if not contraindicated.

Viral surveillance data available from local and state health departments and CDC should be considered when selecting an antiviral for the treatment of seasonal influenza. Strains of circulating influenza viruses and the antiviral susceptibility of these strains constantly evolve, and the possibility that emergence of resistant strains may decrease effectiveness of influenza antivirals should be considered.

CDC issues recommendations concerning the use of antivirals for the treatment of influenza, and these recommendations are updated as needed during each influenza season. Information regarding influenza surveillance and updated recommendations for the treatment of seasonal influenza are available from CDC at https://www.cdc.gov/flu/.

Clinical Experience Efficacy and safety of baloxavir marboxil for the treatment of acute, uncomplicated influenza have been evaluated in 2 randomized, placebo-controlled studies that included otherwise healthy individuals 12–64 years of age. For both studies, enrollment criteria included an axillary temperature of at least 38°C, at least one moderate or severe respiratory symptom (cough, nasal congestion, or sore throat), and at least one moderate or severe systemic symptom (headache, feverishness or chills, muscle or joint pain, or fatigue); patients with severe illness requiring hospitalization, those weighing less than 40 kg, those older than 65 years of age, and pregnant women were excluded. The primary efficacy population was defined as those with a positive rapid influenza diagnostic test (study 1) or with reverse transcriptase-polymerase chain reaction (RT-PCR)-confirmed influenza (study 2). Patients were treated within 48 hours of symptom onset and were required to self-assess the severity of 7 influenza symptoms (cough, sore throat, headache, nasal congestion, feverishness or chills, muscle or joint pain, and fatigue) twice daily on days 1–9 and once daily on days 10–14 and to rate these symptoms as none, mild, moderate, or severe. The primary end point was the time to alleviation of influenza symptoms and was defined as the time when all 7 influenza symptoms were assessed by the study participant as absent or mild for a duration of at least 21.5 hours. The majority of patients enrolled in these studies had infections caused by seasonal influenza A; a smaller number of patients had infections caused by seasonal influenza B.

Study 1 was a phase 2, dose-ranging trial conducted in Japan that included 400 adults 20–64 years of age (62% male, mean age 38 years, 100% Asian) with acute, uncomplicated influenza infection who were randomized in a 1:1:1:1 ratio to receive oral baloxavir marboxil (single 10-, 20-, or 40-mg dose) or placebo administered in an outpatient setting and initiated within 48 hours of onset of symptoms. The median time to alleviation of influenza symptoms was 50 hours in those who received a single 40-mg dose of baloxavir marboxil compared with a duration of 78 hours in those who received placebo. Among study 1 participants treated with baloxavir marboxil who had their influenza strains typed, 63% had influenza A (H1N1), 25% had influenza B, and 12% had influenza A (H3N2). In the subset of patients with influenza B infections, the median time to alleviation of influenza symptoms was 63 hours in those treated with baloxavir marboxil compared with 83 hours in those who received placebo.

Study 2 (CAPSTONE-1) was a phase 3 study conducted in the US and Japan that included 1436 adults and adolescents 12–64 years of age (54% male, mean age 34 years, 78% Asian, 17% white, 4% black) with acute, uncomplicated influenza infection. Study participants 20–64 years of age were randomized in a 2:2:1 ratio to receive oral baloxavir marboxil (single 40-mg dose in those weighing less than 80 kg or single 80-mg dose in those weighing 80 kg or more), oral oseltamivir (75 mg twice daily for 5 days), or placebo administered in an outpatient setting and initiated within 48 hours of onset of symptoms. Adolescents 12–19 years of age were randomized in a 2:1 ratio to receive baloxavir marboxil (single 40-mg oral dose in those weighing less than 80 kg or single 80-mg oral dose in those weighing 80 kg or more) or placebo administered in an outpatient setting and initiated within 48 hours of onset of symptoms. The median time to alleviation of influenza symptoms in those 12–64 years of age treated with baloxavir marboxil or placebo was 54 or 80 hours, respectively. In the subset of patients 12–17 years of age, the median time to alleviation of influenza symptoms was 54 hours in those treated with baloxavir marboxil and 93 hours in those who received placebo. In addition, data from study participants 20–64 years of age indicated that the median time to alleviation of influenza symptoms in patients who received a single weight-based dose of baloxavir marboxil was the same as that reported in patients receiving a 5-day regimen of oseltamivir (54 hours in both groups). Among study 2 participants treated with baloxavir marboxil who had their influenza strains typed, 90% had influenza A (H3N2), 9% had influenza B, and 2% had influenza A (H1N1). In the subset of patients with influenza B infections, the median time to alleviation of influenza symptoms was 93 hours in those treated with baloxavir marboxil compared with 77 hours in those who received placebo; these results may have been affected by the low number of study participants with influenza B infections who received baloxavir marboxil.

Dosage and Administration

■ Administration Baloxavir marboxil is administered orally without regard to meals. However, concomitant administration of baloxavir marboxil and dairy products; calcium-fortified beverages; aluminum-, calcium-, or magnesium-containing antacids; polyvalent cation-containing laxatives; or multivitamins or dietary supplements containing calcium, iron, magnesium, selenium, or zinc should be avoided. (See Drug Interactions: Antacids and Other Preparations Containing Polyvalent Cations.)

■ Dosage ***Adult Dosage*** **Treatment of Seasonal Influenza A and B Virus Infections.** For the treatment of acute, uncomplicated influenza infection in adults, the recommended dosage of oral baloxavir marboxil is a single 40-mg dose in those weighing 40 to less than 80 kg and a single 80-mg dose in those weighing 80 kg or more. The dose should be given within 48 hours after onset of influenza symptoms.

Pediatric Dosage **Treatment of Seasonal Influenza A and B Virus Infections.** For the treatment of acute, uncomplicated influenza infection in adolescents 12 years of age or older, the recommended dosage of oral baloxavir marboxil is a single 40-mg dose in those weighing 40 to less than 80 kg and a single 80-mg dose in those weighing 80 kg or more. The dose should be given within 48 hours after onset of influenza symptoms.

■ Special Populations The manufacturer makes no special population dosage recommendations at this time.

Cautions

■ Contraindications Baloxavir marboxil is contraindicated in individuals with a history of hypersensitivity to the drug or any ingredient in the formulation.

■ Warnings/Precautions ***Bacterial Infections*** When making treatment decisions in patients with suspected influenza, the possibility of primary or concomitant bacterial infection should be considered.

Serious bacterial infections may begin with influenza-like symptoms or may coexist with or occur as complications of influenza. There is no evidence that baloxavir marboxil prevents such complications. If a bacterial infection occurs, it should be treated as appropriate.

There is no evidence that baloxavir marboxil is effective for illness caused by any organisms other than influenza viruses.

Influenza Vaccination Influenza antivirals are not a substitute for annual vaccination with a seasonal influenza vaccine (influenza virus vaccine inactivated, influenza vaccine live intranasal, influenza vaccine recombinant).

Although influenza virus vaccine inactivated or influenza vaccine recombinant may be administered to individuals receiving influenza antivirals, such antivirals may inhibit the vaccine virus contained in influenza vaccine live intranasal and decrease efficacy of this influenza vaccine. (See Influenza Vaccines under Drug Interactions: Vaccines.)

Specific Populations **Pregnancy.** Data are not available regarding use of baloxavir marboxil in pregnant women.

In animal reproduction studies, no adverse embryofetal effects were observed in rats or rabbits receiving oral baloxavir marboxil in dosages resulting in baloxavir exposures approximately 5 or 7 times, respectively, the systemic baloxavir exposures achieved in humans with the maximum recommended human dose.

Pregnant women are at increased risk for severe complications from influenza, which may lead to adverse pregnancy and/or fetal outcomes including maternal death, stillbirths, birth defects, preterm delivery, low birthweight, and small size for gestational age.

The US Centers for Disease Control and Prevention (CDC) states that baloxavir marboxil is not recommended for the treatment of influenza in pregnant women because of the lack of safety and efficacy data in such patients. Oseltamivir is the preferred antiviral for the treatment of suspected or confirmed influenza in women who are pregnant or up to 2 weeks postpartum.

Lactation. It is not known whether baloxavir marboxil is distributed into human milk, affects milk production, or has any effects on breast-fed infants. Baloxavir and its metabolites are distributed into milk in rats.

The manufacturer states that the benefits of breast-feeding and the importance of baloxavir marboxil to the woman should be considered along with the potential adverse effects on the breast-fed child from the drug or from the underlying maternal condition.

CDC states that baloxavir marboxil is not recommended for the treatment of influenza in nursing women because of the lack of safety data in such patients.

Pediatric Use. Safety and efficacy of baloxavir marboxil have not been established in pediatric patients younger than 12 years of age.

Safety and efficacy of baloxavir marboxil for the treatment of influenza in pediatric patients 12 years of age or older weighing 40 kg or more were established in a phase 3, randomized, double-blind, placebo-controlled study. Data from this study indicated that the safety profile of the drug in adolescent patients 12 years of age or older is similar to that reported in adults.

Geriatric Use. Clinical studies of baloxavir marboxil to date have not included individuals 65 years of age or older; data are insufficient to determine whether geriatric patients respond differently than younger adults.

Hepatic Impairment. Baloxavir marboxil has not been evaluated in patients with severe hepatic impairment (Child-Pugh class C).

Population pharmacokinetic analysis indicates there are no clinically important differences in the pharmacokinetics of baloxavir marboxil in individuals with moderate hepatic impairment (Child-Pugh class B) compared with individuals with normal hepatic function.

Renal Impairment. Baloxavir marboxil has not been evaluated in patients with severe renal impairment.

Population pharmacokinetic analysis indicates that there are no clinically important differences in the pharmacokinetics of baloxavir marboxil in individuals with creatinine clearances of 50 mL/minute or greater compared with individuals with normal renal function.

■ Common Adverse Effects Adverse effects reported in 1% or more of patients receiving baloxavir marboxil in clinical studies include GI effects (nausea, diarrhea), bronchitis, nasopharyngitis, and headache.

Drug Interactions

After baloxavir marboxil is converted in vivo to baloxavir, the active metabolite, baloxavir is metabolized principally by uridine diphosphate-glucuronosyltransferase (UGT) 1A3 and, to a minor extent, by cytochrome P-450 (CYP) isoenzyme 3A4.

In vitro studies indicate that baloxavir marboxil and baloxavir do not inhibit CYP isoenzymes 1A2, 2B6, 2C8, 2C9, 2C19, or 2D6 and do not induce CYP isoenzymes 1A2, 2B6, or 3A4.

Baloxavir marboxil and baloxavir are both substrates of P-glycoprotein (P-gp). In vitro studies indicate that baloxavir marboxil and baloxavir do not inhibit UGT1A1, 1A3, 1A4, 1A6, 1A9, 2B7, or 2B15. In addition, baloxavir does not inhibit organic anion transport polypeptide (OATP) 1B1, OATP1B3, organic cation transporter (OCT) 1, OCT2, organic anion transporter (OAT) 1, OAT3, multidrug and toxin extrusion (MATE) 1, or MATE2K.

■ Drugs Affecting or Metabolized by Hepatic Microsomal Enzymes The pharmacokinetics of baloxavir marboxil and baloxavir were not affected when baloxavir marboxil was used concomitantly with a potent CYP3A inhibitor (itraconazole).

Concomitant use of baloxavir marboxil and a CYP3A substrate (midazolam) did not affect the pharmacokinetics of the CYP3A substrate.

■ Drugs Affecting or Affected by the P-glycoprotein Transport System The pharmacokinetics of baloxavir marboxil and baloxavir were not affected when baloxavir marboxil was used concomitantly with a P-gp inhibitor (itraconazole).

Concomitant use of baloxavir marboxil and a P-gp substrate (digoxin) did not affect the pharmacokinetics of the P-gp substrate.

■ Drugs Affected by Other Membrane Transporters The pharmacokinetics of baloxavir marboxil and baloxavir were not affected when baloxavir marboxil was used concomitantly with a UGT inhibitor (probenecid).

Concomitant use of baloxavir marboxil and a breast cancer resistance protein (BCRP) substrate (rosuvastatin) did not affect the pharmacokinetics of the BCRP substrate.

■ **Antacids and Other Preparations Containing Polyvalent Cations** Baloxavir may form a chelate with polyvalent cations (e.g., aluminum, calcium, iron, magnesium). Although specific drug interaction studies have not been performed to evaluate concomitant administration of baloxavir marboxil and food, beverages, drugs, or other preparations containing polyvalent cations, decreased baloxavir exposures were reported in monkeys when baloxavir marboxil was administered concomitantly with aluminum, calcium, iron, or magnesium.

Antacids Concomitant use of baloxavir marboxil and antacids containing aluminum, calcium, or magnesium may decrease baloxavir concentrations and decrease efficacy of baloxavir marboxil.

Concomitant administration of baloxavir marboxil and antacids containing polyvalent cations (e.g., aluminum, calcium, magnesium) should be avoided

Calcium, Iron, and Multivitamins Concomitant use of baloxavir marboxil and calcium supplements, iron preparations, or other oral supplements containing calcium, iron, magnesium, selenium, or zinc (e.g., multivitamins) may decrease baloxavir concentrations and decrease efficacy of baloxavir marboxil.

Concomitant administration of baloxavir marboxil and oral supplements containing polyvalent cations (e.g., calcium, iron, magnesium, selenium, or zinc) should be avoided.

Other Preparations Containing Polyvalent Cations Concomitant use of baloxavir marboxil and drugs containing polyvalent cations (e.g., laxatives) may decrease baloxavir concentrations and decrease efficacy of baloxavir marboxil.

Concomitant administration of baloxavir marboxil and drugs or preparations containing polyvalent cations should be avoided.

■ **Oseltamivir** There was no evidence of pharmacokinetic interactions when baloxavir marboxil (single 40-mg dose) was used concomitantly with oseltamivir (75 mg twice daily for 5 days).

■ **Vaccines** ***Influenza Vaccines*** Although concomitant use of baloxavir marboxil and influenza virus vaccine inactivated (IIV) or influenza vaccine recombinant (RIV) has not been evaluated, the Advisory Committee on Immunization Practices (ACIP) states that antivirals used for the treatment of influenza have no effect on the immune response to inactivated influenza vaccines and these vaccines may be administered concomitantly with or at any time before or after influenza antivirals.

Concomitant use of baloxavir marboxil and influenza vaccine live intranasal (LAIV) has not been evaluated. However, because influenza antivirals, including baloxavir, inhibit replication of influenza viruses, these antivirals potentially could decrease the immune response to LAIV and efficacy of the vaccine. LAIV should not be administered until at least 48 hours after influenza antivirals have been discontinued and, if feasible, influenza antivirals should be avoided until at least 14 days after administration of LAIV. If an influenza antiviral is administered within 2 weeks after administration of LAIV, the LAIV dose should be repeated at least 48 hours after the last antiviral dose. Alternatively, ACIP states that individuals who received an influenza antiviral 2 days before to 14 days after LAIV may be revaccinated using age-appropriate IIV or RIV.

Pharmacokinetics

■ **Absorption** ***Bioavailability*** Following oral administration of baloxavir marboxil, the drug is rapidly and almost completely converted to the active metabolite, baloxavir, by esterases in the GI lumen, liver, and blood.

The median time to peak plasma concentrations of baloxavir after oral administration of baloxavir marboxil is 4 hours.

Following a single 40-mg dose of baloxavir marboxil in individuals weighing less than 80 kg or a single 80-mg dose in those weighing 80 kg or more, mean peak plasma concentrations of baloxavir were 96.4 or 107 ng/mL, respectively.

Food Administration of oral baloxavir marboxil with a meal (approximately 400–500 kcal including 150 kcal from fat) decreases the peak plasma concentration and area under the plasma concentration-time curve (AUC) of baloxavir by approximately 48 and 36%, respectively.

Although specific studies have not been performed, baloxavir may form chelates with polyvalent cations (e.g., aluminum, calcium, iron, magnesium, selenium, zinc). Systemic baloxavir exposures may be decreased if oral baloxavir marboxil is administered with dairy products, calcium-fortified beverages, or other foods, drugs, or preparations containing polyvalent cations. (See Drugs Interactions: Antacids and Other Preparations Containing Polyvalent Cations.)

■ **Distribution** ***Extent*** Baloxavir and its related metabolites are distributed into milk in rats following oral administration of baloxavir marboxil; it is not known whether the drug is distributed into human milk.

Plasma Protein Binding Baloxavir is approximately 93–94% bound to serum proteins in vitro.

■ **Elimination** ***Metabolism*** Following oral administration, baloxavir marboxil is rapidly hydrolyzed by esterases to the active metabolite, baloxavir. Baloxavir is then metabolized principally by uridine diphosphate-glucuronosyltransferase (UGT) 1A3 and, to a minor extent, by cytochrome P-450 (CYP) isoenzyme 3A4.

Elimination Route Approximately 80% of an oral dose of baloxavir marboxil is eliminated in feces as baloxavir and less than 15% is eliminated in urine.

Half-life The mean apparent terminal elimination half-life of baloxavir is approximately 80 hours.

Description

Baloxavir marboxil is a prodrug of baloxavir, a polymerase acidic (PA) endonuclease inhibitor antiviral. Baloxavir marboxil exhibits no antiviral activity until hydrolyzed in vivo to baloxavir, its active metabolite. Baloxavir has a mechanism of action against influenza viruses that differs from that of the neuraminidase inhibitor antivirals (oseltamivir, peramivir, zanamivir) and adamantane derivative antivirals (amantadine, rimantadine).

Baloxavir selectively inhibits the cap-dependent endonuclease activity of the PA subunit of the viral RNA polymerase complex, which is essential for viral replication. Inhibition of the cap-dependent endonuclease activity of the PA subunit prevents transcription of influenza viral messenger RNA, which is required for viral replication.

■ **Spectrum** Baloxavir exhibits potent antiviral activity in vitro against both influenza A and B viruses. In a PA endonuclease assay, the 50% inhibitory concentrations (IC_{50}) of baloxavir for influenza A viruses was 1.4–3.1 nM and the IC_{50} of the drug for influenza B viruses was 4.5–8.9 nM. When susceptibility of laboratory and clinical isolates of influenza A and B viruses was determined in a MDCK cell-based plaque reduction assay, the 50% effective concentration (EC_{50}) of baloxavir was 0.20-1.85 nM for influenza A (H1N1), 0.35-1.87 nM for influenza A (H3N2), and 3.33-13 nM for influenza B.

Baloxavir has been active in vitro in cell culture against some avian influenza A viruses, including some strains of avian influenza A (H5N1) and (H7N9).

Baloxavir is active against some influenza strains resistant to neuraminidase inhibitors (e.g., oseltamivir, peramivir, zanamivir), including influenza A (H1N1) with the H275Y mutation, influenza A (H3N2) with the E119V mutation, influenza B with the D198E mutation, avian influenza A (H5N1) with the H275Y mutation, and avian influenza A (H7N9) with the R292K mutation.

The relationship between in vitro antiviral activity of baloxavir in cell culture and clinical response to treatment with baloxavir marboxil has not been established.

■ **Resistance** Resistance to baloxavir has been produced in vitro by serial passage of influenza A viruses in the presence of increasing concentrations of the drug. In addition, influenza A and B viruses with treatment-emergent amino acid substitutions associated with reduced in vitro susceptibility to baloxavir have been reported in some patients treated with baloxavir marboxil.

Influenza viruses with reduced susceptibility to baloxavir have amino acid substitutions in the PA protein of the viral RNA polymerase complex. Amino acid substitutions that have been associated with reduced in vitro susceptibility to baloxavir include E23K/R and 138F/T (influenza A [H1N1]); E23G/K, A37T, I38F/T, I38M/T, and E199G (influenza A [H3N2]); and I38T (influenza B). Oseltamivir may be active against influenza viruses with reduced susceptibility to baloxavir, including influenza A (H1N1) with amino acid substitutions E23K or I38F/T; influenza A (H3N2) with substitutions E23G/K, A37T, I38M/T, or E199G; and influenza B with the substitution I38T.

Cross-resistance between baloxavir and neuraminidase inhibitors (oseltamivir, peramivir, zanamivir) or adamantane derivatives (amantadine, rimantadine) is not expected since these drugs have different mechanisms of action against influenza viruses. However, influenza viruses with amino acid substitutions in the PA protein of the viral RNA polymerase complex that confer resistance to baloxavir may also have substitutions that confer resistance to neuraminidase inhibitors or adamantane derivatives. The clinical relevance of phenotypic cross-resistance evaluations has not been established.

Advice to Patients

Importance of reading patient information provided by the manufacturer.

Importance of initiating baloxavir marboxil treatment as soon as possible after the first appearance of influenza symptoms (within 48 hours after symptom onset).

Advise patients that baloxavir marboxil may be taken with or without food, but should not be taken with dairy products or calcium-fortified beverages or with antacids, laxatives, multivitamins, or dietary supplements containing polyvalent cations (e.g., calcium, iron, magnesium, selenium, zinc).

Advise patients that influenza antivirals such as baloxavir marboxil may decrease effectiveness of influenza virus vaccine live; importance of consulting clinician before receiving the live intranasal influenza vaccine.

Importance of informing clinicians of existing or contemplated concomitant therapy, including prescription and OTC drugs, as well as any concomitant illnesses.

Importance of women informing clinicians if they are or plan to become pregnant or plan to breast-feed.

Importance of informing patients of other important precautionary information. (See Cautions.)

Overview® (see Users Guide). For additional information on this drug until a more detailed monograph is developed and published, the manu-

facturer's labeling should be consulted. It is *essential* that the manufacturer's labeling be consulted for more detailed information on usual cautions, precautions, contraindications, potential drug interactions, laboratory test interferences, and acute toxicity.

Preparations

Excipients in commercially available drug preparations may have clinically important effects in some individuals; consult specific product labeling for details.

Baloxavir Marboxil

Oral		
Tablets, film-coated	20 mg	**Xofluza®**, Genentech
	40 mg	**Xofluza®**, Genentech

Selected Revisions August 2019, © Copyright, November 2018, American Society of Health-System Pharmacists, Inc.

Foscarnet Sodium

Foscavir, Phosphonoformate, Phosphonoformic Acid Trisodium, Trisodium Phosphonoformate, Trisodium Carboxyphosphate FOS

PFA

■ Foscarnet sodium (phosphonoformic acid), an organic analog of inorganic pyrophosphate, is an antiviral agent active against herpesviruses.

Uses

■ **Treatment of Cytomegalovirus Infection and Disease** ***Cytomegalovirus Retinitis*** Foscarnet sodium is used for initial treatment (induction therapy) and maintenance therapy (secondary prophylaxis) of cytomegalovirus (CMV) retinitis in adults with human immunodeficiency virus (HIV) infection, including those with acquired immunodeficiency syndrome (AIDS). The drug also is used for the management of CMV retinitis in HIV-infected adolescents and children†. Foscarnet can be used in conjunction with ganciclovir for the management of CMV retinitis that relapsed after monotherapy with either drug. Safety and efficacy of foscarnet have not been established for the treatment of CMV retinitis in immunocompetent individuals.

Like other antivirals, foscarnet, is not a cure for CMV retinitis. Although foscarnet can induce stabilization or improvement of ocular manifestations of CMV retinitis, the retinitis may relapse and/or progress during or after discontinuance of the drug. The possibility of foscarnet-resistant CMV should be considered in patients who fail to respond to foscarnet or who experience persistent CMV shedding while receiving maintenance therapy with the drug; some strains resistant to foscarnet may be susceptible to ganciclovir. In some patients whose retinitis progressed with foscarnet or ganciclovir monotherapy, combined therapy with the drugs stabilized progression of the disease.

Retinitis is the most common clinical manifestation of CMV end-organ disease in HIV-infected patients and ideally should be managed in consultation with an ophthalmologist familiar with the diagnosis and treatment of retinal diseases. Antiviral regimens for initial treatment of CMV retinitis in HIV-infected individuals should be selected based on the location and severity of CMV retinal lesions, severity of underlying immunosuppression, concomitant drug therapy, and the patient's ability to adhere to the treatment regimen. The antiviral regimen used for maintenance therapy of CMV retinitis in HIV-infected individuals should be selected with consideration for the location of the CMV retinal lesions, vision in the contralateral eye, the patient's immunologic and virologic status, and the patient's response to antiretroviral therapy.

For the management of immediate sight-threatening CMV retinal lesions (i.e., within 1.5 mm of the fovea) in HIV-infected adults and adolescents, the US Centers for Disease Control and Prevention (CDC), National Institutes of Health (NIH), and HIV Medicine Association of the Infectious Diseases Society of America (IDSA) state that the preferred regimen is initial treatment (induction therapy) with intravitreal ganciclovir or intravitreal foscarnet† (1–4 doses given over a period of 7–10 days) in conjunction with oral valganciclovir (twice daily for 14–21 days) followed by maintenance therapy (secondary prophylaxis) with oral valganciclovir (once daily). One alternative regimen recommended by these experts for management of sight-threatening CMV retinitis in HIV-infected adults and adolescents is intravitreal ganciclovir or intravitreal foscarnet† (1–4 doses given over a period of 7–10 days) in conjunction with IV foscarnet (2 or 3 times daily for 2–3 weeks) followed by maintenance therapy (secondary prophylaxis) with IV foscarnet (once daily). Use of systemic antivirals (without an intravitreal antiviral) usually is adequate for the management of CMV retinitis in patients who have only small peripheral lesions.

For the management of CMV retinitis in HIV-infected pediatric patients, CDC, NIH, IDSA, and others state that IV ganciclovir is the drug of choice for initial treatment (induction therapy) and is one of several options for maintenance therapy (secondary prophylaxis). These experts state that IV foscarnet is a preferred alternative for the management of CMV retinitis in HIV-infected children† and is recommended for infections known or suspected to be caused by ganciclovir-resistant CMV. These experts state that a regimen of IV ganciclovir and IV foscarnet can be considered for initial treatment (induction therapy) in HIV-infected children with sight-threatening CMV retinitis or when the infection failed to respond to or relapsed after monotherapy. Data are limited regarding use of intravitreal antivirals in children, and intravitreal injections are impractical in most children.

Because of the risk of relapse, HIV-infected patients who have received adequate initial treatment of CMV retinitis should receive chronic maintenance therapy (secondary prophylaxis) until immune reconstitution occurs as a result of effective antiretroviral therapy. CDC, NIH, and IDSA state that consideration can be given to discontinuing maintenance therapy of CMV retinitis in HIV-infected adults and adolescents if CMV lesions have been treated for at least 3–6 months and are inactive and there has been a sustained (i.e., 3–6 months) increase in $CD4^+$ T-cell count to greater than 100/mm^3 in response to antiretroviral therapy. The safety of discontinuing maintenance therapy of CMV retinitis in HIV-infected pediatric patients has not been well studied; however, CDC, NIH, IDSA, and others state that consideration can be given to discontinuing such maintenance therapy of CMV retinitis in HIV-infected children who are receiving antiretroviral therapy and have a sustained (i.e., greater than 6 months) increase in $CD4^+$ T-cell percentage to greater than 15% (children younger than 6 years of age) or increase in $CD4^+$ T-cell count to greater than 100/mm^3 (children 6 years of age and older). These experts state that a decision to discontinue maintenance therapy of CMV retinitis should be made in consultation with an ophthalmologist and, if maintenance therapy is discontinued, the patient should continue to receive regular ophthalmologic monitoring (optimally every 3–6 months) for early detection of CMV relapse or immune reconstitution uveitis. If $CD4^+$ T-cell count decreases to less than 100/mm^3 (adults, adolescents, children 6 years of age or older) or if $CD4^+$ T-cell percentage decreases to less than 15% (children younger than 6 years of age), maintenance therapy of CMV retinitis should be reinitiated.

For additional information on the management of CMV retinitis and other CMV infections in HIV-infected individuals, the current clinical practice guidelines from CDC, NIH, and IDSA on the prevention and treatment of opportunistic infections in HIV-infected individuals available at http://www.aidsinfo.nih.gov should be consulted.

Clinical Experience. Efficacy of IV foscarnet sodium for the treatment of CMV retinitis was evaluated in a prospective, randomized, controlled trial in 24 patients with AIDS. Patients received induction treatment with foscarnet sodium (60 mg/kg IV every 8 hours for 3 weeks), followed by maintenance treatment with the drug (90 mg/kg IV once daily until retinitis progression [appearance of a new lesion or advancement of the border of a posterior lesion greater than 750 μm in diameter]). All diagnoses and determinations of retinitis progression were made from masked reading of retinal photographs. The 13 patients randomized to receive IV foscarnet had a delay in progression of CMV retinitis compared with untreated controls. The median time to retinitis progression from study entry was 93 days (range: 21 to greater than 364 days) in those treated with IV foscarnet compared with 22 days (range: 7– 42 days) in untreated controls.

In another prospective trial in AIDS patients with CMV retinitis, 33 patients received induction treatment with IV foscarnet sodium (60 mg/kg IV 3 times daily for 2–3 weeks) and were randomized to receive maintenance therapy with the drug in a dosage of 90 or 120 mg/kg IV once daily. The median time from study entry to retinitis progression was not significantly different between the treatment groups; 96 days (range: 14 to greater than 176 days) in those receiving the lower maintenance dosage and 140 days (range: 16 to greater than 233 days) in those receiving the higher maintenance dosage.

The comparative efficacy of IV foscarnet and IV ganciclovir for the treatment of newly diagnosed CMV retinitis was evaluated in a study that included 107 patients randomized to receive foscarnet sodium (induction treatment with 60 mg/kg IV 3 times daily for 2 weeks followed by maintenance therapy with 90 mg/kg IV once daily) and 127 patients randomized to receive ganciclovir (induction treatment with 5 mg/kg IV twice daily followed by maintenance therapy with 5 mg/kg IV once daily). The median time to retinitis progression was similar with both drugs (59 days in those receiving foscarnet and 56 days in those receiving ganciclovir).

In a study evaluating efficacy of combination therapy with IV foscarnet and IV ganciclovir versus monotherapy with either drug alone for the treatment of persistently active or relapsed CMV retinitis in patients with AIDS, patients who were randomized to combination therapy while receiving IV foscarnet alone continued to receive the usual maintenance dosage of foscarnet sodium (i.e., 90 mg/kg IV once daily) while IV ganciclovir therapy was initiated using usual ganciclovir induction and maintenance dosages (i.e., 5 mg/kg IV every 12 hours for 14 days followed by 5 mg/kg IV once daily). Patients who were randomized to combination therapy while receiving IV ganciclovir alone continued to receive the usual maintenance dosage of ganciclovir (i.e., 5 mg/kg IV once daily) while IV foscarnet therapy was initiated using usual foscarnet sodium induction and maintenance dosages (i.e., 90 mg/kg IV every 12 hours for 14 days followed by 90 mg/kg IV once daily). Therapy was then continued using maintenance dosages of both drugs. Patients who relapsed while receiving combination therapy were reinduced with both drugs using usual induction dosages (i.e., ganciclovir 5 mg/kg IV every 12 hours and foscarnet sodium 90 mg IV every 12 hours for 14 days) followed by usual maintenance dosages (i.e., ganciclovir 5 mg/kg IV once daily and foscarnet sodium 90 mg/kg IV once daily). The median time to retinitis progression in the foscarnet group, ganciclovir group, or combination group was 1.3, 2, or 4.3 months, respectively.

Extraocular Cytomegalovirus Infections Although safety and efficacy of foscarnet sodium have not been established for the treatment of extraocular CMV infections (e.g., pneumonitis, gastroenteritis), the drug has been used for the management of extraocular CMV infections†.

CDC, NIH, and IDSA state that IV ganciclovir usually is the preferred antiviral for initial management of CMV GI disease (e.g., colitis, esophagitis) in HIV-infected adults; however, IV foscarnet is a possible alternative for the management of CMV esophagitis† or colitis† in those who cannot receive ganciclovir or have infections caused by ganciclovir-resistant CMV.

For the management of well-documented CMV pneumonitis† in HIV-infected adults, CDC, NIH, and IDSA state that either IV ganciclovir or IV foscarnet is a reasonable choice.

A combination regimen of IV ganciclovir and IV foscarnet has been used for the management of CMV neurologic disease† (e.g., CMV encephalitis or myelitis) and is recommended by CDC, NIH, IDSA, and others for such infections in HIV-infected individuals.

■ Prevention of Cytomegalovirus Infection and Disease Foscarnet sodium has been used for prophylaxis or preemptive treatment of CMV infection and disease in hematopoietic stem cell transplant (HSCT) recipients†. Although safety and efficacy have not been established, IV foscarnet sodium is considered a second-line or alternative antiviral for prophylaxis or preemptive treatment of CMV infection in HSCT recipients and usually is reserved for resistant and refractory CMV infections or when first-line antivirals cannot be used because of intolerance. Foscarnet also has been recommended as a second-line or alternative antiviral for treatment of CMV infection in solid organ transplant recipients† when first-line antivirals cannot be used because of resistance or intolerance.

CMV infection in transplant recipients can occur either as a primary infection in CMV-seronegative recipients of organs and cells from CMV-positive donors or as reactivation of latent CMV infection in CMV-seropositive recipients. CMV reactivation commonly occurs in CMV-seropositive transplant recipients and can result in severe CMV disease with substantial morbidity and mortality. The risk for CMV infection or reactivation is greatest during the first 3 months after transplantation and depends on several factors, including the serologic status of the recipient and donor and CMV-specific T-cell immunity and immunosuppressive regimens used in the recipient. Certain antiviral strategies have been used to prevent severe, life-threatening CMV disease in HSCT or solid organ transplant patients, including antiviral prophylaxis (initiated posttransplant and continued for at least 3 months) and/or preemptive antiviral treatment (i.e., initiated when CMV infection is detected, but before clinical progression to symptomatic CMV disease). These strategies each have certain advantages and disadvantages.

Specialized references should be consulted for specific information regarding management of CMV infections in HSCT or solid organ transplant recipients.

■ Mucocutaneous Herpes Simplex Virus Infections Foscarnet sodium is used for the management of mucocutaneous infections (e.g., orofacial, genital, digital) caused by acyclovir-resistant herpes simplex virus types 1 and 2 (HSV-1 and HSV-2) in immunocompromised patients, including HIV-infected individuals with AIDS. Safety and efficacy of foscarnet have not been established for the treatment of other HSV infections (e.g., retinitis, encephalitis), congenital or neonatal HSV disease, or HSV infections in immunocompetent individuals.

The drugs of choice for the management of orolabial lesions or initial or recurrent genital lesions caused by HSV are valacyclovir, famciclovir, and acyclovir. For the management of mucocutaneous lesions caused by acyclovir-resistant HSV in HIV-infected adults and adolescents†, CDC, NIH, and IDSA recommend IV foscarnet as the drug of choice. These experts also recommend IV foscarnet as the drug of choice for the management of acyclovir-resistant HSV infections in HIV-infected children†.

Like other antivirals, foscarnet is not a cure for mucocutaneous HSV infections. While complete healing is possible, relapse occurs in most patients. Repeated foscarnet treatment of HSV infections has led to development of resistance that was associated with poor response. If there is a poor therapeutic response to foscarnet therapy, in vitro susceptibility testing of the HSV isolate is advised.

Clinical Experience Efficacy of IV foscarnet sodium for the treatment of mucocutaneous acyclovir-resistant HSV infections was evaluated in a study in AIDS patients that included 8 patients randomized to receive IV foscarnet sodium (40 mg/kg IV 3 times daily), 6 patients randomized to receive vidarabine (15 mg/kg daily; not commercially available in the US), and 11 patients nonrandomly assigned to receive treatment with IV foscarnet sodium because of prior intolerance to vidarabine. HSV lesions in the 8 patients randomized to foscarnet healed after 11–25 days and HSV lesions in 7 of the 11 patients nonrandomly treated with foscarnet healed in 10–30 days. In a second trial, 40 patients with AIDS and 3 bone marrow transplant recipients with mucocutaneous acyclovir-resistant HSV infections were randomized to receive IV foscarnet sodium (40 mg/kg 2 or 3 times daily). HSV lesions in 15 of the 43 patients healed in 11–72 days with no difference in response between the 2 groups.

Foscarnet sodium (40 mg/kg IV every 8 hours until clinical resolution is attained) often is effective in the treatment of acyclovir-resistant genital herpes. Limited data have shown that foscarnet may decrease duration of viral shedding and time required for crusting and healing of lesions, and the duration of positive cultures in AIDS patients with HSV infections that did not respond to oral or parenteral acyclovir therapy. However, eventual recurrence of HSV has been reported in virtually all such patients following discontinuance of foscarnet therapy; median time to recurrence reportedly was 42.5 days (range: 14–191 days) following discontinuance of the drug. Such recurrences may or may not be associated with acyclovir-resistant strains of the virus. In some patients who had received foscarnet (repeated or chronic therapy) for management of acyclovir-resistant HSV infection, foscarnet-resistant strains of the virus were reported. Patients who developed foscarnet-resistant HSV infections subsequently received oral or parenteral acyclovir or, alternatively, concomitant therapy with acyclovir and foscarnet.

■ Varicella-Zoster Virus Infections Foscarnet sodium is used in the management of acyclovir-resistant varicella-zoster virus (VZV) infections† in immunocompromised patients, including those with AIDS.

The preferred antivirals for the management of acute, localized herpes zoster (shingles) in HIV-infected adults and adolescents are acyclovir, famciclovir, and valacyclovir. For the management of proven or suspected acyclovir-resistant VZV infections† in HIV-infected adults or adolescents, CDC, NIH, and IDSA recommend IV foscarnet.

In HIV-infected children, acyclovir is the drug of choice for VZV infections and foscarnet is the preferred alternative for the management of acyclovir-resistant VZV infections†.

Although optimal regimens for the management of progressive outer retinal necrosis caused by VZV† in HIV-infected individuals have not been identified, CDC, NIH, and IDSA recommend treatment with at least one IV antiviral (acyclovir, ganciclovir, foscarnet, cidofovir) used in conjunction with at least one intravitreal antiviral (ganciclovir or foscarnet). Some experts recommend a regimen of IV ganciclovir and/or IV foscarnet used in conjunction with intravitreal ganciclovir and/or intravitreal foscarnet†. The prognosis for visual preservation in patients with progressive outer retinal necrosis caused by VZV is poor and such infections should be managed in consultation with an ophthalmologist.

Dosage and Administration

■ General Renal function *must* be assessed prior to initiation of foscarnet sodium and monitored during therapy with the drug. (See Renal Impairment under Dosage and Administration: Special Populations.)

To reduce the risk of foscarnet-associated nephrotoxicity, patients *must* receive adequate hydration prior to and during foscarnet sodium therapy.

The recommended dosage of foscarnet sodium and recommended frequency and rate of administration of the drug *must* not be exceeded.

Hydration Patients *must* be adequately hydrated before and during administration of foscarnet sodium.

Patients who are clinically dehydrated should have their hydration status corrected before the drug is initiated.

Prior to the first dose of foscarnet, patients should receive IV hydration with 750–1000 mL of 0.9% sodium chloride or 5% dextrose injection to establish diuresis. With each subsequent dose of foscarnet, 750–1000 mL of IV hydration fluid should be administered concurrently with each foscarnet sodium dose of 90–120 mg/kg or 500 mL of IV hydration fluid should be administered concurrently with each foscarnet sodium dose of 40–60 mg/kg. The volume of IV hydration fluid may be decreased if clinically appropriate.

Oral rehydration using similar regimens may be considered in some patients.

■ Administration Foscarnet sodium is administered by slow IV infusion using a controlled-infusion device (e.g., pump). The drug should *not* be administered by rapid IV infusion or direct IV injection since potentially toxic plasma foscarnet concentrations may result.

Foscarnet has been administered by intravitreal injection†; however, a preparation of the drug specifically for intravitreal administration is not commercially available in the US.

IV Infusion IV infusions of foscarnet sodium *must* be administered using a controlled-infusion device (e.g., pump) and the rate of administration carefully controlled to avoid adverse effects and unintentional overdosage.

Foscarnet sodium is commercially available as a solution for IV infusion containing 24 mg/mL.

If a central venous line is used for IV infusion, the commercially available solution of foscarnet sodium can be administered either undiluted or diluted.

If a peripheral vein is used for IV infusion, the commercially available solution of the drug *must* be diluted prior to administration with a compatible infusion solution to a concentration of 12 mg/mL. In addition, care should be taken to select a vein that will provide adequate blood flow for rapid dilution and distribution of the drug.

Foscarnet sodium solution should appear clear and colorless and should not be used if it appears discolored or contains particles.

Commercially available foscarnet sodium solution should be stored at 20–25°C. Precipitates may form if the solution is refrigerated or exposed to freezing temperatures, but may be brought into solution again if kept at room temperature with repeated shaking.

IV solutions of foscarnet sodium should *not* be admixed or administered through the same catheter with other drugs. Foscarnet sodium injection is physically and/or chemically incompatible with certain infusion solutions (e.g., calcium-containing solutions such as Ringer's or lactated Ringer's) and certain drugs (e.g., ganciclovir). Specialized references should be consulted for specific information.

Caution should be exercised when preparing and administering solutions of foscarnet sodium. Accidental skin and eye contact with solutions of the drug may cause local irritation and burning sensation. If accidental contact occurs, the exposed area should be flushed with water.

Dilution. When a diluted solution of foscarnet sodium is indicated for IV infusion (e.g., for infusion via a peripheral vein), the commercially available solution of the drug containing 24 mg/mL *must* be diluted with a compatible infusion solution (i.e., 0.9% sodium chloride injection or 5% dextrose injection) to a concentration of 12 mg/mL.

Diluted solutions of foscarnet sodium should be used within 24 hours after first entry into the sealed bottle.

Rate of Administration. IV infusions of foscarnet sodium should be administered at a constant rate using a controlled-infusion device (e.g., pump) and usually are given over 1–2 hours depending on dosage.

The IV infusion rate *must* not exceed 1 mg/kg per minute.

■ Dosage

Foscarnet is commercially available as the hydrated trisodium salt (i.e., foscarnet sodium); dosage is expressed in terms of foscarnet sodium.

Adult Dosage

Cytomegalovirus Retinitis. For the treatment of cytomegalovirus (CMV) retinitis in adults with human immunodeficiency virus (HIV) infection and normal renal function, the recommended dosage of IV foscarnet sodium for initial treatment (induction therapy) is 60 mg/kg (by IV infusion over at least 1 hour) every 8 hours for 14–21 days or 90 mg/kg (by IV infusion over 1.5–2 hours) every 12 hours for 14–21 days. In patients with immediate sight-threatening CMV retinal lesions (i.e., within 1.5 mm of the fovea), the US Centers for Disease Control and Prevention (CDC), National Institutes of Health (NIH), and HIV Medicine Association of the Infectious Diseases Society of America (IDSA) recommend that initial treatment also include an appropriate intravitreal antiviral. (See Cytomegalovirus Retinitis under Uses: Treatment of Cytomegalovirus Infection and Disease.)

After completion of initial treatment, the recommended dosage of IV foscarnet sodium for maintenance therapy (secondary prophylaxis) of CMV retinitis in adults with normal renal function is 90–120 mg/kg (by IV infusion over 2 hours) once daily. Because superiority of the 120-mg/kg daily dosage has not been established in controlled studies and because such dosage is likely to be associated with an increased risk of toxicity, the manufacturer recommends that most patients initially receive a maintenance dosage of 90 mg/kg IV once daily. However, dosage may be increased up to 120 mg/kg daily in patients in whom early reinduction therapy is required because of progression of CMV retinitis. In addition, some patients exhibiting excellent tolerance to the drug may benefit from early initiation of a maintenance dosage of 120 mg/kg daily.

Patients who experience relapse or progression of CMV retinitis while receiving foscarnet maintenance therapy may be retreated with foscarnet using the usual dosages for initial treatment (induction therapy) and maintenance therapy (secondary prophylaxis) or, alternatively, these patients may receive combination therapy with foscarnet and ganciclovir.

Decisions regarding discontinuance of maintenance therapy of CMV retinitis in HIV-infected individuals who have been treated for at least 3–6 months, have inactive CMV retinal lesions, and have achieved immune reconstitution as the result of antiretroviral therapy should be made in consultation with an ophthalmologist. (See Cytomegalovirus Retinitis under Uses: Treatment of Cytomegalovirus Infection and Disease.)

Cytomegalovirus Esophagitis or Colitis. If IV foscarnet sodium is used as an alternative for the management of CMV esophagitis† or colitis† in HIV-infected adults, CDC, NIH, and IDSA recommend a dosage of 60 mg/kg every 8 hours or 90 mg/kg every 12 hours given for 21–42 days or until signs and symptoms of the infection have resolved. Maintenance therapy (secondary prophylaxis) usually is not necessary, but should be considered if relapse occurs.

Cytomegalovirus Pneumonitis. If IV foscarnet sodium is used as an alternative for the management of well-documented CMV pneumonitis† in HIV-infected adults, CDC, NIH, and IDSA state that the same dosage recommended for the management of CMV retinitis in HIV-infected adults should be used. The optimal duration of treatment in such patients has not been established.

Cytomegalovirus Neurologic Disease. If IV foscarnet sodium is used in conjunction with IV ganciclovir for the management of CMV neurologic disease† in HIV-infected adults, CDC, NIH, and IDSA state that the same dosage recommended for the management of CMV retinitis in HIV-infected adults should be used. The optimal duration of treatment in such patients has not been established.

Mucocutaneous Herpes Simplex Virus Infections. For the management of mucocutaneous herpes simplex virus (HSV) infections known or suspected to be caused by acyclovir-resistant strains in immunocompromised patients, the manufacturer and some clinicians recommend that IV foscarnet sodium be given in a dosage of 40 mg/kg (by IV infusion over at least 1 hour) every 8 or 12 hours for 2–3 weeks or until clinical resolution. For the management of acyclovir-resistant genital herpes, CDC states that foscarnet sodium has been effective when given in a dosage of 40–80 mg/kg IV every 8 hours until clinical resolution.

For the management of acyclovir-resistant mucocutaneous HSV infections in HIV-infected adults, CDC, NIH, and IDSA recommend that IV foscarnet sodium be given in a dosage of 80–120 mg/kg daily in 2 or 3 divided doses until a clinical response is obtained.

Varicella-Zoster Virus Infections. For the management of mucocutaneous varicella-zoster virus (VZV) infections† known or suspected to be caused by acyclovir-resistant strains in immunocompromised patients, some clinicians recommend that IV foscarnet sodium be given in a dosage of 40–60 mg/kg IV every 8 hours for 10–21 days.

For the management of progressive outer retinal necrosis caused by VZV† in HIV-infected adults, CDC, NIH, and IDSA state that a regimen that includes IV foscarnet sodium in a dosage of 90 mg/kg IV every 12 hours (used with or without IV ganciclovir) in conjunction with intravitreal foscarnet† (used with or without intravitreal ganciclovir) can be considered.

Pediatric Dosage

Cytomegalovirus Retinitis. If IV foscarnet sodium is used with or without IV ganciclovir for initial treatment (induction therapy) of CMV retinitis in HIV-infected children†, CDC, NIH, IDSA, and others recommend a dosage of 60 mg/kg IV every 8 hours or 90 mg/kg IV every 12 hours for 14–21 days or until symptomatic improvement.

After completion of initial treatment, the recommended dosage of IV foscarnet sodium for maintenance therapy (secondary prophylaxis) of CMV retinitis in HIV-infected children† is 90–120 mg/kg IV once daily.

Decisions regarding discontinuance of maintenance therapy of CMV retinitis in HIV-infected individuals who have been treated for at least 3–6 months, have inactive CMV retinal lesions, and have achieved immune reconstitution as the result of antiretroviral therapy should be made in consultation with an ophthalmologist. (See Cytomegalovirus Retinitis under Uses: Treatment of Cytomegalovirus Infection and Disease.)

Disseminated Cytomegalovirus Infections. If IV foscarnet sodium is used with or without IV ganciclovir for initial treatment (induction therapy) of disseminated CMV infections in HIV-infected children†, CDC, NIH, IDSA, and others recommend a dosage of 60 mg/kg IV every 8 hours or 90 mg/kg IV every 12 hours until symptomatic improvement.

After completion of initial treatment, the recommended dosage of IV foscarnet sodium for maintenance therapy (secondary prophylaxis) of disseminated CMV infection in HIV-infected children† is 90–120 mg/kg IV once daily.

Mucocutaneous Herpes Simplex Virus Infections. If IV foscarnet sodium is used for the management of mucocutaneous acyclovir-resistant HSV infections in HIV-infected children†, CDC, NIH, IDSA, and others recommend a dosage of 40 mg/kg every 8 hours or 60 mg/kg every 12 hours (by IV infusion over 2 hours).

Varicella-Zoster Virus Infections. If IV foscarnet sodium is used for the management of VZV infections caused by acyclovir-resistant strains in HIV-infected children†, CDC, NIH, IDSA, and others recommend a dosage of 40–60 mg/kg (by IV infusion over 2 hours) given 3 times daily for 7–10 days or until no new lesions have appeared for at least 48 hours.

For the management of progressive outer retinal necrosis caused by VZV† in HIV-infected children, CDC, NIH, IDSA, and others state that a regimen that includes IV foscarnet given in a dosage of 90 mg/kg IV every 12 hours (used with or without IV ganciclovir) in conjunction with intravitreal foscarnet† given in a dosage of 1.2 mg/0.05 mL by intravitreal injection twice weekly (with or without intravitreal ganciclovir) can be considered.

■ Special Populations

Hepatic Impairment

The manufacturer makes no specific dosage recommendations for use of foscarnet sodium in patients with hepatic impairment; some clinicians state that dosage of the drug does not need to be adjusted in such patients.

Renal Impairment

In patients with impaired renal function, dosage of foscarnet sodium *must* be modified based on the degree of impairment. Dosage adjustment may be required in patients with initially normal renal function since most patients will experience a decrease in renal function during foscarnet therapy.

Renal function (i.e., measured and estimated creatinine clearance) should be assessed prior to initiating foscarnet sodium, 2 or 3 times weekly during induction therapy, and at least once every 1 or 2 weeks during maintenance therapy with the drug and dosage should be adjusted accordingly. (See Table 1 and Table 2.)

Dosage of foscarnet sodium should be based on the patient's measured or estimated creatinine clearance. Creatinine clearance (mL/minute per kg) should be calculated even if serum creatinine is within the normal range.

If creatinine clearance declines to less than 0.4 mL/minute per kg during foscarnet therapy, the drug should be discontinued and the patient should be hydrated and monitored daily until resolution of renal impairment is ensured.

To determine dosage of foscarnet sodium in patients with renal impairment, the patient's weight-adjusted 24-hour creatinine clearance (Ccr divided by body weight in kg) is used or Ccr (per kg) can be calculated using the following formulas:

$$Ccr\ (per\ kg)\ male = \frac{(140 - age)}{72 \times serum\ creatinine}$$

$$Ccr\ (per\ kg)\ female = 0.85 \times Ccr\ male$$

where age is in years and serum creatinine is in mg/dL

Table 1. Recommended Foscarnet Sodium Dosage for Initial Treatment (Induction Therapy) of CMV Retinitis or HSV Infections in Adults Based on Patient's Creatinine Clearance.

Creatinine Clearance (mL/minute per kg)	Induction Dosage for CMV (in mg/kg) Equivalent to 60 mg/kg Every 8 Hours	Induction Dosage for CMV (in mg/kg) Equivalent to 90 mg/kg Every 12 Hours	Induction Dosage for HSV (in mg/kg) Equivalent to 40 mg/kg Every 12 Hours	Induction Dosage for HSV (in mg/kg) Equivalent to 40 mg/kg Every 8 Hours
>1.4	60 every 8 hours	90 every 12 hours	40 every 12 hours	40 every 8 hours
>1–1.4	45 every 8 hours	70 every 12 hours	30 every 12 hours	30 every 8 hours
>0.8–1	50 every 12 hours	50 every 12 hours	20 every 12 hours	35 every 12 hours
>0.6–0.8	40 every 12 hours	80 every 24 hours	35 every 24 hours	25 every 12 hours
>0.5–0.6	60 every 24 hours	60 every 24 hours	25 every 24 hours	40 every 24 hours
≥0.4–0.5	50 every 24 hours	50 every 24 hours	20 every 24 hours	35 every 24 hours
<0.4	Not recommended	Not recommended	Not recommended	Not recommended

Table 2. Recommended Foscarnet Sodium Dosage for Maintenance Therapy of CMV Retinitis in Adults Based on Patient's Creatinine Clearance.

Creatinine Clearance (mL/minute per kg)	Maintenance Dosage for CMV (in mg/kg) Equivalent to 90 mg/kg Once Daily	Maintenance Dosage for CMV (in mg/kg) Equivalent to 120 mg/kg Once Daily
>1.4	90 every 24 hours	120 every 24 hours
>1–1.4	70 every 24 hours	90 every 24 hours
>0.8–1	50 every 24 hours	65 every 24 hours
>0.6–0.8	80 every 48 hours	105 every 48 hours
>0.5–0.6	60 every 48 hours	80 every 48 hours
≥0.4–0.5	50 every 48 hours	65 every 48 hours
<0.4	Not recommended	Not recommended

Dosage recommendations are not available for use of foscarnet sodium in patients undergoing hemodialysis. Use of the drug is not recommended in patients undergoing hemodialysis or peritoneal dialysis.

■ **Geriatric Patients** Dosage of foscarnet sodium for geriatric patients should be selected with caution because of age-related decreases in renal function. (See Geriatric Use under Warnings/Precautions: Specific Populations, in Cautions.)

Cautions

■ **Contraindications** Foscarnet sodium is contraindicated in patients with clinically important hypersensitivity to the drug.

■ **Warnings/Precautions** ***Warnings*** **Renal Effects.** Foscarnet appears to be nephrotoxic. Renal impairment and/or failure, manifested mainly as an increase in serum creatinine concentration and/or a decrease in creatinine clearance, is the major toxicity of foscarnet and occurs to some degree in most patients receiving the drug. Renal impairment may be accompanied by polyuria and associated polydipsia and, less frequently, by oliguria. In at least one patient, polyuria and polydipsia were attributed to nephrogenic diabetes insipidus temporally related to foscarnet therapy.

In initial clinical trials in patients with human immunodeficiency virus (HIV) infection and acquired immunodeficiency syndrome (AIDS) who received foscarnet sodium for the treatment of cytomegalovirus (CMV) retinitis, 27% of patients developed abnormal renal function. Approximately 33% of patients who received a dosage of 60 mg/kg 3 times daily *without* adequate hydration developed renal impairment (serum creatinine concentration of 2 mg/dL or greater). In subsequent clinical trials in patients who received 1 L of 0.9% sodium chloride or 5% dextrose injection with each dose of foscarnet, only 12% developed renal impairment.

Based on measurement of serum creatinine, renal impairment is most likely to become clinically evident during the second week of induction therapy in patients receiving foscarnet sodium in a dosage of 180 mg/kg daily; however, renal impairment may occur at any time during therapy with the drug. Foscarnet-induced increases in serum creatinine concentration are usually, but not uniformly, reversible following dosage adjustment or discontinuance of the drug, although maximum deterioration in renal function may not be apparent until several weeks after discontinuance of the drug. Foscarnet is removed by hemodialysis, and some clinicians have suggested that hemodialysis may be useful in the management of foscarnet-induced nephrotoxicity when elevated plasma concentrations of the drug are present and the degree of renal failure is severe.

The risk of foscarnet-induced renal impairment may be decreased by adequate hydration before and during administration of the drug. It is imperative that patients receive adequate hydration to establish diuresis prior to the first dose of foscarnet and also receive a recommended hydration regimen with each subsequent dose of the drug. (See Hydration under Dosage and Administration: General.)

The mechanism of foscarnet-induced nephrotoxicity has not been fully determined. While underlying disease and concomitant therapy may contribute to the development and degree of acute renal impairment in some patients, foscarnet alone appears to be nephrotoxic. Autopsy findings of extensive tubular necrosis have been reported in at least one patient, and clinical and laboratory findings in other patients, as well as evidence of a potential beneficial prophylactic effect of adequate hydration, have been consistent with acute tubulopathy. Biopsy or autopsy findings of tubular interstitial nephritis also have been reported, as well as the presence of crystals within glomerular capillary lumen; while positive identification was not made, the physicochemical characteristics of the crystals were suggestive of foscarnet crystals.

Because renal impairment is the principal toxicity of foscarnet and occurs to some degree in most patients receiving the drug, foscarnet must be used with caution, particularly in patients with a history of renal impairment, and it is imperative that renal function be assessed prior to initiation of foscarnet and continually during therapy with the drug and that dosage be modified as needed based on renal function. In patients with impaired renal function, reduced plasma clearance of foscarnet will result in elevated plasma concentrations of the drug; in addition, foscarnet potentially may further impair renal function in these patients. Therefore, dosage modification based on renal function (i.e., creatinine clearance) is essential.

The manufacturer recommends that creatinine clearance (measured or estimated based on serum creatinine) be determined at baseline prior to initiating foscarnet therapy, 2 or 3 times weekly during induction therapy, and at least once every 1 or 2 weeks during maintenance therapy, and dosage should be adjusted accordingly. More frequent monitoring may be necessary for some patients. It is also recommended that a 24-hour creatinine clearance be determined at baseline and periodically thereafter to ensure appropriate dosing (assuming verification of an adequate urine collection using the creatinine index). If creatinine clearance declines to less than 0.4 mL/minute per kg during foscarnet therapy, the drug should be discontinued and the patient should be hydrated and monitored daily until resolution of renal impairment is ensured. (See Renal Impairment under Dosage and Administration: Special Populations.)

Electrolyte and Metabolic Effects. Foscarnet therapy has been associated with changes in serum electrolyte concentrations, which potentially may contribute to the risk of cardiac disturbances and seizures. Hypocalcemia has occurred in 15–30%, hypophosphatemia in 8–26%, hyperphosphatemia in 6%, hypomagnesemia in 15–30%, and hypokalemia in 16–48% of patients receiving the drug. Hyponatremia, hypercalcemia, decreased body weight, acidosis, cachexia, and thirst (including polydipsia) have been reported in 1–5% of patients receiving foscarnet. The higher incidences of these electrolyte changes were derived from patients receiving hydration. Increased serum creatine kinase (CK; creatine phosphokinase, CPK) concentration, hematuria, and hypoproteinemia have been reported in less than 1% of patients. Rarely, nephrogenic diabetes mellitus has been associated with foscarnet therapy.

Foscarnet has been shown to produce a dose-related decrease in ionized serum calcium concentration that may not be reflected in total serum calcium concentration. Decreased serum concentrations of ionized calcium may result in symptoms such as perioral tingling, numbness in the extremities, or paresthesias. Foscarnet-induced changes in serum concentrations of calcium or other electrolytes most likely result from the drug's ability to chelate divalent metal ions, such as calcium and magnesium, and form stable coordination compounds.

Because foscarnet has a propensity to chelate divalent metal ions and alter serum concentrations of calcium and other electrolytes (including magnesium, potassium, or phosphate), which may contribute to the risk of cardiac disturbances and seizures, patients receiving the drug must be monitored carefully and frequently for such changes and their potential sequelae. The manufacturer recommends that serum calcium (particularly ionized calcium), magnesium, potassium, and phosphorous concentrations be determined on a schedule similar to that recommended for creatinine clearance. Foscarnet should be used with particular caution in patients with altered serum concentrations of calcium or other electrolytes at baseline and especially in those who have neurologic or cardiac abnormalities or are receiving other drugs known to influence electrolytes (especially calcium).

Patients should be advised about the symptoms of low ionized serum calcium concentration (e.g., perioral tingling, numbness in the extremities, paresthesias) and the importance of reporting such symptoms to a clinician. In patients who experience mild (e.g., perioral tingling) or severe (e.g., seizures) symptoms of electrolyte abnormalities, serum electrolyte concentrations should be determined as soon as possible in temporal relation to the symptoms. If adverse nervous system manifestations (e.g., perioral tingling) occur during IV infusion of foscarnet, the infusion should be discontinued, appropriate laboratory samples obtained for assessment of serum electrolyte concentrations, and a clinician consulted before resuming treatment; if the infusion is restarted, the rate of IV infusion should not exceed 1 mg/kg per minute. Clinicians should be prepared to treat manifestations resulting from electrolyte abnormalities, including severe manifestations such as tetany, seizures, or cardiac disturbances. Careful monitoring and appropriate management of serum electrolyte (including calcium and magnesium) concentrations are particularly important in patients with conditions that may predispose to seizures. (See Nervous System Effects under Warning/Precautions: Warnings, in Cautions.) Since the rate of infusion of foscarnet may affect the transient decrease in ionized serum calcium concentrations, a controlled-infusion device (e.g., pump) must be used for administration of foscarnet; in addition, slowing the rate of infusion may decrease or prevent symptoms.

Since foscarnet may decrease serum concentrations of ionized calcium, other drugs known to influence serum calcium concentrations should be administered concomitantly with caution. In addition, elimination of foscarnet may be impaired by drugs that inhibit renal tubular secretion, although no studies have been performed to determine whether this occurs. Because foscarnet may cause renal impairment, concomitant administration with other potentially nephrotoxic drugs (e.g., aminoglycosides, amphotericin B, IV pentamidine) should be avoided unless potential benefits outweigh possible risks. (See Drug Interactions.)

Nervous System Effects. Seizures related to mineral and electrolyte abnormalities have been associated with foscarnet therapy. Several cases of seizures were associated with death. Cases of status epilepticus have been reported. There have been at least 3 reports of seizures associated with overdosage of the drug. In initial clinical studies evaluating foscarnet in patients with AIDS, seizures occurred in 10% of patients; the rate of seizures did not increase with the duration of treatment.

Risk factors associated with seizures during foscarnet therapy have included impaired baseline renal function, low total serum calcium concentration, and underlying CNS conditions. Close monitoring of plasma electrolytes and minerals and appropriate electrolyte and/or mineral supplementation is particularly important in patients predisposed to seizures. (See Electrolyte and Metabolic Effects under Warnings/Precautions: Warnings, in Cautions.)

Cardiovascular Effects. Foscarnet therapy has been associated with prolongation of the QT interval, which may increase the risk of torsades de pointes. There have been postmarketing reports of torsades de pointes in patients receiving foscarnet. Some of these patients had confounding risk factors (e.g., underlying cardiac disease, electrolyte abnormalities, concomitant drug therapy). Foscarnet-associated transient changes in serum concentrations of calcium or other electrolytes may contribute to the risk of cardiac disturbances. (See Electrolyte and Metabolic Effects under Warnings/Precautions: Warnings, in Cautions.)

Foscarnet should be used with caution in patients with a history of QT-interval prolongation and in those receiving other drugs known to prolong the QT interval, those with electrolyte abnormalities, and those with other risk factors for QT-interval prolongation. Electrocardiograms (ECGs) and electrolyte concentrations should be assessed prior to and periodically during foscarnet therapy.

If any cardiovascular adverse effects occur, the foscarnet IV infusion should be stopped, electrolyte concentrations determined, and a clinician consulted before treatment with the drug is resumed.

Selection and Use of Antivirals. Foscarnet is labeled by the FDA *only* for the treatment of CMV retinitis in HIV-infected patients and the treatment of acyclovir-resistant mucocutaneous herpes simplex virus (HSV) infections in immunocompromised patients.

Safety and efficacy of foscarnet have not been established for the treatment of extraocular CMV infections (e.g., pneumonitis, gastroenteritis), congenital or neonatal CMV disease, or CMV disease in individuals not infected with HIV.

Safety and efficacy of foscarnet have not been established for the treatment of systemic HSV infections (e.g., retinitis, encephalitis), congenital or neonatal HSV disease, or HSV infections in immunocompetent individuals.

When used for the management of mucocutaneous HSV infections, repeated treatment with foscarnet has led to the development of resistance associated with poor response. If there is a poor therapeutic response to foscarnet therapy, in vitro susceptibility testing of the HSV isolate is advised.

Sensitivity Reactions

Hypersensitivity Reactions. Serious acute hypersensitivity reactions (e.g., anaphylactic shock, urticaria, angioedema) have been reported in patients receiving foscarnet.

If an acute hypersensitivity reaction occurs, foscarnet therapy should be discontinued and appropriate medical therapy should be immediately initiated.

Other Warnings and Precautions

Administration Precautions. To avoid local irritation, the commercially available preparation of foscarnet sodium containing 24 mg/mL *must* be diluted before IV administration via a peripheral vein. In addition, particular care must be taken to select a vein with adequate blood flow to permit rapid dilution and distribution of the drug. (See Dosage and Administration: Administration.)

Because of the potential for nephrotoxicity, patients *must* receive adequate hydration prior to the initial dose of foscarnet and also receive a recommended hydration regimen with each subsequent dose of the drug. (See Hydration under Dosage and Administration: General.)

To avoid unintentional overdosage, foscarnet *must* be administered by slow IV infusion using a controlled-infusion device (e.g., pump) to carefully control the infusion rate. (See Rate of Administration under Administration: IV Infusion, in Dosage and Administration.)

Genitourinary Effects. Local irritation and ulceration of the penile epithelium (resembling fixed drug eruption grossly but not histologically) have been reported in male patients and vulvovaginal ulceration has been reported in at least one female patient receiving foscarnet. The genital lesions are often painful, erythematous, and erosive and may require discontinuance of the drug. The lesions usually resolve spontaneously within several weeks after discontinuing foscarnet, but may recur when the drug is reinstituted. Occasionally, the lesions may resolve despite continued foscarnet therapy.

The local irritation and ulceration effects may be related to exposure to high concentrations of unchanged foscarnet in the urine; it also has been suggested that precipitation of the drug in arterioles and capillaries may contribute to ulceration. Adequate hydration and close attention to personal hygiene may minimize the risk of genital irritation and lesions associated with foscarnet therapy.

Hematologic Effects. Anemia, manifested as decreased hemoglobin concentration and hematocrit, is the most common adverse hematologic effect of foscarnet and has been reported in 33% of AIDS patients in controlled clinical trials receiving the drug for the treatment of CMV retinitis. The risk of anemia may be increased in patients receiving foscarnet and ganciclovir concomitantly for progressive retinitis.

Granulocytopenia was reported in 17% of AIDS patients with CMV retinitis receiving foscarnet in controlled clinical trials, but resulted in discontinuance of the drug in only 1% of patients. Leukopenia was reported in 5% or more of AIDS patients with CMV retinitis receiving foscarnet, while thrombocytopenia, platelet abnormalities, thrombosis, leukocyte abnormalities, and lymphadenopathy were reported in 1–5% and pancytopenia was reported in less than 1% of patients. Foscarnet generally is not myelosuppressive. Only 1% of patients did not complete clinical studies because of neutropenia.

Sodium Content. Commercially available foscarnet sodium solution containing 24 mg of the drug per mL contains 5.5 mg (0.24 mEq) of sodium per mL.

Foscarnet should be avoided in patients who may not tolerate large amounts of sodium or water (e.g., patients with cardiomyopathy) and in patients on a sodium-controlled diet.

Carcinogenic and Mutagenic Potential. Foscarnet caused genotoxic effects in the BALB/3T3 in vitro transformation assay at concentrations exceeding 0.5 mcg/mL and an increased frequency of chromosomal aberrations in the sister chromatid exchange assay at a concentration of 1 mg/mL. A high dose of foscarnet (350 mg/kg) produced an increase in micronucleated polychromatic erythrocytes in vivo in mice at doses that produced exposures (as measured by the area under the plasma concentration-time curve [AUC]) comparable to that anticipated clinically.

There was no evidence of oncogenicity in studies in rats and mice receiving oral foscarnet dosages of 500 and 250 mg/kg daily, respectively, which resulted in plasma foscarnet concentrations equal to 33 and 20%, respectively, of those in humans (at the maximum recommended human daily dose) as measured by the AUC.

Effects on Fertility. Foscarnet did not adversely affect fertility and general reproductive performance in rats. The results of perinatal and postnatal studies in rats were also negative; however, these studies used exposures that were inadequate to define the potential for impairment of fertility at human foscarnet exposure levels.

Specific Populations

Pregnancy. There are no adequate and well-controlled studies to date using foscarnet sodium in pregnant women. The drug should be used during pregnancy only when clearly needed.

Reproduction studies in female rats given subcutaneous foscarnet sodium in doses up to 75 mg/kg daily prior to and during mating, during gestation, and through 21 days postpartum caused a slight increase (less than 5%) in the number of skeletal anomalies compared with the control group. Daily subcutaneous doses up to 75 mg/kg administered to rabbits and 150 mg/kg administered to rats during gestation also caused an increased frequency of skeletal anomalies and variations. On the basis of estimated drug exposure (as measured by AUC), the 150- and 75-mg/kg doses were approximately one-eighth (rats) and one-third (rabbits) the estimated maximal daily human exposure. These data were inadequate to define the potential teratogenicity of foscarnet at dosages used in humans.

Lactation. It is not known whether foscarnet is distributed into human milk. In lactating rats that received a dose of 75 mg/kg, the drug was distributed in maternal milk at concentrations 3 times higher than peak maternal blood concentrations.

Since there is potential for serious adverse reactions to foscarnet in nursing infants, a decision should be made to discontinue nursing or the drug, taking into consideration the importance of the drug to the woman.

Because of the risk of adverse effects in the infant and the risk of HIV transmission, HIV-infected women should not breast-feed infants.

Pediatric Use. Safety and efficacy of foscarnet sodium have not been established in pediatric patients younger than 18 years of age.

The manufacturer states that the drug should be used in children† *only* after careful evaluation and *only* when potential benefits of the drug outweigh possible risks.

Some experts recommend foscarnet as the preferred alternative for the management of CMV retinitis, acyclovir-resistant mucocutaneous HSV infections, and acyclovir-resistant varicella-zoster virus (VZV) infections in HIV-infected children†.

In animals, foscarnet is deposited in teeth and bone and such deposition is greater in those that are young and growing. Foscarnet adversely affects tooth enamel development in mice and rats; the effects of drug deposition on skeletal development have not been studied. There is evidence that foscarnet accumulates in bone in humans, but the extent to which this occurs has not been studied. Since foscarnet is deposited in human bone, it is likely that it does so to a greater degree in developing bone in children.

Geriatric Use. Safety and efficacy of foscarnet have not been specifically studied in geriatric patients 65 years of age or older.

Adverse effects reported in patients 65 years of age or older have been similar to those reported in younger adults.

Because geriatric patients frequently have decreased renal function and because foscarnet is substantially excreted by the kidneys, particular attention should be paid to evaluating renal function prior to and during foscarnet therapy in this age group. If evidence of renal impairment exists or develops, appropriate dosage adjustments should be made. (See Renal Impairment under Dosage and Administration: Special Populations.)

Renal Impairment. Foscarnet sodium should be used with particular caution in patients with impaired renal function since reduced clearance of the drug will result in increased plasma concentrations and increase the risk of toxicity. In addition, foscarnet has the potential to further impair renal function in patients with preexisting renal impairment. (See Renal Effects under Warnings/Precautions: Warnings, in Cautions.)

Due to the risk of nephrotoxicity, renal function should be assessed at baseline and monitored carefully during foscarnet therapy. Dosage of the drug must be individualized and adjusted as needed based on renal function. (See Renal Impairment under Dosage and Administration: Special Populations.)

If creatinine clearance declines to less than 0.4 mL/minute per kg during foscarnet therapy, the drug should be discontinued and the patient should be hydrated and monitored daily until resolution of renal impairment is ensured.

Only limited safety and efficacy data are available regarding use of foscarnet in patients with baseline serum creatinine concentrations greater than 2.8 mg/dL or measured 24-hour creatinine clearances less than 50 mL/minute.

Foscarnet is not recommended in patients undergoing hemodialysis or peritoneal dialysis. Foscarnet is removed by hemodialysis.

■ **Common Adverse Effects** Adverse effects reported in 10% or more of patients receiving foscarnet include fever, nausea, anemia, diarrhea, abnormal renal function, vomiting, headache, seizures, and marrow suppression.

Drug Interactions

■ **Drugs Affecting Calcium** Because foscarnet sodium can decrease serum concentrations of ionized calcium, possibly because the drug chelates divalent metal ions such as calcium, extreme caution and close monitoring of serum electrolytes is advised if foscarnet is used concomitantly with other drugs known to influence serum calcium concentrations (e.g., IV pentamidine).

■ **Drugs That Prolong QT Interval** Because foscarnet sodium may increase the risk of QT-interval prolongation and the potential for torsades de pointes, concomitant use of foscarnet with drugs known to prolong the QT interval (e.g., class IA antiarrhythmics [procainamide, quinidine], class III antiarrhythmics [amiodarone, dofetilide, sotalol], other antiarrhythmic agents, phenothiazines, tricyclic antidepressants, certain macrolide antibiotics, certain fluoroquinolones) should be avoided. (See Cardiovascular Effects under Warnings/Precautions: Warnings, in Cautions.)

■ **Nephrotoxic Drugs** Concomitant use of foscarnet sodium with potentially nephrotoxic drugs (e.g., acyclovir, aminoglycosides, amphotericin B, cyclosporine, methotrexate, tacrolimus) may increase the risk of nephrotoxicity and should be avoided unless potential benefits outweigh potential risks. If foscarnet is used with another drug known to be nephrotoxic, renal function must be monitored closely.

■ **Antiretroviral Agents** ***Didanosine and Zidovudine*** There are no clinically important pharmacokinetic interactions between foscarnet and didanosine or zidovudine.

Ritonavir Abnormal renal function has been observed when foscarnet was used concomitantly with ritonavir (with or without saquinavir).

■ **Antivirals** ***Acyclovir*** Because acyclovir and foscarnet have both been associated with renal impairment, concomitant use of the drugs should be avoided unless potential benefits outweigh potential risks.

There was no in vitro evidence of antagonistic antiviral effects between acyclovir and foscarnet.

Cidofovir The manufacturer of cidofovir states that concomitant use of cidofovir and foscarnet is contraindicated and foscarnet must be discontinued at least 7 days prior to initiating cidofovir therapy.

Ganciclovir Concomitant use of ganciclovir and foscarnet does not affect the pharmacokinetics of either drug. However, ganciclovir and foscarnet are physically incompatible and *must* not be admixed. (See IV Infusion under Dosage and Administration: Administration.)

There was no in vitro evidence of antagonistic antiviral effects between ganciclovir and foscarnet. Although the clinical importance is unclear, some in vitro studies indicate that the combination of ganciclovir and foscarnet results in synergistic or additive antiviral effects against cytomegalovirus (CMV).

Letermovir In vitro, there was no evidence of antagonistic anti-CMV effects between letermovir and foscarnet.

■ **Diuretics** Concomitant use of foscarnet and loop diuretics may impair elimination of foscarnet due to inhibition of renal tubular excretion, which may lead to toxicity. If concomitant use of foscarnet and a diuretic is required, the manufacturer of foscarnet states that thiazide diuretics are preferred over loop diuretics.

■ **Pentamidine** Concomitant use of IV pentamidine and foscarnet may cause hypocalcemia; severe hypocalcemia resulting in death occurred in at least one patient receiving the drugs concomitantly. Renal impairment also has been observed when IV pentamidine and foscarnet were used concomitantly. Toxicity associated with concomitant use of foscarnet and pentamidine administered by oral inhalation via nebulization (aerosolized pentamidine) has not been reported.

Concomitant use of IV pentamidine and foscarnet should be avoided unless potential benefits outweigh potential risks. If the drugs are used concomitantly, extreme caution is advised and renal function should be monitored closely (e.g., daily assessment of renal function).

■ **Probenecid** There are no clinically important pharmacokinetic interactions between probenecid and foscarnet.

Description

Foscarnet (phosphonoformic acid), an organic analog of inorganic pyrophosphate, is an antiviral agent. The drug is commercially available as the trisodium salt. Foscarnet is structurally unrelated to other currently available antiviral agents. Unlike nucleoside and nucleotide antivirals (e.g., acyclovir, cidofovir, ganciclovir, valganciclovir), foscarnet does not require intracellular enzyme conversion to an active metabolite.

Foscarnet acts as a viral DNA polymerase inhibitor. The mechanism of action of foscarnet against herpesviruses involves selective inhibition of the pyrophosphate binding site on virus-specific DNA polymerases at concentrations that do not affect cellular DNA polymerases.

The pharmacokinetics of foscarnet sodium have been evaluated in patients with human immunodeficiency virus (HIV) infection and acquired immunodeficiency syndrome (AIDS) receiving intermittent IV infusions of the drug for the management of cytomegalovirus (CMV) retinitis. Considerable interindividual variation in plasma concentrations of the drug has been reported. Following a single 90-mg/kg dose of IV foscarnet sodium in one study, plasma concentrations of the drug ranged from 297–1775 mcg/mL. Foscarnet is distributed into CSF; the CSF-to-plasma ratio has been reported to be 0.2–0.7. Postmortem data indicate that foscarnet accumulates in human bones, but the extent to which this occurs has not been determined. In vitro studies indicate that foscarnet is 14–17% bound to plasma proteins. Foscarnet is not substantially metabolized and is principally excreted unchanged in urine by glomerular filtration. Following a single IV infusion of 60 mg/kg of foscarnet sodium, the plasma half-life of the drug was 1.9 hours in adults with normal renal function (creatinine clearance greater than 80 mL/minute) and approximately 3, 13, and 25 hours in those with creatinine clearances of 50–80, 25–49, and 10–24 mL/minute, respectively. However, the terminal half-life of foscarnet determined by urinary excretion has been reported to be 87.5 hours, most likely because of slow release of the drug from bone.

■ **Spectrum** Foscarnet is active in vitro against human herpesviruses, including CMV, herpes simplex virus types 1 and 2 (HSV-1 and HSV-2), and varicella-zoster virus (VZV). Although the clinical importance is unclear, foscarnet has some in vitro activity against Epstein-Barr virus (EBV) and human herpes viruses types 6 and 8 (HHV-6 and HHV-8). Foscarnet also has some in vitro activity against human hepatitis B virus (HBV) and human immunodeficiency virus types 1 and 2 (HIV-1 and HIV-2), but is not used for the treatment of infections caused by these viruses.

■ **Resistance** CMV and HSV isolates with reduced susceptibility to foscarnet have been selected in vitro in cell culture. In CMV strains, foscarnet resistance-associated substitutions are located in the viral DNA polymerase pUL54; in HSV strains, foscarnet resistance-associated substitutions are located in the viral DNA polymerase pUL30. Limited data are available on clinical resistance to foscarnet and several pathways to resistance likely exist.

Certain foscarnet resistance-associated substitutions also result in reduced susceptibility to some other antivirals (e.g., acyclovir, cidofovir, ganciclovir). In CMV strains, foscarnet resistance-associated substitutions associated with cross-resistance to ganciclovir and/or cidofovir have been identified. In HSV-1 and HSV-2 strains, foscarnet resistance-associated substitutions with cross-resistance to acyclovir have been identified; strains marginally cross-resistant to cidofovir also have been identified.

Advice to Patients

Advise patients that foscarnet is not a cure for cytomegalovirus (CMV) retinitis; progression and/or recurrence can occur, particularly during periods of continued immunosuppression. Regular ophthalmologic examinations are necessary.

Advise patients that foscarnet is not a cure for herpes simplex virus (HSV) infections. Although complete healing of HSV lesions is possible, relapse occurs in most patients. Repeated treatment with foscarnet may lead to development of resistance and poor response; in vitro susceptibility testing may be necessary if there is a poor therapeutic response or if relapse occurs.

Inform patients about the major toxicities of foscarnet (e.g., renal impairment, electrolyte disturbances, seizures) and that dosage modifications and possibly discontinuance of the drug may be necessary. The importance of close monitoring during foscarnet therapy must be emphasized.

Advise patients of the importance of adequate hydration to establish and maintain diuresis and minimize the risk of renal impairment during foscarnet therapy.

Advise patients of the importance of promptly informing clinicians if symptoms of electrolyte imbalance (e.g., perioral tingling, numbness in the extremities, paresthesias) or any cardiac symptoms occur during or after IV infusion of foscarnet. If such symptoms occur, the IV infusion should be stopped, electrolyte concentrations determined, and a clinician consulted before treatment with the drug is resumed.

Advise patients that dizziness and convulsions may occur during foscarnet therapy. Patients who experience seizures, dizziness, somnolence, or other adverse reactions that could result in cognitive impairment should avoid driving or operating machinery.

Importance of informing clinicians of existing or contemplated concomitant therapy, including prescription and OTC drugs, as well as any concomitant illnesses.

Importance of women informing clinicians if they are or plan to become pregnant or plan to breast-feed.

Importance of advising patients of other important precautionary information. (See Cautions.)

Overview® (see Users Guide). For additional information on this drug until a more detailed monograph is developed and published, the manufacturer's labeling should be consulted. It is *essential* that the manufacturer's labeling be consulted for more detailed information on usual cautions, precautions, contraindications, potential drug interactions, laboratory test interferences, and acute toxicity.

Preparations

Excipients in commercially available drug preparations may have clinically important effects in some individuals; consult specific product labeling for details.

Foscarnet Sodium

Parenteral		
Injection, for IV infusion only	24 mg/mL	**Foscavir®**, Hospira

†Use is not currently included in the labeling approved by the US Food and Drug Administration

Letermovir

■ Letermovir, an antiviral agent, is a DNA terminase complex inhibitor active against cytomegalovirus (CMV).

Uses

■ Prevention of Cytomegalovirus Infection and Disease Letermovir is used for prophylaxis to prevent cytomegalovirus (CMV) infection and disease in adult CMV-seropositive recipients (R^+) of an allogeneic hematopoietic stem cell transplant (HSCT). The drug has been designated an orphan drug by the US Food and Drug Administration (FDA) for prevention of CMV viremia and disease in at-risk populations.

CMV infection in transplant recipients can occur either as a primary infection in CMV-negative recipients of organs and cells from CMV-positive donors or as reactivation of latent CMV infection in CMV-seropositive recipients. CMV reactivation commonly occurs in CMV-seropositive transplant recipients and can result in severe CMV disease with substantial morbidity and mortality. The risk for CMV reactivation is greatest during the first 3 months after transplantation and depends on several factors, including the serologic status of the recipient and donor, CMV-specific T-cell immunity in the recipient, and immunosuppressive regimens used in the recipient. Certain antiviral strategies have been used to prevent severe, life-threatening CMV disease in transplant recipients, including antiviral prophylaxis (initiated posttransplantation and continued for at least 3 months) and/or preemptive antiviral treatment (i.e., initiated when CMV infection is detected, but before clinical progression to symptomatic CMV disease). These antiviral strategies each have certain advantages and disadvantages.

Safety and efficacy of letermovir for prophylaxis to prevent CMV infection and disease in solid organ transplant recipients or for preemptive treatment of CMV infection or disease in HSCT or solid organ transplant recipients have *not* been established.

Specialized references should be consulted for specific information regarding management of CMV infections in HSCT or solid organ transplant recipients.

Clinical Experience Efficacy and safety of letermovir for prevention of CMV infection and disease following allogeneic HSCT were assessed in a randomized, double-blind, placebo-controlled, phase 3 study that included 565 CMV-seropositive adults (median age 55 years, 57% male, 84% white, 9% Asian, 2% black, 7% Hispanic). The most common reasons for HSCT in these patients were acute myeloid leukemia (38%), myelodysplastic syndrome (16%), and lymphoma (12%). At baseline, 30% of the CMV-seropositive adults had one or more factors associated with increased risk for CMV reactivation and CMV disease (i.e., high-risk stratum) and 70% did not (i.e., low-risk stratum). Although enrolled patients had undetectable plasma CMV DNA levels within 5 days before randomization, 70 patients had detectable CMV viremia at the time study treatment was initiated and were excluded from the efficacy analysis. Patients were randomized in a 2:1 ratio to receive letermovir 480 mg once daily (240 mg once daily if used concomitantly with cyclosporine) or placebo. Letermovir or placebo was initiated within 28 days after HSCT (median time to initiation was 8 days after HSCT) and continued through week 14 (approximately 100 days) posttransplantation. Letermovir was administered orally or IV; dosage was the same for both routes of administration. Plasma CMV DNA levels were assessed once weekly through week 14 posttransplantation and then once every 2 weeks through week 24 and once every other month through week 48. The primary end point was clinically important CMV infection through week 24 posttransplantation (prophylaxis failure) in the primary efficacy population. Clinically important CMV infection was defined as either the occurrence of CMV end-organ disease or use of anti-CMV preemptive therapy initiated based on documented CMV viremia and clinical condition of the patient. Of the 495 patients in the efficacy analysis, 38 or 61% of patients receiving letermovir or placebo, respectively, experienced clinically important CMV infection by week 24.

Dosage and Administration

■ Administration Letermovir is administered orally or by IV infusion.

IV letermovir should be used only in patients unable to receive the drug orally. Patients receiving IV letermovir should be switched to the oral tablet as soon as they are able to receive oral drugs.

Oral Administration Letermovir tablets are administered orally without regard to food. The tablets should be swallowed whole.

IV Infusion Letermovir should be administered by IV infusion through a peripheral catheter or central venous line. The drug should *not* be administered by rapid IV injection.

Letermovir is commercially available as a preservative-free, sterile concentrate for injection that must be diluted prior to IV infusion. The concentrate should appear clear and colorless and should not be used if it appears discolored or contains particles.

Dilution. Letermovir in commercially available single-dose vials containing 240 or 480 mg of the drug (20 mg/mL) must be diluted with 0.9% sodium chloride injection or 5% dextrose injection prior to IV infusion. Letermovir is compatible *only* with 0.9% sodium chloride or 5% dextrose and should *not* be diluted using any other infusion fluids.

To prepare a 240- or 480-mg dose of letermovir, the entire contents of a single-dose vial labeled as containing 240 or 480 mg of the drug, respectively, should be withdrawn and added to a 250-mL prefilled IV bag containing either 0.9% sodium chloride injection or 5% dextrose injection. The bag should be mixed gently and should not be shaken.

The diluted letermovir solution should appear clear and may range from colorless to yellow in color. The solution should be inspected for particulate matter prior to administration and should be discarded if particles are observed.

Letermovir *must* be used only with compatible IV bag materials (e.g., polyvinyl chloride [PVC], ethylene vinyl acetate [EVA], polyolefin [polypropylene and polyethylene]); infusion set materials (e.g., PVC, polyethylene [PE], polybutadiene [PBD], silicone rubber [SR], styrene-butadiene copolymer [SBC], styrene-butadiene-styrene copolymer [SBS], polystyrene [PS]); plasticizers (e.g., diethylhexyl phthalate [DEHP], tris [2-ethylhexyl] trimelliatate [TOTM], benzyl butyl phthalate [BBP]; and catheters (e.g., radiopaque polyurethane). The use of letermovir with polyurethane-containing IV administration set tubing is not recommended.

Following dilution, letermovir solutions for IV infusion are stable at room temperature for up to 24 hours or under refrigeration (2–8°C) for up to 48 hours; this includes storage in the IV bag and the duration of IV infusion.

Rate of Administration. Letermovir solutions should be administered by IV infusion over 1 hour.

■ Dosage Dosage of oral and IV letermovir is identical. Dosage adjustments are not needed when switching from IV to oral administration.

Adult Dosage **Prevention of Cytomegalovirus Infection and Disease.** The recommended dosage of oral or IV letermovir for prevention of cytomegalovirus (CMV) infection and disease in adult CMV-seropositive recipients of an allogeneic hematopoietic stem cell transplant (HSCT) is 480 mg once daily.

Letermovir should be initiated within 28 days after HSCT (before or after engraftment) and should be continued through day 100 posttransplantation. Patients should be monitored for CMV reactivation after letermovir prophylaxis is discontinued.

Prevention of Cytomegalovirus Infection and Disease in Adults Receiving Cyclosporine. The recommended dosage of oral or IV letermovir for prevention of CMV infection and disease in adult CMV-seropositive recipients of an allogeneic HSCT who are receiving concomitant cyclosporine is 240 mg once daily.

If cyclosporine is initiated in a patient receiving letermovir 480 mg once daily, letermovir dosage should be decreased to 240 mg once daily.

If cyclosporine is discontinued in a patient receiving letermovir 240 mg once daily, letermovir dosage should be increased to 480 mg once daily.

If the cyclosporine regimen is interrupted because of high cyclosporine plasma concentrations in a patient receiving letermovir 240 mg once daily, the same letermovir dosage should be continued.

■ Special Populations ***Hepatic Impairment*** Dosage adjustments based on hepatic function are not needed if letermovir is used in patients with mild or moderate hepatic impairment (Child-Pugh class A or B).

Letermovir is not recommended in patients with severe hepatic impairment (Child-Pugh class C).

Renal Impairment Dosage adjustments based on renal function are not needed if letermovir is used in patients with creatinine clearances exceeding 10 mL/minute. Data are insufficient to make dosage recommendations for use of letermovir in patients with creatinine clearances of 10 mL/minute or less, including patients receiving dialysis.

When IV letermovir is used in patients with creatinine clearances less than

50 mL/minute, accumulation of the IV vehicle (i.e., hydroxypropyl betadex) may occur. (See Renal Impairment under Warnings/Precautions: Specific Populations, in Cautions.)

Geriatric Patients Dosage adjustments based on age are not needed.

Cautions

■ Contraindications Concomitant use of letermovir with pimozide or ergot alkaloids is contraindicated. (See Drug Interactions.)

Concomitant use of letermovir with pitavastatin or simvastatin is contraindicated in patients also receiving concomitant cyclosporine. (See Drug Interactions.)

■ Warnings/Precautions *Interactions* Concomitant use of letermovir with certain drugs may result in clinically important drug interactions, which could lead to adverse effects or reduced therapeutic effects of letermovir or the concomitant drug. (See Drug Interactions.)

The potential for drug interactions should be considered prior to and during letermovir therapy. Concomitant drugs should be reviewed and the patient should be monitored for adverse effects associated with letermovir and concomitant drugs.

Specific Populations **Pregnancy.** There are no adequate human data to assess whether letermovir adversely affects pregnancy outcomes.

In animal studies, embryofetal developmental toxicity (including fetal malformations) was observed in rats during organogenesis at letermovir exposures 11 times higher than human exposures at the recommended human dosage. No embryofetal developmental toxicity was observed in rabbits at exposures that were not maternally toxic (letermovir exposures up to 2 times higher than human exposures at the recommended human dosage). In a rat pre- and postnatal development study, total litter loss was observed at maternal letermovir exposures approximately 2 times higher than human exposures at the recommended human dosage.

Lactation. Letermovir is distributed into milk in lactating rats and is present in the blood of nursing pups.

It is not known whether letermovir is distributed into human milk, affects milk production, or affects the breast-fed child.

The developmental and health benefits of breast-feeding should be considered along with the mother's clinical need for letermovir and potential adverse effects on the breast-fed child from letermovir or from the underlying maternal condition.

Pediatric Use. Safety and efficacy of letermovir have not been established in pediatric patients younger than 18 years of age. Pharmacokinetics of the drug have not been evaluated in pediatric patients.

Geriatric Use. Approximately 15% of patients receiving letermovir in a phase 3 clinical study were 65 years of age or older and safety and efficacy of the drug were similar between older and younger adults.

Data indicate that age (18–78 years of age) does not have a clinically important effect on letermovir pharmacokinetics. Dosage adjustments based on age are not needed.

Hepatic Impairment. Letermovir is not recommended in patients with severe hepatic impairment (Child-Pugh class C). Dosage adjustments are not needed in patients with mild or moderate hepatic impairment (Child-Pugh class A or B).

Letermovir exposures are approximately 1.6- or 3.8-fold higher in individuals with moderate or severe hepatic impairment (Child-Pugh class B or C), respectively, compared with healthy individuals.

Renal Impairment. Safety of letermovir in patients with end-stage renal disease (creatinine clearance less than 10 mL/minute), including patients receiving dialysis, is not known. Dosage adjustments are not needed in patients with creatinine clearances exceeding 10 mL/minute.

Letermovir exposures are approximately 1.9- or 1.4-fold higher in individuals with moderate or severe renal impairment, respectively, compared with healthy individuals.

If IV letermovir is used in patients with creatinine clearances less than 50 mL/minute, serum creatinine concentrations should be closely monitored. Decreased elimination of the vehicle used in the IV letermovir preparation (hydroxypropyl betadex) has been reported in patients with severe renal impairment, and accumulation of the vehicle could occur when IV letermovir is used in patients with creatinine clearance less than 50 mL/minute.

It is not known if dialysis removes letermovir from systemic circulation.

■ Common Adverse Effects Adverse effects occurring in 10% or more of adults receiving letermovir and at a frequency at least 2% greater than placebo include nausea, diarrhea, vomiting, peripheral edema, cough, headache, fatigue, and abdominal pain.

Drug Interactions

■ Drugs Affecting or Metabolized by Hepatic Microsomal Enzymes Letermovir is a substrate of cytochrome P-450 (CYP) isoenzymes 3A and 2D6. In vitro, letermovir is not metabolized by CYP1A2, 2A6, 2B6, 2C8, 2C9, 2C18, 2C19, 2E1, or 4A11. The drug does not inhibit CYP1A2, 2A6, 2C9, 2C19, 2D6, or 2E1 and does not induce CYP1A2.

Letermovir is a moderate inhibitor of CYP3A; in vitro, letermovir also induces CYP3A. Concomitant use of letermovir with drugs that are CYP3A substrates (e.g., alfentanil, fentanyl, midazolam, quinidine) may result in clinically important increased plasma concentrations of such drugs. The magnitude of CYP3A-mediated drug interactions may be different when letermovir is used concomitantly with cyclosporine; drug interactions between cyclosporine and other drugs also should be considered.

In vitro, letermovir is a reversible inhibitor of CYP2C8. Concomitant use of letermovir and drugs that are CYP2C8 substrates may increase serum concentrations of such drugs.

Letermovir is expected to induce CYP2C9 and 2C19. Concomitant use of letermovir and drugs that are CYP2C9 or 2C19 substrates may decrease plasma concentrations of such drugs. Although the clinical importance is not known, letermovir induces CYP2B6 in vitro.

■ Drugs Affecting or Affected by Organic Anion Transporters Letermovir is a substrate of organic anion transporter polypeptide (OATP) 1B1 and 1B3. Concomitant use of letermovir with OATP1B1 or 1B3 inhibitors may result in increased letermovir plasma concentrations.

Letermovir inhibits OATP1B1, 1B3, and renal organic anion transporter (OAT) 3. Concomitant use of letermovir with drugs that are OATP1B1 or 1B3 substrates may result in clinically important increased plasma concentrations of such drugs.

The magnitude of OATP1B1- or 1B3-mediated drug interactions may be different when letermovir is used concomitantly with cyclosporine; drug interactions between cyclosporine and other drugs also should be considered.

The transport of letermovir is not mediated by and the drug does not inhibit OATP2B1 or OAT1.

■ Drugs Affecting or Metabolized by Uridine Diphosphate-glucuronosyltransferases Letermovir is metabolized by uridine diphosphate-glucuronosyltransferase (UGT) 1A1 and 1A3 to a minor extent. Clinically important changes in letermovir plasma concentrations are not expected if the drug is used concomitantly with UGT inhibitors.

In vitro, letermovir is not metabolized by UGT1A4, 1A6, 1A7, 1A8, 1A9, 1A10, 2B4, 2B7, 2B15, or 2B17 and does not inhibit UGT1A4, 1A6, 1A9, or 2B7.

■ Drugs Affected by P-glycoprotein Transport Letermovir is a substrate and an inhibitor of P-glycoprotein (P-gp) transport. Clinically important changes in letermovir plasma concentrations are not expected if the drug is used concomitantly with P-gp inhibitors.

■ Drugs Affecting or Affected by Other Membrane Transporters Letermovir inhibits breast cancer resistance protein (BCRP), bile salt export pump (BSEP), and multidrug resistance-associated protein (MRP) 2. The effects of letermovir on drugs that are BCRP, BSEP, and MRP2 substrates have not been evaluated and the clinical importance of any effect of letermovir on such drugs is not known.

In vitro, letermovir does not inhibit renal organic cation transporter (OCT) 1 or 2 and is not transported by OCT1, BCRP, or MRP2.

■ Antiarrhythmic Agents Concomitant use of letermovir and amiodarone is expected to increase amiodarone concentrations. If letermovir and amiodarone are used concomitantly, the patient should be closely monitored for amiodarone-associated adverse effects and amiodarone concentrations should be frequently monitored.

Concomitant use of letermovir and quinidine is expected to result in increased quinidine concentrations due to inhibition of CYP3A by letermovir. If letermovir is used concomitantly with quinidine in a patient also receiving cyclosporine, the magnitude of the CYP3A-mediated drug interaction may be different; drug interactions between cyclosporine and quinidine also should be considered.

■ Anticonvulsants Concomitant use of letermovir and phenytoin is expected to decrease phenytoin concentrations. If letermovir and phenytoin are used concomitantly, phenytoin concentrations should be frequently monitored.

■ Antidiabetic Agents Concomitant use of letermovir and certain antidiabetic agents (e.g., glyburide, repaglinide, rosiglitazone) is expected to increase concentrations of the antidiabetic agent.

If letermovir is used concomitantly with glyburide, repaglinide, or rosiglitazone, the patient's glucose concentrations should be frequently monitored. If the patient is receiving letermovir *and* cyclosporine, concomitant use of repaglinide is not recommended.

■ Antifungal Agents *Fluconazole* Concomitant use of letermovir and fluconazole does not result in clinically important pharmacokinetic interactions. Concomitant use of letermovir (single 480-mg dose) and oral fluconazole (single 400-mg dose) did not affect plasma concentrations or area under the plasma concentration-time curve (AUC) of either drug.

Posaconazole Concomitant use of letermovir and posaconazole does not result in clinically important pharmacokinetic interactions. Concomitant use of letermovir (480 mg once daily) and posaconazole (single 300-mg dose) did not affect plasma concentrations or AUC of posaconazole.

Voriconazole Concomitant use of letermovir (480 mg once daily) and voriconazole (200 mg twice daily) results in decreased voriconazole plasma concentrations and AUC.

If concomitant use of letermovir and voriconazole is required, the patient should be closely monitored for reduced voriconazole efficacy.

■ Antimycobacterial Agents Concomitant use of letermovir and rifampin is expected to decrease letermovir concentrations.

Concomitant use of letermovir and rifampin is not recommended.

■ **Antipsychotic Agents** Concomitant use of letermovir and pimozide is expected to increase pimozide concentrations due to inhibition of CYP3A by letermovir. Increased pimozide concentrations may lead to QT interval prolongation and torsades de pointes.

Concomitant use of letermovir and pimozide is contraindicated.

■ **Antiviral Agents** Concomitant use of letermovir and acyclovir does not result in clinically important pharmacokinetic interactions.

In vitro, there was no evidence of antagonistic anti-CMV effects between letermovir and certain cytomegalovirus (CMV) DNA polymerase inhibitors (i.e., acyclovir, cidofovir, foscarnet, ganciclovir).

■ **Digoxin** Concomitant use of letermovir and digoxin does not result in clinically important pharmacokinetic interactions.

■ **Ergot Alkaloids** Concomitant use of letermovir and ergot alkaloids (e.g., ergotamine, dihydroergotamine) is expected to increase concentrations of the ergot alkaloid due to inhibition of CYP3A by letermovir. Increased ergot alkaloid concentrations may lead to ergotism.

Concomitant use of letermovir and ergot alkaloids is contraindicated.

■ **Estrogens and Progestins** Concomitant use of letermovir and ethinyl estradiol or levonorgestrel does not result in clinically important pharmacokinetic interactions.

■ **HMG-CoA Reductase Inhibitors** ***Atorvastatin*** Concomitant use of letermovir (480 mg once daily) and atorvastatin (single 20-mg dose) results in 3.3- and 2.2-fold increases in atorvastatin AUC and peak plasma concentrations, respectively.

If letermovir and atorvastatin are used concomitantly, atorvastatin dosage should not exceed 20 mg daily and the patient should be closely monitored for myopathy and rhabdomyolysis.

If the patient is receiving letermovir *and* cyclosporine, concomitant use of atorvastatin is not recommended.

Fluvastatin, Lovastatin, Pravastatin, and Rosuvastatin Concomitant use of letermovir and fluvastatin, lovastatin, pravastatin, or rosuvastatin is expected to result in increased concentrations of the HMG-CoA reductase inhibitor (statin).

If letermovir is used concomitantly with fluvastatin, lovastatin, pravastatin, or rosuvastatin, dosage reduction of the statin may be required and the patient should be closely monitored for myopathy and rhabdomyolysis.

If the patient is receiving letermovir *and* cyclosporine, concomitant use of lovastatin is not recommended.

Pitavastatin and Simvastatin Concomitant use of letermovir and pitavastatin or simvastatin is expected to result in increased concentrations of the statin.

Concomitant use of letermovir with pitavastatin or simvastatin is not recommended.

If the patient is receiving letermovir *and* cyclosporine, concomitant use of pitavastatin or simvastatin is contraindicated.

■ **Immunosuppressive Agents** ***Cyclosporine*** Concomitant use of letermovir (240 mg once daily) and a single 200-mg dose of cyclosporine results in 2.1- and 1.5-fold increases in letermovir AUC and peak plasma concentrations, respectively. Concomitant use of letermovir (240 mg once daily) and a single 50-mg dose of cyclosporine results in a 1.7-fold increase in cyclosporine AUC, but does not have a substantial effect on cyclosporine peak plasma concentrations.

If letermovir and cyclosporine are used concomitantly, dosage of letermovir should be decreased to 240 mg once daily. (See Prevention of Cytomegalovirus Infection and Disease in Adults Receiving Cyclosporine under Dosage: Adult Dosage, in Dosage and Administration.) During concomitant use and after letermovir has been discontinued, cyclosporine whole blood concentrations should be frequently monitored and cyclosporine dosage should be adjusted accordingly.

Mycophenolate Mofetil Concomitant use of letermovir and mycophenolate mofetil does not result in clinically important pharmacokinetic interactions.

Sirolimus Concomitant use of letermovir (480 mg once daily) and sirolimus (single 2-mg dose) results in 3.4- and 2.8-fold increases in sirolimus AUC and peak plasma concentrations, respectively.

During concomitant use and after letermovir has been discontinued, sirolimus whole blood concentrations should be frequently monitored and sirolimus dosage should be adjusted accordingly.

Tacrolimus Concomitant use of letermovir (80 mg twice daily) and tacrolimus (single 5-mg dose) does not substantially affect letermovir exposures. Concomitant use of letermovir (480 mg once daily) and a single 5-mg dose of tacrolimus results in 2.4- and 1.6-fold increases in tacrolimus AUC and peak plasma concentrations, respectively.

During concomitant use and after letermovir has been discontinued, tacrolimus whole blood concentrations should be frequently monitored and tacrolimus dosage should be adjusted accordingly.

■ **Midazolam** Concomitant use of letermovir (240 mg once daily) and midazolam (single 1-mg IV dose) results in a 1.5-fold increase in midazolam AUC.

If letermovir is used concomitantly with midazolam in a patients also receiving cyclosporine, the magnitude of the CYP3A-mediated drug interaction may be different; drug interactions between cyclosporine and midazolam also should be considered.

■ **Opiate Agonists** Concomitant use of letermovir and alfentanil or fentanyl is expected to result in increased concentrations of the opiate agonist due to inhibition of CYP3A by letermovir. If letermovir is used concomitantly with alfentanil or fentanyl in a patient also receiving cyclosporine, the magnitude of the CYP3A-mediated drug interaction may be different; drug interactions between cyclosporine and alfentanil or fentanyl also should be considered.

■ **Proton-pump Inhibitors** Concomitant use of letermovir with omeprazole or pantoprazole is expected to decrease omeprazole or pantoprazole exposures.

If letermovir is used concomitantly with omeprazole or pantoprazole, the patient should be clinically monitored and dosage of the proton-pump inhibitor should be adjusted if needed.

■ **Warfarin** Concomitant use of letermovir and warfarin is expected to decrease warfarin concentrations. If letermovir and warfarin are used concomitantly, the international normalized ratio (INR) should be frequently monitored.

Description

Letermovir, a quinazoline antiviral agent, is a cytomegalovirus (CMV) DNA terminase complex inhibitor. CMV DNA terminase complex is a heterodimeric enzyme with several protein subunits (pUL51, pUL56, pUL89) and is required for viral DNA processing and packaging. Letermovir inhibits the terminase complex, thereby interfering with production of proper-length genomes and virion maturation.

Following oral administration of letermovir doses of 240–480 mg (without cyclosporine) in healthy individuals, oral bioavailability of the drug is 94%. In hematopoietic stem cell transplant (HSCT) recipients, oral bioavailability is 35% in those receiving letermovir 480 mg once daily (without cyclosporine) and 85% in those receiving letermovir 240 mg once daily (with cyclosporine). The median time to peak plasma concentrations following an oral dose of letermovir is 0.75–2.25 hours. When the drug is administered with food, peak plasma concentrations are 30% higher and the area under the plasma concentration-time curve (AUC) is similar to that observed when the drug is administered in the fasting state. Following IV infusion of letermovir, peak plasma concentrations occur at the end of the infusion. Steady-state concentrations are achieved within 9–10 days. Letermovir is 99% bound to plasma proteins. Following IV administration of letermovir 480 mg once daily, the mean terminal half-life is 12 hours. Letermovir is metabolized to a minor extent by uridine diphosphate-glucuronosyltransferase (UGT) 1A1 and 1A3 and is eliminated via hepatic uptake by organic anion transporter polypeptide (OATP) 1B1 and 1B3. Following a single oral dose of letermovir, 93% of the dose is excreted in feces (70% as unchanged drug) and less than 2% is excreted in urine.

■ **Spectrum** Letermovir is active in vitro and in vivo against human CMV (HCMV), a human herpesvirus. In vitro studies indicate that letermovir is more potent than ganciclovir against susceptible CMV and has been active against some ganciclovir-resistant strains.

Letermovir has a very limited spectrum of antiviral activity and does not have inhibitory activity in vitro against other herpesviruses or other important human pathogenic viruses tested, including adenovirus type 2, Epstein-Barr virus (EBV), hepatitis B virus (HBV), hepatitis C virus (HCV), herpes simplex virus types 1 and 2 (HSV-1, HSV-2), human herpesvirus type 6 (HHV-6), human immunodeficiency virus type 1 (HIV-1), influenza virus type A, and varicella-zoster virus (VZV).

■ **Resistance** CMV mutants with reduced susceptibility to letermovir have been selected in vitro in cell culture. Most letermovir resistance-associated substitutions reported to date involve pUL56 and positions 231 through 369. In a phase 3 clinical study evaluating letermovir in CMV-seropositive adult recipients of an allogeneic HSCT, viral samples from 2 patients experiencing prophylaxis failure who developed clinically important CMV infection indicated the presence of a letermovir resistance substitution at pUL56 V236M or C325W.

Cross-resistance between letermovir and antivirals in other classes (e.g., DNA polymerase inhibitors) is unlikely. Letermovir has been active against CMV isolates with substitutions conferring resistance to DNA polymerase inhibitors (e.g., cidofovir, foscarnet, ganciclovir) and these DNA polymerase inhibitors have been active against CMV isolates with substitutions conferring resistance to letermovir.

Advice to Patients

Importance of reading the patient information provided by the manufacturer.

Importance of not missing or skipping doses and importance of continuing letermovir for the duration recommended by the clinician.

If a dose of letermovir is missed, advise patients to take the dose as soon as it is remembered. If a dose is missed and not remembered until it is time for the next dose, the missed dose should be skipped and the regular dosing schedule should be resumed. Do not double up on the dose or take more than the prescribed dose.

If using letermovir tablets, advise patients that the tablets may be taken without regard to food and should be swallowed whole.

Advise patients that letermovir may interact with other drugs.

Importance of informing clinicians of existing or contemplated concomitant therapy, including prescription and OTC drugs, as well as any concomitant illnesses.

Importance of women informing clinicians if they are or plan to become pregnant or plan to breast-feed.

Importance of advising patients of other important precautionary information. (See Cautions.)

Overview® (see Users Guide). For additional information on this drug until a more detailed monograph is developed and published, the manufacturer's labeling should be consulted. It is *essential* that the manufacturer's labeling be consulted for more detailed information on usual cautions, precautions, contraindications, potential drug interactions, laboratory test interferences, and acute toxicity.

Preparations

Excipients in commercially available drug preparations may have clinically important effects in some individuals; consult specific product labeling for details.

Letermovir

Oral		
Tablets, film-coated	240 mg	**Prevymis®**, Merck
	480 mg	**Prevymis®**, Merck
Parenteral		
Concentrate, for injection, for IV infusion only	20 mg/mL (240 and 480 mg)	**Prevymis®**, Merck

ANTIPROTOZOALS 8:30

MISCELLANEOUS ANTIPROTOZOALS 8:30.92

Atovaquone

■ Atovaquone, a synthetic hydroxynaphthoquinone derivative, is an antiprotozoal agent.

Uses

■ **Pneumocystis jirovecii Pneumonia** Atovaquone is used as an alternative for treatment of *Pneumocystis jirovecii* (formerly *Pneumocystis carinii*) pneumonia (PCP) and prevention of *P. jirovecii* infections in patients who cannot tolerate co-trimoxazole. Atovaquone is designated an orphan drug by the US Food and Drug Administration (FDA) for treatment of PCP associated with acquired immunodeficiency syndrome (AIDS) and prevention of PCP in high-risk patients with human immunodeficiency virus (HIV) infection (i.e., history of one or more episodes of PCP and/or $CD4^+$ T-cell counts of 200/mm^2 or lower).

Treatment of Pneumocystis jirovecii Pneumonia Atovaquone is used alone as an alternative for treatment of mild to moderate PCP in patients who cannot tolerate co-trimoxazole, including HIV-infected adults, adolescents, and children†. The manufacturer states that clinical experience with atovaquone has been limited to patients with mild to moderate PCP, and use of the drug for treatment of more severe PCP has not been systematically studied.

Co-trimoxazole is the drug of choice for treatment of mild, moderate, or severe PCP, including PCP in HIV-infected adults, adolescents, and children.

The US Centers for Disease Control and Prevention (CDC), National Institutes of Health (NIH), and Infectious Diseases Society of America (IDSA) state that alternative regimens for treatment of mild to moderate PCP in HIV-infected adults and adolescents when co-trimoxazole cannot be used are dapsone in conjunction with trimethoprim, primaquine in conjunction with clindamycin, or atovaquone alone. These experts state that atovaquone may be less effective than co-trimoxazole for treatment of mild to moderate PCP, but has fewer adverse effects. Although efficacy and safety of atovaquone have not been established in pediatric patients and data are limited regarding use of the drug for treatment of PCP in children, CDC, NIH, IDSA, and the American Academy of Pediatrics (AAP) state that the drug also can be considered an alternative for treatment of mild to moderate PCP in HIV-infected children when co-trimoxazole cannot be used. Atovaquone is not included in CDC, NIH, IDSA, and AAP recommendations for treatment of severe PCP.

The indication for use of atovaquone for treatment of mild to moderate PCP is based on data from 2 randomized studies that evaluated efficacy and safety of atovaquone tablets (no longer commercially available in the US) compared with oral co-trimoxazole or IV pentamidine in patients with AIDS and results of comparative pharmacokinetic studies of atovaquone oral suspension and the previously available tablets. Mild to moderate PCP was manifested in these patients by an alveolar-arterial oxygen gradient (P_{A-aD}) of 45 mm Hg or less and an arterial oxygen pressure (PaO_2) on room air of 60 mm Hg or greater.

In the study evaluating comparative efficacy and safety of atovaquone tablets (750 mg 3 times daily for 21 days) or co-trimoxazole (320 mg of trimethoprim [as co-trimoxazole] 3 times daily for 21 days), improvement in clinical and respiratory measures that persisted for at least 4 weeks after discontinuance of treatment was observed in 62 or 64% of patients receiving atovaquone or co-trimoxazole, respectively. While adverse effects were substantially less likely in atovaquone-treated patients, results of this study suggest that failure to respond by day 21 of treatment was more likely in those treated with atovaquone (17%) than in those treated with co-trimoxazole (6%). Mortality rate (intent-to-treat analysis) also was higher in those treated with atovaquone (8%) than in those treated with co-trimoxazole (3.4%). In addition, while most fatalities in atovaquone-treated patients resulted from combined pneumocystis and bacterial infections, bacterial infections did not contribute to death in those receiving co-trimoxazole.

In the study evaluating comparative efficacy and safety of atovaquone tablets (750 mg 3 times daily for 21 days) or pentamidine (3–4 mg/kg given by single IV infusion daily for 21 days) in patients with mild to moderate PCP who could not tolerate co-trimoxazole or sulfonamides, improvement in clinical and respiratory measures that persisted for at least 4 weeks after discontinuance of treatment was observed in 57 or 40% of patients receiving atovaquone or pentamidine, respectively. In this study, failure to respond was more likely in those treated with atovaquone (29%) than in those treated with pentamidine (17%), but adverse effects were less likely with atovaquone (63%) than with pentamidine (72%). Mortality rates were similar (about 14%) in atovaquone- and pentamidine-treated patients.

In both comparative studies, there was a correlation between death and plasma atovaquone concentrations. Patients with lower plasma atovaquone concentrations (e.g., less than 5 mcg/mL on day 4 of treatment) were more likely to die while receiving the drug.

Prevention of Pneumocystis jirovecii Infections Atovaquone is used alone or in conjunction with pyrimethamine (and leucovorin) as an alternative for prevention of *P. jirovecii* infections in HIV-infected adults, adolescents, and children† who cannot tolerate co-trimoxazole.

The indication for use of atovaquone for prevention of PCP is based on data from 2 randomized, open-label studies that evaluated efficacy and safety of atovaquone oral suspension compared with either oral dapsone or aerosolized pentamidine in HIV-infected adults and adolescents at risk for PCP (i.e., $CD4^+$ T-cell counts less than 200/mm^2 or a prior episode of PCP). Results of the study comparing atovaquone (1.5 g once daily) and dapsone (100 mg once daily) indicated that both regimens were similarly effective for prevention of PCP (median duration of follow-up 24 months); this finding was consistent for patients receiving prophylaxis to prevent initial episodes of PCP (primary prophylaxis) and those receiving secondary prophylaxis to prevent recurrence. Results of the study comparing atovaquone oral suspension (750 mg or 1.5 g once daily) and aerosolized pentamidine (300 mg once monthly) indicated that both regimens were similarly effective for prevention of PCP (median duration of follow-up 11.3 months). There were no clinically important differences in mortality rates among any of the treatment groups.

Prevention of Initial Episode (Primary Prophylaxis). CDC, NIH, and IDSA recommend that primary prophylaxis to prevent initial episodes of PCP be initiated in HIV-infected adults and adolescents with $CD4^+$ T-cell counts less than 200/mm^3 or a history of oropharyngeal candidiasis. These experts state that primary PCP prophylaxis should be considered in HIV-infected adults and adolescents with $CD4^+$ T-cell percentages less than 14% or a history of an AIDS-defining illness who would not otherwise qualify for prophylaxis and also should be considered in those with $CD4^+$ T-cell counts greater than 200 but less than 250/ mm^3 if frequent monitoring of $CD4^+$ T-cell counts (e.g., every 3 months) is not possible.

CDC, NIH, and IDSA state that primary PCP prophylaxis should be discontinued in HIV-infected adults and adolescents who have responded to antiretroviral therapy and have $CD4^+$ T-cell counts that have remained greater than 200/mm^3 for longer than 3 months. Discontinuance of primary PCP prophylaxis is recommended in these individuals since it appears to add little benefit in terms of disease prevention (PCP, toxoplasmosis, bacterial infections) and discontinuance reduces the medication burden, cost, and potential for drug toxicity, drug interactions, and selection of drug-resistant pathogens. Primary PCP prophylaxis should be reinitiated if $CD4^+$ T-cell counts decrease to less than 200/mm^3.

Co-trimoxazole is the drug of choice for primary PCP prophylaxis in HIV-infected adults and adolescents. CDC, NIH, and IDSA recommend that co-trimoxazole prophylaxis be continued, if clinically feasible, in individuals who experience adverse reactions to the drug that are not life-threatening; however, co-trimoxazole prophylaxis should be permanently discontinued and an alternative used in those with life-threatening adverse reactions to the drug.

Alternative regimens recommended by CDC, NIH, and IDSA for primary PCP prophylaxis in HIV-infected adults and adolescents who cannot tolerate co-trimoxazole are dapsone alone, dapsone in conjunction with pyrimethamine (and leucovorin), aerosolized pentamidine, atovaquone alone, or atovaquone in conjunction with pyrimethamine (and leucovorin). In HIV-infected adults or adolescents who cannot tolerate co-trimoxazole and are seropositive for *Toxoplasma gondii*, dapsone with pyrimethamine (and leucovorin), atovaquone alone, or atovaquone with pyrimethamine (and leucovorin) would provide prophylaxis against both PCP and toxoplasmosis.

Prevention of Recurrence (Secondary Prophylaxis). CDC, NIH, and IDSA recommend that HIV-infected adults and adolescents who have a history of PCP receive long-term suppressive or chronic maintenance therapy (secondary prophylaxis) to prevent recurrence.

Secondary PCP prophylaxis generally is administered for life, unless immune recovery occurs as a result of antiretroviral therapy. CDC, NIH, and IDSA state that secondary PCP prophylaxis generally can be discontinued in HIV-infected adults and adolescents who have responded to antiretroviral therapy and have CD4+ T-cell counts that have remained greater than 200/mm^3 for longer than 3 months, but should be reinitiated if CD4+ T-cell counts decrease to less than 200/mm^3. In addition, these experts state that it may be prudent to continue secondary PCP prophylaxis for life (regardless of CD4+ T-cell count) if PCP occurred or recurred when CD4+ T-cell counts were greater than 200/mm^3.

Co-trimoxazole is the drug of choice for secondary PCP prophylaxis in HIV-infected adults and adolescents. CDC, NIH, and IDSA recommend that co-trimoxazole prophylaxis be continued, if clinically feasible, in individuals who experience adverse reactions to the drug that are not life-threatening; however, co-trimoxazole prophylaxis should be permanently discontinued and an alternative used in those with life-threatening adverse reactions to the drug.

Alternative regimens recommended by CDC, NIH, and IDSA for secondary PCP prophylaxis in HIV-infected adults and adolescents who cannot tolerate co-trimoxazole are the same as those recommended for primary prophylaxis and include dapsone alone, dapsone in conjunction with pyrimethamine (and leucovorin), aerosolized pentamidine, atovaquone alone, or atovaquone in conjunction with pyrimethamine (and leucovorin). In HIV-infected adults or adolescents who cannot tolerate co-trimoxazole and are seropositive for *T. gondii*, dapsone with pyrimethamine (and leucovorin), atovaquone alone, or atovaquone with pyrimethamine (and leucovorin) would provide prophylaxis against both PCP and toxoplasmosis.

Primary and Secondary Prophylaxis in Children. CDC, NIH, IDSA, and AAP recommend that primary prophylaxis to prevent initial episodes of PCP be initiated in HIV-infected children 1 to less than 6 years of age with CD4+ T-cell counts less than 500/mm^3 or CD4+ T-cell percentages less than 15% and in HIV-infected children 6–12 years of age with CD4+ T-cell counts less than 200/mm^3 or CD4+ T-cell percentages less than 15%. These experts recommend that all HIV-infected infants younger than 1 year of age (regardless of CD4+ T-cell count or percentage) receive primary PCP prophylaxis. In addition, infants born to HIV-infected mothers should be considered for primary PCP prophylaxis beginning at 4–6 weeks of age and those with indeterminate HIV status should continue to receive prophylaxis until they are determined to be non-HIV-infected or presumptively non-HIV-infected. Those found to be HIV-infected should receive primary PCP prophylaxis throughout the first year of life; at 1 year of age, the need for continued PCP prophylaxis should be reassessed based on age-specific CD4+ T-cell thresholds.

HIV-infected children who have a history of PCP should receive long-term suppressive or chronic maintenance therapy (secondary prophylaxis) to prevent recurrence.

CDC, NIH, IDSA, and AAP state that, in HIV-infected children who have received at least 6 months of antiretroviral therapy, discontinuance of primary or secondary PCP prophylaxis should be considered in those 1 to less than 6 years of age if CD4+ T-cell counts have remained at 500/mm^3 or greater or CD4+ T-cell percentages have remained at 15% or greater for more than 3 consecutive months and in those 6–12 years of age if CD4+ T-cell counts have remained at 200/mm^3 or greater or CD4+ T-cell percentages have remained at 15% or greater for more than 3 consecutive months. If primary or secondary PCP prophylaxis is discontinued in HIV-infected children, CD4+ T-cell counts and CD4+ T-cell percentages should be assessed every 3 months and PCP prophylaxis reinitiated if indicated based on age-specific CD4+ T-cell thresholds.

Co-trimoxazole is the drug of choice for primary and secondary PCP prophylaxis in HIV-infected infants and children. CDC, NIH, IDSA, and AAP recommend that co-trimoxazole be continued, if clinically feasible, in individuals who experience adverse reactions to the drug that are not life-threatening; however, co-trimoxazole should be permanently discontinued and an alternative used in those with life-threatening adverse reactions to the drug.

Alternative regimens recommended by CDC, NIH, IDSA, and AAP for primary and secondary PCP prophylaxis in HIV-infected infants and children who cannot tolerate co-trimoxazole are dapsone (1 month of age or older), atovaquone (1 month of age or older†), or aerosolized pentamidine (5 years of age or older).

■ Toxoplasmosis

Atovaquone is used as an alternative for treatment and prevention of toxoplasmosis caused by *Toxoplasma gondii*†, and is designated an orphan drug by FDA for primary prophylaxis in HIV-infected individuals at high risk for developing *T. gondii* encephalitis and for treatment and suppression of *T. gondii* encephalitis.

Treatment of Toxoplasmosis

Atovaquone is used in conjunction with pyrimethamine (and leucovorin), in conjunction with sulfadiazine, or alone as an alternative for treatment of toxoplasmosis†, including *T. gondii* encephalitis in HIV-infected adults and adolescents. Atovaquone regimens have not been evaluated for treatment of toxoplasmosis in HIV-infected infants and children.

CDC, NIH, IDSA, and AAP state that pyrimethamine (and leucovorin) in conjunction with sulfadiazine is the regimen of choice for initial treatment of toxoplasmosis, including toxoplasmosis in HIV-infected adults, adolescents, and children. Pyrimethamine (and leucovorin) in conjunction with clindamycin is the preferred alternative in HIV-infected adults and adolescents who are unable to tolerate sulfadiazine or failed to respond to the regimen of choice. CDC, NIH, and IDSA state that other alternative regimens that have been used for treatment of toxoplasmosis in HIV-infected adults and adolescents include co-trimoxazole alone, atovaquone in conjunction with pyrimethamine (and leucovorin), atovaquone in conjunction with sulfadiazine, atovaquone alone, or pyrimethamine (and leucovorin) in conjunction with azithromycin. Although these alternative regimens have been effective, comparative efficacies with the preferred and preferred alternative regimens have not been established. When a parenteral regimen is required for initial treatment of toxoplasmosis in severely ill HIV-infected adults or adolescents, some experts suggest parenteral co-trimoxazole or a regimen of pyrimethamine (and leucovorin) in conjunction with parenteral clindamycin.

Pregnant HIV-infected women with suspected or confirmed primary *T. gondii* infection should be managed in consultation with a specialist in maternal-fetal medicine or other appropriate specialists. CDC, NIH, and IDSA state that, despite concerns about use of pyrimethamine in pregnant women, treatment of toxoplasmosis in pregnant women generally should be the same as that in nonpregnant adults.

Pyrimethamine (and leucovorin) in conjunction with sulfadiazine also is the regimen of choice for treatment of congenital toxoplasmosis and for treatment of acquired CNS, ocular, or systemic toxoplasmosis in HIV-infected infants and children. The preferred alternative for treatment of toxoplasmosis in neonates and HIV-infected infants and children with sulfonamide sensitivity is pyrimethamine (and leucovorin) in conjunction with clindamycin; other alternative regimens that have been used in adults and adolescents have not been adequately studied in children. Empiric treatment of congenital toxoplasmosis should be strongly considered in infants born to HIV-infected women who had symptomatic or asymptomatic toxoplasmosis during pregnancy, regardless of whether the mother received toxoplasmosis treatment during the pregnancy.

Prevention of Toxoplasmosis

Atovaquone is used in conjunction with pyrimethamine (and leucovorin) or alone for primary prophylaxis to prevent initial episodes of toxoplasmosis† in HIV-infected adults, adolescents, and children† and is used in conjunction with pyrimethamine (and leucovorin), in conjunction with sulfadiazine, or alone for chronic maintenance therapy to prevent relapse of toxoplasmosis (secondary prophylaxis)† in HIV-infected individuals.

Prevention of Initial Episode (Primary Prophylaxis). CDC, NIH, and IDSA recommend primary prophylaxis against *T. gondii* encephalitis in HIV-infected adults and adolescents who are seropositive for *Toxoplasma* IgG antibody and have CD4+ T-cell counts less than 100/mm^3.

CDC, NIH, and IDSA state that primary toxoplasmosis prophylaxis should be discontinued in HIV-infected adults and adolescents who have responded to antiretroviral therapy and have CD4+ T-cell counts that have remained greater than 200/mm^3 for longer than 3 months. Discontinuance of primary toxoplasmosis prophylaxis is recommended in these individuals since it appears to add little benefit in terms of toxoplasmosis disease prevention and discontinuance reduces the medication burden, cost, and potential for toxicity, drug interactions, and selection of drug-resistant pathogens. Primary toxoplasmosis prophylaxis should be reinitiated in HIV-infected adults and adolescents if CD4+ T-cell counts decrease to less than 100–200/mm^3.

Co-trimoxazole is the drug of choice for primary toxoplasmosis prophylaxis in HIV-infected adults and adolescents. Dapsone in conjunction with pyrimethamine (and leucovorin) is the preferred alternative for such prophylaxis in HIV-infected adults and adolescents who cannot tolerate co-trimoxazole. CDC, NIH, and IDSA state that other alternatives for primary toxoplasmosis prophylaxis in those who cannot tolerate co-trimoxazole are atovaquone alone or atovaquone in conjunction with pyrimethamine (and leucovorin).

Prevention of Recurrence (Secondary Prophylaxis). CDC, NIH, and IDSA state that HIV-infected adults and adolescents who have completed initial treatment of *T. gondii* encephalitis should receive chronic maintenance therapy (secondary prophylaxis) to prevent relapse.

CDC, NIH, and IDSA state that secondary toxoplasmosis prophylaxis generally can be discontinued in HIV-infected adults and adolescents who have successfully completed toxoplasmosis treatment, remain asymptomatic with respect to toxoplasmic encephalitis, and have responded to antiretroviral therapy with CD4+ T-cell counts that have remained greater than 200/mm^3 for longer than 6 months. Limited data indicate that such individuals are at low risk for recurrence of toxoplasmic encephalitis. However, some experts would obtain a magnetic resonance image of the brain as part of their evaluation to determine whether discontinuance of secondary toxoplasmosis prophylaxis is appropriate. Secondary toxoplasmosis prophylaxis should be reinitiated in HIV-infected adults and adolescents if CD4+ T-cell counts decrease to less than 200/mm^3.

For secondary toxoplasmosis prophylaxis in HIV-infected adults and adolescents, the regimen of choice is pyrimethamine (and leucovorin) in conjunction with sulfadiazine. CDC, NIH, and IDSA state that alternative regimens for secondary toxoplasmosis prophylaxis in HIV-infected adults and adolescents are pyrimethamine (and leucovorin) in conjunction with clindamycin, atovaquone in conjunction with pyrimethamine (and leucovorin), atovaquone in conjunction with sulfadiazine, or atovaquone alone. Limited data indicate that co-trimoxazole may be another effective alternative for secondary toxoplasmosis prophylaxis in HIV-infected individuals.

Primary and Secondary Prophylaxis in Children. Although specific levels of immunosuppression that increase the risk for *T. gondii* encephalitis in HIV-infected children are less well defined than those for HIV-infected adults and adolescents, CDC, NIH, IDSA, and AAP recommend primary prophylaxis against *T. gondii* encephalitis in toxoplasma-seropositive HIV-infected children younger than 6 years of age who have CD4+ T-cell percentages less than 15% and in toxoplasma-seropositive HIV-infected children 6 years of age or older who have CD4+ T-cell counts less than 100/mm³. In addition, CDC, NIH, IDSA, and AAP state that all HIV-infected infants and children who have completed initial treatment of *T. gondii* encephalitis should receive chronic maintenance therapy (secondary prophylaxis) to prevent relapse.

The safety of discontinuing primary toxoplasmosis prophylaxis in HIV-infected children whose immunologic status improves in response to antiretroviral therapy has not been extensively studied. CDC, NIH, IDSA, and AAP state that primary toxoplasmosis prophylaxis should not be discontinued in HIV-infected children younger than 1 year of age. However, based on data from adults, these experts state that discontinuance of primary toxoplasmosis prophylaxis can be considered in HIV-infected children 1 to less than 6 years of age who have received at least 6 months of antiretroviral therapy and have CD4+ T-cell percentages that have remained at 15% or greater for longer than 3 months. In HIV-infected children 6 years of age or older who have received at least 6 months of antiretroviral therapy, primary toxoplasmosis prophylaxis can be discontinued if CD4+ T-cell counts have remained greater than 200/mm³ for longer than 3 months. Primary toxoplasmosis prophylaxis should be reinitiated if CD4+ T-cell percentages decrease to less than 15% in HIV-infected children younger than 6 years of age or if CD4+ T-cell counts decrease to less than 100–200/mm³ in HIV-infected children 6 years of age or older.

The safety of discontinuing secondary toxoplasmosis prophylaxis in HIV-infected children receiving antiretroviral therapy has not been extensively studied. However, based on data from adults, CDC, NIH, IDSA, and AAP state that discontinuance of secondary toxoplasmosis prophylaxis can be considered in HIV-infected children 1 to less than 6 years of age who have successfully completed toxoplasmosis treatment, remain asymptomatic with respect to toxoplasmic encephalitis, have received more than 6 months of stable antiretroviral therapy, and have CD4+ T-cell percentages that have remained at 15% or greater for more than 6 consecutive months. In HIV-infected children 6 years of age or older who have successfully completed toxoplasmosis treatment, remain asymptomatic with respect to toxoplasmic encephalitis, and have received more than 6 months of antiretroviral therapy, consideration can be given to discontinuing secondary toxoplasmosis prophylaxis if CD4+ T-cell counts have remained greater than 200/mm³ for more than 6 consecutive months. Secondary toxoplasmosis prophylaxis should be reinitiated in HIV-infected children if these age-based parameters are not met.

For primary toxoplasmosis prophylaxis in HIV-infected infants and children, the drug of choice is co-trimoxazole. Dapsone in conjunction with pyrimethamine (and leucovorin) is the preferred alternative for such prophylaxis in those 1 month of age or older who cannot tolerate co-trimoxazole. CDC, NIH, IDSA, and AAP state that atovaquone alone is another alternative for primary toxoplasmosis prophylaxis in HIV-infected children and adolescents 1 month of age or older; those 4–24 months of age can receive atovaquone alone or in conjunction with pyrimethamine (and leucovorin).

For secondary prophylaxis to prevent recurrence of toxoplasmosis in HIV-infected infants and children, the regimen of choice is sulfadiazine in conjunction with pyrimethamine (and leucovorin); pyrimethamine (and leucovorin) in conjunction with clindamycin is the preferred alternative for such prophylaxis in those who cannot tolerate sulfadiazine. CDC, NIH, IDSA, and AAP state that atovaquone alone is another alternative for secondary toxoplasmosis prophylaxis in HIV-infected children and adolescents 1 month of age or older; those 4–24 months of age can receive atovaquone alone or in conjunction with pyrimethamine (and leucovorin). Limited data indicate that co-trimoxazole may be another effective alternative for secondary toxoplasmosis prophylaxis in HIV-infected individuals, but is recommended in children only when pyrimethamine regimens are not tolerated.

■ **Babesiosis** Atovaquone is used in conjunction with azithromycin for treatment of babesiosis† caused by *Babesia microti*.

Although several species of *Babesia* can infect humans, *B. microti* is the most common cause of babesiosis in the US. *B. microti* is transmitted by *Ixodes scapularis* ticks, which also may be simultaneously infected with and transmit *Borrelia burgdorferi* (causative agent of Lyme disease) and *Anaplasma phagocytophilum* (causative agent of human granulocytotropic anaplasmosis [HGA, formerly known as human granulocytic ehrlichiosis]). Therefore, the possibility of coinfection with *B. burgdorferi* and/or *A. phagocytophilum* should be considered in patients who have severe or persistent symptoms despite appropriate anti-infective treatment for babesiosis. (See Lyme Disease in Uses: Spirochetal Infections and see Uses: Ehrlichiosis and Anaplasmosis, in the Tetracyclines General Statement 8:12.24.)

IDSA states that all patients with active babesiosis (i.e., symptoms of viral-like infection and identification of babesial parasites in blood smears or by polymerase chain reaction [PCR] amplification of babesial DNA) should receive anti-infective treatment because of the risk of complications; however, symptomatic patients whose serum contains antibody to babesia but whose blood lacks identifiable babesial parasites on smear or babesial DNA by PCR should not receive treatment. In addition, treatment is not recommended initially for asymptomatic individuals, regardless of the results of serologic examination, blood smears, or PCR, but should be considered if parasitemia persists for longer than 3 months.

When anti-infective treatment of babesiosis is indicated, IDSA and other clinicians recommend either a regimen of clindamycin and quinine or a regimen of atovaquone and azithromycin. The clindamycin and quinine regimen may be preferred in those with severe babesiosis. However, there is some evidence that, in patients with mild or moderate illness, the atovaquone and azithromycin regimen may be as effective and better tolerated than the clindamycin and quinine regimen. Patients with moderate to severe babesiosis should be monitored closely during treatment to ensure clinical improvement. Exchange transfusions have been used successfully in asplenic patients with life-threatening babesiosis, especially in severely ill patients with high levels of parasitemia (10% or more), significant hemolysis, or compromised renal, hepatic, or pulmonary function.

■ **Malaria** Results of studies evaluating use of atovaquone alone for treatment of *Plasmodium falciparum* malaria† indicate that, although an initial clinical response may occur, use of the drug alone is associated with an unacceptable rate of recrudescent parasitemia. Therefore, atovaquone should not be used alone for treatment of malaria.

A fixed-combination preparation containing atovaquone and proguanil hydrochloride (atovaquone/proguanil) is commercially available for treatment and prevention of malaria caused by *P. falciparum*, including chloroquine-resistant *P. falciparum* malaria. (See Atovaquone and Proguanil Hydrochloride 8:30.08.)

Dosage and Administration

■ **Administration** Atovaquone is administered orally.

Atovaquone must be taken with food to optimize GI absorption. (See Pharmacokinetics: Absorption.) Alternative therapy should be considered in patients who have difficulty taking atovaquone with food.

The multiple-dose bottle containing atovaquone oral suspension should be shaken gently before removing a dose.

If a single-dose foil pouch containing atovaquone oral suspension is used, the pouch should be opened by removing the perforated tab and the entire contents of the pouch ingested; the dose can be discharged from the pouch into a dosing spoon or cup or directly into the mouth.

■ **Dosage** ***Pneumocystis jirovecii* Pneumonia** **Treatment of Pneumocystis jirovecii Pneumonia.** When atovaquone monotherapy is used as an alternative for treatment of mild to moderate *Pneumocystis jirovecii* (formerly *Pneumocystis carinii*) pneumonia (PCP) in adults and adolescents 13 years of age or older, including those with human immunodeficiency virus (HIV) infection, the usual dosage is 750 mg twice daily given for 21 days.

When atovaquone monotherapy is used as an alternative for treatment of mild to moderate PCP in HIV-infected children and infants 1 month of age or older†, the US Centers for Disease Control and Prevention (CDC), National Institutes of Health (NIH), Infectious Diseases Society of America (IDSA), American Academy of Pediatrics (AAP), and others recommend a dosage of 30–40 mg/kg once daily in those 1–3 months of age, 45 mg/kg once daily in those 4–24 months of age, and 30–40 mg/kg once daily in those older than 24 months to 12 years of age given for 21 days. Alternatively, some experts recommend that infants 1–3 months of age receive 15–20 mg/kg twice daily, infants 4–24 months of age receive 22.5 mg/kg twice daily, and children older than 24 months to 12 years of age receive 15–20 mg/kg twice daily given for 21 days.

Prevention of Initial Episode (Primary Prophylaxis). When atovaquone is used as an alternative for primary prophylaxis of PCP in adults and adolescents 13 years of age or older, including HIV-infected individuals, the usual dosage is 1.5 g once daily given alone or, alternatively, in conjunction with oral pyrimethamine (25 mg once daily) and oral leucovorin (10 mg once daily). CDC, NIH, and IDSA state that primary PCP prophylaxis should be discontinued in HIV-infected adults and adolescents if CD4+ T-cell counts have remained greater than 200/mm³ for longer than 3 months in response to antiretroviral therapy, but should be reinitiated if CD4+ T-cell counts decrease to less than 200/mm³. (See Prevention of Pneumocystis jirovecii Infections under Uses: Pneumocystis jirovecii Pneumonia.)

When atovaquone monotherapy is used as an alternative for primary PCP prophylaxis in HIV-infected children and infants 1 month of age or older†, CDC, NIH, IDSA, AAP, and others recommend a dosage of 30–40 mg/kg once daily in those 1–3 months of age, 45 mg/kg once daily in those 4–24 months of age, and 30–40 mg/kg once daily in those older than 24 months to 12 years of age. In HIV-infected children 1 year of age or older who have received at least 6 months of antiretroviral therapy, CDC, NIH, IDSA, and AAP state that discontinuance of primary PCP prophylaxis should be considered based on age-related CD4+ T-cell counts or CD4+ T-cell percentages, but should be reinitiated if these parameters decrease below the age-related thresholds. (See Primary and Secondary Prophylaxis in Children under Pneumocystis jirovecii Pneumonia: Prevention of Pneumocystis jirovecii Infections, in Uses.)

Prevention of Recurrence (Secondary Prophylaxis). When atovaquone is used as an alternative for secondary PCP prophylaxis in adults and adolescents 13 years of age or older, including those with HIV infection, the usual dosage is 1.5 g once daily given alone or, alternatively, in conjunction with oral pyrimethamine (25 mg once daily) and oral leucovorin (10 mg once daily). CDC, NIH, and IDSA state that secondary PCP prophylaxis generally can be discontinued in HIV-infected adults and adolescents if CD4+ T-cell counts have remained greater than 200/mm³ for longer than 3 months in response to antiretroviral therapy, but should be reinitiated if CD4+ T-cell counts decrease to less than 200/mm³. However, secondary PCP prophylaxis probably should be continued for life (regardless of CD4+ T-cell count) if PCP occurred or recurred when CD4+ T-cell counts were greater than 200/mm³. (See Prevention of Pneumocystis jirovecii Infections under Uses: Pneumocystis jirovecii Pneumonia.)

When atovaquone monotherapy is used as an alternative for secondary PCP prophylaxis in HIV-infected children and infants 1 month of age or older†, CDC, NIH, IDSA, AAP, and others recommend a dosage of 30–40 mg/kg once daily in those 1–3 months of age, 45 mg/kg once daily in those 4–24 months of age, and 30–40 mg/kg once daily in those older than 24 months to 12 years of age. In HIV-infected children 1 year of age or older who have received at least 6 months of antiretroviral therapy, CDC, NIH, IDSA, and AAP state that discontinuance of secondary PCP prophylaxis should be considered based on age-related CD4+ T-cell counts or CD4+ T-cell percentages, but should be reinitiated if these parameters decrease below the age-related thresholds. (See Primary and Secondary Prophylaxis in Children under Pneumocystis jirovecii Pneumonia: Prevention of Pneumocystis jirovecii Infections, in Uses.)

Toxoplasmosis **Treatment of Toxoplasmosis.** When used as an alternative for treatment of toxoplasmosis† in HIV-infected adults and adolescents, atovaquone is given in a dosage of 1.5 g twice daily in conjunction with oral pyrimethamine (200-mg loading dose, then 50 mg once daily in those weighing less than 60 kg or 75 mg once daily in those weighing 60 kg or more) and oral leucovorin (10–25 mg once daily; may be increased to 50 mg once or twice daily).

Alternatively, HIV-infected adults and adolescents can receive atovaquone in a dosage of 1.5 g twice daily in conjunction with oral sulfadiazine (1 g every 6 hours in those weighing less than 60 kg or 1.5 g every 6 hours in those weighing 60 kg or more) for treatment of toxoplasmosis†.

Alternatively, HIV-infected adults and adolescents can receive atovaquone in a dosage of 1.5 g twice daily alone for treatment of toxoplasmosis†.

The treatment regimen should be continued for at least 6 weeks; a longer duration may be appropriate if clinical or radiologic disease is extensive or there is an incomplete response at 6 weeks.

Prevention of Initial Episode (Primary Prophylaxis). When used as an alternative for primary prophylaxis of toxoplasmosis† in HIV-infected adults and adolescents, CDC, NIH, and IDSA recommend that atovaquone be given in a dosage of 1.5 g once daily either alone or, alternatively, in conjunction with oral pyrimethamine (25 mg once daily) and oral leucovorin (10 mg once daily).

When used as an alternative for primary prophylaxis of toxoplasmosis in HIV-infected children and infants 1 month of age or older†, CDC, NIH, IDSA, and AAP recommend that atovaquone be given alone in a dosage of 30 mg/kg once daily in those 1–3 months of age or older than 24 months of age. In those 4–24 months of age, these experts recommend that atovaquone be given in a dosage of 45 mg/kg once daily alone or, alternatively, in conjunction with oral pyrimethamine (1 mg/kg or 15 mg/m² [up to 25 mg] once daily) and oral leucovorin (5 mg every 3 days).

CDC, NIH, and IDSA state that primary toxoplasmosis prophylaxis should be discontinued in HIV-infected adults and adolescents who have CD4+ T-cell counts that have remained greater than 200/mm³ for longer than 3 months in response to antiretroviral therapy, but should be reinitiated if CD4+ T-cell counts decrease to less than 100–200/mm³. The safety of discontinuing primary toxoplasmosis prophylaxis in HIV-infected children whose immunologic status improves on antiretroviral therapy has not been extensively studied. (See Prevention of Toxoplasmosis under Uses: Toxoplasmosis.)

Prevention of Recurrence (Secondary Prophylaxis). When used as an alternative for long-term suppressive or chronic maintenance therapy (secondary prophylaxis) to prevent recurrence of toxoplasmic encephalitis in HIV-infected adults and adolescents†, CDC, NIH, and IDSA recommend that atovaquone be given in a dosage of 750–1500 mg twice daily in conjunction with oral pyrimethamine (25 mg once daily) and oral leucovorin (10 mg once daily) or, alternatively, in conjunction with oral sulfadiazine (2–4 g daily in 2–4 divided doses). Alternatively, HIV-infected adults and adolescents can receive atovaquone in a dosage of 750–1500 mg twice daily alone.

When used as an alternative for secondary toxoplasmosis prophylaxis in HIV-infected children and infants 1 month of age or older†, CDC, NIH, IDSA, and AAP recommend that atovaquone be given alone in a dosage of 30 mg/kg once daily in those 1–3 months of age or older than 24 months of age. In those 4–24 months of age, these experts recommend that atovaquone be given in a dosage of 45 mg/kg once daily alone or, alternatively, in conjunction with oral pyrimethamine (1 mg/kg or 15 mg/m² [up to 25 mg] once daily) and oral leucovorin (5 mg every 3 days).

CDC, NIH, and IDSA state that secondary toxoplasmosis prophylaxis generally can be discontinued in HIV-infected adults and adolescents who have successfully completed toxoplasmosis treatment, remain asymptomatic with respect to toxoplasmic encephalitis, and have CD4+ T-cell counts that have remained greater than 200/mm³ for longer than 6 months in response to antiretroviral therapy. The safety of discontinuing secondary toxoplasmosis prophylaxis in HIV-infected children receiving antiretroviral therapy has not been extensively studied. (See Prevention of Toxoplasmosis under Uses: Toxoplasmosis.)

Babesiosis For treatment of babesiosis† caused by *Babesia microti*, IDSA recommends that adults receive atovaquone in a dosage of 750 mg twice daily for 7–10 days in conjunction with oral azithromycin (0.5–1 g on day 1, then 250 mg once daily for a total of 7–10 days; immunocompromised patients should receive an azithromycin dosage of 0.6–1 g daily).

For treatment of babesiosis† in pediatric patients. IDSA and other clinicians recommend that atovaquone be given in a dosage of 20 mg/kg (up to 750 mg) twice daily for 7–10 days in conjunction with oral azithromycin (10 mg/kg [up to 500 mg] once on day 1, then 5 mg/kg [up to 250 mg] once daily for a total of 7–10 days).

■ **Dosage in Renal and Hepatic Impairment** The pharmacokinetics of atovaquone in individuals with renal or hepatic impairment and the possible need for caution and/or dosage adjustment remain to be fully determined. The manufacturer states that atovaquone should be used with caution and close monitoring in patients with severe hepatic impairment.

Cautions

Although adverse effects associated with atovaquone therapy are common, the drug generally appears to be well tolerated. The most frequent adverse effects of atovaquone include rash, GI effects, fever, and headache.

In controlled clinical trials that evaluated atovaquone for treatment or prevention of *Pneumocystis jirovecii* (formerly *Pneumocystis carinii*) pneumonia (PCP), adverse effects were severe enough to require discontinuance of the drug in 9 or 25% of patients, respectively; there were no reports of adverse effects that were life-threatening or fatal. Because most HIV-infected patients receiving atovaquone have serious underlying disease with multiple baseline symptomatology and clinical abnormalities, many reported effects may not be directly attributable to the drug. In controlled clinical trials evaluating atovaquone for treatment of PCP, adverse effects were reported in 63% of patients receiving atovaquone and in 65 or 72% of those receiving oral co-trimoxazole or IV pentamidine, respectively. Treatment-limiting adverse effects were substantially less common with atovaquone than with co-trimoxazole or pentamidine. In one comparative study evaluating atovaquone for prevention of PCP, adverse effects were reported in 98 or 89% of individuals receiving atovaquone or aerosolized pentamidine, respectively. In another clinical study, adverse effects were reported in 20.2 or 43.4% of individuals receiving atovaquone or dapsone, respectively.

■ **Dermatologic and Sensitivity Reactions** Rash, which may be maculopapular, erythematous, or bullous, is the most common adverse effect of atovaquone, occurring in up to 39% of patients receiving the drug in controlled clinical trials. Rash generally is mild to moderate in severity, usually does not require discontinuance of the drug, and may resolve despite continued treatment. However, rash occasionally may be severe enough to require discontinuance of atovaquone. In controlled clinical trials, rash required discontinuance of the drug in 4–6% of patients. There is some evidence that rash may be associated with increased steady-state plasma concentrations of atovaquone.

Hypersensitivity reactions have been reported in up to 1% of patients receiving atovaquone in clinical studies. Pruritus was reported in 5% of patients receiving the drug in controlled clinical trials. There have been postmarketing reports of bronchospasm, throat tightness, and urticaria.

Erythema multiforme has occurred rarely in patients receiving atovaquone. Stevens-Johnson syndrome and skin desquamation have been reported in patients receiving a multiple-drug regimen that included atovaquone.

■ **GI Effects** Adverse GI effects are among the most frequently reported effects of atovaquone. Nausea occurred in up to 26%, diarrhea in up to 42%, and vomiting in up to 15% of patients receiving the drug in controlled clinical trials. Vomiting was the only adverse effect besides rash that required discontinuance of atovaquone in more than one patient in controlled clinical trials evaluating the drug for treatment of PCP. Approximately 4 or 3% of patients receiving atovaquone for PCP prophylaxis discontinued the drug because of diarrhea or nausea, respectively. Increased serum amylase concentration (exceeding 1.5 times the upper limit of normal) was reported in 8% of patients receiving the drug in controlled clinical trials. Abdominal pain was reported in up to 20%, constipation in 3%, anorexia in 7%, and dyspepsia in 5% of patients receiving atovaquone in controlled clinical trials. Taste perversion was reported in 3% of patients. Increased appetite has occurred rarely. Absorption of atovaquone may be limited in patients with a GI disorder. (See Cautions: Precautions and Contraindications.)

■ **Nervous System Effects** Headache is the most frequent adverse nervous system effect of atovaquone, occurring in up to 28% of patients receiving the drug in controlled clinical trials. Insomnia occurred in up to 10%, asthenia in up to 22%, dizziness in up to 8%, and anxiety in up to 7% of patients receiving atovaquone in controlled clinical trials. Pain was reported in up to 10% of patients receiving the drug, and dementia has been reported rarely.

■ **Hematologic Effects** The most common adverse hematologic effect of atovaquone is anemia (hemoglobin less than 8 g/dL, a decrease in hemoglobin of at least 2 g/dL, or need for transfusion), which occurred in about 6% of patients receiving the drug in controlled clinical trials. Neutropenia (absolute neutrophil count less than 750/mm³) was reported in 3% of patients receiving atovaquone in controlled clinical trials. Methemoglobinemia or thrombocytopenia has been reported in patients receiving atovaquone.

■ **Hepatic Effects** Increased serum alkaline phosphatase concentrations (exceeding 2.5 times the upper limit of normal) were reported in about 8% of patients receiving atovaquone in controlled clinical trials. Increases (exceeding 5 times the upper limit of normal) in serum concentrations of ALT and AST were reported in 6 and 4% of patients, respectively, receiving the drug in controlled clinical trials. In controlled clinical trials, about 2% of patients discontinued atovaquone because of increased serum ALT or AST concentrations. Increases in serum bilirubin concentrations have occurred rarely in patients receiving the drug.

There have been rare reports of hepatitis and at least one case of fatal liver failure in patients receiving atovaquone. A causal relationship between atovaquone and these events was not established because of confounding medical conditions and concomitant drug therapies.

Pancreatitis has been reported in atovaquone-treated patients.

■ **Renal and Electrolyte Effects** Increased BUN and serum creatinine concentrations have been reported rarely in patients receiving atovaquone and occasionally have required discontinuance of the drug.

Hyponatremia (less than 0.96 times the lower limit of normal range) was reported in up to 10% of patients receiving atovaquone in controlled clinical trials. Acute renal impairment has occurred in patients receiving atovaquone.

■ **Metabolic Effects** Hyperglycemia (exceeding 1.8 times the upper limit of normal) occurred in 9% of patients receiving atovaquone in controlled clinical trials. Hypoglycemia has occurred rarely.

■ **Other Adverse Effects** Fever was reported in up to 40% of patients receiving atovaquone in controlled clinical trials and occasionally has required discontinuance of the drug. Oral candidiasis was reported in 10%, cough in 25%, sweating in 10%, sinusitis in 7%, and rhinitis in 24% of patients receiving atovaquone in controlled clinical trials. Infection or dyspnea has occurred in 22 or 15% of patients receiving atovaquone. Hypotension, vortex keratopathy, transient sinus arrhythmia, increased serum creatine kinase (CK, creatine phosphokinase, CPK) concentrations, and transient conjunctivitis also have been reported rarely.

■ **Precautions and Contraindications** Atovaquone is contraindicated in patients who develop or have had a history of potentially life-threatening hypersensitivity reactions to the drug or any component of the formulation.

Clinical experience with use of atovaquone for treatment of PCP has been limited to patients with mild to moderate infections (alveolar-arterial oxygen diffusion gradient [P_{A-aD}] of 45 mm Hg or less). The drug has not been evaluated systematically for use in patients with more severe PCP or for use in patients who fail to respond to co-trimoxazole treatment. Clinical deterioration during atovaquone treatment of PCP could represent secondary infection with a nonsusceptible pathogen and/or progression of PCP. Atovaquone is not effective therapy for concurrent pulmonary conditions such as bacterial, viral, or fungal pneumonia or mycobacterial diseases. All patients with acute PCP for whom atovaquone treatment is being considered should be evaluated carefully for other possible causes of pulmonary disease and treated with additional agents as appropriate.

Patients should be instructed carefully regarding the importance of taking atovaquone concomitantly with food and the need to follow the prescribed dosage.

If achievement of adequate plasma atovaquone concentrations does not appear likely in any patient for whom therapy with the drug is being considered (e.g., those who have difficulty taking the drug with food), alternatives should be used. Atovaquone should be used with caution in patients with a GI disorder (e.g., chronic diarrhea, malabsorption syndrome), since absorption of the drug may be limited in these patients, possibly resulting in lower plasma concentrations than are required for adequate therapeutic response.

If atovaquone is given to patients with severe hepatic impairment, caution and close monitoring are advised.

■ **Pediatric Precautions** The manufacturer states that safety and efficacy of atovaquone in children have not been established. A relationship between atovaquone plasma concentrations and successful treatment of PCP has been established in adults. One study evaluating the pharmacokinetics and safety of atovaquone in children 4 months of age or older suggested that the drug is well tolerated in this age group. Results of a study using atovaquone oral suspension in HIV-infected, asymptomatic children 1 month to 13 years of age suggest that the pharmacokinetics of the drug is age related. The drug was well tolerated in these children.

■ **Geriatric Precautions** Although studies used to establish efficacy of atovaquone did not include a sufficient number of individuals 65 years of age or older to determine whether geriatric individuals respond differently to the drug than younger individuals, clinical experience to date has not identified differences in response between geriatric and younger adults.

The manufacturer recommends that atovaquone dosage for geriatric patients be selected with caution because of age-related decreases in hepatic, renal, and/or cardiac function and concomitant disease and drug therapy.

■ **Mutagenicity and Carcinogenicity** Atovaquone was not mutagenic in the Ames microbial (*Salmonella*) mutagen test, with or without metabolic activation, or in assays using mouse lymphoma or cultured human lymphocyte cells. The drug was not genotoxic in vivo in the mouse micronucleus assay.

No evidence of carcinogenicity was observed in studies in rats. In 24-month studies in mice, a treatment-related increased incidence in hepatocellular adenoma and hepatocellular carcinoma was observed at all doses evaluated (animal exposure ranged from 1.4–3.6 times the average steady-state atovaquone plasma concentration in humans receiving the drug for treatment of PCP).

■ **Pregnancy, Fertility, and Lactation** Reproduction studies in rats using atovaquone dosages resulting in plasma concentrations up to 2–3 times the estimated human exposure have not revealed evidence of teratogenicity. However, maternal and fetal toxicity (decreased mean fetal body lengths and weights and increased early fetal resorption and postimplantation fetal loss) did occur in rabbits receiving oral atovaquone dosages resulting in plasma concentrations approximately one-half the estimated human exposure. It is not clear whether these effects were caused by atovaquone or resulted from maternal toxicity. Atovaquone concentrations in rabbit fetuses averaged 30% of concurrent maternal plasma concentrations. In another study, atovaquone concentrations in rat fetuses following single ^{14}C-radiolabeled doses were 18% (middle gestation) and 60% (late gestation) of concurrent maternal plasma concentrations. There are no adequate and controlled studies to date using atovaquone in pregnant women, and the drug should be used during pregnancy only when the potential benefits justify the possible risks to the fetus.

Reproduction studies in rats using atovaquone dosages up to 1 g/kg daily (resulting in plasma concentrations up to 5 times the estimated human exposure) have not revealed evidence of impaired fertility.

It is not known whether atovaquone is distributed into human milk. The drug is distributed into breast milk of rats in concentrations 30% of concurrent maternal plasma concentrations. Atovaquone should be used with caution in nursing women.

Drug Interactions

■ **Protein-bound Drugs** Because atovaquone is highly bound to plasma proteins (99.9%), the drug should be used with caution in patients receiving other highly plasma protein-bound drugs with narrow therapeutic indices since competition for binding sites may occur.

■ **Antimycobacterial Agents** In HIV-infected adults, concomitant use of rifampin (600 mg once daily) and atovaquone suspension (750 mg twice daily) resulted in a 52% decrease in average steady-state plasma atovaquone concentrations and about a 40% decrease in the average plasma half-life of the drug; in addition, there was a 37% increase in the average steady-state plasma rifampin concentrations. It has been suggested that alternatives to rifampin be considered in patients receiving atovaquone.

Although specific studies have not been performed, it is possible that similar drug interactions could occur if rifabutin is used concomitantly with atovaquone since the drug is structurally similar to rifampin.

■ **Co-trimoxazole** Concomitant use of atovaquone suspension (500 mg once daily) and co-trimoxazole (800 mg of sulfamethoxazole and 160 mg of trimethoprim twice daily) had no clinically important effect on steady-state plasma concentrations of atovaquone. Although steady-state plasma concentrations of sulfamethoxazole and trimethoprim were decreased slightly, the effect is not expected to be clinically important.

■ **Metoclopramide** Concomitant use of metoclopramide and the fixed combination of atovaquone and proguanil hydrochloride (atovaquone/proguanil) has resulted in decreased bioavailability of atovaquone. Metoclopramide and atovaquone should be used concomitantly only if other antiemetics are not available.

■ **Phenytoin** Plasma protein binding of atovaquone does not appear to be affected by therapeutic concentrations of phenytoin (i.e., 15 mcg/mL) and vice versa.

■ **Tetracycline** Concomitant use of tetracycline and the fixed combination of atovaquone and proguanil hydrochloride (atovaquone/proguanil) has resulted in a 40% decrease in atovaquone plasma concentrations.

■ **Zidovudine** Although concomitant atovaquone can increase oral bioavailability of zidovudine, the clinical importance of this finding is not known. In a study in HIV-infected individuals who received atovaquone (750 mg orally twice daily) and zidovudine (200 mg orally every 8 hours), the apparent oral clearance of zidovudine and the ratio of glucuronide metabolite to parent compound was decreased; however, the effect was minor and would not be expected to produce clinically important effects. Zidovudine has no effect on the pharmacokinetics of atovaquone.

Mechanism of Action

The exact mechanism(s) of antiprotozoal action of hydroxynaphthoquinone derivatives, including atovaquone, has not been fully elucidated. The antiprotozoal activity of the drugs may be related principally to their ability to inhibit selectively mitochondrial electron transport with consequent inhibition of *de novo* pyrimidine synthesis. Unlike mammalian cells, certain protozoa are unable to salvage preformed pyrimidines, thus accounting for the preferential susceptibility (e.g., relative to human cells) of the latter organisms to the toxic effects of the drug. Hydroxynaphthoquinones may act as analogs of ubiquinone, which is involved in mitochondrial electron transport via dihydroorotate dehydrogenase, an important enzyme in pyrimidine synthesis. The site of action in the mitochondrial electron transport chain appears to be the cytochrome bc_1 complex (complex III).

The mechanism of action of atovaquone against *Pneumocystis jirovecii* (formerly *Pneumocystis carinii*) has not been fully elucidated.

Spectrum

Atovaquone is active in vitro and/or in vivo against a variety of protozoa, including *Toxoplasma gondii and Plasmodium*. Atovaquone also is active against the fungus *Pneumocystis jirovecii* (formerly *Pneumocystis carinii*).

Resistance

Pneumocystis jirovecii (formerly *Pneumocystis carinii*) with phenotypic resistance to atovaquone has not been identified in vitro. Although the clinical importance is unknown, clinical isolates of *P. jirovecii* with amino acid substitutions in cytochrome b (a likely target for atovaquone) have been obtained from several patients who developed *P. carinii* pneumonia (PCP) after receiving atovaquone prophylaxis.

Pharmacokinetics

■ **Absorption** Bioavailability of orally administered atovaquone is highly dependent on formulation and diet.

The commercially available oral suspension of atovaquone is approximately twofold more bioavailable in the fasting or fed state compared with the previously available tablet formulation of the drug. In HIV-infected adults, the absolute bioavailability of a 750-mg dose of atovaquone given under fed conditions was approximately 47% when the dose was given as the oral suspension compared with approximately 23% when the dose was given as tablets (no longer commercially available in the US).

Absorption of atovaquone is increased approximately twofold when administered with food. In HIV-infected adults receiving 500 mg of atovaquone daily as the oral suspension, peak plasma concentrations were approximately 15.1 mcg/mL when the drug was administered with food (400 kcal, 23 g fat) compared with approximately 8.8. mcg/mL when administered in the fasting state.

Plasma concentrations of atovaquone do not increase proportionally with the dose. In adults, when atovaquone oral suspension was administered with food in a dosage of 500 mg, 750 mg, or 1 g once daily, peak plasma concentrations of the drug were 15.1, 15.3, or 16.8 mcg/mL, respectively, and average steady-state plasma concentrations were 11.7, 12.5, or 13.5 mcg/mL, respectively.

In a study in HIV-infected, asymptomatic infants and children 1 month to 13 years of age, the pharmacokinetics of atovaquone were age related. When the oral suspension was given once daily with food in a dosage of 30 mg/kg for 12 days, average steady-state plasma concentrations of atovaquone were 27.8, 9.8, or 37.1 mcg/mL in those 1–3 months, older than 3 months to 24 months, or older than 2 years to 13 years of age, respectively,

■ **Distribution** Following IV administration, the volume of distribution of atovaquone at steady state is 0.6 L/kg.

Atovaquone is extensively (99.9%) bound to plasma proteins.

Low concentrations of atovaquone (less than 1% of plasma concentrations) were attained in CSF in 3 HIV-infected children receiving atovaquone tablets (no longer commercially available in the US) in a dosage of 750 mg 4 times daily for 2 weeks.

Animal studies indicate that atovaquone crosses the placenta.

Atovaquone is distributed into milk in rats in concentrations approximately 30% of concurrent maternal plasma concentrations. It is not known whether atovaquone is distributed into human milk.

■ **Elimination** There is some evidence that atovaquone undergoes limited metabolism; however, a specific metabolite has not been identified.

The half-life of atovaquone following administration of the oral suspension has ranged from 67–78 hours.

Atovaquone is presumed to undergo enterohepatic recirculation and is eventually eliminated in feces. More than 94% of an atovaquone dose is excreted unchanged in feces over 21 days; less than 0.6% is eliminated in urine.

Studies using the fixed combination of atovaquone and proguanil hydrochloride (atovaquone/proguanil) indicate that there are no marked differences in the rate or extent of systemic exposure to atovaquone in patients with mild or moderate hepatic impairment, but the elimination half-life of atovaquone is prolonged in those with moderate hepatic impairment.

Studies using atovaquone/proguanil indicate that clearance of atovaquone in patients with mild or moderate renal impairment is similar to that in those with normal renal function, but peak plasma concentrations and area under the plasma concentration-time curve (AUC) of atovaquone are decreased in those with severe renal impairment (creatinine clearance less than 30 mL/minute).

Chemistry and Stability

■ **Chemistry** Atovaquone is a synthetic hydroxynaphthoquinone-derivative antiprotozoal agent. Atovaquone is structurally and pharmacologically related to other hydroxynaphthoquinone derivatives (e.g., lapinone, menoctone, parvaquone, BW 58C), which initially were investigated for antimalarial activity. Various hydroxynaphthoquinones also have been shown to exhibit antiprotozoal activity (e.g., against toxoplasma, trypanosomes).

Atovaquone is commercially available for oral administration as an oral suspension. Atovaquone also is commercially available for oral administration in fixed combination with proguanil hydrochloride (atovaquone/proguanil). (See Atovaquone and Proguanil Hydrochloride 8:30.08.)

■ **Stability** Atovaquone oral suspension should be stored at 15–25°C and should not be frozen.

Preparations

Excipients in commercially available drug preparations may have clinically important effects in some individuals; consult specific product labeling for details.

Atovaquone

Oral		
Suspension	750 mg/5 mL*	Atovaquone Suspension
		Mepron®, GlaxoSmithKline

*available from one or more manufacturer, distributor, and/or repackager by generic (nonproprietary) name

†Use is not currently included in the labeling approved by the US Food and Drug Administration

metroNIDAZOLE
metroNIDAZOLE Hydrochloride

■ Metronidazole is a synthetic, nitroimidazole-derivative antibacterial and antiprotozoal agent.

Uses

■ **Amebiasis** Metronidazole is used orally in the treatment of acute intestinal amebiasis and amebic liver abscess caused by *Entamoeba histolytica*.

The regimen of choice for symptomatic intestinal amebiasis or extraintestinal disease (including liver abscess) is treatment with a nitroimidazole derivative (oral metronidazole or oral tinidazole) followed by treatment with a luminal amebicide (oral iodoquinol or oral paromomycin). The sequential use of these drugs ensures eradication of tissue-invading trophozoites as well as cysts in the intestinal lumen. In patients with severe disease who do not respond to or cannot tolerate these drugs, some clinicians suggest that a regimen of dehydroemetine (available in the US only from CDC) followed by a luminal amebicide be considered. Alternatively, hepatic abscess can be treated with a regimen of chloroquine phosphate and metronidazole (or tinidazole) or, if necessary, dehydroemetine followed by a therapeutic course of a luminal amebicide. However, these alternative regimens are associated with severe adverse effects and generally require hospitalization. Although some clinicians suggest use of oral tetracycline or oral erythromycin followed by a luminal amebicide for the treatment of mild or less severe colitis in patients who cannot tolerate metronidazole, this regimen will not eradicate trophozoites in the liver.

Metronidazole and tinidazole are not recommended for treatment of asymptomatic cyst passers because of limited activity against encysted *E. histolytica*. Asymptomatic cyst passers should be treated with a luminal amebicide such as iodoquinol, paromomycin, or diloxanide furoate (not commercially available in the US). For information on treatment of asymptomatic amebiasis, see Iodoquinol 8:30.04.

■ **Anaerobic and Mixed Aerobic-Anaerobic Bacterial Infections** Metronidazole is used orally or IV in the treatment of serious infections such as intra-abdominal infections (including peritonitis, intra-abdominal abscess, and liver abscess), gynecologic infections (including endometritis, endomyometritis, tubo-ovarian abscess, and postsurgical vaginal cuff infections), skin and skin structure infections, bone and joint infections, lower respiratory infections (including pneumonia, empyema, and lung abscess), CNS infections (including meningitis and brain abscess), septicemia, and endocarditis caused by susceptible anaerobic bacteria. Metronidazole has been effective in some *B. fragilis* infections which failed to respond to clindamycin, chloramphenicol, or penicillin. Prior to and during metronidazole therapy for bacterial infections, the causative organism should be cultured and in vitro susceptibility tests conducted, if possible. *Because metronidazole is inactive against most aerobic bacteria, appropriate anti-infectives should be used in conjunction with metronidazole in the treatment of mixed aerobic-anaerobic bacterial infections.* IV metronidazole is used in conjunction with cefepime for the treatment of complicated intra-abdominal infections caused by *Escherichia coli*, viridans streptococci, *Ps. aeruginosa*, *Klebsiella pneumoniae*, *Enterobacter*, or *Bacteroides fragilis* and is used in conjunction with ciprofloxacin for the treatment of complicated intra-abdominal infections caused by *E. coli*, *Ps. aeruginosa*, *P. mirabilis*, *K. pneumoniae*, or *B. fragilis*. Because brain abscesses often are polymicrobial and can include aerobic bacteria and aerotolerant anaerobes, which usually are resistant to metronidazole, appropriate anti-infectives also should be used in conjunction with the drug in the treatment of this infection. In some studies, IV metronidazole was ineffective in a large percentage of patients when used alone in the treatment of bacterial lung abscess or necrotizing pneumonia; treatment failures in these patients were presumably due to the presence of aerobic bacteria. Use of metronidazole does not replace surgical procedures when indicated.

■ **Bacterial Vaginosis** Metronidazole is used orally (as immediate-release tablets† or as extended-release tablets) or intravaginally (e.g., as a vaginal gel) for the treatment of bacterial vaginosis (formerly called *Haemophilus* vaginitis, *Gardnerella* vaginitis, nonspecific vaginitis, *Corynebacterium* vaginitis, or anaerobic vaginosis).

Bacterial vaginosis is a noninflammatory vaginal syndrome characterized by replacement of the normal vaginal flora (predominantly hydrogen peroxide-producing *Lactobacillus*) with a mixed flora including *Gardnerella vaginalis*, anaerobes (e.g., *Bacteroides ureolyticus, Prevotella, Porphyromonas, Peptostreptococcus, Mobiluncus*), and *Mycoplasma hominis*; vaginal discharge may be an unreliable indicator of infection since many women are asymptomatic. While *Gardnerella* previously was thought to be the sole causative agent of this syndrome, it currently is thought that bacterial vaginosis is a polymicrobial condition in which *Gardnerella* acts synergistically with anaerobic bacteria and genital mycoplasmas. Clinical diagnosis of the syndrome generally is established by characteristic vaginal manifestations rather than bacteriologic determinations. The presence of at least 3 of the following manifestations is considered diagnostic for bacterial vaginosis: a nonirritating, odoriferous, thin, homogeneous, grayish-white, noninflammatory vaginal discharge that smoothly coats the vaginal walls; a vaginal pH exceeding 4.5; the elaboration of malodorous amines ("fishy" odor) from discharge fluid after alkalinization with potassium hydroxide 10% ("whiff test"); and/or microscopic smears containing small coccobacillary organisms adherent to epithelial cells ("clue cells"). The presence of clue cells on wet mount examination of vaginal secretions is one of the most reliable indicators of bacterial vaginosis.

Gram stain results consistent with a diagnosis of bacterial vaginosis include markedly reduced or absent *Lactobacillus* morphology and predominance of *Gardnerella* morphotype. Although Gram stain of vaginal secretions also has been employed as a diagnostic test for bacterial vaginosis, accuracy of this method depends on evaluation by an experienced microbiologist; thus, this technique is used more often in research and hospital settings whereas diagnosis by clinical criteria typically is performed in an office setting. *Gardnerella* can be isolated from vaginal cultures in a large proportion of healthy women; because of this lack of specificity, culture for the organism is not recommended as a diagnostic method for bacterial vaginosis, and it is not used to guide therapy. The possibility of other pathogens commonly associated with vulvovaginitis or cervicitis (e.g., *Trichomonas vaginalis, Chlamydia trachomatis, Neisseria gonorrhoeae, Candida albicans*, herpes simplex viruses) generally should be ruled out, particularly since coinfection with these organisms may occur.

Goals of treatment and recommended therapy for bacterial vaginosis differ for nonpregnant versus pregnant women. However, relief of signs and symptoms of infection is a principal goal of therapy, and all women with *symptomatic* bacterial vaginosis should be treated regardless of pregnancy status.

Nonpregnant Women The principal goal in the treatment of bacterial vaginosis in nonpregnant women is to provide relief of vaginal symptoms and signs of infection. Other potential benefits include a reduction in other infectious complications, including human immunodeficiency virus (HIV) infection and other STDs. The CDC states that treatment of bacterial vaginosis is indicated in all nonpregnant women who are symptomatic. The CDC recommended regimens for treatment of bacterial vaginosis in nonpregnant women are a 7-day regimen of oral metronidazole (500 mg twice daily); a 5-day regimen of intravaginal metronidazole gel; or a 7-day regimen of intravaginal clindamycin cream. Alternative regimens recommended by the CDC for these women are a 7-day regimen of oral clindamycin or a 3-day regimen of intravaginal clindamycin suppositories. (See Uses: Bacterial Vaginosis in Metronidazole 84:04.04 or Clindamycin Phosphate 84:04.04.)

Intravaginal metronidazole results in clinical cure rates comparable to those reported with a 7-day oral metronidazole regimen; intravaginal clindamycin appears to be less effective than the metronidazole regimens. In 2 unpublished comparative studies conducted by the manufacturer of metronidazole extended-release tablets, nonpregnant women with bacterial vaginosis receiving oral metronidazole 750 mg daily (administered as extended-release tablets) for 7 consecutive days had similar (61 versus 59%) or higher (62 versus 43%) clinical cure rates at 28–32 days following completion of therapy than those receiving one applicatorful clindamycin phosphate (2% clindamycin) vaginal cream (100 mg of clindamycin) intravaginally once daily for 7 consecutive days. Regardless of the therapy chosen, relapse or recurrence of bacterial vaginosis is common, and some clinicians suggest that an alternative regimen (e.g., topical therapy when oral therapy was used initially) can be employed in such infections.

A single 2-g dose of oral metronidazole also has been used for the treatment of bacterial vaginosis, and has been recommended for patients who might be noncompliant with multiple-dose regimens. Several comparative studies in women with bacterial vaginosis suggest that a single 2-g dose of oral metronidazole is as effective as 7-day oral regimens of the drug (400 or 500 mg twice daily) when patients are evaluated 7–10 days after completion of therapy. In addition, pooled analysis of data from several randomized, controlled studies indicates that neither efficacy nor recurrence rate differ significantly between the treatment regimens, although analysis of data for recurrence rate was limited by the smaller number of patients evaluated for recurrence of infection. However, efficacy data from several controlled studies indicate an overall cure rate of 84–86% for the single 2-g dose regimen compared with 94–95% for the standard 7-day regimen (500 mg twice daily) and there is some evidence that the recurrence rate several weeks after completion of oral therapy may be higher with the single-dose regimen. Therefore, the CDC states that a 2-g single dose of oral metronidazole is no longer a recommended or alternative regimen for the treatment of bacterial vaginosis.

Pregnant Women An increased risk of obstetric complications, including intraamniotic infection, chorioamnionitis, premature rupture of membranes, preterm delivery, and low-birthweight infants, is associated with the presence of bacterial vaginosis in pregnant women, and the organisms found in increased concentrations in the genital flora of women with bacterial vaginosis are frequently found in patients with postpartum or postcesarean endometritis. Evidence from randomized, controlled trials indicates that systemic treatment of bacterial vaginosis reduces the rate of preterm birth in pregnant women at high risk for complications of pregnancy.

Because of the increased risk of adverse pregnancy outcomes associated with the presence of bacterial vaginosis, the CDC recommends that all *symptomatic* pregnant women be treated for bacterial vaginosis. In addition, because there is evidence from randomized studies that treatment of bacterial vaginosis in *asymptomatic* pregnant women at *high risk* for complications of pregnancy (e.g., those who previously delivered of a premature infant) has reduced preterm delivery, some experts recommend that all women at *high risk* be screened and treated for bacterial vaginosis. The CDC recommends that screening for bacterial vaginosis (if conducted) should be performed at the first prenatal visit and treatment initiated if needed.

The preferred regimens for the treatment of bacterial vaginosis in pregnant women are a 7-day course of oral metronidazole (500 mg twice daily or 250 mg 3 times daily) or a 7-day course of oral clindamycin (300 mg twice daily). (See Uses: Bacterial Vaginosis in Clindamycin 8:12.28.20.) Although some clinicians have recommended single-dose oral metronidazole as another alternative regimen for the treatment of bacterial vaginosis in pregnant women at high risk for complications of pregnancy, the safety and efficacy of this dosage schedule for the treatment of bacterial vaginosis in pregnant women have not been established and the manufacturer and other clinicians state that the single-dose regimen should *not* be used in pregnant women because it may result in slightly higher serum concentrations of the drug, which can reach the fetal circulation.

Although some experts state that intravaginal metronidazole may be used *solely* for symptomatic relief (and *not* for prevention of adverse pregnancy outcomes) in women at low risk for preterm delivery, others prefer use of systemic therapy for all pregnant women, regardless of degree of risk for complications of pregnancy, because systemic treatment may be required to eradicate upper genital tract infection that may be associated with bacterial vaginosis. Because recurrence of bacterial vaginosis is not unusual, and the treatment of this condition may prevent adverse pregnancy outcomes, particularly in women at high risk for complications of pregnancy, follow-up at 1 month to assess for cure and evaluate the need for additional treatment should be considered.

Although analysis of pooled data from case-control and cohort studies indicates that metronidazole therapy during pregnancy (including during the first trimester) is not associated with increased teratogenic risk or mutagenic effects in newborns, systemic therapy with metronidazole is contraindicated in the first trimester of pregnancy.

Women Undergoing Gynecologic Procedures and Surgery The goal of treatment of symptomatic bacterial vaginosis in women undergoing hysterectomy or abortion is to reduce the risk of infectious complications (e.g., pelvic inflammatory disease [PID]) following these procedures.

Treatment of asymptomatic bacterial vaginosis in patients who are about to undergo an invasive gynecologic procedure (e.g., endometrial biopsy, hysteroscopy, hysterosalpingography, hysterectomy, placement of an intrauterine device, uterine curettage), abortion, vaginal surgery, or abdominal surgery may be a reasonable consideration because of the association between this condition and various gynecologic infections (e.g., endometritis, PID, vaginal cuff cellulitis). A reduction in postoperative PID in women with bacterial vaginosis undergoing first-trimester elective abortion has been established in at least one study employing oral metronidazole, but further study is needed to determine the value of treating asymptomatic bacterial vaginosis in patients who are about to undergo other invasive procedures.

HIV-Infected Women Recommendations for treatment and preferred regimens for bacterial vaginosis in patients with concurrent HIV infection are the same as those for patients without HIV infection.

Sexual Contacts Results of several randomized, double-blind, placebo-controlled trials indicate that concurrent treatment of male sexual contacts of a woman with symptomatic bacterial vaginosis generally does not appear to affect the clinical cure rate, including the risk of relapse or recurrence of the syndrome, in the woman. Therefore, routine treatment of male sexual contacts currently is *not* recommended. Further study is needed to elucidate the possible role, if any, of sexual transmission in bacterial vaginosis.

■ **Balantidiasis** Oral metronidazole is recommended as an alternative to tetracycline for the treatment of balantidiasis† caused by *Balantidium coli*.

■ **Blastocystis hominis Infections** Oral metronidazole has been used in the treatment of *Blastocystis hominis* infections†. However, the clinical importance of *B. hominis* as a cause of GI pathology is controversial and it is unclear when treatment of *B. hominis* infection is indicated. If *B. hominis* is identified in stool specimens from symptomatic patients, other causes should be considered before assuming that GI symptoms are related to the organism. Some clinicians suggest that treatment be reserved for certain individuals (e.g., immunocompromised patients) who are symptomatic and in whom no other pathogen or process is found to explain the patient's GI symptoms. Metronidazole, iodoquinol, co-trimoxazole, or nitazoxanide have been used, but metronidazole resistance may be common.

■ Clostridium difficile-Associated Diarrhea and Colitis Oral metronidazole has been used effectively for the treatment of *Clostridium difficile*-associated diarrhea and colitis† (CDAD; also known as antibiotic-associated diarrhea and colitis, *C. difficile* diarrhea, *C. difficile* colitis, and pseudomembranous colitis) and, along with oral vancomycin hydrochloride, is considered the drug of choice for the treatment of *C. difficile*-associated diarrhea and colitis. Most experts and clinicians state that in order to decrease the incidence of vancomycin-resistant enterococci (see Resistance and also Uses in Vancomycin 8:12.28.16), metronidazole therapy should be used first in patients with *C. difficile*-associated diarrhea and colitis, reserving vancomycin therapy for seriously ill patients (i.e. those with severe or potentially life-threatening colitis), patients in whom metronidazole-resistant *C. difficile* is suspected, patients in whom metronidazole therapy is contraindicated or not tolerated, or those who do not respond to metronidazole. Oral metronidazole therapy also generally is preferred because of cost considerations. Diarrhea generally remits gradually over 3–5 days after initiation of oral metronidazole therapy, although resolution occasionally may take a week or longer, probably because of persistent inflammation despite cessation of toxin production.

Oral metronidazole appears to be as effective as oral vancomycin for the treatment of pseudomembranous colitis caused by *C. difficile.* However, the relative efficacy of oral metronidazole for *severe, potentially life-threatening* cases of pseudomembranous colitis remains unclear, and some clinicians continue to prefer vancomycin when anti-infective therapy is indicated for such cases (e.g., in critically ill patients).

Oral therapy is always preferred for the treatment of *C. difficile*-associated diarrhea and colitis, but the oral route may not always be feasible; the drugs should never be administered IV simply for reasons of convenience. Metronidazole has been effective when given IV for the treatment of *C. difficile*-associated diarrhea and colitis in patients in whom oral therapy was not feasible. Although IV therapy with metronidazole may not be as reliable as oral therapy, higher intracolonic drug concentrations are more likely with IV metronidazole than with IV vancomycin, and some clinicians suggest that parenteral metronidazole is the preferred treatment for this disease if oral therapy cannot be used (e.g., in patients with severe ileus or recent surgery). Because treatment failures have been reported with both IV metronidazole and IV vancomycin alone, some clinicians have suggested that both drugs be used if IV therapy is considered necessary (i.e., IV metronidazole combined with IV, enteral, intracolonic, or rectal vancomycin). Alternative approaches have included administration of metronidazole or vancomycin via a nasogastric tube, enterally (e.g., via placement of a tube or pigtail catheter into the small intestine, directly via an ileostomy), intracolonically (e.g., via a pigtail catheter positioned during colonoscopy), or rectally (e.g., via enema). However, the comparative efficacy of these approaches, particularly relative to oral therapy, has not been established.

Although oral metronidazole and intravaginal metronidazole have been associated rarely with causing antibiotic-associated diarrhea and colitis, including pseudomembranous colitis, most clinicians believe this should not discourage use of the drug in the treatment of *C. difficile*-induced diarrhea and/or colitis, especially if the clostridium strain is susceptible to the drug.

Relapse, which usually is apparent within several weeks (occasionally up to several months) and probably is secondary to persistent germinating *C. difficile* spores or reinfection with the same or a different strain, occurs in about 10–35% of patients treated with an effective anti-infective but generally responds to additional therapy with the same or an alternative anti-infective; true treatment failures (i.e., secondary to resistant strains) are rare. Alternative anti-infectives (e.g., bacitracin, fusidic acid, teicoplanin) have been suggested for the treatment of relapses; however, because such relapses rarely are caused by resistant strains, and established evidence of superior efficacy with such alternatives is lacking, treatment with oral metronidazole or oral vancomycin is preferred even in patients who received the respective drug previously. Patients should be advised that while relapses may be common, they do not have a tendency to become more severe, even though they may cause more concern with each episode. Because return of a protective normal fecal flora may be one of the most important factors in preventing relapses, unnecessary use of anti-infectives for prophylaxis or treatment of infections, particularly minor ones, should be avoided for at least 2 months after treatment of an episode of *C. difficile*-associated diarrhea and colitis.

No specific treatment regimen currently available in the US has been established through adequately designed studies to prevent multiple relapses of *C. difficile*-associated diarrhea and colitis, although standard anti-infective therapy (i.e., oral metronidazole or oral vancomycin) usually is effective in treating them even if it does not prevent further recurrences. Some clinicians have suggested that repeated relapses be treated with an intermittent regimen of oral metronidazole (or oral vancomycin when indicated) over several weeks or possibly months, followed by gradual tapering, or with low prophylactic doses of oral metronidazole given daily or on alternate days or weeks; however, while there may be anecdotal evidence of efficacy of such approaches, such positive findings may only have been coincidental rather than the result of the therapy. Anion-exchange resins such as cholestyramine (e.g., combined with the anti-infective regimen) also have been employed in an attempt to reduce the rate of relapse, but an established benefit of this approach is lacking, and these resins can bind to vancomycin in the colon and also can cause constipation and GI obstruction. Various other unproven measures (e.g.,, biotherapies such as *Lactobacillus*, nontoxigenic *C. difficile*, yogurt with live cultures, brewer's yeast) to restore the normal fecal flora also have been employed. One potentially promising approach has been administration of a live yeast preparation (i.e., *Saccharomyces boulardii*, which is different from the species in brewer's yeast) for about 4 weeks beginning several (e.g., 4) days after completion of appropriate anti-infective therapy. Combined oral vancomycin and rifampin also has been used for possible synergistic or other combined activity against the bacteria and/or its spores, but the role, if any, of this approach in the treatment of multiple relapses remains to be established.

Oral metronidazole or oral vancomycin also has been used to *prevent* nosocomial outbreaks of *C. difficile* diarrhea and colitis in institutionalized patients who asymptomatically harbor the organism. However, current evidence suggests that the risks of such prophylactic therapy (e.g., in selecting potentially resistant organisms such as enterococci), particularly with vancomycin, outweigh any possible benefit. Most experts currently recommend that appropriate enteric and barrier precautions (e.g., isolation of patients, private bathroom facilities, strict hygiene) rather than prophylactic anti-infective therapy be implemented to prevent nosocomial transmission of such organisms.

For additional information on *C. difficile*-associated diarrhea and colitis, see Cautions: GI Effects in Clindamycin 8:12.28.20.

■ Crohn's Disease Oral metronidazole (used with or without ciprofloxacin); has been used for the induction of remission of mildly to moderately active Crohn's disease†; the drug also has been used for refractory perianal disease. It appears that the combination of metronidazole and ciprofloxacin is more effective than metronidazole alone. Because the intestinal flora appears to have an association with intestinal inflammation and because metronidazole has a direct anti-inflammatory effect, metronidazole may be useful in the management of Crohn's disease as an adjunct to conventional therapies.

Reports on the efficacy of metronidazole in the management of active Crohn's disease have been equivocal. While results of several open-label, retrospective, comparative, and at least one placebo-controlled study indicate that metronidazole (with or without ciprofloxacin) can result in clinical response (e.g., improvement of clinical condition, clinical remission) in patients with mildly to moderately active Crohn's disease, results of other controlled and uncontrolled studies using metronidazole failed to show evidence of substantial beneficial effects on the clinical condition of the patients. In one double-blind, placebo-controlled study in patients with mildly to moderately active Crohn's disease, oral metronidazole, administered in dosages of 10 or 20 mg/kg daily for 16 weeks, was associated with substantial improvements in disease activity (measured by Crohn's Disease Activity Index [CDAI]); however, remission rates were similar to those reported with placebo. The CDAI score is based on subjective observations by the patient (e.g., the daily number of liquid or very soft stools, severity of abdominal pain, general well-being) and objective evidence (e.g., number of extraintestinal manifestations, presence of an abdominal mass, use or nonuse of antidiarrheal drugs, the hematocrit, body weight). Limited data indicate that metronidazole may be more effective in patients with ileocolitis or colitis rather than in those with ileitis.

Results of a randomized, double-blind, 2-period cross-over trial in 78 patients with active Crohn's disease suggest that oral metronidazole (400 mg twice daily) is at least as effective as sulfasalazine (1.5 g twice daily). Disease activity in this study was monitored by CDAI and serum orosomucoid concentrations. In the first treatment period, there was no significant difference in decreases in CDAI scores between patients receiving metronidazole or sulfasalazine, although decreases in serum orosomucoid concentrations were substantially more pronounced in those receiving metronidazole. After crossover, patients who had responded to the first drug have continued to respond to the other drug. Further studies are needed to determine the long-term efficacy and safety of metronidazole and the role of the drug in the treatment of this condition. Some clinicians suggest that metronidazole be reserved for patients in whom sulfasalazine is ineffective or not tolerated.

Safety and efficacy of concomitant use of metronidazole and ciprofloxacin have been evaluated in a 12-week comparative (versus methylprednisolone) study in 41 patients with active Crohn's disease (CDAI of more than 200 at the time of study entry). Patients were randomized to receive metronidazole 250 mg 4 times daily in conjunction with ciprofloxacin 500 mg twice daily (22 patients) or methylprednisolone (0.7–1 mg/kg daily initially, followed by variable tapering to 40 mg, and subsequent tapering of 4 mg weekly; 19 patients). At 12 weeks of therapy, clinical remission (defined as a CDAI of 150 points or less) has been reported in 63 or 46% of patients receiving the corticosteroid or the combination therapy, respectively. It has been suggested that such combination therapy could be an alternative to corticosteroids, although a high incidence of adverse effects (27% discontinued therapy because of such effects) was associated with the anti-infectives. In addition, results of a multicenter, randomized study in patients with active Crohn's disease indicate that addition of combination therapy with ciprofloxacin and metronidazole to budesonide does not provide greater benefit than budesonide alone; however, it has been suggested that this anti-infective combination may improve outcome in patients with Crohn's disease involving the colon. Results of several small placebo-controlled trials in patients with active Crohn's disease have shown no treatment benefit with metronidazole when compared with placebo. It is not known whether metronidazole is useful for prevention of recurrent disease.

Oral metronidazole has been used effectively for the treatment of refractory perineal Crohn's disease. Nonsuppurative perianal complications of the disease usually respond to metronidazole alone or when used in conjunction with ciprofloxacin. Results of an open-label trial in 21 adults with perineal

Crohn's disease who had an inadequate response to conventional therapies (e.g., corticosteroids, sulfasalazine, antibiotics, antimetabolites) indicate that administration of oral metronidazole (20 mg/kg daily) for 5–21 months decreased pain and tenderness within 1–2 weeks of therapy in 90% (19 out of 21) of patients, while decreases in erythema, drainage, and swelling and beginning of epithelization of open wounds were observed within 2–4 months of therapy in 86% (18 out of 21) patients. Complete healing (e.g., epithelization of ulcerations, closure of draining fistulas) of perianal disease has been reported in about 48% (10 out of 21) of patients; in addition, about 24% (5 out of 21) patients experienced advanced, but not complete healing of the perineum. Results of a follow-up study indicate that discontinuance or dosage reduction of metronidazole has been associated with exacerbation of disease activity in all patients, although perineal manifestations of the disease healed promptly, when full dosage of metronidazole was reinstituted. Although about 28% of patients, who received metronidazole for up to 16 months and in whom metronidazole was gradually discontinued experienced no relapse of the disease, some clinicians state that continuous therapy is needed to prevent recurrence of perineal disease. Because safety and efficacy of long-term metronidazole therapy have not been established, further study is needed to determine the long-term safety and efficacy of the drug in this condition. It has been suggested that patients be monitored for nervous system effects (e.g., peripheral neuropathy) during long-term administration of the drug. Limited data indicate that short-term (8 weeks) combination therapy with metronidazole and ciprofloxacin given with, or followed by, azathioprine (up to about 20 weeks) in patients with perineal Crohn's disease may result in rapid reduction of fistula drainage (induced by the antibiotics) and beneficial maintenance (associated with the azathioprine).

Although the manufacturers state that safe use of oral metronidazole in children for any indication except amebiasis has not been established, some clinicians state that children with mild perianal Crohn's disease† or those intolerant to sulfasalazine or mesalamine may receive oral metronidazole (10–20 mg/kg daily up to 1 g daily). In addition, although the manufacturers state that safe use of IV metronidazole in children for any indication have not been established, IV metronidazole has been used concomitantly with corticosteroids in children with moderately to severely active Crohn's disease† in whom infection or abscess was present.

For further information on the management of Crohn's disease, see Uses; Crohn's Disease, in Mesalamine 56:36.

■ **Dientamoeba fragilis Infections** Oral metronidazole is considered a drug of choice for the treatment of infections caused by *Dientamoeba fragilis*†. Many clinicians recommend iodoquinol, paromomycin, tetracycline, or metronidazole for the treatment of *D. fragilis* infections.

■ **Dracunculiasis** Oral metronidazole has been used in the treatment of dracunculiasis† caused by *Dracunculus medinensis* (guinea worm disease). Slow extraction of the worm and wound care is recommended by some clinicians as the treatment of choice. Although metronidazole therapy is not curative, it decreases inflammation and facilitates removal of the worm.

■ **Giardiasis** Oral metronidazole is used for the treatment of giardiasis† in adults and children.

Drugs of choice for treatment of giardiasis are metronidazole, tinidazole, or nitazoxanide; alternative agents include paromomycin (especially in pregnant women), furazolidone (no longer commercially available in the US), or quinacrine (not commercially available in the US).

Treatment of asymptomatic carriers of giardiasis is controversial. Although some clinicians suggest that asymptomatic carriers be treated if the risk of reinfection is low, the AAP states that treatment of asymptomatic carriers is not generally recommended, except possibly in patients with hypogammaglobulinemia or cystic fibrosis or in an attempt to prevent household transmission of the disease from toddlers to pregnant women. If asymptomatic carriers need to be treated, oral metronidazole may be used for such patients. Oral metronidazole also is used in patients with coexistent giardiasis and amebiasis. (See Giardiasis in Dosage and Administration: Dosage.)

Retreatment for recurrences of giardiasis, either from relapse or reinfection, depends on individual and epidemiologic circumstances. Retreatment with the same initial regimen generally is effective for reinfection; however, use of an alternative agent or combination therapy (e.g., metronidazole and quinacrine hydrochloride) may be necessary in patients who do not respond or relapse following initial therapy. Relapse is common in immunocompromised patients, and these patients may require prolonged therapy and/or use of a combination of agents.

If an outbreak of giardiasis is suspected in a child-care center in the US, the AAP recommends that an epidemiologic investigation be undertaken to identify and treat all symptomatic children, child-care workers, and family members and that all individuals with diarrhea be excluded from the center until they become asymptomatic. The AAP states that treatment of asymptomatic carriers has not been shown to be effective in outbreak control and that exclusion of carriers from child care is not recommended.

■ **Helicobacter pylori Infection and Duodenal Ulcer Disease** Metronidazole is used in combination with tetracycline hydrochloride, bismuth subsalicylate, and an H_2-receptor antagonist for the treatment of *Helicobacter pylori* (formerly *Campylobacter pylori* or *C. pyloridis*) infection in patients with an active duodenal ulcer. Metronidazole also has been used successfully in other multiple-drug regimens (with or without tetracycline hydrochloride, bismuth salts, and/or an H_2-receptor antagonist) for the treatment of *H. pylori* infection† in patients with peptic ulcer disease. Current epidemiologic and clinical evidence supports a strong association between gastric infection with *H. pylori* and the pathogenesis of duodenal and gastric ulcers; long-term *H. pylori* infection also has been implicated as a risk factor for gastric cancer. For additional information on the association of this infection with these and other GI conditions, see Helicobacter pylori Infection, under Uses, in Clarithromycin 8:12.12.92.

Conventional antiulcer therapy with H_2-receptor antagonists, proton-pump inhibitors, sucralfate, and/or antacids heals ulcers but generally is ineffective in eradicating *H. pylori*, and such therapy is associated with a high rate of ulcer recurrence (e.g., 60–100% per year). Several useful therapeutic regimens for *H. pylori*-associated peptic ulcer disease have been identified, and the American College of Gastroenterology (ACG), the National Institutes of Health (NIH), and most clinicians currently recommend that *all* patients with initial or recurrent duodenal or gastric ulcer and documente d*H. pylori* infection receive anti-infective therapy for treatment of the infection.

The optimum regimen for treatment of *H. pylori* infection has not been established; however, combined therapy with 3 drugs that have activity against *H. pylori* (generally a bismuth salt, metronidazole, and tetracycline or amoxicillin) has been effective in eradicating the infection, resolving associated gastritis, healing peptic ulcer, and preventing ulcer recurrence in many patients with *H. pylori*-associated peptic ulcer disease. Although such 3-drug regimens typically have been administered for 10–14 days, current evidence principally from studies in Europe suggests that 1 week of such therapy provides *H. pylori* eradication rates comparable to those of longer treatment periods. Other regimens that combine one or more anti-infective agents (e.g., clarithromycin, amoxicillin) with a bismuth salt and/or an antisecretory agent (e.g., omeprazole, H_2-receptor antagonist) also have been used successfully for *H. pylori* eradication, and the choice of a particular regimen should be based on the rapidly evolving data on optimal therapy, including consideration of the patient's prior exposure to anti-infective agents, the local prevalence of resistance, patient compliance, and costs of therapy. Current data suggest that eradication of *H. pylori* infection using regimens consisting of 1 or 2 anti-infective agents with a bismuth salt and/or an H_2-receptor antagonist or proton-pump inhibitor (e.g., omeprazole, lansoprazole) is cost effective compared with intermittent or continuous maintenance therapy with an H_2-receptor antagonist (considering the costs associated with ulcer recurrence, including endoscopic or other diagnostic procedures, physician visits, and/or hospitalization).

Although high eradication rates have been achieved with standard 3-drug, bismuth-based regimens (e.g., bismuth-metronidazole-tetracycline or bismuth-metronidazole-amoxicillin), such regimens typically involve administration of many tablets/capsules and have been associated with a relatively high (although variable) incidence of adverse effects. In addition, the efficacy of these regimens generally is unacceptable in patients with *H. pylori* strains resistant to the imidazole anti-infective (e.g., metronidazole) component. Current evidence suggests that inclusion of a proton-pump inhibitor (e.g., omeprazole, lansoprazole) in anti-*H. pylori* regimens containing 2 anti-infectives enhances effectiveness, and limited data suggest that such regimens retain good efficacy despite imidazole (e.g., metronidazole) resistance. Therefore, the ACG and many clinicians currently recommend 1 week of therapy with a proton-pump inhibitor and 2 anti-infective agents (usually clarithromycin and amoxicillin or metronidazole), or a 3-drug, bismuth-based regimen (e.g., bismuth-metronidazole-tetracycline) concomitantly with a proton-pump inhibitor, for treatment of *H. pylori* infection. Although few comparative studies have been performed, such regimens appear to provide high (e.g., 85–90%) *H. pylori* eradication rates, are well tolerated, and may be associated with better patient compliance than more prolonged therapy. The ACG states that in a cost-sensitive environment, an alternative regimen consisting of a bismuth salt, metronidazole, and tetracycline for 14 days is a reasonable choice in patients who are compliant and in whom there is a low expectation of metronidazole resistance (no prior exposure to the drug and a low regional prevalence of resistance).

Rapid development of resistance by *H. pylori* to certain drugs (e.g., metronidazole, clarithromycin and other macrolides, quinolones) has occurred when these drugs were used as monotherapy or as the only anti-infective agent in anti-*H. pylori* regimens. Resistance commonly emerges during therapy with metronidazole or clarithromycin when eradication of *H. pylori* is not achieved; therefore, prior exposure to these anti-infectives predicts resistance in individual patients and should be considered when selecting anti-*H. pylori* treatment regimens. Regimens containing metronidazole or clarithromycin should not be used to treat *H. pylori* infection in patients with known or suspected metronidazole- or clarithromycin-resistant isolates because of reduced efficacy in such patients.

For additional discussion of *H. pylori* infection, including details about the efficacy of various regimens and rationale for drug selection, see Helicobacter pylori Infection, under Uses, in Clarithromycin 8:12.12.92.

■ **Nongonococcal Urethritis** Oral metronidazole is used for the treatment of recurrent and persistent urethritis† in patients with nongonococcal urethritis who have already been treated with a recommended regimen. The CDC currently recommends that nongonococcal urethritis in adults be treated with a single oral dose of azithromycin or a 7-day regimen of doxycycline; alternative regimens recommended by the CDC are a 7-day regimen of oral erythromycin base or ethylsuccinate or a 7-day regimen of oral ofloxacin or oral levofloxacin. Patients treated for nongonococcal urethritis should be instructed to abstain from sexual intercourse until 7 days after initiation of treatment and to return for evaluation if symptoms persist or recur after completion of therapy; symptoms alone (without documentation of signs or laboratory evidence of urethral inflammation) are not sufficient basis for retreatment. Patients with persistent or recurrent urethritis who were not compliant with the treatment regimen or were reexposed to untreated sexual partner(s) should be retreated with the initial regimen. If the patient has recurrent and persistent urethritis, was compliant with the regimen, and reexposure can be excluded, the CDC recommends a single 2-g dose of oral metronidazole or oral tinidazole given in conjunction with a single 1-g dose of oral azithromycin (if azithromycin was not used in the initial regimen).

■ **Pelvic Inflammatory Disease** IV or oral metronidazole is used in conjunction with other anti-infectives for the treatment of acute pelvic inflammatory disease (PID).

When a parenteral regimen is indicated for the treatment of PID, the CDC and others generally recommend an initial regimen of IV cefoxitin or IV cefotetan given in conjunction with IV or oral doxycycline or a regimen of IV clindamycin given in conjunction with IV or IM gentamicin; parenteral therapy may be discontinued 24 hours after there is clinical improvement and a regimen of oral doxycycline continued to complete 14 days of therapy. However, if tubo-ovarian abscess is present, many clinicians recommend use of metronidazole or clindamycin with doxycycline for follow-up after the parenteral regimen (rather than doxycycline alone) to provide coverage against anaerobes.

When an oral regimen is indicated for the treatment of PID, the CDC recommends a regimen consisting of a single IM dose of ceftriaxone, cefoxitin (with a single oral dose of probenecid), or other parenteral cephalosporin (e.g., cefotaxime) with a 14-day regimen of oral doxycycline with or without a 14-day regimen of oral metronidazole. If a parenteral cephalosporin is not feasible, a 14-day regimen of oral ofloxacin or oral levofloxacin with or without a 14-day regimen of oral metronidazole can be considered, provided the community prevalence and individual risk of gonorrhea is low.

For further information on the treatment of PID, including regimens recommended by the CDC, see Uses: Pelvic Inflammatory Disease, in the Cephalosporins General Statement 8:12.06.

■ **Rosacea** Oral metronidazole has been used with some success in the treatment of inflammatory lesions (papules and pustules) and erythema associated with rosacea† (acne rosacea) and has decreased total numbers of inflammatory lesions associated with the disease. Metronidazole also is effective in reducing the number of inflammatory lesions and improving erythema associated with rosacea when applied topically to the skin of patients with the disease. Although there are no studies to date comparing efficacy and safety of topical and oral metronidazole therapy in the treatment of rosacea, the topical preparation may be preferred. Long-term therapy generally is required to control the inflammatory lesions of rosacea, and use of oral metronidazole in the disease has been limited by concerns over adverse systemic effects and toxicity of the drug. For information on rosacea and the use of topical metronidazole in the treatment of the disease, see Uses: Rosacea in Metronidazole 84:04.04 and for information on possible mechanism(s) by which metronidazole reduces inflammatory lesions and erythema in patients with rosacea, see Mechanism of Action: Effects on Rosacea in Metronidazole 84:04.04.

■ **Tetanus** Metronidazole is used as an adjunct to tetanus immune globulin (TIG), tetanus toxoid adsorbed, sedatives, and muscle relaxants in the treatment of active tetanus infection caused by *C. tetani*. Anti-infective agents cannot neutralize toxin already formed and cannot eradicate *C. tetani* spores which may revert to toxin-producing vegetative forms. Treatment of a tetanus wound consists of surgical debridement and prevention of associated infections that could create an anaerobic environment and help proliferation of *C. tetani*.

■ **Trichomoniasis** Metronidazole is used orally in the treatment of symptomatic and asymptomatic trichomoniasis in men and women in whom *T. vaginalis* has been demonstrated by an appropriate diagnostic procedure (e.g., wet smear and/or culture, OSOM Trichomonas Rapid Test, Affirm® VP III). Metronidazole also is used orally for the treatment of trichomoniasis in children and adolescents†.

The nitroimidazole derivatives, metronidazole and tinidazole, are the only drugs currently commercially available drugs in the US that are effective in the treatment of this disease. The goal of treatment is to provide symptomatic relief, achieve microbiologic cure, reduce transmission, and prevent reinfection; to achieve this goal, both the index patient and sexual (particularly steady) partner(s) should be treated. Some evidence suggests an association between vaginal trichomoniasis and adverse pregnancy outcomes, particularly premature membrane rupture, preterm delivery, and low birthweight. Trichomoniasis also may be a cofactor for the transmission of human immunodeficiency virus (HIV).

Most infected men are asymptomatic (although some may experience urethritis), while many women with trichomoniasis are symptomatic. *T. vaginalis* infection in women characteristically causes a diffuse, malodorous, yellow-green discharge accompanied by vulvar irritation. Because trichomoniasis is a sexually transmitted disease, the US Centers for Disease Control and Prevention (CDC) and other experts currently recommend that infected individuals and their sexual contacts be treated regardless of symptomatology; therefore, asymptomatic sexual contacts should be treated presumptively even when *T. vaginalis* has not been demonstrated. While trichomoniasis in males generally appears to be transient, some evidence indicates that a large proportion of relapse in females may result from reinfection from untreated male sexual partners; therefore, unless clear evidence accumulates that concomitant treatment of male partners is not beneficial, the current recommendation of concomitantly treating steady male sexual partners should be followed. This strategy is aimed at minimizing the risk of reinfection, curing any symptomatic disease in the male, and diminishing the pool of asymptomatic male carriers. Treatment of female sexual partners of lesbians with trichomoniasis also should be considered since transmission between such women has been reported.

Trichomoniasis cure rates of about 90–95% are achieved with currently recommended metronidazole regimens (2-g single dose or 500 mg twice daily for 7 days); ensuring the treatment of sexual partners may increase the cure rate. Following treatment, test-of-cure is not necessary for females or males who become asymptomatic after treatment or for those who were initially asymptomatic. To minimize the risk of reinfection and transmission, patients should be advised to avoid sex until both the patient and partner(s) are considered cured; in the absence of microbiologic test-of-cure, cure is considered to have been achieved following completion of a recommended regimen and resolution of symptoms. When *T. vaginalis* is associated with endocervicitis, cervicitis, or cervical erosion, the organism may interfere with accurate assessment of cytology smears and additional smears should be obtained after eradication of the infection.

Intravaginal† metronidazole as *sole* therapy for the treatment of trichomoniasis is *not* recommended because of substantially lower efficacy compared with systemic therapy.

For information on the treatment of trichomoniasis during pregnancy and lactation, see Cautions: Pregnancy, Fertility, and Lactation.

Treatment Failure Despite several decades of use of metronidazole for the treatment of trichomoniasis, resistance of *T. vaginalis* to the drug remains relatively uncommon. However, while resistance to metronidazole is not a recent phenomenon, its prevalence appears to be increasing. Most resistant strains exhibit either marginal or very low resistance to the drug. Recent estimates indicate that marginal resistance occurs in about 2% of cases, low to moderate resistance occurs in less than 1% of cases, and high-level resistance occurs rarely (e.g., in about 0.03–0.05% of cases).

In most cases, infection with resistant strains of *T. vaginalis* is cured with repeat courses and/or increased metronidazole dosages. Approximately 85% of marginally resistant cases will be cured by a repeat course at usual dosage, particularly if retreatment is initiated soon after initial failure, when the organism burden is relatively low. If treatment failure occurs following an initial regimen (i.e., a single 2-g dose of oral metronidazole) and reinfection has been excluded, the CDC recommends that the patient be retreated with either oral metronidazole 500 mg twice daily for 7 days or a single 2-g dose of oral tinidazole; if retreatment fails, then the patient should receive oral metronidazole or oral tinidazole in a dosage of 2 g once daily for 5 days. If the multiple-dose regimen is ineffective, consultation with a specialist is recommended and in vitro susceptibility testing of *T. vaginalis* isolates may be indicated. Regimens specific for the level of resistance have been suggested; under aerobic conditions, strains of *T. vaginalis* exhibiting low-level metronidazole resistance (minimum lethal concentration [MLC] less than 100 mcg/mL) can be treated with 2 g daily for 3–5 days, those with moderate (intermediate) resistance (MLC of 100–200 mcg/mL) can be treated with 2–2.5 g daily for 7–10 days, and those with high-level resistance (MLC exceeding 200 mcg/mL) can be treated with 3–3.5 g daily for 14–21 days. However, because infection with strains exhibiting high-level resistance is difficult to treat, CDC currently recommends that patients with culture-documented infection who do not respond to repeat regimens and in whom the possibility of reinfection has been excluded should be managed in consultation with an expert; such consultation is available from CDC. In some such cases, short-course (to minimize the risk of adverse effects) IV metronidazole therapy (e.g., 2 g IV every 6–8 hours for 2–4 days) may be tolerable and effective; however, patients should be advised of the potential risks of such dosages.

Tinidazole (e.g., 2 g daily for 7–14 days), has been effective in for the treatment of trichomoniasis in some patients who did not respond to metronidazole dosages of 3 g or more daily for 14 days. Resistant cases of vaginal trichomoniasis also have been treated in a limited number of patients with combined systemic and intravaginal metronidazole therapy (see Uses: Trichomoniasis, in Metronidazole 84:04.04) or with intravaginal paromomycin (not commercially available). While the choice of treatment of male sexual partners of females with metronidazole-resistant trichomoniasis is not clear, some clinicians treat such males with the same systemic regimen as the female unless the male is tested adequately (cultures of semen, prostatic secretions, and urethra) and shown to be infection free.

Desensitization Because effective alternatives to metronidazole for the treatment of trichomoniasis currently are not available in the US, CDC states that desensitization to the drug can be attempted in patients with metronidazole hypersensitivity†. If desensitization is attempted, the possibility that the procedure may be hazardous should be considered. Adequate procedures (e.g., established IV access, blood pressure monitoring) and therapies (e.g., epinephrine, corticosteroids, antihistamines, oxygen) for the management of an acute hypersensitivity reaction should be readily available. Pretreatment (e.g., with an antihistamine and/or corticosteroid) also should be considered.Desensitization has been performed in a limited number of women by administering increasing IV doses of metronidazole incrementally until a therapeutic dose was achieved, at which time oral dosing was initiated. In this regimen, metronidazole was administered IV beginning with 5 mcg and then the dose was increased at 15- to 20-minute intervals to 15, 50, 150, and 500 mcg and then to 1.5, 5, 15, 30, 60, and 125 mg. Once a dose of 125 mg was achieved IV, incremental increases were switched to oral dosing with 250, 500, and 2 g doses administered at 1-hour intervals. For trichomoniasis, dosing can be stopped after the 2-g dose has been achieved. Monitoring of the patient should continue for at least 4 hours after administration of the last dose (24 hours if there was any evidence of a reaction).

Pediatric Infections The American Academy of Pediatrics (AAP) and other clinicians recommend oral metronidazole for the treatment of trichomoniasis in children†. Because trichomoniasis principally is a sexually transmitted disease, its presence in a prepubertal child should raise the question of sexual abuse. *T. vaginalis* can be acquired by neonates during birth and causes a vaginal discharge in the first weeks of life.

■ **Perioperative Prophylaxis** IV metronidazole is used for perioperative prophylaxis to reduce the incidence of postoperative anaerobic bacterial infections in patients undergoing contaminated or potentially contaminated elective colorectal surgery. For perioperative prophylaxis in patients undergoing colorectal surgery, a regimen of IV cefoxitin alone, IV cefazolin and IV metronidazole, oral erythromycin and oral neomycin, or oral neomycin and oral metronidazole usually is recommended. Although many clinicians use both an oral and a parenteral regimen for perioperative prophylaxis in patients undergoing colorectal surgery; there is controversy about the benefits and risks of this strategy. There is some evidence that a combined oral and parenteral regimen may be more effective than use of an oral or parenteral regimen alone; however, the combined regimen may be associated with a higher incidence of adverse effects (e.g., nausea, vomiting, *Clostridium difficile*-associated diarrhea and colitis).

Metronidazole has been given orally, IV, or rectally for perioperative prophylaxis in patients undergoing appendectomy†. For perioperative prophylaxis in patients undergoing appendectomy (nonperforated), a regimen of IV cefoxitin alone or IV cefazolin and IV metronidazole is recommended.

■ **Prophylaxis in Sexual Assault Victims** Oral metronidazole is used in conjunction with IM ceftriaxone and either oral azithromycin or oral doxycycline for empiric anti-infective prophylaxis in adolescent and adult victims of sexual assault†; postexposure hepatitis B vaccination also is recommended for susceptible victims. Many experts recommend routine empiric prophylactic therapy after a sexual assault, and use of such prophylaxis probably benefits most patients since follow-up of assault victims can be difficult and such prophylaxis allays the patient's concerns about possible infection. The CDC states that trichomoniasis, genital chlamydial infection, gonorrhea, and bacterial vaginosis are the sexually transmitted diseases (STDs) most commonly diagnosed in women following sexual assault; however, the prevalence of these infections is substantial among sexually active women and their presence after assault does not necessarily indicate that the infections were acquired during the assault. Chlamydial and gonococcal infections among females are of special concern because of the possibility of ascending infection.

When empiric anti-infective prophylaxis is indicated in adolescent or adult sexual assault victims, the CDC recommends administration of a single 125-mg IM dose of ceftriaxone given in conjunction with a single 2-g oral dose of metronidazole and a single 1-g oral dose of azithromycin or a 7-day regimen of oral doxycycline (100 mg twice daily). This 3-drug regimen provides coverage against gonorrhea, chlamydia, trichomoniasis, and bacterial vaginosis, but efficacy in preventing these infections after sexual assault has not been specifically studied. Because of possible adverse GI effects with the 3-drug regimen, the CDC suggests that the patient be counseled regarding the possible benefits, as well as the possibility of toxicity of such prophylaxis. Alternative regimens may be required for some patients because of the likelihood of transmission of other STDs from the assailant. CDC states that a recommendation concerning the appropriateness of antiretroviral prophylaxis against HIV cannot be made based on currently available information, and the decision to offer such prophylaxis should be individualized taking into account the probability of HIV transmission from a single act of intercourse and the nature of the assault (e.g., extent and site of physical trauma and exposure to ejaculate). (See Guidelines for Use of Antiretroviral Agents: Antiretroviral Agents for Postexposure Prophylaxis in Sexual Assault Victims or Nonoccupational Exposure to HIV, in the Antiretroviral Agents General Statement 8:18.08.)

There are few data available to establish the risk of a child acquiring a sexually transmitted disease as a result of sexual assault or abuse. The risk is believed to be low in most circumstances, although documentation to support this position is inadequate. The CDC and AAP state that presumptive treatment for children who have been sexually assaulted or abused is not widely recommended because girls appear to be at lower risk for ascending infection than adolescent or adult women, and regular follow-up usually can be ensured. Even if the risk is perceived by the health-care provider to be low, some children or their parents or guardians may have concerns about the possibility of the child contracting a sexually transmitted disease as a result of the assault and these concerns may be an appropriate indication for presumptive treatment in some settings, but only after appropriate specimens for STD testing have been obtained.

For topical and vaginal uses of metronidazole, see 84:04.04.

Dosage and Administration

■ **Reconstitution and Administration** Metronidazole is administered orally or by continuous or intermittent IV infusion; metronidazole hydrochloride is administered by continuous or intermittent IV infusion. Metronidazole has been administered rectally†, but this dosage form is not currently available in the US. The drug also is administered intravaginally or applied topically to the skin. (See Metronidazole 84:04.04.)

While food does not affect the extent of absorption of metronidazole administered as capsules, it does increase the rate of absorption of the drug administered as extended-release tablets. To optimize the pharmacokinetic disposition of the extended-release oral preparation of metronidazole, the manufacturer recommends that metronidazole extended-release tablets be administered during the fasting state (i.e., at least 1 hour before or 2 hours after meals).

Metronidazole and metronidazole hydrochloride should not be mixed with other drugs, and other IV infusions should be discontinued, if possible, while metronidazole or metronidazole hydrochloride is being infused.

Metronidazole injection does not need to be diluted or neutralized prior to IV administration. However, IV infusions of metronidazole hydrochloride must be prepared by reconstituting, diluting, and then neutralizing the commercially available powder for injection. Metronidazole hydrochloride powder for injection is reconstituted by adding 4.4 mL of sterile or bacteriostatic water for injection, 0.9% sodium chloride injection, or bacteriostatic sodium chloride injection to a vial labeled as containing 500 mg of metronidazole. The resultant solution contains approximately 100 mg of metronidazole per mL and must be further diluted with 0.9% sodium chloride injection, 5% dextrose injection, or lactated Ringer's injection to a concentration of 8 mg or less of metronidazole per mL. The reconstituted and diluted metronidazole hydrochloride solution must then be neutralized by adding approximately 5 mEq of sodium bicarbonate injection for each 500 mg of metronidazole. The addition of sodium bicarbonate to the metronidazole hydrochloride solution may generate carbon dioxide gas and it may be necessary to remove gas pressure from the container.

When the commercially available IV infusion solution of metronidazole is used, the accompanying labeling should be consulted for proper methods of administration and associated precautions.

■ **Dosage** Dosage of metronidazole hydrochloride is expressed in terms of metronidazole. Because the pharmacokinetics of metronidazole may be altered in geriatric individuals, monitoring of plasma metronidazole concentrations may be necessary to properly adjust dosage of the drug in such patients.

Amebiasis For the treatment of acute intestinal amebiasis or extraintestinal disease caused by *Entamoeba histolytica*, metronidazole is administered orally and metronidazole therapy is followed by therapy with a luminal amebicide (iodoquinol, paromomycin). (See Uses: Amebiasis.)

The usual adult dosage of metronidazole for acute intestinal disease is 750 mg 3 times daily for 5–10 (usually 10) days. The usual adult dosage for amebic liver abscess is 500–750 mg 3 times daily for 5–10 (usually 10) days. Some clinicians recommend that adults receive 500–750 mg 3 times daily for 7–10 days for mild to moderate intestinal disease or 750 mg 3 times daily for 7–10 days for severe intestinal and extraintestinal disease. Alternatively, amebic liver abscess has been treated in adults with 2.4 g once daily for 1 or 2 days. When oral therapy could not be used, metronidazole has been administered IV in a dosage of 500 mg every 6 hours for 10 days.

For the treatment of mild to moderate intestinal amebiasis, severe intestinal disease, or extraintestinal disease (including amebic liver abscess) in children, the usual dosage of metronidazole is 35–50 mg/kg given in 3 divided doses daily for 7–10 (usually 10) days.

Anaerobic Bacteria Infections For the treatment of serious infections caused by anaerobic bacteria, metronidazole or metronidazole hydrochloride is administered IV initially and oral metronidazole is substituted when the condition of the patient warrants. IV infusions are usually given over 1 hour. Adults should receive an initial IV loading dose of 15 mg/kg followed by IV maintenance doses of 7.5 mg/kg every 6 hours. The usual adult oral dosage is 7.5 mg/kg every 6 hours. The maximum daily adult IV or oral dose recommended by the manufacturers for the treatment of anaerobic bacterial infections is 4 g. The manufacturers state that the usual duration of therapy is 7–10 days; however, most serious anaerobic bacterial infections require 2–3 weeks of therapy.

Bacterial Vaginosis For the treatment of bacterial vaginosis† in nonpregnant women and adolescents, the CDC, AAP, and others recommend an oral metronidazole dosage of 500 mg twice daily for 7 days. Although not recommended by the CDC, alternative regimens that have been used include a single 2-g dose of oral metronidazole (provides improved patient compliance and reduced risk of adverse effects) and 750 mg (as an extended-release tablet) once daily for 7 consecutive days.

For the treatment of bacterial vaginosis in pregnant women, the CDC and other experts currently recommend an oral metronidazole dosage of 500 mg twice daily or 250 mg 3 times daily for 7 days. The manufacturer and some experts state that the single-dose regimen should *not* be used in pregnant women because it may result in slightly higher serum concentrations of the drug, which can reach the fetal circulation. Use of oral metronidazole administered as extended-release tablets for the treatment of bacterial vaginosis currently is being studied in pregnant women.

AAP suggests that prepubertal children weighing less than 45 kg can receive oral metronidazole is a dosage of 15 mg/kg daily (up to 1 g) in 2 divided doses given for 7 days for the treatment of bacterial vaginosis.

Balantidiasis For the treatment of balantidiasis† caused by *Balantidium coli*, many clinicians recommend an oral metronidazole dosage of 750 mg 3 times daily for 5 days in adults and 35–50 mg/kg daily given in 3 divided doses for 5 days in children.

Blastocystis hominis Infections When used in the treatment of symptomatic *Blastocystis hominis* infections†, oral metronidazole has been given in a dosage of 750 mg 3 times daily for 10 days.

Clostridium difficile-Associated Diarrhea and Colitis For the treatment of *Clostridium difficile*-associated diarrhea and colitis† in adults, oral metronidazole dosages of 750 mg to 2 g daily given in 3 or 4 divided doses for 7–14 days have been used. While dose-ranging studies to determine comparative efficacy have not been performed, the most commonly employed oral metronidazole regimens in adults have been 250 mg 4 times daily or 500 mg 3 times daily for 10 days. An IV dosage of 500–750 mg every 6–8 hours has been used in adults when oral therapy was not feasible.

Children have been given oral metronidazole dosages of 30–50 mg/kg daily given in 3 or 4 equally divided doses for 7–10 days, but not to exceed the adult dosage, for the treatment of *C. difficile*-associated diarrhea and colitis†. AAP recommends 30 mg/kg daily (up to 2 g daily) given in 4 divided doses for 7–10 days for initial treatment in most patients with colitis.

Crohn's Disease Optimum metronidazole dosage for the treatment of active Crohn's disease† has not been established, but an oral dosage of 400 mg twice daily or 1 g daily has been effective. For the treatment of refractory perineal disease, an oral dosage of 20 mg/kg (1–1.5 g) given in 3–5 divided doses daily has been employed.

Dientamoeba fragilis Infections For the treatment of infections caused by *Dientamoeba fragilis*†, adults should receive 500–750 mg 3 times daily for 10 days and children should receive 20–40 mg/kg daily given in 3 divided doses for 10 days.

Dracunculiasis For the treatment of dracunculiasis† caused by *Dracunculus medinensis* (guinea worm infection), adults have received oral metronidazole in a dosage of 250 mg 3 times daily for 10 days and children have received 25 mg/kg daily (maximum 750 mg daily) given in 3 divided doses for 10 days. Although not curative, this regimen may decrease inflammation and facilitate worm removal.

Giardiasis For the treatment of giardiasis†, the usual dosage of oral metronidazole for adults is 250 mg 3 times daily for 5–7 days. Adults have been treated successfully with a single daily dose of 2 g for 3 days. For adults with coexistent amebiasis, the usual dosage is 750 mg 3 times daily for 5–10 days.

Some clinicians recommend that children receive 15 mg/kg daily in 3 divided doses for 5–7 days.

Helicobacter pylori Infection For the treatment of *Helicobacter pylori* (formerly *Campylobacter pylori* or *C. pyloridis*) infection† in adults with an active duodenal ulcer, the FDA-labeled dosage of metronidazole is 250 mg in combination with tetracycline hydrochloride (500 mg) and bismuth subsalicylate (525 mg) 4 times daily (at meals and at bedtime) for 14 days; these drugs should be given concomitantly with an H_2-receptor antagonist in recommended dosage. Metronidazole generally has been used in an oral dosage of 250–500 mg 3 times daily in combination with at least one other agent that has activity against *H. pylori* (e.g., bismuth subsalicylate, amoxicillin, tetracycline). (See Helicobacter pylori Infection, in Uses.)

In a limited number of children with *H. pylori*-associated peptic ulcer disease (e.g., gastritis, duodenitis/duodenal ulcer)†, oral metronidazole 15–20 mg/kg daily in 2 divided doses for 4 weeks has been administered as part of a 6-week multiple-drug regimen that included amoxicillin and/or bismuth subsalicylate. Further study is needed to establish an optimal drug regimen for the treatment of *H. pylori* infection in children.

The minimum duration of therapy required to eradicate *H. pylori* infection in peptic ulcer disease has not been fully established. The American College of Gastroenterology (ACG) and many clinicians currently recommend 1 week of therapy with a proton-pump inhibitor and 2 anti-infective agents (usually clarithromycin and amoxicillin or metronidazole), or a 3-drug, bismuth-based regimen (e.g., bismuth-metronidazole-tetracycline) concomitantly with a proton-pump inhibitor, for treatment of *H. pylori* infection. However, the ACG states that in a cost-sensitive environment, an alternative regimen consisting of a bismuth salt, metronidazole, and tetracycline for 14 days is a reasonable choice in patients who are compliant and in whom there is a low expectation of metronidazole resistance (no prior exposure to the drug and a low regional prevalence of resistance). (See Helicobacter pylori Infection in Uses: GI Infections, in the Tetracyclines General Statement 8:12.24.)

Nongonococcal Urethritis For the treatment of recurrent and persistent urethritis† in patients who have already received a regimen recommended for the treatment of nongonococcal urethritis (see Uses: Nongonococcal Urethritis), the CDC recommends a single 2-g dose of oral metronidazole in conjunction with a single 1-g dose of oral azithromycin (if azithromycin was not used in the initial regimen).

Pelvic Inflammatory Disease For the treatment of PID when an oral regimen is indicated, a single IM dose of ceftriaxone (250 mg) or a single IM dose of cefoxitin (2 g with oral probenecid 1 g) is given in conjunction with oral doxycycline (100 mg twice daily for 14 days) with or without oral metronidazole in a dosage of 500 mg twice daily for 14 days.

Alternatively, when a parenteral cephalosporin is not feasible and the community prevalence and individual risk of gonorrhea is low, oral metronidazole is given in a dosage of 500 mg twice daily in conjunction with oral ofloxacin (400 mg twice daily) or oral levofloxacin (500 mg once daily) for 14 days.

Tetanus When used as an adjunct in the treatment of tetanus, some clinicians recommend that IV metronidazole be given in a dosage of 500 mg every 6 hours for 7–10 days. In children, oral or IV metronidazole has been given in a dosage of 30 mg/kg daily in 4 divided doses (maximum 4 g daily).

Trichomoniasis For the initial treatment of symptomatic and asymptomatic trichomoniasis caused by *Trichomonas vaginalis*, metronidazole is administered orally in a single-dose or 7-day regimen; treatment should be individualized. The dosages are the same for sexual contacts. The single-dose regimen can ensure compliance, especially if administered under supervision, in patients who cannot be relied upon to continue the 7-day regimen, and is currently considered the regimen of choice by the US Centers for Disease Control and Prevention (CDC) and other experts. However, the 7-day regimen may minimize reinfection of the woman long enough to treat sexual contacts, and there is some evidence that cure rates as determined by vaginal smears and symptoms may be higher after the 7-day regimen than after the single-dose regimen.

For the single-dose regimen, the dosage for adults and adolescents is 2 g administered as a single dose; alternatively, the dose can be divided and administered in 2 doses on the same day. For the 7-day regimen, the CDC and many clinicians currently recommend an adult dosage of 500 mg twice daily. Alternatively, the manufacturer and some clinicians state that a 375-mg metronidazole capsule can be given twice daily for 7 days; however, this regimen is not included in current CDC guidelines for the treatment of trichomoniasis.

Before repeat courses of therapy are given, the manufacturer states that the presence of the organism should be reconfirmed by wet smear and/or culture and an interval of 4–6 weeks should be allowed between courses of metronidazole. If treatment failure occurs following an initial metronidazole regimen of a single 2-g dose and reinfection has been excluded, the CDC recommends that the patient be retreated with an oral metronidazole regimen of 500 mg twice daily for 7 days or, alternatively, a single 2-g dose of oral tinidazole; if retreatment fails, then 2 g of metronidazole or tinidazole should be given once daily for 5 days. If the multiple-dose regimen is ineffective, consultation with a specialist is recommended and in vitro susceptibility testing of *T. vaginalis* isolates may be indicated. Some clinicians recommend retreatment with a metronidazole regimen of 2–4 g daily for 7–14 days if metronidazole-resistant strains are involved. If treatment of resistant infection is guided by in vitro susceptibility testing under aerobic conditions, some clinicians suggest that strains of *T. vaginalis* exhibiting low-level resistance (minimum lethal concentration [MLC] less than 100 mcg/mL) can be treated orally with 2 g daily for 3–5 days, those with moderate (intermediate) resistance (MLC of 100–200 mcg/mL) can be treated orally with 2–2.5 g daily for 7–10 days, and those with high-level resistance (MLC exceeding 200 mcg/mL) can be treated orally with 3–3.5 g daily for 14–21 days. However, because infection with strains exhibiting high-level resistance is difficult to treat, CDC currently recommends that patients with culture-documented infection who do not respond to repeat regimens at dosages up to 2 g daily for 3–5 days and in whom the possibility of reinfection has been excluded should be managed in consultation with an expert; such consultation is available from CDC.

The AAP and others recommend that children weighing less than 45 kg with trichomoniasis receive 15 mg/kg daily in 3 divided doses (maximum 2 g daily) for 7 days.

Perioperative Prophylaxis When metronidazole is used for perioperative prophylaxis in patients undergoing contaminated or potentially contaminated colorectal surgery, the manufacturers recommend that adults receive 15 mg/kg by IV infusion over 30–60 minutes 1 hour prior to the procedure and, if necessary, 7.5 mg/kg by IV infusion over 30–60 minutes at 6 and 12 hours after the initial dose. The initial preoperative dose must be completely infused approximately 1 hour prior to surgery to ensure adequate serum and tissue concentrations of metronidazole at the time of incision. Prophylactic use of metronidazole should be limited to the day of surgery and should not be continued for more than 12 hours after surgery.

Alternatively, if an oral regimen is used for perioperative prophylaxis in patients undergoing colorectal surgery, adults can receive 2 g of oral metronidazole and 2 g of oral neomycin sulfate at 7 p.m. and 11 p.m. on the day preceding surgery. The oral regimen is used in conjunction with an appropriate diet and catharsis; a minimum residue or clear liquid diet and catharsis usually is prescribed 1–3 days prior to colorectal surgery.

Some clinicians recommend that adults undergoing colorectal surgery receive 0.5 g of metronidazole IV in conjunction with 1–2 g of IV cefazolin just prior to surgery.

Prophylaxis in Sexual Assault Victims If empiric anti-infective prophylaxis is indicated in adolescent or adult victims of sexual assault†, a single 2-g oral dose of metronidazole is given in conjunction with a single 125-mg IM dose of ceftriaxone and either a single 1-g oral dose of azithromycin or a 7-day regimen oral doxycycline given in a dosage of 100 mg twice daily has been recommended. Hepatitis B vaccination also should be initiated in susceptible individuals and completed according to the usual schedule.

If empiric anti-infective prophylaxis is indicated in preadolescent children and use of oral metronidazole for prevention of trichomoniasis and bacterial vaginosis is considered in these children, AAP states that those weighing less than 45 kg can receive metronidazole in a dosage of 15 mg/kg daily given in 3 divided doses for 7 days and those weighing 45 kg or more can receive a single 2-g dose.

■ **Dosage in Hepatic Impairment** In patients with severe hepatic impairment, doses and/or frequency of administration of metronidazole should be modified in response to the degree of hepatic impairment and plasma concentrations of the drug should be monitored.

Cautions

■ **GI Effects** The most frequent adverse reaction to oral metronidazole is nausea, which is sometimes accompanied by headache, anorexia, dry mouth, and a sharp, unpleasant metallic taste. Other occasional adverse GI effects of oral metronidazole include vomiting, diarrhea, epigastric distress, abdominal discomfort, and constipation. Nausea, vomiting, abdominal discomfort, a metallic taste, and diarrhea have also been reported with IV metronidazole. Antibiotic-associated pseudomembranous colitis, presumably caused by toxin-producing clostridia (e.g., *C. difficile*) resistant to metronidazole, has been reported rarely following oral administration of the drug and has also been reported in at least one patient following intravaginal administration of metronidazole. Pancreatitis, which has improved following discontinuance of the drug but recurred upon subsequent rechallenge, has been reported rarely during oral metronidazole therapy.

In clinical trials in which combined therapy with tetracycline hydrochloride, metronidazole, and bismuth subsalicylate was used for the treatment of *H. pylori* infection and associated duodenal ulcer, adverse effects generally were related to the GI tract, were reversible, and infrequently led to discontinuance of therapy. Adverse GI effects reported in at least 1% of patients receiving combined therapy with tetracycline hydrochloride, metronidazole, and bismuth subsalicylate (generally in conjunction with acid-suppression therapy) were nausea (10.2%) diarrhea (5.1%), abdominal pain (3%), melena (2.5%), anal discomfort (1.5%), anorexia (1.5%), vomiting (1.5%), and constipation (1%). Adverse GI effects reported in less than 1% of patients receiving combined therapy with tetracycline hydrochloride-metronidazole-bismuth subsalicylate in clinical trials were dry mouth, dyspepsia, dysphagia, flatulence, GI hemorrhage, glossitis, and stomatitis.

■ **Nervous System Effects** Peripheral neuropathy, characterized by numbness, tingling, or paresthesia of an extremity, and convulsive seizures have been reported rarely with oral or IV metronidazole. Peripheral neuropathy is usually reversible if metronidazole is discontinued but may persist in patients who receive prolonged therapy or higher than recommended dosage of the drug. Dizziness, vertigo, incoordination, ataxia, confusion, irritability, depression, weakness, insomnia, headache, syncope, tinnitus, and hearing loss have also occurred with metronidazole. Headache occurred in 18% of nonpregnant women receiving oral metronidazole (administered as extended-release tablets) for bacterial vaginosis, and among those reporting headache, 10% described it as severe.

Dizziness or paresthesia was reported in 1.5% of patients receiving combined therapy with tetracycline hydrochloride, metronidazole, and bismuth subsalicylate (generally in conjunction with acid-suppression therapy) in clinical trials; asthenia or insomnia was reported in 1% of such patients. Nervousness, malaise, or syncope was reported in less than 1% of patients receiving tetracycline hydrochloride-metronidazole-bismuth subsalicylate therapy in clinical trials.

■ **Hematologic Effects** Mild, transient leukopenia and thrombocytopenia have been reported rarely in patients receiving metronidazole, and bone marrow aplasia has been reported in at least 1 patient.

■ **Genitourinary Effects** Urethral burning or discomfort, dysuria, cystitis, polyuria, incontinence, a sense of pelvic pressure, dryness of the vagina or vulva, dyspareunia, and decreased libido have been reported with oral metronidazole. Urine may be dark or reddish-brown in color following oral or IV administration of metronidazole due to the presence of water-soluble pigments which result from metabolism of the drug. Vulvovaginal candidiasis (or yeast vaginitis) was reported in 15% of nonpregnant women receiving oral metronidazole (administered as extended-release tablets) and in 12% of those receiving clindamycin phosphate (2% clindamycin) vaginal cream in a comparative study for the treatment of bacterial vaginosis. Although a definite causal relationship to the drug has not been established, genital pruritus, dysmenorrhea, and urinary tract infection have been reported in 5, 3, and 2%, respectively, of nonpregnant women receiving oral metronidazole (administered as extended-release tablets) for the treatment of bacterial vaginosis.

■ **Sensitivity Reactions** Hypersensitivity reactions including urticaria, pruritus, erythematous rash, flushing, nasal congestion, fever, and fleeting joint pains sometimes resembling serum sickness have been reported in patients receiving oral metronidazole. Erythematous rash and pruritus have been reported in patients receiving IV metronidazole. Aseptic meningitis, that appeared to be a hypersensitivity reaction, has occurred in at least one patient after administration of oral metronidazole. The reaction consisted of severe headache, fever, arthralgia, myalgia, stiff neck, nausea, and vomiting.

Photosensitivity reaction or rash was reported in less than 1% of patients receiving combined therapy with tetracycline hydrochloride, metronidazole, and bismuth subsalicylate (generally in conjunction with acid-suppression therapy) in clinical trials.

■ **Respiratory Effects** Upper respiratory tract infection, rhinitis, sinusitis, and pharyngitis were each reported in less than 5% of nonpregnant women receiving oral metronidazole (administered as extended-release tablets) for the treatment of bacterial vaginosis.

■ **Other Adverse Effects** Furry tongue, glossitis, and stomatitis have been reported with oral metronidazole and may be due to overgrowth of *Candida* which may occur during metronidazole therapy. Candidiasis was reported in 3% of nonpregnant women receiving oral metronidazole (administered as extended-release tablets) for the treatment of bacterial vaginosis.

Flattening of the T-wave has been reported rarely in ECG tracings of patients receiving oral metronidazole.

Thrombophlebitis has been reported after IV infusion of metronidazole. The manufacturers state that thrombophlebitis may be minimized or avoided by avoiding prolonged use of indwelling IV catheters.

Although a definite causal relationship to the drug has not been established, bacterial infection and flu-like symptoms have been reported in 7 and 6%, respectively, of nonpregnant women receiving oral metronidazole (administered as extended-release tablets) for the treatment of bacterial vaginosis. Myopia in a woman receiving metronidazole for trichomoniasis also has been associated with, but not causally related to, the drug.

Pain or upper respiratory tract infection was reported in 1% of patients receiving combined therapy with tetracycline hydrochloride, metronidazole, and bismuth subsalicylate (generally in conjunction with acid-suppression therapy) in clinical trials, while hypertension, myocardial infarction, or rheumatoid arthritis was reported in less than 1% of such patients.

■ **Precautions and Contraindications** When the commercially available combination preparation containing tetracycline hydrochloride, metronidazole, and bismuth subsalicylate (Helidac® Therapy) is used for the treatment of *Helicobacter pylori* infection and associated duodenal ulcer disease, the cautions, precautions, and contraindications associated with tetracycline hydrochloride and bismuth subsalicylate must be considered in addition to those associated with metronidazole.

If abnormal neurologic symptoms occur during oral or IV metronidazole therapy, such therapy should be discontinued promptly. Metronidazole should be used with caution in patients with CNS diseases.

The manufacturers state that metronidazole should be used with caution in patients with evidence or a history of blood dyscrasias, and total and differential leukocyte counts should be performed before and after treatment with the drug, especially when repeated courses of therapy are necessary.

Patients should be advised to avoid concurrent use of metronidazole and alcoholic beverages. (See Drug Interactions: Alcohol.)

The use of oral or IV metronidazole may result in oral, vaginal, or intestinal candidiasis. If suprainfection or superinfection occurs, appropriate therapy should be instituted.

Metronidazole should be used with caution and in reduced dosage in patients with severe hepatic impairment. The manufacturers recommend that plasma metronidazole concentrations be monitored in patients with severe hepatic impairment. The manufacturers state that commercially available metronidazole injection should be used with caution in patients receiving corticosteroids and in patients predisposed to edema because the injection contains 28 mEq of sodium per gram of metronidazole.

To reduce development of drug-resistant bacteria and maintain effectiveness of metronidazole and other antibacterials, the drug should be used only for the treatment or prevention of infections proven or strongly suspected to be caused by susceptible bacteria. When selecting or modifying anti-infective therapy, results of culture and in vitro susceptibility testing should be used. In the absence of such data, local epidemiology and susceptibility patterns should be considered when selecting anti-infectives for empiric therapy. Patients should be advised that antibacterials (including metronidazole) should only be used to treat bacterial infections and not used to treat viral infections (e.g., the common cold). Patients also should be advised about the importance of completing the full course of therapy, even if feeling better after a few days, and that skipping doses or not completing therapy may decrease effectiveness and increase the likelihood that bacteria will develop resistance and will not be treatable with metronidazole or other antibacterials in the future.

Metronidazole is contraindicated in individuals with a history of hypersensitivity to the drug or other nitroimidazole derivatives. However, cautious desensitization has been employed in some hypersensitive patients in whom metronidazole therapy was considered necessary. (See Trichomoniasis: Desensitization, in Uses.)

■ **Pediatric Precautions** The manufacturers state that safe use of IV metronidazole in children for any indication and safe use of oral metronidazole in children for any indication except amebiasis have not been established; however, oral metronidazole has been used in children for indications other than amebiasis (e.g., trichomoniasis, giardiasis) without unusual adverse effects. The AAP and other clinicians recommend that children with trichomoniasis be treated with oral metronidazole.

■ **Geriatric Precautions** Because of the greater frequency of decreased hepatic function in geriatric patients, the possibility that adjustment of metronidazole dosage may be necessary in this age group should be considered. (See Dosage and Administration: Dosage in Hepatic Impairment.)

■ Mutagenicity and Carcinogenicity In at least 6 different studies in mice, including one in which the animals received metronidazole intermittently (every 4 weeks), the prominent effect of the drug was promotion of pulmonary tumorigenesis. At doses of 1500 mg/m^2 (about 3 times the recommended human dose), there was also a statistically significant increase in the incidence of malignant liver tumors in male mice. In addition, in one study in mice who received lifetime feedings with metronidazole, there was an increase in the incidence of malignant lymphomas as well as pulmonary neoplasms. In long-term studies in rats receiving oral metronidazole, there was a statistically significant increase in the incidence of various neoplasms in the females, particularly mammary and hepatic tumors. Breast and colon cancer have been reported in patients with Crohn's disease who have been treated with high dosages of metronidazole for prolonged periods; however, a direct causal relationship with the drug has not been established and patients with Crohn's disease are known to have an increased incidence of GI and certain extraintestinal cancers.

Metronidazole has shown mutagenic activity in several in vitro studies; however, in vivo studies in mammals failed to demonstrate mutagenic effects.

Oral metronidazole was carcinogenic in mice and rats in chronic studies, but similar studies in hamsters were negative. Long-term, controlled studies are needed to evaluate the carcinogenic and mutagenic effects of metronidazole in humans. The manufacturers state that unnecessary use of metronidazole should be avoided, and the drug should be used only in serious infections where the potential benefit outweighs the possible risk.

■ Pregnancy, Fertility, and Lactation There was no evidence of fetotoxicity when metronidazole was administered orally at a dosage of 20 mg/kg daily (approximately 1.5 times the usual human dosage based on mg/kg of body weight) or at a dosage of 60 mg/m^2 daily (approximately 10% of the usual human dosage) to pregnant mice; however, fetotoxicity did occur when the drug was administered intraperitoneally to pregnant mice at doses approximately equal to the usual human dose. There are no adequate or well-controlled studies to date using metronidazole in pregnant women, and the drug should be used during pregnancy only when clearly needed. The manufacturers, the CDC, and other experts state that use of the drug during the first trimester of pregnancy is contraindicated. Although evidence from case-controlled studies, pooled analysis of cohort and case-controlled studies, and other information, including some experience during first-trimester exposure, suggests that metronidazole is not associated with a clinically important teratogenic or fetotoxic risk, conflicting evidence potentially implicating an association between the drug and certain fetal effects (e.g., cleft palate) also has been reported. Because of conflicting data and theoretical concerns regarding the mutagenic and carcinogenic potentials of the drug, use of metronidazole during the first trimester remains controversial and is considered contraindicated by the manufacturers and others.

Because no therapy other than metronidazole currently has been shown to produce adequate response in the treatment of trichomoniasis, the manufacturers, CDC, and other experts state that oral metronidazole should be used to treat this infection in pregnant women only when severe symptoms cannot be controlled with local palliative treatment and only during the second or third trimester. In addition, the manufacturers state that because the single-dose regimen may result in slightly higher serum concentrations of the drug, the 7-day regimen (see Dosage and Administration: Dosage) should be used to treat trichomoniasis during pregnancy. However, the CDC suggests the single-dose regimen when therapy with the drug is considered necessary. It has been suggested that 100 mg of clotrimazole administered intravaginally at bedtime for 7 days may produce symptomatic improvement but only occasionally cures in pregnant women with trichomoniasis; therefore, such therapy generally should be considered palliative.

Screening and/or treatment for bacterial vaginosis in pregnant women as clinically indicated (see Bacterial Vaginosis: Pregnant Women, in Uses) should be conducted early in the pregnancy (i.e., first prenatal visit for women at high-risk). For the treatment of bacterial vaginosis and reduction in the incidence of adverse pregnancy outcomes associated with bacterial vaginosis (e.g., preterm birth), particularly in pregnant women at high risk for complications of pregnancy, a 7-day regimen of oral metronidazole currently is preferred. the manufacturer and some experts state that the single-dose regimen of metronidazole should *not* be used in pregnant women because it may result in slightly higher serum concentrations of the drug, which can reach the fetal circulation. The safety and efficacy of oral metronidazole administered as extended-release tablets for the treatment of bacterial vaginosis have not been established in pregnant women.

Metronidazole in dosages up to 400 mg/kg daily (approximately 3.5 times the maximum recommended human dosage on a mg/m^2 basis) for 28 days failed to produce any adverse effects on fertility and testicular function in male rats. Reproduction studies in mice using metronidazole doses up to 6 times the human dose on a mg/m^2 basis have not revealed evidence of impaired fertility.

Metronidazole is distributed into milk. Because of the tumorigenic potential of metronidazole in mice and rats, a decision should be made whether to discontinue nursing or the drug, taking into account the importance of the drug to the woman. The AAP states that, if a single 2-g dose of oral metronidazole is indicated in the mother, breast-feeding should be interrupted for 12–24 hours following the dose.

Drug Interactions

■ Coumarin Anticoagulants Oral or IV metronidazole potentiates the effects of oral anticoagulants resulting in prolongation of the prothrombin time, and concurrent administration should be avoided if possible. If metronidazole is used in patients receiving an oral anticoagulant, prothrombin times should be monitored and dosage of the anticoagulant adjusted accordingly.

■ Alcohol Metronidazole appears to inhibit alcohol dehydrogenase and other alcohol oxidizing enzymes. Mild disulfiram-like reactions including flushing, headache, nausea, vomiting, abdominal cramps, and sweating have occurred in some patients who ingested alcohol while receiving oral or IV metronidazole. A disulfiram-like reaction also occurred in one patient who ingested alcohol while receiving intravaginal metronidazole. Patients receiving metronidazole should be warned that this reaction may occur. Studies that investigated the use of metronidazole as an alcohol deterrent in the treatment of chronic alcoholism indicate that these reactions are unpredictable and relatively uncommon. The manufacturers recommend that alcohol not be consumed during or for at least 1 day (or at least 3 days with the oral capsules or extended-release oral tablets) following completion of metronidazole therapy.

■ Disulfiram Administration of disulfiram and metronidazole has been associated with acute psychoses and confusion in some patients; therefore, the drugs should not be used concomitantly and 2 weeks should elapse following discontinuance of disulfiram prior to initiating metronidazole therapy.

■ Phenobarbital Concomitant use of metronidazole and phenobarbital appears to decrease the serum half-life of metronidazole, presumably by increasing metabolism of the anti-infective. Serum concentrations of metronidazole have been decreased and serum concentrations of 2-hydroxymethyl metronidazole increased in patients receiving phenobarbital.

■ Lithium Initiation of short-term metronidazole therapy in patients stabilized on a relatively high dosage of lithium has been reported to increase serum lithium concentrations, resulting in signs of lithium toxicity in several patients; in some cases, signs of renal damage (e.g., persistent elevations in serum creatinine concentration, hypernatremia, abnormally dilute urine) were present. Pending further accumulation of data, caution should be exercised and frequent monitoring of serum lithium and creatinine concentrations should be performed when metronidazole and lithium are administered concurrently.

■ Terfenadine and Astemizole Metronidazole may interact with astemizole (no longer commercially available in the US) and terfenadine (no longer commercially available in the US), resulting in potentially serious adverse cardiovascular effects. Prolongation of the QT interval and QT interval corrected for rate (QT_c) and, rarely, serious cardiovascular effects, including arrhythmias (e.g., ventricular tachycardia, atypical ventricular tachycardia [torsades de pointes], ventricular fibrillation), cardiac arrest, palpitations, hypotension, dizziness, syncope, and death, have been reported in patients receiving the structurally similar antifungal ketoconazole concomitantly with usual dosages of terfenadine or astemizole. Ketoconazole can markedly inhibit the metabolism of astemizole or terfenadine, probably via inhibition of the cytochrome P-450 enzyme system, resulting in increased plasma concentrations of unchanged drug (to measurable levels) and reduced clearance of the active desmethyl or carboxylic acid metabolite, respectively. Such alterations in the pharmacokinetics of these antihistamines may be associated with prolongation of the QT and QT_c intervals. Similar alterations in the pharmacokinetics of these antihistamines and/or adverse cardiac effects have been reported in patients receiving the drugs concomitantly with another structurally related antifungal, itraconazole, although in vitro data suggest that itraconazole may have a less pronounced effect than ketoconazole on the pharmacokinetics of astemizole. Therefore, while astemizole and terfenadine were commercially available in the US, these antihistamines were contraindicated in patients receiving ketoconazole or itraconazole. In addition, it has been recommended that astemizole and terfenadine not be used in patients receiving drugs that are structurally related to itraconazole and ketoconazole, including nitroimidazoles such as metronidazole, imidazoles such as miconazole (systemic form no longer commercially available in the US), and triazoles such as fluconazole. For additional information, see Cautions: Cardiovascular Effects and Precautions and Contraindications, in the Antihistamines General Statement 4:00.

■ Other Drugs In a study in healthy individuals, pretreatment with cimetidine reportedly increased the plasma half-life and decreased total plasma clearance of metronidazole following a single IV dose of the anti-infective, possibly by inhibiting hepatic metabolism of metronidazole. Although further documentation is needed, the possibility of increased adverse effects of metronidazole should be considered if the drugs are administered concomitantly.

Laboratory Test Interferences

Metronidazole interferes with serum AST (SGOT), ALT (SGPT), LDH, triglycerides, or glucose determinations when these determinations are based on the decrease in ultraviolet absorbance which occurs when NADH is oxidized to NAD. Metronidazole interferes with these assays because the drug has an absorbance peak of 322 nm at pH 7 which is close to the 340 nm absorbance peak of NADH; this causes an increase in absorbance at 340 nm resulting in falsely decreased values.

Acute Toxicity

The acute lethal dose of metronidazole in humans is not known. Neurotoxic effects, including seizures and peripheral neuropathy, have occurred in individuals who received 6–10.4 g of metronidazole orally every other day for 5–7 days for the treatment of malignant tumors. Nausea, vomiting, and ataxia without serious resultant toxicity have been reported in individuals who ingested up to 15 g of metronidazole in a single dose. The oral LD_{50} of metronidazole exceeds 5 g/kg in albino rats.

If acute overdosage of metronidazole occurs, symptomatic and supportive treatment should be initiated.

Mechanism of Action

■ **Antimicrobial Effects** Metronidazole is bactericidal, amebicidal, and trichomonacidal in action. The exact mechanism of action of the drug has not been fully elucidated. Metronidazole is un-ionized at physiologic pH and is readily taken up by anaerobic organisms or cells. In susceptible organisms or cells, metronidazole is reduced by low-redox-potential electron transport proteins (e.g., nitroreductases such as ferredoxin) to unidentified polar product(s) which lack the nitro group. The reduction product(s) appears to be responsible for the cytotoxic and antimicrobial effects of the drug which include disruption of DNA and inhibition of nucleic acid synthesis. Metronidazole is equally effective against dividing and nondividing cells.

Metronidazole is referred to as both a luminal or contact amebicide and a tissue amebicide because the drug is active against trophozoites in the intestinal lumen, intestinal wall, and at extraintestinal sites such as the liver and lungs following oral administration. However, because metronidazole is well absorbed from the GI tract, the drug usually has greater activity systemically than locally following oral administration.

■ **Anti-inflammatory and Immunosuppressive Effects** In vitro and in vivo studies indicate that metronidazole has direct anti-inflammatory effects and effects on neutrophil motility, lymphocyte transformation, and some aspects of cell-mediated immunity.

In in vivo studies in rats given metronidazole in dosages of 2–4 mg/100 g of body weight, the drug reportedly inhibited the development of formalin-induced edema in the rat paw. In vitro in neutrophils, metronidazole has a dose-dependent inhibitory effect on generation of hydrogen peroxide and hydroxyl radicals, oxidants that may cause tissue injury at the site of inflammation. This antioxidant effect appears to be caused by a direct effect on neutrophil function and may contribute to the drug's anti-inflammatory effect in vivo.

Results of in vitro studies using leukocytes obtained from patients with Crohn's disease indicate that exposing the cells to metronidazole concentrations of 10 or 50 mcg/mL improved both spontaneous and induced leukocyte migration in cells that previously exhibited reduced migration; the drug had no effect on leukocytes obtained from healthy adults or patients with Crohn's disease when the cells exhibited normal migration prior to exposure to the drug. This effect on leukocyte migration also was observed in vivo in adults with Crohn's disease who received a single 400-mg dose of metronidazole. It has been suggested that metronidazole may increase leukocyte migration by a direct effect on the leukocytes, possibly by causing the release of surface-bound immune complexes from the cell surface.

In in vivo studies in mice, metronidazole given orally in a dosage of 20 or 200 mg/kg daily suppressed granuloma formation around *Schistosoma mansoni* eggs that had been injected IV into the lungs of the mice. In mice sensitized to *S. mansoni* eggs, oral metronidazole (20 mg/kg) inhibited the development of delayed hypersensitivity footpad reactions to soluble schistosome egg antigen. The drug, however, did not affect nonspecific inflammation around divinylbenzene copolymer beads injected in mice and did not suppress skin allograft rejection in mice.

Spectrum

In general, metronidazole is active against most obligately anaerobic bacteria and many protozoa. The drug also is toxic to other anoxic or hypoxic cells. Metronidazole is inactive against fungi, viruses, and most aerobic or facultatively anaerobic bacteria.

When dilution susceptibility testing procedures (e.g., agar or broth dilution) are used to test susceptibility of bacteria to metronidazole, the manufacturer suggests that organisms with an MIC of 8 mcg/mL or less be considered susceptible to metronidazole and those with an MIC of 32 mcg/mL or greater be considered resistant to the drug.

■ **Anaerobic Bacteria** Metronidazole is active in vitro against many anaerobic gram-negative bacilli including *Bacteroides fragilis, B. distasonis, B. ovatus, B. thetaiotaomicron, B. ureolyticus, B. vulgatus, Porphyromonas asaccharolytica, P. gingivalis, Prevotella bivia, P. disiens, P. intermedia, P. melaninogenica, P. oralis, Fusobacterium*, and *Veillonella*. Some strains of *Mobiluncus* (motile, anaerobic, curved rods) are inhibited in vitro by metronidazole; other strains are considered resistant to the drug. The drug also is active against many anaerobic gram-positive cocci including *Clostridium, C. difficile, C. perfringens, Eubacterium, Peptococcus*, and *Peptostreptococcus*. In vitro, the MIC_{90} (minimum inhibitory concentration of the drug at which 90% of strains tested are inhibited) of metronidazole reported for susceptible gram-negative and gram-positive anaerobic bacteria is 0.125–6.25 mcg/mL. *Actinomyces, Lactobacillus, Propionibacterium acnes, P. avidum*, and *P. granulosum* generally are resistant to metronidazole.

■ **Other Bacteria** Most strains of *Gardnerella vaginalis* (formerly *Haemophilus vaginalis*) are susceptible only to relatively high concentrations of metronidazole in vitro. However, the 2-hydroxy metabolite is approximately 4–8 times as active as the parent drug against this organism, and this metabolite may be principally responsible for the activity of metronidazole against *G. vaginalis* in vivo when the drug is administered systemically. Metronidazole has minimal activity against *Lactobacillus* species or other aerobic microorganisms commonly isolated from the vaginal tract.

Metronidazole has some activity in vitro against *Campylobacter fetus*, an organism that can be microaerophilic or anaerobic. In vitro, the MIC_{50} and MIC_{90} of metronidazole reported for *C. fetus* are 3.1 and 25 mcg/mL, respectively.

Limited data indicate that the MIC_{90} of metronidazole for *Helicobacter pylori* (formerly *Campylobacter pylori* or *C. pyloridis*) is 2–4 mcg/mL, although reported MICs of metronidazole for this organism have varied considerably and resistance develops rapidly when the drug is used alone for *H. pylori* infections. The combination of metronidazole and its hydroxy metabolite, or either compound plus tetracycline hydrochloride or amoxicillin, has demonstrated synergism in vitro against *H. pylori*.

■ **Protozoa** Metronidazole is active in vitro and in vivo against *Entamoeba histolytica, Trichomonas vaginalis, Giardia lamblia*, and *Balantidium coli*. In vitro, most strains of *E. histolytica* and *T. vaginalis* are inhibited by metronidazole concentrations less than 3 mcg/mL and most strains of *G. lamblia* are inhibited by metronidazole concentrations of 0.8–32 mcg/mL. Metronidazole acts primarily against the trophozoite forms of *E. histolytica* and has limited activity against the encysted forms.

Metronidazole is believed to exert an anthelmintic effect against the nematode *Dracunculus medinensis* (guinea worm), although this has not been proven to date.

Resistance

Natural and acquired resistances to metronidazole have been reported occasionally in some strains of *Trichomonas vaginalis*. Although the clinical importance is unclear, in vitro studies indicate that while some *T. vaginalis* isolates with reduced susceptibility to metronidazole also have reduced susceptibility to tinidazole, the minimum lethal concentration (MLC) of tinidazole for these strains may be lower than the MLC of metronidazole.

Rarely, resistance to the drug also has been reported in *Bacteroides fragilis* and other anaerobic bacteria following long-term therapy. There has been at least one report of a strain of metronidazole-resistant *B. fragilis* that was cross-resistant in vitro to amoxicillin and clavulanate potassium, imipenem, and tetracycline; the strain was susceptible to chloramphenicol and clindamycin in vitro.

Resistance to metronidazole may be due to poor cell penetration and/or decreased nitroreductase activity.

Pharmacokinetics

■ **Absorption** At least 80% of an oral dose of metronidazole is absorbed from the GI tract. Following oral administration of a single 250-mg, 500-mg, or 2-g dose of metronidazole as immediate-release (conventional) preparations in healthy, fasting adults, peak plasma concentrations of unchanged drug and active metabolites are attained within 1–3 hours and average 4.6–6.5 mcg/mL, 11.5–13 mcg/mL, and 30–45 mcg/mL, respectively. When a single 750-mg dose of metronidazole is administered as two 375-mg capsules or three 250-mg conventional tablets in healthy, fasting adult women, average peak plasma concentrations of unchanged drug and active metabolites of 20.4–21.4 mcg/mL are attained in an average of 1.4–1.6 hours; metronidazole capsules and conventional tablets are bioequivalent at a single dose of 750 mg. The rate of absorption and peak plasma concentrations of metronidazole are decreased when conventional tablets or capsules of the drug are administered with food; however, the total amount of drug absorbed is not affected.

Following oral administration of metronidazole 750 mg once daily as the extended-release tablet for 7 consecutive days in healthy, adult women, steady-state peak plasma concentrations average 12.5 mcg/mL and are attained an average of 6.8 hours after the dose when the drug is given under fasting conditions; when the drug is given at the same dosage under nonfasting conditions, steady-state peak plasma concentrations average 19.4 mcg/mL and are attained an average of 4.6 hours after the dose. Administration of metronidazole extended-release tablets with food increases the rate of absorption and peak plasma concentrations of the drug. According to the manufacturer, metronidazole extended-release and conventional tablets are bioequivalent at a dose of 750 mg given under fasting conditions.

After IV infusion over 1 hour of a loading dose of 15 mg/kg of metronidazole as the hydrochloride followed by IV infusion over 1 hour of 7.5-mg/kg doses every 6 hours in healthy adults, peak steady-state plasma concentrations of unchanged metronidazole average 26 mcg/mL and trough steady-state plasma concentrations of the drug average 18 mcg/mL. In one crossover study in adults, areas under the concentration-time curves (AUCs) were not significantly different following a single 500-mg oral dose of metronidazole as tablets or a single 500-mg IV dose of the drug as metronidazole hydrochloride given over 20 minutes. Small amounts of metronidazole are absorbed systemically when the drug is administered intravaginally.

■ **Distribution** Metronidazole is widely distributed into most body tissues and fluids including bone, bile, saliva, pleural fluid, peritoneal fluid, vaginal secretions, seminal fluid, CSF, and cerebral and hepatic abscesses. Distribution is similar whether the drug is administered orally or by IV infusion. Concentrations of metronidazole in CSF are reported to be 43% of concurrent plasma concentrations in patients with uninflamed meninges and equal to or greater than concurrent plasma concentrations of the drug in patients with inflamed meninges. The drug also distributes into erythrocytes. Limited data suggest that the volume of distribution of metronidazole may be reduced in geriatric individuals as compared with younger individuals, perhaps as a result of decreased erythrocyte uptake of the drug in such patients.

Metronidazole is less than 20% bound to plasma proteins.

Metronidazole readily crosses the placenta. Metronidazole is distributed into milk in concentrations equal to concurrent plasma concentrations of the drug.

■ **Elimination** The plasma half-life of metronidazole is reported to be 6–8 hours in adults with normal renal and hepatic function. In one study using radiolabeled metronidazole hydrochloride, the half-life of unchanged metronidazole averaged 7.7 hours and the half-life of total radioactivity averaged 11.9 hours. The plasma half-life of metronidazole is not affected by changes in renal function; however, the half-life may be prolonged in patients with impaired hepatic function. In one study in adults with alcoholic liver disease and impaired hepatic function, half-life of metronidazole averaged 18.3 hours (range: 10.3–29.5 hours).

Approximately 30–60% of an oral or IV dose of metronidazole is metabolized in the liver by hydroxylation, side-chain oxidation, and glucuronide conjugation. The major metabolite, 2-hydroxy metronidazole, has some antibacterial and antiprotozoal activity. In a group of healthy adults, 19% of a single oral dose of 750-mg of radiolabeled metronidazole was excreted in urine and 3% in feces as unchanged drug and metabolites within 24 hours; 77% of the dose was excreted in urine and 14% in feces as unchanged drug and metabolites within 5 days. Limited data suggest that urinary excretion of unchanged drug and metabolites is decreased in geriatric individuals as compared with younger individuals. Urine may be dark or reddish-brown in color following oral or IV administration of metronidazole or metronidazole hydrochloride due to the presence of water-soluble pigments which result from metabolism of the drug. Metronidazole is removed by hemodialysis but not by peritoneal dialysis.

Chemistry and Stability

■ **Chemistry** Metronidazole is a synthetic, nitroimidazole-derivative antibacterial and antiprotozoal agent. Metronidazole is commercially available as the base and the hydrochloride salt.

The base occurs as white to pale yellow crystals or crystalline powder, is sparingly soluble in water and in alcohol, and has a pK_a of 2.6. Metronidazole injection is a clear, colorless, isotonic solution that has a pH of 4.5–7, an osmolarity of 297–314 mOsm/L, and contains sodium phosphate, citric acid, and sodium chloride. As a result of the excipients, the injection contains 27–28 mEq of sodium per gram of metronidazole, depending on the specific preparation.

Metronidazole hydrochloride is very soluble in water, soluble in alcohol, and is commercially available as an off-white, lyophilized powder for injection which contains mannitol.

■ **Stability** Metronidazole and metronidazole hydrochloride are stable in air but darken following prolonged exposure to light. Metronidazole conventional tablets should be stored in well-closed, light-resistant containers at less than 25°C. Metronidazole capsules should be stored in tight containers at 15–25°C. Metronidazole extended-release tablets should be stored in well-closed containers at approximately 25°C; temporary exposure to temperatures of 15–30°C is acceptable.

Metronidazole hydrochloride powder for injection should be protected from light and stored at less than 30°C. Metronidazole injection should be protected from light and freezing and stored at 15–30°C. The manufacturer (Baxter) of commercially available metronidazole injection RTU® states that this injection has an expiration date of 24 months following the date of manufacture.

Following reconstitution of metronidazole hydrochloride powder for injection with sterile or bacteriostatic water for injection, 0.9% sodium chloride injection, or bacteriostatic sodium chloride injection, solutions containing approximately 100 mg of metronidazole per mL are clear, pale yellow to yellow-green in color, have a pH of 0.5–2, and are chemically stable for 96 hours in room light at less than 30°C. Solutions of metronidazole hydrochloride that have been diluted with 0.9% sodium chloride injection, 5% dextrose injection, or lactated Ringer's injection to a concentration of 8 mg or less of metronidazole per mL and then neutralized with 5 mEq of sodium bicarbonate injection for each 500 mg of metronidazole have a pH of approximately 6–7 and should be stored at room temperature and used within 24 hours. Metronidazole and metronidazole hydrochloride should not be mixed with other drugs.

Because reconstituted metronidazole hydrochloride solution has a low pH, the solution may interact with aluminum resulting in a reddish-brown discoloration of the solution. Therefore, aluminum hub needles should not be used to reconstitute the drug or to transfer the reconstituted solution to the diluting fluid. Metronidazole hydrochloride that has been reconstituted, diluted, and neutralized and metronidazole injection do not interact with aluminum when administered over the time period specified by the manufacturers; however, some discoloration of these solutions may occur when they are in contact with aluminum for periods of 6 hours or longer.

Some commercially available injections of metronidazole (e.g., Baxter's Viaflex® Plus, McGaw's PAB®, Abbott's LifeCare®) are provided in plastic containers. Water can permeate from inside of some plastic containers into the overwrap in amounts insufficient to substantially affect the solutions. Solutions in contact with the plastic containers can leach out some chemical components in very small amounts (e.g., bis(2-ethylhexyl)phthalate [BEHP, DEHP] in up to 5 ppm) within the expiration period of the injections; however, safety of the plastics has been confirmed in tests in animals according to USP biological tests for plastic containers as well as by tissue culture toxicity studies.

Preparations

Excipients in commercially available drug preparations may have clinically important effects in some individuals; consult specific product labeling for details.

metroNIDAZOLE

Oral		
Capsules	375 mg	**Flagyl® 375,** Pfizer
Tablets	250 mg*	**metroNIDAZOLE Tablets**
	500 mg*	**metroNIDAZOLE Tablets**
Tablets, extended-release, film-coated	750 mg	**Flagyl® ER,** Pfizer
Tablets, film-coated	250 mg*	**Flagyl®**, Pfizer
	500 mg*	**Flagyl®**, Pfizer
Parenteral		
Injection, for IV infusion only	5 mg/mL*	**Flagyl® I.V. RTU®** (Viaflex® [Baxter]), SCS Pharmaceuticals
		metroNIDAZOLE Injection (PAB® [Braun]), Various Manufacturers
		metroNIDAZOLE Injection (available in LifeCare® and glass containers), Abbott
		metroNIDAZOLE Injection RTU® (Viaflex® [Baxter]), Various Manufacturers

*available from one or more manufacturer, distributor, and/or repackager by generic (nonproprietary) name

metroNIDAZOLE Combinations

4 Capsules, Tetracycline Hydrochloride 500 mg 4 Tablets, Metronidazole, 250 mg, (with povidone) 8 Tablets, chewable, Bismuth Subsalicylate, 262.4 mg, (with povidone)	**Helidac® Therapy** (available as 14 blister cards), Prometheus

metroNIDAZOLE Hydrochloride

Parenteral		
For injection, for IV infusion only	500 mg (of metronidazole)	**Flagyl I.V.®** (with mannitol 415 mg), SCS Pharmaceuticals

†Use is not currently included in the labeling approved by the US Food and Drug Administration

Miltefosine

HDPC, HePC, Hexadecylphosphocholine

■ Miltefosine, an alkylphosphocholine analog, is an antiprotozoal agent.

Uses

■ **Leishmaniasis** Miltefosine is used for the treatment of cutaneous leishmaniasis caused by *Leishmania braziliensis*, *L. guyanensis*, or *L. panamensis*; mucosal leishmaniasis caused by *L. braziliensis*; and visceral leishmaniasis (also known as kala-azar) caused by *L. donovani*.

The manufacturer states that *Leishmania* species included in clinical studies evaluating efficacy and safety of miltefosine were selected based on epidemiologic data and efficacy of the drug for the treatment of leishmaniasis caused by other species has not been evaluated. When miltefosine is used for the treatment of infections caused by a specific *Leishmania* species, clinicians should consider that clinical response may vary based on geographic location.

Leishmaniasis is caused by more than 15 different species of *Leishmania* that are transmitted to humans by the bite of infected sand flies. *Leishmania* also can be transmitted via blood (e.g., blood transfusions, needles shared by IV drug abusers) and transmitted perinatally from mother to infant. In the Eastern Hemisphere, leishmaniasis is found most frequently in parts of Asia, the Middle East, Africa, and southern Europe; in the Western Hemisphere, the disease is found most frequently in Mexico and Central and South America and has been reported occasionally in Texas and Oklahoma. Leishmaniasis has been reported in short-term travelers to endemic areas and in immigrants and expatriates from such areas, and also has been reported in US military personnel and contract workers serving or working in endemic areas (e.g., Iraq, Afghanistan).

Leishmania infection in humans may cause uncomplicated cutaneous leishmaniasis, diffuse cutaneous leishmaniasis, mucosal leishmaniasis, visceral leishmaniasis, or post-kala-azar leishmaniasis and may be termed Old World (Eastern Hemisphere) or New World (Western Hemisphere). The specific form of leishmaniasis and disease severity depend on the *Leishmania* species involved, geographic area of origin, location of sand fly bite, and patient factors (e.g., nutritional and immune status). Treatment of leishmaniasis (e.g., drug, dosage, duration of treatment) must be individualized based on the region where the disease was acquired, likely infecting species, drug susceptibilities reported in the area of origin, form of the disease, and patient factors (e.g., age, pregnancy, immune status). No single treatment approach is appropriate for all possible clinical presentations. Consultation with clinicians experienced in management of leishmaniasis is recommended.

For assistance with diagnosis or treatment of leishmaniasis in the US, clinicians can contact the US Centers for Disease Control and Prevention (CDC) Parasitic Diseases Hotline at 404-718-4745 from 8:00 a.m. to 4:00 p.m. Eastern Standard Time or CDC Emergency Operation Center at 770-488-7100 after business hours and on weekends and holidays. CDC Drug Service should be contacted at 404-639-3670 for information on how to obtain antiparasitic drugs not commercially available in the US.

Cutaneous Leishmaniasis Although some cases of cutaneous leishmaniasis (usually Old World) may subside or resolve spontaneously over months or years, treatment of cutaneous leishmaniasis is recommended if there are multiple or large lesions, lesions are disabling or disfiguring or fail to heal within 6 months, the patient is immunocompromised, or dissemination to mucosal leishmaniasis is likely (e.g., New World disease caused by *L. braziliensis* or *L. panamensis*). Local treatment (e.g., topical paromomycin [not commercially available in the US], thermotherapy, intralesional pentavalent antimonials [not commercially available in the US], cryotherapy) may be appropriate in selected cases. For systemic treatment of cutaneous leishmaniasis, pentavalent antimonials (i.e., sodium stibogluconate or meglumine antimonate [drugs not commercially available in the US, but may be available from CDC]) usually are used. Other treatment options for cutaneous leishmaniasis include amphotericin B, miltefosine, pentamidine, and ketoconazole, especially when antimonials cannot be used because of tolerance or resistance.

Efficacy and safety of miltefosine for treatment of cutaneous leishmaniasis was evaluated in a randomized, placebo-controlled, double-blind study in Colombia (where *L. braziliensis* and *L. panamensis* are the prevalent infecting species) and Guatemala (where *L. braziliensis* is the prevalent infecting species). Over 130 adults, adolescents, and children 12 years of age and older with newly diagnosed or relapsing cutaneous leishmaniasis (parasitologically confirmed and with at least 1 skin ulcer [minimum area of 50 mm^2] and no mucosal involvement) were randomized in a 2:1 ratio to receive a 28-day treatment regimen of miltefosine given in a dosage based on weight (one 50-mg capsule twice daily in those weighing less than 45 kg or one 50-mg capsule 3 times daily in those weighing 45 kg or more) or placebo. Definite cure was defined as apparent cure (complete epithelialization of all lesions) or partial cure (incomplete epithelialization, no more than 50% lesion enlargement, no appearance of new lesions, and negative parasitology [if done]) at 2 weeks after the end of treatment *and* complete epithelialization of all lesions at 6 months after the end of treatment. The overall definite cure rate was 66% in miltefosine-treated patients (82% in Columbian patients and 48% in Guatemalan patients) compared with 30% in placebo-treated patients (38% in Columbian patients and 20% in Guatemalan patients).

Efficacy of miltefosine also was evaluated in Bahia and Manaus, regions in Brazil where *L. braziliensis* and *L. guyanensis*, respectively, are prevalent. In this study, 80 patients 12–65 years of age received a 28-day treatment regimen of miltefosine given in a dosage based on weight (one 50-mg capsule once daily in those weighing 15–29 kg, one 50-mg capsule twice daily in those weighing 30–45 kg, or one 50-mg capsule 3 times daily in those weighing 46 kg or more). Definite cure (defined as complete healing of lesions at 6 months after completion of therapy) was achieved in 67.5% of patients in Manus, Brazil and 85% of patients in Bahia, Brazil.

Mucocutaneous Leishmaniasis For treatment of mucosal leishmaniasis, pentavalent antimonials (i.e., sodium stibogluconate or meglumine antimonate [drugs not commercially available in the US, but may be available from CDC]), amphotericin B, or miltefosine usually is used. Although data are limited, pentamidine also has been used as an alternative for these infections.

Efficacy of miltefosine for the treatment of mucocutaneous leishmaniasis was evaluated in a single-arm study in Bolivia where *L. braziliensis* is the prevalent species. In this study, 79 adults received a 28-day treatment regimen of miltefosine given in a target dosage of 2.5 mg/kg daily. At 12 months after the end of miltefosine treatment, 62% of patients had complete resolution of edema, erythema, infiltration, and erosion from the involved mucosal sites.

Visceral Leishmaniasis Pentavalent antimonials (i.e., sodium stibogluconate or meglumine antimonate [drugs not commercially available in the US, but may available from CDC]) have historically been considered the drugs of first choice for initial treatment of visceral leishmaniasis; however, drug resistance and treatment failures have become a major concern in some areas (e.g., India, Nepal). Other treatment options for visceral leishmaniasis include amphotericin B, miltefosine, or paromomycin. Relapse of visceral leishmaniasis is common in immunocompromised patients (e.g., patients with human immunodeficiency virus [HIV] infection).

Efficacy of miltefosine for the treatment of visceral leishmaniasis has been evaluated in a phase 3, randomized, open-label, active-controlled study in Bihar, India where *L. donovani* is the prevalent infecting species. Adults, adolescents, and children 12 years of age or older with symptoms compatible with visceral leishmaniasis (e.g., fever, splenomegaly, cytopenia) and confirmed presence of *Leishmania* amastigotes in spleen or bone marrow aspirates were randomized in a 3:1 ratio to receive a 28-day treatment regimen of miltefosine (one 50-mg capsule once daily in those weighing less than 25 kg or one 50-mg capsule twice daily in those weighing 25 kg or more) or a 30-day treatment regimen of amphotericin B deoxycholate (1 mg/kg given IV over 6 hours every other day for 15 doses). Final cure (defined as initial cure at the end of treatment *and* absence of signs and symptoms of visceral leishmaniasis at 6 months after the end of treatment) was achieved in 94% of patients treated with miltefosine and 97% of patients treated with amphotericin B.

■ **Free-living Ameba Infections** Miltefosine has been used in some patients for the treatment of free-living ameba infections†, including primary amebic meningoencephalitis caused by *Naegleria fowleri*† and granulomatous amebic encephalitis or other infections caused by *Balamuthia mandrillaris*† or *Acanthamoeba*†.

CNS infections caused by free-living ameba have a high mortality rate, and only a very limited number of cases have been successfully treated. Early diagnosis and treatment of these infections may increase the chance of survival. Although data are limited, most reported cases of *N. fowleri*, *B. mandrillaris*, or *Acanthamoeba* infection have been treated empirically with multiple-drug regimens. Depending on the specific organism, treatment regimens have included several anti-infectives (e.g., albendazole, amphotericin B, azole antifungals [fluconazole, ketoconazole, itraconazole, or voriconazole], flucytosine, macrolides [azithromycin or clarithromycin], miltefosine, rifampin, pentamidine, sulfonamides [co-trimoxazole or sulfadiazine]) and other therapies (e.g., dexamethasone, phenytoin, therapeutic hypothermia). Miltefosine has been used in the treatment of these infections based on in vitro evidence that the drug has activity against *N. fowleri*, *Balamuthia*, and *Acanthamoeba* and may be amebicidal against some strains.

For assistance with diagnosis or treatment of patients with suspected free-living ameba infections, clinicians can contact the CDC Emergency Operation Center at 770-488-7100. CDC can supply miltefosine for the treatment of infections caused by *N. fowleri*, *B. madrillaris*, or *Acanthamoeba*.

Dosage and Administration

■ **Administration** Miltefosine is administered orally with food to ameliorate adverse GI effects.

Miltefosine capsules should be swallowed whole and should not be broken, chewed, or crushed.

■ **Dosage** ***Leishmaniasis*** For the treatment of cutaneous leishmaniasis caused by *Leishmania braziliensis*, *L. guyanensis*, or *L. panamensis*, mucocutaneous leishmaniasis caused by *L. braziliensis*, or visceral leishmaniasis caused by *L. donovani* in adults, adolescents, and children 12 years of age and older weighing 30 kg or more, dosage of miltefosine is based on weight. (See Table 1.)

Table 1: Dosage of Miltefosine for the Treatment of Cutaneous, Mucocutaneous, or Visceral Leishmaniasis

Body Weight	Miltefosine Dosage
30–44 kg	One 50-mg capsule twice daily (with breakfast and dinner)
45 kg or greater	One 50-mg capsule 3 times daily (with breakfast, lunch, and dinner)

Miltefosine usually is given for 28 consecutive days for the treatment of cutaneous, mucocutaneous, or visceral leishmaniasis.

■ **Special Populations** The manufacturer makes no dosage recommendations for patients with hepatic or renal impairment.

Cautions

■ **Contraindications** Miltefosine is contraindicated in pregnant women; the drug may cause fetal harm. A urine or serum pregnancy test must be obtained prior to prescribing miltefosine for women of reproductive potential.

Miltefosine is contraindicated in patients with known hypersensitivity to the drug or any ingredient in the formulation.

The drug also is contraindicated in patients with Sjögren-Larsson syndrome.

■ **Warnings/Precautions** ***Warnings*** **Fetal/Neonatal Morbidity and Mortality.** Miltefosine may cause fetal harm. Embryofetal toxicity, including fetal death and teratogenicity, has occurred in animals that received miltefosine prior to mating, during early pregnancy, and during organogenesis at doses lower than the maximum recommended human dose.

Miltefosine should *not* be used in pregnant women. Prior to prescribing miltefosine for women of reproductive potential, a urine or serum pregnancy test must be obtained.

Women of reproductive potential should be advised to use effective contraception during and for 5 months after completion of miltefosine treatment. If adverse GI effects occur in such women receiving oral contraceptives, additional nonhormonal or alternative methods of effective contraception should be used. (See GI Effects under Warnings/Precautions: Other Warnings/Precautions, in Cautions.)

Sensitivity Reactions Stevens-Johnson syndrome has been reported during miltefosine therapy.

Miltefosine should be discontinued if an exfoliative or bullous rash occurs during treatment with the drug.

Other Warnings/Precautions **Reproductive Effects.** Impaired fertility was observed in female rats that received miltefosine dosages comparable to the maximum recommended human dose based on body surface area comparisons; reversible follicular atresia and diestrus was observed in female dogs at dosages approximately 0.2 times the maximum recommended human dose. Effects of miltefosine on fertility in female patients have not been adequately studied.

Reduced viable sperm counts and impaired fertility were observed in male rats receiving miltefosine dosages approximately 0.4 times the maximum recommended human dose and testicular atrophy and impaired fertility were observed at dosages comparable to the maximum recommended human dose based on body surface area comparisons. These effects had not fully reversed 10 weeks after discontinuance of the drug.

Scrotal pain and decreased or absent ejaculation have been reported in male patients treated with miltefosine. Effects of miltefosine on fertility in male patients have not been adequately studied.

Patients should be advised of the animal fertility findings and that the potential for impaired fertility in humans receiving miltefosine has not been adequately evaluated.

GI Effects. Vomiting and/or diarrhea commonly occur during miltefosine treatment; vomiting has been reported in up to 48% of patients receiving the drug in clinical trials.

Because vomiting and/or diarrhea may result in volume depletion, fluid intake should be encouraged during miltefosine treatment.

Since GI absorption and efficacy of oral contraceptives may be affected by vomiting and/or diarrhea, women of reproductive potential receiving oral contraceptives should use additional nonhormonal or alternative methods of effective contraception if these adverse GI effects occur. (See Fetal/Neonatal Morbidity and Mortality under Warnings/Precautions: Warnings, in Cautions.)

Hepatic Effects. Elevated hepatic aminotransferase (ALT, AST) and bilirubin concentrations were observed in clinical trials evaluating miltefosine for the treatment of visceral leishmaniasis.

Serum ALT, AST, and bilirubin concentrations should be monitored in patients receiving miltefosine.

Renal Effects. Elevated serum creatinine concentrations were observed in clinical trials evaluating miltefosine for the treatment of cutaneous, mucocutaneous, and visceral leishmaniasis.

Renal function should be monitored weekly during and for 4 weeks after completion of miltefosine treatment.

Hematologic Effects. Thrombocytopenia has been reported in patients receiving miltefosine for the treatment of visceral leishmaniasis. Platelet counts should be monitored in patients receiving the drug for treatment of visceral leishmaniasis.

Specific Populations **Pregnancy.** Category D. (See Users Guide and also see Fetal/Neonatal Morbidity and Mortality under Warnings/Precautions: Warnings, in Cautions.)

Miltefosine should *not* be used in pregnant women.

Embryofetal toxicity, including death and teratogenicity, was observed in rats and rabbits receiving miltefosine during organogenesis, and numerous visceral and skeletal fetal malformations were observed in rats receiving miltefosine prior to mating through day 7 of pregnancy.

Lactation. It is not known whether miltefosine is distributed into human milk.

Because of the potential for serious adverse reactions to miltefosine in nursing infants, a decision should be made whether to discontinue nursing or the drug, taking into account the importance of the drug to the woman. In addition, breast-feeding should be avoided for 5 months after completion of miltefosine treatment.

Pediatric Use. Safety and efficacy of miltefosine have not been established in children younger than 12 years of age.

Animal studies indicate that juvenile rats are more sensitive to miltefosine-induced adverse effects, especially retinal degeneration and kidney effects, than adult rats.

Geriatric Use. Clinical studies of miltefosine did not include sufficient numbers of patients 65 years of age or older to determine whether they respond differently than younger adults.

Hepatic Impairment. Miltefosine pharmacokinetics have not been studied in patients with hepatic impairment. Patients with serum ALT or AST serum concentrations 3 or more times the upper limit of normal (ULN) and bilirubin concentrations 2 or more times the ULN were excluded from miltefosine clinical studies.

Renal Impairment. Miltefosine pharmacokinetics have not been studied in patients with renal impairment. Patients with serum creatinine or BUN concentrations 1.5 or more times the ULN were excluded from miltefosine clinical studies.

■ **Common Adverse Effects** Adverse effects occurring in 2% or more of patients receiving miltefosine for the treatment of cutaneous, mucocutaneous, or visceral leishmaniasis include GI effects (e.g., diarrhea, nausea, vomiting, abdominal pain, epigastralgia, decreased appetite), CNS effects (dizziness, headache, somnolence), motion sickness, asthenia, malaise, pyrexia, pruritus, lymphangitis, increased serum creatinine, increased BUN, and increased hepatic aminotransferase (ALT, AST) concentrations.

Drug Interactions

Miltefosine does not markedly induce or inhibit the activity of cytochrome P-450 (CYP) isoenzymes in vitro or in animal studies.

The potential for miltefosine to interact with drug transporters has not been established.

Description

Miltefosine, an alkylphosphocholine analog, is an antiprotozoal agent with activity against *Leishmania* and some other organisms. Although the precise mechanisms of the drug's antileishmanial effects have not been fully elucidated, the mechanism may involve interaction with phospholipids and sterols (including membrane lipids), inhibition of mitochondrial cytochrome c oxidase (mitochondrial function), and an apoptosis-like effect and cell death.

Miltefosine is active in vitro and in clinical infections against *L. donovani*, *L. braziliensis*, *L. guyanensis*, and *L. panamensis*. The drug also is active in vitro against *L. aethiopica*, *L. amazonensis*, *L. mexicana*, and *L. tropica*. Susceptibility of the different *Leishmania* species to miltefosine varies. In addition, susceptibility of a specific species may vary based on geographic location.

Resistance to miltefosine can occur. Miltefosine-resistant *Leishmania* have been produced in vitro, and strains of *L. braziliensis* with intrinsic resistance to miltefosine have been identified. Resistance to miltefosine may be due to decreased miltefosine accumulation within *Leishmania*, which is thought to be caused by increased drug efflux, mediated by overexpression of the ABC transporter P-glycoprotein, and/or decreased drug uptake due to inactivation of miltefosine transport.

Absolute oral bioavailability of miltefosine has not been determined. Following oral administration of miltefosine in patients with visceral leishmaniasis, peak plasma concentrations of the drug are attained just prior to the next dose in many patients, indicating that absorption of the drug may persist throughout the dosing interval. Distribution of miltefosine in humans has not been evaluated; in rats, the drug is widely distributed following oral administration with highest concentrations in the kidney, liver, and spleen. There is some evidence that miltefosine may be distributed into CSF in some patients. Miltefosine is 98% bound to plasma proteins. In vitro, oxidative metabolism of miltefosine by cytochrome P-450 (CYP) isoenzymes was not observed. Following an oral dose of miltefosine in patients with visceral leishmaniasis, less than 0.2% of the dose is excreted in urine. Results of a study in patients with cutaneous leishmaniasis indicate that miltefosine has a primary elimination half-life of approximately 7 days and a terminal half-life of approximately 31 days.

Advice to Patients

Importance of completing the full course of treatment.

Advise patients to swallow miltefosine capsules whole; the capsules should not be broken, chewed, or crushed.

Importance of taking miltefosine with food to ameliorate adverse GI effects.

Advise patients that abdominal pain, nausea, vomiting, and diarrhea are common adverse effects of miltefosine; importance of informing clinicians if adverse GI effects are severe or persistent.

Instruct patients to consume sufficient fluids to avoid dehydration and, consequently, the risk of kidney injury.

Advise women of reproductive potential to use effective contraception during and for 5 months after miltefosine treatment.

Advise women who use oral contraceptives of the importance of using additional nonhormonal or alternative methods of effective contraception during miltefosine treatment if vomiting and/or diarrhea occurs; these adverse GI effects may decrease effectiveness of oral contraceptives.

Advise men and women that miltefosine has caused infertility in male rats, impaired fertility in female rats, and atresia in ovarian follicles in female dogs. Patients also should be advised that potential effects on fertility in humans have not been adequately evaluated.

Importance of women informing clinicians if they are or plan to become pregnant or plan to breast-feed. Advise nursing mothers not to breast-feed during and for 5 months after miltefosine treatment.

Importance of informing clinicians of existing or contemplated concomitant therapy, including prescription and OTC drugs, as well as any concomitant illnesses.

Importance of informing patients of other important precautionary information. (See Cautions.)

Overview® (see Users Guide). For additional information on this drug until a more detailed monograph is developed and published, the manu-

facturer's labeling should be consulted. It is *essential* that the manufacturer's labeling be consulted for more detailed information on usual cautions, precautions, contraindications, potential drug interactions, laboratory test interferences, and acute toxicity.

Preparations

Excipients in commercially available drug preparations may have clinically important effects in some individuals; consult specific product labeling for details.

Miltefosine

Oral		
Capsules	50 mg	**Impavido®**, Paladin

†Use is not currently included in the labeling approved by the US Food and Drug Administration

Nitazoxanide

■ Nitazoxanide, a synthetic nitrothiazolyl-salicylamide derivative, is an antiprotozoal agent.

Uses

■ **Cryptosporidiosis** Nitazoxanide is used for the treatment of diarrhea caused by *Cryptosporidium parvum* in immunocompetent adults, adolescents, and children 1 year of age or older. The drug is designated an orphan drug by FDA for the treatment of cryptosporidiosis.

Cryptosporidium is an important cause of infectious diarrhea in children and adults in developed and developing countries. Cryptosporidiosis can occur as the result of ingestion of contaminated water, vegetables, fruits, or unpasteurized milk; exposure to infected livestock (e.g., cattle, sheep); or person-to-person transmission via the fecal-oral route. Outbreaks in the US have occurred in child-care centers and have occurred as a result of contaminated municipal water supplies or swimming pools (including chlorinated pools) or infected animals in petting zoos. The duration and severity of clinical symptoms of cryptosporidiosis vary depending on the immune status of the patient. Immunocompetent individuals usually have disease that is asymptomatic or self-limited (i.e., acute, watery diarrhea that persists for up to 2–3 weeks and may be accompanied by nausea, vomiting, abdominal pain, fever); however, immunocompromised individuals can have disease that manifests either as asymptomatic shedding of cryptosporidial oocysts or as transient infection with diarrhea lasting less than 2 months, chronic diarrhea lasting 2 months or longer with persistence of parasites in stool or biopsy specimens, or fulminant cholera-like illness.

Nitazoxanide is considered the drug of choice for the treatment of cryptosporidiosis.

Adults and Adolescents 12 Years of Age or Older Efficacy of nitazoxanide for the treatment of diarrhea caused by *C. parvum* in adults and adolescents 12 years of age or older has been evaluated in several double-blind, controlled studies in Egypt. In one study, patients were randomized to receive nitazoxanide (500 mg as tablets twice daily) or placebo for 3 days; a third group of patients received open label nitazoxanide oral suspension in a dosage of 500 mg twice daily for 3 days. At 4–7 days following the end of treatment, an intent-to-treat analysis in those with *C. parvum* as the sole pathogen indicated that a clinical response (defined as well with no symptoms, no watery stools, and no more than 2 soft stools within the past 24 hours or well with no symptoms and no unformed stools within the past 48 hours) was attained in 96% of those who received nitazoxanide tablets, 87% of those who received nitazoxanide oral suspension, and 41% of those who received placebo.

In another study in Egypt in adults and adolescents with diarrhea caused by *C. parvum* (the sole pathogen), clinical response evaluated 2–6 days following the end of treatment was 71% in those who received nitazoxanide and 43% in those who received placebo.

Although the relevance is unknown, some patients in the above studies categorized as having a clinical response defined as well had *C. parvum* oocysts in their stool at 4–7 days following the end of treatment. Patients should be managed based on clinical response to treatment.

Children 1–11 Years of Age Efficacy of nitazoxanide for the treatment of diarrhea caused by *C. parvum* in children 1–11 years of age has been evaluated in several double-blind, controlled studies. In these studies, clinical response was evaluated 3–7 days following completion of therapy and was defined as well with no symptoms, no watery stools, no more than 2 soft stools, and no hematochezia within the previous 24 hours or well with no symptoms and no unformed stools within the previous 48 hours. In a study in Egypt that included children 1–11 years of age with diarrhea caused by *C. parvum*, clinical response was observed in 88% of those receiving a 3-day regimen of oral nitazoxanide (100 mg twice daily in those 12–47 months of age or 200 mg twice daily in those 4–11 years of age) compared with 38% of those receiving placebo (intent-to-treat analysis).

In a study in malnourished (60% severely underweight, 19% moderately underweight, 17% mildly underweight) hospitalized Zambian children 12–35 months of age with diarrhea caused by *C. parvum*, clinical response was achieved in 56 or 23% of children receiving a 3-day regimen of oral nitazoxanide (100 mg twice daily for 3 days) or placebo, respectively.

HIV-infected Individuals Nitazoxanide has not been shown to be more effective than placebo for the treatment of diarrhea caused by *C. parvum* in immunocompromised patients, including those with human immunodeficiency virus (HIV) infection. Although nitazoxanide has been used for the treatment of cryptosporidiosis in immunocompromised patients, including HIV-infected individuals, no anti-infective has been found to reliably eradicate *Cryptosporidium* in such patients.

In a study in malnourished hospitalized Zambian children with diarrhea caused by *C. parvum*, the clinical response to a 3-day regimen of oral nitazoxanide (100 mg twice daily in those 12–47 months of age or 200 mg twice daily in those 4–11 years of age) in the subgroup of HIV-seropositive patients was no better than that reported for children receiving placebo.

The US Centers for Disease Control and Prevention (CDC), National Institutes of Health (NIH), HIV Medicine Association of the Infectious Diseases Society of America (IDSA), and other clinicians state that the most appropriate treatment for cryptosporidiosis in HIV-infected individuals is the use of potent antiretroviral therapy and supportive care (e.g., aggressive oral and/or IV hydration, correction of electrolyte abnormalities, symptomatic treatment of diarrhea). A highly potent antiretroviral regimen that results in immune restoration ($CD4^+$ T-cell counts exceeding 100/ mm^3) may lead to microbiologic and clinical resolution of *Cryptosporidium* infection. These experts state that adjunctive use of nitazoxanide can be considered for the treatment of cryptosporidiosis in HIV-infected adults, adolescents, or children† receiving effective antiretroviral therapy; however, nitazoxanide should not be used in HIV-infected patients who are not receiving antiretroviral therapy.

■ **Giardiasis** Nitazoxanide is used for the treatment of diarrhea caused by *Giardia intestinalis* (also known as *G. lamblia* or *G. duodenalis*) in immunocompetent adults, adolescents, and children 1 year of age or older. Nitazoxanide is designated an orphan drug by FDA for the treatment of intestinal giardiasis.

Drugs of choice for the treatment of giardiasis are metronidazole, tinidazole, and nitazoxanide; alternative agents include paromomycin (especially in pregnant women), furazolidone (no longer commercially available in the US), or quinacrine (not commercially available in the US).

Adults and Adolescents 12 Years of Age or Older In double-blind controlled studies in Peru and Egypt in adults and adolescents with diarrhea caused by *Giardia*, clinical response was observed in 85–100% of those receiving nitazoxanide tablets (500 mg twice daily for 3 days), 83% of those receiving nitazoxanide oral suspension (500 mg twice daily for 3 days), and in 30–44% of those receiving placebo. Clinical response was evaluated 4–7 days following completion of therapy and was defined as no symptoms, no watery stools, no more than 2 soft stools, and no hematochezia within the previous 24 hours or no symptoms and no unformed stools within the previous 48 hours.

Children 1–11 Years of Age In a controlled study in Peru in children with diarrhea caused by *Giardia*, clinical response rates in children receiving a 3-day regimen of oral nitazoxanide (100 mg twice daily in those 12–47 months of age or 200 mg twice daily in those 4–11 years of age) were similar (80–85%) to response rates achieved in children receiving a 5-day regimen of oral metronidazole (125 mg twice daily in those 2–5 years of age or 250 mg twice daily in those 6–11 years of age). In this study, clinical response was evaluated 7–10 days following initiation of therapy and was defined as no symptoms, no watery stools, no more than 2 soft stools, and no hematochezia within the previous 24 hours or no symptoms and no unformed stools within the previous 48 hours.

HIV-infected Individuals Safety and efficacy of nitazoxanide have not been established for the treatment of diarrhea caused by *Giardia* in HIV-infected patients or other individuals with immunodeficiency. However, CDC, NIH, and IDSA state that tinidazole and nitazoxanide are the drugs of choice for the treatment of giardiasis in HIV-infected infants and children† and metronidazole is the preferred alternative.

■ **Amebiasis** Nitazoxanide has been used for the treatment of amebiasis caused by *Entamoeba*†. The drug is designated an orphan drug by FDA for the treatment of intestinal amebiasis.

The regimen of choice for symptomatic intestinal amebiasis or extraintestinal disease is treatment with a nitroimidazole derivative (tinidazole or metronidazole) followed by treatment with a luminal amebicide (iodoquinol or paromomycin).

Although nitazoxanide has been effective in some patients for the treatment of mild to moderate intestinal amebiasis, data are limited and some clinicians state that additional study is needed to evaluate efficacy of the drug for the treatment of amebiasis.

■ **Isosporiasis (Cystoisosporiasis)** Nitazoxanide has been used in some patients for the treatment of isosporiasis† (also known as cystoisosporiasis) caused by *Isospora belli* (*Cystoisospora belli*).

Co-trimoxazole is the drug of choice for the treatment of infections caused by *I. belli* (*C. belli*); pyrimethamine and ciprofloxacin are recommended as alternatives. Although data are limited, some experts state that nitazoxanide is a potential alternative for the treatment of isosporiasis (cystoisosporiasis) in HIV-infected infants and children† who cannot tolerate co-trimoxazole.

■ **Cestode (Tapeworm) Infections** Nitazoxanide has been used for the treatment of hymenolepiasis caused by *Hymenolepis nana*† (dwarf tapeworm). Praziquantel is considered the drug of choice for the treatment of *H. nana* infections and niclosamide (not commercially available in the US) and nitazoxanide are recommended as alternatives.

In a randomized study comparing efficacy of nitazoxanide and praziquantel for the treatment of hymenolepiasis in children in Peru, nitazoxanide was effective in 82% and praziquantel was effective in 96% of patients.

■ **Nematode (Roundworm) Infections** Nitazoxanide has been used for the treatment of ascariasis† caused by *Ascaris lumbricoides*. Albendazole, mebendazole, and ivermectin are considered the drugs of choice for the treatment of ascariasis. In a randomized study comparing efficacy of nitazoxanide and albendazole for the treatment of ascariasis in children in Peru, nitazoxanide was effective in 89% and albendazole was effective in 91% of patients.

Nitazoxanide has been used for the treatment of trichuriasis† caused by *Trichuris trichiura* (whipworm). Albendazole is considered the drug of choice for treatment of trichuriasis and mebendazole and ivermectin are recommended as alternatives. In a randomized study comparing efficacy of nitazoxanide and albendazole for the treatment of trichuriasis in children in Peru, nitazoxanide was effective in 89% and albendazole was effective in 58% of patients.

■ **Trematode (Fluke) Infections** Nitazoxanide has been used in some patients for the treatment of fascioliasis caused by *Fasciola hepatica*† (sheep liver fluke).

Triclabendazole is considered the drug of choice for the treatment of infections caused by *F. hepatica* and bithionol (not commercially available in the US) and nitazoxanide are recommended as alternatives.

Dosage and Administration

■ **Reconstitution and Administration** Nitazoxanide is administered orally twice daily with food.

Nitazoxanide tablets containing 500 mg of the drug should not be used in pediatric patients 11 years of age or younger since the amount of the drug contained in the tablets exceeds the recommended dosage in this age group.

Nitazoxanide powder for oral suspension should be reconstituted at the time of dispensing by adding 48 mL of water to provide a suspension containing 100 mg/5 mL. After tapping the bottle gently to loosen the powder, the water should be added in 2 portions, and the suspension shaken vigorously after each addition.

Reconstituted nitazoxanide oral suspension may be stored for up to 7 days at room temperature; any unused portion should be discarded after that time.

Prior to administration of each dose, the oral suspension should be shaken well.

■ **Dosage** Nitazoxanide tablets and oral suspension are not bioequivalent. Bioavailability of the oral suspension is 70% relative to that of the tablet.

Adult Dosage **Cryptosporidiosis.** For the treatment of diarrhea caused by *Cryptosporidium parvum* in immunocompetent adults, the usual dosage of nitazoxanide (as tablets or oral suspension) is 500 mg every 12 hours for 3 days.

If nitazoxanide is used for the treatment of cryptosporidiosis in adults with human immunodeficiency virus (HIV) infection† who are receiving an optimized antiretroviral regimen, the US Centers for Disease Control and Prevention (CDC), National Institutes of Health (NIH), and HIV Medicine Association of the Infectious Diseases Society of America (IDSA) recommend a dosage of 0.5–1 g twice daily for 14 days.

Giardiasis. For the treatment of diarrhea caused by *Giardia intestinalis* (also known as *G. lamblia* or *G. duodenalis*) in immunocompetent adults, the recommended dosage of nitazoxanide (as tablets or oral suspension) is 500 mg every 12 hours for 3 days.

Cestode (Tapeworm) Infections. For the treatment of hymenolepiasis caused by *Hymenolepis. nana*† (dwarf tapeworm) in adults, some clinicians recommend a nitazoxanide dosage of 500 mg twice daily for 3 days.

Trematode (Fluke) Infections. If nitazoxanide is used as an alternative for the treatment of fascioliasis caused by *Fasciola hepatica*† (sheep liver fluke) in adults, some clinicians recommend a dosage of 500 mg twice daily for 7 days.

Pediatric Dosage **Cryptosporidiosis.** For the treatment of diarrhea caused by *C. parvum* in immunocompetent children, the recommended dosage of nitazoxanide (as oral suspension) is 100 mg every 12 hours for 3 days for those 1–3 years of age or 200 mg every 12 hours for 3 days for those 4–11 years of age.

For the treatment of diarrhea caused by *C. parvum* in immunocompetent adolescents 12 years of age or older, the usual dosage of nitazoxanide (as tablets or oral suspension) is 500 mg every 12 hours for 3 days.

If nitazoxanide is used for the treatment of cryptosporidiosis in HIV-infected pediatric patients† who are receiving an optimized antiretroviral regimen, CDC, NIH, and IDSA recommend a dosage of 100 mg twice daily in those 1–3 years of age, 200 mg twice daily in those 4–11 years of age, and 500 mg twice daily in those 12 years of age or older. The recommended duration of nitazoxanide treatment in these HIV-infected patients is 3–14 days.

Giardiasis. For the treatment of diarrhea caused by *Giardia* in immunocompetent children, the recommended dosage of nitazoxanide (as oral suspension) is 100 mg every 12 hours for 3 days for those 1–3 years of age or 200 mg every 12 hours for 3 days for those 4–11 years of age.

For the treatment of diarrhea caused by *Giardia* in immunocompetent adolescents 12 years of age or older, the recommended dosage of nitazoxanide (as tablets or oral suspension) is 500 mg every 12 hours for 3 days.

If nitazoxanide is used for the treatment of giardiasis in HIV-infected pediatric patients†, CDC, NIH, and IDSA recommend a dosage of 100 mg every 12 hours in those 1–3 years of age, 200 mg every 12 hours in those 4–11 years of age, and 500 mg every 12 hours in those 12 years of age or older. The recommended duration of nitazoxanide treatment is 3 days.

Isosporiasis (Cystoisosporiasis). If nitazoxanide is used for the treatment of infections caused by *Isospora belli* (*Cystoisospora belli*) in HIV-infected pediatric patients†, CDC, NIH, and IDSA recommend a dosage of 100 mg every 12 hours in those 1–3 years of age, 200 mg every 12 hours in those 4–11 years of age, and 500 mg every 12 hours in those 12 years of age or older. The recommended duration of nitazoxanide treatment in HIV-infected patients is 3 days.

Cestode (Tapeworm) Infections. For the treatment of hymenolepiasis caused by *H. nana*† (dwarf tapeworm) in pediatric patients, some clinicians recommend a nitazoxanide dosage of 100 mg twice daily in those 1–3 years of age, 200 mg twice daily in those 4–11 years of age, and 500 mg twice daily in those 12 years of age or older. The recommended duration of treatment is 3 days.

Nematode (Roundworm) Infections. For the treatment of ascariasis† caused by *Ascaris lumbricoides* in pediatric patients, some clinicians recommend a nitazoxanide dosage of 100 mg twice daily in those 1–3 years of age, 200 mg twice daily in those 4–11 years of age, and 500 mg twice daily in those 12 years of age or older. The recommended duration of treatment is 3 days.

For the treatment of trichuriasis† caused by *Trichuris trichiura* (whipworm) in pediatric patients, some clinicians recommend a nitazoxanide dosage of 100 mg twice daily for 3 days in those 1–3 years of age and 200 mg twice daily for 3 days in those 4–11 years of age.

Trematode (Fluke) Infections. If nitazoxanide is used as an alternative for the treatment of fascioliasis caused by *F. hepatica*† (sheep liver fluke) in pediatric patients, some clinicians recommend a dosage of 100 mg twice daily in those 1–3 years of age, 200 mg twice daily in those 4–11 years of age, and 500 mg twice daily in those 12 years of age or older. The recommended duration of treatment is 7 days.

Cautions

■ **Contraindications** Nitazoxanide is contraindicated in patients hypersensitive to the drug or any ingredient in the formulation.

■ **Warnings/Precautions** ***General Precautions***

Immunodeficiency. Nitazoxanide has not been shown to be more effective than placebo for the treatment of diarrhea caused by *Cryptosporidium parvum* in immunodeficient individuals, including those with human immunodeficiency virus (HIV) infection.

Nitazoxanide has not been evaluated for the treatment of diarrhea caused by *Giardia* in HIV-infected or other immunodeficient individuals.

Specific Populations **Pregnancy.** Data are not available on use of nitazoxanide in pregnant women to inform a drug-associated risk.

In animal reproduction studies, there was no evidence of teratogenicity or fetotoxicity in rats or rabbits when nitazoxanide was given during organogenesis at exposures 30 or 2 times, respectively, the human exposure at the recommended human dosage of 500 mg twice daily based on body surface area.

Lactation. It is not known whether nitazoxanide is distributed into human milk, affects milk production, or affects a breast-fed child.

The developmental and health benefits of breast-feeding should be considered along with the mother's clinical need for nitazoxanide and potential adverse effects on the breast-fed infant from the drug or from the underlying maternal condition.

Pediatric Use. Safety and efficacy of nitazoxanide have not been established in pediatric patients younger than 1 year of age.

Nitazoxanide oral suspension: Safety and efficacy for the treatment of diarrhea caused by *C. parvum* or *G. intestinalis* (also known as *G. lamblia* or *G. duodenalis*) in pediatric patients 1–11 years of age have been established based on results of 3 randomized, controlled studies. Safety and efficacy of the oral suspension for the treatment of diarrhea caused by *C. parvum* or *G. intestinalis* in pediatric patients 12–17 years of age have been established based on results of 2 randomized, controlled studies.

Nitazoxanide tablets: Safety and efficacy for the treatment of diarrhea caused by *C. parvum* or *G. intestinalis* have been established in pediatric patients 12–17 years of age based on results of 3 randomized, controlled studies. The commercially available 500-mg tablets of nitazoxanide should not be used in pediatric patients 11 years of age or younger since the tablets contain a greater amount of the drug than is recommended in this age group.

Geriatric Use. Clinical studies of nitazoxanide did not include a sufficient number of individuals 65 years of age and older to determine whether geriatric adults respond differently than younger individuals. The greater frequency of decreased hepatic, renal, and/or cardiac function and of concomitant disease or drug therapy in this age group should be considered.

Hepatic Impairment. Some clinicians suggest that nitazoxanide should be used with caution in patients with hepatic impairment. Pharmacokinetics of the drug have not been evaluated in patients with hepatic impairment.

Renal Impairment. Some clinicians suggest that nitazoxanide should be used with caution in patients with renal impairment. Pharmacokinetics of the drug have not been evaluated in patients with renal impairment.

■ **Common Adverse Effects** Adverse effects reported in 2% or more of patients receiving nitazoxanide include abdominal pain, headache, chromaturia, and nausea.

Drug Interactions

■ **Protein-bound Drugs** The active metabolite of nitazoxanide (tizoxanide) is highly bound to plasma proteins and pharmacokinetic interactions with other highly protein-bound drugs are possible. Patients should be closely monitored for adverse effects if nitazoxanide is used concomitantly with highly protein-bound drugs that have a narrow therapeutic index (e.g., warfarin).

■ **Drugs Metabolized by Hepatic Microsomal Enzymes** In vitro studies indicate that tizoxanide does not inhibit cytochrome P-450 (CYP) isoenzymes.

■ **Warfarin** Concomitant use of warfarin and nitazoxanide should be avoided. If the drugs are used concomitantly, the patient should be closely monitored for adverse effects.

Description

Nitazoxanide is a synthetic nitrothiazolyl-salicylamide-derivative antiprotozoal agent. Nitazoxanide is rapidly hydrolyzed in vivo to tizoxanide, an active metabolite. Both nitazoxanide and tizoxanide have antiprotozoal activity against the sporozoites and oocysts of *Cryptosporidium parvum* and the trophozoites of *Giardia intestinalis* (also known as *G. lamblia* or *G. duodenalis*). The antiprotozoal activity of nitazoxanide may be related principally to its ability to interfere with the pyruvate:ferredoxin 2-oxidoreductase enzyme-dependent electron transfer reaction essential to anaerobic energy metabolism in susceptible organisms such as *C. parvum* and *Giardia*. Nitazoxanide and tizoxanide also are active against some other protozoa, including *Entamoeba histolytica*, *Trichomonas vaginalis*, *Cyclospora cayetanensis*, and *Isospora belli* (*Cystoisospora belli*).

Nitazoxanide is active against certain helminths, including some cestodes (tapeworms). Although the clinical importance is unclear, nitazoxanide is active in vitro against some anaerobic and microaerophilic gram-positive and gram-negative bacteria, including *Clostridioides difficile* (formerly known as *Clostridium difficile*) and *Helicobacter pylori*, and also is active against some viruses.

Following oral administration, nitazoxanide is rapidly hydrolyzed to tizoxanide (desacetyl-nitazoxanide) and tizoxanide then undergoes conjugation, primarily by glucuronidation. Peak plasma concentrations of tizoxanide and tizoxanide glucuronide usually are attained within 1–5 and 2–8 hours, respectively; nitazoxanide is undetectable in plasma. When nitazoxanide tablets or oral suspension is administered with food, the areas under the plasma concentration-time curves for tizoxanide and tizoxanide glucuronide are increased. Nitazoxanide tablets and oral suspension are not bioequivalent; the relative bioavailability of the oral suspension compared to that of the tablet is 70%. Tizoxanide is more than 99% bound to plasma proteins. The plasma half-life of nitazoxanide is reported to be 6 minutes. The median plasma half-lives of tizoxanide and tizoxanide glucuronide are reported to be 1.2–1.5 and 1.9–2.9 hours, respectively, following a single nitazoxanide dose of 0.5–1 g taken with food and 1.8–6.4 and 3.5–5.6 hours, respectively, following repeated nitazoxanide doses of 0.5–1 g taken with food. Tizoxanide is eliminated in urine, bile, and feces; tizoxanide glucuronide is eliminated in urine and bile. Approximately two-thirds of an oral dose of nitazoxanide is excreted in feces and approximately one-third of the dose is excreted in urine.

Advice to Patients

Advise patients that nitazoxanide tablets or oral suspension should be taken with food.

Advise patients using the oral suspension to keep the container tightly closed and to shake the suspension well prior to each dose. Inform patients that the oral suspension may be stored at room temperature for up to 7 days and any unused portion must be discarded after that time.

Importance of informing clinicians of existing or contemplated concomitant therapy, including prescription and OTC drugs, and any concomitant illnesses. Importance of avoiding concomitant use of warfarin.

Importance of women informing clinicians if they are or plan to become pregnant or to breast-feed.

Importance of informing patients of other important precautionary information. (See Cautions.)

Overview® (see Users Guide). For additional information on this drug until a more detailed monograph is developed and published, the manufacturer's labeling should be consulted. It is *essential* that the manufacturer's labeling be consulted for more detailed information on usual cautions, precautions, contraindications, potential drug interactions, laboratory test interferences, and acute toxicity.

Preparations

Excipients in commercially available drug preparations may have clinically important effects in some individuals; consult specific product labeling for details.

Nitazoxanide

Oral		
For suspension	100 mg/5 mL	**Alinia®**, Romark
Tablets	500 mg	**Alinia®**, Romark

†Use is not currently included in the labeling approved by the US Food and Drug Administration

Pentamidine Isethionate

Pentamidine Diisethionate

■ Pentamidine isethionate, an aromatic diamidine derivative, is an antiprotozoal and antifungal agent.

Uses

■ **Pneumocystis jirovecii Pneumonia** Pentamidine isethionate is used as an alternative for treatment of *Pneumocystis jirovecii* (formerly *Pneumocystis carinii*) pneumonia (PCP) and prevention of *P. jirovecii* infections. Pentamidine is designated an orphan drug by the US Food and Drug Administration (FDA) for treatment and prevention of PCP in patients at high risk for the disease.

Treatment of Pneumocystis jirovecii Pneumonia Parenteral pentamidine is used alone as an alternative for treatment of PCP in patients who cannot tolerate or do not respond to co-trimoxazole, including adults, adolescents, and children with human immunodeficiency virus (HIV) infection. Pentamidine administered by oral inhalation via nebulization (aerosolized pentamidine) should *not* be used for treatment of PCP.

Co-trimoxazole is the drug of choice for treatment of mild, moderate, or severe PCP, including PCP in HIV-infected adults, adolescents, and children.

The US Centers for Disease Control and Prevention (CDC), National Institutes of Health (NIH), and Infectious Diseases Society of America (IDSA) state that alternatives for treatment of moderate to severe PCP in HIV-infected adults and adolescents who cannot tolerate or have not responded to co-trimoxazole are IV pentamidine or a regimen of primaquine in conjunction with clindamycin. Some clinicians prefer the primaquine and clindamycin regimen in such patients since it may be more effective and may be associated with lower toxicity compared with IV pentamidine. For treatment of PCP in HIV-infected children who cannot tolerate co-trimoxazole or have not responded after 5–7 days of co-trimoxazole, CDC, NIH, IDSA, and the American Academy of Pediatrics (AAP) recommend IV pentamidine; these experts state that treatment in such children can be switched to an appropriate oral regimen (e.g., atovaquone) after an initial response is obtained with IV pentamidine.

Parenteral pentamidine is associated with a cure rate of approximately 50–70% in patients with PCP, and has been effective in some patients whose infection did not respond to initial co-trimoxazole treatment. In patients with PCP who respond to pentamidine, a therapeutic clinical response manifested by defervescence and improved respiratory function may be apparent within 24–48 hours, but is generally evident within 2–8 days after initiation of the drug. While improvement in pulmonary radiographic signs generally occurs within several days to a week after the clinical response, complete clearing of radiographic signs may not occur for up to 20–30 days or longer.

Prior to the commercial availability of co-trimoxazole, pentamidine was considered the drug of choice for treatment of PCP; however, because co-trimoxazole has excellent tissue penetration and is associated with rapid clinical response (e.g., 3–5 days in patients with mild to moderate PCP), co-trimoxazole became the drug of choice for treatment of PCP in most patients. Results of limited comparative studies suggest that pentamidine is about as effective as or slightly less effective than co-trimoxazole for treatment of PCP in patients with AIDS and the drugs produce a similar incidence of adverse reactions, including those severe enough to require discontinuance of treatment.

Prevention of Pneumocystis jirovecii Infections Pentamidine administered by oral inhalation via nebulization (aerosolized pentamidine) is used for prevention of initial episodes of PCP (primary prophylaxis) in patients at high risk (e.g., HIV-infected patients with $CD4^+$ T-cell counts of 200/mm^3 or less) and for prevention of recurrence (secondary prophylaxis) in those with a history of PCP.

Prevention of Initial Episode (Primary Prophylaxis). CDC, NIH, and IDSA recommend that primary prophylaxis to prevent initial episodes of PCP be initiated in HIV-infected adults and adolescents with $CD4^+$ T-cell counts less than 200/mm^3 or a history of oropharyngeal candidiasis. These experts state that primary PCP prophylaxis should be considered in HIV-infected adults and adolescents with $CD4^+$ T-cell percentages less than 14% or a history of an AIDS-defining illness who would not otherwise qualify for prophylaxis and also should be considered in those with $CD4^+$ T-cell counts greater than 200/mm^3 but less than 250/mm^3 if frequent monitoring of $CD4^+$ T-cell counts (e.g., every 3 months) is not possible.

CDC, NIH, and IDSA state that primary PCP prophylaxis should be discontinued in HIV-infected adults and adolescents who have responded to antiretroviral therapy and have CD4$^+$ T-cell counts that have remained greater than 200/mm^3 for longer than 3 months. Discontinuance of primary PCP prophylaxis is recommended in these individuals since it appears to add little benefit in terms of disease prevention (PCP, toxoplasmosis, bacterial infections) and discontinuance reduces the medication burden, cost, and potential for drug toxicity, drug interactions, and selection of drug-resistant pathogens. Primary PCP prophylaxis should be reinitiated if CD4$^+$ T-cell counts decrease to less than 200/mm^3.

Co-trimoxazole is the drug of choice for primary PCP prophylaxis in HIV-infected adults and adolescents. CDC, NIH, and IDSA recommend that co-trimoxazole prophylaxis be continued, if clinically feasible, in individuals who experience adverse reactions to the drug that are not life-threatening; however, co-trimoxazole prophylaxis should be permanently discontinued and an alternative used in those with life-threatening adverse reactions to the drug.

Alternative regimens recommended by CDC, NIH, and IDSA for primary PCP prophylaxis in HIV-infected adults and adolescents who cannot tolerate co-trimoxazole are dapsone alone, dapsone in conjunction with pyrimethamine (and leucovorin), aerosolized pentamidine, atovaquone alone, or atovaquone in conjunction with pyrimethamine (and leucovorin). In HIV-infected adults or adolescents who cannot tolerate co-trimoxazole and are seropositive for *Toxoplasma gondii*, dapsone with pyrimethamine (and leucovorin), atovaquone alone, or atovaquone with pyrimethamine (and leucovorin) would provide prophylaxis against both PCP and toxoplasmosis.

In an 18-month, randomized, dose-response study in which 408 HIV-infected patients with or without a history of previous PCP received orally inhaled pentamidine isethionate 30 mg every 2 weeks, 150 mg every 2 weeks, or 300 mg every 4 weeks via a Respirgard® II nebulizer, the risk of developing PCP (either as an initial episode or as recurrence) was reduced by 50–70% in patients receiving the 300-mg dosage regimen compared with patients receiving the 30-mg regimen. Although not statistically significant, a dose-response effect also was apparent in patients receiving the 300-mg regimen versus the 150-mg regimen, and the benefit of the 300-mg dosage was evident even after considering the effect of zidovudine in patients receiving the antiretroviral concurrently. Although the pentamidine dosage had no effect on reduction of overall mortality in this study, mortality was low in all 3 dosage groups. In a study in which oral inhalation therapy with pentamidine isethionate (300 mg every 4 weeks via a Respirgard® II nebulizer) was limited to HIV-infected adults at high risk of PCP (e.g., those with AIDS, advanced AIDS-related complex [ARC], CD4$^+$ T-cell count less than 200/ mm^3) but with no history of previous PCP (primary prevention), the 1-year estimated risk of developing PCP was reduced by about 70% relative to placebo.

Prevention of Recurrence (Secondary Prophylaxis). CDC, NIH, and IDSA recommend that HIV-infected adults and adolescents who have a history of PCP receive long-term suppressive or chronic maintenance therapy (secondary prophylaxis) to prevent recurrence.

Secondary PCP prophylaxis generally is administered for life, unless immune recovery occurs as a result of antiretroviral therapy. CDC, NIH, and IDSA state that secondary PCP prophylaxis generally can be discontinued in HIV-infected adults and adolescents who have responded to antiretroviral therapy and have CD4$^+$ T-cell counts that have remained greater than 200/mm^3 for longer than 3 months, but should be reinitiated if CD4$^+$ T-cell counts decrease to less than 200/mm^3. In addition, these experts state that it may be prudent to continue secondary PCP prophylaxis for life (regardless of CD4$^+$ T-cell count) if PCP occurred or recurred when CD4$^+$ T-cell counts were greater than 200/mm^3.

Co-trimoxazole is the drug of choice for secondary PCP prophylaxis in HIV-infected adults and adolescents. CDC, NIH, and IDSA recommend that co-trimoxazole prophylaxis be continued, if clinically feasible, in individuals who experience adverse reactions to the drug that are not life-threatening; however, co-trimoxazole prophylaxis should be permanently discontinued and an alternative used in those with life-threatening adverse reactions to the drug.

Alternative regimens recommended by CDC, NIH, and IDSA for secondary PCP prophylaxis in HIV-infected adults and adolescents who cannot tolerate co-trimoxazole are the same as those recommended for primary prophylaxis and include dapsone alone, dapsone in conjunction with pyrimethamine (and leucovorin), aerosolized pentamidine, atovaquone alone, or atovaquone in conjunction with pyrimethamine (and leucovorin). In HIV-infected adults or adolescents who cannot tolerate co-trimoxazole and are seropositive for *T. gondii*, dapsone with pyrimethamine (and leucovorin), atovaquone alone, or atovaquone with pyrimethamine (and leucovorin) would provide prophylaxis against both PCP and toxoplasmosis.

Primary and Secondary Prophylaxis in Children. CDC, NIH, IDSA, and AAP recommend that primary prophylaxis to prevent initial episodes of PCP be initiated in HIV-infected children 1 to less than 6 years of age with CD4$^+$ T-cell counts less than 500/mm^3 or CD4$^+$ T-cell percentages less than 15% and in HIV-infected children 6–12 years of age with CD4$^+$ T-cell counts less than 200/mm^3 or CD4$^+$ T-cell percentages less than 15%. These experts recommend that all HIV-infected infants younger than 1 year of age (regardless of CD4$^+$ T-cell count or percentage) receive primary PCP prophylaxis. In addition, infants born to HIV-infected mothers should be considered for primary PCP prophylaxis beginning at 4–6 weeks of age and those with indeterminate HIV status should continue to receive prophylaxis until they are determined to be non-HIV-infected or presumptively non-HIV-infected. Those found to be HIV-infected should receive primary PCP prophylaxis throughout the first year of life; at 1 year of age, the need for continued PCP prophylaxis should be reassessed based on age-specific CD4$^+$ T-cell thresholds.

HIV-infected children who have a history of PCP should receive long-term suppressive or chronic maintenance therapy (secondary prophylaxis) to prevent recurrence.

CDC, NIH, IDSA, and AAP state that, in HIV-infected children who have received at least 6 months of antiretroviral therapy, discontinuance of primary or secondary PCP prophylaxis should be considered in those 1 to less than 6 years of age if CD4$^+$ T-cell counts have remained at 500/mm^3 or greater or CD4$^+$ T-cell percentages have remained at 15% or greater for more than 3 consecutive months and in those 6–12 years of age if CD4$^+$ T-cell counts have remained at 200/mm^3 or greater or CD4$^+$ T-cell percentages have remained at 15% or greater for more than 3 consecutive months. If primary or secondary PCP prophylaxis is discontinued in HIV-infected children, CD4$^+$ T-cell counts and CD4$^+$ T-cell percentages should be assessed every 3 months and PCP prophylaxis reinitiated if indicated based on age-specific CD4$^+$ T-cell thresholds.

Co-trimoxazole is the drug of choice for primary and secondary PCP prophylaxis in HIV-infected infants and children. CDC, NIH, IDSA, and AAP recommend that co-trimoxazole be continued, if clinically feasible, in individuals who experience adverse reactions to the drug that are not life-threatening; however, co-trimoxazole should be permanently discontinued and an alternative used in those with life-threatening adverse reactions to the drug.

Alternative regimens recommended by CDC, NIH, IDSA, and AAP for primary and secondary PCP prophylaxis in HIV-infected infants and children who cannot tolerate co-trimoxazole are dapsone (1 month of age or older), atovaquone (1 month of age or older), or aerosolized pentamidine (5 years of age or older†).

■ **African Trypanosomiasis** Pentamidine is used for treatment of early or first-stage (hemolymphatic) trypanosomiasis caused by *Trypanosoma brucei gambiense*† (West African trypanosomiasis, gambiense sleeping sickness) and has been used as an alternative for treatment of early or first-stage (hemolymphatic) trypanosomiasis caused by *Trypanosoma brucei rhodesiense*† (East African trypanosomiasis, rhodesiense sleeping sickness).

Pentamidine penetrates the CNS poorly and is *not* effective for and should *not* be used for treatment of second-stage (meningoencephalitic) *T. b. gambiense* or *T. b. gambiense* infections when trypanosomes have invaded the CNS.

T. b. gambiense and *T. b. rhodesiense* are transmitted to humans by the bite of infected tsetse flies; transmission via blood or perinatal transmission from mother to infant is rare.

Trypanosoma brucei gambiense Infections *T. b. gambiense* is endemic in West and Central Africa, and more than 95% of reported trypanosomiasis cases involve *T. b. gambiense*. *T. b. gambiense* infection occurs only rarely in short-term travelers to endemic areas, but has been reported in immigrants and expatriates from such areas.

Pentamidine usually is the drug of choice for treatment of first-stage (hemolymphatic) trypanosomiasis caused by *T. b. gambiense*. Suramin (not commercially available in the US, but may be available from CDC) also is effective for these first-stage infections, but is considered an alternative since pentamidine is better tolerated.

For treatment of *T. b. gambiense* infection with CNS involvement, eflornithine (with or without nifurtimox) or melarsoprol (drugs not commercially available in the US, but may be available from CDC) usually is recommended. In untreated patients, CNS invasion and symptoms may not occur for months or years after infection with *T. b. gambiense*.

For assistance with diagnosis or treatment of *T. b. gambiense* trypanosomiasis in the US, clinicians can contact CDC Parasitic Diseases Hotline at 404-718-4745 from 8:00 a.m. to 4:00 p.m. Eastern Standard Time or CDC Emergency Operation Center at 770-488-7100 after business hours and on weekends and holidays. CDC Drug Service should be contacted at 404-639-3670 for information on how to obtain antiparasitic drugs not commercially available in the US.

Trypanosoma brucei rhodesiense Infections *T. b. rhodesiense* is endemic in Eastern and Southern Africa. The disease has been reported occasionally in short-term travelers to endemic areas, especially tourists visiting wildlife reserves in such areas. *T. b. rhodesiense* infections are reported much less frequently than *T. b. gambiense* infections, but usually are associated with more rapidly progressive disease.

For treatment of first-stage (hemolymphatic) trypanosomiasis caused by *T. b. rhodesiense*, suramin (not commercially available in the US, but may be available from CDC) usually is the drug of choice. Pentamidine has been recommended as an alternative to suramin for treatment of first-stage *T. b. rhodesiense* infection because it is better tolerated, but pentamidine may be less active against this infection than against *T. b. gambiense* infection.

Melarsoprol (not commercially available in the US, but may be available from CDC) usually is the drug of choice for treatment of *T. b. rhodesiense* infection with CNS involvement. Clinicians should consider that CNS invasion may occur as soon as 3 weeks to 2 months after infection with *T. b. rhodesiense*.

For assistance with diagnosis or treatment of *T. b. rhodesiense* trypanosomiasis in the US, clinicians can contact CDC Parasitic Diseases Hotline at 404-718-4745 from 8:00 a.m. to 4:00 p.m. Eastern Standard Time or CDC Emergency Operation Center at 770-488-7100 after business hours and on weekends and holidays. CDC Drug Service should be contacted at 404-639-3670 for information on how to obtain antiparasitic drugs not commercially available in the US.

■ **Leishmaniasis** Pentamidine has been used for treatment of cutaneous and mucocutaneous leishmaniasis† caused by various *Leishmania* species and also has been used for treatment of visceral leishmaniasis† (also known as kala-azar).

Leishmaniasis is caused by more than 15 different species of *Leishmania* that are transmitted to humans by the bite of infected sand flies. *Leishmania* also can be transmitted via blood (e.g., blood transfusions, needles shared by IV drug abusers) and transmitted perinatally from mother to infant. In the Eastern Hemisphere, leishmaniasis is found most frequently in parts of Asia, the Middle East, Africa, and southern Europe; in the Western Hemisphere, the disease is found most frequently in Mexico and Central and South America and has been reported occasionally in Texas and Oklahoma. Leishmaniasis has been reported in short-term travelers to endemic areas and in immigrants and expatriates from such areas, and also has been reported in US military personnel and contract workers serving or working in endemic areas (e.g., Iraq, Afghanistan).

Leishmania infection in humans may cause uncomplicated cutaneous leishmaniasis, diffuse cutaneous leishmaniasis, mucosal leishmaniasis, visceral leishmaniasis, or post-kala-azar leishmaniasis and may be termed Old World (Eastern Hemisphere) or New World (Western Hemisphere). The specific form of leishmaniasis and disease severity depend on the *Leishmania* species involved, geographic area of origin, location of sand fly bite, and patient factors (e.g., nutritional and immune status). Treatment of leishmaniasis (e.g., drug, dosage, duration of treatment) must be individualized based on the region where the disease was acquired, likely infecting species, drug susceptibilities reported in the area of origin, form of the disease, and patient factors (e.g., age, pregnancy, immune status). No single treatment approach is appropriate for all possible clinical presentations. Consultation with clinicians experienced in management of leishmaniasis is recommended.

For assistance with diagnosis or treatment of leishmaniasis in the US, clinicians can contact CDC Parasitic Diseases Hotline at 404-718-4745 from 8:00 a.m. to 4:00 p.m. Eastern Standard Time or CDC Emergency Operation Center at 770-488-7100 after business hours and on weekends and holidays. CDC Drug Service should be contacted at 404-639-3670 for information on how to obtain antiparasitic drugs not commercially available in the US.

Cutaneous and Mucocutaneous Leishmaniasis Although some cases of cutaneous leishmaniasis (usually Old World) may subside or resolve spontaneously over months or years, treatment of cutaneous leishmaniasis is recommended if there are multiple or large lesions, lesions are disabling or disfiguring or fail to heal within 6 months, the patient is immunocompromised, or dissemination to mucosal leishmaniasis is likely (e.g., New World disease caused by *L. braziliensis* or *L. panamensis*). Local treatment (e.g., topical paromomycin [not commercially available in the US], thermotherapy, intralesional pentavalent antimonials [not commercially available in the US], cryotherapy) may be appropriate in selected cases. For systemic treatment of cutaneous leishmaniasis, pentavalent antimonials (i.e., sodium stibogluconate or meglumine antimonate [drugs not commercially available in the US, but may be available from CDC]) usually are used. Other treatment options for cutaneous leishmaniasis include amphotericin B, miltefosine, pentamidine, and ketoconazole, especially when antimonials cannot be used because of tolerance or resistance. Pentamidine may be particularly useful for and has been recommended for treatment of New World cutaneous leishmaniasis† caused by *L. guyanensis* or *L. panamensis*. Variable efficacy and potential adverse effects limit usefulness of pentamidine for other types of cutaneous leishmaniasis.

For treatment of mucosal leishmaniasis, pentavalent antimonials (i.e., sodium stibogluconate or meglumine antimonate [drugs not commercially available in the US, but may be available from CDC]), amphotericin B, or miltefosine usually are used. Although data are limited, pentamidine also has been used as an alternative for these infections.

Visceral Leishmaniasis Pentavalent antimonials (i.e., sodium stibogluconate or meglumine antimonate [drugs not commercially available in the US, but may available from CDC]) have historically been considered the drugs of first choice for initial treatment of visceral leishmaniasis; however, drug resistance and treatment failures have become a major concern in some areas (e.g., India, Nepal). Relapse of visceral leishmaniasis is common in immunocompromised patients (e.g., HIV-infected patients), regardless of treatment regimen.

Other treatment options for visceral leishmaniasis include amphotericin B, miltefosine, or paromomycin. Pentamidine has been used for treatment of visceral leishmaniasis, especially when antimonials may be not be effective because of resistance, but pentamidine is not usually recommended for treatment of visceral leishmaniasis, including in HIV-infected individuals, because of variable or suboptimal efficacy and potential adverse effects.

■ **Babesiosis** Because of its activity against *Babesia* infections in animals, pentamidine has been used in a small number of patients for treatment of babesiosis† caused by *B. microti*; however, efficacy has not been established and use of the drug alone has not been shown to be effective. Although parenteral pentamidine used in conjunction with co-trimoxazole has been beneficial for treatment of infection caused by *B. divergens* in at least one patient, potential adverse effects associated with pentamidine limit use of this regimen.

When anti-infective treatment of babesiosis is indicated, IDSA and other clinicians recommend either a regimen of clindamycin and quinine or a regimen of atovaquone and azithromycin.

Dosage and Administration

■ **Reconstitution and Administration** Pentamidine isethionate is administered by deep IM injection or slow IV infusion. The drug should *not* be administered by rapid IV injection or infusion. (See Cautions: Cardiovascular Effects.)

Pentamidine isethionate also is administered by oral inhalation via nebulization (aerosolized pentamidine) using a Respirgard® II jet nebulizer.

IV infusion (not IM injection) is usually recommended for treatment of *Pneumocystis jirovecii* (formerly *Pneumocystis carinii*) pneumonia (PCP); oral inhalation via nebulization is used *only* for prevention of PCP.

Parenteral Administration Because sudden, severe hypotensive reactions can occur following IM or IV administration of pentamidine, the patient should be in a supine position and blood pressure should be monitored closely during administration of the drug and several times thereafter until blood pressure is stable. Equipment and supportive therapy to treat a hypotensive reaction should be readily available. (See Precautions Related to Parenteral Pentamidine under Cautions: Precautions and Contraindications.)

Reconstituted and diluted solutions of pentamidine should be inspected visually for particulate matter and discoloration prior to administration whenever solution and container permit.

IM Injection. For IM injection, a vial of pentamidine isethionate lyophilized powder labeled as containing 300 mg of the drug for IM or IV use should be reconstituted by adding 3 mL of sterile water for injection at 22–30°C to provide a solution containing approximately 100 mg/mL. The powder for IM or IV use should be reconstituted using *only* sterile water for injection; sodium chloride injection should *not* be used since precipitation of the drug will occur.

The desired dose of reconstituted solution should then be withdrawn and administered by deep IM injection. Unused portions of reconstituted solution should be discarded.

Some clinicians suggest that local adverse effects (e.g., sterile abscess, pain) associated with IM administration of pentamidine may be minimized by using the Z-track technique of injection, in which the subcutaneous tissue over the site of injection is firmly pushed aside before inserting the needle at a 90-degree angle, preferably into the upper outer quadrant of the buttock. (See Cautions: Local Effects.)

IV Infusion. For IV infusion, a vial of pentamidine isethionate lyophilized powder labeled as containing 300 mg of the drug for IM or IV use should be reconstituted by adding 3–5 mL of sterile water for injection or 5% dextrose injection at 22–30°C (e.g., using 3, 4, or 5 mL of diluent will provide solutions containing approximately 100, 75, or 60 mg/mL, respectively). The powder for IM or IV use should be reconstituted using *only* sterile water for injection; sodium chloride injection should *not* be used since precipitation of the drug will occur.

The desired dose of reconstituted solution should then be withdrawn and diluted in 50–250 mL of 5% dextrose injection.

The reconstituted and diluted solution of pentamidine should be administered by slow IV infusion over 60–120 minutes. Rapid IV infusion should be avoided. (See Cautions: Cardiovascular Effects.)

The IV needle or catheter should be positioned carefully and closely observed throughout the period of administration. Extravasation should be avoided; if extravasation occurs, the infusion should be immediately discontinued and restarted at another site. (See Cautions: Local Effects.)

Oral Inhalation via Nebulization For oral inhalation via nebulization (aerosolized pentamidine), a vial of pentamidine isethionate lyophilized powder labeled as containing 300 mg of the drug for oral inhalation solution should be reconstituted by adding 6 mL of sterile water for injection. The powder for oral inhalation solution should be reconstituted using *only* sterile water for injection; sodium chloride injection should *not* be used since precipitation of the drug will occur.

Prior to administration of pentamidine oral inhalation solution, the manufacturer's information on administering pentamidine via the Respirgard® II jet nebulizer should be reviewed to assure thorough familiarity with the use and operation of the nebulizer.

The entire contents of the reconstituted vial of pentamidine should be placed into the reservoir of the Respirgard® II jet nebulizer and delivered until the nebulizer chamber is empty (approximately 30–45 minutes) using a flow rate of 5–7 L/minute and an air or oxygen source at 40–50 PSI. Alternatively, an air compressor delivering 40–50 PSI may be used by setting the flowmeter at 5–7 L/minute or the pressure at 22–25 PSI; low-pressure (i.e., less than 20 PSI) air compressors should not be used.

Pentamidine for oral inhalation solution should not be admixed with any other drugs, and the Respirgard® II jet nebulizer should not be used to administer a bronchodilator.

■ **Dosage** ***Pneumocystis jirovecii Pneumonia*** **Treatment of Pneumocystis jirovecii Pneumonia.** When parenteral pentamidine isethionate is used for treatment of PCP in adults and adolescents, including those with human immunodeficiency virus (HIV) infection, the usual dosage is 4 mg/kg once daily given IV or IM. The US Centers for Disease Control and Prevention (CDC), National Institutes of Health (NIH), and Infectious Diseases Society of America (IDSA) recommend that the drug be given IV for treatment of moderate to severe PCP in HIV-infected adults and adolescents and also state that dosage in these patients can be reduced to 3 mg/kg IV once daily if necessary because of toxicity.

When parenteral pentamidine isethionate is used for treatment of PCP in children and infants 4 months of age or older, including those with HIV infection, the usual dosage is 4 mg/kg once daily given IV or IM. CDC, NIH, IDSA, and American Academy of Pediatrics (AAP) recommend that the drug be given IV for treatment of PCP in HIV-infected children and also state that patients who have clinical improvement after 7–10 days of IV pentamidine can be switched to an appropriate oral regimen (e.g., atovaquone) to complete 21 days of treatment.

CDC, NIH, IDSA, and AAP recommend a total treatment duration of 21 days. The manufacturer recommends a treatment duration of 14–21 days and states that parenteral pentamidine has been continued for longer than 21 days, but such treatment may be associated with increased toxicity.

Prevention of Pneumocystis jirovecii Infections. When pentamidine isethionate is administered by oral inhalation via nebulization (aerosolized pentamidine) for prevention of initial episodes (primary prophylaxis) of PCP in adults, adolescents, and children 5 years of age or older†, including HIV-infected individuals, the usual dosage is 300 mg once every 4 weeks (once monthly). CDC, NIH, and IDSA state that primary PCP prophylaxis should be discontinued in HIV-infected adults and adolescents if $CD4^+$ T-cell counts have remained greater than 200/mm^3 for longer than 3 months in response to antiretroviral therapy, but should be reinitiated if $CD4^+$ T-cell counts decrease to less than 200/mm^3. In HIV-infected children who have received at least 6 months of antiretroviral therapy, CDC, NIH, IDSA, and AAP state that discontinuance of primary PCP prophylaxis should be considered based on age-related $CD4^+$ T-cell counts or $CD4^+$ T-cell percentages, but should be reinitiated if these parameters decrease below the age-related thresholds. (See Prevention of Pneumocystis jirovecii Infections under Uses: Pneumocystis jirovecii Pneumonia.)

When pentamidine isethionate is administered by oral inhalation via nebulization (aerosolized pentamidine) for prevention of recurrence (secondary prophylaxis) of PCP in adults, adolescents, and children 5 years of age or older†, including HIV-infected individuals, the usual dosage is 300 mg once every 4 weeks (once monthly). CDC, NIH, and IDSA state that secondary PCP prophylaxis generally can be discontinued in HIV-infected adults and adolescents if $CD4^+$ T-cell counts have remained greater than 200/mm^3 for longer than 3 months in response to antiretroviral therapy, but should be reinitiated if $CD4^+$ T-cell counts decrease to less than 200/mm^3. However, secondary PCP prophylaxis probably should be continued for life (regardless of $CD4^+$ T-cell count) if PCP occurred or recurred when $CD4^+$ T-cell counts were greater than 200/mm^3. In HIV-infected children who have received at least 6 months of antiretroviral therapy, CDC, NIH, IDSA, and AAP state that discontinuance of secondary PCP prophylaxis should be considered based on age-related $CD4^+$ T-cell counts or $CD4^+$ T-cell percentages, but should be reinitiated if these parameters decrease below the age-related thresholds. (See Prevention of Pneumocystis jirovecii Infections under Uses: Pneumocystis jirovecii Pneumonia.)

African Trypanosomiasis For treatment of first-stage (hemolymphatic) trypanosomiasis caused by *Trypanosoma brucei gambiense*† (West African trypanosomiasis, gambiense sleeping sickness), the World Health Organization (WHO) and others recommend that adults and children receive pentamidine isethionate in a dosage of 4 mg/kg once daily for 7–10 days given IM or, alternatively, by IV infusion over 2 hours.

If pentamidine isethionate is used as an alternative for treatment of first-stage (hemolymphatic) trypanosomiasis caused by *T. b. rhodesiense*† (East African trypanosomiasis, rhodesiense sleeping sickness), WHO recommends that adults and children receive 4 mg/kg once daily for 7 days given IM or, alternatively, by IV infusion over 2 hours.

Leishmaniasis For treatment of cutaneous leishmaniasis† caused by various *Leishmania* species, some clinicians recommend that adults and children receive pentamidine isethionate in a dosage of 2–3 mg/kg IM or IV once daily or every other day for 4–7 doses. Others recommend 3–4 mg/kg IM or IV once every other day for 4–10 doses. For treatment of New World cutaneous leishmaniasis caused by *L. guyanensis* or *L. panamensis*, WHO recommends that pentamidine isethionate be given in a dosage of 4 mg/kg IM or IV once every other day for 3 doses.

If pentamidine isethionate is used as an alternative for treatment of visceral leishmaniasis†, some clinicians recommend a dosage of 4 mg/kg IM or IV once every other day or 3 times weekly for 15–20 doses.

■ **Dosage in Renal and Hepatic Impairment** The manufacturer of parenteral pentamidine isethionate states that efficacy and safety of alternative dosage regimens have not been established in patients with impaired renal or hepatic function, and the drug should be used with caution in such patients. (See Precautions Related to Parenteral Pentamidine under Cautions: Precautions and Contraindications.)

When IV pentamidine isethionate is used for treatment of PCP in HIV-infected adults and adolescents with renal impairment, some experts recommend that those with creatinine clearances of 10–50 mL/minute receive a dosage of 3 mg/kg once every 24 hours and that those with creatinine clearances less than 10 mL/minute receive 4 mg/kg once every 48 hours.

Cautions

The most common adverse effects reported with parenteral pentamidine isethionate are nephrotoxic effects; the most common adverse effects reported with pentamidine isethionate administered by oral inhalation via nebulization (aerosolized pentamidine) are cough and bronchospasm.

■ **Renal Effects** Nephrotoxicity is common in patients receiving parenteral pentamidine for treatment of *Pneumocystis jirovecii* (formerly *Pneumocystis carinii*) pneumonia (PCP). Pentamidine-induced nephrotoxicity is manifested by impaired renal function, increased serum creatinine concentration and/or BUN concentrations, and azotemia. Renal impairment usually is mild to moderate in severity and reversible following discontinuance of pentamidine; however, acute renal failure or severe renal insufficiency requiring discontinuance of the drug may occur. Nephrotoxicity and hyperkalemia both may occur more frequently in patients with acquired immunodeficiency syndrome (AIDS) than in other patients treated with parenteral pentamidine; hyperkalemia has been severe in some patients. (See Precautions Related to Parenteral Pentamidine under Cautions: Precautions and Contraindications.) Rarely, pentamidine-induced acute renal failure has been associated with myoglobinuria or gross hematuria. The risk and degree of pentamidine-induced renal impairment may be increased in the presence of dehydration or by concomitant use of other nephrotoxic drugs. (See Drug Interactions: Nephrotoxic Drugs.)

Flank pain, incontinence, increased BUN and serum creatinine concentrations, nephritis, renal failure, renal pain, and syndrome of inappropriate antidiuretic hormone secretion (SIADH) have been reported rarely in patients receiving pentamidine administered by oral inhalation via nebulization.

■ **Cardiovascular Effects** Hypotension, which may develop suddenly and may be moderate to severe (e.g., less than 60 mm Hg systolic), can occur following a single IM or IV dose of pentamidine. Deaths resulting from severe hypotension and cardiac arrhythmias have been reported in patients receiving the drug IM or IV. The risk of hypotensive reactions following IM or IV administration of pentamidine has not been directly compared, but some data suggest that there is no difference in the frequency of these reactions following either route of administration when IV infusions of the drug are administered over a period of at least 60 minutes. Hypotensive reactions may be particularly likely to occur following rapid IV injection or infusion. To minimize the risk of this adverse effect when pentamidine is administered IV, infusions of the drug should be given over a period of 60–120 minutes. In some patients, hypotension was not ameliorated by adjustment of the infusion rate, persisted beyond completion of the infusion, and required volume expansion for correction.

Cardiorespiratory arrest (following rapid IV injection), ventricular tachycardia, atypical ventricular tachycardia (torsades de pointes), ECG abnormalities (abnormal ST segment), facial flushing, cerebrovascular accident, hypertension, palpitations, syncope, vasodilation, and vasculitis have also been reported in patients receiving parenteral pentamidine.

Cerebrovascular accident, hypotension, hypertension, palpitations, poor circulation, syncope, tachycardia, torsades de pointes, vasodilatation, and vasculitis have been reported rarely in patients receiving pentamidine administered by oral inhalation via nebulization.

■ **Hypersensitivity and Dermatologic Effects** There have been rare reports of anaphylaxis and anaphylactoid reactions with shock with parenteral pentamidine. Stevens-Johnson syndrome and toxic epidermal necrolysis have been reported.

Anaphylaxis, allergic reaction, and nonspecific allergy have been reported in patients receiving pentamidine administered by oral inhalation via nebulization.

Pruritus and local or generalized urticaria or rash (e.g., maculopapular, pruritic) occur infrequently in patients receiving parenteral pentamidine.

Rash, including severely pruritic, maculopapular eruption on the upper chest and back, also has occurred when the drug was administered by oral inhalation via nebulization.

Erythema, dry skin, dry and breaking hair, dermatitis, and desquamation have been reported occasionally in patients receiving pentamidine.

■ **Local Effects** Following IM injection of pentamidine, adverse effects at the site of injection, including sterile abscess and/or necrosis, pain, erythema, tenderness, and induration, have been reported in 10–20% of patients. To minimize some of these local adverse effects associated with IM administration of the drug, some clinicians recommend that the Z-track technique of injection be used. (See Parenteral Administration under Dosage and Administration: Reconstitution and Administration.)

Phlebitis may occur following IV administration of pentamidine. Extravasation, sometimes resulting in ulceration, tissue necrosis, and/or sloughing at the injection site, has been reported in patients receiving pentamidine. Surgical debridement and skin grafting have been necessary in a few patients; long-term sequelae have occurred. Because prevention is the most effective means of limiting the severity of pentamidine extravasation, the IV needle or catheter should be properly positioned and closely observed throughout the infusion. If extravasation occurs, the infusion should be discontinued immediately and restarted in another vein; management of the extravasation site is symptomatic.

■ Hypoglycemia and Diabetogenic Effects Hypoglycemia, which may be severe (e.g., blood glucose concentration less than 25 mg/dL) and/or prolonged, appears to occur in at least 5–10% of patients receiving parenteral pentamidine. Hyperglycemia insulin-dependent diabetes mellitus (which appears to be permanent in some cases), with or without preceding hypoglycemia, and ketoacidosis, have also occurred in patients receiving parenteral pentamidine; these adverse effects sometimes occurred several months after discontinuance of parenteral pentamidine. The exact mechanism(s) is not clearly established, but pentamidine-induced hypoglycemia has been associated with pancreatic islet cell necrosis and inappropriately high plasma insulin concentrations and the drug may produce insulin-dependent diabetes mellitus via direct toxic effects on beta cells of the pancreas.

Hypoglycemia, hyperglycemia, and diabetes also have occurred when pentamidine was administered by oral inhalation via nebulization.

Although pentamidine-induced hypoglycemia may occur after initial doses of the drug, it generally occurs after at least 5–7 days of treatment and can even occur up to several days after the drug is discontinued. The duration of hypoglycemia appears to be quite variable, persisting for one or more days up to several weeks. While often asymptomatic, pentamidine-induced hypoglycemia is occasionally severe and has resulted in death. Some data suggest that the occurrence of hypoglycemia caused by the drug in patients with AIDS may be associated with the development of nephrotoxicity. Other apparent risk factors associated with the occurrence of hypoglycemia reportedly include duration of treatment (or total cumulative dosage) and previous treatment with the drug (particularly within the prior 3 months).

Management of pentamidine-induced hypoglycemia depends on the severity and duration of the reaction. Hypoglycemia is usually, but not always, readily controlled by administration of IV dextrose; in some cases, large dosages of IV dextrose and/or supplemental IV dextrose therapy for several days or longer may be required. In a few cases of recurring, severe hypoglycemia, short-term therapy with oral diazoxide was useful.

■ Hematologic Effects Leukopenia (e.g., neutropenia) and thrombocytopenia, which can be severe (e.g., leukocyte count less than 1000/mm^3, platelet count less than 20,000/mm^3), occur occasionally in patients receiving parenteral pentamidine. Leukopenia occurs more frequently than thrombocytopenia. Anemia, defibrination, eosinophilia, pancytopenia, and prolonged clotting time have been reported rarely in patients receiving parenteral pentamidine. Severe thrombocytopenic purpura also has been reported rarely. Although decreased serum folate concentrations (associated with megaloblastic changes in bone marrow in at least one case) have been observed rarely in patients receiving parenteral pentamidine, it is not clear whether the drug can cause folic acid deficiency.

Anemia has been reported occasionally in patients receiving pentamidine by oral inhalation via nebulization; eosinophilia, neutropenia, nonspecific cytopenia, pancytopenia, and thrombocytopenia also have been reported.

■ GI Effects Adverse GI effects reported with parenteral pentamidine or oral inhalation of the drug via nebulization include abdominal cramping or pain, anorexia or decreased appetite, diarrhea, dry mouth, dyspepsia, hematochezia, increased sputum production (hypersalivation), loss of taste, melena, nausea, splenomegaly, and vomiting. An unpleasant (e.g., metallic) taste (dysgeusia) sensation in the mouth or unpleasant feeling on the tongue also have been reported. Dysgeusia may be more severe and persistent with IV than oral inhalation therapy.

Gingivitis, oral ulcer or abscess, gastritis, gastric ulcer, hiatal hernia, esophagitis, constipation, colitis, and numb lips also have been reported in patients receiving pentamidine by oral inhalation via nebulization.

Acute pancreatitis (sometimes fatal) has occurred with parenteral pentamidine; acute pancreatitis also has been reported rarely with pentamidine oral inhalation therapy. (See Cautions: Precautions and Contraindications.)

■ Hepatic Effects Elevated liver function test results, including increased serum AST and ALT concentrations, occur occasionally in patients receiving parenteral pentamidine. Hepatitis, hepatomegaly, and hepatic dysfunction have been reported in patients receiving pentamidine parenterally or by oral inhalation via nebulization.

■ Respiratory Effects Cough and bronchospasm are frequent effects attributed to pentamidine oral inhalation therapy. Cough and bronchospasm also have been reported with parenteral pentamidine.

Cough has occurred in up to 63% of patients receiving pentamidine by oral inhalation via nebulization (38% of patients in initial clinical trials). Cough is most likely in and may be most severe in patients who smoke, and occasionally may be severe enough to require discontinuance of oral inhalation therapy. Bronchospasm has occurred in patients receiving pentamidine oral inhalation via nebulization (15% of patients in initial clinical trials), and is most likely in those with a history of smoking or asthma. Although the exact cause of this bronchospasm has not been elucidated, it has been suggested that it may result, at least in part, from local histamine release and/or anticholinesterase activity induced by the drug.

Cough or bronchospasm occurring during pentamidine oral inhalation therapy can be controlled in most patients by interruption of oral inhalation therapy and administration of a bronchodilator. Coughing also may be controlled by slowing the delivery or intensity of the aerosol stream. In patients who experience cough or bronchospasm with pentamidine oral inhalation, use of an orally inhaled bronchodilator prior to each dose may minimize recurrence of these symptoms. Limited evidence suggests that pretreatment with orally inhaled cromolyn sodium is less effective than bronchodilators in preventing such bronchoconstriction.

Other adverse respiratory effects reported in patients receiving parenteral pentamidine or pentamidine administered by oral inhalation via nebulization include asthma, bronchitis, chest congestion or tightness, coryza, cyanosis, dyspnea, eosinophilic or interstitial pneumonitis, gagging, hemoptysis, hyperventilation, laryngitis (sometimes severe), laryngospasm, nonspecific lung disorder, nasal congestion, pleuritis, pneumothorax, rales, rhinitis, shortness of breath, tachypnea, and wheezing. Bronchial bleeding during bronchoscopy or severe pulmonary hemorrhage following bronchoscopic biopsy also have occurred in association with pentamidine oral inhalation therapy.

■ Nervous System Effects Anxiety, confusion, depression, dizziness, drowsiness, emotional lability, hallucinations, hypesthesia, insomnia, memory loss, nervousness, neuralgia, neuropathy (peripheral or nonspecific), paranoia, paresthesia, seizure, tremors, unsteady gait, and vertigo have been reported in patients receiving parenteral pentamidine and pentamidine oral inhalation therapy.

Fatigue was reported in about 66% of patients receiving pentamidine by oral inhalation via nebulization in initial clinical trials.

■ Other Adverse Effects Other adverse effects reported in patients receiving parenteral pentamidine or pentamidine by oral inhalation via nebulization include arthralgia, body odor, chills, edema (facial or leg), fever, gout, headache, hypocalcemia (sometimes severe), hypomagnesemia, lethargy, low or abnormal body temperature, myalgia, miscarriage, night sweats, nonspecific odor, and extrapulmonary pneumocystosis (sometimes fatal). (See Precautions Related to Pentamidine Oral Inhalation via Nebulization under Cautions: Precautions and Contraindications.)

Blepharitis, blurred vision, conjunctivitis, contact lens discomfort, eye pain or discomfort, hemianopsia, loss of hearing, bad taste, and loss of taste or smell also have been reported in patients receiving pentamidine.

■ Environmental Exposure of Health-care Personnel and Visitors When pentamidine is administered by oral inhalation via nebulization, health-care personnel and visitors or other individuals present during administration of the drug may be at risk of environmental exposure to aerosolized pentamidine and may also be at risk of exposure to pathogens (e.g., *Mycobacterium tuberculosis*) that can be transmitted by patients who cough during the oral inhalation procedure.

There is evidence from several studies that measurable levels of pentamidine can be present in room air when pentamidine is administered by oral inhalation via nebulization. This level may depend on several factors, including room ventilation, proper use of the nebulizer, and variations in treatment practices (e.g., turning off the nebulizer 2–5 minutes before the mouthpiece is removed from the patient). In one study, area air samples were collected using an ambient air sampler over a 4-hour period in an unventilated treatment room where patients received a median dose of 150 mg of aerosolized pentamidine isethionate over 35–40 minutes via a nebulizer (Respirgard® II, which included an expiratory filter); pentamidine concentrations in area air samples averaged about 45 ng/m^{3}during this period. Theoretical estimates based on exposure data from this study indicate that the amount of aerosolized pentamidine isethionate that potentially could be deposited in the lungs of health-care personnel would be 22 ng per 8-hour workday or 4.9 mcg per 225-day workyear, assuming continuous exposure during each 8-hour period. Although it was postulated that the relatively low estimated amounts of drug deposited in the lungs following environmental exposure and the low systemic absorption of pentamidine from the lungs might minimize risk, the potential risk for extrapulmonary toxicity that this or other exposure would represent remains to be established. In another study in a limited number of health-care personnel and other individuals with varying levels of potential exposure to patients receiving the drug via a jet nebulizer (Respirgard® II or AeroTech® II, with expiratory filters), the likelihood of a positive urinary sample for pentamidine appeared to be increased by increasing degrees of potential exposure, with treatment providers being at greatest risk for measurable exposure and personnel simply working in the vicinity of the treatment area or in other areas of the institution being at minimal risk. In this study, approximately 90% of positive samples occurred in treatment providers; urinary concentrations in positive samples ranged from 0.15–8.19 ng/mL, and the number of treatment exposures in providers ranged from 1 monthly in various areas of the institution to 80 monthly in designated rooms with 6 or 35 exchanges of nonrecirculated air per hour.

Adverse effects that have been reported in health-care personnel and others exposed to aerosolized pentamidine in the environment include eye irritation (e.g., conjunctivitis); perioral and perinasal paresthesia; numbness of the mouth and nose; bitter metallic taste; burning sensation of the eyes, nose, and throat; sinus irritation; increased mucous discharge; nasal stuffiness; sneezing; shortness of breath; cough; tightness of the chest; acute bronchospasm; wheezing; hoarseness; fatigue; headache; and light-headedness. Asymptomatic reduction in carbon monoxide diffusion capacity was reported in a nonsmoking, apparently otherwise healthy, respiratory therapist following occupational exposure over a 14-month period to aerosolized pentamidine that was being administered to patients via a Respirgard® II jet nebulizer; this individual's diffusion capacity improved upon removal from exposure and remained stable despite reexposure when ventilation fans were installed in the area used for administration of orally inhaled pentamidine. Reduction in diffusion capacity also has been reported in other health-care personnel.

Because of concerns about the potential risks of environmental exposure to aerosolized pentamidine by health-care personnel and visitors while in contact with patients undergoing oral inhalation therapy with the drug and because of the lack of data on potential effects of pentamidine on the fetus or pregnancy, environmental exposure to aerosolized pentamidine by pregnant women and possibly those planning to become pregnant (e.g., within 8 weeks of potential exposure) should be avoided. (See Pregnancy under Cautions: Pregnancy, Fertility, and Lactation.)

Exposure to tuberculosis is possible in settings where cough-inducing procedures, including administration of aerosolized pentamidine, are performed on patients with undiagnosed *M. tuberculosis* infection. Therefore, it has been suggested that appropriate diagnostic procedures be performed to rule out potentially infectious tuberculosis (e.g., sputum smear, tuberculin skin test, chest radiographs) or other active pulmonary infections prior to initiation of pentamidine oral inhalation therapy. Antituberculosis therapy should be initiated before pentamidine oral inhalation therapy is started in patients with suspected or confirmed potentially infectious tuberculosis. While the risk of tuberculosis transmission to individuals in contact with HIV-infected patients undergoing pentamidine prophylaxis has not been elucidated and some evidence suggests that it may be low overall in some areas (but variable depending on demographics and other factors), epidemiologic studies in one health clinic in which a substantial number of employees developed significant (positive) reactions to a tuberculin skin test (Mantoux) within a 6-month period suggest that occupational exposure to patients with positive *M. tuberculosis* sputum cultures who were receiving pentamidine oral inhalation therapy may have contributed to transmission of the infection. Inadequate fresh air ventilation in this clinic probably contributed substantially to transmission of tuberculosis; several months after installation of adequate ventilation in the facility, no additional significant reactions to a tuberculin skin test were observed. Therefore, adequate air exchange and exhaust to the outside and away from intake vents should be ensured in rooms and booths used for administering aerosolized pentamidine. However, it should be recognized that such ensurance cannot completely eliminate the risk of transmission. Other appropriate preventive measures (e.g., minimizing contact of coughing patients with health-care personnel and others, appropriate use of ultraviolet air disinfection, use of properly constructed and vented and/or filtered [using high-efficiency particulate air filters] administration booths) aimed at reducing the risk of tuberculosis transmission in this setting also should be considered.

The potential risks, particularly long-term and cumulative effects, associated with environmental exposure to aerosolized pentamidine have not been elucidated, and health-care facilities should have procedures to minimize environmental exposure to aerosolized pentamidine. Whenever possible, patients receiving pentamidine oral inhalation via nebulization should be located in rooms where potential exposure to personnel and other patients is minimized (e.g., using separate treatment rooms with closed doors, using properly constructed and vented and/or filtered [with an exhaust HEPA filter] booths or hoods, using nebulizers that have an expiratory filter [e.g., Respirgard® II], instructing the patient to turn off the nebulizer when the mouthpiece is removed). Proper room ventilation can reduce ambient concentrations of the drug. Some clinicians suggest that use of gowns, gloves, goggles, and masks by health-care personnel be considered, although the level of protection provided is not known and some experts state that measures aimed at isolating and engineering out potential exposure generally should be emphasized over *personal* protective apparel and equipment. Use of surgical masks by health-care personnel caring for pentamidine-treated patients probably is unlikely to provide an effective means for reducing environmental exposure to the drug; therefore, if a face mask is used, alternative, appropriately designed (e.g., for adequate particle-size filtration) and well-fitted face masks (e.g., 3M Company model 9970 or 9920) should be employed since they are more likely to substantially reduce respiratory exposure levels. In addition, health-care personnel administering aerosolized pentamidine should be familiar with the manufacturer's instructions for use of the nebulizer delivery system, since improper use of the nebulizer potentially could result in release of substantial amounts of pentamidine into the environment and exposure of health-care personnel to the same risks of adverse effects as patients receiving orally inhaled pentamidine prophylaxis.

■ Precautions and Contraindications

Parenteral pentamidine isethionate is contraindicated in patients with a history of hypersensitivity to the drug.

Pentamidine isethionate administered by oral inhalation via nebulization is contraindicated in patients with a history of anaphylactic reaction following parenteral or oral inhalation of the drug.

Precautions Related to Parenteral Pentamidine Parenteral pentamidine isethionate should be used with caution in patients with hypertension, hypotension, ventricular tachycardia, pancreatitis, Stevens-Johnson syndrome, hyperglycemia, hypoglycemia, hypocalcemia, leukopenia, thrombocytopenia, anemia, or hepatic or renal dysfunction.

Parenteral pentamidine causes adverse effects in a high percentage of patients, and deaths resulting from severe hypotension, hypoglycemia, acute pancreatitis, or cardiac arrhythmias have occurred in patients receiving the drug IM or IV. Therefore, parenteral pentamidine should be used for treatment of PCP only after presence of the organism has been demonstrated. In addition, patients receiving the drug should be closely monitored for the development of severe adverse reactions (e.g., leukopenia, hypoglycemia, nephrotoxicity).

Because sudden, severe hypotension can occur following a single IM or IV dose of pentamidine, patients receiving the drug should be in a supine position and blood pressure should be monitored closely during administration of the drug and several times thereafter until blood pressure is stable. Appropriate equipment for maintenance of an adequate airway and other supportive measures and agents (e.g., IV fluids, vasopressor agents) for the management of hypotensive reactions should be readily available whenever pentamidine is administered parenterally. Since cardiac arrhythmias have been reported in patients receiving pentamidine, the manufacturers recommend that ECGs be performed before, during, and after parenteral therapy with the drug.

Because parenteral pentamidine often causes nephrotoxicity, renal function should be frequently and carefully monitored in patients receiving the drug. Limited evidence suggests that nephrotoxicity associated with parenteral pentamidine may occur more frequently in patients with AIDS than in other patients treated with the drug and may be accompanied by severe, sometimes life-threatening, hyperkalemia despite modest elevations in BUN and/or serum creatinine concentration. Therefore, some clinicians suggest that, in addition to routine monitoring of renal function, serum potassium concentrations should be monitored and patients well hydrated during pentamidine therapy, particularly in AIDS patients. The manufacturers recommend that BUN and serum creatinine concentrations be determined prior to initiation of parenteral pentamidine therapy, daily during therapy with the drug, and after the drug is discontinued.; some clinicians suggest that renal function may be monitored less frequently during therapy (e.g., every other day), unless substantial increases in serum creatinine concentration become evident during treatment and/or other nephrotoxic drugs are administered concomitantly. In addition, to minimize the risk and degree of pentamidine-induced nephrotoxicity, fluid status should be carefully monitored in patients with PCP, particularly patients with AIDS who may be at high risk of dehydration as a result of diarrhea, fever, and poor oral intake. Concurrent administration of IV sodium chloride injection with each dose of parenteral pentamidine has been reported to decrease the incidence and/or severity of adverse effects (e.g., GI symptoms) associated with pentamidine administration.

Since pentamidine commonly causes hypoglycemia (which can occur up to several days after the drug is discontinued) and has diabetogenic effects (which may not be preceded by hypoglycemia and which can sometimes occur several months after therapy with the drug), blood glucose concentration should be frequently and carefully monitored in patients receiving the drug parenterally. The manufacturers recommend that blood glucose concentration be determined before, daily during, and after parenteral pentamidine therapy. Some clinicians suggest that blood glucose concentration may be monitored less frequently during therapy (e.g., every other day), but should be determined daily in patients with a history of diabetes mellitus or hypoglycemia or in those with poor oral intake and should be determined whenever signs and/or symptoms suggestive of hypoglycemia occur.

The manufacturers and some clinicians also recommend that complete blood counts, platelet counts, liver function tests (including serum bilirubin, alkaline phosphatase, AST, and ALT concentrations), and serum calcium concentrations be determined before and at periodic intervals during and after pentamidine therapy.

Because acute pancreatitis has been reported rarely in patients receiving parenteral pentamidine, some clinicians suggest that periodic monitoring of serum amylase concentrations may be warranted in patients receiving the drug. Pentamidine should be discontinued if signs or symptoms of acute pancreatitis develop.

Precautions Related to Pentamidine Oral Inhalation via Nebulization Although pentamidine isethionate administered by oral inhalation via nebulization is generally considered not to be associated with substantial risk of serious adverse effects, the extent and consequences of accumulation of pentamidine following chronic oral inhalation therapy are not known. Therefore, patients receiving pentamidine oral inhalation therapy should be closely monitored for development of serious adverse effects that have been reported with parenteral pentamidine (e.g., hypotension, hypoglycemia, hyperglycemia, hypocalcemia, anemia, thrombocytopenia, leukopenia, hepatic or renal dysfunction, ventricular tachycardia, pancreatitis, Stevens-Johnson syndrome, hyperkalemia, ECG abnormalities [abnormal ST segment]).

Prior to initiating prophylaxis with pentamidine oral inhalation via nebulization, symptomatic patients should be evaluated appropriately to exclude the presence of PCP. Dosage of pentamidine isethionate oral inhalation therapy recommended for prevention of PCP is insufficient for treatment of PCP.

Patients receiving pentamidine oral inhalation via nebulization for prevention of PCP may still develop acute PCP. Relapse of PCP with atypical clinical or radiographic features (e.g., mild disease, granulomatous pulmonary lesions, focal infection confined to the upper lobes of the lung) may occur; such relapses have been treated successfully with parenteral pentamidine, suggesting that inadequate dosage or drug distribution rather than drug resistance is responsible for failure of prophylaxis.

Extrapulmonary and/or disseminated infection caused by *P. jirovecii*, which can be fatal, has been reported occasionally in patients receiving pentamidine oral inhalation therapy for prevention of PCP; most cases have occurred in patients with a history of PCP. The presence of extrapulmonary pneumocystosis should be considered when evaluating patients with unexplained signs and symptoms.

Patients receiving pentamidine by oral inhalation via nebulization for prevention of PCP should be monitored closely for signs and symptoms of pulmonary infection (e.g., fever, cough, dyspnea); those who exhibit such signs or symptoms should have thorough medical evaluations and appropriate diagnostic tests to rule out infection caused by *P. jirovecii* or other opportunistic or nonopportunistic pathogens. If PCP develops in a patient receiving prophylaxis with pentamidine oral inhalation therapy, prophylaxis should be discontinued and treatment with co-trimoxazole, parenteral pentamidine, or other effective treatment regimen should be initiated. Upon completion of treatment, PCP prophylaxis can be reinstituted.

Because acute pancreatitis has been reported rarely in patients receiving orally inhaled pentamidine, some clinicians suggest that periodic monitoring of serum amylase concentrations may be warranted in patients receiving the drug. Pentamidine should be discontinued if signs or symptoms of acute pancreatitis develop.

■ **Pediatric Precautions** Safety and efficacy of parenteral pentamidine isethionate has been established for treatment of PCP in children and infants older than 4 months of age, and there appear to be no unusual risks associated with use of the drug in this age group. Parenteral pentamidine isethionate also has been used effectively and apparently without unusual risks in children for treatment of first-stage (hemolymphatic) African trypanosomiasis† and treatment of leishmaniasis†.

The manufacturer states that safety and efficacy of orally inhaled pentamidine isethionate have not been established in children 16 years of age or younger. The US Centers for Disease Control and Prevention (CDC), National Institutes of Health (NIH), Infectious Diseases Society of America (IDSA), and American Academy of Pediatrics (AAP) recommend pentamidine administered by oral inhalation via nebulization as an alternative for prevention of PCP in children 5 years of age or older† who are capable of effectively using a nebulizer. (See Primary and Secondary Prophylaxis in Children under Pneumocystis jirovecii Pneumonia: Prevention of Pneumocystis jirovecii Infections, in Uses.)

■ **Mutagenicity and Carcinogenicity** Pentamidine was not mutagenic in the Ames bacteria (*Salmonella typhimurium*) test and did not induce an increase in chromosomal aberrations in Chinese hamster ovary (CHO) cells or human lymphocytes in vitro.

Studies have not been performed to date to evaluate the carcinogenic potential of pentamidine isethionate.

■ **Pregnancy, Fertility, and Lactation** ***Pregnancy*** In a study in pregnant rats, IV pentamidine 4 mg/kg daily was embryolethal; teratogenicity was not observed in this study. It is not known whether pentamidine isethionate can cause fetal harm when administered to pregnant women, and parenteral pentamidine or pentamidine administered by oral inhalation via nebulization should be used during pregnancy only when clearly needed.

For treatment of first-stage (hemolymphatic) trypanosomiasis† or treatment of leishmaniasis† in pregnant women, the World Health Organization (WHO) states that parenteral pentamidine should not be used during the first trimester of pregnancy, but may be used after the first trimester.

Although fetal exposure would theoretically not be substantial, some clinicians recommend that pregnant women and possibly those planning to become pregnant (e.g., within 8 weeks of potential exposure) avoid environmental exposure to aerosolized pentamidine. (See Cautions: Environmental Exposure of Health-Care Personnel and Visitors.)

Fertility It is not known whether pentamidine isethionate affects fertility in humans.

Lactation It is not known whether pentamidine isethionate is distributed into milk. Because of the potential for serious adverse reactions to pentamidine isethionate in nursing infants, a decision should be made whether to discontinue nursing or the drug, taking into account the importance of the drug to the woman. The manufacturers state that pentamidine isethionate should not be administered parenterally or by oral inhalation via nebulization in nursing mothers unless potential benefits outweigh potential risks.

Drug Interactions

■ **Nephrotoxic Drugs** Concurrent or sequential use of pentamidine isethionate and other nephrotoxic drugs (e.g., aminoglycosides, amphotericin B, capreomycin, colistin [commercially available in the US as colistimethate sodium], cisplatin, foscarnet, polymyxin B, vancomycin) should be closely monitored or avoided, if possible, since nephrotoxic effects may be additive.

Laboratory Test Interferences

Pentamidine appears to affect the results of bronchoalveolar lavage and induced sputum diagnostic tests for *Pneumocystis jirovecii* (formerly *Pneumocystis carinii*) in patients receiving prophylaxis with the drug administered by oral inhalation via nebulization. The diagnostic yield of bronchoalveolar lavage in patients receiving the drug via oral inhalation was 62% compared with 100% in patients not receiving oral inhalation therapy; similar decreases in diagnostic yield have been observed for induced sputum tests. It is suggested that in the case of bronchoalveolar lavage, both bronchoalveolar and transbronchial biopsy specimens be obtained to optimize the diagnosis of *P. jirovecii* pneumonia (PCP); however, the yield from these tests is still considered high enough to maintain their diagnostic utility in these patients.

Acute Toxicity

Renal and hepatic impairment, hypotension, and cardiopulmonary arrest occurred following inadvertent administration of a 1.6-g dose of IV pentamidine isethionate in a 17-month-old infant. Treatment included cardiopulmonary resuscitation, intubation, epinephrine, atropine, intubation, and 4 hours of charcoal hemoperfusion (resulting in a reduction in serum pentamidine concentrations). The patient recovered from this event, but later died from an unknown cause. One patient with *Pneumocystis jirovecii* (formerly *Pneumocystis carinii*) pneumonia (PCP) inadvertently received a 2-g IM dose of the drug, reportedly without ill effect. In general, overdosage of pentamidine isethionate would be expected to produce effects that are extensions of common adverse reactions.

Overdosage of pentamidine isethionate administered by oral inhalation via nebulization has not been reported to date and the signs and symptoms of such an overdose are not known. Currently available pharmacokinetic data suggest that a dose up to 40 times the recommended dose of orally inhaled pentamidine isethionate would be required to produce plasma concentrations similar to those of a single IV dose of 4 mg/kg; such an overdosage would have the potential of producing adverse effects similar to those seen after parenteral administration of the drug.

In mice, the LD_{50} of pentamidine isethionate has been reported to be 15, 63, or 120 mg/kg following IV, intraperitoneal, or subcutaneous administration, respectively.

Mechanism of Action

■ **Antiprotozoal Effects** The exact mechanism(s) of antiprotozoal action of pentamidine has not been fully elucidated. Several mechanisms of action may be involved, and the role of the mechanism(s) may vary among the different types of protozoa. The effects of pentamidine on various organisms (e.g., bacteria, protozoa) and cells (e.g., murine ascites tumor cells) have been studied to elucidate the mechanism(s) of action, and most information on the antiprotozoal activity of aromatic diamidines such as pentamidine has been derived from studies involving Trypanosomatidae (e.g., *Crithidia*, *Leishmania*, *Trypanosoma*).

In vitro studies indicate that pentamidine interferes with protozoal nuclear metabolism by inhibition of DNA, RNA, phospholipid, and protein synthesis. Mechanisms that may play a role include binding to nucleic acids, disruption of kinetoplast DNA, inhibition of RNA editing in trypanosomes, and inhibition of mRNA trans-splicing. In vitro, pentamidine has been shown to inhibit protein and nucleic acid synthesis in cell-free extracts of *Crithidia oncopelti*. The drug has also been shown to bind to and aggregate ribosomes in cell-free extracts of *C. oncopelti* in vitro, but pentamidine-induced inhibition of protein and nucleic acid synthesis is not associated with marked ribosomal aggregation in intact organisms. In vitro, pentamidine has also been shown to inhibit polyamine synthesis in *Leishmania* spp. and DNA, RNA, protein, and phospholipid synthesis and thymidylate synthetase activity in *C. fasciculata*; in addition, the drug partially inhibits respiration in *C. fasciculata* and in mitochondria-kinetoplast fractions obtained from the organism. The exact mechanism(s) by which pentamidine may impair energy-yielding reactions in trypanosomes is not known, but it has been suggested that the drug may inhibit oxidative phosphorylation. It has also been suggested that the susceptibility of different species of trypanosomes to pentamidine may be related to the relative importance of aerobic and anaerobic glycolysis in their metabolic processes, with the drug being more active against those species that rely more on aerobic glycolysis. There is also some evidence suggesting that susceptibility of different species and subspecies of trypanosomes to pentamidine may be correlated with the rate and/or extent of drug uptake by the organisms. The trypanosomicidal activity of pentamidine and related aromatic diamidine derivatives (e.g., diaminazene, hydroxystilbamidine) may be related in a large part to the ability of the drugs to bind to nucleic acids and DNA, particularly that of mitochondrial kinetoplasts, and thereby produce disruptive effects including inhibition of DNA and RNA synthesis. Ultrastructural studies in various trypanosomes indicate that pentamidine rapidly causes mitochondrial enlargement and fragmentation and condensation of kinetoplast DNA.

■ **Antifungal Effects** In vitro, pentamidine appears to be directly lethal to *Pneumocystis jirovecii* (formerly *Pneumocystis carinii*), although the drug only moderately inhibits glucose metabolism, protein and RNA synthesis, and intracellular amino acid transport in the organism at concentrations attainable in vivo.

■ **Hypotensive Effect** Pentamidine can cause hypotension, which can be severe. (See Cautions: Cardiovascular Effects.) The exact mechanism(s) of pentamidine-induced hypotension is not known, but studies in animals suggest that the drug has a direct vasodilatory action on peripheral small arteries and arterioles. It has also been suggested that histamine release may contribute to the hypotensive effect, since other aromatic diamidine derivatives have been shown to have histamine-releasing activity.

■ **Hypoglycemic and Diabetogenic Effects** Pentamidine can produce hypoglycemia, which may be severe and/or prolonged; in addition, the drug may produce hyperglycemia and insulin-dependent diabetes mellitus, with or without preceding hypoglycemia. (See Cautions: Hypoglycemic and Diabetogenic Effects.) The effect of pentamidine on blood glucose concentration can be multiphasic; an initial increase in blood glucose concentration may occur immediately following administration of the drug (possibly attributed to an adrenergic reaction), followed by a period of hypoglycemia lasting several hours and then hyperglycemia. Although the exact mechanism is not clearly established, pentamidine-induced hypoglycemia has been associated with pancreatic islet cell necrosis and inappropriately elevated plasma insulin concentrations. In vitro studies using pancreatic islet cells and malignant insulinoma cells suggest that pentamidine causes an acute release of insulin from beta cells of the pancreas, possibly via a cytolytic effect, followed by inhibition of insulin release and by cytolysis of the cells. The results of these in vitro studies and in vivo metabolic studies in patients receiving the drug indicate that pentamidine-induced diabetes mellitus probably results from a direct, selective cytotoxic effect of the drug on beta cells of the pancreas.

■ **Other Effects** At concentrations greater than 1 mcg/mL in vitro, pentamidine inhibits platelet aggregation induced by thrombin, epinephrine, adenosine diphosphate (ADP), collagen, and ristocetin in a concentration-dependent manner, with complete inhibition occurring at a concentration of 10 mcg/mL. In vitro, the drug also prolongs thrombin time by a few seconds at a concentration of 5 mcg/mL and slightly prolongs prothrombin and partial thromboplastin times, but only at substantially higher concentrations. At concentrations attained in vivo, pentamidine probably does not affect platelet function or coagulation. Pentamidine also has inhibited cholinesterases in vitro.

Spectrum

■ **Protozoa** Pentamidine is active in vitro and/or in vivo against a variety of protozoa, including Trypanosomatidae that are pathogenic to humans—*Trypanosoma* and *Leishmania*.

Pentamidine is active in vivo against the causative agents of African trypanosomiasis, including most strains of *Trypanosoma brucei gambiense* and some strains of *T. b. rhodesiense*, but is not active against *T. cruzi* (causative agent of American trypanosomiasis [Chagas disease]).

Pentamidine is active in vitro and in vivo against *Leishmania donovani*, including antimony-resistant strains of the organism. In vitro, pentamidine concentrations of 0.05–0.5 mcg/mL result in elimination of 85–90% of *L. donovani* amastigotes in human monocyte-derived macrophages and 20–40% of *L. donovani* promastigotes in cell-free media. The drug is also active in vivo against *L. aethiopica* and has some activity in vitro and possibly in vivo against *L. tropica*. In vitro, pentamidine concentrations of 0.1–0.5 mcg/mL result in elimination of about 85% of *L. tropica* amastigotes in human monocyte-derived macrophages and 10–20% of *L. tropica* promastigotes in cell-free media. Pentamidine also has some activity in vivo against *L. braziliensis* (including *L. b. guyanensis*) and in vitro against *L. mexicana* (including *L. m. amazonensis*) and possibly in vivo against *L. mexicana*.

Pentamidine also is active in vitro against *Crithidia fasciculata* and *C. oncopelti*, which are not pathogenic to humans.

Pentamidine has been shown to have some activity against pathogenic strains of *Acanthamoeba* in vitro, against *Babesia canis* in dogs, and against *B. microti* in rodents. The drug also has some antiplasmodial activity in animals. Pentamidine was inactive in vitro against pathogenic strains of *Naegleria* in one study.

■ **Fungi** Pentamidine is active in vitro and in vivo against *Pneumocystis jirovecii* (formerly *Pneumocystis carinii*). In vitro, the drug appears to be directly lethal to the organism at concentrations attainable in vivo.

Pentamidine is active in vitro and in vivo against some strains of *Candida albicans*. The drug also has some activity in vitro against various *Trichophyton*, *Microsporum*, *Cryptococcus*, *Blastomyces*, and *Histoplasma*, but usually only at very high concentrations.

■ **Other Organisms** In vitro, pentamidine has some antibacterial activity against *Escherichia coli* and *Staphylococcus aureus* and some antiviral activity.

Resistance

Little information is available on natural or acquired resistance of protozoa to pentamidine. Pentamidine resistance can be induced in vitro. Evidence from in vitro studies using *Trypanosoma brucei brucei* and *Crithidia oncopelti* with induced pentamidine resistance and *T. b. brucei* with a degree of natural resistance to the drug suggests that resistance to pentamidine results primarily because of reduced uptake of the drug by the organisms. Studies using trypanosomes indicate that the P2 aminopurine transporter is important for uptake of pentamidine and loss of this transporter results in emergence of resistance. In addition, there is evidence that loss of the P2 transporter and the high-affinity pentamidine transporter appears to be associated with high-level resistance to both pentamidine and melarsoprol (not commercially available in the US, but may be available from the CDC). Trypanosomes resistant to pentamidine are generally cross-resistant to other aromatic diamidine derivatives (e.g., stilbamidine).

Pharmacokinetics

■ **Absorption** Following daily IM administration of single 4-mg/kg doses of pentamidine isethionate (2.3 mg/kg of pentamidine) in an early study in patients with *Pneumocystis jirovecii* (formerly *Pneumocystis carinii*) pneumonia (PCP), plasma pentamidine concentrations (determined using a fluorometric assay) after 1–10 days of therapy averaged 0.3–0.5 mcg/mL (range: 0.3–1.4 mcg/mL). In these patients, plasma drug concentrations did not vary appreciably throughout the day and did not increase with successive doses of the drug. Although plasma pentamidine concentrations generally did not increase immediately after administration of a dose, if an increase did occur, it was usually within 1 hour after administration. Highest plasma drug concentrations occurred in patients with varying degrees of renal impairment.

Following a single 4-mg/kg IM or IV (given as a 2-hour infusion) dose of pentamidine isethionate in patients with acquired immunodeficiency syndrome (AIDS) and PCP, peak plasma pentamidine concentrations (determined using an HPLC assay) averaged 209 ng/mL approximately 40 minutes after the IM dose and 612 ng/mL after completion of the IV infusion. Following IV administration of pentamidine isethionate 3.7–4 mg/kg daily (given as a 4-hour infusion) in HIV-infected patients with PCP, mean peak plasma concentrations were 175.3, 210.9, or 256.7 ng/mL on day 1, 4, or 7, respectively. Data from this study suggest that steady state was not achieved by day 7.

Following oral inhalation of pentamidine isethionate via nebulization (aerosolized pentamidine), bronchoalveolar lavage fluid concentrations of the drug are substantially higher (at least 5–10 times higher) than those attained following IV administration; however, plasma concentrations following oral inhalation are substantially lower than those attained with a comparable IV dose. In a small number of patients with AIDS and suspected PCP, concentrations of pentamidine determined 18–24 hours after oral inhalation of pentamidine isethionate 300 mg via a Respirgard® II jet nebulizer or IV administration of pentamidine isethionate 4 mg/kg averaged 23.2 ng/mL (range: 5.1–43 ng/mL) or 2.6 ng/mL (range: 1.5–4 ng/mL), respectively, in bronchoalveolar lavage fluid and 705 ng/mL (range: 140–1336 ng/mL) or 9.3 ng/mL (range: 6.9–12.8 ng/mL), respectively, in bronchoalveolar lavage sediment; plasma pentamidine concentrations in all but one patient receiving pentamidine by oral inhalation were at or below the level of detection of the HPLC assay (2–3 ng/mL). In other studies in patients receiving orally inhaled pentamidine isethionate 600 mg daily via the Respirgard® II jet nebulizer, mean plasma concentrations after the dose on day 21 reportedly averaged 11.8–13.8 ng/mL. Pentamidine appears to undergo limited absorption from the respiratory tract into systemic circulation; peak plasma concentrations appear to occur at or near completion of oral inhalation administration and appear to be 5% or less of those attained following IV administration. The extent of pentamidine accumulation following chronic oral inhalation therapy is not known.

■ **Distribution** Distribution of pentamidine into human body tissues and fluids has not been well characterized, but the drug appears to be rapidly and extensively distributed and/or bound to tissues. Data from patients with AIDS indicate that following parenteral administration of pentamidine, highest concentrations of the drug (determined using a bioassay) are found in the liver, followed by the kidneys, adrenals, spleen, lungs, and pancreas. Further studies are needed, but these data also suggest that continued parenteral administration beyond the first week of therapy may not substantially increase accumulation of the drug in lung tissue. Since pentamidine is not effective for the treatment of trypanosomiasis involving the CNS, the drug has been believed to poorly penetrate the CNS; this is supported by limited data from patients with AIDS which indicate that pentamidine may distribute into the CNS in some patients, but only in very low concentrations and after prolonged therapy (a month or longer). Following intraperitoneal or IM administration of pentamidine isethionate in mice or rats, respectively, highest concentrations of the drug are found in the kidneys,followed by the liver and lungs. Following IV administration in dogs, highest concentrations of pentamidine are found in the liver, followed by the kidneys, lungs, and spleen; the drug is also distributed into bile and the CNS. IV administration of pentamidine isethionate 5 mg/kg in rats reportedly produced concentrations in the liver and kidney that were 87.5 and 62.3 times higher, respectively, than those produced by an identical dose of pentamidine isethionate administered by oral inhalation.

Deposition of orally inhaled pentamidine shows considerable interindividual variation and appears to depend on several factors, including delivery device, particle size of aerosolized drug, dose, patient position, and nebulization efficiency. Limited data from patients with HIV infections indicate that distribution of the drug in the lungs following oral inhalation via nebulization is more uniform when the patient is in the supine rather than the sitting position. In one study, differences in pulmonary deposition of pentamidine appeared to relate principally to aerosol delivery from the nebulizer system rather than from lung parameters (e.g., breathing pattern, pulmonary function tests, regional ventilation). In this study, the fraction of a dose deposited (amount deposited versus amount inhaled, *not* the amount deposited versus the amount of drug added to the nebulizer) averaged 62% in patients with HIV infection and did not differ substantially as a fraction of that inhaled for the Respirgard® II or AeroTech® II jet nebulizers, although the latter nebulizer was substantially more efficient in delivering the drug to the patient (i.e., the amount inhaled per minute was higher). In an in vitro study simulating clinical conditions, the amount of drug that would be delivered for oral inhalation versus that originally added to the nebulizer (nebulizer efficiency) averaged 4.6, 21, and 16% for the Respirgard® II, AeroTech® II, and FISONeb® nebulizers, respectively, at a simulated tidal volume of 750 cm^3 and a frequency of 20 breaths/minute.

In vitro, pentamidine is reportedly 69% bound to serum proteins. Pentamidine apparently crosses the placenta. In a child delivered by cesarean section from an HIV-infected woman receiving IV pentamidine (3.4 mg/kg daily), concentrations of the drug in cord blood were 13.2 ng/mL; the sample was obtained 16.5 hours after the mother's last dose and blood concentrations of the drug in the mother that day were 81.3 ng/mL. It is not known whether pentamidine isethionate is distributed into milk.

■ **Elimination** Following a single pentamidine isethionate dose of 4 mg/kg given by IM injection or IV infusion over 2 hours in patients with AIDS and PCP who had normal renal function, plasma concentrations of the drug declined in a biphasic manner with a mean half-life of 54 or 18 minutes in the initial phase, respectively, and 9.4 or 6.4 hours in the elimination phase, respectively. Pentamidine appears to be eliminated very slowly from tissues in which the drug principally accumulates (e.g., liver, lungs), and terminal half-lives of 2.8–12 days have been reported with IV dosages of 2–4 mg/kg daily. Following a single pentamidine isethionate dose of 3–4.8 mg/kg given by IV infusion in patients with *Trypanosoma brucei gambiense* infection, the mean terminal elimination half-life was 11 days (range 4–19 days). Limited data suggest that the elimination half-life of pentamidine is not substantially altered in patients with mild to moderate renal impairment but may be prolonged up to 2 days or longer in patients with severe renal impairment.

In mice, pentamidine is excreted in urine and feces in a ratio of about 4:1, respectively; the ratio remains constant for at least 90 hours after administration. In humans, pentamidine is excreted in urine, apparently as unchanged drug; it is not known if the drug is excreted in feces. Following daily IM administration of pentamidine isethionate in a study in patients with PCP who had varying degrees of renal function, 24-hour urinary drug excretion (determined using a fluorometric assay) after 1–10 days of therapy was generally 15–20% (range: 11–29%) of the daily dose; most urinary excretion occurred within the first 6 hours after administration of a dose. In several patients, decreasing amounts of pentamidine were excreted in urine for up to 6–8 weeks after discontinuance of the drug. Following a single 4-mg/kg IM or IV dose of pentamidine isethionate in patients with AIDS and PCP who had normal renal function, about 2.5–5% of the dose (determined using an HPLC assay) was excreted in urine as unchanged drug in 24 hours, mainly within the first 8 hours after administration of the drug; similar amounts (about 1–4% of the dose) were also excreted in urine as unchanged drug in 24 hours in patients with mild to moderate renal impairment. Studies in dogs and humans suggest that renal clearance accounts for about 5% or less of the total body clearance of the drug.

Limited data suggest that pentamidine is not appreciably removed by hemodialysis or peritoneal dialysis.

Data are not available regarding the pharmacokinetics of pentamidine isethionate after oral inhalation via nebulization in patients with hepatic or renal dysfunction.

Chemistry and Stability

■ **Chemistry** Pentamidine isethionate is an aromatic diamidine-derivative antiprotozoal and antifungal agent. The presence of the benzenecarboximidamide (aromatic amidine, benzamidine) group is associated with pentamidine's trypanosomicidal activity, and the presence of both benzenecarboximidamide groups is necessary for this activity.

Pentamidine isethionate is commercially available as a sterile, lyophilized powder for preparation of solutions for IM or IV use and as a sterile, lyophilized powder for preparation of solutions for oral inhalation via nebulization (aerosolized pentamidine). Pentamidine isethionate occurs as white or almost white crystals or powder; the drug is hygroscopic and may be odorless or have a slight butyric odor. The drug is soluble in water, having an aqueous solubility of approximately 100 mg/mL at 25°C, and is slightly soluble in alcohol. Each 1.74 mg of pentamidine isethionate is equivalent to 1 mg of pentamidine. Pentamidine reportedly has a pK_{a1} and pK_{a2} of 11.4.

Following reconstitution with sterile water for injection or 5% dextrose injection, pentamidine isethionate solutions for parenteral use are clear and colorless. After reconstitution with sterile water for injection, solutions of the drug for parenteral use containing 60–100 mg/mL have a pH of approximately 5.4. Following reconstitution with 5% dextrose injection, pentamidine isethionate solutions for parenteral use containing 60 or 100 mg/mL have a pH of 4.09 or 4.38, respectively. Pentamidine isethionate solutions for parenteral use containing 100 mg/mL in sterile water for injection or 5% dextrose injection have osmolalities of 160 or 455 mOsm/kg, respectively.

When pentamidine isethionate lyophilized powder for oral inhalation solution is reconstituted and administered using the Respirgard® II jet nebulizer, the resultant mist contains nebulized particles of the drug with a median mass aerodynamic diameter of 0.8–1.4 μm.

■ **Stability** Prior to reconstitution, pentamidine isethionate lyophilized powders should be stored at 20–25°C and protected from light.

Following reconstitution with sterile water for injection, pentamidine isethionate solutions for parenteral use containing 60–100 mg/mL are stable in the original vial for 48 hours at room temperature if protected from light; to avoid crystallization, reconstituted solutions should be stored at 22–30°C. Unused portions of the reconstituted solutions should be discarded. Reconstituted solutions of the drug for parenteral use that have been further diluted in 5% dextrose injection to a concentration of 1 or 2.5 mg/mL for IV infusion are stable for up to 24 hours at room temperature. Reconstituted solutions that have been diluted to a concentration of 1 or 2 mg/mL in 5% dextrose or 0.9% sodium chloride injection in PVC bags are reportedly stable for 48 hours exposed to normal fluorescent light at 22–26°C; some data suggest that small amounts of the drug may be adsorbed onto PVC infusion sets.

Following reconstitution with sterile water for injection, pentamidine isethionate solutions for oral inhalation are stable in the original vial for 48 hours at room temperature if protected from light.

Preparations

Excipients in commercially available drug preparations may have clinically important effects in some individuals; consult specific product labeling for details.

Pentamidine Isethionate

Oral Inhalation		
For solution, for nebulization	300 mg	**NebuPent®**, APP
Parenteral		
For injection	300 mg*	**Pentam® 300**, APP
		Pentamidine Isethionate for Injection

*available from one or more manufacturer, distributor, and/or repackager by generic (nonproprietary) name

†Use is not currently included in the labeling approved by the US Food and Drug Administration

Selected Revisions October 2014, © Copyright, May 1985, American Society of Health-System Pharmacists, Inc.

Secnidazole

■ Secnidazole, a nitroimidazole derivative, is an antiprotozoal and antibacterial agent.

Uses

■ **Bacterial Vaginosis** Secnidazole is used for the treatment of bacterial vaginosis.

Bacterial vaginosis is a polymicrobial syndrome that can occur when normal hydrogen peroxide-producing *Lactobacillus* in the vagina are replaced by overgrowth of various anaerobic bacteria (e.g., *Atopobium vaginae, Bacteroides, Mobiluncus, Prevotella*), *Gardnerella vaginalis, Ureaplasma urealyticum, Mycoplasma hominis*, or other bacteria. Treatment of bacterial vaginosis is usually recommended in symptomatic women to relieve the signs and symptoms of infection; routine treatment of male sexual partner(s) is not usually recommended. Relapse or recurrence of bacterial vaginosis is common, regardless of the treatment regimen used.

Clinical Experience Efficacy and safety of secnidazole for the treatment of bacterial vaginosis in nonpregnant women were evaluated in 2 similarly designed randomized, placebo-controlled studies (Trial 1 and Trial 2). In both studies, bacterial vaginosis was diagnosed by presence of an off-white (milky or gray), thin, homogeneous vaginal discharge, vaginal pH 4.7 or greater, presence of clue cells as 20% or greater of total epithelial cells on a microscopic examination of vaginal saline wet mount, detection of amine odor on addition of 10% potassium hydroxide (KOH) solution to a sample of vaginal discharge (positive "whiff" test), and a Nugent score 4 or greater. The 144 women enrolled in Trial 1 (19–54 years of age) and 189 women enrolled in Trial 2 (18–54 years of age) were randomized to receive a single 2-g dose of secnidazole oral granules or placebo. The primary end point was clinical response (defined as normal vaginal discharge, negative detection of amine odor on addition of 10% KOH solution, and clue cells less than 20% of total epithelial cells) at the test-of-cure visit (21–30 days after the dose).

In the modified intent-to-treat (MITT) population in Trial 1, clinical response was achieved in 67.7 or 17.7% of patients treated with secnidazole or placebo, respectively; in Trial 2, clinical response was achieved in 53.3 or 19.3% of patients in the MITT population treated with secnidazole or placebo, respectively. In Trial 1, Nugent score cure (i.e., Nugent score 0–3) was achieved in 40.3 or 6.5% of patients treated with secnidazole or placebo, respectively; in Trial 2, Nugent score cure was achieved in 43.9 or 5.3% of patients treated with secnidazole or placebo, respectively.

Dosage and Administration

■ **Administration** Secnidazole is administered orally without regard to meals.

Secnidazole is commercially available as single-dose packets containing oral granules that are taken by sprinkling onto applesauce, yogurt, or pudding. The granules will not dissolve and are not intended to be administered in any liquid.

The entire contents of a single-dose packet of secnidazole granules (2 g of secnidazole) should be sprinkled onto applesauce, yogurt, or pudding and the entire mixture should be consumed within 30 minutes without chewing or crunching the granules. A glass of water may be taken after administration of secnidazole granules to aid in swallowing.

■ **Dosage** ***Bacterial Vaginosis*** For the treatment of bacterial vaginosis in adult women, secnidazole is administered as a single 2-g dose.

■ **Special Populations** The manufacturer makes no specific dosage recommendations for patients with hepatic or renal impairment or for geriatric patients.

Cautions

■ **Contraindications** Secnidazole is contraindicated in patients with known hypersensitivity to secnidazole, other ingredients in the formulation, or other nitroimidazole derivatives.

■ **Warnings/Precautions** ***Vulvovaginal Candidiasis*** The use of secnidazole may result in vulvovaginal candidiasis. In clinical trials in nonpregnant women with bacterial vaginosis, vulvovaginal candidiasis developed in 9.6% of patients who received secnidazole and 2.9% of patients who received placebo. Symptomatic vulvovaginal candidiasis may require treatment with an antifungal.

Carcinogenicity Carcinogenicity has been observed in mice and rats treated chronically with nitroimidazole derivatives structurally related to secnidazole (e.g., metronidazole). In some rodent studies, lifetime exposure to nitroimidazoles was associated with tumors affecting liver, lung, mammary, and lymphatic tissues.

It is not known if positive tumor findings in rodent studies using other nitroimidazoles indicate a risk to patients receiving a single dose of secnidazole to treat bacterial vaginosis. The manufacturer states that chronic use of secnidazole should be avoided.

Selection and Use of Anti-infectives To reduce development of drug-resistant bacteria and maintain effectiveness of secnidazole and other anti-infectives, the drug should be used only for treatment of infections proven or strongly suspected to be caused by susceptible bacteria.

Prescribing secnidazole in the absence of proven or strongly suspected bacterial infection or for prophylaxis is unlikely to provide benefit to the patient and increases the risk of development of drug-resistant bacteria.

When selecting or modifying anti-infective therapy, results of culture and in vitro susceptibility testing should be used. In the absence of such data, local epidemiology and susceptibility patterns should be considered when selecting anti-infectives for empiric therapy.

Specific Populations **Pregnancy.** There are insufficient data on use of secnidazole in pregnant women. In animal reproduction studies, there was no evidence of adverse developmental outcomes when oral secnidazole was administered to pregnant rats and rabbits during organogenesis at doses up to fourfold greater than the recommended human dose.

Lactation. It is not known whether secnidazole is distributed into human milk, affects the breast-fed infant, or affects milk production. Other nitroimidazole derivatives are distributed into human milk.

Due to the potential for serious adverse effects, including tumorigenicity, breast-feeding is not recommended during secnidazole treatment and for 96 hours after administration of the drug. In this situation, a nursing mother may choose to pump and discard her breast milk during and for 96 hours after secnidazole treatment and feed her infant stored human milk or formula during this period.

Pediatric Use. Safety and efficacy of secnidazole have not been established in pediatric patients younger than 18 years of age.

Geriatric Use. Clinical studies of secnidazole did not include a sufficient number of patients 65 years of age and older to determine if geriatric adults respond differently than younger adults.

Hepatic Impairment. Secnidazole has not been studied in patients with hepatic impairment.

Renal Impairment. Secnidazole has not been studied in patients with renal impairment.

■ **Common Adverse Effects** Adverse effects reported in 2% or more of patients receiving secnidazole in clinical trials include vulvovaginal candidiasis, headache, GI effects (nausea, vomiting, diarrhea, dysgeusia, abdominal pain), and vulvovaginal pruritus.

Drug Interactions

■ **Drugs Affecting or Metabolized by Hepatic Microsomal Enzymes** Secnidazole is minimally metabolized by cytochrome P-450 (CYP) isoenzymes and the drug is unlikely to be affected by CYP inducers or inhibitors.

■ **Estrogens and Progestins** Concomitant administration of secnidazole (single 2-g oral dose) and an oral contraceptive containing ethinyl estradiol and norethindrone (single dose) in healthy adult females resulted in a 29% decrease in the mean peak plasma concentration of ethinyl estradiol, but did not affect the area under the plasma concentration-time curve (AUC) of ethinyl estradiol; the mean peak plasma concentration and AUC of norethindrone were increased by 13 and 16%, respectively. However, none of these effects on the oral contraceptive were considered clinically important. Administration of secnidazole (single 2-g dose) 1 day prior to the oral contraceptive did not have a clinically important effect on mean peak plasma concentrations or AUCs of ethinyl estradiol or norethindrone.

Secnidazole may be used concomitantly with oral estrogen-progestin combination contraceptives (e.g., containing ethinyl estradiol and norethindrone).

■ **Ethanol** In vitro studies indicate secnidazole has no effect on aldehyde dehydrogenase activity at clinically important doses.

Description

Secnidazole is a 5-nitroimidazole antiprotozoal and antibacterial agent.

The exact mechanism of action of secnidazole has not been fully elucidated. Secnidazole is a prodrug that is activated after entry into bacterial cells where the nitro group is reduced by bacterial enzymes to form short-lived radical anions. It is believed that these radical anions interfere with DNA synthesis of susceptible bacteria.

Secnidazole is active in vitro against some anaerobic bacteria, including *Bacteroides*, *Gardnerella vaginalis*, *Prevotella*, *Mobiluncus*, and *Megasphaera*-like type I/II. *G. vaginalis* and *Mobiluncus* with reduced in vitro susceptibility or resistance to secnidazole have been reported. Some bacteria with reduced in vitro susceptibility to metronidazole also have reduced susceptibility to secnidazole; the clinical importance of this possible cross-resistance is not known.

Secnidazole is active against some protozoa, including *Giardia duodenalis* (also known as *G. lamblia* or *G. intestinalis*), *Trichomonas vaginalis*, and *Entamoeba histolytica*.

Following oral administration of a single 2-g dose of secnidazole (as granules admixed with applesauce) in healthy, fasting adult females, mean peak plasma concentrations of the drug were 45.4 mcg/mL and the median time to peak plasma concentrations was 4 hours; mean plasma concentrations were 22.1, 9.2, 3.8, and 1.4 mcg/mL at 24, 48, 72, and 96 hours, respectively, after the dose. Peak plasma concentrations and area under the plasma concentration-time curve (AUC) following administration of secnidazole granules admixed in applesauce are similar to those observed when secnidazole granules are admixed in pudding or yogurt. Administration of a single 2-g dose of secnidazole admixed with applesauce followed by a high-fat meal does not affect peak plasma concentrations or AUC of the drug compared with administration in the fasting state. Secnidazole is less than 5% bound to plasma proteins. In vitro studies indicate that no more than 1% of secnidazole is metabolized by cytochrome P-450 (CYP) isoenzymes. Following a single 2-g dose of oral secnidazole, approximately 15% is excreted unchanged in urine. The plasma elimination half-life of secnidazole is approximately 17 hours.

Advice to Patients

Advise patients to read the patient information provided by the manufacturer.

Advise patients that antibacterials (including secnidazole) should only be used to treat bacterial infections and not used to treat viral infections (e.g., the common cold).

Instruct patients that the entire contents of the single-dose packet of secnidazole granules should be sprinkled on applesauce, yogurt, or pudding and the entire mixture should be consumed within 30 minutes (without chewing or crunching the granules). Inform patients that the granules are not intended to be dissolved in any liquid.

Advise patients that secnidazole may be taken without regard to meals.

Advise patients that use of secnidazole may result in vulvovaginal candidiasis that may require treatment with an antifungal.

Importance of informing clinicians of existing or contemplated concomitant therapy, including prescription and OTC drugs and herbal supplements, as well as any concomitant illnesses.

Importance of women informing clinicians if they are or plan to become pregnant or plan to breast-feed. Advise women not to breast-feed during and for 96 hours following administration of secnidazole.

Importance of informing patients of other important precautionary information. (See Cautions.)

Overview® (see Users Guide). For additional information on this drug until a more detailed monograph is developed and published, the manufacturer's labeling should be consulted. It is *essential* that the manufacturer's labeling be consulted for more detailed information on usual cautions, precautions, contraindications, potential drug interactions, laboratory test interferences, and acute toxicity.

Preparations

Excipients in commercially available drug preparations may have clinically important effects in some individuals; consult specific product labeling for details.

Secnidazole

Oral

Granules	2 g	**Solosec®**, Lupin

Tinidazole

■ Tinidazole, a nitroimidazole derivative, is an antiprotozoal and antibacterial agent.

Uses

■ **Amebiasis** Tinidazole is used for the treatment of intestinal amebiasis and amebic liver abscess caused by *Entamoeba histolytica* in adults and children older than 3 years of age. Tinidazole is designated an orphan drug by the US Food and Drug Administration (FDA) for the treatment of amebiasis.

The regimen of choice for symptomatic intestinal amebiasis or extraintestinal disease (including liver abscess) is treatment with a nitroimidazole derivative (oral tinidazole or oral metronidazole) followed by treatment with a luminal amebicide (oral iodoquinol or oral paromomycin). The sequential use of these drugs ensures eradication of tissue-invading trophozoites as well as cysts in the intestinal lumen. In patients with severe disease who do not respond to or cannot tolerate these drugs, some clinicians suggest that a regimen of dehydroemetine (not commercially available in the US) followed by a luminal amebicide can be considered.

Tinidazole and metronidazole should not be used alone for the treatment of asymptomatic cyst passers; these patients require treatment with a luminal amebicide such as iodoquinol, paromomycin, or diloxanide furoate (not commercially available in the US).

Clinical Experience Use of oral tinidazole in patients with intestinal amebiasis is supported by published reports involving more than 1400 patients worldwide. Results of 4 randomized, controlled studies (one single-blind and 3 open-label) in 220 patients have shown that intestinal amebiasis cure rates of 86–93% were achieved with the currently recommended tinidazole regimen (2 g daily for 3 days). A similar cure rate was reported in a clinical series of 40 pediatric patients with intestinal amebiasis treated with the currently recommended pediatric tinidazole regimen (50 mg/kg of tinidazole daily for 3 days).

Use of oral tinidazole in patients with liver abscess is supported by published reports involving more than 470 patients worldwide. Results of 7 randomized, controlled studies (one double-blind, 1 single-blind, and 5 open-label) in 133 patients have shown that liver abscess cure rates of 81–100% were achieved with tinidazole (2 g daily for 2–5 days) accompanied by aspiration of the liver abscess (when clinically necessary).

■ **Giardiasis** Tinidazole is used for the treatment of giardiasis caused by *Giardia duodenalis* (also known as *G. lamblia* or *G. intestinalis*) in adults and children older than 3 years of age. Tinidazole is designated an orphan drug by FDA for the treatment of giardiasis.

Drugs of choice for the treatment of giardiasis are metronidazole, tinidazole, or nitazoxanide; alternative agents include paromomycin (especially in pregnant women), furazolidone (no longer commercially available in the US), or quinacrine (not commercially available in the US). Although tinidazole appears to be as effective or more effective than metronidazole for the treatment of giardiasis and may be better tolerated, limited safety and efficacy information is available in pediatric patients younger than 3 years of age†.

Clinical Experience Use of oral tinidazole in patients with giardiasis is supported by published reports involving more than 1600 adult and pediatric patients worldwide. Results of 8 controlled studies in 619 patients have shown that giardiasis cure rates of about 80–100% were achieved (299 patients received the currently recommended tinidazole regimen, a single 2-g dose in adults and a single 50-mg/kg [up to 2-g] dose in children). In 3 of these studies in which metronidazole was compared with tinidazole, comparative giardiasis cure rates of about 76–93% were achieved with various dosage regimens of metronidazole given for 2–3 days. However, data comparing tinidazole (2-g single dose) with metronidazole (given in the usually recommended dosage of 250 mg 3 times daily for 5–7 days) are limited.

■ **Trichomoniasis** Tinidazole is used for the treatment of symptomatic and asymptomatic trichomoniasis in adults in whom *Trichomonas vaginalis* has been demonstrated by an appropriate diagnostic procedure.

Nitroimidazole anti-infectives (e.g., metronidazole, tinidazole) are the only drugs commercially available in the US that are known to be effective in the treatment of trichomoniasis. The US Centers for Disease Control and Prevention (CDC) and other experts state that the recommended regimen for the treatment of trichomoniasis is either a single 2-g dose of oral metronidazole or a single 2-g dose of oral tinidazole; CDC states that the recommended alternative regimen is a multiple-dose regimen of oral metronidazole (500 mg twice daily for 7 days). In randomized clinical trials, recommended metronidazole regimens have resulted in cure rates of approximately 84–98% and the recommended tinidazole regimen has resulted in cure rates of approximately 92–100%. Although randomized controlled trials comparing single 2-g oral doses of metronidazole and tinidazole suggest that tinidazole is equivalent or superior to metronidazole in achieving parasitologic cure and resolution of symptoms, there is evidence from in vitro studies that some *T. vaginalis* isolates with reduced susceptibility to metronidazole may also have reduced susceptibility to tinidazole.

The goal of treatment of trichomoniasis is to provide symptomatic relief, achieve microbiologic cure, reduce transmission, and prevent reinfection; to achieve this goal, both the index patient and sexual partner(s) should be treated simultaneously. Because trichomoniasis is a sexually transmitted disease with a potential for serious sequelae, individuals known to be infected with *T. vaginalis* should be treated regardless of symptomatology and sexual partners(s) should be treated presumptively to avoid reinfection.

Persistent or recurrent trichomoniasis can occur as the result of infection with resistant *T. vaginalis* or reinfection from an untreated sexual partner(s). In patients with vaginal trichomoniasis, metronidazole resistance reportedly occurs in 4–10% of cases and tinidazole resistance occurs in 1% of cases. Single-dose nitroimidazole regimens are not recommended for retreatment unless the recurrent infection is likely to be caused by reinfection. If treatment failure occurred with a single-dose metronidazole regimen and reinfection has been excluded, CDC recommends that the patient and their sexual partner(s) be treated with a multiple-dose regimen of oral metronidazole (500 mg twice daily for 7 days). If this metronidazole regimen fails, a multiple-dose nitroimidazole regimen using a higher dosage (oral metronidazole or oral tinidazole in a dosage of 2 g daily for 7 days) can be considered.

Persistent trichomoniasis may require treatment with other alternative regimens and should be managed in consultation with an expert. Clinicians can contact CDC at 404-718-4141 or http://cdc.gov/std for assistance regarding in vitro susceptibility testing of *T. vaginalis* and management of persistent infections, including use of alternative regimens.

Clinical Experience Use of oral tinidazole in patients with trichomoniasis is supported by published reports involving more than 2800 patients worldwide. Results of 4 published, blinded, randomized comparative studies in 172 patients have shown that trichomoniasis cure rates of about 92–100% were achieved with the currently recommended tinidazole regimen (single 2-g dose). Test-of-cure in these studies was assessed by culture at time points within 1 week to 1 month post-treatment. In 4 other published, blinded, randomized comparative studies in 116 patients, in which test-of-cure was assessed by wet mount within 7–14 days post-treatment, trichomoniasis cure rates ranged from 80–100%. In these studies, efficacy of tinidazole was superior to placebo and comparable to metronidazole. When efficacy of a single 2-g dose of tinidazole was assessed in 4 open-label trials in 142 men (1 comparative study with metronidazole and 3 single-arm studies), parasitologic evaluation of the urine (pre- and post-treatment) indicated trichomoniasis cure rates of 83–100%.

■ **Bacterial Vaginosis** Tinidazole is used for the treatment of bacterial vaginosis (formerly called *Haemophilus* vaginitis, *Gardnerella* vaginitis, nonspecific vaginitis, *Corynebacterium* vaginitis, or anaerobic vaginosis) in nonpregnant women. Safety and efficacy of tinidazole for the treatment of bacterial vaginosis in pregnant women have not been established.

Bacterial vaginosis is a polymicrobial syndrome that can occur when normal hydrogen peroxide-producing *Lactobacillus* in the vagina are replaced by overgrowth of various anaerobic bacteria (e.g., *Prevotella*, *Mobiluncus*, *Atopobium vaginae*), *G. vaginalis*, *Ureaplasma urealyticum*, *Mycoplasma hominis*, or other bacteria. Treatment of bacterial vaginosis is recommended in symptomatic women to relieve the signs and symptoms of infection. Routine treatment of male sexual partner(s) is not usually recommended.

For the treatment of bacterial vaginosis, CDC and other experts recommend a 7-day regimen of oral metronidazole (500 mg twice daily), a 5-day regimen of intravaginal metronidazole 0.75% gel, or a 7-day regimen of intravaginal clindamycin 2% cream. Alternative regimens include a 2-day regimen of oral tinidazole (2 g once daily), a 5-day regimen of oral tinidazole (1 g once daily), a 7-day regimen of oral clindamycin (300 mg twice daily), or a 3-day regimen of intravaginal clindamycin 100-mg suppositories. The preferred regimens for treatment of bacterial vaginosis in pregnant women are the oral or intravaginal metronidazole or clindamycin regimens.

Relapse or recurrence of bacterial vaginosis is common, regardless of the treatment regimen used. Retreatment with the same regimen or an alternative regimen (e.g., oral therapy when topical therapy was used initially) can be effective for treating persistent or recurrent bacterial vaginosis after the first occurrence. Maintenance suppressive therapy with intravaginal metronidazole (0.75% gel twice weekly for 4–6 months) may reduce recurrences, but this benefit may not persist after suppressive therapy is discontinued.

Clinical Experience Results of clinical studies indicate that tinidazole is effective for the treatment of bacterial vaginosis in nonpregnant women. In one study, nonpregnant women with bacterial vaginosis were randomized to receive tinidazole 1 g daily for 5 days, tinidazole 2 g daily for 2 days, or placebo. Therapeutic cure (clinical cure and microbiologic cure) was reported in approximately 37, 27, or 5% of those receiving tinidazole 1 g daily for 5 days, tinidazole 2 g daily for 2 days, or placebo, respectively, 21–30 days following completion of treatment.

■ **Nongonococcal Urethritis** Tinidazole is used for the treatment of recurrent and persistent urethritis in certain men with nongonococcal urethritis† (NGU) who have already been treated with a recommended regimen.

NGU can be caused by various organisms (e.g., *Chlamydia*, *M. genitalium*, *T. vaginalis*, *Ureaplasma*, enteric bacteria) and is treated presumptively at the time of diagnosis. CDC states that a single dose of oral azithromycin or a 7-day regimen of oral doxycycline are the recommended regimens for the treatment of NGU; a 7-day regimen of oral erythromycin base or ethylsuccinate or a 7-day regimen of oral levofloxacin or ofloxacin are the recommended alternative regimens. To minimize transmission and avoid reinfection, men treated for NGU should abstain from sexual intercourse until they and their sexual partner(s) have been adequately treated (i.e., 7 days after initiation of treatment).

CDC states that men with persistent or recurrent NGU who were not compliant with the treatment regimen or were reexposed to untreated sexual partner(s) can be retreated with the initial regimen. In other patients, symptoms alone (without documentation of signs or laboratory evidence of urethral inflammation) are not a sufficient basis for retreatment and an objective diagnosis of persistent or recurrent NGU should be made before considering additional treatment. Because there is some evidence that *M. genitalium* is the most frequent cause of persistent or recurrent NGU, CDC states that men initially treated with doxycycline should receive retreatment with a single dose of oral azithromycin and those initially treated with azithromycin should receive retreatment with a 7-day regimen of oral moxifloxacin. However, if a patient with persistent or recurrent urethritis has sex with women and is in an area where *T. vaginalis* is prevalent, CDC recommends presumptive retreatment with a single 2-g dose of oral metronidazole or single 2-g dose of oral tinidazole and referral of their sexual partners(s) for evaluation and appropriate treatment.

■ **Prophylaxis in Sexual Assault Victims** A single dose of oral tinidazole (or oral metronidazole) is used in conjunction with a single dose of IM ceftriaxone and a single dose of oral azithromycin for empiric anti-infective prophylaxis in adult or adolescent victims of sexual assault†. Trichomoniasis, bacterial vaginosis, gonorrhea, and genital chlamydial infection are the sexually transmitted diseases most commonly diagnosed in women following sexual assault; however, because of the prevalence of these infections in the general population, their presence after assault does not necessarily imply that the infections were acquired during the assault. Gonococcal and chlamydial infections among females are of particular concern because of the possibility of ascending infection.

CDC recommends routine empiric prophylaxis after a sexual assault, and use of such prophylaxis probably benefits most patients since follow-up of assault victims can be difficult and such prophylaxis allays the patient's concerns about possible infections. The 3-drug empiric anti-infective prophylaxis regimen recommended for adults and adolescents (ceftriaxone, azithromycin, and either metronidazole or tinidazole) provides coverage against gonorrhea, chlamydia, and trichomoniasis, but efficacy in preventing these infections after sexual assault has not been evaluated. Patients should be counseled regarding the potential benefits and toxicities associated with the regimen (e.g., GI effects).

■ **Helicobacter pylori Infection** Tinidazole has been used as a component of various multiple-drug regimens for the treatment of infections caused by *Helicobacter pylori*†. Although safety and efficacy have not been established, tinidazole has been used in 3-drug regimens that include a proton-pump inhibitor, clarithromycin, and tinidazole or 4-drug regimens, including sequential regimens, that include a proton-pump inhibitor, amoxicillin, clarithromycin, and a nitroimidazole (either tinidazole or metronidazole). Tinidazole also has been used in sequential regimens that include a proton-pump inhibitor, bismuth subsalicylate, amoxicillin, and levofloxacin.

Dosage and Administration

■ **Administration** Tinidazole is administered orally with food.

Although food does not affect oral bioavailability of tinidazole, the drug should be given with meals to reduce the incidence of epigastric discomfort and other adverse GI effects.

Alcohol should be avoided during tinidazole treatment and for 3 days after the last dose of the drug. (See Drug Interactions: Alcohol and Propylene Glycol.)

Tinidazole is commercially available as tablets containing 250 or 500 mg of the drug. For children and other patients unable to swallow tablets, the 500-mg tablets can be used to prepare an extemporaneous oral suspension.

Extemporaneous Oral Suspension When an extemporaneous oral suspension is needed for children and other patients unable to swallow tablets, a tinidazole suspension containing 66.7 mg/mL can be prepared by pulverizing 2 g of tinidazole (four 500-mg tablets) to a powder with a mortar and pestle and adding approximately 10 mL of cherry syrup to the powder. After mixing until smooth, the suspension should then be transferred to a graduated amber container. Several small rinses of cherry syrup should be used to transfer any remaining drug in the mortar to the final suspension for a final volume of 30 mL.

The extemporaneous tinidazole oral suspension containing 66.7 mg/mL prepared with cherry syrup is stable for 7 days at room temperature.

The suspension should be shaken well before administration.

■ **Dosage** ***Pediatric Dosage*** **Amebiasis.** The usual dosage of oral tinidazole for the treatment of intestinal amebiasis caused by *Entamoeba histolytica* in pediatric patients older than 3 years of age is 50 mg/kg once daily (up to 2 g daily) for 3 days.

The usual dosage of oral tinidazole for the treatment of amebic liver abscess caused by *E. histolytica* in pediatric patients older than 3 years of age is 50 mg/kg once daily (up to 2 g daily) for 3–5 days. The manufacturer states that only limited data are available regarding use of the drug for longer than 3 days in children. (See Pediatric Use under Warnings/Precautions: Specific Populations, in Cautions.)

Tinidazole treatment should be followed by treatment with a luminal amebicide (oral iodoquinol or oral paromomycin). (See Uses: Amebiasis.)

Giardiasis. The usual dosage of oral tinidazole for the treatment of giardiasis caused by *Giardia duodenalis* (also known as *G. lamblia* or *G. intestinalis*) in children older than 3 years of age is a single dose of 50 mg/kg (up to 2 g).

Trichomoniasis. Although safety and efficacy of oral tinidazole for the treatment of trichomoniasis caused by *Trichomonas vaginalis* have not been established in children†, some clinicians suggest that a single dose of 50 mg/kg (up to 2 g) can be used to treat this infection in pediatric patients.

Adult Dosage **Amebiasis.** The usual dosage of oral tinidazole for the treatment of intestinal amebiasis and amebic liver abscess caused by *E. histolytica* in adults is 2 g once daily. The usual duration of treatment in adults is 3 days for intestinal amebiasis and 3–5 days for amebic liver abscess.

Tinidazole treatment should be followed by treatment with a luminal amebicide (oral iodoquinol or oral paromomycin). (See Uses: Amebiasis.)

Giardiasis. The usual dosage of oral tinidazole for the treatment of giardiasis caused by *Giardia duodenalis* (also known as *G. lamblia* or *G. intestinalis*) in adults is a single 2-g dose.

Trichomoniasis. The usual dosage of oral tinidazole for the treatment of trichomoniasis caused by *T. vaginalis* in adults is a single 2-g dose. Sexual partner(s) of the patient should be treated simultaneously using the same dosage.

If treatment failure occurred following recommended metronidazole treatment regimens (e.g., single 2-g dose of oral metronidazole, 7-day regimen of oral metronidazole 500 mg twice daily), the US Centers for Disease Control and Prevention (CDC) states that retreatment with a regimen of 2 g of oral tinidazole once daily for 7 days can be considered. (See Uses: Trichomoniasis.)

Bacterial Vaginosis. The usual dosage of oral tinidazole for the treatment of bacterial vaginosis in nonpregnant women is 2 g once daily for 2 days or 1 g once daily for 5 days.

Nongonococcal Urethritis. For the treatment of recurrent and persistent urethritis in certain men with nongonococcal urethritis† (NGU) who have already received a recommended treatment regimen (see Uses: Nongonococcal Urethritis), CDC states that presumptive treatment with a single 2-g dose of oral tinidazole can be considered.

Prophylaxis in Sexual Assault Victims. For empiric anti-infective prophylaxis in adult sexual assault victims†, CDC recommends that a single 2-g dose of tinidazole be given in conjunction with ceftriaxone (single 250-mg IM dose) and azithromycin (single 1-g oral dose).

Helicobacter pylori Infection. When used as a component of various multiple-drug regimens for the treatment of infections caused by *Helicobacter pylori*† (see Uses: Helicobacter pylori Infection), tinidazole has been given in a dosage of 500 mg twice daily.

■ **Special Populations** ***Hepatic Impairment*** Data are not available regarding use of tinidazole in patients with hepatic impairment. The manufacturer states that usual dosage of tinidazole should be administered with caution in patients with hepatic impairment. Some clinicians state that tinidazole is not recommended in patients with severe hepatic impairment (Child-Pugh class C). (See Hepatic Impairment under Warnings/Precautions: Specific Populations, in Cautions.)

Renal Impairment No dosage adjustment of tinidazole is necessary in patients with renal impairment, including those with severe renal impairment (creatinine clearance less than 22 mL/minute), unless the patient is undergoing hemodialysis.

In patients undergoing hemodialysis, if tinidazole is administered on the same day as and prior to hemodialysis, the manufacturer states that an additional tinidazole dose (equivalent to 50% of the recommended dose) should be given after the hemodialysis session. (See Renal Impairment under Warnings/Precautions: Specific Populations, in Cautions.)

Geriatric Patients Dosage of tinidazole in geriatric patients generally should be selected with caution because of age-related decreases in hepatic, renal, and/or cardiac function and concomitant disease and drug therapy.

Cautions

■ **Contraindications** Tinidazole is contraindicated in patients with a history of hypersensitivity to tinidazole or other nitroimidazole derivatives.

Tinidazole is contraindicated during the first trimester of pregnancy. (See Pregnancy under Warnings/Precautions: Specific Populations, in Cautions.)

Tinidazole is contraindicated in breast-feeding women. (See Lactation under Warnings/Precautions: Specific Populations, in Cautions.)

■ **Warnings/Precautions** ***Warnings*** **Carcinogenicity.** Carcinogenicity has been observed in mice and rats treated chronically with metronidazole, a nitroimidazole anti-infective chemically related to tinidazole.

Animal studies evaluating the carcinogenicity potential of tinidazole have not been reported to date.

Tinidazole should be reserved for FDA-labeled indications only and unnecessary use should be avoided.

Sensitivity Reactions Hypersensitivity reactions (e.g., urticaria, pruritus, rash, flushing, sweating, mouth dryness, fever, burning sensation, thirst, salivation, angioedema, bronchospasm, dyspnea, Stevens-Johnson syndrome, erythema multiforme) have been reported in patients receiving tinidazole. Anaphylaxis has been reported rarely.

Severe, acute hypersensitivity reactions have been reported with initial or subsequent treatment with tinidazole.

Cross-allergenicity between tinidazole and metronidazole has been reported.

Other Warnings and Precautions **Nervous System Effects.** Convulsive seizures and peripheral neuropathy (characterized by numbness or paresthesia of an extremity) have been reported in patients receiving tinidazole and other nitroimidazoles (e.g., metronidazole).

Other CNS effects reported in patients receiving tinidazole include vertigo, ataxia, giddiness, insomnia, and drowsiness.

If abnormal neurologic signs develop, tinidazole should be promptly discontinued.

History of Blood Dyscrasia. Tinidazole should be used with caution in patients with evidence or history of blood dyscrasia.

As with other nitroimidazoles (e.g., metronidazole), transient leukopenia and neutropenia may occur in patients receiving tinidazole; persistent hematologic abnormalities have not been reported to date.

If retreatment with tinidazole is necessary, total and differential leukocyte counts should be performed.

Vulvovaginal Candidiasis. The use of tinidazole may result in vaginal candidiasis. In a clinical study that included 235 women who received tinidazole for the treatment of bacterial vaginosis, a vaginal fungal infection developed in 11 (4.7%) of study participants.

If vulvovaginal candidiasis occurs, appropriate therapy should be instituted.

Laboratory Test Interferences. Tinidazole, like metronidazole, may interfere with determination of serum AST (SGOT), ALT (SGPT), LDH, triglycerides, or glucose when such determinations are based on the decrease in ultraviolet absorbance that occurs during oxidation of NADH to NAD. Falsely decreased values, including values of zero, may result.

Selection and Use of Anti-infectives. To reduce development of drug-resistant bacteria and maintain effectiveness of tinidazole and other antibacterials, the drug should be used only for the treatment infections proven or strongly suspected to be caused by susceptible organisms.

Prescribing tinidazole in the absence of proven or strongly suspected infection or for a prophylactic indication is unlikely to provide benefit to the patient and increases the risk of development of drug-resistant bacteria.

When selecting or modifying anti-infective therapy, results of culture and in vitro susceptibility testing should be used. In the absence of such data, local epidemiology and susceptibility patterns should be considered when selecting anti-infectives for empiric therapy.

Specific Populations **Pregnancy.** Safety and efficacy of tinidazole have not been evaluated in pregnant women, including use of the drug for the treatment of bacterial vaginosis in pregnant women.

Because tinidazole crosses the placenta and enters fetal circulation, the drug is contraindicated during the first trimester of pregnancy. The US Centers for Disease Control and Prevention (CDC) states that use of tinidazole for the treatment of trichomoniasis or bacterial vaginosis in pregnant women should avoided.

Lactation. Tinidazole is distributed into human milk in concentrations similar to serum concentrations and can be detected in milk for up to 72 hours after administration.

Tinidazole is contraindicated in breast-feeding women. Breast-feeding should be interrupted during tinidazole treatment and for 3 days (72 hours) following the last dose.

Pediatric Use. Safety and efficacy of tinidazole have not been established in pediatric patients 3 years of age or younger. Some data are available regarding safety and efficacy of the drug for the treatment of giardiasis in pediatric patients younger than 3 years of age†.

Safety and efficacy of tinidazole in pediatric patients have been established *only* for the treatment of amebiasis or giardiasis in children older than 3 years of age.

Pediatric patients should be monitored closely when the duration of tinidazole treatment exceeds 3 days (e.g., for treatment of amebic liver abscess). Only limited data are available regarding tinidazole treatment exceeding 3 days in pediatric patients, although the drug has been used for 5 days in a small number of children without an increase in the severity and incidence of adverse effects.

Adverse effects reported in pediatric patients receiving tinidazole are similar in nature and frequency to those reported in adults and include nausea, vomiting, diarrhea, taste change, anorexia, and abdominal pain.

Geriatric Use. Clinical studies of tinidazole did not include a sufficient number of patients 65 years of age or older to determine whether geriatric adults respond differently than younger adults.

Dosage for geriatric patients should be selected with caution because of possible age-related decreases in hepatic, renal, and/or cardiac function and concomitant disease and drug therapy.

Hepatic Impairment. The manufacturer states that usual dosage of tinidazole should be used with caution in patients with hepatic impairment. Some clinicians state that tinidazole is not recommended in patients with severe hepatic impairment (Child-Pugh class C).

The pharmacokinetics of tinidazole have not been evaluated in patients with impaired hepatic function; however, reduced elimination and increased plasma concentrations of metronidazole, a chemically related nitroimidazole, have been reported in patients with hepatic dysfunction.

Renal Impairment. The pharmacokinetics of tinidazole in patients with severe renal impairment (creatinine clearance less than 22 mL/minute) are similar to that reported in healthy individuals and dosage adjustments are not necessary in such patients, unless they are undergoing hemodialysis.

Tinidazole is removed by hemodialysis. The half-life of tinidazole is reduced from 12 hours to 4.9 hours during hemodialysis and approximately 43% of the drug present in the body is eliminated during a 6-hour hemodialysis session. If tinidazole is administered on the same day as and prior to hemodialysis, an additional dose (equivalent to 50% of the recommended dose) is recommended after the hemodialysis session. (See Renal Impairment under Dosage and Administration: Special Populations.)

The effects of continuous ambulatory peritoneal dialysis (CAPD) on the pharmacokinetics of tinidazole have not been studied.

■ **Common Adverse Effects** Adverse effects occurring in 1% or more of patients receiving a single 2-g dose of tinidazole include GI effects (metallic/bitter taste, nausea, anorexia, dyspepsia/cramps/epigastric discomfort, vomiting, constipation) and nervous system effects (weakness/fatigue/malaise, dizziness, headache).

Drug Interactions

Formal drug interaction studies have not been performed to date with tinidazole; however, interactions reported with metronidazole, a nitroimidazole anti-infective chemically related to tinidazole, may also occur in patients receiving tinidazole. For further information on interactions associated with metronidazole, see Drug Interactions, in Metronidazole 8:30.92.

■ **Drugs Affecting or Metabolized by Hepatic Microsomal Enzymes** Metabolism of tinidazole is mediated principally by the cytochrome P-450 (CYP) isoenzyme 3A4. Drugs that induce this isoenzyme (e.g., phenobarbital, rifampin, phenytoin, fosphenytoin) may reduce tinidazole plasma concentrations. Conversely, concomitant use of tinidazole with drugs that inhibit CYP3A4 (e.g., cimetidine, ketoconazole) may increase tinidazole plasma concentrations.

Tinidazole did not inhibit CYP1A2, CYP2B6, CYP2C9, CYP2D6, CYP2E1, or CYP3A4 in an in vitro metabolic drug interaction study.

■ **Alcohol and Propylene Glycol** Disulfiram-like reactions, including abdominal cramps, nausea, vomiting, headaches, and flushing, may occur if alcoholic beverages or preparations containing ethanol or propylene glycol are consumed during or following tinidazole treatment. The manufacturer states that alcohol and preparations containing alcohol or propylene glycol should not be used during tinidazole treatment and for 3 days after the last dose of the drug.

■ **Anticonvulsants** ***Phenobarbital*** Pharmacokinetic interactions may occur between phenobarbital and tinidazole (increased elimination and decreased plasma concentrations of tinidazole).

Phenytoin or Fosphenytoin Pharmacokinetic interactions have been reported between IV phenytoin and oral metronidazole (prolonged half-life and reduced clearance of phenytoin); interactions did not occur between oral phenytoin and metronidazole. It is possible that similar pharmacokinetic interactions may occur if IV phenytoin is used concomitantly with tinidazole.

Pharmacokinetic interactions may occur between tinidazole and phenytoin or fosphenytoin (increased elimination and decreased plasma concentrations of tinidazole).

■ **Antifungal Agents** Pharmacokinetic interactions may occur between ketoconazole and tinidazole (prolonged half-life, decreased clearance, and increased plasma concentrations of tinidazole).

■ **Cholestyramine** Cholestyramine has decreased oral bioavailability of metronidazole by 21%. Because a similar interaction may occur if cholestyramine is used concomitantly with tinidazole, the manufacturer recommends separating doses of tinidazole and cholestyramine to minimize any potential effect on oral bioavailability of the anti-infective.

■ **Cimetidine** Pharmacokinetic interactions may occur between cimetidine and tinidazole (prolonged half-life, decreased clearance, and increased plasma concentrations of tinidazole).

■ **Disulfiram** Psychotic reactions have been reported when metronidazole was used concomitantly with disulfiram. Although such reactions have not been reported to date with tinidazole, the manufacturer states that tinidazole should not be used in patients who have received disulfiram within the last 2 weeks.

■ **Fluorouracil** Pharmacokinetic interactions have been reported when fluorouracil was used concomitantly with metronidazole (decreased fluorouracil clearance) resulting in increased fluorouracil-associated adverse effects without an increase in therapeutic benefits. Because similar interactions may occur between tinidazole and fluorouracil, patients should be monitored for fluorouracil toxicity if concomitant use of tinidazole and fluorouracil cannot be avoided.

■ **Immunosuppressive Agents** Several case reports suggest potential pharmacokinetic interactions between metronidazole and cyclosporine or tacrolimus (increased plasma concentrations of cyclosporine or tacrolimus). Because similar interactions may occur between tinidazole and these immunosuppressive agents, patients should be monitored for cyclosporine or tacrolimus toxicity if tinidazole is used concomitantly with one of these drugs.

■ **Lithium** Pharmacokinetic interactions have been reported between lithium and metronidazole (increased plasma lithium concentration). Although it is not known whether such interactions would also occur with tinidazole, serum lithium and creatinine concentrations should be evaluated after several days of concomitant lithium and tinidazole therapy to detect potential lithium intoxication.

■ **Rifampin** Pharmacokinetic interactions may occur between rifampin and tinidazole (increased elimination and decreased plasma concentrations of tinidazole).

■ **Tetracyclines** Oxytetracycline (no longer commercially available in the US) has been reported to antagonize the therapeutic effects of metronidazole.

■ **Warfarin** Pharmacologic interactions may occur between warfarin and tinidazole (prolonged prothrombin time [PT] and enhanced anticoagulant effects). Warfarin dosage adjustment may be required during tinidazole treatment and for up to 8 days after the last tinidazole dose.

Description

Tinidazole is a 5-nitroimidazole antiprotozoal and antibacterial agent.

Tinidazole is amebicidal, trichomonacidal, and bactericidal in action. Tinidazole is a prodrug that is activated after entry into cells of susceptible organisms where the nitro group is reduced to form short-lived radical anions. Although the exact mechanism of action has not been fully elucidated, it is believed that these free radicals interfere with cellular DNA. Studies using cell extracts of *Trichomonas* indicate that the nitroimidazole group of tinidazole is reduced within the cells and generates the free nitro radical, which appears to be responsible for the drug's anti-infective activity. Similarly, the nitro group is reduced within anaerobic bacteria resulting in reactive intermediates; chemically reduced tinidazole has been shown to release nitrites and cause damage to purified bacterial DNA in vitro. Specific information on the mechanism of tinidazole's activity against *Giardia* and *Entamoeba histolytica* is not available.

Following oral administration, tinidazole is rapidly absorbed and peak plasma concentrations of the drug are attained within about 2 hours. The estimated oral bioavailability of the drug exceeds 90%. Administration with food delays the time to peak plasma concentrations by approximately 2 hours and decreases peak plasma concentrations by 10%, but does not affect the area under the plasma concentration-time curve (AUC) or elimination half-life. Pharmacokinetic parameters reported with an extemporaneous oral suspension of tinidazole containing 66.7 mg/mL (prepared using crushed 500-mg tablets and cherry syrup) in healthy individuals after an overnight fast are similar to those reported with tablets swallowed whole under fasted conditions. Tinidazole is 12% bound to plasma proteins. The drug is widely distributed into body tissues and fluids (e.g., saliva, female reproductive tract, gallbladder, bile, bowel, prostate tissue) and crosses the blood-brain barrier and placenta. Tinidazole is partially metabolized via oxidation, hydroxylation, and conjugation; the drug is metabolized principally by cytochrome P-450 (CYP) isoenzyme 3A4. Approximately 20–50% of an oral dose is excreted unchanged in urine and approximately 12% is excreted in feces. The plasma half-life of tinidazole is approximately 12–14 hours.

■ **Spectrum** Tinidazole is active in vitro and in clinical infections against some protozoa, including *T. vaginalis*, *G. duodenalis* (also known as *G. lamblia* or *G. intestinalis*), and *E. histolytica*. Although the clinical importance is unclear, tinidazole appears to have some in vitro activity against *Dientamoeba fragilis*.

Tinidazole is active in vitro against many anaerobic bacteria, including some *Bacteroides* (e.g., *B. fragilis*, *B. melaninogenicus*), some *Clostridium* (e.g., *C. difficile*, *C. perfringens*), *Fusobacterium*, *Gardnerella vaginalis*, *Peptococcus*, *Peptostreptococcus*, *Prevotella* (including *P. amnii*, *P. timonensis*), and *Veillonella*. Tinidazole also is active in vitro against some strains of *Helicobacter pylori*.

In one study that evaluated in vitro susceptibility of vaginal isolates, *Anaerococcus tetradius*, *Finegoldia magna*, *Megasphaera*-like type I/II, *Megeeibacillus indolicus*, *Peptoniphilus*, and *Porphyromonas* were susceptible to tinidazole; however, *Atopobium vaginae*, *Lactobacillus* (*L. gasseri*, *L. iners*, *L. jensenii*), and *Mobiluncus* (*M. curtisii*, *M. mulieris*) were resistant.

■ **Resistance** The potential for development of tinidazole resistance in *Giardia*, *E. histolytica*, or bacteria associated with bacterial vaginosis has not been evaluated.

In vitro studies indicate that some *T. vaginalis* isolates with reduced susceptibility to metronidazole also have reduced susceptibility to tinidazole; however, the minimum lethal concentration (MLC) of tinidazole for some of these strains may be lower than the MLC of metronidazole.

Although the clinical importance is unclear, *H. pylori* resistant to tinidazole have been reported with increasing frequency in some regions of the world and the rate of resistance to the drug has been reported to be as high as 87% in some areas.

Advice to Patients

Importance of taking with food to reduce the incidence of adverse GI effects (e.g., epigastric discomfort).

Advise patients to avoid alcoholic beverages and preparations containing alcohol or propylene glycol during tinidazole treatment and for at least 3 days after the last dose since abdominal cramps, nausea, vomiting, headaches, and flushing could occur.

Advise patients that antibacterials (including tinidazole) should not be used to treat viral infections (e.g., the common cold).

Importance of completing full course of treatment, even if feeling better after a few days. Advise patients that skipping doses or not completing the full course of treatment may decrease effectiveness and increase the likelihood that bacteria will develop resistance and will not be treatable with tinidazole or other antibacterials in the future.

Advise patients to promptly discontinue tinidazole and contact clinicians if abnormal neurologic signs occur.

Importance of informing clinicians of existing or contemplated concomitant therapy, including prescription and OTC drugs, and any concomitant illnesses.

Importance of women informing clinicians if they are or plan to become pregnant or plan to breast-feed.

Importance of advising patients of other important precautionary information. (See Cautions.)

Overview® (see Users Guide). For additional information on this drug until a more detailed monograph is developed and published, the manufacturer's labeling should be consulted. It is *essential* that the manufacturer's labeling be consulted for more detailed information on usual cautions, precautions, contraindications, potential drug interactions, laboratory test interferences, and acute toxicity.

Preparations

Excipients in commercially available drug preparations may have clinically important effects in some individuals; consult specific product labeling for details.

Tinidazole

Oral		
Tablets, film-coated	250 mg*	**Tindamax®**, Mission
		Tinidazole Tablets
	500 mg*	**Tindamax®**, Mission
		Tinidazole Tablets

*available from one or more manufacturer, distributor, and/or repackager by generic (nonproprietary) name

†Use is not currently included in the labeling approved by the US Food and Drug Administration

10:00 Antineoplastic Agents

§ Omitted from the print version of *AHFS Drug Information* because of space limitations. This monograph is available on the *AHFS Drug Information* web site, http://www.ahfsdruginformation.com. Username: ahfs2020; Password: ASHP94498

ANTINEOPLASTIC AGENTS 10:00

Abemaciclib

■ Abemaciclib, a selective inhibitor of cyclin-dependent kinases 4 (CDK4) and 6 (CDK6), is an antineoplastic agent.

Uses

■ **Breast Cancer** ***Initial Therapy for Advanced Breast Cancer*** Abemaciclib is used in combination with an aromatase inhibitor for the initial treatment of hormone receptor-positive, human epidermal growth factor receptor type 2 (HER2)-negative advanced or metastatic breast cancer in postmenopausal women. A statistically significant progression-free survival benefit has been observed in postmenopausal women with previously untreated, hormone receptor-positive, HER2-negative advanced or metastatic breast cancer receiving combined therapy with abemaciclib and an aromatase inhibitor (i.e., anastrozole or letrozole) compared with patients receiving placebo in combination with an aromatase inhibitor.

The current indication for abemaciclib is based principally on the results of a randomized, double-blind, placebo-controlled phase 3 study (MONARCH-3) in postmenopausal women with previously untreated hormone receptor-positive, HER2-negative advanced or metastatic breast cancer. In this study, 493 patients were randomized (stratified by site of metastases and prior neoadjuvant or adjuvant endocrine therapy) in a 2:1 ratio to receive either abemaciclib (150 mg orally twice daily) in combination with an aromatase inhibitor (letrozole 2.5 mg or anastrozole 1 mg orally once daily) or placebo in combination with an aromatase inhibitor. Treatment was continued until disease progression, death, or unacceptable toxicity occurred or treatment was discontinued for other reasons. Cross over to the opposite treatment arm was not permitted. The primary measure of efficacy was progression-free survival as assessed by the investigator according to Response Evaluation Criteria in Solid Tumors (RECIST). In this study, the median age of patients was 63 years; 58% were white, 30% were Asian, 40% had de novo metastatic disease, 53% had visceral involvement, 22% had bone-only disease, 51% had received prior systemic therapy, and 39% had received prior chemotherapy. All patients enrolled in the study had a baseline ECOG performance status of 0 or 1. Patients who had received prior therapy with a cyclin-dependent kinase (CDK) 4/6 inhibitor or everolimus were excluded from the study.

At the time of analysis, patients receiving abemaciclib in combination with an aromatase inhibitor had a longer median progression-free survival than those receiving placebo in combination with an aromatase inhibitor (28.2 versus 14.8 months; hazard ratio: 0.54). The results of the progression-free survival analysis based on an independent, blinded, central radiologic assessment were consistent with the investigator assessment. Among patients with measurable disease, patients receiving abemaciclib in combination with an aromatase inhibitor also had higher overall response rates compared with those receiving placebo in combination with an aromatase inhibitor (55.4 versus 40.2%). A subset analysis of progression-free survival based on site of metastases and prior neoadjuvant or adjuvant endocrine therapy consistently showed treatment benefit with abemaciclib and an aromatase inhibitor combination therapy compared with placebo in combination with an aromatase inhibitor. Median overall survival had not been reached at the time of the efficacy analysis.

Previously Treated Advanced Breast Cancer Abemaciclib is used alone or in combination with fulvestrant for the treatment of previously treated hormone receptor-positive, HER2-negative advanced or metastatic breast cancer.

Combination Therapy. Abemaciclib is used in combination with fulvestrant for the treatment of hormone receptor-positive, HER2-negative advanced or metastatic breast cancer in women with disease progression following endocrine therapy. A statistically significant progression-free survival benefit has been observed in women with previously treated, hormone receptor-positive, HER2-negative advanced or metastatic breast cancer receiving combined therapy with abemaciclib and fulvestrant compared with patients receiving placebo in combination with fulvestrant.

The current indication for abemaciclib is based principally on the results of a randomized, double-blind, placebo-controlled phase 3 study (MONARCH-2) in women with hormone receptor-positive, HER2-negative metastatic breast cancer. Patients enrolled in this study had disease progression following prior endocrine therapy. In this study, 669 patients were randomized (stratified according to sensitivity to endocrine therapy and site of metastases) in a 2:1 ratio to receive either abemaciclib in combination with fulvestrant or placebo in combination with fulvestrant. Patients randomized to abemaciclib received 200 mg orally twice daily upon initiation of the study, but the protocol was amended to reduce the abemaciclib dosage to 150 mg twice daily following review of safety data and dosage reduction rates. All patients enrolled in the study received fulvestrant 500 mg IM on days 1 and 15 during cycle 1 followed by day 1 of each 28-day cycle thereafter. Patients were treated until disease progression, unacceptable toxicity, or death occurred. Premenopausal or perimenopausal patients received goserelin acetate for at least 4 weeks prior to and during the study. The primary measure of efficacy was progression-free survival as assessed by the investigator according to RECIST. In this study, the median age of patients was 60 years; 56% were Caucasian, 20% had de novo metastatic disease, 56% had visceral disease, 27% had bone-only disease, 25% had primary resistance to endocrine therapy (defined as disease that relapsed during the initial 2 years of adjuvant endocrine therapy or disease progression within the initial 6 months of first-line endocrine therapy for metastatic disease), and 17% were premenopausal or perimenopausal. The majority of patients (99%) had an ECOG performance status of 0 or 1. Patients who had received chemotherapy for metastatic disease or prior therapy with a CDK4/6 inhibitor, fulvestrant, or everolimus were excluded from the study.

At a median follow-up of 19.5 months, patients receiving abemaciclib in combination with fulvestrant had a longer median progression-free survival compared with patients receiving placebo in combination with fulvestrant (16.4 versus 9.3 months; hazard ratio: 0.55). The results of the progression-free survival analysis based on an independent, blinded, central radiologic assessment were consistent with the investigator assessment. Among patients with measurable disease, patients receiving abemaciclib in combination with fulvestrant also had higher overall response rates compared with those receiving placebo in combination with fulvestrant (48.1 versus 21.3%). A subset analysis of progression-free survival based on site of metastases and sensitivity to endocrine therapy consistently showed treatment benefit with abemaciclib and fulvestrant combination therapy compared with placebo and fulvestrant therapy. Median overall survival had not been reached at the time of the efficacy analysis.

Monotherapy. Abemaciclib monotherapy is used for the treatment of hormone receptor-positive, HER2-negative advanced or metastatic breast cancer in adults with disease progression following endocrine therapy and prior chemotherapy for metastatic disease.

The current indication for abemaciclib is based principally on the results of an open-label, noncomparative phase 2 study (MONARCH-1) in women with hormone receptor-positive, HER2-negative metastatic breast cancer. Patients enrolled in this study had received a taxane in any setting and 1–2 prior chemotherapy regimens for metastatic disease and had disease progression during or following prior endocrine therapy. In this study, 132 patients received abemaciclib 200 mg orally twice daily until disease progression or unacceptable toxicity occurred. The primary measure of efficacy was overall response rate as assessed by the investigator according to RECIST. The median age of patients was 58 years and 85% of patients were Caucasian. All patients enrolled in the study had an ECOG performance status of 0 or 1. The median duration of metastatic disease was 27.6 months; 90% had visceral disease and 51% had at least 3 sites of metastases. Approximately one-half (51%) of patients received one prior line of chemotherapy in the metastatic setting; 69% of patients received a taxane-based regimen and 55% received capecitabine. Patients who had received prior therapy with a CDK4/6 inhibitor were excluded from the study.

In this study, the investigator-assessed overall response rate was 19.7%; none of the patients achieved a complete response. At the time of data analysis, the median duration of response was 8.6 months. Effects of abemaciclib on overall response rate as assessed by an independent review facility and investigator-assessed overall response rate were comparable. At the time of the final analysis at a follow-up of 18 months, the median overall survival was 22.3 months.

Dosage and Administration

■ **General** Because abemaciclib may cause neutropenia and hepatotoxicity, the manufacturer states that complete blood cell (CBC) counts and liver function tests should be monitored at baseline, every 2 weeks for the initial 2 months of therapy, monthly for the next 2 months, and then as clinically indicated. (See Hematologic Toxicity and also see Hepatic Toxicity under Dosage: Dosage Modification for Toxicity, in Dosage and Administration.)

Clinicians should consult the respective manufacturers' labelings for information on dosage and administration (including dosage adjustments), adverse effects, and contraindications of other antineoplastic agents used in combination regimens.

■ **Administration** Abemaciclib is administered orally without regard to food at approximately the same time each day. The tablets should be swallowed intact and should *not* be broken, chewed, crushed, or split.

If a dose of abemaciclib is missed or vomited, patients should not take an extra dose. The next dose should be taken at the regularly scheduled time.

■ **Dosage** ***Breast Cancer*** **Initial Therapy for Advanced Breast Cancer.** For the initial treatment of hormone receptor-positive, human epidermal growth factor receptor type 2 (HER2)-negative advanced or metastatic breast cancer in postmenopausal women, the recommended adult dosage of abemaciclib is 150 mg twice daily in combination with an aromatase inhibitor (e.g., anastrozole, letrozole). Therapy should be continued until disease progression or unacceptable toxicity occurs.

Previously Treated Advanced Breast Cancer. For use in combination with fulvestrant in the treatment of hormone receptor-positive, HER2-negative advanced or metastatic breast cancer in women with disease progression following endocrine therapy, the recommended adult dosage of abemaciclib is 150 mg twice daily. Fulvestrant 500 mg is administered IM on days 1, 15, and 29, and then once monthly thereafter. Premenopausal or perimenopausal patients receiving combination therapy with abemaciclib and fulvestrant should be treated with a gonadotropin-releasing hormone (GnRH, luteinizing hormone-releasing hormone) agonist (e.g., goserelin) according to current standards of care.

For use as a single-agent in the treatment of hormone receptor-positive, HER2-negative advanced or metastatic breast cancer in patients with disease progression following endocrine therapy and chemotherapy in the metastatic setting, the recommended adult dosage of abemaciclib is 200 mg twice daily.

Therapy should be continued until disease progression or unacceptable toxicity occurs.

Dosage Modification for Toxicity Dosage interruption and/or reduction or discontinuance of abemaciclib therapy may be necessary based on severity of adverse reactions. The following table on Dosage Modifications for Abemaciclib Toxicity indicates the recommended dosage modifications for abemaciclib during monotherapy or combination therapy with fulvestrant or an aromatase inhibitor.

Table 1: Dosage Modifications for Abemaciclib Toxicity

Toxicity Occurrence	Dosage Modification after Recovery from Toxicity	
	Single-agent Abemaciclib (Starting Dosage = 200 mg twice daily)	Abemaciclib in Combination with Fulvestrant or an Aromatase Inhibitor (Starting Dosage = 150 mg twice daily)
First	Restart at 150 mg twice daily	Restart at 100 mg twice daily
Second	Restart at 100 mg twice daily	Restart at 50 mg twice daily
Third	Restart at 50 mg twice daily	Discontinue abemaciclib
Fourth	Discontinue abemaciclib	

Hematologic Toxicity. For grade 4 hematologic toxicity, abemaciclib therapy should be interrupted until the toxicity improves to grade 2 or less. Upon resumption of therapy, the dosage of abemaciclib should be reduced. Hematopoietic growth factors (e.g., granulocyte colony-stimulating factor [G-CSF]) may be administered if clinically indicated; however, abemaciclib therapy should be withheld for at least 48 hours after the last dose of a hematopoietic growth factor and until the toxicity improves to grade 2 or less. (See Neutropenia under Cautions: Warnings/Precautions.)

For the first occurrence of grade 3 hematologic toxicity, abemaciclib therapy should be interrupted; therapy may be resumed at the same dosage when the toxicity improves to grade 2 or less. If grade 3 hematologic toxicity recurs, abemaciclib therapy should be withheld again; therapy may then be resumed at a reduced dosage when the toxicity improves to grade 2 or less.

For grade 1 or 2 hematologic toxicity, no dosage adjustment is necessary.

Diarrhea. For grade 3 or 4 diarrhea or diarrhea requiring hospitalization, abemaciclib therapy should be interrupted until the toxicity improves to grade 1 or less. Upon resumption of therapy, the dosage of abemaciclib should be reduced. (See Diarrhea under Cautions: Warnings/Precautions.)

For persistent grade 2 diarrhea lasting 24 hours or longer, abemaciclib therapy should be interrupted; therapy may be resumed at the same dosage when the toxicity resolves. If grade 2 diarrhea persists or recurs despite optimal supportive measures, abemaciclib therapy should be withheld again; therapy may then be resumed at a reduced dosage when the toxicity improves to grade 1 or less.

For grade 1 diarrhea, no dosage adjustment is necessary.

Hepatic Toxicity. For grade 4 serum aminotransferase (ALT and/or AST) elevations (i.e., exceeding 20 times the upper limit of normal [ULN]) or serum ALT and/or AST elevations exceeding 3 times the ULN with total bilirubin concentrations exceeding 2 times the ULN in the absence of cholestasis, abemaciclib therapy should be discontinued. (See Hepatic Toxicity under Cautions: Warnings/Precautions.)

For grade 3 serum ALT and/or AST elevations (i.e., exceeding 5 times the ULN, but no more than 20 times the ULN) with total bilirubin concentrations no more than 2 times the ULN, abemaciclib therapy should be interrupted until the toxicity improves to grade 1 or baseline. Upon resumption of therapy, the dosage of abemaciclib should be reduced.

For grade 2 serum ALT and/or AST elevations (i.e., exceeding 3 times the ULN, but no more than 5 times the ULN) with total bilirubin concentrations no more than 2 times the ULN, no dosage adjustment is necessary. If grade 2 serum ALT and/or AST elevations with total bilirubin concentrations no more than 2 times the ULN persist or recur, abemaciclib therapy should be interrupted until the toxicity improves to grade 1 or baseline. Upon resumption of therapy, the dosage of abemaciclib should be reduced.

For grade 1 serum ALT and/or AST elevations (i.e., exceeding the ULN, but no more than 3 times the ULN) with total bilirubin concentrations no more than 2 times the ULN, no dosage adjustment is necessary.

Other Toxicity. For grade 3 or 4 adverse reactions, abemaciclib therapy should be interrupted until the toxicity improves to grade 1 or baseline. Upon resumption of therapy, the dosage of abemaciclib should be reduced.

For grade 2 adverse reactions, abemaciclib therapy may be continued at the same dosage. If grade 2 adverse reactions persist or recur despite optimal supportive measures for up to 7 days, abemaciclib therapy should be interrupted until the toxicity improves to grade 1 or baseline. Upon resumption of therapy, the dosage of abemaciclib should be reduced.

For grade 1 adverse reactions, no dosage adjustment is necessary.

Dosage Modification with Concomitant Drugs or Foods Affecting Hepatic Microsomal Enzymes Concomitant use of abemaciclib with ketoconazole, a potent inhibitor of cytochrome P-450 (CYP) isoenzyme 3A (CYP3A), must be avoided; however, when abemaciclib is used concomitantly with *other* potent CYP3A inhibitors, the manufacturer recommends reducing the initial dosage of abemaciclib (200 or 150 mg twice daily depending on indication) to 100 mg twice daily or, in those already receiving a reduced dosage of abemaciclib (100 mg twice daily), further reducing the dosage of abemaciclib to 50 mg twice daily. When concomitant use of the potent CYP3A inhibitor is discontinued, the abemaciclib dosage should be returned (after at least 3–5 elimination half-lives of the CYP3A inhibitor) to the dosage used prior to initiation of the potent CYP3A inhibitor. (See Inhibitors of CYP3A under Drug Interactions: Drugs and Foods Affecting Hepatic Microsomal Enzymes.)

■ **Special Populations** For patients with severe preexisting hepatic impairment (Child-Pugh class C), the manufacturer recommends reducing the dosage frequency from twice daily to once daily. No dosage adjustment is necessary in patients with mild or moderate preexisting hepatic impairment (Child-Pugh class A or B). (See Hepatic Impairment under Warnings/Precautions: Specific Populations, in Cautions.)

Dosage adjustment is not necessary in patients with mild or moderate renal impairment (creatinine clearance 30–89 mL/minute). The effects of severe renal impairment (creatinine clearance less than 30 mL/minute), end-stage renal disease, or dialysis on the pharmacokinetics of abemaciclib have not been established, and the manufacturer makes no specific dosage recommendations for such patients. (See Renal Impairment under Warnings/Precautions: Specific Populations, in Cautions.)

The manufacturer makes no specific dosage recommendations for geriatric patients. (See Geriatric Use under Warnings/Precautions: Specific Populations, in Cautions.)

Cautions

■ **Contraindications** The manufacturer states there are no known contraindications to the use of abemaciclib.

■ **Warnings/Precautions** ***Diarrhea*** Diarrhea, sometimes resulting in dehydration or infection, occurs frequently in patients receiving abemaciclib, generally during the initial month of therapy. In the MONARCH-3 and MONARCH-2 studies, diarrhea was reported in 81 or 86% of patients receiving abemaciclib in combination with an aromatase inhibitor or fulvestrant, respectively; grade 3 diarrhea occurred in 9 or 13% of patients receiving these respective treatments. In the MONARCH-1 study, diarrhea was reported in 90% of patients receiving single-agent abemaciclib and was grade 3 in 20% of patients. In the MONARCH-3 and MONARCH-2 studies, the median time to first occurrence of diarrhea was 8 or 6 days in patients receiving abemaciclib in combination with an aromatase inhibitor or fulvestrant, respectively. In the MONARCH-3 study, the median duration of grade 2 or 3 diarrhea was 11 or 8 days, respectively, in patients receiving the drug in combination with an aromatase inhibitor; temporary interruption or dosage reduction of abemaciclib was necessary in 19 or 13% of patients, respectively. In the MONARCH-2 study, the median duration of grade 2 or 3 diarrhea was 9 or 6 days, respectively, in patients receiving abemaciclib in combination with fulvestrant;

temporary interruption or dosage reduction of abemaciclib each was necessary in 22% of patients. The median times to onset and resolution of diarrhea were similar in the principal efficacy studies.

Patients receiving abemaciclib should be monitored for development of diarrhea and immediately treated as necessary with appropriate therapy (e.g., antidiarrheal agents, fluid replacement). Temporary interruption, dosage reduction, or discontinuance of abemaciclib may be necessary depending on the severity of the diarrhea. (See Diarrhea under Dosage: Dosage Modification for Toxicity, in Dosage and Administration.)

Neutropenia Neutropenia, including febrile neutropenia and neutropenic sepsis, has occurred in patients receiving abemaciclib. In the MONARCH-3 and MONARCH-2 studies, neutropenia was reported in 41 or 46% of patients receiving abemaciclib in combination with an aromatase inhibitor or fulvestrant, respectively; grade 3 or greater neutropenia occurred in 22 or 32% of patients receiving these respective treatments. In the MONARCH-1 study, neutropenia was reported in 37% of patients receiving single-agent abemaciclib and was grade 3 in 27% of patients. In the MONARCH-3 study, the median time to first occurrence of grade 3 or greater neutropenia was 33 days and the median duration was 11 days. In the MONARCH-2 and MONARCH-1 studies, the median time to first occurrence of grade 3 or greater neutropenia was 29 days and the median duration was 15 days. In the principal efficacy studies, febrile neutropenia was reported in less than 1% of abemaciclib-treated patients. In the MONARCH-2 study, fatal neutropenic sepsis occurred in 2 patients receiving abemaciclib in combination with fulvestrant.

Complete blood cell (CBC) counts should be monitored at baseline, every 2 weeks during the initial 2 months of therapy, monthly during the next 2 months, and then as clinically indicated. Temporary interruption, dosage reduction, or discontinuance of abemaciclib may be necessary if neutropenia occurs during therapy with the drug. (See Hematologic Toxicity under Dosage: Dosage Modification for Toxicity, in Dosage and Administration.)

Hepatic Toxicity Hepatotoxicity has occurred in patients receiving abemaciclib. In the MONARCH-3 study, grade 3 or greater elevations in serum ALT or AST concentrations were reported in 6 or 3%, respectively, of patients receiving combined therapy with abemaciclib and an aromatase inhibitor. In the MONARCH-2 study, grade 3 or greater elevations in serum ALT or AST concentrations were reported in 4 or 2%, respectively, of patients receiving combined therapy with abemaciclib and fulvestrant. In the MONARCH-3 and MONARCH-2 studies, the median time to onset of grade 3 or greater elevations in ALT concentrations was 61 or 57 days in patients receiving abemaciclib in combination with an aromatase inhibitor or fulvestrant, respectively; improvement to less than grade 3 occurred in 14 days. In the MONARCH-3 and MONARCH-2 studies, the median time to onset of grade 3 or greater elevations in AST concentrations was 71 or 185 days in patients receiving abemaciclib in combination with an aromatase inhibitor or fulvestrant, respectively; median time to resolution was 13–15 days.

Liver function tests (i.e., serum ALT, AST, and bilirubin concentrations) should be monitored at baseline, every 2 weeks during the initial 2 months of therapy, monthly during the next 2 months, and then as clinically indicated. Temporary interruption, dosage reduction, or discontinuance of abemaciclib may be necessary if hepatotoxicity occurs during therapy with the drug. (See Hepatic Toxicity under Dosage: Dosage Modification for Toxicity, in Dosage and Administration.)

Thromboembolic Events Venous thromboembolic events (i.e., deep-vein thrombosis, pulmonary embolism, pelvic venous thrombosis, cerebral venous sinus thrombosis, subclavian and axillary vein thrombosis, inferior vena cava thrombosis) have occurred in patients receiving abemaciclib. In the MONARCH-3 study, venous thromboembolism was reported in 5% of patients receiving combined therapy with abemaciclib and an aromatase inhibitor compared with 0.6% of those receiving placebo and an aromatase inhibitor. In the MONARCH-2 study, venous thromboembolism was reported in 5% of patients receiving combined therapy with abemaciclib and fulvestrant compared with 0.9% of those receiving placebo and fulvestrant. Fatal venous thromboembolic events have occurred in clinical trials.

Patients should be monitored for signs or symptoms of venous thromboembolic events, including pulmonary embolism. If a venous thromboembolic event occurs, patients should receive appropriate medical intervention.

Fetal/Neonatal Morbidity and Mortality There are no adequate and well-controlled studies of abemaciclib in pregnant women; however, based on its mechanism of action and animal findings, abemaciclib may cause fetal harm. Embryofetal toxicity (e.g., decreased fetal weight) and teratogenicity (e.g., cardiovascular and skeletal abnormalities) have been demonstrated in rats receiving abemaciclib at exposure levels similar to the human exposure at the maximum recommended dosage.

Pregnancy should be avoided during abemaciclib therapy. The manufacturer recommends confirmation of pregnancy status prior to initiation of abemaciclib, and women of childbearing potential should be advised to use effective contraceptive methods during and for at least 3 weeks after discontinuance of the drug. Patients should be apprised of the potential hazard to the fetus if abemaciclib is used during pregnancy.

Impairment of Fertility Results of animal studies suggest that abemaciclib may impair male fertility.

In a general toxicology study, degeneration of reproductive tissues, decreased reproductive organ weights, intratubular cellular debris, hypospermia, and tubular dilation were observed in male animals receiving abemaciclib at exposure levels as low as 0.02 times the human exposure at the maximum recommended dosage for up to 3 months.

Specific Populations **Pregnancy.** Abemaciclib may cause fetal harm if administered to pregnant women based on its mechanism of action and animal findings. (See Fetal/Neonatal Morbidity and Mortality under Cautions: Warnings/Precautions.)

Confirmation of pregnancy status prior to initiation of abemaciclib therapy is recommended.

Lactation. It is not known whether abemaciclib is distributed into human milk. Because of the potential for serious adverse reactions to abemaciclib in nursing infants, women should be advised to discontinue nursing during and for at least 3 weeks after discontinuance of abemaciclib therapy. The effects of the drug on nursing infants or on milk production are unknown.

Pediatric Use. Safety and efficacy of abemaciclib have not been established in pediatric patients.

Geriatric Use. In the MONARCH-1, MONARCH-2, and MONARCH-3 studies, 38% of patients were 65 years of age or older and 10% were 75 years of age or older. No overall differences in safety and efficacy were observed between geriatric patients and younger adults. Grade 3 or 4 adverse reactions occurring in at least 5% of geriatric patients were neutropenia, diarrhea, fatigue, nausea, dehydration, leukopenia, anemia, infection, and elevated serum ALT concentrations.

Among patients 24–91 years of age, age did not appear to substantially affect systemic exposure to abemaciclib.

Hepatic Impairment. Following administration of a single 200-mg dose of abemaciclib, potency-adjusted total exposure to unbound drug and active metabolites in individuals with mild, moderate, or severe hepatic impairment (Child-Pugh class A, B, or C) increased by 1.2-, 1.1-, or 2.4-fold, respectively, compared with individuals with normal hepatic function; however, the mean elimination half-life of abemaciclib was prolonged by more than twofold in patients with severe hepatic impairment (55 hours) compared with individuals with normal hepatic function (24 hours). Dosage adjustment is required in patients with severe hepatic impairment. (See Dosage and Administration: Special Populations.)

Renal Impairment. Population pharmacokinetic analysis indicated that mild or moderate renal impairment (creatinine clearance 30 to less than 90 mL/minute) did not appear to substantially affect systemic exposure to abemaciclib. (See Dosage and Administration: Special Populations.)

Pharmacokinetics of abemaciclib have not been established in patients with severe renal impairment (creatinine clearance less than 30 mL/minute).

Abemaciclib has been shown to increase serum creatinine concentrations; however, it does not cause a clinically important change in glomerular filtration rate (GFR). Abemaciclib inhibits tubular secretion of creatinine by inhibiting renal organic cation transporter (OCT) 2, multidrug and toxin extrusion transporter (MATE) 1, and MATE2K. (See Drug Interactions.) In clinical studies, the mean increase in serum creatinine concentrations was 0.2–0.3 mg/dL. Elevated concentrations of serum creatinine generally occurred during the initial month of therapy and were reversible after discontinuance of abemaciclib. The manufacturer states that parameters not based on serum creatinine concentrations (e.g., BUN or cystatin C concentrations, estimated GFR) may be considered to evaluate renal function.

■ Common Adverse Effects

Adverse effects reported in 10% or more of patients with advanced breast cancer receiving abemaciclib in combination with an aromatase inhibitor (i.e., anastrozole or letrozole) and at an incidence that is at least 2% higher than that reported with placebo in combination with an aromatase inhibitor in the MONARCH-3 study include diarrhea, neutropenia, fatigue, infection (most commonly upper respiratory tract infection, lung infection, and pharyngitis), nausea, abdominal pain, anemia, vomiting, alopecia, decreased appetite, leukopenia, constipation, rash, cough, pruritus, dyspnea, dizziness, decreased weight, influenza-like illness, and thrombocytopenia. Laboratory abnormalities reported in 10% or more of patients receiving abemaciclib in combination with an aromatase inhibitor (i.e., anastrozole or letrozole) and at an incidence that is at least 2% higher than that reported with placebo in combination with an aromatase inhibitor in the MONARCH-3 study include elevated concentrations of serum creatinine (see Renal Impairment under Warnings/Precautions: Specific Populations, in Cautions), decreased leukocyte count, anemia, decreased neutrophil count, decreased lymphocyte count, elevated concentrations of aminotransferases (i.e., AST, ALT), and decreased platelet count.

Adverse effects reported in 10% or more of patients with advanced breast cancer receiving abemaciclib in combination with fulvestrant and at an incidence that is at least 2% higher than that reported with placebo in combination with fulvestrant in the MONARCH-2 study include diarrhea, fatigue, neutropenia, nausea, infection (includes urinary tract and upper respiratory tract infection, lung infection, pharyngitis, conjunctivitis, sinusitis, vaginal infection, sepsis), abdominal pain, anemia, leukopenia, decreased appetite, vomiting, headache, dysgeusia, alopecia, thrombocytopenia, stomatitis, cough, pruritus, constipation, dizziness, peripheral edema, pyrexia, rash, decreased weight, and myasthenia. Laboratory abnormalities reported in 10% or more of patients receiving abemaciclib in combination with fulvestrant and at an incidence that is at least 2% higher than that reported with placebo in combination with fulvestrant in the MONARCH-2 study include elevated concentrations of serum creatinine (see Renal Impairment under Warnings/Precautions: Specific Populations, in Cautions), decreased leukocyte count, decreased neutrophil count, decreased lymphocyte count, decreased platelet count, and elevated concentrations of aminotransferases (i.e., AST, ALT).

Adverse effects reported in 10% or more of patients with advanced breast cancer receiving abemaciclib as a single-agent in the MONARCH-1 study include diarrhea, fatigue, nausea, decreased appetite, abdominal pain, neutropenia, vomiting, infection, anemia, headache, thrombocytopenia, cough, constipation, leukopenia, arthralgia, decreased weight, dry mouth, stomatitis, alopecia, dysgeusia, dizziness, pyrexia, and dehydration. Laboratory abnormalities reported in 30% or more of patients receiving abemaciclib as a single-agent in the MONARCH-1 study include elevated concentrations of serum creatinine (see Renal Impairment under Warnings/Precautions: Specific Populations, in Cautions), decreased leukocyte count, decreased neutrophil count, decreased lymphocyte count, decreased platelet count, elevated concentrations of aminotransferases (i.e., AST, ALT), hypokalemia, and hyponatremia.

Drug Interactions

Metabolism of abemaciclib to the active *N*-desethyl (M-2), hydroxy-*N*-desethyl (M-18), and hydroxy (M-20) metabolites is mediated principally by cytochrome P-450 (CYP) isoenzyme 3A4.

In vitro studies indicate that abemaciclib and its major active metabolites (M-2 and M-20) do not induce CYP isoenzymes 1A2, 2B6, and 3A at clinically relevant concentrations. In vitro, down-regulation of messenger RNA (mRNA) for CYP isoenzymes 1A2, 2B6, 2C8, 2C9, 2D6, and 3A4 by abemaciclib and its major active metabolites has been observed; however, the mechanism and clinical relevance of this effect are unknown. Autoinhibition of abemaciclib metabolism via CYP3A4 has not been observed.

In vitro studies indicate that abemaciclib inhibits P-glycoprotein (P-gp) and breast cancer resistance protein (BCRP). Abemaciclib and its major active metabolites also inhibit organic cation transporter (OCT) 2, multidrug and toxic compound extrusion protein (MATE) 1, and MATE2K, but do not inhibit OCT1, organic anion transport protein (OATP) 1B1, OATP1B3, organic anion transporter (OAT) 1, and OAT3 at clinically relevant concentrations. In vitro, the drug is a substrate for P-gp and BCRP, but the drug and its major active metabolites are not substrates for OCT1, OATP1B1, or OATP1B3.

■ Drugs and Foods Affecting Hepatic Microsomal Enzymes

Inhibitors of CYP3A Concomitant use of abemaciclib with potent inhibitors of CYP3A may result in increased systemic exposure (area under the concentration-time curve [AUC]) of abemaciclib and its active metabolites and an increased incidence of adverse effects. When the potent CYP3A inhibitor clarithromycin (500 mg twice daily) was administered concomitantly with abemaciclib (single 50-mg dose) in healthy individuals, the potency-adjusted total AUC of unbound abemaciclib and its active metabolites was increased by 1.7-fold compared with cancer patients receiving the drug alone. Simulations using physiologically based pharmacokinetic models suggest that the potent CYP3A inhibitor itraconazole may increase the potency-adjusted total AUC of unbound abemaciclib and its active metabolites by 2.2-fold; however, ketoconazole may increase the AUC of abemaciclib by up to 16-fold. Simulations using physiologically based pharmacokinetic models suggest that the moderate CYP3A inhibitors diltiazem and verapamil may increase the potency-adjusted total AUC of unbound abemaciclib and its active metabolites by 1.7- and 1.3-fold, respectively.

Concomitant use of abemaciclib with the potent CYP3A inhibitor ketoconazole *must* be avoided; however, when abemaciclib is used concomitantly with *other* potent CYP3A inhibitors (e.g., clarithromycin; cobicistat; conivaptan; diltiazem; *ritonavir-boosted* elvitegravir; idelalisib; *ritonavir-boosted* indinavir; itraconazole; ritonavir/lopinavir; nefazodone; nelfinavir; the fixed combination of ombitasvir, paritaprevir, and ritonavir (with or without dasabuvir); posaconazole; ritonavir; *ritonavir-boosted* saquinavir; *ritonavir-boosted* tipranavir; voriconazole), the manufacturer of abemaciclib recommends reducing the initial dosage of abemaciclib (200 or 150 mg twice daily depending on indication) to 100 mg twice daily or, in those already receiving a reduced dosage of abemaciclib (100 mg twice daily), further reducing the dosage of abemaciclib to 50 mg twice daily. When concomitant use of the potent CYP3A inhibitor is discontinued, the abemaciclib dosage should be returned (after at least 3–5 elimination half-lives of the CYP3A inhibitor) to the dosage used prior to initiation of the potent CYP3A inhibitor.

Grapefruit products are CYP3A inhibitors and should be avoided because of the potential for increased systemic exposure of abemaciclib during concurrent use.

Inducers of CYP3A Concomitant use of abemaciclib with potent inducers of CYP3A may result in decreased peak plasma concentrations and AUC of abemaciclib and its active metabolites and reduced abemaciclib efficacy. When the potent CYP3A inducer rifampin (600 mg daily) was administered concomitantly with abemaciclib (single 200-mg dose) in healthy individuals, the potency-adjusted total AUC of unbound abemaciclib and its active metabolites was decreased by 67%. Moderate CYP3A inducers have not been specifically studied in drug interaction studies to date.

Concomitant use of abemaciclib with potent inducers of CYP3A should be avoided, and selection of an alternative drug with less CYP3A induction potential should be considered.

■ Drugs Affected by Transport Systems

Abemaciclib and its active metabolites inhibit OCT2, MATE1, and MATE2K at clinically relevant concentrations. When a single 1-g dose of metformin (a substrate of OCT2, MATE1, and MATE2K) was administered with a single 400-mg dose of abemaciclib, peak plasma concentrations and AUC of metformin increased by 22 and 37%, respectively. Abemaciclib reduced the renal clearance and renal secretion of metformin by 45 and 62%, respectively.

■ Anastrozole

Concomitant administration of abemaciclib and anastrozole did not affect the pharmacokinetics of either drug.

■ Exemestane

Concomitant administration of abemaciclib and exemestane did not affect the pharmacokinetics of either drug.

■ Fulvestrant

Concomitant administration of abemaciclib and fulvestrant did not affect the pharmacokinetics of either drug.

■ Letrozole

Concomitant administration of abemaciclib and letrozole did not affect the pharmacokinetics of either drug.

■ Loperamide

Concomitant administration of loperamide (single 8-mg dose) in healthy individuals receiving abemaciclib (single 400-mg dose) did not have a clinically relevant effect on the pharmacokinetics of abemaciclib and its active metabolites or loperamide.

Description

Abemaciclib, a selective inhibitor of cyclin-dependent kinases 4 (CDK4) and 6 (CDK6), is an antineoplastic agent. Several mechanisms contribute to the dysregulation of the cell cycle during the G1 into S phase, including amplification or overexpression of the cyclin D oncogene or the loss of intrinsic CDK inhibitors (i.e., p16, p15, p18, p19, p21, p27, p57) in breast cancer. Abemaciclib specifically inhibits CDK4 and CDK6 and blocks the interaction of CDK4 and CDK6 with cyclin D, resulting in inhibition of phosphorylation of the tumor suppressor protein retinoblastoma and inhibition of progression of the cell cycle from the G1 into S phase. In vitro, abemaciclib has demonstrated decreased phosphorylation of retinoblastoma protein and reduced cellular proliferation of breast cancer cell lines by inhibiting the G1 into S phase of the cell cycle. The combination of abemaciclib with an antiestrogen agent or as a single-agent demonstrated reduced tumor volume in xenograft models of breast cancer.

Area under the serum concentration-time curve (AUC) and peak plasma concentrations of abemaciclib are dose proportional over a dosage range of 50–200 mg. Peak plasma concentrations of abemaciclib are achieved in a median of 8 hours following oral administration of the drug. Following repeated doses of abemaciclib twice daily, steady-state concentrations of the drug are achieved in 5 days and the mean accumulation ratio for the drug based on AUC or peak plasma concentration is 3.2 or 2.3, respectively. Oral administration of abemaciclib with a high-fat, high-calorie meal (approximately 800–1000 calories with fat accounting for over 50% of the caloric content) increases systemic exposure and peak plasma concentrations of abemaciclib and its active metabolites by 9 and 26%, respectively. Abemaciclib and its active metabolites are highly bound (more than 93%) to plasma proteins, albumin, and α_1-acid glycoprotein. Abemaciclib is metabolized principally by cytochrome P-450 (CYP) isoenzyme 3A4. The main circulating metabolites, M-2 (an *N*-desethyl metabolite), M-18 (a hydroxy-*N*-desethyl metabolite), and M-20 (a hydroxy metabolite) have been shown to be equipotent to abemaciclib, and these metabolites account for 25, 13, and 26%, respectively, of total plasma concentrations of the drug. In patients with advanced cancer, including breast cancer, CSF concentrations of abemaciclib and its active metabolites M-2 and M-20 are similar to unbound plasma concentrations. Following oral administration of a single radiolabeled dose of abemaciclib, approximately 81% of the radioactivity was recovered in feces (mainly as metabolites) and approximately 3% was recovered in urine. The mean plasma elimination half-life of the drug is 18.3 hours.

Population pharmacokinetic analysis indicated that age (24–91 years), gender, and body weight (36–175 kg) do not have clinically important effects on the exposure of abemaciclib.

Advice to Patients

Importance of advising patients to swallow abemaciclib tablets whole and *not* to break, chew, crush, or split the tablets.

If a dose is missed or vomited, importance of administering the next dose at the regularly scheduled time; an additional dose should not be administered to make up for a missed dose.

Risk of diarrhea. Importance of informing patients that early identification and intervention is critical for the optimal management of diarrhea. Importance of informing patients how to manage diarrhea (e.g., oral hydration, antidiarrheal agents) at the first sign of loose stools. Importance of informing clinician if diarrhea occurs.

Risk of neutropenia. Importance of promptly informing clinician if signs or symptoms of neutropenia or infection (e.g., fever) occur.

Risk of hepatotoxicity. Importance of promptly informing clinician if symptoms of hepatotoxicity (e.g., fatigue, anorexia, right upper quadrant pain, bleeding diathesis) occur.

Risk of venous thromboembolic events. Importance of promptly informing clinician if any symptoms suggestive of a thromboembolic event occur (e.g., extremity pain or swelling, chest pain, shortness of breath, tachypnea, tachycardia).

Risk of fetal harm. Necessity of advising women of childbearing potential to use an effective method of contraception during treatment and for at least 3 weeks after discontinuance of therapy. Importance of women informing clinicians if they are or plan to become pregnant. Apprise patient of potential fetal hazard if used during pregnancy.

Importance of advising women to discontinue nursing during therapy and for at least 3 weeks after discontinuance of the drug.

Importance of informing clinicians of existing or contemplated concomitant therapy, including prescription and OTC drugs (e.g., ketoconazole) and dietary (e.g., grapefruit products) or herbal supplements, as well as any concomitant illnesses (e.g., hepatic impairment).

Importance of informing patients of other important precautionary information. (See Cautions.)

Overview® (see Users Guide). For additional information on this drug until a more detailed monograph is developed and published, the manufacturer's labeling should be consulted. It is *essential* that the manufacturer's labeling be consulted for more detailed information on usual cautions, precautions, contraindications, potential drug interactions, laboratory test interferences, and acute toxicity. For further information on the handling of antineoplastic agents, see the ASHP Guidelines on Handling Hazardous Drugs at http://www.ahfsdruginformation.com.

Preparations

Excipients in commercially available drug preparations may have clinically important effects in some individuals; consult specific product labeling for details.

Abemaciclib

Oral		
Tablets	50 mg	Verzenio®, Lilly
	100 mg	Verzenio®, Lilly
	150 mg	Verzenio®, Lilly
	200 mg	Verzenio®, Lilly

Abiraterone Acetate

■ Abiraterone acetate is a prodrug of abiraterone, a potent, selective, and irreversible inhibitor of cytochrome P-450 (CYP) 17α-hydroxylase/C17,20-lyase (also referred to as CYP17); abiraterone is an antineoplastic agent.

Uses

■ **Prostate Cancer** Abiraterone acetate is used in combination with prednisone for the treatment of metastatic castration-resistant prostate cancer previously treated with docetaxel-containing therapy.

The current indication for abiraterone acetate is based principally on the results of a randomized, double-blind, placebo-controlled phase 3 study in patients with metastatic castration-resistant prostate cancer that had progressed following treatment with 1 or 2 cytotoxic regimens, one of which had to contain docetaxel. Patients who previously received ketoconazole for treatment of prostate cancer were excluded from the study. In this study, 1195 patients were randomized in a 2:1 ratio to receive either abiraterone acetate (1 g once daily) in combination with prednisone (5 mg twice daily) or placebo in combination with prednisone (5 mg twice daily). Treatment was continued until disease progression or unacceptable toxicity occurred, new treatment was initiated, or the patient withdrew from the study. The primary measure of efficacy was overall survival. The median age of patients enrolled in the study was 69 years. Most of the patients (70%) had received one prior cytotoxic regimen.

A planned interim analysis indicated that patients receiving abiraterone acetate plus prednisone had a longer median overall survival (14.8 versus 10.9 months) than those receiving placebo plus prednisone. The median follow-up at the time of the interim analysis was 12.8 months, and the median duration of treatment was 8 months for patients receiving abiraterone acetate and prednisone and 4 months for those receiving placebo and prednisone. Because of the survival benefit observed at the interim analysis, study investigators permitted patients previously randomized to receive placebo to cross over to open-label abiraterone acetate therapy. Updated analysis (performed when 97% of the planned number of deaths for final analysis had occurred) confirmed that patients receiving abiraterone acetate plus prednisone had a longer median overall survival (15.8 months) than those who received placebo plus prednisone (11.2 months).

At the interim analysis, patients receiving abiraterone acetate and prednisone also had higher objective response rates (14 versus 3%) and prostate specific antigen (PSA) response rates (29 versus 6%), longer times to PSA progression (10.2 versus 6.6 months), and longer median progression-free survival based on radiographic evidence (5.6 versus 3.6 months) compared with those receiving placebo and prednisone.

Dosage and Administration

■ **General** Because adrenocortical insufficiency has been reported in patients receiving abiraterone acetate when concomitant daily corticosteroid therapy was interrupted and/or during periods of concurrent infection or stress, an increase in corticosteroid dosage may be indicated before, during, and after stressful situations.

Because abiraterone may cause fetal harm, women who are or may be pregnant should not handle abiraterone acetate tablets without protection (e.g., gloves).

■ **Administration** Because administration of abiraterone acetate tablets with food markedly increases exposure to abiraterone, the drug should be administered orally on an empty stomach; no food should be consumed for at least 2 hours before or 1 hour after a dose. (See Description and see Effect of Food on Abiraterone Absorption under Cautions: Warnings/Precautions.) The tablets should be swallowed whole with water.

■ **Dosage** ***Prostate Cancer*** For the treatment of castration-resistant metastatic prostate cancer in patients who previously received a docetaxel-containing regimen, the recommended dosage of abiraterone acetate is 1 g once daily in combination with prednisone 5 mg orally twice daily.

Dosage Modification for Toxicity **Hepatotoxicity.** In patients who exhibit substantial increases in serum transaminase concentrations (ALT and/or AST exceeding 5 times the upper limit of normal [ULN]) or total bilirubin concentrations (exceeding 3 times the ULN), therapy with abiraterone acetate should be withheld until liver function test results return to baseline values or until ALT and AST decrease to no more than 2.5 times the ULN and total bilirubin concentrations decrease to no more than 1.5 times the ULN. Abiraterone acetate therapy may then be resumed at a reduced dosage of 750 mg once daily with monitoring of serum transaminase and bilirubin concentrations at least every 2 weeks for 3 months and monthly thereafter.

If hepatotoxicity recurs at a dosage of 750 mg daily, therapy should be withheld again until liver function test results return to baseline values or until ALT and AST concentrations decrease to no more than 2.5 times the ULN and total bilirubin concentrations decrease to no more than 1.5 times the ULN; therapy may then be resumed at a reduced dosage of 500 mg once daily.

If hepatotoxicity recurs at a dosage of 500 mg daily, treatment with abiraterone acetate should be discontinued.

The safety of reinitiating abiraterone acetate therapy in patients who have exhibited marked elevations in ALT or AST (20 or more times the ULN) and/or bilirubin (10 or more times the ULN) is unknown. (See Hepatic Toxicity under Cautions: Warnings/Precautions.)

■ **Special Populations** Use of abiraterone acetate in patients with severe preexisting hepatic impairment (Child-Pugh class C) is not recommended.

For patients with moderate preexisting hepatic impairment (Child-Pugh class B), the manufacturer recommends an abiraterone acetate dosage of 250 mg once daily with monitoring of serum transaminase and bilirubin concentrations prior to initiation of therapy, every week for the first month of therapy, every 2 weeks during the second and third months of therapy, and then monthly thereafter. Abiraterone acetate should be permanently discontinued in patients with moderate preexisting hepatic impairment if transaminase concentrations (ALT and/or AST) increase above 5 times the ULN or total bilirubin concentrations increase above 3 times the ULN.

Dosage adjustment is not necessary in patients with mild preexisting hepatic impairment.

No dosage adjustment is necessary in patients with renal impairment.

Cautions

■ **Contraindications** Abiraterone acetate is contraindicated in women who are or may become pregnant. (See Fetal/Neonatal Morbidity and Mortality under Cautions: Warnings/Precautions.)

■ **Warnings/Precautions** ***Fetal/Neonatal Morbidity and Mortality*** Abiraterone may cause fetal harm. The drug is contraindicated in women who are or may become pregnant. If used during pregnancy or if the patient becomes pregnant while receiving abiraterone, the patient should be apprised of the potential fetal hazard.

Women who are or may be pregnant should not handle abiraterone acetate tablets without protection (e.g., gloves).

Because it is not known whether abiraterone or its metabolites distribute into semen, men receiving the drug should use a condom during sexual encounters with pregnant women and should use a condom in conjunction with another effective contraceptive method during sexual encounters with women of childbearing potential. These contraceptive measures are required during and for one week following discontinuance of abiraterone therapy.

Excessive Mineralocorticoid Activity Inhibition of the 17α-hydroxylase enzyme results in decreased serum concentrations of cortisol, which leads to stimulation of corticotropin (ACTH) release and a resultant increase in steroids with mineralocorticoid activity upstream of the enzyme blockade. This secondary mineralocorticoid excess commonly is manifested as hypertension, hypokalemia, and fluid retention. The severity and incidence of these mineralocorticoid effects may be reduced by concomitant administration of a glucocorticoid to suppress ACTH release and steroid synthesis upstream of the CYP17 blockade.

Abiraterone acetate should be used with caution in patients with a history of cardiovascular disease or with any underlying medical condition that might be compromised by increases in blood pressure, hypokalemia, or fluid retention (e.g., heart failure, recent myocardial infarction, ventricular arrhythmia). Patients with a left ventricular ejection fraction of less than 50% or with New York Heart Association (NYHA) class III or IV heart failure were excluded from the phase 3 trial evaluating abiraterone in patients with prostate cancer; therefore, safety of the drug in such patients has not been established. Patients should be monitored at least monthly for hypertension, hypokalemia, and fluid retention. Blood pressure should be controlled and hypokalemia should be corrected before and during treatment.

Adrenocortical Insufficiency In patients receiving abiraterone acetate in combination with prednisone, adrenocortical insufficiency has been reported following interruption of the daily corticosteroid regimen and/or during periods of infection or stress. Abiraterone acetate should be used with caution and patients should be monitored for manifestations of adrenocortical insufficiency, especially following dosage reduction or discontinuance of prednisone or when the patient is subjected to unusual stress. An increase in corticosteroid dosage before, during, and after stressful situations may be indicated. Manifestations of adrenocortical insufficiency may be masked by symptoms of mineralocorticoid excess; if clinically indicated, appropriate tests should be performed to confirm the diagnosis of adrenocortical insufficiency.

Hepatic Toxicity Elevations in transaminase (ALT or AST) concentrations exceeding 5 times the upper limit of normal (ULN) have occurred in 2.3% of patients receiving abiraterone acetate , generally during the initial 3 months of therapy. In the phase 3 trial of abiraterone acetate in patients with prostate cancer, elevations in liver function test results were reported more frequently in patients with preexisting ALT or AST elevations than in patients with normal baseline transaminase concentrations.

Serum transaminase (ALT and AST) and bilirubin concentrations should be evaluated prior to initiation of therapy and monitored every 2 weeks for the first 3 months of therapy and then monthly thereafter. For patients with moderate preexisting hepatic impairment, serum transaminase and bilirubin concentrations should be evaluated prior to initiation of therapy and monitored every week for the first month of therapy, every 2 weeks during the second and third months of therapy, and then monthly thereafter. More frequent monitoring is indicated if transaminase or bilirubin concentrations rise above pretreatment levels. If manifestations suggestive of hepatotoxicity develop, liver function tests should be evaluated promptly. If ALT and/or AST elevations exceed 5 times the ULN or total bilirubin elevations exceed 3 times the ULN, treatment should be interrupted and hepatic function monitored closely. Therapy with the drug should be reinitiated at a reduced dosage only after liver function test results have returned to baseline values or after ALT and AST have decreased to no more than 2.5 times the ULN and total bilirubin concentrations have decreased to no more than 1.5 times the ULN. (See Hepatotoxicity under Dosage: Dosage Modification for Toxicity, in Dosage and Administration.) The safety of reinitiating abiraterone acetate therapy in patients who have exhibited marked elevations in ALT or AST (20 or more times the ULN) and/or bilirubin (10 or more times the ULN) is unknown.

Effect of Food on Abiraterone Absorption Systemic exposure and peak plasma concentrations of abiraterone are increased up to tenfold and 17-fold, respectively, when single doses of abiraterone acetate are administered with a meal instead of in the fasted state (see Description). Because of normal variations in the content and composition of meals, administration with food also is likely to result in highly variable exposure to the drug. The safety of administering multiple doses of the drug with food has not been established. Abiraterone acetate must be administered on an empty stomach; no food should be consumed for at least 2 hours before or 1 hour after a dose.

Specific Populations **Pregnancy.** Category X. (See Fetal/Neonatal Morbidity and Mortality under Cautions: Warnings/Precautions.)

Lactation. It is not known whether abiraterone is distributed into milk in humans; because of the potential for serious adverse reactions to abiraterone in nursing infants, a decision should be made whether to discontinue nursing or the drug, taking into account the importance of the drug to the woman.

Pediatric Use. Abiraterone acetate is not indicated for use in children; safety and efficacy have not been established.

Geriatric Use. In the phase 3 clinical trial evaluating abiraterone acetate in men with prostate cancer, 71% of patients were 65 years of age or older and 28% were 75 years of age or older. No overall differences in safety and efficacy were observed between geriatric patients and younger adults.

Hepatic Impairment. Systemic exposure of abiraterone is increased by approximately 1.1- or 3.6-fold in patients with preexisting mild (Child-Pugh class A) or moderate (Child-Pugh class B) hepatic impairment, respectively, compared with individuals with normal hepatic function. Dosage adjustment and careful monitoring of hepatic function are required in patients with moderate hepatic impairment. (See Dosage and Administration: Special Populations.) Safety of the drug has not been established in patients with severe hepatic impairment (Child-Pugh class C), and use of the drug in these patients is not recommended. Patients with active hepatitis, baseline ALT and/or AST concentrations 2.5 or more times the ULN in the absence of liver metastases, or ALT and/or AST concentrations exceeding 5 times the ULN in the presence of liver metastases were excluded from clinical studies of the drug.

Renal Impairment. Following oral administration of a single 1-g dose of abiraterone acetate, pharmacokinetic values in patients with end-stage renal disease requiring hemodialysis were similar to those in individuals with normal renal function; no dosage adjustment is required in patients with renal impairment.

■ **Common Adverse Effects** Adverse effects reported in 5% or more of patients receiving abiraterone acetate in combination with prednisone include joint swelling or discomfort, hypokalemia, edema, muscle discomfort, hot flush, diarrhea, urinary tract infection, cough, hypertension, arrhythmia, urinary frequency, nocturia, dyspepsia, upper respiratory tract infection, hypertriglyceridemia, hypophosphatemia, and elevated transaminase and total bilirubin concentrations.

Drug Interactions

In vitro studies indicate that abiraterone is a potent inhibitor of cytochrome P-450 (CYP) isoenzymes 1A2 and 2D6 and a moderate inhibitor of CYP isoenzymes 2C9, 2C19, and 3A4/5. Abiraterone is a substrate of CYP3A4 in vitro. In vitro studies indicate that neither abiraterone acetate nor abiraterone is a substrate of P-glycoprotein (P-gp) at clinically relevant concentrations; however, abiraterone acetate is an inhibitor of P-gp.

■ **Drugs and Foods Affecting Hepatic Microsomal Enzymes** Concomitant use of abiraterone acetate with potent inhibitors of CYP3A4 (e.g., atazanavir, clarithromycin, grapefruit juice, indinavir, itraconazole, ketoconazole, nefazodone, nelfinavir, ritonavir, saquinavir, telithromycin, voriconazole) may result in increased plasma concentrations of abiraterone and should be avoided, or the drugs should be used concomitantly with caution.

Concomitant use of abiraterone acetate with potent inducers of CYP3A4 (e.g., carbamazepine, phenobarbital, phenytoin, rifabutin, rifampin, rifapentine) may result in decreased plasma concentrations of abiraterone and should be avoided, or the drugs should be used with caution.

■ **Drugs Metabolized by Hepatic Microsomal Enzymes** Concomitant use of abiraterone acetate with CYP2D6 substrates may result in increased serum concentrations of the CYP2D6 substrate drug and possible toxicity. When the CYP2D6 substrate dextromethorphan hydrobromide (single 30-mg dose) was administered concomitantly with abiraterone acetate (1 g daily) and prednisone (5 mg twice daily), peak plasma concentration and systemic exposure of dextromethorphan were increased 2.8- and 2.9-fold, respectively. Concomitant use of abiraterone acetate with CYP2D6 substrates that have a narrow therapeutic index (e.g., thioridazine) should be avoided. If concomitant use cannot be avoided, reduction of the dosage of the CYP2D6 substrate drug should be considered, and the drugs should be used concomitantly with caution.

When the CYP1A2 substrate theophylline (single 100-mg dose) was administered concomitantly with abiraterone acetate (1 g daily) and prednisone (5 mg twice daily), systemic exposure of theophylline was unchanged.

Description

Abiraterone acetate is a prodrug of abiraterone, a potent, selective, and irreversible inhibitor of cytochrome P-450 (CYP) 17α-hydroxylase/C17,20-lyase (also referred to as CYP17); abiraterone is an antineoplastic agent. The CYP17 enzyme is expressed in the testes and adrenal glands, and also is expressed in prostatic tumor tissue. CYP17 catalyzes 2 sequential reactions: 17α-hydroxylase catalyzes the conversion of pregnenolone and progesterone to their 17α-hydroxy derivatives, and C17,20-lyase catalyzes the conversion of these 17α-hydroxy derivatives to dehydroepiandrosterone (DHEA) and androstenedione. DHEA and androstenedione are androgenic precursors of testosterone. Testosterone and dihydrotestosterone bind to and activate the androgen receptor, which is key in the development and progression of prostate cancer. Thus, inhibition of CYP17 activity by abiraterone results in suppression of androgen production. Inhibition of CYP17 activity by abiraterone also can result in increased mineralocorticoid synthesis by the adrenal glands. (See Excessive Mineralocorticoid Activity under Cautions: Warnings/Precautions.) Abiraterone is tenfold to 30-fold more potent than ketoconazole (a nonspecific CYP inhibitor and weak inhibitor of CYP17) in its inhibition of the CYP17 enzyme.

Although decreases in serum testosterone and other androgens have been observed with abiraterone acetate therapy for prostate cancer, it is not necessary to monitor the effect of abiraterone on serum testosterone levels. Changes in serum prostate specific antigen (PSA) concentrations also may be observed, but have not been shown to correlate with clinical benefit in individual patients.

Following oral administration, abiraterone acetate is hydrolyzed, most likely by esterases in non-CYP-dependent pathways, to its active metabolite, abiraterone. Peak plasma concentrations of abiraterone occur 2 hours after administration of the parent drug. Abiraterone is further metabolized to form 2 inactive sulfate conjugates, abiraterone sulfate (formed by SULT2A1, a sulfotransferase that catalyzes the sulfate conjugation of DHEA and other steroids) and *N*-oxide abiraterone sulfate (formed by CYP3A4 and SULT2A1). The mean terminal half-life of abiraterone in patients with metastatic castration-resistant prostate cancer is 12 hours. Following oral administration of a radiolabeled dose of abiraterone acetate, about 88% of the dose is recovered in feces, mainly as abiraterone acetate (55%) and abiraterone (22%), and 5% of the dose is recovered in urine.

Systemic exposure to abiraterone is increased when abiraterone acetate is administered with food. Oral administration of a single 1-g dose of abiraterone acetate with a low-fat or high-fat meal resulted in increases in systemic exposure of approximately fivefold or tenfold, respectively, and increases in peak plasma concentrations of approximately sevenfold or 17-fold, respectively. (See Effect of Food on Abiraterone Absorption under Cautions: Warnings/Precautions.)

Abiraterone is a potent inhibitor of CYP isoenzymes 1A2 and 2D6 and a moderate inhibitor of CYP isoenzymes 2C9, 2C19, and 3A4/5. In vitro studies indicate that neither abiraterone acetate nor abiraterone is a substrate of P-glycoprotein (P-gp); however, abiraterone acetate is an inhibitor of P-gp.

Advice to Patients

Importance of taking the prednisone component of the abiraterone acetate regimen as directed to minimize adverse effects of abiraterone. Importance of advising patients that if a dose of abiraterone acetate or prednisone is missed, the next dose should be taken at the regularly scheduled time; importance of advising clinician if more than one daily dose of abiraterone acetate is missed.

For patients currently receiving gonadotropin-releasing hormone (GnRH) agonist therapy, importance of continuing this therapy during abiraterone acetate therapy.

Risk of increased abiraterone exposure and adverse effects if the drug is taken with food. Importance of swallowing abiraterone acetate tablets whole with water and consuming no food for at least 2 hours before or 1 hour after a dose.

Risk of peripheral edema, hypokalemia, hypertension, and urinary tract infection.

Risk of hepatotoxicity and importance of liver function test monitoring.

Importance of advising patients that abiraterone may cause fetal harm and that it is not known whether the drug distributes into semen. Necessity of advising men to use a condom during sexual encounters with pregnant women and to use a condom in conjunction with another effective contraceptive method during sexual encounters with women of childbearing potential; these contraceptive measures are required during and for 1 week after discontinuance of abiraterone acetate therapy. Importance of advising patients that women who are or may be pregnant should not handle abiraterone acetate tablets without protection (e.g., gloves).

Importance of informing clinicians of existing or contemplated concomitant therapy, including prescription and OTC drugs and herbal supplements, as well as any concomitant illnesses.

Importance of informing patients of other important precautionary information. (See Cautions.)

Overview® (see Users Guide). For additional information on this drug until a more detailed monograph is developed and published, the manufacturer's labeling should be consulted. It is *essential* that the manufacturer's labeling be consulted for more detailed information on usual cautions, precautions, contraindications, potential drug interactions, laboratory test interferences, and acute toxicity. For further information on the handling of antineoplastic agents, see the ASHP Guidelines on Handling Hazardous Drugs at http://www.ahfsdruginformation.com.

Preparations

Excipients in commercially available drug preparations may have clinically important effects in some individuals; consult specific product labeling for details.

Abiraterone Acetate

Oral

Tablets	250 mg	**Zytiga®**, Centocor Ortho Biotech

Acalabrutinib

■ Acalabrutinib, a small-molecule inhibitor of Bruton's tyrosine kinase (BTK), is an antineoplastic agent.

Uses

■ **Mantle Cell Lymphoma** Acalabrutinib is used for the treatment of mantle cell lymphoma in patients who have received at least one prior therapy. The current indication is based on overall response rate; clinical benefit (e.g., increased survival) has not been established. Continued FDA approval for this indication may be contingent on verification and description of clinical benefit in additional trials. Acalabrutinib has been designated an orphan drug by FDA for the treatment of this cancer.

The current indication for acalabrutinib is based principally on the results of an open-label, phase 2 study (ACE-LY-004 trial) in 124 patients with mantle cell lymphoma who had received at least one prior therapy. The primary measure of efficacy was overall response rate (complete plus partial responses) based on the Lugano Classification for non-Hodgkin's lymphoma. The median age of patients enrolled in the study was 68 years (range: 42–90 years), 80% were male, and 74% were Caucasian; most patients (93%) had a baseline ECOG (Eastern Cooperative Oncology Group) performance status of 0 or 1 and the median time since diagnosis of disease was approximately 46 months. Patients in the study had received a median of 2 (range: 1–5) prior therapies for their disease and 18% of patients had previously undergone a stem-cell transplant. Patients who had received prior therapy with a Bruton's tyrosine kinase (BTK) inhibitor (e.g., ibrutinib) were excluded from the study. All patients received acalabrutinib 100 mg orally twice daily in 28-day cycles until disease progression or unacceptable toxicity occurred. The median dose intensity was 98.5%.

Effects of acalabrutinib on investigator-assessed overall response rate and independent review committee-assessed overall response rate were comparable. At a median of 15.2 months' follow-up, the investigator-assessed overall response rate in acalabrutinib-treated patients was 81%; 40% of patients receiving the drug achieved a complete response. At the time of data analysis, the median time to best response was 1.9 months; however, estimated medians for duration of response, progression-free survival, and overall survival had not yet been reached. Following initiation of acalabrutinib therapy, lymphocytosis (i.e., absolute lymphocyte count exceeding 5000/mm³ and an increase of at least 50% from baseline) occurred in 31% of patients; the median time to onset of lymphocytosis was 1.1 weeks and the median duration of lymphocytosis was 6.7 weeks. Acalabrutinib therapy was generally well tolerated; most adverse effects were grade 1 or 2 in severity. Headache, diarrhea, fatigue, and myalgia were the most commonly reported adverse effects in this study. (See Description.)

Dosage and Administration

■ **General** Because acalabrutinib may increase the risk of infectious complications, antimicrobial prophylaxis should be considered in patients at increased risk for opportunistic infections. (See Infectious Complications under Cautions: Warnings/Precautions.)

Restricted Distribution Acalabrutinib is available only through specialty pharmacies and distributors. Clinicians may contact AstraZeneca Access360 at 844-275-2360 or consult the AstraZeneca Access360 website for specific availability information (https://www.myaccess360.com/hcp/hcp-branded-calquence/home.html).

■ **Administration** Acalabrutinib is administered orally twice daily, with doses given approximately 12 hours apart; the drug can be taken without regard to meals. (See Description.)

Acalabrutinib capsules should be swallowed whole with water; they should *not* be opened, broken, or chewed.

If a dose of acalabrutinib is missed by more than 3 hours, the dose should be skipped and the next dose should be taken at the regularly scheduled time. Patients should *not* take extra capsules of the drug to make up for the missed dose.

Concomitant Use with Drugs Affecting Gastric Acidity Because drugs that reduce gastric acidity potentially can decrease plasma concentrations of acalabrutinib and thereby reduce its efficacy, the manufacturer recommends separating administration of acalabrutinib and antacids by at least 2 hours and administering acalabrutinib 2 hours before administration of a histamine H_2-receptor antagonist. The manufacturer recommends avoiding concomitant use of acalabrutinib and proton-pump inhibitors since proton-pump inhibitors have long-lasting gastric acid-reducing effects. (See Drug Interactions: Drugs Affecting Gastric Acidity.)

■ **Dosage** ***Mantle Cell Lymphoma*** For the treatment of mantle cell lymphoma in adults who have received at least one prior therapy, the recommended dosage of acalabrutinib is 100 mg twice daily. Acalabrutinib therapy should be continued until disease progression or unacceptable toxicity occurs.

Dosage Modification for Toxicity Acalabrutinib therapy should be withheld for the occurrence of grade 3 or higher nonhematologic toxicity, grade 3 thrombocytopenia with bleeding, grade 4 thrombocytopenia, or grade 4 neutropenia lasting longer than 7 days. Upon resolution or improvement of the toxicity (i.e., return to baseline or resolution to grade 1), acalabrutinib therapy may be resumed (or discontinued) as described in Table 1.

Table 1: Recommended Dosage Modifications for Acalabrutinib Toxicity

Toxicity Occurrence	Dosage Modification after Recovery from Toxicity (Starting Dosage = 100 mg twice daily)
First	Restart at 100 mg twice daily
Second	Restart at 100 mg twice daily
Third	Restart at 100 mg once daily
Fourth	Discontinue acalabrutinib

Concomitant Use with Drugs Affecting Hepatic Microsomal Enzymes Concomitant use of acalabrutinib and drugs that are *potent* inhibitors of cytochrome P-450 (CYP) isoenzyme 3A (CYP3A) should be avoided. If short-term (e.g., anti-infective therapy for up to 7 days) therapy with a *potent* CYP3A inhibitor is necessary, acalabrutinib should be withheld during such therapy.

If acalabrutinib is used concomitantly with a *moderate* CYP3A inhibitor, the manufacturer recommends reducing the dosage of acalabrutinib to 100 mg once daily. (See Inhibitors of CYP3A under Drug Interactions: Drugs Affecting Hepatic Microsomal Enzymes.)

Concomitant use of acalabrutinib and drugs that are *potent* inducers of CYP3A should be avoided. If therapy with a *potent* CYP3A inducer is necessary, the manufacturer recommends increasing the dosage of acalabrutinib to 200 mg twice daily during such therapy. (See Inducers of CYP3A under Drug Interactions: Drugs Affecting Hepatic Microsomal Enzymes.)

■ **Special Populations** The manufacturer makes no specific dosage recommendations for patients with hepatic or renal impairment. (See Specific Populations under Cautions: Warnings/Precautions.)

The manufacturer makes no special dosage recommendations for geriatric patients; most patients (65%) in the pivotal efficacy study were 65 years of age or older. (See Geriatric Use under Warnings/Precautions: Specific Populations, in Cautions.)

Cautions

■ **Contraindications** The manufacturer states that there are no known contraindications to the use of acalabrutinib.

■ **Warnings/Precautions** ***Hemorrhage*** Serious hemorrhagic events, including fatal events, have occurred in patients with hematologic malignancies treated with acalabrutinib monotherapy (based on the combined safety database). Grade 3 or higher bleeding events (i.e., GI bleeding, intracranial bleeding, epistaxis) were reported in 2% of these patients. Overall, hemorrhagic events, including bruising and petechiae, of any grade of severity occurred in approximately 50% of patients receiving acalabrutinib for hematologic malignancies in clinical trials. The mechanism of bleeding with acalabrutinib therapy is unclear.

Because concomitant use of acalabrutinib with antiplatelet or anticoagulant therapies may further increase the risk of hemorrhagic events, the manufacturer recommends that patients receiving these drugs in combination should be monitored for signs of bleeding.

Because of the risk of bleeding, the potential benefits and risks of withholding acalabrutinib therapy for 3–7 days prior to and following surgery (based on the type of surgery and bleeding risk) should be considered.

Infectious Complications Serious and sometimes fatal infections, including bacterial, fungal, viral, or other opportunistic infections, have been reported in acalabrutinib-treated patients. Grade 3 or higher infections occurred in 18% of patients receiving acalabrutinib monotherapy for hematologic malignancies (based on the combined safety database). The most commonly reported grade 3 or 4 infection was pneumonia. Infections caused by hepatitis B reactivation and progressive multifocal leukoencephalopathy (PML) also have been reported.

Patients receiving acalabrutinib therapy should be monitored for the development of signs and symptoms of infection and treated as medically appropriate. In addition, antimicrobial prophylactic therapy should be considered in patients who are at increased risk for opportunistic infections.

Myelosuppression Cytopenias, including neutropenia, anemia, and thrombocytopenia, have been reported in patients receiving acalabrutinib. Grade 3 or 4 neutropenia, anemia, or thrombocytopenia was reported in 23, 11, or 8%, respectively, of patients with hematologic malignancies treated with acalabrutinib monotherapy (based on the combined safety database).

Complete blood cell (CBC) counts should be monitored monthly during acalabrutinib therapy. Temporary interruption of acalabrutinib therapy or dosage reduction may be necessary if myelosuppression occurs. (See Dosage Modification for Toxicity under Dosage and Administration: Dosage.)

Development of Second Primary Malignancy Second primary malignancies, including non-skin carcinomas, have occurred in 11% of patients with hematologic malignancies treated with acalabrutinib monotherapy (based on the combined safety database). Skin cancer was the most frequently reported second primary malignancy, occurring in 7% of acalabrutinib-treated patients. Patients receiving the drug should therefore be advised to protect themselves from sun exposure.

Atrial Fibrillation and Flutter Atrial fibrillation and atrial flutter of any grade were reported in 3% of patients in the combined safety database of patients treated with acalabrutinib monotherapy for hematologic malignancies. Grade 3 atrial fibrillation and atrial flutter occurred in 1% of such patients.

Patients receiving acalabrutinib should be monitored for the development of atrial fibrillation and flutter and managed appropriately should they occur. (See Advice to Patients.)

Fetal/Neonatal Morbidity and Mortality There are no available data regarding the use of acalabrutinib in pregnant women; however, based on animal findings, the drug may cause fetal harm. Embryofetal toxicity (e.g., decreased fetal body weight, delayed skeletal ossification) has been demonstrated in animals receiving the drug at exposures approximately 4 times the human exposure at the recommended dosage of 100 mg twice daily.

If acalabrutinib is used during pregnancy or if the patient becomes pregnant while receiving the drug, the patient should be apprised of the potential hazard to the fetus.

Specific Populations **Pregnancy.** Acalabrutinib may cause fetal harm if administered to pregnant women based on animal findings. (See Fetal/Neonatal Morbidity and Mortality under Cautions: Warnings/Precautions.)

Lactation. Acalabrutinib and its active metabolite ACP-5862 are distributed into milk in rats. It is not known whether the drug or its active metabolite distributes into human milk or if the drug has any effect on milk production or the nursing infant. Because of the potential for adverse reactions to acalabrutinib in nursing infants, women should be advised not to breast-feed while receiving the drug and for at least 2 weeks after the drug is discontinued.

Pediatric Use. Safety and efficacy of acalabrutinib have not been established in pediatric patients.

Geriatric Use. In clinical studies evaluating acalabrutinib in patients with mantle cell lymphoma, approximately 65% of patients were 65 years of age or older and 26% were 75 years of age or older. No clinically important differences in safety or efficacy were observed between geriatric patients and younger adults in these studies.

Population pharmacokinetic analysis suggests that age does not have a clinically important effect on the pharmacokinetics of acalabrutinib.

Hepatic Impairment. Acalabrutinib is metabolized in the liver. In a hepatic impairment study, acalabrutinib exposure increased by less than twofold in individuals with mild (Child-Pugh class A) or moderate hepatic impairment (Child-Pugh class B). Population pharmacokinetic analysis indicates that there is no clinically important difference in the pharmacokinetics of acalabrutinib in individuals with mild or moderate hepatic impairment (defined as total bilirubin concentrations that are 1.5–3 times the upper limit of normal [ULN] with any AST concentration) compared with individuals with normal hepatic function.

Acalabrutinib has not been studied in patients with severe hepatic impairment (Child-Pugh class C or total bilirubin concentrations 3–10 times the ULN with any AST concentration). (See Dosage and Administration: Special Populations.)

Renal Impairment. Renal elimination of acalabrutinib is minimal (12%). Population pharmacokinetic analysis indicates that there are no clinically important pharmacokinetic differences when acalabrutinib is administered to patients with mild or moderate renal impairment (estimated glomerular filtration rate [eGFR] of at least 30 mL/minute per 1.73 m^2) compared with patients with normal renal function. The manufacturer states that there currently is no experience with acalabrutinib in patients with severe renal impairment (eGFR less than 29 mL/minute per 1.73 m^2) or in patients with renal impairment undergoing dialysis. (See Dosage and Administration: Special Populations.)

■ **Common Adverse Effects** Adverse effects reported in at least 20% of patients receiving acalabrutinib for the treatment of previously treated mantle cell lymphoma in the principal clinical trial include anemia, thrombocytopenia, neutropenia, headache (often transient and usually occurring early during therapy), diarrhea, fatigue, myalgia, and bruising.

Drug Interactions

Acalabrutinib is principally metabolized by cytochrome P-450 (CYP) isoenzyme 3A and, to a minor extent, by glutathione conjugation and amide hydrolysis. Metabolism of acalabrutinib to the principal active metabolite, ACP-5862, is mediated principally by CYP3A.

In vitro studies indicate that acalabrutinib is a weak inhibitor of CYP isoenzymes 3A4/5, 2C8, and 2C9; does not inhibit CYP isoenzymes 1A2, 2B6, 2C19, and 2D6; and is a weak inducer of CYP isoenzymes 3A4, 1A2, and 2B6. In vitro studies also indicate that acalabrutinib's active metabolite, ACP-5862, is a weak inhibitor of CYP isoenzymes 2C8, 2C9, and 2C19; does not inhibit CYP isoenzymes 3A4/5, 1A2, 2B6, and 2D6; and is a weak inducer of CYP3A4.

In vitro studies indicate that acalabrutinib is a substrate of P-glycoprotein (P-gp) and breast cancer resistance protein (BCRP), but is not a substrate of organic anion transporter (OAT) 1, OAT3, organic cation transporter (OCT) 2, and organic anion transport proteins (OATP) 1B1 and OATP1B3. Acalabrutinib does not inhibit P-gp, OAT1, OAT3, OCT2, OATP1B1, and OATP1B3 at clinically relevant concentrations.

■ **Drugs Affecting Hepatic Microsomal Enzymes** ***Inhibitors of CYP3A*** Concomitant use of acalabrutinib with potent or moderate inhibitors of CYP3A may result in substantially increased peak plasma concentrations and systemic exposure (area under the concentration-time curve [AUC]) of acalabrutinib and result in increased toxicity. When the potent CYP3A inhibitor itraconazole (200 mg once daily for 5 days) was administered concomitantly with acalabrutinib in healthy individuals, peak plasma concentration and AUC of acalabrutinib increased by 3.9- and 5.1-fold, respectively. Simulations using physiologically based pharmacokinetic models suggest that moderate inhibitors of CYP3A (e.g., diltiazem, erythromycin, fluconazole) are likely to increase peak plasma concentration and AUC of acalabrutinib by twofold to almost threefold.

Concomitant use of acalabrutinib with *potent* CYP3A inhibitors (e.g., clarithromycin, erythromycin, itraconazole, ketoconazole, posaconazole, voriconazole) should be avoided, if possible. If short-term (7 days or less) therapy with a potent CYP3A inhibitor (e.g., an antifungal [itraconazole, ketoconazole, posaconazole, voriconazole] or anti-infective agent [clarithromycin]) is required, the manufacturer recommends withholding acalabrutinib therapy during administration of the potent CYP3A inhibitor.

If acalabrutinib is used concomitantly with a *moderate* CYP3A inhibitor (e.g., diltiazem, erythromycin, fluconazole), the manufacturer recommends reducing the dosage of acalabrutinib to 100 mg once daily.

Inducers of CYP3A Concomitant use of acalabrutinib with potent inducers of CYP3A may result in decreased peak plasma concentrations and systemic exposure (AUC) of acalabrutinib and therefore reduce its efficacy. When the potent CYP3A inducer rifampin (600 mg once daily for 9 days) was administered concomitantly with acalabrutinib, peak plasma concentration and AUC of acalabrutinib decreased by 68 and 77%, respectively.

Concomitant use of acalabrutinib with potent CYP3A inducers (e.g., carbamazepine, phenytoin, rifampin) should be avoided; if such concomitant use cannot be avoided, the manufacturer recommends increasing the dosage of acalabrutinib to 200 mg twice daily.

■ **Drugs Metabolized by Hepatic Microsomal Enzymes** In vitro studies and simulations using physiologically based pharmacokinetic models indicate that acalabrutinib is unlikely to interact with drugs metabolized by CYP isoenzymes at clinically relevant concentrations.

■ **Substrates of Breast Cancer Resistance Protein** The manufacturer states that acalabrutinib potentially may increase exposure to concurrently administered BCRP substrates (e.g., methotrexate) because of inhibition of intestinal BCRP.

■ **Drugs Affecting Gastric Acidity** The solubility of acalabrutinib decreases with increasing pH; therefore, drugs that reduce gastric acidity such as proton-pump inhibitors, antacids, and histamine H_2-receptor antagonists potentially can decrease plasma concentrations of acalabrutinib and thereby reduce its efficacy. If therapy with an acid suppressive agent is necessary in a patient receiving acalabrutinib, use of a histamine H_2-receptor antagonist (e.g., famotidine, ranitidine) or an antacid (e.g., calcium carbonate) rather than a proton-pump inhibitor should be considered.

Proton-pump Inhibitors When acalabrutinib was administered concomitantly with the proton-pump inhibitor omeprazole (40 mg once daily for 5 days) in healthy individuals, the AUC of acalabrutinib was decreased by 43%.

Because of the long-lasting gastric acid-reducing effect of proton-pump inhibitors, separating doses of acalabrutinib and proton-pump inhibitors may not eliminate the potential pharmacokinetic interaction between these drugs. Therefore, concomitant use of acalabrutinib and proton-pump inhibitors should be avoided, if possible.

Histamine H_2-receptor Antagonists If concurrent use of acalabrutinib and a histamine H_2-receptor antagonist is necessary, acalabrutinib should be taken 2 hours before the histamine H_2-receptor antagonist.

Antacids When acalabrutinib was administered concomitantly with an antacid (calcium carbonate 1 g) in healthy individuals, the AUC of acalabrutinib was decreased by 53%.

If concurrent use of acalabrutinib and an antacid is necessary, dosing of the drugs should be separated by at least 2 hours.

■ **Anticoagulants and Antiplatelet Agents** In the principal efficacy trial (ACE-LY-004 trial), 43% of the patients were concurrently receiving anticoagulants. Because of the increased risk of hemorrhagic events, patients concurrently receiving acalabrutinib and anticoagulants or antiplatelet agents should be monitored for signs of bleeding and hemorrhage. (See Hemorrhage under Cautions: Warnings/Precautions.)

Description

Acalabrutinib is a selective, irreversible, small-molecule inhibitor of Bruton's tyrosine kinase (BTK); the drug is an antineoplastic agent. Acalabrutinib and its active metabolite (ACP-5862) bind covalently with a cysteine residue in the BTK active site, which results in inhibition of BTK enzymatic activity. BTK is an essential signaling molecule of the B-cell antigen receptor (BCR) and cytokine receptor pathways. Within B cells, BTK signaling results in activation of pathways involved in cell proliferation, trafficking, chemotaxis, and adhesion. In nonclinical studies, acalabrutinib inhibited the BTK-mediated activation of downstream signaling proteins CD86 and CD69 resulting in decreased malignant B-cell proliferation and survival. Inhibition of BTK also reduces plasma concentrations of cytokines and chemokines, which may lead to decreased cell adhesion and mobilization of cells from tissues; this redistribution of cells from tissues to peripheral blood may contribute to the transient increase in absolute lymphocyte count (lymphocytosis) that has been observed in patients receiving BTK inhibitors (e.g., acalabrutinib, ibrutinib). (See Uses.) Unlike ibrutinib (another BTK inhibitor used to treat mantle cell lymphoma), acalabrutinib does not appear to irreversibly target kinases other than BTK, including epidermal growth factor receptor (EGFR), tyrosine kinase expressed in hepatocellular carcinoma (TEC), and interleukin 2-inducible T-cell kinase (ITK). The selective targeting of BTK by acalabrutinib may help explain, at least in part, some of the tolerability differences between acalabrutinib and ibrutinib observed in clinical studies to date.

Following oral administration, the mean absolute bioavailability of acalabrutinib is 25%. The median time to achieve peak plasma concentrations of the drug is 0.75 hours. Administration of a high-fat, high-calorie meal did not substantially alter the area under the plasma concentration-time curve (AUC) of acalabrutinib; peak plasma concentrations decreased by 73% and time to achieve peak concentrations was delayed by 1–2 hours compared with administration of the drug under fasting conditions. Acalabrutinib exhibits almost linear pharmacokinetics over a dosage range of 75–250 mg and dose proportionality. Accumulation of the drug does not appear to occur with repeated dosing. In patients with B-cell malignancies receiving acalabrutinib at a dosage of 100 mg twice daily, median steady-state binding of the drug to BTK (BTK occupancy) of 95% or more was maintained over 12 hours, resulting in inactivation of BTK throughout the recommended dosing interval of the drug.

Acalabrutinib is metabolized by the cytochrome P-450 (CYP) microsomal enzyme system, principally by CYP3A, and, to a minor extent, by glutathione conjugation and amide hydrolysis. The principal active metabolite, ACP-5862, is approximately 50% less potent as a BTK inhibitor than acalabrutinib. Acalabrutinib is 97.5% bound to plasma proteins. Following administration of a single radiolabeled dose of acalabrutinib, 84% of the dose was recovered in feces and 12% was recovered in urine; unchanged drug accounted for less than 1% of the recovered dose. The median elimination half-life of acalabrutinib is 0.9 hours (range: 0.6–2.8 hours). The elimination half-life of ACP-5862 is 6.9 hours. The pharmacokinetics of acalabrutinib do not appear to be affected by age (range: 42–90 years), gender, race, or body weight.

Advice to Patients

Importance of instructing patients to read the manufacturer's patient information.

Importance of advising patients to take acalabrutinib as directed by their clinician. If a dose is missed, importance of administering the next dose as soon as it is remembered. However, if it has been more than 3 hours, the missed dose should be skipped and the next dose should be taken at the regularly scheduled time; an extra dose should not be taken to make up for a missed dose.

Importance of advising patients to swallow acalabrutinib capsules whole with a glass of water and not to open, break, or chew the capsules.

Risk of bleeding/hemorrhage. Importance of informing clinician if signs or symptoms of severe bleeding occur (e.g., blood in stool or urine; unexpected, prolonged, or uncontrolled bleeding). Importance of informing patients that acalabrutinib therapy may need to be interrupted for major surgeries.

Risk of serious infection. Importance of promptly reporting signs or symptoms of possible infection (e.g., fever, chills, flu-like symptoms).

Risk of myelosuppression. Importance of informing patients that periodic complete blood cell (CBC) counts are necessary during acalabrutinib therapy.

Possible risk of developing a second primary malignancy (e.g., skin cancer). Importance of advising patients to protect skin from the sun.

Risk of atrial fibrillation and flutter. Importance of informing clinician if palpitations, lightheadedness, dizziness, fainting, shortness of breath, or chest discomfort occurs.

Importance of women informing clinicians if they are or plan to become pregnant or plan to breast-feed. Apprise patient of potential hazard to the fetus if used during pregnancy.

Importance of advising women to avoid breast-feeding while receiving acalabrutinib and for at least 2 weeks after discontinuance of therapy.

Importance of informing clinicians of existing or contemplated concomitant therapy, including prescription and OTC drugs (e.g., anticoagulant or antiplatelet drugs, antacids, histamine H_2-receptor antagonists, proton-pump inhibitors) and dietary or herbal supplements, as well as any concomitant illnesses.

Importance of informing patients of other important precautionary information. (See Cautions.)

Overview® (see Users Guide). For additional information on this drug until a more detailed monograph is developed and published, the manufacturer's labeling should be consulted. It is *essential* that the manufacturer's labeling be consulted for more detailed information on usual cautions, precautions, contraindications, potential drug interactions, laboratory test interferences, and acute toxicity. For further information on the handling of antineoplastic agents, see the ASHP Guidelines on Handling Hazardous Drugs at http://www.ahfsdruginformation.com.

Preparations

Distribution of acalabrutinib is restricted. (See Restricted Distribution under Dosage and Administration: General.)

Excipients in commercially available drug preparations may have clinically important effects in some individuals; consult specific product labeling for details.

Acalabrutinib

Oral

Capsules	100 mg	**Calquence®**, AstraZeneca

Ado-Trastuzumab Emtansine

Trastuzumab-DM1, Trastuzumab Emtansine, Trastuzumab-MCC-DM1, T-DM1

Ado-trastuzumab emtansine (Kadcyla®) should not be confused with trastuzumab (Herceptin®). Ado-trastuzumab emtansine is an anti-human epidermal growth factor receptor type 2 (anti-*HER2*) antibody-drug conjugate; the anti-*HER2* antibody trastuzumab, a humanized immunoglobulin (IgG_1), is conjugated with the microtubule inhibitor DM1 (derivative of maytansine) via the linker MCC (4-[*N*-maleimidomethyl] cyclohexane-1-carboxylate).

The original generic name for Kadcyla®, as established by the US Adopted Name (USAN) Council in 2009, was trastuzumab emtansine. Because of the similarity between the original generic name (trastuzumab emtansine) and the generic name for Herceptin® (trastuzumab), the US Food and Drug Administration (FDA) approved the addition of the prefix "ado" to the generic name for Kadcyla® (i.e., ado-trastuzumab emtansine); however, the potential exists for dispensing or prescribing errors involving these drugs. The manufacturer of ado-trastuzumab emtansine (Kadcyla®) states that this drug should *not* be substituted for or used with trastuzumab (Herceptin®). Therefore, extra care should be exercised to ensure the accuracy of prescriptions for ado-trastuzumab emtansine (Kadcyla®) or trastuzumab (Herceptin®).

To avoid medication errors, the Institute for Safe Medication Practices (ISMP), the FDA, and the manufacturer of ado-trastuzumab emtansine (Kadcyla®) recommend that prescribers communicate both the brand and generic names for ado-trastuzumab emtansine (Kadcyla®) on the prescription order form. (See Dispensing and Administration Precautions under Dosage and Administration: Administration and also under Warnings/Precautions: Warnings, in Cautions.)

■ Ado-trastuzumab emtansine, an anti-human epidermal growth factor receptor type 2 (anti-*HER2*) antibody conjugated with the microtubule inhibitor DM1 (a maytansine derivative), is an antineoplastic agent.

Uses

■ **Breast Cancer** Ado-trastuzumab emtansine is used for the treatment of metastatic breast cancer in patients whose tumors overexpress the human epidermal growth factor receptor type 2 (*HER2*) protein and who have received prior therapy with trastuzumab and a taxane, either separately or in combination. Appropriate candidates for ado-trastuzumab emtansine therapy include those who have received prior therapy for metastatic disease or who developed disease recurrence during or within 6 months of completing adjuvant therapy.

The current indication for ado-trastuzumab emtansine is based principally on the results of a randomized, open-label phase 3 study (EMILIA) in patients with *HER2*-overexpressing metastatic breast cancer. Patients were eligible for enrollment in the study if they had disease demonstrating an immunohistochemistry (IHC) assay score of 3+ or a fluorescent in situ hybridization (FISH) amplification ratio of 2 or higher. In this study, 991 patients were randomized in a 1:1 ratio to receive either ado-trastuzumab emtansine alone (3.6 mg/kg IV every 21 days) or combined therapy with lapatinib (1.25 g once daily, continuously) and capecitabine (2 g/m^2 daily on days 1–14 every 21 days). Treatment was continued until disease progression or unacceptable toxicity occurred, or the patient withdrew from the study. The primary end points of this study were progression-free survival as assessed by an independent review facility (IRF-assessed progression-free survival) and overall survival. The median age of patients enrolled in the study was 53 years; all except 5 of the enrolled patients were women. The majority (88%) of patients had received prior systemic therapy in the metastatic setting and 12% of patients had experienced disease relapse within 6 months of receiving prior adjuvant or neoadjuvant chemotherapy. All except 1 of the enrolled patients had received prior trastuzumab therapy and over 99 or 61% of patients had received prior therapy with a taxane or anthracycline, respectively. Among patients with hormone receptor-positive tumors, approximately 44% of these patients had received prior adjuvant hormonal therapy and approximately 45% had received hormonal therapy for locally advanced or metastatic disease.

At the time of the primary analysis, patients receiving ado-trastuzumab emtansine alone had longer median IRF-assessed progression-free survival compared with patients receiving combined therapy with lapatinib and capecitabine (9.6 versus 6.4 months, respectively). Effects of ado-trastuzumab emtansine on investigator-assessed progression-free survival and IRF-assessed progression-free survival were comparable. A subset analysis of progression-free survival based on clinically relevant baseline patient and disease characteristics consistently showed treatment benefit with ado-trastuzumab emtansine alone compared with combined therapy with lapatinib and capecitabine; however, this benefit was not observed in patients 65 years of age or older and in those with nonmeasurable disease. At the first interim analysis, overall survival did not cross the predefined stopping boundary for significance; however, results of a second interim analysis indicated that median overall survival was prolonged in patients receiving ado-trastuzumab emtansine compared with those receiving combined therapy with lapatinib and capecitabine (30.9 versus 25.1 months, respectively). In addition, patients receiving ado-trastuzumab emtansine appeared to have a higher objective response rate (43.6 versus 30.8%, respectively) and a longer median duration of response (12.6 versus 6.5 months, respectively) compared with those receiving lapatinib and capecitabine. The median follow-up period at the time of the primary analysis for progression-free survival and at the second interim analysis for overall survival was 13 and 19 months, respectively.

Dosage and Administration

■ **General** Ado-trastuzumab emtansine (Kadcyla®) should *not* be substituted for or used with trastuzumab (Herceptin®).

Because infusion or hypersensitivity reactions may occur, patients should be closely observed during infusions and for 90 minutes following the first infusion of ado-trastuzumab emtansine; following subsequent infusions, patients should be observed for 30 minutes. (See Infusion or Hypersensitivity Reactions under Warnings/Precautions: Sensitivity Reactions, in Cautions.)

Ado-trastuzumab emtansine is *not* recommended for use in patients for whom prior therapy with trastuzumab was permanently discontinued because of infusion reactions and/or hypersensitivity to the drug. (See Infusion or Hypersensitivity Reactions under Warnings/Precautions: Sensitivity Reactions, in Cautions.)

Procedures for proper handling (e.g., use of gloves) and disposal of antineoplastic drugs should be followed when preparing or administering ado-trastuzumab emtansine.

■ **Administration** Ado-trastuzumab emtansine is administered by IV infusion through a 0.22-μm polyethersulfone filter. The initial dose of ado-trastuzumab emtansine should be administered as an IV infusion over 90 minutes; if the first infusion is well tolerated, subsequent doses may be administered by IV infusion over 30 minutes. (See Dosage and Administration: General.) *Ado-trastuzumab emtansine solutions should not be administered by rapid IV injection, such as IV push or bolus.*

Unreconstituted vials of ado-trastuzumab emtansine injection should be stored at 2–8°C until use; vials should *not* be frozen or shaken.

Prior to administration, commercially available ado-trastuzumab emtansine powder for injection must be reconstituted and diluted using proper aseptic technique. The powder for injection is reconstituted by adding 5 or 8 mL of sterile water for injection to a vial labeled as containing 100 or 160 mg, respectively, of the drug to provide a solution containing 20 mg/mL. The vial should be gently swirled and inspected visually for particulate matter and discoloration prior to dilution and administration. The resulting solution should *not* be shaken. The solution should be clear to slightly opalescent, colorless to pale brown, and free of visible particulates. The reconstituted ado-trastuzumab emtansine solution may be diluted immediately or stored at 2–8°C for use within 24 hours. The reconstituted solution should *not* be frozen. Any unused solution should be discarded after 24 hours.

For preparation of the final diluted ado-trastuzumab emtansine solution for infusion, the appropriate volume of reconstituted solution should be withdrawn from the vial and further diluted in 250 mL of 0.9% sodium chloride injection. The final diluted ado-trastuzumab emtansine solution for infusion should be mixed by gentle inversion and should *not* be shaken. The solution may be infused immediately or stored at 2–8°C and used within 24 hours following dilution; the solution for infusion should *not* be frozen. Any partially used vials should be discarded. Ado-trastuzumab emtansine solutions for infusion should *not* be diluted in or administered through an IV line containing 5% dextrose injection, and ado-trastuzumab emtansine should *not* be mixed or administered with other drugs.

Dispensing and Administration Precautions Ado-trastuzumab emtansine (Kadcyla®) should not be confused with trastuzumab (Herceptin®). Because of the similarity between the original generic name of Kadcyla® (trastuzumab emtansine) and the generic name for Herceptin® (trastuzumab), the US Food and Drug Administration (FDA) approved the addition of the prefix "ado" to the generic name for Kadcyla® (i.e., ado-trastuzumab emtansine). However, the potential exists for dispensing or prescribing errors involving these drugs. Extra care should be exercised to ensure the accuracy of prescriptions for ado-trastuzumab emtansine (Kadcyla®) or trastuzumab (Herceptin®). To avoid medication errors, the Institute for Safe Medication Practices (ISMP), the FDA, and the manufacturer of ado-trastuzumab emtansine (Kadcyla®) recommend that prescribers communicate both the brand and generic names for ado-trastuzumab emtansine (Kadcyla®) on the prescription order form. (See Special Alerts.)

■ **Dosage** ***Breast Cancer*** For the treatment of metastatic breast cancer that overexpresses the human epidermal growth factor receptor type 2 (*HER2*) protein in patients who have received prior therapy including trastuzumab and a taxane, either separately or in combination, the recommended adult dosage of ado-trastuzumab emtansine is 3.6 mg/kg administered as an IV infusion every 3 weeks. Ado-trastuzumab emtansine should *not* be administered at doses exceeding 3.6 mg/kg. Treatment should be continued until disease progression or unacceptable toxicity occurs.

If a dose is missed or delayed, the dose of ado-trastuzumab emtansine should be administered as soon as possible; waiting until the next scheduled dose is not recommended. The schedule of administration should be adjusted to maintain a 3-week interval between doses.

Dosage Modification for Toxicity When dosage modification is necessary, dosage of ado-trastuzumab emtansine should be reduced by 1 dose level in decrements of 0.6 mg/kg (e.g., from 3.6 to 3 mg/kg, from 3 to 2.4 mg/kg); however, if a dose of 2.4 mg/kg requires further reduction, ado-trastuzumab emtansine should be discontinued.

Dosage of ado-trastuzumab emtansine should *not* be re-escalated following a dosage reduction.

Hepatotoxicity. In patients who exhibit grade 2 serum aminotransferase (ALT and/or AST) elevations (i.e., exceeding 2.5 times the upper limit of normal [ULN], but not more than 5 times the ULN), ado-trastuzumab emtansine therapy may be continued at the same dosage. (See Hepatotoxicity under Warnings/Precautions: Warnings, in Cautions.)

In patients who exhibit grade 2 or 3 elevations in total bilirubin concentrations (i.e., exceeding 1.5 times the ULN, but not more than 10 times the ULN), ado-trastuzumab therapy should be interrupted. If elevations in total bilirubin concentrations decrease to no more than grade 1, therapy with ado-trastuzumab emtansine may be resumed at 1 dose level lower than the previous dosage.

In patients who exhibit grade 3 serum aminotransferase elevations (i.e., exceeding 5 times the ULN, but not more than 20 times the ULN), ado-trastuzumab emtansine therapy should be interrupted. If elevations in ALT and/or AST concentrations decrease to no more than grade 2, therapy with ado-trastuzumab emtansine may be resumed at 1 dose level lower than the previous dosage.

In patients who exhibit grade 4 serum aminotransferase elevations (i.e., exceeding 20 times the ULN) or increased total bilirubin concentrations (i.e., exceeding 10 times the ULN), treatment with ado-trastuzumab emtansine should be permanently discontinued.

In patients who exhibit concurrent increases in serum aminotransferase (exceeding 3 times the ULN) and total bilirubin concentrations (exceeding 2 times the ULN), treatment with ado-trastuzumab emtansine should be permanently discontinued.

If manifestations of nodular regenerative hyperplasia occur, treatment with ado-trastuzumab emtansine should be permanently discontinued.

Infusion or Hypersensitivity Reactions. If infusion reactions occur, the infusion rate should be reduced or ado-trastuzumab emtansine therapy interrupted depending on the severity of the reaction. If life-threatening infusion reactions occur, ado-trastuzumab emtansine should be permanently discontinued. (See Infusion or Hypersensitivity Reactions under Warnings/Precautions: Sensitivity Reactions, in Cautions.)

Left Ventricular Dysfunction. If left ventricular ejection fraction (LVEF) decreases to 45% or less, left ventricular function should be reassessed within 3 weeks. (See Left Ventricular Dysfunction under Warnings/Precautions: Warnings, in Cautions.)

If LVEF decreases to 40–45% with a decrease from baseline of less than 10%, therapy with ado-trastuzumab emtansine may be continued.

If LVEF decreases to 40–45% with a decrease from baseline of 10% or more, ado-trastuzumab emtansine should be withheld for at least 3 weeks. If LVEF has not improved to within 10% of baseline, ado-trastuzumab emtansine should be discontinued.

If LVEF decreases to less than 40%, ado-trastuzumab emtansine should be withheld for at least 3 weeks. If LVEF has not improved or has declined further, ado-trastuzumab emtansine should be permanently discontinued.

If manifestations of congestive heart failure develop, the drug should be discontinued.

Thrombocytopenia. If grade 3 thrombocytopenia (platelet counts of 25,000/mm^3 to less than 50,000/mm^3) occurs, ado-trastuzumab emtansine therapy should be interrupted. Treatment may be resumed at the same dosage if thrombocytopenia resolves to no more than grade 1 (platelet counts reach or exceed 75,000/mm^3). (See Thrombocytopenia under Warnings/Precautions: Other Warnings and Precautions, in Cautions.)

If grade 4 thrombocytopenia (platelet counts less than 25,000/mm^3) occurs, ado-trastuzumab emtansine therapy should be interrupted. If thrombocytopenia resolves to no more than grade 1 (platelet counts of 75,000/mm^3 or more), therapy with ado-trastuzumab emtansine may be resumed at 1 one dose level lower than the previous dosage.

Pulmonary Toxicity. If manifestations of interstitial lung disease or pneumonitis develop, ado-trastuzumab emtansine therapy should be permanently discontinued. (See Pulmonary Effects under Warnings/Precautions: Other Warnings and Precautions, in Cautions.)

Peripheral Neuropathy. If grade 3 or 4 peripheral neuropathy occurs, ado-trastuzumab emtansine therapy should be interrupted until the toxicity resolves to no more than grade 2. (See Peripheral Neuropathy under Warnings/Precautions: Other Warnings and Precautions, in Cautions.)

■ Special Populations

Dosage adjustment is not necessary based on baseline albumin concentrations. (See Description.)

Dosage adjustment is not necessary in patients with mild (creatinine clearance of 60–89 mL/minute) or moderate (creatinine clearance of 30–59 mL/minute) renal impairment. The manufacturer makes no specific dosage recommendations for patients with severe renal impairment (creatinine clearance less than 30 mL/minute) because data are limited in this population. (See Renal Impairment under Warnings/Precautions: Specific Populations, in Cautions.)

The manufacturer makes no specific dosage recommendations for geriatric patients or patients with hepatic impairment. (See Geriatric Use and also Hepatic Impairment under Warnings/Precautions: Specific Populations, in Cautions.)

Cautions

■ Contraindications

The manufacturer states that there are no known contraindications to the use of ado-trastuzumab emtansine.

■ Warnings/Precautions

Warnings

Hepatotoxicity. Hepatotoxicity has been reported in patients receiving ado-trastuzumab emtansine. Hepatotoxicity was mainly manifested by asymptomatic, transient elevations in serum aminotransferase (ALT and/or AST) concentrations. Serious hepatobiliary disorders, including 2 fatal cases of severe drug-induced liver injury and associated hepatic encephalopathy, have been reported in clinical studies. Reported cases of serious hepatobiliary disorders may have been confounded by comorbidities and/or concomitant use of drugs with known hepatotoxic potential.

Nodular regenerative hyperplasia also has been reported and was identified in liver biopsies in 3 of 884 patients receiving ado-trastuzumab emtansine in clinical studies. Nodular regenerative hyperplasia is a rare liver condition that may result in non-cirrhotic portal hypertension; the disease is characterized by widespread benign transformation of hepatic parenchyma into small regenerative nodules. Diagnosis of nodular regenerative hyperplasia must be confirmed by histopathology. Nodular regenerative hyperplasia should be considered in any patient presenting with manifestations of portal hypertension without elevations in serum aminotransferase concentrations or manifestations of cirrhosis. If nodular regenerative hyperplasia occurs, ado-trastuzumab emtansine should be permanently discontinued.

Ado-trastuzumab emtansine has not been studied in patients with active hepatitis B virus or hepatitis C virus infection or in patients with serum aminotransferase concentrations exceeding 2.5 times the upper limit of normal (ULN) or total bilirubin concentrations exceeding 1.5 times the ULN.

Serum aminotransferase and total bilirubin concentrations should be evaluated prior to each dose of ado-trastuzumab emtansine. If serum aminotransferase and/or total bilirubin concentrations are elevated, interruption of ado-trastuzumab emtansine therapy, dosage reduction, or discontinuation of therapy may be necessary. (See Hepatotoxicity under Dosage: Dosage Modification for Toxicity, in Dosage and Administration.)

Left Ventricular Dysfunction. Patients receiving ado-trastuzumab emtansine are at increased risk of developing left ventricular dysfunction. Decreases in left ventricular ejection fraction (LVEF) to less than 40% have been reported in patients receiving ado-trastuzumab emtansine. In the EMILIA study, left ventricular dysfunction occurred in 1.8% of patients receiving ado-trastuzumab emtansine alone and in 3.3% of patients receiving combined therapy with lapatinib and capecitabine.

Ado-trastuzumab emtansine has not been studied in patients with a baseline LVEF less than 50%, history of symptomatic congestive heart failure, or conditions that could impair left ventricular function (e.g., serious cardiac arrhythmia, history of myocardial infarction or unstable angina within 6 months prior to therapy initiation).

LVEF should be assessed prior to initiation of ado-trastuzumab emtansine and at regular intervals (e.g., every 3 months) during treatment. If left ventricular dysfunction occurs, interruption of ado-trastuzumab emtansine therapy and reassessment of left ventricular function within 3 weeks may be necessary; if LVEF has not improved or has declined further, ado-trastuzumab emtansine should be permanently discontinued. (See Left Ventricular Dysfunction under Dosage: Dosage Modification for Toxicity, in Dosage and Administration.)

Fetal/Neonatal Morbidity and Mortality. Ado-trastuzumab emtansine may cause fetal harm if administered to pregnant women. There are no adequate and well-controlled studies to date in pregnant women; however, oligohydramnios, fatal pulmonary hypoplasia, skeletal abnormalities, and neonatal death have been reported in women receiving the anti-human epidermal growth factor receptor type 2 (anti-*HER2*) antibody trastuzumab during pregnancy in postmarketing experience. Based on the mechanism of action of the microtubule inhibitor DM1 (derivative of maytansine), embryotoxic and fetotoxic effects may occur. When trastuzumab was administered to pregnant monkeys at dosages 7 times the human clinical dosage, the drug crossed the placental barrier during early and late phases of gestation. (See Cautions: Pregnancy, Fertility, and Lactation, in Trastuzumab 10:00.)

Pregnancy status should be verified prior to initiation of ado-trastuzumab emtansine, and women of childbearing potential should be advised to use effective contraception during and for 6 months after discontinuance of the drug. If ado-trastuzumab emtansine is used during pregnancy or if the patient becomes pregnant while receiving the drug, the patient should be apprised of the potential fetal hazard. (See Advice to Patients and also see Pregnancy under Warnings/Precautions: Specific Populations, in Cautions.)

Dispensing and Administration Precautions. Ado-trastuzumab emtansine (Kadcyla®) should not be confused with trastuzumab (Herceptin®). Because of the similarity between the original generic name of Kadcyla® (trastuzumab emtansine) and the generic name for Herceptin® (trastuzumab), the US Food and Drug Administration (FDA) approved the addition of the prefix "ado" to the generic name for Kadcyla® (i.e., ado-trastuzumab emtansine). However, the potential exists for dispensing or prescribing errors involving these drugs. Such medication errors may be associated with severe toxicity or lack of appropriate therapy in patients who did not receive the intended drug. The manufacturer of ado-trastuzumab emtansine (Kadcyla®) states that this drug should *not* be substituted for or used with trastuzumab (Herceptin®). Therefore, extra care should be exercised to ensure the accuracy of prescriptions for ado-trastuzumab emtansine (Kadcyla®) and trastuzumab (Herceptin®). (See Special Alerts.)

Sensitivity Reactions

Infusion or Hypersensitivity Reactions. Infusion reactions have been reported in patients receiving ado-trastuzumab emtansine. Infusion reactions were characterized by the presence of 1 or more of the following manifestations: flushing, chills, pyrexia, dyspnea, hypotension, wheezing, bronchospasm, and tachycardia. In the EMILIA study, infusion reactions were reported in 1.4% of patients receiving ado-trastuzumab emtansine; symptoms resolved within several hours to a day following discontinuance of the infusion in most patients. In another clinical study, a serious, allergic anaphylactoid-like reaction was reported in 1 patient.

Ado-trastuzumab emtansine has not been studied in patients for whom prior therapy with trastuzumab was permanently discontinued due to infusion reactions and/or hypersensitivity to the drug; ado-trastuzumab emtansine is not recommended for use in such patients.

Patients should be observed closely for 90 minutes after the first infusion of ado-trastuzumab emtansine and for 30 minutes after subsequent infusions of the drug. If severe or life-threatening infusion reactions occur, temporary or permanent discontinuance of ado-trastuzumab emtansine may be required. (See Infusion or Hypersensitivity Reactions under Dosage: Dosage Modification for Toxicity, in Dosage and Administration.) Appropriate equipment and agents for the treatment of allergic or anaphylactoid-like reactions should be available for immediate use in patients receiving the drug.

Other Warnings and Precautions

Pulmonary Effects. Severe, and sometimes fatal, adverse pulmonary effects, including interstitial lung disease, pneumonitis, and acute respiratory distress syndrome (ARDS), have been reported. In clinical studies, pneumonitis has been reported in 0.8% of patients; grade 3 pneumonitis occurred in 1 of 884 patients receiving ado-trastuzumab emtansine. Patients who have dyspnea at rest resulting from complications of advanced disease or other comorbidities may be at greater risk for pulmonary toxicity. Manifestations of pneumonitis include dyspnea, cough, fatigue, and pulmonary infiltrates; however, these manifestations may also occur as sequelae of infusion reactions.

Ado-trastuzumab emtansine should be permanently discontinued in patients diagnosed with interstitial lung disease or pneumonitis. (See Pulmonary Toxicity under Dosage: Dosage Modification for Toxicity, in Dosage and Administration.)

Thrombocytopenia. Thrombocytopenia is a common dose-limiting adverse effect of ado-trastuzumab emtansine. Thrombocytopenia of any grade was reported in 32% of patients receiving ado-trastuzumab emtansine in clinical trials; grade 3 or greater thrombocytopenia was reported in 11.7% of patients. The incidence of severe hemorrhagic events in patients receiving ado-trastuzumab emtansine was low. In patients with grade 1 or 2 thrombocytopenia, the nadir platelet count occurred around day 8 of each 3-week cycle; thrombocytopenia generally improved to grade 0 or 1 (i.e., platelet counts reach or exceed 75,000/mm³) by the next scheduled dose. In the EMILIA study, thrombocytopenia occurred in 31.2% of patients receiving ado-trastuzumab emtansine alone and in 3.3% of patients receiving combined therapy with lapatinib and capecitabine. The incidence of grade 3 or greater thrombocytopenia was higher in patients receiving ado-trastuzumab emtansine alone compared with those receiving combined therapy with lapatinib and capecitabine (14.5 versus 0.4%, respectively). The first occurrence of grade 3 or 4 thrombocytopenia was reported during the first 2 cycles of therapy with ado-trastuzumab emtansine in most patients enrolled in the EMILIA study; the majority of patients continued treatment following dosage modifications. In the EMILIA study, the incidence and severity of thrombocytopenia was higher in Asian patients; the incidence of grade 3 or greater thrombocytopenia was substantially higher in Asian patients receiving ado-trastuzumab emtansine alone compared with those receiving combined therapy with lapatinib and capecitabine (45.1 versus 1.3%, respectively).

Ado-trastuzumab emtansine has not been studied in patients with baseline platelet counts less than 100,000/mm³.

Platelet counts should be monitored prior to each dose of ado-trastuzumab emtansine. Patients receiving concomitant anticoagulant therapy or those with platelet counts less than 100,000/mm³ should be closely monitored during therapy. Therapy with the drug should be interrupted in patients who experience grade 3 or greater thrombocytopenia until resolution to grade 1 or less. (See Thrombocytopenia under Dosage: Dosage Modification for Toxicity, in Dosage and Administration.)

Peripheral Neuropathy. Peripheral neuropathy of any grade (mainly sensory neuropathy) was reported in 22% of patients receiving ado-trastuzumab emtansine in clinical trials; grade 3 or greater peripheral neuropathy was reported in 1.6% of patients. In the EMILIA study, peripheral neuropathy occurred in 21.2% of patients receiving ado-trastuzumab emtansine alone and in 13.5% of patients receiving combined therapy with lapatinib and capecitabine. The incidence of grade 3 or greater peripheral neuropathy was higher in patients receiving ado-trastuzumab emtansine alone compared with those receiving combined therapy with lapatinib and capecitabine (2.2 versus 0.2%, respectively). Peripheral neuropathy generally was managed with treatment interruption and/or dosage reduction in clinical trials.

Patients receiving ado-trastuzumab emtansine should be monitored for manifestations of neurotoxicity during therapy. The drug should be withheld in patients who experience grade 3 or 4 peripheral neuropathy until it resolves to grade 2 or less. (See Peripheral Neuropathy under Dosage: Dosage Modification for Toxicity, in Dosage and Administration.)

Evaluation of *HER2*. Detection of *HER2* overexpression is necessary prior to initiating therapy because safety and efficacy of ado-trastuzumab emtansine have been established only in patients with *HER2*-overexpressing tumors. In clinical practice and clinical research studies, the methods of *HER2* evaluation most commonly used are immunohistochemistry (IHC) assays, which directly measure overexpression of the *HER2* protein, and fluorescent in situ hybridization (FISH), which measures amplification of the *HER2* oncogene. (See Evaluation of *HER2/neu* in Breast Cancer under Uses: Breast Cancer, in Trastuzumab 10:00.) In the EMILIA study, patients with breast cancer were required to have disease demonstrating an IHC score of 3+ (as determined by the Dako Herceptest®) or a FISH amplification ratio of 2 or higher (as determined by the Dako *HER2* FISH PharmDx® test kit). Limited data are available for patients whose breast tumors are FISH-positive but lack *HER2* overexpression.

Assessment of *HER2* status should be performed by laboratories with demonstrated proficiency in the specific technology being used. Improper assay performance, including use of suboptimally fixed tissue, failure to use specified reagents, deviation from specific assay instructions, and failure to include appropriate controls for assay validation, can lead to unreliable results.

Local Effects. Extravasation of ado-trastuzumab emtansine has resulted in reactions including erythema, tenderness, skin irritation, pain, or swelling at the infusion site; these effects were generally mild and observed more frequently within 24 hours following an infusion. Specific treatment for extravasation following an infusion of ado-trastuzumab emtansine has not been established. The infusion site should be closely monitored for subcutaneous infiltration during administration.

Immunogenicity. As with all therapeutic proteins, there is a potential for immunogenicity. In clinical studies, anti-ado-trastuzumab emtansine antibodies were detected in 44 of 836 patients (5.3%) receiving ado-trastuzumab emtansine. No clinically important effects on safety, efficacy, or pharmacokinetics of the drug were observed in patients who tested positive for anti-ado-trastuzumab emtansine antibodies. Neutralizing antibodies have not been assessed.

The presence of ado-trastuzumab emtansine in the serum sample may interfere with assays used to measure antibodies to the drug. Therefore, data may not accurately reflect the true incidence of anti-ado-trastuzumab emtansine antibody formation.

Specific Populations **Pregnancy.** Category D. (See Fetal/Neonatal Morbidity and Mortality under Warnings/Precautions: Warnings, in Cautions.)

If ado-trastuzumab emtansine is used during pregnancy or if the patient becomes pregnant while receiving the drug, the patient should be apprised of the potential fetal hazard; the patient should be encouraged to enroll in the MotHER Pregnancy Registry (800-690-6720), and clinicians should immediately notify the Genentech Adverse Event Line (888-835-2555).

Lactation. It is not known whether ado-trastuzumab emtansine is distributed into human milk. Trastuzumab is distributed into milk in monkeys; it is not known whether trastuzumab is distributed into milk in humans. (See Cautions: Pregnancy, Fertility, and Lactation, in Trastuzumab 10:00.) Because human immunoglobulin G (IgG) is distributed into milk in humans, and because of the potential for serious adverse reactions to ado-trastuzumab emtansine in nursing infants, a decision should be made whether to discontinue nursing or the drug, taking into account the importance of the drug to the woman.

Pediatric Use. Safety and efficacy of ado-trastuzumab emtansine have not been established in pediatric patients.

Geriatric Use. In the EMILIA study, 13% of patients were 65 years of age or older, and 2% were 75 years of age or older. In a subset analysis, survival benefit (i.e., progression-free survival and overall survival) was not observed in patients 65 years of age or older (hazard ratio 1.06 and 1.05, respectively). In a population pharmacokinetic analysis, no substantial differences in pharmacokinetics were observed between geriatric and younger adults.

Hepatic Impairment. Pharmacokinetic studies have not been conducted in patients with hepatic impairment; however, the microtubule inhibitor DM1 is metabolized by cytochrome P-450 (CYP) isoenzymes 3A4/5.

Ado-trastuzumab emtansine has not been studied in patients with serum aminotransferase concentrations exceeding 2.5 times the upper limit of normal (ULN) or total bilirubin concentrations exceeding 1.5 times the ULN.

Renal Impairment. Formal pharmacokinetic studies have not been conducted in patients with renal impairment. In a population pharmacokinetic analysis, the pharmacokinetics of ado-trastuzumab emtansine were similar between patients with mild (creatinine clearance of 60–89 mL/minute) or moderate (creatinine clearance of 30–59 mL/minute) renal impairment and those with normal renal function. Pharmacokinetic data in patients with severe renal impairment (creatinine clearance less than 30 mL/minute) are limited. (See Dosage and Administration: Special Populations.)

■ **Common Adverse Effects** Adverse effects reported in 10% or more of patients receiving ado-trastuzumab emtansine include stomatitis, dry mouth, abdominal pain, diarrhea, nausea, vomiting, constipation, pyrexia, asthenia, fatigue, myalgia, arthralgia, musculoskeletal pain, dizziness, peripheral neuropathy, headache, insomnia, dyspnea, cough, epistaxis, rash, pain in extremity, infusion reaction, hypokalemia, liver function test (AST, ALT, alkaline phosphatase) abnormalities, anemia, and thrombocytopenia.

Drug Interactions

In vitro studies indicate that DM1, the microtubule-disrupting component of ado-trastuzumab emtansine, is primarily metabolized by cytochrome P-450 (CYP) isoenzyme 3A4 and, to a lesser extent, by CYP3A5. (See Description.) In vitro studies also indicate that DM1 does not inhibit or induce major CYP isoenzymes.

DM1 is a substrate for the efflux transporter P-glycoprotein (P-gp) in vitro.

■ **Drugs Affecting Hepatic Microsomal Enzymes** Concomitant use of ado-trastuzumab emtansine with potent inhibitors of CYP3A4 may result in increased systemic exposure of DM1. Concomitant use with potent CYP3A4 inhibitors (e.g., atazanavir, clarithromycin, indinavir, itraconazole, ketoconazole, nefazodone, nelfinavir, ritonavir, saquinavir, telithromycin, voriconazole) should be avoided, and selection of an alternative drug with no or minimal CYP3A4 inhibition potential is recommended. If concomitant use of the potent CYP3A4 inhibitor is unavoidable, delaying initiation of ado-trastuzumab emtansine therapy until after approximately 3 elimination half-lives of the CYP3A4 inhibitor should be considered. If concomitant use cannot be delayed, patients should be closely monitored for adverse effects.

Description

Ado-trastuzumab emtansine, an anti-human epidermal growth factor receptor type 2 (anti-*HER2*) antibody-drug conjugate, is an antineoplastic agent. The anti-*HER2* antibody, a humanized immunoglobulin (IgG_1), is conjugated with the microtubule inhibitor DM1 (a maytansine derivative). A stable thioether linker (MCC) covalently binds DM1 to the antibody component; the resultant complex, MCC-DM1, is referred to as emtansine. The antibody portion of ado-trastuzumab emtansine binds specifically to the extracellular domain of the *HER2* receptor. Following binding of the antibody portion of ado-trastuzumab emtansine to sub-domain IV of the *HER2* receptor, the resultant complex is internalized by the cell. DM1 is released via lysosomal degradation and binds to tubulin, resulting in cell cycle arrest and apoptosis. In addition, ado-trastuzumab emtansine has been shown to exhibit similar activity (i.e., inhibit *HER2* signaling, mediate antibody-dependent cell-mediated cytotoxicity [ADCC], and inhibit shedding of the *HER2* extracellular domain in breast cancer cells that overexpress the *HER2* protein) and binding affinity to the *HER2* receptor as trastuzumab.

In one in vitro study comparing the relative potency of DM1 and paclitaxel in 6 cell lines in breast cancer, DM1 was approximately 2- to 17-fold more potent than paclitaxel on a molar basis.

The pharmacokinetics of the antibody-drug conjugate following IV administration is characterized by a 2-compartment model with first-order elimination. Peak plasma concentrations of the antibody-drug conjugate and DM1 were observed near the end of IV infusion. Following repeated doses of ado-trastuzumab emtansine administered IV every 3 weeks, systemic accumulation of the antibody-drug conjugate was not observed. Steady-state concentrations are reached by the second cycle of therapy. In vitro studies indicate that DM1 is metabolized by cytochrome P-450 (CYP) 3A4/5 isoenzymes. In vitro, DM1 is 93% bound to plasma proteins. The terminal half-life of the antibody-drug conjugate is approximately 4 days.

Population pharmacokinetic analyses indicate that age, race, and serum albumin concentrations do not have clinically important effects on the pharmacokinetics of the antibody-drug conjugate.

Advice to Patients

Risk of fetal harm (e.g., embryofetal death, birth defects). Necessity of advising women of childbearing potential to use effective contraception during therapy and for 6 months after discontinuance of ado-trastuzumab emtansine. Encourage women who have been exposed to the drug during pregnancy to enroll in the MotHER Pregnancy Registry by contacting 800-690-6720. (See Fetal/Neonatal Morbidity and Mortality under Warnings/Precautions: Warnings, in Cautions.)

Importance of discontinuing breast-feeding during therapy.

Risk of severe hepatotoxicity. Importance of contacting clinician promptly if manifestations of acute hepatitis occur (e.g., nausea, vomiting, abdominal pain [particularly in the right upper quadrant], jaundice, dark urine, generalized pruritus, anorexia).

Importance of contacting clinician promptly if new-onset or worsening shortness of breath, cough, swelling of ankles or legs, palpitations, weight gain exceeding 5 pounds in 24 hours, dizziness, or loss of consciousness occurs.

Importance of informing clinicians of existing or contemplated concomitant therapy, including prescription and OTC drugs, as well as any concomitant illnesses.

Importance of informing patients of other important precautionary information. (See Cautions.)

Overview® (see Users Guide). For additional information on this drug until a more detailed monograph is developed and published, the manufacturer's labeling should be consulted. It is *essential* that the manufacturer's labeling be consulted for more detailed information on usual cautions, precautions, contraindications, potential drug interactions, laboratory test interferences, and acute toxicity. For further information on the handling of antineoplastic agents, see the ASHP Guidelines on Handling Hazardous Drugs at http://www.ahfsdruginformation.com.

Preparations

Ado-trastuzumab emtansine (Kadcyla®) should not be confused with trastuzumab (Herceptin®). (See Special Alerts.)

Excipients in commercially available drug preparations may have clinically important effects in some individuals; consult specific product labeling for details.

Ado-Trastuzumab Emtansine

Parenteral		
For injection, for IV infusion only	100 mg	Kadcyla®, Genentech
	160 mg	Kadcyla®, Genentech

Afatinib Dimaleate

■ Afatinib dimaleate, a second-generation inhibitor of receptor tyrosine kinases, is an antineoplastic agent.

Uses

■ **Non-small Cell Lung Cancer** ***First-line Therapy for Metastatic Non-small Cell Lung Cancer*** Afatinib is used for the first-line treatment of metastatic non-small cell lung cancer (NSCLC) in patients whose tumors harbor nonresistant epidermal growth factor receptor (EGFR) mutations (e.g., exon 19 deletions [del19], exon 21 substitution [L858R]) mutations as detected by an FDA-approved diagnostic test. Nonresistant EGFR mutations are those where efficacy of afatinib may be predicted by a clinically meaningful reduction in tumor size at the recommended dosage of the drug and/or inhibition of cellular proliferation or EGFR tyrosine kinase phosphorylation is expected at the recommended dosage. Afatinib has been designated an orphan drug by FDA for the treatment of EGFR mutation-positive NSCLC.

EGFR-activating mutations are present in approximately 15–22% of NSCLC cases in North America and Europe and are present in up to 30–50% of cases in patients of East Asian descent. The majority of EGFR mutations are exon 19 deletions and an L858R substitution in exon 21, which together account for about 90% of EGFR mutations in patients with NSCLC; less frequently occurring EGFR mutations are a heterogeneous group of molecular alterations within exons 18–21 (i.e., uncommon EGFR mutations), which exhibit variable responses to EGFR tyrosine kinase inhibitor therapy. (See Description.)

The current indication for afatinib in the first-line treatment of metastatic NSCLC is based principally on the results of a randomized, multinational, open-label phase 3 study (LUX-Lung 3) in adults with previously untreated EGFR mutation-positive locally advanced or metastatic (stage IIIB with pleural and/or pericardial effusion or stage IV) NSCLC. In this study, 345 patients were randomized (stratified by type of EGFR mutation and race) in a 2:1 ratio to receive either afatinib (40 mg orally once daily) alone or cisplatin (75 mg/m^2 by IV infusion) in combination with pemetrexed (500 mg/m^2 by IV infusion) once every 3 weeks (for a maximum of 6 cycles) until disease progression. The primary measure of efficacy was progression-free survival as assessed by an independent review committee (IRC); secondary end points included objective response rate (complete plus partial responses) and overall survival. The median age of patients was 61 years. The majority (72%) of patients were of East Asian ancestry. Patients enrolled in the study were required to have evidence of an EGFR mutation as determined by a standardized polymerase chain reaction (PCR) assay; the majority of patients had exon 19 deletions (49%) or exon 21 (L858R) substitution mutations (40%), while the remaining (11%) had other mutations.

At a median follow-up of 16.4 months, patients receiving afatinib had a longer median IRC-assessed progression-free survival compared with patients receiving combined therapy with cisplatin and pemetrexed (11.1 versus 6.9 months). Effects of afatinib on investigator-assessed progression-free survival and IRC-assessed progression-free survival were comparable. Patients receiving afatinib also had a higher objective response rate (50.4 versus 19.1%) and a longer median duration of response (12.5 versus 6.7 months) compared with those receiving combined therapy with cisplatin and pemetrexed. A planned subgroup analysis indicated that the magnitude of progression-free survival benefit from afatinib was greater in patients with common EGFR mutations (del19 and L858R) compared with those in the general study population; among patients with common EGFR mutations, the median IRC-assessed progression-free survival reportedly was 13.6 months in those receiving afatinib and 6.9 months in those receiving combined therapy with cisplatin and pemetrexed. No significant difference in overall survival was observed between patients receiving afatinib and those receiving combined therapy with cisplatin and pemetrexed at the time of final analysis. Another planned subgroup analysis indicated that the magnitude of progression-free survival and overall survival benefit in Japanese patients with common EGFR mutations was greater in those receiving afatinib compared with those receiving combined therapy with cisplatin and pemetrexed; however, no significant difference in overall survival was observed between treatment groups in Japanese patients with L858R mutations. In a pooled analysis of 3 clinical studies involving 32 patients with uncommon EGFR mutations (i.e., S768I; S768I and G719X; S768I and L858R; G719X; G719X and L861Q; L861Q; L861Q and del19 mutations) receiving afatinib (40 or 50 mg orally once daily), responses were observed in 66% of patients. At the time of analysis, 52% of responders maintained a response for 12 months or longer and 33% had ongoing responses.

In a randomized, open-label phase 3 study (LUX-Lung 6) evaluating afatinib or combined therapy with gemcitabine and cisplatin in 364 patients with previously untreated EGFR mutation-positive locally advanced or metastatic (stage IIIB with pleural effusion or stage IV) NSCLC in East Asia (i.e., China, Thailand, South Korea), patients receiving afatinib had longer IRC-assessed progression-free survival (11 versus 5.6 months), higher objective response rates (66.9 versus 23%) and disease control rates (92.6 versus 76.2%), and a longer median duration of response (9.7 versus 4.3 months) compared with those receiving combined therapy with gemcitabine and cisplatin.

Safety and efficacy of afatinib have not been established in patients whose tumors harbor resistant EGFR mutations.

Previously Treated Metastatic Non-small Cell Lung Cancer Afatinib is used for the treatment of metastatic squamous NSCLC that has progressed following therapy with platinum-based chemotherapy. Afatinib has been designated an orphan drug by FDA for the treatment of squamous NSCLC.

The current indication for afatinib in the treatment of previously treated metastatic squamous NSCLC is based principally on the results of a randomized, multicenter, open-label, active-controlled study (LUX-Lung 8) in 795 adults with stage IIIb or IV squamous NSCLC whose disease progressed following a platinum-based doublet chemotherapy regimen for at least 4 cycles. Patients were randomized (stratified by geographic region) in a 1:1 ratio to receive afatinib (40 mg orally once daily) or erlotinib (150 mg orally once daily). Treatment was continued until disease progression, unacceptable toxicity, or study withdrawal occurred. The primary efficacy end point of the study was progression-free survival as assessed by an independent review committee according to Response Evaluation Criteria in Solid Tumors (RECIST 1.1); secondary end points included objective response rate and overall survival. The median age of patients was 64 years; the majority of patients were male (84%), 73% were Caucasian, 24% were of Asian ancestry, 95% were current or former smokers, 96% had squamous cell histology, and 3.5% had mixed cell histology. All patients enrolled in the study had an Eastern Cooperative Oncology Group (ECOG) performance status of 0 or 1.

At a median follow-up of 6.7 months, patients receiving afatinib had a longer median progression-free survival compared with patients receiving erlotinib (2.4 versus 1.9 months). At a median follow-up of 18.4 months, median overall survival also was prolonged in patients receiving afatinib compared with those receiving erlotinib (7.9 versus 6.8 months). The objective response rate was 3 or 2% in afatinib-treated or erlotinib-treated patients, respectively.

Results of subgroup analyses (based on age, gender, ethnicity, response to first-line chemotherapy, interval between first- and second-line therapies, histology, smoking status, ECOG performance status, use of maintenance therapy) suggested that the effect of afatinib on progression-free survival and overall survival was consistent across all subgroups.

Dosage and Administration

■ **General** Confirmation of the diagnosis of nonresistant epidermal growth factor receptor (EGFR) mutation-positive (e.g., exon 19 deletion [del19], exon 21 substitution [L858R]) non-small cell lung cancer (NSCLC) by an FDA-approved diagnostic test is necessary prior to initiating therapy with afatinib for the first-line treatment of metastatic disease.

Antidiarrheal therapy (e.g., loperamide) should be provided for subsequent home use by the patient as needed. (See Diarrhea under Cautions: Warnings/Precautions.)

■ **Administration** Afatinib dimaleate is administered orally once daily. The drug should be administered on an empty stomach, at least 1 hour before or 2 hours after a meal. (See Description and also see Advice to Patients.)

■ **Dosage** Dosage of afatinib dimaleate is expressed in terms of afatinib.

Non-small Cell Lung Cancer For the first-line treatment of metastatic NSCLC in patients whose tumors harbor nonresistant EGFR mutations (e.g., exon 19 deletions or exon 21 substitution [L858R] mutations), the recommended dosage of afatinib in adults is 40 mg once daily. Therapy should be continued until disease progression or unacceptable toxicity occurs. In the LUX-Lung 3 study, afatinib therapy was continued for a median of 11 months. Approximately one-half (53.3%) of patients required dosage reductions within the initial 6 months of therapy; however, median progression-free survival was similar among patients who received a dosage reduction and those who received the recommended dosage.

For the treatment of metastatic squamous NSCLC that has progressed following therapy with platinum-based chemotherapy, the recommended dosage of afatinib in adults is 40 mg once daily. Therapy should be continued until disease progression or unacceptable toxicity occurs. In the LUX-Lung 8 study, afatinib therapy was continued for a median of 2.1 months.

Dosage Modification Afatinib therapy should be *interrupted* in patients who develop any drug-related toxicity of grade 3 or greater, persistent grade 2 diarrhea or grade 3 diarrhea, persistent or intolerable grade 2 cutaneous reactions or grade 3 cutaneous reactions, or renal dysfunction of grade 2 or greater. When the toxicity resolves completely, returns to baseline, or improves to grade 1, afatinib may be resumed at a reduced dosage (i.e., 10 mg less than the daily dosage used prior to the event).

Afatinib should be *permanently discontinued* in patients who develop life-threatening bullous, blistering, or exfoliative skin lesions; interstitial lung disease; severe drug-induced hepatic impairment; persistent ulcerative keratitis; or symptomatic left ventricular dysfunction. (See Cautions: Warnings/Precautions.) The drug also should be permanently discontinued in patients who experience severe or intolerable adverse reactions to an afatinib dosage of 20 mg daily.

Grade 3 or 4 Toxicity. If grade 3 or 4 toxicity occurs, afatinib therapy should be interrupted. When the toxicity resolves completely or improves to grade 1, afatinib may be resumed at a reduced dosage (i.e., 10 mg less than the daily dosage used prior to the event).

Diarrhea. If grade 2 diarrhea persists for more than 48 hours or grade 3 or greater diarrhea occurs, afatinib therapy should be interrupted. When diarrhea improves to grade 1 or less, afatinib may be resumed at a reduced dosage (i.e., 10 mg less than the daily dosage used prior to the event). (See Diarrhea under Cautions: Warnings/Precautions.)

Dermatologic Toxicity. If intolerable or prolonged (lasting more than 7 days) grade 2 cutaneous reactions or grade 3 cutaneous reactions occur, afatinib therapy should be interrupted. When the cutaneous reactions improve to grade 1 or less, afatinib may be resumed at a reduced dosage (i.e., 10 mg less than the daily dosage used prior to the event). (See Dermatologic Effects under Cautions: Warnings/Precautions.)

If life-threatening bullous, blistering, or exfoliating lesions occur, afatinib should be permanently discontinued.

Nephrotoxicity. If renal dysfunction of grade 2 or greater occurs, afatinib therapy should be interrupted. When nephrotoxicity resolves completely, returns to baseline, or improves to grade 1, afatinib may be resumed at a reduced dosage (i.e., 10 mg less than the daily dosage used prior to the event).

Concomitant Use with Drugs Affecting the P-glycoprotein Transport System. If afatinib is used concomitantly with an inhibitor of P-glycoprotein (P-gp), dosage of afatinib should be reduced by 10 mg daily if not tolerated. If concomitant use of the P-gp inhibitor is discontinued, the afatinib dosage should be returned to the dosage used prior to initiation of the P-gp inhibitor as tolerated. (See Drug Interactions: Drugs Affecting the P-glycoprotein Transport System.)

If afatinib is used concomitantly with an inducer of P-gp, dosage of afatinib should be increased by 10 mg daily as tolerated. If concomitant use of the P-gp inducer is discontinued, the afatinib dosage should be returned (2–3 days following discontinuance of the P-gp inducer) to the dosage used prior to initiation of the P-gp inducer. (See Drug Interactions: Drugs Affecting the P-glycoprotein Transport System.)

■ **Special Populations** The manufacturer makes no specific dosage recommendations for geriatric patients.

No initial dosage adjustment is necessary in patients with mild or moderate hepatic impairment (Child-Pugh class A or B). Patients with severe hepatic impairment (Child-Pugh class C) should be closely monitored, and dosage of afatinib should be adjusted if not tolerated. Afatinib has not been studied in patients with severe hepatic impairment.

For patients with severe renal impairment (estimated glomerular filtration rate [eGFR] 15–29 mL/minute per 1.73 m^2), the manufacturer recommends a reduced afatinib dosage of 30 mg once daily. Dosage adjustment is not necessary in patients with mild or moderate renal impairment (eGFR 30–89 mL/minute per 1.73 m^2). Afatinib has not been studied in patients with eGFR less than 15 mL/minute per 1.73 m^2 or in those receiving dialysis.

Cautions

■ **Contraindications** The manufacturer states there are no known contraindications to the use of afatinib.

■ **Warnings/Precautions** ***Diarrhea*** Diarrhea, resulting in dehydration with or without renal impairment, has been reported in patients receiving afatinib; some of these cases were fatal. In clinical studies, grade 3 or 4 diarrhea was reported in 16% of patients receiving afatinib. In the LUX-Lung 3 study in patients with previously untreated metastatic non-small cell lung cancer (NSCLC), diarrhea was reported in 96% of patients receiving afatinib and was grade 3 in 15% of patients; diarrhea occurred within the first 6 weeks of therapy. In the LUX-Lung 8 study in patients with previously treated metastatic squamous NSCLC, diarrhea was reported in 75% of patients receiving afatinib and was grade 3 or 4 in 10 or 0.8%, respectively, of patients. In the LUX-Lung 3 and LUX-Lung 8 studies, renal impairment secondary to diarrhea was reported in 6 and 7% of patients receiving afatinib, respectively, and was grade 3 in 1.3 and 2%, respectively, of patients.

Although the mechanism for development of diarrhea has not been fully determined, an increased incidence and greater severity of diarrhea have been observed with second-generation pan-human epidermal growth factor receptor (pan-HER) inhibitors (e.g., afatinib, dacomitinib) compared with single-target tyrosine kinase inhibitors selective for epidermal growth factor receptor (EGFR) (e.g., erlotinib, gefitinib); therefore, it has been suggested that other members of the HER tyrosine kinase family may have an essential role in the development of diarrhea.

If persistent or severe diarrhea occurs, temporary interruption of therapy followed by dosage reduction may be required. (See Diarrhea under Dosage: Dosage Modification, in Dosage and Administration.) Antidiarrheal therapy (e.g., loperamide) should be provided for subsequent home use by the patient as needed. Patients should be advised to take an antidiarrheal agent at the onset of diarrhea and to continue antidiarrheal therapy until loose bowel movements have ceased for 12 hours.

Dermatologic Effects Cutaneous reactions have been reported frequently in patients receiving afatinib. (See Advice to Patients.) Grade 3 cutaneous reactions (characterized by bullous, blistering, and exfoliating lesions) occurred in 0.2% of 4257 patients receiving afatinib across clinical trials. In the LUX-Lung 3 study in patients with previously untreated metastatic NSCLC, cutaneous reactions (i.e., rash, erythema, acneiform rash) were reported in 90% of patients receiving afatinib, and grade 3 cutaneous reactions were reported in 16% of patients. In the LUX-Lung 8 study in patients with previously treated metastatic squamous NSCLC, cutaneous reactions were reported in 70% of patients receiving afatinib, and grade 3 cutaneous reactions were reported in 7% of patients. In the LUX-Lung 3 and LUX-Lung 8 studies, grade 1–3 palmar-plantar erythrodysesthesia (hand-foot syndrome) was reported in 7 and 1.5%, respectively, of patients receiving afatinib.

Management of afatinib-associated rash may include use of topical or systemic corticosteroids, anti-infectives, or antihistamines. If persistent or severe cutaneous reactions occur, temporary interruption of therapy followed by dosage reduction may be required. (See Dermatologic Toxicity under Dosage: Dosage Modification, in Dosage and Administration.) Afatinib should be permanently discontinued in patients who develop life-threatening bullous, blistering, or exfoliating lesions.

Toxic epidermal necrolysis and Stevens-Johnson syndrome have been reported during postmarketing experience in patients receiving afatinib. Toxic epidermal necrolysis and Stevens-Johnson syndrome bullous cutaneous reactions have occurred from a distinct and separate mechanism of toxicity than bullous lesions secondary to inhibition of EGFR. If toxic epidermal necrolysis or Stevens-Johnson syndrome is suspected, afatinib should be discontinued.

Pulmonary Effects Interstitial lung disease or interstitial lung disease-like events (e.g., lung infiltration, pneumonitis, acute respiratory distress syndrome [ARDS], allergic alveolitis) occurred in 1.6% of 4257 patients receiving afatinib across clinical trials; fatal interstitial lung disease occurred in 0.4% of patients receiving the drug. In the LUX-Lung 3 study in patients with previously untreated metastatic NSCLC, grade 3 or greater interstitial lung disease was reported in 1.3% of patients receiving afatinib and was fatal in 1% of patients. In the LUX-Lung 8 study in patients with previously treated metastatic squamous NSCLC, grade 3 or greater interstitial lung disease was reported in 0.9% of patients receiving afatinib and was fatal in 0.8% of patients. The incidence of interstitial lung disease appears to be higher in Asian patients (2.3%) compared with Caucasian patients (1%).

If interstitial lung disease is suspected, afatinib therapy should be interrupted. If a diagnosis of interstitial lung disease is confirmed, afatinib should be permanently discontinued.

Hepatic Toxicity Abnormal liver function tests were reported in 9.7% of 4257 patients receiving afatinib across clinical trials; fatal hepatic toxicity occurred in 0.2% of patients receiving the drug. In the LUX-Lung 3 study in patients with previously untreated metastatic NSCLC, liver function test abnormalities of any grade were reported in 17.5% of patients receiving afatinib, and were grade 3 or 4 in 3.5% of patients. In the LUX-Lung 8 study in patients with previously treated metastatic squamous NSCLC, liver function test abnormalities of any grade were reported in 6% of patients receiving afatinib, and were grade 3 or 4 in 0.2% of patients.

Liver function tests should be performed periodically during afatinib therapy. Afatinib therapy should be temporarily interrupted in patients who develop worsening of liver function. Afatinib should be permanently discontinued in patients who develop severe hepatic impairment.

Ocular Effects Keratitis (characterized as acute or worsening eye inflammation, lacrimation, light sensitivity, blurred vision, eye pain, and/or red eye) occurred in 0.7% of 4257 patients receiving afatinib across clinical trials; grade 3 keratitis occurred in 0.05% of patients receiving the drug. In the LUX-Lung 3 study in patients with previously untreated metastatic NSCLC, keratitis was reported in 2.2% of patients receiving afatinib; grade 3 keratitis was reported in 0.4% of patients. In the LUX-Lung 8 study in patients with previously treated metastatic squamous NSCLC, keratitis was reported in 0.3% of patients receiving afatinib; grade 3 or greater keratitis was reported in none of the patients.

If keratitis is suspected, afatinib therapy should be interrupted; if a diagnosis of keratitis is confirmed, the potential benefit of the drug to the patient must be carefully weighed against the risks of continued therapy. Afatinib therapy should be temporarily interrupted or discontinued in patients with confirmed ulcerative keratitis; therapy should be permanently discontinued in patients with persistent ulcerative keratitis.

Afatinib should be used with caution in patients with a history of keratitis, ulcerative keratitis, or severe dry eye. Contact lens use is a risk factor for development of keratitis and ulceration.

Fetal/Neonatal Morbidity and Mortality Afatinib may cause fetal harm if administered to pregnant women based on its mechanism of action and animal findings. Embryofetal toxicity (e.g., decreased fetal weight, abortion) and teratogenicity (e.g., skeletal alterations) have been demonstrated in animals. Women of childbearing potential should use effective contraception while receiving afatinib and for at least 2 weeks after the drug is discontinued. Patients should be apprised of the potential fetal hazard if afatinib is used during pregnancy. (See Advice to Patients.)

Cardiovascular Effects Left ventricular dysfunction has been reported in patients receiving afatinib. In the principal efficacy study in patients with previously untreated NSCLC, left ventricular dysfunction was reported in 2.2% of patients receiving afatinib compared with 0.9% of patients receiving combined therapy with cisplatin and pemetrexed. Afatinib therapy should be permanently discontinued if symptomatic left ventricular dysfunction occurs.

Afatinib does not appear to have substantial effects on the corrected QT (QT_c) interval. In an open-label, single-arm study evaluating potential effects of afatinib on the QT_c interval, substantial (i.e., by more 20 msec) increases in the mean QT_c interval were not observed in patients with relapsed or refractory solid tumors who received multiple doses of the drug (50 mg once daily).

Impairment of Fertility Results of animal studies suggest that afatinib may impair female and male fertility; it is not known whether these effects are reversible.

In female rats, administration of afatinib at exposure levels approximately 0.63 times the human exposure at the recommended dosage resulted in decreased corpora lutea and increased postimplantation loss. In a general toxicology study, the effects of afatinib on reduced ovarian weights were not reversible at 2 weeks.

In male rats, administration of afatinib at exposure levels approximately equal to the human exposure at the recommended dosage resulted in reduced or absent sperm count; however overall fertility was not affected. In a general toxicology study, increased apoptosis in the testes and atrophy in seminal vesicles were observed.

Specific Populations **Pregnancy.** Afatinib may cause fetal harm if administered to pregnant women based on its mechanism of action and animal findings. (See Fetal/Neonatal Morbidity and Mortality under Cautions: Warnings/Precautions.)

Lactation. Afatinib is distributed into milk in rats; it is not known whether the drug is distributed into milk in humans or if the drug has any effect on milk production or the nursing infant. Because of the potential for serious adverse reactions to afatinib in nursing infants, women should be advised to discontinue nursing while receiving the drug and for 2 weeks after the drug is discontinued.

Pediatric Use. Safety and efficacy of afatinib have not been established in pediatric patients.

Geriatric Use. The LUX-Lung 3 study evaluating afatinib in patients with previously untreated metastatic NSCLC did not include sufficient numbers of patients 65 years of age and older to determine whether geriatric patients respond differently than younger adults. In subgroup analyses of 3 clinical studies, including LUX-Lung 3, evaluating afatinib as first-line therapy in patients with EGFR mutation-positive NSCLC, efficacy of afatinib in patients 65 years of age and older was consistent with that observed in the overall study population.

In the LUX-Lung 8 study evaluating afatinib in patients with previously treated metastatic squamous NSCLC, 53% of patients were 65 years of age or older and 11% were 75 years of age or older. In an exploratory subgroup analysis, afatinib reduced the risk of death by 5% in patients 65 years of age and older and 32% in those younger than 65 years of age. No overall differences in safety were observed between geriatric patients and younger adults.

Hepatic Impairment. Following administration of a single dose of afatinib, systemic exposure to the drug was not affected by mild or moderate hepatic impairment (Child-Pugh class A or B). Afatinib has not been studied in patients with severe hepatic impairment (Child-Pugh class C); therefore, such patients should be monitored closely. (See Dosage and Administration: Special Populations.)

Renal Impairment. Following administration of a single 40-mg dose of afatinib, peak plasma concentrations and systemic exposure of afatinib in individuals with severe renal impairment (estimated glomerular filtration rate [eGFR] 15–29 mL/minute per 1.73 m^2) were increased by 22 and 50%, respectively, compared with individuals with normal renal function; however, peak plasma concentrations of afatinib in individuals with moderate renal impairment (eGFR 30–59 mL/minute per 1.73 m^2) were similar to those in individuals with normal renal function but systemic exposure was increased by 22%. Dosage adjustment is required in patients with severe renal impairment. Afatinib has not been studied in patients with eGFR less than 15 mL/minute per 1.73 m^2 or in those receiving dialysis. (See Dosage and Administration: Special Populations.)

■ **Common Adverse Effects** Adverse effects reported in 10% or more of patients receiving afatinib for the initial treatment of metastatic NSCLC harboring nonresistant EGFR mutations in the LUX-Lung 3 study include diarrhea, rash/dermatitis acneiform, mucositis or stomatitis, paronychia, dry skin, decreased appetite, pruritus, epistaxis, decreased weight, cystitis, cheilitis, pyrexia, rhinorrhea, conjunctivitis, nausea, vomiting, and fatigue. Laboratory abnormalities reported in 10% or more of patients receiving afatinib for the initial treatment of metastatic NSCLC harboring nonresistant EGFR mutations and at an incidence that is at least 2% higher than that reported with pemetrexed in combination with cisplatin include elevated concentrations of aminotransferases (i.e., ALT, AST), elevated concentrations of alkaline phosphatase, decreased creatinine clearance, lymphopenia, hypokalemia, and elevated concentrations of bilirubin.

Adverse effects reported in 10% or more of patients receiving afatinib for the treatment of previously treated metastatic squamous NSCLC in the LUX-Lung 8 study include diarrhea, rash/dermatitis acneiform, stomatitis, decreased appetite, nausea, fatigue, vomiting, paronychia, and pruritus. Laboratory abnormalities reported in 10% or more of patients receiving afatinib for the treatment of previously treated metastatic squamous NSCLC and at an incidence that is at least 2% higher than that reported with erlotinib include elevated concentrations of alkaline phosphatase, decreased leukocyte counts, and hypokalemia.

Drug Interactions

In vitro studies in human hepatocytes indicate that afatinib does not inhibit or induce cytochrome P-450 (CYP) isoenzyme 1A2, 2B6, 2C8, 2C9, 2C19, or 3A4. CYP-mediated mechanisms play a minor role in the drug's overall metabolism.

In vitro data indicate that afatinib is a substrate and inhibitor of the efflux transporters P-glycoprotein (P-gp) and ABCG2 (breast cancer resistance protein [BCRP]).

■ **Drugs Affecting Hepatic Microsomal Enzymes** Clinically important pharmacokinetic interactions with CYP inhibitors and inducers are unlikely.

■ **Drugs Metabolized by Hepatic Microsomal Enzymes** Clinically important pharmacokinetic interactions with drugs metabolized by CYP isoenzymes are unlikely.

■ **Drugs Affecting the P-glycoprotein Transport System** ***Inhibitors of P-gp*** Concomitant use of afatinib with inhibitors of P-gp may result in increased systemic exposure to afatinib. When the P-gp inhibitor ritonavir (200 mg twice daily for 3 days) was administered 1 hour prior to afatinib (single 20-mg dose) in healthy individuals, area under the plasma concentration-time curve (AUC) and peak plasma concentrations of afatinib were increased by 48 and 39%, respectively. However, AUC of afatinib was not substantially affected when ritonavir (200 mg twice daily for 3 days) was administered concomitantly with or 6 hours following administration of afatinib (single 40-mg dose) in healthy individuals. If afatinib is used concomitantly with a P-gp inhibitor (e.g., amiodarone, cyclosporine, erythromycin, itraconazole, ketoconazole, nelfinavir, quinidine, ritonavir, saquinavir, tacrolimus, verapamil), dosage of afatinib should be reduced by 10 mg daily if not tolerated. If concomitant use of the P-gp inhibitor is discontinued, the afatinib dosage should be returned to the dosage used prior to initiation of the P-gp inhibitor as tolerated.

Inducers of P-gp Concomitant use of afatinib with inducers of P-gp may result in decreased systemic exposure to afatinib. When the potent P-gp inducer rifampin (600 mg once daily for 7 days) was administered concomitantly with afatinib, AUC and peak plasma concentrations of afatinib were decreased by 34 and 22%, respectively. If afatinib is used concomitantly with a P-gp inducer (e.g., carbamazepine, phenobarbital, phenytoin, rifampin, St. John's wort [*Hypericum perforatum*]), dosage of afatinib should be increased by 10 mg daily as tolerated. If concomitant use of the P-gp inducer is discontinued, the afatinib dosage should be returned (2–3 days following discontinuance of the P-gp inducer) to the dosage used prior to initiation of the P-gp inducer.

■ **Antineoplastic Agents** ***Cisplatin*** In patients receiving a cisplatin-containing regimen concomitantly with afatinib, the pharmacokinetics of cisplatin were not substantially altered when cisplatin (50–100 mg/m² as a 1-hour IV infusion) was given 3 or 5 days prior to administration of afatinib (20–50 mg orally once daily).

Paclitaxel In patients receiving a paclitaxel-containing regimen concomitantly with afatinib, the pharmacokinetics of paclitaxel were not substantially altered when paclitaxel (175 mg/m² as a 3-hour IV infusion) was given 3 days prior to administration of afatinib (20–50 mg orally once daily).

Fluorouracil In patients receiving a fluorouracil-containing regimen concomitantly with afatinib, the pharmacokinetics of fluorouracil were not substantially altered when afatinib (20–40 mg orally once daily) was given 1 day after completion of fluorouracil IV infusion (750 or 1000 mg/m² infused over 96 hours).

Description

Afatinib dimaleate, a second-generation inhibitor of receptor tyrosine kinases, is an antineoplastic agent. The drug covalently binds to the kinase domains of epidermal growth factor receptor (EGFR/human epidermal growth factor receptor type 1 [HER1]/ErbB1), HER2/ErbB2, and HER4/ErbB4, and irreversibly inhibits tyrosine kinase phosphorylation, resulting in downregulation of ErbB signaling. Some EGFR-activating mutations, including nonresistant mutations, increase autophosphorylation and activation, sometimes independent of ligand binding, of the tyrosine kinase receptor resulting in increased cell proliferation in non-small cell lung cancer (NSCLC) cells harboring these mutations. Nonresistant EGFR mutations are defined as kinase domain mutations in EGFR that lead to activation of tyrosine kinase activity and where efficacy of afatinib is predicted by a clinically meaningful reduction in tumor size at the recommended dosage of the drug and/or inhibition of cellular proliferation or EGFR tyrosine kinase phosphorylation is expected at afatinib concentrations sustainable at the recommended dosage.

Although first-generation (reversible) EGFR tyrosine kinase inhibitors (e.g., erlotinib, gefitinib) have demonstrated improved outcomes in patients with NSCLC harboring EGFR mutations (e.g., EGFR exon 19 deletion [del19], exon 21 substitution [L858R]), secondary resistance to these agents eventually develops following 9–13 months of treatment. Clinical resistance to first-generation EGFR tyrosine kinase inhibitors has been attributed to several mechanisms, but development of the secondary T790M mutation in exon 20 appears to be the most common, occurring in 50–60% of patients who develop this resistance; this mutation results in production of a bulky methionine side chain in the receptor kinase domain of EGFR that is thought to sterically hinder the binding of first-generation EGFR tyrosine kinase inhibitors to EGFR. It has been suggested that second-generation EGFR tyrosine kinase inhibitors (e.g., afatinib, dacomitinib) may theoretically delay or prevent the emergence of secondary resistance through their irreversible inhibition of EGFR, more complete blockade of the EGFR signaling pathway (i.e., inhibition of EGFR as well as HER2/ErbB2 and HER4/ErbB4), and inhibitory effects against tumors harboring the T790M mutation. Afatinib has been shown to inhibit phosphorylation and in vitro proliferation of cell lines expressing wild-type EGFR and cell lines expressing del19 or L858R mutations, including other less common EGFR-activating (nonresistant) mutations. The drug also has been shown to inhibit in vitro proliferation of cell lines that overexpress HER2. Treatment with afatinib has resulted in inhibition of tumor growth in mice implanted with tumors overexpressing wild-type EGFR, HER2/ErbB2, or the EGFR L858R/T790M mutation. In vitro, afatinib appears to be approximately 100 times more potent than gefitinib against EGFR L858R/T790M EGFR mutations and as potent as lapatinib against HER2.

Following oral administration, peak plasma concentrations of afatinib are achieved within 2–5 hours. The area under the plasma concentration-time curve (AUC) and peak plasma concentration of afatinib increase in a slightly more than dose-proportional manner over a dosage range of 20–50 mg. Administration of afatinib with a high-fat meal decreased the peak plasma concentration and AUC of afatinib by 50 and 39%, respectively, compared with administration in the fasted state. (See Dosage and Administration: Administration.) Cytochrome P-450 (CYP)-mediated mechanisms play a minor role in the drug's overall metabolism; however, in vitro data indicate that afatinib is a substrate for P-glycoprotein (P-gp) and ABCG2 (breast cancer resistance protein [BCRP]). In vitro, afatinib is approximately 95% bound to plasma proteins. Biliary and fecal excretion are the principal routes of elimination of the drug. Following oral administration of a single radiolabeled dose of afatinib as an oral solution (not commercially available in the US), 85% of the dose was recovered in feces and 4% was recovered in urine, mostly (88%) as unchanged drug. Following repeated administration of afatinib in cancer patients, the elimination half-life of afatinib was 37 hours.

Advice to Patients

Importance of advising patients to take afatinib on an empty stomach, at least 1 hour before or 2 hours after a meal. If a dose of afatinib is missed, patients should be instructed to take the missed dose as soon as it is remembered unless it is within 12 hours of the next scheduled dose, in which case they should not take the missed dose. Patients should be informed to not take 2 doses at the same time to make up for a missed dose.

Risk of diarrhea; importance of advising patients about appropriate countermeasures to manage diarrhea. (See Diarrhea under Cautions: Warnings/Precautions.) Importance of informing clinician if diarrhea develops and promptly seeking medical attention if severe or persistent diarrhea occurs.

Risk of cutaneous reactions. Importance of limiting exposure to sunlight by wearing protective clothing and using sunscreen (minimum SPF of 15) during afatinib therapy.

Risk of interstitial lung disease. Importance of immediately informing clinician if new or worsening respiratory symptoms occur or if any combination of the following symptoms occur: difficulty breathing, shortness of breath, cough, and/or fever.

Risk of hepatotoxicity and importance of periodic liver function test monitoring. Importance of immediately reporting any manifestations of hepatotoxicity (e.g., jaundice, unusually dark or "tea-colored" urine, right upper quadrant pain, fatigue, bleeding or bruising more easily than normal).

Risk of ocular effects. Importance of immediately informing clinician if ocular problems (e.g., eye pain, swelling, redness, blurred vision, other vision changes) occur.

Risk of left ventricular dysfunction; importance of immediately informing clinicians if new-onset or worsening shortness of breath, exercise intolerance, cough, fatigue, peripheral edema, palpitations, or sudden weight gain occurs.

Risk of fetal harm. Necessity of advising women of childbearing potential to use adequate methods of contraception while receiving afatinib and for at least 2 weeks after the drug is discontinued. Importance of patients informing their clinicians if they are pregnant or think they may be pregnant.

Risk of impaired female and male fertility.

Importance of advising women to avoid breast-feeding while receiving afatinib therapy and for 2 weeks after discontinuance of therapy.

Importance of informing clinicians of existing or contemplated concomitant therapy, including prescription and OTC drugs and dietary or herbal supplements, as well as any concomitant illnesses.

Importance of informing patients of other important precautionary information. (See Cautions.)

Overview® (see Users Guide). For additional information on this drug until a more detailed monograph is developed and published, the manufacturer's labeling should be consulted. It is *essential* that the manufacturer's labeling be consulted for more detailed information on usual cautions, precautions, contraindications, potential drug interactions, laboratory test interferences, and acute toxicity. For further information on the handling of antineoplastic agents, see the ASHP Guidelines on Handling Hazardous Drugs at http://www.ahfsdruginformation.com.

Preparations

Excipients in commercially available drug preparations may have clinically important effects in some individuals; consult specific product labeling for details.

Afatinib Dimaleate

Oral		
Tablets, film-coated	20 mg (of afatinib)	**Gilotrif®**, Boehringer Ingelheim
	30 mg (of afatinib)	**Gilotrif®**, Boehringer Ingelheim
	40 mg (of afatinib)	**Gilotrif®**, Boehringer Ingelheim

Aldesleukin

Interleukin-2

■ Aldesleukin, a human interleukin-2 derivative, is a biosynthetic (recombinant DNA origin) cytokine (i.e., lymphokine) with antineoplastic and immunomodulating activities.

Uses

■ **Renal Cell Cancer** ***Overview*** Aldesleukin, alone or in combination therapy, is used for the treatment of metastatic renal cell carcinoma in selected patients. There is no generally accepted standard therapy for metastatic renal cell carcinoma.

Surgery. Because of the poor response to systemic therapy, surgical resection often is included in the management of metastatic renal cell carcinoma. Nephrectomy may be performed in selected patients for palliation of symptoms and improvement in the quality of life. Selected patients with a solitary metastasis or a limited number of metastases occurring at a long interval following initial nephrectomy for renal cell carcinoma may achieve prolonged survival with surgical resection of metastases. The benefit of aggressive surgical management in patients with a solitary metastasis found at the time of diagnosis of the primary tumor is less clear; some experts state that nephrectomy and surgical resection of the metastasis provide benefit whereas others observe that outcome is poor in such patients despite surgery.

Although routine surgery to debulk tumors before systemic drug therapy generally is not advised, some evidence suggests that nephrectomy may remove immunosuppressive factors associated with tumor growth, and primary nephrectomy followed by biologic therapy may offer benefit in selected patients with metastatic renal cell carcinoma. In 2 randomized trials, median survival was prolonged in patients with metastatic renal cell cancer who underwent radical nephrectomy followed by interferon alfa compared with patients who received interferon alfa alone. Retrospective analysis of cases from a registry of patients with metastatic renal cell cancer suggests that nephrectomy followed by aldesleukin may achieve similarly prolonged survival. Aldesleukin also has been used prior to surgery in patients with metastatic renal cell cancer; complete responses to therapy have been reported in patients with metastatic renal cell carcinoma undergoing adjunctive nephrectomy (i.e., resection of primary tumor) and/or aggressive surgical resection of residual disease following major response to aldesleukin-based regimens.

Drug Therapy. Various forms of systemic drug therapy, including cytotoxic agents, hormonal agents, and biologic agents (e.g., aldesleukin, interferon alfa), have been studied in patients with metastatic renal cell carcinoma. Response rates with cytotoxic chemotherapy generally have been poor for any regimen that has been studied in adequate numbers of patients with metastatic renal cell carcinoma. Although hormonal therapy (e.g., medroxyprogesterone acetate, tamoxifen) has been studied in the treatment of metastatic renal cell carcinoma, results have been disappointing, and these agents are no longer used.

Immunotherapy with cytokines, such as aldesleukin or interferon alfa, is used for the systemic treatment of metastatic renal cell carcinoma despite low response rates. Both the likelihood and duration of response, including durable complete regression in some cases, appear to be improved compared with those observed with conventional chemotherapy. In addition, a survival benefit has been associated with interferon-alfa-containing regimens in patients with metastatic renal cell carcinoma. Thus, while response rates for this advanced cancer remain disappointing with currently employed therapy, including current aldesleukin regimens, evidence to date indicates that therapy that includes biologic response modifiers such as aldesleukin may provide an option for systemic treatment in some patients. In carefully selected patients with a major response to aldesleukin therapy, nephrectomy and/or surgical resection of residual disease following immunotherapy may prolong disease-free survival.

Whether higher response rates or more durable responses are observed in patients with metastatic renal cell carcinoma receiving immunotherapy with cytokines, such as aldesleukin, than in those receiving supportive care only has not been fully established. Results from a randomized, placebo-controlled trial showed no benefit in overall response rate, rate of durable complete response, time to disease progression, or duration of survival with use of the cytokine interferon gamma-1b for metastatic renal cell carcinoma.

Aldesleukin is labeled for use in the treatment of metastatic renal cell carcinoma based on evidence from noncomparative, phase 2 studies; aldesleukin has not been studied in placebo-controlled trials, and evidence from randomized trials comparing aldesleukin monotherapy or aldesleukin-containing regimens with other agents is limited. Antiangiogenic agents (e.g., sorafenib, sunitinib) are labeled for use in the treatment of advanced renal cell cancer. Studies are under way to establish the role of these agents in the first-line treatment of metastatic renal cell cancer. Because the current prognosis for patients with metastatic renal cell carcinoma is poor and conventional cytokine therapy has minimal activity with substantial toxicity, all patients with this cancer should be considered for inclusion in clinical trials at the time of diagnosis. Supportive care (e.g., adequate analgesia for pain management, surgery for solitary brain metastasis or spinal cord compression, radiation therapy for palliation of metastases, particularly painful bone metastases) remains a mainstay of therapy for patients with metastatic renal cell cancer.

In a phase 3 randomized, controlled trial, the use of aldesleukin as adjuvant therapy following surgical resection of stage III or IV renal cell carcinoma did not affect disease-free or overall survival. Currently, no systemic therapy has been shown to reduce the risk of relapse or prolong survival in patients with localized renal cell carcinoma at high risk of recurrence; preliminary results from a small randomized trial suggest that adjuvant therapy with ex vivo activated T cells (ALT) and high-dose cimetidine delays disease recurrence.

Monotherapy for Metastatic Renal Cell Cancer Aldesleukin is used as monotherapy for the treatment of metastatic renal cell carcinoma. During 7 phase 2 clinical trials in which 255 patients with metastatic renal cell carcinoma received courses of therapy consisting of two 5-day cycles of aldesleukin 600,000 units/kg (5 studies) or 720,000 units/kg (2 studies) given as a 15-minute IV infusion every 8 hours for up to 14 doses per cycle, objective response was observed in 15% (7% complete and 8% partial responses); all patients in these studies were asymptomatic or symptomatic but fully ambulatory (ECOG performance status 0 or 1, respectively). The 95% confidence interval for the objective response rate was 11–20%. Onset of tumor regression has been observed as early as 4 weeks after completion of the first course of treatment, and tumor regression may continue for up to 12 months following initiation of aldesleukin therapy. The median duration of objective response with aldesleukin therapy for those with partial responses is 20 months. The minimum median duration of objective response for those with complete responses is 80 months. The median duration of overall objective response (partial or complete) currently is 54 months (range: 3–131+ months). Continued follow-up shows that complete responses to aldesleukin for metastatic renal cell cancer are durable. Tumor regression was observed in both pulmonary and extrapulmonary sites (e.g., liver, lymph node, renal bed recurrences, soft tissue). Responses also were observed in patients with individual bulky lesions and large cumulative tumor burden.

Objective response rates of 0–50% have been observed in other studies of patients receiving aldesleukin alone or in combination with other agents for metastatic renal cell carcinoma; variability in response rates with aldesleukin therapy is influenced by the small number of patients in many of these studies, study selection criteria (e.g., ECOG performance status), prognostic factors (e.g., prior treatment, site of metastases), dosage schedules, and mode of administration.

Good performance status (i.e., ECOG performance status of 0 corresponding to asymptomatic patients) is associated with higher rates of response and a lower frequency of adverse effects with aldesleukin therapy in patients with metastatic renal cell carcinoma. Although reliable criteria for selecting patients most likely to benefit from cytokine therapy have not been established, prognostic factors have been identified that are associated with poor outcome despite treatment with aldesleukin and/or interferon alfa (e.g., multiple sites of metastasis, metastasis to the liver, metastasis within 1 year following diagnosis of primary tumor).

Evidence from controlled, comparative studies evaluating the efficacy of aldesleukin versus other agents in the treatment of metastatic renal cell carcinoma is limited. Although the overall response rates associated with either aldesleukin or interferon alfa monotherapy appear to be similar at about 15 and 10–15%, respectively, current evidence suggests that the incidence of complete or durable response is greater with aldesleukin therapy (5 versus 1%). However, interferon alfa therapy is less toxic than high-dose aldesleukin therapy, and 2 large randomized trials have demonstrated a survival benefit associated with interferon-alfa-containing regimens in patients with metastatic renal cell carcinoma whereas such data are lacking for aldesleukin.

Combination Therapy for Metastatic Renal Cell Cancer Aldesleukin has been used in various combination regimens with other agents, such as biologic response modifiers (e.g., interferon alfa), or adoptive immunotherapy (e.g., lymphokine-activated killer [LAK] cells, tumor-infiltrating lymphocytes [TILs]), for the treatment of metastatic renal cell carcinoma.

Aldesleukin has been used in combination with interferon alfa, another biologic response modifier, for the treatment of metastatic renal cell carcinoma. A collective response rate of about 20% (5% complete responses, 15% partial responses), similar to the overall response rate of 15% observed with aldesleukin monotherapy, has been observed in patients with metastatic renal cell carcinoma receiving aldesleukin—administered by IV bolus injection, continuous IV infusion, or subcutaneous injection—in combination with interferon alfa. Current evidence has not established whether the combination of aldesleukin and interferon alfa is superior to aldesleukin alone in patients with this cancer. A retrospective analysis indicates that similar efficacy and less toxicity are observed in patients receiving subcutaneous aldesleukin and subcutaneous interferon alfa compared with continuous IV infusion of aldesleukin alone for advanced renal cell carcinoma. In a large, randomized trial, patients receiving continuous IV infusion of aldesleukin combined with subcutaneous interferon alfa-2a had a higher response rate and higher rate of event-free survival at 1 year but no difference in overall survival compared with those receiving either agent alone; greater toxicity was observed in patients receiving aldesleukin, either alone or in combination therapy, than in those receiving interferon alfa. The low response rates observed for monotherapy with aldesleukin or interferon alfa in this trial may have contributed to the differences observed in comparison with the combination therapy.

Limited evidence from a randomized, phase 2 trial suggests that the addition of interferon alfa-2b to a high-dose, intermittent IV infusion regimen of aldesleukin did not improve response rate, and incidence of complete response and duration of response appeared to be more favorable for patients receiving high-dose aldesleukin monotherapy for advanced renal cell carcinoma. At a median follow-up of 72 months in another randomized phase 2 trial, median duration of response was longer (53 versus 14 months) and the rate of progression-free survival at 3 years was higher (13 versus 3%) for patients receiving high-dose IV aldesleukin alone compared with those receiving high-dose IV aldesleukin and IV interferon alfa-2b. In a phase 3 randomized trial, response rates were higher but there was no difference in progression-free survival or overall survival for patients receiving high-dose IV aldesleukin alone versus those receiving an outpatient regimen of subcutaneous aldesleukin and subcutaneous interferon alfa. A phase 2 randomized trial indicates that toxicity is greater but overall survival is not improved when subcutaneous interferon alfa is added to a regimen of subcutaneous aldesleukin. In a randomized trial, no survival difference was observed in patients receiving subcutaneous aldesleukin, subcutaneous interferon alfa, and oral tamoxifen versus oral tamoxifen alone. Large randomized trials comparing various regimens are needed to establish the role of combination therapy with aldesleukin and interferon alfa in patients with metastatic renal cell carcinoma.

Aldesleukin also has been used in combination with other biologic response modifiers (e.g., interferon beta), or adoptive immunotherapy (e.g., LAK cells, TILs), for the treatment of metastatic renal cell carcinoma. Current evidence suggests that the addition of interferon beta does not improve response rate or survival in patients receiving aldesleukin for advanced disease. Concomitant administration of aldesleukin and LAK cells does not provide greater benefit than aldesleukin monotherapy. Although durable antitumor responses have been reported in some patients receiving aldesleukin combined with TILs, with or without interferon alfa, a randomized, phase 3 trial did not show any benefit in response rate or survival duration with the addition of CD8$^+$-selected TILs to low-dose continuous IV infusion of aldesleukin administered following nephrectomy. Further study is needed to establish the role of combination therapy with aldesleukin and adoptive immunotherapy in patients with metastatic renal cell carcinoma.

Further study also is needed to establish the benefit of aldesleukin-containing combination regimens versus aldesleukin monotherapy. Randomized trials are needed to determine the comparative efficacy and safety of an outpatient regimen of subcutaneous aldesleukin and interferon alfa versus high-dose intravenous aldesleukin alone.

Other Considerations Despite initial response to aldesleukin, tumor relapse is common in patients with metastatic renal cell carcinoma, particularly following partial response to therapy. Treatment of relapsed disease with the same aldesleukin-based therapy that produced the initial response rarely is effective. Some secondary responses have been observed in patients receiving an aldesleukin-based regimen different from the regimen that produced the initial response.

■ **Melanoma** ***Overview*** Aldesleukin is used for the palliative treatment of metastatic melanoma in selected patients. Durable complete responses have been observed in a small percentage of patients receiving aldesleukin for metastatic melanoma, including some who have disease with poor prognostic factors (e.g., visceral metastases, ECOG performance status). Because of low response rates and substantial toxicity, use of high-dose aldesleukin therapy is restricted to carefully selected patients receiving treatment from experienced clinicians at established cancer treatment centers. Another established treatment option for patients with metastatic melanoma is dacarbazine monotherapy (see Dacarbazine 10:00). In contrast to other agents or regimens used for the treatment of metastatic melanoma, therapy with aldesleukin appears to offer more complete and durable responses, but comparative studies are lacking. Aldesleukin has been used alone and in combination† with other agents in the palliative treatment of metastatic melanoma.

Monotherapy for Metastatic Melanoma Aldesleukin is used as monotherapy for the treatment of metastatic melanoma. The indication for use of aldesleukin monotherapy for metastatic melanoma is based on evidence from uncontrolled, phase 2 studies; response rates average 16% for aldesleukin as a single agent with a complete response rate of about 6%.

The current indication for use of aldesleukin in the treatment of metastatic melanoma is based on evidence from phase 2 clinical trials in which 270 patients received courses consisting of two 5-day cycles of aldesleukin 600,000 units/kg (4 studies) or 720,000 units/kg (3 studies) given as a 15-minute IV infusion every 8 hours for up to 14 doses per cycle; additional data from a manufacturer-sponsored study involving 5 patients also were included. Objective response was observed in 16% (6% complete and 10% partial responses); all patients in these studies were asymptomatic or symptomatic but fully ambulatory (ECOG performance status 0 or 1, respectively). The 95% confidence interval for the objective response rate was 12–21%.

The median duration of objective response with aldesleukin therapy for those with partial responses is 6 months. The minimum median duration of objective response for those with complete responses is 59 months. The median duration of overall objective response (partial or complete) currently is 9 months (range: 1–122+ months). Tumor regression was observed in both visceral (e.g., lung, liver) and nonvisceral (e.g., lymph nodes, soft tissue, adrenal gland, subcutaneous tissue) sites. Responses also were observed in patients with individual bulky lesions and large cumulative tumor burden. Good performance status (i.e., ECOG performance status of 0 corresponding to asymptomatic patients) is associated with higher rates of response and a lower frequency of adverse effects with aldesleukin therapy in patients with metastatic melanoma.

Combination Therapy for Metastatic Melanoma Aldesleukin has been used in various combination regimens with other agents including biologic response modifiers (e.g., interferon alfa), adoptive immunotherapy (e.g., LAK cells, TILs), and/or conventional chemotherapeutic agents (e.g., cisplatin, dacarbazine) for the treatment of metastatic melanoma. Although higher response rates have been observed with some aldesleukin-containing combination regimens for the treatment of metastatic melanoma, improvement in survival has not been demonstrated and toxicity often is greater. The use of aldesleukin in combination with vaccines containing antigens from melanoma cells is being investigated. The role of aldesleukin in combination regimens for the treatment of metastatic melanoma remains to be established.

Regimens combining aldesleukin with other biologic response modifiers (e.g., interferon alfa) and/or conventional chemotherapeutic agents (cisplatin, dacarbazine) have been studied in randomized trials. Aldesleukin has been used in combination with interferon alfa for the treatment of metastatic melanoma. The addition of interferon alfa did not increase response rate or prolong survival in patients receiving high-dose IV aldesleukin or continuous IV infusion aldesleukin and IV cisplatin. Although favorable response rates have been reported in patients with advanced melanoma receiving aldesleukin and cisplatin in phase 2 studies, the benefit of cisplatin has not been confirmed in randomized trials. A phase 3 randomized trial showed that the addition of cisplatin increased response rate and prolonged progression-free survival but did not prolong overall survival in patients receiving aldesleukin and interferon alfa.

Aldesleukin also has been used, with or without interferon alfa, as a component of biochemotherapy regimens for metastatic melanoma. Although higher objective response rates have been reported in patients who received sequential administration of conventional chemotherapeutic agents (e.g., cisplatin alone; cisplatin and dacarbazine; carmustine, cisplatin, and dacarbazine) followed by aldesleukin with or without interferon alfa, the use of combination therapy with chemotherapy and biologic therapy has not been shown to improve survival and has been associated with substantial toxicity. Analysis of pooled data from randomized studies indicates that the addition of aldesleukin and/or interferon alfa to chemotherapy increases response rates but does not prolong survival in patients with metastatic melanoma. In a phase 3 randomized trial in patients with metastatic melanoma, the addition of biotherapy with IV aldesleukin and subcutaneous interferon alfa following chemotherapy with cisplatin, vincristine, and dacarbazine resulted in high response rates and prolonged time to progression, but there was no difference in survival and toxicity was greater with the biochemotherapy regimen. In a randomized trial, patients receiving combination chemotherapy (cisplatin, dacarbazine, and tamoxifen) followed by high-dose IV aldesleukin and subcutaneous interferon alfa-2b had increased toxicity but no improvement in survival compared with patients receiving chemotherapy alone for metastatic melanoma. In a randomized, phase 2 trial, the addition of immunotherapy with subcutaneous aldesleukin and subcutaneous interferon alfa caused immune activation but greater toxicity and no apparent difference in response rate, progression-free survival, or overall survival in patients receiving chemotherapy with carmustine, cisplatin, dacarbazine, and tamoxifen. Similarly, evidence from uncontrolled studies suggests that concomitant administration of aldesleukin and either cyclophosphamide (as an immunomodulator) or dacarbazine does not offer substantial improvement compared with aldesleukin monotherapy, although toxicity may be reduced with lower doses of aldesleukin used in these regimens.

The timing and sequence of administration of chemotherapy and biotherapy appears to affect efficacy and toxicity, and other regimens (e.g., concurrent biochemotherapy) are being investigated. In a randomized trial in patients with metastatic melanoma, there was no difference in survival for concurrent biochemotherapy with cisplatin, vinblastine, dacarbazine, aldesleukin, and interferon alfa-2b versus combination chemotherapy with cisplatin, vinblastine, and dacarbazine. In another randomized trial in patients with metastatic melanoma, there was no difference in response rates or survival when IV aldesleukin was added following a regimen of dacarbazine, cisplatin, and subcutaneous interferon alfa.

Aldesleukin also has been used in combination with adoptive immunotherapy, such as lymphokine-activated killer (LAK) cells and tumor-infiltrating lymphocytes (TILs), for the management of metastatic melanoma. Evidence to date indicates that, as in metastatic renal cell carcinoma, the efficacy of aldesleukin generally is not improved by the addition of LAK cells to the regimen. The addition of other types of adoptive immunotherapy (e.g., autologous lymphocytes activated by interleukin-2 ex vivo, tumor-infiltrating lymphocytes [TIL]) to aldesleukin for the treatment of metastatic melanoma does not substantially increase response rate or prolong survival, and these methods are associated with considerable complexity and cost compared with other aldesleukin regimens. Additional well-controlled studies are needed to define the role of aldesleukin in the management of metastatic melanoma; response rates, duration of response, toxicity, and careful study of biologic and immunologic mechanisms must be considered in establishing the optimum regimen of the drug in this disease.

Other Considerations Despite initial response to aldesleukin, tumor relapse is common in patients with metastatic melanoma, particularly following partial response to therapy. Treatment of relapsed disease with the same aldesleukin-based therapy that produced the initial response rarely is effective. Some secondary responses have been observed in patients receiving an aldesleukin-based regimen different from the regimen that produced the initial response (e.g., aldesleukin combined with tumor-infiltrating lymphocytes following initial treatment with aldesleukin monotherapy).

Dosage and Administration

■ **Reconstitution and Administration** Aldesleukin is administered by IV infusion; the drug also is administered subcutaneously†.

Aldesleukin powder for injection is reconstituted by adding 1.2 mL of sterile water for injection to a vial labeled as containing 22 million units (1.3 mg) of the drug; the resultant solution contains 18 million units (1.1 mg)/mL. Because aldesleukin is not compatible with bacteriostatic water for injection or sodium chloride injection, use of these diluents should be avoided when preparing aldesleukin solutions. During reconstitution, the water should be directed toward the side of the vial with gentle swirling, not shaking, to avoid excessive foaming of the solution. For rapid IV infusion, the appropriate dose of aldesleukin should then be withdrawn and diluted in 50 mL of 5% dextrose injection, preferably in a plastic (PVC) container, and infused over 15 minutes.

Dilution and delivery of aldesleukin solutions outside the concentration range of 30–70 mcg/mL result in decreased stability and activity of the drug, and use of such solutions for short-duration IV infusion should be avoided. The manufacturer states that a larger or smaller volume of 5% dextrose injection may be used to maintain an aldesleukin concentration of 30–70 mcg/mL.

The use of plastic rather than glass containers reportedly results in more consistent drug delivery because aldesleukin may adhere to glass. Aldesleukin solution should be brought to room temperature prior to IV infusion. Aldesleukin should not be coadministered with other drugs in the same container. **The manufacturer recommends that an inline filter *not* be used during IV administration of the drug.**

Aldesleukin solutions should be inspected visually for discoloration and particulate matter prior to administration whenever solution and container permit.

■ **Dosage** The frequency and severity of adverse effects of aldesleukin generally are dose related. Administration of doses in excess of the recommended dose has been associated with a more rapid onset of anticipated dose-limiting toxicities. Adverse effects of aldesleukin that persist following discontinuance of the drug should be monitored and managed with supportive treatment. Life-threatening toxicities of aldesleukin may be ameliorated by IV administration of dexamethasone, which also may reduce the therapeutic effect of aldesleukin.

Dosage of aldesleukin should be adjusted carefully according to patient tolerance and response. Potency of aldesleukin usually is expressed in international units (IU); because other units also have been reported (e.g., Cetus Units [CU], Roche Units [RU], Biologic Response Modifiers Program Units [BRMPU]) and are not equivalent (e.g., 1 RU = 3 IU, 1 CU = 6 IU), care should be exercised in interpreting published dosages and concentrations. In the dosage section, international units are stated as units rather than as IU in order to minimize medication errors that could have resulted from misinterpretation of written orders employing IU.

When a vial labeled as containing 22 million units of the drug is reconstituted by adding 1.2 mL of sterile water for injection, each mL contains 18 million units of aldesleukin, which is equivalent to 1.1 mg of the drug.

Renal Cell Cancer The optimum dosage and regimen for aldesleukin in the treatment of metastatic renal cell carcinoma have not been established. The course of therapy currently suggested by the manufacturer consists of two 5-day cycles of aldesleukin treatment separated by a 9-day rest period; in each cycle, aldesleukin 600,000 units/kg is given as a 15-minute IV infusion every 8 hours for 14 doses (maximum of 28 doses per course) or until intolerable adverse effects develop.

In clinical trials of high-dose intermittent IV infusion therapy with aldesleukin, individual doses frequently were withheld because of toxicity, with a median of 20 out of 28 doses per course of therapy being administered during the initial course of therapy in patients with metastatic renal cell carcinoma. In practice, greater than 90% of patients had doses of aldesleukin withheld during a course of therapy. Modification of aldesleukin dosage for toxicity should involve withholding or interrupting a dose or doses rather than reducing individual doses. The decision whether to stop, withhold, or restart aldesleukin therapy must be made after global assessment of the patient according to the guidelines outlined in the manufacturer's labeling.

Other dosage schedules and modes of administration for aldesleukin therapy, including administration by continuous IV infusion† over 24 hours and by subcutaneous injection†, have been used in patients with metastatic renal cell carcinoma. Aldesleukin frequently has been administered by continuous IV infusion† in a dosage of 18 million units/m^2 daily for two 5-day cycles, with a drug-free interval of about 5–8 days between cycles. The drug also has been administered by subcutaneousinjection† in a dosage of 18 million units daily for 5 days, followed by a 2-day rest period. For additional cycles, a dosage of 9 million units is given on days 1 and 2, followed by 18 million units daily for the next 3 days. Treatment cycles with subcutaneous therapy have been administered for 6 consecutive weeks separated by a 3-week drug-free period. Additional study is needed to determine the optimum regimen of aldesleukin for patients with metastatic renal cell carcinoma.

Because of errors in dosage calculation and reconstitution, some clinicians have used an aldesleukin dosage of 720,000 units/kg, given as a 15-minute IV infusion every 8 hours for a maximum of 15 doses per cycle, with a rest period of 10 days between the 2 cycles. Alternatively, a low-dose intermittent IV infusion regimen of aldesleukin 72,000 units/kg may be as effective as, and less toxic than, a high-dose intermittent IV infusion regimen of 720,000 units/kg in patients with metastatic renal cell carcinoma. In a randomized trial, higher response rates and trends toward more complete responses and more durable complete responses occurred with high-dose versus low-dose aldesleukin therapy, but there was no difference in overall survival. Limited evidence from a phase 2 study suggests that aldesleukin exhibits a dose-response relationship when used as a single agent for the treatment of metastatic renal cell carcinoma; longer follow-up and further study are needed to establish the effect of dose when aldesleukin is used alone or in combination regimens.

Patients should be evaluated approximately 4 weeks after completion of the initial course of high-dose intermittent IV infusion therapy with aldesleukin and again immediately prior to the scheduled start of the next course. The manufacturer states that further therapy with the drug should be undertaken only if there is some evidence of tumor *regression* following the last course and the patient has *not* developed serious toxicity that would contraindicate continuation of therapy. However, some clinicians believe that *stabilization* of disease alone in the absence of serious toxicity warrants continued therapy with aldesleukin. The manufacturer states that each treatment course should be separated by a drug-free interval of at least 7 weeks from the date of previous hospital discharge; however, some clinicians report use of shorter rest periods (i.e., 2–4 weeks) between courses of treatment with aldesleukin. While the optimum duration of aldesleukin therapy remains to be established, the manufacturer reports that tumor regression has continued for up to at least 12 months after administration of one or more courses of therapy with the drug.

Some evidence suggests that administration of aldesleukin by continuous infusion using a controlled-delivery system results in reduced potency of the drug, and some experts state that aldesleukin should not be administered by continuous IV infusion; manufacturer studies demonstrate that the physical and chemical stability of aldesleukin solutions administered by continuous IV infusion depend on specific conditions including temperature, the concentration of the solution, and the infusion device environment. Subcutaneous administration of aldesleukin, generally in dosages lower than those administered IV, may produce similar response rates but less toxicity than IV infusion; however, additional study and longer follow-up with comparative analysis of overall survival and durability of responses is needed to determine the optimum regimen of aldesleukin for patients with metastatic renal cell carcinoma.

Melanoma The optimum dosage and regimen for aldesleukin in the treatment of metastatic melanoma have not been established. The usual course of therapy consists of two 5-day cycles of aldesleukin treatment separated by a 6- to 9-day rest period; in each cycle, aldesleukin 600,000 units/kg is given as a 15-minute IV infusion every 8 hours for 14 doses (maximum of 28 doses per course) or until intolerable adverse effects develop. Because of errors in dosage calculation and reconstitution, some clinicians used an aldesleukin dosage of 720,000 units/kg, given as a 15-minute IV infusion every 8 hours for a maximum of 15 doses per cycle, with a rest period of 10 days between the 2 cycles.

In clinical trials of high-dose intermittent IV infusion therapy with aldesleukin, individual doses frequently were withheld because of toxicity, with a median of 18 doses out of 28 doses per course of therapy being administered during the initial course of therapy in patients with metastatic melanoma. In practice, greater than 90% of patients had doses of aldesleukin withheld during a course of therapy. Modification of aldesleukin dosage for toxicity should involve withholding or interrupting a dose or doses rather than reducing individual doses. The decision whether to stop, withhold, or restart aldesleukin therapy must be made after global assessment of the patient according to the guidelines outlined in the manufacturer's labeling.

Other aldesleukin dosage regimens, including continuous IV infusion† and subcutaneous administration† of aldesleukin, have been used in patients with metastatic melanoma. Some clinicians report similar efficacy but less toxicity with a low-dose intermittent IV infusion regimen of aldesleukin, but comparative studies are lacking. Therapy with lower doses of aldesleukin also is being investigated in studies of combination regimens including chemotherapy, other biologic agents, or vaccine therapy. Although these alternative methods of administering aldesleukin have been associated with reduced toxicity, further study with comparative analysis of overall survival and durability of responses is needed to establish the comparative efficacy of such regimens in patients with metastatic melanoma.

Patients should be evaluated approximately 4 weeks after completion of the initial aldesleukin course and again immediately prior to the scheduled start of the next course. The manufacturer states that further therapy with the drug should be undertaken only if there is some evidence of tumor *regression* following the last course and the patient has *not* developed serious toxicity that would contraindicate continuation of therapy. However, some clinicians believe that *stabilization* of disease alone in the absence of serious toxicity warrants continued therapy with aldesleukin. The manufacturer states that each treatment course should be separated by a drug-free interval of at least 7 weeks from the date of previous hospital discharge; clinicians report rest periods of 6–12 weeks between courses of treatment with aldesleukin. In clinical trials of aldesleukin used as a single agent for the treatment of metastatic melanoma, therapy typically was limited to 2 or 3 courses in patients experiencing a major response, and a maximum of 5 treatment courses was permitted. While the optimum duration of aldesleukin therapy remains to be established, the manufacturer reports that tumor regression has continued for up to at least 12 months after administration of one or more courses of therapy with the drug.

Dosage Modification for Toxicity and Contraindications for Continued Therapy Toxicities requiring dosage modification should involve withholding or interrupting a dose rather than reducing the individual dose to be given. Most adverse effects are self-limiting and usually reversible after discontinuance of aldesleukin, but adverse effects that persist should be managed with supportive treatment. While glucocorticoids (e.g., IV dexamethasone) have been shown to ameliorate adverse effects of aldesleukin, including fever, renal insufficiency, hyperbilirubinemia, confusion, and dyspnea, concomitant use may reduce the therapeutic effect of aldesleukin and should be avoided except under life-threatening circumstances.

Cardiac Toxicity. Aldesleukin doses should be withheld if atrial fibrillation, supraventricular tachycardia, or bradycardia requiring treatment occurs or is recurrent or persistent; doses of the drug may be administered subsequently if the patient is asymptomatic with complete recovery to normal sinus rhythm.

Aldesleukin doses should be withheld if systolic blood pressure is less than 90 mm Hg with increasing vasopressor requirements; doses of the drug may be administered subsequently if the systolic blood pressure equals or exceeds 90 mm Hg and the requirement for vasopressor therapy is stable or improving.

Aldesleukin doses should be withheld if ECG changes consistent with myocardial infarction, ischemia, or myocarditis, with or without chest pain, occur or if there is suspicion of cardiac ischemia; doses of the drug may be reinstituted subsequently if the patient is asymptomatic, myocardial infarction and myocarditis have been ruled out, the clinical suspicion of angina is minimal, or there is no evidence of ventricular hypokinesia.

Retreatment with aldesleukin is *contraindicated* in patients who developed any of the following cardiac toxicities during a previous course of therapy with the drug: sustained ventricular tachycardia (at least 5 consecutive ventricular beats) or other uncontrolled or treatment-resistant cardiac arrhythmia; chest pain with ECG abnormalities, consistent with angina or myocardial infarction; or cardiac tamponade.

Respiratory Toxicity. Aldesleukin doses should be withheld if oxygen saturation is less than 90%; doses of the drug may be administered subsequently if oxygen saturation equals or exceeds 90%.

Retreatment with aldesleukin is *contraindicated* in patients who developed respiratory dysfunction requiring intubation for longer than 72 hours during a previous course of therapy with the drug. Some clinicians advise that retreatment with aldesleukin not be undertaken in any patient who, during a previous course of therapy, developed respiratory dysfunction requiring intubation, without regard to the duration required for this treatment intervention.

Neurologic Toxicity. Aldesleukin doses should be withheld if changes in mental status, including moderate confusion or agitation, occur; doses of the drug may be administered subsequently if mental status changes resolve completely.

Retreatment with aldesleukin is *contraindicated* in patients who developed repetitive or treatment-resistant seizures, coma, or toxic psychosis persisting longer than 48 hours during a previous course of therapy with the drug.

Renal Toxicity. Aldesleukin doses should be withheld if the serum creatinine concentration equals or exceeds 4.5 mg/dL or is 4 mg/dL or greater in the presence of severe volume overload, acidosis, or hyperkalemia; doses of the drug may be administered subsequently if serum creatinine concentration is less than 4 mg/dL and fluid and electrolyte status is stable.

Aldesleukin doses should be withheld if persistent oliguria is present with urine output of less than 10 mL/hour for 16–24 hours with an increasing serum creatinine concentration; doses of the drug may be administered subsequently if urine output exceeds 10 mL/hour with a decrease in serum creatinine concentration of greater than 1.5 mg/dL or normalization of serum creatinine concentration.

Retreatment with aldesleukin is *contraindicated* in patients who developed renal dysfunction requiring dialysis for longer than 72 hours during a previous course of therapy with the drug. Some clinicians advise that retreatment with aldesleukin not be undertaken in any patient who, during a previous course of therapy, developed renal dysfunction requiring dialysis, without regard to the duration required for this treatment intervention.

Hepatic Toxicity. If signs of hepatic failure occur, including encephalopathy, increasing ascites, liver pain, or hypoglycemia, further treatment with aldesleukin for that course of therapy should be discontinued; consideration may be given to starting a new course of treatment at least 7 weeks after cessation of adverse effects (if all signs of hepatic failure have resolved) and discharge from the hospital. Some clinicians report shorter rest periods (i.e., 2–4 weeks) between courses of treatment with aldesleukin.

GI Toxicity. Aldesleukin doses should be withheld if GI bleeding demonstrated by stool guaiac test is repeatedly positive with a result greater than 3+ or 4+; doses of the drug may be administered subsequently when stool guaiac test results are negative.

Retreatment with aldesleukin is *contraindicated* in patients who developed bowel ischemia or perforation or GI bleeding requiring surgery during a previous course of therapy with the drug.

Infectious Complications. Aldesleukin doses should be withheld if sepsis syndrome occurs and the patient is clinically unstable; doses of the drug may be administered subsequently if sepsis syndrome has resolved, the patient is clinically stable, and the infection is being treated.

Dermatologic Toxicity. Aldesleukin doses should be withheld if bullous dermatitis or marked worsening of preexisting skin condition (topical steroid therapy should be avoided) occurs; doses of the drug may be administered subsequently if all signs of bullous dermatitis resolve.

Cautions

Aldesleukin is a highly toxic drug. The adverse effects of aldesleukin are frequent, often serious, and sometimes fatal. The rate of drug-related death in patients receiving single-agent therapy with aldesleukin for metastatic renal cell carcinoma or metastatic melanoma is 4% (11/255) or 2% (6/270), respectively. The frequency and severity of adverse effects generally are dose related and schedule dependent.Aldesleukin-associated adverse effects appear to be more frequent and severe with high-dose, relatively rapid IV infusion of the drug compared with low-dose, subcutaneous† administration or continuous IV infusion†. Administration of doses in excess of the recommended dose has been associated with a more rapid onset of anticipated dose-limiting toxicities. Most adverse effects of aldesleukin are self-limiting and usually (but not invariably) reverse or improve within 2 or 3 days of discontinuance of the drug because of its short half-life; adverse effects that persist should be monitored and managed with supportive treatment. Adverse effects of aldesleukin resulting in permanent sequelae include myocardial infarction, bowel perforation/infarction, and gangrene.

Data on common adverse effects of aldesleukin are derived from experience with 525 patients receiving the drug as a single agent in clinical trials, including 255 patients with metastatic renal cell carcinoma and 270 patients with metastatic melanoma. The most common adverse effects of aldesleukin include hypotension, diarrhea, renal dysfunction with oliguria, chills, and vomiting. The most frequently reported life-threatening or grade 4 adverse effects of aldesleukin include renal dysfunction with oliguria/anuria, hypotension, respiratory disorder (i.e., ARDS, respiratory failure, intubation), coma, and bilirubinemia. Many adverse effects of aldesleukin, including the most serious, are related to or result from the capillary leak syndrome caused by the drug. Additional adverse effects associated with aldesleukin have been reported in a population of 1800 patients receiving various dosing regimens of the drug (e.g., subcutaneous administration, continuous infusion, administration with LAK cells) and in patients receiving various treatment regimens that included the drug.

Morbidity and mortality associated with aldesleukin treatment of metastatic renal cell carcinoma or metastatic melanoma in clinical trials were related to the ECOG performance status of the patients. Compared with patients who had a performance status of 0, those with a performance status of 1 or higher had a higher rate of aldesleukin-related mortality and a higher incidence of serious adverse effects. Careful patient selection and evaluation and appropriate management of adverse effects can reduce the morbidity and mortality associated with aldesleukin therapy.

■ Flu-like Syndrome

A flu-like syndrome, including fever and/or chills and rigors, develops to some degree in many patients receiving aldesleukin. Chills or fever occurred in 52 or 29%, respectively, of patients with metastatic renal cell carcinoma or metastatic melanoma receiving the recommended dosing regimen of aldesleukin in clinical trials; fever was life-threatening or grade 4 in 1% of patients receiving the drug in clinical trials.Since these signs and symptoms do not occur for a few hours after administration of aldesleukin, they are believed to result from release of pyrogenic factors and/or cytokines. Chills and rigors and/or fever may be accompanied by other symptoms. Pain or abdominal pain occurred in 12 or 11% of patients, respectively; malaise or asthenia (i.e., weakness) occurred in 27 or 23%, respectively, of patients receiving the recommended dosing regimen of aldesleukin in clinical trials. Arthralgia and/or myalgia also may be associated with the syndrome. Chest pain, back pain, and fatigue have been reported in patients receiving aldesleukin.

Treatment with an antipyretic agent or a nonsteroidal anti-inflammatory agent (e.g., ibuprofen, indomethacin), beginning immediately before the initiation of aldesleukin therapy and continuing for 12 hours after the last dose of the drug, may minimize the risk of developing fever and/or its severity, as well as some of the other flu-like symptoms or acute adverse effects. In clinical trials, meperidine was administered to control the rigors associated with fever.

■ Capillary Leak Syndrome

Aldesleukin administration, particularly at dosages currently recommended by the manufacturer, is associated with capillary leak syndrome, which results in hypotension and reduced organ perfusion that may be severe and can result in death. The capillary leak syndrome begins immediately after aldesleukin treatment is initiated and is characterized by increased vascular permeability to proteins and fluids and reduction of vascular tone.

The exact mechanism of increased vascular permeability remains to be established. In most patients, a decrease in mean arterial blood pressure occurs within 2–12 hours after initiation of therapy. With continued aldesleukin treatment, patients will develop clinically important hypotension (i.e., systolic blood pressure less than 90 mm Hg or a decrease of 20 mm Hg from baseline systolic blood pressure) and hypoperfusion. In addition, extravasation of plasma proteins and fluids into the extravascular space leads to formation of edema and, in some patients, development of ascites and/or pleural or pericardial effusions.

Hypotension occurred in 71% of patients with metastatic renal cell carcinoma or metastatic melanoma receiving the recommended dosing regimen of aldesleukin in clinical trials and was life-threatening (grade 4) in 3% of patients. Peripheral edema and edema occurred in 28 and 15%, respectively, of patients receiving the recommended dosing regimen of the drug in clinical trials. Fluid retention associated with capillary leak syndrome can result in substantial increases in body weight; weight gain occurred in 16% of patients receiving the recommended dosing regimen of aldesleukin in clinical trials. Capillary leak syndrome also may be associated with cardiac arrhythmias (supraventricular and ventricular), angina, myocardial infarction, respiratory insufficiency requiring intubation, GI bleeding or infarction, renal insufficiency, and mental status changes.

The management of aldesleukin-induced capillary leak syndrome involves careful monitoring of fluid and organ perfusion status through frequent monitoring of blood pressure, heart rate, and organ function, including assessment of the patient's mental status and urine output. Hypovolemia should be assessed by catheterization and central venous pressure monitoring; administration of IV fluids (e.g., colloid replacement fluids) is recommended for the treatment of hypovolemia. While large volumes of IV fluids may be required to correct hypovolemia, caution is necessary since unrestrained fluid administration may exacerbate complications associated with edema or effusions. Flexibility in fluid and vasopressor management is essential for maintaining organ perfusion and blood pressure; therefore, extreme caution should be used when treating patients with fixed requirements for large volumes of fluid (e.g., those with hypercalcemia). Management of edema and ascites and/or effusions depends on careful balancing of fluid shifts so that the consequences of hypovolemia (e.g., impaired organ perfusion) or fluid accumulation (e.g., pulmonary edema) do not exceed the patient's tolerance.

Based on clinical experience, early administration of IV dopamine 1–5 mcg/kg per minute to patients with manifestations of capillary leak syndrome, before the onset of hypotension, can help maintain organ perfusion, particularly renal perfusion, and thereby preserve urine output. Body weight and urine output should be closely monitored. If blood pressure and organ perfusion are not sustained by the initial dosage of IV dopamine, an increase in the dosage to 6–10 mcg/kg per minute may be beneficial; alternatively, IV phenylephrine hydrochloride 1–5 mcg/kg per minute may be added to the low-dose dopamine infusion. However, caution is required since the prolonged use of vasopressors, alone or in combination, at relatively high doses may be associated with cardiac rhythm disturbances. If adequate organ perfusion is not maintained, as demonstrated by altered mental status, decreased urine output, a decrease in systolic blood pressure to less than 90 mm Hg, or the onset of cardiac arrhythmias, subsequent doses of aldesleukin should be withheld until recovery of organ perfusion and an increase in systolic blood pressure to greater than 90 mm Hg are observed.

Recovery from capillary leak syndrome begins soon after discontinuance of aldesleukin therapy. Usually within a few hours, blood pressure increases, organ perfusion is restored, and reabsorption of extravasated fluid and protein begins. After blood pressure normalizes, administration of diuretics may hasten recovery in patients who experienced excessive weight gain or edema, particularly if these signs are associated with shortness of breath from pulmonary congestion.

■ Cardiovascular Effects Hypotension as a consequence of the capillary leak syndrome is among the most frequent serious adverse effects of aldesleukin, particularly at dosages currently recommended by the manufacturer, and occurs in most patients receiving the drug. (See Cautions: Capillary Leak Syndrome.) Aldesleukin also is associated with a variety of adverse cardiac effects including arrhythmias, myocardial ischemia or infarction, myocarditis, and angina, which appear to result at least in part from the capillary leak syndrome.

Among patients with metastatic renal cell carcinoma or metastatic melanoma receiving the recommended dosing regimen of aldesleukin, tachycardia, occurred in 23% of patients; vasodilation, supraventricular tachycardia, cardiovascular disorder (i.e., fluctuations in blood pressure, asymptomatic ECG changes, congestive heart failure), and arrhythmia occurred in 13, 12, 11, and 10% of patients, respectively. Myocardial infarction and cardiac arrest each occurred in 1% of patients with metastatic renal cell carcinoma or metastatic melanoma receiving the recommended dosing regimen of aldesleukin in clinical trials, and myocardial ischemia occurred in less than 1% of patients. In an additional population of more than 1800 patients receiving various dosing regimens of aldesleukin, fatal myocardial infarction or fatal cardiac arrest occurred in less than 1% of patients. Life-threatening (or grade 4) supraventricular tachycardia, cardiovascular disorder (i.e., fluctuations in blood pressure), or ventricular tachycardia, occurred in 1% of patients with metastatic renal cell carcinoma or metastatic melanoma receiving the recommended dosing regimen of aldesleukin™her adverse cardiovascular effects described as grade 4 or life-threatening in severity, including shock, bradycardia, ventricular extrasystoles, syncope, atrial arrhythmia, phlebitis, second-degree AV block, endocarditis, pericardial effusion, peripheral gangrene, thrombosis, and coronary artery disorder, each were reported in less than 1% of such patients.

Other serious adverse cardiovascular effects, including pericarditis and myocarditis, have been reported in patients receiving various dosing regimens of aldesleukin. Hypertension, cardiomyopathy, and fatal endocarditis each has been reported in patients receiving various treatment regimens that included aldesleukin. Other adverse cardiovascular effects that have been reported in patients receiving aldesleukin include ventricular premature complexes, and atrial premature complexes.

■ Respiratory Effects Dyspnea and lung disorder (i.e., physical findings associated with pulmonary congestion, rales, and rhonchi) are among the most frequent serious adverse effects of aldesleukin, occurring in 43 and 24%, respectively, of patients with metastatic renal cell carcinoma or metastatic melanoma receiving the recommended dosing regimen of the drug in clinical trials. Respiratory disorder, including acute respiratory distress syndrome (ARDS), infiltrates on chest radiograph, or unspecified pulmonary changes, occurred in 11% of patients. These and other adverse respiratory effects of the drug are often associated with the capillary leak syndrome. Pleural effusion may result from accumulation of extravascular fluid caused by aldesleukin-induced capillary leak syndrome.

Life-threatening (or grade 4) respiratory disorder (i.e., ARDS, respiratory failure, intubation), dyspnea, and apnea, have been reported in 3, 1, and 1%, respectively, of patients with metastatic renal cell carcinoma or metastatic melanoma receiving the recommended dosing regimen of aldesleukin; other adverse respiratory effects described as grade 4 or life-threatening in severity, including respiratory acidosis, pulmonary edema, hyperventilation, hypoxia, hemoptysis,hypoventilation, or pneumothorax, each have been reported in less than 1% of such patients. In an additional population of more than 1800 patients receiving various dosing regimens of aldesleukin, fatal pulmonary effects, including pulmonary edema, respiratory arrest, respiratory failure, or pulmonary emboli resulting in death, occurred in less than 1% of patients.

Cough increase and rhinitis occurred in 11 and 10%, respectively, of patients receiving the recommended dosing regimen of aldesleukin in clinical trials. Other serious adverse respiratory effects include tracheoesophageal fistula, reported in patients receiving various dosing regimens of aldesleukin, and pneumonia (bacterial, fungal, viral), reported in patients receiving various treatment regimens that included aldesleukin. Other adverse respiratory effects reported in patients receiving aldesleukin include tachypnea and wheezing.

■ Nervous System Effects Onset of neurologic effects, including changes in mental status, speech difficulties, cortical blindness, limb or gait ataxia, hallucinations, agitation, obtundation, and coma, has been reported following aldesleukin therapy in patients without CNS metastases. Radiologic findings in patients receiving aldesleukin include multiple and, less commonly, single cortical lesions on MRI and evidence of demyelination. Neurologic manifestations associated with aldesleukin usually are reversible with discontinuance of the drug; however, permanent neurologic defects have been reported. At least one case of possible cerebral vasculitis, responsive to dexamethasone, has been reported in a patient receiving aldesleukin.

Changes in mental status (e.g., lethargy, somnolence, confusion, agitation), which are among the most frequent and serious adverse effects of aldesleukin, may be associated with capillary leak syndrome. Confusion occurred in 34% of patients with metastatic renal cell carcinoma or metastatic melanoma receiving the recommended dosing regimen of aldesleukin in clinical trials and was life-threatening or grade 4 in 1% of patients; somnolence was reported in 22% of patients and was life-threatening or grade 4 in less than 1% of patients. Life-threatening or grade 4 adverse nervous system effects, such as coma, stupor, and psychosis, occurred in 2, 1, and 1% of patients, respectively. Life-threatening (or grade 4) agitation, neuropathy, paranoid reaction, seizure, tonic-clonic (grand mal) seizure, or delirium each occurred in less than 1% of patients receiving aldesleukin in clinical trials. Limited data in patients receiving aldesleukin concomitantly with lymphokine-activated killer (LAK) cells suggest that changes in mental status appear to be dose related and tend to occur toward the end of a treatment course. These changes generally are reversible within several days after aldesleukin treatment is discontinued, but occasionally may worsen immediately after cessation of therapy; severe changes may persist longer and require temporary treatment with antipsychotic drugs.

Anxiety and dizziness occurred in 12 and 11%, respectively, of patients with metastatic renal cell carcinoma or metastatic melanoma receiving the recommended dosing regimen of aldesleukin in clinical trials. In an additional population of more than 1800 patients receiving various dosing regimens of aldesleukin, fatal stroke occurred in less than 1% of patients. Other serious adverse nervous system effects reported in patients receiving various dosing regimens of aldesleukin include transient ischemic attacks, meningitis, and cerebral edema; severe depression leading to suicide occurred in less than 1% of patients.

Cerebral lesions, cerebral hemorrhage, encephalopathy, extrapyramidal syndrome, neuralgia, neuritis, neuropathy (i.e., demyelination), and insomnia have been reported in patients receiving various treatment regimens that included aldesleukin. Other adverse neurologic effects reported in patients receiving aldesleukin include headache, sensory dysfunction, and motor dysfunction.

■ Renal and Electrolyte Effects Renal dysfunction with oliguria is one of the most frequent serious adverse effects of aldesleukin, occurring in 63% of patients with metastatic renal cell carcinoma or metastatic melanoma receiving the recommended dosing regimen of the drug in clinical trials; life-threatening or grade 4 oliguria occurred in 6% of patients. Anuria occurred in less than 10% of patients receiving aldesleukin in clinical trials, and life-threatening or grade 4 anuria occurred in 5% of patients. Renal insufficiency may be associated with capillary leak syndrome in patients receiving aldesleukin.Increased serum creatinine concentrations occurred in 33% of patients receiving the recommended dosing regimen of the drug in clinical trials and were life-threatening or grade 4 in 1% of all patients. Grade 4 or life-threatening acute kidney failure occurred in 1% of patients receiving aldesleukin in clinical trials. Increased BUN, increased nonprotein nitrogen (NPN), abnormal kidney function, kidney failure, or acute tubular necrosis was reported as life-threatening or grade 4 in less than 1% of patients receiving aldesleukin in clinical trials. In an additional population of more than 1800 patients receiving various dosing regimens of aldesleukin, renal failure resulting in death occurred in less than 1% of patients.

Other adverse renal effects reported in patients receiving aldesleukin include proteinuria, hematuria, dysuria, renal impairment requiring dialysis, urinary retention, and urinary frequency. Allergic interstitial nephritis has been reported in patients receiving various dosing regimens of aldesleukin.

Aldesleukin-induced renal dysfunction resolves in most patients within 1–2 weeks after discontinuance of the drug, but in some patients recovery may be more prolonged and/or incomplete. Preexisting renal impairment appears to be associated with an increased risk of more severe and prolonged renal dysfunction.

Various electrolyte disturbances may occur in patients receiving aldesleukin. Hypomagnesemia and hypocalcemia occurred in 12 and 11%, respectively, of patients with metastatic renal cell carcinoma or metastatic melanoma receiving the recommended dosing regimen of the drug in clinical trials; grade 4 or life-threatening hypocalcemia occurred in less than 1% of patients. Although intravenous administration of calcium chloride to correct low serum concentrations of ionized calcium has been reported in several patients receiving high-dose intravenous aldesleukin, the intended effects of such treatment on hemodynamic parameters (i.e., mean arterial pressure, systemic vascular resistance) were inconsistent; low serum concentrations of calcium are associated with elevated serum concentrations of parathyroid hormone, which may contribute to the hypotensive effect of aldesleukin therapy. Other electrolyte disturbances reported in patients receiving aldesleukin include hypophosphatemia, hypokalemia, hyponatremia, hyperkalemia, hypercalcemia, hypernatremia, and hyperphosphatemia.

■ **GI Effects** Diarrhea and vomiting occurred in 67 and 50%, respectively, of patients with metastatic renal cell carcinoma or metastatic melanoma receiving the recommended dosing regimen of aldesleukin in clinical trials; grade 4 or life-threatening diarrhea or vomiting were reported in 2 or 1% of all patients, respectively. Nausea or nausea and vomiting occurred in 35 or 19%, respectively, of patients in clinical trials; nausea and vomiting were described as grade 4 or life-threatening in less than 1% of all patients in clinical trials. Stomatitis and anorexia have been reported in 22 and 20%, respectively, of patients receiving the recommended dosing regimen of aldesleukin in clinical trials; stomatitis was described as grade 4 or life-threatening in less than 1% of patients.

GI bleeding or infarction may be associated with capillary leak syndrome in patients receiving aldesleukin; grade 4 or life-threatening GI hemorrhage occurred in less than 1% of patients receiving the recommended dosing regimen of aldesleukin in clinical trials. Adverse GI effects described as grade 4 or life-threatening in severity, including hematemesis, bloody diarrhea, GI disorder, intestinal perforation, or pancreatitis, each were reported in less than 1% of patients receiving aldesleukin in clinical trials. In an additional population of more than 1800 patients receiving various dosing regimens of aldesleukin, other serious adverse GI effects, including duodenal ulceration, and bowel necrosis, have been reported. Intestinal perforation resulting in death has occurred in less than 1% of patients receiving various dosing regimens of aldesleukin.

Other adverse GI effects reported in patients receiving aldesleukin include taste disorders, dyspepsia, and constipation. Colitis, gastritis, intestinal obstruction, and retroperitoneal hemorrhage have been reported in patients receiving various treatment regimens that included aldesleukin. Exacerbation of quiescent Crohn's disease, requiring surgical intervention, has been reported rarely in patients with metastatic renal cell carcinoma following treatment with aldesleukin.

Enlarged abdomen occurred in 10% of patients with metastatic renal cell carcinoma or metastatic melanoma receiving the recommended dosing regimen of aldesleukin in clinical trials.

■ **Hepatic and Biliary Effects** Adverse hepatic effects occur in many patients receiving aldesleukin, perhaps in part because the drug causes substantial, reversible intrahepatic cholestasis. Increased serum concentrations of bilirubin and AST have been reported in 40 and 23%, respectively, of patients with metastatic renal cell carcinoma or metastatic melanoma receiving recommended dosing regimens of aldesleukin in clinical trials; bilirubinemia and increased serum AST concentrations were described as grade 4 or life-threatening in 2 and 1%, respectively, of patients receiving aldesleukin in clinical trials. Increased serum alkaline phosphatase concentration was reported in 10% and described as grade 4 or life-threatening in less than 1% of patients receiving the recommended dosing regimen of aldesleukin in clinical trials. Ascites may result from accumulation of extravascular fluid caused by aldesleukin-induced capillary leak syndrome. Abnormal liver function tests have been reported in less than 1% of patients with metastatic renal cell carcinoma or metastatic melanoma receiving the recommended dosing regimen of the drug in clinical trials.

Adverse hepatic effects generally have been reversible within 5–7 days after discontinuance of aldesleukin therapy. Liver failure resulting in death was reported in less than 1% of patients receiving the drug in various dosing regimens. Jaundice also has been reported in patients receiving aldesleukin. Cholecystitis, hepatitis, and hepatosplenomegaly have been reported in patients receiving various treatment regimens that included aldesleukin.

■ **Dermatologic Effects** The most common adverse dermatologic effects of aldesleukin are rash and pruritus, which occurred in 42 and 24%, respectively, of patients with metastatic renal cell carcinoma or metastatic melanoma receiving the recommended dosing regimen of the drug in clinical trials. Exfoliative dermatitis has been reported in 18% of patients receiving the recommended dosing regimen of the drug in clinical trials.

Erythema has been reported in patients receiving aldesleukin. Aldesleukin-induced dermatologic toxicity commonly is manifested as macular erythema and usually is localized to the head and neck, but occasionally may be generalized. Generalized erythroderma, which has been reported to be dose dependent, may be followed by desquamation within 48–72 hours after drug discontinuance; resolution of these skin changes may require several weeks. Erythrodermic psoriatic exacerbation and localized flare of psoriasis in patients with a history of the disease have been reported during aldesleukin therapy. Persistent but nonprogressive vitiligo has occurred in patients with malignant melanoma treated with the drug. Other adverse dermatologic effects reported in patients receiving aldesleukin include dry skin, purpura or petechiae, and alopecia. Urticaria has been reported in patients receiving aldesleukin or various treatment regimens that included aldesleukin. See Cautions: Sensitivity, Immunologic, and Inflammatory Reactions.

■ **Local Effects** Injection site reactions have been reported in patients receiving the recommended dosing regimen of aldesleukin in clinical trials. Subcutaneous administration of aldesleukin has been commonly associated with the development of nodules or indurations at the injection site. These nodules reportedly are transient and usually disappear within a few months following discontinuance of therapy. The manufacturer states that application of cold compresses to the injection site prior to and following subcutaneous administration of the drug may be used to help reduce pain and swelling. If cold compresses are not effective, moist heat or warm packs may be applied to the injection site before subcutaneous administration of the drug. Cellulitis and injection site necrosis have been reported in patients receiving various treatment regimens that included aldesleukin.

■ **Sensitivity, Immunologic, and Inflammatory Reactions** ***Sensitivity Reactions*** Nonanaphylactic allergic reactions have been reported in patients receiving the recommended dosing regimen of aldesleukin in clinical trials. Treatment with aldesleukin or other interleukin-2 preparations may predispose individuals to acute, atypical adverse reactions to iodinated radiographic contrast media. Approximately 13% of patients (range: 11–28%) receiving various treatment regimens containing interleukin-2 (e.g., aldesleukin) experienced reactions with subsequent administration of iodinated radiographic contrast media, including fever, chills, nausea, vomiting, diarrhea, pruritus, rash, hypotension, edema, and oliguria. (See Drug Interactions: Roentgenographic Agents.) Anaphylaxis has been reported in patients receiving various treatment regimens that included aldesleukin.

Autoimmunity and Inflammatory Reactions Aldesleukin, used alone or in combination with interferon alfa (see Drug Interactions: Interferon Alfa), has been associated with the development or exacerbation of autoimmune disease and inflammatory disorders. Exacerbation of Crohn's disease, scleroderma, thyroiditis, inflammatory arthritis, diabetes mellitus, oculo-bulbar myasthenia gravis, crescentic IgA glomerulonephritis, cholecystitis, cerebral vasculitis, Stevens-Johnson syndrome, or bullous pemphigoid has been reported following aldesleukin therapy. Onset of symptomatic hyperglycemia and/or diabetes has been reported during aldesleukin therapy.

Hypothyroidism, sometimes preceded by hyperthyroidism, has been reported following treatment with aldesleukin, and some patients required thyroid hormone replacement therapy. Hyperthyroidism also has been reported in patients receiving various treatment regimens that included aldesleukin. Aldesleukin-associated changes in thyroid function may be a manifestation of autoimmunity. (See Cautions: Precautions and Contraindications.)

Antibody Formation In patients with metastatic renal cell carcinoma or metastatic melanoma who received the recommended dosing regimen of aldesleukin in clinical trials, 74 or 66%, respectively, developed low titers of non-neutralizing anti-interleukin-2 antibodies. Although neutralizing antibodies were not detected in these patients, they have been detected in 1/106 patients (less than 1%) treated with IV aldesleukin in a wide variety of dosing regimens. The clinical importance of anti-interleukin-2 antibodies is not known.

■ **Infectious Complications** Aldesleukin therapy is associated with impaired neutrophil function (decreased chemotaxis) and an increased risk of disseminated infection (most frequently *Staphylococcus aureus* infection), including sepsis and bacterial endocarditis. (See Cautions: Precautions and Contraindications.) Infections, including infections involving the urinary tract, injection site, indwelling catheter tips, or phlebitis or sepsis, occurred in 13% of patients receiving the recommended dosing regimen of the drug for metastatic renal cell carcinoma or metastatic melanoma in clinical trials and were life-threatening or grade 4 in 1% of patients. Life-threatening sepsis has been reported in 1% of patients receiving aldesleukin in clinical trials. Disseminated infections acquired during aldesleukin therapy contribute substantially to treatment-related morbidity. Antibiotic prophylaxis and aggressive treatment of suspected and documented infections may reduce the morbidity of aldesleukin treatment.

■ **Hematologic Effects** Thrombocytopenia occurred in 37% of patients and was described as grade 4 or life-threatening in severity in 1% of patients with metastatic renal cell carcinoma or metastatic melanoma receiving the recommended dosing regimen of aldesleukin in clinical trials. Anemia and leukopenia occurred in 29 and 16%, respectively, of patients receiving the drug in clinical trials; grade 4 or life-threatening anemia or leukopenia were each reported in less than 1% of patients. Grade 4 or life-threatening coagulation disorder (i.e., intravascular coagulopathy) has been reported in 1% of patients receiving the recommended dosing regimen of aldesleukin in clinical trials. Packed red blood cell and/or platelet transfusions may be necessary in patients receiving the drug. Grade 4 or life-threatening hemorrhage has been reported in less than 1% of patients receiving the recommended dosing regimen of aldesleukin in clinical trials.

Grade 4 or life-threatening leukocytosis occurred in less than 1% of patients receiving the recommended dosing regimen of aldesleukin in clinical trials. Eosinophilia has been reported in patients receiving aldesleukin. Neutropenia has been reported in patients receiving various treatment regimens that included aldesleukin.

■ **Musculoskeletal Effects** Arthralgia and myalgia may be associated with a flu-like syndrome (see Cautions: Flu-like Syndrome) that occurs in patients receiving aldesleukin. Exacerbation or initial presentation of inflammatory arthritis has been reported in patients receiving aldesleukin. Rhabdomyolysis, myopathy, and myositis have been reported in patients receiving various treatment regimens that included aldesleukin. Muscle spasm also has been reported in patients receiving aldesleukin.

■ **Ocular Effects** Optic neuritis resulting in transient or permanent blindness has been reported in patients receiving various dosing regimens of the drug in clinical trials. Mydriasis and pupillary disorder described as grade 4 in severity occurred in less than 1% of patients with metastatic renal cell carcinoma or metastatic melanoma receiving the recommended dosing regimen of aldesleukin in clinical trials. Conjunctivitis has been reported in patients receiving aldesleukin.

■ **Endocrine and Metabolic Effects** Thyroid dysfunction, usually hypothyroidism, sometimes preceded by hyperthyroidism, has been reported in patients receiving aldesleukin. Symptoms of thyroid dysfunction usually have developed within 2 months of initiation of aldesleukin treatment. Some patients have required thyroid hormone replacement therapy. Aldesleukin-associated changes in thyroid function may be a manifestation of autoimmunity. (See Cautions: Precautions and Contraindications.)

Plasma concentrations of cortisol, corticotropin, β-endorphin, epinephrine, and norepinephrine have been reported to be increased during aldesleukin treatment. Adrenal hemorrhage leading to acute adrenal insufficiency during aldesleukin therapy was reported in a patient with renal cell carcinoma with preexisting adrenal metastases.

Metabolic disturbances may occur in patients receiving aldesleukin. Onset of symptomatic hyperglycemia and/or diabetes has been reported during aldesleukin therapy and may be a manifestation of autoimmunity. Acidosis occurred in 12% and was described as grade 4 or life-threatening in severity in 1% of patients with metastatic renal cell carcinoma or metastatic melanoma receiving the recommended dosing regimen of aldesleukin in clinical trials. Grade 4 or life-threatening hyperuricemia has been reported in less than 1% of patients receiving aldesleukin in clinical trials. Other metabolic disturbances reported in patients receiving aldesleukin include hypoalbuminemia, hypoproteinemia, alkalosis, hypoglycemia, and hypocholesterolemia. Rapid and marked reductions in plasma concentrations of ascorbic acid, which appears to be required for optimum cell-mediated immunity, have been reported during adoptive immunotherapy with aldesleukin and lymphokine-activated killer (LAK) cells; ascorbic acid concentrations became undetectable in some patients, and return of these values toward normal was more rapid in patients who had higher baseline ascorbic acid concentrations and who responded to aldesleukin–LAK therapy.

Weight loss of 10% of body weight or greater has been reported in patients receiving the recommended dosing regimen of aldesleukin in clinical trials. Grade 4 or life-threatening hypothermia occurred in less than 1% of patients with metastatic renal cell carcinoma or metastatic melanoma receiving the recommended dosing regimen of aldesleukin in clinical trials. Fatal malignant hyperthermia was reported in less than 1% of patients receiving various dosing regimens of the drug.

■ **Precautions and Contraindications** Because the adverse effects of aldesleukin are frequent, often serious, and sometimes fatal, the potential benefit of the drug to the patient must be weighed carefully against the possible risks involved. The manufacturer states that aldesleukin should be administered in a hospital setting under the supervision of a qualified physician who is experienced in the use of this agent and only when the possible benefits are thought to outweigh the possible risks. In addition, intensive care facilities and specialists in cardiopulmonary or intensive care medicine must be readily available in case certain serious aldesleukin-induced toxicities develop (e.g., capillary leak syndrome and associated cardiac, cardiovascular, pulmonary, and other effects).

Because aldesleukin is a highly toxic drug, careful patient selection, including assessment of cardiac and pulmonary functions, blood chemistry, and blood cell counts, is mandatory prior to initiation of therapy with the drug. Serious, life-threatening, or fatal adverse effects associated with aldesleukin therapy may occur in patients with normal cardiovascular, pulmonary, hepatic, or CNS function. The use of aldesleukin is contraindicated in patients with substantial cardiac, pulmonary, hepatic, renal, or CNS impairment. Treatment with the drug should be limited to patients with normal cardiac and pulmonary functions as determined by thallium stress test and pulmonary function tests, respectively. Patients are eligible for treatment with the drug if their serum creatinine concentration does not exceed 1.5 mg/dL. The performance status of patients also should be considered; experience with aldesleukin in patients with a relatively poor performance status (i.e., an ECOG performance status greater than 1) is extremely limited. Prior to the initiation of aldesleukin therapy and at daily intervals during administration of the drug, hematologic tests (including complete blood count and differential and platelet counts), blood chemistries (including serum electrolyte concentrations and renal and hepatic function tests), and chest radiographs should be performed.

During aldesleukin therapy, vital signs (i.e., temperature, pulse, blood pressure, respiration rate) should be monitored at least every 4 hours and the patient's weight and fluid intake and output should be monitored daily. If systolic blood pressure is decreased, especially to less than 90 mm Hg, constant cardiac rhythm monitoring should be performed. If an abnormal complex or cardiac rhythm occurs, an ECG should be performed. In hypotensive patients, vital signs should be monitored hourly.

Because renal and hepatic function are impaired with aldesleukin therapy, concomitant administration of known nephrotoxic (e.g., aminoglycosides, indomethacin) or hepatotoxic (e.g., methotrexate, asparaginase) drugs may further increase renal or hepatic toxicity, respectively. In addition, decreased renal or hepatic function resulting from aldesleukin therapy may result in delayed elimination of concomitantly administered drugs and increase the risk of toxicity from such drugs. Similarly, concomitant administration of drugs with known cardiotoxic or myelotoxic effects may increase the risk of cardiotoxicity or myelotoxicity, respectively. Safety and efficacy of aldesleukin used in combination with chemotherapeutic agents have not been established. Concomitant administration of β-blocking agents or other antihypertensive agents may potentiate aldesleukin-induced hypotension.

All patients should be thoroughly evaluated and treated for CNS metastases and have a negative CT scan prior to receiving therapy with aldesleukin. New neurologic manifestations and anatomic lesions have been reported following aldesleukin therapy in patients without evidence of CNS metastases. (See Cautions: Nervous System Effects.) Neurologic manifestations associated with aldesleukin usually are reversible with discontinuation of the drug; however, permanent neurologic defects have been reported. In addition, since aldesleukin may cause seizures, the drug should be used with extreme caution in patients with a history of seizure disorder.

Clinicians should keep in mind that mental status changes occurring in patients receiving aldesleukin may be a direct result of CNS toxicity caused by the drug or may be indicative of bacteremia or early bacterial sepsis, hypoperfusion, or occult CNS malignancy. If mental status changes are caused by aldesleukin, they generally reverse within several days after discontinuance of the drug, although they may progress for several days before recovery begins. Rarely, patients have experienced permanent neurologic deficits associated with use of aldesleukin. Aldesleukin therapy should be withheld in patients developing moderate to severe lethargy or somnolence; continued administration of the drug may result in coma. Because aldesleukin can affect CNS function, concomitant administration of drugs that affect the CNS (e.g., opioids, antiemetics, anxiolytics) may increase the risk of CNS effects.

The manufacturer recommends that baseline pulmonary function tests with measurement of arterial blood gases be performed in patients receiving aldesleukin. Adequate pulmonary function (FEV_1 greater than 2 L or exceeding 75% of the predicted value based on height and age) should be documented prior to initiation of therapy with the drug. During treatment, pulmonary function should be monitored regularly by clinical examination, assessment of vital signs, and pulse oximetry. Patients with dyspnea or clinical signs of respiratory impairment (i.e., tachypnea or rales) should be further evaluated with arterial blood gas determinations performed as often as is clinically indicated.

According to the manufacturer, a stress thallium study should be performed in all patients prior to initiation of aldesleukin therapy to document that cardiac ejection fraction is normal and myocardial wall motion is unimpaired. If results of the stress thallium test suggest minor wall motion abnormalities, further testing is suggested to exclude clinically important coronary artery disease. During therapy with aldesleukin, cardiac function should be assessed daily by clinical examination and evaluation of vital signs. Patients with signs or symptoms of chest pain, murmurs, gallops, irregular cardiac rhythm, or palpitation should be further assessed with an ECG examination and evaluation of cardiac enzymes (e.g., determination of serum creatine phosphokinase [CPK] concentration). Evidence of myocardial injury, including findings compatible with myocardial infarction or myocarditis, has been reported in patients receiving aldesleukin. Ventricular hypokinesia caused by myocarditis may persist for several months. If there is evidence of cardiac ischemia or congestive heart failure, aldesleukin therapy should be withheld, and a repeat thallium study should be performed. Aldesleukin should be used with extreme caution in patients with normal thallium stress tests and pulmonary function tests who have a history of prior cardiac or pulmonary disease.

Because aldesleukin treatment is associated with impaired neutrophil function and an increased risk of disseminated infection, including sepsis and bacterial endocarditis, preexisting bacterial infections should be adequately treated prior to initiation of therapy with the drug. In addition, patients with indwelling central catheters should receive prophylaxis with anti-infectives effective against gram-positive microorganisms, particularly *Staphylococcus aureus* (e.g., oxacillin, nafcillin, ciprofloxacin, vancomycin). Such prophylactic regimens have been associated with a reduced incidence of staphylococcal infections in aldesleukin-treated patients. Anti-infective prophylaxis and aggressive treatment of suspected and documented infections may reduce the morbidity of aldesleukin treatment.

Use of aldesleukin, alone or in combination with interferon, may exacerbate preexisting autoimmune disease or inflammatory disorder and also has been associated with the initial presentation of such conditions. (See Autoimmunity and Inflammatory Reactions in Cautions: Sensitivity, Immunologic, and Inflammatory Reactions.) Hypothyroidism, sometimes preceded by hyperthyroidism, has been reported following treatment with aldesleukin, and some patients required thyroid hormone replacement therapy. Changes in thyroid function may be a manifestation of autoimmunity.

Because aldesleukin enhances cellular immune function, the drug may increase the risk of allograft rejection in transplant patients.

Patients receiving aldesleukin experience fever, chills, rigors, pruritus, and/or adverse GI effects, and medical intervention and management of these effects may be beneficial. Administration of standard antipyretic therapy, including a nonsteroidal anti-inflammatory agent (NSAIA), beginning immediately prior to initiation of aldesleukin therapy may reduce fever. Meperidine has been used to control rigors. Histamine H_2-receptor antagonists have been administered for prophylaxis of GI irritation and bleeding, and antiemetics and antidiarrheals have been administered as needed for nausea and diarrhea, respectively. In clinical trials, these medications generally were discontinued 12 hours after the last dose of aldesleukin.Antipruritics (e.g., hydroxyzine) or histamine H_1-receptor antagonists (e.g., diphenhydramine) have been used to control symptoms from pruritic rash and were continued until the condition resolved. Topical creams and ointments may be applied as needed for the symptomatic treatment of aldesleukin-associated skin manifestations; preparations containing a steroid (e.g., hydrocortisone) should be avoided.

Toxicities requiring dosage modification should involve withholding or interrupting a dose of aldesleukin rather than reducing the individual dose to be given. Further therapy with aldesleukin is contraindicated in patients who developed certain toxicities during a previous course of therapy with the drug. (See Dosage Modification for Toxicity and Contraindications for Continued Therapy in Dosage under Dosage and Administration.)

Aldesleukin is contraindicated in patients with a known history of hypersensitivity to interleukin-2 or any component of the formulation. The drug also is contraindicated in patients with an abnormal thallium stress test or pulmonary function test results and in those with organ allografts.

■ **Pediatric Precautions** Safety and efficacy of aldesleukin in children younger than 18 years of age have not been established.

■ **Geriatric Precautions** Safety and efficacy of aldesleukin in geriatric patients have not been studied specifically to date. Twenty-seven patients aged 65 years and older participated in clinical trials of aldesleukin (19 with metastatic renal cell carcinoma and 8 with melanoma). Response rates and median number of courses of therapy were similar between geriatric and younger patients; a trend toward an increased incidence of severe urogenital toxicity and dyspnea was observed among geriatric patients.

Aldesleukin is metabolized principally in the kidney; because geriatric patients may have decreased renal function and because patients with renal impairment may be at increased risk of aldesleukin-induced toxicity, patients in this age group should be monitored closely and dosage adjusted accordingly (see Dosage Modification for Toxicity and Contraindications for Continued Therapy in Dosage under Dosage and Administration).

■ **Mutagenicity and Carcinogenicity** Studies to determine the mutagenic or carcinogenic potential of aldesleukin have not been performed to date.

■ **Pregnancy, Fertility, and Lactation** Although there are no adequate and controlled studies to date in humans, aldesleukin has been shown to have embryolethal effects in rats when given in doses 27 to 36 times the usual human dose. Significant maternal toxicity was observed in pregnant rats receiving aldesleukin by IV injection during a critical period of organogenesis at doses 2.1 to 36 times higher than the usual human dose; no evidence of teratogenicity was observed other than that attributed to maternal toxicity. Aldesleukin should be used during pregnancy only when the potential benefits justify the possible risks to the fetus.

Studies to determine the effects of aldesleukin on fertility have not been performed to date, and it also is not known whether the drug can affect reproductive capacity. It is recommended that aldesleukin not be administered to fertile individuals of either gender who are not practicing effective contraception.

It is not known whether aldesleukin is distributed into human milk. Because of the potential for serious adverse effects in nursing infants if the drug were distributed into milk, a decision should be make whether to discontinue nursing or the drug, taking into account the importance of the drug to the woman.

Drug Interactions

■ **CNS-Active Drugs** Because aldesleukin may affect CNS function, interactions may occur following concomitant administration with CNS-active drugs, such as opiate, analgesic, antiemetic, sedative, or tranquilizing agents.

■ **Nephrotoxic and Hepatotoxic Drugs** Because renal and hepatic function are impaired with aldesleukin therapy, concomitant administration of known nephrotoxic (e.g., aminoglycosides, indomethacin) or hepatotoxic (e.g., methotrexate, asparaginase) drugs may further increase renal or hepatic toxicity, respectively.

■ **Cardiotoxic Drugs** Concomitant administration of known cardiotoxic drugs (e.g., anthracyclines such as doxorubicin) with aldesleukin may increase cardiotoxicity.

■ **Antineoplastic Agents** Concurrent administration of cytotoxic agents that cause myelotoxicity with aldesleukin may increase such toxicity. The safety and efficacy of aldesleukin administered in combination with any chemotherapeutic agent have not been established.

Hypersensitivity reactions, consisting of erythema, pruritus, and hypotension, have been reported in patients receiving combination regimens with sequential administration of high-dose aldesleukin and antineoplastic agents, specifically, dacarbazine, cisplatin, tamoxifen, and interferon alfa. These hypersensitivity reactions occurred within hours of administration of chemotherapy, and medical intervention was required in some patients.

■ **Interferon Alfa** Aldesleukin used in combination with interferon alfa has been associated with the development or exacerbation of autoimmune disease and inflammatory disorders. Development or exacerbation of thyroiditis, inflammatory arthritis, oculo-bulbar myasthenia gravis, crescentic IgA glomerulonephritis, Stevens-Johnson syndrome, or bullous pemphigoid has been reported following concurrent use of aldesleukin and interferon alfa. In one patient who developed rapidly progressive renal failure following combination therapy with aldesleukin and interferon alfa for metastatic renal cell carcinoma, renal biopsy revealed crescentic glomerulonephritis.

The incidence of myocardial injury, including myocardial infarction, myocarditis, ventricular hypokinesia, and severe rhabdomyolysis, appears to be increased in patients receiving concurrent aldesleukin and interferon alfa.

See Drug Interactions: Antineoplastic Agents.

■ **Corticosteroids** Although corticosteroids (i.e., glucocorticoids) have been shown to ameliorate aldesleukin-induced adverse effects, including fever, renal insufficiency, hyperbilirubinemia, confusion, and dyspnea, concomitant use of such agents may reduce the antitumor effectiveness of aldesleukin and should be avoided.

■ **Hypotensive Agents** Concomitant administration of antihypertensive agents (e.g., β-blocking agents) may potentiate aldesleukin-induced hypotension.

■ **Roentgenographic Agents** Treatment with aldesleukin or other interleukin-2 preparations may predispose individuals to acute, atypical adverse reactions to iodinated radiographic contrast media. In a review of reports involving several hundred patients receiving various treatment regimens containing interleukin-2, approximately 13% of patients (range: 11–28%) experienced such reactions with subsequent administration of iodinated radiographic contrast media. The reactions included fever, chills, nausea, vomiting, diarrhea, pruritus, rash, hypotension, edema, and oliguria. The onset of symptoms usually occurred within hours (most often 1–4 hours) after administration of the contrast media. The cause of these reactions is not known, but they are similar to immediate adverse effects caused by interleukin-2. Although most of these reactions were reported to occur when the radiographic contrast media was administered within 4 weeks after the last dose of interleukin-2, some have occurred when the contrast media was administered several months after interleukin-2 treatment.

Pharmacology

Aldesleukin, a biologic response modifier, is a human recombinant interleukin-2 (IL-2) that possesses the biologic activities of endogenous IL-2. Aldesleukin exerts a wide range of regulatory actions on the immune system, including enhancement of lymphocyte mitogenesis and stimulation of long-term growth of human IL-2 dependent cell lines, enhancement of lymphocyte cytotoxicity, induction of lymphokine-activated killer (LAK) cell and natural killer (NK) cell activity, and induction of interferon-gamma production. Administration of aldesleukin in animals and humans produces immune effects in a dose-dependent manner, including activation of cellular immunity with profound lymphocytosis, eosinophilia, and thrombocytopenia; and production of cytokines including tumor necrosis factor, IL-1, and interferon gamma. The precise mechanism of action of aldesleukin is unknown, and how the effects of aldesleukin on the immune system contribute to the antineoplastic activity of the drug have not been established.

Pharmacokinetics

■ **Absorption** Upon completion of IV infusion of aldesleukin, approximately 30% of an administered dose is detectable in plasma.

■ **Distribution** Following IV infusion over short periods, aldesleukin is rapidly distributed into the extravascular space; studies of radiolabeled aldesleukin in rats indicate rapid (less than 1 minute) uptake of the drug into lung, liver, kidney, and spleen.

It is not known whether aldesleukin is distributed into milk.

■ **Elimination** Aldesleukin is cleared from plasma relatively rapidly following IV infusion over a short period. Following a 5-minute IV infusion in cancer patients, the elimination half-life of aldesleukin remaining in plasma was 85 minutes. In cancer patients, clearance of the drug from plasma averaged 268 mL/minute.

Aldesleukin is metabolized principally in the kidney, and the active drug generally is undetectable or present in only trace quantities in the urine. Both glomerular filtration and peritubular extraction contribute to delivery of the drug to the proximal tubule, and clearance of the drug is preserved in patients with rising serum creatinine concentrations. Greater than 80% of the amount of aldesleukin distributed to plasma, cleared from the circulation, and presented to the kidney is metabolized to amino acids in the cells lining the proximal convoluted tubules.

Chemistry and Stability

■ **Chemistry** Aldesleukin, a human interleukin-2 derivative, is a biosynthetic (recombinant DNA origin) cytokine (i.e., lymphokine) that possesses complex antineoplastic and immunomodulating activities. The drug is a biologic response modifier. Aldesleukin, a protein of 132 amino acids, has an amino acid sequence closely related to endogenous human interleukin-2 (HuIL-2), differing from the endogenous glycoprotein only by the absence of an *N*-terminal alanine, the replacement of cysteine with serine at position 125 of the sequence, and the absence of glycosylation.

Potency of aldesleukin is determined by a lymphocyte proliferation bioassay and is expressed in international units (IU) as established by the World Health Organization 1st International Standard for Interleukin-2 (human); because other units also have been reported (e.g., CU, RU, BRMPU) and are not equivalent, care should be exercised in interpreting published dosages and concentrations.

Aldesleukin is commercially available as a sterile, white to off-white, lyophilized cake for injection that contains dibasic and monobasic sodium phosphate as a buffer. Following reconstitution with sterile water for injection, the injection has a pH of about 7.5 (range: 7.2–7.8).

■ **Stability** Aldesleukin lyophilized cake for injection should be refrigerated at 2–8°C with protection from light and should not be used beyond the expiration date printed on the vial. Aldesleukin lyophilized cake for injection or reconstituted or diluted solutions of the drug should not be frozen. Reconstituted or diluted solutions of the drug are stable for up to 48 hours under refrigeration or at room temperature (2–25°C). Reconstituted or diluted solutions of the drug contain no preservative and should be stored in the refrigerator at 2–8°C; the solution should be brought to room temperature prior to infusion. Unused portions of aldesleukin solution should be discarded.

For further information on the handling of antineoplastic agents, see the ASHP Guidelines on Handling Hazardous Drugs at http://www.ahfsdruginformation.com.

Preparations

Excipients in commercially available drug preparations may have clinically important effects in some individuals; consult specific product labeling for details.

Aldesleukin

Parenteral		
For injection, for IV infusion	22 million units	**Proleukin®**, Novartis

†Use is not currently included in the labeling approved by the US Food and Drug Administration

Selected Revisions October 2009, © Copyright, May 1992, American Society of Health-System Pharmacists, Inc.

Alectinib Hydrochloride

■ Alectinib hydrochloride, an inhibitor of several receptor tyrosine kinases including anaplastic lymphoma kinase (ALK), is an antineoplastic agent.

Uses

■ **Non-small Cell Lung Cancer** Alectinib hydrochloride is used for the treatment of anaplastic lymphoma kinase (ALK)-positive metastatic non-small cell lung cancer (NSCLC) following failure (secondary to resistance or intolerance) of prior crizotinib therapy. The drug has been designated an orphan drug by FDA for use in this condition. The accelerated approval of alectinib for this indication is based on tumor response rate and duration of response; continued approval for this indication may be contingent on verification and description of clinical benefit of alectinib in confirmatory studies.

A relatively small subset of patients with NSCLC (approximately 3–7%) have ALK-positive disease, which indicates potential responsiveness to ALK inhibitor therapy (e.g., alectinib, brigatinib, ceritinib, crizotinib). Patients with this form of lung cancer typically are nonsmokers or have a history of light smoking, are female, and are younger in age and often have adenocarcinoma histology. Although crizotinib is highly active in patients with ALK-positive NSCLC, most patients treated with the drug eventually experience disease progression, limiting the drug's long-term therapeutic potential. Disease progression in patients receiving crizotinib can result from acquired resistance mutations in ALK, amplification of gene expression, activation of alternate signaling pathways, and/or progression of brain metastases (because of poor distribution of crizotinib into the CSF). (See Description.)

The current indication for alectinib is based principally on the response rates obtained in 2 noncomparative phase 2 studies that enrolled a total of 225 adults (87 patients in study 1 and 138 in study 2) with locally advanced or metastatic ALK-positive NSCLC (as detected by an FDA-approved diagnostic test) who had experienced disease progression during crizotinib therapy. Most patients enrolled in both studies had received systemic chemotherapy prior to crizotinib therapy for NSCLC, and, among those with CNS metastases, most had received CNS radiation therapy. Patients in both studies received alectinib (600 mg orally twice daily) until disease progression, unacceptable toxicity, death, or study withdrawal occurred. The primary efficacy end point in both studies was the objective response rate according to Response Evaluation Criteria in Solid Tumors (RECIST 1.1) as assessed by an independent review committee (IRC). The objective response rate and duration of response in the CNS in patients with CNS metastases were key secondary end points. IRC-assessed objective response rates with alectinib therapy were 38 and 44% in studies 1 and 2, respectively, and investigator-assessed objective response rates were 46 and 48%, respectively; all responses were partial responses. The median IRC-assessed duration of response was 7.5 and 11.2 months in studies 1 and 2, respectively.

In the subgroup of 51 patients in both studies with baseline measurable CNS metastases according to RECIST 1.1 criteria, the CNS objective response rate with alectinib therapy was 61% (18% complete responses and 43% partial responses) and the median duration of CNS response was 9.1 months. CNS responses were observed irrespective of prior CNS irradiation.

Phase 3 controlled trials comparing alectinib with crizotinib as first-line, single-agent therapy in treatment-naive patients with ALK-positive NSCLC are under way. Alectinib currently is not FDA-labeled for use in patients with treatment-naive ALK-positive NSCLC.

Dosage and Administration

■ **General** ***Restricted Distribution Program*** Alectinib can only be obtained through a limited network of specialty pharmacies. Clinicians may contact the manufacturer by telephone at 888-249-4918 or consult the Genentech Access Solutions® website for specific availability information (http://www.genentech-access.com/alecensa/hcp).

■ **Administration** Alectinib hydrochloride is administered orally twice daily with food. The capsules should be swallowed whole and should *not* be dissolved or opened.

■ **Dosage** Dosage of alectinib hydrochloride is expressed in terms of alectinib.

Non-small Cell Lung Cancer The recommended adult dosage of alectinib for the treatment of anaplastic lymphoma kinase (ALK)-positive metastatic non-small cell lung cancer (NSCLC) following failure (secondary to resistance or intolerance) of prior crizotinib therapy is 600 mg twice daily. Alectinib therapy should be continued until disease progression or unacceptable toxicity occurs.

Dosage Modification for Toxicity In the principal efficacy studies, at least one dosage reduction from the recommended initial alectinib dosage (600 mg twice daily) was necessary in 23% of patients (most commonly for hepatic toxicity, serum creatine kinase [CK, creatine phosphokinase, CPK] elevation, or vomiting); the median time to the first dosage reduction was 48 days.

When dosage reduction is necessary, an initial dosage reduction to 450 mg twice daily is recommended. If further dosage reduction is necessary, the dosage should be reduced to 300 mg twice daily. If a dosage of 300 mg twice daily is not tolerated, alectinib should be discontinued.

Hepatic Toxicity. If an elevation in serum ALT or AST concentrations exceeding 5 times the upper limit of normal (ULN) occurs with a total bilirubin concentration of no more than 2 times the ULN, alectinib therapy should be withheld until liver function test results return to baseline values or decrease to no more than 3 times the ULN. Alectinib therapy may then be resumed at a reduced dosage.

If an elevation in ALT or AST concentrations exceeding 3 times the ULN occurs with an elevation in total bilirubin concentrations exceeding 2 times the ULN in the absence of cholestasis or hemolysis, therapy with alectinib should be permanently discontinued.

If an elevation in total bilirubin concentrations exceeding 3 times the ULN occurs, alectinib therapy should be withheld until total bilirubin concentrations return to baseline values or decrease to no more than 1.5 times the ULN. Alectinib therapy may then be resumed at a reduced dosage. (See Hepatic Toxicity under Cautions: Warnings/Precautions.)

Interstitial Lung Disease/Pneumonitis. If treatment-related interstitial lung disease/pneumonitis of any grade occurs, alectinib therapy should be permanently discontinued. (See Interstitial Lung Disease/Pneumonitis under Cautions: Warnings/Precautions.)

Bradycardia. If symptomatic, but non-life-threatening, bradycardia occurs, therapy with alectinib should be withheld until recovery to asymptomatic bradycardia or to a heart rate of at least 60 beats/minute. If concomitant drugs known to cause bradycardia or hypotension are identified and the dosage of the concomitant drug can be adjusted or the drug can be discontinued, alectinib therapy can be resumed at the previous dosage upon recovery to asymptomatic bradycardia or to a heart rate of at least 60 beats/minute. If dosage adjustment or discontinuance of such concomitant drugs is not possible, or if no concomitant contributory drugs are identified, alectinib should be resumed at a reduced dosage upon recovery to asymptomatic bradycardia or to a heart rate of at least 60 beats/minute. (See Drug Interactions: Drugs Associated with Bradycardia.)

If life-threatening bradycardia or bradycardia requiring urgent intervention occurs in patients receiving concomitant drugs known to cause bradycardia or hypotension, therapy with alectinib should be withheld until recovery to asymptomatic bradycardia or to a heart rate of at least 60 beats/minute. If the dosage of the concomitant drug can be adjusted or the drug can be discontinued, alectinib therapy may then be resumed at a reduced dosage with frequent monitoring; alectinib therapy should be permanently discontinued in case of recurrence.

If life-threatening bradycardia or bradycardia requiring urgent intervention occurs in patients not receiving concomitant therapy with drugs known to cause bradycardia or hypotension, alectinib therapy should be permanently discontinued. (See Bradycardia under Cautions: Warnings/Precautions.)

Creatine Kinase Elevation. If an elevation in serum CK concentrations exceeding 5 times the ULN occurs, alectinib therapy should be withheld until serum CK concentrations return to baseline values or decrease to no more than 2.5 times the ULN. Alectinib therapy may then be resumed at the previous dosage. If an elevation in serum CK concentrations exceeding 5 times the ULN *recurs*, alectinib therapy should be withheld until serum CK concentrations return to baseline values or decrease to no more than 2.5 times the ULN; alectinib therapy may then be resumed at a reduced dosage.

If an elevation in serum CK concentrations exceeding 10 times the ULN occurs, alectinib therapy should be withheld until serum CK concentrations return to baseline values or decrease to no more than 2.5 times the ULN. Alectinib therapy may then be resumed at a reduced dosage.

■ **Special Populations** The manufacturer makes no specific dosage recommendations for geriatric patients. (See Geriatric Use under Warnings/Precautions: Specific Populations, in Cautions.)

No initial dosage adjustment is necessary in patients with mild hepatic impairment (total bilirubin concentrations not exceeding the ULN with AST concentrations exceeding the ULN, or total bilirubin concentrations exceeding 1 but not exceeding 1.5 times the ULN with any AST concentration). Pharmacokinetics and safety of alectinib have not been established in patients with moderate or severe hepatic impairment. (See Hepatic Impairment under Warnings/Precautions: Specific Populations, in Cautions.)

No initial dosage adjustment is necessary in patients with mild or moderate renal impairment (creatinine clearance of 30–89 mL/minute). Pharmacokinetics and safety of alectinib have not been established in patients with severe renal impairment (creatinine clearance less than 30 mL/minute) or end-stage renal disease. (See Renal Impairment under Warnings/Precautions: Specific Populations, in Cautions.)

Cautions

■ Contraindications The manufacturer states that there are no known contraindications to the use of alectinib.

■ Warnings/Precautions ***Hepatic Toxicity*** Drug-induced hepatotoxicity, including elevations in ALT, AST, and total bilirubin concentrations and biopsy-confirmed liver injury, has occurred in patients receiving alectinib. Elevations in ALT or AST concentrations exceeding 5 times the upper limit of normal (ULN) were reported in 4.8 or 3.6%, respectively, of alectinib-treated patients in the primary efficacy studies; elevations in bilirubin concentrations exceeding 3 times the ULN were reported in 2.8% of alectinib-treated patients. These elevations generally occurred during the first 2 months of treatment. Permanent discontinuance of the drug because of grade 3 or 4 aminotransferase elevations or grade 3 bilirubin elevations was necessary in 7 patients in the primary efficacy studies.

The manufacturer states that liver function tests, including ALT, AST, and total bilirubin concentrations, should be monitored every 2 weeks for the first 2 months of alectinib therapy and periodically thereafter, with more frequent testing in patients who develop aminotransferase or bilirubin elevations during therapy. Temporary interruption followed by dosage reduction or permanent discontinuance of alectinib may be necessary depending on the severity of the hepatic toxicity. (See Hepatic Toxicity under Dosage: Dosage Modification for Toxicity, in Dosage and Administration.)

Interstitial Lung Disease/Pneumonitis Severe interstitial lung disease (ILD)/pneumonitis may occur in patients receiving alectinib. In the primary efficacy studies, grade 3 ILD occurred in 1 of 253 patients (0.4%) receiving alectinib.

Patients receiving alectinib should be monitored for pulmonary symptoms indicative of ILD or pneumonitis (see Advice to Patients), and other potential causes of ILD or pneumonitis should be excluded. Alectinib should be permanently discontinued in patients who are diagnosed with treatment-related ILD or pneumonitis of any grade.

Bradycardia Alectinib may cause bradycardia. In the primary efficacy studies, bradycardia (defined as a heart rate of less than 60 beats/minute) was reported in 7.5% of alectinib-treated patients; a heart rate of less than 50 beats/minute was reported in 20% of patients in whom serial ECGs were obtained.

Heart rate and blood pressure should be monitored regularly in all patients receiving alectinib. If symptomatic bradycardia occurs, temporary interruption of alectinib therapy, subsequent dosage reduction, or permanent discontinuance of the drug may be necessary depending on the severity of the bradycardia, the concomitant use of drugs known to cause bradycardia or hypotension, and the feasibility of modifying such concomitant therapy. Any concomitantly used drugs that may cause bradycardia or hypotension should be identified and the dosage should be adjusted or the drug should be discontinued if possible. (See Bradycardia under Dosage: Dosage Modification for Toxicity, in Dosage and Administration.)

Severe Myalgia and Creatine Kinase Elevation In the primary efficacy studies, myalgia or musculoskeletal pain was reported in 29% of alectinib-treated patients; 1.2% of patients receiving the drug experienced grade 3 myalgia/musculoskeletal pain. Elevated serum creatine kinase (CK, creatine phosphokinase, CPK) concentrations were reported in 43% of patients receiving alectinib; 4.6% of patients receiving the drug had grade 3 elevations in CK concentrations. Median time to grade 3 CK elevations was 14 days. Dosage modification because of elevated serum CK concentrations was required in 5% of patients.

The manufacturer states that serum CK concentrations should be monitored every 2 weeks for the first month of alectinib therapy and as clinically indicated in patients reporting muscle symptoms (e.g., unexplained or persistent muscle pain, tenderness, or weakness). Temporary interruption followed by dosage reduction or permanent discontinuance of alectinib may be necessary depending on the severity of the CK elevation. (See Creatine Kinase Elevation under Dosage: Dosage Modification for Toxicity, in Dosage and Administration.)

Fetal/Neonatal Morbidity and Mortality Based on its mechanism of action, alectinib may cause fetal harm if administered to pregnant women. There are no adequate and well-controlled studies in humans; developmental toxicity, abortion, and embryolethality were observed when alectinib was administered to pregnant animals at maternally toxic dosages. Pregnancy should be avoided during therapy. Women of childbearing potential should use effective methods of contraception while receiving the drug and for at least 1 week after the drug is discontinued. If alectinib is used during pregnancy or if the patient becomes pregnant while receiving the drug, the patient should be apprised of the potential fetal hazard.

In addition, based on genotoxicity findings, men with female partners of childbearing potential should use effective methods of contraception while receiving the drug and for at least 3 months after the drug is discontinued.

Specific Populations **Pregnancy.** Based on animal studies and its mechanism of action, alectinib may cause fetal harm if administered to pregnant women. (See Fetal/Neonatal Morbidity and Mortality under Cautions: Warnings/Precautions.)

Lactation. It is not known whether alectinib or its metabolites are distributed into human milk. Because of the potential for serious adverse reactions to alectinib in nursing infants, women should be advised not to breast-feed while receiving the drug and for at least 1 week after the drug is discontinued.

Pediatric Use. Safety and efficacy of alectinib have not been established in pediatric patients. In animal toxicology studies, alectinib has been associated with changes in growing teeth (discoloration, changes in tooth size, histopathologic disarrangement of ameloblast and odontoblast layers) and bones (decreases in trabecular bone, increased osteoclast activity).

Geriatric Use. Clinical studies of alectinib did not include sufficient numbers of patients 65 years of age and older to determine whether geriatric patients respond differently than younger adults. In the primary efficacy studies evaluating alectinib in patients with locally advanced or metastatic anaplastic lymphoma kinase (ALK)-positive non-small cell lung cancer (NSCLC), 10–18% of patients were 65 years of age or older.

In pharmacokinetic population analyses, age did not have a clinically important effect on systemic exposure to alectinib and its major active metabolite (M4).

Hepatic Impairment. Mild hepatic impairment (total bilirubin concentrations not exceeding the ULN with AST concentrations exceeding the ULN, or total bilirubin concentrations exceeding 1 but not exceeding 1.5 times the ULN with any AST concentration) did not have clinically important effects on systemic exposure to alectinib and its M4 metabolite. Pharmacokinetics and safety of alectinib have not been established in patients with moderate or severe hepatic impairment.

Renal Impairment. Mild to moderate renal impairment (creatinine clearance of 30–89 mL/minute) did not have clinically important effects on systemic exposure to alectinib and its M4 metabolite. Pharmacokinetics and safety of alectinib have not been established in patients with severe renal impairment (creatinine clearance less than 30 mL/minute) or end-stage renal disease.

Hemodialysis is not expected to enhance clearance of alectinib because the drug and its M4 metabolite are extensively bound to plasma proteins.

■ Common Adverse Effects Adverse effects reported in 10% or more of patients receiving alectinib in the primary clinical studies include fatigue/asthenia, constipation, edema (including peripheral, generalized, eyelid, and periorbital edema), myalgia/musculoskeletal pain, cough, rash (including acneiform dermatitis, erythema, and generalized, papular, pruritic, maculopapular, and macular rashes), nausea, headache, diarrhea, dyspnea, back pain, vomiting, increased weight, and vision disorder (including blurred vision, vitreous floaters, visual impairment, reduced visual acuity, asthenopia, and diplopia).

Laboratory abnormalities reported in more than 20% of patients receiving alectinib in the primary clinical studies include anemia, increased concentrations of aminotransferases (i.e., ALT, AST), increased concentrations of alkaline phosphatase, increased concentrations of CK, hyperbilirubinemia, hyperglycemia, hypocalcemia, hypokalemia, increased concentrations of creatinine, lymphopenia, hypophosphatemia, and hyponatremia.

Drug Interactions

Clinically important drug interactions with alectinib have not been identified to date.

Alectinib is metabolized by cytochrome P-450 (CYP) isoenzyme 3A4 to its major active metabolite, M4. In vitro studies suggest that M4, but not alectinib, is a substrate of P-glycoprotein (P-gp); neither alectinib nor M4 is a substrate of breast cancer resistance protein (BCRP), organic anion transport protein (OATP) 1B1, or OATP1B3.

In vitro studies indicate that alectinib and M4 do not inhibit CYP isoenzymes 1A2, 2B6, 2C9, 2C19, or 2D6. Alectinib also does not inhibit OATP1B1 or OATP1B3, organic anion transporter (OAT) 1 and OAT3, or organic cation transporter (OCT) 2 in vitro.

In vitro studies suggest that alectinib and M4 inhibit P-gp and BCRP.

■ Drugs Affecting or Metabolized by Hepatic Microsomal Enzymes Clinically important drug interactions with alectinib have not been identified to date. Concomitant administration of alectinib and posaconazole (a potent CYP3A inhibitor) or rifampin (a potent CYP3A inducer) did not have a clinically important effect on the combined systemic exposure to alectinib and its M4 metabolite. Clinically important pharmacokinetic interactions between alectinib and midazolam (a CYP3A substrate) or repaglinide (a CYP2C8 substrate) are unlikely.

■ Drugs Associated with Bradycardia Alectinib has been associated with bradycardia. If clinically important bradycardia occurs with concomitant use of alectinib and other drugs known to cause bradycardia (including hypotensive agents), the dosage of the concomitant drug should be adjusted or the concomitant drug should be discontinued, if possible. (See Bradycardia under Cautions: Warnings/Precautions.)

■ Drugs Affecting Gastric Acidity Concomitant administration of alectinib and esomeprazole did not have a clinically important effect on the combined systemic exposure to alectinib and its M4 metabolite.

Description

Alectinib hydrochloride, an inhibitor of receptor tyrosine kinases, including anaplastic lymphoma kinase (ALK) and ret proto-oncogene (RET), is an antineoplastic agent. The drug inhibits ALK phosphorylation and ALK-mediated activation of the downstream signaling proteins signal transducer and activator of transcription 3 (STAT3) and AKT serine/threonine kinase. The drug also inhibits leukocyte tyrosine kinase receptor (LTK) and cyclin-G-associated kinase (GAK).

Activating mutations or translocations of the ALK gene have been identified in several malignancies and can result in the expression of oncogenic fusion proteins (e.g., echinoderm microtubule-associated protein-like 4 [EML4]-ALK). Such ALK gene rearrangements have been identified in approximately 3–7% of patients with non-small cell lung cancer (NSCLC). Formation of ALK fusion proteins such as EML4-ALK results in activation and dysregulation of the gene's expression and signaling, which can contribute to increased cell proliferation and survival in tumors expressing these proteins.

Although the ALK inhibitor crizotinib has demonstrated improved outcomes in patients with NSCLC harboring ALK mutations, secondary resistance to crizotinib eventually develops, generally within the first 1–2 years of treatment. Clinical resistance to crizotinib has been attributed to several possible mechanisms, including acquired resistance mutations of ALK, amplification of gene expression, and activation of alternate signaling pathways. Secondary mutations of ALK are responsible for about 30% of cases of acquired crizotinib resistance and gene amplification is implicated in 9% of these cases.

In vitro, alectinib is approximately fivefold more potent than crizotinib in its activity against ALK. Alectinib demonstrated dose-dependent antitumor activity and increased survival in mice bearing NSCLC tumor xenografts that expressed EML4-ALK, including several cell lines with demonstrated resistance to crizotinib. In preclinical studies in vitro and in vivo, alectinib was active against several crizotinib-resistant ALK mutations (e.g., L1196M, C1156Y, F1174L, G1269A).

The CNS is a common site of disease progression in crizotinib-treated patients because of poor distribution of crizotinib into CSF; development and/or progression of brain metastases occurs in approximately one-half of patients during crizotinib treatment. Alectinib crosses the blood-brain barrier, distributing into CSF at concentrations similar to estimated alectinib free plasma concentrations; the drug demonstrated antitumor activity and increased survival in mice bearing intracranial ALK-positive NSCLC tumor xenografts. In clinical studies, alectinib demonstrated antitumor activity in patients with crizotinib-resistant disease and baseline CNS metastases.

Exposure to alectinib is dose proportional over the oral dose range of 460–900 mg in the fed state. Following oral administration under fed conditions, peak plasma concentrations of alectinib are achieved within 4 hours. Steady-state concentrations of alectinib and its major active metabolite (M4) are achieved within 7 days. The absolute oral bioavailability of alectinib under fed conditions is 37%. Oral administration of a single 600-mg dose of the drug with a high-calorie, high-fat meal increases total systemic exposure to alectinib and M4 by 3.1-fold compared with administration in the fasting state. Alectinib and M4 are more than 99% bound to plasma proteins; the drug distributes into CSF at concentrations similar to estimated alectinib free plasma concentrations. Alectinib is metabolized by cytochrome P-450 (CYP) isoenzyme 3A4 to its major active metabolite, M4, which also is metabolized by CYP3A4. M4 exhibits in vitro potency and activity similar to those of alectinib. Following oral administration of radiolabeled alectinib, 98% of the dose is eliminated in feces, mainly as unchanged drug (84%) and, to a lesser extent, as M4 (6%); less than 0.5% of the dose is eliminated in urine. The mean elimination half-lives of alectinib and M4 in patients with ALK-positive NSCLC are 33 and 31 hours, respectively.

Advice to Patients

Importance of instructing patients to read the manufacturer's patient information.

Importance of advising patients to take alectinib exactly as prescribed and of not altering the dosage or discontinuing therapy unless advised to do so by their clinician. Importance of advising patients to swallow alectinib capsules whole with food and not to dissolve or open the capsules. If a dose is missed or if vomiting occurs after a dose is administered, the next dose should be taken at the regularly scheduled time; the missed dose should not be taken, and an extra dose should not be administered to replace the vomited dose.

Risk of hepatotoxicity; importance of liver function test monitoring. Importance of advising patients to immediately report possible manifestations of hepatotoxicity (e.g., fatigue, anorexia, nausea, vomiting, right upper quadrant pain, jaundice, dark urine, generalized pruritus, unusual bleeding or bruising) to their clinician.

Risk of severe or fatal interstitial lung disease/pneumonitis. Importance of advising patients that symptoms may be similar to those of lung cancer and to contact their clinician immediately if they experience any new or worsening pulmonary symptoms (e.g., dyspnea, shortness of breath, cough, fever).

Risk of bradycardia. Importance of advising patients to contact their clinician immediately if they experience dizziness, lightheadedness, or faintness during therapy.

Risk of muscle problems or myalgia; importance of creatine kinase (CK, creatine phosphokinase, CPK) monitoring. Importance of advising patients to promptly inform clinicians if they experience any unexplained or persistent muscle pain, tenderness, or weakness.

Risk of photosensitivity. Importance of advising patients to avoid prolonged sun exposure while receiving alectinib and for at least 7 days after the drug is discontinued and to use a broad-spectrum sunscreen and lip balm (minimum SPF of 50) during alectinib therapy.

Risk of fetal harm. Necessity of advising women of childbearing potential that they should use effective methods of contraception while receiving alectinib and for at least 1 week after discontinuance of therapy. Importance of advising men who are partners of such women that they should use adequate methods of contraception while receiving the drug and for at least 3 months after the drug is discontinued.

Importance of women informing their clinicians if they are or plan to become pregnant. If pregnancy occurs, the patient should be advised of the potential risk to the fetus.

Importance of advising women to avoid breast-feeding while receiving alectinib and for at least 1 week after discontinuance of therapy.

Importance of informing clinicians of existing or contemplated concomitant therapy, including prescription and OTC drugs (e.g., cardiac or hypotensive agents) and dietary or herbal supplements, as well as any concomitant illnesses (e.g., hepatic impairment).

Importance of informing patients of other important precautionary information. (See Cautions.)

Overview® (see Users Guide). For additional information on this drug until a more detailed monograph is developed and published, the manufacturer's labeling should be consulted. It is *essential* that the manufacturer's labeling be consulted for more detailed information on usual cautions, precautions, contraindications, potential drug interactions, laboratory test interferences, and acute toxicity. For further information on the handling of antineoplastic agents, see the ASHP Guidelines on Handling Hazardous Drugs at http://www.ahfsdruginformation.com.

Preparations

Distribution of alectinib is restricted. (See Restricted Distribution Program under Dosage and Administration: General.)

Excipients in commercially available drug preparations may have clinically important effects in some individuals; consult specific product labeling for details.

Alectinib Hydrochloride

Oral

Capsules	150 mg (of alectinib)	**Alecensa®**, Genentech

Apalutamide

■ Apalutamide, a nonsteroidal antiandrogen, is an antineoplastic agent.

Uses

■ **Prostate Cancer** Apalutamide is used for the treatment of nonmetastatic castration-resistant prostate cancer.

The current indication for apalutamide is based principally on the results of a randomized, double-blind, placebo-controlled phase 3 study (SPARTAN) in 1207 patients with nonmetastatic castration-resistant prostate cancer who were at high risk for metastasis (i.e., prostate specific antigen [PSA] doubling time of 10 months or less despite continuous androgen deprivation therapy). Patients were randomized in a 2:1 ratio to receive either apalutamide (240 mg once daily) or placebo; androgen deprivation therapy was continued in all patients. Patients were stratified by PSA doubling time, use of bone resorption inhibitors, and presence of locoregional nodal disease. Treatment was continued until disease progression or unacceptable toxicity occurred, new treatment was initiated, or the patient withdrew from the study. The primary measure of efficacy was metastasis-free survival; secondary end points included time to metastasis, progression-free (including locoregional or distant metastatic progression) survival, time to symptomatic progression, and overall survival. The median age of patients enrolled in the study was 74 years; 26% of patients were 80 years of age or older. Most patients (77%) had undergone prior surgery or radiation therapy of the prostate; 78% had a Gleason score of 7 or higher, 73% had received prior treatment with a nonsteroidal antiandrogen (69% had received bicalutamide and 10% had received flutamide), and all had an Eastern Cooperative Oncology Group (ECOG) performance status of 0 or 1.

At a median follow-up of 20.3 months, metastasis-free survival was substantially longer in apalutamide-treated patients compared with those who received placebo (40.5 and 16.2 months, respectively). Results of a subgroup analysis (based on PSA doubling time, baseline PSA concentration, number of prior hormonal therapies, use of bone resorption inhibitors, locoregional nodal disease, age, race, ECOG performance status, and geographic region) suggested that the drug's effect on metastasis-free survival was consistent across all subgroups. Patients receiving apalutamide also had longer time to metastasis, progression-free survival, and time to symptomatic progression compared with those receiving placebo. Overall survival had not been reached at the time of primary analysis; the study was terminated early because clinical benefit of apalutamide had been demonstrated.

Dosage and Administration

■ **General** Patients receiving apalutamide should receive concurrent therapy with a gonadotropin-releasing hormone (GnRH) analog unless they have undergone bilateral orchiectomy.

Restricted Distribution Apalutamide is available only through specialty pharmacies. Clinicians may contact Janssen CarePath at 877-227-3728 or consult the Janssen CarePath website for specific availability information (https://www.janssencarepath.com/hcp/erleada).

■ **Administration** Apalutamide is administered orally once daily without regard to food. The tablets should be swallowed whole.

■ **Dosage** ***Prostate Cancer*** For the treatment of nonmetastatic castration-resistant prostate cancer, the recommended dosage of apalutamide is 240 mg once daily. In the principal efficacy study, therapy was continued until disease progression or unacceptable toxicity occurred.

Dosage Modification for Toxicity **General Toxicity.** If an intolerable adverse effect or grade 3 or greater toxicity occurs, apalutamide therapy should be interrupted until symptoms improve to grade 1 or less or return to baseline. Apalutamide therapy may then be resumed with or without a dosage reduction. If a dosage reduction is warranted, the dosage of apalutamide may be reduced to 180 or 120 mg daily.

■ **Special Populations** Initial dosage adjustment is not necessary in patients with mild or moderate hepatic impairment (Child-Pugh class A or B). (See Hepatic Impairment under Warnings/Precautions: Specific Populations, in Cautions.)

Initial dosage adjustment is not necessary in patients with mild or moderate renal impairment (estimated glomerular filtration rate [eGFR] of 30–89 mL/minute per 1.73 m^2). (See Renal Impairment under Warnings/Precautions: Specific Populations, in Cautions.)

The manufacturer makes no special dosage recommendations for geriatric patients; most patients (87%) in the principal efficacy study were 65 years of age or older. (See Geriatric Use under Warnings/Precautions: Specific Populations, in Cautions.)

Cautions

■ **Contraindications** Apalutamide is contraindicated in pregnant women. (See Pregnancy under Warnings/Precautions: Specific Populations, in Cautions.)

■ **Warnings/Precautions** ***Falls and Fractures*** Falls and fractures have occurred in patients receiving apalutamide. In the principal efficacy study in patients with nonmetastatic castration-resistant prostate cancer, falls were reported in 16% of patients receiving apalutamide compared with 9% of those receiving placebo and were not associated with loss of consciousness or seizure. Fractures were reported in 12% of apalutamide-treated patients compared with 7% of those receiving placebo; grade 3 or 4 fractures occurred in 3% of patients receiving the drug compared with 1% of those receiving placebo. The median time to onset of fracture was 314 days (range: 20–953 days) in patients receiving apalutamide. Routine bone density assessments were not performed during the study. In addition, patients receiving bone resorption inhibitors (e.g., denosumab, zoledronic acid) at dosages recommended for prevention of tumor-related skeletal events were excluded from the study, and relatively few patients received these agents at dosages recommended for prevention of bone loss in the setting of osteoporosis.

Patients receiving apalutamide should be evaluated for fracture and fall risk. Patients at risk for fractures should be monitored and managed according to established treatment guidelines; therapy with bone resorption inhibitors should be considered.

Seizures Seizures have occurred in patients receiving apalutamide. In the principal efficacy study in patients with nonmetastatic castration-resistant prostate cancer, seizure was reported in 0.2% of patients receiving apalutamide compared with none of those receiving placebo. Patients with predisposing factors for seizures (e.g., history of seizure, concomitant use of drugs that lower the seizure threshold or induce seizures) were excluded from the study. Time to onset of seizures ranged from 354–475 days following initiation of the drug.

It is not known whether anticonvulsants will prevent seizures in patients receiving apalutamide. The safety of resuming apalutamide therapy in patients who experienced a seizure while receiving the drug has not been established. Apalutamide should be permanently discontinued in patients who develop a seizure during treatment. (See Advice to Patients.)

Fetal/Neonatal Morbidity and Mortality Based on its mechanism of action, apalutamide may cause fetal harm. The drug is contraindicated in pregnant women. Based on findings in an animal reproduction and fertility study, men with female partners of childbearing potential should use effective methods of contraception during apalutamide therapy and for 3 months after the last dose of the drug; in addition, men should not donate sperm while receiving the drug and for 3 months after the drug is discontinued. Patients receiving the drug should use a condom during sexual encounters with pregnant women.

Impairment of Male Fertility Based on animal studies, apalutamide may impair male fertility. In male rats, apalutamide was associated with decreased sperm concentration and motility, increased abnormal sperm morphology, reduced epididymis and secondary sex gland weights, lower copulation and fertility rates upon pairing with untreated females, and a reduced number of live fetuses secondary to increased pre- and/or post-implantation loss; effects on male rats were reversible following discontinuance of drug administration.

Specific Populations **Pregnancy.** Based on its mechanism of action, apalutamide can cause fetal harm and potential loss of pregnancy if administered to pregnant women. The drug is contraindicated in pregnant women. (See Fetal/Neonatal Morbidity and Mortality under Cautions: Warnings/Precautions.)

Lactation. It is not known whether apalutamide or its metabolites are distributed into milk; the drug is not indicated for use in women. The effects of apalutamide on nursing infants or on milk production are not known.

Pediatric Use. Safety and efficacy of apalutamide have not been established in pediatric patients.

Geriatric Use. In the principal efficacy study evaluating apalutamide in men with nonmetastatic castration-resistant prostate cancer, 87% of patients were 65 years of age or older and 49% were 75 years of age or older. No overall differences in efficacy were observed between geriatric patients and younger adults. Among patients 65 years of age or older, grade 3 or 4 adverse reactions were reported in 46% of apalutamide-treated patients compared with 35% of placebo recipients; among patients 75 years of age or older, the respective frequencies were 51 and 37%.

Hepatic Impairment. No clinically important differences in systemic exposure of apalutamide or *N*-desmethylapalutamide were observed in patients with mild or moderate hepatic impairment (Child-Pugh class A or B) compared with individuals with normal hepatic function. The unbound fraction of apalutamide or *N*-desmethylapalutamide was not affected by hepatic impairment.

Pharmacokinetics of apalutamide have not been established in patients with severe hepatic impairment (Child-Pugh class C).

Renal Impairment. Renal impairment is not expected to affect the elimination of apalutamide or *N*-desmethylapalutamide. No clinically important differences in systemic exposure of apalutamide or *N*-desmethylapalutamide were observed in patients with mild or moderate renal impairment (estimated glomerular filtration rate [eGFR] of 30–89 mL/minute per 1.73 m^2) compared with individuals with normal renal function.

Pharmacokinetics of apalutamide have not been established in patients with severe renal impairment (eGFR of 29 mL/minute or less per 1.73 m^2).

■ **Common Adverse Effects** Adverse effects reported in 10% or more of patients receiving apalutamide and at an incidence at least 2% higher than that reported with placebo include fatigue/asthenia, hypertension, rash, diarrhea, nausea, weight loss, arthralgia, falls, hot flush, decreased appetite, fracture, and peripheral edema.

Laboratory abnormalities reported in 15% or more of patients receiving apalutamide and at an incidence more than 5% higher than that reported with placebo include hypercholesterolemia, hyperglycemia, anemia, hypertriglyceridemia, leukopenia, lymphopenia, and hyperkalemia.

Drug Interactions

Apalutamide is metabolized principally by cytochrome P-450 (CYP) isoenzymes 2C8 and 3A4 to form its major active metabolite, *N*-desmethylapalutamide.

Apalutamide is a potent inducer of CYP3A4 and 2C19 and a weak inducer of CYP2C9 in humans. In addition, in vitro studies indicate that apalutamide and *N*-desmethylapalutamide are moderate to potent inducers of CYP3A4 and 2B6, moderate inhibitors of CYP2B6 and 2C8, and weak inhibitors of CYP2C9, 2C19, and 3A4. Apalutamide and *N*-desmethylapalutamide neither inhibit nor induce CYP1A2 or 2D6 at clinically relevant concentrations.

Apalutamide and *N*-desmethylapalutamide are substrates of P-glycoprotein (P-gp) in vitro; however, apalutamide absorption is not limited by P-gp. Apalutamide and *N*-desmethylapalutamide are not substrates of breast cancer resistance protein (BCRP), organic anion transport protein (OATP) 1B1, or OATP1B3.

Apalutamide is a weak inducer of P-gp, BCRP, and OATP1B1 in humans. In vitro, apalutamide and *N*-desmethylapalutamide inhibit organic cation transporter 2 (OCT2), organic anion transporter 3 (OAT3), and multidrug and toxin extrusion (MATE) transporters. Apalutamide may induce uridine diphosphate-glucuronosyltransferase (UGT). Apalutamide and *N*-desmethylapalutamide do not inhibit organic anion transporter 1 (OAT1).

■ **Drugs Affecting Hepatic Microsomal Enzymes** Concomitant use of apalutamide with potent inhibitors of CYP2C8 or 3A4 may result in increased steady-state exposure of the total active forms of apalutamide (i.e., unbound apalutamide plus potency-adjusted unbound *N*-desmethylapalutamide). No initial dosage adjustment is necessary; however, reduction of apalutamide dosage may be necessary based on tolerability. (See General Toxicity under Dosage: Dosage Modification for Toxicity, in Dosage and Administration.)

Mild or moderate inhibitors of CYP2C8 or 3A4 are not expected to affect the exposure of apalutamide.

Concomitant use of apalutamide with inducers of CYP2C8 and/or 3A4 may decrease steady-state apalutamide concentrations.

■ **Drugs Metabolized by Hepatic Microsomal Enzymes** Concomitant use of apalutamide with drugs that are principally metabolized by

CYP3A4, 2C9, or 2C19 may result in decreased exposure of the CYP substrate. The manufacturer of apalutamide recommends that concomitant use be avoided when possible (e.g., by switching to an alternative drug that is not metabolized by these isoenzymes); if concomitant use cannot be avoided, patients should be monitored for decreased therapeutic effect of the CYP substrate.

Concomitant administration of apalutamide with a CYP2C8 substrate did not result in clinically important changes in exposure of the CYP2C8 substrate. (See Drug Interactions: Pioglitazone.)

■ **Drugs Affecting or Affected by P-glycoprotein Transport** Inhibition or induction of P-gp is not expected to affect the bioavailability of apalutamide.

Concomitant use of apalutamide and P-gp substrates may result in decreased exposure of the P-gp substrate. If concomitant use is necessary, caution should be exercised and patients should be monitored for decreased therapeutic effect of the P-gp substrate.

■ **Drugs Affected by Breast Cancer Resistance Protein and/or Organic Anion Transport Polypeptide 1B1** Concomitant use of apalutamide with drugs that are substrates of BCRP or OATP1B1 may result in decreased exposure of the BCRP or OATP1B1 substrate. If concomitant use is necessary, caution should be exercised and patients should be monitored for decreased therapeutic effect of the BCRP or OATP1B1 substrate.

■ **Drugs Metabolized by Uridine Diphosphate-glucuronosyltransferase** Concomitant use of apalutamide with drugs that are substrates of UGT may result in decreased exposure of the UGT substrate. If concomitant use is necessary, caution should be exercised and patients should be monitored for decreased therapeutic effect of the UGT substrate.

■ **Drugs Affected by Other Transporters** In vitro, apalutamide and *N*-desmethylapalutamide inhibit OCT2, OAT3, and MATE transporters, but do not inhibit OAT1. Apalutamide is not expected to cause clinically important changes in exposure of OAT3 substrates (e.g., penicillin G).

■ **Drugs Affecting Gastric Acidity** Because apalutamide remains unionized at physiologic pH, concomitant administration of apalutamide and drugs that increase gastric pH (e.g., proton-pump inhibitors, histamine H_2-receptor antagonists, antacids) are not expected to have a clinically important effect on the solubility and bioavailability of apalutamide.

■ **Antifungal Agents** ***Itraconazole*** Concomitant administration of the potent CYP3A4 inhibitor itraconazole (200 mg daily for 32 days) and apalutamide (single 240-mg dose) decreased peak plasma concentrations of apalutamide and *N*-desmethylapalutamide by 22 and 15%, respectively; areas under the concentration-time curve (AUCs) were not affected.

No initial dosage adjustment is necessary; however, reduction of apalutamide dosage may be necessary based on tolerability in patients receiving concomitant itraconazole therapy. (See General Toxicity under Dosage: Dosage Modification for Toxicity, in Dosage and Administration.)

Ketoconazole Based on pharmacokinetic modeling, concomitant use of ketoconazole (a potent CYP3A4 inhibitor) and apalutamide is expected to increase AUC of single-dose apalutamide by 24% with no change in apalutamide peak plasma concentration, and to increase steady-state AUC and peak plasma concentration of apalutamide by 51 and 38%, respectively. At steady state, AUC and peak plasma concentration of the total active forms of apalutamide (i.e., unbound apalutamide plus potency-adjusted unbound *N*-desmethylapalutamide) are expected to increase by 28 and 23%, respectively.

No initial dosage adjustment is necessary; however, reduction of apalutamide dosage may be necessary based on tolerability in patients receiving concomitant ketoconazole therapy. (See General Toxicity under Dosage: Dosage Modification for Toxicity, in Dosage and Administration.)

■ **Abiraterone** In an open-label phase 1b trial in patients with progressive metastatic castration-resistant prostate cancer treated with abiraterone acetate (1 g daily) and prednisone (5 mg twice daily), addition of apalutamide (240 mg daily) did not result in clinically important changes in the pharmacokinetics of apalutamide or abiraterone.

■ **Fexofenadine** Concomitant administration of the P-gp substrate fexofenadine (single dose) and apalutamide (240 mg daily at steady state) decreased fexofenadine AUC by 30%. If concomitant use of fexofenadine and apalutamide is necessary, caution should be exercised and patients should be monitored for decreased therapeutic effect of fexofenadine.

■ **Gemfibrozil** Concomitant administration of the potent CYP2C8 inhibitor gemfibrozil (600 mg twice daily for 32 days) and apalutamide (single 240-mg dose) decreased peak plasma concentration of apalutamide by 21% and increased AUC of apalutamide by 68%. Based on pharmacokinetic modeling, gemfibrozil is expected to increase steady-state AUC and peak plasma concentrations of apalutamide by 44 and 32%, respectively, and to increase steady-state AUC and peak plasma concentrations of the total active forms of apalutamide (i.e., unbound apalutamide plus potency-adjusted unbound *N*-desmethylapalutamide) by 23 and 19%, respectively.

No initial dosage adjustment is necessary; however, reduction of apalutamide dosage may be necessary based on tolerability in patients receiving concomitant gemfibrozil therapy. (See General Toxicity under Dosage: Dosage Modification for Toxicity, in Dosage and Administration.)

■ **Midazolam** Concomitant administration of the CYP3A4 substrate midazolam (single oral dose) and apalutamide (240 mg daily) decreased midazolam AUC by 92%. Concomitant use of apalutamide and midazolam should be avoided when possible (e.g., by switching to an alternative drug that is not metabolized by CYP3A4); if concomitant use cannot be avoided, patients should be monitored for decreased therapeutic effect of midazolam.

■ **Omeprazole** Concomitant administration of the CYP2C19 substrate omeprazole (single dose) and apalutamide (240 mg daily) decreased omeprazole AUC by 85%. Concomitant use of apalutamide and omeprazole should be avoided when possible (e.g., by switching to an alternative drug that is not metabolized by CYP2C19); if concomitant use cannot be avoided, patients should be monitored for decreased therapeutic effect of omeprazole.

■ **Pioglitazone** Concomitant administration of the CYP2C8 substrate pioglitazone (single dose) and apalutamide (240 mg daily) decreased pioglitazone AUC by 18%.

■ **Prednisone** In an open-label phase 1b trial in patients with progressive metastatic castration-resistant prostate cancer treated with abiraterone acetate (1 g daily) and prednisone (5 mg twice daily), addition of apalutamide (240 mg daily) did not result in clinically important changes in the pharmacokinetics of apalutamide or abiraterone.

■ **Rifampin** Based on pharmacokinetic modeling, concomitant use of the potent CYP3A4 and moderate CYP2C8 inducer rifampin (600 mg daily) and apalutamide is expected to decrease steady-state AUC and peak plasma concentrations of apalutamide by 34 and 25%, respectively, and to decrease steady-state AUC and peak plasma concentrations of the total active forms of apalutamide (i.e., unbound apalutamide plus potency-adjusted unbound *N*-desmethylapalutamide) by 19 and 15%, respectively. However, no pharmacokinetic interactions were observed between apalutamide and CYP3A4 inducers in a population pharmacokinetic analysis based on limited data.

■ **Rosuvastatin** Concomitant administration of the BCRP and OATP1B1 substrate rosuvastatin (single dose) and apalutamide (240 mg daily) decreased rosuvastatin AUC by 41% with no change in rosuvastatin peak plasma concentration. If concomitant use of rosuvastatin and apalutamide is necessary, caution should be exercised and patients should be monitored for decreased therapeutic effect of rosuvastatin.

■ **Warfarin** Concomitant administration of the CYP2C9 substrate warfarin (single dose) and apalutamide (240 mg daily) decreased AUC of *S*-warfarin by 46%. If apalutamide is used concomitantly with warfarin, international normalized ratio (INR) should be monitored at initiation of concomitant therapy and upon discontinuance of apalutamide.

Description

Apalutamide, a nonsteroidal antiandrogen, is an antineoplastic agent. The drug competitively inhibits androgen binding to androgen receptors; its mechanisms of action are similar to those of enzalutamide. Apalutamide binds directly to the ligand-binding domain of the androgen receptor and inhibits nuclear translocation of the activated androgen receptor, androgen-dependent binding of the androgen receptor complex to DNA, and androgen receptor-mediated gene transcription in cells that overexpress the androgen receptor. Apalutamide reduced tumor growth and induced apoptosis of tumor cells, leading to decreased tumor volume, in xenograft models of castration-resistant prostate cancer in mice.

In castration-resistant prostate cancer, alterations in androgen receptor signaling (e.g., androgen receptor gene mutation or amplification, androgen receptor overexpression) have been shown to result in persistence of androgen receptor signaling and to contribute to disease progression despite castrate levels of androgens. Resistance to conventional antiandrogens (e.g., bicalutamide, flutamide, nilutamide) in castration-resistant prostate cancer has been associated with paradoxical agonistic effects of these drugs and continued androgen receptor signaling. Unlike these conventional antiandrogens but similar to enzalutamide, apalutamide does not exhibit agonistic activity in cells that overexpress the androgen receptor.

The binding affinity of apalutamide at the androgen receptor is 7–10 times greater than that of bicalutamide. Although apalutamide and enzalutamide exhibit similar antiandrogenic activity in vitro, apalutamide demonstrated greater activity than enzalutamide in xenograft models of castration-resistant prostate cancer. At equivalent dosages, steady-state concentrations of apalutamide and enzalutamide in xenograft tumors in mice were similar, but steady-state plasma and CNS concentrations of apalutamide were twofold to fourfold lower and fourfold lower, respectively, compared with concentrations of enzalutamide. Whether these higher murine tumor-to-plasma and tumor-to-CNS ratios for apalutamide translate into a lower risk of adverse effects, including seizures and other CNS toxicity, remains to be established.

Apalutamide exhibits dose-proportional pharmacokinetics over a dosage range of 30–480 mg once daily. Following oral administration, the median time to peak plasma concentrations is 2 hours; the mean absolute bioavailability of apalutamide is approximately 100%. Steady-state concentrations of apalutamide are achieved after 4 weeks of once-daily dosing and the mean accumulation ratio is approximately fivefold. Administration of apalutamide with a high-fat meal delays time to peak plasma concentration by approximately 2 hours but has no clinically important effects on peak plasma concentration or area under the concentration-time curve (AUC). Apalutamide is metabolized principally by cytochrome P-450 (CYP) isoenzymes 2C8 and 3A4 to form its major active metabolite, *N*-desmethylapalutamide, which exhibits antiandrogenic activity at one-third the potency of the parent drug in vitro. The contributions of CYP2C8 and 3A4 to the metabolism of apalutamide are approximately 58 and 13%, respectively, following a single dose and 40 and 37%, respectively, at steady state. Apalutamide and *N*-desmethylapalutamide account for 45 and 44%, respectively, of the total drug exposure following a single 240-mg dose of apalutamide.

Apalutamide and *N*-desmethylapalutamide are 96 and 95% bound, respectively, to plasma proteins; the extent of binding is independent of plasma concentration. Clearance of apalutamide is increased at steady state, suggesting that the drug may induce its own metabolism by CYP3A4. The mean steady-state half-life of apalutamide is approximately 3 days. Following oral administration of a single radiolabeled dose of apalutamide, 65% of the dose was recovered in urine (1.2% as unchanged drug and 2.7% as *N*-desmethylapalutamide) and 24% of the dose was recovered in feces (1.5% as unchanged drug and 2% as *N*-desmethylapalutamide).

Advice to Patients

Importance of reading the manufacturer's patient information.

For patients currently receiving gonadotropin-releasing hormone (GnRH) analog therapy, importance of continuing this therapy during apalutamide therapy.

Importance of advising patients to take apalutamide at the same time each day without regard to food and to swallow tablets whole. If a dose is missed, importance of taking the missed dose as soon as possible on the same day and taking the next dose at the regularly scheduled time on the following day. Extra tablets should not be taken to make up for a missed dose.

Risk of falls and fractures.

Risk of seizures. Importance of informing patients of the risk of engaging in activities where sudden loss of consciousness could cause serious harm to themselves or others. Importance of patients immediately informing their clinician if a seizure occurs.

Importance of patients notifying their clinician if a rash develops during apalutamide therapy.

Risk of fetal harm. Necessity of advising patients with female partners of childbearing potential to use effective methods of contraception during apalutamide therapy and for 3 months after the last dose of the drug. In addition, patients receiving the drug should be advised to use a condom during sexual encounters with pregnant women.

Importance of advising patients that apalutamide may impair male fertility and that they should not donate sperm during apalutamide therapy and for 3 months after the last dose of the drug.

Importance of informing clinicians of existing or contemplated concomitant therapy, including prescription and OTC drugs and dietary or herbal supplements, as well as any concomitant illnesses (e.g., seizures).

Importance of informing patients of other important precautionary information. (See Cautions.)

Overview® (see Users Guide). For additional information on this drug until a more detailed monograph is developed and published, the manufacturer's labeling should be consulted. It is *essential* that the manufacturer's labeling be consulted for more detailed information on usual cautions, precautions, contraindications, potential drug interactions, laboratory test interferences, and acute toxicity. For further information on the handling of antineoplastic agents, see the ASHP Guidelines on Handling Hazardous Drugs at http://www.ahfsdruginformation.com.

Preparations

Distribution of apalutamide is restricted. (See Restricted Distribution under Dosage and Administration: General.)

Excipients in commercially available drug preparations may have clinically important effects in some individuals; consult specific product labeling for details.

Apalutamide

Oral		
Tablets, film-coated	60 mg	Erleada®, Janssen

Arsenic Trioxide

■ Arsenic trioxide is an antineoplastic agent.

Uses

■ **Acute Myeloid Leukemia** ***Refractory or Relapsed Acute Promyelocytic Leukemia*** Arsenic trioxide is used for remission-induction and consolidation of the acute promyelocytic (M3) subtype of acute myeloid (myelogenous, nonlymphocytic) leukemia (AML, ANLL) that is refractory to retinoid and anthracycline therapy or has relapsed despite such therapy. Arsenic trioxide is used in patients whose disease is characterized by the presence of the t(15;17) translocation or promyelocytic leukemia-retinoic acid receptor (PML-RAR)-α gene expression.

The current indication for use of arsenic trioxide in the treatment of refractory or relapsed acute promyelocytic leukemia (APL) is based principally on the results of an open-label, single-arm study in 40 patients previously treated with an anthracycline and a retinoid regimen. In this study, arsenic trioxide was administered IV at a dosage of 0.15 mg/kg over 1–2 hours daily until clearing of leukemic cells in bone marrow occurred or up to a maximum of 60 days. A complete response, defined as the absence of visible leukemic cells in bone marrow and peripheral recovery of platelets and leukocytes with a confirmatory bone marrow at least 30 days later, was reported in 70% of patients receiving the drug. The median time to bone marrow remission was 44 days, and the median time to onset of complete response was 53 days. In 31 patients, consolidation therapy consisting of the same daily dosage of arsenic trioxide used for induction was administered for 25 additional days (over a period of up to 5 weeks) 3–6 weeks following bone marrow remission. Eighteen patients received additional maintenance treatment consisting of up to four 25-day cycles of arsenic trioxide 0.15 mg/kg given over 1–2 hours, while 15 patients underwent bone marrow transplantation. At a median follow-up of 484 days (range: 280–755 days), 68% of patients were alive while 58% remained in complete remission at a median follow-up of 483 days (range: 280–755 days). Among the 28 patients who achieved a complete response to arsenic trioxide therapy, cytogenetic response (consisting of conversion to no detection of APL chromosome rearrangement) was observed in 86% while conversion based on reverse transcriptase polymerase chain reaction (RT-PCR) was seen in 79%.

Newly Diagnosed Acute Promyelocytic Leukemia Arsenic trioxide is used as a component of therapy for newly diagnosed APL†. In a small randomized study, 61 patients (including adults and children older than 14 years of age) with newly diagnosed APL receiving arsenic trioxide, tretinoin, or a combination of the 2 agents, followed by similar regimens of consolidation chemotherapy but differing regimens of maintenance therapy, had a similar rate of complete response (90% or greater), but time to complete response was shorter and durability of complete response (at a median follow-up of 18 months) was superior in patients receiving combination therapy. In a phase III randomized trial using tretinoin, cytarabine, and daunorubicin as induction therapy for newly diagnosed APL, the addition of 2 courses of arsenic trioxide preceding consolidation therapy with tretinoin and daunorubicin increased the rates of event-free survival and overall survival in adults.

Combination therapy with arsenic trioxide and tretinoin has been used as an alternative to standard chemotherapy for induction and postremission therapy in patients with newly diagnosed APL. Durable remissions and mostly mild toxicity have been reported in patients receiving arsenic trioxide as a single agent for previously untreated APL. Further study is needed, but these regimens may be considered for selected patients who cannot tolerate standard anthracycline-containing chemotherapy as a component of induction therapy for newly diagnosed APL, such as patients with cardiac dysfunction or geriatric patients with poor performance status.

■ **Other Uses** Arsenic trioxide is being investigated for use in the treatment of multiple myeloma†. In small uncontrolled phase II studies, arsenic trioxide demonstrated clinical activity in the treatment of relapsed or refractory multiple myeloma.

Arsenic trioxide also is being investigated for use in the treatment of myelodysplastic syndrome†.

Dosage and Administration

■ **General** ***Reconstitution and Administration*** Arsenic trioxide is administered by IV infusion over 1–2 hours; if acute vasomotor reactions occur, the drug may be administered over longer infusion periods (e.g., up to 4 hours). Arsenic trioxide injection should be diluted prior to administration. Contents of an ampul labeled as containing 10 mg of arsenic trioxide should be diluted with 100–250 mL of 5% dextrose injection or 0.9% sodium chloride injection, immediately after withdrawing the appropriate dose of the drug from the ampul. Proper aseptic technique must be observed since the drug contains no preservatives and unused portions of each ampul should be discarded. The diluted solutions of arsenic trioxide are physically and chemically stable for 24 hours at room temperature or 48 hours when refrigerated. The manufacturer states that arsenic trioxide should not be mixed with other drugs.

Dosage For remission induction in the management of acute promyelocytic leukemia (APL) that is refractory to retinoid and anthracycline therapy, or has relapsed despite such therapy, the recommended dosage of arsenic trioxide in adults and children 5 years of age and older is 0.15 mg/kg daily given by IV infusion. Arsenic trioxide therapy should be continued until bone marrow remission occurs or for a maximum of 60 doses. When used for consolidation therapy, arsenic trioxide (0.15 mg/kg daily for 25 doses, administered over a period up to 5 weeks) should be initiated 3–6 weeks after completion of induction therapy.

■ **Special Populations** No special population dosage recommendations at this time.

Cautions

■ **Contraindications** Known hypersensitivity to arsenic.

■ **Warnings/Precautions** ***Warnings*** Arsenic trioxide should be used under the supervision of a qualified clinician experienced in the management of patients with acute leukemia.

Acute Promyelocytic Leukemia (APL) Differentiation Syndrome. Manifestations (e.g., fever, dyspnea, weight gain, pulmonary infiltrates, pleural or pericardial effusions [with or without leukocytosis]) similar to those associated with the potentially fatal APL differentiation syndrome (also known as the retinoic acid-APL [RA-APL] syndrome) have been reported in about 23% of patients receiving arsenic trioxide for the management of APL in one clinical trial. If signs or symptoms suggestive of the syndrome (e.g., unexplained fever, dyspnea, weight gain, abnormal chest auscultatory findings, radiographic abnormalities) occur, high-dose corticosteroid therapy (e.g., dexamethasone 10 mg IV twice daily for 3 days or longer until symptoms resolve) should be initiated *immediately* regardless of the patient's leukocyte count; discontinuance of arsenic trioxide generally is not required.

Cardiovascular Effects. Arsenic trioxide has been shown to prolong the QT and QT interval corrected for rate (QT_c), which may predispose the patient to potentially fatal atypical ventricular tachycardia (torsades de pointes) and produce complete atrioventricular block. The risk of arsenic trioxide-induced torsades de pointes is related to increases in the QT interval, concomitant administration of drugs that might prolong the QT interval or those (e.g., potassium-wasting diuretics) that could produce electrolyte abnormalities such as hypokalemia or hypomagnesemia, a history of torsades de pointes, congestive heart failure, and preexisting QT interval prolongation.

In one clinical trial in patients receiving arsenic trioxide (Trisenox®) for the management of acute promyelocytic leukemia (APL) that was refractory to retinoid and anthracycline therapy or had relapsed despite such therapy, 40% (16 out of 40 patients) had at least one ECG tracing with QT_c interval greater than 500 msec, and torsades de pointes was observed in one patient. Prolongation of the QT_c interval was observed between 1–5 weeks after initiation of arsenic trioxide therapy and returned toward baseline values by the end of 8 weeks of drug treatment. In this study, age and gender did not correlate with extent of QT_c interval prolongation. In another study in patients receiving arsenic trioxide for management of acute myeloid leukemia (AML), prolongation of QT interval and torsades de pointes was reported in 3 patients. In one patient, torsades de pointes resolved upon correction of serum potassium and magnesium concentrations while the other 2 patients died of cardiac arrhythmia; all 3 patients had been intubated because of respiratory distress. In a phase I study, 3 sudden unexplained deaths occurred among 10 patients receiving arsenic trioxide (as an extemporaneously prepared IV solution) for acute promyelocytic leukemia. The manufacturer of Trisenox® states that no sudden deaths have been reported in clinical trials to date. The manufacturer also states that no cardiac deaths have been reported in clinical trials or during postmarketing surveillance to date, and data from more than 360 patients receiving arsenic trioxide in clinical trials indicate that safe administration of the drug may be optimized by appropriate monitoring and management of abnormalities.

The manufacturer states that prior to initiation of arsenic trioxide therapy, ECG evaluation and serum electrolyte (potassium, calcium, and magnesium) and creatinine concentrations should be determined. Preexisting electrolyte abnormalities should be corrected, and drugs known to prolong the QT interval should be discontinued, if possible. If the QT_c interval exceeds 500 msec, appropriate corrective measures should be completed and the QT_c interval reassessed with serial ECG determinations prior to considering arsenic trioxide therapy. During arsenic trioxide therapy, serum potassium and magnesium concentrations should be maintained above 4 mEq/L and 1.8 mg/dL, respectively; ECGs should be performed weekly and more frequently in clinically unstable patients. If QT interval exceeds 500 msec, any concomitant risk factors should be corrected immediately and the benefit of continued therapy must be weighed against the risk of developing serious cardiac adverse effects. If syncope and/or rapid or irregular heartbeat occurs, the patient should be hospitalized and carefully monitored; arsenic trioxide therapy should be discontinued until the QT_c interval decreases to below 460 msec, electrolyte abnormalities are corrected, and syncope and irregular heartbeat resolve. Health-care providers are encouraged to report any adverse effect associated with arsenic trioxide to the manufacturer by phone (800-368-1377) or fax (206-270-8418) or to the FDA Medwatch program by phone (800-FDA-1088) or by fax (800-FDA-0178), or by internet (https://www.accessdata.fda.gov/scripts/medwatch).

Hyperleukocytosis. In one clinical study, hyperleukocytosis (leukocyte counts of 10,000/mm³ or more), which was reported in 50% of patients receiving arsenic trioxide, was not treated with additional chemotherapy. Leukocyte counts during consolidation therapy were not as high as those observed during induction therapy.

Carcinogenicity. Carcinogenicity studies have not been performed using IV arsenic trioxide; however, arsenic trioxide is a human carcinogen.

Fetal/Neonatal Morbidity and Mortality. May cause fetal harm; inorganic arsenical preparations cross the placental barrier in animals receiving the drugs orally or parenterally. Teratogenicity demonstrated in animals receiving arsenic trioxide orally or sodium arsenite parenterally. No studies to date in humans. It is recommended that pregnancy be avoided during therapy. If used during pregnancy or patient becomes pregnant, apprise of potential fetal hazard. One patient who became pregnant while receiving arsenic trioxide therapy had a miscarriage.

General Precautions **Adequate Patient Monitoring.** The manufacturer recommends that hematologic and coagulation tests and serum electrolyte concentrations be determined at least twice weekly during induction therapy with arsenic trioxide (more frequently in clinically unstable patients) and at least weekly during consolidation therapy. In addition, the manufacturer recommends that ECG be monitored weekly (more frequently in clinically unstable patients) during induction and consolidation therapy.

Specific Populations **Pregnancy.** Category D. (See Users Guide, and see Fetal/Neonatal Morbidity and Mortality under Warnings/Precautions: Warnings, in Cautions.)

Lactation. Arsenic is distributed in milk in humans. Discontinue nursing or the drug, taking into account the importance of the drug to the woman.

Pediatric Use. Safety and efficacy of arsenic trioxide not established in children younger than 5 years of age. Arsenic trioxide (at dosages of 0.15 mg/kg daily) was used in 7 children (5–16 years of age) with acute promyelocytic leukemia (APL); 5 (71%) of these children achieved a complete response. In another study, complete response was observed in 11 (85%) of 13 children and young adults (4–21 years of age) receiving arsenic trioxide 0.15 mg/kg daily (5 consecutive days per week for 20 doses followed by a 2-week break between treatment cycles for up to 70 doses total) for refractory or relapsed APL.

Renal Impairment. Arsenic is excreted principally in urine; use with caution in patients with renal failure.

■ **Common Adverse Effects** Adverse effects occurring in 10% or more of patients include fatigue, fever, edema, rigors, chest pain, reactions at the injection site (i.e., pain, erythema, edema), weakness, weight gain, nausea, anorexia, decreased appetite, diarrhea or loose stools, vomiting, abdominal pain, dyspepsia, sore throat, constipation, hypokalemia, hypomagnesemia, hyperglycemia, increases in serum AST (SGOT) and/or ALT (SGPT), hyperkalemia, hypocalcemia, headache, insomnia, paresthesia, dizziness, tremor, cough, dyspnea, epistaxis, hypoxia, pleural effusion, postnasal drip, wheezing, decreased breath sounds, crepitations, rales, dermatitis, pruritus, ecchymosis, dry skin, erythema, sweating, tachycardia, ECG abnormalities, sinusitis, herpes simplex, upper respiratory infection, arthralgia, myalgia, bone pain, back pain, neck pain, limb pain, leukocytosis, anemia, thrombocytopenia, neutropenia (may be febrile), hypotension, hypertension, flushing, pallor, anxiety, depression, ocular irritation, blurred vision, and vaginal hemorrhage.

Drug Interactions

No formal drug interaction studies have been performed.

■ **Drugs That Prolong the QT Interval or May Be Associated with Electrolyte Abnormalities** Arsenic trioxide should not be used concomitantly with ziprasidone or pimozide because of potentially additive effects on prolongation of the QT interval.

The manufacturer states that arsenic trioxide should be administered with caution in patients receiving drugs that may prolong the QT interval (e.g., certain antiarrhythmics, thioridazine) or those that may cause electrolyte abnormalities (e.g., potassium-wasting diuretics, amphotericin B).

Pharmacokinetics

Pharmacokinetics of trivalent arsenic have not been characterized.

■ **Distribution** ***Extent*** Arsenic is stored mainly in liver, kidney, heart, lung, hair, and nails.

Inorganic arsenical preparations cross the placenta in animals.

■ **Elimination** ***Metabolism*** Arsenic trioxide is extensively metabolized via reduction by arsenate reductase and methylation (mainly in the liver) by methyltransferases.

Elimination Route Trivalent arsenic is excreted in urine.

Description

Arsenic trioxide is an antineoplastic agent. Although the mechanism of action of arsenic trioxide has not been fully elucidated, results from in vitro studies using NB4 human promyelocytic leukemia cells suggest that arsenic trioxide may cause morphologic changes and DNA fragmentation, which are characteristic of apoptosis (programmed cell death). The drug also causes damage or degradation of the fusion gene PML-RAR-α which results from the fusion of the promyelocytic leukemia (PML) gene (which encodes a transcription factor located on chromosome 15) and the retinoic acid receptor (RAR)-α gene (on chromosome 17) and is characteristic of acute promyelocytic leukemia (APL).

Arsenic trioxide undergoes extensive hepatic metabolism and is eliminated principally by metabolism and urinary excretion.

Advice to Patients

Importance of informing clinicians if patients develop unexplained fever, dyspnea, and/or weight gain. Importance of women informing clinicians if they are or plan to become pregnant or breast-feed. Importance of informing clinicians of existing or contemplated concomitant therapy, including prescription and OTC drugs.

Overview (see Users Guide). For additional information until a more detailed monograph is developed and published, the manufacturer's labeling should be consulted. It is *essential* that the manufacturer's labeling be consulted for more detailed information on usual cautions, precautions, contraindications, potential drug interactions, laboratory test interferences, and acute toxicity. For further information on the handling of antineoplastic agents, see the ASHP Guidelines on Handling Hazardous Drugs at http://www.ahfsdruginformation.com.

Preparations

Excipients in commercially available drug preparations may have clinically important effects in some individuals; consult specific product labeling for details.

Arsenic Trioxide

Parenteral

For injection, for IV use only	1 mg/mL (10 mg)	**Trisenox®**, Cephalon

†Use is not currently included in the labeling approved by the US Food and Drug Administration

Asparaginase (Erwinia chrysanthemi)

Crisantaspasum, Cristantaspase, Erwinia L-asparginase, Erwinia ASNase

■ Asparaginase (Erwinia chrysanthemi), an asparaginase enzyme derived from *Erwinia chrysanthemi* (formerly *Erwinia carotovora*; also known as *Pectobacterium chrysanthemi*), is an antineoplastic agent.

Uses

■ **Acute Lymphocytic Leukemia** ***Acute Lymphocytic Leukemia and Hypersensitivity to Escherichia coli-derived Asparaginase*** Asparaginase (Erwinia chrysanthemi) is used as a component of combination chemotherapy for the treatment of acute lymphocytic (lymphoblastic) leukemia (ALL) in patients who are hypersensitive to *E. coli*-derived asparaginase (native [nonconjugated] asparaginase [Escherichia coli] or pegaspargase; asparaginase [Escherichia coli] no longer commercially available in the US). Asparaginase (Erwinia chrysanthemi) has been designated an orphan drug by the US Food and Drug Administration (FDA) for this use. For additional information on other asparaginase preparations and the treatment of ALL, see Pegaspargase 10:00.

The current indication for asparaginase (Erwinia chrysanthemi) is based on an open-label, noncomparative safety and clinical pharmacology study in patients on National Cancer Institute (NCI)-sponsored cooperative group ALL protocols who were unable to continue pegaspargase therapy because of hypersensitivity reactions. Patients received asparaginase (Erwinia chrysanthemi) 25,000 units/m^2 by IM injection on a Monday, Wednesday, and Friday schedule for 2 weeks (total of 6 doses) as a replacement for each scheduled dose of pegaspargase remaining on their original treatment protocol. The primary outcome measure was the proportion of patients who achieved sustained asparaginase activity at a level predicted to result in clinical efficacy (i.e., serum trough asparaginase activity of 0.1 units/mL or greater, which has been demonstrated to correlate with asparagine depletion [asparagine concentration of less than 0.4 mcg/mL]). Of the 58 patients enrolled in the study, 48 were evaluated for the primary outcome measure based on availability of pharmacokinetic samples; the median age of patients in the study was 10 years (range: 2–18 years of age). The proportion of patients who achieved serum trough asparaginase activity of 0.1 units/mL or greater was 100% at either 48 hours (35 of 35 patients) or 72 hours (13 of 13 patients) following the third dose of asparaginase (Erwinia chrysanthemi). Because some clinicians suggest that serum trough asparaginase activity of 0.4 units/mL or greater is a better predictor of clinical efficacy, an exploratory analysis was performed using this outcome measure. The proportion of patients who achieved serum trough asparaginase activity of 0.4 units/mL or greater was 80% at 48 hours (28 of 35 patients) and 38% at 72 hours (5 of 13 patients) following the third dose of asparaginase (Erwinia chrysanthemi).

Dosage and Administration

■ **Reconstitution and Administration** Asparaginase (Erwinia chrysanthemi) is administered by IM injection. Asparaginase (Erwinia chrysanthemi) should be administered in a setting with resuscitation equipment and other agents necessary to treat anaphylaxis. (See Hypersensitivity Reactions under Warnings/Precautions: Sensitivity Reactions, in Cautions.)

Asparaginase (Erwinia chrysanthemi) lyophilized powder for injection should be inspected visually for foreign particulate matter and discoloration prior to reconstitution and discarded if either is present.

Asparaginase (Erwinia chrysanthemi) sterile lyophilized powder for injection is reconstituted by adding 1 or 2 mL of sterile, preservative-free 0.9% sodium chloride injection to a vial labeled as containing 10,000 units of asparaginase (Erwinia chrysanthemi) to provide a solution containing 10,000 or 5000 units/mL, respectively. Based on the indicated dosage of asparaginase (Erwinia chrysanthemi), the appropriate number of vials of the drug should be reconstituted. During reconstitution, the sterile, preservative-free 0.9% sodium chloride injection should be injected slowly against the inner wall of the vial and should not be forcefully injected directly onto or into the powder. The contents of the vial should be dissolved by gently mixing or swirling the vial; the vial should not be shaken or inverted. The reconstituted solution should be clear and colorless and should be discarded if any visible particles or protein aggregates are present. The appropriate dose of asparaginase (Erwinia chrysanthemi) should be withdrawn from the vial into a polypropylene syringe within 15 minutes of reconstitution. Unused portions of the injection should be discarded and should not be saved for later administration. The reconstituted solution should be administered within 4 hours or discarded and should not be frozen or refrigerated.

The manufacturer recommends that not more than 2 mL of reconstituted asparaginase (Erwinia chrysanthemi) solution be administered at any one injection site; if the total volume exceeds 2 mL, the dose should be divided and administered at separate sites.

Asparaginase (Erwinia chrysanthemi) lyophilized powder for injection in unopened vials and cartons should be stored at 2–8°C and protected from light.

Procedures for proper handling and disposal of antineoplastic drugs should be followed when preparing or administering asparaginase preparations.

■ **Dosage** Dosage of asparaginase (Erwinia chrysanthemi) is expressed in international units (IU, units) and must be individualized according to body surface area. Clinicians should consult published protocols for the dosage of asparaginase (Erwinia chrysanthemi) and other chemotherapeutic agents and the method and sequence of administration.

Acute Lymphocytic Leukemia **Acute Lymphocytic Leukemia and Hypersensitivity to Escherichia coli-derived Asparaginase.** When asparaginase (Erwinia chrysanthemi) is substituted for a dose of pegaspargase, the recommended dosage of asparaginase (Erwinia chrysanthemi) is 25,000 units/m^2 administered IM 3 times weekly (Monday, Wednesday, Friday) for 6 doses for each planned dose of pegaspargase.

When asparaginase (Erwinia chrysanthemi) is substituted for a dose of native (nonconjugated) asparaginase (Escherichia coli) (no longer commercially available in the US), the recommended dosage of asparaginase (Erwinia chrysanthemi) is 25,000 units/m^2 administered IM for each scheduled dose of native asparaginase (Escherichia coli).

Dosage Modification for Toxicity and Contraindications to Continued Therapy **Anaphylaxis and Allergic Reactions.** Asparaginase (Erwinia chrysanthemi) therapy should be discontinued in patients with serious allergic reactions.

Thrombosis and Hemorrhage. Asparaginase (Erwinia chrysanthemi) therapy should be withheld in patients experiencing thrombotic or hemorrhagic events until the symptoms resolve; after resolution, therapy may be resumed. (See Cautions: Contraindications.)

Pancreatitis. Asparaginase (Erwinia chrysanthemi) therapy should be discontinued permanently in patients who experience severe pancreatitis. (See Pancreatitis under Cautions: Warnings/Precautions.) In patients with mild pancreatitis, the drug should be withheld until the signs and symptoms resolve and amylase concentrations return to normal; after resolution, therapy may be resumed.

■ **Special Populations** The manufacturer makes no specific dosage recommendations for patients with hepatic or renal impairment. Safety and efficacy of asparaginase (Erwinia chrysanthemi) have not been established in geriatric patients.

Cautions

■ **Contraindications** Asparaginase (Erwinia chrysanthemi) is contraindicated in patients with a history of serious pancreatitis, serious thrombosis, or serious hemorrhagic events associated with prior asparaginase therapy or a history of serious hypersensitivity reactions (including anaphylaxis) to asparaginase (Erwinia chrysanthemi).

■ **Warnings/Precautions** ***Sensitivity Reactions*** **Hypersensitivity Reactions.** Serious hypersensitivity reactions, including anaphylaxis, have occurred in 5% of patients receiving asparaginase (Erwinia chrysanthemi) in clinical studies. Systemic allergic reactions (anaphylaxis, hypersensitivity, urticaria) have occurred in 17% of patients receiving the drug in clinical studies. In one small series, allergic reactions to asparaginase (Erwinia chrysanthemi) were reported in 33% of patients switching to asparaginase (Erwinia chrysanthemi) following clinical hypersensitivity to native (nonconjugated) asparaginase (Escherichia coli).

Asparaginase (Erwinia chrysanthemi) should be administered in a setting with resuscitation equipment and other agents necessary to treat anaphylaxis. If a serious hypersensitivity reaction occurs, asparaginase (Erwinia chrysanthemi) therapy should be discontinued and appropriate therapy should be initiated.

Pancreatitis Pancreatitis has been reported in 4% of patients receiving asparaginase (Erwinia chrysanthemi) in clinical studies. Grade 3 or 4 pancreatitis has been reported in 0.6% of patients receiving the drug in clinical studies. Patients experiencing symptoms compatible with pancreatitis should be evaluated to establish a diagnosis. In patients with severe or hemorrhagic pancreatitis associated with abdominal pain for longer than 72 hours and amylase concentrations 2 or more times the upper limit of normal (ULN), asparaginase (Erwinia chrysanthemi) therapy should be discontinued. Severe pancreatitis is a contraindication to continued asparaginase (Erwinia chrysanthemi) therapy. In patients with mild pancreatitis, asparaginase (Erwinia chrysanthemi) therapy should be withheld until the signs and symptoms resolve and amylase concentrations return to normal; after resolution, therapy may be resumed.

Hyperglycemia Glucose intolerance, sometimes irreversible, has been reported in 2% of patients receiving asparaginase (Erwinia chrysanthemi) in clinical studies. Hyperglycemia was grade 3 or 4 in 1.7% of patients receiving the drug in clinical studies. Glucose concentrations should be monitored at baseline and periodically during therapy. Insulin therapy should be administered as necessary in patients with hyperglycemia.

Thrombosis and Hemorrhage Serious thrombotic events, including sagittal sinus thrombosis, have been associated with both *E. coli*- and *Erwinia chrysanthemi*-derived asparaginase therapy. Grade 3 or 4 thrombosis has been reported in about 1% of patients receiving asparaginase (Erwinia chrysanthemi) in clinical studies, and grade 3 or 4 hemorrhage has been reported in 0.2% of patients. Coagulation proteins (i.e., antithrombin III, fibrinogen, protein C activity, protein S activity) were decreased in most patients after 2 weeks of asparaginase (Erwinia chrysanthemi) therapy. Asparaginase (Erwinia chrysanthemi) therapy should be withheld in patients experiencing thrombotic or hemorrhagic events until the symptoms resolve; after resolution, therapy may be resumed.

Immunogenicity There is potential for immunogenicity with the use of therapeutic proteins such as asparaginase (Erwinia chrysanthemi). Insufficient data are available to characterize the incidence of antibody formation to asparaginase (Erwinia chrysanthemi).

Specific Populations **Pregnancy.** Category C. (See Users Guide.)

Lactation. It is not known whether asparaginase (Erwinia chrysanthemi) is distributed into milk. A decision should be made whether to discontinue nursing or the drug, taking into account the importance of the drug to the woman.

Pediatric Use. Safety and efficacy of asparaginase (Erwinia chrysanthemi) as a component of combination chemotherapy for the treatment of acute lymphocytic (lymphoblastic) leukemia (ALL) have been evaluated in a safety and clinical pharmacology study in patients 2–18 years of age (median: 10 years of age) who were hypersensitive to *E. coli*-derived asparaginase. (See Acute Lymphocytic Leukemia and Hypersensitivity to Escherichia coli-derived Asparaginase under Uses: Acute Lymphocytic Leukemia.)

Geriatric Use. Safety and efficacy of asparaginase (Erwinia chrysanthemi) have not been established in geriatric patients.

■ **Common Adverse Effects** Adverse effects reported in more than 1% of patients receiving asparaginase (Erwinia chrysanthemi) include serious hypersensitivity reactions (e.g., anaphylaxis, urticaria), pancreatitis, abnormal transaminases, thrombosis, fever, hyperglycemia, nausea, and vomiting.

Drug Interactions

No formal drug interaction studies have been performed with asparaginase (Erwinia chrysanthemi) to date.

Description

Asparaginase (Erwinia chrysanthemi) catalyzes the deamidation of the amino acid asparagine to aspartic acid and ammonia, resulting in reduced concentrations of circulating asparagine. Because of a lack of asparagine synthetase, some leukemic cells cannot synthesize asparagine and depend on an exogenous source of the amino acid for protein synthesis and cell survival. Because normal cells are able to synthesize asparagine, they are less affected by asparaginase-induced depletion of the amino acid.

The pharmacokinetics of asparaginase (Erwinia chrysanthemi) have not been fully characterized. However, the half-life of asparaginase (Erwinia chrysanthemi) reportedly is approximately 0.65 days and appears to be shorter than that of native (nonconjugated) asparaginase (Escherichia coli) or pegaspargase (conjugate of polyethylene glycol [PEG] and *E. coli*-derived asparaginase). Asparaginase (Erwinia chrysanthemi) is antigenically distinct from asparaginase (Escherichia coli).

Advice to Patients

Risk of hypersensitivity reactions, including the possibility of anaphylaxis. Importance of informing patients of the symptoms of allergic reactions, including anaphylaxis, and instructing them to immediately contact clinicians if such symptoms occur.

Risk of pancreatitis. Importance of immediately informing clinicians if abdominal pain occurs.

Risk of glucose intolerance. Importance of informing clinicians if excessive thirst or any increase in the volume or frequency of urination occurs.

Risk of thrombosis and hemorrhage. Importance of immediately informing clinicians if headache, arm or leg swelling, shortness of breath, or chest pain occurs.

Importance of informing clinicians of existing or contemplated concomitant therapy, including prescription and OTC drugs, as well as any concomitant illnesses.

Importance of women informing clinicians if they are or plan to become pregnant or plan to breast-feed.

Importance of informing patients of other important precautionary information. (See Cautions.)

Overview® (see Users Guide). For additional information on this drug until a more detailed monograph is developed and published, the manufacturer's labeling should be consulted. It is *essential* that the manufacturer's labeling be consulted for more detailed information on usual cautions, precautions, contraindications, potential drug interactions, laboratory test interferences, and acute toxicity. For further information on the handling of antineoplastic agents, see the ASHP Guidelines on Handling Hazardous Drugs.

Preparations

Excipients in commercially available drug preparations may have clinically important effects in some individuals; consult specific product labeling for details.

Asparaginase (Erwinia chrysanthemi)

Parenteral

For injection, for IM use	10,000 units	**Erwinaze®**, EUSA

Atezolizumab

■ Atezolizumab, a humanized anti-programmed-death ligand-1 (anti-PD-L1) monoclonal antibody, is an antineoplastic agent.

Uses

■ **Urothelial Carcinoma** Atezolizumab is used for the treatment of locally advanced or metastatic urothelial carcinoma that has progressed during or following platinum-containing therapy for advanced disease or within 12 months of neoadjuvant or adjuvant chemotherapy. Atezolizumab also is used for the treatment of locally advanced or metastatic urothelial carcinoma in patients with high programmed-death ligand-1 (PD-L1) expression (defined as PD-L1 staining in tumor-infiltrating immune cells covering at least 5% of the tumor area) who are not candidates for cisplatin-containing therapy; an FDA-approved diagnostic test is required to confirm the presence of PD-L1 expression prior to initiation of therapy in patients who are not candidates for cisplatin-containing therapy. Atezolizumab also is used for the treatment of locally advanced or metastatic urothelial carcinoma in patients who are not candidates for platinum-containing chemotherapy regardless of PD-L1 expression. The accelerated approval of atezolizumab for these indications is based on objective response rate and duration of response. Continued approval for these indications may be contingent on verification and description of clinical benefit of atezolizumab in confirmatory studies.

The current indications for atezolizumab in the treatment of locally advanced or metastatic urothelial carcinoma are based principally on the results of an open-label, multicenter, noncomparative, 2-cohort, phase 2 study (IMvigor210). The first cohort (cohort 1) included 119 patients with locally advanced or metastatic urothelial carcinoma that was previously untreated or that had progressed following neoadjuvant or adjuvant chemotherapy who were not candidates for cisplatin-containing therapy. The second cohort (cohort 2) included 310 patients with previously treated locally advanced or metastatic urothelial carcinoma that had progressed during or following platinum-containing therapy for advanced disease or within 12 months of platinum-containing therapy in the neoadjuvant or adjuvant setting. The primary measure of efficacy was objective response rate as assessed by an independent review facility according to Response Evaluation Criteria in Solid Tumors (RECIST). Patients received atezolizumab 1.2 g administered as an IV infusion every 3 weeks until disease progression or unacceptable toxicity occurred. Patients with a history of autoimmune disease; those with active or corticosteroid-dependent brain metastases; those who had received a live, attenuated vaccine within 28 days prior to enrollment; and those who had received systemic immunostimulatory agents within 6 weeks or immunosuppressive agents within 2 weeks prior to enrollment were excluded from the study.

In the cisplatin-ineligible cohort (cohort 1), the median age of patients was 73 years; 91% were Caucasian, 81% were male, 80% had a baseline Eastern Cooperative Oncology Group (ECOG) performance status of 0 or 1, 66% had visceral metastases, 35% had non-bladder urothelial carcinoma, and 20% had disease progression following platinum-containing therapy in the neoadjuvant or adjuvant setting. Most patients (73%) had low expression of PD-L1 (defined as PD-L1 staining in tumor-infiltrating immune cells covering less than 5% of the tumor area) as detected by an immunohistochemistry assay (Ventana PD-L1 [SP142]). Approximately 27% of patients had high expression of PD-L1 (defined as PD-L1 staining in tumor-infiltrating immune cells covering 5% or more of the tumor area). The median age of patients with high expression of PD-L1 was 67 years; 88% were Caucasian, 81% were male, 72% had a baseline ECOG performance status of 0 or 1, 56% had visceral metastases, 28% had non-bladder urothelial carcinoma, and 31% had disease progression following platinum-containing therapy in the neoadjuvant or adjuvant setting. Reasons for cisplatin ineligibility included baseline renal impairment (creatinine clearance 30–59 mL/minute), poor performance status (ECOG performance status of 2), hearing loss (25-decibel or more loss at 2 contiguous frequencies), or baseline grade 2–4 peripheral neuropathy in 70, 20, 14, or 6%, respectively, of patients in the entire cohort and in 66, 28, 16, or 9%, respectively, of those in the subset with high PD-L1 expression. The objective response rate for patients in the cisplatin-ineligible cohort of this study was 23.5%; complete response was achieved in 6.7% of patients in this cohort. Among patients who had disease progression following therapy in the neoadjuvant or adjuvant setting, the objective response rate was 33%. Objective response rates in patients with high or low levels of PD-L1 expression were 28.1 or 21.8%, respectively; complete response was achieved in 6.3 or 6.9% of patients, respectively. At a median follow-up of 14.4 months, the median duration of response had not been reached.

In the cohort previously treated with platinum-containing therapy (cohort 2), the median age of patients was 66 years; 91% were Caucasian, 78% were male, 78% had visceral metastases, 62% had a baseline ECOG performance status of 1, 35% had a baseline creatinine clearance less than 60 mL/minute, and 26% had non-bladder urothelial carcinoma. Approximately one-half (41%) of patients enrolled in this cohort had received at least 2 prior therapies for metastatic disease and 19% had disease progression following platinum-containing therapy in the neoadjuvant or adjuvant setting; 73, 26, or 1% of patients had received prior treatment with cisplatin-, carboplatin-, or other platinum-based regimens, respectively. Most patients (68%) had low expression of PD-L1 (defined as PD-L1 staining in tumor-infiltrating immune cells covering less than 5% of the tumor area) and 32% had high expression of PD-L1 (defined as PD-L1 staining in tumor-infiltrating immune cells covering 5% or more of the tumor area) as detected by an immunohistochemistry assay (Ventana PD-L1 [SP142]). The objective response rate for patients in the previously treated cohort of this study was 14.8%; complete response was achieved in 5.5% of patients in this cohort. Among patients who had disease progression following therapy in the neoadjuvant or adjuvant setting, the objective response rate was 22%. At a median follow-up of 32.9 months, the median duration of response for patients in the previously treated cohort was 27.7 months. Median progression-free and overall survival times were 2.1 and 7.9 months, respectively. A planned subgroup analysis indicated that patients with high levels of PD-L1 expression had higher objective response rates compared with those with low levels of PD-L1 expression (26 versus 9.5%); the median duration of response was 29.7 or 20.9 months, respectively, and complete response was achieved in 12 or 2.4% of patients, respectively.

Decreased survival with atezolizumab monotherapy compared with platinum-based therapy has been reported in an ongoing clinical trial (IMvigor130) in patients with previously untreated metastatic urothelial carcinoma with low PD-L1 expression; atezolizumab monotherapy is *not* currently FDA-labeled for use in such patients. In this trial, patients with previously untreated metastatic urothelial carcinoma who were eligible for platinum-containing therapy were randomized to receive atezolizumab monotherapy, atezolizumab in combination with platinum-based therapy (cisplatin or carboplatin in combination with gemcitabine), or platinum-based therapy alone. A preliminary data analysis showed decreased survival of patients with low PD-L1 expression who were receiving atezolizumab monotherapy compared with those receiving platinum-based therapy. Therefore, at the request of the independent data monitoring committee, enrollment in the atezolizumab monotherapy group was halted for patients with low expression of PD-L1 (defined as PD-L1 staining in tumor-infiltrating immune cells covering less than 5% of the tumor area) as detected by an immunohistochemistry assay (Ventana PD-L1 [SP142]).

■ **Non-small Cell Lung Cancer** ***Combination Therapy for Previously Untreated Metastatic Nonsquamous Non-small Cell Lung Cancer*** Atezolizumab is used in combination with bevacizumab, carboplatin, and paclitaxel for the initial treatment of metastatic nonsquamous non-small cell lung cancer (NSCLC) without epidermal growth factor receptor (EGFR) or anaplastic lymphoma kinase (ALK) genomic aberrations.

The current indication for atezolizumab in combination with bevacizumab, carboplatin, and paclitaxel for the initial treatment of metastatic nonsquamous NSCLC is based principally on the results of a randomized, open-label, phase 3 study (IMpower150). In this study, 1202 adults with metastatic NSCLC with nonsquamous histology who had not received prior chemotherapy for metastatic disease were randomized (stratified by sex, presence of liver metastases, and PD-L1 expression) in a 1:1:1 ratio to receive 4 or 6 cycles of therapy with atezolizumab in combination with carboplatin and paclitaxel (atezolizumab-carboplatin-paclitaxel); atezolizumab in combination with bevacizumab, carboplatin, and paclitaxel (atezolizumab-bevacizumab-carboplatin-paclitaxel); or bevacizumab, carboplatin, and paclitaxel alone (bevacizumab-carboplatin-paclitaxel). Following the initial 4 or 6 cycles of therapy, carboplatin and paclitaxel were discontinued and patients continued receiving atezolizumab and/or bevacizumab as initially assigned until disease progression or unacceptable toxicity occurred; however, atezolizumab-treated patients with disease progression could continue receiving treatment if they were considered to be deriving clinical benefit. The treatment regimens were administered in 3-week cycles at the following dosages: atezolizumab 1.2 g every 3 weeks, bevacizumab 15 mg/kg every 3 weeks, carboplatin at the dose required to obtain an area under the concentration-time curve (AUC) of 6 mg/mL per minute every 3 weeks, and paclitaxel 200 mg/m^2 (175 mg/m^2 in patients of Asian ancestry) every 3 weeks. The primary measures of efficacy were overall survival in patients with wild-type EGFR and ALK expression (wild-type population) and progression-free survival as assessed by investigators according to RECIST in the wild-type population and in the subset of the wild-type population with high expression of an effector T-cell (Teff) gene signature.

The median age of patients receiving atezolizumab-bevacizumab-carboplatin-paclitaxel or bevacizumab-carboplatin-paclitaxel in the IMpower150 study was 63 years; within these 2 treatment groups, 82% of patients were Caucasian, 80% were current or prior smokers, 60% were male, 49% had negative PD-L1 expression (defined as PD-L1 expression on less than 1% of tumor cells and tumor-infiltrating immune cells, as detected by the Ventana PD-L1 [SP142] immunohistochemistry assay), 39% had high Teff gene-signature expression (defined as a score of −1.91 or greater based on PD-L1, CXCL9, and interferon gamma mRNA expression in tumor tissue, as detected by a clinical trial assay), 14% had liver metastases at baseline, 13% were of Asian ancestry, and 10% were Hispanic. All patients had a baseline ECOG performance status of 0 or 1. The study excluded patients with a history of autoimmune disease; those with active or untreated CNS metastases; those who had received a live, attenuated vaccine within 28 days prior to randomization; those who had received systemic immunostimulatory agents within 4 weeks or systemic immunosuppressive agents within 2 weeks prior to randomization; and those with tumor infiltration into the thoracic great vessels or cavitation of pulmonary lesions. Neoadjuvant or adjuvant chemotherapy must have been completed at least 6 months before randomization into the IMpower150 study.

In the subset of patients with wild-type EGFR and ALK expression, median progression-free survival was prolonged in those receiving atezolizumab-bevacizumab-carboplatin-paclitaxel compared with those receiving bevacizumab-carboplatin-paclitaxel (8.5 versus 7 months; hazard ratio: 0.71). At a median follow-up of approximately 20 months, median overall survival also was prolonged in those receiving atezolizumab-bevacizumab-carboplatin-paclitaxel compared with those receiving bevacizumab-carboplatin-paclitaxel (19.2 versus 14.7 months; hazard ratio: 0.78). However, neither progression-free survival (6.7 or 7 months, respectively; hazard ratio: 0.94) nor overall survival (19.4 or 14.7 months, respectively; hazard ratio: 0.84) was prolonged in those receiving atezolizumab-carboplatin-paclitaxel compared with those receiving bevacizumab-carboplatin-paclitaxel. In patients with wild-type EGFR and ALK expression, the objective response rate was 55% in those receiving atezolizumab-bevacizumab-carboplatin-paclitaxel, 43% in those receiving atezolizumab-carboplatin-paclitaxel, and 42% in those receiving bevacizumab-carboplatin-paclitaxel; complete responses were achieved in 4, 3, or 1% of patients receiving these respective treatments. The median duration of response was 10.8 months in patients receiving atezolizumab-bevacizumab-carboplatin-paclitaxel, 9.5 months in those receiving atezolizumab-carboplatin-paclitaxel, and 6.5 months in those receiving bevacizumab-carboplatin-paclitaxel. In patients with wild-type EGFR and ALK expression, subset analyses indicated a progression-free survival benefit for atezolizumab-bevacizumab-carboplatin-paclitaxel compared with bevacizumab-carboplatin-paclitaxel regardless of level of PD-L1 or Teff gene-signature expression and across subgroups based on sex, age, ECOG performance status, smoking status, presence of liver metastases, and KRAS mutation status.

In the subset of patients with wild-type EGFR and ALK expression and high Teff gene-signature expression, median progression-free survival was prolonged in patients receiving atezolizumab-bevacizumab-carboplatin-paclitaxel compared with those receiving bevacizumab-carboplatin-paclitaxel; however, progression-free survival was not prolonged in patients receiving atezolizumab-carboplatin-paclitaxel compared with those receiving bevacizumab-carboplatin-paclitaxel.

In an exploratory analysis, efficacy in patients receiving atezolizumab-bevacizumab-carboplatin-paclitaxel appeared to be similar in those who tested positive for anti-atezolizumab antibodies by week 4 compared with those who did not develop anti-atezolizumab antibodies by week 4. (See Immunogenicity under Cautions: Warnings/Precautions.)

Monotherapy for Previously Treated Metastatic Non-small Cell Lung Cancer Atezolizumab is used for the treatment of metastatic NSCLC that has progressed during or following platinum-based chemotherapy. Patients with EGFR- or ALK-positive tumors also should have documented disease progression during or following an FDA-labeled anti-EGFR or anti-ALK therapy prior to initiating therapy with atezolizumab.

The current indication for atezolizumab in the treatment of previously treated NSCLC is based principally on the results of a randomized, open-label phase 3 study (OAK), with supporting data from a similarly designed phase 2 study (POPLAR), in patients with locally advanced or metastatic NSCLC that had progressed during or following platinum-based chemotherapy. Patients in these studies were randomized (stratified by level of PD-L1 expression in tumor-infiltrating immune cells, number of prior chemotherapy regimens, and histology) in a 1:1 ratio to receive either atezolizumab (1.2 g IV every 3 weeks) or docetaxel (75 mg/m^2 IV every 3 weeks). Treatment was continued until disease progression or unacceptable toxicity occurred; however, atezolizumab-treated patients with disease progression could continue receiving treatment if they were considered to be deriving clinical benefit. The studies excluded patients with a history of autoimmune disease; those with symptomatic or corticosteroid-dependent brain metastases; and those who received systemic immunosuppressive agents within 2 weeks prior to enrollment. In both studies, the primary measure of efficacy was overall survival.

In the OAK study, the primary efficacy population consisted of the initial 850 patients randomized in the study. In the primary efficacy population, the median age of patients was 64 years; 94% had metastatic disease, 74% had nonsquamous histology, 70% were Caucasian, 67% were former smokers, 61% were male, 55% had positive PD-L1 expression, 47% were 65 years of age or older, 21% were of Asian ancestry, 15% were current smokers, 10% had EGFR mutation-positive disease, 7% had KRAS mutation-positive disease, and less than 1% had ALK-positive disease. All patients had a baseline ECOG performance status of 0 or 1. Most patients (75%) had received one prior platinum-based chemotherapy regimen. In the primary efficacy population, patients receiving atezolizumab had longer median overall survival (13.8 versus 9.6 months; hazard ratio: 0.74) compared with patients receiving docetaxel; however, progression-free survival appeared to be shorter in patients receiving atezolizumab compared with those receiving docetaxel (2.8 versus 4 months). At the time of analysis, no difference in objective response rates was observed between patients receiving atezolizumab and those receiving docetaxel (14 and 13%, respectively); however, median response duration was prolonged in patients receiving atezolizumab compared with those receiving docetaxel (16.3 versus 6.2 months). Effects of atezolizumab on overall survival in the total patient population were comparable to those observed in the primary efficacy population. In the primary efficacy population, a planned subgroup analysis indicated that the risk of death was decreased with atezolizumab compared with docetaxel regardless of PD-L1 expression; however, survival benefit for atezolizumab compared with docetaxel was more pronounced in patients with high levels of PD-L1 expression (defined as PD-L1 expression on 50% or more of tumor cells or 10% or more of tumor-infiltrating immune cells) as detected by an immunohistochemistry assay (Ventana PD-L1 [SP142]) (hazard ratio: 0.41) compared with those with lower levels of PD-L1 expression (hazard ratio: 0.82). In an exploratory analysis, efficacy appeared to be reduced in patients who tested positive for anti-atezolizumab antibodies by week 4 compared with those who did not develop anti-atezolizumab antibodies by week 4. (See Immunogenicity under Cautions: Warnings/Precautions.)

In the POPLAR study, the median age of patients was 62 years. All patients enrolled in the study had a baseline ECOG performance status of 0 or 1, 66% had nonsquamous histology, 7% had EGFR mutation-positive disease, and 1% had ALK-positive disease. Approximately 67% had received one prior platinum-based chemotherapy regimen. After a median follow-up of 22 months, patients receiving atezolizumab had longer median overall survival (12.6 versus 9.7 months) compared with patients receiving docetaxel. Although objective response rates were similar between both treatment groups, patients receiving atezolizumab had a longer median duration of response (18.6 versus 7.2 months) compared with those receiving docetaxel. A subgroup analysis also indicated that increasing levels of PD-L1 expression were associated with an overall survival benefit for atezolizumab compared with docetaxel. Overall survival benefit for atezolizumab compared with docetaxel also was apparent regardless of histology and prior tobacco use.

Dosage and Administration

■ **General** ***Restricted Distribution*** Atezolizumab can only be obtained through a limited network of specialty distributors. Clinicians may contact the manufacturer (Genentech) by telephone at 800-551-2231 or consult the Tecentriq® website for specific availability information (https://www.genentech-access.com/hcp/brands/tecentriq/learn-about-our-services/product-distribution.html).

■ **Administration** Atezolizumab is administered by IV infusion. The initial dose of atezolizumab should be administered as an IV infusion over 60 minutes; if the first infusion is tolerated, subsequent doses may be administered by IV infusion over 30 minutes. *The drug should not be administered by rapid IV injection, such as IV push or bolus.*

Unopened vials of atezolizumab injection concentrate should be protected from light, stored at 2–8°C, and should *not* be frozen or shaken.

Atezolizumab injection concentrate must be diluted prior to administration. Prior to dilution and administration, atezolizumab injection concentrate should be inspected visually for particulate matter and discoloration. The undiluted solution should be colorless to slightly yellow; the solution should *not* be used if it is cloudy or discolored or if particulate matter is present. Atezolizumab is diluted by adding 20 mL of atezolizumab injection concentrate (containing 60 mg/mL) to a polyvinyl chloride (PVC), polyethylene, or polyolefin infusion bag containing 250 mL of 0.9% sodium chloride injection. No other diluent should be used. The diluted solution should be mixed by gentle inversion and should *not* be shaken. The manufacturer recommends immediate administration of diluted solutions of the drug. If immediate administration is not possible, the diluted solution of the drug should be stored at room temperature for up to 6 hours from the time of preparation (including infusion time) or 2–8°C for up to 24 hours from time of preparation; diluted solutions of the drug should *not* be frozen.

Atezolizumab should *not* be administered simultaneously through the same IV line with any other drug. Use of a low-protein-binding 0.2- to 0.22-μm inline filter is optional. Atezolizumab injection concentrate contains no preservatives and is intended for single use only; any partially used vials should be discarded.

■ **Dosage** ***Urothelial Carcinoma*** For the treatment of locally advanced or metastatic urothelial carcinoma that has progressed during or following platinum-containing therapy for advanced disease or within 12 months of chemotherapy in the neoadjuvant or adjuvant setting, the recommended adult dosage of atezolizumab is 1.2 g as an IV infusion every 3 weeks. Therapy should be continued until disease progression or unacceptable toxicity occurs.

For the treatment of locally advanced or metastatic urothelial carcinoma in patients with high programmed-death ligand-1 (PD-L1) expression (defined as PD-L1 staining in tumor-infiltrating immune cells covering at least 5% of the tumor area) who are not candidates for cisplatin-containing therapy, and in those who are not candidates for platinum-containing chemotherapy regardless of PD-L1 expression, the recommended adult dosage of atezolizumab is 1.2 g as an IV infusion every 3 weeks. Therapy should be continued until disease progression or unacceptable toxicity occurs.

Selection of atezolizumab for the treatment of previously untreated locally advanced or metastatic urothelial carcinoma in patients who are not candidates for cisplatin-containing therapy should be based on the presence of PD-L1 expression. (See Uses: Urothelial Carcinoma.)

Non-small Cell Lung Cancer For the initial treatment of metastatic nonsquamous non-small cell lung cancer (NSCLC) without epidermal growth factor receptor (EGFR) or anaplastic lymphoma kinase (ALK) genomic aberrations, the recommended adult dosage of atezolizumab is 1.2 g as an IV infusion every 3 weeks in combination with bevacizumab, carboplatin, and paclitaxel. Atezolizumab should be administered before bevacizumab, carboplatin, and paclitaxel. Carboplatin and paclitaxel should be administered for a maximum of 4–6 cycles; therapy with atezolizumab and bevacizumab should be continued until disease progression or unacceptable toxicity occurs.

For the treatment of metastatic NSCLC that has progressed during or following platinum-based chemotherapy, the recommended adult dosage of atezolizumab is 1.2 g as an IV infusion every 3 weeks. Therapy should be continued until disease progression or unacceptable toxicity occurs.

Therapy Interruption for Toxicity If immune-mediated adverse effects occur, temporary or permanent discontinuance of atezolizumab may be required based on severity of the reaction.

Atezolizumab should be permanently discontinued in patients experiencing persistent grade 2 or 3 immune-mediated adverse effects (except for endocrinopathies) that do not recover to grade 0 or 1 within 12 weeks of the last dose of atezolizumab. Therapy with the drug also should be permanently discontinued in patients unable to reduce corticosteroid dosage to 10 mg or less of prednisone daily (or equivalent) within 12 weeks of the last dose of atezolizumab.

Therapy with the drug also should be permanently discontinued if any grade 3 or 4 immune-mediated adverse effects recur.

Immune-mediated Pneumonitis. If grade 2 immune-mediated pneumonitis occurs, atezolizumab therapy should be interrupted until the toxicity resolves to grade 0 or 1 *and* the corticosteroid dosage has been reduced to 10 mg or less of prednisone daily (or equivalent). (See Immune-mediated Pneumonitis under Cautions: Warnings/Precautions.)

If grade 3 or 4 immune-mediated pneumonitis occurs, atezolizumab therapy should be permanently discontinued.

Immune-mediated Hepatic Effects. For grade 2 immune-mediated hepatitis, serum aminotransferase (ALT or AST) elevations exceeding 3 times but not more than 8 times the upper limit of normal (ULN), or total bilirubin concentrations exceeding 1.5 times but not more than 3 times the ULN, atezolizumab therapy should be interrupted until the toxicity resolves to grade 0 or 1 *and* the corticosteroid dosage has been reduced to 10 mg or less of prednisone daily (or equivalent). (See Immune-mediated Hepatic Effects under Cautions: Warnings/Precautions.)

For grade 3 or 4 immune-mediated hepatitis, ALT or AST elevations exceeding 8 times the ULN, or total bilirubin concentrations exceeding 3 times the ULN, atezolizumab therapy should be permanently discontinued.

Immune-mediated GI Effects. If grade 2 or 3 immune-mediated colitis or diarrhea occurs, atezolizumab therapy should be interrupted until the toxicity resolves to grade 0 or 1 *and* the corticosteroid dosage has been reduced to 10 mg or less of prednisone daily (or equivalent). (See Immune-mediated GI Effects under Cautions: Warnings/Precautions.)

If grade 4 immune-mediated colitis or diarrhea occurs, atezolizumab therapy should be permanently discontinued.

Immune-mediated Endocrine Effects. If grade 2–4 immune-mediated endocrinopathies (e.g., hypophysitis, adrenal insufficiency, hyperthyroidism, type 1 diabetes mellitus) occur, atezolizumab therapy should be interrupted until the toxicity resolves to grade 0 or 1 *and* the patient's condition is stable on replacement therapy, if needed. (See Immune-mediated Endocrine Effects under Cautions: Warnings/Precautions.)

Other Immune-mediated Adverse Effects. If any other grade 3 immune-mediated adverse effects involving a major organ occur, atezolizumab therapy should be interrupted until the toxicity resolves to grade 0 or 1 *and* the corticosteroid dosage has been reduced to 10 mg or less of prednisone daily (or equivalent). (See Other Immune-mediated Effects under Cautions: Warnings/Precautions.)

If any other grade 4 immune-mediated adverse effects involving a major organ occur, atezolizumab therapy should be permanently discontinued.

Infusion-related Reactions. If grade 1 or 2 infusion-related reactions occur, the infusion should be interrupted or the infusion rate should be reduced. (See Infusion-related Effects under Cautions: Warnings/Precautions.)

If grade 3 or 4 infusion-related reactions occur, atezolizumab therapy should be permanently discontinued.

Infectious Complications. If grade 3 or 4 infection occurs, atezolizumab therapy should be interrupted until the infection resolves to grade 0 or 1. (See Infectious Complications under Cautions: Warnings/Precautions.)

■ **Special Populations** The manufacturer makes no special dosage recommendations for patients with hepatic or renal impairment or for geriatric patients. (See Specific Populations under Cautions: Warnings/Precautions.)

Cautions

■ **Contraindications** The manufacturer states there are no known contraindications to the use of atezolizumab.

■ **Warnings/Precautions** ***Immune-mediated Pneumonitis*** Immune-mediated pneumonitis or interstitial lung disease (defined as pneumonitis or interstitial lung disease requiring corticosteroid therapy), sometimes fatal, has occurred in patients receiving atezolizumab therapy.

In clinical studies, immune-mediated pneumonitis occurred in 2.5% of patients receiving atezolizumab as a single agent and was grade 3 or greater in approximately 0.8% of patients receiving the drug. The median time to onset of immune-mediated pneumonitis was 3.6 months (range: 3 days to 20.5 months) and the median duration was 1.4 months (range: 1 day to 15.1 months). Systemic corticosteroid therapy was required for treatment of immune-mediated pneumonitis in 1.5% of patients receiving atezolizumab; 0.8% of patients receiving atezolizumab received high-dose corticosteroid therapy (40 mg or more of prednisone daily [or equivalent]) for a median duration of 4 days (range: 1–45 days) for treatment of immune-mediated pneumonitis, followed by tapering of the corticosteroid dosage. Atezolizumab was discontinued because of immune-mediated pneumonitis in 0.4% of patients receiving the drug. Immune-mediated pneumonitis resolved in 67% of patients.

In the IMpower150 study, immune-mediated pneumonitis occurred in 4.5% of patients receiving atezolizumab in combination with carboplatin and paclitaxel with or without bevacizumab, and was grade 3 or 4 in 1.8% of patients receiving atezolizumab combination therapy. Systemic corticosteroid therapy was required for treatment of immune-mediated pneumonitis in 4% of patients receiving atezolizumab combination therapy; 2.8% of patients receiving atezolizumab combination therapy received high-dose corticosteroid therapy (40 mg or more of prednisone daily [or equivalent]) for a median duration of 3 days (range: 1–43 days) for treatment of immune-mediated pneumonitis, followed by tapering of the corticosteroid dosage.

Patients receiving atezolizumab should be monitored for manifestations of pneumonitis. If pneumonitis is suspected, patients should be evaluated using radiographic imaging. Temporary interruption or discontinuance of atezolizumab may be necessary if immune-mediated pneumonitis occurs during therapy with the drug. (See Immune-mediated Pneumonitis under Dosage: Therapy Interruption for Toxicity, in Dosage and Administration.) If grade 2 or greater pneumonitis occurs, systemic corticosteroid therapy should be initiated (1–2 mg/kg of prednisone daily [or equivalent]) followed by tapering of the corticosteroid dosage.

Immune-mediated Hepatic Effects Immune-mediated hepatitis (defined as hepatitis requiring corticosteroid therapy), sometimes fatal, and liver function test abnormalities have occurred in patients receiving atezolizumab therapy.

In clinical studies, immune-mediated hepatitis occurred in 9% of patients receiving atezolizumab as a single agent and was grade 3 or greater in approximately 3% of patients receiving the drug. The median time to onset of immune-mediated hepatitis was 1.4 months (range: 1 day to 25.8 months) and the median duration was 24 days (range: 1 day to 13 months). Systemic corticosteroid therapy was required for treatment of immune-mediated hepatitis in 2% of patients receiving atezolizumab; 1.3% of patients receiving atezolizumab received high-dose corticosteroid therapy for a median duration of 3 days (range: 1–35 days) for treatment of immune-mediated hepatitis, followed by tapering of the corticosteroid dosage. Atezolizumab was discontinued because of immune-mediated hepatitis in 0.4% of patients receiving the drug. Immune-mediated hepatitis resolved in 71% of patients.

In the IMpower150 study, immune-mediated hepatitis occurred in 12.1% of patients receiving atezolizumab in combination with carboplatin and paclitaxel with or without bevacizumab, and was grade 3 or 4 in 4% of patients receiving atezolizumab combination therapy. Systemic corticosteroid therapy was required for treatment of immune-mediated hepatitis in 3.8% of patients receiving atezolizumab combination therapy; 2.6% of patients receiving atezolizumab combination therapy received high-dose corticosteroid therapy for a median duration of 7 days (range: 1–68 days) for treatment of immune-mediated hepatitis, followed by tapering of the corticosteroid dosage.

Patients receiving atezolizumab should be monitored for signs and symptoms of hepatitis (including liver chemistry tests) during atezolizumab therapy and following discontinuance of the drug. Temporary interruption or discontinuance of atezolizumab may be necessary if immune-mediated hepatitis or liver function test abnormalities occur during therapy with the drug. (See Immune-mediated Hepatic Effects under Dosage: Therapy Interruption for Toxicity, in Dosage and Administration.) If grade 2 or greater serum ALT, AST, and/or total bilirubin elevations occur, systemic corticosteroid therapy should be initiated (1–2 mg/kg of prednisone daily [or equivalent]) followed by tapering of the corticosteroid dosage.

Immune-mediated GI Effects Immune-mediated colitis or diarrhea (defined as colitis or diarrhea requiring corticosteroid therapy) has occurred in patients receiving atezolizumab therapy.

In clinical studies, immune-mediated colitis or diarrhea occurred in 20% of patients receiving atezolizumab as a single agent and was grade 3 in 1.4% of patients receiving the drug. The median time to onset of immune-mediated colitis or diarrhea was 1.5 months (range: 1 day to 41 months). Systemic corticosteroid therapy was required for treatment of immune-mediated colitis or diarrhea in 1.1% of patients receiving atezolizumab; 0.4% of patients receiving atezolizumab received high-dose corticosteroid therapy for a median duration of 3 days (range: 1–11 days) for treatment of immune-mediated colitis or diarrhea, followed by tapering of the corticosteroid dosage. Atezolizumab was discontinued because of immune-mediated colitis or diarrhea in 0.2% of patients receiving the drug. Immune-mediated colitis or diarrhea resolved in 85% of patients.

In the IMpower150 study, immune-mediated colitis or diarrhea occurred in 27% of patients receiving atezolizumab in combination with carboplatin and paclitaxel with or without bevacizumab, and was grade 3 or 4 in 4.3% of patients receiving atezolizumab combination therapy. Systemic corticosteroid therapy was required for treatment of immune-mediated colitis or diarrhea in 4.5% of patients receiving atezolizumab combination therapy; 3.2% of patients receiving atezolizumab combination therapy received high-dose corticosteroid therapy for a median duration of 5 days (range: 1–103 days) for treatment of immune-mediated hepatitis, followed by tapering of the corticosteroid dosage.

Patients receiving atezolizumab should be monitored for signs and symptoms of colitis or diarrhea. Temporary interruption or discontinuance of atezolizumab may be necessary if immune-mediated colitis or diarrhea occurs during therapy with the drug. (See Immune-mediated GI Effects under Dosage: Therapy Interruption for Toxicity, in Dosage and Administration.) If grade 2 or 3 colitis or diarrhea occurs, atezolizumab therapy should be temporarily withheld. If grade 2 colitis or diarrhea recurs or persists for longer than 5 days, systemic corticosteroid therapy should be initiated (1–2 mg/kg of prednisone daily [or equivalent]) followed by tapering of the corticosteroid dosage. If grade 4 immune-mediated colitis or diarrhea occurs, atezolizumab therapy should be permanently discontinued.

Immune-mediated Endocrine Effects Immune-mediated endocrinopathies, such as thyroid dysfunction (i.e., hypothyroidism, hyperthyroidism), adrenal insufficiency, hypophysitis/hypopituitarism, and diabetes mellitus (including ketoacidosis), have occurred in patients receiving atezolizumab therapy.

Thyroid Dysfunction. In clinical studies, immune-mediated hypothyroidism occurred in 4.6% of patients receiving atezolizumab as a single agent; thyroid hormone replacement was required in 3.8% of patients receiving atezolizumab. Immune-mediated hyperthyroidism occurred in 1.6% of patients receiving atezolizumab. Acute immune-mediated thyroiditis occurred rarely in clinical studies.

In the IMpower150 study, immune-mediated hypothyroidism occurred in 11.3% of patients receiving atezolizumab in combination with carboplatin and paclitaxel with or without bevacizumab; thyroid hormone replacement was required in 8.6% of patients receiving atezolizumab combination therapy. Immune-mediated hyperthyroidism or thyroiditis occurred in 3.4 or 0.1%, respectively, of patients receiving atezolizumab combination therapy.

Thyroid function should be evaluated prior to initiation of atezolizumab therapy and periodically during therapy. In patients who develop immune-mediated hypothyroidism, thyroid hormone replacement therapy should be initiated as clinically indicated. If immune-mediated hyperthyroidism occurs, temporary interruption of atezolizumab may be necessary and appropriate medical therapy should be initiated as clinically indicated. (See Immune-mediated Endocrine Effects under Dosage: Therapy Interruption for Toxicity, in Dosage and Administration.)

Adrenal Insufficiency. In clinical studies, immune-mediated adrenal insufficiency occurred in 0.4% of patients receiving atezolizumab as a single agent and was grade 3 in less than 0.1% of patients receiving the drug. The median time to onset of immune-mediated adrenal insufficiency was 5.7 months (range: 3 days to 19 months). Data were insufficient to evaluate the median duration of immune-mediated adrenal insufficiency. Systemic corticosteroid therapy was required for treatment of immune-mediated adrenal insufficiency in 0.3% of patients receiving atezolizumab; 0.1% of patients receiving atezolizumab received high-dose corticosteroid therapy for treatment of immune-mediated adrenal insufficiency. Immune-mediated adrenal insufficiency resolved in 27% of patients.

In the IMpower150 study, immune-mediated adrenal insufficiency occurred in 0.8% of patients receiving atezolizumab in combination with carboplatin and paclitaxel with or without bevacizumab.

Patients receiving atezolizumab should be monitored for signs and symptoms of adrenal insufficiency. Temporary interruption of atezolizumab may be necessary if immune-mediated adrenal insufficiency occurs during therapy with the drug. (See Immune-mediated Endocrine Effects under Dosage: Therapy Interruption for Toxicity, in Dosage and Administration.) If grade 2 or greater immune-mediated adrenal insufficiency occurs, systemic corticosteroid therapy (1–2 mg/kg of prednisone daily [or equivalent] followed by tapering of the corticosteroid dosage) and replacement therapy should be initiated as clinically indicated.

Hypophysitis. In clinical studies, grade 2 immune-mediated hypophysitis occurred in less than 0.1% of patients receiving atezolizumab as a single agent.

In the IMpower150 study, immune-mediated hypophysitis occurred in 0.4% of patients receiving atezolizumab in combination with carboplatin and paclitaxel with or without bevacizumab.

Patients receiving atezolizumab should be monitored for signs and symptoms of hypophysitis. If immune-mediated hypophysitis occurs, temporary interruption of atezolizumab may be necessary. (See Immune-mediated Endocrine Effects under Dosage: Therapy Interruption for Toxicity, in Dosage and Administration.) If grade 2 or greater immune-mediated hypophysitis occurs, systemic corticosteroid therapy (1–2 mg/kg of prednisone daily [or equivalent] followed by tapering of the corticosteroid dosage) and hormone replacement therapy should be initiated as clinically indicated.

Diabetes Mellitus. In clinical studies, immune-mediated type 1 diabetes mellitus occurred in less than 0.1% of patients receiving atezolizumab as a single agent. Insulin therapy was required in one patient.

In the IMpower150 study, new-onset immune-mediated type 1 diabetes mellitus occurred in 0.1% of patients receiving atezolizumab in combination with carboplatin and paclitaxel with or without bevacizumab.

Patients receiving atezolizumab should be monitored for signs and symptoms of diabetes mellitus (e.g., hyperglycemia). If immune-mediated type 1 diabetes mellitus occurs, temporary interruption of atezolizumab may be necessary and insulin therapy should be initiated as clinically indicated. (See Immune-mediated Endocrine Effects under Dosage: Therapy Interruption for Toxicity, in Dosage and Administration.)

Other Immune-mediated Effects Other immune-mediated adverse effects, including myocarditis, dermatologic effects (i.e., bullous dermatitis, pemphigoid, erythema multiforme, Stevens-Johnson syndrome, toxic epidermal necrolysis), pancreatitis, systemic inflammatory response syndrome, histiocytic necrotizing lymphadenitis, autoimmune hemolytic anemia, immune thrombocytopenic purpura, myositis, rhabdomyolysis, Guillain-Barré syndrome, myasthenic syndrome/myasthenia gravis, demyelination, meningoencephalitis, aseptic meningitis, encephalitis, facial and abducens nerve paresis, polymyalgia rheumatica, autoimmune neuropathy, Vogt-Koyanagi-Harada syndrome, uveitis, iritis, nephrotic syndrome, nephritis, and vasculitis, have occurred rarely in patients receiving atezolizumab or other anti-programmed-death ligand-1 (anti-PD-L1) or anti-programmed-death receptor-1 (anti-PD-1) antibodies. Some cases have resulted in death. Immune-mediated adverse effects generally occur during atezolizumab therapy, but also may occur following discontinuance of the drug.

Temporary interruption or discontinuance of atezolizumab may be necessary if immune-mediated adverse effects occur during therapy with the drug. (See Therapy Interruption for Toxicity under Dosage and Administration: Dosage.) If a grade 2 immune-mediated adverse effect is suspected, adequate evaluation should be performed to exclude other causes and systemic corticosteroid therapy should be initiated as clinically indicated. If severe (grade 3 or 4) immune-mediated adverse effects occur, systemic corticosteroid therapy (1–2 mg/kg of prednisone daily [or equivalent]) followed by tapering of the corticosteroid dosage should be initiated.

If uveitis occurs in conjunction with other immune-mediated adverse effects, Vogt-Koyanagi-Harada syndrome (which has been observed in patients receiving other anti-PD-L1 or anti-PD-1 antibodies) should be considered. Systemic corticosteroid therapy may be required to reduce the risk of permanent vision loss.

Infectious Complications Serious infections, sometimes fatal, have occurred in patients receiving atezolizumab therapy.

In clinical studies, infections occurred in 42% of patients receiving atezolizumab as a single agent; grade 3 or greater infections occurred in 11.2% of patients receiving the drug. The most common grade 3 or greater infection in patients receiving atezolizumab for the treatment of urothelial carcinoma or non-small cell lung cancer (NSCLC) was urinary tract infection (6.5%) or pneumonia (3.8%), respectively.

In the IMpower150 study, infections occurred in 50% of patients receiving atezolizumab in combination with carboplatin and paclitaxel with or without bevacizumab; grade 3 or greater infections occurred in approximately 14.3% of patients receiving atezolizumab combination therapy. The most common grade 3 or greater infection was pneumonia (4.8%).

Patients should be monitored for signs and symptoms of infection. If grade 3 or greater infection occurs, atezolizumab therapy should be temporarily withheld until the patient's condition is stable. (See Infectious Complications under Dosage: Therapy Interruption for Toxicity, in Dosage and Administration.)

Infusion-related Effects Severe or life-threatening infusion-related reactions may occur in patients receiving atezolizumab therapy. In clinical studies, infusion-related reactions occurred in 1.3% of patients receiving atezolizumab as a single agent and were grade 3 in 0.2% of patients receiving the drug.

In the IMpower150 study, infusion-related reactions occurred in 3.8% of patients receiving atezolizumab in combination with carboplatin and paclitaxel with or without bevacizumab, and were grade 3 or 4 in 0.8% of patients receiving atezolizumab combination therapy.

Patients receiving atezolizumab should be monitored for signs and symptoms of infusion-related reactions. In patients experiencing infusion-related reactions, interruption of the infusion, reduction in the infusion rate, or discontinuance of atezolizumab may be necessary. (See Infusion-related Reactions under Dosage: Therapy Interruption for Toxicity, in Dosage and Administration.) For patients experiencing grade 1 or 2 infusion-related reactions, premedication may be considered prior to subsequent atezolizumab infusions.

Fetal/Neonatal Morbidity and Mortality Atezolizumab may cause fetal harm if administered to pregnant women. Blockade of signaling of the PD-1 and PD-L1 pathway in animals has been shown to disrupt maternal immune tolerance to the fetus and has been associated with increased fetal loss (e.g., abortion, stillbirth) and immune-mediated disorders; however, teratogenicity has not been observed.

Pregnancy should be avoided during atezolizumab therapy. The manufacturer states that pregnancy status should be confirmed prior to initiation of atezolizumab. Women of childbearing potential should be advised to use an effective method of contraception while receiving atezolizumab and for at least 5 months after discontinuance of therapy. Women of childbearing potential should be apprised of the potential fetal hazard if atezolizumab is used during pregnancy.

Immunogenicity There is a potential for immunogenicity with atezolizumab therapy. In the OAK study in patients with NSCLC and in cohorts 1 and 2 of the IMvigor210 study in patients with urothelial carcinoma, development of anti-atezolizumab antibodies was detected at one or more postdose time points in 30, 48, and 42%, respectively, of patients receiving atezolizumab. In the IMpower150 study in patients with nonsquamous NSCLC, development of anti-atezolizumab antibodies was detected at one or more postdose time points in 36% of evaluable patients receiving atezolizumab in combination with bevacizumab, carboplatin, and paclitaxel; anti-atezolizumab antibodies were detected prior to the second dose of the drug in 83% of these patients. In the OAK study, the median time to onset of development of anti-atezolizumab antibodies was 3 weeks. The neutralizing capacity of anti-atezolizumab antibodies has not been established.

In patients receiving atezolizumab in the OAK study and in those receiving atezolizumab in combination with bevacizumab, carboplatin, and paclitaxel in the IMpower150 study, clearance of atezolizumab increased by 25 and 18%, respectively, in the presence of anti-atezolizumab antibodies. Systemic exposure of atezolizumab was decreased in patients who developed anti-atezolizumab antibodies in the OAK, IMvigor210, and IMpower150 studies. No clinically important effects on safety were observed in patients who developed anti-atezolizumab antibodies in the OAK and IMvigor210 studies.

Exploratory analysis of the OAK study suggested reduced efficacy in patients who were positive for anti-atezolizumab antibodies by week 4 compared with those who did not develop anti-atezolizumab antibodies by week 4. Survival of patients who developed anti-atezolizumab antibodies by week 4 appeared to be similar to that of docetaxel-treated patients. In another exploratory analysis comparing matched populations of atezolizumab- and docetaxel-treated patients, the risk of death in atezolizumab-treated patients was reduced by 11 or 32% in the presence or absence of anti-atezolizumab antibodies, respectively, compared with a matched control population of docetaxel-treated patients.

Exploratory analysis of the IMpower150 study suggested that efficacy of atezolizumab in combination with bevacizumab, carboplatin, and paclitaxel was similar in patients who were positive or negative for anti-atezolizumab antibodies by week 4. In an exploratory analysis comparing matched populations of patients receiving atezolizumab in combination with bevacizumab, carboplatin, and paclitaxel and those receiving bevacizumab, carboplatin, and paclitaxel alone, the risk of death in patients receiving the atezolizumab-containing regimen was reduced by 31 or 36% in the presence or absence of anti-atezolizumab antibodies, respectively, compared with a matched control population of patients receiving bevacizumab, carboplatin, and paclitaxel alone.

Impairment of Fertility Results of animal studies suggest that atezolizumab may impair female fertility. In a 26-week general toxicology study, irregular menstrual cycle patterns and absence of corpora lutea were observed in female animals receiving atezolizumab at exposure levels approximately 6 times the human exposure at the recommended dosage; however, these adverse effects were reversible. Adverse reproductive effects in male animals were not observed.

Specific Populations **Pregnancy.** Atezolizumab may cause fetal harm if administered to pregnant women based on its mechanism of action and animal findings. (See Fetal/Neonatal Morbidity and Mortality under Cautions: Warnings/Precautions.)

Pregnancy status should be confirmed prior to initiation of atezolizumab.

Lactation. It is not known whether atezolizumab is distributed into human milk. Because human immunoglobulin G (IgG) is distributed into milk and because of the potential for serious adverse reactions to atezolizumab in nursing infants, women should be advised to discontinue nursing during atezolizumab therapy and for at least 5 months after discontinuance of therapy. The effects of the drug on nursing infants or on milk production are unknown.

Pediatric Use. Safety and efficacy of atezolizumab have not been established in pediatric patients.

Geriatric Use. In the OAK study in patients with locally advanced or metastatic NSCLC and in cohort 2 (previously treated patients) of the IMvigor210 study in patients with locally advanced or metastatic urothelial carcinoma, 50% of patients receiving atezolizumab as a single agent were 65 years of age or older. In the IMpower150 study in patients with locally advanced or metastatic urothelial carcinoma, 46% of those receiving atezolizumab in combination with bevacizumab, carboplatin, and paclitaxel were 65 years of age or older, while 9% were 75 years of age or older. In these studies, no overall differences in safety or efficacy were observed between patients 65 years of age or older and younger adults.

In cohort 1 (cisplatin-ineligible patients) of the IMvigor210 study, 83% of patients with locally advanced or metastatic urothelial carcinoma who received atezolizumab as a single agent were 65 years of age or older, while 41% were 75 years of age or older. No overall differences in safety or efficacy were observed between these patients and younger adults.

Hepatic Impairment. The effects of hepatic impairment on the pharmacokinetics of atezolizumab have not been formally studied. Analysis of population pharmacokinetic data indicates that clearance and systemic exposure of atezolizumab are similar between patients with mild hepatic impairment (total bilirubin concentration not exceeding the ULN with AST concentration exceeding the ULN, or total bilirubin concentration more than 1 times but no more than 1.5 times the ULN with any AST concentration) and those with normal hepatic function. Pharmacokinetic data in patients with moderate or severe hepatic impairment are lacking.

Renal Impairment. The effects of renal impairment on the pharmacokinetics of atezolizumab have not been formally studied. Analysis of population pharmacokinetic data indicates that atezolizumab clearance is not substantially affected by mild or moderate renal impairment (estimated glomerular filtration rate [GFR] 30–89 mL/minute per 1.73 m^2). Pharmacokinetic data in patients with severe renal impairment are limited.

■ **Common Adverse Effects** Adverse effects reported in 10% or more of patients receiving atezolizumab as a single agent for the treatment of locally advanced or metastatic urothelial carcinoma in cohort 1 (cisplatin-ineligible patients) of the IMvigor210 study include fatigue, diarrhea, decreased appetite, nausea, back or neck pain, pruritus, peripheral edema, rash, urinary tract infection, vomiting, abdominal pain, constipation, cough, pyrexia, arthralgia, and dyspnea. Grade 3 or 4 laboratory abnormalities reported in 5% or more of patients receiving atezolizumab include hyponatremia, hyperglycemia, lymphopenia, anemia, elevated concentrations of alkaline phosphatase, and elevated concentrations of serum creatinine.

Adverse effects reported in 10% or more of patients receiving atezolizumab as a single agent for the treatment of relapsed or refractory locally advanced or metastatic urothelial carcinoma in cohort 2 of the IMvigor210 study include fatigue, loss of appetite, nausea, urinary tract infection, constipation, pyrexia, diarrhea, peripheral edema, abdominal pain, vomiting, dyspnea, back/neck pain, rash, arthralgia, cough, hematuria, and pruritus. Grade 3 or 4 laboratory abnormalities reported in 5% or more of patients receiving atezolizumab include lymphopenia, hyponatremia, anemia, and hyperglycemia.

Adverse effects reported in 15% or more of patients receiving atezolizumab in combination with bevacizumab, carboplatin, and paclitaxel for the initial treatment of metastatic nonsquamous NSCLC in the IMpower150 study include neuropathy, fatigue/asthenia, alopecia, myalgia/pain, nausea, diarrhea, constipation, decreased appetite, arthralgia, hypertension, rash, cough, pyrexia, vomiting, epistaxis, headache, and proteinuria. Laboratory abnormalities reported in 20% or more of patients receiving atezolizumab in combination with bevacizumab, carboplatin, and paclitaxel include anemia, hyperglycemia, increased BUN, neutropenia, lymphopenia, hypomagnesemia, hypoalbuminemia, elevated concentrations of alkaline phosphatase, elevated concentrations of aminotransferases (i.e., ALT, AST), hyponatremia, increased thyrotropin (thyroid-stimulating hormone, TSH) concentration, hyperkalemia, elevated concentrations of serum creatinine, hypocalcemia, hypophosphatemia, hypokalemia, and hyperphosphatemia.

Adverse effects reported in 10% or more of patients receiving atezolizumab as a single agent for the treatment of previously treated metastatic NSCLC in the OAK study include fatigue, cough, decreased appetite, dyspnea, musculoskeletal pain, constipation, nausea, pyrexia, diarrhea, arthralgia, and rash. Laboratory abnormalities reported in 20% or more of patients receiving atezolizumab include anemia, lymphocytopenia, hypoalbuminemia, hyponatremia, elevated concentrations of alkaline phosphatase, elevated concentrations of aminotransferases (i.e., ALT, AST), hypophosphatemia, hypomagnesemia, and elevated concentrations of serum creatinine.

Drug Interactions

No formal drug interaction studies have been performed to date.

Description

Atezolizumab, a humanized anti-programmed-death ligand-1 (anti-PD-L1) monoclonal antibody, is an antineoplastic agent. The drug is an IgG_1 kappa immunoglobulin.

The immune-checkpoint receptor PD-1 is expressed on activated T-cells, monocytes, B-cells, natural killer (NK) T-cells, and dendritic cells. Overexpression of PD-1 ligands on the surface of tumor cells results in activation of PD-1 and B7.1 and suppression of cytotoxic T-cell activity, T-cell proliferation, and cytokine production. Atezolizumab blocks the interaction between PD-L1 and the receptors PD-1 and B7.1, resulting in activation of the antitumor immune response without inducing antibody-dependent cell-mediated cytotoxicity (ADCC). The drug also has been shown to reduce tumor growth in syngeneic mouse tumor models.

Systemic exposure to atezolizumab is proportional to dose over the dose range of 1–20 mg/kg, including the fixed dosage of 1.2 g every 3 weeks. Following repeated doses of atezolizumab 1.2 g every 3 weeks, steady-state concentrations are reached by 6–9 weeks; systemic accumulation of the drug is 1.9-fold. Atezolizumab clearance decreases over time by approximately 17% from baseline values; however, this difference is not considered clinically important. The terminal half-life of atezolizumab is 27 days.

Systemic exposure to atezolizumab does not appear to be affected by age (range of 21–89 years), body weight, sex, serum albumin concentration, tumor burden, geographic region, race, PD-L1 expression, or performance status.

Advice to Patients

Importance of advising patients to read the manufacturer's medication guide.

Risk of immune-mediated pneumonitis. Importance of informing clinician immediately if new or worsening cough, chest pain, or shortness of breath occurs.

Risk of immune-mediated hepatitis. Importance of informing clinician immediately if signs and symptoms of liver damage (e.g., jaundice, severe nausea or vomiting, abdominal pain [particularly in the right upper quadrant], lethargy, easy bruising or bleeding, lack of appetite, dark urine, drowsiness) occur.

Risk of immune-mediated colitis. Importance of informing clinician immediately if diarrhea or severe abdominal pain occurs or if mucus or blood is present in stool.

Risk of immune-mediated endocrine effects. Importance of informing clinician immediately if manifestations of hypophysitis, hyperthyroidism, hypothyroidism, adrenal insufficiency, or diabetes mellitus (including ketoacidosis) occur.

Risk of other immune-mediated adverse effects. Importance of informing clinician immediately if manifestations of other potential immune-mediated adverse effects occur.

Risk of infections. Importance of informing clinician if fever, flu-like symptoms, cough, or painful or frequent urination occurs.

Risk of infusion-related reactions. Importance of informing clinician if signs and symptoms of such reactions, including dizziness, chills, fever, breathing difficulty (i.e., shortness of breath, wheezing), pruritus, flushing, feeling of faintness, back or neck pain, and angioedema, occur.

Risk of fetal harm. Necessity of advising women of childbearing potential that they should use an effective method of contraception while receiving atezolizumab and for at least 5 months after discontinuance of therapy. Importance of women informing clinicians if they are or plan to become pregnant. If pregnancy occurs, advise pregnant women of potential risk to the fetus.

Importance of advising women to avoid breast-feeding while receiving atezolizumab and for at least 5 months after discontinuance of therapy.

Importance of informing clinicians of existing or contemplated concomitant therapy, including prescription and OTC drugs and dietary or herbal supplements, as well as any concomitant illnesses.

Importance of informing patients of other important precautionary information. (See Cautions.)

Overview® (see Users Guide). For additional information on this drug until a more detailed monograph is developed and published, the manufacturer's labeling should be consulted. It is *essential* that the manufacturer's labeling be consulted for more detailed information on usual cautions, precautions, contraindications, potential drug interactions, laboratory test interferences, and acute toxicity. For further information on the handling of antineoplastic agents, see the ASHP Guidelines on Handling Hazardous Drugs at http://www.ahfsdruginformation.com.

Preparations

Distribution of atezolizumab is restricted. (See Restricted Distribution under Dosage and Administration: General.)

Excipients in commercially available drug preparations may have clinically important effects in some individuals; consult specific product labeling for details.

Atezolizumab

Parenteral		
Concentrate, for injection, for IV infusion	60 mg/mL (1.2 g)	**Tecentriq®**, Genentech

Avelumab

■ Avelumab, a fully human anti-programmed-death ligand-1 (anti-PD-L1) monoclonal antibody, is an antineoplastic agent. The drug is an IgG_1 lambda immunoglobulin.

Uses

■ **Merkel Cell Carcinoma** Avelumab is used for the treatment of metastatic Merkel cell carcinoma; avelumab has been designated an orphan drug by FDA for the treatment of this cancer. The accelerated approval of avelumab for this indication is based on objective response rate and duration of response. Continued approval for this indication may be contingent on verification and description of clinical benefit of avelumab in confirmatory studies.

The current indication for avelumab is based principally on the results of an open-label, multicenter, noncomparative phase 2 study (JAVELIN Merkel 200) in 88 adults with metastatic Merkel cell carcinoma that had progressed during or following cytotoxic chemotherapy for metastatic disease. The primary measure of efficacy was objective response rate as assessed by a blinded independent review committee according to Response Evaluation Criteria in Solid Tumors (RECIST). In this study, the median age of patients was 73 years; 92% were Caucasian, 74% were male, 53% had visceral metastases, 65% had received one prior chemotherapy regimen for metastatic disease, and 35% had received 2 or more prior therapies. All patients enrolled in the study had an ECOG performance status of 0 or 1. Most patients (66%) had positive programmed-death ligand-1 (PD-L1) expression (defined as PD-L1 expression of any intensity in at least 1% of tumor cells) and 18% had negative PD-L1 expression as detected by an immunohistochemistry assay. Among 77 patients with evaluable tumor samples, Merkel cell polyomavirus was detected in 52% of patients. Patients received avelumab 10 mg/kg administered as an IV infusion every 2 weeks until disease progression or unacceptable toxicity occurred; however, patients with radiologic evidence of disease progression in the absence of substantial clinical deterioration (defined as new or worsening symptoms, change in performance status for more than 2 weeks, necessity of salvage therapy) could continue receiving avelumab therapy. Patients with a history of autoimmune disease; those with brain metastases or hematologic malignancies; those with human immunodeficiency virus

(HIV), hepatitis B virus (HBV), or hepatitis C virus (HCV) infection; those with a history of allogeneic stem-cell or solid organ transplant; those with conditions requiring therapy with immunosuppressive agents; those who had received any vaccine within 4 weeks prior to administration of avelumab; and those who had received prior therapy with other anti-programmed-death 1 (anti-PD-1), anti-PD-L1, or anti-cytotoxic T-lymphocyte-associated antigen 4 (anti-CTLA-4) antibodies were excluded from the study.

At a minimum follow-up of 12 months, the objective response rate was 33%; complete responses were achieved in 11.4% of patients. At the time of analysis, the median duration of response had not been reached; however, 45% of patients had durable responses of 12 months or more. After a median follow-up of 10.4 months, median progression-free and overall survival were 2.7 and 11.3 months, respectively. Objective responses were observed regardless of PD-L1 expression or presence of Merkel cell polyomavirus.

■ **Urothelial Carcinoma** Avelumab is used for the treatment of locally advanced or metastatic urothelial carcinoma that has progressed during or following platinum-containing therapy or within 12 months of platinum-containing therapy in the neoadjuvant or adjuvant setting. The accelerated approval of avelumab for this indication is based on objective response rate and duration of response. Continued approval for this indication may be contingent on verification and description of clinical benefit of avelumab in confirmatory studies.

The current indication for avelumab in the treatment of locally advanced or metastatic urothelial carcinoma is based principally on the results for a cohort of patients with urothelial carcinoma in an open-label, multicenter, noncomparative, phase 1 study (JAVELIN Solid Tumor); the cohort of patients with urothelial carcinoma included 242 adults with locally advanced or metastatic urothelial carcinoma that had progressed during or following platinum-containing therapy or within 12 months of platinum-containing therapy in the neoadjuvant or adjuvant setting. The primary measure of efficacy was objective response rate as assessed by an independent review committee according to RECIST. In this study, the median age of patients in the urothelial carcinoma cohort was 68 years; 80% were Caucasian, 83% had visceral metastases, 72% were male, and 44% had nonbladder urothelial carcinoma (23% had upper urinary tract disease). All patients enrolled in the study had an ECOG performance status of 0 or 1. In the cohort of patients with urothelial carcinoma, 47, 32, or 20% of patients had received prior treatment with cisplatin-, carboplatin-, or both cisplatin- and carboplatin-based regimens, respectively; 4% of patients had disease progression following platinum-containing therapy in the neoadjuvant or adjuvant setting only. Patients received avelumab 10 mg/kg administered as an IV infusion every 2 weeks until disease progression or unacceptable toxicity occurred. Patients with a history of autoimmune disease (except for type 1 diabetes mellitus, vitiligo, psoriasis, or thyroid disease not requiring immunosuppressive therapy); those with active brain metastases or a history of brain metastases; those with HIV, HBV, or HCV infection; those with a history of allogeneic stem-cell or solid organ transplant; those diagnosed with other malignancies within the past 5 years; and those with conditions requiring therapy with immunosuppressive agents were excluded from the study. Patients were eligible for enrollment in the study regardless of their PD-L1 status.

At a minimum follow-up of 13 weeks or 6 months, the objective response rate for patients in the urothelial carcinoma cohort of this study was 13.3 or 16.1%, respectively; complete responses were achieved in 4 or 5.6%, respectively, of patients. At a minimum follow-up of 6 months, the median duration of response had not been reached. The median time to response was 2 months (range: 1.3–11 months). Among patients with evaluable data on PD-L1 expression, there were no clear differences in objective response rates based on PD-L1 expression.

Dosage and Administration

■ **General** Because infusion-related events may occur, the manufacturer recommends a premedication regimen (i.e., acetaminophen and an antihistamine) prior to the initial 4 infusions of avelumab. Premedication also may be administered as clinically indicated prior to subsequent infusions of the drug based on the occurrence and severity of previous infusion reactions. In the JAVELIN Solid Tumor study, patients received an antihistamine (e.g., diphenhydramine hydrochloride 25–50 mg) and IV acetaminophen 500–650 mg (or oral equivalent) 30–60 minutes prior to each infusion of avelumab.

Restricted Distribution Program Avelumab can only be obtained through specialty distributors. Clinicians may consult the Bavencio® website for specific availability information (https://www.bavencio.com).

■ **Administration** Avelumab is administered by IV infusion over 60 minutes. Avelumab should be administered through a sterile, nonpyrogenic, low-protein-binding 0.2-μm inline filter.

Avelumab injection concentrate must be diluted prior to IV administration. Prior to dilution, the injection concentrate should be inspected visually for particulate matter and discoloration. The solution should be clear and colorless to pale yellow; the solution should not be used if it is cloudy or discolored or contains a precipitate. The appropriate dose (10 mg/kg) of avelumab injection concentrate (containing 20 mg/mL) should be withdrawn and injected into an infusion bag containing 250 mL of 0.45 or 0.9% sodium chloride injection. This diluted solution should be mixed by gentle inversion and should *not* be shaken. Diluted solutions of the drug should be clear, colorless, and free of visible particulate matter.

Diluted solutions of the drug are stable for up to 4 hours after dilution when stored at room temperature or up to 24 hours after dilution when stored under refrigeration (2–8°C), and should be protected from light; diluted solutions of the drug should be brought to room temperature prior to administration. Diluted solutions of the drug should *not* be frozen.

Any unused portion in the vial should be discarded since avelumab injection concentrate contains no preservative.

Avelumab should *not* be administered simultaneously through the same IV line with any other drug.

■ **Dosage** ***Merkel Cell Carcinoma*** For the treatment of metastatic Merkel cell carcinoma in adults and adolescents (12 years of age and older), the recommended dosage of avelumab is 10 mg/kg administered as a 60-minute IV infusion every 2 weeks. Therapy should be continued until disease progression or unacceptable toxicity occurs.

Urothelial Carcinoma For the treatment of locally advanced or metastatic urothelial carcinoma that has progressed during or following therapy with platinum-containing chemotherapy or within 12 months of platinum-containing chemotherapy in the neoadjuvant or adjuvant setting, the recommended adult dosage of avelumab is 10 mg/kg administered as a 60-minute IV infusion every 2 weeks. Therapy should be continued until disease progression or unacceptable toxicity occurs.

Therapy Interruption for Toxicity If immune-mediated adverse effects occur, temporary or permanent discontinuance of avelumab may be required based on the severity of the reaction.

Immune-mediated Pneumonitis. If grade 2 immune-mediated pneumonitis occurs, avelumab therapy should be interrupted. Once the toxicity has resolved to grade 0 or 1, avelumab may be restarted following completion of the corticosteroid taper. If pneumonitis recurs, avelumab therapy should be permanently discontinued. (See Immune-mediated Pneumonitis under Cautions: Warnings/Precautions.)

If grade 3 or 4 immune-mediated pneumonitis occurs, avelumab therapy should be permanently discontinued.

Immune-mediated Hepatic Effects. For serum aminotransferase (ALT or AST) elevations exceeding 3 times but not more than 5 times the upper limit of normal (ULN) or total bilirubin concentrations exceeding 1.5 times but not more than 3 times the ULN, avelumab therapy should be interrupted. Once the toxicity has resolved to grade 0 or 1, avelumab may be restarted following completion of the corticosteroid taper. (See Immune-mediated Hepatic Effects under Cautions: Warnings/Precautions.)

For ALT or AST elevations exceeding 5 times the ULN or total bilirubin concentrations exceeding 3 times the ULN, avelumab therapy should be permanently discontinued.

Immune-mediated GI Effects. If grade 2 or 3 immune-mediated colitis or diarrhea occurs, avelumab therapy should be interrupted. Once the toxicity has resolved to grade 0 or 1, avelumab may be restarted following completion of the corticosteroid taper. If grade 3 colitis or diarrhea recurs, avelumab therapy should be permanently discontinued. (See Immune-mediated GI Effects under Cautions: Warnings/Precautions.)

If grade 4 immune-mediated colitis or diarrhea occurs, avelumab therapy should be permanently discontinued.

Immune-mediated Endocrine Effects. If grade 3 or 4 immune-mediated endocrinopathies (e.g., hypothyroidism, hyperthyroidism, adrenal insufficiency, diabetes mellitus) occur, avelumab therapy should be interrupted. Once the toxicity has resolved to grade 0 or 1, avelumab may be restarted following completion of the corticosteroid taper. (See Immune-mediated Endocrine Effects under Cautions: Warnings/Precautions.)

Immune-mediated Renal Effects. For serum creatinine concentrations exceeding 1.5 times but not more than 6 times the ULN, avelumab therapy should be interrupted. Once the toxicity has resolved to grade 0 or 1, avelumab may be restarted following completion of the corticosteroid taper. (See Immune-mediated Renal Effects under Cautions: Warnings/Precautions.)

For serum creatinine concentrations exceeding 6 times the ULN, avelumab therapy should be permanently discontinued.

Other Immune-mediated Adverse Effects. If any other immune-mediated adverse effects with moderate or severe signs or symptoms occur, avelumab therapy should be interrupted while an evaluation is performed to exclude other causes. Once the toxicity has resolved to grade 0 or 1, avelumab may be restarted following completion of the corticosteroid taper. (See Other Immune-mediated Effects under Cautions: Warnings/Precautions.)

Avelumab should be permanently discontinued in patients experiencing persistent grade 2 or 3 immune-mediated adverse effects lasting 12 weeks or longer and in those unable to reduce corticosteroid dosage to less than 10 mg of prednisone daily (or equivalent) within 12 weeks.

Avelumab should be permanently discontinued in patients experiencing life-threatening immune-mediated adverse effects (except for endocrinopathies). Therapy with the drug also should be permanently discontinued if severe immune-mediated adverse effects recur.

Infusion-related Reactions. If grade 1 or 2 infusion-related reactions occur, the infusion should be interrupted or the infusion rate should be reduced. (See Infusion-related Effects under Cautions: Warnings/Precautions.)

If grade 3 or 4 infusion-related reactions occur, avelumab therapy should be permanently discontinued.

■ **Special Populations** The manufacturer makes no special population dosage recommendations at this time. (See Specific Populations under Cautions: Warnings/Precautions.)

Cautions

■ **Contraindications** The manufacturer states there are no known contraindications to the use of avelumab.

■ **Warnings/Precautions** ***Immune-mediated Pneumonitis*** Immune-mediated pneumonitis, sometimes fatal, has occurred in patients receiving avelumab therapy. Immune-mediated pneumonitis was reported in 21 of 1738 patients (1.2%) receiving avelumab in clinical studies and was fatal in one patient. The median time to occurrence of immune-mediated pneumonitis was 2.5 months (range: 3 days to 11 months) and the median duration was 7 weeks (range: 4 days to more than 4 months). Corticosteroid therapy was administered in all 21 patients and avelumab therapy was permanently discontinued in 6 patients. Most patients (81%) experiencing immune-mediated pneumonitis received high-dose corticosteroid therapy for a median duration of 8 days. At the time of analysis, immune-mediated pneumonitis had resolved in 12 of 21 patients (57%).

Patients receiving avelumab should be monitored for manifestations of pneumonitis, and those with suspected pneumonitis should be evaluated with radiographic imaging. Temporary interruption or discontinuance of avelumab may be necessary if immune-mediated pneumonitis occurs during therapy with the drug. (See Immune-mediated Pneumonitis under Dosage: Therapy Interruption for Toxicity, in Dosage and Administration.) If grade 2 or greater pneumonitis occurs, systemic corticosteroid therapy should be initiated (1–2 mg/kg of prednisone daily [or equivalent]) followed by tapering of the corticosteroid dosage.

Immune-mediated Hepatic Effects Immune-mediated hepatitis, sometimes fatal, has occurred in patients receiving avelumab therapy. Immune-mediated hepatitis occurred in 16 of 1738 patients (0.9%) receiving avelumab in clinical studies and was fatal in 2 patients. The median time to occurrence of immune-mediated hepatitis was 3.2 months (range: 1 week to 15 months) and the median duration was 2.5 months (range: 1 day to more than 7.4 months). Corticosteroid therapy was administered in all 16 patients and avelumab therapy was permanently discontinued in 9 patients. Most patients (94%) experiencing immune-mediated hepatitis received high-dose corticosteroid therapy for a median duration of 14 days. At the time of analysis, immune-mediated hepatitis had resolved in 9 of 16 patients (56%).

Patients receiving avelumab should be monitored for manifestations of hepatitis. Liver function tests should be assessed prior to initiation of avelumab therapy and then monitored periodically during treatment. Temporary interruption or discontinuance of avelumab may be necessary if immune-mediated hepatitis occurs during therapy with the drug. (See Immune-mediated Hepatic Effects under Dosage: Therapy Interruption for Toxicity, in Dosage and Administration.) If grade 2 or greater hepatitis occurs, systemic corticosteroid therapy should be initiated (1–2 mg/kg of prednisone daily [or equivalent]) followed by tapering of the corticosteroid dosage.

Immune-mediated GI Effects Immune-mediated colitis has occurred in patients receiving avelumab therapy. Immune-mediated colitis occurred in 26 of 1738 patients (1.5%) receiving avelumab in clinical studies and was grade 3 in 7 patients. The median time to occurrence of immune-mediated colitis was 2.1 months (range: 2 days to 11 months) and the median duration was 6 weeks (range: 1 day to more than 14 months). Corticosteroid therapy was administered in all 26 patients and avelumab therapy was permanently discontinued in 9 patients. Approximately one-half of patients (58%) experiencing immune-mediated colitis received high-dose corticosteroid therapy for a median duration of 19 days. At the time of analysis, immune-mediated colitis had resolved in 18 of 26 patients (70%).

Patients receiving avelumab should be monitored for manifestations of colitis. Temporary interruption or discontinuance of avelumab may be necessary if immune-mediated colitis occurs during therapy with the drug. (See Immune-mediated GI Effects under Dosage: Therapy Interruption for Toxicity, in Dosage and Administration.) If grade 2 or greater colitis occurs, systemic corticosteroid therapy should be initiated (1–2 mg/kg of prednisone daily [or equivalent]) followed by tapering of the corticosteroid dosage.

Immune-mediated Endocrine Effects Immune-mediated endocrinopathies, such as thyroid dysfunction (i.e., hypothyroidism, hyperthyroidism), adrenal insufficiency, and diabetes mellitus (including ketoacidosis), have occurred in patients receiving avelumab therapy.

Adrenal Insufficiency. Immune-mediated adrenal insufficiency occurred in 8 of 1738 patients (0.5%) receiving avelumab in clinical studies; grade 3 immune-mediated adrenal insufficiency occurred in one patient. The median time to occurrence of immune-mediated adrenal insufficiency was 2.5 months (range: 1 day to 8 months). Corticosteroid therapy was administered in all 8 patients and avelumab therapy was permanently discontinued in 2 patients. One-half of patients experiencing immune-mediated adrenal insufficiency received high-dose corticosteroid therapy for a median duration of one day.

Patients receiving avelumab should be monitored for manifestations of adrenal insufficiency. Temporary interruption of avelumab may be necessary if immune-mediated adrenal insufficiency occurs during therapy with the drug. (See Immune-mediated Endocrine Effects under Dosage: Therapy Interruption for Toxicity, in Dosage and Administration.) Systemic corticosteroid therapy should be initiated as appropriate.

Thyroid Dysfunction. Immune-mediated thyroid dysfunction occurred in 98 of 1738 patients (6%) receiving avelumab in clinical studies and was grade 3 in 3 patients. Immune-mediated hypothyroidism occurred in 90 of 1738 patients (5%), immune-mediated hyperthyroidism occurred in 7 patients (0.4%), and immune-mediated thyroiditis occurred in 4 patients (0.2%). The median time to occurrence of thyroid dysfunction was 2.8 months (range: 2 weeks to 13 months); however, thyroid dysfunction may occur at any time during treatment. The median duration of thyroid dysfunction was not estimable (range: 6 days to more than 26 months). Avelumab therapy was discontinued in 2 patients. Immune-mediated thyroid dysfunction resolved in 7 of 98 patients (7%).

Patients receiving avelumab should be monitored for manifestations of thyroid dysfunction. Thyroid function should be evaluated prior to initiation of avelumab therapy, periodically during therapy, and as clinically indicated. Temporary interruption of avelumab may be necessary if immune-mediated thyroid dysfunction occurs during therapy with the drug. (See Immune-mediated Endocrine Effects under Dosage: Therapy Interruption for Toxicity, in Dosage and Administration.) In patients who develop immune-mediated hypothyroidism, thyroid hormone replacement therapy should be initiated. If immune-mediated hyperthyroidism occurs, appropriate medical therapy should be initiated.

Diabetes Mellitus. Immune-mediated type 1 diabetes mellitus and ketoacidosis have occurred in patients receiving avelumab therapy. Type 1 diabetes mellitus of no clear alternate etiology occurred in 2 of 1738 patients (0.1%) receiving avelumab in clinical studies and was grade 3 in both patients. Avelumab therapy was permanently discontinued in both patients.

Patients receiving avelumab should be monitored for manifestations of type 1 diabetes mellitus. If severe or life-threatening (grade 3 or greater) immune-mediated type 1 diabetes mellitus occurs, avelumab therapy should be temporarily interrupted and antidiabetic agents (i.e., insulin therapy) should be initiated. Avelumab may be resumed once blood glucose concentrations have stabilized on antidiabetic therapy.

Immune-mediated Renal Effects Immune-mediated nephritis has occurred in patients receiving avelumab therapy. Immune-mediated nephritis occurred in 1 of 1738 patients (0.1%) in clinical studies and avelumab therapy was permanently discontinued in this patient.

Patients receiving avelumab should be monitored for manifestations of renal dysfunction. Serum creatinine concentrations should be assessed prior to initiation of avelumab therapy and then monitored periodically during treatment. Temporary interruption or discontinuance of avelumab may be necessary if immune-mediated nephritis occurs during therapy with the drug. (See Immune-mediated Renal Effects under Dosage: Therapy Interruption for Toxicity, in Dosage and Administration.) If grade 2 or greater nephritis occurs, systemic corticosteroid therapy should be initiated (1–2 mg/kg of prednisone daily [or equivalent]) followed by tapering of the corticosteroid dosage.

Other Immune-mediated Effects Other immune-mediated adverse effects, sometimes severe or fatal, have occurred in patients receiving avelumab therapy. In clinical studies, immune-mediated adverse effects such as myocarditis, myositis, psoriasis, arthritis, exfoliative dermatitis, erythema multiforme, pemphigoid, hypopituitarism, uveitis, Guillain-Barré syndrome, and systemic inflammatory responses were each observed in less than 1% of patients receiving avelumab. Additional immune-mediated adverse effects, including bullous dermatitis, Stevens-Johnson syndrome, toxic epidermal necrolysis, pancreatitis, rhabdomyolysis, myasthenia gravis, histiocytic necrotizing lymphadenitis, demyelination, vasculitis, hemolytic anemia, hypophysitis, iritis, and encephalitis, have been reported with other anti-programmed-death 1 (anti-PD-1) and anti-PD ligand 1 (anti-PD-L1) antibodies. Immune-mediated adverse effects may initially occur during avelumab therapy, but may also occur following discontinuance of the drug.

If an immune-mediated adverse effect is suspected, adequate evaluation should be performed to exclude other causes. Depending on the severity of the immune-mediated adverse effect, avelumab therapy should be temporarily interrupted or discontinued and high-dose corticosteroid therapy initiated; hormone replacement therapy also should be initiated, if indicated. (See Other Immune-mediated Effects under Dosage: Therapy Interruption for Toxicity, in Dosage and Administration.)

Infusion-related Effects Infusion-related reactions, sometimes severe or life-threatening, have occurred in patients receiving avelumab therapy; infusion-related reactions also have occurred following completion of the infusion. Infusion-related reactions occurred in 25% of patients receiving avelumab in clinical studies. Grade 3 or 4 infusion-related reactions occurred in 0.5 or 0.2% of avelumab-treated patients, respectively; 92% of patients experiencing grade 3 or 4 infusion-related reactions received IV corticosteroid therapy. Most patients (93%) receiving avelumab were premedicated with an antihistamine and acetaminophen. Infusion-related effects may include pyrexia, chills, flushing, hypotension, dyspnea, wheezing, back pain, abdominal pain, and urticaria.

Patients receiving avelumab should be premedicated with acetaminophen and an antihistamine prior to the initial 4 infusions of the drug. (See Dosage and Administration: General.) Patients should be monitored for manifestations of infusion-related reactions. In patients experiencing infusion-related reactions, interruption of the infusion, reduction in the infusion rate, or permanent discontinuance of the drug may be necessary. (See Infusion-related Reactions under Dosage: Therapy Interruption for Toxicity, in Dosage and Administration.)

Fetal/Neonatal Morbidity and Mortality Avelumab may cause fetal harm if administered to pregnant women. Blockade of signaling of the programmed death 1 (PD-1) and ligand 1 (PD-L1) pathway in animals has been shown to disrupt maternal immune tolerance to the fetus and has been associated with increased fetal loss (e.g., abortion, stillbirth) and immune-mediated disorders; however, teratogenicity has not been observed.

Pregnancy should be avoided during avelumab therapy. Women of childbearing potential should be advised to use an effective method of contraception while receiving avelumab and for at least 1 month after discontinuance of therapy. If avelumab is used during pregnancy or if the patient becomes pregnant while receiving the drug, the patient should be apprised of the potential fetal hazard.

Immunogenicity There is a potential for immunogenicity with avelumab therapy. Development of anti-avelumab antibodies was detected in 64 of 1558 patients (4.1%) receiving avelumab. No effects on safety (including risk of infusion-related reactions) or pharmacokinetics of the drug were observed in clinical studies.

Specific Populations **Pregnancy.** Avelumab may cause fetal harm if administered to pregnant women based on its mechanism of action and animal findings. (See Fetal/Neonatal Morbidity and Mortality under Cautions: Warnings/Precautions.)

Lactation. It is not known whether avelumab is distributed into human milk. Because many drugs and human immunoglobulin G (IgG) are distributed into human milk and because of the potential for serious adverse reactions to avelumab in nursing infants, women should be advised to discontinue nursing during avelumab therapy and for at least 1 month after discontinuance of therapy. The effects of the drug on nursing infants or on milk production are unknown.

Pediatric Use. Safety and efficacy of avelumab have not been established in pediatric patients younger than 12 years of age.

Because the clinical course and treatment of Merkel cell carcinoma are similar in adults and pediatric patients, safety and efficacy of avelumab for the treatment of metastatic Merkel cell carcinoma in adolescents 12 years of age or older are supported by extrapolation of data from clinical studies evaluating avelumab in adults, population pharmacokinetic analyses indicating that age (range of 20–91 years) and body weight (range of 30–90 kg) do not have clinically important effects on systemic exposure to the drug, and evidence that exposure to monoclonal antibodies generally is similar in adults and adolescents.

In one case, a 10-year-old girl with metastatic Merkel cell carcinoma experienced pain, nausea, and vomiting during and following avelumab therapy. The child initially received 6 cycles of cisplatin and etoposide and experienced disease progression following 3 doses of avelumab 10 mg/kg.

Geriatric Use. Clinical studies evaluating avelumab in patients with metastatic Merkel cell carcinoma did not include sufficient numbers of patients 65 years of age and older to determine whether geriatric patients respond differently than younger adults.

In the JAVELIN Solid Tumor study, 68% of patients receiving avelumab for the treatment of locally advanced or metastatic urothelial carcinoma were 65 years of age or older, while 29% were 75 years of age or older; among 153 patients 65 years of age or older who were assessed for a minimum of 13 weeks, 14% responded to avelumab and 58% experienced a grade 3 or 4 adverse effect. In this study, no overall differences in safety or efficacy were observed between geriatric patients and younger adults.

Hepatic Impairment. Analysis of population pharmacokinetic data indicates that the pharmacokinetics of avelumab are not influenced by mild (total bilirubin concentration not exceeding the ULN *with* AST concentration exceeding the ULN, or total bilirubin concentration between 1–1.5 times the ULN) or moderate (total bilirubin concentration between 1.5–3 times the ULN) hepatic impairment. Pharmacokinetic data in patients with severe hepatic impairment (total bilirubin concentration exceeding 3 times the ULN) are limited.

Renal Impairment. Analysis of population pharmacokinetic data indicates that the pharmacokinetics of avelumab are not influenced by mild, moderate, or severe renal impairment (creatinine clearance 15–89 mL/minute).

■ **Common Adverse Effects** Adverse effects reported in 10% or more of patients receiving avelumab for the treatment of metastatic Merkel cell carcinoma include fatigue, musculoskeletal pain, diarrhea, infusion-related reactions, nausea, rash, loss of appetite, peripheral edema, cough, constipation, abdominal pain, arthralgia, decreased weight, dizziness, hypertension, vomiting, dyspnea, headache, and pruritus. Laboratory abnormalities reported in 10% or more of patients receiving avelumab include lymphopenia, anemia, elevated concentrations of aminotransferases (i.e., ALT, AST), thrombocytopenia, and elevated concentrations of lipase.

Adverse effects reported in 10% or more of patients receiving avelumab for the treatment of locally advanced or metastatic urothelial carcinoma include fatigue, infusion-related reactions, musculoskeletal pain, nausea, loss of appetite, urinary tract infection, abdominal pain, decreased weight, constipation, diarrhea, dyspnea (including dyspnea on exertion), peripheral edema, elevated concentrations of serum creatinine/renal failure, pyrexia, rash, cough, vomiting/retching, hypertension (including hypertensive crisis), and pruritus. Grade 3 or 4 laboratory abnormalities reported in 5% or more of patients receiving avelumab include hyponatremia, elevated concentrations of γ-glutamyltransferase (γ-glutamyltranspeptidase, GGT, GGTP), lymphopenia, hyperglycemia, elevated concentrations of alkaline phosphatase, anemia, and elevated concentrations of lipase.

Drug Interactions

No formal drug interaction studies have been performed to date.

Description

Avelumab, a fully human anti-programmed-death ligand-1 (anti-PD-L1) monoclonal antibody, is an antineoplastic agent. The drug is an IgG_1 lambda immunoglobulin.

The immune-checkpoint receptor PD-1 is expressed on activated T-cells, monocytes, B-cells, natural killer (NK) T-cells, and dendritic cells. Overexpression of PD-1 ligands on the surface of tumor cells results in activation of PD-1 and B7.1 and suppression of cytotoxic T-cell activity, T-cell proliferation, and cytokine production. Avelumab blocks the interaction between PD-L1 and the receptors PD-1 and B7.1, resulting in restoration of immune responses, including activation of the antitumor immune response. In vitro, avelumab has been shown to induce antibody-dependent cell-mediated cytotoxicity (ADCC). The drug also has been shown to reduce tumor growth in syngeneic mouse tumor models.

Systemic exposure to avelumab is proportional to dose over the dosage range of 3–20 mg/kg every 2 weeks. When avelumab is administered every 2 weeks, steady-state concentrations are reached by 4–6 weeks, and systemic accumulation of the drug is approximately 1.3-fold. Following completion of a 1-hour IV infusion of avelumab, peak plasma concentrations of the drug are reached within 1 hour. Avelumab is metabolized by proteolytic degradation. The terminal half-life of avelumab is 6.1 days.

The pharmacokinetics of avelumab does not appear to be affected by age (range of 20–91 years), gender, race, PD-L1 status, or tumor burden.

Advice to Patients

Importance of advising patients to read the manufacturer's medication guide.

Risk of immune-mediated pneumonitis. Importance of informing clinician immediately if new or worsening cough, chest pain, or shortness of breath occurs.

Risk of immune-mediated hepatitis. Importance of informing clinician immediately if signs and symptoms of liver damage (e.g., jaundice, severe nausea or vomiting, abdominal pain [particularly in the right upper quadrant], lethargy, easy bruising or bleeding) occur.

Risk of immune-mediated colitis. Importance of informing clinician immediately if diarrhea or severe abdominal pain occurs.

Risk of immune-mediated endocrinopathies. Importance of informing clinician immediately if signs and symptoms of adrenal insufficiency, hypothyroidism, hyperthyroidism, or diabetes mellitus occur.

Risk of immune-mediated nephritis or renal dysfunction. Importance of informing clinician immediately if signs and symptoms of nephritis (e.g., decreased urine output, hematuria, peripheral edema, lack of appetite) occur.

Risk of infusion-related reactions. Importance of informing clinician immediately if signs and symptoms of such reactions, including chills, fever, breathing difficulty (i.e., shortness of breath, wheezing), urticaria, flushing, hypotension, and back or abdominal pain, occur.

Risk of fetal harm. Necessity of advising women of childbearing potential that they should use a highly effective method of contraception while receiving the drug and for at least 1 month after discontinuance of therapy. Importance of women informing clinicians if they are or plan to become pregnant. If pregnancy occurs, importance of advising pregnant women of potential risk to the fetus.

Importance of advising women to avoid breast-feeding while receiving the drug and for at least 1 month after discontinuance of therapy.

Importance of informing clinicians of existing or contemplated concomitant therapy, including prescription and OTC drugs, as well as any concomitant illnesses.

Importance of informing patients of other important precautionary information. (See Cautions.)

Overview® (see Users Guide). For additional information on this drug until a more detailed monograph is developed and published, the manufacturer's labeling should be consulted. It is *essential* that the manufacturer's labeling be consulted for more detailed information on usual cautions, precautions, contraindications, potential drug interactions, laboratory test interferences, and acute toxicity. For further information on the handling of antineoplastic agents, see the ASHP Guidelines on Handling Hazardous Drugs at http://www.ahfsdruginformation.com.

Preparations

Distribution of avelumab is restricted. (See Restricted Distribution Program under Dosage and Administration: General.)

Excipients in commercially available drug preparations may have clinically important effects in some individuals; consult specific product labeling for details.

Avelumab

Parenteral		
Injection concentrate, for IV infusion only	20 mg/mL (200 mg)	**Bavencio®**, EMD Serono (comarketed with Pfizer)

Axitinib

■ Axitinib is a second-generation tyrosine kinase inhibitor that selectively inhibits vascular endothelial growth factor receptors (VEGFR)-1, VEGFR-2, and VEGFR-3; the drug is an antineoplastic agent.

Uses

■ **Renal Cell Carcinoma** Axitinib is used for the treatment of advanced renal cell carcinoma following failure of one prior systemic therapy.

The current indication for axitinib is based principally on the results of a randomized, open-label, multicenter, phase 3 study (AXIS) in adults with advanced renal cell carcinoma whose disease progressed during or following treatment with one prior systemic therapy, including sunitinib-, bevacizumab plus interferon alfa-, temsirolimus-, or cytokine-based therapy. In the AXIS study, 723 patients were randomized in a 1:1 ratio to receive either axitinib (5 mg orally twice daily initially with dosage adjustment as needed) or sorafenib (400 mg orally twice daily initially with dosage adjustment as needed). Patients were treated until disease progression, unacceptable toxicity, death, or withdrawal of patient consent. The primary end point of this study was progression-free survival; secondary endpoints included overall survival, objective response rate, duration of response, and time to deterioration. The median age of patients enrolled in the study was 61 years; enrolled patients had received one prior therapy for their disease, including regimens consisting of sunitinib (54% of patients), cytokines (35%), bevacizumab (8%), and temsirolimus (3%). The majority of enrolled patients (99%) had clear-cell carcinoma histology.

Patients receiving axitinib in the AXIS study had a substantially longer median progression-free survival than those receiving sorafenib (6.7 versus 4.7 months). In the patients treated with axitinib, median progression-free survival was longer in those who had previously been treated with a cytokine (12.1 months) than in those previously treated with sunitinib (4.8 months). Improved progression-free survival was observed in the axitinib-treated patients regardless of their Memorial Sloan-Kettering Cancer Center (MSKCC) risk category, gender, age, or region. Patients receiving axitinib also had higher objective response rates (19 versus 9%) with a median response duration of 11 months for those receiving axitinib and 10.6 months for those receiving sorafenib; there were no complete responses in the axitinib treatment group. Median overall survival was 20.1 months with axitinib and 19.2 months with sorafenib, which was not a statistically significant difference. Treatment was discontinued because of adverse effects in 4% of patients receiving axitinib compared with 8% of those receiving sorafenib.

Use of axitinib also was investigated in an open-label, multicenter, phase 2 study in 62 adults with sorafenib-refractory metastatic renal cell carcinoma whose disease had progressed following at least one prior systemic therapy, including sorafenib. All patients enrolled in this study had undergone nephrectomy and approximately 95% of patients had clear-cell and/or mixed histology. All patients received axitinib at an initial dosage of 5 mg orally twice daily with subsequent dosage adjustments made based on tolerability. Most patients (74.2%) in this study had been treated with at least 2 prior systemic therapies. In addition, most patients (85.5%) also had received sorafenib as the only or final treatment before beginning axitinib therapy. The primary end point of this study was objective response rate. The objective response rate with axitinib therapy was 22.6% with a median response duration of 17.5 months; there were no complete responses. At a median follow-up of 22.7 months, the study revealed a median progression-free survival of 7.4 months and median overall survival of 13.6 months with axitinib therapy.

Dosage and Administration

■ **General** Axitinib can only be obtained through a limited network of specialty pharmacies. Clinicians may contact the manufacturer (Pfizer) by telephone at 877-744-5675 or consult the Inlyta® website for specific ordering and availability information (http://www.inlytahcp.com).

■ **Administration** Axitinib is administered orally twice daily (in doses given approximately 12 hours apart). The drug may be given without regard to meals. Axitinib tablets should be swallowed whole with a glass of water; the tablets should *not* be crushed or split.

If a dose of axitinib is missed or vomited, patients should *not* double the dosage or take extra doses. The next dose should be taken at the regularly scheduled time.

For patients unable to swallow tablets in clinical trials, axitinib tablets have been dissolved (without crushing) in 15 mL of USP-grade water in an amber-colored syringe and administered through a nasogastric tube; use of tap or bottled water was avoided. The nasogastric tube should be flushed with 15 mL of USP-grade water prior to and following administration of the dose. The prepared dose should not be exposed to direct light and should be prepared just prior to administration.

Procedures for proper handling of antineoplastic drugs should be followed when preparing doses of axitinib for nasogastric administration.

■ **Dosage** ***Renal Cell Carcinoma*** For the treatment of advanced renal cell carcinoma in adults, the recommended initial dosage of axitinib is 5 mg twice daily, with doses administered approximately 12 hours apart. In the principal efficacy study, therapy was continued until disease progression or unacceptable toxicity occurred. Patients in this study received axitinib for a median duration of 6.4 months. (See Dosage Modification for Toxicity under Dosage and Administration: Dosage.)

During the course of therapy, patients who tolerate axitinib for at least 2 consecutive weeks without adverse effects greater than grade 2, are normotensive, and are not receiving antihypertensive agents may have their axitinib dosage increased. When a dosage increase from 5 mg twice daily is recommended, the dosage may be increased to 7 mg twice daily, and then further increased to 10 mg twice daily using the same criteria.

Dosage Modification for Toxicity Upward or downward adjustment of axitinib dosage is recommended based on individual safety and tolerability.

Over the course of treatment, management of some adverse effects may require temporary interruption, permanent discontinuance, and/or dosage reduction of axitinib therapy. If dosage reduction from 5 mg twice daily is necessary, the recommended dosage is 3 mg twice daily. If further dosage reduction is required, the recommended axitinib dosage is 2 mg twice daily.

Concomitant Use with Drugs Affecting Hepatic Microsomal Enzymes Concomitant use of axitinib with drugs that are potent inhibitors of cytochrome P-450 (CYP) isoenzymes 3A4 or 3A5 should be *avoided.* (See Drug Interactions: Drugs Affecting Hepatic Microsomal Enzymes.) If concomitant use of a potent CYP3A4/5 inhibitor cannot be avoided, the manufacturer recommends reducing the axitinib dosage by approximately 50% (i.e., one half). This dosage is predicted to adjust the area under the plasma concentration-time curve (AUC) of axitinib to the range observed in the absence of CYP3A4/5 inhibitors. However, there are no clinical studies to date evaluating this reduced dosage in patients concomitantly receiving potent CYP3A4/5 inhibitors. Subsequent increases or decreases in axitinib dosage may be made based on individual safety and tolerability. If concurrent administration of the potent inhibitor is discontinued, the axitinib dosage should be returned (after 3–5 elimination half-lives of the CYP3A4/5 inhibitor) to the dosage used prior to initiation of the potent CYP3A4/5 inhibitor.

■ **Special Populations** No dosage adjustment is necessary in geriatric patients. (See Geriatric Use under Warnings/Precautions: Specific Populations, in Cautions.)

Dosage adjustment is not necessary in patients with mild preexisting hepatic impairment (Child-Pugh class A). In patients with moderate preexisting hepatic impairment (Child-Pugh class B), the initial dosage of axitinib should be reduced by approximately 50% (i.e., to 2.5 mg twice daily); subsequent dosage may be increased or decreased based on individual safety and tolerability. Axitinib has not been studied in patients with severe hepatic impairment (Child-Pugh class C). (See Hepatic Impairment under Warnings/Precautions: Specific Populations, in Cautions.)

Initial dosage adjustment is not necessary in patients with mild to severe preexisting renal impairment (creatinine clearance of 15 to less than 89 mL/minute). Axitinib should be used with caution in patients with end-stage renal disease (creatinine clearance less than 15 mL/minute). (See Renal Impairment under Warnings/Precautions: Specific Populations, in Cautions.)

Cautions

■ **Contraindications** The manufacturer states there are no known contraindications to the use of axitinib.

■ **Warnings/Precautions** ***Hypertension and Hypertensive Crisis*** In the AXIS clinical trial evaluating axitinib and sorafenib for advanced renal cell carcinoma, hypertension was reported in 40% (grade 3 or 4 in 16%) of patients receiving axitinib compared with 29% (grade 3 or 4 in 11%) of those receiving sorafenib. Hypertensive crisis was reported in less than 1% of patients receiving axitinib compared with none of those receiving sorafenib. Median time to development of hypertension (systolic blood pressure exceeding 150 mm Hg or diastolic blood pressure exceeding 100 mm Hg) was within the first month of axitinib therapy, and blood pressure increases were observed as early as 4 days after initiating the drug. Hypertension necessitated discontinuance of therapy in less than 1% of axitinib-treated patients.

Blood pressure should be well controlled prior to initiating axitinib therapy. Patients should be monitored for the development of hypertension during therapy and treated as needed with standard antihypertensive therapy. Axitinib-associated hypertension usually responds well to antihypertensive treatment. However, if hypertension persists despite antihypertensive therapy, the dosage of axitinib should be reduced. (See Dosage Modification for Toxicity under Dosage and Administration: Dosage.) Axitinib therapy should be discontinued if severe and persistent hypertension occurs despite dosage reduction and antihypertensive therapy. Discontinuance of the drug also should be considered if there is evidence of hypertensive crisis. If axitinib therapy is interrupted, patients continuing to receive antihypertensive therapy should be monitored for hypotension.

Arterial Thromboembolic Events Arterial thromboembolic events, including fatal cases, have been reported in axitinib-treated patients. In the phase 3 clinical study, grade 3 or 4 arterial thromboembolic events were reported in 1% of patients receiving axitinib and 1% of those receiving sorafenib. Fatal cerebrovascular accident occurred in less than 1% of patients receiving axitinib compared with none of those receiving sorafenib. In clinical trials, arterial thromboembolic events (including transient ischemic attack, cerebrovascular accident, myocardial infarction, and retinal artery occlusion) were reported in 2% of axitinib-treated patients, including 2 deaths secondary to cerebrovascular accident.

The manufacturer states that axitinib should be used with caution in patients who are at risk for, or have a history of, arterial thromboembolic events. Axitinib has not been evaluated in patients who had an arterial thromboembolic event within the past 12 months.

Venous Thromboembolic Events Venous thromboembolic events, including fatal cases, have been reported in axitinib-treated patients in clinical trials. In the phase 3 clinical study, venous thromboembolic events occurred in 3% of patients receiving axitinib and 1% of patients receiving sorafenib. Grade 3 or 4 venous thromboembolic events (including pulmonary embolism, deep-vein thrombosis, retinal vein occlusion, and retinal vein thrombosis) were reported in 3% of patients receiving axitinib and 1% of those receiving sorafenib. Fatal pulmonary embolism occurred in less than 1% of patients receiving axitinib compared with none of those receiving sorafenib. In clinical trials with axitinib, venous thromboembolic events were reported in 3% of patients, including 2 deaths secondary to pulmonary embolism.

The manufacturer states that axitinib should be used with caution in patients who are at risk for, or have a history of, venous thromboembolic events. Axitinib has not been evaluated in patients who had a venous thromboembolic event within the past 6 months.

Hemorrhage In the phase 3 clinical trial (AXIS), hemorrhagic events were reported in 16 and 18% of patients receiving axitinib and sorafenib, respectively. Grade 3 or 4 hemorrhagic events (including cerebral hemorrhage, hematuria, hemoptysis, lower GI hemorrhage, and melena) were reported in 1% of axitinib-treated patients compared with 3% of those receiving sorafenib. Fatal hemorrhage occurred in less than 1% of patients receiving axitinib (gastric hemorrhage) and in 1% of those receiving sorafenib.

Axitinib has not been evaluated in patients with evidence of untreated brain metastasis or recent, active GI bleeding; the manufacturer states that axitinib should not be used in such patients. If any bleeding requires medical intervention, axitinib therapy should be temporarily interrupted.

GI Perforation and Fistula Formation GI perforation occurred in less than 1% of patients receiving axitinib and none of those receiving sorafenib in the phase 3 trial. In clinical trials with axitinib, GI perforation and fistula formation were each reported in approximately 1% of patients; one death from GI perforation also was reported.

Axitinib should be used with caution in patients at risk for GI perforation or fistula. Patients receiving the drug should be monitored for symptoms of GI perforation and fistula formation periodically during treatment. (See Advice to Patients.)

Thyroid Dysfunction Thyroid dysfunction (hypothyroidism or hyperthyroidism), which may require thyroid hormone replacement therapy, commonly occurs during treatment with certain tyrosine kinase inhibitors, including axitinib. In the phase 3 clinical study, hypothyroidism was reported in 19 and 8% of patients receiving axitinib and sorafenib, respectively; hyperthyroidism occurred at a similar rate (1%) between the 2 treatment groups. In patients with baseline thyrotropin (thyroid-stimulating hormone, TSH) concentrations of less than 5 microunits/mL, elevations in thyrotropin concentration to 10 microunits/mL or greater occurred in 32% of patients receiving axitinib and 11% of those receiving sorafenib.

Baseline thyroid function should be assessed prior to initiation of axitinib therapy and then monitored periodically during treatment. Hypothyroidism and hyperthyroidism should be treated according to standard medical practice to maintain a euthyroid state.

Wound Healing Complications The effect of axitinib on wound healing has not been specifically studied; however, inhibitors of vascular endothelial growth factor receptor (VEGFR) may impair wound healing.

The manufacturer recommends that axitinib be discontinued at least 24 hours prior to scheduled surgery. The decision to resume therapy postoperatively should be based on clinical assessment of the adequacy of wound healing.

Reversible Posterior Leukoencephalopathy Syndrome Reversible posterior leukoencephalopathy syndrome (RPLS) has occurred in patients receiving axitinib. This complication occurred in one patient (less than 1%) treated with axitinib in the phase 3 clinical study; 2 additional cases of RPLS have been reported in other clinical trials with the drug. RPLS is a neurologic disorder that may manifest with headache, seizures, lethargy, confusion, blindness, and other visual and neurologic disturbances. Mild to severe hypertension may also be present. Magnetic resonance imaging (MRI) is necessary to confirm the diagnosis of RPLS.

Axitinib should be discontinued in patients who develop signs or symptoms of RPLS. The safety of reinitiating axitinib therapy in patients previously experiencing RPLS is not known.

Proteinuria Proteinuria was reported in 11% (grade 3 in 3%) of patients receiving axitinib compared with 7% (grade 3 in 2%) of those receiving sorafenib in the phase 3 clinical trial for renal cell carcinoma. The manufacturer recommends that patients be evaluated for proteinuria prior to initiation of axitinib therapy and monitored for proteinuria periodically during treatment with the drug. In patients who develop moderate to severe proteinuria, the dosage of axitinib should be reduced or therapy with the drug temporarily interrupted. (See Dosage Modification for Toxicity under Dosage and Administration: Dosage.)

Hepatic Effects In the phase 3 clinical trial, elevations in serum concentrations of alanine aminotransferase (ALT [SGPT]) occurred in 22% of patients receiving either axitinib or sorafenib, with grade 3 or 4 elevations reported in less than 1% of patients receiving axitinib and 2% of patients receiving sorafenib. Serum aminotransferase (ALT and AST [SGOT]) and bilirubin concentrations should be monitored prior to initiation of, and periodically during, treatment with axitinib.

Fetal/Neonatal Morbidity and Mortality Axitinib may cause fetal harm in humans based on its mechanism of action; the drug has been shown to be teratogenic, embryotoxic, and fetotoxic in animals. There are no adequate and well-controlled studies in pregnant women. Pregnancy should be avoided during therapy. If axitinib is used during pregnancy or if the patient becomes pregnant while receiving the drug, the patient should be apprised of the potential fetal hazard. (See Advice to Patients.)

Specific Populations **Pregnancy.** Category D. (See Fetal/Neonatal Morbidity and Mortality under Cautions: Warnings/Precautions and also see Users Guide.)

Lactation. It is not known whether axitinib is distributed into human milk. Because many drugs are distributed into human milk and because of the potential for serious adverse reactions to axitinib in nursing infants, a decision should be made whether to discontinue nursing or the drug, taking into account the importance of the drug to the woman.

Pediatric Use. Safety and efficacy of axitinib have not been established in pediatric patients younger than 18 years of age. The pharmacokinetics of axitinib also have not been studied in pediatric patients.

Toxicities in bone (e.g., thickened growth plates) and teeth (e.g., abnormalities in growing incisor teeth, including dental caries, malocclusions, broken and/or missing teeth) have been observed in immature animals receiving oral axitinib for one month or longer. Other toxicities of potential concern in pediatric patients have not been evaluated to date in juvenile animal studies.

Geriatric Use. In a controlled clinical study evaluating axitinib in patients with renal cell carcinoma, 34% of patients were 65 years of age or older. Although no overall differences in safety and efficacy were observed between geriatric and younger patients, the possibility of increased sensitivity to the drug in some geriatric patients cannot be ruled out. (See Dosage and Administration: Special Populations.)

Hepatic Impairment. Following a single dose of axitinib, systemic exposure of the drug in patients with mild hepatic impairment (Child-Pugh class A) was similar to that in individuals with normal hepatic function. However, systemic exposure of axitinib was increased in individuals with moderate hepatic impairment (Child-Pugh class B) compared with individuals with normal hepatic function. Initial dosage reduction is therefore recommended in patients with moderate hepatic impairment. Axitinib has not been studied in patients with severe hepatic impairment (Child-Pugh class C) to date. (See Dosage and Administration: Special Populations and see also Hepatic Effects under Cautions.)

Renal Impairment. A dedicated renal impairment trial for axitinib has not been conducted to date. Population pharmacokinetic analyses indicate that preexisting mild to severe renal impairment does not substantially alter the pharmacokinetics of axitinib. However, data in patients with end-stage renal disease are very limited, and axitinib should therefore be used with caution in such patients. (See Dosage and Administration: Special Populations.)

■ **Common Adverse Effects** Adverse effects occurring in 20% or more of patients receiving axitinib for advanced renal cell carcinoma in the randomized trial were diarrhea, hypertension, fatigue, decreased appetite, nausea, dysphonia, palmar-plantar erythrodysesthesia (hand-foot syndrome), weight loss, vomiting, asthenia, and constipation.

Laboratory abnormalities reported in 20% or more of patients receiving axitinib include decreased hemoglobin, decreased lymphocytes, increased creatinine concentrations, decreased serum bicarbonate concentrations, hypocalcemia, hyperglycemia, elevated concentrations of pancreatic enzymes (e.g., amylase, lipase), and elevated concentrations of hepatic enzymes (e.g., AST, ALT, alkaline phosphatase).

Drug Interactions

Axitinib is metabolized principally by the cytochrome P-450 (CYP) isoenzyme 3A4/5 and, to a lesser extent, by CYP1A2, CYP2C19, and uridine diphosphate-glucurosyltransferase (UGT) 1A1 in vitro.

In vitro studies demonstrate that axitinib has the potential to inhibit CYP isoenzymes 1A2 and 2C8.

In vitro studies indicate that axitinib does not inhibit CYP2A6, 2C9, 2C19, 2D6, 2E1, 3A4/5, or UGT1A1 at therapeutic plasma concentrations.

Axitinib inhibits P-glycoprotein (P-gp) in vitro; however, the drug is not expected to inhibit P-gp at therapeutic plasma concentrations.

Axitinib does not induce CYP1A1, CYP1A2, or CYP3A4/5 in human hepatocytes in vitro.

■ **Drugs Affecting Hepatic Microsomal Enzymes** ***Potent Inhibitors of CYP3A4/5*** Concomitant administration of axitinib with potent inhibitors of CYP3A4/5 may result in increased plasma concentrations of axitinib. When the potent CYP3A4/5 inhibitor ketoconazole (400 mg once daily for 7 days) was administered concomitantly with axitinib (single 5-mg dose) in healthy individuals, mean peak plasma concentrations and systemic exposure of axitinib increased by approximately 1.5- and twofold, respectively.

Concomitant use of axitinib with potent CYP3A4/5 inhibitors (e.g., atazanavir, clarithromycin, indinavir, itraconazole, ketoconazole, nefazodone, nelfinavir, ritonavir, saquinavir, telithromycin, voriconazole) should be avoided, and selection of an alternative drug with no or minimal CYP3A4/5 inhibition potential is recommended. If concomitant use with a potent CYP3A4/5 inhibitor cannot be avoided, the manufacturer recommends reducing the axitinib dosage by approximately 50%; subsequent axitinib dosages may be increased or decreased based on individual safety and tolerability. (See Concomitant Use with Drugs Affecting Hepatic Microsomal Enzymes under Dosage and Administration: Dosage.) If concomitant use of the potent CYP3A4/5 inhibitor is discontinued, the axitinib dosage should be returned (after 3–5 elimination half-lives of the CYP3A4/5 inhibitor) to the dosage used prior to initiation of the potent CYP3A4/5 inhibitor. (See Drug Interactions: Grapefruit.)

Inducers of CYP3A4/5 Concomitant administration of axitinib with inducers of CYP3A4/5 may result in decreased plasma concentrations of axitinib. When the potent CYP3A4/5 inducer rifampin (600 mg once daily for 9 days) was administered concomitantly with axitinib (single 5-mg dose), mean peak plasma concentrations and systemic exposure of axitinib decreased by 71 and 79%, respectively. When the potent CYP3A4/5 inducer phenytoin was administered concomitantly with axitinib in one patient, peak plasma concentrations and systemic exposure of axitinib decreased approximately tenfold.

Concomitant use of axitinib with potent CYP3A4/5 inducers (e.g., carbamazepine, dexamethasone, rifabutin, rifampin, rifapentine, phenobarbital, phenytoin, St. John's wort [*Hypericum perforatum*]) should be avoided, and selection of an alternative drug with no or minimal CYP3A4/5 induction potential is recommended. Concomitant use of axitinib with moderate CYP3A4/5 inducers (e.g., bosentan, efavirenz, etravirine, modafinil, nafcillin) also should be avoided if possible.

■ **Drugs Metabolized by Hepatic Microsomal Enzymes** In vitro studies indicate that axitinib has the potential to inhibit CYP isoenzymes 1A2 and 2C8. However, when the CYP2C8 substrate paclitaxel was administered concomitantly with axitinib, plasma concentrations of paclitaxel were unchanged.

■ **Drugs Affecting Gastric Acidity** Because the aqueous solubility of axitinib is dependent on pH, drugs that increase the pH of the upper GI tract (e.g., antacids, histamine H_2-receptor antagonists, proton-pump inhibitors) may potentially decrease the solubility of axitinib and subsequently reduce its bioavailability. However, when the proton-pump inhibitor rabeprazole (20 mg once daily) was administered concomitantly with axitinib, the peak plasma concentration of axitinib was decreased and changes in systemic exposure of axitinib were not considered clinically important. The manufacturer states that dosage adjustment is not necessary when axitinib is administered concurrently with drugs affecting gastric acidity, including antacids and proton-pump inhibitors.

■ **Antineoplastic Agents** Concomitant administration of axitinib and bevacizumab in combination with FOLFIRI (irinotecan/fluorouracil/leucovorin) or FOLFOX (oxaliplatin/fluorouracil/leucovorin) did not substantially alter the pharmacokinetics of axitinib or the other antineoplastic agents.

Concurrent administration of axitinib and a standard regimen of paclitaxel plus carboplatin did not substantially affect the pharmacokinetics of axitinib or the other antineoplastic agents.

Concomitant administration of axitinib and gemcitabine plus cisplatin did not substantially affect the pharmacokinetics of axitinib, gemcitabine, or cisplatin.

■ **Grapefruit** Grapefruit products are CYP3A4/5 inhibitors and should be avoided during axitinib therapy because of the potential for increased plasma axitinib concentrations.

■ **Warfarin** Because warfarin is a substrate of CYP1A2, axitinib may increase plasma warfarin concentrations; however, this potential interaction has not been systematically evaluated to date and its clinical importance is unclear. Pending further accumulation of data, clinicians should consider that hemorrhagic events have been reported in some patients receiving axitinib therapy alone. (See Hemorrhage under Cautions: Warnings/Precautions.)

Description

Axitinib is a selective, second-generation inhibitor of receptor tyrosine kinases, including vascular endothelial growth factor receptors (VEGFR)-1, VEGFR-2, and VEGFR-3; the drug is an antineoplastic agent. Chemically, axitinib is a substituted indazole derivative. Receptor tyrosine kinases (TKs) are involved in the initiation of various cascades of intracellular signaling events that lead to cell proliferation and/or influence processes critical to cancer cell survival and tumor progression (e.g., angiogenesis, metastasis, inhibition of apoptosis), based on the respective kinase. Axitinib potently and selectively inhibits VEGFR-1, VEGFR-2, and VEGFR-3 at therapeutic plasma concentrations. The VEGFR signaling pathway plays an important role in the pathogenesis and progression of several types of tumors since it is a pivotal mediator of tumor angiogenesis; the pathway also regulates tumor growth and metastatic spread. Axitinib appears to be 50–450 times more potent at blocking VEGFR receptors than first-generation VEGFR inhibitors (e.g., sorafenib, sunitinib, pazopanib). Axitinib exhibits eightfold to tenfold lower inhibitory activity against platelet-derived growth factor receptor beta (PDGFR-β) and stem cell factor receptor (c-Kit); the drug also has minimal inhibitory effects on other receptor kinases, including colony stimulating factor receptor type 1 (CSF-1R), fms-like tyrosine kinase 3 (Flt-3), fibroblast growth factor receptor (FGFR)-1, ret proto-oncogene (RET), epidermal growth factor receptor (EGFR), and met proto-oncogene encoding hepatocyte growth factor (c-MET). Axitinib has been shown to inhibit VEGF-mediated endothelial cell proliferation and survival in vitro and in mice. The drug has also demonstrated inhibition of tumor growth and VEGFR-2 phosphorylation in mice bearing tumor xenografts.

Following oral administration, axitinib is readily absorbed with peak plasma concentrations occurring within 2.5–4.1 hours. When axitinib is administered orally twice daily, accumulation of the drug is approximately 1.4-fold higher compared with administration of a single dose. At steady state, axitinib exhibits approximately linear pharmacokinetics within a dosage range of 1–20 mg. Steady-state concentrations of the drug are expected within 2–3 days. Axitinib is metabolized in the liver principally by cytochrome P-450 (CYP) 3A4/5 and, to a lesser extent, by CYP1A2, CYP2C19, and uridine diphosphate-glucuronosyl transferase (UGT) 1A1. (See Drug Interactions.) Axitinib is highly bound (more than 99%) to plasma proteins. The elimination half-life of axitinib ranges from 2.5–6.1 hours. Following oral administration of a radiolabeled dose of axitinib, approximately 41% of the dose is recovered in the feces (mainly as unchanged drug) and approximately 23% of the dose is recovered in urine (mainly as carboxylic acid and sulfoxide metabolites). In vitro, the sulfoxide and *N*-glucuronide metabolites are more than 400 times less potent against VEGFR-2 compared with axitinib.

Advice to Patients

Importance of reading the manufacturer's patient information prior to beginning axitinib therapy and rereading it each time the prescription is refilled.

Importance of swallowing axitinib tablets whole with a glass of water. Importance of avoiding grapefruit or grapefruit juice while taking the drug.

If a dose is missed or vomited, importance of administering the next dose at the regularly scheduled time; an additional dose should not be administered to make up for a missed dose.

Risk of hypertension developing during therapy. Importance of regular monitoring of blood pressure during treatment.

Risk of arterial and venous thromboembolic events. Importance of getting emergency help and contacting clinician if any symptoms suggestive of a thromboembolic event occur (e.g., chest pain or pressure, shortness of breath, unilateral numbness or weakness, difficulty talking, headache, vision changes, or arm, back, neck, or jaw pain).

Increased risk of bleeding. Importance of promptly informing clinician of any episodes of bleeding (e.g., unusual bleeding, bruising).

Risk of GI disorders. Importance of advising patients that GI disorders such as diarrhea, nausea, vomiting, and constipation may develop during axitinib therapy and to seek immediate medical attention if they experience symptoms of GI perforation or fistula (e.g., persistent or severe abdominal pain, vomiting blood, red or black stools).

Risk of thyroid dysfunction. Importance of informing clinician if symptoms of abnormal thyroid function occur (e.g., persistent or worsening fatigue, deepened voice, hair loss, weight gain or loss, myalgia, feeling hot or cold).

Risk of wound healing complications. Importance of informing clinician of any scheduled surgery or wounds that do not heal.

Risk of reversible posterior leukoencephalopathy syndrome (RPLS). Importance of immediately informing clinician if headache, seizures, weakness, lethargy, confusion, hypertension, blindness, or other visual and neurologic disturbances occur during axitinib therapy.

Risk of fetal harm and fetal loss. Importance of women informing their clinicians if they are or plan to become pregnant. Importance of advising men who are receiving axitinib to inform their clinician if their female partner becomes pregnant. Necessity of advising women to avoid pregnancy during therapy. Necessity of advising women and men receiving axitinib to use effective methods of contraception during axitinib therapy. Advise women of the potential risk to the fetus (e.g., birth defects) and/or the potential risk for loss of the pregnancy.

Importance of advising women to avoid breast-feeding while receiving axitinib therapy.

Risk of proteinuria. Importance of informing patients that they will be monitored for proteinuria before and during axitinib therapy.

Risk of hepatotoxicity; importance of informing patients about need for liver function test monitoring during axitinib therapy.

Importance of informing clinicians of existing or contemplated concomitant therapy, including prescription and OTC drugs and dietary or herbal supplements (e.g., St. John's wort), as well as any concomitant illnesses (e.g., hypertension or other cardiovascular disease, cerebrovascular disease, thyroid disease, hepatic disease, bleeding disorders).

Importance of informing patients of other important precautionary information. (See Cautions.)

Overview® (see Users Guide). For additional information on this drug until a more detailed monograph is developed and published, the manufacturer's labeling should be consulted. It is *essential* that the manufacturer's labeling be consulted for more detailed information on usual cautions, precautions, contraindications, potential drug interactions, laboratory test interferences, and acute toxicity. For further information on the handling of antineoplastic agents, see the ASHP Guidelines on Handling Hazardous Drugs at http://www.ahfsdruginformation.com.

Preparations

Excipients in commercially available drug preparations may have clinically important effects in some individuals; consult specific product labeling for details.

Axitinib

Oral		
Tablets, film-coated	1 mg	**Inlyta®**, Pfizer
	5 mg	**Inlyta®**, Pfizer

Selected Revisions August 2014, © Copyright, October 2012, American Society of Health-System Pharmacists, Inc.

Belinostat

■ Belinostat, a histone deacetylase (HDAC) inhibitor, is an antineoplastic agent.

Uses

■ **Peripheral T-cell Lymphoma** Belinostat is used for the treatment of relapsed or refractory peripheral T-cell lymphoma (PTCL); the drug is designated an orphan drug by the US Food and Drug Administration (FDA) for the treatment of this cancer. The current indication is based on overall response rate and duration of response; there currently are no controlled trials demonstrating a clinical benefit (e.g., improvement in disease-related symptoms, increased survival).

The current indication for belinostat is based principally on the results of an open-label, noncomparative, nonrandomized study (BELIEF) in 129 patients with relapsed or refractory PTCL. The primary measure of efficacy was overall response rate (complete plus partial responses) as assessed by an independent review committee using the International Workshop Criteria (IWC). The median age of patients was 64 years; the patients had received a median of 2 prior therapies for their disease. In this study, all patients received belinostat (1 g/m^2 IV daily on days 1–5 every 3 weeks) until disease progression or unacceptable toxicity occurred. The overall response rate was 25.8%; 10.8% of patients receiving the drug achieved a complete response. At the time of analysis, the median duration of response for all responders was 5.6 weeks (range: 4.3–50.4 weeks); the median duration of response based on the first date of response to disease progression or death was 8.4 months. Following therapy with belinostat, 7.5% of patients underwent stem cell transplantation.

Dosage and Administration

■ **General** Complete blood cell counts (CBCs) should be obtained prior to initiation of belinostat therapy and monitored weekly during therapy. In addition, serum chemistry tests, including hepatic and renal function tests, should be performed before administration of the first belinostat dose of each treatment cycle.

Procedures for proper handling (e.g., use of gloves or protective clothing) and disposal of antineoplastic agents should be followed.

■ **Administration** Belinostat is administered by IV infusion over 30 minutes. If infusion site reactions (e.g., pain) occur, the infusion time may be extended to 45 minutes.

Prior to administration, commercially available belinostat powder for injection must be reconstituted and diluted using proper aseptic technique. The lyophilized powder is reconstituted by adding 9 mL of sterile water for injection to a vial labeled as containing 500 mg of the drug to provide a solution containing 50 mg/mL. The vial should be swirled until complete dissolution of the powder occurs. The solution should be inspected visually for particulate matter and discoloration prior to dilution and administration. The reconstituted belinostat solution may be stored at 15–25°C for up to 12 hours.

For preparation of the final diluted belinostat solution for infusion, the required dose of reconstituted belinostat solution should be injected into an infusion bag containing 250 mL of 0.9% sodium chloride injection. The final diluted solution may be stored at 15–25°C for up to 36 hours (including infusion time). Belinostat should be administered through a 0.22-μm inline filter.

■ **Dosage** ***Peripheral T-cell Lymphoma*** For the treatment of relapsed or refractory peripheral T-cell lymphoma (PTCL), the recommended adult dosage of belinostat is 1 g/m^2 administered as a 30-minute IV infusion daily on days 1–5 of each 21-day cycle. Therapy should be continued until disease progression or unacceptable toxicity occurs.

Dosage Modification **Hematologic Toxicity.** Dosage adjustments for thrombocytopenia or neutropenia should be based on nadir blood cell counts during the previous treatment cycle.

If the absolute neutrophil count (ANC) decreases to no less than 500/mm^3 and platelet counts decrease to no less than 25,000/mm^3, belinostat therapy should be withheld until ANC reaches or exceeds 1000/mm^3 and platelet counts reach or exceed 50,000/mm^3. Therapy may then be resumed at the same dosage.

If ANC decreases to less than 500/mm^3 with any platelet count, belinostat therapy should be withheld until ANC reaches or exceeds 1000/mm^3 and platelet counts reach or exceed 50,000/mm^3. Upon resumption of therapy, the belinostat dosage should be reduced by 25%.

If platelet counts decrease to less than 25,000/mm^3 with any ANC, belinostat therapy should be withheld until ANC reaches or exceeds 1000/mm^3 and platelet counts reach or exceed 50,000/mm^3. Upon resumption of therapy, the belinostat dosage should be reduced by 25%.

If ANC less than 500/mm^3 and/or platelet count less than 25,000/mm^3 recurs following 2 dosage reductions, belinostat therapy should be discontinued.

Nonhematologic Toxicity. If prolonged grade 3 or 4 nausea, vomiting, and/or diarrhea (i.e., lasting more than 7 days despite initiation of supportive management) or if other grade 3 or 4 nonhematologic toxicity occurs, belinostat therapy should be withheld until the toxicity resolves to grade 2 or less. Upon resumption of therapy, the belinostat dosage should be reduced by 25%.

If grade 3 or 4 nonhematologic toxicity recurs following 2 dosage reductions, belinostat therapy should be discontinued.

Reduced Uridine Diphosphate-glucuronosyltransferase (UGT) 1A1 Activity. In patients who are homozygous for the UGT1A1*28 allele, the initial dose of belinostat should be reduced to 750 mg/m^2. (See Description.)

■ **Special Populations** The manufacturer states that insufficient data are available to provide dosage recommendations for patients with moderate or severe hepatic impairment or for patients with a creatinine clearance of 39 mL/minute or less. The manufacturer makes no specific dosage recommendations for geriatric patients. (See Specific Populations under Cautions: Warnings/Precautions.)

Cautions

■ **Contraindications** The manufacturer states there are no known contraindications to the use of belinostat.

■ **Warnings/Precautions** ***Hematologic Effects*** Thrombocytopenia, leukopenia (neutropenia and lymphopenia), and/or anemia may occur. In the principal efficacy study of belinostat in patients with peripheral T-cell lymphoma (PTCL), thrombocytopenia or anemia occurred in 16 or 32% of patients, respectively; grade 3 or 4 thrombocytopenia occurred in 7% of patients, and grade 3 or 4 anemia occurred in 11% of patients. Complete blood cell counts (CBCs) should be monitored weekly during therapy and the dosage of belinostat should be adjusted if necessary. (See Hematologic Toxicity under Dosage: Dosage Modification, in Dosage and Administration.)

Infectious Complications Serious and sometimes fatal infections, including pneumonia and sepsis, have been reported in patients receiving belinostat. Patients with a history of extensive or intensive chemotherapy may be at greater risk for life-threatening infections. Belinostat should *not* be administered to patients with an active infection.

Hepatic Toxicity Fatal hepatotoxicity and liver function test abnormalities may occur. In the principal efficacy study of belinostat in patients with PTCL, fatal hepatic failure was reported in one patient. Liver function tests should be performed prior to initiation of belinostat therapy and prior to each treatment cycle. In patients who develop hepatotoxicity, temporary interruption of therapy, dosage reduction, or drug discontinuance may be required. (See Nonhematologic Toxicity under Dosage: Dosage Modification, in Dosage and Administration.)

Tumor Lysis Syndrome Tumor lysis syndrome has been reported in patients receiving belinostat for the treatment of relapsed or refractory PTCL. In the principal efficacy study of belinostat in patients with PTCL, grade 4 tumor lysis syndrome resulting in death occurred in one patient with baseline hyperuricemia and bulky disease during the first cycle of therapy. The risk of tumor lysis syndrome is increased in patients with advanced stage disease and/or a large tumor burden; such patients should be monitored closely and appropriate precautions should be taken.

GI Effects Nausea, vomiting, and diarrhea occur frequently in patients receiving belinostat. In the principal efficacy study of belinostat in patients with PTCL, nausea, vomiting, and diarrhea were reported in 42, 29, and 23% of patients, respectively. Antiemetic and antidiarrheal therapy may be necessary in patients receiving belinostat therapy.

Fetal/Neonatal Morbidity and Mortality Belinostat may cause fetal harm if administered to pregnant women. Based on its mechanism of action, teratogenicity and embryo and fetal lethality may occur. Pregnancy should be avoided during belinostat therapy. If belinostat is used during pregnancy or if the patient becomes pregnant while receiving the drug, the patient should be apprised of the potential fetal hazard.

Impairment of Fertility Results of animal studies suggest that belinostat may impair male fertility. The effect of belinostat on fertility in humans is not known.

Specific Populations **Pregnancy.** Category D. (See Users Guide and see Fetal/Neonatal Morbidity and Mortality under Cautions: Warnings/Precautions.)

Lactation. It is not known whether belinostat is distributed into milk in humans; because of the potential for serious adverse reactions to belinostat in nursing infants, a decision should be made whether to discontinue nursing or the drug, taking into account the importance of the drug to the woman.

Pediatric Use. Safety and efficacy of belinostat have not been established in pediatric patients.

Geriatric Use. In the principal efficacy study evaluating belinostat in patients with PTCL, 48% of patients were 65 years of age or older and 10% were 75 years of age or older. In patients with PTCL, the overall response rate was 36% in those 65 years of age and older compared with 16% in those younger than 65 years of age. No meaningful differences in overall response rate were observed between patients 75 years of age and older and those younger than 75 years of age. No clinically important differences in safety were observed between geriatric patients and younger adults. (See Dosage and Administration: Special Populations.)

Hepatic Impairment. Data are lacking on use of belinostat in patients with moderate or severe hepatic impairment (total bilirubin concentrations exceeding 1.5 times the upper limit of normal [ULN]); however, since belinostat is eliminated principally by hepatic metabolism, hepatic impairment may result in increased plasma belinostat concentrations. (See Dosage and Administration: Special Populations.)

Renal Impairment. Systemic exposure to belinostat was not altered in patients with creatinine clearance exceeding 39 mL/minute. Data are lacking on use of belinostat in patients with creatinine clearance of 39 mL/minute or less. (See Dosage and Administration: Special Populations.)

■ **Common Adverse Effects** Adverse effects reported in 10% or more of patients receiving belinostat include nausea, fatigue, pyrexia, vomiting, constipation, diarrhea, dyspnea, rash, peripheral edema, cough, pruritus, chills, decreased appetite, headache, infusion site pain, prolonged QT interval, abdominal pain, hypotension, phlebitis, and dizziness. Laboratory abnormalities reported in 10% or more of patients receiving belinostat include anemia, thrombocytopenia, elevated serum LDH concentrations, and hypokalemia.

Drug Interactions

Belinostat is metabolized principally (80–90%) by uridine diphosphate-glucuronosyltransferase (UGT) 1A1. In vitro studies indicate that belinostat and its metabolites, including belinostat glucuronide, belinostat amide, and methyl belinostat, are inhibitors of cytochrome P-450 (CYP) isoenzymes 2C8 and 2C9; other metabolites, including 3-(anilinosulfonyl)-benzenecarboxylic acid (3-ASBA) and belinostat acid, are inhibitors of CYP2C8 in vitro.

Belinostat is a likely substrate, but an unlikely inhibitor, of P-glycoprotein (P-gp).

■ **Drugs Affecting Uridine Diphosphate-glucuronosyltransferase (UGT)** Concomitant use of belinostat with potent inhibitors of UGT1A1 may result in increased systemic exposure to belinostat. Concomitant use of belinostat with potent UGT1A1 inhibitors should be avoided.

■ **Warfarin** In cancer patients receiving warfarin sodium (5 mg), a CYP2C9 substrate, concomitantly with belinostat (1 g/m²), the area under the concentration-time curve (AUC) and peak plasma concentrations of the *R*- and *S*-enantiomers of warfarin were not substantially altered.

Description

Belinostat, a histone deacetylase (HDAC) inhibitor, is an antineoplastic agent. HDAC enzymes catalyze the removal of acetyl groups from the lysine residues of proteins, including histones and transcription factors. Overexpression of HDAC enzymes or aberrant recruitment of HDAC enzymes to oncogenic transcription factors causing hypoacetylation of core nucleosomal histones has been observed in some cancer cells. Hypoacetylation of histones is associated with a condensed chromatin structure and repression of gene transcription. Inhibition of HDAC activity allows for the accumulation of acetyl groups on the histone lysine residues, resulting in an open chromatin structure and transcriptional activation. In vitro, belinostat causes the accumulation of acetylated histones and induces cell cycle arrest and/or apoptosis of some transformed cells. Belinostat inhibits the enzymatic activity of histone deacetylases and exhibits cytotoxic activity and induces apoptosis in various tumor cell lines at nanomolar concentrations.

Belinostat is metabolized principally (80–90%) by uridine diphosphate-glucuronosyltransferase (UGT) 1A1; the drug also is metabolized by cytochrome P-450 (CYP) isoenzymes 2A6, 2C9, and 3A4 to form the metabolites belinostat amide and belinostat acid. Other metabolites of the drug include methyl belinostat and 3-(anilinosulfonyl)-benzenecarboxylic acid (3-ASBA); the enzymes responsible for the formation of these metabolites have not been determined. Belinostat is a likely substrate, but an unlikely inhibitor, of P-glycoprotein (P-gp). The main circulating metabolites are excreted in urine, with 2 metabolites predominating (3-ASBA and belinostat glucuronide, which account for 4.61 and 30.5%, respectively, of an administered dose); only a small portion (less than 2%) of a dose is excreted in urine as unchanged drug. Belinostat is 92.9–95.8% bound to plasma proteins. Following administration of belinostat (150–1200 mg/m²), the elimination half-life of the drug was 1.1 hours.

In patients with genetic polymorphisms associated with reduced UGT1A1 activity (e.g., individuals who are homozygous for the UGT1A1*28 allele), clearance of belinostat may be reduced and dosage adjustment may be required. (See Reduced Uridine Diphosphate-glucuronosyltransferase [UGT] 1A1 Activity under Dosage: Dosage Modification, in Dosage and Administration.)

Advice to Patients

Importance of instructing patients to read the manufacturer's patient information carefully before starting belinostat therapy and to reread it before each treatment.

Importance of informing patients that nausea, vomiting, and diarrhea occur frequently with belinostat therapy and that treatment with antiemetic and/or antidiarrheal agents may be necessary. Importance of informing clinicians if nausea, vomiting, or diarrhea occurs.

Risk of cytopenias. Importance of informing clinician immediately if unusual bleeding or bruising, tiredness, pallor, shortness of breath, or infection occurs.

Risk of infections. Importance of informing clinician if fever, flu-like symptoms, cough, shortness of breath, burning on urination, muscle aches, or worsening skin problems occur.

Risk of fetal harm. Importance of women informing clinicians if they are or plan to become pregnant or plan to breast-feed. Apprise patient of potential hazard to the fetus if used during pregnancy; women of childbearing potential should avoid becoming pregnant.

Risk of hepatotoxicity and importance of liver function test monitoring. Importance of informing clinician if icteric changes, dark urine, pruritus, or abdominal pain (particularly in the right upper quadrant) occurs.

Risk of tumor lysis syndrome.

Importance of informing clinicians of existing or contemplated concomitant therapy, including prescription and OTC drugs and herbal supplements, as well as any concomitant illnesses (e.g., hepatic impairment).

Importance of informing patients of other important precautionary information. (See Cautions.)

Overview® (see Users Guide). For additional information on this drug until a more detailed monograph is developed and published, the manufacturer's labeling should be consulted. It is *essential* that the manufacturer's labeling be consulted for more detailed information on usual cautions, precautions, contraindications, potential drug interactions, laboratory test interferences, and acute toxicity. For further information on the handling of antineoplastic agents, see the ASHP Guidelines on Handling Hazardous Drugs at http://www.ahfsdruginformation.com.

Preparations

Excipients in commercially available drug preparations may have clinically important effects in some individuals; consult specific product labeling for details.

Belinostat

Parenteral

For injection, for IV infusion	500 mg	**Beleodaq®**, Spectrum

Bendamustine Hydrochloride

■ Bendamustine, a bifunctional nitrogen mustard-derivative alkylating agent and purine analog, is an antineoplastic agent.

Uses

■ **Chronic Lymphocytic Leukemia** Bendamustine hydrochloride is used for the treatment of chronic lymphocytic leukemia (CLL) and has been designated an orphan drug by the US Food and Drug Administration (FDA) for use in this condition.

The current indication for use of bendamustine in the treatment of CLL is based principally on the results of a randomized, controlled, multicenter, open-label, phase 3 study comparing bendamustine with chlorambucil in 301 patients with previously untreated, Binet stage B or C (Rai stages I–IV) CLL. Criteria for treatment included hematopoietic insufficiency, constitutional ("B") symptoms (e.g., weight loss of 10% or more, drenching night sweats, extreme fatigue, unexplained fever of 38°C or greater), rapidly progressive disease, or risk of complications from bulky lymphadenopathy. Patients with autoimmune hemolytic anemia, autoimmune thrombocytopenia, Richter's syndrome, or transformation to prolymphocytic leukemia were excluded. In this study, patients were randomized to receive up to 6 cycles of therapy with bendamustine hydrochloride (100 mg/m² IV daily on days 1 and 2 of each 28-day treatment cycle) or chlorambucil (0.8 mg/kg orally on days 1 and 15 of each 28-day cycle). The overall response rate, assessed according to National Cancer Institute (NCI) Working Group criteria for CLL, was 59% for bendamustine versus 26% for chlorambucil, with 8% of patients receiving bendamustine and less than 1% of those receiving chlorambucil achieving complete responses. In addition, median progression-free survival was longer (18 versus 6 months) in patients receiving bendamustine than in those receiving chlorambucil. The incidence of adverse effects (most commonly neutropenia, leukopenia, thrombocytopenia, anemia, pyrexia, nausea, and vomiting) generally was higher with bendamustine than with chlorambucil therapy.

Efficacy of bendamustine relative to first-line therapies other than chlorambucil in the treatment of CLL has not been established.

■ **Non-Hodgkin's Lymphoma** ***Rituximab-refractory, Indolent, B-cell Non-Hodgkin's Lymphoma*** Bendamustine hydrochloride is used for the treatment of rituximab-refractory, indolent, B-cell non-Hodgkin's lymphoma (NHL).

The current indication for use of bendamustine in the treatment of rituximab-refractory, indolent, B-cell NHL is based principally on the results of an open-label, single-arm, phase 3 study in 100 patients with indolent B-cell NHL that had progressed during or within 6 months following the first dose of rituximab induction therapy (monotherapy) or completion of a rituximab maintenance regimen or a rituximab-containing combination regimen. Patients received bendamustine hydrochloride 120 mg/m^2 IV daily on days 1 and 2 of each 21-day cycle, for up to 8 cycles. The overall response rate was 74%; 13% of patients achieved a complete response. At a median follow-up of 11.8 months, median progression-free survival was 9.3 months. Median progression-free survival was longer in patients whose disease was sensitive to their last prior chemotherapy regimen than in those whose disease was refractory to their last prior chemotherapy regimen (11.8 versus 7.5 months).

In a phase 2 study of bendamustine therapy in patients with rituximab-refractory NHL, median progression-free survival was shorter in patients with indolent disease that had transformed into a more aggressive subtype (i.e., Richter's transformation) than in those without evidence of such transformation (4.2 versus 8.3 months). In this study, thrombocytopenia requiring discontinuance of bendamustine therapy occurred disproportionately in patients who had received prior therapy with a radioimmunoconjugate (i.e., in 6 of 9 such patients); however, 8 of the 9 patients responded to the drug.

Previously Untreated, Indolent Non-Hodgkin's Lymphoma or Mantle Cell Lymphoma Efficacy and safety of bendamustine in combination with rituximab† for the treatment of previously untreated† advanced-stage indolent NHL or previously untreated advanced-stage mantle cell lymphoma† have been studied in two phase 3 studies (Study Group Indolent Lymphomas [StiL] NHL 1-2003 study and BRIGHT).

The first study (StiL NHL 1-2003) was a phase 3, open-label, randomized, noninferiority study in which 514 patients received up to 6 cycles of therapy with either bendamustine in combination with rituximab or rituximab plus cyclophosphamide, doxorubicin, vincristine, and prednisone (R-CHOP). Patients with previously untreated mantle cell lymphoma or indolent NHL, including the CD20-positive histologic subtypes follicular lymphoma (grade 1 or 2), Waldenstrom macroglobulinemia, small lymphocytic lymphoma, and marginal-zone lymphoma, were eligible for enrollment in the study. Patients receiving the bendamustine-rituximab regimen received rituximab 375 mg/m^2 IV on day 1 and bendamustine hydrochloride 90 mg/m^2 IV daily on days 1 and 2 of each 28-day cycle. Those receiving R-CHOP received rituximab 375 mg/m^2 IV, cyclophosphamide 750 mg/m^2 IV, doxorubicin hydrochloride 50 mg/m^2 IV, and vincristine sulfate 1.4 mg/m^2 (up to 2 mg) IV on day 1, followed by prednisone 100 mg orally daily on days 1–5 of each 21-day cycle. The median patient age was about 64 years (range: 31–83), about 78% of patients had stage IV disease, 19% had stage III disease, 54% had follicular lymphoma, and 18% had mantle cell lymphoma. The primary measure of efficacy was progression-free survival. Tumor responses were assessed using the World Health Organization (WHO) criteria.

At a median follow-up of 45 months, bendamustine in combination with rituximab was noninferior to R-CHOP in terms of progression-free survival; median progression-free survival was 69.5 and 31.2 months in patients receiving bendamustine in combination with rituximab and those receiving R-CHOP, respectively. A progression-free survival benefit was observed for the bendamustine-rituximab regimen compared with R-CHOP in subset analyses in patients with mantle cell lymphoma, follicular lymphoma, and Waldenstrom macroglobulinemia, but not in those with marginal-zone lymphoma. Overall response rates were similar in patients receiving bendamustine in combination with rituximab and those receiving R-CHOP (93 versus 91%, respectively); however, the complete response rate was higher in the bendamustine-rituximab group (40 versus 30%). Although median overall survival had not been reached in either group at the time of analysis, substantial differences were not observed between the treatment groups. Subgroup analysis suggested that the progression-free survival benefit observed for the bendamustine-rituximab regimen was independent of age, serum LDH concentration, and Follicular Lymphoma International Prognostic Index (FLIPI) score; however, statistical significance was not reached for elevated serum LDH concentration or unfavorable FLIPI score. Although erythematous (16 versus 9%) or allergic (15 versus 6%) skin reactions occurred more frequently in patients receiving bendamustine in combination with rituximab, serious adverse effects (19 versus 29%), grade 3 or 4 leukopenia (37 versus 72%), grade 3 or 4 neutropenia (29 versus 69%), alopecia (0 versus 100%), paresthesia (7 versus 29%), stomatitis (6 versus 19%), infection (37 versus 50%), and sepsis (less than 1 versus 3%) occurred more frequently in those receiving R-CHOP.

The second study (BRIGHT) was a phase 3, open-label, randomized, noninferiority study in which 447 patients received 6–8 cycles of therapy with either bendamustine in combination with rituximab or standard combination chemotherapy (R-CHOP or rituximab plus cyclophosphamide, vincristine, and prednisone [R-CVP]). Patients with previously untreated mantle cell lymphoma or CD20-positive indolent NHL, including the histologic subtypes follicular lymphoma (grade 1 or 2), Waldenstrom macroglobulinemia, and marginal-zone lymphoma, were eligible for enrollment in the study. Patients receiving the bendamustine-rituximab regimen received rituximab 375 mg/m^2 IV on day 1 and bendamustine hydrochloride 90 mg/m^2 IV daily on days 1 and 2 of each 28-day cycle. Those receiving R-CHOP received rituximab 375 mg/m^2 IV, cyclophosphamide 750 mg/m^2 IV, doxorubicin hydrochloride 50 mg/m^2 IV, and vincristine sulfate 1.4 mg/m^2 (up to 2 mg) IV on day 1, followed by prednisone 100 mg daily on days 1–5 of each 21-day cycle, while those receiving R-CVP received rituximab 375 mg/m^2 IV, cyclophosphamide 750 mg/m^2 (option of 1 g/m^2) IV, and vincristine sulfate 1.4 mg/m^2 (up to 2 mg) IV on day 1, followed by prednisone 100 mg daily on days 1–5 of each 21-day cycle. The median patient age was about 60 years (range: 25–86); about 68% of patients had stage IV disease, 22% had stage III disease, 70% had follicular lymphoma, and 17% had mantle cell lymphoma. The primary measure of efficacy was the rate of complete response, as defined by the International Working Group (IWG) criteria and assessed by a blinded independent review committee.

Bendamustine in combination with rituximab was noninferior to R-CHOP and R-CVP for attainment of complete response; complete response was achieved in 31% of patients receiving bendamustine in combination with rituximab compared with 25% of those receiving R-CHOP or R-CVP. Although complete response rates in patients with indolent NHL (mainly follicular lymphoma) tended to favor the bendamustine-rituximab regimen over R-CHOP or R-CVP, subset analysis failed to establish noninferiority of the bendamustine-rituximab regimen in patients with indolent NHL or follicular lymphoma. In the subset of patients with mantle cell lymphoma, complete response rates were higher in patients receiving bendamustine in combination with rituximab compared with those receiving R-CHOP or R-CVP. Overall response rates were higher in patients receiving bendamustine in combination with rituximab compared with those receiving R-CHOP or R-CVP (97 versus 91%). Follow-up to establish long-term efficacy is ongoing for this study. Hypersensitivity reactions, vomiting, and nausea occurred more frequently in patients receiving bendamustine in combination with rituximab, while peripheral neuropathy, paresthesia, alopecia, constipation, and grade 3 or 4 leukopenia or neutropenia occurred more frequently in patients receiving R-CHOP and/or those receiving R-CVP. Although use of type 3 serotoninergic (5-HT_3) receptor antagonists was similar in all treatment groups, concomitant use of aprepitant was more common in patients receiving R-CHOP than in those receiving bendamustine in combination with rituximab or those receiving R-CVP.

Based on current evidence, use of bendamustine in combination with rituximab may be considered a reasonable choice (accepted, with possible conditions) for the treatment of previously untreated advanced-stage indolent NHL or mantle cell lymphoma; however, the histologic subtype of NHL should be considered when selecting a combination chemotherapy regimen.

Relapsed or Refractory Non-Hodgkin's Lymphoma or Mantle Cell Lymphoma Efficacy and safety of bendamustine in combination with rituximab† for the treatment of relapsed or refractory† indolent NHL or relapsed or refractory mantle cell lymphoma† in patients who had received up to 3 prior treatment regimens has been studied in 2 open-label, phase 2 studies.

In the first study, 63 patients received rituximab 375 mg/m^2 as an IV infusion on day 1, followed by bendamustine hydrochloride 90 mg/m^2 daily as an IV infusion on days 2 and 3, administered on a 28-day cycle for a total of 4 cycles. An additional dose of rituximab was administered one week prior to the first bendamustine-rituximab treatment cycle and repeated at 28 days following the last bendamustine-rituximab treatment cycle. Patients with relapsed or refractory mantle cell lymphoma or indolent NHL, including the histologic subtypes follicular lymphoma (grade 1 or 2), Waldenstrom macroglobulinemia, and marginal-zone lymphoma, were eligible for enrollment in the study. Patients who previously received immunotherapy (i.e., rituximab) were excluded from the study. The median patient age was 64 years; 38% of patients had follicular lymphoma, 27% had Waldenstrom macroglobulinemia, and 25% had mantle cell lymphoma. Most patients (68%) enrolled in the study had received 1 prior therapy for their disease and 30% of patients were refractory to their last prior therapy. The primary efficacy end point was progression-free survival. At a median follow-up of 20 months, median progression-free survival was 24 months. Overall response rate was 90%; 60% of patients achieved complete response. Median progression-free survival for the 16 patients with mantle cell lymphoma was 18 months and overall response rate was 75%; 50% of patients with mantle cell lymphoma achieved complete response. Median overall survival had not been reached at the time of analysis; however, the actuarial 48-month survival rate was 55%. Grade 3 or 4 leukopenia, thrombocytopenia, and anemia occurred during 16, 3, and 1% of treatment cycles, respectively.

In the second study, 66 patients received rituximab 375 mg/m^2 on day 1, followed by bendamustine hydrochloride 90 mg/m^2 daily as an IV infusion on days 2 and 3, administered on a 28-day cycle for a total of 4 cycles. An additional dose of rituximab was administered one week prior to the first bendamustine-rituximab treatment cycle and repeated at 28 days following the last bendamustine-rituximab treatment cycle. Patients achieving a response between the second and fourth treatment cycles were permitted to receive an additional 2 cycles of bendamustine-rituximab treatment. Patients with relapsed, CD20-positive mantle cell lymphoma or indolent NHL, including the histologic subtypes follicular lymphoma, small lymphocytic lymphoma, Waldenstrom macroglobulinemia, and marginal-zone lymphoma, were eligible for enrollment in the study. Patients who received prior radioimmunotherapy or high-dose chemotherapy with allogeneic stem-cell transplantation, those receiving concurrent therapy with therapeutic dosages of systemic corticosteroids, and those with rituximab-refractory disease were excluded from the study. The median patient age was 60 years; 61% of patients had follicular lymphoma, and 18% had mantle cell lymphoma. All patients enrolled in the study had a World Health Organization (WHO) performance status of 0–2. The primary efficacy end point was overall response rate. At a median follow-up of 20 months, the overall response rate was 92%; 41% of patients achieved complete response. The median duration of response for all responders was 21 months (range: 18–24 months). Among patients who received prior therapy with rituximab or those who were rituximab-naive, the overall response rate was 86 or 100%, respectively, and the complete response rate was 35 or 48%, respectively. At the time of analysis, median progression-free survival was 23 months. Overall response rate for the 12 patients with mantle cell lymphoma was 92% with a median duration of response of 19 months; 42% of patients with mantle cell lymphoma achieved complete response. Grade 3 or 4 leukopenia, neutropenia, febrile neutropenia, thrombocytopenia, and anemia occurred in 30, 36, 6, 9, and 2% of patients, respectively.

Based on current evidence and because of the favorable toxicity profile, combination therapy with bendamustine and rituximab is recommended (accepted) for use in the treatment of relapsed or refractory indolent NHL or mantle cell lymphoma.

Dosage and Administration

■ **Administration** Bendamustine hydrochloride is commercially available as an injection concentrate (Bendeka®, Treanda®) and as a lyophilized powder (Treanda®). Treanda® is administered by IV infusion over 30 minutes in patients with chronic lymphocytic leukemia (CLL) or over 60 minutes in patients with rituximab-refractory, indolent, B-cell non-Hodgkin's lymphoma (NHL). Bendeka® is administered by IV infusion over 10 minutes in patients with either CLL or rituximab-refractory, indolent, B-cell NHL. Care should be taken to avoid extravasation of the drug. (See Local Effects under Cautions: Warnings/Precautions.) Appropriate measures (e.g., adequate hydration) should be taken during therapy to prevent tumor lysis syndrome. Although allopurinol has been used during the initiation of bendamustine therapy to prevent hyperuricemia, such use may increase the risk of severe skin reactions. (See Dermatologic Reactions under Cautions: Warnings/Precautions.) In patients who have experienced grade 1 or 2 infusion reactions to the drug, a premedication regimen (e.g., antihistamine, antipyretic, and corticosteroid) should be considered during subsequent treatment cycles. (See Dosage and Administration: Dosage.)

Reconstitution and Dilution The usual precautions for handling and preparing solutions of cytotoxic drugs should be observed with bendamustine. The manufacturer recommends use of gloves and safety glasses when handling the drug. If bendamustine comes in contact with skin or mucosa, affected areas of skin should be washed immediately and thoroughly with soap and water and affected mucosa should be rinsed thoroughly with water. If the undiluted 90-mg/mL injection concentrate comes in contact with gloves, the manufacturer states that the gloves should be removed and discarded according to usual procedures for handling cytotoxic drugs.

Bendamustine hydrochloride is commercially available as an injection concentrate (Bendeka®, Treanda®) and as a lyophilized powder (Treanda®). The lyophilized powder must be reconstituted and then diluted to prepare a final bendamustine infusion solution. Bendamustine hydrochloride injection concentrate must be diluted prior to IV administration. Bendamustine hydrochloride injection concentrate is commercially available as a 25-mg/mL (Bendeka®) or 90-mg/mL (Treanda®) solution, but the concentration of reconstituted bendamustine hydrochloride lyophilized powder is 5 mg/mL. The injection concentrate and lyophilized powder formulations should *not* be mixed or combined.

Treanda® injection concentrate contains propylene glycol and *N*, *N*-dimethylacetamide (DMA), while Bendeka® injection concentrate contains propylene glycol, monothioglycerol, and polyethylene glycol and may contain sodium hydroxide to adjust the pH. DMA is incompatible with devices containing polycarbonate or acrylonitrile butadiene styrene (ABS). Device failure (e.g., leaking, breaking, operational failure of closed-system transfer device [CSTD] components), contamination of the drug solution, and occupational exposure resulting in serious adverse effects or skin reactions may occur when Treanda® injection concentrate is used with incompatible devices. Small blood vessel blockage may occur if patients receive diluted Treanda® solutions contaminated with dissolved ABS or polycarbonate. CSTDs, adapters, and syringes containing polycarbonate or ABS have been shown to dissolve when contact with DMA occurs; therefore, devices containing polycarbonate or ABS must *not* be used to withdraw and transfer Treanda® injection concentrate from the vial into the infusion bag. However, devices, including infusion sets, that contain polycarbonate or ABS may be used with the final diluted infusion solution.

Devices that are compatible with Treanda® injection concentrate are commercially available; prior to preparing infusion solutions from Treanda® injection concentrate, users should verify with the manufacturers that the device to be used is compatible with this injection concentrate. If a CSTD or adapter that contains polycarbonate or ABS will be used for supplemental protection during preparation of Treanda® infusion solutions, bendamustine hydrochloride powder for injection must be used. When a syringe is used to withdraw and transfer Treanda® injection concentrate from the vial into the infusion bag, *only* a polypropylene syringe with metal needle and polypropylene hub should be used. Treanda® injection concentrate must be diluted in a biosafety cabinet or containment isolator.

Because bendamustine hydrochloride injection concentrates (Bendeka®, Treanda®) and powder for injection contain no preservatives, infusion solutions should be prepared as close as possible to the time of administration. Any unused portions of Treanda® solutions or diluted solutions of Bendeka® should be discarded. Because Bendeka® injection concentrate is bacteriostatic, partially used vials may be stored at 2–8°C for up to 28 days in the original package for protection from light; however, the manufacturer does not recommend more than 6 withdrawals per vial.

Dilution of Bendamustine Hydrochloride Injection Concentrate (Treanda®). CSTDs, adapters, or syringes containing polycarbonate or ABS must *not* be used to withdraw and transfer Treanda® injection concentrate from the vial into the infusion bag. Prior to preparing infusion solutions, users should verify with the manufacturers that the device to be used is compatible with this injection concentrate. When a syringe is used to withdraw and transfer Treanda® injection concentrate from the vial into the infusion bag, *only* a polypropylene syringe with metal needle and polypropylene hub should be used. The injection concentrate must be diluted in a biosafety cabinet or containment isolator.

Treanda® injection concentrate is diluted by withdrawing the appropriate dose of bendamustine hydrochloride injection concentrate (containing 90 mg/mL) into a polypropylene syringe with metal needle and polypropylene hub and immediately adding the concentrate to an infusion bag containing 500 mL of either 0.9% sodium chloride or 2.5% dextrose and 0.45% sodium chloride injection, to yield a final concentration of 0.2–0.7 mg/mL. The injection concentrate and diluted solutions of the drug should be inspected visually for particulate matter and discoloration. Diluted bendamustine hydrochloride solutions should be clear and colorless to yellow. When prepared as directed using Treanda® injection concentrate, infusion solutions of bendamustine hydrochloride are stable for 24 hours when stored at 2–8°C and for *2 hours* when stored at room temperature under normal room light conditions. Administration of the drug must be completed within these time periods.

Dilution of Bendamustine Hydrochloride Injection Concentrate (Bendeka®). Bendeka® injection concentrate is diluted by withdrawing the appropriate dose of bendamustine hydrochloride injection concentrate (containing 25 mg/mL) and immediately adding the concentrate to an infusion bag containing 50 mL of 0.9% sodium chloride, 2.5% dextrose and 0.45% sodium chloride, or 5% dextrose injection to yield a final concentration of 1.85–5.6 mg/mL. The injection concentrate should be allowed to reach room temperature prior to dilution. The injection concentrate and final diluted solutions of the drug should be inspected visually for particulate matter and discoloration. The contents of the vials may partially freeze during refrigeration; the injection concentrate should be discarded if particulate matter is visible after the solution has reached room temperature. Diluted bendamustine hydrochloride solutions should be clear and colorless to yellow. When prepared as directed using Bendeka® injection concentrate in 0.9% sodium chloride or 2.5% dextrose and 0.45% sodium chloride injection, infusion solutions of bendamustine hydrochloride are stable for 24 hours when stored at 2–8°C and for *6 hours* when stored at room temperature under normal room light conditions. When prepared as directed using Bendeka® injection concentrate in 5% dextrose injection, infusion solutions of bendamustine hydrochloride are stable for 24 hours when stored at 2–8°C and for *3 hours* when stored at room temperature under normal room light conditions. Administration of the drug must be completed within these time periods. Any unused portions of the final diluted solution should be discarded.

Reconstitution and Dilution of Bendamustine Hydrochloride Lyophilized Powder (Treanda®). Bendamustine hydrochloride powder for injection is reconstituted by adding 5 or 20 mL of sterile water for injection to a vial labeled as containing 25 or 100 mg, respectively, of the drug to provide a solution containing 5 mg/mL. The lyophilized powder should dissolve within 5 minutes; the vial should be shaken well to facilitate dissolution. Within 30 minutes of reconstitution, the appropriate volume of reconstituted solution should be withdrawn from the vial and further diluted immediately in 500 mL of either 0.9% sodium chloride injection or 2.5% dextrose and 0.45% sodium chloride injection, to yield a final concentration of 0.2–0.6 mg/mL. The diluted bendamustine hydrochloride solution should be mixed thoroughly. Reconstituted and diluted solutions of the drug should be inspected visually for particulate matter and discoloration. Reconstituted and diluted bendamustine hydrochloride solutions should be clear and colorless to slightly yellow. When prepared as directed using the lyophilized powder, infusion solutions of bendamustine hydrochloride are stable for 24 hours when stored at 2–8°C and for *3 hours* when stored at room temperature under normal room light conditions. Administration of the drug must be completed within these time periods.

■ **Dosage** Appropriate measures (e.g., adequate hydration) should be taken during therapy to prevent hyperuricemia. (See Tumor Lysis Syndrome under Cautions: Warnings/Precautions.) Although measures to prevent infusion reactions are not routinely recommended by the manufacturer prior to the initial dose of bendamustine, a premedication regimen (e.g., antihistamine, antipyretic, and corticosteroid) should be considered during subsequent treatment cycles in patients who have experienced grade 1 or 2 infusion reactions to the drug. Discontinuance of bendamustine therapy should be considered in patients who experience grade 3 or 4 infusion reactions. (See Infusion Reactions under Cautions: Warnings/Precautions.)

Adults **Chronic Lymphocytic Leukemia.** The recommended adult dosage of bendamustine hydrochloride for the treatment of CLL is 100 mg/m² administered by IV infusion over 10 minutes (Bendeka®) or over 30 minutes (Treanda®) on days 1 and 2 of each 28-day cycle, for up to 6 cycles.

Dosage reduction and/or interruption of bendamustine therapy may be necessary in patients experiencing hematologic toxicity. Dose delays may be required if blood counts have not recovered to recommended values (absolute neutrophil count [ANC] of at least 1000/mm³ and platelet count of at least 75,000/mm³) prior to initiation of a new treatment cycle. Therapy should be interrupted in patients with grade 4 hematologic toxicity. Once blood counts have improved and the ANC is at least 1000/mm³ and the platelet count is at least 75,000/mm³, therapy with bendamustine can be resumed at the discretion of the clinician. In patients who experience grade 3 or 4 hematologic toxicity, dosage of the drug should be reduced to 50 mg/m² on days 1 and 2 of each treatment cycle; if grade

3 or 4 toxicity recurs, dosage should be further reduced to 25 mg/m² on days 1 and 2 of each cycle. In patients who have required dosage reductions for toxicity, re-escalation of dosage in subsequent cycles may be considered.

Dosage reduction and/or interruption of bendamustine therapy also may be necessary in patients experiencing nonhematologic toxicity. Therapy should be interrupted in patients with clinically important nonhematologic toxicity of grade 2 or greater. Once nonhematologic toxicity has improved to grade 1 or better, therapy with bendamustine can be resumed at the discretion of the clinician. In patients with clinically important nonhematologic toxicity of grade 3 or greater, dosage of the drug should be reduced to 50 mg/m² on days 1 and 2 of each treatment cycle. In patients who have required dosage reductions for toxicity, re-escalation of dosage in subsequent cycles may be considered.

Non-Hodgkin's Lymphoma. The recommended adult dosage of bendamustine hydrochloride for the treatment of rituximab-refractory, indolent, B-cell NHL is 120 mg/m² administered by IV infusion over 10 minutes (Bendeka®) or over 60 minutes (Treanda®) on days 1 and 2 of each 21-day cycle, for up to 8 cycles.

Dosage reduction and/or interruption of bendamustine therapy may be necessary in patients experiencing hematologic toxicity. Dose delays may be required if blood counts have not recovered to recommended values (ANC of at least 1000/mm³ and platelet count of at least 75,000/mm³) prior to initiation of a new treatment cycle. Therapy should be interrupted in patients with grade 4 hematologic toxicity. Once blood counts have improved and the ANC is at least 1000/mm³ and the platelet count is at least 75,000/mm³, therapy with bendamustine can be resumed at the discretion of the clinician. In patients who experience grade 4 hematologic toxicity, dosage of the drug should be reduced to 90 mg/m² on days 1 and 2 of each treatment cycle; if grade 4 toxicity recurs, dosage should be further reduced to 60 mg/m² on days 1 and 2 of each cycle.

Dosage reduction and/or interruption of bendamustine therapy also may be necessary in patients experiencing nonhematologic toxicity. Therapy should be interrupted in patients with clinically important nonhematologic toxicity of grade 2 or greater. Once nonhematologic toxicity has improved to grade 1 or better, therapy with bendamustine can be resumed at the discretion of the clinician. In patients with nonhematologic toxicity of grade 3 or greater, dosage of the drug should be reduced to 90 mg/m² on days 1 and 2 of each treatment cycle; if grade 3 or greater toxicity recurs, dosage should be further reduced to 60 mg/m² on days 1 and 2 of each cycle.

When bendamustine has been used in combination with rituximab† in adults with previously untreated† advanced-stage indolent NHL or in adults with previously untreated advanced-stage mantle cell lymphoma†, rituximab 375 mg/m² has been administered by IV infusion on day 1, followed by IV infusion (over 30–60 minutes) of bendamustine hydrochloride 90 mg/m² on days 1 and 2. The bendamustine-rituximab regimen has been administered on a 28-day cycle for up to 8 cycles.

When bendamustine has been used in combination with rituximab† in adults with relapsed or refractory† indolent NHL or in adults with relapsed or refractory mantle cell lymphoma†, rituximab 375 mg/m² has been administered by IV infusion on day 1, followed by IV infusion (over 30–60 minutes) of bendamustine hydrochloride 90 mg/m² on days 2 and 3. The bendamustine-rituximab regimen has been administered on a 28-day cycle for a total of 4–6 cycles. An additional dose of rituximab has been administered one week prior to the first bendamustine-rituximab treatment cycle and repeated at 28 days following the last bendamustine-rituximab treatment cycle.

■ **Special Populations** The pharmacokinetics of bendamustine have not been formally studied in patients with renal or hepatic impairment. The drug should not be used in patients with severe renal impairment (creatinine clearance of less than 30 mL/minute) or moderate (serum AST or ALT concentration of 2.5–10 times the upper limit of normal [ULN] and total serum bilirubin concentration of 1.5–3 times the ULN) or severe (total bilirubin concentration exceeding 3 times the ULN) hepatic impairment. (See Renal Impairment and also see Hepatic Impairment under Warnings/Precautions: Specific Populations, in Cautions.)

Cautions

■ **Contraindications** Known history of hypersensitivity (e.g., anaphylactic or anaphylactoid reaction) to bendamustine or any ingredient in the formulation.

■ **Warnings/Precautions** ***Myelosuppression*** In clinical trials in patients with rituximab-refractory, indolent, B-cell non-Hodgkin's lymphoma (NHL), grade 3 or 4 myelosuppression occurred in 98% of patients receiving bendamustine, and 2% of patients receiving the drug died from related complications (i.e., neutropenic sepsis, diffuse alveolar hemorrhage, cytomegalovirus [CMV] pneumonia). Leukocytes, platelets, hemoglobin, and neutrophils should be monitored frequently. In clinical trials of the drug, blood counts have been monitored weekly initially. Data from these studies indicate that blood counts may be expected to reach a nadir during the third week of the treatment cycle; dose delays and/or dosage reductions may be required if recovery to recommended values (i.e., absolute neutrophil count [ANC] of at least 1000/mm³ and platelet count of at least 75,000/mm³) has not occurred prior to initiation of the next cycle of therapy. (See Dosage and Administration: Dosage.)

Infectious Complications Infections, including pneumonia, sepsis, and hepatitis, have been reported in adults and pediatric patients receiving bendamustine and have been associated with septic shock and death in clinical trials and during postmarketing surveillance. Patients with myelosuppression have increased susceptibility to infection and should be advised to contact their clinician immediately if signs or symptoms of infection occur. Bendamustine may increase the risk of reactivation of infections, including hepatitis B virus (HBV) infection, CMV infection, tuberculosis, and herpes zoster. Appropriate monitoring and measures to prevent reactivation of infections should be instituted prior to initiation of bendamustine therapy. If reactivation of an infection occurs, patients should receive appropriate anti-infective therapy.

Infusion Reactions Infusion reactions, including fever, chills, pruritus, and rash, occur commonly in patients receiving bendamustine. Severe anaphylactic and anaphylactoid reactions have occurred rarely, mainly in the second and subsequent cycles of therapy. Patients should be monitored clinically and bendamustine should be discontinued if a severe reaction occurs. Patients should be asked about symptoms suggestive of infusion reactions after their first cycle of therapy. A premedication regimen (e.g., antihistamine, antipyretic, and corticosteroid) should be considered during subsequent treatment cycles in patients who experience grade 1 or 2 infusion reactions. Bendamustine therapy should be discontinued in patients who experience grade 4 infusion reactions. If clinically appropriate, discontinuance of bendamustine therapy also may be considered in patients who experience grade 3 infusion reactions. Patients who experience grade 3 or worse allergic-type reactions should not be rechallenged with the drug.

Tumor Lysis Syndrome Tumor lysis syndrome has been reported in patients receiving bendamustine in clinical trials and during postmarketing surveillance. The onset generally occurs during the first cycle of bendamustine therapy; without appropriate intervention, acute renal failure and death may occur. Appropriate measures (e.g., adequate hydration; close monitoring of blood chemistries, particularly potassium and uric acid concentrations) should be used to prevent tumor lysis syndrome. Allopurinol has been used during initiation of bendamustine therapy to prevent hyperuricemia; however, concomitant allopurinol therapy may increase the risk of severe skin reactions. (See Dermatologic Reactions under Cautions: Warnings/Precautions.)

Dermatologic Reactions Serious or fatal dermatologic reactions, including rash, toxic skin reactions (e.g., Stevens-Johnson syndrome, toxic epidermal necrolysis, drug reaction with eosinophilia and systemic symptoms [DRESS]), and bullous exanthema, have been reported in patients receiving bendamustine as a single agent, in combination with other antineoplastic agents, or concomitantly with allopurinol. Dermatologic reactions in patients receiving the drug may be progressive and increase in severity with continued therapy. Patients receiving bendamustine who experience dermatologic reactions should be monitored closely. If the reaction is severe or progressive, bendamustine should be withheld or discontinued.

Hepatic Toxicity Liver injury, sometimes fatal or serious, has been reported in patients receiving bendamustine, although confounding factors (e.g., concomitant use of other antineoplastic agents, progressive disease, reactivation of HBV) may have been present in some cases. Liver injury generally occurred within the initial 3 months of bendamustine therapy. Liver function tests should be monitored prior to and during therapy.

Development of Other Malignancies Development of premalignant (e.g., myelodysplastic syndrome, myeloproliferative disorders) and malignant diseases (e.g., acute myelogenous leukemia, bronchial carcinoma) has been reported in patients treated with bendamustine.

Local Effects Extravasation of bendamustine has resulted in pain, erythema, and marked swelling that required hospitalization. Care should be taken to avoid extravasation of the drug (e.g., by ensuring good venous access prior to administration); the infusion site should be monitored for erythema, swelling, pain, infection, and necrosis during and after administration.

Fetal/Neonatal Morbidity and Mortality Bendamustine can cause fetal harm; single intraperitoneal doses of bendamustine in mice and rats administered during organogenesis caused an increase in resorptions, skeletal and visceral malformations, and decreased fetal body weights. Women should avoid becoming pregnant during and for 3 months after discontinuance of bendamustine therapy (see Advice to Patients). Men with partners of childbearing potential should be advised to use a reliable method of contraception during and for 3 months after discontinuance of bendamustine therapy. If bendamustine is used during pregnancy or if the patient becomes pregnant, the patient should be apprised of the potential fetal hazard.

Specific Populations **Pregnancy.** Category D. (See Fetal/Neonatal Morbidity and Mortality under Cautions: Warnings/Precautions.)

Lactation. It is not known whether bendamustine is distributed into milk. The manufacturer states that a decision should be made whether to discontinue nursing or the drug, taking into account the importance of the drug to the woman.

Pediatric Use. Pharmacokinetic and adverse effect profiles of bendamustine in pediatric patients (1–19 years of age) with relapsed or refractory acute leukemia are similar to those in adults.

Efficacy of bendamustine has not been established in pediatric patients. Bendamustine hydrochloride (90 or 120 mg/m² IV daily on days 1 and 2 of each 21-day cycle) was evaluated in a phase 1–2 study in pediatric patients with relapsed or refractory acute leukemia. No responses were observed in 32 patients evaluated in the phase 2 portion of the study; however, complete responses were observed in 2 patients with acute lymphocytic leukemia (ALL) receiving bendamustine hydrochloride 90 mg/m² during the phase 1 portion of the study.

Geriatric Use. Pharmacokinetic and adverse effect profiles are similar to those in younger adults. In the phase 3 study in chronic lymphocytic leukemia (CLL), overall response rates for bendamustine and chlorambucil were 47 and

22%, respectively, in patients 65 years of age or older versus 70 and 30%, respectively, in those younger than 65 years of age. Median durations of progression-free survival with bendamustine and chlorambucil were 12 and 8 months, respectively, in patients 65 years of age or older versus 19 and 8 months, respectively, in those younger than 65 years of age.

Among patients with rituximab-refractory, indolent, B-cell NHL, overall response rate and duration of response in individuals 65 years of age or older were similar to results in younger adults.

Hepatic Impairment. Population pharmacokinetic analyses indicate that the pharmacokinetics of bendamustine are not substantially altered in patients with mild hepatic impairment; effects of moderate or severe hepatic impairment on the pharmacokinetics of the drug have not been evaluated to date. Use of bendamustine is not recommended in moderate (serum AST or ALT concentration of 2.5–10 times the upper limit of normal [ULN] and total serum bilirubin concentration of 1.5–3 times the ULN) or severe (total bilirubin concentration exceeding 3 times the ULN) hepatic impairment.

Renal Impairment. Population pharmacokinetic analyses indicate that the pharmacokinetics of bendamustine are not substantially altered in patients with mild or moderate renal impairment (creatinine clearance of 30–80 mL/minute); effects of severe renal impairment on the pharmacokinetics of the drug have not been evaluated to date. Use of bendamustine is not recommended in patients with severe renal impairment (creatinine clearance of less than 30 mL/minute).

Race. Limited data suggest that exposure to bendamustine may be increased in Japanese individuals; however, clinical importance in terms of safety and efficacy has not been established.

Gender. Pharmacokinetic and adverse effect profiles are not affected substantially by gender in patients with either CLL or indolent NHL. No clinically important differences in efficacy between men and women were observed in patients with rituximab-refractory, indolent B-cell NHL. In the phase 3 study in CLL, overall response rates for bendamustine and chlorambucil were 60 and 24%, respectively, in men versus 57 and 28%, respectively, in women. Median durations of progression-free survival with bendamustine and chlorambucil were 19 and 6 months, respectively, in men versus 13 and 8 months, respectively, in women.

■ **Common Adverse Effects** Adverse effects reported in 15% or more of patients with rituximab-refractory, indolent, B-cell NHL or with CLL receiving bendamustine therapy include neutropenia, thrombocytopenia, anemia, leukopenia, pyrexia, nausea, vomiting, and decreased lymphocyte counts. Elevated bilirubin concentrations also have been reported in more than 15% of patients with CLL receiving the drug, and fatigue, diarrhea, constipation, decreased weight, anorexia, dyspnea, cough, headache, rash, and stomatitis also have been reported in 15% or more of patients with rituximab-refractory, indolent, B-cell NHL receiving the drug. Adverse effects are similar following administration of bendamustine as a 10-minute IV infusion (Bendeka®) or following IV infusion over 30–60 minutes (Treanda®).

Drug Interactions

No formal drug interaction studies have been performed to date.

■ **Drugs Affecting Hepatic Microsomal Enzymes** In vitro data indicate that bendamustine is metabolized mainly via hydrolysis to form metabolites with low cytotoxic activity and, to a lesser extent, via cytochrome P-450 (CYP) isoenzyme 1A2 to form 2 minor active metabolites, γ-hydroxybendamustine (M3) and *N*-desmethylbendamustine (M4).

CYP1A2 inhibitors (e.g., fluvoxamine, ciprofloxacin): Potential pharmacokinetic interaction (increased plasma concentrations of bendamustine and decreased plasma concentrations of γ-hydroxybendamustine and *N*-desmethylbendamustine). Use concomitantly with caution or consider alternative therapy.

CYP1A2 inducers (e.g., omeprazole, cigarette smoking): Potential pharmacokinetic interaction (decreased plasma concentrations of bendamustine and increased plasma concentrations of γ-hydroxybendamustine and *N*-desmethylbendamustine). Use concomitantly with caution or consider alternative therapy.

■ **Drugs Metabolized by Hepatic Microsomal Enzymes** In vitro data indicate that bendamustine is unlikely to inhibit CYP isoenzymes 1A2, 2C9/10, 2D6, 2E1, or 3A4/5, or to induce CYP isoenzymes 1A2, 2A6, 2B6, 2C8, 2C9, 2C19, 2E1, or 3A4/5.

■ **Drugs that Affect Transport Systems** In vitro data suggest that P-glycoprotein, breast cancer resistance protein (BCRP), and/or other efflux transporters may have a role in bendamustine transport; however, the effect of active transport systems on bendamustine has not been fully evaluated to date.

Description

Bendamustine, a bifunctional nitrogen mustard-derivative alkylating agent and purine analog, is an antineoplastic agent. Bendamustine is structurally related to chlorambucil, with the molecules differing only in the central ring structure; whereas chlorambucil contains a benzene ring, bendamustine contains a purine-like benzimidazole ring.

The exact mechanism(s) of action of bendamustine has not been conclusively established. As an alkylating agent, bendamustine interferes with DNA replication and transcription of RNA, ultimately resulting in disruption of nucleic acid function. In vitro data suggest that bendamustine activates different DNA repair pathways compared with conventional alkylating agents. In addition, other effects of bendamustine may contribute to its antineoplastic activity, including induction of p53-dependent genes that activate apoptosis and inhibition of several mitotic checkpoints. As a consequence of the latter effect, DNA-damaged cells entering the M phase of the cell cycle may undergo a premature form of necrotic cell death known as mitotic catastrophe. The drug is active against both quiescent and dividing cells. Cross-resistance between bendamustine and other alkylating agents or fludarabine appears to be incomplete.

Following IV infusion of bendamustine hydrochloride over 10 minutes (Bendeka®) or over 60 minutes (Treanda®), systemic exposure to the drug is equivalent although peak plasma concentrations are higher following the shorter infusion. Bendamustine is metabolized extensively by hydrolysis, oxidation, and conjugation. In vitro data indicate that bendamustine is metabolized mainly via hydrolysis to form 2 metabolites with low cytotoxic activity, monohydroxybendamustine (HP1) and dihydroxybendamustine (HP2), and to a lesser extent via cytochrome P-450 (CYP) isoenzyme 1A2 to form 2 active metabolites, γ-hydroxybendamustine (M3) and *N*-desmethylbendamustine (M4). However, because plasma concentrations of γ-hydroxybendamustine and *N*-desmethylbendamustine are only 10 and 1%, respectively, that of the parent drug, the cytotoxic activity of bendamustine appears to result mainly from the parent drug. Following administration of radiolabeled bendamustine hydrochloride, plasma radioactivity levels were more sustained than plasma concentrations of the drug and its active metabolites, suggesting the presence of bendamustine-derived compounds with longer half-lives. Approximately 50% of the radiolabeled dose was recovered in urine (approximately 3.3% of the dose as unchanged drug, less than 6% as the dihydroxy, γ-hydroxy, and *N*-desmethyl metabolites) and 25% was recovered in feces. Following IV administration of bendamustine hydrochloride as a single 120-mg/m^2 dose over 1 hour, the intermediate half-life of the parent drug was approximately 40 minutes. Little or no accumulation of bendamustine in plasma is expected when the drug is administered on days 1 and 2 of a 28-day treatment cycle.

Advice to Patients

Risk of allergic reactions; importance of immediately reporting rash, facial swelling, or difficulty breathing during or soon after bendamustine infusion.

Importance of immediately reporting severe or worsening rash or itching to clinician.

Risk of leukopenia, thrombocytopenia, and anemia; importance of frequent monitoring of blood cell counts; importance of reporting any shortness of breath, marked fatigue, bleeding, or fever or other manifestations of infection.

Risk of hepatic toxicity; importance of immediately reporting signs and symptoms of hepatic failure (e.g., jaundice, anorexia, bleeding, bruising).

Importance of women informing clinicians if they are or plan to become pregnant or plan to breast-feed; necessity for clinicians to advise women of childbearing potential and men with partners of childbearing potential to avoid pregnancy and to use effective contraceptive methods during therapy and for 3 months following discontinuance of therapy. Importance of advising male patients that alkylating agents may impair spermatogenesis.

Risk of increased fatigue; importance of avoiding driving a vehicle or operating machinery if fatigue occurs.

Risk of nausea, vomiting, and diarrhea; importance of reporting these adverse GI effects so that symptomatic treatment may be provided.

Importance of informing clinicians of existing or contemplated concomitant therapy, including prescription and OTC drugs, as well as any concomitant illnesses.

Importance of informing patients of other important precautionary information. (See Cautions.)

Overview® (see Users Guide). For additional information on this drug until a more detailed monograph is developed and published, the manufacturer's labeling should be consulted. It is *essential* that the manufacturer's labeling be consulted for more detailed information on usual cautions, precautions, contraindications, potential drug interactions, laboratory test interferences, and acute toxicity. For further information on the handling of antineoplastic agents, see the ASHP Guidelines on Handling Hazardous Drugs at http://www.ahfsdruginformation.com.

Preparations

Excipients in commercially available drug preparations may have clinically important effects in some individuals; consult specific product labeling for details.

Bendamustine Hydrochloride

Parenteral		
Concentrate for injection, for IV infusion only	25 mg/mL (100 mg)	**Bendeka®**, Teva
	90 mg/mL (45 and 180 mg)	**Treanda®**, Teva
For injection, for IV infusion only	25 mg	**Treanda®**, Teva
	100 mg	**Treanda®**, Teva

†Use is not currently included in the labeling approved by the US Food and Drug Administration

Bevacizumab

■ Bevacizumab, a recombinant humanized monoclonal antibody, is an antineoplastic agent.

Uses

■ **Colorectal Cancer** ***First-line Treatment of Metastatic Cancer of the Colon or Rectum*** Bevacizumab is used in combination with IV fluorouracil-based chemotherapy for the first-line treatment of metastatic cancer of the colon or rectum.

The indication for use of bevacizumab in combination with IV fluorouracil-based chemotherapy for the first-line treatment of metastatic cancer of the colon or rectum is based mainly on the results of 2 randomized, controlled clinical studies (one phase 2 and one phase 3).

In the phase 3, randomized, double-blind, active-controlled study, 813 patients received either a placebo (administered every 2 weeks) or bevacizumab (5 mg/kg administered by IV infusion every 2 weeks until disease progression occurred) in conjunction with a combination irinotecan/fluorouracil/leucovorin regimen. The combination regimen consisted of irinotecan 125 mg/m^2, fluorouracil 500 mg/m^2, and leucovorin 20 mg/m^2, administered as an IV bolus injection once weekly for 4 out of every 6 weeks. Patients who received bevacizumab in combination with the irinotecan/fluorouracil/leucovorin regimen had a higher median overall response rate (45 versus 35%, respectively) and prolonged median overall survival (20.3 versus 15.6 months, respectively), median progression-free survival (10.6 versus 6.2 months, respectively), and median duration of response (10.4 versus 7.1 months, respectively) than patients receiving placebo in conjunction with the same combination regimen. Grade 3–4 adverse effects, including leukopenia (37 versus 31%), diarrhea (34 versus 25%), neutropenia (21 versus 14%), hypertension (12 versus 2%), asthenia (10 versus 7%), deep-vein thrombosis (9 versus 5%), pain (8 versus 5%), abdominal pain (8 versus 5%), constipation (4 versus 2%), intra-abdominal thrombosis (3 versus 1%), and syncope (3 versus 1%), occurred more frequently in patients receiving bevacizumab rather than placebo in conjunction with the irinotecan/fluorouracil/leucovorin regimen.

This phase 3 study also included initial enrollment of patients by random assignment into a third group receiving fluorouracil/leucovorin and bevacizumab to establish a comparison group for determining the toxicity of bevacizumab combined with irinotecan. When the toxicity of bevacizumab with the irinotecan/fluorouracil/leucovorin regimen was deemed acceptable, enrollment of patients into this treatment group was discontinued. Among 110 patients receiving bevacizumab (5 mg/kg administered by IV infusion every 2 weeks) with fluorouracil and leucovorin (each 500 mg/m^2 IV once weekly for 6 out of every 8 weeks), the objective response rate was 39%, median overall survival was 18.3 months, median progression-free survival was 8.8 months, and median duration of response was 8.5 months.

In the phase 2, open-label, dose-ranging study, 104 patients with previously untreated metastatic colorectal cancer were randomized to receive a combination regimen of fluorouracil and leucovorin (leucovorin 500 mg/m^2 administered by IV infusion over 2 hours, followed by fluorouracil 500 mg/m^2 administered by slow IV injection [1 hour after initiation of leucovorin] given once weekly for the first 6 weeks out of every 8-week cycle) alone or in conjunction with either low-dose bevacizumab (5 mg/kg every 2 weeks) or high-dose bevacizumab (10 mg/kg every 2 weeks); bevacizumab was given for a total of 6 cycles (i.e., 48 weeks) or until disease progression occurred. Results of this study suggest that patients receiving combination therapy with bevacizumab and the fluorouracil-containing regimen may have a higher overall response rate and prolonged median overall survival and median progression-free survival than those receiving the fluorouracil-containing regimen alone. Although progression-free survival was longer in patients receiving low-dose bevacizumab in conjunction with the fluorouracil-containing regimen than in those receiving the fluorouracil-containing regimen alone, overall survival and overall response rate were similar between the 2 groups. In addition, overall outcomes for patients receiving high-dose bevacizumab in conjunction with the fluorouracil-containing regimen were similar to outcomes in those receiving the fluorouracil-containing regimen alone. In this study, median overall survival was 13.6, 17.7, or 15.2 months in patients receiving the fluorouracil-containing combination alone, with the 5 mg/kg-bevacizumab regimen, or with the 10 mg/kg-bevacizumab regimen, respectively. Median survival was 13.8, 21.5, or 16.1 months in patients receiving the fluorouracil-containing combination alone, in conjunction with the 5-mg/kg bevacizumab regimen, or in conjunction with the 10-mg/kg bevacizumab regimen, respectively. Median progression-free survival was 5.2, 9, or 7.2 months in patients receiving the fluorouracil-containing combination alone, in conjunction with the 5-mg/kg bevacizumab regimen, or in conjunction with the 10-mg/kg bevacizumab regimen, respectively. In addition, the overall response rate was 17, 40, or 24% among patients receiving the fluorouracil-containing combination alone, in conjunction with the 5-mg/kg bevacizumab regimen, or in conjunction with the10-mg/kg bevacizumab regimen, respectively.

The combination of bevacizumab with fluorouracil/leucovorin for previously untreated metastatic colorectal cancer also has been studied in patients who were not optimal candidates for first-line irinotecan-containing therapy (i.e., 65 years of age or older, ECOG performance status of 1 or 2, serum albumin concentration of 3.5 g/dL or less, or prior pelvic or abdominal radiation therapy). In a phase 2 randomized trial involving 209 patients with previously untreated metastatic colorectal cancer who were not considered optimal candidates for irinotecan-containing therapy, median progression-free survival was prolonged (9.2 versus 5.5 months) but median overall survival was similar (16.6 versus 12.9 months) in patients receiving bevacizumab/fluorouracil/leucovorin compared with those receiving fluorouracil/leucovorin. Grade 3 or 4 toxicity occurred more frequently in patients receiving bevacizumab versus placebo (87 versus 71%) in combination with fluorouracil/leucovorin, including grade 3 hypertension (16 versus 3%). Proteinuria (38 versus 19%) and arterial thrombotic events (10 versus 5%) also occurred more often in patients receiving bevacizumab. Combined analysis of pooled individual data from this trial as well as the 2 primary efficacy studies suggests that survival is prolonged when bevacizumab is added to the fluorouracil/leucovorin regimen for the first-line treatment of metastatic colorectal cancer.

Bevacizumab also has been used in combination with oxaliplatin-containing regimens† as first-line therapy for metastatic colorectal cancer. In a randomized phase 3 trial, the addition of bevacizumab to oxaliplatin-containing chemotherapy (either capecitabine and oxaliplatin [XELOX] or fluorouracil/leucovorin and oxaliplatin [FOLFOX4]) in first-line therapy for metastatic colorectal cancer prolonged median progression-free survival, but no difference in overall survival was observed.

Second-line Treatment of Metastatic Cancer of the Colon or Rectum Bevacizumab is used in combination with IV fluorouracil-based chemotherapy for the second-line treatment of metastatic cancer of the colon or rectum.

The indication for use of bevacizumab in combination with IV fluorouracil-based chemotherapy for the second-line treatment of metastatic cancer of the colon or rectum is based mainly on the results of a randomized, controlled clinical study and an open-access single-arm study.

In an open-label, randomized, 3-arm, active-controlled, multicenter clinical study, 829 patients received bevacizumab in combination with FOLFOX4 (i.e., fluorouracil/leucovorin and oxaliplatin), FOLFOX4 alone, or bevacizumab alone, for the second-line treatment of metastatic carcinoma of the colon or rectum. Patients had received prior treatment with irinotecan, with or without fluorouracil, as initial therapy for metastatic disease (99%) or irinotecan and fluorouracil as adjuvant therapy (1%). The FOLFOX4 regimen consisted of oxaliplatin 85 mg/m^2 and leucovorin 200 mg/m^2 concurrently IV, then fluorouracil 400 mg/m^2 by IV bolus, followed by fluorouracil 600 mg/m^2 by continuous IV infusion on day 1; and leucovorin 200 mg/m^2 IV, then fluorouracil 400 mg/m^2 by IV bolus, followed by fluorouracil 600 mg/m^2 by continuous IV infusion on day 2; with treatment cycles repeated every 2 weeks. Bevacizumab was administered at a dose of 10 mg/kg every 2 weeks. For patients receiving the combination of the 2 regimens, bevacizumab was administered prior to the FOLFOX4 regimen on day 1 of the treatment cycle. The median age of patients was 61 years, 40% were female, 87% were Caucasian, and 49% had an ECOG performance status of 0. Most patients (80%) had received adjuvant chemotherapy, and 26% had received prior radiation therapy.

Following an interim analysis that showed decreased survival in patients receiving bevacizumab alone compared with those receiving FOLFOX4 alone, the bevacizumab monotherapy arm was closed to accrual after enrollment of 244 of the planned 290 patients. In patients receiving bevacizumab in combination with FOLFOX4, median overall survival was prolonged (13 versus 10.8 months), and progression-free survival and overall response rate based on investigator assessment were higher than in patients receiving FOLFOX4 alone. Grade 3–5 nonhematologic and grade 3–4 hematologic adverse effects, including fatigue (19 versus 13%), diarrhea (18 versus 13%), sensory neuropathy (17 versus 9%), nausea (12 versus 5%), vomiting (11 versus 4%), dehydration (10 versus 5%), hypertension (9 versus 2%), abdominal pain (8 versus 5%), hemorrhage (5 versus 1%), other neurologic adverse effects (5 versus 3%), ileus (4 versus 1%), and headache (3 versus 0%), occurred more frequently in patients receiving bevacizumab with FOLFOX4 compared with those receiving FOLFOX4 alone. Because of the reporting mechanisms used in this study, the manufacturer states that the true incidence of adverse effects associated with bevacizumab therapy may have been underestimated.

In a multicenter, single-arm, open-access protocol, 339 patients received bevacizumab in combination with fluorouracil/leucovorin (administered by either IV infusion or rapid IV injection) for metastatic colorectal cancer with disease progression following both irinotecan-containing and oxaliplatin-containing regimens. Most patients (73%) received concurrent fluorouracil and leucovorin according to a rapid IV injection ("bolus") regimen. Among the first 100 evaluable patients, there was one objective partial response for an overall response rate of 1%. The median progression-free survival of the first 100 evaluable patients was 3.5 months, and the median overall survival was 9 months. Among 322 patients evaluated for toxicity, 47% had at least one grade 3 or higher adverse event, and 14% discontinued treatment because of adverse effects.

Adjuvant Therapy for Early-stage Colon Cancer Bevacizumab has been investigated for use in combination with fluorouracil, leucovorin, and oxaliplatin (modified FOLFOX6)† as adjuvant therapy following surgery for early-stage (i.e., stage II or III)† colon cancer. Results of a phase 3, randomized, open-label study (National Surgical Adjuvant Breast and Bowel Project [NSABP] C-08) demonstrated no improvement in disease-free survival following use of bevacizumab (5 mg/kg administered by IV infusion every 2 weeks for 1 year) in combination with modified FOLFOX6 (leucovorin 400 mg/m^2 IV on day 1, fluorouracil 400 mg/m^2 by IV injection on day 1 followed by fluorouracil 2400 mg/m² by continuous IV infusion over 46 hours, and oxaliplatin 85 mg/m² IV on day 1; regimen administered every 2 weeks for 6 months). The 3-year disease-survival rate was 77.4% in patients with stage II or III colon adenocarcinoma who received bevacizumab in combination with modified FOLFOX6 compared with 75.5% in those who received modified FOLFOX6 alone. Because of the lack of improvement in disease-free survival, investigators of this study recommended that bevacizumab *not* be used in combination with modified FOLFOX6 as adjuvant therapy for stage II or III colon cancer.

■ **Non-small Cell Lung Cancer** Bevacizumab is used in combination with carboplatin and paclitaxel for the first-line treatment of unresectable, locally advanced, recurrent or metastatic nonsquamous non-small cell lung cancer.

This indication is based on the results of a randomized, active-controlled, open-label, multicenter study (supported by a randomized, dose-ranging, active-controlled phase 2 study) in which 878 chemotherapy-naive patients with locally advanced, metastatic, or recurrent nonsquamous non-small cell lung cancer were randomized to receive paclitaxel and carboplatin either with or without bevacizumab. Patients received paclitaxel 200 mg/m² and carboplatin (dose required to obtain an area under the plasma concentration-time curve [AUC] of 6 mg/mL per minute) both by IV infusion on day 1 with bevacizumab 15 mg/kg by IV infusion on day 1 or the same regimen of paclitaxel/carboplatin alone (without bevacizumab); each regimen was administered every 21 days for up to 6 cycles. Upon completion or discontinuance of chemotherapy, patients receiving bevacizumab continued to receive bevacizumab alone until disease progression or intolerable toxicity occurred. Most of the patients (89%) had newly diagnosed disease (stage IV in 76%), 46% were female, 43% were 65 years of age or older (median age: 63 years), and 28% of the patients had at least a 5% weight loss at the time of entry to the study. Excluded from the study were patients with disease of predominantly squamous histology, CNS metastasis, gross hemoptysis (0.5 teaspoon of red blood or more), unstable angina, and those receiving anticoagulant therapy.

The median overall survival was prolonged (12.3 versus 10.3 months) in patients receiving chemotherapy (paclitaxel and carboplatin) and bevacizumab compared with those receiving chemotherapy alone for advanced nonsquamous non-small cell lung cancer. Subgroup analysis suggested that the benefit of the addition of bevacizumab to this chemotherapy regimen was less certain in women, patients 65 years of age or older, and patients with at least a 5% weight loss at study entry. Grade 3–5 nonhematologic and grade 4–5 hematologic adverse effects, including neutropenia (27 versus 17%), fatigue (16 versus 13%), hypertension (8 versus 0.7%), infection without neutropenia (7 versus 3%), venous thrombosis or embolism (5 versus 3%), febrile neutropenia (5 versus 2%), pneumonitis or pulmonary infiltrates (5 versus 3%), infection with grade 3 or 4 neutropenia (4 versus 2%), hyponatremia (4 versus 1%), headache (3 versus 1%), and proteinuria (3 versus 0%), occurred more frequently in patients receiving bevacizumab and chemotherapy than in those receiving chemotherapy alone.

Bevacizumab has been investigated for use in combination with cisplatin and gemcitabine† for the first-line treatment of locally advanced, metastatic, or recurrent nonsquamous non-small cell lung cancer. In a randomized, double-blind, active-controlled study, 1043 patients with locally advanced, metastatic, or recurrent nonsquamous non-small cell lung cancer were randomized to receive bevacizumab 7.5 mg/kg in combination with cisplatin and gemcitabine, bevacizumab 15 mg/kg in combination with cisplatin and gemcitabine, or cisplatin and gemcitabine with placebo. Most of the patients (77%) had stage IV disease, 8% had recurrent disease, 36% were female, and 29% were 65 years of age or older. Patients receiving bevacizumab 7.5 or 15 mg/kg in combination with cisplatin and gemcitabine had longer progression-free survival, but not a significantly longer overall survival, compared with patients receiving cisplatin and gemcitabine alone.

■ **Glioblastoma** Bevacizumab is used as a single agent for the treatment of glioblastoma (also known as glioblastoma multiforme) in patients whose disease has progressed following radiation therapy and chemotherapy (i.e., temozolomide). Labeling for use of bevacizumab for the management of previously treated glioblastoma was approved under the principles and procedures of the US Food and Drug Administration's (FDA's) accelerated review process that allows approval based on analysis of surrogate markers of response. As a result of the accelerated review, labeling of bevacizumab for management of previously treated glioblastoma was based on improvement in objective response rate; currently, there are no data demonstrating amelioration of disease-related symptoms or prolonged survival with use of the drug for this condition.

The current indication for use of bevacizumab in the management of previously treated glioblastoma is based principally on the results of 2 studies (one open-label, multicenter, randomized, noncomparative study and one single-arm, single-institution study).

In the phase 2, open-label, multicenter, randomized, noncomparative study (AVF3708g, BRAIN), 167 patients with previously treated glioblastoma were randomized to receive either bevacizumab (10 mg/kg administered by IV infusion every 2 weeks) alone or bevacizumab in combination with irinotecan (340 mg/m² in patients receiving enzyme-inducing antiepileptic drugs or 125 mg/m² in those not receiving enzyme-inducing antiepileptic drugs, administered by IV infusion over 90 minutes every 2 weeks); treatment was continued until disease progression or unacceptable toxicity occurred, up to a maximum of 104 weeks. Because this study design did not permit isolation of the contribution of each drug to the efficacy of the bevacizumab plus irinotecan regimen, efficacy data for the combination regimen could not be used to support drug approval and were not analyzed by FDA; only efficacy data for bevacizumab monotherapy were evaluated. Patients enrolled in this study had received prior radiation therapy (completed at least 8 weeks prior to receiving bevacizumab) and chemotherapy (i.e., temozolomide); patients with active brain hemorrhage were excluded. Of the 85 patients randomized to receive bevacizumab monotherapy, the median age was 54 years (range: 23–78 years), 32% were female, 81% were in first relapse, and 45 or 55% had a Karnofsky performance status of 90–100 or 70–80, respectively; the mean treatment duration was 4.8 months (range: 0–12.9 months). Response to bevacizumab was determined by magnetic resonance imagery (MRI) (using WHO radiographic criteria) and by evaluation of corticosteroid usage (i.e., stabilization or reduction of corticosteroid dosage). Analysis of efficacy data differed between FDA and the manufacturer; only FDA's analysis is discussed. Treatment with bevacizumab monotherapy resulted in an objective response rate of 25.9% (partial responses only), a median duration of response of 4.2 months, a 6-month progression-free survival rate of 36%, and a median overall survival of 9.3 months. In addition, corticosteroid dosage decreased by a median of 37.5% at the time of response compared with baseline. The most common adverse effects reported with bevacizumab monotherapy included infection (55%), fatigue (45%), headache (37%), hypertension (30%), epistaxis (19%), and diarrhea (21%). Serious (grade 3 or greater) adverse effects included infection (10%), fatigue (4%), headache (4%), hypertension (8%), and diarrhea (1%). Two deaths (one from retroperitoneal hemorrhage and one from neutropenic infection), possibly associated with bevacizumab, also have been reported in patients receiving bevacizumab monotherapy. Other serious (grade 3–5) adverse effects reported in patients receiving bevacizumab alone or in combination with irinotecan included bleeding or hemorrhage (2%), CNS hemorrhage (1%), venous thromboembolic events (7%), arterial thromboembolic events (3%), wound healing complications (3%), proteinuria (1%), and GI perforation (2%); because some of these adverse effects (i.e., CNS hemorrhage, wound healing complications, venous thromboembolic events) are inherent in patients with glioblastoma and associated with prior surgery and radiation therapy, a causal relationship of such adverse effects to bevacizumab has not been established.

In the single-arm, single-institution study (study NCI 06-C-0064E), 56 patients with previously treated glioblastoma received bevacizumab (10 mg/kg administered by IV infusion every 2 weeks) until disease progression or unacceptable toxicity occurred. All patients had documented disease progression after receiving temozolomide and radiation therapy. The median age was 54 years, 54% were male, 68% had a Karnofsky performance status of 90–100, and 54% were receiving corticosteroids. Treatment with bevacizumab resulted in an objective response rate of 19.6% (partial responses only) and a median duration of response of 3.9 months. Although evaluation of corticosteroid usage was not a required efficacy end point, it was noted that 58% of patients were able to reduce their corticosteroid dosage during treatment with bevacizumab; the average reduction in corticosteroid dosage was 59%. Grade 3 or greater adverse effects associated with bevacizumab included thromboembolic events (12.7%), hypertension (3.6%), arterial thromboembolic events (1.8%), GI perforation (1.8%), and wound healing complications (1.8%).

■ **Renal Cell Carcinoma** Bevacizumab is used in combination with interferon alfa for the first-line treatment of metastatic renal cell carcinoma and is designated an orphan drug by FDA for use in this condition.

The current indication for use of bevacizumab in combination with interferon alfa in patients with metastatic renal cell carcinoma is based principally on the results of a multicenter, randomized, double-blind, placebo-controlled study (AVOREN).

In the AVOREN study, 649 patients with previously untreated metastatic renal cell carcinoma (predominantly [more than 50%] clear-cell histology) who had undergone nephrectomy (or partial nephrectomy) were randomized to receive bevacizumab (10 mg/kg administered by IV infusion every 2 weeks) in combination with interferon alfa-2a (9 million units by subcutaneous injection 3 times weekly) or interferon alfa-2a in combination with placebo; treatment was continued until disease progression or unacceptable toxicity occurred (up to a maximum of 52 weeks for interferon alfa-2a). The median age of the patients was 60 years (range: 18–82 years), and 70% were male; 28, 56, or 8% of patients had Motzer scores of 0 (favorable risk), 1–2 (intermediate risk), or 3–5 (poor risk), respectively. In this study, patients receiving bevacizumab in combination with interferon alfa-2a had prolonged median progression-free survival (10.2 versus 5.4 months) and a higher overall response rate (30 versus 12%), but similar median overall survival (23 versus 21 months), compared with those receiving interferon alfa-2a alone. Grade 3–5 adverse effects occurring at a higher incidence (2% or greater) in patients receiving bevacizumab in combination with interferon alfa-2a than in those receiving interferon alfa-2a monotherapy included fatigue (13 versus 8%), asthenia (10 versus 7%), proteinuria (7 versus 0%), hypertension (6 versus 1%), and hemorrhage (3 versus 0.3%).

■ **Breast Cancer** ***First-line Treatment of Metastatic Breast Cancer*** Although bevacizumab in combination with paclitaxel previously was labeled for use as first-line treatment of metastatic HER2-negative breast cancer†, FDA concluded that such use has not been shown in postmarketing studies to prolong overall survival or provide sufficient clinical benefit (e.g., prolongation of progression-free survival, amelioration of disease-related symptoms, improvement in quality of life) to outweigh the risk of severe, potentially fatal, adverse effects (e.g., myocardial infarction [MI], heart failure, severe hypertension, bleeding or hemorrhage, perforation and fistula/abscess formation, wound healing complications). On November 18, 2011, the agency rescinded approval of bevacizumab for use (in combination with paclitaxel) as first-line treatment of metastatic HER2-negative breast cancer; as a result, this indication no longer appears in bevacizumab's current approved labeling. (See FDA Decisions Regarding Breast Cancer Indication under Breast Cancer: First-line Treatment of Metastatic Breast Cancer, in Uses.) Following FDA's decision, Health Canada, but not the European Medicines Agency (EMA), took similar action. The United Kingdom's National Institute for Health and Clinical Excellence (NICE) reached similar conclusions about the lack of evidence of clinical benefit and has not supported this use. The AHFS Oncology Expert Committee concluded that use of bevacizumab in combination with paclitaxel for the first-line treatment of metastatic breast cancer currently is not fully established because of equivocal evidence; additional studies are needed to identify subgroups of patients who might derive clinical benefit from bevacizumab treatment. (See AHFS Oncology Expert Committee Decision Regarding Use as First-line Therapy under Breast Cancer: First-line Treatment of Metastatic Breast Cancer, in Uses.)

Patients currently receiving bevacizumab for breast cancer should consult their clinician about whether to continue bevacizumab therapy or consider other treatment options. Clinicians should use clinical judgment in deciding whether patients should continue receiving bevacizumab in combination with paclitaxel, receive paclitaxel monotherapy, or consider other treatment options.

FDA Decisions Regarding Breast Cancer Indication. Bevacizumab (in combination with paclitaxel) received approval for use as first-line treatment of metastatic HER2-negative breast cancer in February 2008 under the principles and procedures of FDA's accelerated review process that allows approval based on analysis of surrogate markers of response (i.e., prolongation of progression-free survival) rather than clinical endpoints (e.g., prolongation of overall survival, amelioration of disease-related symptoms). Approval for this indication was based principally on the results of a single multicenter, open-label, randomized study (E2100) in which 722 patients received bevacizumab and paclitaxel or paclitaxel alone as first-line therapy for locally recurrent or metastatic breast cancer. Patients with HER2-overexpressing breast cancer were not eligible for the study unless they had received previous therapy with trastuzumab. Patients who had received hormonal therapy for metastatic disease or adjuvant therapy (chemotherapy or hormonal therapy) for breast cancer were eligible for the study. Patients who had received adjuvant taxane therapy were eligible for the study if they had completed treatment at least 12 months prior to entry to the study. Patients with CNS metastasis were excluded from the study. The median age of patients was 55 years (range: 27–85 years), 76% were white, about 55% were postmenopausal, and 64% had estrogen receptor-positive and/or progesterone receptor-positive disease; 36% had received hormonal therapy for advanced disease and 66% had received adjuvant therapy for breast cancer, including 20% with previous taxane use and 50% with previous anthracycline use. Treatment consisted of paclitaxel 90 mg/m^2 IV once weekly for 3 out of 4 weeks, with or without bevacizumab 10 mg/kg by IV infusion every 2 weeks, until disease progression or unacceptable toxicity occurred. Among patients randomized to receive the combination regimen in whom paclitaxel was withheld or discontinued, bevacizumab monotherapy was allowed to continue until disease progression or unacceptable toxicity occurred.

Because study E2100 was open-label and included patients without measurable disease, efficacy data from a planned interim analysis were subjected to independent, retrospective, blinded review. Although some data points were missing, this analysis of interim data confirmed a higher response rate (48.9 versus 22.2%, partial responses only) and a progression-free survival benefit (11.3 versus 5.8 months) for combined therapy with bevacizumab and paclitaxel compared with paclitaxel alone, and achieved 76–80% concordance with investigator assessments of individual patient results. Final analyses performed by the investigators indicated that patients receiving bevacizumab and paclitaxel had longer progression-free survival (11.8 versus 5.9 months), similar overall survival (26.7 versus 25.2 months), and a higher response rate (36.9 versus 21.2%) compared with those receiving paclitaxel alone as first-line therapy for metastatic breast cancer. Grade 3–4 adverse effects, including sensory neuropathy (24 versus 18%), hypertension (15 versus 0%), fatigue (9 versus 5%), infection (9 versus 3%), proteinuria (4 versus 0%), nausea (3 versus 1%), arthralgia (3 versus 1%), headache (2 versus 0%), and cerebrovascular ischemia (2 versus 0%)occurred more frequently in patients receiving bevacizumab and paclitaxel than in those receiving paclitaxel alone.

As a condition of the accelerated approval process, the manufacturer of bevacizumab was required to submit data from 2 controlled clinical studies (AVADO and RIBBON1) to confirm the progression-free survival benefit that was observed with use of bevacizumab in study E2100 and to provide additional information regarding effects of the drug on overall survival of patients with metastatic HER2-negative breast cancer. In the AVADO study, 736 patients were randomized to receive bevacizumab (7.5 or 15 mg/kg) plus docetaxel (100 mg/m^2) or docetaxel (100 mg/m^2) plus placebo every 3 weeks as first-line therapy for metastatic or locally recurrent HER2-negative breast cancer; bevacizumab or placebo was continued until disease progression or unacceptable toxicity occurred, while docetaxel was administered for up to 9 cycles. In the RIBBON1 study, 1237 patients were randomized to receive either bevacizumab (15 mg/kg every 3 weeks) or placebo in conjunction with a taxane- or anthracycline-based regimen or in conjunction with capecitabine as first-line therapy for metastatic or locally recurrent HER2-negative breast cancer; treatment was continued until disease progression or unacceptable toxicity occurred.

In the AVADO study, objective response rates were higher for patients receiving bevacizumab 7.5 or 15 mg/kg plus docetaxel (55.2 or 64.1%, respectively) compared with those receiving docetaxel alone (46.4%). Inclusion of bevacizumab in the treatment regimen prolonged median progression-free survival by 0.8–1.9 months but did not prolong overall survival. Among patients receiving bevacizumab 7.5 mg/kg plus docetaxel, bevacizumab 15 mg/kg plus docetaxel, or docetaxel alone, median progression-free survival was 9, 10.1, or 8.2 months, respectively, and median overall survival was 30.8, 30.2, or 31.9 months, respectively.

In the RIBBON1 study, patients receiving bevacizumab in conjunction with capecitabine or in conjunction with a taxane- or anthracycline-based regimen had higher objective response rates and longer progression-free survival than did those receiving either capecitabine or a taxane- or anthracycline-based regimen alone; inclusion of bevacizumab in the treatment regimen did not significantly prolong overall survival. Patients receiving bevacizumab and capecitabine had a higher objective response rate (35.4 versus 23.6%) and longer median progression-free survival (8.6 versus 5.7 months), but not a significantly longer median overall survival (25.7 versus 22.8 months), compared with patients receiving capecitabine alone. Similarly, patients receiving bevacizumab in conjunction with a taxane- or anthracycline-based regimen had a higher objective response rate (51.3 versus 37.9%) and longer median progression-free survival (9.2 versus 8 months) compared with patients receiving a taxane- or anthracycline-based regimen alone; inclusion of bevacizumab in these regimens did not provide an overall survival benefit (hazard ratio of 1.11 favoring the use of a taxane- or anthracycline-based regimen).

In both the AVADO and RIBBON1 studies, adverse effects described as grade 3–5 in severity and serious adverse effects (i.e., those requiring medical intervention or hospitalization or resulting in death) were more common in patients receiving bevacizumab-containing regimens compared with those receiving comparator regimens. In the AVADO study, patients were more likely to experience adverse effects requiring docetaxel modification (discontinuance, interruption, dosage reduction) if they received concomitant therapy with bevacizumab.

The FDA Oncologic Drugs Advisory Committee (ODAC) reviewed data from the AVADO and RIBBON1 studies in July 2010 and concluded that these studies did not provide evidence of an overall survival benefit for bevacizumab in patients with metastatic HER2-negative breast cancer; the committee also concluded that the increases in progression-free survival observed in the confirmatory studies were marginal compared with that observed in study E2100 and not clinically meaningful. The committee recommended that the current indication for use of bevacizumab in combination with paclitaxel in the first-line treatment of metastatic HER2-negative breast cancer be removed from the drug's approved labeling.

In December 2010, after reviewing the committee's recommendation and data from 4 clinical studies (i.e., E2100, AVADO, RIBBON1, AVF2119g), FDA's Center for Drug Evaluation and Research (CDER) concurred with the committee, stating that bevacizumab does not prolong overall survival in patients with metastatic HER2-negative breast cancer or provide a sufficient benefit in slowing disease progression to outweigh the substantial risk of serious adverse effects (e.g., hypertension, bleeding or hemorrhage, wound healing complications or wound dehiscence, perforation and fistula/abscess formation, MI, heart failure). Because bevacizumab (in combination with paclitaxel) has not been shown to be safe and effective for first-line treatment of metastatic HER2-negative breast cancer, CDER recommended that this indication be removed from the drug's approved labeling. A public hearing on this recommendation was held on June 28–29, 2011.

On November 18, 2011, after reviewing submissions from the manufacturer and CDER, recommendations from ODAC, and public comments, the FDA Commissioner issued a final decision to rescind approval of bevacizumab for use in combination with paclitaxel as first-line treatment of metastatic HER2-negative breast cancer, citing 3 main reasons for the decision: lack of clinical benefit, unfavorable benefit-to-risk ratio, and lack of other compelling reasons (i.e., special circumstances) to support continued accelerated approval. In evaluating clinical benefit, the commissioner noted that confirmatory studies (AVADO and RIBBON1) failed to verify the magnitude of effect on progression-free survival observed in study E2100, and that none of the 5 studies submitted by the manufacturer (E2100, AVADO, RIBBON1, AVF2119g, RIBBON2) demonstrated an overall survival benefit or an improvement in quality of life. In evaluating the regimen's safety profile, it was noted that the addition of bevacizumab to chemotherapy resulted in an increased risk of severe (grade 3 or greater) adverse effects (e.g., neutropenia, sensory neuropathy, hypertension, febrile neutropenia, proteinuria, arterial thromboembolic events, left ventricular systolic dysfunction, hemorrhage, wound healing complications, fistula formation, GI perforation) that was considered unacceptable for a regimen that has not demonstrated clinical benefit. In evaluating special circumstances that may justify continuing accelerated approval (e.g., until clinical benefit is fully established or until a subset of patients likely to benefit from therapy is identified), the commissioner concluded that continuing an approval that is no longer supported by current data and allowing a substantial length of time for additional studies to be completed would be inconsistent with the protection of public health. The commissioner noted that because FDA does not regulate the practice of medicine, clinicians may continue to prescribe bevacizumab for the treatment of metastatic breast cancer (i.e., unlabeled [off-label] use) despite withdrawal of approval for this use.

AHFS Oncology Expert Committee Decision Regarding Use as First-line Therapy. The AHFS Oncology Expert Committee was concerned that the E2100 study failed to demonstrate an overall survival benefit despite showing prolonged disease-free survival in patients receiving combined therapy with bevacizumab and paclitaxel, and also was concerned by the failure of the confirmatory studies (AVADO and RIBBON1) to verify the same magnitude of effect on progression-free survival as observed in the E2100 study. These studies provide a basis for assessing tolerability of bevacizumab in patients with previously untreated metastatic breast cancer, but the results provide equivocal evidence of the drug's efficacy for this use. In the absence of additional data, attempts to identify subgroups of patients in whom bevacizumab might provide clinical benefit (e.g., prolonged progression-free survival, prolonged overall survival, improved quality of life) and achieve a favorable benefit-to-risk ratio are speculative; additional studies are needed to identify subgroups of patients with previously untreated metastatic breast cancer who might derive clinical benefit from bevacizumab treatment. Therefore, the committee concluded that use of bevacizumab in combination with paclitaxel for the first-line treatment of metastatic breast cancer currently is not fully established because of equivocal evidence.

Previously Treated Metastatic Breast Cancer The efficacy and safety of bevacizumab for the treatment of metastatic breast cancer† previously treated with cytotoxic chemotherapy has been studied in several randomized studies.

The first study (AVF2119g) was an open-label, randomized study in which 462 patients received either bevacizumab and capecitabine or capecitabine alone. Patients with metastatic breast cancer who had received prior therapy with both an anthracycline (or anthracenedione) and a taxane and had received 1 or 2 prior chemotherapy regimens for metastatic disease were eligible to enroll in the study; patients who relapsed within 12 months of completing adjuvant anthracycline (or anthracenedione) and taxane therapy also were eligible to enroll in the study without having received additional chemotherapy. Patients with HER2-overexpressing breast cancer were not eligible for the study unless their disease had progressed following treatment with trastuzumab. Patients with CNS disease and those who had received prior therapy with bevacizumab or capecitabine were excluded from the study. The mean age of patients was about 51 years (range: 29–78 years), about 81% were white, 47% had estrogen receptor-positive disease, and 37% had progesterone receptor-positive disease. Treatment consisted of capecitabine (1.25 g/m^2 orally twice daily on days 1–14 of each 3-week cycle) given alone or in combination with bevacizumab (15 mg/kg by IV infusion on day 1 of each 3-week cycle) for a maximum of 35 cycles or until disease progression or unacceptable toxicity occurred. Patients without disease progression following 35 cycles of therapy could continue to receive their assigned treatment in an extension study. Patients randomized to receive bevacizumab and capecitabine could continue to receive bevacizumab either alone or in combination with other therapies following initial disease progression.

Patients receiving bevacizumab and capecitabine had higher response rates (19.8 versus 9.1%) but similar median progression-free survival (4.9 versus 4.2 months) and overall survival (15.1 months versus 14.5 months) compared with those receiving capecitabine alone. Hypertension (23.6 versus 2.3%, frequently grade 3), proteinuria (22.3 versus 7.4%, mostly grade 1 or 2), and hemorrhage (28.8 versus 11.2%, mostly grade 1) occurred more frequently in patients receiving bevacizumab and capecitabine than in those receiving capecitabine alone.

The second study (AVF3693g, RIBBON2) was a double-blind, placebo-controlled trial evaluating safety and efficacy of bevacizumab in combination with taxanes (paclitaxel, albumin-bound paclitaxel, or docetaxel), capecitabine, gemcitabine, or vinorelbine as second-line therapy for locally recurrent or metastatic breast cancer in 684 patients who had received one prior cytotoxic chemotherapy regimen for metastatic disease. Patients with HER2-overexpressing breast cancer, those with untreated CNS metastases, and those who had received prior therapy with bevacizumab or other vascular endothelial growth factor (VEGF) inhibitors were not eligible to enroll in the study. The median age of patients was 55 years (range: 23–90 years) and about 72% had hormone receptor-positive disease. Patients were randomized in a 2:1 ratio to receive either bevacizumab (15 mg/kg every 3 weeks or 10 mg/kg every 2 weeks depending on the chemotherapy regimen) or placebo in combination with the investigator-selected chemotherapy regimen. Most patients received a taxane (44.4%), gemcitabine (23.4%), or capecitabine (21.1%). Bevacizumab could be continued until disease progression or unacceptable toxicity occurred, up to a maximum of 36 months of therapy; the chemotherapy regimen could be continued until disease progression or unacceptable toxicity occurred. If chemotherapy was discontinued before disease progression occurred, patients could continue receiving bevacizumab (or placebo, as assigned) as monotherapy.

At a median follow-up of 15 months, combined therapy with bevacizumab and chemotherapy prolonged median progression-free survival (7.2 versus 5.1 months) but was not associated with an overall survival benefit compared with chemotherapy alone; in patients receiving bevacizumab and chemotherapy, median overall survival was 18 months and the one-year survival rate was 69.5%, compared with 16.4 months and 66.2%, respectively, for those receiving chemotherapy alone. No significant difference in objective response rate was observed between patients receiving bevacizumab in combination with chemotherapy and those receiving chemotherapy alone (39.5 and 29.6%, respectively). Subgroup analysis showed that the progression-free survival benefit observed when bevacizumab and chemotherapy were given in combination was not uniform across all 4 chemotherapy regimens. When bevacizumab was used in combination with capecitabine, gemcitabine, or a taxane, median progression-free survival was prolonged by 0.5–2.8 months (depending on the regimen) compared with the chemotherapy regimen alone; however, when bevacizumab was used in combination with vinorelbine, median progression-free survival was 1.3 months shorter than when vinorelbine was used alone. Grade 3 or greater hypertension (9 versus 0.5%), neutropenia (17.7 versus 14.5%), proteinuria (3.1 versus 0.5%), and hemorrhage (1.7 versus 0%) occurred more frequently in patients receiving bevacizumab in combination with chemotherapy than in those receiving chemotherapy alone. In each chemotherapy subgroup, the incidence of adverse effects requiring study drug discontinuance was higher when the chemotherapy regimen was given in combination with bevacizumab.

Although combined therapy with bevacizumab and chemotherapy prolonged progression-free survival in the RIBBON2 study, the same benefit was not observed in the AVF2119g study; in addition, combined therapy did not prolong overall survival in either study. Therefore, usefulness of the drug in combination with chemotherapy for the treatment of metastatic breast cancer previously treated with cytotoxic chemotherapy is unclear. Use of bevacizumab in combination with chemotherapy for the treatment of metastatic breast cancer previously treated with cytotoxic chemotherapy currently is not fully established because of equivocal evidence.

■ **Other Uses** Bevacizumab has been investigated for use in the treatment of ovarian cancer†. Results of two phase 3 randomized trials indicate that addition of bevacizumab to chemotherapy (carboplatin and paclitaxel) prolonged progression-free survival by approximately 1.5–4 months in patients with advanced ovarian epithelial cancer, primary peritoneal cancer, or fallopian-tube cancer. Effects on overall survival have not been fully elucidated (i.e., no difference in overall survival reported in one study, final overall survival data not yet available for the second study). Bevacizumab in combination with chemotherapy was associated with an increased risk of hypertension and GI perforation compared with chemotherapy alone. Further study is needed to determine the optimal timing and duration of bevacizumab therapy and to identify patient populations most likely to benefit from this drug.

Intravitreal injection† of bevacizumab has been used for the treatment of neovascular age-related macular degeneration†. Results of several randomized controlled studies suggest that intravitreal bevacizumab has similar efficacy as ranibizumab in improving visual acuity. In one study, the incidence of serious systemic adverse effects (primarily hospitalizations) appeared to be higher with bevacizumab compared with ranibizumab; however, other studies, including a systematic review of 9 randomized controlled studies, directly comparing intravitreal injections of bevacizumab and ranibizumab in patients with neovascular age-related macular degeneration have found no such difference. Patient-specific factors, which may vary the level of risk associated with these VEGF antagonists, should be considered prior to the use of intravitreal bevacizumab. (See Ocular Effects under Warnings/Precautions: Other Warnings and Precautions, in Cautions.)

Intravitreal injection† of bevacizumab also has been used for the treatment of diabetic macular edema†. Results of a study comparing intravitreal ranibizumab, aflibercept, and bevacizumab for the treatment of diabetic macular edema suggest that the relative treatment effect of these drugs may be dependent upon a patient's baseline visual acuity. (See Uses: Diabetic Macular Edema, in Aflibercept 52:92.) Further study is needed to establish the role of bevacizumab in the treatment of diabetic macular edema.

Dosage and Administration

■ **Administration** Bevacizumab is administered by IV infusion. The drug should *not* be administered by rapid IV injection, such as IV push or bolus. The initial dose of bevacizumab should be infused over 90 minutes (following other antineoplastic agents); if the infusion is well tolerated, the second dose may be infused over 60 minutes. If this second infusion also is well tolerated, subsequent doses may be infused over 30 minutes. One institution has reported use of shorter infusion times for bevacizumab at an infusion rate of 0.5 mg/kg per minute.

For IV infusion, the appropriate dose of bevacizumab should be withdrawn into a syringe and diluted in a total volume of 100 mL of 0.9% sodium chloride using aseptic technique. Bevacizumab infusions should not be administered or mixed with dextrose solutions. Bevacizumab injection should be inspected visually for particulate matter and discoloration prior to administration. Any unused portion left in the vial should be discarded since the injection contains no preservative. The diluted drug may be stored at 2–8°C for up to 8 hours.

The manufacturer states that no incompatibilities between bevacizumab and polyvinylchloride or polyolefin bags have been observed.

Bevacizumab injection should be protected from light and stored in the original carton at 2–8°C until use; freezing should be avoided. The injection should not be shaken prior to use.

■ **General Dosage** Bevacizumab therapy should *not* be initiated for at least 28 days following major surgery, and the surgical incision should be fully healed prior to initiation of the drug. (See Surgery and Wound Healing Complications under Warnings/Precautions: Warnings, in Cautions.)

Clinicians should consult the respective manufacturers or published protocols for information on the dosage, method of administration, and administration sequence of other antineoplastic agents used in combination regimens.

First-line Treatment for Metastatic Colorectal Cancer For the first-line treatment of metastatic cancer of the colon or rectum in adults, a bevacizumab dosage of 5 mg/kg, administered by IV infusion every 2 weeks, is used in combination with IV irinotecan/fluorouracil/leucovorin. Bevacizumab therapy should be continued until disease progression or unacceptable toxicity occurs.

Second-line Treatment for Metastatic Colorectal Cancer For the second-line treatment of metastatic cancer of the colon or rectum in adults, a bevacizumab dosage of 10 mg/kg, administered by IV infusion every 2 weeks, is used in combination with FOLFOX4 (IV fluorouracil/leucovorin and oxaliplatin). Bevacizumab therapy should be continued until disease progression or unacceptable toxicity occurs.

First-line Treatment for Advanced Nonsquamous Non-small Cell Lung Cancer For the first-line treatment of unresectable, locally advanced, recurrent or metastatic nonsquamous non-small cell lung cancer, the recommended dosage of bevacizumab is 15 mg/kg by IV infusion on day 1 every 3 weeks. In the pivotal study, bevacizumab was administered in combination with paclitaxel and carboplatin. Bevacizumab therapy should be continued until disease progression or unacceptable toxicity occurs.

Second-line Treatment for Glioblastoma For the second-line treatment of glioblastoma in adults whose disease has progressed following radiation therapy and chemotherapy, the recommended dosage of bevacizumab is 10 mg/kg by IV infusion every 2 weeks. Bevacizumab therapy should be continued until disease progression or unacceptable toxicity occurs.

First-line Treatment for Renal Cell Carcinoma For the first-line treatment of metastatic renal cell carcinoma in adults, a bevacizumab dosage of 10 mg/kg, administered by IV infusion every 2 weeks, is used in combination with interferon alfa. Bevacizumab therapy should be continued until disease progression or unacceptable toxicity occurs.

First-line Treatment for Metastatic Breast Cancer For the first-line treatment of metastatic breast cancer†, a bevacizumab dosage of 10 mg/kg, administered by IV infusion every 2 weeks, has been used in combination with IV paclitaxel. However, this combination regimen has not been shown to prolong overall survival or provide sufficient clinical benefit to outweigh the risk of severe, potentially fatal, adverse effects. (See Uses: Breast Cancer.)

Dosage Modification for Toxicity Bevacizumab dosage reductions are not recommended in any patient; instead, the drug should either be temporarily suspended or permanently discontinued, according to causality.

Bevacizumab should be *permanently discontinued* in patients who develop GI perforation (GI perforation, fistula formation in the GI tract, and/or intra-abdominal abscess), non-GI fistula formation involving an internal organ, wound dehiscence and wound healing complications requiring medical intervention, severe hemorrhage requiring medical intervention, severe arterial thromboembolic events, hypertensive crisis, hypertensive encephalopathy, or nephrotic syndrome.

Bevacizumab therapy also should be *permanently discontinued* in patients who develop reversible posterior leukoencephalopathy syndrome (RPLS). Treatment of hypertension should be initiated as clinically indicated. The risk of reinitiating bevacizumab therapy in patients previously experiencing RPLS is not known.

Temporary suspension is recommended in patients who develop moderate to severe proteinuria (pending further evaluation) and in those with severe hypertension (not controlled by medical management). The risk of continuing bevacizumab therapy in patients with moderate to severe proteinuria is not known. Bevacizumab infusion should be interrupted in patients with severe infusion reactions, and appropriate medical therapy should be initiated. Adequate information regarding rechallenge with bevacizumab is unavailable; whether therapy with the drug may be safely resumed following resolution of a severe bevacizumab-induced infusion reaction has not been determined. Bevacizumab therapy should be suspended at least 28 days prior to elective surgery and should not be resumed until at least 28 days following major surgery and after the surgical incision has fully healed.

■ **Special Populations** No special populations dosage recommendations at this time.

Cautions

■ **Contraindications** The manufacturer states that there are no contraindications to the use of bevacizumab.

■ **Warnings/Precautions** ***Warnings*** Because the bevacizumab therapeutic regimen may include the use of other antineoplastic agents, the usual cautions, precautions, and contraindications of these drugs also should be considered.

GI Perforation. Severe GI perforation, sometimes fatal, occurs more frequently in patients receiving bevacizumab than in those receiving placebo or active controls. GI perforation has been reported in 0.3–2.4% of patients receiving bevacizumab in clinical studies. Manifestations may include abdominal pain, nausea, emesis, constipation, and fever. GI perforation can be complicated by intra-abdominal abscess and fistula formation. The majority of cases occurred within the first 50 days of initiation of bevacizumab.

Bevacizumab should be *permanently discontinued* in patients with GI perforation (GI perforation, fistula formation in the GI tract, and/or intra-abdominal abscess).

Surgery and Wound Healing Complications. Wound healing and bleeding complications (including wound dehiscence) have occurred in patients who underwent surgery during bevacizumab therapy. In a randomized trial involving patients with metastatic colorectal cancer, wound healing and/or bleeding complications, including serious and fatal complications, occurred in 15% (6/39) of patients undergoing surgery during or within 60 days following therapy with bevacizumab and chemotherapy compared with 4% (1/25) of patients undergoing surgery within the same time period following chemotherapy alone; the incidence of wound dehiscence was also higher in the patients receiving bevacizumab (1 versus 0.5%). In one patient, dehiscence occurred 56 days after the last dose of bevacizumab.

Bevacizumab therapy should not be initiated until at least 28 days following major surgery and after the surgical incision has fully healed.

The appropriate interval between discontinuance of bevacizumab and subsequent elective surgery has not been established, but the long half-life of the drug (approximately 20 days) should be considered. The manufacturer recommends that bevacizumab be suspended at least 28 days prior to elective surgery and not resumed until the surgical incision has fully healed.

Bevacizumab should be *permanently discontinued* if wound dehiscence and wound healing complications requiring medical intervention occur.

Hemorrhage. Severe or fatal hemorrhages, including hemoptysis, GI bleeding, hematemesis, CNS hemorrhage, epistaxis, and vaginal bleeding, occurred up to fivefold more frequently in patients receiving bevacizumab and chemotherapy than in those receiving chemotherapy alone.

Grade 3 or greater hemorrhagic events have been reported in 1.2–4.6% of patients receiving bevacizumab in clinical studies. Serious or fatal pulmonary hemorrhage occurred in 31% (4/13) of patients with squamous cell carcinoma of the lung and 4% (2/53) of patients with nonsquamous non-small cell lung cancer receiving bevacizumab with chemotherapy compared with 0% (0/32) of patients receiving chemotherapy alone. Symptomatic grade 2 CNS hemorrhage occurred in 1.2% (1/83) of patients with non-small cell lung cancer with CNS metastases receiving bevacizumab in clinical studies. Intracranial hemorrhage (including grade 3–4 hemorrhage) has been reported in 4.9% (8/163) of patients with previously treated glioblastoma receiving bevacizumab.

Mild to moderate hemorrhagic events also have been reported more frequently in patients receiving bevacizumab. Grade 1 epistaxis was common in clinical studies and occurred in up to 35% of patients receiving bevacizumab in conjunction with other antineoplastic agents for metastatic colorectal cancer. Epistaxis generally was mild and resolved without medical intervention. Other grade 1–2 hemorrhagic events reported more frequently in patients receiving bevacizumab in conjunction with other antineoplastic agents for metastatic colorectal cancer when compared with those not receiving bevacizumab included GI hemorrhage (24 versus 6%, respectively), minor gum bleeding (2 versus 0%, respectively), and vaginal hemorrhage (4 versus 2%, respectively).

Patients with a history of recent hemoptysis (0.5 teaspoon of red blood or more) should not receive bevacizumab. Bevacizumab should be *permanently discontinued* in patients with severe hemorrhage requiring medical intervention.

Sensitivity Reactions **Infusion Reactions.** In clinical studies, infusion reactions with the first bevacizumab dose were uncommon (less than 3%). Severe infusion reactions occurred in 0.2% of patients receiving bevacizumab. Infusion reactions include hypertension, hypertensive crises associated with neurologic manifestations, wheezing, oxygen desaturation, grade 3 hypersensitivity, chest pain, headaches, rigors, and diaphoresis.

Initial doses of bevacizumab should be infused slowly; if well tolerated, the rate of IV infusion may be increased during administration of subsequent doses. (See Dosage and Administration: Administration.)

Bevacizumab infusion should be interrupted if severe infusion reaction occurs, and appropriate medical therapy should be initiated.

Other Warnings and Precautions **Non-GI Fistula Formation.** Severe, sometimes fatal, non-GI fistula formation involving tracheo-esophageal, bronchopleural, biliary, vaginal, renal, and bladder sites has been reported more frequently in patients receiving bevacizumab compared with those receiving controls. Non-GI fistula formation was reported in 0.3% or less of patients in controlled clinical studies and typically occurred within the first 6 months of bevacizumab therapy.

Bevacizumab should be *permanently discontinued* in patients with non-GI fistula formation involving an internal organ.

Thromboembolism. Severe, sometimes fatal, arterial thromboembolic events (e.g., cerebral infarction, transient ischemic attacks [TIAs], myocardial infarction [MI], angina) occurred at a higher incidence in patients receiving bevacizumab in combination with chemotherapy compared with those receiving chemotherapy alone. In clinical studies, grade 3 or greater arterial thromboembolic events have been reported in 2.6% of patients receiving bevacizumab in combination with chemotherapy compared with 0.8% of those receiving chemotherapy alone. The relative risk of arterial thromboembolic events in patients receiving bevacizumab in combination with chemotherapy was increased in patients with a history of arterial thromboembolism and in patients older than 65 years of age.

Whether bevacizumab therapy can be safely resumed following resolution of an arterial thromboembolic event has not been studied. Bevacizumab should be *permanently discontinued* in patients who experience severe arterial thromboembolic events.

Grade 3 or 4 venous thromboembolic events, such as deep-vein thrombosis and intra-abdominal venous thrombosis, occurred more often in patients receiving bevacizumab with chemotherapy than in those receiving chemotherapy alone for metastatic colorectal cancer or advanced non-small cell lung cancer. In addition, the risk of developing a second thromboembolic event was increased in patients receiving bevacizumab with chemotherapy compared with those receiving chemotherapy alone for metastatic colorectal cancer despite the use of full-dose warfarin therapy following an initial venous thromboembolic event.

Hypertension. The incidence of severe hypertension was increased in patients receiving bevacizumab in combination with chemotherapy compared with those receiving chemotherapy alone. Grade 3 or 4 hypertension occurred in 5–18% of patients receiving bevacizumab in clinical studies. Hypertension was more common in patients with previous history of hypertension and may respond to antihypertensive therapy. Hypertension also occurred more frequently in patients who received higher dosages of bevacizumab (e.g., 10 mg/kg).

Blood pressure should be monitored every 2–3 weeks during bevacizumab therapy. If hypertension occurs, patients should be treated with appropriate antihypertensive therapy, and blood pressure should be monitored regularly.

Temporary suspension of bevacizumab therapy is recommended in patients with severe hypertension that is not controlled with medical management. Bevacizumab should be *permanently discontinued* in patients who develop hypertensive crisis or hypertensive encephalopathy. If bevacizumab is discontinued because of hypertension, blood pressure should be monitored at regular intervals thereafter.

Reversible Posterior Leukoencephalopathy Syndrome. Reversible posterior leukoencephalopathy syndrome (RPLS) has occurred in patients receiving bevacizumab. This complication occurred in less than 0.1% of patients receiving bevacizumab in clinical studies.

RPLS, a brain-capillary leak syndrome associated with hypertension, fluid retention, and the cytotoxic effects of immunosuppressive drugs on the vascular endothelium, is a neurological disorder that may manifest with headache, seizure, lethargy, confusion, blindness, and other visual and neurologic disturbances. Mild to severe hypertension may occur, but it is not necessary for the diagnosis of RPLS. Magnetic resonance imaging is necessary to confirm the diagnosis of RPLS. The onset of symptoms has occurred from 16 hours to 1 year after initiation of bevacizumab therapy.

Blood pressure should be closely monitored and strictly controlled during and following bevacizumab infusion. If RPLS develops, bevacizumab should be *permanently discontinued*, and treatment of hypertension should be initiated as clinically indicated. Symptoms of RPLS usually lessen or resolve within days of discontinuance of bevacizumab, but some patients have experienced ongoing neurologic sequelae. The risk of reinitiating bevacizumab therapy in patients previously experiencing RPLS is not known.

Proteinuria. Increased incidence and severity of proteinuria have been reported in patients receiving bevacizumab. In clinical trials, proteinuria ranged in severity from clinically silent to nephrotic syndrome. Grade 3 or 4 proteinuria (defined as greater than 3.5 g of protein in the urine collected over 24 hours) occurred in 0.7–7.4% of patients receiving bevacizumab for colorectal cancer, non-small cell lung cancer, or renal cell carcinoma. In the randomized clinical study in patients with metastatic renal cell carcinoma, proteinuria (all grades) was reported in 20% of those receiving bevacizumab. In this study, the median onset of proteinuria was 5.6 months (range: 15 days to 37 months) after initiation of bevacizumab; median time to resolution was 6.1 months. Proteinuria did not resolve in 40% of patients after a median follow-up of 11.2 months, and 30% of patients required permanent discontinuance of bevacizumab. Proteinuria with findings of thrombotic microangiopathy on renal biopsy has been reported in patients receiving bevacizumab alone or in combination with other antineoplastic agents for various cancers. Nephrotic syndrome, sometimes fatal, occurred in less than 1% of patients receiving bevacizumab in clinical studies.

Patients receiving bevacizumab should be monitored for the development or worsening of proteinuria. Patients with a 2+ or greater urine dipstick reading should undergo further assessment with a 24-hour urine collection.

Bevacizumab therapy should be interrupted for proteinuria of or exceeding 2 g per 24 hours and resumed when proteinuria declines below this level. The safety of continued treatment in patients with moderate to severe proteinuria has not been evaluated.

Bevacizumab should be *permanently discontinued* in patients with nephrotic syndrome.

Ovarian Failure. Ovarian failure has been reported more frequently in premenopausal women receiving bevacizumab in combination with chemotherapy (i.e., fluorouracil, leucovorin, and oxaliplatin [modified FOLFOX6]†) (34%) compared with those receiving chemotherapy alone (2%) for adjuvant treatment of colorectal cancer. Following discontinuance of bevacizumab, recovery of ovarian function occurred in 22% of patients. The long-term effects of bevacizumab exposure on fertility are unknown.

Women of childbearing potential should be informed of the risk of ovarian failure prior to initiating bevacizumab therapy.

Neutropenia and Infection. Increased rates of severe (grade 3 or 4) neutropenia, febrile neutropenia, infection with severe neutropenia (sometimes fatal), and serious infections (e.g., pneumonia, catheter infections, wound infections) have been observed in patients receiving bevacizumab and chemotherapy compared with those receiving chemotherapy alone.

Congestive Heart Failure. Congestive heart failure has been reported in patients receiving bevacizumab. Grade 3 or greater left ventricular dysfunction was reported in 1% of patients receiving bevacizumab in clinical studies. Among patients receiving bevacizumab and paclitaxel for metastatic breast cancer† in a randomized trial, grade 3 or 4 congestive heart failure occurred in 2.2%; of these patients, those who had received previous anthracycline therapy had a higher rate of congestive heart failure (3.8%). The safety of continuation or resumption of bevacizumab in patients who develop cardiac dysfunction has not been studied.

Microangiopathic Hemolytic Anemia. Cases of microangiopathic hemolytic anemia have been reported in patients with solid tumors receiving bevacizumab and sunitinib†. In a phase 1 study involving 25 patients receiving bevacizumab at a fixed dose and sunitinib at escalating dose levels, 5 of 12 patients receiving bevacizumab with the highest dose level of sunitinib had laboratory findings consistent with microangiopathic hemolytic anemia. Of these 5 patients, 2 patients had evidence of severe microangiopathic hemolytic anemia, including thrombocytopenia, anemia, reticulocytosis, reduced serum haptoglobin concentrations, schistocytes on peripheral smear, modest increases in serum creatinine concentrations, severe hypertension, RPLS, and proteinuria. These findings were reversed within 3 weeks following discontinuance of both drugs without other interventions. Use of bevacizumab in combination with sunitinib is *not* recommended. Clinicians should report cases of microangiopathic hemolytic anemia associated with bevacizumab therapy to the manufacturer or the US Food and Drug Administration (FDA).

Immunogenicity. As with all therapeutic proteins, there is a potential for immunogenicity. The incidence of antibody formation to bevacizumab has not been established.

Ocular Effects. Permanent loss of vision, endophthalmitis (infectious and sterile), intraocular inflammation, retinal detachment, increased intraocular pressure, hemorrhage (including conjunctival, vitreous, or retinal hemorrhage), vitreous floaters, ocular hyperemia, and ocular pain or discomfort have been reported during postmarketing experience in patients receiving intravitreal injection† of bevacizumab for treatment of various ocular disorders†.

Specific Populations **Pregnancy.** Category C. (See Users Guide.)

Lactation. It is not known whether bevacizumab is distributed into milk. Human immunoglobulin G_1 (IgG_1) is distributed into milk; however, published data suggest that antibodies in breast milk do not enter the neonatal and infant circulations in substantial amounts. Because many drugs are distributed into milk and because of the potential for serious adverse reactions in nursing infants from bevacizumab, a decision should be made whether to discontinue nursing or the drug, taking into account the long half-life (approximately 20 days [range: 11–50 days]) and the importance of the drug to the woman.

Pediatric Use. Safety and efficacy of bevacizumab have not been established in children younger than 18 years of age.

Geriatric Use. No difference in overall survival relative to younger adults was observed in patients receiving bevacizumab and chemotherapy (irinotecan, fluorouracil, and leucovorin) for metastatic colorectal cancer; experience in those 65 years of age and older is insufficient to determine whether overall adverse effect profile differs compared with younger adults. Severe adverse effects reported more frequently among patients 65 years of age and older than among younger adults receiving bevacizumab and chemotherapy for metastatic colorectal cancer included asthenia, sepsis, deep thrombophlebitis, hypertension, hypotension, myocardial infarction, congestive heart failure, diarrhea, constipation, anorexia, leukopenia, anemia, dehydration, hypokalemia, and hyponatremia. Geriatric patients receiving bevacizumab and chemotherapy (fluorouracil, leucovorin, and oxaliplatin) for metastatic colorectal cancer also may be at greater risk for nausea, vomiting (emesis), ileus, or fatigue. Geriatric patients receiving bevacizumab and chemotherapy (carboplatin and paclitaxel) for advanced non-small cell lung cancer may be at greater risk for proteinuria than younger patients. Other adverse effects reported more frequently among patients 65 years of age and older included dyspepsia, GI hemorrhage, edema, epistaxis, increased cough, and voice alteration.

Analysis of pooled data from 5 randomized controlled trials involving 1745 patients (35% aged 65 years or older) showed that arterial thromboembolic events occurred more frequently in all patients receiving bevacizumab with chemotherapy compared with those receiving chemotherapy alone, regardless of age. However, the increase in the incidence of arterial thromboembolic events associated with concomitant bevacizumab therapy was greater in patients 65 years of age or older (8.5 versus 2.9%) compared with those younger than 65 years of age (2.1 versus 1.4%). (See Thromboembolism under Warnings/Precautions: Other Warnings and Precautions, in Cautions.)

■ **Common Adverse Effects** Adverse effects reported in more than 10% of patients receiving bevacizumab and at a frequency at least twice that reported among patients receiving controls include epistaxis, headache, hypertension, rhinitis, proteinuria, taste alteration, dry skin, rectal hemorrhage, lacrimation disorder, back pain, and exfoliative dermatitis.

Drug Interactions

■ **Carboplatin** Pharmacokinetic interaction is unlikely (no effect on mean carboplatin exposure). (See Drug Interactions: Paclitaxel.)

■ **Interferon Alfa** Pharmacokinetic interaction is unlikely (no effect on mean interferon alfa exposure).

■ **Irinotecan** Pharmacokinetic interaction is unlikely (no effect on pharmacokinetics of irinotecan or the active metabolite of irinotecan [SN38]).

■ **Paclitaxel** Limited data indicate that although mean paclitaxel exposure was not altered following concomitant use of bevacizumab with carboplatin and paclitaxel, paclitaxel exposure after 4 treatment cycles decreased in patients receiving concomitant therapy (lower paclitaxel exposure observed on day 63 than on day 0) compared with that in patients receiving carboplatin and paclitaxel alone (higher paclitaxel exposure observed on day 63 than on day 0).

■ **Sunitinib** Cases of microangiopathic hemolytic anemia have been reported. (See Microangiopathic Hemolytic Anemia under Warnings/Precautions: Other Warnings and Precautions, in Cautions.) Use of bevacizumab in combination with sunitinib is *not* recommended.

Description

Bevacizumab, a recombinant humanized monoclonal antibody, is an antineoplastic agent. The drug is an IgG_1 antibody that contains human framework regions and murine complementarity-determining regions.

Bevacizumab binds to human vascular endothelial growth factor (VEGF) and prevents interaction of VEGF with its receptors (Flt-1, KDR) on the surface of endothelial cells. In vitro models of angiogenesis have shown that interaction of VEGF with its receptors may lead to endothelial cell proliferation and new blood vessel formation. Evidence from animal models has suggested that administration of an anti-VEGF monoclonal antibody (e.g., bevacizumab) may inhibit angiogenesis and thus may reduce microvascular growth of tumors and inhibit metastatic disease progression. Bevacizumab is metabolized and eliminated via the reticuloendothelial system.

Advice to Patients

Importance of understanding potential risks associated with therapy, including severe hypertension, wound healing complications, arterial thromboembolic events, and ovarian failure.

Importance of routine monitoring of blood pressure and informing clinician if blood pressure is elevated.

Importance of immediately informing clinician if unusual bleeding, high fever, rigors, sudden worsening of neurologic function, persistent or severe abdominal pain, severe constipation, or vomiting occurs.

Risk of fetal toxicity. Necessity of advising women to use an effective method of contraception during and for at least 6 months after the last dose of bevacizumab.

Importance of informing clinicians of existing or contemplated concomitant therapy, including prescription and OTC drugs, as well as any concomitant illnesses.

Importance of informing patients of other important precautionary information. (See Cautions.)

Overview (see Users Guide). For additional information until a more detailed monograph is developed and published, the manufacturer's labeling should be consulted. It is *essential* that the manufacturer's labeling be consulted for more detailed information on usual cautions, precautions, contraindications, potential drug interactions, laboratory test interferences, and acute toxicity.

Preparations

Excipients in commercially available drug preparations may have clinically important effects in some individuals; consult specific product labeling for details.

Bevacizumab (Recombinant)

Parenteral

For injection, concentrate, for IV infusion	25 mg/mL (100 and 400 mg)	**Avastin®**, Genentech

†Use is not currently included in the labeling approved by the US Food and Drug Administration

Bicalutamide

■ Bicalutamide, a nonsteroidal antiandrogen, is an antineoplastic agent.

Uses

■ **Prostate Cancer** Bicalutamide is used in combination with a gonadotropin-releasing hormone (GnRH) luteinizing hormone-releasing hormone analog (e.g., goserelin or leuprolide acetate) for the palliative treatment of metastatic (stage D2) prostate cancer. In a double-blind, multicenter, randomized study in 813 patients with previously untreated advanced prostate cancer, similar survival rate, time to progression, and quality-of-life measurements were reported for bicalutamide (50 mg daily) and flutamide (250 mg 3 times daily) combined with a GnRH analog (goserelin acetate implant or leuprolide acetate depot). For additional information on combined antiandrogenic and GnRH analog therapy, see Uses: Prostate Cancer in Leuprolide Acetate 68:18.08.

Prostate specific antigen (PSA) concentrations should be determined periodically during bicalutamide therapy to monitor therapeutic response, including successful remission or possible progression of cancer. If PSA concentrations increase substantially and consistently during bicalutamide therapy, the possibility of clinical progression should be evaluated. For patients with objective progression of disease and an elevated serum PSA, temporary withdrawal of bicalutamide therapy may be considered. Withdrawal of bicalutamide in such patients can be associated with a decrease in PSA. The mechanism of this response to bicalutamide withdrawal has not been determined, but may involve the development of mutations at the androgen receptor.

Dosage and Administration

Patients should be advised of the possibility of facial flushing during bicalutamide therapy and that alcohol could exacerbate this effect. Patients who experience such intolerance during therapy with the drug should avoid alcohol consumption.

■ **Administration** Bicalutamide is administered orally without regard to meals.

Dispensing and Administration Precautions Dispensing errors have occurred because of similarity in spelling between Casodex® (the trade name for bicalutamide) and Kapidex® (the former trade name for dexlansoprazole, a proton-pump inhibitor). Therefore, in April 2010, the manufacturer of Kapidex® changed the trade name for dexlansoprazole from Kapidex® to Dexilant® to avoid future dispensing errors. The potential exists for serious adverse effects to occur if patients receive the incorrect drug (see Dosage and Administration: Dosage). Some experts recommend that pharmacists assess measures of avoiding dispensing errors and implement them as appropriate (e.g., by using computerized name alerts, matching the prescribed drug with the patient's medical history, verifying orders for these drugs) and that clinicians consider including the intended use of the drug on the prescription.

■ **Dosage** The safety and efficacy of bicalutamide have not been established in women or children. Bicalutamide is not intended for use in women and should not be used in women, particularly for nonserious or nonlife-threatening conditions. In addition, bicalutamide is contraindicated in women who are or may became pregnant.

Prostate Cancer For use in combination with a gonadotropin-releasing hormone (GnRH) analog in the palliative treatment of metastatic (stage D2) prostate cancer, the usual dosage of bicalutamide is 50 mg once daily in the morning or evening. Treatment with bicalutamide and the GnRH analog should be initiated concomitantly, and bicalutamide should be taken at the same time each day. The duration of combined therapy with bicalutamide and a GnRH analog depends on the clinical response of the patient. Periodic monitoring of serum prostate specific antigen (PSA) may be useful for assessing the patient's response to therapy. For patients with objective progression of disease and an elevated serum PSA, temporary withdrawal of bicalutamide therapy while continuing therapy with the GnRH analog may be considered.

Discontinuance of Therapy for Hepatic Toxicity Severe liver injury, in some cases leading to hospitalization and/or death, has been reported rarely in association with bicalutamide therapy. Hepatotoxicity generally occurred within the first 3–4 months of bicalutamide therapy. Hepatitis or marked increases in serum concentrations of hepatic transaminases leading to discontinuance of bicalutamide therapy were reported in 1% of patients receiving the drug in controlled clinical trials.

Serum transaminase concentrations should be measured prior to initiation of bicalutamide therapy, at regular intervals during the first 4 months of treatment, and periodically thereafter. If clinical signs or symptoms suggestive of liver dysfunction (e.g., nausea, vomiting, abdominal pain, fatigue, anorexia, "flu-like" symptoms, dark urine, jaundice, or right upper quadrant tenderness) occur, serum transaminase (especially ALT) concentrations should be measured immediately. Bicalutamide should be discontinued immediately in any patient who develops jaundice or an increase in serum ALT concentration to greater than 2 times the upper limit of normal, and liver function should be monitored closely.

■ **Dosage in Renal and Hepatic Impairment** No adjustment of bicalutamide dosage is necessary in patients with renal impairment. Bicalutamide is extensively metabolized in the liver; however, the pharmacokinetics of the drug do not appear to be altered in patients with mild to moderate hepatic impairment, and no dosage adjustment is required in such patients. Limited pharmacokinetic data indicate that bicalutamide elimination may be delayed in patients with severe hepatic impairment, and the manufacturer states that the drug should be used with caution in patients with moderate to severe hepatic impairment. While no specific recommendations are made regarding modification of bicalutamide dosage in patients with moderate to severe hepatic impairment, the manufacturer states that periodic tests of liver function should be considered in patients with hepatic impairment receiving long-term therapy with the drug. Serum transaminase concentrations should be measured prior to initiation of bicalutamide therapy, at regular intervals during the first 4 months of treatment, and periodically thereafter in all patients receiving bicalutamide. (See Dosage: Discontinuance of Therapy for Hepatic Toxicity under Dosage and Administration.)

Description

Bicalutamide is a nonsteroidal antiandrogen that is structurally and pharmacologically related to flutamide and nilutamide.

Bicalutamide inhibits the action of androgens by competitively blocking nuclear androgen receptors in target tissues such as the prostate, seminal vesicles, and adrenal cortex; blockade of androgen receptors in the hormone-sensitive tumor cells may result in growth arrest or transient tumor regression through inhibition of androgen-dependent DNA and protein synthesis. Bicalutamide is a selective antiandrogen with no androgenic or progestational activity in various animal models. The relative binding affinity of bicalutamide at the androgen receptor is more than that of nilutamide and approximately 4 times that of hydroxyflutamide, the active metabolite of flutamide.

Common pharmacologic therapies for prostate cancer (i.e., gonadotropin-releasing hormone [GnRH] analogs, nonsteroidal antiandrogens) when used as monotherapy initially result in increased serum testosterone concentrations, which may limit the effects of the drugs. Androgen receptors in the hypothalamus are blocked by bicalutamide, which disrupts the inhibitory feedback of testosterone on luteinizing hormone (LH) release, resulting in a temporary increase in secretion of LH; the increase in LH stimulates an increase in the production of testosterone. As GnRH analogs have potent GnRH agonist properties, testicular steroidogenesis continues during the first few weeks after initiating therapy. However, the combination of orchiectomy or GnRH analog therapy to suppress testicular androgen production and an antiandrogen to block response of remaining adrenal androgens provides maximal androgen blockade. Concomitant administration of antiandrogens such as bicalutamide in patients initiating therapy with a GnRH analog can inhibit initial androgenic stimulation and potential exacerbation of symptoms (e.g., bone pain, urinary obstruction, liver pain, impending spinal cord compression) that may occur during the first month of GnRH analog therapy. (See Cautions in Leuprolide Acetate 68:18.08.)

SumMon® (see Users Guide). For additional information on this drug until a more detailed monograph is developed and published, the manufacturer's labeling should be consulted. It is *essential* that the labeling be consulted for detailed information on the usual cautions, precautions, and contraindications. For further information on the handling of antineoplastic agents, see the ASHP Guidelines on Handling Hazardous Drugs at http://www.ahfsdruginformation.com.

Preparations

Excipients in commercially available drug preparations may have clinically important effects in some individuals; consult specific product labeling for details.

Bicalutamide

Oral

Tablets, film-coated	50 mg	**Casodex®**, AstraZeneca

Binimetinib

■ Binimetinib, a reversible inhibitor of mitogen-activated extracellular signal-regulated kinase (MEK) 1 and MEK2, is an antineoplastic agent.

Uses

■ **Melanoma** Binimetinib is used in combination with encorafenib for the treatment of unresectable or metastatic melanoma with b-Raf serine-threonine kinase (BRAF) V600E or V600K mutation. Binimetinib has been designated an orphan drug by FDA for the treatment of this cancer. An FDA-approved diagnostic test (e.g., bioMerieux THxID® BRAF V600 mutation test) is required to confirm the presence of the BRAF V600E or V600K mutation prior to initiation of therapy. In patients with unresectable or metastatic melanoma with BRAF V600E or V600K mutation, combined therapy with binimetinib and encorafenib has been shown to prolong progression-free survival and overall survival, and increase response rate compared with vemurafenib alone.

The current indication for binimetinib is based principally on the results of a randomized, open-label, phase 3 study (COLUMBUS) in patients with unresectable locally advanced or metastatic melanoma positive for V600E or V600K BRAF mutation as detected by the bioMerieux THxID® BRAF V600 mutation test. In this study, 577 patients were randomized (stratified by disease stage, Eastern Cooperative Oncology Group [ECOG] performance status, and prior immunotherapy use) in a 1:1:1 ratio to receive binimetinib 45 mg twice daily with encorafenib 450 mg once daily (binimetinib-encorafenib), encorafenib 300 mg once daily alone, or vemurafenib 960 mg twice daily. Treatment was continued until disease progression or unacceptable toxicity occurred or the patient withdrew from the study. The primary measure of efficacy was progression-free survival (as evaluated by a blinded independent central review committee). The median age of patients randomized to the binimetinib-encorafenib or vemurafenib treatment groups was 56 years; 91% of patients were Caucasian, 59% were male, 95% had metastatic disease, 65% had stage M1c disease, 72% had a baseline ECOG performance status of 0, 28% had elevated LDH concentrations, 45% had tumor involvement in at least 3 organs, and 3% of patients had brain metastases. Approximately 4% of patients enrolled in the binimetinib-encorafenib or vemurafenib treatment groups received prior therapy with an anti-programmed-death 1 (anti-PD-1), anti-programmed-death ligand-1 (anti-PD-L1), or anti-cytotoxic T-lymphocyte-associated antigen 4 (anti-CTLA-4) antibody. Most patients (88%) randomized to receive binimetinib-encorafenib or vemurafenib had BRAF V600E mutation; 11% had V600K mutation and less than 1% had both BRAF V600E and V600K mutations. Patients who had received immunotherapy in the adjuvant setting or one prior immunotherapy regimen for unresectable locally advanced or metastatic melanoma were eligible for this study; however, patients with prior exposure to BRAF or mitogen-activated extracellular signal-regulated kinase (MEK) inhibitors were not eligible to enroll in the study.

At a median follow-up of 16.7 or 14.4 months in patients receiving binimetinib-encorafenib or vemurafenib alone, respectively, median progression-free survival was 14.9 months in patients receiving binimetinib-encorafenib compared with 7.3 months in those receiving vemurafenib. The objective response rate was 63% for patients receiving binimetinib-encorafenib and 40% for those receiving vemurafenib; complete response was achieved in 8% of patients receiving binimetinib-encorafenib and 6% of those receiving vemurafenib. The median duration of response in patients receiving binimetinib-encorafenib or vemurafenib alone was 16.6 or 12.3 months, respectively. At the time of the interim analysis for overall survival at a median follow-up of 36.8 months for the overall study population, the median overall survival was 33.6 or 16.9 months in patients receiving binimetinib-encorafenib or vemurafenib alone, respectively. Results of a subgroup analysis (based on age, gender, race, ECOG performance status, geographic region, baseline serum LDH concentration, BRAF mutation status, disease stage, organ involvement, presence of brain metastases, prior use of first-line immunotherapy or adjuvant therapy) suggested that the effect of binimetinib in combination with encorafenib was consistent across most subgroups; an overall survival benefit for combination therapy with binimetinib and encorafenib versus vemurafenib was not apparent in the small subgroup of patients with brain metastases (hazard ratio: 1.34).

Dosage and Administration

■ **General** Presence of the b-Raf serine-threonine kinase (BRAF) V600E or V600K mutation must be confirmed prior to initiation of therapy with binimetinib in combination with encorafenib. (See Uses: Melanoma.)

Clinicians should consult the manufacturer's labeling for information on the dosage and administration of encorafenib.

Restricted Distribution Program Binimetinib can only be obtained through select specialty pharmacies. Clinicians may contact the manufacturer (Array BioPharma) by telephone at 844-492-7729 or consult the Braftovi® and Mektovi® website for specific availability information (https://www.braftovimektovi.com/hcp/).

■ **Administration** Binimetinib is administered orally twice daily, with doses given approximately 12 hours apart; the drug can be taken without regard to meals. (See Description.)

If a dose of binimetinib is missed by more than 6 hours, the missed dose should be skipped and the next dose should be taken at the regularly scheduled time. Patients should *not* take extra tablets of the drug to make up for the missed dose.

If vomiting occurs following administration of binimetinib, a replacement dose should *not* be administered, and the next dose should be taken at the regularly scheduled time.

■ **Dosage** ***Melanoma*** For use in combination with encorafenib in the treatment of unresectable or metastatic melanoma with BRAF V600E or V600K mutation, the recommended adult dosage of binimetinib is 45 mg twice daily. Therapy should be continued until disease progression or unacceptable toxicity occurs.

If encorafenib therapy is permanently discontinued, binimetinib also should be discontinued. Clinicians should consult the manufacturer's labeling for information on recommended dosage modifications for encorafenib.

Dosage Modification for Toxicity If adverse reactions occur, interruption of therapy, dosage reduction, and/or permanent discontinuance of binimetinib may be required based on severity of the reaction. If dosage modification of binimetinib is necessary, a dosage reduction to 30 mg twice daily is recommended. If a dosage of 30 mg twice daily is not tolerated, binimetinib should be permanently discontinued.

Cardiovascular Toxicity. If an asymptomatic absolute decrease in left ventricular ejection fraction (LVEF) from baseline of more than 10% and to a level below the lower limit of normal (LLN) occurs, binimetinib therapy should be withheld for up to 4 weeks and left ventricular function should be reassessed every 2 weeks; therapy may be resumed at a reduced dosage when an asymptomatic absolute decrease in LVEF from baseline improves to 10% or less and to a level at least the LLN. If the toxicity does not improve within 4 weeks of withholding binimetinib, the drug should be permanently discontinued. (See Cardiac Effects under Cautions: Warnings/Precautions.)

If symptomatic congestive heart failure or an absolute decrease in LVEF from baseline of more than 20% and to a level below the LLN occurs, binimetinib therapy should be permanently discontinued.

If prolongation of QT interval occurs during combination therapy with binimetinib and encorafenib, no dosage modification of binimetinib is necessary.

Venous Thromboembolism. If uncomplicated deep-vein thrombosis (DVT) or pulmonary embolism (PE) occurs, binimetinib therapy should be withheld; therapy may be resumed at a reduced dosage when the toxicity improves to grade 1 or less. If the toxicity does not improve, the drug should be permanently discontinued. (See Venous Thromboembolism under Cautions: Warnings/Precautions.)

If life-threatening PE occurs, binimetinib therapy should be permanently discontinued.

Ocular Effects. If symptomatic serous retinopathy or retinal pigment epithelial detachment occurs, binimetinib therapy should be withheld for up to 10 days; therapy may be resumed at the same dosage when the toxicity improves and the patient becomes asymptomatic. If the toxicity does not improve within 10 days of withholding therapy, therapy may be resumed at a reduced dosage or permanently discontinued. (See Ocular Effects under Cautions: Warnings/Precautions.)

If grade 1 or 2 uveitis unresponsive to ocular therapy occurs, binimetinib therapy should be withheld for up to 6 weeks. If the toxicity improves within 6 weeks of withholding therapy, therapy may be resumed at the same or reduced dosage. If the toxicity does not improve within 6 weeks of withholding therapy, binimetinib therapy should be permanently discontinued.

If grade 3 uveitis occurs, binimetinib therapy should be withheld for up to 6 weeks. If grade 3 uveitis improves within 6 weeks of withholding therapy, therapy may be resumed at the same or reduced dosage. If grade 3 uveitis does not improve within 6 weeks of withholding therapy, binimetinib therapy should be permanently discontinued.

If retinal vein occlusion or grade 4 uveitis occurs, binimetinib therapy should be permanently discontinued.

Pulmonary Effects. If grade 2 interstitial lung disease occurs, binimetinib therapy should be withheld for up to 4 weeks; therapy may be resumed at a reduced dosage when the toxicity improves to grade 1 or less. If grade 2 interstitial lung disease does not improve within 4 weeks of withholding therapy, the drug should be permanently discontinued. (See Pulmonary Effects under Cautions: Warnings/Precautions.)

If grade 3 or 4 interstitial lung disease occurs, binimetinib therapy should be permanently discontinued.

Hepatotoxicity. In patients who develop grade 2 elevations of serum aminotransferases (ALT or AST), binimetinib therapy may be continued at the same dosage for up to 2 weeks. If the toxicity persists, binimetinib therapy should be withheld; therapy may be resumed at the same dosage when the toxicity improves to grade 1 or less or to baseline. (See Hepatic Toxicity under Cautions: Warnings/Precautions.)

For the first occurrence of grade 3 elevations of serum ALT or AST, binimetinib therapy should be withheld for up to 4 weeks; therapy may be resumed at a reduced dosage when the toxicity improves to grade 1 or less or to baseline. If the toxicity does not improve to grade 1 or less or to baseline within 4 weeks of withholding therapy, the drug should be permanently discontinued. If grade 3 elevations of serum ALT or AST recur, permanent discontinuance of binimetinib should be considered.

For the first occurrence of grade 4 elevations of serum ALT or AST, binimetinib therapy may be permanently discontinued or temporarily interrupted. If binimetinib therapy is temporarily interrupted, the drug should be withheld for up to 4 weeks; therapy may be resumed at a reduced dosage when the toxicity improves to grade 1 or less or to baseline. If the toxicity does not improve to grade 1 or less or to baseline within 4 weeks of withholding therapy, the drug should be permanently discontinued. For recurrent grade 4 serum ALT or AST elevations, binimetinib therapy should be permanently discontinued.

Musculoskeletal Effects. In patients who exhibit asymptomatic grade 4 creatine kinase (CK, creatine phosphokinase, CPK) elevations or any grade of CK elevation with symptoms or concomitant renal impairment, binimetinib therapy should be withheld for up to 4 weeks; therapy may be resumed at a reduced dosage when the toxicity improves to grade 1 or less. If the toxicity does not improve within 4 weeks of withholding therapy, the drug should be permanently discontinued. (See Musculoskeletal Effects under Cautions: Warnings/Precautions.)

Dermatologic Effects. For the first occurrence of grade 2 dermatologic reactions, binimetinib therapy should be continued at the same dosage. If the toxicity does not improve within 2 weeks, binimetinib therapy should be withheld; therapy may be resumed at the same dosage when the toxicity improves to grade 1 or less. If grade 2 dermatologic reactions recur and do not improve within 2 weeks, binimetinib therapy should be withheld; therapy may be resumed at a reduced dosage when the toxicity improves to grade 1 or less.

For the first occurrence of grade 3 dermatologic reactions, binimetinib therapy should be withheld; therapy may be resumed at the same dosage when the toxicity improves to grade 1 or less. If grade 3 dermatologic reactions recur, binimetinib therapy should be withheld; therapy may be resumed at a reduced dosage when the toxicity improves to grade 1 or less.

If grade 4 dermatologic reactions occur, binimetinib therapy should be permanently discontinued.

If palmar-plantar erythrodysesthesia syndrome (hand-foot syndrome) develops during combination therapy with binimetinib and encorafenib, no dosage modification of binimetinib is necessary.

Development of New Primary Malignancies. No dosage adjustment of binimetinib is necessary in patients who develop new primary RAS mutation-positive, noncutaneous malignancies during combination therapy with binimetinib and encorafenib. (See Development of New Primary Malignancies under Cautions: Warnings/Precautions.)

Other Toxicity. If grade 2 adverse reaction recurs, binimetinib therapy should be withheld for up to 4 weeks; therapy may be resumed at a reduced dosage when the toxicity improves to grade 1 or less or to baseline. If the toxicity does not improve to grade 1 or less or to baseline within 4 weeks of withholding therapy, the drug should be permanently discontinued.

For the first occurrence of grade 3 adverse reaction, binimetinib therapy should be withheld for up to 4 weeks; therapy may be resumed at a reduced dosage when the toxicity improves to grade 1 or less or to baseline. If the toxicity does not improve to grade 1 or less or to baseline within 4 weeks of withholding therapy, the drug should be permanently discontinued. If grade 3 adverse reaction recurs, permanent discontinuance of binimetinib should be considered.

For the first occurrence of grade 4 adverse reaction, binimetinib therapy may be permanently discontinued or temporarily interrupted. If binimetinib therapy is temporarily interrupted, the drug should be withheld for up to 4 weeks; therapy may be resumed at a reduced dosage when the toxicity improves to grade 1 or less or to baseline. If the grade 4 adverse reaction does not improve to grade 1 or less or to baseline within 4 weeks of withholding therapy, the drug should be permanently discontinued. For recurrent grade 4 adverse reactions, binimetinib therapy should be permanently discontinued.

■ **Special Populations** In patients with moderate (total bilirubin concentration exceeding 1.5 times the upper limit of normal [ULN], but no more than 3 times the ULN, with any AST concentration) or severe (total bilirubin concentration exceeding 3 times the ULN, with any AST concentration) preexisting hepatic impairment, the manufacturer recommends a reduced binimetinib dosage of 30 mg twice daily. No dosage adjustment is necessary in patients with mild hepatic impairment (total bilirubin concentration not exceeding the ULN with AST concentration exceeding the ULN or total bilirubin concentration exceeding the ULN, but no more than 1.5 times the ULN, with any AST concentration). (See Hepatic Impairment under Warnings/Precautions: Specific Populations, in Cautions.)

The manufacturer makes no specific dosage recommendations for patients with renal impairment. (See Renal Impairment under Warnings/Precautions: Specific Populations, in Cautions.)

The manufacturer makes no specific dosage recommendations for geriatric patients. (See Geriatric Use under Warnings/Precautions: Specific Populations, in Cautions.)

Cautions

■ **Contraindications** The manufacturer states there are no known contraindications to the use of binimetinib.

■ **Warnings/Precautions** ***Combination Therapy*** When binimetinib is used in combination with encorafenib, the usual cautions, precautions, and contraindications associated with encorafenib must be considered in addition to those associated with binimetinib. For further information regarding warnings and precautions associated with encorafenib, see Cautions in Encorafenib 10:00.

Cardiac Effects Cardiomyopathy, which may manifest as a symptomatic or asymptomatic decrease in left ventricular ejection fraction (LVEF), has been reported in patients receiving binimetinib in combination with encorafenib. In the COLUMBUS study, cardiomyopathy (defined as an absolute decrease in LVEF from baseline of more than 10% and to a level below the lower limit of normal [LLN]) occurred in 7% of patients receiving binimetinib in combination with encorafenib; grade 3 left ventricular dysfunction occurred in 1.6% of patients receiving combination therapy. The median time to first onset of left ventricular dysfunction was 3.6 months (range: 0–21 months). Cardiomyopathy resolved in 87% of patients receiving combination therapy with binimetinib and encorafenib.

Safety of combination therapy with binimetinib and encorafenib has not been established in patients with a baseline LVEF below the LLN or less than 50%.

LVEF should be assessed using echocardiogram or multigated radionuclide angiography (MUGA) prior to and 1 month after initiation of binimetinib and then every 2–3 months during therapy. Close monitoring during therapy is indicated in patients with preexisting cardiovascular risk factors. If left ventricular dysfunction occurs, temporary interruption followed by dosage reduction or discontinuance of binimetinib may be necessary. (See Cardiovascular Toxicity under Dosage: Dosage Modification for Toxicity, in Dosage and Administration.)

Venous Thromboembolism Venous thromboembolism (VTE) has been reported in patients receiving binimetinib in combination with encorafenib. In the COLUMBUS study, VTE occurred in 6% of patients receiving binimetinib in combination with encorafenib; 3.1% of patients receiving combination therapy developed pulmonary embolism (PE).

If deep-vein thrombosis (DVT) or PE occurs, temporary interruption followed by dosage reduction or discontinuance of binimetinib may be necessary. (See Venous Thromboembolism under Dosage: Dosage Modification for Toxicity, in Dosage and Administration.)

Ocular Effects Serous retinopathy, retinal vein occlusion, retinal pigment epithelial detachment, and macular edema have been reported in patients receiving binimetinib in combination with encorafenib. Uveitis, including iritis and iridocyclitis, also has occurred in patients receiving binimetinib in combination with encorafenib.

In the COLUMBUS study, serous retinopathy occurred in 20% of patients receiving combination therapy with binimetinib and encorafenib; macular edema and retinal detachment were reported in 6 and 8%, respectively, of patients receiving combination therapy. Symptomatic serous retinopathy occurred in 8% of patients receiving combination therapy with binimetinib and encorafenib; blindness was not reported in these patients. The median time to initial onset of serous retinopathy was 1.2 months (range: 0–17.5 months). Discontinuance of binimetinib therapy was not necessary in patients experiencing serous retinopathy; however, dosage modification or interruption of binimetinib therapy was necessary in 6% of patients.

Retinal vein occlusion is a known risk of mitogen-activated extracellular signal-regulated kinase (MEK) inhibitors. In clinical trials evaluating combination therapy with binimetinib and encorafenib, retinal vein occlusion occurred in 1 of 690 patients (0.1%) with b-Raf serine-threonine kinase (BRAF) mutation-positive melanoma. In the COLUMBUS study, uveitis was reported in 4% of patients receiving binimetinib in combination with encorafenib.

Safety of binimetinib has not been established in patients with a history of or predisposition to retinal vein occlusion, including those with uncontrolled glaucoma or a history of hyperviscosity or hypercoagulability syndromes.

Ophthalmologic examinations should be performed regularly and as clinically indicated (i.e., if new or worsening visual disturbances occur; to follow new or persistent ophthalmologic findings) during binimetinib therapy. Patients should be monitored for visual symptoms at each visit. If visual disturbances are reported, ophthalmologic evaluations should be performed urgently (within 24 hours). Temporary interruption, dosage reduction, or discontinuance of binimetinib may be necessary if ocular toxicities occur during therapy with the drug. (See Ocular Effects under Dosage: Dosage Modification for Toxicity, in Dosage and Administration.)

Pulmonary Effects Interstitial lung disease or pneumonitis has been reported in patients receiving combination therapy with binimetinib and encorafenib. In clinical trials evaluating combination therapy with binimetinib and encorafenib, interstitial lung disease and pneumonitis occurred in 2 of 690 patients (0.3%) with BRAF mutation-positive melanoma.

Patients presenting with manifestations of interstitial lung disease (e.g., new or progressive pulmonary symptoms) should be evaluated. If a diagnosis of interstitial lung disease is confirmed, temporary interruption followed by dosage reduction or discontinuance of binimetinib may be necessary. (See Pulmonary Effects under Dosage: Dosage Modification for Toxicity, in Dosage and Administration.)

Hepatic Toxicity Liver function test abnormalities have been reported in patients receiving combination therapy with binimetinib and encorafenib. In the COLUMBUS study, grade 3 or 4 elevations in ALT, AST, or alkaline phosphatase concentrations occurred in 6, 2.6, or 0.5%, respectively, of patients receiving combination therapy with binimetinib and encorafenib; grade 3 or 4 elevations in serum bilirubin were not reported.

Liver function tests should be performed prior to initiation of binimetinib therapy and then monthly, or more frequently as clinically indicated, during therapy with the drug. Temporary interruption, dosage reduction, or discontinuance of binimetinib may be necessary if liver function test abnormalities occur during therapy with the drug. (See Hepatotoxicity under Dosage: Dosage Modification for Toxicity, in Dosage and Administration.)

Musculoskeletal Effects Rhabdomyolysis has been reported in patients receiving combination therapy with binimetinib and encorafenib. In clinical trials evaluating combination therapy with binimetinib and encorafenib, rhabdomyolysis occurred in 1 of 690 patients (0.1%) with BRAF mutation-positive melanoma. In the COLUMBUS study, elevations of serum creatine kinase (CK, creatine phosphokinase, CPK) occurred in 58% of patients receiving combination therapy with binimetinib and encorafenib.

Serum CK and creatinine concentrations should be evaluated at baseline, periodically during binimetinib therapy, and as clinically indicated. If elevated CK concentrations occur, therapy interruption followed by dosage reduction or discontinuance of binimetinib may be necessary. (See Musculoskeletal Effects under Dosage: Dosage Modification for Toxicity, in Dosage and Administration.)

Hemorrhage Hemorrhage has been reported in patients receiving combination therapy with binimetinib and encorafenib. In the COLUMBUS study, hemorrhage occurred in 19% of patients and was grade 3 or greater in 3.2% of patients receiving binimetinib in combination with encorafenib. The most common hemorrhagic events in patients receiving binimetinib in combination with encorafenib were GI hemorrhage, including rectal hemorrhage (4.2%), hematochezia (3.1%), and hemorrhoidal hemorrhage (1%). Intracranial hemorrhage was fatal in 1.6% of patients with new or progressive brain metastases receiving combination therapy with binimetinib and encorafenib.

If hemorrhagic events occur, therapy interruption followed by dosage reduction or discontinuance of binimetinib may be necessary. (See Other Toxicity under Dosage: Dosage Modification for Toxicity, in Dosage and Administration.)

Fetal/Neonatal Morbidity and Mortality Binimetinib may cause fetal harm in humans based on its mechanism of action and animal findings; the drug has been shown to be embryotoxic, fetotoxic, and teratogenic in animals. There are no available data regarding the risk of binimetinib use in pregnant women to date. In animal reproduction studies, embryofetal toxicity (i.e., decreases in fetal body weight, postimplantation loss, abortion) and teratogenic effects were observed in rabbits receiving binimetinib at exposure levels of approximately 5 times the human exposure at the recommended dosage; fetal ventricular septal defects and pulmonary trunk alterations were increased at exposure levels less than 8 times the human exposure. Skeletal anomalies also were observed in rats receiving binimetinib at exposure levels of approximately 37 times the human exposure at the recommended dosage.

Pregnancy should be avoided during binimetinib therapy. The manufacturer states that pregnancy status should be verified prior to initiation of binimetinib therapy in women of childbearing potential and that such women should be advised to use effective contraception while receiving binimetinib and for at least 30 days after the last dose. Patients should be apprised of the potential hazard to the fetus if the drug is used during pregnancy.

Development of New Primary Malignancies New primary cutaneous and noncutaneous malignancies are a known class effect of BRAF inhibitors (i.e., dabrafenib, encorafenib, vemurafenib). In the COLUMBUS study, cutaneous squamous cell carcinoma (including keratoacanthoma) or basal cell carcinoma occurred in 2.6 or 1.6%, respectively, of patients receiving binimetinib in combination with encorafenib. In the COLUMBUS study, noncutaneous malignancy was reported in 3 of 192 patients (1.6%) receiving single-agent encorafenib compared with 2 of 192 patients (1%) receiving combination therapy with encorafenib and binimetinib.

Although the mechanism for development of cutaneous squamous cell carcinoma has not been fully determined, it has been suggested that BRAF inhibitors may cause paradoxical activation of mitogen-activated protein kinase (MAPK) signaling, which may lead to accelerated growth of such skin lesions as well as development of other primary malignancies. Some data suggest that MEK inhibitors (i.e., binimetinib, cobimetinib, trametinib) block the paradoxical activation of the MAPK pathway induced by BRAF inhibitors; therefore, combination therapy with a BRAF inhibitor and an MEK inhibitor may reduce the risk of developing cutaneous squamous cell carcinoma. Findings from a meta-analysis of randomized controlled studies that assessed the relative risk of development of cutaneous squamous cell carcinoma in cancer patients receiving a BRAF inhibitor indicate that the risk of cutaneous squamous cell carcinoma is higher in patients receiving a BRAF inhibitor than in patients receiving combination therapy with a BRAF inhibitor and an MEK inhibitor.

Specific Populations **Pregnancy.** Binimetinib may cause fetal harm if administered to pregnant women based on its mechanism of action and animal findings. (See Fetal/Neonatal Morbidity and Mortality under Cautions: Warnings/Precautions.)

Pregnancy status should be verified in women of childbearing potential prior to initiation of binimetinib therapy.

Lactation. It is not known whether binimetinib or its metabolites are distributed into human milk. Because of the potential for serious adverse reactions to binimetinib in nursing infants, women should be advised not to breast-feed while receiving the drug and for 3 days after the last dose. The effects of the drug on nursing infants or on the production of milk are unknown.

Pediatric Use. Safety and efficacy of binimetinib have not been established in pediatric patients.

Geriatric Use. In clinical trials evaluating binimetinib (45 mg twice daily) in combination with encorafenib (300–600 mg once daily) in patients with BRAF mutation-positive melanoma, 20% of patients were 65–74 years of age and 8% were 75 years of age or older. No overall differences in safety or efficacy were observed between geriatric patients and younger adults.

Hepatic Impairment. Systemic exposure of binimetinib is increased by 80 or 110% in individuals with moderate (total bilirubin concentration exceeding 1.5 times the ULN, but not more than 3 times the ULN, with any AST concentration) or severe (total bilirubin concentration exceeding 3 times the ULN, with any AST concentration) hepatic impairment, respectively, compared with individuals with normal hepatic function; therefore, dosage adjustment is recommended in patients with moderate or severe hepatic impairment. (See Dosage and Administration: Special Populations.)

No clinically important differences in systemic exposure of binimetinib were observed between individuals with mild hepatic impairment (total bilirubin concentration not exceeding the ULN with AST concentration exceeding the ULN or total bilirubin concentration exceeding the ULN, but no more than 1.5 times the ULN, with any AST concentration) and those with normal hepatic function; no dosage adjustment is necessary in patients with mild hepatic impairment.

Renal Impairment. No clinically important differences in systemic exposure of binimetinib were observed between individuals with severe renal impairment (estimated glomerular filtration rate not more than 29 mL/minute per 1.73 m^2) and those with normal renal function.

■ Common Adverse Effects

Adverse effects reported in 20% or more of patients receiving binimetinib in combination with encorafenib for the treatment of unresectable or metastatic melanoma with BRAF V600E or V600K mutation include fatigue, nausea, diarrhea, vomiting, abdominal pain, constipation, arthralgia, hyperkeratosis, myopathy, headache, rash, asthenia, visual impairment, serous retinopathy/retinal pigment epithelial detachment (RPED), and pyrexia. Laboratory abnormalities reported in 20% or more of patients receiving binimetinib in combination with encorafenib include elevated concentrations of serum creatinine, elevated concentrations of CK, elevated concentrations of γ-glutamyltransferase (γ-glutamyltranspeptidase, GGT, GGTP), anemia, elevated concentrations of aminotransferases (i.e., AST, ALT), and elevated concentrations of alkaline phosphatase.

Drug Interactions

Binimetinib is metabolized principally by uridine diphosphate-glucuronosyltransferase (UGT) 1A1 and, to a lesser extent, by cytochrome P-450 (CYP) isoenzymes 1A2 and 2C19 to form a minor active metabolite (M3). Binimetinib is a weak inhibitor of UGT1A. The drug does not demonstrate time-dependent inhibition of CYP isoenzymes 1A2, 2C9, 2D6, and 3A, and shows little to no induction of CYP2C9.

In vitro studies indicate that binimetinib is a substrate of P-glycoprotein (P-gp) and breast cancer resistance protein (BCRP); the drug is not a substrate of organic cation transporter (OCT) 1 or organic anion transport protein (OATP) 1B1, OATP1B3, and OATP2B1. In vitro, binimetinib is a weak inhibitor of OCT2, but does not inhibit OCT1.

■ **Drugs Metabolized by Hepatic Microsomal Enzymes** Concomitant administration of binimetinib (30 mg orally twice daily for 7 or 15 days) with the CYP3A4 substrate midazolam (single oral dose of 4 mg) did not substantially alter systemic exposure of midazolam.

■ **Drugs Affecting Uridine Diphosphate-glucuronosyltransferase** Binimetinib is a substrate of UGT1A1; however, in vitro studies indicate that binimetinib is unlikely to interact with drugs affecting UGT1A1.

Concomitant administration of binimetinib with the UGT1A1 inhibitor encorafenib did not substantially alter systemic exposure of binimetinib. Pharmacokinetic simulations also suggest that concomitant administration of atazanavir (single 400-mg dose), a UGT1A1 inhibitor, and binimetinib (single 45-mg dose) does not substantially alter peak plasma concentrations of binimetinib.

Cigarette smoking has been shown to induce UGT1A1; however, cigarette smoking did not have a clinically important effect on systemic exposure of binimetinib.

■ **Drugs Transported by Organic Cation Transporters** Clinically important pharmacokinetic interactions between drugs that are substrates of OCT1 or OCT2 and binimetinib are not expected during concurrent use.

■ **Drugs Affecting Gastric Acidity** Concomitant administration of the proton-pump inhibitor rabeprazole (20 mg once daily for 4 days) with binimetinib (single 45-mg dose) did not result in clinically important changes in peak plasma concentrations and systemic exposure of binimetinib and M3.

Description

Binimetinib, a reversible inhibitor of mitogen-activated extracellular signal-regulated kinase (MEK) 1 and MEK2, is an antineoplastic agent. MEK proteins are upstream regulators of the extracellular signal-related kinase (ERK) pathway, which promotes cellular proliferation. Approximately 40–60% of cutaneous melanomas carry a b-Raf serine-threonine kinase (BRAF) mutation. The most common BRAF mutation is the substitution of glutamic acid for valine at codon 600 in exon 15 (BRAF V600E); a less frequently occurring BRAF mutation is the substitution of lysine for valine at codon 600 in exon 15 (BRAF V600K). BRAF V600 mutations result in activation of the BRAF pathway that includes MEK 1 and 2. The mutation of BRAF V600E activates the mitogen-activated protein kinase (MAPK) and ERK signal transduction pathway, which enhances cell proliferation and tumor progression (e.g., metastasis). In vitro studies have demonstrated that binimetinib inhibits phosphorylation of ERK in cell-free assays and MEK-dependent phosphorylation of melanoma cells harboring BRAF mutation. The drug also has demonstrated inhibition of ERK phosphorylation and tumor growth in xenograft models of melanoma harboring BRAF mutation in mice.

Clinical resistance to monotherapy with a BRAF inhibitor, generally occurring 6–7 months following initiation of therapy, has been attributed to several possible resistance mechanisms mostly relying on reactivation of the MAPK/ERK pathway. Complete inhibition of the MAPK/ERK pathway resulting in durable responses may be achieved with the use of combination therapy with a BRAF inhibitor (i.e., dabrafenib, encorafenib, vemurafenib) and an MEK inhibitor (i.e., binimetinib, cobimetinib, trametinib). In vitro, use of binimetinib in combination with encorafenib resulted in increased antiproliferative activity compared with either drug alone in BRAF mutation-positive cell lines. The combination of binimetinib and encorafenib also has demonstrated increased inhibition of tumor growth and delayed emergence of resistance compared with either drug alone in xenograft models of melanoma harboring BRAF V600E mutation in mice.

Following oral administration of binimetinib 45 mg twice daily, at least 50% of the dose is rapidly absorbed with peak plasma concentrations occurring in 1.6 hours. Peak plasma concentrations and systemic exposure of binimetinib and its active metabolite (M3) are proportional to dose following single or repeated administration of the drug over the dosage range of 5–80 mg or 5–60 mg once daily, respectively. Repeated administration of binimetinib 45 mg twice daily resulted in a 1.5-fold binimetinib accumulation ratio. Administration of a single 45-mg dose of binimetinib with a high-fat, high-calorie meal (approximately 150 calories from protein, 350 calories from carbohydrates, 500 calories from fat) did not affect systemic exposure (area under the serum concentration-time curve [AUC]) of the drug in healthy individuals. Binimetinib is highly bound (97%) to plasma proteins. The mean terminal half-life of binimetinib is 3.5 hours. Binimetinib is metabolized principally by uridine diphosphate-glucuronosyltransferase (UGT) 1A1 and, to a lesser extent, by *N*-dealkylation and amide hydrolysis by cytochrome P-450 (CYP) isoenzymes 1A2 and 2C19 to form its minor active metabolite (M3). Following oral administration of a single radiolabeled dose of binimetinib, 62% of the radioactivity was recovered in feces (32% of the dose as unchanged drug) and 31% was recovered in urine (6.5% of the dose as unchanged drug).

The pharmacokinetics of binimetinib do not appear to be affected substantially by age (20–94 years), gender, body weight, or UGT1A1 genotype.

Advice to Patients

Importance of reading the manufacturer's patient information.

If a dose of binimetinib is missed by more than 6 hours or vomited, importance of administering the next dose at the regularly scheduled time; an additional dose should not be administered to replace the missed or vomited dose.

Risk of hemorrhage. Importance of contacting a clinician promptly and seeking immediate medical attention if signs and/or symptoms of unusual bleeding (e.g., headache, dizziness, weakness, blood in stool, coughing up blood, vomiting blood) occur.

Risk of venous thromboembolism (VTE). Importance of contacting a clinician promptly and seeking immediate medical attention if sudden onset of breathing difficulty, chest pain, leg pain, or swelling occurs.

Risk of cardiomyopathy. Importance of contacting a clinician promptly if manifestations of heart failure (e.g., tachycardia, shortness of breath, peripheral edema, feeling lightheaded) occur.

Risk of serous retinopathy or retinal vein occlusion. Importance of contacting a clinician promptly if ocular pain, swelling, redness, changes in vision, or blurred vision occurs.

Risk of interstitial lung disease. Importance of contacting a clinician if new or progressive pulmonary symptoms (e.g., cough, dyspnea) occur.

Risk of hepatotoxicity. Importance of liver function test monitoring before and during binimetinib therapy. Importance of reporting any possible manifestations of hepatotoxicity (e.g., jaundice, dark or tea-colored urine, nausea, vomiting, fatigue, loss of appetite, bruising, bleeding).

Risk of rhabdomyolysis. Importance of monitoring creatine kinase (CK, creatine phosphokinase, CPK) concentrations before and during binimetinib therapy. Importance of immediately reporting any possible manifestations of rhabdomyolysis (e.g., dark or red urine, muscle pain, unusual or new-onset weakness).

Risk of fetal harm. Necessity of advising women of childbearing potential that they should use an effective method of contraception while receiving the drug and for at least 30 days after the last dose. Importance of women informing clinicians if they are or plan to become pregnant. Apprise patient of potential fetal hazard if used during pregnancy. (See Fetal/Neonatal Morbidity and Mortality under Cautions: Warnings/Precautions.)

Importance of advising women to avoid breast-feeding while receiving binimetinib and for 3 days after the last dose.

Importance of informing clinicians of existing or contemplated concomitant therapy, including prescription and OTC drugs and herbal supplements, as well as any concomitant illnesses.

Importance of informing patients of other important precautionary information. (See Cautions.)

Overview® (see Users Guide). For additional information on this drug until a more detailed monograph is developed and published, the manufacturer's labeling should be consulted. It is *essential* that the manufacturer's labeling be consulted for more detailed information on usual cautions, precautions, contraindications, potential drug interactions, laboratory test interferences, and acute toxicity. For further information on the handling of antineoplastic agents, see the ASHP Guidelines on Handling Hazardous Drugs at http://www.ahfsdruginformation.com.

Preparations

Distribution of binimetinib is restricted. (See Restricted Distribution Program under Dosage and Administration: General.)

Excipients in commercially available drug preparations may have clinically important effects in some individuals; consult specific product labeling for details.

Binimetinib

Oral

Tablets, film-coated	15 mg	**Mektovi®**, Array BioPharma

Bleomycin Sulfate

■ Bleomycin sulfate, a mixture of basic cytotoxic glycopeptide antibiotics produced by *Streptomyces verticillus* (bleomycin A_2 and bleomycin B_2 are the major components), is an antineoplastic agent.

Uses

■ **Hodgkin's Disease** Bleomycin is used in combination chemotherapy for the treatment of Hodgkin's disease. Combination therapy for induction of remissions in Hodgkin's disease is superior to single-drug therapy. Various regimens have been used in combination therapy and comparative efficacy is continually being evaluated.

Bleomycin is used with doxorubicin, vinblastine, and dacarbazine (known as the ABVD regimen) for the treatment of Hodgkin's disease. Use of the ABVD regimen for 6–8 months is as effective and less myelotoxic than use of an alternating schedule of ABVD with the MOPP regimen (mechlorethamine, vincristine, procarbazine, and prednisone) for 12 months for the treatment of advanced Hodgkin's disease.

Bleomycin also has been used in hybrid regimens in which 7 or 8 active antineoplastic agents are given during the same course of treatment; however, a large randomized trial comparing the ABVD regimen with the MOPP/ABV hybrid regimen in patients with stage III or IV Hodgkin's disease or recurrent Hodgkin's disease following radiation therapy shows equivalent rates of complete response, failure-free survival, and overall survival, but greater incidence of toxicity, including life-threatening hematologic toxicity and secondary hematologic malignancies, in those receiving the hybrid regimen.

■ **Testicular Cancer** Bleomycin is labeled for use in the treatment of testicular embryonal cell carcinoma, choriocarcinoma, and teratocarcinoma.

For the treatment of advanced nonseminomatous testicular carcinoma, combination chemotherapy with bleomycin, cisplatin, and etoposide is a regimen of choice; this regimen also is used for the treatment of disseminated seminoma testis. Although testicular cancer often is curable, all newly diagnosed patients may be considered for enrollment in clinical trials investigating therapies to improve cure rates and reduce treatment-related morbidity.

■ **Pleural Effusions** Bleomycin is used by intracavitary injection as a sclerosing agent for the management of pleural effusions and for prevention of recurrent pleural effusions caused by metastatic tumors. Patients with pleural effusions frequently have symptoms of dyspnea, cough, and chest pain and heaviness. Although thoracentesis (needle aspiration) may provide temporary relief of such symptoms, the effusion often reaccumulates rapidly; surgical insertion of a thoracostomy tube with subsequent intrapleural instillation of a sclerosing agent generally is considered the treatment of choice for such effusions in patients with neoplasms unresponsive to systemic antineoplastic or radiation therapy. When instilled into the pleural space, sclerosing agents cause inflammation that results in fibrosis and adherence of serosal surfaces (pleurodesis), thereby obliterating the pleural space and reducing the chance of fluid reaccumulation; however, most current pleurodesis procedures for malignant pleural effusion appear to be associated with a substantial risk of recurrence.

Bleomycin appears to be at least as effective as and possibly better tolerated than tetracycline in the treatment of these effusions. Therefore, bleomycin has been suggested as a suitable alternative to tetracycline, which no longer is commercially available in the US as a parenteral preparation, for pleural effusions when intracavitary therapy is indicated.

In a randomized, multicenter clinical study in patients with malignant pleural effusions, intracavitary administration of 60 units of bleomycin was associated with substantial lower recurrence rate and longer time to recurrence compared to those associated with intracavitary administration of 1 g of tetracycline; toxicity and overall survival were similar in both groups. Recurrence rates within 30 days of drug administration were 36 or 67% for patients receiving bleomycin or tetracycline, respectively, while corresponding recurrence rates within 90 days of drug administration were 30 or 53% for patients receiving bleomycin or tetracycline, respectively. In addition, the median time to recurrence was at least 46 days in patients receiving bleomycin and 32 days in patients receiving tetracycline.

The efficacy and safety of intrapleural bleomycin compared with intrapleural administration of doxycycline, minocycline, talc slurry, or other therapies (e.g., talc insufflation during thoracoscopy or open thoracotomy) for the management of malignant pleural effusions remain to be determined. In one randomized trial, similar response rates were observed in patients receiving bleomycin or doxycycline sclerotherapy for the treatment of malignant pleural effusions. Limited evidence from small randomized studies suggests that talc slurry, a less costly drug, is as effective as bleomycin as a sclerosing agent administered via bedside thoracostomy for the treatment of malignant pleural effusions, but further study is needed to establish these findings. A large, randomized trial comparing the safety and efficacy of bleomycin, doxycycline, or talc administered via an indwelling pleural catheter for the treatment of malignant pleural effusions is under way.

■ **Head and Neck Cancer** Bleomycin is labeled for use in the palliative treatment of squamous cell carcinomas of the head and neck (including mouth, tongue, tonsils, nasopharynx, oropharynx, sinuses, palate, lip, buccal mucosa, gingiva, epiglottis, larynx, skin). A poorer response to bleomycin has been reported in patients who have received prior radiation therapy for the treatment of head and neck cancer.

Bleomycin has been used in the treatment of advanced head and neck cancer. In a randomized trial, patients receiving bleomycin, cisplatin, methotrexate, and vincristine for recurrent or metastatic head and neck cancer had higher rates of complete response than those receiving cisplatin and fluorouracil. Although both combination regimens produced a higher rate of objective response than cisplatin alone, no difference in survival was detected among the treatment groups.

■ **Cervical Cancer** Bleomycin is labeled for use in the palliative treatment of squamous cell carcinoma of the cervix.

Although bleomycin has been shown to be an active agent in cervical cancer and has been used in various combination chemotherapy regimens (bleomycin, cisplatin, and ifosfamide with mesna [BIP]; bleomycin, cisplatin, mitomycin, and vincristine [BOMP]) for the treatment of metastatic or recurrent cervical cancer, most experts currently do not consider it a drug of choice for the treatment of advanced cervical cancer. The benefit of combination cisplatin-based chemotherapy regimens versus cisplatin alone has not been fully established, and further study is needed to determine the role of bleomycin, which can cause pulmonary toxicity, in the treatment of advanced cervical cancer. (See Uses: Cervical Cancer in Cisplatin 10:00 for overview of treatment for cervical cancer.)

■ **AIDS-related Kaposi's Sarcoma** Bleomycin sulfate is used in combination chemotherapy for the palliative treatment of AIDS-related Kaposi's sarcoma†. Combination chemotherapy with the drug (e.g., bleomycin, doxorubicin, and a vinca alkaloid [vinblastine or vincristine]) has been considered a regimen of choice, but many clinicians currently consider a liposomal anthracycline (doxorubicin or daunorubicin) the first-line therapy of choice for advanced AIDS-related Kaposi's sarcoma (see Uses: AIDS-related Kaposi's Sarcoma in Doxorubicin 10:00 for overview and further discussion of therapy; also see Daunorubicin 10:00).

Combination chemotherapy with conventional antineoplastic agents (e.g., bleomycin, conventional doxorubicin, etoposide, vinblastine, vincristine) usually has been used for more advanced disease (e.g., extensive mucocutaneous disease, lymphedema, symptomatic visceral disease). However, the results of several randomized, multicenter trials indicate that patients receiving a liposomal anthracycline for the treatment of advanced AIDS-related Kaposi's sarcoma experience similar or higher response rates with a more favorable toxic effects profile than those receiving combination therapy with conventional chemotherapeutic agents.

Bleomycin sulfate also has been used alone for the palliative treatment of AIDS-related Kaposi's sarcoma. Response rates observed with bleomycin monotherapy in early stage AIDS-related Kaposi's sarcoma appear to be similar to those observed with other single-agent chemotherapy (e.g., conventional doxorubicin, etoposide, vinblastine, vincristine). Although single-agent therapy usually has not been used in the management of advanced stages of AIDS-related Kaposi's sarcoma, in one study in patients with advanced-stage disease who received a 72-hour continuous IV infusion of bleomycin (20 units/m^2daily) every 3 weeks, partial response was reported in up to 65% of patients.

■ **Other Uses** Bleomycin is labeled for use in the palliative treatment of squamous cell carcinomas of the penis and vulva. Bleomycin has been used in combination with other antineoplastic agents for the treatment of advanced or recurrent penile cancer.

Bleomycin has been used in the treatment of non-Hodgkin's lymphoma; however, several randomized controlled trials and an analysis of pooled data from several randomized studies indicate that second- or third-generation combination regimens containing bleomycin are no more effective than the standard CHOP regimen (cyclophosphamide, doxorubicin, vincristine, and prednisone) for the treatment of advanced intermediate-grade or high-grade non-Hodgkin's lymphoma.

Bleomycin is used in combination with cisplatin and etoposide for the treatment of ovarian germ cell tumors†.

Bleomycin in combination with cisplatin and vinblastine has been used for the treatment of intracranial germ cell tumors†.

Bleomycin has been used intrapleurally for sclerotherapy in the management of pneumothorax† in a limited number of patients (e.g., pneumothorax associated with acquired immunodeficiency syndrome [AIDS] and *Pneumocystis jiroveci* [formerly *Pneumocystis carinii*] pneumonia).

Dosage and Administration

■ **Reconstitution and Administration** Bleomycin sulfate is administered by IV, IM, subcutaneous, or intrapleural (intracavitary) injection.

For IM or subcutaneous administration, the drug is reconstituted by adding 1–5 or 2–10 mL of sterile water for injection, 0.9% sodium chloride injection, or bacteriostatic water for injection to the vial labeled as containing 15 or 30 units of bleomycin, respectively, to provide solutions containing 3–15 units/mL. For IV administration, a minimum of 5 or 10 mL of 0.9% sodium chloride injection is added to the vial labeled as containing 15 or 30 units of bleomycin, respectively, to provide a solution containing not more than 3 units/mL. IV administration of bleomycin should be made slowly over a 10-minute period. For intrapleural administration, 60 units of bleomycin should be dissolved in 50–100 mL of 0.9% sodium chloride injection and administered through a thoracostomy tube.

Parenteral drug products should be inspected visually for particulate matter and discoloration whenever solution and container permit.

■ **Dosage** Dosage of bleomycin sulfate is expressed in terms of bleomycin. Dosage of bleomycin must be based on the tolerance and clinical response of the patient in order to obtain optimum therapeutic results with minimum adverse effects. Clinicians should consult published protocols for the dosage of bleomycin and other chemotherapeutic agents and the method and sequence of administration.

Hodgkin's Disease Because of an increased possibility of anaphylactoid reactions in lymphoma patients, these patients should receive test doses of 2 units of bleomycin or less for the first 2 doses. If no acute reaction occurs, the recommended adult dosage may then be administered.

For the treatment of Hodgkin's disease in adults, the manufacturer recommends weekly or twice weekly IV, IM, or subcutaneous bleomycin doses of 0.25–0.5 units/kg (10–20 units/m^2). Following a 50% regression of tumor size in adults with Hodgkin's disease, a maintenance IM or IV dose of 1 unit of bleomycin daily or 5 units weekly can be given. If improvement occurs in patients with Hodgkin's disease, it is usually evident within 2 weeks.

Testicular Cancer For the treatment of testicular cancer in adults, the manufacturer recommends weekly or twice weekly IV, IM, or subcutaneous bleomycin doses of 0.25–0.5 units/kg (10–20 units/m^2). If improvement occurs in patients with testicular cancer, it is usually evident within 2 weeks.

Pleural Effusions Drainage of the pleural fluid is necessary prior to instillation of bleomycin.When used as a sclerosing agent to control pleural effusions caused by metastatic tumors in adults, 50–60 units (but generally not exceeding 1 unit/kg or 40 units/m^2 in geriatric patients) of bleomycin usually should be diluted with 50–100 mL of 0.9% sodium chloride and instilled into the chest through a thoracostomy tube followed by clamping of the tube, periodic rotation (from the supine to the left and right lateral position) of the patient during the next 4 hours, and subsequent removal of the fluid. Some clinicians state that periodic rotation of patients is not necessary since repositioning is unlikely to increase efficacy of sclerotherapy.

Prior to instillation of bleomycin in patients with effusions, the pleural cavity should be drained via the thoracostomy by gravity or suction; confirmation of complete expansion of the lungs is recommended. Complete drainage of the pleural fluid and reestablishment of negative intrapleural pressure prior to instillation of sclerotherapy is considered necessary for successful pleurodesis; therefore, the amount of drainage from the chest tube should be as minimal as possible prior to the instillation of bleomycin. Efficacy may be reduced if the solution were introduced into the pleural cavity while fluid drainage continued to exceed 100 mL per 24 hours. However, the manufacturer states that intrapleural administration of bleomycin sulfate may be initiated when drainage is 100–300 mL in 24 hours provided that the patient's clinical condition requires sclerotherapy.

The manufacturer states that the length of time the chest tube remains in the pleural space after instillation of the drug should be individualized depending on the clinical status of the patient; some clinicians recommend that the chest tube remain for at least 4 days after instillation, in order to prevent pneumothorax.

Squamous Cell Carcinomas For the treatment of squamous cell carcinoma in adults, the manufacturer recommends weekly or twice weekly IV, IM, or subcutaneous bleomycin doses of 0.25–0.5 units/kg (10–20 units/m^2). Three weeks of bleomycin therapy may be required before improvement is seen in patients with squamous cell carcinoma.

Dosage Modification for Toxicity and Contraindications to Continued Therapy Because of the increased incidence of toxicity, especially pulmonary toxicity, associated with large cumulative dosages, cumulative dosages exceeding 400 units of bleomycin in adults should be given with great caution. When bleomycin is used in conjunction with other antineoplastic agents, pulmonary toxicity may occur at lower cumulative dosages of bleomycin.

Pulmonary Toxicity. Bleomycin therapy should be promptly discontinued with the appearance of clinical manifestations or radiologic evidence of pulmonary toxicity until it can be determined whether it is drug related. Bleomycin should be discontinued when the pulmonary diffusion capacity for carbon monoxide (DL_{co}) is less than 30–35% of the pretreatment value.

Monitoring of pulmonary function tests for alteration in the pulmonary status, such as decreased total lung volume and decreased vital capacity, is not reliable for predicting the development of pulmonary fibrosis. Some clinicians suggest that bleomycin should be discontinued if forced vital capacity decreases rapidly.

Reduction in the infusion rate of bleomycin or discontinuance of the drug is advised in patients experiencing acute chest pain syndrome suggestive of pleuropericarditis. (See Dosage Modification for Toxicity and Contraindications to Continued Therapy: Cardiac Toxicity, under Dosage and Administration: Dosage.)

Cardiac Toxicity. Reduction in the infusion rate of bleomycin or discontinuance of the drug is advised in patients experiencing acute chest pain syndrome suggestive of pleuropericarditis. (See Cautions: Respiratory Effects.) The manufacturer states that further courses of bleomycin therapy do not appear to be contraindicated, although careful evaluation of the patient must precede continuation of therapy. Some clinicians recommend discontinuance of the drug in patients with intractable pain or ECG changes suggestive of pericarditis.

Dermatologic and Mucocutaneous Toxicity. Discontinuance of therapy because of mucocutaneous toxicity may be required in patients receiving bleomycin.

■ Dosage in Renal Impairment Clearance of bleomycin may be reduced in patients with renal impairment; there are no guidelines for dosage adjustments in such patients, but the manufacturer states that the drug should be used with extreme caution in patients with severe renal impairment.

Cautions

■ Respiratory Effects The most serious toxic effect of bleomycin is pulmonary reactions, usually presenting as interstitial pneumonitis, which occurs in approximately 10% of patients receiving the drug. Bleomycin pneumonitis occasionally progresses to pulmonary fibrosis and has resulted in death in approximately 1% of patients receiving the drug. Pulmonary toxicity generally appears to be dose and age related, occurring most frequently in patients older than 70 years of age and those receiving a total dosage of more than 400 units; however, pulmonary toxicity is unpredictable and reportedly has developed in younger patients receiving lower doses (e.g., after a total dosage of less than 200 units). Fatal pulmonary fibrosis occurred in a geriatric patient who received a total dosage of only 20 units of the drug.

Dyspnea and fine rales are early manifestations of pulmonary toxicity. Because of the nonspecific signs and symptoms, identification of patients with bleomycin-induced pulmonary toxicity has been extremely difficult. Radiographic changes associated with bleomycin-induced pneumonitis consist of nonspecific patchy opacities, usually in the lower lung fields. Microscopic tissue changes also are nonspecific and are similar to the alterations seen with radiation pneumonitis or pneumocystic pneumonitis. The acute pulmonary tissue changes may include capillary changes and subsequent fibrinous exudation into the alveoli (similar to hyaline membrane formation), which may progress to diffuse interstitial fibrosis resembling Hamman-Rich syndrome. Other microscopic tissue changes include bronchiolar squamous metaplasia, reactive macrophages, atypical alveolar epithelial cells, and fibrinous edema.

Appropriate anti-infectives are indicated if bleomycin-induced pneumonitis proves to be infectious. Although it has been suggested that the use of corticosteroids in patients with bleomycin pneumonitis may prevent the development of pulmonary fibrosis or reverse pulmonary toxicity, some clinicians report that this measure has little value.

Rarely, sudden onset of an acute chest pain syndrome suggestive of pleuropericarditis has been reported during continuous infusions of bleomycin. Improvement of this syndrome may be noted with slower infusion rates of the drug and patients may require analgesics for treatment of pain; total recovery usually occurs after discontinuance of the drug.

In at least one patient, cavitary pulmonary nodules associated with granuloma developed after combination therapy containing bleomycin; spontaneous resolution of these lesions occurred despite continuation of therapy.

Careful monitoring for clinical manifestations and evidence of pulmonary toxicity is required in patients receiving bleomycin. (See Cautions: Precautions and Contraindications.) Dosage modification or discontinuance of the drug may be necessary in patients experiencing pulmonary toxicity. (See Dosage Modification for Toxicity and Contraindications for Continued Therapy in Dosage and Administration: Dosage.)

■ Dermatologic and Mucocutaneous Effects Mucocutaneous toxicity is the most frequent adverse effect of bleomycin, occurring in at least 50% of patients receiving the drug. Adverse mucocutaneous effects, including erythema, rash, striae, vesiculation, hyperpigmentation, and tenderness of the skin, usually develop in the second or third week of bleomycin therapy. Mucocutaneous effects appear to be related to total dosage, usually occurring after 150–200 units of bleomycin have been administered. Discontinuance of therapy because of mucocutaneous toxicity has been required in 2% of patients receiving bleomycin.

The onset of skin toxicity may be accompanied by hypoesthesia which may progress to hyperesthesia; paresthesia has also been reported. Skin toxicity may be initially manifested as urticaria or erythematous swelling; lesions may then become tender and pruritic. Hyperpigmentation is a frequently reported adverse effect, occurring particularly in those areas subject to friction or pressure and in skin folds, nail cuticles, scars, and IM injection sites. Hyperkeratosis, nail changes, and pruritus also have been reported. Diffuse alopecia of varying degrees may occur in patients receiving bleomycin therapy. Other reported skin reactions include ichthyosis, peeling, and bleeding. Scleroderma-like skin changes have been reported in patients receiving bleomycin. Mucosal lesions, including stomatitis and ulcerations of the tongue and lips also may occur.

■ Sensitivity Reactions Anaphylactoid reactions, consisting of hypotension, fever, chills, mental confusion, and wheezing, have occurred in approximately 1% of patients with lymphomas receiving bleomycin. This idiosyncratic reaction may be immediate or delayed for several hours, and usually occurs after the first or second dose. The reaction has resulted in death. Treatment of anaphylactoid reactions is supportive and symptomatic and may include volume expansion, vasopressor therapy, antihistamines, and corticosteroids.

■ Cardiovascular Effects Sudden onset of an acute chest pain syndrome suggestive of pleuropericarditis has been reported rarely during continuous infusions of bleomycin. (See Cautions: Respiratory Effects.)

Rarely, vascular toxicities have been associated with the use of bleomycin-containing combination chemotherapy. The adverse vascular effects are clinically heterogeneous and may include myocardial infarction, cerebrovascular accident, thrombotic microangiopathy, or cerebral arteritis. Various mechanisms have been suggested, including endothelial cell damage.

Raynaud's phenomenon has occurred in patients receiving bleomycin and vinblastine, with or without cisplatin, and in a few patients receiving bleomycin as a single agent. Cisplatin-induced hypomagnesemia may be an additional, although not essential, factor associated with its occurrence in patients receiving combination regimens including bleomycin and cisplatin. (For further information on hypomagnesemia associated with the use of cisplatin, see Hypomagnesemia and Other Electrolyte Effects in Cautions: Renal and Electrolyte Effects in Cisplatin 10:00.) The cause of Raynaud's phenomenon in these cases, however, is not clearly established and may involve the underlying disease or vascular compromise, bleomycin, vinblastine, hypomagnesemia, or some combination of these factors.

■ **Renal Effects** Renal toxicity, initially manifested by abnormal renal function test results, has been reported infrequently in patients receiving bleomycin. Renal toxicity may occur at any time following initiation of bleomycin therapy.

■ **Febrile Reactions** Fever and chills frequently follow parenteral administration of bleomycin. Febrile reactions have been reported to occur most frequently with large single doses within a few hours after bleomycin administration and last for 4–12 hours. Usually, febrile reactions become less frequent with continued use of the drug; however, they may occur sporadically and recur later in the course of therapy. Salicylates and antihistamines have not produced uniform results in reducing the fever associated with bleomycin administration. Fever is one of the most common adverse effects of intracavitary administration of sclerosing agents (e.g., bleomycin).

■ **GI Effects** Vomiting frequently occurs in patients receiving bleomycin; nausea also has been reported.

■ **Metabolic Effects** Anorexia and weight loss are common and may persist after discontinuance of bleomycin.

■ **Intrapleural Administration–related Effects** Because bleomycin is well absorbed systemically following intrapleural instillation, the possibility of systemic toxicity, particularly in patients receiving systemic chemotherapy, immunocompromised patients, or those with impaired renal function, should be considered. In most patients, however, evidence of systemic toxicity is minimal.

The most common adverse effects reported with intracavitary administration of sclerosing agents into the pleural space are chest pain and fever. Opiate analgesics may be administered prior to the procedure to relieve pain associated with pleurodesis; lidocaine also has been instilled into the chest tube prior to pleurodesis to help alleviate discomfort. The manufacturer states that the intrapleural injection of local anesthetics or systemic administration of opiates generally is not necessary. Mild analgesics and/or antipyretics also may be used for management of pain and fever.

Intrapleural administration of bleomycin sulfate has been associated infrequently with hypotension requiring symptomatic treatment. Other adverse effects associated with intrapleural administration of bleomycin sulfate include nausea, vomiting, diarrhea, hemoptysis, fluid accumulations, septic shock, rash, and alopecia. Adverse pulmonary effects possibly related to the intrapleural administration of bleomycin have been reported rarely. Death attributed to bleomycin pleurodesis has been reported rarely.

■ **Hematologic Effects** Unlike many other antineoplastic agents, bleomycin does not frequently produce serious bone marrow toxicity. The adverse hematologic effects of bleomycin therapy that have been reported include thrombocytopenia, leukopenia, and slight depression of hemoglobin levels. In one study, all of these levels reached a nadir by the twelfth day and returned to pretreatment levels by the seventeenth day of continued daily IV bleomycin doses of 0.25 units/kg.

■ **Hepatic Effects** Hepatic toxicity, initially manifested by abnormalities in liver function test results, has been reported infrequently in patients receiving bleomycin. Hepatotoxicity may occur at any time following initiation of bleomycin therapy.

■ **Genitourinary Effects** Hematuria, cystitis, and hemorrhagic cystitis have been reported rarely in patients receiving bleomycin.

■ **Other Adverse Effects** Pain at the tumor site and local reactions (e.g., phlebitis) at the injection site have been reported infrequently. Malaise and general weakness also have been reported. Rarely, disorientation and aggressive behavior have been reported.

■ **Precautions and Contraindications** Bleomycin is a toxic drug with a low therapeutic index. The drug should be used only under constant supervision by physicians experienced in cancer chemotherapy, and it should be administered only in settings where adequate diagnostic and treatment facilities are readily available for management of therapy and potential complications. Patients receiving bleomycin must be monitored carefully and frequently during and after therapy.

Bleomycin should be administered with extreme caution to patients with clinically important impairment of renal function or compromised pulmonary function. Some clinicians recommend that use of bleomycin as a sclerosing agent be avoided in patients with underlying lung disease or lung metastases.

Patients receiving bleomycin should be closely monitored for signs of pulmonary toxicity and chest radiographs should be taken every 1–2 weeks. Sequential measurement of pulmonary diffusion capacity for carbon monoxide (DL_{co}) performed monthly during bleomycin therapy may be of value in predicting pulmonary toxicity. (Also see Pulmonary Toxicity in Dosage and Administration: Dosage: Dosage Modification for Toxicity and Contraindications to Continued Therapy.)

Because of bleomycin's effects on lung tissue, patients who have received the drug are at increased risk of developing pulmonary toxicity when oxygen is administered during surgery. Long exposure to very high concentrations of oxygen is a known cause of lung damage, but after administration of bleomycin, lung damage can occur at oxygen concentrations lower than those usually considered safe. To minimize the risk in patients undergoing surgery who have received bleomycin, the FI O_2 concentration should be maintained at approximately that of room air (25%) during surgery and the postoperative period; in addition, fluid replacement should be carefully monitored, with emphasis on administration of colloid rather than crystalloid.

Limited data indicate that risk of bleomycin-induced pulmonary toxicity may be increased in patients receiving filgrastim or other cytokines concomitantly. However, increased risk of pulmonary toxicity was not reported in randomized clinical studies in patients receiving bleomycin concomitantly with filgrastim.

All lymphoma patients should receive test doses of bleomycin before initiating full-dose therapy. (See Dosage and Administration: Dosage.) Careful monitoring of patients with lymphoma is essential after administration of the first and second doses of bleomycin since that is when severe idiosyncratic reactions have most commonly occurred.

Bleomycin is contraindicated in patients with known hypersensitivity or idiosyncrasy to the drug.

■ **Pediatric Precautions** The manufacturer states that safety and efficacy of bleomycin in children have not been established.

■ **Geriatric Precautions** The risk of pulmonary toxicity associated with bleomycin is greater in patients older than 70 years of age than in younger patients. While clinical experience has not revealed other age-related differences in response or tolerance, the possibility that some older patients may exhibit increased sensitivity to the drug cannot be ruled out. Because geriatric patients may have decreased renal function and because patients with renal impairment may be at increased risk of bleomycin-induced toxicity, patients in this age group should be monitored closely and dosage adjusted accordingly.

■ **Mutagenicity and Carcinogenicity** Bleomycin has been shown to be mutagenic in vitro and in vivo. It is not known if bleomycin is carcinogenic in humans. However, an increased incidence of nodular hyperplasia was observed in F344/N male rats that received bleomycin following nitrosamine-induced lung carcinogenesis. In another study, necropsy findings included dose-related injection site fibrosarcomas and various renal tumors in rats receiving subcutaneous bleomycin dosages of 0.35 mg/kg weekly (3.82 units/m^2 weekly, about 30% of the recommended human dosage).

■ **Pregnancy, Fertility, and Lactation** Bleomycin sulfate can cause fetal toxicity when administered to pregnant women. The drug has been shown to be teratogenic in rats receiving intraperitoneal dosages of 1.5 mg/kg daily (about 1.6 times the recommended human dosage on a units/m^2 basis) on days 6–15 of gestation. Fetal malformations included skeletal defects, shortened innominate artery, and hydroureter. The drug has been shown to be abortifacient, but not teratogenic in rabbits receiving IV dosages of 1.2 mg/kg daily (about 2.4 times the recommended human dosage on a units/m^2 basis) on days 6–18 of gestation. There are no adequate and controlled studies to date using bleomycin sulfate in pregnant women. When the drug is administered during pregnancy or if the patient becomes pregnant while receiving the drug, the patient should be informed of the potential hazard to the fetus. Women of childbearing potential should be advised to avoid becoming pregnant during bleomycin sulfate therapy.

The effects of bleomycin on fertility have not been studied.

It is not known whether bleomycin is excreted in human milk. Because of the potential for serious adverse reactions to bleomycin in nursing infants if it were distributed, the manufacturer recommends that women receiving bleomycin discontinue nursing.

Drug Interactions

Vitamins may decrease the activity of certain antibiotics; bleomycin has been shown to be inactivated in vitro by ascorbic acid and riboflavin.

Pharmacology

Bleomycin is an antineoplastic antibiotic. The drug is active against gram-positive and gram-negative bacteria and fungi, but its cytotoxicity precludes its use as an anti-infective agent. The precise mechanism(s) of action of bleomycin is not fully known. Several studies in *Escherichia coli* and HeLa cells suggest that the drug inhibits the incorporation of thymidine into DNA. In these in vitro studies, DNA synthesis was inhibited to a greater extent than was RNA or protein synthesis. Bleomycin also appears to labilize the DNA structure, resulting in scission of both single- and double-stranded DNA. The drug has no immunosuppressive activity in mice.

Pharmacokinetics

■ **Absorption** Bleomycin sulfate is not significantly absorbed from the GI tract and the drug must be administered parenterally. Bleomycin is absorbed systemically following intrapleural or intraperitoneal administration. Systemic absorption of 45% has been reported following intrapleural administration of bleomycin.

■ **Distribution** Following parenteral administration of bleomycin in animals, the drug is distributed mainly into the skin, lungs, kidneys, peritoneum, and lymphatics. Concentrations of the drug in tumor cells of the skin and lungs are higher than those in hematopoietic tissue. The low concentrations of bleomycin found in bone marrow may be related to the high concentrations of bleomycin degradative enzymes present in that tissue. Results of an animal study suggest that the concentration of bleomycin in chemically induced squamous cell carcinomas is higher than that in sarcomas, partially as a result of a lower concentration of bleomycin degradative enzymes in squamous cell carcinomas than in sarcomas.

■ **Elimination** In patients with creatinine clearance exceeding 35 mL/minute, the serum or plasma terminal half-life of bleomycin is about 2 hours. In patients with creatinine clearances less than 35 mL/minute, the terminal half-life of the drug is inversely related to creatinine clearance.

The metabolic fate of bleomycin has not been determined. In patients with normal renal function, 60–70% of a parenterally administered dose is excreted in the urine as active drug. In patients with moderately severe renal impairment (creatinine clearance of less than 35 mL/minute), less than 20% of a parenterally administered dose is excreted in urine as active drug, indicating that accumulation of the drug may occur in patients with severe renal impairment.

Chemistry and Stability

■ **Chemistry** Bleomycin sulfate is a mixture of basic cytotoxic glycopeptide antibiotics produced by *Streptomyces verticillus;* bleomycin A_2 and bleomycin B_2 are the major components. Bleomycin sulfate occurs as a cream-colored, amorphous powder and is very soluble in water and sparingly soluble in alcohol. The potency of bleomycin is assayed microbiologically; the activity of 1 unit of bleomycin is equivalent to the formerly used reference standard, the activity of 1 mg of bleomycin A_2. The previously used term mg activity has been replaced with the more precise term of units. Following reconstitution, bleomycin sulfate injection has a pH of 4.5–6, depending upon the diluent used.

■ **Stability** In vitro, bleomycin is inactivated by agents containing sulfhydryl groups, hydrogen peroxide, and ascorbic acid. Bleomycin sulfate sterile powder is stable under refrigeration at 2–8°C and should not be used after the expiration date is reached.

Following reconstitution with 0.9% sodium chloride injection, the manufacturer states that bleomycin sulfate solutions are stable for 24 hours at room temperature. The manufacturer states that 5% dextrose injection or other diluents containing dextrose should not be used to reconstitute bleomycin sulfate injection since losses of potency (determined by high-performance liquid chromatography [HPLC]) of bleomycin A_2 and bleomycin B_2 have been reported when 5% dextrose was used as diluent. It has been suggested that loss of bleomycin potency in dextrose solutions probably results from formation of Schiff base-type adducts with dextrose. Although reconstituted solutions of bleomycin sulfate are reportedly stable for 2 weeks at room temperature and 4 weeks at 2–8°C, the reconstituted solutions contain no preservatives and the manufacturer recommends that they be used within 24 hours of reconstitution; unused portions should be discarded.

For further information on the handling of antineoplastic agents, see the ASHP Guidelines on Handling Hazardous Drugs at http://www.ahfsdruginformation.com.

Preparations

Excipients in commercially available drug preparations may have clinically important effects in some individuals; consult specific product labeling for details.

Bleomycin Sulfate

Parenteral		
For injection	15 units (of bleomycin)*	**Blenoxane®**, Bristol-Myers Squibb
		Bleomycin Sulfate for Injection
	30 units (of bleomycin)*	**Blenoxane®**, Bristol-Myers Squibb
		Bleomycin Sulfate for Injection

*available from one or more manufacturer, distributor, and/or repackager by generic (nonproprietary) name

†Use is not currently included in the labeling approved by the US Food and Drug Administration

Blinatumomab

■ Blinatumomab, a CD3 T-cell-engaging anti-CD19 monoclonal antibody, is an antineoplastic agent; the drug also is referred to as a bispecific T-cell-engager (BiTE) monoclonal antibody.

REMS

FDA approved a REMS for blinatumomab to ensure that the benefits outweigh the risks. The REMS may apply to one or more preparations of blinatumomab and consists of the following: communication plan. See the FDA REMS page (https://www.accessdata.fda.gov/scripts/cder/rems/index.cfm).

Uses

■ **Philadelphia Chromosome-Negative Precursor B-Cell Acute Lymphoblastic Leukemia** Blinatumomab is used for the treatment of Philadelphia chromosome-negative (Ph⁻) relapsed or refractory precursor B-cell acute lymphoblastic leukemia (pre-B-ALL). The drug has been designated an orphan drug by FDA for use in this condition. Continued approval for this indication may be contingent on verification of clinical benefit of blinatumomab in confirmatory studies.

The current indication for blinatumomab is based principally on the results of an open-label, noncomparative, phase 2 study in 185 adults with Ph⁻ relapsed or refractory pre-B-ALL. Patients were enrolled if their disease was primary refractory following induction therapy, had relapsed or was refractory following first salvage therapy, or had relapsed within 12 months of first remission or following allogeneic stem cell transplantation. Patients enrolled in the study also were required to have at least 10% blast cells in bone marrow. In this study, patients received a target blinatumomab dosage of 28 mcg daily by continuous IV infusion for 4 weeks followed by a 2-week rest period; dosage was escalated to the target level during cycle 1 (blinatumomab 9 mcg daily was given by continuous IV infusion for the first week of cycle 1 with a subsequent increase to 28 mcg daily by continuous IV infusion for the remaining 3 weeks of treatment during cycle 1) to reduce the risk of cytokine release syndrome. The primary measure of efficacy was complete remission (CR) or complete remission with partial hematologic recovery (CRh) within the first 2 treatment cycles; CR was defined as the presence of 5% or less blasts in bone marrow without evidence of disease and with full recovery of peripheral blood cell counts (platelet count exceeding 100,000/mm³ and absolute neutrophil count [ANC] exceeding 1000/mm³), and CRh was defined as the presence of 5% or less blasts in bone marrow without evidence of disease and with partial recovery of peripheral blood cell counts (platelet count exceeding 50,000/mm³ and ANC exceeding 500/mm³). The median age of patients was 39 years; 34% of the patients had undergone allogeneic stem cell transplantation prior to study entry and 17% of patients had received more than 2 prior salvage therapies for their disease. Overall, CR or CRh was reported in 41.6% of patients within the first 2 treatment cycles; most (81%) of these patients achieved a response within the first treatment cycle. At the time of analysis, the median duration of response for all responders was 5.9 months (range: 0.13–16.5 months); the median duration of response was 6.7 months for patients achieving CR and 5 months for those achieving CRh. Minimal residual disease (defined as the presence of less than 0.01% blasts using a polymerase chain reaction [PCR] assay) was reported in 80 or 58.8% of patients who achieved CR or CRh, respectively.

Dosage and Administration

■ **General** The manufacturer recommends that blinatumomab be administered in a hospital setting for days 1–9 of cycle 1 and days 1–2 of cycle 2; administration of the drug under the supervision of a clinician or in a hospital setting also is recommended during initiation of all subsequent cycles and for reinitiation of therapy (i.e., following interruption of therapy for 4 or more hours).

Premedication with IV dexamethasone 20 mg should be administered 1 hour prior to the first infusion of blinatumomab in each cycle, prior to a dosage escalation (i.e., from 9 mcg daily to 28 mcg daily), and when reinitiating therapy following an interruption lasting 4 or more hours.

■ **Reconstitution and Administration** Procedures for proper handling (e.g., use of gloves and protective clothing) and disposal of antineoplastic agents should be followed.

Blinatumomab is administered by continuous IV infusion. Prior to administration, blinatumomab lyophilized powder for injection must be reconstituted and diluted. The manufacturer states that strict aseptic technique must be observed in preparing and administering blinatumomab solutions since the powder for injection contains no preservative.

Final diluted solutions of the drug should be prepared in polyolefin, non-diethylhexylphthalate (non-DEHP) plasticized polyvinyl chloride (PVC), or ethyl vinyl acetate (EVA) infusion bags or pump cassettes and administered through polyolefin, non-DEHP plasticized PVC, or EVA administration sets. Final diluted solutions of the drug may be administered via a programmable, non-elastomeric ambulatory infusion pump equipped with an alarm and locking mechanism. The administration set tubing should be attached to the infusion bag with a sterile, nonpyrogenic, low-protein-binding 0.2-μm inline filter. Any air remaining in the infusion bag should be removed and the administration set tubing should be primed with the final diluted solution of blinatumomab. The administration set tubing should *not* be primed with 0.9% sodium chloride injection.

The proper procedure for preparing a final blinatumomab infusion solution from the reconstituted solution varies according to the dosage (9 or 28 mcg daily), infusion time for the IV bag (24 or 48 hours), and rate of infusion (5 or 10 mL/hour). The manufacturer's labeling should be consulted for detailed information on the preparation of blinatumomab. The IV solution stabilizer provided by the manufacturer is added to the infusion bag containing 0.9% sodium chloride injection prior to addition of the reconstituted blinatumomab solution to minimize adsorption of the drug to the infusion bag and administration set tubing; the stabilizer contains citric acid monohydrate, lysine hydrochloride, polysorbate 80, and sodium hydroxide (to adjust pH to 7) in sterile water for injection. The IV solution stabilizer should *not* be used to reconstitute blinatumomab powder for injection.

Reconstituted and diluted solutions of the drug should be inspected visually for particulate matter and discoloration. Solutions of the drug should be clear to slightly opalescent and colorless to slightly yellow; the drug should be discarded if the solution is cloudy or contains a precipitate.

Blinatumomab should be administered through a dedicated lumen. Flushing the IV administration line may result in the patient receiving an excess dosage of blinatumomab; therefore, the IV administration line should *not* be flushed following completion of an infusion or when changing infusion bags.

Reconstituted blinatumomab solutions are stable for up to 4 hours when stored at room temperature (23–27°C) or up to 24 hours when stored under refrigeration (2–8°C), and should be protected from light until time of use. Final diluted solutions of the drug are stable for up to 8 days after dilution when stored under refrigeration or up to 48 hours (including infusion time) after dilution when stored at room temperature. Diluted solutions of the drug should *not* be frozen. Any unused portion in a vial, an infusion bag, or administration set tubing should be discarded.

Reconstitution and Dilution for Administration of Blinatumomab 9 mcg Daily at an IV Infusion Rate of 10 mL/hour for 24 Hours To minimize adsorption of blinatumomab to infusion bags and administration set tubing, 5.5 mL of the manufacturer-provided IV solution stabilizer should be withdrawn into a 10-mL syringe and added to a prefilled infusion bag labeled as containing 250 mL of 0.9% sodium chloride injection. Instructions for preparation of final diluted blinatumomab solutions for infusion account for an overfill of 15–25 mL (total volume of 265–275 mL) in 250-mL prefilled infusion bags; therefore, the volume of the prefilled infusion bag should be adjusted, if necessary, to achieve an initial volume of 265–275 mL prior to addition of the solution stabilizer. The solution should be gently mixed to avoid foaming.

Blinatumomab powder for injection is reconstituted by adding 3 mL of preservative-free sterile water for injection using a 5-mL syringe to a vial labeled as containing 35 mcg of the drug to provide a solution containing 12.5 mcg/mL. The diluent should be directed toward the wall of the vial and not directly at the blinatumomab cake or powder. The vial should be gently swirled to avoid excess foaming. The resulting solution should *not* be shaken.

For preparation of the final diluted blinatumomab solution for infusion, 0.83 mL of reconstituted blinatumomab solution should be withdrawn into a 1-mL syringe and injected into the 250-mL prefilled infusion bag containing 265–275 mL of 0.9% sodium chloride injection and IV solution stabilizer. The resulting solution should be gently mixed to avoid foaming.

Reconstitution and Dilution for Administration of Blinatumomab 9 mcg Daily at an IV Infusion Rate of 5 mL/hour for 48 Hours To minimize adsorption of blinatumomab to infusion bags and administration set tubing, 5.5 mL of the manufacturer-provided IV solution stabilizer should be withdrawn into a 10-mL syringe and added to a prefilled infusion bag labeled as containing 250 mL of 0.9% sodium chloride injection. Instructions for preparation of final diluted blinatumomab solutions for infusion account for an overfill of 15–25 mL (total volume of 265–275 mL) in 250-mL prefilled infusion bags; therefore, the volume of the prefilled infusion bag should be adjusted, if necessary, to achieve an initial volume of 265–275 mL prior to addition of the solution stabilizer. The solution should be gently mixed to avoid foaming.

Blinatumomab powder for injection is reconstituted by adding 3 mL of preservative-free sterile water for injection using a 5-mL syringe to a vial labeled as containing 35 mcg of the drug to provide a solution containing 12.5 mcg/mL. The diluent should be directed toward the wall of the vial and not directly at the blinatumomab cake or powder. The vial should be gently swirled to avoid excess foaming. The resulting solution should *not* be shaken.

For preparation of the final diluted blinatumomab solution for infusion, 1.7 mL of reconstituted blinatumomab solution should be withdrawn into a 3-mL syringe and injected into the 250-mL prefilled infusion bag containing 265–275 mL of 0.9% sodium chloride injection and IV solution stabilizer. The resulting solution should be gently mixed to avoid foaming.

Reconstitution and Dilution for Administration of Blinatumomab 28 mcg Daily at an IV Infusion Rate of 10 mL/hour for 24 Hours To minimize adsorption of blinatumomab to infusion bags and administration set tubing, 5.6 mL of the manufacturer-provided IV solution stabilizer should be withdrawn into a 10-mL syringe and added to a prefilled infusion bag labeled as containing 250 mL of 0.9% sodium chloride injection. Instructions for preparation of final diluted blinatumomab solutions for infusion account for an overfill of 15–25 mL (total volume of 265–275 mL) in 250-mL prefilled infusion bags; therefore, the volume of the prefilled infusion bag should be adjusted, if necessary, to achieve an initial volume of 265–275 mL prior to addition of the solution stabilizer. The solution should be gently mixed to avoid foaming.

Blinatumomab powder for injection is reconstituted by adding 3 mL of preservative-free sterile water for injection using a 5-mL syringe to a vial labeled as containing 35 mcg of the drug to provide a solution containing 12.5 mcg/mL. The diluent should be directed toward the wall of the vial and not directly at the blinatumomab cake or powder. The vial should be gently swirled to avoid excess foaming. The resulting solution should *not* be shaken.

For preparation of the final diluted blinatumomab solution for infusion, 2.6 mL of reconstituted blinatumomab solution should be withdrawn into a 3-mL syringe and injected into the 250-mL prefilled infusion bag containing 265–275 mL of 0.9% sodium chloride injection and IV solution stabilizer. The resulting solution should be gently mixed to avoid foaming.

Reconstitution and Dilution for Administration of Blinatumomab 28 mcg Daily at an IV Infusion Rate of 5 mL/hour for 48 Hours To minimize adsorption of blinatumomab to infusion bags and administration set tubing, 5.6 mL of the manufacturer-provided IV solution stabilizer should be withdrawn into a 10-mL syringe and added to a prefilled infusion bag labeled as containing 250 mL of 0.9% sodium chloride injection. Instructions for preparation of final diluted blinatumomab solutions for infusion account for an overfill of 15–25 mL (total volume of 265–275 mL) in 250-mL prefilled infusion bags; therefore, the volume of the prefilled infusion bag should be adjusted, if necessary, to achieve an initial volume of 265–275 mL prior to addition of the solution stabilizer. The solution should be gently mixed to avoid foaming.

For reconstitution of blinatumomab for IV infusion at a dosage of 28 mcg daily for 48 hours, 2 vials of blinatumomab powder for injection labeled as containing 35 mcg of the drug should be reconstituted. The powder is reconstituted by adding 3 mL of preservative-free sterile water for injection using a 5-mL syringe to each vial labeled as containing 35 mcg of the drug to provide a solution containing 12.5 mcg/mL. The diluent should be directed toward the wall of the vial and not directly at the blinatumomab cake or powder. The vials should be gently swirled to avoid excess foaming. The resulting solution should *not* be shaken.

For preparation of the final diluted blinatumomab solution for infusion, 2.7 mL of reconstituted blinatumomab solution should be withdrawn from one vial and 2.5 mL withdrawn from the other vial using a 3-mL syringe and injected into the 250-mL prefilled infusion bag containing 265–275 mL of 0.9% sodium chloride injection and IV solution stabilizer. The resulting solution should be gently mixed to avoid foaming.

Preparation and Administration Precautions Medication errors resulting in underdosage or overdosage of blinatumomab have occurred in patients receiving the drug. Extra care should be exercised to ensure proper preparation and administration of blinatumomab. (See Preparation and Administration Errors under Warnings/Precautions: Other Warnings and Precautions, in Cautions.)

■ **Dosage** ***Philadelphia Chromosome-Negative Precursor B-Cell Acute Lymphoblastic Leukemia*** For the treatment of Philadelphia chromosome-negative (Ph^-) relapsed or refractory precursor B-cell acute lymphoblastic leukemia (pre-B-ALL) in adults weighing at least 45 kg, the recommended dosage of blinatumomab during cycle 1 is 9 mcg daily by continuous IV infusion on days 1–7, followed by 28 mcg daily by continuous IV infusion on days 8–28, then followed by a 2-week rest period. For subsequent cycles, the recommended adult dosage is 28 mcg daily by continuous IV infusion on days 1–28 of each 6-week treatment cycle. A treatment course consists of induction therapy with blinatumomab for up to 2 cycles followed by consolidation therapy for 3 additional cycles (total of up to 5 cycles).

Dosage Modification for Toxicity If toxicity requires interruption of blinatumomab therapy for no more than 7 days, the current cycle should be continued for a total of 28 days of blinatumomab treatment (including the days prior to and after the interruption in therapy). If blinatumomab therapy is interrupted for more than 7 days, a new cycle should be started.

Grade 3 or 4 Toxicity. If grade 3 toxicity occurs, blinatumomab therapy should be withheld until the toxicity has resolved to grade 0 or 1; if the toxicity resolves within 14 days, therapy may then be resumed at a reduced dosage of 9 mcg daily. If the toxicity does not recur within 7 days, blinatumomab may be re-escalated to a dosage of 28 mcg daily. If the toxicity persists for more than 14 days following interruption of therapy, blinatumomab therapy should be permanently discontinued.

If grade 4 toxicity occurs, permanent discontinuance of blinatumomab therapy should be considered.

Cytokine Release Syndrome. If grade 3 cytokine release syndrome occurs, blinatumomab therapy should be withheld until the toxicity has resolved. Blinatumomab therapy may then be resumed at a reduced dosage of 9 mcg daily. If the toxicity does not recur within 7 days, blinatumomab may be re-escalated to a dosage of 28 mcg daily. (See Cytokine Release Syndrome under Warnings/Precautions: Warnings, in Cautions.)

If grade 4 cytokine release syndrome occurs, blinatumomab therapy should be permanently discontinued.

Neurologic Toxicity. If grade 3 neurologic toxicity occurs, blinatumomab therapy should be withheld until the toxicity has resolved to grade 0 or 1 for at least 3 days; therapy may then be resumed at a reduced dosage of 9 mcg daily. If the toxicity does not recur within 7 days, blinatumomab may be re-escalated to a dosage of 28 mcg daily. If the toxicity occurred at a dosage of 9 mcg daily or persisted for more than 7 days following interruption of therapy, blinatumomab therapy should be permanently discontinued. (See Neurologic Toxicity under Warnings/Precautions: Warnings, in Cautions.)

If more than one seizure occurs or if grade 4 neurologic toxicity occurs, blinatumomab therapy should be permanently discontinued.

■ **Special Populations** Blinatumomab has not been studied in patients with hepatic impairment, and the manufacturer provides no specific dosage recommendations for such patients.

Blinatumomab has not been formally studied in patients with renal impairment; however, no dosage adjustment is necessary in patients with creatinine clearance of 30 mL/minute or more. The manufacturer provides no specific dosage recommendations for patients with creatinine clearance less than 30 mL/minute or in patients receiving hemodialysis. (See Renal Impairment under Warnings/Precautions: Specific Populations, in Cautions.)

The manufacturer makes no specific dosage recommendations for geriatric patients. (See Geriatric Use under Warnings/Precautions: Specific Populations, in Cautions.)

Cautions

■ **Contraindications** Blinatumomab is contraindicated in patients with known hypersensitivity to the drug or any ingredient in the formulation.

■ **Warnings/Precautions** ***Warnings*** **Cytokine Release Syndrome.** Cytokine release syndrome, sometimes life-threatening or fatal, has been reported in patients receiving blinatumomab. Peak cytokine release has been observed within 2 days following initiation of blinatumomab infusion. In clinical studies of blinatumomab in patients with relapsed or refractory acute lymphoblastic leukemia (ALL), cytokine release syndrome occurred in 11% of patients receiving blinatumomab; grade 3 or greater cytokine release syndrome was reported in 1% of patients receiving the drug. Disseminated intravascular coagulation, capillary leak syndrome, and hemophagocytic lymphohistiocytosis/macrophage activation syndrome have been reported in some patients with cytokine release syndrome. Serious adverse effects that may be associated with cytokine release syndrome include pyrexia, headache, nausea, asthenia, hypotension, and elevated serum aminotransferase (ALT and AST) and bilirubin concentrations; however, discontinuance of therapy was not necessary in most patients experiencing these adverse effects. Infusion-related reactions observed with blinatumomab may be clinically indistinguishable from manifestations of cytokine release syndrome.

Patients receiving blinatumomab should be monitored closely for signs and symptoms of cytokine release syndrome. Temporary interruption or discontinuance of blinatumomab may be necessary if cytokine release syndrome occurs during therapy with the drug. (See Cytokine Release Syndrome under Dosage: Dosage Modification for Toxicity, in Dosage and Administration.)

Neurologic Toxicity. Neurologic toxicities occur frequently (approximately 50%) in patients receiving blinatumomab and may be severe, life-threatening, or fatal. In clinical studies, grade 3 or greater neurologic toxicities (e.g., encephalopathy, seizures, speech impairment, disturbances in consciousness, confusion and disorientation, coordination and balance disorders) occurred in approximately 15% of patients following initiation of blinatumomab therapy. The median time to onset of neurologic toxicity was 7 days. Neurologic toxicity generally resolved following treatment interruption; however, discontinuance of blinatumomab was necessary in some patients. In the principal efficacy study, most neurologic toxicities were grade 1 or 2 in severity and were managed with dexamethasone without treatment interruption.

Patients receiving blinatumomab should be monitored for manifestations of neurologic toxicities. Temporary interruption or discontinuance of blinatumomab may be necessary if neurologic toxicities occur during therapy with the drug. (See Neurologic Toxicity under Dosage: Dosage Modification for Toxicity, in Dosage and Administration.)

Because neurologic toxicities resulting in loss of consciousness or seizures may occur, patients receiving blinatumomab should be advised to avoid driving a motor vehicle or engaging in hazardous occupations or activities (e.g., operating hazardous machinery) while receiving the drug.

Other Warnings and Precautions **Infectious Complications.** Serious infections, such as sepsis, pneumonia, bacteremia, opportunistic infections, and catheter-site infections, have been reported in approximately 25% of patients receiving blinatumomab in clinical studies and may be life-threatening or fatal.

Prophylactic anti-infective therapy should be initiated as appropriate and surveillance testing should be employed during blinatumomab therapy. Patients should be monitored for signs and symptoms of infection and should receive appropriate anti-infective treatment as clinically indicated.

Tumor Lysis Syndrome. Tumor lysis syndrome, sometimes life-threatening or fatal, has been reported in patients receiving blinatumomab. In clinical studies of blinatumomab in patients with relapsed or refractory ALL, tumor lysis syndrome occurred in 4% of patients receiving the drug.

The manufacturer states that patients should be monitored for signs and symptoms of tumor lysis syndrome during blinatumomab therapy and, if present, interruption or discontinuance of blinatumomab therapy may be necessary. Appropriate prophylactic measures (e.g., pretreatment nontoxic cytoreduction, adequate hydration during therapy) should be used.

Neutropenia and Febrile Neutropenia. Neutropenia and febrile neutropenia, sometimes life-threatening, have been reported in patients receiving blinatumomab. In clinical studies of blinatumomab in patients with relapsed or refractory ALL, neutropenia or febrile neutropenia occurred in 16 or 25%, respectively, of patients receiving blinatumomab. Grade 3 or greater neutropenia or febrile neutropenia was reported in 15 or 23%, respectively, of patients receiving the drug.

Complete blood cell (CBC) counts, including differential, should be monitored during blinatumomab therapy. Therapy should be interrupted if prolonged neutropenia occurs.

Hepatic Effects. Transient increases in hepatic enzyme concentrations have occurred in patients receiving blinatumomab. Elevations in hepatic enzyme concentrations mostly occur in association with cytokine release syndrome; however, grade 3 or greater elevations in liver enzymes were reported in approximately 6% of patients without cytokine release syndrome and resulted in discontinuance of blinatumomab is less than 1% of patients. The median time to onset of elevated hepatic enzyme concentrations was 15 days.

Serum aminotransferase (ALT and AST), γ-glutamyltransferase (γ-glutamyltranspeptidase, GGT, GGTP), and total bilirubin concentrations should be evaluated prior to and during blinatumomab therapy. If ALT and/or AST concentrations exceed 5 times the upper limit of normal (ULN) or total bilirubin concentrations exceed 3 times the ULN, treatment should be interrupted.

Leukoencephalopathy. Cranial magnetic resonance imaging (MRI) changes showing leukoencephalopathy have been observed in patients receiving blinatumomab, particularly in those who previously received cranial irradiation and antileukemic chemotherapy (including systemic high-dose methotrexate or intrathecal cytarabine). The clinical importance of these changes is not known.

Preparation and Administration Errors. Medication errors resulting in underdosage or overdosage of blinatumomab have occurred in patients receiving the drug. The proper procedure for preparing a final blinatumomab infusion solution from the reconstituted solution varies according to the dosage, infusion time of the IV bag, and rate of infusion. Extra care should be exercised to ensure proper preparation and administration of blinatumomab. (See Dosage and Administration: Reconstitution and Administration.)

Immunogenicity. As with all therapeutic proteins, there is a potential for immunogenicity. In clinical studies, anti-blinatumomab antibody formation occurred in less than 1% of patients receiving blinatumomab; neutralizing antibodies were detected in all of these patients. Pharmacokinetics of blinatumomab may be affected by anti-blinatumomab antibody formation. No clinically important effects on safety of the drug were observed in patients who tested positive for anti-blinatumomab antibodies.

Specific Populations **Pregnancy.** Category C. (See Users Guide.)

There are no adequate and well-controlled studies of blinatumomab in pregnant women; however, because of its mechanism of action, blinatumomab may cause fetal harm, including B-cell lymphocytopenia, if administered to pregnant women. Embryofetal toxicity and teratogenicity were not observed when a murine surrogate molecule was administered IV to pregnant mice; however, the surrogate molecule crossed the placenta. Administration of the surrogate molecule to pregnant mice caused B-cell and T-cell depletion in pregnant mice, but hematologic effects were not assessed in fetuses.

Blinatumomab should be used during pregnancy only if the potential benefit justifies the potential risk to the fetus.

Lactation. It is not known whether blinatumomab is distributed into human milk. Because many drugs are distributed into human milk and because of the potential for serious adverse reactions to blinatumomab in nursing infants, a decision should be made whether to discontinue nursing or the drug, taking into account the importance of the drug to the woman.

Pediatric Use. Clinical experience with use of blinatumomab in pediatric patients is limited. In a phase 1 dose-escalation study, 41 pediatric patients 2–17 years of age with relapsed or refractory precursor B-cell acute lymphoblastic leukemia (pre-B-ALL) received blinatumomab in dosages ranging from 5–30 mcg/m^2 daily. Cytokine release syndrome was a dose-limiting toxicity associated with blinatumomab therapy; however, stepwise dosing of blinatumomab (5 mcg/m^2 daily for 7 days, then 15 mcg/m^2 daily) reduced the occurrence of cytokine release syndrome. Fatal respiratory failure and grade 4 cytokine release syndrome resulting in fatal cardiac failure and life-threatening GI hemorrhage occurred in 3 patients following administration of blinatumomab 15–30 mcg/m^2 daily. Pharmacokinetic parameters (i.e., steady-state concentrations, clearance, half-life) of blinatumomab were similar to values reported in adults with relapsed or refractory pre-B-ALL who received equivalent dosages based on body surface area (BSA).

Based on the results of this dose-escalation study, a blinatumomab dosage of 5 mcg/m^2 daily on days 1–7 followed by 15 mcg/m^2 daily on days 8–28 for cycle 1, and then 15 mcg/m^2 daily on days 1–28 for subsequent cycles, has been recommended for phase 2 studies in pediatric patients.

Geriatric Use. In clinical studies evaluating blinatumomab for relapsed or refractory ALL, approximately 13% of patients were 65 years of age or older. Although efficacy and safety of blinatumomab generally were similar regardless of patient age in these studies, neurologic toxicities (e.g., cognitive disorder, encephalopathy, confusion) and serious infections occurred more frequently in patients 65 years of age or older compared with younger patients.

Hepatic Impairment. The pharmacokinetics of blinatumomab have not been studied in patients with hepatic impairment. (See Dosage and Administration: Special Populations.)

Renal Impairment. Formal pharmacokinetic studies have not been conducted in patients with renal impairment. Analysis of available pharmacokinetic data indicates an approximately twofold difference in mean blinatumomab clearance between patients with moderate renal impairment (creatinine clearance of 30–59 mL/minute) and those with normal renal function. However, high interpatient variability was apparent and clearance values for patients with renal impairment were within the range observed in patients with normal renal function. The effects of severe renal impairment (creatinine clearance less than 30 mL/minute) or hemodialysis on the pharmacokinetics of blinatumomab have not been established.

■ **Common Adverse Effects** Adverse effects reported in 20% or more of patients receiving blinatumomab for the treatment of relapsed or refractory ALL include pyrexia, infection, headache, peripheral edema, febrile neutropenia, nausea, hypokalemia, rash, constipation, diarrhea, and tremor.

Drug Interactions

No formal drug interaction studies have been performed to date.

■ **Drugs Metabolized by Hepatic Microsomal Enzymes** Following initiation of blinatumomab therapy, a transient release of cytokines may result in suppression of cytochrome P-450 (CYP) isoenzymes and potentially increase serum concentrations of other drugs metabolized by CYP isoenzymes.

Risk of drug interactions is highest during days 1–9 of cycle 1 and days 1–2 of cycle 2 in patients receiving drugs metabolized by CYP isoenzymes, particularly those with a low therapeutic index that require individualized dosing (e.g., warfarin, cyclosporine). Patients receiving certain drugs metabolized by CYP isoenzymes should be monitored for toxicity and/or changes in serum concentrations, and dosages of these drugs should be adjusted as needed.

Description

Blinatumomab, a CD3 T-cell-engaging anti-CD19 monoclonal antibody, is an antineoplastic agent; the drug also is referred to as a bispecific T-cell-engager (BiTE) monoclonal antibody. The drug is a single-chain antibody composed of the variable fragments of antibodies to CD3 and CD19. The 2 antibodies are connected by a nonglycosylated, nonimmunogenic linker protein, which allows for rotational flexibility and close proximity of malignant $CD19^+$ B cells to $CD3^+$ T cells. Blinatumomab binds specifically to the CD3 signaling chain of the T-cell receptor (TCR) complex and to antigen CD19, a transmembrane glycoprotein expressed on the surface of normal and malignant B lymphocytes, including precursor B-cell acute lymphoblastic leukemia cells. Following activation of endogenous T cells, proinflammatory cytokines (interleukin-2 [IL-2], interleukin-4 [IL-4], interleukin-6 [IL-6], interleukin-10 [IL-10], tumor necrosis factor [TNF; TNF-α], interferon gamma) are released and upregulation of cell adhesion molecules induces the release of cytotoxic granules containing perforins and granzymes, which results in activation of caspases and apoptosis (programmed cell death) of $CD19^+$ B cells.

Initial redistribution of peripheral T cells, a decrease in peripheral B-cell counts, and transient release of proinflammatory cytokines are observed in patients receiving blinatumomab therapy. Redistribution of peripheral T cells occurred following initiation of blinatumomab infusion or dosage escalation. In most patients, T-cell counts decreased during the initial 1–2 days of therapy and returned to baseline levels within 7–14 days; however, elevation of T-cell counts above baseline was observed in some patients. Blinatumomab decreased peripheral B-cell counts to 10 cells/mm^3 or less during the first treatment cycle in most patients receiving blinatumomab 5 mcg/m^2 or more daily or 9 mcg or more daily. Peripheral B-cell recovery was not observed during the 2-week rest period between treatment cycles. Following administration of blinatumomab, the proinflammatory cytokines IL-2, IL-4, IL-6, IL-10, TNF-α, and interferon gamma are released; levels of IL-6, IL-10, and interferon gamma increase immediately following initiation of an infusion in most patients. Cytokine levels are highest 1–2 days following initiation of the blinatumomab infusion and return to baseline within 24–48 hours during the infusion. (See Drug Interactions: Drugs Metabolized by Hepatic Microsomal Enzymes.) The incidence and intensity of elevated cytokine levels are decreased in subsequent treatment cycles compared with elevations observed during the initial 48 hours of the first treatment cycle.

In patients receiving blinatumomab by continuous IV infusion, steady-state concentrations are reached within 1 day and remain stable over time. Steady-state concentrations of blinatumomab are proportional to dose over the dosage range of 5–90 mcg/m^2 daily. The metabolic pathway of blinatumomab has not been characterized. As with other therapeutic proteins, the drug is expected to be degraded into small peptides and amino acids via catabolic pathways. Following administration of blinatumomab 60 mcg/m^2 daily, negligible amounts of the drug were detectable in urine at steady state. The mean elimination half-life of blinatumomab is 2.11 hours.

Pharmacokinetic parameters of blinatumomab do not appear to be affected by age (range of 18–80 years), gender, body weight (44–134 kg), and body surface area (1.39–2.57 m^2).

Advice to Patients

Importance of advising patients to read the manufacturer's medication guide before beginning treatment and each time blinatumomab is administered.

Risk of cytokine release syndrome and infusion-related reactions. Importance of immediately reporting signs and symptoms of such reactions (e.g., pyrexia, fatigue, dizziness, headache, nausea, vomiting, chills, hypotension, rash, facial swelling, wheezing).

Risk of neurologic toxicity. Importance of informing clinician immediately if signs and symptoms of neurologic toxicity (e.g., seizures, speech impairment, loss of consciousness, confusion, loss of balance) occur. Necessity of advising patients to avoid driving or engaging in hazardous occupations or activities (e.g., operating hazardous machinery) while receiving the drug.

Risk of infections. Importance of instructing patients to immediately contact their clinician if symptoms suggestive of an infection develop. Importance of advising patients to keep the IV injection site clean in order to reduce the risk of catheter-related infection.

Risk of tumor lysis syndrome.

Risk of neutropenia and importance of monitoring of blood cell counts.

Risk of hepatotoxicity and importance of liver function test monitoring.

Necessity of advising patients to avoid adjusting settings on the infusion pump. Importance of informing clinician immediately if a problem with the infusion pump occurs or if the pump alarm sounds.

Importance of women informing clinicians if they are or plan to become pregnant or plan to breast-feed. Importance of advising women not to breast-feed during therapy.

Importance of informing clinicians of existing or contemplated concomitant therapy, including prescription and OTC drugs, as well as any concomitant illnesses.

Importance of informing patients of other important precautionary information. (See Cautions.)

Overview® (see Users Guide). For additional information on this drug until a more detailed monograph is developed and published, the manufacturer's labeling should be consulted. It is *essential* that the manufacturer's labeling be consulted for more detailed information on usual cautions, precautions, contraindications, potential drug interactions, laboratory test interferences, and acute toxicity. For further information on the handling of antineoplastic agents, see the ASHP Guidelines on Handling Hazardous Drugs at http://www.ahfsdruginformation.com.

Preparations

Excipients in commercially available drug preparations may have clinically important effects in some individuals; consult specific product labeling for details.

Blinatumomab

Parenteral

For injection, for IV infusion	35 mcg	**Blincyto®** (with IV solution stabilizer in 10-mL single-use glass vial), Amgen

Bortezomib

■ Bortezomib, an inhibitor of the 26S proteasome, is an antineoplastic agent.

Uses

■ **Multiple Myeloma** ***Previously Untreated Multiple Myeloma*** Bortezomib is used in combination with melphalan and prednisone for the treatment of previously untreated multiple myeloma.

The current indication for bortezomib in patients with previously untreated multiple myeloma is based principally on the results of a phase 3, open-label, randomized study (Velcade as Initial Standard Therapy in Multiple Myeloma: Assessment with Melphalan and Prednisone [VISTA]) involving 682 patients with newly diagnosed multiple myeloma who were considered ineligible (e.g., because of a coexisting medical condition, an age of 65 years or older) for high-dose chemotherapy followed by stem cell transplantation. Patients were assigned to receive either melphalan plus prednisone (MP) or bortezomib plus melphalan and prednisone (VMP). Patients were stratified according to their baseline β_2-microglobulin concentration (less than 2.5, 2.5–5.5, or above 5.5 mg/L), baseline serum albumin concentration (below 3.5 g/dL, equal to or above 3.5 g/dL), and the geographic region where they received treatment. The planned course of therapy for both regimens was 9 six-week courses for a total treatment duration of 54 weeks. Patients in the control group received melphalan 9 mg/m^2 orally plus prednisone 60 mg/m^2 orally (both administered once daily on days 1–4). Patients in the study group received the same regimen of melphalan plus prednisone with the addition of bortezomib (1.3 mg/m^2 by IV injection) on days 1, 4, 8, 11, 22, 25, 29, and 32 during cycles 1–4; during cycles 5–9, bortezomib was administered on days 1, 8, 22, and 29.

At the time of the initial interim analysis (median follow-up of 16.3 months), the complete response rates, defined by immunofixation negativity and using the European Group for Blood and Marrow Transplantation (EBMT) response criteria, were 30 and 4% for VMP and MP, respectively; rates for partial response or better (i.e., partial plus complete) were 69 and 34%, respectively. Using the International Uniform Response criteria, rates for partial response or better (i.e., partial response plus very good partial response plus complete response) were 74 and 39%, respectively, for VMP and MP. The median time to disease progression (20.7 months versus 15 months) and median progression-free survival (18.3 versus 14 months) were prolonged with VMP compared with MP. This study was terminated prematurely at the request of the independent data monitoring committee because of improved time to disease progression, tumor response rate, and progression-free and overall survival observed during the initial prespecified interim analysis in patients receiving VMP. Updated analysis of overall survival after a median follow-up of 36.7 months indicated a survival benefit (hazard ratio of 0.65) in patients receiving VMP despite subsequent therapies, including bortezomib-based regimens. After a median follow-up of 60.1 months, analysis of data also indicated that median overall survival was prolonged in patients receiving VMP compared with those receiving MP (56.4 versus 43.1 months, respectively; hazard ratio of 0.7). No important differences in the complete response rates, time to progression, or overall survival were reported for patients with impaired renal function (i.e., creatinine clearance less than 60 mL/minute) compared with patients with normal renal function in the VMP group. Similar complete response rates (28%), time to progression, and overall survival rates were reported for patients with high-risk cytogenetic features (e.g., t(4;14), t(14;16) translocation; a 17p or 13q deletion) receiving VMP compared with standard-risk patients.

Results from this study demonstrated superiority of the VMP regimen compared with the MP regimen for previously untreated patients ineligible for peripheral blood stem cell transplantation and for patients older than 65 years of age.

Relapsed Multiple Myeloma Bortezomib is used alone for the treatment of relapsed multiple myeloma in patients who have received at least one prior therapy, including those who previously responded to bortezomib-containing therapy and relapsed at least 6 months following completion of therapy.

The current indication for bortezomib in patients with relapsed multiple myeloma is based principally on the results of a phase 3, randomized, open-label study involving 669 patients and several open-label studies in more than 250 patients with multiple myeloma.

In the prospective phase 3 open-label study, random assignment of patients with progressive multiple myeloma was stratified according to number of lines of prior therapy (1 versus greater than 1 line), time of progression relative to prior treatment (during or within 6 months of stopping most recent therapy versus greater than 6 months following completion of most recent therapy), and screening β_2-microglobulin concentration (2.5 mg/L or less versus greater than 2.5 mg/L). Exclusion criteria included disease refractory to prior therapy with high-dose dexamethasone, grade 2 or higher peripheral neuropathy at baseline, or platelet count less than 50,000/mm^3. Treatment regimens consisted of either bortezomib or high-dose dexamethasone according to the following schedules: bortezomib (1.3 mg/m^2 by IV bolus injection) administered in a 3-week standard treatment cycle (twice weekly for 2 weeks on days 1, 4, 8, and 11 followed by a 10-day rest period) for 8 cycles followed by 5-week maintenance treatment cycles (once weekly for 4 weeks on days 1, 8, 15, and 22 followed by a 13-day rest period) for 3 cycles; or dexamethasone (40 mg orally) administered in a 5-week standard treatment cycle (once daily on days 1–4, 9–12, and 17–20, followed by a 15-day rest period) for 4 cycles followed by 4-week maintenance treatment cycles (once daily on days 1–4 followed by a 24-day rest period) for 5 cycles. Patients experiencing progression of disease during dexamethasone therapy were offered enrollment in a companion study allowing crossover to bortezomib therapy. Bortezomib was administered for a maximum of 11 cycles (9 months). Responses and disease progression were assessed according to EBMT response criteria. A complete response was defined as less than 5% plasma cells in the bone marrow, 100% reduction in serum myeloma (M) protein, and a negative immunofixation test; a partial response was defined as reductions in myeloma protein concentrations of at least 50% in serum and at least 90% in urine on at least 2 occasions for a minimum of 6 weeks, and stable bone disease and normal serum calcium concentrations.

At a planned interim analysis, the study was terminated early and patients receiving dexamethasone were offered therapy with bortezomib. At the time of early termination of the study, at a median follow-up of 8.3 months, prolonged median time to progression of disease (6.2 versus 3.5 months), prolonged survival (hazard ratio of 0.57), and higher response rates (complete plus partial responses) (38 versus 18%) were observed in patients receiving bortezomib compared with those receiving dexamethasone. Overall survival was prolonged in patients receiving bortezomib, both for those who had received one prior treatment (hazard ratio of 0.39) and for those who had received more than one prior treatment (hazard ratio of 0.65). The median duration of response was 8 months in patients receiving bortezomib and 5.6 months in patients receiving dexamethasone. A higher response rate was observed in patients receiving bortezomib regardless of baseline β_2-microglobulin concentration. Limitations of the study that may have affected the outcome include previous corticosteroid therapy in most patients, higher dose intensity for bortezomib than dexamethasone, and the short period of follow-up. Patients receiving bortezomib experienced a greater frequency of grade 3 toxicity (61 versus 44%) than patients receiving dexamethasone.

The primary phase 2 efficacy study enrolled 202 patients with multiple myeloma who had received at least 2 prior chemotherapy regimens and had experienced disease progression following the most recent regimen; patients in this study had received a median of 6 prior chemotherapy regimens, and 64% of patients had received prior stem cell transplantation or other high-dose therapy. Ninety-eight percent of enrolled patients received the standard 21-day regimen of bortezomib (1.3 mg/m^2 by IV injection twice weekly for 2 weeks on days 1, 4, 8, and 11, followed by a 10-day rest period) with subsequent doses adjusted as needed if serious adverse effects occurred; patients exhibiting progressive disease after 2 cycles or stable disease after 4 cycles were eligible to receive oral dexamethasone (20 mg) on the day of and the day after each dose of bortezomib. A mean of 6 treatment cycles was administered.

Using the EBMT response criteria, complete responses or partial responses were observed in 3 or 25%, respectively, of 188 evaluable patients receiving bortezomib. Clinical remission, as determined by the Southwest Oncology Group (SWOG) criteria (defined as reductions in serum M protein concentrations of at least 75% in serum and/or 90% in urine on at least 2 occasions for a minimum of at least 6 weeks, and stable bone disease and normal serum calcium concentrations), was observed in 18% of these patients. Among the 202 enrolled patients, the median time to first response was 38 days, and median survival was 17 months. In this study, response to bortezomib was not influenced by gender, type of myeloma, serum concentrations of β_2-microglobulin, or number or types of prior chemotherapy treatments. However, the likelihood of attaining a response was reduced in patients with more than 50% plasma cells or abnormal cytogenetics in the bone marrow. Responses were observed in patients with or without chromosome 13 abnormalities.

In a small dose-response phase 2 study in 54 patients with relapsed multiple myeloma, the overall response rate (complete plus partial responses) was approximately 30 or 38% in patients receiving bortezomib 1 or 1.3 mg/m^2, respectively, by IV injection twice weekly for 2 weeks on days 1, 4, 8, and 11, followed by a 10-day rest period. A mean of 7 or 6 treatment cycles was administered in patients receiving the 1- or 1.3-mg/m^2 dose, respectively.

Patients from the two phase 2 studies who were expected to benefit from extended therapy were able to continue receiving bortezomib therapy beyond 8 cycles in an extension study. A total of 63 patients from the phase 2 multiple myeloma studies were enrolled and received a median of 7 additional cycles of bortezomib therapy for a total median of 14 cycles (range: 7–32 cycles). The overall median dosing intensity in this study was similar to that in the phase 2 studies. In this study, 67% of patients initiated bortezomib at the same or higher dose intensity compared with that used at the end of the phase 2 studies, and 89% of patients maintained the standard 3-week dosing schedule during the study. No new cumulative or long-term toxicities were observed with prolonged bortezomib treatment.

Efficacy and safety of retreatment with bortezomib (with or without dexamethasone) is based principally on the results of a phase 2 open-label study involving 130 adults with multiple myeloma who had previously achieved at least a partial response to bortezomib-based therapy but had relapsed 6 or more months following completion of therapy. In this study, patients received the last tolerated dose of bortezomib (up to 1.3 mg/m^2 by IV injection) on days 1, 4, 8, and 11 of each 21-day cycle for up to 8 cycles; however, lower doses of bortezomib could be increased to 1.3 mg/m^2. Patients who had received treatment for multiple myeloma (except for maintenance therapy with an immunomodulatory agent or corticosteroid) following the prior course of bortezomib therapy and those with baseline grade 2 or greater peripheral neuropathy or neuropathic pain were excluded from the study. The primary measure of efficacy was best confirmed response according to EBMT response criteria. The overall best confirmed response rate was 38.5%; complete response was achieved in 1 patient. At the time of analysis, the median duration of response for all responders was 6.5 months (range: 0.6–19.3 months). Results of a subgroup analysis suggested that the drug's effect on overall response rate decreased with increasing number of prior therapies. The overall response rate with bortezomib retreatment appeared to be higher in patients who had achieved a complete response rather than a partial response to prior bortezomib-based therapy.

Subcutaneous Versus IV Administration. Efficacy and safety of bortezomib administered by subcutaneous injection are based principally on the results of an open-label, randomized, phase 3 study (MMY-3021) in patients with relapsed multiple myeloma who had not previously received bortezomib. Patients with baseline grade 2 or greater peripheral neuropathy or neuropathic pain or platelet count less than 50,000/mm^3 were excluded from the study. In this study, 222 patients were randomized in a 2:1 ratio to receive bortezomib 1.3 mg/m^2 by either subcutaneous or IV injection on days 1, 4, 8, and 11 of each 21-day cycle for up to 8 cycles. The median number of cycles of bortezomib administered by either route was 8. Patients with a suboptimal response (less than a complete response, without disease progression) after 4 cycles could receive oral dexamethasone (20 mg on the day of and the day after bortezomib administration); approximately one-half of patients in both treatment groups received oral dexamethasone. The primary objective of the study was to show that single-agent bortezomib administered by subcutaneous injection retains at least 60% of the overall response rate attained after 4 cycles with single-agent IV bortezomib.

At a median follow-up of 11.8 months, no significant difference in median time to progression (10.4 versus 9.4 months, respectively), median progression-free survival (10.2 versus 8 months, respectively), and 1-year overall survival (72.6 versus 76.7%, respectively) were observed in patients receiving bortezomib by subcutaneous injection compared with those receiving the drug by IV injection. The overall response rates with subcutaneous and IV injection were 43 and 42%, respectively, following 4 cycles of bortezomib and 53 and 51%, respectively, following 8 cycles; complete response rates following 8 cycles of bortezomib were 11 and 12%, respectively. Overall response rates, median time to progression, median progression-free survival, and overall survival remained similar in both groups at the time of the final analysis after a median follow-up of 17.3 or 17.8 months for patients receiving subcutaneous or IV bortezomib, respectively. Adverse effects generally were similar in both treatment groups, although grade 3 or 4 neuralgia (3 versus 9%), peripheral neuropathy (6 versus 15%), neutropenia (13 versus 18%), and thrombocytopenia (8% versus 16%) occurred less frequently in patients receiving bortezomib by subcutaneous injection compared with those receiving the drug by IV injection.

Induction Therapy Prior to Stem Cell Transplantation in Newly Diagnosed Multiple Myeloma Bortezomib has been studied as a component of various induction regimens for newly diagnosed multiple myeloma in transplant-eligible patients†.

Bortezomib and Dexamethasone. Efficacy and safety of bortezomib in combination with dexamethasone† as induction therapy for newly diagnosed multiple myeloma in transplant-eligible patients† have been studied in an open-label, randomized phase 3 study (IFM 2005-01).

In the IFM 2005-01 study, 482 patients with previously untreated multiple myeloma were randomized to receive bortezomib in combination with dexamethasone (bortezomib-dexamethasone) or the combination of vincristine, doxorubicin, and dexamethasone (vincristine-doxorubicin-dexamethasone) as an induction regimen; both regimens were administered with or without dexamethasone, cyclophosphamide, etoposide, and cisplatin (DCEP) consolidation therapy. Patients receiving the bortezomib-dexamethasone induction regimen received bortezomib 1.3 mg/m^2 as an IV injection on days 1, 4, 8, and 11 of each 3-week cycle for 4 cycles along with dexamethasone 40 mg orally on days 1–4 and 9–12 during cycles 1 and 2 and then on days 1–4 of cycles 3 and 4. Those receiving the vincristine-doxorubicin-dexamethasone induction regimen received vincristine sulfate 0.4 mg and doxorubicin hydrochloride 9 mg/m^2 per day by continuous IV infusion on days 1–4 of each 4-week cycle for 4 cycles along with dexamethasone 40 mg orally on days 1–4, 9–12, and 17–20 during cycles 1 and 2 and then on days 1–4 of cycles 3 and 4. The median age of patients enrolled in the study was 57.1 years; 22% had International Staging System (ISS) stage III disease, 57.5% had a baseline β_2-microglobulin concentration exceeding 3 mg/L, 42.3% had chromosome 13 deletion (del(13)), and 14.3% had t(4;14) translocation with or without chromosome 17p deletion (del(17p)).

The primary measure of efficacy was complete plus near-complete response rate following induction therapy. Tumor responses were assessed using EBMT response criteria. The postinduction complete plus near-complete response rate (14.8 versus 6.4%) and the postinduction overall response rate (78.5 versus 62.8%) were higher in patients receiving bortezomib-dexamethasone compared with those receiving vincristine-doxorubicin-dexamethasone. The complete plus near-complete response rate also was higher following initial transplantation (35 versus 18.4%) and overall (39.5 versus 22.5%), including responses following second transplants when required, in patients receiving bortezomib-dexamethasone compared with those receiving vincristine-doxorubicin-dexamethasone. Postinduction response rates were higher in patients receiving bortezomib-dexamethasone compared with those receiving vincristine-doxorubicin-dexamethasone regardless of disease stage or presence of high-risk cytogenetic features (i.e., del(13), t(4;14) translocation and/or del(17p) chromosomal abnormality). Among patients who received bortezomib-dexamethasone induction therapy, rates of attaining a very good partial response or better were similar regardless of disease stage, use of consolidation therapy, or presence of the t(4;14) translocation with or without del(17p), but were slightly higher in patients with del(13) compared with those without this chromosomal abnormality. Following initial autologous stem cell transplantation, 38.6% of patients who had received bortezomib-dexamethasone induction therapy required a second stem cell transplant compared with 56% of those who had received vincristine-doxorubicin-dexamethasone. Although median overall survival had not been reached at a median follow-up of 32.2 months, median progression-free survival at a median follow-up of 31.2 months was numerically, but not significantly, longer in patients who received induction therapy with bortezomib-dexamethasone compared with those who received vincristine-doxorubicin-dexamethasone (36 versus 29.7 months).

Infection (48.1 versus 38.1%), peripheral neuropathy (45.6 versus 28%), thrombocytopenia (10.9 versus 4.6%), and herpes zoster infection (9.2 versus 2.1%) occurred more frequently in patients receiving bortezomib-dexamethasone, while neutropenia (13.8 versus 8%) and thrombosis (12.1 versus 4.6%) occurred more frequently in patients receiving vincristine-doxorubicin-dexamethasone.

Based on current evidence, use of bortezomib in combination with dexamethasone may be considered a reasonable choice (accepted, with possible conditions) as induction therapy for newly diagnosed multiple myeloma in transplant-eligible patients; factors that should be considered when selecting a combination chemotherapy regimen for use as induction therapy include performance status and preexisting conditions (e.g., peripheral neuropathy).

Bortezomib, Dexamethasone, and Thalidomide. Efficacy and safety of bortezomib in combination with thalidomide and dexamethasone† (bortezomib-thalidomide-dexamethasone) as induction therapy for newly diagnosed multiple myeloma in transplant-eligible patients† have been studied in several phase 3, open-label, randomized studies.

The GIMEMA and PETHEMA/GEM studies compared bortezomib-thalidomide-dexamethasone with the combination of thalidomide and dexamethasone (thalidomide-dexamethasone). In the GIMEMA study, 480 patients were randomized to receive bortezomib-thalidomide-dexamethasone or thalidomide-dexamethasone; both induction regimens were followed by tandem autologous stem cell transplantation and consolidation therapy with the same drug combination used for induction therapy. Patients receiving bortezomib-thalidomide-dexamethasone induction therapy received bortezomib 1.3 mg/m^2 as an IV injection on days 1, 4, 8, and 11 along with thalidomide 200 mg orally daily (after initial dose escalation during cycle 1) and dexamethasone 40 mg orally on days 1, 2, 4, 5, 8, 9, 11, and 12 of each 21-day cycle. Those receiving thalidomide-dexamethasone induction therapy received the same dosage of thalidomide; however, dexamethasone 40 mg was administered orally on days 1–4 and 9–12 of each 21-day cycle. Both regimens were continued for a total of 3 cycles. In the PETHEMA/GEM study, 386 patients were randomized to receive bortezomib-thalidomide-dexamethasone, thalidomide-dexamethasone, or alternating cycles of vincristine, carmustine, melphalan, cyclophosphamide, and prednisone (VBMCP) and vincristine, carmustine, doxorubicin, and dexamethasone (VBAD) followed by bortezomib as induction therapy. Patients receiving bortezomib-thalidomide-dexamethasone received bortezomib 1.3 mg/m^2 as an IV injection on days 1, 4, 8, and 11 along with thalidomide 200 mg orally daily (after initial dose escalation during cycle 1) and dexamethasone 40 mg orally on days 1–4 and 9–12 of each 4-week cycle for 6 cycles. Patients receiving thalidomide-dexamethasone received the same dosages of thalidomide and dexamethasone. Those receiving VBMCP/VBAD received each regimen in alternating cycles for 4 cycles followed by two 3-week cycles of bortezomib 1.3 mg/m^2 administered as an IV injection on days 1, 4, 8, and 11. In the GIMEMA study, the primary measure of efficacy was postinduction complete plus near-complete response rate. In the PETHEMA/GEM study, the primary measures of efficacy were postinduction and posttransplant complete response rates. In both studies, responses were assessed according to EBMT response criteria. In both studies, a higher postinduction response rate and prolonged progression-free survival were observed in patients who received bortezomib-thalidomide-dexamethasone compared with those who received the comparator regimens; however, addition of bortezomib to thalidomide and dexamethasone induction therapy did not provide an overall survival benefit in either study.

In the GIMEMA study, postinduction complete plus near-complete response rate was 31% in patients receiving bortezomib-thalidomide-dexamethasone compared with 11% in those receiving thalidomide-dexamethasone; improved responses also were observed with bortezomib-thalidomide-dexamethasone following first (52 versus 31%) and second (55 versus 41%) autologous stem cell transplants and subsequent consolidation therapy (62 versus 45%). The median time to best complete or near-complete response was shorter in patients receiving bortezomib-thalidomide-dexamethasone compared with those receiving thalidomide-dexamethasone (9 versus 14 months). At a median follow-up of 36 months, progression-free survival was prolonged in patients who received bortezomib-thalidomide-dexamethasone compared with those who received thalidomide-dexamethasone (hazard ratio 0.63); however, no difference in estimated 3-year overall survival (86 versus 84%, respectively) was observed between the groups. Subgroup analysis based on poor prognostic factors (i.e., older than 60 years of age, advanced disease stage, elevated serum LDH concentration, high infiltration of bone marrow plasma cells, del(13q), t(4;14) translocation with or without del(17p) chromosomal abnormality) suggested that the progression-free survival benefit of bortezomib-thalidomide-dexamethasone was consistent across these subgroups; however, because the proportion of patients with the del(17p) chromosomal abnormality was substantially smaller than the proportion of patients with other high-risk cytogenetic abnormalities, the effect of bortezomib-thalidomide-dexamethasone on progression-free survival in patients with the del(17p) chromosomal abnormality was not evaluated.

In the PETHEMA/GEM study, the complete response rate (35 versus 14%) was higher following induction therapy with bortezomib-thalidomide-dexamethasone compared with thalidomide-dexamethasone; improved complete response rates also were maintained following autologous stem cell transplantation (46 versus 24%). Among patients evaluated for high-risk cytogenetic features, 21% had high-risk features (i.e., t(4;14), t(14;16), and/or del(17p) chromosomal abnormalities); 64 or 31% of these patients had t(4;14) or del(17p) chromosomal abnormalities, respectively. Among the patients with high-risk cytogenetic features, complete response rate was substantially higher in patients who received bortezomib-thalidomide-dexamethasone compared with those who received thalidomide-dexamethasone (35 versus 0%); complete responses were achieved in 38 or 58% of patients receiving bortezomib-thalidomide-dexamethasone who had t(4;14) or del(17p) chromosomal abnormalities, respectively, compared with 0% of patients receiving thalidomide-dexamethasone who had either chromosomal abnormality. At a median follow-up of 35.2 months, median progression-free survival was prolonged in patients who received bortezomib-thalidomide-dexamethasone compared with those who received thalidomide-dexamethasone (56.2 versus 28.2 months); however, no difference in estimated 4-year overall survival (74 versus 65%, respectively) was observed between the treatment groups.

In both the GIMEMA and PETHEMA/GEM studies, grade 3 or 4 peripheral neuropathy occurred more frequently in patients receiving bortezomib-thalidomide-dexamethasone (10 and 14%, respectively) compared with those receiving thalidomide-dexamethasone (2 and 5%, respectively).

In the third study (IFM2013-04), 340 patients were randomized to receive bortezomib by subcutaneous injection in combination with thalidomide and dexamethasone or in combination with cyclophosphamide and dexamethasone. Patients receiving bortezomib-thalidomide-dexamethasone received bortezomib 1.3 mg/m^2 by subcutaneous injection on days 1, 4, 8, and 11 along with thalidomide 100 mg orally daily and dexamethasone 40 mg orally on days 1–4 and 9–12 of each 3-week cycle. Those receiving bortezomib-cyclophosphamide-dexamethasone received the same dosages of bortezomib and dexamethasone along with cyclophosphamide 500 mg/m^2 orally on days 1, 8, and 15 of each 3-week cycle. Both induction regimens were continued for a total of 4 cycles. The median age of patients enrolled in the study was approximately 60 years; 22% had ISS stage III disease, and 18% had t(4;14) translocation and/or del(17p) chromosomal abnormalities. The primary measure of efficacy was the rate of very good partial response or better, as assessed according to the International Myeloma Working Group Uniform Response criteria, following induction therapy. Overall response rate (92.3 versus 83.4%) and the rate of very good partial response or better (66.3 versus 56.2%) based on intent-to-treat analysis were higher following induction therapy with bortezomib-thalidomide-dexamethasone compared with bortezomib-cyclophosphamide-dexamethasone; however, no significant difference in complete response rate was observed between the treatment groups. Grade 2 or greater peripheral neuropathy (21.9 versus 12.9%) occurred more frequently in patients receiving bortezomib-thalidomide-dexamethasone, while grade 3 or 4 neutropenia (33.1 versus 18.9%), thrombocytopenia (10.6 versus 4.7%), and anemia (9.5 versus 4.1%) occurred more frequently in patients receiving bortezomib-cyclophosphamide-dexamethasone.

Because peripheral neuropathy occurs frequently with bortezomib- and thalidomide-based induction regimens, a modified bortezomib-thalidomide-dexamethasone induction regimen was compared with bortezomib-dexamethasone in another phase 3 study in 199 patients. Patients receiving bortezomib-dexamethasone received bortezomib 1.3 mg/m² as an IV injection on days 1, 4, 8, and 11 of each 3-week cycle for 4 cycles along with dexamethasone 40 mg orally on days 1–4 and 9–12 during cycles 1 and 2 and then on days 1–4 during cycles 3 and 4. Patients receiving the modified bortezomib-thalidomide-dexamethasone regimen received the same dosage of dexamethasone along with bortezomib 1 mg/m² as an IV injection on days 1, 4, 8, and 11 and thalidomide 100 mg orally daily during each 3-week cycle for 4 cycles. In patients with an inadequate (less than partial) response after 2 cycles of the modified bortezomib-thalidomide-dexamethasone regimen (7% of patients receiving the regimen), the dose of bortezomib was increased to 1.3 mg/m² and the dosage of thalidomide was increased to 200 mg daily during subsequent cycles. The median age of patients enrolled in the study was approximately 58 years; 22% had ISS stage III disease and, among those with cytogenetic test results, 20% had t(4;14) translocation or del(17p) chromosomal abnormalities. The primary measure of efficacy was complete response rate, as assessed according to the International Myeloma Working Group Uniform Response criteria, following induction therapy. The rate of very good partial response or better following induction therapy was higher with bortezomib-thalidomide-dexamethasone compared with bortezomib-dexamethasone (49 versus 36%); however, postinduction complete response (13 and 12%, respectively) and overall response (88 and 81%, respectively) rates were similar for both treatment groups. At a median follow-up of 32 months, median progression-free survival was similar in patients who received bortezomib-thalidomide-dexamethasone compared with those who received bortezomib-dexamethasone (26 versus 30 months, respectively). Peripheral neuropathy occurred more frequently in patients receiving bortezomib-dexamethasone compared with those receiving bortezomib-thalidomide-dexamethasone (70 versus 53%).

Use of bortezomib in combination with thalidomide and dexamethasone also was investigated in an open-label, noncomparative phase 2 study in 98 patients randomized to receive bortezomib-thalidomide-dexamethasone with or without cyclophosphamide. Patients receiving bortezomib-thalidomide-dexamethasone received bortezomib 1.3 mg/m² as an IV injection on days 1, 4, 8, and 11 along with thalidomide 100 mg orally daily and dexamethasone 40 mg orally on days 1–4 and 9–12 of each 21-day cycle. Patients receiving bortezomib-thalidomide-dexamethasone-cyclophosphamide received the same dosages of bortezomib, thalidomide, and dexamethasone along with cyclophosphamide 400 mg/m² IV on days 1 and 8 of each 21-day cycle. Both induction regimens were continued for a total of 4 cycles. Postinduction rates of overall response and complete plus near-complete response were 100 and 51%, respectively, in patients receiving bortezomib-thalidomide-dexamethasone and 94 and 43%, respectively, in those receiving bortezomib-thalidomide-dexamethasone-cyclophosphamide. At a median follow-up of 64.8 months, median progression-free survival was 56.3 months with bortezomib-thalidomide-dexamethasone and 36.3 months with bortezomib-thalidomide-dexamethasone-cyclophosphamide; the difference was not statistically significant and was largely related to an imbalance between treatment groups in the number of patients receiving subsequent therapy for relapsed disease prior to meeting the specified criteria for disease progression. A trend toward improved quality of life (assessed using the European Organisation for Research and Treatment of Cancer Quality of Life Questionnaire C30 [EORTC QLQ-C30] and EuroQoL EQ-5D health status questionnaire) was observed following the first posttransplantation follow-up visit in patients who received bortezomib-thalidomide-dexamethasone compared with those who received bortezomib-thalidomide-dexamethasone-cyclophosphamide.

Use of bortezomib-thalidomide-dexamethasone as induction therapy for newly diagnosed multiple myeloma in transplant-eligible patients has improved postinduction response rates and prolonged progression-free survival in several randomized controlled studies; however, the same benefits were not observed in a study evaluating a modified bortezomib-thalidomide-dexamethasone regimen (i.e., reduced bortezomib and thalidomide dosages). Therefore, the role of a modified bortezomib-thalidomide-dexamethasone regimen using reduced dosages of bortezomib and thalidomide is unclear. In addition, in the absence of studies including adequate numbers of patients with the del(17p) chromosomal abnormality, attempts to identify whether these patients might derive clinical benefit (e.g., prolonged progression-free survival) from bortezomib-thalidomide-dexamethasone induction therapy are speculative; additional studies are needed to identify subgroups of patients with high-risk cytogenetic features who might benefit from such therapy. The AHFS Oncology Expert Committee concluded that use of bortezomib in combination with thalidomide and dexamethasone as induction therapy for newly diagnosed multiple myeloma in transplant-eligible patients may be considered a reasonable choice (accepted; with possible conditions); however, use of a modified bortezomib-thalidomide-dexamethasone regimen using reduced dosages of bortezomib and thalidomide is not fully established because of unclear risk/benefit and/or inadequate experience. Factors that should be considered when selecting a combination chemotherapy regimen for use as induction therapy for newly diagnosed multiple myeloma in transplant-eligible patients include performance status and preexisting conditions (e.g., peripheral neuropathy).

Bortezomib, Dexamethasone, and Doxorubicin (or Pegylated Liposomal Doxorubicin). Efficacy and safety of bortezomib in combination with dexamethasone and conventional doxorubicin† (bortezomib-doxorubicin-dexamethasone) as induction therapy for newly diagnosed multiple myeloma in transplant-eligible patients† have been studied in an open-label, randomized phase 3 study (HOVON-65/GMMG-HD4).

In the HOVON-65/GMMG-HD4 study, 827 patients with newly diagnosed multiple myeloma were randomized to receive conventional doxorubicin and dexamethasone in combination with either bortezomib or vincristine as an induction regimen. Patients receiving the bortezomib-doxorubicin-dexamethasone induction regimen received bortezomib 1.3 mg/m² as an IV injection on days 1, 4, 8, and 11 along with doxorubicin hydrochloride 9 mg/m² IV per day on days 1–4 and dexamethasone 40 mg orally on days 1–4, 9–12, and 17–20 during each 28-day cycle for 3 cycles. Those receiving the vincristine-doxorubicin-dexamethasone induction regimen received vincristine sulfate 0.4 mg and doxorubicin hydrochloride 9 mg/m² IV per day on days 1–4 and dexamethasone 40 mg orally on days 1–4, 9–12, and 17–20 during each 28-day cycle for 3 cycles. Patients who received bortezomib-doxorubicin-dexamethasone induction therapy received 2 years of maintenance therapy with bortezomib (1.3 mg/m² every 2 weeks) following stem cell transplantation, while those who received vincristine-doxorubicin-dexamethasone induction therapy received thalidomide (50 mg daily) as maintenance therapy. The median age of patients enrolled in the study was 57 years; 87% had World Health Organization (WHO) performance status of 0 or 1, and 23% had ISS stage III disease. Among patients for whom cytogenetic tests were performed, 43, 14, or 11% had del(13q), t(4;14) translocation, or del(17p13) chromosomal abnormalities, respectively.

The primary measure of efficacy in the HOVON-65/GMMG-HD4 study was progression-free survival. Tumor responses were assessed using EBMT response criteria. At a median follow-up of 41 months, patients who received bortezomib-doxorubicin-dexamethasone had prolonged progression-free survival (35 versus 28 months; hazard ratio: 0.75) and higher postinduction (11 versus 5%) and posttransplant (31 versus 15%) complete plus near-complete response rates compared with those who received vincristine-doxorubicin-dexamethasone. Median overall survival had not been reached at a median follow-up of 66 months; however, no significant difference in 5-year overall survival was observed between the groups. Subgroup analyses based on presence of renal insufficiency or high-risk cytogenetic features (i.e., del(13q14), t(4;14), del(17p13) chromosomal abnormalities) suggested prolonged progression-free and overall survival with bortezomib-doxorubicin-dexamethasone compared with vincristine-doxorubicin-dexamethasone induction therapy in patients with serum creatinine concentrations exceeding 2 mg/dL and in those with del(17p13) chromosomal abnormality, as well as an overall survival benefit for bortezomib-doxorubicin-dexamethasone compared with vincristine-doxorubicin-dexamethasone in patients with del(13q14) chromosomal abnormality. Herpes zoster (2 versus 0%) and grade 3 or 4 thrombocytopenia (10 versus 5%), GI toxicity (11 versus 7%), and peripheral neuropathy (24 versus 10%) occurred more frequently in patients receiving bortezomib-doxorubicin-dexamethasone compared with those receiving vincristine-doxorubicin-dexamethasone.

Use of bortezomib and dexamethasone also has been studied in combination with pegylated liposomal doxorubicin† (bortezomib-pegylated liposomal doxorubicin-dexamethasone) as induction therapy for previously untreated multiple myeloma† in 2 open-label, noncomparative phase 2 studies.

In the first study, 40 patients with newly diagnosed multiple myeloma received bortezomib 1.3 mg/m² as an IV injection on days 1, 4, 8, and 11 along with pegylated liposomal doxorubicin hydrochloride 30 mg/m² IV on day 4 and dexamethasone 40 mg orally on days 1, 2, 4, 5, 8, 9, 11, and 12 during cycle 1. During cycles 2–6, the same dosages of bortezomib and pegylated liposomal doxorubicin were administered, but the dexamethasone dosage was 20 mg orally daily. Treatment cycles were repeated every 3 weeks for a total of 6 cycles. Overall response rate and complete plus near-complete response rate were 85 and 38%, respectively, following 6 cycles of induction therapy with bortezomib-pegylated liposomal doxorubicin-dexamethasone. Among patients who underwent stem cell transplantation, the complete plus near-complete response rate increased to 57% following transplantation, but the overall response rate did not improve substantially. At a median follow-up of 45.1 months, median progression-free survival had not been reached; however, among patients who underwent stem cell transplantation, actuarial 2- and 4-year progression-free survival rates were 93 and 65%, respectively, and actuarial 2- and 4-year overall survival rates were 97 and 67%, respectively. Grade 1 or 2 peripheral neuropathy, fatigue, palmar-plantar erythrodysesthesia (hand-foot syndrome), and constipation occurred in 90, 88, 75, and 70% of patients, respectively.

Because bortezomib and pegylated liposomal doxorubicin frequently cause adverse effects, another phase 2 study evaluated a modified bortezomib-pegylated liposomal doxorubicin-dexamethasone regimen in 35 patients with previously untreated multiple myeloma. Patients received bortezomib 1 mg/m² as an IV injection, pegylated liposomal doxorubicin hydrochloride 5 mg/m² IV, and dexamethasone phosphate 40 mg IV on days 1, 4, 8, and 11 of each 28-day cycle for a maximum of 8 cycles. Overall response rate was 86%; complete response was achieved in 20% of patients. At a median follow-up of 17.7 months, median time to progression, duration of response, and overall survival had not been reached. Constipation, fatigue, peripheral neuropathy, insomnia, and nausea occurred in 51, 46, 34, 29, and 26%, respectively, of patients.

Based on current evidence, use of bortezomib in combination with doxorubicin (or pegylated liposomal doxorubicin) and dexamethasone as induction therapy for newly diagnosed multiple myeloma in transplant-eligible patients may be considered a reasonable choice (accepted; with possible conditions);

however, in the absence of longer follow-up data, use of a modified bortezomib-pegylated liposomal doxorubicin-dexamethasone regimen (i.e., reduced dosages of bortezomib and pegylated liposomal doxorubicin) is not fully established because of unclear risk/benefit and/or inadequate experience. Factors that should be considered when selecting a combination chemotherapy regimen for use as induction therapy include performance status and preexisting conditions (e.g., peripheral neuropathy).

Bortezomib, Dexamethasone, and Cyclophosphamide. Efficacy and safety of bortezomib in combination with cyclophosphamide and dexamethasone† (bortezomib-cyclophosphamide-dexamethasone) as induction therapy for newly diagnosed multiple myeloma in transplant-eligible patients† have been studied in 2 noncomparative phase 2 studies and an open-label, randomized phase 3 study (GMMG-MM5).

In the first phase 2 study, patients with newly diagnosed multiple myeloma receiving bortezomib in combination with cyclophosphamide and dexamethasone were compared with a historical control group (34 patients who received lenalidomide 25 mg orally on days 1–21 and dexamethasone 40 mg orally on days 1–4, 9–12, and 17–20 during each 28-day cycle for 4 cycles). In this study, 33 patients received bortezomib 1.3 mg/m^2 as an IV injection twice weekly (days 1, 4, 8, and 11) along with cyclophosphamide 300 mg/m^2 orally on days 1, 8, 15, and 22 and dexamethasone 40 mg orally on days 1–4, 9–12, and 17–20 during each 28-day cycle for 4 cycles. The mean age of patients enrolled in the study was 60 years; 48% were female and 30% had ISS stage III disease. Among patients for whom cytogenetic tests were performed, 50, 18, or 13% had del(13q), t(4;14) translocation, or del(17) chromosomal abnormalities, respectively. The overall response rate and rate of very good partial response or better after 4 cycles of therapy were 88 and 61%, respectively, in patients who received bortezomib-cyclophosphamide-dexamethasone compared with 91 and 44%, respectively, in the historical control group based on intent-to-treat analysis. Among patients who underwent stem cell transplantation following bortezomib-cyclophosphamide-dexamethasone induction therapy, the posttransplant complete or near-complete response rate was 70%.

Patients from this study (twice-weekly bortezomib; cohort 1) also were compared with a subsequent cohort of 30 patients who received bortezomib 1.5 mg/m^2 as an IV injection once weekly (days 1, 8, 15, and 22) along with cyclophosphamide (same dosage as in cohort 1) and dexamethasone (same dosage as in cohort 1 during cycles 1 and 2, followed by 40 mg once weekly during cycles 3 and 4). Comparison of the 2 cohorts suggested that overall response rates and rates of very good partial response or better for the regimens containing once-weekly (93 and 60%, respectively) or twice-weekly (88 and 61%, respectively) bortezomib were similar; however, the incidences of grade 3 or 4 thrombocytopenia (0 versus 25%), neutropenia (7 versus 13%), anemia (0 versus 12%), and peripheral neuropathy (0 versus 7%) were lower in patients receiving the regimen containing once-weekly bortezomib compared with those receiving the regimen containing twice-weekly bortezomib. Analysis of pooled data for the 2 cohorts indicated a median progression-free survival of 40 months; in addition, 5-year progression-free and overall survival rates for the 2 cohorts combined were 42 and 70%, respectively. Although the overall response rate was similar in patients with high-risk cytogenetic features and those with standard-risk cytogenetic features, median progression-free survival was shorter and 5-year progression-free and overall survival rates were lower in patients with high-risk cytogenetic features (27.6 months, 33%, and 54%, respectively) compared with those with standard-risk cytogenetic features (55.7 months, 48%, and 81%, respectively).

In another phase 2 study, patients with newly diagnosed multiple myeloma received the combination of bortezomib-cyclophosphamide-dexamethasone followed by bortezomib-thalidomide-dexamethasone to determine if sequential combination therapy could improve response rates and tolerability. In this study, 44 patients received bortezomib 1.3 mg/m^2 as an IV injection on days 1, 4, 8, and 11 along with cyclophosphamide 300 mg/m^2 IV on days 1 and 8 and dexamethasone 40 mg orally on days 1, 2, 4, 5, 8, 9, 11, and 12 during each 21-day cycle for 3 cycles (cycles 1–3) followed by bortezomib 1 mg/m^2 as an IV injection on days 1, 4, 8, and 11 along with thalidomide 100 mg orally daily and dexamethasone 40 mg orally on days 1, 2, 4, 5, 8, 9, 11, and 12 during each 21-day cycle for 3 cycles (cycles 4–6). The median age of patients enrolled in the study was 58 years, and the median Karnofsky performance status was 90%; 60% of patients had ISS stage II or III disease, 49% had a baseline β_2-microglobulin concentration of 3.5 mg/L or greater, and 7 patients had cytogenetic abnormalities, including t(4;14) translocation, del(17p), and/or del(13) chromosomal abnormalities. Very good partial response or better was observed in 31 or 57% of 42 evaluable patients following 3 cycles of bortezomib-cyclophosphamide-dexamethasone or 6 cycles of sequential combination therapy, respectively; near-complete response or better was observed following 3 or 6 cycles of therapy in 2 or 36% of patients, respectively. At a median follow-up of 20.9 months, median event-free and overall survival had not been reached; however, estimated 1-year event-free and overall survival rates were 81 and 91%, respectively.

In the GMMG-MM5 study, 502 patients with newly diagnosed multiple myeloma were randomized to receive bortezomib in combination with either cyclophosphamide and dexamethasone or doxorubicin and dexamethasone. Patients receiving bortezomib-cyclophosphamide-dexamethasone received bortezomib 1.3 mg/m^2 as an IV injection on days 1, 4, 8, and 11 along with cyclophosphamide 900 mg/m^2 IV on day 1 and dexamethasone 40 mg orally on days 1, 2, 4, 5, 8, 9, 11, and 12 during each 21-day cycle. Those receiving bortezomib-doxorubicin-dexamethasone received the same dosage of bortezomib along with doxorubicin hydrochloride 9 mg/m^2 IV per day on days 1–4 and dexamethasone 20 mg orally on days 1–4, 9–12, and 17–20 of each 28-day cycle. Both regimens were continued for a total of 3 cycles. The route of administration for bortezomib was changed from IV to subcutaneous injection when data from a prior study in patients with relapsed multiple myeloma demonstrated no apparent loss in efficacy or increase in toxicity with subcutaneous administration. The median age of patients enrolled in the GMMG-MM5 study was 59 years, and 29% had ISS stage III disease. Among patients for whom cytogenetic tests were performed, 11, 11, or 40% had del(17p), t(4;14) translocation, or chromosome 1q21 duplication (i.e., 1q21 gain) abnormalities, respectively. The primary measure of efficacy was the rate of very good partial response or better, as assessed according to the International Myeloma Working Group Uniform Response criteria, following induction therapy.

Rates of overall response (78.1 versus 72.1%, respectively) and very good partial response or better (37 versus 34.3%, respectively) in the GMMG-MM5 study did not differ significantly between patients receiving bortezomib-cyclophosphamide-dexamethasone and those receiving bortezomib-doxorubicin-dexamethasone. In subgroups of patients with poor prognostic factors (i.e., t(4;14) translocation, del(17p), and/or 1q21 gain; renal impairment [serum creatinine concentration of 2 mg/dL or higher]), response rates attained with bortezomib-cyclophosphamide-dexamethasone appeared to be at least as high as those attained with bortezomib-doxorubicin-dexamethasone; the rate of progressive disease in patients with high-risk cytogenetic features, ISS stage III disease, or renal impairment appeared to be higher in those receiving bortezomib-doxorubicin-dexamethasone compared with those receiving bortezomib-cyclophosphamide-dexamethasone. In an exploratory analysis, overall response rates were similar with IV or subcutaneous injection of bortezomib, including in patients with poor prognostic factors. Grade 3 or greater leukopenia and/or neutropenia (35.2 versus 11.3%) occurred more frequently in patients receiving bortezomib-cyclophosphamide-dexamethasone, while grade 2 or greater neuropathy (14.9 versus 8.4%) occurred more frequently in patients receiving bortezomib-doxorubicin-dexamethasone.

Based on current evidence, use of bortezomib in combination with cyclophosphamide and dexamethasone may be considered a reasonable choice (accepted, with possible conditions) as induction therapy for newly diagnosed multiple myeloma in transplant-eligible patients; factors that should be considered when selecting a combination chemotherapy regimen for use as induction therapy include cytogenetic features, performance status, preexisting conditions (e.g., peripheral neuropathy), and tolerability.

■ **Non-Hodgkin's Lymphoma** ***Previously Untreated Mantle Cell Lymphoma*** Bortezomib is used in combination with rituximab, cyclophosphamide, doxorubicin, and prednisone for the treatment of previously untreated mantle cell lymphoma.

The current indication for bortezomib in patients with previously untreated mantle cell lymphoma is based principally on the results of a phase 3, open-label, randomized study (LYM-3002) in patients with newly diagnosed stage II–IV mantle cell lymphoma who were considered ineligible for or were not considered for stem cell transplantation. In this study, 487 patients were randomized (stratified by International Prognostic Index [IPI] score and disease stage) in a 1:1 ratio to receive either rituximab plus cyclophosphamide, doxorubicin, vincristine, and prednisone (R-CHOP) or bortezomib plus rituximab, cyclophosphamide, doxorubicin, and prednisone (VR-CAP). The planned course of therapy for both regimens was six 21-day cycles; patients were permitted to receive up to 2 additional cycles if a response was first observed at cycle 6. Patients in the control group received rituximab 375 mg/m^2 IV, cyclophosphamide 750 mg/m^2 IV, doxorubicin hydrochloride 50 mg/m^2 IV, and vincristine sulfate 1.4 mg/m^2 (maximum dose of 2 mg) IV on day 1 plus prednisone 100 mg/m^2 orally on days 1–5 of each 21-day cycle. Patients in the study group received the same dosages of rituximab, cyclophosphamide, doxorubicin hydrochloride, and prednisone with the addition of bortezomib 1.3 mg/m^2 by IV injection on days 1, 4, 8, and 11 of each 21-day cycle. The median number of cycles for patients receiving R-CHOP or VR-CAP was 6; 17 or 14% of patients receiving R-CHOP or VR-CAP, respectively, received up to 2 additional cycles of their respective chemotherapy regimen. The primary end point of this study was progression-free survival as assessed by an independent review committee. The median age of patients enrolled in the study was 66 years; 74% of patients were male, 66% were white, 54% had an IPI score of 3 or greater, 76% had stage IV disease, and 69% had a positive bone marrow aspirate and/or bone marrow biopsy for mantle cell lymphoma.

At a median follow-up of 40 months, median progression-free survival was prolonged in patients who received VR-CAP compared with those who received R-CHOP (25 versus 14 months; hazard ratio of 0.63). The overall response rates with VR-CAP and R-CHOP were 88 and 85%, respectively, with 44% of patients receiving VR-CAP and 34% of those receiving R-CHOP achieving complete responses. Median overall survival had not been reached at the time of the analysis.

Relapsed Mantle Cell Lymphoma Bortezomib is used for treatment of mantle cell lymphoma in patients who have received at least one prior therapy. The current indication for bortezomib in patients with relapsed mantle cell lymphoma is based principally on the results of a phase 2, open-label, single-arm, clinical study involving 155 patients (median age: 65 years; range: 42–89 years). Patients received bortezomib 1.3 mg/m^2 by IV injection administered in 21-day treatment cycles (on days 1, 4, 8, and 11 followed by a 10-day rest period on days 12–21) for a maximum of 17 cycles; patients achieving a complete response or an unconfirmed complete response were treated for 4 cycles beyond the first evidence of complete response or unconfirmed complete response. Therapy was discontinued if progressive disease or unacceptable toxicity occurred or based on a decision by the patient and clinician. The median number of cycles administered in all patients was 4; in responding patients, the median number of cycles was 8.

Responses were assessed according to International Workshop Response Criteria (IWRC) based on independent review of CT scans. The median time to response was 40 days (range: 31–204 days). The overall response rate (complete responses, unconfirmed complete responses, and partial responses) was 31%, and the median duration of response was 9.3 months. A complete response or an unconfirmed complete response was reported in 8%.

Other Non-Hodgkin's Lymphomas Bortezomib is being investigated for use in the treatment of other non-Hodgkin's lymphomas†. In small phase 2 uncontrolled studies, bortezomib has shown activity in the treatment of relapsed or refractory B-cell lymphomas.

Dosage and Administration

■ **General** Clinicians should consult the respective manufacturers' labelings for information on the dosage and method of administration of other antineoplastic agents used in combination regimens.

Because reactivation of latent varicella zoster virus infection has been reported in bortezomib-treated patients, the manufacturer recommends that antiviral prophylaxis be considered in patients receiving the drug.

■ **Reconstitution and Administration** Bortezomib is administered by IV injection (over 3–5 seconds) or by subcutaneous injection; the drug should *not* be administered by any other route. (See Cautions: Contraindications.) A sticker indicating the route of administration is provided by the manufacturer and should be affixed directly to the syringe following reconstitution. Subcutaneous administration of bortezomib may be considered in patients with preexisting peripheral neuropathy and those at high risk for developing peripheral neuropathy. (See Relapsed Multiple Myeloma under Uses: Multiple Myeloma.) Recommended sites for subcutaneous injection of bortezomib include the thigh and abdominal region. Injection sites should be rotated, with new injections administered at least one inch from the previous injection site; any area that is tender, erythematous, bruised, or indurated should be avoided.

The manufacturer recommends that procedures for proper handling (e.g., use of gloves or protective clothing) and disposal of bortezomib be used.

Prior to administration, bortezomib powder for injection must be reconstituted using proper aseptic technique. The manufacturer states that only 0.9% sodium chloride injection should be used to reconstitute the lyophilized powder. The reconstituted bortezomib solution should be inspected visually for particulate matter and/or discoloration prior to administration and should be discarded if either is present.

For IV injection, bortezomib sterile powder for injection is reconstituted by adding 3.5 mL of 0.9% sodium chloride injection to a vial labeled as containing 3.5 mg of the drug to yield a final concentration of 1 mg/mL.

For subcutaneous injection, bortezomib sterile powder for injection is reconstituted by adding 1.4 mL of 0.9% sodium chloride injection to a vial labeled as containing 3.5 mg of the drug to yield a final concentration of 2.5 mg/mL. If local injection site reactions occur following subcutaneous administration of the drug at a reconstituted concentration of 2.5 mg/mL, the manufacturer states that the solution may be reconstituted to a lower concentration of 1 mg/mL; however, administration of subsequent doses of the drug by IV injection also should be considered.

Unreconstituted bortezomib powder for injection should be stored in unopened vials at a controlled room temperature of 25°C but may be exposed to temperatures ranging from 15–30°C. Unopened vials should be retained in the original package to protect from light. The reconstituted drug may be stored at 25°C in the original vial and/or syringe but should be administered within 8 hours after reconstitution.

■ **Dosage** The amount of bortezomib contained in one 3.5-mg vial may exceed the usual single dose required. Because the final concentration of reconstituted bortezomib solutions varies depending on the route of administration, caution should be exercised in calculating the dose and respective volume of bortezomib to be administered to prevent overdosage.

Previously Untreated Multiple Myeloma For the treatment of previously untreated multiple myeloma, bortezomib is administered in combination with melphalan and prednisone as part of the VMP regimen. The recommended adult dosage of bortezomib during cycles 1–4 (of the recommended nine 6-week cycles) is 1.3 mg/m^2 by IV injection over 3–5 seconds or by subcutaneous injection twice weekly during weeks 1, 2, 4, and 5 (days 1, 4, 8, 11, 22, 25, 29, and 32 of the 6-week cycle) followed by a 10-day rest period (days 33–42). For cycles 5–9, the same dosage of bortezomib is administered once weekly during weeks 1, 2, 4, and 5 (days 1, 8, 22, and 29) followed by a 13-day rest period. In all 9 cycles, melphalan 9 mg/m^2 and prednisone 60 mg/m^2 are administered orally once daily on days 1–4. The manufacturer states that at least 72 hours should elapse between consecutive doses of bortezomib.

Previously Untreated Mantle Cell Lymphoma For the treatment of previously untreated mantle cell lymphoma, bortezomib is administered in combination with rituximab, cyclophosphamide, doxorubicin, and prednisone as part of the VR-CAP regimen in 3-week cycles for 6 cycles. The recommended adult dosage of bortezomib is 1.3 mg/m^2 by IV injection over 3–5 seconds twice weekly for 2 weeks (days 1, 4, 8, and 11), followed by a 10-day rest period (days 12–21). Rituximab 375 mg/m^2, cyclophosphamide 750 mg/m^2, and doxorubicin hydrochloride 50 mg/m^2 are administered IV on day 1 and prednisone 100 mg/m^2 is administered orally on days 1–5 of each 3-week cycle. For patients in whom a response is first observed at cycle 6, the manufacturer recommends 2 additional cycles of the VR-CAP regimen. The manufacturer states that at least 72 hours should elapse between consecutive doses of bortezomib.

Relapsed Multiple Myeloma and Mantle Cell Lymphoma For the treatment of relapsed multiple myeloma and mantle cell lymphoma, the recommended adult dosage of bortezomib for the standard schedule is 1.3 mg/m^2 by IV injection over 3–5 seconds or by subcutaneous injection twice weekly for 2 weeks (days 1, 4, 8, and 11), followed by a 10-day rest period (days 12–21). For extended therapy of more than 8 treatment cycles, bortezomib may be administered on the standard schedule or, for patients with relapsed multiple myeloma, on a maintenance schedule consisting of bortezomib 1.3 mg/m^2 by IV injection or by subcutaneous injection once weekly for 4 weeks (days 1, 8, 15, and 22), followed by a 13-day rest period (days 23–35). The manufacturer states that at least 72 hours should elapse between consecutive doses of bortezomib.

For the retreatment of multiple myeloma in patients who previously responded to bortezomib-based therapy and relapsed at least 6 months following therapy, the last tolerated dose of bortezomib is administered twice weekly for 2 weeks (days 1, 4, 8, and 11), followed by a 10-day rest period (days 12–21) for up to 8 cycles. Bortezomib may be reinitiated with or without dexamethasone. The manufacturer states that at least 72 hours should elapse between consecutive doses of bortezomib.

Induction Therapy Prior to Stem-Cell Transplantation in Newly Diagnosed Multiple Myeloma **Bortezomib and Dexamethasone.** When bortezomib has been used in combination with dexamethasone† as induction therapy for newly diagnosed multiple myeloma in transplant-eligible patients†, bortezomib 1.3 mg/m^2 has been administered by IV injection twice weekly for 2 weeks (days 1, 4, 8, and 11) followed by a 10-day rest period (days 12–21) of each 21-day cycle for 4 cycles. In cycles 1 and 2, dexamethasone 40 mg was administered orally on days 1–4 and 9–12; in cycles 3 and 4, dexamethasone 40 mg was administered orally on days 1–4.

Bortezomib, Dexamethasone, and Thalidomide. Bortezomib has been used in several regimens in combination with thalidomide and dexamethasone† as induction therapy for newly diagnosed multiple myeloma in transplant-eligible patients†.

When bortezomib has been used in combination with thalidomide and dexamethasone as induction therapy for newly diagnosed multiple myeloma in transplant-eligible patients, bortezomib 1.3 mg/m^2 has been administered by IV injection twice weekly for 2 weeks (days 1, 4, 8, and 11) along with dexamethasone 40 mg orally on days 1, 2, 4, 5, 8, 9, 11, and 12 and thalidomide 200 mg orally daily (after initial dosage escalation during cycle 1 with 100 mg orally on days 1–14 followed by 200 mg orally daily thereafter). Treatment cycles were repeated every 21 days for 3 cycles.

Bortezomib 1.3 mg/m^2 also has been administered by IV injection twice weekly for 2 weeks (days 1, 4, 8, and 11) along with dexamethasone 40 mg orally on days 1–4 and 9–12 and thalidomide 200 mg orally daily (after initial dosage escalation during cycle 1 with 50 mg orally on days 1–14 followed by 100 mg orally on days 15–28). Treatment cycles were repeated every 4 weeks for 6 cycles.

Bortezomib 1.3 mg/m^2 also has been administered by subcutaneous or IV injection twice weekly for 2 weeks (days 1, 4, 8, and 11) along with dexamethasone 40 mg orally on days 1–4 and 9–12 and thalidomide 100 mg orally daily. Treatment cycles were repeated every 3 weeks for 4 cycles.

A modified regimen using reduced dosages of bortezomib and thalidomide is not fully established.

Bortezomib, Dexamethasone, and Doxorubicin (or Pegylated Liposomal Doxorubicin). Bortezomib has been used in several regimens in combination with doxorubicin (or pegylated liposomal doxorubicin) and dexamethasone† as induction therapy for newly diagnosed multiple myeloma in transplant-eligible patients†.

When bortezomib has been used in combination with doxorubicin and dexamethasone as induction therapy for newly diagnosed multiple myeloma in transplant-eligible patients, bortezomib 1.3 mg/m^2 has been administered by IV injection twice weekly for 2 weeks (days 1, 4, 8, and 11) along with doxorubicin hydrochloride 9 mg/m^2 IV per day on days 1–4 and dexamethasone 40 mg orally on days 1–4, 9–12, and 17–20 of each 28-day cycle for 3 cycles.

Bortezomib 1.3 mg/m^2 also has been administered by IV injection twice weekly for 2 weeks (days 1, 4, 8, and 11) along with pegylated liposomal doxorubicin hydrochloride 30 mg/m^2 IV on day 4 and dexamethasone 40 mg orally on days 1, 2, 4, 5, 8, 9, 11, and 12 during cycle 1. During cycles 2–6, the same dosages of bortezomib and pegylated liposomal doxorubicin were administered along with dexamethasone 20 mg orally daily. Treatment cycles were repeated every 3 weeks for a total of 6 cycles.

A modified regimen using reduced dosages of bortezomib and pegylated liposomal doxorubicin is not fully established.

Bortezomib, Dexamethasone, and Cyclophosphamide. Bortezomib has been used in several regimens in combination with cyclophosphamide and dexamethasone† as induction therapy for newly diagnosed multiple myeloma in transplant-eligible patients†.

When bortezomib has been used in combination with cyclophosphamide and dexamethasone as induction therapy for newly diagnosed multiple myeloma in transplant-eligible patients, bortezomib 1.3 mg/m^2 has been administered by IV injection twice weekly for 2 weeks (days 1, 4, 8, and 11) along with cyclophosphamide 300 mg/m^2 orally on days 1, 8, 15, and 22 and dexamethasone 40 mg orally on days 1–4, 9–12, and 17–20 of each 28-day cycle for 4 cycles.

Bortezomib 1.5 mg/m^2 also has been administered by IV injection once weekly (days 1, 8, 15, and 22) along with cyclophosphamide 300 mg/m^2 orally on days 1, 8, 15, and 22 of each 28-day cycle for 4 cycles, with dexamethasone 40 mg administered orally on days 1–4, 9–12, and 17–20 during cycles 1 and 2 and then once weekly during cycles 3 and 4.

Bortezomib 1.3 mg/m^2 also has been administered by IV injection twice weekly for 2 weeks (days 1, 4, 8, and 11) along with cyclophosphamide 300 mg/m^2 IV on days 1 and 8 and dexamethasone 40 mg orally on days 1, 2, 4, 5, 8, 9, 11, and 12 of each 21-day cycle for 3 cycles (cycles 1–3) followed by bortezomib 1 mg/m^2 by IV injection twice weekly for 2 weeks (days 1, 4, 8, and 11) along with thalidomide 100 mg orally daily and dexamethasone 40 mg orally on days 1, 2, 4, 5, 8, 9, 11, and 12 of each 21-day cycle for 3 cycles (cycles 4–6).

Bortezomib 1.3 mg/m^2 also has been administered by subcutaneous or IV injection twice weekly for 2 weeks (days 1, 4, 8, and 11) along with cyclophosphamide 900 mg/m^2 IV on day 1 and dexamethasone 40 mg orally on days 1, 2, 4, 5, 8, 9, 11, and 12 of each 21-day cycle for 3 cycles.

■ **Dosage Modification for Toxicity** ***Dosage Modification in Patients with Newly Diagnosed Multiple Myeloma Receiving Bortezomib with Melphalan and Prednisone (VMP)*** The manufacturer of bortezomib states that before administration of any cycle of VMP, platelet counts should be 70,000/mm^3 or higher and the absolute neutrophil count (ANC) should be 1000/mm^3 or above. In addition, any nonhematologic toxicities should have resolved to grade 1 or baseline before any VMP cycle is administered.

Hematologic Toxicity. If prolonged grade 4 neutropenia or thrombocytopenia, or thrombocytopenia with bleeding, was observed in the previous VMP cycle, reduction of the melphalan dose by 25% in the next cycle should be considered.

If the platelet count is 30,000/mm^3 or less or if the ANC is 750/mm^3 or less on a day when bortezomib is to be administered (other than on day 1), the dose of bortezomib should be withheld. If several doses of bortezomib were withheld because of toxicity in consecutive cycles, it is recommended that the dose of bortezomib be reduced by one dose level (i.e., a dose of 1.3 mg/m^2 reduced to 1 mg/m^2; a dose of 1 mg/m^2 reduced to 0.7 mg/m^2).

Nonhematologic Effects. If nonhematologic toxicities (other than neuropathy) of grade 3 or more in severity occur during VMP therapy, bortezomib therapy should be withheld until symptoms of the toxicity have resolved to grade 1 or baseline. Bortezomib may then be reinitiated with a reduction of one dose level (i.e., a dose of 1.3 mg/m^2 reduced to 1 mg/m^2; a dose of 1 mg/m^2 reduced to 0.7 mg/m^2).

If neuropathic pain and/or peripheral neuropathy occurs during VMP therapy, bortezomib should be withheld or the dose reduced as recommended in patients with relapsed multiple myeloma or mantle cell lymphoma who develop such manifestations. (See Peripheral Neuropathy under Dosage Modification for Toxicity: Dosage Modification in Patients with Relapsed Multiple Myeloma or Mantle Cell Lymphoma, in Dosage and Administration.)

Dosage Modification in Patients with Newly Diagnosed Mantle Cell Lymphoma Receiving Bortezomib with Rituximab, Cyclophosphamide, Doxorubicin, and Prednisone (VR-CAP) The manufacturer of bortezomib states that before administration of cycles 2–6 of VR-CAP therapy, platelet counts should be at least 100,000/mm^3, ANC should be at least 1500/mm^3, hemoglobin concentration should be at least 8 g/dL, and any nonhematologic toxicities should have resolved to grade 1 or baseline.

Hematologic Toxicity. If neutropenia of grade 3 or more in severity or platelet count less than 25,000/mm^3 occurs on a day when bortezomib is to be administered (other than on day 1 of the cycle), the dose of bortezomib should be withheld for up to 2 weeks until ANC reaches or exceeds 750/mm^3 and platelet count reaches or exceeds 25,000/mm^3; bortezomib may then be resumed at one dose level lower than the previous dosage (i.e., a dose of 1.3 mg/m^2 reduced to 1 mg/m^2; a dose of 1 mg/m^2 reduced to 0.7 mg/m^2). If hematologic toxicity has not resolved after withholding bortezomib for 2 weeks, bortezomib therapy should be discontinued.

Nonhematologic Effects. If nonhematologic toxicities (other than neuropathy) of grade 3 or more in severity occur during VR-CAP therapy on a day when bortezomib is to be administered (other than on day 1 of the cycle), bortezomib therapy should be withheld until symptoms of the toxicity have resolved to grade 2 or less. Bortezomib may then be reinitiated with a reduction of one dose level (i.e., a dose of 1.3 mg/m^2 reduced to 1 mg/m^2; a dose of 1 mg/m^2 reduced to 0.7 mg/m^2).

If neuropathic pain and/or peripheral neuropathy occurs during VR-CAP therapy, bortezomib should be withheld or the dose reduced as recommended in patients with relapsed multiple myeloma or mantle cell lymphoma who develop such manifestations. (See Peripheral Neuropathy under Dosage Modification for Toxicity: Dosage Modification in Patients with Relapsed Multiple Myeloma or Mantle Cell Lymphoma, in Dosage and Administration.)

Dosage Modification in Patients with Relapsed Multiple Myeloma or Mantle Cell Lymphoma **Peripheral Neuropathy.** Adjustment of the dose and/or frequency of administration of bortezomib may be required in patients who develop new or worsening peripheral neuropathy. In patients who develop grade 1 peripheral neuropathy (asymptomatic, loss of deep tendon reflexes or paresthesia) *without* pain or loss of function, no dosage modification is necessary. However, in patients who develop grade 1 peripheral neuropathy *with* pain or grade 2 peripheral neuropathy (moderate symptoms resulting in interference with instrumental activities of daily living), the dose of bortezomib should be reduced to 1 mg/m^2. In patients who develop grade 2 peripheral neuropathy with pain or grade 3 peripheral neuropathy (severe symptoms resulting in interference with self-care activities of daily living), bortezomib therapy should be temporarily discontinued; once manifestations of toxicity have resolved, the drug may be reinitiated at a dosage of 0.7 mg/m^2 once weekly. Bortezomib therapy should be discontinued in patients who develop grade 4 peripheral neuropathy (sensory neuropathy that is disabling or motor neuropathy that is life threatening or leads to paralysis). The manufacturer states that bortezomib should be used in patients with preexisting severe neuropathy only after careful assessment of the risks and benefits for the individual patient.

Other Nonhematologic or Hematologic Effects. Bortezomib therapy should be temporarily discontinued in patients who develop any grade 3 nonhematologic or grade 4 hematologic toxicities (e.g., grade 4 thrombocytopenia [platelet count less than 25,000/mm^3]). Once manifestations of toxicity have resolved, bortezomib may be reinitiated but dosage of the drug should be reduced by 25% (i.e., a dose of 1.3 mg/m^2 reduced to 1 mg/m^2; a dose of 1 mg/m^2 reduced to 0.7 mg/m^2).

■ **Special Populations** Bortezomib is metabolized by hepatic enzymes, and exposure to the drug is increased in patients with moderate hepatic impairment (defined as bilirubin concentrations ranging from more than 1.5 to 3 times the upper limit of normal with any AST concentrations) or severe hepatic impairment (defined as bilirubin concentrations exceeding 3 times the upper limit of normal with any AST concentrations). The manufacturer recommends that doses of bortezomib during the first cycle of treatment be reduced to 0.7 mg/m^2 in patients with moderate or severe hepatic impairment. Based on patient tolerance, dosage in subsequent cycles may be increased to 1 mg/m^2 or further reduced to 0.5 mg/m^2. The manufacturer states that no adjustment in the initial dose is needed in patients with mild hepatic impairment (defined as bilirubin concentrations at or below the upper limit of normal with AST concentrations exceeding the upper limit of normal *or* bilirubin concentrations ranging from more than 1 to 1.5 times the upper limit of normal with any AST concentrations); such patients should be treated with the usual recommended initial dosage.

The pharmacokinetics of bortezomib are not influenced by the degree of renal impairment; therefore, dosage adjustment is not necessary in such patients. Because dialysis may decrease bortezomib concentrations, the drug should be administered after a dialysis procedure. (See Renal Impairment under Warnings/Precautions: Specific Populations, in Cautions.)

Cautions

■ **Contraindications** Bortezomib is contraindicated in patients with known hypersensitivity (except for local reactions) to bortezomib, boron, or mannitol. Anaphylactic reactions have been reported in patients receiving bortezomib.

Intrathecal administration of bortezomib is contraindicated. Intrathecal administration of bortezomib has resulted in death.

■ **Warnings/Precautions** ***Peripheral Neuropathy*** Bortezomib mainly causes sensory peripheral neuropathy, but severe motor peripheral neuropathy also has been reported. Patients with preexisting manifestations of peripheral neuropathy (e.g., numbness, pain, or burning sensation in feet or hands) may experience worsening peripheral neuropathy (including grade 3 or higher) during therapy with bortezomib.

In clinical studies in patients with relapsed multiple myeloma or mantle cell lymphoma, peripheral neuropathy occurred in 38% of patients receiving IV bortezomib and was grade 3 or higher in approximately 11% of patients receiving the drug. In the phase 3 randomized study in patients with relapsed multiple myeloma, dosage adjustments resulted in amelioration or resolution of peripheral neuropathy in 48% of patients with grade 2 or higher peripheral neuropathy within a median of 3.8 months from onset. In the phase 2 trials in patients with relapsed multiple myeloma, amelioration or resolution of peripheral neuropathy occurred in 73% of patients who discontinued bortezomib therapy because of grade 2 peripheral neuropathy or who had grade 3 or 4 peripheral neuropathy; the median time to improvement of one grade or more from the last dose of bortezomib was 47 days. The long-term outcome of peripheral neuropathy has not been elucidated in patients with mantle cell lymphoma. About 8% of patients with multiple myeloma or mantle cell lymphoma discontinued IV bortezomib therapy because of peripheral neuropathy.

In the phase 3 study evaluating subcutaneous administration of bortezomib in patients with relapsed multiple myeloma, grade 2 or higher peripheral neuropathy occurred in 39% of patients receiving bortezomib by IV injection compared with 24% of those receiving subcutaneous bortezomib. Grade 3 or higher peripheral neuropathy occurred more frequently in patients receiving bortezomib by IV injection compared with those receiving subcutaneous bortezomib (15 versus 6%). (See Dosage and Administration: Reconstitution and Administration.)

Patients receiving bortezomib should be monitored for manifestations of neuropathy (e.g., burning sensation, hyperesthesia, hypoesthesia, paresthesia, discomfort, neuropathic pain or weakness). Adjustment of the dose and/or frequency of administration of bortezomib may be required in patients who experience new onset or exacerbation of peripheral neuropathy. (See Dosage and Administration: Dosage Modification for Toxicity.)

Hypotension In clinical studies in patients with relapsed multiple myeloma or mantle cell lymphoma, hypotension, including orthostatic hypotension, was reported in 8% of patients receiving IV bortezomib; grade 3 or higher hypotension occurred in approximately 2% of patients receiving the drug. Hypotension was reported as a serious adverse event in 2% of patients receiving bortezomib, and 1% of patients discontinued bortezomib therapy because of hypotension. In addition, less than 1% of patients who developed hypotension also experienced a concurrent syncopal event.

The manufacturer states that bortezomib should be used with caution in patients with a history of syncope, in patients receiving drugs known to be associated with hypotension, and in patients who are dehydrated. Orthostatic hypotension may be managed with adjustment of antihypertensive therapy, hydration, and administration of mineralocorticoids and/or sympathomimetic agents.

Cardiovascular Effects Death from cardiogenic shock, congestive heart failure, or cardiac arrest has occurred in patients receiving bortezomib. Acute development or exacerbation of congestive heart failure and new onset of decreased left ventricular ejection fraction have been reported in association with bortezomib therapy, including in patients who had no risk factors for decreased left ventricular ejection fraction. Patients with existing heart disease and patients with increased risk for heart disease should be monitored closely during bortezomib therapy. In the phase 3 study in patients with relapsed multiple myeloma, the incidence of any treatment-emergent cardiac disorder was 8 or 5% in patients receiving bortezomib or dexamethasone, respectively. The incidence of cardiac failure and congestive cardiac failure was similar in patients receiving bortezomib versus dexamethasone (less than 1%); however, acute pulmonary edema, cardiogenic shock, and pulmonary edema each occurred in less than 1% of patients receiving bortezomib compared with none of those receiving dexamethasone. Isolated cases of prolonged QT interval have been reported; a causal relationship to bortezomib has not been established.

Pulmonary Effects Death from respiratory insufficiency has occurred in patients receiving bortezomib. Acute diffuse infiltrative pulmonary disease of unknown etiology (e.g., pneumonitis, interstitial pneumonia, lung infiltration) and acute respiratory distress syndrome, sometimes fatal, have been reported in patients receiving bortezomib. Pulmonary hypertension in the absence of left heart failure or substantial pulmonary disease also has been reported. If new or worsening cardiopulmonary symptoms occur, a prompt comprehensive diagnostic evaluation should be conducted; temporary interruption of therapy should be considered pending evaluation of symptoms.

Reversible Posterior Leukoencephalopathy Syndrome Reversible posterior leukoencephalopathy syndrome (RPLS) has occurred in patients receiving bortezomib. RPLS may manifest with seizures, hypertension, headache, lethargy, confusion, blindness, and other visual and neurologic disturbances. Brain imaging, preferably magnetic resonance imaging, is used to confirm the diagnosis. Bortezomib should be discontinued in patients who develop RPLS. The safety of reinitiating bortezomib in patients previously experiencing RPLS has not been established.

GI Effects Nausea, diarrhea, constipation, vomiting, loss of appetite, dyspepsia, and dysgeusia can occur in patients receiving bortezomib therapy; ileus also may occur. In clinical studies in patients with relapsed multiple myeloma or mantle cell lymphoma, 75% of patients receiving IV bortezomib experienced at least one GI disorder; grade 3 or higher adverse GI effects occurred in approximately 14% of patients receiving the drug, and serious adverse GI effects occurred in 7% of patients. About 4% of patients receiving bortezomib discontinued therapy because of adverse GI effects.

Because adverse GI effects may be severe and sometimes may require use of antiemetics and antidiarrheals, the manufacturer states that fluid and electrolyte replacement should be used in patients receiving bortezomib therapy to prevent dehydration. If severe adverse GI effects occur, temporary interruption of therapy is recommended.

Hematologic Effects In clinical studies in patients with relapsed multiple myeloma or mantle cell lymphoma, thrombocytopenia was reported in 32% of patients receiving IV bortezomib and was grade 3 or higher in 26% of patients receiving the drug. Neutropenia was reported in 15% of patients receiving bortezomib and was grade 3 or higher in approximately 10% of patients receiving the drug. Thrombocytopenia or neutropenia was reported as a serious adverse event in 2 or less than 1%, respectively, of patients receiving bortezomib. In these studies, thrombocytopenia or neutropenia occurred during days 1–11 of each cycle and platelet and neutrophil counts returned toward baseline during the 10-day rest period.

Dose-related decreases in absolute neutrophil count (ANC) and platelet count followed a cyclical pattern with nadirs occurring following the last dose of each cycle and typically recovering prior to initiation of the subsequent cycle. The pattern of ANC and platelet count decreases and recovery remained consistent with no evidence of cumulative neutropenia or thrombocytopenia in the regimens evaluated for the treatment of multiple myeloma or mantle cell lymphoma.

In the phase 3 randomized study in patients with relapsed multiple myeloma, the platelet count nadir in patients receiving bortezomib averaged approximately 40% of the baseline platelet count. The severity of thrombocytopenia associated with bortezomib was related to pretreatment platelet count. In this study, platelet count less than 10,000/mm^3 occurred in 1 (14%) of 7 patients with a baseline platelet count of 10,000–49,999/mm^3, in 2 (14%) of 14 patients with a baseline platelet count of 50,000–74,999/mm^3, and in 8 (3%) of 309 patients with a baseline platelet count of at least 75,000/mm^3; platelet count of 10,000–25,000/mm^3 occurred in 5 (71%) of 7 patients with a baseline platelet count of 10,000–49,999/mm^3, in 11 (79%) of 14 patients with a baseline platelet count of 50,000–74,999/mm^3, and in 36 (12%) of 309 patients with a baseline platelet count of at least 75,000/mm^3. Grade 3 or higher bleeding events occurred in 2% of patients receiving bortezomib compared with less than 1% of patients receiving dexamethasone. GI and intracerebral hemorrhage associated with thrombocytopenia have been reported in patients receiving bortezomib.

In the phase 3 clinical study evaluating bortezomib in combination with rituximab, cyclophosphamide, doxorubicin, and prednisone (VR-CAP) in patients with previously untreated mantle cell lymphoma, grade 4 or higher thrombocytopenia or neutropenia was reported in 32 or 70%, respectively, of patients receiving VR-CAP compared with 1 or 52%, respectively, of those receiving rituximab plus cyclophosphamide, doxorubicin, vincristine, and prednisone (R-CHOP). Grade 3 or higher bleeding events or grade 4 or higher febrile neutropenia occurred in 1 or 5%, respectively, of patients receiving VR-CAP compared with less than 1 or 6%, respectively, of those receiving R-CHOP. Platelet transfusions were administered in 23 or 3% of patients receiving VR-CAP or R-CHOP, respectively. Granulocyte colony-stimulating factor or granulocyte-macrophage colony-stimulating factor support was administered in 78 or 61% of patients receiving VR-CAP or R-CHOP, respectively.

The manufacturer states that complete blood cell counts should be performed frequently in patients receiving bortezomib therapy. Platelet counts should be monitored prior to the administration of each dose of bortezomib. Depending on the severity of thrombocytopenia or neutropenia, temporary interruption of bortezomib followed by dosage reduction may be required. (See Dosage and Administration: Dosage Modification for Toxicity.) Supportive care (e.g., transfusions) should be administered according to published guidelines.

Tumor Lysis Syndrome Tumor lysis syndrome has been reported in patients receiving bortezomib. The risk of tumor lysis syndrome is increased in patients with a large tumor burden; such patients should be monitored closely and appropriate precautions should be taken.

Hepatic Effects Acute liver failure has been reported in patients with serious underlying medical conditions who were receiving bortezomib with multiple concomitant drugs. Increases in hepatic enzyme concentrations, hyperbilirubinemia, and hepatitis also have been reported. If such effects occur, the manufacturer recommends interrupting therapy with the drug to assess reversibility of adverse hepatic effects. Information on the results of rechallenge with the drug in these patients is limited.

Fetal/Neonatal Morbidity and Mortality There are no adequate and well-controlled studies of bortezomib in pregnant women; however, based on animal findings, bortezomib may cause fetal harm. Embryofetal toxicity (i.e., decreased fetal weight) and lethality were observed in pregnant animals receiving bortezomib at a dosage approximately 0.5 times the recommended human dosage; no evidence of teratogenicity was observed.

Pregnancy should be avoided during therapy. (See Advice to Patients.) If bortezomib is used during pregnancy or if the patient becomes pregnant while receiving the drug, the patient should be apprised of the potential hazard to the fetus.

Herpes Virus Infections In randomized studies in patients with previously untreated or relapsed multiple myeloma, reactivation of varicella zoster virus infection was more common in patients receiving bortezomib (6–11%) compared with those receiving other therapies (3–4%). The frequency of herpes simplex virus infection was similar in patients receiving bortezomib and those receiving other therapies (1–3%). In the phase 3 study in patients with previously untreated multiple myeloma, reactivation of latent varicella zoster virus infection occurred less frequently in patients receiving bortezomib plus melphalan and prednisone (VMP) with prophylactic antiviral therapy (3%) compared with patients receiving VMP without antiviral prophylaxis (17%).

Specific Populations **Pregnancy.** Category D. (See Fetal/Neonatal Morbidity and Mortality under Cautions: Warnings/Precautions.)

Lactation. It is not known whether bortezomib is distributed into milk. Because of the potential for serious adverse reactions to bortezomib in nursing infants, a decision should be made whether to discontinue nursing or the drug, taking into account the importance of the drug to the woman.

Pediatric Use. Efficacy of bortezomib has not been established in pediatric patients with relapsed pre-B acute lymphoblastic leukemia (ALL). In a study evaluating the activity and safety of bortezomib (1.3 mg/m^2 IV) in combination with intensive reinduction chemotherapy in pediatric patients and young adults with lymphoid malignancies, bortezomib did not alter complete remission rates at day 36 in the subset of patients with pre-B ALL compared with a historical control. No new safety concerns were identified in this study.

In pediatric patients, clearance of bortezomib normalized to body surface area (BSA) was comparable to that observed in adults.

Geriatric Use. Although no overall differences in efficacy or safety were observed between geriatric and younger patients receiving bortezomib, the possibility that some older patients may exhibit increased sensitivity to the drug cannot be ruled out. Exposure to bortezomib may be increased in geriatric patients compared with younger adults.

Of the 669 patients with relapsed multiple myeloma enrolled in the phase 3 randomized trial, 245 (37%) were 65 years of age or older. Among geriatric patients, longer median time to progression (5.5 versus 4.3 months), longer median duration of response (8 versus 4.9 months), and higher rates of overall response (40 versus 18%) were observed for those receiving bortezomib versus dexamethasone. Among patients receiving bortezomib, grade 3 or 4 adverse effects were reported in 64% of patients 50 years of age or younger, 78% of patients 51–64 years of age, and 75% of patients 65 years of age or older.

In patients with multiple myeloma, exposure to bortezomib (based on dose-normalized area under the concentration-time curve [AUC] and peak plasma concentrations) following the first 1- or 1.3-mg/m² IV dose of the drug was 25% lower in patients younger than 65 years of age compared with older adults.

Renal Impairment. In a pharmacokinetic study in patients with normal renal function or with varying degrees of renal impairment, exposure to bortezomib (based on dose-normalized AUC and peak plasma concentrations) was comparable among all the groups. However, because dialysis may decrease bortezomib concentrations, the drug should be administered after a dialysis procedure. (See Dosage and Administration: Special Populations.)

Hepatic Impairment. Bortezomib is metabolized by hepatic enzymes (e.g., cytochrome P-450 [CYP] microsomal enzymes), and exposure to the drug is increased in patients with moderate or severe hepatic impairment. In a pharmacokinetic study in cancer patients, exposure to bortezomib (based on dose-normalized AUC) was increased by approximately 60% in patients with moderate or severe hepatic impairment compared with patients with normal hepatic function; mild hepatic impairment did not alter the dose-normalized AUC of bortezomib. Patients with moderate or severe hepatic impairment should receive reduced initial dosages of bortezomib and be closely monitored for adverse effects. (See Dosage and Administration: Special Populations.)

■ **Common Adverse Effects** Adverse effects reported in 10% or more of patients with previously untreated multiple myeloma receiving IV bortezomib plus melphalan and prednisone (VMP) include thrombocytopenia, neutropenia, peripheral neuropathy, nausea, diarrhea, neuralgia, anemia, leukopenia, vomiting, fatigue, constipation, lymphopenia, anorexia, asthenia, pyrexia, paresthesia, herpes zoster, rash, abdominal pain (upper quadrant), and insomnia. Serious (grade 3 or higher) adverse effects reported in 5% or more of patients receiving VMP include neutropenia, leukopenia, thrombocytopenia, lymphopenia, anemia, peripheral neuropathy, neuralgia, diarrhea, fatigue, asthenia, hypokalemia, and pneumonia.

Adverse effects reported in 10% or more of patients with relapsed multiple myeloma receiving IV bortezomib include nausea, diarrhea, fatigue, peripheral neuropathy, thrombocytopenia, constipation, vomiting, anorexia, pyrexia, paresthesia, anemia, headache, neutropenia, rash, decreased appetite, dyspnea, abdominal pain, dizziness (excluding vertigo), and weakness. Serious (grade 3 or higher) adverse effects reported in 5% or more of patients receiving bortezomib include thrombocytopenia, neutropenia, diarrhea, peripheral neuropathy, anemia, and fatigue.

Adverse effects reported in 10% or more of patients with relapsed multiple myeloma receiving bortezomib by subcutaneous injection include peripheral neuropathy, thrombocytopenia, neuralgia, neutropenia, anemia, diarrhea, leukopenia, nausea, pyrexia, vomiting, asthenia, weight loss, constipation, and fatigue. Serious (grade 3 or higher) adverse effects reported in 5% or more of patients receiving bortezomib by subcutaneous injection include neutropenia, anemia, leukopenia, peripheral neuropathy, thrombocytopenia, and pneumonia.

Adverse effects reported in 10% or more of patients with previously untreated mantle cell lymphoma receiving IV bortezomib plus rituximab, cyclophosphamide, doxorubicin, and prednisone (VR-CAP) include neutropenia, thrombocytopenia, leukopenia, anemia, peripheral neuropathy, lymphopenia, diarrhea, nausea, pyrexia, cough, constipation, fatigue, febrile neutropenia, loss of appetite, peripheral edema, alopecia, asthenia, pneumonia, neuralgia, and vomiting. Serious (grade 3 or higher) adverse effects reported in 5% or more of patients receiving VR-CAP include thrombocytopenia, leukopenia, neutropenia, anemia, febrile neutropenia, lymphopenia, peripheral neuropathy, pneumonia, diarrhea, and fatigue.

Adverse effects reported in 10% or more of patients with relapsed mantle cell lymphoma receiving IV bortezomib include peripheral neuropathy, fatigue, diarrhea, nausea, constipation, rash, vomiting, dizziness (excluding vertigo), thrombocytopenia, anorexia, anemia, weakness, headache, and pyrexia. Serious (grade 3 or higher) adverse effects reported in 5% or more of patients receiving bortezomib include peripheral neuropathy, fatigue, thrombocytopenia, and diarrhea.

Drug Interactions

Bortezomib is metabolized principally by cytochrome P-450 (CYP) isoenzymes 1A2, 2C19, and 3A4 and, to a lesser extent, by CYP2C9 and 2D6. In vitro, bortezomib may inhibit CYP2C19. However, bortezomib is a poor inhibitor of CYP1A2, 2C9, 2D6, and 3A4 and does not induce CYP1A2 or CYP3A4 in vitro.

■ **Drugs Affecting Hepatic Microsomal Enzymes** ***Inhibitors of CYP3A4*** Concomitant use of bortezomib with potent inhibitors of CYP3A4 may result in increased systemic exposure of bortezomib. Concomitant administration of the potent CYP3A4 inhibitor ketoconazole with bortezomib increased systemic exposure of bortezomib by 35%.

If bortezomib is used concomitantly with a potent CYP3A4 inhibitor, patients should be monitored for bortezomib-associated toxicity and a reduced dosage of bortezomib should be considered.

Inducers of CYP3A4 Concomitant use of bortezomib with potent inducers of CYP3A4 may result in decreased systemic exposure and reduced efficacy of bortezomib. Concomitant administration of the potent CYP3A4 inducer rifampin with bortezomib is expected to decrease bortezomib exposure by at least 45%, although larger reductions in exposure may occur. Concomitant use with St. John's wort (*Hypericum perforatum*) may result in unpredictable decreases in bortezomib exposure. Concomitant use of bortezomib with potent inducers of CYP3A4 (e.g., rifampin, St. John's wort) should be avoided.

Concomitant administration of the weak CYP3A4 inducer dexamethasone with bortezomib did not alter systemic exposure of bortezomib.

Inhibitors of CYP2C19 Concomitant administration of the potent CYP2C19 inhibitor omeprazole with bortezomib did not alter systemic exposure of bortezomib.

■ **Melphalan and Prednisone** Concomitant administration of melphalan and prednisone with bortezomib resulted in a 17% increase in systemic exposure of bortezomib. However, the manufacturer states that this increase is unlikely to be clinically relevant.

■ **Oral Antidiabetic Agents** In clinical studies, hypoglycemia and hyperglycemia have been reported in patients with diabetes mellitus who received bortezomib concomitantly with oral antidiabetic agents. If bortezomib is used concomitantly with oral antidiabetic agents, blood glucose concentrations should be monitored carefully and dosage of the antidiabetic agent adjusted as necessary.

■ **Hypotensive Agents** Concomitant use of bortezomib with drugs that can cause hypotension may result in an increased risk of hypotension. Dosage adjustment of hypotensive agents may be necessary.

Description

Bortezomib, a modified dipeptidyl boronic acid, is an antineoplastic agent. The drug reversibly inhibits the 26S proteasome, a large protein complex that degrades ubiquitinated proteins. The ubiquitin-proteasome pathway plays an essential role in regulating the intracellular concentration of specific proteins, thereby maintaining homeostasis within cells. Inhibition of the 26S proteasome by bortezomib prevents targeted proteolysis and causes disruption of normal homeostatic mechanisms, which can lead to cell death. In vitro studies indicate that bortezomib is cytotoxic to a variety of cancer cell types. Bortezomib has been shown to cause a delay in tumor growth in vivo in tumor models, including multiple myeloma.

Systemic exposure to bortezomib was similar following IV or subcutaneous administration in patients with multiple myeloma receiving repeated 1.3-mg/m² doses of the drug. Bortezomib is approximately 83% bound to plasma proteins. In vitro studies indicate that bortezomib is metabolized by the cytochrome P-450 (CYP) enzyme system, principally by isoenzymes 1A2, 2C19, and 3A4, to inactive metabolites; metabolism by isoenzymes 2C9 and 2D6 is minor. Following repeated IV administration of bortezomib 1 or 1.3 mg/m² in patients with multiple myeloma, the mean terminal half-life of the drug was 40–193 or 76–108 hours, respectively. Exposure to bortezomib is increased in patients with moderate or severe hepatic impairment and in patients 65 years of age or older; pharmacokinetics of bortezomib are not influenced by renal impairment or gender. (See Dosage and Administration: Special Populations and see Specific Populations under Cautions: Warnings/Precautions.)

Advice to Patients

Risk of fatigue, dizziness, syncope, or orthostatic hypotension; do not drive a motor vehicle or operate machinery if any of these symptoms are experienced.

Risk of dehydration secondary to vomiting and/or diarrhea. Importance of advising patients regarding appropriate measures (e.g., adequate fluid intake) to avoid dehydration. Importance of advising patients to inform a clinician if dizziness, lightheadedness, fainting spells, or muscle cramps develop.

Necessity of advising women to use an effective method of contraception and to avoid breast-feeding while receiving bortezomib therapy. Importance of women informing a clinician immediately if they are or plan to become pregnant or plan to breast-feed. Advise pregnant women of risk to the fetus.

If used concomitantly with oral antidiabetic agents, importance of frequent monitoring of blood glucose concentrations and informing a clinician of any unusual change.

Risk of peripheral neuropathy. Importance of informing a clinician of new-onset or worsening symptoms of peripheral neuropathy (e.g., tingling, numbness, pain, burning sensation in hands or feet, weakness in arms or legs).

Risk of reversible posterior leukoencephalopathy syndrome (RPLS). Importance of reporting any possible manifestations of RPLS (e.g., seizure, persistent headache, reduced eyesight, blurred vision, confusion, lethargy, inability to think, difficulty walking).

Risk of cardiac effects. Importance of informing clinician if swelling (of the feet, ankles, or legs) or other cardiac-related problems occur.

Risk of pulmonary effects. Importance of informing clinician if shortness of breath, cough, or other pulmonary problems occur.

Risk of hepatotoxicity. Importance of reporting any possible manifestations of hepatotoxicity (e.g., jaundice, abdominal pain [particularly in the right upper quadrant]).

Importance of informing clinician if rash, severe injection site reactions, or dermatologic pain occurs.

Risk of reactivation of latent varicella zoster virus infection. Importance of discussing with clinician whether antiviral prophylaxis should be initiated.

Importance of informing clinician if increase in blood pressure, bleeding, fever, constipation, or loss of appetite occurs.

Importance of informing clinicians of existing or contemplated concomitant therapy, including prescription and OTC drugs and dietary or herbal supplements (e.g., St. John's wort), as well as any concomitant illnesses.

Importance of informing patients of other important precautionary information. (See Cautions.)

Overview (see Users Guide). For additional information until a more detailed monograph is developed and published, the manufacturer's labeling should be consulted. It is *essential* that the manufacturer's labeling be consulted for more detailed information on usual cautions, precautions, contraindications, potential drug interactions, laboratory test interferences, and acute toxicity. For further information on handling of antineoplastic agents, see the ASHP Guidelines on Handling Hazardous Drugs at http://www.ahfsdruginformation.com.

Preparations

Excipients in commercially available drug preparations may have clinically important effects in some individuals; consult specific product labeling for details.

Bortezomib

Parenteral		
For injection, for IV or subcutaneous use	3.5 mg	**Velcade®**, Millennium

†Use is not currently included in the labeling approved by the US Food and Drug Administration

Selected Revisions August 2018,

Bosutinib

■ Bosutinib, an inhibitor of multiple tyrosine kinases, is an antineoplastic agent.

Uses

■ **Chronic Myelogenous Leukemia** Bosutinib is used for the treatment of chronic, accelerated, or blast phase Philadelphia chromosome-positive (Ph^+) chronic myelogenous leukemia (CML) after failure (secondary to resistance or intolerance) of prior therapy. Bosutinib is designated an orphan drug by the US Food and Drug Administration (FDA) for use in the treatment of CML.

The current indication for bosutinib is based principally on the results of an open-label, single-arm, multicenter, phase 1/phase 2 study in adults with chronic, accelerated, or blast phase CML following therapy with either imatinib alone or imatinib followed by dasatinib and/or nilotinib; patients were intolerant of or had disease that was resistant to imatinib. In this study, 546 patients received bosutinib 500 mg once daily (increased to 600 mg daily if complete hematologic or cytogenetic response was not achieved by week 8 or 12, respectively). The median duration of therapy with bosutinib was 22 months in patients with chronic phase CML previously treated with only imatinib; patients previously treated with imatinib followed by dasatinib and/or nilotinib received therapy with bosutinib for a median duration of 8 months.

At the time of data analysis, patients with chronic phase CML previously treated with imatinib alone or imatinib followed by dasatinib and/or nilotinib had been followed for at least 23 or 13 months, respectively. The primary efficacy end point of this study was major cytogenetic response (defined as elimination or substantial reduction [by at least 65%] of Ph+ hematopoietic cells) at 24 weeks. In this study, resistance to imatinib was defined as failure to achieve or maintain any hematologic improvement within 4 weeks of therapy; or failure to achieve a complete hematologic response by 3 months, a cytogenetic response by 6 months, or a major cytogenetic response by 12 months; or disease progression after a previous cytogenetic or hematologic response; or evidence of the genetic mutation in the Bcr-Abl gene associated with imatinib resistance. Imatinib intolerance was defined as inability to tolerate imatinib because of toxicity, or disease progression with imatinib and inability to receive a higher dosage because of toxicity. Definitions of resistance and intolerance to both dasatinib and nilotinib were similar to those for imatinib. Major cytogenetic response was achieved at 24 weeks in 34% of patients in chronic phase CML who were previously treated with imatinib alone and in 27% of those previously treated with imatinib followed by dasatinib or nilotinib. At the time of data analysis, median durations of response had not been reached. Disease progression (i.e., transformation from chronic phase to accelerated or blast phase CML) occurred in 4.3% of patients with chronic phase CML. In an exploratory analysis, treatment with bosutinib resulted in confirmed complete hematologic responses at 48 weeks in 30 or 15% of patients in accelerated or blast phase CML, respectively; the median duration of therapy with bosutinib for these patients previously treated with at least imatinib who were in the accelerated or blast phase of the disease was 10 or 3 months, respectively.

Dosage and Administration

■ **General** Procedures for proper handling and disposal of antineoplastic drugs should be followed when preparing and administering bosutinib.

A complete blood cell count (CBC) should be performed weekly for the first month of therapy and monthly (or as clinically indicated) thereafter.

Liver function tests should be monitored monthly for the first 3 months of therapy and then as clinically indicated; more frequent monitoring is recommended if increased transaminase concentrations occur.

■ **Administration** Bosutinib is administered orally once daily with food; tolerability of the drug was increased when taken with food.

Bosutinib tablets should *not* be crushed or cut. Touching or handling of crushed or broken tablets should be avoided.

■ **Dosage** Bosutinib is commercially available as the monohydrate; dosage is expressed in terms of anhydrous bosutinib.

Chronic Myelogenous Leukemia The recommended initial adult dosage of bosutinib for the treatment of Philadelphia chromosome-positive (Ph^+) chronic, accelerated, or blast phase chronic myelogenous leukemia (CML) is 500 mg once daily. Patients who do not reach complete hematologic response by 8 weeks or complete cytogenetic response by 12 weeks may receive an increased dosage of 600 mg once daily if they did not experience grade 3 or higher adverse effects while receiving the original starting dosage (500 mg daily). Therapy should be continued for as long as the patient derives clinical benefit from the drug or until unacceptable toxicity occurs.

If a dose of bosutinib is missed by more than 12 hours, the dose should be omitted, and the next dose should be taken at the regularly scheduled time. A double dose should *not* be administered to make up for a missed dose.

Dosage Modification for Toxicity **Myelosuppression.** In patients who experience neutropenia (i.e., absolute neutrophil counts [ANC] less than 1000/mm³) or thrombocytopenia (i.e., platelet counts less than 50,000/mm³) unrelated to the underlying CML, therapy with bosutinib should be withheld until ANC reaches or exceeds 1000/mm³ and platelet counts reach or exceed 50,000/mm³. Bosutinib therapy may then be resumed at the original starting dosage if recovery occurs within 2 weeks; if recovery is delayed (exceeding 2 weeks), the dosage of bosutinib should be reduced by 100 mg (i.e., a dose of 500 mg reduced to 400 mg) upon resumption of therapy. If neutropenia or thrombocytopenia recurs, bosutinib therapy should be withheld until recovery, then reinitiated at a reduced dosage of 300 mg once daily. Dosages less than 300 mg daily have not been evaluated.

Hepatotoxicity. In patients who exhibit increases in serum aminotransferase concentrations (ALT or AST exceeding 5 times the upper limit of normal [ULN]), therapy with bosutinib should be withheld until serum aminotransferase concentrations decrease to no more than 2.5 times the ULN. Bosutinib therapy may then be resumed at a reduced dosage of 400 mg once daily. If recovery is delayed (exceeding 4 weeks), treatment with bosutinib should be discontinued.

In patients who exhibit increases in aminotransferase concentrations (ALT or AST 3 or more times the ULN) concurrently with total bilirubin concentrations exceeding 2 times the ULN and alkaline phosphatase concentrations less than 2 times the ULN, treatment with bosutinib should be discontinued.

Diarrhea. In patients with grade 3 or 4 diarrhea (7 or more stools per day over baseline), therapy with bosutinib should be withheld until diarrhea resolves to no more than grade 1. Bosutinib therapy may then be resumed at a reduced dosage of 400 mg once daily.

Other Nonhematologic Effects. In patients who exhibit other clinically important, moderate or severe nonhematologic toxicity, therapy with bosutinib should be withheld until the toxicity has resolved. Bosutinib therapy may then be resumed at a reduced dosage of 400 mg once daily. If clinically appropriate, bosutinib may be re-escalated to a dosage of 500 mg once daily.

■ **Special Populations** For patients with mild to severe preexisting hepatic impairment, the manufacturer recommends a bosutinib dosage of 200 mg daily. (See Hepatic Impairment under Warnings/Precautions: Specific Populations, in Cautions.)

For patients with severe preexisting renal impairment (creatinine clearance less than 30 mL/minute), the manufacturer recommends a bosutinib dosage of 300 mg daily. (See Renal Impairment under Warnings/Precautions: Specific Populations, in Cautions.)

The manufacturer makes no specific dosage recommendations for geriatric patients. (See Geriatric Use under Warnings/Precautions: Specific Populations, in Cautions.)

Cautions

■ **Contraindications** Known hypersensitivity to bosutinib.

■ **Warnings/Precautions** ***GI Toxicity*** Nausea, vomiting, and diarrhea occur frequently in patients receiving bosutinib. In the principal efficacy study, nausea, vomiting, and diarrhea were reported in 46, 39, and 82% of patients. The median time to onset of diarrhea was 2 days and the median duration of each episode of diarrhea was 1 day. Among patients who experienced diarrhea, the median number of episodes of diarrhea per patient during therapy with bosutinib was 3 (range: 1–221 episodes).

Temporary interruption, dosage reduction, or discontinuance of bosutinib may be necessary if GI toxicity occurs during therapy with the drug. (See Dosage Modification for Toxicity under Dosage and Administration.)

Myelosuppression Cytopenias, including thrombocytopenia, anemia, and neutropenia, have been reported in patients receiving bosutinib. Complete blood cell (CBC) counts should be monitored weekly for the first month of therapy and monthly thereafter, or as clinically indicated.

Temporary interruption, dosage reduction, or discontinuance of bosutinib may be necessary if myelosuppression occurs during therapy with the drug. (See Myelosuppression under Dosage: Dosage Modification for Toxicity, in Dosage and Administration.)

Hepatic Toxicity Elevations in aminotransferase (ALT or AST) concentrations have occurred in patients receiving bosutinib, generally occurring early during therapy with a median duration of 21 days; the median time to onset of elevated ALT and AST concentrations was 30 and 33 days, respectively.

One case of drug-induced hepatic injury has occurred in a patient receiving bosutinib in combination with letrozole; hepatotoxicity occurred within the first week of therapy and resolved following discontinuance of bosutinib.

Liver function tests should be monitored monthly for the first 3 months of therapy and then as clinically indicated. More frequent monitoring is recommended if elevations in aminotransferase concentrations occur. Temporary interruption, dosage reduction, or discontinuance of bosutinib may be necessary if hepatic toxicity occurs during therapy with the drug. (See Hepatotoxicity under Dosage: Dosage Modification for Toxicity, in Dosage and Administration.)

Fluid Retention Fluid retention has occurred in patients receiving bosutinib and may manifest as pericardial effusion, pleural effusion, pulmonary edema, and/or peripheral edema. In the principal efficacy study, grade 3 or 4 fluid retention, including pleural effusion, pleural and pericardial effusions, peripheral and pulmonary edema, and edema, was reported in 3% of patients. If fluid retention occurs, patients should be monitored and managed according to current standards of care. Temporary interruption, dosage reduction, or discontinuance of bosutinib therapy may be necessary. (See Other Nonhematologic Effects under Dosage: Modification for Toxicity, in Dosage and Administration.)

Fetal/Neonatal Morbidity and Mortality Bosutinib may cause fetal harm when administered to pregnant women; the drug has been shown to be embryotoxic and fetotoxic in animals. There are no adequate and well-controlled studies in pregnant women. Pregnancy should be avoided during therapy. If used during pregnancy or if the patient becomes pregnant while receiving the drug, the patient should be apprised of the potential fetal hazard. (See Advice to Patients.)

Interactions with Cytochrome P-450 Isoenzyme 3A Inhibitors and Inducers Concomitant use of bosutinib with moderate or potent cytochrome P-450 (CYP) 3A inhibitors (e.g., ketoconazole) may substantially increase systemic exposure of bosutinib. Therefore, concomitant use of bosutinib with moderate or potent CYP3A inhibitors should be avoided. (See Drug Interactions.)

Concomitant use of bosutinib with moderate or potent CYP3A inducers (e.g., rifampin) may substantially decrease systemic exposure of bosutinib. Therefore, concomitant use of bosutinib with moderate or potent CYP3A inducers should be avoided. (See Drug Interactions.)

Specific Populations **Pregnancy.** Category D. (See Fetal/Neonatal Morbidity and Mortality, under Cautions: Warnings/Precautions.)

Lactation. It is not known whether bosutinib is distributed into milk in humans. Because of the potential for serious adverse reactions to bosutinib in nursing infants, a decision should be made whether to discontinue nursing or the drug, taking into account the importance of the drug to the woman.

Pediatric Use. Safety and efficacy of bosutinib in pediatric patients younger than 18 years of age have not been established.

Geriatric Use. In clinical trials evaluating bosutinib in patients with Philadelphia chromosome-positive (Ph^+) chronic myelogenous leukemia (CML), 20% of patients were 65 years of age or older and 4% were 75 years of age or older. No overall differences in safety or efficacy were observed between geriatric and younger adults. However, the possibility of increased sensitivity to the drug in some geriatric patients cannot be ruled out. (See Dosage and Administration: Special Populations.)

Hepatic Impairment. Following oral administration of a single 200-mg dose of bosutinib with food, peak plasma concentrations of bosutinib were increased by 2.4-, 2-, or 1.5-fold in patients with preexisting mild (Child-Pugh class A), moderate (Child-Pugh class B), or severe (Child-Pugh class C) hepatic impairment, respectively, compared with healthy individuals with normal hepatic function. In the same study, systemic exposure of bosutinib was increased by 2.3-, 2-, and 1.9-fold, respectively. Systemic exposure following administration of bosutinib 200 mg daily in patients with hepatic impairment is expected to be similar to that observed in those with normal hepatic function receiving bosutinib 500 mg once daily; however, efficacy of bosutinib 200 mg once daily in patients with hepatic impairment and CML is unknown. In addition, the elimination half-life of bosutinib was prolonged in patients with preexisting mild to severe hepatic impairment compared with healthy individuals with normal hepatic function. The incidence of QT interval prolongation (i.e., QT interval corrected for rate [QT_c] exceeding 450 msec or increased by more than 30 msec compared with baseline) increased with declining hepatic function; QT_c interval prolongation was observed in all patients with severe (Child-Pugh class C) hepatic impairment enrolled in the study. Dosage adjustment is required in patients with preexisting mild, moderate, or severe hepatic impairment. (See Dosage and Administration: Special Populations.)

Renal Impairment. Following oral administration of a single 200-mg dose of bosutinib with food, systemic exposure of bosutinib was increased by 35 or 60% in patients with preexisting moderate (creatinine clearance of 30–50 mL/minute) or severe (creatinine clearance of less than 30 mL/minute) renal impairment, respectively, compared with healthy individuals with normal renal function. Systemic exposure following administration of bosutinib 300 mg daily in patients with severe renal impairment is expected to be similar to that observed in those with normal renal function receiving bosutinib 500 mg once daily; however, efficacy of bosutinib 300 mg once daily in patients with renal impairment and CML is unknown. Systemic exposure of bosutinib was not affected by mild (creatinine clearance of 51–80 mL/minute) renal impairment. The elimination half-life of bosutinib in patients with renal impairment and in healthy individuals is similar. Bosutinib has not been studied in patients receiving hemodialysis. Dosage adjustment is required in patients with preexisting severe renal impairment. (See Dosage and Administration: Special Populations.)

■ **Common Adverse Effects** Adverse effects reported in 20% or more of patients receiving bosutinib include diarrhea, nausea, abdominal pain, vomiting, thrombocytopenia, anemia, fatigue, pyrexia, headache, cough, and rash.

Drug Interactions

Bosutinib is principally metabolized by cytochrome P-450 (CYP) isoenzyme 3A4.

In vitro studies indicate that bosutinib is a substrate and inhibitor of P-glycoprotein (P-gp).

■ **Drugs and Foods Affecting Hepatic Microsomal Enzymes**

Inhibitors of CYP3A Concomitant use of bosutinib with moderate or potent inhibitors of CYP3A may result in increased plasma concentrations of bosutinib. When the potent CYP3A inhibitor ketoconazole (400 mg once daily for 5 days) was administered concomitantly with bosutinib (single 100-mg dose) under fasting conditions, peak plasma concentrations and systemic exposure of bosutinib were increased 5.2- and 8.6-fold, respectively; however, in another study, adverse effects generally were mild in severity when a single bosutinib dose ranging from 100–600 mg was administered with ketoconazole (400 mg once daily for 5 days).

Concomitant use of bosutinib with moderate (e.g., amprenavir, aprepitant, atazanavir, ciprofloxacin, crizotinib, darunavir, diltiazem, erythromycin, fluconazole, fosamprenavir, grapefruit products, imatinib, verapamil) or potent inhibitors of CYP3A (e.g., boceprevir, clarithromycin, conivaptan, indinavir, itraconazole, ketoconazole, nefazodone, nelfinavir, posaconazole, ritonavir, saquinavir, telaprevir, telithromycin, voriconazole) should be avoided.

Inducers of CYP3A Concomitant use of bosutinib with moderate or potent inducers of CYP3A may decrease bosutinib exposure. When the potent CYP3A inducer rifampin (600 mg once daily for 6 days) was administered concomitantly with bosutinib (single 500-mg dose) with meals, peak plasma concentrations and systemic exposure of bosutinib were decreased by 86 and 94%, respectively.

Concomitant use of bosutinib with moderate (e.g., bosentan, efavirenz, etravirine, modafinil, nafcillin) or potent inducers of CYP3A (e.g., carbamazepine, phenobarbital, phenytoin, rifabutin, rifampin, St. John's wort [*Hypericum perforatum*]) should be avoided.

■ **Substrates or Inhibitors of P-glycoprotein Transport Systems** Bosutinib inhibits the efflux transporter P-gp. If bosutinib is administered with drugs that are substrates of P-gp (e.g., digoxin), increased concentrations of the substrate drug may occur.

Bosutinib also is a P-gp substrate. If bosutinib is administered with drugs that inhibit P-gp, increased concentrations of bosutinib may occur. Concomitant use of bosutinib with moderate or potent inhibitors of P-gp should be avoided.

■ **Drugs that Prolong the QT Interval** In a study of the effects of bosutinib on the QT interval in healthy individuals, bosutinib (single 500-mg dose) was administered alone and concomitantly with ketoconazole and compared with placebo and the active control (moxifloxacin 400 mg). Clinically important changes in the baseline-corrected QT_c interval were not observed.

■ **Proton-pump Inhibitors** When bosutinib (single 400-mg dose) was administered in combination with lansoprazole (multiple 60-mg doses) under fasting conditions, peak plasma concentrations and area under the concentration-time curve (AUC) of bosutinib were reduced by 46 and 26%, respectively. Concomitant use of bosutinib and proton-pump inhibitors is not recommended. Instead, use of histamine H_2-receptor antagonists or short-acting antacids, administered at least 2 hours before or after a dose of bosutinib, should be considered.

Description

Bosutinib, an inhibitor of multiple tyrosine kinases (including Bcr-Abl and the Src family [Src, Lyn, Hck]), is an antineoplastic agent; the drug has minimal inhibitory activity against c-Kit or platelet-derived growth factor (PDGF)-β.

The Philadelphia chromosome, characteristic of chronic myelogenous leukemia (CML), is created by a reciprocal translocation between chromosomes 9 and 22. Translocation between these chromosomes results in production of an abnormal protein (Bcr-Abl tyrosine kinase) that exhibits enhanced tyrosine kinase activity (i.e., increased phosphorylation of tyrosine residues); phosphorylation of tyrosine residues on growth factor receptors is thought to be important in stimulating cell proliferation and inhibiting cell death (apoptosis). Bosutinib competitively and selectively inhibits Bcr-Abl tyrosine kinase, thereby inhibiting tyrosine phosphorylation of proteins involved in Bcr-Abl signal transduction. In vitro studies show the drug inhibits the growth of leukemic cell lines expressing Bcr-Abl.

Clinical resistance to imatinib in CML has been attributed to several mechanisms, but point mutations in the Bcr-Abl kinase domain appear to be the most common, occurring in 30–90% of patients who develop resistance. In preclinical studies in cell-line models, bosutinib inhibited most (16 of 18) imatinib-resistant Bcr-Abl kinase domain mutant forms except for T315I and V299L mutant cells. Data from preclinical and clinical studies also implicate signaling pathways involving the Src family kinases (Lyn, Hck) in imatinib resistance.

Bosutinib is 94–96% bound to plasma proteins in vitro. In a dose escalation study, bosutinib exhibited linear and dose proportional pharmacokinetics under fed conditions; area under the serum concentration-time curve (AUC) and peak plasma concentrations of the drug are dose proportional over the bosutinib dosage range of 200–800 mg. Administration of bosutinib (500 mg) with a high-fat meal resulted in increases in systemic exposure and peak plasma concentrations of 1.7- and 1.8-fold, respectively. Bosutinib is extensively metabolized by the cytochrome P-450 (CYP) microsomal enzyme system, principally by the isoenzyme 3A4 to inactive metabolites. In vitro studies indicate that bosutinib is a substrate and inhibitor of P-glycoprotein (P-gp). Following administration of a single radiolabeled dose of bosutinib, 91.3% of the dose was recovered in feces and 3% was recovered in urine. Following administration of single 500-mg doses of bosutinib with food, the elimination half-life of bosutinib was 22.5 hours.

Advice to Patients

Importance of not altering the dosage or discontinuing bosutinib therapy without first consulting clinician.

If a dose is missed by more than 12 hours, importance of advising patients to take the next dose at the regularly scheduled time; the dose should *not* be doubled.

Importance of advising patients to swallow bosutinib tablets whole and not to crush or cut the tablets. Importance of not touching or handling crushed or broken tablets.

Importance of advising patients to take bosutinib tablets with food and not to drink grapefruit juice or consume grapefruit products while taking the drug.

Risk of diarrhea, nausea, vomiting, abdominal pain, or bloody stools. Importance of promptly seeking medical attention if any of these symptoms occur.

Risk of cytopenias. Importance of informing clinician if fever, easy bruising, or other signs and symptoms of infection or bleeding occur.

Risk of liver function abnormalities. Importance of contacting clinician promptly if jaundice or dark urine occurs.

Risk of fluid retention. Importance of contacting clinician promptly if swelling, weight gain, shortness of breath, coughing, or chest pain occurs.

Necessity of advising women of childbearing potential to use an effective method of contraception while receiving bosutinib and for at least 30 days after discontinuance of therapy. Necessity of advising women to avoid pregnancy during therapy.

Importance of women informing clinicians if they become pregnant. Bosutinib may cause fetal harm. Advise pregnant women of risk to the fetus.

Necessity of advising women to avoid breast-feeding during therapy. Importance of women informing clinicians if they plan to breast-feed. If a woman wishes to resume breast-feeding following therapy, importance of advising the woman to discuss the appropriate timing with her clinician.

Importance of informing patients of other important precautionary information.

Importance of informing clinicians of existing or contemplated concomitant therapy, including prescription and OTC drugs and herbal supplements (e.g., St. John's wort), as well as any concomitant illnesses.

Overview® (see Users Guide). For additional information on this drug until a more detailed monograph is developed and published, the manufacturer's labeling should be consulted. It is *essential* that the manufacturer's labeling be consulted for more detailed information on usual cautions, precautions, contraindications, potential drug interactions, laboratory test interferences, and acute toxicity. For further information on the handling of antineoplastic agents, see the ASHP Guidelines on Handling Hazardous Drugs at http://www.ahfsdruginformation.com.

Preparations

Excipients in commercially available drug preparations may have clinically important effects in some individuals; consult specific product labeling for details.

Bosutinib

Oral

Tablets, film-coated	100 mg	**Bosulif®**, Pfizer
	500 mg	**Bosulif®**, Pfizer

Selected Revisions April 2016, © Copyright, October 2013, American Society of Health-System Pharmacists, Inc.

Brentuximab Vedotin

■ Brentuximab vedotin, a chimeric human-murine anti-CD30 antibody conjugated with the microtubule inhibitor monomethyl auristatin E (MMAE), is an antineoplastic agent.

Uses

■ **Hodgkin Lymphoma** Brentuximab vedotin is used for the treatment of Hodgkin lymphoma following failure of autologous stem cell transplantation (ASCT) or following failure of 2 or more multiple-agent chemotherapy regimens in patients who are not ASCT candidates; brentuximab vedotin is designated an orphan drug by the US Food and Drug Administration (FDA) for the treatment of this cancer. The current indication is based on objective response rate; there currently are no controlled trials demonstrating a clinical benefit (e.g., improvement in disease-related symptoms, increased survival).

The current indication for brentuximab vedotin is based principally on the results of an open-label, noncomparative, phase 2 study in 102 patients with Hodgkin lymphoma who relapsed following ASCT. The primary measure of efficacy was overall response rate (complete plus partial responses). The median age of patients was 31 years; the patients had received a median of 5 prior therapies for their disease. In this study, all patients received brentuximab vedotin (1.8 mg/kg IV every 3 weeks) for a maximum of 16 cycles or until disease progression or unacceptable toxicity occurred. The overall response rate was 73%; 32% of patients receiving the drug achieved a complete response. At the time of analysis, the median duration of response for all responders was 6.7 months (range: 1.3–21.9 months); the median duration of response was 20.5 months for patients achieving a complete response but only 3.5 months for those achieving a partial response.

■ **Anaplastic Large Cell Lymphoma** Brentuximab vedotin is used for the treatment of systemic anaplastic large cell lymphoma (sALCL) following failure of 1 or more multiple-agent chemotherapy regimens; brentuximab vedotin is designated an orphan drug by FDA for the treatment of this cancer. The current indication is based on objective response rate; there currently are no controlled trials demonstrating a clinical benefit (e.g., improvement in disease-related symptoms, increased survival).

The current indication for brentuximab vedotin is based principally on the results of an open-label, noncomparative, phase 2 study in 58 patients with sALCL who relapsed following prior therapy. The primary measure of efficacy was overall response rate (complete plus partial responses). The median age of patients was 52 years; the patients had received a median of 2 prior therapies, 26% of the patients had received prior ASCT for their disease, and 72% of the patients had anaplastic lymphoma kinase (ALK)-negative disease, which is associated with a worse prognosis. In this study, all patients received brentuximab vedotin (1.8 mg/kg IV every 3 weeks) for a maximum of 16 cycles or until disease progression or unacceptable toxicity occurred. The overall response rate was 86%; 57% of patients receiving the drug achieved a complete response. At the time of analysis, the median duration of response for all responders was 12.6 months (range: 0.1–15.9 months); the median duration of response was 13.2 months for patients achieving a complete response but only 2.1 months for those achieving a partial response.

Dosage and Administration

■ **General** Because brentuximab vedotin may cause neutropenia, the manufacturer states that complete blood cell (CBC) counts should be obtained prior to each dose; more frequent monitoring should be considered in patients with evidence of grade 3 or 4 neutropenia.

Patients who experience an infusion-related reaction to brentuximab vedotin should receive a premedication regimen (e.g., a corticosteroid, an antihistamine, and acetaminophen) prior to each subsequent dose of the drug. (See Sensitivity Reactions under Warnings/Precautions: Other Warnings and Precautions, in Cautions.)

■ **Administration** Procedures for proper handling (e.g., use of gloves or protective clothing) and disposal of antineoplastic agents should be followed.

Brentuximab vedotin is administered by IV infusion over 30 minutes. *The drug should not be administered by rapid IV injection, such as IV push or bolus.*

Unreconstituted brentuximab vedotin powder for injection should be stored in unopened vials at 2–8°C. Unopened vials should be retained in the original package for protection from light.

Prior to administration, commercially available brentuximab vedotin powder for injection must be reconstituted and diluted using proper aseptic technique. The powder is reconstituted by adding 10.5 mL of sterile water for injection to a vial labeled as containing 50 mg of the drug to provide a solution containing 5 mg/mL. The diluent should be directed toward the wall of the vial and not directly at the brentuximab vedotin cake or powder. The vial should be gently swirled and inspected visually for particulate matter and discoloration prior to dilution and administration. The resulting solution should *not* be shaken. The solution should be clear to slightly opalescent, colorless, and free of visible particulates. The reconstituted brentuximab vedotin solution may be diluted immediately or stored at 2–8°C for use within 24 hours, and should be protected from direct sunlight until time of use. The reconstituted solution should not be frozen.

For preparation of the final diluted brentuximab vedotin solution for infusion, the required amount of reconstituted brentuximab vedotin solution should be injected into an infusion bag containing a minimum volume of 100 mL of 0.9% sodium chloride injection, 5% dextrose injection, or lactated Ringer's injection to produce a final solution with brentuximab vedotin concentration of 0.4–1.8 mg/mL. The final diluted brentuximab vedotin solution for infusion should be mixed by gentle inversion. The solution may be infused immediately or stored at 2–8°C and used within 24 hours following reconstitution; the solution for infusion should not be frozen and should be protected from direct sunlight until use. Any partially used vials should be discarded. Brentuximab vedotin should not be admixed with any other drug, nor should any other drug be administered simultaneously in the same IV line with brentuximab vedotin infusion.

■ **Dosage** In patients who weigh 100 kg or less, dosage of brentuximab vedotin should be based on actual body weight; however, in patients who weigh more than 100 kg, dosage should be calculated based on a weight of 100 kg.

Hodgkin Lymphoma For the treatment of Hodgkin lymphoma following failure of autologous stem cell transplantation (ASCT) or following failure of 2 or more multiple-agent chemotherapy regimens in patients who are not ASCT candidates, the recommended adult dosage of brentuximab vedotin is 1.8 mg/kg administered as a 30-minute IV infusion every 3 weeks. Therapy should be continued until disease progression or unacceptable toxicity occurs.

Systemic Anaplastic Large Cell Lymphoma For the treatment of systemic anaplastic large cell lymphoma (sALCL) following failure of 1 or more multiple-agent chemotherapy regimens, the recommended adult dosage of brentuximab vedotin is 1.8 mg/kg administered as a 30-minute IV infusion every 3 weeks. Therapy should be continued until disease progression or unacceptable toxicity occurs.

Dosage Modification for Toxicity **Peripheral Neuropathy.** If grade 2 or 3 peripheral neuropathy occurs, brentuximab vedotin therapy should be interrupted until the toxicity resolves to grade 1 or to baseline; therapy may then be resumed at a reduced dosage of 1.2 mg/kg every 3 weeks. (See Peripheral Neuropathy under Warnings/Precautions: Other Warnings and Precautions, in Cautions.) If grade 4 peripheral neuropathy occurs, treatment with brentuximab vedotin should be discontinued.

Neutropenia. If grade 3 or 4 neutropenia occurs, brentuximab vedotin therapy should be interrupted until the toxicity resolves to grade 2 or less or to baseline, and use of a granulocyte colony-stimulating factor (G-CSF) during subsequent cycles should be considered. If grade 4 neutropenia recurs despite the use of a G-CSF, drug discontinuance or dosage reduction (i.e., reduced brentuximab vedotin dosage of 1.2 mg/kg every 3 weeks) may be considered. (See Hematologic Effects under Warnings/Precautions: Other Warnings and Precautions, in Cautions.)

■ **Special Populations** For patients with mild, moderate, or severe hepatic impairment (Child-Pugh class A, B, or C, respectively), the manufacturer recommends an initial brentuximab vedotin dosage of 1.2 mg/kg every 3 weeks with close monitoring for adverse effects. (See Hepatic Impairment under Warnings/Precautions: Specific Populations, in Cautions.)

For patients with severe renal impairment (creatinine clearance less than 30 mL/minute), the manufacturer recommends an initial brentuximab vedotin dosage of 1.2 mg/kg every 3 weeks with close monitoring for adverse effects. (See Renal Impairment under Warnings/Precautions: Specific Populations, in Cautions.)

The manufacturer makes no specific dosage recommendations for geriatric patients. (See Geriatric Use under Warnings/Precautions: Specific Populations, in Cautions.)

Cautions

■ **Contraindications** Concomitant use with bleomycin. (See Respiratory Effects under Warnings/Precautions: Other Warnings and Precautions, in Cautions.)

■ **Warnings/Precautions** ***Warnings*** **Progressive Multifocal Leukoencephalopathy.** JC virus infection causing progressive multifocal leukoencephalopathy (PML), sometimes fatal, has been reported in patients receiving brentuximab vedotin. Other factors that might increase the risk for PML include prior therapies and underlying disease that may cause immunosuppression. Signs and symptoms of PML may develop over several weeks or months.

The possible diagnosis of PML should be considered in any patient receiving brentuximab vedotin who experiences new neurologic manifestations suggestive of PML (e.g., changes in mood or behavior, confusion, changes in thinking, memory loss, vision changes, changes in speech or walking, decreased strength or weakness on one side of the body). If PML is suspected, the drug should be withheld and diagnostic evaluation, including consultation with a neurologist, brain magnetic resonance imaging (MRI) scan, and lumbar puncture or brain biopsy, should be considered as clinically indicated. If PML is confirmed, brentuximab vedotin should be permanently discontinued.

Other Warnings and Precautions **Respiratory Effects.** Concomitant use of brentuximab vedotin and bleomycin may increase the risk of pulmonary toxicity; such concomitant use is contraindicated. In a clinical trial, the incidence of noninfectious pulmonary reactions (e.g., cough, dyspnea, interstitial infiltration, inflammation) in patients receiving brentuximab vedotin in combination with chemotherapy containing bleomycin (40%) was higher than the historical incidence of pulmonary reactions in patients receiving bleomycin-based regimens (e.g., doxorubicin, bleomycin, vinblastine, and dacarbazine [ABVD]) (10–25%). Most patients responded to corticosteroid therapy.

Peripheral Neuropathy. Peripheral neuropathy occurred in 54% of patients with Hodgkin lymphoma or systemic anaplastic large cell lymphoma (sALCL) receiving brentuximab vedotin in clinical trials. Brentuximab vedotin mainly causes sensory neuropathy, but motor neuropathy also has been reported. In phase 2 clinical trials, the median time to onset of peripheral neuropathy was approximately 12.4 weeks (range: 0.1–41.3 weeks), and the median time to resolution or improvement was 6.6 weeks. Peripheral neuropathy was managed with treatment delays and/or dosage reductions; 49% of patients had complete resolution, 31% had partial improvement, and 20% had no improvement. The median delay in treatment was 17 days in patients with Hodgkin lymphoma and 8.5 days in patients with sALCL.

Patients receiving brentuximab vedotin should be monitored for manifestations of neuropathy (e.g., hypoesthesia, hyperesthesia, paresthesia, discomfort, burning sensation, neuropathic pain, weakness). Dosage reduction, treatment delay, or drug discontinuance may be required in patients who experience new or worsening neuropathic symptoms. (See Peripheral Neuropathy under Dosage: Dosage Modification for Toxicity, in Dosage and Administration.)

Sensitivity Reactions. Infusion-related reactions, including anaphylaxis, have been reported in patients receiving brentuximab vedotin. In phase 2 clinical trials, infusion-related reactions, including chills, nausea, dyspnea, pruritus, pyrexia, and/or cough, occurred in 12% of patients; no grade 3 or 4 infusion-related reactions were reported. In a phase 2 trial in patients with Hodgkin lymphoma, one patient discontinued treatment because of grade 1 throat tightness during the sixth cycle of brentuximab vedotin administration. In a phase 1 trial, 2 patients experienced anaphylaxis during the second treatment cycle within 30 minutes following initiation of the brentuximab vedotin infusion. Patients should be monitored during infusions of the drug for manifestations of infusion-related reactions.

In patients experiencing infusion-related reactions, the brentuximab vedotin infusion should be interrupted and appropriate therapy should be instituted. The drug should be immediately and permanently discontinued in patients who experience anaphylaxis. The manufacturer states that patients who experience an infusion-related reaction to brentuximab vedotin should be premedicated (e.g., with a corticosteroid, an antihistamine, and acetaminophen) prior to each subsequent dose of the drug.

Hematologic Effects. Severe and prolonged (lasting 1 week or longer) neutropenia, grade 3 or 4 anemia, or thrombocytopenia may occur. Febrile neutropenia has been reported during postmarketing experience. Complete blood cell (CBC) counts should be monitored prior to each dose of brentuximab vedotin; if grade 3 or 4 neutropenia occurs, more frequent monitoring should be considered. Patients should be monitored closely for fever. In patients who develop grade 3 or 4 neutropenia, use of a granulocyte colony-stimulating factor (G-CSF), temporary interruption of therapy, dosage reduction, or drug discontinuance may be required. (See Neutropenia under Dosage: Dosage Modification for Toxicity, in Dosage and Administration.)

Infectious Complications. Serious infections and opportunistic infections, such as pneumonia, bacteremia, and sepsis/septic shock, sometimes fatal, have been reported in patients receiving brentuximab vedotin.

Patients receiving brentuximab vedotin should be monitored closely for signs and symptoms of bacterial, fungal, or viral infections.

Tumor Lysis Syndrome. Tumor lysis syndrome may occur following rapid lysis of malignant cells. The risk of tumor lysis syndrome is increased in patients with a large tumor burden; such patients should be monitored closely and appropriate precautions should be taken.

Dermatologic Effects. Stevens-Johnson syndrome has been reported in patients receiving brentuximab vedotin. If Stevens-Johnson syndrome occurs, brentuximab vedotin should be discontinued and appropriate treatment should be provided.

Fetal/Neonatal Morbidity and Mortality. Brentuximab vedotin may cause fetal harm if administered to pregnant women; the drug has been shown to be embryotoxic, fetotoxic, and teratogenic in animals. If brentuximab vedotin is used during pregnancy or if the patient becomes pregnant while receiving the drug, the patient should be apprised of the potential fetal hazard.

Immunogenicity. Antibodies to brentuximab vedotin have been detected in patients receiving the drug; the clinical relevance of such antibodies is not known. In phase 2 clinical trials, testing for anti-brentuximab vedotin antibodies was performed every 3 weeks using a sensitive electrochemiluminescent immunoassay; test results were persistently (at more than 2 time points) or transiently (at 1 or 2 postbaseline time points) positive in approximately 7 or 30%, respectively, of patients. A higher incidence of infusion-related reactions was observed in patients who persistently tested positive for anti-brentuximab vedotin antibodies. Neutralizing antibodies were detected in 62% of patients who tested positive (either transiently or persistently) for anti-brentuximab vedotin antibodies.

Specific Populations **Pregnancy.** Category D. (See Users Guide and see Fetal/Neonatal Morbidity and Mortality under Warnings/Precautions: Other Warnings and Precautions, in Cautions.)

Lactation. It is not known whether brentuximab vedotin is distributed into milk in humans; because of the potential for serious adverse reactions to brentuximab vedotin in nursing infants, a decision should be made whether to discontinue nursing or the drug, taking into account the importance of the drug to the woman.

Pediatric Use. Safety and efficacy of brentuximab vedotin have not been established in pediatric patients. Clinical studies of brentuximab vedotin did not include sufficient numbers of pediatric patients to determine whether pediatric patients respond differently than adults.

Geriatric Use. Safety and efficacy have not been established in patients 65 years of age and older. Clinical studies of brentuximab vedotin did not include sufficient numbers of patients 65 years of age and older to determine whether geriatric patients respond differently than younger adults. (See Dosage and Administration: Special Populations.)

Hepatic Impairment. Following administration of brentuximab vedotin (1.2 mg/kg), systemic exposure of the microtubule disrupting component (monomethyl auristatin E [MMAE]) of the drug was increased by approximately 2.3-fold in individuals with mild, moderate, or severe hepatic impairment (Child-Pugh class A, B, or C, respectively) compared with individuals with normal hepatic function. (See Dosage and Administration: Special Populations.)

Renal Impairment. Following administration of brentuximab vedotin (1.2 mg/kg), systemic exposure of the microtubule disrupting component (MMAE) of the drug was increased by approximately 1.9-fold in individuals with severe renal impairment (creatinine clearance less than 30 mL/minute) compared with individuals with normal renal function. (See Dosage and Administration: Special Populations.)

■ **Common Adverse Effects** Adverse effects reported in 20% or more of patients receiving brentuximab vedotin include neutropenia, peripheral sensory neuropathy, fatigue, nausea, anemia, upper respiratory tract infection, diarrhea, pyrexia, rash, thrombocytopenia, cough, and vomiting.

Drug Interactions

In vitro studies indicate that monomethyl auristatin E (MMAE), the microtubule-disrupting component of brentuximab vedotin, is a substrate and an inhibitor of cytochrome P-450 (CYP) isoenzymes 3A4/5. (See Description.) In vitro studies also indicate that MMAE does not inhibit other CYP isoenzymes at clinically relevant concentrations and does not induce major CYP isoenzymes. MMAE is a substrate of P-glycoprotein (P-gp) and is not a potent inhibitor of P-gp.

■ **Drugs Affecting Hepatic Microsomal Enzymes** Concomitant use of brentuximab vedotin with potent inhibitors of CYP3A4 may result in increased systemic exposure of MMAE and possible adverse effects. When the potent CYP3A4 inhibitor ketoconazole (400 mg once daily from day 19 of cycle 1 to day 21 of cycle 2) was administered concomitantly with brentuximab vedotin (1.2 mg/kg on day 1 of each cycle), the systemic exposure of MMAE was increased by approximately 34%. The manufacturer states that patients receiving brentuximab vedotin concomitantly with potent CYP3A4 inhibitors should be closely monitored for adverse effects.

When the potent CYP3A4 inducer rifampin (600 mg once daily from day 14 of cycle 1 to day 21 of cycle 2) was administered concomitantly with brentuximab vedotin (1.8 mg/kg on day 1 of each cycle), the systemic exposure of MMAE was decreased by approximately 46%. However, dosage adjustment is not necessary. Clinically important effects on MMAE concentrations are not expected when other inducers of CYP3A4 (i.e., carbamazepine, dexamethasone, phenobarbital, phenytoin) are used concomitantly with brentuximab vedotin.

■ **Drugs Metabolized by Hepatic Microsomal Enzymes** Brentuximab vedotin is not expected to alter the systemic exposure of drugs that are metabolized by CYP3A4. When the CYP3A4 substrate midazolam was administered 2 days after brentuximab vedotin (at approximately peak MMAE concentrations), systemic exposure of midazolam was unchanged.

■ **Drugs Affecting Efflux Transport Systems** Concomitant use of brentuximab vedotin with inhibitors of P-gp may result in increased systemic exposure of MMAE and possible adverse effects. The manufacturer states that patients receiving brentuximab vedotin concomitantly with P-gp inhibitors should be monitored closely for adverse effects.

■ **Bleomycin** The incidence of noninfectious pulmonary reactions (e.g., cough, dyspnea, interstitial infiltration, inflammation) in patients receiving brentuximab vedotin in combination with chemotherapy containing bleomycin was higher than the historical incidence of pulmonary reactions in patients receiving bleomycin-based regimens. Concomitant use of brentuximab vedotin and bleomycin is contraindicated. (See Respiratory Effects under Warnings/Precautions: Other Warnings and Precautions, in Cautions.)

Description

Brentuximab vedotin, an anti-CD30 antibody-drug conjugate, is an antineoplastic agent. The anti-CD30 antibody, a chimeric human-murine IgG_1 immunoglobulin, is conjugated with the microtubule inhibitor monomethyl auristatin E (MMAE), a synthetic analog of dolastatin 10, a naturally occurring product isolated from the sea hare *Dolabella auriculara*. A dipeptide bond covalently links MMAE to the antibody component; on average, 4 molecules of MMAE are attached to each antibody molecule. The antibody portion of brentuximab vedotin binds specifically to antigen CD30, a membrane glycoprotein and member of the tumor necrosis factor (TNF) family that is expressed on malignant cells in 98.4% of Hodgkin lymphoma cases. The CD30 antigen also is expressed in other hematologic malignancies, including anaplastic large cell lymphoma, but has limited expression in normal tissue. Following binding of the antibody portion of brentuximab vedotin to antigen CD30, the resultant complex is internalized by the cell. MMAE is released via proteolytic cleavage of the dipeptide bond and binds to tubulin, resulting in cell cycle arrest and apoptosis.

Areas under the serum concentration-time curve (AUCs) of the antibody-drug conjugate and free MMAE are dose proportional over the brentuximab vedotin single-dose range of 1.2–2.7 mg/kg. Peak MMAE concentrations are achieved about 1–3 days following an IV dose of brentuximab vedotin. When brentuximab vedotin is administered IV every 3 weeks, minimal systemic accumulation of the antibody-drug conjugate occurs, and MMAE exposure is decreased to about 50–80% of the exposure achieved following the initial dose. A small fraction of free MMAE is metabolized, mainly via oxidation by the cytochrome P-450 (CYP) 3A4/5 isoenzyme. Elimination of MMAE appears to be limited by the rate of release from the antibody-drug conjugate. Following administration of a single 1.8-mg/kg dose of brentuximab vedotin, approximately 24% of the total administered dose of MMAE is excreted over a 1-week period in feces (72%) and to a lesser extent in urine, mainly as unchanged drug. The terminal half-lives of the antibody-drug conjugate and MMAE are 4–6 and 3–4 days, respectively.

Advice to Patients

Risk of progressive multifocal leukoencephalopathy (PML). Importance of patients, family, and caregivers being alert to and immediately reporting emergence of signs and symptoms suggestive of PML (e.g., changes in mood, unusual changes in behavior, confusion, changes in thinking, memory loss, vision changes, changes in speech or walking, decreased strength or weakness on one side of the body).

Risk of infusion-related reactions. Importance of reporting signs and symptoms of such reactions, including fever, chills, rash, or breathing difficulty, that occur within 24 hours of an infusion of the drug.

Risk of peripheral neuropathy. Importance of informing clinician of new or worsening symptoms of peripheral neuropathy (e.g., tingling or numbness of the hands or feet, any muscle weakness).

Risk of neutropenia. Importance of informing clinician of fever or other signs and symptoms of infection (e.g., chills, cough, painful urination).

Necessity of advising women to avoid pregnancy and breast-feeding while receiving therapy. Importance of women informing clinicians immediately if they are pregnant. Advise pregnant women of risk to the fetus.

Risk of pancreatitis. Importance of informing clinician of severe abdominal pain.

Importance of informing clinicians of existing or contemplated concomitant therapy, including prescription and OTC drugs, as well as any concomitant illnesses.

Importance of informing patients of other important precautionary information. (See Cautions.)

Overview® (see Users Guide). For additional information on this drug until a more detailed monograph is developed and published, the manufacturer's labeling should be consulted. It is *essential* that the manufacturer's labeling be consulted for more detailed information on usual cautions, precautions, contraindications, potential drug interactions, laboratory test interferences, and acute toxicity. For further information on the handling of antineoplastic agents, see the ASHP Guidelines on Handling Hazardous Drugs at http://www.ahfsdruginformation.com.

Preparations

Excipients in commercially available drug preparations may have clinically important effects in some individuals; consult specific product labeling for details.

Brentuximab Vedotin

Parenteral

For injection, for IV infusion only	50 mg	**Adcetris®**, Seattle Genetics

Brigatinib

■ Brigatinib, an inhibitor of multiple tyrosine kinases, including anaplastic lymphoma kinase (ALK), is an antineoplastic agent.

Uses

■ **Non-small Cell Lung Cancer** Brigatinib is used for the treatment of anaplastic lymphoma kinase (ALK)-positive metastatic non-small cell lung cancer (NSCLC) following failure (secondary to resistance or intolerance) of prior crizotinib therapy. The accelerated approval of brigatinib for this indication is based on tumor response rate and duration of response; continued approval for this indication may be contingent on verification and description of clinical benefit of brigatinib in a confirmatory study. Brigatinib has been designated an orphan drug by the FDA for the treatment of ALK-positive, c-ros oncogene-1 (ROS-1)-positive, or epidermal growth factor receptor (EGFR) mutation-positive NSCLC.

A relatively small subset of patients with NSCLC (approximately 3–7%) have ALK-positive disease, which indicates potential responsiveness to ALK inhibitor therapy (e.g., alectinib, brigatinib, ceritinib, crizotinib). Patients with this form of lung cancer typically are nonsmokers or have a history of light smoking, are female, and are younger in age and often have adenocarcinoma histology. Although crizotinib is highly active in patients with ALK-positive NSCLC, most patients treated with the drug eventually experience disease progression, limiting the drug's long-term therapeutic potential. Disease progression in patients receiving crizotinib can result from acquired resistance mutations in ALK, amplification of gene expression, activation of alternate signaling pathways, and/or progression of brain metastases (because of poor distribution of crizotinib into the CSF). (See Description.)

The current indication for brigatinib is based principally on the results of a multicenter, two-arm, open-label, phase 2 study (ALTA) that enrolled a total of 222 adults with locally advanced or metastatic ALK-positive NSCLC who had experienced disease progression while receiving crizotinib therapy. ALK rearrangement was required for study entry and was confirmed by an FDA-approved diagnostic test or a different test with adequate archival tissue to confirm ALK rearrangement by the Vysis® ALK Break Apart fluorescence in situ hybridization (FISH) Probe Kit test. Patients were randomized in a 1:1 ratio to initially receive brigatinib in a dosage of 90 mg once daily (arm A) or 180 mg once daily (following an initial dosage of 90 mg once daily for 7 days) (arm B) until disease progression, unacceptable toxicity, or consent withdrawal occurred. Patients in arm A could receive brigatinib 180 mg once daily after objective progression occurred on a dosage of 90 mg once daily. The primary efficacy end point was confirmed overall response rate according to the Response Evaluation Criteria in Solid Tumors (RECIST 1.1) as evaluated by a central independent review committee (IRC); additional outcome measures included investigator-assessed overall response rate, duration of response, overall response rate in patients with CNS metastases, and duration of response in patients with CNS metastases. The median age of patients enrolled in the study was 54 years (range: 18–82 years); 67% of enrolled patients were white and 31% were Asian; and 57% were female. Stage IV disease was present in 98% of the patients and 97% had adenocarcinoma histology, 74% of the patients had received prior systemic chemotherapy, and 64% of patients had an objective response to prior crizotinib treatment. CNS metastases were present in 69% of patients and 61% had previously received radiation to the brain.

The median duration of follow-up in the ALTA study was 8 months (range: 0.1–20.2 months). The IRC-assessed overall response rate in patients receiving brigatinib 180 mg daily was 53%; partial responses were achieved in 48% of patients and 4.5% had a complete response. The investigator-assessed overall response rate in patients receiving brigatinib 180 mg daily was 54%; partial responses were achieved in 50% of patients and 3.6% had a complete response. Patients receiving brigatinib 90 mg daily had IRC- or investigator-assessed overall response rates of 48 or 45%, respectively; IRC- or investigator-assessed partial responses were achieved in 45 or 44% of patients, respectively, and complete responses were achieved in 3.6 or 0.9% of patients, respectively. The median IRC-assessed duration of response was 13.8 months in both dosage groups and the median investigator-assessed duration of response was 13.8 months in the 90-mg dosage group and 11.1 months in the 180-mg dosage group.

In the subgroup of 44 patients with measurable brain metastases at baseline in the ALTA study, the IRC-assessed intracranial overall response rate was 67% (all partial responses) in patients receiving brigatinib 180 mg daily and 42% (7.7% complete responses and 35% partial responses) in patients receiving brigatinib 90 mg daily. The median duration of intracranial response was 5.6 months in the 180-mg dosage group and could not be estimated at the time of analysis in the 90-mg dosage group. Among the 23 patients who demonstrated an intracranial response to brigatinib therapy, 78% of the patients receiving 90 mg once daily and 68% of the patients receiving 180 mg once daily maintained a response for at least 4 months.

A phase 3 controlled trial (ALTA-1L) comparing brigatinib and crizotinib in patients with ALK-positive advanced NSCLC who have not previously been treated with an ALK inhibitor (i.e., ALK-inhibitor naive)† currently is under way. Brigatinib currently is not indicated for use in ALK inhibitor-naive patients with NSCLC.

Dosage and Administration

■ **General** Because brigatinib may cause hypertension, blood pressure should be controlled prior to initiating therapy and then monitored 2 weeks after starting therapy and at least monthly thereafter. (See Hypertension under Dosage: Dosage Modification for Toxicity, in Dosage and Administration.) Brigatinib also can cause bradycardia; therefore, heart rate and blood pressure should be monitored during treatment with the drug. (See Bradycardia under Dosage: Dosage Modification for Toxicity, in Dosage and Administration.)

Because brigatinib may cause elevations in serum creatine kinase (CK, creatine phosphokinase, CPK) and pancreatic enzyme concentrations, the manufacturer states that CK concentrations as well as lipase and amylase concentrations should be monitored during therapy. (See Creatine Kinase Elevation and also see Pancreatic Enzyme Elevation under Dosage: Dosage Modification for Toxicity, in Dosage and Administration.)

Because brigatinib may cause hyperglycemia, the manufacturer states that fasting serum glucose concentrations should be assessed prior to initiating therapy and then periodically monitored during therapy. (See Hyperglycemia under Dosage: Dosage Modification for Toxicity, in Dosage and Administration.)

Restricted Distribution Brigatinib can only be obtained through a limited network of specialty pharmacies. Clinicians may consult the Alunbrig® website (https://www.alunbrig.com) for specific information regarding distribution of the drug.

■ **Administration** Brigatinib is administered orally once daily without regard to food. (See Description.) The tablets should be swallowed whole and should *not* be crushed or chewed.

If a dose of brigatinib is missed or vomiting occurs after taking a dose, the next dose should be taken at the regularly scheduled time; an additional dose should not be taken.

■ **Dosage** ***Non-small Cell Lung Cancer*** The recommended adult dosage of brigatinib for the treatment of anaplastic lymphoma kinase (ALK)-positive metastatic non-small cell lung cancer (NSCLC) following failure (secondary to resistance or intolerance) of prior crizotinib therapy is 90 mg once daily for the first 7 days. If the 90-mg daily dosage is tolerated during the first 7 days, the dosage should be increased to 180 mg once daily. Brigatinib therapy should be continued until disease progression or unacceptable toxicity occurs.

Following treatment interruptions of 14 or more days for reasons other than adverse reactions, brigatinib should be resumed at a dosage of 90 mg once daily for 7 days, then increased to the previously tolerated dosage.

Dosage Modification for Toxicity Dosing interruption and/or dosage reduction of brigatinib may be necessary based on individual safety and tolerability.

In the principal efficacy study, dosage reduction because of adverse effects was necessary in 7.3 or 20% of patients receiving brigatinib 90 mg daily or 180 mg daily, respectively (most commonly for serum CK elevations).

If dosage reduction is necessary in a patient receiving 90 mg of brigatinib once daily, the dosage should be reduced to 60 mg once daily. If further dosage reduction is necessary, the drug should be permanently discontinued.

If dosage reduction is necessary in a patient receiving 180 mg of brigatinib once daily, an initial dosage reduction to 120 mg once daily is recommended. If further dosage reduction is necessary, the dosage should be reduced to 90 mg once daily. If dosage reduction from 90 mg once daily is necessary, a dosage of 60 mg once daily is recommended. If a dosage of 60 mg once daily is not tolerated, brigatinib should be permanently discontinued.

Once the dosage of brigatinib has been reduced because of adverse reactions, the dosage should not be subsequently increased.

Interstitial Lung Disease/Pneumonitis. If new grade 1 pulmonary symptoms occur *during* the first 7 days of treatment, brigatinib should be withheld until recovery to baseline. Therapy may then be resumed at the same dosage; dosage should *not* be increased to 180 mg once daily if interstitial lung disease (ILD)/pneumonitis is suspected.

If new grade 1 pulmonary symptoms occur *after* the first 7 days of treatment, brigatinib should be withheld until recovery to baseline. Therapy may then be resumed at the same dosage.

If new grade 2 pulmonary symptoms occur *during* the first 7 days of treatment, brigatinib should be withheld until recovery to baseline. Therapy may then be resumed at the next lower dosage; dosage should *not* be increased if ILD/pneumonitis is suspected.

If new grade 2 pulmonary symptoms occur *after* the first 7 days of treatment, brigatinib should be withheld until recovery to baseline. If ILD/pneumonitis is suspected, therapy may be resumed at the next lower dosage; otherwise, therapy may be resumed at the same dosage.

If grade 1 or 2 ILD/pneumonitis *recurs*, brigatinib therapy should be permanently discontinued.

If grade 3 or 4 ILD/pneumonitis occurs, brigatinib therapy should be permanently discontinued. (See Interstitial Lung Disease/Pneumonitis under Cautions: Warnings/Precautions.)

Hypertension. If grade 3 hypertension (i.e., systolic blood pressure of 160 mm Hg or greater or diastolic blood pressure of 100 mm Hg or greater requiring medical intervention and more than one antihypertensive agent or more intensive therapy than previously used) occurs, brigatinib should be withheld until recovery to grade 1 or less hypertension (i.e., systolic blood pressure less than 140 mm Hg and diastolic blood pressure less than 90 mm Hg). Therapy may then be resumed at the next lower dosage.

If grade 3 hypertension *recurs*, brigatinib should be withheld until recovery to grade 1 or less; therapy should then be resumed at the next lower dosage *or* permanently discontinued.

If grade 4 hypertension (i.e., life-threatening consequences, requiring urgent intervention) occurs, brigatinib should be withheld until recovery to grade 1 or less; therapy may then be resumed at the next lower dosage or permanently discontinued.

If grade 4 hypertension *recurs*, brigatinib therapy should be permanently discontinued. (See Hypertension under Cautions: Warnings/Precautions.)

Bradycardia. If symptomatic, but non-life-threatening, bradycardia occurs, therapy with brigatinib should be withheld until recovery to asymptomatic bradycardia or to a resting heart rate of at least 60 beats/minute. If concomitant drugs known to cause bradycardia are identified and discontinued or their dosage is adjusted, brigatinib therapy may be resumed at the same dosage upon recovery to asymptomatic bradycardia or to a resting heart rate of at least 60 beats/minute. If no concomitant drugs known to cause bradycardia are identified or if discontinuance or dosage adjustment of such concomitant drugs is not possible, brigatinib should be resumed at the next lower dosage upon recovery to asymptomatic bradycardia or to a resting heart rate of at least 60 beats/minute.

If life-threatening bradycardia requiring urgent intervention occurs in patients receiving concomitant contributory drugs, brigatinib should be withheld until recovery to asymptomatic bradycardia or to a resting heart rate of at least 60 beats/minute. If such concomitant drugs are discontinued or the dosage adjusted, brigatinib therapy may be resumed at the next lower dosage with frequent monitoring as clinically indicated. Brigatinib should be permanently discontinued in case of recurrence.

If life-threatening bradycardia requiring urgent intervention occurs in patients not receiving concomitant contributory drugs, brigatinib should be permanently discontinued. (See Bradycardia under Cautions: Warnings/Precautions.)

Visual Disturbances. If grade 2 or 3 visual disturbance occurs, brigatinib should be withheld until recovery to grade 1 or baseline. Therapy may then be resumed at the next lower dosage.

If grade 4 visual disturbance occurs, brigatinib therapy should be permanently discontinued. (See Visual Disturbances under Cautions: Warnings/Precautions.)

Creatine Kinase Elevation. If an elevation in serum CK concentrations exceeding 5 times the upper limit of normal (ULN; i.e., grade 3) occurs, brigatinib therapy should be withheld until CK concentrations return to baseline values or decrease to no more than 2.5 times the ULN (i.e., grade 1 or less). Brigatinib may then be resumed at the same dosage. If an elevation in serum CK concentrations exceeding 5 times the ULN *recurs*, brigatinib therapy should be withheld until CK concentrations return to baseline values or decrease to grade 1 or less; brigatinib therapy may then be resumed at the next lower dosage.

If an elevation in serum CK concentrations exceeding 10 times the ULN (i.e., grade 4) occurs, brigatinib therapy should be withheld until serum CK concentrations return to baseline values or decrease to grade 1 or less. Brigatinib therapy should then be resumed at the next lower dosage. (See Creatine Kinase Elevation under Cautions: Warnings/Precautions.)

Pancreatic Enzyme Elevation. If an elevation in serum amylase or lipase concentrations exceeding 2 times the ULN (i.e., grade 3) occurs, brigatinib therapy should be withheld until amylase or lipase concentrations return to baseline values or decrease to no more than 1.5 times the ULN (i.e., grade 1 or less). Brigatinib may then be resumed at the same dosage. If grade 3 elevation in serum amylase or lipase concentrations *recurs*, brigatinib should be withheld until amylase or lipase concentrations return to baseline values or decrease to grade 1 or less; brigatinib therapy may then be resumed at the next lower dosage.

If an elevation in serum amylase or lipase concentrations exceeding 5 times the ULN (i.e., grade 4) occurs, brigatinib therapy should be withheld until amylase or lipase concentrations return to baseline values or decrease to grade 1 or less. Brigatinib therapy may then be resumed at the next lower dosage. (See Pancreatic Enzyme Elevation under Cautions: Warnings/Precautions.)

Hyperglycemia. If hyperglycemia with serum glucose concentrations exceeding 250 mg/dL (i.e., grade 3) occurs and adequate hyperglycemic control cannot be achieved despite optimal antidiabetic agent therapy, brigatinib should be withheld until adequate control of the hyperglycemia is achieved. Resumption of brigatinib at the next lower dosage or permanent discontinuance of brigatinib should then be considered. (See Hyperglycemia under Cautions: Warnings/Precautions.)

Other Toxicity. If any other grade 3 adverse reaction occurs, brigatinib therapy should be withheld until recovery to baseline. Brigatinib therapy may then be resumed at the same dosage. If the grade 3 adverse reaction *recurs*, brigatinib therapy should be withheld until recovery to baseline; brigatinib may then be resumed at the next lower dosage or the drug discontinued.

If any other grade 4 adverse reaction occurs, brigatinib therapy should be withheld until recovery to baseline. Brigatinib therapy may then be resumed at the next lower dosage or permanently discontinued. If the grade 4 adverse reaction *recurs*, brigatinib therapy should be permanently discontinued.

Concomitant Use of Drugs Affecting Hepatic Microsomal Enzymes Concomitant use of brigatinib with drugs that are potent inhibitors of cytochrome P-450 (CYP) isoenzyme 3A should be avoided. If concomitant use of a potent CYP3A inhibitor cannot be avoided, the manufacturer recommends reducing the daily dosage of brigatinib by approximately 50% (e.g., from 180 mg to 90 mg once daily or from 90 mg to 60 mg once daily). If concomitant use of the potent CYP3A inhibitor is discontinued, the brigatinib dosage should be returned to the dosage that was tolerated prior to initiation of the potent CYP3A inhibitor. (See Inhibitors of CYP3A under Drug Interactions: Drugs and Foods Affecting Hepatic Microsomal Enzymes.)

■ **Special Populations** The manufacturer makes no specific dosage recommendations for geriatric patients. (See Geriatric Use under Warnings/Precautions: Specific Populations, in Cautions.)

No dosage adjustment is necessary in patients with mild hepatic impairment (total bilirubin concentrations not exceeding the ULN with AST concentrations exceeding the ULN, or total bilirubin concentrations exceeding 1 but not exceeding 1.5 times the ULN with any AST concentration). Pharmacokinetics and safety of brigatinib have not been established in patients with moderate or severe hepatic impairment. (See Hepatic Impairment under Warnings/Precautions: Specific Populations, in Cautions.)

No dosage adjustment is necessary in patients with mild or moderate renal impairment (creatinine clearance of 30–89 mL/minute). Pharmacokinetics and safety of brigatinib have not been established in patients with severe renal impairment (creatinine clearance less than 30 mL/minute). (See Renal Impairment under Warnings/Precautions: Specific Populations, in Cautions.)

Cautions

■ **Contraindications** The manufacturer states that there are no known contraindications to the use of brigatinib.

■ **Warnings/Precautions** ***Interstitial Lung Disease/Pneumonitis*** Severe, life-threatening, or fatal adverse pulmonary reactions consistent with interstitial lung disease (ILD)/pneumonitis may occur in patients receiving brigatinib. In the principal efficacy study, ILD or pneumonitis occurred in 3.7% of patients receiving brigatinib 90 mg once daily and in 9.1% of patients receiving the recommended dosage regimen (180 mg once daily with a 7-day lead-in at 90 mg once daily), and grade 3 or 4 adverse reactions consistent with possible ILD or pneumonitis occurred in 2.7% of patients receiving the drug. Adverse pulmonary symptoms consistent with possible ILD/pneumonitis occurred early (i.e., within 9 days of initiation of therapy; median onset was 2 days) in 6.4% of patients in this study, and all patients were receiving brigatinib 90 mg once daily at the time of symptom onset.

Patients receiving brigatinib should be monitored for new or worsening respiratory symptoms (e.g., dyspnea, cough), particularly during the first week of initiating therapy. (See Advice to Patients.) If such respiratory manifestations occur, brigatinib therapy should be interrupted and patients should be promptly evaluated for ILD/pneumonitis or other causes of respiratory symptoms (e.g., pulmonary embolism, tumor progression, pneumonia). If ILD/pneumonitis is confirmed, dosage reduction or discontinuance of therapy may be necessary depending on the severity or for recurrent ILD/pneumonitis. (See Interstitial Lung Disease/Pneumonitis under Dosage: Dosage Modification for Toxicity, in Dosage and Administration.)

Hypertension Hypertension occurred in 21% of patients and grade 3 or 4 hypertension occurred in 6.4% of patients receiving the recommended dosage regimen of brigatinib (180 mg once daily with a 7-day lead-in at 90 mg once daily) in the principal efficacy study. Among patients receiving brigatinib 90 mg once daily, hypertension occurred in 11% and grade 3 or 4 hypertension occurred in 5.5%.

Blood pressure should be controlled prior to initiating therapy with brigatinib. Blood pressure should be monitored 2 weeks after treatment initiation and at least monthly during therapy with the drug. If severe hypertension (i.e., grade 3) occurs despite optimal antihypertensive therapy, brigatinib therapy should be interrupted until blood pressure is controlled. Dosage reduction or discontinuance of therapy may be necessary depending on the severity or for recurrent hypertension. (See Hypertension under Dosage: Dosage Modification for Toxicity, in Dosage and Administration.)

The manufacturer recommends using caution when brigatinib is administered concurrently with antihypertensive agents that cause bradycardia. (See Drug Interactions: Drugs Associated with Bradycardia.)

Bradycardia Brigatinib may cause bradycardia. In the principal efficacy study, bradycardia with a heart rate of less than 50 beats/minute was reported in 7.6 or 5.7% of patients receiving brigatinib 180 mg once daily (with a 7-day lead-in at 90 mg once daily) or 90 mg once daily, respectively. Grade 2 bradycardia occurred in one patient (0.9%) receiving the 90-mg daily dosage.

Heart rate and blood pressure should be monitored periodically during brigatinib therapy. (See Hypertension under Cautions: Warnings/Precautions.) More frequent monitoring is recommended if concomitant use of a drug known to cause bradycardia cannot be avoided. If symptomatic or life-threatening bradycardia occurs, brigatinib therapy should be interrupted; dosage reduction or discontinuance of therapy may be necessary depending on concomitant use of other drugs known to cause bradycardia. (See Bradycardia under Dosage: Dosage Modification for Toxicity, in Dosage and Administration.)

Visual Disturbances In the principal efficacy study, adverse reactions leading to visual disturbances, including blurred vision, diplopia, and reduced visual acuity, were reported in 10 or 7.3% of patients receiving brigatinib 180 mg once daily (with a 7-day lead-in at 90 mg once daily) or 90 mg once daily, respectively. Grade 3 macular edema and cataract each occurred in one patient receiving brigatinib 180 mg once daily (with a 7-day lead-in at 90 mg once daily).

In patients who report new or worsening visual symptoms of grade 2 or higher severity, brigatinib therapy should be interrupted and an ophthalmologic evaluation performed. Dosage reduction or drug discontinuance may be required depending on the severity. (See Visual Disturbances under Dosage: Dosage Modification for Toxicity, in Dosage and Administration and see also Advice to Patients.)

Creatine Kinase Elevation In the principal efficacy study, elevated serum creatine kinase (CK, creatine phosphokinase, CPK) concentrations were reported in 48% and were grade 3 or 4 in 12% of patients receiving brigatinib 180 mg once daily (with a 7-day lead-in at 90 mg once daily). Among patients receiving brigatinib 90 mg once daily, elevated serum CK concentrations were reported in 27% of patients; 2.8% of these patients had grade 3 or 4 elevations in CK concentrations. Dosage modification because of elevated serum CK concentrations was required in 4.5 or 1.8% of patients receiving brigatinib 180 or 90 mg daily, respectively.

Serum CK concentrations should be monitored periodically during brigatinib therapy. (See Advice to Patients.) Temporary interruption followed by resumption of therapy at the same or at a reduced dosage of brigatinib may be necessary, depending on the severity of the CK elevation. (See Creatine Kinase Elevation under Dosage: Dosage Modification for Toxicity, in Dosage and Administration.)

Pancreatic Enzyme Elevation In the principal efficacy study, elevated serum amylase concentrations and grade 3 or 4 elevated serum amylase concentrations were reported in 39 and 2.7% of patients receiving brigatinib 180 mg once daily (with a 7-day lead-in at 90 mg once daily), respectively. Elevated serum lipase concentrations and grade 3 or 4 elevated serum lipase concentrations were reported in 45 and 5.5% of patients receiving the 180-mg daily dosage, respectively. Among patients receiving brigatinib 90 mg once daily, elevated serum amylase concentrations and grade 3 or 4 elevated serum amylase concentrations were reported in 27 and 3.7% of patients, respectively. Elevated serum lipase concentrations and grade 3 or 4 elevated serum lipase concentrations were reported in 21 and 4.6% of patients receiving the 90-mg daily dosage of brigatinib, respectively.

Serum amylase and lipase concentrations should be monitored periodically during brigatinib therapy. Temporary interruption followed by resumption of therapy at the same or a reduced dosage of brigatinib may be necessary, depending on the severity of the amylase and/or lipase elevation. (See Pancreatic Enzyme Elevation under Dosage: Dosage Modification for Toxicity, in Dosage and Administration.)

Hyperglycemia Hyperglycemia may occur in patients receiving brigatinib. In the principal efficacy study, new or worsening hyperglycemia occurred in 43% of brigatinib-treated patients; grade 3 hyperglycemia (based on fasting serum glucose concentrations) occurred in 3.7% of patients receiving the drug. Among patients with diabetes mellitus or glucose intolerance at baseline, 10% required initiation of insulin during brigatinib therapy.

Fasting serum glucose concentrations should be assessed prior to initiation of brigatinib and monitored periodically during treatment. Antidiabetic agents should be initiated or optimized as necessary. If adequate glycemic control cannot be achieved despite optimal medical management, brigatinib therapy should be interrupted until hyperglycemia is adequately controlled. Dosage reduction or discontinuance of therapy may be necessary depending on the severity of hyperglycemia. (See Hyperglycemia under Dosage: Dosage Modification for Toxicity, in Dosage and Administration.)

Fetal/Neonatal Morbidity and Mortality Brigatinib may cause fetal harm if administered to pregnant women based on its mechanism of action and animal findings. There are no clinical data on the use of brigatinib in pregnant women. Dose-related skeletal abnormalities were observed when the drug was administered to pregnant animals during the period of organogenesis at dosages equivalent to approximately 0.7 times the human exposure achieved with the recommended dosage. In addition, increased post-implantation loss, malformations, and decreased fetal body weight were observed in animals at dosages equivalent to approximately 1.26 times the human exposure achieved at the recommended dosage.

Pregnancy should be avoided during brigatinib therapy. Women of childbearing potential should use effective nonhormonal contraception during brigatinib therapy and for at least 4 months after the drug is discontinued. (See Drug Interactions: Hormonal Contraceptives and see also Advice to Patients.) In addition, men with female partners of childbearing potential should use effective methods of contraception while receiving brigatinib therapy and for at least 3 months after the drug is discontinued. If brigatinib is used during pregnancy or if the patient becomes pregnant while receiving the drug, the patient should be apprised of the potential fetal hazard.

Impairment of Fertility Based on findings in male reproductive organs in animal studies, brigatinib may impair male fertility.

Specific Populations **Pregnancy.** Although there are no clinical data in pregnant women to date, animal studies and its mechanism of action suggest that brigatinib may cause fetal harm. (See Fetal/Neonatal Morbidity and Mortality under Cautions: Warnings/Precautions.)

Lactation. It is not known whether brigatinib is distributed into human milk or if the drug has any effect on milk production or the nursing infant. Because of the potential for adverse reactions to brigatinib in nursing infants, women should be advised not to breast-feed while receiving the drug and for at least 1 week after the drug is discontinued.

Pediatric Use. Safety and efficacy of brigatinib have not been established in pediatric patients.

Geriatric Use. Clinical studies of brigatinib did not include sufficient numbers of patients 65 years of age and older to determine whether geriatric patients respond differently than younger adults. In the principal efficacy study evaluating brigatinib in patients with NSCLC, approximately 19% of patients were 65–74 years of age and 4% were 75 years of age or older. No clinically important differences in safety or efficacy were observed between geriatric patients and younger adults in this study.

Age does not have a clinically important effect on the pharmacokinetics of brigatinib.

Hepatic Impairment. In a population pharmacokinetic analysis, mild hepatic impairment (total bilirubin concentrations not exceeding the upper limit of normal [ULN] with AST concentrations exceeding the ULN, or total bilirubin concentrations exceeding 1 but not exceeding 1.5 times the ULN with any AST concentration) did not affect systemic exposure to brigatinib. Pharmacokinetics and safety of brigatinib have not been studied in patients with moderate or severe hepatic impairment.

Renal Impairment. In a population pharmacokinetic analysis, mild or moderate renal impairment (creatinine clearance of 30–89 mL/minute) did not affect systemic exposure to brigatinib. Pharmacokinetics and safety of brigatinib have not been studied in patients with severe renal impairment (creatinine clearance less than 30 mL/minute); such patients were excluded from clinical trials.

■ **Common Adverse Effects** Adverse effects reported in 10% or more of patients receiving the recommended dosage regimen of brigatinib in the principal efficacy study include nausea, vomiting, diarrhea, fatigue/asthenia, cough, headache, rash (including acneiform dermatitis and exfoliative, pruritic, or pustular rash), dyspnea, hypertension, muscle spasms, decreased appetite, constipation, back pain, myalgia/musculoskeletal pain, arthralgia, peripheral neuropathy (including paresthesia), abdominal pain, visual disturbances (including diplopia, photophobia, blurred vision, reduced visual acuity, visual impairment, vitreous floaters, visual field defect, macular edema, and vitreous detachment), and pneumonia.

Laboratory abnormalities reported in at least 20% of patients receiving the recommended dosage regimen of brigatinib in the principal efficacy study include increased concentrations of aminotransferases (i.e., ALT, AST), increased concentrations of alkaline phosphatase, increased concentrations of CK, hyperglycemia, increased concentrations of lipase and/or amylase, anemia, lymphopenia, hypophosphatemia, and prolonged activated partial thromboplastin time.

Drug Interactions

Brigatinib is metabolized principally by cytochrome P-450 (CYP) isoenzymes 2C8 and 3A4. In vitro studies indicate that brigatinib is a substrate of P-glycoprotein (P-gp) and breast cancer resistance protein (BCRP), but not a substrate of organic anion transport protein (OATP) 1B1, OATP1B3, organic anion transporter (OAT) 1, OAT3, organic cation transporter (OCT) 1, OCT2, multidrug and toxin extrusion transporter (MATE) 1, MATE2K, or bile salt export pump (BSEP).

In vitro studies indicate that brigatinib inhibits P-gp, BCRP, OCT1, MATE1, and MATE2K. Brigatinib does not inhibit OATP1B1, OATP1B3, OAT1, OAT3, OCT2, or BSEP.

Brigatinib induces CYP3A and also may induce CYP2C isoenzymes via activation of the pregnane X receptor (PXR). Brigatinib and its principal metabolite do not inhibit CYP isoenzymes 1A2, 2B6, 2C8, 2C9, 2C19, 2D6, or 3A4/5 at clinically relevant concentrations.

■ **Drugs and Foods Affecting Hepatic Microsomal Enzymes**

Inhibitors of CYP3A Concomitant use of brigatinib with potent inhibitors of CYP3A may increase plasma concentrations of brigatinib, which may result in increased adverse effects. Concurrent administration of itraconazole (200 mg twice daily) and brigatinib (single 90-mg dose) increased peak plasma concentrations and area under the concentration-time curve (AUC) of brigatinib by 21 and 101%, respectively, compared with administration of brigatinib alone.

The manufacturer states that concomitant use of potent CYP3A inhibitors, including certain antiretrovirals (e.g., indinavir, lopinavir, nelfinavir, ritonavir, saquinavir), macrolide antibiotics (e.g., clarithromycin), antifungals (e.g., itraconazole, ketoconazole, posaconazole, voriconazole), cobicistat, conivaptan, and products containing grapefruit, should be avoided during brigatinib therapy. If concomitant use of a potent CYP3A inhibitor cannot be avoided, the manufacturer recommends reducing the daily dosage of brigatinib by approximately 50%. If concomitant use of the potent CYP3A inhibitor is discontinued, the brigatinib dosage should be returned to the dosage that was tolerated prior to initiation of the potent CYP3A inhibitor. (See Concomitant Use of Drugs Affecting Hepatic Microsomal Enzymes under Dosage: Dosage and Administration.)

Inhibitors of CYP2C8 Concomitant administration of the potent CYP2C8 inhibitor gemfibrozil (600 mg twice daily) and brigatinib (single 90-mg dose) decreased peak plasma concentrations and the AUC of brigatinib by 41 and 12%, respectively. The manufacturer states that the effect of gemfibrozil on the pharmacokinetics of brigatinib is not considered clinically important and that the underlying mechanism for the decreased exposure of brigatinib is not known.

Inducers of CYP3A Concomitant use of brigatinib with potent inducers of CYP3A (e.g., carbamazepine, phenytoin, rifampin) may decrease plasma concentrations and reduce efficacy of brigatinib and should be avoided. When the potent CYP3A inducer rifampin (600 mg daily) was administered concomitantly with brigatinib (single 180-mg dose), peak plasma concentrations and AUC of brigatinib decreased by 60 and 80%, respectively.

Use of St. John's wort (*Hypericum perforatum*), a potent CYP3A inducer, also should be avoided during brigatinib therapy.

■ **Drugs Metabolized by Hepatic Microsomal Enzymes** Brigatinib induces CYP3A in vitro; therefore, concomitant use of brigatinib and drugs metabolized by CYP3A may result in decreased concentrations and loss of efficacy of the CYP3A substrate. (See Drug Interactions: Hormonal Contraceptives.)

■ **Substrates of Drug Transport Systems** Brigatinib inhibits P-gp, BCRP, OCT1, MATE1, and MATE2K in vitro and potentially may increase concentrations of drugs that are substrates of these transport systems.

■ **Drugs Associated with Bradycardia** Because brigatinib has been associated with bradycardia, caution is advised when brigatinib is used concurrently with other drugs known to cause bradycardia. Heart rate should be monitored more frequently if such concomitant use cannot be avoided. If clinically important bradycardia occurs with concomitant use of brigatinib and drugs known to cause bradycardia (including antihypertensive agents), the dosage of the concomitant drug should be adjusted or the concomitant drug should be discontinued, if possible. (See Bradycardia under Cautions: Warnings/Precautions.)

■ **Hormonal Contraceptives** Concomitant use of brigatinib and hormonal contraceptives, which are CYP3A substrates, may result in decreased plasma concentrations and reduced efficacy of the hormonal contraceptive. Women of childbearing potential should therefore use effective nonhormonal contraception during brigatinib therapy and for at least 4 months after the drug is discontinued. (See Fetal/Neonatal Morbidity and Mortality under Cautions: Warnings/Precautions.)

■ **Grapefruit** Grapefruit products are CYP3A inhibitors and should be avoided because of the potential for increased plasma brigatinib concentrations during concurrent use.

Description

Brigatinib, an inhibitor of multiple tyrosine kinases, including anaplastic lymphoma kinase (ALK), c-ros oncogene-1 (ROS-1), insulin-like growth factor receptor-1 (IGFR-1), and fms-like tyrosine kinase 3 (FLT-3) as well as epidermal growth factor receptor (EGFR) deletion and point mutations, is an antineoplastic agent. The drug inhibits autophosphorylation of ALK and ALK-mediated phosphorylation of the downstream signaling proteins signal transducer and activator of transcription 3 (STAT3), AKT serine/threonine kinase, extracellular signal-regulated kinase (ERK) 1/2, and ribosomal protein S6 in vitro and in vivo.

Activating mutations or translocations of the ALK gene have been identified in several malignancies and can result in the expression of oncogenic fusion proteins (e.g., echinoderm microtubule-associated protein-like 4 [EML4]-ALK). Such ALK gene rearrangements have been identified in approximately 3–7% of patients with non-small cell lung cancer (NSCLC). Formation of ALK fusion proteins such as EML4-ALK results in activation and dysregulation of the gene's expression and signaling, which can contribute to increased cell proliferation and survival in tumors expressing these proteins.

Although the ALK inhibitor crizotinib has demonstrated improved outcomes in patients with NSCLC harboring ALK mutations, secondary resistance to crizotinib eventually develops, generally within the first 1–2 years of treatment. Clinical resistance to crizotinib has been attributed to several possible mechanisms, including acquired resistance mutations of ALK, amplification of gene expression, and activation of alternate signaling pathways. Secondary mutations of ALK are responsible for about 30% of cases of acquired crizotinib resistance and gene amplification is implicated in 9% of these cases. The CNS is a common site of disease progression in crizotinib-treated patients because of poor distribution of the drug into CSF; development and/or progression of brain metastases occurs in approximately one-half of patients during crizotinib treatment.

In vitro, brigatinib is approximately 12-fold more potent than crizotinib in its activity against native ALK-positive cell lines and is active against cell lines expressing EML4-ALK and nucleophosmin (NPM)-ALK fusion proteins and many mutant forms associated with resistance to alectinib, ceritinib, and/or crizotinib, as well as EGFR-Del (E746-A750), ROS1-L2026M, FLT3-F691L, and FLT3-D835Y. Brigatinib also demonstrated dose-dependent antitumor activity in mice bearing NSCLC tumor xenografts that expressed EML4-ALK, including those with the crizotinib resistance-conferring L1196M mutation and the G1202R mutation that also confers resistance to ceritinib and alectinib. In addition, brigatinib reduced tumor burden and prolonged survival in mice bearing intracranial ALK-positive NSCLC tumor xenografts. Brigatinib also has demonstrated antitumor activity in patients with crizotinib-resistant disease and baseline CNS metastases.

Systemic exposure to brigatinib is dose proportional over the oral dosage range of 60–240 mg following single or multiple doses. Following oral administration, peak plasma concentrations of brigatinib are achieved in 1–4 hours. Administration of brigatinib with a high-fat meal decreases peak plasma concentrations of brigatinib by 13% but has no effect on systemic exposure compared with administration in the fasting state. Brigatinib is 66% bound to plasma proteins and binding is independent of drug concentration. Brigatinib is primarily metabolized by cytochrome P-450 (CYP) isoenzymes 2C8 and 3A4; its major active metabolite, AP26123, inhibits ALK with approximately threefold lower potency than the parent drug. Steady-state systemic exposure of AP26123 is less than 10% of the parent drug. Following oral administration of radiolabeled brigatinib, 65% of the dose is eliminated in feces (41% as unchanged drug) and 25% of the dose is eliminated in urine (86% as unchanged drug). The mean elimination half-life of brigatinib is 25 hours. Age, gender, race, body weight, and serum albumin concentration do not have clinically important effects on the pharmacokinetics of brigatinib.

Advice to Patients

Importance of instructing patients to read the manufacturer's patient information.

Importance of advising patients to take brigatinib exactly as prescribed and of not altering the dosage or discontinuing therapy unless advised to do so by their clinician. Importance of advising patients to swallow brigatinib tablets whole without regard to food and not to crush or chew the tablets. If a dose is missed or if vomiting occurs after a dose is administered, the next dose should be taken at the regularly scheduled time; the missed dose should not be taken, and an additional dose should not be administered to replace the vomited dose.

Importance of informing patients of the symptoms and risks of serious adverse pulmonary reactions such as interstitial lung disease/pneumonitis, which occur particularly during the first week of brigatinib therapy. Importance of advising patients to immediately report any new or worsening pulmonary symptoms (e.g., dyspnea or shortness of breath, cough with or without mucus, chest pain, fever) to their clinician and informing them that such symptoms may be similar to those of lung cancer.

Risk of muscle problems or myalgia; importance of creatine kinase (CK, creatine phosphokinase, CPK) monitoring. Importance of advising patients to promptly inform clinicians if they experience any new or worsening signs and symptoms of muscle problems, including unexplained or persistent muscle pain, tenderness, or weakness.

Risk of hypertension. Importance of promptly reporting signs or symptoms of hypertension (e.g., headache, dizziness, blurred vision, chest pain, shortness of breath).

Risk of bradycardia. Importance of patients immediately contacting their clinician if they experience dizziness, lightheadedness, or faintness during therapy.

Risk of visual disturbances. Importance of informing clinician of any new or worsening visual symptoms (e.g., diplopia, blurred vision, flashes of light, photophobia, new or increased floaters).

Risk of elevated concentrations of pancreatic enzymes and importance of monitoring amylase and lipase concentrations. Importance of patients immediately contacting their clinician if they experience manifestations of pancreatitis (e.g., upper abdominal pain that may spread to the back and get worse with eating, weight loss, nausea).

Risk of new or worsening hyperglycemia and importance of periodically monitoring blood glucose concentrations. Importance of immediately informing clinician if manifestations of hyperglycemia occur (e.g., increased thirst, increased urination, increased appetite, nausea, weakness, fatigue, confusion). Patients with diabetes mellitus or glucose intolerance may require dosage adjustment of antidiabetic therapy during brigatinib treatment.

Risk of fetal harm. Necessity of advising women of childbearing potential that they should use effective, nonhormonal methods of contraception while receiving brigatinib and for at least 4 months after discontinuance of therapy and of also advising such women that oral contraceptives and other hormonal forms of contraception may not be effective during brigatinib therapy. Importance of advising men with female partners of childbearing potential to use effective methods of contraception while receiving the drug and for at least 3 months after the drug is discontinued. Importance of also advising men that brigatinib may cause fertility problems and to discuss any concerns about fertility with their clinician.

Importance of women informing their clinicians if they are or plan to become pregnant. If pregnancy occurs, the patient should be advised of the potential risk to the fetus.

Importance of advising women to avoid breast-feeding while receiving brigatinib and for at least 1 week after discontinuance of therapy.

Importance of informing clinicians of existing or contemplated concomitant therapy, including prescription and OTC drugs (e.g., cardiac or antihypertensive agents, antidiabetic agents) and dietary or herbal supplements (e.g., St. John's wort, grapefruit-containing products), as well as any concomitant illnesses (e.g., cardiovascular disease, diabetes mellitus, pancreatitis).

Importance of advising patients to avoid grapefruit and grapefruit juice while taking brigatinib.

Importance of informing patients of other important precautionary information. (See Cautions.)

Overview® (see Users Guide). For additional information on this drug until a more detailed monograph is developed and published, the manufacturer's labeling should be consulted. It is *essential* that the manufacturer's labeling be consulted for more detailed information on usual cautions, precautions, contraindications, potential drug interactions, laboratory test interferences, and acute toxicity. For further information on the handling of antineoplastic agents, see the ASHP Guidelines on Handling Hazardous Drugs at http://www.ahfsdruginformation.com.

Preparations

Brigatinib can only be obtained through select specialty distributors. (See Restricted Distribution under Dosage and Administration: General.)

Excipients in commercially available drug preparations may have clinically important effects in some individuals; consult specific product labeling for details.

Brigatinib

Oral		
Tablets, film-coated	30 mg	**Alunbrig®**, Ariad
	90 mg	**Alunbrig®**, Ariad
	180 mg	**Alunbrig®**, Ariad

†Use is not currently included in the labeling approved by the US Food and Drug Administration

Busulfan

Busulphan

■ Busulfan, a bifunctional alkylating agent, is an antineoplastic agent.

Uses

■ **Chronic Myelogenous Leukemia** ***Allogeneic Hematopoietic Stem Cell Transplantation*** Busulfan is used in combination with cyclophosphamide as a conditioning regimen prior to allogeneic hematopoietic progenitor cell transplantation in patients with chronic myelogenous leukemia (CML) and is designated an orphan drug by the US Food and Drug Administration (FDA) for the treatment of this disease. Although a preparative regimen of high-dose chemotherapy followed by allogeneic stem cell transplantation currently is the only consistently curative treatment for CML, the selection of candidates is limited by age restrictions and the availability of ideal donors (i.e., HLA-matched siblings). Survival rates and duration are most favorable for patients undergoing transplantation during the chronic phase of CML and progressively worse for those in the accelerated or blastic phases.

The current indication for the use of IV busulfan as a component of a conditioning regimen prior to allogeneic hematopoietic stem cell transplantation is based on data from an uncontrolled, phase 2 trial of IV busulfan and from previously published randomized, controlled studies of high-dose oral busulfan. In an open-label, uncontrolled trial, 61 patients received busulfan 0.8 mg/kg as a 2-hour IV infusion every 6 hours for 4 days for a total of 16 doses, followed by cyclophosphamide 60 mg/kg once a day for 2 days; after one day of rest, allogeneic hematopoietic stem cells were infused. The study patients had various hematologic malignancies, including acute leukemia (relapsed, refractory, or high-risk first remission), chronic myelogenous leukemia (chronic phase, accelerated phase, or blast crisis), Hodgkin's disease or non-Hodgkin's lymphoma (primary refractory or resistant relapsed disease), and myelodysplastic syndrome. Approximately half (48%) of the patients were heavily pretreated, defined as one or more of the following: prior radiation therapy, 3 or more prior chemotherapy regimens, or prior hematopoietic stem cell transplantation.

Myeloablation (defined as at least one of the following: absolute neutrophil count below 0.5×10^9/L, absolute lymphocyte count below 0.1×10^9/L, platelet count below 20,000/mm^3, or a requirement for platelet transfusion) was achieved in all patients. Onset of neutropenia occurred at a median of 4 days; prophylactic granulocyte colony-stimulating factor was administered in the majority of patients. Engraftment was achieved in all 60 evaluable patients and occurred at a median of 13 days after transplant (range: 9–29 days). Relapse occurred in 38% of patients at a median of 183 days after transplant (range: 36–406 days). A total of 62% of patients were free from disease with a median follow-up of 269 days after transplant (range: 20–583 days). A survival rate of 70% with a median follow-up of 288 days after transplant (range: 51–583 days) was reported.

Busulfan also has been administered orally† as a component of a conditioning regimen prior to allogeneic transplantation. In 4 randomized, controlled studies in patients undergoing allogeneic bone marrow transplantation for CML or other hematologic malignancies, patients randomized to the busulfan-containing regimen generally received oral busulfan 4 mg/kg daily for 4 days and cyclophosphamide 60 mg/kg daily for 2 days. The results of these studies indicated that the efficacy of the busulfan and cyclophosphamide regimen was similar to the comparator regimens, which included cyclophosphamide plus total body irradiation and etoposide plus total body irradiation. Based on the clinical trial using IV busulfan and on the available literature on oral busulfan, the FDA Oncologic Drugs Advisory Committee concluded that the 2 dosage forms are comparably safe and effective as part of a conditioning regimen prior to allogeneic stem cell transplants.

Conventional Chemotherapy Busulfan rarely is used as an alternative agent for the palliative treatment of chronic myelogenous leukemia (CML). Interferon alfa, with or without cytarabine, is a first-line therapy for the palliative treatment of CML in patients who cannot undergo allogeneic hematopoietic progenitor cell transplantation, which is the only therapy known to be curative for this leukemia. In a randomized trial, median survival was longer in patients receiving interferon alfa versus busulfan for CML. Unlike interferon alfa, busulfan has not been associated with prolonged cytogenetic response (i.e., suppression of Philadelphia chromosome-positive cells) in patients with Philadelphia chromosome (Ph)-positive CML. Hydroxyurea, an alternative agent for the palliative treatment of CML, is superior to busulfan; in a randomized trial, patients receiving hydroxyurea experienced prolonged median survival and less toxicity compared with those receiving busulfan.

Busulfan is not curative, but approximately 90% of patients in the chronic phase of CML treated with the drug obtain remissions. Subjective response generally starts within 1–3 weeks, and remissions are characterized by a decrease in the leukocyte count and spleen size, disappearance of sternal tenderness, and an increase in hemoglobin. Duration of therapy required to bring the leukocyte count to normal depends mainly on the level of the leukocyte count when therapy was begun, the daily dose, and the sensitivity of the patient. Approximately 2 months of continuous therapy is required in most patients to reduce the leukocyte count to desired levels. In about half the patients with CML, busulfan induces an initial remission of 9–12 months or longer. During remissions, the patient's quality of life is reportedly improved due to increased comfort, appetite, sense of well-being, and general ability to function. Resistance to busulfan develops progressively. Subsequent remissions usually become shorter and more difficult to achieve, but may be maintained for months or even years with busulfan therapy. Busulfan is an alternative agent for the palliative treatment of the accelerated phase of CML. The drug does not prevent, and is ineffective during, the blastic phase of CML.

Busulfan is less effective in the management of patients with CML who lack the Philadelphia (Ph[1]) chromosome. In addition, the juvenile type of CML responds poorly to busulfan.

Chemotherapy typically is used to reduce leukocyte count and stabilize hematologic status prior to allogeneic bone marrow transplantation. Retrospective analysis indicates that probability of disease-free survival at 3 years is higher in patients receiving hydroxyurea rather than busulfan for CML in chronic phase prior to allogeneic transplant.

■ **Other Uses** Busulfan has been used as a component of pretransplant conditioning regimens in patients undergoing bone marrow transplantation for acute myeloid leukemia and nonmalignant diseases (e.g., sickle cell disease)†.

Dosage and Administration

■ **Reconstitution and Administration** Busulfan tablets are administered orally.

Busulfan for injection concentrate is administered by IV infusion. The manufacturer states that rapid infusion of busulfan has not been evaluated and is *not* recommended.

Commercially available busulfan for injection concentrate must be diluted prior to IV infusion. The manufacturer recommends diluting busulfan for injection concentrate in 0.9% sodium chloride injection or 5% dextrose injection with approximately 10 times the volume of the calculated dose of busulfan to achieve a final busulfan concentration of approximately 0.5 mg/mL. A 5-μm nylon filter is provided with each ampul of busulfan and should be used to withdraw the calculated volume of busulfan for injection concentrate from the ampul. If using the provided syringe filter in the forward flow direction, the calculated volume of busulfan for injection concentrate should allow for approximately 0.16 mL of residual busulfan for injection concentrate that will remain in the filter. The use of filters other than the specific type of filter provided with the busulfan ampul is *not* recommended. A new needle should then be used to inject the drug into an IV bag (or large-volume syringe) that contains the calculated volume of diluent; according to the manufacturer, the busulfan always must be added to the diluent rather than the diluent being added to the drug. The manufacturer states that polycarbonate syringes or polycarbonate filter needles should *not* be used for the preparation or administration of busulfan solutions. The diluted busulfan infusion should be inverted several times to ensure thorough mixing.

Caution should be exercised in handling and preparing solutions of busulfan. Busulfan solutions should be prepared under a vertical laminar-flow safety hood. Because dermatologic reactions may occur with accidental exposure to the drug, the manufacturer recommends the use of protective gloves and clothing during the preparation and administration of busulfan infusions. Skin or mucosa accidentally exposed to the drug should be washed immediately and thoroughly with water.

Busulfan for injection concentrate and diluted solutions of the drug should be inspected visually for particulate matter whenever solution and container permit. If particulate matter is observed in the ampul of busulfan, it should not be used.

According to the manufacturer, an administration set with minimal residual hold-up volume (2–5 mL) should be used to administer the drug. Diluted IV solutions of busulfan should be administered via a central venous catheter over 2 hours using a controlled-infusion device (e.g., pump). The catheter line should be flushed with about 5 mL of 0.9% sodium chloride or 5% dextrose injection before and after each busulfan infusion. Busulfan solutions should *not* be mixed or administered with other IV solutions of unknown compatibility.

For additional administration instructions related to therapeutic drug monitoring and adjust dosage of IV busulfan in children, see Pediatric Dosage in Dosage and Administration: Dosage: Chronic Myelogenous Leukemia: Allogeneic Hematopoietic Stem Cell Transplantation.

■ **Dosage** ***Chronic Myelogenous Leukemia*** **Allogeneic Hematopoietic Stem Cell Transplantation: Adult Dosage.** When used in combination with cyclophosphamide as a conditioning regimen prior to allogeneic hematopoietic progenitor cell transplantation in adult patients with chronic myelogenous leukemia, the recommended dose of IV busulfan is 0.8 mg/kg of ideal body weight or actual body weight (whichever is lower) every 6 hours for 4 consecutive days (for a total of 16 doses). In obese patients, busulfan dosage should be based on adjusted ideal body weight (ideal body weight plus 0.25 times the difference between actual weight and ideal body weight). The manufacturer states that all patients should receive premedication with phenytoin for seizure prophylaxis; in addition, all patients should receive antiemetics prior to the first dose of IV busulfan and on a fixed schedule throughout busulfan therapy. Cyclophosphamide should be administered (at a dose of 60 mg/kg IV over 1 hour daily for 2 days) starting 6 hours after the 16th dose of IV busulfan (i.e., on bone marrow transplant day 3). When available, monitoring of the busulfan area under the plasma concentration-time curve (AUC) may be considered to optimize dosage adjustment for busulfan.

When administered orally† as a component of a conditioning regimen prior to allogeneic transplantation, a busulfan dosage of 4 mg/kg per day for 4 days most commonly has been used.

Allogeneic Hematopoietic Stem Cell Transplantation: Pediatric Dosage. When used in combination with cyclophosphamide as a conditioning regimen prior to allogeneic hematopoietic progenitor cell transplantation in pediatric patients, the manufacturer suggests an initial IV busulfan dosage (based on actual body weight) of 1.1 mg/kg in children weighing 12 kg or less, and 0.8 mg/kg in children weighing more than 12 kg. Simulations based on a pharmacokinetic model of a pediatric population indicate that about 60% of children will achieve a target busulfan area under the plasma concentration-time curve (AUC) of 900–1350 μM•minute with the first dose of IV busulfan using these recommended initial dosages. Therapeutic drug monitoring and dosage adjustment following the first dose of IV busulfan is recommended.

Dosage Adjustment Based on Therapeutic Drug Monitoring. The manufacturer suggests the use of therapeutic drug monitoring to adjust the dosage of IV busulfan in children following administration of the initial dose.

The busulfan AUC should be calculated based on blood samples collected at specified time points; actual sampling times should be recorded. When measuring serum busulfan concentrations with the initial dose of the drug, blood samples should be collected at 2 hours (the end of the infusion), 4 hours, and 6 hours (immediately prior to the next scheduled busulfan dose). For doses other than the first dose, blood samples should be collected prior to the infusion (baseline), and then at 2 hours (the end of the infusion), 4 hours, and 6 hours (immediately prior to the next scheduled busulfan dose). Calculations based on fewer samples than specified may result in inaccurate AUC determinations.

Special instructions for drug administration and blood sample collection should be followed to ensure accurate therapeutic drug monitoring. An administration set with minimal residual hold-up (priming) volume (1–3 mL) should be used for drug infusion to ensure accurate delivery of the entire prescribed dose and to ensure accurate collection of blood samples for the measurement of serum busulfan concentrations. The administration set tubing should be primed with drug solution to allow accurate documentation of the start time of the busulfan infusion. The blood sample should be collected from a peripheral IV line to avoid contamination with the infusing drug solution. If the blood sample is taken directly from the existing central venous catheter, it is important that the blood sample *not* be collected while the drug is infusing to ensure that the end of the infusion sample is not contaminated with any residual drug. At the end of the infusion (2 hours), the administration tubing should be disconnected and the central venous catheter line should be flushed with 5 mL of normal saline prior to the collection of the blood sample from the central venous catheter port. The blood samples should be collected from a different port than that used for the busulfan infusion. The time required to flush the indwelling catheter line should not be included when recording the busulfan infusion stop time. The administration tubing should be discarded at the end of the 2-hour infusion.

Collection of the blood samples should be performed by collecting 1–3 mL of blood into heparinized (Na or Li heparin) Vacutainer® tubes. The blood samples should be placed on wet ice immediately after collection and should be centrifuged (at 4°C) within 1 hour. The plasma should be harvested into appropriate cryovial storage tubes and frozen immediately at −20°C. All plasma samples should be sent in a frozen state (i.e., on dry ice) to the assay laboratory for the determination of plasma busulfan concentrations.

Busulfan AUC following the initial dose may be calculated using the following equation where $AUC_{0\text{–}6hr}$ is estimated using the linear trapezoidal rule and $AUC_{extrapolated}$ is the ratio of the busulfan concentration at hour 6 and the terminal elimination rate constant, λ_z. The terminal elimination rate constant must be calculated from the terminal elimination phase of the busulfan concentration versus time curve. A pre-dose busulfan concentration of zero is assumed and should be used in calculating the AUC.

$$\text{busulfan } AUC_{\infty} \text{ for dose } 1 = AUC_{0\text{-}6hr} + AUC_{extrapolated}$$

When busulfan AUC for dose 1 has been calculated, the following formula may be used for the adjustment of subsequent busulfan doses to achieve the target busulfan AUC of 1125 μM•minute:

$$\text{adjusted dose (mg)} = \text{actual dose (mg)} \times \frac{\text{target AUC } (\mu M\text{·minute})}{\text{actual AUC } (\mu M\text{·minute})}$$

For the determination of AUC following subsequent doses of IV busulfan, determination of steady-state busulfan AUC ($AUC_{0\text{–}6hr}$) should be estimated from the trough, 2 hour, 4 hour, and 6 hour concentrations using the linear trapezoidal rule.

Conventional Chemotherapy. Dosage of oral busulfan must be individualized based on clinical and hematologic response and tolerance of the patient in order to obtain optimum therapeutic results with minimum adverse effects.

For remission induction in the management of chronic myelogenous leukemia, the usual adult dosage of busulfan is 4–8 mg daily, but dosages ranging from 1–12 mg daily have been used. The manufacturer states that dosing on a weight basis is the same for both children and adults, and recommends daily dosages of approximately 0.06 mg/kg or 1.8 mg/m². Some clinicians have recommended dosages of 0.065–0.1 mg/kg daily. The manufacturer states that dosages exceeding 4 mg daily are especially likely to reduce the leukocyte count rapidly and should be used only in patients with severely symptomatic disease; higher dosages increase the risk of inducing bone marrow aplasia. A reduction in the leukocyte count is not usually seen during the first 10–15 days of busulfan therapy; the leukocyte count may actually increase during this period and should not be interpreted as resistance to the drug nor should the dosage be increased. Since the leukocyte count may continue to fall for more than 1 month after discontinuing the drug, the manufacturer states that therapy with busulfan should be discontinued before the leukocyte count falls to normal levels. The manufacturer states that busulfan should be discontinued when the leukocyte count has decreased to approximately 15,000/mm³. Some authorities believe dosage should be continued until the leukocyte count falls below 10,000/mm³, while others prefer to discontinue the drug when leukocyte count reaches 15,000 to 25,000/mm³; still others propose decreasing dosage in proportion to the decrease in leukocyte count. During remissions induced by intermittent treatment regimens, the patient should be examined at monthly intervals and busulfan therapy should be resumed when the leukocyte count reaches 50,000/mm³.

There is little agreement on whether busulfan should be administered continually or intermittently. Although many clinicians use maintenance doses, others believe toxicities occur less frequently on intermittent therapy and maintenance dosage should be reserved for patients who cannot sustain a remission without the drug. When remission is not sustained for longer than 3 months, the manufacturer states that maintenance therapy of 1–3 mg daily may be advisable in order to prevent rapid relapses. Other suggested maintenance dosages range from 2 mg/week to 4 mg/day.

Pediatric busulfan dosage recommendations range from 0.06–0.12 mg/kg daily. Alternatively, 1.8–4.6 mg/m² daily has been recommended. Dosage should be titrated to maintain a leukocyte count of about 20,000/mm³.

Cautions

Information on the adverse effects of IV busulfan is based mainly on data from an uncontrolled clinical trial involving 61 patients with various hematologic malignancies who received the drug as part of a conditioning regimen for allogeneic hematopoietic stem cell transplantation. In this study, 2 deaths occurred during the 28 days following the allogeneic transplant, and 6 deaths occurred between day 29 and day 100 following transplant. Additional information on adverse effects of the drug in this setting is derived from randomized trials using high-dose oral busulfan as part of a conditioning regimen for bone marrow transplant in patients with CML or other types of leukemia.

Dimethylacetamide, a solvent that previously was studied as a potential chemotherapy agent, is present in the daily recommended dosage of IV busulfan in an amount equivalent to 42% of the maximum tolerated dose on a mg/m² basis. The dose-limiting toxicities of dimethylacetamide are hepatotoxicity, including increased serum AST concentrations, and neurotoxicity, including hallucinations, somnolence, lethargy, and confusion; the relative contribution of the solvent (and/or other concomitantly administered medications) to adverse hepatic and neurologic effects observed in patients receiving IV busulfan is not known.

■ **Hematologic Effects and Infectious Complications** The major adverse effect of busulfan is hematologic toxicity, which is usually dose related and reversible after discontinuance of the drug. Myelosuppression may manifest as leukopenia, thrombocytopenia, anemia, or any combination of these.

In patients receiving oral busulfan, pancytopenia generally occurs with failure to adequately monitor hematologic status and promptly discontinue the drug in response to a large or rapid decrease in leukocyte or platelet counts. Although individual variation in response to the drug does not appear to be an important contributing factor, some patients may be especially sensitive to busulfan and experience abrupt onset of neutropenia or thrombocytopenia. Busulfan-induced pancytopenia may be more prolonged than that induced by other alkylating agents; although recovery may take 1 month to 2 years, the toxicity is potentially reversible and patients should be vigorously supported through any period of severe pancytopenia. Some patients develop bone marrow fibrosis or chronic aplasia which is probably due to busulfan toxicity. Aplastic anemia, sometimes irreversible, has been reported rarely in patients receiving oral busulfan; aplastic anemia usually has occurred following high doses of the drug or long-term administration of conventional doses.

Profound myelosuppression occurs in all patients receiving the recommended dosage of IV busulfan, with absolute neutrophil counts decreasing to below 0.5 x 10^9/L at a median of 4 days after allogeneic transplant. Recovery of the absolute neutrophil count occurred at a median of 13 days after transplantation; prophylactic granulocyte colony-stimulating factor was administered in the majority of patients. Thrombocytopenia (platelet count below 25,000/mm³ or requiring platelet transfusion; median onset of 5–6 days) was reported in 98% of patients receiving IV busulfan, and a median of 6 platelet transfusions and 4 red blood cell transfusions per patient were required. Anemia (hemoglobin less than 8 g/dL) occurred in 69% of patients. Prolonged prothrombin time was reported in 1 patient receiving IV busulfan.

Infections, including sepsis and pneumonia, have been reported in patients receiving oral or IV busulfan. Infections were reported in 51% of patients receiving IV busulfan. Life-threatening pneumonia occurred in 3% of patients and was fatal in at least one patient.

■ **Pulmonary Effects** Fatal pulmonary effects have occurred in patients receiving oral or intravenous busulfan.

A rare but serious syndrome which usually occurs only after long-term busulfan therapy with onset of symptoms at an average of 4 years following initiation of therapy (range: 4 months to 10 years) is "busulfan lung." The syndrome is manifested by bronchopulmonary dysplasia with a diffuse interstitial pulmonary fibrosis and is characterized by persistent cough, fever, rales, and dyspnea. Histologically, the syndrome mimics findings associated with pulmonary irradiation. Pulmonary function studies have shown diminished diffusion capacity and decreased pulmonary compliance. Diagnosis of "busulfan lung" may be confounded by the presence of common underlying conditions (e.g., opportunistic infections, pulmonary leukemic infiltrates). If diagnostic measures such as sputum cultures, virologic studies, and exfoliative cytology fail to establish the etiology of pulmonary infiltrates, lung biopsy may be necessary to establish the diagnosis. There is no specific therapy for "busulfan lung," and the drug should be discontinued immediately if this toxicity develops; although corticosteroids have been used, their efficacy seems equivocal. In some patients, "busulfan lung" has been relieved by discontinuance of the drug and administration of corticosteroids; in most patients, however, the syndrome has progressed to respiratory insufficiency despite the discontinuance of busulfan, and deaths have usually occurred within 6 months of diagnosis of the syndrome.

In patients receiving IV busulfan in combination with cyclophosphamide prior to allogeneic hematopoietic stem cell transplantation, lung disorders were reported in 34% of patients. Alveolar hemorrhage requiring mechanical ventilation and resulting in death was reported in 3 patients (5%) receiving IV busulfan. Dyspnea occurred in 27% of patients and was severe in 2% of patients, and cough occurred in 28% of patients and was mild to moderate. Mild or moderate asthma was reported in 8% of patients receiving IV busulfan. Hyperventilation was reported in 5% of patients and was severe in one patient.

Rhinitis, epistaxis, and pharyngitis were reported in 44, 25, and 18% of patients receiving IV busulfan. Additional adverse pulmonary effects reported in less than 5% of patients receiving IV busulfan were mild to moderate and included atelectasis, pleural effusion, hypoxia, sinusitis, and hemoptysis.

Interstitial pneumonitis and pulmonary fibrosis, which rarely were fatal, also have been reported in patients receiving high oral doses of busulfan as a component of a conditioning regimen prior to allogeneic bone marrow transplantation. Nonspecific interstitial fibrosis was diagnosed by lung biopsy in one patient receiving IV busulfan who subsequently died from respiratory failure.

■ **Hepatic Effects** Life-threatening hepatic veno-occlusive disease has occurred in patients receiving busulfan (usually in combination with cyclophosphamide or other antineoplastic agents as a component of marrow-ablative therapy prior to bone marrow transplantation). The manufacturer states that a clear causal relationship to busulfan has not been demonstrated. Hepatic veno-occlusive disease diagnosed by clinical examination and laboratory findings occurred in 8% (5/61) of patients receiving IV busulfan in the allogeneic transplant clinical trial and was fatal in 40% (2/5) of cases. Overall mortality from hepatic veno-occlusive disease was 3% for the entire study population. Retrospectively, 3 of the 5 patients diagnosed with hepatic veno-occlusive disease were found to meet the Jones' criteria for this condition. In patients receiving high-dose oral busulfan as a component of a conditioning regimen prior to bone marrow transplant in randomized, controlled studies, the incidence of hepatic veno-occlusive disease was 7.7–12%.

Other adverse hepatic effects reported in patients receiving oral busulfan include cholestatic jaundice, centrilobular sinusoidal fibrosis, and hepatocellular atrophy or necrosis.

Hyperbilirubinemia has been reported in patients receiving oral or IV busulfan. In patients receiving IV busulfan prior to allogeneic hematopoietic stem cell transplant, hyperbilirubinemia occurred in 49% of patients; hyperbilirubinemia was grade 3 or 4 in severity in 30% of patients and was life-threatening in 5% of these patients. Hyperbilirubinemia was associated with graft-versus-host disease in 6 patients and with hepatic veno-occlusive disease in 5 patients. Jaundice and hepatomegaly were reported in 12 and 6% of patients, respectively, and were mild or moderate in severity. Increases in serum ALT occurred in 31% of patients and were grade 3 or 4 in severity in 7% of patients, and mild or moderate increases in alkaline phosphatase concentrations were reported in 15% of patients.

■ **Nervous System Effects** Busulfan has been associated with adverse nervous system effects, including dizziness, blurred vision, loss of consciousness, intermittent muscle twitching, myoclonic seizures, and generalized tonic-clonic (grand mal) seizures.

Seizures have been reported in patients receiving busulfan orally, including administration of the drug at high doses (resulting in plasma concentrations similar to those achieved with the recommended dose of IV busulfan) as part of a conditioning regimen prior to bone marrow transplant. In addition, despite the use of prophylactic phenytoin therapy, a seizure was reported in a patient receiving IV busulfan. According to the manufacturers, prophylactic anticonvulsant therapy should be started prior to treatment with IV busulfan and also may be considered in patients receiving oral busulfan. (See Precautions and Contraindications.)

Additional adverse neurologic effects reported in patients receiving IV busulfan include insomnia, anxiety, headache, dizziness, and depression, which were reported in 84, 75, 69, 30, and 23% of patients, respectively. Confusion and hallucinations were observed in 11 and 5%, respectively, of patients receiving IV busulfan, and lethargy was reported in 7% of patients. Delirium, agitation, somnolence, and encephalopathy each occurred in 2% of patients.

■ **Cardiovascular Effects** Cardiac tamponade, often fatal, has been reported in a small number of pediatric patients with thalassemia who received oral busulfan and cyclophosphamide as the preparatory regimen for bone marrow transplantation; abdominal pain and vomiting preceded the tamponade in most cases. Cardiac tamponade was not reported in a clinical study of patients receiving IV busulfan.

One case of endocardial fibrosis has been reported in a patient receiving long-term therapy with oral busulfan.

In patients receiving IV busulfan, mild or moderate tachycardia was reported in 44% of patients; in 11% of patients, the tachycardia was first reported during administration of the drug. Mild or moderate thrombosis involving a central venous catheter was reported in 33% of patients receiving IV busulfan. Hypertension occurred in 36% of patients and was grade 3 or 4 in severity in 7% of patients, and hypotension occurred in 11% of patients and was grade 3 or 4 in severity in 3% of patients. Mild vasodilation, manifested as flushing and hot flushes (flashes), was observed in 25% of patients. Edema and chest pain were reported in 36 and 26% of patients, respectively. Other adverse cardiovascular effects reported in 5% or fewer of patients receiving IV busulfan included mild or moderate arrhythmia, mild or moderate atrial fibrillation, and mild or moderate ventricular extrasystoles. Mild or moderate third degree heart block also has occurred in patients receiving IV busulfan. Cardiomegaly, mild ECG abnormality, grade 3 or 4 left-sided heart failure, and moderate pericardial effusion were reported in 5% or fewer of patients receiving IV busulfan, but were reported principally in the post-cyclophosphamide phase.

Some form of mild or moderate edema was reported in 79% of patients receiving IV busulfan for allogeneic progenitor cell transplant. Hypervolemia also was reported, and documented weight increase occurred in 8% of patients.

■ **GI Effects** Adverse GI effects occur frequently in patients receiving IV busulfan. Nausea was reported in 98% of patients receiving IV busulfan in clinical trials and was severe in 7% of patients, and vomiting occurred in 95% of patients. The incidence of vomiting during administration of IV busulfan was 43%. Stomatitis occurred in 97% of patients and was grade 3 or 4 in severity in 26% of patients. Diarrhea was mild to moderate in 75% of patients and grade 3 or 4 in 5% of patients. Anorexia was reported in 85% of patients and was severe in 21% of patients, and abdominal pain was reported in 72% of patients. Mild to moderate constipation occurred in 38% of patients, and ileus occurred in 8% of patients and was severe in 2% of patients. Dyspepsia and rectal discomfort were reported in 44 and 24%, respectively, of patients receiving IV busulfan and were mild or moderate. Dry mouth and abdominal enlargement occurred in 26 and 23% of patients, respectively. Pancreatitis, grade 3 esophagitis, and mild hematemesis each was reported in 2% of patients.

GI distress, nausea, vomiting, diarrhea, anorexia, and weight loss have been reported in patients receiving oral busulfan. Cheilosis, mucositis, and glossitis also have been reported in patients receiving oral busulfan.

■ **Metabolic Effects** As a result of extensive purine catabolism accompanying rapid cellular destruction, hyperuricemia may occur in patients receiving busulfan, especially those with widespread disease. In some patients, uric acid nephropathy, renal stones, and acute renal failure may result. These effects may be minimized by adequate hydration, alkalinization of the urine, and/or administration of a xanthine oxidase inhibitor, such as allopurinol.

A wasting or Addison-like syndrome has occurred in a small number of patients, usually after long-term busulfan therapy. The wasting syndrome is generally characterized by melanoderma, asthenia, hypotension, nausea, vomiting, diarrhea, anorexia, weight loss, fatigue, apathy, and confusion. Patients with this syndrome do not usually exhibit a corresponding deficit in adrenocorticoid function; however, the pituitary response to metyrapone may be decreased (i.e., decreased urinary excretion of 17-hydroxycorticosteroids). Symptoms of this syndrome have occasionally resolved when busulfan was discontinued.

In a clinical trial, hyperglycemia was reported in 67% of patients receiving IV busulfan, and was of grade 3 or 4 severity in 15% of patients. Hypomagnesemia was reported in 77% of patients and was mild to moderate in severity. Mild or moderate hypokalemia was observed in 62% of patients, and severe hypokalemia occurred in 2% of patients. Hypocalcemia occurred in 49% of patients and was severe in 3% of patients, and mild or moderate hypophosphatemia was reported in 17% of patients. Hyponatremia was reported in 2% of patients.

■ **Immunologic Reactions** Graft-versus-host disease, in some cases fatal, has occurred in patients receiving busulfan as a component of a conditioning regimen prior to allogeneic transplant. In patients receiving IV busulfan in a clinical trial, graft-versus-host disease occurred in 18% of patients, was severe in 3% of patients, and resulted in death in 5% of patients (i.e., 3 patients).

■ **Dermatologic Effects** Adverse dermatologic effects reported in patients receiving busulfan include rash, pruritus, and alopecia. An increased incidence of local cutaneous reactions has been reported in patients receiving radiation therapy soon after busulfan therapy.

In a clinical trial, rash and pruritus occurred in 57 and 28%, respectively, of patients receiving IV busulfan. Alopecia was reported to be mild in 15% of patients and moderate in 2% of patients. Mild vesicular rash and vesiculobullous rash each occurred in 10% of patients, and mild to moderate maculopapular rash occurred in 8% of patients. Skin discoloration, acne, and exfoliative dermatitis were reported in 8, 7, and 5% of patients, respectively, and erythema nodosum occurred in 2% of patients.

Hyperpigmentation has been reported in 5–10% of patients receiving oral busulfan and appears to occur more frequently in patients with a dark complexion. Erythema nodosum, erythema multiforme, urticaria, porphyria cutanea tarda, dryness of the skin and mucous membranes, and anhidrosis also have been reported in patients receiving the drug orally.

Renal Effects Mild to moderate increases in serum creatinine concentrations were reported in 21% of patients receiving IV busulfan in a clinical trial. In addition, elevated BUN was reported in 3% of patients and was grade 3 or 4 in 2% of patients. Oliguria, hematuria, and dysuria occurred in 15, 8, and 7% of patients, respectively, and grade 3 or 4 hemorrhagic cystitis was reported in 7% of patients.

Genitourinary Effects Use of busulfan has been associated with hemorrhagic cystitis; grade 3 or 4 hemorrhagic cystitis was reported in 7% of patients receiving IV busulfan in a clinical trial.

Ocular Effects Cataracts rarely have occurred in patients receiving oral busulfan. Corneal thinning and lens changes also have been reported in patients receiving oral busulfan.

Musculoskeletal Effects Back pain, mild or moderate myalgia, and mild or moderate arthralgia was reported in 23, 16, and 13%, respectively, of patients receiving IV busulfan in a clinical trial. Myasthenia gravis has been reported in patients receiving oral busulfan.

Sensitivity Reactions Allergic reactions occurred in 26% of patients receiving IV busulfan in a clinical trial and were severe in 2% of patients. Erythema nodosum occurred in 2% of patients receiving IV busulfan in a clinical trial and also has been reported in patients receiving oral busulfan.

Local Effects Inflammation and mild or moderate pain at the injection site occurred in 25 and 15%, respectively, of patients receiving IV busulfan in a clinical trial.

Other Adverse Effects Fever has been reported in 80% of patients receiving IV busulfan and was severe in 3%. Other adverse effects reported in patients receiving IV busulfan include asthenia in 51%, chills in 46%, pain in 44%, hiccup in 18%, and otic disorder in 3%. Gynecomastia has been reported in patients receiving oral busulfan.

Cellular dysplasia characterized by giant, hyperchromic nuclei has occurred in the cells of many organs, including lymph nodes, pancreas, thyroid, adrenal glands, liver, and bone marrow. Cytologic dysplasia may be severe enough to make interpretation of exfoliative cytologic examinations of cells from lung, bladder, breast, and cervix difficult.

Precautions and Contraindications Busulfan is a highly toxic drug with a low therapeutic index, and a therapeutic response is not likely to occur without some evidence of toxicity. The drug must be used only under constant supervision by clinicians experienced in therapy with cytotoxic agents. Clinicians supervising the administration of IV busulfan also should be experienced in hematopoietic stem cell transplantation and the management of patients with severe pancytopenia.

Patients who receive myelosuppressive drugs experience an increased incidence of infections as well as possible hemorrhagic complications. Because these complications are potentially fatal, the patient should be instructed to notify the physician if fever, sore throat, unusual bleeding or bruising, or symptoms suggestive of anemia occur.

Patients beginning oral busulfan therapy should be informed of the importance of having periodic blood counts. The patient's hematologic status must be monitored carefully, and blood counts (hemoglobin or hematocrit, leukocyte and differential counts, and quantitative platelet count) should be performed at least once a week during oral busulfan therapy. Since the maximum effect on bone marrow function may be delayed, therapy should be discontinued temporarily or dosage reduced at the first sign of abnormal bone marrow depression. In some cases, bone marrow examination may be necessary in addition to blood counts. The decision to adjust dosage and/or continue therapy must be based on the rapidity of hematologic changes as well as on absolute hematologic values. Dosage of busulfan may need to be reduced when the drug is administered concomitantly with other drugs whose principal toxicity is myelosuppression. Busulfan should not be used when facilities for performing complete blood counts, including quantitative platelet counts, at weekly (or more frequent) intervals are not available. Busulfan should be used with extreme caution and particular vigilance in patients whose bone marrow reserve may have been compromised by other myelosuppressive drugs or radiation therapy, or whose marrow function is recovering from previous cytotoxic therapy.

Profound myelosuppression occurs universally in patients receiving IV busulfan at the recommended dose as part of a preparatory regimen prior to allogeneic hematopoietic stem cell transplant (see Cautions: Hematologic Effects and Infectious Complications). Daily complete blood cell counts, including leukocyte cell differentials, and platelet counts should be monitored during therapy and until recovery occurs. Anti-infective therapy and platelet and red blood cell transfusions should be administered when needed.

Patients receiving busulfan should be informed that diffuse pulmonary fibrosis is an infrequent but serious and potentially life-threatening complication of long-term therapy with the drug. Patients should be instructed to report any difficulty in breathing or persistent cough or congestion. If interstitial pulmonary fibrosis occurs during busulfan therapy, the drug should be discontinued immediately. (See Cautions: Pulmonary Effects.)

Patients receiving busulfan must not be allowed to take the drug without close medical supervision. In addition to warnings about the potential hematologic and pulmonary toxicities, patients should be instructed to report any signs of abrupt weakness, unusual fatigue, anorexia, weight loss, nausea and vomiting, and melanoderma that could be associated with a wasting or Addison-like syndrome. Patients also should be informed that other adverse effects of busulfan may include infertility, amenorrhea, skin hyperpigmentation, hypersensitivity, dryness of the mucous membranes, and, rarely, cataract formation.

Because life-threatening hepatic veno-occlusive disease has occurred in patients receiving busulfan (usually in combination with cyclophosphamide or other antineoplastic agents prior to bone marrow transplantation), the manufacturer recommends that serum alkaline phosphatase, bilirubin, and aminotransferase concentrations be determined periodically during oral busulfan therapy (and daily through bone marrow transplant day +28 in patients receiving IV busulfan) so that possible hepatotoxicity can be detected early. Possible risk factors for the development of hepatic veno-occlusive disease include a total busulfan dose exceeding 16 mg/kg based on ideal body weight and concurrent use of multiple alkylating agents. The incidence of hepatic veno-occlusive disease is higher (about 33% versus 3%) in those with an average busulfan concentration at steady state exceeding 900 ng/mL and/or an area under the plasma concentration-time curve (AUC) exceeding 1500 μM•minute than in those with lesser values for these parameters. A reduced incidence of hepatic veno-occlusive disease has been observed in patients receiving high-dose oral busulfan and cyclophosphamide when the first dose of cyclophosphamide was delayed for more than 24 hours following the last dose of busulfan. In addition, the manufacturer of busulfan for injection concentrate states that the risk of hepatic veno-occlusive disease associated with busulfan may be increased in patients who have received prior radiation therapy, 3 or more cycles of chemotherapy, or a prior progenitor cell transplant. A busulfan AUC of 1500 μM•minute or greater also is thought to be associated with a greater risk of hepatic veno-occlusive disease in patients receiving IV busulfan. A busulfan AUC below 1500 μM•minute measured at the time of dose 9 was reported in almost all (i.e., 93%) of evaluable patients receiving IV busulfan in clinical trials.

Concomitant therapy with busulfan and cyclophosphamide should be administered with caution in the treatment of patients with thalassemia; cardiac tamponade, often fatal, has been reported in a small number (2% in one series) of patients with thalassemia who received busulfan and cyclophosphamide as the preparatory regimen for bone marrow transplantation. Abdominal pain and vomiting preceded the occurrence of cardiac tamponade in most of these patients.

Oral busulfan should be administered with caution and administration of prophylactic anticonvulsant therapy may be considered in patients with a history of seizures or head trauma or those receiving other potentially epileptogenic drugs, since seizures have been reported in patients receiving busulfan. Prophylactic administration of phenytoin is recommended in all patients receiving IV busulfan, and caution is advised when administering the recommended dose of IV busulfan to patients with a history of seizures or head trauma or those receiving other potentially epileptogenic drugs. (See Dosage: Allogeneic Hematopoietic Stem Cell Transplantation under Dosage and Administration.)

Patients receiving busulfan should be informed of the increased risk of a secondary malignancy associated with use of the drug. (See Cautions: Mutagenicity and Carcinogenicity.)

Busulfan is contraindicated in patients with chronic myelogenous leukemia whose disease was resistant to prior therapy with the drug. Busulfan is contraindicated in patients in whom a definitive diagnosis of chronic myelogenous leukemia has not been firmly established. Busulfan also is contraindicated in patients who are hypersensitive to busulfan or any ingredient in the respective formulation.

Pediatric Precautions Safety and efficacy of IV busulfan for the treatment of chronic myelogenous leukemia in children have not been studied specifically to date.

The pharmacokinetics of IV busulfan have been evaluated in an uncontrolled study involving 24 children (age range 5 months to 16 years, median age 3 years) receiving the drug as part of a conditioning regimen prior to hematopoietic progenitor cell transplantation for various malignant hematologic or non-malignant diseases. Following an initial IV busulfan dose (based on actual body weight) of 1 mg/kg in patients 4 years of age or younger or 0.8 mg/kg in patients older than 4 years of age, subsequent doses were adjusted based on plasma busulfan concentration to achieve a target AUC of 900–1350 μM•minute. Busulfan doses were administered as a 2-hour IV infusion every 6 hours for 4 days (for a total of 16 doses), followed by cyclophosphamide 50 mg/kg once daily for 4 days. After one rest day, hematopoietic progenitor cells were infused. Phenytoin was administered to all patients for seizure prophylaxis. The target busulfan AUC was achieved with the first dose in 71% of patients. Steady-state pharmacokinetic analysis was performed at doses 9 and 13, and serum busulfan concentrations were within the target range for 21 of 23 evaluable patients. Based on the results of this study, the manufacturer has developed a suggested dosing regimen for IV busulfan in children. (See Pediatric Dosage in Dosage and Administration: Dosage: Chronic Myelogenous Leukemia: Allogeneic Hematopoietic Stem Cell Transplantation.)

Myeloablation consisting of neutropenia (absolute neutrophil count less than 500/mm^3) and thrombocytopenia (platelet transfusions or platelet count below 20,000/mm^3) was observed in all 24 patients, and lymphopenia (absolute lymphocyte count less than 100/mm^3) occurred in 79% of patients. Absolute neutrophil count recovered to above 500/mm^3 in 23 patients at a median of bone marrow transplant (BMT) day +13 (range, BMT day +9 to +22). Absolute neutrophil count had not recovered to above 500/mm^3 in one patient who died on BMT day +28.

The mortality rate in the study was 17% (4 deaths). Two patients died within

28 days of the transplant, one due to pneumonia and capillary leak syndrome and the other due to pneumonia and hepatic veno-occlusive disease. Two more patients died before day 100, one due to progressive disease and one due to multiorgan failure. Adverse effects reported during or after the study period (up to BMT day +100) included vomiting (100%), nausea (83%), stomatitis (79%), hepatic veno-occlusive disease (21%), graft-versus-host disease (25%), and pneumonia (21%).

According to the manufacturer, the recommended weight-adjusted dosage of oral busulfan for remission induction in chronic myelogenous leukemia is the same for children and adults; however, alternative dosing regimens have been suggested because of the higher clearance of the drug observed in children.

Poor response to oral busulfan has been reported in patients with the "juvenile" type of chronic myelogenous leukemia, which typically occurs in young children and is characterized by the absence of a Philadelphia chromosome.

■ **Geriatric Precautions** Safety and efficacy of busulfan in geriatric patients have not been studied specifically to date. Clinical studies of busulfan did not include sufficient numbers of patients 65 years of age and older to determine whether geriatric patients respond differently than younger patients. While other clinical experience has not revealed age-related differences in response, drug dosage generally should be titrated carefully in geriatric patients, usually initiating therapy at the low end of the dosage range. The greater frequency of decreased hepatic, renal, and/or cardiac function and of concomitant disease and drug therapy observed in the elderly also should be considered.

In a phase 2 clinical trial using IV busulfan as part of a conditioning regimen prior to allogeneic hematopoietic stem cell transplantation, the 5 patients (out of a total of 61 patients) who were older than 55 years of age (range: 57–64) all achieved myeloablation and engraftment.

■ **Mutagenicity and Carcinogenicity** Busulfan is potentially mutagenic in humans. Busulfan has caused chromosomal aberrations in patients receiving the drug and has been shown to be mutagenic in mice.

Busulfan is a presumed human carcinogen. Malignant tumors and acute leukemias have occurred in patients receiving the drug. Although the exact mechanism has not been determined, busulfan is thought to be leukemogenic. A few cases of acute leukemia, becoming clinically apparent 5–8 years after pancytopenia had developed during busulfan therapy, have been reported in patients who received the drug as adjunctive therapy following surgical resection of bronchogenic carcinoma. The World Health Organization has determined that sufficient evidence exists to support a causal relationship between busulfan exposure and the development of secondary cancers. The increased risk of a secondary malignancy with busulfan therapy should be explained to patients receiving the drug.

■ **Pregnancy, Fertility, and Lactation** Busulfan may cause fetal harm when administered to pregnant women, but potential benefits from use of the drug may be acceptable in certain conditions despite the possible risks to the fetus. Fetal malformation early in pregnancy, bone marrow depression late in gestation, fetal growth retardation, and fetal deaths have been reported in pregnant women who received therapeutic doses of busulfan or other alkylating agents. Mild anemia and neutropenia were present in one neonate whose mother had received busulfan from the eighth week of pregnancy until parturition.

Busulfan has been shown to be teratogenic in mice, rats, and rabbits; teratogenic effects included abnormalities in the musculoskeletal system, body weight, and size. Sterility in male and female offspring secondary to an absence of germinal cells in the testes and ovaries also was observed in reproduction studies in rats.

Dimethylacetamide (DMA), the solvent used in commercially available busulfan for injection concentrate, also may cause fetal harm when administered to pregnant women. When administered to pregnant rats at a dose of 400 mg/kg daily (about 40% of the amount present on a mg/m^2 basis in the recommended daily dose of IV busulfan), dimethylacetamide caused developmental abnormalities, including anasarca, cleft palate, vertebral anomalies, rib malformation, and serious anomalies of the vessels of the heart.

There are no adequate and well-controlled studies using busulfan or dimethylacetamide in pregnant women. Busulfan should be used during pregnancy only in conditions such as life-threatening situations or severe disease for which safer drugs cannot be used or are ineffective. Women of childbearing potential should be advised to avoid becoming pregnant during busulfan therapy. If the drug is administered during pregnancy or if the patient becomes pregnant while receiving the drug, the patient should be informed of the potential hazard to the fetus.

Busulfan can impair fertility. Busulfan produces sterility in male and female offspring of drug-exposed pregnant rats resulting from germinal cell aplasia in testes and ovaries. Germinal cell aplasia and sterility have *not* been reported in human offspring of mothers who received busulfan during pregnancy. Ovarian suppression and amenorrhea with menopausal symptoms commonly occur during long-term busulfan therapy in premenopausal women; ovarian fibrosis and atrophy have also occurred. Failure to achieve puberty due to ovarian failure also has been reported in female patients receiving busulfan. Busulfan interferes with spermatogenesis in animals, and there have been reports of impotence, sterility, azoospermia, and testicular atrophy in men who received the drug.

Dimethylacetamide (DMA), the solvent used in commercially available busulfan for injection concentrate, also may impair fertility. When administered to rats at a dose of approximately 0.5 g/kg daily (about 44% of the amount present in the recommended daily dose of IV busulfan on a mg/m^2 basis) for 9 days, dimethylacetamide caused decreases in spermatogenesis. In addition, administration of a single subcutaneous dose of 2.2 g/kg (about 27% of the amount present in the recommended daily dose of IV busulfan on a mg/m^2 basis) to hamsters 4 days after insemination resulted in termination of pregnancy in all of the hamsters tested.

It is not known whether busulfan is distributed into milk. Because of the potential for serious adverse reactions from busulfan in nursing infants, a decision should be made whether to discontinue nursing or the drug, taking into account the importance of the drug to the woman.

Drug Interactions

Additive myelosuppression may occur with concomitant administration of busulfan with other myelosuppressive agents. In addition, additive pulmonary toxicity may occur when busulfan is administered in combination with other cytotoxic agents.

■ **Cyclophosphamide** Concomitant use of cylcophosphamide may result in reduced clearance of busulfan, presumably due to competition for glutathione. A reduced incidence of hepatic veno-occlusive disease and other toxicities has been observed in patients receiving high-dose busulfan and cyclophosphamide when the first dose of cyclophosphamide was delayed for longer than 24 hours following the last dose of busulfan.

■ **Thioguanine** Hepatotoxicity, esophageal varices, and portal hypertension were reported in some patients receiving long-term therapy with busulfan and thioguanine concomitantly; hepatotoxicity was manifested by elevations of hepatic enzyme concentrations and nodular regenerative hyperplasia of the liver. Similar effects were not reported in patients receiving busulfan therapy alone. Although further studies are needed to establish a causal relationship between these adverse effects and concomitant use of busulfan and thioguanine, the manufacturer of busulfan states that caution should be exercised during such long-term concomitant therapy.

■ **Itraconazole** Itraconazole may reduce the clearance of busulfan by up to 25% in patients receiving oral or IV busulfan therapy. Administration of itraconazole with IV busulfan may result in a busulfan AUC exceeding 1500 *μM*•minute (which may be associated with an increased risk of hepatic veno-occlusive disease). Patients receiving busulfan and concomitant itraconazole therapy should be monitored carefully for busulfan toxicity.

■ **Anticonvulsant Agents** Concomitant use of phenytoin increases clearance of busulfan and cyclophosphamide, which may lead to decreased serum concentrations of both drugs.

Phenytoin has been reported to increase busulfan clearance by 15% or more, possibly by induction of glutathione-*S*-transferase. Because the patients included in pharmacokinetic evaluations of IV busulfan also were receiving phenytoin (which is recommended for seizure prophylaxis), administration of the recommended dose of IV busulfan without concomitant phenytoin therapy may result in reduced busulfan clearance and greater exposure to the drug. The manufacturer recommends monitoring busulfan plasma concentrations in patients who must receive anticonvulsants other than phenytoin with IV busulfan.

■ **Acetaminophen** Use of acetaminophen in combination with or within 72 hours prior to busulfan therapy may cause a decrease in busulfan clearance by reducing glutathione concentrations in the blood and tissues.

Acute Toxicity

Limited information is available on the acute toxicity of busulfan. Without subsequent hematopoietic progenitor cell transplantation, the recommended dosage of IV busulfan used prior to transplantation would constitute an overdose of the drug.

■ **Pathogenesis** The single-dose LD_{50} of busulfan in mice is 120 mg/kg. At median lethal doses administered intraperitoneally in animals, two distinct types of toxic responses are observed. Within hours of administration, there are signs of CNS stimulation with seizures and death on the first day; mice are more sensitive to this effect than rats. At the LD_{50} dose, delayed death secondary to bone marrow damage also occurs. At doses 3 times the LD_{50}, atrophy of the large intestine mucosa is evident after a week, but the mucosa of the small intestine is minimally affected.

■ **Manifestations** The principal toxic effect of busulfan is on the bone marrow, including myelosuppression and pancytopenia, but the CNS, liver, lungs, and GI tract also may be affected. A 4-year-old child was reported to survive an acute ingestion of 140 mg (approximately 8 mg/kg). Accidental administration of a dose of 2.1 mg/kg of busulfan orally (total dose: 23.3 mg/kg) in a 2-year-old patient prior to bone marrow transplant resulted in no adverse sequelae. A fatal overdose of 2.4 g of busulfan has been reported in a 10-year-old boy.

■ **Treatment** There is no specific antidote for busulfan intoxication (other than hematopoietic stem cell transplantation). If acute overdosage occurs, the hematologic status of the patient should be closely monitored and vigorous supportive measures instituted if necessary.

Following recent acute ingestion of oral busulfan, the stomach should be emptied immediately by inducing emesis or by gastric lavage. If the patient is comatose, having seizures, or lacks the gag reflex, gastric lavage may be performed if an endotracheal tube with cuff inflated is in place to prevent aspiration of gastric contents. Following emesis or gastric lavage, activated charcoal may be administered.

Because at least one report has suggested that busulfan is dialyzable, dialysis should be considered in the event of busulfan overdose. (See Pharmacokinetics: Elimination.) In addition, administration of glutathione may be considered since busulfan is metabolized by conjugation with glutathione.

Pharmacology

Busulfan, as an alkylating agent, interferes with DNA replication and transcription of RNA and ultimately results in the disruption of nucleic acid function. Busulfan contains 2 labile methanesulfonate groups attached to opposite ends of a 4-carbon alkyl chain; in aqueous media, busulfan is hydrolyzed, releasing the methanesulfonate groups and producing reactive carbonium ions capable of alkylating DNA. Damage to DNA is considered largely responsible for the cytotoxic activity of the drug. Busulfan exhibits little immunosuppressive activity.

Pharmacokinetics

Based on currently available data, the US Food and Drug Administration (FDA) Oncologic Drugs Advisory Committee concluded that similar variability in pharmacokinetics is exhibited with both IV busulfan and oral busulfan. The pharmacokinetics of busulfan have not been evaluated separately by gender, ethnic group, or hepatic or renal impairment.

■ **Absorption** Busulfan is rapidly and completely absorbed from the GI tract after oral administration of the drug. The effect of food on the bioavailability of busulfan is not known.

For adults receiving busulfan 2, 4, or 6 mg orally as a single dose on consecutive days, the drug exhibits linear kinetics for both the maximum plasma concentration and the area under the concentration-time curve (AUC); a mean peak plasma concentration (normalized to a dose of 2 mg) of about 30 ng/mL was observed. In a study of 12 patients receiving single oral busulfan doses of 4–8 mg, a mean peak plasma concentration (normalized to a dose of 4 mg) of about 68 ng/mL was reported; the time to peak plasma concentration was about 0.9 hours.

In patients receiving busulfan (0.8 mg/kg IV every 6 hours for 4 days) in combination with cyclophosphamide prior to allogeneic hematopoietic progenitor stem cell transplantation, a mean peak plasma concentration of 1222 ng/mL (range: 496–1684 ng/mL) and a mean area under the plasma concentration-time curve (AUC) of 1167 μM•minute (range: 556–1673 μM•minute) were reported at steady state.

■ **Distribution** Busulfan, a small and highly lipophilic molecule, easily crosses the blood-brain barrier. Busulfan concentrations in the CSF are approximately equal to concurrent busulfan plasma concentrations. It is not known whether the drug is distributed into milk.

Irreversible binding of the drug to plasma proteins (mainly albumin) is reported to be about 32%.

The pharmacokinetic disposition of busulfan differs in children versus adults. The mean bioavailability of busulfan is lower in children than in adults; the interindividual variation in bioavailability for oral busulfan is large, particularly in children. In a pharmacokinetic study in children receiving IV busulfan (0.8 or 1 mg/kg based on actual body weight), an estimated volume of distribution of 0.64 L/kg (with an interpatient variability of 11%) was reported.

■ **Elimination** The elimination half-life is about 2.6 hours in adults receiving oral busulfan.

In patients receiving busulfan (0.8 mg/kg IV every 6 hours for 4 days) in combination with cyclophosphamide prior to allogeneic hematopoietic progenitor stem cell transplantation, a mean clearance of 2.52 mL/minute per kg (range: 1.49–4.31 mL/minute per kg) was reported.

Busulfan is rapidly eliminated from the plasma. The drug is reported to be extensively metabolized by the liver; at least 12 metabolites have been isolated, including methanesulfonic acid and 3-hydroxytetrahydrothiophene-1,1-dioxide, and these metabolites do not have cytotoxic activity. Busulfan is metabolized in the liver mainly by glutathione conjugation (spontaneous and glutathione *S*-transferase-mediated). The glutathione conjugate is then further metabolized in the liver by oxidation. Busulfan is slowly excreted in urine, as metabolites. About 30–60% of a dose of busulfan is excreted in the urine within 48 hours. Less than 2% of a dose of busulfan is excreted in the urine unchanged within 24 hours. Negligible amounts of busulfan are excreted in the feces.

Because it is poorly soluble in water and rapidly metabolized, it is expected that dialysis would remove minimal amounts of unreacted busulfan.

The effect of hemodialysis on the oral clearance of busulfan has been reported in one patient with chronic renal failure who was undergoing autologous peripheral stem cell transplantation. An increase of about 65% in the apparent oral clearance of busulfan was observed following 4 hours of hemodialysis; however, the mean 24-hour oral clearance of the drug was increased by only 11%.

Busulfan clearance is higher in children than in adults. In a pharmacokinetic study in children receiving IV busulfan (0.8 or 1 mg/kg based on actual body weight) in combination with cyclophosphamide, an estimated clearance of 3.37 mL/minute per kg (with an interpatient variability of 23%) was reported.

Chemistry and Stability

■ **Chemistry** Busulfan, an alkylsulfonate, is a bifunctional alkylating agent. The drug occurs as a white, crystalline powder and is very slightly soluble in water and slightly soluble in alcohol. Because busulfan is only very slightly soluble in water, the commercially available for injection concentrate, which occurs as a sterile, colorless, clear solution, is a nonaqueous solution of the drug in *N,N*-dimethylacetamide (DMA) and polyethylene glycol 400. Solutions of busulfan containing a drug concentration of approximately 0.5 mg/mL have a pH of 3.4–3.9, depending on the diluent used (i.e., 0.9% sodium chloride injection or 5% dextrose injection).

■ **Stability** Commercially available busulfan tablets should be stored in well-closed containers at 25°C but may be exposed to temperatures ranging from 15–30°C.

Commercially available busulfan for injection concentrate should be stored in unopened ampuls at 2–8°C. The manufacturer states that, when diluted as directed in 0.9% sodium chloride injection or 5% dextrose injection, busulfan solutions are stable for up to 8 hours when stored at room temperature (approximately 25°C), and the busulfan infusion must be completed during the 8-hour time period. Solutions of busulfan diluted in 0.9% sodium chloride injection also have been shown to be stable when refrigerated at 2–8°C for up to 12 hours, during which time the infusion must be completed.

For further information on the handling of antineoplastic agents, see the ASHP Guidelines on Handling Hazardous Drugs at http://www.ahfsdruginformation.com.

Preparations

Excipients in commercially available drug preparations may have clinically important effects in some individuals; consult specific product labeling for details.

Busulfan

Oral		
Tablets, film-coated	2 mg	**Myleran®**, GlaxoSmithKline
Parenteral		
For injection concentrate, for IV infusion only	6 mg/mL (60 mg)	**Busulfex®**, Otsuka Pharmaceutical

†Use is not currently included in the labeling approved by the US Food and Drug Administration

Cabazitaxel

■ Cabazitaxel, a semisynthetic taxoid derived from the major natural taxoid (10-deacetyl baccatin III) extracted from the needles of various species of yew trees (*Taxus* species), is an antineoplastic agent.

Uses

■ **Prostate Cancer** Cabazitaxel is used in combination with prednisone for the treatment of hormone-refractory metastatic prostate cancer in patients with disease that has progressed following prior treatment with docetaxel-based therapy.

The current indication for cabazitaxel is based principally on the results of a randomized, multicenter, phase 3 study (TROPIC) in 755 men with hormone-refractory metastatic prostate cancer who had experienced disease progression during or after completion of a docetaxel-containing regimen. Approximately 92% of patients had received a cumulative docetaxel dose of at least 225 mg/m^2 at time of study entry. Patients with measurable disease who were enrolled in the study had disease progression documented by Response Evaluation Criteria in Solid Tumors (RECIST) with at least one visceral or soft-tissue metastatic lesion, while those with nonmeasurable disease were required to have either rising serum prostate specific antigen (PSA) concentrations or the presence of at least one new radiographic lesion. Patients were randomized to receive either cabazitaxel and prednisone or mitoxantrone and prednisone. Treatment consisted of cabazitaxel 25 mg/m^2 administered IV over 1 hour or mitoxantrone 12 mg/m^2 administered IV over 15–30 minutes on day 1 of each 21-day treatment cycle; prednisone 10 mg daily (or an equivalent dosage of prednisolone) was administered orally throughout both treatment courses. Patients receiving cabazitaxel were premedicated with an antihistamine, a histamine H_2-receptor antagonist (excluding cimetidine), and a corticosteroid at least 30 minutes prior to cabazitaxel administration. Treatment duration in both groups was limited to 10 cycles to minimize the risk of mitoxantrone-induced cardiotoxicity. Prophylactic use of granulocyte colony-stimulating factors was not permitted during the first cycle of treatment, but use of these agents was allowed after the first occurrence of prolonged neutropenia (i.e., lasting 7 days or longer) or neutropenia associated with fever or infection.

At a median follow-up of 12.8 months, patients receiving cabazitaxel and prednisone had longer median overall survival (15.1 versus 12.7 months) and progression-free survival (2.8 versus 1.4 months) compared with those receiving mitoxantrone and prednisone. A subset analysis of overall survival based on prognostic features at baseline consistently favored the cabazitaxel regimen over the mitoxantrone regimen. Patients receiving cabazitaxel and prednisone also had higher objective tumor response rates (14.4 versus 4.4%) and PSA response rates (39.2 versus 17.8%) and longer median times to tumor progression (8.8 versus 5.4 months) and PSA progression (6.4 versus 3.1 months), but had similar times to pain progression, compared with those receiving mitoxantrone and prednisone. In both treatment groups, the most common reason for drug discontinuance was disease progression; discontinuance because of disease progression was more common (71 versus 48%) in patients receiving mitoxantrone and prednisone, whereas discontinuance because of adverse effects was more common (18 versus 8%) in patients receiving cabazitaxel and prednisone.

Higher frequencies of severe (grade 3 or greater) neutropenia (82 versus 58%), severe febrile neutropenia (7 versus 1%), diarrhea (47 versus 11%, severe in 6 versus less than 1%), and peripheral neuropathy (13 versus 3%) were observed in patients receiving cabazitaxel and prednisone compared with those receiving mitoxantrone and prednisone. The frequency of peripheral edema was similar in both treatment groups (9%). About 5% of cabazitaxel-treated patients compared with 2% of mitoxantrone-treated patients died within 30 days of the last dose of the drug; disease progression was the most common cause of early death among patients receiving mitoxantrone, whereas adverse reactions, including neutropenic complications and renal failure, were the most frequent causes of early death among patients receiving cabazitaxel.

Dosage and Administration

■ General Cabazitaxel should administered under the supervision of a qualified clinician experienced in therapy with cytotoxic agents; appropriate diagnostic and treatment facilities should be readily available for the management of treatment-related complications.

To minimize the risk and/or severity of hypersensitivity reactions, patients should be premedicated with an IV antihistamine (diphenhydramine hydrochloride 25 mg or equivalent), IV histamine H_2-receptor antagonist (ranitidine 50 mg or equivalent [except cimetidine]), and IV corticosteroid (dexamethasone 8 mg or equivalent) at least 30 minutes prior to each cabazitaxel infusion.

Antiemetic prophylaxis, administered orally or IV as needed, also is recommended in patients receiving cabazitaxel.

■ Reconstitution and Administration Cabazitaxel is administered by IV infusion over 1 hour.

Caution should be exercised when preparing and handling cabazitaxel solutions, and the use of protective equipment (e.g., gloves) is recommended. If the drug (as a concentrate or diluted solution) comes into contact with mucous membranes, the affected area should be flushed immediately and thoroughly with water. Skin accidentally exposed to the drug should be washed immediately and thoroughly with soap and water.

Cabazitaxel injection concentrate must be diluted prior to IV infusion. First, the cabazitaxel injection concentrate is diluted to prepare the initial diluted cabazitaxel solution and then the initial diluted cabazitaxel solution is further diluted to prepare the final dilution of cabazitaxel solution for infusion. Both the cabazitaxel injection concentrate and diluent vials contain an overfill to compensate for the loss of liquid during preparation.

For preparation of the *initial* diluted solution, the entire contents of the diluent vial supplied by the manufacturer (approximately 5.7 mL of 13% [w/w] ethanol in water for injection) is withdrawn and transferred to a vial labeled as containing cabazitaxel 60 mg in 1.5 mL; the resultant solution contains cabazitaxel 10 mg/mL. The diluent should be directed toward the wall of the vial and injected slowly to minimize foaming. The vial should be inverted repeatedly for at least 45 seconds to fully mix the injection concentrate and diluent; the vial should not be shaken. The solution should be allowed to stand for a few minutes to let any foam dissipate; then preparation may continue even if some foam remains. The initial diluted cabazitaxel solution should be further diluted within 30 minutes of preparation.

For preparation of the *final* diluted cabazitaxel solution, the required amount of the initial diluted cabazitaxel solution (cabazitaxel 10 mg/mL) should be injected into a 250-mL non-PVC infusion bag or bottle containing 0.9% sodium chloride injection or 5% dextrose injection to produce a final solution with a cabazitaxel concentration of 0.1–0.26 mg/mL. If the required dose exceeds 65 mg, the volume of IV solution should be increased accordingly so that a cabazitaxel concentration of 0.26 mg/mL is not exceeded. The final diluted cabazitaxel solution for infusion should be mixed thoroughly by gently inverting the bag or bottle. Infusion of the final diluted cabazitaxel solution should be completed within 8 hours if stored at room temperature or within 24 hours if stored under refrigeration. The infusion solution should be at room temperature for administration. Any unused portion should be discarded. Cabazitaxel should not be admixed with other drugs.

Because both the initial and final diluted cabazitaxel solutions are supersaturated, crystallization may occur over time. Diluted solutions of the drug should be inspected visually for particulate matter, including crystals, and discoloration; the drug should be discarded if either the initial or final diluted solution is cloudy or contains a precipitate. Cabazitaxel should be administered through a 0.22-μm in-line filter.

Cabazitaxel injection concentrate contains polysorbate 80, which can cause leaching of diethylhexyl phthalate (DEHP) from PVC containers. PVC infusion containers and polyurethane administration sets should not be used during preparation or administration of the drug.

■ Dosage ***Prostate Cancer*** The recommended adult dosage of cabazitaxel for the treatment of hormone-refractory metastatic prostate cancer in patients previously treated with a docetaxel-containing regimen is 25 mg/m^2 administered as a 1-hour IV infusion every 3 weeks. Prednisone (10 mg orally once daily) is administered continuously throughout cabazitaxel treatment. In the phase 3 clinical trial supporting use of cabazitaxel for this indication, treatment duration was limited to 10 cycles because of the potential for cumulative cardiotoxicity with the comparator regimen (mitoxantrone). Although no cumulative dose-limiting toxicities have been described with cabazitaxel use, the manufacturer states there are no data to support use of the drug beyond 10 cycles.

Dosage Modification for Toxicity **Dosage Modification for Hematologic Toxicity.** Complete blood cell counts should be monitored weekly during the first cycle of cabazitaxel therapy and prior to *each* treatment cycle thereafter. In patients who experience severe prolonged neutropenia (i.e., grade 3 or greater neutropenia lasting longer than one week) despite appropriate use of a granulocyte colony-stimulating factor (e.g., filgrastim, pegfilgrastim), cabazitaxel therapy should be interrupted until the neutrophil count exceeds 1500/mm^3; upon resumption of therapy, the cabazitaxel dosage should be reduced to 20 mg/m^2 every 3 weeks. In patients who experience an episode of febrile neutropenia, therapy should be interrupted until improvement or resolution occurs and the neutrophil count exceeds 1500/mm^3; upon resumption of therapy, the cabazitaxel dosage should be reduced to 20 mg/m^2 every 3 weeks. The manufacturer recommends use of a granulocyte colony-stimulating factor for secondary prophylaxis in patients who have experienced severe prolonged neutropenia or an episode of febrile neutropenia. Cabazitaxel therapy should be discontinued if severe prolonged neutropenia or febrile neutropenia recurs following reduction of the cabazitaxel dosage to 20 mg/m^2 every 3 weeks.

Dosage Modification for GI Toxicity. In patients who experience severe diarrhea (grade 3 or greater) or persistent diarrhea despite use of appropriate medical therapy (e.g., antidiarrheals, fluid and electrolyte replacement), cabazitaxel therapy should be interrupted until the diarrhea improves or resolves; upon resumption of therapy, the cabazitaxel dosage should be reduced to 20 mg/m^2 every 3 weeks. Cabazitaxel therapy should be discontinued if severe or persistent diarrhea recurs following reduction of the cabazitaxel dosage to 20 mg/m^2 every 3 weeks.

■ Special Populations The manufacturer makes no special population dosage recommendations at this time. The manufacturer states that cabazitaxel should *not* be used in patients with hepatic impairment (serum AST and/or ALT concentrations of 1.5 or more times the upper limit of normal [ULN] or total serum bilirubin concentrations at or above the ULN). (See Specific Populations under Cautions: Warnings/Precautions.)

Cautions

■ Contraindications Known severe hypersensitivity reaction to cabazitaxel or other formulations containing polysorbate 80.

Baseline neutrophil count of 1500/mm^3 or less.

■ Warnings/Precautions ***Warnings*** **Neutropenia.** Neutropenia, including fatal neutropenic episodes, have been reported in patients receiving cabazitaxel. In the TROPIC study in patients with prostate cancer, grade 3 or 4 neutropenia was reported in 82% and febrile neutropenia was reported in 7% of patients receiving cabazitaxel and prednisone. Five deaths due to sepsis or septic shock were reported with this regimen in the TROPIC study; all 5 patients had severe (grade 4) neutropenia, and one patient had febrile neutropenia. One additional death was attributed to neutropenia without documented infection.

Granulocyte colony-stimulating factors (G-CSF) (e.g., filgrastim, pegfilgrastim) may be used to reduce the risk of neutropenic complications associated with cabazitaxel. The manufacturer recommends that primary prophylaxis with G-CSF be considered in patients with high-risk clinical features that could potentially increase the risk of complications associated with prolonged neutropenia, including patients older than 65 years of age and those with poor performance status, prior episodes of febrile neutropenia, extensive prior radiation, poor nutritional status, or other serious comorbidities. The manufacturer recommends that therapeutic use of G-CSF and secondary prophylaxis be considered in all patients at increased risk for neutropenic complications.

Complete blood cell counts should be monitored weekly during the first treatment cycle and prior to *each* treatment cycle thereafter. After administration of the recommended dosage for the initial cycle, dosage for each subsequent cycle should be adjusted as needed based on hematologic recovery. Cabazitaxel should *not* be administered until neutrophil counts exceed 1500/mm^3. In patients who experience severe prolonged neutropenia despite appropriate treatment (e.g., G-CSF) or febrile neutropenia, temporary interruption of cabazitaxel therapy followed by dosage reduction or discontinuance of cabazitaxel therapy may be required. (See Dosage Modification for Hematologic Toxicity under Dosage: Dosage Modification for Toxicity, in Dosage and Administration.)

Sensitivity Reactions. Cabazitaxel can cause severe hypersensitivity reactions (e.g., generalized rash/erythema, hypotension, bronchospasm), and all patients receiving the drug should be premedicated to minimize the risk and/or severity of these reactions. (See Dosage and Administration: General.) Patients should be observed closely for hypersensitivity reactions, especially during the first and second infusions of the drug. Appropriate facilities and equipment for the treatment of hypotension and bronchospasm should be readily available, since hypersensitivity reactions may occur within minutes following initiation of a cabazitaxel infusion. If a severe hypersensitivity reaction develops, the infusion should be discontinued immediately and appropriate supportive treatment instituted. Cabazitaxel injection concentrate contains polysorbate 80 and should *not* be used in patients with a history of severe hypersensitivity to cabazitaxel or to other formulations containing polysorbate 80.

Other Warnings and Precautions **GI Effects.** Cabazitaxel can cause nausea, vomiting, and severe diarrhea. Death related to diarrhea and associated dehydration and electrolyte imbalance has been reported in a patient who received the drug. Antiemetic prophylaxis, administered orally or IV as needed, is recommended in patients receiving cabazitaxel. Rehydration therapy and antidiarrheal and antiemetic agents should be used as needed; intensive measures may be required for the management of severe diarrhea and electrolyte imbalance. In patients with severe or persistent diarrhea, temporary interruption of therapy followed by dosage reduction, or discontinuance of cabazitaxel therapy, may be required. (See Dosage Modification for GI Toxicity under Dosage: Dosage Modification for Toxicity, in Dosage and Administration.)

Renal Effects. Renal failure, sometimes fatal, has been reported in patients receiving cabazitaxel, generally in association with sepsis, dehydration, or obstructive uropathy; some deaths due to renal failure did not have a clear etiology. If renal failure develops during cabazitaxel therapy, appropriate measures should be taken to identify the cause and the renal failure should be treated aggressively.

Fetal/Neonatal Morbidity and Mortality. Cabazitaxel may cause fetal harm if administered to pregnant women; the drug has been shown to be embryotoxic, fetotoxic, and abortifacient in animals. Pregnancy should be avoided during therapy. If cabazitaxel is used during pregnancy or if the patient becomes pregnant while receiving the drug, the patient should be apprised of the potential fetal hazard.

Specific Populations **Pregnancy.** Category D. (See Fetal/Neonatal Morbidity and Mortality under Warnings/Precautions: Other Warnings and Precautions, in Cautions.) (See Users Guide.)

Lactation. Cabazitaxel or its metabolites are distributed into milk in lactating rats. It is not known whether cabazitaxel or its metabolites are distributed into human milk. Because of the potential for serious adverse reactions to cabazitaxel in nursing infants, a decision should be made whether to discontinue nursing or the drug, taking into account the importance of the drug to the woman.

Pediatric Use. Safety and efficacy of cabazitaxel have not been established in pediatric patients.

Geriatric Use. In the TROPIC study in patients with prostate cancer, 65% of patients receiving cabazitaxel and prednisone were 65 years of age or older, while 19% were 75 years of age or older. Although no substantial differences in efficacy or pharmacokinetics of cabazitaxel were observed between individuals 65 years of age or older and younger adults, reported frequencies of neutropenia, fatigue, asthenia, pyrexia, dizziness, urinary tract infection, and dehydration were at least 5 percentage points higher in patients 65 years of age or older compared with younger adults. In addition, 6% of patients 65 years of age or older, compared with 2% of patients younger than 65 years of age, died within 30 days of the last cabazitaxel dose from a cause other than disease progression.

Hepatic Impairment. Safety and efficacy of cabazitaxel have not been established in patients with hepatic impairment. Patients with serum transaminase (AST, ALT) concentrations of 1.5 or more times the upper limit of normal (ULN) or serum bilirubin concentrations at or above the ULN were excluded from the TROPIC study.

Because cabazitaxel is extensively metabolized in the liver, hepatic impairment is expected to result in increased serum concentrations of the drug. Hepatic impairment increases the risk of severe or life-threatening complications of other taxanes (e.g., docetaxel). The manufacturer states that cabazitaxel should *not* be used in patients with hepatic impairment (i.e., AST and/or ALT concentrations of 1.5 or more times the ULN or total serum bilirubin concentrations at or above the ULN).

Renal Impairment. Safety and efficacy of cabazitaxel in patients with renal impairment have not been studied specifically to date. Only minimal amounts of cabazitaxel (3.7%) are excreted as unchanged drug or metabolites in urine. A population pharmacokinetic analysis indicated that mild to moderate renal impairment (creatinine clearance of 30 to less than 80 mL/minute) did not substantially alter cabazitaxel clearance. However, no data are available for patients with severe renal impairment (creatinine clearance less than 30 mL/minute) or end-stage renal disease, and the manufacturer states that cabazitaxel should be used with caution in patients with severe renal impairment or end-stage renal disease.

■ **Common Adverse Effects** Adverse effects reported in 10% or more of patients receiving cabazitaxel in combination with prednisone include neutropenia, leukopenia, anemia, thrombocytopenia, diarrhea, fatigue, nausea, vomiting, constipation, asthenia, abdominal pain, anorexia, back pain, hematuria, peripheral neuropathy, pyrexia, dyspnea, cough, dysgeusia, arthralgia, and alopecia. Serious (grade 3 or 4) adverse effects reported in 5% or more of patients receiving cabazitaxel in combination with prednisone include neutropenia, leukopenia, anemia, febrile neutropenia, diarrhea, fatigue, and asthenia.

Drug Interactions

No formal drug interaction studies have been performed to date.

The manufacturer states that cabazitaxel is unlikely to inhibit multidrug resistance proteins MRP1 and MRP2, the efflux transporter P-glycoprotein (P-gp, ABCB1), or breast cancer resistance protein (BCRP) in vivo following administration of the drug at a dose of 25 mg/m^2. In vitro data indicate that cabazitaxel does not inhibit MRP1 or MRP2; although in vitro inhibition of P-gp transport and BCRP has been observed, inhibition occurred at concentrations at least 38 times those achieved clinically.

In vitro data indicate that cabazitaxel is a substrate of P-gp, but not a substrate of MRP1, MRP2, or BCRP.

■ **Drugs Affecting or Metabolized by Hepatic Microsomal Enzymes** Because cabazitaxel is extensively metabolized by cytochrome P-450 (CYP) isoenzyme 3A (CYP3A), potent inhibitors or inducers of this isoenzyme are expected to alter the drug's pharmacokinetics. Cabazitaxel does not induce CYP isoenzymes in vitro. In vitro data also indicate that cabazitaxel is unlikely to inhibit metabolism of drugs that are substrates of CYP isoenzymes 1A2, 2B6, 2C8, 2C9, 2C19, 2D6, 2E1, or 3A4/5.

Concomitant use of cabazitaxel with potent inhibitors of CYP3A (e.g., atazanavir, clarithromycin, indinavir, itraconazole, ketoconazole, nefazodone, nelfinavir, ritonavir, saquinavir, telithromycin, voriconazole) is expected to result in increased plasma cabazitaxel concentrations and should be avoided. Moderate CYP3A inhibitors should be used concomitantly with caution.

Concomitant use of cabazitaxel with potent inducers of CYP3A (e.g., carbamazepine, phenobarbital, phenytoin, rifampin, rifabutin, rifapentine) is expected to result in decreased plasma cabazitaxel concentrations and should be avoided. Concomitant use of St. John's wort (*Hypericum perforatum*) also should be avoided.

■ **Corticosteroids** Administration of prednisone or prednisolone at a dosage of 10 mg daily did not affect the pharmacokinetics of cabazitaxel.

Description

Cabazitaxel, a semisynthetic taxoid derived from the major natural taxoid (10-deacetyl baccatin III) extracted from the needles of various species of yew trees (*Taxus* species), is an antimicrotubule antineoplastic agent. Cabazitaxel is the 7,10-dimethoxy analog of docetaxel. Like other taxanes (e.g., docetaxel, paclitaxel), cabazitaxel binds to β-tubulin subunits on microtubules and stabilizes and suppresses microtubule activity, thereby resulting in mitotic arrest and cell death.

In preclinical studies, cabazitaxel was active against some cell lines that are resistant to other antineoplastic agents, including anthracyclines, vinca alkaloids, and other taxanes (i.e., docetaxel, paclitaxel). Cabazitaxel, a weak substrate for the efflux transporter P-glycoprotein (P-gp), has demonstrated activity in cell lines with acquired resistance to docetaxel resulting from P-gp overexpression and in cell lines with primary resistance to taxanes resulting from increased expression of the multidrug resistance (MDR) gene and its product P-gp. Cabazitaxel has demonstrated activity against some taxane-resistant tumors in vivo, including activity against docetaxel-resistant prostate cancer.

Evidence from animal studies suggests that cabazitaxel may cross the blood-brain barrier to a greater extent than docetaxel or paclitaxel, possibly because of cabazitaxel's lower affinity for P-gp, which is expressed in the blood-brain barrier. Animal data suggest that P-gp-mediated transport across the blood-brain barrier can be saturated, resulting in nonlinear accumulation of the drug in the brain. The clinical relevance of these findings to neurotoxicity or antitumor effects of the drug in humans is unknown.

Cabazitaxel is extensively metabolized in the liver, primarily by cytochrome P-450 (CYP) isoenzyme 3A4/5 and to a lesser extent by CYP isoenzyme 2C8. About 76% of a dose of cabazitaxel is eliminated in feces as metabolites, and about 3.7% is eliminated in urine as unchanged drug or metabolites; about 20 metabolites of the drug have been identified in urine or feces. The terminal elimination half-life of cabazitaxel is 95 hours.

Advice to Patients

Risk of hypersensitivity reactions. Importance of informing clinician immediately if manifestations of severe hypersensitivity (e.g., rash, itching, dizziness or faintness, difficulty breathing, chest or throat tightness, facial swelling) occur. Importance of informing clinician of any history of hypersensitivity to cabazitaxel or other formulations containing polysorbate 80.

Risk of infection, including severe or potentially fatal infection. Importance of routine monitoring of blood cell counts. Importance of patients monitoring their temperature frequently and immediately notifying their clinician if fever or other manifestations of infection (e.g., cough, burning on urination, myalgia) occur.

Risk of dehydration and renal failure. Importance of informing clinician if substantial vomiting or diarrhea occurs, decreased urine output occurs, or edema develops.

Importance of informing geriatric patients that certain adverse effects may be more frequent or severe in older patients. (See Geriatric Use under Warnings/Precautions: Specific Populations, in Cautions.)

Importance of taking the oral prednisone component of the cabazitaxel/prednisone regimen for prostate cancer as directed. Importance of informing clinician if not adherent to the oral prednisone regimen.

Importance of women informing clinicians if they are or plan to become pregnant or plan to breast-feed. Apprise patient of potential hazard to the fetus if used during pregnancy; women of childbearing potential should avoid becoming pregnant.

Importance of informing clinician of existing or contemplated concomitant therapy, including prescription and OTC drugs and herbal supplements, as well as any concomitant illnesses.

Importance of informing patients of other important precautionary information. (See Cautions.)

Overview® (see Users Guide). For additional information on this drug until a more detailed monograph is developed and published, the manufacturer's labeling should be consulted. It is *essential* that the manufacturer's labeling be consulted for more detailed information on usual cautions, precautions, contraindications, potential drug interactions, laboratory test interferences, and acute toxicity. For further information on the handling of antineoplastics agents, see the ASHP Guidelines on Handling Hazardous Drugs at http://www.ahfsdruginformation.com.

Preparations

Excipients in commercially available drug preparations may have clinically important effects in some individuals; consult specific product labeling for details.

Cabazitaxel

Parenteral

Injection concentrate, for IV infusion only	40 mg/mL (60 mg)	**Jevtana®** (with water for injection containing alcohol 13% w/w diluent), Sanofi-Aventis

Cabozantinib *S*-malate

■ Cabozantinib *S*-malate, an inhibitor of multiple receptor tyrosine kinases, is an antineoplastic agent.

Uses

■ **Medullary Thyroid Cancer** Cabozantinib *S*-malate is used for the treatment of progressive, metastatic medullary thyroid cancer. Cabozantinib has been designated an orphan drug by the US Food and Drug Administration (FDA) for the treatment of this cancer.

The current indication for cabozantinib is based principally on the results of a randomized, multicenter, double-blind, placebo-controlled, phase 3 study (EXAM) in patients with unresectable, locally advanced or metastatic medullary thyroid cancer who had evidence of actively progressive disease within 14 months prior to study entry according to Response Evaluation Criteria in Solid Tumors (RECIST). In the EXAM study, 330 patients were randomized in a 2:1 ratio to receive either cabozantinib (140 mg) or placebo orally once daily, without food, until disease progression or intolerable toxicity occurred. The primary efficacy end point of this study was progression-free survival according to RECIST; secondary endpoints included overall survival, objective response rate, and duration of response. The median age of patients enrolled in the study was 55 years; 25% of the patients had received 2 or more prior systemic therapies and 21% had previously received a tyrosine kinase inhibitor. Rearranged during transfection (RET) mutation status was positive, negative, or unknown in 48, 12, or 39% of the enrolled patients, respectively.

Patients receiving cabozantinib in the EXAM study demonstrated a longer median progression-free survival than those receiving placebo (11.2 versus 4 months, respectively). The favorable treatment effect of cabozantinib on progression-free survival was consistent across patient subgroups, including RET mutation status and previous therapy with a tyrosine kinase inhibitor. Patients receiving cabozantinib also had higher overall response rates (all were partial responses) compared with those receiving placebo (27 versus 0%), and their median duration of response was 14.7 months. Overall survival was not substantially different between the cabozantinib and placebo groups in a planned interim analysis and later in an unplanned analysis requested by the FDA.

Dosage and Administration

■ **General** ***Restricted Distribution*** Cabozantinib *S*-malate can only be obtained through a specialty pharmacy. Specific information regarding distribution of the drug is available by telephone at 855-253-3273 or at http://www.cometriq.com/hcp/index.php).

■ **Administration** Cabozantinib *S*-malate is administered orally once daily. The drug should *not* be administered with food; patients should not eat for at least 2 hours before and at least 1 hour after taking cabozantinib. (See Description.)Cabozantinib capsules should be swallowed whole with a full glass of water; the capsules should *not* be opened or crushed.

If a dose of cabozantinib is missed, the missed dose should not be taken within 12 hours of the next dose. (See Advice to Patients.)

■ **Dosage** Dosage of cabozantinib, which is commercially available as cabozantinib *S*-malate, is expressed in terms of cabozantinib.

Medullary Thyroid Cancer The recommended adult dosage of cabozantinib for the treatment of progressive, metastatic medullary thyroid cancer is 140 mg (one 80-mg and three 20-mg capsules) once daily. Therapy should be continued until disease progression or unacceptable toxicity occurs.

Dosage Modification for Toxicity Cabozantinib therapy should be *withheld* if grade 4 hematologic adverse effects, grade 3 or greater nonhematologic adverse effects, or intolerable grade 2 adverse effects (as defined by the National Cancer Institute [NCI] Common Terminology Criteria for Adverse Events [CTCAE]) occur. Upon resolution or improvement of the adverse effect (i.e., return to baseline or resolution to grade 1), the dosage of cabozantinib should be reduced as follows: in patients previously receiving 140 mg daily, cabozantinib therapy should be resumed at a dosage of 100 mg daily (one 80-mg and one 20-mg capsule); in patients previously receiving 100 mg daily, cabozantinib therapy should be resumed at a dosage of 60 mg daily (three 20-mg capsules); and in patients previously receiving 60 mg daily, cabozantinib therapy should be resumed at a dosage of 60 mg daily, if tolerated. Otherwise, cabozantinib therapy should be discontinued.

Cabozantinib should be *permanently discontinued* in patients who develop visceral perforation or fistula formation, severe hemorrhage, serious arterial thromboembolic events (e.g., myocardial infarction, cerebral infarction), nephrotic syndrome, malignant hypertension, hypertensive crisis, persistent uncontrolled hypertension despite optimal medical management, osteonecrosis of the jaw, or reversible posterior leukoencephalopathy syndrome. (See Cautions: Warnings/Precautions.)

Concomitant Use with Drugs Affecting Hepatic Microsomal Enzymes Concomitant use of cabozantinib with drugs that are potent inhibitors of cytochrome P-450 (CYP) isoenzyme 3A4 should be *avoided*. (See Drug Interactions: Drugs and Foods Affecting Hepatic Microsomal Enzymes.)If concomitant use of a potent CYP3A4 inhibitor cannot be avoided, the manufacturer recommends reducing the daily dosage of cabozantinib by 40 mg (e.g., from 140 mg daily to 100 mg daily or from 100 mg daily to 60 mg daily). If concomitant use of the potent CYP3A4 inhibitor is discontinued, the cabozantinib dosage should be returned to the dosage used prior to initiation of the potent CYP3A4 inhibitor 2–3 days following discontinuance of the potent CYP3A4 inhibitor.

Chronic concomitant use of potent CYP3A4 inducers should be *avoided* in patients receiving cabozantinib if alternative therapy is available. (See Drug Interactions: Drugs and Foods Affecting Hepatic Microsomal Enzymes.)Foods or nutritional supplements (e.g., St. John's wort [*Hypericum perforatum*]) that are known to induce CYP450 activity should *not* be ingested during therapy with the drug. If concomitant use of a potent CYP3A4 inducer cannot be avoided, the manufacturer recommends increasing the daily dosage of cabozantinib by 40 mg (e.g., from 140 mg daily to 180 mg daily or from 100 mg daily to 140 mg daily) as tolerated. If concomitant use of the potent CYP3A4 inducer is discontinued, the cabozantinib dosage should be returned to the dosage used prior to initiation of the potent CYP3A4 inducer 2–3 days following discontinuance of the potent CYP3A4 inducer. The daily dosage of cabozantinib should not exceed 180 mg.

■ **Special Populations** Cabozantinib is *not* recommended for use in patients with moderate or severe hepatic impairment because safety and efficacy have not been established in these patients. (See Hepatic Impairment under Warnings/Precautions: Specific Populations, in Cautions.)

Dosage adjustment is not necessary in patients with mild or moderate renal impairment. The manufacturer states that there is no experience with cabozantinib in patients with severe renal impairment and does not make specific dosage recommendations for such patients. (See Renal Impairment under Warnings/Precautions: Specific Populations, in Cautions.)

The manufacturer makes no specific dosage recommendations for geriatric patients. (See Geriatric Use under Warnings/Precautions: Specific Populations, in Cautions.)

Cautions

■ **Contraindications** The manufacturer states there are no known contraindications to the use of cabozantinib *S*-malate.

■ **Warnings/Precautions** ***Warnings*** **Perforations and Fistulas.** GI perforations and fistulas were reported in 3 and 1%, respectively, of cabozantinib-treated patients. All cases were serious and one GI fistula was fatal. Non-GI fistulas, including tracheal/esophageal fistulas, were reported in 4% of patients receiving the drug, and were fatal in two (1%) of these cases.

Patients receiving cabozantinib should be monitored for symptoms of perforations and fistulas. Cabozantinib should be permanently discontinued in patients who develop a visceral perforation or fistula.

Hemorrhage. Serious, sometimes fatal, hemorrhage, including hemoptysis and GI hemorrhage, has been reported with cabozantinib. The incidence of grade 3 or greater adverse hemorrhagic events was higher in patients receiving cabozantinib compared with those receiving placebo (3 versus 1%, respectively).

Patients receiving cabozantinib should be monitored for signs and symptoms of bleeding. The drug should not be used in patients with severe hemorrhage or a recent history of hemorrhage or hemoptysis. Cabozantinib should be permanently discontinued if severe hemorrhage occurs.

Other Warnings and Precautions **Thromboembolic Events.** Cabozantinib therapy is associated with an increased incidence of thromboembolic events. Venous thromboembolism was reported in 6 or 3% of patients receiving cabozantinib or placebo, respectively, and arterial thromboembolism was reported in 2 or 0% of patients receiving cabozantinib or placebo, respectively.

Cabozantinib should be permanently discontinued in patients who develop an acute myocardial infarction, cerebral infarction, or any other serious or clinically important arterial thromboembolic event.

Wound-healing Complications. Inhibitors of vascular endothelial growth factor receptor (VEGFR) may impair wound healing (see Description), and wound-healing complications have been reported in patients receiving cabozantinib.

The manufacturer recommends that cabozantinib be discontinued at least 28 days prior to scheduled surgery. Therapy with the drug may be resumed following surgery based on clinical judgment of adequate wound healing. Cabozantinib should be withheld in patients with dehiscence or other wound healing complications requiring medical intervention.

Hypertension. Cabozantinib is associated with an increased incidence of treatment-induced hypertension. Nearly all cabozantinib-treated patients experienced elevated blood pressure; stage 1 or 2 hypertension occurred in 61% of patients receiving cabozantinib compared with 30% of those receiving placebo in the phase 3 clinical study. None of the patients in this study developed malignant hypertension.

Blood pressure should be monitored prior to initiation of cabozantinib and periodically during therapy. Cabozantinib should be temporarily withheld for hypertension that is not adequately controlled with medical management; when controlled, cabozantinib therapy should be resumed at a reduced dosage. Cabozantinib should be permanently discontinued for malignant hypertension, hypertensive crisis, or persistent uncontrolled hypertension despite optimal medical management (i.e., antihypertensive therapy).

Osteonecrosis of the Jaw. Osteonecrosis of the jaw (ONJ) occurred in 1% of cabozantinib-treated patients. The condition may manifest as jaw pain, osteomyelitis, osteitis, bone erosion, tooth or periodontal infection, toothache, gingival ulceration or erosion, persistent jaw pain, or delayed healing of the mouth or jaw following dental surgery.

An oral examination should be performed prior to initiation of cabozantinib and periodically during therapy. Patients should be advised to maintain good oral hygiene during treatment. (See Advice to Patients.)For patients requiring invasive dental procedures, cabozantinib therapy should be withheld for at least 28 days prior to scheduled surgery, if possible. Cabozantinib should be permanently discontinued in patients who develop ONJ.

Palmar-plantar Erythrodysesthesia Syndrome. Palmar-plantar erythrodysesthesia syndrome (hand-foot syndrome) occurred in 50% of cabozantinib-treated patients, and was severe (grade 3 or greater) in 13% of patients. In addition, a hand-foot skin reaction with subungual splinter hemorrhages and hypertension has been reported in at least one patient receiving the drug.

Cabozantinib should be withheld in patients who develop intolerable grade 2 or grade 3–4 palmar-plantar erythrodysesthesia syndrome until improvement to grade 1 has occurred; cabozantinib should then be resumed at a reduced dosage. (See Dosage Modification for Toxicity under Dosage and Administration: Dosage.)

Proteinuria. Proteinuria was observed in 4 patients (2%) receiving cabozantinib, including one patient with nephrotic syndrome, compared with none of those receiving placebo. Urine protein should be monitored regularly during cabozantinib therapy. Cabozantinib should be permanently discontinued in patients who develop nephrotic syndrome.

Reversible Posterior Leukoencephalopathy Syndrome. Reversible posterior leukoencephalopathy syndrome (RPLS) has occurred in one (less than 1%) cabozantinib-treated patient. RPLS is a syndrome of subcortical vasogenic edema that may manifest with seizures, headache, visual disturbances, confusion, or altered mental function. Magnetic resonance imaging (MRI) is necessary to confirm the diagnosis of RPLS.

The possible diagnosis of RPLS should be considered in any patient receiving cabozantinib who presents with neurologic manifestations suggestive of RPLS. Cabozantinib should be permanently discontinued in patients who develop RPLS.

Interactions. Concomitant use of cabozantinib with potent inducers or inhibitors of cytochrome P-450 (CYP) isoenzyme 3A4 should be avoided. (See Concomitant Use with Drugs Affecting Hepatic Microsomal Enzymes under Dosage and Administration: Dosage and also see Drug Interactions: Drugs and Foods Affecting Hepatic Microsomal Enzymes.)

Fetal/Neonatal Morbidity and Mortality. Cabozantinib may cause fetal harm if administered to pregnant women; the drug has been shown to be embryotoxic, fetotoxic, and teratogenic in animals (e.g., fetal loss, skeletal variations, visceral variations, malformations).

Women of childbearing potential and men who are partners of such women should be advised to use an effective method of contraception while receiving cabozantinib and for at least 4 months after discontinuance of therapy. If cabozantinib is used during pregnancy or if the patient becomes pregnant while receiving the drug, the patient should be apprised of the potential fetal hazard. (See Advice to Patients.)

Impairment of Fertility. The manufacturer states that there are no data on the effect of cabozantinib on human fertility. However, cabozantinib impaired male and female fertility in animal studies.

Specific Populations **Pregnancy.** Category D. (See Users Guide and see Fetal/Neonatal Morbidity and Mortality under Warnings/Precautions: Other Warnings and Precautions, in Cautions.)

Lactation. It is not known whether cabozantinib or its metabolites are distributed into human milk. Because of the potential for serious adverse reactions to cabozantinib in nursing infants, a decision should be made whether to discontinue nursing or the drug, taking into account the importance of the drug to the woman.

Pediatric Use. Safety, efficacy, and pharmacokinetics of cabozantinib have not been established in pediatric patients.

Geriatric Use. Clinical studies of cabozantinib did not include sufficient numbers of patients 65 years of age and older to determine whether geriatric patients respond differently than younger adults. The pharmacokinetics of cabozantinib do not appear to be affected by age in adults (20–86 years of age).

Hepatic Impairment. The pharmacokinetics of cabozantinib have not been studied in patients with hepatic impairment. There are limited data in patients with serum bilirubin concentrations exceeding 1.5 times the upper limit of normal (ULN). Cabozantinib is not recommended in patients with moderate or severe hepatic impairment since safety and efficacy of the drug have not been established in such patients.

Renal Impairment. Formal pharmacokinetic studies of cabozantinib have not been conducted in patients with renal impairment. A population pharmacokinetic analysis suggests that mild to moderate renal impairment (creatinine clearance of 30 mL/minute or greater) does not have a clinically important effect on the clearance of cabozantinib. Dosage adjustment is not recommended in patients with mild or moderate renal impairment. The manufacturer states that there is no experience with cabozantinib in patients with severe renal impairment.

■ Common Adverse Effects

Adverse effects reported in 25% or more of patients receiving cabozantinib include diarrhea, stomatitis, palmar-plantar erythrodysesthesia syndrome (hand-foot syndrome), weight loss, decreased appetite, nausea, fatigue, oral pain, hair color changes, dysgeusia, hypertension, abdominal pain, and constipation.

Laboratory abnormalities reported in 25% or more of patients receiving cabozantinib include increased AST concentrations, increased ALT concentrations, lymphopenia, increased alkaline phosphatase concentrations, hypocalcemia, neutropenia, thrombocytopenia, hypophosphatemia, and hyperbilirubinemia.

Drug Interactions

Cabozantinib is metabolized in the liver by cytochrome P-450 (CYP) isoenzyme 3A4. Inhibition of CYP3A4 reduced the formation of the drug's *N*-oxide metabolite by more than 80%. Inhibition of CYP2C9 had minimal effects on cabozantinib metabolite formation (i.e., less than a 20% reduction). Inhibition of CYP isoenzymes 1A2, 2A6, 2B6, 2C8, 2C19, 2D6, and 2E1 had no effect on cabozantinib metabolite formation.

Cabozantinib is a noncompetitive inhibitor of CYP2C8, a mixed-type inhibitor of CYP2C9 and CYP2C19, and a weak competitive inhibitor of CYP3A4 in human liver microsomal preparations. Cabozantinib is not expected to inhibit CYP isoenzymes 1A2, 2D6, or 3A4 to a clinically important degree in patients receiving 140 mg of the drug daily.

Cabozantinib is an inducer of CYP1A1 messenger RNA (mRNA) in human hepatocyte incubations, but does not induce CYP1A2, CYP2B6, CYP2C8, CYP2C9, CYP2C19, or CYP3A4 mRNA or isoenzyme-associated enzyme activities.

Cabozantinib is an inhibitor, but not a substrate, of P-glycoprotein (P-gp) transport activities in a bi-directional assay system.

■ Drugs and Foods Affecting Hepatic Microsomal Enzymes

Inhibitors of CYP3A4 and Other CYP450 Isoenzymes Concomitant use of cabozantinib with potent inhibitors of CYP3A4 may increase systemic exposure of cabozantinib. When the potent CYP3A4 inhibitor ketoconazole (400 mg daily for 27 days) was administered concomitantly with cabozantinib (as a single 140-mg dose) in healthy individuals, plasma cabozantinib exposure increased by 38%.

Concomitant use of cabozantinib with potent CYP3A4 inhibitors (e.g., atazanavir, clarithromycin, indinavir, itraconazole, ketoconazole, nefazodone, nelfinavir, ritonavir, saquinavir, telithromycin, voriconazole) should be *avoided.* If concomitant use of a potent CYP3A4 inhibitor cannot be avoided, the manufacturer recommends reducing the daily dosage of cabozantinib by 40 mg (e.g., from 140 mg daily to 100 mg daily or from 100 mg daily to 60 mg daily). If concomitant use of the potent CYP3A4 inhibitor is discontinued, the cabozantinib dosage should be returned (2–3 days following discontinuance of the potent CYP3A4 inhibitor) to the dosage used prior to initiation of the potent CYP3A4 inhibitor.

The manufacturer states that foods (e.g., grapefruit, grapefruit juice) or nutritional supplements that are known to inhibit CYP isoenzymes, including CYP3A4, should *not* be ingested during cabozantinib therapy. (See Drug Interactions: Grapefruit.)

Inducers of CYP3A4 and Other CYP450 Isoenzymes Chronic concomitant use of potent inducers of CYP3A4 with cabozantinib may reduce systemic exposure of cabozantinib. When the potent CYP3A4 inducer rifampin (600 mg daily for 31 days) was administered concomitantly with cabozantinib (as a single 140-mg dose) in healthy individuals, plasma cabozantinib exposure decreased by 77%.

Chronic concurrent use of potent CYP3A4 inducers (e.g., carbamazepine, dexamethasone, rifabutin, rifampin, rifapentine, phenobarbital, phenytoin, St. John's wort [*Hypericum perforatum*]) with cabozantinib should be *avoided* if alternative therapy is available. If concomitant use with a potent CYP3A4 inducer cannot be avoided, the manufacturer recommends increasing the daily dosage of cabozantinib by 40 mg (e.g., from 140 mg daily to 180 mg daily or from 100 mg daily to 140 mg daily) as tolerated. If concomitant use of the potent CYP3A4 inducer is discontinued, the cabozantinib dosage should be returned (2–3 days following the discontinuance of the potent CYP3A4 inducer) to the dosage used prior to initiation of the potent CYP3A4 inducer. The daily dosage of cabozantinib should not exceed 180 mg.

The manufacturer states that foods or nutritional supplements (e.g., St. John's wort [*Hypericum perforatum*]) that are known to induce CYP activity, including CYP3A4, should *not* be ingested during cabozantinib therapy.

■ **Drugs Affected by the P-glycoprotein Transport System** Cabozantinib is an inhibitor, but not a substrate, of P-gp transport activities in a bidirectional assay system. Therefore, cabozantinib may have the potential to increase plasma concentrations of concomitantly administered substrates of P-gp.

■ **Grapefruit** Grapefruit products are CYP3A4 inhibitors and should be avoided during cabozantinib therapy because of the potential for increased cabozantinib concentrations.

■ **Rosiglitazone** Cabozantinib at steady-state plasma concentrations (100 mg or more daily for a minimum of 21 days) did not affect single-dose rosiglitazone (a CYP2C8 substrate) plasma exposure (peak concentration and area under the concentration-time curve [AUC]) in patients with solid tumors. A clinically important pharmacokinetic interaction with these drugs therefore appears unlikely.

Description

Cabozantinib *S*-malate, an inhibitor of multiple receptor tyrosine kinases, is an antineoplastic agent. Receptor tyrosine kinases (RTKs) are involved in the initiation of various cascades of intracellular signaling events that lead to cell proliferation and/or influence processes critical to cell survival and tumor progression (e.g., angiogenesis, metastasis, inhibition of apoptosis), based on the respective kinase. Various tyrosine kinases and pathways are abnormally activated in medullary thyroid carcinoma cells (e.g., rearranged during transfection [RET] proto-oncogene mutations are associated with the development of hereditary medullary thyroid cancer). In vitro biochemical and/or cellular assays have shown that cabozantinib inhibits the activity of multiple receptor tyrosine kinases, including RET; met proto-oncogene encoding hepatocyte growth factor (c-MET); vascular endothelial growth factor receptors (VEGFR)-1, VEGFR-2, and VEGFR-3; stem cell factor receptor (c-Kit); tropomyosin receptor kinase B (trkB); fms-like tyrosine kinase 3 (Flt-3); AXL; and TIE-2. These receptor tyrosine kinases are involved in both normal cellular function and pathologic processes (e.g., oncogenesis, metastasis, tumor angiogenesis, and maintenance of the tumor microenvironment).

The absolute oral bioavailability of cabozantinib has not been established. Following oral administration, median time to peak plasma concentrations of cabozantinib ranged from 2–5 hours. Repeated administration of cabozantinib 140 mg daily for 19 days resulted in fourfold to fivefold mean cabozantinib accumulation (based on area under the concentration-time curve [AUC]) compared with single-dose administration; steady-state concentrations of the drug were achieved in 15 days. A high-fat meal increased the peak plasma concentration and AUC of cabozantinib by 41 and 57%, respectively, relative to fasted conditions following administration of a single 140-mg oral dose of the drug in healthy individuals. (See Dosage and Administration: Administration.)Cabozantinib is highly bound (99.7% or more) to plasma proteins. Cabozantinib is metabolized in the liver by cytochrome P-450 (CYP) isoenzyme 3A4, and is a substrate of CYP3A4 in vitro. Inhibition of CYP3A4 reduced the formation of the cabozantinib *N*-oxide metabolite by greater than 80%; inhibition of CYP2C9 had minimal effects on cabozantinib metabolite formation (i.e., less than a 20% reduction). Inhibition of CYP isoenzymes 1A2, 2A6, 2B6, 2C8, 2C19, 2D6, and 2E1 had no effect on cabozantinib metabolite formation. (See Drug Interactions.)Following administration of a single dose of radiolabeled cabozantinib in healthy individuals, approximately 81% of the total administered radioactivity was recovered with 54% in feces and 27% in urine within 48 days. The elimination half-life of cabozantinib is approximately 55 hours.

Advice to Patients

Importance of informing patients that cabozantinib should *not* be taken with food; importance of instructing patients not to eat for at least 2 hours before and at least 1 hour after taking the drug. Importance of swallowing cabozantinib capsules whole with a full glass (at least 240 mL [8 ounces]) of water and not to open or crush the capsules. Importance of avoiding grapefruit or grapefruit juice while taking the drug.

If a dose of cabozantinib is missed and it is 12 hours or more before the next scheduled dose, the dose should be taken as soon as it is remembered, and the next dose should be taken at the regularly scheduled time. If a dose is missed and there are less than 12 hours before the next scheduled dose, the next dose should be taken at the regularly scheduled time; the missed dose should not be replaced.

Importance of informing patients that cabozantinib often causes diarrhea, which may be severe in some cases. Importance of contacting clinician if severe diarrhea occurs during therapy.

Risk of palmar-plantar erythrodysesthesia syndrome. Importance of contacting clinician if progressive or intolerable rash occurs. Importance of advising patients to protect their skin to avoid subclinical vascular damage and subsequent adverse cutaneous effects that may interrupt ongoing therapy.

Risk of mouth sores, oral pain, taste changes, nausea, or vomiting. Importance of contacting clinician if any of these symptoms are severe or prevent eating or drinking.

Risk of weight loss, which may be substantial in some cases. Importance of informing clinician if substantial weight loss occurs.

Risk of osteonecrosis of the jaw; symptoms may include jaw pain, toothache, or sores on the gums. Importance of advising patient that their clinician should examine their mouth before and during cabozantinib therapy. Importance of informing dentist about therapy with the drug. Importance of maintaining good oral hygiene during treatment.

Importance of contacting clinician before any planned surgeries, including dental procedures.

Risk of fetal harm. Necessity of advising women of childbearing potential and men who are partners of such women that they must use an effective method of contraception while receiving cabozantinib and for at least 4 months after discontinuance of therapy. Importance of patients informing their clinicians if they or their partners become pregnant. If pregnancy occurs, apprise patient of potential hazard to the fetus. Importance of discontinuing nursing while receiving cabozantinib therapy.

Importance of informing clinician of existing or contemplated concomitant therapy, including prescription and OTC drugs and herbal supplements (e.g., St. John's wort), as well as any concomitant illnesses (e.g., hypertension, bleeding or wound disorders, hepatic impairment).

Importance of informing patients of other important precautionary information. (See Cautions.)

Overview® (see Users Guide). For additional information on this drug until a more detailed monograph is developed and published, the manufacturer's labeling should be consulted. It is *essential* that the manufacturer's labeling be consulted for more detailed information on usual cautions, precautions, contraindications, potential drug interactions, laboratory test interferences, and acute toxicity. For further information on the handling of antineoplastic agents, see the ASHP Guidelines on Handling Hazardous Drugs at http://www.ahfsdruginformation.com.

Preparations

Distribution of cabozantinib *S*-malate is restricted. (See Restricted Distribution under Dosage and Administration: General.)

Excipients in commercially available drug preparations may have clinically important effects in some individuals; consult specific product labeling for details.

Cabozantinib *S*-malate

Oral

Capsules	20 mg (of cabozantinib)	**Cometriq®**, Exelixis
Kit	84 Capsules, Cabozantinib *S*-malate 20 mg (of cabozantinib) (Cometriq®)	**Cometriq® 60 mg Daily Dose Blister Cards** (available in a package containing 4 blister cards), Exelixis
	28 Capsules, Cabozantinib *S*-malate 20 mg (of cabozantinib) (Cometriq®) 28 Capsules, Cabozantinib *S*-malate 80 mg (of cabozantinib) (Cometriq®)	**Cometriq® 100 mg Daily Dose Blister Cards** (available in a package containing 4 blister cards), Exelixis
	84 Capsules, Cabozantinib *S*-malate 20 mg (of cabozantinib) (Cometriq®) 28 Capsules, Cabozantinib *S*-malate 80 mg (of cabozantinib) (Cometriq®)	**Cometriq® 140 mg Daily Dose Blister Cards** (available in a package containing 4 blister cards), Exelixis

Capecitabine

■ Capecitabine, a prodrug that has little pharmacologic activity until it is converted to fluorouracil (an antimetabolite) in tumor tissue, is an antineoplastic agent.

Uses

■ **Breast Cancer** *Combination Therapy* Capecitabine is used in combination with docetaxel for the treatment of metastatic breast cancer in patients with disease that failed to respond to, or recurred or relapsed during or following, anthracycline-containing chemotherapy. In addition to their individual antineoplastic effects, combination therapy with these agents appears to have a synergistic effect because docetaxel acts to increase the expression of an enzyme found at higher concentrations in many tumor cells that is involved in converting capecitabine to its active drug, fluorouracil.

The current indication for capecitabine as a component of combination chemotherapy is based principally on the results of an open-label, multicenter, randomized trial involving 511 patients with metastatic breast cancer resistant to or recurring during or following anthracycline-containing therapy, or relapsing during or recurring within 2 years of completion of anthracycline-containing adjuvant therapy. Patients received either combination therapy with capecitabine 1250 mg/m^2 twice daily for 14 days followed by 1 week without treatment and docetaxel 75 mg/m^2 as a 1-hour IV infusion administered on the first day of each 3-week cycle or monotherapy with docetaxel 100 mg/m^2 as a 1-hour IV infusion administered on the first day of each 3-week cycle. Patients receiving combination therapy with capecitabine and docetaxel had increased overall median survival (442 versus 352 days), longer median time to disease progression (186 versus 128 days), and higher objective response rate (32 versus 22%) than those receiving docetaxel alone.

Adverse GI effects and hand-foot syndrome occurred more frequently in patients receiving capecitabine and docetaxel whereas myalgia and arthralgia were more common in those receiving docetaxel alone. Dose reduction (typically involving both drugs) for adverse effects was frequently required in patients receiving combination therapy with capecitabine and docetaxel.

Monotherapy Capecitabine is used as monotherapy for the palliative treatment of metastatic breast cancer in patients with disease resistant to both paclitaxel and an anthracycline-containing chemotherapy regimen or in patients with disease resistant to paclitaxel who are not candidates for further anthracycline therapy (e.g., those who have received cumulative doses of 400 mg/m^2 of doxorubicin or doxorubicin equivalents). Resistance to paclitaxel or an anthracycline agent is defined as progressive disease during treatment (regardless of initial response) with the respective agent or relapse within 6 months of completing adjuvant therapy with a regimen containing the respective agent. Capecitabine became commercially available in the US under the principles and procedures of the accelerated review policy of the US Food and Drug Administration (FDA), which allows approval based on analysis of surrogate markers of response (e.g., tumor shrinkage) rather than clinical end points such as improvement in disease-related symptoms, disease progression, or survival. The principal goal of therapy in patients with metastatic breast cancer generally has been palliative with an emphasis on extension of survival and improvement in the quality of life.

The current indication for capecitabine monotherapy is based principally on the results of a multicenter, open-label, single-arm phase 2 trial in 162 patients (135 patients with measurable disease) with previously treated stage IV breast cancer. Patients in the trial received 3-week treatment cycles of capecitabine 1255 mg/m^2 twice daily for 2 weeks followed by a 1-week rest period. Most patients in the study had 3 or more sites of metastatic disease and predominantly visceral metastases (i.e., lung, pleura, liver, peritoneum). All patients had received prior paclitaxel treatment, and almost all (i.e., greater than 80%) patients also had previous treatment with anthracyclines and fluorouracil; 77% of patients in the study had disease that was resistant to paclitaxel, 41% had disease that was resistant to an anthracycline, and 31% had disease that was resistant to both paclitaxel and an anthracycline.

For the subgroup of 43 patients whose disease was resistant to both paclitaxel and an anthracycline, objective response rate was 25.6% (all partial responses), median time to progression was 102 days (3.4 months), and median survival was 255 days (8.5 months). For the 135 patients with measurable disease, objective response rate was 18.5% (0.7% complete responses, 17.8% partial responses), median time to progression was 90 days (3 months), and median survival was 306 days (10.2 months). Among patients with disease that responded to the drug, onset of response typically occurred within 6–12 weeks of capecitabine therapy.

Comparative studies are under way to confirm the clinical efficacy of capecitabine in patients with metastatic breast cancer. The role of capecitabine in the initial treatment of advanced breast cancer also is being studied.

■ **Colorectal Cancer** ***Adjuvant Therapy for Colon Cancer*** Capecitabine is used alone as adjuvant therapy following the complete resection of primary tumor in patients with stage III (Dukes' C) colon cancer when treatment with fluoropyrimidine therapy alone is preferred. Capecitabine also has been used in combination with oxaliplatin† as adjuvant therapy following the complete resection of the primary tumor in patients with stage III colon cancer.

Monotherapy. The current indication for use of capecitabine alone as adjuvant therapy in patients with stage III (Dukes' C) colon cancer is based principally on the results of a multicenter, randomized, controlled, phase 3 clinical study (X-ACT) in patients with stage III colon cancer who received capecitabine or IV fluorouracil and leucovorin following complete resection of the primary tumor.

In this study, 1987 patients were randomized to receive either capecitabine 1250 mg/m^2 orally twice daily for 2 weeks followed by a 1-week rest period, administered in 3-week cycles for a total of 8 cycles (24 weeks), or rapid IV injection ("bolus") fluorouracil 425 mg/m^2 and IV leucovorin 20 mg/m^2 on days 1–5, administered as 4-week cycles for a total of 6 cycles (24 weeks). The starting dose of capecitabine was reduced in patients with moderate renal impairment (i.e., creatinine clearance 30–50 mL/minute calculated with the formula of Cockroft-Gault) at baseline. For all patients, doses were reduced or interrupted according to toxicity. The median age of patients in this study was 62–63 years.

At a median follow-up of 83 months, the 5-year disease-free (59 versus 55%, respectively; hazard ratio 0.88) and overall (71 versus 68%, respectively; hazard ratio 0.86) survival rates in patients receiving capecitabine were at least equivalent to those in patients receiving fluorouracil and leucovorin as adjuvant therapy for colon cancer. These results indicate that capecitabine is noninferior to fluorouracil and leucovorin as adjuvant therapy for stage III colon cancer. While patients receiving either capecitabine or fluorouracil and leucovorin frequently required dose reductions (42 versus 44%, respectively), delay of treatment cycles (46 versus 29%) and treatment interruption (15 versus 5%) occurred more frequently in patients receiving capecitabine. Subgroup analysis based on prognostic factors (e.g., age, regional lymph node involvement, baseline carcinoembryonic antigen [CEA] concentration) suggested that capecitabine's effect on disease-free and overall survival was consistent across the subgroups, including those 70 years of age or older.

The onset of grade 3 or 4 adverse events was delayed in patients receiving capecitabine compared with those receiving fluorouracil and leucovorin. Hand-foot syndrome (all grades: 60 versus 9%, severe: 17 versus <1%) and grade 3 or 4 hyperbilirubinemia (defined as 1.5 or more times the upper limit of normal) occurred more frequently in patients receiving capecitabine (20 versus 6%), while diarrhea (65 versus 47%), stomatitis (60 versus 22%), nausea (47 versus 34%), alopecia (22 versus 6%), and neutropenia (8 versus 2%) occurred more frequently in patients receiving fluorouracil and leucovorin.

Combination Therapy. Capecitabine has been used in combination with oxaliplatin† (CapeOx) as adjuvant therapy in patients with stage III colon cancer who have undergone complete resection of the primary tumor.

Adjuvant therapy with oxaliplatin in combination with IV fluorouracil and leucovorin has been shown to increase disease-free and overall survival in patients with stage III colon cancer who have undergone complete resection of the primary tumor. Therefore, efficacy and safety of oxaliplatin in combination with capecitabine as adjuvant therapy in patients with stage III colon cancer have been evaluated in an open-label, randomized phase 3 study (NO16968; XELOXA).

In this study, 1886 patients were randomized to receive either combination therapy with oxaliplatin (130 mg/m^2 administered by IV infusion over 2 hours on day 1) and capecitabine (1 g/m^2 administered orally twice daily on days 1–14) on a 3-week cycle for 8 cycles or combination therapy with IV fluorouracil and leucovorin (Mayo Clinic or Roswell Park regimen). The Mayo Clinic regimen consisted of fluorouracil 425 mg/m^2 administered by rapid IV injection ("bolus") and leucovorin 20 mg/m^2 administered by rapid IV infusion on days 1–5 of each 4-week cycle for a total of 6 cycles (24 weeks), and the Roswell Park regimen consisted of fluorouracil 500 mg/m^2 administered by rapid IV injection ("bolus") and leucovorin 500 mg/m^2 administered as a 2-hour IV infusion on day 1 of weeks 1–6 of each 8-week cycle for a total of 4 cycles (32 weeks). Patients were enrolled no more than 8 weeks following surgery with curative intent, by which time full recovery from surgery was required. The median age of patients was 61–62 years. Most patients (99%) enrolled in the study had a baseline ECOG performance status of 0 or 1. The primary measure of efficacy was disease-free survival. At a median follow-up of 74 months, patients who received capecitabine in combination with oxaliplatin had higher disease-free (66.1 versus 59.8%; hazard ratio: 0.8) and relapse-free (69.3 versus 62.2%; hazard ratio: 0.78) survival rates compared with patients who received fluorouracil and leucovorin.

At a median follow-up of 83 months, patients who received capecitabine in combination with oxaliplatin also had a higher overall survival rate (74.4 versus 69.6%; hazard ratio: 0.83) compared with those who received fluorouracil and leucovorin. Subgroup analysis based on prognostic factors (e.g., age, regional lymph node involvement, baseline CEA concentration) suggested that the effect of capecitabine in combination with oxaliplatin on disease-free and overall survival was consistent across the subgroups, including those 70 years of age or older; however, the effect size appeared to be reduced in patients 70 years of age or older compared with younger patients. Neurosensory toxicity (any grade: 78 versus 8%; grade 3 or 4: 11 versus less than 1%), grade 3 or 4 hand-foot syndrome (5 versus less than 1%), and grade 3 or 4 thrombocytopenia (5% versus less than 1%) occurred more frequently in patients receiving capecitabine in combination with oxaliplatin, while grade 3 or 4 neutropenia (9 versus 16%), febrile neutropenia (less than 1 versus 4%), and stomatitis (less than 1 versus 9%) occurred more frequently in those receiving fluorouracil and leucovorin.

Use of combination therapy with oxaliplatin and capecitabine also was investigated in a randomized, multicenter, phase 3 study in patients with high-risk stage II or stage III colorectal cancer who had undergone complete resection of the primary tumor; however, interpretation of the results is limited by the failure to meet the planned accrual of 800 patients in the study to demonstrate superiority. In this study, 408 patients were randomized to receive either combination therapy with oxaliplatin (130 mg/m^2 on day 1) and capecitabine (1 g/m^2 twice daily on days 1–14) on a 3-week cycle for 8 cycles or combination therapy with an oxaliplatin, fluorouracil, and leucovorin (modified FOLFOX6) regimen on a 2-week cycle for 12 cycles. At a median follow-up of 74.7 months, median disease-free and overall survival had not been reached; however, 3-year disease-free and overall survival rates were similar between patients receiving capecitabine in combination with oxaliplatin (79.5 and 86.9%, respectively) compared with patients receiving modified FOLFOX6 (79.8 and 87.2%, respectively).

Based on current evidence, combination therapy with oxaliplatin and capecitabine is a reasonable choice (accepted, treatment option) for use as adjuvant therapy in patients with stage III colon cancer who have undergone complete resection of the primary tumor.

First-line Therapy for Metastatic Colorectal Cancer Capecitabine is used for the first-line treatment of metastatic colorectal cancer when treatment with fluoropyrimidine therapy alone is preferred. Analysis of data from two phase 3 randomized trials indicates that higher response rates but similar duration of progression-free survival are observed for capecitabine compared with fluorouracil and leucovorin (IV loading "bolus" schedule) in previously untreated advanced or metastatic colorectal cancer; no difference in overall survival between the groups was demonstrated.

In 2 randomized trials involving a total of 1207 patients with previously untreated advanced or metastatic colorectal cancer, those receiving capecitabine 1250 mg/m^2 twice daily for 2 weeks followed by a 1-week rest period in 3-week cycles had higher overall objective response rates (21 versus 11% and 21 versus 14%) than those receiving fluorouracil and leucovorin (20 mg/m^2 IV leucovorin followed by 425 mg/m^2 rapid IV injection ["bolus"] fluorouracil, on days 1–5, every 28 days). Median time to progression (128 versus 131 days and 137 versus 131 days) and median survival (380 versus 407 days and 404 versus 369 days) were similar for patients receiving capecitabine versus fluorouracil and leucovorin. Pooled data from the two studies is consistent with capecitabine showing retention of at least 50% of the survival effect of fluorouracil and leucovorin; these results do not exclude the possibility of true equivalence of capecitabine to this schedule of fluorouracil and leucovorin.

Hand-foot syndrome and hyperbilirubinemia were more common and greater in severity in those receiving capecitabine, whereas stomatitis and neutropenia occurred more frequently and with greater severity in patients receiving fluorouracil and leucovorin. In both randomized trials, data analysis showed later onset of serious adverse reactions and longer median time to dose reduction in patients receiving capecitabine compared with those receiving fluorouracil and leucovorin as the IV loading rapid IV ("bolus") schedule. The comparative efficacy and toxicity of capecitabine compared with other parenteral fluorouracil regimens (e.g., weekly "bolus" fluorouracil and leucovorin, continuous IV infusion fluorouracil) is not known. In addition to its equivalent efficacy and differing toxicity profile from the schedule of parenteral fluorouracil used in these randomized trials, the convenience of capecitabine, a prodrug of fluorouracil that is administered orally, may be a factor in choice of drug therapy.

A survival benefit has been demonstrated for the use of fluorouracil and leucovorin in combination with other agents compared with fluorouracil and leucovorin alone for advanced colorectal cancer. A survival benefit for the use of capecitabine alone versus fluorouracil and leucovorin has not been demonstrated. The comparative safety and efficacy of combination regimens using capecitabine as a substitute for fluorouracil and leucovorin is being investigated.

■ **Other Uses** Capecitabine also has been used for treatment of gastric cancer†. Interim results of phase 3 randomized trials suggest that capecitabine is noninferior with regard to progression-free survival or overall survival when used in place of fluorouracil in combination regimens for advanced gastric cancer.

Dosage and Administration

■ **Administration** Capecitabine is administered orally. Capecitabine tablets should be swallowed whole with water within 30 minutes after the end of a meal; the tablets should not be cut or crushed. Although some clinicians state that capecitabine may be administered concomitantly with antacids containing aluminum and magnesium hydroxide, other clinicians advise delay of administration of antacids for at least 2 hours following induction of capecitabine therapy.

Individual adjustment of capecitabine dosage may be necessary for optimal management.

■ **Dosage** ***Breast Cancer*** **Combination Therapy.** When used in combination therapy with docetaxel for the treatment of metastatic breast cancer in patients with disease that failed to respond to or recurred following anthracycline-containing chemotherapy, the recommended initial dosage of capecitabine is 1250 mg/m^2 twice daily (morning and evening), equivalent to a total daily dose of 2500 mg/m^2, for 2 weeks followed by a 1-week rest period; courses of therapy are given in 3-week cycles. Docetaxel 75 mg/m^2 is administered as a 1-hour IV infusion on the first day of each 3-week cycle. Patients should be premedicated prior to docetaxel administration (see Dosage and Administration: Dosage in Docetaxel 10:00). Treatment with the combination regimen was continued for at least 6 weeks in the randomized trial.

Treatment interruptions and dosage reductions because of adverse effects were required in 79 and 65%, respectively, of patients receiving capecitabine and docetaxel for metastatic breast cancer.

Monotherapy. For the palliative treatment of metastatic breast cancer in patients with disease resistant to both paclitaxel and an anthracycline-containing chemotherapy regimen or in patients with disease resistant to paclitaxel who are not candidates for further anthracycline therapy (e.g., those who have received cumulative doses of 400 mg/m^2 of doxorubicin or doxorubicin equivalents), the recommended initial dosage of capecitabine is 1250 mg/m^2 twice daily (morning and evening), equivalent to 2500 mg/m^2 total daily dose, for 2 weeks followed by a 1-week rest period; courses of therapy are given in 3-week cycles. Some experts suggest that a trial of 2 cycles (i.e., 6 weeks) of capecitabine therapy is adequate to assess response to the drug. During a clinical trial of patients with metastatic breast cancer, onset of response typically occurred within 6–12 weeks of capecitabine therapy.

Colorectal Cancer **Adjuvant Therapy for Colon Cancer.** For adjuvant therapy following the complete resection of primary tumor in patients with stage III (Dukes' C) colon cancer when treatment with fluoropyrimidine therapy alone is preferred, the recommended dosage of capecitabine is 1250 mg/m^2 twice daily (morning and evening) for 2 weeks followed by a 1-week rest period; courses of therapy are given in 3-week cycles for a total of 8 cycles and a treatment period of 6 months.

When capecitabine has been used in combination with oxaliplatin† (CapeOx) as adjuvant therapy following the complete resection of the primary tumor in patients with stage III colon cancer, capecitabine 1 g/m^2 has been administered orally twice daily on days 1–14 and oxaliplatin 130 mg/m^2 has been administered by IV infusion over 2 hours on day 1 of each 3-week cycle. Treatment has been continued for 8 cycles of therapy.

First-line Therapy for Metastatic Colorectal Cancer. For the first-line treatment of metastatic colorectal cancer when treatment with fluoropyrimidine therapy alone is preferred, the recommended initial dosage of capecitabine is 1250 mg/m^2 twice daily (morning and evening), equivalent to 2500 mg/m^2 total daily dose, for 2 weeks followed by a 1-week rest period; courses of therapy are given in 3-week cycles.

Other Dosage Considerations The following Recommended Initial Dosage table indicates the recommended initial dosage of capecitabine according to body surface area.

Table 1. Recommended Initial Dosage of Capecitabine: 1250 mg/m^2 twice daily

Body Surface Area (m^2)	Total Daily Dose (mg) [a]
≤1.25	3000
1.26–1.37	3300
1.38–1.51	3600
1.52–1.65	4000
1.66–1.77	4300
1.78–1.91	4600
1.92–2.05	5000
2.06–2.17	5300
≥2.18	5600

[a] divide into 2 equal doses given morning and evening

Therapy with capecitabine should not be initiated in patients with baseline neutrophil counts of less than 1500/mm^3 and/or baseline platelet counts of less than 100,000/mm^3.

Dosage Modification for Age-related Effects. Some clinicians recommend that capecitabine dosage be reduced (e.g., initial dosage reduced by up to 20%) in patients older than 80 years of age receiving capecitabine monotherapy. Because of decreased tolerance of the combination regimen of capecitabine and docetaxel for advanced breast cancer in patients 60 years of age or older, a 25% reduction of the initial capecitabine dose (to 950 mg/m^2) should be considered. (See Cautions: Geriatric Precautions.)

Dosage Modification for Toxicity. After the initial dose of capecitabine, subsequent doses should be modified as necessary based on individual patient tolerance with careful monitoring to obtain optimal therapeutic response with minimal toxicity. (See Cautions and the following table on Criteria for Selected Toxicities Commonly Associated with Capecitabine Therapy for information on specific adverse effects of capecitabine.) The dose-limiting toxicities of capecitabine include diarrhea, nausea, vomiting, abdominal pain, palmar-plantar erythrodysesthesia (hand-foot syndrome), and leukopenia.

If a patient experiences a grade 4 toxicity, the drug should be discontinued or therapy interrupted until the toxicity resolves or decreases in intensity to grade 1; if capecitabine therapy is resumed, the dose should be decreased to 50% of the original dose. If a patient experiences a grade 2 or 3 toxicity, capecitabine therapy should be interrupted until the toxicity resolves or decreases in severity to grade 1.

At the start of the next treatment cycle, subsequent doses should be reduced according to the severity and number of appearances of the toxicity as shown in the following table on Recommended Dosage Modifications for Toxicity of Capecitabine. The manufacturer states that once the capecitabine dosage has been reduced, the dosage should not be increased at a later time.

When capecitabine therapy is interrupted because of toxicity, therapy should be resumed according to planned treatment cycles; doses of the drug omitted because of toxicity should not be replaced.

If a patient experiences either no toxicity or NCIC grade 1 toxicity within a course of treatment, the current capecitabine dose level may be maintained for subsequent courses of therapy until more serious toxicity occurs.

In patients receiving capecitabine in combination with docetaxel, modification of the docetaxel dosage also may be required, as shown in the table on Recommended Dosage Modifications for Docetaxel During Capecitabine and Docetaxel Combination Therapy. If initiation of a treatment cycle must be delayed because of toxicity associated with either capecitabine or docetaxel, administration of both drugs should be delayed until the criteria for reinitiating therapy with both drugs are met.

Table 2. Criteria for Selected Toxicities Commonly Associated with Capecitabine Therapy[a]

Toxicity	Grade	Criteria
Diarrhea	1	2–3 stools daily > pretreatment
	2	4–6 stools daily > pretreatment or nocturnal stools
	3	7–9 stools daily > pretreatment or incontinence and malabsorption
	4	>10 stools daily > pretreatment, grossly bloody diarrhea, or need for parenteral support
Nausea	1	able to eat reasonable intake of food
	2	significant decrease in intake of food but able to eat intermittently
	3	no significant intake of food
Vomiting	1	1 episode in 24 hours
	2	2–5 episodes in 24 hours
	3	6–10 episodes in 24 hours
	4	>10 episodes in 24 hours, dehydration, or need for parenteral support
Abdominal pain	1	pain but no treatment required
	2	pain controlled with nonopiates
	3	pain controlled with opiates
	4	uncontrollable pain
Palmar-plantar erythrodysesthesia (hand-foot syndrome)	1	numbness, dysesthesia/paresthesia, tingling, painless swelling, or erythema of the hands and/or feet that causes discomfort but does not disrupt normal activities of daily living
	2	painful erythema and swelling of the hands and/or feet that results in discomfort affecting the normal activities of daily living
	3	moist desquamation, ulceration, blistering, and severe pain of the hands and/or feet and/or severe discomfort that causes inability to work or perform activities of daily living
Lymphopenia	1	lymphocyte count 1500–1999/mm^3
	2	lymphocyte count 1000–1499/mm^3
	3	lymphocyte count 500–999/mm^3
	4	lymphocyte count <500/mm^3

[a] NCIC Common Toxicity Criteria except for hand-foot syndrome, which is defined according to a grading system incorporated by Roche and accepted by the FDA; consult NCIC Common Toxicity Criteria for grading of other toxicities.

Table 3. Recommended Dosage Modifications for Toxicity of Capecitabine

NCIC Grade of Toxicity[a]	Number of Appearances	During a Course of Therapy[b]	Dose Adjustment for Next Cycle (% of Initial Dose)
No toxicity		Maintain dose level	Maintain dose level
Grade 1	Any appearance	Maintain dose level	Maintain dose level
Grade 2	1st appearance	Interrupt therapy until resolved to grade 0–1	100%
	2nd appearance	Interrupt therapy until resolved to grade 0–1	75%
	3rd appearance	Interrupt therapy until resolved to grade 0–1	50%
	4th appearance	Discontinue drug permanently	
Grade 3	1st appearance	Interrupt therapy until resolved to grade 0–1	75%
	2nd appearance	Interrupt therapy until resolved to grade 0–1	50%
	3rd appearance	Discontinue drug permanently	
Grade 4	1st appearance	Discontinue drug permanently *or* If deemed in best interest of patient to continue therapy, interrupt therapy until resolved to grade 0–1	50%

[a] NCIC Common Toxicity Criteria except for hand-foot syndrome, which is defined according to a grading system incorporated by Roche and accepted by the FDA.

[b] All dose modifications should be based on the worst preceding toxicity.

Table 4. Recommended Dosage Modifications for Docetaxel During Capecitabine and Docetaxel Combination Therapy[a]

NCIC Grade of Toxicity[b]	Number of Appearances	Dosage Modification
Grade 2	1st appearance	Interrupt therapy until resolved to grade 0–1, then resume therapy at 100% of the original dose of docetaxel (75 mg/m^2)
	2nd appearance	Interrupt therapy until resolved to grade 0–1, then resume therapy with docetaxel 55 mg/m^2
	3rd appearance	Discontinue docetaxel therapy
Grade 3	1st appearance	Interrupt therapy until resolved to grade 0–1, then resume therapy with docetaxel 55 mg/m^2
	2nd appearance	Discontinue docetaxel therapy
Grade 4	1st appearance	Discontinue docetaxel therapy

[a] Prophylaxis for toxicity should be instituted whenever possible; all dosage modifications should be based on the worst preceding toxicity.

[b] NCIC Common Toxicity Criteria except for hand-foot syndrome, which is defined according to a grading system incorporated by Roche and accepted by the FDA.

■ **Dosage in Renal and Hepatic Impairment** Capecitabine is *contraindicated* in patients with severe renal impairment (i.e., creatinine clearance less than 30 mL/minute calculated with the formula of Cockroft-Gault). In patients with moderate renal impairment (i.e., creatinine clearance 30–50 mL/minute calculated with the formula of Cockroft-Gault), a dosage reduction to 75% of the initial capecitabine dose when used as monotherapy or in combination with docetaxel (i.e., from 1250 to 950 mg/m^2 twice daily) is recommended. No adjustment in starting dose is recommended in patients with mild renal impairment. Careful monitoring is required in patients with mild or moderate renal impairment receiving capecitabine because the frequency and/or severity of adverse effects of capecitabine may be increased. If the patient develops a grade 2, 3, or 4 adverse effect, treatment with capecitabine should be discontinued promptly, and subsequent dose modification for toxicity should be made. (See table on Recommended Dosage Modifications for Toxicity of Capecitabine in Dosage and Administration: Dosage.)

The effects of hepatic impairment on the pharmacokinetics of capecitabine have not been fully evaluated. The manufacturer states that no adjustment in initial dosage of capecitabine is necessary in patients with mild to moderate hepatic dysfunction secondary to liver metastases. However, caution is advised and patients with mild to moderate hepatic dysfunction should be monitored carefully during capecitabine therapy. The safety and efficacy of capecitabine in patients with severe hepatic impairment have not been evaluated.

Cautions

Most adverse effects associated with capecitabine are reversible and do not necessitate discontinuance of the drug; however, depending on the severity and recurrence of the adverse effect, capecitabine doses may need to be withheld or reduced.

The incidence of adverse effects associated with capecitabine therapy for metastatic disease is derived principally from data for patients receiving the drug as a single agent in clinical trials for metastatic breast cancer (162 patients, mean duration of treatment of 114 days) or metastatic colorectal cancer (596 patients, median duration of treatment of 139 days) or in combination with docetaxel for metastatic breast cancer (251 patients, mean duration of treatment of 129 days). Unless otherwise specified, the incidence of adverse effects in patients with metastatic disease reflects the use of capecitabine alone or in combination with docetaxel. Information on adverse effects occurring in fewer than 5% of patients receiving capecitabine monotherapy for metastatic breast cancer or metastatic colorectal cancer is derived from a clinical trial safety database reporting on 875 patients. The severity of adverse effects was graded according to toxicity criteria established by the National Cancer Institute of Canada (NCIC). Among patients receiving capecitabine in clinical trials, 8–13% or 26% of patients receiving the drug as a single agent for metastatic breast cancer or metastatic colorectal cancer, or in combination therapy for metastatic breast cancer, respectively, discontinued treatment because of adverse effects or intercurrent illness. Abdominal pain, diarrhea, and hand-foot syndrome were among the most common adverse events leading to withdrawal from the study among patients receiving capecitabine for metastatic breast cancer in clinical trials. Among patients with metastatic colorectal cancer, death due to all causes occurred during the study or within 28 days of receiving the study drug in 50 patients (8.4%) randomized to receive capecitabine compared with 32 patients (5.4%) randomized to receive 5-fluorouracil and leucovorin.

The incidence of adverse effects associated with capecitabine as adjuvant therapy for colon cancer is derived principally from data for patients receiving the drug as a single agent in a phase 3 study for stage III colon cancer (995 patients, median duration of treatment of 164 days). Among patients receiving capecitabine as adjuvant therapy for stage III colon cancer in a clinical trial, 11% discontinued treatment because of adverse effects and 0.8% died during the study or within 28 days of receiving the study drug.

■ GI Effects Diarrhea, a dose-limiting and common adverse effect of capecitabine, occurs in 55–67% of patients receiving the drug for metastatic breast cancer or metastatic colorectal cancer, and is severe or life-threatening in 15% of patients. Nausea and vomiting occur in 43–53% and 27–37%, respectively, of patients receiving capecitabine for metastatic breast cancer or metastatic colorectal cancer. Among patients with metastatic breast cancer who developed severe nausea and/or vomiting associated with capecitabine monotherapy, onset of these adverse GI effects was early, usually occurring during the first month of treatment.

Among patients receiving capecitabine alone as adjuvant therapy for stage III colon cancer, diarrhea occurred in 47% of patients and was severe or life-threatening (grade 3 or 4) in 12%; nausea occurred in 34%, and vomiting in 15%, of patients.

Severe adverse GI effects associated with capecitabine may occur more frequently in geriatric patients. Among 21 patients aged 80 years or older receiving capecitabine monotherapy for metastatic breast cancer or metastatic colorectal cancer in clinical trials, severe or life-threatening (grade 3 or 4) diarrhea, nausea, or vomiting occurred in 29, 14, or 10%, respectively. Among 10 patients aged 70–80 years receiving capecitabine in combination with docetaxel for metastatic breast cancer, grade 3 or 4 diarrhea and stomatitis each occurred in 30%.

The median time to onset of grade 2 to 4 diarrhea was 34 days (range: 1–369 days) following initiation of capecitabine therapy for metastatic breast cancer or metastatic colorectal cancer, and the median duration of grade 3 to 4 diarrhea was 5 days. According to NCIC toxicity criteria, grade 1 diarrhea is defined as an increase of 2–3 stools daily; grade 2 diarrhea, an increase of 4–6 stools daily or nocturnal stools; grade 3 diarrhea, an increase of 7–9 stools daily or incontinence and malabsorption; and grade 4 diarrhea, an increase of 10 or more stools daily, grossly bloody diarrhea, or the need for parenteral support. If grade 2, 3, or 4 diarrhea occurs, administration of capecitabine should be discontinued immediately until the diarrhea resolves or decreases in intensity to grade 1. The manufacturer recommends use of standard antidiarrheal therapy (e.g., loperamide) in patients experiencing diarrhea. Patients with severe diarrhea should be closely monitored and given fluid and electrolyte replacement for dehydration as indicated. Subsequent doses of capecitabine should be decreased in patients who have experienced grade 3 or 4 diarrhea or recurring episodes of grade 2 diarrhea. (See table on Recommended Dosage Modifications for Toxicity of Capecitabine in Dosage and Administration: Dosage.)

Abdominal pain has been reported in 20–35% of patients receiving capecitabine monotherapy for metastatic breast cancer or metastatic colorectal cancer or capecitabine and docetaxel for metastatic breast cancer. Among patients receiving capecitabine alone as adjuvant therapy for stage III colon cancer, abdominal pain occurred in 14%, and upper abdominal pain in 7%, of patients. Stomatitis has occurred in about 25% of patients receiving capecitabine monotherapy for metastatic breast cancer or metastatic colorectal cancer; a higher incidence of stomatitis (67%), including severe or life-threatening stomatitis (approximately 20%), was reported in patients receiving capecitabine and docetaxel for metastatic breast cancer. Among patients receiving capecitabine alone as adjuvant therapy for stage III colon cancer, stomatitis occurred in 22% of patients. Constipation has been reported in 14–20% of patients receiving the drug for metastatic breast cancer or metastatic colorectal cancer and in 9% of patients receiving capecitabine alone as adjuvant therapy for stage III colon cancer. Among patients receiving capecitabine for metastatic colorectal cancer, GI motility disorder or oral discomfort each occurred in 10%, upper GI inflammatory disorders in 8%, and GI hemorrhage in 6%. Taste disturbance, which was reported in 6% of patients receiving capecitabine alone for metastatic colorectal cancer, occurred in about 15% of patients receiving either capecitabine and docetaxel or docetaxel alone for metastatic breast cancer.

Among patients receiving capecitabine for metastatic breast cancer, dyspepsia was reported in 8–14% of those receiving the drug alone or in combination therapy; dry mouth was reported in 6% of those receiving the drug in combination therapy. Among patients receiving capecitabine alone as adjuvant therapy for stage III colon cancer, dyspepsia occurred in 6% of patients.

Adverse GI effects occurring in less than 5% of patients receiving capecitabine monotherapy for metastatic breast cancer or metastatic colorectal cancer in clinical trials include abdominal distention, dysphagia, proctalgia, ascites, gastric ulcer, ileus, toxic dilation of the intestine, and gastroenteritis. Ileus, necrotizing enterocolitis, esophageal ulcer, and hemorrhagic diarrhea have been reported in less than 5% of patients receiving capecitabine and docetaxel for metastatic breast cancer; intestinal obstruction, rectal bleeding, esophagitis, gastritis, colitis, duodenitis, and hematemesis also have been reported in patients receiving capecitabine.

■ Hematologic Effects and Infectious Complications Among those receiving capecitabine as a single agent or in combination therapy for metastatic breast cancer, lymphopenia is a common adverse effect, occurring in 94–99% of patients; grade 3 or grade 4 lymphopenia has been reported in approximately 60–90% of such patients. Among patients receiving capecitabine alone as adjuvant therapy for stage III colon cancer, grade 3 or 4 decreased lymphocyte concentrations occurred in 13% of patients. Leukopenia, which was reported in less than 5% of patients receiving capecitabine monotherapy for metastatic breast cancer or metastatic colorectal cancer, occurred in about 90% of patients receiving either capecitabine and docetaxel or docetaxel alone for metastatic breast cancer and was often severe or life-threatening. Thrombocytopenia has been reported in 41% of patients receiving capecitabine and docetaxel for metastatic breast cancer, and in 24% of patients receiving capecitabine alone, for metastatic breast cancer. Among patients receiving capecitabine alone as adjuvant therapy for stage III colon cancer, grade 3 or 4 decreased platelet concentrations occurred in 1% of patients.

Anemia occurred in 72–80% of patients receiving capecitabine alone for metastatic breast cancer or metastatic colorectal cancer. Anemia occurred in 80% of patients receiving capecitabine and docetaxel for metastatic breast cancer and was severe or life-threatening in 10%. Among patients receiving capecitabine alone as adjuvant therapy for stage III colon cancer, grade 3 or 4 decreased hemoglobin concentrations occurred in 1% of patients.

Neutropenia has been reported in 13–26% of patients receiving capecitabine as a single agent for metastatic breast cancer or metastatic colorectal cancer; neutropenia/granulocytopenia, often severe or life-threatening, occurred frequently in patients receiving either capecitabine and docetaxel (86%) or docetaxel alone (87%) for metastatic breast cancer. Severe or life-threatening neutropenic fever was reported in 16% of patients receiving capecitabine and docetaxel and in 21% of patients receiving docetaxel alone for metastatic breast cancer. Among patients receiving capecitabine alone as adjuvant therapy for stage III colon cancer, neutropenia occurred in 2% of patients.

Adverse hematologic effects reported in less than 5% of patients receiving capecitabine monotherapy for metastatic breast cancer or metastatic colorectal cancer in clinical trials include hemorrhage, coagulation disorder, idiopathic thrombocytopenic purpura, pancytopenia, and bone marrow depression. Agranulocytosis and decreased prothrombin time have been reported in less than 5% of patients receiving capecitabine and docetaxel for metastatic breast cancer.

Oral candidiasis (7%) or urinary tract infection (6%) occurred in patients receiving capecitabine and docetaxel for metastatic breast cancer; similar rates of such infections were observed in patients receiving docetaxel alone. Urinary tract infection also has been reported in patients receiving capecitabine as a single agent. Unspecified viral infection occurred in 5% of patients receiving capecitabine monotherapy for metastatic colorectal cancer. Infectious complications reported in less than 5% of patients receiving capecitabine monotherapy for metastatic breast cancer or metastatic colorectal cancer in clinical trials include sepsis, gastroenteritis, bronchitis, pneumonia, bronchopneumonia, laryngitis, keratoconjunctivitis, influenza-like illness, and fungal infections (including candidiasis). Upper respiratory tract infection has been reported in patients receiving capecitabine as a single agent or in combination with docetaxel; neutropenic sepsis also has been reported in patients receiving capecitabine and docetaxel for metastatic breast cancer.

■ Dermatologic and Sensitivity Reactions Palmar-plantar erythrodysesthesia or chemotherapy-induced acral erythema (commonly referred to as hand-foot syndrome) is a cutaneous toxicity ranging in severity from grade 1 to grade 3 that occurs in 54–63% of patients receiving capecitabine for metastatic breast cancer or metastatic colorectal cancer and is severe (grade 3) in 11–24% of patients. Among patients receiving capecitabine alone as adjuvant therapy for stage III colon cancer, hand-foot syndrome occurred in 60% of patients and was severe (grade 3 or 4) in 17% of patients. Grade 1 hand-foot syndrome is defined as numbness, dysesthesia/paresthesia, tingling, painless swelling, and/or erythema of the hands and/or feet that causes discomfort but does not disrupt the patient's normal activities of daily living; grade 2 hand-foot syndrome is defined as painful erythema and swelling of the hands and/or feet that results in discomfort affecting the patient's activities of daily living; grade 3 hand-foot syndrome is defined as moist desquamation, ulceration, blistering, or severe pain of the hands and/or feet and/or severe discomfort that causes the patient to be unable to work or perform activities of daily living. The median time to onset of hand-foot syndrome was 79 days (range: 11–360 days) in patients receiving capecitabine monotherapy for metastatic breast cancer or metastatic colorectal cancer in clinical trials.

Severe adverse dermatologic effects associated with capecitabine may occur more frequently in geriatric patients. Among 21 patients aged 80 years or older receiving capecitabine for metastatic breast cancer or metastatic colorectal cancer in clinical trials, severe (grade 3) hand-foot syndrome occurred in 14%. Among 10 patients aged 70–80 years receiving capecitabine in combination with docetaxel for metastatic breast cancer, grade 3 hand-foot syndrome occurred in 40%.

If grade 2 or 3 hand-foot syndrome occurs, administration of capecitabine should be interrupted until manifestations resolve or decrease in intensity to grade 1. Subsequent doses of capecitabine should be decreased in patients experiencing grade 3 hand-foot syndrome or recurring episodes of grade 2 hand-foot syndrome. (See table on Recommended Dosage Modifications for Toxicity of Capecitabine in Dosage and Administration: Dosage.) In addition to dose interruption and subsequent dose reductions, topical emollients (e.g., hand creams, udder balm) or oral pyridoxine therapy may ameliorate the manifestations of hand-foot syndrome in patients receiving capecitabine.

Severe, sometimes fatal, mucocutaneous reactions such as Stevens-Johnson syndrome and toxic epidermal necrolysis also can occur in patients receiving capecitabine. If such reactions occur and are potentially related to capecitabine, therapy with the drug should be permanently discontinued.

Capecitabine-induced dermatitis has been reported in 27–37% of patients receiving the drug alone for metastatic breast cancer or metastatic colorectal cancer and in 8% of patients receiving capecitabine and docetaxel for metastatic breast cancer. Alopecia, which was reported in 6% of patients receiving capecitabine alone for metastatic colorectal cancer or as adjuvant therapy for stage III colon cancer, occurred in about 40% of those receiving either capecitabine and docetaxel or docetaxel alone for metastatic breast cancer. Skin discoloration was reported in 7% of patients receiving capecitabine for metastatic colorectal cancer. Nail disorder, which was reported in less than 5% of patients receiving capecitabine alone for metastatic breast cancer or metastatic colorectal cancer, occurred in about 15% of patients receiving either capecitabine and docetaxel or docetaxel alone for metastatic breast cancer. Erythematous rash, nail discoloration, and onycholysis have been reported in 9, 6, and 5%, respectively, of patients receiving capecitabine and docetaxel for metastatic breast cancer. Among patients receiving capecitabine alone as adjuvant therapy for stage III colon cancer, rash occurred in 7%, and erythema in 6%, of patients. Adverse dermatologic effects reported in less than 5% of patients receiving capecitabine monotherapy for metastatic breast cancer or metastatic colorectal cancer in clinical trials include increased sweating, photosensitivity, skin ulceration, pruritus, and radiation recall syndrome.

Hypersensitivity reactions, including bronchospasm, have been reported in patients receiving capecitabine.

■ **Nervous System Effects** Fatigue/weakness has been reported in about 40% of patients receiving capecitabine monotherapy for metastatic breast cancer or metastatic colorectal cancer and 16–22% of those receiving capecitabine and docetaxel for metastatic breast cancer in clinical trials. Among patients receiving capecitabine alone as adjuvant therapy for stage III colon cancer, fatigue occurred in 16%, and lethargy in 10%, of patients. Asthenia was reported in about 25% of patients receiving either capecitabine and docetaxel or docetaxel alone for metastatic breast cancer and in 10% of patients receiving capecitabine alone as adjuvant therapy for stage III colon cancer. The incidence of pain was higher in the subset of patients receiving capecitabine for metastatic colorectal cancer than in the overall database of patients receiving capecitabine monotherapy for metastatic colorectal cancer or metastatic breast cancer (12% versus less than 5%).

Paresthesia occurred in 12–21% of patients receiving capecitabine alone or in combination with docetaxel for metastatic breast cancer. Headache was reported in 9–15% of patients receiving capecitabine alone for metastatic breast cancer or metastatic colorectal cancer or in combination with docetaxel for metastatic breast cancer. Dizziness occurred in approximately 10% of patients receiving capecitabine for metastatic breast cancer or metastatic colorectal cancer in clinical trials. Among patients receiving capecitabine alone as adjuvant therapy for stage III colon cancer, dizziness occurred in 6%, dysgeusia in 6%, and headache in 5%, of patients. Peripheral neuropathy has occurred in patients receiving capecitabine as a single agent for metastatic colorectal cancer (10%) and in patients receiving capecitabine and docetaxel for metastatic breast cancer (6%). Mood alteration was reported in 5% of patients receiving capecitabine for metastatic colorectal cancer.

Insomnia, ataxia, tremor, dysphasia, encephalopathy, abnormal coordination, dysarthria, loss of consciousness, vertigo, impaired balance, irritability, sedation, mental depression, and confusion have been reported in less than 5% of patients receiving capecitabine monotherapy for metastatic breast cancer or metastatic colorectal cancer in clinical trials. Depressed level of consciousness and syncope also have been reported in patients receiving capecitabine. Hypoesthesia, ataxia, syncope, taste loss, polyneuropathy, and migraine headache have been reported in less than 5% of patients receiving capecitabine and docetaxel for metastatic breast cancer. Lethargy also has been reported in patients receiving combined therapy with the drugs.

■ **Hepatic Effects** Adverse hepatobiliary effects associated with capecitabine include elevations in serum concentrations of bilirubin, alkaline phosphatase, and hepatic aminotransferases (i.e., AST and/or ALT).

Hyperbilirubinemia was reported in 48% of patients receiving capecitabine as a single agent for metastatic colorectal cancer, and was severe or life-threatening in 18 or 5%, respectively. Among patients receiving capecitabine alone as adjuvant therapy for stage III colon cancer, grade 3 or 4 hyperbilirubinemia occurred in 20% of patients. Hyperbilirubinemia occurred in about 20% of patients receiving capecitabine alone or in combination with docetaxel for metastatic breast cancer, and was severe or life-threatening in about 8 or 2%, respectively. According to the overall database of 875 patients with metastatic colorectal cancer or metastatic breast cancer receiving at least one twice-daily dose of capecitabine, severe (grade 3) or life-threatening (grade 4) hyperbilirubinemia occurred in 15 or 4%, respectively. In patients with metastatic colorectal cancer, the median time to onset of grade 3 or 4 hyperbilirubinemia was 64 days, and the median total serum bilirubin concentration increased from 8 μm/L at baseline to 13 μm/L during capecitabine therapy.

According to NCIC version 1 toxicity criteria, grade 2 hyperbilirubinemia is defined as an elevated serum bilirubin concentration of up to 1.5 times the normal value; grade 3 hyperbilirubinemia, 1.5–3 times the normal value; and grade 4 hyperbilirubinemia, greater than 3 times the normal value. If grade 2, 3, or 4 elevations in serum bilirubin concentration occur, administration of capecitabine should be discontinued until the hyperbilirubinemia resolves or decreases in intensity to grade 1.

Severe or life-threatening hyperbilirubinemia associated with capecitabine therapy occurs more frequently in patients with hepatic metastases; among 566 patients with hepatic metastases and 309 patients without hepatic metastases at baseline of a total of 875 patients with metastatic breast cancer or metastatic colorectal cancer, hyperbilirubinemia (grade 3 or 4) occurred in 23 and 12%, respectively. Liver function should be monitored carefully during capecitabine therapy in patients with mild to moderate hepatic impairment secondary to liver metastases.

Among patients with metastatic breast cancer or metastatic colorectal cancer who had grade 3 or 4 hyperbilirubinemia, both prebaseline and postbaseline elevations in serum concentrations of alkaline phosphatase or hepatic aminotransferase occurred in 58 or 35%, respectively. Among patients with metastatic breast cancer or metastatic colorectal cancer who had grade 3 or 4 hyperbilirubinemia, postbaseline only (but not necessarily concurrent) elevations in alkaline phosphatase or hepatic aminotransferase concentrations occurred in 19 or 28% and were severe/life-threatening in 8 or 3%, respectively; a majority of these patients had hepatic metastases.

Hepatic failure, hepatic fibrosis, cholestatic hepatitis, hepatitis, and abnormal liver function test results have been reported in less than 5% of patients receiving capecitabine monotherapy for metastatic breast cancer or metastatic colorectal cancer in clinical trials. Jaundice, abnormal liver function test results, hepatic failure, hepatic coma, and hepatotoxicity have been reported in less than 5% of patients receiving capecitabine and docetaxel for metastatic breast cancer.

Among patients receiving capecitabine alone as adjuvant therapy for stage III colon cancer, grade 3 or 4 increased serum ALT concentrations occurred in 1.6% of patients.

■ **Cardiovascular Effects** Myocardial infarction/ischemia, angina, dysrhythmias, cardiac arrest, cardiac failure, sudden death, ECG changes, and cardiomyopathy have occurred in patients receiving capecitabine. The incidence of these adverse cardiovascular effects may be increased in patients with a history of coronary artery disease.

The incidence of edema was higher in the subsets of patients receiving capecitabine as a single agent for metastatic colorectal cancer (15%) or metastatic breast cancer (9%) than in the overall database of patients receiving capecitabine monotherapy for metastatic colorectal cancer or metastatic breast cancer (less than 5%); edema was reported in about 35% of those receiving either capecitabine and docetaxel or docetaxel alone for metastatic breast cancer. Venous thrombosis was reported in 8% of patients receiving capecitabine monotherapy for metastatic colorectal cancer. Other adverse cardiovascular effects, including tachycardia, bradycardia, atrial fibrillation, ventricular extrasystoles, extrasystoles, myocarditis, pericardial effusion, hypotension, hypertension, lymphedema, pulmonary embolism, hot flushes, and cerebrovascular accident, have been reported in less than 5% of patients receiving capecitabine monotherapy for metastatic breast cancer or metastatic colorectal cancer in clinical trials. Supraventricular tachycardia, venous phlebitis and thrombophlebitis, and postural hypotension have been reported in less than 5% of patients receiving capecitabine and docetaxel for metastatic breast cancer; flushing also has been reported in patients receiving combined therapy with the drugs. Deep-vein thrombosis also has been reported in patients receiving capecitabine.

■ **Metabolic Effects** Decreased appetite was reported in 26% of patients receiving capecitabine alone for metastatic colorectal cancer and in 10% of patients receiving capecitabine and docetaxel for metastatic breast cancer. Anorexia occurred in 13–23% of patients receiving capecitabine alone or in combination with docetaxel for metastatic breast cancer. Among patients receiving capecitabine alone as adjuvant therapy for stage III colon cancer, anorexia occurred in 9% of patients. Dehydration was reported in 7–10% of patients receiving capecitabine alone for metastatic breast cancer or metastatic colorectal cancer or in combination with docetaxel for metastatic breast cancer. Decreased weight occurred in 7% of patients receiving capecitabine and docetaxel for metastatic breast cancer. Increased weight, cachexia, hypertriglyceridemia, hypokalemia, and hypomagnesemia occurred in less than 5% of patients receiving capecitabine monotherapy for metastatic breast cancer or metastatic colorectal cancer in clinical trials.

Dehydration can develop rapidly in patients with anorexia, asthenia, nausea, vomiting, or diarrhea. Acute renal failure secondary to dehydration, which can be fatal, can occur; patients with preexisting renal impairment and those receiving concomitant therapy with nephrotoxic agents are at increased risk. Dehydration should be corrected at its onset. In patients with grade 2 or greater dehydration, capecitabine therapy should interrupted immediately, and treatment should not be restarted until the patient is rehydrated and any precipitating causes have been corrected or controlled; any necessary dosage modifications for the precipitating adverse event should be made. (See Dosage Modification for Toxicity under Dosage: Other Dosage Considerations, in Dosage and Administration.)

■ **Ocular Effects** Ocular irritation occurred in 5–15% of patients receiving capecitabine for metastatic breast cancer or metastatic colorectal cancer. Abnormal vision occurred in 5% of patients receiving capecitabine monotherapy for metastatic colorectal cancer. Severe ocular irritation and corneal deposits were reported in 2 patients with a history of keratoconjunctivitis sicca who received higher doses of capecitabine for metastatic breast cancer or metastatic colon cancer. Ophthalmic examination is recommended for patients receiving capecitabine who experience severe ocular symptoms or decreased visual acuity. Increased lacrimation was reported in 12% of patients receiving capecitabine and docetaxel and in 7% of those receiving docetaxel alone for metastatic breast cancer. Among patients receiving capecitabine alone as adjuvant therapy for stage III colon cancer, conjunctivitis occurred in 5% of patients. Conjunctivitis and lacrimal duct stenosis each occurred in less than 5% of patients receiving capecitabine monotherapy for metastatic breast cancer or metastatic colorectal cancer in clinical trials.

■ **Musculoskeletal Effects** Back pain was reported in 10–12% and arthralgia was reported in 8–15% of patients receiving capecitabine as a single agent for metastatic colorectal cancer or in combination with docetaxel for metastatic breast cancer. The incidence of myalgia was higher in the subset of patients receiving capecitabine as a single agent for metastatic breast cancer (9%) than in the overall database of patients receiving capecitabine monotherapy for metastatic colorectal cancer or metastatic breast cancer (less than 5%); myalgia was reported in 15% of those receiving capecitabine and docetaxel, and in 25% of those receiving docetaxel alone, for metastatic breast cancer. Limb pain has been reported in 6–13% of patients receiving capecitabine alone or in combination with docetaxel for metastatic breast cancer. Adverse musculoskeletal effects reported in less than 5% of patients receiving capecitabine monotherapy for metastatic breast cancer or metastatic colorectal cancer in clinical trials include bone pain, arthritis, and muscle weakness. Joint stiffness also has been reported in patients receiving capecitabine.

■ **Respiratory Effects** The incidence of dyspnea was higher in the subset of patients receiving capecitabine as a single agent for metastatic colorectal cancer (14%) than in the overall database of patients receiving capecitabine monotherapy for metastatic colorectal cancer or metastatic breast cancer (less than 5%); dyspnea was reported in about 15% of those receiving either capecitabine and docetaxel or docetaxel alone for metastatic breast cancer. Cough was reported in 13% of patients receiving capecitabine and docetaxel for metastatic breast cancer and in less than 5% of patients receiving capecitabine monotherapy for metastatic breast cancer or metastatic colorectal cancer. Sore throat was reported in 11–12% of patients receiving either capecitabine and docetaxel or docetaxel alone for metastatic breast cancer and in 2% of patients receiving capecitabine as a single agent for metastatic colorectal cancer. Other reported adverse respiratory effects include pharyngeal disorder (5%) in patients receiving capecitabine for metastatic colorectal cancer, and rhinorrhea (5%) and pleural effusion (2%) in patients receiving capecitabine and docetaxel for metastatic breast cancer. Among patients receiving capecitabine alone as adjuvant therapy for stage III colon cancer, epistaxis occurred in 2% of patients. Epistaxis, asthma, hemoptysis, and respiratory distress each has been reported in less than 5% of patients receiving capecitabine monotherapy for metastatic breast cancer or metastatic colorectal cancer in clinical trials. Bronchospasm also has been reported in patients receiving capecitabine as a single agent.

■ **Renal Effects** Renal impairment has been reported in less than 5% of patients receiving capecitabine monotherapy for metastatic breast cancer or metastatic colorectal cancer in clinical trials. Renal failure has been reported in less than 5% of patients receiving capecitabine and docetaxel for metastatic breast cancer. Nocturia also has been reported in patients receiving capecitabine.

■ **Electrolyte Effects** Among patients receiving capecitabine alone as adjuvant therapy for stage III colon cancer, grade 3 or 4 decreased serum calcium concentrations occurred in about 2% of patients, and grade 3 or 4 increased serum calcium concentrations occurred in approximately 1% of patients.

■ **Other Adverse Effects** Pyrexia (fever) occurred in 12–18% of patients receiving capecitabine alone for metastatic breast cancer or metastatic colorectal cancer and in 28% of patients receiving capecitabine and docetaxel for metastatic breast cancer. Among patients receiving capecitabine alone as adjuvant therapy for stage III colon cancer, pyrexia occurred in 7% of patients. Other adverse effects, including chest pain, hoarseness, difficulty in walking, thirst, chest mass, collapse, fibrosis, and drug hypersensitivity, have been reported in less than 5% of patients receiving capecitabine monotherapy for metastatic breast cancer or metastatic colorectal cancer in clinical trials.

■ **Precautions and Contraindications** Capecitabine should be used under the supervision of a qualified clinician experienced in therapy with cytotoxic agents.

Patients and their caregivers should be informed of the expected adverse effects of capecitabine, particularly nausea, vomiting, diarrhea, and hand-foot syndrome; in addition, patients should understand that dosage adjustments during therapy are expected and necessary. Patients also should be instructed to recognize the common toxicities associated with capecitabine therapy and know when to discontinue the drug depending on the severity of symptoms. Patients experiencing any of the following adverse effects of capecitabine at the severity described should immediately discontinue capecitabine therapy and promptly notify their clinician:

- nocturnal stools or an increase of 4–6 stools daily or greater
- severe bloody diarrhea with severe abdominal pain and fever
- grade 2 or greater dehydration
- nausea with a substantial decrease in food intake
- frequent vomiting (i.e., 2–5 or more episodes of vomiting in a 24-hour period)
- painful erythema and swelling of the hands and/or feet that results in discomfort affecting activities of daily living
- painful erythema, edema, or ulcers of the mouth or tongue

Symptomatic treatment of such adverse effects (e.g., with antidiarrheals or antiemetics) is recommended. Patients who develop a fever of 100.5°F or greater or other evidence of potential infection should promptly notify their clinician.

Patients receiving capecitabine should be monitored to prevent and promptly correct dehydration, which can develop rapidly in patients with anorexia, asthenia, nausea, vomiting, or diarrhea, and can result in acute renal failure; patients with preexisting renal impairment and those receiving concomitant therapy with nephrotoxic agents are at increased risk.

Geriatric patients, particularly those 80 years of age and older, may be at increased risk for severe or life-threatening adverse effects of capecitabine and should be monitored closely. (See Cautions: Geriatric Precautions.)

In patients with mild to moderate hepatic impairment secondary to hepatic metastases, capecitabine should be used with caution and liver function should be monitored carefully during therapy; use of the drug in patients with severe hepatic impairment has not been studied.

Because the incidence of adverse cardiovascular effects associated with fluorinated pyrimidines (e.g., myocardial infarction/ischemia, angina, dysrhythmias, cardiac arrest, cardiac failure, sudden death, ECG changes) may be increased in patients with a history of coronary artery disease, such patients should be monitored carefully during capecitabine therapy (e.g., ECG for patients experiencing chest pain).

Patients who develop severe ocular symptoms or decreased visual acuity while receiving capecitabine should undergo ophthalmologic examination.

If capecitabine is used in patients receiving a coumarin-derivative anticoagulant, prothrombin time (PT) or international normalized ratio (INR) should be monitored *frequently*, and adjustment of the anticoagulant dose should be made accordingly. (See Drug Interactions: Anticoagulants.)

If capecitabine is used in patients receiving phenytoin, serum phenytoin concentrations must be monitored carefully, and reduction in the phenytoin dosage may be necessary. (See Drug Interactions: Phenytoin.)

In patients with moderate renal impairment (i.e., creatinine clearance 30–50 mL/minute calculated with the formula of Cockroft-Gault) at baseline, dosage reduction for capecitabine is required. (See: Dosage in Renal and Hepatic Impairment.) In patients with mild or moderate renal impairment receiving capecitabine, careful monitoring is necessary; prompt interruption of treatment is recommended if the patient develops a grade 2, 3, or 4 adverse effect, and subsequent dose adjustments should be made accordingly. (See table on Recommended Dosage Modifications for Toxicity of Capecitabine in Dosage and Administration: Dosage.).

Capecitabine is contraindicated in patients with severe renal impairment (i.e., creatinine clearance less than 30 mL/min calculated with the formula of Cockroft-Gault).

Capecitabine should be withheld or permanently discontinued in patients experiencing acute early-onset or unusually severe toxicity, which may indicate near complete or total absence of dihydropyrimidine dehydrogenase (DPD) activity. Patients with certain homozygous or certain compound heterozygous mutations in the DPD gene resulting in complete or near complete absence of DPD activity are at increased risk for acute early-onset toxicity and severe, life-threatening, or fatal toxicity (e.g., mucositis, diarrhea, neutropenia, neurotoxicity); patients with partial DPD activity also may be at increased risk for severe, life-threatening, or fatal toxicity. No dosage of capecitabine has been proven safe for patients with complete absence of DPD activity, and there are insufficient data to support dosage recommendations for those with partial DPD activity. Patients should be advised to inform their clinician if they are known to have deficient DPD activity.

The use of capecitabine in combination with irinotecan has not been adequately studied.

Capecitabine is contraindicated in patients with known hypersensitivity to capecitabine (including any component of the commercially available tablets) or fluorouracil.

■ **Pediatric Precautions** The manufacturer states that safety and efficacy of capecitabine in children younger than 18 years of age have not been established.

■ **Geriatric Precautions** Although the safety and efficacy of capecitabine in geriatric patients have not been specifically studied to date, the manufacturer reports that elderly individuals may experience increased frequency and severity of the toxic effects of capecitabine and its metabolites. Among 21 patients aged 80 years or older receiving capecitabine for metastatic breast cancer or metastatic colorectal cancer in clinical trials, 62% experienced a grade 3 or 4 adverse effect. In particular, severe adverse GI effects (grade 3 or 4 diarrhea, nausea, or vomiting) or severe hand-foot syndrome associated with capecitabine may occur more frequently in such patients. (See Cautions: GI Effects.) (See Cautions: Dermatologic and Sensitivity Reactions.) Among 67 patients aged 60 years or older receiving capecitabine in combination with docetaxel for metastatic breast cancer, a higher incidence of grade 3 or 4 adverse effects, serious adverse effects, withdrawals due to adverse effects, treatment discontinuations due to adverse effects, and treatment discontinuations within the first 2 treatment cycles was reported than in those less than 60 years of age.

Among 398 patients aged 65 years or older receiving capecitabine as adjuvant therapy for stage III colon cancer, 41% experienced a grade 3 or 4 adverse effect. Geriatric patients appeared to have similar or slightly higher rates of severe adverse effects, such as hand-foot syndrome, diarrhea, stomatitis, neutropenia/granulocytopenia, vomiting, and nausea, compared with the total patient population in this clinical trial. The hazard ratio for disease recurrence for capecitabine versus fluorouracil/leucovorin in patients 65 years of age or older was 1.01 compared with 0.87 for the total patient population.

According to the manufacturer, insufficient data are available to recommend adjustment of capecitabine dosage for age in geriatric patients; however, the greater frequency of decreased hepatic and/or renal function in the elderly should be considered, and some experts recommend dosage reduction for geriatric patients. (See Dosage Modification for Age-related Effects, under Dosage: Breast Cancer.) Geriatric patients should be monitored closely for the occurrence of capecitabine-induced adverse effects.

■ **Mutagenicity and Carcinogenicity** Capecitabine was clastogenic to human peripheral blood lymphocytes in vitro but was not clastogenic to mouse bone marrow (micronucleus test) in vivo. Capecitabine was not mutagenic in the Ames test or the Chinese hamster V79/HPRT gene mutation assay. Fluorouracil, the biologically active form of capecitabine, has been shown to be mutagenic in some bacteria and yeast. Fluorouracil also causes chromosomal aberrations in the micronucleus test in mice in vivo.

Adequate studies evaluating the carcinogenic potential of capecitabine have not been performed to date.

■ **Pregnancy, Fertility, and Lactation** Capecitabine may cause fetal harm when administered to pregnant women, but potential benefits from use of the drug may be acceptable in certain conditions despite the possible risks to the fetus.

Capecitabine has been shown to be embryotoxic and teratogenic in animal studies. Fetal death was observed in monkeys receiving capecitabine 90 mg/kg daily (a dosage producing an AUC value for capecitabine metabolite 5′-deoxy-5-fluorouridine [5′-DFUR] in monkeys about 0.6 times the corresponding value in humans receiving the recommended daily dosage) during organogenesis. Embryocidal and teratogenic effects, including cleft palate, anophthalmia, microphthalmia, oligodactyly, polydactyly, syndactyly, kinky tail, and dilation of cerebral ventricles, were observed in the offspring of mice receiving capecitabine doses of 198 mg/kg daily (a dosage producing an AUC value for capecitabine metabolite 5′-DFUR in mice about 0.2 times the corresponding value in humans receiving the recommended daily dosage) during organogenesis. There are no adequate and well-controlled studies using capecitabine in pregnant women.

Capecitabine should be used during pregnancy only in life-threatening situations or severe disease for which safer drugs cannot be used or are ineffective. If the drug is used during pregnancy or if the patient becomes pregnant while receiving the drug, the patient should be informed of the potential hazard to the fetus. Women of childbearing potential should be advised to avoid becoming pregnant during therapy with capecitabine.

In reproduction studies in mice, oral capecitabine dosages of 760 mg/kg daily (a dosage producing an AUC value for capecitabine metabolite 5′-DFUR in mice about 0.7 times the corresponding value in humans receiving the recommended daily dosage) caused a reversible disturbance in estrus and a consequent decrease in fertility; no fetuses survived in mice that became pregnant. Administration of the same dosage of capecitabine to male mice resulted in degenerative changes in the testes, including a decrease in the number of spermatocytes and spermatids.

In lactating mice receiving a single dose of capecitabine, significant amounts of capecitabine metabolites were distributed into milk. Because of the potential for serious adverse reactions to capecitabine in nursing infants, nursing should be discontinued during capecitabine therapy.

Drug Interactions

■ **Drugs Affecting Hepatic Microsomal Enzymes** Capecitabine and/or its metabolites inhibit the metabolism of warfarin, probably through inhibition of the cytochrome P-450 (CYP) 2C9 isoenzyme. (See Drug Interactions: Anticoagulants.) No formal drug-drug interaction studies between capecitabine and CYP2C9 substrates other than warfarin have been performed. Caution is advised when capecitabine is administered concomitantly with other CYP2C9 substrates (e.g., phenytoin) (see Drug Interactions: Phenytoin), and the need for dosage adjustment should be considered.

Results of in vitro studies indicate that capecitabine and its metabolites do not inhibit the metabolism of substrates of the major cytochrome P-450 isoenzymes.

■ **Antacids** In a small number of patients, administration of an antacid containing aluminum hydroxide and magnesium hydroxide (Maalox®, 20 mL) immediately following capecitabine (1250 mg/m²) resulted in an increased rate and extent of absorption of capecitabine; AUC and peak plasma concentration increased by 16 and 35%, respectively, for capecitabine and by 18 and 22%, respectively, for 5′-deoxy-5-fluorocytidine (5′-DFCR). Antacid administration had no effect on the other 3 major metabolites of capecitabine (i.e., 5′-deoxy-5-fluorouridine [5′-DFUR], fluorouracil, and α-fluoro-β-alanine [FBAL]).

Some experts state that the effects of concomitant administration of capecitabine with an antacid containing aluminum hydroxide and magnesium hydroxide are not clinically important, and adjustments in the dosage or timing of capecitabine are not necessary. In a clinical study of patients receiving capecitabine for metastatic breast cancer, administration of antacids was delayed for at least 2 hours following induction of capecitabine therapy.

■ **Anticoagulants** Altered coagulation parameters and/or bleeding, sometimes fatal, have been reported in patients receiving capecitabine and concomitant therapy with coumarin anticoagulants (e.g., warfarin, phenprocoumon). In patients receiving coumarin anticoagulants, altered coagulation parameters (e.g., increased prothrombin time, increased international normalized ratio) and/or bleeding episodes have occurred within several days to months following initiation of capecitabine therapy; similar events have been reported in at least a few patients within 1 month following discontinuance of capecitabine therapy. Alterations in anticoagulant effect associated with capecitabine therapy have been reported in patients with or without liver metastases. Age exceeding 60 years and diagnosis of cancer are independent variables predisposing patients to an increased risk of coagulopathy.

In 4 patients receiving chronic administration of capecitabine 1250 mg/m² twice daily with a single dose of warfarin 20 mg, the mean area under the concentration-time curve (AUC) of *S*-warfarin was increased by 57% and clearance was decreased by 37%. The baseline corrected AUC of INR in these patients increased by 2.8-fold, and the maximum observed mean INR increased by 91%. The mechanism for this interaction probably involves inhibition of cytochrome P-450 (CYP) 2C9 isoenzyme by capecitabine and/or its metabolites. Because the decreased rate of anticoagulant metabolism may increase patient response to coumarin and indandione derivatives, capecitabine and these agents should be used concomitantly with great caution. If capecitabine is used concomitantly with a coumarin anticoagulant, prothrombin time (PT) or international normalized ratio (INR) should be monitored *frequently*, and the anticoagulant dose should be adjusted accordingly.

■ **Phenytoin** Concomitant use of phenytoin and capecitabine may result in toxicity from increased serum phenytoin concentrations. The mechanism of interaction is presumed to be inhibition of the metabolism of phenytoin by capecitabine and/or its metabolites through inhibition of the cytochrome P-450 (CYP) 2C9 isoenzyme. In patients receiving capecitabine, serum concentrations of phenytoin must be monitored carefully, and reduction in the phenytoin dosage may be necessary.

■ **Leucovorin** Leucovorin potentiates the antineoplastic activity of fluorouracil (the active drug of capecitabine) and also may increase its toxicity. Deaths from severe enterocolitis, diarrhea, and dehydration have been reported in geriatric patients receiving a weekly regimen of combination therapy with leucovorin and fluorouracil.

Leucovorin potentiated the antitumor activity of capecitabine in some xenograft tumors in mice but did not increase the toxicity of the drug; however, evidence from an open-label, randomized trial in patients with advanced colorectal cancer demonstrated comparable efficacy but greater toxicity for combination therapy with capecitabine and leucovorin compared with capecitabine alone.

■ **Food** Food decreases the rate and extent of absorption of capecitabine. (See Pharmacokinetics: Absorption.) Administration with food causes decreases in peak plasma concentration and AUC and an increase in time to peak plasma concentration for capecitabine and its metabolites. According to data in 11 adult cancer patients, the magnitude of the effect of food on the pharmacokinetic parameters was most pronounced for capecitabine and decreased with the order of formation of its metabolites. Because food had only a minor effect on the AUC of the major metabolites of capecitabine, the investigators concluded that the effect of food on the pharmacokinetics of capecitabine probably is not clinically important. However, because current safety and efficacy data are based on administration with food (i.e., within 30 minutes following a meal), it is recommended that capecitabine be administered with food.

Acute Toxicity

■ **Pathogenesis** Limited information is available on the acute toxicity of capecitabine. The acute lethal dose of capecitabine in humans is not known. Single doses of capecitabine of up to 2 g/kg were not lethal to mice, rats, or monkeys (2.4, 4.8, or 9.6 times the recommended human daily dosage on a mg/m² basis, respectively).

■ **Manifestations** Overdosage of capecitabine would be expected to cause nausea, vomiting, diarrhea, GI irritation and bleeding, and bone marrow depression. Patients receiving capecitabine 1657 mg/m² daily (as 2 divided doses) in a continuous daily regimen for at least 6 weeks experienced severe palmar-plantar erythrodysesthesia, mucositis, and diarrhea.

■ **Treatment** Management of capecitabine toxicity and overdosage generally consists of discontinuance of the drug and initiation of supportive measures appropriate for the type of toxicity observed. For information on the emergency treatment of capecitabine toxicity or overdosage with uridine triacetate, see Uridine Triacetate 92.12.

Pharmacology

Capecitabine is a prodrug and has little pharmacologic activity until it is converted to fluorouracil, an antimetabolite. Because capecitabine is converted to fluorouracil by enzymes that are expressed at higher concentrations in many tumors than in adjacent normal tissues or plasma, it is thought that high tumor concentrations of the active drug may be achieved with less systemic toxicity. (See Distribution and also Elimination, in Pharmacokinetics.) Fluorouracil is metabolized in both normal and tumor cells to 5-fluoro-2′-deoxyuridine 5′-monophosphate (FdUMP) and 5-fluorouridine triphosphate (FUTP). Although the precise mechanisms of action of fluorouracil have not been fully elucidated, the main mechanism is thought to be the binding of the deoxyribonucleotide of the drug (FdUMP) and the folate cofactor (N^{5-10}-methylenetetrahydrofolate) to thymidylate synthase (TS) to form a covalently bound ternary complex, which inhibits the formation of thymidylate from 2′-deoxyuridylate, thereby interfering with DNA synthesis. In addition, FUTP can be incorporated into RNA in place of uridine triphosphate (UTP), producing a fraudulent RNA and interfering with RNA processing and protein synthesis. Capecitabine has been shown to be active in xenograft tumors that are resistant to fluorouracil indicating incomplete cross-resistance between the drugs.

An animal study using human cancer xenografts suggests that the antitumor activity of capecitabine may correlate with the ratio of thymidine phosphorylase (an enzyme that catalyzes the conversion of a capecitabine metabolite to the active drug, fluorouracil) and dihydropyrimidine dehydrogenase (an enzyme that catabolizes fluorouracil to a less active metabolite) in tumor tissue; however, the clinical importance of this observation is unknown, and further study is needed to determine whether measurements of enzyme concentrations in tumor tissue can predict the efficacy of capecitabine. In another animal study involving human cancer xenografts, paclitaxel, docetaxel, and mitomycin caused up-regulation of thymidine phosphorylase in tumors; in a large randomized trial, the addition of docetaxel had a synergistic antitumor effect when combined with capecitabine for the treatment of advanced breast cancer.

Pharmacokinetics

The pharmacokinetic behavior of capecitabine may be influenced by race or age. Limited evidence from population analysis of pooled data from 2 large controlled studies in 505 patients (303 males, 202 females; 455 white, 22 black, 28 other race) receiving capecitabine 1250 mg/m^2 twice daily for metastatic colorectal cancer does not reveal any influence of gender or race on the pharmacokinetics of the intermediate metabolite of capecitabine, 5′-deoxy-5-fluorouridine (5′-DFUR), the active drug fluorouracil, or its catabolite, α-fluoro-β-alanine (FBAL). However, data from a study in 18 Japanese patients and 22 white patients receiving capecitabine 825 mg/m^2 twice daily for 14 days shows differences in the pharmacokinetic disposition of capecitabine and its catabolite, FBAL. Peak plasma concentration and the area under the concentration-time curve (AUC) of capecitabine were reduced by about 36 and 24%, respectively, and peak plasma concentration and AUC of FBAL were about 25 and 34% lower, respectively, in the Japanese patients than in the white patients. The clinical importance of these differences is not known. Among patients aged 27 to 86 years, age does not appear to affect the pharmacokinetic disposition of 5′-DFUR or fluorouracil, but a 20% increase in age is associated with a 15% increase in the AUC of FBAL.

The following discussion of the pharmacokinetics of capecitabine and its metabolites is based on data from approximately 200 cancer patients receiving the drug at dosages of 500–3514 mg/m^{2}daily.

■ **Absorption** Capecitabine is readily absorbed from the GI tract; on average, at least 70% of an oral dose of the drug is absorbed. Although in vitro studies have shown that capecitabine is unstable under highly acidic conditions, the drug appears to be absorbed intact immediately upon dissolution without degradation secondary to the acidic pH of the stomach. According to the manufacturer, peak plasma concentrations of capecitabine occur in about 1.5 hours, and peak plasma concentrations of fluorouracil, its active drug, occur slightly later at 2 hours. In adults with cancer who received a capecitabine dosage of 2510 mg/m^2 daily in 2 divided doses, administered approximately 12 hours apart within 30 minutes following the end of a meal, blood samples drawn on day 1 of the treatment cycle showed that peak plasma concentrations of 3.93 and 0.66 mcg/mL for capecitabine and fluorouracil, respectively, were achieved in about 2 hours. Considerable interindividual variations (i.e., exceeding 85%) in peak plasma concentrations and areas under the concentration-time curves (AUCs) have been reported following oral administration of capecitabine.

Presence of food in the GI tract decreases the rate and extent of absorption of capecitabine and, to a lesser extent, decreases the peak plasma concentration and AUC of its metabolites. Peak plasma concentrations and AUC were decreased by 60 and 35%, respectively, for capecitabine and by 43 and 21%, respectively, for fluorouracil when the drug was administered with food. Times to peak plasma concentration for both capecitabine and fluorouracil were delayed by 1.5 hours when capecitabine was administered with food. (See Drug Interactions: Food.)

Over a dosage range of 500–3500 mg/m^2 daily, the pharmacokinetics of capecitabine and its metabolite, 5′-deoxy-5-fluorocytidine (5′-DFCR), were dose proportional and did not change over time. However, the manufacturer reports that increases in AUCs of metabolites 5′-deoxy-5-fluorouridine (5′-DFUR) and fluorouracil were greater than proportional to the increase in dose, and the AUC of fluorouracil was 34% higher on day 14 than on day 1. In one study of adults with cancer at a capecitabine dosage of 2510 mg/m^2 daily, no change was observed in the pharmacokinetics of capecitabine metabolite 5′-DFUR over time, but concentrations of fluorouracil were 22% higher on day 14 than on day 1.

■ **Distribution** Distribution of capecitabine and its metabolites into body tissues and fluids has not been fully characterized. Capecitabine or its metabolites are distributed into tumors, intestinal mucosa, plasma, liver, and other tissues. Animal studies show that capecitabine and its metabolites do not readily penetrate the blood-brain barrier; it is not known whether capecitabine or its metabolites distribute into CSF and brain tissue in humans.

Studies in animals and humans receiving capecitabine have shown a higher concentration of fluorouracil, its active drug, in tumor than in surrounding normal tissue, plasma, or muscle. In patients with colorectal cancer receiving capecitabine for 5–7 days prior to surgery, the median ratio of fluorouracil concentration in colorectal tumors to adjacent tissues was 2.9 (range: 0.9–8), and the median ratio of fluorouracil concentration in tumor to plasma was 16.6. The relative concentration of fluorouracil in tumor to that in normal tissues or plasma has not been evaluated in patients with breast cancer receiving oral capecitabine or in patients receiving fluorouracil by IV infusion. In studies of human colon cancer xenografts, higher concentrations of fluorouracil in tumor were observed in mice receiving oral capecitabine than in those receiving IV fluorouracil. Whereas fluorouracil concentrations were higher in tumor than in plasma or muscle in mice receiving oral capecitabine, similar fluorouracil concentrations in tumor, plasma, or muscle were observed in mice receiving IV fluorouracil.

Plasma protein binding (mainly to albumin) of capecitabine and its metabolites is less than 60% and is not concentration dependent.

It is not known whether capecitabine or its metabolites cross the placenta. It is not known whether capecitabine or its metabolites are distributed into milk.

■ **Elimination** Capecitabine is extensively metabolized in the liver and tumors. The plasma elimination half-life of capecitabine and its metabolites, including the active drug, fluorouracil, is about 45–60 minutes, except for α-fluoro-β-alanine (FBAL), a catabolite of fluorouracil, which has an initial half-life of about 3 hours.

Because it is designed to be converted to the active drug fluorouracil preferentially in tumor tissue, capecitabine is described as a tumor-activated, tumor-selective antineoplastic agent. Capecitabine and its intermediate metabolites have minimal cytotoxic activity. In the liver, capecitabine is largely hydrolyzed to 5′-deoxy-5-fluorocytidine (5′-DFCR) by carboxylesterase, an enzyme almost exclusively located in the liver and hepatoma. 5′-DFCR subsequently is converted to another noncytotoxic intermediate, 5′-deoxy-5-fluorouridine (5′-DFUR), by cytidine deaminase, an enzyme found in most tissues but with high concentrations in the liver and various solid tumors. Hydrolysis of 5′-DFUR to the active drug fluorouracil is catalyzed by thymidine phosphorylase, an enzyme found in many body tissues that also is an angiogenic factor found in higher concentrations in tumor tissue. Once capecitabine is converted to the active drug fluorouracil mainly in tumor tissue, fluorouracil is anabolized to 5-fluoro-2′-deoxyuridine-5′-monophosphate (FdUMP) and 5-fluorouridine triphosphate (FUTP), the active metabolites of the drug.

Fluorouracil is catabolized to dihydrofluorouracil (FUH_2), a much less toxic metabolite, by dihydropyrimidine dehydrogenase. Dihydropyrimidinase cleaves the pyrimidine ring of dihydrofluorouracil, yielding 5-fluoro-ureidopropionic acid (FUPA), which is then cleaved by β-ureido-propionase to form α-fluoro-β-alanine (FBAL). Capecitabine and its metabolites are excreted predominantly in urine (95.5%); fecal excretion is minimal (2.6%). Greater than 70% of a dose of capecitabine is excreted in urine within 24 hours. Most of the capecitabine dose is excreted in urine as metabolites, principally FBAL, a catabolite of fluorouracil (57% of an administered dose); about 3% of an administered dose is excreted in urine as unchanged drug.

The effect of renal impairment on the elimination of capecitabine has been evaluated in cancer patients. Renal impairment causes increased systemic exposure to capecitabine and its metabolites. Following oral administration of capecitabine 1250 mg/m^2 twice daily, systemic exposure to FBAL on day 1 was 85% higher in patients with moderate renal impairment (creatinine clearance of 30–50 mL/min) and 258% higher in patients with severe renal impairment (creatinine clearance <30 mL/min) than in patients with normal renal function (creatinine clearance >80 mL/min). Systemic exposure to 5′-DFUR was 42 and 71% greater in patients with moderate or severe renal impairment, respectively, than in those with normal renal function. Systemic exposure to capecitabine was about 25% greater in patients with moderate or severe renal impairment than in those with normal renal function.

The effect of hepatic impairment on the elimination of capecitabine has not been fully established. In a small number of patients with mild to moderate hepatic impairment secondary to liver metastases, nonsignificant increases in AUC and peak plasma concentration of capecitabine and fluorouracil were reported following a single dose of capecitabine 1255 mg/m^2. The effect of severe hepatic dysfunction on the pharmacokinetics of capecitabine and its metabolites has not been evaluated.

The effect of dialysis on the elimination of capecitabine has not been determined; however, the manufacturer reports that dialysis may reduce circulating concentrations of 5′-DFUR, a low molecular weight metabolite of the drug.

Chemistry and Stability

■ **Chemistry** Capecitabine, a fluoropyrimidine carbamate, is an antineoplastic agent. Capecitabine is a prodrug of 5′-deoxy-5-fluorouridine (doxifuridine, 5′-DFUR) and has little pharmacologic activity until it is converted to fluorouracil, a fluorinated pyrimidine antagonist, in tumor tissue. The drug occurs as a white to off-white crystalline powder and has a solubility of 26 mg/mL in water at 20°C.

■ **Stability** Capecitabine tablets should be stored in tightly closed containers at 25°C but may be exposed to temperatures of 15–30°C. Capecitabine tablets reportedly are stable for at least 9 months when stored in tightly closed containers at room temperature.

For further information on the handling of antineoplastic agents, see the ASHP Guidelines on Handling Hazardous Drugs at http://www.ahfsdruginformation.com.

Preparations

Excipients in commercially available drug preparations may have clinically important effects in some individuals; consult specific product labeling for details.

Capecitabine

Oral		
Tablets	150 mg	**Xeloda®**, Roche
	500 mg	**Xeloda®**, Roche

†Use is not currently included in the labeling approved by the US Food and Drug Administration

CARBOplatin

■ Carboplatin is a platinum-containing antineoplastic agent.

Uses

While the relative efficacy of carboplatin and cisplatin in the treatment of specific malignancies remains to be more fully elucidated, the drugs appear to have similar efficacy in platinum-responsive ovarian tumors, lung cancers, and certain head and neck cancers, but carboplatin is less effective than cisplatin in certain testicular cancers. Carboplatin and cisplatin are associated with different toxicity profiles and carboplatin may be effective in patients with platinum-responsive tumors who are unable to tolerate cisplatin because of renal impairment, refractory nausea, hearing impairment, or neuropathy. It has been suggested that while carboplatin may be preferred in patients with renal failure or patients at high risk for ototoxicity or neurotoxicity, cisplatin may be preferred in patients who have decreased bone marrow reserve or a high risk of sepsis, or who require anticoagulation therapy.

■ **Ovarian Cancer** Carboplatin is used alone or in combination therapy for the treatment of ovarian cancer.

First-line Therapy for Advanced Ovarian Epithelial Cancer

Combination Chemotherapy. Carboplatin in combination with paclitaxel† is a preferred regimen for the initial treatment of advanced ovarian epithelial cancer. The best combination or sequential therapy with multiple agents in the treatment of advanced ovarian tumors has not been established, and comparative efficacy is continually being evaluated.

*Carboplatin versus Cisplatin:*Randomized trials have demonstrated that carboplatin is as effective as but less toxic than cisplatin when used in combination with either paclitaxel or cyclophosphamide for the initial treatment of advanced ovarian cancer. Further study is needed to determine optimal dosing for carboplatin.

Carboplatin has been substituted for cisplatin in combination therapy with paclitaxel. In randomized trials in advanced ovarian cancer, carboplatin was as effective as cisplatin when combined with paclitaxel but was better tolerated.

In a randomized trial designed to establish noninferiority of the studied carboplatin-containing regimen, 792 women with small-volume stage III ovarian cancer (i.e., no tumor nodule greater than 1 cm in diameter following the initial surgery) received either carboplatin/paclitaxel or cisplatin/paclitaxel. The treatment regimens consisted of carboplatin at the dose required to obtain an area under the plasma concentration-time curve (AUC) of 7.5 mg/mL per minute (using the Calvert formula in which creatinine clearance, calculated using the Jellife formula, was substituted for GFR) and paclitaxel 175 mg/m^2 as a 3-hour IV infusion; or cisplatin 75 mg/m^2 IV administered at 1 mg per minute and paclitaxel 135 mg/m^2 as a 24-hour continuous IV infusion every 3 weeks for a total of six courses. Based on median overall survival and median progression-free survival, carboplatin with paclitaxel was as effective as cisplatin with paclitaxel for small-volume stage III ovarian epithelial cancer. Grade 2 to 4 thrombocytopenia and grade 1 to 2 pain occurred more frequently in patients receiving the carboplatin regimen, whereas leukopenia and GI, renal (genitourinary), and metabolic toxicities (e.g., hypomagnesemia or abnormal electrolytes) occurred more frequently in patients receiving the cisplatin regimen. Grade 2 to 4 neurologic toxicity, mainly peripheral neuropathy, occurred with similar frequency (about 30%) in both groups.

In another randomized trial designed to establish noninferiority of carboplatin, 798 women with FIGO stage IIb–IV ovarian cancer received either carboplatin/paclitaxel or cisplatin/paclitaxel. The treatment regimens consisted of paclitaxel 185 mg/m^2 administered IV over 3 hours followed by carboplatin at the dose required to obtain an AUC of 6 mg/mL per minute (using the Calvert formula in which GFR was estimated using the Jellife formula) administered IV over 30–60 minutes; or paclitaxel 185 mg/m^2 administered IV over 3 hours followed by cisplatin 75 mg/m^2 administered IV over 30 minutes. Regardless of calculated doses, the maximal absolute doses administered for each drug were paclitaxel 400 mg, carboplatin 880 mg, and cisplatin 165 mg. Based on the proportion of patients without disease progression at 2 years, median overall survival, and median progression-free survival, carboplatin with paclitaxel was as effective as cisplatin with paclitaxel for FIGO stage IIa–IV ovarian epithelial cancer. Grade 3 or 4 hematologic toxicity and grade 3 or 4 non-neutropenic infections occurred more frequently in patients receiving the carboplatin regimen, whereas certain grade 3 or 4 nonhematologic toxicities, including nausea, vomiting, and peripheral sensory neuropathy, occurred more frequently in patients receiving the cisplatin regimen.

Carboplatin also has been substituted for cisplatin in combination therapy with cyclophosphamide. In randomized trials comparing the use of carboplatin versus cisplatin in combination with cyclophosphamide for advanced ovarian cancer, similar efficacy was observed but carboplatin appeared to have a more favorable therapeutic index than cisplatin.

Because carboplatin is as effective as cisplatin in combination regimens for advanced ovarian cancer, it is preferred except in patients who are unable to tolerate carboplatin (e.g., those who have decreased bone marrow reserve, a high risk of sepsis, or imperative need for anticoagulation therapy).

*Platinum-containing Agent with Paclitaxel Versus Platinum-containing Agent with Cyclophosphamide:*Evidence from randomized trials indicates that combined therapy with a platinum-containing agent and paclitaxel is superior to therapy with cyclophosphamide and a platinum-containing agent for the initial treatment of advanced epithelial ovarian carcinoma and therefore is the preferred regimen. In a comparative study of patients with suboptimally debulked (greater than 1 cm residual tumor mass) stage III or IV ovarian cancer who had no prior chemotherapy, combined therapy with cisplatin and paclitaxel produced higher rates of overall objective response (73 versus 60%), increased disease-free survival (median: 18 versus 13 months), and increased overall survival (median: 38 versus 24 months) compared with a combined regimen of cisplatin and cyclophosphamide. A higher frequency of neutropenia, fever, alopecia, and allergic reactions was observed in patients receiving cisplatin and paclitaxel compared with those receiving cisplatin and cyclophosphamide. In another randomized trial, a higher rate of complete response and prolonged overall survival was observed in patients receiving paclitaxel and cisplatin versus cyclophosphamide and cisplatin for advanced epithelial ovarian cancer. At a follow-up of 6.5 years, the survival benefit associated with the cisplatin and paclitaxel regimen in both randomized trials has been maintained.

*Carboplatin and Docetaxel:*Carboplatin in combination with docetaxel† has been used for the first-line treatment of ovarian cancer. In a phase III randomized trial, response rates, progression-free survival, and 2-year survival rates were similar in patients receiving docetaxel and carboplatin versus paclitaxel and carboplatin for stage Ic–IV epithelial ovarian cancer or primary peritoneal cancer. Severe or life-threatening neutropenia and neutropenic complications occurred more frequently in patients receiving docetaxel and carboplatin, whereas neurotoxicity was more common in patients receiving paclitaxel and carboplatin.

Monotherapy. Carboplatin also has been used as a single agent in the first-line treatment of advanced ovarian cancer†. However, the specific role of carboplatin monotherapy for this advanced cancer remains to be established.

In a large randomized trial known as the ICON3 (International Collaborative Ovarian Neoplasm 3) trial, 2074 patients with invasive ovarian cancer were randomly assigned to receive carboplatin alone, carboplatin and paclitaxel, or cyclophosphamide/doxorubicin/cisplatin (also known as CAP). About 95% of the patients were randomly assigned to a control group (carboplatin alone or CAP) or the standard regimen (carboplatin and paclitaxel) on a 2:1 basis favoring the control group. Patients enrolled in the study had invasive ovarian cancer that was FIGO stage I (9%), FIGO stage II (11%), FIGO stage III (64%), or FIGO stage IV (16%). Treatment regimens consisted of carboplatin at the dose required to obtain an AUC of 5–6 mg/mL per minute; paclitaxel 175 mg/m^2 IV over 3 hours followed by carboplatin (at the same dose used for carboplatin monotherapy); or cyclophosphamide 500 mg/m^2, doxorubicin 50 mg/m^2, and cisplatin 50 mg/m^2. At least 80% of the patients received 6 cycles of chemotherapy, and approximately one-third of patients receiving a control regimen (carboplatin alone or CAP) received taxane-based therapy as second-line treatment upon progression of disease.

At a median follow-up of 4.25 years, median overall survival and median progression-free survival were similar among the treatment groups. Alopecia, fever, and sensory neuropathy occurred more frequently in patients receiving carboplatin combined with paclitaxel than in those receiving carboplatin alone. Sensory neuropathy also occurred more frequently in patients receiving carboplatin and paclitaxel than in those receiving CAP. Fever occurred more frequently in patients receiving CAP than in those receiving carboplatin and paclitaxel.

The combination regimen of carboplatin plus paclitaxel generally remains preferred for the initial treatment of advanced ovarian cancer. However, because of the comparable efficacy and lesser toxicity demonstrated in this randomized trial, some clinicians consider single-agent carboplatin a reasonable option for the first-line treatment of advanced ovarian cancer.

Second-line Therapy for Advanced Ovarian Epithelial Cancer

Combination Chemotherapy. Carboplatin is being studied for use in combination regimens for the second-line treatment of advanced ovarian epithelial cancer†. Most experience to date has been with platinum-based regimens that included paclitaxel.

Combined analysis of data from 2 randomized trials in which a total of 802 patients with platinum-responsive ovarian cancer received either paclitaxel with platinum-based chemotherapy or conventional platinum-based chemotherapy for relapsed disease suggested a survival benefit associated with combination therapy. The median age of the patients was 59–60 years, and 75% of the patients did not experience relapse of ovarian cancer until at least 12 months following prior therapy. About 92% of patients had received only 1 prior line of treatment, and prior therapy included a taxane in only 43% of patients.

Inclusion criteria and treatment regimens differed among the 3 protocols used in the 2 randomized trials.

In all 3 protocols, courses of treatment were administered every 3 weeks. Treatment regimens included carboplatin alone in 71% of patients receiving a platinum-based regimen alone and paclitaxel combined with carboplatin in 80% of patients receiving combination therapy. Dosages for the agents were paclitaxel 175 mg/m² or 185 mg/m² administered as a 3-hour IV infusion; cisplatin 75 mg/m² as monotherapy or 50 mg/m² in combination; carboplatin at the dose required to obtain a minimum AUC of 5–6 mg/mL per minute.

At a median follow-up of 3.5 years, median overall survival and median progression-free survival were prolonged in patients receiving paclitaxel and platinum-based chemotherapy versus platinum-based chemotherapy alone. Grade 2–4 neurologic toxicity (20 versus 1%) and alopecia (86 versus 25%) occurred more frequently in patients receiving combination therapy with paclitaxel and a platinum agent than in those receiving a platinum agent alone.

Carboplatin also is being studied in combination with other agents for the treatment of relapsed ovarian cancer. In a phase III randomized trial, patients with platinum-responsive recurrent ovarian cancer receiving combination therapy with carboplatin and gemcitabine appear to have prolonged progression-free survival compared with those receiving carboplatin alone; combination therapy was associated with a higher frequency of grade 3 or 4 hematologic toxicity.

Monotherapy. Carboplatin is used alone as second-line (salvage) therapy for the palliative treatment of patients with advanced ovarian carcinoma who have recurrence following an initial chemotherapy regimen, including ones that had cisplatin as a component. Either cisplatin or carboplatin can be used when retreatment is indicated in patients with platinum-responsive disease who relapse; however, some clinicians suggest that carboplatin may be preferred because it is associated with a more favorable toxicity profile than cisplatin.

Although some patients who failed to respond to cisplatin or had a response of only short duration have responded to carboplatin, nonplatinum-based regimens generally are preferred for retreatment of patients with platinum-refractory disease.

Adjuvant Therapy for Early-stage Ovarian Epithelial Cancer Carboplatin also has been used alone or in combination therapy for the adjuvant treatment of early-stage ovarian cancer†. In 2 large randomized trials, patients receiving adjuvant therapy with single-agent or combination platinum-based therapy experienced prolonged overall survival and/or prolonged recurrence-free survival compared with patients undergoing observation (i.e., no adjuvant chemotherapy until chemotherapy was clinically indicated). However, evidence from one study (EORTC–ACTION trial) suggests that survival benefit may be limited to patients whose early-stage disease is associated with a poorer prognosis.

In a large randomized trial known as the EORTC–ACTION trial (i.e., European Organisation for Research and Treatment of Cancer–Adjuvant ChemoTherapy in Ovarian Neoplasm trial), 448 patients who underwent appropriate surgery and had disease identified with surgical staging as any of the qualifying FIGO stages (i.e., stages Ia–Ib, grade II–III; all stages Ic and IIa; and all stages I–IIa with clear-cell epithelial cancer of the ovary) were randomly assigned to either adjuvant chemotherapy or observation. The median age of patients in the study was 54–55 years.

Adjuvant chemotherapy consisted of at least 4 courses (but preferably 6 courses) of a platinum-based regimen following surgery. Platinum-based therapy included single-agent therapy or combination therapy with either carboplatin (at a required dose of 350 mg/m²) or cisplatin (at a required dose of 75 mg/m²). Most patients in the chemotherapy arm received cisplatin combined with cyclophosphamide (about half of the patients) or single-agent carboplatin (about one third of the patients).

At a median follow-up of 5.5 years, patients receiving adjuvant chemotherapy had similar 5-year overall survival (85 versus 78%) and prolonged recurrence-free survival (76 versus 68%) compared with patients under observation. About 66% of the patients in the trial had undergone nonoptimal surgical staging, and completeness of surgical staging was identified as an independent prognostic factor. Optimal surgical staging of ovarian cancer minimizes the likelihood of undetected residual disease. Subgroup analysis showed that overall survival and recurrence-free survival were prolonged in patients with nonoptimally staged disease who received adjuvant chemotherapy, but not in patients with optimally staged disease who received adjuvant chemotherapy. The results of this analysis suggest that the observed benefit of adjuvant therapy may be limited to patients with inadequately staged epithelial ovarian cancer who are likely to have appreciable residual disease.

In another large randomized trial known as the ICON1 (International Collaborative Ovarian Neoplasm 1) trial, 477 patients with early-stage ovarian cancer were randomly assigned to either adjuvant chemotherapy or observation. The adequacy of surgical staging was not monitored; 93% of the patients had FIGO stage I disease, and most patients had well differentiated (32%) or moderately differentiated (41%) tumors. The median age of patients in the study was 55 years.

Recommended adjuvant chemotherapy following surgery consisted of 6 courses of a platinum-based regimen administered at 3-week intervals. Platinum-based therapy included either carboplatin or cisplatin, as single-agent therapy or in combination therapy (e.g., cyclophosphamide, doxorubicin, and cisplatin, also known as CAP). Using the Calvert formula, the recommended dose of carboplatin when used as a single agent was based on the dose required to obtain an area under the plasma concentration-time curve (AUC) of 5 mg/mL per minute; the recommended dose of carboplatin when used in combination was based on the dose required to obtain an AUC of 4 mg/mL per minute. The recommended dose of cisplatin when used as a single agent was 70 mg/m². The recommended doses for the CAP regimen were cyclophosphamide 500 mg/m², doxorubicin 50 mg/m², and cisplatin 50 mg/m².

Of the 241 patients assigned to adjuvant chemotherapy, 197 patients received chemotherapy that was documented; among these patients, 171 (87%) received single-agent carboplatin, 21 (11%) received cisplatin-based combination therapy, 3 (2%) received carboplatin-based combination therapy, 1 (less than 1%) received single-agent cisplatin, and 1 (less than 1%) received an unspecified regimen. Among the patients receiving adjuvant chemotherapy, a total of 168 patients (85%) received all 6 cycles of chemotherapy but 65 patients required delayed doses or reduced dosage typically because of treatment toxicity.

At a median follow-up of 4.25 years, patients receiving adjuvant chemotherapy had prolonged 5-year overall survival (79 versus 70%; hazard ratio: 0.66) and prolonged 5-year recurrence-free survival (73 versus 62%; hazard ratio: 0.65) compared with patients under observation.

Interpretation of the results of each of the 2 randomized trials is limited by the small sample size; enrollment in both studies was stopped before the planned number of patients (i.e., at least 1000 patients in the ACTION trial and 2000 patients in the ICON1 trial) was accrued. Although the outcomes of the 2 randomized trials were similar, some important differences between the studies include the broader inclusion criteria and lack of strict surgical staging in the ICON1 trial. Combined analysis of the data from the ACTION and the ICON1 trials showed that at a median follow-up of at least 4 years, patients receiving adjuvant chemotherapy had prolonged 5-year overall survival (82 versus 74%; hazard ratio: 0.67) and prolonged 5-year recurrence-free survival (76 versus 65%; hazard ratio: 0.64) compared with patients under observation. Subgroup analyses of the combined data from the 2 trials according to age, tumor stage, histologic cell type, and cell differentiation did not identify any prognostic factor for the effect of adjuvant chemotherapy; subgroup analysis according to the completeness of surgical staging was not done because information about surgical staging was not collected in the ICON1 trial.

In patients with FIGO stage Ia or Ib ovarian epithelial cancer, surgery alone generally is adequate. However, some prognostic factors, including grade III tumor, densely adherent tumor, or FIGO stage Ic disease, are associated with higher risk of recurrence of the disease, and additional treatment options may be considered. The results of these 2 randomized trials, individually or combined, suggest that adjuvant chemotherapy may benefit some patients with early-stage (FIGO stage I or II) ovarian epithelial cancer. However, further study is needed to differentiate patients with good-prognosis early-stage ovarian epithelial cancer who can be treated with surgery alone from patients with poor-prognosis early-stage disease who may benefit from surgery with immediate adjuvant chemotherapy. Various regimens were used for adjuvant chemotherapy in the 2 trials, and further study also is needed to compare the efficacy and toxicity of different regimens.

■ **Lung Cancer** ***Small Cell Lung Cancer*** Carboplatin is used as a component of combination regimens for the treatment of small cell lung cancer†. Combination chemotherapy regimens are superior to single-agent therapy for the treatment of small cell lung cancer and moderately intensive drug doses are superior to doses that produce minimal toxicity. Various regimens have been used in combination therapy and many 2- to 4-drug combination regimens, including carboplatin-containing regimens, have produced objective response rates of 65–90 or 70–85% and complete response rates of 45–75 or 20–30% in patients with limited-stage or extensive-stage disease, respectively.

Carboplatin-containing regimens are used in chemotherapy for extensive-stage small cell lung cancer and in combined modality treatment (i.e., combination chemotherapy with concurrent thoracic irradiation administered early in the course of treatment) for limited-stage disease. In the treatment of small cell lung cancer, carboplatin has been used in conjunction with etoposide with or without ifosfamide. In a randomized study, patients with small cell lung cancer receiving carboplatin and etoposide had similar response rates and median survival but less toxicity than those receiving cisplatin and etoposide.

Although optimum duration of chemotherapy has not been clearly defined, additional improvement in survival has not been observed when the duration of drug administration exceeds 3–6 or 6 months in patients with limited-stage or extensive-stage small cell lung cancer, respectively. While efficacy of the various available regimens is continually being evaluated, combination chemotherapy regimens containing carboplatin and etoposide (with or without ifosfamide) currently are considered preferred or alternative regimens for the treatment of small cell lung carcinoma.

Because the current prognosis for small cell lung carcinoma is unsatisfactory regardless of stage and despite considerable diagnostic and therapeutic advances, all patients with this cancer are candidates for inclusion in clinical trials at the time of diagnosis.

Non-small Cell Lung Cancer Carboplatin is an active agent in non-small cell lung carcinoma†. A small survival benefit has been demonstrated for the use of platinum-based (cisplatin) chemotherapy alone or combined with radiation therapy in selected patients with metastatic or unresectable, locally advanced non-small cell lung cancer who have a good performance status.

Carboplatin in combination with paclitaxel is used as an alternative to cisplatin-containing regimens in the treatment of advanced non-small cell lung cancer. Similar response rates and median survival were observed in a randomized trial in which patients received carboplatin and paclitaxel versus regimens of cisplatin in combination with paclitaxel, gemcitabine, or docetaxel for advanced non-small cell lung cancer. However, in another randomized trial, response rates were similar but median survival was shorter for patients receiving carboplatin and paclitaxel than for those receiving cisplatin and paclitaxel for advanced non-small cell lung cancer. In other randomized trials, response rates and median survival were similar in patients receiving either carboplatin and paclitaxel or cisplatin and vinorelbine for advanced non-small cell lung cancer; grade 3 peripheral neurotoxicity occurred more frequently in patients receiving paclitaxel and carboplatin whereas leukopenia/neutropenia and nausea and vomiting were more frequent in patients receiving vinorelbine and cisplatin.

Carboplatin also is used as an alternative to cisplatin in combination with docetaxel for the treatment of advanced non-small cell lung cancer. In a randomized phase III trial comparing a platinum agent and docetaxel with cisplatin and vinorelbine for the treatment of locally advanced, recurrent, or metastatic non-small cell lung cancer, patients receiving carboplatin and docetaxel had similar response rates and median survival as those receiving cisplatin and vinorelbine; higher response rates and a trend toward prolonged median survival were observed in patients receiving cisplatin and docetaxel compared with those receiving cisplatin and vinorelbine.

Various chemotherapy regimens used alone or in combination with other treatment modalities, such as radiation therapy, are continually being evaluated for the treatment of advanced non-small cell lung cancer. Because current treatment is not satisfactory for almost all patients with non-small cell lung cancer except selected patients with early-stage, resectable disease, all patients may be considered for enrollment in clinical trials at the time of diagnosis.

■ Cervical Cancer The role of carboplatin in the treatment of cervical cancer† remains to be established. (See Uses: Cervical Cancer in Cisplatin 10:00 for an overview of treatment for cervical cancer.)

Concurrent Chemotherapy and Radiation Therapy for Invasive Cervical Cancer Concurrent platinum (i.e., cisplatin)-containing chemotherapy and radiation therapy is recommended in women with invasive cervical cancer (FIGO stage IB2 through IVA disease or FIGO stage IA2, IB, or IIA disease with poor prognostic factors). Although carboplatin often is used as a less toxic substitute for cisplatin, current evidence supports the use of cisplatin in chemotherapy regimens given concurrently with radiation therapy in patients with locally advanced cervical cancer, and similar benefit with the use of carboplatin-containing chemotherapy cannot be assumed.

Metastatic or Recurrent Cervical Cancer Carboplatin is an active agent in the treatment of metastatic or recurrent cervical cancer†. Objective response rates of 15% have been reported with the use of carboplatin as a single agent for the treatment of metastatic or recurrent squamous cervical cancer. Because of its lesser toxicity, carboplatin may be considered as an alternative to cisplatin, particularly in patients with nephrotoxicity or neurotoxicity caused by advanced cervical tumor who are not suitable candidates for cisplatin therapy. However, randomized controlled trials comparing carboplatin and cisplatin have not been performed to date, and because of superior response rates and lesser hematologic toxicity, most experts consider cisplatin the current drug of choice in the treatment of advanced cervical cancer, particularly in patients who have received radiation therapy. Some experts suggest that study of higher dosages and various dosage schedules is needed to fully establish the activity of carboplatin in advanced cervical cancer.

Various single agents and combination regimens for the treatment of advanced cervical cancer have been evaluated mostly in phase II studies, and optimal treatment has not been established. Combination regimens have not been consistently shown to be superior to the use of single agents, such as cisplatin, one of the most active drugs in the treatment of metastatic or recurrent cervical cancer. In addition, the benefit of chemotherapy versus best supportive care has not been studied in patients with metastatic or recurrent cervical cancer. Because the prognosis of patients with advanced cervical cancer remains poor and optimal therapy has not been established, all such patients may be considered for enrollment in clinical trials investigating new agents or combination regimens.

■ Head and Neck Cancer Carboplatin may be useful in the treatment of recurrent or metastatic squamous cell carcinoma of the head and neck†. Therapy that includes carboplatin has been suggested as one of several alternatives to various cisplatin-containing regimens for recurrent or metastatic squamous cell carcinoma of the head and neck, but experience with carboplatin is less extensive than with cisplatin. In a randomized study, patients with recurrent or metastatic squamous cell carcinoma of the head and neck who received cisplatin and fluorouracil, carboplatin and fluorouracil, or methotrexate alone had objective response rates of 32, 21, and 10%, respectively. Median survival was similar among the groups. Combination chemotherapy was associated with increased toxicity (particularly hematologic toxicity for cisplatin and carboplatin and renal toxicity for cisplatin).

In males younger than 50 years of age with metastatic squamous neck cancer who have a poorly differentiated tumor, an occult primary, and elevated β-human chorionic gonadotropin (β-hCG) and α-fetoprotein (AFP), chemotherapy with a platinum-containing regimen should be considered because these tumors may respond to such therapy in a manner similar to extragonadal germ cell malignancies. Although surgical resection, radiation therapy, or both are preferred therapy for the initial management of cancer of the head and neck, chemotherapy before or after surgery or radiation therapy can be considered for such tumors.

■ Wilms' Tumor Carboplatin has shown activity in the management of Wilms' tumor†. Second-line (salvage) therapy with ifosfamide, carboplatin, and etoposide may be considered for patients with recurrent tumors of unfavorable histology, abdominal recurrence after radiation therapy, or recurrence within 6 months of nephrectomy or after initial 3-drug combination chemotherapy (e.g., vincristine, dactinomycin, and doxorubicin); however, this regimen is associated with substantial hematologic toxicity. Cyclophosphamide and etoposide alternating with carboplatin and etoposide has been used as an induction regimen preceding surgery and then as maintenance chemotherapy for patients with high-risk, relapsed Wilms' tumor. Patients with recurrent disease failing to respond to such attempts with salvage therapy should be offered treatment under protocol conditions in ongoing clinical trials.

■ Brain Tumors Carboplatin has been used for the palliative treatment of various primary brain tumors†. Regimens that include carboplatin have been used principally in the treatment of germ cell tumors. Most primary brain tumors are treated with surgery and/or radiation therapy, but adjuvant chemotherapy may prolong survival in some tumor types and has increased disease-free survival in patients with medulloblastoma, certain germ cell tumors, and gliomas.

Malignant Gliomas **Astrocytic Tumors.** Carboplatin has shown activity in the treatment of progressive or recurrent low-grade gliomas in children†. Use of carboplatin in combination with vincristine for the treatment of progressive low-grade gliomas in children is being investigated.

Responses to IV carboplatin have been observed in adults with recurrent gliomas, including those who had received previous chemotherapy with nitrosoureas.

Medulloblastoma. Carboplatin has shown activity in the treatment of recurrent medulloblastoma†. The use of carboplatin in myeloablative chemotherapy regimens (e.g., carboplatin, thiotepa, and etoposide) with autologous bone marrow or stem cell rescue has been studied in a limited number of children with recurrent medulloblastoma. In children with newly diagnosed medulloblastoma, combination regimens containing carboplatin are being investigated for use as neoadjuvant therapy preceding radiation therapy or as a component of intensive chemotherapy accompanied by autologous bone marrow rescue to avoid the need for radiotherapy in young children. Further study is needed to compare the efficacy and toxicity of carboplatin versus cisplatin in the treatment of medulloblastoma. (For further discussion of the treatment of medulloblastoma, see Uses: Brain Tumors in Cisplatin 10:00.)

Intracranial Germ Cell Tumors Combination therapy with a platinum-containing agent (i.e., cisplatin or carboplatin) and etoposide is used in the treatment of intracranial germ cell tumors†.

■ Neuroblastoma Carboplatin is used as a component of combination therapy for neuroblastoma†. Combination chemotherapy with moderate doses of carboplatin, cyclophosphamide, doxorubicin, and etoposide is used in conjunction with surgery (with or without radiation therapy) for the treatment of neuroblastoma in patients with intermediate-risk tumors or, in some cases, low-risk tumors. Although surgery alone typically is adequate for the treatment of low-risk tumors, combination chemotherapy is administered if surgical resection is incomplete (less than 50% of the primary tumor is resected) or if life-threatening or organ-threatening symptomatic disease is present (e.g., spinal cord compression). In patients with high-risk tumors, aggressive chemotherapy using higher doses of these drugs and additional drugs (e.g., ifosfamide, high-dose cisplatin, vincristine) is used. If high-risk disease responds to the initial regimen of chemotherapy, further therapy consists of surgical resection of the primary tumor, myeloablative therapy and autologous stem cell transplantation (bone marrow transplantation or peripheral blood stem cell transplantation), and radiation therapy (radiation to the primary tumor site and sometimes total-body irradiation); following recovery, 6 months of therapy with oral 13-*cis*-retinoic acid (isotretinoin) is administered.

■ Testicular Cancer Randomized trials indicate that a cisplatin-based regimen (i.e., cisplatin/etoposide or cisplatin/etoposide/bleomycin) is more effective than a carboplatin-based regimen (i.e., carboplatin/etoposide or carboplatin/etoposide/bleomycin) in the initial treatment of good-prognosis metastatic nonseminomatous germ cell tumors, and treatment with a carboplatin regimen generally is reserved for patients who do not tolerate or who refuse cisplatin. Limited data suggest that high-dose carboplatin and etoposide may be effective in the treatment of relapsed or refractory germ cell tumors† in some patients. High-dose carboplatin and etoposide with autologous bone marrow transplant has been associated with complete remission in 10–20% of patients with cisplatin-resistant germ cell tumors. Even higher rates of durable complete response (exceeding 50%) have been observed when high-dose carboplatin and etoposide, followed by peripheral blood stem cell transplantation or autologous bone marrow transplantation, is used as initial salvage therapy in patients with relapsed testicular cancer.

■ Bladder Cancer Carboplatin has been substituted as a less toxic alternative to cisplatin in some patients receiving combination chemotherapy for advanced bladder cancer†. Inadequate dosing of carboplatin may have contributed to its lesser efficacy compared with cisplatin in earlier studies of platinum-based regimens for the treatment of advanced or metastatic bladder cancer.

Combination therapy with paclitaxel followed by carboplatin is being investigated as a tolerable and active regimen in patients with advanced bladder cancer, including patients with abnormal renal function. In a phase III randomized trial, 80 patients received paclitaxel 225 mg/m^2 IV over 3 hours, followed by carboplatin (at the dose required to obtain an AUC of 6 mg/mL per minute)

IV over 30 minutes, every 21 days, or the standard MVAC regimen (i.e., cisplatin, methotrexate, vinblastine, and doxorubicin) every 28 days, for a maximum of 6 treatment cycles. The response rates were similar; at a median follow-up of 2.7 years, patients receiving paclitaxel and carboplatin had similar median overall survival as patients receiving MVAC. Severe neutropenia occurred more frequently in patients receiving MVAC than in those receiving paclitaxel and carboplatin. Interpretation of the results is limited by the failure to meet the planned accrual of 330 patients in the trial.

■ **Retinoblastoma** Carboplatin has been used in combination with etoposide in a limited number of children† with recurrent or progressive retinoblastoma†. While regimens including doxorubicin, cyclophosphamide, and/or vincristine have been used, some clinicians consider carboplatin one of several alternative agents that can be used in children with extraocular retinoblastoma. Therapy with carboplatin in combination with etoposide has been associated with partial or complete responses in up to 85% of children with recurrent disease; the role of carboplatin-containing regimens as adjuvant therapy after enucleation or as neoadjuvant therapy of ocular tumors remains to be determined.

■ **Other Uses** Carboplatin has been used for the treatment of breast cancer†. In a phase III randomized trial, higher response rates and prolonged median progression-free survival were observed with the addition of carboplatin to trastuzumab and paclitaxel for the treatment of HER2-overexpressing metastatic breast cancer; grade 4 neutropenia occurred more frequently in patients receiving carboplatin with trastuzumab and paclitaxel.

Carboplatin is being studied for use in the treatment of endometrial cancer†. A phase III randomized trial comparing carboplatin and paclitaxel versus doxorubicin, cisplatin, paclitaxel and filgrastim (G-CSF) for advanced or recurrent endometrial cancer is under way.

Dosage and Administration

■ **Reconstitution and Administration** Carboplatin is administered by IV infusion. Infusions of the drug usually are administered IV over a period of 15 minutes or longer; carboplatin has been administered by continuous IV infusion over 24 hours. Unlike precautions required during cisplatin administration, pretreatment and posttreatment hydration and/or diuresis are *not* necessary when carboplatin is administered. Carboplatin also has been administered intraperitoneally†. Needles, syringes, catheters, and IV administration sets that contain aluminum parts which may come in contact with carboplatin should *not* be used for preparation or administration of the drug. (See Chemistry and Stability: Stability.) The usual precautions for handling and preparing cytotoxic drugs should be observed when preparing or administering carboplatin.

Commercially available carboplatin injection is a premixed aqueous solution containing 10 mg of carboplatin per mL. The manufacturer states that carboplatin aqueous solution may be further diluted with 0.9% sodium chloride injection or 5% dextrose injection to a concentration as low as 0.5 mg/mL. Prior to administration, carboplatin solutions should be inspected visually for particulate matter and discoloration.

■ **Dosage** Dosage of carboplatin must be based on the clinical, renal, and hematologic response and tolerance of the patient in order to obtain optimum therapeutic response with minimum adverse effects. While initial carboplatin dosage can be based on body surface area, dosage may be more accurately calculated using formula dosing methods based on the patient's renal function. Because renal function often is reduced in geriatric patients, the manufacturer recommends that dosing formulas incorporating estimates of glomerular filtration rate be used in geriatric patients to help minimize the risk of toxicity. (See Dosage: Individualization of Dosage.) The manufacturer recommends that carboplatin generally be given no more frequently than once every 4 weeks at usual dosage. *A repeat course of carboplatin should not be administered until the patient's hematologic functions are within acceptable limits, and precautions must always be taken to treat a hypersensitivity reaction if it occurs.* (See Cautions: Precautions and Contraindications.) When carboplatin is used as a component of a multiple-drug regimen, clinicians should consult published protocols for the dosage of each chemotherapeutic agent and the method and sequence of administration.

Because carboplatin is an antineoplastic agent of moderate emetic risk, antiemetic therapy is recommended. (See Cautions: GI Effects.)

Ovarian Cancer For the treatment of advanced ovarian carcinoma (stage III and IV) in combination chemotherapy regimens (i.e., with cyclophosphamide), an initial IV carboplatin dose of 300 mg/m² can be used in adults. Subsequent dosage of the drug should be adjusted according to the patient's hematologic tolerance of the previous dose (e.g., as described below); doses should not be administered until the patient's hematologic function is within acceptable limits. Alternatively, carboplatin dosage can be calculated using formula dosing methods based on renal function. (See Dosage: Individualization of Dosage.) A course of carboplatin consists of single doses administered once every 4 weeks (or longer if delayed for hematologic toxicity) for a total of 6 cycles.

When carboplatin is used alone in the treatment of recurrent ovarian carcinoma, an initial dose of 360 mg/m² can be used, administering the drug once every 4 weeks (or longer if delayed for hematologic toxicity). Doses of carboplatin generally should not be repeated until the patient's hematologic function is within acceptable limits, adjusting dosage according to the patient's hematologic tolerance of the most recent dose (e.g., as described in the following paragraph).

For patients who experience no hematologic toxicity (i.e., platelet counts greater than 100,000/mm³ and neutrophil counts greater than 2000/mm³) with the previous dose, dosage of carboplatin in single or combination therapy may be increased by 25%. In studies used to establish efficacy of carboplatin in combination with cyclophosphamide, dosage escalation above 25% of the initial dose was not evaluated. For patients who experience only mild to moderate hematologic toxicity (i.e., platelet counts of 50,000–100,000 mm³ or neutrophil counts of 500–2000/mm³, respectively) with the previous dose, dosage adjustment is not necessary in single agent or combination regimens. For patients who experience moderate to severe hematologic toxicity (e.g., platelet counts lower than 50,000 mm³ or neutrophil counts lower than 500/mm³, respectively) with the previous dose, the dosage of carboplatin in single agent or combination regimens should be reduced by 25%. In studies used to establish efficacy of carboplatin in stage III and IV ovarian carcinoma, carboplatin therapy was continued only at the investigator's discretion in patients who experienced hematologic toxicity following 2 dosage reductions (i.e., while receiving a carboplatin dosage equivalent to 50% of the initial dosage). Some authorities suggest that, rather than compromise carboplatin's efficacy by dosage reduction in patients who experience substantial hematologic toxicity, carboplatin therapy should be replaced with cisplatin (which is less myelosuppressive) therapy if possible. Whether concomitant hematopoietic agents (colony-stimulating factor) can obviate carboplatin dosage reduction in patients who experience substantial hematologic toxicity remains to be established.

Other Neoplasms Dosage of carboplatin used in the treatment of other malignant neoplasms† generally has been similar to that used in the treatment of ovarian carcinoma; however, various dosage schedules and regimens of carboplatin alone or in conjunction with other antineoplastic agents have been used. Clinicians should consult published protocols for dosages and the method and sequence of administration. In general, escalation of carboplatin dosages above 400 mg/m² results in substantial hematologic toxicity, but high-dose carboplatin (900–2000 mg/m²) has been used with colony-stimulating factors, autologous bone marrow rescue, and/or peripheral stem cell rescue.

Individualization of Dosage Several alternative methods for calculating initial carboplatin dosage have been suggested based on the patient's pretreatment renal function or pretreatment renal function and desired platelet nadir. These methods, compared with empiric dosage calculations based only on body surface area, compensate for patient variations in pretreatment renal function that may otherwise result in carboplatin underdosing (e.g., in patients with above average renal function) or overdosing (e.g., in patients with impaired renal function). The methods incorporate considerations about the direct relationship between renal clearance of carboplatin and glomerular filtration rate (GFR) over widely ranging renal function and about the predictive relationship between the area under the plasma concentration-time curve (AUC) of ultrafilterable platinum and the degree of subsequent thrombocytopenia and neutropenia.

One commonly employed method for carboplatin dosage calculation in adults is the Calvert formula based on the patient's GFR (in mL/minute) and the target AUC (in mg/mL per minute). *Using the Calvert formula, carboplatin dosage is calculated in mg, not mg/m².* Because the predictability of this calculation has been established using chromic edetate Cr 51 (^{51}Cr-EDTA) clearance to establish GFR, some clinicians have recommended that other methods for estimating creatinine clearance (e.g., Cockcroft-Gault equation, Jelliffe equation) not be substituted for this determination since carboplatin dosing based on such estimates may not be predictive. However, other clinicians have successfully employed such methods for estimating creatinine clearance because of their simplicity and/or unavailability of ^{51}Cr-EDTA clearance, although they may not be as precisely predictive.

Calvert Formula for Carboplatin Dosing:

total dose (mg) =

target AUC (in mg/mL per min) x [GFR (in mL/min) + 25]

In studies used to derive the Calvert formula, the GFR was measured by ^{51}Cr-EDTA, which correlates well with creatinine clearance. A target AUC of 5 (range: 4–6) mg/mL per minute appears to provide the most appropriate dosage range for use of carboplatin alone in patients previously treated with chemotherapeutic agents. Analysis of toxicity in previously treated patients receiving carboplatin alone indicates that substantial thrombocytopenia (grade 3 or 4 [platelet counts less than 50,000/ mm³]) occurs in 16% and leukopenia (grade 3 or 4 [leukocyte counts less than 200,000/ mm³]) occurs in 13% of patients with target AUCs of 4–5 mg/mL per minute. A higher incidence of myelotoxicity was reported in patients with target AUCs of 6–7 mg/mL per minute with thrombocytopenia (grade 3 or 4) occurring in 33% and leukopenia (grade 3 or 4) occurring in 34% of patients. For patients who previously did not receive chemotherapy, a target AUC of 7 (range: 6–8) mg/mL per minute has been recommended when carboplatin is used alone. Higher target AUCs (e.g., 7.5 mg/mL) also have been used (e.g., when carboplatin was used as a component of high-intensity dosing with paclitaxel and a hematopoietic agent for non-small cell lung carcinoma). Subsequent carboplatin dosage has been adjusted according to hematologic tolerance to the previous dose (e.g., reducing the dose by 25% for moderate to severe hematologic toxicity).

The Calvert formula is not sufficiently accurate to determine carboplatin dosage for children or for adults with severe renal impairment (i.e., GFR less than 20 mL/minute); therefore, this formula should *not* be used in such patients. An alternative pediatric formula has been suggested, but specialized references should be consulted.

Another method (the Chatelut or French formula) for carboplatin dosage calculation in adults that is simplified by not requiring determination of GFR has been suggested. While this method is more recent and therefore has not been employed as extensively as the Calvert method, it offers a means of estimating carboplatin clearance that relies only on patient age, gender, and serum creatinine concentration. *Using the Chatelut formula, carboplatin dosage is calculated in mg, not mg/m².*

Chatelut (French) Formula for Carboplatin Dosing:

total dose (mg) = target AUC (in mg/mL/min) × carboplatin clearance (in mL/min)

When carboplatin clearance is calculated as follows:
Carboplatin clearance (mL/min) =

$$[0.134 \times \text{wt}] + \frac{[218 \times \text{wt} \times (1 - \{0.00457 \times \text{age}\})] \times [1 - \{0.314 \times \text{gender}\}]}{\text{serum creatinine } (\mu\text{mol/L})}$$

where weight is in kg, age is in years, and gender is 0 for males and 1 for females

This formula should *not* be used for calculating carboplatin dosage in pediatric patients or those undergoing hemodialysis.

■ Dosage in Renal Impairment Dosage of carboplatin should be reduced in patients with impaired renal function. Because patients with creatinine clearances less than 60 mL/minute are at increased risk of myelosuppression during carboplatin therapy, dosage in such patients should be adjusted according to the degree of renal impairment. When carboplatin is used alone in the treatment of recurrent ovarian carcinoma in patients with renal impairment, the manufacturer recommends that those with creatinine clearances of 41–59 mL/minute receive an initial dose of 250 mg/m² and those with creatinine clearances of 16–40 mL/minute receive an initial dose of 200 mg/m². The incidence of severe leukopenia, neutropenia, or thrombocytopenia in these patients at these dosages is about 25%. Subsequent carboplatin dosage should be adjusted according to the patient's hematologic tolerance to the previous dose. Although carboplatin has been used in a limited number of patients with creatinine clearances less than 15 mL/minute, the manufacturer states that experience in these patients is too limited to make dosage recommendations.

Cautions

Although carboplatin and cisplatin are both platinum-coordination compounds and have similar mechanism(s) of action, they have different toxicologic profiles, with carboplatin being better tolerated overall. While the major dose-limiting adverse effects associated with cisplatin therapy include nonhematologic toxicities such as nephrotoxicity, ototoxicity, neurotoxicity, and emesis, the major dose-limiting adverse effects associated with carboplatin therapy are hematologic toxicities such as thrombocytopenia and leukopenia. The improved overall toxicity profile of carboplatin relative to cisplatin appears to result at least partly from the presence of a cyclobutane dicarboxylate ligand on carboplatin which results in a more stable compound; decreased reactivity with macromolecules and differences in renal handling appear to be important factors in this improvement. Differences in the toxicity and pharmacokinetic profiles of the drugs may be important determinants in the selection of carboplatin versus cisplatin for specific patients. In addition, differences in toxicity profile may make it possible to escalate carboplatin dosages beyond those usually recommended particularly when autologous bone marrow transplantation (ABMT), peripheral stem cell transplantation, and/or hematopoietic agents (colony-stimulating factors) are used concomitantly.

Information on safety and efficacy of carboplatin has been obtained from clinical studies in patients with malignancy who received the drug alone or in conjunction with other antineoplastic agents (i.e., cyclophosphamide).

■ Hematologic Effects The major and dose-limiting adverse effect of carboplatin is bone marrow suppression, which is manifested as thrombocytopenia, leukopenia, neutropenia, and/or anemia and is more pronounced than that with cisplatin. Carboplatin-induced myelosuppression is dose related and appears to be most common and more severe in patients who have received prior antineoplastic therapy (especially cisplatin-containing regimens), those who are receiving concurrently or have received recently other myelosuppressive drugs or radiation therapy, and those who have renal impairment. The correlation between renal function and degree of thrombocytopenia and neutropenia is related to the pharmacokinetic characteristics of carboplatin and has resulted in the development of individualized dosing schedules based on glomerular filtration rate. (See Dosage: Individualization of Dosage, in Dosage and Administration.) Patients with poor performance status also appear to be at increased risk for severe leukopenia and thrombocytopenia during carboplatin therapy.

At usual dosages, carboplatin-induced thrombocytopenia is more common and pronounced than leukopenia. Thrombocytopenia (platelet counts less than 100,000/mm³) occurred in about 60–70% of patients receiving usual dosages of carboplatin alone or in conjunction with cyclophosphamide in clinical trials; more severe thrombocytopenia (platelet counts less than 50,000/mm³) occurred in 22–41% of patients. Thrombocytopenia may be cumulative and occasionally require platelet transfusions. Leukopenia (leukocyte count less than 4000/mm³) was reported in up to 85–98% of patients receiving usual dosages of the drug alone or in conjunction with cyclophosphamide in clinical trials. Leukopenia was pronounced (leukocyte count less than 2000/mm³) in 15–26% of patients receiving usual dosages of carboplatin alone and in 68–76% of patients receiving the drug in conjunction with cyclophosphamide. In patients who received carboplatin alone, neutrophil counts less than 2000/mm³ occurred in 67% and neutrophil counts less than 1000/mm³ occurred in 16–21% of patients. When the drug was used in conjunction with cyclophosphamide, neutrophil counts less than 2000/mm³ occurred in 95–97% and counts less than 1000/mm³ occurred in up to 84% of patients. At high doses (i.e., 1.2 g/m² or greater), more than 90% of patients reportedly experience grade IV thrombocytopenia and neutropenia (platelet counts less than 25,000/mm³ and neutrophil counts less than 500/mm³, respectively), and decreases in hemoglobin concentrations of 3–3.5 g/dL.

When carboplatin is administered alone, leukocyte and platelet nadirs generally occur 21 days (range: 14–28 days) following administration of the drug, and recovery of platelet counts (exceeding 100,000/mm³), leukocyte counts (exceeding 4000/mm³, and neutrophil counts (exceeding 2000/mm³) occurs within 28 days in 90, 67, and 74% of patients, respectively. In most patients, recovery generally is adequate to permit a repeat carboplatin dose 4 weeks after a previous dose. In clinical studies, at least one episode of infection occurred in 5% of patients receiving carboplatin alone and in 14–18% of patients receiving the drug in conjunction with cyclophosphamide.

Anemia (hemoglobin less than 11 g/dL), which may be symptomatic (e.g., accompanied by asthenia), occurred in 71–91% of patients receiving usual dosages of carboplatin alone or in conjunction with cyclophosphamide in clinical trials, and anemia was severe (hemoglobin less than 8 g/dL) in 8–21% of such patients. The incidence of anemia appears to increase with increased exposure to carboplatin. Since anemia may be cumulative, transfusions may be needed during carboplatin therapy, particularly in patients receiving prolonged (e.g., more than 6 cycles) therapy. In clinical studies, bleeding was reported in 5–10% and transfusions were administered to 25–44% of patients.

While hematologic toxicity associated with the standard dosages of carboplatin usually is not of sufficient magnitude to warrant routine administration of hematopoietic agents, autologous bone marrow transplant (ABMT), peripheral stem cell transplantation, and/or colony-stimulating factors (e.g., granulocyte colony-stimulating factor) have been used in patients receiving high-dose carboplatin or carboplatin in conjunction with other myelosuppressive therapy.

■ GI Effects Nausea and/or vomiting, which generally are mild to moderate in severity, have occurred in 65–94% of patients receiving carboplatin alone or in conjunction with cyclophosphamide. Carboplatin is classified as an antineoplastic agent of *moderate emetic risk* (i.e., incidence of emesis without antiemetics exceeds 30% but does not exceed 90%). Although nausea and/or vomiting occur in most patients receiving carboplatin, the drug is substantially less emetogenic and better tolerated than cisplatin. When carboplatin is used alone, nausea occurs in 10–15% and vomiting occurs in 65–81% of patients. Nausea and vomiting usually begin within 6–12 hours after administration of carboplatin and may persist up to 24 hours or longer; in some patients, vomiting may persist for up to 3 days. Delayed vomiting beginning 24 hours or longer after chemotherapy also has occurred in some patients. The incidence and severity of emesis may be reduced by pretreatment with antiemetics, although nausea and vomiting rarely may be refractory to antiemetic therapy. Carboplatin-induced acute vomiting episodes appear to be mediated by local GI and central mechanisms involving serotonin, and are most common in patients who have received prior emetogenic antineoplastic regimens (especially cisplatin-containing regimens) and in those who are receiving other emetogenic agents concurrently.

There is some evidence that the incidence of nausea and vomiting is reduced when carboplatin is given as a 24-hour continuous IV infusion or administered IV in divided doses over 5 consecutive days rather than as a single IV infusion; however, efficacy of these administration schedules in the treatment of ovarian carcinoma has not been established. For the prevention of *acute* emesis, the American Society of Clinical Oncology (ASCO) currently recommends a 2-drug antiemetic regimen consisting of a 5-HT_3 serotonin receptor antagonist and dexamethasone given before the administration of carboplatin or other chemotherapy with moderate emetic risk. Delayed or anticipatory vomiting is more difficult to manage. For the prevention of *delayed* emesis, ASCO currently recommends single-agent therapy with dexamethasone or a 5-HT_3 serotonin receptor antagonist following the administration of carboplatin or other chemotherapy regimens with moderate emetic risk. Because anticipatory vomiting is a learned response conditioned by the severity and duration of previous emetic reactions to chemotherapy, optimal use of antiemetics for prevention of acute and delayed emesis during early courses of therapy is the most important means for preventing this effect; behavioral modification, hypnosis, and drug therapy (e.g., a benzodiazepine such as alprazolam or lorazepam [for anxiolytic, sedative, amnesic, and possibly antiemetic effects] with or without conventional antiemetics) also may be useful. For additional information on the mechanisms and management of nausea and vomiting induced by platinum compounds, see Cautions: GI Effects in Cisplatin 10:00.

Adverse GI effects other than nausea and vomiting have been reported in 21% of patients receiving carboplatin alone and in 40–50% of patients receiving carboplatin in conjunction with cyclophosphamide. When carboplatin is used alone, GI pain, diarrhea, and constipation have been reported in 6–17% of patients. Anorexia also has been reported in patients receiving carboplatin.

Mucositis (i.e., oral ulceration) has been reported in 1% of patients receiving carboplatin alone and in 6–10% of patients receiving the drug in conjunction with cyclophosphamide.

Nervous System Effects Carboplatin-containing regimens are associated with a lower incidence of, and less severe, neurotoxicity than cisplatin-containing regimens. Neurotoxicity associated with carboplatin usually is characterized by peripheral neuropathies, which generally are sensory in nature (e.g., paresthesia). Peripheral neuropathies have occurred in 4–6% of patients receiving carboplatin alone and in 13–16% of patients receiving the drug in conjunction with cyclophosphamide. Carboplatin-induced peripheral neuropathy appears to be more common in patients older than 65 years of age than in younger adults. In addition, carboplatin-induced peripheral neuropathies appear to be cumulative occurring most commonly in patients receiving prolonged therapy and/or those who have received prior cisplatin therapy; in some cases, the neurotoxicity may be a delayed effect of cisplatin rather than secondary to carboplatin. Patients with preexisting cisplatin-induced peripheral neurotoxicity generally do not experience additional neurologic deterioration during carboplatin therapy.

Adverse sensory effects, including otic and ocular effects (see Cautions: Otic and Ocular Effects) and taste abnormalities, have been reported in up to 13% of patients receiving usual dosages of carboplatin. Central neurotoxicity has been reported in 5% of patients receiving carboplatin alone and in 23–28% of patients receiving carboplatin in conjunction with cyclophosphamide. It has been suggested that central neurotoxicity in many of these patients may have been related to concomitant antiemetic therapy. Fatigue was one of the most common nonhematologic effects reported in patients receiving carboplatin concomitantly with paclitaxel.

Otic and Ocular Effects Ototoxicity has been reported in 12–13% of patients receiving usual dosages of carboplatin in conjunction with cyclophosphamide. When carboplatin has been used alone, ototoxicity and adverse sensory effects have been reported in only 1% of patients. While carboplatin is associated with a low incidence of hearing loss at usual dosages, ototoxicity may be dose-limiting at carboplatin doses of 2 g/m^2 or greater. The risk of ototoxicity also may be increased by concomitantly administered ototoxic drugs (e.g., aminoglycosides, furosemide, ifosfamide). (See Drug Interactions: Other Drugs.) Clinically important hearing loss has occurred in pediatric patients receiving carboplatin at higher than recommended doses in combination with other ototoxic agents.

Other adverse sensory effects, including visual abnormalities, have been reported in 4–6% of patients receiving usual dosages of carboplatin in conjunction with cyclophosphamide. Loss of vision (which can be complete for light and colors) has been reported rarely in patients receiving carboplatin doses higher than those usually recommended; improvement and/or total recovery of vision occurred within weeks after the drug was discontinued.

Renal and Electrolyte Effects Mild and transient elevations of serum creatinine and BUN concentrations have occurred in 6–22% of patients receiving carboplatin alone or in conjunction with cyclophosphamide. Acute renal failure has been reported rarely. Nephrotoxicity is less common and severe than that associated with cisplatin, and concomitant IV hydration and diuresis generally are not necessary with carboplatin. As a result, administration regimens and monitoring requirements with carboplatin generally are less complex, and outpatient therapy is easier to accomplish. However, the risk of carboplatin-induced nephrotoxicity (e.g., impaired creatinine clearance) becomes more prominent at relatively high dosages. Animal studies indicate that carboplatin's reduced nephrotoxic potential relative to cisplatin may relate to differences in renal handling of the drugs and reactivity with macroglobulins; differences in risk do not appear to correlate with renal platinum concentrations.

Carboplatin may cause electrolyte abnormalities, principally hyponatremia, hypokalemia, hypocalcemia, and/or hypomagnesemia. Such electrolyte changes, unlike those reported with cisplatin, usually are not symptomatic and do not require administration of supplemental electrolytes. Hyponatremia, hypocalcemia, and hypokalemia have been reported in 10–47% and hypomagnesemia has been reported in 29–62% of patients receiving carboplatin alone or in conjunction with cyclophosphamide.

Hepatic Effects Mild and usually transient elevations of serum alkaline phosphatase, aspartate aminotransferase (AST, SGOT), or bilirubin concentrations have been reported in 24–37, 15–23, or 5% of patients, respectively, receiving carboplatin alone or in conjunction with cyclophosphamide. Substantial abnormalities in liver function test results have been reported in a few patients receiving high doses of carboplatin (more than 4 times higher than the usually recommended dosage) and autologous bone marrow transplantation.

Sensitivity Reactions Allergic reactions have been reported in 2% of patients receiving carboplatin alone and in 10–12% of patients receiving carboplatin in conjunction with other antineoplastic agents. Allergic reactions associated with carboplatin are similar in nature and severity to those associated with other platinum-containing antineoplastic agents (e.g., cisplatin) and have included anaphylaxis and anaphylactoid reactions. Although allergic reactions usually have occurred following multiple courses of platinum-containing therapy, such reactions can occur with the initial dose. The risk of allergic reactions, including anaphylaxis, is increased in patients who previously have received treatment with platinum-containing agents. Rash, perioral tingling, urticaria, erythema, pruritus, bronchospasm, hypotension, and hypoxia have occurred within a few minutes after IV administration of carboplatin in patients who previously received a platinum-containing antineoplastic agent. Exfoliative dermatitis has been reported rarely.

In many cases, allergic reactions appear to be immediate type I IgE-mediated hypersensitivity reactions, although some reactions may result from direct, nonimmunologic histamine release. In addition, some reactions may have been secondary to mannitol (which was present in the previous formulation) hypersensitivity rather than to carboplatin. Hypersensitivity reactions may be alleviated by IV epinephrine, corticosteroids, and/or antihistamines; in some cases, continued therapy with carboplatin may be possible with prophylactic corticosteroid and antihistamine therapy. While the manufacturer states that carboplatin is contraindicated in patients with a history of sensitivity reactions to other platinum-containing compounds, switching to cisplatin may be tolerated by some, but not all, patients who have experienced hypersensitivity reactions to carboplatin and vice versa.

Other Adverse Effects Although alopecia is uncommon in patients receiving carboplatin alone, occurring in about 2–3% of such patients, it occurs in 43–50% of patients receiving carboplatin in conjunction with cyclophosphamide. In patients receiving concurrent cyclophosphamide, the frequency and severity of alopecia was attributed to the cyclophosphamide dosage.

Pain, most likely related to tumor size, has been reported in 36–54% of patients receiving carboplatin in conjunction with cyclophosphamide. In addition, asthenia, presumably secondary to carboplatin-induced anemia, has occurred in 40–43% of patients receiving carboplatin in conjunction with cyclophosphamide. Malaise also has been reported in patients receiving the drug. Adverse respiratory and genitourinary effects have occurred in 2–6% of patients receiving carboplatin alone and in 8–12% of patients receiving the drug in conjunction with cyclophosphamide. Hemolytic uremic syndrome has occurred rarely. Myalgias/arthralgias were one of the most common nonhematologic adverse effects reported in patients receiving carboplatin concomitantly with paclitaxel; these effects were cumulative with repeated cycles.

Although not attributed to antineoplastic therapy, adverse cardiovascular effects, including cardiac failure, embolism, and cerebrovascular accident, have been reported in up to 23% of patients receiving carboplatin. Fatalities associated with cardiovascular events occurred in less than 1% of patients receiving the drug. Hypertension also has been reported in patients receiving carboplatin.

Precautions and Contraindications Carboplatin is a highly toxic drug with a low therapeutic index, and a therapeutic response is not likely to occur without some evidence of toxicity. The drug should be used under the supervision of physicians experienced in therapy with cytotoxic agents. In addition, the manufacturer states that carboplatin should be used only when adequate treatment facilities for appropriate management of therapy and complications are readily available.

Patients receiving carboplatin should be observed closely for possible hypersensitivity reactions, and appropriate equipment for maintenance of an adequate airway and other supportive measures and agents for the treatment of such reactions (e.g., antihistamines, epinephrine, oxygen, corticosteroids) should be readily available whenever carboplatin is administered. Patients with prior exposure to other platinum-containing agents are at increased risk for carboplatin-induced allergic reactions, including anaphylaxis. The manufacturer states that carboplatin is contraindicated in patients with a history of sensitivity reactions to the drug or other platinum-containing compounds (e.g., cisplatin); however, cross-sensitivity is not absolute, and occasionally with appropriate precautions patients sensitive to one platinum-containing compound have tolerated another. Exposure (e.g., industrial) to platinum-containing compounds can cause asthma and immediate and delayed hypersensitivity reactions, and the possibility that patients with a history of such exposure may be cross-sensitive to carboplatin should be considered.

The emetogenic potential of carboplatin should be considered. (See Cautions: GI Effects.) The neurotoxic potential of the drug also should be considered, particularly in geriatric patients older than 65 years of age and patients previously treated with cisplatin. (See Cautions: Nervous System Effects.) Vision loss is possible in patients receiving carboplatin, particularly at high doses. (See Cautions: Otic and Ocular Effects.)

Because patients who receive myelosuppressive drugs experience an increased frequency of infection and/or bleeding, hematologic status must be carefully monitored. While the hematologic toxicity of carboplatin usually is moderate and reversible, severe myelosuppression may occur in patients who received prior antineoplastic therapy (especially cisplatin-containing regimens), those who are receiving concurrently or have received recently other myelosuppressive drugs or radiation therapy, and those with renal impairment. To monitor for the occurrence of carboplatin-induced bone marrow suppression, the manufacturer recommends that peripheral blood counts be performed at frequent intervals in all patients receiving the drug. In studies used to establish efficacy of carboplatin, peripheral blood counts were determined weekly. Carboplatin usually should not be administered to patients with severe bone marrow depression or substantial bleeding. Pretreatment platelet counts and performance status are important prognostic factors for severity of myelosuppression in previously treated patients. In patients who experience myelosuppression following a dose of carboplatin, the manufacturer recommends that subsequent cycles of the drug be withheld until neutrophil counts exceed 2000/mm^3 and platelet counts exceed 100,000/mm^3. Treatment of severe hematologic toxicity may consist of supportive care, anti-infective agents for complicating infections, blood product transfusions, autologous bone marrow rescue, peripheral stem cell transplantation, and hematopoietic agents (colony-stimulating factors).

Because patients with renal impairment are at risk for severe bone marrow depression, renal function must be monitored carefully in patients receiving carboplatin. Creatinine clearance appears to most accurately reflect kidney function in patients receiving the drug. Although carboplatin has a low nephrotoxic potential, concomitant administration of an aminoglycoside has been associated with an increased risk of nephrotoxicity and/or ototoxicity. The possibility that carboplatin's nephrotoxicity may be potentiated by other nephrotoxic drugs also should be considered. (See Drug Interactions: Other Drugs.)

■ **Pediatric Precautions** The manufacturer states that safety and efficacy of carboplatin in children have not been established. Although experience is limited, carboplatin has been used in the treatment of germ cell tumors in adolescents 16 year of age or older, in the treatment of various brain tumors or neuroblastoma in children and adolescents 6 months to 19 years of age, and in the treatment of Wilms' tumor in children 2–15 years of age. Adverse effects reported to date in children are similar to those reported in adults and include hematologic toxicity (principally thrombocytopenia), adverse GI effects such as nausea and vomiting, and hypersensitivity reactions such as urticaria, facial swelling, abdominal pain, coryza, and cough. Hearing loss also has been reported in children receiving carboplatin. (See Cautions: Otic and Ocular Effects.)

■ **Geriatric Precautions** While the safety and efficacy of carboplatin in geriatric patients have not been established specifically, a substantial number of patients who received the drug in clinical trials as part of combination therapy for ovarian cancer were elderly (i.e., 36% were 65 years of age or older and 6% were 75 years of age or older). Age was not found to be a prognostic factor for survival in these studies.

Severe thrombocytopenia associated with carboplatin therapy occurred more frequently in geriatric patients than in younger patients. In addition, carboplatin-induced peripheral neuropathy appears to be more common in adults older than 65 years of age than in younger patients. Among a total of 1942 patients (21% of whom were 65 years of age or older) receiving carboplatin monotherapy for different tumor types, a similar incidence of adverse effects was observed in older and younger patients; other clinical experience has not revealed age-related differences among patients receiving the drug. However, the possibility of greater sensitivity of some older patients and increased risk for other effects of carboplatin related to age cannot be ruled out.

Because dosage of carboplatin generally is based on the clinical and hematologic response, renal function, and tolerance of the patient, the fact that geriatric patients may have decreased renal function as well as decreased hematopoietic function should be considered. The manufacturer recommends that dosing formulas based on estimates of glomerular filtration rate be used to determine the appropriate dosage of carboplatin in geriatric patients.

■ **Mutagenicity and Carcinogenicity** Carboplatin is mutagenic in both in vitro and in vivo experimental models.

Although the carcinogenic potential of carboplatin has not been fully studied, the manufacturer states that drugs with similar mechanisms of action and evidence of mutagenic effects have been reported to be carcinogenic. Secondary malignancies have been reported in patients receiving carboplatin in combination with other agents.

■ **Pregnancy, Fertility, and Lactation** Carboplatin can cause fetal toxicity when administered to pregnant women, but potential benefits from use of the drug may be acceptable in certain conditions despite possible risks to the fetus. Carboplatin has been shown to be embryotoxic and teratogenic in rats. Reproductive studies in rats receiving carboplatin during organogenesis revealed evidence of embryotoxicity and teratogenicity. There are no adequate or controlled studies to date using carboplatin in pregnant women. Carboplatin should be used during pregnancy only in life-threatening situations or for disease for which safer drugs cannot be used or are ineffective. If the drug is administered during pregnancy or if the patient becomes pregnant while receiving carboplatin, the patient should be informed of the potential hazard to the fetus. Women of childbearing potential should be advised to avoid becoming pregnant during carboplatin therapy.

The effects of carboplatin on the gonads and fertility have not been fully determined.

It is not known whether carboplatin or its platinum-containing products are distributed into human milk. Because of the potential for serious adverse reactions to carboplatin in nursing infants if the drug were distributed into milk, nursing should be discontinued during carboplatin therapy.

Drug Interactions

■ **Myelosuppressive Therapy** Concomitant use of carboplatin and other myelosuppressive agents or radiation therapy may potentiate the hematologic toxicity of the other agents and vice versa. Patients receiving concurrently or who have received recently such therapy should be monitored carefully, and dosage of the drugs and time of administration should be managed to minimize additive toxic effects. In addition, the fact that use of carboplatin in individuals who have received prior antineoplastic therapy is associated with an increased risk of bone marrow suppression should be considered.

■ **Other Drugs** Concomitant administration of carboplatin and aminoglycosides results in an increased risk of nephrotoxicity and/or ototoxicity, and the drugs should be used concurrently with caution. Clinically important hearing loss has been reported in children receiving carboplatin at higher than recommended doses in combination with other ototoxic medications. The manufacturer states that the renal effects of other nephrotoxic drugs may be potentiated by carboplatin.

Concomitant use of carboplatin and other emetogenic drugs or use of carboplatin in individuals who previously received emetogenic therapy is associated with an increased incidence of emesis.

Acute Toxicity

■ **Manifestations** Limited information is available on the acute toxicity of carboplatin. Overdosage of the drug would be expected to produce complications secondary to bone marrow suppression and/or hepatotoxicity. In addition, typical nonhematologic toxicity associated with platinum-containing antineoplastic agents (e.g., nephrotoxicity, neurotoxicity, ototoxicity) would be expected to become prominent with carboplatin overdosage. Carboplatin is substantially less toxic on a mg-for-mg basis than cisplatin, and inadvertent substitution of *cisplatin* (which usually is administered at substantially lower dosages) for carboplatin has resulted in massive cisplatin overdosage, including fatalities. (See Acute Toxicity in Cisplatin 10:00.)

■ **Treatment** There currently is no established specific antidote for carboplatin overdosage. Management of overdosage currently consists principally in discontinuance of the drug and initiation of supportive measures appropriate for the type of toxicity observed. The use of colony-stimulating factors (CSFs), platelet transfusions, and/or red blood cell transfusions should be considered in patients experiencing substantial myelosuppression. Whether measures suggested for the management of cisplatin overdosage, including the possible merits of chemoprotectants,would be of benefit in the event of massive carboplatin overdosage remains to be established. (For additional information on acute toxicity associated with platinum compounds, see Acute Toxicity in Cisplatin 10:00.)

Although carboplatin is removed by hemodialysis, it is not known whether this procedure would enhance elimination of the drug following overdosage. Plasmapheresis has been used effectively in the management of cisplatin overdosage, and the possibility that it may be useful in the management of massive carboplatin overdosage should be considered.

Pharmacology

The exact mechanism(s) of action of carboplatin has not been conclusively determined. Platinum-containing antineoplastic agents such as carboplatin and cisplatin appear to exert their effects by binding to DNA, thereby inhibiting DNA synthesis. The drugs are cycle-phase nonspecific. Carboplatin and cisplatin appear to act on tumor cells by the same general molecular mechanisms and, once bound to DNA, have virtually the same action. Although the principal mechanism of action of the drugs appears to be inhibition of DNA synthesis, other mechanisms also are involved in their antineoplastic activity.

Carboplatin, like cisplatin, must undergo activation before antineoplastic activity occurs. The bidentate dicarboxylate ligands of carboplatin presumably are displaced by water (aquation), forming positively charged platinum complexes that react with nucleophilic sites on DNA. Although both carboplatin and cisplatin are activated by an initial aquation reaction, carboplatin is a more stable compound and is activated more slowly than cisplatin.

Carboplatin produces predominantly DNA intrastrand interstrand cross-links rather than DNA-protein cross-links. The relative importance of intrastrand or interstrand DNA cross-linking in the antineoplastic activity of carboplatin remains to be clearly determined; however, interstrand cross-linking appears to correlate well with the cytotoxicity of the drug. Intrastrand cross-links result from the formation of adducts between the activated platinum complexes of the drug and (but not exclusively) the N-7 atom on guanine to produce 1,2-intrastrand links between adjacent guanosine molecules, between neighboring guanosine and adenosine molecules, or between neighboring guanosine molecules. Interstrand cross-linking within the DNA helix also occurs. The resultant interstrand intrastrand cross-links are stable bonds that do not dissociate easily. While the mechanism through which DNA adducts exert their cytotoxic effects has not been determined, limited evidence indicates that platinum adducts may inhibit DNA replication, transcription, and ultimately cell division.

Higher concentrations of carboplatin than cisplatin are required to produce equivalent levels of DNA binding. In one in vitro study comparing the relative potency of the drugs in L1210 cells, carboplatin was 45 times less cytotoxic than cisplatin on a molar basis and peak levels of cross-linking occurred 6-12 hours later with carboplatin than with cisplatin. These differences are believed to result from the difference in rates of aquation or activation of the drugs. When the drugs are compared at concentrations that produce equivalent levels of DNA binding, however, both drugs induce equal numbers of drug-DNA cross-links, resulting in equivalent lesions and biologic activity. In various studies in mice, the antitumor activity of carboplatin was comparable to or slightly less than that of cisplatin.

Further study is needed to elucidate more fully the extent of cross-resistance between cisplatin and carboplatin. Although some cisplatin-refractory tumors may respond to carboplatin, a high degree of cross-resistance appears to occur between the drugs. The mechanisms of cellular resistance to platinum-containing antineoplastic agents have not been fully elucidated, but studies using cisplatin indicate that resistance can be related to decreased cellular uptake of the drug or enhanced DNA repair and may be related to elevated cellular levels of sulfhydryl (thiol) compounds including glutathione or metallothionein. Glutathione appears to play an essential role in protecting cells from the effects of certain toxins including certain antineoplastic agents, and increased levels of this sulfhydryl compound have been demonstrated in certain cell lines resistant to cisplatin and other analogs. Increased repair of platinum complex-induced DNA adducts also has been demonstrated in certain resistant cell lines. The relative roles of these mechanisms of resistance and their relationship to treatment failure in patients who do not respond to platinum-containing antineoplastic agents has not been fully determined.

Pharmacokinetics

The pharmacokinetics of carboplatin are complex and involve the parent compound as well as total platinum and ultrafilterable platinum. Total platinum consists of both protein-bound and nonprotein-bound platinum, while ultrafilterable platinum consists of carboplatin and nonprotein-bound carboplatin metabolites. Measurement of ultrafilterable platinum is commonly used in pharmacokinetic studies of carboplatin since only nonprotein-bound platinum or its platinum-containing products are cytotoxic.

The pharmacokinetics of carboplatin have been studied principally in adults with various malignancies who received the drug IV either alone or in conjunction with other antineoplastic agents. The pharmacokinetics of the drug are similar to those of cisplatin; however, a smaller percentage of carboplatin's total platinum is protein-bound, carboplatin has a longer initial distribution half-life ($t_{1/2\alpha}$), and carboplatin undergoes more extensive renal excretion.

■ **Absorption** Following IV infusion of a single dose of carboplatin in adults with malignancies, peak plasma concentrations of carboplatin, total platinum, and ultrafilterable platinum occur immediately. When a single carboplatin dose of 290–370 mg/m² is administered IV over 30–40 minutes in cancer patients with normal renal function, peak plasma concentrations of carboplatin, total platinum, and ultrafilterable platinum range from 84–140, 84–134, and 90–130 μmol/L, respectively; these plasma concentrations are essentially the same over the first 6 hours. Over a dosage range of 20–500 mg/m², peak plasma concentrations of carboplatin and free platinum and area under the plasma concentration-time curve (AUC) of the drug increase linearly with dose.

Carboplatin is absorbed following intraperitoneal administration†, and peak concentrations of total platinum, free platinum, and carboplatin are attained within 2–4 hours following instillation. In a limited number of patients receiving intraperitoneal carboplatin dosages of 200–300 mg/m², approximately 65% of the dose was absorbed over a 4-hour dwell period. Although peak concentrations of ultrafilterable platinum in peritoneal fluid substantially exceed those achieved in plasma, penetration of platinum from the peritoneal cavity into tumor tissue is limited. While the clinical importance is unclear, data from studies in rats indicate that cisplatin is able to penetrate tumor tissue more effectively than carboplatin following intraperitoneal administration.

■ **Distribution** Following IV administration of carboplatin, platinum is widely distributed into body tissues and fluids, with highest concentrations in the kidney, liver, skin, and tumor tissue. Lower concentrations are found in fat and brain. Platinum also is distributed into erythrocytes, with maximum platinum concentrations of 2.5 μmol/L obtained 6 hours after IV infusion of a carboplatin dose of 290–370 mg/m². Following IV administration, the initial distribution half-lives of carboplatin, total platinum, and ultrafilterable platinum are essentially the same; the $t_{1/2\alpha}$ of carboplatin has been reported to be 1–2 hours. The volumes of distribution at steady-state of carboplatin, total platinum, and ultrafilterable platinum average 9–25, 23–117, and 10–20 L/m² respectively.

In vitro studies indicate that carboplatin is not bound to plasma proteins, but degrades to platinum-containing products which rapidly bind to protein. In vivo, protein binding increases over time as the platinum-containing products of carboplatin become bound to tissue and plasma proteins. During the first 4 hours following IV administration of carboplatin, less than 24% of platinum is bound to plasma proteins; however, within 24 hours, 87% of platinum is protein-bound.

It is not known whether carboplatin or its platinum-containing products cross the placenta or are distributed into milk.

■ **Elimination** Following IV administration of carboplatin, plasma concentrations of carboplatin and ultrafilterable platinum has been reported to decline in a biphasic manner, while plasma concentrations of total platinum reportedly decline in a triphasic manner. In adults with malignancy and normal renal function, plasma elimination half-lives ($t_{1/2\beta}$) of 2–3 hours have been reported for carboplatin and ultrafilterable platinum. A terminal elimination half-life ($t_{1/2\gamma}$) of 4–6 days has been reported for total platinum. Small amounts of total platinum can be detected in plasma 4 weeks after administration of carboplatin, indicating that the rate of elimination of total platinum may decrease with time.

The mean elimination half-life of total platinum from erythrocytes reportedly is about 12 days following IV administration of the drug. Following intraperitoneal administration of carboplatin, the peritoneal elimination half-life of ultrafilterable platinum is about 4.2 hours.

Renal clearance and total body clearance of platinum are reduced in patients with impaired renal function. In patients undergoing hemodialysis, the $t_{1/2\beta}$ of total and ultrafilterable platinum is increased compared with values reported in individuals with normal renal function.

The metabolic fate of carboplatin has not been completely elucidated. There is no evidence to date that the drug undergoes enzymatic biotransformation; the bidentate dicarboxylate ligands of carboplatin are believed to be displaced by water, forming positively charged platinum complexes that react with nucleophilic sites on DNA.

Carboplatin and its platinum-containing product(s) are excreted principally in urine; there are insufficient data to date to determine whether intestinal secretion or fecal elimination occurs. Renal excretion predominantly occurs via glomerular filtration. The clearance of carboplatin is directly affected by the glomerular filtration rate (GFR), and this parameter of renal function often is decreased in geriatric patients. Dosing formulas that incorporate estimates of GFR to provide predictable areas under the plasma concentration-time curve (AUCs) for carboplatin should be used in geriatric patients to minimize the risk of toxicity. The relationship between GFR and AUC of ultrafilterable platinum has been used to develop several formulas for calculating carboplatin dosage. (See Dosage: Individualization of Dosage, in Dosage and Administration.) In patients with malignancy and normal renal function, about 65% of an IV dose of carboplatin is eliminated in urine within 12 hours and 71% is eliminated within 24 hours; a substantial portion of the amount excreted is unchanged carboplatin. Carboplatin (as ultrafilterable carboplatin) is removed extensively by hemodialysis.

Chemistry and Stability

■ **Chemistry** Carboplatin is a platinum-containing antineoplastic agent. Carboplatin, like cisplatin, is a platinum coordination compound composed of a platinum atom surrounded in a plane by 2 ammonia groups and 2 other ligands in the *cis* position; presence of the ammonia groups, the *cis* configuration, and neutrality in plasma are necessary for the activity of both drugs. However, the other 2 ligands in carboplatin are present in a bidentate dicarboxylate chelate ring structure rather than as 2 chloride atoms present in cisplatin. The cyclobutane dicarboxylate moiety has greater chemical stability than the chlorides contained in cisplatin and this difference results in a less reactive compound that is associated with reduced toxicity (e.g., nephrotoxicity) but with antineoplastic activity that may be comparable to or slightly less than that of cisplatin.

Carboplatin occurs as a white to off-white crystalline powder. The drug has a solubility of 14 mg/mL in water and is insoluble in alcohol. A 1% solution of carboplatin has a pH of 5–7. Carboplatin is commercially available as a sterile, pyrogen-free, aqueous solution containing 10 mg of carboplatin per mL.

■ **Stability** Commercially available carboplatin aqueous solution in unopened vials is stable until the date indicated on the package when protected from light and stored as directed; the solution should be stored at 25°C, but may be exposed to temperatures ranging from 15–30°C. Carboplatin injection in multidose vials is stable for up to 14 days at 25°C.

Carboplatin aqueous solution may be further diluted in 5% dextrose injection or 0.9% sodium chloride injection to concentrations as low as 0.5 mg/mL, and these dilutions are stable for 8 hours at 25°C; because there is no preservative in the formulation, the manufacturer states that unused portions of diluted carboplatin solution for infusion should be discarded 8 hours after preparation.

Because some platinum coordination compounds (e.g., cisplatin) are unstable in certain sodium chloride solutions and because there is evidence that carboplatin dissolved in sodium chloride solutions is converted partially in vitro to cisplatin, it previously was suggested that these solutions not be used to dilute carboplatin. However, while the rate of carboplatin decomposition in 0.9% sodium chloride or 5% dextrose and 0.9% sodium chloride is greater than that in sterile water for injection (i.e., 4% loss in 7 days at 27°C), it still does not exceed 10% per day at room temperature (i.e., 4-5% loss in 24 hours at 25°C). In addition, while the process responsible for the loss of carboplatin potency in these solutions has not been fully characterized, a study using carboplatin solutions containing 1 mg/mL in 0.9% sodium chloride indicates that only a minimal amount of carboplatin (less than 0.7%) is converted to cisplatin within 24 hours at 25°C. Therefore, previous recommendations not to use sodium chloride solutions to dilute carboplatin no longer appear to be justified.

Aluminum displaces platinum from the carboplatin molecule, resulting in the formation of a black precipitate and loss of potency. Carboplatin solutions should not be prepared or administered with needles, syringes, catheters, or IV administration sets containing aluminum parts that might come in contact with the drug.

For further information on the handling of antineoplastic agents, see the ASHP Guidelines on Handling Hazardous Drugs at http://www.ahfsdruginformation.com.

Preparations

Excipients in commercially available drug preparations may have clinically important effects in some individuals; consult specific product labeling for details.

CARBOplatin

Parenteral

For injection, concentrate, for IV infusion	10 mg/mL (50, 150, 450, or 600 mg)*	**CARBOplatin for Injection**
		Paraplatin®, Bristol-Myers Squibb
For injection, for IV infusion	50 mg*	**CARBOplatin for Injection**
		Paraplatin®, Bristol-Myers Squibb
	150 mg*	**CARBOplatin for Injection**
		Paraplatin®, Bristol-Myers Squibb
	450 mg*	**CARBOplatin for Injection**
		Paraplatin®, Bristol-Myers Squibb

*available from one or more manufacturer, distributor, and/or repackager by generic (nonproprietary) name

†Use is not currently included in the labeling approved by the US Food and Drug Administration

Carfilzomib

■ Carfilzomib, an inhibitor of the 20S proteasome, is an antineoplastic agent.

Uses

■ **Multiple Myeloma** Carfilzomib is used alone for the treatment of multiple myeloma in patients who have received at least 2 prior therapies including bortezomib and an immunomodulatory agent (e.g., lenalidomide, thalidomide) and have demonstrated disease progression during or within 60 days following completion of their last therapy. Carfilzomib is designated an orphan drug by the US Food and Drug Administration (FDA) for use in multiple myeloma. The current indication is based on overall response rate; there currently are no clinical trials demonstrating a clinical benefit (e.g., improvement in disease-related symptoms, increased survival).

The current indication for carfilzomib is based principally on the results of an open-label, noncomparative, multicenter, phase 2 study in 266 adults with relapsed multiple myeloma who had received at least 2 prior therapies, including bortezomib and an immunomodulatory agent (e.g., lenalidomide, thalidomide, pomalidomide). Other prior therapies included high-dose corticosteroids, alkylating agents, anthracyclines, and stem cell transplantation. Patients were enrolled if their disease was refractory to their most recent therapy (i.e., response of no more than 25% or disease progression during or within 60 days following completion of their most recent therapy). Patients received IV carfilzomib on 2 consecutive days each week for 3 weeks followed by a 12-day rest period (28-day treatment cycle) until disease progression, unacceptable toxicity, or for a maximum of 12 cycles. Treatment consisted of carfilzomib 20 mg/m^2 for each dose during the first cycle and 27 mg/m^2 in subsequent cycles. The primary end point of this study was overall response rate, which was assessed according to the International Myeloma Working Group Uniform Response criteria; secondary end points included progression-free survival, overall survival, clinical benefit rate, and duration of response.

The median age of enrolled patients in this study was 63 years, and patients had received a median of 5 prior therapies for multiple myeloma. All except one of the enrolled patients had previously received bortezomib; a majority of these patients were refractory to bortezomib in any prior line of therapy and 45% were refractory to bortezomib in their most recent therapy. The overall response rate with carfilzomib was 22.9% with a median duration of response of 7.8 months; one patient (0.4%) achieved a complete response. In 257 response-evaluable patients, median progression-free survival and overall survival were 3.7 and 15.6 months, respectively; median overall survival was slightly shorter in patients refractory or intolerant to both bortezomib and lenalidomide and in those refractory to both drugs (13.2 and 11.9 months, respectively).

Longer-term maintenance therapy (i.e., more than 12 cycles) with carfilzomib has been shown to be effective and well tolerated in patients with relapsed and/or refractory multiple myeloma in an extension study.

The overall tolerability profile of carfilzomib appears to compare favorably with that of other drugs used in the treatment of multiple myeloma (e.g., bortezomib, lenalidomide, thalidomide). In particular, carfilzomib appears to be less likely than bortezomib and thalidomide to cause peripheral neuropathy; the incidence of new-onset or worsening peripheral neuropathy in the carfilzomib-treated patients in the main efficacy study was 12.4%. In addition, carfilzomib appears to be well tolerated when used in multiple myeloma patients with preexisting peripheral neuropathy. (See Description.) The incidence of thrombocytopenia appears to be similar between carfilzomib and bortezomib, and carfilzomib appears to cause minimal neutropenia; however, additional studies, including comparative trials, are needed to confirm these initial findings.

Dosage and Administration

■ **General** To minimize the risk of nephrotoxicity and tumor lysis syndrome associated with carfilzomib treatment, patients should be hydrated. Adequate fluid volume status should be maintained throughout therapy and blood chemistries should be monitored closely. The manufacturer recommends that 250–500 mL of 0.9% sodium chloride injection or other appropriate IV fluid be given prior to each dose of carfilzomib in cycle 1. An additional 250–500 mL of IV fluids may be given as needed following administration of the drug. In subsequent cycles, IV hydration may be continued as needed. Patients also should be monitored for fluid overload during this period. (See Tumor Lysis Syndrome under Cautions: Warnings/Precautions.)

To reduce the incidence and/or severity of infusion-related reactions, patients should be premedicated with dexamethasone 4 mg orally or IV prior to each dose of carfilzomib in cycle 1 and prior to each dose during the first cycle of dosage escalation to 27 mg/m^2. If an infusion-related reaction develops or reappears during subsequent cycles, dexamethasone premedication (4 mg orally or IV) should be reinstated. (See Infusion Reactions under Cautions: Warnings/Precautions.)

Because reactivation of herpes zoster was reported in 2% of carfilzomib-treated patients, the manufacturer and some clinicians recommend that antiviral prophylaxis (e.g., acyclovir) be considered in patients receiving the drug who have a history of herpes zoster infection.

Routine antiemetic and antidiarrheal prophylaxis is not necessary in patients receiving carfilzomib therapy.

Restricted Distribution Carfilzomib is currently available through select specialty distributors and wholesalers. Specific information regarding distribution of the drug is available from the manufacturer at http://www.kyprolis.com.

■ **Administration** Carfilzomib is administered IV over 2–10 minutes. The drug should *not* be administered by rapid IV injection, such as IV push or bolus. Immediately prior to and following carfilzomib administration, the IV administration line should be flushed with 0.9% sodium chloride injection or 5% dextrose injection.

Unreconstituted carfilzomib powder for injection should be stored in unopened vials at 2–8°C. Unopened vials should be retained in the original package for protection from light.

Prior to administration, commercially available carfilzomib powder for injection must be reconstituted and the reconstituted solution of the drug may be diluted using proper aseptic technique. The powder is reconstituted by adding 29 mL of sterile water for injection to a vial labeled as containing 60 mg of the drug to provide a solution containing 2-mg/mL. The diluent should be directed toward the inside wall of the vial to minimize foaming. The vial should then be gently swirled and/or inverted for approximately 1 minute, or until complete dissolution of the cake or powder occurs, and inspected visually for particulate matter and discoloration prior to dilution and administration. The resulting solution should *not* be shaken. If foaming occurs, the solution should be allowed to stand for about 2–5 minutes until foaming subsides. The solution should be clear, colorless, and free of visible particulates.

The desired dose of the carfilzomib reconstituted solution may be given by IV injection or may be further diluted with 5% dextrose injection for IV infusion. The reconstituted solution is diluted by adding an appropriate volume of carfilzomib 2-mg/mL solution to a 50-mL infusion bag containing 5% dextrose injection. Reconstituted and diluted solutions of the drug are stable for up to 4 or 24 hours at room temperature (15–30°C) or under refrigeration (2–8°C), respectively, regardless of container (e.g., vial, syringe, IV bag).

Carfilzomib should *not* be admixed with or administered as an infusion with any other drug. Commercially available carfilzomib for injection contains no preservatives and is intended for single use; vials containing the unused portion of the reconstituted solution should be immediately discarded.

■ **Dosage** ***Multiple Myeloma*** Carfilzomib dosage is calculated according to the patient's actual body surface area (BSA) at baseline. In patients with a BSA greater than 2.2 m^2, dosage of carfilzomib should be based on a BSA of 2.2 m^2. No dosage adjustment is necessary for weight changes of 20% or less.

For the treatment of multiple myeloma following failure of 2 or more chemotherapy regimens including bortezomib and an immunomodulatory agent and disease progression during or within 60 days following completion of the last therapy, the recommended adult dosage of carfilzomib during cycle 1 is 20 mg/m^2 administered IV over 2–10 minutes on 2 consecutive days each week for 3 weeks (days 1, 2, 8, 9, 15, and 16) followed by a 12-day rest period (days 17 through 28) of a 28-day cycle. If the dosage in cycle 1 is tolerated, the recommended dosage for cycle 2 and subsequent cycles is 27 mg/m^2. Therapy should be continued until disease progression or unacceptable toxicity occurs. In the principal efficacy study, therapy was continued for a maximum of 12 cycles.

The amount of carfilzomib contained in one 60-mg, single-use vial may exceed the single dose required. Caution should therefore be exercised in calculating the dose to prevent overdosage.

Dosage Modification for Toxicity **Dosage Modification for Hematologic Toxicity.** Platelet counts should be monitored frequently during carfilzomib therapy. If grade 3 or 4 neutropenia or grade 4 thrombocytopenia occurs, carfilzomib therapy should be withheld. If full recovery occurs prior to the next scheduled dose, carfilzomib may be resumed at the same dosage level. If the toxicity resolves to grade 2 neutropenia or grade 3 thrombocytopenia, the dosage of carfilzomib may be reduced by one dose level (i.e., a dose of 27 mg/m^2 reduced to 20 mg/m^2; a dose of 20 mg/m^2 reduced to 15 mg/m^2). If the reduced dosage is tolerated, the dosage may be escalated back to the previous dosage at the discretion of the clinician. (See Thrombocytopenia under Cautions: Warnings/Precautions.)

Dosage Modification for Cardiac Toxicity. If grade 3 or 4 new onset or worsening of congestive heart failure, decreased left ventricular function, or myocardial ischemia occurs, carfilzomib therapy should be withheld until the toxicity resolves or returns to baseline. Following resolution, it should be considered whether resuming carfilzomib therapy at a reduced dosage (i.e., a dose of 27 mg/m^2 reduced to 20 mg/m^2; a dose of 20 mg/m^2 reduced to 15 mg/m^2) is appropriate based on assessment of potential risks and benefits. If the reduced dosage is tolerated, the dosage may be escalated back to the previous dosage at the discretion of the clinician. (See Cardiac Effects under Cautions: Warnings/Precautions.)

Dosage Modification for Pulmonary Hypertension. If pulmonary arterial hypertension (PAH) occurs, carfilzomib therapy should be withheld until the toxicity resolves or returns to baseline. Following resolution, therapy may then be resumed at either the previous dosage or at a dosage reduced by one dose level (i.e., a dose of 27 mg/m^2 reduced to 20 mg/m^2; a dose of 20 mg/m^2 reduced to 15 mg/m^2) at the discretion of the clinician. If the reduced dosage is tolerated, the dosage may be escalated back to the previous dosage at the discretion of the clinician. (See Pulmonary Hypertension under Cautions: Warnings/Precautions.)

Dosage Modification for Pulmonary Complications. If grade 3 or 4 pulmonary complications (e.g., dyspnea) occur, carfilzomib therapy should be withheld until the toxicity resolves or returns to baseline. Resumption of therapy at a dosage reduced by one dose level (i.e., a dose of 27 mg/m² reduced to 20 mg/m²; a dose of 20 mg/m² reduced to 15 mg/m²) may then be considered. If the reduced dosage is tolerated, the dosage may be escalated back to the previous dosage at the discretion of the clinician. (See Pulmonary Complications under Cautions: Warnings/Precautions.)

Dosage Modification for Hepatic Toxicity. In patients who develop grade 3 or 4 elevations of serum aminotransferases (ALT or AST), bilirubin, or other liver abnormalities, carfilzomib therapy should be withheld until the toxicity resolves or returns to baseline. Following resolution, it should be considered whether resuming therapy is appropriate. Therapy may be resumed at a reduced dosage (i.e., a dose of 27 mg/m² reduced to 20 mg/m²; a dose of 20 mg/m² reduced to 15 mg/m²) with frequent monitoring of liver function tests. If the reduced dosage is tolerated, the dosage may be escalated back to the previous dosage at the discretion of the clinician. (See Hepatic Toxicity and Hepatic Failure under Cautions: Warnings/Precautions.)

Dosage Modification for Nephrotoxicity. In patients who develop elevated serum creatinine concentrations of 2 or more times the baseline value, carfilzomib therapy should be withheld until renal function recovers to grade 1 or baseline and renal function should be monitored. If nephrotoxicity is attributable to carfilzomib, therapy may then be resumed at a reduced dosage (i.e., a dose of 27 mg/m² reduced to 20 mg/m²; a dose of 20 mg/m² reduced to 15 mg/m²). If nephrotoxicity is not attributable to carfilzomib, therapy may be resumed at the dosage used prior to the event. If the reduced dosage is tolerated, the dosage may be escalated back to the previous dosage at the discretion of the clinician.

Dosage Modification for Peripheral Neuropathy. If grade 3 or 4 peripheral neuropathy occurs, carfilzomib therapy should be withheld until the condition resolves or returns to baseline. Therapy may then be resumed at the dosage used prior to the event or at a reduced dosage (i.e., a dose of 27 mg/m² reduced to 20 mg/m²; a dose of 20 mg/m² reduced to 15 mg/m²). If the reduced dosage is tolerated, the dosage may be escalated back to the previous dosage at the discretion of the clinician.

Dosage Modification for Other Nonhematologic Toxicity. If other grade 3 or 4 nonhematologic toxicity occurs, carfilzomib therapy should be withheld until the toxicity resolves or returns to baseline. Resumption of therapy at a dosage reduced by one dose level (i.e., a dose of 27 mg/m² reduced to 20 mg/m²; a dose of 20 mg/m² reduced to 15 mg/m²) may then be considered. If the reduced dosage is tolerated, the dosage may be escalated back to the previous dosage at the discretion of the clinician.

■ **Special Populations** Carfilzomib has not been studied in patients with preexisting hepatic impairment. The manufacturer does not provide specific dosage recommendations for such patients. (See Hepatic Impairment under Warnings/Precautions: Specific Populations, in Cautions.)

The pharmacokinetics and safety of carfilzomib are not influenced by the degree of preexisting renal impairment; therefore, dosage adjustment is not necessary in patients with renal impairment. However, because clearance of carfilzomib by hemodialysis has not been studied, the drug should be administered after the dialysis procedure. (See Renal Impairment under Warnings/Precautions: Specific Populations, in Cautions.)

Dosage adjustment is not necessary in geriatric patients. (See Geriatric Use under Warnings/Precautions: Specific Populations, in Cautions.)

Cautions

■ **Contraindications** The manufacturer states there are no known contraindications to the use of carfilzomib.

■ **Warnings/Precautions** ***Cardiac Effects*** Death from cardiac arrest has occurred within 24 hours of carfilzomib administration. New onset or worsening of preexisting congestive heart failure with decreased left ventricular function or myocardial ischemia also has been reported following administration of the drug. Heart failure-related events (e.g., congestive heart failure, pulmonary edema, decreased left ventricular ejection fraction) have been reported in 7% of patients receiving carfilzomib. Patients with New York Heart Association (NYHA) class III or IV heart failure, history of myocardial infarction in the preceding 6 months, or conduction abnormalities not controlled by medication were excluded from clinical trials; these patients may be at greater risk for cardiac complications.

Patients receiving carfilzomib should be monitored for the development of cardiac complications and managed promptly if they occur. If grade 3 or 4 cardiac toxicity occurs, therapy should be withheld until the toxicity resolves or returns to baseline. If resumption of therapy is considered appropriate based on assessment of potential risks and benefits, therapy may be resumed at a reduced dosage. (See Dosage Modification for Cardiac Toxicity under Dosage: Dosage Modification for Toxicity, in Dosage and Administration.)

Pulmonary Hypertension Pulmonary arterial hypertension (PAH) has been reported in 2% of patients receiving carfilzomib in clinical trials, and was grade 3 or greater in less than 1% of patients. Patients should be evaluated for PAH using cardiac imaging and/or other tests as indicated. If PAH is suspected, carfilzomib therapy should be withheld until signs and symptoms resolve or return to baseline. If resumption of therapy is considered appropriate based on assessment of potential risks and benefits, therapy may be resumed at either the previous dosage or at a reduced dosage. (See Dosage Modification for Pulmonary Hypertension under Dosage: Dosage Modification for Toxicity, in Dosage and Administration.)

Pulmonary Complications Dyspnea was reported in approximately 35% of patients receiving carfilzomib in clinical trials. Grade 3 dyspnea occurred in 5% of patients; no grade 4 cases and one fatal case of dyspnea were reported. In the main clinical trial, dyspnea generally occurred early in therapy and was transient, did not increase with cumulative exposure to the drug, and was not associated with progressive lung injury.

Patients should be monitored for dyspnea during carfilzomib therapy, and dyspnea should be managed immediately if it occurs. If grade 3 or 4 pulmonary toxicity (i.e., dyspnea) occurs, carfilzomib therapy should be withheld until the symptoms resolve or return to baseline; resumption of therapy at a reduced dosage may then be considered. (See Dosage Modification for Pulmonary Complications under Dosage: Dosage Modification for Toxicity, in Dosage and Administration.)

Infusion Reactions Infusion-related reactions characterized by a spectrum of systemic symptoms, including pyrexia, chills, arthralgia, myalgia, flushing, facial edema, emesis, weakness, dyspnea, hypoxia, hypotension, syncope, chest tightness, or angina, have been reported in patients receiving carfilzomib. These reactions can occur immediately following or up to 24–48 hours following IV administration of the drug.

To minimize the incidence and/or severity of infusion reactions, patients should be premedicated with dexamethasone prior to each dose of carfilzomib in cycle 1 and prior to each dose during the first cycle of dosage escalation to 27 mg/m². (See Dosage and Administration: General and also see Advice to Patients.)

Tumor Lysis Syndrome Tumor lysis syndrome has been reported rarely in patients receiving carfilzomib. In the principal phase 2 clinical trial, tumor lysis syndrome occurred in one patient (0.4%) who received the drug. Patients with multiple myeloma and a high tumor burden should be considered to be at greater risk for the syndrome. Patients should be well hydrated prior to administration of carfilzomib. Some clinicians also administer allopurinol to reduce the risk of tumor lysis syndrome. The manufacturer states that patients should be monitored for signs and symptoms of tumor lysis syndrome during carfilzomib therapy and, if present, they should be managed promptly. Carfilzomib therapy should be interrupted until tumor lysis syndrome has resolved. (See Dosage and Administration: General.)

Thrombocytopenia Thrombocytopenia, which in rare cases has required dosage reduction or discontinuance of therapy, has been reported in patients receiving carfilzomib. Among patients receiving carfilzomib for multiple myeloma, thrombocytopenia occurred in 36% of patients, including grade 4 thrombocytopenia in 10% of patients. Thrombocytopenia associated with the drug usually is transient; the nadir platelet count occurs around day 8 of each 4-week cycle, and recovery to baseline typically occurs by the start of the subsequent cycle.

The manufacturer states that platelet counts should be monitored frequently in patients receiving carfilzomib therapy. If thrombocytopenia occurs, the dosage of carfilzomib should be reduced or treatment interrupted as clinically indicated. (See Dosage Modification for Hematologic Toxicity under Dosage: Dosage Modification for Toxicity, in Dosage and Administration.)

Hepatic Toxicity and Hepatic Failure Hepatic failure, including fatal cases, has been reported in less than 1% of patients receiving carfilzomib. The drug also may cause elevations in serum aminotransferase (ALT or AST) and bilirubin concentrations. In the phase 2 clinical trial, 2 patients with normal baseline aminotransferase concentrations died from hepatic failure following carfilzomib therapy; aminotransferase elevations were reversible in the other patients in this study.

Liver enzymes should be monitored frequently in patients receiving carfilzomib. In patients who develop grade 3 or greater elevations of liver function tests, including serum aminotransferase or bilirubin concentrations, therapy with the drug should be withheld until the toxicity resolves or returns to baseline. Following resolution, it should be considered whether resuming carfilzomib therapy is appropriate. (See Dosage Modification for Hepatic Toxicity under Dosage: Dosage Modification for Toxicity, in Dosage and Administration.)

Fetal/Neonatal Morbidity and Mortality Carfilzomib may cause fetal harm if administered to pregnant women based on its mechanism of action and animal findings. There are no adequate and well-controlled studies in humans. The drug has been shown to be embryotoxic and fetotoxic in animals. Pregnancy should be avoided during carfilzomib therapy. Women of childbearing potential should use effective contraception while receiving the drug. If carfilzomib is used during pregnancy or if the patient becomes pregnant while receiving the drug, the patient should be apprised of the potential fetal hazard. (See Advice to Patients.)

Specific Populations **Pregnancy.** Category D. (See Users Guide and see Fetal/Neonatal Morbidity and Mortality under Cautions: Warnings/Precautions.)

Lactation. It is not known whether carfilzomib is distributed into human milk. Because many drugs are distributed into human milk and because of the potential for serious adverse reactions to carfilzomib in nursing infants, a decision should be made whether to discontinue nursing or the drug, taking into account the importance of the drug to the woman.

Pediatric Use. Safety and efficacy of carfilzomib have not been established in pediatric patients.

Geriatric Use. In a population pharmacokinetic analysis, carfilzomib exposure in patients 65 years of age and older did not differ substantially from that in adult patients younger than 65 years of age following a single 20–mg/m^2 IV dose of the drug. In clinical studies, no clinically important differences in safety or efficacy were observed between patients 65 years of age and older and younger adults. (See Dosage and Administration: Special Populations.)

Hepatic Impairment. The efficacy, safety, and pharmacokinetics of carfilzomib have not been studied in patients with baseline hepatic impairment. Patients with baseline serum aminotransferase (e.g., ALT, AST) concentrations 3 or more times the upper limit of normal (ULN) or bilirubin concentrations 2 or more times the ULN were excluded from carfilzomib clinical trials. (See Dosage and Administration: Special Populations.)

Renal Impairment. In a phase 2 study evaluating the pharmacokinetics and safety of carfilzomib in multiple myeloma patients with normal renal function and those with mild, moderate, and severe renal impairment, including patients on chronic hemodialysis, patients were treated with the drug for an average of 5.5 cycles in a dosage of 15 mg/m^2 in cycle 1, 20 mg/m^2 in cycle 2, and 27 mg/m^2 in cycle 3 and beyond. The pharmacokinetics and safety of carfilzomib were not affected by the degree of baseline renal impairment, including in patients who were receiving hemodialysis. However, because dialysis clearance of carfilzomib has not been specifically studied, the drug should be administered after the hemodialysis session. (See Dosage and Administration: Special Populations.)

Gender. A population pharmacokinetic analysis indicated that the area under the plasma concentration-time curve (AUC) and peak plasma concentrations of carfilzomib were not substantially affected by gender.

■ **Common Adverse Effects** Adverse effects reported in 30% or more of multiple myeloma patients receiving carfilzomib include fatigue, anemia, nausea, dyspnea, diarrhea, and pyrexia. Serious adverse effects occurred in 45% of patients, and included pneumonia, acute renal failure, pyrexia, and congestive heart failure.

Laboratory abnormalities reported in 10% or more of patients receiving carfilzomib include anemia, thrombocytopenia, increased creatinine concentrations, lymphopenia, neutropenia, hypokalemia, hypomagnesemia, leukopenia, increased AST concentrations, hyperglycemia, hypercalcemia, hypophosphatemia, and hyponatremia.

Drug Interactions

Carfilzomib appears to be metabolized principally by extrahepatic peptidase cleavage and epoxide hydrolysis. Cytochrome P-450 (CYP)-mediated mechanisms play a minor role in the drug's overall metabolism. In an in vitro study, carfilzomib demonstrated a modest inhibitory effect on CYP3A4/5. The drug does not induce CYP1A2 and CYP3A4 in human hepatocytes in vitro. Carfilzomib is a substrate of P-glycoprotein (P-gp). The drug has shown marginal inhibitory effects on P-gp in a Caco-2 monolayer system.

■ **Drugs Affecting Hepatic Microsomal Enzymes** Clinically important pharmacokinetic interactions with CYP inhibitors and inducers are unlikely.

■ **Drugs Metabolized by Hepatic Microsomal Enzymes** Clinically important pharmacokinetic interactions are not expected with concurrent use of drugs metabolized by CYP3A4/5.

When the CYP3A substrate midazolam was administered concomitantly with carfilzomib, the pharmacokinetics of midazolam were not affected.

■ **Drugs Affecting the P-glycoprotein Transport System** Carfilzomib is a substrate of P-gp and has demonstrated marginal inhibitory effects on P-gp. However, because carfilzomib is administered IV and extensively metabolized, the pharmacokinetics of carfilzomib are unlikely to be substantially affected by concurrent use of either P-gp inhibitors or inducers.

Description

Carfilzomib, a tetrapeptide epoxyketone proteasome inhibitor, is an antineoplastic agent. The drug selectively and irreversibly binds to the NH_2-terminal threonine active sites of the 20S proteolytic core particle within the 26S proteasome. The 26S proteasome is a large protein complex composed of the 20S proteolytic core, which contains the proteolytic active sites, and 19S regulatory complexes. Ubiquitinated proteins targeted for degradation by the 19S regulatory particles are cleaved by catalytic activities in the 20S proteolytic core; major catalytic activities of the 20S proteolytic core include chymotrypsin-like activity, trypsin-like activity, and caspase-like activity. The ubiquitin-proteasome pathway plays an essential role in regulating the intracellular concentration of specific proteins, thereby maintaining homeostasis within cells; cancer cells appear to be particularly dependent on proteasome-mediated homeostatic pathways. Carfilzomib potently and selectively inhibits chymotrypsin-like activity of the 20S proteasome, which results in accumulation of ubiquitinated proteins and causes proteotoxic stress and leads to cell cycle arrest and apoptosis. In vitro studies indicate that carfilzomib has antiproliferative and proapoptotic activities in solid and hematologic tumor cells, including in some bortezomib-resistant cell lines. In animal studies, carfilzomib inhibits proteasome activity in blood and tissue and delayed tumor growth in models of multiple myeloma, hematologic, and solid tumors.

Carfilzomib differs structurally from bortezomib; unlike bortezomib, carfilzomib contains an epoxyketone pharmacophore which is selective for the NH_2-terminal threonine active sites unique to the 20S proteolytic core of the 26S proteasome. The mechanism by which carfilzomib maintains activity in some bortezomib-resistant tumor cells has not been fully elucidated; however, studies suggest that carfilzomib produces more selective, potent, and durable proteasome inhibition than bortezomib. Although the exact mechanism for peripheral neuropathy resulting from proteasome inhibitor therapy has not been fully elucidated, it has been suggested that the selectivity of carfilzomib for the 26S proteasome and its weak activity on other protease classes may explain the lower incidence of neurotoxicity observed with the drug in animal and clinical studies. Neurodegeneration independent of proteasome inhibition also has been proposed as a mechanism for this class adverse effect associated with proteasome inhibitors; despite equivalent levels of proteasome inhibition with carfilzomib and bortezomib in vitro, only bortezomib reduced neurite length and neuronal cell survival.

Carfilzomib is approximately 97–98% bound to plasma proteins. Metabolism is thought to occur primarily by extrahepatic peptidase cleavage and epoxide hydrolysis to inactive metabolites; peptide fragments of carfilzomib (i.e., M14, M15) and carfilzomib diol (M16) are the major metabolites found in plasma and urine. Following initial IV doses of carfilzomib of 15 mg/m^2 or more, carfilzomib was rapidly cleared from plasma with an elimination half-life of no more than 1 hour.

Advice to Patients

Importance of informing clinician if fever, chills, rigors, chest pain, cough, or swelling of the feet or legs occurs.

Risk of fatigue, dizziness, syncope, and/or hypotension; importance of advising patients to avoid driving or operating machinery if these effects occur.

Risk of dyspnea, which generally occurs within a day of dosing. Importance of informing clinician if shortness of breath occurs.

Importance of advising patients to avoid dehydration since carfilzomib therapy may cause vomiting and/or diarrhea. Importance of advising patients to inform a clinician if dizziness, lightheadedness, or fainting spells occur.

Risk of fetal harm. Necessity of advising women of childbearing potential to avoid pregnancy and to use effective methods of contraception while receiving carfilzomib therapy. Importance of women informing clinicians immediately if they become pregnant during therapy. If pregnancy occurs, advise pregnant women of potential risk to the fetus.

Importance of advising women to avoid breast-feeding while receiving carfilzomib therapy. If patient wishes to resume breast-feeding following therapy, importance of discussing the appropriate timing with clinician.

Importance of informing clinicians of existing or contemplated concomitant therapy, including prescription and OTC drugs and dietary or herbal supplements, as well as any concomitant illnesses (e.g., congestive heart failure, history of myocardial infarction, conduction abnormalities).

Importance of informing patients of other important precautionary information. (See Cautions.)

Overview® (see Users Guide). For additional information on this drug until a more detailed monograph is developed and published, the manufacturer's labeling should be consulted. It is *essential* that the manufacturer's labeling be consulted for more detailed information on usual cautions, precautions, contraindications, potential drug interactions, laboratory test interferences, and acute toxicity. For further information on the handling of antineoplastic agents, see the ASHP Guidelines on Handling Hazardous Drugs at http://www.ahfsdruginformation.com.

Preparations

Carfilzomib is currently available through select specialty distributors and most wholesalers. Specific information regarding distribution of carfilzomib is available from the manufacturer at http://www.kyprolis.com.

Excipients in commercially available drug preparations may have clinically important effects in some individuals; consult specific product labeling for details.

Carfilzomib

Parenteral

For injection, for IV use only	60 mg	**Kyprolis®**, Onyx

Cemiplimab-rwlc

■ Cemiplimab, a fully human anti-programmed-death receptor-1 (anti-PD-1) monoclonal antibody, is an antineoplastic agent.

Uses

■ **Cutaneous Squamous Cell Carcinoma** Cemiplimab-rwlc is used for the treatment of metastatic or locally advanced cutaneous squamous cell carcinoma in patients who are not candidates for curative surgery or radiation therapy.

The current indication for cemiplimab-rwlc is based principally on the combined results of an open-label, multicenter, nonrandomized, phase 1 study (Study 1423) and an open-label, multicenter, nonrandomized, multicohort phase 2 study (Study 1540) in 108 adults with metastatic or locally advanced cutaneous squamous cell carcinoma who were not candidates for curative surgery or radiation therapy. In these studies, patients received cemiplimab-rwlc 3 mg/kg administered as an IV infusion every 2 weeks for up to 48 or 96 weeks. Treatment was continued for the specified duration or until the occurrence of unacceptable toxicity or disease progression. The primary measures of efficacy were objective response rate and duration of response as evaluated by an independent central review committee. Response was evaluated according to Response Evaluation Criteria in Solid Tumors (RECIST) in patients without externally visible target lesions or by a composite end point that included radiographic assessment according to RECIST and digital medical images according to World Health Organization (WHO) criteria in patients with externally visible target lesions.

The median age of patients in the combined analysis of Study 1423 and Study 1540 was 71 years (range: 38–96 years); 97% were white, 85% were male, 50% had received at least one prior systemic therapy, 96% had previously undergone surgery, and 79% had received prior radiation therapy. All patients enrolled in the studies had an Eastern Cooperative Oncology Group (ECOG) performance status of 0 or 1. Most patients (69%) had metastatic cutaneous squamous cell carcinoma and 31% had locally advanced disease. Among patients with metastatic cutaneous squamous cell carcinoma, 69% had distant metastases and 31% had nodal metastases only. These studies excluded patients with active autoimmune disease that required systemic therapy in the past 5 years; those who had received a solid organ transplant; those who had received prior therapy with other anti-programmed-death 1 (anti-PD-1) or anti-PD ligand 1 (anti-PD-L1) antibodies or other immune-checkpoint inhibitors; those with an ECOG performance status of 2 or greater; and those with human immunodeficiency virus (HIV), hepatitis B virus (HBV), or hepatitis C virus (HCV) infection.

At a median follow-up of 8.9 months, the objective response rate was 47.2%; complete responses were achieved in 3.7% of patients. In the cohort of patients with metastatic cutaneous squamous cell carcinoma at a median follow-up of 8.1 months, the objective response rate was 46.7%; complete responses were achieved in 5.3% of patients. In the cohort of patients with locally advanced cutaneous squamous cell carcinoma at a median follow-up 10.2 months, the objective response rate was 48.5%; there were no complete responses. At the time of analysis, the overall median duration of response had not been reached; however, 60 or 63% of patients with metastatic or locally advanced cutaneous squamous cell carcinoma, respectively, had durable responses of 6 months or more.

Dosage and Administration

■ General

Because immune-mediated adverse effects may occur in any organ system or tissue, the manufacturer states that blood chemistries and liver and thyroid function tests should be assessed prior to initiation of cemiplimab therapy and periodically during therapy.

Restricted Distribution Cemiplimab-rwlc can only be obtained through a limited network of speciality distributors or pharmacies. Clinicians may contact the manufacturer (Regeneron) at 877-542-8296 or consult the Libtayo® website (https://www.libtayohcp.com) for specific ordering and availability information.

■ Administration

Cemiplimab-rwlc is administered by IV infusion over 30 minutes.

Unopened vials of cemiplimab-rwlc injection concentrate should be stored at 2–8°C in the original carton to protect the drug from light, and should *not* be frozen or shaken.

Cemiplimab-rwlc injection concentrate must be diluted prior to administration. Prior to administration, cemiplimab-rwlc injection concentrate should be inspected visually for particulate matter and discoloration. The undiluted solution should be clear to slightly opalescent and colorless to pale yellow; the solution should *not* be used if it is cloudy or discolored or if foreign particles other than translucent to white particles are present. Cemiplimab-rwlc is diluted by adding 7 mL of cemiplimab-rwlc injection concentrate (containing 50 mg/mL) to an appropriate volume of 0.9% sodium chloride or 5% dextrose injection to a final concentration of 1–20 mg/mL. The diluted solution should be mixed by gentle inversion and should *not* be shaken. Cemiplimab-rwlc should be administered through a sterile, 0.2- to 5-μm inline or add-on filter.

Diluted solutions of the drug are stable for up to 8 hours after dilution (including infusion time) when stored at room temperature (up to 25°C) or up to 24 hours after dilution (including infusion time) when stored under refrigeration (2–8°C); diluted solutions of the drug should be brought to room temperature prior to administration. Diluted solutions of the drug should *not* be frozen.

Cemiplimab-rwlc injection concentrate is intended for single use only; any unused portion in the vial should be discarded.

■ Dosage

Cutaneous Squamous Cell Carcinoma For the treatment of metastatic or locally advanced cutaneous squamous cell carcinoma, the recommended adult dosage of cemiplimab-rwlc is 350 mg administered every 3 weeks. Therapy should be continued until disease progression or unacceptable toxicity occurs.

Therapy Interruption for Toxicity If immune-mediated adverse effects occur, temporary or permanent discontinuance of cemiplimab may be required based on the severity of the reaction.

Cemiplimab should be *permanently discontinued* in patients experiencing recurrent grade 3 or 4 immune-mediated adverse effects or persistent grade 2 or 3 immune-mediated adverse effects lasting 12 weeks or longer, and in those requiring a corticosteroid dosage of 10 mg or more of prednisone daily (or equivalent) for 12 weeks or longer.

Immune-mediated Pneumonitis. If grade 2 immune-mediated pneumonitis occurs, cemiplimab therapy should be interrupted. Once the toxicity has resolved to grade 0 or 1, cemiplimab therapy may be resumed following completion of the corticosteroid taper. (See Immune-mediated Pneumonitis under Cautions: Warnings/Precautions.)

If grade 3 or 4 immune-mediated pneumonitis occurs, cemiplimab therapy should be permanently discontinued.

Immune-mediated GI Effects. If grade 2 or 3 immune-mediated colitis occurs, cemiplimab therapy should be interrupted. Once the toxicity has resolved to grade 0 or 1, cemiplimab therapy may be resumed following completion of the corticosteroid taper. (See Immune-mediated GI Effects under Cautions: Warnings/Precautions.)

If grade 4 immune-mediated colitis occurs, cemiplimab therapy should be permanently discontinued.

Immune-mediated Hepatic Effects. For serum aminotransferase (ALT or AST) elevations exceeding 3 times but not more than 10 times the upper limit of normal (ULN) or total bilirubin concentrations exceeding the ULN but not more than 3 times the ULN, cemiplimab therapy should be interrupted. Once the toxicity has resolved to grade 0 or 1, cemiplimab therapy may be resumed following completion of the corticosteroid taper. (See Immune-mediated Hepatic Effects under Cautions: Warnings/Precautions.)

For ALT or AST elevations exceeding 10 times the ULN or total bilirubin concentrations exceeding 3 times the ULN, cemiplimab therapy should be permanently discontinued.

Immune-mediated Endocrine Effects. If grade 2–4 endocrinopathies (e.g., adrenal insufficiency, hypophysitis, hypothyroidism, hyperthyroidism, diabetes mellitus) occur, cemiplimab therapy should be interrupted if clinically necessary. (See Immune-mediated Endocrine Effects under Cautions: Warnings/Precautions.)

Other Immune-mediated Adverse Effects. If any other grade 3 immune-mediated adverse effects involving a major organ occur, cemiplimab therapy should be interrupted. Once the toxicity has resolved to grade 0 or 1, cemiplimab therapy may be resumed following completion of the corticosteroid taper. (See Other Immune-mediated Effects under Cautions: Warnings/Precautions.)

If any other grade 4 immune-mediated adverse effects involving a major organ occur, cemiplimab therapy should be permanently discontinued.

Infusion-related Reactions. If grade 1 or 2 infusion-related reactions occur, the infusion should be interrupted or the infusion rate should be reduced. (See Infusion-related Effects under Cautions: Warnings/Precautions.)

If grade 3 or 4 infusion-related reactions occur, cemiplimab therapy should be permanently discontinued.

■ Special Populations

The manufacturer makes no special population dosage recommendations at this time. (See Specific Populations under Cautions: Warnings/Precautions.)

Cautions

■ Contraindications

The manufacturer states there are no known contraindications to the use of cemiplimab.

■ Warnings/Precautions

Immune-mediated Pneumonitis Immune-mediated pneumonitis, sometimes fatal, has occurred in patients receiving cemiplimab therapy. Immune-mediated adverse effects generally occur during therapy with anti-programmed-death 1 (anti-PD-1) and anti-PD ligand 1 (anti-PD-L1) antibodies, but also may occur following discontinuance of the drug.

In clinical trials, immune-mediated pneumonitis occurred in 2.4% of 534 patients receiving cemiplimab-rwlc and was fatal in 0.2% of patients. Grade 2 or 3 immune-mediated pneumonitis was reported in 2% of patients. Cemiplimab-rwlc was permanently discontinued because of immune-mediated pneumonitis in 1.3% of patients receiving the drug. All patients experiencing immune-mediated pneumonitis received systemic corticosteroid therapy and 85% received high-dose corticosteroid therapy (40 mg or more of prednisone daily [or equivalent]). Immune-mediated pneumonitis resolved in 62% of patients.

Patients receiving cemiplimab should be monitored for manifestations of pneumonitis. Temporary interruption or discontinuance of cemiplimab may be necessary if immune-mediated pneumonitis occurs during therapy with the drug. (See Immune-mediated Pneumonitis under Dosage: Therapy Interruption for Toxicity, in Dosage and Administration.) In patients who develop grade 2 or greater pneumonitis, systemic corticosteroid therapy should be initiated (1–2 mg/kg of prednisone daily [or equivalent]) followed by tapering of the corticosteroid dosage over 1 month once symptoms improve to grade 0 or 1. Systemic immunosuppressive therapy may be considered in patients experiencing immune-mediated pneumonitis inadequately controlled with systemic corticosteroid therapy.

Immune-mediated GI Effects Immune-mediated colitis has occurred in patients receiving cemiplimab therapy. Immune-mediated adverse effects generally occur during therapy with anti-PD-1 and anti-PD-L1 antibodies, but also may occur following discontinuance of the drug.

In clinical trials, grade 2 or 3 immune-mediated colitis occurred in 0.9% of 534 patients receiving cemiplimab-rwlc. Cemiplimab-rwlc was permanently discontinued because of immune-mediated colitis in 0.2% of patients. All patients experiencing immune-mediated colitis received systemic corticosteroid therapy and 60% received high-dose corticosteroid therapy (40 mg or more of prednisone daily [or equivalent]). Immune-mediated colitis resolved in 80% of patients.

Patients receiving cemiplimab should be monitored for manifestations of colitis. Temporary interruption or discontinuance of cemiplimab may be necessary if immune-mediated colitis occurs during therapy with the drug. (See Immune-mediated GI Effects under Dosage: Therapy Interruption for Toxicity, in Dosage and Administration.) In patients who develop grade 2 or greater colitis, systemic corticosteroid therapy should be initiated (1–2 mg/kg of prednisone daily [or equivalent]) followed by tapering of the corticosteroid dosage over 1 month once symptoms improve to grade 0 or 1. Systemic immunosuppressive therapy may be considered in patients experiencing immune-mediated colitis inadequately controlled with systemic corticosteroid therapy.

Immune-mediated Hepatic Effects Immune-mediated hepatitis, sometimes fatal, has occurred in patients receiving cemiplimab therapy. Immune-mediated adverse effects generally occur during therapy with anti-PD-1 and anti-PD-L1 antibodies, but also may occur following discontinuance of the drug.

In clinical trials, immune-mediated hepatitis occurred in 2.1% of 534 patients receiving cemiplimab-rwlc and was fatal in 0.2% of patients. Grade 3 or 4 immune-mediated hepatitis was reported in 1.9% of patients. Cemiplimab-rwlc was permanently discontinued because of immune-mediated hepatitis in 0.9% of patients receiving the drug. All patients experiencing immune-mediated hepatitis received systemic corticosteroid therapy and 91% received high-dose corticosteroid therapy (40 mg or more of prednisone daily [or equivalent]). Immune-mediated hepatitis resolved in 64% of patients.

Patients receiving cemiplimab should be monitored for manifestations of hepatitis. Liver function tests should be assessed prior to initiation of cemiplimab therapy and periodically during therapy. Temporary interruption or discontinuance of cemiplimab may be necessary if immune-mediated hepatitis occurs during therapy with the drug. (See Immune-mediated Hepatic Effects under Dosage: Therapy Interruption for Toxicity, in Dosage and Administration.) If serum aminotransferase (ALT or AST) elevations exceeding 3 times the upper limit of normal (ULN) (i.e., grade 2 or greater) or total bilirubin concentrations exceeding the ULN occur, systemic corticosteroid therapy should be initiated (1–2 mg/kg of prednisone daily [or equivalent]) followed by tapering of the corticosteroid dosage over 1 month once the toxicity improves to grade 0 or 1. Systemic immunosuppressive therapy may be considered in patients experiencing immune-mediated hepatitis inadequately controlled with systemic corticosteroid therapy.

Immune-mediated Endocrine Effects Immune-mediated endocrinopathies, such as adrenal insufficiency, hypophysitis (including hypopituitarism), thyroid dysfunction (i.e., hypothyroidism, hyperthyroidism), and diabetes mellitus (including ketoacidosis), have occurred in patients receiving cemiplimab therapy. Immune-mediated adverse effects generally occur during therapy with anti-PD-1 and anti-PD-L1 antibodies, but also may occur following discontinuance of the drug.

Temporary interruption or discontinuance of cemiplimab may be necessary if immune-mediated endocrinopathies occur during therapy with the drug. (See Immune-mediated Endocrine Effects under Dosage: Therapy Interruption for Toxicity, in Dosage and Administration.) Certain grade 2 or greater endocrinopathies may require initiation of systemic corticosteroid therapy (1–2 mg/kg of prednisone daily [or equivalent]) followed by tapering of the corticosteroid dosage over 1 month once the toxicity improves to grade 0 or 1. Systemic immunosuppressive therapy may be considered in patients experiencing certain immune-mediated endocrinopathies inadequately controlled with systemic corticosteroid therapy. Hormone replacement therapy, including antidiabetic therapy (e.g., insulin), also should be administered as clinically indicated.

Adrenal Insufficiency. In clinical trials, grade 2 or 3 immune-mediated adrenal insufficiency occurred in 0.4% of 534 patients receiving cemiplimab-rwlc.

Patients receiving cemiplimab should be monitored for signs and symptoms of adrenal insufficiency.

Hypophysitis. In clinical trials, grade 3 immune-mediated hypophysitis occurred in 1 of 534 patients (0.2%) receiving cemiplimab-rwlc.

Patients receiving cemiplimab should be monitored for manifestations of hypophysitis.

Thyroid Dysfunction. In clinical trials, immune-mediated hypothyroidism occurred in 6% of 534 patients receiving cemiplimab-rwlc therapy and was grade 3 in 0.2% of patients. None of the patients experiencing immune-mediated hypothyroidism were able to discontinue thyroid hormone replacement therapy.

In clinical trials, immune-mediated hyperthyroidism occurred in 1.5% of 534 patients receiving cemiplimab-rwlc and was grade 2 or 3 in 0.6% of patients. Immune-mediated hyperthyroidism resolved in 38% of patients.

Patients receiving cemiplimab should be monitored for manifestations of thyroid dysfunction. Thyroid function should be evaluated prior to initiation of cemiplimab therapy and periodically during therapy.

Diabetes Mellitus. In clinical trials, grade 3 or 4 immune-mediated type 1 diabetes mellitus and ketoacidosis occurred in 0.7% of 534 patients receiving cemiplimab-rwlc. Cemiplimab-rwlc was permanently discontinued because of immune-mediated type 1 diabetes mellitus in 0.2% of patients receiving the drug.

Patients should be monitored for manifestations of diabetes mellitus. Blood glucose concentrations should be assessed prior to initiation of cemiplimab therapy and periodically during therapy.

Immune-mediated Renal Effects Immune-mediated nephritis has occurred in patients receiving cemiplimab therapy. Immune-mediated adverse effects generally occur during therapy with anti-PD-1 and anti-PD-L1 antibodies, but also may occur following discontinuance of the drug.

In clinical trials, grade 2 or 3 immune-mediated nephritis occurred in 0.6% of 534 patients receiving cemiplimab-rwlc. Cemiplimab-rwlc was permanently discontinued because of immune-mediated nephritis in 0.2% of patients receiving the drug. All patients experiencing immune-mediated nephritis received systemic corticosteroid therapy and 67% received high-dose corticosteroid therapy (40 mg or more of prednisone daily [or equivalent]). Complete resolution of immune-mediated nephritis occurred in all patients.

Patients receiving cemiplimab should be monitored for changes in renal function. Serum creatinine should be assessed prior to initiation of cemiplimab therapy and periodically during therapy. Temporary interruption or discontinuance of cemiplimab may be necessary if immune-mediated nephritis occurs. (See Other Immune-mediated Adverse Effects under Dosage: Therapy Interruption for Toxicity, in Dosage and Administration.) If grade 2 or greater nephritis occurs, systemic corticosteroid therapy should be initiated (1–2 mg/kg of prednisone daily [or equivalent]) followed by tapering of the corticosteroid dosage over 1 month once the toxicity improves to grade 0 or 1. Systemic immunosuppressive therapy may be considered in patients experiencing immune-mediated nephritis inadequately controlled with systemic corticosteroid therapy.

Immune-mediated Dermatologic Effects Immune-mediated dermatologic reactions, including Stevens-Johnson syndrome, toxic epidermal necrolysis, erythema multiforme, and pemphigoid, have occurred in patients receiving cemiplimab therapy. Immune-mediated adverse effects generally occur during therapy with anti-PD-1 and anti-PD-L1 antibodies, but also may occur following discontinuance of the drug.

In clinical trials, grade 2 or 3 immune-mediated dermatologic reactions, including erythema multiforme and pemphigoid, occurred in 1.7% of 534 patients receiving cemiplimab-rwlc. Stevens-Johnson syndrome and toxic epidermal necrolysis also have occurred in patients receiving anti-PD-1 and anti-PD-L1 antibodies, including cemiplimab-rwlc. All patients experiencing immune-mediated dermatologic reactions received systemic corticosteroid therapy and 89% received high-dose corticosteroid therapy (40 mg or more of prednisone daily [or equivalent]). Immune-mediated dermatologic reactions resolved in 33% of patients. Following reinitiation of cemiplimab-rwlc, immune-mediated dermatologic reactions recurred in approximately 22% of patients.

Patients receiving cemiplimab should be monitored for dermatologic reactions. Temporary interruption or discontinuance of cemiplimab may be necessary if immune-mediated dermatologic reactions occur. (See Other Immune-mediated Adverse Effects under Dosage: Therapy Interruption for Toxicity, in Dosage and Administration.) If grade 2 or greater dermatologic reactions occur, systemic corticosteroid therapy should be initiated (1–2 mg/kg of prednisone daily [or equivalent]) followed by tapering of the corticosteroid dosage over 1 month once the toxicity improves to grade 0 or 1. Systemic immunosuppressive therapy may be considered in patients experiencing immune-mediated dermatologic reactions inadequately controlled with systemic corticosteroid therapy.

Other Immune-mediated Effects Other immune-mediated adverse effects, sometimes severe or fatal, including meningitis, encephalitis, myelitis and demyelination, myasthenic syndrome/myasthenia gravis, Guillain-Barré syndrome, nerve paresis, autoimmune neuropathy, myocarditis, pericarditis, vasculitides, pancreatitis (including elevations in serum amylase and lipase concentrations), gastritis, duodenitis, myositis, rhabomyolysis and associated sequelae (e.g., renal failure), arthritis, polymyalgia rheumatica, hemolytic anemia, aplastic anemia, hemophagocytic lymphohistiocytosis, systemic inflammatory response syndrome, histiocytic necrotizing lymphadenitis, sarcoidosis, and immune thrombocytopenic purpura, were observed in less than 1% of 534 patients receiving cemiplimab-rwlc in clinical trials or have been reported in patients receiving other anti-PD-1 or anti-PD-L1 antibodies. Immune-mediated rejection of solid organ transplants also was reported in patients who received cemiplimab. Immune-mediated adverse effects generally occur during therapy with anti-PD-1 and anti-PD-L1 antibodies, but also may occur following discontinuance of the drug.

Ocular inflammatory toxicity (e.g., uveitis, iritis), sometimes associated with retinal detachment, visual impairment, or blindness, also has been reported rarely in patients receiving cemiplimab-rwlc in clinical trials. If uveitis occurs in conjunction with other immune-mediated adverse effects, a Vogt-Koyanagi-Harada-like syndrome should be considered. Systemic corticosteroid therapy may be required to reduce the risk of permanent vision loss.

Patients receiving cemiplimab should be monitored for immune-mediated adverse effects. Temporary interruption or discontinuance of cemiplimab may be necessary if immune-mediated adverse effects occur. (See Other Immune-mediated Adverse Effects under Dosage: Therapy Interruption for Toxicity, in Dosage and Administration.) If grade 2 or greater adverse effects occur, systemic corticosteroid therapy should be initiated (1–2 mg/kg of prednisone daily [or equivalent]) followed by tapering of the corticosteroid dosage over 1 month once the toxicity improves to grade 0 or 1. Systemic immunosuppressive therapy may be considered in patients experiencing immune-mediated adverse effects inadequately controlled with systemic corticosteroid therapy.

Infusion-related Effects Severe infusion-related reactions have occurred in 0.2% of patients receiving cemiplimab-rwlc.

Patients receiving cemiplimab should be monitored for manifestations of infusion-related reactions. In patients experiencing infusion-related reactions, interruption of the infusion, reduction in the infusion rate, or permanent discontinuance of the drug may be necessary. (See Infusion-related Reactions under Dosage: Therapy Interruption for Toxicity, in Dosage and Administration.)

Fetal/Neonatal Morbidity and Mortality Cemiplimab may cause fetal harm if administered to pregnant women. Blockade of signaling of the PD-1 and PD-L1 pathway in animals has been shown to disrupt maternal immune tolerance to the fetus and has been associated with increased fetal loss and immune-mediated disorders. Therefore, inhibition of this pathway by cemiplimab may increase the risk of fetal loss (e.g., abortion, stillbirth). Human immunoglobulin G_4 (IgG_4) has been shown to cross the placenta; therefore, fetal exposure to cemiplimab may occur and increase the risk of immune-mediated disorders or alter normal immune response of the developing fetus.

Pregnancy should be avoided during cemiplimab therapy. The manufacturer recommends confirmation of pregnancy status prior to initiation of cemiplimab. Women of childbearing potential should be advised to use an effective method of contraception while receiving cemiplimab and for at least 4 months after the last dose. If cemiplimab is used during pregnancy or if the patient becomes pregnant while receiving the drug, the patient should be apprised of the potential fetal hazard.

Immunogenicity There is a potential for immunogenicity with cemiplimab therapy. Development of anti-cemiplimab antibodies was detected by electrochemiluminescence (ECL) in 5 of 398 patients (1.3%) receiving cemiplimab-rwlc. Among the 5 patients who tested positive for antibody formation during treatment, one patient had persistently positive test results and none of the patients had evidence of neutralizing antibodies to the drug. Data are insufficient to determine the clinical importance of such anti-drug antibodies; however, no effects of antibody formation on pharmacokinetics or safety (i.e., infusion-related reactions) of the drug were observed.

Specific Populations **Pregnancy.** Cemiplimab may cause fetal harm if administered to pregnant women based on its mechanism of action and animal findings. (See Fetal/Neonatal Morbidity and Mortality under Cautions: Warnings/Precautions.)

Lactation. It is not known whether cemiplimab is distributed into human milk. Because many drugs are distributed into human milk and because of the potential for serious adverse reactions to cemiplimab in nursing infants, women should be advised to discontinue nursing during cemiplimab therapy and for at least 4 months after the last dose. The effects of the drug on nursing infants or on milk production are unknown.

Pediatric Use. Safety and efficacy of cemiplimab have not been established in pediatric patients.

Geriatric Use. In clinical trials evaluating cemiplimab-rwlc for metastatic or locally advanced cutaneous squamous cell carcinoma, 72% of patients were 65 years of age or older and 37% were 75 years of age or older. No overall differences in safety or efficacy were observed between geriatric patients and younger adults.

Hepatic Impairment. Systemic exposure of cemiplimab-rwlc was unaffected following administration of the drug in individuals with total bilirubin concentrations of 0.02–2.63 mg/dL. Cemiplimab has not been studied in patients with moderate or severe hepatic impairment.

Renal Impairment. Systemic exposure of cemiplimab-rwlc was unaffected following administration of the drug in individuals with creatinine clearance of 25 mL/minute or greater.

■ **Common Adverse Effects** Adverse effects reported in 10% or more of patients receiving cemiplimab-rwlc for the treatment of metastatic or locally advanced cutaneous squamous cell carcinoma include fatigue, rash, diarrhea, nausea, musculoskeletal pain, pruritus, cough, headache, constipation, dry skin, vomiting, and decreased appetite. Grade 3 or 4 laboratory abnormalities reported in 1% or more of patients receiving cemiplimab-rwlc for the treatment of metastatic or locally advanced cutaneous squamous cell carcinoma include lymphopenia, hypophosphatemia, elevated concentrations of aspartate aminotransferase (AST), hyponatremia, increased international normalized ratio (INR), anemia, hypoalbuminemia, and hypercalcemia.

Drug Interactions

No formal drug interaction studies have been performed to date.

Description

Cemiplimab, a fully human anti-programmed-death receptor-1 (anti-PD-1) monoclonal antibody, is an antineoplastic agent. The drug is an IgG_4 immunoglobulin.

Cemiplimab is highly selective for PD-1, an immune-checkpoint receptor expressed on activated T cells, monocytes, B cells, natural killer (NK) T cells, and dendritic cells. Overexpression of PD-1 ligands on the surface of tumor cells results in activation of PD-1 and suppression of cytotoxic T-cell activity. Cemiplimab blocks the interaction between PD-1 and its ligands, resulting in enhanced immune response, including enhanced antitumor immune response. The drug also has been shown to reduce tumor growth in syngeneic mouse tumor models.

Cemiplimab-rwlc exhibits linear and dose-proportional pharmacokinetics over the dosage range of 1–10 mg/kg IV every 2 weeks and at a dosage of 350 mg IV every 3 weeks. Following repeated doses of cemiplimab-rwlc 350 mg IV every 3 weeks, steady-state concentrations are reached by approximately 4 months. Clearance of cemiplimab-rwlc is approximately 34% lower at steady state than following the initial dose. The elimination half-life of cemiplimab-rwlc is 19 days.

Systemic exposure to cemiplimab-rwlc does not appear to be affected by age (range: 27–96 years), gender, body weight (range: 31–156 kg), race, cancer type, or serum albumin concentration (2.2–4.8 g/dL).

Advice to Patients

Importance of advising patients to read the manufacturer's medication guide.

Risk of immune-mediated pneumonitis. Importance of informing clinician immediately if new or worsening cough, chest pain, or shortness of breath occurs.

Risk of immune-mediated colitis. Importance of informing clinician immediately if diarrhea, severe abdominal pain, or changes in stool occur.

Risk of immune-mediated hepatitis. Importance of informing clinician immediately if signs and symptoms of liver damage (e.g., jaundice, severe nausea or vomiting, abdominal pain [particularly in the right upper quadrant], drowsiness, dark urine, easy bruising or bleeding, lack of appetite) occur.

Risk of immune-mediated endocrine effects. Importance of informing clinician immediately if signs and symptoms of hypothyroidism, hyperthyroidism, adrenal insufficiency, hypophysitis, or diabetes mellitus occur.

Risk of immune-mediated nephritis or renal dysfunction. Importance of informing clinician immediately if signs and symptoms of nephritis (e.g., decreased urine output, hematuria, peripheral edema, lack of appetite) occur.

Risk of immune-mediated rash. Importance of informing clinician immediately if a new rash develops.

Risk of infusion-related reactions. Importance of informing clinician immediately if signs and symptoms of such reactions (e.g., chills, pruritus, flushing, difficulty breathing, dizziness, fever, feeling of faintness, back or neck pain, angioedema) occur.

Risk of fetal harm. Necessity of advising women of childbearing potential that they should use an effective method of contraception while receiving the drug and for at least 4 months after the last dose. Importance of women informing clinicians if they are or plan to become pregnant. If pregnancy occurs, advise pregnant women of potential risk to the fetus.

Importance of advising women to avoid breast-feeding while receiving cemiplimab therapy and for at least 4 months after the last dose.

Importance of informing clinicians of existing or contemplated concomitant therapy, including prescription and OTC drugs, as well as any concomitant illnesses (e.g., autoimmune disorders, history of solid organ transplantation, hepatic or renal dysfunction, pulmonary disorders, diabetes mellitus).

Importance of informing patients of other important precautionary information. (See Cautions.)

Overview® (see Users Guide). For additional information on this drug until a more detailed monograph is developed and published, the manufacturer's labeling should be consulted. It is *essential* that the manufacturer's labeling be consulted for more detailed information on usual cautions, precautions, contraindications, potential drug interactions, laboratory test interferences, and acute toxicity. For further information on the handling of antineoplastic agents, see the ASHP Guidelines on Handling Hazardous Drugs at http://www.ahfsdruginformation.com.

Preparations

Cemiplimab-rwlc can only be obtained through a limited network of specialty distributors or specialty pharmacies. (See Restricted Distribution under Dosage and Administration: General.)

Excipients in commercially available drug preparations may have clinically important effects in some individuals; consult specific product labeling for details.

Cemiplimab-rwlc

Parenteral

Concentrate, for injection, for IV infusion	50 mg/mL (350 mg)	**Libtayo®**, Regeneron (comarketed by Sanofi-Aventis)

Ceritinib

■ Ceritinib, an inhibitor of several receptor tyrosine kinases including anaplastic lymphoma kinase (ALK), is an antineoplastic agent.

Uses

■ **Non-small Cell Lung Cancer** Ceritinib is used for the treatment of adults with anaplastic lymphoma kinase (ALK)-positive metastatic non-small cell lung cancer (NSCLC) following failure (secondary to resistance or intolerance) of prior crizotinib therapy. The drug has been designated an orphan drug by the FDA for use in this condition. The accelerated approval of ceritinib for this indication is based on tumor response rate and duration of response; there currently are no clinical data demonstrating an improvement in survival or disease-related symptoms with the drug. Continued approval for this indication may be contingent on verification and description of clinical benefit of ceritinib in confirmatory studies.

A relatively small subset of patients with NSCLC (approximately 3–7%) have ALK-positive disease, which indicates potential responsiveness to ALK inhibitor therapy (e.g., alectinib, brigatinib, ceritinib, crizotinib). Patients with this form of lung cancer typically are nonsmokers or have a history of light smoking, are female, and are younger in age and often have adenocarcinoma histology. Although crizotinib is highly active in patients with ALK-positive NSCLC, most patients treated with the drug eventually experience disease progression, limiting the drug's long-term therapeutic potential. Disease progression in patients receiving crizotinib can result from acquired resistance mutations in ALK, amplification of gene expression, activation of alternate signaling pathways, and/or progression of brain metastases (because of poor distribution of crizotinib into the CSF). (See Description.)

The current indication for ceritinib is based principally on the results of a multicenter, single-arm, open-label study that enrolled 163 adult patients with metastatic ALK-positive NSCLC whose cancer had progressed with or who were intolerant of crizotinib. All patients in this study received an initial ceritinib dosage of 750 mg once daily. The primary efficacy end point was overall response rate (as evaluated by both investigators and a Blinded Independent Central Review Committee [BIRC]); an additional outcome measure was duration of response. The median age of patients enrolled in the study was 52 years; 91% of the patients had progressed during crizotinib therapy and 93% had adenocarcinoma histology. In the efficacy analysis, the BIRC-assessed overall response rate with ceritinib was 43.6%; partial responses were achieved in 41.1% of patients and 2.5% had a complete response. The investigator-assessed overall response rate with ceritinib was comparable (54.6%), with partial responses achieved in 53.4% of patients and complete responses achieved in 1.2% of patients. The median BIRC-assessed duration of response was 7.1 months, and the median investigator-assessed duration of response was similar (7.4 months).

Phase 3 controlled trials comparing ceritinib as single-agent therapy with standard-of-care chemotherapy in patients with treatment-naive, or previously treated, ALK-positive NSCLC are underway. Ceritinib currently is not indicated for use in patients with treatment-naive ALK-positive NSCLC†.

Dosage and Administration

■ **General** Because ceritinib may cause hepatotoxicity, the manufacturer states that liver function tests should be monitored monthly and as clinically indicated. More frequent repeat testing is recommended in patients who develop elevated serum transaminase concentrations during therapy. (See Hepatic Toxicity under Dosage: Dosage Modification, in Dosage and Administration.)

Because ceritinib may cause hyperglycemia, the manufacturer states that serum glucose concentrations should be monitored during therapy as clinically indicated. (See Hyperglycemia under Dosage: Dosage Modification, in Dosage and Administration.)

Restricted Distribution Program Ceritinib can only be obtained through a limited network of specialty pharmacies. Clinicians may contact the manufacturer (Novartis) by telephone at 888-669-6682 or consult the Zykadia® website for specific availability information (http://www.zykadia.com/healthcare-professional/pharmacy-network.jsp).

■ **Administration** Ceritinib is administered orally once daily on an empty stomach (i.e., the drug should be taken at least 2 hours before or after a meal). Systemic exposure when the drug is administered with a meal may exceed that of a typical dose taken in a fasted state and result in increased adverse effects. (See Description.)

■ **Dosage** ***Non-small Cell Lung Cancer*** The recommended adult dosage of ceritinib for the treatment of anaplastic lymphoma kinase (ALK)-positive metastatic non-small cell lung cancer (NSCLC) following failure (secondary to resistance or intolerance) of prior crizotinib therapy is 750 mg (five 150-mg capsules) once daily. Ceritinib therapy should be continued until disease progression or unacceptable toxicity occurs.

Dosage Modification for Toxicity In the principal efficacy study, at least one dosage reduction from the recommended initial ceritinib dosage (750 mg once daily) was necessary in approximately 60% of patients (most commonly for GI toxicity); the median time to the first dosage reduction was 7 weeks.

When dosage modification is necessary, the daily dosage of ceritinib should be reduced in decrements of 150 mg; however, if a dosage of 300 mg daily requires further reduction, ceritinib should be discontinued.

Hepatic Toxicity. If an elevation in serum alanine aminotransferase (ALT) or aspartate aminotransferase (AST) concentrations exceeding 5 times the upper limit of normal (ULN) occurs with an elevation in total bilirubin concentrations no more than 2 times the ULN, ceritinib therapy should be withheld until the liver function test results return to baseline values or decrease to no more than 3 times the ULN. Ceritinib therapy may then be resumed with a 150-mg dosage reduction.

If an elevation in ALT or AST concentrations exceeding 3 times the ULN occurs with an elevation in total bilirubin concentrations exceeding 2 times the ULN in the absence of cholestasis or hemolysis, therapy with ceritinib should be permanently discontinued. (See Hepatic Toxicity under Cautions: Warnings/Precautions.)

Interstitial Lung Disease/Pneumonitis. If treatment-related interstitial lung disease/pneumonitis of any grade occurs, ceritinib therapy should be permanently discontinued. (See Interstitial Lung Disease/Pneumonitis under Cautions: Warnings/Precautions.)

Cardiovascular Toxicity. If corrected QT (QT_c) interval exceeds 500 msec on at least 2 separate ECGs, ceritinib therapy should be withheld until the QT_c interval is less than 481 msec or returns to baseline (if baseline QT_c interval is 481 msec or more). Ceritinib therapy may then be resumed with a 150-mg dosage reduction.

If QT_c-interval prolongation occurs concurrently with torsades de pointes, polymorphic ventricular tachycardia, or signs and/or symptoms of serious arrhythmia, ceritinib therapy should be permanently discontinued. (See Prolongation of QT Interval under Cautions: Warnings/Precautions.)

If symptomatic, but non-life-threatening, bradycardia occurs, therapy with ceritinib should be withheld until recovery to asymptomatic bradycardia or to a heart rate of 60 beats per minute or more occurs. Concomitant medications known to cause bradycardia should be evaluated, and the dosage of ceritinib should be adjusted. (See Drug Interactions: Drugs Associated with Bradycardia.)

If clinically significant bradycardia requiring intervention or life-threatening bradycardia occurs in patients receiving concomitant medications known to cause bradycardia or hypotension, therapy with ceritinib should be withheld until recovery to asymptomatic bradycardia or to a heart rate of 60 or more beats per minute occurs. If therapy with the concomitant medication can be adjusted or discontinued, ceritinib therapy may then be resumed with a 150-mg dosage reduction and frequent monitoring.

If life-threatening bradycardia occurs in patients not receiving concomitant medications known to cause bradycardia or hypotension, ceritinib therapy should be permanently discontinued. (See Bradycardia under Cautions: Warnings/Precautions.)

GI Toxicity. In patients experiencing severe or intolerable nausea, vomiting, or diarrhea despite appropriate medical therapy (e.g., antiemetics, antidiarrhea agents), ceritinib therapy should be withheld until the GI symptoms have improved. Ceritinib may then be resumed with a 150-mg dosage reduction. (See Severe or Persistent GI Toxicity under Cautions: Warnings/Precautions.)

Hyperglycemia. If persistent hyperglycemia with serum glucose concentrations exceeding 250 mg/dL occurs despite optimal antidiabetic agent therapy, ceritinib therapy should be withheld until adequate control of the hyperglycemia is achieved. Ceritinib therapy may then be resumed with a 150-mg dosage reduction. However, if hyperglycemia persists despite optimal medical management, ceritinib therapy should be discontinued. (See Hyperglycemia under Cautions: Warnings/Precautions.)

Concomitant Use of Drugs Affecting Hepatic Microsomal Enzymes Concomitant use of ceritinib with drugs that are potent inhibitors of cytochrome P-450 (CYP) isoenzyme 3A should be avoided. If concomitant use of a potent CYP3A inhibitor cannot be avoided, the manufacturer recommends reducing the daily dosage of ceritinib by approximately 33% and rounding dosage to the nearest 150-mg strength of ceritinib capsules (e.g., from 750 mg daily to 450 mg daily). If concomitant use of the potent CYP3A inhibitor is discontinued, the ceritinib dosage should be returned to the dosage used prior to initiation of the potent CYP3A inhibitor. (See Inhibitors of CYP3A under Drug Interactions: Drugs Affecting Hepatic Microsomal Enzymes.)

■ **Special Populations** Patients with hepatic impairment may have an increased exposure to ceritinib. No dosage adjustment is necessary in patients with mild hepatic impairment. The manufacturer states that the recommended dosage of ceritinib in patients with moderate or severe hepatic impairment has not been determined. (See Hepatic Impairment under Warnings/Precautions: Specific Populations, in Cautions.)

There are currently no special dosage recommendations for geriatric patients or patients with renal impairment. (See Geriatric Use and also see Renal Impairment under Warnings/Precautions: Specific Populations, in Cautions.)

Cautions

■ **Contraindications** The manufacturer states that there are no known contraindications to the use of ceritinib.

■ **Warnings/Precautions** ***Severe or Persistent GI Toxicity*** Diarrhea, nausea, vomiting, or abdominal pain occurred in 96% of patients receiving the recommended dosage of ceritinib (750 mg once daily) in the principal efficacy study, with severe cases reported in 14% of the patients. Over one-third (38%) of patients in this study required dosage modification.

Patients receiving ceritinib should be monitored for development of GI toxicity and treated as necessary with appropriate therapy (e.g., antidiarrhea agents, antiemetics, fluid replacement). Temporary interruption, followed by dosage reduction or discontinuance of ceritinib may be necessary depending on the severity of the GI toxicity. (See GI Toxicity under Dosage: Dosage Modification for Toxicity, in Dosage and Administration.)

Hepatic Toxicity Drug-induced hepatotoxicity has occurred in patients receiving ceritinib. Elevations in alanine aminotransferase (ALT) exceeding 5 times the upper limit of normal (ULN) were reported in 27% of ceritinib-treated patients in the primary efficacy study; permanent discontinuance of the drug due to transaminase elevations and jaundice was necessary in 1 of 255 patients (0.4%) in this study.

The manufacturer states that liver function tests, including ALT, aspartate aminotransferase (AST), and total bilirubin, should be monitored once every month and as clinically indicated during ceritinib therapy, with more frequent testing in patients who develop transaminase elevations during therapy. Temporary interruption, followed by dosage reduction or permanent discontinuance of ceritinib may be necessary depending on the severity of the hepatic toxicity. (See Hepatic Toxicity under Dosage: Dosage Modification for Toxicity, in Dosage and Administration.)

Interstitial Lung Disease/Pneumonitis Severe, life-threatening, or fatal interstitial lung disease (ILD)/pneumonitis may occur in patients receiving ceritinib. In the primary efficacy study, pneumonitis occurred in 4% of ceritinib-treated patients, grade 3 or 4 ILD or pneumonitis occurred in 3% of patients, and fatal ILD/pneumonitis was reported in one patient (0.4%). Discontinuance of ceritinib due to ILD or pneumonitis occurred in 1% of ceritinib-treated patients.

Patients receiving ceritinib should be monitored for pulmonary symptoms indicative of ILD or pneumonitis (see Advice to Patients), and other potential causes of ILD or pneumonitis should be excluded. Ceritinib should be permanently discontinued in patients who are diagnosed with treatment-related ILD or pneumonitis. (See Interstitial Lung Disease/Pneumonitis under Dosage: Dosage Modification for Toxicity, in Dosage and Administration.)

Prolongation of QT Interval Prolongation of the corrected QT (QT_c) interval has been reported in patients receiving ceritinib. The prolongation appears to occur in a plasma concentration-dependent manner. An increase in the QT_c interval exceeding 60 msec from baseline occurred in 3% of patients receiving ceritinib in the primary efficacy study. In the clinical development program, a QT_c interval exceeding 500 msec occurred in one of 304 ceritinib-treated patients (less than 1%) and 3% of ceritinib-treated patients had an increase exceeding 60 msec from baseline; dosages in these studies ranged from 50–750 mg daily.

Ceritinib should be avoided in patients with congenital long QT syndrome, if possible. The manufacturer recommends periodic monitoring of ECGs and serum electrolytes during ceritinib therapy in patients with congestive heart failure, bradyarrhythmias, or electrolyte abnormalities and in those who are receiving drugs known to prolong the QT interval. (See Drug Interactions: Drugs that Prolong the QT Interval.)

Temporary interruption, followed by dosage reduction of ceritinib is necessary when the QT_c interval exceeds 500 msec on at least 2 separate ECGs. When QT_c-interval prolongation occurs concurrently with torsades de pointes, polymorphic ventricular tachycardia, or signs and/or symptoms of serious arrhythmia, ceritinib therapy should be permanently discontinued. (See Cardiovascular Toxicity under Dosage: Dosage Modification for Toxicity, in Dosage and Administration.)

Hyperglycemia Hyperglycemia has been reported in patients receiving ceritinib. In the primary efficacy study, grade 3 or 4 hyperglycemia occurred in 13% of ceritinib-treated patients. The risk of grade 3 or 4 hyperglycemia was increased by sixfold in patients with diabetes or glucose intolerance and by twofold in those concurrently receiving corticosteroids.

Serum glucose concentrations should be monitored in patients receiving ceritinib as clinically indicated. Antidiabetic agents should be initiated or optimized as necessary. Temporary interruption, followed by dosage reduction or discontinuance of ceritinib may be necessary depending on the severity of the hyperglycemia. (See Hyperglycemia under Dosage: Dosage Modification for Toxicity, in Dosage and Administration.)

Bradycardia Ceritinib may cause bradycardia. In the primary efficacy study, sinus bradycardia (defined as a heart rate of less than 50 beats per minute) was reported as a new finding in 1% of ceritinib-treated patients; bradycardia was reported as an adverse drug reaction in 3% of patients in this study.

Ceritinib should be avoided in patients who are receiving other drugs known to cause bradycardia when possible. (See Drug Interactions: Drugs Associated with Bradycardia.)

Heart rate and blood pressure should be monitored regularly in all patients receiving ceritinib.

Temporary interruption, followed by dosage reduction is necessary if non-life-threatening, symptomatic bradycardia occurs. If life-threatening bradycardia occurs in patients who are not concomitantly receiving medications known to cause bradycardia or hypotension, ceritinib therapy should be permanently discontinued. However, if associated with a concomitant medication known to cause bradycardia or hypotension, ceritinib should be withheld until recovery to asymptomatic bradycardia or to a heart rate of 60 beats per minute or more occurs. If the concomitant medication can be adjusted or discontinued, ceritinib therapy can be resumed at a reduced dosage upon recovery to asymptomatic bradycardia or to a heart rate of 60 beats per minute or more occurs; such patients should be monitored frequently. (See Cardiovascular Toxicity under Dosage: Dosage Modification for Toxicity, in Dosage and Administration.)

Fetal/Neonatal Morbidity and Mortality Based on its mechanism of action, ceritinib may cause fetal harm if administered to pregnant women. Ceritinib produced developmental toxicity, including dose-related skeletal abnormalities (e.g., delayed or incomplete ossification, skeletal variations) and a low incidence of visceral abnormalities, when administered to pregnant animals in dosages associated with exposure levels lower than those associated with the recommended human dosage; maternal toxicity, abortion, and embryolethality also were observed. Pregnancy should be avoided during therapy. Women of childbearing potential should use effective methods of contraception while receiving the drug and for at least 2 weeks after the drug is discontinued. If ceritinib is used during pregnancy or if the patient becomes pregnant while receiving the drug, the patient should be apprised of the potential fetal hazard. (See Advice to Patients.)

Specific Populations **Pregnancy.** Category D. (See Users Guide and also see Fetal/Neonatal Morbidity and Mortality under Cautions: Warnings/Precautions.)

Lactation. It is not known whether ceritinib or its metabolites are distributed into human milk. Because many drugs are distributed into human milk and because of the potential for serious adverse reactions to ceritinib in nursing infants, a decision should be made whether to discontinue nursing or the drug, taking into account the importance of the drug to the woman.

Pediatric Use. Safety, efficacy, and pharmacokinetics of ceritinib have not been established in pediatric patients.

Geriatric Use. Clinical studies of ceritinib did not include sufficient numbers of patients 65 years of age and older to determine whether geriatric patients respond differently than younger adults. In the primary efficacy trial evaluating ceritinib in patients with metastatic anaplastic lymphoma kinase (ALK)-positive non-small cell lung cancer (NSCLC), 16% of patients receiving ceritinib at the recommended dosage were 65 years of age or older.

In pharmacokinetic population analyses, age did not have a clinically important effect on the systemic exposure of ceritinib in adults.

Hepatic Impairment. Formal pharmacokinetic studies of ceritinib have not been conducted in patients with hepatic impairment. However, ceritinib is eliminated principally by the liver and increased exposure to the drug may occur in patients with hepatic impairment.

In a population pharmacokinetic analysis, the systemic exposure to ceritinib was similar in patients with mild hepatic impairment (total bilirubin concentration no more than the ULN with AST concentration exceeding the ULN or total bilirubin concentration exceeding 1–1.5 times the ULN with any AST concentration) and those with normal hepatic function. Ceritinib dosage adjustment is not recommended in patients with mild hepatic impairment.

Because the pharmacokinetics of ceritinib have not been studied in patients with moderate to severe hepatic impairment, the recommended dosage of the drug has not yet been determined in such patients.

Renal Impairment. Formal pharmacokinetic studies of ceritinib have not been conducted in patients with renal impairment. In a population pharmacokinetic analysis, the pharmacokinetics of ceritinib were similar in patients with mild (creatinine clearance of 60–89 mL/minute) or moderate (creatinine clearance of 30–59 mL/minute) renal impairment compared with patients with normal renal function. Patients with severe renal impairment (creatinine clearance less than 30 mL/minute) were not included in the clinical trials.

■ **Common Adverse Effects** Adverse effects reported in more than 10% of patients receiving ceritinib in the main efficacy trial include diarrhea, nausea, vomiting, abdominal pain, constipation, esophageal disorder (including dyspepsia, gastroesophageal reflux disease, and dysphagia), fatigue, decreased appetite, neuropathy (including paresthesia, muscular weakness, gait disturbance, peripheral neuropathy, hypoesthesia, peripheral sensory neuropathy, dysesthesia, neuralgia, peripheral motor neuropathy, hypotonia, and polyneuropathy), and rash.

Laboratory abnormalities reported in more than 10% of patients receiving ceritinib in the main efficacy trial include anemia, elevated concentrations of transaminases (i.e., ALT, AST), elevated concentrations of serum creatinine, hyperglycemia, hypophosphatemia, increased lipase concentrations, and hyperbilirubinemia.

Drug Interactions

Ceritinib is metabolized principally by cytochrome P-450 (CYP) isoenzyme 3A4. In vitro, ceritinib is a substrate of CYP3A and P-glycoprotein (P-gp). In vitro studies also indicate that ceritinib may inhibit CYP isoenzymes 3A and 2C9 at clinically relevant concentrations. In vitro, ceritinib induces CYP3A4, but does not induce CYP isoenzymes 1A2, 2B6, or 2C9.

In vitro, ceritinib is not a substrate or inhibitor of breast cancer resistance protein (BCRP), multidrug resistance protein (MRP) 2, organic cation transporter (OCT) 1, organic anion transporter (OAT) 2, or organic anion transport protein (OATP) 1B1. Ceritinib also does not inhibit apical efflux transporters, P-gp, OATP1B3, renal organic anion transporters (OAT) 1 and OAT3, or OCT2 in vitro at clinically relevant concentrations.

■ **Drugs Affecting Hepatic Microsomal Enzymes** ***Inhibitors of CYP3A*** Concomitant use of ceritinib with potent inhibitors of CYP3A is likely to increase systemic exposure of ceritinib. When the potent CYP3A inhibitor ketoconazole (200 mg twice daily for 14 days) was administered concomitantly with ceritinib (as a single 450-mg dose) in healthy individuals, AUC and peak plasma concentrations of ceritinib increased by 2.9-fold and 22%, respectively. The steady-state AUC of ceritinib following concurrent administration of ketoconazole (200 mg twice daily for 14 days) with reduced dosages of ceritinib is expected to be similar to the steady-state AUC of ceritinib alone.

Concomitant use of potent CYP3A inhibitors, including certain antivirals (e.g., ritonavir), macrolide antibiotics (e.g., telithromycin), antifungals (e.g., ketoconazole), and nefazodone, should be avoided during ceritinib therapy. If concomitant use of a potent CYP3A inhibitor cannot be avoided, the manufacturer recommends reducing the daily dosage of ceritinib by approximately 33% and rounding to the nearest 150-mg strength of ceritinib capsules (e.g., from 750 mg daily to 450 mg daily). If concomitant use of the potent CYP3A inhibitor is discontinued, the ceritinib dosage should be returned to the dosage used prior to initiation of the potent CYP3A4 inhibitor.

Inducers of CYP3A Concomitant use of ceritinib with potent inducers of CYP3A (e.g., carbamazepine, phenytoin, rifampin) may result in decreased systemic exposure of ceritinib and should be avoided. When the potent CYP3A4 inducer rifampin (600 mg daily for 14 days) was administered concomitantly with ceritinib (as a single 750-mg dose) in healthy individuals, AUC and peak plasma concentrations of ceritinib decreased by 70 and 44%, respectively.

Use of St. John's wort (*Hypericum perforatum*), a potent CYP3A inducer, also should be avoided during ceritinib therapy.

■ **Drugs Metabolized by Hepatic Microsomal Enzymes** ***Substrates of CYP3A*** Ceritinib may inhibit CYP3A at clinically relevant concentrations and potentially can increase plasma concentrations of other drugs metabolized by CYP3A. Concomitant use of ceritinib with CYP3A substrates with a narrow therapeutic index (e.g., alfentanil, cyclosporine, dihydroergotamine, ergotamine, fentanyl, pimozide, quinidine, sirolimus, tacrolimus) or substrates primarily metabolized by CYP3A should be avoided. If concomitant use of CYP3A substrates with a narrow therapeutic index cannot be avoided, a dosage reduction of the CYP3A substrate should be considered.

Substrates of CYP2C9 Ceritinib may inhibit CYP2C9 at clinically relevant concentrations and potentially can increase plasma concentrations of other drugs metabolized by CYP2C9. Concomitant use of ceritinib with CYP2C9 substrates that have a narrow therapeutic index (e.g., phenytoin, warfarin) or substrates principally metabolized by CYP2C9 should be avoided. If concomitant use of CYP2C9 substrates with a narrow therapeutic index cannot be avoided, a dosage reduction of the CYP2C9 substrate should be considered.

■ **Drugs Affecting the P-glycoprotein Transport System** Ceritinib is a substrate of the efflux transporter P-glycoprotein (P-gp). If ceritinib is administered with drugs that inhibit P-gp (e.g., ketoconazole), increased concentrations of ceritinib may occur.

■ **Drugs that Prolong the QT Interval** Because ceritinib has been associated with QT-interval prolongation, the manufacturer recommends periodic monitoring of ECGs and electrolytes in ceritinib-treated patients concurrently receiving other drugs known to prolong the QT interval, including class IA antiarrhythmics (e.g., quinidine, procainamide), class III antiarrhythmics (e.g., amiodarone, sotalol), some antipsychotic agents (e.g., chlorpromazine, haloperidol, pimozide, thioridazine), citalopram, and clarithromycin. (See Prolongation of QT Interval under Cautions: Warnings/Precautions.)

■ **Drugs Associated with Bradycardia** Because ceritinib has been associated with bradycardia, the manufacturer recommends that concurrent use with other drugs known to cause bradycardia (e.g., β-adrenergic blocking agents, nondihydropyridine calcium-channel blocking agents [e.g., diltiazem, verapamil], clonidine, digoxin) be avoided, if possible. (See Bradycardia under Cautions: Warnings/Precautions.)

■ **Drugs Affecting Gastric Acidity** Although formal studies with ceritinib have not been conducted to date, the possibility exists that drugs that increase gastric pH (e.g., antacids, histamine H_2-receptor antagonists, proton-pump inhibitors) may decrease the solubility of ceritinib and subsequently reduce its bioavailability.

■ **Grapefruit** Grapefruit products are CYP3A inhibitors and should be avoided because of the potential for increased plasma ceritinib concentrations during concurrent use.

Description

Ceritinib, an inhibitor of receptor tyrosine kinases, including anaplastic lymphoma kinase (ALK), insulin-like growth factor receptor-1 (IGFR-1), insulin receptor, and c-ros oncogene-1 (ROS-1), is an antineoplastic agent. Among these tyrosine kinases, ceritinib is most active against ALK.

Activating mutations or translocations of the ALK gene have been identified in several malignancies and can result in the expression of oncogenic fusion proteins (e.g., echinoderm microtubule-associated protein-like 4 [EML4]-ALK). Such ALK gene rearrangements have been identified in approximately 3–7% of patients with NSCLC. Formation of ALK fusion proteins such as EML4-ALK results in activation and dysregulation of the gene's expression and signaling, which can contribute to increased cell proliferation and survival in tumors expressing these proteins. In vitro and in vivo, ceritinib has demonstrated inhibition of ALK phosphorylation, ALK-mediated phosphorylation of the downstream signaling protein signal transducer and activator of transcription-3 (STAT-3), and proliferation of ALK-dependent cancer cells. In vitro, ceritinib inhibited proliferation of cell lines that expressed EML4-ALK and nucleophosmin (NPM)-ALK fusion proteins. The drug also has demonstrated dose-dependent inhibition of EML4-ALK in mice and rats bearing NSCLC tumor xenografts that expressed EML4-ALK. In vitro, ceritinib is approximately 20-fold more potent than crizotinib in its activity against ALK.

At clinically relevant concentrations, ceritinib has demonstrated dose-dependent antitumor activity in mice bearing NSCLC tumor xenografts that expressed EML4-ALK with demonstrated resistance to crizotinib. Clinical resistance to crizotinib has been attributed to several possible mechanisms, including acquired resistance mutations of ALK, amplification of gene expression, and activation of alternate signaling pathways. Limited data to date suggest that secondary mutations of ALK (e.g., L1196M, G1269A) are responsible for only about 30% of cases of acquired crizotinib resistance. The CNS is a common site of disease progression in crizotinib-treated patients because of poor distribution of the drug into CSF; development and/or progression of brain metastases occurs in approximately one-half of patients during crizotinib treatment. In preclinical studies in cell-line models, ceritinib inhibited several crizotinib-resistant ALK kinase domain mutant forms.

The absolute bioavailability of ceritinib has not been established. Peak plasma concentrations of ceritinib are achieved about 4–6 hours following single-dose, oral administration of the drug. Following repeated administration of ceritinib 50–750 mg once daily, systemic exposure increases in a greater than dose-proportional manner. Following multiple-dose administration of ceritinib 750 mg daily, steady-state concentrations of the drug were achieved in approximately 15 days. Systemic exposure to ceritinib is increased when the drug is administered with food. Oral administration of a single 500-mg dose of ceritinib with a low-fat (approximately 330 calories and 9 g of fat) or high-fat meal (approximately 1000 calories and 58 g of fat) resulted in increases in systemic exposure of 58 or 73%, respectively, and increases in peak plasma concentrations by 43 or 41%, respectively, compared with the fasted state. Administration of a 600 mg or higher dose of ceritinib with a meal is expected to result in an increase in systemic exposure exceeding that of a 750-mg dose taken in a fasted state. Ceritinib is predominantly metabolized by the cytochrome P-450 (CYP) isoenzyme 3A4. The drug is 97% bound to plasma proteins. Following oral administration of a single 750-mg radiolabeled dose of ceritinib, 92.3% of the dose was recovered in feces and 1.3% was recovered in urine; unchanged drug accounted for 68% of the dose recovered in feces. The mean terminal half-life of ceritinib is 41 hours.

Advice to Patients

Importance of instructing patients to read the manufacturer's patient information.

If a dose is missed, importance of advising patients to take it as soon as they remember unless it is less than 12 hours before the next dose, in which case they should not take the missed dose.

Importance of informing patients that ceritinib should be taken on an empty stomach since taking the drug with food may increase blood concentrations and the risk of adverse effects; importance of instructing patients not to eat for at least 2 hours before and after taking the drug. Importance of also advising patients to avoid grapefruit and grapefruit juice while taking ceritinib.

Importance of informing patients that nausea, vomiting, diarrhea, and abdominal pain are the most common adverse effects associated with ceritinib therapy, as well as supportive treatment options (e.g., antiemetic and/or antidiarrhea agents). Importance of contacting clinician if severe or persistent adverse GI effects occur.

Risk of hepatotoxicity; importance of liver function test monitoring. Importance of informing patients of the signs and symptoms of hepatotoxicity (e.g., fatigue, anorexia, nausea, vomiting, abdominal pain [especially right upper quadrant pain], jaundice, dark or "tea-colored" urine, generalized pruritus, unusual bleeding or bruising) and advising them to immediately report possible symptoms of hepatotoxicity to their clinician.

Risk of severe or fatal interstitial lung disease/pneumonitis. Importance of advising patients that pneumonitis symptoms may be similar to those of lung cancer and to contact their clinician immediately if they experience any new or worsening pulmonary symptoms (e.g., dyspnea, shortness of breath, cough with or without mucus, chest pain, fever).

Risk of QT_c-interval prolongation and bradycardia. Importance of informing clinicians immediately if new chest pain or discomfort, changes in heartbeat, palpitations, dizziness, lightheadedness, faintness, or changes in or new use of cardiovascular or antihypertensive therapy occurs.

Risk of hyperglycemia, particularly in patients with diabetes or glucose intolerance and in those receiving corticosteroid medications. Importance of informing patients of the signs and symptoms of hyperglycemia (e.g., increased thirst, increased urination, increased appetite, fatigue, blurred vision, headache, difficulty thinking or concentrating, breath that smells like fruit) and advising patients to immediately contact their clinician if they experience such signs and symptoms.

Risk of fetal harm. Necessity of advising women of childbearing potential that they should use effective methods of contraception while receiving ceritinib and for at least 2 weeks after discontinuance of therapy. Importance of patients informing their clinicians if they are pregnant or plan to become pregnant. If pregnancy occurs, advise patient of potential risk to the fetus.

Importance of advising women to avoid breast-feeding while receiving ceritinib therapy.

Importance of informing clinicians of existing or contemplated concomitant therapy, including prescription and OTC drugs and dietary or herbal supplements (e.g., St. John's wort), as well as any concomitant illnesses (e.g., hepatic impairment, cardiovascular disease [including congenital long QT syndrome], diabetes mellitus or hyperglycemia).

Importance of informing patients of other important precautionary information. (See Cautions.)

Overview® (see Users Guide). For additional information on this drug until a more detailed monograph is developed and published, the manufacturer's labeling should be consulted. It is *essential* that the manufacturer's labeling be consulted for more detailed information on usual cautions, precautions, contraindications, potential drug interactions, laboratory test interferences, and acute toxicity. For further information on the handling of antineoplastic agents, see the ASHP Guidelines on Handling Hazardous Drugs at http://www.ahfsdruginformation.com.

Preparations

Distribution of ceritinib is restricted. (See Restricted Distribution under Dosage and Administration: General.)

Excipients in commercially available drug preparations may have clinically important effects in some individuals; consult specific product labeling for details.

Ceritinib

Oral

Capsules	150 mg	**Zykadia®**, Novartis

†Use is not currently included in the labeling approved by the US Food and Drug Administration

Cetuximab

■ Cetuximab, a recombinant chimeric (human-murine) monoclonal antibody that binds to epidermal growth factor receptors (EGFR), is an antineoplastic agent.

Uses

■ **Colorectal Cancer** Patients enrolled in clinical studies for the use of cetuximab for colorectal cancer were required to have immunohistochemical (IHC) evidence of epidermal growth factor receptor (EGFR) expression; however, response rates in these clinical studies did not correlate with either the percentage of positive cells or the intensity of EGFR expression. In addition, responses to cetuximab therapy have been observed in patients with EGFR-negative colorectal cancer. Some authorities state that routine EGFR expression testing is not recommended in patients with colorectal cancer and that patients should not be included or excluded from cetuximab therapy based solely on EGFR test results.

Because retrospective stratified analyses of metastatic colorectal cancer trials have not shown a treatment benefit for cetuximab in patients whose tumors had *KRAS* mutations in codon 12 or 13, use of the drug is *not* recommended for the treatment of colorectal cancer with such mutations. (See *KRAS* Testing in Patients Receiving Cetuximab for Colorectal Cancer under Uses: Colorectal Cancer.)

Cetuximab Monotherapy for Advanced Colorectal Cancer Cetuximab is used as a single agent for the treatment of EGFR-expressing metastatic colorectal cancer in patients with disease that has failed treatment with both irinotecan-based and oxaliplatin-based regimens. Cetuximab also is used as a single agent for the treatment of EGFR-expressing, metastatic colorectal cancer in patients who are intolerant of irinotecan-based chemotherapy.

The current indication for cetuximab monotherapy for recurrent EGFR-expressing metastatic colorectal cancer is based mainly on the results of a multicenter, open-label, randomized trial in 572 patients receiving either cetuximab and best supportive care or best supportive care alone for EGFR-expressing metastatic colorectal cancer. All patients had progression of disease following previous treatment with an irinotecan-containing regimen and an oxaliplatin-containing regimen or had contraindications to treatment with these agents. The treatment regimen consisted of an initial dose of cetuximab 400 mg/m^2 as a 2-hour IV infusion followed by cetuximab 250 mg/m^2 as a 1-hour IV infusion weekly until disease progression or unacceptable toxicity occurred. The median age of the patients was 63 years, 64% were male, and most of the patients (89%) were Caucasian; 77% had a baseline ECOG performance status of 0–1.

Median overall survival was prolonged in patients receiving cetuximab and best supportive care compared with those receiving best supportive care alone (6.1 versus 4.6 months; hazard ratio for death 0.77 with a 95% confidence interval of 0.64–0.92). Adverse effects were more frequent in patients receiving cetuximab therapy and best supportive care than in those receiving best supportive care alone, particularly rash/desquamation (89 versus 16%, grade 3 or 4 in 12 versus less than 1%).

Cetuximab and Irinotecan for Advanced Colorectal Cancer Cetuximab is used in combination with irinotecan for the treatment of EGFR-expressing metastatic colorectal cancer that is refractory to irinotecan-based chemotherapy. The indication for cetuximab in combination with irinotecan for EGFR-expressing, metastatic colorectal cancer is based on objective response rates; there currently are no data demonstrating a clinical benefit (e.g., improvement in disease-related symptoms, increased survival).

The current indication for cetuximab in combination with irinotecan is based principally on the results of a phase 2, multicenter, randomized, controlled study that compared safety and efficacy of cetuximab monotherapy with the combination regimen of cetuximab and irinotecan.

This phase 2 study enrolled 329 patients with EGFR-expressing, metastatic colorectal cancer refractory to irinotecan-based chemotherapy; approximately two thirds of enrolled patients had previously failed oxaliplatin therapy. In this study, 111 patients were randomized to receive cetuximab monotherapy (400 mg/m^2 initially, followed by 250 mg/m^2 weekly until disease progression or unacceptable toxicity occurred), and 218 patients were randomized to receive cetuximab (at the same dosage) in combination with irinotecan (350 mg/m^2 every 3 weeks, 180 mg/m^2 every 2 weeks, *or* 125 mg/m^2 weekly for 4 doses every 6 weeks).

The overall response rate (complete plus partial responses) was higher in patients receiving the combination regimen (about 23%) than in those receiving cetuximab monotherapy (about 11%). In addition, median time to radiographic disease progression and median duration of response were longer in patients receiving the combination regimen (4.1 and 5.7 months, respectively) than in those receiving cetuximab alone (1.5 and 4.2 months, respectively). Median survival was not substantially different between the 2 groups (8.6 months for the combination regimen versus 6.9 months for cetuximab monotherapy).

Cetuximab and Combination Chemotherapy as First-line Therapy for Metastatic Colorectal Cancer Cetuximab has been used with combination chemotherapy regimens for the first-line treatment of metastatic colorectal cancer.

In a phase 3 randomized trial that enrolled 238 patients with previously untreated metastatic colorectal cancer before closing early because of slow accrual, the addition of cetuximab to either FOLFIRI (irinotecan/fluorouracil/leucovorin) or FOLFOX (oxaliplatin/fluorouracil/leucovorin) appeared to increase response rates; at a median follow-up of about 1 year, analysis of the data did not show any effect of the addition of cetuximab on progression-free survival or duration of response. A phase 3 randomized trial comparing the addition of cetuximab, bevacizumab, or both to combination chemotherapy (FOLFOX or FOLFIRI) for the first-line treatment of metastatic colorectal cancer is under way.

KRAS Testing in Patients Receiving Cetuximab for Colorectal Cancer The presence of mutations in the *KRAS* (also called *K-ras*) gene in codon 12 or 13 in colorectal cancer tumor tissue has been associated with a lack of benefit from therapy with anti-EGFR monoclonal antibodies (e.g., cetuximab, panitumumab); such mutations appear to be present in approximately 30–50% of primary colorectal tumors. Retrospective subset analyses from 7 randomized clinical studies evaluating cetuximab or panitumumab either as monotherapy or in combination with chemotherapy in metastatic colorectal cancer suggest that these anti-EGFR monoclonal antibodies are not effective for the treatment of patients with colorectal cancer containing *KRAS* mutations in codon 12 or 13. The American Society of Clinical Oncology (ASCO) and some clinicians recommend that all patients with metastatic colorectal cancer who are potential candidates for EGFR inhibitor therapy (e.g., cetuximab, panitumumab) have their tumor tested for *KRAS* mutations in a Clinical Laboratory Improvement Amendments (CLIA)-accredited laboratory. If *KRAS* mutation in codon 12 or 13 is detected, the use of cetuximab is *not* recommended.

■ **Head and Neck Cancer** Because expression of EGFR has been detected in nearly all head and neck cancers, patients enrolled in the studies on which the labeled indications for cetuximab for this neoplasm were based were not required to have immunohistochemical evidence of EGFR expression.

Cetuximab and Radiation Therapy for Locally or Regionally Advanced Disease Cetuximab is used in combination with radiation therapy for the initial treatment of locally or regionally advanced squamous cell carcinoma of the head and neck, particularly for patients who cannot tolerate platinum-based chemotherapy with radiation therapy.

In a multicenter randomized controlled trial, 424 patients with stage III or IV squamous cell carcinoma of the oropharynx (60%), larynx (25%), or hypopharynx (15%) received initial treatment with either cetuximab and radiation therapy or radiation therapy alone. Stratification factors were Karnofsky performance status (60–80 versus 90–100), nodal stage (N0 versus N+), tumor stage (T1–3 versus T4 according to AJCC 1998 staging criteria), and radiation therapy fractionation (concomitant boost, once daily, or twice daily).

Patients receiving cetuximab were given premedication with IV diphenhydramine hydrochloride 50 mg or an equivalent histamine H_1-receptor antagonist to reduce the risk of infusion-related reactions. Patients receiving cetuximab were given a 20-mg test dose of the drug on day 1; an initial dose of cetuximab 400 mg/m^2 was administered by 2-hour IV infusion 1 week before the initiation of radiation therapy followed by cetuximab 250 mg/m^2 by 1-hour IV infusion 1 hour prior to radiation therapy once weekly for 6–7 weeks. Radiation therapy was administered for 6–7 weeks as concomitant boost (56%), once daily fractionation (26%), or twice daily fractionation (18%). For patients with stage N1 or higher neck disease, neck dissection at 4–8 weeks following completion of radiation therapy was recommended. The patients enrolled in the trial were mostly Caucasian men with a baseline Karnofsky performance status of at least 80; the median age of the patients was 57 years.

Patients with locally or regionally advanced squamous cell carcinoma of the head and neck receiving cetuximab and radiation therapy had prolonged median duration of locoregional control (24 versus 15 months, hazard ratio for locoregional progression or death: 0.68) and prolonged median overall survival (49 versus 29 months, hazard ratio for death: 0.74) compared with those receiving radiation therapy alone. Subgroup analysis according to tumor type suggested efficacy of cetuximab and radiation therapy for oropharyngeal tumors, but not for hypopharyngeal or laryngeal tumors. Acneiform rash (all grades: 87 versus 10%, grade 3 or 4: 17 versus 1%) and infusion reactions (all grades: 15 versus 2%, grade 3 or 4: 3 versus 0%) occurred more frequently in patients receiving cetuximab and radiation therapy than in those receiving radiation therapy alone.

The use of platinum-based chemotherapy with radiation therapy is the current standard of care for the treatment of advanced head and neck cancer. Further study is needed to compare the efficacy and toxicity for cetuximab and radiation therapy versus platinum-based chemotherapy and radiation therapy.

Monotherapy for Advanced Disease Cetuximab is used alone for the treatment of recurrent or metastatic squamous cell carcinoma of the head and neck in patients with disease that has failed platinum-based therapy.

The current indication for use of cetuximab as a single agent for the treatment of recurrent or metastatic squamous cell carcinoma of the head and neck is based principally on the results of a single-arm, multicenter clinical trial involving 103 patients with disease that progressed within 30 days following 2–6 cycles of platinum-based chemotherapy. Patients received a 20-mg test dose of cetuximab on day 1, an initial dose of cetuximab 400 mg/m^2, and then cetuximab 250 mg/m^2 once weekly until disease progression or unacceptable toxicity. The patients enrolled in the trial were mostly Caucasian men, and 62% of the patients had a baseline Karnofsky performance status of at least 80; the median age of the patients was 57 years.

The objective response rate was 13% and the median duration of response was 5.8 months for patients receiving cetuximab monotherapy for recurrent or metastatic head and neck cancer.

Cetuximab and Chemotherapy With or Without Radiation Therapy for Advanced Disease Cetuximab has been used in combination with chemotherapy, with or without radiation therapy†, for the treatment of recurrent or metastatic squamous cell carcinoma of the head and neck.

In two phase 2 studies, cetuximab with platinum-based chemotherapy demonstrated activity in the treatment of recurrent or metastatic platinum-refractory squamous cell carcinoma of the head and neck. In a phase 3 randomized trial, the addition of cetuximab to cisplatin improved response rates but did not affect progression-free survival or overall survival in patients receiving first-line treatment for recurrent or metastatic squamous cell carcinoma of the head and neck. In another phase 3 randomized trial, the addition of cetuximab to a platinum agent (cisplatin or carboplatin) and fluorouracil prolonged median overall survival (10.1 versus 7.4 months) and median progression-free survival (5.6 versus 3.3 months) and increased the response rate (36 versus 20%) in the first-line treatment of recurrent and/or metastatic squamous cell cancer of the head and neck. Grade 3 or 4 adverse effects that occurred more frequently in patients receiving cetuximab with a platinum agent and fluorouracil than in those receiving a platinum agent and fluorouracil included skin reactions (grade 3 only, in 9 versus less than 1%), hypomagnesemia and anorexia (each in 5 versus 1%), and sepsis, including septic shock (in 4 versus less than 1%).

In a pilot study, cetuximab and cisplatin were administered with delayed, accelerated (concomitant boost) fractionation radiation therapy for the treatment of locoregionally advanced squamous cell head and neck cancer. The study was closed early because of safety concerns regarding fatalities and serious adverse events. Of the 21 patients enrolled in the study, one patient died from pneumonia and one patient died of an unknown cause. Four patients discontinued treatment because of adverse events; adverse cardiac events were the reason for discontinuation of treatment in two of these patients with myocardial infarction in one patient and arrhythmia, diminished cardiac output, and hypotension in another patient. Although use of this regimen is not recommended outside of a clinical trial because of safety concerns, high rates of response and high 3-year survival rates suggest that further study of cetuximab in combined modality treatment for advanced head and neck cancer is warranted.

A phase 3 randomized trial studying the effect of the addition of cetuximab to a regimen of concurrent accelerated fractionated radiation therapy and cisplatin for stage III or IV squamous cell carcinoma of the oropharynx, hypopharynx, or larynx is under way.

■ **Non-small Cell Lung Cancer** Efficacy and safety of cetuximab in combination with various chemotherapy regimens as first-line therapy for advanced (stage IIIB [with malignant pleural effusion] or IV [metastatic]) non-small cell lung cancer (NSCLC)† has been studied in several randomized studies.

Use of cetuximab either concurrently with or following carboplatin and paclitaxel therapy was investigated in a randomized phase 2 study (S0342) in 242 patients with previously untreated stage IIIB or IV NSCLC. Patients in both treatment groups received carboplatin (at the dose required to obtain an area under the plasma concentration-time curve [AUC] of 6 mg/mL per minute) and paclitaxel (225 mg/m^2 by IV infusion) in 21-day cycles for 4 cycles; cetuximab (initial dose of 400 mg/m^2 by IV infusion followed by 250 mg/m^2 by IV infusion once weekly) was initiated either concurrently with or following completion of carboplatin and paclitaxel therapy and was continued until disease progression, unacceptable toxicity, or withdrawal of patient consent. At a median follow-up of 32 months, overall survival (10.9 versus 10.7 months), progression-free survival (4.3 versus 4.4 months), and response rates (32 versus 30%) were similar in both treatment groups; however, the incidence of grade 3/4 sensory neuropathy was higher in patients receiving concurrent therapy compared with those receiving sequential therapy (15 versus 5%, respectively). About one-third of patients underwent EGFR testing (using fluorescent in situ hybridization [FISH] methodology); those with EGFR-positive tumors had longer median progression-free survival (6 versus 3 months) and overall survival (15 versus 7 months) compared with those with EGFR-negative tumors. Overall survival favored EGFR-positive patients receiving cetuximab concurrently with chemotherapy.

Efficacy and safety of cetuximab administered concurrently with up to 6 cycles of chemotherapy and then continued alone as maintenance therapy have been evaluated in two phase 3, open-label, randomized studies (First-line Erbitux in Lung Cancer [FLEX] and BMS-099) in patients with previously untreated stage IIIB or IV NSCLC. Patients in these studies received either cetuximab and chemotherapy (either cisplatin and vinorelbine or carboplatin and a taxane) or chemotherapy alone. The studies included patients with any histologic cell type but excluded those with metastatic CNS disease and those who had received prior anti-EGFR therapy. Patient enrollment in the BMS-099 study was independent of EGFR expression status, while enrollment in the FLEX study required immunohistochemical (IHC) evidence of EGFR expression (using the Dako EGFR pharmDx® test kit). In the BMS-099 study, patients were stratified according to their baseline ECOG performance status (0 or 1), intended taxane (paclitaxel or docetaxel), and study site.

In the FLEX study, 1125 patients were randomized to receive vinorelbine (25 mg/m^2 by IV infusion on days 1 and 8) and cisplatin (80 mg/m^2 by IV infusion on day 1) in 21-day cycles either alone or in combination with cetuximab (initial dose of 400 mg/m^2 as a 2-hour IV infusion on day 1 followed by 250 mg/m^2 by IV infusion over 1 hour once weekly); cetuximab was continued until disease progression or unacceptable toxicity occurred, while vinorelbine and cisplatin were administered for up to 6 cycles. In the BMS-099 study, 676 patients were randomized to receive carboplatin (administered on day 1 at the dose required to obtain an AUC of 6 mg/mL per minute) and a taxane (paclitaxel 225 mg/m^2 as a 3-hour IV infusion or docetaxel 75 mg/m^2 as a 1-hour IV infusion on day 1) in 21-day cycles either alone or in combination with cetuximab (initial dose of 400 mg/m^2 as a 2-hour IV infusion followed by 250 mg/m^2 by IV infusion over 1 hour once weekly); cetuximab was continued until disease progression or unacceptable toxicity occurred, while carboplatin and a taxane were administered for up to 6 cycles.

In the FLEX study, the primary measure of efficacy was overall survival. At a median follow-up of 23.8 months, median overall survival was 1.2 months longer (11.3 versus 10.1 months; hazard ratio of 0.87) and the rate of survival at 1 year was higher (47 versus 42%) for patients receiving cetuximab in combination with cisplatin and vinorelbine compared with those receiving cisplatin and vinorelbine alone. Median progression-free survival was 4.8 months in both treatment groups. The overall response rate was 36% for patients receiving cetuximab in combination with chemotherapy and 29% for those receiving chemotherapy alone. Subset analysis suggested that ECOG performance status, smoking status, histologic type, gender, and age did not influence the treatment effect on overall survival.

Subset analysis of the FLEX study results based on ethnicity indicated that characteristics associated with a more favorable prognosis (i.e., adenocarcinoma histology, female gender, never smoked) were more common in Asian patients than in Caucasian patients and that the median survival of Asian patients was 10 months longer than that of Caucasian patients. However, a higher proportion of Asian patients received oral tyrosine kinase inhibitors following their assigned study treatment, and the possibility that additional EGFR-targeted therapy might have contributed to an improved survival rate for these patients cannot be ruled out. The addition of cetuximab to chemotherapy did not significantly improve survival of Asian patients or other non-Caucasian patients. In contrast, median overall survival of Caucasian patients (84% of patients in the study) was longer for those receiving cetuximab in combination with chemotherapy compared with those receiving chemotherapy alone (10.5 versus 9.1 months). Subset analysis based on tumor histology indicated that median survival times for patients receiving cetuximab in combination with chemotherapy compared with those receiving chemotherapy alone were 12 versus 10.3 months, respectively, for patients with adenocarcinoma and 10.2 versus 8.9 months, respectively, for those with squamous cell carcinoma.

In the FLEX study, grade 3 or 4 febrile neutropenia (22 versus 15%), acneiform rash (10 versus less than 1%), infusion-related reactions (4 versus 1%), and diarrhea (5 versus 2%) occurred more frequently in patients receiving cetuximab in combination with cisplatin and vinorelbine than in those receiving cisplatin and vinorelbine alone.

In the BMS-099 study, the primary measure of efficacy was progression-free survival assessed by an independent radiologic review committee. The addition of cetuximab to carboplatin and taxane therapy improved the overall response rate (25.7 versus 17.2%) but did not substantially improve median progression-free survival (4.4 versus 4.2 months) or median overall survival (9.7 versus 8.4 months). Subgroup analyses suggested that the addition of cetuximab to chemotherapy had a greater effect on progression-free survival in certain subgroups of patients (those with an ECOG performance status of 0, those receiving docetaxel, and those with squamous cell histology) than in the overall study population; however, similar trends were not observed for overall survival. Grade 3 or 4 acneiform rash (10.5 versus 0%), infusion-related reactions (4.6 versus 0.9%), hypomagnesemia (8.8 versus 0.7%), diarrhea (5.2 versus 2.5%), dehydration (8.6 versus 4.7%), and neutropenia (62.5 versus 56%) occurred more frequently in patients receiving cetuximab in combination with carboplatin and a taxane than in those receiving carboplatin and a taxane alone.

Post-hoc analyses of the FLEX and BMS-099 studies were performed in an attempt to identify tumor markers that would predict which patients might benefit from the addition of cetuximab to chemotherapy as first-line treatment for advanced NSCLC. Comparisons of outcomes between treatment groups according to tumor marker status revealed no significant associations between efficacy (i.e., overall survival, progression-free survival, tumor response) and *KRAS* mutation status, EGFR mutation status, EGFR gene copy number (assessed by FISH methodology), or phosphatase and tensin homolog (PTEN) gene expression (assessed by IHC methodology) that would identify patients who might benefit from receiving cetuximab in addition to chemotherapy. In the BMS-099 study, EGFR expression (assessed by IHC methodology and described as either positive or negative) was not associated with improved efficacy for cetuximab and chemotherapy compared with chemotherapy alone. However, in the FLEX study, addition of cetuximab to chemotherapy was associated with a survival benefit in patients with high EGFR expression (IHC score of 200 or greater on a scale of 0–300); among patients with high EGFR expression, overall survival was 12 months for those receiving cetuximab and chemotherapy compared with 9.6 months for those receiving chemotherapy alone.

Although combined therapy with cetuximab and chemotherapy prolonged overall survival in the FLEX study, the magnitude of the benefit was modest and the same benefit was not observed in the BMS-099 study; in addition, combined therapy did not prolong progression-free survival in either study. Therefore, the role of the drug in combination with chemotherapy for the treatment of previously untreated advanced NSCLC is unclear. In addition, although exploratory analyses in the FLEX and BMS-099 studies suggested that overall survival results were generally consistent across most patient subgroups, exploratory analyses of progression-free survival in the BMS-099 study suggested some differences in treatment effect in certain patient subgroups (as compared with the overall population). Additional studies are needed to validate predictive tumor biomarkers and identify subgroups of patients with previously untreated advanced NSCLC who might derive clinical benefit (e.g., prolonged progression-free survival, prolonged overall survival, improved quality of life) from the addition of cetuximab to chemotherapy. The AHFS Oncology Expert Committee concluded that use of cetuximab in combination with various chemotherapy regimens as first-line therapy for advanced (stage IIIB [with malignant pleural effusion] or IV [metastatic]) NSCLC currently is not fully established because of equivocal evidence.

Dosage and Administration

■ **Administration** Cetuximab is administered by IV infusion. *The drug should not be administered by rapid IV injection, such as IV push or bolus.* The initial dose of cetuximab is administered over 2 hours, and the subsequent weekly dose is administered over 1 hour. The maximum infusion rate should not exceed 10 mg/minute.

Cetuximab injection should be inspected visually for particulate matter and discoloration whenever solution and container permit. Cetuximab injection for IV infusion should be clear and colorless and may contain a small amount of easily visible, white, amorphous cetuximab particulates. Cetuximab injection for IV infusion should not be diluted, and vials should not be shaken.

Cetuximab may be administered using either an infusion pump or a syringe pump. The drug must be administered through a low-protein-binding 0.22-μm inline filter. Patients should be monitored for signs of infusion reactions during and for 1 hour following cetuximab infusion. For patients experiencing infusion reactions requiring treatment, monitoring should be continued until the event is resolved. (See Infusion-related Effects under Warnings/Precautions: Warnings, in Cautions.)

Cetuximab solution should be stored in unopened vials under refrigeration at 2–8°C and protected from freezing. Preparations of cetuximab solution in infusion containers are chemically and physically stable for up to 12 hours at 2–8°C and up to 8 hours at controlled room temperature (20–25°C); any solution remaining in the infusion container after 8 hours (if stored at room temperature) or after 12 hours (if refrigerated) should be discarded. Cetuximab contains no preservatives; any unused portion of the vial should be discarded.

■ **General Dosage** ***Premedication*** To minimize the risk of infusion-related reactions associated with cetuximab, premedication with an antihistamine (e.g., 50 mg of IV diphenhydramine hydrochloride 30–60 minutes prior to the first dose of cetuximab) is recommended. Based on the occurrence and severity of previous infusion reactions, premedication with an antihistamine may be administered for subsequent cetuximab doses as clinically indicated.

Colorectal Cancer For the management of previously treated EGFR-expressing metastatic colorectal cancer, either as monotherapy or in combination therapy with irinotecan, an initial dose of cetuximab 400 mg/m² is administered by IV infusion over 2 hours, followed by cetuximab 250 mg/m² as a 1-hour IV infusion once weekly until disease progression or unacceptable toxicity occurs; the maximum infusion rate should not exceed 10 mg/minute.

Head and Neck Cancer For use in combination with radiation therapy for the treatment of locally or regionally advanced squamous cell cancer of the head and neck, an initial dose of cetuximab 400 mg/m² is administered by IV infusion over 2 hours at 1 week prior to the initiation of a course of radiation therapy. For the duration of radiation therapy (6–7 weeks), cetuximab 250 mg/m² is administered by 1-hour IV infusion once weekly. Administration of cetuximab should be completed 1 hour prior to radiation therapy. The maximum infusion rate for cetuximab should not exceed 10 mg/minute. In a randomized trial for locally or regionally advanced head and neck cancer, a median of 8 doses of cetuximab was administered in patients receiving cetuximab and radiation therapy.

For use as monotherapy for the treatment of recurrent or metastatic squamous cell cancer of the head and neck, an initial dose of cetuximab 400 mg/m² is administered as a 2-hour IV infusion followed by cetuximab 250 mg/m² as a 1-hour IV infusion once weekly (maximum infusion rate of 10 mg/min for initial and subsequent doses) until disease progression or unacceptable toxicity occurs.

■ **Dosage Modification for Toxicity and Contraindications for Continued Therapy** ***Infusion-related Reactions*** In patients who develop grade 1 or 2 or nonserious grade 3 or 4 infusion-related reactions, the infusion rate should be reduced by 50%. In patients who develop serious infusion-related reactions, requiring medical intervention and/or hospitalization, cetuximab therapy should be immediately and permanently discontinued. (See Infusion-related Effects under Warning/Precautions: Warnings, in Cautions.)

Dermatologic Toxicity In patients who experience severe acneiform rash, cetuximab therapy should be temporarily delayed, and subsequent doses should be reduced or therapy discontinued depending on the patient's response (see Table 1).

Table 1. Cetuximab Dosage Modification for Severe Acneiform Rash

Occurrence of Severe Acneiform Rash	Intervention	Outcome	Cetuximab Dosage
First occurrence	Delay cetuximab infusion for 1–2 weeks	Improvement	Continue subsequent weekly dose of 250 mg/m²
		No improvement	Discontinue cetuximab therapy
Second occurrence	Delay cetuximab infusion for 1–2 weeks	Improvement	Reduce subsequent weekly dose to 200 mg/m²
		No improvement	Discontinue cetuximab therapy
Third occurrence	Delay cetuximab infusion for 1–2 weeks	Improvement	Reduce subsequent weekly dose to 150 mg/m²
		No improvement	Discontinue cetuximab therapy
Fourth occurrence	Discontinue cetuximab therapy		

Pulmonary Toxicity If acute onset or worsening of pulmonary symptoms occurs, cetuximab therapy should be interrupted. If interstitial lung disease is confirmed, cetuximab therapy should be permanently discontinued.

■ **Special Populations** No special population dosage recommendations at this time.

Cautions

■ **Contraindications** The manufacturer states that there are no contraindications to the use of cetuximab.

■ **Warnings/Precautions** ***Warnings*** **Infusion-related Effects.** Infusion-related effects (e.g., chills, fever, rigors, dyspnea, bronchospasm, angioedema, urticaria, hypertension, hypotension) have been reported in 15–21% of patients receiving cetuximab in clinical trials. Serious infusion-related effects, requiring medical intervention and immediate, permanent discontinuance of cetuximab, have included rapid airway obstruction (bronchospasm, stridor, hoarseness), hypotension, shock, loss of consciousness, myocardial infarction, and cardiac arrest. Severe (grade 3 or 4) infusion reactions occurred in 2–5% of 1373 patients in clinical trials; one patient died. Approximately 90% of severe infusion reactions occurred in association with the initial infusion of cetuximab despite premedication with antihistamines.

Patients should be monitored for signs of infusion reactions during and for 1 hour following cetuximab infusion in a setting where resuscitation equipment and agents necessary to treat anaphylaxis are readily available. For patients experiencing infusion reactions requiring treatment, monitoring should be continued until the event is resolved.

If grade 1 or 2 or nonserious grade 3 or 4 infusion-related reactions occur, the infusion rate for cetuximab should be reduced by 50%. If serious infusion-related effects occur, cetuximab therapy should be immediately and permanently discontinued, and appropriate therapy (e.g., epinephrine, corticosteroids, IV antihistamines, bronchodilators, oxygen) initiated. Patients should be monitored until all infusion-related manifestations have completely resolved.

Cardiac Effects. Cardiopulmonary arrest and/or sudden death occurred in 4 (2%) of 208 patients receiving cetuximab and radiation therapy compared with none of 212 patients receiving radiation therapy alone for squamous cell carcinoma of the head and neck in a randomized, controlled trial. One patient with no history of coronary artery disease died 1 day following the last dose of cetuximab. Three patients with histories of coronary artery disease died at home at 27, 32, and 43 days following the last dose of cetuximab; myocardial infarction was the presumed cause of death. One of these patients had arrhythmia and one patient had congestive heart failure.

Cetuximab and radiation therapy for the treatment of head and neck cancer should be used with caution in patients with a history of coronary artery disease, congestive heart failure, or arrhythmias. Serum concentrations of electrolytes, including magnesium, potassium, and calcium, should be monitored closely during and following cetuximab therapy.

Adverse cardiac events—myocardial infarction in one patient and arrhythmia, diminished cardiac output, and hypotension in another patient—caused discontinuation of treatment in patients with head and neck cancer receiving cetuximab with cisplatin and radiation therapy in a clinical trial. The safety of cetuximab in combination with cisplatin and radiation therapy has not been established.

Pulmonary Effects. Interstitial lung disease, interstitial pneumonitis (fatal in one case), and exacerbation of preexisting fibrotic lung disease have been reported in patients receiving cetuximab alone or in combination with other antineoplastic agents (e.g., cisplatin, irinotecan). Interruption or discontinuance of cetuximab therapy may be required in patients with pulmonary symptoms. (See Pulmonary Toxicity under Dosage Modification for Toxicity and Contraindications for Continued Therapy, in Dosage and Administration.)

Electrolyte Effects. Electrolyte abnormalities, sometimes severe, including hypomagnesemia, hypocalcemia, and hypokalemia, have occurred in patients receiving cetuximab. Hypomagnesemia occurred in 199 (55%) of 365 patients receiving cetuximab in clinical trials and was severe (grade 3 or 4) in 6–17% of patients. The onset of hypomagnesemia and accompanying electrolyte abnormalities may occur from days to months following initiation of cetuximab therapy. Manifestations of hypomagnesemia may include fatigue and hypocalcemia. Patients should be monitored for hypomagnesemia, hypocalcemia, and hypokalemia during and for at least 8 weeks following completion of cetuximab therapy. Electrolyte repletion therapy should be administered as necessary and, in severe cases, intravenous replacement therapy is required.

Sensitivity Reactions **Dermatologic Effects.** Acneiform rash occurred in 76–88% of 1373 patients receiving cetuximab in clinical trials and was severe in 1–17% of patients. Acneiform rash generally appears within the first 2 weeks of cetuximab therapy and may resolve following discontinuance of cetuximab; however, manifestations have persisted beyond 28 days in nearly 50% of cases.

Other adverse dermatologic effects, including skin drying/fissuring, paronychial inflammation, infectious sequelae (e.g., abscess formation, blepharitis, conjunctivitis, keratitis, cheilitis, cellulitis, *Staphylococcus aureus* sepsis), and hypertrichosis also have been reported. Fatal toxic epidermal necrolysis has been reported in a patient receiving cetuximab for colorectal cancer. Abnormal hair growth has been reported in a patient receiving cetuximab for head and neck cancer.

Reduction of dosage or discontinuance of therapy is required in patients who develop severe acneiform rash. (See Dermatologic Toxicity under Dosage Modification for Toxicity and Contraindications for Continued Therapy, in Dosage and Administration.)

Major Toxicities **Serious Adverse Effects.** Other serious adverse effects associated with cetuximab include radiation dermatitis, sepsis, renal failure, and pulmonary embolus. Sepsis occurred in 1–4% of patients receiving cetuximab. Renal failure was reported in 1% of patients receiving cetuximab for colorectal cancer. Across all studies, cetuximab therapy was discontinued in 3–10% of patients because of adverse effects. (See Warnings under Cautions: Warnings/Precautions.)

General Precautions **EGFR Testing.** In clinical trials for colorectal cancer, testing for evidence of EGFR expression was required. However, some authorities state that routine EGFR expression testing is not recommended in patients with colorectal cancer and that patients should not be included or excluded from cetuximab therapy based solely on EGFR test results.

Because expression of EGFR has been detected in nearly all head and neck cancers, EGFR testing was not required in these clinical trials.

Therapy Monitoring. Patients receiving cetuximab should be monitored for dermatologic toxicity and infectious sequelae.

Patients should be monitored periodically for hypomagnesemia, and accompanying hypocalcemia and hypokalemia, during and following the completion of cetuximab therapy. Monitoring should be continued for at least 8 weeks following completion of therapy.

Immunologic Effects. Non-neutralizing anticetuximab antibodies were detected in about 5% of patients (49/1001) receiving cetuximab; although the incidence of antibody development to cetuximab has not been fully established, there appears to be no effect on the safety and efficacy of the drug.

Specific Populations **Pregnancy.** Category C. (See Users Guide.)

Lactation. It is not known whether cetuximab is distributed into milk; however, human immunoglobulin G_1 (IgG_1) is distributed into milk. Because of the potential for distribution of IgG antibodies such as cetuximab into milk and the risks for serious adverse reactions from cetuximab in nursing infants, a decision should be made whether to discontinue nursing or the drug, taking into account the importance of the drug to the woman. Based on the long half-life of cetuximab, women should be advised to discontinue nursing while receiving cetuximab therapy and for at least 60 days following the last dose of the drug (see Description).

Pediatric Use. Safety and efficacy of cetuximab have not been established in pediatric patients.

Geriatric Use. Approximately 34% of the 1062 patients receiving cetuximab (alone or in combination with irinotecan) in clinical studies for advanced colorectal cancer were 65 years of age or older. No overall differences in safety and efficacy relative to younger adults were observed.

Clinical studies of cetuximab for head and neck cancer did not include sufficient numbers of patients 65 years of age and older to determine whether geriatric patients respond differently than younger patients. Of 208 patients with advanced head and neck cancer receiving cetuximab and radiation therapy in a clinical trial, 45 patients (22%) were 65 years of age or older.

■ **Common Adverse Effects** The most common adverse effects, observed in at least 25% of patients receiving cetuximab, are adverse dermatologic effects (including rash, pruritus, and nail changes), headache, diarrhea, and infection. Across studies, infection occurred in 13–35% of patients receiving cetuximab.

The most common adverse effects in patients receiving cetuximab in combination with irinotecan for advanced colorectal cancer include acneiform rash (88%), asthenia/malaise (73%), diarrhea (72%), and nausea (55%); the most common grade 3 or 4 adverse effects include diarrhea (22%), leukopenia (17%), asthenia/malaise (16%), and acneiform rash (14%).

The most common adverse effects in patients receiving cetuximab and best supportive care for advanced colorectal cancer include rash/desquamation (89%), fatigue (89%), abdominal pain (59%), pain (51%), dry skin (49%), dyspnea (48%), and constipation (46%).

The most common adverse effects in patients receiving cetuximab in combination with radiation therapy for advanced head and neck cancer include acneiform rash (87%); radiation dermatitis (86%); weight loss (84%); asthenia (56%); nausea (49%); and elevated serum ALT (43%), AST (38%), and alkaline phosphatase concentrations (33%).

Drug Interactions

■ **Antineoplastic Agents** Pharmacokinetic interaction with irinotecan unlikely.

■ **Radiation Therapy** Potential pharmacologic interaction (death, cardiotoxicity, increased risk of adverse dermatologic effects). Death and serious cardiotoxicity occurred in patients with locally advanced squamous cell head and neck cancer receiving cetuximab, cisplatin, and radiation therapy. Rash was reported in 87% of patients with locally advanced squamous cell head and neck cancer who received cetuximab concomitantly with radiation therapy. The incidence of late radiation toxicities was higher in patients receiving cetuximab and radiation therapy than in those receiving radiation therapy alone.

Description

Cetuximab, a recombinant chimeric (human-murine) monoclonal antibody, is an antineoplastic agent. The drug is an immunoglobulin containing human framework (i.e., IgG_1 heavy and kappa light constant regions) and murine Fv regions.

Cetuximab binds specifically to the extracellular domain of the human epidermal growth factor receptor (EGFR, HER1, c-erbB-1) on both normal and tumor cells and competitively blocks the cellular action of EGF and other ligands (e.g., transforming growth factor [TGF]-α). EGFR is a transmembrane glycoprotein that belongs to the subfamily of type I receptor tyrosine kinases, which includes EGFR (HER1), HER2, HER3, and HER4. While EGFR is expressed in many normal epithelial tissues (e.g., skin, hair follicle), overexpression of the glycoprotein is detected in human carcinomas (e.g., colon, rectum, head and neck). In vitro assays and in vivo animal studies have shown that binding of cetuximab to EGFR blocks phosphorylation and activation of receptor-associated kinases; this results in inhibition of cell growth, induction of apoptosis (programmed cell death), and decreased matrix metalloproteinase and vascular endothelial growth factor production. Signal transduction through EGFR leads to activation of the wild-type (nonmutated) *KRAS* gene. However, the presence of an activating somatic mutation of the *KRAS* gene (mutated *KRAS*) in a cancer cell can lead to dysregulation of signaling pathways and resistance to EGFR inhibitor therapy (e.g., cetuximab, panitumumab). In vitro, cetuximab can mediate antibody-dependent cellular cytotoxicity against certain types of human tumors.

In vitro tests and in vivo animal studies have suggested that cetuximab inhibits growth and survival of tumor cells that express EGFR, while such antitumor effects were not observed in human cancer xenografts that lacked EGFR expression. In xenograft models for human tumors in mice, addition of cetuximab to radiation therapy or irinotecan resulted in an increased antitumor effect when compared with radiation therapy or chemotherapy alone.

The pharmacokinetic disposition of cetuximab was similar in patients receiving the drug for head and neck cancer or colorectal cancer. Following administration of the recommended regimen of cetuximab (initial dose, followed by subsequent weekly doses), steady-state cetuximab concentrations are achieved by the third weekly infusion; the mean half-life of cetuximab following multiple dosing is approximately 112 hours. The major route of clearance from the circulation is believed to be through internalization of the cetuximab EGFR complex on hepatocytes and skin.

Advice to Patients

Risk of infusion-related effects and adverse pulmonary and dermatologic effects. Advise patients to report signs or symptoms of infusion reactions, such as fever, chills, or breathing problems.

Importance of advising patients to use sunscreen and hats and limit sun exposure during and for 2 months following discontinuance of cetuximab therapy to avoid exacerbation of adverse dermatologic effects.

Necessity of advising men and women to use an effective method of contraception during and for 6 months following the last dose of cetuximab therapy. Advise pregnant women of risk to the fetus. Advise women to avoid breast-feeding during and for 2 months following the last dose of cetuximab.

Importance of informing clinicians of existing or contemplated concomitant therapy, including prescription and OTC drugs, as well as any concomitant illnesses.

Overview (see Users Guide). For additional information until a more detailed monograph is developed and published, the manufacturer's labeling should be consulted. It is *essential* that the manufacturer's labeling be consulted for more detailed information on usual cautions, precautions, contraindications, potential drug interactions, laboratory test interferences, and acute toxicity.

Preparations

Excipients in commercially available drug preparations may have clinically important effects in some individuals; consult specific product labeling for details.

Cetuximab (Recombinant)

Parenteral

Injection, for IV infusion only	2 mg/mL (100 and 200 mg)	**Erbitux®**, Bristol-Myers Squibb

†Use is not currently included in the labeling approved by the US Food and Drug Administration

CISplatin

DDP, *cis*-DDP

■ Cisplatin is a platinum-containing antineoplastic agent.

Uses

Cisplatin is often used as a component of combination chemotherapeutic regimens because of its relative lack of hematologic toxicity.

■ Testicular Cancer Cisplatin is used as a component of various chemotherapeutic regimens for the treatment of metastatic testicular tumors, including nonseminomatous testicular carcinoma, seminoma testis, and extragonadal germ-cell tumors, in patients who have already received appropriate surgery and/or radiation therapy.

Nonseminomatous Testicular Carcinoma In the treatment of disseminated nonseminomatous testicular carcinoma (stage III), cisplatin is one of the most active single agents; however, combination chemotherapy for induction of remissions is superior to single-agent therapy. Various regimens have been evaluated in combination therapy, and comparative efficacy is continually being evaluated. Most clinicians use cisplatin in combination with other antineoplastic agents as initial therapy in patients with stage III or unresectable stage II nonseminomatous testicular carcinoma; if the patient has persistent, localized tumor following chemotherapy, the residual tumor is removed surgically, and if the residual disease contains malignant elements, additional chemotherapy is administered.

Cisplatin has been used in combination with bleomycin and vinblastine, with or without other antineoplastic agents, for the induction of remissions. Cisplatin also has been used in combination with bleomycin and etoposide for the treatment of disseminated disease. These chemotherapy regimens usually produce a complete remission in 60–70% of patients with disseminated disease. Response rates generally are higher in patients with minimal stage III disease and less advanced disease and lower in patients with advanced stage III disease. An additional 10–20% of patients can attain a complete remission following surgical removal of localized residual disease after chemotherapy-induced partial remissions. Most patients who attain a complete remission remain disease free, and those patients who have continuous disease-free remission for longer than 2 years generally are considered cured. Maintenance chemotherapy does not appear to be necessary following the attainment of a complete remission. Although not clearly established, patients with embryonal carcinoma may have a better response to chemotherapy than do patients with choriocarcinoma or teratocarcinoma.

For the initial treatment of advanced nonseminomatous testicular carcinoma, most clinicians recommend regimens containing cisplatin and bleomycin, in combination with etoposide rather than vinblastine, particularly because of the reduced neuromuscular toxicity and evidence suggesting greater efficacy in poor-risk patients. In addition, while a regimen of etoposide, cisplatin, and bleomycin appears to be as effective overall as a regimen of vinblastine, cisplatin, and bleomycin, the etoposide-containing regimen may be more effective than the vinblastine-containing regimen in a subgroup of patients with advanced disease (i.e., high tumor load). However, the best combination or sequential therapy in the treatment of advanced nonseminomatous testicular tumors has not been established, and comparative efficacy is continually being evaluated.

A regimen of cisplatin, ifosfamide with mesna, and either vinblastine or etoposide has induced complete responses in 20–45% of patients who previously received other cisplatin-based chemotherapy regimens, and is considered by most clinicians to be the standard initial salvage (i.e., second-line) regimen in patients with recurrent testicular cancer. Patients with minimal or moderate disease have a more favorable outcome with this salvage regimen than those with extensive disease. In a clinical study in patients with recurrent germ cell tumors (who had previously received at least 2 cisplatin-based chemotherapy regimens and were considered to have cisplatin-responsive disease), a regimen of cisplatin, ifosfamide, and either vinblastine or etoposide resulted in disease-free status in 36% of patients (with or without surgery) and median duration of disease control ranged from 3 to more than 42 weeks, median survival was 53 weeks, and 20% of patients had survival of 2 years or longer. In patients with refractory disease, high-dose chemotherapy with autologous bone marrow transplant (ABMT) or peripheral stem cell rescue may produce durable complete remissions in some patients. Patients with progressive tumors during initial or salvage therapy and those with refractory mediastinal germ cell tumors generally appear to benefit less from high-dose chemotherapy and ABMT or peripheral stem cell rescue than those whose disease relapses after a response. Salvage surgery also may be considered for certain highly selected patients (e.g., those with chemorefractory disease confined to a single site).

The role of chemotherapy in the treatment of stage I and resectable stage II nonseminomatous testicular carcinoma has not been clearly established. Although most patients with stage I disease are cured by surgery alone, cisplatin-containing combination chemotherapy regimens have been used successfully to induce complete remissions in a limited number of these patients whose disease relapsed following surgical treatment. Cisplatin-containing combination chemotherapy regimens have also been used successfully as an adjuvant to surgery (orchiectomy and retroperitoneal lymphadenectomy) to induce complete remissions in patients with resectable stage II disease. Although the precise role of chemotherapy as an adjuvant to surgery in the treatment of stage II disease remains to be clearly established, such therapy with cisplatin-containing combination regimens is effective in preventing tumor recurrence in patients with such disease. When surgery, follow-up, and chemotherapy are optimal in patients with stage II disease who have no postoperative evidence of residual or recurrent disease, including absence of elevated tumor markers, cure rates appear to be similar whether cisplatin-containing chemotherapy is administered as an adjuvant to surgery (i.e., beginning postoperatively) or is withheld and used to treat relapse in closely monitored patients. In patients with residual gross disease or residual elevated tumor markers following retroperitoneal lymphadenopathy, some clinicians recommend that all such patients receive cisplatin-containing combination chemotherapy.

Seminoma Testis Cisplatin-containing combination chemotherapy regimens have been used successfully in the treatment of disseminated seminoma testis, with complete remission rates comparable to those in patients with disseminated nonseminomatous disease. Further evaluation is needed to determine the optimum therapy.

Extragonadal Germ-Cell Tumors Although data are limited and some reports indicate a low response rate, cisplatin-containing combination chemotherapy regimens (followed by surgery when feasible) have reportedly been successful in the treatment of advanced extragonadal germ-cell tumors, with complete remission rates comparable to those in patients with nonseminomatous tumors of similar advanced stages. Cisplatin-containing combination chemotherapy regimens have also been reported to be successful in a few cases for the treatment of extragonadal endodermal sinus tumor (yolk-sac carcinoma) in males, although this tumor is generally considered poorly responsive to chemotherapy.

■ Ovarian Cancer Cisplatin is used alone or in combination therapy for the treatment of ovarian cancer.

Adjuvant Therapy for Early-stage Ovarian Epithelial Cancer Platinum-based therapy has been used for adjuvant treatment following surgery in early-stage ovarian epithelial cancer†. (See Uses: Ovarian Cancer: Adjuvant Therapy for Early-stage Ovarian Epithelial Cancer in Carboplatin 10:00.)

First-line Therapy for Advanced Ovarian Epithelial Cancer A platinum-containing agent in combination with paclitaxel is a preferred regimen for the treatment of advanced ovarian epithelial cancer. The best combination or sequential therapy with multiple agents in the treatment of advanced ovarian tumors has not been established, and comparative efficacy is continually being evaluated.

Combination chemotherapy regimens containing platinum are associated with higher response rates and improved survival compared with non-platinum-containing regimens as first-line treatment for advanced ovarian cancer. The benefit of cisplatin used in combination therapy rather than as monotherapy has not been fully established. In a large randomized trial, cisplatin combined with paclitaxel produced higher response rates than paclitaxel alone and similar response rates but less toxicity than cisplatin alone; median survival did not differ among the groups.

Carboplatin versus Cisplatin. Randomized trials have demonstrated that carboplatin is as effective as but less toxic than cisplatin when used in combination with either paclitaxel or cyclophosphamide for the initial treatment of advanced ovarian cancer. Carboplatin in combination with paclitaxel currently is a preferred regimen for the initial treatment of advanced ovarian epithelial cancer. (See Uses: Ovarian Cancer: First-line Therapy for Advanced Ovarian Epithelial Cancer in Carboplatin 10:00.)

Platinum-Containing Agent with Paclitaxel Versus Platinum-containing Agent with Cyclophosphamide. The combination of IV cisplatin and IV paclitaxel has been used for the initial treatment of advanced epithelial ovarian carcinoma, and evidence from randomized trials indicates that this combination is superior to combined cisplatin and cyclophosphamide for initial treatment. In a comparative study of patients with suboptimally debulked (greater than 1 cm residual tumor mass) stage III or IV ovarian cancer who had no prior chemotherapy, combined therapy with paclitaxel and cisplatin produced higher rates of overall objective response (73 versus 60%), increased disease-free survival (median: 18 versus 13 months), and increased overall survival (median: 38 versus 24 months) compared with a combined regimen of cisplatin and cyclophosphamide. A higher frequency of neutropenia, fever, alopecia, and allergic reactions was observed in patients receiving cisplatin and paclitaxel compared with those receiving cisplatin and cyclophosphamide. In another randomized trial, higher rates of overall and complete response (59 versus 45% and 41 versus 27%, respectively) and prolonged median overall survival (36 versus 26 months) were observed in patients receiving paclitaxel and cisplatin versus cyclophosphamide and cisplatin for advanced epithelial ovarian cancer. At a follow-up of 6.5 years, the survival benefit associated with the cisplatin and paclitaxel regimen in both randomized trials has been maintained.

Intraperitoneal Cisplatin and Paclitaxel. Combined IV and intraperitoneal therapy with IV paclitaxel, intraperitoneal cisplatin, and intraperitoneal paclitaxel† has been used for the treatment of optimally debulked stage III epithelial ovarian cancer.

The National Cancer Institute (NCI) recommends use of a combined IV and intraperitoneal regimen for eligible patients with advanced epithelial ovarian cancer because of a substantial survival benefit. Based on clinical trials, NCI recommends that use of a regimen containing intraperitoneal cisplatin (100 mg/m^2) and a taxane (either IV only or IV plus intraperitoneal) should be strongly considered following primary surgery in patients with optimally debulked stage III epithelial ovarian cancer. Although an optimal intraperitoneal chemotherapy regimen has not been established, favorable results were observed following sequential administration of IV paclitaxel, intraperitoneal cisplatin, and intraperitoneal paclitaxel in the Gynecologic Oncology Group (GOG)-172 study.

In this randomized phase 3 trial (GOG-172), 429 patients with previously untreated stage III epithelial ovarian cancer or primary peritoneal cancer, with no residual mass exceeding 1 cm in diameter following surgery, received either combined IV and intraperitoneal therapy or IV therapy. All patients enrolled in this study had good baseline GOG performance status (0–2) and adequate bone marrow, renal, and hepatic function. Most patients (88%) had ovarian cancer, and serous adenocarcinoma was the most common histologic type (79% of patients). The primary end points of the study were progression-free survival and overall survival. Combined IV and intraperitoneal therapy consisted of IV paclitaxel 135 mg/m^2 by 24-hour infusion on day 1, followed by intraperitoneal cisplatin 100 mg/m^2 on day 2 and intraperitoneal paclitaxel 60 mg/m^2 on day 8. IV therapy consisted of IV paclitaxel 135 mg/m^2 by 24-hour infusion on day 1 followed by IV cisplatin 75 mg/m^2 on day 2. Both regimens were repeated every 21 days for up to 6 cycles. Patients who received combined IV and intraperitoneal therapy had longer median progression-free (23.8 versus 18.3 months) and overall (65.6 versus 49.7 months) survival compared with patients who received IV therapy.

Most (83%) of the patients receiving IV therapy completed 6 cycles of their assigned chemotherapy regimen; however, only 42% of patients receiving combined IV and intraperitoneal therapy completed 6 cycles of assigned chemotherapy; patients who could not complete the intraperitoneal regimen received IV therapy for the remaining treatment cycles. The most common reason for discontinuance of intraperitoneal therapy was catheter-related complications. Grade 3 or 4 leukopenia (76 versus 64%), GI effects (46 versus 24%), metabolic effects (27 versus 7%), fatigue (18 versus 4%), neurologic effects (19 versus 9%), infection (16 versus 6%), thrombocytopenia (12 versus 4%), and pain (11 versus 1%) occurred more frequently in patients receiving combined IV and intraperitoneal therapy than in those receiving IV therapy. Although patients receiving combined IV and intraperitoneal therapy reported less improvement in abdominal discomfort before cycle 4, improvement in abdominal discomfort was similar in both treatment groups 1 year after completion of therapy. Among patients who received combined IV and intraperitoneal therapy, quality of life was worse during and shortly after completion of therapy (before cycle 4 and at 3–6 weeks following therapy) compared with those who received IV therapy. Quality-of-life scores were similar for the groups at 1 year after completion of treatment, except for greater persistence of moderate paresthesias in patients receiving combined IV and intraperitoneal therapy.

Retrospective review of baseline data (patient and disease characteristics) from two phase 3 clinical trials (including GOG-172) for patients receiving intraperitoneal therapy for optimally debulked stage III epithelial ovarian cancer suggested that extent of residual tumor mass, histology, and age were important predictors of survival in such patients. Patients with clear cell histology appeared to derive less benefit from intraperitoneal therapy compared with those with serous histology (hazard ratio for progression-free and overall survival of 2.66 and 3.88, respectively). In addition, each additional year of age was associated with a 1% increase in the risk of death. Although patients enrolled in the studies had optimally debulked (1 cm or less residual tumor mass) disease, survival was greater in patients with only microscopic residual disease.

Retrospective analysis of data from patients receiving a modified IV and intraperitoneal regimen suggests that a reduced dosage of intraperitoneal cisplatin administered in conjunction with a shortened IV paclitaxel infusion time may result in less toxicity and produce a survival benefit similar to that reported in the GOG-172 study (67 months versus 65.6 months reported in GOG-172). The modified IV and intraperitoneal regimen consisted of IV paclitaxel 135 mg/m^2 by 3-hour infusion on day 1, followed by intraperitoneal cisplatin 75 mg/m^2 on day 2 and intraperitoneal paclitaxel 60 mg/m^2 on day 8 of each 21-day cycle. Most patients (80%) completed 4 or more cycles of therapy and 55% completed 6 cycles. The frequency of grade 3 or 4 neutropenia (12%), GI effects (8%), metabolic effects (5%), neurologic effects (6%), infection (2%), fatigue (2%), and thrombocytopenia (0%) in this series of patients receiving the modified IV and intraperitoneal regimen appeared to be lower than toxicity rates reported in the GOG-172 study. By shortening the infusion time for IV paclitaxel to 3 hours, the modified regimen also may provide an outpatient alternative to inpatient administration over 24 hours. However, randomized controlled trials are needed to establish comparative safety and efficacy of this modified regimen. The modified IV and intraperitoneal schedule containing the lower intraperitoneal cisplatin dosage and the 3-hour IV paclitaxel infusion also has been studied in conjunction with a third cytotoxic drug, but with evidence of excessive toxicity.

Based on current evidence, combined IV and intraperitoneal therapy with IV paclitaxel, intraperitoneal cisplatin, and intraperitoneal paclitaxel is recommended (accepted) for use as initial adjuvant treatment of optimally debulked stage III epithelial ovarian cancer in patients with good performance status (GOG performance status of 0–2).

Second-line Therapy for Advanced Ovarian Epithelial Cancer

Either cisplatin or carboplatin can be used when retreatment is indicated in patients with platinum-sensitive disease who relapse; however, some clinicians suggest that carboplatin may be preferred because it is associated with a more favorable toxicity profile than cisplatin. Although some patients who failed to respond to cisplatin or had a response of only short duration have responded to carboplatin, nonplatinum-based regimens (e.g., paclitaxel) generally are preferred for retreatment of patients with platinum-resistant disease. Responses to cisplatin also have been observed in patients with disease resistant to initial treatment with paclitaxel monotherapy.

Dosage and Other Therapeutic Considerations While some evidence indicates that dose intensity (i.e., amount of platinum per unit time) is an important factor in achieving optimum results in patients with stage III or IV ovarian carcinoma, other evidence suggests that total platinum dose or duration of exposure is a more important factor in improving progression-free survival in responding patients. However, no improvement in response appears to occur with increased dose intensity or increased total dose once a certain threshold is reached. Although optimum duration of chemotherapy has not been clearly defined, there currently is no evidence of improved response and/or survival when the duration of drug administration exceeds 6 cycles. Despite the fact that platinum-containing combination chemotherapy regimens are associated with high response rates, no regimen has been found that is sufficiently active to prevent disease progression and/or recurrence in most women with stage III or IV ovarian carcinoma.

Other therapeutic techniques, such as interval debulking surgery, may improve survival in patients with advanced ovarian carcinoma. In a randomized study involving patients with residual lesions (greater than 1 cm) following primary surgery for advanced ovarian cancer (stages IIB through IV) who responded to cisplatin-based induction chemotherapy, those who received interval debulking surgery accompanied by subsequent chemotherapy had improved survival compared with those who received chemotherapy alone.

Ovarian Germ Cell Tumors Cisplatin-containing chemotherapy regimens are used in the treatment of ovarian germ-cell tumors, including endodermal sinus tumors. Combination chemotherapy with cisplatin, bleomycin, and etoposide currently is a regimen of choice for the adjuvant therapy of ovarian germ-cell tumors.

■ **Bladder Cancer** Cisplatin is used widely in the treatment of muscle-invasive and advanced bladder cancer. Approximately 20–25% of patients with bladder cancer are initially diagnosed with invasive tumors. Radical cystectomy is the standard therapy for muscle-invasive bladder cancer; however, because of the high rate of metastasis following local therapy, combined modality treatment including chemotherapy (neoadjuvant or adjuvant), radiation therapy, and surgery is being evaluated for the management of invasive disease and also has been used to allow bladder preservation in selected patients. Combination chemotherapy alone or as an adjunct to local therapy with surgery and/or radiation therapy is used for the palliative and occasionally curative treatment of locally advanced (unresectable) or metastatic bladder cancer.

Over 90% of bladder tumors are transitional cell carcinomas originating from the uroepithelium. Other histologic types of bladder cancer, such as squamous cell carcinoma (6–8%) and adenocarcinoma (2%), are associated with greater resistance to treatment and a more aggressive pattern of local spread than transitional cell carcinoma. Bladder carcinoma is clinically staged according to the TNM classification. Major prognostic factors in patients with carcinoma of the bladder include the depth of tumor invasion into the bladder wall and the degree of differentiation or grade of the tumor.

Muscle-invasive Bladder Carcinoma **Overview.** Choice of therapy in muscle-invasive cancer must be individualized according to prognostic factors, the patient's medical condition, expected benefits and risks of therapy, and patient preference. Important prognostic factors used to guide selection of therapy for invasive bladder cancer include stage of tumor, particularly whether the tumor is organ-confined (stage 2 or T3a) or not organ-confined (stage T3b, 4, 4a, or 4b); presence of lymph node involvement, and lymphatic or vascular invasion of the tumor.

There is a 30–50% risk of nodal or distant metastases in patients with muscle-invasive bladder carcinoma. Radical cystectomy (i.e., removal of the bladder, prostate, and seminal vesicles in men or removal of the bladder, uterus, fallopian tubes, ovaries, and upper vagina in women) with pelvic lymphadenectomy is considered standard therapy in the US; depending on the location of the tumor, partial cystectomy rarely may be adequate in some patients. A retrospective analysis demonstrated that radical cystectomy with urinary diversion is well tolerated and effective for the definitive treatment of muscle-invasive bladder cancer in geriatric patients (70 years of age or older) in good health (i.e., good cardiac performance and absence of cardiovascular or pulmonary problems) in comparison with younger patients (younger than 70 years).

Rarely, transurethral resection (TUR) alone has been effective in selected patients with a small (less than 2 cm), solitary papillary tumor that is minimally invasive into muscle and is not associated with carcinoma in situ, a palpable mass, or hydronephrosis; however, in the treatment of muscle-invasive bladder carcinoma, TUR more often is used to debulk tumors prior to the administration of systemic therapy with chemotherapy and/or radiation therapy in selected patients receiving combined modality treatment with bladder preservation. Some clinicians perform a second TUR in selected patients to further reduce tumor burden or to pursue findings (e.g., progression of disease, absence of residual tumor) that may influence treatment strategy.

The addition of preoperative radiation has not been shown to affect overall survival in patients undergoing radical cystectomy for muscle-invasive bladder cancer and is not standard care in the US; however, limited evidence from a matched analysis suggests that preoperative radiation therapy may reduce the rate of local recurrence in patients with T3b tumors. Although overall survival in patients receiving sole treatment with radiation for invasive disease is inferior to that obtained with radical cystectomy, treatment with radiation therapy alone with external beam radiation may be considered in patients who refuse or are unable to tolerate surgery. Treatment with radiation therapy followed by salvage cystectomy does not appear to adversely affect survival or rate of metastasis compared with immediate cystectomy in patients with muscle-invasive bladder cancer.

Despite treatment with radical cystectomy, 50% of patients with muscle-invasive bladder cancer will develop metastases within 18 months. Because of the high rates of metastasis following local therapy with cystectomy and/or radiation therapy, the addition of chemotherapy to the treatment regimen for muscle-invasive bladder cancer is being investigated. Randomized trials are being conducted to determine the benefit of chemotherapy (adjuvant or neoadjuvant) added to cystectomy or used in conjunction with radiation therapy for muscle-invasive bladder carcinoma; studies to date have shown no effect on overall survival. Combined modality therapy with combination chemotherapy, radiation therapy, and conservative surgery (aggressive transurethral resection or partial cystectomy) has been used to allow organ preservation in selected patients with muscle-invasive bladder cancer; however, the effect on survival with use of organ-sparing treatment versus standard therapy with radical cystectomy is not known.

Neoadjuvant or Adjuvant Chemotherapy. In patients with muscle-invasive bladder cancer, chemotherapy has been given prior to (i.e., as neoadjuvant therapy) or following (i.e., as adjuvant therapy) local treatment with surgery and/or radiation therapy. The benefit of adjuvant or neoadjuvant chemotherapy has not been established, and use of chemotherapy as a component of therapy currently is considered investigational in the treatment of muscle-invasive bladder cancer.

Although no survival benefit has been conclusively demonstrated with the use of adjuvant chemotherapy, some experts recommend systemic therapy following either cystectomy or aggressive transurethral resection in patients with adverse prognostic factors (e.g., stage T3b or greater, node-positive disease, lymphatic or vascular invasion of the tumor). Use of adjuvant chemotherapy may be unnecessary or excessive treatment, particularly in patients with muscle-invasive bladder cancer that is organ-confined (e.g., stage T2 or T3a) and node-negative.

Trials evaluating the use of single chemotherapeutic agents as adjuvant therapy have not shown any benefit, and combination regimens consisting of cisplatin, methotrexate, and vinblastine with or without doxorubicin (abbreviated as M-VAC or CMV, respectively) currently are used for the adjuvant treatment of muscle-invasive bladder cancer. Combination chemotherapy used as adjuvant treatment has been demonstrated to delay progression of disease and decrease local recurrence of tumor in patients with muscle-invasive bladder cancer. When chemotherapy is administered in the adjuvant setting, it is recommended that a minimum of 4 cycles (at full doses) be given; however, the optimal dose, schedule, and number of courses for adjuvant chemotherapy in the treatment of muscle-invasive bladder carcinoma has not been determined. Additional study in randomized trials is needed to determine the benefit of adjuvant chemotherapy for invasive bladder cancer.

Single-agent cisplatin or cisplatin-containing combination chemotherapy has been used as neoadjuvant therapy preceding cystectomy and/or radiation therapy or as concurrent therapy with definitive or preoperative radiation therapy in patients with muscle-invasive bladder cancer. The addition of neoadjuvant chemotherapy to local treatment appears to cause regression of existing tumor, decrease local recurrence of tumor, and increase time to relapse of disease in patients with muscle-invasive bladder cancer; however, no effect on overall survival has been conclusively demonstrated. Results of a pooled analysis that mostly included randomized trials of single-agent cisplatin did not demonstrate a difference in survival with the addition of chemotherapy (neoadjuvant or concurrent) in patients undergoing cystectomy and/or radiation therapy for muscle-invasive bladder cancer; however, based on experience with treatment of advanced bladder cancer, single-agent cisplatin is considered less effective than combination cisplatin-based chemotherapy.

Results from large randomized trials of neoadjuvant therapy with cisplatin-based combination regimens (e.g., cisplatin, methotrexate, and vinblastine; cisplatin and doxorubicin) have not shown a survival benefit in patients with muscle-invasive bladder cancer. Subgroup analysis suggests a possible effect of neoadjuvant chemotherapy on overall survival in patients with cancers of histologic grade G3 or stage T3 or T4a disease, and further randomized trials may identify prognostic factors that allow selection of a subgroup of patients with locally advanced bladder cancer who are likely to benefit from neoadjuvant chemotherapy. Because a conclusive survival benefit has not been shown, routine use of neoadjuvant therapy with combination chemotherapy regimens (e.g., cisplatin, methotrexate, and vinblastine with or without doxorubicin) for muscle-invasive bladder cancer is *not* recommended, and such therapy is considered investigational. Longer periods of follow-up in ongoing randomized trials are needed to establish the benefit (if any) of neoadjuvant chemotherapy in patients undergoing cystectomy and/or radiation therapy for muscle-invasive bladder cancer.

The effect of sequence of therapy when chemotherapy is used in conjunction with local treatment (i.e., cystectomy and/or radiation therapy) for invasive bladder cancer is not known. Interim analysis of a randomized trial of patients with stage T3b or T4a tumors receiving either adjuvant or neoadjuvant chemotherapy did not detect any difference in survival. Further study is needed to establish the benefit of adding chemotherapy (adjuvant or neoadjuvant) to cystectomy and/or radiation therapy for the treatment of muscle-invasive bladder cancer.

Neoadjuvant chemotherapy for muscle-invasive bladder cancer typically is administered IV. In a limited number of patients with muscle-invasive bladder cancer, neoadjuvant chemotherapy has been administered intra-arterially; however, this method of administration is associated with substantial toxicity, and the comparative efficacy of intra-arterial chemotherapy versus IV chemotherapy for the neoadjuvant treatment of muscle-invasive bladder cancer is not known.

Combined Modality Therapy with Bladder Preservation. Single-agent cisplatin or cisplatin-containing combination chemotherapy (e.g., cisplatin with methotrexate and vinblastine [CMV]) has been used in conjunction with radiation therapy and conservative surgery as a bladder-sparing approach for the treatment of selected patients with muscle-invasive bladder cancer. Clinical trials are under way to investigate whether bladder preservation is a reasonable goal in patients with small-volume, organ-confined (stage T2 or T3a) disease when total eradication of the tumor can be achieved; patients with bulky tumors, tumors with overexpression of p53 nuclear protein, nontransitional or mixed histology carcinoma, hydronephrosis, and/or ureteral obstruction are at high risk for relapse of invasive bladder tumor and generally are not good candidates for clinical trials of organ-preserving therapy.

Following aggressive transurethral resection (TUR), use of chemotherapy with radiation therapy appears to produce survival rates comparable to those reported for radical cystectomy in patients with muscle-invasive bladder cancer. In one case series, patients with muscle-invasive bladder cancer (stages T2 through T4, node-negative disease) underwent TUR followed by combination chemotherapy with cisplatin, methotrexate, and vinblastine (CMV) and then radiation therapy with concurrent cisplatin therapy. At 5 years, the overall survival rate was 52%, and 43% of all patients who entered the study had survived with a functioning bladder. However, in a randomized trial of patients with muscle-invasive bladder cancer (stages T2 through T4, node-negative disease) undergoing aggressive TUR followed by radiation therapy with concurrent cisplatin therapy, with or without the addition of neoadjuvant combination chemotherapy with cisplatin, methotrexate, and vinblastine (CMV) preceding concurrent chemoradiation therapy, neoadjuvant chemotherapy caused substantial toxicity (particularly severe neutropenia and sepsis) and did not provide additional benefit in rate of overall survival (48 versus 49%), rate of survival with a functioning bladder (36 versus 40%), or rate of distant metastases (33 versus 39%). Combination chemotherapy with cisplatin, methotrexate, vinblastine, and doxorubicin (M-VAC) followed by partial cystectomy also has been used as an organ-preserving approach to the treatment of muscle-invasive bladder cancer. Response to induction chemotherapy and/or radiation therapy confirmed by cystoscopy and/or bladder biopsy is an important predictor of survival in patients with muscle-invasive bladder cancer.

Bladder preservation is attempted only in patients with disease that responds to induction chemotherapy and/or radiation therapy. Patients with disease that does not demonstrate a complete response to chemotherapy and/or radiation therapy are immediately referred for radical cystectomy; further study is needed to determine whether delay of cystectomy adversely affects outcome in such patients. All patients who receive organ-sparing therapy must be carefully monitored for tumor recurrence and/or occurrence of new tumors; local therapy (e.g., intravesical instillation) and/or cystectomy eventually is required in some patients. Combined modality treatment with conservative surgery and radiation therapy with concurrent cisplatin-containing chemotherapy may be a reasonable alternative in patients with muscle-invasive bladder cancer who refuse or are unable to tolerate radical cystectomy, and clinical trials are under way to investigate this approach; however, unless randomized trials demonstrate that survival is comparable to that achieved with radical cystectomy, organ-preserving treatment cannot be routinely recommended in patients with muscle-invasive bladder cancer.

Advanced Bladder Carcinoma Combination chemotherapy is used alone or as an adjunct to local therapy with surgery and/or radiation therapy for the palliative treatment of advanced (unresectable) or metastatic bladder carcinoma. The prognosis for patients with advanced or metastatic bladder cancer generally is poor, particularly in patients with bony or hepatic metastases. Although complete response to combination chemotherapy has been observed in some patients with metastatic bladder cancer, median survival with current treatment is only 12 months.

Combination Cisplatin-based Chemotherapy. Cisplatin-based combination chemotherapy regimens (e.g., cisplatin, methotrexate, and vinblastine with or without doxorubicin, abbreviated as M-VAC or CMV, respectively; cisplatin and gemcitabine) currently are used for the palliative treatment of advanced or metastatic bladder cancer. In patients with metastatic bladder cancer, the potential benefit must be weighed against the substantial toxicity associated with aggressive chemotherapy. The activity of new agents and optimal regimens for the treatment of advanced or metastatic bladder cancer are continually being evaluated.

Combination cisplatin-based therapy is superior to single-agent cisplatin, and combination chemotherapy regimens consisting of 3 or 4 drugs are considered standard therapy for patients with metastatic bladder cancer. Overall response rates with cisplatin-based combination regimens range from 40–70%, with complete responses rates of 10–20%.

In randomized trials, patients with advanced or metastatic bladder cancer receiving combination chemotherapy with cisplatin, methotrexate, vinblastine, and doxorubicin (M-VAC) had higher response rates and more prolonged survival compared with single-agent cisplatin or combination therapy with cisplatin, doxorubicin, and cyclophosphamide. The use of M-VAC also is associated with greater toxicity than single-agent cisplatin, particularly leukopenia, mucositis, granulocytopenia, and drug-related mortality. At 6 years of follow-up, patients receiving M-VAC have more prolonged survival than those receiving cisplatin, but despite the superior efficacy of this regimen, only 3.7% of patients receiving M-VAC are alive and continuously disease-free.

Combination therapy with cisplatin and gemcitabine is an alternative to M-VAC for the treatment of advanced or metastatic bladder cancer. In a large randomized trial of patients receiving either M-VAC or cisplatin and gemcitabine for the treatment of advanced or metastatic bladder cancer, overall median survival (14.8 versus 13.8 months, respectively), median time to progressive disease (7.4 months for each regimen), and response rates (38 versus 44%, respectively, using intent-to-treat analysis) were similar. Prophylactic hematopoietic agents (growth factors) were not administered to either group; grade 3 or 4 neutropenia, neutropenic sepsis, grade 3 or 4 mucositis, and alopecia occurred more frequently in patients receiving M-VAC whereas grade 3 or 4 anemia or grade 3 or 4 thrombocytopenia were observed more often in patients receiving cisplatin and gemcitabine.

Patients receiving combination chemotherapy with cisplatin, methotrexate, and vinblastine (CMV) had a higher rate of survival at 1 year (29 versus 16%) but experienced more toxicity than those receiving methotrexate and vinblastine for advanced or metastatic bladder cancer. The comparative efficacy of M-VAC and CMV has not been investigated in randomized trials; some clinicians favor M-VAC as the established regimen of choice for the treatment of advanced or metastatic bladder cancer whereas others prefer CMV because of decreased toxicity associated with this regimen. Because of the cardiac toxicity associated with doxorubicin, CMV generally is preferable to M-VAC in patients with cardiac dysfunction. Non-transitional cell bladder cancers are less sensitive to standard cisplatin-based chemotherapy regimens than is transitional cell bladder carcinoma, and most clinicians recommend that standard regimens such as M-VAC or CMV not be used in patients with metastatic adenocarcinoma or squamous cell carcinoma of the bladder.

Because of the substantial toxicity and poor survival associated with current regimens, optimal therapy for advanced bladder cancer continually is being evaluated and all eligible candidates should be considered for entry into clinical trials; randomized trials are under way to compare the efficacy and toxicity of M-VAC with other regimens (e.g., paclitaxel and carboplatin) for the treatment of advanced or metastatic bladder cancer.

Dosage Considerations. The usual dosage schedule for the M-VAC regimen is a monthly cycle consisting of IV cisplatin 70 mg/m² (administered on day 2), IV methotrexate 30 mg/m² (administered on days 1, 15, and 22), IV vinblastine 3 mg/m² (administered on days 2, 15, and 22), and IV doxorubicin 30 mg/m² (administered on day 2).

Higher doses of cisplatin are administered in the CMV regimen. The usual dosage schedule for the CMV regimen is a 21-day cycle consisting of IV cisplatin 100 mg/m² (administered on day 2), IV methotrexate 30 mg/m² (administered on days 1 and 8), and IV vinblastine 4 mg/m² (administered on days 1 and 8).

Escalated doses in the M-VAC regimen with concomitant administration of hematopoietic therapy (GM-CSF or G-CSF) have been used in patients with advanced urothelial carcinoma. In a randomized, phase III trial, a higher rate of complete response but no difference in overall survival was observed in patients receiving high-dose M-VAC with G-CSF versus classic M-VAC alone (without G-CSF) for advanced bladder cancer.

Treatment with cisplatin-based regimens should be discontinued if objective response is not observed following 2 or 3 cycles of therapy. Although the optimal duration of therapy has not been fully determined, some experts recommend 4–6 cycles of therapy as tolerated for patients showing clinical response; additional cycles of therapy do not appear to improve outcome. Surgical resection, when indicated, generally is considered after 4 cycles of therapy; additional cycles of chemotherapy following surgery have not been shown to provide benefit.

Administration of cisplatin in divided doses may be necessary in patients with renal impairment receiving cisplatin-based regimens for the treatment of advanced bladder cancer.

Adverse Effects and Other Considerations. Substantial toxicity, including myelosuppression and mucositis, is associated with use of the M-VAC regimen in patients with advanced or metastatic bladder cancer. The administration of hematopoietic agents (e.g., G-CSF, GM-CSF) has been used to reduce the incidence and severity of myelosuppression in patients receiving M-VAC for advanced bladder cancer. Prophylactic use of G-CSF should be strongly considered in patients receiving M-VAC.

Carboplatin has been substituted as a less toxic alternative to cisplatin in some patients receiving combination chemotherapy for advanced bladder cancer. Inadequate dosing of carboplatin may have contributed to its lesser efficacy compared with cisplatin in earlier studies of platinum-based regimens for the treatment of advanced or metastatic bladder cancer. Combination therapy with paclitaxel followed by carboplatin is being investigated as an active regimen in patients with advanced bladder cancer, including patients with abnormal renal function.

■ Head and Neck Cancer

Cisplatin is commonly used in combination with fluorouracil for the palliative treatment of recurrent or metastatic head and neck cancer†. Combination therapy with cisplatin, methotrexate, bleomycin, and vincristine also has been used for the treatment of recurrent or metastatic squamous cell carcinoma of the head and neck. Methotrexate alone also may be used for the treatment of recurrent or metastatic head and neck cancer, particularly in patients who cannot tolerate aggressive chemotherapy.

Cisplatin-containing combination therapy is superior to single-agent therapy in producing higher response rates; however, no effect on overall survival has been demonstrated. In a randomized study, patients with recurrent or metastatic squamous cell carcinoma of the head and neck who received cisplatin and fluorouracil, carboplatin and fluorouracil, or methotrexate alone had objective response rates of 32, 21, and 10%, respectively. Although the objective response rate achieved with cisplatin and fluorouracil was greater than that observed with methotrexate alone, combination chemotherapy was associated with increased toxicity (particularly hematologic and renal toxicity), and no difference in survival was observed. Patients receiving cisplatin and fluorouracil for advanced head and neck cancer had a higher response rate and delayed progression of disease but no difference in survival compared with those receiving either cisplatin or fluorouracil alone. In another randomized trial, patients receiving cisplatin, methotrexate, bleomycin, and vincristine for recurrent or metastatic head and neck cancer had higher rates of complete response than those receiving cisplatin and fluorouracil; although both combination regimens produced a higher rate of objective response than cisplatin alone, no difference in survival was detected among the treatment groups.

Cisplatin has been administered concurrently with radiation therapy for the palliative treatment of head and neck cancer in patients with locally advanced disease that is unresectable. The use of cisplatin-containing chemotherapy administered concurrently with radiation therapy is being investigated as an approach to resectable disease in cases where surgical resection would lead to functional deficit. Cisplatin also has been used in combination with docetaxel and fluorouracil as induction therapy prior to radiotherapy or chemoradiotherapy in the treatment of locally advanced squamous cell carcinoma of the head and neck. (See Uses: Head and Neck Cancer, in Docetaxel 10:00.)

In males younger than 50 years of age with metastatic squamous neck cancer who have a poorly differentiated tumor, an occult primary tumor, and elevated β-human chorionic gonadotropin (β-hCG) and α-fetoprotein (AFP), chemotherapy with a platinum-containing regimen should be considered because these tumors may respond to such therapy in a manner similar to extragonadal germ cell malignancies.

■ Cervical Cancer

Cisplatin is used, alone or in combination therapy, concurrently with radiation therapy for the treatment of invasive cervical cancer† (FIGO stages IB2 through IVA cervical cancer or FIGO stage IA2, IB, or IIA cervical cancer with poor prognostic factors, such as metastatic disease in pelvic lymph nodes, parametrial disease, or positive surgical margins, identified at the time of primary surgery). Cisplatin also is used in the treatment of metastatic or recurrent cervical cancer†.

Overview About 13,000–16,000 new cases of invasive cervical cancer and 5,000 deaths from this disease occur in the US each year. The most common histologic types of cervical cancer are squamous cell carcinoma (approximately 80–90%) and adenocarcinoma (approximately 10–20%); adenosquamous carcinoma and small cell carcinoma of the cervix occur less frequently, and other types of cancers of the cervix are relatively rare. The principal risk factor for the development of preinvasive cervical lesions or invasive cervical cancer is infection with certain subtypes of human papilloma virus (HPV).

Procedures routinely used to determine the clinical stage of cervical cancer include physical examination, radiologic studies, and cervical biopsy; although they are not included in the process of clinical staging, imaging procedures, such as computed tomography (CT) or magnetic resonance imaging (MRI), and/or lymphangiography with fine-needle aspiration may be used to establish the extent of invasive disease. HIV testing should be considered, particularly in younger (less than 50 years of age), at-risk patients diagnosed with invasive cervical cancer, because of the higher prevalence of HIV infection, often asymptomatic, in these women compared with women in the general population. Prognostic factors for cervical cancer include the stage of disease, the volume and grade of tumor, histologic type, spread of disease to pelvic or para-aortic lymph nodes, and vascular invasion. Controversy exists regarding whether adenocarcinoma of the cervix carries a worse prognosis than squamous cell carcinoma of the cervix, and most treatment recommendations for cervical cancer are based on experience in patients with squamous cell carcinoma. The clinical staging system established by the Federation Internationale de Gynecologie et d'Obstetrique (FIGO) is commonly used to classify cervical cancer.

The earliest stage of invasive cervical cancer (FIGO stage IA1) may be treated surgically. Other early-stage, small-volume cervical cancer (FIGO stage IA2, IB1, or IIA) may be treated initially with surgery or radiation therapy. According to the findings from randomized trials, strong consideration should be given to the concurrent administration of cisplatin-based chemotherapy to prolong overall survival and progression-free survival in women who require postoperative radiation therapy for the treatment of stage IA2, IB1, or IIA cervical cancer with poor prognostic factors identified at the time of primary surgery or in women who require primary radiation therapy for the treatment of stage IB1 or IIA cervical cancer with poor prognostic factors.

For the initial treatment of early stages of cervical cancer, surgery is preferred for younger women who have concerns about preservation of the ovaries and avoidance of vaginal atrophy and stenosis; radiation therapy is advisable in women who have bulky disease, women who have disease with poor prognostic factors (e.g., metastasis to pelvic lymph nodes), or women who are not suitable candidates for surgery. Although randomized controlled studies are needed, some evidence suggests that survival may be prolonged in patients receiving primary treatment with surgery rather than radiation therapy for early stages of adenocarcinoma of the cervix. Patients initially treated with surgery may require postoperative radiation therapy to reduce the risk of local recurrence if tumor is present in the margins of the surgical specimen or has metastasized to pelvic or para-aortic lymph nodes. Because the combination of radical surgery and adjuvant radiation therapy increases both morbidity and the cost of treatment, careful staging and identification of prognostic factors are important in the selection of the optimal mode of initial treatment.

Although controversy exists regarding the optimal treatment of stage IB2 cervical cancer, many experts prefer the use of primary radiation therapy. Initial treatment with radiation therapy generally is recommended in women with stages IIB through IVA cervical cancer. According to the findings from randomized trials, strong consideration should be given to the concurrent administration of cisplatin-based chemotherapy to prolong overall survival and progression-free survival in women receiving primary radiation therapy for the treatment of stage IB2 or stages IIB through IVA cervical cancer. Results of randomized trials and pooled data from randomized trials did *not* demonstrate prolonged survival or improved local control of disease with use of neoadjuvant chemotherapy followed by radiation therapy in locally advanced cervical cancer; evidence from at least 2 randomized trials suggests that use of neoadjuvant chemotherapy may adversely affect survival in patients receiving radiation therapy for locally advanced cervical cancer.

Palliative treatment with radiation and/or chemotherapy has been used in patients with metastatic or recurrent cervical cancer. The benefit of chemotherapy and/or radiation therapy versus best supportive care has not been established in patients with advanced cervical cancer.

FIGO Stage IA1 Cervical Cancer. Chemotherapy currently is not usually recommended for FIGO stage IA1 cervical cancer. Instead, simple hysterectomy or cone biopsy are initial treatments of choice. The use of conservative surgical management of adenocarcinoma in situ of the uterine cervix with conization has not been established. Radiation therapy alone (intracavitary insertion only) may be used to treat stage IA1 disease in women who are not suitable candidates for surgery.

FIGO Stage IA2 Cervical Cancer. In patients with FIGO stage IA2 cervical cancer, surgery or pelvic radiation therapy is the initial treatment of choice. Concurrent cisplatin-based chemotherapy may be strongly considered for certain women with this stage of the cancer.

Primary surgical treatment for FIGO stage IA2 cervical cancer generally consists of radical hysterectomy with pelvic lymph node dissection. The use of conservative surgical management with cone biopsy alone is not established as an appropriate treatment option for stage IA2 cervical cancer. Postoperative radiation therapy is required in women with stage IA2 cervical cancer with poor prognostic factors (i.e., metastatic disease in pelvic lymph nodes, parametrial disease, positive surgical margins) identified at the time of primary surgery. According to the findings from randomized trials, strong consideration should be given to the concurrent administration of cisplatin-based chemotherapy in women who require postoperative radiation therapy for the treatment of stage IA2 cervical cancer with poor prognostic factors.

Primary radiation therapy for FIGO stage IA2 cervical cancer consists of intracavitary brachytherapy with or without external-beam radiation therapy.

FIGO Stage IB1 or IIA Cervical Cancer. In patients with FIGO stage IB1 or IIA cervical cancer, the use of surgery or pelvic radiation therapy as initial treatment appears to produce equivalent results. Concurrent cisplatin-based chemotherapy may be strongly considered for certain women with this stage of the cancer.

Primary surgical treatment for FIGO stage IB1 or IIA cervical cancer generally consists of radical hysterectomy with pelvic lymph node dissection (with or without para-aortic lymph node dissection); depending on the extent of vaginal involvement in patients with stage IIA disease, a more extensive upper vaginectomy also is performed. Postoperative radiation therapy is required in women with stage IB1 or IIA cervical cancer with poor prognostic factors (i.e., metastatic disease in pelvic or para-aortic lymph nodes, parametrial disease, or positive surgical margins) identified at the time of primary surgery. According to the findings from randomized trials, strong consideration should be given to the concurrent administration of cisplatin-based chemotherapy in women who require postoperative radiation therapy for the treatment of stage IB1 or IIA cervical cancer with poor prognostic factors.

Primary radiation therapy for stage IB1 or IIA cervical cancer consists of a combination of external-beam radiation and intracavitary implants. Some evidence suggests that the use of prophylactic radiation of the para-aortic nodes may prolong overall survival in patients receiving pelvic radiation therapy for bulky stage IIA cervical cancer. According to the findings from randomized trials, strong consideration should be given to the concurrent administration of cisplatin-based chemotherapy in women who require primary radiation therapy for the treatment of stage IB1 or IIA cervical cancer with poor prognostic factors.

FIGO Stage IB2 Cervical Cancer. The treatment of stage IB2 cervical cancer is controversial, and numerous methods have been used including surgery alone, radiation therapy alone, surgery with adjuvant radiation therapy, radiation therapy with adjuvant surgery, and neoadjuvant chemotherapy and surgery.

Many experts currently prefer initial treatment with pelvic radiation therapy consisting of a combination of external-beam radiation and intracavitary implants for bulky stage IB cervical tumors. According to the findings from randomized trials, strong consideration should be given to the concurrent administration of cisplatin-based chemotherapy in women receiving primary radiation therapy for the treatment of stage IB2 cervical cancer. Some evidence suggests that the use of prophylactic radiation of the para-aortic nodes may prolong overall survival in patients receiving pelvic radiation therapy for stage IB2 cervical cancer. Although it does not improve survival and many experts discourage its routine practice, extrafascial hysterectomy has been performed following primary radiation therapy for stage IB2 cervical tumors to reduce the risk of recurrence of central pelvic disease. In a randomized controlled trial, the addition of neoadjuvant chemotherapy did not improve control of local disease or prolong disease-free survival in patients receiving radiation therapy for invasive cervical cancer, including those with bulky stage IB tumors.

Primary surgery for bulky stage IB cervical cancer consists of radical hysterectomy with pelvic node and para-aortic lymph node dissection. The addition of adjuvant radiation therapy to primary surgery increases morbidity in patients with stage IB cervical cancer, including those with bulky tumors, and routine use of this combination is not advised in such patients. Long-term follow-up from a randomized controlled trial involving patients with stage IB squamous carcinoma of the cervix suggests that the addition of neoadjuvant cisplatin-containing chemotherapy reduces tumor volume, improves tumor operability, and consequently prolongs survival and disease-free survival in patients receiving surgery and adjuvant pelvic radiation therapy for bulky tumors.

FIGO Stages IIB–IVA Cervical Cancer. Because of high rates of local relapse, extensive locoregional disease (FIGO stages IIB through IVA) generally is treated with pelvic radiation therapy consisting of external-beam radiation therapy and brachytherapy. According to the findings from randomized trials, strong consideration should be given to the concurrent administration of cisplatin-based chemotherapy in women receiving radiation therapy for the treatment of stages IIB through IVA cervical cancer. Some evidence suggests that the use of prophylactic radiation of the para-aortic nodes may prolong overall survival in patients receiving pelvic radiation therapy for stage IIB cervical cancer.

FIGO Stage IVB Cervical Cancer. Patients with distant metastases (FIGO stage IVB) may receive chemotherapy for control of systemic disease; such patients also may benefit from palliative treatment with radiation therapy for symptoms from pelvic disease and/or distant metastases. The benefit of chemotherapy and/or radiation therapy versus best supportive care has not been established in patients with metastatic cervical cancer.

Recurrent Cervical Cancer. Depending on the initial treatment of cervical cancer, local recurrence of disease is treated with the treatment modality the patient did not previously receive. Radiation therapy can prolong survival and improve local control of disease in patients with locally recurrent cervical cancer following hysterectomy. In patients with local recurrence of disease following primary radiation therapy for cervical cancer, the overall survival rate following pelvic exenteration is 30–60%.

Most patients with recurrent cervical cancer have disease at local and distant sites. Palliative treatment with chemotherapy may be considered in patients with recurrent cervical cancer, but responses to treatment typically are short-lived. Radiation therapy may be useful in the palliation of symptoms in such patients, although many patients are symptomatic from recurrence of disease in a previously irradiated field where additional radiation may be contraindicated. The benefit of palliative chemotherapy versus best supportive care has not been established in patients with recurrent cervical cancer.

Treatment of Cervical Cancer during Pregnancy. Treatment for preinvasive cervical lesions (i.e., CIN 2, CIN 3, cervical carcinoma in situ) in pregnant women may be delayed and followed up with reevaluation in the postpartum period, but expert colposcopy and cervical biopsy should be performed promptly to confirm the absence of invasive disease. Diagnostic cone biopsy should be performed when microinvasive or invasive cervical carcinoma is suspected; cone biopsy is associated with substantial morbidity, such as excessive blood loss and increased risk of miscarriage, in pregnant women.

Most patients with cervical cancer during pregnancy are diagnosed with early-stage disease. The prognosis of early-stage cervical cancer appears to be similar in pregnant and nonpregnant women receiving standard treatment. Although surgery and radiation therapy are equally effective for the treatment of early-stage cervical cancer, surgical treatment is preferred in pregnant women because it allows preservation of ovarian and sexual function in this younger patient population.

The choice and timing of treatment of invasive cervical cancer during pregnancy depend on the stage of disease, duration of the pregnancy (i.e., gestational age of the fetus) at the time of diagnosis, risk to the mother and the fetus, and the wishes of the patient. The treatment of invasive cervical cancer diagnosed before fetal maturity (less than 20 weeks' gestation) is controversial; although many experts traditionally have recommended immediate treatment (according to stage of disease) with loss of the pregnancy, some clinicians support longer delays in treatment for patients with early-stage, nonbulky cervical tumors who desire completion of the pregnancy. If invasive cervical cancer is detected later in pregnancy when the fetus is viable (generally at greater than 20 weeks' gestation), planned delay of treatment is offered to appropriate candidates (according to stage and extent of disease, histology, and lesion size) who are placed under close surveillance for progression of disease, and delivery of the fetus by cesarean section is followed by surgery or radiation therapy for invasive cervical cancer according to the stage of disease. Most experts agree that planned delay of treatment to improve fetal viability is a reasonable option in women with early-stage cervical cancer (FIGO stage IA or IB1) detected in the third trimester or late second trimester of pregnancy.

Treatment of Cervical Cancer in HIV-infected Women. The prevalence of cervical squamous intraepithelial lesions and HPV infection with oncogenic genotypes is high among women with human immunodeficiency virus (HIV) infection, and the US Centers for Disease Control and Prevention (CDC) has designated invasive cervical cancer in HIV-positive women as an acquired immunodeficiency syndrome (AIDS)-defining illness. Some evidence suggests that antiretroviral therapy (triple-drug therapy including an HIV protease inhibitor) may reduce the prevalence and/or lower the grade of cervical lesions in HIV-infected women despite the persistence of HPV infection. Women with HIV infection who are diagnosed with invasive cervical cancer often have more aggressive and advanced disease with a poorer prognosis. The same standard treatment for preinvasive cervical lesions or invasive cervical cancer used in non-HIV-infected women generally is recommended in HIV-infected women, but response to treatment may be poor; close surveillance is required, and repetitive treatment of cervical intraepithelial neoplasia (CIN) may be necessary in HIV-infected women to prevent progression of disease. Evidence from a phase III, nonblinded, randomized trial indicates that the recurrence rate of CIN is reduced and time to recurrence is prolonged in women with HIV infection receiving adjunctive therapy with vaginal fluorouracil† versus observation only following excisional or ablative treatment of high-grade cervical dysplasia (i.e., CIN 2 or 3).

Concurrent Chemotherapy and Radiation Therapy for Invasive Cervical Cancer Results from 3 large randomized, controlled, phase III trials at 3 years or more of follow-up show that the addition of cisplatin-based chemotherapy given concurrently with radiation therapy decreases the risk of death by 40–50% in women receiving primary radiation therapy for FIGO stages IB2 through IVA cervical cancer and in women receiving postoperative radiation therapy for FIGO stage IA2, IB, or IIA cervical cancer with poor prognostic factors (i.e., metastatic disease in pelvic lymph nodes, parametrial disease, positive surgical margins) identified at the time of primary surgery. Results from 2 other large randomized trials show that in patients receiving concomitant chemotherapy and radiation therapy for FIGO stages IIB through IVA cervical cancer, risk of death is decreased by about 30–40% among those receiving cisplatin-containing versus non-cisplatin-containing chemotherapeutic regimens.

Because of the findings from these randomized trials, NCI recommends that strong consideration be given to the concurrent administration of cisplatin-based chemotherapy in women who require radiation therapy for the treatment of cervical cancer. Substitution of carboplatin for cisplatin is not recommended because of the lack of evidence supporting comparable efficacy of this agent for cervical cancer. Further study is needed to establish the magnitude of benefit when chemotherapy is given concurrently with optimal-dose radiation therapy in patients with locally advanced cervical cancer.

Clinical Trials. In addition to its cytotoxic effects, chemotherapy is believed to have a synergistic antineoplastic effect with radiation therapy by mechanisms that include increased sensitivity of tumor to radiation and inhibition of the repair of sublethal damage to tumor induced by radiation. The current recommendation for concurrent cisplatin-containing chemotherapy and radiation therapy in women with invasive cervical cancer (FIGO stage IB2 through IVA disease or FIGO stage IA2, IB, or IIA disease with poor prognostic factors) is based principally on the findings from 5 large, randomized trials (3 randomized trials showing prolonged survival with the concurrent use of chemotherapy and radiation therapy versus radiation therapy alone and 2 randomized trials showing the superiority of cisplatin-containing regimens versus non-cisplatin-containing regimens for concurrent use with radiation therapy).

In a randomized trial of 403 patients (386 evaluable patients) with advanced squamous cell carcinoma, adenocarcinoma, or adenosquamous carcinoma of the cervix confined to the pelvis (FIGO stages IIB through IVA or FIGO stage IB or IIA with a tumor diameter of at least 5 cm or involvement of the pelvic lymph nodes), the estimated overall rate of survival at 5 years (calculated at a median follow-up of 43 months) was higher (73 versus 58%) among those receiving concurrent chemotherapy (with cisplatin and fluorouracil) and pelvic radiation therapy than among those receiving radiation therapy alone (consisting of pelvic radiation therapy and irradiation of the para-aortic lymph nodes). The estimated rate of disease-free survival at 5 years was 67% among patients who received combined therapy with chemotherapy and radiation and 40% among those who received radiation therapy alone. According to stage of disease, overall survival was prolonged with the addition of chemotherapy to radiation therapy in patients with FIGO stage IB, IIA, or IIB cervical cancer but not in patients with stage III or IVA disease; however, the study was not designed to test for differences in survival within these subgroups. The rates of distant or locoregional metastases were lower among patients receiving combined modality treatment (14 versus 33% and 19 versus 35%, respectively); a higher rate of reversible adverse hematologic effects was observed in patients receiving combined chemotherapy and radiation therapy, but the severity of late adverse effects was similar between the groups.

In a randomized trial of 374 patients (369 evaluable patients) with bulky or barrel-shaped stage IB (i.e., FIGO stage IB2) squamous cell carcinoma, adenocarcinoma, or adenosquamous carcinoma of the cervix, higher rates of overall survival (83 versus 74% at 3 years) and progression-free survival were observed at 4 years in those receiving concurrent chemotherapy (with cisplatin) and radiation therapy with adjuvant hysterectomy than in those receiving radiation therapy with adjuvant hysterectomy. The relative risks of progression of disease and death among women receiving combined chemotherapy and radiation therapy were 0.51 and 0.54, respectively, compared with those receiving radiation therapy alone. Higher frequencies of adverse hematologic effects (21 versus 2%) and adverse GI effects (14 versus 5%) were observed in patients receiving combined chemotherapy and radiation therapy than in those receiving radiation therapy alone.

At a median follow-up of 42 months in a randomized trial of 268 patients (243 evaluable patients) with clinical stage IA2, IB, or IIA cervical cancer initially treated with radical hysterectomy and pelvic node dissection, higher rates of overall survival (estimated 4-year survival of 81 versus 71%) and progression-free survival (estimated 4-year progression-free survival of 80 versus 63%) were observed in those receiving concurrent chemotherapy (with cisplatin and fluorouracil) and pelvic radiation therapy versus pelvic radiation therapy alone for high risk factors, such as positive pelvic lymph nodes, positive surgical margins, and/or microscopic involvement of the parametrium, identified at the time of primary surgery.

Optimal chemotherapy regimens for the treatment of invasive cervical cancer have not been established. Current evidence from large, randomized, phase III trials indicates that cisplatin is a drug of choice for chemotherapy to be used concomitantly with radiation therapy for locally advanced cervical cancer. Cisplatin may be used alone or in combination therapy (e.g., cisplatin and fluorouracil) as an adjunct to radiation therapy in patients with locally advanced cervical cancer; however, results from at least one randomized trial suggest that cisplatin alone is as effective but less toxic than cisplatin-containing combination regimens for concomitant use with radiation therapy. Improvement in survival with the combination of chemotherapy and radiation therapy in patients with locally advanced cervical cancer has been observed only with *concurrent* administration of chemotherapy. Analysis of pooled data from several randomized trials did *not* demonstrate prolonged survival or improved local control of disease with use of neoadjuvant chemotherapy followed by radiation therapy in locally advanced cervical cancer.

In a randomized trial of 575 patients (526 evaluable patients) receiving concurrent chemotherapy and radiation therapy for stage IIB, III, or IVA squamous cell carcinoma, adenocarcinoma, or adenosquamous carcinoma of the cervix without involvement of the para-aortic lymph nodes, follow-up at a median duration of 35 months showed higher rates of survival and progression-free survival among those receiving cisplatin alone or a combination regimen of cisplatin, fluorouracil, and hydroxyurea than among those receiving hydroxyurea alone. The rates of progression-free survival at 24 months were 67, 64, and 47% in patients receiving radiation therapy and concomitant chemotherapy with cisplatin alone; cisplatin, fluorouracil, and hydroxyurea; and hydroxyurea alone, respectively. Relative risk of death was 0.61 or 0.58 in those receiving cisplatin alone or combination therapy with cisplatin, fluorouracil, and hydroxyurea, respectively, compared with those receiving hydroxyurea alone. The rate of local recurrences was lower in patients receiving radiation therapy with cisplatin or cisplatin-containing combination therapy (19 and 20%, respectively) than in those receiving radiation therapy with hydroxyurea alone (30%); the rate of distant metastases (i.e., lung metastases) also was lower in patients receiving radiation therapy with cisplatin alone or radiation therapy with cisplatin in combination chemotherapy (3 and 4%, respectively) than in those receiving radiation therapy with hydroxyurea alone (10%). Compared with patients receiving either cisplatin or hydroxyurea alone, the frequency of moderate or severe leukopenia was more than double and the frequency of moderate or severe granulocytopenia was approximately double in patients receiving the 3-drug regimen (cisplatin, fluorouracil, and hydroxyurea).

In a randomized trial of 388 patients (368 evaluable patients) receiving concomitant chemotherapy and radiation therapy for FIGO stage IIB, III, or IVA squamous cell carcinoma, adenocarcinoma, or adenosquamous carcinoma of the cervix without involvement of the para-aortic lymph nodes, follow-up at a median duration of 8.7 years showed higher rates of survival (55 versus 43%) and progression-free survival in those receiving cisplatin and fluorouracil than in those receiving hydroxyurea alone. Relative risk of progression of disease or death was 0.79 and relative risk of death was 0.74 in those receiving cisplatin and fluorouracil compared with those receiving hydroxyurea. Severe (grade 3) or life-threatening (grade 4) leukopenia occurred less frequently in patients receiving combination therapy with cisplatin and fluorouracil (4%) than in those receiving hydroxyurea alone (24%).

The results of these randomized trials suggest that agents other than hydroxyurea, particularly cisplatin (alone or in combination with other agents), are preferred for concurrent use with radiation therapy in the treatment of locally advanced cervical cancer. Fluorouracil is used in combination with cisplatin for concurrent chemotherapy and radiation therapy in patients with locally advanced cervical cancer, but randomized controlled studies are needed to determine if this combination regimen is superior to cisplatin alone. Although carboplatin often is used as a less toxic substitute for cisplatin, current evidence supports the use of cisplatin-containing chemotherapy given concurrently with radiation therapy in patients with locally advanced cervical cancer, and similar benefit with carboplatin-containing chemotherapy cannot be assumed. Additional comparative studies are needed to determine the optimal chemotherapy regimens and schedules to be used concurrently with radiation therapy for the treatment of locally advanced cervical cancer.

Chemotherapy for Metastatic or Recurrent Cervical Cancer Cisplatin is used in the palliative treatment of metastatic or recurrent squamous cell carcinoma of the cervix†. The drug is considered one of the most active agents in the treatment of cervical neoplasms. Response rates of 18–31% have been reported with use of cisplatin as a single agent in advanced cervical cancer.

Cisplatin also has been used as a component of various combination chemotherapeutic regimens (e.g., bleomycin, cisplatin and ifosfamide [BIP]; bleomycin, cisplatin, mitomycin, and vincristine [BOMP]) for the treatment of metastatic or recurrent cervical cancer. Limited evidence from a small randomized trial of patients with advanced cervical cancer suggests that cisplatin-based chemotherapy is superior to hydroxyurea, which has minimal activity as a single agent in the treatment of metastatic or recurrent cervical cancer. Combination regimens have not been consistently shown to be superior to the use of single agents, such as cisplatin, one of the most active drugs in the treatment of metastatic or recurrent cervical cancer. Although relatively high response rates have been reported with cisplatin-containing combination chemotherapy regimens, these regimens generally are more toxic and do not appear to be superior to cisplatin alone in the treatment of metastatic or recurrent cervical cancer. For example, high objective response rates have been observed with the combination regimen of bleomycin, ifosfamide, and cisplatin in women with metastatic or recurrent cervical cancer, but toxicity is greater and survival is not improved in women receiving the combination regimen rather than cisplatin alone. Similarly, higher response rates and prolonged progression-free survival but greater toxicity and no difference in overall survival has been observed with use of the combination of cisplatin and ifosfamide (with mesna) compared with cisplatin alone in patients with metastatic or recurrent squamous cell carcinoma of the cervix.

Because of its lesser toxicity, carboplatin may be considered as an alternative to the parent compound cisplatin, particularly in patients with nephrotoxicity or neurotoxicity caused by advanced cervical tumor who are not suitable candidates for cisplatin therapy; however, randomized controlled trials comparing carboplatin and cisplatin have not been performed to date, and because of superior response rates and lesser hematologic toxicity, most experts consider cisplatin the current drug of choice in the treatment of advanced cervical cancer, particularly in patients who have received radiation therapy.

Various single agents and combination regimens for the treatment of advanced cervical cancer have been evaluated mostly in phase II studies, and optimal treatment has not been established. In addition, the benefit of chemotherapy versus best supportive care has not been studied in patients with metastatic or recurrent cervical cancer. Because the prognosis of patients with advanced cervical cancer remains poor and optimal therapy has not been established, all such patients may be considered for enrollment in clinical trials investigating new agents or combination regimens. The use of cisplatin with other agents (e.g., paclitaxel, gemcitabine, fluorouracil, vinorelbine) or in other combination regimens (e.g., cisplatin, methotrexate, vinblastine, and doxorubicin [MVAC]) is being evaluated in patients with metastatic or recurrent cervical cancer.

■ **Non-small Cell Lung Cancer** ***Overview*** Cisplatin is used as a component of various chemotherapeutic regimens for advanced non-small cell lung cancer†. Non-small cell lung cancer, which includes squamous cell carcinoma, adenocarcinoma, and large cell carcinoma, accounts for approximately 80% of all lung cancers; the prognosis for this neoplasm is poor with a 5-year survival of less than 10% in patients with advanced disease.

Cisplatin-containing chemotherapy is used for the treatment of advanced non-small cell lung cancer. A small survival benefit has been demonstrated for the use of platinum-based (cisplatin) chemotherapy alone or combined with radiation therapy in selected patients with unresectable, locally advanced or metastatic non-small cell lung cancer who have a good performance status. Analysis of pooled data from individual patients enrolled in published and unpublished randomized trials or from published randomized trials indicates a 13% reduction in risk of death and an absolute increase in survival rate of 4% at 2 years for cisplatin-based chemotherapy combined with radiation therapy compared with radiation therapy alone in the treatment of unresectable, locally advanced non-small cell lung cancer. The optimal timing of chemotherapy used in conjunction with radiation therapy (sequential, concurrent, or alternating) has not been established. Analysis of pooled data from individual patients enrolled in published and unpublished randomized trials indicates that the addition of cisplatin-containing chemotherapy to supportive care in patients with advanced non-small cell lung cancer provides a small survival advantage (i.e., absolute increase in survival rate of approximately 10% at 1 year or increased median survival of about 1.5 months). Results from two small randomized trials suggest that the administration of cisplatin-containing chemotherapy preceding surgery prolongs survival in patients with resectable, locally advanced non-small cell lung cancer although further study is needed to confirm these findings.

Because many patients with earlier stages of disease treatable with surgical resection subsequently develop metastases, the use of adjuvant chemotherapy and/or radiotherapy is being investigated. Current evidence does not show improvement in survival with radiation therapy and/or chemotherapy administered following surgery in patients with resectable non-small cell lung cancer. Although limited by the inclusion of mostly studies involving now-obsolete equipment, analysis of pooled data from individual patients enrolled in published and unpublished randomized trials indicates that postoperative treatment with conventional radiation therapy reduces local recurrence of disease but adversely affects survival in patients with completely resected stage I and II non-small cell lung cancer. The effect of postoperative radiation therapy in patients with later stages of non-small cell lung cancer (e.g., stage IIIA with N2) has not been established. Differing regimens of radiation therapy (e.g., accelerated versus conventional radiation therapy) also are being investigated.

Combination Chemotherapy for Advanced Non-small Cell Lung Cancer Platinum-based chemotherapy regimens currently are preferred for the treatment of non-small cell lung cancer. A detrimental effect on survival has been observed for patients with non-small cell lung cancer receiving treatment based on alkylating agents, such as busulfan and cyclophosphamide, and such regimens are *not* recommended. Currently preferred regimens for the treatment of advanced non-small cell lung cancer include the combination of cisplatin with another agent, such as paclitaxel, vinorelbine, gemcitabine, or docetaxel.

In randomized trials, patients with advanced non-small cell lung cancer receiving cisplatin combined with paclitaxel or gemcitabine had higher response rates and similar median survival compared with those receiving combination therapy with cisplatin and etoposide; consequently, paclitaxel-containing regimens or other platinum-based regimens currently are preferred in the treatment of patients with advanced non-small cell lung cancer. (See Uses: Non-small Cell Lung Carcinoma in Paclitaxel 10:00 or Gemcitabine 10:00.) Cisplatin combined with gemcitabine is associated with improved survival (estimated median survival of 9.1 versus 7.6 months) and higher response rates (30 versus 11%) compared with cisplatin alone in patients with advanced non-small cell lung cancer. Patients with stage IIIB or IV non-small cell lung carcinoma receiving cisplatin and vinorelbine had a longer median survival, higher survival rate at 1 year, a longer median progression-free survival, and higher response rate than those receiving cisplatin alone. (See Uses: Non-small Cell Lung Carcinoma in Vinorelbine 10:00.)

Use of chemotherapy for the treatment of advanced non-small cell lung cancer generally is advised only in patients with good performance status (ECOG performance status of 0 or 1, and 2 in selected patients) and evaluable lesions so that treatment can be discontinued if the disease does not respond. The decision to use chemotherapy must be individualized according to several factors, including patient preference, toxicity, survival benefit, quality of life, and cost of treatment. Once the decision is made to use chemotherapy, treatment should begin promptly to allow for optimal response in patients receiving chemotherapy combined with radiation therapy for unresectable stage III disease and to allow treatment before deterioration of performance status in patients with stage IV disease. Although the optimal duration of chemotherapy has not been fully established, treatment with 2–8 cycles generally is advised in patients with stage IV or unresectable stage III non-small cell lung cancer; periodic imaging studies are used to monitor response and determine whether to continue treatment.

Cisplatin, an active agent in the treatment of non-small cell lung carcinoma, produces an objective response in about 10–20% of patients, No single chemotherapy regimen currently can be recommended as superior in the treatment of non-small cell lung cancer. Analysis of pooled data from published randomized trials involving patients with advanced non-small cell lung cancer indicates higher response rates and a small increase in survival rates at 6 months and 1 year but greater toxicity in patients receiving combination chemotherapy versus single-agent chemotherapy. A large randomized trial showed a higher response rate but no difference in median survival in patients receiving combination therapy with cisplatin and paclitaxel for advanced non-small cell lung cancer compared with those receiving high-dose cisplatin alone.

Various chemotherapy regimens used alone or in combination with other treatment modalities, such as radiation therapy, are continually being evaluated for the treatment of advanced non-small cell lung cancer. Because current treatment is not satisfactory for almost all patients with non-small cell lung cancer except selected patients with early-stage, resectable disease, all patients may be considered for enrollment in clinical trials at the time of diagnosis.

■ **Small Cell Lung Cancer** Cisplatin is used in combination chemotherapy for the treatment of small cell lung cancer†. Combination chemotherapy regimens are superior to single-agent therapy for the treatment of small cell lung cancer and moderately intensive drug doses are superior to doses that produce minimal toxicity. Various regimens have been used in combination therapy, and many 2- to 4-drug combination regimens, including cisplatin-containing regimens, have produced response rates of 65–90 or 70–85% and complete response rates of 45–75 or 20–30% in patients with limited-stage or extensive-stage disease, respectively; however, comparative efficacy is continually being evaluated. While efficacy of the various available regimens is continually being evaluated, combination chemotherapy containing cisplatin and etoposide currently is considered a preferred regimen for the treatment of small cell lung carcinoma. Combination therapy with cisplatin and etoposide used in combined modality treatment with concurrent thoracic irradiation that is administered early in the course of treatment is a preferred regimen for limited-stage small cell lung cancer. Cisplatin in conjunction with etoposide also is used in the treatment of extensive-stage small cell lung cancer.

In a randomized study, patients with previously untreated extensive-stage small cell lung cancer receiving combination therapy with cisplatin and etoposide (PE); cyclophosphamide, doxorubicin, and vincristine (CAV); or an alternation of these regimens (PE/CAV) had similar objective response rates, complete response rates, and median survival; because of a higher frequency of severe thrombocytopenia associated with the alternation of regimens, therapy with PE/CAV generally is not recommended. Cisplatin in combination with etoposide and ifosfamide with mesna is used as an alternative regimen for the treatment of small cell lung cancer. Second-line therapy with combination regimens (e.g., cisplatin and etoposide) or single agents (e.g., paclitaxel, topotecan) may be of some value for the treatment of small cell lung cancer refractory to other chemotherapy regimens (particularly when relapse occurs more than 6 months following completion of initial treatment).

Although optimum duration of chemotherapy has not been clearly defined, additional improvement in survival has not been observed when the duration of drug administration exceeds 3–6 or 6 months in patients with limited-stage or extensive-stage small cell lung cancer, respectively. Because the current prognosis for small cell lung carcinoma is unsatisfactory regardless of stage and despite considerable diagnostic and therapeutic advances, all patients with this cancer are candidates for inclusion in clinical trials at the time of diagnosis.

■ **Malignant Pleural Mesothelioma** Cisplatin is used in combination with pemetrexed for the treatment of malignant pleural mesothelioma in patients who are not eligible for surgery. (See Uses: Malignant Pleural Mesothelioma in Pemetrexed 10:00.)

Cisplatin alone or in combination with other agents (e.g., doxorubicin, mitomycin) is used in the palliative treatment of advanced malignant pleural mesothelioma†. Combination chemotherapy regimens are associated with greater toxicity and do not appear to prolong survival or improve control of symptoms in patients with unresectable malignant pleural mesothelioma.

■ **Esophageal Cancer** Cisplatin has been used alone and in combination therapy for the treatment of localized or advanced esophageal cancer†. Optimum therapy for esophageal cancer has not been established, and new therapies are continually being evaluated. Because the prognosis for most patients with esophageal cancer remains poor, all newly diagnosed patients should be considered for enrollment in clinical trials comparing various treatment modalities.

Localized Esophageal Cancer For the treatment of patients with localized esophageal cancer, combined modality treatment consisting of combination chemotherapy with cisplatin and fluorouracil and concurrent radiation therapy may be used prior to surgery (as neoadjuvant therapy) or as an alternative to surgery (i.e., in patients who are not considered suitable surgical candidates or in an attempt to avoid perioperative mortality [less than 10%] and to relieve dysphagia).

Combined modality therapy consisting of combination chemotherapy with cisplatin and fluorouracil and concurrent radiation therapy is more effective than radiation therapy alone in patients with localized esophageal carcinoma. Patients with locally advanced esophageal cancer (most patients had squamous cell carcinoma) who received combined modality therapy with cisplatin and fluorouracil and concurrent radiation therapy had longer survival (12.5 versus 8.9 months) and higher survival rates (38 versus 10% at 24 months) than patients who received radiation therapy alone. Cisplatin 75 mg/m^2 (up to a maximum dose of 150 mg) was administered IV on day 1 and fluorouracil 1 g/m^2 (up to a maximum dose of 8 g) was administered by 96-hour continuous IV infusion on days 1–4 every 4 weeks during concurrent radiation therapy and every 3 weeks following the completion of radiation therapy. At 5 years, 26% of patients who received combined modality therapy were alive compared with none of the patients who received radiation therapy alone. In patients with localized esophageal cancer, particularly squamous cell carcinoma, who are not considered suitable candidates for surgery, combined modality treatment with cisplatin and fluorouracil and concurrent radiation therapy may be used as an alternative therapy. Although the comparative benefit of combined chemotherapy and radiation versus surgery has not been established, some experts recommend combined modality treatment with combination chemotherapy (e.g., cisplatin and fluorouracil) and concurrent radiation therapy with or without surgery as primary treatment for localized, resectable esophageal cancer.

Because of high rates of distant metastasis or locoregional recurrence of disease in patients undergoing surgery for localized esophageal cancer, the addition of systemic therapy was proposed to provide early treatment of disseminated but undetected disease and to reduce the risk of recurrent locoregional disease. Neoadjuvant therapy may reduce tumor size and increase the chances of complete resection in patients with locally advanced esophageal cancer. Variable results have been observed in studies of induction therapy with cisplatin-based chemotherapy and concurrent radiation therapy followed by surgery in patients with squamous cancer or adenocarcinoma of the esophagus. In a large, randomized trial, surgery combined with preoperative and postoperative chemotherapy with cisplatin and fluorouracil did not improve survival compared with surgery alone in patients with localized, operable esophageal carcinoma. Combined modality treatment of esophageal cancer may be associated with substantial toxicity, and choice of therapy must be individualized. Histologic type also influences choice of therapy for esophageal carcinoma. Clinical trials for esophageal cancer have included mostly patients with squamous cell carcinomas, and surgical resection remains standard therapy for esophageal adenocarcinoma. Further study is needed to determine the role of neoadjuvant or adjuvant therapy in combination with surgery in the treatment of localized esophageal cancer.

Advanced Esophageal Cancer Combination therapy with cisplatin and fluorouracil is used for the palliative treatment of metastatic (local or distant) disease or recurrent or locally advanced disease that is not amenable to surgery or radiation therapy, and such combined therapy currently is considered a regimen of choice. Cisplatin also has been used alone in the palliative treatment of advanced esophageal cancer. Although higher response rates are achieved with cisplatin and fluorouracil than with cisplatin alone in patients with metastatic disease, no overall difference in survival has been observed. Combination therapy with cisplatin and other active agents for advanced esophageal cancer (e.g., paclitaxel) is being investigated.

■ **Biliary Tract Cancer** Cisplatin has been used in combination with gemcitabine for the treatment of unresectable locally advanced or metastatic biliary tract cancer† (intrahepatic or extrahepatic cholangiocarcinoma, gallbladder cancer, or ampullary cancer), including unresectable recurrent disease following surgical resection.

Experts state that, in patients with biliary tract adenocarcinoma (the most common type of biliary tract cancer), chemotherapy can be recommended in individuals with unresectable locally advanced or metastatic disease and in those with recurrent disease following surgical resection. Chemotherapy is recommended in such individuals with good performance status (ECOG performance status of 0 or 1). However, in patients with poor performance status (ECOG performance status of 2 or 3) or insufficient biliary decompression, the benefits of chemotherapy are limited and use of alternative therapy for palliation of associated symptoms (e.g., pain) and improvement in quality of life is recommended.

In a phase 3 trial in 410 patients with unresectable locally advanced or metastatic biliary tract carcinoma, including unresectable recurrent disease following surgical resection, patients who received cisplatin in combination with gemcitabine had longer median overall (11.7 versus 8.1 months) and progression-free (8 versus 5 months) survival, a higher 6-month progression-free survival rate (59.3 versus 42.5%), and higher rates of tumor control (complete or partial responses or stable disease) (81.4 versus 71.8%) compared with those who received gemcitabine alone. Only one patient in each treatment group achieved a complete response. Patients enrolled in the study generally had good baseline performance status (ECOG performance status of 0 or 1 in 88% of patients). Based on current evidence, combination therapy with cisplatin and gemcitabine is recommended (accepted) for use in the treatment of unresectable locally advanced or metastatic biliary tract cancer (intrahepatic or extrahepatic cholangiocarcinoma, gallbladder cancer, or ampullary cancer), including unresectable recurrent disease following surgical resection, in patients with good performance status (ECOG performance status of 0 or 1).

For further information on the treatment of unresectable locally advanced or metastatic biliary tract cancer, including use of combination therapy with cisplatin and gemcitabine, see Uses: Biliary Tract Cancer, in Gemcitabine 10:00.

■ **Melanoma** Cisplatin and other platinum analogs, such as carboplatin, have minimal activity but substantial toxicity in metastatic melanoma†. Although cisplatin has been used in combination therapy (e.g., carmustine, cisplatin, dacarbazine, and tamoxifen) for the palliative treatment of metastatic melanoma, evidence suggests that the addition of cisplatin to dacarbazine-containing regimens increases toxicity but does not improve survival. Evidence from large, randomized trials has not established the superiority of combination regimens compared with dacarbazine alone, and dacarbazine monotherapy currently is a systemic treatment of choice for metastatic melanoma (see Uses: Melanoma in Dacarbazine 10:00 for an overview of therapy for melanoma). The use of cisplatin-containing chemotherapy in combination with biologic therapy using aldesleukin and interferon alfa is being investigated for the treatment of metastatic melanoma.

Intra-arterial† infusions of cisplatin have been used in the treatment of regionally confined metastases from malignant melanoma. Cisplatin also has been used for hyperthermic isolated limb perfusion for recurrent melanoma of the extremity.

■ **Brain Tumors** Cisplatin has been used for the palliative treatment of various primary brain tumors†. Regimens that include cisplatin have been used principally in the treatment of medulloblastoma and germ cell tumors. Most primary brain tumors are treated with surgery and/or radiation therapy, but adjuvant chemotherapy may prolong survival in some tumor types and has increased disease-free survival in patients with medulloblastoma, certain germ cell tumors, and gliomas.

Malignant Gliomas **Astrocytic Tumors.** Cisplatin has been used as an adjunct for the treatment of astrocytic tumors†, such as anaplastic astrocytoma and glioblastoma multiforme. Although brief in duration, responses to high-dose IV cisplatin have been observed in patients with malignant glioma that recurred following previous chemotherapy with nitrosoureas. (For further discussion of the treatment of astrocytic tumors, see Uses: Brain Tumors in Carmustine 10:00.)

The use of cisplatin and carmustine as adjuvant and/or neoadjuvant therapy in conjunction with radiation therapy for the treatment of high-grade gliomas† is being investigated. In a large randomized trial, cisplatin and carmustine administered by continuous IV infusion prior to postoperative radiation therapy in patients with newly diagnosed glioblastoma multiforme did not increase survival and was associated with greater toxicity than standard adjuvant therapy consisting of IV carmustine administered concurrently with radiation therapy.

Medulloblastoma. Cisplatin is used in combination with lomustine and vincristine as adjuvant therapy following surgical resection and radiation therapy for the treatment of medulloblastoma†, the most common malignant childhood brain tumor. Such adjuvant chemotherapy is associated with improved progression-free survival in patients with poor prognostic factors (i.e., younger than 3 years of age, metastatic disease and/or subtotal resection with >1.5 cm^3 of residual disease and/or nonposterior fossa location), but the role of adjuvant chemotherapy in children with average-risk medulloblastoma has not been established.

The use of adjuvant chemotherapy coupled with reduced-dose radiation therapy in children with average-risk medulloblastoma (i.e., older than 3 years of age, total or near-total resection with <1.5 cm^3 of residual disease, no dissemination) is being investigated. Because of the debilitating effects of radiation on growth and neurologic development, the use of postoperative chemotherapy (e.g., induction therapy with cyclophosphamide and vincristine followed by cisplatin and etoposide, with or without bone marrow rescue) to delay, modify, or possibly avoid the need for radiation therapy in children younger than 3–6 years of age is being studied.

Cisplatin is an active agent in the treatment of recurrent medulloblastoma in children; response to chemotherapy is observed in more than 50% of patients with disease that recurs following treatment with surgery and radiation therapy, but long-term control of the disease is rare.

Oligodendroglioma. Cisplatin also has been used, alone or in combination with other agents (e.g., cisplatin and etoposide) as salvage therapy for recurrent oligodendroglioma†, a uniquely chemosensitive form of glioma.

Intracranial Germ Cell Tumors Combination therapy with a platinum-containing agent (i.e., cisplatin or carboplatin) and etoposide is used in the treatment of intracranial germ cell tumors†. Other combination chemotherapy regimens (e.g., cisplatin, vinblastine, bleomycin) also have been used. The role of adjuvant chemotherapy in addition to radiation therapy for the treatment of such tumors remains to be established.

Intra-arterial Therapy Intra-arterial† administration of cisplatin, alone or in combination with other agents, has been investigated in the treatment of newly diagnosed or recurrent gliomas; severe adverse effects, including renal, otologic, neurologic, and retinal toxicity, have been reported in patients receiving such therapy, and the role of intra-arterial cisplatin in the treatment of primary brain tumors has not been established.

■ **Neuroblastoma** Cisplatin is used as a component of combination therapy for high-risk neuroblastoma†. Combination chemotherapy with moderate doses of carboplatin, cyclophosphamide, doxorubicin, and etoposide is used in conjunction with surgery (with or without radiation therapy) for the treatment of neuroblastoma in patients with intermediate-risk tumors or, in some cases, low-risk tumors. Although surgery alone typically is adequate for the treatment of low-risk tumors, combination chemotherapy is administered if surgical resection is incomplete (less than 50% of the primary tumor is resected) or if life-threatening or organ-threatening symptomatic disease is present (e.g., spinal cord compression). In patients with high-risk tumors, aggressive chemotherapy using higher doses of these drugs and additional drugs (e.g., ifosfamide, high-dose cisplatin, vincristine) is used. If high-risk disease responds to the initial regimen of chemotherapy, further therapy consists of surgical resection of the primary tumor, myeloablative therapy and autologous stem cell transplantation (bone marrow transplantation or peripheral blood stem cell transplantation), and radiation therapy (radiation to the primary tumor site and sometimes total-body irradiation); following recovery, 6 months of therapy with oral 13-*cis*-retinoic acid (isotretinoin) is administered.

■ **Other Uses** Cisplatin is used in the treatment of adrenocortical cancer†, anal cancer†, GI carcinoid tumors†, choriocarcinoma†, endometrial cancer†, gastric cancer†, hepatoblastoma†, liver cancer†, certain types of non-Hodgkin's lymphoma†, osteosarcoma†, and soft-tissue sarcomas in adults†. Cisplatin also is used in the treatment of penile cancer†, malignant thymoma†, and anaplastic thyroid cancer†. Cisplatin has been used in the treatment of rhabdoid tumor of the kidney†, a highly malignant form of childhood kidney cancer. The drug also has shown some activity in the palliative treatment of advanced medullary thyroid cancer†.

Intra-arterial† infusions of cisplatin have been used with some success in the treatment of regionally confined malignancies, including osteogenic sarcomas. Cisplatin has also been administered intraperitoneally† alone or in conjunction with IV sodium thiosulfate in patients with various tumors (e.g., adenocarcinoma of the breast, carcinoid, mesothelioma) that were associated with malignant ascites and/or were confined to the peritoneal cavity. (See also Intraperitoneal Cisplatin and Paclitaxel under Ovarian Cancer: First-line Therapy for Advanced Ovarian Epithelial Cancer, in Uses.)

Dosage and Administration

■ **Reconstitution and Administration** Cisplatin is administered by IV infusion. The drug has also been administered intra-arterially† and intraperitoneally†. Needles, syringes, catheters, or IV administration sets that contain aluminum parts which may come in contact with cisplatin should *not* be used for preparation or administration of the drug. (See Chemistry and Stability: Stability.)

The manufacturer recommends that protective gloves be used during handling of commercially available cisplatin injection and during preparation of cisplatin solutions, since skin reactions associated with accidental exposure to the drug may occur. If cisplatin solution comes in contact with the skin or mucosa, the affected area should be washed with soap and water (skin) or flushed with water (mucosa) immediately and thoroughly. Rarely, adverse local effects have occurred following extravasation of cisplatin during administration. (See Cautions: Local Effects.)

Patients should be adequately hydrated before and for 24 hours after administration of cisplatin to ensure good urinary output and minimize nephrotoxicity. (See Cautions: Renal and Electrolyte Effects.) Various regimens of IV hydration, with or without mannitol and/or furosemide diuresis, and various rates of administration of cisplatin have been employed. The clinician should consult published protocols for information related to specific regimens. The manufacturer and many clinicians recommend IV infusion of 1–2 L of fluid over 8–12 hours prior to administration of the drug. In adults, unless contraindicated, IV fluids are usually administered alone or with mannitol and/or furosemide at an initial rate sufficient to maintain hydration and a diuresis of 150–400 mL/hour during and for at least 4–6 hours after administration of cisplatin, and then a diuresis of 100–200 mL or more per hour for the next 18–24 hours or until vomiting stops and oral fluids are tolerated. Patients must be closely monitored for fluid and serum electrolyte disturbances. (See Cautions: Renal and Electrolyte Effects.) Potassium chloride is often added (e.g., 10–20 mEq/L) to IV fluids infused during and/or following administration of cisplatin to replace losses and prevent deficiencies.

IV Infusion For IV infusion, the manufacturer recommends that the required dose of cisplatin (as the commercially available injection) be diluted in 2 L of 5% dextrose and 0.33 or 0.45% sodium chloride injection containing 18.75 g of mannitol per liter (i.e., 37.5 g in 2 L), and infused IV over 6–8 hours. Various other methods of dilution and/or rates of administration are used, and the clinician should consult published protocols for information related to specific regimens. IV infusions over 15 minutes to 2 hours are commonly employed and have been used with minimal adverse renal effects. Continuous 24-hour or 5-day IV infusions of the drug have also been used. While cisplatin has been administered by rapid IV injection (e.g., over 1–5 minutes), such rapid administration may be associated with increased nephrotoxicity or ototoxicity compared with slower IV infusion of the drug.

Intra-arterial Infusion For intra-arterial† infusion, cisplatin has been administered via an appropriately placed catheter using a controlled-infusion device. The cisplatin dose has generally been diluted in 0.9% sodium chloride injection (300 mL for doses less than 300 mg and 450 mL for doses greater than 300 mg) containing small amounts of heparin sodium (e.g., 3000 units) and infused over 2–4 hours (range 1–24 hours).

Intraperitoneal Instillation For intraperitoneal† administration in the Gynecologic Oncology Group (GOG)-172 study in patients with advanced epithelial ovarian cancer, the cisplatin dose was diluted in 2 L of 0.9% sodium chloride solution that was warmed to 37°C and administered as rapidly as possible through a surgically implanted peritoneal catheter. Following peritoneal infusion, patients were asked to roll into a different position every 15 minutes for the next 2 hours to disperse the drug throughout the peritoneal cavity. In this study, the paclitaxel dose was diluted in a liter of saline solution that was warmed to 37°C and infused through the intraperitoneal catheter, followed by intraperitoneal infusion of an additional liter of warmed saline solution. Some clinicians have recommended that intraperitoneal chemotherapeutic agents be mixed in 1 L of 0.9% sodium chloride solution warmed to 37°C and administered by gravity flow as rapidly as possible; after infusion and in the absence of pain, an additional 1 L of 0.9% sodium chloride solution may be administered to ensure adequate distribution within the peritoneal cavity.

Cisplatin also has been diluted in 2 L of lactated Ringer's injection and administered by gravity flow over 10–12 minutes; after a 15- to 20-minute dwell, the peritoneal cavity was drained as completely as possible. Alternatively, the cisplatin dose has been diluted in 500 mL of 0.9% sodium chloride solution and administered by gravity flow over 15–20 minutes; after 24 hours, paracentesis was begun. There is some evidence that the risk of systemic anaphylactoid reactions may be increased when doses of 100 mg/m^2 are administered relatively rapidly into the peritoneal cavity; therefore, some clinicians have recommended that intraperitoneal administration of such doses be over 45 minutes or longer.

Various implanted access ports and connecting catheters have been used for intraperitoneal administration of chemotherapeutic agents. The intraperitoneal catheter may be placed at the time of primary (cytoreductive) surgery as long as contamination of the peritoneal cavity has not occurred. Timing of placement of the intraperitoneal catheter (at the time of primary surgery versus delayed insertion) does not appear to affect tolerance of intraperitoneal therapy or treatment completion rates. The intraperitoneal catheter should be removed as soon as intraperitoneal therapy is completed to avoid catheter-related complications. Further study is needed to optimize techniques for intraperitoneal therapy to minimize the risk of complications (e.g., infection, catheter obstruction, catheter retraction, bowel perforation, pain, leakage, port access problems). Specialized sources should be consulted for guidance on how to administer intraperitoneal therapy.

Supportive therapy should include hydration and antiemetic therapy for the intraperitoneal infusion of cisplatin.

■ **Dosage** Dosage of cisplatin must be based on the clinical, renal, hematologic, and otic response and tolerance of the patient in order to obtain optimum therapeutic results with minimum adverse effects. The clinician should consult published protocols for the dosage of cisplatin and other chemotherapeutic agents and the method and sequence of administration. At the usual dosage, courses of cisplatin therapy should not be given more frequently than once every 3–4 weeks. *A repeat course of cisplatin should not be administered until the patient's renal, hematologic, and otic functions are within acceptable limits, and precautions must always be taken to treat an anaphylactoid reaction if it occurs.* (See Cautions: Precautions and Contraindications.)

Inadvertent substitution of cisplatin for carboplatin can result in potentially fatal overdosage. Therefore, care should be taken to ensure that such mix-ups do not occur. In addition, care should be taken to avoid prescribing practices by clinicians that fail to differentiate between daily doses of cisplatin and a total cisplatin dosage used in one course of therapy. To minimize the risk of overdosage, the manufacturer recommends that an alerting mechanism be instituted to verify any prescription or order for cisplatin doses exceeding 100 mg/m^2 per course. IV dosages exceeding 100 mg/m^2 per course once every 3–4 weeks are rarely used. Other safeguard procedures to minimize the risk of accidental overdosage of cisplatin (e.g., overdosage resulting from inadvertent administration of the drug when carboplatin was intended) also should be considered.

Because cisplatin is considered an antineoplastic agent of high emetic risk, antiemetic therapy for the prevention of acute and delayed emesis is recommended. (See Emetogenic Effects in Cautions: GI Effects.)

Testicular Cancer For remission induction in the treatment of metastatic testicular neoplasms, the usual dosage of cisplatin in combination chemotherapy regimens (e.g., with bleomycin and etoposide) is 20 mg/m^2 IV daily for 5 consecutive days every 3 weeks for 3 or 4 courses of therapy. Randomized trials indicate that 3 cycles of therapy are sufficient for favorable-prognosis germ cell tumors since similar results are achieved with either 3 or 4 cycles of therapy in such patients. Use of high-dose cisplatin in combination chemotherapy for poor-risk germ cell tumors results in increased toxicity without additional clinical benefit.

Ovarian Cancer For the treatment of advanced ovarian carcinoma, a cisplatin dosage of 75 mg/m^2 IV once every 3 weeks has been used in combination therapy with paclitaxel. The usual dosage of cisplatin when used in combination with cyclophosphamide is 50–100 mg/m^2 IV once every 3–4 weeks. In combination therapy, cisplatin and cyclophosphamide are administered sequentially. When cisplatin is used as a single agent, the manufacturer's recommended dosage is 100 mg/m^2 IV once every 4 weeks, but some experts recommend dosages of 50–100 mg/m^2 IV once every 3 weeks, and dosages of 30–120 mg/m^2 IV once every 3–4 weeks have been used.

Bladder Cancer For the treatment of advanced bladder cancer, the usual dosage of cisplatin is 50–70 mg/m^2 IV once every 3–4 weeks, depending on the extent of prior radiation therapy and/or chemotherapy. For patients who have been extensively pretreated, the recommended initial dosage is 50 mg/m^2 IV once every 4 weeks. For additional information, see Advanced Bladder Carcinoma: Dosage Considerations, under Uses: Bladder Cancer.

Head and Neck Cancer When used alone in the treatment of recurrent or advanced head and neck cancer†, cisplatin has been given in a dosage of 80–120 mg/m^2 IV once every 3 weeks or 50 mg/m^2 IV on the first and eighth days of every 4 weeks. In combination chemotherapy regimens, the usual dose of cisplatin has generally been 50–120 mg/m^2 IV, with the frequency of administration depending on the specific regimen employed. When used as induction chemotherapy in combination with docetaxel and fluorouracil, cisplatin 75–100 mg/m^2 has been administered IV once every 3 weeks. (See Head and Neck Cancer under Dosage and Administration: Dosage, in Docetaxel 10:00.)

Cervical Cancer **Invasive Cervical Cancer.** For the treatment of invasive cervical cancer† (FIGO stages IB2 through IVA or FIGO stages I through IIA with poor prognostic factors), cisplatin doses of 40–75 mg/m^2 have been given concurrently with radiation therapy. Weekly or daily infusions of cisplatin have been used concomitantly with radiation therapy in patients with invasive cervical cancer. When used alone for the treatment of invasive cervical cancer, cisplatin 40 mg/m^2 IV once weekly has been administered concurrently with radiation therapy up to a maximum of 6 doses. When used in combination chemotherapy regimens (e.g., cisplatin and fluorouracil) for the treatment of invasive cervical cancer, cisplatin 50–75 mg/m^2 has been administered IV concurrently with radiation therapy according to various dosage schedules. Various regimens, doses, and dosage schedules have been used for concurrent cisplatin-based chemotherapy and radiation therapy, and the optimal treatment for locally advanced cervical cancer has not been established.

Metastatic or Recurrent Cervical Cancer. For the treatment of metastatic or recurrent cervical carcinoma†, the usual dosage of cisplatin used alone or in combination therapy is 50 mg/m^2 IV once every 3 weeks up to a maximum of 6 courses. Higher dosages of cisplatin (e.g., 100 mg/m^2 IV once every 3 weeks) produce higher response rates in patients with advanced cervical cancer, but duration of response, survival, and progression-free survival are similar to those observed with the usual dosage, and toxicity is greater.

Non-small Cell Lung Cancer When used in combination chemotherapy for the treatment of non-small cell lung carcinoma†, cisplatin typically has been given in a dosage of 75–100 mg/m^2 IV once every 3–4 weeks depending on the specific regimen used.

Esophageal Cancer When used alone in the treatment of advanced esophageal cancer†, cisplatin has been given in a dosage of 50–120 mg/m^2 IV once every 3–4 weeks. In combination chemotherapy regimens for esophageal cancer, the usual dosage of cisplatin is 75–100 mg/m^2 IV once every 3–4 weeks.

Biliary Tract Cancer When cisplatin has been used in combination with gemcitabine for the treatment of unresectable locally advanced or metastatic biliary tract cancer† in adults, including treatment of unresectable recurrent disease following surgical resection, cisplatin 25 mg/m^2 has been administered by 1-hour IV infusion on days 1 and 8 of each 21-day cycle, and gemcitabine 1 g/m^2 has been administered by 30-minute IV infusion on days 1 and 8 after cisplatin administration. Treatment has been continued for 24 weeks (8 cycles of therapy) in the absence of disease progression or unacceptable toxicity.

Intra-arterial Dosage When cisplatin has been administered intra-arterially† for the treatment of regionally confined malignancies, including advanced bladder cancer, metastases from malignant melanoma, and osteogenic sarcomas, a dose of 75–150 mg/m^2 at intervals ranging from 2–5 weeks for at least 1–4 courses of therapy has been used.

Intraperitoneal Dosage For the management of intraperitoneal tumors (e.g., advanced ovarian carcinoma, carcinoid, mesothelioma) that are confined to the peritoneal cavity and/or are associated with malignant ascites, cisplatin has been administered intraperitoneally† in doses of 60–100 mg/m^2.

When combined therapy with intraperitoneal cisplatin and IV and intraperitoneal paclitaxel† has been used for the initial adjuvant treatment of optimally debulked stage III epithelial ovarian cancer, IV paclitaxel 135 mg/m^2 by 24-hour infusion on day 1, followed by intraperitoneal cisplatin 100 mg/m^2 on day 2 and intraperitoneal paclitaxel 60 mg/m^2 on day 8, has been administered every 21 days for up to 6 cycles. Modified IV and intraperitoneal regimens are being investigated. (See Uses: Ovarian Cancer.)

Pediatric Dosage Pediatric dosage of cisplatin has not been fully established. For the treatment of osteogenic sarcoma† or neuroblastoma†, cisplatin has been given in a dosage of 90 mg/m^2 IV once every 3 weeks or 30 mg/m^2 IV once weekly. For the treatment of recurrent brain tumors†, cisplatin has been given in a dosage of 60 mg/m^2 IV once daily for 2 consecutive days every 3–4 weeks.

■ **Dosage in Renal Impairment** Cisplatin therapy is contraindicated in patients with preexisting renal impairment. Because cisplatin-induced renal toxicity may become more prolonged and severe with repeated doses of the drug, the manufacturer states that cisplatin therapy should be resumed only when the patient has recovered normal renal function. (See Cautions: Precautions and Contraindications.)

Cautions

Cisplatin is a highly toxic drug, and generally is more poorly tolerated overall compared with carboplatin, another platinum-coordination compound. While the major dose-limiting adverse effects associated with cisplatin therapy include nonhematologic toxicities such as nephrotoxicity, ototoxicity, neurotoxicity, and emesis, the major dose-limiting adverse effects associated with carboplatin therapy are hematologic toxicities such as thrombocytopenia and leukopenia. Differences in the toxicity and pharmacokinetic profiles of the drugs may be important determinants in the selection of cisplatin versus carboplatin for specific patients.

■ **Renal and Electrolyte Effects** ***Renal Effects*** Nephrotoxicity, which is dose related and can be severe, may occur in patients receiving cisplatin and is more common and severe than that associated with carboplatin. Geriatric patients may be at increased risk for nephrotoxicity associated with cisplatin therapy. (See Cautions: Geriatric Precautions.) When cisplatin formerly was administered without concomitant IV hydration and diuresis, nephrotoxicity was clearly cumulative and was the major dose-limiting adverse effect. Renal toxicity has occurred in 28–36% of patients receiving a single dose of cisplatin 50 mg/m^2. Renal toxicity is manifested by an increase in serum creatinine, BUN, serum uric acid, and/or a decrease in creatinine clearance and glomerular filtration rate.

Cisplatin-induced renal impairment has been associated with renal tubular damage as evidenced by renal pathologic changes and by increased urinary excretion of β_2-microglobulin and enzymes such as *N*-acetyl-β-glucosaminidase (NAG), leucine aminopeptidase (LAP), and β-glucuronidase. Focal acute tubular necrosis may occur, with tubular degeneration, interstitial edema and fibrosis, dilation of convoluted tubules, and cast formation. Both proximal and distal tubules are affected, but glomeruli appear intact. While the exact mechanism(s) is not known, renal toxicity may be caused by the positively charged products of cisplatin that are formed in vivo.

If renal toxicity occurs in patients receiving cisplatin, it generally appears during the second week after administration of the drug; with high-dose regimens, it may occur within several days. Renal insufficiency is usually mild to moderate and reversible with usual doses of the drug; however, high or repeated doses can increase the severity and duration of renal impairment and may produce irreversible renal insufficiency (sometimes fatal). The risk and degree of renal impairment may be increased by concomitant use of other nephrotoxic drugs. (See Drug Interactions: Nephrotoxic Drugs.) There is some evidence that cisplatin-induced renal impairment is not age dependent and that nephrotoxic effects may actually be less severe in patients with a single functional kidney.

Regimens of IV hydration, diuresis, and 6- to 8-hour infusions of cisplatin are used to decrease the incidence and severity of nephrotoxicity (see Dosage and Administration: Reconstitution and Administration), possibly by decreasing renal and urinary concentrations of the drug or its platinum-containing product(s). While several regimens have been shown to be very effective in reducing and minimizing renal toxicity, the most effective regimen remains to be established. The value of diuretics in minimizing nephrotoxicity is not clearly defined, and hydration alone may be equally effective. There is some evidence that intensive IV hydration with 0.9% sodium chloride injection and administration of cisplatin in 3% sodium chloride injection may substantially reduce the risk of nephrotoxicity, possibly by providing a chloride concentration that minimizes the formation and renal tubular concentration of nephrotoxic product(s) of the drug. Use of prophylactic amifostine (ethiofos), a phosphorylated sulfhydryl compound, reduces the incidence and severity of cisplatin-induced nephrotoxicity in patients with advanced ovarian cancer. (See Amifostine 92:56.) There is also some evidence that concurrent administration of IV sodium thiosulfate with cisplatin may reduce the risk of nephrotoxicity, but further studies are needed to determine whether the therapeutic efficacy of cisplatin is also affected; although the exact mechanism in preventing nephrotoxicity is not known, sodium thiosulfate may be concentrated in renal tubules, where it could react covalently with cisplatin to form an inactive compound and thereby protect the kidneys.

The effect of the rate of administration of cisplatin on the incidence and severity of nephrotoxicity has not been fully elucidated. While there is some evidence that 6- to 8-hour infusions are less nephrotoxic than rapid IV administration, infusions over 15 minutes to 2 hours are commonly employed and have been used with minimal adverse renal effects. Continuous 24-hour or 5-day IV infusions of the drug have generally not been associated with a reduction in renal toxicity compared with shorter periods of drug administration; while there is some evidence that continuous 5-day IV infusions with IV hydration and diuresis may be employed with minimal adverse renal effects, a relative therapeutic advantage has not been established.

The value of plasma platinum concentrations for predicting or monitoring nephrotoxicity has not been defined, but there is some evidence that patients who eventually develop cisplatin-induced renal toxicity may have elevated plasma platinum concentrations early in the course of 24-hour IV infusions of the drug.

Recovery of renal function generally occurs within 2–4 weeks after administration of cisplatin, but may be delayed or rarely not occur. The long-term effects of the drug on renal function are not fully known. In patients who received cisplatin without concomitant hydration and diuresis, decreases in creatinine clearance have been reported to persist for up to 1–2 years after discontinuance of the drug. While subclinical renal impairment (which may be detected only by measurement of creatinine clearance) may develop and persist even when regimens of hydration and diuresis are employed, the evidence to date suggests that clinically important chronic renal failure or cumulative, delayed nephrotoxicity does not occur following discontinuance of therapy with usual doses of the drug (total cumulative doses of about 300–700 mg/m^2) and regimens of hydration and diuresis.

Hypomagnesemia and Other Electrolyte Effects Cisplatin may cause serious electrolyte disturbances, principally hypomagnesemia, hypocalcemia, and hypokalemia; hypophosphatemia may also occur, and hyponatremia has occurred in some patients receiving cisplatin-containing combination chemotherapy. The disturbances in serum electrolytes have been associated principally with cisplatin-induced renal tubular dysfunction. The drug markedly increases urinary excretion of magnesium and calcium; urinary excretion of potassium, zinc, copper, and amino acids is also increased. Although the exact mechanism(s) is not known, the renal tubular dysfunction caused by cisplatin may result from a specific drug-induced membrane or transport-system defect.

Hypomagnesemia and hypocalcemia may develop during cisplatin therapy or following discontinuance of the drug; although these electrolyte disturbances may occur within several days after an initial dose of the drug, hypomagnesemia usually develops within 3–4 weeks after therapy is initiated and appears to increase in severity with progressive courses of treatment. Children may be particularly susceptible to the development of cisplatin-induced hypomagnesemia. Hypomagnesemia and/or hypocalcemia may become symptomatic, with muscle irritability or cramps, clonus, tremor, carpopedal spasm, and/or tetany. Generally, these manifestations are managed and normal serum electrolyte concentrations may be restored by administration (usually parenteral) of appropriate supplemental electrolytes and discontinuance of the drug; however, hypomagnesemia may persist for several months to years after cisplatin therapy is discontinued and, in some patients, has persisted for longer than 3 years. The long-term effects of the drug on renal tubular dysfunction remain to be fully evaluated. The severity of hypomagnesemia has been associated with an increased risk of subsequently developing Raynaud's phenomenon, but a causal relationship has not been clearly established. (See Cautions: Cardiovascular Effects.)

Methods of preventing cisplatin-induced hypomagnesemia and optimum management of persistent hypomagnesemia have not been fully established. In patients with advanced ovarian cancer, use of prophylactic amifostine reduces the incidence and severity of cisplatin-induced hypomagnesemia. (See Amifostine 92:56.) Although not universally recommended, prophylactic administration of magnesium supplements during cisplatin therapy to patients without renal insufficiency has been suggested. Specific dosage recommendations have not been established, but some clinicians have given 3 g of magnesium sulfate IV during a 6-hour IV infusion of cisplatin in each course of therapy with the drug, or 1 g of magnesium sulfate IV daily for 5 days with each 5-day course of cisplatin when the serum magnesium concentration was less than 1.2 mEq/L. However, some data indicate that hypomagnesemia may develop despite replacement therapy. The value of oral magnesium supplements in the management of asymptomatic cisplatin-induced hypomagnesemia has not been established; chronic oral magnesium supplements do not appear to increase serum magnesium concentrations or hasten the resolution of such hypomagnesemia. It is also uncertain whether continuous administration of oral magnesium supplements is of value in preventing the development of symptomatic hypomagnesemia; however, to minimize the risk of recurrent, symptomatic episodes, adequate magnesium intake is generally recommended in patients who become symptomatic.

■ **GI Effects** ***Emetogenic Effects*** Cisplatin, one of the most emetogenic antineoplastic agents, induces marked nausea and vomiting in virtually all patients. Because of its universal emetogenic potential, cisplatin is classified as an antineoplastic agent of *high emetic risk* (i.e., incidence of emesis exceeds 90% if no antiemetic agents are administered). In the absence of effective antiemetic therapy, patients develop an average of 10–12 vomiting episodes within the first 24 hours after an initial dose. Although cisplatin-induced nausea and vomiting generally are self-limited and seldom life-threatening, they occasionally are severe enough to require discontinuance of the drug. In addition, of all the adverse effects of cisplatin, patients often are most fearful of the emetogenic effects and may develop anticipatory nausea and vomiting and/or refuse further therapy with the drug.

Nausea and vomiting, which appear to be mediated via local GI stimulation of central mechanisms, generally begin within 1–6 (usually 2–3) hours after administration of cisplatin; this early period of emesis after a dose is the most severe and generally persists for about 8 hours with repeating emetic episodes but may persist up to 24 hours or longer. Various degrees of nausea, vomiting, and anorexia may persist for up to 5–10 days. Delayed nausea and vomiting beginning or persisting 24 hours or longer (although occasionally beginning 16–20 hours) following chemotherapy has occurred in patients who had attained complete emetic control on the day of cisplatin therapy. The incidence and severity of cisplatin-induced nausea and vomiting appear to be increased in females, in young patients, and in patients receiving the drug in high doses, by rapid infusion, and/or in combination with other emetogenic drugs such as anthracyclines (e.g., doxorubicin); patients with a history of chronic heavy alcohol use appear to experience less frequent and severe emetogenic effects.

Mechanism. The role of serotonin as a mediator of acute cisplatin-induced emesis has been strongly suggested by the temporal relationship between the emetogenic action of the drug and the release (e.g., from GI enterochromaffin cells) of serotonin (e.g., as reflected by increases in plasma and urine concentrations of the serotonin metabolite 5-hydroxyindoleacetic acid (5-HIAA)] as well as by the clinical efficacy of antiemetic agents that act as inhibitors of the type 3 (5-HT$_3$) serotonin receptor (e.g., dolasetron, granisetron, ondansetron, palonosetron, tropisetron [not commercially available in the US]). In addition, the severity of emetogenic activity and degree of serotonin release appear to be dose related and increased with repeated cisplatin courses. Studies in animals have shown that cisplatin-induced emesis can be prevented completely by ablation of the area postrema (the locus of the chemoreceptor trigger zone [CTZ]) or depletion of serotonin from this area; in addition, high levels of 5-HT_3 receptors have been demonstrated in this area, and direct injection of 5-HT_3 receptor antagonists into the area postrema also can prevent cisplatin-induced emesis. Therefore, current evidence suggests that the emetogenic action of cisplatin may be initiated by degenerative changes in the GI tract (e.g., small intestine) induced by the drug and associated increases in endogenous serotonin release; serotonin then stimulates vagal and splanchnic nerve receptors that project to the medullary vomiting (emetic) center of the brain and also appears to stimulate 5-HT_3 receptors in the area postrema. Thus, 5-HT_3 receptor antagonists appear to prevent or ameliorate acute cisplatin-induced emesis by inhibiting visceral (from the GI tract) afferent stimulation of the vomiting center probably indirectly at the level of the area postrema and by directly inhibiting serotonin activity within the area postrema and CTZ.

Alternative mechanisms appear to be principally responsible for delayed nausea and vomiting induced by cisplatin, since similar temporal relationships between serotonin and emesis beyond the first day after a dose have not been established, and inhibitors of 5-HT_3 receptors do not appear to be effective alone in preventing or ameliorating delayed effects. Antagonists at substance P/neurokinin 1 (NK_1) receptors represent another class of antiemetic agents. The binding of the tachykinin substance P to NK_1 receptors in the GI tract and the brainstem emetic center appears to cause emesis. Substance P/NK_1 receptor antagonists, such as aprepitant, block the binding of substance P and therefore prevent acute and delayed emesis. (See Aprepitant 56:22.92.) Anticipatory vomiting is a learned response conditioned by the severity and duration of previous emetic reactions to chemotherapy.

Management. There is some evidence that the incidence and/or severity of nausea and vomiting may be reduced with 5-day continuous IV infusions of cisplatin compared with rapid, intermittent IV administration.

For the prevention of *acute* emesis, the American Society of Clinical Oncology (ASCO) currently recommends a 3-drug antiemetic regimen consisting of a type 3 serotonin receptor antagonist, dexamethasone, and aprepitant given before the administration of cisplatin or other chemotherapy regimens with high emetic risk. (See Aprepitant 56:22.92.) Currently available selective 5-HT_3 receptor antagonists (e.g., dolasetron, granisetron, ondansetron, palonosetron, or tropisetron [not commercially available in the US], are comparably effective in preventing acute chemotherapy-induced nausea and vomiting. (For additional information, see the individual monographs for 5-HT_3 receptor antagonists in 56:22.20.)

For the prevention of *delayed* emesis, ASCO currently recommends a 2-drug regimen of dexamethasone and aprepitant following the administration of cisplatin or other chemotherapy associated with high emetic risk.

Antiemetic agents with a lower therapeutic index (i.e., less efficacious and generally associated with more frequent adverse effects), including cannabinoids (e.g., dronabinol, nabilone), metoclopramide, butyrophenones, and phenothiazines, are *not* considered by ASCO to be appropriate first-line antiemetics for chemotherapy of high emetic risk; these drugs should be reserved for patients with refractory emesis or unacceptable toxicity from first-line agents. Although antihistamines (e.g., diphenhydramine) and benzodiazepines (e.g., alprazolam, lorazepam) may be useful as adjunctive antiemetic agents, they should *not* be used as monotherapy.

Aggressive antiemetic therapy for the prevention of acute and delayed emesis during early courses of emetogenic chemotherapy is the best way to prevent *anticipatory* nausea and vomiting; behavioral modification and hypnosis also may be useful. Although evidence is lacking, many clinicians also find benzodiazepines useful in the management of anticipatory emesis.

Other GI Effects Diarrhea also has occurred in patients receiving cisplatin.

■ Otic Effects

Ototoxicity, manifested as tinnitus, with or without clinical hearing loss, and occasional deafness, may occur in patients receiving cisplatin and may be more severe in children than in adults. Rarely, temporary unilateral otalgia and recruitment have also occurred.

Tinnitus has occurred in about 9% of patients receiving cisplatin and is usually reversible; it is not clear whether tinnitus is dose related. The most common cisplatin-induced hearing changes are audiogram abnormalities, which occur in about 24% of patients receiving usual doses of the drug, but high-frequency loss on audiograms has been reported in up to 74–100% of patients receiving cumulative doses of 200 mg/m² or more. Audiogram abnormalities usually appear within 4 days after administration of the drug, consist of at least a 15-dB loss in pure-tone threshold, and are principally bilateral but can be unilateral. Cisplatin-induced audiogram abnormalities are dose related (increasing with higher single doses and total cumulative dosage) and cumulative; there is also some evidence that audiogram abnormalities may occur more frequently when the drug is administered by rapid IV injection compared with infusion over 1–3 hours or 24 hours. The audiogram abnormalities appear to be most severe in older adults and in children, especially young children. Although not clearly established, patients with preexisting hearing impairment may be more susceptible to cisplatin-induced ototoxicity. The long-term effects have not been fully determined, but the audiogram abnormalities generally appear to be irreversible; however, partial or complete recovery has been reported.

Cisplatin-induced audiogram abnormalities are most common and usually most severe in the high frequency range (4000–8000 Hz); however, audiogram abnormalities may occur at frequencies up to 20,000 Hz, and with increasing cumulative dosage, abnormalities may become evident at lower frequencies (1000–4000 Hz) and result in clinical hearing loss. About 6% of patients receiving the drug have developed clinical hearing loss, manifested as decreased hearing acuity. Although audiogram abnormalities and clinical hearing loss usually develop gradually, rapid-onset clinical hearing loss has occurred rarely. Rarely, deafness after the initial dose of cisplatin has been reported. Clinically important hearing loss may occasionally require dosage reduction or discontinuance of cisplatin therapy.

Although the exact mechanism of cisplatin-induced ototoxicity is not known, the drug has been shown to cause loss of hair cells of the organum spirale in animals and there are limited data to suggest that a similar effect occurs in humans. Electrophysiologic studies have shown the site of principal damage to be the apical stereocilia on the hair cell surface. The possibility that concomitant administration of other potentially ototoxic drugs (e.g., aminoglycosides) may increase the risk of ototoxicity in patients receiving cisplatin should be considered. (See Drug Interactions: Ototoxic Drugs.) In addition, ototoxicity may be enhanced in patients with prior or simultaneous cranial irradiation.

Rarely, cisplatin has been reported to cause vestibular ototoxicity, manifested as vertigo or vestibular dysfunction. Although data are limited, cisplatin-induced vestibular ototoxicity may increase with increasing cumulative dosage and may be most likely to occur in patients with preexisting vestibular dysfunction.

■ Nervous System Effects

Neurotoxicity produced by cisplatin usually is characterized by peripheral neuropathies, which are generally sensory in nature (e.g., paresthesias of the upper and lower extremities)but can also include motor (especially gait) difficulties; reduced or absent deep-tendon reflexes and leg weakness may also occur. A myasthenic-like syndrome characterized by ptosis and proximal muscle weakness also has been associated with cisplatin. Geriatric patients may be at increased risk for peripheral neuropathy associated with cisplatin therapy. (See Cautions: Geriatric Precautions.) Cisplatin-containing regimens are associated with a higher incidence of, and more severe, neurotoxicity than carboplatin-containing regimens, and neurotoxic effects of cisplatin have become the principal dose-limiting toxicity of the drug subsequent to institution of more effective means of controlling renal and GI toxicities.

Cisplatin-induced peripheral neuropathies occur infrequently with usual doses of the drug and usually only with prolonged therapy (4–7 months) or high cumulative doses; however, neurologic manifestations have been reported after a single dose of the drug, and some evidence suggests that both cumulative-dose intensity and single-dose intensity may be risk factors in the development of neurotoxicity.Manifestations of cisplatin-induced neuropathy usually develop during treatment; rarely, neurologic manifestations may occur 3–8 weeks or longer after the last dose of cisplatin.

The incidence of peripheral neuropathy may be increased when cisplatin is administered concurrently with other potentially neurotoxic agents (e.g., altretamine, paclitaxel, vincristine). Peripheral nerve damage caused by cisplatin has been documented by sensory and motor nerve conduction studies. Sural nerve biopsies from patients with cisplatin-induced paresthesias of the upper and lower extremities and gait disturbances have shown microscopic features consistent with a segmented demyelination pattern of peripheral nerve injury; loss of axons may also be present. In one case of cisplatin neurotoxicity, the spinal cord showed loss of myelinated fibers and gliosis of the dorsal columns at autopsy. Muscle cramps, defined as localized, painful, involuntary skeletal muscle contractions of sudden onset and short duration, have been reported and usually occurred in patients with symptomatic peripheral neuropathy who received relatively high cumulative doses of cisplatin.

Lhermitte's sign (a sensation during neck flexion resembling electric shock) often is present with cisplatin-induced neuropathy. The occurrence of Lhermitte's sign may be particularly likely to coincide with the onset of peripheral neuropathy. Lhermitte's sign has persisted for 2–8 months. As the neuropathy progresses, the sense of joint position also becomes impaired, and severely affected patients may become markedly impaired by sensory ataxia. Temperature and pain sensations remain relatively preserved.

Dorsal column myelopathy and autonomic neuropathy have occurred in some patients receiving cisplatin. Transient partial (focal) or tonic-clonic (grand mal) seizures have also occurred in some patients receiving the drug. Other manifestations of focal neurologic deficits induced by the drug have included cortical blindness and aphasia with seizures or with homonymous hemianopia. Other reported adverse nervous system effects include slurred speech, loss of taste, memory loss, and intention tremor. Postmortem findings of leukoencephalopathy also have been reported.

If manifestations of neuropathy occur, cisplatin therapy should immediately be discontinued; however, neuropathy may worsen even after discontinuance of the drug. Peripheral neuropathy may be irreversible in some patients but has been partially or completely reversible in others following discontinuance of cisplatin therapy.

Management The role, if any, of neurotrophic peptides (e.g., Org 2766, an analog of corticotropin devoid of glucocorticoid activity) or other drugs on neurotoxic effects of cisplatin remains to be more fully elucidated. There is limited evidence from a study in women receiving cisplatin (75 mg/m² every 3 weeks) and cyclophosphamide (750 mg/m² every 3 weeks) for ovarian cancer that Org 2766 (1 mg/m² administered subcutaneously before and after each cycle of chemotherapy) can prevent or attenuate cisplatin-induced neuropathy, as determined by effects on the threshold value for vibration perception, without apparently affecting the cytotoxic effects of the drugs adversely; fewer neurologic manifestations relative to placebo also were observed in patients receiving Org 2766. However, the drug does not appear to prevent delayed neurotoxic effects several months after discontinuance of cisplatin and Org 2766 therapy; therefore, it has been suggested that continued therapy with this drug may be necessary for up to several months after discontinuance of cisplatin. Although the mechanism of possible neuroprotection by Org 2766 is unclear, the drug is a melanocortin and has been postulated to trigger or facilitate peripheral-nerve repair. Amifostine (ethiofos), a phosphorylated sulfhydryl compound, and glutathione, another sulfhydryl compound, also have exhibited neuroprotective effects. In a randomized study of patients with advanced ovarian cancer, the incidence and severity of cisplatin-induced neurotoxicity appeared to be reduced in patients who received prophylactic amifostine. Additional study and experience are needed to determine the usefulness of potential neuroprotectant compounds in patients receiving cisplatin.

■ **Hematologic Effects** The hematologic toxicity of cisplatin is usually moderate and reversible and affects all 3 blood lineages. Myelosuppression, which is manifested as leukopenia, thrombocytopenia, and anemia (a decrease in hemoglobin of greater than 2 g/dL), occurs in about 25–30% of patients receiving the drug. Geriatric patients may be at increased risk for myelosuppression associated with cisplatin therapy. (See Cautions: Geriatric Precautions.) Bone marrow suppression associated with cisplatin is less pronounced than that associated with carboplatin.

Cisplatin-induced myelosuppression may be cumulative and may be more severe in patients previously treated with other antineoplastic agents or radiation therapy. Leukopenia and thrombocytopenia are dose related and more pronounced at doses exceeding 50 mg/m². Leukocyte and platelet nadirs generally occur 18–23 days (range: 7.2–45 days) following a single dose of cisplatin, with levels returning to pretreatment values in most patients within 39 days (range: 13–62 days). The incidence and severity of cisplatin-induced anemia are not clearly related to dose. The anemia is usually normochromic and normocytic and generally occurs over the same time course as leukopenia and thrombocytopenia; occasionally, the anemia may be severe, and patients may require transfusions.

The etiology of cisplatin-induced anemia appears to be complex and several mechanisms may be involved. It has been suggested that anemia caused by cisplatin may result from a drug-induced decrease in erythropoietin or erythroid stem cells. There is also some evidence that both hemolysis and decreased erythropoiesis may contribute to the anemia. Rarely, cisplatin has reportedly caused hemolytic anemia; in a few of these cases, positive direct antiglobulin (Coombs') test results were observed, but it is not clear if this effect is immunologically mediated. Positive direct antiglobulin test results can apparently occur without evidence of hemolysis in patients receiving cisplatin.

■ **Sensitivity Reactions** Anaphylactoid reactions consisting principally of facial edema, flushing, bronchoconstriction, wheezing or respiratory difficulty (e.g., dyspnea), tachycardia, and hypotension have occurred within a few minutes after IV administration of cisplatin in patients who previously received the drug; diaphoresis, nasal stuffiness, rhinorrhea, conjunctivitis, generalized erythema, apprehension, and sensation of chest constriction also may occur. Anaphylactoid reactions also have occurred following intravesical† or intraperitoneal† administration of the drug. Cisplatin-induced anaphylactoid reactions usually have occurred only after multiple cycles (e.g, at least 5 doses) of the drug, but also can occur after the initial dose. The exact mechanism(s) is not known, but the reactions may be immune mediated in some patients. The reactions may be controlled by IV epinephrine, corticosteroids, and/or antihistamines as clinically indicated. Occasionally, patients who experienced anaphylactoid reactions reportedly have been safely retreated with cisplatin following pretreatment with corticosteroids and/or antihistamines; however, such prophylaxis is not uniformly effective in preventing recurrence.

Rarely, urticarial or nonspecific maculopapular rashes, recurrent dermatitis, exfoliative dermatitis, and erythema have been reported in patients receiving cisplatin. In at least one patient, severe exfoliative dermatitis (diffuse erythroderma, desquamation, and eosinophilia) occurred after the second cycle of carboplatin and recurred with subsequent administration of cisplatin despite antihistamine and corticosteroid prophylaxis; with cisplatin, the dermatitis was associated with fever, facial edema, hypotension, tachycardia, and edema and cyanosis of the hands (as well as hypoesthesia and pain consistent with local ischemia).

■ **Ocular Effects** Optic neuritis (principally retrobulbar), papilledema, and cerebral (cortical) blindness have been reported infrequently in patients receiving recommended dosages of cisplatin. Improvement and/or total recovery usually occur after discontinuance of the drug. Corticosteroids, with or without mannitol, have been used in the management of these adverse ocular effects; however, the efficacy of such treatment has not been established.

■ **Cardiovascular Effects** Rarely, bradycardia, left bundle-branch block, and ST-T-wave changes with congestive heart failure have been associated with cisplatin therapy. Postural hypotension, which has been attributed to cisplatin-induced neurotoxicity, has also occurred. Hypertension, which persisted for up to 6 months and in some cases required treatment, has occurred following intra-arterial† infusion of the drug.

Rarely, vascular toxicities have been associated with the use of cisplatin-containing combination chemotherapy. The adverse vascular effects are clinically heterogeneous and may include thrombotic microangiopathy, renovascular lesions, severe coronary artery disease, myocardial infarction, cerebrovascular accident, or cerebral arteritis. Various mechanisms have been suggested, including endothelial cell damage. Raynaud's phenomenon has also occurred in patients receiving bleomycin and vinblastine, with or without cisplatin. It has been suggested that cisplatin-induced hypomagnesemia may be an additional, although not essential, factor associated with its occurrence. (See Hypomagnesemia and Other Electrolyte Effects in Cautions: Renal and Electrolyte Effects.) The cause of Raynaud's phenomenon in these cases, however, is not clearly established and may involve the underlying disease or vascular compromise, bleomycin, vinblastine, hypomagnesemia, or some combination of these factors.

■ **Hepatic Effects** Mild and transient elevations of serum AST (SGOT), ALT (SGPT), and bilirubin concentrations may occur in patients receiving cisplatin. There has been one report of acute, reversible liver toxicity, manifested by transient elevations of serum bilirubin and hepatic enzymes, associated with cisplatin therapy.

■ **Local Effects** Rarely, local phlebitis has been associated with IV administration of cisplatin. There also have been rare reports of severe cellulitis with residual fibrosis and full-thickness skin necrosis following extravasation of the drug. Severity of local tissue toxicity appears to be related to the concentration of the cisplatin solution. Infusion of solutions with a cisplatin concentration exceeding 0.5 mg/mL may result in tissue cellulitis, fibrosis, and necrosis. Intra-arterial† infusion of cisplatin may result in local pain, edema, and erythema.

■ **Other Adverse Effects** Hyperuricemia may occur in patients receiving cisplatin, principally as a result of drug-induced nephrotoxicity. Hyperuricemia is more pronounced with doses greater than 50 mg/m², and peak serum concentrations of uric acid generally occur 3–5 days after administration of the drug. Allopurinol has been given to reduce serum uric acid concentrations.

Elevated serum amylase concentrations have been reported infrequently in patients receiving cisplatin. Other adverse effects associated with cisplatin include mild alopecia or thinning of the hair, malaise, asthenia, hiccups, myalgia, pyrexia, and gingival platinum line. Although the exact mechanism(s) has not been determined, gynecomastia has occurred in some males with testicular carcinomas treated with cisplatin-containing combination chemotherapy; a direct causal relationship to cisplatin has not been established. Cisplatin has also been associated with the occurrence of syndrome of inappropriate antidiuretic hormone secretion (SIADH).

■ **Precautions and Contraindications** Cisplatin is a highly toxic drug with a low therapeutic index, and a therapeutic response is not likely to occur without some evidence of toxicity. The drug must be used only under constant supervision by clinicians experienced in therapy with cytotoxic agents.

Patients receiving cisplatin should be observed closely for possible anaphylactoid reactions, and appropriate equipment for maintenance of an adequate airway and other supportive measures and agents for the treatment of anaphylactoid reactions (e.g., antihistamines, epinephrine, oxygen, corticosteroids) should be readily available whenever cisplatin is administered. The manufacturer states that cisplatin is contraindicated in patients with a history of sensitivity reactions to the drug or other platinum-containing compounds; however, cross-sensitivity is not absolute, and occasionally with appropriate precautions patients sensitive to one platinum-containing compound have tolerated another. Exposure (e.g., industrial) to platinum-containing compounds can cause asthma and immediate and delayed hypersensitivity reactions, and the possibility that patients with a history of such exposure may be cross-sensitive to cisplatin should be considered.

Renal, hematologic, otic, and neurologic function must be frequently and carefully monitored in patients receiving cisplatin; hepatic function should also be monitored periodically. Patients receiving the drug should be adequately hydrated, and serum electrolyte concentrations and fluid requirements carefully monitored; if serum electrolyte and/or fluid disturbances occur, appropriate treatment should be instituted.

Cisplatin therapy is contraindicated in patients with preexisting renal impairment. The manufacturer recommends that serum magnesium, sodium, potassium, calcium, and creatinine concentrations and creatinine clearance and BUN be determined prior to beginning cisplatin therapy and prior to each additional course of therapy. While creatinine clearance appears to most accurately reflect the degree of renal insufficiency produced by the drug, some clinicians suggest that it is usually necessary to repeat measurement of creatinine clearance during cisplatin therapy only when the serum creatinine concentration increases by more than 33% over the baseline value. Since renal toxicity may become more prolonged and severe with repeated doses of cisplatin, the manufacturer states that another cisplatin dose should not be given until serum creatinine concentration is less than 1.5 mg/dL and/or BUN is less than 25 mg/dL. Cisplatin has been used successfully, however, in some patients with obstructive uropathy caused by tumors sensitive to the drug; in some of these patients, renal function improved following treatment with the drug. The drug has also been used successfully in some patients with a single functional kidney.

The manufacturer recommends that peripheral blood cell counts be monitored weekly in patients receiving cisplatin; some clinicians suggest that blood counts can be monitored less frequently (e.g., every 2 weeks). While the hematologic toxicity of the drug is usually moderate and reversible, treatment of severe hematologic toxicity may consist of supportive therapy, anti-infectives for complicating infections, and blood product transfusions. The manufacturer states that a repeat dose of cisplatin should not be administered unless circulating blood elements are at an acceptable level (i.e., leukocyte count of at least 4000/mm^3 and platelet count of at least 100,000/mm^3). Fever and infection have been reported in patients with neutropenia. In the presence of cisplatin-induced hemolytic anemia, a further course of treatment may be accompanied by increased hemolysis, and the risk should be considered. The manufacturer states that cisplatin is contraindicated in patients with myelosuppression.

Since cisplatin-induced ototoxicity is cumulative, the manufacturer recommends that audiometry be performed prior to initiating cisplatin therapy and prior to each additional course of therapy and that additional doses be withheld until audiometric determinations indicate that auditory acuity is within normal limits. Many clinicians believe that repeat audiograms are of limited value in the routine management of most patients receiving the drug and suggest that repeat audiometry be performed only when auditory symptoms occur or clinical hearing changes become apparent. Clinically important hearing changes may require dosage modification or discontinuance of therapy. The manufacturer states that cisplatin is contraindicated in patients with hearing impairment.

Neurologic examinations should be performed regularly in patients receiving cisplatin, and the manufacturer recommends discontinuing therapy when symptoms of neurotoxicity first appear.

■ **Pediatric Precautions** Safety and efficacy of cisplatin in children have not been established. The drug has been used in the treatment of osteogenic sarcoma†, neuroblastoma†, and brain tumors† in children, but additional evaluation is needed. Some adverse effects (e.g., ototoxicity) appear to be more severe in children.

■ **Geriatric Precautions** While the safety and efficacy of cisplatin in geriatric patients have not been established specifically, data from 4 clinical trials involving a total of 1484 patients (29% of whom were older than 65 years of age) receiving cisplatin in combination with cyclophosphamide or paclitaxel for advanced ovarian cancer indicate that a higher incidence and greater severity of certain adverse effects may occur in older patients. Although age was not found to be a prognostic factor for survival in these studies, secondary analysis of data from one of these clinical trials demonstrated shorter survival in older patients compared with younger patients. Data from clinical trials involving the use of cisplatin in the treatment of metastatic testicular cancer or advanced bladder cancer are insufficient to determine whether elderly patients respond to the drug differently than younger patients.

In all 4 clinical trials, severe neutropenia associated with cisplatin-containing chemotherapy occurred more frequently in geriatric patients than in younger patients; higher incidences of severe thrombocytopenia and leukopenia were observed in elderly patients receiving some cisplatin-containing regimens. A numerically higher incidence of peripheral neuropathy was observed in geriatric patients in 2 of the clinical trials, which evaluated nonhematologic toxicity according to age. Other clinical experience suggests that geriatric patients are at increased risk for myelosuppression, infectious complications, and nephrotoxicity associated with cisplatin therapy.

Cisplatin is excreted mainly by the kidney and is contraindicated in patients with preexisting renal impairment. Because geriatric patients may have decreased renal function, careful dosage selection and monitoring of renal function are advised.

■ **Mutagenicity and Carcinogenicity** In vitro, cisplatin has been shown to be mutagenic in bacteria and has produced chromosomal aberrations in animal cells in tissue culture.

Cisplatin has been shown to be carcinogenic in mice and rats. In studies in BD IX rats receiving intraperitoneal cisplatin at a dosage of 1 mg/kg body weight weekly for 3 weeks, 66% of the animals died within 450 days following the first application of the drug; approximately 40% of the deaths were related to malignancies (i.e., predominantly leukemias and 1 renal fibrosarcoma). Cisplatin-containing combination chemotherapy has been associated with the development of bladder cancer in a patient treated for nonseminomatous testicular carcinoma; however, other drugs and radiation therapy were used in this patient, and a direct causal relationship to cisplatin has not been established. Rarely, acute leukemia (e.g., lymphocytic, myeloid) has developed in patients receiving cisplatin therapy; in such patients, cisplatin generally has been given in combination with other leukemogenic agents and/or radiation.

■ **Pregnancy, Fertility, and Lactation** Cisplatin and/or its platinum-containing products appear to cross the placenta. Cisplatin may cause fetal harm when administered to a pregnant woman, but potential benefits from use of the drug may be acceptable in certain conditions despite possible risks to the fetus. Cisplatin has been shown to be teratogenic in mice and embryotoxic in mice and rats. Cisplatin should be used during pregnancy only in life-threatening situations or severe disease for which safer drugs cannot be used or are ineffective. When the drug is administered during pregnancy or if the patient becomes pregnant while receiving the drug, the patient should be informed of the potential hazard to the fetus. Patients should be advised to avoid becoming pregnant during the period in which they are receiving cisplatin therapy.

The effects of cisplatin on the gonads and fertility have not been fully determined. Since the drug has produced testicular atrophy in animals and platinum is distributed in high concentration into testes, a risk of adverse testicular effects in humans exists. Although impairment of spermatogenesis is present in many males with testicular carcinomas prior to treatment, most males with these tumors become aspermic during and after treatment with cisplatin-containing combination chemotherapy; however, in some of these males, disease- and drug-induced impairment of spermatogenesis are apparently reversible. In one study in males with disseminated nonseminomatous testicular carcinoma treated with cisplatin, bleomycin, and vinblastine, with or without doxorubicin, 77% were initially oligospermic and 96% became aspermic within 2 months after initiation of therapy; however, there appears to be a high degree of reversibility as evidenced by a return of spermatogenesis with normal sperm counts 2–3 years after initiation of therapy. In addition, some of the males with recovery of spermatogenesis successfully impregnated their wives, resulting in 5 normal births, 3 ongoing pregnancies at the time of the study, and 1 spontaneous abortion. While recovery of spermatogenesis may occur, abnormal sperm may be present.

Cisplatin is distributed into milk. Because of the potential for serious adverse reactions to cisplatin in nursing infants, nursing should not be undertaken by women receiving the drug.

Drug Interactions

■ **Nephrotoxic Drugs** Cisplatin produces cumulative nephrotoxicity that is potentiated by aminoglycoside antibiotics. Concurrent administration of the drugs or administration of an aminoglycoside within 1–2 weeks after cisplatin therapy has been associated with an increased risk of nephrotoxicity and acute renal failure (sometimes severe). Aminoglycosides should be used with extreme caution, if at all, during or shortly after cisplatin therapy. Some clinicians suggest that the risk of this drug interaction may be reduced if the aminoglycoside is administered at least 2 weeks after cisplatin. Concomitant use of other potentially nephrotoxic drugs (e.g., amphotericin B) should probably also be avoided during cisplatin therapy.

■ **Ototoxic Drugs** Patients receiving cisplatin and other potentially ototoxic drugs such as aminoglycoside antibiotics or loop diuretics (e.g., ethacrynic acid, furosemide) concomitantly should be carefully monitored for signs of ototoxicity. A study in guinea pigs has shown that cisplatin and ethacrynic acid potentiate the ototoxic effects of each other.

■ **Antineoplastic Agents** Studies in animals and clinical trials in humans indicate that the antineoplastic activity of cisplatin and etoposide may be synergistic against some tumors. In mice implanted with P388 or L1210 leukemia or B16 melanoma, a combination of cisplatin and etoposide was shown to act synergistically in reducing the body burden of tumor cells and/or increasing survival. Response rates in humans receiving combination chemotherapy with cisplatin and etoposide suggest that the combination has synergistic antineoplastic activity against testicular carcinomas, small cell carcinoma of the lung, or non-small cell carcinoma of the lung. Studies in animals also indicate that the antineoplastic activity of cisplatin and some other antineoplastic agents (e.g., bleomycin, doxorubicin, fluorouracil, methotrexate, vinblastine, vincristine) is potentially synergistic.

Limited data indicate that elimination of etoposide may be impaired in patients previously treated with cisplatin. In a randomized trial in patients with advanced ovarian cancer, response duration was adversely affected when pyroxidine was used in combination with altretamine (hexamethylmelamine) and cisplatin.

■ **Renally Excreted Drugs** Limited data suggest that cisplatin may alter the renal elimination of bleomycin and methotrexate, possibly as a result of cisplatin-induced nephrotoxicity. Although further documentation is needed, the possibility that cisplatin may affect the elimination of renally excreted drugs should be considered.

■ **Phenytoin** In patients receiving cisplatin and phenytoin, serum concentrations of phenytoin may be decreased, possibly as a result of decreased absorption and/or increased metabolism of phenytoin. In patients receiving cisplatin therapy, serum concentrations of phenytoin should be monitored and dosage adjustments made as necessary.

Acute Toxicity

■ **Manifestations** **Overdosage of cisplatin may be fatal.** In some cases, cisplatin overdosage resulted from inadvertent substitution of the drug for carboplatin; the latter drug is substantially less toxic than cisplatin and generally is administered at much higher dosages. Caution should be exercised to avoid inadvertent overdosage with cisplatin. (See Dosage and Administration: Dosage.)

Acute overdosage with cisplatin may result in acute renal failure, ototoxicity that can progress to irreversible deafness, severe myelosuppression, intractable nausea and vomiting, and neuritis. Less commonly, hepatotoxicity (e.g., hepatic failure manifested as increased serum transaminase concentrations and elevations in clotting times, prothrombin time, and partial thromboplastin time), central neurotoxicity (e.g., manifested as generalized seizures and hallucinations), and ocular toxicity (e.g., manifested as visual changes such as blurring and altered color perception that are attributable to retinal damage, including retinal detachment) can occur. Other manifestations of neurotoxicity have included dysarthria, paresthesias, and impaired taste perception. Myelosuppression, nephrotoxicity, ocular toxicity, and neuropathy may be partially or totally reversible. However, ototoxicity (e.g., bilateral sensorineural hearing loss) often is irreversible and, in patients whose overdosage was not accompanied by IV hydration (e.g., when cisplatin inadvertently was given instead of carboplatin), renal failure also may be irreversible.

■ **Treatment** Although there currently is no established antidote for cisplatin overdosage, nucleophilic (reducing) sulfhydryl (thiol) compounds (e.g., glutathione, acetylcysteine, mesna) can inactivate cisplatin and act as chemoprotectants (e.g., protecting against nephrotoxicity). However, the potential benefits of such therapy in the management of cisplatin overdosage remain to be established, and many of these compounds would be of limited, if any, benefit if administration were delayed for several hours after cisplatin administration since most platinum would be protein bound and not in its reactive form. Theoretically offering potentially greater usefulness would be dithiocarbamates (e.g., dithiocarb [diethyldithiocarbamate, DDTC], amifostine [ethiofos]) since the drugs can react with platinum even after protein binding has occurred and can stimulate substantial biliary excretion of the metal. *Since most experience to date with the effects of various chemoprotectants on cisplatin toxicity has been in animal or in vitro studies or in preliminary studies in humans, the role, if any, of these agents in treating cisplatin toxicity remains to be elucidated. The role, if any, of neurotrophic peptides (e.g., Org 2766, an analog of corticotropin devoid of glucocorticoid activity) on neurotoxic effects of cisplatin also remains to be elucidated.*

Management of cisplatin overdosage currently consists principally of discontinuance of the drug and general supportive measures to sustain the patient throughout any period of toxicity that may occur. Hemodialysis, even when initiated within 4 hours following overdosage of cisplatin, appears to have little effect on removing platinum from the body because of cisplatin's rapid and high degree of protein binding. However, limited evidence suggests that aggressive plasmapheresis may be useful in removing protein-bound platinum and thus ameliorating toxicity. Antiemetics that are recommended for the prevention of acute or delayed emesis associated with cisplatin (type 3 serotonin receptor antagonists, dexamethasone and aprepitant) may be useful for managing acute intractable nausea and vomiting. Hematopoietic agents (e.g., sargramostim [GM-CSF]) may be useful in managing myelosuppression, and hemodialysis may be required for the management of renal failure.

Pharmacology

The exact mechanism(s) of action of cisplatin has not been conclusively determined, but the drug has biochemical properties similar to those of bifunctional alkylating agents. Platinum-containing antineoplastic agents appear to exert their effects by binding to DNA, thereby inhibiting DNA synthesis. Cisplatin is cycle-phase nonspecific. Although the principal mechanism of action of cisplatin appears to be inhibition of DNA synthesis, other mechanisms, possibly including enhancement of tumor immunogenicity, are involved in its antineoplastic activity.

Neutrality of charge and the *cis* configuration are necessary for the cisplatin complex to exert antineoplastic activity. In the relatively high chloride concentration of plasma, the cisplatin complex is believed to be un-ionized, allowing passage of the drug through cell membranes. Intracellularly, in the presence of a low chloride concentration, the chloride ligands of the complex are displaced by water (aquation), resulting in formation of positively charged platinum complexes that are toxic and react with the nucleophilic sites on DNA. Cisplatin binds to DNA and inhibits DNA synthesis; protein and RNA synthesis also are inhibited but less extensively. The drug produces predominately DNA intrastrand and interstrand cross-links, with intrastrand cross-links resulting from the formation of adducts between activated platinum complexes of the drug and areas of specific base sequences; DNA-protein cross-links also are formed. The relative importance of intrastrand or interstrand DNA cross-links in the antineoplastic activity of cisplatin remains to be clearly determined; however, interstrand cross-linking appears to correlate well with the cytotoxicity of the drug. Interstrand cross-linking within the DNA helix also occurs. The resultant interstrand and intrastrand cross-links are stable bonds that do not dissociate easily. While the mechanism through which DNA adducts exert their cytotoxic effects has not been determined, limited evidence indicates that platinum adducts may inhibit DNA replication, transcription, and ultimately cell division.

Cisplatin also has immunosuppressive, radiosensitizing, and antimicrobial properties.

Further study is needed to elucidate more fully the extent of cross-resistance between cisplatin and carboplatin. Although some cisplatin-refractory tumors may respond to carboplatin, a high degree of cross-resistance appears to occur between the drugs. The mechanisms of cellular resistance to platinum-containing antineoplastic agents have not been fully elucidated, but resistance can be related to decreased cellular uptake of the drug or enhanced DNA repair and may be related to elevated cellular levels of sulfhydryl (thiol) compounds including glutathione or metallothionein. Glutathione appears to play an essential role in protecting cells from the effects of certain toxins including certain antineoplastic agents, and increased levels of this sulfhydryl compound have been demonstrated in certain cell lines resistant to cisplatin and other analogs. Increased repair of platinum complex-induced DNA adducts also has been demonstrated in certain resistant cell lines. The relative roles of these mechanisms of resistance and their relationship to treatment failure in patients who do not respond to platinum-containing antineoplastic agents have not been fully determined.

Pharmacokinetics

The pharmacokinetics of cisplatin are complex and have been studied principally by using assays for elemental platinum or by using preparations of the drug containing radioactive platinum; only a few studies have used analytical methods capable of measuring intact cisplatin. Published studies on the pharmacokinetics of cisplatin have varied widely in the doses administered, the rate of administration, the use of IV hydration, and the concurrent use of diuretics; the effects of these factors, if any, on the pharmacokinetics of the drug and their clinical importance remain to be fully elucidated. The chemical identities of platinum-containing products of cisplatin that are formed in vivo have not been definitely determined. In addition, relationships between therapeutic activity or toxicity and plasma concentrations of cisplatin or platinum have not been clearly established; however, results of in vitro studies have suggested that only nonprotein-bound cisplatin or its platinum-containing products are cytotoxic.

■ **Absorption** Following rapid IV injection of cisplatin over 1–5 minutes or rapid IV infusion over 15 minutes or 1 hour, peak plasma drug and platinum concentrations occur immediately. Following rapid IV injection of a 50-mg/m² dose of cisplatin over 3–5 minutes to patients with normal renal function in one study, peak plasma concentrations of intact cisplatin, total platinum, and nonprotein-bound platinum averaged 2.3, 4.7, and 2.7 mcg/mL, respectively; after a 100-mg/m² dose, peak plasma concentrations averaged 3.3, 6.2, and 4.5 mcg/mL, respectively. Following rapid IV infusion of a 100-mg/m² dose of the drug over 15 minutes to patients with normal renal function in another study, peak plasma concentrations of nonprotein-bound platinum averaged 2.73 mcg/mL. Following 1-hour IV infusions of 50 and 70 mg/m² to patients with normal renal function, peak plasma total platinum concentrations of 2.26–2.45 and 4.25–7.02 mcg/mL, respectively, have been reported.

When cisplatin is administered by IV infusion over 6 or 24 hours, plasma concentrations of total platinum increase gradually during the infusion and peak immediately following the end of the infusion. Following 6-hour IV infusions of 100 mg/m² to patients with normal renal function, peak plasma total and nonprotein-bound platinum concentrations ranging from 2.5–5.3 and 0.22–0.73 mcg/mL, respectively, have been reported. Following a 24-hour IV infusion of 80 mg/m² in one study, peak plasma total platinum concentrations ranged from 1.03–1.90 mcg/mL. When equal doses of cisplatin are administered by rapid IV infusion or infusion over 2–3 or 24 hours in patients with normal renal and hepatic function, the areas under the plasma nonprotein-bound platinum concentration-time curves (AUCs) appear to be equivalent.

Concomitant IV administration of cisplatin and mannitol appeared to increase peak plasma concentrations of nonprotein-bound platinum in one study, but in another study mannitol appeared to have no effect on plasma concentrations of intact cisplatin, total platinum, or nonprotein-bound platinum. In one study comparing the effects of IV furosemide or mannitol on the pharmacokinetics of cisplatin, plasma concentrations of total platinum and nonprotein-bound platinum were similar following administration of either diuretic.

Following intra-arterial† infusion of cisplatin, local tumor exposure to the drug is increased compared with IV administration as evidenced by increased plasma platinum concentrations in local veins draining the infused region compared with systemic veins and by increased AUCs calculated for local versus systemic exposure. Following local infusion, systemic plasma platinum concentrations are similar to those attained following IV administration of comparable doses of the drug. Local venous plasma platinum concentrations are reportedly lower following infusion of cisplatin into the hepatic artery compared with other arteries (e.g., brachial, femoral), suggesting that the drug is highly extracted by the liver.

Cisplatin is rapidly and well absorbed systemically following intraperitoneal administration†, resulting in 50–100% of the degree of systemic exposure compared with IV administration when comparable doses are given; however, peak intraperitoneal fluid concentrations of nonprotein-bound platinum are greatly increased, and intraperitoneal exposure to nonprotein-bound platinum is increased by about 15- to 30-fold compared with IV administration.

■ **Distribution** Following IV administration of cisplatin, platinum is widely distributed into body fluids and tissues, with highest concentrations in the kidneys, liver, and prostate. Lower concentrations are found in the bladder, muscle, testes,pancreas, and spleen; platinum is also distributed into the small and large intestines, adrenals, heart, lungs, lymph nodes, thyroid, gallbladder, thymus, cerebrum, cerebellum, ovaries, and uterus. Platinum appears to accumulate in body tissues following administration of cisplatin and has been detected in many of these tissues for up to 6 months after the last dose of the drug. Platinum is also distributed minimally into leukocytes and erythrocytes.

The volume of distribution of platinum in adults following IV administration of cisplatin has been reported to range from 20–80 L and averaged 41 L/m² in one study. Platinum is rapidly distributed into pleural effusions and ascitic fluid following IV administration of cisplatin. The manufacturer states that small amounts of platinum have been detected in the bile and large intestine following administration of cisplatin, but fecal excretion of platinum appears to be insignificant. Cisplatin is distributed into milk, and limited evidence indicates that the drug and/or its platinum-containing products cross the placenta.

Although there is some evidence to the contrary, cisplatin and/or its platinum-containing products apparently do not readily penetrate the CNS. Following IV administration of cisplatin, platinum is distributed into intracerebral tumor tissue and edematous brain tissue adjacent to tumor; however, only low concentrations of platinum have been detected in healthy brain tissue. In one study in patients with brain tumors, platinum was barely or not detectable in CSF following IV administration of cisplatin, but, in other reports, platinum was detected in the CSF of patients with or without brain tumors following IV administration of the drug. When platinum has been detected in CSF, peak CSF platinum concentrations occurred within 30–60 minutes after IV administration of cisplatin and CSF platinum concentrations ranged from less than 5% to up to 100% of concurrent plasma concentrations.

Cisplatin does not undergo the instantaneous and reversible binding to plasma proteins that is characteristic of typical drug-protein binding. The platinum from cisplatin, but not cisplatin itself, is rapidly and extensively bound to tissue and plasma proteins, including albumin, γ-globulins, and transferrin. Binding to tissue and plasma proteins appears to be essentially irreversible.Protein binding increases with time, and less than 2–10% of platinum in blood remains unbound several hours after IV administration of cisplatin.

■ **Elimination** Following rapid IV injection or infusion of cisplatin, plasma concentrations of intact cisplatin, total platinum, and nonprotein-bound platinum have generally been reported to decline in a monophasic, biphasic, and biphasic manner, respectively; however, some reports indicate that plasma concentrations of nonprotein-bound platinum decline in a monophasic manner and that plasma concentrations of total platinum may exhibit triphasic or quadraphasic elimination with a prolonged terminal phase. In adults with normal renal function, the following plasma elimination half-lives have been reported after rapid IV injection or infusion of cisplatin: intact cisplatin, about 20–30 minutes; total platinum, 8.1–49 minutes in the initial phase and 30.5–107 hours or possibly longer in the terminal phase; and nonprotein-bound platinum, 2.7–30 minutes in the initial phase and 32–53.5 minutes in the terminal phase. Concomitant administration of IV mannitol does not alter the terminal plasma half-life of nonprotein-bound platinum. Following 6-hour IV infusions of cisplatin in patients with normal renal function, a terminal plasma elimination half-life for total platinum of 73–290 hours has been reported. Some data suggest that the rate of elimination of total plasma platinum in patients with normal renal function may decrease with time. In one patient with acute oliguric renal failure requiring hemodialysis, the terminal plasma half-life of total platinum was approximately 10 days.

In children with normal renal function, the serum elimination half-lives of total platinum reportedly average about 25 minutes in the initial phase and 44 hours in the terminal phase, and the serum elimination half-life of nonprotein-bound platinum averages 1.3 hours.

Following IV administration of cisplatin, the elimination half-lives of total platinum from CSF and pleural effusion fluid are reportedly about 0.75–1.5 hours and 22 days, respectively. Following IV administration of the drug, a mean elimination half-life of total platinum from erythrocytes of about 30 hours has been reported, suggesting that cisplatin may increase the breakdown of erythrocytes. Following intraperitoneal administration of cisplatin, the peritoneal elimination half-lives of total platinum and nonprotein-bound platinum are about 33 hours and 1 hour, respectively.

The metabolic fate of cisplatin has not been completely elucidated. There is no evidence to date that the drug undergoes enzymatic biotransformation; the chloride ligands of the cisplatin complex are believed to be displaced by water, forming positively charged platinum complexes that react with nucleophilic sites. The chemical identities of platinum-containing products of the drug that are formed in vivo have not been definitely determined. Intact cisplatin and its platinum-containing product(s) are excreted principally in urine; fecal elimination of platinum appears to be insignificant. The presence of a secondary peak in plasma platinum concentration during the principal elimination phase of platinum has been reported, suggesting that cisplatin or its platinum-containing products may undergo enterohepatic circulation.

Renal excretion appears to occur predominantly via glomerular filtration, but there is some evidence that secretion and possibly reabsorption of cisplatin or a platinum-containing product(s) also occurs. Following a 6-hour IV infusion of the drug, the renal clearance of total platinum decreases substantially to a relatively low, constant value about 6–12 hours after the end of the infusion; this appears to be consistent with a relatively high, initial renal clearance of intact cisplatin and nonprotein-bound platinum, followed by clearance of nonprotein-bound platinum-containing product(s). The urinary excretion of 2 platinum-containing compounds has been partially characterized. The first, a water-elutable compound believed to be intact cisplatin, represents most of the platinum initially excreted in urine but rapidly decreases to represent a very small fraction of excreted platinum. The second, a hydrochloric acid-elutable compound believed to be a positively charged complex formed by replacement of one of cisplatin's chloride ligands with water, initially represents a small fraction of platinum excreted in urine but rapidly increases to represent a large fraction of urinary platinum. A third, unidentified platinum-containing compound also appears to be excreted in urine.

Following rapid IV injection or infusion of cisplatin in patients with normal renal function, approximately 15–50% of a dose is excreted in urine within 24–48 hours; most urinary excretion occurs within the first 4–6 hours following administration of the drug, apparently principally as intact cisplatin.Following IV infusion of the drug over 6 hours in patients with normal renal function, 24-hour urinary excretion has generally ranged from about 10–35% of a dose; however, in some reports as much as 65–80% of the dose administered was excreted within 24 hours. Concomitant IV administration of mannitol and a 15-minute or 6-hour IV infusion of cisplatin reportedly results in substantially decreased 24-hour urinary excretion of platinum. An average of 14% of the administered dose was excreted in urine within 24 hours in one study when cisplatin was given as a 24-hour IV infusion to patients with normal renal function. There is some evidence that the circadian timing of cisplatin administration has a pronounced effect on urinary platinum excretion, with evening administration of the drug resulting in greater urine output and lower peak urinary platinum concentrations than morning administration.

The effects of renal impairment on the elimination of cisplatin and its platinum-containing products have not been fully evaluated; individuals with decreased renal function may have impaired elimination. There is also some evidence that patients with impaired renal function may have elevated plasma concentrations of nonprotein-bound platinum.

Limited data indicate that cisplatin and/or its platinum-containing products are minimally removed by hemodialysis. In one patient, 4- to 5.5-hour periods of hemodialysis removed into the dialysate about 8% of individual doses of cisplatin given by IV infusion over 0.75–1.5 hours immediately prior to dialysis; about 3% of a dose was removed into the dialysate per period during periods of hemodialysis 24 and 48 hours after the first period.

Chemistry and Stability

■ **Chemistry** Cisplatin is a platinum-containing antineoplastic agent. The drug is an inorganic complex that contains a platinum atom surrounded in a plane by 2 chloride atoms and 2 ammonia molecules in the *cis* position. Cisplatin occurs as a yellow to orange crystalline powder and has a solubility of 1 mg/mL in water or in 0.9% sodium chloride solution.

Commercially available cisplatin injection is a clear, colorless solution and contains hydrochloric acid and/or sodium hydroxide to adjust pH and sodium chloride. The commercially available injection has a pH of 3.7–6, an osmolality of about 285–286 mOsm/kg, and contains a sodium chloride concentration of 0.9%.

Cisplatin powder for injection (no longer commercially available in the US; see Preparations) occurs as a white, lyophilized powder and contains sodium chloride and mannitol, and hydrochloric acid to adjust pH. Following reconstitution of the powder for injection with sterile water for injection as recommended (see Dosage and Administration: Reconstitution and Administration), solutions containing 1 mg of cisplatin per mL are clear and colorless and have a pH of 3.5–5.5 and sodium chloride and mannitol concentrations of 0.9 and 1%, respectively.

■ **Stability** Commercially available cisplatin injection should be protected from light. The injection should be stored at 15–25°C and refrigeration avoided (since precipitation of the drug may occur); however, if cisplatin injection is inadvertently refrigerated, the precipitate will dissolve at room temperature, without loss of potency. If freezing occurs, cisplatin injection may be thawed at room temperature until precipitate dissolves; the manufacturer states that the chemical or physical stability of the injection is not affected. When stored under recommended conditions, commercially available cisplatin injection is stable for 17 months following the date of manufacture; cisplatin injection remaining in the amber vial following initial entry is stable for 28 days when protected from light or for 7 days when stored under fluorescent room light. Cisplatin powder for injection should be stored at room temperature. Unopened vials of the powder for injection are stable for 2 years at room temperature (27°C).

The manufacturer states that, when reconstituted as directed from cisplatin powder for injection, cisplatin solutions are stable for 20 hours when stored at 27°C. Following reconstitution of the powder for injection with bacteriostatic water for injection containing benzyl alcohol or parabens, cisplatin solutions containing 1 mg/mL are reportedly stable for at least 72 hours at 25°C. Reconstituted solutions of cisplatin removed from the amber vial should be protected from light if they are not to be used within 6 hours. Reconstituted solutions of cisplatin should be stored at room temperature and should *not* be refrigerated, since precipitation may occur; a precipitate reportedly forms within 1 hour when solutions containing 1 mg of cisplatin per mL of 0.9% sodium chloride injection are refrigerated (2–6°C). Redissolution of the precipitate may occur very slowly when the solution is warmed to room temperature, but such warming to effect redissolution is not recommended and cisplatin solutions containing a precipitate should be discarded.

In aqueous solutions or solutions containing less than 0.2% sodium chloride, cisplatin is decomposed with displacement of chloride ions by water. Increasing the chloride concentration in the solvent up to 0.9% improves the stability of cisplatin in solution. The stability of cisplatin in various IV solutions and admixtures is reported as follows:

IV Solution	Cisplatin Concentration (mg/mL)	Duration of Stability (time and temperature)
5% Dextrose and 0.45 or 0.9% Sodium Chloride	0.05, 0.5	at least 24 h at room temperature
5% Dextrose and 0.33% Sodium Chloride with 1.875% Mannitol (with or without 0.15% Potassium Chloride)	0.05, 0.1, 0.2	at least 72 h at 4 or 25°C
5% Dextrose and 0.45% Sodium Chloride with 1.875% Mannitol	0.05, 0.1, 0.2	at least 72 h at 4 or 25°C
0.2% Sodium Chloride	0.2	at least 24 h at room temperature
0.225% Sodium Chloride	0.05, 0.1, 0.2	at least 72 h at 4 or 25°C
0.3% Sodium Chloride	0.05, 0.1, 0.2	at least 72 h at 4 or 25°C
0.45% Sodium Chloride	0.2	at least 24 h at room temperature
	0.05, 0.5	at least 24 h at 25°C
0.9% Sodium Chloride	0.2	at least 24 h at room temperature
	0.05, 0.5	at least 24 h at 25°C

The stability of cisplatin in solution is reportedly not adversely affected by the presence of up to 5% mannitol; however, cisplatin-mannitol complexes may form after several days, and advanced preparation and storage of such admixtures should be avoided. Cisplatin solutions should generally not be diluted in sodium bicarbonate or other alkaline solutions because of enhanced decomposition of cisplatin; formation of a bright gold precipitate has occurred after admixture of 5% sodium bicarbonate and a cisplatin solution. Cisplatin may react covalently with sodium thiosulfate to form a pharmacologically inactive compound and may also react with sodium bisulfite. Specialized references should be consulted for specific stability and compatibility information.

Aluminum displaces platinum from the cisplatin molecule, causing the formation of a black precipitate and loss of potency. Cisplatin solutions should not be prepared or administered with needles or IV administration sets containing aluminum parts that might come in contact with the drug. Stainless steel needles and plated brass hubs do not react with cisplatin within 24 hours.

For further information on the handling of antineoplastic agents, see the ASHP Guidelines on Handling Hazardous Drugs at http://www.ahfsdruginformation.com.

Preparations

Excipients in commercially available drug preparations may have clinically important effects in some individuals; consult specific product labeling for details.

CISplatin

Parenteral		
Injection, for IV infusion	1 mg/mL (50 or 100 mg)*	**Cisplatin Injection**
		Platinol®-AQ, Bristol-Myers Squibb

*available from one or more manufacturer, distributor, and/or repackager by generic (nonproprietary) name

†Use is not currently included in the labeling approved by the US Food and Drug Administration

Cladribine

Chlorodeoxyadenosine, CdA, 2-CdA

■ Cladribine, a synthetic purine nucleoside, is an antimetabolite antineoplastic agent.

Uses

■ **Hairy Cell Leukemia** Cladribine is used for the treatment of active hairy cell leukemia (leukemic reticuloendotheliosis). Active hairy cell leukemia is defined as disease involving clinically important anemia, neutropenia, thrombocytopenia, or other disease-related symptoms.

The current indication for cladribine is based principally on limited data from 2 single-center, open-label studies in patients with hairy cell leukemia and evidence of active disease requiring therapy. During these open-label studies, overall responses (complete, good partial, or partial responses) determined by intent-to-treat analysis were observed in approximately 85–90% of patients. Among evaluable patients, overall responses were observed in about 86–89% of patients.

A complete response to cladribine therapy generally was defined as clearing of the peripheral blood and bone marrow of hairy cells and recovery of hemoglobin concentration to at least 12 g/dL, platelet count to at least 100,000/mm^3, and absolute neutrophil count to at least 1500/mm^3. For evaluation of the data using intent-to-treat analysis, an additional criterion for complete response was absence of evidence of splenomegaly indicated by absence of palpable spleen on physical examination and spleen size not exceeding 13 cm on CT scan. A good partial response was defined as a decrease to fewer than 5% hairy cells in bone marrow; hematologic parameters for a good partial response were the same as those for a complete response. A partial response was defined as a decrease of at least 50% in the number of hairy cells in bone marrow; hematologic parameters for a partial response also were the same as those for a complete response.

A pathologic relapse was defined as an increase in the number of hairy cells in bone marrow to at least 25% of pretreatment levels. A clinical relapse was defined as the recurrence of cytopenias, specifically, decreases in hemoglobin concentration of at least 2 g/dL, decreases in absolute neutrophil count of at least 25%, and/or decreases in platelet count of at least 50,000/mm^3. Patients who met the criteria for a complete response but subsequently were found to have evidence of hairy cells in bone marrow (less than 25% of pretreatment levels) were reclassified as exhibiting partial responses and were not considered to exhibit complete responses with relapse.

Complete responses to cladribine were observed in 65–68% of evaluable patients but in only 54% of patients when determined according to intent-to-treat analysis. The median time to response in these patients reportedly was about 4 months. The median duration of complete response to cladribine therapy exceeded 8 months and in some patients ranged to longer than 25 months.

In these studies, 60% of patients had not received prior chemotherapy for hairy cell leukemia or had undergone splenectomy as the only prior treatment and were receiving cladribine as initial systemic antineoplastic therapy. The remaining 40% of the patients had been treated previously with other agents,

including interferon alfa and/or pentostatin. The overall response rate for patients without prior chemotherapy was 92% compared with 84% for previously treated patients.

In a large case series, long-term follow-up of 358 patients receiving cladribine for hairy cell leukemia showed an overall response rate of 95% and a complete response rate of 89% according to intention-to-treat analysis at a median follow-up of approximately 4 years. An increased risk of secondary malignancies (observed to expected ratio of 1.88) was reported in this series. Under a group C protocol, follow-up of 979 patients receiving cladribine for hairy cell leukemia for at least 4 years showed an overall response rate of 76% and a complete response rate of 44% according to intention-to-treat analysis. A high rate of secondary malignancies was observed in this protocol also. It is unclear whether the high rate of secondary malignancy associated with cladribine therapy is attributable to the drug or to the underlying disease itself.

Additional data from other case series or open-label studies in small numbers of patients with hairy cell leukemia receiving cladribine demonstrate a consistently high rate of response to the drug. Although durable complete responses to cladribine therapy have been observed in many patients, longer follow-up is needed to determine the curative potential of the drug. To date, extended follow-up shows high rates of overall survival in a subset of 207 patients from a large case series (97% at 9 years) and in a case series of 86 patients (87% at 12 years).

Because of their apparent greater efficacy (i.e., higher complete response rate) compared with interferon alfa, cladribine or pentostatin is considered *first-line* therapy for most patients with hairy cell leukemia who require treatment. Similar response rates have been reported for cladribine and pentostatin, but the comparative efficacy and safety of these agents have not been studied in phase III randomized trials. Common toxicities of cladribine therapy include infection, fever, and neutropenia. Some evidence suggests that prior treatment with splenectomy and/or interferon alfa, or with pentostatin, does not alter response to cladribine in patients with hairy cell leukemia; however, conflicting data exist.

Cladribine typically is administered by continuous IV infusion (0.1 mg/kg daily) as a single course of therapy given over 7 consecutive days. In some patients, a second course of cladribine therapy may be required to achieve a desirable response. Cladribine also may be administered as daily subcutaneous injections for 7 consecutive days†. In an open-label study of 73 patients receiving cladribine 3.4 mg/m^2 SC once daily for 7 days, the rate of overall response was 96% and the rate of complete response was 81%.

Among patients with active hairy cell leukemia that responds to initial treatment with cladribine, retreatment with cladribine or another purine analogue often induces another response.

■ **Other Uses** Cladribine is used in the treatment of chronic lymphocytic leukemia,† low-grade non-Hodgkin's lymphoma,† and cutaneous T-cell lymphoma.†

Dosage and Administration

■ **Reconstitution and Administration** Cladribine is administered by continuous IV infusion as a single course of therapy given over 7 consecutive days. *Cladribine for injection concentrate must be diluted prior to IV infusion.*

For IV infusion, the calculated single daily dose of cladribine for injection concentrate is added to a polyvinyl chloride infusion bag containing 500 mL of 0.9% sodium chloride injection. Such solutions are infused IV continuously over 24 hours. Subsequent doses are repeated as 24-hour infusions daily for a total of 7 consecutive days. Dextrose 5% injection should *not* be used because cladribine degradation is accelerated in this diluent.

Alternatively, if the entire 7-day course of cladribine is to be administered as a single continuous IV infusion, the manufacturer recommends that the entire dose for this period be diluted in bacteriostatic 0.9% sodium chloride injection containing benzyl alcohol as a preservative. To minimize the risk of microbial contamination, first the calculated 7-day dose of cladribine concentrate for injection (0.63 mg/kg total) and then the calculated amount of diluent needed to bring the total volume of the solution to 100 mL should be passed through a sterile 0.22-μm disposable hydrophilic syringe filter as each solution is being introduced into the infusion reservoir. Solutions of cladribine prepared with bacteriostatic sodium chloride injection for individuals weighing more than 85 kg may have reduced preservative effectiveness because of greater dilution of the benzyl alcohol.

Cladribine IV infusion solutions that have been prepared with bacteriostatic sodium chloride injection containing benzyl alcohol should *not* be used in neonates. (See Cautions: Pediatric Precautions.)

The manufacturer's labeling should be consulted for additional information on proper techniques for dilution, storage, and administration of cladribine as well as measures to avoid precipitation of the drug.

■ **Dosage** The usual adult dosage of cladribine for the treatment of active hairy cell leukemia is 0.09 mg/kg daily repeated for 7 consecutive days for a total dosage of 0.63 mg/kg. The manufacturer states that if the patient fails to respond to the initial course of therapy, additional courses of cladribine are unlikely to provide any benefit. The drug can be infused IV over 7 consecutive 24-hour periods as repeated 0. 09-mg/kg daily doses or as a continuous 7-day infusion of the total 0. 63-mg/kg dose. The manufacturer states that deviations from this dosage regimen are not advised.

Because cladribine is a highly toxic drug (consult the manufacturer's labeling), patients undergoing therapy should be observed closely for signs of hematologic and nonhematologic toxicity. (See Cautions: Precautions and Contraindications.) Discontinuance or interruption of cladribine therapy should be considered in patients who experience neurotoxicity and/or renal toxicity.

■ Dosage in Renal and Hepatic Impairment The effects of renal or hepatic impairment on the elimination of cladribine have not been elucidated. The manufacturer recommends monitoring of renal and hepatic function during cladribine therapy, especially in patients with renal and/or hepatic impairment, but makes no specific recommendations for dosage adjustment. Cladribine should be used with caution in patients with known or suspected renal and/or hepatic insufficiency.

Cautions

Cladribine is a toxic drug and has been associated with severe, irreversible neurotoxicity, acute nephrotoxicity, and severe bone marrow suppression at high doses. Specific risk factors predisposing patients to increased toxicity from cladribine have not been defined.

The most common adverse effects of cladribine in patients with hairy cell leukemia during the first month after initiation of therapy in clinical trials were severe neutropenia, fever (often culture negative), and documented infection. Myelosuppression, which may be severe, usually is reversible, and appears to be dose dependent, should be anticipated with use of the drug. At recommended doses, cladribine appears to be rarely associated with many adverse effects that frequently occur with antineoplastic therapy (e.g., nausea, vomiting, hair loss, abnormal renal or hepatic function). The most frequent adverse nonhematologic effects of the drug that occur during the first 2 weeks after initiation of therapy are fatigue, nausea, rash, headache, and reactions at the injection site. Most adverse nonhematologic effects are mild to moderate in severity.

■ Hematologic Effects Severe bone marrow suppression resulting in neutropenia, anemia, and thrombocytopenia occurs frequently in patients with hairy cell leukemia receiving cladribine, especially at high doses or in patients with preexisting pancytopenia. Most patients with hairy cell leukemia receiving cladribine in clinical trials had hematologic impairment as a manifestation of the disease. Following cladribine treatment, further hematologic impairment occurred before recovery of peripheral blood counts began. Prolonged pancytopenia including aplastic anemia and hemolytic anemia (reported in patients with lymphoid malignancies within the first few weeks following cladribine therapy) has been reported in postmarketing surveillance of patients usually receiving multiple courses of the drug.

Myelosuppression occurred frequently during the first month after initiation of cladribine therapy in patients with hairy cell leukemia in clinical trials; 44% of patients received red blood cell transfusions and 14% received platelet transfusions. During the first 2 weeks after treatment was initiated, mean platelet count, absolute neutrophil count (ANC), and hemoglobin concentration declined and subsequently increased with normalization of mean counts by day 12, week 5, and week 8, respectively. Platelet recovery may be delayed in patients with severe baseline thrombocytopenia. During the first month after treatment initiation, severe neutropenia (ANC less than 500/mm^3) occurred in 70% of patients; it was present in 26% of patients before treatment. The time of maximum cladribine-induced neutropenia appears to correspond with an increased risk of serious infection. (See Cautions: Infectious Complications.) Severe anemia (hemoglobin less than 8.5 g/dL), which was present in 10% of patients before treatment, developed in 37% of patients, and thrombocytopenia (platelet count less than 20,000/mm^3), which was present in 4% of patients before treatment, developed in 12% of patients. Hematologic function must be monitored carefully in patients receiving cladribine, particularly during the first 4–8 weeks after therapy is initiated. (See Cautions: Precautions and Contraindications.) Multiple cycles of cladribine therapy may be associated with cumulative myelotoxicity and prolonged thrombocytopenia. Thrombocytopenia was the limiting toxicity in 20–30% of patients with chronic lymphocytic leukemia† or lymphomas† after repeated courses of cladribine therapy.

Prolonged bone marrow hypocellularity was observed in patients with hairy cell leukemia treated with cladribine in clinical trials, but its clinical importance is not known. Bone marrow hypocellularity of less than 35% was observed after 4 months in 34% of patients and was observed as late as 33 months after treatment was initiated. It is not known whether the hypocellularity results from disease-related marrow fibrosis or cladribine toxicity. No apparent clinical effect on peripheral blood counts was observed.

Purpura was reported in 10%, petechiae in 8%, and epistaxis in 5% of patients with hairy cell leukemia during the first 2 weeks after initiation of cladribine therapy in clinical trials. Erythroid macrocytosis that persisted for 6 months or longer in patients with cutaneous T-cell lymphomas† who received as many as 6 courses of cladribine therapy also has been reported.

In patients with normal bone marrow function, only lymphopenia and transient profound monocytopenia as well as neutropenia and thrombocytopenia may be observed after cladribine therapy.

Based on analysis of lymphocyte subsets from patients with hairy cell leukemia, cladribine therapy is associated with prolonged depression of helper/inducer (CD4$^+$, T4$^+$) T-cell counts. Prior to treatment, the mean CD4$^+$ T-cell count was 766/mm^3; the mean CD4$^+$ T-cell count nadir, which occurred 4–6 months following treatment, was 272/mm^3. Fifteen months after treatment, mean CD4$^+$ T-cell counts remained below 500/mm^3. The effect on cytotoxic/suppressor (CD8$^+$, T8$^+$) T-cell counts was similar, although increasing counts were observed after 9 months. The clinical importance of the prolonged depression of the helper/inducer (CD4$^+$, T4$^+$) T-cell subset is not known. No associated opportunistic infections were reported during this period.

■ Nervous System Effects High doses of cladribine (4–9 times the currently recommended dose for hairy cell leukemia), in conjunction with cyclophosphamide and total body irradiation as preparation for bone marrow transplantation, have been associated with severe, irreversible neurologic toxicity (paraparesis/quadriparesis) in 35% of patients. In most patients, the neurotoxicity was characterized by progressive, irreversible motor weakness of the upper and/or lower extremities and its onset was delayed, with manifestations first noted 35–84 days after the initiation of therapy with the drug. Results of electromyography and nerve conduction studies were consistent with demyelinating disease. Severe neurologic toxicity also has been observed with high doses of another drug in the same class as cladribine. Similar neurotoxicity has been reported rarely in patients with hairy cell leukemia receiving the currently recommended cladribine dosage regimen (0.09 mg/kg daily for 7 consecutive days). Axonal peripheral polyneuropathy was observed in a dose-escalation study at the highest dose levels (about 4 times the currently recommended dose for hairy cell leukemia) in patients not receiving cyclophosphamide or total body irradiation therapy. Mild neurotoxicity has been reported in postmarketing surveillance of patients usually receiving multiple courses of the drug.

Fatigue and headache are among the most frequent adverse effects of cladribine and are the most frequent adverse nervous system effects of the drug, occurring in 45 and 22% of patients with hairy cell leukemia, respectively, during the first 2 weeks after initiation of therapy in clinical trials. After this period, fatigue and headache were reported in 11 and 7% of patients, respectively. Dizziness was reported in 9%, asthenia in 9%, trunk pain in 6%, and insomnia in 7% of patients with hairy cell leukemia during the first 2 weeks after initiation of cladribine therapy in clinical trials. Confusion and paresthesias also have been reported rarely.

■ Renal Effects High doses of cladribine (4–9 times the currently recommended dose for hairy cell leukemia), in conjunction with cyclophosphamide and total body irradiation as preparation for bone marrow transplantation, have been associated with manifestations of acute renal insufficiency (e.g., acidosis, anuria, elevated serum creatinine concentration) in 19% of patients within 1–2 weeks after starting treatment. Several of the patients also were receiving other potentially nephrotoxic drugs. Most of the patients developing acute renal insufficiency required dialysis. Renal dysfunction was reversible in some of the patients. In several patients in whom renal function had not recovered by the time of death, evidence of renal tubular damage was found. Similar nephrotoxicity has not been reported in patients with hairy cell leukemia receiving the currently recommended cladribine dosage regimen (0.09 mg/kg daily for 7 consecutive days).

■ Infectious Complications Infectious complications, including those associated with immunosuppression (e.g., fungal, viral), were documented in 28% of patients with hairy cell leukemia during the first month after initiation of cladribine treatment and in 6% of patients during the second month after initiation of treatment in clinical trials. Opportunistic infections also have been reported in postmarketing surveillance of patients usually receiving multiple courses of the drug. Serious infections (e.g., septicemia, pneumonia) were reported in 6% of patients and occurred only during the first month after initiation of cladribine treatment; the remaining infections were mild or moderate in severity. Several deaths were attributed to infection and/or complications related to the underlying disease. (See Cautions: Precautions and Contraindications.) During the second month, documented infections were mild to moderate in severity and no severe systemic infections occurred. Approximately 10% of the patients with hairy cell leukemia in clinical trials had a documented infection in the month prior to cladribine treatment. After the third month, the incidence of monthly infections was less than or equal to that of the months immediately preceding cladribine therapy. This trend toward a reduced incidence of infection corresponded to normalization of the ANC.

Of the documented infections occurring in the first month following cladribine therapy, 42% were bacterial, 20% were fungal, and 20% were viral. The most frequently reported infection associated with a fatal outcome following cladribine therapy was *Candida* sepsis, although a number of other bacterial, fungal, and viral infections were reported. Most of the documented episodes of herpes zoster infections occurred during the first month following treatment, and almost all of the documented fungal infections occurred during the first 2 months after treatment.

During the first 2 weeks after initiation of cladribine treatment in clinical trials, approximately two-thirds of patients with hairy cell leukemia developed fever, and during the first month, 11% of patients developed severe fever (temperature greater than or equal to 40°C); virtually all patients developing fever were treated empirically with parenteral anti-infectives. Overall, 47% of patients had fever in the presence of neutropenia (ANC less than or equal to 1000/mm^3), including 32% with severe neutropenia (ANC less than or equal to 500/mm^3). Less than one-third of the febrile events were associated with documented infection. In many cases, fever probably was related to the release of pyrogens from tumor cells.

■ GI and Hepatic Effects Nausea is among the most frequent adverse effects of cladribine and is the most frequent adverse GI effect of the drug, occurring in 28% of patients with hairy cell leukemia during the first 2 weeks after initiation of therapy in clinical trials. Most episodes of nausea were mild, were not accompanied by vomiting, and did not require treatment with antiemetics. In those patients requiring antiemetics, nausea was readily controlled, most often with chlorpromazine. Decreased appetite was reported in 17%, vomiting in 13%, diarrhea in 10%, constipation in 9%, and abdominal pain in 6% of patients with hairy cell leukemia during the first 2 weeks after initiation of cladribine therapy in clinical trials.

In a study using high doses of cladribine (4–9 times the recommended dose for hairy cell leukemia) in conjunction with cyclophosphamide and total body irradiation as preparation for bone marrow transplantation, 26% of patients experienced adverse GI effects during infusion of the drug.

Reversible increases in serum concentrations of aminotransferases and bilirubin have been reported in postmarketing surveillance of patients usually receiving multiple courses of the drug. Several patients with advanced hematologic malignancy who had abnormal liver function tests prior to treatment with cladribine were reported to have mild and transient increases in serum AST (SGOT) concentrations during infusion of the drug.

■ **Dermatologic and Local Reactions** Rash is among the most frequent adverse effects of cladribine and is the most frequent adverse dermatologic effect of the drug, occurring in 27% of patients with hairy cell leukemia during the first 2 weeks after initiation of therapy in clinical trials. After this period, rash was reported in 10% of patients. Most rashes were mild and occurred in patients who were receiving or had recently been treated with other drugs known to cause rash (e.g., allopurinol, antibiotics).

Urticaria and hypereosinophilia also have been reported, mainly in patients who have received multiple courses of cladribine therapy. In isolated cases, Stevens-Johnson syndrome and toxic epidermal necrolysis have been reported in patients receiving cladribine who also were receiving or recently had received other medications (e.g., allopurinol, anti-infectives) known to cause these conditions.

Reactions at the injection site (i.e., erythema, swelling, pain) were reported in 19% of patients and pruritus, pain, and erythema were each reported in 6% of patients with hairy cell leukemia during the first 2 weeks after initiation of cladribine therapy in clinical trials. Thrombosis and phlebitis were each reported in 2% and a broken catheter in 1% of patients receiving the drug, but these effects appeared to be related to the infusion procedure and/or indwelling catheter.

■ **Cardiovascular Effects** Edema and tachycardia were each reported in 6% of patients with hairy cell leukemia during the first 2 weeks after initiation of cladribine therapy in clinical trials. Peripheral vein phlebitis has been reported rarely.

■ **Respiratory Effects** Abnormal breath sounds were reported in 11%, cough in 10%, abnormal chest sounds in 9%, and shortness of breath in 7% of patients with hairy cell leukemia during the first 2 weeks after initiation of cladribine therapy in clinical trials. After this period, cough was reported in 7% of patients. Pulmonary interstitial infiltrates, resulting mainly from infectious etiology, have been reported in postmarketing surveillance of patients usually receiving multiple courses of the drug.

■ **Musculoskeletal Effects** Myalgia was reported in 7% and arthralgia in 5% of patients with hairy cell leukemia during the first 2 weeks after initiation of cladribine therapy in clinical trials.

■ **Metabolic Effects** Tumor lysis syndrome has been reported rarely in patients with other hematologic malignancies with large tumor burdens who were receiving cladribine; hyperuricemia also may occur in patients with large tumor burdens who receive the drug. Empiric therapy with allopurinol was used in studies of cladribine in patients with active hairy cell leukemia, and no episodes of tumor lysis were reported.

■ **Other Adverse Effects** Chills and sweating were each reported in 9% of patients with hairy cell leukemia during the first 2 weeks after initiation of cladribine therapy in clinical trials.

■ **Precautions and Contraindications** Cladribine is a toxic drug with a low therapeutic index, and a therapeutic response is not likely to occur without evidence of toxicity. The drug must be used only under constant supervision by clinicians experienced in therapy with cytotoxic agents. Suppression of bone marrow function should be anticipated. Cladribine-induced bone marrow suppression usually is reversible and appears to be dose dependent; it is frequently severe, especially at high doses. Patients receiving the drug should be observed closely for signs of hematologic and nonhematologic toxicity. High doses of cladribine (4–9 times the currently recommended dose for hairy cell leukemia), in conjunction with cyclophosphamide and total body irradiation as preparation for bone marrow transplantation, have been associated with severe, irreversible neurotoxicity (e.g., paraparesis/quadriparesis) and/or acute renal insufficiency in 45% of patients treated for 7–14 days. (See Cautions: Nervous System Effects and also Renal Effects.) Discontinuance or interruption of cladribine therapy should be considered in patients who experience neurotoxicity and/or renal toxicity. No specific antidote for cladribine overdosage is known. Management of overdosage consists of discontinuance of the drug, careful monitoring of the patient, and institution of appropriate supportive treatment. It is not known whether cladribine is removed from circulation by dialysis or hemofiltration.

In clinical trials involving 196 patients with hairy cell leukemia receiving currently recommended dosages of cladribine, 8 deaths occurred following treatment with the drug. Six of these deaths resulted from infectious etiology (including three pneumonias), and two occurred in the first month after therapy with the drug was initiated. Six of the deaths occurred in previously treated patients who were refractory to interferon alfa.

Hematologic function must be monitored frequently and carefully during and after cladribine therapy. Peripheral blood cell counts should be performed, particularly during the first 4–8 weeks after treatment, to detect the development of anemia, neutropenia, and thrombocytopenia and for early detection of any potential sequelae (e.g., infection, bleeding). After peripheral blood counts have returned to within normal limits, bone marrow aspiration and biopsy should be performed to confirm the response to cladribine therapy. The drug should be used with caution in patients with severe bone marrow impairment regardless of etiology.

Because fever occurs frequently during the first month of cladribine therapy, mainly in neutropenic patients, patients receiving the drug should be monitored carefully during this period. (See Cautions: Infectious Complications.) Febrile episodes should be evaluated with appropriate laboratory and radiologic studies, and empiric anti-infective therapy should be initiated as clinically indicated. Because of the myelosuppressive effects of cladribine, clinicians should weigh carefully the risks and benefits of administering the drug to patients with active infections. In addition, caution should be exercised if cladribine is administered before, after, or in conjunction with other drugs known to cause immunosuppression or myelosuppression.

Renal and hepatic function should be monitored periodically in patients treated with cladribine, especially in those with underlying renal or hepatic dysfunction and in patients receiving other potentially nephrotoxic agents. Cladribine should be used with caution in patients with known or suspected renal and/or hepatic insufficiency. (See Cautions: Renal Effects.) There are inadequate data on dosing in patients with renal or hepatic insufficiency.

The possibility of tumor lysis syndrome and hyperuricemia, which have been reported rarely in patients with large tumor burdens receiving cladribine, should be considered. Empiric therapy with allopurinol appears to reduce the risk of tumor lysis syndrome in cladribine-treated patients with active hairy cell leukemia.

Cladribine is contraindicated in patients with known hypersensitivity to the drug or any of its components.

■ **Pediatric Precautions** Safety and efficacy of cladribine in children have not been established. When cladribine was administered by continuous IV infusion at dosages of 3–10.7 mg/m^2 daily for 5 days in patients 1–21 years of age with relapsed acute leukemia, the dose-limiting toxicity was severe myelosuppression with profound neutropenia and thrombocytopenia. At the highest dosage, several patients developed irreversible myelosuppression and fatal systemic bacterial or fungal infections. No unique toxicities were reported in these patients. Children may tolerate cladribine better than adults.

Cladribine IV infusion solutions that have been prepared with bacteriostatic sodium chloride injection containing benzyl alcohol should *not* be used in neonates. Although a causal relationship has not been established, administration of injections preserved with benzyl alcohol has been associated with toxicity in neonates.

■ **Geriatric Precautions** Clinical studies of cladribine did not include sufficient numbers of patients 65 years of age and older to determine whether geriatric patients respond differently than younger patients. While other clinical experience has not revealed age-related differences in response, drug dosage generally should be titrated carefully in geriatric patients, usually initiating therapy at the low end of the dosage range. The greater frequency of decreased hepatic, renal, and/or cardiac function and of concomitant disease and drug therapy observed in the elderly also should be considered.

■ **Mutagenicity and Carcinogenicity** Like other cytotoxic agents in its class, cladribine has been shown to cause DNA damage. In vitro studies with mammalian cells demonstrated that cladribine causes the accumulation of DNA strand breaks. In addition, cladribine was incorporated into the DNA of human lymphoblastic leukemia cells. In vitro tests have not shown cladribine to be mutagenic, and the drug did not induce unscheduled DNA synthesis in primary rat hepatocyte cultures. However, cladribine was demonstrated to be clastogenic in both in vitro tests (chromosome aberrations in Chinese hamster ovary cells) and in vivo tests (mouse bone marrow micronucleus test).

Studies in animals to determine the carcinogenic potential of cladribine have not been performed to date. However, based on the demonstrated genotoxicity of the drug, the carcinogenic potential of cladribine in humans cannot be ruled out.

■ **Pregnancy, Fertility, and Lactation** Cladribine may cause fetal harm when administered to pregnant women. Although there is no evidence of teratogenicity in humans caused by cladribine, other drugs that inhibit DNA synthesis (e.g., methotrexate, aminopterin) have been reported to be teratogenic in humans, and cladribine has been shown to be teratogenic in mice and rabbits. A substantial increase in fetal variations occurred in mice receiving cladribine 1.5 mg/kg (4.5 mg/m^2) daily, and increased resorptions, reduced litter size, and increased fetal malformations occurred at a dosage of 3 mg/kg (9 mg/m^2) daily. Fetal death and malformations were observed in rabbits receiving 3 mg/kg (33 mg/m^2) daily. No fetal effects occurred in mice at a dosage of 0.5 mg/kg (1.5 mg/m^2) daily or in rabbits at a dosage of 1 mg/kg (11 mg/m^2) daily. Cladribine was embryotoxic in mice at doses equivalent to the recommended human dose. Women of childbearing potential should be advised to avoid becoming pregnant while receiving cladribine. The drug should not be used during pregnancy. When cladribine is used during pregnancy or if the patient becomes pregnant while receiving the drug, the patient should be informed of the potential hazard to the fetus.

Following IV administration in cynomolgus monkeys, cladribine has been shown to cause suppression of rapidly generating cells, including testicular cells. The effect of the drug on fertility in humans is not known.

It is not known whether cladribine is distributed into human milk. Because of the potential for serious adverse reactions to cladribine in nursing infants if the drug were distributed into milk, a decision should be made whether to discontinue nursing or the drug, taking into account the importance of the drug to the woman.

Description

Cladribine (chlorodeoxyadenosine, 2-CdA), a synthetic purine nucleoside, is an antineoplastic agent. Cladribine differs structurally from deoxyadenosine only by the presence of a chlorine atom at position 2 of the purine ring, which results in resistance to enzymatic degradation by adenosine deaminase. Because of its resistance to deamination, cladribine exhibits a more prolonged cytotoxic effect than deoxyadenosine against resting and proliferating lymphocytes.

The precise mechanism(s) of antileukemic action of cladribine has not been fully elucidated. Cladribine is phosphorylated by deoxycytidine kinase to the nucleotide cladribine triphosphate (CdATP; 2-chloro-2′-deoxyadenosine 5′-triphosphate), which accumulates and is incorporated into DNA in cells such as lymphocytes that have high levels of deoxycytidine kinase and low levels of deoxynucleotidase. High intracellular concentrations of cladribine triphosphate appear to inhibit ribonucleotide reductase, causing an imbalance in triphosphorylated deoxynucleotide (dNTP) pools and subsequent DNA strand breaks, inhibition of DNA synthesis and repair, nicotinamide adenine dinucleotide (NAD) and ATP depletion, and cell death. Incorporation of accumulated cladribine triphosphate into DNA also may contribute to DNA strand breakage and inhibition of DNA synthesis and repair. Unlike other commonly used antineoplastic drugs that affect purine and pyrimidine metabolism, cladribine has cytotoxic effects on resting as well as proliferating lymphocytes and monocytes.

SumMon® (see Users Guide). For additional information on this drug until a more detailed monograph is developed and published, the manufacturer's labeling should be consulted. It is *essential* that the labeling be consulted for detailed information on the usual cautions, precautions, and contraindications concerning potential drug interactions and/or laboratory test interferences and for information on acute toxicity. For further information on the handling of antineoplastic agents, see the ASHP Guidelines on Handling Hazardous Drugs at http://www.ahfsdruginformation.com.

Preparations

Excipients in commercially available drug preparations may have clinically important effects in some individuals; consult specific product labeling for details.

Cladribine

Parenteral

For injection concentrate, for IV infusion only	1 mg/mL*	**Cladribine for Injection Concentrate**
		Leustatin®, Janssen Biotech (formerly Centocor Ortho Biotech)

*available from one or more manufacturer, distributor, and/or repackager by generic (nonproprietary) name

†Use is not currently included in the labeling approved by the US Food and Drug Administration

Cobimetinib Fumarate

■ Cobimetinib, a potent, selective, and reversible inhibitor of mitogen-activated extracellular signal-regulated kinase (MEK) 1 and MEK2, is an antineoplastic agent.

Uses

■ **Melanoma** Cobimetinib is used in combination with vemurafenib for the treatment of unresectable or metastatic melanoma with b-Raf serine-threonine kinase (BRAF) V600E or V600K mutation. Cobimetinib has been designated an orphan drug by FDA for the treatment of this cancer. An FDA-approved diagnostic test (e.g., cobas® 4800 BRAF V600 mutation test) is required to confirm the presence of the BRAF V600E or V600K mutation prior to initiation of therapy. In patients with previously untreated, unresectable or metastatic melanoma with BRAF V600E or V600K mutation, combined therapy with cobimetinib and vemurafenib has been shown to prolong progression-free survival and increase response rate compared with vemurafenib alone.

The current indication for cobimetinib is based principally on the results of a randomized, double-blind, placebo-controlled phase 3 study (coBRIM) in patients with previously untreated, unresectable or metastatic melanoma with BRAF V600E or V600K mutation as detected by the cobas® 4800 BRAF V600 mutation test. In this study, 495 patients were randomized (stratified by disease stage and geographic region) in a 1:1 ratio to receive either cobimetinib (60 mg once daily for 21 days followed by a 7-day rest period) in combination with vemurafenib (960 mg twice daily) or placebo in combination with vemurafenib (960 mg twice daily). Treatment was continued until disease progression or unacceptable toxicity occurred or the patient withdrew from the study. Patients randomized to receive placebo were not permitted to cross over to open-label cobimetinib therapy upon disease progression. The primary end point of this study was progression-free survival as assessed by the investigator according to Response Evaluation Criteria in Solid Tumors (RECIST). The median age of patients enrolled in the study was 55 years; 93% of patients were white, 60% had stage M1c disease, 72% had a baseline ECOG performance status of 0, 45% had elevated LDH concentrations, 10% had previously received adjuvant therapy, and less than 1% of patients had previously received therapy for brain metastases. Most patients (86% of those with known mutation status) had BRAF V600E mutations. Median progression-free survival was 12.3 months in patients receiving cobimetinib and vemurafenib compared with 7.2 months in those receiving placebo and vemurafenib. A progression-free survival benefit for cobimetinib and vemurafenib was confirmed by independent blinded review. In addition, patients receiving cobimetinib and vemurafenib had higher objective response rates (70 versus 50%) compared with those receiving placebo and vemurafenib. The median duration of response in patients receiving cobimetinib and vemurafenib or receiving placebo and vemurafenib was 13 or 9.2 months, respectively. Median overall survival had not been reached at the time of the analysis. Results of a subgroup analysis (based on age, gender, disease stage, geographic region, ECOG performance status, LDH concentration, use of prior adjuvant therapy, and BRAF V600 mutation status) suggested that the drug's effect on progression-free survival was consistent across all subgroups.

Use of cobimetinib in combination with vemurafenib also was investigated in a phase 1b study in 129 patients with advanced melanoma with BRAF V600 mutation. Patients enrolled in the study were either BRAF inhibitor therapy naive (BRAF inhibitor-naive) or had experienced disease progression during prior vemurafenib therapy. At a median follow-up of 21 or 8 months for these respective subgroups, patients who were BRAF inhibitor-naive had prolonged median progression-free survival (13.8 versus 2.8 months), prolonged median overall survival (28.5 versus 8.4 months), and higher objective response rates (87 versus 15%) compared with patients who had disease progression during prior vemurafenib therapy.

Dosage and Administration

■ **General** Presence of the b-Raf serine-threonine kinase (BRAF) V600E or V600K mutation must be confirmed prior to initiation of therapy with cobimetinib in combination with vemurafenib. (See Uses: Melanoma.)

■ **Administration** Cobimetinib fumarate is administered orally without regard to meals.

■ **Dosage** Dosage of cobimetinib fumarate is expressed in terms of cobimetinib.

Melanoma For use in combination with vemurafenib in the treatment of unresectable or metastatic melanoma with BRAF V600E or V600K mutation, the recommended adult dosage of cobimetinib is 60 mg once daily for 21 days followed by a 7-day rest period; courses of therapy are given in 28-day cycles. Therapy should be continued until disease progression or unacceptable toxicity occurs.

Dosage Modification If adverse reactions occur, interruption of therapy, dosage reduction, and/or permanent discontinuance of cobimetinib should be considered. If dosage modification of cobimetinib is necessary, an initial dosage reduction to 40 mg once daily is recommended. If further dosage reduction is necessary, the dosage should be reduced to 20 mg once daily. Dosages less than 20 mg once daily are not recommended; the drug should be permanently discontinued if the 20-mg daily dosage is not tolerated.

Hemorrhage. If grade 3 hemorrhage occurs, cobimetinib therapy should be withheld for up to 4 weeks; therapy may be resumed at a reduced dosage when the toxicity improves to grade 1 or less. If the toxicity does not improve within 4 weeks of withholding cobimetinib, the drug should be permanently discontinued. (See Hemorrhage under Cautions: Warnings/Precautions.)

If grade 4 hemorrhage occurs, cobimetinib therapy should be permanently discontinued.

Cardiovascular Toxicity. If an asymptomatic absolute decrease in left ventricular ejection fraction (LVEF) from baseline of more than 10% and to a level below the lower limit of normal (LLN) occurs, cobimetinib therapy should be withheld for 2 weeks and left ventricular function should be reassessed; therapy may be resumed at a reduced dosage when LVEF recovers to at least the LLN *and* the absolute decrease in LVEF from baseline is 10% or less. (See Cardiac Effects under Cautions: Warnings/Precautions.)

If a symptomatic decrease in LVEF from baseline occurs, cobimetinib therapy should be withheld for up to 4 weeks and left ventricular function should be reassessed; therapy may be resumed at a reduced dosage when symptoms resolve, LVEF recovers to at least the LLN, *and* the absolute decrease from baseline is 10% or less.

If LVEF remains below the LLN, the absolute decrease from baseline remains above 10%, or symptoms persist, cobimetinib therapy should be permanently discontinued.

If QT-interval prolongation occurs during combination therapy with cobimetinib and vemurafenib, dosage modifications for vemurafenib may be required. (See Dosage and Administration: Dosage, in Vemurafenib 10:00.) Cobimetinib may be continued without dosage modification.

Dermatologic Effects. If intolerable grade 2 dermatologic reactions or grade 3 or 4 dermatologic reactions occur, cobimetinib therapy should be withheld or the dosage should be reduced. (See Dermatologic Effects under Cautions: Warnings/Precautions.)

Ocular Effects. If serous retinopathy occurs, cobimetinib therapy should be withheld for up to 4 weeks; therapy may be resumed at a reduced dosage when visual manifestations improve. If the toxicity does not improve or if symptoms recur within 4 weeks of resuming therapy at a reduced dosage, the drug should be permanently discontinued. (See Ocular Effects under Cautions: Warnings/Precautions.)

If retinal vein occlusion occurs, cobimetinib therapy should be permanently discontinued.

Hepatotoxicity. For the first occurrence of grade 4 liver function test abnormalities, cobimetinib therapy should be withheld for up to 4 weeks; therapy may be resumed at a reduced dosage when the toxicity improves to grade 1 or less. If liver function test abnormalities do not improve to grade 1 or less within 4 weeks of withholding therapy, the drug should be permanently discontinued. (See Hepatic Toxicity under Cautions: Warnings/Precautions.)

If grade 4 liver function test abnormalities recur, cobimetinib therapy should be permanently discontinued.

Musculoskeletal Effects. In patients who exhibit grade 4 creatine kinase (CK, creatine phosphokinase, CPK) elevations or any grade of CK elevation with concomitant myalgia, cobimetinib therapy should be withheld for up to 4 weeks; therapy may be resumed at a reduced dosage when the toxicity improves to grade 3 or less. If the toxicity does not improve within 4 weeks of withholding therapy, the drug should be permanently discontinued.

Photosensitivity Reactions. If intolerable grade 2 photosensitivity or grade 3 or 4 photosensitivity occurs, cobimetinib therapy should be withheld for up to 4 weeks; therapy may be resumed at a reduced dosage when the toxicity improves to grade 1 or less. If the toxicity does not improve within 4 weeks of withholding therapy, the drug should be permanently discontinued. (See Photosensitivity Reactions under Warnings/Precautions: Sensitivity Reactions, in Cautions.)

Development of New Primary Malignancies. No dosage adjustment is necessary in patients who develop new primary cutaneous or noncutaneous malignancies.

Other Toxicity. If an intolerable grade 2 or any grade 3 adverse reaction occurs, cobimetinib therapy should be withheld for up to 4 weeks; therapy may be resumed at a reduced dosage when the toxicity improves to grade 1 or less. If the toxicity does not improve within 4 weeks of withholding therapy, the drug should be permanently discontinued.

For the first occurrence of any grade 4 adverse reaction, cobimetinib therapy may be permanently discontinued *or* withheld; therapy may be resumed at a reduced dosage when the toxicity improves to grade 1 or less. If the grade 4 adverse reaction recurs, cobimetinib therapy should be permanently discontinued.

Concomitant Use with Drugs and Foods Affecting Hepatic Microsomal Enzymes. Concomitant use of cobimetinib with drugs that are moderate or potent inhibitors of cytochrome P-450 (CYP) isoenzyme 3A should be avoided. If concomitant short-term (14 days or less) therapy with a moderate CYP3A inhibitor cannot be avoided, the manufacturer recommends reducing the dosage of cobimetinib from 60 mg once daily to 20 mg once daily. When concomitant use of the moderate CYP3A inhibitor is discontinued, the prior cobimetinib dosage of 60 mg once daily should be resumed. In patients receiving a reduced dosage of cobimetinib (40 or 20 mg once daily), an alternative drug with no or only mild CYP3A inhibitory activity should be selected. (See Inhibitors of CYP3A under Drug Interactions: Drugs and Foods Affecting Hepatic Microsomal Enzymes.)

■ **Special Populations** No dosage adjustment is necessary in patients with mild, moderate, or severe preexisting hepatic impairment (Child-Pugh class A, B, or C). (See Hepatic Impairment under Warnings/Precautions: Specific Populations, in Cautions.)

No dosage adjustment is necessary in patients with mild or moderate renal impairment (creatinine clearance of 30–89 mL/minute). The manufacturer states that an appropriate dosage for patients with severe renal impairment has not been established. (See Renal Impairment under Warnings/Precautions: Specific Populations, in Cautions.)

The manufacturer makes no specific dosage recommendations for geriatric patients. (See Geriatric Use under Warnings/Precautions: Specific Populations, in Cautions.)

Cautions

■ **Contraindications** The manufacturer states that there are no known contraindications to the use of cobimetinib.

■ **Warnings/Precautions** ***Sensitivity Reactions*** **Photosensitivity Reactions.** Photosensitivity reactions, sometimes severe, have been reported in patients receiving cobimetinib. In the coBRIM study, photosensitivity reactions occurred in 47% of patients receiving combination therapy with cobimetinib and vemurafenib; grade 3 reactions occurred in 4% of patients receiving combined therapy. The median time to first onset of photosensitivity reactions in patients receiving combined therapy was 2 months (range: 1 day to 14 months). The median duration of photosensitivity reactions was 3 months (range: 2 days to 14 months). Most patients (63%) had resolution of photosensitivity reactions.

The manufacturer recommends that patients avoid exposure to sunlight during cobimetinib therapy. (See Advice to Patients.) Temporary interruption, dosage reduction, or discontinuance of cobimetinib may be necessary if photosensitivity reactions occur during therapy with the drug. (See Photosensitivity Reactions under Dosage: Dosage Modification, in Dosage and Administration.)

Combination Therapy When cobimetinib in used in combination with vemurafenib, the usual cautions, precautions, and contraindications associated with vemurafenib must be considered in addition to those associated with cobimetinib. For further information regarding warnings and precautions associated with vemurafenib, see Cautions: Warnings/Precautions, in Vemurafenib 10:00.

Development of New Primary Malignancies New primary cutaneous or noncutaneous malignancies have been reported in patients receiving cobimetinib.

In the coBRIM study, cutaneous squamous cell carcinoma or keratoacanthoma, basal cell carcinoma, or new primary melanoma occurred in 6, 4.5, or 0.8%, respectively, of patients receiving cobimetinib in combination with vemurafenib compared with 20, 2.4, or 2.4%, respectively, of those receiving vemurafenib alone. In this study, the median time to detection of cutaneous squamous cell carcinoma, including keratoacanthoma, or basal cell carcinoma was 4 months in patients receiving combination therapy with cobimetinib and vemurafenib. Development of new primary melanoma occurred 9 and 12 months after initiation of combination therapy with cobimetinib and vemurafenib in 2 patients.

In the coBRIM study, noncutaneous malignancies were reported in 0.8% of patients receiving cobimetinib in combination with vemurafenib compared with 1.2% of those receiving vemurafenib alone.

Although the mechanism for development of cutaneous squamous cell carcinoma has not been fully determined, it has been suggested that b-Raf serine-threonine kinase (BRAF) inhibitors (i.e., dabrafenib, encorafenib, vemurafenib) may cause paradoxical activation of mitogen-activated protein kinase (MAPK) signaling, which may lead to accelerated growth of such skin lesions as well as development of other primary malignancies. Some data suggest that mitogen-activated extracellular signal-regulated kinase (MEK) inhibitors (i.e., binimetinib, cobimetinib, trametinib) block the paradoxical activation of the MAPK pathway induced by BRAF inhibitors; therefore, combination therapy with a BRAF inhibitor and an MEK inhibitor may reduce the risk of developing cutaneous squamous cell carcinoma. Findings from a meta-analysis of randomized controlled studies that assessed the relative risk of development of cutaneous squamous cell carcinoma in cancer patients receiving a BRAF inhibitor indicate that the risk of cutaneous squamous cell carcinoma is higher in patients receiving a BRAF inhibitor than in patients receiving combination therapy with a BRAF inhibitor and an MEK inhibitor. For further information regarding the development of new primary malignancies during vemurafenib therapy, see Cautions: Development of New Primary Malignancies, in Vemurafenib 10:00.

A dermatologic evaluation should be performed at baseline and every 2 months during therapy. Monitoring should be continued for 6 months following discontinuance of cobimetinib and vemurafenib. Suspicious cutaneous lesions should be treated as appropriate and excised for pathologic evaluation. Monitoring for new noncutaneous malignancies also should be performed when cobimetinib is used in combination with vemurafenib.

Hemorrhage Hemorrhage, including major hemorrhagic events (defined as symptomatic bleeding in a critical area or organ), has been reported in patients receiving cobimetinib. In the coBRIM study, hemorrhage occurred in 13% of patients receiving cobimetinib in combination with vemurafenib compared with 7% of those receiving vemurafenib alone. Grade 3 or 4 hemorrhage was reported in 1.2% of patients receiving combination therapy compared with 0.8% of those receiving vemurafenib alone. An increased incidence of GI hemorrhage, reproductive system hemorrhage, or hematuria was observed in patients receiving combination therapy with cobimetinib and vemurafenib (3.6, 2, or 2.4%, respectively) compared with those receiving vemurafenib alone (1.2, 0.4, or 0.8%, respectively). Cerebral hemorrhage occurred in 0.8% of patients receiving combination therapy compared with none of those receiving vemurafenib alone.

Temporary interruption, dosage reduction, or discontinuance of cobimetinib may be necessary if hemorrhagic events occur during therapy with the drug. (See Hemorrhage under Dosage: Dosage Modification, in Dosage and Administration.)

Cardiac Effects Cardiomyopathy (defined as a symptomatic or asymptomatic decrease in left ventricular ejection fraction [LVEF]) has been reported in patients receiving cobimetinib. In the coBRIM study, grade 2 or 3 decreases in LVEF occurred in 26% of patients receiving combination therapy with cobimetinib and vemurafenib and in 19% of those receiving vemurafenib alone; temporary interruption and/or dosage modification or permanent discontinuance of therapy was necessary in 22 or 14%, respectively, of those with left ventricular dysfunction. The median time to first onset of left ventricular dysfunction was 4 months (range: 23 days to 13 months). Left ventricular dysfunction resolved (i.e., LVEF improved to above the lower limit of normal [LLN] or to within 10% of baseline) in 62% of patients receiving combination therapy with cobimetinib and vemurafenib; the median time to resolution was 3 months (range: 4 days to 12 months).

Safety of cobimetinib has not been established in patients with a baseline LVEF below the LLN or less than 50%.

LVEF should be assessed prior to and 1 month after initiation of cobimetinib therapy and then every 3 months during therapy. If left ventricular dysfunction occurs, temporary interruption, dosage reduction, or discontinuance of cobimetinib may be necessary; LVEF should be reassessed at approximately 2, 4, 10, and 16 weeks following reinitiation of the drug and then as clinically indicated. (See Cardiovascular Toxicity under Dosage: Dosage Modification, in Dosage and Administration.)

Dermatologic Effects Severe dermatologic reactions, sometimes requiring hospitalization, have been reported in patients receiving cobimetinib. In the coBRIM study, grade 3 or 4 rash occurred in 16% (grade 4 in 1.6%) of patients receiving combination therapy with cobimetinib and vemurafenib and in 17% (grade 4 in 0.8%) of those receiving vemurafenib alone; hospitalization was required in 3.2 or 2% of patients receiving combination therapy with cobimetinib and vemurafenib or vemurafenib alone, respectively. The median time to onset of grade 3 or 4 rash in patients receiving combination therapy with cobimetinib and vemurafenib was 11 days (range: 3 days to 2.8 months). Complete resolution occurred in 95% of patients with grade 3 or 4 rash; the median time to resolution was 21 days (range: 4 days to 17 months).

Temporary interruption, dosage reduction, or discontinuance of cobimetinib may be necessary if dermatologic reactions occur during therapy with the drug. (See Dermatologic Effects under Dosage: Dosage Modification, in Dosage and Administration.)

Ocular Effects Ocular toxicities, such as serous retinopathy, have been reported in patients receiving cobimetinib. In the coBRIM study, symptomatic or asymptomatic serous retinopathy occurred in 26% of patients receiving combination therapy with cobimetinib and vemurafenib; the most common events were chorioretinopathy and retinal detachment. The time to initial onset of serous retinopathy ranged from 2 days to 9 months and the duration ranged from 1 day to 15 months. Retinal vein occlusion occurred in one patient in each treatment group.

Ophthalmologic examinations should be performed regularly and as clinically indicated (i.e., if new or worsening visual disturbances occur) during cobimetinib therapy. Temporary interruption, dosage reduction, or discontinuance of cobimetinib may be necessary if ocular toxicities occur during therapy with the drug. (See Ocular Effects under Dosage: Dosage Modification, in Dosage and Administration.)

Hepatic Toxicity Liver function test abnormalities have been reported in patients receiving cobimetinib. In the coBRIM study, grade 3 or 4 elevations in ALT, AST, total bilirubin, or alkaline phosphatase concentrations occurred in 11, 8, 1.6, or 7%, respectively, of patients receiving combination therapy with cobimetinib and vemurafenib and in 5, 2.1, 1.2, or 3.3%, respectively, of patients receiving vemurafenib alone. Concurrent elevations in ALT (exceeding 3 times the upper limit of normal [ULN]) and total bilirubin concentrations (exceeding 2 times the ULN) with normal alkaline phosphatase concentrations (not exceeding 2 times the ULN) occurred in 1 of 247 patients (0.4%) receiving combination therapy with cobimetinib and vemurafenib and in none of those receiving vemurafenib alone.

Liver function tests should be performed prior to initiation of cobimetinib therapy and then monthly, or more frequently as clinically indicated, during therapy with the drug. Temporary interruption, dosage reduction, or discontinuance of cobimetinib may be necessary if liver function test abnormalities occur during therapy with the drug. (See Hepatotoxicity under Dosage: Dosage Modification, in Dosage and Administration.)

Musculoskeletal Effects Rhabdomyolysis has been reported in patients receiving cobimetinib. In the coBRIM study, grade 3 or 4 elevations of serum creatine kinase (CK, creatine phosphokinase, CPK), including asymptomatic elevations over baseline, occurred in 14% of patients receiving combination therapy with cobimetinib and vemurafenib and in 0.5% of patients receiving vemurafenib alone. The median time to first occurrence of grade 3 or 4 elevations in CK concentrations was 16 days (range: 12 days to 11 months) in patients receiving combination therapy with cobimetinib and vemurafenib. The median time to complete resolution of elevated CK concentrations was 15 days (range: 9 days to 11 months). Concurrent elevations in CK concentrations (exceeding 10 times the baseline value) and serum creatinine concentrations (1.5 or more times the baseline value) occurred in 3.6% of patients receiving combination therapy with cobimetinib and vemurafenib and in 0.4% of patients receiving vemurafenib alone.

Serum CK and creatinine concentrations should be evaluated at baseline, periodically during cobimetinib therapy, and as clinically indicated. Patients with elevated CK concentrations should be evaluated for manifestations of rhabdomyolysis and for other potential causes. Temporary interruption, dosage reduction, or discontinuance of cobimetinib may be necessary if increased CK concentrations occur during therapy with the drug. (See Musculoskeletal Effects under Dosage: Dosage Modification, in Dosage and Administration.)

Fetal/Neonatal Morbidity and Mortality There are no adequate and well-controlled studies of cobimetinib in pregnant women; however, based on its mechanism of action and animal findings, cobimetinib may cause fetal harm. Embryotoxicity (i.e., post-implantation loss) and teratogenicity (i.e., great vessel and eye socket abnormalities) were observed in pregnant animals receiving cobimetinib at exposure levels equivalent to 0.9–1.4 times the human exposure at the recommended dosage.

Pregnancy should be avoided during cobimetinib therapy. Women of childbearing potential should be advised to use an effective method of contraception while receiving cobimetinib and for at least 2 weeks after discontinuance of therapy. Patients should be apprised of the potential hazard to the fetus if the drug is used during pregnancy.

Impairment of Fertility Results of animal studies suggest that cobimetinib may impair female and male fertility. In a general toxicology study, degeneration of reproductive tissues was observed in female (apoptosis and necrosis of corpora lutea and vaginal epithelial cells) and male (testicular degeneration) animals receiving cobimetinib at exposure levels approximately 2 and 0.1 times, respectively, the human exposure at the recommended dosage.

Specific Populations **Pregnancy.** Cobimetinib may cause fetal harm if administered to pregnant women based on its mechanism of action and animal findings. (See Fetal/Neonatal Morbidity and Mortality under Cautions: Warnings/Precautions.)

Lactation. It is not known whether cobimetinib is distributed into milk. Because of the potential for serious adverse reactions to cobimetinib in nursing infants, women should be advised to discontinue nursing during cobimetinib therapy. Women may begin nursing 2 weeks after discontinuance of therapy. The effects of the drug on nursing infants or on the production of milk are unknown.

Pediatric Use. Safety and efficacy of cobimetinib have not been established in pediatric patients.

Mortality from unknown cause has been observed in immature rats receiving cobimetinib (exposure level on postnatal days 10–17 of approximately 0.13–0.5 times the area under the concentration-time curve [AUC] at the recommended human adult dosage).

Geriatric Use. Clinical studies of cobimetinib did not include sufficient numbers of patients 65 years of age and older to determine whether geriatric patients respond differently than younger adults.

Hepatic Impairment. Following administration of a single 10-mg dose of cobimetinib, systemic exposure to cobimetinib was similar in individuals with mild or moderate hepatic impairment and those with normal hepatic function, but systemic exposure to cobimetinib was decreased by 31% in individuals with severe hepatic impairment. Cobimetinib dosage adjustment is not necessary in patients with hepatic impairment.

Renal Impairment. Formal pharmacokinetic studies of cobimetinib have not been conducted in patients with renal impairment; however, cobimetinib undergoes minimal renal elimination.

In a population pharmacokinetic analysis, systemic exposure to cobimetinib was similar in patients with mild (creatinine clearance of 60–89 mL/minute) or moderate (creatinine clearance of 30–59 mL/minute) renal impairment compared with patients with normal renal function. Cobimetinib dosage adjustment is not necessary in patients with mild to moderate renal impairment. Cobimetinib has not been studied in patients with severe renal impairment; therefore, the manufacturer states that an appropriate dosage for these patients has not been established.

■ Common Adverse Effects

Adverse effects reported in 10% or more of patients receiving cobimetinib in combination with vemurafenib for the treatment of unresectable or metastatic melanoma with BRAF V600E or V600K mutation and at an incidence that is at least 5% higher than that reported with vemurafenib alone include diarrhea, photosensitivity reaction, nausea, pyrexia, vomiting, acneiform rash, hypertension, vision impairment, stomatitis, chorioretinopathy, hemorrhage, retinal detachment, chills, and arthralgia. Laboratory abnormalities reported in more than 10% of patients receiving cobimetinib in combination with vemurafenib include elevated concentrations of serum creatinine, elevated concentrations of CK, elevated concentrations of aminotransferases (i.e., AST, ALT), lymphopenia, elevated concentrations of alkaline phosphatase, anemia, hypophosphatemia, elevated concentrations of γ-glutamyltransferase (γ-glutamyltranspeptidase, GGT, GGTP), hypoalbuminemia, hyponatremia, hyperkalemia, hypokalemia, hypocalcemia, and thrombocytopenia.

Drug Interactions

Cobimetinib is metabolized principally by cytochrome P-450 (CYP) isoenzyme 3A and uridine diphosphate-glucuronosyltransferase (UGT) 2B7. In vitro, cobimetinib is a substrate of CYP3A and P-glycoprotein (P-gp). In vitro studies also indicate that cobimetinib may inhibit CYP isoenzymes 3A and 2D6. In vitro, cobimetinib does not inhibit CYP isoenzymes 1A2, 2B6, 2C8, 2C9, and 2C19 or induce CYP isoenzymes 1A2, 2B6, and 3A4 at clinically relevant concentrations. Cobimetinib also does not inhibit P-gp in vitro at clinically relevant concentrations.

In vitro studies indicate that cobimetinib is not a substrate or inhibitor of breast cancer resistance protein (BCRP), organic cation transporter (OCT) 1, OCT2, organic anion transport protein (OATP) 1B1, OATP1B3, organic anion transporter (OAT) 1, and OAT3 at clinically relevant concentrations.

■ Drugs and Foods Affecting Hepatic Microsomal Enzymes

Inhibitors of CYP3A Concomitant use of cobimetinib with potent or moderate inhibitors of CYP3A may result in increased systemic exposure (area under the concentration-time curve [AUC]) of cobimetinib. Concomitant administration of the potent CYP3A inhibitor itraconazole (200 mg daily for 14 days) with cobimetinib (single 10-mg dose) in healthy individuals increased the peak plasma concentration and AUC of cobimetinib by 3.2- and 6.7-fold, respectively. Simulations suggest that steady-state concentrations of cobimetinib following concomitant administration of a reduced dosage of cobimetinib (20 mg once daily) with a moderate CYP3A inhibitor for less than 14 days are similar to steady-state concentrations attained with cobimetinib alone at a dosage of 60 mg once daily.

Concomitant use of cobimetinib with potent (e.g., clarithromycin, cobicistat, grapefruit juice, itraconazole, lopinavir, nefazodone, posaconazole, ritonavir, telithromycin, voriconazole) or moderate (e.g., amiodarone, ciprofloxacin, delavirdine, diltiazem, erythromycin, fluconazole, fosamprenavir, imatinib, verapamil) inhibitors of CYP3A should be avoided. If concomitant short-term (14 days or less) therapy with a moderate CYP3A inhibitor (e.g., an anti-infective agent [e.g., erythromycin, ciprofloxacin]) cannot be avoided, the manufacturer recommends reducing the dosage of cobimetinib from 60 mg once daily to 20 mg once daily. When concomitant use of the moderate CYP3A inhibitor is discontinued, the prior cobimetinib dosage of 60 mg once daily should be resumed. In patients receiving a reduced dosage of cobimetinib (40 or 20 mg once daily), an alternative drug with no or only mild CYP3A inhibitory activity should be selected.

Inducers of CYP3A Concomitant use of cobimetinib with potent or moderate inducers of CYP3A may result in decreased systemic exposure and reduced efficacy of cobimetinib. Simulations suggest that concomitant administration of a potent or moderate CYP3A inducer and cobimetinib may decrease systemic exposure of cobimetinib by 83 or 73%, respectively.

Concomitant use of cobimetinib with potent or moderate inducers of CYP3A (e.g., carbamazepine, efavirenz, phenytoin, rifampin, St. John's wort [*Hypericum perforatum*]) should be avoided.

■ **Drugs Metabolized by Hepatic Microsomal Enzymes** Concomitant administration of cobimetinib (60 mg once daily for 15 days) with the CYP2D6 substrate dextromethorphan (single 30-mg dose) or the CYP3A substrate midazolam (single 2-mg dose) in patients with solid tumors did not substantially alter systemic exposure to dextromethorphan or midazolam.

■ **Drugs Affecting Efflux Transport Systems** Cobimetinib is a substrate of the efflux transporter P-gp. Concomitant use of cobimetinib with drugs that inhibit P-gp may result in increased concentrations of cobimetinib.

■ **Drugs Affecting Gastric Acidity** Concomitant administration of the proton-pump inhibitor rabeprazole (20 mg once daily for 5 days) with cobimetinib (single 20-mg dose) under fed and fasted conditions did not result in clinically important changes in systemic exposure of cobimetinib.

■ **Vemurafenib** Concomitant use of cobimetinib (60 mg once daily) with vemurafenib (960 mg twice daily) did not result in clinically important pharmacokinetic interactions.

Description

Cobimetinib, a potent, selective, and reversible inhibitor of mitogen-activated extracellular signal-regulated kinase (MEK) 1 and MEK2, is an antineoplastic agent. MEK proteins are upstream regulators of the extracellular signal-related kinase (ERK) pathway, which promotes cellular proliferation. Approximately 40–60% of cutaneous melanomas carry a BRAF mutation. The most common BRAF mutation is the substitution of glutamic acid for valine at codon 600 in exon 15 (BRAF V600E); a less frequently occurring BRAF mutation is the substitution of lysine for valine at codon 600 in exon 15 (BRAF V600K). BRAF V600 mutations result in activation of the BRAF pathway that includes MEK 1 and 2. The mutation of BRAF V600E activates the mitogen-activated protein kinase (MAPK) and ERK signal transduction pathway, which enhances cell proliferation and tumor progression (e.g., metastasis). Cobimetinib has demonstrated antitumor activity in mice bearing tumor xenografts that expressed BRAF V600E.

Clinical resistance to monotherapy with a BRAF inhibitor, generally occurring 6–7 months following initiation of therapy, has been attributed to several possible resistance mechanisms mostly relying on reactivation of the MAPK/ERK pathway. Complete inhibition of the MAPK/ERK pathway resulting in durable responses may be achieved with the use of combination therapy with a BRAF inhibitor (i.e., dabrafenib, encorafenib, vemurafenib) and an MEK inhibitor (i.e., binimetinib, cobimetinib, trametinib). In vitro, use of cobimetinib in combination with vemurafenib resulted in increased apoptosis and reduced tumor growth of melanoma cell lines testing positive for BRAF V600E compared with either drug alone. In addition, cobimetinib prevented vemurafenib-mediated growth enhancement of a wild-type BRAF tumor cell line in mice bearing tumor xenografts.

Following oral administration of cobimetinib in healthy individuals, the absolute bioavailability of the drug is 46%. Cobimetinib exhibits linear pharmacokinetics over a dose range of 3.5–100 mg. Following oral administration in cancer patients, median time to peak plasma concentrations of cobimetinib is 2.4 hours. Repeated administration of cobimetinib 60 mg daily resulted in a 2.4-fold mean cobimetinib accumulation ratio. Steady-state concentrations are reached within 9 days. Administration of a single 20-mg dose of cobimetinib with a high-fat meal did not affect systemic exposure (area under the serum concentration-time curve [AUC]) and peak plasma concentration of the drug in healthy individuals. Cobimetinib is highly bound (95%) to plasma proteins. Following oral administration of cobimetinib 60 mg once daily in cancer patients, the mean terminal half-life of cobimetinib was 44 hours. Cobimetinib is metabolized mainly by cytochrome P-450 (CYP) isoenzyme 3A and uridine diphosphate-glucuronosyltransferase (UGT) 2B7. Following oral administration of a single radiolabeled dose of cobimetinib, 76% of the radioactivity was recovered in feces (6.6% of the dose as unchanged drug) and 17.8% was recovered in urine (1.6% of the dose as unchanged drug).

The pharmacokinetics of cobimetinib do not appear to be affected substantially by age (19–88 years), gender, or ethnicity.

Advice to Patients

If a dose of cobimetinib is missed or vomited, importance of administering the next dose at the regularly scheduled time; an additional dose should not be administered to replace the missed or vomited dose.

Risk of new primary cutaneous malignancies. Importance of contacting a clinician promptly if dermatologic changes (e.g., new wart, skin sore or reddish bump that bleeds or does not heal, mole that changes in size or color) occur.

Risk of hemorrhage. Importance of contacting a clinician promptly and seeking immediate medical attention if signs and/or symptoms of unusual bleeding (e.g., blood in stool or urine, unusual vaginal bleeding) occur.

Risk of cardiomyopathy. Importance of cardiac monitoring before and during cobimetinib therapy. Importance of contacting a clinician promptly if manifestations of left ventricular dysfunction (e.g., shortness of breath, persistent coughing or wheezing, fatigue, peripheral edema, tachycardia) occur.

Risk of serious adverse dermatologic effects. Importance of contacting a clinician promptly if a serious reaction (e.g. rash affecting a large area, blistering or peeling of the skin) occurs.

Risk of serous retinopathy or retinal vein occlusion. Importance of contacting a clinician promptly if visual disturbances (i.e., blurred, distorted, partial, or halo vision) occur.

Risk of hepatotoxicity. Importance of liver function test monitoring before and during cobimetinib therapy. Importance of immediately reporting any possible manifestations of hepatotoxicity (e.g., jaundice, dark or tea-colored urine, nausea, vomiting, fatigue, loss of appetite).

Risk of rhabdomyolysis. Importance of monitoring creatine kinase (CK, creatine phosphokinase, CPK) concentrations before and during cobimetinib therapy. Importance of immediately reporting any possible manifestations of rhabdomyolysis (e.g., dark or red urine; muscle pain, spasms, or weakness).

Risk of photosensitivity reactions. Importance of using a broad-spectrum sunscreen and lip balm (minimum SPF of 30), wearing protective clothing, and avoiding exposure to sunlight during therapy. Importance of contacting a clinician if skin becomes red, painful, itchy, or warm; irritated; or thick, dry, or wrinkled; if bumps or small papules develop; or if a rash from sunlight exposure occurs.

Risk of fetal harm. Necessity of advising women of childbearing potential that they should use an effective method of contraception while receiving the drug and for at least 2 weeks after discontinuance of therapy. Importance of women informing clinicians if they are or plan to become pregnant. If pregnancy occurs, advise pregnant women of potential risk to the fetus.

Importance of advising women to avoid breast-feeding while receiving cobimetinib and for 2 weeks after discontinuance of therapy.

Importance of informing clinicians of existing or contemplated concomitant therapy, including prescription and OTC drugs and dietary or herbal supplements (e.g., St. John's wort), as well as any concomitant illnesses.

Importance of informing patients of other important precautionary information. (See Cautions.)

Overview® (see Users Guide). For additional information on this drug until a more detailed monograph is developed and published, the manufacturer's labeling should be consulted. It is *essential* that the manufacturer's labeling be consulted for more detailed information on usual cautions, precautions, contraindications, potential drug interactions, laboratory test interferences, and acute toxicity. For further information on the handling of antineoplastic agents, see the ASHP Guidelines on Handling Hazardous Drugs at http://www.ahfsdruginformation.com.

Preparations

Excipients in commercially available drug preparations may have clinically important effects in some individuals; consult specific product labeling for details.

Cobimetinib Fumarate

Oral

Tablets, film-coated	20 mg (of cobimetinib)	**Cotellic®**, Genentech

Crizotinib

■ Crizotinib, an inhibitor of several receptor tyrosine kinases including anaplastic lymphoma kinase (ALK), is an antineoplastic agent.

Uses

■ **Non-small Cell Lung Cancer** Crizotinib is used for the treatment of locally advanced or metastatic non-small cell lung cancer (NSCLC) in adults whose cancer is anaplastic lymphoma kinase (ALK) positive as detected by a US Food and Drug Administration (FDA)-approved companion diagnostic test. The drug has been designated an orphan drug by the FDA for use in this condition. The manufacturer states that this indication is based on overall response rate; there are currently no clinical data demonstrating an improvement in patient-reported outcomes or overall survival with the drug.

A relatively small subset of patients with NSCLC (approximately 3–7%) have ALK-positive disease, which indicates potential responsiveness to ALK inhibitor therapy (e.g., alectinib, brigatinib, ceritinib, crizotinib). Patients with this form of lung cancer typically are nonsmokers or have a history of light smoking, are female, and are younger in age and often have adenocarcinoma histology. Although crizotinib is highly active in patients with ALK-positive NSCLC, most patients treated with the drug eventually experience disease progression, limiting the drug's long-term therapeutic potential. Disease progression in patients receiving crizotinib can result from acquired resistance mutations in ALK, amplification of gene expression, activation of alternate signaling pathways, and/or progression of brain metastases (because of poor distribution of crizotinib into the CSF). (See Anaplastic Lymphoma Kinase Testing under Cautions: Warnings/Precautions and see also Description.)

The current indication for crizotinib as single-agent therapy is based on the response rates obtained in 2 multicenter, single-arm studies that enrolled a total of 255 patients with late-stage (locally advanced or metastatic), ALK-positive NSCLC. Study A (called PROFILE 1005) was a phase 2 trial conducted in 136 patients with ALK-positive NSCLC, which was identified using the Vysis ALK Break Apart FISH Probe Kit. Study B (called study 1001) was a phase 1 trial in 119 patients with ALK-positive NSCLC, which was identified using several local clinical trial assays. Most patients enrolled in both studies had received prior systemic therapy for NSCLC. Patients in both studies received 250 mg of crizotinib orally twice daily. The primary efficacy end point in both studies was the objective response rate according to Response Evaluation Criteria in Solid Tumors (RECIST); duration of response was also evaluated.

The objective response rates with crizotinib therapy were 50% in study A and 61% in study B. Response to therapy usually was rapid, with objective tumor responses achieved within 8 weeks of treatment initiation in 79 and 55% of patients in studies A and B, respectively. The median duration of response was approximately 42 and 48 weeks in studies A and B, respectively. A preliminary median progression-free survival of 10 months was estimated in study B, but median overall survival was not yet reached. In addition, a substantial reduction in NSCLC-related symptoms (e.g., dyspnea, pain, cough, fatigue, insomnia, alopecia) was observed in study A.

Two phase 3 controlled trials comparing crizotinib as single-agent therapy with standard-of-care chemotherapy (e.g., docetaxel, pemetrexed disodium either alone or in combination with cisplatin or carboplatin) are currently under way to further evaluate the drug's efficacy and safety in patients with advanced ALK-positive NSCLC. Crizotinib currently is not indicated for use in combination with other antineoplastic agents for the treatment of ALK-positive NSCLC.

Dosage and Administration

■ **General** Crizotinib can only be obtained through a limited network of specialty pharmacies. Clinicians may contact the manufacturer (Pfizer) by telephone at 877-744-5675 or consult the Xalkori® website for specific availability information (http://www.pfizerpro.com/resources/minisites/xalkori_home/docs/Specialty_Pharmacy.pdf).

Confirmation of the diagnosis of anaplastic lymphoma kinase (ALK)-positive non-small cell lung cancer (NSCLC) by an FDA-approved companion diagnostic test is necessary prior to initiating therapy with crizotinib. (See Anaplastic Lymphoma Kinase Testing under Cautions: Warnings/Precautions.)

Because crizotinib may cause hepatotoxicity and hematologic toxicity, the manufacturer states that liver function tests and complete blood cell counts (CBCs) including differential counts should be monitored monthly and as clinically indicated. More frequent repeat testing is recommended in patients with evidence of grade 2–4 (as defined by the National Cancer Institute [NCI] Common Terminology Criteria for Adverse Events [CTCAE]) hepatotoxicity, patients with grade 3 or 4 (NCI) hematologic toxicity, or if fever or infection occurs. (See Dosage Modification for Toxicity under Dosage and Administration: Dosage.)

■ **Administration** Crizotinib is administered orally twice daily without regard to meals. The capsules should be swallowed whole and should *not* be crushed, dissolved, or opened.

■ **Dosage** ***Non-small Cell Lung Cancer*** The recommended adult dosage of crizotinib for the treatment of locally advanced or metastatic NSCLC that is ALK-positive is 250 mg twice daily. Therapy should be continued for as long as the patient derives clinical benefit from the drug. The median durations of therapy in studies A and B were 22 and 32 weeks, respectively.

Dosage Modification for Toxicity Dosing interruption and/or dosage reduction of crizotinib may be necessary based on individual safety and tolerability. If dosage reduction is necessary, the dosage should be reduced to 200 mg twice daily. If further dosage reduction is necessary, the dosage should be reduced to 250 mg once daily based on individual safety and tolerability.

Hematologic Toxicity. Dosage of crizotinib should be modified based on grade 3 or 4 hematologic toxicity. However, dosage modification is not recommended for lymphopenia unless it is associated with clinical events (e.g., opportunistic infections).

If grade 3 hematologic toxicity occurs, crizotinib therapy should be withheld until the hematologic toxicity resolves to grade 2 or less, then therapy with the drug may be resumed at the same dosage schedule.

If grade 4 hematologic toxicity occurs, crizotinib therapy should be withheld until the hematologic toxicity resolves to grade 2 or less, then therapy may be resumed at a reduced dosage of 200 mg twice daily. If hematologic toxicity recurs at a dosage of 200 mg twice daily, treatment with crizotinib should be withheld until resolution to grade 2 or less, then therapy may be resumed at a further reduced dosage of 250 mg once daily. If grade 4 hematologic toxicity recurs at this dosage, crizotinib treatment should be permanently discontinued.

Hepatic Toxicity. If grade 3 or 4 elevation in serum alanine aminotransferase (ALT) or aspartate aminotransferase (AST) concentrations occurs with a total bilirubin elevation of grade 1 or less, crizotinib therapy should be withheld until the liver function test results return to grade 1 or less or to baseline values. Crizotinib therapy may then be resumed at a reduced dosage of 200 mg twice daily. If hepatotoxicity recurs at a dosage of 200 mg twice daily, therapy should be withheld again until liver function test results improve to grade 1 or less, then therapy may be resumed at a further reduced dosage of 250 mg once daily. If grade 3 or 4 hepatotoxicity subsequently recurs, treatment with crizotinib should be permanently discontinued.

If grade 2–4 elevation in ALT or AST with concurrent grade 2–4 elevation in total bilirubin concentration occurs in the absence of cholestasis or hemolysis, therapy with crizotinib should be permanently discontinued. (See Hepatic Toxicity under Cautions: Warnings/Precautions.)

Pneumonitis. If pneumonitis of any grade occurs that is not attributable to disease progression, other pulmonary disease, infection, or radiation effect, crizotinib therapy must be permanently discontinued. (See Pneumonitis under Cautions: Warnings/Precautions.)

Cardiovascular Toxicity. If grade 3 corrected QT (QT_c)-interval prolongation occurs, therapy with crizotinib should be withheld until the QT_c-interval prolongation improves to grade 1 or less. Crizotinib therapy may then be resumed at a reduced dosage of 200 mg twice daily. If grade 3 QT_c-interval prolongation recurs at a dosage of 200 mg twice daily, therapy should be withheld again until the QT_c-interval prolongation improves to grade 1 or less; therapy may then be resumed at a further reduced dosage of 250 mg once daily. If grade 3 or 4 QT_c-interval prolongation recurs at a dosage of 250 mg once daily, therapy with the drug should be permanently discontinued.

If grade 4 QT_c-interval prolongation occurs, crizotinib therapy should be permanently discontinued.

■ **Special Populations** The manufacturer does not make any specific dosage recommendations for geriatric patients. (See Geriatric Use under Warnings/Precautions: Specific Populations, in Cautions.)

Although the manufacturer does not make specific dosage recommendations for patients with preexisting hepatic impairment, increased plasma concentrations of crizotinib are likely and the drug should be used with caution in such patients. (See Hepatic Impairment under Warnings/Precautions: Specific Populations, in Cautions.)

No initial dosage adjustment is necessary in patients with mild (creatinine clearance 60–90 mL/minute) or moderate (creatinine clearance 30–60 mL/minute) renal impairment. The manufacturer states that the potential need for initial dosage adjustment in patients with severe renal impairment or end-stage renal disease cannot be determined because of very limited data in these populations. (See Renal Impairment under Warnings/Precautions: Specific Populations, in Cautions.)

Cautions

■ **Contraindications** The manufacturer states there are no known contraindications to the use of crizotinib.

■ **Warnings/Precautions** ***Hepatic Toxicity*** Drug-induced hepatotoxicity with fatal outcome has occurred; such cases were reported in less than 1% of patients in clinical trials. Concurrent elevations in alanine aminotransferase (ALT) exceeding 3 times the upper limit of normal and total bilirubin exceeding 2 times the upper limit of normal with normal alkaline phosphatase occurred in less than 1% of crizotinib-treated patients in clinical trials. ALT elevations exceeding 5 times the upper limit of normal occurred in 4–7% of patients receiving crizotinib in the 2 main clinical trials. The elevations usually occurred within the first 2 months of treatment and generally were asymptomatic and reversible upon dosage interruption.

The manufacturer states that liver function tests, including ALT and total bilirubin, should be monitored once every month and as clinically indicated. More frequent repeat testing for increased transaminases, alkaline phosphatase, or total bilirubin is necessary in patients who develop transaminase elevations during therapy. In clinical studies, patients who developed liver function test elevations usually were able to resume crizotinib therapy at a lower dosage without recurrence; however, permanent discontinuance of the drug was necessary in several patients. (See Hepatic Toxicity under Dosage: Dosage Modification for Toxicity, in Dosage and Administration.)

Pneumonitis Severe, life-threatening, or fatal pneumonitis occurred in 1.6% of patients receiving crizotinib in clinical studies. All of these cases occurred within the first 2 months of therapy. Patients receiving the drug should be monitored for pulmonary symptoms indicative of pneumonitis (see Advice to Patients), and other causes of pneumonitis should be excluded (e.g., disease progression, other pulmonary disease, infection, radiation therapy). Crizotinib should be permanently discontinued in patients who are diagnosed with treatment-related pneumonitis.

Prolongation of QT Interval Prolongation of the corrected QT (QT_c) interval has been observed in crizotinib-treated patients. The prolongation appears to occur in a plasma concentration-dependent manner. An increase in the QT_c interval (corrected for heart rate using Fridericia's formula [QT_cF]) of 60 msec or more from baseline occurred in 3.5% of patients receiving crizotinib 250 mg twice daily, and QT_cF intervals of 500 msec or more occurred in 1.3% of crizotinib-treated patients.

Crizotinib should be avoided in patients with congenital long QT syndrome. Periodic monitoring of ECGs and serum electrolytes should be considered in patients with congestive heart failure, bradyarrhythmias, or electrolyte abnormalities and in those who are receiving drugs known to prolong the QT interval.

Dosing interruption and/or dosage reduction of crizotinib is necessary when grade 3 QT_c-interval prolongation occurs. When grade 4 QT_c-interval prolongation occurs, the drug must be permanently discontinued. (See Cardiovascular Toxicity under Dosage: Dosage Modification for Toxicity, in Dosage and Administration.)

Anaplastic Lymphoma Kinase Testing Detection of anaplastic lymphoma kinase (ALK)-positive NSCLC using an FDA-approved companion diagnostic test (Vysis ALK Break Apart FISH Probe Kit from Abbott) indicated for this use is necessary for selecting patients for crizotinib therapy. Approximately 3–7% of patients with NSCLC express the ALK gene abnormality, which indicates potential responsiveness to crizotinib and other ALK inhibitors. (See Description.)

This assessment should be performed by laboratories with demonstrated proficiency in the specific technology being used. Improper assay performance may lead to unreliable results. Clinicians should refer to the FDA-approved test's package insert for instructions on the identification of patients eligible for crizotinib therapy.

Fetal/Neonatal Morbidity and Mortality Crizotinib may cause fetal harm if administered to pregnant women; the drug has been shown to be embryotoxic and fetotoxic in animals. There are no adequate and well-controlled studies in humans. Pregnancy should be avoided during therapy. Women of childbearing potential and men who are partners of such women should use adequate methods of contraception while receiving the drug and for at least 90 days after the drug is discontinued. If crizotinib is used during pregnancy or if the patient or their partner becomes pregnant during therapy, the patient should be apprised of the potential fetal hazard.

Specific Populations **Pregnancy.** Category D. (See Users Guide and see Fetal/Neonatal Morbidity and Mortality under Cautions: Warnings/Precautions.)

Lactation. It is not known whether crizotinib is distributed into human milk. Because of the potential for serious adverse reactions to crizotinib in nursing infants, a decision should be made whether to discontinue nursing or the drug, taking into account the importance of the drug to the woman.

Pediatric Use. Safety and efficacy of crizotinib have not been established in pediatric patients.

Decreased bone formation in growing long bones has been observed in immature rats receiving crizotinib for 28 days (approximately 10 times the area under the concentration-time curve [AUC] in adult patients at the recommended human dosage); other toxicities of potential concern in pediatric patients have not been evaluated to date in juvenile animal studies.

Geriatric Use. In clinical studies, 13–14% of patients receiving crizotinib were 65 years of age or older. No overall differences in safety or efficacy were observed between geriatric patients and younger adults.

Hepatic Impairment. Crizotinib has not been studied in patients with hepatic impairment. However, crizotinib is extensively metabolized in the liver and increased plasma concentrations of the drug are likely in such patients. Crizotinib should therefore be used with caution in patients with hepatic impairment. (See Dosage and Administration: Special Populations.)

Renal Impairment. A dedicated renal impairment trial for crizotinib has not been conducted to date. In study B, steady-state trough concentrations of crizotinib were similar in patients with mild (creatinine clearance 60–90 mL/minute) and moderate (creatinine clearance 30–60 mL/minute) renal impairment compared with patients with normal renal function. There are limited data in patients with severe (creatinine clearance less than 30 mL/minute) renal impairment and no data in patients with end-stage renal disease. Therefore, crizotinib should be used in caution in patients with severe renal impairment or end-stage renal disease. (See Dosage and Administration: Special Populations.)

■ **Common Adverse Effects** Adverse effects reported in 10% or more of patients receiving crizotinib include visual disturbances (including diplopia, photopsia, photophobia, blurred vision, visual field defect, visual impairment, vitreous floaters, visual brightness, and reduced visual acuity), nausea, diarrhea, vomiting, constipation, esophageal disorder, abdominal pain, stomatitis, edema (including localized edema and peripheral edema), fatigue, chest pain/discomfort, fever, upper respiratory infection, increased ALT concentrations, increased aspartate aminotransferase (AST) concentrations, decreased appetite, arthralgia, back pain, dizziness, neuropathy, headache, dysgeusia, insomnia, dyspnea, cough, and rash.

Drug Interactions

In vitro and in vivo studies suggest that crizotinib is a moderate inhibitor of cytochrome P-450 (CYP) isoenzyme 3A. In vitro studies indicate that the drug also is an inhibitor and substrate of P-glycoprotein (P-gp).

■ **Drugs Affecting Hepatic Microsomal Enzymes** ***Inhibitors of CYP3A*** Crizotinib plasma concentrations may be increased during concomitant use with potent CYP3A inhibitors (e.g., atazanavir, clarithromycin, indinavir, itraconazole, ketoconazole, nefazodone, nelfinavir, ritonavir, saquinavir, telithromycin, voriconazole); concomitant use of crizotinib with these drugs should therefore be avoided. Concurrent administration of ketoconazole (200 mg twice daily), a potent CYP3A inhibitor, and a single 150-mg dose of crizotinib resulted in increased crizotinib systemic exposure; area under the concentration-time curve (AUC) and peak plasma concentrations of crizotinib increased by approximately 3.2- and 1.4-fold, respectively, compared with crizotinib administration alone.

Caution should be exercised with concomitant use of crizotinib and moderate CYP3A inhibitors. The magnitude of effect of CYP3A inhibitors on steady-state crizotinib exposure has not been studied to date.

Inducers of CYP3A Concomitant use of crizotinib with potent inducers of CYP3A (e.g., carbamazepine, phenobarbital, phenytoin, rifabutin, rifampin) decreases plasma concentrations of crizotinib and should be avoided. Concurrent administration of rifampin (600 mg daily), a potent CYP3A inducer, and a single 250-mg dose of crizotinib decreased crizotinib AUC and peak plasma concentrations by 82 and 69%, respectively, compared with crizotinib administration alone. However, the effect of CYP3A inducers on steady-state crizotinib exposure has not been studied to date.

Use of St. John's wort (*Hypericum perforatum*), a potent CYP3A inducer, should be avoided during crizotinib therapy.

■ **Drugs Metabolized by Hepatic Microsomal Enzymes** ***Substrates of CYP3A*** Crizotinib inhibits CYP3A both in vitro and in vivo and potentially can increase plasma concentrations of other drugs metabolized by CYP3A. When the CYP3A substrate midazolam was administered concomitantly with crizotinib (250 mg twice daily for 28 days), mean oral AUC of midazolam was 3.7-fold higher compared with midazolam administration alone. Dosage reduction may be necessary for concurrently administered drugs that are predominantly metabolized by CYP3A. Concomitant use of crizotinib with CYP3A substrates that have a narrow therapeutic index (e.g., alfentanil, cyclosporine, dihydroergotamine, ergotamine, fentanyl, pimozide, quinidine, sirolimus, tacrolimus) should be avoided.

Other CYP Substrates In vitro studies indicate that clinically important pharmacokinetic interactions are not expected with concurrent use of crizotinib and drugs metabolized by CYP1A2, 2B6, 2C8, 2C9, 2C19, or 2D6.

■ **Drugs Affecting Gastric Acidity** Although formal drug interaction studies have not been conducted to date, drugs that increase gastric pH (e.g., antacids, histamine H_2-receptor antagonists, proton-pump inhibitors) may decrease the solubility of crizotinib and subsequently reduce its bioavailability.

■ **Drugs that Prolong the QT Interval** Because crizotinib has been associated with QT-interval prolongation, the manufacturer states that periodic monitoring of ECGs and electrolytes should be considered in crizotinib-treated patients concurrently receiving other drugs known to prolong the QT interval, including class IA antiarrhythmics (e.g., quinidine, procainamide), class III antiarrhythmics (e.g., amiodarone, sotalol), some antipsychotic agents (e.g., chlorpromazine, haloperidol, mesoridazine, pimozide, thioridazine), citalopram, and clarithromycin. (See Prolongation of QT Interval under Cautions: Warnings/Precautions.)

■ **Substrates of P-glycoprotein Transport Systems** Crizotinib inhibits the efflux transporter P-glycoprotein (P-gp) in vitro. If crizotinib is administered with drugs that are substrates of P-gp, increased concentrations of the P-gp substrate may result.

■ **Substrates of Organic Anion-transporting Polypeptide 1B1 and 1B3** Crizotinib did not inhibit the human hepatic uptake transport proteins OATP1B1 or OATP1B3 at therapeutic concentrations in vitro. Clinically important interactions are therefore unlikely to occur with concomitant use of crizotinib and substrates of these transporters.

■ **Grapefruit** Grapefruit products are CYP3A inhibitors and should be avoided because of the potential for increased plasma crizotinib concentrations during concurrent use.

Description

Crizotinib, an inhibitor of receptor tyrosine kinases, including anaplastic lymphoma kinase (ALK), hepatocyte growth factor receptor (HGFR, c-Met), and recepteur d'origine nantais (RON), is an antineoplastic agent. Activating mutations or translocations of the ALK gene have been identified in several malignancies and can result in the expression of oncogenic fusion proteins (e.g., echinoderm microtubule-associated protein-like 4 [EML4]-ALK). Such ALK gene rearrangements have been identified in approximately 3–7% of patients with non-small cell lung cancer (NSCLC). Formation of ALK fusion proteins such as EML4-ALK results in activation and dysregulation of the gene's expression and signaling, which can contribute to increased cell proliferation and survival in tumors expressing these proteins. In vitro, crizotinib has demonstrated concentration-dependent inhibition of ALK and c-Met phosphorylation. The drug has also demonstrated antitumor activity in mice bearing tumor xenografts that expressed EML4-ALK or nucleophosmin (NPM)-ALK fusion proteins or c-Met.

Although crizotinib has demonstrated improved outcomes in patients with

NSCLC harboring ALK mutations, secondary resistance to crizotinib eventually develops, generally within the first 1–2 years of treatment. Clinical resistance to crizotinib has been attributed to several possible mechanisms, including acquired resistance mutations of ALK, amplification of gene expression, and activation of alternate signaling pathways. Secondary mutations of ALK are responsible for about 30% of cases of acquired crizotinib resistance and gene amplification is implicated in 9% of these cases. The CNS is a common site of disease progression in crizotinib-treated patients because of poor distribution of the drug into CSF; development and/or progression of brain metastases occurs in approximately one-half of patients during crizotinib treatment.

Crizotinib is predominantly metabolized by the cytochrome P-450 (CYP) isoenzymes 3A4/5. Following oral administration of a single 250-mg radiolabeled dose of crizotinib, approximately 63% of the radioactivity was recovered in feces and 22% was recovered in urine; unchanged drug accounted for 53% of the dose recovered in feces and 2.3% of the dose recovered in urine. The mean terminal half-life of crizotinib is 42 hours. Area under the concentration-time curve (AUC) and peak plasma concentrations were reduced by approximately 14% when crizotinib was administered with a high-fat meal. (See Dosage and Administration: Administration.) Following administration of 250 mg twice daily, peak plasma concentrations and AUCs of the drug were 1.57- and 1.5-fold higher, respectively, in Asian patients compared with non-Asian patients; body size may play a role in this observed pharmacokinetic difference.

Advice to Patients

Importance of instructing patients to read the manufacturer's patient information before starting crizotinib therapy and each time their prescription is refilled.

Importance of anaplastic lymphoma kinase (ALK) testing for therapy with crizotinib.

Importance of advising patients to take crizotinib exactly as prescribed and of not altering the dosage or discontinuing the therapy unless advised to do so by their clinician. Importance of advising patients to swallow crizotinib capsules whole and not to crush, dissolve, or open the capsules.

If a dose is missed, importance of advising patients to take it as soon as they remember unless it is less than 6 hours before the next dose, in which case they should not take the missed dose. Patients should be informed to not take 2 doses at the same time to make up for a missed dose.

Importance of advising patients to avoid grapefruit and grapefruit juice while taking crizotinib.

Risk of fetal harm. Necessity of advising women of childbearing potential and men who are partners of such women that they should use adequate methods of contraception while receiving the drug and for at least 90 days after the drug is discontinued. Importance of patients informing their clinicians if they or their partners are pregnant or think they may be pregnant. If pregnancy occurs, advise patient of potential risk to fetus.

Importance of advising women to avoid breast-feeding while receiving crizotinib therapy.

Risk of hepatotoxicity; importance of liver function test monitoring. Importance of advising patients to immediately report possible symptoms of hepatotoxicity (e.g., weakness, fatigue, anorexia, nausea, vomiting, abdominal pain [especially right upper quadrant pain], jaundice, dark urine, generalized pruritus, bleeding diathesis), particularly in combination with fever and rash, to their clinician.

Importance of informing patients that nausea, vomiting, diarrhea, and constipation are the most common adverse GI effects associated with crizotinib therapy, and that treatment with antiemetic and/or antidiarrheal agents or laxatives may be necessary.

Risk of pneumonitis. Importance of advising patients that pneumonitis symptoms may be similar to those of lung cancer and to contact their clinician immediately if they experience any new or worsening pulmonary symptoms (e.g., dyspnea, shortness of breath, cough with or without mucus, fever).

Risk of QT-interval prolongation. Importance of informing clinicians immediately if an abnormal heartbeat or feelings of dizziness or faintness occur.

Importance of informing patients that visual changes such as perceived flashes of light, blurred vision, photosensitivity, and floaters commonly occur during crizotinib therapy, usually during the first 2 weeks of treatment. Importance of advising patients to report flashes or floaters to their clinicians.

Although the effect of crizotinib on the ability to drive and use machinery has not yet been studied, importance of advising patients experiencing visual changes, dizziness, or fatigue to exercise caution when driving or operating machinery.

Importance of informing clinicians of existing or contemplated concomitant therapy, including prescription and OTC drugs and herbal supplements (e.g., St. John's wort), as well as any concomitant illnesses (e.g., hepatic or renal impairment, cardiovascular disease [including congenital long QT syndrome]).

Importance of informing patients of other important precautionary information. (See Cautions.)

Overview® (see Users Guide). For additional information on this drug until a more detailed monograph is developed and published, the manufacturer's labeling should be consulted. It is *essential* that the manufacturer's labeling be consulted for more detailed information on usual cautions, precautions, contraindications, potential drug interactions, laboratory test interferences, and acute toxicity. For further information on the handling of antineoplastic agents, see the ASHP Guidelines on Handling Hazardous Drugs at http://www.ahfsdruginformation.com.

Preparations

Excipients in commercially available drug preparations may have clinically important effects in some individuals; consult specific product labeling for details.

Crizotinib

Oral

Capsules	200 mg	**Xalkori®**, Pfizer
	250 mg	**Xalkori®**, Pfizer

Cyclophosphamide

CPM, CTX, CYT

■ Cyclophosphamide, a nitrogen mustard-derivative, polyfunctional alkylating agent, is an antineoplastic agent and immunosuppressant.

Uses

■ **Hodgkin's Disease** Cyclophosphamide is used in combination regimens (e.g., bleomycin, etoposide, doxorubicin, cyclophosphamide, vincristine, procarbazine, and prednisone [BEACOPP]) for the treatment of Hodgkin's disease.

■ **Non-Hodgkin's Lymphoma** Cyclophosphamide is used in combination therapy for the treatment of non-Hodgkin's lymphoma, including high-grade lymphomas, such as Burkitt's lymphoma and lymphoblastic lymphoma, as well as intermediate- and low-grade lymphomas. For example, cyclophosphamide is commonly used with doxorubicin, vincristine, and prednisone (known as the CHOP regimen), with or without other agents, in the treatment of various types of intermediate-grade non-Hodgkin's lymphoma. Cyclophosphamide also has been used as a single agent in the treatment of low-grade lymphomas.

■ **Multiple Myeloma** Cyclophosphamide is used in combination with prednisone, or as a component of combination chemotherapy (i.e., vincristine, carmustine, melphalan, cyclophosphamide, and prednisone [VBMCP]) for the treatment of multiple myeloma. Comparative studies have shown the effectiveness of cyclophosphamide in the treatment of multiple myeloma to be equivalent to that of melphalan, and the combination of either agent with prednisone is considered a treatment of choice. Some authorities prefer melphalan to cyclophosphamide because of the lesser severity of adverse effects; in the presence of severe thrombocytopenia, others prefer cyclophosphamide because of its relative platelet-sparing effect.

Use of cyclophosphamide in combination with bortezomib and dexamethasone (bortezomib-cyclophosphamide-dexamethasone) as induction therapy for newly diagnosed multiple myeloma in transplant-eligible patients may be considered a reasonable choice (accepted, with possible conditions) based on current evidence from 2 noncomparative phase 2 studies and an open-label, randomized phase 3 study (GMMG-MM5); factors that should be considered when selecting a combination chemotherapy regimen for use as induction therapy include cytogenetic features, performance status, preexisting conditions (e.g., peripheral neuropathy), and tolerability.

In the first phase 2 study, the overall response rate and rate of very good partial response or better after 4 cycles of therapy were 88 and 61%, respectively, in the study group (cohort of 33 patients with newly diagnosed multiple myeloma who received cyclophosphamide in combination with bortezomib [twice weekly] and dexamethasone) compared with 91 and 44%, respectively, in a historical control group (34 patients who received lenalidomide and dexamethasone). Among patients who underwent stem cell transplantation following bortezomib-cyclophosphamide-dexamethasone induction therapy, the post-transplant complete or near-complete response rate was 70%. A subsequent cohort of 30 patients who received cyclophosphamide with bortezomib (once weekly) and dexamethasone achieved similar overall response rates and rates of very good partial response or better (93 and 60%, respectively). Median progression-free survival for the 2 cohorts combined was 40 months, and 5-year progression-free and overall survival rates for the 2 cohorts were 42 and 70%, respectively. Although the overall response rate was similar in patients with high-risk cytogenetic features and those with standard-risk cytogenetic features, median progression-free survival was shorter and 5-year progression-free and overall survival rates were lower in patients with high-risk cytogenetic features (27.6 months, 33%, and 54%, respectively) compared with those with standard-risk cytogenetic features (55.7 months, 48%, and 81%, respectively).

In another phase 2 study in 44 patients with newly diagnosed multiple myeloma who received 3 cycles of bortezomib-cyclophosphamide-dexamethasone followed by 3 cycles of bortezomib-thalidomide-dexamethasone, very good partial response or better was observed in 31 or 57% of 42 evaluable patients following 3 or 6 treatment cycles, respectively; near-complete response or better was observed following 3 or 6 cycles in 2 or 36% of patients, respectively. At a median follow-up of 20.9 months, estimated 1-year event-free and overall survival rates were 81 and 91%, respectively.

In the GMMG-MM5 study in 502 patients with newly diagnosed multiple myeloma, rates of overall response (78.1 versus 72.1%, respectively) and very good partial response or better (37 versus 34.3%, respectively) did not differ significantly between patients receiving bortezomib-cyclophosphamide-dexamethasone and those receiving bortezomib-doxorubicin-dexamethasone. In subgroups of patients with poor prognostic factors (i.e., t(4;14) translocation, chromosome 17p deletion [del(17p)], and/or chromosome 1q21 duplication [1q21 gain]; renal impairment), response rates attained with bortezomib-cyclophosphamide-dexamethasone appeared to be at least as high as those attained with bortezomib-doxorubicin-dexamethasone; the rate of progressive disease in patients with high-risk cytogenetic features, International Staging System (ISS) stage III disease, or renal impairment appeared to be higher in those receiving bortezomib-doxorubicin-dexamethasone compared with those receiving bortezomib-cyclophosphamide-dexamethasone.

For further information on the use of combination therapy with cyclophosphamide, bortezomib, and dexamethasone as induction therapy for newly diagnosed multiple myeloma in transplant-eligible patients, see Induction Therapy Prior to Stem Cell Transplantation in Newly Diagnosed Multiple Myeloma under Uses: Multiple Myeloma, in Bortezomib 10:00.

■ **Leukemias** In the treatment of chronic lymphocytic (lymphoblastic) leukemia, cyclophosphamide is considered one of the drugs of choice. Cyclophosphamide is used in combination with busulfan as a conditioning regimen prior to allogeneic hematopoietic progenitor cell transplantation in patients with chronic myelogenous leukemia.

Cyclophosphamide is used in the treatment of acute lymphoblastic leukemia, especially in children.

In the treatment of acute myeloid (myelogenous, nonlymphocytic) leukemia (AML, ANLL), cyclophosphamide has been used as an additional drug for induction or post induction therapy.

Although cyclophosphamide and its metabolites appear in the brain and CSF, concentrations are probably insufficient to treat meningeal leukemia.

■ **Cutaneous T-cell Lymphoma** Cyclophosphamide is used alone or in combination regimens for the treatment of advanced mycosis fungoides, a form of cutaneous T-cell lymphoma.

■ **Neuroblastoma** In the treatment of disseminated neuroblastoma, cyclophosphamide used alone has been reported to produce objective responses in up to 65% of patients; used in combinations, the response rate and duration of survival may increase. Combination chemotherapy that includes cyclophosphamide is a treatment of choice for this neoplasm.

■ **Ovarian Cancer** Cyclophosphamide is used in combination chemotherapy (vincristine, dactinomycin, and cyclophosphamide [VAC]) as an alternative regimen for the treatment of ovarian germ cell tumors†.

Although cyclophosphamide has been used in combination with a platinum-containing agent for the treatment of advanced (stage III or IV) epithelial ovarian cancer, evidence from randomized trials indicates that combined therapy with paclitaxel and a platinum-containing agent is superior (higher response rates, prolonged overall survival) and therefore is the preferred regimen. (See Uses: Ovarian Cancer, in Carboplatin 10:00 and Cisplatin 10:00.)

■ **Retinoblastoma** Cyclophosphamide is used in combination therapy for the treatment of retinoblastoma.

■ **Breast Cancer** In the treatment of breast cancer, cyclophosphamide used alone has been reported to produce objective responses in about 35% of patients. Used in combination regimens, objective responses have been reported in up to 90% of patients, and cyclophosphamide-containing combinations are believed by some experts to be the treatment of choice.

Combination chemotherapy used as an adjunct to surgery has been shown to increase both disease-free (i.e., decreased recurrence) and overall survival in premenopausal and postmenopausal women with node-negative or -positive early (TNM stage I or II) breast cancer. Adjuvant combination chemotherapy has produced overall reductions in the annual rates of recurrence and death of 28 and 16%, respectively, with overall 5-year disease-free survival rates of 58.8 versus 49.6% for patients receiving combination chemotherapy versus those who did not. Adjuvant combination chemotherapy that includes cyclophosphamide, methotrexate, and fluorouracil has been used extensively and is considered a regimen of choice. Although adjuvant hormonal therapy with tamoxifen (with or without combination chemotherapy) generally is used for node-positive, estrogen-receptor-positive postmenopausal women, adjuvant combination chemotherapy (with or without tamoxifen) also can be used in such patients, but differences in toxicity profiles may influence the choice of regimen. For node-positive premenopausal women, adjuvant combination chemotherapy (with or without tamoxifen) generally is used. Adjuvant therapy with combination chemotherapy and/or tamoxifen has been used in women with node-negative disease.

Controversy currently exists regarding which patients with node-negative and estrogen-receptor-negative breast cancer are most likely to benefit from such adjuvant therapy following surgery (see Uses: Breast Cancer, in Fluorouracil 10:00), but such patients with poor prognosis are reasonable candidates for adjuvant chemotherapy with an effective regimen (e.g., 6–12 months of cyclophosphamide, methotrexate, and fluorouracil initiated within 6 weeks of surgery); other node-negative patients also may be suitable candidates, but toxicities, costs, and other quality-of-life considerations should be weighed in assessing potential benefit. All patients with node-negative breast cancer are at some risk of recurrence, and effective adjuvant combination chemotherapy can increase both disease-free and overall survival, albeit less markedly than in patients with node-positive disease.

In patients with node-positive early breast cancer (i.e., stage II), an effective regimen of adjuvant combination chemotherapy (e.g., cyclophosphamide, methotrexate, and fluorouracil; cyclophosphamide, doxorubicin, and fluorouracil; cyclophosphamide and doxorubicin with or without tamoxifen) is used to reduce the rate of recurrence and improve survival in both premenopausal and postmenopausal patients once treatment to control local disease (surgery, with or without radiation therapy) has been undertaken. These combinations have been tested and established as providing therapeutic benefit, and are superior to single-agent therapy with conventional agents; numerous other combination regimens providing apparently similar outcomes also have been used but are less common or have been studied less extensively. Although long-term (e.g., 6 months or longer) chemotherapy with adjuvant regimens is clinically superior to short-term (e.g., preoperative and perioperative) adjuvant regimens, clinical superiority between 6- versus 12-month regimens has not been demonstrated. There is some evidence that the addition of doxorubicin to a regimen of cyclophosphamide, methotrexate, and fluorouracil can improve outcome further in patients with more than 3 positive axillary lymph nodes, and that sequential (i.e., administering several courses of doxorubicin first) regimens are more effective than alternating regimens in such patients; in patients with fewer positive nodes, no additional benefit from doxorubicin has been demonstrated. The dose intensity of adjuvant combination chemotherapy also appears to be an important factor influencing clinical outcome in patients with early node-positive breast cancer, with response increasing with increasing dose intensity; therefore, arbitrary reductions in dose intensity should be avoided.

In stage III (locally advanced) breast cancer, combination chemotherapy (with or without hormonal therapy) is used sequentially following surgery and radiation therapy for operable disease and following biopsy and radiation therapy for inoperable disease; commonly employed effective regimens include cyclophosphamide, methotrexate, and fluorouracil; cyclophosphamide, doxorubicin, and fluorouracil; and cyclophosphamide, methotrexate, fluorouracil, and prednisone. These and other regimens also have been used in the treatment or more advanced (stage IV) and recurrent disease.

■ **Small Cell Lung Cancer** Cyclophosphamide is used in combination chemotherapy regimens (e.g., cyclophosphamide, doxorubicin, and vincristine [CAV]; cyclophosphamide, doxorubicin, and etoposide [CAE]) for the treatment of extensive-stage small cell lung cancer†. Survival outcomes are similar in patients with extensive-stage small cell lung cancer receiving CAV or cisplatin/etoposide. Combination chemotherapy regimens have produced response rates of 70–85% and complete response rates of 20–30% in patients with extensive-stage disease; however, comparative efficacy is continually being evaluated. Because the current prognosis for small cell lung cancer is unsatisfactory regardless of stage and despite considerable diagnostic and therapeutic advances, all patients with this cancer are candidates for inclusion in clinical trials at the time of diagnosis.

■ **Sarcomas** Cyclophosphamide has been used in combination regimens (usually with dactinomycin and vincristine) and as an adjunct to surgery and radiation therapy in the treatment of rhabdomyosarcoma†. In children in groups I and II, 2-year relapse-free survival rates of 80–90% have been reported. Intensive regimens of dactinomycin, cyclophosphamide, and vincristine (with or without doxorubicin) followed by radiation therapy have produced an objective response in 80% of patients having residual tumor following surgery (group III) or with metastatic tumor (group IV). Cyclophosphamide used in combination regimens as an adjunct to surgery and radiation therapy is considered one of the treatments of choice for Ewing's sarcoma†.

■ **Other Uses** Cyclophosphamide is used in selected cases of biopsy-proven minimal change nephrotic syndrome in children; the drug should not be used as initial therapy in such patients. Cyclophosphamide has induced remission in patients whose disease has not responded to appropriate corticosteroid therapy or in whom such therapy produces intolerable adverse effects (e.g., growth failure).

Cyclophosphamide is used in combination with vincristine and dacarbazine for the treatment of pheochromocytoma†. Cyclophosphamide also is used in the treatment of brain tumors†, choriocarcinoma†, and Wilms' tumor†.

As an immunosuppressant, cyclophosphamide has been used to control rejection following kidney, heart, liver, and bone marrow transplants†. Some experts consider cyclophosphamide as effective as azathioprine for the maintenance of renal allografts and superior to azathioprine for the maintenance of hepatic allografts. Cyclophosphamide has also been used with some success in the treatment of severe, active and progressive rheumatoid disorders†. In the treatment of glomerulonephritis,† especially in children, cyclophosphamide alone or in conjunction with corticosteroids has been useful. Other disorders of altered immune reactivity in which cyclophosphamide has been used with some success include Wegener's granulomatosis†, idiopathic pulmonary hemosiderosis†, myasthenia gravis†, multiple sclerosis†, polymyositis†, pyoderma gangrenosum†, bullous pemphigoid†, pemphigus vulgaris†, autoallergic ocular disease†, uveitis†, orbital pseudotumor†, scleromalacia perforans†, thyroid exophthalmopathy†, corneal transplant rejection†, systemic lupus erythematosus†, lupus nephritis†, autoimmune hemolytic anemia†, idiopathic thrombocytic purpura†, macroglobulinemia†, cryoglobulinemia†, and antibody-induced pure red cell aplasia†. The drug has also been used for the treatment of bleeding syndromes in patients with acquired antibodies to clotting factors†. Because of the potential for serious adverse effects, cyclophosphamide must be used as an immunosuppressant† with caution, and some experts advocate reserving use of cyclophosphamide for patients who become refractory to corticosteroids or other less toxic agents, or limiting it to short-term use whenever feasible.

Dosage and Administration

■ **Reconstitution and Administration** Cyclophosphamide is administered orally or by IV injection or infusion. Less frequently, the drug has been administered IM and by intracavitary (e.g., intrapleural, intraperitoneal) injection and direct perfusion, but some experts believe the drug should not be administered via routes which bypass activation in the liver.

The choice of diluent for reconstituting cyclophosphamide powder for injection containing cyclophosphamide monohydrate depends on the route of administration to be used. If the solution is to be used for direct injection, cyclophosphamide powder for injection (containing cyclophosphamide monohydrate) is reconstituted by adding 0.9% sterile sodium chloride solution. If the solution is to be used for IV infusion, cyclophosphamide powder for injection (containing cyclophosphamide monohydrate) is reconstituted by adding sterile water for injection. Cyclophosphamide powder for injection (containing cyclophosphamide monohydrate) reconstituted in water is *hypotonic* and should *not* be injected directly. Cyclophosphamide powder for injection (containing cyclophosphamide monohydrate) is reconstituted by adding 25 mL of diluent to the vial labeled as containing 500 mg, 50 mL to the vial labeled as containing 1 g, or 100 mL to the vial labeled as containing 2 g. After adding the diluent to the vial, the vial should be shaken vigorously to dissolve the drug. If the powder fails to dissolve immediately and completely, the vial should be allowed to stand for a few minutes.

Reconstituted solutions of cyclophosphamide to be used for IV infusion may be diluted in one of the following compatible solutions: 5% dextrose injection, 5% dextrose and 0.9% sodium chloride injection, 5% dextrose and Ringer's injection, lactated Ringer's injection, 0.45% sodium chloride injection, or ⅙ *M* sodium lactate injection.

Cyclophosphamide solutions should be inspected visually for particulate matter and discoloration prior to administration whenever solution and container permit.

Extemporaneous liquid preparations of the drug for oral administration may be prepared by dissolving cyclophosphamide powder for injection in aromatic elixir. The manufacturer states that such solutions should be stored under refrigeration in glass containers and used within 14 days.

■ **Dosage** Because of the risk of certain toxicities (e.g., cardiotoxicity) and overdosage with high doses of cyclophosphamide, particular care should be taken to ensure that correct dosages and administration schedules have been prescribed and appropriate monitoring instituted when higher than usual dosages (e.g., those employed under protocol conditions) are encountered.

Clinicians should consult published protocols for the dosage of cyclophosphamide and other chemotherapeutic agents in combination regimens and the method and sequence of administration.

General Dosage The manufacturers state that, in patients with no hematologic deficiencies receiving cyclophosphamide monotherapy, induction therapy in adults and children is usually initiated with an IV cyclophosphamide loading dose of 40–50 mg/kg administered in divided doses over 2–5 days. Other regimens for IV administration include 10–15 mg/kg every 7–10 days or 3–5 mg/kg twice weekly.

If cyclophosphamide is administered orally, the usual dose for induction or maintenance therapy is 1–5 mg/kg daily, depending on the tolerance of the patient.

Various other regimens for IV or oral cyclophosphamide have been reported. Dosage of cyclophosphamide must be adjusted according to tumor response and/or leukopenia. The total leukocyte count is used as a guide for regulating cyclophosphamide dosage. Transient decreases in the total leukocyte count to 2000/mm^3 (following short courses of therapy) or more persistent reduction to 3000/mm^3 (with continuing therapy) may be tolerated without serious risk of infection if there is no marked granulocytopenia.

When cyclophosphamide is included in combination regimens with other cytotoxic agents, dosage reduction for cyclophosphamide as well as for the other agents may be necessary.

Breast Cancer Various cyclophosphamide-containing combination chemotherapy regimens have been used in the treatment of breast cancer, and published protocols should be consulted for dosages and the method and sequence of administration. The dose intensity of adjuvant combination chemotherapy appears to be an important factor influencing clinical outcome in patients with early node-positive breast cancer, with response increasing with increasing dose intensity; therefore, *arbitrary* reductions in dose intensity should be avoided.

One commonly employed regimen for the treatment of early breast cancer includes a cyclophosphamide dosage of 100 mg/m^2 orally on days 1 through 14 of each cycle combined with methotrexate 40 mg/m^2 IV on days 1 and 8 of each cycle and fluorouracil 600 mg/m^2 IV on days 1 and 8 of each cycle. In patients older than 60 years of age, the initial methotrexate dosage was reduced to 30 mg/m^2 IV and the initial fluorouracil dosage was reduced to 400 mg/m^2 IV. Dosage also was reduced if myelosuppression developed. Cycles generally were repeated monthly (i.e., allowing a 2-week rest period between cycles) for a total of 6–12 cycles (i.e., 6–12 months of therapy). Clinical superiority between 6- versus 12-month regimens has not been demonstrated.

There is some evidence that the addition of doxorubicin to a regimen of cyclophosphamide, methotrexate, and fluorouracil can improve outcome further in patients with early breast cancer and more than 3 positive axillary lymph nodes, and that sequential (i.e., administering several courses of doxorubicin first) regimens are more effective than alternating regimens in such patients; in patients with fewer positive nodes, no additional benefit from doxorubicin has been demonstrated. In the sequential regimen, 4 doses of doxorubicin hydrochloride 75 mg/m^2 IV were administered initially at 3-week intervals followed by 8 cycles of cyclophosphamide 600 mg/m^2 IV, methotrexate 40 mg/m^2 IV, and fluorouracil 600 mg/m^2 IV at 3-week intervals for a total of approximately 9 months of therapy. If myelosuppression developed with this sequential regimen, the subsequent cycle generally was delayed rather than reducing dosage.

Nephrotic Syndrome In the treatment of minimal change nephrotic syndrome in children, an oral dosage of 2.5–3 mg/kg daily for 60–90 days has been recommended. In males, treatment for longer than 60 days increases the incidence of oligospermia and azoospermia; treatment for longer than 90 days increases the risk of sterility. Corticosteroid therapy may be tapered and discontinued during the course of cyclophosphamide therapy.

Multiple Myeloma Cyclophosphamide has been used in several regimens in combination with bortezomib and dexamethasone as induction therapy for newly diagnosed multiple myeloma in transplant-eligible patients.

When cyclophosphamide has been used in combination with bortezomib and dexamethasone as induction therapy for newly diagnosed multiple myeloma in transplant-eligible patients, cyclophosphamide 300 mg/m^2 has been administered orally on days 1, 8, 15, and 22 along with bortezomib 1.3 mg/m^2 by IV injection twice weekly for 2 weeks (days 1, 4, 8, and 11) and dexamethasone 40 mg orally on days 1–4, 9–12, and 17–20 of each 28-day cycle for 4 cycles.

Cyclophosphamide 300 mg/m^2 also has been administered orally on days 1, 8, 15, and 22 along with bortezomib 1.5 mg/m^2 by IV injection once weekly (days 1, 8, 15, and 22) during each 28-day cycle for 4 cycles. In this regimen, dexamethasone 40 mg has been administered orally on days 1–4, 9–12, and 17–20 during cycles 1 and 2 and then once weekly during cycles 3 and 4.

Cyclophosphamide 300 mg/m^2 also has been administered IV on days 1 and 8 along with bortezomib 1.3 mg/m^2 by IV injection twice weekly for 2 weeks (days 1, 4, 8, and 11) and dexamethasone 40 mg orally on days 1, 2, 4, 5, 8, 9, 11, and 12 of each 21-day cycle for 3 cycles (cycles 1–3) followed by bortezomib 1 mg/m^2 by IV injection twice weekly for 2 weeks (days 1, 4, 8, and 11) along with thalidomide 100 mg orally daily and dexamethasone 40 mg orally on days 1, 2, 4, 5, 8, 9, 11, and 12 of each 21-day cycle for 3 cycles (cycles 4–6).

Cyclophosphamide 900 mg/m^2 also has been administered IV on day 1 along with bortezomib 1.3 mg/m^2 by subcutaneous or IV injection twice weekly for 2 weeks (days 1, 4, 8, and 11) and dexamethasone 40 mg orally on days 1, 2, 4, 5, 8, 9, 11, and 12 of each 21-day cycle for 3 cycles.

■ **Dosage in Renal and Hepatic Impairment** The effects of renal or hepatic impairment on the elimination of cyclophosphamide have not been elucidated. The manufacturers recommend caution and careful monitoring for toxicity in patients with renal and/or hepatic impairment, but makes no specific recommendations for adjustment of cyclophosphamide dosage. Measurable changes in pharmacokinetic parameters for cyclophosphamide may be observed in patients with renal impairment, but there is no consistent evidence demonstrating the need for dosage adjustment.

Cautions

■ **Hematologic Effects** One of the major and dose-limiting adverse effects of cyclophosphamide is hematologic toxicity, which is usually reversible after discontinuance of the drug. Hematopoietic adverse effects include leukopenia, thrombocytopenia, hypothrombinemia, and anemia. Leukopenia is considered to be an expected effect of cyclophosphamide therapy and may be severe. Leukopenia nadirs generally occur at 8–15 days following a single dose of cyclophosphamide and recovery usually occurs within 17–28 days. Fever in the absence of documented infection has been reported in some patients with neutropenia. Thrombocytopenia reportedly is less common, with nadirs occurring 10–15 days after administration of the drug. Anemia, particularly after large doses or prolonged therapy, and rarely, hypoprothrombinemia have been reported. Rarely, cyclophosphamide has been reported to produce positive direct antiglobulin (Coombs') test results and hemolytic anemia.

■ **GI and Hepatic Effects** Anorexia, nausea, and vomiting occur commonly with cyclophosphamide, especially at high doses; some clinicians reported that these effects respond to treatment with antiemetics. Occasionally, diarrhea, hemorrhagic colitis, mucosal irritation, and oral ulceration have been reported. Rarely, aphthous stomatitis, enterocolitis, and hepatotoxicity as evidenced by jaundice and hepatic dysfunction have occurred.

■ **Genitourinary Effects** Sterile hemorrhagic cystitis has been reported to occur in up to 20% of patients (especially children) on long-term cyclophosphamide therapy. This effect, which rarely can be severe and even fatal, is attributed to chemical irritation by active metabolites of cyclophosphamide that accumulate in concentrated urine. Hematuria usually resolves spontaneously within a few days after discontinuance of cyclophosphamide therapy but may persist for several months. Fibrosis of the bladder (sometimes extensive), with or without cystitis, also has occurred, but less frequently. Atypical epithelial cells may be found in the urinary sediment. These adverse effects appear to be related to the dosage and duration of cyclophosphamide therapy. Nephrotoxicity, including hemorrhagic ureteritis and renal tubular necrosis, has been reported; such lesions reportedly resolve in most instances following discontinuance of cyclophosphamide therapy.

Although the incidence of hemorrhagic cystitis associated with cyclophosphamide therapy appears to be lower than that associated with ifosfamide therapy, mesna (sodium 2-mercaptoethanesulfonate) has been used prophylactically as a uroprotective agent in some patients receiving cyclophosphamide. (See Drug Interactions: Mesna.) Evidence from animal and clinical studies suggests that prophylactic mesna therapy, when used concomitantly with cyclophosphamide, can substantially decrease the incidence and severity of, or prevent, cyclophosphamide-induced urothelial toxicity (e.g., hemorrhagic cystitis). Mesna also has uroprotective activity in preventing or ameliorating recurrent or worsening bladder toxicity during subsequent cyclophosphamide therapy in patients with a history of such toxicity induced by the drug or other oxazaphosphorine derivatives (e.g., ifosfamide). Clinical studies indicate that mesna generally is more effective than, but at least as effective as, standard prophylactic measures (e.g., forced diuresis, hydration) in preventing bladder toxicity (e.g., hematuria, hemorrhagic cystitis) commonly associated with cyclophosphamide therapy, although prophylactic mesna therapy is not effective in all patients.

■ **Dermatologic Effects** Alopecia occurs frequently in patients who receive cyclophosphamide, and patients should be forewarned of this possibility. In usual doses, about 33% of patients who receive the drug experience alopecia, generally beginning about 3 weeks after initiation of therapy; the condition is usually reversible, but new hair may be a different color or texture. Transverse ridging, retarded growth, and/or pigmentation of fingernails may occur, as well as skin pigmentation. Nonspecific dermatitis has also been reported.

Stevens-Johnson syndrome and toxic epidermal necrolysis have been reported rarely in patients receiving cyclophosphamide; a causal relationship to the drug has not been established.

■ **Respiratory Effects** Patients who receive high doses of cyclophosphamide over prolonged periods may develop interstitial pulmonary fibrosis, which can be fatal. In some cases, discontinuance of the drug and administration of corticosteroids has failed to reverse this syndrome. Interstitial pneumonitis also has been reported in patients receiving cyclophosphamide.

■ **Metabolic Effects** As a result of extensive purine catabolism accompanying rapid cellular destruction, hyperuricemia may occur in some patients receiving cyclophosphamide, especially those with non-Hodgkin's lymphomas or leukemias. Hyperuricemia may be minimized by adequate hydration, alkalinization of the urine, and/or administration of allopurinol. If allopurinol is administered, the patient should be watched carefully for cyclophosphamide toxicity. (See Drug Interactions: Drugs Affecting Hepatic Microsomal Enzymes.) Hyperkalemia has been reported in patients receiving cyclophosphamide. Hyperkalemia probably is related to rapid lysis of tumor cells which occurs especially in connection with lymphomas or leukemias.

A syndrome of inappropriate antidiuretic hormone secretion has occurred during cyclophosphamide therapy. Hyponatremia resulting from impaired excretion of water associated with progressive weight gain without edema occurs. The tendency toward water retention in these patients is aggravated by the common practice of encouraging fluid intake to prevent formation of uric acid calculi and the occurrence of chemical cystitis.

■ **Cardiac Effects** Cardiotoxicity, which is uncommon at usual dosages, has been reported in patients receiving high doses of cyclophosphamide (120 [i.e., 60 mg/kg daily] to 270 mg/kg over a period of a few days), generally as part of an intensive, multiple-drug antineoplastic regimen or in conjunction with transplantation procedures. Potentially fatal cardiotoxicity also has occurred when cyclophosphamide (given concomitantly with mesna and followed with autologous bone marrow transplant) was administered inadvertently in a dosage of 4 g/m^2 daily for 4 doses rather than in a total dosage of 4 g/m^2 administered over 4 days in equally divided doses of 1 g/m^2 daily as part of a phase I protocol. Deaths have occurred from diffuse hemorrhagic myocardial necrosis and from a syndrome of acute myopericarditis when cyclophosphamide was used in high doses alone or in combination regimens; severe, sometimes fatal congestive heart failure has occurred rarely within a few days after the first dose of cyclophosphamide in such cases. Hemopericardium secondary to hemorrhagic myocarditis and myocardial necrosis, and pericarditis without evidence of hemopericardium, also have been reported. Acute myocardial infarction occurred in a patient with no history of cardiac conditions who received conventional doses of cyclophosphamide in conjunction with vincristine.

The precise mechanism of cyclophosphamide-induced cardiotoxicity is not known, but it has been postulated that the drug and/or its metabolites may affect the endothelium directly with secondary extravasation of blood containing high concentrations of cyclophosphamide. The antidiuretic effect of cyclophosphamide observed with high doses also may contribute to cardiopulmonary manifestations. Although clear risk factors have not been established, patients who have received or are receiving concomitantly radiation therapy and/or other potentially cardiotoxic drugs (e.g., anthracyclines) appear to be at increased risk. Some indicators of cyclophosphamide-induced cardiotoxicity include sudden weight gain, ECG abnormalities, dyspnea, and/or other signs of congestive heart failure, and patients receiving higher than usual dosages of the drug should be monitored for such effects. In addition to death, possible consequences of the cardiotoxicity include debilitating heart failure, arrhythmias, and potentially irreversible cardiomyopathy and/or pericarditis.

■ **Other Adverse Effects** Malaise and asthenia have been reported in patients receiving cyclophosphamide. Other reported adverse effects of cyclophosphamide include headache, dizziness, and myxedema. Faintness, facial flushing, diaphoresis, and oropharyngeal sensation have occurred following IV administration. Rarely, decreased serum cholinesterase concentrations, especially following IV administration of cyclophosphamide, have been reported. The drug may interfere with normal wound healing.

Anaphylactic reaction, including fatality, has been reported with cyclophosphamide therapy. Possible cross-sensitivity with other alkylating agents also has been reported. Positive reactions to skin test antigens (e.g., tuberculin purified protein derivative, mumps, trichophyton, candida) are reported to be frequently suppressed in patients receiving cyclophosphamide.

■ **Precautions and Contraindications** Cyclophosphamide is a highly toxic drug with a low therapeutic index, and a therapeutic response is not likely to occur without some evidence of toxicity. The drug must be used only under constant supervision by clinicians experienced in therapy with cytotoxic agents.

Patients who receive myelosuppressive drugs experience an increased frequency of infections, as well as possible hemorrhagic complications. Because these complications are potentially fatal, the patient should be instructed to notify the clinician if fever, sore throat, or unusual bleeding or bruising occurs. The patient's hematologic status must be carefully monitored, at least weekly for the first few months of therapy or until the maintenance dosage is determined, and then at intervals of 2–3 weeks. Leukopenia is dose-related and can be used as a guide to adjusting dosage of cyclophosphamide. A reduction in leukocyte count to less than 2000/mm^3 occurs commonly with initial loading doses of the drug, and less frequently in patients maintained on smaller doses. Transient decreases in leukocyte count to 2000/mm^3(during short courses of treatment) or more persistent reductions to 3000/mm^3 (with continuing therapy) reportedly are tolerated without serious risk of infection if marked granulocytopenia is not present.

To prevent the occurrence of hemorrhagic cystitis in patients receiving cyclophosphamide, many experts recommend adequate hydration and frequent voiding. Patients should be instructed to increase their fluid intake for 24 hours before, during, and for at least 24 hours after receiving cyclophosphamide and to void frequently for 24 hours after receiving the drug. Urine also should be examined regularly for the presence of red cells, which may precede hemorrhagic cystitis. Since hemorrhagic cystitis can be severe and even fatal, the drug should be discontinued and not resumed if possible in patients who develop this complication. In severe cases, replacement of blood may be needed. Protracted cases have been treated with 1–10% formaldehyde irrigations, electrocautery to the telangiectatic areas of the bladder, diversion of urine flow, and cryosurgery.

Because of the immunosuppressive activity of cyclophosphamide, interruption or reduction of dosage should be considered for patients who develop bacterial, fungal, protozoan, helminthic, or viral infections, especially those patients who are receiving or perhaps in those who have recently received corticosteroid therapy. Infections in some of these patients have been fatal; varicella-zoster infections appear to be particularly dangerous. Cyclophosphamide has been reported to be more toxic in adrenalectomized dogs, and adjustment of both replacement corticosteroids and cyclophosphamide may be necessary in adrenalectomized patients.

Cyclophosphamide should be administered with caution to patients with severe leukopenia, thrombocytopenia, tumor cell infiltration of bone marrow, previous therapy with radiation or other cytotoxic agents, impaired hepatic function, or impaired renal function. The drug is contraindicated in patients with severely depressed bone marrow function and in those who have demonstrated hypersensitivity to cyclophosphamide.

Patients should be informed that exposure to large doses of cyclophosphamide causes gonadal toxicity (see Cautions: Pregnancy, Fertility, and Lactation); counseling on fertility options, prior to such therapy whenever possible for young patients, and long-term follow-up for evaluation of gonadal function is advised.

■ **Pediatric Precautions** According to the manufacturers, the safety profile of cyclophosphamide in children is similar to that observed in adult patients. Children receiving large doses of cyclophosphamide are at high risk for long-term gonadal damage and infertility. (See Cautions: Pregnancy, Fertility, and Lactation.)

■ **Geriatric Precautions** Safety and efficacy of cyclophosphamide in geriatric patients have not been studied specifically to date. Clinical studies of cyclophosphamide for malignant lymphoma, multiple myeloma, leukemia, mycosis fungoides, neuroblastoma, retinoblastoma, and breast cancer did not include sufficient numbers of patients 65 years of age and older to determine whether geriatric patients respond differently than younger patients. In 2 clinical trials in which cyclophosphamide and cisplatin were compared with paclitaxel and cisplatin for the treatment of advanced ovarian cancer, 154 (28%) of 552 patients receiving cyclophosphamide and cisplatin were 65 years or older. Subset analyses according to age (younger than 65 years versus 65 years or older) from these trials, published reports of clinical trials of cyclophosphamide-containing regimens in breast cancer and non-Hodgkin's lymphoma, and postmarketing experience suggest that geriatric patients may be more susceptible to cyclophosphamide-induced toxicity. In general, dosage should be titrated carefully in geriatric patients, usually initiating therapy at the low end of the dosage range.

■ **Carcinogenicity** Some patients who have received cyclophosphamide alone, as part of a combination regimen, or as adjunctive therapy have developed secondary malignancies, most frequently urinary bladder, myeloproliferative, and lymphoproliferative malignancies. Although a causal relationship has not been definitely established, the possibility of development of a secondary malignancy should be considered in weighing the possible benefit from the drug against the potential risk. Secondary malignancies have occurred most frequently in patients who have been treated with cyclophosphamide for primary myeloproliferative and lymphoproliferative malignancies and primary nonmalignant diseases in which immune processes are believed to be involved. Secondary urinary bladder malignancies generally have occurred in patients who previously developed hemorrhagic cystitis. In some cases, the secondary malignancy was not detected until several years after discontinuance of cyclophosphamide therapy. In one study in patients with breast cancer who received 2–4 times the standard dose of cyclophosphamide in conjunction with doxorubicin, cases of secondary acute myeloid leukemia were reported within 2 years of treatment initiation. Long-term follow-up of women who received cyclophosphamide-containing adjuvant chemotherapy regimens for the treatment of early breast cancer indicates that the incidence of other solid tumors and secondary leukemia in these women is not substantially greater than that in the general population.

■ **Pregnancy, Fertility, and Lactation** Cyclophosphamide can cause fetal toxicity when administered to pregnant women, but potential benefits from use of the drug may be acceptable in certain conditions despite the possible risks to the fetus. Abnormalities, including ectrodactylia, have occurred in infants born to women treated with the drug during pregnancy. Normal infants also have been born to women who received cyclophosphamide, including during the first trimester. Cyclophosphamide should be used during pregnancy only in life-threatening situations or severe disease for which safer drugs cannot be used or are ineffective. When the drug is administered during pregnancy or if the patient becomes pregnant while receiving cyclophosphamide, the patient should be informed of the potential hazard to the fetus. Women of childbearing potential should be advised to avoid becoming pregnant.

Gonadal suppression, which appears to be related to dose and duration of therapy, has been reported in patients who received cyclophosphamide. The drug interferes with oogenesis and spermatogenesis. Amenorrhea, azoospermia, oligospermia, and ovarian fibrosis have been reported in patients who receive cyclophosphamide. Sterility may occur in both men and women and may be permanent. Although the full effect of cyclophosphamide on prepubertal gonads has not been established, ovarian failure and testicular atrophy have occurred. Male patients who receive high-dose cyclophosphamide for childhood cancer, including treatment prior to the onset of puberty, are at high risk for long-term, irreversible gonadal damage, such as infertility and subclinical Leydig cell insufficiency.

Cyclophosphamide is distributed into milk. Because of the potential for serious adverse reactions to cyclophosphamide in nursing infants, a decision should be made whether to discontinue nursing or the drug, taking into account the importance of the drug to the woman.

Drug Interactions

■ **Mesna** Mesna (sodium 2-mercaptoethanesulphonate) is a synthetic sulfhydryl compound that can chemically interact with urotoxic metabolites (and/or their precursors) of cyclophosphamide (e.g., acrolein, 4-hydroxycyclophosphamide) and other oxazaphosphorine derivatives (e.g., ifosfamide) to decrease the incidence and severity of, or prevent, bladder toxicity (e.g., hemorrhagic cystitis) induced by these drugs. (See Mesna 92:56.)

Mesna is rapidly oxidized in systemic circulation to dimesna (mesna disulfide), which is substantially less chemically reactive than mesna; following glomerular filtration, dimesna is reduced to mesna by the glutathione system in the renal tubular epithelium and is excreted by the kidneys. In urine, mesna reacts chemically (e.g., binding with 4-hydroxycyclophosphamide to form 4-sulfoethylthiocyclophosphamide and/or binding with double-bonds of acrolein) with the urotoxic metabolites (and/or their precursors) of cyclophosphamide thought to be principally responsible for drug-induced hematuria and hemorrhagic cystitis and thus detoxifies these metabolites. In addition, mesna enhances urinary excretion of cysteine, which also can react chemically with acrolein, and this effect may contribute to the uroprotective activity of mesna. While limited evidence in animals suggests that mesna also may enhance systemic deactivation of cyclophosphamide to some extent, pharmacokinetic characteristics of mesna may differ in mice compared with humans, and the poor lipophilicity of mesna and dimesna (resulting in poor distribution into tumor cells in humans), evidence from in vitro and in vivo tumor models, and clinical evidence in humans indicate that mesna does not substantially deactivate active cyclophosphamide metabolites in tumor cells or interfere with the systemic antineoplastic activity of the drug.

■ **Cardiotoxic Drugs** Because potentiation of cardiotoxic effects may result, caution should be exercised in the concomitant administration of cyclophosphamide and other cardiotoxic drugs such as doxorubicin.

■ **Drugs Affecting Hepatic Microsomal Enzymes** Barbiturates and other drugs which induce liver microsomal enzymes may result in an increased pharmacologic effect and increased toxicity of cyclophosphamide because of increased conversion of the drug to active metabolites. Although the full clinical importance of this interaction has not been assessed, it is advisable to monitor patients who receive both drugs closely for cyclophosphamide toxicity.

Although it has been proposed that corticosteroids and sex hormones may inhibit liver microsomal enzymes and that discontinuance or reduction in steroid dosage can cause an increase in the toxicity of previously well-tolerated doses of cyclophosphamide, the clinical importance of this effect has not been established. Other drugs which may inhibit microsomal enzyme activity in the liver and therefore interfere with the metabolism of cyclophosphamide include allopurinol, chloramphenicol, chloroquine, imipramine, phenothiazines, potassium iodide, and vitamin A. In one controlled study, concomitant administration of cyclophosphamide and allopurinol increased the incidence of bone marrow depression as compared to cyclophosphamide alone, but the mechanism or clinical importance of the interaction has not been established.

■ **Succinylcholine** Cyclophosphamide reportedly reduces serum pseudocholinesterase concentrations and may prolong the neuromuscular blocking activity of succinylcholine, especially in very ill patients who are receiving large IV doses of cyclophosphamide. Although the clinical importance has not been established, it has been suggested that succinylcholine be administered with caution in patients receiving cyclophosphamide and that succinylcholine or cyclophosphamide be avoided in patients with substantially depressed pseudocholinesterase concentrations. The anesthesiologist should be informed before general anesthesia is administered if a patient has received cyclophosphamide within the previous 10 days.

Acute Toxicity

Limited information is available on acute overdosage of cyclophosphamide.

■ **Manifestations** Overdosage with cyclophosphamide would be expected to produce effects that are mainly extensions of common adverse reactions, particularly severe leukopenia and thrombocytopenia; cardiotoxicity also may be prominent. In patients who received 4- to 10-day courses of cyclophosphamide with total dosage of the drug per course exceeding 140 mg/kg (5.2 g/m^2), cardiac damage manifested by heart failure occurred within 15 days of the initial dose. Impairment of water excretion with hyponatremia, weight gain, and inappropriately concentrated urine has been reported after cyclophosphamide doses exceeding 50 mg/kg (2 g/m^2).

Overdosage, which was fatal in at least one case, also has occurred in several patients who were enrolled in high-dose protocols in which cyclophosphamide (given concomitantly with mesna and followed with autologous bone marrow transplant) was administered inadvertently in a dosage of 4 g/m^2 daily for 4 doses rather than in a total dosage of 4 g/m^{2}administered over 4 days in equally divided doses of 1 g/m^2 daily; potentially irreversible or fatal cardiotoxicity was the most serious consequence of overdosage in these patients. Potentially fatal cardiotoxicity, manifested as congestive heart failure, ECG abnormalities, cardiomyopathy, and/or pericarditis, also has been reported in other patients receiving high doses of cyclophosphamide (120 mg/kg [60 mg/kg daily] or more over several days), and the risk of such toxicity appears to be increased in patients who have received or are receiving concomitantly radiation therapy or other potentially cardiotoxic drugs (e.g., anthracyclines). (See Cautions: Cardiac Effects.)

■ **Treatment** If overdosage of cyclophosphamide is known or suspected, the patient should be hospitalized for general supportive therapy. There is no known specific antidote. Although cyclophosphamide theoretically is dialyzable, no studies have been performed to date to evaluate efficacy of dialysis in the treatment of acute overdosage of the drug.

Pharmacology

Following conversion to active metabolites in the liver, cyclophosphamide functions as an alkylating agent, interfering with DNA replication and transcription of RNA, and ultimately resulting in the disruption of nucleic acid function. The drug exhibits phosphorylating properties that also enhance its cytotoxicity. Cyclophosphamide also possesses potent immunosuppressive activity.

Pharmacokinetics

■ **Absorption** Cyclophosphamide appears to be well absorbed following oral administration, with a reported bioavailability greater than 75%. Maximum plasma concentrations of cyclophosphamide occur at about 1 hour. Concentrations of cyclophosphamide metabolites reportedly reach maximum levels 2–3 hours after an IV dose of the drug.

■ **Distribution** Cyclophosphamide and its metabolites appear to be distributed throughout the body, including the brain and CSF, but probably not in concentrations sufficient to treat meningeal leukemia. It is assumed that cyclophosphamide crosses the placenta. The drug is distributed into milk.

Although in vitro binding of cyclophosphamide to plasma proteins has not been demonstrated, in vivo binding generally has been reported to range from 0–10% and protein binding for some alkylating metabolites has been reported to exceed 60%.

■ **Elimination** The serum half-life after IV administration of cyclophosphamide has been reported to range from 3–12 hours; however, the drug and/or its metabolites can be detected in the serum up to 72 hours after administration.

Cyclophosphamide is metabolized in the liver by the enzymatic mixed-function oxidase system of liver microsomes to 4-hydroxycyclophosphamide, which is in equilibrium with aldophosphamide, the acyclic tautomer. 4-Hydroxycyclophosphamide may be enzymatically metabolized to 4-ketocyclophosphamide, and aldophosphamide may be enzymatically metabolized to carboxyphosphamide, phosphoramide mustard, and acrolein. Some authorities believe that phosphoramide mustard and acrolein account for the cytotoxic properties of the drug, and that 4-ketocyclophosphamide and carboxyphosphamide do not possess substantial biologic activity. However, there is controversy regarding the toxicity of 4-ketocyclophosphamide.

Cyclophosphamide and its metabolites are excreted principally in urine, with about 36–99% of a dose being eliminated within 48 hours; of the amount excreted, about 5–30% is unchanged drug.

Chemistry and Stability

■ **Chemistry** Cyclophosphamide is a nitrogen mustard-derivative, polyfunctional alkylating agent. The drug occurs as a monohydrate, white, crystalline powder and is soluble in water and in alcohol. Potency of cyclophosphamide is calculated on the anhydrous basis.

Cyclophosphamide is commercially available as cyclophosphamide tablets containing anhydrous cyclophosphamide. Cyclophosphamide for injection is commercially available as a sterile white powder containing cyclophosphamide monohydrate.

When reconstituted as directed with sterile 0.9% sodium chloride solution (for direct injection), solutions of cyclophosphamide monohydrate (Cytoxan®) have an osmolarity of 374 mOsm/L. When reconstituted as directed with sterile water for injection (for IV infusion), solutions of cyclophosphamide monohydrate (Cytoxan®) have an osmolarity of 74 mOsm/L and are hypotonic.

■ **Stability** Commercially available cyclophosphamide tablets should be stored at a temperature not exceeding 25°C; the tablets will withstand brief exposure to temperatures up to 30°C, but should be protected from temperatures exceeding 30°C.

Commercially available cyclophosphamide powder for injection containing cyclophosphamide monohydrate should be stored at a temperature not exceeding 25°C. During storage or transport, exposure of the vials to temperature fluctuations may result in melting of the contents; vials should be visually inspected, and any vials with signs of melting of the cyclophosphamide monohydrate into a clear or yellowish viscous liquid, in droplets or as a connected phase, should be discarded.

Following reconstitution as directed with sterile 0.9% sodium chloride solution or sterile water for injection, solutions of cyclophosphamide powder for injection containing cyclophosphamide monohydrate are stable for 24 hours at room temperature or 6 days when refrigerated. Reconstituted solutions of the drug to be used for IV infusion are compatible with 5% dextrose, 5% dextrose and 0.9% sodium chloride, 5% dextrose and Ringer's, lactated Ringer's, 0.45% sodium chloride, or ⅙ *M* sodium lactate injection.

Extemporaneous oral liquid preparations of cyclophosphamide, prepared by dissolving the powder for injection in aromatic elixir, are stable for 14 days in glass containers when refrigerated.

For further information on the handling of antineoplastic agents, see the ASHP Guidelines on Handling Hazardous Drugs at http://www.ahfsdruginformation.com.

Preparations

Excipients in commercially available drug preparations may have clinically important effects in some individuals; consult specific product labeling for details.

Cyclophosphamide

Oral		
Tablets	25 mg (of anhydrous cyclophosphamide)*	**Cyclophosphamide Tablets**
		Cytoxan®, Bristol-Myers Squibb
	50 mg (of anhydrous cyclophosphamide)*	**Cyclophosphamide Tablets**
		Cytoxan®, Bristol-Myers Squibb
Parenteral		
For injection	500 mg (of anhydrous cyclophosphamide)*	**Cyclophosphamide for Injection**
		Cytoxan®, Bristol-Myers Squibb
	1 g (of anhydrous cyclophosphamide)*	**Cyclophosphamide for Injection**
		Cytoxan®, Bristol-Myers Squibb
	2 g (of anhydrous cyclophosphamide)*	**Cyclophosphamide for Injection**
		Cytoxan®, Bristol-Myers Squibb

*available from one or more manufacturer, distributor, and/or repackager by generic (nonproprietary) name

†Use is not currently included in the labeling approved by the US Food and Drug Administration

Cytarabine

1-β-Arabinofuranosylcytosine, Arabinosylcytosine, Cytosine Arabinoside, Ara-C

■ Cytarabine, a synthetic pyrimidine antagonist, is an antimetabolite antineoplastic agent.

Uses

■ **Conventional Cytarabine** ***Acute Myeloid Leukemia*** Cytarabine is used principally as a component of various chemotherapeutic regimens for remission induction in acute myeloid (myelogenous, nonlymphocytic) leukemia (AML, ANLL). AML includes acute promyelocytic, monocytic, myelomonocytic, megakaryoblastic, and erythroid leukemias. Induction regimens are used to rapidly reduce the tumor burden in order to achieve complete remission, which generally is defined as less than 5% leukemic blast cells in the bone marrow and normalization of peripheral blood counts (including hemoglobin concentration, hematocrit, granulocyte count, and platelet count). Cytarabine used alone has produced complete remissions in 25–40% of patients, but combination therapy for induction of remissions is superior to single-agent therapy and is preferred. Although maintenance regimens (with lower doses) previously were administered for prolonged periods (e.g., years) in the treatment of AML, most current treatment regimens in the US no longer employ maintenance therapy but instead use intensive consolidation therapy that is administered for a shorter period of time at higher doses and then discontinued since there is no evidence of superior disease-free survival with prolonged maintenance.

Remission rates in adult AML are inversely related to age, with expected rates exceeding 65% in those younger than 60 years of age. In addition, some evidence suggests that, once attained, duration of remission may be shorter in older patients, and increased morbidity and mortality during induction also appear to be directly related to age. Other adverse prognostic factors include leukemic CNS involvement, systemic infection at diagnosis, elevated leukocyte count (exceeding 100,000/ mm^3) treatment-induced AML, and a history of myelodysplastic syndrome. In addition, leukemias that express the progenitor cell antigen CD34 and/or P-glycoprotein (MDR-1 gene product) have an inferior outcome. Cytogenetic analysis, although not readily available, provides the strongest prognostic information for newly diagnosed AML, with abnormalities that indicate a good prognosis including t(8;21), inv(16), and t(15; 17); normal cytogenetics generally indicate average-risk AML. Patients with AML that is characterized by deletions of the long arms or monosomies of chromosomes 5 or 7; by translocations or inversions of chromosome 3, t(6;9),t(9; 22); or by abnormalities of 11q23 exhibit particularly poor prognoses with chemotherapy.

Cytarabine and an anthracycline (usually daunorubicin) have been principal components of induction regimens, but various regimens have been used in combination therapy and comparative efficacy is continually being evaluated. Cytarabine has been used with agents such as daunorubicin, doxorubicin, idarubicin, thioguanine, or vincristine. The 2-drug regimen of cytarabine and daunorubicin generally results in a complete response rate of approximately 65% in patients with previously untreated AML. The results of randomized trials comparing combined mitoxantrone and cytarabine therapy with combined daunorubicin and cytarabine therapy have shown the two regimens to have similar efficacy and toxicity as induction therapy in patients with previously untreated AML. There is some evidence that dose intensity of cytarabine as a component of induction therapy may affect disease-free survival. In one study, high-dose rapid cytarabine administration combined with daunorubicin and etoposide produced similar complete response rate but superior disease-free survival compared with conventional-dose continuous-infusion cytarabine combined with these drugs. In another study in which the second course of induction therapy was administered after hematopoietic recovery or in a planned sequence beginning on day 10 of therapy (i.e., during aplasia), both regimens produced similar remission rates but the timed sequential regimen produced superior disease-free survival regardless of the postremission therapy (e.g., consolidation chemotherapy, allogeneic or autologous bone marrow transplantation). Some clinicians have used thioguanine or mercaptopurine in addition to intensive therapy with cytarabine and daunorubicin for remission induction; complete remissions occurred in 60–85% of patients.

Cytarabine has also been used with other antineoplastic agents in regimens of consolidation therapy for AML following induction of a complete remission; however, the role of such therapy in the prolongation of remissions is not firmly established. Cytarabine-containing consolidation chemotherapy regimens that do not employ bone marrow transplantation are associated with treatment-related death rates that usually are less than 10–20% and have produced disease-free survival rates of 20–50%. There is some evidence that high-dose cytarabine consolidation regimens provide a clear benefit in survival in patients younger than 60 years of age,but dose-intensive cytarabine-based chemotherapy can be complicated by severe neurologic and/or pulmonary toxicity and therefore should be administered under the direction of clinicians experienced in the use of such regimens in facilities equipped to manage potential complications. Consolidation therapy has ranged in duration from one to 4 or more cycles, but the optimal doses, schedules, and duration of consolidation chemotherapy remain to be established.

Cytarabine also has been used with other antineoplastic agents in the treatment of erythroleukemia.

Cytarabine has been used alone in high-dose† regimens to induce remissions in some patients with refractory acute myeloid leukemia, or with secondary acute myeloid leukemia.

Acute Lymphocytic Leukemia Cytarabine has been used alone or with other antineoplastic agents for remission induction in acute lymphocytic (lymphoblastic) leukemia (ALL); however, combinations containing other antineoplastic agents are more effective. Cytarabine has generally been limited to use with other antineoplastic agents for remission induction in some patients who do not achieve a complete remission with combinations containing other agents or who relapse during maintenance therapy. Cytarabine has also been used occasionally in regimens of consolidation and/or maintenance therapy following induction of a complete remission by combinations containing other agents. Although long-term survivors may eventually experience a recurrence or relapse, a substantial number of children with acute lymphocytic leukemia have achieved long-term complete remissions following induction and maintenance combination therapy.

Cytarabine has been used alone in high-dose regimens to induce remissions in some patients with refractory ALL.

Meningeal Leukemia and Other Meningeal Neoplasms Cytarabine has been used effectively alone or with other chemotherapeutic agents in the treatment and maintenance therapy of meningeal leukemia and other meningeal neoplasms (e.g., lymphoma). Although therapeutic concentrations of cytarabine in the CSF have apparently been attained during continuous IV or subcutaneous infusions of the drug, cytarabine is usually administered intrathecally to ensure therapeutic concentrations of the drug. Many clinicians consider intrathecal cytarabine and intrathecal methotrexate to have similar efficacy in the treatment of these conditions; however, intrathecal cytarabine produces less systemic toxicity than intrathecal methotrexate. Intrathecal cytarabine may be useful in patients whose CNS disease does not respond to intrathecal methotrexate or in patients with methotrexate-related neurotoxicity. Focal leukemic involvement of the CNS may not respond to intrathecal cytarabine or intrathecal methotrexate and may better be treated with radiation therapy. The value of intrathecal cytarabine in the prophylaxis of meningeal leukemia has not been established.

Chronic Myelogenous Leukemia IV cytarabine is used with other antineoplastic agents (e.g., daunorubicin) in the treatment of patients with chronic myelogenous leukemia (CML) who are in the accelerated or blastic phase of the disease; however, the prognosis for patients receiving standard therapy remains poor and other therapies are continually being evaluated.

Cytarabine also is used in combination with interferon alfa for the treatment of the chronic phase of CML. Concomitant administration of cytarabine with interferon alfa-2b has been associated with increased survival in patients with CML. Results of a randomized controlled study in previously untreated patients with CML demonstrate a longer survival in patients receiving interferon alfa-2b (5 million units/m^2 given subcutaneously daily) in combination with cytarabine (20 mg/m^2 daily for 10 days given subcutaneously 2 weeks after initiation of interferon alfa-2b therapy and monthly thereafter) versus those receiving interferon alfa-2b without cytarabine; patients from both groups also received hydroxyurea 50 mg/kg daily until a complete hematologic remission was achieved. After 3 years, median survival rate of about 86 or 79%, respectively, reportedly was observed in patients receiving combined interferon alfa-2b therapy with cytarabine or interferon alfa-2b without cytarabine while overall hematologic response rate was 66 or 55% in patients receiving combined interferon alfa-2b therapy with cytarabine or interferon alfa-2b without cytarabine, respectively. Major cytogenetic response rate after 12 months was 41 or 24% in patients receiving combined interferon alfa-2b therapy with cytarabine or interferon alfa-2b without cytarabine, respectively. Longer survival was observed in patients with cytogenetic response. Some patients underwent allogeneic or autologous bone marrow transplantation, and the 2-year survival rate after allogeneic bone marrow transplantation was 56 or 59% in patients receiving combined interferon alfa-2b therapy with cytarabine or interferon alfa-2b without cytarabine, respectively, while 2-year survival rate after autologous bone marrow transplantation was 61 or 68% in patients receiving combined interferon alfa-2b therapy with cytarabine or interferon alfa-2b without cytarabine, respectively. Patients who did not have complete hematologic or major cytogenetic responses within 6 or 12 months, respectively, were allowed to cross over to combined treatment with interferon alfa-2b and cytarabine. Among patients who received initial therapy with interferon alfa-2b without cytarabine, but then crossed over to receive combined treatment with interferon alfa-2b and cytarabine, complete and partial responses of 2 and 6%, respectively, were observed.

Other Uses Cytarabine has been used with other antineoplastic agents in regimens of maintenance therapy in the treatment of non-Hodgkin's lymphomas in children. Cytarabine has also been used with other antineoplastic agents for remission induction and/or maintenance therapy in adults with non-Hodgkin's lymphomas†, principally advanced diffuse histiocytic lymphoma. It has been suggested, but is not clearly established, that cytarabine decreases the incidence of CNS relapse in patients with advanced diffuse histiocytic lymphoma because the drug crosses the blood-brain barrier. However, the best combination or sequential therapy in the treatment of advanced diffuse histiocytic lymphoma has not been established and comparative efficacy is continually being evaluated. Cytarabine has also been used alone in high-dose† regimens with some success for the treatment of refractory non-Hodgkin's lymphomas.

■ **Liposomal Cytarabine** ***Lymphomatous Meningitis*** Liposomal cytarabine is used for the intrathecal treatment of lymphomatous meningitis. This indication is based on a controlled study showing an increased complete response rate for liposomal cytarabine compared with conventional (unencapsulated) cytarabine in patients with lymphomatous meningitis. There are no controlled trials that demonstrate a clinical benefit (e.g., amelioration of disease-related symptoms, increased time to disease progression, prolonged survival) for the use of intrathecal therapy with liposomal cytarabine for lymphomatous meningitis.

In a multicenter randomized trial, 99 patients with neoplastic meningitis caused by solid tumors, lymphoma (33 patients), or leukemia, received either liposomal cytarabine or conventional (unencapsulated) cytarabine. The patients with lymphoma received either liposomal cytarabine 50 mg intrathecally once every 2 weeks or conventional (unencapsulated) cytarabine 50 mg intrathecally twice weekly. According to the study protocol, patients were to receive concurrent treatment with dexamethasone to minimize symptoms associated with chemical arachnoiditis, a known toxicity associated with intrathecal therapy with cytarabine and methotrexate. Patients with disease that did not achieve a complete response at 4 weeks discontinued treatment with the study drug.

Among the 33 patients with lymphoma in the randomized trial, complete response rates were 41% (7/17) in those receiving liposomal cytarabine and 6% (1/16) in those receiving conventional cytarabine. For 4 of the 7 patients with a complete response to liposomal cytarabine, the study protocol was violated when response was determined by the reading of an unblinded pathologist rather than by central pathology review of the data. The median overall survival was 99.5 days in those receiving liposomal cytarabine and 63 days in those receiving conventional cytarabine; the majority of patients in the study died from progressive systemic disease and not neoplastic meningitis.

Seizures occurred more frequently in patients receiving liposomal cytarabine (24%) than in those receiving conventional cytarabine (6%).

Dosage and Administration

■ **Reconstitution and Administration** Cytarabine as a single-entity preparation is not interchangeable with the fixed liposomal combination of daunorubicin and cytarabine (daunorubicin/cytarabine liposomal; Vyxeos®). To avoid dosing errors, clinicians should confirm the correct drug name, formulation, and dose prior to preparation and administration.

Conventional Cytarabine Conventional (unencapsulated) cytarabine may be administered IV by rapid injection or continuous infusion, or by subcutaneous or intrathecal injection.

For IV, intrathecal, or subcutaneous injection or IV infusion, commercially available conventional (unencapsulated) cytarabine injection may be diluted with a compatible IV solution (e.g., water for injection, 5% dextrose injection, 0.9% sodium chloride injection). Only the preservative-free preparation of conventional (unencapsulated) cytarabine injection is suitable for intrathecal administration; conventional (unencapsulated) cytarabine injection containing benzyl alcohol should be used only for IV or subcutaneous administration. (See Chemistry and Stability: Stability.) Alternatively, conventional (unencapsulated) cytarabine sterile powder can be used for IV or subcutaneous administration by reconstituting it with bacteriostatic water for injection containing 0.945% benzyl alcohol. The sterile powder is usually reconstituted by adding 5 mL of diluent to the vial labeled as containing 100 mg, 10 mL of diluent to the vial labeled as containing 500 mg, 10 mL of diluent to the vial labeled as containing 1 g, or 20 mL of diluent to the vial labeled as containing 2 g of the drug. The resultant solutions contain 20, 50, 100, or 100 mg of cytarabine per mL, respectively. The desired dose of the reconstituted solution may be given IV rapidly or may be further diluted with 5% dextrose or 0.9% sodium chloride injection for IV infusion. Because of the potential toxicity of large amounts of benzyl alcohol, the manufacturers warn that diluents containing this preservative should *not* be used to reconstitute cytarabine if high-dose† regimens of the drug are employed.

The manufacturers state that diluents containing benzyl alcohol should *not* be used when conventional (unencapsulated) cytarabine is administered intrathecally. Cytarabine that has been reconstituted with bacteriostatic water for injection containing benzyl alcohol should *not* be used in neonates. (See Cautions: Pediatric Precautions.) Many clinicians recommend that conventional (unencapsulated) cytarabine sterile powder be reconstituted with preservative-free 0.9% sodium chloride injection, Elliott's B solution or other isotonic buffered diluents which do not contain a preservative (e.g., lactated Ringer's injection), or the patient's spinal fluid. Cytarabine is usually administered in 5–15 mL of solution, after an equivalent volume of CSF is removed.

Conventional (unencapsulated) cytarabine injection that is commercially available in pharmacy bulk packages is *not* intended for direct IV infusion; individual doses can be withdrawn and used undiluted or further diluted in a compatible IV solution. The manufacturer states that pharmacy bulk packages are *not* intended for preparation of doses intended for intrathecal administration.

Liposomal Cytarabine Cytarabine liposome injection is administered intrathecally *only*.

For intrathecal administration, commercially available cytarabine liposome injection is suitable; no reconstitution or dilution of the injection is required. Dilution of the cytarabine liposome injection is *not* recommended. Particles of liposomal cytarabine have a greater density than the diluent and may settle with time. Vials of cytarabine liposome injection should be allowed to warm to room temperature and then the vials should be gently agitated or inverted to resuspend the particles immediately prior to withdrawal of the injection from the vial. Aggressive agitation of the vials should be avoided. Cytarabine liposome injection is a potentially toxic compound that should be handled with caution; the use of gloves is recommended. If liposomal cytarabine suspension contacts the skin, wash immediately with soap and water; if it contacts mucous membranes, flush thoroughly with water.

Cytarabine liposome injection should be withdrawn from the vial immediately before administration. The single-use vial does not contain any preservative; cytarabine liposome injection must be used within 4 hours of withdrawal from the vial. Unused portions of the injection should be discarded properly, and unused portions of the drug should *not* be saved for later administration. Cytarabine liposome injection should not be mixed with any other medications.

In-line filters should *not* be used when administering cytarabine liposome injection. Liposomal cytarabine should be administered directly into the CSF via an intraventricular reservoir or by direct injection into the lumbar sac. Liposomal cytarabine should be injected slowly over a period of 1–5 minutes. Following administration of the drug by lumbar puncture, the patient should be instructed to lie flat for 1 hour. Following administration of the drug, patients should be observed by the clinician for immediate toxic reactions.

■ **Dosage** Dosage of conventional (unencapsulated) cytarabine must be based on the clinical and hematologic response and tolerance of the patient to obtain optimum therapeutic results with minimum adverse effects. Although higher total doses of cytarabine can be given by rapid IV injection compared with continuous IV infusion with similar hematologic toxicity, the most effective dosage schedule and method of administration have not been established. Clinicians should consult published protocols for the dosage of cytarabine and other chemotherapeutic agents and the method and sequence of administration.

IV Dosage **Acute Myeloid Leukemia.** In combination chemotherapy, the usual dosage of conventional (unencapsulated) cytarabine for induction therapy in acute myeloid leukemia is 2–6 mg/kg daily or 100–200 mg/m² daily by continuous IV infusion or in 2 or 3 divided doses by rapid IV injection or IV infusion, for 5–10 days in a course of therapy or daily until a remission is attained.

Non-Hodgkin's Lymphomas. For the treatment of refractory non-Hodgkin's lymphomas, conventional (unencapsulated) cytarabine has been administered by IV infusion in a dosage of 3 g/m² every 12 hours for up to 12 doses†; IV infusions generally were made over 1–3 hours.

Intrathecal Dosage **Meningeal Leukemia and Other Meningeal Neoplasms.** In the treatment and maintenance therapy of meningeal leukemia and other meningeal neoplasms, conventional (unencapsulated) cytarabine has been given by intrathecal injection in doses of 5–75 mg/m² or 30–100 mg once every 2–7 days to once daily for 4 or 5 days. The dosage schedule is usually determined by the type and severity of CNS manifestations and the patient's response to prior therapy. A frequently used intrathecal cytarabine dosage has been 30 mg/m² once every 4 days until CSF findings are normal, followed by one additional dose. If systemic toxicity occurs with intrathecal cytarabine, modification of other therapy may be necessary.

Lymphomatous Meningitis. Intrathecal therapy with liposomal cytarabine can cause serious toxicity, such as chemical arachnoiditis (see Cautions: Adverse Effects Associated With Intrathecal Administration: Liposomal Cytarabine) or neurotoxicity. All patients receiving liposomal cytarabine should receive dexamethasone concurrently to lessen the manifestations of chemical arachnoiditis, and patients should be monitored carefully throughout therapy for drug-related neurotoxicity. Therapy with oral or IV dexamethasone 4 mg twice daily for 5 days should be initiated on the day of intrathecal administration of liposomal cytarabine in each 14-day treatment cycle.

For the treatment of lymphomatous meningitis, induction therapy with liposomal cytarabine 50 mg is administered intrathecally (by intraventricular delivery or lumbar puncture) once every 14 days for 2 doses (weeks 1 and 3). Consolidation therapy with liposomal cytarabine 50 mg is administered intrathecally (by intraventricular delivery or lumbar puncture) once every 14 days for 3 doses (weeks 5, 7 and 9) followed by one additional dose at week 13. Maintenance therapy with liposomal cytarabine 50 mg is administered intrathecally (by intraventricular delivery or lumbar puncture) once every 28 days for 4 doses (weeks 17, 21, 25, and 29).

Dosage Modification for Toxicity and Contraindications for Continued Therapy **Hematologic Toxicity.** *Conventional Cytarabine:* Suspension or modification of therapy should be considered if the polymorphonuclear granulocyte count falls below 1000/mm³ or the platelet count falls below 50,000/mm³; however, during remission induction therapy in acute leukemia, the drug is usually administered in a short course and therapy is not discontinued or adjusted based on peripheral blood counts. If therapy has been discontinued, definite signs of bone marrow recovery appear, and granulocyte and platelet counts are at least 1000/mm³ and 50,000/mm³, respectively, cytarabine therapy should be resumed if indicated. If therapy is withheld until peripheral counts of blood elements return to normal, cytarabine may not be effective. Treatment of severe hematologic toxicity may consist of supportive therapy, antibiotics for complicating infections, and blood product transfusions.

Neurotoxicity. *Conventional Cytarabine:* Patients receiving high-dose cytarabine should be monitored carefully for signs of neuropathy; dosage schedule adjustment may be required to avoid irreversible neurotoxicity.

Liposomal Cytarabine: Patients receiving intrathecal therapy with liposomal cytarabine should be monitored continuously for the development of neurotoxicity. If the patient develops neurotoxicity, subsequent doses of liposomal cytarabine should be reduced to 25 mg. If toxicity persists, therapy with liposomal cytarabine should be discontinued.

■ **Dosage in Renal and Hepatic Impairment** Reduction of cytarabine dosage in patients with impaired renal function does not appear to be necessary. The manufacturers state that cytarabine should be used with caution and in reduced dosage in patients with poor hepatic function, but some clinicians believe that dosage adjustment is not necessary in patients with impaired hepatic function.

Cautions

For patients receiving liposomal cytarabine for lymphomatous meningitis, adverse effects are reported as the rate per cycle occurring in at least 10% of patients in the randomized study comparing intrathecal administration of liposomal cytarabine with intrathecal administration of conventional cytarabine or methotrexate.

■ **Hematologic Effects and Infectious Complications** ***Conventional Cytarabine*** The major adverse effect of conventional (unencapsulated) cytarabine is hematologic toxicity; the severity depends on the dose of the drug and schedule of administration. Myelosuppression is manifested by megaloblastosis, reticulocytopenia, leukopenia, thrombocytopenia, and anemia. Leukopenia results mainly from granulocyte depression; lymphocytes are minimally affected. The incidence and severity of hematologic toxicity is minimal after a single IV dose of cytarabine, but myelosuppression, anemia, and thrombocytopenia occur in almost all patients with daily IV injections or continuous IV infusions of the drug. Myelosuppression after subcutaneous injection is similar to that which occurs after IV injection. Following 5-day constant IV infusions or rapid IV injections of cytarabine 50–600 mg/m², the leukocyte count decreases in a biphasic manner. There is an initial decrease beginning in the first 24 hours after the drug is administered, with a nadir at 7–9 days. This nadir is followed by a brief rise in the leukocyte count with a peak at about 12 days. The second leukocyte count nadir, which is greater than the first, occurs at 15–24 days and is followed by a rapid rise to above baseline levels in the next 10 days. The platelet count begins to decrease by 5 days after beginning cytarabine therapy with the nadir at 12–15 days; platelet levels rise rapidly to above baseline levels in the next 10 days.

Liposomal Cytarabine Adverse hematologic or lymphatic effects occurred in 19% of treatment cycles, and were severe in 11% of treatment cycles, in patients receiving liposomal cytarabine for lymphomatous meningitis, including neutropenia in 9% (severe in 8%), thrombocytopenia in 8% (severe in 5%), and anemia in 1% (severe in 1%), of treatment cycles. Transient elevations in CSF protein and white blood cell counts have been observed in patients following intrathecal therapy with methotrexate or (conventional or liposomal) cytarabine.

■ **Nervous System Effects** ***Conventional Cytarabine*** Severe, sometimes fatal, neurologic toxicity has occurred in patients receiving high-dose regimens of conventional (unencapsulated) cytarabine. (See Cautions: Adverse Effects Associated With High-Dose Regimens.) Neuritis, neural toxicity, headache, and dizziness have been reported in patients receiving cytarabine.

Liposomal Cytarabine Adverse neurologic effects occurred in 45% of treatment cycles, and were severe in 18% of treatment cycles, in patients receiving liposomal cytarabine for lymphomatous meningitis, including confusion in 14% (severe in 4%), somnolence in 12% (severe in 4%), and abnormal gait in 4% (severe in 1%) of treatment cycles.

Headache, associated with chemical arachnoiditis, occurred in 28% of treatment cycles, and was severe in 5% of treatment cycles, in patients receiving liposomal cytarabine for lymphomatous meningitis. In the controlled lymphoma study, seizures occurred in 24% of patients receiving liposomal cytarabine. Infectious meningitis may be associated with intrathecal drug therapy. Hydrocephalus, possibly precipitated by arachnoiditis, also has been reported.

Intrathecal administration of cytarabine may cause myelopathy or other neurologic toxicity and, rarely, can lead to a permanent neurologic deficit. Administration of intrathecal cytarabine in combination with other chemotherapeutic agents or with cranial/spinal irradiation may increase the risk of neurotoxicity. Blockage to CSF flow may increase free cytarabine concentrations in the CSF and increase the risk of neurotoxicity. Following intrathecal administration of liposomal cytarabine, CNS toxicity, including persistent extreme somnolence, hemiplegia, visual disturbances including blindness, deafness, and cranial nerve palsies have been reported. Manifestations of peripheral neuropathy, such as pain, numbness, paresthesia, weakness, and impaired bowel and bladder control, also have been observed in patients receiving liposomal cytarabine.

■ **GI Effects** ***Conventional Cytarabine*** Severe, sometimes fatal, GI toxicity has occurred in patients receiving high-dose regimens of conventional (unencapsulated) cytarabine. (See Cautions: Adverse Effects Associated With High-Dose Regimens.)

Nausea and vomiting may occur in patients receiving conventional cytarabine and generally occur more frequently and are more severe following rapid IV administration than with continuous IV infusion of the drug. After intrathecal administration of cytarabine, the most common adverse effects are nausea, vomiting, and fever. Antiemetics may be effective in treating nausea and vomiting.

Other adverse GI effects include diarrhea, anorexia, and oral and anal inflammation or ulceration; less frequently, abdominal pain, sore throat, esophagitis, esophageal ulceration, bowel necrosis, and GI hemorrhage may occur. In one study, conventional cytarabine reportedly induced severe intestinal toxicity when used in several sequential chemotherapeutic regimens. Toxic effects on GI mucosa included cellular atypia, immaturity, and necrosis, and were associated with diarrhea, ileus, abdominal pain, hematemesis, melena, hypokalemia, hypocalcemia, protein-losing enteropathy, transient weight gain, and intestinal infections.

Liposomal Cytarabine Adverse GI effects occurred in 27% of treatment cycles, and were severe in 7% of treatment cycles, in patients receiving liposomal cytarabine for lymphomatous meningitis, including nausea and vomiting associated with chemical arachnoiditis in 11 and 12%, respectively, and constipation in 7%, of treatment cycles.

■ **Respiratory Effects** Severe, sometimes fatal, pulmonary toxicity has occurred in patients receiving high-dose regimens of conventional (unencapsulated) cytarabine. (See Cautions: Adverse Effects Associated With High-Dose Regimens.) Pneumonia and shortness of breath have been reported in patients receiving conventional cytarabine.

■ **Hepatic Effects** Hepatic dysfunction is a frequent adverse effect of cytarabine therapy. Jaundice and elevations in serum bilirubin, transaminases, and alkaline phosphatase have occurred in patients receiving cytarabine alone or with other antineoplastic agents. Veno-occlusive hepatic disease also reportedly developed in 2 men and 4 children who were receiving chemotherapy for acute myelogenous leukemia; all patients had received prior cytarabine therapy but were receiving thioguanine alone or with other agents when they became symptomatic.

■ **Adverse Effects Associated with Intrathecal Administration**

Conventional Cytarabine Intrathecal administration of conventional (unencapsulated) cytarabine infrequently causes systemic toxicity, but the patient's hematologic status must be carefully monitored. Dosage adjustment of concurrently administered antineoplastic agents may be necessary.

The most frequent adverse effects of intrathecally administered conventional cytarabine are nausea, vomiting, fever, and transient headaches; these effects generally are mild and self-limiting. Meningism, paresthesia, paraplegia, spastic paraparesis, and seizures have been reported rarely.

Neurotoxicity following intrathecal injection of conventional cytarabine has been associated with diluents containing preservatives, and many clinicians recommend that preserved diluents not be used. The manufacturers state that diluents containing benzyl alcohol should *not* be used if the drug is administered intrathecally. (See Dosage and Administration: Reconstitution and Administration.) Blindness occurred in 2 leukemic patients in remission who had received systemic combination chemotherapy, prophylactic CNS irradiation, and intrathecal conventional cytarabine. Necrotizing leukoencephalopathy also occurred in 5 children who had received intrathecal conventional cytarabine, methotrexate, and hydrocortisone sodium succinate and CNS irradiation.

The manufacturer states that administration of cytarabine both IV and intrathecally within a period of a few days may be associated with an increased risk of neurotoxicity (i.e., spinal cord toxicity).

Progressive ascending paralysis, resulting in death in one patient, occurred in 2 children 4–6 months after receiving intrathecal and IV conventional cytarabine at usual doses in combination with other drugs and CNS irradiation.

Liposomal Cytarabine Chemical arachnoiditis, a syndrome manifested mainly by nausea, vomiting, headache, and fever, is a common adverse effect of intrathecal therapy with liposomal cytarabine and appears to be more common with this formulation than with the conventional (unencapsulated) formulation. Toxic effects may occur following a single dose or cumulative doses of liposomal cytarabine. Although toxicity is most likely to occur within 5 days of administration of the drug, adverse effects can occur at any time during therapy, and patients receiving intrathecal therapy with liposomal cytarabine should be monitored continuously. If it is not treated, chemical arachnoiditis may be fatal. Concurrent administration of dexamethasone may reduce the incidence and severity of chemical arachnoiditis associated with intrathecal administration of liposomal cytarabine.

Arachnoiditis is a common adverse effect of neoplastic meningitis, and it may be difficult to distinguish the disease-related syndrome from drug-related, or chemical, arachnoiditis. In clinical studies of liposomal cytarabine, chemical arachnoiditis was defined as the occurrence of neck rigidity, neck pain, or meningism, or any two of the following manifestations: nausea, vomiting, headache, fever, back pain, or CSF pleocytosis; the grade of severity of chemical arachnoiditis was based on the most severe manifestation. More than 90% of the cases of chemical arachnoiditis occurred within 48 hours of the intrathecal administration of liposomal cytarabine. The duration of manifestations was 1–5 days.

Concurrent administration of dexamethasone may reduce the incidence and severity of chemical arachnoiditis associated with intrathecal administration of liposomal cytarabine. In an early study of liposomal cytarabine, chemical arachnoiditis was observed in 100% of treatment cycles in patients who did not receive prophylactic treatment with dexamethasone, and in 33% of treatment cycles in patients who did receive prophylactic treatment with dexamethasone. In the randomized study, a greater number of episodes of chemical arachnoiditis, including grade 3 or 4 chemical arachnoiditis, occurred in patients receiving liposomal cytarabine compared with those receiving conventional cytarabine for lymphomatous meningitis.

Deaths have occurred in patients receiving intrathecal liposomal cytarabine during clinical studies. One patient developed encephalopathy and died 36 hours after an intraventricular dose of liposomal cytarabine 125 mg. This patient was receiving concurrent whole-brain irradiation and had previously received cyclophosphamide, doxorubicin, and fluorouracil, as well as intraventricular methotrexate. Another patient developed focal seizures and progressed to status epilepticus after receiving liposomal cytarabine 50 mg by the intraventricular route. This patient died approximately 8 weeks following the last dose of the drug. A patient with extensive lymphoma involving the nasopharynx, brain, and meninges with multiple neurologic deficits died of apparent disease progression 4 days after his second dose of liposomal cytarabine.

■ **Metabolic Effects** ***Conventional Cytarabine*** As a result of extensive purine catabolism accompanying rapid cellular destruction, hyperuricemia may occur in patients receiving cytarabine, and serum uric acid concentrations should be monitored. Hyperuricemia may be minimized or prevented by adequate hydration, alkalinization of the urine, and/or administration of allopurinol.

Liposomal Cytarabine Adverse metabolic or nutritional effects occurred in 16% of treatment cycles in patients receiving liposomal cytarabine for lymphomatous meningitis, including peripheral edema in 7% of treatment cycles.

■ **Dermatologic and Sensitivity Reactions** Anaphylactic reactions have been reported following IV administration of conventional cytarabine. Anaphylaxis with acute cardiopulmonary arrest that required resuscitation occurred in one patient immediately after IV administration of conventional (unencapsulated) cytarabine.

Allergic edema, pruritus, and urticaria have been reported with conventional (unencapsulated) cytarabine. Alopecia, freckling, rash (occasionally associated with conjunctivitis), and skin ulceration also have been reported. A corticosteroid-responsive syndrome that includes maculopapular rash may occur. (See Cautions: Other Adverse Effects.)

■ **Genitourinary Effects** ***Conventional Cytarabine*** Urinary retention has been reported in patients receiving cytarabine.

Liposomal Cytarabine Adverse genitourinary effects occurred in 11% of treatment cycles, and were severe in 3% of treatment cycles, in patients receiving liposomal cytarabine for lymphomatous meningitis. Urinary incontinence occurred in 3% of treatment cycles.

■ **Local Effects** Reactions at the injection site including pain, inflammation, thrombophlebitis, or cellulitis have been reported in patients receiving conventional (unencapsulated) cytarabine. Rarely, pain and inflammation have occurred at sites of subcutaneous injection.

■ **Other Adverse Effects** ***Conventional Cytarabine*** Other reported adverse effects of cytarabine include fever, sepsis, conjunctivitis (may occur with rash), chest pain, pericarditis, pancreatitis, renal dysfunction. A cytarabine syndrome manifested as fever, myalgia, bone pain, maculopapular rash, conjunctivitis, malaise, and occasionally chest pain, has been reported. The syndrome usually occurs 6–12 hours after administration of the drug; corticosteroids are beneficial in the treatment and prevention of the syndrome. If symptoms of the syndrome require treatment, administration of corticosteroids should be considered as well as continuation of cytarabine therapy.

Liposomal Cytarabine Asthenia, adverse effects of the special senses, and pain were reported in 19, 16, and 11% of treatment cycles, and were severe in 5, 1, and 3% of treatment cycles, respectively, in patients receiving liposomal cytarabine for lymphomatous meningitis. Fever and back pain, associated with chemical arachnoiditis, occurred in 11 and 7% of treatment cycles, and were severe in 4 and 0% of treatment cycles, respectively, in patients receiving liposomal cytarabine for lymphomatous meningitis.

■ **Adverse Effects Associated with High-Dose Regimens** Severe and sometimes fatal CNS, GI, and pulmonary toxicity, which differs from that seen with usual dosages, has been associated with high-dose† cytarabine regimens for refractory or secondary acute leukemia or refractory non-Hodgkin's lymphomas. Adverse effects associated with these regimens include cerebral and cerebellar dysfunction (e.g., somnolence, coma, personality changes), which are usually reversible; hemorrhagic conjunctivitis and reversible corneal toxicity (e.g., keratitis), which may be minimized or prevented by prophylaxis with ophthalmic corticosteroid preparations; one case of syndrome of inappropriate secretion of antidiuretic hormone (SIADH); severe GI ulceration, including pneumatosis cystoides intestinalis leading to peritonitis; bowel necrosis; necrotizing colitis; sepsis and liver abscess; liver damage with increased hyperbilirubinemia; pericarditis with tamponade; and pulmonary edema. Reversible, acute aseptic meningitis, combined with cerebellar dysfunction, has been reported in at least one patient. Rarely, severe rash leading to desquamation has occurred. Complete alopecia occurs more commonly with high-dose regimens than with usual dosage regimens of the drug. A syndrome of sudden respiratory distress, rapidly progressing to pulmonary edema and radiographically pronounced cardiomegaly and which was sometimes fatal, has been reported in patients with refractory acute leukemia receiving high-dose therapy. Cases of cardiomyopathy with subsequent death also have been reported in patients receiving high-dose cytarabine in combination with cyclophosphamide in preparation for bone marrow transplantation; this cardiac toxicity may be schedule dependent.

Peripheral motor and sensory neuropathies also have occurred occasionally in patients receiving high-dose cytarabine therapy. Neuropathies have involved the lower and/or upper extremities, and have been manifested as muscle weakness, gait disturbances, walking difficulties, handwriting difficulties, paresthesia, numbness, hypoalgesia, hypoesthesia, and myalgia. Patients receiving high-dose cytarabine should be observed for signs of neuropathy; dosage schedule adjustment may be necessary to avoid irreversible neurologic toxicity. According to the manufacturer, patients with renal or hepatic impairment may be at increased risk of CNS toxicity associated with high-dose cytarabine therapy.

Diffuse interstitial pneumonitis, possibly related to cytarabine therapy, has been reported occasionally in patients receiving relatively high doses (e.g., 1 g/m^2) of cytarabine alone or in combination with other antineoplastic agents. Pancreatitis also has occurred in patients receiving high-dose cytarabine therapy. Cases of acute pancreatitis have been reported in patients receiving cytarabine who were previously treated with asparaginase.

There is some evidence to suggest that the incidence of cerebellar dysfunction (e.g., ataxia, dysarthria, dysdiadochokinesia, dysmetria, tremor, nystagmus) associated with high-dose† (1–3 g/m^2 given by IV infusion over 1 hour twice daily for 2–6 days) regimens of cytarabine may be increased when drug manufactured by Quad (no longer commercially available in the US) is used compared with that when cytarabine manufactured by Upjohn is used. A causal relationship of this apparent increased incidence of cerebellar dysfunction associated with the Quad preparation has not been established, but results of a retrospective analysis conducted by FDA of a limited number of case histories (25 received Quad's product and 34 received Upjohn's product) revealed that cerebellar dysfunction occurred in 32% of patients receiving the high-dose regimen with cytarabine manufactured by Quad compared with 9% in those receiving the Upjohn preparation. While both preparations meet USP compendial standards, there are small differences in impurities and potency of the sterile powders manufactured by these companies; however, the clinical importance of these differences has not been established, but it is possible that such differences are of no consequence with usual regimens but may be important at very high dosages. Quad recommends that any remaining cytarabine manufactured by them be used *only* at the *labeled* dosages, and that their preparation *not* be used for *high-dose* regimens.

■ Precautions and Contraindications

Cytarabine is a highly toxic drug with a low therapeutic index, and a therapeutic response is not likely to occur without some evidence of toxicity. The drug must be used only under constant supervision by clinicians experienced in therapy with cytotoxic agents. Liposomal cytarabine must be used only by clinicians experienced in intrathecal therapy with cytotoxic agents. Adequate diagnostic and treatment facilities are required for the management of complications associated with cytarabine therapy.

Hematologic Toxicity **Conventional Cytarabine.** Treatment with conventional (unencapsulated) cytarabine should be initiated only with extreme caution in patients with preexisting drug-induced bone marrow suppression. Patients who receive myelosuppressive drugs experience an increased frequency of infections (e.g., viral, bacterial, fungal, parasitic, or saprophytic) as well as possible hemorrhagic complications. Because these complications are potentially fatal, the patient should be instructed to notify the clinician if fever, sore throat, or unusual bleeding or bruising occurs.

The patient's hematologic status must be carefully monitored during conventional cytarabine therapy. Leukocyte and platelet counts should be performed frequently during therapy. Leukocyte and platelet counts should be determined daily during remission induction therapy of acute leukemia. Frequent bone marrow examinations should be performed after blast cells have disappeared from the peripheral blood. Patients should receive conventional cytarabine therapy only in facilities where seriously, and possibly fatal, complications of bone marrow suppression can be adequately managed (e.g., infection secondary to granulocytopenia or other impaired body defenses, hemorrhage secondary to thrombocytopenia).

Liposomal Cytarabine. Although systemic exposure to free cytarabine is expected to be minimal following intrathecal administration of liposomal cytarabine, the possibility of hematologic toxicity, including leukopenia, thrombocytopenia, and anemia, cannot be ruled out. Patients should be monitored carefully for hematologic toxicity during therapy with liposomal cytarabine.

Renal or Hepatic Toxicity Periodic determinations of renal function should be performed in patients receiving cytarabine. Periodic determinations of hepatic function also should be performed in patients receiving cytarabine, and the drug should be used with caution and in reduced dosage in patients with poor hepatic function.

Neurotoxicity **Conventional Cytarabine.** Patients receiving high-dose† cytarabine therapy should be monitored closely for signs of neurotoxicity (e.g., peripheral neuropathy, cerebellar dysfunction). (See Cautions: Adverse Effects Associated with High-Dose Regimens.)

Liposomal Cytarabine. Patients receiving intrathecal therapy with liposomal cytarabine should be monitored continuously for the development of neurotoxicity. If neurotoxicity occurs, dosage reduction or discontinuance of therapy is required. (See Dosage Modification for Toxicity and Contraindications for Continued Therapy: Neurotoxicity in Dosage and Administration: Dosage.)

Toxicity Associated with Intrathecal Administration of Liposomal Cytarabine Patients should be informed about the expected adverse effects of intrathecal therapy with liposomal cytarabine, including headache, nausea, vomiting, and fever. Patients should be informed about early signs and symptoms of neurotoxicity. The importance of concurrent dexamethasone administration should be emphasized when each cycle of therapy with liposomal cytarabine is initiated. Patients should be instructed to notify the clinician if signs or symptoms of neurotoxicity develop, or if oral dexamethasone is not well tolerated.

Other Toxicity Serum uric acid concentrations should be monitored in patients receiving conventional cytarabine; rapid lysis of neoplastic cells can lead to hyperuricemia.

Lack of Interchangeability with the Fixed Liposomal Combination of Daunorubicin and Cytarabine The pharmacokinetic properties, formulation, and dosage of cytarabine as a single-entity preparation differ from those of the fixed liposomal combination of daunorubicin and cytarabine (Vyxeos®); these preparations are *not* interchangeable.

Contraindications Conventional cytarabine is contraindicated in patients with known hypersensitivity to the drug. Liposomal cytarabine is contraindicated in patients who are hypersensitive to cytarabine or any component of the formulation, and in patients with active meningeal infection.

■ Pediatric Precautions

Benzyl alcohol is associated with a fatal "gasping syndrome" in premature infants. Conventional (unencapsulated) cytarabine that has been reconstituted with bacteriostatic water for injection containing benzyl alcohol should *not* be used in neonates. Administration of injections preserved with benzyl alcohol has been associated with toxicity in neonates. Toxicity appears to have resulted from administration of large amounts (i.e., 100–400 mg/kg daily) of benzyl alcohol in these neonates.

Safety and efficacy of liposomal cytarabine in children have not been established.

■ Mutagenicity and Carcinogenicity

Cytarabine is mutagenic and potentially carcinogenic. Studies have not been performed to date to evaluate the mutagenic or carcinogenic potential of liposomal cytarabine, but its active ingredient is cytarabine. Cytarabine was mutagenic in in vitro tests. Cytarabine was clastogenic, exhibiting chromosomal aberrations and sister chromatid exchange, in in vitro tests in human leukocytes and in in vivo tests in rodent bone marrow; clastogenicity also was demonstrated using the mouse micronucleus assay. In in vitro tests, cytarabine caused the transformation of hamster embryo cells and rat H43 cells. Cytarabine was clastogenic to meiotic cells; a dose-dependent increase in sperm-head abnormalities and chromosomal aberrations were observed in mice given cytarabine intraperitoneally.

■ Pregnancy, Fertility, and Lactation

Cytarabine can cause fetal toxicity when administered to pregnant women, but potential benefits from use of the drug may be acceptable in certain conditions despite the possible risks to the fetus. Because systemic exposure to cytarabine is negligible during intrathecal therapy with liposomal cytarabine, the risk of fetal toxicity is thought to be low. However, there are no formal studies assessing the reproductive toxicity of liposomal cytarabine.

Congenital abnormalities have been reported, particularly when the fetus has been exposed to systemic therapy with cytarabine during the first trimester. There is a definite, but considerably reduced risk to the fetus when therapy is initiated during the second or third trimester. At least 3 cases of major limb malformations have been reported in infants of mothers who received IV cytarabine, alone or in combination with other agents, during the first trimester. One infant had extremity and ear deformities, and another infant had upper and lower distal limb defects. A few women have received cytarabine with other antineoplastic agents during the second and third trimesters (20th–28th week of gestation) and delivered apparently normal infants. However, in one patient a trisomy C chromosomal abnormality was found in the chorionic tissue following a therapeutic abortion at 24 weeks of gestation after 4 weeks of therapy with cytarabine and thioguanine; the fetus appeared to have no congenital abnormalities.

In animal studies, cytarabine has been shown to cause abnormal cerebellar development in the neonatal hamster. Cytarabine has been shown to be teratogenic in mice and rats. Abnormalities including cleft palate, phocomelia, deformed appendages, and skeletal abnormalities have been observed in the offspring of mice given cytarabine doses of at least 2 mg/kg daily (about 0.2 times the recommended human dose on a mg/m^2 basis) administered intraperitoneally during the period of organogenesis. Deformed appendages have been observed in the offspring of rats given cytarabine 20 mg/kg (about 4 times the recommended human dose on a mg/m^2 basis) as a single intraperitoneal dose on day 12 of gestation. Reduced prenatal and postnatal brain size and permanent impairment of learning ability were observed in rats given single intraperitoneal doses of cytarabine 50 mg/kg (about 10 times the recommended human dose on a mg/m^2 basis) on day 14 of gestation.

Cytarabine was embryotoxic in mice when given during the period of organogenesis. Decreased fetal weight was observed in mice given cytarabine 0.5 mg/kg daily (about 0.05 times the recommended human dose on a mg/m^2 basis), and increased early and late resorptions and decreased live litter sizes were observed in mice given cytarabine 8 mg/kg daily (approximately equal to the recommended human dose on a mg/m^2 basis).

There are no adequate and well-controlled studies to date using conventional or liposomal cytarabine in pregnant women. Cytarabine should be used during pregnancy only in life-threatening situations or severe disease for which safer drugs cannot be used or are ineffective. When the drug is administered during pregnancy or if the patient becomes pregnant while receiving the drug, the patient should be informed of the potential hazard to the fetus. Women receiving systemic therapy with cytarabine, particularly during the first trimester, should be counseled on the advisability of continuing the pregnancy. The manufacturers suggest that infants delivered by women who received cytarabine therapy during pregnancy receive follow-up monitoring. Women of childbearing potential should be advised to avoid becoming pregnant while receiving the drug.

There are no adequate studies on the effects of cytarabine on fertility. Because systemic exposure to free cytarabine is expected to be minimal following intrathecal administration of liposomal cytarabine, the risk of impaired fertility is thought to be low.

It is not known whether cytarabine is distributed into human milk. Because of the potential for serious adverse reactions to conventional cytarabine in nursing infants, a decision should be made whether to discontinue nursing or the drug, taking into account the importance of the drug to the woman. Systemic exposure to free cytarabine following intrathecal administration of liposomal cytarabine is negligible, so the risk of the drug being distributed into human milk is thought to be low. However, because many drugs are distributed into human milk and because of the potential for serious adverse reactions in nursing infants, the use of liposomal cytarabine is not recommended in nursing women.

Drug Interactions

Formal studies of drug interactions have not been conducted for liposomal cytarabine.

■ **Cardiac Glycosides** GI absorption of oral digoxin tablets may be substantially reduced in patients receiving combination chemotherapy regimens (including regimens containing cytarabine), possibly as a result of temporary damage to intestinal mucosa caused by the cytotoxic agents. Plasma concentrations of digoxin should be carefully monitored in patients receiving such combination chemotherapy regimens. Use of digoxin oral elixir or liquid-filled capsules may minimize the potential interaction, since the drug is rapidly and extensively absorbed from these dosage forms. Limited data suggest that the extent of GI absorption of digitoxin (no longer commercially available in the US) is not substantially affected by concomitant administration of combination chemotherapy regimens known to decrease absorption of digoxin.

■ **Anti-infective Agents** One in vitro study indicates that cytarabine may antagonize the activity of gentamicin against *Klebsiella pneumoniae*. Patients receiving concurrent cytarabine and aminoglycoside therapy for the treatment of infections caused by *K. pneumoniae* should be closely monitored; if therapeutic response is not achieved, reevaluation of anti-infective therapy may be necessary.

Limited data suggest that cytarabine may antagonize the anti-infective activity of flucytosine, possibly by competitive inhibition of the anti-infective's uptake by fungi.

■ **Antineoplastic Agents** The incidence of toxicity may be increased when liposomal cytarabine is used concurrently with systemic chemotherapy in patients with neoplastic meningitis. Increased neurotoxicity has been observed in patients receiving concomitant intrathecal administration of conventional cytarabine and other cytotoxic agents.

■ **Radiation Toxicity** The incidence of toxicity may be increased when cytarabine is used concurrently with radiation therapy in patients with neoplastic meningitis.

Laboratory Test Interferences

Because particles of liposomal cytarabine are similar in size and appearance to white blood cells, CSF examinations must be interpreted carefully following administration of the drug.

Acute Toxicity

Limited information is available on the acute toxicity of conventional (unencapsulated) cytarabine. IV doses of cytarabine 4.5 g/m^2 administered over 1 hour every 12 hours for 12 doses caused excessive toxicity, including irreversible CNS toxicity and death. Single doses of cytarabine up to 3 g/m^2 IV have been administered by rapid IV infusion without apparent toxicity. There is no known antidote for overdosage of conventional (unencapsulated) cytarabine.

Limited information is available on the acute toxicity of liposomal cytarabine. Overdosage of liposomal cytarabine may be associated with severe chemical arachnoiditis, including encephalopathy. In an uncontrolled study, single doses of liposomal cytarabine up to 125 mg were administered without dexamethasone prophylaxis. One patient died of encephalopathy 36 hours after receiving an intraventricular dose of liposomal cytarabine 125 mg. This patient also was receiving concomitant whole brain irradiation and had previously received intraventricular methotrexate. There is no known antidote for overdosage of liposomal cytarabine by intrathecal administration or free (unencapsulated) cytarabine released from the drug. In a case of overdosage of free cytarabine administered intrathecally, exchange of CSF with isotonic saline solution was performed; this method may be considered in case of overdosage with liposomal cytarabine. Treatment of toxicity is mainly supportive and should be directed at maintaining vital functions.

Pharmacology

Cytarabine is converted intracellularly to the nucleotide, cytarabine triphosphate (ara-CTP, cytosine arabinoside triphosphate). Although the exact mechanism(s) of action of cytarabine has not been fully elucidated, cytarabine triphosphate appears to inhibit DNA polymerase by competing with the physiologic substrate, deoxycytidine triphosphate, resulting in the inhibition of DNA synthesis. Although limited, incorporation of cytarabine triphosphate into DNA and RNA may also contribute to the cytotoxic effects of the drug.

Cytarabine is a potent immunosuppressant which can suppress humoral and/or cellular immune responses; however, the drug does not decrease preexisting antibody titers and has no effect on established delayed hypersensitivity reactions.

Pharmacokinetics

The effects of gender, race, or renal or hepatic impairment on the pharmacokinetics of liposomal cytarabine have not been studied.

■ **Absorption** Less than 20% of a dose of conventional (unencapsulated) cytarabine is absorbed from the GI tract, and the drug is not effective when administered orally. Following subcutaneous or IM† injection of radiolabeled cytarabine (as the conventional formulation), peak plasma concentrations of radioactivity occur within 20–60 minutes and are considerably lower than those attained after IV administration. Continuous IV infusions of conventional cytarabine produce relatively constant plasma concentrations of the drug in 8–24 hours.

Cytarabine liposome injection is a sustained-release formulation of the drug that is designed for intrathecal administration. According to preliminary analysis of pharmacokinetic data, peak concentrations of free cytarabine occur within 5 hours in both the ventricle and the lumbar sac following intrathecal administration of liposomal cytarabine into the lumbar sac or an intraventricular reservoir.

■ **Distribution** Conventional (unencapsulated) cytarabine is rapidly and widely distributed into tissues and fluids, including liver, plasma, and peripheral granulocytes. Following rapid IV injection of conventional cytarabine in one study, approximately 13% of the drug was bound to plasma proteins.

Cytarabine crosses the blood-brain barrier to a limited extent. During a continuous IV infusion or subcutaneous infusion†, cytarabine concentrations in the CSF are higher than those attained after rapid IV injection and are about 40–60% of plasma concentrations. Most of an intrathecal dose of conventional cytarabine diffuses into the systemic circulation but is rapidly metabolized and usually only low plasma concentrations of unchanged drug occur.

Following intrathecal administration of 50 or 75 mg of liposomal cytarabine, systemic exposure to cytarabine is negligible. Cytarabine apparently crosses the placenta. It is not known if cytarabine or ara-U is distributed into milk.

■ **Elimination** After rapid IV injection of cytarabine, plasma drug concentrations appear to decline in a biphasic manner with a half-life of about 10 minutes in the initial phase and about 1–3 hours in the terminal phase. Cytarabine reportedly undergoes triphasic elimination in some patients. After intrathecal injection, cytarabine concentrations in the CSF reportedly decline with a half-life of about 2 hours.

Following intrathecal administration of 12.5–75 mg of liposomal cytarabine, CSF concentrations of the drug decline in a biphasic manner with a terminal phase half-life of 100–263 hours.

Cytarabine is rapidly and extensively metabolized mainly in the liver but also in kidneys, GI mucosa, granulocytes, and to a lesser extent in other tissues by the enzyme cytidine deaminase, producing the inactive metabolite 1-β-d-arabinofuranosyluracil (ara-U, uracil arabinoside). After the initial distribution phase, more than 80% of the drug in plasma is present as ara-U. In the CSF, only minimal amounts of cytarabine are converted to ara-U because of low CSF concentrations of cytidine deaminase. The clearance rate of cytarabine in CSF is similar to the CSF bulk flow rate of 0.24 mL/minute. Intracellularly, cytarabine is metabolized by deoxycytidine kinase and other nucleotide kinases to cytarabine triphosphate, the active metabolite of the drug. Cytarabine triphosphate is inactivated by a pyrimidine nucleoside deaminase, which produces the uracil derivative.

Cytarabine and ara-U are excreted in urine. After rapid IV, IM† , subcutaneous, or intrathecal injection or continuous IV infusion of cytarabine, about 70–80% of the dose is excreted in urine within 24 hours. Approximately 90% of the urinary drug excretion occurs as ara-U and about 10% as unchanged cytarabine.

Chemistry and Stability

■ **Chemistry** Cytarabine is a synthetic pyrimidine nucleoside. Cytarabine differs from the physiological nucleosides, cytidine and deoxycytidine, in that the sugar moiety is arabinose instead of ribose or deoxyribose. Cytarabine is a pyrimidine antagonist antimetabolite. The drug occurs as an odorless, white to off-white, crystalline powder, is very slightly soluble in alcohol and has a solubility of 100 mg/mL in water. Cytarabine has a pK_a of 4.35. Hydrochloric acid and/or sodium hydroxide may be added to the commercially available lyophilized product to adjust the pH. Commercially available cytarabine injection 100 mg/5 mL (20 mg/mL) occurs as a sterile, isotonic solution of the drug in 0.68% sodium chloride; hydrochloric acid and/or sodium hydroxide may be added to adjust the pH to 7.4; this preparation also is available in a pharmacy bulk package that is restricted to use in the preparation of admixtures for IV infusion. Each mL of the cytarabine injection contains approximately 0.12 mEq of sodium. Commercially available cytarabine injection 2 g/20 mL occurs as a sterile solution in water for injection; hydrochloric acid and/or sodium hydroxide may be added to adjust the pH to 7.7. Commercially available cytarabine injection 500 mg/25 mL (20 mg/mL) contains benzyl alcohol as a preservative and hydrochloric acid and/or sodium hydroxide may be added to adjust the pH to 7.6.

Commercially available cytarabine liposome injection is a sterile, preservative-free injectable suspension of cytarabine encapsulated in multivesicular lipid-based particles. The injection is a sterile, nonpyrogenic, white to off-white suspension of cytarabine in 0.9% sodium chloride in water for injection that has a pH of 5.5–8.5. Each mL of the cytarabine liposome injection contains 10 mg of cytarabine encapsulated in lipid-based particles.

■ **Stability** ***Conventional Cytarabine*** Conventional (unencapsulated) cytarabine sterile powder should be stored at 25°C but may be exposed to temperatures of 15–30°C. Commercially available conventional cytarabine injection should be stored at controlled room temperature (15–30°C); the injection should be stored in the manufacturer's carton until time of use and should be protected from light.

Following reconstitution of the sterile powder with bacteriostatic water for injection containing 0.945% benzyl alcohol, solutions containing 20, 50, or 100 mg of cytarabine per mL have a pH of about 5 and are stable for 48 hours at 20–25°C; solutions that develop a slight haze should not be used. The manufacturer states that following dilution of the reconstituted solution with water for injection, 5% dextrose injection, or 0.9% sodium chloride injection, solutions containing 0.5 mg of cytarabine per mL are stable for at least 8 days at room temperature. In a study of solutions for intrathecal injection, those containing 5 mg of cytarabine per mL in Elliott's B solution (an investigational electrolyte solution containing sodium bicarbonate as a buffer), 0.9% sodium chloride injection, or lactated Ringer's injection were stable for 7 days at room temperature. However, when cytarabine is reconstituted with a diluent that does not contain a preservative or when reconstituted solutions of the drug are diluted in compatible IV solutions, the possibility of contamination should be considered. Although commercially available cytarabine injection is stable for 8 days at room temperature when diluted with sterile water for injection, 5% dextrose injection, or 0.9% sodium chloride injection, the manufacturer states that good professional practice suggests that these admixtures be used as soon after preparation as possible; in addition, any unused portions should be discarded. The manufacturer also recommends that any unused portion of cytarabine injection in pharmacy bulk packages be discarded within 4 hours after initial entry through the closure into the container.

Solutions of cytarabine have been reported to be incompatible with various drugs, but the incompatibility depends on several factors (e.g., concentration of the drugs, specific diluents used, resulting pH, temperature). Specialized references should be consulted for specific compatibility information.

Liposomal Cytarabine Cytarabine liposome injection should be stored at 2–8°C; freezing should be avoided and the vial should be protected from aggressive agitation. Cytarabine liposome injection contains no preservative and should be used within 4 hours of withdrawal from the vial; unused portions should be discarded. When stored according to manufacturer recommendations, cytarabine liposome injection may be used up to the expiration date printed on the label. Cytarabine liposome injection should not be mixed with any other medications.

For further information on the handling of antineoplastic agents, see the ASHP Guidelines on Handling Hazardous Drugs at http://www.ahfsdruginformation.com.

Preparations

Excipients in commercially available drug preparations may have clinically important effects in some individuals; consult specific product labeling for details.

Cytarabine

Parenteral		
Injection	20 mg/mL (500 mg)	**Cytarabine Injection**

Cytarabine (Preservative-free)

Parenteral		
For injection	100 mg	**Cytarabine for Injection**
		Cytosar-U®, Pfizer
	500 mg	**Cytarabine for Injection**
		Cytosar-U®, Pfizer
	1 g	**Cytarabine for Injection**
		Cytosar-U®, Pfizer
	2 g	**Cytarabine for Injection**
		Cytosar-U®, Pfizer
Injection	20 mg/mL (100 mg)	**Cytarabine Injection**
	100 mg/mL (2 g)	**Cytarabine Injection**
	1 g (20 mg/mL) pharmacy bulk package	**Cytarabine Injection**

Cytarabine Liposomal

Parenteral		
Injectable suspension, extended-release, for intrathecal use only	10 mg/mL	**DepoCyt®**, SkyePharma

†Use is not currently included in the labeling approved by the US Food and Drug Administration

Selected Revisions October 2018, © Copyright, August 1981, American Society of Health-System Pharmacists, Inc.

Dabrafenib Mesylate

■ Dabrafenib, an inhibitor of b-Raf serine-threonine kinase (BRAF) with V600E or V600K mutation, is an antineoplastic agent.

Uses

■ **Melanoma** ***Adjuvant Therapy for Melanoma*** Dabrafenib is used in combination with trametinib as adjuvant therapy following complete resection of melanoma with b-Raf serine-threonine kinase (BRAF) V600E or V600K mutation and nodal involvement. An FDA-approved diagnostic test (e.g., THxID® BRAF kit) is required to confirm the presence of the BRAF V600E or V600K mutation prior to initiation of therapy.

The current indication for dabrafenib in combination with trametinib as adjuvant therapy following complete resection of melanoma with BRAF V600E or V600K mutation and nodal involvement is based principally on the results of a randomized, double-blind, placebo-controlled phase 3 study (COMBI-AD) in patients who had undergone complete resection of stage III melanoma with BRAF V600E or V600K mutation (as detected by the bioMerieux THxID® BRAF V600 mutation test) and involvement of regional lymph nodes. In this study, 870 patients were randomized (stratified by disease stage and BRAF mutation status) in a 1:1 ratio to receive dabrafenib 150 mg twice daily with trametinib 2 mg once daily or placebo for up to 12 months. Patients enrolled in this study must have had undergone complete resection of melanoma with complete lymphadenectomy within 12 weeks of randomization. The primary measure of efficacy was relapse-free survival. The median age of patients enrolled in the study was 51 years; 99% of patients were Caucasian, 55% were male, 91% had a baseline Eastern Cooperative Oncology Group (ECOG) performance status of 0, 65% had macroscopic lymph node involvement, 41% had tumor ulceration, 41% had stage IIIb disease, and 40% had stage IIIc disease. The majority (91%) of patients had BRAF V600E mutation and 9% had a V600K mutation. Patients who had mucosal or ocular melanoma, unresectable in-transit metastases, or distant metastatic disease and those who had previously received systemic therapy (including radiation therapy) were not eligible to enroll in the study.

After a median follow-up of 2.8 years, median relapse-free survival had not been reached in patients receiving dabrafenib in combination with trametinib and was 16.6 months in those receiving placebo; however, dabrafenib in combination with trametinib reduced the risk of relapse by 53% compared with placebo. In an updated analysis at a median follow-up of 44 or 42 months for patients receiving dabrafenib in combination with trametinib or those receiving placebo, respectively, relapse-free survival remained similar to the primary results. Dabrafenib in combination with trametinib was associated with a numerically, but not significantly, higher estimated 3-year overall survival rate as compared with placebo. Results of a subgroup analysis (based on disease stage, lymph node involvement, presence of tumor ulceration) suggested that the effect of dabrafenib in combination with trametinib was consistent across all subgroups.

The safety and efficacy of dabrafenib in patients with wild-type BRAF melanoma have not been established; use of dabrafenib is *not* recommended by the manufacturer for these patients. (See Tumor Promotion in Wild-Type BRAF Tumors under Cautions: Warnings/Precautions.)

Unresectable or Metastatic Melanoma Dabrafenib, alone or in combination therapy, is used for the treatment of unresectable or metastatic melanoma in selected patients.

Monotherapy. Dabrafenib is used as monotherapy for the treatment of unresectable or metastatic melanoma with BRAF V600E mutation. Dabrafenib has been designated an orphan drug by the FDA as monotherapy for the treatment of this cancer. An FDA-approved diagnostic test (e.g., THxID® BRAF kit) is required to confirm the presence of the BRAF V600E mutation prior to initiation of monotherapy.

The current indication for dabrafenib monotherapy is based principally on the results of an open-label, randomized, phase 3 study (BREAK-3) in patients with previously untreated stage IV or unresectable stage III melanoma positive for BRAF V600E mutation. Patients receiving dabrafenib experienced longer progression-free survival when compared with those receiving dacarbazine. In the BREAK-3 study, 250 adults (median 52 years of age, 60% male, 99% white, 67% with ECOG performance status of 0, 66% with stage M1c disease, 62% with normal LDH) were randomized in a 3:1 ratio to receive oral dabrafenib 150 mg twice daily or IV dacarbazine 1 g/m² every 3 weeks; treatment was continued until disease progression, death, or study withdrawal occurred. Patients who experienced disease progression while receiving dacarbazine were allowed to cross over to dabrafenib treatment. The median duration of follow-up was 5.1 and 3.5 months in those receiving dabrafenib and dacarbazine, respectively. The median progression-free survival assessed radiographically or photographically by the investigator was 5.1 and 2.7 months for those receiving dabrafenib and dacarbazine, respectively. An independent review committee assessed progression-free survival as 6.7 and 2.9 months for patients receiving dabrafenib and dacarbazine, respectively. The independent review committee reported a confirmed objective response in 50% of patients receiving dabrafenib compared with 6% of those receiving dacarbazine. The estimated median duration of response was 5.5 months for those receiving dabrafenib and was not yet reached for those receiving dacarbazine.

Dabrafenib treatment has been shown to be effective in patients with melanoma with brain metastasis. Dabrafenib was evaluated in a single-arm, open-label, phase 2 study (BREAK-MB) of 139 adults with melanoma positive for BRAF mutation (V600E) and at least one asymptomatic brain metastasis. Patients received oral dabrafenib 150 mg twice daily until disease progression, death, or unacceptable toxicity occurred. Up to 2 previous treatment regimens for extracranial metastatic melanoma were allowed, but patients could not have received prior treatment with a BRAF inhibitor or a mitogen-activated extracellular signal regulated kinase (MEK) inhibitor. The BREAK-MB study consisted of 2 cohorts: patients with no prior treatment for brain metastasis (median 50 years of age, 72% male, 59% with ECOG performance status of 0, 57% with elevated LDH) and those with prior local treatment for brain metastasis (median 51 years of age, 63% male, 66% with ECOG performance status of 0, 54% with elevated LDH). Among 139 patients with melanoma positive for BRAF V600E mutation, 18% in each cohort achieved an overall intracranial response (i.e., best intracranial response was a complete or partial response) as assessed by an independent review committee. The median duration of overall intracranial response was 4.6 months in both cohorts.

The safety and efficacy of dabrafenib in patients with wild-type BRAF melanoma have not been established; use of dabrafenib is *not* recommended by the manufacturer for these patients. (See Tumor Promotion in Wild-Type BRAF Tumors under Cautions: Warnings/Precautions.)

Combination Therapy. Dabrafenib is used in combination with trametinib for the treatment of unresectable or metastatic melanoma with BRAF V600E or V600K mutation. Dabrafenib has been designated an orphan drug by the FDA when used in combination with trametinib for the treatment of this cancer. When dabrafenib is used in combination with trametinib, the presence of BRAF V600E or V600K mutation should be confirmed using an FDA-approved diagnostic test (e.g., THxID® BRAF kit) prior to initiation of therapy.

The current indication for dabrafenib in combination with trametinib in the treatment of unresectable or metastatic melanoma with BRAF V600E or V600K mutation is based principally on the results of 2 randomized phase 3 studies (COMBI-D and COMBI-V) in patients with previously untreated stage IIIc or IV cutaneous melanoma with BRAF V600E or V600K mutation. In the COMBI-D and COMBI-V studies, the primary measures of efficacy were progression-free survival and overall survival, respectively.

In the COMBI-D study, 423 patients were randomized in a 1:1 ratio to receive either dabrafenib (150 mg twice daily) in combination with trametinib (2 mg once daily) or dabrafenib in combination with placebo. Treatment was continued until disease progression or unacceptable toxicity occurred or the patient withdrew from the study; however, patients with disease progression could continue receiving treatment if they met prespecified criteria for continuation. The median age of patients was 56 years; greater than 99% were Caucasian, 72% had an ECOG performance status of 0, 66% had stage M1c disease, 65% had normal LDH concentrations, and 2 patients had a history of brain metastases. Most patients (85%) had BRAF V600E mutation and 15% had a V600K mutation. At a median follow-up of 9 months, median progression-free survival or overall survival was 9.3 or 25.1 months, respectively, in patients receiving dabrafenib and trametinib compared with 8.8 or 18.7 months, respectively, in those receiving placebo and dabrafenib. An updated progression-free survival analysis confirmed prolonged median progression-free survival (11 versus 8.8 months; hazard ratio for death or disease progression: 0.67) in patients receiving dabrafenib in combination with trametinib compared with those receiving placebo and dabrafenib. A final analysis for overall survival estimated a prolonged median overall survival (25.1 versus 18.7 months) and a reduction in the risk of death (29%) in patients receiving dabrafenib in combination with trametinib. In addition, patients receiving dabrafenib and trametinib had higher overall response rates (66 versus 51%) compared with those receiving placebo and dabrafenib; complete responses were achieved in 10 or 8% of patients receiving dabrafenib in combination with trametinib or placebo in combination with dabrafenib, respectively. The median duration of response in patients receiving dabrafenib and trametinib or those receiving placebo and dabrafenib was 9.2 or 10.2 months, respectively. Results of a subgroup analysis (based on age, gender, disease stage, baseline ECOG performance status, baseline serum LDH concentration, visceral involvement, number of disease sites, and BRAF V600 mutation status) suggested that the effects of combination therapy with dabrafenib and trametinib on progression-free survival and overall survival were consistent across all subgroups.

In the COMBI-V study, 704 patients were randomized in a 1:1 ratio to receive either dabrafenib (150 mg twice daily) in combination with trametinib (2 mg once daily) or vemurafenib (960 mg twice daily). The median age of patients was 55 years; 96% were Caucasian, 70% had an ECOG performance status of 0, 67% had normal LDH concentrations, 61% had stage M1c disease, 6% had stage IIIc disease, and one patient had a history of brain metastases. Most patients (89%) had BRAF V600E mutation and 10% had a V600K mutation. The median follow-up period at the time of the interim analysis was 11 months for those receiving dabrafenib in combination with trametinib and 10 months for those receiving vemurafenib alone. Median overall survival had not been reached in patients receiving dabrafenib in combination with trametinib and was 17.2 months in those receiving vemurafenib alone; however, dabrafenib in combination with trametinib reduced the risk of death by 31% compared with vemurafenib alone. Patients receiving dabrafenib in combination with trametinib also had longer median progression-free survival (11.4 versus 7.3 months) and higher overall response rates (64 versus 51%) compared with patients receiving vemurafenib alone. Because of the survival benefit observed at the interim analysis, study investigators permitted patients previously randomized to receive vemurafenib alone to cross over to combination therapy with dabrafenib and trametinib. Results of a subgroup analysis (based on age, gender, BRAF mutation status, ECOG performance status, and baseline LDH concentration) suggested that the effect of dabrafenib in combination with trametinib was consistent across most subgroups; an overall survival benefit for combination therapy with dabrafenib and trametinib versus vemurafenib was not apparent in the subgroup of patients with an ECOG performance status of 1 (hazard ratio: 1.03).

The safety and efficacy of dabrafenib in patients with wild-type BRAF melanoma have not been established; use of dabrafenib is *not* recommended by the manufacturer for these patients. (See Tumor Promotion in Wild-Type BRAF Tumors under Cautions: Warnings/Precautions.)

■ **Non-small Cell Lung Cancer** Dabrafenib is used in combination with trametinib for the treatment of metastatic non-small cell lung cancer (NSCLC) with BRAF V600E mutation. Dabrafenib has been designated an orphan drug by the FDA when used in combination with trametinib for the treatment of this cancer. An FDA-approved diagnostic test (e.g., THxID® BRAF kit) is required to confirm the presence of the BRAF V600E mutation prior to initiation of therapy.

The current indication for dabrafenib in combination with trametinib in the treatment of metastatic NSCLC with BRAF V600E mutation is based principally on the results of an open-label, multicenter, nonrandomized, 3-cohort, phase 2 study (BRF113928). Patients in the BRF113928 study were enrolled into 2 cohorts: those previously treated with 1–3 systemic therapies with disease progression following at least one platinum-containing regimen and those with treatment-naive metastatic NSCLC. The cohort of patients with previously treated disease received either single-agent dabrafenib (150 mg twice daily) or dabrafenib (150 mg twice daily) in combination with trametinib (2 mg once daily). The cohort of patients with previously untreated disease received dabrafenib (150 mg twice daily) in combination with trametinib (2 mg once daily). Treatment was continued until disease progression or unacceptable toxicity occurred or the patient withdrew from the study. Patients with prior exposure to BRAF or mitogen-activated extracellular signal-regulated kinase (MEK) inhibitors were not eligible to enroll in the study; however, prior exposure to epidermal growth factor receptor (EGFR) or anaplastic lymphoma kinase (ALK) inhibitors was permitted in patients with EGFR- or ALK-positive tumors. The primary measure of efficacy was objective response rate as assessed by an independent review committee according to Response Evaluation Criteria in Solid Tumors (RECIST) and duration of response. The median age of patients was 66 years; 98% had squamous cell histology, 90% had an ECOG performance status of 0 or 1, 81% were Caucasian, 60% had a history of smoking, 48% were male, 32% were nonsmokers, 14% were Asian, 11% had received adjuvant chemotherapy, 8% were current smokers, 3% were black, and 2% were Hispanic. The majority (99%) of patients had metastatic disease; brain or liver metastases were present in 6 or 14% of these patients, respectively. Among the cohort of patients with previously treated disease, 58% had received only one prior systemic therapy for metastatic disease.

In the cohort of patients with previously treated disease, the objective response rate was 27 or 63% in patients receiving single-agent dabrafenib or combination therapy with dabrafenib and trametinib, respectively, and the median duration of response was 9.9 or 12.6 months, respectively. In the cohort of patients receiving dabrafenib in combination with trametinib for treatment-naive disease, the objective response rate was 61%. In the overall study population, 52 or 59–64% of the patients who responded to single-agent dabrafenib or dabrafenib and trametinib combination therapy, respectively, had durable responses of 6 months or more.

The safety and efficacy of dabrafenib in patients with wild-type BRAF NSCLC have not been established; use of dabrafenib is *not* recommended by the manufacturer for these patients. (See Tumor Promotion in Wild-Type BRAF Tumors under Cautions: Warnings/Precautions.)

■ **Anaplastic Thyroid Cancer** Dabrafenib is used in combination with trametinib for the treatment of locally advanced or metastatic anaplastic thyroid cancer with BRAF V600E mutation when no satisfactory locoregional treatment options are available. Dabrafenib has been designated an orphan drug by the FDA when used in combination with trametinib for the treatment of this cancer. An FDA-approved diagnostic test (e.g., THxID® BRAF kit) is required to confirm the presence of the BRAF V600E mutation prior to initiation of therapy.

The current indication for dabrafenib in combination with trametinib in the treatment of anaplastic thyroid cancer with BRAF V600E mutation is based principally on the results of an activity-estimating, open-label, multicenter, nonrandomized, 9-cohort, phase 2 trial (BRF117019) in patients with rare BRAF V600E mutation-positive malignancies, including anaplastic thyroid cancer. In this trial, a cohort of 26 patients with locally advanced, unresectable, or metastatic anaplastic thyroid cancer received dabrafenib (150 mg twice daily) in combination with trametinib (2 mg once daily). Treatment was continued until disease progression or unacceptable toxicity occurred or the patient withdrew from the study. Patients with prior exposure to BRAF or MEK inhibitors, symptomatic or untreated CNS metastases, airway obstruction, or inability to swallow or retain oral drugs were not eligible to enroll in the study. The primary measure of efficacy was objective response rate as assessed by an independent review committee according to RECIST and duration of response. The median age of patients enrolled in the anaplastic thyroid cancer cohort was 70 years; 50% were male, 50% were Caucasian, 46% were Asian, and 54% had a history of differentiated thyroid cancer. All patients had an ECOG performance status of 0 or 1. The majority (92%) of patients had previously undergone surgery, 81% had received prior external beam radiation therapy, and 54% had received systemic therapy. The objective response rate in 23 evaluable patients in the anaplastic thyroid cancer cohort was 61%; complete response was achieved in 4% of the evaluable patients. Durable responses of 6 months or more were observed in 64% of responders.

The safety and efficacy of dabrafenib in patients with wild-type BRAF anaplastic thyroid cancer have not been established; use of dabrafenib is *not* recommended by the manufacturer for these patients. (See Tumor Promotion in Wild-Type BRAF Tumors under Cautions: Warnings/Precautions.)

Dosage and Administration

■ General An FDA-approved diagnostic test (e.g., THxID® BRAF kit) is required to confirm the presence of the b-Raf serine-threonine kinase (BRAF) V600E mutation prior to initiation of dabrafenib monotherapy for the treatment of unresectable or metastatic melanoma or combination therapy with dabrafenib and trametinib for the treatment of metastatic non-small cell lung cancer (NSCLC) or locally advanced or metastatic anaplastic thyroid cancer; the presence of BRAF V600E or V600K mutation must be confirmed prior to initiation of combination therapy with dabrafenib and trametinib for the treatment of unresectable or metastatic melanoma or for the adjuvant treatment of melanoma.

■ Administration Dabrafenib should be administered orally twice daily, approximately every 12 hours, at least 1 hour before or 2 hours after a meal. Dabrafenib capsules should not be opened, crushed, or broken.

If a dose of dabrafenib is missed, the dose may be taken as soon as it is remembered, but only if it can be taken at least 6 hours prior to the next scheduled dose. Patients should *not* take extra capsules of the drug to make up for the missed dose.

■ Dosage Dosage of dabrafenib mesylate is expressed in terms of dabrafenib.

Melanoma **Adjuvant Therapy for Melanoma.** For use in combination with trametinib as adjuvant treatment following complete resection of melanoma with BRAF V600E or V600K mutation and nodal involvement, the recommended adult dosage of dabrafenib is 150 mg twice daily. Therapy should be continued for up to 1 year or until disease progression or unacceptable toxicity occurs.

Monotherapy for Unresectable or Metastatic Melanoma. For use as a single-agent for the treatment of unresectable or metastatic melanoma with BRAF V600E mutation, the recommended adult dosage of dabrafenib is 150 mg twice daily. Therapy should be continued until disease progression or unacceptable toxicity occurs.

Combination Therapy for Unresectable or Metastatic Melanoma. For use in combination with trametinib for the treatment of unresectable or metastatic melanoma with BRAF V600E or V600K mutation, the recommended adult dosage of dabrafenib is 150 mg twice daily. Therapy should be continued until disease progression or unacceptable toxicity occurs.

Non-small Cell Lung Cancer For use in combination with trametinib for the treatment of metastatic NSCLC with BRAF V600E mutation, the recommended adult dosage of dabrafenib is 150 mg twice daily. Therapy should be continued until disease progression or unacceptable toxicity occurs.

Anaplastic Thyroid Cancer For use in combination with trametinib for the treatment of locally advanced or metastatic anaplastic thyroid cancer with BRAF V600E mutation when no satisfactory locoregional treatment options are available, the recommended adult dosage of dabrafenib is 150 mg twice daily. Therapy should be continued until disease progression or unacceptable toxicity occurs.

Dosage Modification for Toxicity Dosage of dabrafenib may be reduced or therapy temporarily interrupted in patients who develop adverse effects. Up to 3 dosage reductions for toxicity may be made. If dosage modification of dabrafenib is necessary, an initial dosage reduction to 100 mg twice daily is recommended. If further dosage modification is necessary, dosage reduction to 75 mg twice daily or subsequently to 50 mg twice daily may be considered. For patients unable to tolerate a dosage of dabrafenib 50 mg twice daily, the drug should be permanently discontinued.

For further information regarding dosage modification when dabrafenib is used in combination with trametinib, including information regarding trametinib dosage modification for toxicity, see Dosage and Administration: Dosage Modification for Toxicity, in Trametinib 10:00.

Dosage Modification for New Primary Cutaneous Malignancies. If new primary cutaneous malignancies occur, no dosage modification of dabrafenib is recommended.

Dosage Modification for New Primary Noncutaneous Malignancies. If new RAS mutation-positive, noncutaneous malignancies occur, dabrafenib should be permanently discontinued.

Dosage Modification for Febrile Drug Reactions. If fever (temperature of 38.5–40°C) occurs, dabrafenib treatment should be interrupted until the adverse reaction resolves. Once fever resolves, dabrafenib may be resumed at the same or a reduced dosage.

If a higher fever (temperature exceeding 40°C) or fever complicated by rigors, hypotension, dehydration, or renal failure occurs, dabrafenib treatment should be permanently discontinued or interrupted until such adverse reactions resolve. Once fever resolves, dabrafenib may be resumed at a reduced dosage.

Dosage Modification for Dermatologic Effects. If grade 2 skin toxicity develops and is intolerable, dabrafenib should be withheld for up to 3 weeks. If grade 2 toxicity improves within 3 weeks of withholding dabrafenib, the drug should be resumed at a reduced dosage. If grade 2 skin toxicity does not improve within 3 weeks of withholding dabrafenib, the drug should be permanently discontinued.

If grade 3 or 4 skin toxicity occurs, dabrafenib should be withheld for up to 3 weeks. If grade 3 or 4 skin toxicity improves within 3 weeks of withholding dabrafenib, the drug may be resumed at a reduced dosage. If grade 3 or 4 skin toxicity does not improve within 3 weeks of withholding dabrafenib, the drug should be permanently discontinued.

Dosage Modification for Cardiac Effects. If symptomatic congestive heart failure (CHF) or an asymptomatic decrease in LVEF from baseline exceeding 20% and to a level below the lower limit of normal (LLN) occurs, dabrafenib therapy should be withheld; therapy may be resumed at the same dosage when LVEF is at or above the LLN and no more than 10% below the baseline value.

Dosage Modification for Hemorrhage. If grade 3 hemorrhagic events occur, dabrafenib therapy should be withheld. If improvement is observed, dabrafenib may be resumed at a reduced dosage. If grade 3 hemorrhagic events do not improve, dabrafenib should be permanently discontinued.

If any grade 4 hemorrhagic events occur, dabrafenib should be permanently discontinued.

Dosage Modification for Venous Thromboembolism. If uncomplicated venous thromboembolism (VTE) occurs in patients receiving dabrafenib in combination with trametinib, no dosage modification of dabrafenib is recommended.

Dosage Modification for Ocular Effects. If retinal pigment epithelial detachment or retinal vein occlusion occurs in patients receiving combination therapy with trametinib, no dosage modification of dabrafenib is needed.

If iritis occurs, dabrafenib therapy may be continued at the same dosage and ocular therapy should be initiated.

If grade 2 or 3 uveitis occurs and is unresponsive to ocular therapy, dabrafenib treatment should be interrupted for up to 6 weeks. If improvement to grade 0 or 1 is observed within 6 weeks, dabrafenib therapy may be resumed at the same or a reduced dosage. If no improvement is observed within 6 weeks, dabrafenib therapy should be permanently discontinued.

If severe uveitis or iridocyclitis occurs, dabrafenib treatment should be interrupted for up to 6 weeks and ocular therapy should be initiated as clinically indicated. If improvement to grade 0 or 1 is observed within 6 weeks, dabrafenib therapy may be resumed at the same or a reduced dosage. If no improvement is observed within 6 weeks, dabrafenib therapy should be permanently discontinued.

Dosage Modification for Pulmonary Effects. If interstitial lung disease or pneumonitis occurs during combination therapy with dabrafenib and trametinib, no dosage modification of dabrafenib is needed.

Dosage Modification for Other Toxicity. If an intolerable grade 2 adverse reaction or any grade 3 adverse reaction occurs, dabrafenib treatment should be interrupted until the adverse reaction resolves to grade 1 or less. Once the adverse reaction has resolved, dabrafenib may be resumed at a reduced dosage. If no improvement is observed, dabrafenib should be permanently discontinued.

For a first occurrence of any grade 4 adverse reaction, dabrafenib treatment should be permanently discontinued or interrupted until the adverse reaction resolves to grade 1 or less. Once the adverse reaction has resolved, dabrafenib may be resumed at a reduced dosage. If a grade 4 adverse reaction recurs, dabrafenib therapy should be permanently discontinued.

■ Special Populations In patients with mild hepatic impairment, dosage adjustments are not necessary. However, appropriate dosage has not been established in patients with moderate to severe hepatic impairment.

In patients with mild or moderate renal impairment, dosage adjustments are not necessary. However, appropriate dosage has not been established in patients with severe renal impairment.

Cautions

■ Contraindications The manufacturer states there are no known contraindications to the use of dabrafenib.

■ Warnings/Precautions ***Combination Therapy*** When combination therapy with dabrafenib includes the use of trametinib, the manufacturer's prescribing information for trametinib should be consulted for detailed information on the usual cautions, precautions, and contraindications of this drug. For further information regarding warnings and precautions associated with trametinib, also see Cautions: Warnings/Precautions, in Trametinib 10:00.

Development of New Primary Malignancies New primary cutaneous or noncutaneous malignancies have been reported in patients receiving b-Raf serine-threonine kinase (BRAF) inhibitors, including dabrafenib.

In the BREAK-3 study, cutaneous squamous cell carcinoma and keratoacanthoma occurred in 7% of patients receiving dabrafenib. Among patients receiving single-agent dabrafenib during clinical trials, the overall incidence of cutaneous squamous cell carcinoma and keratoacanthoma was 11%. Approximately one-third of patients experiencing cutaneous squamous cell carcinoma and keratoacanthoma had additional occurrences with continued dabrafenib treatment.

In the COMBI-D study, basal cell carcinoma occurred in 3.3% of patients receiving dabrafenib in combination with trametinib compared with 6% of those receiving dabrafenib monotherapy. Additional occurrences of basal cell carcinoma were reported in 2 of the 7 patients who developed basal cell carcinoma following combination therapy with dabrafenib and trametinib. Cutaneous squamous cell carcinoma or new primary melanoma occurred in 3 or 0.5%, respectively, of patients receiving dabrafenib in combination with trametinib.

In the COMBI-AD study, cutaneous squamous cell carcinoma or new primary melanoma occurred in 1 or less than 1%, respectively, of patients receiving dabrafenib in combination with trametinib. In the BRF113928 study, cutaneous cell carcinoma occurred in 3.2% of patients receiving dabrafenib in combination with trametinib.

In the COMBI-D, COMBI-AD, and BRF113928 studies, noncutaneous malignancies occurred in 1.4, 1, and 1.1%, respectively, of patients receiving dabrafenib in combination with trametinib.

Although the mechanism for development of cutaneous squamous cell carcinoma has not been fully determined, it has been suggested that paradoxical activation of mitogen-activated protein kinase (MAPK) signaling may lead to accelerated growth of such skin lesions as well as development of other primary malignancies. MAPK-mediated events in wild-type BRAF cells have been observed in a study evaluating the pathology and immunohistochemistry of normal and proliferating skin lesions in patients receiving the weak b-Raf kinase inhibitor sorafenib. Another study performed a molecular analysis of DNA extracted from tumor specimens of patients receiving the BRAF inhibitor vemurafenib; results indicated that these patients have a secondary mutation (in addition to the BRAF V600E mutation) that appears to be activated by vemurafenib treatment. Some clinicians suggest that advanced age (i.e., 65 years of age or older), history of skin cancer, and chronic sun exposure may be risk factors for developing cutaneous squamous cell carcinoma. Some data suggest that mitogen-activated extracellular signal-regulated kinase (MEK) inhibitors (i.e., binimetinib, cobimetinib, trametinib) block the paradoxical activation of the MAPK pathway induced by BRAF inhibitors (i.e., dabrafenib, encorafenib, vemurafenib); therefore, combination therapy with a BRAF inhibitor and an MEK inhibitor may reduce the risk of developing cutaneous squamous cell carcinoma. Findings from a meta-analysis of randomized controlled studies that assessed the relative risk of development of cutaneous squamous cell carcinoma in cancer patients receiving a BRAF inhibitor indicate that the risk of cutaneous squamous cell carcinoma is higher in patients receiving a BRAF inhibitor than in patients receiving combination therapy with a BRAF inhibitor and an MEK inhibitor.

Dermatologic evaluations should be performed prior to initiation of therapy, every 2 months during therapy, and for up to 6 months following discontinuance of dabrafenib monotherapy or combination therapy with trametinib. Monitoring for signs and symptoms of new noncutaneous malignancies should be performed. If new primary RAS mutation-positive, noncutaneous malignancies occur, dabrafenib therapy should be permanently discontinued. In patients who develop new primary cutaneous malignancies during combination therapy with dabrafenib and trametinib, the manufacturer states that no dosage adjustment of dabrafenib is necessary.

Tumor Promotion in Wild-Type BRAF Tumors In vitro evidence of increased MAPK signaling and cell proliferation in wild-type BRAF cells exposed to BRAF inhibitors has been observed.

Presence of BRAF V600E or V600K mutation should be confirmed prior to initiating dabrafenib monotherapy or combination therapy with trametinib. Use of dabrafenib is not recommended in patients with wild-type BRAF melanoma.

Hemorrhage Hemorrhage, including major hemorrhagic events (i.e., symptomatic bleeding in a critical area or organ), has occurred when dabrafenib is used in combination with trametinib. In the COMBI-D study, hemorrhage occurred in 19% of patients receiving dabrafenib in combination with trametinib compared with 15% of those receiving dabrafenib monotherapy. Gastric hemorrhage occurred in 6% of patients receiving dabrafenib in combination with trametinib compared with 3% of those receiving dabrafenib monotherapy. Intracranial hemorrhage was fatal in 1.4% of those receiving dabrafenib as combination therapy. In the BRF113928 study, retroperitoneal and subarachnoid hemorrhage were fatal in 2.2% of patients receiving dabrafenib in combination with trametinib. In the COMBI-AD study, no fatal hemorrhagic events were observed in patients receiving combination therapy with dabrafenib and trametinib.

If hemorrhagic events occur, dosage modification and/or treatment discontinuance may be necessary. (See Dosage Modification for Hemorrhage under Dosage: Dosage Modification for Toxicity, in Dosage and Administration.)

Cardiac Effects Cardiomyopathy has been reported in patients receiving dabrafenib monotherapy or combination therapy with trametinib.

In the COMBI-D study, 6 or 2.9% of patients receiving dabrafenib in combination with trametinib or dabrafenib monotherapy, respectively, experienced an absolute decrease in left ventricular ejection fraction (LVEF) from baseline of 10% or more and to a level below institution-specific lower limit of normal. Dosage interruption or discontinuance of dabrafenib was necessary in 4.4 or 1%, respectively, of patients receiving dabrafenib in combination with trametinib. Dosage interruption, dosage reduction, or discontinuance of dabrafenib was necessary in 2.4, 0.5, or 1%, respectively, of patients receiving dabrafenib monotherapy. Cardiomyopathy resolved in 83 or 50% of these patients receiving combination therapy with dabrafenib and trametinib or dabrafenib monotherapy, respectively.

In the COMBI-AD study, 3% of patients receiving dabrafenib in combination with trametinib experienced an absolute decrease in LVEF from baseline exceeding 10% and to a level below institution-specific lower limit of normal. Dosage interruption, dosage reduction, or discontinuance of dabrafenib was necessary in 2.1, 1.6, or 0.2%, respectively, of patients receiving combination therapy with dabrafenib and trametinib. Cardiomyopathy resolved in 86% of these patients.

In the BRF113928 study, 9% of patients receiving dabrafenib in combination with trametinib experienced an absolute decrease in LVEF from baseline exceeding 10% and to a level below institution-specific lower limit of normal. Dosage interruption or discontinuance of dabrafenib therapy was necessary in 3.2 or 2.2%, respectively, of patients receiving combination therapy with dabrafenib and trametinib. Cardiomyopathy resolved in 50% of these patients.

LVEF should be assessed using echocardiogram or multigated radionuclide angiography (MUGA) prior to and 1 month after initiation of dabrafenib and then every 2–3 months during therapy. If left ventricular dysfunction occurs, temporary interruption of dabrafenib may be necessary. (See Dosage Modification for Cardiac Effects under Dosage: Dosage Modification for Toxicity, in Dosage and Administration.)

Ocular Effects Uveitis has occurred in patients receiving dabrafenib monotherapy or combination therapy with trametinib. In clinical trials, uveitis has been reported in 1% of patients receiving dabrafenib and in 2% of patients receiving dabrafenib in combination with trametinib. Symptomatic treatment (e.g., ophthalmic corticosteroid or mydriatic preparations) was used during clinical trials for management of this condition.

Patients receiving dabrafenib should be monitored for signs and symptoms of uveitis (e.g., vision change, photophobia, eye pain). Temporary interruption, dosage reduction, or discontinuance of dabrafenib and/or initiation of ocular therapy may be necessary if ocular toxicities occur during therapy with the drug. (See Dosage Modification for Ocular Effects under Dosage: Dosage Modification for Toxicity, in Dosage and Administration.)

Febrile Drug Reactions Serious febrile drug reactions (including fever accompanied by hypotension, rigors/chills, dehydration, or renal failure) have occurred in patients receiving dabrafenib as monotherapy or as combination therapy with trametinib. Increased incidence and severity of pyrexia have been observed during combination therapy with dabrafenib and trametinib compared with dabrafenib alone. In the BREAK-3 study, serious febrile reactions and fever of any severity complicated by hypotension, rigors, or chills occurred in 3.7% of patients receiving dabrafenib alone. Fever (any grade) occurred in 28% of patients receiving dabrafenib alone and 10% of those receiving dacarbazine. In the COMBI-D and COMBI-V studies, pyrexia occurred in 54% of patients receiving dabrafenib in combination with trametinib; approximately 50% of these patients experienced at least 3 discrete episodes.

Across clinical trials evaluating dabrafenib in combination with trametinib in patients with unresectable or metastatic melanoma, the incidence of serious febrile reactions or fever of any severity complicated by severe rigors or chills, hypotension, dehydration, renal failure, or syncope was 17%. Fever was complicated by severe chills or rigors, dehydration, syncope, or renal failure in 0.4, 1.8, 0.7, or 0.5%, respectively, of patients receiving dabrafenib in combination with trametinib.

If any serious febrile reaction or fever complicated by hypotension, rigors/chills, dehydration, or renal failure occurs, dabrafenib treatment should be interrupted and the patient evaluated for manifestations of infection. If severe pyrexia occurs, renal function should be monitored (e.g., serum creatinine) during and following severe pyrexia. Dosage modification or treatment discontinuance may be necessary. (See Dosage Modification for Febrile Drug Reactions under Dosage: Dosage Modification for Toxicity, in Dosage and Administration.) Prophylactic antipyretics should be administered in patients resuming dabrafenib following a serious febrile reaction or fever associated with complications. For second or subsequent occurrences of prolonged fever (lasting longer than 3 days) or fever associated with complications (e.g., dehydration, hypotension, renal failure, severe chills/rigors) without evidence of an active infection, corticosteroids (e.g., prednisone 10 mg daily) should be administered for at least 5 days.

Dermatologic Effects Serious dermatologic toxicity has occurred in patients receiving dabrafenib in combination with trametinib. Across clinical trials, serious dermatologic toxicity occurred in 0.7% of patients with unresectable or metastatic melanoma receiving dabrafenib in combination with trametinib.

Dosage modification or treatment discontinuance may be necessary if dermatologic toxicity occurs. (See Dosage Modification for Dermatologic Effects under Dosage: Dosage Modification for Toxicity, in Dosage and Administration.)

Hyperglycemia Hyperglycemia requiring increased dosage of insulin or oral hypoglycemic agents or requiring initiation of these antidiabetic agents has occurred in patients receiving dabrafenib as monotherapy or as combination therapy with trametinib. In the BREAK-3 study, grade 3 hyperglycemia occurred in 6% of patients receiving dabrafenib. Of the 12 patients with a history of diabetes mellitus, 5 required intensification of hypoglycemic therapy during dabrafenib treatment. In the COMBI-D study, grade 3 or 4 hyperglycemia occurred in 5 or 0.5%, respectively, of patients receiving dabrafenib in combination with trametinib, and in 4.3 or 0%, respectively, of patients receiving dabrafenib monotherapy. In this study, intensification of hypoglycemic therapy was required in 13 or 27% of patients with a history of diabetes mellitus receiving dabrafenib as monotherapy or in combination with trametinib, respectively.

Serum glucose concentrations should be monitored prior to initiation of therapy and as clinically appropriate in patients with preexisting diabetes mellitus or hyperglycemia.

Hemolytic Anemia Dabrafenib contains a sulfonamide moiety and has the potential to induce hemolytic anemia in patients with glucose-6-phosphate dehydrogenase (G-6-PD) deficiency.

Patients with G-6-PD deficiency should be monitored for manifestations of hemolytic anemia.

Fetal/Neonatal Morbidity and Mortality Dabrafenib may cause fetal harm in humans based on its mechanism of action and animal findings; the drug has been shown to be teratogenic and embryotoxic in rats given dabrafenib dosages equivalent to 3 times the human exposure achieved with recommended dosages.

Since hormonal contraceptives may be ineffective when used concomitantly with dabrafenib, female patients of childbearing potential should use an effective nonhormonal method of contraception during treatment and for 2 weeks after the last dose. (See Drug Interactions: Hormonal Contraceptives.)

Women should be advised to contact their clinician if pregnancy is suspected or confirmed. If dabrafenib is used during pregnancy, the patient should be informed of the potential hazard to the fetus.

Impairment of Fertility Results of animal studies suggest that dabrafenib may reduce male and female fertility. In fertility studies, impairment of fertility (reduced corpora lutea in females and impaired spermatogenesis in males) was observed in animals receiving dabrafenib at exposure levels approximately or up to 3 times the human exposure at the recommended dosage.

Specific Populations **Pregnancy.** Dabrafenib may cause fetal harm if administered to pregnant women based on its mechanism of action and animal findings. (See Fetal/Neonatal Morbidity and Mortality under Cautions: Warnings/Precautions.)

Lactation. It is not known whether dabrafenib is distributed into human milk. Because of the potential for serious adverse reactions to dabrafenib in breast-fed infants, women should be advised not to breast-feed while receiving the drug and for 2 weeks after the last dose. The effects of the drug on breast-fed infants or on the production of milk are unknown.

Pediatric Use. Safety and efficacy of dabrafenib have not been established in pediatric patients.

Geriatric Use. No substantial differences in safety and efficacy of dabrafenib monotherapy have been observed in those 65 years of age or older relative to younger adults.

In the COMBI-D, COMBI-V, and COMBI-AD studies evaluating dabrafenib in combination with trametinib in patients with melanoma, 21% of patients were 65 years of age or older and 5% were 75 years of age or older. No overall differences in efficacy were observed between geriatric patients and younger adults, but some adverse effects (i.e., peripheral edema, anorexia) occurred more frequently in geriatric patients with metastatic melanoma.

Clinical experience with dabrafenib and trametinib combination therapy in patients 65 years of age or older with non-small cell lung cancer (NSCLC) is insufficient to determine whether geriatric patients respond differently than younger adults.

Hepatic Impairment. In population pharmacokinetic analyses, systemic exposure of dabrafenib and its metabolites was not affected in patients with mild hepatic impairment. (See Dosage and Administration: Special Populations.)

The pharmacokinetic profile of dabrafenib has not been established in patients with moderate or severe hepatic impairment; however, since dabrafenib is eliminated principally by hepatic metabolism, moderate to severe hepatic impairment may result in increased systemic exposure of dabrafenib.

Renal Impairment. In population pharmacokinetic analyses, systemic exposure of dabrafenib and its metabolites was not affected in patients with mild to moderate renal impairment (glomerular filtration rate [GFR] 30–89 mL/minute per 1.73 m^2). (See Dosage and Administration: Special Populations.)

The pharmacokinetic profile of dabrafenib has not been established in patients with severe renal impairment.

■ **Common Adverse Effects** Adverse effects reported in 20% or more of patients receiving dabrafenib monotherapy for the treatment of unresectable or metastatic melanoma with BRAF V600E mutation in the BREAK-3 study include hyperkeratosis, headache, pyrexia, arthralgia, papilloma, alopecia, and palmar-plantar erythrodysesthesia syndrome (hand-foot syndrome). Laboratory abnormalities reported in 10% or more of patients receiving dabrafenib monotherapy for the treatment of unresectable or metastatic melanoma with BRAF V600E mutation and at an incidence that is at least 5% higher than that reported with dacarbazine include hyperglycemia, hypophosphatemia, and elevated concentrations of alkaline phosphatase.

Adverse effects reported in 20% or more of patients receiving dabrafenib in combination with trametinib for the treatment of previously untreated unresectable or metastatic melanoma with BRAF V600E or V600K mutation in the COMBI-D and COMBI-V studies include pyrexia, diarrhea, fatigue, nausea, rash, chills, headache, vomiting, arthralgia, hypertension, and cough. Laboratory abnormalities reported in 20% or more of patients receiving dabrafenib in combination with trametinib for the treatment of previously untreated unresectable or metastatic melanoma with BRAF V600E or V600K mutation include hyperglycemia, elevated concentrations of alkaline phosphatase, hypophosphatemia, and hyponatremia.

Adverse effects reported in 20% or more of patients receiving dabrafenib in combination with trametinib for the adjuvant treatment of melanoma with BRAF V600E or V600K mutation in the COMBI-AD study include pyrexia, fatigue, nausea, headache, chills, rash, diarrhea, arthralgia, vomiting, and myalgia. Laboratory abnormalities reported in 20% or more of patients receiving dabrafenib in combination with trametinib for the adjuvant treatment of melanoma with BRAF V600E or V600K mutation include hyperglycemia, elevated concentrations of aminotransferases (i.e., AST, ALT), neutropenia, hypophosphatemia, elevated concentrations of alkaline phosphatase, lymphopenia, anemia, and hypoalbuminemia.

Adverse effects reported in 20% or more of patients receiving dabrafenib in combination with trametinib for the treatment of metastatic NSCLC with BRAF V600E mutation in the BRF113928 study include pyrexia, fatigue, nausea, vomiting, diarrhea, dry skin, decreased appetite, edema, rash, chills, hemorrhage, cough, and dyspnea. Laboratory abnormalities reported in 20% or more of patients receiving dabrafenib in combination with trametinib for the treatment of metastatic NSCLC with BRAF V600E mutation include hyperglycemia, elevated concentrations of alkaline phosphatase, elevated concentrations of aminotransferases (i.e., AST, ALT), hyponatremia, leukopenia, anemia, neutropenia, lymphopenia, hypophosphatemia, and elevated concentrations of serum creatinine.

Adverse effects reported in the BRF117019 study in patients receiving dabrafenib in combination with trametinib for the treatment of locally advanced or metastatic anaplastic thyroid cancer were similar to those reported in other studies in patients receiving combination therapy with dabrafenib and trametinib for the treatment of melanoma or NSCLC.

Drug Interactions

■ **Drugs Affecting Hepatic Microsomal Enzymes** Dabrafenib is metabolized by cytochrome P-450 (CYP) isoenzymes 3A4 and 2C8.

Potential pharmacokinetic interactions may occur when dabrafenib is used concomitantly with potent inhibitors of CYP isoenzymes 3A4 or 2C8 (e.g., gemfibrozil, ketoconazole) resulting in increased dabrafenib concentrations. In a pharmacokinetic study, concomitant administration of dabrafenib 75 mg twice daily and ketoconazole 400 mg once daily (a potent CYP3A4 inhibitor) for 4 days resulted in a 71% increase in area under the concentration-time curve (AUC) of dabrafenib, an 82% increase in the AUC of hydroxy-dabrafenib, and a 68% increase in the AUC of desmethyl-dabrafenib. In another study, concomitant administration of dabrafenib 75 mg twice daily and gemfibrozil 600 mg twice daily (a potent CYP2C8 inhibitor) for 4 days resulted in a 47% increase in the AUC of dabrafenib with no change in the AUC of dabrafenib's metabolites. Alternative therapy to potent inhibitors of CYP3A4 or 2C8 is recommended. If concomitant use is unavoidable, the patient should be monitored closely for dabrafenib-associated adverse reactions.

Potential pharmacokinetic interactions may occur when dabrafenib is used concomitantly with potent inducers of CYP3A4 or moderate inducers of CYP2C8 (e.g., rifampin) resulting in decreased dabrafenib concentrations. In a pharmacokinetic study, concomitant administration of dabrafenib 150 mg twice daily and rifampin 600 mg once daily (a potent CYP3A4 and moderate CYP2C8 inducer) for 10 days resulted in a 34% decrease in AUC of dabrafenib, a 30% decrease in the AUC of desmethyl-dabrafenib, and no change in the AUC of hydroxy-dabrafenib.

■ **Drugs Metabolized by Hepatic Microsomal Enzymes** Dabrafenib is an inducer of CYP isoenzymes 3A4 and 2C9. In vitro studies show that dabrafenib induces CYP3A4 and CYP2B6 via activation of the pregnane X receptor and constitutive androstane receptor. Dabrafenib also may induce CYP2C isoenzymes via this same mechanism of action. In a pharmacokinetic study, concomitant use of dabrafenib 150 mg twice daily for 15 days and a single dose of midazolam 3 mg (a CYP3A4 substrate) resulted in a 65% decrease in midazolam AUC. In another study, concomitant administration of dabrafenib 150 mg twice daily for 15 days and a single dose of warfarin sodium 15 mg resulted in a 37% decrease in the AUC of *S*-warfarin (a CYP2C9 substrate) and a 33% reduction in the AUC of *R*-warfarin (a CYP3A4/CYP1A2 substrate). International normalized ratio (INR) should be monitored frequently in patients receiving warfarin during initiation or discontinuance of dabrafenib.

Potential pharmacokinetic interactions may occur when dabrafenib is used concomitantly with substrates of CYP isoenzymes 3A4, 1A2, 2B6, 2C8, 2C9, or 2C19 (e.g., dexamethasone, hormonal contraceptives, midazolam, warfarin sodium) possibly resulting in decreased concentrations and reduced efficacy of the substrate drug. Alternative therapy to the substrate drug is recommended. If concomitant use is unavoidable, the patient should be monitored closely for reduced efficacy of the substrate drug.

■ **Drugs Metabolized by Uridine Diphosphate-glucuronosyltransferase** Dabrafenib may induce uridine diphosphate-glucuronosyltransferase (UGT).

Potential pharmacokinetic interactions may occur when dabrafenib is used concomitantly with substrates of UGT (decreased concentrations of the substrate drug). Alternative therapy to the substrate drug should be considered. If concomitant use is unavoidable, the patient should be monitored for reduced efficacy of the substrate drug.

■ **Drugs Transported by Organic Anion-Transporting Polypeptide and Organic Anion Transporters** Dabrafenib and its hydroxy, carboxy, and desmethyl metabolites are inhibitors of organic anion-transporting polypeptide (OATP) 1B1 and 1B3 as well as organic anion transporters (OAT) 1 and 3 in vitro. Potential pharmacokinetic interactions may occur when dabrafenib is used concomitantly with drugs transported by OATP1B1, OATP1B3, OAT1, or OAT3. Concomitant administration of a single dose of the sensitive OATP1B1 and OATP1B3 substrate rosuvastatin with dabrafenib (150 mg twice daily) resulted in a 2.6-fold increased in peak plasma concentrations of rosuvastatin and no change in AUC of rosuvastatin.

■ **Drugs Affecting Gastric Acidity** Concomitant use of dabrafenib (150 mg twice daily) with the proton-pump inhibitor rabeprazole (40 mg once daily for 4 days) resulted in no clinically important changes in peak plasma concentration or systemic exposure of dabrafenib or its metabolites.

■ **Hormonal Contraceptives** Dabrafenib is an inducer of CYP isoenzymes 3A4, 1A2, and 2C9. Concomitant use of dabrafenib with hormonal contraceptives that are metabolized by CYP3A4, 1A2, or 2C9 may result in decreased systemic exposure to the substrate drug and reduced contraceptive efficacy. (See Drug Interactions: Drugs Metabolized by Hepatic Microsomal Enzymes.) Alternative nonhormonal contraception is recommended. If concomitant use is unavoidable, the patient should be monitored closely for reduced efficacy of the hormonal contraceptive.

■ **Trametinib** Concomitant administration of dabrafenib 150 mg twice daily with trametinib 2 mg once daily resulted in a 23% increase in AUC of dabrafenib, a 33% increase in AUC of desmethyl-dabrafenib, and no change in AUC of hydroxy-dabrafenib compared with administration of dabrafenib alone.

■ **Warfarin** Dabrafenib is an inducer of CYP isoenzymes 3A4, 1A2, and 2C9. Concomitant use of dabrafenib with warfarin may result in decreased systemic exposure to *S*-warfarin (a CYP2C9 substrate) and *R*-warfarin (a CYP3A4/CYP1A2 substrate). (See Drug Interactions: Drugs Metabolized by Hepatic Microsomal Enzymes.) International normalized ratio (INR) should be monitored frequently in patients receiving warfarin during initiation or discontinuance of dabrafenib.

Description

Dabrafenib, a potent inhibitor of b-Raf serine-threonine kinase (BRAF) with V600E or V600K mutation, is an antineoplastic agent. Approximately 50% of cutaneous melanomas carry a BRAF mutation. The most common BRAF mutation is the substitution of glutamic acid for valine at codon 600 in exon 15 (BRAF V600E); a less frequently occurring BRAF mutation is the substitution of lysine for valine at codon 600 in exon 15 (BRAF V600K). The mutation of BRAF V600E activates the mitogen-activated protein kinase (MAPK) and extracellular signal-regulated kinase (ERK) signal transduction pathway, which enhances cell proliferation and tumor progression (e.g., metastasis). In vitro studies indicate that dabrafenib also inhibits BRAF with V600D mutation. Paradoxical activation of MAPK and increased cell proliferation have been observed in BRAF wild-type cells exposed to BRAF inhibitors.

Clinical resistance to monotherapy with a BRAF inhibitor, generally occurring 6–7 months following initiation of therapy, has been attributed to several possible resistance mechanisms mostly relying on reactivation of the MAPK/ERK pathway. Complete inhibition of the MAPK/ERK pathway resulting in durable responses may be achieved with the use of combination therapy with a BRAF inhibitor (i.e., dabrafenib, encorafenib, vemurafenib) and an MEK inhibitor (i.e., binimetinib, cobimetinib, trametinib). Use of dabrafenib and trametinib in combination resulted in greater growth inhibition of melanoma cell lines testing positive for BRAF V600 mutations in vitro. In addition, combination therapy was associated with prolonged inhibition of tumor growth in melanoma xenografts testing positive for BRAF V600 mutations compared with either drug alone.

Following oral administration, the absolute bioavailability of dabrafenib is 95%. Peak plasma concentrations of dabrafenib occur within 2 hours after oral administration. Following administration of a single dose of dabrafenib within the dosage range of 12–300 mg, the drug exhibits dose-proportional increases in peak plasma concentrations and area under the concentration-time curve (AUC); however, these increases are less than dose proportional after repeated twice-daily dosing. Administration of a single dose of dabrafenib with a high-fat meal (approximately 1000 calories) decreased peak plasma concentrations and AUC of the drug by 51 and 31%, respectively, and delayed the rate of absorption (time to reach peak concentrations delayed by 3.6 hours). (See Dosage and Administration: Administration.) Dabrafenib is more than 99% bound to plasma proteins; in vitro studies suggest that dabrafenib is a substrate of P-glycoprotein (P-gp) and breast cancer resistance protein (BCRP). Dabrafenib is principally metabolized by cytochrome P-450 (CYP) isoenzymes 3A4 and 2C8. Dabrafenib is an inducer of CYP3A4 and 2C19 and may induce other CYP isoenzymes. Dabrafenib also may induce uridine diphosphate glucuronosyltransferase (UGT). The metabolites hydroxy- and desmethyl-dabrafenib are likely to contribute to the clinical activity of dabrafenib. The mean terminal half-life of dabrafenib is 8 hours. Following oral administration of a radiolabeled dose of dabrafenib, about 71% of the dose is recovered in feces and 23% is recovered in urine.

Advice to Patients

Importance of advising patient to read the manufacturer's medication guide before beginning treatment and each time the prescription is refilled.

Importance of taking dabrafenib exactly as prescribed and of not altering the dosage or discontinuing therapy unless advised to do so by their clinician.

Importance of taking dabrafenib at least 1 hour before or 2 hours after a meal and of not opening, crushing, or breaking the capsules.

Importance of taking a missed dose as soon as it is remembered, but only if it can be taken at least 6 hours prior to the next scheduled dose. Patients should be informed not to take 2 doses at the same time to make up for a missed dose.

Risk of new primary cutaneous and noncutaneous malignancies. Importance of contacting a clinician promptly if dermatologic changes (i.e., new lesions or changes to existing lesions) or signs and/or symptoms of other malignancies occur.

Risk of intracranial and GI hemorrhage. Importance of contacting a clinician promptly if signs and/or symptoms of unusual bleeding or hemorrhage occur.

Risk of cardiomyopathy. Importance of contacting a clinician promptly if signs and/or symptoms of heart failure occur.

Risk of serious febrile drug reactions. Patients should be informed that the incidence and severity of pyrexia are increased when dabrafenib is used in combination with trametinib. Importance of contacting a clinician if fever occurs.

Risk of serious skin toxicities. Importance of contacting a clinician if progressive or intolerable rash occurs.

Risk of impaired glucose control in patients with diabetes mellitus resulting in the need for more intensive antidiabetic treatment. Importance of contacting a clinician if symptoms of severe hyperglycemia occur.

Risk of hemolytic anemia in patients with glucose-6-phosphate dehydrogenase (G-6-PD) deficiency. Importance of contacting a clinician if manifestations of anemia or hemolysis occur in patients with known G-6-PD deficiency.

Risk of fetal harm. Necessity of advising women to avoid pregnancy by using effective nonhormonal contraception during dabrafenib treatment and for 2 weeks after the last dose. Importance of women informing their clinicians if they become pregnant or suspect they may be pregnant during therapy.

Importance of advising women to avoid breast-feeding while receiving dabrafenib and for 2 weeks after the last dose.

Importance of advising men and women of reproductive potential that dabrafenib may reduce male and female fertility.

Risk of uveitis, iritis, and iridocyclitis. Importance of contacting a clinician promptly if any vision changes or other ocular effects (e.g., ocular pain, swelling, redness, blurred vision) occur.

Importance of informing clinicians of existing or contemplated concomitant therapy, including prescription and OTC drugs and dietary or herbal supplements, as well as any concomitant illnesses (e.g., diabetes mellitus).

Importance of informing patients of other important precautionary information. (See Cautions.)

Overview® (see Users Guide). For additional information on this drug until a more detailed monograph is developed and published, the manufacturer's labeling should be consulted. It is *essential* that the manufacturer's labeling be consulted for more detailed information on usual cautions, precautions, contraindications, potential drug interactions, laboratory test interferences, and acute toxicity. For further information on the handling of antineoplastic agents, see the ASHP Guidelines on Handling Hazardous Drugs at http://www.ahfsdruginformation.com.

Preparations

Excipients in commercially available drug preparations may have clinically important effects in some individuals; consult specific product labeling for details.

Dabrafenib Mesylate

Oral

Capsules	50 mg (of dabrafenib)	**Tafinlar®**, Novartis
	75 mg (of dabrafenib)	**Tafinlar®**, Novartis

Dacarbazine

Dimethyl Triazeno Imidazol Carboxamide, Imidazole Carboxamide, DIC, DTIC

■ Dacarbazine, a synthetic analog of a naturally occurring purine precursor, is an antimetabolite antineoplastic agent.

Uses

■ **Melanoma** Dacarbazine monotherapy currently is a systemic treatment of choice for metastatic melanoma. Although dacarbazine also has been used in various combination regimens† for the treatment of this disease, randomized trials currently have not shown that combination regimens are superior to dacarbazine alone, and the optimal regimen remains to be established.

Overview Localized melanoma is highly curable with surgical excision. In some patients with spread of melanoma to regional lymph nodes, wide surgical excision and removal of the involved lymph nodes may be curative. Adjuvant therapy with interferon alfa following resection of melanoma at high risk for recurrence has been shown to prolong disease-free but not overall survival, particularly in patients with node-positive disease. (See Uses: Melanoma in Interferon Alfa 10:00.) The role of adjuvant therapy following surgical resection of localized melanoma without nodal involvement has not been fully established, and eligible candidates should continue to be enrolled in clinical trials. Adjuvant therapy with conventional antineoplastic agents (e.g., dacarbazine, melphalan), nonspecific immunotherapy (e.g., BCG), or cell-based melanoma vaccine has not been shown to increase survival in patients with localized melanoma at high risk for recurrence, and inconclusive results have been reported with the use of levamisole, a nonspecific immunomodulating agent.

Locally recurrent or in-transit metastatic melanoma of the extremities has been treated with surgical resection, local injection of lesions (e.g., BCG), or isolated limb perfusion (e.g., melphalan) (see Uses: Melanoma in Melphalan 10:00); for patients rendered free of disease following treatment, enrollment in a clinical trial for adjuvant therapy may be considered. Primary or recurrent disseminated (i.e., metastatic) melanoma generally is incurable, and palliative treatment may include surgery (e.g., regional lymphadenectomy, metastasectomy), radiation therapy, and/or systemic therapy with chemotherapy and/or biologic therapy. Surgical resection of isolated metastases may prolong disease-free or overall survival in some patients with metastatic or recurrent melanoma; for patients rendered free of disease following treatment, enrollment in a clinical trial for adjuvant therapy may be considered. Radiation therapy may provide symptomatic relief for brain, bone, and visceral metastases.

Advanced melanoma is relatively resistant to systemic therapy, and combination chemotherapy regimens have not been shown to be superior to dacarbazine used as a single agent, the current standard of care to which all experimental therapies for metastatic melanoma should be compared. Palliative treatment with aldesleukin or interferon alfa provides durable remissions in about 5% of selected patients with advanced melanoma. (See Uses: Metastatic Melanoma in Aldesleukin 10:00 or Uses: Melanoma in Interferon Alfa 10:00.)The use of vaccines, monoclonal antibodies, and gene therapy also is being investigated in patients with metastatic melanoma. Because the prognosis for patients with advanced melanoma is poor, all patients should be considered for enrollment in clinical trials at the time of diagnosis.

Metastatic Melanoma Dacarbazine monotherapy is used for the palliative treatment of metastatic melanoma. Overall response rates of about 10–15% have been reported in patients receiving dacarbazine as a single agent in randomized trials; although durable complete responses have occurred in some patients (less than 5%), the duration of response usually is short (e.g., 3–6 months). Dacarbazine also has been used with other agents, but randomized trials currently have not shown that combination regimens are superior to dacarbazine alone in the treatment of metastatic melanoma. The use of dacarbazine-containing chemotherapy in combination with biologic therapy using aldesleukin and interferon alfa is being investigated for the treatment of metastatic melanoma; a large randomized trial is under way to investigate the comparative efficacy and toxicity of concurrent biochemotherapy with interferon alfa-2b, aldesleukin, cisplatin, vinblastine, and dacarbazine versus combination chemotherapy with cisplatin, vinblastine, and dacarbazine in patients with metastatic melanoma.

In phase II, single-institution studies, some combination chemotherapy regimens (e.g., dacarbazine, carmustine, cisplatin, and tamoxifen) for metastatic melanoma showed higher response rates than those observed in other studies using single-agent therapy, but evidence from large, randomized trials has not shown combination therapy to be superior to dacarbazine alone. In a multicenter, phase III, randomized trial, toxicity was greater but response rate and survival time did not differ among patients receiving combination therapy with dacarbazine, carmustine, cisplatin, and tamoxifen versus dacarbazine alone.

Evidence suggests that the addition of cisplatin to dacarbazine-containing regimens increases toxicity but does not improve survival. The addition of tamoxifen and/or interferon alfa to dacarbazine (used alone or in combination regimens) has not been shown to improve efficacy in patients with metastatic melanoma. Interpretation of the results from a randomized trial suggesting that the combination of dacarbazine and tamoxifen was superior to dacarbazine alone in patients with metastatic melanoma was limited by design flaws (e.g., small sample size, imbalance in prognostic factors), and other studies have not confirmed the benefit of tamoxifen. In a phase III, randomized trial, response rates, progression-free survival, or overall survival did not differ among patients receiving combination chemotherapy with dacarbazine, cisplatin, and carmustine, with or without tamoxifen. In another phase III, randomized trial, the addition of tamoxifen to combination therapy with dacarbazine, cisplatin, and carmustine did not improve response rates in patients with metastatic melanoma. In a large randomized trial, the addition of tamoxifen, with or without interferon, to dacarbazine did not increase the response rate, time to treatment failure, or duration of survival. Results from a small randomized trial suggested that the combination of dacarbazine and interferon alfa was superior to dacarbazine alone, but other studies did not confirm these findings. Although duration of response was prolonged with the addition of interferon alfa-2a to dacarbazine in patients with advanced melanoma, no difference was observed in objective response rate or overall survival. In a large randomized trial, the addition of interferon alfa, with or without tamoxifen, to dacarbazine did not increase the response rate, time to treatment failure, or duration of survival, but significantly increased toxicity.

Further study is needed to establish the optimal regimen for the treatment of metastatic melanoma.

■ **Hodgkin's Disease** Dacarbazine is used in combination with other antineoplastic agents in the treatment of advanced Hodgkin's disease. Combination therapy for Hodgkin's disease is clearly superior to single-agent therapy. Various regimens have been used in combination therapy and comparative efficacy is continually being evaluated. Dacarbazine is often used with doxorubicin, bleomycin, and vinblastine (known as the ABVD regimen) for the treatment of patients with advanced Hodgkin's disease. The ABVD regimen also is used in an alternating schedule with the MOPP regimen (mechlorethamine, vincristine, procarbazine, and prednisone) for the treatment of advanced Hodgkin's disease.

■ **Other Uses** Dacarbazine has been used with some success alone or in conjunction with other antineoplastic agents in the treatment of soft-tissue sarcomas† (e.g., leiomyosarcoma, fibrosarcoma, rhabdomyosarcoma) and neuroblastomas†. Dacarbazine alone has reportedly been beneficial in the treatment of a few cases of malignant glucagonoma†.

Dosage and Administration

■ **Reconstitution and Administration** Dacarbazine is administered by IV injection or infusion. *Care should be taken to avoid extravasation of the drug.* (See Cautions: Local Effects.) The powder for injection is reconstituted by adding 19.7 mL of sterile water for injection to a vial labeled as containing 200 mg of the drug. The resultant solution contains 10 mg of dacarbazine per mL. Reconstituted solutions may be administered by IV push over a 1-minute period. Alternatively, the reconstituted solution may be further diluted with up to 250 mL of 5% dextrose or 0.9% sodium chloride injection and infused IV over a 15- to 30-minute period. The manufacturer's labeling should be consulted for information on reconstitution and further dilution of other strengths of the powder for injection.

■ **Dosage** Dosage of dacarbazine must be based on the clinical and hematologic response and tolerance of the patient in order to obtain optimum therapeutic results with minimum adverse effects. Clinicians should consult published protocols for the dosage of dacarbazine and other chemotherapeutic agents and the method and sequence of administration.

Because dacarbazine is considered an antineoplastic agent of high emetic risk, antiemetic therapy for the prevention of acute and delayed emesis is recommended. (See Cautions: GI Effects.)

Melanoma For the treatment of metastatic melanoma, the manufacturer states that the recommended adult dosage of dacarbazine is 2–4.5 mg/kg daily for 10 days. It appears that the drug may be equally efficacious at the lower dosage. This regimen may be repeated at 4-week intervals. Alternatively, 250 mg/m^2 may be given daily for 5 days. This treatment course may be repeated every 3 weeks.

In the treatment of melanoma, dacarbazine has also been administered by regional intra-arterial† infusion to increase the concentration of drug delivered directly into the tumor.

Hodgkin's Disease For the treatment of Hodgkin's disease, the usual adult dosage of dacarbazine is 150 mg/m^2 daily for 5 days in combination with other antineoplastic agents; the regimen may be repeated every 4 weeks. Alternatively, a dacarbazine dose of 375 mg/m^{2}is administered on the first day, in combination with other antineoplastic agents, and repeated every 15 days.

Cautions

■ **GI Effects** GI symptoms of nausea, vomiting, and anorexia occur in over 90% of patients treated with dacarbazine. Because of its emetogenic potential, dacarbazine is classified as an antineoplastic agent of *high emetic risk* (i.e., incidence of emesis exceeds 90% if no antiemetic agents are administered). GI symptoms generally occur within 1 hour after the initial dose and may persist up to 12 hours. Rapid tolerance to adverse GI effects develops in most patients with symptoms subsiding after 1–2 days of treatment, suggesting that a CNS mechanism may be involved. Rarely, diarrhea, stomatitis, or intractable nausea and vomiting which necessitated discontinuance of dacarbazine therapy have occurred.

For the prevention of *acute* emesis, the American Society of Clinical Oncology (ASCO) currently recommends that a 3-drug antiemetic regimen consisting of a type 3 serotonin receptor antagonist, dexamethasone, and aprepitant be given before the administration of dacarbazine or other chemotherapy regimens with high emetic risk. (See Aprepitant 56:22.92.) Currently available selective 5-HT_3 receptor antagonists (e.g., dolasetron, granisetron, ondansetron, palonosetron, or tropisetron [not commercially available in the US]) are comparably effective in preventing acute chemotherapy-induced nausea and vomiting. (For additional information, see the individual monographs for 5-HT_3 receptor antagonists in 56:22.20.)

For the prevention of *delayed* emesis, ASCO currently recommends a 2-drug regimen of dexamethasone and aprepitant following the administration of chemotherapy associated with high emetic risk, such as dacarbazine.

Aggressive antiemetic therapy for the prevention of acute and delayed emesis during early courses of emetogenic chemotherapy is the best way to prevent *anticipatory* nausea and vomiting; behavioral therapy also may be useful. Although evidence is lacking, many clinicians also find benzodiazepines useful in the management of anticipatory emesis. For further discussion of the mechanism and management of emesis for antineoplastic agents of high emetic risk, see Emetogenic Effects in Cautions: GI Effects in Cisplatin 10:00.

■ **Hematologic Effects** The predominant manifestations of hematologic toxicity produced by dacarbazine are leukopenia and thrombocytopenia. These effects generally appear 2–4 weeks after the last dose of the drug; rarely, deaths have occurred. The patient's hematologic status must be carefully monitored. (See Cautions: Precautions and Contraindications.) Eosinophilia has also been reported in one patient receiving the drug.

■ **Hepatic Effects** Hepatotoxicity accompanied by hepatic vein thrombosis and potentially fatal hepatocellular necrosis has been reported in approximately 0.01% of in patients receiving dacarbazine therapy. Adverse hepatic effects have occurred more frequently when dacarbazine was administered concomitantly with other antineoplastic agents; however, these effects have also been reported in some patients receiving dacarbazine alone.

■ **Local Effects** Administration of concentrated dacarbazine solutions may cause severe pain along the injected vein. For this reason, it has been recommended that the drug be diluted and administered by infusion. Extravasation of dacarbazine must be avoided as it may cause tissue damage and severe pain. Local pain, burning sensation, and irritation at the injection site may be relieved by local application of hot packs.

■ **Other Adverse Effects** A flu-like syndrome, consisting of fever, myalgia, and malaise, may occur during or after treatment with dacarbazine. This flu-like syndrome, although infrequent, may recur with successive treatments.

Facial flushing and paresthesia have been reported occasionally, but appear to be transitory. Alopecia has also occurred. Rarely, transient elevations in serum alkaline phosphatase, AST (SGOT), ALT (SGPT), and BUN concentrations have been reported. CNS symptoms such as confusion, lethargy, blurred vision, seizures, and headache also have occurred during dacarbazine therapy. Dermatologic reactions, including erythematous, macular, papular, and/or urticarial rashes, have been reported infrequently, and photosensitivity reactions have occurred rarely.

■ **Precautions and Contraindications** Dacarbazine should be used only under constant supervision by clinicians experienced in cancer chemotherapy. The drug can produce severe, possibly fatal, hematologic or hepatic toxicity and severe GI reactions, and should be administered to patients who are preferably hospitalized and receive frequent determinations of hematopoietic function. In the treatment of each patient, the clinician must carefully weigh the possibility of achieving therapeutic benefits against the risks of toxicity.

Leukocyte, erythrocyte, and platelet counts should be performed prior to and at regular intervals during dacarbazine therapy. Hematopoietic toxicity (generally a leukocyte count of less than 3000/mm^3 and a platelet count of less than 100,000/mm^3) may require temporary suspension or cessation of the drug.

Dacarbazine can cause anaphylactic reactions and is contraindicated in patients who have demonstrated hypersensitivity to the drug.

■ **Carcinogenicity** Dacarbazine has carcinogenic effects in animals; however, the importance of these effects in humans has not been determined.

■ **Pregnancy, Fertility, and Lactation** Although there are no adequate and controlled studies to date in humans, dacarbazine has been shown to be teratogenic in rats when given at dosages 20 times the usual human dosage. Dacarbazine should be used during pregnancy only when the potential benefits justify the possible risks to the fetus.

The effect of dacarbazine on fertility in humans is not known. Reproduction studies in male rats using dacarbazine dosages 10 times the usual human dosage have not revealed evidence of impaired fertility; however, in female rats receiving dacarbazine, fetal resorptions occurred more frequently than in rats receiving placebo.

It is not known whether dacarbazine is distributed into milk. Because of the carcinogenic potential of dacarbazine in nursing infants, a decision should be made whether to discontinue nursing or the drug, taking into account the importance of the drug to the woman.

Pharmacology

The precise mechanism(s) of action of dacarbazine has not been determined, but it appears that the drug exerts its cytotoxic effect by acting as an alkylating agent. Dacarbazine is probably not a cell cycle-phase specific agent; it exhibits no specific dose-response relationship or schedule dependency. The drug possesses minimal immunosuppressive activity.

Pharmacokinetics

■ **Absorption** Dacarbazine is poorly absorbed from the GI tract. Peak plasma concentrations of about 8 mcg/mL are reached immediately following administration of dacarbazine 4.5 mg/kg by IV push.

■ **Distribution** The volume of distribution of dacarbazine exceeds total body water content, suggesting localization in some body tissue, probably the liver. The drug is only slightly bound to plasma proteins. Dacarbazine crosses the blood-brain barrier to a limited extent; CSF concentrations are reported to be about 14% of plasma concentrations. It is not known if dacarbazine crosses the placenta or distributes into milk.

■ **Elimination** Plasma concentrations of dacarbazine appear to decline in a biphasic manner. In individuals with normal renal function, the half-life in the initial phase ($t_{1/2\alpha}$) averages 19 minutes and the half-life in the terminal phase ($t_{frac12;\beta}$) averages 5 hours. The manufacturer states that in one patient with renal and hepatic dysfunction, the $t_{1/2\alpha}$ was 55 minutes and the $t_{1/2\beta}$ was 7.2 hours.

Dacarbazine is extensively metabolized. Dacarbazine is N-demethylated by liver microsomal enzymes to 5-(3-monomethyl-1-triazenyl)-1*H*-imidazole-4-carboxamide (MIC) which spontaneously decomposes to form AIC plus an unidentified alkylating or methylating moiety. Small amounts of the drug may also be converted to the diazonium salt of AIC (Diazo-ICA), which undergoes spontaneous intramolecular coupling to form 2-azahypoxanthine. Some dacarbazine metabolites may contribute to the antineoplastic effect of the drug. Metabolism of dacarbazine may be enhanced by agents such as phenobarbital and phenytoin which induce liver microsomal enzymes.

Dacarbazine is excreted in the urine by tubular secretion; 30–46% of an administered dose is excreted in the urine within 6 hours. About half of the drug excreted is recovered as unchanged dacarbazine and half as AIC.

Chemistry and Stability

■ **Chemistry** Dacarbazine, a synthetic analog of the naturally occurring purine precursor 5-amino-1*H*-imidazole-4-carboxamide (AIC), is an antineoplastic agent. Dacarbazine occurs as a colorless to ivory-colored crystalline solid. The drug is slightly soluble in water and in alcohol. Protonated dacarbazine has a pK_a of 4.42. Commercially available dacarbazine powder for injection also contains anhydrous citric acid and mannitol. When reconstituted with sterile water for injection to a concentration of 10 mg/mL, dacarbazine solutions have a pH of 3–4.

■ **Stability** Dacarbazine is sensitive to light and heat; elevated temperatures may cause a color change from ivory to pink which is indicative of some decomposition. Commercially available dacarbazine powder for injection must be protected from light and should be refrigerated at 2–8°C.

Dacarbazine solutions containing 10 mg/mL in sterile water for injection are stable for up to 72 hours when stored at 4°C or up to 8 hours at room temperature. Solutions further diluted with up to 500 mL of 5% dextrose or 0.9% sodium chloride injection are stable for at least 24 hours when stored at 2–8°C or up to 8 hours at room temperature (under normal room light conditions). Dacarbazine solutions are physically incompatible with solutions of hydrocortisone sodium succinate.

For further information on the handling of antineoplastic agents, see the ASHP Guidelines on Handling Hazardous Drugs at http://www.ahfsdruginformation.com.

Preparations

Excipients in commercially available drug preparations may have clinically important effects in some individuals; consult specific product labeling for details.

Dacarbazine

Parenteral

For injection, for IV use	100 mg*	**Dacarbazine for Injection**
	200 mg*	**Dacarbazine for Injection**
		DTIC-Dome®, Bayer
	500 mg*	**Dacarbazine for Injection**

*available from one or more manufacturer, distributor, and/or repackager by generic (nonproprietary) name

†Use is not currently included in the labeling approved by the US Food and Drug Administration

Dacomitinib

■ Dacomitinib, an epidermal growth factor receptor (EGFR) tyrosine kinase inhibitor, is an antineoplastic agent.

Uses

■ **Non-small Cell Lung Cancer** Dacomitinib is used for the first-line treatment of metastatic non-small cell lung cancer (NSCLC) in patients whose tumors harbor epidermal growth factor receptor (EGFR) exon 19 deletions (del19) or exon 21 (L858R) substitution mutations as detected by an FDA-approved diagnostic test (e.g., *therascreen*® EGFR RGQ PCR Kit, cobas® EGFR Mutation Test). Information on FDA-approved companion diagnostic tests for the detection of EGFR mutations in NSCLC is available at http://www.fda.gov/CompanionDiagnostics. Dacomitinib has been designated an orphan drug by FDA for use in this condition. A progression-free survival benefit has been observed in adults with previously untreated EGFR mutation-positive metastatic NSCLC receiving dacomitinib compared with patients receiving gefitinib.

EGFR-activating mutations are present in approximately 15–22% of NSCLC cases in North America and Europe and are present in up to 30–50% of cases in patients of East Asian descent. The majority of EGFR mutations are exon 19 deletions and an L858R substitution in exon 21, which together account for about 90% of EGFR mutations in patients with NSCLC. (See Description.)

The current indication for dacomitinib in the treatment of metastatic NSCLC is based principally on the results of a randomized, multinational, open-label phase 3 study (ARCHER-1050) in adults with newly diagnosed locally advanced or metastatic NSCLC. Patients who received systemic therapy in the adjuvant or neoadjuvant setting were enrolled in this study if disease progression occurred at least 12 months following adjuvant or neoadjuvant therapy. In this study, 452 patients were randomized (stratified by ethnicity and type of EGFR mutation) in a 1:1 ratio to receive either dacomitinib (45 mg orally once daily) or gefitinib (250 mg orally once daily) until disease progression or unacceptable toxicity occurred. The primary measure of efficacy was progression-free survival (as evaluated by a blinded independent central review committee according to Response Evaluation Criteria in Solid Tumors [RECIST]). The median age of patients was 62 years (range: 28–87 years); most patients (92%) had metastatic disease, 77% were of Asian ancestry, 70% had a baseline Eastern Cooperative Oncology Group (ECOG) performance status of 1, 64% had never smoked, and 1% had received prior adjuvant or neoadjuvant therapy. All patients enrolled in the study were required to have evidence of an EGFR mutation (confirmed by the *therascreen*® EGFR RGQ PCR Kit); 59% of patients had exon 19 deletions and 41% had exon 21 (L858R) substitution mutations.

At a median follow-up of 22.1 months, patients receiving dacomitinib had a longer median progression-free survival compared with patients receiving gefitinib (14.7 versus 9.2 months; hazard ratio of 0.59). Although objective response rates were similar between both treatment groups, patients receiving dacomitinib had a longer median duration of response (14.8 versus 8.3 months) compared with those receiving gefitinib. At a median follow-up of approximately 31 months, median overall survival was prolonged in patients receiving dacomitinib compared with those receiving gefitinib (34.1 months versus 26.8 months; hazard ratio of 0.76). Results of a subgroup analysis (based on age, gender, ECOG performance status, race, smoking status, EGFR mutation) suggested that the effect of dacomitinib on progression-free survival was evident across all subgroups; however, subgroup analysis according to race (Asian versus non-Asian) suggested that dacomitinib had a greater effect on progression-free survival in Asian patients relative to non-Asian patients (hazard ratio: 0.51 and 0.89, respectively).

Dosage and Administration

■ General Confirmation of the presence of epidermal growth factor receptor (EGFR) exon 19 deletions (del19) or exon 21 (L858R) substitution mutations in the tumors of patients with metastatic non-small cell lung cancer (NSCLC) by an FDA-approved diagnostic test is necessary prior to initiating first-line therapy with dacomitinib. (See Uses: Non-small Cell Lung Cancer.)

To minimize the incidence and severity of treatment-related rash or exfoliative skin reactions, patients should routinely moisturize their skin and limit exposure to sunlight by wearing protective clothing and/or using a sunscreen upon initiation of and during dacomitinib therapy. (See Dermatologic Effects under Cautions: Warnings/Precautions.)

■ Administration Dacomitinib is administered orally once daily at approximately the same time each day; the drug can be taken without regard to meals. (See Description.)

If a dose of dacomitinib is missed or vomited, patients should not double the dose or take extra doses. The next dose should be taken at the regularly scheduled time.

■ Dosage ***Non-small Cell Lung Cancer*** For the first-line treatment of metastatic NSCLC in patients whose tumors harbor EGFR del19 or L858R substitution mutations, the recommended dosage of dacomitinib in adults is 45 mg once daily. Therapy should be continued until disease progression or unacceptable toxicity occurs. In the principal efficacy study (ARCHER-1050), dacomitinib therapy was continued for a median duration of 15 months.

Dosage Modification for Toxicity Dosage interruption and/or reduction or discontinuance of dacomitinib therapy may be necessary based on severity of adverse reactions. If dosage reduction from 45 mg once daily is necessary, the dosage should be reduced to 30 mg once daily. If the toxicity recurs at a dosage of 30 mg once daily, the dosage should be reduced to 15 mg once daily. The manufacturer provides no specific recommendations for further dosage reductions.

Pulmonary Effects. If interstitial lung disease occurs, dacomitinib therapy should be permanently discontinued. (See Pulmonary Effects under Cautions: Warnings/Precautions.)

GI Toxicity. If grade 2 diarrhea occurs, dacomitinib therapy should be withheld. When the toxicity improves to grade 1 or less, dacomitinib therapy may be resumed at the same dosage. If grade 2 diarrhea recurs, dacomitinib therapy should be withheld; therapy may be resumed at a reduced dosage when the toxicity improves to grade 1 or less. (See Diarrhea under Cautions: Warnings/Precautions.)

If grade 3 or 4 diarrhea occurs, dacomitinib therapy should be withheld. When the toxicity improves to grade 1 or less, dacomitinib therapy may be resumed at a reduced dosage.

Dermatologic Toxicity. If grade 2 dermatologic reactions occur and persist during dacomitinib therapy, the drug should be withheld. When the toxicity improves to grade 1 or less, dacomitinib therapy may be resumed at the same dosage. If grade 2 dermatologic reactions recur and persist during dacomitinib therapy, the drug should be withheld; therapy may be resumed at a reduced dosage when the toxicity improves to grade 1 or less. (See Dermatologic Effects under Cautions: Warnings/Precautions.)

If grade 3 or 4 dermatologic reactions occur, dacomitinib therapy should be withheld. When the toxicity improves to grade 1 or less, dacomitinib therapy may be resumed at a reduced dosage.

Other Toxicity. If any other grade 3 or 4 adverse reaction occurs, dacomitinib therapy should be interrupted. When the toxicity improves to grade 2 or less, dacomitinib may be resumed at a reduced dosage.

■ Special Populations No dosage adjustment is necessary in patients with mild (total bilirubin concentration not exceeding the upper limit of normal [ULN] with AST concentration exceeding the ULN *or* total bilirubin concentration exceeding the ULN, but not more than 1.5 times the ULN, with any AST concentration) or moderate (total bilirubin concentration exceeding 1.5 times the ULN, but not more than 3 times the ULN, with any AST concentration) hepatic impairment. There are limited data in patients with severe hepatic impairment (total bilirubin concentration exceeding 3 times the ULN, but not more than 10 times the ULN, with any AST concentration); the manufacturer provides no specific dosage recommendations for such patients. (See Hepatic Impairment under Warnings/Precautions: Specific Populations, in Cautions.)

No dosage adjustment is necessary in patients with mild or moderate renal impairment (creatinine clearance 30–89 mL/minute). There are limited data in patients with severe renal impairment (creatinine clearance less than 30 mL/minute); the manufacturer provides no specific dosage recommendations for such patients. (See Renal Impairment under Warnings/Precautions: Specific Populations, in Cautions.)

The manufacturer makes no specific dosage recommendations for geriatric patients. (See Geriatric Use under Warnings/Precautions: Specific Populations, in Cautions.)

Cautions

■ Contraindications The manufacturer states there are no known contraindications to the use of dacomitinib.

■ Warnings/Precautions ***Pulmonary Effects*** Interstitial lung disease or pneumonitis, sometimes fatal, has been reported in patients receiving dacomitinib. In clinical trials, severe or fatal interstitial lung disease or pneumonitis occurred in 0.5% of 394 patients receiving dacomitinib; fatal interstitial lung disease or pneumonitis occurred in 0.3% of patients. In the principal efficacy study in patients with previously untreated metastatic non-small cell lung cancer (NSCLC) (ARCHER-1050), interstitial lung disease occurred in 1.3% of patients receiving dacomitinib and 1% of those receiving gefitinib; interstitial lung disease was fatal in one patient receiving dacomitinib. Temporary interruption or discontinuance of dacomitinib therapy was necessary because of interstitial lung disease in 1 or 1.8%, respectively, of patients receiving the drug.

Patients receiving dacomitinib should be monitored for manifestations of interstitial lung disease or pneumonitis. In patients experiencing progressive pulmonary symptoms (e.g., dyspnea, cough, fever), dacomitinib therapy should be withheld and the patient promptly evaluated. If a diagnosis of interstitial lung disease is confirmed, dacomitinib should be permanently discontinued.

Diarrhea Diarrhea has been reported frequently in patients receiving dacomitinib. Some cases have resulted in death. In clinical trials, diarrhea was reported in 86% of patients receiving dacomitinib; grade 3 or 4 diarrhea occurred in 11% of patients and diarrhea was fatal in 0.3% of patients. In the ARCHER-1050 study, diarrhea was reported in 87% of patients receiving dacomitinib compared with 56% of those receiving gefitinib; grade 3 or 4 diarrhea occurred in 8% of patients receiving dacomitinib compared with 0.9% of those receiving gefitinib. Temporary interruption, dosage reduction, or discontinuance of dacomitinib therapy was necessary because of diarrhea in 10, 8, or 0.9%, respectively, of patients receiving the drug.

Although the mechanism for development of diarrhea has not been fully determined, an increased incidence and greater severity of diarrhea have been observed with second-generation pan-human epidermal growth factor receptor (pan-HER) inhibitors (e.g., dacomitinib, afatinib) compared with single-target tyrosine kinase inhibitors selective for epidermal growth factor receptor (EGFR) (e.g., erlotinib, gefitinib); therefore, it has been suggested that other members of the HER tyrosine kinase family may have an essential role in the development of diarrhea.

If diarrhea occurs, appropriate therapy (e.g., loperamide, diphenoxylate hydrochloride in fixed combination with atropine sulfate, fluid replacement) should be promptly initiated as necessary. Dosage modification of dacomitinib therapy may be necessary depending on the severity of the diarrhea. (See GI Toxicity under Dosage: Dosage Modification for Toxicity, in Dosage and Administration.)

Dermatologic Effects Dermatologic toxicity has been reported frequently in patients receiving dacomitinib. In clinical trials, rash or exfoliative skin reactions were reported in 78 or 7% of patients receiving dacomitinib, respectively; grade 3 or 4 rash or exfoliative skin reactions were reported in 21 or 1.8%, respectively, of patients receiving dacomitinib. In the ARCHER-1050 study, rash was reported in 69% of patients receiving dacomitinib compared with 47% of those receiving gefitinib; grade 3 or 4 rash occurred in 23% of patients receiving dacomitinib compared with 0.4% of those receiving gefitinib. Temporary interruption, dosage reduction, or discontinuance of dacomitinib therapy was necessary because of rash in 23, 29, or 2.6%, respectively, of patients receiving the drug. Paronychia also was reported in 64% of patients receiving dacomitinib compared with 21% of those receiving gefitinib in the ARCHER-1050 study; temporary interruption or dosage reduction of dacomitinib therapy was necessary because of paronychia in 13 or 17%, respectively, of patients receiving the drug.

The incidence and severity of rash and exfoliative skin reactions may increase with sun exposure. Patients should be advised to routinely moisturize their skin and limit exposure to sunlight during dacomitinib therapy. (See Advice to Patients.) Some clinicians state that prophylaxis with a systemic anti-infective may be helpful in some cases. Dosage modification of dacomitinib therapy may be necessary if grade 2 or greater rash occurs during therapy with the drug; systemic anti-infective therapy also should be initiated. (See Dermatologic Toxicity under Dosage: Dosage Modification for Toxicity, in Dosage and Administration.) If grade 1 rash occurs, topical anti-infective and corticosteroid therapy should be initiated.

Fetal/Neonatal Morbidity and Mortality Dacomitinib may cause fetal harm in humans based on its mechanism of action and animal findings; the drug has been shown to be embryotoxic and fetotoxic in animals. There are no available data regarding the risk of dacomitinib use in pregnant women to date. Disruption or blockade of signaling of the EGFR pathway in animals has been associated with preimplantation loss, increased embryofetal loss, postnatal death, developmental anomalies, and visceral abnormalities. Embryofetal toxicity (e.g., decreased fetal body weight, postimplantation loss) has been demonstrated in animals receiving the drug at exposure levels equivalent to approximately 1.2 times the human exposure at the recommended dacomitinib dosage.

Pregnancy should be avoided during dacomitinib therapy. The manufacturer states that pregnancy status should be confirmed prior to initiation of dacomitinib therapy in women of childbearing potential and that such women should be advised to use effective contraception while receiving dacomitinib and for at least 17 days after the last dose of the drug. Women of childbearing potential should be apprised of the potential hazard to the fetus if the drug is used during pregnancy. (See Advice to Patients.)

Specific Populations **Pregnancy.** Dacomitinib may cause fetal harm if administered to pregnant women based on its mechanism of action and animal findings. (See Fetal/Neonatal Morbidity and Mortality under Cautions: Warnings/Precautions.)

Lactation. It is not known whether dacomitinib or its metabolites distribute into human milk or if the drug or its metabolites have any effect on milk production or the nursing infant. Because of the potential for adverse reactions to dacomitinib in nursing infants, women should be advised not to breast-feed while receiving the drug and for at least 17 days after the last dose of the drug.

Pediatric Use. Safety and efficacy of dacomitinib have not been established in pediatric patients.

Geriatric Use. In clinical trials, 40% of patients receiving dacomitinib were 65 years of age or older. Patients 65 years of age or older had higher incidences of grade 3 or 4 adverse reactions, dosage interruptions, and discontinuance of dacomitinib due to adverse reactions compared with younger adults.

Hepatic Impairment. In a hepatic impairment study, peak plasma concentrations and systemic exposure of dacomitinib in individuals with mild hepatic impairment (Child-Pugh class A) were similar to those in individuals with normal hepatic function but decreased by 20 and 15%, respectively, in those with moderate hepatic impairment (Child-Pugh class B). (See Dosage and Administration: Special Populations.)

Population pharmacokinetic analyses suggest that clearance of dacomitinib is not altered to a clinically important extent in individuals with mild (total bilirubin concentration not exceeding the upper limit of normal [ULN] with AST concentration exceeding the ULN *or* total bilirubin concentration exceeding the ULN, but not more than 1.5 times the ULN, with any AST concentration) or moderate (total bilirubin concentration exceeding 1.5 times, but not more than 3 times the ULN, with any AST concentration) hepatic impairment.

The pharmacokinetic profile of dacomitinib has not been established in patients with severe hepatic impairment (total bilirubin concentration exceeding 3 times the ULN, but not more than 10 times the ULN, with any AST concentration).

Renal Impairment. Population pharmacokinetic analyses suggest that there is no clinically important difference in the pharmacokinetics of dacomitinib in individuals with mild or moderate renal impairment (creatinine clearance 30 to less than 90 mL/minute) compared with individuals with normal renal function. (See Dosage and Administration: Special Populations.)

The pharmacokinetic profile of dacomitinib has not been established in patients with severe renal impairment (creatinine clearance less than 30 mL/minute) and in those receiving dialysis.

■ **Common Adverse Effects** Adverse effects reported in the ARCHER-1050 study in at least 20% of patients receiving dacomitinib for the treatment of previously untreated metastatic NSCLC harboring EGFR exon 19 deletions (del19) or exon 21 (L858R) substitution mutations include diarrhea, rash, paronychia, stomatitis, decreased appetite, dry skin, decreased weight, alopecia, cough, and pruritus. Laboratory abnormalities reported in at least 20% of patients receiving dacomitinib for the treatment of previously untreated metastatic NSCLC include anemia, hypobilirubinemia, lymphopenia, elevated concentrations of aminotransferases (i.e., ALT, AST), hyperglycemia, hypocalcemia, hypokalemia, hyponatremia, elevated concentrations of serum creatinine, elevated concentrations of alkaline phosphatase, and hypomagnesemia.

Drug Interactions

Dacomitinib is principally metabolized by oxidation and glutathione conjugation. Dacomitinib also is metabolized by cytochrome P-450 isoenzyme 2D6 (CYP2D6) to form its major metabolite, *O*-desmethyldacomitinib, and by CYP3A4 to form other minor oxidative metabolites.

In vitro studies indicate that dacomitinib is a potent inhibitor and substrate of CYP2D6; dacomitinib does not induce CYP isoenzymes 1A2, 2B6, or 3A4. In vitro studies show that dacomitinib and its principal active metabolite do not inhibit CYP isoenzymes 1A2, 2B6, 2C8, 2C9, 2C19, or 3A4/5. Dacomitinib also is an inhibitor of uridine diphosphate-glucuronosyltransferase (UGT) 1A1, but does not inhibit UGT1A4, 1A6, 1A9, 2B7, or 2B15.

In vitro studies indicate that dacomitinib is a substrate of P-glycoprotein (P-gp) and breast cancer resistance protein (BCRP). In vitro, dacomitinib is an inhibitor of P-gp, BCRP, and organic cation transporter (OCT) 1, but does not inhibit organic anion transporter (OAT) 1, OAT3, OCT2, organic anion transport protein (OATP) 1B1, or OATP1B3.

■ **Drugs Affecting Hepatic Microsomal Enzymes** ***Potent Inhibitors of CYP2D6*** Although dacomitinib is a substrate of CYP2D6, CYP2D6-mediated mechanisms play a minor role in the drug's overall metabolism. Concomitant use of dacomitinib (single 45-mg dose) with the potent CYP2D6 inhibitor paroxetine (30 mg once daily) did not result in clinically important changes in area under the concentration-time curve (AUC) of the total active forms of the drug (i.e., dacomitinib plus *O*-desmethyldacomitinib); no initial dosage adjustment is necessary.

■ **Drugs Metabolized by Hepatic Microsomal Enzymes** Concomitant use of dacomitinib with drugs that are metabolized by CYP2D6 may result in increased exposure of the substrate drug and an increased incidence of drug toxicity. When the CYP2D6 substrate dextromethorphan (single 30-mg dose) was administered concomitantly with dacomitinib (single 45-mg dose), the peak plasma concentration and AUC of dextromethorphan were increased by 9.7- and 9.6-fold, respectively. Concomitant use of dacomitinib with sensitive CYP2D6 substrates or CYP2D6 substrates with a narrow therapeutic index should be avoided.

■ **Drugs Affecting Gastric Acidity** The solubility of dacomitinib decreases with increasing pH; therefore, drugs that reduce gastric acidity such as proton-pump inhibitors, antacids, and histamine H_2-receptor antagonists potentially can decrease plasma concentrations of dacomitinib and thereby reduce its efficacy. Concomitant use of dacomitinib and proton-pump inhibitors should be avoided. If therapy with an acid suppressive agent is necessary in a patient receiving dacomitinib, use of a histamine H_2-receptor antagonist (e.g., cimetidine, famotidine, nizatidine, ranitidine) or an antacid (e.g., magnesium oxide) rather than a proton-pump inhibitor should be considered. The manufacturer states that dacomitinib should be administered at least 6 hours prior to or 10 hours following administration of a histamine H_2-receptor antagonist.

Proton-pump Inhibitors When dacomitinib (single 45-mg dose) was administered concomitantly with the proton-pump inhibitor rabeprazole sodium (40 mg once daily for 7 days) in healthy individuals, the AUC and peak plasma concentration of dacomitinib were decreased by 39 and 51%, respectively.

Concomitant use of dacomitinib and proton-pump inhibitors should be avoided.

Histamine H_2-receptor Antagonists No formal drug interaction studies have been performed to date; however, if concurrent use of dacomitinib and a histamine H_2-receptor antagonist is necessary, dacomitinib should be taken at least 6 hours prior to or 10 hours following administration of the histamine H_2-receptor antagonist.

Antacids Concomitant use of dacomitinib (single 45-mg dose) with magnesium oxide (single 1.6-g dose) did not result in clinically important changes in AUC or peak plasma concentrations of dacomitinib.

Description

Dacomitinib, a selective and irreversible inhibitor of epidermal growth factor receptor (EGFR/human epidermal growth factor receptor type 1 [HER1]/ErbB1), HER2/ErbB2, HER4/ErbB4, and mutated EGFR (e.g., exon 19 deletion [del19], exon 21 substitution [L858R]) tyrosine kinases, is an antineoplastic agent. EGFR is expressed on the cell surface of many cancer cells, as well as many normal cells; activation of EGFR tyrosine kinase is thought to initiate a cascade of intracellular signaling events leading to cell proliferation and influencing processes critical to cell survival and tumor progression (e.g., angiogenesis, apoptosis, metastasis). Some EGFR-activating mutations, such as exon 19 deletion (del19) and exon 21 (L858R) substitution mutation, contribute to increased cell proliferation and survival in non-small cell lung cancer (NSCLC) cells harboring these mutations.

Although first-generation (reversible) EGFR tyrosine kinase inhibitors (e.g., erlotinib, gefitinib) have demonstrated improved outcomes in patients with NSCLC harboring EGFR mutations (e.g., EGFR exon 19 deletion [del19], exon 21 substitution [L858R]), secondary resistance to these agents eventually develops following 9–13 months of treatment. Clinical resistance to first-generation EGFR tyrosine kinase inhibitors has been attributed to several mechanisms, but development of the secondary T790M mutation in exon 20 appears to be the most common, occurring in 50–60% of patients who develop this resistance; this mutation results in production of a bulky methionine side chain in the receptor kinase domain of EGFR that is thought to sterically hinder the binding of first-generation EGFR tyrosine kinase inhibitors to EGFR. It has been suggested that second-generation EGFR tyrosine kinase inhibitors (e.g., dacomitinib, afatinib) may theoretically delay or prevent the emergence of secondary resistance through their irreversible inhibition of EGFR, more complete blockade of the EGFR signaling pathway (i.e., inhibition of EGFR as well as HER2/ErbB2 and HER4/ErbB4), and inhibitory effects against tumors harboring the T790M mutation. Dacomitinib has demonstrated dose-dependent inhibition of phosphorylation of wild-type EGFR and HER2 and tumor growth in xenograft models of human NSCLC or ovarian cancer cell lines that harbored HER2 or EGFR (i.e., del19, L858R, T790M) mutations in mice. The drug also has demonstrated antitumor activity in xenograft models of human glioblastoma cells driven by EGFR gene amplifications, including EGFR variant III (EGFRvIII, EGFR exon 2–7 deletion [del2–7]), in mice. In vitro, dacomitinib also has been shown to inhibit DDR1, DDR2, EPHA6, LCK, MNK1 at clinically relevant concentrations.

Dacomitinib exhibits dose-proportional pharmacokinetics over a dosage range of 2–60 mg once daily. Following oral administration, the median time to peak plasma concentrations is approximately 6 hours; the mean absolute bioavailability of dacomitinib is 80%. Steady-state concentrations of dacomitinib are achieved within 14 days of repeated dosing and the mean accumulation ratio is 5.7. Based on dose-exposure safety relationships, higher dacomitinib exposures at the recommended dacomitinib dosage have been associated with an increased incidence of grade 3 or greater adverse effects, particularly dermatologic toxicities (e.g., rash, dermatitis acneiform) and diarrhea. (See Cautions.) Administration with a high-fat, high-calorie meal did not substantially alter the pharmacokinetics of dacomitinib. Dacomitinib is approximately 98% bound to plasma proteins. Dacomitinib is principally metabolized by oxidation and glutathione conjugation. Cytochrome P-450 (CYP) isoenzyme 2D6 metabolizes dacomitinib to its major metabolite, *O*-desmethyldacomitinib, which has similar activity inhibiting EGFR tyrosine kinase as dacomitinib in vitro. Pharmacokinetics of dacomitinib are not substantially different between poor and extensive metabolizers of CYP2D6. *O*-desmethyldacomitinib accounts for 7.4–19% of the total trough concentrations at steady state. The mean terminal half-lives of dacomitinib and *O*-desmethyldacomitinib are 70.3 and 72.8 hours, respectively. Following oral administration of a radiolabeled dose of dacomitinib, 79% of the dose is recovered in feces (approximately 20% of the dose as unchanged drug) and 3% is recovered in urine (less than 1% of the dose as unchanged drug).

Analysis of population pharmacokinetic data indicates that age (range: 20–92 years), body weight, gender, race (Asian versus non-Asian), EGFR mutation status, and baseline albumin concentrations have no clinically important effects on clearance of dacomitinib.

Advice to Patients

Importance of instructing patients to read the manufacturer's patient information.

If a dose is missed or vomited, importance of administering the next dose at the regularly scheduled time; an additional dose should not be administered to make up for a missed dose.

Risk of interstitial lung disease. Importance of immediately informing clinician if new or worsening respiratory symptoms occur (e.g., dyspnea, cough, fever).

Risk of diarrhea. Importance of informing clinician at the first sign of loose stools.

Risk of dermatologic reactions. Importance of routinely moisturizing skin and limiting exposure to sunlight by wearing protective clothing and using sunscreen during dacomitinib therapy. Importance of immediately informing clinician if new or worsening rash or erythematous or exfoliative reactions occur.

Risk of fetal harm. Necessity of advising women of childbearing potential that they should use effective methods of contraception while receiving dacomitinib and for at least 17 days after the last dose of the drug. Importance of women informing their clinicians if they are or plan to become pregnant. If pregnancy occurs, advise pregnant women of potential risk to the fetus.

Importance of advising women to avoid breast-feeding while receiving dacomitinib and for at least 17 days after the last dose of the drug.

Importance of informing clinician of existing or contemplated concomitant therapy, including prescription and OTC drugs (e.g., antacids, histamine H_2-receptor antagonists, proton-pump inhibitors) and herbal supplements, as well as any concomitant illnesses.

Importance of informing patients of other important precautionary information. (See Cautions.)

Overview® (see Users Guide). For additional information on this drug until a more detailed monograph is developed and published, the manufacturer's labeling should be consulted. It is *essential* that the manufacturer's labeling be consulted for more detailed information on usual cautions, precautions, contraindications, potential drug interactions, laboratory test interferences, and acute toxicity. For further information on the handling of antineoplastic agents, see the ASHP Guidelines on Handling Hazardous Drugs at http://www.ahfsdruginformation.com.

Preparations

Excipients in commercially available drug preparations may have clinically important effects in some individuals; consult specific product labeling for details.

Dacomitinib

Oral		
Tablets, film-coated	15 mg	**Vizimpro®**, Pfizer
	30 mg	**Vizimpro®**, Pfizer
	45 mg	**Vizimpro®**, Pfizer

Daratumumab

■ Daratumumab, a recombinant humanized anti-CD38 monoclonal antibody, is an antineoplastic agent.

Uses

■ **Multiple Myeloma** Daratumumab is used for the treatment of multiple myeloma in patients who have received at least 3 prior therapies including a proteasome inhibitor and an immunomodulatory agent or in those with disease refractory to a proteasome inhibitor and an immunomodulatory agent. Daratumumab is designated an orphan drug by the FDA for use in multiple myeloma. The accelerated approval of daratumumab for this indication is based on overall response rate. Continued approval for this indication may be contingent on verification and description of clinical benefit of daratumumab in confirmatory studies.

The current indication for daratumumab is based principally on the results of an open-label, multicenter phase 2 study (SIRIUS) in 106 adults with relapsed or refractory multiple myeloma, with supporting data from an open-label, multicenter phase 1/2 study. In the SIRIUS study, 106 patients with relapsed or refractory multiple myeloma received IV daratumumab 16 mg/kg once a week for 8 weeks (cycles 1 and 2), then every 2 weeks for 16 weeks (cycles 3–6), then every 4 weeks thereafter until disease progression or unacceptable toxicity occurred. The median age of patients enrolled in the study was 63.5 years, and patients had received a median of 5 prior therapies for their disease, including bortezomib (99%), lenalidomide (99%), pomalidomide (63%), carfilzomib (50%), and thalidomide (44%). The majority of patients were refractory to their last line of therapy (97%), a proteasome inhibitor and an immunomodulatory agent (95%), or an alkylating agent (77%). Most patients (80%) had received an autologous stem-cell transplant. The primary end point of this study was overall response rate as assessed by an independent review committee according to the International Myeloma Working Group Uniform Response criteria; secondary end points included progression-free survival, overall survival, clinical benefit rate, and duration of response. The overall response rate with daratumumab was 29.2% with a median duration of response of 7.4 months; 3 patients (2.8%) achieved a stringent complete response. The clinical benefit rate (defined as overall response rate and minimal response) was 34%. The median time to initial response was 1 month. Median progression-free survival was 3.7 months; however, median overall survival had not been reached in patients who achieved a response, but was 13.7 months in nonresponders.

In the phase 1/2 study, 42 patients with relapsed or refractory multiple myeloma received IV daratumumab 16 mg/kg once a week for 7 weeks, then every 2 weeks for 14 weeks, then every 4 weeks thereafter until disease progression or unacceptable toxicity occurred. The median age of patients enrolled in the study was 64 years, and patients had received a median of 4 prior therapies for their disease, including bortezomib (100%), lenalidomide (95%), pomalidomide (36%), and carfilzomib (19%). Most patients were refractory to their last line of therapy (76%), a proteasome inhibitor and an immunomodulatory agent (64%), or an alkylating agent (60%). Most patients (74%) had received an autologous stem-cell transplant. The overall response rate with daratumumab was 36% with a median time to response of 1 month; 1 patient achieved a complete response. The median duration of response had not been reached at the time of the analysis.

Dosage and Administration

■ **General** Daratumumab should be administered only in settings where emergency equipment and appropriate medical support is available for management of potential infusion-related reactions. (See Infusion-related Effects under Cautions: Warnings/Precautions.)

To minimize the risk of infusion-related reactions associated with daratumumab, a premedication regimen consisting of a corticosteroid, antihistamine, and antipyretic should be administered prior to each daratumumab infusion. An intermediate- or long-acting IV corticosteroid (e.g., methylprednisolone 100 mg or equivalent), oral antipyretic (e.g., acetaminophen 650 mg or 1 g), and oral or IV antihistamine (e.g., diphenhydramine hydrochloride 25–50 mg or equivalent) should be administered approximately 1 hour prior to each infusion of daratumumab; however, the IV corticosteroid dosage may be reduced (e.g., methylprednisolone from 100 mg to 60 mg or equivalent) following the second infusion. (See Infusion-related Effects under Cautions: Warnings/Precautions.)

Because of the potential for delayed infusion-related reactions associated with daratumumab, an oral corticosteroid (e.g., methylprednisolone 20 mg or equivalent) should be administered on the first and second days following each daratumumab infusion. Therapy with short- and long-acting bronchodilators and inhaled corticosteroids should be considered for patients with a history of chronic obstructive pulmonary disease; if major infusion-related reactions do not occur during or following the first 4 infusions, such inhaled therapy may be discontinued. (See Infusion-related Effects under Cautions: Warnings/Precautions.)

Because herpes zoster was reported in 3% of daratumumab-treated patients, antiviral prophylaxis (e.g., acyclovir) to prevent reactivation of latent virus should be administered within 1 week of initiating daratumumab and continued for 3 months following discontinuance of the drug.

■ **Administration** Daratumumab is administered by IV infusion. Daratumumab infusion solution should be administered using polyurethane, polybutadiene, polyvinyl chloride (PVC), polypropylene, or polyethylene administration sets fitted with a flow regulator and a low-protein-binding 0.2- or 0.22-μm inline polyethersulfone filter.

Other drugs should *not* be administered simultaneously through the same IV line with daratumumab infusion.

Unopened vials of daratumumab injection concentrate should be protected from light and stored at 2–8°C, and should not be frozen or shaken.

Dilution Prior to administration, commercially available daratumumab injection concentrate must be diluted using proper aseptic technique.

Daratumumab injection concentrate should be inspected visually for particulate matter and discoloration; the injection concentrate should be colorless to pale yellow and should *not* be used if it is discolored or if particulate matter is present.

The manufacturer states that daratumumab should be diluted in PVC, polypropylene, polyethylene, or polyolefin bags.

For the first dose, daratumumab injection concentrate should be diluted in 0.9% sodium chloride injection to provide a total volume of 1 L. For subsequent doses, daratumumab injection concentrate should be diluted in 0.9% sodium chloride injection to provide a total volume of 500 mL. A volume of diluent equal to the total required volume of daratumumab injection concentrate should be removed from the infusion bag prior to addition of the injection concentrate. The total required volume of daratumumab injection concentrate should then be added slowly to the diluent in the infusion bag.

Diluted solutions of daratumumab should be mixed by gentle inversion and should *not* be shaken. Diluted solutions of daratumumab should be inspected visually for particulate matter and discoloration prior to administration; the solution may contain small translucent-to-white proteinaceous particulates and should *not* be administered if visibly opaque particles, foreign particles, or discoloration is observed. The diluted drug should be protected from light and stored at 2–8°C for up to 24 hours; the solution should be brought to room temperature and then administered immediately. Infusion of diluted daratumumab solutions should be completed within 15 hours.

Any unused portion of injection concentrate left in the vial or diluted solution should be discarded since the injection contains no preservative.

Rate of Administration The first 2 infusions of daratumumab should be infused IV at an initial rate of 50 mL/hour. If infusion-related reactions do not occur, the infusion rate may be increased in increments of 50 mL/hour every hour to a maximum rate of 200 mL/hour. The infusion rate for the second infusion should only be increased if grade 1 or greater infusion-related reactions did *not* occur during the first 3 hours of the first infusion. Subsequent infusions of daratumumab should be infused at an initial rate of 100 mL/hour; if infusion-related reactions do not occur, the infusion rate may be increased in increments of 50 mL/hour every hour to a maximum rate of 200 mL/hour. The infusion rate for subsequent infusions should only be increased if grade 1 or greater infusion-related reactions did *not* occur during a final infusion rate of 100 mL/hour or greater during the first 2 infusions.

If infusion-related reactions occur, the infusion should be interrupted and the infusion rate should be reduced or therapy with the drug permanently discontinued depending on the severity of the reaction. If the infusion-related reaction is grade 4 in severity, therapy with daratumumab should be permanently discontinued. For the first or second occurrence of grade 3 infusion-related reactions, the daratumumab infusion should be interrupted; once the reaction has improved to grade 2 or less, the infusion may be resumed but the rate of infusion should be reduced by at least 50%. If no further infusion-related reactions occur, the infusion rate may be increased in increments and intervals appropriate for the treatment dose. For the third occurrence of grade 3 infusion-related reactions, treatment with daratumumab should be permanently discontinued. For grade 1 and 2 infusion-related reactions, the daratumumab infusion should be interrupted; once the reaction has resolved, the infusion may be resumed but the rate of infusion should be reduced by at least 50%. If no further infusion-related reactions occur, the infusion rate may be increased in increments and intervals appropriate for the treatment dose. (See Infusion-related Effects under Cautions: Warnings/Precautions.)

■ **Dosage** ***Multiple Myeloma*** For the treatment of multiple myeloma in patients who have received at least 3 prior therapies including a proteasome inhibitor and an immunomodulatory agent or in those with disease refractory to a proteasome inhibitor and an immunomodulatory agent, the recommended adult dosage of daratumumab is 16 mg/kg once a week for 8 weeks (weeks 1–8), followed by every 2 weeks for 16 weeks (weeks 9–24), then every 4 weeks thereafter (from week 25 onward). Therapy should be continued until disease progression or unacceptable toxicity occurs.

If a dose is missed or delayed, the dose of daratumumab should be administered as soon as possible. The schedule of administration should be adjusted to maintain the appropriate treatment interval between doses.

■ **Special Populations** No dosage adjustment is necessary in patients with mild hepatic impairment (total bilirubin concentrations 1–1.5 times the upper limit of normal [ULN] or AST concentrations exceeding the ULN). (See Hepatic Impairment under Warnings/Precautions: Specific Populations, in Cautions.)

No dosage adjustment is necessary in patients with renal impairment. (See Renal Impairment under Warnings/Precautions: Specific Populations, in Cautions.)

The manufacturer makes no specific dosage recommendations for geriatric patients. (See Geriatric Use under Warnings/Precautions: Specific Populations, in Cautions.)

Cautions

■ **Contraindications** The manufacturer states there are no known contraindications to the use of daratumumab.

■ **Warnings/Precautions** ***Infusion-related Effects*** Infusion-related reactions (sometimes serious) have been reported frequently in patients receiving daratumumab. In clinical studies of daratumumab in patients with relapsed or refractory multiple myeloma, infusion-related reactions occurred in 46% of patients during the first infusion; however, the incidence declined to 4–5% with subsequent infusions. Infusion-related reactions generally have occurred during or within 4 hours following completion of the daratumumab infusion. In clinical trials, the median time to onset of an infusion-related reaction was 1.5 hours (range: 0.02–9.3 hours). Prior to routine use of post-infusion medication in clinical studies, delayed infusion-related reactions occurred up to 48 hours following completion of the daratumumab infusion. Serious infusion-related reactions including bronchospasm, hypoxia, dyspnea, and hypertension have been reported. Signs or symptoms of such reactions may include respiratory effects (e.g., cough, wheezing, larynx and throat tightness and irritation, laryngeal edema, pulmonary edema, nasal congestion, allergic rhinitis). Hypotension, headache, rash, urticaria, pruritus, nausea, vomiting, and chills have occurred less frequently.

Patients should be monitored frequently for signs or symptoms of infusion reactions during each daratumumab infusion in a setting where resuscitation equipment and agents necessary to treat infusion reactions are readily available. To minimize the risk of infusion-related reactions, patients receiving daratumumab should receive premedication with an antihistamine, antipyretic, and corticosteroid prior to each infusion of the drug. Because delayed infusion-related reactions may occur, patients also should receive therapy with an oral corticosteroid on the first and second days following each infusion to reduce the risk of such reactions. Patients with a history of chronic obstructive pulmonary disorders may require an inhaled bronchodilator or corticosteroid following the infusion. (See Dosage and Administration: General.) If infusion-related reactions occur, reduction in infusion rate or temporary interruption or permanent discontinuance of daratumumab may be required; medical management also should be instituted as necessary. (See Rate of Administration under Dosage and Administration: Administration.) For patients experiencing a life-threatening infusion-related reaction, the manufacturer recommends permanent discontinuance of therapy.

Interference with Serologic Testing Because daratumumab binds to CD38, a protein expressed on the surface of erythrocytes, positive indirect antiglobulin (Coombs') test results have occurred in patients receiving the drug. Pan-agglutination resulting in positive indirect antiglobulin test results may persist for up to 6 months after the last infusion of daratumumab. Daratumumab masks the detection of antibodies to minor antigens in serum; however, determination of ABO and Rh blood type is not affected.

Blood typing and screening should be performed prior to initiation of daratumumab. If blood transfusion is required, clinicians must notify the blood center of the serologic test interference and inform them that the patient has received daratumumab. If blood typing and screening occur after initiation of daratumumab, genotyping or treatment of reagent erythrocytes with the reducing agent dithiothreitol (DTT) should be used to disrupt daratumumab binding. DTT also denatures a limited number of other blood group antigens, including Kell antigens; therefore, patients receiving daratumumab who require a blood transfusion should receive K-negative units after ruling out or identifying alloantibodies using erythrocytes treated with DTT. If an immediate transfusion is required because of emergency, non-cross-matched ABO/RhD blood type-compatible red blood cell (RBC) units can be administered according to local blood center practices.

Interference with Serum Protein Electrophoresis and Immunofixation Electrophoresis Assays Daratumumab is a human IgG kappa immunoglobulin; therefore, the drug may be detected as an individual monoclonal band on serum protein electrophoresis (SPEP) and immunofixation electrophoresis (IFE) assays used for clinical monitoring of endogenous monoclonal immunoglobulins such as myeloma (M) protein. Daratumumab also comigrates with IgG kappa M-protein; therefore, a daratumumab-specific IFE reflex assay (DIRA) has been used to separate the migration of daratumumab and endogenous M-protein. Daratumumab also may mask clearance of endogenous M-protein resulting in false-positive IFE assay results and misinterpretation of tumor response.

The manufacturer recommends considering other methods to evaluate the level of tumor response in patients who have persistently achieved very good partial responses. Some experts recommend use of DIRA in patients with IgG kappa M-protein who have achieved a very good response to therapy; however, if a complete response has been demonstrated utilizing DIRA, patients should undergo further examination with bone marrow biopsy and free-light chain measurements to confirm a complete response.

Immunogenicity As with all therapeutic proteins, there is a potential for immunogenicity. In a clinical trial, testing for anti-daratumumab antibodies was performed during therapy and up to 8 weeks following discontinuance of the drug using electrochemiluminescence (ECL); none of the 111 patients tested positive for anti-daratumumab antibodies. However, the ability of the ECL assay to detect anti-daratumumab antibodies is limited by the presence of circulating drug.

Specific Populations **Pregnancy.** There are no adequate and well-controlled studies of daratumumab in pregnant women; however, based on its mechanism of action, daratumumab may cause fetal harm. Because human immunoglobulin G (IgG) crosses the placenta in humans, and because of the potential for serious adverse reactions to daratumumab (e.g., myeloid- or lymphoid-cell depletion, decreased bone density) in infants born to pregnant women treated with daratumumab, pregnancy should be avoided during daratumumab therapy. Women of childbearing potential should be advised to use an effective method of contraception while receiving daratumumab and for at least 3 months after discontinuance of therapy. Patients should be apprised of the potential hazard to the fetus if the drug is used during pregnancy.

Because myeloid- or lymphoid-cell depletion may occur in infants born to pregnant women treated with daratumumab, administration of live vaccines should be avoided in these infants until a hematologic evaluation has been completed.

Lactation. It is not known whether daratumumab is distributed into human milk; however, human IgG is distributed into milk. The effects of the drug on nursing infants or on the production of human milk are unknown.

The benefits of breast-feeding and the importance of daratumumab to the woman should be considered along with the potential adverse effects on the breast-fed child from the drug or from the underlying maternal condition.

Pediatric Use. Safety and efficacy of daratumumab have not been established in pediatric patients.

Geriatric Use. In clinical studies, 45% of patients with relapsed or refractory multiple myeloma receiving daratumumab were 65 years of age or older, and 10% were 75 years of age or older. No overall differences in safety or efficacy were observed between geriatric and younger adults.

Hepatic Impairment. In a population pharmacokinetic analysis, no clinically meaningful differences in exposure of daratumumab were observed between patients with mild (total bilirubin concentrations 1–1.5 times the upper limit of normal [ULN] or AST concentrations exceeding the ULN) hepatic impairment and those with normal hepatic function. Formal pharmacokinetic studies have not been conducted in patients with moderate (total bilirubin concentrations exceeding 1.5 times, but not more than 3 times, the ULN and any AST concentrations) or severe (total bilirubin concentrations exceeding 3 times the ULN and any AST concentrations) hepatic impairment. (See Dosage and Administration: Special Populations.)

Renal Impairment. In a population pharmacokinetic analysis, no clinically meaningful differences in exposure of daratumumab were observed between patients with mild (creatinine clearance of 60–89 mL/minute), moderate (creatinine clearance of 30–59 mL/minute), or severe renal impairment or end-stage renal disease (creatinine clearance less than 30 mL/minute) and those with normal renal function. (See Dosage and Administration: Special Populations.)

■ **Common Adverse Effects** Adverse effects reported in 10% or more of patients with relapsed or refractory multiple myeloma receiving daratumumab in clinical trials include infusion-related reactions, fatigue, nausea, back pain, cough, pyrexia, upper respiratory tract infection, arthralgia, nasal congestion, diarrhea, constipation, dyspnea, loss of appetite, nasopharyngitis, pain in extremity, vomiting, headache, musculoskeletal chest pain, pneumonia, chills, and hypertension. Laboratory abnormalities reported in more than 10% of patients receiving daratumumab include lymphopenia, neutropenia, thrombocytopenia, and anemia.

Drug Interactions

No formal drug interaction studies have been performed to date.

Description

Daratumumab, a recombinant humanized anti-CD38 monoclonal antibody, is an antineoplastic agent. The drug is an IgG_1 kappa immunoglobulin produced by recombinant DNA technology in mammalian cell (Chinese hamster ovary) culture. Daratumumab binds specifically to antigen CD38, a glycoprotein expressed on the surface of normal and malignant hematopoietic stem cells, including multiple myeloma and other cell types and tissues of nonhematopoietic origin. Following binding of daratumumab to antigen CD38, the Fc domain triggers host immune responses (i.e., antibody-dependent cell-mediated cytotoxicity [ADCC], antibody-dependent cellular phagocytosis [ADCP], complement-dependent cytotoxicity [CDC]) causing cell lysis. Myeloid-derived suppressor cells, a subset of regulatory T cells, and natural killer (NK) cells expressing CD38 are also susceptible to daratumumab-mediated cell lysis.

Decreased absolute counts and percentages of total NK cells ($CD16/56^+$) and activated NK cells ($CD16^+/56^{dim}$) in peripheral blood and bone marrow have been observed following daratumumab therapy. Absolute $CD4^+$ and $CD8^+$ T-cell counts, including the percentage of total lymphocytes, increased in peripheral blood and bone marrow following daratumumab therapy.

Areas under the serum concentration-time curve (AUCs) of daratumumab are more than dose proportional over the dosage range of 1–24 mg/kg. Clearance decreased with increasing dose and following repeated administration, indicating target-mediated pharmacokinetics. Steady-state concentrations are reached by approximately 5 months following administration every 4 weeks. The estimated terminal half-life associated with linear clearance of daratumumab is 18 days. Data from a population pharmacokinetic analysis indicate that age (31–84 years) and gender do not have clinically important effects on the pharmacokinetics of daratumumab.

Advice to Patients

Importance of reading the manufacturer's patient information before beginning treatment and each time the drug is administered.

Risk of infusion-related reactions. Importance of immediately reporting signs or symptoms of such reactions (e.g., nasal itching, congestion, or rhinitis; chills, nausea, throat irritation, cough, headache, breathing difficulty, shortness of breath).

Importance of advising patients about the possibility for serologic test interference in the event of a planned blood transfusion and of the need to inform clinicians, including blood center personnel, that they are receiving daratumumab.

Importance of advising patients that daratumumab may affect the results of some tests used to determine complete response to the drug and that additional tests may be needed to evaluate the response.

Risk of fetal harm. Necessity of advising women of childbearing potential to use an effective method of contraception while receiving the drug and for at least 3 months after the last dose. If pregnancy occurs, advise pregnant women of potential fetal risk.

Importance of women informing clinicians if they are or plan to become pregnant or plan to breast-feed.

Importance of advising women who received daratumumab during pregnancy that infants exposed to the drug in utero should have a hematologic evaluation performed before they receive live vaccines.

Importance of informing clinicians of existing or contemplated concomitant therapy, including prescription and OTC drugs, as well as any concomitant illnesses (e.g., respiratory problems, history of herpes zoster).

Importance of informing patients of other important precautionary information. (See Cautions.)

Overview® (see Users Guide). For additional information on this drug until a more detailed monograph is developed and published, the manufacturer's labeling should be consulted. It is *essential* that the manufacturer's labeling be consulted for more detailed information on usual cautions, precautions, contraindications, potential drug interactions, laboratory test interferences, and acute toxicity. For further information on the handling of antineoplastic agents, see the ASHP Guidelines on Handling Hazardous Drugs at http://www.ahfsdruginformation.com.

Preparations

Excipients in commercially available drug preparations may have clinically important effects in some individuals; consult specific product labeling for details.

Daratumumab

Parenteral

Concentrate, for injection, for IV infusion	20 mg/mL (100 and 400 mg)	**Darzalex®**, Janssen Biotech

Dasatinib

■ Dasatinib, a kinase inhibitor, is an antineoplastic agent.

Uses

■ **Chronic Myelogenous Leukemia** Dasatinib is used for the treatment of newly diagnosed Philadelphia chromosome-positive (Ph$^+$) chronic myelogenous leukemia (CML) in adults who are in the chronic phase of the disease. Dasatinib also is used for the treatment of Ph$^+$ CML in adults who are in myeloid or lymphoid blast crisis, in the accelerated phase, or in the chronic phase of the disease after failure (secondary to resistance or intolerance) of prior therapy including imatinib. Dasatinib is designated an orphan drug by the US Food and Drug Administration (FDA) for use in the treatment of CML.

Treatment of Newly Diagnosed Chronic Phase CML The current indication for use of dasatinib in the treatment of newly diagnosed chronic phase CML is based on complete cytogenetic response rates obtained within 12 months of treatment initiation from an ongoing open-label, randomized phase 3 study (Dasatinib versus Imatinib Study in Treatment-Naive CML Patients [DASISION]) in patients with newly diagnosed chronic phase Ph$^+$ CML. Additional follow-up data are needed to establish long-term efficacy of dasatinib for this use.

In this study, 519 patients who had been diagnosed with chronic phase Ph$^+$ CML within the previous 3 months and who had received no prior therapies for CML (except hydroxyurea or anagrelide) were randomized to receive either dasatinib (100 mg once daily) or imatinib (400 mg once daily) until disease progression or unacceptable toxicity occurred. The interim analysis was performed after a minimum follow-up of 12 months. At the time of the analysis, patients in both treatment groups had received a median of 14 months of treatment.

Confirmed complete cytogenetic response (defined as 2 consecutive assessments at least 28 days apart documenting complete eradication of Ph$^+$ metaphases in cells from a bone marrow sample) was the primary efficacy end point. Confirmed complete cytogenetic responses or major molecular responses (defined as a Bcr-Abl transcript level of 0.1% or less in peripheral blood) were reported within 12 months of treatment initiation in 77 or 46%, respectively, of patients receiving dasatinib and 66 or 28%, respectively, of those receiving imatinib. The median time to a confirmed complete cytogenetic response or a major molecular response was 3.1 or 6.3 months, respectively, for those receiving dasatinib and 5.6 or 9.2 months, respectively, for those receiving imatinib. Disease progression (i.e., transformation from chronic phase to accelerated or blast phase CML) occurred by the data cutoff in 1.9% of those receiving dasatinib and 3.5% of those receiving imatinib.

When results were stratified by prognosis (according to Hasford risk score, a CML-specific prognostic indicator based on age, spleen size, and platelet, basophil, eosinophil, and peripheral blast counts), dasatinib or imatinib therapy resulted in complete cytogenetic response within 12 months of treatment initiation in 94 or 76%, respectively, of low-risk patients and 78 or 64%, respectively, of high-risk patients.

Nausea, vomiting, rash, myalgia, muscle inflammation, and grade 3 or 4 hypophosphatemia occurred more frequently in patients receiving imatinib, whereas grade 3 or 4 thrombocytopenia occurred more frequently in those receiving dasatinib. Fluid retention (including superficial edema) also occurred more frequently in patients receiving imatinib, although pleural effusion was reported only in patients receiving dasatinib.

Treatment of Chronic Phase CML Following Prior Treatment Failure Initial FDA approval of dasatinib for the treatment of chronic phase CML after failure of prior therapy including imatinib was based principally on results of phase 2 studies evaluating safety and efficacy of the drug at a dosage of 70 mg twice daily. In a subsequent phase 3 randomized, open-label study, safety and efficacy of dasatinib administered at various dosages once or twice daily were evaluated in 670 patients with chronic phase CML following failure of imatinib therapy. Major cytogenetic response (defined as elimination or substantial reduction [by at least 65%] of Ph$^+$ hematopoietic cells) was the primary efficacy end point in these studies. In the phase 3 study, resistance to imatinib was defined as failure to achieve a complete hematologic response after 3 months, major cytogenetic response after 6 months, complete cytogenetic response after 12 months, and a reduction in leukocyte count after 4 or more weeks of therapy; loss of a previous major cytogenetic response, molecular response (with concurrent increase of 10% or more in Ph$^+$ metaphases), or complete hematologic response; or evidence of a new mutation in the Bcr-Abl kinase domain. In the phase 3 study, imatinib intolerance was defined as toxicity (grade 3 or worse) that occurred at an imatinib dosage of 400 mg or more daily and resulted in discontinuance of the drug.

In the phase 3 study, patients were randomized to receive dasatinib 100 mg once daily, 140 mg once daily, 50 mg twice daily, or 70 mg twice daily; the median duration of treatment was 22 months. The 4 dasatinib dosing regimens had similar efficacy, but patients receiving dasatinib 100 mg once daily experienced less toxicity than did those receiving dasatinib 70 mg twice daily. Among patients receiving dasatinib 100 mg once daily, 92% achieved a complete hematologic response, 63% achieved a major cytogenetic response, and 50% achieved a complete cytogenetic response; the median time to achieve a major cytogenetic response was 2.9 months. The estimated 2-year progression-free and overall survival rates for patients treated with dasatinib 100 mg once daily were 80 and 91%, respectively. Severe myelosuppression and drug discontinuance or dosage reduction because of adverse reactions were reported less frequently with dasatinib 100 mg once daily than with other dosing regimens.

In one phase 2 open-label, noncomparative study in patients with chronic phase CML following failure of imatinib therapy, complete hematologic, major cytogenetic, and complete cytogenetic responses were reported with dasatinib therapy (70 mg twice daily) in 91, 59, and 49%, respectively, of patients at a median follow-up of approximately 15 months; the median 15-month progression-free and overall survival rates were 90 and 96%, respectively. In a phase 2 open-label, randomized study, patients with chronic phase CML whose disease was resistant to conventional doses of imatinib (400–600 mg daily) were randomized to receive dasatinib 70 mg twice daily or imatinib 400 mg twice daily. At 15 months' follow-up, complete hematologic, major cytogenetic, and complete cytogenetic responses were reported in 93, 52, and 40%, respectively, of patients receiving dasatinib compared with 82, 33, and 16%, respectively, of those receiving high-dose imatinib.

Treatment of Accelerated Phase or Blast Phase CML Following Prior Treatment Failure Initial FDA approval of dasatinib for the treatment of accelerated phase CML or CML in myeloid or lymphoid blast crisis after failure of prior therapy including imatinib was based principally on results of phase 2 studies evaluating safety and efficacy of the drug at a dosage of 70 mg twice daily. In a subsequent phase 3, multicenter, randomized, open-label study, safety and efficacy of dasatinib administered once or twice daily were evaluated in 611 adults with CML in accelerated, myeloid blast, or lymphoid blast phase who were intolerant of or had disease that was resistant to prior therapy including imatinib. Major hematologic response, a primary efficacy end point in the studies, was defined as complete hematologic response or no evidence of leukemia; major cytogenetic response included complete and partial responses.

In the phase 3 study, patients were randomized to receive dasatinib 140 mg once daily or 70 mg twice daily; the median duration of treatment was approximately 6 months. The once-daily and twice-daily regimens had comparable efficacy as measured by rates of major hematologic response. Major hematologic and cytogenetic responses were reported with dasatinib 140 mg once daily in 66 and 39%, respectively, of patients in the accelerated phase of CML; 28 and 28%, respectively, of those in the myeloid blast phase; and 42 and 52%, respectively, of those in the lymphoid blast phase. The median time to achieve a major hematologic response with dasatinib 140 mg once daily was 1.9 months for those in the accelerated or myeloid blast phase of CML and 1.8 months for those in the lymphoid blast phase.

In a phase 2 open-label, noncomparative study in patients in the accelerated phase of the disease, major hematologic and cytogenetic responses were reported with dasatinib therapy (70 mg twice daily) in 64 and 33%, respectively, of patients at 8 months' follow-up. In phase 2 open-label, noncomparative studies in patients in blast crisis, major hematologic and cytogenetic responses were reported with dasatinib therapy (70 mg twice daily) in 34 and 33%, respectively, of patients in the myeloid blast phase and in 35 and 52%, respectively, of patients in the lymphoid blast phase after at least 12 months' follow-up; median overall survival and progression-free survival were 11.8 and 6.7 months, respectively, for patients in the myeloid blast phase and 5.3 and 3 months, respectively, for those in the lymphoid blast phase.

■ **Philadelphia Chromosome-Positive Acute Lymphocytic Leukemia** Dasatinib is used for the treatment of Ph$^+$ acute lymphocytic (lymphoblastic) leukemia (ALL) in adults following failure (secondary to resistance or intolerance) of prior therapy. Dasatinib is designated an orphan drug by FDA for use in this condition.

Safety and efficacy of dasatinib for this indication have been evaluated in a phase 2 open-label, noncomparative study and a phase 3 randomized study in patients with Ph$^+$ ALL who were intolerant of or had disease that was resistant to prior therapy including imatinib. A total of 130 patients were enrolled in the 2 studies, and the median duration of therapy was about 3 months. Major hematologic response, the primary efficacy end point in the 2 studies, was defined as complete hematologic response or no evidence of leukemia.

In the phase 2 study, treatment with dasatinib 70 mg twice daily resulted in a major hematologic response in 42% of patients. With minimum follow-up of 8 months, median duration of major hematologic response had not yet been reached (range: 1.9 to more than 8.7 months). Median progression-free survival was 3.3 months.

In the phase 3 study, patients were randomized to receive either once-daily or twice-daily dasatinib therapy (140 mg once daily or 70 mg twice daily). Major hematologic response was reported in 38% of patients receiving dasatinib 140 mg once daily; the median duration of response was 4.6 months. Median progression-free survival was 4 months for those receiving the once-daily regimen and 3.5 months for those receiving the twice-daily regimen.

Dosage and Administration

■ **General** Dasatinib is administered orally once daily. The drug should be administered at about the same time each day, either in the morning or evening, and may be administered without regard to food. Dasatinib tablets should be swallowed whole and should not be cut, chewed, or crushed.

Because dasatinib may cause fetal harm, women who are pregnant should not handle crushed or broken dasatinib tablets.

■ **Dosage** ***Chronic Myelogenous Leukemia*** The currently recommended adult dosage of dasatinib for the treatment of chronic myelogenous leukemia (CML) in the chronic phase is 100 mg once daily. In patients who do not achieve a hematologic or cytogenetic response at the recommended initial dosage, dosage may be increased to 140 mg once daily.

The currently recommended adult dosage of dasatinib for the treatment of advanced (e.g., accelerated phase, myeloid or lymphoid blast phase) CML after failure of prior therapy (including imatinib) is 140 mg once daily. In patients who do not achieve a hematologic or cytogenetic response at the recommended initial dosage, dosage may be increased to 180 mg once daily.

The optimal duration of dasatinib therapy has not been clearly established. In clinical trials, treatment generally was continued until evidence of disease progression or until no longer tolerated by the patient. The effect of discontinuance of treatment after achievement of a complete cytogenetic response has not been established.

Philadelphia Chromosome-Positive Acute Lymphocytic Leukemia The currently recommended adult dosage of dasatinib for the treatment of Philadelphia chromosome-positive (Ph$^+$) acute lymphocytic leukemia (ALL) after failure of prior therapy is 140 mg once daily. In patients who do not achieve a hematologic or cytogenetic response at the recommended initial dosage, dosage may be increased to 180 mg once daily.

The optimal duration of dasatinib therapy has not been clearly established. In clinical trials, treatment generally was continued until evidence of disease progression or unacceptable toxicity was observed. The effect of discontinuance of treatment after achievement of a complete cytogenetic response has not been established.

■ **Dose Modification** ***Myelosuppression*** Temporary interruption, dosage reduction, or discontinuance of dasatinib therapy is indicated in patients experiencing severe neutropenia and/or thrombocytopenia. Hematopoietic growth factor has been used in patients with resistant myelosuppression associated with dasatinib therapy.

Chronic Phase CML. Dasatinib therapy should be withheld in patients in the *chronic phase* of CML if absolute neutrophil counts (ANC) decrease to less than 500/mm^3 and/or platelet counts decrease to less than 50,000/mm^3. Treatment may be resumed at the original starting dosage of 100 mg once daily if ANC reaches or exceeds 1000/mm^3 and platelet counts reach or exceed 50,000/mm^3 in 7 days or less.

Following a second episode of neutropenia or thrombocytopenia, in which ANC decreases to less than 500/mm^3 for longer than 7 days or platelet counts decrease to less than 25,000/mm^3, treatment should again be withheld. Treatment may be resumed at a reduced dosage of 80 mg once daily when ANC reaches or exceeds 1000/mm^3 and platelet counts reach or exceed 50,000/mm^3.

Following a third episode of neutropenia or thrombocytopenia, in which ANC decreases to less than 500/mm^3 for longer than 7 days or platelet counts decrease to less than 25,000/mm^3, treatment should again be withheld in patients receiving dasatinib for newly diagnosed disease; treatment in these patients may be resumed at a reduced dosage of 50 mg once daily when ANC reaches or exceeds 1000/mm^3 and platelet counts reach or exceed 50,000/mm^3. However, dasatinib should be discontinued following a third such episode in patients receiving the drug following failure of prior therapy including imatinib.

Accelerated Phase or Blast Phase CML. Dasatinib therapy should be withheld in patients in the *accelerated phase* or *blast phase* of CML if ANC decreases to less than 500/mm^3 or platelet counts decrease to less than 10,000/mm^3 and the cytopenia is *unrelated* to leukemia (as determined by bone marrow aspirate or biopsy). Treatment may be resumed at the original starting dosage of 140 mg once daily when ANC reaches or exceeds 1000/mm^3 and platelet counts reach or exceed 20,000/mm^3. Treatment should again be withheld if the ANC decreases to less than 500/mm^3 or platelet counts decrease to less than 10,000/mm^3. Treatment may be resumed at a reduced dosage of 100 mg once daily (following a second episode) or 80 mg once daily (following a third episode) when ANC reaches or exceeds 1000/mm^3 and platelet counts reach or exceed 20,000/mm^3.

If patients in the *accelerated phase* or *blast phase* of CML have reductions in ANC to less than 500/mm^3 or reductions in platelet counts to less than 10,000/mm^3 and the cytopenia is *related* to leukemia (as determined by marrow aspirate or biopsy), the manufacturer recommends that an escalation in dasatinib dosage to 180 mg once daily be considered.

Philadelphia Chromosome-Positive ALL. Dasatinib therapy should be withheld in patients with Ph$^+$ ALL if ANC decreases to less than 500/mm^3 or platelet counts decrease to less than 10,000/mm^3 and the cytopenia is *unrelated* to leukemia (as determined by marrow aspirate or biopsy). Treatment may be resumed at the original starting dosage of 140 mg once daily when ANC reaches or exceeds 1000/mm^3 and platelet counts reach or exceed 20,000/mm^3. Treatment should again be withheld if ANC decreases to less than 500/mm^3 or platelet counts decrease to less than 10,000/mm^3. Treatment may be resumed at a reduced dosage of 100 mg once daily (following a second episode) or 80 mg once daily (following a third episode) when ANC reaches or exceeds 1000/mm^3 and platelet counts reach or exceed 20,000/mm^3.

If patients with Ph$^+$ ALL have reductions in ANC to less than 500/mm^3 or reductions in platelet counts to less than 10,000/mm^3 and the cytopenia is *related* to leukemia (as determined by marrow aspirate or biopsy), the manufacturer recommends that an increase in dasatinib dosage to 180 mg once daily be considered.

Nonhematologic Effects Dasatinib therapy should be withheld in patients experiencing severe adverse nonhematologic reactions; once the adverse reaction has resolved or improved, treatment may be resumed as appropriate at a reduced dosage depending on the initial severity of the event.

Concomitant Use with Drugs Affecting Hepatic Microsomal Enzymes Concomitant use of dasatinib with potent inhibitors of cytochrome P-450 (CYP) isoenzyme 3A4 should be avoided. (See Inhibitors of Cytochrome P-450 [CYP] 3A4 Isoenzyme under Drug Interactions: Drugs Affecting or Metabolized by Hepatic Microsomal Enzymes.) If such concomitant therapy cannot be avoided, reduction of dasatinib dosage should be considered. Based on pharmacokinetic considerations, the manufacturer recommends that a dosage of 20 mg daily be considered for patients currently receiving dasatinib 100 mg daily and that a dosage of 40 mg daily be considered for those receiving dasatinib 140 mg daily; no clinical data with these dosage adjustments currently are available. If dasatinib is not tolerated following dosage reduction, either the CYP3A4 inhibitor must be discontinued or dasatinib therapy must be interrupted until treatment with the CYP3A4 inhibitor is completed. Upon discontinuance of the CYP3A4 inhibitor, approximately 1 week should elapse before the dasatinib dosage is increased.

Concomitant use of dasatinib with potent CYP3A4 inducers should be avoided. (See Inducers of CYP3A4 under Drug Interactions: Drugs Affecting or Metabolized by Hepatic Microsomal Enzymes.) If such concomitant therapy cannot be avoided, an increase in dasatinib dosage should be considered based on pharmacokinetic considerations. If the dosage is increased, the patient should be monitored closely for toxicity.

■ **Special Populations** Dosage adjustment is not necessary in patients with hepatic impairment. The manufacturer makes no special dosage recommendations for geriatric patients or patients with renal impairment at this time. (See Specific Populations under Cautions: Warnings/Precautions.)

Cautions

■ **Contraindications** The manufacturer states that there are no known contraindications to the use of dasatinib.

■ **Warnings/Precautions** ***Fetal/Neonatal Morbidity and Mortality*** Dasatinib may cause fetal harm; teratogenicity and embryolethality have been demonstrated in animals. There are no studies to date in humans. Pregnancy should be avoided during therapy. If dasatinib is used during pregnancy or the patient becomes pregnant while receiving the drug, the patient should be apprised of the potential fetal hazard.

Women who are pregnant should not handle crushed or broken dasatinib tablets.

Hematologic Effects Dasatinib is commonly associated with grade 3 or 4 neutropenia, anemia, and thrombocytopenia. These effects are more frequent in patients in the accelerated phase or blast phase of CML and in those with Ph$^+$ ALL than in patients in the chronic phase of CML. In patients with chronic phase CML, grade 3 or 4 myelosuppression has been reported less frequently with once-daily dosing (100 mg once daily) than with other (e.g., twice-daily) dosing regimens. Complete blood cell counts (CBCs) should be monitored weekly during the first 2 months of therapy and monthly (or as clinically indicated) thereafter. If hematologic toxicity occurs, dasatinib should be withheld (see Myelosuppression under Dosage and Administration: Dose Modification).

Hemorrhage Severe hemorrhage, usually associated with severe thrombocytopenia, has occurred in patients receiving dasatinib. Severe CNS hemorrhage, in some cases fatal, has been reported in 1% of patients. Severe GI hemorrhage, in some cases fatal, has been reported in 4% of patients and generally has required treatment interruption and transfusions. Other cases of severe hemorrhage have been reported in 2% of patients. Caution should be used in patients receiving anticoagulants or drugs that inhibit platelet function (see Drug Interactions: Drugs Affecting Coagulation).

Fluid Retention or Edema Severe fluid retention occurred in 10% of patients receiving dasatinib in clinical trials. Severe pulmonary edema was reported in 1% and ascites and generalized edema each were reported in less than 1% of patients. Fluid retention has been reported less frequently with once-daily dosing compared with other (e.g., twice-daily) dosing regimens. Patients developing symptoms suggestive of pleural effusion (e.g., dyspnea, dry cough) should be evaluated by chest radiograph. Severe pleural effusion may require thoracentesis and oxygen therapy. Fluid retention associated with dasatinib usually can be managed with supportive care (e.g., diuretics, short course of corticosteroids).

Cardiac Effects Dasatinib may cause prolongation of the QT interval. The drug should be used with caution in patients who have or may develop prolongation of the QT interval (e.g., hypokalemia, hypomagnesemia, congenital long QT syndrome, use of drugs known to prolong QT interval, cumulative high-dose anthracycline therapy). Hypokalemia or hypomagnesemia should be corrected prior to administration of dasatinib.

Other adverse cardiac effects, including cardiomyopathy, congestive heart failure, diastolic dysfunction, fatal myocardial infarction, and left ventricular dysfunction, have occurred in 5.8% of patients receiving dasatinib. Patients should be monitored for manifestations of cardiac dysfunction, and appropriate treatment should be provided if cardiac dysfunction occurs.

Pulmonary Arterial Hypertension Dasatinib may increase the risk for development of pulmonary arterial hypertension (PAH). Cases of PAH, including some cases attributed to dasatinib and confirmed by cardiac catheterization, have been reported during postmarketing experience in patients receiving the drug. Development of PAH has been reported at various time intervals (e.g., 8–60 months) after initiation of dasatinib therapy. The mechanism of this adverse effect is unknown; however, reported cases of PAH have occurred most often in patients with comorbidities or receiving other drugs concomitantly. In some cases, improvement in hemodynamic and clinical parameters was observed following discontinuance of dasatinib therapy. In one case, PAH recurred following treatment with another tyrosine kinase inhibitor, nilotinib.

Patients should be evaluated for manifestations of underlying cardiopulmonary disease before and during dasatinib therapy. PAH should be considered in any patient presenting with dyspnea, fatigue, hypoxia, and fluid retention; however, other etiologies of dyspnea should be excluded prior to initiating invasive diagnostic procedures for PAH. Since PAH may be reversible following discontinuance of dasatinib, interruption of therapy accompanied by monitoring for improvement may be considered if PAH is suspected. If a diagnosis of PAH is confirmed (e.g., by cardiac catheterization), the drug should be permanently discontinued.

Lactose-intolerant Patients Each 140-mg daily dosage contains 189 mg of lactose monohydrate and each 100-mg daily dosage contains 135 mg of lactose monohydrate.

Specific Populations **Pregnancy.** Category D. (See Fetal/Neonatal Morbidity and Mortality under Warnings/Precautions.)

Lactation. It is not known whether dasatinib is distributed into milk. Because of the potential for serious adverse reactions from dasatinib in nursing infants, a decision should be made whether to discontinue nursing or the drug, taking into account the importance of the drug to the woman.

Pediatric Use. Safety and efficacy of dasatinib have not been established in patients younger than 18 years of age.

Geriatric Use. When the total number of patients studied in clinical trials of dasatinib is considered, 10% of those with newly diagnosed chronic phase CML were 65 years of age or older and 3% were 75 years of age or older, while 25% of those receiving dasatinib following failure of prior therapy were 65 years of age or older and 5% were 75 years of age or older. Although no overall differences in efficacy were observed between geriatric and younger patients, patients 65 years of age or older are more likely to experience toxicity.

Hepatic Impairment. Although peak plasma concentration and AUC (normalized for differences in administered doses) were lower in patients with moderate or severe hepatic impairment (Child-Pugh class B or C) than in healthy individuals, the differences were not considered clinically important. Dosage adjustment is not necessary in patients with hepatic impairment. However, the drug should be used with caution in hepatic impairment.

Renal Impairment. Dasatinib has not been studied in patients with renal impairment; however, renal excretion of unchanged dasatinib and its metabolites is minimal (less than 4%).

■ **Common Adverse Effects** Adverse effects reported in 10% or more of patients receiving dasatinib as first-line therapy include neutropenia, thrombocytopenia, anemia, fluid retention (e.g., pleural effusion or superficial localized edema), diarrhea, headache, musculoskeletal pain, and rash.

Adverse effects reported in 10% or more of patients receiving dasatinib following failure of prior therapy include fluid retention (e.g., superficial and/or localized edema, generalized edema, pleural effusion, pericardial effusion, congestive heart failure or cardiac dysfunction, pulmonary edema), neutropenia, thrombocytopenia, anemia, hemorrhage (e.g., GI or CNS hemorrhage), diarrhea, vomiting, abdominal pain, nausea, headache, fatigue, pyrexia, musculoskeletal pain, myalgia, arthralgia, rash, dyspnea, hypophosphatemia, hypokalemia, hypocalcemia, febrile neutropenia, and infection (e.g., bacterial, viral, fungal).

Drug Interactions

■ **Drugs Affecting or Metabolized by Hepatic Microsomal Enzymes** ***Inhibitors of Cytochrome P-450 (CYP) 3A4 Isoenzyme*** Pharmacokinetic interactions (increased plasma dasatinib concentrations) may occur during concomitant use of dasatinib and atazanavir, clarithromycin, erythromycin, indinavir, itraconazole, ketoconazole, nefazodone, nelfinavir, ritonavir, saquinavir, telithromycin, or voriconazole; concomitant use of dasatinib (20 mg once daily) and ketoconazole (200 mg twice daily) increased peak plasma concentrations and area under the plasma concentration-time curve (AUC) of dasatinib by fourfold and fivefold, respectively. Concomitant use of dasatinib with these drugs or with grapefruit juice should be avoided. Close monitoring for toxicity and reduction of dasatinib dosage should be considered if concomitant therapy with a potent CYP3A4 inhibitor and dasatinib is needed. (See Concomitant Use with Drugs Affecting Hepatic Microsomal Enzymes under Dosage and Administration: Dose Modification.)

Inducers of CYP3A4 Pharmacokinetic interactions (decreased plasma dasatinib concentrations) may occur during concomitant use of dasatinib and carbamazepine, dexamethasone, phenobarbital, phenytoin, rifabutin, rifampin, or St. John's wort (*Hypericum perforatum*). When a single dose of dasatinib was administered following 8 days of rifampin administration (600 mg daily), the mean peak plasma concentration and AUC of dasatinib were decreased by 81 and 82%, respectively. If administration with a CYP3A4 inducer is indicated, drugs with less enzyme induction potential should be used; close monitoring for toxicity and an increase in dasatinib dosage should be considered. Since St. John's wort may cause unpredictable decreases in plasma dasatinib concentrations, such concomitant use should be avoided.

CYP3A4 Substrates Dasatinib, a weak time-dependent inhibitor of CYP3A4, may decrease the metabolic clearance of drugs that are metabolized mainly by CYP3A4. At clinically relevant concentrations, dasatinib does not inhibit CYP isoenzymes 1A2, 2A6, 2B6, 2C8, 2C9, 2C19, 2D6, or 2E1. Pharmacokinetic interactions (increased plasma CYP3A4-substrate concentrations) are possible when dasatinib is used with CYP3A4 substrates. Concomitant administration of simvastatin (a CYP3A4 substrate) and dasatinib (single 100-mg dose) increased the mean peak plasma concentration and AUC of simvastatin by 37 and 20%, respectively. Therefore, CYP3A4 substrates known to have a narrow therapeutic index (e.g., alfentanil, astemizole [no longer commercially available in the US], terfenadine [no longer commercially available in the US], cisapride, cyclosporine, fentanyl, pimozide, quinidine, simvastatin, sirolimus, tacrolimus, ergot alkaloids [ergotamine, dihydroergotamine]) should be used with caution in patients receiving dasatinib.

■ **Drugs Affecting Coagulation** Since dasatinib may cause severe thrombocytopenia and bleeding, anticoagulants and drugs that inhibit platelet function should be used concomitantly with caution. Patients receiving anticoagulants or drugs that inhibit platelet function were excluded from initial clinical trials of dasatinib; however, use of anticoagulants, aspirin, and nonsteroidal anti-inflammatory agents (NSAIAs) was permitted in subsequent clinical trials if the patient's platelet count exceeded 50,000–75,000/mm^3.

■ **Antacids** Because solubility of dasatinib is pH dependent, concomitant administration of dasatinib and antacids may reduce plasma dasatinib concentrations. Administration of an antacid containing aluminum and magnesium hydroxides (Maalox® 30 mL) 2 hours before dasatinib (single 50-mg dose) increased peak plasma dasatinib concentrations by 26% but did not substantially alter the AUC of the drug; however, when the antacid and dasatinib were administered concomitantly, peak plasma concentrations and AUC of dasatinib were reduced by 58 and 55%, respectively. Concomitant administration should be avoided. If antacid therapy is needed, the antacid dose should be administered at least 2 hours before or after a dose of dasatinib.

■ **Histamine H_2-receptor Antagonists, Proton-pump Inhibitors** Long-term suppression of gastric acid secretion by histamine H_2-receptor antagonists or proton-pump inhibitors is likely to reduce dasatinib exposure. When dasatinib 50 mg was administered 10 hours after famotidine (single 40-mg dose), peak plasma concentrations and AUC of dasatinib were reduced by 63 and 61%, respectively. When dasatinib (single 100-mg dose) was administered 22 hours after omeprazole (40 mg) at steady state, peak plasma concentrations and AUC of dasatinib were reduced by 42 and 43%, respectively. Concomitant use of dasatinib and histamine H_2-receptor antagonists or proton-pump inhibitors is not recommended. Instead, use of antacids (administered at least 2 hours before or after a dose of dasatinib) should be considered.

Description

Dasatinib, an inhibitor of multiple tyrosine kinases (including Bcr-Abl, the Src family [Src, Lck, Yes, Fyn], c-Kit, EphA-2, and platelet-derived growth factor [PDGF]-β), is an antineoplastic agent. Dasatinib is a thiazolecarboxamide that is structurally unrelated to imatinib.

The Philadelphia chromosome, characteristic of chronic myelogenous leukemia (CML) and Philadelphia chromosome-positive (Ph$^+$) acute lymphocytic leukemia (ALL), is created by a reciprocal translocation between chromosomes 9 and 22. Translocation between these chromosomes results in production of an abnormal protein (Bcr-Abl tyrosine kinase) that exhibits enhanced tyrosine kinase activity (i.e., increased phosphorylation of tyrosine residues); phosphorylation of tyrosine residues on growth factor receptors is thought to be important in stimulating cell proliferation and inhibiting cell death (apoptosis). Dasatinib inhibits Bcr-Abl tyrosine kinase, thereby inhibiting tyrosine phosphorylation of proteins involved in Bcr-Abl signal transduction. In vitro, the drug has been shown to inhibit the growth of CML and ALL cell lines overexpressing Bcr-Abl.

Data from in vitro studies indicate that dasatinib may overcome imatinib resistance resulting from Bcr-Abl kinase domain mutations, activation of alternate signaling pathways involving the Src family kinases (Lyn, Hck), and multi-drug-resistance gene overexpression.

In preclinical studies in cell-line models, dasatinib inhibited most (18 of 19) imatinib-resistant Bcr-Abl kinase domain mutant forms.

Dasatinib is extensively metabolized by the cytochrome P-450 (CYP) microsomal enzyme system, principally by the isoenzyme 3A4. An active metabolite, formed principally by CYP3A4, is approximately equipotent to dasatinib but accounts for only about 5% of total plasma concentrations of the drug. Following oral administration of a single radiolabeled dose of dasatinib, approximately 85% of the radioactivity was recovered in feces and 4% was recovered in urine within 10 days; unchanged drug accounted for 19% of the dose recovered in feces and 0.1% of the dose recovered in urine, with the remainder being metabolites.

Advice to Patients

Importance of advising patients to take dasatinib at about the same time each day.

Importance of advising patients to swallow dasatinib tablets whole with water and not to break, chew, cut, or crush the tablets. Importance of not drinking grapefruit juice while taking the drug.

Importance of not discontinuing dasatinib therapy without first consulting clinician.

Importance of informing clinician immediately if patient accidentally ingested more than the prescribed dose.

Importance of advising patient that if a dose of dasatinib is missed, the next dose should be taken at the regularly scheduled time; the dose should not be doubled.

Importance of informing clinicians if patient is lactose intolerant.

Importance of informing clinician if fever or other symptom of infection, any bleeding or bruising, difficulty in breathing, swelling, weight gain, or increasing shortness of breath occurs.

Importance of advising patients of other common adverse effects, including diarrhea, rash, headache, musculoskeletal pain, fatigue, and nausea.

Necessity of monitoring blood cell counts.

Importance of advising women to use an effective method of contraception and to avoid breast-feeding while undergoing dasatinib therapy. Importance of women informing a clinician immediately if they are or plan to become pregnant or plan to breast-feed. Importance of advising patients that women who are pregnant should not handle crushed or broken dasatinib tablets.

Importance of advising patients to avoid taking antacids within 2 hours of dasatinib administration and to avoid taking histamine H_2-receptor antagonists or proton-pump inhibitors while undergoing dasatinib therapy.

Importance of informing clinicians of existing or contemplated concomitant therapy, including prescription and OTC drugs and herbal supplements, as well as any concomitant illnesses.

Importance of informing patients of other important precautionary information. (See Cautions.)

Overview® (see Users Guide). For additional information on this drug until a more detailed monograph is developed and published, the manufacturer's labeling should be consulted. It is *essential* that the manufacturer's labeling be consulted for more detailed information on usual cautions, precautions, contraindications, potential drug interactions, laboratory test interferences, and acute toxicity.

Preparations

Excipients in commercially available drug preparations may have clinically important effects in some individuals; consult specific product labeling for details.

Dasatinib

Oral

Tablets, film-coated	20 mg	**Sprycel®**, Bristol Myers-Squibb
	50 mg	**Sprycel®**, Bristol Myers-Squibb
	70 mg	**Sprycel®**, Bristol Myers-Squibb
	80 mg	**Sprycel®**, Bristol Myers-Squibb
	100 mg	**Sprycel®**, Bristol Myers Squibb
	140 mg	**Sprycel®**, Bristol Myers Squibb

DAUNOrubicin

Daunomycin, Rubidomycin

■ Daunorubicin is an anthracycline glycoside antineoplastic antibiotic produced by *Streptomyces coeruleorubidus*.

Uses

■ **Leukemias** ***Acute Myeloid Leukemia*** Daunorubicin hydrochloride is used in combination with other antineoplastic agents for the treatment of acute myeloid (myelogenous, nonlymphocytic) leukemia (AML, ANLL) in adults. Cytarabine with either daunorubicin or idarubicin is a regimen of choice for remission induction in AML. Induction regimens are used to rapidly reduce the tumor burden in order to achieve complete remission, which generally is defined as less than 5% leukemic blast cells in the bone marrow, and normalization of peripheral blood counts (including hemoglobin concentration, hematocrit, granulocyte count, and platelet count), and absence of any evidence of extramedullary disease. Optimal postremission therapy has not been established, but current approaches include consolidation chemotherapy with cytarabine-based regimens similar to standard induction regimens, consolidation chemotherapy with high-dose cytarabine-based regimens (for younger adults), high-dose chemotherapy or chemoradiotherapy with autologous bone marrow rescue, or high-dose marrow-ablative therapy with allogeneic bone marrow rescue. There is no evidence of benefit from prolonged administration of chemotherapy in the treatment of AML, and most current treatment regimens in the US no longer employ maintenance therapy.

The 2-drug regimen of daunorubicin hydrochloride and cytarabine generally results in a complete response rate of approximately 65% in patients with previously untreated AML. There is some evidence that dose intensity of cytarabine as a component of induction therapy may affect disease-free survival. (See Acute Myeloid Leukemia under Uses: Conventional Cytarabine, in Cytarabine 10:00.) Some clinicians have used thioguanine in addition to intensive therapy with daunorubicin and cytarabine for remission induction.

Patients with AML who have complete remission of disease following induction therapy generally receive consolidation chemotherapy. The optimal regimen has not been established, but consolidation chemotherapy typically consists of a cytarabine-based regimen similar to that used in induction therapy administered over a short-term period. Consolidation therapy has ranged in duration from one to 4 or more cycles, but the optimal doses, schedules, and duration of consolidation chemotherapy remain to be established. Maintenance therapy for AML generally is *not* recommended.

Acute Lymphocytic Leukemia Daunorubicin hydrochloride is used as a component of combination chemotherapeutic regimens for the induction of remissions of childhood or adult acute lymphocytic (lymphoblastic) leukemia (ALL). Combination therapy with an asparaginase preparation, a corticosteroid (dexamethasone or prednisone), and vincristine is used as an induction regimen for non-high-risk childhood ALL. (For additional information on the asparaginase component of ALL regimens, see Asparaginase [Erwinia chrysanthemi] 10:00.) The use of intensive induction regimens with 4 or more drugs, including an anthracycline (e.g., daunorubicin), an asparaginase preparation, a corticosteroid (e.g., prednisone), and vincristine, with or without cyclophosphamide, may improve the rate of event-free survival but is associated with greater toxicity. An induction regimen containing 4 or more drugs does not appear to be necessary to achieve favorable outcomes in patients at low or standard risk of treatment failure provided adequate intensification therapy is provided following achievement of remission. Therefore, some clinicians reserve such regimens for patients with high-risk childhood ALL. However, other clinicians have elected to use a 4- or 5-drug induction regimen for all patients with childhood ALL regardless of presenting features. Induction regimens for adult ALL typically include an anthracycline, prednisone, and vincristine; some regimens also add other drugs, such as an asparaginase preparation or cyclophosphamide.

Various drugs have been used for combination chemotherapy of childhood and adult ALL, and comparative efficacy of these regimens is continually being evaluated. Other regimens are preferred in certain subsets of patients with ALL (e.g., B-cell ALL, T-cell ALL, Philadelphia chromosome-positive ALL); specialized references and experts should be consulted for additional information.

Chronic Myelogenous Leukemia Daunorubicin hydrochloride is used with other antineoplastic agents in the treatment of the accelerated or blastic phase of chronic myelogenous leukemia†.

■ **AIDS-related Kaposi's Sarcoma** Daunorubicin citrate encapsulated in liposomes is used as first-line therapy for advanced AIDS-related Kaposi's sarcoma. The encapsulated drug is not recommended for patients with early stages of the disease. Administration of daunorubicin citrate encapsulated in liposomes (see Chemistry and Stability: Chemistry) allows the drug-containing liposomes to remain circulating in plasma for prolonged periods and reduces extravasation of the drugwhile substantially increasing concentrations of daunorubicin in the lesions of Kaposi's sarcoma compared with administration of comparable doses of conventional (nonencapsulated) daunorubicin hydrochloride injections (see Pharmacokinetics: Distribution). Liposomal anthracycline (daunorubicin or doxorubicin) is the first-line therapy of choice for advanced AIDS-related Kaposi's sarcoma. (See Uses: AIDS-related Kaposi's Sarcoma in Doxorubicin 10:00 for overview and further discussion of therapy.) The comparative efficacy of daunorubicin citrate encapsulated in liposomes relative to liposomal doxorubicin has not been established, but liposomal daunorubicin appears to be better tolerated than and comparably effective to combination chemotherapy (e.g., conventional doxorubicin, bleomycin, and vincristine) for the management of advanced AIDS-related Kaposi's sarcoma.

Results of an open-label, randomized, multicenter, controlled clinical study in patients with advanced AIDS-related Kaposi's sarcoma (e.g., those with extensive mucocutaneous disease, lymphedema, symptomatic visceral disease) who had not received prior systemic chemotherapy, response rates (using the National Institute of Allergy and Infectious Diseases [NIAID] AIDS Clinical Trials Group [ACTG] criteria for response) and quality-of-life scores were similar in patients receiving daunorubicin citrate liposomal injection (40 mg/m^2 every 2 weeks) to those receiving combination chemotherapy every 2 weeks with conventional antineoplastic agents (e.g., conventional doxorubicin 10 mg/m^2, bleomycin 15 units, vincristine 1 mg). In this study, response rates of about 23–25 or 28–30%, respectively, reportedly were observed in patients receiving daunorubicin citrate liposomal injection or combination chemotherapy with conventional antineoplastic agents while median duration of response was 110–175 or 113–168 days in patients receiving daunorubicin citrate liposomal injection or combination chemotherapy with conventional antineoplastic agents, respectively. Median time to progression of the disease was 92–115 or 99–105 days, respectively, in patients receiving daunorubicin citrate liposomal injection or combination chemotherapy with conventional antineoplastic agents while median survival was 342–369 or 291–342 days in patients receiving daunorubicin citrate liposomal injection or combination chemotherapy with conventional antineoplastic agents, respectively. It should be considered, however, that no treatment has been shown conclusively to alter the natural history of AIDS-related Kaposi's sarcoma. Daunorubicin citrate liposomal injection also has been used as second-line treatment of advanced AIDS-related Kaposi's sarcoma that has progressed or relapsed with anthracycline or other systemic chemotherapy; responses have been reported in some patients, including partial responses in a limited number of patients who previously have received conventional (nonencapsulated) doxorubicin and in at least one patient who previously has received liposomal doxorubicin. However, limited evidence suggests that cross-resistance between liposomal daunorubicin and prior anthracycline therapy may occur.

Toxicity, including cardiotoxicity and myelosuppression, has occurred in patients receiving liposomal daunorubicin; therefore, the usual precautions of conventional (nonencapsulated) anthracycline therapy should be observed when the liposomal formulation of daunorubicin is used.

■ **Other Uses** Daunorubicin possesses activity against a wide range of grafted or spontaneous animal tumors; however, in contrast to doxorubicin, daunorubicin hydrochloride has not been extensively studied in the treatment of solid tumors in humans.

Dosage and Administration

■ **Reconstitution and Administration** Daunorubicin hydrochloride is administered IV into a rapidly flowing IV infusion. The drug is extremely irritating to tissues and, therefore, should *not* be given IM or subcutaneously. *Care should be taken to avoid extravasation of the drug.* (See Cautions: Local Effects.)

If daunorubicin contacts the skin or mucosa, the area should be washed promptly and thoroughly with soap and water.

Daunorubicin hydrochloride powder for injection is reconstituted by adding 4 mL of sterile water for injection to the vial labeled as containing 20 mg of daunorubicin. The vial should be gently agitated until the contents are completely dissolved. The resultant solution contains 5 mg of daunorubicin per mL. The manufacturer recommends that the desired dose of the reconstituted solution be withdrawn into a syringe containing 10–15 mL of 0.9% sodium chloride injection and then injected over 2–3 minutes into the tubing or sidearm of a freely flowing IV infusion of 0.9% sodium chloride or 5% dextrose injection. Small veins, swollen or edematous extremities, and areas overlying joints and tendons should be avoided as injection sites. The IV injection site and surrounding area should be observed for infiltration and vein irritation during administration of the drug. Patients should be instructed to immediately report any stinging or burning; if either occurs, the infusion should be stopped and restarted at another site, preferably in a different extremity. Following injection of daunorubicin, some clinicians recommend flushing the vein with the running IV infusion for 2–5 minutes and/or injecting 5–10 mL of IV solution into the sidearm to flush any remaining drug from the tubing. Daunorubicin hydrochloride has also been diluted in 100 mL of 0.9% sodium chloride or 5% dextrose injection and infused over 30–45 minutes.

Commercially available daunorubicin hydrochloride injection containing 5 mg/mL should be diluted prior to IV administration. The appropriate dose of the injection should be withdrawn into a syringe containing 10–15 mL of 0.9% sodium chloride injection and then injected into the tubing or sidearm of a rapidly flowing IV infusion of 5% dextrose or 0.9% sodium chloride injection. The injection should not be admixed with other drugs or heparin.

Solutions of liposomal daunorubicin citrate injection should be diluted in 5% dextrose injection and infused slowly over 60 minutes.

Although tissue necrosis associated with extravasation of the liposomally encapsulated drug has not been reported to date, liposomal daunorubicin should be considered an irritant, and the usual precautions to avoid extravasation of the drug should be followed. When extravasation of liposomal daunorubicin citrate occurs, application of ice packs over the site of extravasation and local infiltration of dexamethasone or hydrocortisone may help alleviate the local reaction.

Commercially available liposomal daunorubicin citrate injection for IV infusion containing 2 mg of the drug per mL must be diluted prior to administration. The appropriate dose of liposomal daunorubicin citrate should be withdrawn from the vial with a sterile syringe and transferred unto a small-volume PVC container containing an equivalent volume of dextrose 5% injection to provide a solution containing 1 mg of the drug per mL; strict aseptic technique must be observed since the injection does not contain any preservative or bacteriostatic agent. The manufacturer states that diluents containing preservatives (e.g., benzyl alcohol) or other diluents should not be used and other drugs should not be mixed with the solution. Because liposomal daunorubicin citrate occurs as a liposomal dispersion of the drug, inline filters should not be used. The manufacturer recommends that diluted liposomal daunorubicin citrate solutions be used immediately; however, if not used immediately, the manufacturer states that diluted solutions of liposomal daunorubicin are stable for up to 6 hours when refrigerated at 2–8°C.

Parenteral daunorubicin hydrochloride solutions should be inspected visually for particulate matter prior to administration whenever solution and container permit. Because liposomal daunorubicin citrate occurs as a liposomal dispersion, the injection is not clear but rather is translucent and red; the injection should not be used if precipitation or foreign matter is evident or if the injection appears opaque.

Daunorubicin as a single-entity preparation is not interchangeable with the fixed liposomal combination of daunorubicin and cytarabine (daunorubicin/cytarabine liposomal; Vyxeos®). To avoid dosing errors, clinicians should confirm the correct drug name, formulation, and dose prior to preparation and administration.

■ **Dosage** Dosage of daunorubicin hydrochloride is expressed in terms of daunorubicin. Dosage of daunorubicin must be based on the clinical and hematologic response and tolerance of the patient and whether or not other chemotherapy or radiation therapy has been or is also being used in order to obtain optimum therapeutic results with minimum adverse effects. Clinicians should consult published protocols for the dosage of daunorubicin and other chemotherapeutic agents and the method and sequence of administration.

Conventional Daunorubicin Hydrochloride **Acute Myeloid Leukemia.** In combination chemotherapy for remission induction in acute myeloid leukemia, the usual dosage of daunorubicin for adults younger than 60 years of age is 45 mg/m^2 (30 mg/m^2 for adults 60 years of age and older) administered daily on 3 successive days of the first course of induction therapy, and daily on 2 successive days of subsequent courses. Up to 3 courses of induction therapy may be required for optimal response.

Acute Lymphocytic Leukemia. In combination chemotherapy for remission induction in acute lymphocytic leukemia in adults, the usual dose of daunorubicin is 45 mg/m^2 administered daily on the first 3 days of a course of induction therapy.

In combination chemotherapy for remission induction in acute lymphocytic leukemia in children, the usual dose of daunorubicin is 25 mg/m^2 administered on the first day of each week. A complete remission generally will be obtained within 4 courses of therapy; if a partial remission is obtained following 4 courses of therapy, 1 or 2 additional courses of therapy may be administered in an effort to achieve a complete remission.

In children younger than 2 years of age or with a body surface area of less than 0.5 m^2, the manufacturer states that daunorubicin dosage should be calculated on the basis of body weight (1 mg/kg) rather than body surface area.

Consolidation and Cumulative Dosage. Appropriate consolidation therapy may be initiated after induction of a complete remission.

Total daunorubicin dosage should not exceed 550 mg/m^2 in adults because of the risk of cumulative cardiotoxicity. Cardiotoxicity may occur more frequently and at lower cumulative dosages of daunorubicin in children than in adults. In both adults and children, the total daunorubicin dosage administered should take into account previous or concomitant therapy with other potentially cardiotoxic agents or with related drugs such as doxorubicin. (See Cautions: Cardiac Effects and Precautions and Contraindications.) In adults who received irradiation of the cardiac region, congestive heart failure may occur at a lower cumulative dosage, and total daunorubicin dosage in these patients should be limited to 400 mg/m^2.

Liposomal Daunorubicin Citrate **Kaposi's Sarcoma.** The usual adult dosage of liposomal daunorubicin citrate for the first-line treatment of advanced AIDS-related Kaposi's sarcoma is 40 mg/m^2 administered as a 60-minute IV infusion once every 2 weeks. Blood cell counts should be performed prior to each dose of liposomal daunorubicin citrate. If absolute granulocyte count is less than 750/ mm^3, therapy with the drug should be withheld until the counts exceed this level. Treatment should be continued until there is evidence of progressive disease (e.g., based on best response achieved, new visceral sites of involvement or progression of visceral disease, development of 10 or more new cutaneous lesions or a 25% increase in the number of lesions compared with baseline, a change in the character of 25% or more of all previously counted flat lesions to raised lesions, increased surface area of the indicator lesions) or until other complications of HIV disease preclude continuation of therapy.

■ **Dosage in Renal and Hepatic Impairment** Doses of conventional or liposomal daunorubicin should be reduced in patients with hepatic or renal impairment. The manufacturers recommend that patients with serum bilirubin concentrations of 1.2–3 mg/dL receive 75% of the usual dose and those with serum bilirubin concentrations exceeding 3 mg/dL receive 50% of the usual dose of daunorubicin. The manufacturers recommend that patients with serum creatinine concentrations exceeding 3 mg/dL receive 50% of the usual dose of daunorubicin.

Cautions

■ **Hematologic Effects** Hematologic toxicity occurs in all patients receiving daunorubicin. Severe myelosuppression occurs when daunorubicin is used in therapeutic dosages; this may cause infection or hemorrhage. Myelosuppression is manifested primarily by leukopenia, which is usually severe, and thrombocytopenia; anemia may also occur.

The principal dose-limiting toxicity of liposomal daunorubicin in patients with AIDS-related Kaposi's sarcoma has been myelosuppression, mainly granulocytopenia, which may be severe and associated with fever, and may result in infection; liposomal daunorubicin has a lesser effect on platelets and erythroid cells. Neutropenia (neutrophil count of less than 1000/mm^3) has been reported in 51% (15% having a neutrophil count of less than 500/mm^3) of patients receiving the liposomal preparation. However, experience with liposomal daunorubicin has been principally in patients who had baseline myelosuppression secondary to their underlying human immunodeficiency virus (HIV) infection and/or numerous concomitant drug therapy. Opportunistic infections, probably associated with severe myelosuppression, have been reported in 40% of patients receiving liposomal daunorubicin. Filgrastim (a granulocyte colony-stimulating factor, G-CSF) has been used with some success in a limited number of AIDS patients who developed severe neutropenia during liposomal daunorubicin therapy. Hematologic status must be monitored carefully in patients receiving daunorubicin. (See Cautions: Precautions and Contraindications.) Following administration of conventional (nonencapsulated) daunorubicin hydrochloride, leukocyte and platelet nadirs usually occur within 10–14 days, and leukocyte and platelet counts generally return to normal levels during the third week.

■ **Cardiac Effects** As with doxorubicin, 3 types of cardiotoxicity may occur in patients receiving daunorubicin: an acute, transient type; a chronic, subacute type, which is related to cumulative dose and has a later, more indolent onset; and a late-onset type that manifests years after anthracycline therapy and occurs mainly in patients exposed to the drugs as children.

Acute anthracycline-induced cardiotoxicity is uncommon. It occurs immediately after a single dose or a single course of anthracycline therapy and may involve abnormal ECG findings including ST-T wave changes (e.g., T-wave flattening and ST-segment depression), prolongation of the QT interval, and arrhythmias (e.g., sinus tachycardia; ventricular, supraventricular, and junctional tachycardia). Conduction disturbances (including atrioventricular [AV] and bundle-branch block) have been reported rarely in acute anthracycline-induced cardiotoxicity; such disturbances usually are associated more with late-onset anthracycline-induced cardiotoxicity. Although acute cardiotoxicity generally is transient, rarely, pericarditis-myocarditis syndrome (e.g., pericardial effusion and/or decreased myocardial contractility) that is not dose-related, and possible cardiac failure, may occur.

Chronic cardiotoxicity may occur as total dosage of conventional (nonencapsulated) daunorubicin approaches 400–550 mg/m^2. Time of onset of chronic cardiotoxicity may vary but usually is manifested within 1 year of anthracycline therapy. In one study, onset of congestive heart failure developed 0–231 days after discontinuance of anthracycline therapy. Chronic cardiotoxicity reflects a progressive injury and loss of cardiac myocyte, with increasing cumulative anthracycline doses resulting in thinning of ventricular walls and decreased systolic performance. Initially, there is functional compensation by the remaining myocytes allowing overall cardiac function to appear normal despite histologic damage, which can be demonstrated by endomyocardial biopsy. However, as cumulative doses of anthracycline increase, there is a decrease in systolic performance, as measured by a decrease in fractional shortening (FS) and left-ventricular ejection fraction (LVEF) with eventual progression to symptomatic congestive heart failure, if cardiac reserve is exhausted, and cardiorespiratory decompensation.

Symptoms of the described rapidly progressing syndrome may include tachycardia, tachypnea, dilation of the heart, exercise intolerance, pulmonary and venous congestion, poor perfusion, and pleural effusion; these manifestations may respond to cardiac supportive therapy and may be self-limiting, or, alternatively, may be irreversible and unresponsive to therapy and fatal. Early diagnosis of daunorubicin-induced congestive heart failure and prompt initiation of treatment is essential for optimizing response to supportive therapy.

Congestive heart failure occurs in approximately 1–2% of adults at a total conventional daunorubicin dosage of 550 mg/m^2, but the incidence increases after this cumulative dosage is exceeded. In adults who received radiation therapy that encompassed the heart, congestive heart failure may occur at a lower total dosage of conventional (nonencapsulated) daunorubicin (400 mg/m^2). The incidence of daunorubicin-induced myocardial toxicity increases after a cumulative dosage of conventional (nonencapsulated) daunorubicin exceeding 400–550 mg/m^2 in adults, 300 mg/m^2 in children older than 2 years of age, or 10 mg/kg in children younger than 2 years of age. In both adults and children, the total dose of daunorubicin administered should take into account any previous or concomitant therapy with other anthracyclines, such as doxorubicin, or with other potentially cardiotoxic drugs.

Infants and children appear to be more susceptible to anthracycline-induced cardiotoxicity than adults, in whom cardiotoxicity is more clearly dose related. Impaired left ventricular systolic performance, reduced contractility, and congestive heart failure, sometimes resulting in death, have occurred in pediatric patients months to years following discontinuance of therapy with anthracyclines such as daunorubicin. These conditions appear to be dose dependent and are more likely to occur in patients who receive radiation therapy of the thorax. Such patients should receive long-term periodic evaluation of cardiac function.

Late-onset anthracycline-induced cardiotoxicity, which may include late-onset ventricular dysfunction, heart failure, conduction disturbances, and arrhythmias (e.g., nonsustained ventricular tachycardia), which may be life-threatening, occurs several years or even decades after discontinuance of anthracycline therapy, and it may develop after a prolonged asymptomatic interval. In one study in patients with solid tumors or leukemia, those who were followed for 4 to less than 10 or 10–20 years after discontinuance of anthracycline therapy had an 18 or 38% incidence, respectively, of abnormal FS in echocardiograms. It has been suggested that myocyte damage and ventricular dysfunction progress after the initial myocardial insult and may lead to late-onset cardiac decompensation. Some clinicians state that late-onset cardiotoxicity can manifest clinically in response to stressful situations (e.g., surgery, pregnancy), exercise (e.g., weight lifting), and acute viral infection.

Cardiotoxicity also has been reported in patients receiving daunorubicin encapsulated in liposomes. Congestive heart failure was reported in a patient with AIDS-related Kaposi's sarcoma at a cumulative dose of 340 mg/m^2. Among 8 patients with AIDS-related Kaposi's sarcoma, decreases in LVEF occurred at a median cumulative dose of 320 mg/m^2 (range, 200–2100 mg/m^2). Congestive heart failure has been reported at a cumulative dose as low as 200 mg/m^2 in patients with other malignancies receiving liposomal daunorubicin at doses exceeding the recommended dose of 40 mg/m^2 in clinical studies; decreases in LVEF occurred in 7 patients. The incidence of cardiotoxicity in patients receiving liposomal daunorubicin has not been established. Other serious adverse cardiac effects reported in patients receiving liposomal daunorubicin in clinical trials for AIDS-related Kaposi's sarcoma or other malignancies include pericardial effusion, pericardial tamponade, ventricular extrasystoles, cardiac arrest, sinus tachycardia, atrial fibrillation, pulmonary hypertension, myocardial infarction, supraventricular tachycardia, and angina pectoris. Further study and experience are needed to determine the relative risk of anthracycline-induced cardiotoxicity associated with liposomal versus conventional preparations.

Hot flushes, hypertension, palpitation, syncope, and tachycardia have been reported in 5% of patients or less receiving liposomal daunorubicin. Edema and chest pain have been reported in patients receiving liposomal daunorubicin.

For additional information on the cardiotoxicity of anthracyclines, see Cautions: Cardiac Effects in Doxorubicin Hydrochloride 10:00.

■ **Infusion-related Effects** Back pain accompanied by flushing and chest tightness has been reported in about 14% of patients receiving liposomal daunorubicin in a phase III trial; these symptoms generally occur during the first 5 minutes of drug infusion, usually resolve if the infusion is stopped, and typically do not recur when the infusion is resumed at a slower rate. Similar manifestations also have been reported with other liposomal preparations and appear to be related to the lipid component of liposomal daunorubicin.

■ **GI Effects** Mucositis or stomatitis may occur as early as 3–7 days after administration of daunorubicin. Stomatitis usually begins as a burning sensation with erythema of the oral mucosa leading to ulceration in 2–3 days. Esophagitis may occur in some patients. Acute nausea and vomiting, usually mild, occur in patients receiving daunorubicin. Nausea and vomiting may occur soon after administration of the drug and last for 24–48 hours. Antiemetics may be of some help in preventing or treating nausea and vomiting. Diarrhea, abdominal pain, anorexia, and constipation have occasionally been reported.

Increased appetite, dysphagia, GI hemorrhage, gastritis, gingival bleeding, hemorrhoids, melena, dry mouth, taste perversion, thirst, hiccups, or tooth caries have been reported in 5% of patients or less receiving liposomal daunorubicin. Constipation and tenesmus have been reported in patients receiving liposomal daunorubicin.

■ **Nervous System Effects** Neuropathy was reported in 13% of patients and amnesia, anxiety, ataxia, confusion, emotional lability, hallucination, abnormal thinking, hyperkinesia, hypertonia, tremor, somnolence, or seizures have been reported in 5% of patients or less receiving liposomal daunorubicin. Fatigue, headache, increased sweating, rigors, depression, malaise, dizziness, and insomnia have been reported in patients receiving liposomal daunorubicin.

■ **Dermatologic and Sensitivity Reactions** Reversible alopecia occurs in most patients receiving conventional (nonencapsulated) daunorubicin. Complete alopecia involving the scalp, axillary, and pubic hair almost always occurs with daunorubicin therapy, and patients should be advised of this effect. Growth of hair usually resumes 5 or more weeks after daunorubicin is discontinued. Limited data indicate that mild or moderate alopecia occurred in 6 or 2%, respectively, of patients with AIDS-related Kaposi's sarcoma receiving liposomal daunorubicin.

Transverse pigmentation of fingernails and toenails has occurred in a patient receiving the drug. Rarely occurring adverse dermatologic effects include rash, contact dermatitis, and urticaria. Daunorubicin may also reactivate skin lesions produced by previous radiation therapy in some patients. Anaphylactoid reaction has been reported rarely in patients receiving daunorubicin. Folliculitis, seborrhea, or dry skin has been reported in 5% of patients or less receiving liposomal daunorubicin; allergic reactions and pruritus occurred in patients receiving the drug.

■ **Local Effects** Extravasation of daunorubicin can produce severe local tissue necrosis, severe cellulitis, thrombophlebitis, or painful induration. Extravasation is usually accompanied by an immediate burning sensation at the site. Slow, progressive necrosis of skin can develop, leading to deep, painful ulceration which can require multiple surgical debridements and skin grafting. Although injection site inflammation rarely has been reported in patients receiving liposomal daunorubicin citrate, tissue necrosis associated with extravasation of the liposomally encapsulated drug has not been reported to date; however, liposomal daunorubicin also should be considered an irritant, and the usual precautions to avoid extravasation of the drug should be followed. If extravasation occurs, as much infiltrated drug as possible should be aspirated. Although no specific treatments are of proven value in preventing or reducing tissue damage, the local reaction may be minimized by promptly infiltrating the area with hydrocortisone sodium succinate injection (50–100 mg of hydrocortisone) and/or sodium bicarbonate (5 mL of 8.4% injection) and applying cold compresses. Extensive necrosis of the hand, without evidence of infiltration or cellulitis at the infusion site, occurred in one patient following infusion of conventional (nonencapsulated) daunorubicin distal to an arteriovenous fistula.

■ **Metabolic Effects** As a result of extensive purine catabolism accompanying rapid destruction of leukemic cells, hyperuricemia may occur in patients receiving daunorubicin; serum uric acid concentrations should be monitored, and appropriate therapy should be initiated as necessary. To minimize or prevent hyperuricemia, allopurinol typically is started prior to the initiation of antileukemic therapy.

■ **Other Adverse Effects** Transient fever and chills occur rarely after administration of daunorubicin, but the drug has been associated with one case of fulminant hyperpyrexia. Transient elevations in serum bilirubin, AST (SGOT), and alkaline phosphatase concentrations and hepatomegaly have occurred in patients receiving daunorubicin.

Dehydration, lymphadenopathy, abnormal gait, hemoptysis, pulmonary infiltration, increased sputum, conjunctivitis, ocular pain, loss of hearing, earache, tinnitus, dysuria, nocturia, and polyuria have been reported in 5% of patients or less receiving liposomal daunorubicin. Cough, dyspnea, rhinitis, sinusitis, flu-like symptoms, arthralgia, myalgia, and abnormal vision also have been reported in patients receiving liposomal daunorubicin.

■ **Precautions and Contraindications** The usual precautions and contraindications of daunorubicin apply to both the conventional and liposomally encapsulated formulations.

Daunorubicin is a highly toxic drug with a low therapeutic index, and a therapeutic response is not likely to occur without some evidence of toxicity. Conventional (nonencapsulated) daunorubicin should be administered only by clinicians experienced in using chemotherapeutic agents for leukemia in facilities with adequate laboratory and supportive resources for monitoring and treating drug toxicity. The clinician and staff must be prepared to rapidly respond to and comprehensively treat severe hemorrhagic conditions and/or overwhelming infections in patients receiving daunorubicin. Liposomal daunorubicin must be used only under constant supervision by clinicians experienced in therapy with cytotoxic agents.

Myelosuppression Daunorubicin therapy should not be initiated in patients with preexisting drug-induced bone marrow suppression unless the potential benefit from such treatment outweighs the risk.

The manufacturers state that appropriate measures must be taken to control systemic infections before beginning daunorubicin therapy; however, in some patients with acute leukemia, treatment of the underlying malignancy in addition to other therapy (e.g., anti-infective) may be necessary before systemic infections can be controlled.

One of the main dose-limiting toxicities of daunorubicin is myelosuppression. (See Cautions: Hematologic Effects.) Patients who receive myelosuppressive drugs experience an increased frequency of infections as well as hemorrhagic complications. Because these complications are potentially fatal, the patient should be instructed to notify the clinician if fever, sore throat, or unusual bleeding or bruising occurs.

The patient's hematologic status must be carefully monitored. Leukocyte, platelet, and erythrocyte counts should be determined prior to and at frequent intervals during daunorubicin therapy. Evaluation of bone marrow function is necessary to guide treatment, and sufficient time should elapse between courses of daunorubicin therapy to allow for bone marrow recovery. Treatment of severe hematologic toxicity may consist of supportive therapy, antibiotics for complicating infections, and blood product transfusions.

Cardiotoxicity Because of the increased risk of cardiotoxicity, daunorubicin should *not* be used in patients who have already received the recommended maximum cumulative dose of doxorubicin or daunorubicin. (See Drug Interactions: Cardiotoxic Drugs.)

Preexisting cardiac disease or previous therapy with doxorubicin or other anthracyclines increases the risk of daunorubicin-induced cardiotoxicity, and the risk-benefit ratio should be considered carefully before initiating daunorubicin therapy in patients with these risk factors.

Cardiotoxicity is a dose-limiting adverse effect associated with the use of daunorubicin. (See Cautions: Cardiac Effects.)

Previous therapy with anthracyclines (doxorubicin exceeding 300 mg/m^2 or equivalent) may predispose a patient to an increased risk of cardiotoxicity with liposomal daunorubicin and this must be carefully considered before beginning therapy with the drug. Infants and children are at greater risk of daunorubicin-induced cardiotoxicity. (See Pediatric Precautions.)

The manufacturer recommends that cardiac function be monitored carefully in patients receiving liposomal doxorubicin because of the risk of cardiac toxicity and congestive heart failure. Cardiac monitoring is necessary for all patients receiving liposomal daunorubicin and is particularly important in patients with preexisting cardiac disease, prior therapy with anthracyclines, or prior radiation therapy encompassing the heart.

Because cardiotoxicity may occur months to years following discontinuance of daunorubicin therapy, long-term periodic evaluation of cardiac function should be performed. There is no completely reliable method for predicting which patients will develop congestive heart failure with daunorubicin. Endomyocardial biopsy, ejection fractions determined from echocardiograms or first-pass radionuclide angiography, systolic time intervals derived from phonocardiograms, and ECGs have been used serially to monitor the cardiac effects of the drug and may help identify patients at greatest risk of developing congestive heart failure. However, in most patients, routine serial ECG determinations or noninvasive studies of left ventricular function are not of proven value to predict the development of congestive heart failure.

The manufacturers of conventional (nonencapsulated) doxorubicin recommend that an ECG and/or determination of ejection fraction be performed before each course of daunorubicin therapy; if a decrease of 30% or greater in limb lead QRS voltage in the ECG or a decrease in the systolic ejection fraction from pretreatment baseline occurs, the benefit of therapy must be weighed against the risk of cardiac damage. The manufacturer of liposomal daunorubicin recommends that cardiac function be evaluated (e.g., history of previous cardiac disease, physical examination) before each course of liposomal daunorubicin therapy; in addition, determination of left ventricular ejection fraction (LVEF) should be performed at a total cumulative dose of 320 mg/m^2 and at every 160-mg/m^2 increment thereafter. The manufacturer states that regular cardiac monitoring is advised, particularly in patients who have received prior anthracycline therapy, who have preexisting cardiac disease, or who have had prior radiation therapy encompassing the heart; because these patients may be at greater risk for cardiotoxicity associated with daunorubicin therapy, monitoring of LVEF should be performed before the initiation of therapy, at a total cumulative dose of 160 mg/m^2, and at every 160-mg/m^2 increment thereafter.

Hepatic and Renal Impairment Hepatic or renal impairment may enhance the toxicity of usual doses of daunorubicin. The patient's hepatic and renal function should be evaluated prior to administration of daunorubicin, and the dosage of the drug should be reduced in patients with hepatic or renal impairment. (See Dosage in Renal and Hepatic Impairment in Dosage and Administration.)

Other Precautions and Contraindications To minimize or prevent hyperuricemia, allopurinol typically is started prior to the initiation of antileukemic therapy and serum uric acid concentrations should be monitored.

Conventional (nonencapsulated) daunorubicin may transiently impart a red color to the urine, and patients should be advised to expect this during therapy.

Use of conventional (nonencapsulated) daunorubicin is contraindicated in patients with known hypersensitivity to the drug.

Interruption of therapy and slowing of the infusion rate may be required in patients experiencing adverse infusion-related effects during liposomal daunorubicin therapy. (See Cautions: Infusion-related Effects.)

In addition to the usual precautions and contraindications associated with daunorubicin therapy, use of liposomal daunorubicin citrate is contraindicated in patients who are hypersensitive to daunorubicin or to any component in the liposomal formulation.

The pharmacokinetic properties, formulation, and dosage of daunorubicin as a single entity preparation differ from those of the fixed liposomal combination of daunorubicin and cytarabine (Vyxeos®); these preparations are *not* interchangeable.

■ **Pediatric Precautions** Safety and efficacy of conventional (nonencapsulated) daunorubicin in children have not been specifically studied to date. The risk of cardiotoxicity should be weighed carefully before initiating daunorubicin therapy, particularly in infants and children. The manufacturers report that cardiotoxicity may occur more frequently and at lower cumulative doses of daunorubicin in children than in adults. (See Cautions: Cardiac Effects.)

Safety and efficacy of liposomal daunorubicin in children have not been established.

■ **Geriatric Precautions** The manufacturer states that safety and efficacy of liposomal daunorubicin citrate in geriatric patients have not been established.

Safety and efficacy of conventional (nonencapsulated) daunorubicin in geriatric patients have not been specifically studied to date. The manufacturers report that cardiotoxicity may occur more frequently in geriatric patients than in younger patients receiving daunorubicin. Daunorubicin should be administered with caution in patients who have inadequate bone marrow reserves because of old age. In addition, because geriatric patients may have decreased renal function, reduction of daunorubicin dosage may be necessary.

■ **Mutagenicity and Carcinogenicity** Daunorubicin is potentially mutagenic and carcinogenic. Conventional (nonencapsulated) daunorubicin was mutagenic when tested in vitro with the Ames test and V79 hamster cell assay. In addition, conventional (nonencapsulated) daunorubicin was clastogenic in vitro in human lymphoblasts (CCRF-CEM) and in vivo mouse bone marrow (SCE) tests.

Secondary leukemias have been reported in patients receiving topoisomerase II inhibitors in combination with other antineoplastic agents or radiation therapy. In male rats receiving conventional (nonencapsulated) daunorubicin 3 times weekly for 6 months at 1/70th the recommended human dose based on body surface area, peritoneal sarcomas were found at 18 months. A high incidence of mammary tumors was seen in female rats 120 days after receiving a single 12.5-mg/kg IV dose (about twice the daily recommended human dose on a mg/m^2 basis) of conventional (nonencapsulated) daunorubicin. Mammary adenocarcinomas appeared at 1 year in rats receiving a single IV dose of conventional (nonencapsulated) daunorubicin (at about 1.6 times the recommended human dose based on body surface area). Fibrosarcomas have developed at the injection site following subcutaneous injection of the conventional (nonencapsulated) form of the drug in mice. When conventional (nonencapsulated) daunorubicin was administered intraperitoneally 3 times weekly in mice, no carcinogenic effect was observed after 18 months.

Studies to determine the mutagenic and carcinogenic potential of liposomal daunorubicin have not been performed to date.

■ **Pregnancy, Fertility, and Lactation** Conventional (nonencapsulated) daunorubicin can cause fetal toxicity when administered to pregnant women, but potential benefits from use of the drug may be acceptable in certain conditions despite possible risks to the fetus. An increased incidence of fetal abnormalities (parieto-occipital cranioschisis, umbilical hernias, or rachischisis) and abortions was observed in rabbits receiving conventional (nonencapsulated) daunorubicin at doses of 0.05 mg/kg daily (approximately 1/100th of the highest recommended human dose based on body surface area). An increased incidence of esophageal, cardiovascular, and urogenital abnormalities as well as rib fusions were observed in rats receiving conventional (nonencapsulated) daunorubicin at doses of 4 mg/kg daily (approximately one-half the human dose based on body surface area). Decreased fetal birthweight and post-delivery growth rate were observed following administration of the drug to mice.

Encapsulated daunorubicin citrate in liposomes also can cause fetal toxicity when administered to pregnant women. Reproduction studies in rats given liposomal daunorubicin dosages of 2 mg/kg daily (approximately ⅓ of the recommended human dosage on a mg/m² basis) revealed evidence of severe maternal toxicity and embryolethality, while dosages of 0.3 mg/kg daily (approximately 120th of the recommended human dosage on a mg/m² basis) were associated with embryotoxicity (e.g., increased embryofetal deaths, reduction in the number of offspring per litter, decreased litter sizes) and fetal malformations (characterized by anophthalmia, microphthalmia, and incomplete ossification).

There are no adequate and well-controlled studies using conventional or liposomal daunorubicin in pregnant women. Conventional or liposomal daunorubicin should be used during pregnancy only in life-threatening situations or severe disease for which safer drugs cannot be used or are ineffective. If the drug is administered during pregnancy or if the patient becomes pregnant while receiving the drug, the patient should be informed of the potential hazard to the fetus. Women of childbearing potential should be advised to avoid becoming pregnant while receiving the drug.

Following IV administration of daunorubicin in male dogs at a dosage of 0.25 mg/kg daily (about 8 times the human dose on a mg/m² basis), testicular atrophy and total aplasia of the spermatocyte series in the seminiferous tubules with complete aspermatogenesis were observed. The effects of liposomal daunorubicin on fertility have not been adequately studied.

It is not known whether daunorubicin is distributed into milk. Because of the potential for serious adverse reactions to daunorubicin in nursing infants, nursing should be discontinued during daunorubicin therapy.

Drug Interactions

Liposomal daunorubicin citrate has been studied mainly in patients with Kaposi's sarcoma; such patients usually receive a variety of concomitant drugs (e.g., antiretroviral agents, antiviral agents, anti-infective agents). Although interactions of daunorubicin citrate liposomal injection with other drugs have not been reported, no formal drug interaction studies employing liposomal daunorubicin citrate have been performed to date.

■ Cardiotoxic Drugs The risk of cardiotoxicity is increased if daunorubicin is used in a patient who has received previous therapy with doxorubicin. Daunorubicin therapy should *not* be used in patients who have received the recommended maximum cumulative dose of doxorubicin or daunorubicin. Because potentiation of cardiotoxic effects may result, caution is advised when daunorubicin is used concurrently with other cardiotoxic drugs, such as cyclophosphamide.

■ Myelosuppressive Drugs Because potentiation of hematologic toxicity may result, caution is advised when daunorubicin is used concurrently with other myelosuppressive agents; reduction of daunorubicin dosage may be required.

■ Hepatotoxic Drugs Concurrent use of hepatotoxic therapy, such as high-dose methotrexate, may cause hepatic impairment and interfere with the metabolism of daunorubicin, resulting in increased risk of toxicity.

Pharmacology

Daunorubicin is an antineoplastic antibiotic. Daunorubicin has antimitotic and cytotoxic activity. Daunorubicin forms a complex with DNA by intercalation between base pairs. By stabilizing the complex between DNA and topoisomerase II, daunorubicin inhibits the activity of this enzyme, resulting in single-strand and double-strand breaks in DNA. Daunorubicin also may inhibit polymerase activity, affect regulation of gene expression, and be involved in free radical damage to DNA. Although daunorubicin is maximally cytotoxic in the S phase, the drug is not cycle-phase specific. Daunorubicin also has antibacterial and immunosuppressive properties.

Pharmacokinetics

Encapsulation of daunorubicin citrate in liposomes substantially alters the pharmacokinetics of the drug relative to conventional IV formulations (i.e., nonencapsulated drug) with resultant decreased distribution into the peripheral compartment, increased distribution into Kaposi's lesions, and decreased plasma clearance. The pharmacokinetics of the drug encapsulated in liposomes have not been evaluated separately by gender, ethnic group, or hepatic or renal impairment. In the Pharmacokinetics section, liposomal daunorubicin citrate was administered as the drug encapsulated in liposomes composed of a phospholipid bilayer of distearoylphosphatidylcholine (DSPC) and cholesterol.

■ Absorption Daunorubicin hydrochloride is extremely irritating to tissues and, therefore, must be administered IV. Following IV infusion of a single 40-mg/m² dose of liposomal daunorubicin citrate as a liposomal injection in patients with AIDS-related Kaposi's sarcoma, mean peak plasma daunorubicin (mostly bound to liposomes) concentrations are approximately 18 mcg/mL following a 30–60 minute infusion. Peak plasma concentrations of daunorubicin are higher following IV administration of liposomal daunorubicin citrate than those attained following IV administration of conventional (nonencapsulated) daunorubicin hydrochloride. In one study in patients with disseminated malignancies receiving a single 80-mg/m² IV dose of nonencapsulated daunorubicin, peak plasma concentrations of the drug were 0.4 mcg/mL while in patients with solid tumors (including those with Kaposi's sarcoma) who received a single 80-mg/m² IV dose of liposomal daunorubicin, peak plasma concentrations of daunorubicin were about 44 mcg/mL (about 100-fold greater than those receiving a comparable dose of the nonencapsulated drug); area under the plasma concentration-time curve (AUC) was about 36-fold greater than that observed with conventional daunorubicin hydrochloride. Following IV administration of liposomal daunorubicin, peak plasma concentrations and AUCs of daunorubicin generally increase linearly with increasing doses (at doses of 10–80 mcg/mL).

■ Distribution Daunorubicin administered as a conventional (nonencapsulated) injection is rapidly and widely distributed in tissues, with highest levels in the spleen, kidneys, liver, lungs, and heart. The drug is absorbed by cells and binds to cellular components, particularly nucleic acids. The volume of distribution of daunorubicin hydrochloride administered IV as a conventional (nonencapsulated) injection is about 1006–1055 L. Noncapsulated daunorubicin is approximately 63% bound to serum proteins, principally albumin; the protein binding of liposomally encapsulated drug is minimal.

Encapsulation of daunorubicin in liposomes substantially slows the rate of distribution of the drug into the extravascular space. As a result, the liposomally encapsulated daunorubicin citrate does not distribute into plasma and tissues as widely as daunorubicin hydrochloride administered as the conventional injection; liposomal daunorubicin distributes mainly into intravascular fluid, whereas nonencapsulated daunorubicin distributes widely into extravascular fluids and tissues. Animal studies indicate that liposomally encapsulated daunorubicin citrate distributes from blood vessels into tumors, and once distributed into the tissue compartment, the drug is released. The exact mechanism of drug release from liposomal encapsulation is not known; however, it has been suggested that liposomes penetrate the tumor cells by endocytosis where the entrapped daunorubicin gradually is released directly within cells to exert its antineoplastic effects. Because of the gradual release and higher intracellular concentrations of liposomal daunorubicin when compared with the nonencapsulated drug, liposomally encapsulated daunorubicin is more cytotoxic over time than the conventional (nonencapsulated) drug. The volume of distribution of daunorubicin following IV administration of a single 40-mg/m² dose of the drug as a liposomal injection in patients with AIDS-related Kaposi's sarcoma is about 6.4 L.

Daunorubicin citrate administered IV as an injection encapsulated in liposomes distributes into Kaposi's sarcoma lesions to a greater extent than into healthy skin. Following IV administration of a single 20- or 40-mg/m² dose of daunorubicin citrate as liposomal injections in patients with Kaposi's sarcoma, distribution of daunorubicin into Kaposi's sarcoma lesions was about 4- to 12-fold higher than that observed in healthy skin; 24 hours after such administration, daunorubicin concentrations in Kaposi's sarcoma lesions were 1.07 or 1.06 mcg/g, respectively, while daunorubicin was not detected in healthy skin. In addition, animal studies indicate that accumulation of daunorubicin in solid tumors following IV administration of the liposomally encapsulated drug was tenfold greater than that following IV administration of comparable doses of a conventional (nonencapsulated) injection.

There is no evidence that daunorubicin administered as a conventional injection crosses the blood-brain barrier.

Although preclinical data suggest that liposomal daunorubicin crosses the blood-brain barrier in animals, it is not known whether liposomal daunorubicin crosses the blood-brain barrier in humans. It appears that daunorubicin crosses the placenta. It is not known if daunorubicin is distributed into milk.

■ Elimination Following rapid IV administration of conventional daunorubicin hydrochloride injection, total plasma concentrations of daunorubicin and its metabolites decline in a triphasic manner, and plasma concentrations of unchanged daunorubicin decline in a biphasic manner. The plasma half-life of nonencapsulated daunorubicin averages 45 minutes in the initial phase and 18.5 hours in the terminal phase. By 1 hour after administration of nonencapsulated daunorubicin, the predominant form of the drug in plasma is the active metabolite daunorubicinol, which has an average terminal plasma half-life of 26.7 hours.

Plasma concentrations of liposomally encapsulated daunorubicin citrate appear to decline principally in a monoexponential fashion, although biexponential elimination from plasma has been described occasionally in some patients. In a few patients receiving 60-mg/m² IV doses of daunorubicin liposomal injection, evidence of saturable clearance mechanisms has been reported. Following IV administration of a single 40-mg/m² dose as liposomal daunorubicin injection in patients with AIDS-related Kaposi's sarcoma, the apparent elimination half-life of daunorubicin averaged 4.4 hours, which is shorter than that of conventional daunorubicin and probably represents a distribution half-life.

Daunorubicin hydrochloride is extensively metabolized in the liver and other tissues, mainly by cytoplasmic aldo-keto reductases, producing daunorubicinol, the major metabolite which has antineoplastic activity. Approximately 40% of the drug in the plasma is present as daunorubicinol within 30 minutes and 60% in 4 hours after a dose of nonencapsulated daunorubicin. Daunorubicinol has been detected only in low concentrations in the plasma following IV administration of daunorubicin citrate liposomal injection. In patients with AIDS-associated Kaposi's sarcoma receiving IV administration of liposomal daunorubicin doses of 40 mg/m², the AUC of daunorubicinol represented only 2% of the total daunorubicin AUC. Additional metabolism by reductive cleavage of the glycosidic bond produces aglycones, which have little or no cytotoxic activity and are demethylated and conjugated with sulfate and glucuronide by microsomal enzymes.

Daunorubicin and its metabolites are excreted in urine and bile. Following administration of nonencapsulated daunorubicin, urinary excretion of the drug and its metabolites is reported to be 14–23% of the dose, with most urinary excretion of the drug occurring within 3 days. After the first 24 hours, the drug is excreted in urine mainly as daunorubicinol. An estimated 40% of a dose is eliminated by biliary excretion. In one study in patients with disseminated solid malignancies who received a single 80-mg/m² IV dose of nonencapsulated daunorubicin, plasma clearance of the drug was about 236 mL/minute. Plasma clearance of daunorubicin encapsulated in liposomes appears to be substantially slower. In adults with AIDS-related Kaposi's sarcoma, plasma clearance of liposomal daunorubicin following administration of a single 40-mg/m² IV dose averaged 17.3 mL/minute. This reduction in plasma clearance with the liposomal injection results in a substantial increase in the AUC compared with that of nonencapsulated drug.

Chemistry and Stability

■ **Chemistry** Daunorubicin is an anthracycline glycoside antibiotic produced by *Streptomyces coeruleorubidus.* The drug is structurally related to doxorubicin and epirubicin. Daunorubicin differs structurally from doxorubicin in that daunorubicin contains an acetyl group instead of a hydroxyacetyl group in the 8-position.

As a conventional injection, daunorubicin is commercially available as the hydrochloride salt which occurs as a hygroscopic, reddish, lyophilized crystalline powder; the commercially available product also contains mannitol. Daunorubicin hydrochloride is soluble in water, slightly soluble in alcohol, and has a pK_a of 10.3. Following reconstitution of the commercially available powder for injection with sterile water for injection as directed, daunorubicin hydrochloride solutions have a pH of 4.5–6.5.

A conventional injection also is commercially available as a deep red sterile solution with a pH of 3–4.

As an injection, daunorubicin also is available in a liposomal formulation. In the liposomal injection, an aqueous solution of the citrate salt of daunorubicin is encapsulated in lipid vesicles (liposomes). Liposomes are spherical, microscopic vesicles composed of a phospholipid bilayer that is capable of encapsulating the drug. These liposomes contain distearoylphosphatidylcholine (DSPC) and cholesterol in the phospholipid bilayer in a 2:1 molar ratio and have a mean diameter of 45 nm (range: 35–65 nm). The total lipid-to-daunorubicin base weight ratio is 18.7:1 equivalent to a 10:5:1 molar composition of DSPC:cholesterol:daunorubicin.

The physicochemical properties of liposomes (e.g., size, fluidity of the membrane, surface charge) depend on the lipid composition and method of preparation of the liposomes. The selection of appropriate lipid components and ratios ensures the formation of stable vesicles that retain the pharmacologically active drug in the presence of serum at body temperature and also controls the length of time these vesicles remain intact in systemic circulation. It has been suggested that liposomes can penetrate the altered and often compromised vasculature of tumors because of their small size (usually less than 100 nm in diameter; preferably 30–80 nm) and persistence in blood circulation. The ability to achieve sustained high plasma concentrations of the drug encapsulated in liposomes is related to the stability of such liposomes; the addition of cholesterol strengthens the bilayers of the liposomes, particularly in the presence of serum by controlling loss of DSPC to high-density lipoproteins. Animal studies indicate that the net neutral surface charge also may contribute to the stability of the liposomes in vivo; the leakage of daunorubicin from the liposomes appears to be less than 1% over 24 hours.

Daunorubicin citrate liposomal injection is a sterile, pyrogen-free, translucent red liposomal dispersion and has a pH of 4.9–6. Daunorubicin citrate liposomal injection also contains sucrose for isotonicity, glycine as a stabilizing agent, and calcium chloride dihydrate.

■ **Stability** Daunorubicin hydrochloride powder for injection should be stored at 15–30°C, protected from light, and stored in the carton until time of use.

Following reconstitution as directed, daunorubicin hydrochloride solutions are stable for 24 hours at room temperature or 48 hours when refrigerated at 2–8°C. The reconstituted solution should be protected from sunlight. Daunorubicin hydrochloride is unstable in solutions with a pH greater than 8; decomposition is indicated by a color change from red to blue-purple. A precipitate may form immediately if daunorubicin hydrochloride solution is mixed with heparin sodium injection or dexamethasone sodium phosphate injection. The manufacturer states that daunorubicin hydrochloride injection should not be mixed with other drugs or heparin.

Commercially available daunorubicin hydrochloride injection should be protected from light in the carton until time of use and refrigerated at 2–8°C. Following further dilution in 0.9% sodium chloride injection, resultant solutions are stable for 24 hours at room temperatures of 15–30°C; these solutions contain no preservatives, and unused portions should be discarded after this period.

Commercially available daunorubicin citrate liposomal injection should be refrigerated at 2–8°C and protected from light and freezing; the shelf-life of the injection is 24 weeks when stored as recommended. When diluted as directed with dextrose 5% injection, solutions of daunorubicin citrate liposomal injection are stable for up to 6 hours when refrigerated at 2–8°C.

For further information on the handling of antineoplastic agents, see the ASHP Guidelines on Handling Hazardous Drugs at http://www.ahfsdruginformation.com.

Preparations

Excipients in commercially available drug preparations may have clinically important effects in some individuals; consult specific product labeling for details.

DAUNOrubicin Citrate Liposomal

Parenteral		
Injection, for IV infusion	2 mg (of daunorubicin) per mL (50 mg)	**DaunoXome®**, Gilead

DAUNOrubicin Hydrochloride

Parenteral		
For injection	20 mg (of daunorubicin)	**Cerubidine®**, Bedford
Injection	5 mg (of daunorubicin) per mL*	**DAUNOrubicin Hydrochloride Injection**

*available from one or more manufacturer, distributor, and/or repackager by generic (nonproprietary) name

†Use is not currently included in the labeling approved by the US Food and Drug Administration

Selected Revisions October 2018, © Copyright, May 1981, American Society of Health-System Pharmacists, Inc.

DAUNOrubicin and Cytarabine

DAUNOrubicin/cytarabine Liposomal1-β-Arabinofuranosylcytosine, Arabinosylcytosine, Cytosine Arabinoside, Ara-C

■ The fixed liposomal combination of daunorubicin and cytarabine (daunorubicin/cytarabine liposomal) contains 2 antineoplastic agents coencapsulated in liposomes; daunorubicin is an anthracycline and cytarabine is an antimetabolite.

Uses

■ **Acute Myeloid Leukemia** The fixed liposomal combination of daunorubicin and cytarabine (daunorubicin/cytarabine liposomal; Vyxeos®) is used for the treatment of newly diagnosed therapy-related acute myeloid leukemia (t-AML; secondary AML) or AML with myelodysplasia-related changes (AML-MRC). Daunorubicin/cytarabine liposomal has been designated an orphan drug by FDA for the treatment of this cancer. Evidence supporting the use of daunorubicin/cytarabine liposomal is based principally on a study performed in a subset of patients with high-risk AML (i.e., patients older than 60 years of age with t-AML or AML-MRC). In these patients, daunorubicin/cytarabine liposomal induction therapy followed by use as consolidation therapy substantially prolonged survival compared with a standard combination of the 2 drugs.

AML is generally regarded as a disease of the elderly with a median age at diagnosis of 67 years; however, patients older than 60 years of age usually have a poor prognosis due to unfavorable cytogenetics or poor compliance due to treatment-related adverse effects. The specific type of AML can also affect prognosis; t-AML and AML-MRC are subtypes that are less likely to respond to standard induction therapy with cytarabine and an anthracycline. Several strategies (e.g., modified treatment intensity or duration of treatment, new formulations of standard drugs) have been employed to improve overall efficacy and tolerability of combination chemotherapy.

Combination chemotherapy is widely used in an effort to delay the emergence of resistance to antineoplastic agents and to obtain an additive or synergistic therapeutic effect with minimum toxicity; however, in vitro data indicate that the synergistic, additive, or antagonistic interaction of a drug combination is dependent on the ratio of the individual drugs in cancer cells. In vivo, maintenance of an optimal drug ratio is precluded by independent and dissimilar pharmacokinetics of individual drugs administered as conventional aqueous-based drug combinations. The rationale for use of a liposomal delivery system is to control the release of drug combinations such that fixed synergistic drug ratios established in vitro are maintained in vivo following drug administration; this strategy, known as "ratiometric dosing," has been employed to optimize therapeutic efficacy of antineoplastic drug combinations including the combination of daunorubicin and cytarabine. (See Description.)

The current indication for daunorubicin/cytarabine liposomal is based principally on the results of a randomized, multicenter, open-label phase 3 trial in patients 60–75 years of age with newly diagnosed t-AML or AML-MRC. A total of 309 patients were randomized in a 1:1 ratio to receive induction and consolidation therapy with either daunorubicin/cytarabine liposomal or a standard combination of daunorubicin and cytarabine administered as single-entity preparations (standard combination therapy). Daunorubicin (44 mg/m²) in fixed combination with cytarabine (100 mg/m²) encapsulated in liposomes was administered by IV infusion on days 1, 3, and 5 during the first induction cycle and, if necessary, on days 1 and 3 during the second induction cycle. During consolidation therapy, daunorubicin (29 mg/m²) in fixed combination with cytarabine (65 mg/m²) encapsulated in liposomes was administered by IV infusion on days 1 and 3 for up to 2 cycles. Induction therapy with standard combination therapy consisted of daunorubicin 60 mg/m² daily by IV infusion on days 1–3 and cytarabine 100 mg/m² daily by continuous IV infusion on days 1–7 of the first induction cycle; if necessary, a second induction cycle consisting of daunorubicin 60 mg/m² daily by IV infusion on days 1–2 and cytarabine 100 mg/m² daily by continuous IV infusion on days 1–5 was administered. Consolidation therapy with standard combination therapy consisted of daunorubicin 60 mg/m² daily by IV infusion on days 1–2 and cytarabine 100 mg/m² daily by continuous IV infusion on days 1–5 for up to 2 cycles. In all patients, a second cycle of induction therapy was administered if a reduction in leukemic blast cells exceeding 50% was achieved and was strongly recommended if complete remission was not achieved. Stem cell transplantation was permitted as consolidation therapy or post-consolidation therapy. The primary measure of efficacy was overall survival. In this trial, 100 or 97% of patients in the daunorubicin/cytarabine liposomal or standard combination therapy groups, respectively, received at least one cycle of induction therapy, and 32 or 21% of patients in the respective treatment groups received at least one cycle of consolidation therapy. Following initial complete remission, induction failure, or salvage therapy after relapse, 34% of daunorubicin/cytarabine liposomal-treated patients and 25% of those who received standard combination therapy underwent stem cell transplantation.

The median age of patients enrolled in the study was 68 years (range: 60–75 years); 61% were male, 88% had an Eastern Cooperative Oncology Group (ECOG) performance status of 0 or 1, 54% had AML with an antecedent hematologic disorder, 25% had de novo AML with myelodysplasia-related cytogenetic abnormalities, and 20% had t-AML. Approximately one-third of patients previously received a hypomethylating agent for myelodysplastic syndrome (MDS). Fms-like tyrosine kinase-3 (Flt-3) mutation was present in 43 of 279 patients (15%) evaluated for this mutation. In addition, nucleophosmin 1 (NPM1) mutation was present in 25 of 283 patients (9%) evaluated for this mutation. Baseline characteristics were generally balanced between treatment groups.

At the time of analysis, patients receiving daunorubicin/cytarabine liposomal had a longer median overall survival (9.6 versus 5.9 months; hazard ratio: 0.69) than those receiving standard combination therapy. In addition, patients receiving the fixed-combination liposomal preparation had higher complete remission rates compared with those receiving the standard combination regimen (38 versus 26%).

Dosage and Administration

■ **General** The commercially available fixed liposomal combination of daunorubicin and cytarabine (daunorubicin/cytarabine liposomal; Vyxeos®) is *not* interchangeable with other daunorubicin- and/or cytarabine-containing preparations. To avoid dosing errors, clinicians should confirm the drug name, formulation, and dose prior to preparation and administration. (See Lack of Interchangeability with Other Daunorubicin and Cytarabine Preparations under Warnings/Precautions: Warnings, in Cautions.)

Cardiac, hepatic, and renal function should be assessed prior to initiation of induction therapy and prior to each cycle of consolidation therapy. In addition, complete blood cell counts (CBCs) should be monitored prior to each cycle of consolidation therapy. The manufacturer states that consolidation therapy should not be administered until neutrophil counts exceed 500/mm³ and platelet counts exceed 50,000/mm³.

Because daunorubicin/cytarabine liposomal contains the anthracycline daunorubicin, the lifetime cumulative anthracycline exposure should be calculated prior to each cycle; the fixed-combination preparation should not be used in patients who have reached the maximum cumulative limit. (See Cardiac Effects under Warnings/Precautions: Other Warnings and Precautions, in Cautions.)

Because nausea occurs frequently in patients receiving daunorubicin/cytarabine liposomal, premedication with an antiemetic agent should be administered prior to therapy.

■ **Reconstitution and Administration** Procedures for proper handling and disposal of antineoplastic drugs should be followed when preparing or administering daunorubicin/cytarabine liposomal.

Daunorubicin/cytarabine liposomal is administered *only* by IV infusion over 90 minutes through a central venous line (e.g., central venous catheter or peripherally inserted central catheter [PICC]) using an infusion pump. Because the daunorubicin component may cause severe tissue necrosis if extravasation occurs, the fixed-combination preparation must *not* be given by IM or subcutaneous injection. (See Local Effects under Warnings/Precautions: Other Warnings and Precautions, in Cautions.) The manufacturer states that an inline filter should *not* be used. The infusion line should be flushed with 0.9% sodium chloride injection or 5% dextrose injection after the drug is administered.

Unopened vials of daunorubicin/cytarabine liposomal powder for injection should be stored upright at 2–8°C in the original package for protection from light. Prior to administration, the lyophilized powder must be reconstituted and diluted using proper aseptic technique. The number of vials needed should be determined based on the indicated dose of the daunorubicin component. The vials should be removed from the refrigerator and allowed to come to room temperature for 30 minutes prior to reconstitution. The lyophilized powder is reconstituted by adding 19 mL of sterile water for injection to a vial labeled as containing 44 mg of daunorubicin and 100 mg of cytarabine to provide a colloidal dispersion containing 2.2 mg of daunorubicin and 5 mg of cytarabine per mL. Using a timer, each vial should be swirled for 5 minutes, including gentle inversion every 30 seconds. The resulting dispersion should not be heated, vortexed, or shaken vigorously. The vials should be allowed to rest for 15 minutes and then gently inverted an additional 5 times prior to dilution. The reconstituted daunorubicin/cytarabine liposomal colloidal dispersion should be opaque, purple, homogeneous, and free of visible particulates. Following reconstitution, the drug may be diluted immediately for preparation of the final infusion solution or stored at 2–8°C for up to 4 hours.

To prepare the final diluted daunorubicin/cytarabine liposomal solution for infusion, the required amount of reconstituted drug should be withdrawn from the vials and transferred to an infusion bag containing 500 mL of 0.9% sodium chloride injection or 5% dextrose injection. The diluted solution should be mixed by gentle inversion. The final diluted daunorubicin/cytarabine liposomal solution should be a translucent, deep purple, homogeneous dispersion that is free of visible particulates. The solution may be infused immediately or stored at 2–8°C for up to 4 hours.

Daunorubicin/cytarabine liposomal solutions should be inspected visually for particulate matter and discoloration prior to administration whenever solution and container permit; the solution should *not* be used if particulate matter is present.

Daunorubicin/cytarabine liposomal should not be admixed with or infused simultaneously with any other drug. Any unused portions in the vials or infusion bag should be discarded since the daunorubicin/cytarabine liposomal product contains no preservative.

■ **Dosage** Daunorubicin/cytarabine liposomal is a fixed-combination preparation containing a 1:5 molar ratio of daunorubicin to cytarabine coencapsulated in liposomes. Each single-dose vial of daunorubicin/cytarabine liposomal contains 44 mg of daunorubicin and 100 mg of cytarabine coencapsulated in liposomes. Dosage of the fixed-combination preparation should be calculated based on the daunorubicin component.

Acute Myeloid Leukemia A complete course of daunorubicin/cytarabine liposomal therapy consists of 1–2 cycles of induction therapy and 1–2 cycles of consolidation therapy.

The recommended adult dosage of daunorubicin/cytarabine liposomal as induction therapy for newly diagnosed therapy-related acute myeloid leukemia (t-AML) or AML with myelodysplasia-related changes (AML-MRC) is daunorubicin 44 mg/m² and cytarabine 100 mg/m² on days 1, 3, and 5; if complete remission is not achieved following the first induction cycle and the fixed drug combination is well tolerated, a second induction cycle may be administered 2–5 weeks after the first induction cycle on days 1 and 3 at the same dosage.

Consolidation therapy should be administered 5–8 weeks after the start of the last induction cycle. (See Dosage and Administration: General.) The recommended adult dosage of daunorubicin/cytarabine liposomal as consolidation therapy is daunorubicin 29 mg/m² and cytarabine 65 mg/m² on days 1 and 3; a second consolidation cycle should be administered 5–8 weeks following initiation of the first consolidation cycle in the absence of disease progression or unacceptable toxicity.

If a dose of daunorubicin/cytarabine liposomal is missed, the dose should be administered as soon as possible. The schedule of administration should be adjusted to maintain the treatment interval between cycles.

Dosage Modification for Toxicity **Hypersensitivity Reactions.** If mild hypersensitivity reactions occur, the daunorubicin/cytarabine liposomal infusion should be interrupted immediately and supportive treatment should be initiated; upon resolution of symptoms, the infusion may be resumed but the rate of infusion should be reduced by 50%. Premedication with an antihistamine and/or corticosteroid should be considered prior to subsequent infusions. (See Hypersensitivity Reactions under Warnings/Precautions: Sensitivity Reactions, in Cautions.)

If moderate hypersensitivity reactions occur, the daunorubicin/cytarabine liposomal infusion should be interrupted immediately and supportive treatment should be initiated; the infusion should *not* be resumed upon resolution of symptoms. Subsequent infusions of daunorubicin/cytarabine liposomal may be administered at the same rate following administration of a premedication regimen (i.e., antihistamine and/or corticosteroid).

If severe or life-threatening hypersensitivity reactions occur, daunorubicin/cytarabine liposomal therapy should be permanently discontinued. Supportive treatment should be initiated and the patient should be monitored until symptoms resolve.

■ **Special Populations** No adjustment of daunorubicin/cytarabine liposomal dosage is necessary in patients with serum bilirubin concentrations of 3 mg/dL or less. (See Hepatic Impairment under Warnings/Precautions: Specific Populations, in Cautions.)

No adjustment of daunorubicin/cytarabine liposomal dosage is necessary in patients with mild or moderate renal impairment (creatinine clearance of 30–89 mL/minute). (See Renal Impairment under Warnings/Precautions: Specific Populations, in Cautions.)

The manufacturer makes no specific dosage recommendations for geriatric patients. (See Geriatric Use under Warnings/Precautions: Specific Populations, in Cautions.)

Cautions

■ **Contraindications** History of serious hypersensitivity reactions to cytarabine, daunorubicin, or any component of the formulation.

■ **Warnings/Precautions** ***Warnings*** **Lack of Interchangeability with Other Daunorubicin and Cytarabine Preparations.** The fixed liposomal combination of daunorubicin and cytarabine (daunorubicin/cytarabine liposomal) is *not* interchangeable with other daunorubicin- and/or cytarabine-containing preparations (e.g., daunorubicin hydrochloride injection, daunorubicin citrate liposomal injection, cytarabine injection, cytarabine liposomal injection). The pharmacokinetic properties of the fixed-combination liposomal preparation differ from those of the single-entity preparations of each drug (including their liposomal and nonliposomal forms), and dosage for each product is specific to the formulation. Clinicians should confirm the correct drug, formulation, and dosage prior to preparation and administration of daunorubicin/cytarabine liposomal.

Sensitivity Reactions **Hypersensitivity Reactions.** Serious or fatal hypersensitivity reactions, including anaphylactic reactions, have been reported in patients receiving daunorubicin and cytarabine as single agents.

Patients should be monitored for manifestations of hypersensitivity reactions. If a hypersensitivity reaction occurs, appropriate treatment and supportive care should be initiated. Reduction in infusion rate, temporary interruption, or discontinuance of therapy may be required depending on the severity of the reaction. (See Hypersensitivity Reactions under Dosage: Dosage Modification for Toxicity, in Dosage and Administration.) If a severe or life-threatening hypersensitivity reaction occurs, daunorubicin/cytarabine liposomal should be permanently discontinued.

Other Warnings and Precautions **Hemorrhage.** Serious or fatal hemorrhage associated with prolonged severe thrombocytopenia has been reported in patients receiving daunorubicin/cytarabine liposomal. In the principal efficacy trial in patients with therapy-related acute myeloid leukemia (t-AML) or AML with myelodysplasia-related changes (AML-MRC), hemorrhage occurred in 74% of patients receiving daunorubicin/cytarabine liposomal compared with 56% of those receiving a standard combination of daunorubicin and cytarabine. Grade 3 or greater hemorrhage was reported in 12% of patients receiving daunorubicin/cytarabine liposomal compared with 8% of those receiving standard combination therapy. Fatal CNS hemorrhage in the absence of disease progression occurred in 2% of patients receiving daunorubicin/cytarabine liposomal compared with 0.7% of those receiving standard combination therapy. The most common hemorrhagic event reported in the trial was epistaxis.

If hemorrhage occurs, complete blood cell counts (CBCs) should be monitored until resolution and platelet transfusions should be administered if necessary.

Cardiac Effects. The daunorubicin component of daunorubicin/cytarabine liposomal is an anthracycline, and cardiotoxicity is a known risk of anthracycline therapy. Among patients receiving daunorubicin/cytarabine liposomal in the principal efficacy study, cardiotoxicity, including acute coronary syndrome, acute myocardial infarction, decreased left ventricular ejection fraction (LVEF), congestive heart failure, cardiac failure or arrest, cardiomyopathy, endocarditis, pericarditis, and valvular abnormalities, was reported in 20% of patients, which was comparable to the incidence of cardiotoxicity in patients receiving a standard combination of daunorubicin and cytarabine. Arrhythmias occurred in 30% of patients receiving the fixed-combination preparation. The cumulative dosage of daunorubicin/cytarabine liposomal administered in the study ranged from 44–337 mg/m^2 (of daunorubicin). Patients with baseline LVEF less than 50% and a lifetime cumulative exposure of 368 mg/m^2 or more of daunorubicin (or equivalent) were not included in the study.

Factors that may increase the risk of daunorubicin-induced cardiotoxicity include previous therapy with other anthracycline agents, preexisting heart disease, previous radiation therapy to the mediastinal region, or concomitant use of other cardiotoxic drugs. With conventional daunorubicin, the incidence of heart failure increases with cumulative dosages exceeding 550 mg/m^2 (or 400 mg/m^2 in patients who have received radiation therapy to the mediastinal region). The lifetime cumulative anthracycline exposure should be calculated prior to each cycle of daunorubicin/cytarabine liposomal; the total cumulative dosage should include any previous or concomitant therapy with other anthracycline agents, such as doxorubicin, or related compounds. Daunorubicin/cytarabine liposomal should not be used in patients who have reached the maximum cumulative limit.

Cardiac function should be evaluated prior to initiating daunorubicin/cytarabine liposomal therapy; the assessment should include an ECG and baseline determination of LVEF with an echocardiogram or multigated radionuclide angiography (MUGA). Patients with baseline LVEF below the lower limit of normal should not receive daunorubicin/cytarabine liposomal therapy. A repeat echocardiogram or MUGA should be performed prior to initiation of consolidation therapy and as clinically indicated. Daunorubicin/cytarabine liposomal should be discontinued in patients with impaired cardiac function unless the potential benefits outweigh the risks.

For additional information on the cardiotoxicity of daunorubicin, see Cautions: Cardiac Effects, in Daunorubicin Hydrochloride 10:00.

Copper Overload. The reconstituted daunorubicin/cytarabine liposomal dispersion contains 5 mg/mL of copper gluconate (14% of which is elemental copper). Clinical studies of daunorubicin/cytarabine liposomal did not include patients with Wilson disease or other copper-related metabolic disorders. The maximum theoretical total exposure of copper based on the recommended dosage of daunorubicin/cytarabine liposomal for induction and consolidation therapy is 106 mg/m^2.

In patients with Wilson disease, daunorubicin/cytarabine liposomal should be used only if the potential benefit outweighs the risk. If the drug is used in such patients, total serum copper, serum non-ceruloplasmin-bound copper, and 24-hour urine copper excretion should be monitored and neuropyschological assessments should be performed periodically. Consultation with a clinician who has expertise in managing acute copper toxicity is recommended in patients with Wilson disease who are treated with daunorubicin/cytarabine liposomal. If manifestations of acute copper toxicity occur in any patient, daunorubicin/cytarabine liposomal therapy should be discontinued.

Local Effects. Extravasation of daunorubicin, a component of daunorubicin/cytarabine liposomal, can produce severe local tissue necrosis. Daunorubicin/cytarabine liposomal must *not* be given by IM or subcutaneous injection.

For additional information on the local effects of daunorubicin, see Cautions: Local Effects, in Daunorubicin Hydrochloride 10:00.

Fetal/Neonatal Morbidity and Mortality. Daunorubicin/cytarabine liposomal may cause fetal harm in humans based on animal findings and anecdotal reports with the individual drugs in pregnant women; liposomal daunorubicin and conventional cytarabine have been shown to be teratogenic, embryotoxic, and fetotoxic in animals. There are no adequate and well-controlled studies using the fixed liposomal combination of daunorubicin and cytarabine or the individual drugs in pregnant women; however, 4 cases of major limb malformations have been reported in infants of mothers who received IV cytarabine, alone or in combination with other agents, during the first trimester.

Severe maternal toxicity and embryolethality have been demonstrated in animals receiving liposomal daunorubicin at doses approximately 0.3 times the recommended human dose on a mg/m^2 basis, while embryofetal toxicity (e.g., abortion, reduced number of offspring per litter, decreased litter sizes) and fetal malformations (i.e., anophthalmia, microphthalmia, incomplete ossification) have been observed at doses approximately 0.04 times the recommended human dose on a mg/m^2 basis. Abnormalities including cleft palate, phocomelia, deformed appendages, and skeletal abnormalities have been observed in the offspring of mice given intraperitoneal cytarabine during the period of organogenesis at doses approximately 0.06 times the recommended human dose on a mg/m^2 basis. Deformed appendages or reduced prenatal and postnatal brain size and permanent impairment of learning ability have been observed in the offspring of rats given cytarabine during the gestational period as a single intraperitoneal dose equivalent to approximately 1.2 or 3 times, respectively, the recommended human dose on a mg/m^2 basis. Embryofetal toxicity (i.e., decreased fetal weight, increased early or late resorptions) and decreased live litter sizes have been observed in animals receiving cytarabine at doses as low as approximately 0.02 times the recommended human dose on a mg/m^2 basis.

Pregnancy should be avoided during daunorubicin/cytarabine liposomal therapy. The manufacturer recommends confirmation of pregnancy status prior to initiation of therapy, and women of childbearing potential should be advised to use effective contraceptive methods during and for at least 6 months after discontinuance of the drug. In addition, men with female partners of childbearing potential should use effective methods of contraception during and for at least 6 months after discontinuance of the drug. Patients should be apprised of the potential hazard to the fetus if daunorubicin/cytarabine liposomal is used during pregnancy.

Impairment of Fertility. Results of animal studies suggest that daunorubicin administered as a single agent may cause reversible or permanent impairment of male fertility. In these animal studies, degeneration of reproductive tissues (testicular degeneration) and total aplasia of spermatocytes were observed in male dogs given IV daunorubicin at doses approximately 0.12 times the recommended human dose on a mg/m^2 basis.

There are no available data regarding the effect of cytarabine on fertility to date; however, a dose-dependent increase in sperm-head abnormalities and chromosomal aberrations were observed in animals receiving intraperitoneal cytarabine.

Specific Populations **Pregnancy.** Daunorubicin/cytarabine liposomal may cause fetal harm if administered to pregnant women based on animal findings and anecdotal reports in pregnant women. (See Fetal/Neonatal Morbidity and Mortality under Warnings/Precautions: Other Warnings and Precautions, in Cautions.)

Lactation. It is not known whether daunorubicin, cytarabine, or their metabolites are distributed into human milk. Because of the potential for serious adverse reactions to daunorubicin/cytarabine liposomal in nursing infants, women should be advised to discontinue nursing during and for at least 2 weeks after discontinuance of daunorubicin/cytarabine liposomal therapy. The effects of the fixed-combination preparation on nursing infants or on milk production are unknown.

Pediatric Use. Safety and efficacy of daunorubicin/cytarabine liposomal have not been established in pediatric patients.

Geriatric Use. In clinical trials, 57% of patients receiving daunorubicin/cytarabine liposomal were 65 years of age or older. No overall differences in safety were observed between geriatric patients and younger adults; however, hemorrhagic events occurred more frequently in geriatric patients compared with younger adults (77 versus 59%).

Hepatic Impairment. Pharmacokinetics of total (encapsulated plus unencapsulated) daunorubicin and cytarabine were not altered following administration of the fixed liposomal combination in patients with serum bilirubin concentrations of 3 mg/dL or less. Patients with serum bilirubin concentrations exceeding 3 mg/dL were not evaluated.

Renal Impairment. Pharmacokinetics of total (encapsulated plus unencapsulated) daunorubicin and cytarabine were not altered following administration of the fixed liposomal combination in patients with mild or moderate renal impairment (creatinine clearance of 30–89 mL/minute). Patients with severe renal impairment (creatinine clearance of 15–29 mL/minute) or end-stage renal disease were not evaluated.

■ **Common Adverse Effects** Adverse effects reported in 20% or more of adults receiving daunorubicin/cytarabine liposomal as induction therapy for newly diagnosed t-AML or AML-MRC include hemorrhage, febrile neutropenia, rash, edema, nausea, diarrhea/colitis, mucositis, constipation, musculoskeletal pain, abdominal pain, cough, headache, dyspnea, fatigue, arrhythmia, loss of appetite, pneumonia (excluding fungal pneumonia), sleep disorders, bacteremia (excluding sepsis), vomiting, chills, hypotension, and non-conduction cardiotoxicity. Similar adverse effects were observed with daunorubicin/cytarabine liposomal in the consolidation phase; however, adverse effects with the exception of chills, dizziness, and pyrexia were reported at a lower incidence during consolidation therapy.

Laboratory abnormalities reported in 10% or more of patients with newly diagnosed t-AML and AML-MRC receiving daunorubicin/cytarabine liposomal during induction and consolidation therapy include prolonged (defined as persisting beyond 42 days in the absence of active leukemia) thrombocytopenia and neutropenia; however, hyponatremia also occurred in patients receiving daunorubicin/cytarabine liposomal during induction therapy.

Drug Interactions

Specific drug interaction studies have not been performed to date with daunorubicin/cytarabine liposomal; however, interactions mediated by inhibitors or inducers of cytochrome P-450 (CYP) isoenzymes or common transporters are not likely based on available clinical data with other liposomal or nonliposomal cytarabine and daunorubicin preparations.

■ **Cardiotoxic Drugs** Concomitant use of daunorubicin/cytarabine liposomal with other cardiotoxic drugs may increase the risk of cardiotoxicity. If concomitant use cannot be avoided, the manufacturer recommends more frequent assessment of cardiac function. (See Cardiac Effects under Warnings/Precautions: Other Warnings and Precautions, in Cautions.)

■ **Hepatotoxic Drugs** Concomitant use of daunorubicin/cytarabine liposomal with hepatotoxic drugs may cause hepatic impairment and increase the incidence of adverse effects. If concomitant use cannot be avoided, the manufacturer recommends more frequent monitoring of hepatic function.

Description

The fixed liposomal combination of daunorubicin and cytarabine (daunorubicin/cytarabine liposomal) contains 2 antineoplastic agents in a fixed molar ratio coencapsulated in liposomes. Daunorubicin is an anthracycline antineoplastic antibiotic produced by *Streptomyces coeruleorubidus* that exhibits antimitotic and cytotoxic activity. The drug forms a complex with DNA by intercalation between base pairs. By stabilizing the complex between DNA and topoisomerase II, daunorubicin inhibits the activity of this enzyme, resulting in single-strand and double-strand breaks in DNA. Daunorubicin also may inhibit polymerase activity, affect regulation of gene expression, and be involved in free radical damage to DNA. Cytarabine is a cycle-phase specific antineoplastic agent, inducing G1-phase arrest and preferentially killing cells in the S phase. Although the exact mechanism(s) of action of cytarabine has not been fully elucidated, the drug appears to act primarily through inhibition of DNA polymerase.

In vitro studies indicate that efficacy of combination chemotherapy is dependent on the molar ratio of the component drugs. The fixed liposomal combination of daunorubicin and cytarabine is formulated in a 1:5 molar ratio, which has been shown to provide the greatest synergistic effect with the least antagonism. (See Uses: Acute Myeloid Leukemia.) The liposomes encapsulating the drug combination are composed of distearoylphosphatidylcholine (DSPC), distearoylphosphatidylglycerol (DSPG), and cholesterol in a molar ratio of 7:2:1. In addition to maintaining favorable drug ratios in the plasma after administration, preclinical studies also indicate that liposomes can penetrate and sustain higher concentrations of the drugs at the tumor site (specifically the bone marrow). Following administration of daunorubicin/cytarabine liposomal in leukemia-bearing mice, the liposomes are preferentially internalized by leukemic cells. Following cellular internalization and degradation of the liposomes, daunorubicin and cytarabine are released into the intracellular environment.

Following IV infusion of daunorubicin/cytarabine liposomal over 90 minutes on days 1, 3, and 5 in adults, the accumulation ratio of daunorubicin and cytarabine is 1.3 and 1.4, respectively. The pharmacokinetics of the drugs are dose proportional over the dose range of 1.3–59 mg/m^2 for daunorubicin and 3–134 mg/m^2 for cytarabine. Following release from liposomes, daunorubicin is mainly catalyzed by aldo-keto reductase and carbonyl reductase enzymes to the active metabolite daunorubicinol, and cytarabine is metabolized by the enzyme cytidine deaminase to the inactive metabolite 1-β-D-arabinofuranosyluracil (ara-U, uracil arabinoside). Following administration of daunorubicin/cytarabine liposomal, approximately 9% of the daunorubicin dose is eliminated as unchanged drug and daunorubicinol in urine, and approximately 71% of the cytarabine dose is eliminated as unchanged drug and 1-β-D-arabinofuranosyluracil in urine. When administered as the daunorubicin/cytarabine liposomal combination, the half-lives of the drugs are prolonged (to 31.5 hours for daunorubicin and 40.4 hours for cytarabine) with more than 99% of daunorubicin and cytarabine in plasma remaining encapsulated in liposomes.

Data from a population pharmacokinetic analysis indicate that age, gender, race, body weight, body mass index, and leukocyte count do not have clinically important effects on the systemic exposure of total daunorubicin or cytarabine.

Advice to Patients

Risk of hemorrhage. Importance of monitoring complete blood cell counts (CBCs). Importance of contacting a clinician if manifestations of infection (e.g., fever), unusual bleeding, or bruising occurs.

Risk of cardiotoxicity. Importance of informing clinicians if manifestations of heart failure occur.

Risk of hypersensitivity reactions, including anaphylaxis. Importance of seeking immediate medical attention if manifestations of a hypersensitivity reaction or anaphylaxis occur.

Risk of impaired fertility in men.

Risk of fetal harm. Necessity of advising women of childbearing potential and men who are partners of such women that they should use an effective method of contraception while receiving the drug and for at least 6 months after discontinuance of therapy. Importance of women informing clinicians if they are or plan to become pregnant. If pregnancy occurs, advise pregnant women of potential risk to the fetus.

Importance of advising women to avoid breast-feeding while receiving the drug and for at least 2 weeks after discontinuance of therapy.

Importance of informing clinicians of existing or contemplated concomitant therapy, including prescription and OTC drugs, as well as any concomitant illnesses.

Importance of informing patients of other important precautionary information. (See Cautions.)

Overview® (see Users Guide). For additional information on this drug until a more detailed monograph is developed and published, the manufacturer's labeling should be consulted. It is *essential* that the manufacturer's labeling be consulted for more detailed information on usual cautions, precautions, contraindications, potential drug interactions, laboratory test interferences, and acute toxicity. For further information on the handling of antineoplastic agents, see the ASHP Guidelines on Handling Hazardous Drugs at http://www.ahfsdruginformation.com.

Preparations

Excipients in commercially available drug preparations may have clinically important effects in some individuals; consult specific product labeling for details.

DAUNOrubicin and Cytarabine Liposomal

Parenteral

For injection, for IV infusion only	Daunorubicin 44 mg and Cytarabine 100 mg	**Vyxeos® (combination),** Jazz

Denileukin Diftitox

■ Denileukin diftitox, a recombinant DNA-derived cytotoxic protein, is an antineoplastic agent.

Uses

■ **Cutaneous T-cell Lymphoma** Denileukin diftitox is used for the treatment of persistent or recurrent cutaneous T-cell lymphoma (CTCL; e.g., mycosis fungoides, Sézary syndrome) in patients whose malignant cells express the CD25 component of the IL-2 receptor. Denileukin diftitox is designated an orphan drug by the US Food and Drug Administration (FDA) for use in this condition. Clinicians interested in the performance of such an assay for CD25 expression may obtain information by contacting the testing service at 800-964-5836. The manufacturer states that safety and efficacy of denileukin diftitox in patients with CTCL whose malignant cells do not express the CD25 component of the IL-2 receptor remains to be elucidated, but currently is being studied.

Efficacy of denileukin diftitox was evaluated in a phase III, randomized, double-blind clinical trial in 71 patients with recurrent or persistent stage Ib to IVa biopsy-proven CTCL that expressed CD25 in at least 20% of tumor cells or lymphocytes (see Description and opening paragraph in Uses). Enrolled patients have received a median number of 5 prior therapies (range: 1–12) and 63% of those had stage IIB or more advanced disease. Patients were randomized (stratified according to disease stage) to receive IV infusion of denileukin diftitox (9 or 18 mcg/kg daily for 5 consecutive days, every 3 weeks for up to 8 cycles). Overall, objective response (50% reduction in tumor burden sustained for at least 6 weeks) was observed in 30% (10% complete and 20% partial responses) of patients. The median time to first response in these patients reportedly was about 6 weeks (range: 3–27 weeks) and the median duration of objective response with denileukin diftitox therapy was 6.9 months (range: 2.7 to more than 46.1 months). No substantial differences in response rates were observed between the 2 denileukin diftitox dosage groups. However, there was a trend suggesting a dose effect for patients with more advanced disease (minimal stage IIb); objective response was observed in 2 of 21 (10%) or 9 of 34 (38%) of these patients receiving denileukin diftitox dosages of 9 or 18 mcg/kg daily, respectively. Limited data suggest that pretreatment with corticosteroids may be associated with increased response rate because of less frequent discontinuance of denileukin diftitox due to adverse effects; however, additional study is needed to confirm these results.

Dosage and Administration

■ **Reconstitution and Administration** Denileukin diftitox is administered by IV infusion over at least 15 minutes. The drug should not be administered by bolus IV injection. If infusion-related adverse effects occur, infusion should be discontinued or the rate reduced by administering the drug over longer periods (e.g., up to 80 minutes), depending on the severity of symptoms.

Prior to administration, commercially available denileukin diftitox concentrate for injection must be thawed at room temperature for 1–2 hours or under refrigeration (2–8°C) for up to 24 hours; denileukin diftitox solution should not be heated. The solution may be mixed by gentle swirling and should not be shaken vigorously. The manufacturer states that after thawing, a haze might develop in the solution that should clear upon reaching room temperature; only clear, colorless solutions without particulate matter should be used. Once thawed, solutions should not be refrozen.

Prior to IV infusion, commercially available denileukin diftitox concentrate for injection in single-use vials containing 150 mcg/mL *must* be diluted with preservative-free 0.9% sodium chloride injection to provide a solution containing at least 15 mcg/mL, a concentration that must be maintained during all steps of the preparation of the solution. Strict aseptic technique must be observed in preparing the solution, and only plastic syringes and plastic IV bags should be used, since adsorption of the drug to glass containers may occur. The appropriate volume of denileukin diftitox concentrate for injection is added to an empty IV infusion bag and each mL of the concentrate should be diluted with no more than 9 mL of the 0.9% sodium chloride injection. The diluted solutions should be used within 6 hours and unused portions of the solution should be discarded immediately. Denileukin diftitox should not be mixed with other drugs. The manufacturer recommends that an inline filter not be used during IV administration of the drug.

■ **General Dosage** ***Cutaneous T-cell Lymphoma*** The recommended dosage of denileukin diftitox for the treatment of persistent or recurrent cutaneous T-cell lymphoma (CTCL) is 9 or 18 mcg/kg daily for 5 consecutive days and repeated every 21 days. While the optimum duration of therapy remains to be established, the manufacturer reports that only 2% of patients who did not experience at least a 25% decrease in tumor burden prior to the fourth course of treatment subsequently responded.

■ **Special Populations** No special population recommendations at this time.

Cautions

■ **Contraindications** Known hypersensitivity to denileukin diftitox, diphtheria toxin, aldesleukin interleukin-2), or any other ingredient in the formulation.

■ **Warnings/Precautions** ***Warnings*** Denileukin diftitox should be used under the supervision of a qualified clinician experienced in therapy with antineoplastic agents. In addition, the patient should be closely monitored in a setting equipped and staffed by health-care personnel appropriately trained in cardiopulmonary resuscitation.

Capillary Leak Syndrome. Capillary leak syndrome, associated with at least 2 characteristic manifestations (e.g., hypotension, edema, hypoalbuminemia) has been reported in 38 of 143 patients (27%) in clinical trials and in some cases has been fatal. Onset of manifestations usually occurs within the first 2 weeks of the infusion and may persist or worsen after completion of the treatment cycle. Management of denileukin-induced capillary leak syndrome involves careful monitoring of weight, edema, blood pressure, and serum albumin concentrations. Manifestations usually are self-limiting and treatment should be initiated only if clinically indicated (e.g., careful use of diuretics for edema, slow hydration for hypotension); however, manifestations may be severe enough in some patients to require hospitalization. Generally, denileukin should be used with caution in patients with preexisting cardiovascular disease and/or low serum albumin concentrations, since they appear to be at increased risk of developing this syndrome.

Visual Loss. Decreased visual acuity, typically with loss of color vision, with or without retinal pigment mottling, has been reported in patients receiving denileukin. Although this condition was reversible in some patients, most patients reported persistent visual impairment.

Sensitivity Reactions The 2 distinct clinical syndromes associated with infusion of denileukin diftitox are an acute hypersensitivity symptom complex and a flu-like syndrome.

Hypersensitivity. Death during infusion has been reported. Acute hypersensitivity reactions, characterized by hypotension, back pain, dyspnea, vasodilation, rash, chest pain or tightness, tachycardia, dysphagias, syncope, allergic reactions, or anaphylaxis, have been reported in 98 of 143 patients (about 69%). Denileukin diftitox-induced hypersensitivity reactions almost always occur during or within 24 hours of administration of the infusion and in about 50% of cases on the first day of dosing, regardless of the treatment cycle. In clinical trials, severe hypersensitivity reactions requiring discontinuance or reduction in infusion rate were reported in 3 or 4% of patients, respectively.

Depending on the severity of the symptoms, appropriate treatment for sensitivity reactions associated with denileukin diftitox may include a decrease in the rate of the infusion, immediate interruption of the infusion, and/or IV administration of an antihistamine (with or without a corticosteroid and/or epinephrine), as needed. These drugs and resuscitative equipment should be immediately available during denileukin diftitox therapy. Limited data suggest that pretreatment with corticosteroids (e.g., oral prednisone 20 mg administered prior to each IV denileukin diftitox infusion, 8 mg of IV dexamethasone administered on day 1 and prior to each subsequent IV denileukin diftitox infusion) may be associated with decreased incidence of acute hypersensitivity reactions.

Flu-like Syndrome. A flu-like syndrome developed in about 91% of patients within several hours to days after denileukin diftitox infusion. The syndrome is characterized by fever and/or chills, asthenia, GI effects, myalgia, or arthralgia. In most patients, these symptoms were mild to moderate and generally responded to treatment with antipyretics, antiemetics, or antidiarrhea agents. However, it is not known if prophylactic administration of these drugs would ameliorate or decrease the incidence of such symptoms.

General Precautions **Adequate Patient Evaluation and Monitoring.** The manufacturer states that prior to initiation of denileukin diftitox therapy and at weekly intervals during administration of the drug, complete blood cell counts (CBCs), blood chemistries, and renal and hepatic function tests should be performed.In addition, prior to initiation of denileukin therapy, patients' malignant cells should be tested for CD25 expression. (See Uses: Cutaneous T-cell Lymphoma.)

Immunologic Reactions. Prior to denileukin therapy, enzyme-linked immunoassay (ELISA) testing showed that 39% (51/131) of patients with lymphoma had antibodies to the intact denileukin diftitox molecule (presumably associated with prior diphtheria immunization), and 18% (24/131) had antibodies directed against the IL-2 portion of the molecule. Analysis using a cellular assay indicated that 45% (27/60) of patients tested had evidence of an immune response inhibiting functional activity of denileukin diftitox prior to initiation of therapy with the drug. After one cycle of therapy, antibodies against the intact denileukin diftitox molecule or the IL-2 portion were detected in 76 or 35% of patients, respectively, using the ELISA assay, and a positive immune response was detected in 73% of patients, using the cellular assay. After 3 cycles of therapy, development of antibodies to denileukin diftitox was observed in 97% of patients for both the ELISA and the cellular assay. Following formation of these antibodies, there was a substantial increase (twofold to threefold) in drug clearance which resulted in a 75% lower systemic exposure to denileukin diftitox. The manufacturer states that presence or absence of antibodies did not correlate with the risk of immediate hypersensitivity reactions associated with IV infusion of the drug.

Infectious Complications. Patients should be monitored carefully for development of infections, since patients with CTCL may be predisposed to cutaneous infection. In addition, binding of denileukin diftitox to activated lymphocytes and macrophages may lead to cell death and thus impair immune function. Infections were reported in 48% (69 out of 143) of patients (23% of which were severe).

Hypoalbuminemia. Hypoalbuminemia (sometimes associated with capillary leak syndrome) has been reported in 83% (118 out of 143) of patients with lymphoma and was considered moderate or severe in 17% of such patients.(1,4,6) In most patients, hypoalbuminemia occurred 1 or 2 weeks after administration of denileukin diftitox. Serum albumin concentrations should be monitored prior to initiating each course of therapy. Administration of denileukin diftitox should be delayed until serum albumin concentrations are at least 3 g/dL.

Specific Populations **Pregnancy.** Category C. See Users Guide.

Lactation. Not known whether denileukin diftitox is distributed in milk. Discontinue nursing because of potential risk in nursing infants.

Pediatric Use. Safety and efficacy not established in children.

Geriatric Use. No substantial differences in efficacy relative to younger adults. However, in geriatric patients older than 65 years of age, higher incidence and greater severity of anorexia, hypotension, anemia, confusion, rash, nausea, and/or vomiting have been observed following administration of denileukin diftitox.

■ **Common Adverse Effects** Adverse effects occurring in 5% or more of patients include nausea/vomiting, anorexia, diarrhea, constipation, dyspepsia, dysphagia, anemia, thrombocytopenia, leukopenia, thrombotic complications, hematuria, albuminuria, pyuria, increase in serum creatinine concentration, increase in serum aminotransferase concentrations, dizziness, nervousness, confusion, insomnia, paresthesia, pain, headache, sweating, weight loss, dehydration, hypocalcemia, hypokalemia, cough, pulmonary effects, pharyngitis, rhinitis, arrhythmia, hypertension, rash, pruritus, and reactions at the injection site.

Drug Interactions

No formal drug interaction studies have been performed. In a single animal study, denileukin diftitox had no effect on the cytochrome P-450 enzyme system.

Description

Denileukin diftitox, a recombinant DNA-derived cytotoxic protein, is an antineoplastic agent. The amino acid sequence of the drug is composed of the domains of diphtheria toxin fragments A and B (Met1 to Thr387)-His and of interleukin-2 (IL-2; Ala1-Thr133). Denileukin diftitox is prepared from cultures of genetically modified *Escherichia coli* using recombinant DNA technology. The commercially available preparation of denileukin diftitox is purified using reverse phase chromatography followed by a multistep diafiltration process.

Denileukin diftitox is a fusion protein designed to direct the cytocidal activity of diphtheria toxin to cells that express the interleukin-2 (IL-2) receptor. The human IL-2 receptor is present in 3 forms (i.e., a low-affinity [containing 1 protein; CD2], an intermediate-affinity [containing 2 proteins; CD122 and CD132], and a high-affinity [containing 3 proteins; CD25, CD122, and CD132]) receptor. The low-affinity receptor is not capable of mediating endocytosis of bound ligand, while the intermediate- or high-affinity complex rapidly internalizes bound IL-2. The high-affinity receptor usually is found on activated T lymphocytes, activated B cells, and activated macrophages. Malignant cells expressing 1 or more of the subunits type of the IL-2 receptors are present in certain leukemias and lymphomas (e.g., cutaneous T-cell lymphoma [CTCL]). Although the exact mechanism of action of denileukin diftitox in the treatment of CTCL has not been fully elucidated, ex vivo studies suggest that the drug interacts with the high affinity IL-2 receptor on the cell surface and inhibits cellular protein synthesis, which results in cell death within hours.

Denileukin diftitox is metabolized by proteolytic degradation. Clearance of the drug may be substantially increased (twofold to threefold) by the formation of anti-denileukin diftitox antibodies which may result in lower systemic exposure to denileukin diftitox. (See Immunologic Reactions under Warnings/Precautions: Warnings in Cautions.)

Advice to Patients

Importance of women informing clinicians if they are or plan to become pregnant or to breast-feed.

Importance of informing clinicians of existing or contemplated concomitant therapy, including prescription and OTC drugs.

Overview® (see Users Guide). For additional information on this drug until a more detailed monograph is developed and published, the manufacturer's labeling should be consulted. Is is *essential* that the manufacturer's labeling be consulted for more detailed information on usual cautions, precautions, contraindications, potential drug interactions, laboratory test interferences, and acute toxicity. For further information on the handling of antineoplastic agents, see the ASHP Guidelines on Handling Hazardous Drugs at http://www.ahfsdruginformation.com.

Preparations

Excipients in commercially available drug preparations may have clinically important effects in some individuals; consult specific product labeling for details.

Denileukin Diftitox

Parenteral

For injection concentrate (frozen), for IV infusion	150 mcg per mL (300 mcg)	**Ontak®**, Ligand

Selected Revisions January 2007, © Copyright, January 2003, American Society of Health-System Pharmacists, Inc.

Dinutuximab

■ Dinutuximab, a chimeric human-murine anti-glycolipid disialoganglioside (anti-GD2) monoclonal antibody, is an antineoplastic agent.

Uses

■ **Neuroblastoma** Dinutuximab is used in combination with granulocyte-macrophage colony-stimulating factor (GM-CSF), interleukin-2 (IL-2), and isotretinoin for the treatment of high-risk neuroblastoma in pediatric patients who previously achieved at least a partial response to first-line antineoplastic therapy and multimodality therapy. The drug has been designated an orphan drug by FDA for use in this condition.

The current indication for dinutuximab is based principally on the results of a randomized, open-label, multicenter study in 226 pediatric patients with high-risk neuroblastoma. The primary measure of efficacy was event-free survival as assessed by the investigator. All patients had received prior therapy consisting of induction combination chemotherapy, maximum feasible surgical resection, myeloablative consolidation chemotherapy followed by autologous stem cell transplantation, and radiation therapy to residual soft tissue disease. Patients were enrolled if they achieved at least a partial response prior to undergoing autologous stem cell transplantation and if there was no evidence of disease progression following completion of first-line multimodality therapy. Patients enrolled in the study also were required to have adequate pulmonary (no dyspnea at rest and peripheral arterial oxygen saturation of at least 94% on room air), cardiac (shortening fraction of more than 30% by echocardiogram [ECHO] or ejection fraction of 55% by gated radionuclide study), hematologic (platelet count of 20,000/mm^3 or more and total absolute phagocyte count [APC] of 1000/mm^3 or more), hepatic (total bilirubin concentrations less than 1.5 times the upper limit of normal [ULN] and ALT concentrations less than 5 times the ULN), and renal (glomerular filtration rate [GFR] of at least 70 mL/minute per 1.73 m^2) function. The median age of patients was 3.8 years (range: 0.9 months to 15 years), 82% of patients were white, and 80% had stage 4 disease according to the International Neuroblastoma Staging System (INSS); 35, 43, and 23% of these patients achieved a complete response, a very good partial response, and a partial response, respectively, to therapy they received prior to undergoing autologous stem cell transplantation.

In this study, patients were randomized in a 1:1 ratio between days 50–77 following autologous stem cell transplantation to receive either dinutuximab in combination with isotretinoin and alternating cycles of sargramostim (GM-CSF) and aldesleukin (IL-2) or isotretinoin alone. Patients in the control group received isotretinoin 160 mg/m^2 (for patients weighing more than 12 kg) or 5.33 mg/kg (for patients weighing 12 kg or less) daily administered orally in 2 divided doses for 14 consecutive days for six 28-day cycles. Patients in the dinutuximab group received the same dosage of isotretinoin administered on days 11–24 of a 24-day cycle during cycles 1, 3, and 5 and on days 15–28 of a 32-day cycle during cycles 2 and 4 with the addition of dinutuximab (dosage equivalent to 17.5 mg/m^2 of the commercially available preparation [i.e., 25 mg/m^2 of drug product lots used during the clinical trial] administered by IV infusion) on days 4–7 and sargramostim (250 mcg/m^2 administered by subcutaneous injection or IV infusion over 2 hours) on days 1–14 during cycles 1, 3, and 5; during cycles 2 and 4, dinutuximab was administered on days 8–11 and aldesleukin was administered by continuous IV infusion on days 1–4 (dosage of 3 million units/m^2 daily) and days 8–11 (dosage of 4.5 million units/m^2 daily). During cycle 6, patients received isotretinoin alone at the same dosage as in cycles 1–5. Patients with systemic infections and those requiring concomitant systemic corticosteroids or immunosuppressive agents were excluded from the study. (See Drug Interactions: Immunosuppressive Therapy.)

Although median event-free survival for patients receiving the combination regimen had not been reached at the time of the primary analysis, median event-free survival appeared to be prolonged in patients receiving dinutuximab in combination with sargramostim, aldesleukin, and isotretinoin compared with those receiving isotretinoin alone. At the time of the primary analysis, median overall survival had not been reached in either group; however, overall survival also appeared to be prolonged in patients receiving dinutuximab in combination with sargramostim, aldesleukin, and isotretinoin compared with those receiving isotretinoin alone.

Dosage and Administration

■ **General** Adequate pulmonary, hematologic, hepatic, and renal function should be confirmed before administration of the first dinutuximab dose of each treatment cycle. (See Uses: Neuroblastoma.)

To minimize the risk of infusion-related adverse events associated with dinutuximab, a premedication regimen consisting of an antihistamine and acetaminophen should be administered prior to each dinutuximab infusion. An antihistamine (e.g., IV diphenhydramine hydrochloride 0.5–1 mg/kg [up to a maximum dose of 50 mg] over 10–15 minutes) should be administered beginning 20 minutes prior to each infusion of dinutuximab and every 4–6 hours as tolerated during the infusion. Acetaminophen 10–15 mg/kg (up to a maximum dose of 650 mg) should be administered orally 20 minutes prior to each infusion of dinutuximab and then every 4–6 hours as needed for fever or pain. If persistent fever or pain occurs, ibuprofen 5–10 mg/kg may be administered every 6 hours as needed. (See Infusion-related Effects under Warnings/Precautions: Warnings, in Cautions.)

To reduce pain associated with dinutuximab, the manufacturer recommends IV administration of morphine sulfate 50 mcg/kg immediately before each dinutuximab infusion. Morphine sulfate should be continued at an infusion rate of 20–50 mcg/kg per hour during and for 2 hours following completion of the dinutuximab infusion. Additional doses of IV morphine sulfate 25–50 mcg/kg may be administered as needed for pain every 2 hours followed by an increase in the morphine sulfate infusion rate in clinically stable patients. Fentanyl citrate or hydromorphone hydrochloride may be considered if morphine sulfate is not tolerated. If pain persists despite use of opiate analgesics, the manufacturer recommends that use of gabapentin or lidocaine in conjunction with IV morphine sulfate be considered. (See Pain under Warnings/Precautions: Warnings, in Cautions.)

Because of the potential for hypotension, adequate IV fluids should be administered prior to each infusion of dinutuximab. The manufacturer recommends IV hydration with 0.9% sodium chloride injection 10 mL/kg over 1 hour immediately before each dinutuximab infusion.

Clinicians should consult the respective manufacturers' labelings or published protocols for information on the dosage, method of administration, and administration sequence of other antineoplastic agents used in combination regimens.

Restricted Distribution Program Dinutuximab can only be obtained through a specialty pharmacy. Clinicians may consult the Unituxin® website for specific availability information (https://www.unituxin.com/pharmacist-information/ordering-distribution).

■ **Administration** Dinutuximab is administered by IV infusion over 10–20 hours. *The drug should not be administered by rapid IV injection, such as IV push or bolus.*

Dinutuximab should be infused at an initial rate of 0.875 mg/m² per hour for 30 minutes. The rate of infusion may be gradually increased as tolerated to a maximum infusion rate of 1.75 mg/m² per hour.

Dinutuximab injection concentrate must be diluted prior to administration. Prior to dilution, the injection concentrate should be inspected visually for particulate matter and discoloration. The solution should be clear to slightly opalescent and colorless; the solution should not be used if it is cloudy or discolored or if particulate matter is present. The appropriate dose (17.5 mg/m² per treatment day) of dinutuximab injection concentrate (containing 3.5 mg/mL) should be withdrawn and added to an infusion bag containing 100 mL of 0.9% sodium chloride injection. This diluted solution should be mixed by gentle inversion and should not be shaken.

Diluted solutions of the drug should be stored under refrigeration (2–8°C). Infusion of the drug should be initiated within 4 hours of dilution, and the drug should be discarded 24 hours after dilution.

Any unused portion left in the vial should be discarded since dinutuximab injection concentrate contains no preservative.

■ **Dosage** ***Neuroblastoma*** For the treatment of high-risk neuroblastoma in pediatric patients who previously achieved at least a partial response to first-line therapy, the recommended dosage of dinutuximab is 17.5 mg/m² daily by IV infusion over 10–20 hours on days 4–7 of a 24-day cycle during cycles 1, 3, and 5; granulocyte-macrophage colony-stimulating factor (GM-CSF) and isotretinoin also are administered during these cycles. For cycles 2 and 4, the same dosage of dinutuximab is administered on days 8–11 of a 32-day cycle; interleukin-2 (IL-2) and isotretinoin also are administered during these cycles. In the principal efficacy study, dinutuximab therapy was continued for a maximum of 5 cycles. During cycle 6, isotretinoin is administered alone. (See Uses: Neuroblastoma.)

Dosage Modification for Toxicity If toxicity occurs, temporary or permanent discontinuance of dinutuximab may be required based on causality.

Dinutuximab should be permanently discontinued in patients experiencing grade 3 or 4 anaphylaxis, grade 3 or 4 serum sickness, grade 3 pain unresponsive to optimal pain management, grade 4 peripheral sensory neuropathy, grade 3 peripheral sensory neuropathy that interferes with daily activities for more than 2 weeks, grade 2 peripheral motor neuropathy, subtotal or total loss of vision, grade 4 hyponatremia despite appropriate fluid management, or hemolytic uremic syndrome. (See Cautions: Warnings/Precautions.)

Infusion-related Reactions. If mild or moderate infusion-related reactions (e.g., transient rash, fever, rigors, localized urticaria) occur, appropriate symptomatic therapy should be provided and the rate of infusion should be reduced by 50%. If the patient responds promptly to symptomatic therapy, the infusion rate may be gradually increased following resolution of the reaction up to a maximum infusion rate of 1.75 mg/m² per hour. (See Infusion-related Effects under Warnings/Precautions: Warnings, in Cautions.)

If prolonged or severe infusion-related reactions (e.g., mild bronchospasm without other symptoms, angioedema that does not affect the airway) occur, the dinutuximab infusion should be interrupted immediately; if the reaction resolves rapidly, the infusion may be resumed but the rate of infusion should be reduced by 50%.

Following a second episode of prolonged or severe infusion-related reactions, the dinutuximab infusion should be interrupted until the next day. If continued therapy is warranted and the reaction has resolved, premedication with IV hydrocortisone 1 mg/kg (up to a maximum dose of 50 mg) should be administered and dinutuximab should be administered at a rate of 0.875 mg/m² per hour in an intensive care unit (ICU).

Following a third episode of prolonged or severe infusion-related reaction or following a life-threatening infusion-related reaction, dinutuximab therapy should be permanently discontinued.

Capillary Leak Syndrome. If moderate or severe capillary leak syndrome occurs, dinutuximab therapy should be interrupted immediately. Once the toxicity has resolved, the infusion may be resumed but the rate of infusion should be reduced by 50%. (See Capillary Leak Syndrome under Warnings/Precautions: Other Warnings and Precautions, in Cautions.)

If life-threatening capillary leak syndrome occurs, dinutuximab therapy should be discontinued for the current cycle. Once the toxicity has resolved, the rate of infusion should be reduced by 50% for subsequent cycles. If life-threatening capillary leak syndrome recurs, dinutuximab therapy should be permanently discontinued.

Hypotension. If symptomatic hypotension, systolic blood pressure less than the lower limit of normal (LLN) for age, or a reduction in systolic blood pressure by more than 15% compared with baseline occurs, therapy with dinutuximab should be interrupted. Once the toxicity has resolved, the infusion may be resumed but the rate of infusion should be reduced by 50%. If blood pressure remains stable for at least 2 hours, the infusion rate may be increased as tolerated up to a maximum infusion rate of 1.75 mg/m² per hour. (See Hypotension under Warnings/Precautions: Other Warnings and Precautions, in Cautions.)

Infectious Complications. If severe systemic infection or sepsis occurs, dinutuximab therapy should be interrupted until the infection resolves. (See Infectious Complications under Warnings/Precautions: Other Warnings and Precautions, in Cautions.)

Ocular Effects. In patients with dilated pupils with sluggish light reflex or other visual disturbances that do not cause vision loss, dinutuximab therapy should be withheld until resolution. If continued therapy is warranted, the dinutuximab dosage should be reduced by 50%. (See Ocular Effects under Warnings/Precautions: Other Warnings and Precautions, in Cautions.)

Following a second episode of ocular toxicity, dinutuximab therapy should be permanently discontinued.

If ocular toxicity is accompanied by visual impairment, dinutuximab therapy should be permanently discontinued.

Pain. If severe pain occurs, the rate of infusion should be reduced to 0.875 mg/m² per hour. If pain persists despite optimal medical management and reduction of the infusion rate, dinutuximab therapy should be discontinued. (See Pain under Warnings/Precautions: Warnings, in Cautions.)

■ **Special Populations** There are no special population dosage recommendations at this time. Dinutuximab has not been studied in patients with hepatic or renal impairment or in geriatric patients.

Cautions

■ **Contraindications** Dinutuximab is contraindicated in patients with a history of anaphylaxis to the drug.

■ **Warnings/Precautions** ***Warnings*** **Infusion-related Effects.** Serious infusion-related reactions have been reported in patients receiving dinutuximab. Serious infusion-related reactions including facial and upper airway edema, dyspnea, bronchospasm, stridor, urticaria, and hypotension requiring urgent intervention (i.e., blood pressure support, bronchodilator or corticosteroid therapy, a reduction in the infusion rate, temporary interruption or permanent discontinuance of dinutuximab therapy) may occur. Infusion-related reactions generally have occurred during or within 24 hours following completion of the dinutuximab infusion. Infusion-related reactions and hypersensitivity reactions have been indistinguishable in some patients. In the principal efficacy study in pediatric patients with high-grade neuroblastoma, grade 3 or 4 infusion-related reactions or serious urticaria occurred in 26 or 13%, respectively, of patients receiving dinutuximab in combination with sargramostim, aldesleukin, and isotretinoin compared with 1 or 0%, respectively, of those receiving isotretinoin alone. Serious adverse reactions that were consistent with anaphylaxis and required permanent discontinuance of dinutuximab therapy occurred in 2 of 134 dinutuximab-treated patients. In another clinical study, death from cardiac arrest occurred in 1 of 783 patients within 24 hours of dinutuximab administration.

Patients should be monitored closely for signs of infusion reactions during and for at least 4 hours following each dinutuximab infusion in a setting where resuscitation equipment and agents necessary to treat infusion-related reactions are readily available. To minimize the risk of infusion-related reactions, patients receiving dinutuximab should receive IV fluids and premedication with an antihistamine, analgesic, and antipyretic prior to each infusion of the drug. (See Dosage and Administration: General.) If infusion-related reactions occur, reduction in infusion rate or temporary or permanent discontinuance of dinutuximab may be required. (See Infusion-related Reactions under Dosage: Dosage Modification for Toxicity, in Dosage and Administration.) For patients experiencing a life-threatening infusion-related reaction, the manufacturer recommends permanent discontinuance of therapy. Appropriate treatment and supportive care should be provided for severe, prolonged, or life-threatening infusion-related reactions.

Peripheral Neuropathy. Peripheral neuropathy has been reported in patients receiving dinutuximab. (See Description.) In the principal efficacy study in pediatric patients with high-grade neuroblastoma, grade 3 peripheral sensory and motor neuropathy each occurred in 1% of patients receiving dinutuximab in combination with sargramostim, aldesleukin, and isotretinoin compared with none of those receiving isotretinoin alone. In another clinical study, peripheral sensory or motor neuropathy of any grade occurred in 9 or 0%, respectively, of dinutuximab-treated patients; the median duration of peripheral sensory neuropathy was 9 days (range: 3–163 days).

In a study of a similar anti-glycolipid disialoganglioside (anti-GD2) monoclonal antibody in adults with metastatic melanoma, severe peripheral motor neuropathy occurred in 2 of 12 patients. One patient experienced lower extremity weakness resulting in an inability to ambulate that persisted for approximately 6 weeks. The other patient experienced neurogenic bladder, which persisted for approximately 3 weeks, and lower extremity weakness resulting in an inability to ambulate without assistance, which persisted for approximately 16 weeks; complete resolution of peripheral motor neuropathy was not documented in this patient.

Dinutuximab should be permanently discontinued in patients who develop grade 2 peripheral motor neuropathy, grade 3 peripheral sensory neuropathy that interferes with daily activities for more than 2 weeks, or grade 4 peripheral sensory neuropathy.

Pain. Pain despite premedication with analgesics, including IV morphine sulfate, occurs commonly in dinutuximab-treated patients and was reported in 85% of patients receiving the drug in the principal efficacy study in pediatric patients with high-grade neuroblastoma; abdominal pain, generalized pain, extremity pain, back pain, neuralgia, musculoskeletal chest pain, and arthralgia were most commonly reported. Grade 3 pain was reported in 51% of patients receiving dinutuximab in combination with sargramostim, aldesleukin, and isotretinoin compared with 5% of those receiving isotretinoin alone. Grade 3 or

4 pain occurred more frequently during administration of dinutuximab in cycle 1 and often subsided during subsequent cycles.

To reduce pain during administration of dinutuximab, patients should receive premedication with analgesics, including an IV opiate analgesic initiated prior to each dinutuximab infusion and continued until 2 hours following completion of the infusion. (See Dosage and Administration: General.) If severe pain occurs, the infusion rate of dinutuximab should be reduced. (See Pain under Dosage: Dosage Modification for Toxicity, in Dosage and Administration.) Dinutuximab should be discontinued if pain persists despite reduction of the infusion rate and optimal pain management.

Other Warnings and Precautions **Capillary Leak Syndrome.** Capillary leak syndrome has been reported in patients receiving dinutuximab during any treatment cycle, but has occurred more commonly during cycles containing IL-2. In the principal efficacy study in pediatric patients with high-grade neuroblastoma, grade 3–5 capillary leak syndrome occurred in 23% of patients receiving dinutuximab in combination with sargramostim, aldesleukin, and isotretinoin compared with none of those receiving isotretinoin alone.

If capillary leak syndrome occurs, supportive treatment (i.e., respiratory support, albumin replacement therapy) should be provided. Temporary interruption of dinutuximab therapy followed by a reduction in the infusion rate or discontinuance of therapy may be necessary depending on the severity of the toxicity. (See Capillary Leak Syndrome under Dosage: Dosage Modification for Toxicity, in Dosage and Administration.)

Hypotension. Hypotension has been reported in patients receiving dinutuximab. In the principal efficacy study in pediatric patients with high-risk neuroblastoma, grade 3 or 4 hypotension occurred in 16% of patients receiving dinutuximab in combination with sargramostim, aldesleukin, and isotretinoin compared with none of those receiving isotretinoin alone.

Blood pressure should be closely monitored during therapy. Adequate IV fluids should be administered immediately before each dinutuximab infusion. (See Dosage and Administration: General.) In patients who develop symptomatic hypotension, systolic blood pressure less than the lower limit of normal (LLN) for age, or a reduction in systolic blood pressure by more than 15% compared with baseline, supportive treatment should be provided. Temporary interruption of dinutuximab therapy followed by a reduction in the infusion rate or discontinuance of therapy may be necessary if hypotension occurs during therapy with the drug. (See Hypotension under Dosage: Dosage Modification for Toxicity, in Dosage and Administration.)

Infectious Complications. Serious infections, such as bacteremia and sepsis, have been reported in patients receiving dinutuximab. In the principal efficacy study in pediatric patients with high-risk neuroblastoma, grade 3 or 4 bacteremia requiring urgent medical intervention (i.e., IV antibiotics) or sepsis occurred in 13 or 18%, respectively, of patients receiving dinutuximab in combination with sargramostim, aldesleukin, and isotretinoin compared with 5 or 9%, respectively, of those receiving isotretinoin alone.

Patients should be monitored for signs and symptoms of systemic infection. If a systemic infection develops, dinutuximab therapy should be temporarily interrupted until the infection has resolved.

Ocular Effects. Adverse ocular effects including blurred vision, photophobia, mydriasis, fixed or unequal pupils, optic nerve disorder, eyelid ptosis, and papilledema have occurred in patients receiving dinutuximab. Ocular effects generally have resolved over time. In the principal efficacy study in pediatric patients with high-risk neuroblastoma, blurred vision occurred in 2% of patients receiving dinutuximab in combination with sargramostim, aldesleukin, and isotretinoin compared with none of those receiving isotretinoin alone. Diplopia, mydriasis, and unequal pupillary size were reported rarely in the dinutuximab treatment group. In a noncomparative study evaluating the safety of dinutuximab in combination with GM-CSF, IL-2, and isotretinoin, ocular disorders were reported in 15% of patients with a median duration of 4 days (range: 0–221 days) among those with documented resolution.

In patients who develop ocular toxicities, temporary interruption of therapy followed by dosage reduction or drug discontinuance may be required. (See Ocular Effects under Dosage: Dosage Modification for Toxicity, in Dosage and Administration.)

Hematologic Effects. Severe thrombocytopenia, anemia, neutropenia, and febrile neutropenia have been reported in patients receiving dinutuximab. In the principal efficacy study in pediatric patients with high-risk neuroblastoma, grade 3 or 4 thrombocytopenia, anemia, neutropenia, or febrile neutropenia occurred in 39, 34, 34, or 4%, respectively, of patients receiving dinutuximab in combination with sargramostim, aldesleukin, and isotretinoin compared with 25, 16, 13, or 0%, respectively, of those receiving isotretinoin alone.

Peripheral blood cell counts should be monitored closely during therapy.

Electrolyte Abnormalities. Electrolyte abnormalities (i.e., hyponatremia, hypokalemia, hypocalcemia) have been reported in patients receiving dinutuximab. In the principal efficacy study in pediatric patients with high-risk neuroblastoma, grade 3 or 4 hypokalemia or hyponatremia occurred in 37 or 23%, respectively, of patients receiving dinutuximab in combination with sargramostim, aldesleukin, and isotretinoin compared with 2 or 4%, respectively, of those receiving isotretinoin alone. In a study of a similar anti-GD2 monoclonal antibody in adults with metastatic melanoma, severe hyponatremia caused by syndrome of inappropriate secretion of antidiuretic hormone (SIADH) occurred in 2 of 12 patients.

Serum electrolytes should be monitored daily during therapy. If grade 4 hyponatremia occurs despite appropriate fluid management, dinutuximab therapy should be permanently discontinued.

Atypical Hemolytic Uremic Syndrome. Hemolytic uremic syndrome occurring in the absence of a documented infection and resulting in renal insufficiency, electrolyte abnormalities, anemia, and hypertension has been reported in 2 patients, approximately 4 days following the first treatment cycle, in an expanded access study. Hemolytic uremic syndrome recurred following reinitiation of dinutuximab in one patient.

In patients who develop hemolytic uremic syndrome, dinutuximab therapy should be permanently discontinued and appropriate treatment should be provided.

Fetal/Neonatal Morbidity and Mortality. Dinutuximab may cause fetal harm if administered to pregnant women. A linear relationship between placental transfer of human immunoglobulin G (IgG) and gestational age appears to exist; therefore, fetal exposure to dinutuximab may be highest during the third trimester of pregnancy.

Pregnancy should be avoided during dinutuximab therapy. Women of childbearing potential should be advised to use an effective method of contraception while receiving dinutuximab and for at least 2 months after discontinuance of therapy. Patients should be apprised of the potential hazard to the fetus if the drug is used during pregnancy.

Immunogenicity. As with all therapeutic proteins, there is a potential for immunogenicity. In clinical studies, anti-dinutuximab antibody formation occurred in 16.8% of patients receiving dinutuximab. Neutralizing antibodies were detected in 3.6% of patients who tested positive for anti-dinutuximab antibodies.

Specific Populations **Pregnancy.** Dinutuximab may cause fetal harm if administered to pregnant women based on its mechanism of action. The effects of dinutuximab may be greater during the third trimester of pregnancy. (See Fetal/Neonatal Morbidity and Mortality under Warnings/Precautions: Other Warnings and Precautions, in Cautions.)

Lactation. It is not known whether dinutuximab is distributed into human milk; however, human IgG is distributed into milk. Because of the potential for serious adverse reactions to dinutuximab in nursing infants, women should be advised to discontinue nursing during dinutuximab therapy. Women may begin nursing 6 months after discontinuance of therapy. The effects of the drug on nursing infants or on the production of human milk are unknown.

Pediatric Use. Safety and efficacy of dinutuximab have not been established in infants younger than 11 months of age.

Geriatric Use. Safety and efficacy of dinutuximab have not been established in geriatric patients.

Hepatic Impairment. Pharmacokinetics of dinutuximab have not been evaluated in patients with hepatic impairment.

Renal Impairment. Pharmacokinetics of dinutuximab have not been evaluated in patients with renal impairment.

■ **Common Adverse Effects** Adverse effects reported in 25% or more of patients receiving dinutuximab in combination with sargramostim, aldesleukin, and isotretinoin include pain, pyrexia, thrombocytopenia, lymphopenia, infusion-related reactions, hypotension, hyponatremia, elevated aminotransferase (i.e., AST, ALT) concentration, anemia, vomiting, diarrhea, hypokalemia, capillary leak syndrome, neutropenia, urticaria, hypoalbuminemia, hypocalcemia, and infection.

Drug Interactions

No formal drug interaction studies have been performed to date.

■ **Immunosuppressive Therapy** Concomitant immunosuppressive therapy may interfere with the mechanism of action of dinutuximab. Patients requiring concomitant therapy with systemic corticosteroids or other immunosuppressive agents were excluded from the principal efficacy study of dinutuximab in pediatric patients with high-grade neuroblastoma. Concomitant use of systemic corticosteroids with dinutuximab is not recommended unless required for the management of toxicity (e.g., serious hypersensitivity or infusion-related reactions).

Immune globulin IV also may interfere with the mechanism of action of dinutuximab and should not be administered within 2 weeks before or 1 week after each course of dinutuximab.

Description

Dinutuximab, a chimeric human-murine anti-glycolipid disialoganglioside (anti-GD2) monoclonal antibody, is an antineoplastic agent. The drug is an IgG_1 kappa immunoglobulin. Dinutuximab is selective for GD2, a glycolipid minimally expressed on the surface of normal cells of neuroectodermal origin, including central neurons, peripheral nerve fibers, and melanocytes. Overexpression of GD2 has been identified in several malignancies, including neuroblastoma and most melanomas. Following binding of dinutuximab to antigen GD2, cell lysis occurs through complement-dependent cytotoxicity (CDC) and antibody-dependent cell-mediated cytotoxicity (ADCC). In the presence of human effector cells, including peripheral blood mononuclear cells (PBMCs) and granulocytes, dinutuximab has demonstrated dose-dependent cytotoxicity of neuroblastoma cells; enhanced cell lysis has been observed with the addition of granulocyte-macrophage colony-stimulating factor (GM-CSF) and interleukin-2 (IL-2). Dinutuximab also has been shown to reduce tumor growth of GD2-expressing cell lines in xenograft models.

Nonclinical studies suggest that dinutuximab-induced peripheral neuropathy may be a pharmacologic consequence of dinutuximab binding to antigen GD2 on the surface of peripheral nerve fibers and/or myelin. Decreases in mechanical pain thresholds have been demonstrated in animal studies beginning shortly after administration of anti-GD2 monoclonal antibodies, including dinutuximab, and persisting for up to 48 hours after completion of drug administration. (See Peripheral Neuropathy and also see Pain under Warnings/Precautions: Warnings, in Cautions.)

The elimination half-life of dinutuximab is 10 days.

Advice to Patients

Risk of serious infusion-related reactions and anaphylaxis. Importance of informing clinician immediately if signs and symptoms of such reactions, including facial swelling, urticaria, breathing difficulty, and lightheadedness or dizziness, occur during or within 24 hours of an infusion of the drug.

Risk of severe pain and peripheral sensory and motor neuropathy. Importance of promptly informing clinician if severe or worsening pain or signs and symptoms of neuropathy (e.g., numbness, tingling, burning, weakness) occur.

Risk of capillary leak syndrome. Importance of informing clinician immediately if signs and symptoms of capillary leak syndrome (e.g., hypotension, generalized edema, dyspnea) occur.

Risk of hypotension during infusion of the drug. Importance of informing clinician immediately if signs and symptoms of hypotension occur.

Risk of infection. Importance of informing clinician immediately if signs and symptoms of infection occur.

Risk of adverse ocular effects. Importance of promptly informing clinician if signs and symptoms of ocular toxicity (e.g., blurred vision, photophobia, ptosis, diplopia, unequal pupil size) occur.

Risk of myelosuppression. Importance of promptly informing clinician if signs and symptoms of anemia, thrombocytopenia, or infection occur.

Risk of electrolyte abnormalities (i.e., hypokalemia, hyponatremia, hypocalcemia). Importance of informing clinician if signs and symptoms of electrolyte abnormalities (e.g., seizures, palpitations, muscle cramping) occur.

Risk of atypical hemolytic uremic syndrome. Importance of informing clinician if signs and symptoms of hemolytic uremic syndrome (e.g., fatigue, dizziness, fainting, pallor, edema, decreased urination, hematuria) occur.

Risk of fetal harm. Necessity of advising women of childbearing potential that they should use an effective method of contraception while receiving the drug and for at least 2 months after discontinuance of therapy. If pregnancy occurs, advise pregnant women of potential risk to the fetus.

Importance of advising women not to breast-feed during therapy.

Importance of informing clinicians of existing or contemplated concomitant therapy, including prescription and OTC drugs, as well as any concomitant illnesses.

Importance of informing patients of other important precautionary information. (See Cautions.)

Overview® (see Users Guide). For additional information on this drug until a more detailed monograph is developed and published, the manufacturer's labeling should be consulted. It is *essential* that the manufacturer's labeling be consulted for more detailed information on usual cautions, precautions, contraindications, potential drug interactions, laboratory test interferences, and acute toxicity. For further information on the handling of antineoplastic agents, see the ASHP Guidelines on Handling Hazardous Drugs at http://www.ahfsdruginformation.com.

Preparations

Distribution of dinutuximab is restricted. (See Restricted Distribution Program under Dosage and Administration: General.)

Excipients in commercially available drug preparations may have clinically important effects in some individuals; consult specific product labeling for details.

Dinutuximab

Parenteral

For injection concentrate, for IV infusion	3.5 mg/mL	**Unituxin®**, United Therapeutics

DOCEtaxel

■ Docetaxel, a semisynthetic taxoid produced from the needles of the European yew (*Taxus baccata*) tree, is an antineoplastic agent.

Uses

■ **Breast Cancer** ***Adjuvant Therapy for Early-stage Breast Cancer*** Docetaxel is used in combination with doxorubicin and cyclophosphamide for the adjuvant treatment of operable node-positive breast cancer.

The current indication is based on a multicenter, open-label, randomized trial (the BCIRG 001 trial) in which 1491 patients with axillary node-positive breast cancer and no evidence of metastatic disease received either doxorubicin and cyclophosphamide followed by docetaxel (TAC) or doxorubicin followed by fluorouracil and cyclophosphamide (FAC). The median age of women participating in this study was 49 years. Treatment regimens consisted of doxorubicin 50 mg/m^2 as a 15-minute IV infusion and cyclophosphamide 500 mg/m^2 IV administered over 1–5 minutes followed by a 1-hour interval and then docetaxel 75 mg/m^2 as a 1-hour IV infusion on day 1 (TAC regimen), or doxorubicin 50 mg/m^2 followed by fluorouracil 500 mg/m^2 each administered as a 15-minute IV infusion and then cyclophosphamide 500 mg/m^2 as a 1- to 5-minute IV infusion on day 1 (FAC regimen); each regimen was administered once every 3 weeks for up to 6 cycles. Stratification was performed according to the number of positive lymph nodes (1–3, 4+). Following the completion of chemotherapy, patients with hormone receptor-positive disease received tamoxifen 20 mg daily for up to 5 years. About 70% of patients in each group received adjuvant radiation therapy.

Results of a second interim analysis of the data at a median follow-up of 55 months indicate that disease-free survival was prolonged in patients receiving the docetaxel-containing regimen. The estimated rate of disease-free survival at 5 years was 75% in patients receiving the TAC regimen compared with 68% in those receiving the FAC regimen. An overall reduction of about 26% in risk of relapse, including local or distant recurrence, contralateral breast cancer, and death from any cause, was observed in patients receiving the TAC regimen. At the time of this interim analysis, overall survival also was prolonged in patients receiving the docetaxel-containing regimen. Subgroup analysis suggests that those most likely to benefit from docetaxel-containing adjuvant treatment are patients with 1–3 positive nodes. Because this trial was restricted to women who were 70 years of age or younger, the benefit and risk associated with use of the TAC regimen as adjuvant therapy for breast cancer in older patients is not known.

Patients receiving TAC generally experienced increased toxicity compared with those receiving FAC. A higher rate of severe nonhematologic treatment-emergent adverse events occurred in patients receiving TAC (36%) than in those receiving FAC (27%). Treatment was discontinued because of adverse effects in 6% of patients receiving TAC compared with about 1% of those receiving FAC. Fever in the absence of infection and allergy were the most common reasons for withdrawal from the study among patients receiving TAC. Anemia (92 versus 72%), stomatitis (69 versus 53%), grade 3 or 4 neutropenia (66 versus 49%), fever in the absence of infection (46 versus 17%), fluid retention (35 versus 15%) including peripheral edema (27 versus 7%), myalgia (27 versus 10%), sensory neuropathy (26 versus 10%), and febrile neutropenia (25 versus 2%) occurred more frequently in patients receiving TAC. Neutropenia of any grade (82 versus 71%) and vomiting (59 versus 44%) occurred more frequently in those receiving FAC. The most frequent adverse effects in patients receiving TAC included alopecia (98%), hematologic toxicity (anemia [92%], neutropenia [71%], grade 3 or 4 neutropenia [66%]), asthenia (81%), GI toxicity (nausea [80%], stomatitis [69%], vomiting [44%]), amenorrhea (62%), and fever in the absence of infection (46%).

In this trial (BCIRG 001), patients receiving TAC experienced a higher rate of febrile neutropenia than those receiving FAC (25 versus 2.5%). Primary prophylaxis with granulocyte colony-stimulating factor (G-CSF) was not allowed, but use of G-CSF was mandatory in subsequent cycles for any patient experiencing febrile neutropenia or infection. Another randomized trial (RAPP-01), which compared doxorubicin and docetaxel versus doxorubicin and cyclophosphamide as adjuvant therapy for intermediate-risk breast cancer, was prematurely terminated because of serious adverse events, including 2 deaths, associated with febrile neutropenia in patients receiving the docetaxel-containing regimen. Some clinicians, including the investigators in these trials (BCIRG 001 and RAPP-01), currently recommend primary prophylaxis with G-CSF in patients receiving docetaxel with an anthracycline agent as adjuvant therapy for early-stage breast cancer.

Other docetaxel-containing regimens are being investigated as adjuvant therapy for early-stage breast cancer, including nonanthracycline-containing regimens†. In a randomized trial involving 1016 patients, patients receiving docetaxel and cyclophosphamide as adjuvant therapy for operable breast cancer had prolonged disease-free survival and similar overall survival compared with those receiving doxorubicin and cyclophosphamide. Grade 1 or 2 edema, myalgia, and arthralgia occurred more frequently in patients receiving docetaxel and cyclophosphamide whereas grade 1 to 4 nausea and vomiting were more frequent in patients receiving doxorubicin and cyclophosphamide.

Docetaxel and Doxorubicin as First-line Therapy for Advanced Breast Cancer Docetaxel is used in combination with doxorubicin for the first-line treatment of metastatic breast cancer†.

In a multicenter, randomized, phase 3 trial, 429 patients received either doxorubicin and docetaxel or doxorubicin and cyclophosphamide for the initial treatment of metastatic breast cancer. Treatment consisted of doxorubicin 50 mg/m^2 as a 15-minute IV infusion followed 1 hour later by docetaxel 75 mg/m^2 as a 1-hour IV infusion, or doxorubicin 60 mg/m^2 as a 15-minute IV infusion followed by cyclophosphamide 600 mg/m^2 as a 15-minute IV infusion, on day 1 once every 3 weeks for up to 8 cycles. Among patients receiving doxorubicin and docetaxel, median time to progression was prolonged (37 versus 32 weeks), overall response rate was higher (59 versus 47%), and overall survival was similar compared with those receiving doxorubicin and cyclophosphamide as initial treatment for metastatic breast cancer. Diarrhea, febrile neutropenia, edema, neurosensory toxicity, nail changes, rashes, and grade 3 or 4 infections occurred more frequently in patients receiving doxorubicin and docetaxel whereas nausea and vomiting were more frequent in patients receiving doxorubicin and cyclophosphamide.

Other dosage schedules have been investigated for the use of doxorubicin and docetaxel as first-line therapy for metastatic breast cancer. In a multicenter, randomized, phase 3 trial involving 144 patients, sequential administration of doxorubicin and docetaxel was shown to be as effective but less toxic than concomitant administration of these drugs for the first-line treatment of metastatic breast cancer. Patients who had not received previous treatment with anthracycline agents received either 3 cycles of doxorubicin 75 mg/m^2 every 21 days followed by 3 cycles of docetaxel 100 mg/m^2 every 21 days (sequential treatment) or 6 cycles of doxorubicin 50 mg/m^2 and docetaxel 75 mg/m^2 every 21 days (concomitant treatment). Dosage adjustments were made for patients who had received previous treatment with anthracycline agents, so these patients received either 2 cycles of doxorubicin 75 mg/m^2 every 21 days followed by 4 cycles of docetaxel 100 mg/m^2 every 21 days (sequential treatment) or 3 cycles of doxorubicin 50 mg/m^2 and docetaxel 75 mg/m^2 every 21 days followed by 3 cycles of docetaxel 100 mg/m^2 every 21 days (concomitant treatment). Patients received premedication with a corticosteroid regimen and prophylactic antiemetic therapy. The use of granulocyte colony-stimulating factor (G-CSF) was not allowed as primary prophylaxis but was allowed following a first episode of febrile neutropenia. Patients receiving sequential treatment with doxorubicin and docetaxel had a higher rate of completion of 6 cycles of therapy (81 versus 67%) and a lower rate of withdrawal from the study because of adverse events (1 versus 14.5%) compared with those receiving concomitant treatment with doxorubicin and docetaxel. Efficacy was similar between the groups, but febrile neutropenia was less frequent (29 versus 48%) in patients receiving sequential administration of doxorubicin and docetaxel than in those receiving concomitant administration of these agents.

Because of the higher rate of febrile neutropenia and increased risk of life-threatening sepsis associated with the use of doxorubicin in combination with docetaxel as adjuvant or neoadjuvant therapy for early-stage breast cancer, some clinicians recommend use of G-CSF and/or antibiotics as primary prophylaxis in patients receiving these agents for metastatic breast cancer.

Second-line Therapy for Advanced Breast Cancer **Docetaxel and Capecitabine.** Docetaxel is used in combination with capecitabine for the treatment of metastatic breast cancer in patients with disease that has failed anthracycline-containing chemotherapy. In a randomized trial, patients receiving combination therapy with docetaxel and capecitabine for metastatic breast cancer had longer time to disease progression, prolonged survival, and higher objective response rate than those receiving docetaxel alone. (See Uses: Breast Cancer: Combination Therapy in Capecitabine 10:00.)

Docetaxel Monotherapy. Docetaxel is used as monotherapy for the second-line treatment of locally advanced or metastatic breast cancer after failure of prior chemotherapy. As with paclitaxel, clinical cross-resistance with anthracyclines is incomplete with docetaxel, and patients with metastatic breast cancer refractory to treatment with anthracycline antineoplastic agents (e.g., doxorubicin) may respond to docetaxel therapy.

The current indication for docetaxel is based principally on the results of 2 large randomized trials in patients with locally advanced or metastatic breast cancer that failed to respond to prior chemotherapy regimens.

Docetaxel (100 mg/m^2 IV over 1 hour every 3 weeks) was compared with a combination of mitomycin (12 mg/m^2 IV every 6 weeks) and vinblastine (6 mg/m^2 IV every 3 weeks) in an open-label, multicenter, randomized phase 3 study in 392 patients with a history of treatment failure with an anthracycline regimen. Most patients in the study had received prior anthracycline-based chemotherapy for the treatment of metastatic disease (rather than as adjuvant therapy) and 75% had measurable, visceral metastases; only 15% of patients at study entry were those whose disease had relapsed after adjuvant therapy. Patients receiving docetaxel experienced a longer median survival duration (11.4 versus 8.7 months), longer median time to progression (4.3 versus 2.5 months), and higher overall and complete response rates (28.1 versus 9.5% overall and 3.4 versus 1.6% complete) compared with patients receiving mitomycin and vinblastine. Grade 3 or 4 neutropenia, asthenia, stomatitis, neurosensory toxicity, nail disorder, diarrhea, skin toxicity, grade 3 or 4 infections, and febrile neutropenia occurred more frequently in patients receiving docetaxel whereas thrombocytopenia and constipation occurred more frequently in those receiving mitomycin and vinblastine.

In a second open-label, multicenter phase 3 trial, 326 patients with metastatic breast cancer and a history of treatment failure with an alkylating agent-containing chemotherapy regimen were randomized to receive either docetaxel (100 mg/m^2 IV over 1 hour every 3 weeks) or doxorubicin (75 mg/m^2 IV over 15–20 minutes every 3 weeks). Prior chemotherapy was administered for metastatic disease in about half of the patients studied and as adjuvant therapy in the other half of the patients, and 75% of patients had measurable, visceral metastases. Higher overall and complete response rates (45.3 versus 29.7% overall and 6.8 versus 4.2% complete) were observed in patients receiving docetaxel, and a similar median survival (14.7 and 14.3 months) and median time to progression (6.5 and 5.3 months) were reported with docetaxel and doxorubicin, respectively. Fluid retention, diarrhea, nail disorder, neurosensory toxicity, skin toxicity, allergy, and neuromotor toxicity occurred more frequently in patients receiving docetaxel whereas nausea, vomiting, stomatitis, thrombocytopenia, cardiac toxicity, grade 3 or 4 anemia, red blood cell transfusions, febrile neutropenia, and grade 3 or 4 infections were more frequent in patients receiving doxorubicin.

In another randomized trial, 527 patients with advanced breast cancer that had progressed or relapsed after 1 prior chemotherapy regimen received docetaxel at dose levels of 60, 75, or 100 mg/m^2. Most patients (94%) had metastatic disease and 79% had received prior anthracycline-containing therapy. Response rate and toxicity increased with increase in dose. Patients receiving docetaxel 100 mg/m^2 had a higher response rate (30 versus 20%) than those receiving docetaxel 60 mg/m^2. Grade 3 or 4 adverse events occurred in 49% of patients receiving docetaxel 60 mg/m^2, 55% of those receiving docetaxel 75 mg/m^2, and 66% of those receiving docetaxel 100 mg/m^2. Discontinuance of therapy because of toxicity was reported in 5% of patients receiving docetaxel 60 mg/m^2 compared with 16.5% of patients receiving docetaxel 100 mg/m^2. Adverse effects that occurred at higher frequency in respective order with increasing docetaxel dose (60, 75, and 100 mg/m^2) included neutropenia (92, 94, and 97%), anemia (87, 94, and 97%), fluid retention (26, 38, and 46%), thrombocytopenia (7, 11, and 12%), febrile neutropenia (5, 7, and 14%), and treatment-related grade 3 or 4 infection (2, 3, and 7%).

In phase 2 studies, docetaxel has been evaluated in patients with locally advanced or metastatic breast cancer, including those with disease resistant to treatment with anthracycline antineoplastic agents. Anthracycline resistance was defined as progression of disease while undergoing anthracycline-containing therapy for advanced disease or disease relapse while undergoing anthracycline-containing adjuvant therapy. Among 309 patients receiving a docetaxel dose of 100 mg/m^2 as second-line therapy for metastatic breast cancer in 6 single-arm studies, 190 patients had anthracycline-resistant disease. Among patients with anthracycline-resistant disease, the overall response rate was about 38% with a complete response rate of 2%. A similar rate of overall response (about 35%) was observed in 26 patients with anthracycline-resistant disease among a total of 174 patients receiving a docetaxel dose of 60 mg/m^2 as second-line therapy for locally advanced or metastatic breast cancer in 3 single-arm studies conducted in Japan.

■ **Non-small Cell Lung Cancer** ***Docetaxel and Cisplatin as First-line Therapy for Advanced Disease*** Docetaxel is used in combination with cisplatin as first-line therapy for unresectable, locally advanced or metastatic non-small cell lung cancer.

The current indication is based on a randomized trial in which 1218 patients with unresectable stage IIIB or stage IV non-small cell lung cancer received initial treatment with docetaxel and cisplatin, vinorelbine and cisplatin, or docetaxel and carboplatin. Treatment regimens consisted of docetaxel 75 mg/m^2 as a 1-hour IV infusion immediately followed by cisplatin 75 mg/m^2 IV over 30–60 minutes on day 1 once every 3 weeks; vinorelbine 25 mg/m^2 IV over 6–10 minutes on days 1, 8, 15, and 22 followed by cisplatin 100 mg/m^2 IV on day 1 in 4-week cycles; or docetaxel 75 mg/m^2 IV as a 1-hour IV infusion and carboplatin IV at the dose required to obtain an area under the concentration-time curve (AUC) of 6 mg/mL per minute on day 1 once every 3 weeks.

Median survival was similar in patients receiving docetaxel and cisplatin compared with those receiving vinorelbine and cisplatin. Among patients receiving docetaxel and cisplatin, at least 62% of the known survival effect of adding vinorelbine to cisplatin was maintained. The use of the docetaxel/carboplatin regimen did not prolong survival compared with the vinorelbine/cisplatin regimen, and less than 50% of the known survival effect of adding vinorelbine to cisplatin was maintained.

Hematologic toxicity was frequent for all 3 regimens. Alopecia (75 versus 42%), fluid retention (54 versus 42%) including peripheral edema (34 versus 18%), diarrhea (47 versus 25%), and nail disorders (14 versus less than 1%) occurred more frequently in patients receiving docetaxel and cisplatin. Grade 3 or 4 anemia (25 versus 7%), grade 3 or 4 nausea (17 versus 10%), and grade 3 or 4 vomiting (16 versus 8%) were more common in patients receiving vinorelbine and cisplatin.

Docetaxel as Second-line Therapy for Locally Advanced or Metastatic Disease Docetaxel is used alone as second-line therapy for locally advanced or metastatic non-small cell lung cancer in patients with disease that has recurred or progressed following prior treatment with platinum-based chemotherapy.

A small survival benefit has been demonstrated for the use of platinum-based (cisplatin) chemotherapy in selected patients with unresectable, locally advanced or metastatic non-small cell lung cancer who have a good performance status. Platinum-based chemotherapy regimens currently are preferred for the treatment of non-small cell lung cancer. (See Uses: Non-small Cell Lung Cancer in Cisplatin 10:00 for comprehensive discussion.) Use of chemotherapy for the treatment of advanced non-small cell lung cancer generally is advised only in patients with good performance status (ECOG performance status of 0 or 1, and 2 in selected patients) and evaluable lesions so that treatment can be discontinued if the disease does not respond. The decision to use chemotherapy must be individualized according to several factors, including patient preference, toxicity, survival benefit, quality of life, and cost of treatment.

The current indication is based on the results of 2 randomized trials that established the use of docetaxel 75 mg/m^2 as a tolerable dose level for patients who had previously received platinum-based chemotherapy for advanced non-small cell lung cancer. In a randomized trial, median survival was prolonged and the 1-year survival rate was higher in patients receiving docetaxel (75 mg/m^2) versus best supportive care for the treatment of unresectable locally advanced or metastatic (stage IIIB or IV) non-small cell lung cancer that had previously been treated with platinum-containing chemotherapy. In another randomized trial, patients receiving docetaxel (75 mg/m^2) experienced higher response rates (all partial responses) and a higher 1-year survival rate but similar median survival compared with those receiving a control regimen of vinorelbine or ifosfamide for advanced non-small cell lung cancer previously treated with platinum-containing chemotherapy. In both randomized trials, the optimum dosage of docetaxel was 75 mg/m^2 by 1-hour IV infusion once every 3 weeks; higher doses of docetaxel (100 mg/m^2) were associated with excessive toxicity. Docetaxel at a dose of 100 mg/m^2 caused unacceptable hematologic toxicity, infections, and treatment-related mortality, and the use of this higher dose in this patient population is not recommended. Of the 5 patients who died from treatment-related toxicity while receiving docetaxel 75 mg/m^2 in the 2 randomized trials, 3 had a performance status of 2 upon entry to the study.

■ Prostate Cancer Docetaxel is used in combination with prednisone for the treatment of androgen-independent (hormone-refractory) metastatic prostate cancer.

The current indication is based on the results of a multicenter, randomized, active-control trial involving 1006 patients with androgen-independent metastatic prostate cancer receiving prednisone with either docetaxel or the active control, mitoxantrone. Treatment consisted of docetaxel 75 mg/m^2 as a 1-hour IV infusion once every 3 weeks for up to 10 cycles or docetaxel 30 mg/m^2 as a 30-minute IV infusion once weekly for the first 5 weeks in a 6-week cycle for up to 5 cycles. The active control regimen was mitoxantrone 12 mg/m^2 as a 30-minute IV infusion once every 3 weeks for 10 cycles. Each patient also received prednisone 5 mg orally twice daily continually.

Median survival was prolonged (18.9 versus 16.5 months) in patients receiving the docetaxel once-every-3-weeks regimen and prednisone compared with those receiving mitoxantrone and prednisone. No difference in survival was observed for patients receiving the docetaxel once-weekly regimen and prednisone compared with those receiving mitoxantrone and prednisone.

Anemia (66 versus 58%), alopecia (65 versus 13%), fatigue (53 versus 35%), grade 3 or 4 neutropenia (32 versus 22%), infection (32 versus 20%), diarrhea (32 versus 10%), nail changes (30 versus 8%), sensory neuropathy (30 versus 7%), fluid retention (24 versus 4%) including peripheral edema (18 versus 2%), stomatitis (20 versus 8%), and taste disturbance (18 versus 7%) occurred more frequently in patients receiving docetaxel and prednisone. Left ventricular cardiac dysfunction (22 versus 10%) was more frequent in patients receiving mitoxantrone and prednisone. The most frequent adverse effects in patients receiving docetaxel and prednisone included anemia (66%), alopecia (65%), fatigue (53%), neutropenia (41%), and nausea (41%).

■ Gastric Cancer Docetaxel is used in combination with cisplatin and fluorouracil for the initial treatment of advanced gastric adenocarcinoma, including adenocarcinoma of the gastroesophageal junction.

The current indication is based on the results of a multicenter, open-label, randomized trial in which 445 patients received either docetaxel/cisplatin/fluorouracil or cisplatin/fluorouracil for the initial treatment of advanced gastric adenocarcinoma, including gastric adenocarcinoma of the gastroesophageal junction. Treatment regimens consisted of docetaxel 75 mg/m^2 as a 1-hour IV infusion on day 1 in combination with cisplatin 75 mg/m^2 as a 1-hour to 3-hour IV infusion on day 1 and fluorouracil 750 mg/m^2 as a continuous IV infusion daily for 5 days (on days 1–5) in 3-week cycles; or cisplatin 100 mg/m^2 on day 1 and fluorouracil 1000 mg/m^2 daily for 5 days (on days 1–5) in 4-week cycles. Most (71%) of the patients were Caucasian males, and the median age was 55 years; 19% of the patients had undergone prior curative surgery and 12% of patients had undergone palliative surgery. The median number of cycles of therapy administered per patient was 6 cycles (range: 1–16 cycles) for those receiving docetaxel/cisplatin/fluorouracil and 4 cycles (range: 1–12 cycles) for those receiving cisplatin/fluorouracil.

Patients receiving docetaxel, cisplatin, and fluorouracil had longer median time to progression (5.6 versus 3.7 months) and prolonged survival (9.2 versus 8.6 months) compared with those receiving cisplatin and fluorouracil as first-line therapy for advanced gastric cancer.

Neutropenia (96 versus 83%) including severe neutropenia (82 versus 57%), diarrhea (78 versus 50%) including severe diarrhea (20 versus 8%), alopecia (66 versus 41%), neurosensory toxicity (38 versus 25%), fever in the absence of infection (36 versus 23%), febrile neutropenia (16 versus 4%), and fluid retention (15 versus 4%) occurred more frequently in patients receiving docetaxel with cisplatin and fluorouracil. Thrombocytopenia (39 versus 26%) occurred more frequently in patients receiving cisplatin and fluorouracil. The most frequent adverse effects in patients receiving docetaxel with cisplatin and fluorouracil for advanced gastric cancer were anemia (97%), neutropenia (96%) including severe neutropenia (82%), diarrhea (78%), nausea (73%), vomiting (66%), alopecia (66%), lethargy (63%), stomatitis (59%), and anorexia (51%).

■ Head and Neck Cancer Docetaxel is used in combination with cisplatin and fluorouracil as induction chemotherapy for locally advanced squamous cell carcinoma of the head and neck.

The current indication is based on the results of 2 randomized trials in which patients received induction chemotherapy with cisplatin and fluorouracil, with or without docetaxel, followed by radiotherapy or chemoradiotherapy for locally advanced squamous cell carcinoma of the head and neck.

In the first randomized trial (TAX323), a multicenter, open-label study, 358 patients with inoperable locally advanced squamous cell carcinoma of the head and neck received induction chemotherapy with either docetaxel/cisplatin/fluorouracil or cisplatin/fluorouracil. All patients had a WHO performance status of 0 or 1. The median age of patients in the study was 53 years.

Treatment regimens consisted of docetaxel 75 mg/m^2 as a 1-hour IV infusion on day 1, followed by cisplatin 75 mg/m^2 as a 1-hour IV infusion on day 1, followed by fluorouracil 750 mg/m^2 daily as a continuous IV infusion on days 1–5 (the TPF regimen); or cisplatin 100 mg/m^2 as a 1-hour IV infusion on day 1, followed by fluorouracil 1000 mg/m^2 daily as a continuous IV infusion on days 1–5 (the PF regimen). Each regimen was administered every 3 weeks for up to 4 cycles. At an interval of 4–7 weeks following completion of chemotherapy, patients with disease that did not progress also received locoregional radiation therapy with either a conventional fraction regimen (1.8–2 Gy once daily for 5 days per week for a total dose of 66–70 Gy) or an accelerated or hyperfractionated regimen (twice daily with a minimum interfraction interval of 6 hours for 5 days per week for a total dose of 70 Gy or 74 Gy, respectively). Surgical resection was allowed following completion of chemotherapy, preceding or following radiation therapy.

At a median follow-up of 34 months, patients receiving docetaxel in combination with cisplatin and fluorouracil for inoperable locally advanced squamous cell carcinoma of the head and neck had prolonged median progression-free survival (11 versus 8 months) compared with those receiving cisplatin and fluorouracil. At a median follow-up of 51 months, patients receiving the docetaxel-containing regimen also had prolonged median overall survival (19 versus 14 months).

Alopecia (81 versus 43%), grade 3 or 4 neutropenia (76 versus 53%), and grade 3 or 4 leukopenia (42 versus 23%) occurred more frequently in patients receiving docetaxel/cisplatin/fluorouracil. Thrombocytopenia (47 versus 24%) including grade 3 or 4 thrombocytopenia (18 versus 5%), vomiting (39 versus 26%), toxic death (6 versus 2%), and hearing loss (3 versus 0%) occurred more frequently in patients receiving cisplatin/fluorouracil. The most frequent adverse effects in patients receiving docetaxel with cisplatin and fluorouracil as induction chemotherapy for locally advanced head and neck cancer followed by radiotherapy were neutropenia (93%) including grade 3 or 4 neutropenia (76%), anemia (89%), alopecia (81%), nausea (47%), stomatitis (42%), and lethargy (41%).

In the second randomized trial (TAX324), a multicenter, open-label study, 501 patients with locally advanced squamous cell carcinoma of the head and neck who had unresectable disease or disease with low chance of surgical cure, or who were candidates for organ preservation received induction chemotherapy with either docetaxel/cisplatin/fluorouracil or cisplatin/fluorouracil. All patients had a WHO performance status of 0 or 1. The median age of patients in the study was 55–56 years.

Treatment regimens consisted of docetaxel 75 mg/m^{2}as a 1-hour IV infusion on day 1, followed by cisplatin 100 mg/m^2 as a 30-minute to 3-hour IV infusion on day 1, followed by fluorouracil 1000 mg/m^2 daily as a continuous IV infusion on days 1–4 (the TPF regimen); or cisplatin 100 mg/m^2 as a 30-minute to 3-hour IV infusion on day 1, followed by fluorouracil 1000 mg/m^2 daily as a continuous IV infusion on days 1–5 (the PF regimen). Each regimen was administered every 3 weeks for up to 3 cycles. At 3–8 weeks following the start of the last cycle of induction chemotherapy, patients with disease that did not progress received 7 weeks of chemoradiotherapy. Radiotherapy was administered with megavoltage equipment as once daily fractionation (2 Gy daily for 5 days per week for 7 weeks for a total dose of 70–72 Gy). During radiotherapy, carboplatin (at the dose required to obtain an AUC of 1.5 mg/mL per minute) was administered once weekly as a 1-hour IV infusion for up to 7 doses. Surgical resection was allowed at any time following the completion of chemoradiotherapy.

Patients receiving docetaxel/cisplatin/fluorouracil had prolonged overall survival (71 versus 30 months, hazard ratio for death: 0.70) compared with those receiving cisplatin/fluorouracil as induction chemotherapy for locally advanced squamous cell carcinoma of the head and neck.

Neutropenia of grade 3 or 4 in severity (84 versus 56%) and alopecia (68 versus 44%) occurred more frequently in patients receiving docetaxel/cisplatin/fluorouracil. Constipation (38 versus 27%) was more frequent in patients receiving cisplatin/fluorouracil. The most frequent adverse effects in patients receiving docetaxel with cisplatin and fluorouracil as induction chemotherapy for locally advanced head and neck cancer followed by chemoradiotherapy were neutropenia (95%) including grade 3 or 4 neutropenia (84%), anemia (90%), nausea (76%), alopecia (68%), stomatitis (66%), lethargy (61%), vomiting (56%), diarrhea (48%), and anorexia (40%).

■ Ovarian Cancer Docetaxel in combination with carboplatin is used as an alternative regimen for the first-line treatment of ovarian epithelial cancer†.

In a randomized trial involving 1077 patients with stage Ic–IV ovarian epithelial cancer, patients received either docetaxel/carboplatin or paclitaxel/carboplatin. Treatment regimens consisted of docetaxel 75 mg/m^2 as a 1-hour IV infusion followed by carboplatin (at the dose required to obtain an AUC of 5 mg/mL per minute) as a 1-hour IV infusion; or paclitaxel 175 mg/m^2 as a 3-hour IV infusion followed by carboplatin (at the dose required to obtain an AUC of 5 mg/mL per minute) as a 1-hour IV infusion. The treatment regimens were repeated every 3 weeks for 6 cycles of therapy; patients who responded to combination therapy then could receive an additional 3 cycles of carboplatin alone. Median progression-free survival was similar (about 15 months) between the groups. Grade 3 or 4 neutropenia (94 versus 84%) and complicated neutropenia (25 versus 5%) occurred more frequently in patients receiving docetaxel and carboplatin. GI toxicity, peripheral edema, allergic reactions, and nail changes also were more frequent in patients receiving docetaxel and carboplatin. Neurotoxicity, including neurosensory toxicity (78 versus 45%) and neuromotor toxicity (16 versus 9%), occurred more frequently in patients receiving paclitaxel and carboplatin. Arthralgia, myalgia, alopecia, and abdominal pain also were more frequent in patients receiving paclitaxel and carboplatin.

Docetaxel also is used for the treatment of recurrent or persistent ovarian epithelial cancer that is platinum-resistant or platinum-refractory†.

Dosage and Administration

■ **Reconstitution and Administration** Docetaxel is administered by IV infusion over a 1-hour period under ambient room temperature and lighting conditions. Infusion of the drug over longer periods (e.g., 6 or 24 hours) or the use of frequently repeated infusions (e.g., over 5 days) was associated with clinically important and dose-limiting mucositis in phase 1 studies.

Caution should be exercised when preparing and handling docetaxel solutions, and the use of protective gloves is recommended. Skin accidentally exposed to the drug should be immediately and thoroughly washed with soap and water. If the drug comes into contact with mucous membranes, the affected area should be flushed immediately and thoroughly with water.

Docetaxel is commercially available as an injection concentrate and as a lyophilized powder. The lyophilized powder must be reconstituted and then diluted to prepare a final docetaxel infusion solution. *Docetaxel injection concentrate must be diluted prior to IV administration.* The proper procedure for preparing a final docetaxel infusion solution from an injection concentrate may vary by manufacturer (i.e., some manufacturers' preparations may require one dilution step, whereas other manufacturers' preparations may require 2 dilution steps). Taxotere® injection concentrate has been reformulated to require one dilution step rather than 2 dilution steps. In addition, injection concentrates available from various manufacturers may contain different concentrations of the drug. *The manufacturer's instructions for the specific formulation should be consulted to ensure that the correct preparation procedure is followed.* Formulations requiring 2 dilution steps should not be used with formulations requiring one dilution step.

Because reconstituted and diluted docetaxel solutions are supersaturated, crystallization may occur over time. Docetaxel injection concentrate and reconstituted and diluted solutions of the drug should be inspected visually for particulate matter and discoloration whenever solution and container permit. If the solution is not clear or appears to have precipitation, the solution should be discarded.

Contact of docetaxel injection concentrate or reconstituted docetaxel solution with plasticized polyvinyl chloride (PVC) equipment or devices used to prepare solutions for infusion is *not* recommended. Polysorbate 80 can cause leaching of diethylhexyl phthalate (DEHP) from PVC containers and, following dilution of docetaxel injection concentrate in PVC containers, substantial leaching of DEHP occurs in a time-dependent and concentration-dependent manner. To minimize exposure of the patient to leached DEHP, final diluted docetaxel solutions for infusion preferably should be stored in glass or polypropylene containers or in plastic (polypropylene or polyolefin) bags and administered through polyethylene-lined administration sets.

Dilution of Docetaxel Injection Concentrate Requiring One Dilution Step If the vial containing docetaxel injection concentrate has been stored in the refrigerator, it should be allowed to stand at room temperature for approximately 5 minutes prior to dilution. When the docetaxel injection concentrate is a formulation that requires one dilution step, the required amount of docetaxel injection concentrate should be withdrawn from the vial using a syringe with a 21-gauge needle and injected into a 250-mL infusion bag or bottle containing either 0.9% sodium chloride injection or 5% dextrose injection to produce a final solution with a docetaxel concentration of 0.3–0.74 mg/mL. If doses larger than 200 mg of docetaxel are required, the volume of IV solution should be increased accordingly so that the docetaxel concentration does not exceed 0.74 mg/mL. The final diluted docetaxel solution for infusion should be mixed thoroughly by gentle manual rotation.

Dilution of Docetaxel Injection Concentrate Requiring Two Dilution Steps When the docetaxel injection concentrate is a formulation that requires 2 dilution steps, the docetaxel injection concentrate is first diluted with the diluent supplied by the manufacturer (13% w/v polyethylene glycol 400 in water for injection) to prepare the initial diluted docetaxel solution, and then the initial diluted docetaxel solution is further diluted to make the final dilution of docetaxel solution for infusion.

For preparation of the initial diluted docetaxel solution, the entire contents of the vial of diluent supplied by the manufacturer (approximately 1.95 mL of diluent for docetaxel 20 mg and approximately 7.2 mL of diluent for docetaxel 80 mg) should be added to the appropriate vial of docetaxel injection concentrate to create an initial diluted solution of docetaxel 10 mg/mL. The vial should be inverted repeatedly for at least 45 seconds to fully mix the concentrate and the diluent; the vial should not be shaken. The initial diluted docetaxel solution should be clear but there may be some foam on top because of the presence of polysorbate 80. The solution should be allowed to stand for a few minutes to let the foam dissipate, and then preparation may continue even if some foam remains. The initial diluted docetaxel solution may be used immediately to prepare the final diluted docetaxel solution for infusion or it may be stored either in the refrigerator or at room temperature for up to 8 hours.

For preparation of the final diluted docetaxel solution for infusion, the required amount of the initial diluted docetaxel solution (docetaxel 10 mg/mL) should be injected into a 250-mL infusion bag or bottle containing either 0.9% sodium chloride injection or 5% dextrose injection to produce a final solution with a docetaxel concentration of 0.3–0.74 mg/mL. If doses larger than 200 mg of docetaxel are required, the volume of IV solution should be increased accordingly so that the docetaxel concentration does not exceed 0.74 mg/mL. The final diluted docetaxel solution for infusion should be mixed thoroughly by manual rotation.

Reconstitution and Dilution of Docetaxel Lyophilized Powder Commercially available docetaxel powder for injection must be reconstituted and diluted prior to IV infusion. The drug should be reconstituted with the diluent supplied by the manufacturer (ethanol 35.4% w/w and polysorbate 80). The appropriate number of diluent vials and vials containing docetaxel lyophilized powder should be removed from the refrigerator and allowed to stand at room temperature for approximately 5 minutes prior to reconstitution. The powder is reconstituted by withdrawing 1 mL of diluent using a 1-mL syringe with an 18- or 21-gauge needle and adding the diluent to a vial labeled as containing docetaxel 20 mg to provide a solution containing 20 mg in 0.8 mL or by withdrawing 4 mL of diluent using a 4-mL syringe with an 18- or 21-gauge needle and adding the diluent to a vial labeled as containing docetaxel 80 mg to provide a solution containing 24 mg/mL of the drug. The vial should be shaken well to ensure complete dissolution of the drug. The resulting solution should be clear but may contain some air bubbles because of the presence of polysorbate 80. The solution should be allowed to stand for a few minutes to let the bubbles dissipate. The reconstituted docetaxel solution may be used immediately to prepare the final diluted docetaxel solution for infusion or it may be stored either in a refrigerator or at room temperature for up to 8 hours.

For preparation of the final diluted docetaxel solution for infusion, the required amount of reconstituted docetaxel solution should be injected into a 250-mL infusion bag or bottle containing 0.9% sodium chloride injection or 5% dextrose injection to produce a final solution with a docetaxel concentration of 0.3–0.74 mg/mL. If doses larger than 200 mg of docetaxel are required, the volume of IV solution should be increased accordingly so that the docetaxel concentration does not exceed 0.74 mg/mL. The final diluted docetaxel solution for infusion should be mixed thoroughly by manual rotation.

Dispensing and Administration Precautions The manufacturer states that formation of particulate matter in docetaxel solutions has not been observed when the drug has been administered at recommended doses; therefore, the use of inline filters with docetaxel infusion solutions is neither required nor recommended. Medication errors have occurred that involved confusion between docetaxel (Taxotere®) and paclitaxel (Taxol®). Two pharmacists should provide independent confirmation that the correct drug is being ordered before chemotherapy is dispensed, and two nurses should confirm that the correct drug has been dispensed for the correct patient before administering the medication. (See Cautions: Precautions and Contraindications.)

■ **Dosage** The incidence of mortality associated with docetaxel therapy is higher in patients with hepatic impairment (see Dosage and Administration: Dosage in Renal and Hepatic Impairment) and in patients receiving higher doses of the drug.

Concomitant use of potent inhibitors of cytochrome P-450 (CYP) isoenzyme 3A4 (CYP3A4) (e.g., atazanavir, clarithromycin, indinavir, itraconazole, ketoconazole, nefazodone, nelfinavir, ritonavir, saquinavir, telithromycin, voriconazole) may increase docetaxel exposure and should be avoided. If such concomitant use cannot be avoided, a reduction in docetaxel dosage with careful monitoring for toxicity should be considered. Based on limited pharmacokinetic data, the manufacturers state that a 50% reduction in docetaxel dosage may be considered in patients requiring concomitant therapy with a potent CYP3A4 inhibitor; however, there are no clinical data with use of this adjusted docetaxel dosage. (See Drug Interactions: Drugs Affecting or Metabolized by Hepatic Microsomal Enzymes.)

Premedication Regimen All patients should be premedicated with oral corticosteroids before docetaxel administration to reduce the severity of hypersensitivity reactions and to reduce the incidence and severity of fluid retention. For patients receiving docetaxel for hormone-refractory metastatic prostate cancer, the manufacturers recommend a regimen of oral dexamethasone 8 mg at 12 hours, 3 hours, and 1 hour prior to the infusion of docetaxel. For patients receiving docetaxel for other cancers, the manufacturer recommends a regimen of oral dexamethasone 8 mg twice daily for 3 days, starting 1 day prior to docetaxel administration.

Breast Cancer The manufacturers state that prophylaxis with granulocyte colony-stimulating factor (G-CSF) may be used to reduce the risk of hematologic toxicity associated with docetaxel therapy. Some clinicians recommend primary prophylaxis with G-CSF in patients receiving docetaxel with an anthracycline agent for breast cancer.

Adjuvant Therapy for Breast Cancer. For the adjuvant treatment of operable node-positive breast cancer, the recommended dosage is docetaxel 75 mg/m^2 as a 1-hour IV infusion administered 1 hour following doxorubicin 50 mg/m^2 IV and cyclophosphamide 500 mg/m^2 IV; this regimen is administered once every 3 weeks for up to 6 courses of therapy.

Advanced Breast Cancer. Optimum dosage of docetaxel for the treatment of advanced or metastatic breast cancer has not been established. The manufacturers currently recommend a docetaxel regimen of 60–100 mg/m^2 infused IV over 1 hour and repeated every 3 weeks as tolerated in patients with locally advanced or metastatic breast cancer after failure of prior chemotherapy.

Among patients who are dosed initially at docetaxel 60 mg/m^2 and who do not experience severe adverse effects (e.g., febrile neutropenia, severe neutropenia for more than 1 week, severe or cumulative cutaneous reactions, or severe peripheral neuropathy), higher doses of docetaxel may be tolerated.

In phase 2 studies, patients received a median of 4 or 5 cycles of docetaxel therapy; however, the usual course of therapy remains to be established.

Non-small Cell Lung Cancer **First-line Therapy for Advanced Disease.** For the first-line treatment of unresectable, locally advanced or metastatic non-small cell lung cancer, the recommended dosage is docetaxel 75 mg/m^2 administered as a 1-hour IV infusion followed by cisplatin 75 mg/m^2 IV administered over 30–60 minutes; this regimen is administered once every 3 weeks.

Second-line Therapy for Advanced Disease. When used as monotherapy for the second-line treatment of non-small cell lung cancer, docetaxel 75 mg/m^2 IV is administered as a 1-hour infusion once every 3 weeks; higher doses of docetaxel are associated with excessive toxicity in this patient population, including increased rates of hematologic toxicity, infection, and treatment-related mortality, and are *not* recommended.

Prostate Cancer For the treatment of hormone-refractory metastatic prostate cancer, the recommended dosage is docetaxel 75 mg/m^2 administered as a 1-hour IV infusion once every 3 weeks. Prednisone 5 mg orally twice daily is administered continually.

Gastric Cancer Premedication with antiemetic agents and adequate hydration for cisplatin administration are required. Primary prophylaxis with G-CSF should be considered.

For the first-line treatment of gastric adenocarcinoma, the recommended dosage is docetaxel 75 mg/m^2 as a 1-hour IV infusion on day 1 followed by cisplatin 75 mg/m^2 as a 1-hour to 3-hour IV infusion on day 1 followed by fluorouracil 750 mg/m^2 as a 24-hour continuous IV infusion daily for 5 days (days 1–5) initiated upon completion of the cisplatin infusion; this regimen is repeated every 3 weeks.

Head and Neck Cancer Premedication with antiemetic agents and adequate hydration preceding and following cisplatin administration are required. Prophylaxis for neutropenic infections also should be administered. In the randomized trials, all patients receiving the docetaxel-containing regimen were given prophylactic antibiotic therapy.

Induction Chemotherapy Followed by Radiotherapy. For induction chemotherapy of inoperable locally advanced squamous cell carcinoma of the head and neck, the recommended dosage is docetaxel 75 mg/m^2 as a 1-hour IV infusion (day 1) followed by cisplatin 75 mg/m^2 as a 1-hour IV infusion (day 1) followed by fluorouracil 750 mg/m^2 as a 24-hour continuous IV infusion daily for 5 days (days 1–5) initiated upon completion of the cisplatin infusion; this regimen is administered once every 3 weeks for up to 4 cycles. Following the completion of chemotherapy, patients should receive radiotherapy.

Induction Chemotherapy Followed by Chemoradiotherapy. For induction chemotherapy of locally advanced squamous cell carcinoma of the head and neck in patients who have unresectable disease or disease with low chance of surgical cure, or who are candidates for organ preservation, the recommended dosage is docetaxel 75 mg/m^2 as a 1-hour IV infusion (day 1) followed by cisplatin 100 mg/m^2 as a 30-minute to 3-hour IV infusion (day 1) followed by fluorouracil 1000 mg/m^2 as a 24-hour continuous IV infusion daily for 4 days (days 1–4); this regimen is administered once every 3 weeks for up to 3 cycles. Following the completion of chemotherapy, patients should receive chemoradiotherapy.

Dosage Modification for Toxicity and Contraindications for Continued Therapy Adjustment of docetaxel dosage may be required according to toxicity. When docetaxel is used in combination regimens, adjustment of dosage for the other drugs may be necessary. In addition to the dosage adjustments for cisplatin and fluorouracil described here, also see the manufacturers' labelings.

Hematologic Toxicity. For patients who experience neutropenia and/or thrombocytopenia, docetaxel doses should be withheld until neutrophil counts are at least 1500/mm^3 and platelet counts exceed 100,000/mm^3.

For patients who have experienced severe neutropenia (neutrophil count less than 500/mm^3) for at least 7 days, febrile neutropenia, or a grade 4 infection during a cycle of therapy, a 25% reduction in the dose of docetaxel is recommended for subsequent cycles.

Among patients receiving docetaxel monotherapy for breast cancer who are dosed initially at 100 mg/m^2 and who experience either febrile neutropenia or severe neutropenia (neutrophil count less than 500/mm^3) for more than 1 week, the manufacturer recommends a 25% reduction in the dose (from 100 to 75 mg/m^2) for subsequent courses of therapy. If the patient continues to experience these reactions, either the dose of docetaxel should be reduced further to 55 mg/m^2 or the drug should be discontinued.

Among patients receiving docetaxel with doxorubicin and cyclophosphamide for the adjuvant treatment of breast cancer who are dosed initially at 75 mg/m^2, those who experience febrile neutropenia should receive G-CSF for all subsequent cycles of therapy. If febrile neutropenia persists, G-CSF should be continued and the docetaxel dose should be reduced to 60 mg/m^2.

Among patients receiving docetaxel monotherapy for advanced non-small cell lung cancer who are dosed initially at 75 mg/m^2 and who experience severe neutropenia (neutrophil count less than 500/mm^3) for more than 1 week or febrile neutropenia, treatment with the drug should be interrupted. Upon resolution of the toxicity, therapy may be resumed at a reduced dose of docetaxel 55 mg/m^2.

Among patients receiving docetaxel in combination with cisplatin for advanced non-small cell lung cancer who are dosed initially at 75 mg/m^2 and who experience a nadir platelet count of less than 25,000/mm^3 during the previous course of therapy or febrile neutropenia, the docetaxel dose should be reduced to 65 mg/m^2 for subsequent cycles. If toxicity persists, further reduction to a docetaxel dose of 50 mg/m^2 is recommended. For recommendations for cisplatin dosage reduction, consult the manufacturer's labeling.

Among patients receiving docetaxel with prednisone for advanced prostate cancer who have experienced severe neutropenia (less than 500/mm^3) for at least 7 days or febrile neutropenia, the docetaxel dose should be reduced from 75 mg/m^2 to 60 mg/m^2. If these reactions persist at a docetaxel dose of 60 mg/m^2, treatment should be discontinued.

Among patients receiving docetaxel in combination with cisplatin and fluorouracil for either advanced gastric cancer or locally advanced head and neck cancer who experience neutropenia lasting more than 7 days, febrile neutropenia, or documented infection with neutropenia, the use of G-CSF during the second or subsequent cycles of therapy is recommended. If the patient experiences an episode of prolonged neutropenia, febrile neutropenia, or neutropenic infection despite use of G-CSF, the docetaxel dose should be reduced from 75 mg/m^2 to 60 mg/m^2. If the patient experiences subsequent episodes of complicated neutropenia, the docetaxel dose should be reduced from 60 mg/m^2 to 45 mg/m^2. If toxicity persists, treatment should be discontinued.

Among patients receiving docetaxel in combination with cisplatin and fluorouracil for either advanced gastric cancer or locally advanced head and neck cancer who experience grade 4 thrombocytopenia, the docetaxel dose should be reduced from 75 mg/m^2 to 60 mg/m^2. If toxicity persists, treatment should be discontinued.

Hypersensitivity. If signs or symptoms of a severe reaction (e.g., hypotension requiring treatment, bronchospasm/dyspnea requiring bronchodilators, generalized rash/erythema, anaphylaxis) occur during administration of the drug, the infusion should be discontinued immediately and aggressive symptomatic therapy instituted as necessary. Docetaxel therapy should *not* be reinitiated in patients experiencing severe hypersensitivity reactions.

Mild manifestations, such as pruritus, flushing, or localized skin reactions, do not require interruption of therapy; however, decreasing the infusion rate until recovery from symptoms may be considered.

Dermatologic Toxicity. Among patients receiving docetaxel monotherapy for breast cancer who are dosed initially at 100 mg/m^2 and who experience severe or cumulative cutaneous reactions, the manufacturer recommends a 25% reduction in the dose (from 100 mg/m^2 to 75 mg/m^2) for subsequent courses of therapy. If the patient continues to experience these reactions, either the docetaxel dose should be reduced further to 55 mg/m^2 or the drug should be discontinued.

Among patients receiving docetaxel with doxorubicin and cyclophosphamide for the adjuvant treatment of breast cancer who experience severe or cumulative cutaneous reactions, the docetaxel dose should be reduced from 75 to 60 mg/m^2. If these reactions persist at docetaxel dose 60 mg/m^2, treatment should be discontinued.

Among patients receiving docetaxel monotherapy for advanced non-small cell lung cancer who are dosed initially at 75 mg/m^2 and who experience severe or cumulative cutaneous reactions, treatment with the drug should be interrupted. Upon resolution of the toxicity, therapy may be resumed at a reduced dose of docetaxel 55 mg/m^2.

Among patients receiving docetaxel with prednisone for advanced prostate cancer who experience severe or cumulative cutaneous reactions, the docetaxel dose should be reduced from 75 mg/m^2 to 60 mg/m^2. If these reactions persist at a docetaxel dose of 60 mg/m^2, treatment should be discontinued.

Among patients receiving docetaxel in combination with cisplatin and fluorouracil who experience palmar-plantar toxicity (hand-foot syndrome) that is grade 2 or higher in severity, fluorouracil should be stopped until recovery and then the fluorouracil dose should be reduced by 20%. This dose modification is based on the adjustment used for the advanced gastric cancer study.

Neurologic Toxicity. Among patients receiving docetaxel monotherapy for advanced breast cancer or advanced non-small cell lung cancer who develop grade 3 or higher peripheral neuropathy, docetaxel therapy should be discontinued.

Among patients receiving docetaxel with doxorubicin and cyclophosphamide for the adjuvant treatment of breast cancer or docetaxel with prednisone for advanced prostate cancer who experience moderate neurosensory manifestations, the docetaxel dose should be reduced from 75 mg/m^2 to 60 mg/m^2. If these reactions persist at a docetaxel dose of 60 mg/m^2, treatment should be discontinued.

Among patients receiving docetaxel in combination with cisplatin and fluorouracil who experience grade 2 peripheral neuropathy, the cisplatin dose should be reduced by 20%. For patients who experience grade 3 peripheral neuropathy, treatment should be discontinued. These dose modifications are based on the adjustments used for the advanced gastric cancer study.

GI Toxicity. Among patients receiving docetaxel with doxorubicin and cyclophosphamide for the adjuvant treatment of breast cancer who experience grade 3 or 4 stomatitis, the docetaxel dose should be reduced from 75 mg/m^2 to 60 mg/m^2.

Among patients receiving docetaxel in combination with cisplatin and fluorouracil for either advanced gastric cancer or locally advanced head and neck cancer who experience grade 3 diarrhea, the guidelines for dosage reduction are as follows: after the first episode, the fluorouracil dose should be reduced by 20%; after the second episode, the docetaxel dose should be reduced by 20%. For patients who experience grade 4 diarrhea, the guidelines for dosage reduction are as follows: after the first episode, both the docetaxel dose and the fluorouracil dose should be reduced by 20%; after the second episode, treatment should be discontinued.

Among patients receiving docetaxel in combination with cisplatin and fluorouracil for either advanced gastric cancer or locally advanced head and neck cancer who experience grade 3 stomatitis/mucositis, the guidelines for dosage reduction are as follows: after the first episode, the fluorouracil dose should be reduced by 20%; after the second episode, fluorouracil should be discontinued for all subsequent cycles; after the third episode, the docetaxel dose should be reduced by 20%. For patients who experience grade 4 stomatitis/mucositis, the guidelines for dosage reduction are as follows: after the first episode, fluorouracil should be discontinued for all subsequent cycles; after the second episode, the docetaxel dose should be reduced by 20%.

Hepatic Toxicity. Among patients receiving docetaxel in combination with cisplatin and fluorouracil for advanced gastric cancer who exhibit increases in serum AST and/or ALT exceeding 2.5 times the upper limit of normal (up to 5 times the upper limit of normal) and alkaline phosphatase up to 2.5 times the upper limit of normal, the docetaxel dose should be reduced by 20%. For patients with serum AST and/or ALT exceeding 1.5 times the upper limit of normal (up to 5 times the upper limit of normal) and alkaline phosphatase exceeding 2.5 times the upper limit of normal (up to 5 times the upper limit of normal), the docetaxel dose should be reduced by 20%. For patients with serum AST and/or ALT exceeding 5 times the upper limit of normal and/or alkaline phosphatase exceeding 5 times the upper limit of normal, docetaxel should be discontinued.

Nephrotoxicity. Among patients receiving docetaxel in combination with cisplatin and fluorouracil who experience a rise in serum creatinine concentration that is grade 2 or higher in severity (greater than 1.5 times the normal value) despite adequate hydration, the creatinine clearance should be determined before each subsequent cycle of therapy and the following dose reductions should be considered. These dose modifications are based on the adjustments used for the advanced gastric cancer study.

For patients with a creatinine clearance of 60 mL/minute or higher, the full dose of cisplatin may be given for the subsequent cycle, and the creatinine clearance should be measured prior to each treatment cycle.

For patients with a creatinine clearance of 40–59 mL/minute, the cisplatin dose should be reduced by 50% for the subsequent cycle. If the creatinine clearance exceeds 60 mL/minute at the end of the cycle using the 50% cisplatin dose, the full cisplatin dose may be given for the next cycle. If recovery does not occur at the end of the cycle using the 50% cisplatin dose, cisplatin should be omitted from the next treatment cycle.

For patients with a creatinine clearance less than 40 mL/minute, the cisplatin dose should be omitted for that treatment cycle only. If the creatinine clearance remains low (less than 40 mL/minute) at the end of the treatment cycle omitting the cisplatin dose, cisplatin should be discontinued. If the creatinine clearance exceeds 40 mL/minute but is less than 60 mL/minute at the end of the treatment cycle omitting the cisplatin dose, a 50% cisplatin dose may be given for the next cycle. If the creatinine clearance exceeds 60 mL/minute at the end of the treatment cycle using the 50% cisplatin dose, the full cisplatin dose may be given for the next cycle.

Ototoxicity. Among patients receiving docetaxel in combination with cisplatin and fluorouracil who experience grade 3 ototoxicity, treatment should be discontinued. This dose modification is based on the adjustment used for the advanced gastric cancer study.

Ocular Toxicity. If cystoid macular edema is diagnosed, docetaxel therapy should be discontinued and appropriate treatment initiated. Alternative therapy with a nontaxane antineoplastic agent should be considered.

Other Toxicity. For patients receiving docetaxel alone or in combination with cisplatin for advanced non-small cell lung cancer who experience grade 3 or 4 nonhematologic toxicities, the same recommendations for reduction of the docetaxel dose should be followed as for patients experiencing hematologic toxicities. (See Hematologic Toxicity under Dosage: Dosage Modification for Toxicity and Contraindications for Continued Therapy, in Dosage and Administration.)

Among patients receiving docetaxel in combination with cisplatin and fluorouracil who experience toxicity (except alopecia and anemia) that is higher than grade 3 in severity, chemotherapy should be delayed for up to 2 weeks from the planned date of infusion until resolution of the toxicity to grade 1 or less in severity occurs and then resumption of chemotherapy may be considered. These dose modifications are based on the adjustments used for the advanced gastric cancer study.

■ **Dosage in Renal and Hepatic Impairment** Urinary excretion of docetaxel has been reported to be low (less than 10%), and reduction of dosage in patients with impaired renal function does not appear to be necessary.

Docetaxel clearance appears to be reduced in patients with abnormal liver function, and an increased incidence of adverse effects (including treatment-related mortality) has been reported in patients with moderate to severe hepatic impairment. Therefore, patients with serum total bilirubin exceeding the upper limit of normal, and patients with serum AST and/or ALT exceeding 1.5 times the upper limit of normal concomitant with alkaline phosphatase exceeding 2.5 times the upper limit of normal, generally should not receive docetaxel.

For further information on the handling of antineoplastic agents, see the guidelines at the end of Antineoplastic Agents 10:00.

Cautions

The principal, dose-limiting adverse effect of docetaxel is bone marrow suppression, manifested by neutropenia, leukopenia, thrombocytopenia, and anemia.

The incidence of treatment-related adverse effects associated with docetaxel therapy is increased in patients with abnormal liver function and in those receiving higher doses. (See Cautions: Precautions and Contraindications.) The incidence of adverse effects reported here is based principally upon data from 2045 patients with normal liver function receiving docetaxel 100 mg/m² for various solid tumors, including a subset of 965 patients with locally advanced or metastatic breast cancer and a subset of 61 patients with various tumor types and hepatic dysfunction manifested by elevated results of liver function tests. The incidence of selected adverse effects is reported for differing dose levels (e.g., 60 mg/m² in 174 patients with metastatic breast cancer), combination regimens, and/or patient populations receiving docetaxel for specific cancers when the rates or types of adverse effects differed substantially from the patterns of toxicity reported for the 2045 patients with various solid tumors. This information may include selected adverse effects for patients receiving docetaxel every 3 weeks as follows: at doses of 60, 75, and 100 mg/m² for advanced breast cancer; or at a dose of 75 mg/m² as adjuvant therapy for breast cancer (with doxorubicin and cyclophosphamide), as second-line therapy for advanced non-small cell lung cancer, as first-line therapy for advanced non-small cell lung cancer (with cisplatin), for androgen-independent (hormone-refractory) metastatic prostate cancer (with prednisone), as first-line therapy for advanced gastric cancer (with cisplatin and fluorouracil), and as induction chemotherapy for advanced head and neck cancer (with cisplatin and fluorouracil). Additional incidence data for adverse effects and information on the comparative toxicity of chemotherapy regimens evaluated in clinical trials is discussed in the corresponding Uses section for each cancer. In general, the safety profile of docetaxel in patients being treated for breast cancer or other types of solid tumors is similar. The most common adverse effects of docetaxel across all labeled indications for the drug are infection, neutropenia, anemia, febrile neutropenia, hypersensitivity, thrombocytopenia, neuropathy, dysgeusia, dyspnea, constipation, anorexia, nail disorders, fluid retention, asthenia, pain, nausea, diarrhea, vomiting, mucositis, alopecia, skin reactions, and myalgia.

Death possibly or probably related to treatment occurred in 2% of patients with normal hepatic function receiving docetaxel 100 mg/m² for metastatic breast cancer and in 11.5% of patients receiving docetaxel 100 mg/m² for various tumor types who had hepatic dysfunction. Among patients receiving docetaxel 60 mg/m² for breast cancer, treatment-related mortality occurred in about 1% of patients with normal liver function and in 3 of 7 patients with hepatic dysfunction. Approximately half of these deaths occurred during the first treatment cycle, and sepsis accounted for a majority of the deaths.

■ **Hematologic Effects and Infectious Complications** The frequency and severity of docetaxel-induced hematologic toxicity, febrile reactions and infections, and rates of death caused by sepsis increase with dose and in the presence of hepatic dysfunction. As with paclitaxel, docetaxel-induced myelosuppression may be more severe in patients who have received prior radiation therapy.

Docetaxel-induced neutropenia generally is reversible. Neutropenia secondary to docetaxel, in contrast to that caused by paclitaxel, is not schedule-dependent. Neutropenia (neutrophil count less than 2000/mm³) occurred in almost all patients (96%) receiving docetaxel for solid tumors. Severe (grade 4) neutropenia (less than 500/mm³) occurred in 75% of patients with solid tumors and lasted more than 7 days in about 3% of treatment cycles. Severe neutropenia occurred at a higher rate among the subsets of patients receiving docetaxel for locally advanced or metastatic breast cancer (86%) or patients with hepatic dysfunction (88%). Similarly high rates of neutropenia were reported in patients receiving docetaxel in combination therapy for other cancers except for advanced prostate cancer (41%, grade 3 or 4 in 32%).

The onset of neutropenia is rapid, with neutrophil nadirs generally occurring 7–8 days following docetaxel administration; the median duration of severe (grade 4) neutropenia is about 7 days. Subsequent courses of docetaxel therapy generally do not result in lower neutrophil nadirs than in the initial course, suggesting that the drug may not be irreversibly toxic to stem cells.

Leukopenia (leukocyte count less than 4000/mm³) occurred in almost all patients (96%) receiving docetaxel for solid tumors. Severe leukopenia (less than 1000/mm³) occurred in 32% of patients with solid tumors and at a higher rate among the subsets of patients receiving docetaxel for locally advanced or metastatic breast cancer (44%) or patients with hepatic dysfunction (47%).

Anemia (hemoglobin less than 11 g/dL) occurred in 90% of patients receiving docetaxel for solid tumors. Severe anemia (hemoglobin less than 8 g/dL) occurred in 9% of patients with solid tumors and in 31% of the subset of patients with hepatic dysfunction. Similarly high rates of anemia were reported in patients receiving docetaxel in combination therapy for other cancers except advanced prostate cancer (66%). A lower rate of anemia was reported in patients receiving docetaxel 60 mg/m² for advanced breast cancer (65%). Packed red blood cell transfusions may be required in some patients.

Fever in the absence of infection occurred in 31% of patients receiving docetaxel for solid tumors and in 41% (severe in 8%) of the subset of patients with hepatic dysfunction. Fever in the absence of infection was reported in

46% of patients receiving docetaxel with doxorubicin and cyclophosphamide as adjuvant therapy for breast cancer.

Febrile neutropenia (neutrophil count less than 500/mm^3 with fever greater than 38°C and IV anti-infectives and/or hospitalization required) occurred in 11% of patients receiving docetaxel for solid tumors and in 26% of the subset of patients with hepatic dysfunction. Patients with isolated elevations of serum aminotransferase concentrations (more than 1.5 times the upper limit of normal) had a higher rate of grade 4 febrile neutropenia but the incidence of toxic death was not increased in these patients. Febrile neutropenia (grade 3 or 4 neutropenia with fever greater than 38.1°C) occurred in none of 174 patients receiving docetaxel 60 mg/m^2 for advanced breast cancer. Febrile neutropenia was reported in 25% of patients receiving docetaxel with doxorubicin and cyclophosphamide as adjuvant therapy for breast cancer. Among patients receiving docetaxel with cisplatin and fluorouracil for gastric cancer, febrile neutropenia and/or neutropenic infection occurred in 28% of patients who did not receive granulocyte colony-stimulating factor (G-CSF) versus 12% of patients who did receive G-CSF.

Infection occurred in 22% of patients receiving docetaxel for solid tumors and was severe in 6%. The rate of infection (33%) and severe infection (16%) was higher in the subset of patients with hepatic dysfunction. Fatal sepsis occurred in about 2% of patients receiving docetaxel for solid tumors and in 5% of the subset of patients with hepatic dysfunction. Higher rates of infection were reported in patients receiving docetaxel in combination therapy for the adjuvant treatment of breast cancer (39%), for advanced non-small cell lung cancer (35%), for advanced prostate cancer (32%), and for advanced gastric cancer (29%, grade 3 or 4 in 16%). Neutropenic infection was reported in patients receiving docetaxel in combination regimens for gastric cancer (16%), head and neck cancer (14 or 12%), and adjuvant treatment of breast cancer (12%). Infection occurred in 1% of patients receiving docetaxel 60 mg/m^2 for advanced breast cancer.

Thrombocytopenia (platelet count less than 100,000/mm^3) occurred in 8% of patients receiving docetaxel for solid tumors and in 25% of the subset of patients with hepatic dysfunction. A higher rate of thrombocytopenia (44%), including grade 4 thrombocytopenia (17%), was reported in 18 patients with hepatic dysfunction receiving docetaxel 100 mg/m^2 for metastatic breast cancer. Higher rates of thrombocytopenia also were reported in patients receiving docetaxel in combination therapy for the adjuvant treatment of breast cancer (39%), for advanced gastric cancer (26%), for locally advanced head and neck cancer (24 or 28%), and for advanced non-small cell lung cancer (15%).

Bleeding episodes have occurred in patients receiving docetaxel in clinical trials, including 3 breast cancer patients with severe liver impairment (serum total bilirubin value exceeding 1.7 times the upper limit of normal) who developed fatal GI hemorrhage associated with severe docetaxel-induced thrombocytopenia. GI bleeding also was reported in patients receiving docetaxel with cisplatin and fluorouracil as induction chemotherapy for locally advanced head and neck cancer (approximately 5%). Epistaxis occurred in 6% of patients receiving docetaxel and prednisone for advanced prostate cancer. Disseminated intravascular coagulation, often associated with sepsis or multiorgan failure, has occurred in patients receiving docetaxel.

■ Sensitivity Reactions Docetaxel frequently causes hypersensitivity reactions, which can be severe, and all patients receiving the drug should be premedicated to reduce the severity of these reactions. (See Dosage and Administration: Dosage.) Severe hypersensitivity reactions, characterized by generalized rash/erythema, hypotension and/or bronchospasm, or rarely, fatal anaphylaxis, have occurred in patients receiving docetaxel who received the recommended premedication regimen. Discontinuance of therapy and aggressive management is required in patients experiencing severe hypersensitivity reactions associated with docetaxel. (See Hypersensitivity under Dosage: Dosage Modification for Toxicity and Contraindications for Continued Therapy, in Dosage and Administration.)

Hypersensitivity reactions occurred in 21% of patients receiving docetaxel for solid tumors and were severe in 4%; in the subset of 92 patients receiving the 3-day premedication regimen, hypersensitivity reactions occurred in 15% and were severe in 2%. In the subset of patients with hepatic dysfunction, severe hypersensitivity reactions occurred in 10%. Hypersensitivity reactions or allergic reactions were reported in patients receiving docetaxel in combination therapy for adjuvant treatment of breast cancer (13%), for advanced non-small cell lung cancer (12%), for advanced gastric cancer (10%), and for advanced prostate cancer (8%) and in patients receiving docetaxel alone for non-small cell lung cancer (6%). Allergy (6 or 2%) was reported in patients receiving docetaxel with cisplatin and fluorouracil as induction chemotherapy for locally advanced head and neck cancer. A lower rate of hypersensitivity reactions (about 1%, none severe) was reported in patients receiving docetaxel 60 mg/m^2 for advanced breast cancer.

Docetaxel-induced hypersensitivity reactions almost always occur with the first or second cycle of therapy, usually within a few minutes following initiation of docetaxel infusion. In clinical trials, mild reactions (e.g., flushing, localized skin reactions) generally did not require interruption of docetaxel administration or prevent completion of treatment with the drug. Some mild adverse effects, such as flushing, rash with or without pruritus, chest tightness, back pain, dyspnea, drug fever, or chills, resolved after completion of the infusion and appropriate therapy.

The exact cause of hypersensitivity reactions associated with docetaxel therapy is not known, but they may result from the polysorbate 80 in commercially available docetaxel injection concentrate and/or from docetaxel itself. Both docetaxel and paclitaxel can cause hypersensitivity reactions, despite the fact that the vehicles used for formulation are different; the Cremophor® EL in paclitaxel concentrate for injection has been suggested as a possible cause of hypersensitivity reactions with paclitaxel therapy.

■ Nervous System Effects Because of the alcohol content of parenteral formulations of docetaxel, alcohol intoxication has been reported during postmarketing experience in patients receiving the drug. After a review of the Adverse Event Reporting System (AERS) database and case reports, the US Food and Drug Administration (FDA) identified 3 cases of alcohol intoxication following administration of docetaxel. In these cases, onset of alcohol intoxication occurred during administration or within 24 hours of administration of the drug. Symptoms of alcohol intoxication were transient in one patient. In another patient, symptoms subsided and the infusion was completed at a slower infusion rate.

Adverse neurosensory effects occurred in 49% of patients receiving docetaxel for solid tumors and were severe in 4%. The rate of adverse neurosensory effects was 58% in the subset of patients receiving docetaxel for locally advanced or metastatic breast cancer and 20% in patients receiving docetaxel 60 mg/m^2 for advanced breast cancer. Severe neurosensory effects (i.e., paresthesia, dysesthesia, pain) were reported in 5.5% of patients receiving docetaxel for metastatic breast cancer in clinical trials and required treatment discontinuance in 6.1% of these patients. Adverse neurosensory effects were reported in patients receiving docetaxel in combination therapy for advanced non-small cell lung cancer (47%), advanced gastric cancer (38%), and locally advanced head and neck cancer (18 or 14%) and in patients receiving docetaxel alone for advanced non-small cell lung cancer (23%). Sensory neuropathy was reported in patients receiving docetaxel in combination therapy for advanced prostate cancer (30%) and the adjuvant treatment of breast cancer (26%).

Docetaxel can cause a predominantly sensory neuropathy similar to that reported with paclitaxel administration. The neuropathy usually is characterized by paresthesia or dysesthesia with numbness and tingling in a stocking-and-glove distribution. Some patients also have experienced pain (including burning sensation) in the hands and/or feet.

The frequency and severity of docetaxel-induced neurotoxicity increase with cumulative dose, especially at cumulative doses exceeding 400–600 mg/m^2. Sensory manifestations usually improve or resolve following discontinuance of docetaxel, with most patients experiencing improvement within 9 weeks from onset (range: 0–106 weeks); however, neuropathy may continue to worsen after stopping docetaxel in some patients.

Neuromotor toxicity also has been reported with docetaxel. Motor involvement is less frequent than sensory involvement and is usually only seen in patients who experience relatively severe neuropathy secondary to docetaxel therapy. Neuromotor toxicity has been manifested principally as both proximal and distal muscle weakness in the extremities, predominantly in the legs. Neuromotor toxicity was reported in patients receiving docetaxel in combination therapy for advanced non-small cell lung cancer (19%), advanced gastric cancer (9%), advanced prostate cancer (7%), and locally advanced head and neck cancer (2 or 9%) and in patients receiving docetaxel alone for advanced non-small cell lung cancer (16%). Severe peripheral neuromotor toxicity, consisting principally of distal extremity weakness, was reported in about 4% of patients receiving docetaxel for breast cancer in clinical trials. Although docetaxel-induced neuropathy has been reported in some patients with prior cisplatin therapy, no apparent relationship between docetaxel-induced neuropathy and prior treatment with cisplatin has been observed, and prior neurotoxic therapy may not necessarily predispose patients to docetaxel neuropathy. Neurocortical (5%), neuromotor (4%), and neurocerebellar (2%) toxicity were reported in patients receiving docetaxel with doxorubicin and cyclophosphamide for the adjuvant treatment of breast cancer.

Asthenia occurred in 62% of patients receiving docetaxel for solid tumors and was severe in 13%. Severe asthenia occurred in 25% of the subset of patients with hepatic dysfunction. Severe asthenia was reported in about 15% of patients with metastatic breast cancer treated with docetaxel in clinical trials and required discontinuance of the drug in approximately 2% of patients. Higher rates of asthenia were reported in patients receiving docetaxel in combination therapy for the adjuvant treatment of breast cancer (81%) and for advanced non-small cell lung cancer (74%). Symptoms of fatigue and weakness may persist for a few days to several weeks and may be associated with a deterioration in performance status in patients with progressive disease. Among patients receiving docetaxel in combination therapy, lethargy was reported in patients with advanced gastric cancer (63%, grade 3 or 4 in 21%) and in patients with locally advanced head and neck cancer (41% in TAX323 and 61% in TAX324), and fatigue was reported in patients with advanced prostate cancer (53%).

Dizziness occurred in patients receiving docetaxel in combination therapy for advanced gastric cancer (16%) and locally advanced head and neck cancer (2% in TAX323 and 16% in TAX324). Confusion has been reported in patients receiving docetaxel. Seizures or transient loss of consciousness has been reported rarely in patients receiving docetaxel, sometimes occurring during infusion of the drug.

■ Cardiovascular Effects Hypotension associated with severe hypersensitivity reactions has occurred in patients receiving docetaxel. (See Cautions: Sensitivity Reactions.)

Hypotension was reported in about 3% of patients receiving docetaxel for solid tumors in clinical trials, with approximately 1% of such patients requiring treatment. In selected phase 1 studies of docetaxel therapy in which continuous Holter monitoring was used, no clinically relevant bradycardia or cardiac rhythm disturbances were observed. However, adverse cardiovascular events such as heart failure, sinus tachycardia, atrial flutter, dysrhythmia, unstable angina, pulmonary edema, and hypertension have been reported rarely in patients receiving the drug. A deterioration in left-ventricular ejection fraction (LVEF) by 10% or more associated with a decline to below the institutional lower limit of normal occurred in 8% of patients with metastatic breast cancer receiving docetaxel 100 mg/m^2.

Fluid retention, sometimes severe, has occurred in patients receiving docetaxel despite premedication with dexamethasone. Fluid retention generally is manifested by peripheral edema and weight gain; less frequently, pleural or pericardial effusion and/or ascites may occur. During docetaxel therapy, pleural effusion has been reported in patients with non-small cell lung cancer and lymphedema has been reported in patients with breast cancer.

The exact mechanism by which docetaxel causes fluid retention is unknown; renal, hepatic, cardiac, or endocrinologic abnormalities have not been documented. However, limited data based on capillary filtration tests with technetium-99m albumin and capillaroscopy suggest that an abnormality in capillary permeability may be the cause of the fluid retention. Docetaxel-induced fluid retention usually starts in the lower extremities but may become generalized and appears to be completely (although sometimes slowly) reversible; a median weight gain of 2 kg has been reported with resolution of fluid retention after a median of 16 weeks (range: 0–42+ weeks) from the last infusion of docetaxel. Peripheral edema can be treated with standard measures (e.g., sodium restriction, diuretics).

Fluid retention occurred in 47% of patients receiving docetaxel for solid tumors and was severe in 7%; in the subset of 92 patients receiving the 3-day premedication regimen, fluid retention occurred in 64% and was severe in 6.5%. In the subset of patients receiving docetaxel for locally advanced or metastatic breast cancer, fluid retention occurred in 60% and was severe in 9%. Among patients receiving docetaxel in combination therapy, rates reported for fluid retention were 54% for advanced non-small cell lung cancer, 35% for adjuvant treatment of breast cancer (including peripheral edema in 27% and weight gain in 13%), 15% for advanced gastric cancer (plus edema in 13%), 24% for advanced prostate cancer (including peripheral edema in 18% and weight gain in 7.5%), and 20% (TAX323) or 13% (TAX324) for locally advanced head and neck cancer. Fluid retention was reported in 13% of patients receiving docetaxel 60 mg/m^2 for advanced breast cancer.

The incidence and severity of fluid retention appear to be related to the cumulative dose of docetaxel, increasing in incidence with cumulative doses of 400 mg/m^2 or greater. Premedication with oral corticosteroids has been reported to delay the onset and decrease the severity of fluid retention. In a phase 2 clinical trial of docetaxel as first-line therapy in patients with breast cancer in whom no routine premedication was used, 76% of responding patients discontinued treatment because of fluid retention after a median cumulative dose of 574 mg/m^2. In 92 patients with metastatic breast cancer receiving docetaxel in clinical trials with the recommended 3-day corticosteroid premedication regimen, moderate or severe fluid retention occurred in 27 or 6.5%, respectively; the median cumulative dose associated with the onset of moderate or severe fluid retention was 819 mg/m^2. Severe fluid retention, characterized by poorly tolerated peripheral edema, generalized edema, pleural effusion requiring urgent drainage, dyspnea at rest, cardiac tamponade, and/or pronounced abdominal distention (caused by ascites), may lead to discontinuance of docetaxel therapy. Discontinuance of docetaxel therapy secondary to fluid retention was required in about 10% of these patients; median cumulative dose to treatment discontinuance was 1021 mg/m^2.

Vasodilatation was reported in 27% of patients receiving docetaxel with doxorubicin and cyclophosphamide for the adjuvant treatment of breast cancer. Left ventricular cardiac dysfunction was reported in 10% of patients receiving docetaxel and prednisone for advanced prostate cancer. Cardiac dysrhythmias were reported in patients receiving docetaxel in combination therapy for the adjuvant treatment of breast cancer (8%), for advanced gastric cancer (4%), and for locally advanced head and neck cancer (2% in TAX323 and 6% in TAX324). Congestive heart failure (CHF) was reported in 2% of patients receiving docetaxel with doxorubicin and cyclophosphamide for the adjuvant treatment of breast cancer in the randomized trial, including fatal CHF in 1 patient.

Venous thromboembolic events, including superficial and deep-vein thrombosis and pulmonary embolism, were reported in patients receiving docetaxel with cisplatin and fluorouracil as induction chemotherapy for locally advanced head and neck cancer (3 or 4%). Other adverse cardiovascular effects that have been reported in patients receiving docetaxel include ECG abnormalities, atrial fibrillation, tachycardia, thrombophlebitis, acute pulmonary edema, myocardial ischemia, myocardial infarction, and syncope.

■ **GI Effects** Fatal GI hemorrhage associated with thrombocytopenia has been reported in patients receiving docetaxel for locally advanced or metastatic breast cancer. GI bleeding was reported in 4 or 5% of patients receiving docetaxel in combination therapy for locally advanced head and neck cancer. Colitis/enteritis/large intestine perforation was reported in 7 patients receiving docetaxel with doxorubicin and cyclophosphamide for the adjuvant treatment of breast cancer; discontinuance of therapy was required in 5 of these patients.

Pronounced abdominal distention caused by ascites may be a manifestation of severe fluid retention in patients receiving docetaxel. (See Cautions: Cardiovascular Effects.)

Nausea occurred in 39%, diarrhea in 39%, and vomiting in 22% of patients receiving docetaxel for solid tumors; these adverse GI effects generally are mild to moderate in severity in most patients but were severe in 3–5% of patients. Higher rates of nausea, typically ranging from 70–80%, were reported in patients receiving docetaxel in combination therapy for other cancers in some randomized trials, such as advanced non-small cell lung cancer, gastric cancer (grade 3 or 4 in 16%), locally advanced head and neck cancer (grade 3 or 4 in 14% in TAX324), and breast cancer (adjuvant treatment). Higher rates of vomiting and diarrhea also have been reported in patients receiving docetaxel in combination therapy, particularly when docetaxel is used in combination with cisplatin. Among patients receiving docetaxel with cisplatin and fluorouracil, vomiting occurred in 66% (grade 3 or 4 in 15%) of patients with advanced gastric cancer and 56% of patients with locally advanced head and neck cancer in TAX324. Among patients receiving docetaxel with cisplatin and fluorouracil, diarrhea occurred in 78% (grade 3 or 4 in 20%) of patients with advanced gastric cancer and 48% of patients with locally advanced head and neck cancer in TAX324. Among patients receiving docetaxel and cisplatin for advanced non-small cell lung cancer, vomiting was reported in 55% and diarrhea in 47% of patients. Among patients receiving docetaxel in combination therapy for the adjuvant treatment of breast cancer, vomiting occurred in 44% and diarrhea in 35% of patients.

Stomatitis occurred in 42% of patients receiving docetaxel for solid tumors and was severe in 5.5%. Stomatitis occurred in 52% of the subset of patients receiving docetaxel for locally advanced or metastatic breast cancer, and severe stomatitis was more frequent (13%) in the subset of patients with hepatic dysfunction. Stomatitis was reported at various rates in patients receiving docetaxel in combination therapy for the adjuvant treatment of breast cancer (69%), for locally advanced head and neck cancer (42% in TAX323; 66% in TAX324, grade 3 or 4 in 21%), and for advanced gastric cancer (59%, grade 3 or 4 in 21%). Similar rates of stomatitis were reported in patients receiving docetaxel for advanced non-small cell lung cancer as monotherapy (26%) or in combination therapy (24%). Stomatitis/pharyngitis was reported in 20% of patients receiving docetaxel and prednisone for advanced prostate cancer. Lower rates of stomatitis (19%) and severe stomatitis (about 1%) were reported in patients receiving docetaxel 60 mg/m^2 for advanced breast cancer.

Docetaxel-induced stomatitis (mucositis), is characterized by diffuse ulceration of the lips, tongue, and oral cavity. Mucositis reportedly is schedule-dependent and was observed more commonly in patients receiving longer infusions of docetaxel; radiation-recall mucositis also has been reported with docetaxel therapy.

Anorexia was reported in patients receiving docetaxel in combination therapy for gastric cancer (51%, grade 3 or 4 in 13%), advanced non-small cell lung cancer (42%), adjuvant treatment of breast cancer (22%), advanced prostate cancer (17%), and locally advanced head and neck cancer (16% in TAX323 and 40% in TAX324). Constipation was reported in patients receiving docetaxel in combination therapy for the adjuvant treatment of breast cancer (34%), for advanced gastric cancer (25%), and for locally advanced head and neck cancer (17% in TAX323 and 27% in TAX324). Taste perversion/disturbance was reported in patients receiving docetaxel in combination therapy for the adjuvant treatment of breast cancer (28%) and advanced prostate cancer (18%) and in patients receiving docetaxel alone for non-small cell lung cancer (6%). Altered taste or sense of smell was reported in patients receiving docetaxel with cisplatin and fluorouracil as induction chemotherapy for locally advanced head and neck cancer (10% in TAX323 and 20% in TAX324). Esophagitis/dysphagia/odynophagia was reported in patients receiving docetaxel in combination therapy for advanced gastric cancer (16%) and locally advanced head and neck cancer (13% in TAX323 and 25% in TAX324). Also reported in patients receiving docetaxel in combination therapy were abdominal pain (11% of patients receiving adjuvant treatment for breast cancer), GI pain/cramping (11% of patients with advanced gastric cancer; 8% of patients in TAX323 and 15% of patients in TAX324 for locally advanced head and neck cancer), and heartburn (6% of patients in TAX323 and 13% of patients in TAX324 for locally advanced head and neck cancer).

Other adverse GI effects reported in patients receiving docetaxel include duodenal ulcer, ischemic colitis, intestinal obstruction, ileus, and dehydration caused by adverse GI events. In addition, at least one case of typhlitis (neutropenic enterocolitis) and fatal sepsis secondary to *Clostridium septicum* has been reported with docetaxel.

■ **Dermatologic Effects** Alopecia occurred in 76% of patients receiving docetaxel for solid tumors and at similar rates in patients receiving the drug in combination regimens for other cancers. Alopecia occurred in almost all patients (98%) receiving docetaxel with doxorubicin and cyclophosphamide as adjuvant therapy for breast cancer. A lower rate of alopecia was reported in patients receiving docetaxel alone for advanced non-small cell lung cancer (56%).

Alopecia has a sudden onset and occurs 14–21 days after administration of docetaxel. Patients often experience loss of all body hair, including axillary and pubic hair and that on the extremities, eyelashes, and eyebrows. Alopecia is dose-related and generally occurs at docetaxel doses exceeding 55 mg/m^2. Docetaxel-induced alopecia is fully reversible after treatment discontinuance. Limited data suggest that the use of a cold cap during docetaxel infusion may lessen the incidence and severity of alopecia.

Adverse cutaneous reactions occurred in 48% of patients receiving docetaxel for solid tumors and were severe in 5%. In the subset of patients receiving docetaxel for locally advanced or metastatic breast cancer, 1.6% of patients discontinued therapy because of skin toxicity. A lower rate of cutaneous toxicity (30.5%) was reported in patients receiving docetaxel 60 mg/m^2 for advanced breast cancer. Skin toxicity was reported in patients receiving docetaxel in combination therapy for the adjuvant treatment of breast cancer (26%) and for advanced non-small cell lung cancer (16%) and in patients receiving docetaxel alone for advanced non-small cell lung cancer (20%). Also reported in patients receiving docetaxel in combination therapy were rash/itch (12% of patients with advanced gastric cancer; 12% of patients in TAX323 and 20% of patients in TAX324 for locally advanced head and neck cancer), rash/desquamation (6% of patients with advanced prostate cancer), dry skin (6 or 5% of patients with locally advanced head and neck cancer), and desquamation (4 or 2% of patients with locally advanced head and neck cancer; 2% of patients with advanced gastric cancer).

Generalized rash/erythema associated with severe hypersensitivity reactions have occurred in patients receiving docetaxel. (See Cautions: Sensitivity Reactions.) As with paclitaxel, transient skin changes have been observed in patients experiencing hypersensitivity reactions to docetaxel. In addition, cutaneous reactions, which occasionally are severe, appear to occur more frequently with docetaxel than with paclitaxel therapy. Reversible cutaneous reactions, characterized by rash, including localized eruptions (usually on the feet and/or hands, and less commonly on the arms, face, or trunk) usually associated with pruritus, occur frequently in patients receiving docetaxel. Such eruptions generally occurred within 1 week after docetaxel administration, resolved before the next infusion, and were not disabling. Severe cutaneous toxicity, such as localized erythema and edema of the extremities followed by desquamation, has been observed in patients receiving docetaxel.

Other skin reactions such as macular erythema have been observed at sites of previous tissue injury in patients receiving docetaxel. Cutaneous reactions are dose-dependent and cumulative and rarely have been seen at doses less than 85 mg/m^2. A syndrome of erythrodysesthesia, characterized by a painful, tender, erythematous eruption, frequently followed by tingling and decreased sensation, has been reported with docetaxel therapy. In addition, there have been reports of scleroderma-like changes, usually preceded by peripheral lymphedema and affecting the lower extremities, associated with docetaxel therapy.

In cases of severe skin toxicity, the dosage of docetaxel should be reduced or therapy with the drug should be discontinued. (See Dermatologic Toxicity under Dosage: Dosage Modification for Toxicity and Contraindications for Continued Therapy, in Dosage and Administration.)

Treatment of docetaxel-induced cutaneous reactions, when necessary, generally has been symptomatic. Cutaneous reactions in some patients have been successfully treated with an ointment consisting of glycerin and chlorhexidine. Topical corticosteroids and cool compresses also have been used, especially in patients with erythrodysesthesia. A decreased incidence and severity of cutaneous reactions to docetaxel with recommended corticosteroid premedication has been reported by some clinicians, while others have found no benefit. A severe case of erythrodysesthesia that occurred despite pretreatment with corticosteroids and failed to respond to oral pyridoxine treatment reportedly was treated successfully with localized hypothermia during docetaxel infusion.

Nail changes occurred in 31% of patients receiving docetaxel for solid tumors and were severe in 2.5%. Severe nail disorders were characterized by hypopigmentation or hyperpigmentation and, occasionally, onycholysis and pain; onycholysis occurred in about 1% of patients receiving docetaxel for solid tumors. Nail disorders were reported in patients receiving docetaxel in combination therapy for advanced prostate cancer (30%), adjuvant treatment of breast cancer (18%), advanced non-small cell lung cancer (14%), and advanced gastric cancer (8%) and in patients receiving docetaxel alone for advanced non-small cell lung cancer (11%). Thinning and ridging of the nail plates as well as subungual erythema and subungual hemorrhage also have been reported in patients receiving docetaxel. Nail toxicity appears to be related to the cumulative dose of docetaxel.

Cutaneous lupus erythematosus and bullous eruptions, such as erythema multiforme, Stevens-Johnson syndrome, and toxic epidermal necrolysis, have occurred rarely in patients receiving docetaxel.

■ **Musculoskeletal Effects** Musculoskeletal effects, including arthralgia and/or myalgia, have been reported with docetaxel therapy but appear to be less common than with paclitaxel. Myalgia occurred in 19% of patients receiving docetaxel for solid tumors and was severe in 1.5%; arthralgia occurred in 9%. A similar rate of myalgia was reported in patients receiving docetaxel in combination therapy for advanced non-small cell lung cancer. Myalgia was reported in 27% and arthralgia in 19% of patients receiving docetaxel with doxorubicin and cyclophosphamide for the adjuvant treatment of breast cancer. Lower rates of adverse musculoskeletal effects were reported in patients receiving docetaxel in combination therapy for locally advanced head and neck cancer (myalgia in 10 or 7%), patients receiving docetaxel alone for advanced non-small cell lung cancer (myalgia in 6%, arthralgia in 3%), and patients receiving docetaxel 60 mg/m^2 for advanced breast cancer (myalgia in 3%). Musculoskeletal manifestations usually are mild and transient, occurring within a few days after docetaxel administration and lasting about 4 days, and have been reported to respond to mild analgesics (e.g., acetaminophen) when needed.

■ **Hepatic Effects** Hepatitis, sometimes fatal, has been reported rarely in patients receiving docetaxel. Fatal hepatitis occurred mainly in patients with pre-existing liver disorders. Abnormalities in liver function test results have occurred in patients receiving docetaxel. In clinical trials in the US and Europe in patients with normal liver function test results at baseline, serum total bilirubin values exceeding the upper limit of normal occurred in 8.9% of patients. Increases in serum AST (SGOT) or ALT (SGPT) values to greater than 1.5 times the upper limit of normal were observed in 18.9% of patients, and serum alkaline phosphatase concentrations exceeding 2.5 times normal were observed in 7.3% of patients. In clinical trials, increases in AST or ALT to greater than 1.5 times the upper limit of normal concomitant with increases in serum alkaline phosphatase to greater than 2.5 times the normal value were reported in 4.3% of patients with normal liver function test results at baseline.

■ **Respiratory Effects** Bronchospasm associated with severe hypersensitivity reactions has occurred in patients receiving docetaxel. (See Cautions: Sensitivity Reactions.) Pleural effusion requiring urgent drainage or dyspnea at rest may be manifestations of severe fluid retention in patients receiving docetaxel. (See Cautions: Cardiovascular Effects.)

Adverse pulmonary effects occurred in patients receiving docetaxel (41%), best supportive care (49%), or either vinorelbine or ifosfamide (45%) for advanced non-small cell lung cancer in randomized trials. Dyspnea was reported in 15% of patients receiving docetaxel and prednisone for advanced prostate cancer.

Other adverse pulmonary effects reported in patients receiving docetaxel include acute pulmonary edema, acute respiratory distress syndrome/pneumonitis, interstitial lung disease, and interstitial pneumonia. Pulmonary fibrosis has been reported rarely. Radiation pneumonitis has been reported rarely in patients receiving concomitant radiation therapy.

■ **Local Effects** Local reactions at the injection site occurred in about 4% of patients receiving docetaxel for solid tumors and generally were mild and consisted of hyperpigmentation, inflammation, erythema or dryness of the skin, phlebitis, extravasation, or venous swelling. Extravasation of docetaxel has led to localized pain, discoloration, and erythema, and desquamation has continued for up to 6 weeks in some cases. Specific treatment for docetaxel-induced extravasation reactions currently has not been fully determined. However, the manufacturer recommends using general conservative measures and avoiding the application of warm compresses (which may result in skin discoloration, blistering, and peeling) in the treatment of docetaxel extravasation. Reversible peripheral vein inflammation has been reported rarely with docetaxel administration.

■ **Ocular Effects** Cystoid macular edema has been reported in patients receiving docetaxel.

Lacrimation disorder occurred in 11% and conjunctivitis in 5% of patients receiving docetaxel in combination therapy as adjuvant treatment for breast cancer. Conjunctivitis was reported in 1% of patients receiving docetaxel in combination therapy for locally advanced head and neck cancer. Tearing was reported in patients receiving docetaxel in combination therapy for advanced prostate cancer (10%), advanced gastric cancer (8%), and locally advanced head and neck cancer (2%). Excessive tearing may be caused by lacrimal duct obstruction. Transient visual disturbances, such as flashes, flashing lights, and scotomata, have been reported rarely in patients receiving docetaxel; these visual disturbances typically occurred during the infusion in association with hypersensitivity reactions and were reversible upon discontinuance of the drug.

■ **Otic Effects** Adverse otic effects, including ototoxicity, hearing disorders, and/or hearing loss, have been reported in patients receiving docetaxel, including some cases associated with other ototoxic agents. Altered hearing was reported in patients receiving docetaxel with cisplatin and fluorouracil for advanced gastric cancer (6%) or locally advanced head and neck cancer (6% in TAX323 and 13% in TAX324).

■ **Other Adverse Effects** Amenorrhea was reported in patients receiving either docetaxel (62%) or fluorouracil (52%) (each in combination with doxorubicin and cyclophosphamide) for the adjuvant treatment of breast cancer. Weight loss (21 or 14%) and cancer pain (21 or 17%) were reported in patients receiving docetaxel with cisplatin and fluorouracil as induction chemotherapy for locally advanced head and neck cancer. Cough was reported in patients receiving docetaxel in combination therapy for the adjuvant treatment of breast cancer (14%) and for advanced prostate cancer (12%).

Other adverse effects reported in patients receiving docetaxel include diffuse pain, chest pain, radiation recall phenomenon, and hyponatremia. Renal insufficiency and renal failure also have been reported, generally in patients receiving docetaxel concomitantly with nephrotoxic drugs.

■ **Precautions and Contraindications** Docetaxel is a toxic drug with a low therapeutic index at the maximum recommended dose of 100 mg/m^2. Appropriate diagnostic and treatment facilities must be readily available in case the patient develops any severe adverse effects, such as severe hypersensitivity reactions to docetaxel (e.g., hypotension requiring treatment, bronchospasm/dyspnea requiring bronchodilators, generalized rash/erythema, anaphylaxis). Patients who respond to docetaxel may not experience an improvement and/or may experience worsening in performance status while receiving the drug. The relationship between changes in performance status, response to therapy, and treatment-related adverse effects has not been established.

Docetaxel should *not* be given to patients with baseline neutrophil counts less than 1500/mm^3. Bone marrow suppression with docetaxel is dose-dependent and is the dose-limiting toxicity. To monitor for the occurrence of docetaxel-induced bone marrow suppression, mainly neutropenia, which may be severe and result in infection, it is recommended that frequent peripheral blood cell counts be performed in all patients receiving the drug. Patients receiving docetaxel with cisplatin and fluorouracil should be monitored closely for the occurrence of febrile neutropenia and neutropenic infection.

Because of the alcohol content of parenteral formulations of docetaxel, patients should be advised that alcohol-induced CNS effects (e.g., intoxication) can occur during or following infusions of the drug. Patients should be advised to avoid driving, operating machinery, or performing other dangerous activities for 1–2 hours following administration of the drug. Patients also should be instructed to inform a clinician of symptoms of alcohol intoxication (e.g., confusion, stumbling, drowsiness) during or after docetaxel administration. Clinicians should consider the alcohol content of docetaxel formulations available from various manufacturers, especially when administering the drug to patients with hepatic impairment, patients in whom alcohol intake should be avoided or minimized, patients who experienced alcohol intoxication with a previous infusion of docetaxel, and those receiving concomitant therapy with drugs with CNS depressant effects (see Drug Interactions: CNS Depressants). Patients should be monitored for symptoms of alcohol intoxication during and following infusions of the drug. If such symptoms occur, reduction of the infusion rate may resolve symptoms. For patients who experience alcohol intoxication, use of a formulation of docetaxel containing the least amount of alcohol should be considered. The manufacturer's labeling should be consulted for the alcohol content of the specific formulation, as formulations of docetaxel available from various manufacturers may contain different amounts of alcohol.

Patients experiencing impaired vision during docetaxel therapy should promptly receive a comprehensive ophthalmologic examination. If cystoid macular edema is diagnosed, docetaxel therapy should be discontinued and appropriate treatment initiated. Alternative therapy with a nontaxane antineoplastic agent should be considered.

Fluid retention, generally manifested by peripheral edema and weight gain, occurs frequently in patients receiving docetaxel. Patients with preexisting effusions should be monitored closely beginning with the first dose of docetaxel to detect possible exacerbation of effusions.

Among patients receiving docetaxel with doxorubicin and cyclophosphamide as adjuvant therapy for breast cancer, continued hematologic monitoring is required because of the risk of delayed myelodysplasia or treatment-related acute myeloid leukemia. (See Cautions: Mutagenicity and Carcinogenicity.)

Among patients receiving docetaxel in combination with cisplatin and fluorouracil for advanced gastric cancer in the randomized trial, neurologic examination was performed before entry into the study, periodically during the study (at least after every 2 cycles of therapy), and at the completion of treatment. In patients experiencing peripheral neuropathy or other neurologic manifestations, examinations should be performed more frequently and dosage reduction and/or discontinuance of the drug may be required. (See Neurologic Toxicity under Dosage: Dosage Modification for Toxicity and Contraindications for Continued Therapy, in Dosage and Administration.)

Docetaxel injection concentrate contains polysorbate 80 and should *not* be used in patients with known severe hypersensitivity to polysorbate 80 or to the drug. To reduce the severity of hypersensitivity reactions and to reduce the incidence and severity of fluid retention, the manufacturers recommend that all patients be pretreated with oral corticosteroids. (See Premedication Regimen under Dosage and Administration: Dosage.) Patients should be observed closely for hypersensitivity reactions, particularly during the first and second infusions of docetaxel. Docetaxel therapy should not be undertaken in any patient who experienced a severe hypersensitivity reaction during a previous course of therapy with the drug.

Medication errors have occurred that involved confusion between docetaxel (Taxotere®) and paclitaxel (Taxol®). To avoid medication errors, the prescriber should print both the brand and generic names for docetaxel on the prescription order form. If a handwritten prescription is difficult to read, the pharmacist should confirm the drug name with the prescriber. If the prescription is confirmed verbally, the drug names should be spelled out. Pharmacy labels and preprinted order forms should list both the generic and brand names using upper-case and lower-case fonts (i.e., DOCEtaxel and TaxoTERE). Two pharmacists should provide independent confirmation that the correct drug is being ordered before chemotherapy is dispensed, and two nurses should confirm that the correct drug has been dispensed for the correct patient before administering the medication.

Docetaxel generally should not be given to patients with serum total bilirubin concentrations exceeding the upper limit of normal, or to patients with serum AST (SGOT) and/or ALT (SGPT) concentrations exceeding 1.5 times the upper limit of normal concomitant with serum alkaline phosphatase concentrations exceeding 2.5 times the upper limit of normal. Patients with elevations of serum bilirubin or abnormalities of serum transaminases concurrent with serum alkaline phosphatase are at increased risk for the development of severe or life-threatening complications, including severe neutropenia, febrile neutropenia, infections, severe thrombocytopenia, severe stomatitis, severe skin toxicity, and toxic death. Determinations of serum bilirubin, AST and/or ALT, and alkaline phosphatase concentrations should be obtained prior to each cycle of docetaxel therapy and reviewed by the clinician.

The incidence of mortality was higher in patients with non-small cell lung cancer previously treated with platinum-based chemotherapy who received docetaxel as a single agent at a dose of 100 mg/m^2. Because of excessive toxicity with higher doses, such patients should receive the recommended dosage of (i.e., docetaxel 75 mg/m^2 once every 3 weeks). (See Non-small Cell Lung Cancer under Dosage and Administration: Dosage.)

The patient should be instructed to notify a clinician immediately about difficulty breathing or swallowing, facial swelling, or rash during or shortly after the infusion of docetaxel because this may indicate an allergic reaction to the drug. The patient should be informed of the importance of routine monitoring of blood cell counts and should be advised to notify a clinician immediately if he or she develops a fever, because this may be an early sign of infection. The patient should be instructed to monitor for signs of fluid retention (e.g., edema in the lower extremities, weight gain, dyspnea) and should be advised of the importance of taking the corticosteroid premedication as directed to lessen fluid retention and to reduce the severity of hypersensitivity reactions. Patients also should be instructed to inform a clinician of excessive or persistent fatigue, muscle pain, rash, or sensations (numbness, tingling, or burning) in the hands and/or feet after treatment with docetaxel.

■ **Pediatric Precautions** Clinicians should consider the alcohol content of docetaxel formulations available from various manufacturers when administering the drug to pediatric patients. (See Cautions: Nervous System Effects and Cautions: Precautions and Contraindications.)

Efficacy of docetaxel administered as monotherapy or in combination chemotherapy regimens has not been established in pediatric patients. In clinical trials to date, the safety profile of docetaxel in pediatric patients has been similar to that in adults. Clearance of the drug (adjusted for body surface area) also has been similar in pediatric patients and adults.

In a dose-finding study in 61 patients 1–22 years of age (median age: 12.5 years) with various refractory solid tumors, the primary dose-limiting toxicity of docetaxel was neutropenia. The dosage identified in this study (125 mg/m^2 IV every 21 days) subsequently was evaluated in a phase 2 noncomparative trial in 178 patients 1–26 years of age (median age: 12 years) with various recurrent or refractory solid tumors. This phase 2 trial failed to establish efficacy of docetaxel monotherapy in pediatric patients; tumor responses in this trial included one complete response in a patient with undifferentiated sarcoma and 4 partial responses, one each in patients with Ewing's sarcoma, neuroblastoma, osteosarcoma, and squamous cell carcinoma.

In a study in 75 patients 9–21 years of age (median age: 16 years) with nasopharyngeal carcinoma, 1 of 50 patients receiving an induction regimen of docetaxel, cisplatin, and fluorouracil prior to chemoradiation consolidation achieved a complete response following the induction regimen compared with none out of 25 patients receiving an induction regimen of cisplatin and fluorouracil.

■ **Geriatric Precautions** Certain toxicities associated with docetaxel therapy may occur more frequently and with greater severity in geriatric patients. Because of the greater frequency of decreased hepatic, renal, and/or cardiac function and of concomitant disease and drug therapy observed in the elderly, caution is advised in dose selection for geriatric patients.

Among patients receiving docetaxel and cisplatin as first-line treatment of advanced non-small cell lung cancer in the randomized trial, 36% were 65 years of age or older. Geriatric patients experienced similar survival but greater toxicity than younger patients. Among patients receiving docetaxel and cisplatin, median survival was 12 months in geriatric patients compared with about 10 months in younger patients. Adverse effects that occurred more frequently in geriatric patients than in younger patients receiving docetaxel and cisplatin include diarrhea (55 versus 43%), infections (42 versus 31%), peripheral edema (39 versus 31%), and stomatitis (28 versus 21%). Among geriatric patients, diarrhea (55 versus 24%), peripheral edema (39 versus 20%), and stomatitis (28 versus 20%) occurred more frequently in those receiving docetaxel and cisplatin than in those receiving vinorelbine and cisplatin. Among patients receiving docetaxel and carboplatin as first-line treatment of advanced non-small cell lung cancer in the same randomized trial, 28% were 65 years of age or older. Among geriatric patients, those receiving docetaxel and carboplatin had a higher frequency of infection than those receiving docetaxel and cisplatin and a higher frequency of diarrhea, infection, and peripheral edema than those receiving vinorelbine and cisplatin.

Among patients receiving docetaxel and prednisone for the treatment of androgen-independent (hormone-refractory) advanced prostate cancer in the randomized trial, 63% were 65 years of age or older and 20% were older than 75 years of age. Treatment-emergent adverse effects that occurred more frequently in geriatric patients than in younger patients receiving docetaxel and prednisone included anemia (71 versus 59%), infection (37 versus 24%), nail changes (34 versus 23%), anorexia (21 versus 10%), and weight loss (15 versus 5%).

Among patients receiving docetaxel with cisplatin and fluorouracil for advanced gastric cancer in the randomized trial, 24% were 65 years of age or older. Although this trial did not include sufficient numbers of elderly patients to determine whether geriatric patients respond differently than younger patients, the incidence of serious adverse effects was higher. The incidence rates of lethargy, stomatitis, diarrhea, dizziness, edema, and febrile neutropenia/neutropenic infection were at least 10% higher in geriatric patients than in younger patients, and close monitoring is advised for elderly patients.

Among patients receiving docetaxel with cisplatin and fluorouracil as induction therapy for advanced head and neck cancer in randomized trials, the number of patients 65 years of age or older (10% in TAX323 and 13% in TAX324) was not sufficient to determine whether geriatric patients respond differently than younger patients. Other clinical experience has not revealed age-related differences in response for patients receiving this regimen.

Among patients receiving docetaxel with doxorubicin and cyclophosphamide as adjuvant therapy for breast cancer in the randomized trial, the number of patients 65 years of age or older (6%) was not sufficient to determine age-related differences in response or tolerance.

■ **Mutagenicity and Carcinogenicity** Docetaxel has been shown to be clastogenic in the in vitro chromosome aberration test in CHO-K1 cells and in the in vivo micronucleus test in mice; however, the drug was not mutagenic in the Ames test or the CHO/HGPRT gene mutation assay.

Studies to determine the carcinogenic potential of docetaxel have not been performed to date.

Acute myeloid leukemia and myelodysplastic syndrome have been reported in patients receiving docetaxel in combination therapy with other antineoplastic agents with or without radiation therapy. Acute myeloid leukemia (AML) or myelodysplasia related to treatment has occurred in patients receiving anthracycline agents and/or cyclophosphamide, including those receiving these drugs as adjuvant therapy for breast cancer. In the randomized trial, AML occurred in 3 of 744 patients receiving docetaxel, doxorubicin, and cyclophosphamide and in 1 of 736 patients receiving fluorouracil, doxorubicin, and cyclophosphamide as adjuvant therapy for breast cancer.

■ **Pregnancy, Fertility, and Lactation** Docetaxel may cause fetal harm when administered to pregnant women, but potential benefits may be acceptable in certain conditions despite possible risks to the fetus. Reproduction studies in rats and rabbits given docetaxel doses greater than or equal to 0.3 and 0.03 mg/kg (about 1/50 and 1/300 the maximum daily recommended human dose on a mg/m^2 basis), respectively, during organogenesis revealed evidence of maternal toxicity, embryotoxicity, and fetotoxicity; fetotoxicity was characterized by intrauterine mortality, increased resorption, reduced fetal weight, and fetal ossification delay. There are no adequate and well-controlled studies to date using docetaxel in pregnant women. Docetaxel should be used during pregnancy only in life-threatening situations or in diseases for which safer drugs cannot be used or are ineffective. Women of childbearing potential should be advised to avoid becoming pregnant during therapy with docetaxel. When docetaxel is used during pregnancy or if the patient becomes pregnant while receiving the drug, the patient should be apprised of the potential hazard to the fetus.

When administered in multiple IV doses of up to 0.3 mg/kg (about 1/50 of the recommended human dose on a mg/m^2 basis), docetaxel produced no impairment of fertility in rats, but decreased testicular weights were reported. These findings correlate with those of a 10-cycle toxicity study (dosing once every 21 days for 6 months) in rats and dogs in which testicular atrophy or degeneration was observed at IV doses of 5 mg/kg in rats and 0.375 mg/kg in dogs (about 1/3 and 1/15 the recommended human dose on a mg/m^2 basis, respectively). An increased frequency of dosing in rats produced similar effects at lower dose levels.

It is not known whether docetaxel is distributed into milk. Because of the potential for serious adverse reactions to docetaxel in nursing infants, a decision should be made whether to discontinue nursing or the drug, taking into account the importance of the drug to the woman.

Drug Interactions

Formal drug interaction studies of docetaxel have not been conducted.

■ **Drugs Affecting or Metabolized by Hepatic Microsomal Enzymes** Results of in vitro studies show that the metabolism of docetaxel may be altered by the concomitant administration of drugs that induce, inhibit, or are metabolized by cytochrome P-450 isoenzyme 3A4 (CYP3A4). In a limited number of patients, administration of ketoconazole (200 mg orally once daily for 3 days) concomitantly with docetaxel (10 mg/m^2 IV) resulted in a 2.2-fold increase in exposure and a 49% reduction in clearance of docetaxel. Concomitant use of potent CYP3A4 inhibitors (e.g., atazanavir, clarithromycin, indinavir, itraconazole, ketoconazole, nefazodone, nelfinavir, ritonavir, saquinavir, telithromycin, voriconazole) with docetaxel should be avoided. If such concomitant use cannot be avoided, a reduction in docetaxel dosage with careful monitoring for toxicity should be considered. Based on extrapolation of limited pharmacokinetic data for ketoconazole, the manufacturers state that a 50% reduction in docetaxel dosage may be considered in patients requiring concomitant therapy with a potent CYP3A4 inhibitor; however, there are no clinical data with use of this adjusted docetaxel dosage in patients receiving potent CYP3A4 inhibitors.

■ **CNS Depressants** Because of the alcohol content of parenteral formulations of docetaxel, concomitant use of drugs with CNS depressant effects (e.g., opiate analgesics, sedatives) may worsen the effects of alcohol. (See Cautions: Nervous System Effects.)

Acute Toxicity

Limited information is available on the acute toxicity of docetaxel. In male and female rats, lethality occurred at a dose of 20 mg/kg (comparable to a human dose of 100 mg/m^2 on a mg/m^2 basis) and was associated with abnormal mitosis and necrosis of multiple organs. In mice, lethality was observed following single IV doses of 154 mg/kg (about 4.5 times a human dose of 100 mg/m^2 on a mg/m^2 basis) or greater. In mice, at a dose of 48 mg/kg (about 1.5 times a human dose of 100 mg/m^2 on a mg/m^2 basis), neurotoxicity associated with paralysis, nonextension of hind limbs, and myelin degeneration was observed.

Overdosage of docetaxel produces symptoms that are mainly extensions of common adverse reactions, including bone marrow suppression, peripheral neurotoxicity, and mucositis. In 2 reports of overdosage, one in a patient receiving docetaxel 150 mg/m^2 and another in a patient receiving docetaxel 200 mg/m^2 (both as 1-hour IV infusions), both patients experienced severe neutropenia, mild asthenia, cutaneous reactions, and mild paresthesias. These patients recovered without incident.

There is no known antidote for docetaxel overdosage. In case of overdosage, the patient should be moved to a specialized unit that allows close monitoring of vital functions. As soon as possible after the discovery of docetaxel overdosage, therapeutic G-CSF should be administered. Other supportive and symptomatic treatment should be initiated as clinically indicated.

Pharmacology

Like paclitaxel, docetaxel is an antimicrotubule antineoplastic agent. Unlike some other common antimicrotubule agents (e.g., vinca alkaloids, colchicine, podophyllotoxin), however, docetaxel and paclitaxel *promote* rather than inhibit microtubule assembly while simultaneously preventing microtubule disassembly. Microtubules are organelles that exist in a state of dynamic equilibrium with their components, tubulin dimers. They are an essential part of the mitotic spindle and also are involved in maintenance of cell shape and motility, and transport between organelles within the cell.

Docetaxel enhances the polymerization of tubulin, the protein subunit of the spindle microtubules, even in the absence of factors that are normally required for microtubule assembly (e.g., guanosine triphosphate [GTP]); as a result, the drug induces the formation of stable, nonfunctional microtubules. While the precise mechanism of action of the drug is not understood fully, docetaxel disrupts the dynamic equilibrium within the microtubule system and arrests the cell cycle in the late G_2 and M phases, inhibiting cell replication.

Docetaxel results in the formation of tubulin polymers that differ structurally from those generated by paclitaxel and, unlike paclitaxel, does not alter the number of protofilaments in the microtubules. As an inhibitor of microtubule depolymerization, docetaxel is approximately twice as potent as paclitaxel; the increased potency of docetaxel may be related to its higher affinity for microtubules, its higher achievable intracellular concentration, and its slower cellular efflux. In addition, higher radiosensitivity effects have been observed with docetaxel as compared with paclitaxel (at equimolar concentrations). Preclinical evidence suggests that cross-resistance between docetaxel and paclitaxel is incomplete; a lack of cross-resistance between docetaxel and fluorouracil or cisplatin also has been noted.

Docetaxel is a schedule-independent antineoplastic agent. Preclinical studies using different dosage schedules revealed no alteration in antitumor activity with splitting of the total dose of docetaxel.

Pharmacokinetics

■ **Absorption** Docetaxel exhibits linear, dose-dependent pharmacokinetics. The area under the concentration-time curve (AUC) was dose-proportional following docetaxel doses of 70–115 mg/m^2 IV administered over 1–2 hours.

■ **Distribution** The pharmacokinetic disposition of docetaxel is consistent with a 3-compartment model with initial rapid decline indicating distribution to peripheral compartments and a late (terminal) phase with a half-life of about 11 hours suggesting relatively slow efflux of docetaxel from the peripheral compartment. Following docetaxel doses of 70–115 mg/m^2 IV administered over 1–2 hours, the steady-state volume of distribution averaged 113 L.

About 94% of docetaxel is bound to plasma proteins (97% in patients with cancer). It is not known whether docetaxel is distributed into milk.

■ **Elimination** Following docetaxel doses of 70–115 mg/m^2 IV administered over 1–2 hours, total body clearance averaged 21 L/hour per m^2.

Docetaxel is metabolized in the liver and undergoes oxidative metabolism of the *tert*-butyl ester group. (See Drug interactions: Drugs Affecting or Metabolized by Hepatic Microsomal Enzymes.) Docetaxel is excreted mainly in the feces (75% of the dose) with minimal excretion (about 6% of the dose) in the urine. Following the administration of a radioactive dose, about 80% of the dose is excreted in the feces during the first 48 hours as a major metabolite and 3 minor metabolites with small amounts (less than 8% of the dose) excreted as unchanged drug.

In patients with mild to moderate hepatic impairment (serum AST and/or ALT concentration exceeding 1.5 times the upper limit of normal and serum alkaline phosphatase concentration exceeding 2.5 times the upper limit of normal), total body clearance was lowered by an average of 27% and resulted in a 38% increase in systemic exposure (AUC) for docetaxel. Docetaxel has not been studied in patients with severe hepatic impairment.

The pharmacokinetics of docetaxel do not appear to be influenced by age or gender.

Chemistry and Stability

■ **Chemistry** Docetaxel, a semisynthetic taxoid produced from the needles of the European yew (*Taxus baccata*) tree, is an antineoplastic agent. The drug is derived from a noncytotoxic precursor (10-deacetyl baccatin III) and is structurally and pharmacologically similar to paclitaxel.

Docetaxel is a complex diterpene with a taxane ring system linked at positions 4 and 5 to a four-membered oxetane ring and at position 13 to an ester side chain. The taxane nucleus is important for binding of docetaxel to microtubules, and this binding is stabilized by the ester side chain at position 13 of the taxane ring, which is required for the drug's cytotoxic activity. Docetaxel differs structurally from paclitaxel by the presence of a hydroxyl group rather than an acetyl group on position 10 of the baccatin III ring and by a trimethylmethoxy moiety instead of a benzamide phenyl group on the 3′ position of the side chain at position 13 of the taxane ring.

Docetaxel occurs as a white to almost-white powder. Docetaxel is highly lipophilic and practically insoluble in water; however, docetaxel is more water soluble than paclitaxel, permitting its formulation in polysorbate (Tween®) 80 rather than Cremophor® EL (polyoxyl 35 castor oil).

Commercially available docetaxel injection concentrate (Taxotere®) is a sterile solution of the drug in a 50/50 v/v mixture of polysorbate 80 and dehydrated alcohol. The injection concentrate is a pale yellow to brownish-yellow solution. The injection concentrate must be diluted with an appropriate infusion solution prior to administration (one dilution step).

Commercially available docetaxel injection concentrate (Hospira) is a sterile solution of the drug in a vehicle containing polysorbate 80, citric acid, polyethylene glycol 300, and dehydrated alcohol 23% v/v. The injection concentrate is a clear, colorless to pale yellow solution. The injection concentrate must be diluted with an appropriate infusion solution prior to administration (one dilution step).

Commercially available docetaxel injection concentrate requiring one dilution step (one-vial formulation, Accord) is a sterile solution of the drug in a vehicle containing polysorbate 80, citric acid, and dehydrated alcohol. The injection concentrate is a pale yellow to brownish-yellow solution. The injection concentrate must be diluted with an appropriate infusion solution prior to administration (one dilution step).

Commercially available docetaxel injection concentrate requiring 2 dilution steps (2-vial formulation, Accord) is a sterile solution of the drug in polysorbate 80 and dehydrated alcohol with an accompanying diluent of 13% w/v polyethylene glycol 400 in water for injection; citric acid may be added to adjust the pH. The injection concentrate is a clear yellow to brownish-yellow viscous solution. The injection concentrate must be diluted with the diluent supplied by the manufacturer, followed by dilution with an appropriate infusion solution prior to administration (2 dilution steps).

Docetaxel also is commercially available as a lyophilized powder (Docefrez®) with an accompanying diluent of ethanol 35.4% w/w and polysorbate 80. The lyophilized powder must be reconstituted with the diluent supplied by the manufacturer, followed by dilution with an appropriate infusion solution.

■ **Stability** Commercially available docetaxel injection concentrate (Taxotere®) should be stored in unopened vials at 2–25°C and retained in the original package for protection from light. Freezing does not adversely affect docetaxel for injection concentrate. The final diluted docetaxel solution for infusion (prepared by mixing the required amount of the injection concentrate with either 0.9% sodium chloride injection or 5% dextrose injection) is stable for up to 6 hours at 2–25°C. The infusion solution should be used within 6 hours, so it may be stored for up to 5 hours at 2–25°C before initiating the 1-hour IV infusion. When prepared as directed and stored in non-PVC bags at 2–8°C, the final diluted docetaxel infusion solution is stable for up to 48 hours.

Commercially available docetaxel injection concentrate (Hospira) should be stored in unopened vials at 20–25°C and retained in the original package for protection from light. Between uses, multiple-dose vials of the injection concentrate are stable for up to 28 days when stored at 2–8°C and protected from light. Freezing does not adversely affect docetaxel for injection concentrate. The final diluted docetaxel solution for infusion (prepared by mixing the required amount of the injection concentrate with either 0.9% sodium chloride injection or 5% dextrose injection) is stable for up to 4 hours at 2–25°C. The infusion solution should be used within 4 hours, so it may be stored for up to 3 hours at 2–25°C before initiating the 1-hour IV infusion.

Commercially available docetaxel injection concentrate requiring one dilution step (one-vial formulation, Accord) should be stored in unopened vials at 15–25°C and protected from light. Between uses, multiple-dose vials of the injection concentrate are stable for up to 28 days when stored at room temperature and protected from light. Freezing does not adversely affect this formulation. The final diluted docetaxel solution for infusion (prepared by mixing the required amount of the injection concentrate with either 0.9% sodium chloride injection or 5% dextrose injection) is stable for up to 4 hours at 2–25°C. The infusion solution should be used within 4 hours, so it may be stored for up to 3 hours at 2–25°C before initiating the 1-hour IV infusion.

Commercially available docetaxel injection concentrate requiring 2 dilution steps (2-vial formulation, Accord) should be stored in unopened vials at 25°C (but may be exposed to temperatures ranging from 15–30°C) and protected from light. The initial diluted docetaxel solution (prepared by mixing the contents of the diluent vial with the docetaxel injection concentrate) may be used immediately to prepare the final diluted docetaxel solution for infusion or it may be stored either in the refrigerator or at room temperature for up to 8 hours. The final diluted docetaxel solution for infusion (prepared by mixing the required amount of the initial diluted docetaxel solution with either 0.9% sodium chloride injection or 5% dextrose injection) is stable for up to 4 hours at 2–25°C. The final diluted docetaxel solution for infusion should be used within 4 hours, so it may be stored for up to 3 hours at 2–25°C before initiating the 1-hour IV infusion.

Commercially available docetaxel lyophilized powder (Docefrez®) should be stored at 2–8°C and retained in the original package for protection from bright light. The reconstituted docetaxel solution may be used immediately to prepare the final diluted docetaxel solution for infusion or it may be stored either in the refrigerator or at room temperature for up to 8 hours. The final diluted docetaxel solution for infusion (prepared by mixing the required amount of the reconstituted docetaxel solution with either 0.9% sodium chloride injection or 5% dextrose injection) is stable for up to 6 hours at 2–25°C. The final diluted docetaxel solution for infusion should be used within 6 hours, so it may be stored for up to 5 hours at 2–25°C before initiating the 1-hour IV infusion. When prepared as directed and stored in non-PVC bags at 2–8°C, the final diluted docetaxel infusion solution is stable for up to 48 hours.

For further information on the handling of antineoplastic agents, see the ASHP Guidelines on Handling Hazardous Drugs at http://www.ahfsdruginformation.com.

Preparations

Excipients in commercially available drug preparations may have clinically important effects in some individuals; consult specific product labeling for details.

DOCEtaxel

Parenteral

For injection, for IV infusion	20 mg	**Docefrez®** (with ethanol 35.4% w/w in polysorbate 80 diluent), Sun
	80 mg	**Docefrez®** (with ethanol 35.4% w/w in polysorbate 80 diluent), Sun
Injection concentrate, for IV infusion	10 mg (of anhydrous docetaxel) per mL (20, 80, or 160 mg)	**Docetaxel Injection**
	20 mg (of anhydrous docetaxel) per mL (20, 80, or 160 mg)*	**Taxotere®**, Sanofi-Aventis
	40 mg (of anhydrous docetaxel) per mL (20 or 80 mg)	**Docetaxel Injection** (with 13% w/v polyethylene glycol 400 in water for injection diluent)

*available from one or more manufacturer, distributor, and/or repackager by generic (nonproprietary) name

†Use is not currently included in the labeling approved by the US Food and Drug Administration

DOXOrubicin Hydrochloride

Hydroxydaunomycin Hydrochloride, Hydroxydaunorubicin Hydrochloride

■ Doxorubicin is an anthracycline glycoside antineoplastic antibiotic produced by *Streptomyces peucetius* var. *caesius*.

Uses

Since doxorubicin does not cross the blood-brain barrier or achieve a measurable concentration in CSF, there is a possibility of metastases to the brain and meninges from potentially metastatic tumors.

■ **Breast Cancer** Doxorubicin hydrochloride is used in the treatment of breast cancer. Use of the drug in combination with other chemotherapeutic agents and/or surgery in the early stage of breast cancer has produced clinically important responses in both quantity and duration. Combination chemotherapy used as an adjunct to surgery has been shown to increase both disease-free (i.e., decreased recurrence) and overall survival in premenopausal and postmenopausal women with node-negative or node-positive early (TNM stage I or II) breast cancer. Although adjuvant combination chemotherapy that includes cyclophosphamide, methotrexate, and fluorouracil has been used most extensively and is considered a regimen of choice for early breast cancer, doxorubicin-containing regimens (e.g., combined cyclophosphamide and doxorubicin with or without fluorouracil; combined cyclophosphamide and doxorubicin with or without tamoxifen) appear to be comparably effective and also are considered regimens of choice, but differences in toxicity profiles may influence the choice of regimen. There is some evidence that the addition of doxorubicin to a regimen of cyclophosphamide, methotrexate, and fluorouracil can improve outcome further in patients with early breast cancer and more than 3 positive axillary lymph nodes, and that sequential (i.e., administering several courses of doxorubicin first) regimens are more effective than alternating regimens in such patients; in patients with fewer positive nodes, no additional benefit from doxorubicin has been demonstrated. The dose intensity of adjuvant combination chemotherapy also appears to be an important factor influencing clinical outcome in patients with early node-positive breast cancer, with response increasing with increasing dose intensity; therefore, arbitrary reductions in dose intensity should be avoided. In stage III (locally advanced) breast cancer, combination chemotherapy (with or without hormonal therapy) is used sequentially following surgery and radiation therapy for operable disease and following biopsy and radiation therapy for inoperable disease; commonly employed effective regimens include cyclophosphamide, methotrexate, and fluorouracil; cyclophosphamide, doxorubicin, and fluorouracil; and cyclophosphamide and doxorubicin.

Patients refractory to cyclophosphamide, vincristine sulfate, dactinomycin, or daunorubicin have responded to doxorubicin hydrochloride; however, apparent cross-resistance between doxorubicin and daunorubicin has been noted in some patients with neuroblastoma. Cross-resistance between doxorubicin and vincristine sulfate or dactinomycin in animals or cell cultures has been reported, but clinical evidence of these cross-resistances in humans is lacking.

■ **AIDS-related Kaposi's Sarcoma** ***Overview*** Doxorubicin hydrochloride as conventional (nonencapsulated) injections has been used alone or in combination chemotherapy for the palliative treatment of AIDS-related Kaposi's sarcoma†, and combination chemotherapy that includes the drug (e.g., doxorubicin, bleomycin, and vincristine) has been a preferred regimen; but many clinicians currently consider a liposomal anthracycline (doxorubicin or daunorubicin) the first-line therapy of choice for advanced AIDS-related Kaposi's sarcoma (see also Uses: AIDS-related Kaposi's Sarcoma in Daunorubicin 10:00).

Although single-agent therapy with conventional (i.e., nonencapsulated) cytotoxic agents generally has been used in the early stage of disease, Kaposi's sarcoma in patients with human immunodeficiency virus (HIV) infection often is rapidly progressive. AIDS-related Kaposi's sarcoma often progresses to multifocal, widespread lesions that may involve the skin, oral mucosa, and lymph nodes as well as visceral organs such as the GI tract, lung, liver, and spleen; such lesions often are numerous and may be cosmetically unattractive or disfiguring and accompanied by lymphedema. Appropriate evaluation of the effects of drug therapies on survival in patients with Kaposi's sarcoma must include assessment of the effects of such therapies on the development of infection as well as on tumor regression.Although treatment may result in disappearance or reduction in the size of Kaposi's sarcoma skin lesions and thereby alleviate the discomfort associated with chronic edema and ulcerations that often accompany multiple skin lesions on the lower extremities and in symptomatic control of mucosal and visceral lesions, there currently are no data demonstrating unequivocal evidence of improved survival with any therapy. Small localized Kaposi's sarcoma lesions may be treated with electrodesiccation and curettage cryotherapy or by surgical excision; the lesions also generally are responsive to local radiation, and excellent palliation often can be achieved. Localized palatal lesions have been treated effectively with intralesional injections of vinblastine or bleomycin.

Alitretinoin gel (Panretin®, Ligand Pharmaceuticals), a topical retinoid, is used for the treatment of localized cutaneous lesions in patients with AIDS-related Kaposi's sarcoma; responses of cutaneous lesions to topical therapy with alitretinoin have been reported in patients who have received prior systemic and/or topical therapy for Kaposi's sarcoma as well as in those with previously untreated disease.

Liposomal Agents Pegylated liposomal doxorubicin is labeled for use in the palliative treatment of AIDS-related Kaposi's sarcoma in adults intolerant to combination chemotherapy or whose disease has progressed while receiving such therapy. Liposomal daunorubicin citrate is labeled for use as first-line therapy for advanced AIDS-related Kaposi's sarcoma. (See Daunorubicin 10:00.) The results of several randomized, multicenter trials indicate that patients receiving a liposomal anthracycline for the treatment of advanced AIDS-related Kaposi's sarcoma experience similar or higher response rates with a more favorable toxic effects profile than those receiving combination therapy with conventional chemotherapeutic agents.

Administration of doxorubicin hydrochloride encapsulated in PEG-stabilized liposomes (see Chemistry and Stability: Chemistry) allows the drug-containing liposomes to remain circulating in plasma for prolonged periods and reduces extravascular circulation of the drug while substantially increasing concentrations of the drug in the lesions of Kaposi's sarcoma compared with administration of equivalent doses of conventional (nonencapsulated) doxorubicin hydrochloride injections (see Pharmacokinetics: Distribution).

In an open-label, single-arm, multicenter study in patients with moderate to severe AIDS-related Kaposi's sarcoma whose disease had progressed on prior combination chemotherapy (consisting of at least 2 cycles of a regimen containing bleomycin, a vinca alkaloid [vincristine or vinblastine], and/or doxorubicin) or who were intolerant of such therapy, response rates were analyzed according to the investigator assessment of changes in lesions over the entire body or according to changes in indicator lesions; in this study, liposomal doxorubicin was administered IV in doses of 20-mg/m² once every 3 weeks, generally until disease progression or intolerance to doxorubicin therapy occurred. According to investigator assessment of changes, partial response, stable disease, or progressive disease was observed in 27, 29, or 44% of patients, respectively, while duration of partial response or time to partial response was 73 (range: 42–210) days or 43 (range: 15–133) days, respectively. According to indicator lesion assessment, partial response, stable disease, or progressive disease was observed in 48, 26, or 26%, respectively, while duration of partial response or time to partial response was 71 (range: 22–210) days or 22 (range: 15–109) days, respectively.

In a large, randomized trial, patients with AIDS-related Kaposi's sarcoma receiving liposomal doxorubicin (20 mg/m² by IV infusion over 30 minutes) had a higher objective response rate (58.7 versus 23.3%) than those receiving a combination regimen of bleomycin (15 mg/m² by IV infusion over 30 minutes) and vincristine (1.4 mg/m² or a maximum of 2 mg by IV bolus); each regimen was administered every 3 weeks for a maximum of 6 cycles. Treatment with liposomal doxorubicin was associated with greater improvement in signs and symptoms of pulmonary Kaposi's sarcoma (e.g., dyspnea, cough, chest pain, effusions) and GI Kaposi's sarcoma (e.g., GI bleeding, early satiety, dysphagia). Early termination from the study, withdrawal because of adverse effects, and withdrawal because of progressive disease occurred less frequently in patients receiving liposomal doxorubicin than in those receiving combination chemotherapy with bleomycin and vincristine. The incidence of paresthesia, peripheral neuropathy, and constipation was higher in patients receiving bleomycin and vincristine, whereas leukopenia and opportunistic infections (particularly oral candidiasis) occurred more frequently in those receiving liposomal doxorubicin. In another large, randomized trial involving 258 patients with advanced AIDS-related Kaposi's sarcoma, a higher rate of objective response (45.9 versus 24.8%) and less toxicity were reported in those receiving liposomal doxorubicin (20 mg/m² IV over 30 minutes) versus the ABV regimen, consisting of conventional doxorubicin (20 mg/m²), bleomycin (10 mg/m²), and vincristine (1 mg); each regimen was administered every 14 days for a maximum of 6 cycles. Treatment was discontinued because of adverse effects more frequently among those receiving the ABV regimen (37%) than among those receiving liposomal doxorubicin (11%). A higher incidence of nausea and vomiting, alopecia, and peripheral neuropathy was reported in patients receiving the ABV regimen, whereas stomatitis and rash were reported more frequently in patients receiving liposomal doxorubicin.

Preliminary evidence suggests that the mean survival period in patients with pulmonary AIDS-related Kaposi's sarcoma receiving liposomal doxorubicin may be increased compared with those receiving conventional chemotherapy (bleomycin and/or vincristine). Similar response rates, time to treatment failure, and overall survival, with less toxicity, were observed in patients receiving liposomal daunorubicin versus combination chemotherapy with bleomycin, conventional doxorubicin, and vincristine for advanced AIDS-related Kaposi's sarcoma. The comparative efficacy of liposomal doxorubicin relative to liposomal daunorubicin has not been established.

Although treatment may result in the reduction in size or disappearance of specific skin lesions and alleviation of the associated symptoms, no treatment has been shown conclusively to alter the natural history of AIDS-related Kaposi's sarcoma and additional study and experience are needed to establish the optimal regimen.

Conventional Chemotherapy Response rates observed with single-agent chemotherapy (e.g., doxorubicin, etoposide, vinblastine, vincristine) appear to be similar to those observed with interferon alfa; however, studies directly comparing the efficacy of doxorubicin alone with that of interferon alfa have not been performed. The wide variation in response rates reported in clinical studies generally appear to reflect differences in patient selection and in the heterogeneity of criteria used to evaluate response rather than in drug activity. Combined treatment with chemotherapy (e.g., vinblastine or etoposide) and interferon alfa generally appears to result in enhanced systemic toxicity without added therapeutic benefits.

Combination chemotherapy with conventional antineoplastic agents (e.g., conventional doxorubicin, etoposide, vinblastine, vincristine) has been used for advanced disease (e.g., extensive mucocutaneous disease, lymphedema, symptomatic visceral disease). Evidence from a study in patients with advanced Kaposi's sarcoma indicates that combined therapy with low-dose conventional (nonencapsulated) doxorubicin, bleomycin, and vincristine is more effective than low-dose doxorubicin alone in inducing response and prolonging disease-free survival, although overall survival with either regimen was comparable. In this study, complete and partial tumor remissions as well as disease-free survival were higher in patients receiving combination therapy with low-dose conventional doxorubicin (20 mg/m²), bleomycin (10 units/m²), and vincristine (1.4 mg/m²; up to 2 mg) every 2 weeks than in those receiving low-dose doxorubicin (20 mg/m²) alone every 2 weeks; complete and partial remissions occurred in 88 or 48% of patients receiving combination or single-agent chemotherapy, respectively, while a median survival of 9 months was observed with both therapies.

■ **Ovarian Cancer** ***Liposomal Doxorubicin*** Pegylated liposomal doxorubicin is used for the treatment of ovarian cancer that has progressed or recurred following platinum-based chemotherapy.

The current indication for use of liposomal doxorubicin in platinum-refractory ovarian cancer is based principally on data from a subset of patients involved in 3 uncontrolled studies and a randomized trial. In these clinical trials, liposomal doxorubicin was administered at an initial dosage of 50 mg/m² IV over 1 hour every 3–4 weeks for 3–6 cycles or more. Among 145 patients with metastatic ovarian carcinoma refractory to paclitaxel- and platinum-based chemotherapy regimens who received liposomal doxorubicin in 3 open-label, phase II studies, the objective response rate was 13.8% (range: 0–22%), the median time to response was 17.6 weeks, the median duration of response was 39.4 weeks, and the median time to progression was 15.9 weeks. In a randomized, open-label trial involving 474 patients with epithelial ovarian cancer (mostly stage III–IV disease) who had received platinum-based chemotherapy, similar median time to progression (4 months), median overall survival (14 months) and response rates (20 versus 17%) were observed in those receiving liposomal doxorubicin or topotecan. Hand-foot syndrome (51 versus 1%), stomatitis (41 versus 15%), and rash (28 versus 12%) occurred more frequently in patients receiving liposomal doxorubicin, whereas nausea (63 versus 46%), alopecia (52 versus 19%), and constipation (46 versus 30%) occurred more frequently in those receiving topotecan. Severe hematologic toxicity, including neutropenia, anemia, and thrombocytopenia, occurred more frequently in patients receiving topotecan than in those receiving liposomal doxorubicin. Severe neutropenia (less than 500/mm³) was reported in 4% of patients receiving liposomal doxorubicin compared with 62% of patients receiving topotecan.

Conventional Doxorubicin Although conventional doxorubicin is labeled for use in the treatment of ovarian carcinoma and has been used in combination regimens for the treatment of this cancer, other agents currently are preferred.

■ **Bladder Cancer** Doxorubicin has been used intravesically† for the treatment of residual tumor and/or as adjuvant therapy for prophylaxis of superficial bladder carcinoma†.

Complete response rates of about 40–50% have been observed in patients receiving intravesical doxorubicin for the treatment of papillary tumors; complete responses to intravesical doxorubicin also have been reported in a small number of patients with carcinoma in situ. No additional benefit has been shown for the use of maintenance therapy with intravesical doxorubicin. Treatment with intravesical doxorubicin generally is well tolerated; the most common adverse effect observed is chemical cystitis, usually reversible, in approximately 20–30% of patients. Systemic toxicity, including hypersensitivity reactions and cardiovascular events, have been reported in patients receiving intravesical doxorubicin for the prophylaxis or treatment of superficial bladder cancer.

Although evidence from comparative studies is limited, other agents (e.g. mitomycin, epirubicin) that appear to be similar in efficacy but less toxic than doxorubicin generally are preferred for the prophylaxis or treatment of superficial bladder cancer. (See Uses: Bladder Cancer in Mitomycin 10:00 for further discussion of intravesical chemotherapy for superficial bladder cancer.)

Doxorubicin is used in combination regimens with cisplatin, methotrexate, and vinblastine for the treatment of invasive and advanced bladder carcinoma. (See Uses: Bladder Cancer in Cisplatin 10:00.)

■ **Small Cell Lung Cancer** Doxorubicin is used in combination chemotherapy regimens (e.g., cyclophosphamide, doxorubicin, and vincristine [CAV]; cyclophosphamide, doxorubicin, and etoposide [CAE]) for the treatment of extensive-stage small cell lung cancer†. Survival outcomes are similar in patients with extensive-stage small cell lung cancer receiving CAV or cisplatin/etoposide. Combination chemotherapy regimens have produced response rates of 70–85% and complete response rates of 20–30% in patients with extensive-stage disease; however, comparative efficacy is continually being evaluated. Because the current prognosis for small cell lung carcinoma is unsatisfactory regardless of stage and despite considerable diagnostic and therapeutic advances, all patients with this cancer are candidates for inclusion in clinical trials at the time of diagnosis.

■ **Multiple Myeloma** ***Induction Therapy Prior to Stem Cell Transplantation*** **Conventional Doxorubicin.** Use of conventional doxorubicin in combination with bortezomib and dexamethasone† (bortezomib-doxorubicin-dexamethasone) as induction therapy for newly diagnosed multiple myeloma in transplant-eligible patients† may be considered a reasonable choice (accepted; with possible conditions) based on current evidence from an open-label, randomized phase 3 study (HOVON-65/GMMG-HD4). Factors that should be considered when selecting a combination chemotherapy regimen for use as induction therapy include performance status and preexisting conditions (e.g., peripheral neuropathy).

In the HOVON-65/GMMG-HD4 study in 827 patients with newly diagnosed multiple myeloma, patients who received bortezomib-doxorubicin-dexamethasone had prolonged progression-free survival (35 versus 28 months; hazard ratio: 0.75) and higher postinduction (11 versus 5%) and posttransplant (31 versus 15%) complete plus near-complete response rates compared with those who received vincristine-doxorubicin-dexamethasone at a median follow-up of 41 months. Median overall survival had not been reached at a median follow-up of 66 months; however, no significant difference in 5-year overall survival was observed between the groups. Subgroup analyses based on presence of renal insufficiency or high-risk cytogenetic features (i.e., chromosome 13q14 deletion [del(13q14)], t(4;14) translocation, chromosome 17p13 deletion [del(17p13)]) suggested prolonged progression-free and overall survival with bortezomib-doxorubicin-dexamethasone compared with vincristine-doxorubicin-dexamethasone induction therapy in patients with serum creatinine concentrations exceeding 2 mg/dL and in those with del(17p13) chromosomal abnormality, as well as an overall survival benefit for bortezomib-doxorubicin-dexamethasone compared with vincristine-doxorubicin-dexamethasone in patients with del(13q14) chromosomal abnormality.

For further information on the use of combination therapy with conventional doxorubicin, bortezomib, and dexamethasone as induction therapy for newly diagnosed multiple myeloma in transplant-eligible patients, see Induction Therapy Prior to Stem Cell Transplantation in Newly Diagnosed Multiple Myeloma under Uses: Multiple Myeloma, in Bortezomib 10:00.

Liposomal Doxorubicin. Use of pegylated liposomal doxorubicin also has been studied in combination with bortezomib and dexamethasone† (bortezomib-liposomal doxorubicin-dexamethasone) as induction therapy for previously untreated multiple myeloma† in 2 open-label, noncomparative phase 2 studies. Based on current evidence, use of liposomal doxorubicin in combination with bortezomib and dexamethasone as induction therapy for newly diagnosed multiple myeloma in transplant-eligible patients may be considered a reasonable choice (accepted; with possible conditions); however, in the absence of longer follow-up data, use of a modified bortezomib-liposomal doxorubicin-dexamethasone regimen (i.e., reduced dosages of liposomal doxorubicin and bortezomib) is not fully established because of unclear risk/benefit and/or inadequate experience (see Liposomal Doxorubicin Hydrochloride under Dosage and Administration: Dosage). Factors that should be considered when selecting a combination chemotherapy regimen for induction therapy include performance status and preexisting conditions (e.g., peripheral neuropathy).

In the first study in 40 patients with newly diagnosed multiple myeloma, overall response rate and complete plus near-complete response rate were 85 and 38%, respectively, following 6 cycles of induction therapy with bortezomib-liposomal doxorubicin-dexamethasone. Among patients who underwent stem cell transplantation, the complete plus near-complete response rate increased to 57% following transplantation, but the overall response rate did not improve substantially. At a median follow-up of 45.1 months, median progression-free survival had not been reached; however, among patients who underwent stem cell transplantation, actuarial 2- and 4-year progression-free survival rates were 93 and 65%, respectively, and actuarial 2- and 4-year overall survival rates were 97 and 67%, respectively.

Because liposomal doxorubicin and bortezomib frequently cause adverse effects, another phase 2 study evaluated a modified bortezomib-liposomal doxorubicin-dexamethasone regimen (i.e., reduced dosages of liposomal doxorubicin and bortezomib) in 35 patients with previously untreated multiple myeloma. Overall and complete response rates were 86 and 20%, respectively. At a median follow-up of 17.7 months, median time to progression, duration of response, and overall survival had not been reached.

For further information on the use of combination therapy with liposomal doxorubicin, bortezomib, and dexamethasone as induction therapy for newly diagnosed multiple myeloma in transplant-eligible patients, see Induction Therapy Prior to Stem Cell Transplantation in Newly Diagnosed Multiple Myeloma under Uses: Multiple Myeloma, in Bortezomib 10:00.

Refractory Multiple Myeloma Doxorubicin is used in combination therapy for refractory multiple myeloma†. A regimen employing continuous IV infusions of doxorubicin and vincristine and high-dose dexamethasone is used in patients with advanced multiple myeloma refractory to alkylating agents and in patients with relapsing disease.

■ **Other Uses** Doxorubicin hydrochloride is used in the treatment of solid tumors including thyroid cancer, gastric cancer, soft-tissue and osteogenic sarcomas, neuroblastoma, and Wilms' tumor; malignant lymphomas of both Hodgkin and non-Hodgkin type; and acute lymphocytic leukemia.

Doxorubicin is used in the treatment of Ewing's sarcoma†, squamous cell carcinomas of the cervix† and prostate†, and uterine cancer†.

Doxorubicin also is used in the treatment of adrenocortical cancer†, carcinoid tumors†, endometrial cancer†, islet cell carcinoma†, chronic lymphocytic leukemia†, liver cancer†, and mesothelioma†.

Although doxorubicin is labeled for use in the treatment of acute myeloid leukemia, other agents are preferred.

Dosage and Administration

■ **Reconstitution and Administration** Doxorubicin hydrochloride conventional and PEG-stabilized liposomal for injection concentrate are administered IV. The drug is extremely irritating to tissues and, therefore, must not be given IM or subcutaneously. (See Cautions: Local Effects.) *Care should be taken to avoid extravasation of the drug.*

Because doxorubicin may cause adverse local dermatologic reactions, commercially available conventional and liposomal doxorubicin hydrochloride for injection concentrate, the powder for injection, and solutions of the drug must be prepared and handled cautiously and the use of latex gloves is recommended. If the powder or solutions of the drug contact the skin or mucous membranes, the affected area should be immediately and thoroughly washed with soap and water. Parenteral doxorubicin hydrochloride solutions should be inspected visually for particulate matter and discoloration prior to administration whenever solution and container permit. However, because PEG-stabilized liposomal doxorubicin hydrochloride occurs as a liposomal dispersion, the for injection concentrate is not clear but rather is translucent and red.

Conventional Doxorubicin Hydrochloride The lyophilized drug is reconstituted by adding 5, 10, 25, 50, or 75 mL of 0.9% sodium chloride injection to a vial labeled as containing 10, 20, 50, 100, or 150 mg of doxorubicin hydrochloride, respectively. The vial should then be shaken and the contents allowed to dissolve. When reconstituted as directed above, the resultant solution contains 2 mg of doxorubicin hydrochloride per mL. Diluents containing preservatives should not be used to reconstitute the powder for injection. Alternatively, to avoid the potential risks associated with reconstitution of the powder, the commercially available injection can be used; however, handling of the solution is *not* without risk.

Solutions of the conventional doxorubicin hydrochloride injection should be administered slowly into the tubing of a freely running IV infusion of 0.9% sodium chloride or 5% dextrose injection, preferably via a Butterfly® needle inserted into a large vein. When possible, veins over joints or in extremities with compromised venous or lymphatic drainage should *not* be used. The rate of the conventional doxorubicin hydrochloride injection depends on the size of the vein and the dose, but the dose should be administered over at least 3–5 minutes. Local erythematous streaking along the vein and/or facial flushing may be indicative of too rapid an administration rate.

Although a stinging or burning sensation may be a symptom of extravasation during IV administration of conventional doxorubicin hydrochloride, extravasation may occur without these symptoms and even when blood returns well during initial aspiration of the infusion needle. If any signs or symptoms of extravasation occur, the injection or infusion of conventional doxorubicin hydrochloride should be immediately stopped and restarted at another site. When extravasation of the conventional injection occurs or is suspected, intermittent application of ice packs to the site for 15 minutes four times daily for

3 days may be helpful in reducing the local reaction. The benefit of local administration of drugs to the extravasation site has not been established. Because of the progressive nature of extravasation reactions, the affected area should be examined frequently and consultation with a specialist in plastic surgery should be obtained. If blistering, ulceration, and/or persistent pain occurs, wide excision of the affected area followed by split-thickness skin grafting should be considered.

Liposomal Doxorubicin Hydrochloride *PEG-stabilized liposomal doxorubicin hydrochloride for injection concentrate must be diluted prior to IV infusion.* The concentrate should be diluted in 5% dextrose injection *only*, and no other diluent should be used. Doses of PEG-stabilized liposomal doxorubicin hydrochloride for injection concentrate up to 90 mg should be diluted in 250 mL of 5% dextrose injection. Doses of PEG-stabilized liposomal doxorubicin hydrochloride for injection concentrate exceeding 90 mg should be diluted in 500 mL of 5% dextrose injection. Strict aseptic technique must be observed because the liposomal doxorubicin for injection concentrate does not contain any preservative or bacteriostatic agent. Diluents containing preservatives (e.g., benzyl alcohol) should *not* be used to dilute the liposomal for injection concentrate, and other drugs should *not* be mixed with the solution. Because PEG-stabilized liposomal doxorubicin hydrochloride occurs as a liposomal dispersion of the drug, inline filters should *not* be used. Rapid flushing of the infusion line should be avoided.

The diluted solution of liposomal doxorubicin hydrochloride should be infused at an initial rate of 1 mg/minute in patients receiving the drug for ovarian cancer or AIDS-related Kaposi's sarcoma to reduce the risk of infusion-related reactions; if no infusion-related reactions occur, the rate of infusion may be increased to complete administration of the infusion over a 1-hour period. If infusion reactions manifested as flushing, shortness of breath, facial edema, headache, chills, chest pain, back pain, tightness of the chest or throat, fever, tachycardia, pruritus, rash, cyanosis, syncope, bronchospasm, asthma, apnea, and/or hypotension occur, the rate of infusion should be slowed or the infusion stopped. Because rapid infusion may increase the risk of such reactions, the liposomal injection should *not* be administered by rapid direct injection nor as an undiluted solution.

Although a stinging or burning sensation may be a symptom of extravasation during IV administration of liposomal doxorubicin hydrochloride, extravasation may occur without these symptoms and even when blood returns well during initial aspiration of the infusion needle. If any signs or symptoms of extravasation occur, the injection or infusion of liposomal doxorubicin hydrochloride should be immediately stopped and restarted at another site. When extravasation of liposomal doxorubicin hydrochloride occurs, applying ice packs over the site of extravasation for about 30 minutes may help alleviate the local reaction.

■ **Dosage** To obtain optimum therapeutic results with minimum adverse effects, dosage of doxorubicin hydrochloride must be based on the clinical, cardiac, hepatic, renal, and hematologic response and tolerance of the patient and on other chemotherapy or irradiation being used. Dosage reduction may be necessary in patients who have received extensive prior radiation therapy or in those whose bone marrow has been infiltrated with malignant cells, since severe myelosuppression is likely to occur. Clinicians should consult published protocols for the dosage of doxorubicin hydrochloride and other chemotherapeutic agents and the method and sequence of administration. Dosage of doxorubicin hydrochloride is based indirectly on body weight; if the patient has abnormal fluid retention, the patient's ideal weight is used to calculate body surface area.

Accidental substitution of liposomal doxorubicin for conventional doxorubicin hydrochloride injection has resulted in severe adverse effects. Liposomal doxorubicin hydrochloride should *not* be substituted for conventional doxorubicin hydrochloride, and the drugs are not equivalent on a mg per mg basis.

The total cumulative dose of doxorubicin hydrochloride should not exceed 550 mg/m^2 because of the risk of potentially irreversible cardiotoxicity, but higher cumulative doses may be tolerated when dexrazoxane (Zinecard®) is used concomitantly as a cardioprotectant. (See Cautions: Cardiac Effects.) If previous or concomitant therapy includes the use of other potentially cardiotoxic agents, such as cyclophosphamide, or irradiation of the cardiac region, total doxorubicin hydrochloride dosage should not exceed 400 mg/m^2. The total dosage of doxorubicin hydrochloride should include any previous or concomitant therapy with other anthracycline agents or related compounds.

Conventional Doxorubicin Hydrochloride The usual adult dosage of conventional (nonencapsulated) doxorubicin hydrochloride is 60–75 mg/m^2, administered as a single dose at 21-day intervals; the lower dose should be considered for patients with poor performance status, inadequate bone marrow reserves secondary to old age, prior therapy, or marrow infiltration with malignant cells. Alternatively, a dosage of 20 mg/m^2 once weekly may be used; this dosage schedule has been reported to produce a lower incidence of congestive heart failure. A dosage of 30 mg/m^2 daily on 3 successive days every 4 weeks has also been used; this dosage schedule is usually associated with a higher incidence of stomatitis. When used in combination with other chemotherapy, doxorubicin hydrochloride commonly has been used in a dosage of 40–60 mg/m^2 given as a single IV dose and repeated at 21- to 28-day intervals.

When doxorubicin hydrochloride has been used in combination with bortezomib and dexamethasone† as induction therapy for newly diagnosed multiple myeloma in transplant-eligible patients†, doxorubicin hydrochloride 9 mg/m^2 per day has been administered IV on days 1–4 along with bortezomib 1.3 mg/m^2 by IV injection twice weekly for 2 weeks (days 1, 4, 8, and 11) and dexamethasone 40 mg orally on days 1–4, 9–12, and 17–20 of each 28-day cycle for 3 cycles.

Liposomal Doxorubicin Hydrochloride For the treatment of AIDS-related Kaposi's sarcoma, the usual adult dosage of pegylated liposomal doxorubicin hydrochloride is 20 mg/m^2 once every 3 weeks, administered at an initial rate of 1 mg/minute. If no infusion-related adverse effects occur, the rate of infusion may be increased to complete administration of the infusion over a 1-hour period. The duration of therapy depends on response and tolerance of the patient.

When used for the treatment of ovarian cancer that has progressed or recurred following platinum-based chemotherapy, the manufacturer recommends a pegylated liposomal doxorubicin hydrochloride dosage of 50 mg/m^2 IV once every 4 weeks, administered at an initial rate of 1 mg/minute. If no infusion-related adverse effects occur, the rate of infusion may be increased to complete administration of the infusion over a 1-hour period. In patients without disease progression or intolerable toxicity, the manufacturer recommends a minimum of 4 courses of therapy because the median time to response with liposomal doxorubicin therapy in clinical trials for metastatic ovarian cancer was approximately 4 months.

When pegylated liposomal doxorubicin hydrochloride has been used in combination with bortezomib and dexamethasone† as induction therapy for newly diagnosed multiple myeloma in transplant-eligible patients†, pegylated liposomal doxorubicin hydrochloride 30 mg/m^2 has been administered IV on day 4 along with bortezomib 1.3 mg/m^2 by IV injection twice weekly for 2 weeks (days 1, 4, 8, and 11) and dexamethasone 40 mg orally on days 1, 2, 4, 5, 8, 9, 11, and 12 during cycle 1. During cycles 2–6, the same dosages of pegylated liposomal doxorubicin hydrochloride and bortezomib were administered along with dexamethasone 20 mg orally daily. Treatment cycles were repeated every 3 weeks for a total of 6 cycles.

Although a modified regimen using reduced dosages of both pegylated liposomal doxorubicin hydrochloride and bortezomib given in combination with dexamethasone† also has been used as induction therapy for newly diagnosed multiple myeloma in transplant-eligible patients†, use of this regimen is not fully established.

The management of certain adverse effects (e.g., hand-foot syndrome, hematologic toxicity, stomatitis) in patients receiving liposomal doxorubicin hydrochloride may require reduction in dosage and/or delay of doses. The manufacturer recommends the following dosage modifications for liposomal doxorubicin hydrochloride based on drug-induced adverse effects (see Dosage Modification tables). Once the dose of liposomal doxorubicin hydrochloride has been reduced because of drug-related toxicity, such as hand-foot syndrome or stomatitis, the dose should not be increased. For the management of nausea and vomiting associated with liposomal doxorubicin therapy, pretreatment with or concomitant use of antiemetic therapy should be considered.

Table 1. Dosage Modification for Hand-Foot Syndrome

Toxicity Grade	Symptoms	Dose Modification
0	No symptoms	None
1	Mild erythema, swelling, or desquamation not interfering with daily activities	Redose unless patient has experienced previous grade 3 or 4 skin toxicity in which case delay dose up to 2 weeks and decrease dose by 25%; then return to original dose interval
2	Erythema, desquamation, or swelling interfering with, but not precluding, normal physical activities; small blisters or ulcerations <2 cm in diameter	Delay dosing up to 2 weeks or until toxicity resolved to grade 0–1; if no resolution after 2 weeks, discontinue liposomal doxorubicin; if resolved to grade 0–1 within 2 weeks and no previous grade 3–4 toxicity, continue treatment at previous dose and return to original dose interval; if patient experienced previous grade 3–4 toxicity, decrease dose by 25% and return to original dose interval
3	Blistering, ulceration, or swelling interfering with walking or normal daily activities; cannot wear regular clothing	Delay dosing up to 2 weeks or until toxicity resolved to grade 0–1, then decrease dose by 25% and return to original dose interval; if no resolution after 2 weeks, discontinue liposomal doxorubicin
4	Diffuse or local process causing infectious complications, or a bedridden state or hospitalization	Delay dosing up to 2 weeks or until toxicity resolved to grade 0–1, then decrease dose by 25% and return to original dose interval; if no resolution after 2 weeks, discontinue liposomal doxorubicin

For further information on reduced dosage of Doxil® (liposomal doxorubicin hydrochloride) based on drug-induced adverse effects, consult the manufacturer at (415) 617-3078.

Table 2. Dosage Modification for Hematologic Toxicity

Toxicity Grade	ANC (per mm³)	Platelets (per mm³)	Dose Modification
1	1500–1900	75,000–150,000	None
2	1000–1499	50,000–74,999	Wait until ANC ≥1500 and platelets ≥75,000, then redose with no dose reduction
3	500–999	25,000–49,999	Wait until ANC ≥1500 and platelets ≥75,000, then redose with no dose reduction
4	<500	<25,000	Wait until ANC ≥1500 and platelets ≥75,000, then redose at 25% dose reduction or continue full dose with cytokine support

Table 3. Dosage Modification for Stomatitis

Toxicity Grade	Symptoms	Dose Modification
1	Painless ulcers, erythema, or mild soreness	Redose unless patient has experienced previous grade 3 or 4 toxicity, in which case delay up to 2 weeks and decrease dose by 25%, returning to original dose interval
2	Painful erythema, edema, or ulcers, but can eat	Delay dosing up to 2 weeks or until resolved to grade 0–1; if no improvement after 2 weeks, discontinue liposomal doxorubicin; if resolved to grade 0–1 within 2 weeks and no previous grade 3–4 toxicity, continue treatment at previous dose and return to original dose interval; if patient experienced previous grade 3–4 toxicity, decrease dose by 25% and return to original dose interval
3	Painful erythema, edema, or ulcers, and cannot eat	Delay dosing up to 2 weeks or until resolution to grade 0–1, then redose at 25% dose reduction and return to original dose interval; if no improvement after 2 weeks, discontinue liposomal doxorubicin
4	Requires parenteral or enteral support	Delay dosing up to 2 weeks or until resolution to grade 0–1, then redose at 25% dose reduction and return to original dose interval; if no improvement after 2 weeks, discontinue liposomal doxorubicin

■ **Dosage in Hepatic Impairment** In adults with impairment of hepatic function, conventional or liposomal doxorubicin dosage *must* be reduced. Patients with serum bilirubin concentrations of 1.2–3 mg/dL should receive 50% of the usual dose of doxorubicin hydrochloride and those with serum bilirubin concentrations exceeding 3 mg/dL should receive 25% of the usual dose.

Cautions

■ **Hematologic Effects** Because of the risk of myelosuppression, hematologic status must be monitored carefully in patients receiving conventional or liposomal doxorubicin.

Conventional Doxorubicin Leukopenia (principally granulocytopenia) is the predominant manifestation of hematologic toxicity, the severity of which depends on the dose of the drug and on the regenerative capacity of the bone marrow. Leukocyte counts as low as 1000/mm³ should be anticipated during therapy with appropriate doses of doxorubicin, although severe myelosuppression can occur. Thrombocytopenia and anemia may also occur. Deaths from septicemia have been associated with severe leukopenia. Maximum leukopenia, thrombocytopenia, and anemia generally occur during the second week (nadir at 10–14 days) following administration of the drug and generally return to normal by the third week.

Liposomal Doxorubicin The principal dose-limiting toxicity of pegylated liposomal doxorubicin in patients with AIDS-related Kaposi's sarcoma has been myelosuppression, commonly manifested by leukopenia and neutropenia; anemia and thrombocytopenia also occur frequently. Among 720 patients with AIDS-related Kaposi's sarcoma receiving liposomal doxorubicin in clinical trials, neutropenia less than 2000/mm³ was reported in 85% of patients, neutropenia less than 1000/mm³ was reported in about 49% of patients, and severe or life-threatening neutropenia (less than 500/mm³) occurred in 13% of patients. Leukopenia less than 4000/mm³ was reported in about 91% of patients, and leukopenia less than 1000/mm³ occurred in 11.5% of patients. Anemia was reported in 55.4% of patients and was severe or life-threatening in 18.2% of patients. Hypochromic anemia was reported in about 10% of patients. Thrombocytopenia was reported in 61% of patients and was life-threatening in 4% of patients.

Patients receiving pegylated liposomal doxorubicin for AIDS-related Kaposi's sarcoma often have baseline myelosuppression secondary to their underlying human immunodeficiency virus (HIV) infection and/or numerous concomitant drug therapy. With the recommended dosage schedule, leukopenia associated with liposomal doxorubicin usually is transient, but hematologic toxicity occasionally may be severe enough to require dose reduction or delay or suspension of therapy with the drug. Persistent, severe myelosuppression may result in superinfection or hemorrhage. In patients with AIDS-related Kaposi's sarcoma receiving liposomal doxorubicin, sepsis occurred in 5% of patients and was considered possibly or probably related to the drug in 0.7% of patients. Discontinuance of liposomal doxorubicin because of myelosuppression or neutropenia was required in 1.6% of patients with AIDS-related Kaposi's sarcoma. The development of neutropenic sepsis rarely has resulted in death.

Adverse hematologic effects reported in 1–5% of patients receiving pegylated liposomal doxorubicin for AIDS-related Kaposi's sarcoma include hemolysis and increased prothrombin time.

In patients with relapsed ovarian cancer, myelosuppression associated with pegylated liposomal doxorubicin generally has been moderate and reversible. Anemia was the most common adverse hematologic effect in patients with relapsed ovarian cancer, occurring in about 53% of patients receiving liposomal doxorubicin in 3 single-arm clinical trials. Neutropenia with an absolute neutrophil count less than 2000/mm³ was reported in 52%, and neutropenia with an absolute neutrophil count less than 1000/mm³ was reported in 19%, of patients with relapsed ovarian cancer receiving liposomal doxorubicin. Leukopenia (white blood cell count less than 4000/mm³) was reported in 42%, and thrombocytopenia was reported in 24%, of patients with relapsed ovarian cancer receiving liposomal doxorubicin. In the randomized trial, anemia occurred in 40%, leukopenia in 37%, neutropenia (absolute neutrophil count less than 1000/mm³) in 35%, and thrombocytopenia in 13%, of patients receiving liposomal doxorubicin for ovarian cancer. Granulocyte colony-stimulating factor or granulocyte-macrophage colony-stimulating factor was used in 4.6% of patients receiving liposomal doxorubicin for relapsed ovarian cancer to reduce the severity of myelosuppression associated with therapy.

■ **Cardiac Effects** ***Types of Cardiotoxicity*** Three types of cardiotoxicity may occur in patients receiving an anthracycline (e.g., doxorubicin): an acute transient type; a chronic, subacute type, which is related to cumulative dose and has a later, more indolent onset; and a late-onset type that manifests years after anthracycline therapy and occurs mainly in patients exposed to the drugs as children. The use of conventional or liposomal doxorubicin may cause cardiac toxicity.

Acute anthracycline-induced cardiotoxicity usually is uncommon. It occurs immediately after a single dose or a single course of anthracycline therapy and may involve abnormal ECG findings including ST-T wave changes (e.g., T-wave flattening and ST-segment depression), prolongation of the QT interval, and arrhythmias (e.g., sinus tachycardia; ventricular, supraventricular, and junctional tachycardia). Conduction disturbances (including atrioventricular [AV] and bundle-branch block) have been reported rarely in acute anthracycline-induced cardiotoxicity (they are more usually associated with late-onset anthracycline-induced cardiotoxicity). Although acute cardiotoxicity generally is transient, rarely, pericarditis-myocarditis syndrome (e.g., pericardial effusion and/or decreased myocardial contractility) and possible cardiac failure may occur.

Chronic cardiotoxicity, such as congestive heart failure or cardiomyopathy, usually occurs within 1 year after discontinuance of anthracycline therapy, is more common than acute cardiotoxicity, and is considered clinically the most important anthracycline-associated toxicity. Chronic cardiotoxicity, such as heart failure, may occur as total cumulative dosage of doxorubicin hydrochloride approaches or exceeds 550 mg/m². Heart failure may occur at a lower total cumulative dosage (i.e., 400 mg/m²) in patients who have received radiotherapy to the mediastinal region or in patients receiving concomitant therapy with other potentially cardiotoxic agents, such as cyclophosphamide. Time of onset of chronic cardiotoxicity may vary but usually is manifested within 1 year of anthracycline therapy. In one study, onset of congestive heart failure developed 0–231 days after discontinuance of anthracycline therapy.

Chronic cardiotoxicity reflects a progressive injury and loss of cardiac myocytes, with increasing cumulative anthracycline doses resulting in thinning of ventricular walls and decreased systolic performance. Initially, there is functional compensation by the remaining myocytes allowing overall cardiac function to appear normal despite histologic damage, which can be demonstrated by endomyocardial biopsy. However, as cumulative doses of anthracycline increase, there is a decrease in systolic performance, as measured by a decrease in fractional shortening (FS) and in left-ventricular ejection fraction (LVEF) with eventual progression to symptomatic congestive heart failure, if cardiac reserve is exhausted, and to cardiorespiratory decompensation. Symptoms of the described rapidly progressing syndrome may include tachycardia, tachypnea, dilation of the heart, exercise intolerance, pulmonary and venous congestion, poor perfusion, and pleural effusion; these manifestations may respond to cardiac supportive therapy and may be self-limiting, or, alternatively, may be irreversible and unresponsive to therapy and fatal.

Sensitivity to anthracycline-induced cardiotoxicity exhibits interindividual variation, with some patients occasionally tolerating cumulative doxorubicin hydrochloride doses exceeding 1 g/m² while other patients exhibit histopathologic changes characteristic of doxorubicin-induced cardiotoxicity, decreases in LVEF, and even congestive heart failure at cumulative doses of less than 300 mg/m². Despite such interindividual variation, the risk of developing doxorubicin-induced impairment in myocardial function (based on a combined index of signs, symptoms, and decline in LVEF) increases with increasing cumulative dose, occurring in 1–2% of patients receiving cumulative doses of 300 mg/m^2 and increasing to 3–5, 5–8, and 6–20% in those receiving cumulative doses of 400, 450, or 500 mg/m^2 in schedules of rapid IV doses given once every 3 weeks. In one retrospective review, congestive heart failure developed in 3, 7, or 21% of patients at cumulative doses of 430, 575, or 728 mg/m^2, and the slope of the probability curve for developing congestive heart failure increased at around 550 mg/m^2. However, in a prospective study in which doxorubicin was administered concomitantly with cyclophosphamide, fluorouracil, and/or vincristine in patients with breast cancer or small cell lung cancer, the risk of congestive heart failure was 1.5, 4.9, 7.7, or 20.5% at cumulative doses of 300, 400, 450, or 500 mg/m^2.

Adverse cardiac effects occurred in 9.6% of patients with AIDS-related Kaposi's sarcoma receiving pegylated liposomal doxorubicin in clinical trials and were considered possibly or probably related to the drug in 4.3% of patients. Cardiomyopathy and congestive heart failure have been reported in patients receiving liposomal doxorubicin for AIDS-related Kaposi's sarcoma. Severe adverse cardiac effects, including arrhythmia, cardiomyopathy, heart failure, pericardial effusion, and tachycardia, were reported in 1% of patients receiving liposomal doxorubicin for AIDS-related Kaposi's sarcoma. The manufacturer reports that therapy with liposomal doxorubicin was discontinued because of adverse cardiac events in 3 patients with AIDS-related Kaposi's sarcoma receiving the drug in clinical trials.

In 250 patients with advanced breast cancer receiving pegylated liposomal doxorubicin hydrochloride at a starting dose of 50 mg/m^2 every 4 weeks, the incidence of cardiac toxicity was 11% at cumulative doses of 450–500 mg/m^2 and 500–550 mg/m^2.

Factors reported to increase the risk of anthracycline-induced cardiotoxicity (some of which may cause such toxicity at lower cumulative doxorubicin doses) include irradiation to the mediastinal region, concomitant cyclophosphamide, preexisting heart disease (e.g., occult hypertension, subclinical coronary artery disease), extremes in age, liver disease, whole body hyperthermia, and female gender (mainly in children). In one study in women with early breast cancer receiving cyclophosphamide-based adjuvant chemotherapy following either surgery alone or surgery and mediastinal irradiation, cardiac abnormalities (e.g., ECG changes) developed in about 5% of all (both those who did and did not receive irradiation) patients and about 70% of these cases of cardiac abnormalities occurred in patients receiving irradiation of the left breast; all cases of congestive heart failure (which was fatal in several patients) reported in irradiated patients occurred at cumulative doxorubicin hydrochloride doses that did not exceed 315 mg/m^2. This and other evidence suggest that irradiation of the left breast may be a more important cardiotoxic cofactor than concomitant alkylating chemotherapy. Anthracycline therapy may potentiate cardiotoxicity caused by high-dose cyclophosphamide therapy used for bone marrow ablation and transplantation. It is unclear if lower doses of cyclophosphamide interact with anthracyclines in the development of cardiotoxicity. Some evidence also suggests that the risk of cardiotoxicity may be increased in patients receiving calcium-channel blocking agents concomitantly. The cardiotoxic risk associated with cumulative doses of doxorubicin also should take into account previous or concomitant therapy with related drugs such as daunorubicin, idarubicin, and mitoxantrone.

Late-onset anthracycline-induced cardiotoxicity, which may include late-onset ventricular dysfunction, heart failure, conduction disturbances, and arrhythmias (e.g., nonsustained ventricular tachycardia) which may be life-threatening, occurs several years or even decades after discontinuance of anthracycline therapy and it may develop after a prolonged asymptomatic interval. In one study in patients with solid tumors or leukemia, those who were followed for 4 to less than 10 or 10–20 years after discontinuance of anthracycline therapy had an 18 or 38% incidence, respectively, of abnormal FS in echocardiograms. In another study in children with acute lymphoblastic leukemia who were followed for up to 15 years after discontinuance of anthracycline therapy, increases in myocardial afterload and/or decreases in myocardial contractility were reported in 65% of patients receiving cumulative doses of at least 228 mg/m^2; these cardiac abnormalities appeared to be progressive and were predictive of future cardiac decompensation. It has been suggested that myocyte damage and ventricular dysfunction progress after the initial myocardial insult and may lead to late-onset cardiac decompensation.Some clinicians state that late-onset cardiotoxicity can be clinically manifest in response to stressful situations (e.g., surgery, pregnancy), exercise (e.g., weight lifting), and acute viral infection. In at least one patient, postpartum-associated congestive heart failure occurred 7 years after discontinuance of doxorubicin therapy. Some clinicians suggested that the postpartum effects of anemia, hypertension, and fluid mobilization on subclinical doxorubicin fibrosis resulted in reversible cardiac decompensation. The incidence of late-onset cardiotoxicity may be increased with increasing cumulative doses of anthracyclines, high rates of administration, or irradiation to the mediastinal region; young age at the time of anthracycline therapy and female gender may be contributing factors to such cardiotoxicity, but further study is needed.

Late-onset anthracycline toxicity can be expected to be observed more frequently with the growing census of long-term survivors (e.g., survivors of childhood cancers) who have received anthracyclines. It also is expected that this cardiotoxicity will be associated with increased morbidity and mortality. Substantial cardiac injury may occur even with low-dose anthracycline therapy. Since the observed incidence of severe anthracycline-induced cardiotoxicity appears to increase (especially after irradiation to the mediastinal region) with duration of long-term monitoring, the full extent of late-onset anthracycline toxicity in asymptomatic patients remains to be elucidated since data currently are inadequate regarding cardiotoxicity occurring 15 years or more after discontinuance of anthracycline therapy. Long-term follow-up shows that overt cardiac failure occurs in about 4.5–7% of patients receiving anthracycline therapy.

Assessment of Cardiotoxicity Clinical manifestations found on physical examination (e.g., shortness of breath, pulmonary rales) and/or changes detected on electrocardiographic monitoring (e.g., sinus tachycardia) are not specific enough to diagnose anthracycline-induced cardiotoxicity. More sensitive methods are needed to detect early signs of cardiac damage so that the potential benefits from larger than usual dosages of anthracyclines in cancer therapy may be weighed against the possible risks of drug-induced cardiotoxicity. Monitoring of the left-ventricular ejection fraction with serial echocardiographic studies is a sensitive, noninvasive method for the detection and follow-up of anthracycline-induced cardiomyopathy.Radionuclide angiography also has been used to monitor the ejection fraction, but this procedure exposes the patient to ionizing radiation. The combination of exercise stress testing and ejection-fraction studies is a more sensitive indicator for detecting early signs of subclinical cardiomyopathy associated with anthracycline therapy. Endomyocardial biopsy (using a semiquantitative histologic scoring system) currently is considered the most sensitive and specific method for diagnosing and determining the degree of anthracycline-induced cardiotoxicity; however, this invasive procedure is not routinely used. Concerns for safety, especially in children requiring multiple biopsies, and in those with thrombocytopenia, and the lack of experience in obtaining and scoring biopsies have limited the use of endomyocardial biopsy; the correlation between biopsy scores and the long-term effects of anthracycline cardiotoxicity has not been established, and underestimation of cardiac damage may occur. Guidelines for cardiac monitoring of children receiving anthracycline therapy have been published, although their general acceptance remains to be established. Guidelines also have been published for adults using multigated radionuclide angiography (MUGA scans).

Anthracycline-induced cardiomyopathy usually is associated with characteristic histopathologic changes on endomyocardial (EM) biopsy (e.g., fibrosis, myofibrillar dropout, intracellular vacuolar degeneration) and with decreased LVEF, as determined by multi-gated radionuclide angiography (MUGA scans) and/or echocardiogram (ECHO), relative to baseline values. In adults, a 10% decline in LVEF to below the lower limit of normal, a 20% decline in LVEF at any level, or an absolute LVEF of 45% is indicative of a deterioration in cardiac function. Although monitoring the ejection fraction has not been shown to be predictive of impending maximal tolerance of the cumulative doxorubicin dose, the benefits of continued therapy with the drug should be weighed carefully against the risk of irreversible cardiotoxicity whenever test results indicate a deterioration in cardiac function.

Mechanism of Cardiotoxicity Several anthracycline-induced effects may contribute to the development of cardiotoxicity. In animals, anthracyclines cause a selective inhibition of cardiac muscle gene expression for α-actin, troponin, myosin light-chain 2, and the M isoform of creatine kinase, which may result in myofibrillar loss associated with anthracycline-induced cardiotoxicity. Other potential causes of anthracycline-induced cardiotoxicity include myocyte damage from calcium overload, altered myocardial adrenergic function, release of vasoactive amines, and proinflammatory cytokines. Limited data indicate that calcium-channel blocking agents (e.g., prenylamine) or β-adrenergic blocking agents may prevent calcium overload; however, the cardioprotective effects of β-adrenergic blocking agents have not been studied. It has been suggested that the principal cause of anthracycline-induced cardiotoxicity is associated with free radical damage to DNA.

Anthracyclines intercalate DNA, chelate metal ions to produce drug-metal complexes, and generate oxygen free radicals via oxidation-reduction reactions. Anthracyclines contain a quinone structure that may undergo reduction via NADPH-dependent reactions to produce a semiquinone free radical that initiates a cascade of oxygen-free radical generation. It appears that the metabolite, doxorubicinol, may be the moiety responsible for cardiotoxic effects, and the heart may be particularly susceptible to free-radical injury because of relatively low antioxidant concentrations. Initial attempts at preventing anthracycline-induced cardiotoxicity by administering antioxidants (e.g., vitamin E) to act as free-radical scavengers were not successful. Limited animal data indicate that probucol (no longer commercially available in the US), an antilipemic agent structurally similar to vitamin E, may prevent anthracycline-induced cardiotoxicity without interfering with the antineoplastic effect of doxorubicin. Chelation of metal ions, particularly iron, by the drug results in a doxorubicin-metal complex that catalyzes the generation of reactive oxygen free radicals, and the complex is a powerful oxidant that can initiate lipid peroxidation in the absence of oxygen free radicals. This reaction is not blocked by free-radical scavengers, and probably is the principal mechanism of anthracycline-induced cardiotoxicity. As a result, administration of dexrazoxane (ICRF-187), a cyclic derivative of EDTA that is converted intracellularly to a ring-opened chelating agent, can prevent anthracycline-induced cardiotoxicity, at least in part, by chelating free iron and thus preventing the formation of the anthracycline-iron complex and resultant free radical generation.

Management of Cardiotoxicity Effective management of anthracycline-induced cardiotoxicity requires early diagnosis and intervention by identifying patients with existing risk factors for cardiotoxicity.

Dexrazoxane has been shown to prevent or reduce the incidence and severity of anthracycline-induced cardiotoxicity, although some, but not all, evidence suggests that the drug also may interfere with the antineoplastic efficacy of certain chemotherapeutic regimens (e.g., when initiated concurrently with cyclophosphamide, doxorubicin, and fluorouracil therapy). This potentially detrimental effect was not observed when dexrazoxane therapy was withheld until several initial courses of chemotherapy could be administered, and results from most clinical studies have failed to demonstrate interference by dexrazoxane with the antineoplastic efficacy of chemotherapeutic regimens. Therefore, the manufacturer of dexrazoxane currently recommends that cardioprotectant therapy with the drug *not* be initiated at the time doxorubicin-containing chemotherapy is initiated but instead be delayed until patients have received a cumulative doxorubicin dose of 300 mg/m². Although patients receiving dexrazoxane generally can tolerate higher cumulative doses of doxorubicin before experiencing cardiotoxicity, the cardioprotectant will not eliminate the risk of cardiotoxicity in patients who have already received cumulative doxorubicin hydrochloride doses of 300 mg/m². Therefore, cardiac function should be monitored carefully even when dexrazoxane is used. Use of dexrazoxane is associated with severe myelosuppression, which is potentiated by doxorubicin, and the long-term effect of the drug on the prevention of doxorubicin-induced cardiotoxicity is not known.

In one study in women receiving doxorubicin with cyclophosphamide and fluorouracil for advanced breast cancer, patients receiving concomitant cardioprotection with dexrazoxane tolerated higher cumulative doxorubicin hydrochloride doses (median: 500 mg/m²) than those who did not receive the cardioprotectant (median: 441 mg/m²), and one-third of cardioprotected patients were able to tolerate cumulative doxorubicin doses of at least 700 mg/m² (about 40% of whom received cumulative doses of 1 g/m² or more) whereas only 4% of unprotected patients could tolerate such doses. There also was some evidence that dexrazoxane may reduce the risk of doxorubicin-induced cardiotoxicity in patients with other contributing risk factors (e.g., mediastinal irradiation).

Doxorubicin-induced cardiotoxicity also has reportedly been reduced by administration of low doses of doxorubicin at weekly intervals or by administration of the drug by prolonged, continuous IV infusion (e.g., over 48–96 hours) via a central venous catheter; the comparative efficacy of these dosage schedules in various cancers and the long-term effects on the development of anthracycline-induced cardiotoxicity have not been established.

Management of doxorubicin-induced congestive heart failure should include cardiac glycosides, inotropic agents (e.g., dobutamine), diuretics, after-load reduction (e.g., with vasodilators), angiotensin-converting enzyme (ACE) inhibitors, restricted sodium intake, and bed rest. β-Blocking agents (β_1-selective adrenergic blocking agents) also have been used in conjunction with other treatment for anthracycline-induced congestive heart failure. Early treatment of subclinical anthracycline-induced systolic dysfunction, possibly with an ACE inhibitor, may reduce mortality rates in these patients. Although such interventions may provide symptomatic relief and improvement in the functional status of the patient, myocardial toxicity can be poorly responsive and irreversible; prognosis for patients with anthracycline-induced cardiomyopathic failure is poor. (See Cautions: Precautions and Contraindications.) Heart transplantation may be a consideration for some patients with cardiac decompensation.

Other Cardiovascular Effects Adverse cardiovascular effects reported in 1–5% of patients receiving pegylated liposomal doxorubicin for AIDS-related Kaposi's sarcoma include chest pain, hypotension, and tachycardia.

Adverse cardiovascular effects reported in 1–10% of patients receiving pegylated liposomal doxorubicin for ovarian cancer include vasodilation, tachycardia, deep thrombophlebitis, hypotension, pallor, and cardiac arrest.

■ GI Effects ***Conventional Doxorubicin*** Stomatitis and esophagitis (mucositis) may occur in patients receiving doxorubicin, especially when the drug is administered daily on several successive days. Stomatitis usually begins as a burning sensation accompanied by erythema of the oral mucosa, which in 2–3 days may progress to ulceration, particularly in the sublingual and lateral tongue margins and on the palate. Ulceration is sometimes severe enough to result in difficulty in swallowing, but seldom requires cessation of therapy. Stomatitis is maximal during the second week of therapy and lasts an additional 3–7 days. GI toxicity (evidenced frequently by nausea and vomiting and occasionally by anorexia and diarrhea) may occur, usually on the day of drug administration. Nausea and vomiting can be severe but may be alleviated by antiemetic therapy.

Ulceration and necrosis of the colon, particularly the cecum, leading to bleeding or severe and possibly fatal infection, have occurred in patients with acute myelogenous leukemia who received combined doxorubicin and cytarabine therapy.

Liposomal Doxorubicin Among patients receiving pegylated liposomal doxorubicin for AIDS-related Kaposi's sarcoma in randomized trials, nausea occurred in 17%, vomiting in 8%, diarrhea in 8%, and stomatitis in 7%, of patients. Oral moniliasis was reported in 5.5% of these patients. Adverse GI effects reported in 1–5% of patients receiving liposomal doxorubicin for AIDS-related Kaposi's sarcoma include mouth ulceration, glossitis, constipation, aphthous stomatitis, anorexia, dysphagia, and abdominal pain.

Among patients receiving pegylated liposomal doxorubicin for ovarian cancer in the randomized trial, nausea occurred in 46%, stomatitis in 41%, and vomiting in 33%, of patients. Abdominal pain occurred in 33.5% of these patients. Constipation was reported in 30%, and diarrhea and anorexia each were reported in about 20% of these patients. Dyspepsia occurred in 12%, and intestinal obstruction in 11%, of patients receiving liposomal doxorubicin for ovarian cancer in the randomized trial. Adverse GI effects reported in 1–10% of patients receiving liposomal doxorubicin for ovarian cancer include oral moniliasis, mouth ulceration, dry mouth, gingivitis, esophagitis, dysphagia, flatulence, rectal bleeding, ileus, enlarged abdomen, and ascites.

■ Dermatologic Effects ***Conventional Doxorubicin*** Complete alopecia almost always accompanies doxorubicin therapy, and patients should be advised of this effect. Regrowth of hair usually begins 2–3 months after doxorubicin is discontinued. The degree of doxorubicin-induced alopecia has been reduced by use of scalp hypothermia before and for 30 minutes after administration of the drug. Hyperpigmentation of nailbeds, pigmented banding of fingernails, and phalangeal and other dermal creases may occur in patients receiving doxorubicin. One clinician reported that pigment changes appeared 6 or more weeks following initiation of doxorubicin administration. Onycholysis, plantar callus formation, and epidermolysis also have been reported in patients receiving the drug.

Like dactinomycin, doxorubicin has reactivated latent effects of previous irradiation in some patients, producing erythema with vesiculation, nonpitting edema, severe pain, and moist desquamation in sites which were previously subjected to radiation therapy and which had subsequently returned to normal appearance. The reaction occurred from 4–7 days after each doxorubicin hydrochloride dose was administered and lasted an average of 7 days thereafter.

Liposomal Doxorubicin Palmar-plantar erythrodysesthesia (PPE), or hand-foot syndrome, characterized by swelling, pain, erythema, and occasionally desquamation of the hands and feet, has been reported in patients receiving pegylated liposomal doxorubicin for ovarian cancer or AIDS-related Kaposi's sarcoma. In patients receiving liposomal doxorubicin for ovarian cancer in the randomized trial, hand-foot syndrome occurred in 51% of patients and was severe (grade 3 or 4) in 24% of patients; 4.2% of patients discontinued therapy with the drug because of hand-foot syndrome or other dermatologic toxicity. In patients receiving liposomal doxorubicin 20 mg/m² every 2 weeks for AIDS-related Kaposi's sarcoma, 3.4% developed palmar-plantar skin eruptions, and 0.9% of patients discontinued therapy with the drug because of such effects.

Hand-foot syndrome generally developed after 2 or 3 cycles (i.e., 6 or more weeks) of therapy but occasionally occurred sooner. Although the reaction generally is mild and resolves within 1–2 weeks so that prolonged delay of therapy usually is not necessary, dose modification may be necessary (see Dosage Modification for Hand-Foot Syndrome table in Dosage section), and discontinuance of liposomal doxorubicin therapy may be required in some patients because of severe and debilitating effects.

Among patients receiving pegylated liposomal doxorubicin for AIDS-related Kaposi's sarcoma in randomized trials, alopecia was reported in about 9% of patients. Adverse dermatologic effects reported in 1–5% of patients receiving liposomal doxorubicin for AIDS-related Kaposi's sarcoma include herpes simplex, rash, and itching.

Among patients receiving pegylated liposomal doxorubicin for ovarian cancer in the randomized trial, rash occurred in 28.5%, and alopecia in 19%, of patients. Adverse dermatologic effects reported in 1–10% of patients receiving liposomal doxorubicin for ovarian cancer include pruritus, skin discoloration, vesiculobullous rash, maculopapular rash, exfoliative dermatitis, herpes zoster, sweating, dry skin, herpes simplex, fungal dermatitis, furunculosis, and acne.

■ Infusion-related Effects Acute infusion-related reactions in patients receiving pegylated liposomal doxorubicin were characterized by one or more of the following manifestations: flushing, shortness of breath, facial edema, headache, chills, chest pain, back pain, tightness of the chest and throat, fever, tachycardia, pruritus, rash, cyanosis, syncope, bronchospasm, asthma, apnea, and hypotension. Allergic or anaphylactoid-like reactions, sometimes life-threatening or fatal, also have been reported.

Acute infusion-related reactions occurred in 7% of patients with ovarian cancer receiving pegylated liposomal doxorubicin in the randomized trial; 2 patients (0.8%) discontinued therapy because of infusion-related reactions. Discontinuance of therapy with liposomal doxorubicin because of infusion-related reactions was required in 1.7% of patients receiving drug for solid tumors and in 0.9% of patients receiving the drug for AIDS-related Kaposi's sarcoma.

Infusion-related reactions typically occur during the first infusion and usually resolve over the course of several hours to a day once the infusion is stopped. Occasionally, the reactions may resolve simply by slowing the rate of infusion. The manufacturer recommends an initial infusion rate of 1 mg/minute to minimize the risk of infusion-related reactions in patients receiving liposomal doxorubicin. Medications and emergency equipment for the treatment of allergic or anaphylactoid-like reactions should be available for immediate use in patients receiving liposomal doxorubicin. Similar reactions have not been reported with conventional doxorubicin and therefore have been attributed to the liposomes or one of their surface components.

■ Local Effects ***Conventional Doxorubicin*** Extravasation of conventional doxorubicin produces severe local tissue necrosis, as well as possible cellulitis, vesication, thrombophlebitis, lymphangitis, or painful induration and may result in limitation of mobility of the adjacent joints. Erythematous streaking along the vein proximal to the site of injection has been reported. Phlebosclerosis may also occur, especially when conventional doxorubicin is administered into small vein or repeatedly into a single vein.

Liposomal Doxorubicin Although animal evidence suggests that lesions associated with extravasation of pegylated liposomal doxorubicin may be minor and reversible relative to more severe and irreversible lesions associated with conventional doxorubicin, liposomal doxorubicin also should be considered an irritant, and the usual precautions to avoid extravasation of the drug should be followed. For information on the management of extravasation of conventional or liposomal doxorubicin, see Dosage and Administration: Reconstitution and Administration.

■ **Sensitivity Reactions** ***Conventional Doxorubicin*** Fever, chills, and urticaria have been reported occasionally in patients receiving conventional doxorubicin. Anaphylaxis may occur, and a case of apparent cross-sensitivity to lincomycin has been reported.

Liposomal Doxorubicin Allergic or anaphylactoid-like reactions, sometimes life-threatening or fatal, have been reported in patients receiving liposomal doxorubicin. Among patients receiving pegylated liposomal doxorubicin for AIDS-related Kaposi's sarcoma, allergic reactions were reported in 1–5% of patients.

■ **Respiratory Effects** Pulmonary embolism, sometimes fatal, has occurred rarely in patients receiving pegylated liposomal doxorubicin.

Dyspnea and pneumonia were each reported in 1–5% of patients receiving pegylated liposomal doxorubicin for AIDS-related Kaposi's sarcoma.

Pharyngitis occurred in 16%, dyspnea in 15%, and increased cough in about 10%, of patients receiving pegylated liposomal doxorubicin for ovarian cancer in the randomized trial. Adverse respiratory effects reported in 1–10% of patients receiving liposomal doxorubicin for ovarian cancer include rhinitis, pneumonia, pleural effusion, sinusitis, apnea, and epistaxis.

■ **Nervous System Effects** ***Conventional Doxorubicin*** Peripheral neurotoxicity, manifested as local-regional sensory and/or motor disturbances, has been reported in patients receiving conventional doxorubicin by intra-arterial administration; in most cases, patients also were receiving cisplatin. Seizures and coma have been reported in patients receiving doxorubicin in combination with cisplatin or vincristine. Seizures also have been reported in a patient receiving doxorubicin at 2–3 times the recommended dosage in combination with high-dose cyclophosphamide.

Liposomal Doxorubicin Adverse neurologic effects reported in 1–5% of patients receiving pegylated liposomal doxorubicin for AIDS-related Kaposi's sarcoma include headache, dizziness, and somnolence.

Among patients receiving pegylated liposomal doxorubicin for ovarian cancer in the randomized trial, paresthesia and headache each occurred in about 10%, and dizziness occurred in 4%, of patients. Adverse neurologic effects reported in 1–10% of patients receiving liposomal doxorubicin for ovarian cancer include somnolence, dizziness, depression, insomnia, anxiety, confusion, neuropathy, hypertonia, agitation, neuralgia, peripheral neuritis, and vertigo.

■ **Metabolic and Electrolyte Effects** ***Conventional Doxorubicin*** As a result of extensive purine catabolism accompanying rapid cellular destruction, hyperuricemia may occur in patients receiving conventional doxorubicin, and serum uric acid concentrations should be monitored. Hyperuricemia and its potential adverse effects may be minimized or prevented by adequate hydration, alkalinization of the urine, and/or administration of allopurinol.

Liposomal Doxorubicin Adverse metabolic and electrolyte effects reported in 1–5% of patients receiving pegylated liposomal doxorubicin for AIDS-related Kaposi's sarcoma include weight loss, hypocalcemia, and hyperglycemia.

Adverse metabolic and electrolyte effects reported in 1–10% of patients receiving pegylated liposomal doxorubicin for ovarian cancer include dehydration, weight loss, hypokalemia, hypercalcemia, edema, cachexia, hyperglycemia, and hyponatremia.

■ **Genitourinary Effects** Albuminuria was reported in 1–5% of patients receiving pegylated liposomal doxorubicin for AIDS-related Kaposi's sarcoma.

Adverse genitourinary effects reported in 1–10% of patients receiving pegylated liposomal doxorubicin for ovarian cancer include urinary tract infection, dysuria, leukorrhea, urinary frequency, cystitis, hematuria, urinary incontinence, urinary urgency, vaginal moniliasis, vaginal bleeding, and pelvic pain.

■ **Musculoskeletal Effects** Adverse musculoskeletal effects reported in 1–10% of patients receiving pegylated liposomal doxorubicin for ovarian cancer include myalgia, arthralgia, and pathological fracture. Muscle spasms have been reported rarely in patients receiving liposomal doxorubicin.

■ **Ocular Effects** ***Conventional Doxorubicin*** Conjunctivitis and lacrimation occur rarely in patients receiving doxorubicin.

Liposomal Doxorubicin Retinitis was reported in 1–5% of patients receiving pegylated liposomal doxorubicin for AIDS-related Kaposi's sarcoma.

Adverse ocular effects reported in 1–10% of patients receiving pegylated liposomal doxorubicin for ovarian cancer include conjunctivitis and dry eyes.

■ **Hepatic Effects** Among patients receiving pegylated liposomal doxorubicin for AIDS-related Kaposi's sarcoma in randomized trials, increased serum concentrations of alkaline phosphatase occurred in 8% of patients. Other adverse hepatic effects reported in 1–5% of patients receiving liposomal doxorubicin for AIDS-related Kaposi's sarcoma include increased serum concentrations of ALT (SGPT) and hyperbilirubinemia.

Among patients receiving pegylated liposomal doxorubicin for ovarian cancer, hyperbilirubinemia was reported in 1–10% of patients.

■ **Other Adverse Effects** ***Conventional Doxorubicin*** Other reported adverse effects of doxorubicin include facial flushes (especially when doxorubicin is injected rapidly) and rarely conjunctivitis and lacrimation.

Acute "recall" pneumonitis, occurring at variable times after local radiation therapy, has been reported in children receiving concomitant doxorubicin and dactinomycin. Prepubertal growth failure and gonadal impairment, usually reversible, have occurred in children receiving doxorubicin-containing regimens.

Liposomal Doxorubicin Among patients receiving pegylated liposomal doxorubicin for AIDS-related Kaposi's sarcoma in randomized trials, asthenia occurred in 10%, and fever occurred in 9%, of patients. Other adverse effects reported in 1–5% of patients receiving liposomal doxorubicin for AIDS-related Kaposi's sarcoma include back pain, infection, chills, and emotional lability.

Among patients receiving pegylated liposomal doxorubicin for ovarian cancer in the randomized trial, asthenia occurred in 40%, fever in 21%, pain in 21%, mucous membrane disorder in 14%, back pain in 12%, infection in 12%, and peripheral edema in 11%, of patients. Other adverse effects reported in 1–10% of patients receiving liposomal doxorubicin for ovarian cancer include ecchymosis, taste perversion, and ear pain.

■ **Precautions and Contraindications** The usual precautions and contraindications of doxorubicin apply to both the conventional and liposomal formulations.

Doxorubicin hydrochloride is a toxic drug with a low therapeutic index. A therapeutic response is not likely to occur without some evidence of toxicity. The major toxic effects of the drug are on the normal, rapidly proliferating tissues, particularly those of the bone marrow, GI and oral mucosa, and hair follicles. Patients receiving doxorubicin should be under constant supervision by clinicians experienced in cancer chemotherapy and should be hospitalized during the initial phase of treatment. If feasible, subsequent therapy and patient evaluation may be performed on an outpatient basis. Determinations of hepatic, hematopoietic, and cardiac function should be performed prior to and at regular intervals during doxorubicin therapy. Possible synergism of therapeutic response and toxicity with other antineoplastic agents used in concomitant chemotherapy should be considered.

Medications and emergency equipment for the treatment of allergic or anaphylactoid-like reactions should be available for immediate use in patients receiving liposomal doxorubicin.

Myelosuppression Leukocyte, erythrocyte, and platelet counts should be performed prior to and at frequent intervals during doxorubicin therapy. Hematopoietic toxicity may require dosage reduction or suspension of the drug until blood cell counts return to normal or may be severe enough to require discontinuance of therapy. If a profound drop in blood cell count occurs, the patient should be closely observed and anti-infective therapy initiated if there are signs of infection; suspension of doxorubicin therapy may be necessary during this period. Platelet and leukocyte transfusions have proved beneficial in patients with severe bone marrow depression; use of hematopoietic agents (colony-stimulating factors) also can be considered. Doxorubicin is contraindicated in patients with preexisting myelosuppression.

Cardiotoxicity Early recognition of drug-induced cardiac failure appears essential for successful treatment with cardiac glycosides, diuretics, sodium intake restriction, and rest. Cardiac evaluation employing ECGs and determination of left-ventricular ejection fraction with echocardiogram (ECHO) should be performed prior to initiation of doxorubicin therapy and subsequently prior to each dose or course of therapy after a total cumulative dosage of 400 mg/m^2 has been given. Such evaluation is particularly important in patients with preexisting risk factors for cardiotoxicity (e.g., those with heart disease or who received mediastinal irradiation or cyclophosphamide). Although T-wave flattening, ST depression, and arrhythmias may occur and last up to 2 weeks after a dose or course of doxorubicin, these effects currently are not considered indications for suspension of doxorubicin therapy.

Doxorubicin-induced cardiomyopathy has been reported to be associated with persistent reduction in QRS voltage, prolongation of the systolic time interval, and reduction of the ejection fraction (as determined by echocardiography or radionuclide angiography), but none of these tests has been shown to consistently identify those patients who are approaching their maximally tolerated cumulative dose of doxorubicin. If these or other test results indicate changes in cardiac function associated with doxorubicin, the benefit of continued therapy must be carefully weighed against the risk of irreversible cardiac damage. Fatal cardiotoxicity can occur without antecedent ECG alterations.

Administration of low doses of doxorubicin at weekly intervals or administration of the drug by continuous IV infusion (e.g., over 48–96 hours) reportedly has reduced anthracycline-associated cardiotoxicity. Consideration also can be given to cardioprotectant therapy with dexrazoxane, which can reduce substantially but not eliminate fully, the risk of doxorubicin-induced cardiotoxicity. Because anthracycline-induced cardiotoxicity may develop long after discontinuance of therapy with the drug, periodic monitoring of cardiac function with evaluation of ejection fraction should be continued throughout the patient's lifetime.

Patients with a history of cardiovascular disease should receive doxorubicin only when the potential benefit outweighs the risk. Doxorubicin is contraindicated in patients with impaired cardiac function and in patients who have been treated previously with complete cumulative doses of doxorubicin, daunorubicin, and/or epirubicin. In patients who have received anthracyclines previously, addition of further anthracycline therapy can be contemplated *only* after careful assessment of the cardiac status of the patient with noninvasive and/or invasive procedures. However, it also should be considered that functional impairment can be masked by compensatory hypertrophy and patients with previous abnormal test results should still be considered at risk. The potential benefit of additional anthracycline therapy must be weighed carefully against the possible risks of cardiotoxicity associated with such therapy.

Hepatic Impairment Prolonged and elevated plasma concentrations of doxorubicin and its metabolites in patients with impaired hepatic function have resulted in increased toxicity. Prior to each dose of doxorubicin, it is recommended that liver function tests be performed, including serum AST (SGOT), ALT (SGPT), alkaline phosphatase, and bilirubin concentrations. Dosage of doxorubicin hydrochloride should be reduced in patients with impaired hepatic function.

Advice to Patients Conventional doxorubicin often imparts a red color to the urine for 1–2 days after administration, and patients should be advised to expect this effect during therapy.

Patients receiving pegylated liposomal doxorubicin should be informed to notify the clinician if they experience signs or symptoms of any of the expected adverse effects of the drug, including hand-foot syndrome (tingling or burning, redness, flaking, bothersome swelling, small blisters, or small sores on the palms of the hands or soles of the feet), stomatitis (painful redness, swelling, or sores in the mouth), fever of 100.5°F or higher, nausea, vomiting, tiredness, weakness, rash, or mild hair loss. Patients should be informed that urine or other body fluids may appear reddish-orange in color during therapy with liposomal doxorubicin; this is a nontoxic reaction and the color will dissipate as the drug is eliminated from the body.

Other Precautions and Contraindications Clearance of doxorubicin is reduced in obese women (actual body weight exceeding 130% of ideal body weight).

In addition to the usual precautions and contraindications associated with doxorubicin therapy, use of liposomal doxorubicin hydrochloride is contraindicated in patients who are hypersensitive to conventional doxorubicin preparations or to any component in the liposomal formulation.

■ **Pediatric Precautions** ***Cardiotoxicity*** Doxorubicin-induced cardiomyopathy impairs myocardial growth as children mature. Therefore, pediatric patients appear to be at particular risk for developing delayed cardiac toxicity with the drug, with possible subsequent development of congestive heart failure during early adulthood.

Results of studies to date are inconclusive concerning the relative risk of children for developing acute or chronic anthracycline-induced cardiotoxicity. Children are at increased risk for developing late-onset anthracycline toxicity since such cardiotoxicity is expected to increase with the growing census of long-term survivors (e.g., survivors of childhood cancers). Children who have received doxorubicin therapy develop subclinical cardiac dysfunction including abnormal fractional shortening (FS) in 23% of patients and abnormal afterload and/or contractility in 65% of patients. Overt congestive heart failure has been reported in about 5% of patients during long-term follow-up with a median length of follow-up of 9 years; 5–10% develop overt congestive heart failure during long-term follow-up. This late cardiotoxicity may be dose related, and the rate of detection increases with increased duration of follow-up. Therefore, periodic long-term follow-up is recommended for children treated with doxorubicin. In children, deterioration in cardiac function during or after therapy with the drug is indicated by a decrease in fractional shortening (FS) that declines by an absolute value of 10 or more percentile units or to less than 29%, and by a decrease in left-ventricular ejection fraction (LVEF) of 10 percentile units or an LVEF less than 55%. Although monitoring the ejection fraction has not been shown to be predictive of impending maximal tolerance of the cumulative doxorubicin dose, the benefits of continued therapy with the drug should be weighed carefully against the risk of irreversible cardiotoxicity whenever test results indicate a deterioration in cardiac function.

Other Precautions Doxorubicin, when administered as a component of intensive chemotherapy regimens in children, may contribute to prepubertal growth failure. Gonadal impairment, which usually is reversible, also may occur.

The use of doxorubicin or other topoisomerase II inhibitors in children is associated with increased risk of acute myelogenous leukemia and other secondary malignancies.

Caregivers of children receiving doxorubicin should be advised to take precautions (e.g., wearing latex gloves) to prevent contact with the patient's urine and other body fluids for at least 5 days after administration of doxorubicin.

The manufacturer states that safety and efficacy of pegylated liposomal doxorubicin hydrochloride in children have not been established.

■ **Geriatric Precautions** Safety and efficacy of liposomal doxorubicin in geriatric patients have not been specifically studied to date. In single-arm studies of pegylated liposomal doxorubicin for ovarian cancer, 29% of patients were 60–69 years of age, and 23% were 70 years of age or older. In the randomized trial of pegylated liposomal doxorubicin for ovarian cancer, 35% of patients were 65 years of age or older. No overall differences in efficacy or safety were observed between geriatric and younger patients.

■ **Mutagenicity and Carcinogenicity** Doxorubicin has been shown to be mutagenic and carcinogenic in experimental models. Secondary acute myeloid (myelogenous) leukemia, sometimes fatal, has been reported in adults and children receiving topoisomerase II inhibitors, including rare cases in patients receiving liposomal doxorubicin. The extent of increased risk of developing secondary malignancies associated with the use of doxorubicin has not been fully established. There was no evidence of mutagenic potential when Stealth® liposomes (see Chemistry and Stability: Chemistry) that were devoid of doxorubicin hydrochloride were tested in vitro in the Ames, mouse lymphoma, and chromosomal aberration assays or in vivo in the mammalian micronucleus assay.

■ **Pregnancy, Fertility, and Lactation** ***Pregnancy*** Doxorubicin can cause fetal toxicity when administered to pregnant women, but potential benefits from use of the drug may be acceptable in certain conditions despite the possible risks to the fetus. The drug is embryotoxic and teratogenic in rats and embryotoxic and abortifacient in rabbits, and trace amounts of drug have been found in mouse fetuses and in one aborted human fetus following administration of conventional (nonencapsulated) doxorubicin. Liposomal doxorubicin is embryotoxic at doses of 1 mg/kg daily (about one-eighth the 50 mg/m² human dose on a mg/m² basis) in rats and is embryotoxic and abortifacient at doses of 0.5 mg/kg daily (about one-eighth the 50 mg/m² human dose on a mg/m² basis) in rabbits. Embryotoxicity consisted of increased embryo-fetal deaths and reduced live litter sizes.

There are no adequate and well-controlled studies to date using conventional or liposomal doxorubicin in pregnant women. Doxorubicin should be used during pregnancy only in life-threatening situations or for disease for which safer drugs cannot be used or are ineffective. When conventional or liposomal doxorubicin is used during pregnancy, or if the patient becomes pregnant while receiving the drug, the patient should be apprised of the potential hazard to the fetus. If a patient becomes pregnant during the first few months following liposomal doxorubicin therapy, the prolonged elimination half-life of the drug must be taken into account. Women of childbearing potential should be advised to avoid becoming pregnant during doxorubicin therapy.

Fertility Information on whether conventional or liposomal doxorubicin affects fertility has not been evaluated adequately. Liposomal doxorubicin hydrochloride has been associated with mild to moderate ovarian and testicular atrophy in mice after a single 36-mg/kg dose (about 2 times the 50-mg/m² human dose on a mg/m² basis), decreased testicular weight and hypospermia in rats after repeated dosages of 0.25 mg/kg or more daily (about one-thirtieth of the 50-mg/m² human dosage on a mg/m² basis), and diffuse degeneration of the seminiferous tubules and marked decreases in spermatogenesis in dogs after repeated dosages of 1 mg/kg daily (about one-half the 50-mg/m² human dosage on a mg/m² basis).

Lactation Conventional (nonencapsulated) doxorubicin is distributed into milk. It is not known whether liposomal doxorubicin is distributed into milk. Because of the potential for serious adverse reactions to doxorubicin in nursing infants, nursing should be discontinued during doxorubicin therapy. Liposomal doxorubicin is contraindicated in nursing women.

Drug Interactions

Formal drug interaction studies employing liposomal doxorubicin have not been performed to date; therefore, pending further accumulation of data, drugs known to interact with conventional (nonencapsulated) doxorubicin should be considered to also interact with the liposomal formulation. In addition, although most patients who have received liposomal doxorubicin to date were receiving antiviral therapy concomitantly, the potential for interactions with these drugs has not been evaluated.

■ **Antineoplastic Agents** Doxorubicin has been used in combination with other antineoplastic agents. Although combination chemotherapy has been shown to be more effective than single-agent therapy in some types of neoplasms, the benefits and risks of such therapy have not been fully elucidated.

Compared with administration of doxorubicin followed by paclitaxel, initial administration of paclitaxel (by IV infusion over 24 hours) followed by doxorubicin (administered over 48 hours) was shown to result in a decrease in doxorubicin clearance and an increase in the severity of neutropenia and stomatitis.

Doxorubicin may potentiate the toxicity of other antineoplastic therapies and vice versa. Doxorubicin reportedly has exacerbated cyclophosphamide-induced hemorrhagic cystitis and enhanced mercaptopurine-induced hepatotoxicity. Concomitant or previous administration with cyclophosphamide, irradiation of the cardiac region, daunorubicin, idarubicin, or mitoxantrone may potentiate the cardiotoxic effects of doxorubicin, and the maximum cumulative dose of doxorubicin should be reduced. (See Dosage and Administration: Dosage.) Combined therapy with other myelosuppressive agents may increase the severity of hematologic toxicity. Acute "recall" pneumonitis, occurring at variable times after local radiation therapy, has been reported in children receiving concomitant doxorubicin and dactinomycin. Seizures and/or coma have occurred in patients receiving doxorubicin and vincristine concomitantly. Seizures also have been reported in a patient receiving doxorubicin at 2–3 times the recommended dosage in combination with high-dose cyclophosphamide.

■ **Cyclosporine** The use of cyclosporine in combination with doxorubicin may result in an increase in the area under the plasma concentration-time curve for both doxorubicin and doxorubicinol, possibly due to a decrease in doxorubicin clearance and a decrease in the metabolism of doxorubicinol. Evidence suggests that concomitant use of cyclosporine may result in more severe and prolonged hematologic toxicity associated with doxorubicin. In addition, seizures and/or coma have occurred in patients receiving doxorubicin and cyclosporine concomitantly.

■ **Other Drugs** Some evidence suggests that doxorubicin-induced cardiotoxicity may be potentiated by concomitant use of calcium-channel blocking agents.

Exacerbation of doxorubicin-induced neutropenia and thrombocytopenia has been reported in patients with advanced malignancies receiving high doses of progesterone (up to 10 g IV over 24 hours) concomitantly with doxorubicin (60 mg/m² by IV bolus).

Phenobarbital has increased the elimination of doxorubicin, doxorubicin has decreased serum phenytoin concentrations, and streptozocin may inhibit hepatic metabolism of doxorubicin.

Acute Toxicity

Overdosage with doxorubicin exacerbates known adverse effects of the drug, including mucositis, leukopenia, and thrombocytopenia.

Management of acute doxorubicin overdosage consists of hospitalization of the severely myelosuppressed patient, anti-infective therapy, platelet and granulocyte transfusions, and symptomatic treatment of mucositis. The use of hematopoietic growth factor (granulocyte colony-stimulating factor or granulocyte-macrophage colony-stimulating factor) to reduce the severity of myelosuppression may be considered.

Pharmacology

Doxorubicin hydrochloride is an antineoplastic antibiotic with pharmacologic actions similar to those of daunorubicin. Although the drug has anti-infective properties, its cytotoxicity precludes its use as an anti-infective agent. The precise and/or principal mechanism(s) of the antineoplastic action of doxorubicin is not fully understood. It appears that the cytotoxic effect of the drug results from a complex system of multiple modes of action related to free radical formation secondary to metabolic activation of the doxorubicin by electron reduction, intercalation of the drug into DNA, induction of DNA breaks and chromosomal aberrations, and alterations in cell membranes induced by the drug. Evidence from in vitro studies in cells treated with doxorubicin suggests that apoptosis (programmed cell death) also may be involved in the drug's mechanism of action. These and other mechanisms (chelation of metal ions to produce drug-metal complexes) also may contribute to the cardiotoxic effects of the drug. (See Cautions: Cardiac Effects.)

Doxorubicin undergoes enzymatic 1- and 2-electron reduction to the corresponding semiquinone and dihydroquinone. 7-Deoxyaglycones are formed enzymatically by 1-electron reduction, and the resulting semiquinone free radical reacts with oxygen to produce the hydroxyl radical in a cascade of reactions; this radical may lead to cell death by reacting with DNA, RNA, cell membranes, and proteins. The dihydroquinone that results from 2-electron reduction of doxorubicin also can be formed by the reaction of 2 semiquinones. In the presence of oxygen, dihydroquinone reacts to form hydrogen peroxide, and in its absence, loses its sugar and gives rise to the quinone methide, a monofunctional alkylating agent with low affinity for DNA. The contribution of dihydroquinone and the quinone methide to the cytotoxicity of doxorubicin is unclear. Experimental evidence indicates that doxorubicin forms a complex with DNA by intercalation between base pairs, causing inhibition of DNA synthesis and DNA-dependent RNA synthesis by the resulting template disordering and steric obstruction. Doxorubicin also inhibits protein synthesis. Doxorubicin is active throughout the cell cycle including the interphase.

Of the cell types tested in vitro, cardiac cells are the most sensitive to the effects of doxorubicin, followed by sarcoma and melanoma cells, normal muscle fibroblasts, and normal skin fibroblasts. Normal, rapidly proliferating tissues such as those of bone marrow, GI and oral mucosa, and hair follicles are also affected to varying degrees. Doxorubicin hydrochloride also has immunosuppressive activity.

Pharmacokinetics

Nonencapsulated (conventional) doxorubicin hydrochloride exhibits linear pharmacokinetics; PEG-stabilized liposomal doxorubicin hydrochloride also exhibits dose-proportional, linear pharmacokinetics over a dosage range of 10–20 mg/m². The pharmacokinetics of liposomally encapsulated doxorubicin at a dose of 50 mg/m² have been reported to be nonlinear. At a dose of 50 mg/m², a longer elimination half-life and lower clearance compared to those observed with a 20 mg/m² dose are expected, with greater-than-proportional increases in area under the plasma concentration-time curve. Encapsulation of doxorubicin hydrochloride in PEG-stabilized (Stealth®) liposomes substantially alters the pharmacokinetics of the drug relative to conventional IV formulations (i.e., nonencapsulated drug), with resultant decreased distribution into the peripheral compartment, increased distribution into Kaposi's lesions, and decreased plasma clearance. The pharmacokinetics of the drug encapsulated in PEG-stabilized liposomes have not been evaluated separately by gender, ethnic group, or hepatic or renal impairment. In the Pharmacokinetics section, liposomal doxorubicin hydrochloride was administered as the drug encapsulated in PEG-stabilized liposomes.

■ **Absorption** Nonencapsulated doxorubicin hydrochloride is not stable in gastric acid, and animal studies indicate that the drug undergoes little, if any, absorption from the GI tract. The drug is extremely irritating to tissues and, therefore, must be administered IV. Following IV infusion of a single 10- or 20-mg/m² dose of liposomal doxorubicin hydrochloride in patients with AIDS-related Kaposi's sarcoma, average peak plasma doxorubicin (mostly bound to liposomes) concentrations are 4.33 or 10.1 mcg/mL, respectively, following a 15-minute infusion and 4.12 or 8.34 mcg/mL, respectively, following a 30-minute infusion. Following IV infusion over 15 minutes of a 40-mg/m² dose of liposomal doxorubicin hydrochloride in adults with AIDS-related Kaposi's, peak plasma concentrations averaged 20.1 mcg/mL.

■ **Distribution** Doxorubicin administered as a conventional injection is widely distributed in the plasma and in tissues. As early as 30 seconds after IV administration, doxorubicin is present in the liver, lungs, heart, and kidneys. Doxorubicin is absorbed by cells and binds to cellular components, particularly to nucleic acids. The volume of distribution of doxorubicin hydrochloride administered IV as a conventional injection is about 700–1100 L/m². Nonencapsulated doxorubicin is approximately 50–85% bound to plasma proteins; the protein binding of liposomally encapsulated drug has not been determined.

Encapsulation in PEG-stabilized liposomes substantially slows the rate of distribution of doxorubicin into the extravascular space. As a result, the liposomally encapsulated drug does not distribute into plasma and tissues as widely as doxorubicin hydrochloride administered as the conventional injection; doxorubicin hydrochloride encapsulated in liposomes distributes mainly in intravascular fluid, whereas nonencapsulated drug distributes widely into extravascular fluids and tissues. Animal studies indicate that liposomally encapsulated doxorubicin hydrochloride distributes from blood vessels into tumors, and once distributed into the tissue compartment, the drug is released; the exact mechanism of drug release from liposomal encapsulation is not known. The steady-state volume of distribution of doxorubicin following IV administration of a single 10–40-mg/m² dose of the drug as a PEG-stabilized liposomal for injection concentrate in patients with AIDS-related Kaposi's sarcoma ranges from 2.2–4.4 L/m².

Doxorubicin hydrochloride administered IV as the liposomally encapsulated drug distributes into Kaposi's sarcoma lesions to a greater extent than into healthy skin. Following IV administration of a single 20-mg/m² dose of liposomal doxorubicin hydrochloride, doxorubicin concentrations in Kaposi's sarcoma lesions were 19 (range: 3–53)-fold higher than those observed in healthy skin; however, blood concentrations in the lesions or in healthy skin were not considered. In addition, distribution of doxorubicin into Kaposi's sarcoma lesions following IV administration of liposomally encapsulated drug was 5.2–11.4 times greater than that following IV administration of comparable doses of a conventional (nonencapsulated) injection. The mechanism by which liposomal encapsulation enhances doxorubicin distribution into Kaposi's sarcoma lesions has not been elucidated fully, but similar PEG-stabilized liposomes containing colloidal gold as a marker have been shown to enter Kaposi's sarcoma-like lesions in animals. Extravasation of the liposomes also may occur by passage of the particles through endothelial cell gaps present in Kaposi's sarcoma. Once within the lesions, the drug presumably is released locally as the liposomes degrade and become permeable *in situ*.

Doxorubicin does not cross the blood-brain barrier or achieve a measurable concentration in the CSF.

Trace amounts of doxorubicin have been found in fetal mice whose mothers received the drug during pregnancy, and there are limited data to indicate that nonencapsulated doxorubicin crosses the human placenta. Nonencapsulated doxorubicin is distributed into milk, achieving concentrations that often exceed those in plasma; doxorubicinol (the major metabolite) also distributes into milk.

■ **Elimination** Plasma concentrations of nonencapsulated doxorubicin and its metabolites decline in a biphasic or triphasic manner. In the first phase of the triphasic model, nonencapsulated doxorubicin is rapidly metabolized, presumably by a first-pass effect through the liver. It appears that most of this metabolism is completed before the entire dose is administered. In the triphasic model, nonencapsulated doxorubicin and its metabolites are rapidly distributed into the extravascular compartment with a plasma half-life of approximately 0.2–0.6 hours for doxorubicin and 3.3 hours for its metabolites. This is followed by relatively prolonged plasma concentrations of doxorubicin and its metabolites, probably resulting from tissue binding. During the second phase, the plasma half-life of nonencapsulated doxorubicin is 16.7 hours and that of its metabolites is 31.7 hours. In the biphasic model, the initial distribution $t_{1/2}$ has been reported to average about 5–10 minutes, and the terminal elimination $t_{1/2}$ has been reported to average about 30 hours.

In patients with impaired hepatic function, particularly those who are hyperbilirubinemic, clearance of doxorubicin is reduced and plasma concentrations of both the drug and its metabolites are elevated; doxorubicin dosage must be reduced in patients with hepatic impairment. (See: Dosage and Administration: Dosage in Hepatic Impairment.)

Plasma clearance of nonencapsulated doxorubicin (when administered as a conventional injection) ranges from 8–20 mL/minute per kilogram (or 324–809 mL/minute per m²). Systemic clearance of doxorubicin is reduced in obese women (actual body weight exceeding 130% of ideal body weight). Clearance of doxorubicin was reduced without any change in volume of distribution in obese patients compared with patients with an actual body weight less than 115% of ideal body weight. Limited evidence suggests that the pharmacokinetics of nonencapsulated doxorubicin is influenced by gender. In a clinical study involving 6 men and 21 women with no history of prior anthracycline treatment, doxorubicin clearance was higher in men than in women (1883 versus 750 mL/min, respectively). However, the terminal elimination half-life of the drug was longer in men than in women (54 versus 35 hours, respectively).

The pharmacokinetics of nonencapsulated doxorubicin also appears to be influenced by age. In a pharmacokinetic study in 60 children and adolescents (aged 2 months to 20 years) receiving 10–75 mg/m² nonencapsulated doxorubicin, a mean clearance of 1443 mL/min per m^2 was reported. Further analysis indicated that doxorubicin clearance in 52 children older than 2 years of age (1540 mL/minute per m^2) was increased compared with clearance reported for adults. In contrast, clearance of the drug in children younger than 2 years of age (813 mL/minute per m^2) was decreased compared with that in older children and approached the range of clearance values reported for adults.

Plasma concentrations of liposomally encapsulated doxorubicin hydrochloride appear to decline in a biphasic manner. Following IV administration of a single 10- to 40-mg/m^2 dose of doxorubicin hydrochloride as a liposomal injection in patients with AIDS-related Kaposi's sarcoma, the initial plasma half-life ($t_{1/2\alpha}$) of doxorubicin averaged 3.76–5.2 hours while the terminal elimination half-life ($t_{1/2\beta}$) averaged 39.1–55 hours.

Plasma clearance of doxorubicin encapsulated in PEG-stabilized liposomes appears to be substantially slower than that of nonencapsulated doxorubicin. In adults with AIDS-related Kaposi's sarcoma, plasma clearance of PEG-stabilized liposomal doxorubicin hydrochloride following a single IV dose of 10–40 mg/m^2 averaged 0.57–1.8 mL/minute per m^2. This reduction in plasma clearance with liposomal doxorubicin results in a substantial increase in the area under the plasma concentration-time curve (AUC) compared with that of nonencapsulated drug.

Nonencapsulated doxorubicin is metabolized by NADPH-dependent aldoketoreductases to the hydrophilic 13-hydroxyl metabolite doxorubicinol, which exhibits antineoplastic activity and is the major metabolite; these reductases are present in most if not all cells, but particularly in erythrocytes, liver, and kidney. Although not clearly established, doxorubicinol also appears to be the moiety responsible for the cardiotoxic effects of the drug. Undetectable or low plasma concentrations (i.e., 0.8–26.2 ng/mL) of doxorubicinol have been reported following IV administration of a single 10- to 50-mg/m^2 dose of doxorubicin hydrochloride as a PEG-stabilized liposomal injection; it remains to be established whether such liposomally encapsulated anthracyclines are less cardiotoxic than conventional (nonencapsulated) drug, and the usual precautions for unencapsulated drug currently also should be observed for the liposomal preparation. (See Cautions: Cardiac Effects.) Substantially reduced or absent plasma concentrations of the usual major metabolite of doxorubicin observed with the PEG-stabilized liposomal injection suggests that either the drug is not released appreciably from the liposomes as they circulate or that some doxorubicin may be released but that the rate of doxorubicinol elimination greatly exceeds the release rate; doxorubicin hydrochloride encapsulated in liposomes that have *not* been PEG-stabilized is metabolized to doxorubicinol.

Other metabolites, which are therapeutically inactive, include the poorly water-soluble aglycones, doxorubicinone (adriamycinone) and 7-deoxydoxorubicinone (17-deoxyadriamycinone), and conjugates. The aglycones are formed in microsomes by NADPH-dependent, cytochrome reductase-mediated cleavage of the amino sugar moiety. The enzymatic reduction of doxorubicin to 7-deoxyaglycones is important to the cytotoxic effect of the drug since it results in hydroxyl radicals that cause extensive cell damage and death. (See Pharmacology.) With nonencapsulated doxorubicin, more than 20% of the total drug in plasma is present as metabolites as soon as 5 minutes after a dose, 70% in 30 minutes, 75% in 4 hours, and 90% in 24 hours.

Nonencapsulated doxorubicin and its metabolites are excreted predominantly in bile; about 10–20% of a single dose is excreted in feces in 24 hours, and 40–50% of a dose is excreted in bile or feces within 7 days. About 50% of the drug in bile is unchanged drug, 23% is doxorubicinol, and the remainder is other metabolites including aglycones and conjugates. About 4–5% (range: 0.7–23%) of the administered dose is excreted in urine after 5 days, principally as unchanged doxorubicin. It appears that very little further urinary excretion of the drug occurs after 5 days. Although only small urinary concentrations of the drug usually are achieved, doxorubicin often imparts a red color to the urine for the first hours to days after administration, and patients should be advised to expect this effect during therapy.

Chemistry and Stability

■ Chemistry Doxorubicin is an anthracycline glycoside antibiotic produced by *Streptomyces peucetius* var. *caesius*. The drug is structurally related to daunorubicin and epirubicin. Doxorubicin differs structurally from daunorubicin in that doxorubicin contains a hydroxyacetyl group instead of an acetyl group in the 8-position. Epirubicin is the 4′-epimer of doxorubicin.

Doxorubicin is commercially available as the hydrochloride salt. Commercially available doxorubicin hydrochloride powder for injection occurs as a sterile, lyophilized, crystalline, red-orange or red powder; the powder for injection also may contain lactose and methylparaben to enhance dissolution. Doxorubicin hydrochloride is freely soluble in water, slightly soluble in 0.9% sodium chloride solution, and very slightly soluble in alcohol. When doxorubicin hydrochloride powder for injection is reconstituted with 0.9% sodium chloride injection, the pH of the resulting solution is 3.8–6.5.

Doxorubicin hydrochloride also is commercially available as a sterile, isotonic, aqueous solution of the drug. Hydrochloric acid is added during manufacture of the injection to adjust the pH to approximately 3 (range: 2.5–3.5); the injection also contains 0.9% sodium chloride.

As an injection, doxorubicin hydrochloride also is available in a liposomal formulation. In the liposomal doxorubicin hydrochloride for injection concentrate, an aqueous core of doxorubicin hydrochloride is encapsulated in Stealth® liposomes; approximately 90% of the drug present in the commercially available liposomal doxorubicin hydrochloride is encapsulated. Liposomes are microscopic vesicles composed of a phospholipid bilayer that is capable of encapsulating drugs; the lipid bilayer separates the internal aqueous core, which for doxorubicin hydrochloride liposomal for injection concentrate contains the drug, from the external environment. Stealth® liposomes, which contain hydrogenated soy phosphatidylcholine (HSPC) and cholesterol in the phospholipid bilayer, are formulated with methoxypolyethylene glycol (MPEG, a hydrophilic polymer) combined with distearoyl-*sn*-glycerophosphoethanolamine (DSPE) on their surface (combined as MPEG-DSPE). Formulating the liposomes with surface-bound MPEG has been referred to as "pegylation," and the resulting polymer coating protects the liposomes from opsonization by plasma proteins and subsequent detection as a foreign protein by the mononuclear phagocyte system (MPS) and rapid clearance from circulation (e.g., by fixed macrophages in the liver and spleen); as a result, the blood circulation time of the liposomes is prolonged. The Stealth® liposomes also have been referred to as PEG-stabilized; the MPEG groups extend 5 nm from the liposome surface creating a protective wall that inhibits interaction between the lipid bilayer membrane and plasma components. It has been suggested that liposomes can penetrate the altered and often compromised vasculature of tumors because of their small size (about 100 nm) and persistence in the blood circulation. Doxorubicin hydrochloride liposomal for injection concentrate is a sterile, translucent red liposomal dispersion. Hydrochloric acid and/or sodium hydroxide is added during manufacture of the for injection concentrate to adjust the pH to approximately 6.5. Doxorubicin hydrochloride liposomal for injection concentrate also contains sucrose for isotonicity, histidine as a buffer, and ammonium sulfate. During manufacturing, inclusion of sucrose in the external phase and ammonium sulfate in the internal phase creates the chemical gradient needed for promoting diffusion of doxorubicin hydrochloride from the external phase into the aqueous core of the liposomes.

■ Stability Commercially available doxorubicin hydrochloride lyophilized powder for injection should be stored in a dry place protected from sunlight. When stored at 15–30°C, Adriamycin RDF® or Rubex® has an expiration date of 3 or 2 years, respectively, following the date of manufacture. Doxorubicin hydrochloride conventional (nonencapsulated) injection should be protected from light and refrigerated at 2–8°C; when stored under these conditions, the injection is stable for 18 months.

Solutions of doxorubicin hydrochloride should be protected from exposure to sunlight. When reconstituted as directed, solutions prepared from the single-dose or multiple-dose vial of the powder for injection can be stored for up to 7 days at room temperature and under normal room light (100 foot-candles) or for up to 15 days when refrigerated at 2–8°C; unused portions should be discarded after these storage periods. Doxorubicin hydrochloride is unstable in solutions with a pH less than 3 or greater than 7. Acids split the glycosidic bond in doxorubicin, yielding a red-colored, water insoluble aglycone (doxorubicinone, also known as adriamycinone) and a water soluble, reducing amino sugar (daunosamine). Doxorubicin hydrochloride solution is chemically incompatible with heparin sodium injection, and a precipitate may form if the solutions are mixed. Doxorubicin hydrochloride solution also is reportedly incompatible with fluorouracil, and a precipitate may form if the solutions are mixed. The manufacturers recommend that doxorubicin hydrochloride solutions or doxorubicin liposomal dispersion generally *not* be mixed with other drugs; specialized references should be consulted for specific compatibility information.

Commercially available doxorubicin hydrochloride liposomal for injection concentrate should be refrigerated at 2–8°C and protected from freezing. The manufacturer states that prolonged freezing may adversely affect stability of liposomal doxorubicin hydrochloride; however, short-term freezing (less than 1 month) does not appear to affect stability of liposomal doxorubicin hydrochloride. During shipping, vials of doxorubicin hydrochloride for injection concentrate are packaged with a gel refrigerant ("blue ice") to maintain a temperature of 2–8°C. When diluted as directed with 5% dextrose injection, solutions of liposomal doxorubicin hydrochloride are stable for 24 hours when refrigerated at 2–8°C.

For further information on the handling of antineoplastic agents, see the ASHP Guidelines on Handling Hazardous Drugs at http://www.ahfsdruginformation.com.

Preparations

Excipients in commercially available drug preparations may have clinically important effects in some individuals; consult specific product labeling for details.

DOXOrubicin Hydrochloride

Parenteral

For injection, for IV use only	10 mg*	**Adriamycin®**, Bedford
		Adriamycin RDF®, Pfizer
		Doxorubicin Hydrochloride for Injection
	20 mg*	**Adriamycin®**, Bedford
		Adriamycin RDF®, Pfizer
		Doxorubicin Hydrochloride for Injection
	50 mg*	**Adriamycin®**, Bedford
		Adriamycin RDF®, Pfizer
		Doxorubicin Hydrochloride for Injection
		Rubex®, Bristol-Myers Squibb

	100 mg	Rubex®, Bristol-Myers Squibb
	150 mg	Adriamycin RDF®, Pfizer
Injection, for IV use only	2 mg/mL (10, 20, 50, 75, 150, and 200 mg)*	Adriamycin®, Bedford
		Adriamycin PFS® (available in Cytosafe® and glass vials), Pfizer
		Doxorubicin Hydrochloride Injection (available in polymer vials)

*available from one or more manufacturer, distributor, and/or repackager by generic (nonproprietary) name

DOXOrubicin Hydrochloride Liposomal

Parenteral		
For injection concentrate, for IV infusion only	2 mg/mL (20 and 50 mg)	Doxil®, Janssen Therapeutics (formerly Tibotec Therapeutics)

†Use is not currently included in the labeling approved by the US Food and Drug Administration

Selected Revisions August 2018, © Copyright, October 1975, American Society of Health-System Pharmacists, Inc.

Durvalumab

■ Durvalumab, a recombinant fully human anti-programmed-death ligand-1 (anti-PD-L1) monoclonal antibody, is an antineoplastic agent. The drug is an IgG_1 kappa immunoglobulin.

Uses

■ **Urothelial Carcinoma** Durvalumab is used for the treatment of locally advanced or metastatic urothelial carcinoma that has progressed following therapy with platinum-containing chemotherapy or has progressed within 12 months of neoadjuvant or adjuvant treatment with platinum-containing chemotherapy. The accelerated approval of durvalumab for this indication is based on overall tumor response rate and duration of response; there currently are no controlled trials demonstrating a clinical benefit (e.g., improvement in disease-related symptoms, increased survival). Continued approval for this indication may be contingent on verification and description of clinical benefit of durvalumab in confirmatory studies.

The current indication for durvalumab in the treatment of locally advanced or metastatic urothelial carcinoma is based principally on the results for a cohort of previously treated patients in an open-label, multicenter, noncomparative, multi-cohort, phase ½ study; the cohort of previously treated patients included 182 adults with locally advanced or metastatic urothelial carcinoma that had progressed during or following platinum-containing therapy for advanced disease or within 12 months of platinum-containing therapy in the neoadjuvant or adjuvant setting. The primary measure of efficacy was objective response rate as assessed by an independent review facility according to Response Evaluation Criteria in Solid Tumors (RECIST).

In this study, the median age of patients in the previously treated cohort was 67 years; 64% were Caucasian; 72% were male; 66% had visceral metastases; 66% had a baseline Eastern Cooperative Oncology Group (ECOG) performance status of 1; and 41% had a baseline creatinine clearance less than 60 mL/minute. Approximately one-third (35%) of patients enrolled in this cohort had received at least 2 prior therapies for metastatic disease and 20% had disease progression following platinum-containing therapy in the neoadjuvant or adjuvant setting; 70 or 30% of patients had received prior treatment with cisplatin- or carboplatin-based regimens, respectively. Most patients (52%) had high expression of programmed-death ligand-1 (PD-L1), 40% of patients had low PD-L1 expression, and samples from 8% of patients were not evaluable. High PD-L1 expression was defined as 25% or more of tumor cells or immune cells expressing PD-L1 if immune cells involve more than 1% of the tumor area *or* defined as 25% or more of tumor cells or 100% of immune cells if the immune cells involve 1% or less of the tumor area, as detected by an immunohistochemistry assay (Ventana PD-L1 [SP263]). Patients received durvalumab 10 mg/kg administered as an IV infusion every 2 weeks for up to 12 months or until disease progression or unacceptable toxicity occurred. This study excluded patients with a history of immunodeficiency or severe autoimmune disease; those with medical conditions requiring systemic immunosuppression; those with untreated brain metastases; and those with human immunodeficiency virus (HIV) infection, active tuberculosis, or hepatitis B virus (HBV) or hepatitis C virus (HCV) infection.

The overall response rate for patients in the previously treated cohort of this study was 17%; complete response was achieved in 2.7% of patients in this cohort. At a median follow-up of 5.6 months, the median duration of response had not been reached. A subgroup analysis indicated that patients with high levels of PD-L1 expression had higher objective response rates compared with those having low levels of PD-L1 expression (26.3 versus 4.1%).

■ **Non-small Cell Lung Cancer** Durvalumab is used for the treatment of unresectable stage III non-small cell lung cancer (NSCLC) that has not progressed following platinum-based chemotherapy combined with radiation therapy.

The current indication for durvalumab in the treatment of unresectable NSCLC that has not progressed following platinum-based chemotherapy combined with radiation therapy is based principally on the results of a multicenter, double-blind, randomized, placebo-controlled, phase 3 trial (PACIFIC). In this study, 713 patients with unresectable stage III NSCLC that had not progressed following at least 2 cycles of platinum-based chemotherapy and concurrent radiation therapy within 42 days of study initiation, were randomized (stratified by gender, age, and smoking history) in a 2:1 ratio to receive either durvalumab (10 mg/kg by IV infusion every 2 weeks) or placebo. Treatment was continued for up to 12 months or until disease progression or unacceptable toxicity occurred. The median age of patients in this study was 64 years; 69% were Caucasian; 27% were Asian; 70% were male; 75% were former smokers and 16% were current smokers; and 51% had a baseline ECOG performance status of 1. All patients had received radiation therapy and 99% of patients had received concomitant platinum-based chemotherapy; 55 or 42% of patients had received prior treatment with cisplatin- or carboplatin-based regimens, respectively, and 2% switched between cisplatin and carboplatin. This study excluded patients whose disease progressed during platinum-containing chemotherapy and radiation therapy, those with autoimmune disease within the previous 2 years, and those receiving immunosuppressive agents. The primary measures of efficacy were progression-free survival and overall survival (as evaluated by a blinded independent central review committee according to RECIST); an additional outcome measure was overall response rate.

In the PACIFIC study, patients receiving durvalumab had a longer median progression-free survival compared with patients receiving placebo (16.8 months versus 5.6 months; hazard ratio of 0.52). Median overall survival had not been reached at the time of the interim analysis (at a median follow-up of 14.5 months). At the time of the interim analysis, patients receiving durvalumab had higher overall response rates compared with those receiving placebo (26 versus 14%); complete responses were achieved in 1 or 0% of patients receiving durvalumab or placebo, respectively.

Dosage and Administration

■ **General** ***Restricted Distribution*** Durvalumab can only be obtained through a limited network of specialty distributors. Clinicians may contact the manufacturer (AstraZeneca) by telephone at 844-275-2360 or consult the Imfinzi® website for specific availability information (https://www.imfinzihcp.com/imfinzi-durvalumab-resources.html#how-to-order).

■ **Administration** Durvalumab is administered by IV infusion over 60 minutes.

For IV infusion, the appropriate dose (10 mg/kg) of durvalumab injection concentrate (containing 50 mg/mL) should be diluted with an appropriate volume of 0.9% sodium chloride or 5% dextrose injection to a final concentration of 1–15 mg/mL. Prior to dilution, the injection should be inspected visually for particulate matter and discoloration. The solution should be clear to opalescent and colorless to slightly yellow; the solution should not be used if it is cloudy or discolored or if foreign particles are present. The diluted solution should be mixed by gentle inversion and should *not* be shaken. Durvalumab should be administered through a sterile, low-protein-binding 0.2- or 0.22-μm inline filter.

Diluted solutions of durvalumab should be administered immediately after preparation. If the diluted solution is not administered immediately, it may be stored for up to 4 hours at room temperature or up to 24 hours at 2–8°C (total storage time from initial vial entry for preparation of the dilution until start of the IV infusion.) Diluted solutions of the drug should *not* be frozen.

Any unused portion in the vial or infusion bag should be discarded since durvalumab injection contains no preservative.

Durvalumab should *not* be administered simultaneously through the same IV line with any other drug.

■ **Dosage** ***Urothelial Carcinoma*** For the treatment of locally advanced or metastatic urothelial carcinoma that has progressed following therapy with platinum-containing chemotherapy or within 12 months of neoadjuvant or adjuvant treatment with platinum-containing chemotherapy, the recommended adult dosage of durvalumab is 10 mg/kg administered as a 60-minute IV infusion once every 2 weeks. Therapy should be continued until disease progression or unacceptable toxicity occurs.

Non-small Cell Lung Cancer For the treatment of unresectable non-small cell lung cancer (NSCLC) that has not progressed following platinum-based chemotherapy combined with radiation therapy, the recommended adult dosage of durvalumab is 10 mg/kg administered as a 60-minute IV infusion once every 2 weeks. Therapy should be continued until disease progression or unacceptable toxicity occurs, or for up to 12 months.

Therapy Interruption for Toxicity If immune-mediated adverse effects or certain other adverse effects occur, temporary or permanent discontinuance of durvalumab may be required based on severity of the reaction. Dosage reductions of durvalumab are not recommended.

Durvalumab should be permanently discontinued in patients experiencing persistent grade 2 or 3 adverse effects (except for endocrinopathies) that do not recover to grade 0 or 1 within 12 weeks of the last dose of durvalumab. Therapy with the drug also should be permanently discontinued in patients unable to reduce corticosteroid dosage to 10 mg or less of prednisone daily (or equivalent) within 12 weeks of the last dose of durvalumab.

Durvalumab should be permanently discontinued in patients experiencing recurrent grade 3 or 4 (severe or life-threatening) adverse effects.

Immune-mediated Pneumonitis. If grade 2 immune-mediated pneumonitis occurs, durvalumab therapy should be interrupted until the toxicity resolves to grade 0 or 1 and the patient is receiving 10 mg or less of prednisone daily (or equivalent). (See Immune-mediated Pneumonitis under Cautions: Warnings/Precautions.)

If grade 3 or 4 immune-mediated pneumonitis occurs, durvalumab therapy should be permanently discontinued.

Immune-mediated Hepatic Effects. For serum aminotransferase (ALT or AST) elevations exceeding 3 times but not more than 8 times the upper limit of normal (ULN) or total bilirubin concentrations exceeding 1.5 times but not more than 5 times the ULN, durvalumab therapy should be interrupted until the toxicity resolves to grade 0 or 1 and the patient is receiving 10 mg or less of prednisone daily (or equivalent). (See Immune-mediated Hepatic Effects under Cautions: Warnings/Precautions.)

For ALT or AST elevations exceeding 8 times the ULN or total bilirubin concentrations exceeding 5 times the ULN, durvalumab therapy should be permanently discontinued.

For ALT or AST elevations exceeding 3 times the ULN *and* total bilirubin concentrations exceeding 2 times the ULN with no other cause, durvalumab therapy should be permanently discontinued.

Immune-mediated GI Effects. If grade 2 immune-mediated colitis or diarrhea occurs, durvalumab therapy should be interrupted until the toxicity resolves to grade 0 or 1 and the patient is receiving 10 mg or less of prednisone daily (or equivalent). (See Immune-mediated GI Effects under Cautions: Warnings/Precautions.)

If grade 3 or 4 immune-mediated colitis or diarrhea occurs, durvalumab therapy should be permanently discontinued.

Immune-mediated Endocrine Effects. If grade 2–4 immune-mediated adrenal insufficiency, hyperthyroidism, hypophysitis, hypopituitarism, or type 1 diabetes mellitus occurs, durvalumab should be interrupted until the patient is clinically stable. (See Immune-mediated Endocrine Effects under Cautions: Warnings/Precautions.)

Immune-mediated Renal Effects. For serum creatinine elevations exceeding 1.5 times but not more than 3 times the ULN (i.e., grade 2 toxicity), durvalumab therapy should be interrupted until the toxicity resolves to grade 0 or 1 and the patient is receiving 10 mg or less of prednisone daily (or equivalent). (See Immune-mediated Renal Effects under Cautions: Warnings/Precautions.)

For serum creatinine concentrations exceeding 3 times the ULN (i.e., grade 3 or 4 toxicity), durvalumab therapy should be permanently discontinued.

Immune-mediated Dermatologic Effects. If grade 2 immune-mediated rash or dermatitis occurs and persists for more than 1 week or if grade 3 immune-mediated rash or dermatitis occurs, durvalumab therapy should be interrupted until the toxicity resolves to grade 0 or 1 and the patient is receiving 10 mg or less of prednisone daily (or equivalent). (See Immune-mediated Dermatologic Effects under Cautions: Warnings/Precautions.)

If grade 4 immune-mediated rash or dermatitis occurs, durvalumab therapy should be permanently discontinued.

Other Immune-mediated Adverse Effects. If any other grade 3 immune-mediated adverse effects occur, durvalumab therapy should be interrupted until the toxicity resolves to grade 0 or 1 and the patient is receiving 10 mg or less of prednisone daily (or equivalent). (See Other Immune-mediated Effects under Cautions: Warnings/Precautions.)

If any other grade 4 immune-mediated adverse effects occur, durvalumab therapy should be permanently discontinued.

Infectious Complications. If grade 3 or 4 infection occurs, durvalumab therapy should be interrupted until the patient is clinically stable. (See Infectious Complications under Cautions: Warnings/Precautions.)

Infusion-related Reactions. If grade 1 or 2 infusion-related reactions occur, the infusion rate of durvalumab should be decreased or durvalumab therapy should be interrupted. (See Infusion-related Reactions under Cautions: Warnings/Precautions.)

If grade 3 or 4 infusion-related reactions occur, durvalumab therapy should be permanently discontinued.

■ **Special Populations** No dosage adjustment of durvalumab is necessary in patients with mild preexisting hepatic impairment. Durvalumab has not been studied in patients with moderate or severe preexisting hepatic impairment, and the manufacturer provides no specific dosage recommendations for such patients. (See Hepatic Impairment under Warnings/Precautions: Specific Populations, in Cautions.)

No dosage adjustment of durvalumab is necessary in patients with mild or moderate preexisting renal impairment. Durvalumab has not been studied in patients with severe preexisting renal impairment, and the manufacturer provides no specific dosage recommendations for such patients. (See Renal Impairment under Warnings/Precautions: Specific Populations, in Cautions.)

Dosage adjustments of durvalumab based on age, race, gender, or weight are not necessary.

Cautions

■ **Contraindications** The manufacturer states there are no known contraindications to the use of durvalumab.

■ **Warnings/Precautions** ***Immune-mediated Pneumonitis*** Pneumonitis, including interstitial lung disease and immune-mediated pneumonitis (requiring corticosteroid therapy), sometimes fatal, has occurred in patients receiving durvalumab therapy.

In a combined safety database that included 1889 clinical study patients with urothelial carcinoma, non-small cell lung cancer (NSCLC), or other cancers who were receiving durvalumab 10 mg/kg every 2 weeks, pneumonitis (not specific to immune-mediated pneumonitis) occurred in 5% of patients; grade 3, 4, or 5 immune-mediated pneumonitis was reported in 0.8, less than 0.1, or 0.3% of patients, respectively. The median time to onset and the median time to resolution of pneumonitis were 1.8 months (range: 1 day to 13.9 months) and 4.9 months (range: 0 days to 13.7 months), respectively. Overall, 3.5% of patients required systemic corticosteroid therapy and 2.5 or 0.1% of these patients required high-dose corticosteroid therapy (40 mg or more of prednisone daily [or equivalent]) or infliximab, respectively. Pneumonitis led to discontinuance of durvalumab in 1.5% of patients in the combined safety database. Resolution of pneumonitis occurred in 54% of patients.

In the PACIFIC study evaluating durvalumab in 475 patients with NSCLC, pneumonitis of any grade, including radiation pneumonitis, was reported in 34% of patients who received radiation therapy within 42 days prior to initiation of durvalumab therapy compared with 2.3% of patients in other clinical studies who did not receive radiation therapy immediately prior to initiation of the drug. Grade 3 or 5 pneumonitis was reported in 3.4 or 1.1% of patients, respectively. The median time to onset and the median duration of pneumonitis in this study were 1.8 and 2.1 months, respectively. In addition, 21% of patients with pneumonitis required systemic corticosteroids with 12 or 0.1% of these patients requiring high-dose corticosteroids or infliximab, respectively. In this study, durvalumab was discontinued in 6.3% of patients because of pneumonitis. Resolution of pneumonitis occurred in 47% of patients experiencing this adverse effect.

Patients receiving durvalumab should be monitored for pulmonary symptoms indicative of pneumonitis, and those with suspected pneumonitis, should be evaluated with radiographic imaging. Temporary interruption or discontinuance of durvalumab may be necessary if immune-mediated pneumonitis occurs during therapy with the drug. In patients who develop grade 2 immune-mediated pneumonitis, durvalumab should be temporarily interrupted and systemic corticosteroid therapy should be initiated (1–2 mg/kg of prednisone daily [or equivalent]) followed by tapering of the corticosteroid dosage. For toxicity not resulting in permanent discontinuance of the drug, durvalumab therapy may be resumed when the toxicity resolves to grade 0 or 1 and the corticosteroid dosage is reduced to less than 10 mg of prednisone daily (or equivalent). In patients who develop grade 3 or 4 immune-mediated pneumonitis, durvalumab therapy should be permanently discontinued and systemic corticosteroid therapy should be initiated (1–4 mg/kg of prednisone daily [or equivalent]) followed by tapering of the corticosteroid dosage.

Immune-mediated Hepatic Effects Immune-mediated hepatitis (requiring corticosteroid therapy) and hepatotoxicity (i.e., elevations in serum ALT or AST, alkaline phosphatase, or total bilirubin concentrations), sometimes fatal, have occurred in patients receiving durvalumab therapy.

In the combined safety database, immune-mediated hepatitis occurred in 12% of 1889 patients; grade 3, 4, or 5 hepatitis was reported in 4.4, 0.4, or 0.2% of patients, respectively. The median time to onset was 1.2 months (range: 1 day to 13.6 months). Overall, 2.7% of patients required systemic corticosteroid therapy; 1.7 or 0.1% of these patients required high-dose corticosteroid therapy (40 mg or more of prednisone daily [or equivalent]) or mycophenolate treatment, respectively. Hepatitis resulted in discontinuance of durvalumab therapy in 0.7% of patients in the combined safety database. Resolution of immune-mediated hepatitis occurred in 49% of patients.

Patients receiving durvalumab should be monitored for signs and symptoms of hepatitis; liver function tests should be performed during and following discontinuation of durvalumab therapy. In patients who develop immune-mediated hepatitis, temporary interruption of therapy or drug discontinuance may be required. If ALT or AST concentrations exceed 3 times but not more than 8 times the ULN or total bilirubin concentrations exceed 1.5 times but not more than 5 times the ULN, durvalumab should be temporarily interrupted and systemic corticosteroid therapy at a dosage of 1–2 mg/kg of prednisone daily (or equivalent) should be initiated followed by tapering of the corticosteroid dosage. For toxicity not resulting in permanent discontinuance of the drug, durvalumab therapy may be resumed when the toxicity resolves to grade 0 or 1 and the corticosteroid dosage is reduced to less than 10 mg of prednisone daily (or equivalent). If ALT or AST elevations exceeding 8 times the ULN or total bilirubin concentrations exceeding 5 times the ULN occur *or* if AST or ALT concentrations exceeding 3 times the ULN occur with total bilirubin concentrations exceeding 2 times the ULN, durvalumab should be permanently discontinued and systemic corticosteroid therapy at a dosage of 1–2 mg/kg of prednisone daily (or equivalent) should be initiated followed by tapering of the corticosteroid dosage.

Immune-mediated GI Effects Diarrhea or colitis, including immune-mediated colitis (requiring corticosteroid therapy), has occurred in patients receiving durvalumab therapy.

In the combined safety database, immune-mediated colitis or diarrhea occurred in 18% of 1889 patients; grade 3 and 4 immune-mediated colitis was reported in 1 and 0.1% of patients, respectively. The median time to onset was 1.4 months (range: 1 day to 14 months). In addition, 1.9% of patients required systemic corticosteroid therapy; 1 or 0.1% of patients required high-dose corticosteroid therapy (40 mg or more of prednisone daily [or equivalent]) or nonsteroidal immunosuppressants (e.g., infliximab, mycophenolate), respectively. Diarrhea or colitis resulted in discontinuance of durvalumab therapy in

0.4% of patients in the combined safety database. Resolution of immune-mediated GI effects occurred in 78% of patients.

Patients receiving durvalumab should be monitored for manifestations of colitis or diarrhea. Temporary interruption or discontinuance of durvalumab may be necessary if immune-mediated colitis occurs during therapy with the drug. In patients who develop grade 2 immune-mediated colitis or diarrhea, durvalumab should be temporarily interrupted and systemic corticosteroid therapy (1–2 mg/kg of prednisone daily [or equivalent]) should be initiated followed by tapering of the corticosteroid dosage. For toxicity not resulting in permanent discontinuance of the drug, durvalumab therapy may be resumed when the toxicity resolves to grade 0 or 1 and the corticosteroid dosage is reduced to less than 10 mg of prednisone daily (or equivalent). In patients who develop grade 3 or 4 immune-mediated colitis or diarrhea, durvalumab should be permanently discontinued and systemic corticosteroid therapy at a dosage of 1–2 mg/kg of prednisone daily (or equivalent) should be initiated followed by tapering of the corticosteroid dosage.

Immune-mediated Endocrine Effects Immune-mediated endocrinopathies, including hypothyroidism, hyperthyroidism, adrenal insufficiency, type 1 diabetes mellitus, hypophysitis, and hypopituitarism, have occurred in patients receiving durvalumab therapy.

Thyroid Dysfunction. In the combined safety database, hypothyroidism or hyperthyroidism occurred in 11 or 7% of 1889 patients, respectively. Thyroiditis occurred in 0.9% of patients; grade 3 thyroiditis was reported in 0.1% of these patients. Thyroiditis or hyperthyroidism preceded hypothyroidism in 25% of patients.

Thyroid function should be evaluated prior to initiation of durvalumab therapy and periodically during therapy. In patients who develop immune-mediated hypothyroidism, durvalumab therapy may be continued and thyroid hormone replacement therapy should be initiated as clinically indicated. If immune-mediated hyperthyroidism occurs, appropriate medical therapy should be initiated and durvalumab therapy should be interrupted until the patient is clinically stable.

Adrenal Insufficiency, Hypophysitis, and Hypopituitarism. In the combined safety database, adrenal insufficiency occurred in 0.7% of 1889 patients; grade 3 adrenal insufficiency was reported in less than 0.1% of these patients. In addition, 0.4% of patients required systemic corticosteroids and 0.1% of patients required high-dose corticosteroid therapy.

In the combined safety database, hypopituitarism leading to adrenal insufficiency and diabetes insipidus occurred in less than 0.1% of 1889 patients.

Patients should be monitored for signs and symptoms of adrenal insufficiency, hypophysitis, and hypopituitarism. If grade 2 or greater adrenal insufficiency, hypophysitis, or hypopituitarism occurs, systemic corticosteroid therapy at a dosage of 1–2 mg/kg of prednisone daily (or equivalent) should be initiated followed by tapering of the corticosteroid dosage; hormone replacement therapy should be initiated as clinically indicated. Durvalumab therapy should be interrupted until the patient is clinically stable.

Diabetes Mellitus. In the combined safety database, new-onset type 1 diabetes mellitus occurred in less than 0.1% of 1889 patients. The median time to onset of type 1 diabetes mellitus was 1.4 months.

Patients should be monitored for hyperglycemia or other signs and symptoms of diabetes. If grade 2 or greater type 1 diabetes mellitus occurs, insulin should be initiated as clinically indicated and durvalumab therapy should be interrupted until the patient is clinically stable.

Immune-mediated Renal Effects Immune-mediated nephritis (evidence of renal dysfunction and requiring corticosteroid therapy), including elevations in serum creatinine or urea concentrations, decreased creatinine clearance, acute kidney injury, renal failure, decreased glomerular filtration rate, tubulointerstitial nephritis, or glomerulonephritis, sometimes fatal, have occurred in patients receiving durvalumab therapy.

In the combined safety database, nephritis occurred in 6.3% of 1889 patients; grade 3, 4, or 5 nephritis was reported in 1.1, 0.2, or 0.1% of patients, respectively. The median time to onset of nephritis was 2 months (range: 1 day to 14.2 months). In addition, 0.6% of patients required systemic corticosteroid therapy; 0.4% of patients received high-dose corticosteroid therapy (40 mg or more of prednisone daily [or equivalent]). Nephritis resulted in discontinuance of durvalumab therapy in 0.3% of patients in the combined safety database. Resolution of nephritis occurred in 50% of patients.

Renal function should be evaluated prior to initiation of durvalumab therapy and periodically during therapy. In patients who experience grade 2 elevations in serum creatinine concentrations (elevations exceeding 1.5 times but not more than 3 times the ULN), durvalumab should be temporarily interrupted and systemic corticosteroid therapy should be initiated at a dosage of 1–2 mg/kg of prednisone daily (or equivalent) followed by tapering of the corticosteroid dosage. In patients who develop grade 3 or 4 elevations in serum creatinine concentrations (elevations exceeding 3 times the ULN), durvalumab should be permanently discontinued and systemic corticosteroid therapy at a dosage of 1–2 mg/kg of prednisone daily (or equivalent) should be initiated followed by tapering of the corticosteroid dosage. For toxicity not resulting in permanent discontinuance of the drug, durvalumab therapy may be resumed when the adverse reaction resolves to grade 0 or 1 and the corticosteroid dosage is reduced to less than 10 mg of prednisone daily (or equivalent).

Immune-mediated Dermatologic Effects Immune-mediated rash (e.g., bullous dermatitis, Stevens-Johnson syndrome/toxic epidermal necrolysis) has occurred in patients receiving durvalumab therapy.

In the combined safety database, rash or dermatitis occurred in 26% of 1889 patients and 0.4% of patients developed vitiligo. In addition, 2% of patients required systemic corticosteroid therapy; 1% of patients received high-dose corticosteroid therapy (40 mg or more of prednisone daily [or equivalent]). Rash or dermatitis resulted in discontinuance of durvalumab therapy in 0.1% of patients in the combined safety database. Resolution of immune-mediated rash occurred in 62% of patients.

Patients should be monitored for signs and symptoms of rash. Temporary interruption or discontinuance of durvalumab may be necessary if immune-mediated dermatologic effects occur during therapy with the drug. If grade 2 rash that persists more than 1 week or any grade 3 rash occurs, durvalumab should be temporarily interrupted and systemic corticosteroid therapy should be initiated at a dosage of 1–2 mg/kg of prednisone daily (or equivalent) followed by tapering of the corticosteroid dosage. For toxicity not resulting in permanent discontinuance of the drug, durvalumab therapy may be resumed when the toxicity resolves to grade 0 or 1 and the corticosteroid dosage is reduced to less than 10 mg of prednisone daily (or equivalent). If grade 4 rash or dermatitis occurs, durvalumab therapy should be permanently discontinued and systemic corticosteroid therapy at a dosage of 1–2 mg/kg of prednisone daily (or equivalent) should be initiated followed by tapering of the corticosteroid dosage.

Other Immune-mediated Effects Other immune-mediated adverse effects, including aseptic meningitis, hemolytic anemia, thrombocytopenic purpura, myocarditis, myositis, and ocular inflammatory toxicity (e.g., uveitis, keratitis), have occurred in less than 1% of patients in the combined safety database receiving durvalumab therapy. Immune-mediated adverse effects may be severe and result in death. Immune-mediated adverse effects may occur in any organ system and may occur following discontinuance of durvalumab therapy.

If a grade 2 immune-mediated adverse effect is suspected, adequate evaluation should be performed to exclude other causes and corticosteroid therapy should be initiated as clinically indicated. In patients who experience such grade 3 immune-mediated toxicity, durvalumab should be temporarily interrupted and initiation of systemic corticosteroid therapy at a dosage of 1–4 mg/kg of prednisone daily (or equivalent) should be considered followed by tapering of the corticosteroid dosage. For toxicity not resulting in permanent discontinuance of the drug, durvalumab therapy may be resumed when the toxicity resolves to grade 0 or 1 and the corticosteroid dosage is reduced to less than 10 mg of prednisone daily (or equivalent). In patients who develop grade 4 immune-mediated toxicity, durvalumab should be permanently discontinued and initiation of systemic corticosteroid therapy at a dosage of 1–4 mg/kg of prednisone daily (or equivalent) should be considered followed by tapering of the corticosteroid dosage.

If uveitis occurs in conjunction with other immune-mediated adverse effects, Vogt-Koyanagi-Harada syndrome should be considered. Systemic corticosteroid therapy may be required to reduce the risk of permanent vision loss.

Infectious Complications Severe infections, sometimes fatal, including sepsis and pneumonia, have occurred in patients receiving durvalumab therapy.

In the combined safety database, infections occurred in 43% of 1889 patients; grade 3, 4, or 5 infections were reported in 8, 1.9, or 1% of patients, respectively. In the study evaluating durvalumab in patients with urothelial carcinoma, urinary tract infections were the most common cause of grade 3 or higher infection, occurring in 4% of patients. In the study evaluating durvalumab in patients with NSCLC, pneumonia was the most common cause of grade 3 or higher infection, occurring in 5% of patients.

Patients should be monitored for signs and symptoms of infection. In patients experiencing grade 3 or higher infection, durvalumab should be temporarily interrupted until the patient is clinically stable.

Infusion-related Reactions Severe or life-threatening infusion-related reactions have been reported in patients receiving durvalumab therapy.

In the combined safety database, infusion-related reactions occurred in 2.2% of 1889 patients; grade 3 reactions were reported in 0.3% of patients.

Patients should be monitored for signs and symptoms of infusion-related reactions. In patients with grade 1 or 2 infusion-related reactions, durvalumab therapy should be interrupted or the rate of infusion should be decreased; the manufacturer states that use of appropriate premedications (e.g., corticosteroids) should be considered with subsequent infusions. In patients experiencing grade 3 or 4 infusion-related reactions, durvalumab therapy should be permanently discontinued.

Fetal/Neonatal Morbidity and Mortality Durvalumab may cause fetal harm if administered to pregnant women. Blockade of signaling of the programmed-death receptor-1 (PD-1) and programmed-death ligand-1 (PD-L1) pathway in animals has been shown to disrupt maternal immune tolerance to the fetus and has been associated with increased fetal loss and immune-mediated disorders. Therefore, inhibition of this pathway by durvalumab may increase the risk of fetal loss (e.g., abortion, stillbirth) or neonatal death. In cynomolgus monkeys receiving durvalumab (at exposure levels of 6–20 times the human exposure at the recommended dosage), increased premature delivery, fetal loss, and premature neonatal death occurred. Human immunoglobulin G_1 (IgG_1) has been shown to cross the placenta; therefore, fetal exposure to durvalumab may occur.

Pregnancy should be avoided during durvalumab therapy. Women of childbearing potential should be advised to use an effective method of contraception while receiving durvalumab and for at least 3 months after discontinuance of therapy. If durvalumab is used during pregnancy or if the patient becomes pregnant while receiving the drug, the patient should be apprised of the potential fetal hazard.

Immunogenicity There is a potential for immunogenicity with durvalumab therapy. Development of anti-durvalumab antibodies was detected in 45 of 1570 patients (2.9%) receiving durvalumab. The presence of anti-durvalumab antibodies does not appear to have clinically important effects on the pharmacokinetic profile of the drug. However, the number of patients with anti-durvalumab antibodies is insufficient to determine whether such antibodies affect efficacy or safety of the drug.

Specific Populations **Pregnancy.** Durvalumab may cause fetal harm if administered to pregnant women based on its mechanism of action and animal findings. (See Fetal/Neonatal Morbidity and Mortality under Cautions: Warnings/Precautions.)

Lactation. It is not known whether durvalumab is distributed into human milk. Human IgG_1 is distributed into human milk. Because of the potential for serious adverse reactions to durvalumab in nursing infants, women should be advised to discontinue nursing during durvalumab therapy and for at least 3 months after discontinuance of therapy.

Pediatric Use. Safety and efficacy of durvalumab have not been established in pediatric patients.

Geriatric Use. In the study evaluating durvalumab in patients with urothelial carcinoma, 112 of 182 patients (61.5%) were 65 years of age or older and 34 patients (18.7%) were 75 years of age or older. In these respective age groups, the overall response rates were 15 and 12%. Grade 3 or 4 adverse reactions occurred in 38% of patients 65 years of age or older and 35% of patients 75 years of age or older.

In the study evaluating durvalumab in patients with NSCLC, 214 of 476 patients (45%) were 65 years of age or older and 36 patients (7.6%) were 75 years of age or older. In this study, the number of patients 75 years of age or older was insufficient to determine whether they respond differently than younger adults.

No overall differences in safety and efficacy were observed between geriatric patients 65 years of age or older and younger adults.

Hepatic Impairment. Analysis of population pharmacokinetic data indicates that durvalumab clearance in patients with mild hepatic impairment (total bilirubin concentrations not exceeding the ULN *with* AST concentrations exceeding the ULN, or total bilirubin concentrations greater than 1 to 1.5 times the ULN *with* any AST concentrations) is similar to that in patients with normal hepatic function. Data are not available for patients with moderate or severe hepatic impairment (total bilirubin concentrations exceeding 1.5 times the ULN *with* any AST concentrations).

Renal Impairment. Analysis of population pharmacokinetic data indicates that durvalumab clearance in patients with mild or moderate renal impairment (creatinine clearance 30–89 mL/minute per 1.73 m^2) is similar to that in patients with normal renal function. Data are not available for patients with severe renal impairment (creatinine clearance 15–29 mL/minute per 1.73 m^2).

■ **Common Adverse Effects** Adverse effects reported in 10% or more of patients receiving durvalumab for the treatment of urothelial carcinoma include fatigue, musculoskeletal pain, constipation, decreased appetite/hypophagia, nausea, peripheral edema, urinary tract infection, abdominal pain, pyrexia/tumor-associated fever, diarrhea/colitis, dyspnea/exertional dyspnea, rash, and cough/productive cough. Grade 3 or 4 laboratory abnormalities reported in 10% or more of patients receiving durvalumab for the treatment of urothelial carcinoma include hyponatremia and lymphopenia.

Adverse effects reported in 10% or more of patients receiving durvalumab for the treatment of NSCLC include cough/productive cough, pneumonitis/radiation pneumonitis, fatigue, upper respiratory infections, dyspnea, rash, diarrhea, pneumonia, pyrexia, hypothyroidism, pruritus, and abdominal pain. Laboratory abnormalities reported in 20% or more of patients receiving durvalumab for the treatment of NSCLC include hyperglycemia, hypocalcemia, lymphopenia, elevated ALT and AST concentrations, hyponatremia, hyperkalemia, and elevated concentrations of γ-glutamyltransferase (GGT).

Drug Interactions

No formal drug interaction studies have been performed to date.

Description

Durvalumab, a recombinant fully human anti-programmed-death ligand-1 (anti-PD-L1) monoclonal antibody, is an antineoplastic agent. The drug is an IgG_1 kappa immunoglobulin that binds to PD-L1.

The immune-checkpoint receptor programmed-death receptor-1 (PD-1) is expressed on activated T cells, B cells, macrophages, and dendritic cells. Overexpression of PD-1 ligands on the surface of tumor cells results in activation of PD-1 and CD80 (i.e., B7.1) and suppression of cytotoxic T-cell activity, T-cell proliferation, and cytokine production. Durvalumab blocks the interaction between PD-L1 and the receptors PD-1 and CD80, resulting in activation of the antitumor immune response without inducing antibody-dependent cell-mediated cytotoxicity (ADCC). The drug also has been shown to reduce tumor growth in mouse tumor models.

Systemic exposure of durvalumab is dose proportional over the dosage range of 3–20 mg/kg. Following repeated doses of durvalumab every 2, 3, or 4 weeks, steady-state concentrations are reached by approximately 16 weeks. The mean terminal half-life of durvalumab is approximately 18 days.

Pharmacokinetics of durvalumab do not appear to be affected by age (range of 19–96 years), body weight (34–149 kg), gender, race, albumin concentrations, LDH concentrations, creatinine concentrations, PD-L1 expression, or ECOG performance status.

Advice to Patients

Importance of advising patients to read the manufacturer's medication guide.

Risk of immune-mediated pneumonitis. Importance of informing clinician immediately if new or worsening cough, chest pain, or shortness of breath occurs.

Risk of immune-mediated hepatitis. Importance of informing clinician immediately if signs and symptoms of liver damage (e.g., jaundice, severe nausea or vomiting, abdominal pain [particularly in the right upper quadrant], lethargy, easy bruising or bleeding) occur.

Risk of immune-mediated colitis. Importance of informing clinician immediately if diarrhea, severe abdominal pain, or changes in stool occur.

Risk of immune-mediated endocrine effects. Importance of informing clinician immediately if manifestations of hypophysitis, hyperthyroidism, hypothyroidism, adrenal insufficiency, or type 1 diabetes mellitus occur.

Risk of immune-mediated nephritis. Importance of informing clinician immediately if signs or symptoms of nephritis occur.

Risk of immune-mediated dermatologic effects. Importance of informing clinician immediately if signs or symptoms of severe dermatologic reactions occur.

Risk of other immune-mediated adverse effects. Importance of informing clinician immediately if manifestations of aseptic meningitis, thrombocytopenic purpura, myocarditis, hemolytic anemia, myositis, uveitis, or keratitis occur.

Risk of infections. Importance of informing clinician if fever, flu-like symptoms, cough, or painful or frequent urination occurs.

Risk of infusion-related reactions. Importance of informing clinician if signs and symptoms of such reactions, including dizziness, chills, fever, breathing difficulty (e.g., shortness of breath, wheezing), pruritus, flushing, feeling of faintness, back or neck pain, and angioedema, occur.

Risk of fetal harm. Necessity of advising women of childbearing potential that they should use an effective method of contraception while receiving the drug and for at least 3 months after discontinuance of therapy. Importance of women informing clinicians if they are or plan to become pregnant. If pregnancy occurs, advise pregnant women of potential risk to the fetus.

Importance of advising women to avoid breast-feeding while receiving the drug and for at least 3 months after discontinuance of therapy.

Importance of informing clinicians of existing or contemplated concomitant therapy, including prescription and OTC drugs and dietary or herbal supplements, as well as any concomitant illnesses (e.g., autoimmune disorders, history of organ transplantation, liver damage, pulmonary disorders).

Importance of informing patients of other important precautionary information. (See Cautions.)

Overview® (see Users Guide). For additional information on this drug until a more detailed monograph is developed and published, the manufacturer's labeling should be consulted. It is *essential* that the manufacturer's labeling be consulted for more detailed information on usual cautions, precautions, contraindications, potential drug interactions, laboratory test interferences, and acute toxicity. For further information on the handling of antineoplastic agents, see the ASHP Guidelines on Handling Hazardous Drugs at http://www.ahfsdruginformation.com.

Preparations

Distribution of durvalumab is restricted. (See Restricted Distribution under Dosage and Administration: General.)

Excipients in commercially available drug preparations may have clinically important effects in some individuals; consult specific product labeling for details.

Durvalumab

Parenteral

Concentrate, for injection, for IV infusion	50 mg/mL (120 and 500 mg)	**Imfinzi®**, AstraZeneca

Duvelisib

■ Duvelisib, an inhibitor of phosphatidylinositol-3-kinase (PI3K) with inhibitory activity mainly against PI3K-δ and PI3K-γ isoforms, is an antineoplastic agent.

REMS

FDA approved a REMS for duvelisib to ensure that the benefits outweigh the risks. The REMS may apply to one or more preparations of duvelisib and consists of the following: communication plan. See the FDA REMS page (http://www.accessdata.fda.gov/scripts/cder/rems/index.cfm) or the ASHP REMS Resource Center (https://www.ashp.org/REMS).

Uses

■ Chronic Lymphocytic Leukemia/Small Lymphocytic Lymphoma Duvelisib is used for the treatment of relapsed or refractory chronic lymphocytic leukemia (CLL) or small lymphocytic lymphoma (SLL) in patients who previously received at least 2 therapies; duvelisib has been designated an orphan drug by FDA for the treatment of these cancers.

The current indication for duvelisib in the treatment of relapsed or refractory CLL and SLL is based principally on the results for a subset of patients enrolled in a randomized, open-label phase 3 study (DUO) evaluating duvelisib compared with ofatumumab in 319 patients with CLL or SLL that had progressed during or had relapsed following at least one prior therapy; the subset analysis included 196 patients in the study who had previously received at least 2 therapies for CLL or SLL. In this study, patients were randomized in a 1:1 ratio to receive either duvelisib (25 mg orally twice daily) or ofatumumab (300 mg administered by IV infusion initially, followed one week later by 2 g by IV infusion once weekly for 7 doses and then every 4 weeks for an additional 4 doses). Patients received duvelisib until disease progression or unacceptable toxicity occurred. Patients who had received prior therapy with a phosphatidylinositol-3-kinase (PI3K) inhibitor or Bruton tyrosine kinase inhibitor, had undergone prior allogeneic stem-cell transplantation, had undergone autologous stem-cell transplantation within the previous 6 months, or had a history of Richter transformation were excluded from the study. The primary end point of this study was progression-free survival as assessed by an independent review committee; secondary end points included overall response rate as assessed using 2008 updated International Workshop on CLL (IWCLL) National Cancer Institute-sponsored Working Group Guidelines or the 2007 revised International Working Group (IWG) criteria for malignant lymphoma, with modification for treatment-related lymphocytosis.

In the DUO study, the median age of patients who had received at least 2 prior therapies for CLL or SLL was 69 years (range: 40–90 years); 59% of these patients were male, 97% had CLL, 88% had a baseline Eastern Cooperative Oncology Group (ECOG) performance status of 0 or 1, 54% had received at least 3 prior therapies, 52% had at least one tumor measuring at least 5 cm, and 22% had tumors harboring the 17p deletion chromosomal abnormality. The median duration of duvelisib treatment in patients who had received at least 2 prior therapies was 13 months; 80 or 52% of these patients received duvelisib for at least 6 or 12 months, respectively. In the subset of patients who had received at least 2 prior therapies, patients who received duvelisib had longer median progression-free survival compared with those who received ofatumumab (16.4 versus 9.1 months). The overall response rates for duvelisib and ofatumumab were 78 and 39%, respectively; there were no complete responses in either treatment group. Although duvelisib provided a modest progression-free survival benefit compared with ofatumumab in the overall study population (13.3 versus 9.9 months), duvelisib is associated with serious, sometimes fatal adverse effects; therefore, FDA considered the benefit-to-risk ratio to be more favorable in patients with CLL or SLL who had received at least 2 prior therapies.

■ Follicular Lymphoma Duvelisib is used for the treatment of relapsed or refractory follicular lymphoma in patients who previously received at least 2 systemic therapies; duvelisib has been designated an orphan drug by FDA for the treatment of this cancer. The accelerated approval of duvelisib for the treatment of relapsed or refractory follicular lymphoma is based on overall response rate. Continued approval for this indication may be contingent on verification and description of clinical benefit in confirmatory studies.

The current indication for duvelisib in the treatment of relapsed or refractory follicular lymphoma is based principally on the results for a subset of patients enrolled in a noncomparative, open-label phase 2 study (DYNAMO) evaluating duvelisib in 129 adults with indolent lymphoma that had not responded to or that had progressed within 6 months following rituximab therapy and either chemotherapy or radioimmunotherapy; the subset analysis included 83 patients in the study with refractory follicular lymphoma. In this study, all patients received duvelisib 25 mg orally twice daily until disease progression or unacceptable toxicity occurred. Patients with grade 3b follicular lymphoma or large cell transformation were excluded from the study. In addition, patients who had received prior therapy with a PI3K inhibitor or Bruton tyrosine kinase inhibitor or had undergone allogeneic stem-cell transplantation were excluded. The primary end point was overall response rate as assessed by an independent review committee using the 2007 revised IWG criteria for malignant lymphoma.

In the DYNAMO study, the median age of patients with follicular lymphoma was 64 years (range: 30–82 years); 68% of these patients were male, 93% had a baseline ECOG performance status of 0 or 1; and 37% had bulky disease (defined as nodal target lesion at least 5 cm in diameter). Patients with follicular lymphoma had received a median of 3 (range: 1–10) prior therapies; 94% of patients with follicular lymphoma were refractory to their most recent therapy and 81% were refractory to at least 2 prior therapies. The median duration of duvelisib therapy in patients with follicular lymphoma was 5 months; treatment was continued for at least 6 or 12 months in 41 or 10% of patients, respectively. At the time of data analysis, the overall response rate in patients with follicular lymphoma was 42%; complete response was achieved in 1% of patients. The median duration of response was not evaluable; however, 43% of patients with follicular lymphoma who responded to duvelisib maintained a response at 6 months, and 17% maintained a response at 12 months.

Dosage and Administration

■ General To minimize the risk of *Pneumocystis jiroveci* (formerly *Pneumocystis carinii*) pneumonia (PCP), the manufacturer states that anti-infectives should be given as prophylaxis upon initiation of duvelisib and continued until completion of therapy *and* until the CD4$^+$ T-cell count exceeds 200/mm^3. To minimize the risk of cytomegalovirus (CMV) infection and/or reactivation, the manufacturer recommends that antiviral prophylaxis be considered. (See Infectious Complications under Warnings/Precautions: Warnings, in Cautions.)

■ Administration Duvelisib is administered orally twice daily without regard to meals. The capsules should be swallowed whole and should not be opened, broken, or chewed.

■ Dosage ***Chronic Lymphocytic Leukemia/Small Lymphocytic Lymphoma*** For the treatment of relapsed or refractory chronic lymphocytic leukemia (CLL) or small lymphocytic lymphoma (SLL) in patients who have received at least 2 prior therapies, the recommended adult dosage of duvelisib is 25 mg twice daily. In the phase 3 study (DUO) in patients with relapsed or refractory CLL or SLL, therapy was continued until disease progression or unacceptable toxicity occurred; the median duration of duvelisib therapy in patients who had received at least 2 prior therapies was 13 months.

Follicular Lymphoma For the treatment of relapsed or refractory follicular lymphoma in patients who have received at least 2 prior systemic therapies, the recommended adult dosage of duvelisib is 25 mg twice daily. In the phase 2 study (DYNAMO) evaluating such use, therapy was continued until disease progression or unacceptable toxicity occurred; the median duration of duvelisib therapy in patients with follicular lymphoma was 5 months.

Dosage Modification for Toxicity Temporary interruption of therapy, dosage reduction, and/or permanent discontinuance of duvelisib may be necessary in patients experiencing certain adverse effects.

When dosage modification is necessary, the dosage of duvelisib should be reduced from 25 mg twice daily to 15 mg twice daily; if a dosage of 15 mg twice daily is not tolerated, duvelisib should be discontinued.

Infections. If grade 3 or 4 infection occurs, duvelisib therapy should be withheld until the infection resolves. Duvelisib may then be resumed at the previous dosage or at a reduced dosage of 15 mg twice daily.

If CMV infection or viremia (confirmed by polymerase chain reaction [PCR] or antigen assay) occurs, duvelisib therapy should be withheld until the infection or viremia resolves. Duvelisib may then be resumed at the previous dosage or at a reduced dosage; following resumption of therapy, patients should be monitored at least monthly for reactivation of CMV infection by PCR or antigen assay.

If PCP of any grade is suspected, duvelisib therapy should be withheld. If PCP is confirmed, duvelisib should be permanently discontinued. (See Infectious Complications under Warnings/Precautions: Warnings, in Cautions.)

Noninfectious Diarrhea or Colitis. In patients with mild or moderate noninfectious diarrhea (grade 1 or 2; up to 6 stools per day over baseline) that is responsive to antidiarrheal therapy or in those with asymptomatic (grade 1) colitis, duvelisib therapy may be continued at the same dosage, and patients should be monitored at least weekly until diarrhea or colitis resolves. If mild or moderate noninfectious diarrhea is not responsive to antidiarrheal therapy, duvelisib therapy should be withheld, supportive therapy with enteric-acting corticosteroids (e.g., budesonide) should be initiated, and patients should be monitored at least weekly. When diarrhea resolves, duvelisib therapy may be resumed at a reduced dosage.

In patients with severe noninfectious diarrhea (grade 3; more than 6 stools per day over baseline), abdominal pain, blood or mucus in stools, change in bowel habits, or peritoneal signs, duvelisib therapy should be withheld, supportive therapy with enteric-acting (e.g., budesonide) or systemic-acting corticosteroids should be initiated, and patients should be monitored at least weekly. When diarrhea or colitis resolves, duvelisib may be resumed at a reduced dosage. In patients with recurrent severe diarrhea or recurrent colitis of any grade, therapy with duvelisib should be permanently discontinued. (See Diarrhea or Colitis under Warnings/Precautions: Warnings, in Cautions.)

In patients with life-threatening diarrhea or colitis, therapy with duvelisib should be permanently discontinued.

Dermatologic Toxicity. If grade 1 or 2 dermatologic reactions occur, duvelisib therapy may be continued at the same dosage, supportive care (e.g., emollients, antihistamines for relief of pruritus, topical corticosteroids) should be initiated, and patients should be monitored closely.

If severe (grade 3) dermatologic reactions occur, duvelisib therapy should be withheld until toxicity resolves, supportive care (e.g., emollients, antihistamines for relief of pruritus, topical or systemic corticosteroids) should be initiated, and patients should be monitored at least weekly. When toxicity resolves, duvelisib may be resumed at a reduced dosage. If severe toxicity does not improve, worsens, or recurs, duvelisib therapy should be permanently discontinued.

If life-threatening dermatologic toxicity occurs, duvelisib therapy should be permanently discontinued.

If Stevens-Johnson syndrome, toxic epidermal necrolysis, or drug reaction with eosinophilia and systemic symptoms (DRESS) occurs, duvelisib therapy should be permanently discontinued. (See Dermatologic Effects under Warnings/Precautions: Warnings, in Cautions.)

Noninfectious Pneumonitis. If grade 2 noninfectious pneumonitis occurs, duvelisib therapy should be withheld and systemic corticosteroid therapy should be initiated. When symptoms resolve to grade 1 or less, duvelisib may be resumed at a reduced dosage. If noninfectious pneumonitis recurs or is not responsive to corticosteroid therapy, duvelisib should be permanently discontinued.

If grade 3 or life-threatening noninfectious pneumonitis occurs, duvelisib should be permanently discontinued and systemic corticosteroid therapy should be initiated. (See Pneumonitis under Warnings/Precautions: Warnings, in Cautions.)

Hepatotoxicity. For grade 2 serum aminotransferase (ALT and/or AST) elevations (i.e., concentrations 3–5 times the upper limit of normal [ULN]), duvelisib therapy may be continued at the same dosage. Liver function tests should be monitored at least weekly until ALT and AST concentrations return to less than 3 times the ULN.

For the first occurrence of grade 3 ALT and/or AST elevations (i.e., concentrations exceeding 5 times but not exceeding 20 times the ULN), therapy with duvelisib should be withheld and liver function tests should be monitored at least weekly until ALT and AST concentrations return to less than 3 times the ULN; duvelisib may then be resumed at the previous dosage. If grade 3 toxicity recurs, therapy with duvelisib should be withheld again and liver function tests should be monitored at least weekly until ALT and AST concentrations return to less than 3 times the ULN; duvelisib may then be resumed at a reduced dosage.

For grade 4 ALT and/or AST elevations (i.e., concentrations exceeding 20 times the ULN), therapy with duvelisib should be permanently discontinued. (See Hepatotoxicity under Warnings/Precautions: Other Warnings and Precautions, in Cautions.)

Hematologic Toxicity. In patients with grade 3 neutropenia (i.e., absolute neutrophil count [ANC] of 500–1000/mm^3), duvelisib therapy may be continued at the same dosage, and ANC should be monitored at least weekly.

For the first occurrence of grade 4 neutropenia (i.e., ANC less than 500/mm^3), therapy with duvelisib should be withheld and ANC should be monitored. When ANC reaches or exceeds 500/mm^3, duvelisib may be resumed at the previous dosage. If grade 4 neutropenia recurs, duvelisib should be withheld again; when ANC reaches or exceeds 500/mm^3, the drug may be resumed at a reduced dosage. (See Neutropenia under Warnings/Precautions: Other Warnings and Precautions, in Cautions.)

In patients with grade 3 thrombocytopenia (i.e., platelet counts of 25,000/mm^3 to less than 50,000/mm^3) and grade 1 bleeding, duvelisib therapy may be continued at the same dosage, and platelet counts should be monitored at least weekly.

For the first occurrence of grade 3 thrombocytopenia and grade 2 bleeding, therapy with duvelisib should be withheld and platelet counts should be monitored. When platelet counts reach or exceed 25,000/mm^3 *and* bleeding resolves, duvelisib may be resumed at the previous dosage. If toxicity recurs, therapy with duvelisib should be withheld again. When platelet counts reach or exceed 25,000/mm^3, duvelisib may be resumed at a reduced dosage.

For the first occurrence of grade 4 thrombocytopenia (i.e., platelet counts less than 25,000/mm^3), therapy with duvelisib should be withheld and platelet counts should be monitored. When platelet counts reach or exceed 25,000/mm^3, duvelisib may be resumed at the previous dosage. If grade 4 thrombocytopenia recurs, therapy with duvelisib should be withheld again. When platelet counts reach or exceed 25,000/mm^3, duvelisib may be resumed at a reduced dosage.

Concomitant Use with Drugs Affecting Hepatic Microsomal Enzymes Concomitant use of duvelisib and drugs that are potent inhibitors of cytochrome P-450 (CYP) isoenzyme 3A may result in increased duvelisib exposure and may increase the risk of toxicity. If concomitant use of duvelisib and potent CYP3A inhibitors cannot be avoided, the manufacturer recommends that the duvelisib dosage be reduced to 15 mg twice daily. (See Drug Interactions: Drugs Affecting Hepatic Microsomal Enzymes.)

■ **Special Populations** The manufacturer makes no specific dosage recommendations for geriatric patients; however, 61% of patients enrolled in clinical studies of the drug were 65 years of age or older. The manufacturer also makes no specific dosage recommendations for patients with renal or hepatic impairment. (See Specific Populations under Cautions: Warnings/Precautions.)

Cautions

■ **Contraindications** The manufacturer states that there are no known contraindications to the use of duvelisib.

■ **Warnings/Precautions** ***Warnings*** **Infectious Complications.** Serious infections, sometimes fatal, have been reported in 31% of patients receiving duvelisib in clinical trials. Pneumonia, sepsis, and lower respiratory infections were the most frequently reported serious infections. The median time to occurrence of infection of any grade was 3 months (range: 1 day to 32 months); 75% of infections occurred within 6 months.

Serious *Pneumocystis jiroveci* (formerly *Pneumocystis carinii*) pneumonia (PCP), sometimes fatal, has been reported in 1% of patients receiving duvelisib in clinical trials. PCP prophylaxis is recommended for all patients during duvelisib therapy; after duvelisib therapy is discontinued, PCP prophylaxis should be continued until the absolute CD4$^+$ T-cell count exceeds 200/mm^3. The drug should be withheld in patients with suspected PCP of any grade. If PCP is confirmed, duvelisib should be permanently discontinued.

Cytomegalovirus [CMV] infection and/or reactivation has been reported in 1% of patients receiving duvelisib in clinical trials. Antiviral prophylaxis should be considered during duvelisib therapy to prevent CMV infection and/or reactivation. If CMV infection or viremia occurs, duvelisib treatment should be interrupted until infection or viremia resolves. Duvelisib may then be resumed at the previous dosage or at a reduced dosage, and patients should be monitored at least monthly for CMV reactivation by polymerase chain reaction (PCR) or antigen assay.

Preexisting infections should be treated prior to initiating duvelisib therapy. Patients receiving duvelisib should be monitored for signs and symptoms of infection. The drug should be withheld in those who develop grade 3 or greater infection. (See Infections under Dosage: Dosage Modification for Toxicity, in Dosage and Administration.)

Diarrhea or Colitis. Serious diarrhea or colitis, sometimes fatal, has been reported in 18% of patients receiving duvelisib in clinical trials. The median time to occurrence of diarrhea or colitis was 4 months (range: 1 day to 33 months); 75% of cases of diarrhea or colitis occurred within 8 months of initiation of therapy, and the median duration was 0.5 month (range: 1 day to 29 months).

Patients receiving duvelisib should be monitored for the development of severe diarrhea or colitis. If mild or moderate noninfectious diarrhea or asymptomatic colitis occurs, duvelisib may be continued at the same dosage, antidiarrheal therapy should be initiated as needed, and patients should be monitored at least weekly until diarrhea or colitis resolves. If diarrhea is not responsive to antidiarrheal therapy, temporary interruption of therapy, supportive therapy with enteric-acting corticosteroids, and/or dosage reduction may be necessary. (See Noninfectious Diarrhea or Colitis under Dosage: Dosage Modification for Toxicity, in Dosage and Administration.)

If severe diarrhea (grade 3 or greater) or colitis with abdominal pain, blood or mucus in stool, change in bowel habits, or peritoneal signs occurs, duvelisib treatment should be interrupted, supportive therapy with enteric-acting or systemic corticosteroids should be initiated, and a diagnostic evaluation, including colonoscopy, should be performed to determine the etiology. Patients should be monitored at least weekly until diarrhea or colitis resolves. Dosage reduction or discontinuance of the drug may be necessary. (See Noninfectious Diarrhea or Colitis under Dosage: Dosage Modification for Toxicity, in Dosage and Administration.)

Dermatologic Effects. Serious dermatologic reactions, sometimes fatal, have been reported in 5% of patients receiving duvelisib in clinical trials. Serious dermatologic reactions have included erythroderma, exfoliative dermatitis, desquamation, pruritus, keratinocyte necrosis, and rash (including exanthem and erythematous, papular, or maculopapular rash); fatal dermatologic reactions, including drug reaction with eosinophilia and systemic symptoms (DRESS) and toxic epidermal necrolysis, have been reported. The median time to occurrence of dermatologic reactions of any grade was 3 months (range: 1 day to 29 months), and the median duration was 1 month (range: 1 day to 37 months).

If dermatologic reactions occur, all concomitant therapy should be reviewed and drugs that may be contributing to dermatologic reactions should be discontinued. Supportive care (e.g., emollients, antihistamines for relief of pruritus, topical or systemic corticosteroids) should be initiated, and patients should be monitored closely. Temporary interruption of duvelisib therapy and/or dosage reduction or discontinuance of therapy may be necessary depending on the severity of dermatologic reactions. (See Dermatologic Toxicity under Dosage: Dosage Modification for Toxicity, in Dosage and Administration.)

Pneumonitis. Serious noninfectious pneumonitis, sometimes fatal, has been reported in 5% of patients receiving duvelisib in clinical trials. The median time to occurrence of noninfectious pneumonitis was 4 months (range: 9 days to 27 months); 75% of cases of noninfectious pneumonitis occurred within 9 months. The median duration of noninfectious pneumonitis was 1 month; 75% of the cases of noninfectious pneumonitis resolved within 2 months.

Patients receiving duvelisib should be monitored for respiratory symptoms and presence of interstitial infiltrates. If new or progressive respiratory signs and symptoms (e.g., cough, dyspnea, hypoxia, interstitial infiltrates, decrease in oxygen saturation of more than 5%) occur, duvelisib therapy should be interrupted and the etiology should be evaluated. If infectious pneumonitis is confirmed, duvelisib therapy may be resumed at the previous dosage when infection and respiratory manifestations resolve. For grade 2 or greater noninfectious pneumonitis, systemic corticosteroid therapy should be initiated; temporary interruption of duvelisib therapy and/or dosage reduction or discontinuance of therapy may be necessary depending on the severity and persistence of pneumonitis. (See Noninfectious Pneumonitis under Dosage: Dosage Modification for Toxicity, in Dosage and Administration.)

Other Warnings and Precautions **Hepatotoxicity.** Grade 3 or 4 elevations in aminotransferases (ALT and/or AST) have been reported in 8 or 2%, respectively, of patients receiving duvelisib in clinical trials. Elevations in both aminotransferase (ALT or AST) and total bilirubin concentrations exceeding 3 and 2 times the upper limit of normal (ULN), respectively, have been reported in 2% of patients receiving duvelisib. The median time to occurrence of elevated ALT or AST concentrations of any grade was 2 months (range: 3 days to 26 months); the median duration was 1 month (range: 1 day to 16 months).

Liver function tests, including ALT and AST concentrations, should be monitored periodically during therapy, with more frequent monitoring in patients who develop aminotransferase elevations during therapy. Temporary interruption of duvelisib therapy and/or dosage reduction or discontinuance of therapy may be necessary depending on the severity of hepatotoxicity. (See Hepatotoxicity under Dosage and Administration: Dosage Modification for Toxicity, in Dosage and Administration.)

Neutropenia. Severe (grade 3 or 4) neutropenia has been reported in 42% of patients receiving duvelisib in clinical trials; grade 4 neutropenia has been reported in 24% of patients receiving the drug. The median time to onset of severe neutropenia was 2 months (range: 3 days to 31 months); 75% of cases of severe neutropenia occurred within 4 months.

Absolute neutrophil count (ANC) should be monitored at least every 2 weeks during the first 2 months of therapy. If ANC decreases to less than 1000/mm^3, ANC should be monitored at least every week. Temporary interruption of duvelisib therapy and/or dosage reduction may be necessary depending on the severity of neutropenia. (See Hematologic Toxicity under Dosage: Dosage Modification for Toxicity, in Dosage and Administration.)

Fetal/Neonatal Morbidity and Mortality. Data are lacking on use of duvelisib in pregnant women; however, based on its mechanism of action and animal findings, duvelisib may cause fetal harm. Embryofetal death, teratogenicity (e.g., fetal malformations), and decreased fetal weight have been demonstrated in rats and rabbits receiving duvelisib at dosages approximately 10 and 39 times, respectively, the maximum recommended human dosage.

Pregnancy should be avoided during duvelisib therapy. The manufacturer states that a pregnancy test should be performed prior to initiation of duvelisib therapy in women of childbearing potential and that such women and men who are partners of such women should be advised to use effective contraceptive methods while receiving duvelisib and for at least one month after discontinuance of therapy. If duvelisib is used during pregnancy or if the patient becomes pregnant while receiving the drug, the patient should be apprised of the potential fetal hazard.

Impairment of Fertility. Results of animal studies suggest that duvelisib may impair male fertility. In repeat-dose toxicity studies, testicular and epididymal changes (i.e., seminiferous epithelial atrophy, decreased testicular weight, soft testes, small epididymis, oligospermia, aspermia) were observed in male rats.

Specific Populations **Pregnancy.** Duvelisib may cause fetal harm if administered to pregnant women based on animal findings and its mechanism of action. (See Fetal/Neonatal Morbidity and Mortality under Warnings/Precautions: Other Warnings and Precautions, in Cautions.)

Lactation. It is not known whether duvelisib and/or its metabolites distribute into human milk or if the drug has any effect on milk production or on the nursing infant. Because of the potential for serious adverse reactions to duvelisib in nursing infants, women should be advised not to breast-feed while receiving the drug and for at least one month after the drug is discontinued.

Pediatric Use. Safety and efficacy of duvelisib have not been established in pediatric patients.

Geriatric Use. In clinical studies evaluating duvelisib, 61% of patients were 65 years of age or older, while 24% were 75 years of age or older. No substantial differences in efficacy or safety were observed between geriatric patients and younger adults.

Hepatic Impairment. Systemic exposure to duvelisib does not appear to be altered in patients with hepatic impairment (Child-Pugh class A, B, or C).

Renal Impairment. Systemic exposure to duvelisib does not appear to be altered in patients with creatinine clearance of at least 23 mL/minute.

■ Common Adverse Effects

Adverse effects reported in at least 10% of patients receiving duvelisib include diarrhea or colitis, rash, pyrexia, fatigue, upper or lower respiratory tract infection, pneumonia, cough, nausea, musculoskeletal pain, abdominal pain, vomiting, constipation, decreased appetite, edema, mucositis, dyspnea, headache, decreased weight, and arthralgia. Laboratory abnormalities reported in at least 20% of patients receiving duvelisib include neutropenia, anemia, thrombocytopenia, elevated concentrations of aminotransferases (i.e., AST, ALT) and alkaline phosphatase, elevated serum lipase concentrations, hypophosphatemia, lymphocytosis, elevated serum amylase concentrations, hyponatremia, hyperkalemia, hypoalbuminemia, elevated concentrations of serum creatinine, leukopenia, hypocalcemia, lymphopenia, and hypokalemia.

Drug Interactions

Duvelisib is metabolized principally by cytochrome P-450 (CYP) isoenzyme 3A4.

In vitro, duvelisib is a substrate of the efflux transporters P-glycoprotein (P-gp) and breast cancer resistance protein (BCRP). In vitro studies indicate that duvelisib does not inhibit renal organic anion transporter (OAT) 1, OAT3, organic cation transporter (OCT) 1, OCT2, organic anion transport protein (OATP) 1B1, OATP1B3, BCRP, or P-gp.

■ Drugs Affecting Hepatic Microsomal Enzymes

Inhibitors of CYP3A Isoenzymes Concomitant use of duvelisib with potent inhibitors of CYP3A may increase systemic exposure to duvelisib and increase the risk of toxicity. When the potent CYP3A inhibitor ketoconazole (200 mg orally once daily for 5 days) was administered concomitantly with duvelisib (single 10-mg oral dose) in healthy individuals, area under the plasma concentration-time curve (AUC) and peak plasma concentration of duvelisib were increased by 4- and 1.7-fold, respectively. Simulations suggest that concomitant use of duvelisib and a potent CYP3A inhibitor (e.g., ketoconazole) would result in a twofold increase in exposure to duvelisib at steady state. Simulations also suggest that concomitant use of duvelisib with mild or moderate inhibitors of CYP3A4 would not affect systemic exposure to duvelisib.

If duvelisib is used concomitantly with a potent CYP3A inhibitor (e.g., ketoconazole), the manufacturer recommends that the dosage of duvelisib be reduced from 25 mg twice daily to 15 mg twice daily.

Inducers of CYP3A Isoenzymes Concomitant use of duvelisib with potent inducers of CYP3A may result in decreased systemic exposure to duvelisib and decrease therapeutic efficacy of the drug. When the potent CYP3A inducer rifampin (600 mg once daily for 7 days) was administered concomitantly with duvelisib (single 25-mg oral dose) in healthy individuals, AUC and peak plasma concentration of duvelisib were decreased by 82 and 66%, respectively. Concomitant use of duvelisib with potent CYP3A inducers (e.g., rifampin) should be avoided. The potential for moderate CYP3A inducers to alter duvelisib exposure has not been established.

■ Drugs Metabolized by Hepatic Microsomal Enzymes

Substrates of CYP3A Isoenzymes Duvelisib may increase systemic exposure to and risk of adverse effects of other drugs metabolized by CYP3A. When the CYP3A substrate midazolam (single 2-mg oral dose) was administered concomitantly with duvelisib (25 mg twice daily for 5 days) in healthy individuals, AUC and peak plasma concentration of midazolam were increased by 4.3- and 2.2-fold, respectively. If duvelisib is used concomitantly with a CYP3A substrate (e.g., midazolam), reduction in the dosage of the CYP3A substrate should be considered, and the patient should be monitored for CYP3A substrate-related toxicity.

Description

Duvelisib, an inhibitor of phosphatidylinositol-3-kinase (PI3K), is an antineoplastic agent. Phosphatidylinositol-3-kinases are lipid kinases consisting of a catalytic subunit that exists in 4 different isoforms (α, β, γ, δ). Duvelisib is predominantly active against the PI3K-δ and PI3K-γ isoforms, which are expressed in hematopoietic cells and mediate B-cell and T-cell receptor signaling critical for B-cell and T-cell homeostasis and function. Duvelisib has been shown to induce tumor cell death by apoptosis and to inhibit proliferation of primary malignant B-cell lines. Duvelisib has demonstrated inhibition of several important cell signaling pathways, including B-cell receptor (BCR) signaling and CXCR12-mediated chemotaxis of malignant B cells. The drug also has demonstrated inhibition of CXCL12-induced T-cell migration and macrophage colony-stimulating factor- and interleukin-4-driven M2 polarization of macrophages.

Systemic exposure to duvelisib increases in a dose-proportional manner over a dosage range of 8–75 mg twice daily. Following oral administration of a single 25-mg dose of duvelisib, the absolute oral bioavailability was 42%; peak plasma concentrations of the drug were achieved within 1–2 hours. Administration of a single dose of duvelisib with a high-fat meal decreased peak plasma concentrations and area under the concentration-time curve (AUC) of the drug by 37 and 6%, respectively, compared with administration in the fasted state. Duvelisib is more than 98% bound to plasma proteins. Duvelisib is metabolized principally by cytochrome P-450 (CYP) isoenzyme 3A4. The mean terminal half-life of duvelisib is 4.7 hours. Following oral administration of a single 25-mg dose of radiolabeled duvelisib, 79% of the dose was recovered in feces (11% as unchanged drug) and 14% was recovered in urine (less than 1% as unchanged drug).

Advice to Patients

Importance of instructing patients to read the manufacturer's patient information (medication guide) before initiating duvelisib therapy and each time the prescription is refilled.

Importance of advising patients to take duvelisib exactly as prescribed and of not altering the dosage or discontinuing therapy unless advised to do so by their clinician. Importance of advising patients to swallow duvelisib capsules whole and not to open, break, or chew the capsules.

Importance of advising patients to take a missed dose as soon as it is remembered unless the dose was missed by more than 6 hours, in which case they should not take the missed dose.

Risk of serious infections such as pneumonia. Importance of immediately reporting fever or any other signs of infection.

Risk of severe diarrhea or colitis. Importance of immediately informing clinician if mucus or blood is present in stool or if abdominal pain or new or worsening diarrhea occurs.

Risk of severe dermatologic reactions. Importance of immediately informing clinician if dermatologic reactions (e.g., new or worsening rash; rash accompanied by itching or peeling skin, blisters, or fever; painful sores) occur.

Risk of pneumonitis. Importance of informing clinician if new or worsening respiratory symptoms (e.g., cough, dyspnea) occur.

Risk of hepatotoxicity; importance of regular liver function test monitoring. Importance of immediately informing clinician if possible signs or symptoms of hepatotoxicity (e.g., abdominal pain, jaundice, bruising, bleeding diathesis) occur.

Risk of neutropenia; importance of periodic monitoring of blood cell counts during duvelisib therapy. Importance of immediately informing clinician if fever or other signs of infection occur.

Risk of fetal harm. Necessity of advising women of childbearing potential to avoid pregnancy and to use effective contraceptive methods while receiving duvelisib and for at least one month following discontinuance of therapy. Importance of advising men who are partners of such women that they should use effective methods of contraception while receiving the drug and for at least one month after the drug is discontinued. Importance of women informing clinicians immediately if they become pregnant during therapy or think they may be pregnant. If pregnancy occurs, advise pregnant women of potential risk to the fetus.

Importance of advising women to avoid breast-feeding while receiving duvelisib and for at least one month after discontinuance of therapy.

Importance of informing clinicians of existing or contemplated concomitant therapy, including prescription and OTC drugs and dietary or herbal supplements, as well as any concomitant illnesses.

Importance of informing patients of other important precautionary information. (See Cautions.)

Overview® (see Users Guide). For additional information on this drug until a more detailed monograph is developed and published, the manufacturer's labeling should be consulted. It is *essential* that the manufacturer's labeling be consulted for more detailed information on usual cautions, precautions, contraindications, potential drug interactions, laboratory test interferences, and acute toxicity. For further information on the handling of antineoplastic agents, see the ASHP Guidelines on Handling Hazardous Drugs at http://www.ahfsdruginformation.com.

Preparations

Excipients in commercially available drug preparations may have clinically important effects in some individuals; consult specific product labeling for details.

Duvelisib

Oral		
Capsules	15 mg	**Copiktra®**, Verastem
	25 mg	**Copiktra®**, Verastem

Elotuzumab

■ Elotuzumab, a recombinant humanized monoclonal antibody that is an antagonist of signaling lymphocytic activation molecule (SLAM) family member 7 (SLAMF7), is an antineoplastic agent; the drug also is referred to as an anti-CS1 (anti-CD2 subset 1) monoclonal antibody.

Uses

■ Multiple Myeloma Elotuzumab is used in combination with lenalidomide and dexamethasone for the treatment of multiple myeloma in patients who have received 1–3 prior therapies. Elotuzumab has been designated an orphan drug by FDA for the treatment of this cancer. In patients with relapsed or refractory multiple myeloma, combined therapy with elotuzumab, lenalidomide, and dexamethasone has been shown to prolong progression-free survival and increase response rate compared with lenalidomide and dexamethasone alone.

The current indication for elotuzumab is based principally on the results of a randomized, open-label, multicenter, phase 3 study (ELOQUENT-2) in adults with relapsed or refractory multiple myeloma who had received 1–3 prior therapies. Patients were enrolled if they had documented disease progression following their most recent therapy. In this study, 646 adults were randomized in a 1:1 ratio to receive either elotuzumab (10 mg/kg IV on days 1, 8, 15, and 22 during cycles 1 and 2, followed by 10 mg/kg on days 1 and 15 during cycle 3 and onward) in combination with lenalidomide (25 mg orally on days 1–21) and dexamethasone (28 mg of dexamethasone orally *plus* 8 mg of dexamethasone phosphate IV on days 1, 8, 15, and 22 during cycles 1 and 2, followed by 28 mg orally *plus* 8 mg IV on days 1 and 15 and 40 mg orally on days 8 and 22 during cycle 3 and onward) *or* lenalidomide (25 mg orally on days 1–21) in combination with dexamethasone (40 mg orally on days 1, 8, 15, and 22). Therapy was administered in 4-week cycles until disease progression or unacceptable toxicity occurred. Prior to each elotuzumab infusion, patients also received acetaminophen, a histamine H_2-receptor antagonist, and a histamine H_1-receptor antagonist as prophylaxis for infusion-related reactions. All enrolled patients were required to receive thromboprophylaxis. The primary end points of this study were progression-free survival and overall response rate, which was assessed by a blinded independent review committee according to the European Group for Blood and Marrow Transplantation (EBMT) response criteria.

The median age of patients enrolled in the ELOQUENT-2 study was 66 years (range: 37–91 years); 84% of patients were white, 91% had an ECOG (Eastern Cooperative Oncology Group) performance status of 0 or 1, 43% had stage I disease according to the International Staging System (ISS), 32% had stage II disease, and 21% had stage III disease. Patients enrolled in the study had received a median of 2 prior therapies; 70% of patients had previously received bortezomib, 65% had received melphalan, 48% had received thalidomide, 6% had received lenalidomide, and 55% had undergone stem cell transplantation. Approximately 65 or 35% of patients had relapsed or refractory disease, respectively. High-risk cytogenetic features, t(4;14) translocation or 17p deletion, were present in 9 or 32% of patients, respectively.

At a median follow-up of 24.5 months, median progression-free survival was prolonged in patients who received elotuzumab in combination with lenalidomide and dexamethasone compared with those who received lenalidomide and dexamethasone alone (19 versus 15 months; hazard ratio: 0.7). The rates of 1- and 2-year progression-free survival were higher in patients receiving elotuzumab in combination with lenalidomide and dexamethasone (68 and 41%, respectively) compared with those receiving lenalidomide and dexamethasone alone (57 and 27%, respectively). In addition, patients receiving elotuzumab in combination with lenalidomide and dexamethasone had higher overall response rates (79 versus 66%) and more-durable responses (21 versus 17 months) compared with those receiving lenalidomide and dexamethasone alone. Median overall survival had not been reached at the time of the analysis. Results of a subgroup analysis (based on age, disease stage, baseline β_2-microglobulin concentration, response to most recent line of therapy, prior exposure to bortezomib or an immunomodulatory agent, prior stem cell transplantation, presence of high-risk cytogenetic features, baseline creatinine clearance) suggested that the drug's effect on progression-free survival was consistent across all subgroups.

Dosage and Administration

■ General Clinicians should consult the respective manufacturers' labelings for information on the dosage and method of administration of other antineoplastic agents used in combination regimens.

To minimize the risk of infusion-related events associated with elotuzumab, the manufacturer recommends premedication with oral acetaminophen 650 mg to 1 g, an oral or IV histamine H_2-receptor antagonist (e.g., ranitidine 50 mg IV or 150 mg orally or equivalent), an oral or IV histamine H_1-receptor antagonist (e.g., diphenhydramine hydrochloride 25–50 mg or equivalent), and IV dexamethasone phosphate 8 mg administered 45–90 minutes prior to each elotuzumab infusion.

Restricted Distribution Program Elotuzumab can only be obtained through select specialty distributors. Clinicians may consult the Empliciti® website for specific availability information (http://www.emplicitihcp.com/ordering).

■ Administration Elotuzumab is administered by IV infusion using a sterile, nonpyrogenic, low-protein-binding, 0.2- to 1.2-μm inline filter. Solutions of the drug should be administered via an infusion pump. Other drugs should not be administered simultaneously through the same IV line with elotuzumab infusion.

Prior to administration, commercially available elotuzumab lyophilized powder for injection must be reconstituted and diluted using proper aseptic technique.

Unreconstituted elotuzumab lyophilized powder for injection should be stored in unopened vials at 2–8°C, and should not be frozen or shaken. Unopened vials should be retained in the original package for protection from light.

Reconstitution The manufacturer recommends use of a 15- to 18-gauge needle for preparation. The lyophilized powder is reconstituted by adding 13 mL of sterile water for injection to a vial labeled as containing 300 mg of elotuzumab or by adding 17 mL of sterile water for injection to a vial labeled as containing 400 mg of elotuzumab to provide a solution containing 25 mg/mL. The 300- and 400-mg vials are formulated to provide a slight overfill when reconstituted as directed. Slight back pressure may occur when injecting the diluent into the vial. The vials should be held upright and swirled to facilitate dissolution of the lyophilized powder, which should dissolve in less than 10 minutes, and then inverted a few times to facilitate dissolution of lyophilized powder that may be present on top of the vial or on the stopper. The vials should not be shaken or vigorously agitated. The contents of the reconstituted vials should not be removed until all of the solids have completely dissolved and the solution has been allowed to stand for about 5–10 minutes. The reconstituted solution should be inspected visually for particulate matter and discoloration prior to dilution and should not be used if particles are present or if the solution appears discolored. The resulting solution should be colorless to slightly yellow and clear to slightly opalescent.

Commercially available elotuzumab lyophilized powder for injection contains no preservatives and is intended for single use; any partially used vials should be discarded.

Dilution The appropriate dose (10 mg/kg) of reconstituted elotuzumab solution (containing 25 mg/mL) should be withdrawn and added to a polyvinylchloride (PVC) or non-PVC (polyolefin) infusion bag containing 230 mL of 0.9% sodium chloride or 5% dextrose injection. The volume of 0.9% sodium chloride or 5% dextrose injection may be adjusted to avoid exceeding 5 mL of fluid per kg of patient weight.

If immediate administration is not possible, diluted solutions of the drug should be protected from light and stored at 2–8°C for up to 24 hours; however, diluted solutions of the drug may be stored at 20–25°C under room light for up to 8 hours during the 24-hour period. Infusion of diluted elotuzumab solutions should be completed within 24 hours of reconstitution.

Elotuzumab should not be admixed with any other drug.

Rate of Administration The initial elotuzumab dose (day 1 of cycle 1) should be infused IV at an initial rate of 0.5 mL/minute; if infusion-related reactions do not occur, the infusion rate may be doubled every 30 minutes up to a maximum rate of 2 mL/minute. The second dose of elotuzumab (day 8 of cycle 1) should be infused at an initial rate of 1 mL/minute; if infusion-related reactions do not occur within 30 minutes of initiating the infusion, the infusion rate may be increased to 2 mL/minute. Subsequent doses of elotuzumab should be infused at a rate of 2 mL/minute. The maximum infusion rate should not exceed 2 mL/minute; however, in patients who have received 4 cycles of elotuzumab, the infusion rate may be increased to a maximum infusion rate of 5 mL/minute.

If infusion-related reactions occur, elotuzumab therapy should be interrupted and the infusion rate should be reduced depending on the severity of the reaction, and appropriate symptomatic and supportive therapy should be provided as clinically indicated. If the infusion-related reaction is grade 2 or greater in severity, therapy with elotuzumab should be interrupted and appropriate medical treatment should be provided; once the reaction has resolved to grade 1 or less, the infusion may be resumed at a rate of 0.5 mL/minute and may be increased as tolerated in increments of 0.5 mL/minute every 30 minutes to the rate at which the infusion-related reaction occurred. If infusion-related reactions do not recur, the infusion rate may be increased in increments and intervals appropriate for the treatment cycle dose (as described in the previous paragraph). (See Infusion-related Effects under Cautions: Warnings/Precautions.) If infusion-related reactions recur, elotuzumab therapy should be interrupted and not restarted on that same day. If severe infusion-related reactions occur, permanent discontinuance of elotuzumab therapy may be necessary and emergency treatment should be provided.

■ **Dosage** ***Multiple Myeloma*** For use in combination with lenalidomide and dexamethasone in the treatment of multiple myeloma in adults who have received 1–3 prior therapies, the recommended dosage of elotuzumab is 10 mg/kg administered IV once weekly (days 1, 8, 15, and 22) with lenalidomide 25 mg administered orally once daily on days 1–21 and dexamethasone 28 mg administered orally on days 1, 8, 15, and 22 of each 28-day cycle during cycles 1 and 2. During cycle 3 and onward, the recommended dosage of elotuzumab is 10 mg/kg administered IV every 2 weeks (days 1 and 15) with lenalidomide 25 mg administered orally once daily on days 1–21 and dexamethasone 28 mg administered orally on days 1 and 15 and 40 mg administered orally on days 8 and 22 of each 28-day cycle. The oral dexamethasone dose (28 versus 40 mg) varies according to whether elotuzumab is administered that day. On days that elotuzumab is not administered but dexamethasone is scheduled, a 40-mg oral dexamethasone dose is administered. On days that elotuzumab is administered, dexamethasone 28 mg is administered orally 3–24 hours prior to administration of elotuzumab, with an additional 8-mg IV dose of dexamethasone phosphate given as premedication. To minimize the risk of infusion-related events associated with elotuzumab, appropriate premedications (including IV dexamethasone phosphate) should be administered 45–90 minutes prior to administration of elotuzumab. (See Dosage and Administration: General.)

Therapy should be continued until disease progression or unacceptable toxicity occurs.

Dosage Modification If administration of one drug in the combination regimen is delayed, interrupted, or discontinued, therapy with the other drugs may be continued; however, since dexamethasone also is used to reduce the risk of infusion-related events associated with elotuzumab, clinical judgment should be used in deciding whether elotuzumab should be continued without dexamethasone. Clinicians should consult the respective manufacturers' labelings for information on recommended dosage modifications for lenalidomide and dexamethasone.

■ **Special Populations** The manufacturer makes no special population dosage recommendations at this time. (See Specific Populations under Cautions: Warnings/Precautions.)

Cautions

■ **Contraindications** The manufacturer states there are no known contraindications to the use of elotuzumab.

■ **Warnings/Precautions** ***Combination Therapy*** When elotuzumab is used in combination with lenalidomide and dexamethasone, the usual cautions, precautions, and contraindications associated with lenalidomide and dexamethasone must be considered in addition to those associated with elotuzumab. For further information regarding warnings and precautions associated with lenalidomide and dexamethasone, see Cautions in Lenalidomide 10:00 and also in the Corticosteroids General Statement 68:04.

Infusion-related Effects Infusion-related reactions have been reported in patients receiving elotuzumab in combination with lenalidomide and dexamethasone. Infusion-related reactions generally occurred more frequently during the first infusion. In the ELOQUENT-2 study, infusion reactions were reported in approximately 10% (grade 3 in 1%) of patients receiving elotuzumab in combination with lenalidomide and dexamethasone; the most common infusion-related reactions were pyrexia, chills, and hypertension. Infusion-related reactions also have included bradycardia and hypotension. Infusion-related reactions requiring temporary interruption or discontinuance of elotuzumab therapy occurred in 5 or 1%, respectively, of patients; the median time for temporarily interrupting elotuzumab therapy was 25 minutes.

To minimize the risk of infusion-related reactions, patients receiving elotuzumab should be premedicated with acetaminophen, a histamine H_2-receptor antagonist, histamine H_1-receptor antagonist, and dexamethasone prior to administration of the drug. (See Dosage and Administration: General.)

If infusion-related reactions occur, elotuzumab therapy should be interrupted and the infusion rate should be reduced depending on the severity of the reaction, and appropriate symptomatic and supportive therapy should be provided as clinically indicated. (See Rate of Administration under Dosage and Administration: Administration.) In patients who experience infusion-related reactions, vital signs should be monitored every 30 minutes for 2 hours following the end of the infusion. If severe infusion-related reactions occur, permanent discontinuance of elotuzumab therapy may be necessary and emergency treatment should be provided.

Infectious Complications Infections, sometimes fatal or requiring discontinuance of therapy, have been reported in patients receiving elotuzumab in combination with lenalidomide and dexamethasone. In the ELOQUENT-2 study, infection was reported in 81.4% (grade 3 or 4 in 28%) of patients receiving elotuzumab in combination with lenalidomide and dexamethasone compared with 74.4% (grade 3 or 4 in 24.3%) of those receiving lenalidomide and dexamethasone alone. Opportunistic infections, fungal infections, and herpes zoster occurred in 22, 9.7, and 13.5%, respectively, of elotuzumab-treated patients compared with 12.9, 5.4, and 6.9%, respectively, of patients receiving lenalidomide and dexamethasone alone. Fatal infections occurred in 2.5% of elotuzumab-treated patients compared with 2.2% of patients receiving lenalidomide and dexamethasone alone.

Patients should be monitored for signs and symptoms of infection. If an infection develops, therapy should be initiated promptly.

Development of Second Primary Malignancy Second primary malignancies have been reported in patients receiving elotuzumab in combination with lenalidomide and dexamethasone. In the ELOQUENT-2 study, invasive second primary malignancies were reported more frequently in patients receiving elotuzumab in combination with lenalidomide and dexamethasone compared with those receiving lenalidomide and dexamethasone alone (9.1 versus 5.7%). In this study, solid tumors and skin cancer occurred in 3.5 and 4.4%, respectively, of elotuzumab-treated patients compared with 2.2 and 2.8%, respectively, of those receiving lenalidomide and dexamethasone alone; however, the incidence of hematologic malignancies was similar between elotuzumab-treated patients and those receiving lenalidomide and dexamethasone alone (1.6%).

Patients should be monitored for development of second primary malignancies.

Hepatic Effects Liver function test abnormalities have been reported in patients receiving elotuzumab in combination with lenalidomide and dexamethasone. In the ELOQUENT-2 study, concurrent elevations in ALT or AST (exceeding 3 times the upper limit of normal [ULN]) and total bilirubin concentrations (exceeding 2 times the ULN) with normal alkaline phosphatase concentrations (less than 2 times the ULN) occurred in 2.5% of patients receiving elotuzumab in combination with lenalidomide and dexamethasone and in 0.6% of those receiving lenalidomide and dexamethasone alone. Hepatotoxicity resolved in 6 of 8 elotuzumab-treated patients and resulted in permanent discontinuance of therapy in 2 patients.

Liver function tests should be evaluated periodically during therapy with the drug. If grade 3 or greater elevations in ALT or AST occur, elotuzumab therapy should be interrupted. Once the toxicity has completely resolved, resumption of elotuzumab therapy may be considered.

Interference with Serum Protein Electrophoresis and Immunofixation Assays Elotuzumab is a human IgG kappa immunoglobulin; therefore, the drug may be detected on serum protein electrophoresis (SPEP) and immunofixation (IFE) assays, particularly in patients with IgA, IgM, IgD, or lambda light chain-restricted endogenous monoclonal immunoglobulins (M-protein). Elotuzumab also comigrates with IgG kappa M-protein; therefore, the drug may mask clearance of endogenous M-protein resulting in false-positive SPEP and IFE assay results and misinterpretation of tumor response.

Immunogenicity There is potential for immunogenicity with the use of therapeutic proteins such as elotuzumab. Anti-elotuzumab antibodies were detected by electrochemiluminescent immunoassay in 72 of 390 patients (18.5%) treated with elotuzumab in clinical studies. In 63 (88%) of these patients, anti-elotuzumab antibodies developed during the first 2 months of elotuzumab therapy; anti-elotuzumab antibodies were resolved by 2–4 months in 49 (78%) of these patients. In the ELOQUENT-2 study, neutralizing antibodies were detected in 19 of 299 patients (6%).

Specific Populations **Pregnancy.** There are no adequate and well-controlled studies of elotuzumab in pregnant women. Animal reproduction studies have not been performed to date with the drug.

Because elotuzumab is administered in combination with lenalidomide and dexamethasone, clinicians *must* consider that lenalidomide is contraindicated in pregnant women. (See Combination Therapy under Cautions: Warnings/Precautions.)

Lactation. It is not known whether elotuzumab is distributed into milk. Because of the potential for serious adverse reactions in nursing infants, women should be advised to discontinue nursing during combination therapy with elotuzumab, lenalidomide, and dexamethasone. The effects of elotuzumab on nursing infants or on milk production are unknown.

Pediatric Use. Safety and efficacy of elotuzumab have not been established in pediatric patients.

Geriatric Use. In the phase 3 clinical trial evaluating elotuzumab in combination with lenalidomide and dexamethasone for the treatment of relapsed or refractory multiple myeloma, 57% of patients were 65 years of age or older. No overall differences in safety or efficacy were observed between geriatric patients and younger adults.

Hepatic Impairment. The pharmacokinetic profile of elotuzumab has not been established in patients with moderate to severe hepatic impairment.

In a population pharmacokinetic analysis, systemic exposure to elotuzumab in patients with mild hepatic impairment was similar to that observed in patients with normal hepatic function.

Renal Impairment. In a population pharmacokinetic analysis, systemic exposure to elotuzumab in patients with severe renal impairment (creatinine clearance less than 30 mL/minute) or end-stage renal disease requiring dialysis was similar to that observed in patients with normal renal function.

■ **Common Adverse Effects** Adverse effects reported in 10% or more of patients receiving elotuzumab in combination with lenalidomide and dexamethasone for the treatment of previously treated multiple myeloma and at an incidence that is at least 5% higher than that reported with lenalidomide and dexamethasone alone include fatigue, diarrhea, pyrexia, constipation, cough, peripheral neuropathy, nasopharyngitis, upper respiratory tract infection, loss of appetite, pneumonia, extremity pain, headache, vomiting, weight loss, lymphopenia, cataracts, and oropharyngeal pain.

Laboratory abnormalities reported in 10% or more of patients receiving elotuzumab in combination with lenalidomide and dexamethasone and at an incidence that is at least 5% higher than that reported with lenalidomide and dexamethasone alone include lymphopenia, leukopenia, thrombocytopenia, hypoalbuminemia, elevated concentrations of alkaline phosphatase, hyperglycemia, hypocalcemia, decreased serum bicarbonate concentrations, and hyperkalemia.

Drug Interactions

No formal drug interactions studies have been performed to date.

Description

Elotuzumab, a recombinant humanized monoclonal antibody that is an antagonist of signaling lymphocytic activation molecule (SLAM) family member 7 (SLAMF7), is an antineoplastic agent; the drug also is referred to as an anti-CS1 (anti-CD2 subset 1) monoclonal antibody. The drug is an IgG_1 kappa immunoglobulin produced by recombinant DNA technology in NS0 mouse myeloma-based cell culture. Elotuzumab binds specifically to SLAMF7, a glycoprotein expressed on the surface of normal and malignant plasma cells, natural killer (NK) cells, and, at lower levels, specific immune cell subsets of differentiated cells within the hematopoietic lineage (e.g., $CD8^+$ T cells). Following binding of elotuzumab to SLAMF7 on myeloma cells and direct activation of NK cells via the SLAMF7 pathway, the Fc domain triggers host immune responses (i.e., antibody-dependent cell-mediated cytotoxicity [ADCC]) causing lysis of myeloma cells. In preclinical models, concomitant use of elotuzumab and lenalidomide enhanced activation of NK cells compared with either drug alone and also demonstrated increased antitumor activity in vitro and in vivo.

Areas under the serum concentration-time curve (AUCs) of elotuzumab are more than dose proportional over the dose range of 0.5–20 mg/kg, indicating target-mediated clearance. Pharmacokinetic simulations indicate that following administration of elotuzumab 10 mg/kg IV once weekly for two 28-day cycles followed by 10 mg/kg IV every 2 weeks thereafter, plasma concentrations of elotuzumab increase for approximately 8 weeks after initiation of elotuzumab administration and steady-state concentrations are reached by 2–4 weeks following initiation of administration every 2 weeks. Within about 3 months (geometric mean: 82.4 days) following discontinuance of combination therapy with elotuzumab, lenalidomide, and dexamethasone, elotuzumab concentrations are predicted to decline by approximately 97% from peak steady-state values.

Data from a population pharmacokinetic analysis indicate that age (25–88 years), gender, race, baseline LDH concentrations, and albumin concentrations do not have clinically important effects on the pharmacokinetics of elotuzumab.

Advice to Patients

Risk of infusion-related reactions; importance of reporting signs and symptoms of such reactions, including fever, chills, rash, or breathing difficulty, that occur during or within 24 hours of an infusion of the drug. Importance of taking premedications as directed to minimize risk of infusion-related reactions.

Risk of fetal harm when used in combination with lenalidomide. Importance of advising women of childbearing potential and men who are partners of such women to take precautions to avoid fetal exposure to lenalidomide. (See Combination Therapy under Cautions: Warnings/Precautions.) Importance of women informing a clinician immediately if they are or plan to become pregnant.

Importance of advising women to avoid breast-feeding while receiving elotuzumab. Importance of women informing a clinician if they plan to breast-feed.

Risk of infection. Importance of reporting signs or symptoms of infection (e.g., cough, fever, flu-like symptoms, shortness of breath, painful rash, burning on urination).

Risk of developing a second primary malignancy.

Risk of hepatotoxicity and importance of periodic liver function test monitoring. Importance of reporting any manifestations of hepatotoxicity (e.g., jaundice, weakness, loss of appetite, fatigue, confusion, abdominal swelling, unusually colored stool).

Importance of informing clinicians of existing or contemplated concomitant therapy, including prescription and OTC drugs and dietary or herbal supplements, as well as any concomitant illnesses.

Importance of informing patients of other important precautionary information. (See Cautions.)

Overview® (see Users Guide). For additional information on this drug until a more detailed monograph is developed and published, the manufacturer's labeling should be consulted. It is *essential* that the manufacturer's labeling be consulted for more detailed information on usual cautions, precautions, contraindications, potential drug interactions, laboratory test interferences, and acute toxicity. For further information on the handling of antineoplastic agents, see the ASHP Guidelines on Handling Hazardous Drugs at http://www.ahfsdruginformation.com.

Preparations

Distribution of elotuzumab is restricted. (See Restricted Distribution Program under Dosage and Administration: General.)

Excipients in commercially available drug preparations may have clinically important effects in some individuals; consult specific product labeling for details.

Elotuzumab

Parenteral

For injection, for IV infusion	300 mg	**Empliciti®**, Bristol-Myers Squibb
	400 mg	**Empliciti®**, Bristol-Myers Squibb

Enasidenib Mesylate

■ Enasidenib, a potent and selective inhibitor of isocitrate dehydrogenase-2 (IDH2), is an antineoplastic agent.

Uses

■ **Acute Myeloid Leukemia** Enasidenib mesylate is used for the treatment of relapsed or refractory acute myeloid leukemia (AML) with isocitrate dehydrogenase-2 (IDH2) mutation. Enasidenib has been designated an orphan drug by FDA for the treatment of this cancer. An FDA-approved diagnostic test (e.g., Abbott RealTi*me*® IDH2 assay) is required to confirm the presence of IDH2 mutation (peripheral blood or bone marrow) prior to initiation of therapy. The current indication is based on complete remission (CR) or complete remission with partial hematologic recovery (CRh) and improvement of hematologic deficits (determined by rate of conversion from transfusion dependence to transfusion independence).

The current indication for enasidenib is based principally on the results of an open-label, multicenter, 2-cohort, single-arm study (AG221-C-001) in adults with relapsed or refractory AML with IDH2 mutation as detected by the Abbott RealTi*me*® IDH2 mutation test. The primary measures of efficacy were CR and CRh, duration of response, and loss of transfusion dependence (red blood cells [RBCs] and/or platelets). CR was defined as the presence of less than 5% blasts in bone marrow without evidence of disease and with full recovery of peripheral blood cell counts (platelet count exceeding 100,000/mm^3 and absolute neutrophil count [ANC] exceeding 1000/mm^3), and CRh was defined as the presence of less than 5% blasts in bone marrow without evidence of disease and with partial recovery of peripheral blood cell counts (platelet count exceeding 50,000/mm^3 and ANC exceeding 500/mm^3). Overall, the median age of patients was 68 years (range: 19–100 years); 77% were Caucasian, 62% were 65 years of age or older, 52% were male, 62% had an Eastern Cooperative Oncology Group (ECOG) performance status of 1, 52% had refractory AML, 49% had intermediate-risk cytogenetics, 27% had poor-risk cytogenetics, 79% were transfusion dependent at baseline, and 13% had previously undergone stem cell transplantation. Patients enrolled in this study had received a median of 2 prior antineoplastic chemotherapy regimens. IDH2 mutations at codon R140 or R172 were present in 78 or 22% of patients, respectively; mutations detected in peripheral blood were reported if bone marrow and peripheral blood mutations were inconsistent. In this study, 199 adults received an enasidenib dosage of 100 mg orally once daily. Therapy was continued until disease progression or unacceptable toxicity occurred. At a median follow-up of 6.6 months, CR or CRh was achieved in 23% of patients with a median response duration of 8.2 months; 19% of patients achieved CR. The median time to initial CR or CRh was 1.9 months. The median time to best response (CR or CRh) was 3.7 months; the majority (85%) of these patients achieved a best response within 6 months of initiating enasidenib therapy. Approximately one-third (34%) of patients who were transfusion dependent at baseline became transfusion independent during any 56-day period during the study. The majority (76%) of patients who were transfusion independent at baseline remained transfusion independent during any 56-day period during the study.

Dosage and Administration

■ **General** Presence of the isocitrate dehydrogenase-2 (IDH2) mutation (peripheral blood or bone marrow) must be confirmed prior to initiation of therapy with enasidenib. (See Uses: Acute Myeloid Leukemia.)

Because leukocytosis or tumor lysis syndrome may occur, complete blood cell (CBC) counts and blood chemistries should be monitored prior to initiation of enasidenib therapy and at least every 2 weeks for at least the initial 3 months of therapy. Laboratory abnormalities should be managed promptly. (See Dosage: Dosage Modification for Toxicity.)

Restricted Distribution Program Enasidenib mesylate can only be obtained through designated specialty pharmacies and distributors. Clinicians may consult the Idhifa® website for specific ordering and availability information (https://idhifapro.com/).

■ **Administration** Enasidenib mesylate is administered orally without regard to meals. The drug should be taken at approximately the same time each day. The tablets should be swallowed whole with water; they should *not* be chewed, crushed, or split.

■ **Dosage** Dosage of enasidenib mesylate is expressed in terms of enasidenib.

Acute Myeloid Leukemia For the treatment of relapsed or refractory acute myeloid leukemia (AML) with IDH2 mutation, the recommended adult dosage of enasidenib is 100 mg once daily. Therapy should be continued until disease progression or unacceptable toxicity occurs. In the principal efficacy study, most patients achieved best response within 6 months of initiating enasidenib; therefore, the manufacturer states that therapy should be continued for at least 6 months to allow time for response.

In patients who present with leukocytosis (leukocyte counts exceeding 30,000/mm^3) in the absence of infection, hydroxyurea therapy should be initiated according to standard practices. If leukocytosis persists, temporary interruption of enasidenib therapy may be necessary. (See Leukocytosis under Dosage: Dosage Modification for Toxicity, in Dosage and Administration.)

Dosage Modification for Toxicity **Differentiation Syndrome.** If severe pulmonary symptoms requiring respiratory support (i.e., intubation, assisted respiration) occur and/or renal dysfunction persists for more than 48 hours despite systemic corticosteroid therapy, enasidenib should be withheld until the toxicity improves to grade 2 or less. (See Differentiation Syndrome under Warnings/Precautions: Warnings, in Cautions)

Leukocytosis. If leukocytosis persists despite hydroxyurea therapy, enasidenib therapy should be withheld until leukocyte counts decrease to less than 30,000/mm^3; therapy may then be resumed at the initial dosage (100 mg daily). (See Acute Myeloid Leukemia under Dosage and Administration: Dosage.)

Hepatotoxicity. In patients who exhibit increases in serum bilirubin concentrations exceeding 3 times the upper limit of normal (ULN) for 2 weeks or more (in the absence of elevated aminotransferase [ALT/AST] concentrations or other hepatic disorders), enasidenib therapy may be continued at a reduced dosage of 50 mg daily. When serum bilirubin concentrations improve to less than 2 times the ULN, the dosage of enasidenib should be re-escalated to 100 mg daily. (See Hepatic Effects under Warnings/Precautions: Other Warnings and Precautions, in Cautions.)

Tumor Lysis Syndrome. In patients who develop grade 3 or greater tumor lysis syndrome, therapy with enasidenib should be withheld. When tumor lysis syndrome improves to grade 2 or less, enasidenib may be resumed at a reduced dosage of 50 mg daily; the dosage of enasidenib may be re-escalated to 100 mg daily when tumor lysis syndrome improves to grade 1 or less.

If grade 3 or greater tumor lysis syndrome recurs, enasidenib therapy should be discontinued.

Other Toxicity. If a grade 3 or greater adverse reaction occurs, therapy with enasidenib should be withheld. When the toxicity improves to grade 2 or less, enasidenib may be resumed at a reduced dosage of 50 mg daily; the dosage of enasidenib may be re-escalated to 100 mg daily when the toxicity improves to grade 1 or less.

If the grade 3 or greater adverse reaction recurs, enasidenib therapy should be discontinued.

■ **Special Populations** No dosage adjustment is necessary in patients with mild hepatic impairment (total bilirubin concentration not exceeding the ULN with AST concentration exceeding the ULN *or* total bilirubin concentration 1–1.5 times the ULN with any AST concentration). (See Hepatic Impairment under Warnings/Precautions: Specific Populations, in Cautions.)

No dosage adjustment is necessary in patients with renal impairment. (See Renal Impairment under Warnings/Precautions: Specific Populations, in Cautions.)

No dosage adjustment is necessary in geriatric patients. (See Geriatric Use under Warnings/Precautions: Specific Populations, in Cautions.)

Cautions

■ **Contraindications** The manufacturer states that there are no known contraindications to the use of enasidenib.

■ **Warnings/Precautions** ***Warnings*** **Differentiation Syndrome.** Differentiation syndrome, which may be life-threatening or fatal, occurred in 14% of patients receiving enasidenib in the principal efficacy study; approximately one-half of these patients continued therapy without interruption. Differentiation syndrome following therapy with an isocitrate dehydrogenase-2 (IDH2) inhibitor, including enasidenib, is associated with rapid proliferation and differentiation of myeloid cells. Differentiation syndrome has been characterized by acute respiratory distress (dyspnea and/or hypoxia), hypoxia requiring supplemental oxygen, pulmonary infiltrates, renal or hepatic impairment, multiorgan dysfunction, pyrexia, lymphadenopathy, bone pain, peripheral edema, rapid weight gain, rash, and pleural or pericardial effusions in patients receiving enasidenib. Differentiation syndrome has been observed with or without concomitant leukocytosis as early as 10 days or up to 5 months after initiation of enasidenib.

The risk of developing differentiation syndrome associated with IDH2 inhibitor therapy is increased in patients with bone marrow blast counts exceeding 20% and those who have received fewer prior antileukemic therapies. High peripheral blast counts and high serum concentrations of LDH are less predictive of the development of differentiation syndrome associated with IDH2 inhibitor therapy than they are of the development of acute promyelocytic leukemia (APL) differentiation syndrome (also known as retinoic acid-APL [RA-APL] syndrome).

Manifestations of differentiation syndrome may be clinically indistinguishable from manifestations of disease progression or other acute comorbidities; therefore, differentiation syndrome should be suspected if there is no clear alternate etiology. If signs or symptoms suggestive of differentiation syndrome occur, IV or oral corticosteroid therapy (e.g., dexamethasone 10 mg every 12 hours) should be initiated and hemodynamic parameters should be monitored until symptoms improve. Because enasidenib has a long half-life (see Description), signs or symptoms of differentiation syndrome may recur if systemic corticosteroid therapy is discontinued prematurely; therefore, corticosteroid therapy should be continued until symptoms resolve followed by tapering of the corticosteroid dosage. If severe pulmonary symptoms requiring respiratory support (i.e., intubation, assisted respiration) occur and/or renal dysfunction persists for more than 48 hours despite corticosteroid therapy, enasidenib should be temporarily interrupted until symptoms improve. (See Differentiation Syndrome under Dosage: Dosage Modification for Toxicity, in Dosage and Administration.) The manufacturer recommends close monitoring in a hospital setting in patients with pulmonary and/or renal manifestations of differentiation syndrome.

Other Warnings and Precautions **Fetal/Neonatal Morbidity and Mortality.** Enasidenib may cause fetal harm in humans based on animal findings; the drug has been shown to be teratogenic, embryotoxic, and fetotoxic in animals. There are no available data regarding the risk of enasidenib use in pregnant women to date. In animal reproduction studies, postimplantation loss, increased rate of resorption, decreased fetal body weight, and skeletal anomalies were observed in rats receiving enasidenib at a maternally toxic dosage (exposure level equivalent to approximately 1.6 times the human exposure at the recommended human dosage). The drug also was abortifacient in rabbits receiving enasidenib at exposure levels below the human exposure at the recommended dosage.

Pregnancy should be avoided during enasidenib therapy. The manufacturer recommends confirmation of pregnancy status prior to initiation of enasidenib, and women of childbearing potential and men who are partners of such women should use adequate methods of contraception while receiving the drug and for at least 1 month after the drug is discontinued. (See Drug Interactions: Hormonal Contraceptives.) If enasidenib is used during pregnancy or if the patient or their partner becomes pregnant during therapy, the patient should be apprised of the potential fetal hazard.

Hepatic Effects. Enasidenib has been shown to increase serum bilirubin concentrations. Enasidenib may interfere with bilirubin metabolism by inhibiting uridine diphosphate-glucuronosyl transferase (UGT) 1A1. (See Drug Interactions.) In the principal efficacy study, 37% of patients had at least one elevated total bilirubin measurement (2 times the ULN or more). Elevated concentrations of total bilirubin occurred during the initial month of therapy in 35% of patients. Concomitant elevations in aminotransferases or other severe adverse reactions associated with hepatic disorders were not present in 89% of patients. Dosage reduction was not necessary in enasidenib-treated patients experiencing hyperbilirubinemia; however, the drug was permanently discontinued in 1.4% of patients or temporarily interrupted in 3.7% of patients for a median duration of 6 days. (See Hepatotoxicity under Dosage: Dosage Modification for Toxicity, in Dosage and Administration.)

Impairment of Fertility. Results of animal studies suggest that enasidenib may impair female and male fertility.

Fertility studies have not been conducted with enasidenib in animals. In a general toxicology study, decreased corpora lutea, uterine degeneration, and increased ovarian atretic follicles were observed in female animals and seminiferous tubular degeneration, seminal vesicle and prostate atrophy, and hypospermia were observed in male animals receiving enasidenib twice daily for up to 90 days.

Specific Populations **Pregnancy.** Enasidenib may cause fetal harm if administered to pregnant women based on animal findings. (See Fetal/Neonatal Morbidity and Mortality under Warnings/Precautions: Other Warnings and Precautions, in Cautions.)

Pregnancy status should be confirmed prior to initiation of enasidenib therapy.

Lactation. It is not known whether enasidenib or its metabolites are distributed into milk. Because of the potential for serious adverse reactions to enasidenib in nursing infants, women should be advised to discontinue nursing during enasidenib therapy. Women may begin nursing 1 month after discontinuance of therapy. The effects of the drug on nursing infants or on the production of milk are unknown.

Pediatric Use. Safety and efficacy of enasidenib have not been established in pediatric patients.

Geriatric Use. In the principal efficacy study, 61% of patients receiving enasidenib were 65 years of age or older and 24% were 75 years of age or older. No overall differences in safety and efficacy were observed between these geriatric patients and younger adults.

In a pharmacokinetic population analysis, age (range of 19–100 years) did not have a substantial effect on the pharmacokinetics of enasidenib.

Hepatic Impairment. In a population pharmacokinetic analysis, mild hepatic impairment (total bilirubin concentration not exceeding the upper limit of normal [ULN] with AST concentration exceeding the ULN or total bilirubin concentration 1–1.5 times the ULN with any AST concentration) did not have a substantial effect on the systemic exposure of enasidenib. However, since enasidenib is eliminated principally by hepatic metabolism, hepatic impairment may result in increased exposure to the drug and increased potential for adverse reactions. (See Dosage and Administration: Special Populations.)

Renal Impairment. Formal pharmacokinetic studies of enasidenib have not been conducted in patients with renal impairment; however, enasidenib undergoes minimal renal elimination.

In a population pharmacokinetic analysis, renal impairment (estimated glomerular filtration rate [GFR] of 30 mL/minute or more) did not have a substantial effect on the systemic exposure of enasidenib. (See Dosage and Administration: Special Populations.)

■ Common Adverse Effects

Adverse effects reported in at least 10% of patients receiving enasidenib for the treatment of relapsed or refractory acute myeloid leukemia (AML) in the principal efficacy study include nausea, diarrhea, decreased appetite, vomiting, differentiation syndrome, dysgeusia, noninfectious leukocytosis (may present as a rapid rise in leukocyte count), and tumor lysis syndrome. Laboratory abnormalities reported in at least 20% of enasidenib-treated patient include hyperbilirubinemia, hypocalcemia, hypokalemia, and hypophosphatemia.

Drug Interactions

Metabolism of enasidenib to the active AGI-16903 metabolite is mediated by cytochrome P-450 (CYP) isoenzymes 1A2, 2B6, 2C8, 2C9, 2C19, 2D6, and 3A4 and by uridine diphosphate-glucuronosyl transferases (UGT) 1A1, 1A3, 1A4, 1A9, 2B7, and 2B15. AGI-16903 is subsequently metabolized by CYP isoenzymes 1A2, 2C19, and 3A4 and by UGT1A1, 1A3, and 1A9.

In vitro, enasidenib inhibits CYP isoenzymes 1A2, 2B6, 2C8, 2C9, 2C19, 2D6, and 3A4; enasidenib also inhibits UGT1A1. In vitro, AGI-16903 inhibits CYP isoenzymes 1A2, 2B6, 2C8, 2C9, 2C19, and 2D6. In vitro studies show that enasidenib induces CYP isoenzymes 2B6 and 3A4.

In vitro studies indicate that enasidenib inhibits P-glycoprotein (P-gp), breast cancer resistance protein (BCRP), organic anion transporter (OAT) 1, organic anion transport protein (OATP) 1B1, OATP1B3, and organic cation transporter (OCT) 2, but does not inhibit multidrug resistance protein 2 (MRP2) or OAT3. In vitro, AGI-16903 inhibits BCRP, OAT1, OAT3, OATP1B1, and OCT2, but does not inhibit P-gp, MRP2, or OATP1B3. In vitro, AGI-16903 is a substrate of efflux transporters P-gp and BCRP; enasidenib is not a substrate of these transporters. Neither enasidenib nor AGI-16903 is a substrate of MRP2, OATP1B1, OATP1B3, OAT1, OAT3, or OCT2.

■ Hormonal Contraceptives

Concomitant use of enasidenib with combination hormonal contraceptives (e.g,. estrogen-progestin combination contraceptives) may result in increased or decreased plasma concentrations of the combination hormonal contraceptive. The clinical relevance of this drug interaction is unknown.

Description

Enasidenib, a potent and selective inhibitor of isocitrate dehydrogenase-2 (IDH2), is an antineoplastic agent. Isocitrate dehydrogenases (IDH) are metabolic enzymes in the citric acid cycle responsible for the oxidative decarboxylation of isocitrate to α-ketoglutarate, which is essential for normal cellular processes. Approximately 15–20% of acute myeloid leukemia (AML) cases carry IDH2 mutations. The most common IDH2 mutation is a point mutation at codon R140Q; a less frequently occurring IDH2 mutation is a point mutation at codon R172K. IDH2 mutations cause a reduction of α-ketoglutarate to the oncometabolite 2-hydroxyglutarate, which competitively inhibits α-ketoglutarate-dependent dioxygenases resulting in epigenetic dysregulation and subsequent histone and DNA hypermethylation and differentiation arrest of hematopoietic stem cells. In vitro studies indicate that enasidenib inhibits IDH2 with R140Q, R172S, or R172K mutation at approximately 40-fold lower concentrations than IDH2 wild-type enzymes. Enasidenib has demonstrated decreased 2-hydroxyglutarate levels and induction of myeloid cell differentiation in vitro and in mice bearing tumor xenografts that expressed IDH2 mutation. Enasidenib also has demonstrated decreased 2-hydroxyglutarate levels, reduced blast cell counts, and increased percentages of mature myeloid cells in patients with AML that expressed IDH2 mutation. In the phase 1/2 study evaluating enasidenib in patients with relapsed or refractory AML, mature granulocytes retained baseline IDH2 mutations and cytogenetic abnormalities in patients who achieved remission, indicating continued differentiation of abnormal myeloblast cells into mature granulocytes.

Following oral administration of enasidenib, the absolute bioavailability of the drug is 57%. Area under the serum concentration-time curve (AUC) of enasidenib is dose proportional over the enasidenib dosage range of 50–450 mg daily. Following oral administration of a single dose, median time to peak plasma concentrations of enasidenib is 4 hours. Repeated administration of enasidenib resulted in an approximately tenfold mean enasidenib accumulation ratio. Steady-state concentrations are reached within 29 days. Systemic exposure of enasidenib was increased by 50% when enasidenib was administered with a high-fat meal; however, this effect is not considered clinically important. (See Dosage and Administration: Administration.) Enasidenib is metabolized to the active AGI-16903 metabolite by cytochrome P-450 (CYP) isoenzymes 1A2, 2B6, 2C8, 2C9, 2C19, 2D6, and 3A4 and by uridine diphosphate-glucuronosyl transferases (UGT) 1A1, 1A3, 1A4, 1A9, 2B7, and 2B15. AGI-16903 is subsequently metabolized by CYP isoenzymes 1A2, 2C19, and 3A4 and by UGT1A1, 1A3, and 1A9. Enasidenib and AGI-16903 are highly bound (98.5 and 96.6%, respectively) to plasma proteins. The terminal half-life of enasidenib is 137 hours. Following administration of a radiolabeled dose of enasidenib, 89% of the radioactivity was recovered in feces (34% of the dose as unchanged drug) and 11% was recovered in urine (0.4% of the dose as unchanged drug).

The pharmacokinetics of enasidenib do not appear to be affected substantially by age (19–100 years), gender, race, body weight (39–136 kg), or body surface area.

Advice to Patients

Importance of advising patients to swallow enasidenib tablets whole with a full glass of water and *not* to chew, crush, or split the tablets.

Importance of advising patients to take enasidenib as directed by their clinician and at approximately the same time each day. If a dose is missed or vomited, importance of administering the missed dose on the same day as soon as it is remembered. Patients should be advised not to take 2 doses on the same day to make up for a missed dose.

Risk of developing differentiation syndrome. Importance of advising patients to immediately report possible symptoms of differentiation syndrome (e.g., pyrexia, cough, difficulty breathing, bone pain, rapid weight gain, peripheral edema) to their clinician.

Risk of tumor lysis syndrome. Importance of monitoring blood chemistry and maintaining adequate hydration during enasidenib therapy.

Risk of diarrhea, nausea, vomiting, decreased appetite, and taste changes. Importance of contacting clinician if any of these adverse reactions occur.

Risk of elevated serum bilirubin concentrations. Importance of contacting clinician if jaundice occurs.

Risk of fetal harm. Necessity of advising women of childbearing potential and men who are partners of such women that they should use adequate methods of contraception while receiving the drug and for at least 1 month after the drug is discontinued. Importance of informing patients of potential pharmacokinetic interaction between enasidenib and combination hormonal contraceptives. Importance of patients informing their clinicians if they or their partners are pregnant or think they may be pregnant. If pregnancy occurs, advise patient of potential risk to fetus.

Importance of advising women to discontinue nursing during therapy and for at least 1 month after discontinuance of the drug.

Importance of informing clinicians of existing or contemplated concomitant therapy, including prescription and OTC drugs (e.g,. combination hormonal contraceptives) and dietary or herbal supplements, as well as any concomitant illnesses.

Importance of informing patients of other important precautionary information. (See Cautions.)

Overview® (see Users Guide). For additional information on this drug until a more detailed monograph is developed and published, the manufacturer's labeling should be consulted. It is *essential* that the manufacturer's labeling be consulted for more detailed information on usual cautions, precautions, contraindications, potential drug interactions, laboratory test interferences, and acute toxicity. For further information on the handling of antineoplastic agents, see the ASHP Guidelines on Handling Hazardous Drugs at http://www.ahfsdruginformation.com.

Preparations

Enasidenib mesylate can only be obtained through select specialty distributors. (See Restricted Distribution under Dosage and Administration: General.)

Excipients in commercially available drug preparations may have clinically important effects in some individuals; consult specific product labeling for details.

Enasidenib Mesylate

Oral

Tablets, film-coated	50 mg (of enasidenib)	**Idhifa®**, Celgene
	100 mg (of enasidenib)	**Idhifa®**, Celgene

Encorafenib

■ Encorafenib, an inhibitor of b-Raf serine-threonine kinase (BRAF) V600E or V600K mutation, is an antineoplastic agent.

Uses

■ **Melanoma** Encorafenib is used in combination with binimetinib for the treatment of unresectable or metastatic melanoma with b-Raf serine-threonine kinase (BRAF) V600E or V600K mutation. Encorafenib has been designated an orphan drug by FDA for the treatment of this cancer. An FDA-approved diagnostic test (e.g., bioMerieux THxID® BRAF V600 mutation test) is required to confirm the presence of the BRAF V600E or V600K mutation prior to initiation of therapy. In patients with unresectable or metastatic melanoma with BRAF V600E or V600K mutation, combined therapy with encorafenib and binimetinib has been shown to prolong progression-free survival and overall survival, and increase response rate compared with vemurafenib alone.

The current indication for encorafenib is based principally on the results of a randomized, open-label, phase 3 study (COLUMBUS) in patients with unresectable locally advanced or metastatic melanoma positive for V600E or V600K BRAF mutation as detected by the bioMerieux THxID® BRAF V600 mutation test. In this study, 577 patients were randomized (stratified by disease stage, Eastern Cooperative Oncology Group [ECOG] performance status, and prior immunotherapy use) in a 1:1:1 ratio to receive encorafenib 450 mg once daily with binimetinib 45 mg twice daily (encorafenib-binimetinib), encorafenib 300 mg once daily alone, or vemurafenib 960 mg twice daily. Treatment was continued until disease progression or unacceptable toxicity occurred or the patient withdrew from the study. The primary measure of efficacy was progression-free survival (as evaluated by a blinded independent central review committee). The median age of patients randomized to the encorafenib-binimetinib or vemurafenib treatment groups was 56 years; 91% of patients were Caucasian, 59% were male, 95% had metastatic disease, 65% had stage M1c disease, 72% had a baseline ECOG performance status of 0, 28% had elevated LDH concentrations, 45% had tumor involvement in at least 3 organs, and 3% of patients had brain metastases. Approximately 4% of patients enrolled in the encorafenib-binimetinib or vemurafenib treatment groups received prior therapy with an anti-programmed-death 1 (anti-PD-1), anti-programmed-death ligand-1 (anti-PD-L1), or anti-cytotoxic T-lymphocyte-associated antigen 4 (anti-CTLA-4) antibody. Most patients (88%) randomized to receive encorafenib-binimetinib or vemurafenib had BRAF V600E mutation; 11% had V600K mutation and less than 1% had both BRAF V600E and V600K mutations. Patients who had received immunotherapy in the adjuvant setting or one prior immunotherapy regimen for unresectable locally advanced or metastatic melanoma were eligible for this study; however, patients with prior exposure to BRAF or mitogen-activated extracellular signal-regulated kinase (MEK) inhibitors were not eligible to enroll in the study.

At a median follow-up of 16.7 or 14.4 months in patients receiving encorafenib-binimetinib or vemurafenib alone, respectively, median progression-free survival was 14.9 months in patients receiving encorafenib-binimetinib compared with 7.3 months in those receiving vemurafenib. The objective response rate was 63% for patients receiving encorafenib-binimetinib and 40% for those receiving vemurafenib; complete response was achieved in 8% of patients receiving encorafenib-binimetinib and 6% of those receiving vemurafenib. The median duration of response in patients receiving encorafenib-binimetinib or vemurafenib alone was 16.6 or 12.3 months, respectively. At the time of the interim analysis for overall survival at a median follow-up of 36.8 months for the overall study population, the median overall survival was 33.6 or 16.9 months in patients receiving encorafenib-binimetinib or vemurafenib alone, respectively. Results of a subgroup analysis (based on age, gender, race, ECOG performance status, geographic region, baseline serum LDH concentration, BRAF mutation status, disease stage, organ involvement, presence of brain metastases, prior use of first-line immunotherapy or adjuvant therapy) suggested that the effect of encorafenib in combination with binimetinib was consistent across most subgroups; an overall survival benefit for combination therapy with encorafenib and binimetinib versus vemurafenib was not apparent in the small subgroup of patients with brain metastases (hazard ratio: 1.34).

The safety and efficacy of encorafenib in patients with wild-type BRAF melanoma have not been established; use of encorafenib is not indicated for use in these patients. (See Tumor Promotion in Wild-type BRAF Tumors under Cautions: Warnings/Precautions.)

Dosage and Administration

■ **General** Presence of the b-Raf serine-threonine kinase (BRAF) V600E or V600K mutation must be confirmed prior to initiation of therapy with encorafenib in combination with binimetinib. (See Uses: Melanoma.)

Clinicians should consult the manufacturer's labeling for information on the dosage and administration of binimetinib.

Restricted Distribution Program Encorafenib can only be obtained through select specialty pharmacies. Clinicians may contact the manufacturer (Array BioPharma) by telephone at 844-492-7729 or consult the Braftovi® and Mektovi® website for specific availability information (https://www.braftovimektovi.com/hcp/).

■ **Administration** Encorafenib is administered orally once daily without regard to meals. (See Description.)

If a dose of encorafenib is missed by more than 12 hours, the missed dose should be skipped and the next dose should be taken at the regularly scheduled time. Patients should *not* take extra capsules of the drug to make up for the missed dose.

If vomiting occurs following administration of encorafenib, a replacement dose should *not* be administered, and the next dose should be taken at the regularly scheduled time.

■ **Dosage** ***Melanoma*** For use in combination with binimetinib in the treatment of unresectable or metastatic melanoma with BRAF V600E or V600K mutation, the recommended adult dosage of encorafenib is 450 mg once daily. Therapy should be continued until disease progression or unacceptable toxicity occurs.

If binimetinib therapy is temporarily interrupted, the dosage of encorafenib should be reduced to a maximum dosage of 300 mg once daily until binimetinib therapy is resumed.

Dosage Modification for Toxicity If adverse reactions occur, interruption of therapy, dosage reduction, and/or permanent discontinuance of encorafenib may be required based on severity of the reaction. If dosage modification of encorafenib is necessary, an initial dosage reduction to 300 mg once daily is recommended. If further dosage reduction is necessary, the dosage should be reduced to 200 mg once daily. Dosages less than 200 mg once daily are not recommended; the drug should be permanently discontinued if the 200-mg once daily dosage is not tolerated.

If concomitant therapy with binimetinib is temporarily interrupted or permanently discontinued, therapy with encorafenib may be continued at a reduced dosage. (See Melanoma under Dosage and Administration: Dosage.)

No dosage adjustment of encorafenib is necessary in patients who experience interstitial lung disease, pneumonitis, cardiac dysfunction, increased creatine kinase (CK, creatine phosphokinase, CPK) concentrations, rhabdomyolysis, or venous thromboembolism during combination therapy with encorafenib and binimetinib.

For further information regarding dosage modification when encorafenib is used in combination with binimetinib, including information regarding binimetinib dosage modification for toxicity, see Dosage Modification for Toxicity under Dosage and Administration: Dosage, in Binimetinib 10:00.

Development of New Primary Malignancies. If new primary RAS mutation-positive, noncutaneous malignancies occur, encorafenib therapy should be permanently discontinued. (See Development of New Primary Malignancies under Cautions: Warnings/Precautions.)

No dosage adjustment of encorafenib is necessary in patients who develop new primary cutaneous malignancies during combination therapy with encorafenib and binimetinib.

Ocular Effects. If grade 1 or 2 uveitis unresponsive to ocular therapy occurs, encorafenib therapy should be withheld for up to 6 weeks. If the toxicity improves within 6 weeks of withholding therapy, therapy may be resumed at the same or reduced dosage. If the toxicity does not improve within 6 weeks of withholding therapy, encorafenib therapy should be permanently discontinued. (See Ocular Effects under Cautions: Warnings/Precautions.)

If grade 3 uveitis occurs, encorafenib therapy should be withheld for up to 6 weeks. If grade 3 uveitis improves within 6 weeks of withholding therapy, therapy may be resumed at the same or reduced dosage. If the toxicity does not improve within 6 weeks of withholding therapy, encorafenib therapy should be permanently discontinued.

If grade 4 uveitis occurs, encorafenib therapy should be permanently discontinued.

If adverse ocular reactions other than uveitis, iritis, or iridocyclitis occur during combination therapy with encorafenib and binimetinib, no dosage modification of encorafenib is necessary.

Prolongation of QT Interval. For the first occurrence of corrected QT (QT_c)-interval prolongation during which the QT_c interval exceeds 500 msec and increases by no more than 60 msec from baseline, encorafenib therapy should be withheld; therapy may be resumed at a reduced dosage of 300 mg once daily when the QT_c interval decreases to 500 msec or less. (See Prolongation of QT Interval under Cautions: Warnings/Precautions.)

For the second occurrence of QT_c-interval prolongation during which the QT_c interval exceeds 500 msec and increases by no more than 60 msec from baseline, encorafenib therapy should be withheld; therapy may be resumed at a reduced dosage of 200 mg once daily when the QT_c interval decreases to 500 msec or less.

For the third occurrence of QT_c-interval prolongation during which the QT_c interval exceeds 500 msec and increases by no more than 60 msec from baseline, encorafenib therapy should be permanently discontinued.

If the QT_c interval exceeds 500 msec and increases more than 60 msec from baseline, encorafenib therapy should be permanently discontinued.

Hepatotoxicity. In patients who develop grade 2 elevations of serum aminotransferases (ALT or AST), encorafenib therapy may be continued at the same dosage for up to 4 weeks. If the toxicity persists, encorafenib therapy should be withheld; therapy may be resumed at the same dosage when the toxicity improves to grade 1 or less or to baseline. If grade 2 elevations of ALT or AST concentrations recur, encorafenib therapy should be withheld for up to 4 weeks; therapy may be resumed at a reduced dosage when the toxicity improves to grade 1 or less or to baseline. If recurrent grade 2 elevations of ALT or AST concentrations do not improve within 4 weeks of withholding therapy, the drug should be permanently discontinued.

For the first occurrence of grade 3 elevations of serum ALT or AST, encorafenib therapy should be withheld for up to 4 weeks; therapy may be resumed at a reduced dosage when the toxicity improves to grade 1 or less or to baseline. If the toxicity does not improve to grade 1 or less or to baseline within 4 weeks of withholding therapy, the drug should be permanently discontinued. If recurrent grade 3 hepatic toxicity occurs, permanent discontinuance of encorafenib should be considered.

For the first occurrence of grade 4 elevations of serum ALT or AST, encorafenib therapy may be permanently discontinued or temporarily interrupted. If encorafenib therapy is temporarily interrupted, the drug should be withheld for up to 4 weeks; therapy may be resumed at a reduced dosage when the toxicity improves to grade 1 or less or to baseline. If the toxicity does not improve to grade 1 or less or to baseline within 4 weeks of withholding therapy, the drug should be permanently discontinued. If recurrent grade 4 hepatic toxicity occurs, the drug should be permanently discontinued.

Dermatologic Effects. If grade 2 dermatologic reactions occur, encorafenib therapy may be continued at the same dosage for up to 2 weeks. If the toxicity persists, encorafenib therapy should be withheld; therapy may be resumed at the same dosage when the toxicity improves to grade 1 or less

For the first occurrence of grade 3 dermatologic reactions, encorafenib therapy should be withheld; therapy may be resumed at the same dosage when the toxicity improves to grade 1 or less. If grade 3 dermatologic reactions recur, encorafenib therapy should be withheld; therapy may be resumed at a reduced dosage when the toxicity improves to grade 1 or less.

If grade 4 dermatologic reactions occur, encorafenib therapy should be permanently discontinued.

Other Toxicity. For recurrent grade 2 adverse reaction, encorafenib therapy should be withheld for up to 4 weeks; therapy may be resumed at a reduced dosage when the toxicity improves to grade 1 or less or to baseline. If the toxicity does not improve to grade 1 or less or to baseline within 4 weeks of withholding therapy, the drug should be permanently discontinued.

For the first occurrence of grade 3 adverse reaction, encorafenib therapy should be withheld for up to 4 weeks; therapy may be resumed at a reduced dosage when the toxicity improves to grade 1 or less or to baseline. If the toxicity does not improve to grade 1 or less or to baseline within 4 weeks of withholding therapy, the drug should be permanently discontinued. If grade 3 adverse reaction recurs, permanent discontinuance of encorafenib should be considered.

For the first occurrence of grade 4 adverse reaction, encorafenib therapy may be permanently discontinued or temporarily interrupted. If encorafenib therapy is temporarily interrupted, the drug should be withheld for up to 4 weeks; therapy may be resumed at a reduced dosage when the toxicity improves to grade 1 or less or to baseline. If the grade 4 adverse reaction does not improve to grade 1 or less or to baseline within 4 weeks of withholding therapy, the drug should be permanently discontinued. For recurrent grade 4 adverse reaction, encorafenib therapy should be permanently discontinued.

Concomitant Use with Drugs and Foods Affecting Hepatic Microsomal Enzymes Concomitant use of encorafenib with moderate or potent inhibitors of cytochrome P-450 (CYP) isoenzyme 3A4 should be avoided; however, if such concomitant use cannot be avoided, the manufacturer recommends reducing the dosage of encorafenib to one-third of the dose given prior to initiation of the *potent* CYP3A4 inhibitor (e.g., a dose of 450 mg reduced to 150 mg) or to one-half of the dose given prior to initiation of the *moderate* CYP3A4 inhibitor (e.g., a dose of 450 mg reduced to 225 mg). If concomitant use of the potent or moderate CYP3A4 inhibitor is discontinued, the encorafenib dosage should be returned (after 3–5 terminal half-lives of the CYP3A4 inhibitor) to the dosage used prior to initiation of the potent or moderate CYP3A4 inhibitor. (See Drug Interactions: Drugs and Foods Affecting Hepatic Microsomal Enzymes.)

■ **Special Populations** Dosage adjustment is not necessary in patients with mild hepatic impairment (Child-Pugh class A). Use of encorafenib in patients with moderate or severe (Child-Pugh class B or C) hepatic impairment has not been studied, and the manufacturer provides no specific dosage recommendations for such patients. (See Hepatic Impairment under Warnings/Precautions: Specific Populations, in Cautions.)

Dosage adjustment is not necessary in patients with mild or moderate renal impairment (creatinine clearance of 30 to less than 90 mL/minute). Use of encorafenib in patients with severe renal impairment (creatinine clearance of less than 30 mL/minute) has not been studied, and the manufacturer provides no specific dosage recommendations for such patients. (See Renal Impairment under Warnings/Precautions: Specific Populations, in Cautions.)

The manufacturer makes no specific dosage recommendations for geriatric patients. (See Geriatric Use under Warnings/Precautions: Specific Populations, in Cautions.)

Cautions

■ **Contraindications** The manufacturer states there are no known contraindications to the use of encorafenib.

■ **Warnings/Precautions** ***Combination Therapy*** When encorafenib is used in combination with binimetinib, the usual cautions, precautions, and contraindications associated with binimetinib must be considered in addition to those associated with encorafenib. For further information regarding warnings and precautions associated with binimetinib, see Cautions in Binimetinib 10:00.

Some adverse effects may occur less frequently during combination therapy with encorafenib and binimetinib compared to single-agent encorafenib. Grade 3 or 4 dermatologic reactions occurred in 21 or 2% of patients receiving single-agent encorafenib or combination therapy with encorafenib and binimetinib, respectively.

Development of New Primary Malignancies New primary cutaneous or noncutaneous malignancies have been reported in patients receiving b-Raf serine-threonine kinase (BRAF) inhibitors, including encorafenib.

In the COLUMBUS study, cutaneous squamous cell carcinoma (including keratoacanthoma) or basal cell carcinoma occurred in 8 or 1%, respectively, of patients receiving single-agent encorafenib compared with 2.6 or 1.6%, respectively, of those receiving encorafenib in combination with binimetinib. New primary melanoma also was reported in 5% of patients receiving single-agent encorafenib. The median time to first onset of cutaneous squamous cell carcinoma or keratoacanthoma in patients receiving encorafenib in combination with binimetinib was 5.8 months (range: 1–9 months).

In the COLUMBUS study, noncutaneous malignancy was reported in 3 of 192 patients (1.6%) receiving single-agent encorafenib compared with 2 of 192 of patients (1%) receiving combination therapy with encorafenib and binimetinib.

Although the mechanism for development of cutaneous squamous cell carcinoma has not been fully determined, it has been suggested that paradoxical activation of mitogen-activated protein kinase (MAPK) signaling may lead to accelerated growth of such skin lesions as well as development of other primary malignancies. MAPK-mediated events in wild-type BRAF cells have been observed in a study evaluating the pathology and immunohistochemistry of normal and proliferating skin lesions in patients receiving the weak b-Raf kinase inhibitor sorafenib. Another study performed a molecular analysis of DNA extracted from tumor specimens of patients receiving the BRAF inhibitor vemurafenib; results indicated that these patients have a secondary mutation (in addition to the BRAF V600E mutation) that appears to be activated by vemurafenib treatment. Some clinicians suggest that advanced age (i.e., 65 years of age or older), history of skin cancer, and chronic sun exposure may be risk factors for developing cutaneous squamous cell carcinoma. Some data suggest that mitogen-activated extracellular signal-regulated kinase (MEK) inhibitors (i.e., binimetinib, cobimetinib, trametinib) block the paradoxical activation of the MAPK pathway induced by BRAF inhibitors; therefore, combination therapy with a BRAF inhibitor and an MEK inhibitor may reduce the risk of developing cutaneous squamous cell carcinoma. Findings from a meta-analysis of randomized controlled studies that assessed the relative risk of development of cutaneous squamous cell carcinoma in cancer patients receiving a BRAF inhibitor indicate that the risk of cutaneous squamous cell carcinoma is higher in patients receiving a BRAF inhibitor than in patients receiving combination therapy with a BRAF inhibitor and an MEK inhibitor.

A dermatologic evaluation should be performed at baseline, every 2 months during therapy, and for up to 6 months following discontinuance of therapy. Suspicious cutaneous lesions should be treated as appropriate and excised for pathologic evaluation. Monitoring for signs and symptoms of new noncutaneous malignancies should be performed. If new primary RAS mutation-positive, noncutaneous malignancies occur, encorafenib therapy should be permanently discontinued. In patients who develop new primary cutaneous malignancies during combination therapy with encorafenib and binimetinib, the manufacturer states that no dosage adjustment of encorafenib is necessary.

Tumor Promotion in Wild-type BRAF Tumors In vitro, paradoxical activation of MAPK signaling and increased cell proliferation have been observed in wild-type BRAF cells exposed to BRAF inhibitors. Presence of BRAF V600E or V600K mutation must be confirmed prior to initiation of therapy. (See Uses: Melanoma)

Hemorrhage Hemorrhage has been reported in patients receiving combination therapy with encorafenib and binimetinib. In the COLUMBUS study, hemorrhage occurred in 19% of patients and was grade 3 or greater in 3.2% of patients receiving encorafenib in combination with binimetinib. The most common hemorrhagic events in patients receiving encorafenib in combination with binimetinib were GI hemorrhage, including rectal hemorrhage (4.2%), hematochezia (3.1%), and hemorrhoidal hemorrhage (1%). Intracranial hemorrhage was fatal in 1.6% of patients with new or progressive brain metastases receiving combination therapy with encorafenib and binimetinib.

If hemorrhagic events occur, therapy interruption followed by dosage reduction or discontinuance of encorafenib may be necessary. (See Other Toxicity under Dosage: Dosage Modification for Toxicity, in Dosage and Administration.)

Ocular Effects Uveitis, including iritis and iridocyclitis, have occurred in patients receiving encorafenib in combination with binimetinib. In the COLUMBUS study, uveitis occurred in 4% of patients receiving encorafenib in combination with binimetinib.

Ophthalmologic examinations should be performed regularly and as clinically indicated (i.e., if new or worsening visual disturbances occur; to follow new or persistent ophthalmologic findings) during encorafenib therapy. Patients should be monitored for visual symptoms at each visit. Temporary interruption, dosage reduction, or discontinuance of encorafenib may be necessary if ocular toxicities occur during therapy with the drug. (See Ocular Effects under Dosage: Dosage Modification for Toxicity, in Dosage and Administration.)

Prolongation of QT Interval Encorafenib is associated with dose-dependent prolongation of the QT interval. In the COLUMBUS study, a QT interval (corrected for heart rate using Fridericia's formula [QT_cF]) exceeding 500 msec was observed in 1 of 192 patients (0.5%) receiving encorafenib in combination with binimetinib. Analysis of central tendency showed a peak mean QT_cF interval change from baseline of 18 msec in adult patients with melanoma receiving encorafenib in combination with binimetinib.

Patients at an increased risk for QT_c-interval prolongation, including those with a history of long QT syndromes, clinically important bradyarrhythmias, or severe or uncontrolled heart failure, and those concurrently receiving other drugs known to prolong the QT interval should be monitored. Hypokalemia and hypomagnesemia should be corrected prior to administration of encorafenib and as clinically indicated during therapy. If prolongation of the QT interval occurs, therapy interruption followed by dosage reduction or discontinuance of encorafenib may be necessary. (See Prolongation of QT Interval under Dosage: Dosage Modification Toxicity, in Dosage and Administration.)

Fetal/Neonatal Morbidity and Mortality Encorafenib may cause fetal harm in humans based on its mechanism of action and animal findings; the drug has been shown to be embryotoxic, fetotoxic, and teratogenic in animals. There are no available data regarding the risk of encorafenib use in pregnant women to date. In animal reproduction studies, embryofetal toxicity (i.e., decreases in fetal body weight) and teratogenic effects (i.e., skeletal anomalies) have been demonstrated in pregnant rats receiving encorafenib at exposure levels equivalent to approximately 26 times the human exposure at the recommended human dosage. Postimplantation loss and abortion also were observed in rabbits receiving encorafenib at exposure levels of approximately 178 times the human exposure at the recommended human dosage. Although formal placental transfer studies have not been conducted, encorafenib has been detected in fetal plasma of rats and rabbits at concentrations up to 1.7 and 0.8%, respectively, of maternal plasma concentrations.

Pregnancy should be avoided during encorafenib therapy. The manufacturer states that pregnancy status should be verified prior to initiation of encorafenib therapy in women of childbearing potential and that such women should be advised to use an effective nonhormonal method of contraception while receiving encorafenib and for 2 weeks after the last dose. (See Drug Interactions: Hormonal Contraceptives.) Patients should be apprised of the potential hazard to the fetus if the drug is used during pregnancy.

Impairment of Fertility Results of animal studies suggest that encorafenib may reduce male fertility. The effect of the drug on fertility in humans is not known.

Specific Populations **Pregnancy.** Encorafenib may cause fetal harm if administered to pregnant women based on its mechanism of action and animal findings. (See Fetal/Neonatal Morbidity and Mortality under Cautions: Warnings/Precautions.)

Pregnancy status should be verified in women of childbearing potential prior to initiation of encorafenib therapy.

Lactation. It is not known whether encorafenib or its metabolites are distributed into human milk. Because of the potential for serious adverse reactions to encorafenib in breast-fed infants, women should be advised not to breast-feed while receiving the drug and for 2 weeks after the last dose. The effects of the drug on breast-fed infants or on the production of milk are unknown.

Pediatric Use. Safety and efficacy of encorafenib have not been established in pediatric patients.

Geriatric Use. In the clinical trials evaluating encorafenib (300–600 mg once daily) in combination with binimetinib (45 mg twice daily) in patients with BRAF mutation-positive melanoma, 20% of patients were 65–74 years of age and 8% were 75 years of age or older. No overall differences in safety or efficacy were observed between geriatric patients and younger adults.

Hepatic Impairment. In population pharmacokinetic analyses, systemic exposure of encorafenib was similar in patients with mild hepatic impairment (Child-Pugh class A) and those with normal hepatic function. (See Dosage and Administration: Special Populations.)

The pharmacokinetic profile of encorafenib has not been established in patients with moderate or severe hepatic impairment (Child-Pugh class B or C).

Renal Impairment. In population pharmacokinetic analyses, systemic exposure of encorafenib was similar in patients with mild or moderate renal impairment (creatinine clearance of 30–89 mL/minute) and those with normal renal function. (See Dosage and Administration: Special Populations.)

The pharmacokinetic profile of encorafenib has not been established in patients with severe renal impairment (creatinine clearance less than 30 mL/minute).

■ **Common Adverse Effects** Adverse effects reported in 20% or more of patients receiving encorafenib in combination with binimetinib for the treatment of unresectable or metastatic melanoma with BRAF V600E or V600K mutation include fatigue, nausea, diarrhea, vomiting, abdominal pain, constipation, arthralgia, hyperkeratosis, myopathy, headache, rash, asthenia, visual impairment, serous retinopathy/retinal pigment epithelial detachment (RPED), and pyrexia. Laboratory abnormalities reported in 20% or more of patients receiving encorafenib in combination with binimetinib include elevated concentrations of serum creatinine, elevated concentrations of creatine kinase (CK, creatine phosphokinase, CPK) elevated concentrations of γ-glutamyltransferase (γ-glutamyltranspeptidase, GGT, GGTP), anemia, elevated concentrations of aminotransferases (i.e., AST, ALT), and elevated concentrations of alkaline phosphatase.

Drug Interactions

Encorafenib is metabolized principally by cytochrome P-450 (CYP) isoenzyme 3A4 and, to a lesser extent, by CYP isoenzymes 2C19 and 2D6. In vitro studies also indicate that encorafenib is a reversible inhibitor of uridine diphosphate-glucuronosyltransferase (UGT) 1A1 and CYP isoenzymes 1A2, 2B6, 2C8, 2C9, 2D6, and 3A. The drug has demonstrated time-dependent inhibition of CYP3A4 at clinically relevant concentrations. In vitro, encorafenib induces CYP isoenzymes 2B6, 2C9, and 3A4 at clinically relevant concentrations.

Encorafenib is an inhibitor of P-glycoprotein (P-gp), breast cancer resistance protein (BCRP), organic cation transporter (OCT) 2, organic anion transporter (OAT) 1, OAT3, organic anion transporting polypeptide (OATP) 1B1, and OATP1B3, but does not inhibit OCT1 or multidrug resistance-associated protein (MRP) 2 at clinically relevant concentrations.

In vitro studies indicate that encorafenib is a substrate of P-gp, but is not a substrate for BCRP, MRP2, OATP1B1, OATP1B3, or OCT1 at clinically relevant concentrations.

■ **Drugs and Foods Affecting Hepatic Microsomal Enzymes**

Inhibitors of CYP3A4 Concomitant use of encorafenib with potent or moderate inhibitors of CYP3A4 may result in increased peak plasma concentrations and systemic exposure (area under the concentration-time curve [AUC]) of encorafenib and an increased incidence of adverse effects. When the potent CYP3A4 inhibitor posaconazole (400 mg twice daily) was administered concomitantly with encorafenib (single 50-mg dose), the peak plasma concentration and AUC of encorafenib were increased by 1.7- and 2.8-fold, respectively. When the moderate CYP3A4 inhibitor diltiazem hydrochloride (240 mg [as an extended-release formulation] on days 1 and 7) was administered concomitantly with encorafenib (single 50-mg dose), the peak plasma concentration and AUC of encorafenib were increased by 1.4- and 1.8-fold, respectively.

Concomitant use of encorafenib with potent (e.g., posaconazole) or moderate (e.g., diltiazem) inhibitors of CYP3A4 should be avoided. (See Drug Interactions: Grapefruit.) If concomitant use of a *potent* CYP3A4 inhibitor cannot be avoided, the manufacturer recommends dosage reduction of encorafenib to one-third of the dose given prior to initiation of the potent CYP3A4 inhibitor (e.g., a dose of 450 mg reduced to 150 mg). If concomitant use of a *moderate* CYP3A4 inhibitor cannot be avoided, the manufacturer recommends dosage reduction of encorafenib to one-half of the dose given prior to initiation of the moderate CYP3A4 inhibitor (e.g., a dose of 450 mg reduced to 225 mg). If concomitant use of the potent or moderate CYP3A4 inhibitor is discontinued, the encorafenib dosage should be returned (after 3–5 terminal half-lives of the CYP3A4 inhibitor) to the dosage used prior to initiation of the potent or moderate CYP3A4 inhibitor.

Inducers of CYP3A4 Concomitant use of encorafenib with potent or moderate inducers of CYP3A4 may result in decreased systemic exposure and reduced efficacy of encorafenib. There are data suggesting that encorafenib induces CYP3A4 resulting in autoinduction of its own metabolism. In a physiologically based pharmacokinetic model, systemic exposure of encorafenib was lower at steady state compared to systemic exposure following the initial dose. (See Description.)

Because formal drug interaction studies with potent or moderate CYP3A4 inducers have not been performed, the manufacturer states that concomitant use of encorafenib with potent or moderate inducers of CYP3A4 should be avoided.

■ **Drugs Metabolized by Hepatic Microsomal Enzymes** Concomitant administration of encorafenib with sensitive CYP3A4 substrates may result in an increased incidence of adverse effects or reduced efficacy of the substrate drug. (See Drug Interactions: Hormonal Contraceptives.)

■ **Drugs Metabolized by Uridine Diphosphate-glucuronosyltransferase** Concomitant administration of encorafenib with the UGT1A1 substrate binimetinib did not substantially alter systemic exposure of binimetinib.

■ **Drugs that Prolong the QT Interval** Because encorafenib has been associated with QT-interval prolongation, concomitant use of encorafenib with drugs known to prolong the QT interval should be avoided. (See Prolongation of QT Interval under Cautions: Warnings/Precautions.)

■ **Drugs Affecting Gastric Acidity** Concomitant administration of encorafenib (single 100-mg dose) with the proton-pump inhibitor rabeprazole (20 mg once daily for 5 days) resulted in no clinically important changes in peak plasma concentration or systemic exposure of encorafenib.

■ **Grapefruit** Concomitant use of encorafenib with grapefruit products (CYP3A4 inhibitor) may result in increased peak plasma concentrations and systemic exposure of encorafenib. Patients receiving encorafenib should be advised to avoid consuming grapefruit products.

■ **Hormonal Contraceptives** Concomitant use of encorafenib with hormonal contraceptives that are metabolized by CYP3A4 may result in decreased systemic exposure to the substrate drug and reduced contraceptive efficacy. Concomitant use of encorafenib with hormonal contraceptives should be avoided. (See Fetal/Neonatal Morbidity and Mortality under Cautions: Warnings/Precautions.)

Description

Encorafenib, an inhibitor of b-Raf serine-threonine kinase (BRAF) with V600E or V600K mutation, is an antineoplastic agent. Approximately 40–60% of cutaneous melanomas carry a BRAF mutation. The most common BRAF mutation is the substitution of glutamic acid for valine at codon 600 in exon 15 (BRAF V600E); a less frequently occurring BRAF mutation is the substitution of lysine for valine at codon 600 in exon 15 (BRAF V600K). The mutation of BRAF V600E activates the mitogen-activated protein kinase (MAPK) and extracellular signal-regulated kinase (ERK) signal transduction pathway, which enhances cell proliferation and tumor progression (e.g., metastasis). Encorafenib induced tumor regression associated with inhibition of the MAPK/ERK signal transduction pathway in xenograft models of tumor cells with BRAF V600E mutation in mice. In vitro studies have demonstrated that encorafenib inhibited tumor growth of cell lines testing positive for BRAF with V600E, V600D, or V600K mutation. Encorafenib also inhibits wild-type b-Raf and other kinases such as c-Raf, JNK1, JNK2, JNK3, LIMK1, LIMK2, MEK4, and STK36 and substantially reduces ligand binding to these kinases at clinically relevant concentrations.

Clinical resistance to monotherapy with a BRAF inhibitor, generally occurring 6–7 months following initiation of therapy, has been attributed to several possible resistance mechanisms mostly relying on reactivation of the MAPK/ERK pathway. Complete inhibition of the MAPK/ERK pathway resulting in durable responses may be achieved with the use of combination therapy with a BRAF inhibitor (i.e., dabrafenib, encorafenib, vemurafenib) and an MEK inhibitor (i.e., binimetinib, cobimetinib, trametinib). In vitro, use of encorafenib in combination with binimetinib resulted in increased antiproliferative activity compared with either drug alone in BRAF mutation-positive cell lines. The combination of encorafenib and binimetinib also has demonstrated increased inhibition of tumor growth and delayed emergence of resistance compared with either drug alone in xenograft models of melanoma harboring BRAF V600E mutations in mice.

Following oral administration of encorafenib, at least 86% of the dose is rapidly absorbed with peak plasma concentrations occurring in 2 hours. Systemic exposure of encorafenib is proportional to dose following single administration of the drug over the dosage range of 50–700 mg, but less than proportional to dose following repeated administration of the drug over the dosage range of 50–800 mg once daily. Steady-state concentrations are achieved within 15 days. In a physiologically based pharmacokinetic model, systemic exposure of encorafenib at steady state was 50% lower compared to the systemic exposure following the initial dose, suggesting that encorafenib causes autoinduction of its own metabolism; however, intersubject variability ranged from 12–69%. Administration of a single 100-mg dose of encorafenib with a high-fat, high-calorie meal (approximately 150 calories from protein, 350 calories from carbohydrates, 500 calories from fat) decreased mean peak plasma concentrations of the drug by 36%, but did not affect the extent of absorption (area under the concentration-time curve [AUC]). (See Dosage and Administration: Administration.) Encorafenib is 86% bound to plasma proteins. Encorafenib is metabolized principally by cytochrome P-450 (CYP) isoenzyme 3A4 and, to a lesser extent, by CYP2C19 and CYP2D6. The mean terminal half-life of encorafenib is 3.5 hours. Following oral administration of a radiolabeled dose of encorafenib, 47% of the dose is recovered in feces (5% of the dose as unchanged drug) and 47% is recovered in urine (2% of the dose as unchanged drug).

The pharmacokinetics of encorafenib do not appear to be affected substantially by age (19–89 years), gender, or body weight.

Advice to Patients

Importance of reading the manufacturer's patient information.

If a dose of encorafenib is missed by more than 12 hours or vomited, importance of administering the next dose at the regularly scheduled time; an additional dose should not be administered to replace the missed or vomited dose.

Risk of new primary cutaneous malignancies. Importance of contacting a clinician promptly if dermatologic changes (e.g., new wart, skin sore or reddish bump that bleeds or does not heal, mole that changes in size or color).

Risk of hemorrhage. Importance of contacting a clinician promptly and seeking immediate medical attention if signs and/or symptoms of unusual bleeding (e.g., headache, dizziness, weakness, blood in stool, coughing up blood, vomiting blood) occur.

Risk of QT-interval prolongation. Importance of contacting a clinician promptly if syncope, abnormal heartbeat, or feelings of dizziness or faintness occur.

Risk of uveitis. Importance of contacting a clinician promptly if ocular pain, swelling, redness, changes in vision, or blurred vision occurs.

Risk of fetal harm. Necessity of advising women of childbearing potential that they should use an effective nonhormonal method of contraception while receiving the drug and for 2 weeks after the last dose. Importance of women informing clinicians if they are or plan to become pregnant. Apprise patient of potential fetal hazard if used during pregnancy. (See Fetal/Neonatal Morbidity and Mortality under Cautions: Warnings/Precautions.)

Importance of advising women to avoid breast-feeding while receiving encorafenib and for 2 weeks after the last dose.

Importance of advising men of reproductive potential that encorafenib may reduce male fertility.

Importance of informing clinicians of existing or contemplated concomitant therapy, including prescription and OTC drugs and herbal supplements, as well as any concomitant illnesses.

Importance of informing patients of other important precautionary information. (See Cautions.)

Overview® (see Users Guide). For additional information on this drug until a more detailed monograph is developed and published, the manufacturer's labeling should be consulted. It is *essential* that the manufacturer's labeling be consulted for more detailed information on usual cautions, precautions, contraindications, potential drug interactions, laboratory test interferences, and acute toxicity. For further information on the handling of antineoplastic agents, see the ASHP Guidelines on Handling Hazardous Drugs at http://www.ahfsdruginformation.com.

Preparations

Distribution of encorafenib is restricted. (See Restricted Distribution Program under Dosage and Administration: General.)

Excipients in commercially available drug preparations may have clinically important effects in some individuals; consult specific product labeling for details.

Encorafenib

Oral		
Capsules	50 mg	Braftovi®, Array BioPharma
	75 mg	Braftovi®, Array BioPharma

Enzalutamide

■ Enzalutamide, a nonsteroidal antiandrogen, is an antineoplastic agent.

Uses

■ **Prostate Cancer** Enzalutamide is used for the treatment of castration-resistant prostate cancer.

The current indication for enzalutamide for the treatment of castration-resistant prostate cancer is based principally on the results of 3 randomized, double-blind, placebo-controlled phase 3 studies (AFFIRM, PREVAIL, and PROSPER) and results of a multicenter, double-blind, randomized phase 2 study (TERRAIN).

In the AFFIRM study, 1199 patients with metastatic castration-resistant prostate cancer that had progressed following treatment with 1 or 2 cytotoxic regimens, at least one of which had to contain docetaxel, were randomized in a 2:1 ratio to receive either enzalutamide (160 mg once daily) or placebo; androgen deprivation therapy was continued in all patients. Treatment was continued until disease progression or unacceptable toxicity occurred, new treatment was initiated, or the patient withdrew from the study. Continuation or initiation of glucocorticoid therapy was permitted but not required; 48 or 46% of patients receiving enzalutamide or placebo, respectively, received glucocorticoids. The primary measure of efficacy was overall survival. The median age of patients enrolled in the study was 69 years; 93% of the patients were Caucasian, 91% had bone metastases, 59% had disease progression based on radiographic evidence, 41% had prostate specific antigen (PSA)-only progression, 24% had received 2 prior cytotoxic regimens, and 23% had visceral (lung and/or liver) involvement. The majority (92%) of patients had an Eastern Cooperative Oncology Group (ECOG) performance status of 0 or 1, and 28% of patients had a mean Brief Pain Inventory score of 4 or greater.

In the AFFIRM study, a planned interim analysis after a specified number of deaths occurred indicated that patients receiving enzalutamide had a longer median overall survival (18.4 versus 13.6 months) than those receiving placebo. The median follow-up at the time of the interim analysis was 14.4 months, and the median duration of treatment was 8.3 months for patients receiving enzalutamide and 3 months for those receiving placebo. Because of the survival benefit observed at the interim analysis, study investigators permitted patients previously randomized to receive placebo to cross over to open-label enzalutamide therapy. At the interim analysis, patients receiving enzalutamide also had higher PSA response rates (54 versus 2%), higher soft tissue response rates (29 versus 4%), higher quality-of-life response rates (43 versus 18%), longer median time to PSA progression (8.3 versus 3 months), longer median progression-free survival based on radiographic evidence (8.3 versus 2.9 months), and longer median time to the first skeletal-related event (16.7 versus 13.3 months) compared with those receiving placebo.

In the PREVAIL study, 1717 patients with chemotherapy-naive metastatic castration-resistant prostate cancer were randomized in a 1:1 ratio to receive either enzalutamide (160 mg once daily) or placebo; androgen deprivation therapy was continued in all patients. Treatment was continued until disease progression or unacceptable toxicity occurred, new treatment was initiated, or the patient withdrew from the study. Continuation or initiation of glucocorticoid therapy was permitted but not required; 27 or 30% of patients receiving enzalutamide or placebo, respectively, received glucocorticoids. The primary measures of efficacy were overall survival and progression-free survival based on radiographic evidence (as evaluated by a central review committee according to Prostate Cancer Clinical Trials Working Group [PCCTWG] criteria for bone lesions and/or Response Evaluation Criteria in Solid Tumors [RECIST] for soft tissue lesions). The median age of patients enrolled in the study was 71 years; 77% of patients were Caucasian, 54% had radiographic evidence of disease progression, 43% had PSA-only progression, and 12% had visceral (lung and/or liver) involvement. Baseline pain assessment indicated the presence of mild or no pain in 32 or 67%, respectively, of patients enrolled in the study. All patients enrolled in the study had an ECOG performance status of 0 or 1.

At a median follow-up of approximately 22 months in the PREVAIL study, patients receiving enzalutamide had longer median overall survival (32.4 versus 30.2 months) and progression-free survival based on radiographic evidence (20 versus 5.4 months) than those receiving placebo. Overall survival for enzalutamide-treated patients at the time of updated analysis (at a median follow-up of 31 months) remained similar to the interim results. At the time of the updated analysis, 52% of enzalutamide-treated patients and 81% of placebo recipients had received subsequent antineoplastic therapy associated with overall survival benefit; 29% of patients randomized to receive placebo crossed over to receive enzalutamide therapy. Results of a subgroup analysis (based on age, geographic region, ECOG performance status, Gleason score, PSA-only progression, disease progression based on radiographic evidence, visceral involvement, baseline PSA concentration, baseline LDH concentration, baseline hemoglobin concentration) suggested that the drug's effect on overall survival was consistent across all subgroups. Patients receiving enzalutamide also had longer median time to initiation of antineoplastic chemotherapy and first skeletal-related event (i.e., radiation therapy or surgery for prostate cancer-related bone metastases, pathologic bone fracture, spinal cord compression, subsequent antineoplastic therapy for the treatment of prostate cancer-related bone pain) compared with those receiving placebo.

In the TERRAIN study, 375 patients with chemotherapy-naive metastatic castration-resistant prostate cancer were randomized in a 1:1 ratio to receive either enzalutamide (160 mg once daily) or bicalutamide (50 mg once daily); androgen deprivation therapy was continued in all patients. Treatment was continued until disease progression or unacceptable toxicity occurred, new treatment was initiated, or the patient withdrew from the study. The primary measure of efficacy was progression-free survival based on radiographic evidence (as evaluated by an independent central review committee according to PCCTWG criteria and/or RECIST for soft tissue lesions). The median age of patients enrolled in the study was 71 years; 93% of patients were Caucasian, 98% had radiographic evidence of disease progression, and 46% had received prior therapy with bicalutamide. Baseline pain assessment indicated the presence of mild or no pain in 36 or 58%, respectively, of patients enrolled in the study. All patients enrolled in the study were enzalutamide-naive and had an ECOG performance status of 0 or 1. Patients were excluded from the study if disease progression occurred during prior treatment with an antiandrogen (e.g., bicalutamide). Patients receiving enzalutamide had longer median progression-free survival based on radiographic evidence than those receiving bicalutamide (19.5 versus 13.4 months).

In the PROSPER study, 1401 patients with nonmetastatic castration-resistant prostate cancer were randomized (stratified by PSA doubling time and use of bone resorption inhibitors) in a 2:1 ratio to receive either enzalutamide (160 mg once daily) or placebo; androgen deprivation therapy was continued in all patients. Treatment was continued until disease progression or unacceptable toxicity occurred, new treatment was initiated, or the patient withdrew from the study. The primary measure of efficacy was metastasis-free survival. Patients were enrolled in the study if they had a PSA doubling time of 10 months or less and serum PSA concentration of 2 ng/mL or greater. The median age of patients enrolled in the study was 74 years; 77% had a Gleason score of 7 or higher, 71% were Caucasian, and 54% had undergone prior surgery or radiation therapy of the prostate. The majority (63%) of patients had received therapy with an antiandrogen; 56 or 11% had received bicalutamide or flutamide, respectively. All patients enrolled in the study had an ECOG performance status of 0 or 1.

At a median follow-up of 18.5 or 15.1 months in patients receiving enzalutamide or placebo, respectively, in the PROSPER study, patients receiving enzalutamide had longer median metastasis-free survival than those receiving placebo (36.6 versus 14.7 months). Overall survival had not been reached at the time of analysis. Results of a subgroup analysis (based on PSA doubling time and previous therapy with a bone resorption inhibitor) suggested that the drug's effect on metastasis-free survival was consistent across all subgroups. Patients receiving enzalutamide also had longer median time to initiation of antineoplastic chemotherapy (39.6 versus 17.7 months) and longer median time to PSA progression (37.2 versus 3.9 months) compared with those receiving placebo.

Dosage and Administration

■ **General** Patients receiving enzalutamide should receive concurrent therapy with a gonadotropin-releasing hormone (GnRH) analog unless they have undergone bilateral orchiectomy.

Restricted Distribution Enzalutamide can only be obtained through designated specialty pharmacies. Clinicians may contact the manufacturer (Astellas) at 855-898-2634 or consult the Xtandi® website for specific ordering and availability information (https://www.xtandi.com).

■ **Administration** Enzalutamide is administered orally without regard to meals. The capsules should be swallowed whole and should *not* be chewed, dissolved, or opened.

■ **Dosage** ***Prostate Cancer*** For the treatment of castration-resistant prostate cancer, the recommended dosage of enzalutamide is 160 mg once daily.

Dosage Modification **General Toxicity.** If an intolerable adverse effect or grade 3 or greater toxicity occurs, enzalutamide therapy should be interrupted for one week or until symptoms improve to grade 2 or less. Enzalutamide therapy may then be resumed with or without a dosage reduction. If a dosage reduction is necessary, the dosage of enzalutamide should be reduced to 120 or 80 mg daily.

Concomitant Use with Drugs Affecting or Metabolized by Hepatic Microsomal Enzymes. Concomitant use with drugs that affect or are metabolized by certain hepatic microsomal enzymes may alter systemic exposure to enzalutamide or the concomitantly administered drug. For specific recommendations regarding concomitant use of such drugs (including any recommendations for dosage adjustment when concomitant use cannot be avoided), see Drug Interactions.

■ **Special Populations** Initial dosage adjustment is not necessary in patients with mild, moderate, or severe hepatic impairment (Child-Pugh class A, B, or C). (See Hepatic Impairment under Warnings/Precautions: Specific Populations, in Cautions.)

Initial dosage adjustment is not necessary in patients with mild or moderate renal impairment (creatinine clearance 30–89 mL/minute). (See Renal Impairment under Warnings/Precautions: Specific Populations, in Cautions.)

Cautions

■ **Contraindications** The manufacturer states that there are no known contraindications to the use of enzalutamide.

■ **Warnings/Precautions** ***Sensitivity Reactions*** Hypersensitivity reactions, including angioedema, have occurred in patients receiving enzalutamide. In clinical trials, edema of the face, tongue, or lip was reported in 0.5, 0.1, or 0.1%, respectively, of patients receiving enzalutamide. Pharyngeal edema also has been reported during postmarketing experience.

Enzalutamide should be permanently discontinued in patients who develop a serious hypersensitivity reaction during treatment.

Seizures Seizures have occurred in patients receiving enzalutamide. In clinical trials, seizure was reported in 0.4% of patients receiving enzalutamide; seizures resolved following permanent discontinuance of the drug. Time to onset of seizures ranged from 13–604 days following initiation of enzalutamide therapy.

Patients with predisposing factors for seizures generally were excluded from clinical trials. However, in a trial designed to assess the risk of seizures in such patients, seizure was reported in 8 of 366 enzalutamide-treated patients (2.2%) with predisposing factors for seizures (i.e., concomitant use of drugs that lower seizure threshold; history of cerebrovascular accident, transient ischemic attack, head trauma, seizure, cerebral arteriovenous malformation, or CNS infection; Alzheimer's disease; meningioma; prostate cancer with leptomeningeal involvement; unexplained loss of consciousness within the past 12 months; presence of space-occupying brain lesion). Enzalutamide therapy was resumed in all patients experiencing seizure; seizure recurred in 3 patients following resumption of the drug. Approximately 17% of patients had more than one risk factor for developing seizure. It is not known whether anticonvulsants will prevent seizures in patients receiving enzalutamide.

Enzalutamide should be permanently discontinued in patients who develop a seizure during treatment.

Reversible Posterior Leukoencephalopathy Syndrome Reversible posterior leukoencephalopathy syndrome (RPLS) has occurred in patients receiving enzalutamide. RPLS is a neurologic disorder that may manifest with seizure, headache, lethargy, confusion, blindness, or other visual and neurologic disturbances. Hypertension may occur, but it is not necessary for the diagnosis of RPLS. Brain imaging, preferably magnetic resonance imaging (MRI), is used to confirm the diagnosis. Enzalutamide therapy should be discontinued in patients who develop RPLS.

Cardiovascular Effects Ischemic heart disease, sometimes fatal, has occurred in patients receiving enzalutamide. In the AFFIRM, PREVAIL, and PROSPER studies in patients with castration-resistant prostate cancer, ischemic heart disease was reported in 2.7% of patients receiving enzalutamide compared with 1.2% of those receiving placebo; grade 3 or 4 ischemic events occurred in 1.2% of patients receiving the drug compared with 0.5% of those receiving placebo. Fatal ischemic events occurred in 0.4% of patients receiving enzalutamide and 0.1% of those receiving placebo.

Patients receiving enzalutamide therapy should be monitored for signs or symptoms of ischemic heart disease, and management of preexisting cardiovascular risk factors (e.g., hypertension, diabetes mellitus, dyslipidemia) should be optimized. Enzalutamide therapy should be discontinued in patients who develop grade 3 or 4 ischemic heart disease.

In the AFFIRM, PREVAIL, and PROSPER studies, an increased incidence of hypertension was observed during therapy with enzalutamide compared with placebo. In the AFFIRM and PREVAIL studies, less than 1% of both enzalutamide- and placebo-treated patients withdrew from the study because of hypertension.

Falls and Fractures Falls and fractures have occurred in patients receiving enzalutamide. In the AFFIRM, PREVAIL, and PROSPER studies in patients with castration-resistant prostate cancer, falls were reported in 10% of patients receiving enzalutamide compared with 4% of those receiving placebo and were not associated with loss of consciousness or seizure. Fractures were reported in 8% of patients receiving enzalutamide compared with 3% of those receiving placebo; grade 3 or 4 fractures occurred in 2% of patients receiving the drug compared with less than 1% of those receiving placebo. The median time to occurrence of fracture was 337 days (range: 2–996 days) in patients receiving enzalutamide. Routine bone density assessments were not performed during these studies. In addition, bone-targeting agents for the prevention of bone loss in the setting of osteoporosis were not administered.

Patients receiving enzalutamide should be evaluated for fracture and fall risk. Patients at risk for fractures should be monitored and managed according to established treatment guidelines; therapy with bone-targeting agents should be considered.

Fetal/Neonatal Morbidity and Mortality Enzalutamide may cause fetal harm in humans based on its mechanism of action and animal findings; the drug has been shown to be teratogenic, embryotoxic, and fetotoxic in animals. Safety and efficacy of enzalutamide have not been established in females. Reproduction studies in mice revealed post-implantation loss and resorption, decreased anogenital distance, cleft palate, and absent palatine bone at dosages below the maximum recommended human dosage. However, there was no evidence of developmental toxicity in rabbits at exposure levels approximately 0.4 times the human exposure. If used during pregnancy or if the patient becomes pregnant while receiving enzalutamide, the patient should be apprised of the potential hazard to the fetus and the potential risk for loss of the pregnancy.

Women who are or may be pregnant should *not* handle enzalutamide capsules.

Because it is not known whether enzalutamide or its metabolites distribute into semen, men receiving the drug should use a condom during sexual encounters with pregnant women and should use a condom in conjunction with another effective contraceptive method during sexual encounters with women of childbearing potential. These contraceptive measures are required during enzalutamide therapy and for 3 months after the last dose of the drug.

Impairment of Fertility Results of animal studies suggest that enzalutamide may impair male fertility. In repeat-dose toxicity studies, hypospermatogenesis and atrophy of seminal vesicles, prostate, and epididymis were observed in male rats and dogs.

Specific Populations **Pregnancy.** Based on its mechanism of action and animal findings, enzalutamide can cause fetal harm and potential loss of pregnancy if administered to pregnant women. (See Fetal/Neonatal Morbidity and Mortality under Cautions: Warnings/Precautions.)

Women who are or may become pregnant should *not* handle enzalutamide capsules.

Lactation. Enzalutamide and/or its metabolites are distributed into milk in rats; peak concentrations in milk (achieved 4 hours following oral administration of the drug) are 4 times higher than plasma concentrations. It is not known whether the drug distributes into human milk or if the drug has any effect on milk production or on the nursing infant.

Pediatric Use. Safety and efficacy of enzalutamide have not been established in pediatric patients.

Geriatric Use. In clinical trials evaluating enzalutamide in men with castration-resistant prostate cancer, 79% of patients were 65 years of age or older and 36% were 75 years of age or older. No overall differences in safety and efficacy were observed between geriatric patients and younger adults. However, the possibility of increased sensitivity to the drug in some geriatric patients cannot be ruled out.

Hepatic Impairment. Following a single 160-mg dose of enzalutamide, systemic exposure to the major active forms of the drug (i.e., enzalutamide plus *N*-desmethylenzalutamide) in individuals with mild, moderate, or severe hepatic impairment (Child-Pugh class A, B, or C) was similar to that in individuals with normal hepatic function. (See Dosage and Administration: Special Populations.)

Renal Impairment. The effect of renal impairment on the pharmacokinetic disposition of enzalutamide has not been specifically studied to date. In a population pharmacokinetic analysis, clearance of enzalutamide in patients with mild to moderate renal impairment (creatinine clearance 30–89 mL/minute) was similar to that in individuals with normal renal function. Enzalutamide has not been evaluated systematically in patients with severe renal impairment (creatinine clearance less than 30 mL/minute) or end-stage renal disease. (See Dosage and Administration: Special Populations.)

■ **Common Adverse Effects** Adverse effects reported in 10% or more of patients receiving enzalutamide for the treatment of castration-resistant prostate cancer and at an incidence that is at least 2% higher than that reported with placebo in the AFFIRM, PREVAIL, and PROSPER studies include asthenia/fatigue, decreased appetite, hot flush, arthralgia, dizziness/vertigo, hypertension, headache, and decreased weight. Laboratory abnormalities reported in 5% or more of patients receiving enzalutamide for the treatment of castration-resistant prostate cancer and at an incidence that is at least 2% higher than that reported with placebo include hyperglycemia, hypermagnesemia, hyponatremia, and neutropenia.

Adverse effects reported in 10% or more of patients receiving enzalutamide for the treatment of castration-resistant prostate cancer and at an incidence that is at least 2% higher than that reported with bicalutamide in the TERRAIN study include asthenia/fatigue, musculoskeletal pain, hot flush, hypertension, diarrhea, upper respiratory tract infection, and decreased weight.

Drug Interactions

In vivo studies indicate that enzalutamide is a potent inducer of cytochrome P-450 (CYP) isoenzyme 3A4 and a moderate inducer of CYP isoenzymes 2C9 and 2C19; enzalutamide does not induce CYP1A2 at clinically relevant concentrations. Enzalutamide also induces CYP2B6 in vitro. In vitro studies show that enzalutamide and its 2 major metabolites (an active *N*-desmethyl metabolite and an inactive carboxylic acid metabolite) are inhibitors of CYP isoenzymes 2B6, 2C8, 2C9, 2C19, 2D6, and 3A4/5; enzalutamide also causes time-dependent inhibition of CYP1A2 in vitro. In vitro, *N*-desmethylenzalutamide is not a substrate of CYP isoenzymes 1A1, 1A2, 2A6, 2B6, 2C8, 2C9, 2C18, 2C19, 2D6, 2E1, or 3A4/5. In vitro studies indicate that neither enzalutamide nor its 2 major metabolites are substrates of P-glycoprotein (P-gp); however, both enzalutamide and *N*-desmethylenzalutamide are inhibitors of P-gp. Enzalutamide is metabolized by CYP isoenzymes 2C8 and 3A4; formation of the active *N*-desmethyl metabolite is mediated principally by CYP2C8.

■ **Drugs Affecting Hepatic Microsomal Enzymes** ***Potent Inhibitors of CYP2C8*** Concomitant use of enzalutamide with potent inhibitors of CYP2C8 may result in increased systemic exposure to enzalutamide and its active *N*-desmethyl metabolite. When the potent CYP2C8 inhibitor gemfibrozil (600 mg twice daily) was administered concomitantly with enzalutamide (single 160-mg dose) in healthy individuals, systemic exposure to the major active forms of the antiandrogen (i.e., enzalutamide plus *N*-desmethylenzalutamide) was increased by approximately 2.2-fold; however, peak plasma concentrations of these active forms of the drug were not substantially affected. Concomitant use of enzalutamide with potent CYP2C8 inhibitors should be avoided if possible. If concomitant use cannot be avoided, the dosage of enzalutamide should be reduced to 80 mg once daily. If concomitant use of the potent CYP2C8 inhibitor is discontinued, the enzalutamide dosage should be returned to the dosage used prior to initiation of the potent CYP2C8 inhibitor.

Potent Inhibitors of CYP3A4 When the potent CYP3A4 inhibitor itraconazole (200 mg once daily) was administered concomitantly with enzalutamide (single 160-mg dose) in healthy individuals, systemic exposure to the major active forms of the antiandrogen (i.e., enzalutamide plus *N*-desmethylenzalutamide) was increased by approximately 1.3-fold; peak plasma concentrations of these active forms of the drug were not affected. Initial dosage adjustment is not necessary.

Inducers of CYP3A4 Concomitant use of enzalutamide with potent inducers of CYP3A4 (e.g., carbamazepine, phenobarbital, phenytoin, rifabutin, rifampin, rifapentine) may result in decreased systemic exposure to enzalutamide. When the combined potent CYP3A4 and moderate CYP2C8 inducer rifampin (600 mg once daily) was administered concomitantly with enzalutamide (single 160-mg dose) in healthy individuals, systemic exposure to the major active forms of the antiandrogen (i.e., enzalutamide plus *N*-desmethylenzalutamide) was decreased by 37%; however, peak plasma concentrations of these active forms of the drug were not affected.

Concomitant use of enzalutamide with potent CYP3A4 inducers should be avoided if possible. If concomitant use cannot be avoided, the dosage of enzalutamide should be increased from 160 mg to 240 mg once daily. If concomitant use of the potent CYP3A4 inducer is discontinued, the enzalutamide dosage should be returned to the dosage used prior to initiation of the potent CYP3A4 inducer.

St. John's wort (*Hypericum perforatum*) is an inducer of CYP3A4 and can decrease systemic exposure to enzalutamide. Concomitant use of enzalutamide with St. John's wort should be avoided.

■ **Drugs Metabolized by Hepatic Microsomal Enzymes** Concomitant use of enzalutamide with drugs that are metabolized by CYP isoenzymes 3A4, 2C9, or 2C19 may result in decreased systemic exposure to the substrate drug. When the CYP3A4 substrate midazolam (single 2-mg dose), CYP2C9 substrate warfarin sodium (single 10-mg dose), and CYP2C19 substrate omeprazole (single 20-mg dose) were administered concomitantly with enzalutamide (160 mg daily), systemic exposure and peak plasma concentrations of midazolam were decreased by 86 and 77%, respectively; systemic exposure to *S*-warfarin was decreased by 56%; and systemic exposure and peak plasma concentrations of omeprazole were decreased by 70%. Concomitant use of enzalutamide with CYP 3A4, 2C9, or 2C19 substrates that have a narrow therapeutic index (e.g., alfentanil, clopidogrel, cyclosporine, dihydroergotamine, ergotamine, fentanyl, phenytoin, pimozide, quinidine, sirolimus, tacrolimus, warfarin) should be avoided. If concomitant use with warfarin cannot be avoided, additional monitoring of the international normalized ratio (INR) is recommended.

When the CYP2C8 substrate pioglitazone (single 30-mg dose) was administered concomitantly with enzalutamide (160 mg daily), clinically important changes in systemic exposure to pioglitazone were not observed; therefore, dosage adjustment is not necessary.

When the CYP1A2 substrate caffeine (single 100-mg dose) and CYP2D6 substrate dextromethorphan (single 30-mg dose) were administered concomitantly with enzalutamide (160 mg daily), clinically important changes in systemic exposure to caffeine and dextromethorphan were not observed; therefore, dosage adjustment is not necessary.

■ **Protein-bound Drugs** Because enzalutamide and *N*-desmethylenzalutamide are highly protein bound (97–98 and 95%, respectively), the drug could be displaced from binding sites by, or could displace from binding sites, other protein-bound drugs. In vitro data indicate that displacement between enzalutamide and other highly protein-bound drugs (i.e., salicylates, ibuprofen) is unlikely at clinically relevant concentrations.

Description

Enzalutamide, a nonsteroidal antiandrogen, is an antineoplastic agent. Like conventional nonsteroidal antiandrogens (e.g., bicalutamide, flutamide, nilutamide), enzalutamide competitively inhibits androgen binding to androgen receptors; blockade of androgen receptors may result in growth arrest or apoptosis of prostate cancer cells through inhibition of nuclear translocation of the activated androgen receptor and through inhibition of androgen-dependent binding of the androgen receptor complex to DNA. In vitro, enzalutamide has been shown to reduce tumor growth and induce apoptosis of tumor cells; the drug also has been shown to induce tumor regression in mouse models of castration-resistant prostate cancer. The binding affinity of enzalutamide at the androgen receptor is 5–8 times greater than that of bicalutamide. The main circulating metabolite of enzalutamide, an *N*-desmethyl derivative, has been shown to have activity similar to that of the parent drug in vitro.

In castration-resistant prostate cancer, alterations in androgen receptor signaling (e.g., androgen receptor gene mutation or amplification and androgen receptor overexpression) have been shown to result in persistence of androgen receptor signaling and to contribute to disease progression despite castrate levels of androgens. Androgen receptor overexpression has been associated with resistance to conventional antiandrogens. In cells that overexpress the androgen receptor, conventional antiandrogens (e.g., bicalutamide, flutamide, nilutamide) have been shown to have partial agonistic effects on the androgen receptor, which results in continued activation of the androgen receptor signaling axis despite castrate levels of androgens; this paradoxical effect has been attributed to alterations in the androgen signaling cascade (e.g., androgen receptor gene amplification or mutation). Unlike these conventional antiandrogens, enzalutamide appears to lack agonistic effects in cells that overexpress the androgen receptor, which may result in retained antagonism of the androgen receptor despite overexpression of the receptor.

Pharmacokinetics of enzalutamide are dose proportional over a dosage range of 30–360 mg daily. Following oral administration, the median time to peak plasma concentrations is 1 hour. Steady-state concentrations of enzalutamide are achieved after 28 days of once-daily dosing and the accumulation ratio is approximately 8.3-fold. Administration of enzalutamide with a high-fat meal did not affect the extent of absorption. Enzalutamide is metabolized by cytochrome P-450 (CYP) isoenzymes 2C8 and 3A4. Major metabolites of the drug include an active *N*-desmethyl derivative and an inactive carboxylic acid derivative; formation of *N*-desmethylenzalutamide is mediated principally by CYP2C8. Enzalutamide and *N*-desmethylenzalutamide are 97–98 and 95% bound, respectively, to plasma proteins. The terminal half-lives of enzalutamide and *N*-desmethylenzalutamide following a single oral dose of the drug are 5.8 and approximately 7.8–8.6 days, respectively. Following oral administration of a radiolabeled dose of enzalutamide, about 71% of the dose is recovered in urine (including only trace amounts of unchanged drug and *N*-desmethylenzalutamide) and 14% of the dose is recovered in feces (0.4% as unchanged drug and 1% as *N*-desmethylenzalutamide).

In a dose-finding study, the maximum tolerated dosage of enzalutamide was 240 mg daily; decreases in serum prostate specific antigen (PSA) concentrations were dose dependent at dosages of 30–150 mg daily, but reached a plateau at dosages between 150–240 mg daily.

The pharmacokinetics of enzalutamide do not appear to be affected by age, body weight, or race (Asian versus non-Asian).

Advice to Patients

Importance of advising patients to take enzalutamide as directed by their clinician and at the same time each day. If a dose is missed, importance of administering the missed dose on the same day as soon as it is remembered. Patients should be informed to not take 2 doses on the same day to make up for a missed dose.

Importance of advising patients to swallow enzalutamide capsules whole and not to chew, dissolve, or open the capsules. Importance of advising patients that women who are or may be pregnant should not handle enzalutamide capsules.

For patients currently receiving gonadotropin-releasing hormone (GnRH) agonist therapy, importance of continuing this therapy during enzalutamide therapy.

Risk of seizures. Importance of advising patients to avoid activities where sudden loss of consciousness could cause serious harm to themselves or others. Importance of informing clinician immediately if loss of consciousness or seizure occurs.

Risk of reversible posterior leukoencephalopathy syndrome (RPLS). Importance of informing clinician immediately if rapidly worsening symptoms suggestive of RPLS (e.g., seizure, headache, decreased alertness, confusion, visual disturbances) occur.

Risk of hypersensitivity reactions, including angioedema. Importance of seeking immediate medical care if signs or symptoms of hypersensitivity reactions (e.g., edema of the face, lip, tongue, or throat) occur.

Risk of ischemic heart disease. Importance of seeking immediate medical care if signs or symptoms of a cardiovascular event (e.g., angina, shortness of breath) occur.

Risk of dizziness, vertigo, falls, and fractures. Importance of informing clinician if these adverse effects occur.

Risk of hypertension.

Risk of impairment of male fertility.

Importance of advising patients that enzalutamide may cause fetal harm. Necessity of advising men receiving the drug to use a condom during sexual encounters with pregnant women and to use a condom in conjunction with another effective contraceptive method during sexual encounters with women of childbearing potential; these contraceptive measures are required during enzalutamide therapy and for 3 months after the last dose of the drug.

Importance of informing clinicians of existing or contemplated concomitant therapy, including prescription (e.g., drugs that lower seizure threshold) and OTC drugs and herbal supplements, as well as any concomitant illnesses or conditions that might predispose to seizures.

Importance of informing patients of other important precautionary information. (See Cautions.)

Overview® (see Users Guide). For additional information on this drug until a more detailed monograph is developed and published, the manufacturer's labeling should be consulted. It is *essential* that the manufacturer's labeling be consulted for more detailed information on usual cautions, precautions, contraindications, potential drug interactions, laboratory test interferences, and acute toxicity. For further information on the handling of antineoplastic agents, see the ASHP Guidelines on Handling Hazardous Drugs at http://www.ahfsdruginformation.com.

Preparations

Enzalutamide can only be obtained through designated specialty pharmacies. (See Restricted Distribution under Dosage and Administration: General.)

Excipients in commercially available drug preparations may have clinically important effects in some individuals; consult specific product labeling for details.

Enzalutamide

Oral

Capsules, liquid-filled	40 mg	**Xtandi®**, Astellas

epiRUBicin Hydrochloride

■ Epirubicin, the 4′-epimer of doxorubicin, is an anthracycline glycoside antineoplastic antibiotic.

Uses

■ **Breast Cancer** Epirubicin is used as a component of adjuvant therapy in patients with evidence of axillary node tumor involvement following resection of primary breast carcinoma. Efficacy as adjuvant therapy in the treatment of breast cancer (axillary node-positive with no evidence of distant metastatic disease [stage II or II]) was established in 2 randomized phase III clinical studies; one a comparative study and the other a dose-ranging study. Patients in one arm of the comparative study received cyclophosphamide, fluorouracil, and epirubicin hydrochloride (120 mg/m² per cycle [60 mg/m² on days 1 and 8 of each cycle] for 6 cycles); patients in the second arm received cyclophosphamide, fluorouracil, and methotrexate. Patients studied were premenopausal and perimenopausal women. Relapse-free (RFS) and overall (OS) survival were the clinical end points. The epirubicin-containing regimen was statistically superior to the methotrexate-containing regimen with respect to 5-year RFS (62 versus 53%) and OS (77 versus 70%). The dose-ranging study randomized premenopausal and postmenopausal women, with both groups receiving cyclophosphamide and fluorouracil, along with either 50 or 100 mg/m² of epirubicin hydrochloride on day 1 of each cycle for 6 cycles. The 100-mg/m² dose of epirubicin hydrochloride was more effective than the 50-mg/m² dose with respect to 5-year RFS (65 versus 52%) and OS (76 versus 65%). Similar improvements in RFS and OS were observed in both premenopausal and postmenopausal women treated with the 100-mg/m² epirubicin hydrochloride dose.

Dosage and Administration

■ **Administration** Epirubicin hydrochloride is administered IV. The drug is extremely irritating to tissues and, therefore, must not be given IM or subcutaneously. *Care should be taken to avoid extravasation of the drug.* It is recommended that solutions of the drug be administered slowly into the tubing of a freely running IV infusion of 0.9 % sodium chloride or 5% dextrose injection. Direct IV injection of epirubicin hydrochloride is *not* recommended because of the risk of extravasation even in the presence of adequate blood return upon needle aspiration. When possible, veins over joints or in extremities with compromised venous or lymphatic drainage should not be used. The rate of injection depends on the volume of the infusion solution and the dosage, but usually ranges from 3–20 minutes. Local erythematous streaking along the vein and/or facial flushing may be indicative of too rapid an administration rate, and may be followed by local phlebitis or thrombophlebitis.

Although a stinging or burning sensation may be a symptom of extravasation during IV administration of epirubicin hydrochloride, extravasation may occur without these symptoms and even when blood returns well during initial aspiration of the infusion needle. If any signs or symptoms of extravasation occur, the injection or infusion should be immediately stopped and restarted at another site. For information on the management of extravasation, see Dosage and Administration: Reconstitution and Administration, in Doxorubicin 10:00.

Epirubicin hydrochloride is incompatible with any alkaline pH solution; hydrolysis of the drug will occur with prolonged contact. The drug also is incompatible with heparin or fluorouracil; precipitation may occur. The manufacturer recommends that epirubicin hydrochloride not be mixed with other drugs in the same syringe.

Epirubicin hydrochloride injection and solutions of the drug must be prepared and handled cautiously by trained nonpregnant personnel, and the use of protective equipment (e.g., latex gloves) is recommended. Hands must be washed after removal of the latex gloves. Accidental contact with the skin, mucous membranes, or eyes should be treated immediately by copious lavage with water, soap and water, or sodium bicarbonate solution; abrasion of the skin by use of a scrub brush should be avoided, and prompt medical attention is necessary. Parenteral epirubicin hydrochloride solutions should be inspected visually for particulate matter and discoloration prior to administration whenever solution and container permit.

■ **Dosage** To obtain optimum therapeutic results with minimum adverse effects, dosage of epirubicin hydrochloride must be based on the clinical, cardiac, hepatic, renal, and hematologic response and tolerance of the patient and on other chemotherapy or irradiation being used.

Breast Cancer The recommended initial dosage of epirubicin hydrochloride as a component of adjuvant therapy for axillary node-positive breast cancer is 100–120 mg/m^2. Doses of the anthracycline are given in repeated 3- to 4-week cycles, with the total dose for each cycle given as a single dose on day 1 *or* as 2 equally divided doses on days 1 and 8. In clinical trials, the 100-mg epirubicin hydrochloride regimen (FEC-100) included fluorouracil 500 mg/m^2 and cyclophosphamide 500 mg/m^2, with all drugs administered IV on day 1 of a 21-day cycle and repeated for 6 cycles. In clinical trials, the 120-mg epirubicin hydrochloride regimen (CEF-120) was given IV as 60 mg/m^2 of the anthracycline and fluorouracil 500 mg/m^2 on days 1 and 8 of each cycle combined with oral cyclophosphamide 75 mg/m^2 on days 1–14 of each cycle, with the cycles being repeated at 28-day intervals; for 6 cycles. Prophylactic anti-infective therapy with co-trimoxazole or a fluoroquinolone was used concomitantly for the duration of chemotherapy.

Dose Modification for Toxicity. Dosage adjustments after the first treatment cycle should be made based on hematologic and nonhematologic toxicities. Patients experiencing (during the current treatment cycle) nadir platelet counts less than 50,000/mm^3, absolute neutrophil counts (ANC) less than 250/mm^3, neutropenic fevers, or grade 3 or 4 nonhematologic toxicity should have the day-1 dose of each antineoplastic agent in subsequent cycles reduced to 75% of the day-1 dose given in the current cycle. Day-1 chemotherapy in subsequent cycles should be delayed until platelet counts are at least 100,000/mm^3, ANCs are at least 1500/mm^3, and nonhematologic toxicities have recovered to grade 1 or better. For patients receiving a divided dose of epirubicin hydrochloride (days 1 and 8), the day-8 dose of the anthracycline, fluorouracil, and cyclophosphamide should be 75% of the day-1 dose if platelet counts and ANCs are 75,000–100,000 and 1000–1499/mm^3, respectively. If day-8 platelet counts or ANCs are less than 75,000 or 1000/mm^3, respectively, or grade 3 or 4 nonhematologic toxicity has occurred, the day-8 dose of each drug should be omitted.

Radiation Therapy. Radiation therapy in combination with epirubicin may result in additive cytotoxicity, and generally is not administered concurrently with antineoplastic agents. In adjuvant trials with the drug, radiation was delayed until after completion of chemotherapy; such delay did not appear to result in any appreciable increase in local breast cancer recurrence. In the limited number of patients who received concomitant radiation, chemotherapy was interrupted to avoid overlapping toxicities. Epirubicin is likely to sensitize tissues to the cytotoxic effects of radiation, and administration of the drug after radiation may induce an inflammatory recall reaction at the site of irradiation.

■ **Special Populations** ***Bone Marrow Impairment*** For patients with bone marrow impairment (e.g., those extensively pretreated or with preexisting myelosuppression or neoplastic bone marrow infiltration), decreasing the epirubicin hydrochloride dosage for the initial cycle to 75–90 mg/m^2 should be considered.

Renal or Hepatic Impairment Although the manufacturer does not provide definitive recommendations for dosage adjustment in patients with hepatic or renal impairment, reduced dosage should be given to those with hepatic impairment and considered for those with renal impairment. In clinical trials, patients with a serum bilirubin concentration of 1.2–3 mg/dL or AST concentration 2–4 times the upper limit of normal (ULN) received 50% of the recommended initial epirubicin hydrochloride dosage, and patients with bilirubin exceeding 3 mg/dL or AST exceeding 4 times the ULN received 25% of the initial dosage. Patients with severe hepatic impairment have not been evaluated; therefore, epirubicin should not be used in this population. Patients with severe renal impairment (serum creatinine concentration exceeding 5 mg/dL) may require dosage reductions; the drug has not been studied in those undergoing dialysis

Cautions

■ **Contraindications** Known hypersensitivity to epirubicin, other anthracyclines, anthracenediones, or any ingredient in the formulation.

Baseline neutrophil count less than 1500/mm^3; severe myocardial or hepatic impairment or recent myocardial infarction; previous anthracycline therapy up to the maximum cumulative dose.

■ **Warnings/Precautions** ***Warnings*** **Adequate Patient Evaluation and Monitoring.** Epirubicin should be administered only under the supervision of qualified clinicians experienced in the use of cytotoxic therapy. Patients must have recovered from acute toxicities (e.g., stomatitis, neutropenia, thrombocytopenia, generalized infections) of prior cytotoxic therapy before starting treatment with epirubicin. Prior to and during therapy, determination of hematopoietic, hepatic, renal, and cardiac (left ventricular ejection fraction [LVEF]) function should be performed. Monitor for clinical complications associated with myelosuppression (e.g., granulocytopenia and infections) and potential cardiotoxicity (e.g., congestive heart failure [CHF]), especially with increasing cumulative exposure to anthracyclines. Supportive care may be necessary for the treatment of toxicity (e.g., severe neutropenia, severe infectious complications, cardiotoxicity).

Hematologic Effects. Dose-dependent, reversible leukopenia and/or granulocytopenia is the principal manifestation of hematologic toxicity and is the most common acute dose-limiting toxicity. Leukocyte nadir at day 10–14; return to baseline by day 21. Severe myelosuppression may occur.

Cardiac Effects. Cardiotoxicity is a known risk of anthracycline therapy; toxicity may be manifested by early (acute) or late (delayed) events.

Early cardiotoxicity of epirubicin consists of sinus tachycardia and/or ECG abnormalities such as nonspecific ST-T wave changes, but more serious signs (e.g., AV block, ventricular tachycardia) also have been reported. Early effects generally do not predict subsequent development of delayed cardiotoxicity, are rarely of clinical importance, and generally are not an indication for suspension of epirubicin therapy.

Delayed cardiotoxicity (cardiomyopathy) is manifested by reduced LVEF and CHF, which may be life-threatening in its most severe form. Active or occult cardiovascular disease, prior or concomitant irradiation to the mediastinal/pericardial area, previous therapy with other anthracyclines or anthracenediones, or concomitant use of other cardiotoxic drugs may increase the risk of cardiotoxicity.

Risk of serious cardiotoxicity may be decreased by regular monitoring of LVEF during therapy, and prompt discontinuance of epirubicin at the first sign of impaired cardiac function. In patients with risk factors for cardiotoxicity, monitoring of cardiac function must be particularly strict; risk versus benefit of continued therapy with impaired cardiac function must be carefully evaluated.

Cardiotoxicity depends on the cumulative dose of epirubicin and represents the cumulative dose-limiting toxicity of the drug. Probability of developing clinically evident CHF is estimated as: 0.9, 1.6, and 3.3% at cumulative epirubicin hydrochloride dosages of 550, 700, and 900 mg/m^2, respectively. The risk of developing CHF increases rapidly with increasing total cumulative doses exceeding 900 mg/m^2; this cumulative dosage should only be exceeded with extreme caution. Toxicity may occur at lower cumulative doses, regardless of whether cardiac risk factors are present. It is probable that the cardiac effects of epirubicin and other anthracyclines or anthracenediones are additive.

Thrombophlebitis and thromboembolic phenomena, including pulmonary embolism, sometimes fatal, also have been reported in patients receiving epirubicin.

For a more complete discussion of the cardiotoxic effects of anthracyclines, see Cautions: Cardiac Effects, in Doxorubicin 10:00.

Carcinogenicity. Secondary acute myelogenous leukemia (AML) has been reported in patients treated with anthracyclines; risk of refractory AML increases when epirubicin is combined with other DNA-damaging antineoplastics, when patients have had extensive exposure to cytotoxic drugs, or when anthracycline doses have been escalated. The cumulative risk for adjuvant epirubicin therapy-related leukemia is estimated as 0.2 and 0.8% at 3 and 5 years, respectively.

Epirubicin is mutagenic, clastogenic, and carcinogenic in animals. Although experimental data are not available, epirubicin could induce chromosomal damage in human spermatozoa. Males should utilize effective contraceptive methods. Epirubicin may induce irreversible amenorrhea in premenopausal women.

Hepatic Effects. See Dosage and Administration: Special Populations, and Cautions: Specific Populations. Contraindicated in patients with severe hepatic impairment.

Local Effects. Severe local necrosis if extravasation during administration occurs. Must *not* be given by IM or subcutaneous injection. (See Cautions: General Precautions, and Dosage and Administration: Administration.)

Other Adverse Effects. As a result of extensive purine catabolism accompanying rapid cellular destruction, hyperuricemia, including tumor lysis syndrome, may occur in patients receiving epirubicin; serum uric acid concentrations should be monitored. Hyperuricemia and its potential adverse effects may be minimized or prevented by adequate hydration, alkalinization of the urine, and/or administration of allopurinol.

General Precautions **Local Effects.** Venous sclerosis may result from injection into a small vessel or repeated injections into the same vein. Extravasation during infusion may cause local pain, severe tissue lesions, and necrosis. (See Cautions: Warnings/Precautions, and Dosage and Administration: Administration.)

GI Effects. Epirubicin is emetogenic; prophylaxis with antiemetics should be considered prior to administration.

Irradiation. Epirubicin, like other anthracyclines, may induce an inflammatory recall reaction at the site of prior irradiation. (See Dosage and Administration: Dosage.)

Specific Populations **Pregnancy.** Category D. (See Users' Guide.)

Lactation. It is unknown whether epirubicin is distributed in milk. Because other anthracyclines are distributed in milk, and because of the potential for serious adverse reactions in nursing infants from epirubicin, nursing should be discontinued prior to therapy.

Pediatric Use. Safety and efficacy have not been established in children; children may be at greater risk for anthracycline-induced acute manifestations of cardiotoxicity and for chronic CHF.

Geriatric Use. Although a reduced initial dosage was not used in clinical trials in women 70 years of age and older, careful monitoring for toxicity should be employed in this age group.

Hepatic Impairment. Use is not recommended in severe impairment. Dosage adjustment for mild-to-moderate impairment.

Renal Impairment. Dosage reductions should be considered for severe impairment. (See Dosage and Administration: Special Populations.)

Bone Marrow Impairment. Dosage reductions should be considered. (See Dosage and Administration: Special Populations.)

■ **Common Adverse Effects** Epirubicin hydrochloride is a toxic drug with a low therapeutic index. A therapeutic response is not likely to occur without some evidence of toxicity. The major toxic effects of the drug are on the normal, rapidly proliferating tissues, particularly those of the bone marrow, GI and oral mucosa, and hair follicles. Alopecia, nausea/vomiting, myelosuppression (leukopenia, neutropenia, anemia, thrombocytopenia), amenorrhea, mucositis, lethargy, hot flushes (flashes), diarrhea, infection, local effects (e.g., venous irritation), conjunctivitis/keratitis, rash/pruritus, skin and nail changes (e.g., hyperpigmentation) , fever, and anorexia occur commonly. Urticaria, photosensitivity, and anaphylaxis (including shock) also have occurred.

Drug Interactions

■ **Antineoplastic Agents** Potential pharmacodynamic interaction; additive pharmacologic and toxic effects.

■ **Cardiotoxic Drugs** Cardioactive drugs that may precipitate CHF (e.g., calcium-channel blocking agents such as verapamil); close cardiac function monitoring required.

■ **Radiation** Potential additive toxicities and inflammatory recall reactions at the site of irradiation. (See Dosage and Administration: Dosage.)

■ **Cimetidine** Potential pharmacokinetic interaction (increased epirubicin concentrations); discontinue during epirubicin therapy.

■ **Hepatoactive Drugs** Because of epirubicin's extensive hepatic metabolism, changes in hepatic function induced by concomitant therapy may affect metabolism, pharmacokinetics, efficacy, and/or toxicity.

Description

Epirubicin, the 4′-epimer of doxorubicin, is an anthracycline glycoside antineoplastic antibiotic that is a semisynthetic derivative of daunorubicin. The spacial orientation of the hydroxyl group at carbon 4′ of the sugar moiety results in epirubicin being a weaker base and more lipophilic than doxorubicin, which may result in an improved therapeutic index for epirubicin; however, substantial differences in the *types* of biochemical interactions involved in the mechanism(s) of action and toxicity of the epimeric analogs do not appear to exist. As a result, the spectrum of pharmacologic, antineoplastic, and toxic effects of the drugs are*qualitatively* identical, but at equimolar doses, epirubicin appears to be less toxic with regard to both general toxicity and cardiotoxicity. The spacial orientation of the hydroxyl group also allows glucuronide conjugation of epirubicin, which is unique among currently available anthracyclines, and may be responsible for the relatively high plasma clearance and faster elimination of the drug.

Epirubicin exhibits pharmacologic actions similar to those of daunorubicin and doxorubicin. The precise and/or principal mechanism(s) of antineoplastic action of anthracyclines is not fully understood. Experimental evidence indicates that epirubicin, like other anthracyclines, forms a complex with DNA by intercalation between base pairs, causing inhibition of DNA synthesis and DNA-dependent RNA synthesis by the resulting template disordering and steric obstruction. Protein synthesis also is inhibited. Such intercalation triggers DNA cleavage by topoisomerase II, resulting in cytocidal activity. DNA helicase also is inhibited, resulting in interference with replication and transcription; epirubicin also generates cytotoxic free radicals. For additional information, see Pharmacology in Doxorubicin 10:00. Because of the shared mechanisms between doxorubicin and epirubicin, the drugs appear to exhibit a similar spectrum of activity against a wide variety of solid tumors and hematologic malignancies, and complete cross-resistance between the 2 anthracyclines has been documented in vitro.

Epirubicin undergoes extensive hepatic metabolism, and is eliminated principally by metabolism and biliary excretion; urinary excretion is only a minor elimination pathway.

Advice to Patients

Importance of recognizing and reporting adverse effects of epirubicin, including GI and myelosuppressive effects (and related precautions), infectious complications, CHF symptoms, and injection site pain.

Risk of irreversible myocardial toxicity and leukemia.

Apprise patient of potential hazard to the fetus if used during pregnancy; women of childbearing potential should avoid becoming pregnant. Males must utilize effective contraception during therapy. (See Carcinogenicity in Cautions: Warnings.) Inform women of risk of irreversible amenorrhea or premature menopause.

Importance of informing clinicians of existing or contemplated concomitant therapy, including prescription and OTC drugs, as well as concomitant illnesses.

Advise patients on alopecia, and reddish appearance of urine for 1–2 days (harmless).

Overview (see Users Guide). For additional information until a more detailed monograph is developed and published, the manufacturer's labeling should be consulted. It is *essential* that the manufacturer's labeling be consulted for more detailed information on usual cautions, precautions, contraindications, potential drug interactions, laboratory test interferences, and acute toxicity. For further information on the handling of antineoplastic agents, see the ASHP Guidelines on Handling Hazardous Drugs at http://www.ahfsdruginformation.com.

Preparations

Excipients in commercially available drug preparations may have clinically important effects in some individuals; consult specific product labeling for details.

epiRUBicin Hydrochloride

Parenteral

Injection, for IV use only	2 mg/mL (50 and 200 mg)	**Ellence®**, Pfizer

eriBULin Mesylate

■ Eribulin mesylate, a synthetic analog of halichondrin B and nontaxane microtubule dynamics inhibitor, is an antineoplastic agent.

Uses

■ **Breast Cancer** Eribulin mesylate is used for the treatment of metastatic breast cancer in patients who have previously received at least 2 chemotherapeutic regimens for the treatment of metastatic disease; prior therapy should have included an anthracycline and a taxane in either the adjuvant or metastatic setting.

The current indication for eribulin is based principally on the results of an open-label, randomized, multicenter phase 3 trial (the EMBRACE trial) conducted in 762 extensively pretreated women with metastatic or locally recurrent breast cancer. This study compared eribulin monotherapy to any single-agent treatment of the physician's choice, which served as a control designed to represent actual clinical options available for the management of metastatic breast cancer. Patients who had received from 2 to 5 previous chemotherapy regimens, including an anthracycline- and a taxane-based regimen for adjuvant or metastatic disease (unless contraindicated), and whose disease had progressed within 6 months of their last treatment were enrolled in the study. Median age of the patients was 55 years (range: 27–85 years), 92% were Caucasian, and 91% had an ECOG performance status of 0–1. Tumor prognostic characteristics, including hormone receptor status, expression of HER2, and site and extent of disease, were similar between the 2 treatment groups. Patients were randomized in a 2:1 ratio to receive eribulin (1.4 mg/m^2 IV on days 1 and 8 of a 21-day treatment cycle) or any single-agent chemotherapy, hormonal therapy, biologic therapy, radiotherapy, or symptomatic treatment alone. The majority of patients in the control group received a chemotherapeutic agent (vinorelbine [26%], gemcitabine [18%], capecitabine [18%], a taxane [16%], an anthracycline [9%], or other chemotherapy [10%]) and the remainder received hormonal therapy (3%). Therapy was continued until disease progression, intolerable toxicity, or patient withdrawal for other reasons occurred.

Overall survival, which was the primary efficacy end point of the EMBRACE trial, was prolonged in patients receiving eribulin compared with those receiving a control therapy (median overall survival of 13.1 and 10.6 months, respectively). Patients treated with eribulin had an objective response rate of 11% and a median duration of response of 4.2 months. Progression-free survival, a secondary outcome of the study, also was prolonged in the eribulin group compared with the control group, but the difference was less than that observed for overall survival and did not reach statistical significance by independent (versus investigator) review. Eribulin was relatively well tolerated; grade 3 or 4 adverse effects that occurred more often with eribulin than with comparator regimens included neutropenia, leukopenia, and peripheral neuropathy.

Although several drugs (e.g., capecitabine, eribulin, gemcitabine, ixabepilone, vinorelbine) have been used in the treatment of anthracycline- and taxane-refractory metastatic breast cancer, there currently is no generally accepted standard of care for the management of patients with such advanced and heavily pretreated disease. Some clinicians recommend that choice of therapy should therefore be individualized based on factors such as the patient's disease stage and tumor type, performance status, quality of life, preferences, treatment history including toxicity, underlying medical conditions, and the expected benefits and risks of each treatment option.

Dosage and Administration

■ **General** Patients receiving eribulin mesylate should be assessed for peripheral neuropathy and a complete blood cell count (CBC) should be performed prior to administration of each dose of the drug. The dose of eribulin should be modified or temporarily withheld for hematologic and non-hematologic toxicities according to the degree of the toxicities. (See Dosage and Administration: Dosage Modification for Toxicity.)

Because eribulin may cause nausea and vomiting, use of prophylactic antiemetics, including corticosteroids, may be considered.

Routine premedication to prevent hypersensitivity reactions is not necessary with eribulin.

■ **Administration** Eribulin mesylate is administered IV, either as an injection or short infusion, over 2–5 minutes. The drug should be given *only* by IV administration. In clinical trials, the drug was given IV over 1–60 minutes† either directly or diluted in 0.9% sodium chloride injection to a concentration of 0.01–0.1 mg/mL; the infusion time was independent of whether the injection was diluted or undiluted.

Good peripheral venous access or a patent central line should be ensured prior to administration. The injection does not appear to be a vesicant or irritant; if extravasation occurs, there is no specific antidote and treatment should be symptomatic.

Eribulin mesylate injection is commercially available as a ready-to-use solution containing 0.5 mg of eribulin mesylate per mL in single-use vials. The appropriate dose of the drug should be withdrawn from the vial and administered either undiluted or diluted with 100 mL of 0.9% sodium chloride injection. The manufacturer states that eribulin injection should not be diluted or administered with dextrose solutions; the injection also should not be administered in the same IV line with other drugs.

Undiluted solutions of eribulin may be stored in the syringe for up to 4 hours at room temperature or up to 24 hours under refrigeration (4°C). Diluted solutions also may be stored for up to 4 hours at room temperature or up to 24 hours under refrigeration. Any unused portions of the vial should be discarded.

Procedures for proper handling and disposal of antineoplastic drugs should be followed when preparing or administering eribulin. For additional information on proper procedures for handling antineoplastic agents, see the ASHP Guidelines on Handling Hazardous Drugs at http://www.ahfsdruginformation.com.

Unopened vials of eribulin mesylate injection should be stored in their original cartons at 25°C, but may be exposed to temperatures ranging from 15–30°C. Freezing of the vials should be avoided.

■ **Dosage** Eribulin is commercially available as eribulin mesylate; dosage of eribulin mesylate is expressed in terms of the mesylate salt.

Dosage of eribulin mesylate is based on the patient's body surface area.

For the treatment of metastatic breast cancer in patients who have received at least 2 prior chemotherapeutic regimens (including an anthracycline and a taxane), the recommended dosage of eribulin mesylate in adults is 1.4 mg/m^2 administered IV over 2–5 minutes on days 1 and 8 of a 21-day treatment cycle. Patients should have an absolute neutrophil count (ANC) of at least 1000/mm^3 and a platelet count of at least 75,000/mm^3 prior to each dose. In addition, any nonhematologic toxicities should have resolved to grade 2 in severity or less before a dose is administered. Dose delays and reductions are required in patients who experience severe hematologic and/or nonhematologic toxicities during therapy. (See Dosage and Administration: Dosage Modification for Toxicity.)

In the principal efficacy study, eribulin was continued until disease progression, intolerable toxicity, or patient withdrawal for other reasons occurred; patients received a median of 5 cycles (range: 1–23 cycles) of therapy with the drug.

■ **Dosage Modification for Toxicity** The dose of eribulin mesylate on day 1 or day 8 of the treatment cycle should be withheld if ANC counts are less than 1000/mm^3, platelet counts are less than 75,000/mm^3, or grade 3 or 4 nonhematologic toxicities are present. The dose on day 8 may be delayed for a maximum of 1 week for these toxicities. If toxicities resolve or improve to grade 2 in severity or less by day 15, eribulin therapy may be resumed at a reduced dosage (see Table 1) and the next treatment cycle should be initiated no sooner than 2 weeks later. If toxicities do not resolve or improve to grade 2 or less within this 1-week time period, the dose should be omitted.

Table 1. Recommended Dosage Reductions for Hematologic and Nonhematologic Toxicities

Permanently Reduce Dosage in Patients Initially Dosed with 1.4 mg/m^2 for Any of the Following Toxicities:	Recommended Dosage on Days 1 and 8 of 21-Day Cycle
ANC <500/mm^3 for >7 days	1.1 mg/m^2
ANC <1000/mm^3 with fever or infection	1.1 mg/m^2
Platelets <25,000/mm^3	1.1 mg/m^2
Platelets <50,000/mm^3 requiring transfusion	1.1 mg/m^2
Nonhematologic grade 3 or 4 toxicities	1.1 mg/m^2
Omission or delay of day 8 dose in previous cycle for toxicity	1.1 mg/m^2
If any of the above events occurs while receiving 1.1 mg/m^2, reduce dosage to 0.7 mg/m^2.	
If any of the above events occurs while receiving 0.7 mg/m^2, discontinue therapy.	

■ **Special Populations** The manufacturer recommends that the dosage of eribulin mesylate be reduced to 1.1 mg/m^2 on days 1 and 8 of a 21-day cycle in patients with mild (Child-Pugh class A) hepatic impairment and to 0.7 mg/m^2 on days 1 and 8 of a 21-day cycle in those with moderate (Child-Pugh class B) hepatic impairment. Eribulin has not been studied in patients with severe (Child-Pugh class C) hepatic impairment and the manufacturer does not make specific dosage recommendations for such patients. (See Hepatic Impairment under Warnings/Precautions: Specific Populations, in Cautions.)

No dosage adjustment is necessary in patients with mild renal impairment (creatinine clearance of 50–80 mL/minute). The manufacturer recommends that the initial dosage of eribulin mesylate be reduced to 1.1 mg/m^2 on days 1 and 8 of a 21-day cycle in patients with moderate renal impairment (creatinine clearance of 30–50 mL/minute). Eribulin has not been studied in patients with severe renal impairment (creatinine clearance less than 30 mL/minute) and the manufacturer does not make specific dosage recommendations for such patients. (See Renal Impairment under Warnings/Precautions: Specific Populations, in Cautions.)

Cautions

■ **Contraindications** The manufacturer states that there are no known contraindications to the use of eribulin mesylate.

■ **Warnings/Precautions** ***Neutropenia*** Neutropenia is the most common adverse effect associated with eribulin mesylate therapy, occurring in 82% of patients in the EMBRACE trial; grade 3 or 4 neutropenia was reported in 28 or 29% of patients receiving the drug, respectively. Febrile neutropenia occurred in 5% of patients, and 2 patients (0.4%) died from complications of febrile neutropenia. Severe neutropenia (absolute neutrophil count [ANC] less than 500/mm^3) lasting more than 1 week was reported in 12% of the patients in this study. Patients with serum AST or ALT concentrations exceeding 3 times the upper limit of normal or serum bilirubin concentrations exceeding 1.5 times the upper limit of normal had higher incidences of grade 4 neutropenia and febrile neutropenia than those with normal aminotransferase concentrations. In patients with grade 3 or 4 neutropenia, the mean time to nadir neutrophil count within a treatment cycle was approximately 13 days, and the mean time to recovery from severe neutropenia was approximately 8 days.

A complete blood cell count (CBC) should be obtained prior to administering each dose of eribulin and more frequently in patients who develop grade 3 or 4 cytopenias. Administration should be delayed and subsequent doses reduced in patients with febrile neutropenia or grade 4 neutropenia lasting longer than 7 days. (See Dosage and Administration: Dosage Modification for Toxicity.) In the EMBRACE trial, granulocyte colony-stimulating factor or granulocyte-macrophage colony-stimulating factor was used in 19% of the eribulin-treated patients who developed cytopenias.

Peripheral Neuropathy Peripheral neuropathy is a common dose-limiting adverse effect of microtubule inhibitors, including eribulin. Peripheral neuropathy of any grade (motor neuropathy, polyneuropathy, sensory neuropathy, paresthesias) was reported in 35% of patients receiving eribulin in the EMBRACE study and was the most common adverse effect resulting in discontinuance of the drug. Grade 3 and 4 peripheral neuropathy occurred in 8 and 0.4%, respectively, of patients receiving eribulin in the study; in those who continued therapy, peripheral neuropathy improved to grade 2 or less after the dose was delayed and reduced. About 5% of patients experienced neuropathy that lasted for more than 1 year, and 22% developed new-onset or worsening neuropathy that persisted for at least a median follow-up period of 269 days.

Patients receiving eribulin should be closely monitored for manifestations of peripheral motor and sensory neuropathy (e.g., numbness, tingling, or burning sensation in the hands and/or feet) prior to each dose of eribulin. The drug should be withheld in patients who experience grade 3 or 4 peripheral neuropathy until it resolves to grade 2 or less; therapy may then be resumed at a reduced dosage. (See Dosage and Administration: Dosage Modification for Toxicity.)

Fetal/Neonatal Morbidity and Mortality There are no adequate and well-controlled studies of eribulin in pregnant women. Because eribulin is a microtubule inhibitor, it is expected to cause fetal harm when administered to pregnant women. Embryofetal toxicity and teratogenicity (e.g., increased abortion, increased resorption and death, decreased fetal weight, severe external or soft tissue malformations) have been demonstrated in animals. If eribulin is used during pregnancy or the patient becomes pregnant while receiving the drug, the patient should be apprised of the potential fetal hazard. (See Advice to Patients.)

Prolongation of QT Interval Eribulin has been associated with QT-interval prolongation, which appears to be a delayed effect of the drug. In an uncontrolled, open-label study, prolongation of the QT interval (maximum QTc change from baseline of 11.4 msec) was observed on day 8 of the treatment cycle, independent of eribulin concentration, in patients receiving the drug; QT-interval prolongation was not observed on day 1.

Eribulin should be avoided in patients with congenital long QT syndrome. Hypokalemia or hypomagnesemia should be corrected prior to initiating eribulin therapy and serum potassium and magnesium concentrations should be monitored periodically during therapy with the drug. The manufacturer recommends that ECG monitoring for QT-interval prolongation in patients with congestive heart failure, bradyarrhythmias, and electrolyte abnormalities and in those receiving drugs known to prolong the QT interval (e.g., class Ia and III antiarrhythmic agents). (See Drug Interactions: Drugs that Prolong the QT Interval.)

Specific Populations **Pregnancy.** Category D. (See Fetal/Neonatal Morbidity and Mortality under Cautions: Warnings/Precautions.)

Lactation. Not known whether eribulin mesylate is distributed into human milk. Because of the potential for serious adverse reactions to eribulin in nursing infants, a decision should be made whether to discontinue nursing or the drug, taking into account the importance of the drug to the woman.

Pediatric Use. Safety and effectiveness of eribulin in pediatric patients younger than 18 years of age have not been established.

Geriatric Use. The EMBRACE study did not include sufficient numbers of patients 65 years of age and older to determine whether geriatric patients respond differently to eribulin than younger patients. Among 827 patients who received eribulin in clinical studies, 121 (15%) were 65 years of age or older and 17 (2%) were 75 years of age or older. No overall differences in safety were observed in these patients compared with those younger than 65 years of age.

Hepatic Impairment. In an open-label study, systemic exposure to eribulin was increased by approximately 1.8- or 2.5-fold in those with mild (Child-Pugh class A) or moderate (Child-Pugh class B) hepatic impairment, respectively. Dosage of eribulin should therefore be reduced in patients with mild or moderate hepatic impairment. The drug has not been studied in patients with severe (Child-Pugh class C) hepatic impairment. (See Dosage and Administration: Special Populations.)

Renal Impairment. Formal pharmacokinetic studies have not been conducted in patients with renal impairment. Available data suggest that dosage adjustment is not required in patients with mild renal impairment (creatinine clearance of 50–80 mL/minute). However, a twofold increase in eribulin exposure has been observed in patients with moderate renal impairment (creatinine clearance of 30–50 mL/minute); therefore, a lower initial dosage is recommended in such patients. (See Dosage and Administration: Special Populations.)The safety of eribulin in patients with severe renal impairment (creatinine clearance less than 30 mL/minute) has not been studied.

■ **Common Adverse Effects** Adverse effects reported in 25% or more of patients receiving eribulin mesylate in clinical studies included neutropenia, anemia, asthenia or fatigue, alopecia, peripheral neuropathy, nausea, and constipation.

Among patients with grade 0 or 1 ALT levels at baseline, 18% of eribulin-treated patients experienced grade 2 or greater ALT elevation.

Drug Interactions

■ **Drugs Affecting or Metabolized by Hepatic Microsomal Enzymes** Eribulin mesylate is minimally metabolized by cytochrome P-450 (CYP) 3A4 isoenzyme; clinically important pharmacokinetic interactions are not expected with concomitant use of drugs that inhibit CYP3A4.

In vitro studies indicate that eribulin does not substantially inhibit CYP1 isoenzymes A2, 2C9, 2C19, 2D6, 2E1, or 3A4 and does not induce CYP1 isoenzymes A2, 2C9, 2C19, or 3A4; therefore, eribulin is not expected to alter plasma concentrations of drugs metabolized by these CYP isoenzymes. Although eribulin demonstrated some CYP3A4-inhibitory activity in human liver microsomes in one study, the drug did not appear to inhibit the metabolism of several substrates of CYP3A4 (carbamazepine, diazepam, paclitaxel, midazolam, tamoxifen, terfenadine [no longer commercially available in the US]) at clinically relevant concentrations.

■ **Drugs Affecting the P-glycoprotein Transport System** Eribulin is both a substrate and weak inhibitor of the efflux transporter P-glycoprotein in vitro. Clinically important pharmacokinetic interactions are not expected with concurrent use of drugs that inhibit P-glycoprotein (e.g., ketoconazole). (See Drug Interactions: Ketoconazole.)

■ **Drugs that Prolong the QT Interval** Potential pharmacologic interaction (additive effect on QT-interval prolongation). ECG monitoring is recommended in patients concurrently receiving other drugs known to prolong the QT interval, including class Ia (e.g., quinidine, procainamide) and class III (e.g., amiodarone, sotalol) antiarrhythmic agents, some antipsychotic agents (e.g., chlorpromazine, thioridazine, haloperidol, asenapine, olanzapine, paliperidone, pimozide, quetiapine, ziprasidone), some antibiotics (e.g., gatifloxacin, moxifloxacin), and tetrabenazine. (See Prolongation of QT Interval under Cautions: Warnings/Precautions.)

Certain type 3 serotonin (5-HT_3) receptor antagonists used as antiemetic agents (e.g., dolasetron, ondansetron, palonosetron) are associated with QT-interval prolongation. If a 5-HT_3 receptor antagonist is clinically necessary, granisetron, which has not been associated with QT-interval prolongation, is recommended by some clinicians.

■ **Carboplatin** Pharmacokinetic interaction has not been observed with concomitant use of eribulin and carboplatin.

■ **Ketoconazole** Pharmacokinetic interaction unlikely. Concomitant administration of ketoconazole, a potent CYP3A4 and P-glycoprotein inhibitor, did not substantially affect AUC values of eribulin in patients with advanced solid tumors in an open-label crossover study.

■ **Palifermin** Increased severity and duration of oral mucositis has been observed in patients receiving palifermin within 24 hours of myelotoxic chemotherapy administration, presumably because of increased sensitivity of the rapidly dividing epithelial cells to chemotherapy after palifermin treatment. Because eribulin can be myelotoxic, palifermin should *not* be administered during or within 24 hours before or after eribulin administration.

Description

Eribulin mesylate is a nontaxane microtubule dynamics inhibitor antineoplastic agent. The drug is a synthetic analog of halichondrin B, which is a naturally occurring product originally isolated from the marine sponge *Halichondria okadai* and has been shown to possess potent antitumor activity. Eribulin appears to have a distinct mechanism of action from that of other currently available antimicrotubule agents (e.g., epothilones, taxanes, vinca alkaloids). Similar to these agents, eribulin binds to a unique site on tubulin and blocks cell cycle progression at the G_2/M phase, resulting in irreversible mitotic arrest and apoptosis. However, unlike these agents, eribulin inhibits the growth of microtubules without affecting the shortening phase and also causes sequestration of tubulin into nonfunctional aggregates. In preclinical studies, eribulin demonstrated antitumor activity in paclitaxel-resistant cell lines.

Eribulin exhibits linear, dose-proportional pharmacokinetics. Eribulin exposure after multiple dosing is similar to that following a single dose of the drug; no accumulation of eribulin has been observed with weekly administration. Plasma concentrations of the drug decline in a triphasic manner with an initial rapid distribution phase followed by a slower elimination phase with a mean terminal elimination half-life of approximately 40 hours. Eribulin is principally excreted in feces; following IV administration, approximately 82% of the dose is eliminated in feces and 9% in urine, mainly as unchanged drug. About 49–65% of the drug is bound to plasma proteins. Eribulin is primarily metabolized by cytochrome P-450 (CYP) isoenzyme 3A4; however, no major human metabolites of the drug have been detected. In vitro studies using human liver microsomes indicate that eribulin does not substantially inhibit CYP isoenzymes 1A2, 2C9, 2C19, 2D6, 2E1, and 3A4 nor induce CYP1 isoenzymes A2, 2C9, 2C19, and 3A4. Eribulin is a substrate and weak inhibitor of P-glycoprotein.

Advice to Patients

Importance of instructing patients to carefully read the manufacturer's patient information before initiating eribulin therapy and also before receiving each injection of the drug.

Risk of myelosuppression; importance of patients immediately informing a clinician if they develop any symptoms of an infection (e.g., fever of 100.5°F or higher, chills, cough, burning or pain upon urination). Necessity of obtaining complete blood cell counts (CBCs) periodically.

Risk of peripheral neuropathy. Importance of patients informing a clinician if they develop any numbness, tingling, or burning in their hands or feet.

Importance of informing clinicians of existing or contemplated concomitant therapy, including prescription and OTC drugs and herbal supplements, as well as any concomitant illnesses (e.g., liver and kidney disease, heart problems including congenital long QT syndrome).

Necessity of advising women to use an effective method of contraception and to avoid breast-feeding while receiving eribulin therapy. Advise pregnant women of potential risk to the fetus. Importance of women informing a clinician immediately if they are or plan to become pregnant or plan to breast-feed.

Importance of informing patients of other important precautionary information. (See Cautions.)

Overview® (see Users Guide). For additional information on this drug until a more detailed monograph is developed and published, the manufacturer's labeling should be consulted. It is *essential* that the manufacturer's labeling be consulted for more detailed information on usual cautions, precautions, contraindications, potential drug interactions, laboratory test interferences, and acute toxicity. For further information on the handling of antineoplastic agents, see the ASHP Guidelines on Handling Hazardous Drugs at http://www.ahfsdruginformation.com.

Preparations

Excipients in commercially available drug preparations may have clinically important effects in some individuals; consult specific product labeling for details.

eriBULin Mesylate

Parenteral

Injection, for IV use only	0.5 mg/mL (1 mg)	**Halaven® (available in single-use vials),** Eisai

†Use is not currently included in the labeling approved by the US Food and Drug Administration

Erlotinib Hydrochloride

■ Erlotinib hydrochloride, an epidermal growth factor receptor (EGFR) tyrosine kinase inhibitor, is an antineoplastic agent.

Uses

■ **Non-small Cell Lung Cancer** Erlotinib hydrochloride is used for the first-line or maintenance treatment of metastatic non-small cell lung cancer (NSCLC) in patients whose tumors harbor epidermal growth factor receptor (EGFR) exon 19 deletions (del19) or exon 21 (L858R) substitution mutations as detected by an FDA-approved diagnostic test (e.g., cobas® EGFR Mutation Test); the drug also is used for second-line or subsequent treatment in such patients whose disease progressed following at least one chemotherapy regimen. Information on FDA-approved companion diagnostic tests for the detection of EGFR mutations in NSCLC is available at http://www.fda.gov/CompanionDiagnostics.

Data from 2 multicenter, randomized, placebo-controlled studies in over 1000 patients did not demonstrate any clinical benefit from concurrent administration of erlotinib with carboplatin and paclitaxel or with gemcitabine and cisplatin in the first-line setting. Therefore, the manufacturer states that use of erlotinib in combination with platinum-based chemotherapy is not recommended.

The manufacturer states that the safety and efficacy of erlotinib have not been established in patients with NSCLC whose tumors harbor EGFR mutations other than exon 19 deletions or exon 21 substitution mutations.

EGFR-activating mutations are present in approximately 15–22% of NSCLC cases in North America and Europe and are present in up to 30–50% of cases in patients of East Asian descent. The majority of EGFR mutations are exon 19 deletions and an L858R substitution in exon 21, which together account for about 90% of EGFR mutations in patients with NSCLC. (See Description.)

First-line Treatment of Metastatic Non-small Cell Lung Cancer The current indication for erlotinib in the first-line treatment of metastatic NSCLC is based principally on the results of a randomized, multicenter, open-label phase 3 study (EURTAC) in adults with newly diagnosed locally advanced or metastatic NSCLC. In this study, 174 patients were randomized (stratified by type of EGFR mutation and Eastern Cooperative Oncology Group [ECOG] performance status) in a 1:1 ratio to receive either erlotinib (150 mg orally once daily until disease progression occurred) or investigator's choice of platinum-based chemotherapy (cisplatin 75 mg/m^2 and docetaxel 75 mg/m^2 on day 1 of each 3-week cycle for 4 cycles; gemcitabine 1.25 g/m^2 on days 1 and 8 and cisplatin 75 mg/m^2 on day 1 of each 3-week cycle for 4 cycles; carboplatin at the dose required to obtain an area under the concentration-time curve [AUC] of 6 mg/mL per minute and docetaxel 75 mg/m^2 on day 1 of each 3-week cycle for 4 cycles; gemcitabine 1 g/m^2 on days 1 and 8 and carboplatin at the dose required to obtain an AUC of 5 mg/mL per minute on day 1 of each 3-week cycle for 4 cycles). The primary measure of efficacy was progression-free survival. The median age of patients was 65 years (range: 24–82 years); most patients (99%) were Caucasian, 93% had metastatic disease, 93% had adenocarcinoma histology, 72% were female, 86% had a baseline ECOG performance status of 0 or 1, 69% had never smoked, 20% were former smokers, and 11% were current smokers. The majority (66%) of patients had exon 19 deletions and 34% of patients had L858R substitution mutations as determined by a clinical trial assay. The majority (84%) of patients randomized to investigator's choice of platinum-based chemotherapy received at least one subsequent therapy; 97% of these patients received an EGFR tyrosine kinase inhibitor. Approximately 66% of patients randomized to erlotinib received at least one subsequent therapy.

In the EURTAC study, patients receiving erlotinib had longer median progression-free survival compared with patients receiving platinum-based chemotherapy (10.4 versus 5.2 months; hazard ratio of 0.34). Effects of erlotinib on investigator-assessed progression-free survival and progression-free survival as assessed by an independent review committee were comparable. Patients receiving erlotinib also had a higher objective response rate compared with those receiving platinum-based chemotherapy (65 versus 16%). At the time of analysis, no significant difference in overall survival was observed between patients receiving erlotinib and those receiving platinum-based chemotherapy. An exploratory subgroup analysis based on EGFR mutation (del19 or L858R substitution mutations) indicated that the magnitude of progression-free survival benefit from erlotinib was greater in patients with exon 19 deletions than in those with L858R substitution mutations (hazard ratio: 0.27 and 0.52, respectively); however, an overall survival benefit for the drug in patients with exon 19 deletions or L858R substitution mutations was not apparent. Subgroup analysis suggested that erlotinib had a greater effect on progression-free survival relative to platinum-based chemotherapy in patients who had never smoked than in those who were current smokers (hazard ratio: 0.24 and 0.56, respectively) and in those who had not received prior surgery or radiation therapy than in those who had previously undergone surgery (hazard ratio: 0.32 and 0.61, respectively) or radiation therapy (hazard ratio: 0.31 and 0.79, respectively); a progression-free survival benefit for the drug versus platinum-based chemotherapy was not apparent in patients who were former smokers or those who previously had received chemotherapy.

Second-line or Subsequent Treatment of Metastatic Non-small Cell Lung Cancer Safety and efficacy of erlotinib in the second-line or subsequent treatment of patients with metastatic NSCLC were established in a randomized, double-blind, placebo-controlled study in 731 patients with locally advanced or metastatic non-small cell lung cancer after failure of at least one prior chemotherapy regimen. In this study, patients were randomized on a 2:1 basis to receive either erlotinib (150 mg) or placebo, respectively, orally once daily until disease progression or unacceptable toxicity occurred; therapy was continued for a median of 9.6 weeks. The objective response rate was higher in patients receiving erlotinib (8.9%) than in those receiving placebo (0.9%). In addition, median overall survival and progression-free survival were longer in patients receiving erlotinib (6.7 and 2.3 months, respectively) than in those receiving placebo (4.7 and 1.8 months, respectively).

Maintenance Therapy The current indication for maintenance therapy with erlotinib is based principally on the results of a randomized, double-blind, placebo-controlled phase 3 study (Sequential Tarceva® in Unresectable NSCLC [SATURN]) in adults with metastatic NSCLC who did not experience disease progression following prior platinum-based chemotherapy. In this study, 889 patients were randomized in a 1:1 ratio to receive either erlotinib (150 mg orally once daily) or placebo until disease progression or unacceptable toxicity occurred. The primary measure of efficacy was progression-free survival. The median age of patients was 60 years (range: 30–83 years); most patients (84%) were Caucasian, 74% were male, 55% were current smokers, 27% were former smokers, 17% had never smoked, and 15% of patients were of Asian ancestry. The majority (75%) of patients had metastatic disease and 25% of patients had stage IIIB disease with pleural effusion; approximately one-half (45%) of patients had adenocarcinoma/bronchoalveolar carcinoma, 40% had squamous histology, and 5% had large cell carcinoma. The majority (70%) of patients had positive EGFR expression as detected by an immunohistochemistry assay; 14% of patients had negative EGFR expression.

In the SATURN study, the risk of disease progression or death was reduced by 29 or 19%, respectively, in patients receiving erlotinib maintenance therapy compared with those receiving placebo. Progression-free survival and overall survival benefits were observed in the overall study population and in patients with positive EGFR expression. Results of a subgroup analysis (based on age, gender, ethnicity, ECOG performance status, disease stage, histology) suggested that the effect of erlotinib on progression-free survival and overall survival was evident across all subgroups.

The manufacturer states that the safety and efficacy of erlotinib have not been established in patients with NSCLC whose tumors harbor EGFR mutations other than exon 19 deletions or exon 21 substitution mutations. In a multicenter, randomized, placebo-controlled study, clinical benefit was not demonstrated in 643 patients with advanced NSCLC without exon 19 deletions or exon 21 (L858R) substitution mutations who received erlotinib maintenance therapy.

■ **Pancreatic Cancer** Erlotinib is used in combination with gemcitabine for the first-line treatment of locally advanced, unresectable or metastatic pancreatic cancer.

The safety and efficacy of erlotinib and gemcitabine as first-line therapy for locally advanced, unresectable or metastatic pancreatic cancer was evaluated in a randomized, double-blind, placebo-controlled trial in 569 patients. Patients received either erlotinib (100 mg or 150 mg) or placebo orally once daily in combination with gemcitabine 1 g/m^2 IV once weekly (for 7 consecutive weeks of an 8-week cycle and thereafter for 3 consecutive weeks of a 4-week cycle) until disease progression or unacceptable toxicity. Because of the small number of patients receiving erlotinib 150 mg or placebo (24 patients in each group), efficacy and safety results are reported only for the patients receiving erlotinib 100 mg (261 patients) or placebo (260 patients). These groups were comparable except there were more females in the group receiving erlotinib 100 mg (51%) than in the group receiving placebo (44%). Upon entry to the study, most of the patients (about 76%) had metastatic disease as the initial manifestation of pancreatic cancer.

Patients receiving erlotinib and gemcitabine had longer median overall survival (6.5 versus 6 months) and median progression-free survival (3.8 versus 3.6 months) than those receiving placebo and gemcitabine as first-line therapy for locally advanced, unresectable or metastatic pancreatic cancer. The objective response rate was 8.6 or 7.9% in patients receiving erlotinib and gemcitabine or placebo and gemcitabine, respectively. Among the most common adverse effects, rash (70 versus 30%) and diarrhea (48 versus 36%) occurred more frequently in patients receiving erlotinib and gemcitabine than in those receiving placebo and gemcitabine.

Dosage and Administration

■ **General** Confirmation of the presence of epidermal growth factor receptor (EGFR) exon 19 deletions (del19) or exon 21 (L858R) substitution mutations in tumor or plasma specimens of patients with metastatic non-small cell lung cancer (NSCLC) by an FDA-approved diagnostic test is necessary prior to initiating therapy with erlotinib. Patients with a negative plasma del19 or L858R mutation result should be reevaluated for the feasibility of a tumor biopsy. (See Uses: Non-small Cell Lung Cancer.)

■ **Administration** Erlotinib hydrochloride is administered orally once daily. The drug should be administered on an empty stomach (e.g., at least 1 hour before or 2 hours after ingestion of food).

■ **Dosage** Dosage of erlotinib hydrochloride is expressed in terms of erlotinib.

Non-small Cell Lung Cancer For the first-line or subsequent treatment or maintenance treatment of metastatic NSCLC in patients whose tumors harbor EGFR del19 or L858R substitution mutations and progressed following at least one chemotherapy regimen, the usual adult dosage of erlotinib is 150 mg once daily. Treatment should be continued until disease progression or unacceptable toxicity occurs.

Pancreatic Cancer For the first-line treatment of locally advanced, unresectable or metastatic pancreatic cancer, erlotinib 100 mg once daily, is used in combination with gemcitabine. In the randomized trial, patients received erlotinib in combination with gemcitabine 1 g/m^2 IV once weekly (for 7 consecutive weeks of an 8-week cycle and thereafter for 3 consecutive weeks of a 4-week cycle). Treatment should be continued until disease progression or unacceptable toxicity occurs.

Dosage Modification for Toxicity and Contraindications for Continued Therapy Dosage interruption and/or reduction, or discontinuance of erlotinib therapy, may be necessary based on severity of adverse reactions. When dosage reduction is required, the erlotinib dose should be reduced in 50-mg decrements.

Pulmonary Toxicity. In patients who experience acute onset of new or progressive pulmonary manifestations (e.g., dyspnea, cough, fever), treatment with erlotinib should be interrupted pending diagnostic evaluation. If interstitial lung disease is diagnosed, erlotinib should be permanently discontinued. If interstitial lung disease is excluded, erlotinib may be resumed at a reduced dosage when the pulmonary manifestations resolve completely or improve to grade 1 or less. (See Pulmonary Toxicity under Cautions: Warnings/Precautions.)

Renal Toxicity. If severe (grade 3 or 4) renal toxicity occurs, discontinuance of erlotinib therapy should be considered. Alternatively, erlotinib therapy may be interrupted; when the toxicity resolves completely or improves to grade 1 or less, erlotinib may be resumed at a reduced dosage. (See Renal Failure under Cautions: Warnings/Precautions.)

Hepatotoxicity. If total bilirubin concentrations increase to 2 times baseline values or serum aminotransferase concentrations increase to 3 times baseline values in patients with preexisting hepatic impairment or biliary obstruction, discontinuance of erlotinib therapy should be considered. Alternatively, erlotinib therapy may be interrupted; when hepatic impairment resolves or improves to grade 1 or less, erlotinib may be resumed at a reduced dosage. (See Hepatic Toxicity under Cautions: Warnings/Precautions.)

If elevated total bilirubin concentrations greater than 3 times the upper limit of normal (ULN) or serum aminotransferase concentrations greater than 5 times the ULN occur in patients without preexisting hepatic impairment, discontinuance of erlotinib therapy should be considered. Alternatively, erlotinib therapy may be interrupted; when hepatic impairment resolves or improves to grade 1 or less, erlotinib may be resumed at a reduced dosage.

If severe hepatotoxicity occurs and does not improve substantially or resolve within 3 weeks, erlotinib should be discontinued.

GI Toxicity. In patients with severe and persistent diarrhea that is unresponsive to medical management (e.g., loperamide), erlotinib therapy should be interrupted. When the toxicity resolves completely or improves to grade 1 or less, erlotinib may be resumed at a reduced dosage. (See Diarrhea under Cautions: Warnings/Precautions.)

If GI perforation occurs, erlotinib therapy should be permanently discontinued. (See GI Perforation under Cautions: Warnings/Precautions.)

Dermatologic Toxicity. If severe rash unresponsive to medical management occurs, erlotinib therapy should be interrupted. When the rash resolves completely or improves to grade 1 or less, erlotinib may be resumed at a reduced dosage.

In patients with severe skin reactions, such as severe bullous, blistering, or exfoliative conditions, erlotinib therapy should be discontinued. (See Bullous and Exfoliative Skin Disorders under Cautions: Warnings/Precautions.)

Ocular Toxicity. In patients who experience acute or worsening ocular toxicity, such as eye pain, discontinuance of erlotinib therapy should be considered. Alternatively, erlotinib therapy may be interrupted; when the toxicity resolves completely or improves to grade 1 or less, erlotinib may be resumed at a reduced dosage.

If grade 3 or 4 keratitis or persistent (lasting longer than 2 weeks) grade 2 keratitis occurs, erlotinib therapy should be interrupted. When toxicity resolves completely or improves to grade 1 or less, erlotinib may be resumed at a reduced dosage.

In patients who experience corneal perforation or severe corneal ulceration, erlotinib therapy should be discontinued. (See Corneal Ulceration or Perforation under Cautions: Warnings/Precautions.)

Concomitant Use with Drugs and Foods Affecting Hepatic Microsomal Enzymes. Concomitant use with potent inhibitors of cytochrome P-450 (CYP) isoenzyme 3A4 (e.g., atazanavir, clarithromycin, conivaptan, indinavir, itraconazole, ketoconazole, lopinavir/ritonavir, nefazodone, nelfinavir, posaconazole, ritonavir, saquinavir, telithromycin, voriconazole) or combined inhibitors of CYP3A4 and CYP1A2 (e.g., ciprofloxacin) should be avoided. If concomitant use cannot be avoided, the manufacturer recommends reducing the dosage of erlotinib in 50-mg decrements. (See Drug Interactions: Drugs and Foods Affecting Hepatic Microsomal Enzymes.)

Concomitant use with an inducer of CYP3A4 (e.g., carbamazepine, phenobarbital, phenytoin, rifabutin, rifampin, rifapentine, St. John's wort [*Hypericum perforatum*]) should be avoided. If concomitant use cannot be avoided, the manufacturer recommends increasing the dosage of erlotinib in 50-mg increments (not to exceed 450 mg daily) as tolerated at 2-week intervals. (See Drug Interactions: Drugs and Foods Affecting Hepatic Microsomal Enzymes.)

Concomitant use with moderate inducers of CYP1A2 (e.g., phenytoin, rifampin, teriflunomide) should be avoided. If concomitant use cannot be avoided, the manufacturer recommends increasing the dosage of erlotinib. (See Drug Interactions: Drugs and Foods Affecting Hepatic Microsomal Enzymes.)

Cigarette Smoking. Because cigarette smoking reduces systemic exposure to erlotinib, patients should be advised to stop smoking. In patients who continue to smoke, the manufacturer recommends increasing the dosage of erlotinib in 50-mg increments (not to exceed 300 mg daily) at 2-week intervals. Upon cessation of smoking, the erlotinib dose should be reduced immediately to the recommended starting dose. (See Drug Interactions: Cigarette Smoking.)

Grapefruit. Concomitant use with grapefruit or grapefruit juice, a potent inhibitor of CYP3A4, should be avoided. If concomitant use cannot be avoided, the manufacturer recommends reducing the dosage of erlotinib in 50-mg decrements.

■ **Special Populations** Dosage interruption or discontinuance of erlotinib therapy should be considered if abnormal liver function tests occur in patients with preexisting hepatic impairment. (See Hepatic Impairment under Warnings/Precautions: Specific Populations, in Cautions.)

The manufacturer currently makes no special dosage recommendations for geriatric patients or patients with renal impairment. (See Geriatric Use and also see Renal Impairment under Warnings/Precautions: Specific Populations, in Cautions.)

Cautions

■ **Contraindications** The manufacturer states that there are no known contraindications to the use of erlotinib.

■ **Warnings/Precautions** ***Pulmonary Toxicity*** Serious, sometimes fatal, interstitial lung disease has occurred in patients receiving erlotinib. Interstitial lung disease has been reported in approximately 1.1% of patients receiving erlotinib in controlled and uncontrolled studies. Onset of manifestations occurred from 5 days to more than 9 months (median: 39 days) after initiating erlotinib therapy.

Interruption or discontinuance of erlotinib therapy may be required in patients experiencing pulmonary toxicity. (See Pulmonary Toxicity under Dosage: Dosage Modification for Toxicity and Contraindications for Continued Therapy, in Dosage and Administration.)

Renal Failure Hepatorenal syndrome or acute renal failure, sometimes fatal, and renal insufficiency have been reported in patients receiving erlotinib. Factors contributing to these adverse renal effects included baseline hepatic impairment and severe dehydration. In clinical studies for non-small cell lung cancer (NSCLC), severe renal impairment occurred in 0.5% of patients receiving erlotinib monotherapy compared with 0.8% of those assigned to the control groups. In the principal efficacy study for pancreatic cancer, renal impairment occurred in 1.4% of patients receiving erlotinib and gemcitabine versus 0.4% of those receiving placebo and gemcitabine.

Renal function and serum electrolytes should be monitored periodically.

If severe (grade 3 or 4) renal impairment occurs, erlotinib therapy should be interrupted or discontinued. (See Renal Toxicity under Dosage: Dosage Modification for Toxicity and Contraindications for Continued Therapy, in Dosage and Administration.)

Hepatic Toxicity Hepatic failure and hepatorenal syndrome, sometimes fatal, have occurred in patients receiving erlotinib, particularly in patients with hepatic impairment prior to treatment. In clinical studies for NSCLC, which excluded patients with baseline moderate to severe hepatic impairment, hepatic failure occurred in 0.4% of patients receiving erlotinib monotherapy compared with none of those assigned to the control groups. In the principal efficacy study for pancreatic cancer, the reported incidence of hepatic failure (0.4%) was similar between patients receiving erlotinib and gemcitabine and those receiving placebo and gemcitabine.

In a small subset of 15 patients with substantial tumor burden in the liver and moderate hepatic impairment (Child-Pugh class B), 10 patients died within 30 days of the last dose of erlotinib; 6 of the 10 patients had baseline total bilirubin concentrations greater than 3 times the upper limit of normal (ULN). Hepatorenal syndrome and rapidly progressing hepatic failure were the cause of death in 2 patients; the remaining 8 patients died from disease progression.

Liver function tests (i.e., serum concentrations of aminotransferases, bilirubin, and alkaline phosphatase) should be monitored periodically during therapy and more frequently in patients with preexisting hepatic impairment (e.g., total bilirubin concentrations greater than 3 times the ULN) or biliary obstruction. Erlotinib therapy should be interrupted or discontinued if changes in liver function are severe. (See Hepatotoxicity under Dosage: Dosage Modification for Toxicity and Contraindications for Continued Therapy, in Dosage and Administration.)

GI Perforation GI perforation, sometimes fatal, has been reported in patients receiving erlotinib. Patients with a history of peptic ulcer disease or diverticulitis and those who are receiving concomitant therapy with antiangiogenesis drugs, corticosteroids, nonsteroidal anti-inflammatory agents (NSAIAs), and/or taxane-based chemotherapy are at increased risk for perforation while receiving erlotinib therapy. In clinical studies for NSCLC, GI perforation occurred in 0.2% of patients receiving erlotinib monotherapy compared with 0.1% of those assigned to the control groups. In the principal efficacy study for pancreatic cancer, GI perforation occurred in 0.4% of patients receiving erlotinib and gemcitabine compared with none of those receiving placebo and gemcitabine. If GI perforation occurs, erlotinib therapy should be permanently discontinued.

Bullous and Exfoliative Skin Disorders Bullous, blistering, and exfoliative skin reactions, including cases suggestive of Stevens-Johnson syndrome or toxic epidermal necrolysis, have been reported in patients receiving erlotinib therapy; some cases have been fatal. In clinical studies for NSCLC, bullous and exfoliative skin reactions occurred in 1.2% of patients receiving erlotinib monotherapy compared with none of those assigned to the control groups. In the principal efficacy study for pancreatic cancer, GI perforation occurred in 0.4% of patients receiving erlotinib and gemcitabine compared with none of those receiving placebo and gemcitabine. If severe dermatologic reactions occur, erlotinib therapy should be interrupted or discontinued. (See Dermatologic Toxicity under Dosage: Dosage Modification for Toxicity and Contraindications for Continued Therapy, in Dosage and Administration.)

Cerebrovascular Accident In the principal efficacy study for pancreatic cancer, cerebrovascular accidents occurred in 7 patients (2.5%) receiving erlotinib and gemcitabine compared with none of those receiving placebo and gemcitabine; one of these events was a hemorrhagic stroke and the patient died. In clinical studies for NSCLC, cerebrovascular accident occurred in 0.6% of patients receiving erlotinib monotherapy.

Microangiopathic Hemolytic Anemia with Thrombocytopenia In clinical studies for NSCLC, microangiopathic hemolytic anemia with thrombocytopenia occurred in none of the patients receiving erlotinib monotherapy compared with 0.1% of those assigned to the control groups. In the principal efficacy study for pancreatic cancer, microangiopathic hemolytic anemia with thrombocytopenia occurred in 1.4% of patients receiving erlotinib and gemcitabine compared with none of those receiving placebo and gemcitabine.

Corneal Ulceration or Perforation Abnormal eyelash growth, keratoconjunctivitis sicca (i.e., dry eye), keratitis, and decreased lacrimation may occur in patients receiving erlotinib and are considered risk factors for corneal ulceration or perforation. In clinical studies for NSCLC, ocular disorders occurred in 17.8% of patients receiving erlotinib monotherapy compared with 4% of those assigned to the control groups. In the principal efficacy study for pancreatic cancer, ocular disorders occurred in 12.8% of patients receiving erlotinib and gemcitabine compared with 11.4% of those receiving placebo and gemcitabine. If patients experience ocular toxicity, erlotinib therapy should be interrupted or discontinued. (See Ocular Toxicity under Dosage: Dosage Modification for Toxicity and Contraindications for Continued Therapy, in Dosage and Administration.)

Fetal/Neonatal Morbidity and Mortality Erlotinib may cause fetal harm in humans based on its mechanism of action and animal findings; the drug has been shown to be embryotoxic and fetotoxic in animals. Limited data are available regarding use of erlotinib in pregnant women; data are insufficient to inform a drug-associated risk of adverse developmental outcomes or miscarriage. Embryofetal toxicity (e.g., embryofetal lethality, abortion) has been demonstrated in animals receiving the drug at exposure levels equivalent to approximately 3 times the human exposure at the recommended erlotinib dosage of 150 mg daily. In a fertility study, increased early resorptions were observed in animals receiving the drug at exposure levels equivalent to 0.3 or 0.7 times the human exposure at the recommended daily dosage.

Pregnancy should be avoided during erlotinib therapy. Women of childbearing potential should be advised to use effective contraception while receiving erlotinib and for 1 month after the last dose of the drug. Patients should be apprised of the potential fetal hazard or potential risk for loss of the pregnancy if erlotinib is used during pregnancy.

Dermatologic Effects Among patients receiving erlotinib monotherapy for NSCLC in controlled studies, rash was reported in 60–85% of patients, with the highest incidence occurring in patients receiving erlotinib as first-line therapy for NSCLC; grade 3 or 4 rash was reported in 9–14% of patients. The median time to onset of rash was 15 days in those receiving erlotinib as first-line therapy, 10 days in those receiving the drug as maintenance therapy, and 8 days in those receiving the drug as second- or third-line therapy. In studies of erlotinib monotherapy for NSCLC, dosage modification was required because of rash in 13% of patients receiving the drug as first-line therapy, 5% of those receiving the drug as maintenance therapy, and 6% of those receiving the drug as second- or third-line therapy; in addition, 1% of patients receiving erlotinib as maintenance therapy or as second- or third-line therapy withdrew from the studies because of rash.

Among patients receiving erlotinib and gemcitabine for pancreatic cancer in a randomized trial, rash was reported in 70% of patients; grade 3 or 4 rash was reported in 5% of patients. The median time to onset of rash was 10 days. Approximately 3% of patients receiving erlotinib and gemcitabine required dosage reduction or withdrew from the study because of rash.

Hyperpigmentation or dry skin, with or without digital skin fissures, may occur. Rash may occur or worsen in sun-exposed areas of the skin. (See Advice to Patients.) Dosage modification of erlotinib therapy may be necessary depending on the severity of the rash. (See Dermatologic Toxicity under Dosage: Dosage Modification for Toxicity and Contraindications for Continued Therapy, in Dosage and Administration.)

Diarrhea Among patients receiving erlotinib monotherapy for NSCLC in controlled studies, diarrhea occurred in 20–62%, with the highest incidence occurring in patients receiving erlotinib as first-line therapy for NSCLC; grade 3 or 4 diarrhea was reported in 2–7% of patients. The median time to onset of diarrhea was 32 days in those receiving erlotinib as first-line therapy, 15 days in those receiving the drug as maintenance therapy, and 12 days in those receiving the drug as second- or third-line therapy. In studies of erlotinib monotherapy for NSCLC, dosage modification was required because of diarrhea in 10% of patients receiving the drug as first-line therapy, 3% of those receiving the drug as maintenance therapy, and 1% of those receiving the drug as second- or third-line therapy; in addition, 0.5% of patients receiving erlotinib as maintenance therapy and 1% of those receiving the drug as second- or third-line therapy withdrew from the studies because of diarrhea.

Among patients receiving erlotinib and gemcitabine for pancreatic cancer in a randomized trial, diarrhea occurred in 48% and stomatitis in 22%; grade 3 or 4 diarrhea was reported in approximately 6% of patients. The median time to onset of diarrhea was 15 days. Approximately 3% of patients receiving erlotinib and gemcitabine required dosage reduction or withdrew from the study because of diarrhea. (See GI Toxicity under Dosage: Dosage Modification for Toxicity and Contraindications for Continued Therapy, in Dosage and Administration.)

Diarrhea usually can be managed with loperamide. However, if diarrhea becomes severe and is unresponsive to loperamide, temporary interruption of therapy and dosage reduction may be required.

Elevated International Normalized Ratio (INR) and Bleeding Increased INR and hemorrhagic events, sometimes fatal, have been reported in clinical studies; some of these patients were receiving erlotinib concomitantly with warfarin or a nonsteroidal anti-inflammatory agent (NSAIA). (See Drug Interactions.) GI bleeding included peptic ulcer bleeding (gastritis, gastroduodenal ulcers), hematemesis, hematochezia, melena, and hemorrhage from possible colitis.

Specific Populations **Pregnancy.** Erlotinib may cause fetal harm if administered to pregnant women based on its mechanism of action and animal findings. (See Fetal/Neonatal Morbidity and Mortality under Cautions: Warnings/Precautions.)

Lactation. It is not known whether erlotinib is distributed into human milk or if the drug or its metabolites have any effect on milk production or the nursing infant. Because of the potential for serious adverse reactions to erlotinib in nursing infants, women should be advised not to breast-feed while receiving the drug and for 2 weeks after the last dose of the drug.

Pediatric Use. Safety and efficacy of erlotinib have not been established in pediatric patients.

In a clinical trial, 25 patients 3–20 years of age with recurrent or refractory ependymoma received erlotinib (85 mg/m^2 orally daily). No overall difference in safety relative to adults was observed.

Among patients 2–21 years of age, age did not appear to substantially affect erlotinib clearance normalized to body surface area in a population pharmacokinetic analysis.

Geriatric Use. In clinical studies in patients with NSCLC or pancreatic cancer, 40% of patients receiving erlotinib were 65 years of age or older and 10% were 75 years of age or older. No overall differences in safety and efficacy relative to younger adults were observed.

Hepatic Impairment. Although erlotinib is eliminated mainly by the liver, systemic exposure was not substantially altered in patients with Child-Pugh class B hepatic impairment relative to those with adequate hepatic function (including individuals with primary liver cancer or hepatic metastases); however, because hepatic failure and hepatorenal syndrome, sometimes fatal, have been reported in patients with normal hepatic function, the risk of hepatotoxicity is increased in patients with preexisting hepatic impairment. Close monitoring is required during erlotinib therapy in patients with hepatic impairment (total bilirubin concentrations greater than the upper limit of normal [ULN] or Child-Pugh class A, B, or C); patients with biliary obstruction or total bilirubin concentrations greater than 3 times the ULN should be monitored more frequently. If worsening of liver dysfunction occurs, interruption of erlotinib therapy or reduction of erlotinib dosage accompanied by frequent monitoring of liver function tests should be considered before changes in liver function become severe. If severe changes in liver function test results, such as doubling of total bilirubin and/or tripling of serum aminotransferase concentrations, occur in patients with hepatic dysfunction prior to treatment, erlotinib therapy should be interrupted or discontinued. (See Hepatotoxicity under Dosage: Dosage Modification for Toxicity and Contraindications for Continued Therapy, in Dosage and Administration.)

Renal Impairment. Safety and efficacy of erlotinib have not been established in patients with renal impairment.

■ **Common Adverse Effects** Adverse effects occurring in 10% or more of patients receiving erlotinib monotherapy as first-line therapy for NSCLC harboring EGFR exon 19 deletions (del19) or exon 21 (L858R) substitution mutations and at an incidence at least 5% greater than with platinum-based chemotherapy include rash, diarrhea, cough, dyspnea, dry skin, back pain, chest pain, conjunctivitis, mucosal inflammation, pruritus, paronychia, arthralgia, and musculoskeletal pain.

Adverse effects occurring in 10% or more of patients receiving erlotinib monotherapy as second-line or subsequent therapy for NSCLC harboring EGFR del19 or L858R substitution mutations and at an incidence at least 5% greater than with placebo include rash, diarrhea, anorexia, fatigue, dyspnea, nausea, infection, stomatitis, pruritus, dry skin, conjunctivitis, and keratoconjunctivitis sicca.

Adverse effects occurring in 10% or more of patients receiving erlotinib monotherapy as maintenance therapy for NSCLC harboring EGFR del19 or L858R substitution mutations and at an incidence at least 5% greater than with placebo include rash and diarrhea.

Adverse effects occurring in 10% or more of patients receiving erlotinib in combination with gemcitabine for pancreatic cancer and at an incidence at least 5% greater than with placebo and gemcitabine include rash, diarrhea, decreased weight, infection, pyrexia, stomatitis, depression, cough, and headache.

Drug Interactions

Erlotinib is metabolized principally by cytochrome P-450 (CYP) isoenzyme 3A4 and, to a lesser extent, CYP1A1 and CYP1A2.

■ Drugs and Foods Affecting Hepatic Microsomal Enzymes

Inhibitors of CYP3A4 Concomitant use of erlotinib with potent inhibitors of CYP3A4 may result in increased erlotinib exposure. When the potent CYP3A4 inhibitor ketoconazole was administered concomitantly with erlotinib, the area under the concentration-time curve (AUC) of erlotinib was increased by 67%. Concomitant use of erlotinib with potent CYP3A4 inhibitors (e.g., atazanavir, clarithromycin, conivaptan, indinavir, itraconazole, ketoconazole, lopinavir/ritonavir, nefazodone, nelfinavir, posaconazole, ritonavir, saquinavir, telithromycin, voriconazole, grapefruit or grapefruit juice) should be avoided. If concomitant use cannot be avoided, the manufacturer recommends reducing the dosage of erlotinib in 50-mg decrements.

Combined Inhibitors of CYP3A4 and 1A2 Concomitant use of erlotinib with combined inhibitors of CYP3A4 and 1A2 may result in increased peak plasma concentrations and systemic exposure of erlotinib. When the combined CYP3A4 and CYP1A2 inhibitor ciprofloxacin was administered concomitantly with erlotinib, the peak plasma concentration and AUC of erlotinib was increased by 17 and 39%, respectively. Concomitant use of erlotinib with combined CYP3A4 and CYP1A2 inhibitors (e.g., ciprofloxacin) should be avoided. If concomitant use cannot be avoided, the manufacturer recommends reducing the dosage of erlotinib in 50-mg decrements.

Inducers of CYP3A4 Concomitant use of erlotinib with inducers of CYP3A4 may result in decreased erlotinib exposure. When the CYP3A4 inducer rifampin was administered 7–11 days prior to erlotinib, the AUC of erlotinib was decreased by 58–80%. Concomitant use of erlotinib with CYP3A4 inducers (e.g., carbamazepine, phenobarbital, phenytoin, rifabutin, rifampin, rifapentine, St. John's wort [*Hypericum perforatum*]) should be avoided. If concomitant use with these agents cannot be avoided, the manufacturer recommends increasing the dosage of erlotinib in 50-mg increments (not to exceed 450 mg daily) as tolerated at 2-week intervals.

Inducers of CYP1A2 Concomitant use of erlotinib with moderate inducers of CYP1A2 may result in decreased erlotinib exposure. Concomitant use with moderate CYP1A2 inducers (e.g., phenytoin, rifampin, teriflunomide) should be avoided. If concomitant use with these agents cannot be avoided, the manufacturer recommends increasing the dosage of erlotinib.

■ Cigarette Smoking

Because cigarette smoking moderately induces CYP1A2, concomitant cigarette smoking may result in decreased systemic exposure to erlotinib. Patients should be advised to stop smoking. Cigarette smoking decreases the AUC of erlotinib by approximately 64%. In a clinical trial, clearance of erlotinib was increased by 24% resulting in steady-state plasma trough concentrations of erlotinib approximately twofold less in current smokers compared with those who never smoked or were former smokers. In a pharmacokinetic analysis in current smokers, steady-state exposure of erlotinib increased in a dose-proportional manner following an increase in erlotinib dosage from 150 to 300 mg.

If patients continue to smoke, the manufacturer recommends increasing the dosage of erlotinib in 50-mg increments (not to exceed 300 mg daily) at 2-week intervals. Upon cessation of smoking, the erlotinib dose should be reduced immediately to the recommended starting dose.

■ Drugs Affecting Gastric Acidity

Drugs that increase the pH of the upper GI tract decrease the solubility of erlotinib and reduce its bioavailability. Concomitant administration of omeprazole, a proton-pump inhibitor, decreased the peak plasma concentration and AUC of erlotinib by 61 and 46%, respectively. Increasing the dose level of erlotinib is not likely to compensate for the loss of exposure, and separation of doses may not eliminate the interaction because proton-pump inhibitors have an extended effect on the pH of the upper GI tract. If possible, the concomitant use of erlotinib and proton-pump inhibitors should be avoided.

If use of a histamine H_2-receptor antagonist (e.g., ranitidine) is necessary, the H_2-receptor antagonist should be administered 10 hours before or at least 2 hours after a dose of erlotinib. Concomitant administration of ranitidine (300 mg) administered 2 hours prior to erlotinib decreased the peak plasma concentration and AUC of erlotinib by 54 and 33%, respectively; however, when ranitidine (150 mg twice daily) was administered at least 10 hours before or 2 hours after erlotinib, the peak plasma concentration and AUC of erlotinib decreased by 17 and 15%, respectively.

The effect of antacids on the pharmacokinetics of erlotinib has not been studied. If use of an antacid is necessary, the antacid dose and the erlotinib dose should be separated by several hours.

■ Antineoplastic Agents

Concomitant use of erlotinib with gemcitabine did not affect the clearance of erlotinib.

Concomitant use of erlotinib with paclitaxel and carboplatin in patients with cancers other than non-small cell lung cancer (NSCLC) did not substantially alter the pharmacokinetics of these antineoplastic agents.

Concomitant use of erlotinib with gemcitabine and cisplatin in patients with cancers other than NSCLC did not substantially alter the pharmacokinetics of these antineoplastic agents.

Concomitant use of erlotinib with capecitabine and docetaxel in patients with cancers other than NSCLC did not substantially alter the pharmacokinetics of these antineoplastic agents.

Concomitant use of erlotinib with docetaxel in patients with cancers other than NSCLC did not substantially alter the pharmacokinetics of either drug.

Concomitant use of erlotinib with capecitabine in patients with pancreatic cancer did not substantially alter the pharmacokinetics of either drug.

■ Crizotinib

Concomitant use of erlotinib with crizotinib 150 or 200 mg twice daily in patients with NSCLC increased the AUC of erlotinib by 1.5- or 1.8-fold, respectively.

■ Warfarin

Increased international normalized ratio [INR] and hemorrhagic events, sometimes fatal, have been reported in patients receiving erlotinib concomitantly with coumarin-derivative anticoagulants, including warfarin. Prothrombin time (PT) or INR should be monitored regularly in patients receiving erlotinib concomitantly with warfarin or other coumarin-derivative anticoagulants. Dosage adjustment of erlotinib is not necessary.

Description

Erlotinib, a reversible inhibitor of epidermal growth factor receptor (EGFR/human epidermal growth factor receptor type 1 [HER1]/ErbB1) and mutated EGFR (e.g., exon 19 deletion [del19], exon 21 substitution [L858R]) tyrosine kinases, is an antineoplastic agent. EGFR is expressed on the cell surface of many cancer cells, as well as many normal cells; activation of EGFR tyrosine kinase is thought to initiate a cascade of intracellular signaling events leading to cell proliferation and influencing processes critical to cell survival and tumor progression (e.g., angiogenesis, apoptosis, metastasis). Some EGFR-activating mutations, such as exon 19 deletion (del19) and exon 21 (L858R) substitution mutation, contribute to increased cell proliferation and survival in non-small cell lung cancer (NSCLC) cells harboring these mutations. The drug binds to the kinase domains of EGFR and reversibly inhibits tyrosine kinase phosphorylation, resulting in downregulation of EGFR signaling. Erlotinib has demonstrated a greater affinity for cell lines expressing del19 or L858R mutations than for wild-type EGFR. Specificity with regard to other tyrosine kinase receptors has not been fully characterized.

Approximately 60% of an oral dose of erlotinib is absorbed from the GI tract; presence of food in the GI tract increases oral bioavailability to approximately 100%. (See Dosage and Administration: Administration.) Peak plasma concentrations of erlotinib occur at 4 hours following oral administration. Steady-state concentrations of erlotinib are achieved within 7–8 days. Erlotinib is 93% bound to plasma proteins (mainly to albumin and α_1-acid glycoprotein). Erlotinib is extensively metabolized via the cytochrome P-450 (CYP) enzyme system, mainly by CYP3A4 and, to a lesser extent, by CYP1A1 (principally an extrahepatic enzyme) and CYP1A2. The half-life of erlotinib is approximately 36 hours; the clearance is approximately 24% higher in smokers. Following a 100-mg oral dose, erlotinib is excreted mainly as metabolites in feces (83%) and urine (8%).

Systemic exposure of erlotinib does not appear to be affected substantially by age, body weight, or gender in patients receiving the drug as a single agent for maintenance or second- or third-line therapy in NSCLC or in combination with gemcitabine for the treatment of pancreatic cancer.

Advice to Patients

Importance of skin care, including alcohol-free emollient cream and use of sunscreen or avoidance of sun exposure, to minimize the risk of skin reactions during erlotinib therapy.

Risk of serious dermatologic reactions. Importance of immediately informing clinician if severe dermatologic reactions occur.

Risk of diarrhea. Importance of informing clinician if severe or persistent diarrhea occurs.

Risk of interstitial lung disease. Importance of immediately informing clinician if new or worsening respiratory symptoms (e.g., dyspnea, cough) occur.

Risk of renal failure and importance of periodic monitoring.

Risk of hepatotoxicity and importance of periodic liver function test monitoring. Importance of reporting any manifestations of hepatotoxicity.

Risk of GI perforation and fistula formation. Importance of advising patients to seek immediate medical attention if they experience symptoms of GI perforation (e.g., severe abdominal pain).

Risk of cerebrovascular accident. Importance of advising patients to seek immediate medical attention if they experience symptoms of cerebrovascular accident.

Risk of ocular disorders. Importance of promptly informing clinician if ocular problems (e.g., lacrimation, sensitivity to light, eye pain, redness, blurred vision, other vision changes) occur.

Risk of hair or nail disorders (e.g., hirsutism, brittle or loose nails).

Importance of advising smokers to stop smoking during erlotinib therapy because plasma concentrations of the drug and therapeutic efficacy may be reduced.

Importance of women using an effective method of contraception while receiving erlotinib therapy and for one month after discontinuance of therapy. If pregnancy occurs, advise patient of risk to the fetus.

Importance of women informing clinicians if they plan to breast-feed. Importance of advising women to avoid breast-feeding while receiving erlotinib and for 2 weeks after discontinuance of therapy.

Importance of informing clinicians of existing or contemplated concomitant therapy, including prescription and OTC drugs (e.g., warfarin), as well as any concomitant illnesses.

Importance of informing patients of other important precautionary information. (See Cautions.)

Overview® (see Users Guide). For additional information on this drug until a more detailed monograph is developed and published, the manufacturer's labeling should be consulted. It is *essential* that the manufacturer's labeling be consulted for more detailed information on usual cautions, precautions, contraindications, potential drug interactions, laboratory test interferences, and acute toxicity. For further information on the handling of antineoplastic agents, see the ASHP Guidelines on Handling Hazardous Drugs at http://www.ahfsdruginformation.com.

Preparations

Excipients in commercially available drug preparations may have clinically important effects in some individuals; consult specific product labeling for details.

Erlotinib Hydrochloride

Oral		
Tablets	25 mg (of erlotinib)	**Tarceva®**, Genentech
	100 mg (of erlotinib)	**Tarceva®**, Genentech
	150 mg (of erlotinib)	**Tarceva®**, Genentech

Etoposide

■ Etoposide is a semisynthetic podophyllotoxin-derivative antineoplastic agent.

Uses

■ **Testicular Neoplasms** Etoposide or etoposide phosphate may be used IV as a component of various chemotherapeutic regimens for the treatment of refractory testicular tumors in patients who have already received appropriate surgery, chemotherapy, and radiation therapy. Adequate data on the use of oral etoposide for the treatment of testicular tumors are currently not available.

Nonseminomatous Testicular Carcinoma In the treatment of disseminated nonseminomatous testicular carcinoma (Stage III), etoposide alone produces an objective response in about 35% of patients and is active in some patients whose disease is refractory to cisplatin-containing combination chemotherapy; however, combination chemotherapy for induction of remissions is superior to single-agent therapy. Various regimens have been used in combination therapy, and comparative efficacy is continually being evaluated. Most clinicians use cisplatin-containing combination chemotherapy regimens as initial therapy in patients with Stage III or unresectable Stage II nonseminomatous testicular carcinoma; if the patient has persistent, localized tumor following chemotherapy, the residual tumor is removed surgically, and if the disease contains malignant elements, additional chemotherapy is administered. Combination chemotherapy regimens containing etoposide and cisplatin have been evaluated in the treatment of disseminated nonseminomatous testicular carcinomas. For the initial treatment of advanced nonseminomatous testicular carcinoma, most clinicians recommend regimens containing cisplatin and bleomycin, in combination with etoposide rather than vinblastine, particularly because of the reduced neuromuscular toxicity and evidence suggesting greater efficacy in poor-risk patients. In addition, while a regimen of etoposide, cisplatin, and bleomycin appears to be as effective overall as a regimen of vinblastine, cisplatin, and bleomycin, the etoposide-containing regimen may be more effective than the vinblastine-containing regimen in a subgroup of patients with advanced disease (i.e., high tumor load). However, the best combination or sequential therapy in the treatment of advanced nonseminomatous testicular tumors has not been established, and comparative efficacy is continually being evaluated.

Although studied less extensively than cisplatin-containing regimens, etoposide in combination with carboplatin with or without bleomycin has produced clinical response in the treatment of stage II or stage III nonseminomatous testicular cancer†. However, there is evidence that a regimen of etoposide and cisplatin is more effective than standard dosages of etoposide and carboplatin in the initial treatment of germ cell tumors, and treatment with a carboplatin regimen generally is reserved for patients who do not tolerate or refuse cisplatin. Limited data suggest that high-dose etoposide and carboplatin may be effective in the treatment of relapsed or refractory germ cell tumors in some patients. High-dose etoposide and carboplatin with autologous bone marrow transplant has been associated with complete remission in 10–20% of patients with cisplatin-resistant germ cell tumors.

Etoposide also is used effectively in cisplatin-containing combination chemotherapy regimens for the treatment of those patients whose disease is refractory to chemotherapy, with or without surgery; a complete remission has been produced in about 50% of such patients treated with regimens that include etoposide and cisplatin, followed by surgery when feasible. Some data suggest that combination chemotherapy containing etoposide and cisplatin is effective in the treatment of refractory disease principally in those patients whose disease relapses after having achieved a complete remission with cisplatin-containing chemotherapy, followed by surgery when necessary. This combination does not appear to be very effective in patients with multiple tumor sites, increasing tumor markers, and refractory disease (as evidenced by incomplete response to conventional chemotherapy). Intensive combination chemotherapy regimens containing etoposide and high-dose cisplatin are currently being evaluated for the initial treatment of patients with disseminated disease associated with a poor prognosis.

Etoposide also is used as a component of various other chemotherapeutic regimens for salvage therapy in patients with recurrent or refractory germ cell testicular cancer. A regimen of ifosfamide, cisplatin, and either etoposide or vinblastine has induced complete responses in 20–45% of patients who previously received other cisplatin-based chemotherapy regimens, and is considered by most clinicians to be the standard initial salvage (i.e., second-line) regimen in patients with recurrent testicular cancer. Patients with minimal or moderate disease have a more favorable outcome with this salvage regimen than those with extensive disease. In a clinical study in patients with recurrent germ cell tumors (who had previously received at least 2 cisplatin-based chemotherapy regimens and were considered to have cisplatin-responsive disease), a regimen of ifosfamide, cisplatin, and either etoposide or vinblastine resulted in disease-free status in 36% of patients (with or without surgery) and median duration of disease control ranged from 3 to more than 42 weeks, median survival was 53 weeks, and 20% of patients had survival of 2 years or longer. In patients with refractory disease, high-dose chemotherapy (e.g., etoposide and carboplatin with or without ifosfamide) with autologous bone marrow transplant (ABMT) or peripheral stem cell rescue may produce durable complete remissions in some patients. Patients with progressive tumors during initial or salvage therapy and those with refractory mediastinal germ cell tumors generally appear to benefit less from high-dose chemotherapy and ABMT or peripheral stem cell rescue than those whose disease relapses after a response. Salvage surgery also may be considered for certain highly selected patients (e.g., those with chemorefractory disease confined to a single site).

The role of chemotherapy in the treatment of Stage I and resectable Stage II nonseminomatous testicular carcinoma has not been clearly established. Although most patients with Stage I disease are cured by surgery alone, combination chemotherapy regimens containing etoposide and cisplatin have been used successfully to induce complete remissions in a limited number of patients whose disease relapsed following surgical treatment.

Seminoma Testis Etoposide has been used successfully as a component of cisplatin-containing combination chemotherapy regimens in a limited number of patients for the initial treatment of disseminated seminoma testis and for the treatment of disseminated disease refractory to initial chemotherapy regimens, with complete remission rates comparable to those in patients with disseminated nonseminomatous disease. Further evaluation is needed to determine the optimum therapy.

Extragonadal Germ-Cell Tumors Data are limited, but etoposide-containing combination chemotherapy regimens (usually also containing cisplatin), followed by surgery when feasible, have reportedly been successful in the initial treatment of advanced extragonadal germ-cell tumors, but have generally produced only partial responses in the treatment of advanced extragonadal germ-cell tumors refractory to initial chemotherapy regimens.

■ **Lung Cancer** Etoposide has been widely used for the treatment of lung cancer, principally as a component of chemotherapeutic regimens in the treatment of small cell lung carcinoma.

Small Cell Lung Cancer Etoposide is used IV (either as etoposide or etoposide phosphate) in combination chemotherapy regimens for the treatment of small cell lung carcinoma; etoposide also has been used orally, either alone or as a component of combination therapy for this cancer. Combination chemotherapy regimens are superior to single-agent therapy in the treatment of this tumor and moderately intensive drug doses are superior to doses that produce minimal toxicity. Staging the cancer provides useful prognostic information and has implications for the specific course of therapy employed; all patients with small cell lung cancer generally should receive combination chemotherapy initially regardless of the extent of tumor dissemination since this cancer is the most aggressive form of lung cancer and some degree of metastasis is present in most patients regardless of whether it is detected at initial diagnosis.

Various regimens have been used in combination therapy, and many 2- to 4-drug regimens, including etoposide-containing regimens, have produced response rates of 65–90 or 70–85% and complete response rates of 45–75 or 20–30% in patients with limited-stage or extensive-stage disease, respectively; however, comparative efficacy is continually being evaluated. Etoposide-containing regimens are used in chemotherapy for extensive-stage small cell lung cancer and in combined modality treatment (i.e., combination chemotherapy with concurrent thoracic irradiation administered early in the course of treatment) for limited-stage disease.

Etoposide used in combination with cisplatin or carboplatin is a preferred regimen for the treatment of small cell lung cancer; this combination also may be of some value for the treatment of small cell lung carcinoma refractory to other chemotherapy regimens (particularly when relapse occurs more than 6 months following completion of initial treatment). Etoposide also has been employed in conjunction with a platinum agent (i.e., cisplatin or carboplatin) and ifosfamide with mesna. Other etoposide-containing combination chemotherapy regimens (e.g., etoposide, cyclophosphamide, and doxorubicin; etoposide, cyclophosphamide, and vincristine) have been used less commonly for the treatment of extensive-stage small cell lung cancer.

Concomitant administration of granulocyte colony-stimulating factor has been used in some patients with small cell lung carcinoma but is not routinely used to reduce the incidence and severity of myelosuppression associated with therapy.

Monotherapy with oral etoposide is inferior to combination therapy, and even geriatric and/or debilitated patients should be offered standard IV combination chemotherapy regimens for the treatment of advanced small cell lung cancer. In a randomized trial involving patients with poor-prognosis extensive-stage small cell lung cancer and geriatric patients (older than 75 years of age) with any stage of small cell lung cancer, fewer complete responses, reduced survival, and comparable or worse toxicity were observed among patients who received oral etoposide alone compared with those who received IV combination chemotherapy with alternating cycles of cisplatin/etoposide and cyclophosphamide/doxorubicin/vincristine. A randomized trial involving patients with previously untreated extensive-stage small cell lung cancer and poor performance status (WHO grade performance status 2–4) was stopped when interim analysis showed reduced survival and increased hematologic toxicity for those receiving oral etoposide alone compared with those receiving IV combination chemotherapy with etoposide/vincristine or cyclophosphamide/doxorubicin/vincristine.

Etoposide currently is considered one of the most active antineoplastic agents in the treatment of small cell lung carcinoma, producing an objective response in about 35–40% of previously untreated patients when used alone†.Although results of initial studies suggested that etoposide alone had substantial activity in patients whose disease was refractory to initial combination chemotherapy, more extensive studies have shown that monotherapy with the drug generally is of little benefit in these patients.

Although optimum duration of chemotherapy has not been clearly defined, additional improvement in survival has not been observed when the duration of drug administration exceeds 3–6 or 6 months in patients with limited-stage or extensive-stage small cell lung cancer, respectively. Because the current prognosis for small cell lung carcinoma is unsatisfactory regardless of stage and despite considerable diagnostic and therapeutic advances, all patients with this cancer are candidates for inclusion in clinical trials at the time of diagnosis.

Non-small Cell Lung Carcinoma In the treatment of non-small cell lung carcinoma†, etoposide alone appears to be of little benefit. A small survival benefit has been demonstrated for the use of platinum-based (cisplatin) chemotherapy in selected patients with unresectable, locally advanced or metastatic non-small cell lung cancer who have a good performance status. Etoposide has been used in combination with cisplatin for the treatment of advanced non-small cell lung cancer. However, in randomized trials, patients with stage IIIB or IV non-small cell lung cancer receiving paclitaxel combined with cisplatin or gemcitabine combined with cisplatin had higher response rates and similar median survival compared with those receiving combination therapy with etoposide and cisplatin; consequently, paclitaxel-containing regimens or other platinum-based regimens currently are preferred in the treatment of patients with advanced non-small cell lung cancer. Some clinicians consider etoposide and cisplatin an alternative regimen for the treatment of advanced non-small cell lung cancer.

Various chemotherapy regimens used alone or in combination with other treatment modalities, such as radiation therapy, are continually being evaluated for the treatment of advanced non-small cell lung cancer. A randomized trial is under way to determine the comparative efficacy and toxicity of combination therapy with etoposide and cisplatin versus paclitaxel and carboplatin in patients with advanced non-small cell lung cancer. Because current treatment is not satisfactory for almost all patients with non-small cell lung cancer except selected patients with early-stage, resectable disease, all patients may be considered for enrollment in clinical trials at the time of diagnosis.

■ **Malignant Lymphomas and Hodgkin's Disease** Etoposide appears to be one of the more active antineoplastic agents in the treatment of advanced non-Hodgkin's lymphomas†. The drug appears to be particularly effective for the treatment of advanced diffuse lymphomas of unfavorable histology such as diffuse histiocytic lymphoma, producing an objective response in about 30–40% of previously treated patients. Etoposide has been used in effective combination chemotherapy regimens (e.g., etoposide, ifosfamide, and methotrexate) for the treatment of refractory advanced diffuse lymphomas of unfavorable histology. Etoposide has also been used in effective alternating combination chemotherapy regimens for the initial treatment of advanced diffuse lymphomas of unfavorable histology.

Data are limited, but etoposide has produced transient responses in a few patients with mycosis fungoides†.

Etoposide has shown some activity in the treatment of advanced Hodgkin's disease†, and combination chemotherapy regimens containing the drug are currently being evaluated in the treatment of refractory disease.

■ **Leukemias** Although the exact role of etoposide has not been established, the drug has been shown to be active in the treatment of refractory acute myeloid (myelogenous, nonlymphocytic) leukemia (AML, ANLL)† in adults and children. When used alone in patients whose disease is refractory to initial chemotherapy, etoposide induces complete remission in about 10–15% of patients; response rates appear to be higher in patients with acute monocytic and myelomonocytic leukemias. Since etoposide appears to be particularly effective for the treatment of acute monocytic and myelomonocytic leukemias, the drug may be useful when monocytoid cells are not cleared with conventional combination chemotherapy. Because of its antileukemic activity, etoposide also has been employed in various combination chemotherapy regimens for remission induction in adults and children with refractory AML; while some of these regimens are effective (e.g., etoposide and azacitidine), the role of etoposide in these regimens remains to be clearly established. Additional studies are needed to evaluate the role of etoposide as a single agent and in combination chemotherapy for the treatment of AML.

Data are limited, but etoposide has shown activity alone and in combination chemotherapy for remission induction in the treatment of refractory acute lymphocytic (lymphoblastic) leukemia† in children; in adults with acute lymphocytic leukemia, etoposide appears to have little, if any, activity.

■ **Wilms' Tumor** Etoposide has shown activity in the management of Wilms' tumor and has been used with encouraging results in conjunction with carboplatin in a limited number of children with recurrent (relapsed or refractory) disease. Etoposide also has been used as an alternative to standard preferred regimens (e.g., combined vincristine and dactinomycin with or without doxorubicin) in patients with less severe stages of Wilms' tumor. Second-line (salvage) therapy with etoposide and carboplatin may be considered for patients with recurrent tumors of unfavorable histology, abdominal recurrence after radiation therapy, or recurrence within 6 months of nephrectomy or after initial 3-drug combination chemotherapy (e.g., vincristine, dactinomycin, and doxorubicin). In a study in a limited number of children with recurrent Wilms' tumor, most of whose tumors were of favorable histology, second-line therapy (2 courses separated by 21 days) with etoposide (100 mg/m^2 daily for 5 days) and carboplatin (160 mg/m^2 daily for 5 days) resulted in complete or partial responses in 73% of patients; complete response was maintained for a median follow-up of 40 months (range: 24–56 months) in about 30% of patients. The principal toxicity in these children was high-grade hematologic toxicity, particularly thrombocytopenia. Second-line therapy with high-dose chemotherapy followed by autologous bone marrow transplantation also has been used effectively in patients with recurrent disease, occasionally resulting in long-term survival. Patients with recurrent disease failing to respond to such attempts with salvage therapy should be offered treatment under protocol conditions in ongoing clinical trials.

■ **Neuroblastoma** Etoposide also has been used in the treatment of disseminated neuroblastoma†, and combination regimens using cyclophosphamide, doxorubicin, cisplatin, and/or etoposide or teniposide generally are preferred in children with this tumor. For localized resectable neuroblastoma, complete gross surgical excision produces disease-free survival that is indistinguishable from that obtained with surgery and adjuvant chemotherapy or adjuvant radiation therapy and therefore is preferred; however, the importance of certain tumor biologic properties (e.g., N-myc amplification and DNA ploidy) and other prognostic factors should be considered in evaluating the possible need for adjuvant therapy. For localized unresectable tumor, subtotal resection followed by chemotherapy is used for initial treatment, and short-term treatment (e.g., 4–6 months) usually is adequate. For regional neuroblastoma in children younger than 1 year of age, chemotherapy generally is limited to relatively resistant tumors since prognosis in less resistant tumors treated with surgery alone is good. In older children with regional neuroblastoma, chemotherapy may be employed for tumor reduction prior to surgery or may be employed aggressively following surgery; the role of aggressive therapy that includes high-dose chemotherapy, radiation therapy, and bone marrow transplant is being evaluated for children older than 1 year of age and/or those with poor prognostic characteristics (e.g., N-myc amplification). For disseminated neuroblastoma, intensive conventional chemotherapy, with or without surgery and radiation therapy (depending on clinical presentation and course), currently is the preferred initial therapy, although the relative efficacy of such therapy compared with myeloablative chemotherapy and autologous bone marrow transplant is being evaluated. For infants with stage IVS (special) neuroblastoma, chemotherapy often is unnecessary, but the management course should be individualized.

■ **AIDS-related Kaposi's Sarcoma** Etoposide has been used alone or in combination chemotherapy for the palliative treatment of AIDS-related Kaposi's sarcoma†. Single-agent therapy with etoposide is an alternative regimen for treatment of such sarcoma. Combination chemotherapy that includes bleomycin, doxorubicin, and a vinca alkaloid (vinblastine or vincristine) has been considered a regimen of choice for the disease, but many clinicians currently consider a liposomal anthracycline (doxorubicin or daunorubicin) the first-line therapy of choice for advanced AIDS-related Kaposi's sarcoma (see Uses: AIDS-related Kaposi's Sarcoma in Doxorubicin 10:00 or Daunorubicin 10:00).

Although single-agent therapy with conventional (i.e., nonencapsulated) cytotoxic agents generally has been used in the early stage of disease, Kaposi's sarcoma in patients with human immunodeficiency virus (HIV) infection often is rapidly progressive. AIDS-related Kaposi's sarcoma often progresses to multifocal, widespread lesions that may involve the skin, oral mucosa, and lymph nodes as well as visceral organs such as the GI tract, lung, liver, and spleen; such lesions often are numerous and may be cosmetically unattractive or disfiguring and accompanied by lymphedema. Appropriate evaluation of the effects of drug therapies on survival in patients with Kaposi's sarcoma must include assessment of the effects of such therapies on the development of infection as well as on tumor regression. Although treatment may result in disappearance or reduction in the size of Kaposi's sarcoma skin lesions and thereby alleviate the discomfort associated with chronic edema and ulcerations that often accompany multiple skin lesions on the lower extremities and in symptomatic control of mucosal and visceral lesions, there currently are no data demonstrating unequivocal evidence of improved survival with any therapy. Small localized Kaposi's sarcomalesions may be treated with electrodesiccation and curettage cryotherapy or by surgical excision; the lesions also generally are responsive to local radiation, and excellent palliation often can be achieved. Localized palatal lesions have been treated effectively with intralesional† injections of vinblastine. Alitretinoin gel (Panretin®, Ligand Pharmaceuticals), a topical retinoid, is used for the treatment of localized cutaneous lesions in patients with AIDS-related Kaposi's sarcoma; responses of cutaneous lesions to topical therapy with alitretinoin have been reported in patients who have received prior systemic and/or topical therapy for Kaposi's sarcoma as well as in those with previously untreated disease.

Response rates observed with single-agent chemotherapy (e.g., doxorubicin, etoposide, vinblastine, vincristine) appear to be similar to those observed with interferon alfa; however, studies directly comparing the efficacy of doxorubicin alone with that of interferon alfa have not been performed. Any differences in response rates reported in clinical studies generally appear to reflect differences in patient selection and in the criteria used to evaluate response rather than in drug activity. In one study in patients with AIDS-related Kaposi's sarcoma who received etoposide in an IV dosage of 150 mg/m^2 daily for 3 consecutive days at the beginning of a 28-day cycle for a median of 6 or 7 cycles (range: 2–26 cycles), complete or partial response was observed in about 30 or 46% of evaluable patients, respectively. Combined treatment with etoposide and interferon alfa generally appears to result in enhanced systemic toxicity without added therapeutic benefit.

Combination chemotherapy with conventional antineoplastic agents (e.g., bleomycin, conventional doxorubicin, etoposide, vinblastine, vincristine) usually has been used for more advanced disease (e.g., extensive mucocutaneous disease, lymphedema, symptomatic visceral disease). Doxorubicin hydrochloride liposomal injection (Doxil® by Alza Pharmaceuticals) is approved for use in the palliative treatment of AIDS-related Kaposi's sarcoma in adults who are intolerant to combination chemotherapy or whose disease has progressed while receiving such therapy. Liposomal daunorubicin citrate (DaunoXome®by NeXstar) is approved for use as first-line therapy for advanced AIDS-related Kaposi's sarcoma. The results of several randomized, multicenter trials indicate that patients receiving a liposomal anthracycline for the treatment of advanced AIDS-related Kaposi's sarcoma experience similar or higher response rates with a more favorable toxic effects profile than those receiving combination therapy with conventional chemotherapeutic agents. Preliminary evidence suggests that the mean survival period in patients with AIDS-related pulmonary Kaposi's sarcoma receiving liposomal doxorubicin may be increased compared with those receiving conventional chemotherapy (bleomycin and/or vincristine). The comparative efficacy of liposomal daunorubicin relative to liposomal doxorubicin has not been established.

Although treatment may result in the reduction or disappearance of lesions and alleviation of the associated symptoms, no treatment has been shown conclusively to alter the natural history of AIDS-related Kaposi's sarcoma and additional study and experience are needed to establish the optimal regimen.

■ **Ovarian Neoplasms** ***Epithelial Ovarian Cancer*** Etoposide currently is being investigated as an active agent for use in the treatment of advanced epithelial ovarian cancer†. In phase II studies, objective responses were observed in 6–26% of patients receiving low-dose oral etoposide as salvage therapy for previously treated advanced epithelial ovarian cancer; responses occurred in patients with platinum- and paclitaxel-resistant disease.

Ovarian Germ Cell Tumors Etoposide is used in combination with cisplatin and bleomycin for the treatment of ovarian germ cell tumors†.

■ **Other Uses** The use of high-dose† etoposide regimens in conjunction with autogenous (autologous) bone marrow transplantation is currently being evaluated for the treatment of various refractory advanced malignant neoplasms (e.g., nonseminomatous testicular carcinoma). Etoposide has been used with encouraging results in the treatment of gestational trophoblastic tumors† (choriocarcinoma and chorioadenoma destruens) in women. The drug has also shown some activity in the treatment of hepatoma†, Ewing's sarcoma†, rhabdomyosarcoma†, and brain tumors†. The role of etoposide in the treatment of these neoplasms has not been fully elucidated.

Dosage and Administration

■ **Administration** Etoposide is administered orally and by slow IV infusion. Etoposide phosphate is administered by IV infusion.

Etoposide solutions should not be administered by rapid IV injection. (See Cautions: Cardiovascular Effects.) *Because delayed, severe (sometimes fatal) toxicity has occurred in animals following intraperitoneal and intrapleural administration of etoposide, it is recommended that the drug not be administered by these routes.*

The toxicity of rapidly infused etoposide phosphate in patients with impaired renal or hepatic function has not been adequately evaluated, and the toxicity profile of etoposide phosphate when infused at doses exceeding 175 mg/m^2 has not been delineated.

To minimize the risk of hypotensive reactions, IV infusions of etoposide should be administered over a period of at least 30–60 minutes. The manufacturer states that a longer duration of administration may be used if the volume of fluid to be infused is a concern. Patients should be observed closely for possible hypotensive or anaphylactoid reactions during administration of the drug. (See Cautions: Precautions and Contraindications.) When a hypotensive reaction occurs and the infusion is discontinued and then restarted after appropriate treatment of the reaction, a slower rate of infusion should be employed. Etoposide has been administered by continuous IV infusion over 5 days, but this method of administration has not been shown to date to have any therapeutic advantage over intermittent IV infusions of the drug.

Etoposide phosphate solutions may be administered over 5–210 minutes.

The manufacturer recommends that protective gloves be used during handling of etoposide concentrate for injection and preparation of etoposide and etoposide phosphate solutions, since skin reactions associated with accidental exposure to the drug may occur. If etoposide concentrate for injection or a solution of the drug comes in contact with the skin, the affected area should be washed immediately and thoroughly with soap and water. If solutions of etoposide phosphate come in contact with the skin or mucosa, the affected skin should be washed immediately and thoroughly with soap and water, and the affected mucosa should be rinsed thoroughly with water.

Etoposide concentrate for injection must be diluted before administration. It is recommended that syringes with Luer-Lok® fittings be used for handling of etoposide concentrate for injection; when under pressure, needles have become displaced from etoposide-containing syringes without Luer-Lok® fittings, an effect which may be related to the drug's vehicle. The manufacturer recommends that the required dose of etoposide concentrate for injection be diluted to a final concentration of 0.2 or 0.4 mg/mL in 0.9% sodium chloride or 5% dextrose injection prior to slow IV infusion. (See Chemistry and Stability: Stability.) Etoposide concentrate for injection and the diluted solution for infusion should be inspected visually for particulate matter and discoloration prior to administration whenever solution and container permit.

Etoposide phosphate powder for injection should be reconstituted with 5 or 10 mL of sterile water for injection, 5% dextrose injection, 0.9% sodium chloride, bacteriostatic water for injection (with benzyl alcohol), or bacteriostatic sodium chloride for injection (with benzyl alcohol), resulting in a concentration equivalent to 20 or 10 mg of etoposide per mL (22.7 or 11.4 mg of etoposide phosphate per mL), respectively. Following reconstitution, the solution may be administered without further dilution, or it may be further diluted to concentrations as low as 0.1 mg of etoposide per mL with either 5% dextrose injection or 0.9% sodium chloride injection.

■ **Dosage** Dosage of etoposide must be based on the clinical and hematologic response and tolerance of the patient and whether or not other chemotherapy or radiation therapy has been or is also being used in order to obtain optimum therapeutic results with minimum adverse effects. Clinicians should consult published protocols for the dosage of etoposide and other chemotherapeutic agents and the method and sequence of administration. *A repeat course of etoposide should not be administered until the patient's hematologic function is within acceptable limits.* (See Cautions: Precautions and Contraindications.) When etoposide phosphate is used, dosage is expressed in terms of etoposide; 113.6 mg of etoposide phosphate is equivalent to 100 mg of etoposide.

Testicular Neoplasms For remission induction in the treatment of refractory testicular neoplasms, the usual IV dosage of etoposide in combination chemotherapy regimens is 50–100 mg/m^2 daily for 5 consecutive days every 3–4 weeks or 100 mg/m^2 daily on days 1, 3, and 5 every 3–4 weeks, for 3 or 4 courses of therapy. When the consecutive-day dosage regimen is employed, some clinicians administer etoposide for 3–5 days, depending on the patient's hematologic tolerance.

Small Cell Lung Carcinoma For the treatment of small cell lung carcinoma, the usual IV dosage of etoposide in combination chemotherapy regimens ranges from 35 mg/m^2 daily for 4 consecutive days to 50 mg/m^2 daily for 5 consecutive days, every 3–4 weeks. The recommended oral dosage of the drug is twice the IV dosage rounded to the nearest 50 mg.

Other Malignant Neoplasms For the treatment of other malignant neoplasms†, the optimum dosage of etoposide remains to be clearly established. Various dosage schedules and regimens of etoposide, alone or in combination with other antineoplastic agents, have been used. While the dosage of etoposide employed for the treatment of other malignant neoplasms has generally been similar to that used for the treatment of refractory testicular neoplasms, dosage has varied widely. Some high-dose† IV etoposide regimens (e.g., 400–800 mg/m^2 daily for 3 consecutive days for 1 or 2 courses of therapy in conjunction with autogenous bone marrow transplantation for the treatment of various advanced malignant neoplasms) have been investigated. Clinicians should consult published protocols for the dosage of etoposide and other chemotherapeutic agents and the method and sequence of administration.

For the treatment of Kaposi's sarcoma† in patients with AIDS, etoposide has been given in an IV dosage of 150 mg/m^2 daily for 3 consecutive days every 4 weeks, with cycles of therapy repeated as necessary depending on the patient's response and dosage reduced as necessary depending on the myelosuppressive effect of the drug.

■ Dosage in Renal and Hepatic Impairment The effects of renal or hepatic impairment on the elimination of etoposide have not been fully evaluated. Because a substantial fraction of the drug is excreted unchanged in urine, it is suggested that dosage reductions be considered in patients with impaired renal function. In patients with a measured creatinine clearance of greater than 50 mL/minute, no initial dose modification is required. In patients with a measured creatinine clearance of 15–50 mL/minute, 75% of the initial recommended etoposide dose should be administered. Although specific data are not available in patients with a measured creatinine clearance less than 15 mL/minute, further dose reduction should be considered. Subsequent etoposide dosing should be based on patient tolerance and clinical effect. Since etoposide-induced hematologic toxicity appeared to be more severe in patients with elevated serum bilirubin concentrations in one study and there is some evidence that total plasma clearance and elimination of the drug may be reduced in patients with impaired hepatic function, etoposide should probably be used with caution and the need for dosage reduction considered in patients with hepatic impairment.

Cautions

Because etoposide phosphate is converted rapidly and completely in vivo to etoposide, the adverse effects associated with etoposide can be expected to occur with etoposide phosphate.

■ Hematologic Effects The major and dose-limiting adverse effect of etoposide is hematologic toxicity. Myelosuppression, which is dose related, is manifested mainly by leukopenia (principally granulocytopenia). Myelosuppression resulting in death has been reported in patients receiving etoposide. Thrombocytopenia occurs less frequently, and anemia may also occur; pancytopenia has occurred in some patients. Myelosuppression apparently is not cumulative but may be more severe in patients previously treated with other antineoplastic agents or radiation therapy. Leukopenia has reportedly occurred in 60–91% of patients receiving etoposide and was severe (leukocyte count less than 1000/mm^3) in 3–17% of patients. Neutropenia (less than 2000/mm^3) occurred in 88% of patients treated with etoposide phosphate; severe neutropenia (less than 500/mm^3) occurred in 37% of patients treated. Thrombocytopenia has reportedly occurred in 22–41% of patients receiving the drug and was severe (platelet count less than 50,000/mm^3) in 1–20% of patients. Anemia has occurred in up to 33% of patients receiving etoposide. Anemia (hemoglobin less than 11 g/dL) occurred in 72% of patients treated with etoposide phosphate; severe anemia (hemoglobin less than 8 g/dL) occurred in 19% of patients treated. Granulocyte and platelet nadirs usually occur within 7–14 and 9–16 days, respectively, after administration of etoposide, and within 12–19 and 10–15 days, respectively, after administration of etoposide phosphate; leukocyte nadir has been reported to occur within 15–22 days after administration of etoposide, phosphate. Bone marrow recovery is usually complete within 20 days after administration, but may occasionally require longer periods. Fever and infection have been reported in patients with drug-induced neutropenia.

■ GI Effects Nausea and vomiting are the principal adverse GI effects of etoposide, occurring in about 30–40% of patients receiving the drug. Etoposide-induced nausea and vomiting do not appear to be dose related and are usually mild to moderate in severity and readily controlled by conventional antiemetics. Nausea and vomiting have required discontinuance of the drug in about 1% of patients. There is some evidence that the incidence of nausea and vomiting may be reduced with 5-day continuous IV infusions of etoposide compared with intermittent IV administration.

Other adverse GI effects of etoposide include abdominal pain, anorexia, and diarrhea, which have occurred in up to 7%, about 10–16%, and about 1–13% of patients, respectively. Stomatitis has reportedly occurred in about 1–6% of patients receiving usual dosages of etoposide and may be more likely to occur and/or be more severe in patients previously treated with radiation therapy to the head and neck region; in studies evaluating high-dose† etoposide regimens, stomatitis occurred more frequently and was found to be the dose-limiting adverse effect. Mucositis, constipation, and taste alteration have been reported in 11%, 8%, and 6%, respectively, of patients treated with etoposide phosphate. Aftertaste, dysphagia, and parotitis have also been reported rarely.

Adverse GI effects appear to occur slightly more frequently following oral administration of etoposide than following IV administration.

■ Cardiovascular Effects Transient hypotension has occurred in about 1–2% of patients following rapid IV administration of etoposide, but has not been associated with cardiotoxicity or ECG changes to date. Hypotension also has been reported following administration of etoposide phosphate solution. While delayed hypotension has not been reported with recommended doses and rates of administration, it has occurred following slow IV infusion of higher than recommended doses. Geriatric patients may be particularly susceptible to etoposide-induced hypotension. While etoposide does not consistently induce hypotension following rapid IV administration, to minimize the risk of this adverse effect, etoposide solutions should be infused slowly over a period of at least 30–60 minutes. If hypotension occurs during administration of etoposide or etoposide phosphate solutions, it usually subsides with discontinuance of the infusion and administration of IV fluids or other supportive therapy as necessary. In some patients, etoposide and etoposide phosphate have reportedly caused a transient increase in blood pressure. Blood pressure usually normalizes within a few hours after discontinuance of the infusion.

Etoposide has been associated with myocardial infarction or congestive heart failure in a small number of patients; however, these effects occurred almost exclusively in patients receiving etoposide by continuous IV infusion over 5 days, some of whom had preexisting cardiovascular disease, and were attributed to the large volumes of sodium chloride injection used as the diluent for administration of the drug.

■ Sensitivity Reactions Anaphylactoid reactions consisting principally of chills, rigors, diaphoresis, pruritus, loss of consciousness, nausea, vomiting, fever, bronchospasm, dyspnea, tachycardia, hypertension, and/or hypotension have occurred during or immediately after administration of etoposide or etoposide phosphate in 0.7–3% of patients receiving the drug. Other manifestations have included flushing, rash, substernal chest pain, lacrimation, sneezing, coryza, throat pain, back pain, generalized body pain, abdominal cramps, and auditory impairment. Anaphylactoid reactions have occurred during the initial infusion of etoposide in some patients. Facial/lingual swelling, coughing, diaphoresis, cyanosis, tightness in the throat, laryngospasm, back pain, and/or loss of consciousness have sometimes occurred in association with the above reactions in patients receiving etoposide. Rarely, an apparent hypersensitivity-associated apnea has been reported. Anaphylactoid reactions are usually controlled by discontinuance of the drug infusion and administration of vasopressors, corticosteroids, antihistamines, and/or plasma volume expanders as necessary; however, these reactions can be fatal. In one patient who had experienced several acute anaphylactoid reactions to the drug, prolonging the infusion over 4–6 hours prevented further occurrences of the reactions.

Bronchospasm with severe wheezing, responsive to antihistamine therapy, has been reported, and at least one fatal acute reaction associated with etoposide-induced bronchospasm has occurred. Acute pulmonary dysfunction, with or without hypertension, which may progress to pulmonary edema has also occurred.

■ Dermatologic and Local Effects Reversible alopecia, sometimes progressing to complete baldness, has occurred in 8–66% of patients receiving etoposide. The degree of alopecia may be dose related. Stevens-Johnson syndrome has been reported infrequently in patients receiving etoposide.Rash, pigmentation, urticaria, and severe pruritus have occurred infrequently, and cutaneous radiation-recall reactions associated with etoposide have been reported. At investigational doses, a generalized pruritic erythematous maculopapular rash, consistent with perivasculitis, has been reported. Localized herpes zoster infections have occurred in a few patients with AIDS during therapy with the drug.

Swelling of the forearm and upper arm with erythema was reported in one patient receiving an IV infusion of etoposide via a hand vein. Phlebitis has occurred following IV administration of undiluted etoposide concentrate for injection, and local pain has occurred following rapid IV injection of the drug diluted with 0.9% sodium chloride injection to a final concentration of 10 mg/mL; these irritant effects may be related to the solubilizing agents in the drug's vehicle. While etoposide and its vehicle have been shown to produce ulceration in mice following intradermal injection, only one case of soft-tissue ulceration following extravasation of an etoposide infusion has been reported to date. In mice, local infiltration of 0.9% sodium chloride injection or hyaluronidase was an effective local antidote, probably by diluting the local tissue concentration of the drug.

■ Nervous System Effects Peripheral neuropathy has occurred in about 1–2% of patients receiving etoposide. Although not clearly established, it has been suggested that the risk and/or severity of peripheral neuropathy may be increased when etoposide is administered concurrently with other potentially neurotoxic agents (e.g., vincristine).

Adverse CNS effects, including somnolence and fatigue, have been reported to occur in up to 3% of patients receiving etoposide. Seizure, occasionally associated with allergic reactions, has been reported infrequently in patients receiving etoposide. Headache, transient cortical blindness, optic neuritis, and transient vertigo have been reported rarely. Transient mental confusion during administration of etoposide has been reported in a few patients receiving high-dose regimens of the drug; this effect appeared to be consistent with alcohol intoxication resulting from the large volume of the drug's vehicle necessary to administer the dose.

■ Other Adverse Effects Hepatotoxicity has been reported in patients receiving etoposide. Hepatic toxicity generally has occurred in those patients receiving doses of the drug higher than recommended. Metabolic acidosis also has been reported in patients receiving such doses of etoposide.

Interstitial pneumonitis or pulmonary fibrosis has been reported infrequently in patients receiving etoposide.Fever and intermittent muscle cramps have been reported rarely in patients receiving etoposide. Although a causal relationship has not been established, etoposide has been associated with increases in serum bilirubin (sometimes resulting in jaundice), AST (SGOT), and alkaline phosphatase concentrations; these effects were transient and resolved without sequelae and occurred almost exclusively in patients in studies evaluating high-dose† regimens of the drug. Transient compensated metabolic acidosis has also occurred in patients receiving high-dose† etoposide regimens and was presumably caused by the agents contained in the drug's vehicle.

■ Precautions and Contraindications Etoposide is a toxic drug with a low therapeutic index, and a therapeutic response is not likely to occur without evidence of toxicity. The drug must be used only under constant supervision by clinicians experienced in therapy with cytotoxic agents and only when the potential benefits of etoposide therapy are thought to outweigh the possible risks. Most adverse effects of etoposide are reversible if detected promptly. When severe adverse effects occur during etoposide therapy, the drug should be discontinued or dosage reduced and appropriate measures instituted as necessary. Etoposide therapy should be reinstituted with caution, with adequate consideration of further need for the drug and awareness of possible recurrence of toxicity.

Patients receiving etoposide should be observed closely for possible hypotensive or anaphylactoid reactions, and appropriate equipment for maintenance of an adequate airway and other supportive measures and agents for the treatment of these reactions should be readily available whenever etoposide is administered. Higher rates of anaphylactoid reactions have been reported in children who received etoposide infusions at concentrations higher than those recommended. The role that the concentration of the infusion (or rate of infusion) plays in the development of anaphylactoid reactions is uncertain. If hypotension occurs during administration of etoposide, it usually subsides with discontinuance of the infusion and administration of IV fluids or other supportive therapy as necessary. If an anaphylactoid reaction occurs during administration of the drug, the infusion should be discontinued and appropriate therapy (e.g., antihistamines, epinephrine, oxygen, corticosteroids) instituted as necessary. Etoposide and etoposide phosphate are contraindicated in patients who are hypersensitive to either etoposide or etoposide phosphate or any ingredient in the formulation.

Hematologic function must be frequently and carefully monitored during and after etoposide therapy. The manufacturer states that complete blood cell counts (leukocyte count with differential, platelet count, hemoglobin) should be performed prior to initiation of etoposide therapy, at appropriate intervals during the course of treatment (e.g., twice weekly), and before each subsequent course of treatment with the drug. The manufacturer also states that therapy should be suspended if the platelet count is less than 50,000/mm^3 or the absolute neutrophil count is less than 500/mm^3; when blood counts have returned to an acceptable level, therapy may be resumed if indicated. Severe myelosuppression with resulting infection or bleeding may occur in patients receiving the drug. Treatment of severe hematologic toxicity may consist of supportive therapy, antibiotics for complicating infections, and blood product transfusions.

■ **Pediatric Precautions** Safety and efficacy of etoposide in children have not been established. The drug has been used with encouraging results in children for the treatment of refractory acute myelogenous leukemia†, principally in combination chemotherapy regimens, and has shown some activity in the treatment of refractory acute lymphocytic leukemia† and other pediatric malignancies†, but additional evaluation is needed.

Higher rates of anaphylactoid reactions have been reported in children who received infusions of etoposide at higher-than-recommended concentrations. The role that the concentration or rate of infusion plays in the development of anaphylactoid reactions is uncertain.

Each mL of etoposide concentrate for injection and etoposide for injection pharmacy bulk package contains 30 mg of benzyl alcohol as a preservative. Although a causal relationship has not been established, administration of injections preserved with benzyl alcohol has been associated with toxicity in neonates. Toxicity appears to have resulted from administration of large amounts (i.e., 100–400 mg/kg daily) of benzyl alcohol in these neonates. Although use of drugs preserved with benzyl alcohol should be avoided in neonates whenever possible, the American Academy of Pediatrics states that the presence of small amounts of the preservative in a commercially available injection should not proscribe its use when indicated in neonates.

A complex, potentially fatal syndrome including thrombocytopenia, ascites, and renal, pulmonary, and hepatic failure has occurred in several premature infants who received IV therapy with an injectable vitamin E product containing polysorbate 80; etoposide injection contains polysorbate 80.

■ **Mutagenicity and Carcinogenicity** Etoposide is mutagenic and potentially carcinogenic; the occurrence of acute leukemia (with or without a preleukemic phase) has been reported rarely in patients receiving etoposide in association with other antineoplastic agents. Etoposide has been shown to induce chromosomal aberrations in embryonic murine cells and in human hematopoietic cell lines in vitro; gene mutations in Chinese hamster ovary cells; and DNA damage via strand breakage and DNA-protein crosslinks in mouse leukemia cells. The drug also caused a dose-related increase in sister chromatid exchanges in Chinese hamster ovary cells. Although etoposide phosphate was nonmutagenic in the in vitro Ames microbial mutagenicity assay and the *E. coli* WP2 uvrA reverse mutation assay, because it is rapidly and completely converted to etoposide in vivo, etoposide phosphate also should be considered as a potential mutagen.

Studies in animals to determine the carcinogenic potential of etoposide have not been performed to date; however, because of its mechanism of action, the drug should be considered a potential carcinogen.

■ **Pregnancy, Fertility, and Lactation** Etoposide may cause fetal harm when administered to pregnant women, but potential benefits from use of the drug may be acceptable in certain conditions despite possible risks to the fetus. Etoposide has been shown to be teratogenic and embryocidal in mice and rats at doses of 1–5% of the recommended human dose based on body surface area. In rats, etoposide caused dose-related maternal toxicity, embryotoxicity, and teratogenicity with IV dosages of 0.4–3.6 mg/kg daily. Embryonic resorptions, decreased fetal weights, and fetal abnormalities including major skeletal anomalies, exencephaly, encephalocele, and anophthalmia, were observed; even at an IV dosage of 0.13 mg/kg daily, a substantial increase in retarded ossification occurred. In mice, intraperitoneal etoposide doses of 1–2 mg/kg caused dose-related embryotoxicity, cranial abnormalities, and major skeletal malformations. There are no adequate and controlled studies to date using etoposide in pregnant women. Women of childbearing potential should be advised to avoid becoming pregnant while receiving the drug. Etoposide should be used during pregnancy only in life-threatening situations or severe disease for which safer drugs cannot be used or are ineffective. When the drug is administered during pregnancy or if the patient becomes pregnant while receiving the drug, the patient should be informed of the potential hazard to the fetus.

The effect of etoposide on fertility in humans is not known. In rats, oral doses of etoposide phosphate at 86 mg (of etoposide) per kg daily (approximately 10 times the human dosage based on body surface area) or greater for 5 consecutive days resulted in irreversible testicular atrophy also was observed in rats given IV etoposide phosphate at a dosage of 5.11 mg (of etoposide) per kg daily for 30 days (approximately 50% the human dosage based on body surface area).

It is not known whether etoposide is distributed into milk. Because of the potential for serious adverse reactions to etoposide in nursing infants, a decision should be made whether to discontinue nursing or the drug, taking into account the importance of the drug to the woman.

Drug Interactions

■ **Antineoplastic Agents** Studies in animals and clinical trials in humans indicate that the antineoplastic activity of etoposide and cisplatin may be synergistic against some tumors. In mice implanted with P388 or L1210 leukemia or B16 melanoma, a combination of etoposide and cisplatin was shown to act synergistically in reducing the body burden of tumor cells and/or increasing survival. Response rates in humans receiving combination chemotherapy with etoposide and cisplatin suggest that the combination has synergistic antineoplastic activity against testicular carcinomas, small cell carcinoma of the lung, or non-small cell carcinoma of the lung. Studies in animals also indicate that the antineoplastic activity of etoposide and some other antineoplastic agents (e.g., carmustine, cytarabine, cyclophosphamide) is potentially additive or synergistic.

Limited data indicate that patients previously treated with cisplatin may have impaired elimination of etoposide. Although further documentation is needed, the potential effect should be considered when etoposide is administered to patients who received prior cisplatin therapy.

■ **Other Drugs** Caution should be exercised when administering etoposide phosphate with drugs that are known to inhibit phosphatase activity (e.g., levamisole hydrochloride).

High-dose cyclosporine administration, resulting in blood cyclosporine concentrations greater than 2000 ng/mL, with concomitant oral etoposide administration, resulted in an 80% increase in etoposide exposure with a 38% decrease in total body clearance of etoposide compared with etoposide alone.

Pharmacology

The exact mechanism(s) of action of etoposide is not known, but the drug appears to produce its cytotoxic effects by damaging DNA and thereby inhibiting or altering DNA synthesis. Although the in vitro cytotoxicity of etoposide phosphate is significantly less than that seen with etoposide, once the drug has undergone dephosphorylation in vivo to the active etoposide moiety, the mechanism of action is believed to be the same as that of etoposide. Etoposide appears to be cell-cycle dependent and cycle-phase specific, inducing G_2-phase arrest and preferentially killing cells in the G_2 and late S phases.

Etoposide has been shown to arrest metaphase in chick fibroblasts, but its principal effect in mammalian cells appears to be in the G_2 phase. At etoposide concentrations of 0.3–10 mcg/mL in vitro, cells are inhibited from entering prophase; at concentrations of 10 mcg/mL or higher, lysis of cells entering mitosis occurs. Unlike podophyllotoxin, etoposide does not inhibit microtubule assembly. Etoposide has been shown to induce single-stranded DNA breaks in HeLa cells and in murine leukemia L1210 cells in vitro; the drug also induces double-stranded DNA breaks and DNA-protein crosslinks in L1210 cells. Etoposide-induced DNA damage appears to correlate well with the cytotoxicity of the drug. While the exact mechanism remains to be determined, etoposide appears to induce single-stranded DNA breaks indirectly, possibly through endonuclease activation, inhibition of intranuclear type II topoisomerase, or formation of a free-radical metabolite via an enzymatic reaction involving the hydroxyl group at the C-4′ position of the E ring. Etoposide also reversibly inhibits the facilitated diffusion of nucleosides into HeLa cells in a concentration-dependent manner in vitro; however, the relative importance of this effect to the cytotoxicity of the drug is unclear.

Pharmacokinetics

Although some minor differences in etoposide pharmacokinetic parameters between age and gender have been observed, these differences were not considered clinically important.

■ **Absorption** Etoposide is variably absorbed following oral administration. The extent of absorption of etoposide is not affected by food. Several oral dosage preparations of the drug have been evaluated. Lipophilic capsules containing etoposide were found to be erratically absorbed and produced dose-limiting adverse GI effects. An oral solution of the drug (known as the "drink ampul") was about 50–90% absorbed but was unpalatable. The absolute bioavailability of the currently available hydrophilic liquid-filled soft gelatin capsules containing the drug averages about 50% (range: 25–75%). Following oral administration of the commercially available capsules, peak plasma etoposide concentrations are generally attained within 1–1.5 hours (range: 0.75–4 hours) and peak plasma concentration and area under the plasma concentration-time curve (AUC) exhibit marked intraindividual and interindividual variation. However, peak plasma concentrations and AUCs for a given oral dose consistently fall in the same range as those following an IV dose one half as large. There is some evidence that the extent of absorption of etoposide does not increase proportionately with doses greater than 200 mg and may plateau at doses of 400 mg or more, but further studies are needed to evaluate the dose-bioavailability relationship of the drug. Following oral administration of 160 or 200 mg/m^2 as the commercially available capsules, peak plasma etoposide concentrations of 9 mcg/mL (range: 3–19 mcg/mL) and 9.6 mcg/mL (range: 2.1–15.9 mcg/mL), respectively, were attained. There is no evidence that the drug undergoes first-pass metabolism.

Following IV administration of etoposide phosphate, the drug is rapidly and completely converted to etoposide in plasma. A direct comparison of the pharmacokinetic parameters (area under the plasma concentration-time curve [AUC] and maximum plasma concentration) of etoposide following IV administration of molar equivalent doses of etoposide phosphate and etoposide was made in 2 randomized, crossover studies in patients with a variety of malignancies. Results from both studies demonstrated no statistically significant differences in the AUC and maximum plasma concentration of etoposide when administered as either etoposide phosphate or etoposide. Therefore, the pharmacokinetic data reported for etoposide apply also to etoposide phosphate.

Peak plasma concentrations and AUCs following IV administration of etoposide exhibit marked interindividual variation, but possibly less intraindividual variation than after oral administration. Over the dose range of 100–600 mg/m^2, peak plasma concentration and AUC increase linearly with dose. Following IV infusion of an 80-mg/m^2 dose of etoposide over 1 hour in adults with normal renal and hepatic function, peak plasma drug concentrations occurred at the end of the infusion and averaged 14.9 mcg/mL (range: 7.8–19.3 mcg/mL). Following 500-mg/hour IV infusions of 400, 500, or 600 mg/m^2 in adults with normal renal function in one study, peak plasma etoposide concentrations of 26–53, 27–73, and 42–114 mcg/mL, respectively, were attained. When etoposide was administered as a 72-hour continuous IV infusion in a dosage of 100 mg/m^2 daily in several patients with normal renal and hepatic function, plasma drug concentrations of about 2–5 mcg/mL were attained 2–3 hours after beginning the infusion and were maintained until the end of the infusion. In a limited number of children 3 months to 16 years of age with normal renal and hepatic function who were given IV infusions of 200–250 mg/m^2 over 0.5–2.25 hours, peak serum etoposide concentrations ranged from 17–88 mcg/mL.

■ **Distribution** Distribution of etoposide into human body tissues and fluids has not been fully characterized. Following IV administration of etoposide in mice and rats, highest concentrations of the drug are attained in the small intestine, kidneys, and liver, with lower concentrations in the lungs, stomach, pancreas, spleen, heart, and skin.

Following IV administration in humans, etoposide undergoes rapid distribution. The apparent steady-state volume of distribution of the drug averages 20–28% of body weight or 18–29 L or 7–17 L/m^2 in adults and 5–10 L/m^2 in children. The major metabolite of etoposide appears to be distributed into a volume approximately equal to total body water. Following IV administration, etoposide is distributed minimally into pleural fluid and has been detected in the saliva, liver, spleen, kidney, myometrium, healthy brain tissue, and brain tumor tissue. Limited data suggest that distribution of the drug into bile is minimal. It is not known if etoposide is distributed into milk. The drug apparently crosses the placenta in animals.

Etoposide and its metabolites apparently do not readily penetrate the CNS. While variable, CSF etoposide concentrations generally range from undetectable to less than 5% of concurrent plasma concentrations during the initial 24 hours after IV administration of the drug, even after administration of very high doses. Limited data suggest that etoposide distributes into brain tumor tissue more readily than into healthy brain tissue. Concentrations of the drug are higher in healthy lung tissue than in lung metastases but those achieved in primary myometrial tumors are similar to those achieved in healthy myometrial tissues.

In vitro, etoposide is approximately 94% bound to serum proteins at a concentration of 10 mcg/mL.

■ **Elimination** Following IV infusion of etoposide, plasma concentrations of the drug have generally been reported to decline in a biphasic manner; however, some data indicate that the drug may exhibit triphasic elimination with a prolonged terminal phase. In adults with normal renal and hepatic function, the half-life of etoposide averages 0.6–2 hours (range: 0.2–2.5 hours) in the initial phase and 5.3–10.8 hours (range: 2.9–19 hours) in the terminal phase. In one adult with impaired hepatic function, the terminal elimination half-life was reportedly 78 hours. In children with normal renal and hepatic function, the half-life of etoposide averages 0.6–1.4 hours in the initial phase and 3–5.8 hours in the terminal phase.

The metabolic fate of etoposide has not been completely determined. Etoposide appears to be metabolized principally at the D ring to produce the resulting hydroxy acid (probably the *trans*-hydroxy acid); this metabolite appears to be pharmacologically inactive. The picrolactone isomer of etoposide has been detected in low concentrations in the plasma and urine of some patients but not in others. The aglycone of etoposide and/or its conjugates have not been detected to date in patients receiving the drug. In vitro, the picrolactone isomer and aglycone of etoposide have minimal cytotoxic activity.

Metabolism and excretion of etoposide appear to be similar following oral or IV administration of the drug. Etoposide and its metabolites are excreted principally in urine; fecal excretion of the drug is variable. Following IV infusion of etoposide in patients with normal renal and hepatic function, approximately 40–60% of a dose is excreted in urine as unchanged drug and metabolites within 48–72 hours and from less than 2 to 16% is excreted in feces within 72 hours; about 20–30% of the dose is excreted in urine unchanged within 24 hours and 30–45% within 48 hours. The principal urinary metabolite is the hydroxy acid of the drug. Following oral administration in patients with normal renal and hepatic function, about 5–25% of the dose is excreted in urine within 24–48 hours.

Total plasma clearance of etoposide reportedly averages 19–28 mL/minute per m^2 in adults and 18–39 mL/minute per ^{2} in children with normal renal and hepatic function; renal clearance of the drug is approximately 30–40% of the total plasma clearance. The effects of renal impairment on the elimination of the drug and its metabolites have not been fully evaluated; individuals with decreased renal function may have impaired elimination. Patients with impaired renal function receiving etoposide have exhibited reduced total body clearance, increased AUC, and a lower volume of distribution at steady state. Limited evidence suggests that total plasma clearance and elimination of etoposide may be reduced in patients with impaired hepatic function.

Limited data suggest that etoposide is not appreciably dialyzable.

Chemistry and Stability

■ **Chemistry** Etoposide is a semisynthetic podophyllotoxin-derivative antineoplastic agent. Etoposide differs structurally from podophyllotoxin by having a glucoside moiety and the epimeric configuration at the C-4 position of the C ring and by the presence of a hydroxyl group, rather than a methoxy group, at the C-4′ position of the E ring. The presence of the hydroxyl group at the C-4′ position is associated with the drug's ability to induce single-stranded DNA breaks, and the presence of the glucoside moiety is associated with the drug's inability to inhibit microtubule assembly. Etoposide also is commercially available as etoposide phosphate, a water-soluble ester; this chemical modification decreases the potential for precipitation following dilution of the drug in aqueous solution, while maintaining pharmacologic activity in vivo. Etoposide phosphate undergoes dephosphorylation in vivo to etoposide, the active moiety. Each single-dose vial of etoposide phosphate contains 100 mg of etoposide, equivalent to 113.6 mg of etoposide phosphate.

Etoposide occurs as a white to yellow-brown crystalline powder and is sparingly soluble in water (approximately 0.03 mg/mL) and slightly soluble in alcohol (approximately 0.76 mg/mL); the water miscibility of the drug is increased by the presence of organic solvents. Etoposide phosphate occurs as a white to off-white crystalline powder and is freely soluble in water (exceeding 100 mg/mL) and slightly soluble in alcohol. Etoposide concentrate for injection is a sterile, nonaqueous solution of the drug in a vehicle consisting of dehydrated alcohol, benzyl alcohol, citric acid, polyethylene glycol 300, and polysorbate (Tween®) 80. Etoposide phosphate for injection is a sterile, nonpyrogenic, lyophilized powder containing sodium citrate and dextran 40; following reconstitution of etoposide phosphate with water for injection to a concentration of 1 mg/mL, the solution has a pH of 2.9. The concentrate for injection occurs as a clear, yellow solution and has a pH of 3–4. Etoposide is also commercially available as soft gelatin capsules containing the drug in a vehicle consisting of citric acid, glycerin, purified water, and polyethylene glycol 400; the soft gelatin capsules contain gelatin, glycerin, sorbitol, purified water, and parabens.

■ **Stability** Etoposide concentrate for injection should be stored at room temperature. Unopened vials of the drug are stable for 2 years when stored at room temperature (25°C). Etoposide phosphate powder for injection should be stored in unopened vials at 2–8°C and retained in the original package to protect from light; such unopened vials of the drug are stable at least 36 months when refrigerated at 2–8°C. Etoposide liquid-filled capsules should be refrigerated at 2–8°C. The capsules are stable for 2 years when refrigerated at 2–8°C.

Etoposide concentrate for injection must be diluted before administration. The manufacturer states that, following dilution in 0.9% sodium chloride or 5% dextrose injection, etoposide solutions containing 0.2 or 0.4 mg/mL are stable for 96 or 24 hours, respectively, at room temperature (25°C) in glass or plastic (PVC) containers under exposure to normal room fluorescent light; following dilution in lactated Ringer's or 10% mannitol injection, solutions of the drug containing 0.2 or 0.4 mg/mL are stable for 8 hours at 25°C in glass containers under exposure to normal room fluorescent light. Because etoposide is sparingly soluble in water, the drug may crystallize following dilution in the above diluents; if crystallization occurs, the solution should be discarded. Crystallization of etoposide in aqueous solutions appears to be concentration dependent. At a concentration of 1 mg/mL in 0.9% sodium chloride or 5% dextrose injection, crystallization has occurred within 5 minutes upon stirring the solution or within 30 minutes upon allowing the solution to stand; therefore, this concentration is *not* recommended for IV administration. If solutions of etoposide are prepared at concentrations above 0.4 mg/mL, precipitation may occur, and the manufacturer recommends that the concentration not exceed 0.4 mg/mL.

Etoposide solutions containing 0.1–0.4 mg/mL in 0.9% sodium chloride or 5% dextrose injection have been filtered through several commercially available filters (e.g., 0.22-μm Millex®-GS or Millex®-GV) without filter decomposition.

Plastic devices composed of acrylic or ABS (a polymer composed of acrylonitrile, butadiene, and styrene) have been reported to crack and leak when used with undiluted etoposide injection.

When reconstituted and/or diluted as directed, solutions of etoposide phosphate can be stored in glass or plastic containers at controlled room temperature (20–25°C) or under refrigeration (2–8°C) for 24 hours. Refrigerated solutions of etoposide phosphate should be used immediately following return to room temperature.

For further information on the handling of antineoplastic agents, see the ASHP Guidelines on Handling Hazardous Drugs at http://www.ahfsdruginformation.com.

Preparations

Excipients in commercially available drug preparations may have clinically important effects in some individuals; consult specific product labeling for details.

Etoposide

Oral		
Capsules, liquid-filled	50 mg	**Etoposide Capsules** **VePesid®**, Bristol-Myers Squibb
Parenteral		
For injection concentrate, for IV infusion only	20 mg/mL (100, 150, 200, 250, and 500 mg)*	**Etoposide for Injection** **Toposar®**, Pfizer **VePesid®**, Bristol-Myers Squibb
	20 mg/mL (1 g) pharmacy bulk package*	**Etoposide for Injection** **VePesid®**, Bristol-Myers Squibb

*available from one or more manufacturer, distributor, and/or repackager by generic (nonproprietary) name

Etoposide Phosphate

Parenteral		
For injection	500 mg (of etoposide) pharmacy bulk package	**Etopophos®**, Bristol-Myers Squibb
	1 g (of etoposide) pharmacy bulk package	**Etopophos®**, Bristol-Myers Squibb
For injection, for IV infusion	100 mg (of etoposide)	**Etopophos®**, Bristol-Myers Squibb

†Use is not currently included in the labeling approved by the US Food and Drug Administration

Everolimus

RAD001

■ Everolimus, an inhibitor of mammalian target of rapamycin (mTOR) kinase, is an antineoplastic agent and macrolide immunosuppressive agent.

Uses

■ **Breast Cancer** Everolimus (Afinitor®) is used in combination with exemestane for the treatment of advanced hormone receptor-positive, human epidermal growth factor receptor type 2 (*HER2*)-negative breast cancer in postmenopausal women following failure of prior therapy with letrozole or anastrozole.

The current indication for everolimus in breast cancer is based principally on the results of a randomized, double-blind, placebo-controlled, phase 3 study (Breast Cancer Trials of Oral Everolimus-2 [BOLERO-2]) in postmenopausal women with hormone receptor-positive, *HER2*-negative advanced or metastatic breast cancer whose disease was refractory to previous letrozole or anastrozole therapy. Patients had at least 1 measurable lesion or mainly lytic bone lesions in the absence of measurable disease. In addition, patients had to have an ECOG performance status of 2 or less. In this study, 724 patients were randomized (stratified by documented prior sensitivity to hormonal therapy and the presence of visceral metastasis) in a 2:1 ratio to receive either everolimus (10 mg daily) or placebo in combination with exemestane (25 mg daily). Treatment was continued until disease progression, unacceptable toxicity occurred, or withdrawal of patient consent. The primary end point of efficacy was progression-free survival (assessed using Response Evaluation Criteria in Solid Tumors [RECIST]) evaluated by local investigators; secondary end points included overall survival, objective response rate, clinical benefit rate, time to deterioration of ECOG performance status, safety, and quality of life. The median age of patients enrolled in the study was 62 years (range: 28–93). Of the enrolled patients, 56% had visceral involvement, 76% had bone metastasis, and 69% had measurable disease. All patients had received prior therapy for breast cancer, including regimens consisting of letrozole or anastrozole (100%), tamoxifen (48%), fulvestrant (16%), and chemotherapy (68%).

Patients receiving everolimus in combination with exemestane in the BOLERO-2 study had a longer median progression-free survival than those receiving placebo in combination with exemestane (7.8 and 3.2 months, respectively). The results of the progression-free survival analysis based on an independent, blinded, central radiological assessment were consistent with the investigator assessment. In addition, patients receiving everolimus in combination with exemestane had a higher objective response rate than those receiving placebo (12.6 versus 1.7%, respectively). There were 3 complete responses (0.6%) and 58 partial responses (12%) in patients receiving everolimus in combination with exemestane compared with no complete responses and 4 partial responses (1.7%) in patients receiving placebo in combination with exemestane. Median overall survival had not been reached at the time of the interim analysis; however, no substantial difference in overall survival was observed between the treatment groups.

In a health-related quality of life analysis of the BOLERO-2 study data, median time to definitive deterioration in global health status was prolonged in patients receiving everolimus in combination with exemestane compared with those receiving placebo in combination with exemestane (8.3 versus 5.8 months, respectively).

■ **Neuroendocrine Tumors of Pancreatic Origin** Everolimus (Afinitor®) is used for the treatment of progressive neuroendocrine tumors of pancreatic origin (PNET) in adults with unresectable, locally advanced, or metastatic disease. Everolimus has been designated an orphan drug by the US Food and Drug Administration (FDA) for the treatment of this cancer. The manufacturer states that the safety and efficacy of everolimus in the treatment of patients with carcinoid tumors† have not been established.

The use of everolimus in patients with advanced neuroendocrine tumors of pancreatic origin was mainly established in a randomized, double-blind, placebo-controlled, multicenter, phase 3 study (RAD001 in Advanced Neuroendocrine Tumors, Third Trial [RADIANT-3]) conducted in 410 adults with advanced, low- or intermediate-grade pancreatic neuroendocrine tumors with radiologic documentation of disease progression within the previous 12 months. Patients had measurable disease, as assessed by RECIST, and a World Health Organization (WHO) performance status of 2 or less. Patients were randomized in a 1:1 ratio to receive either everolimus (10 mg once daily) or placebo, along with best supportive care (including somatostatin analogues [e.g., octreotide]). Treatment was continued until disease progression, unacceptable toxicity, drug interruption for 3 weeks or longer, or withdrawal of consent; upon disease progression, patients previously randomized to receive placebo were permitted to cross over to open-label everolimus therapy. The primary end point was progression-free survival (assessed using RECIST) evaluated by local investigators; secondary end points included safety, objective response rate, response duration, and overall survival. Median duration of treatment was approximately 8.8 months in patients receiving everolimus compared with approximately 3.7 months in those receiving placebo.

Patients randomized to receive everolimus along with best supportive care in the RADIANT-3 study demonstrated a substantial improvement in progression-free survival (11 months) compared with patients receiving placebo and best supportive care (4.6 months). At 18 months, the estimated proportion of patients who were alive and free of disease progression was 34% in patients receiving everolimus compared with 9% in patients receiving placebo. Confirmed objective responses (i.e., partial responses) were observed in 5 or 2% of patients receiving everolimus or placebo, respectively; there were no complete responses. Median overall survival had not been reached at the time of the interim analysis; however, no substantial difference in overall survival was observed between the treatment groups.

■ **Renal Cell Carcinoma** Everolimus (Afinitor®) is used for the treatment of advanced renal cell carcinoma in adults following failure of sunitinib and/or sorafenib therapy.

The current indication for everolimus is based principally on the results of a randomized, double-blind, placebo-controlled, multicenter, phase 3 study (RECORD-1) in 416 patients 18 years of age and older with metastatic clear-cell renal cell carcinoma that had progressed during or within 6 months following discontinuance of therapy with sunitinib, sorafenib, or both (given sequentially); patients who previously received aldesleukin, bevacizumab, or interferon alfa also were permitted to enroll in the study. Patients were randomized in a 2:1 ratio to receive either everolimus (10 mg daily) or placebo, along with best supportive care. Treatment in both groups was continued until disease progression, unacceptable toxicity, death, or discontinuance of therapy for other reasons occurred; upon radiographic progression, patients previously randomized to receive placebo were permitted to cross over to open-label everolimus. A planned second interim analysis indicated that patients receiving everolimus had longer median progression-free survival (4 months) compared with those receiving placebo (1.9 months). Following these favorable results, the independent data monitoring committee recommended early termination of the trial, and *all* patients previously randomized to receive placebo crossed over to receive open-label everolimus. Updated analysis confirmed that patients receiving everolimus (following a median duration of treatment of 141 days) had longer median progression-free survival (4.9 months) compared with those receiving placebo (1.9 months); improved progression-free survival was observed across all Memorial Sloan-Kettering Cancer Center (MSKCC) risk categories. Objective responses (i.e., partial responses) were observed in 2 or 0% of patients receiving everolimus or placebo, respectively. Final overall survival data did not show a substantial difference between the treatment groups; however, planned crossover between treatments at the time of disease progression may have confounded interpretation of the survival data.

■ **Renal Angiomyolipoma with Tuberous Sclerosis Complex** Everolimus (Afinitor®) is used in adults for the treatment of renal angiomyolipoma and tuberous sclerosis complex (TSC) not requiring immediate surgery. Everolimus has been designated an orphan drug by the FDA for the treatment of this cancer. The efficacy of everolimus in the treatment of renal angiomyolipoma is based on an analysis of durable objective responses in patients treated for a median of 8.3 months; further follow-up of patients is needed to determine long-term outcomes with everolimus therapy.

The current indication for everolimus in renal angiomyolipoma with TSC is based principally on the results of a randomized, double-blind, placebo-controlled, phase 3 study (EXIST-2) conducted in 118 adults with renal angiomyolipoma as a feature of TSC or sporadic lymphangioleiomyomatosis. The median age of enrolled patients was 31 years (age range: 18–61 years) and eligibility requirements for the study included at least one angiomyolipoma (3 cm or larger in its longest diameter) and no immediate indication for surgery. Patients were randomized (stratified by enzyme-inducing anticonvulsant use at randomization and presence of sporadic lymphangioleiomyomatosis) in a 2:1 ratio to receive either everolimus (10 mg daily) or placebo. Treatment was continued until disease progression or unacceptable toxicity occurred. The primary efficacy end point was the angiomyolipoma response rate based on independent central radiology review (defined as a 50% or greater reduction in angiomyolipoma volume, absence of new angiomyolipoma lesions of 1 cm or greater, absence of kidney volume increase of 20% or greater, and no angiomyolipoma-related bleeding of grade 2 or greater). The median duration of follow-up was 8.3 months (range: 0.7–24.8 months).

In the EXIST-2 study, the renal angiomyolipoma response rate was substantially higher in patients receiving everolimus (41.8%) than in those receiving placebo (0%). Responses were ongoing, with a median response duration of at least 5.3 months (range: 2.3–19.6 months at the time of analysis). Angiomyolipoma progression was documented in 3 patients receiving everolimus and in 8 patients receiving placebo, according to central radiologic review. The response rate of skin lesions, assessed by local investigators, also was substantially higher in patients receiving everolimus compared with patients receiving placebo (26 and 0%, respectively); all of the skin responses in the everolimus treatment group were partial responses. Everolimus demonstrated an acceptable safety profile in this study.

■ **Subependymal Giant Cell Astrocytoma with Tuberous Sclerosis Complex** Everolimus tablets (Afinitor®) and everolimus tablets for oral suspension (Afinitor® Disperz®) are used in pediatric patients (1 year of age or older) and adults with tuberous sclerosis complex (TSC) for the treatment of subependymal giant cell astrocytoma (SEGA) that requires therapeutic intervention but cannot be curatively resected. Everolimus has been designated an orphan drug by the FDA for the treatment of this cancer. The efficacy of everolimus in the treatment of SEGA is based on demonstration of a durable objective response, as evidenced by reduction in SEGA tumor volume; improvement in disease-related symptoms and overall survival in patients with SEGA and TSC has not been demonstrated.

The current indication for everolimus in SEGA with TSC is based principally on the results of 2 clinical trials. In a double-blind, placebo-controlled phase 3 study (EXIST-1) conducted in 117 pediatric and adult patients (median age: 9.5 years; age range: 0.8–26 years) with SEGA and TSC, patients were randomized to receive everolimus (Afinitor®) at an initial dosage of 4.5 mg/m^2 daily (with subsequent dosage adjustments to achieve and maintain everolimus trough blood concentrations of 5–15 ng/mL as tolerated) or placebo. Treatment was continued until disease progression or unacceptable toxicity occurred. The median duration of treatment was 41.9 weeks (range: 24–78.9 weeks) in patients receiving everolimus and 36.1 weeks (range: 13.9–79.7 weeks) in patients receiving placebo. The primary efficacy outcome was the proportion of patients with confirmed tumor response (defined as reduction in the total volume of all target SEGAs of 50% or more relative to baseline, in the absence of worsening of non-target SEGAs, new lesions of 1 cm or greater in diameter, and new or worsening hydrocephalus). Patients receiving everolimus had a substantially higher SEGA response rate (35%) than patients receiving placebo (0%). With a median follow-up of 8.4 months, SEGA progression was observed in 15.4% of the placebo recipients and in none (0%) of the everolimus recipients.

The second trial was open-label and single-arm in design and was conducted in 28 patients 3 years of age and older (median age: 11 years; age range: 3–34 years) with SEGA and TSC and serial radiologic evidence of SEGA growth; patients who previously underwent surgical resection of their SEGA lesions were permitted to enroll in the study. Patients received everolimus for a core treatment phase of 6 months; after the core phase, patients could continue to receive everolimus as part of an extension treatment phase. After the initial 6 months of everolimus treatment, 50% or greater reduction in tumor volume of the patient's largest SEGA lesion (assessed via independent central radiology review) was observed in 32% of patients. In a longer-term extension phase in 27 of these patients, the tumor volume of the patient's largest SEGA lesion was reduced by 50% or greater in 50, 41.2, and 55.6% of patients at 24, 30, and 36 months, respectively. The median duration of treatment in these patients was 34.2 months (range: 4.7–47.1 months), and the median duration of response was 11.8 months (range: 3.2–39.1 months). Development of new SEGA lesions was not observed in any of the patients receiving everolimus. Reduction in volume of the largest SEGA lesion of 50% or greater was reported in 3 of 4 patients who had prior surgical resection; of the 3 patients who responded, one responded by month 6 of everolimus therapy.

■ **Renal Allotransplantation** Everolimus (Zortress®) is used in combination with basiliximab induction and concurrently with corticosteroids and reduced dosages of cyclosporine for the prevention of rejection of renal allografts in adults with low to moderate immunologic risk. In a clinical trial in renal transplant patients, a regimen consisting of everolimus, reduced-dose cyclosporine, and corticosteroids was similarly effective compared with a regimen consisting of mycophenolate sodium, cyclosporine, and corticosteroids in preventing acute rejection, graft loss, and death at 12 months following transplantation. The manufacturer recommends therapeutic drug monitoring of everolimus and cyclosporine in all patients. Standard dosages of cyclosporine in combination with everolimus are associated with an increased risk of nephrotoxicity and should *not* be used. (See Renal Allotransplantation under Dosage and Administration: Dosage.) Safety and efficacy of everolimus have *not* been established in renal transplant recipients with high immunologic risk or in recipients of transplanted organs other than kidney and liver.

The current indication for everolimus in the prevention of renal allograft rejection is based principally on the results of an open-label, randomized, multicenter controlled study involving 833 patients 18–70 years of age with low to moderate immunologic risk receiving their first renal allograft. Low to moderate immunologic risk was defined as an ABO blood type-compatible first organ or tissue transplant recipient with an anti-human leukocyte antigen (HLA) Class I Panel Reactive Antibody (PRA) of less than 20% by a complement-dependent cytotoxicity-based assay, or less than 50% by a flow cytometry or enzyme-linked immunosorbent assay (ELISA), and with a negative T-cell cross-match. In this study, everolimus was given in 2 different concentration-controlled dosages (initial dosage of 1.5 mg daily targeting an everolimus trough concentration of 3–8 ng/mL using a liquid chromatography-tandem mass spectrometry [LC/MS/MS] assay method or initial dosage of 3 mg daily targeting an everolimus trough concentration of 6–12 ng/mL using an LC/MS/MS assay method) in immunosuppressive regimens that included reduced-exposure cyclosporine and corticosteroids. Everolimus was compared with mycophenolate sodium (mycophenolic acid 1.44 g daily) in combination with standard-exposure cyclosporine and corticosteroids. All patients also received basiliximab induction therapy. The primary efficacy end point was the rate of treatment failure, defined as the first occurrence of a treated episode of biopsy-proven acute rejection, death, graft loss, or loss to follow-up for any reason without a prior biopsy-proven acute rejection episode, at 12 months after transplantation. Results of this study indicate that everolimus (with corticosteroids and reduced-exposure cyclosporine) was similarly effective compared with mycophenolate sodium (with corticosteroids and standard-exposure cyclosporine) in reducing the incidence of treatment failure at 12 months following transplantation. The treatment failure rates at 12 months for everolimus 1.5 mg daily, everolimus 3 mg daily, and mycophenolate sodium (mycophenolic acid 1.44 g daily) were 25, 22, and 24%, respectively. Incidence rates of treated biopsy-proven acute rejection, graft loss, and death at 12 months in patients receiving everolimus 1.5 mg daily or mycophenolate sodium (mycophenolic acid 1.44 g daily) were 16.2 or 17%, 4.3 or 3.2%, and 2.5 or 2.2%, respectively. Estimated glomerular filtration rates (GFRs) were similar at 12 months in patients receiving everolimus 1.5 mg daily or mycophenolate sodium (mycophenolic acid 1.44 g daily).

Two earlier randomized, double-blind, multicenter controlled trials compared fixed dosages of everolimus 1.5 or 3 mg daily, without therapeutic drug monitoring, combined with standard exposures of cyclosporine and corticosteroids to mycophenolate mofetil 2 g daily combined with corticosteroids in de novo renal transplant recipients. In both studies, increased rates of renal impairment (based on calculated GFR) at 12 months were observed in both everolimus groups compared with the mycophenolate mofetil groups. Reduced-exposure cyclosporine and therapeutic drug monitoring targeting everolimus trough concentrations of 3–8 ng/mL should be used with everolimus regimens for renal allograft recipients.

■ **Hepatic Allotransplantation** Everolimus (Zortress®) is used in combination with tacrolimus (in reduced dosages) and corticosteroids for the prevention of rejection of hepatic allografts in adults. Everolimus should be administered no earlier than 30 days posttransplantation. In a clinical trial in hepatic transplant recipients, a regimen consisting of everolimus, reduced-exposure tacrolimus, and corticosteroids was similarly effective compared with a regimen consisting of standard-exposure tacrolimus and corticosteroids in preventing acute rejection, graft loss, death, or loss to follow-up at 12 months following transplantation. The manufacturer recommends therapeutic drug monitoring of everolimus and tacrolimus in all patients. Safety and efficacy of everolimus have *not* been established in recipients of transplanted organs other than kidney and liver.

The current indication for everolimus in the prevention of hepatic allograft rejection is based principally on the results of a randomized, open-label, controlled, multicenter study in 719 patients 18–70 years of age receiving their first transplant. Patients were initiated on an immunosuppressive regimen consisting of tacrolimus (trough concentrations of at least 8 ng/mL in the week prior to randomization) and corticosteroids, with or without mycophenolate mofetil. No induction antibody was administered. At randomization, mycophenolate mofetil was discontinued and patients were randomized to one of 3 treatment groups: everolimus (initially, 1 mg twice daily and adjusted to achieve target trough concentrations of 3–8 ng/mL using an LC/MS/MS assay) in conjunction with either reduced-exposure tacrolimus (target trough whole blood concentrations of 3–5 ng/mL) or tacrolimus elimination (at month 4 posttransplant, reduced-exposure tacrolimus was eliminated once everolimus trough concentrations were within the target range of 6–10 ng/mL) or a control group. In the control group, patients received standard-exposure tacrolimus (tacrolimus trough concentrations of 8–12 ng/mL tapered to 6–10 ng/mL by month 4 posttransplant). The tacrolimus elimination group was terminated prematurely because of a higher incidence of acute rejection and adverse reactions leading to discontinuance of therapy reported during the elimination phase of tacrolimus; therefore, an immunosuppressive regimen of everolimus in conjunction with tacrolimus elimination is *not* recommended. All patients received corticosteroids during the study.

The primary efficacy end point in this study was the composite efficacy failure rate of treated biopsy-proven acute rejection, graft loss, death, or loss to follow-up at 12 months posttransplant. At 12 months, everolimus with reduced-exposure tacrolimus was comparable to standard-exposure tacrolimus with respect to efficacy failure. The treatment failure rates at 12 months for everolimus with reduced-exposure tacrolimus and standard-exposure tacrolimus were 9 and 13.6%, respectively. Incidence rates of treated biopsy-proven acute rejection, death, and graft loss at 12 months were 2.9, 5.3, and 2.4%, respectively, in patients receiving everolimus with reduced-exposure tacrolimus and 7, 2.9, and 1.2%, respectively, in those receiving standard-exposure tacrolimus. The estimated mean GFR was 80.9 mL/min per 1.73 m^2 in patients receiving everolimus with reduced-exposure tacrolimus and 70.3 mL/min per 1.73 m^2 in those receiving standard-exposure tacrolimus at 12 months.

Dosage and Administration

■ **Administration** Everolimus is administered orally as tablets (Afinitor®, Zortress®) and as tablets for oral suspension (Afinitor® Disperz®). Afinitor® Disperz® is recommended for use only for the treatment of subependymal giant cell astrocytoma (SEGA) with tuberous sclerosis complex (TSC) in conjunction with therapeutic drug monitoring. The different formulations of Afinitor® are *not* interchangeable, and they should not be combined to achieve the desired dose.

Tablets Everolimus tablets (Afinitor® and Zortress®) are administered orally once or twice daily. The tablets should be administered at the same time every day (or approximately 12 hours apart when given twice daily), either consistently with food or consistently without food. In patients with renal or hepatic allografts, everolimus should be administered at the same time as cyclosporine or tacrolimus, respectively.

Everolimus tablets should be swallowed whole with a glass of water; the tablets should not be broken or crushed.

Tablets for Oral Suspension Everolimus tablets for oral suspension (Afinitor® Disperz®) are administered orally once daily. The drug should be administered at the same time every day, either consistently with food or consistently without food.

Everolimus tablets for oral suspension should only be used as a suspension. The oral suspension should be prepared in water only and administered immediately after preparation; if not administered within 60 minutes of preparation, the suspension should be discarded.

If the tablets for oral suspension are to be administered using an oral syringe, the prescribed dose (up to 10 mg) should then be placed in a 10-mL syringe; the tablets should not be crushed or broken. Approximately 5 mL of water and 4 mL of air should be drawn into the syringe. The syringe containing the mixture should then be placed in a container (tip up) for 3 minutes, until the tablets are in suspension. Immediately prior to administration, the syringe should be gently inverted 5 times. Following administration, the syringe should be refilled with 5 mL of water and 4 mL of air, swirled to suspend remaining particles, and the entire contents of the syringe administered. If a dose of more than 10 mg is required, an additional syringe should be prepared.

If the tablets for oral suspension are to be administered using a small drinking glass (maximum size 100 mL), the prescribed dose (up to 10 mg) should be placed into a glass containing approximately 25 mL of water; the tablets should not be crushed or broken. The mixture should be allowed to suspend for 3 minutes. Immediately prior to administration, the contents of the drinking glass should be stirred gently with a spoon. Following administration of the prepared suspension, 25 mL of water should be added to the glass and the mixture should be stirred with the same spoon to resuspend remaining particles. The entire contents of the glass should then be swallowed. If a dose of more than 10 mg is required, an additional glass should be prepared.

■ **Dosage** ***Breast Cancer*** The recommended adult dosage of everolimus for the treatment of advanced hormone receptor-positive, *HER2*-negative breast cancer in combination with exemestane therapy following failure of letrozole or anastrozole therapy is 10 mg once daily. Therapy should be continued until disease progression or unacceptable toxicity occurs. Dosage adjustments may be required based on tolerability or change in concomitant drug therapy. (See Drug Interactions.)

Neuroendocrine Tumors of Pancreatic Origin The recommended adult dosage of everolimus for the treatment of advanced neuroendocrine tumors of pancreatic originis 10 mg once daily. Therapy should be continued until disease progression or unacceptable toxicity occurs. Dosage adjustments may be required based on tolerability or change in concomitant drug therapy. (See Drug Interactions.)

Renal Cell Carcinoma The recommended adult dosage of everolimus for the treatment of advanced renal cell carcinoma following failure of sunitinib or sorafenib therapy is 10 mg once daily. Therapy should be continued until disease progression or unacceptable toxicity occurs. Dosage adjustments may be required based on tolerability or change in concomitant drug therapy. (See Drug Interactions.)

Renal Angiomyolipoma with TSC The recommended adult dosage of everolimus for the treatment of renal angiomyolipoma with TSCis 10 mg once daily. Therapy should be continued until disease progression or unacceptable toxicity occurs. Dosage adjustments may be required based on tolerability or change in concomitant drug therapy. (See Drug Interactions.)

SEGA with TSC The recommended initial dosage of everolimus for the treatment of SEGA with TSC in adult and pediatric patients 1 year of age or older is 4.5 mg/m^2 once daily. The dosage should be rounded to the nearest strength of either everolimus tablets (Afinitor®) or everolimus tablets for oral suspension (Afinitor® Disperz®). Subsequent dosing should be guided by therapeutic drug monitoring. Dosage adjustments should be made at 2-week intervals as needed to achieve and maintain everolimus trough concentrations of 5–15 ng/mL.

Higher everolimus trough concentrations appear to be associated with larger reductions in SEGA volume. However, responses have been observed at trough concentrations as low as 5 ng/mL; therefore, additional dosage increases may not be necessary once acceptable efficacy has been achieved. Treatment with everolimus should be continued until disease progression or unacceptable toxicity occurs; the optimal duration of therapy is not known.

Therapeutic Drug Monitoring and Dosage Adjustment in SEGA with TSC. Routine monitoring of everolimus whole blood trough drug concentrations is recommended for all patients receiving everolimus for the treatment of SEGA with TSC. The same assay and laboratory should be used for therapeutic drug monitoring throughout treatment when possible. Trough concentrations should be measured approximately 2 weeks after initiation of treatment. Trough concentrations also should be measured approximately 2 weeks after any change in everolimus dosage, a change in concomitant treatment with inducers or inhibitors of cytochrome P-450 (CYP) isoenzyme 3A4 and/or P-glycoprotein, a change in hepatic function, or a change in dosage form between everolimus tablets (Afinitor®) and everolimus tablets for oral suspension (Afinitor® Disperz®).

Dosage should be titrated to attain trough everolimus concentrations of 5–15 ng/mL. In patients with trough concentrations below 5 ng/mL, daily everolimus dosage may be increased by 2.5 mg in patients receiving everolimus tablets or by 2 mg in patients receiving everolimus tablets for oral suspension. In patients with trough everolimus concentrations exceeding 15 ng/mL, daily everolimus dosage may be decreased by 2.5 mg in patients receiving everolimus tablets or by 2 mg in patients receiving everolimus tablets for oral suspension. If dosage reduction is required in patients receiving the lowest available strength, alternate day dosing should be used.

Once a stable dosage of everolimus has been attained, trough concentrations should be monitored every 3–6 months in patients with changing body surface area and every 6–12 months in patients with stable body surface area for the duration of everolimus treatment.

Renal Allotransplantation For the prevention of renal allograft rejection in adults, the usual initial dosage of everolimus is 0.75 mg orally twice daily (1.5 mg/day). Everolimus is used in combination with basiliximab induction and concurrently with *reduced-dosage* cyclosporine and corticosteroids, and should be initiated as soon as possible after transplantation.

Patients receiving everolimus may require dosage adjustments based on everolimus blood concentrations, tolerability, individual response, change in concomitant drug therapy, and the clinical situation. Everolimus maintenance dosage should preferably be adjusted based on trough concentrations obtained 4–5 days after a change in dosage of either everolimus or cyclosporine (since reduced cyclosporine exposure may result in decreased everolimus concentrations). (See Drug Interactions.)

Oral prednisone also should be administered once oral medications are tolerated. Tapering of steroid dosages should be individualized based on the patient's clinical status and function of the allograft.

Therapeutic Drug Monitoring and Dosage Adjustment of Everolimus for Renal Allotransplantation. Routine monitoring of trough whole blood everolimus concentrations is recommended for all renal transplant patients. The recommended therapeutic range is 3–8 ng/mL. In clinical trials, a lower incidence of treated biopsy-proven acute rejection was observed in renal allograft recipients with whole blood trough everolimus concentrations of 3 ng/mL or greater compared with patients whose trough concentrations were less than 3 ng/mL. Similar efficacy and an increased incidence of adverse effects were observed in patients with trough everolimus concentrations of 6–12 ng/mL compared with patients with trough concentrations of 3–8 ng/mL. Clinical signs and symptoms, tissue biopsies, and laboratory parameters should be carefully monitored.

The recommended trough concentration range of 3–8 ng/mL for everolimus is based on a liquid chromatography-tandem mass spectrometry (LC/MS/MS) assay method. In clinical practice, everolimus whole blood concentrations may be measured by chromatographic or immunoassay methodologies. However, the measured concentrations of everolimus in whole blood depend on the type of assay used, and the individual patient sample concentration values from different assay methodologies may not be interchangeable. Consideration of assay results should be made with knowledge of the specific assay that was used. Therefore, it is essential that communication be maintained with the laboratory performing the everolimus assays.

Blood everolimus concentrations should be monitored carefully in patients with hepatic impairment, patients receiving concomitant treatment with inducers or inhibitors of CYP3A4, when switching cyclosporine formulations, and/or when cyclosporine dosages are reduced according to recommended target concentrations.

Therapeutic Drug Monitoring and Dosage Adjustment of Cyclosporine for Renal Allotransplantation. Cyclosporine dosages and target concentrations should both be *reduced* when cyclosporine is used in combination with everolimus to minimize the risk of nephrotoxicity. When administered with everolimus, the recommended therapeutic ranges for cyclosporine are 100–200 ng/mL through month 1 posttransplant, 75–150 ng/mL at months 2 and 3, 50–100 ng/mL at month 4, and 25–50 ng/mL from month 6 through month 12. Cyclosporine (USP modified) should be administered as oral capsules twice daily unless administration of oral solution or IV cyclosporine cannot be avoided. Cyclosporine should be initiated as soon as possible and no later than 48 hours after reperfusion of the graft, and the dosage should be adjusted to target concentrations from day 5 onward. The treatment regimen should be adjusted if progressive impairment of renal function occurs. Cyclosporine dosage should be adjusted based on whole blood trough concentrations.

Data regarding everolimus dosages with reduced cyclosporine trough concentrations of 25–50 ng/mL after 12 months are limited. Everolimus has not been evaluated in clinical trials with other formulations of cyclosporine. Prior to dosage reduction of cyclosporine, steady-state everolimus whole blood trough concentrations of 3 ng/mL or greater should be verified. Everolimus concentrations may decrease if cyclosporine exposure is reduced.

Hepatic Allotransplantation For the prevention of hepatic allograft rejection in adults, the usual initial dosage of everolimus is 1 mg orally twice daily (2 mg/day). Everolimus is used in combination with *reduced-dosage* tacrolimus and corticosteroids, and should be initiated at least 30 days following transplantation. Tapering of steroid dosages should be individualized based on the patient's clinical status and function of the allograft.

Patients receiving everolimus for prevention of hepatic allograft rejection may require dosage adjustment based on everolimus blood concentrations, tolerability, individual response, change in concomitant drug therapy, and the clinical situation. (See Drug Interactions.) Everolimus maintenance dosage should preferably be adjusted based on trough everolimus concentrations obtained 4–5 days after a change in dosage of everolimus.

Therapeutic Drug Monitoring and Dosage Adjustment of Everolimus for Hepatic Allotransplantation. Routine monitoring of whole blood everolimus concentrations is recommended for all hepatic transplant patients. The recommended therapeutic range is 3–8 ng/mL. Clinical signs and symptoms, tissue biopsies, and laboratory parameters should be carefully monitored.

The recommended trough concentration range of 3–8 ng/mL for everolimus is based on an LC/MS/MS assay method. In clinical practice, everolimus whole blood concentrations may be measured by chromatographic or immunoassay methodologies. However, the measured concentrations of everolimus in whole blood depend on the type of assay used, and the individual patient sample concentration values from different assay methodologies may not be interchangeable. Consideration of assay results should be made with knowledge of the specific assay that was used. Therefore, it is essential that communication be maintained with the laboratory performing the everolimus assays.

Blood everolimus concentrations should be monitored carefully in patients with hepatic impairment and patients receiving concomitant treatment with inducers or inhibitors of CYP3A4.

Therapeutic Drug Monitoring and Dosage Adjustment of Tacrolimus for Hepatic Allotransplantation. Tacrolimus dosages and the target concentrations should both be *reduced* when tacrolimus is used in combination with everolimus to minimize the risk of nephrotoxicity. When administered with everolimus, the recommended therapeutic range for whole blood trough tacrolimus concentrations is 3–5 ng/mL by 3 weeks after the first dose of everolimus (approximately month 2 posttransplant) and through month 12 posttransplant. Tacrolimus should be administered as oral capsules twice daily unless administration of IV tacrolimus cannot be avoided. Tacrolimus dosage should be adjusted based on whole blood trough concentrations.

Data regarding everolimus dosages with reduced tacrolimus trough concentrations of 3–5 ng/mL after 12 months are limited. Prior to dosage reduction of tacrolimus, steady-state everolimus whole blood trough concentration of 3 ng/mL or greater should be verified. Tacrolimus does not affect everolimus trough concentrations, and everolimus concentrations do not decrease if tacrolimus exposure is reduced.

Dosage Modification for Toxicity Management of severe or intolerable adverse effects in patients receiving everolimus for breast cancer, neuroendocrine tumors of pancreatic origin, renal cell carcinoma, renal angiomyolipoma, or SEGA with TSC may require temporary dosage reduction and/or interruption of everolimus therapy. If dosage reduction is required, the manufacturer recommends an everolimus dosage approximately 50% lower than the previously administered daily dosage.

If dosage reduction is required for patients with SEGA with TSC receiving the lowest available strength of everolimus, alternate-day dosing should be used.

Noninfectious Pneumonitis. In patients with grade 1 noninfectious pneumonitis (i.e., asymptomatic, radiographic changes only), everolimus dosage adjustment is not necessary but appropriate monitoring should be initiated.

In patients experiencing grade 2 noninfectious pneumonitis (i.e., symptomatic, does not interfere with activities of daily living), consideration should be given to interrupting everolimus therapy until symptoms improve; possible infection should be ruled out and initiation of corticosteroid therapy should be considered until symptoms improve to grade 0 or 1. Everolimus may then be resumed at a lower dosage.. If recovery does not occur within 4 weeks, everolimus should be discontinued.

In patients with grade 3 noninfectious pneumonitis (i.e., symptomatic, interferes with activities of daily living, oxygen is necessary), everolimus therapy should then be interrupted until symptoms resolve to grade 1 or less, infection should be ruled out, and corticosteroid therapy should be considered. Resuming everolimus therapy at a reduced dosage should be considered. If toxicity recurs at grade 3, discontinuance of the drug should be considered.

In patients experiencing grade 4 noninfectious pneumonitis (i.e., life-threatening, ventilatory support necessary), everolimus therapy should be discontinued, infection should be ruled out, and initiation of corticosteroid therapy should be considered. (See Interstitial Lung Disease/Noninfectious Pneumonitis under Cautions: Other Warnings and Precautions.)

Stomatitis. In patients with breast cancer, neuroendocrine tumors of pancreatic origin, renal cell carcinoma, SEGA, or renal angiomyolipoma, everolimus therapy may be continued without any dosage adjustment in patients with grade 1 stomatitis (minimal symptoms, normal diet). In patients experiencing grade 2 stomatitis (symptomatic but can eat and swallow modified diet), everolimus therapy should be temporarily interrupted until recovery to grade 1 or less; everolimus may be reinitiated at the same dosage following recovery. If stomatitis recurs at grade 2, therapy should then be interrupted until recovery to grade 1 or less; everolimus should be reinitiated at a reduced dosage.

In patients with grade 3 stomatitis (symptomatic and unable to adequately aliment or hydrate orally), everolimus therapy should be temporarily interrupted until recovery to grade 1 or less; everolimus therapy should then be reinitiated at a reduced dosage. In patients with grade 4 stomatitis (symptoms associated with life-threatening consequences), everolimus should be discontinued. (See Oral Ulceration under Cautions: Other Warnings and Precautions.)

Other Nonhematologic Toxicity. In patients with breast cancer, neuroendocrine tumors of pancreatic origin, renal cell carcinoma, SEGA, or renal angiomyolipoma who develop grade 1 or 2 nonhematologic toxicities, everolimus therapy may be continued without any dosage adjustment if the toxicity is tolerable. If grade 2 toxicity becomes intolerable, everolimus therapy should be temporarily interrupted until recovery to grade 1 or less; everolimus may then be reinitiated at the same dosage following recovery. If grade 2 nonhematologic toxicity recurs, therapy should be interrupted until recovery to grade 1 or less; everolimus should then be reinitiated at a reduced dosage.

In patients with grade 3 nonhematologic toxicity, everolimus therapy should be temporarily interrupted until recovery to grade 1 or less; reinitiation of everolimus therapy at a reduced dosage should be considered. If grade 3 toxicity recurs, discontinuance of everolimus should be considered. In patients with grade 4 nonhematologic toxicity, everolimus should be discontinued.

Metabolic Events. In patients with breast cancer, neuroendocrine tumors of pancreatic origin, renal cell carcinoma, SEGA, or renal angiomyolipoma, everolimus therapy may be continued without any dosage adjustment in patients with grade 1 or 2 metabolic events (e.g., hyperglycemia, dyslipidemia). In patients experiencing grade 3 metabolic events, everolimus therapy should be temporarily interrupted; everolimus therapy should then be reinitiated at a reduced dosage. In patients experiencing grade 4 metabolic events, everolimus should be discontinued.

■ **Special Populations** In patients with breast cancer, neuroendocrine tumors of pancreatic origin, renal cell carcinoma, or renal angiomyolipoma, the manufacturer recommends an everolimus dosage of 7.5 mg daily in patients with mild (Child-Pugh class A) hepatic impairment; the dosage may be further reduced to 5 mg daily based on patient tolerability. The manufacturer recommends a dosage of 5 mg daily in patients with moderate (Child-Pugh class B) hepatic impairment; the dosage may be further reduced to 2.5 mg daily based on patient tolerability. In patients with severe (Child-Pugh class C) hepatic impairment, the manufacturer recommends a maximum dosage of 2.5 mg daily, if the potential benefit of therapy outweighs the risk. If the patient's hepatic status changes during everolimus treatment, adjustments to the dosage should be made.

In patients who are receiving everolimus for the prevention of renal or liver allograft rejection with mild (Child-Pugh class A) hepatic impairment, the manufacturer recommends that the usual recommended initial dosage of everolimus be reduced by approximately 33%. The manufacturer recommends that the usual recommended initial dosage of everolimus be reduced by approximately 50% in patients with moderate or severe (Child-Pugh class B or C) hepatic impairment. Further dosage adjustments should be made if a patient's whole blood trough concentration of everolimus is not within the target therapeutic range of 3–8 ng/mL.

The manufacturer states that adjustment of the initial dosage of everolimus (Afinitor® or Afinitor® Disperz®) in patients with SEGA with TSC who have mild or moderate (Child-Pugh class A or B) hepatic impairment may not be required. The manufacturer recommends that the initial daily dosage be reduced by approximately 50% in patients with SEGA who have severe (Child-Pugh class C) hepatic impairment. Subsequent dosage should be based on therapeutic drug monitoring. (See Hepatic Impairment under Warnings/Precautions: Specific Populations, in Cautions.)

The manufacturer states that no dosage adjustment is required in patients with renal impairment. (See Renal Impairment under Warnings/Precautions: Specific Populations, in Cautions.)

The manufacturer states that no adjustment of the initial dosage is required in geriatric patients; however, close monitoring and appropriate dosage adjustments for adverse effects are recommended for Afinitor® and Afinitor® Disperz®. (See Geriatric Use under Warnings/Precautions: Specific Populations, in Cautions.)

Cautions

■ **Contraindications** Known hypersensitivity to everolimus, other rapamycin derivatives (e.g., sirolimus, temsirolimus), or any ingredient in the everolimus formulations.

■ **Warnings/Precautions** ***Warnings*** *Everolimus (Zortress®) should be used only by clinicians experienced in immunosuppressive therapy and the management of transplant patients. Patients receiving the drug should* *be managed in facilities equipped and staffed with adequate laboratory and supportive medical resources, and the clinician responsible for maintenance therapy should have complete information requisite for follow-up of the patient.*

Malignancies and Serious Infections. Everolimus has immunosuppressive properties and may predispose patients to bacterial, fungal, viral, or protozoal infections, including opportunistic infections. Some of these infections have been severe (e.g., resulting in respiratory or hepatic failure) or fatal.

Localized and systemic infections (e.g., pneumonia and other bacterial infections, mycobacterial infections, invasive fungal infections such as aspergillosis or candidiasis) have been reported in 37% of patients with advanced renal cell carcinoma receiving everolimus; grade 3 or 4 infections have been reported in 7 or 3% of patients, respectively. Viral infections, including reactivation of hepatitis B virus, also have been reported. Infections have been reported in 64% of patients receiving a regimen containing everolimus for prevention of rejection of renal allografts. Respiratory tract infections have been reported in 31% of patients with subependymal giant cell astrocytoma (SEGA) receiving everolimus.

The manufacturer states that antimicrobial prophylaxis for *Pneumocystis jiroveci* (formerly *Pneumocystis carinii*) pneumonia and cytomegalovirus (CMV) is recommended in transplant recipients.

Clinicians should be vigilant for signs and symptoms of infection; if infection develops, appropriate treatment should be promptly instituted and interruption or discontinuance of everolimus therapy should be considered. If invasive systemic fungal infection occurs, everolimus should be discontinued and appropriate antifungal therapy initiated. Treatment of a preexisting invasive fungal infection should be completed prior to initiating everolimus therapy.

Patients receiving immunosuppressive therapy, including everolimus, are at increased risk of developing malignancies, such as lymphomas and other malignancies, particularly of the skin. The risk of malignancy appears to be related to the intensity and duration of immunosuppression rather than to the use of any specific drug. (See Advice to Patients.)

Kidney Graft Thrombosis. An increased risk of kidney arterial and venous thrombosis, resulting in graft loss and occurring primarily within the first 30 days posttransplantation, has been reported with the use of everolimus in renal transplantation.

Renal Effects. Increases in serum creatinine concentrations and proteinuria have been reported in clinical trials with everolimus (Afinitor®). Cases of renal failure (including acute renal failure), some with a fatal outcome, also have been observed in everolimus-treated patients. Renal function (including BUN, urinary proteins, and/or serum creatinine) should be monitored prior to and periodically during therapy.

Increased nephrotoxicity resulting in a lower glomerular filtration rate can occur with the use of standard dosages of cyclosporine concurrently with everolimus (Zortress®) in renal transplant patients. Therefore, reduced dosages of cyclosporine should be administered when the drug is used in combination with everolimus, and cyclosporine and everolimus whole blood trough concentrations should be monitored. (See Drug Interactions: Cyclosporine.) In hepatic transplant recipients, everolimus has not been studied with standard dosages of tacrolimus. Reduced dosages of tacrolimus should be used in combination with everolimus to minimize the potential risk of nephrotoxicity with this combination. (See Drug Interactions: Tacrolimus.) Renal function should be monitored during everolimus therapy in all transplant patients. Clinicians should consider switching to other immunosuppressive therapies if renal function does not improve after dosage adjustments or if the renal dysfunction is thought to be drug related.

An increased risk of proteinuria has been reported in transplant patients receiving everolimus (Zortress®), with a higher risk observed in patients with higher everolimus whole blood trough concentrations. Transplant patients receiving everolimus should therefore be monitored for proteinuria.

Increased Mortality in Cardiac Transplantation. In a clinical trial of de novo cardiac transplant patients, everolimus (Zortress®) in an immunosuppressive regimen with or without induction therapy resulted in increased mortality, often associated with serious infections, in the first 3 months posttransplantation compared with the control regimen (containing mycophenolate mofetil). Therefore, use of everolimus in cardiac transplantation is *not* recommended by the manufacturer.

Sensitivity Reactions

Hypersensitivity Reactions. Hypersensitivity reactions including anaphylaxis, dyspnea, flushing, chest pain, and/or angioedema (e.g., swelling of the airways or tongue, with or without respiratory impairment) have been reported with everolimus and other rapamycin derivatives. (See Angioedema under Cautions: Other Warnings and Precautions and also see Drug Interactions: Angiotensin-converting Enzyme Inhibitors.)

Other Warnings and Precautions

Interstitial Lung Disease/Noninfectious Pneumonitis. Noninfectious pneumonitis, which is a class effect of rapamycin derivatives, has been reported in up to 19% of patients receiving everolimus (Afinitor®) in clinical trials (including at reduced dosages) and was described as a grade 3 or 4 event in up to 4 or 0.2%, respectively, of patients receiving the drug. Fatal noninfectious pneumonitis also has been reported with everolimus.

A diagnosis of noninfectious pneumonitis should be considered in patients presenting with nonspecific respiratory signs and symptoms (e.g., hypoxia, pleural effusion, cough, dyspnea) and in whom other causes (e.g., infection, cancer) have been excluded. If moderate or severe symptoms of noninfectious pneumonitis develop in patients with breast cancer, neuroendocrine tumors of pancreatic origin, renal cell carcinoma, renal angiomyolipoma, or SEGA, everolimus therapy should be temporarily interrupted or discontinued and subsequent dosage reduced. (See Noninfectious Pneumonitis under Dosage and Administration: Dosage Modification for Toxicity.) Corticosteroids may be indicated until symptoms resolve in patients with grade 2 or greater noninfectious pneumonitis.

A diagnosis of interstitial lung disease should be considered in patients presenting with symptoms consistent with infectious pneumonia but not responding to antibiotic therapy and in whom other causes (e.g., infection, cancer, other non-drug causes) have been excluded. In renal or hepatic transplant patients, cases of interstitial lung disease generally resolve following interruption of everolimus therapy with or without glucocorticoid therapy; however, fatal cases have been reported.

Oral Ulceration. Oral ulcerations are a common adverse effect associated with everolimus and other mammalian target of rapamycin (mTOR) inhibitors; such ulcerations usually appear as aphthous-like ulcerations rather than the mucositis typically observed with conventional chemotherapy. Mouth ulcers, stomatitis, and oral mucositis have been reported in 44–86% of patients treated with everolimus (Afinitor®) in clinical trials. Grade 3 or 4 stomatitis was reported in 4–9% of patients.

Topical therapy is recommended for patients experiencing such oral ulcerations; however, alcohol-, peroxide-, iodine-, and thyme-containing mouthwashes should be *avoided* because they may exacerbate the condition. Grade 1 stomatitis can be managed with nonalcoholic or salt water (0.9%) mouthwash several times daily. Grade 2 and 3 stomatitis can be managed with topical analgesic mouth treatments (e.g., benzocaine, butyl aminobenzoate, tetracaine hydrochloride, menthol or phenol) with or without topical corticosteroids (e.g., triamcinolone oral paste). Because of the high potential for drug interactions, systemic antifungal therapy should *not* be used unless fungal infection has been diagnosed. (See Drug Interactions.)

For additional recommendations concerning temporary interruption of therapy, dosage reduction, and/or discontinuance of therapy based on the severity of stomatitis, see Stomatitis under Dosage and Administration: Dosage Modification for Toxicity.

Hepatic Artery Thrombosis. mTOR inhibitors are associated with an increased risk of hepatic artery thrombosis (HAT). Most cases of HAT have occurred within the first 30 days posttransplantation and most resulted in graft loss or death. Therefore, the manufacturer states that everolimus should not be administered earlier than 30 days following liver transplantation.

Polyoma Virus Infections. Patients receiving immunosuppressants, including everolimus, are at an increased risk for opportunistic infections, including polyoma virus infections. Polyoma virus infections in transplant recipients may have serious, sometimes fatal outcomes. These include polyoma virus-associated neuropathy (PVAN), mostly due to BK virus infection, and JC virus-associated progressive multiple leukoencephalopathy (PML). PVAN has been reported in patients receiving immunosuppressants, including everolimus, and may lead to deteriorating renal function and renal graft loss. Patient monitoring may help detect patients at risk of PVAN.

Decreasing total immunosuppression should be considered in patients who develop evidence of PVAN or PML. Clinicians should also consider the potential risk that reduced immunosuppression represents to the functioning allograft. (For further information about these latent viral infections, see Latent Viral Infections under Cautions: Other Warnings and Precautions, in Sirolimus 92:44.)

Immunization. Use of live vaccines (e.g., influenza virus vaccine live intranasal, measles virus vaccine live, mumps virus vaccine live, rubella virus vaccine live, poliovirus vaccine live oral [OPV; no longer commercially available in the US], BCG vaccine, yellow fever vaccine, varicella vaccine live, typhoid vaccine live oral) and close contact with individuals who have received live vaccines should be *avoided* during everolimus therapy.

The manufacturer recommends that for pediatric patients with SEGA who do not require immediate treatment, the recommended childhood series of live virus vaccinations according to the US Public Health Service Advisory Committee on Immunization Practices (ACIP) guidelines should be completed prior to initiation of everolimus therapy. The manufacturer also states that an accelerated vaccination schedule may be appropriate.

Angioedema. Everolimus and other mTOR inhibitors are associated with the development of angioedema. The concomitant use of everolimus with other drugs known to cause angioedema such as angiotensin-converting enzyme (ACE) inhibitors may increase the risk of developing angioedema. Patients receiving everolimus should be monitored for possible symptoms of angioedema; if angioedema occurs, prompt treatment is necessary. (See Hypersensitivity Reactions under Warnings/Precautions: Sensitivity Reactions, in Cautions and also see Drug Interactions: Angiotensin-converting Enzyme Inhibitors.)

Delayed Wound Healing and Fluid Accumulation. Everolimus increases the risk of delayed wound healing and increases the incidence of wound-related complications, including wound dehiscence, wound infection, incisional hernia, lymphocele, and seroma. Surgical intervention may be required to treat these wound-related complications. Generalized fluid accumulation, including peripheral edema (e.g., lymphedema), and other types of localized fluid accumulation, such as pericardial and pleural effusions and ascites, also have been reported.

Patients receiving everolimus should be monitored for possible symptoms of delayed wound healing and fluid accumulation, and the conditions should be treated promptly to minimize potential complications. (See Advice to Patients.)

Hyperglycemia and Diabetes Mellitus. Hyperglycemia has been reported in everolimus-treated patients. Fasting glucose concentrations should be monitored prior to and periodically during everolimus (Afinitor®) therapy; when possible, optimal glycemic control should be achieved prior to initiation of everolimus therapy.

An increased risk of developing new-onset diabetes mellitus has been observed with everolimus (Zortress®) therapy following transplantation. Glucose concentrations should be monitored closely in patients receiving everolimus following renal and hepatic allotransplantation.

Hyperlipidemia. Hyperlipidemia (e.g., hypercholesterolemia, hypertriglyceridemia) has been reported in patients receiving everolimus (Afinitor®, Zortress®) and may require treatment. Risk of hyperlipidemia is increased in patients with higher whole blood trough everolimus concentrations. Fasting lipid profile should be monitored prior to and periodically during therapy. When possible, optimal lipid control should be achieved prior to initiation of everolimus therapy.

Patients who develop hyperlipidemia while receiving everolimus (Zortress®) should be treated according to current standards of care. Normalization of serum lipids with antihyperlipidemic agents may not be possible in patients receiving everolimus. The risk/benefit of everolimus therapy should be considered prior to initiating therapy in patients with baseline hyperlipidemia and should be reevaluated in patients who develop severe refractory hyperlipidemia while receiving the drug. Safety and efficacy of everolimus in patients with baseline cholesterol concentrations above 350 mg/dL have not been evaluated.

Patients with Hereditary Disorders. Everolimus may cause diarrhea and malabsorption in patients with rare hereditary problems of galactose intolerance, the Lapp lactase deficiency, or glucose-galactose malabsorption; everolimus should not be used in such patients.

Hematologic Effects. Anemia, lymphopenia, neutropenia, and thrombocytopenia have been reported with everolimus therapy. A complete blood count (CBC) should therefore be monitored prior to and periodically during therapy.

Increased Risk of Thrombotic Microangiopathy/Thrombotic Thrombocytopenic Purpura/Hemolytic Uremic Syndrome. Concurrent use of everolimus and cyclosporine may increase the risk of thrombotic microangiopathy (TMA)/thrombotic thrombocytopenic purpura (TTP)/hemolytic uremic syndrome (HUS). Hematologic parameters should be monitored in patients concurrently receiving everolimus and cyclosporine.

CYP3A4- and P-glycoprotein-mediated Interactions. Concomitant use of everolimus with certain drugs (e.g., moderate or potent inhibitors of cytochrome P-450 [CYP] isoenzyme 3A4 [CYP3A4], potent inducers of CYP3A4, moderate inhibitors of P-glycoprotein) or foods (e.g., grapefruit juice) is not recommended or requires close monitoring of whole blood trough everolimus concentrations and/or adjustment of everolimus dosage. (See Drug Interactions.)

Fetal/Neonatal Morbidity and Mortality. Everolimus can cause fetal harm; teratogenicity and embryolethality have been demonstrated in animals. There are no adequate and well-controlled studies in humans. Women of childbearing potential should be advised to use a highly effective method of contraception during and for up to 8 weeks following discontinuance of everolimus. If everolimus is used during pregnancy or if the patient becomes pregnant while receiving the drug, the patient should be apprised of the potential hazard to the fetus.

Impairment of Male Fertility. Male infertility may be observed with mTOR inhibitors, including everolimus. Everolimus may impair male fertility (decreased fertility was observed in male rats) through its effects on rapidly dividing cells (e.g., germ cells); azoospermia or oligospermia may be observed.

Adequate Patient Evaluation and Monitoring. Fasting glucose and lipid profiles, CBCs, and renal function tests should be monitored prior to and periodically during everolimus therapy.

Specific Populations

Pregnancy. Afinitor® and Afinitor® Disperz®: Category D. Zortress®: Category C. (See Fetal/Neonatal Morbidity and Mortality under Warnings/Precautions: Other Warnings and Precautions, in Cautions, and also see Users Guide.)

The National Transplantation Pregnancy Registry (NTPR) is a pregnancy registry for pregnant women receiving immunosuppressants following any solid organ transplantation; the NTPR encourages reporting of all immunosuppressant exposures during pregnancy in transplant patients by telephone at 877-955-6877 or via their website: http://ntpr.giftoflifeinstitute.org.

Lactation. Everolimus and/or its metabolites readily distribute into milk in lactating rats at a concentration 3.5 times higher than in maternal serum. It is not known whether everolimus is distributed into human milk. Because many drugs are distributed into human milk and because of the potential for serious adverse reactions to everolimus in nursing infants, patients receiving everolimus for breast cancer, progressive neuroendocrine tumors of pancreatic origin, renal angiomyolipoma, renal cell carcinoma, or SEGA should make a decision whether to discontinue nursing or the drug, taking into account the importance of the drug to the woman. Renal and hepatic transplant patients receiving everolimus should avoid breast-feeding during treatment with the drug.

Pediatric Use. Safety and efficacy of everolimus for the treatment of SEGA associated with tuberous sclerosis complex (TSC) have been evaluated in pediatric patients 1 year of age and older. Safety and efficacy have not been established in pediatric patients younger than 1 year of age with SEGA. Safety and efficacy of everolimus for the treatment of renal angiomyolipoma with TSC in the absence of SEGA have not been established in pediatric patients.

Clearance of everolimus normalized to body surface area was higher in pediatric patients compared with adults with SEGA.

Safety and efficacy of everolimus for the prevention of renal or hepatic allograft rejection have not been established in pediatric patients younger than 18 years of age.

In pediatric patients with SEGA who do not require immediate everolimus treatment, the recommended childhood series of live virus vaccinations should be completed prior to initiation of everolimus therapy. The manufacturer also states that an accelerated vaccination schedule may be appropriate. (See Immunization under Warnings/Precautions: Other Warnings and Precautions, in Cautions.)

The manufacturer states that the long-term effects of everolimus on growth and pubertal development are not known.

Geriatric Use. In a randomized clinical study evaluating everolimus in patients with advanced hormone receptor-positive, *HER2*-negative breast cancer, 40% of patients receiving everolimus were 65 years of age or older, and 15% were 75 years of age or older. No overall differences in efficacy relative to younger adults were observed. The incidence of deaths due to any cause within 28 days of the last everolimus dose in patients younger than 65 years of age was 2% compared with 6% in patients 65 years of age or older. Adverse effects leading to permanent treatment discontinuance occurred in 33% of patients aged 65 or older compared with 17% of patients younger than 65 years of age.

In 2 other randomized clinical studies in patients with advanced renal cell carcinoma and advanced neuroendocrine tumors of pancreatic origin, 41 and 30% of patients receiving everolimus were 65 years of age or older, respectively, and 7% were 75 years of age or older in both studies. No overall differences in safety and efficacy relative to younger adults were observed in these studies. Other clinical experience with everolimus (Afinitor®) has not revealed differences in response between geriatric and younger patients, but increased sensitivity cannot be ruled out.

Although routine initial dosage adjustment does not appear to be necessary, the manufacturer of Afinitor® and Afinitor® Disperz® recommends close monitoring and appropriate dosage adjustments in geriatric patients receiving the drug.

Clinical experience with the use of everolimus (Zortress®) following transplantation in patients 65 years of age or older is limited to date.

Hepatic Impairment. Following administration of a single oral dose of everolimus, exposure (i.e., average area under the plasma concentration-time curve [AUC]) was increased by 1.6-, 3.2-, or 3.6-fold in patients with mild, moderate, or severe hepatic impairment, respectively, compared with individuals with normal hepatic function. In another study, the average AUC of everolimus in individuals with moderate hepatic impairment reportedly was twice that observed in those with normal hepatic function.

In patients with mild, moderate, or severe (Child-Pugh class A, B, or C) hepatic impairment with breast cancer, neuroendocrine tumors of pancreatic origin, advanced renal cell carcinoma, or renal angiomyolipoma, or who have received a renal or hepatic allotransplant, everolimus dosage reduction is recommended. In patients with mild or moderate (Child-Pugh class A or B) hepatic impairment with SEGA, the everolimus dosage should be adjusted based on therapeutic drug monitoring. In patients with severe hepatic impairment (Child-Pugh class C) with SEGA, a reduction in the initial dosage is recommended and subsequent dosage adjustment should be based on therapeutic drug monitoring. (See Dosage and Administration: Special Populations.)

Renal Impairment. Safety and efficacy of everolimus in patients with renal impairment have not been studied specifically to date. However, a population pharmacokinetic analysis demonstrated no significant correlation between creatinine clearance (range: 25–178 mL/minute) and everolimus clearance. In renal transplant patients, creatinine clearance (range: 11–107 mL/minute) did not affect the pharmacokinetics of everolimus. Because renal impairment is not expected to influence drug exposure, the manufacturer states that no dosage adjustment is necessary in patients with renal impairment.

■ Common Adverse Effects

Adverse effects reported in 10% or more of patients receiving everolimus for the treatment of advanced hormone receptor-positive, *HER2*-negative breast cancer and more frequently with the drug than with placebo include stomatitis (including mouth ulceration, aphthous stomatitis, glossodynia, gingival pain, glossitis, and lip ulceration), infections, rash, fatigue or asthenia, diarrhea, decreased appetite, nausea, weight loss, cough, dysgeusia, headache, dyspnea, arthralgia, peripheral edema, pneumonitis (including interstitial lung disease, lung infiltration, and pulmonary fibrosis), epistaxis, vomiting, pyrexia, back pain, constipation, pruritus, insomnia, dry mouth, and alopecia. Laboratory abnormalities reported in 10% or more of patients and more frequently than with placebo include hypercholesterolemia, hyperglycemia, increased AST concentrations, anemia, leukopenia, thrombocytopenia, lymphopenia, increased ALT concentrations, hypertriglyceridemia, decreased albumin concentrations, neutropenia, hypokalemia, and increased creatinine concentrations.

Adverse effects reported in 10% or more of patients receiving everolimus for the treatment of advanced neuroendocrine tumors of pancreatic origin and more frequently with the drug than with placebo include stomatitis, rash, diarrhea, fatigue/malaise, edema (peripheral or generalized), abdominal pain, fever, headache/migraine, decreased appetite, vomiting, weight loss, nasopharyngitis/rhinitis/upper respiratory tract infection, cough, nail disorders, epistaxis, pruritus, dyspnea, dysgeusia, pneumonitis, urinary tract infection, arthralgia, back pain, pain in extremity, insomnia, constipation, dry skin, hypertension, dizziness, dry mouth, oropharyngeal pain, diabetes mellitus, and muscle spasms. Laboratory abnormalities reported in 10% or more of patients and more frequently than with placebo include anemia, increased alkaline phosphatase concentrations, hyperglycemia, hypercholesterolemia, decreased bicarbonate concentrations, increased AST concentrations, increased ALT concentrations, lymphopenia, thrombocytopenia, leukopenia, hypophosphatemia, hypertriglyceridemia, hypocalcemia, neutropenia, hypokalemia, increased creatinine concentrations, and hypoalbuminemia.

Adverse effects reported in 10% or more of patients receiving everolimus for the treatment of advanced renal cell carcinoma and more frequently with the drug than with placebo include stomatitis, infections, asthenia, fatigue, diarrhea, cough, rash, nausea, peripheral edema, anorexia, dyspnea, vomiting, pyrexia, mucosal inflammation, headache, epistaxis, pneumonitis, pruritus, dry skin, dysgeusia, and pain in extremity.

Adverse effects reported in 10% or more of patients receiving everolimus for the treatment of renal angiomyolipoma with tuberous sclerosis complex (TSC) and more frequently with the drug than with placebo include stomatitis, acne, cough, vomiting, diarrhea, arthralgia, amenorrhea, peripheral edema, and upper respiratory tract infection. Hypercholesterolemia, hypertriglyceridemia, and anemia also were commonly reported.

Adverse effects reported in 10% or more of patients receiving everolimus for the treatment of subependymal giant cell astrocytoma (SEGA) with TSC include stomatitis (including mouth and lip ulceration), respiratory tract infection, elevated cholesterol concentrations, increased AST concentrations, increased ALT concentrations, elevated partial thromboplastin time, neutropenia, reduced hemoglobin concentrations, pyrexia, fatigue, vomiting, diarrhea, constipation, gastroenteritis, psychiatric disorders (including anxiety, aggression, or other behavioral disturbances), hyperglycemia, cellulitis, rash, acne, increased creatinine concentrations, hypertriglyceridemia, and pharyngitis.

Adverse effects reported in 10% or more of patients receiving everolimus in combination with reduced-exposure cyclosporine for prevention of organ rejection after renal transplantation include infections, peripheral edema, constipation, hypertension, nausea, anemia, urinary tract infection, hyperlipidemia, diarrhea, pyrexia, headache, hyperkalemia, increased creatinine concentrations, hypercholesterolemia, insomnia, incision site pain, upper respiratory tract infection, dyslipidemia, procedural pain, vomiting, abdominal pain, hypomagnesemia, hypophosphatemia, extremity pain, hematuria, hyperglycemia, hypokalemia, back pain, and dysuria.

Adverse effects reported in 10% or more of patients receiving everolimus in combination with reduced-exposure tacrolimus for prevention of organ rejection after hepatic transplantation include infections, diarrhea, headache, peripheral edema, hypertension, nausea, leukopenia, abdominal pain, and pyrexia.

Drug Interactions

Everolimus is a substrate of cytochrome P-450 (CYP) isoenzyme 3A4; the drug is a competitive inhibitor of CYP3A4 and a mixed inhibitor of CYP2D6 in vitro. Everolimus also is a substrate and moderate inhibitor of the efflux transporter P-glycoprotein.

■ Drugs and Foods Affecting or Metabolized by Hepatic Microsomal Enzymes ***CYP3A4 Inhibitors*** Pharmacokinetic interactions have been observed during concomitant use with ketoconazole, erythromycin, or verapamil (increased peak plasma concentrations and area under the plasma concentration-time curve [AUC] of everolimus). Concomitant use of everolimus with potent CYP3A4 inhibitors (e.g., atazanavir, boceprevir, clarithromycin, grapefruit or grapefruit juice, indinavir, itraconazole, ketoconazole, nefazodone, nelfinavir, ritonavir, saquinavir, telaprevir, telithromycin, voriconazole) should be *avoided.*

Everolimus should be used with caution with moderate inhibitors of CYP3A4 (e.g., aprepitant, diltiazem, erythromycin, fluconazole, fosamprenavir, verapamil).

If erythromycin or verapamil is used concurrently with everolimus in transplant patients, blood everolimus concentrations should be monitored and everolimus dosage adjusted accordingly.

If coadministration of a moderate inhibitor of CYP3A4 is required in patients with breast cancer, neuroendocrine tumors of pancreatic origin, advanced renal cell carcinoma, or renal angiomyolipoma, everolimus dosage should be reduced to 2.5 mg daily, which is predicted to adjust everolimus AUC to the range observed without coadministration of a CYP3A4 inhibitor. An increase in everolimus dosage from 2.5 mg to 5 mg daily may be considered based on patient tolerance. However, if the moderate CYP3A4 inhibitor is discontinued, a washout period of approximately 2–3 days should be allowed before the everolimus dosage is increased. If the moderate CYP3A4 inhibitor is discontinued, the everolimus dosage should be returned to the dosage used prior to initiation of the moderate CYP3A4 inhibitor.

If coadministration of a moderate inhibitor of CYP3A4 is required in patients with subependymal giant cell astrocytoma (SEGA), the initial recommended everolimus dosage is 2.5 mg/m^2 daily. If a moderate inhibitor of CYP3A4 is initiated during everolimus therapy, everolimus dosage should be reduced by approximately 50%. If dosage reduction is required in patients receiving the lowest available strength, alternate-day dosing should be considered. Subsequent dosing should be individualized based on therapeutic drug monitoring. Trough everolimus concentrations should be assessed approximately 2 weeks after dosage reduction. If the moderate CYP3A4 inhibitor is discontinued, the everolimus dosage should be returned to the dosage used prior to initiation of the moderate CYP3A4 inhibitor 2–3 days after discontinuance of the moderate inhibitor; trough everolimus concentration should be reassessed approximately 2 weeks later.

In patients with SEGA, foods and nutritional supplements known to inhibit CYP or P-glycoprotein activity (e.g., grapefruit, grapefruit juice) should *not* be consumed.

CYP3A4 Inducers Pharmacokinetic interactions have been observed during concomitant use with rifampin (decreased peak plasma concentrations and AUC of everolimus). Concomitant use with potent CYP3A4 inducers (e.g., carbamazepine, phenobarbital, phenytoin, rifabutin, rifampin, rifapentine) should be *avoided* if alternative therapy is available.

If concomitant use with a potent CYP3A4 inducer cannot be avoided in patients with breast cancer, neuroendocrine tumors of pancreatic origin, renal cell carcinoma, or renal angiomyolipoma, an increase in everolimus dosage (from 10 mg daily up to 20 mg daily, titrated in 5-mg increments) should be considered based on pharmacokinetic considerations; however, no clinical data on this dosage adjustment in this patient population are available. If the potent CYP3A4 inducer is discontinued, dosage of everolimus should be returned to the dosage used prior to initiation of the potent CYP3A4 inducer.

If concomitant use with a potent CYP3A4 inducer cannot be avoided in patients with SEGA, the recommended initial dosage of everolimus is 9 mg/m^2 once daily. If a potent CYP3A4 inducer is initiated during everolimus therapy, dosage of everolimus should be doubled. Trough everolimus concentrations should be assessed approximately 2 weeks after doubling the dosage, and the dosage should be adjusted if necessary to maintain a trough concentration of 5–15 ng/mL. If the potent CYP3A4 inducer is discontinued, dosage of everolimus should be reduced to the dosage used prior to initiation of the potent CYP3A4 inducer and everolimus trough concentrations should be reassessed approximately 2 weeks later. Foods or nutritional supplements known to induce CYP activity (e.g., St. John's wort) should not be consumed.

St. John's Wort St. John's wort (*Hypericum perforatum*) may decrease everolimus exposure unpredictably, and its use should be avoided in patients receiving everolimus.

Substrates of CYP3A4 and CYP2D6 Everolimus is unlikely to affect the metabolism of CYP3A4 or CYP2D6 substrates. However, everolimus increased concentrations of these substrates in vitro. Everolimus should therefore be used with caution with CYP3A4 or CYP2D6 substrates.

■ Drugs Affecting the P-Glycoprotein Transport System Pharmacokinetic interactions have been observed during concomitant use of everolimus with inhibitors of P-glycoprotein (P-gp; e.g., erythromycin, ketoconazole, verapamil) that resulted in increased peak plasma concentrations and AUC of everolimus. Everolimus should therefore be used with caution with P-gp inhibitors (e.g., cyclosporine, digoxin, erythromycin, verapamil). If erythromycin or verapamil is used concurrently with everolimus in renal or hepatic transplant patients, blood everolimus concentrations should be monitored and everolimus dosage adjusted as necessary.

If coadministration of a P-gp inhibitor is required in patients with advanced renal cell carcinoma, everolimus dosage should be reduced to 2.5 mg daily, which is predicted to adjust everolimus AUC to the range observed without coadministration of a P-gp inhibitor. An increase in everolimus dosage from 2.5 mg to 5 mg daily may be considered based on patient tolerance. However, if the P-gp inhibitor is discontinued, a washout period of approximately 2–3 days should be allowed before the everolimus dosage is increased. If the P-gp inhibitor is discontinued, the everolimus dosage should be returned to the dosage used prior to initiation of the P-gp inhibitor.

If coadministration of a P-gp inhibitor is required in patients with SEGA, everolimus dosage should be reduced by approximately 50% to maintain trough everolimus concentrations of 5–10 ng/mL. If dosage reduction is required in patients receiving 2.5 mg daily, alternate-day dosing should be considered. Subsequent dosing should be individualized based on therapeutic drug monitoring. Trough everolimus concentrations should be assessed approximately 2 weeks after the addition of the P-gp inhibitor. If the P-gp inhibitor is discontinued, the everolimus dosage should be returned to the dosage used prior to initiation of the P-gp inhibitor and the trough everolimus concentration should be reassessed approximately 2 weeks later.

■ Angiotensin-converting Enzyme Inhibitors Concomitant use of angiotensin-converting enzyme (ACE) inhibitors with everolimus may increase the risk of angioedema. The use of alternative antihypertensive agents should be considered in everolimus-treated patients, if necessary.

■ Antilipemic Agents Studies in healthy individuals indicate that there are no clinically important pharmacokinetic interactions between single-dose everolimus and atorvastatin (a CYP3A4 substrate) or pravastatin (a non-CYP3A4 substrate and P-gp substrate); HMG-CoA reductase bioactivity in plasma also was not substantially affected. Therefore, dosage adjustments are not necessary when everolimus and atorvastatin or pravastatin are used concurrently. In a population pharmacokinetic analysis, simvastatin (a CYP3A4 substrate) did not affect clearance of everolimus. The manufacturer of Zortress® cautions that these results cannot be extrapolated to other HMG-CoA reductase inhibitors.

Use of HMG-CoA reductase inhibitors such as lovastatin or simvastatin was strongly discouraged in clinical trials of everolimus with cyclosporine in renal transplant patients because of an interaction between HMG-CoA reductase inhibitors and cyclosporine. The manufacturer of Zortress® recommends that patients receiving everolimus and cyclosporine therapy who are concurrently receiving an HMG-CoA reductase inhibitor and/or fibric acid derivative be monitored for the possible development of rhabdomyolysis and other adverse effects, which are described in the prescribing information for these antilipemic agents.

■ Cyclosporine Administration of a single dose of cyclosporine resulted in increased steady-state peak plasma concentrations and AUC of everolimus.

Use of standard-dose cyclosporine therapy with everolimus results in increased risk of nephrotoxicity and decreased glomerular filtration rate. Renal transplant patients receiving everolimus should receive reduced-dose cyclosporine therapy, and renal function should be monitored. Adjustment of everolimus dosage may be required if cyclosporine dosage is altered. Switching to alternative immunosuppressive therapies should be considered if renal function does not improve after dosage adjustments or if renal dysfunction is thought to be drug-related.

Concomitant use of everolimus and cyclosporine may increase the risk of thrombotic microangiopathy/thrombotic thrombocytopenic purpura/hemolytic uremic syndrome. Hematologic parameters should be monitored in patients receiving everolimus and cyclosporine concurrently.

■ **Exemestane** Concomitant use of everolimus and exemestane increased exemestane trough plasma concentrations by 45% and plasma concentrations at 2 hours by 64%. However, corresponding estradiol concentrations at steady state (4 weeks) were not different in patients receiving exemestane and everolimus compared with patients receiving exemestane and placebo. In addition, no increase in adverse effects related to exemestane was observed in patients with hormone receptor-positive, *HER2*-negative advanced breast cancer who received combined everolimus and exemestane therapy.

■ **Immunosuppressive Agents** Caution is recommended when other immunosuppressive agents are used with everolimus because of the risk of increased immunosuppression and increased risk of lymphoma, other malignancies, and infection.

■ **Midazolam** Concurrent administration of single-dose midazolam (4 mg as oral solution), a CYP3A4/5 substrate, with steady-state everolimus (10 mg daily for 5 days) in healthy males increased peak plasma concentrations and AUC of midazolam by 25 and 30%, respectively. The elimination half-life of midazolam and the metabolic AUC ratio (i.e., the ratio of 1-hydroxymidazolam AUC to midazolam AUC) were not altered. Dosage adjustment of midazolam or other CYP3A4/5 substrates is not necessary when used concomitantly with everolimus.

■ **Nephrotoxic Agents** Caution is recommended when other nephrotoxic agents are used with everolimus because of the risk of increased nephrotoxicity.

■ **Octreotide** Concurrent use of everolimus and the long-acting parenteral formulation of octreotide acetate increased trough plasma concentrations of octreotide by approximately 50%.

■ **Tacrolimus** There is little to no pharmacokinetic effect of tacrolimus on everolimus; therefore, dosage adjustment of everolimus is generally not necessary when used concomitantly with tacrolimus.

In hepatic transplant recipients, everolimus has not been studied with standard-dose tacrolimus. Reduced dosages of tacrolimus should be used in combination with everolimus to minimize the potential risk of nephrotoxicity with this combination. Renal function should be monitored during combined therapy, and clinicians should consider switching to other immunosuppressive therapies if renal function does not improve after dosage adjustments or if the renal dysfunction is thought to be drug related.

■ **Vaccines** The manufacturer states that live vaccines (including influenza virus vaccine live intranasal, measles virus vaccine live, mumps virus vaccine live, rubella virus vaccine live, poliovirus vaccine live oral [OPV; no longer commercially available in the US], BCG vaccine, yellow fever vaccine, varicella virus vaccine live, typhoid vaccine live oral) should be avoided in patients receiving everolimus therapy. (See Immunization under Warnings/Precautions: Other Warnings and Precautions, in Cautions.)

Description

Everolimus, an inhibitor of mammalian target of rapamycin (mTOR), is an antineoplastic agent and macrolide immunosuppressive agent. Everolimus inhibits antigenic and interleukin (IL-2 and IL-15) stimulated activation and proliferation of T and B lymphocytes. Serine/threonine kinases, such as mTOR, are involved in various cascades of intracellular signaling events that regulate cell growth and proliferation and/or influence processes critical to cell survival and tumor progression (e.g., angiogenesis, metastasis). Everolimus binds with high affinity to the intracellular protein FK506 binding protein-12 (FKBP-12), forming a drug-protein complex with mTOR complex 1 (mTORC1 or everolimus:FKBP-12) that binds to and inhibits the activation of mTOR. This disruption of mTOR reduces the activity of downstream effectors (i.e., S6 ribosomal protein kinase [S6K1], eukaryotic elongation factor 4E-binding protein [4E-BP1]), thereby blocking progression of cells from G1 into S phase and, subsequently, inducing cell growth arrest and apoptosis. S6K1 is a substrate of mTORC1 and phosphorylates the activation domain 1 of the estrogen receptor, resulting in ligand-independent activation of the receptor. The everolimus:FKBP-12 complex has no effect on calcineurin activity. Everolimus also inhibits expression of hypoxia-inducible factor (e.g., HIF-1α), thereby reducing the expression of vascular endothelial growth factor (VEGF). Inhibition of mTOR by everolimus has been shown to reduce cell proliferation, angiogenesis, and glucose uptake *in vitro* and/or *in vivo*.

Constitutive activation of the phosphoinositide 3-kinase inhibitor (PI3K)/Akt/mTOR pathway can lead to endocrine resistance in breast cancer. Estrogen-dependent and *HER2*-positive breast cancer cells are sensitive to the inhibitory effects of everolimus in vitro. Concomitant use of everolimus with Akt, *HER2*, or aromatase inhibitors (e.g., anastrozole, exemestane, letrozole) enhances the anti-tumor activity of everolimus in a synergistic manner.

Loss or inactivation of tuberin-sclerosis complexes 1 and 2 (*TSC1* and *TSC2*), oncogene suppressors that are two of the regulators of mTORC1 signaling, leads to activation of downstream signaling. In the genetic disorder tuberous sclerosis, inactivating mutations in the *TSC1* or *TSC2* gene leads to hematoma formation throughout the body; subependymal giant cell astrocytomas (SEGA) may develop in patients with tuberous sclerosis.

Following oral administration of doses ranging from 5–70 mg in patients with advanced solid tumors, peak everolimus concentrations are attained within 1–2 hours. Steady-state concentrations are achieved within 2 weeks of once-daily dosing in patients with advanced solid tumors. In patients with SEGA, intrapatient steady-state trough everolimus concentrations were dose-proportional at daily dosages of 1.5–14.6 mg/m^2. In renal allograft patients, steady-state peak plasma concentrations and area under the concentration-time curve (AUC) values were dose-proportional at dosages of 0.5–2 mg twice daily; steady-state concentrations were achieved by day 4, with an accumulation in blood concentrations of twofold to threefold compared with exposure following the first dose. In healthy individuals, administration of 10-mg tablets with a high-fat meal reduces peak plasma concentrations and AUC of everolimus by 54 and 22%, respectively; administration with a light-fat meal reduces peak plasma concentration and AUC by 42 and 32%, respectively. However, food has no effect on the post-absorption phase concentration-time profile of everolimus. In healthy individuals and in those with moderate hepatic impairment, everolimus is approximately 74% bound to plasma proteins. The drug has been shown to cross the placenta and distribute into milk in rats. Everolimus is metabolized by the cytochrome P-450 (CYP) microsomal enzyme system, principally by isoenzyme 3A4. The mean elimination half-life of everolimus is approximately 30 hours. Following administration of a single 3-mg dose in patients receiving concomitant cyclosporine, approximately 80 and 5% of the dose is excreted in feces and urine, respectively, as inactive metabolites.

The AUC of everolimus tablets for oral suspension (Afinitor® Disperz®) was equivalent to the AUC of everolimus tablets (Afinitor®); peak plasma concentrations were 20–36% lower for everolimus tablets for oral suspension compared with everolimus tablets. Following daily administration, predicted steady-state trough concentrations were similar in patients receiving everolimus tablets for oral suspension and everolimus tablets.

A cross-study comparison of pharmacokinetic data reported higher exposure to everolimus among Japanese patients compared with non-Japanese patients. Data from a population pharmacokinetic analysis indicate that clearance of everolimus is 20% higher in black patients than in Caucasian patients. The relevance of these differences to the safety and efficacy of everolimus in Japanese or black patients has not been established.

Advice to Patients

Importance of providing patient a copy of manufacturer's patient information (Afinitor® and Afinitor® Disperz®) or medication guide (Zortress®).

Importance of taking everolimus tablets at about the same time each day (or twice daily approximately 12 hours apart), either consistently with food or consistently without food. Importance of swallowing the tablets (Afinitor® or Zortress®) whole with a glass of water and not crushing or chewing the tablets.

Importance of informing patients that everolimus tablets for oral suspension (Afinitor® Disperz®) should be taken as a suspension only and should not be swallowed whole. The suspension should be taken orally once daily at the same time each day, either consistently with food or consistently without food. Procedures for preparation of everolimus tablets for oral suspension (Afinitor® Disperz®) should be reviewed with patients.

Importance of storing everolimus (Afinitor® or Afinitor® Disperz®) tablets in the original package and keeping the blister package and tablets dry and protected from light. Importance of opening the blister package (scissors may be used to avoid spillage) immediately prior to taking everolimus. Importance of keeping everolimus (Zortress®) tablets dry and protecting the tablets from light.

If a dose of everolimus (Afinitor® or Afinitor® Disperz®) is missed by 6 hours or less, the dose should be taken as soon as it is remembered, and the next dose should be taken at the regularly scheduled time; if a dose is missed by more than 6 hours, the dose should be omitted, and the next dose should be taken at the regularly scheduled time. A double dose should not be administered to make up for a missed dose.

Risk of serious allergic reactions, including anaphylaxis; importance of immediately reporting any facial swelling or difficulty breathing.

Risk of noninfectious pneumonitis, which may be fatal; importance of promptly reporting any new or worsening respiratory symptoms (e.g., cough, shortness of breath, difficulty breathing, wheezing).

Risk of increased susceptibility to infection, which may be fatal; importance of promptly reporting any signs or symptoms of infection (e.g., fever, chills).

Risk of reactivation of hepatitis B virus infection. Importance of promptly reporting any signs and symptoms of possible hepatitis B virus infection (e.g., loss of appetite, pale stools or dark urine, yellowing of the skin, pain in upper right side of the abdomen).

Risk of malignancy, including lymphoma and skin cancer. Importance of limiting exposure to sunlight and ultraviolet light by wearing protective clothing and using sunscreen with a high protection factor.

Risk of new-onset diabetes mellitus; importance of reporting any signs or symptoms of diabetes mellitus (e.g., frequent urination, increased thirst or hunger).

Risk of mouth ulcers, stomatitis, and oral mucositis. Importance of reporting any signs or symptoms of oral ulceration (e.g., pain, discomfort, or open sores in the mouth). Use of mouthwashes and/or topical treatments is recommended to treat oral ulceration; however, alcohol-, peroxide-, iodine-, or thyme-containing preparations should be *avoided* since they may exacerbate the condition.

Risk of kidney arterial and venous thrombosis leading to graft loss in renal transplant recipients; usually occurs within first 30 days after transplantation. Importance of promptly reporting any signs and symptoms of possible kidney thrombosis (e.g., pain in groin, lower back, side, or stomach, decreased urination, blood in urine or dark colored urine, fever, nausea, vomiting).

Risk of polyoma virus-associated nephropathy (PVAN), which may result in deteriorating renal function and renal graft loss.

Risk of proteinuria in patients receiving everolimus following transplantation.

Risk of angioedema; risk may be increased by concomitant use of other drugs known to cause angioedema (e.g., angiotensin-converting enzyme inhibitors). Importance of seeking prompt medical attention in case of symptoms of angioedema (e.g., sudden swelling of face, mouth, throat, tongue, or hands; hives or welts; itchy or painful swollen skin; trouble breathing).

Risk of impaired wound healing and fluid accumulation. Importance of careful observation of incision site in patients who have undergone renal or hepatic allotransplantation. Importance of promptly informing healthcare provider if incision is red, warm, or painful; if there is blood, fluid, or pus in incision; if incision opens up; or in case of swelling of incision.

Risk of increased blood glucose, triglyceride, and/or cholesterol concentrations; risk of adverse renal and hematologic effects. Fasting glucose and lipid profiles, complete blood counts (CBCs), and renal and liver function tests are required; importance of adherence to laboratory appointment schedules.

Need for therapeutic drug monitoring in patients receiving everolimus for the treatment of subependymal giant cell astrocytoma (SEGA) or for the prevention of rejection of renal or hepatic allografts; importance of adherence to laboratory appointment schedules.

Importance of avoiding use of live vaccines and close contact with those who have received live vaccines.

Importance of avoiding grapefruit and grapefruit juice while receiving everolimus therapy.

Importance of informing clinicians of hereditary disorders of galactose intolerance (Lapp lactase deficiency or glucose-galactose malabsorption); Zortress® therapy should be avoided in patients with these conditions.

Importance of informing clinicians of existing or contemplated concomitant therapy, including prescription and OTC drugs (e.g., antifungals, antivirals, anticonvulsants [carbamazepine, phenytoin, barbiturates]) and herbal products (e.g., St. John's wort), as well as any concomitant illnesses (e.g., hepatic impairment, diabetes mellitus or hyperglycemia, hyperlipidemia, infection, history of hepatitis B virus infection, personal or family history of skin cancer).

Importance of women informing clinicians if they are or plan to become pregnant or plan to breast-feed; necessity for clinicians to advise women of childbearing potential to avoid pregnancy and to use a highly effective contraceptive method during therapy and for 8 weeks following discontinuance of therapy. Necessity of advising women to avoid breastfeeding while receiving everolimus therapy. Risk of male infertility (low or no sperm count). Everolimus tablets for oral suspension (Afinitor® Disperz®) can cause fetal harm; the suspension should be prepared by an adult who is not pregnant or planning to become pregnant. Anyone who prepares everolimus tablets for suspension (Afinitor® Disperz®) for another person should wear gloves to avoid possible contact with the drug.

Importance of informing patients of other important precautionary information. (See Cautions.)

Overview® (see Users Guide). For additional information on this drug until a more detailed monograph is developed and published, the manufacturer's labeling should be consulted. It is *essential* that the manufacturer's labeling be consulted for more detailed information on usual cautions, precautions, contraindications, potential drug interactions, laboratory test interferences, and acute toxicity.

Preparations

Excipients in commercially available drug preparations may have clinically important effects in some individuals; consult specific product labeling for details.

Everolimus

Oral		
Tablets	0.25 mg	**Zortress®**, Novartis
	0.5 mg	**Zortress®**, Novartis
	0.75 mg	**Zortress®**, Novartis
	2.5 mg	**Afinitor®**, Novartis
	5 mg	**Afinitor®**, Novartis
	7.5 mg	**Afinitor®**, Novartis
	10 mg	**Afinitor®**, Novartis
Tablets for oral suspension	2 mg	**Afinitor® Disperz®**, Novartis
	3 mg	**Afinitor® Disperz®**, Novartis
	5 mg	**Afinitor® Disperz®**, Novartis

†Use is not currently included in the labeling approved by the US Food and Drug Administration

Fludarabine Phosphate

2-Fluoro-ara-A Monophosphate, 2-Fluoro-ara AMP, FAMP

■ Fludarabine phosphate, a synthetic purine antagonist, is an antimetabolite antineoplastic agent.

Uses

■ **Chronic Lymphocytic Leukemia** Fludarabine is used for the palliative treatment of chronic lymphocytic leukemia (CLL) in patients whose disease does not respond adequately to or progresses during treatment with at least one standard alkylating agent-containing regimen (e.g., chlorambucil with or without prednisone).

While it has been suggested that chronic lymphocytic leukemia can principally involve T-cell proliferation in some patients and fludarabine is active against T cells, some experts currently believe that all cases of chronic lymphocytic leukemia principally involve monoclonal proliferation of B cells. Controlled clinical studies establishing efficacy of fludarabine in the treatment of this leukemia have been limited to a clinical diagnosis of disease phenotypically characterized as B-cell chronic lymphocytic leukemia. The role of fludarabine in the treatment of chronic T-cell lymphocytosis remains to be established.

Fludarabine also has been used in previously untreated patients† and in those whose leukemia contemporaneously was responsive to standard therapy†. While the manufacturer states that safety and efficacy of the drug in such patients remain to be established, some experts believe that use of the drug in this patient population is clinically reasonable. Fludarabine also has been used in the treatment of prolymphocytic leukemia and prolymphocytoid variant of chronic lymphocytic leukemia. (See Uses: Prolymphocytic Leukemia and Prolymphocytoid Variant.)

Because chronic lymphocytic leukemia generally is not curable, occurs principally in geriatric patients, and often progresses slowly, the disease generally is treated conservatively unless there is a clear indication for immediate, aggressive therapy. Therefore, antineoplastic chemotherapy usually is reserved for patients with progressive, symptomatic disease (e.g., those with disease-related symptoms such as fever, night sweats, or weight loss; progressive bone marrow failure; acquired autoimmune hemolytic anemia or thrombocytopenia; enlarged or painful lymph nodes or spleen; disease-related recurrent infections; or progressive lymphocytosis). Most clinicians currently consider chlorambucil, alone or combined with prednisone, the *initial* treatment of choice for chronic lymphocytic leukemia when antineoplastic therapy is indicated and fludarabine the treatment of choice for refractory disease. However, some clinicians currently consider fludarabine an alternative to chlorambucil as initial therapy. Current chemotherapy regimens are only palliative in this leukemia.

In clinical studies employing fludarabine dosages of 15–40 mg/m^2 daily for 5 days every 28 days in patients with refractory chronic lymphocytic leukemia, clinical response rates (including complete remissions and partial responses as defined by the National Cancer Institute Chronic Lymphocytic Leukemia Working Group [NCIWG]) ranged from 32–57%, with up to 13% being complete remissions. The drug has been reported to induce a complete remission with residual nodular or focal lymphoid infiltration of bone marrow in up to another 16–20% of patients. In clinical studies, the median time to response ranged from 7–21 weeks, the median duration of disease control ranged from 65–91 weeks, and the median survival of all patients with refractory disease treated with fludarabine ranged from 43–52 weeks. Survival of 36 months or longer has been reported in patients with complete remission or complete remission with residual nodular or focal lymphoid infiltration of bone marrow. Rai stage (a clinical staging system for CLL based on groupings of prognostic variables) improved to stage II or better in 58–71% of patients whose disease was stage III or IV at baseline but returned to stage 0 in only 43 or 19% of those with stage I–III or IV disease, respectively, at baseline. Survival appears to correlate with final Rai stage achieved, and patients diagnosed with earlier Rai stage disease are more likely to achieve complete remissions compared with patients with later-stage disease. In patients who were anemic and/or thrombocytopenic at baseline, mean hemoglobin concentration improved from 9 to 11.8 g/dL and/or mean platelet count improved from 65,500 to 103,300/mm^3, respectively, at the time of response.

The ability of fludarabine to induce responses in chronic lymphocytic leukemia that was refractory to standard therapy suggests minimal cross-resistance with other agents commonly used in the treatment of this leukemia. Because of an increased incidence of infections with opportunistic pathogens in patients receiving purine analogs in combination with corticosteroids, prednisone should be omitted from regimens containing fludarabine or other purine analogs.

Fludarabine also has been used in patients with previously untreated† chronic lymphocytic leukemia. In a large randomized trial comparing fludarabine, chlorambucil, and fludarabine plus chlorambucil for the initial treatment of CLL, patients receiving fludarabine had higher rates of complete and overall (complete or partial) response (20 and 63%, respectively) than those receiving chlorambucil (4 and 37%, respectively), but no difference was observed in median survival (66 versus 56 months). Both the median duration of response and the median time to progression of disease were longer with fludarabine (25 and 20 months, respectively) than with chlorambucil (14 months for both). The combination of fludarabine and chlorambucil was associated with similar response rates as fludarabine alone, but caused excessive toxicity. Although either single-drug regimen was considered tolerable, higher rates of infections and severe or life-threatening neutropenia were observed in patients receiving fludarabine. Further study is needed to establish the role of fludarabine in patients with previously untreated or nonrefractory disease†.

■ **Non-Hodgkin's Lymphoma** Fludarabine is used alone or in combination regimens for the treatment of low-grade, advanced (stage III or IV) adult non-Hodgkin's lymphoma† that failed or relapsed after previous therapy. Optimal therapy for advanced stages of low-grade adult non-Hodgkin's lymphoma remains controversial, in part because eventual relapse is common regardless of the therapy employed.

Overall response rates with fludarabine have ranged from 45–67% for patients with low-grade histologies. Response may be particularly likely in follicular small-cleaved cell lymphoma (a low-grade lymphoma). Fludarabine in combination with mitoxantrone, with or without dexamethasone, is used in the treatment of advanced, low-grade non-Hodgkin's lymphoma.

■ **Acute Leukemias** Fludarabine has been used in a limited number of patients with either acute myeloid (myelogenous, nonlymphocytic) leukemia† (AML, ANLL) or acute lymphocytic leukemia† (ALL) whose disease failed to respond adequately to conventional therapy or relapsed following remission; the drug was used at dosages substantially higher than those used in the treatment of chronic lymphocytic leukemia. While fludarabine exhibits some activity against these acute leukemias, severe toxicity (e.g., neurotoxicity) associated with the relatively high dosages that would appear necessary for adequate response are thought to preclude the usefulness of the drug as monotherapy for remission induction in these leukemias. Whether fludarabine would be beneficial at lower dosages as an adjunct to other antineoplastic agents to reduce leukemic cell burden in these leukemias remains to be established.

■ **Prolymphocytic Leukemia and Prolymphocytoid Variant** Fludarabine has been used in a limited number of patients for the palliative treatment of prolymphocytic leukemia† (PLL) or prolymphocytoid chronic lymphocytic leukemia† (CLL-Pro) that was refractory to standard chemotherapy (e.g., chlorambucil and prednisone). The drug occasionally has produced complete remissions or partial responses in such patients.Responses in peripheral blood were most common, with those in bone marrow and the spleen being less common. In one small group of patients with these leukemias, complete remissions or partial responses each occurred in 18% of patients (overall response rate of 35%), most of whose disease was refractory at the time fludarabine (alone or combined with prednisone) was initiated. Response to previous therapy with other drugs appeared to be an indicator of the likelihood of response to fludarabine, with those whose disease responded initially to other therapy and then relapsed being more likely to respond to fludarabine than those whose disease was resistant to previous therapy. While the modest response to fludarabine therapy is encouraging in these poorly responsive leukemias, additional study and experience are needed to establish the role of fludarabine in the treatment of these leukemias, particularly concerning whether efficacy can be improved with combination regimens.

■ **Hairy Cell Leukemia** While other drugs (e.g., cladribine, pentostatin) are considered the initial therapies of choice in the treatment of hairy cell leukemia† (leukemic reticuloendotheliosis), limited evidence suggests that fludarabine may be useful in selected patients with this disease. At least partial responses have been reported in several patients with hairy cell leukemia whose disease was refractory to interferon alfa or pentostatin. Additional study and experience are needed to define further the role of fludarabine in the treatment of hairy cell leukemia.

■ **Waldenstrom's Macroglobulinemia** Fludarabine has been shown to be somewhat effective in the treatment of refractory macroglobulinemia† in a limited number of patients. In one study, 45% of patients responded with a greater than 50% reduction of immunoglobulin M (IgM) tumor mass for a projected median duration of greater than one year. Onset of remission was slow; the median time to decrease tumor mass by 50% was greater than 5 months. Further study of fludarabine in the treatment of macroglobulinemia, including study of the drug in combination therapy with other treatment modalities, is needed.

■ **Other Uses** Fludarabine is used in the treatment of mycosis fungoides, a form of cutaneous T-cell lymphoma†.

Dosage and Administration

■ **Reconstitution and Administration** Fludarabine phosphate is administered by IV infusion. The drug also has been administered by rapid IV injection† and by continuous† IV infusion (e.g., over 48 hours), but the manufacturer recommends that fludarabine phosphate be administered by IV infusion over 30 minutes. While the risk of certain toxic effects (e.g., neurotoxicity) is increased with increasing dosage, it remains to be established whether the rate of IV administration of the drug affects the risk of such toxicity, and neurotoxicity has occurred when the drug either was administered by rapid IV injection or slow IV infusion.

Fludarabine phosphate powder for injection is reconstituted by adding 2 mL of sterile water for injection to a vial labeled as containing 50 mg of the drug to provide a solution containing 25 mg/mL. With agitation, the drug should dissolve completely within 15 seconds or less. Alternatively, the commercially available aqueous injection containing 25 mg/mL can be used. The appropriate dose of the drug should then be withdrawn from the vial and added to a compatible IV fluid; in clinical studies, the drug was administered in 100 or 125 mL of 5% dextrose or 0.9% sodium chloride injection.

Fludarabine phosphate solutions contain no preservatives and should be used within 8 hours after reconstitution. (See Chemistry and Stability: Stability.) Care must be taken to ensure the sterility of prepared solutions. The commercially available injection and reconstituted and diluted solutions of fludarabine phosphate should be inspected visually for particulate matter and/or discoloration prior to administration.

Because of the carcinogenic potential of fludarabine (see Cautions: Mutagenicity and Carcinogenicity), the usual cautions for handling and preparing solutions of cytotoxic drugs should be exercised. The manufacturer recommends the use of latex gloves and protective eyewear to avoid exposure to the drug in case of breakage of the container or other accidental spillage; exposure to the drug via inhalation or direct contact with the skin or mucous membranes should be avoided. If fludarabine phosphate powder for injection or a solution of the drug comes in contact with the skin or mucosa, the affected area should be washed immediately and thoroughly with soap and water. If the drug comes in contact with the eyes, the affected eye(s) should be flushed thoroughly with water or saline.

■ **Dosage** ***Chronic Lymphocytic Leukemia*** The recommended initial IV dosage of fludarabine phosphate for the treatment of chronic lymphocytic leukemia in adults is 25 mg/m^2, administered as single daily doses for 5 consecutive days; dosages up to 30 mg/m^2, administered as single daily doses for 5 consecutive days, also have been used. The possible need for dosage adjustment in patients who may be predisposed to fludarabine-induced toxicity (e.g., geriatric patients, those with impaired renal or bone marrow function) should be considered.

Each 5-day course of fludarabine phosphate therapy should begin at 28-day intervals. Some clinicians initially administer the drug for at least 2 or 3 courses to determine patient response, unless unacceptable toxicity or disease progression occurs. Although the optimum duration of therapy remains to be established, it currently is recommended that fludarabine phosphate be continued until a maximal response is achieved or dose-limiting toxicity develops; once a maximal response is achieved in the absence of such toxicity, 3 additional courses of therapy are administered and the drug then is discontinued. Dosage may be decreased or therapy temporarily withheld if evidence of hematologic or nonhematologic toxicity is observed. Therapy should be delayed or discontinued permanently if neurologic toxicity develops. Some patients have received up to at least 15 courses of therapy.

Other Neoplasms Relatively low fludarabine phosphate dosages similar to those currently recommended for the treatment of chronic lymphocytic leukemia also have been used for the treatment of other neoplasms† (e.g., 18–30 mg/m^2 daily for 5 consecutive days at 28-day intervals), but studies currently are ongoing to establish optimum dosages in these conditions.

Maximum Dosage While the maximum safe dosage of fludarabine phosphate for the treatment of chronic lymphocytic leukemia or other neoplasms in adults has not been elucidated fully, severe and potentially irreversible or fatal toxicity (e.g., neurotoxicity) has been observed at dosages of 96 mg/m^2 or more daily for 5–7 days; such relatively high dosages currently are not recommended. Limited data suggest that maximum dosages of up to 40 mg/m^2 daily for 5 days may be well tolerated in adults, but the relative risk to benefit of dosages exceeding those currently recommended remains to be established, and such dosages currently are not recommended except under controlled clinical conditions (e.g., in investigational protocols).

■ **Dosage in Renal Impairment** Because fludarabine (2-fluoro-ara-A), the principal systemically circulating form of fludarabine phosphate, appears to be eliminated mainly unchanged in urine, with total body clearance of this metabolite being directly correlated with creatinine clearance, the drug should be administered cautiously in patients with impaired renal function, including geriatric patients. Close monitoring for potential excessive toxicity is necessary; dosage should be adjusted accordingly. The manufacturer recommends a 20% reduction in fludarabine dosage and close monitoring in adults with moderate renal impairment (creatinine clearance 30–70 mL/minute per 1.73 m^2). Use of fludarabine is *not* recommended in patients with severe renal impairment (creatinine clearance less than 30 mL/minute per 1.73 m^2).

Cautions

Fludarabine is a highly toxic drug. (See Cautions: Precautions and Contraindications.) Many toxic effects of the drug are dose dependent, and the risk of severe and potentially irreversible or fatal toxicity (e.g., neurotoxicity) is increased substantially at relatively high dosages. (See Chronic Toxicity.)

The most common adverse effects of fludarabine include dose-related myelosuppression (e.g., neutropenia, thrombocytopenia, and anemia), fever and chills, infection, and nausea/vomiting. In clinical trials, myelosuppression was the most frequently reported dose-limiting toxicity. Other common adverse effects of the drug include malaise, fatigue, anorexia, and weakness. Serious opportunistic infections also have occurred in patients receiving the drug for chronic lymphocytic leukemia, but infections are common complications of the disease itself. (See Cautions: Infectious Complications.)

Much of the information reported by the manufacturer regarding the adverse effect profile of fludarabine was compiled from single-arm, open-label studies of the drug in several hundred patients with chronic lymphocytic leukemia; however, the manufacturer states that the spectrum of these effects is similar to that observed in other populations involving several thousand patients who were receiving the drug for other neoplastic diseases (e.g., other leukemias, lymphomas, solid tumors). Adverse effects other than myelosuppression and neurotoxicity also may be dose related.

■ **Hematologic Effects** The major and dose-limiting toxicity of fludarabine is hematologic toxicity. The drug can severely suppress bone marrow function and result in anemia, thrombocytopenia, and neutropenia, even at currently recommended, relatively low dosages (e.g., 25 mg/m^2). The possibility that certain hematologic effects may partly represent manifestations of the underlying disease (e.g., immune-mediated cytopenias in patients with chronic lymphocytic leukemia) should be considered.

In clinical trials in patients with chronic lymphocytic leukemia, evidence of hematologic toxicity was present in up to 75% of patients receiving fludarabine, and peripheral blood cell counts eventually decreased in most patients with adequate baseline counts. Neutropenia and thrombocytopenia were the most frequent myelosuppressive effects, but thrombocytopenia was responsible for most cases of severe and life-threatening hematologic toxicity.

Approximately 60% of patients with chronic lymphocytic leukemia in one study experienced decreases in absolute neutrophil counts to less than 500/mm^3 and/or decreases in hemoglobin concentration of at least 2 g/dL from baseline; platelet count in 55% of these patients decreased by at least 50% from baseline. Absolute T-cell counts have been observed to decrease by 90% and B-cell counts by 50%, but, in part, such reductions in lymphocyte counts represent therapeutic responses to the drug in this leukemia. In a study in patients with solid tumors, the median time to nadir granulocyte or platelet count was 13 (range: 3–25) or 16 (range: 2–32) days, respectively. Many of these patients had baseline abnormalities in hematologic indices either as a result of the disease process or from prior myelosuppressive therapy.

Several cases of trilineage bone marrow hypoplasia or aplasia resulting in pancytopenia, sometimes fatal, have been reported in patients receiving fludarabine. Cases have occurred in both previously treated and untreated patients. The duration of clinically significant cytopenia ranged from about 2 months to 1 year.

Life-threatening and sometimes fatal autoimmune hemolytic anemia has been reported after one or more courses of fludarabine therapy in patients with or without a history of autoimmune hemolytic anemia or a positive Coombs' test and whose disease may or may not be in remission. It is not known if administration of corticosteroids is beneficial for management of these hemolytic episodes. Hemolytic anemia recurred following rechallenge with the drug. The mechanisms that predispose patients to the development of hemolytic anemia are not known, and patients receiving fludarabine should be evaluated and monitored closely for hemolysis. Severe anemia requiring hospitalization and transfusion, including fatality, reportedly has occurred.

Fludarabine-induced myelosuppression can be severe, cumulative, and may affect multiple cell lines. While myelosuppression usually is reversible, careful hematologic monitoring is necessary during fludarabine therapy. Depending on the severity of hematologic toxicity, dosage adjustment, interruption of therapy, and/or transfusions may be necessary. Recovery of neutrophil and platelet count usually is complete within 5–7 weeks after discontinuance of fludarabine therapy, but occasionally may require longer periods. Bone marrow fibrosis has occurred rarely.

■ **Nervous System Effects** In early, dose-ranging studies in patients with acute leukemias, relatively high dosages of fludarabine (e.g., 96–150 mg/m^2 daily for 5–7 days, which are approximately 4–6 times the currently recommended dosage for chronic lymphocytic leukemia) were associated with severe, potentially irreversible or fatal neurologic effects (e.g., delayed, progressive encephalopathy and blindness, coma) in approximately 36% of such treated patients. (See Chronic Toxicity.)Fludarabine-induced neurotoxicity is a delayed effect, with manifestations usually appearing 21–60 days after completion of the course.

While the risk of such toxicity clearly appears to be dose related, similar neurotoxic effects have been reported rarely in patients receiving relatively low dosages (e.g., equivalent to those currently recommended for chronic lymphocytic leukemia) of the drug. The relationship, if any, of neurotoxicity to peak plasma concentrations of the drug or cumulative dose remains unclear; such toxicity has been associated with rapid IV administration as well as with slow IV infusion, and the risk of its development appears to be substantially lower with equal cumulative doses that are administered as repeated low doses rather than as high-dose schedules. Rarely, neurotoxicity has been reversible.

While it has been suggested that the presence of underlying meningeal mycosis fungoides and/or vitamin B_{12} deficiency may have predisposed to neurotoxicity in at least one patient receiving relatively low dosages of fludarabine, factors other than dosage that may predispose to the development of fludarabine-induced neurotoxicity remain to be established. The neurotoxicity appears to be leukoencephalopathic and/or myelinoclastic, and may have a predilection for optic fibers. Autopsy findings have revealed diffuse, necrotizing leukoencephalopathy characterized by demyelination, vacuolization, and axonal swelling with spheroid formation. Demyelination of the optic nerves also has been observed. Progressive demyelination in the CNS appears to be principally responsible for, or at least principally contributory to, fatal outcome.

Adverse nervous system effects reportedly occur in 21–69% of patients receiving fludarabine at currently recommended dosages. Objective weakness has been reported in up to 65%, pain in up to 44%, malaise in up to 22%, fatigue in up to 38%, paresthesia in up to 12%, visual disturbances in up to 15%, hearing disturbances (e.g., hearing loss, auditory hallucinations) in up to 6%, and sleep disorder or headache in up to 3% of patients receiving the drug at such dosages. Agitation, confusion, coma, peripheral neuropathy, depression, cerebellar syndrome, ambulatory equilibrium disturbance, fatigue, somnolence, and impaired mentation also have been reported in patients receiving fludarabine at dosages recommended for chronic lymphocytic leukemia. Wrist drop has been reported rarely.

The effect of chronic administration of fludarabine on the risk of adverse nervous system effects currently is not known; however, some patients have received the currently recommended dosage for chronic lymphocytic leukemia for up to at least 15 courses of therapy. Further study and experience are necessary to elucidate further the risks and mechanisms of fludarabine-induced neurotoxicity and possibly better predict and avoid its development. While some clinicians recommended during early studies with the drug that even patients receiving relatively low dosages (e.g., those currently recommended for chronic lymphocytic leukemia) be monitored closely with frequent neurologic evaluation and tests for possible neurotoxic effects, most clinicians currently suggest that such evaluation would not be cost-effective and that visual changes generally can be monitored as evidence of neurotoxicity.

■ **Infectious Complications** Infection has been reported in up to 44% of patients receiving fludarabine for CLL. Infection is a common complication of CLL, in part secondary to associated hypogammaglobulinemia, and the frequency of infection in several clinical trials with fludarabine reportedly was comparable to that associated with the disease. However, in addition to the underlying immunodysfunction associated with this leukemia, it has been suggested that fludarabine may contribute to this dysfunction by depleting helper/inducer (CD4$^+$, T4$^+$) T cells. Prophylactic immune globulin or anti-infective therapy has been suggested for selected patients with CLL considered at risk for infectious complications of the disease (e.g., patients with documented recurrent bacterial infections or low titers of IgG or of antibodies to encapsulated organisms); however, the costs and potential benefits of such therapy must be weighed carefully.

Whereas bacterial infections frequently occur in patients receiving treatment with conventional alkylating agents for CLL, bacterial infections and infections with opportunistic pathogens are common in patients receiving fludarabine. Concomitant therapy with corticosteroids increases the risk of infections with opportunistic pathogens, such as *Pneumocystis carinii* and *Listeria*, in patients receiving purine analogs such as fludarabine and should be avoided. Herpesvirus infections, particularly with varicella zoster virus, frequently occur in patients receiving fludarabine.

In a large randomized trial, patients with CLL receiving fludarabine had a greater frequency of infections (77 versus 61%) and major infections (29 versus 17%) than those receiving chlorambucil. Infection with varicella zoster virus, which usually is not fatal but may cause substantial morbidity, occurred more frequently in patients receiving fludarabine rather than chlorambucil.

■ **Respiratory Effects** Severe pulmonary toxicity, including ARDS, respiratory distress, pulmonary hemorrhage, pulmonary fibrosis, and respiratory failure, has been reported in patients receiving fludarabine. Following exclusion of an infectious etiology, administration of corticosteroids has resulted in symptomatic improvement in some patients.

Adverse respiratory effects have been observed in 14–69% of patients receiving fludarabine therapy for chronic lymphocytic leukemia. Pneumonia, which is a frequent manifestation of infection in patients with this leukemia (see Cautions: Infectious Complications), has been observed in 9–22% of patients receiving the drug. In some cases, infection with an opportunistic pathogen (e.g., *Pneumocystis carinii*, cytomegalovirus) may be responsible for the pneumonia.

Cough has been reported in up to 44%, dyspnea in up to 22%, upper respiratory infection in up to 16%, pharyngitis in up to 9%, allergic pneumonitis or hemoptysis in up to 6%, and sinusitis bronchitis, epistaxis, hypoxia, and pulmonary hypersensitivity (e.g., diffuse interstitial pneumonitis characterized by dyspnea, hypoxia, cough, and pulmonary infiltrates) in 5% or less of patients receiving fludarabine. This drug-induced interstitial pneumonitis appears to be a delayed effect, usually manifesting 3–28 days after administration of the third or later course of therapy. Subsequent lung biopsy in one patient showed an interstitial mononuclear cell infiltrate consistent with this diagnosis. Administration of corticosteroid therapy has resulted in prompt resolution of symptoms in several patients; however, the symptoms may recur following discontinuance of the steroid. In some cases, respiratory dysfunction may resolve spontaneously. The precise contribution of fludarabine to the development of this pneumonitis remains to be elucidated further since this effect is a well-documented complication of chemotherapy for chronic lymphocytic leukemia, particularly with alkylating agents, and most such patients receiving fludarabine were exposed previously to such agents. In addition, in some cases, an underlying disease-related process, infection, or exposure to some other pulmonotoxic agent may have contributed to the observed effect.

■ **GI Effects** Adverse GI effects reportedly occur in 46–63% of patients receiving fludarabine for chronic lymphocytic leukemia. Nausea and/or vomiting, which generally are mild but occasionally may be severe, are reported in up to 36%, anorexia in up to 34%, diarrhea in up to 15%, GI bleeding in up to 13%, stomatitis in up to 9%, and esophagitis, constipation, mucositis, and dysphagia in less than 5% of treated patients. Altered taste sensation also has been reported.

■ **Cardiovascular Effects** Adverse cardiovascular effects have been reported in 12–38% of patients receiving fludarabine for chronic lymphocytic leukemia. Edema has been reported in up to 19%, angina in up to 6%, and congestive heart failure, arrhythmia, supraventricular tachycardia, myocardial infarction, deep vein thrombosis,phlebitis, transient ischemic attack, and aneurysm in less than 5% of treated patients, but these effects have not been attributed directly to the drug. At least one patient developed a pericardial effusion, which possibly was related to fludarabine therapy. Chest pain also has been reported rarely.

■ **Genitourinary Effects** Adverse genitourinary effects reportedly occur in 12–22% of patients receiving fludarabine for chronic lymphocytic leukemia.

Urinary tract infection has been reported in up to 15%, and dysuria , urinary hesitancy, hematuria, renal failure, abnormal renal function tests, and proteinuria in less than 5% of treated patients. In some cases, tumor lysis syndrome may have been responsible for the observed genitourinary effect (e.g., renal dysfunction, hematuria). (See Cautions: Metabolic Effects.) Increased serum creatinine concentration also has been reported in patients receiving the drug at doses higher than those recommended for chronic lymphocytic leukemia. Hemorrhagic cystitis has been reported rarely in patients receiving fludarabine.

■ **Metabolic Effects** Although rapid tumor lysis occurs rarely in patients with chronic lymphocytic leukemia receiving conventional chemotherapy, presumably because of the slow proliferative rate that usually characterizes this neoplasm and the corresponding slow cytolysis induced by such agents, the syndrome may be more likely in patients receiving fludarabine for the treatment of this leukemia, especially in those with large initial tumor burdens. Patients with advanced lymphoproliferative disease, including those with chronic lymphocytic leukemia accompanied by generalized lymphadenopathy and substantial splenomegaly and lymphocytosis, may be at particular risk of developing this syndrome following initiation of fludarabine therapy secondary to the rapid cytolysis induced by the drug. Such patients should be observed closely during initiation of fludarabine therapy, and the potential benefit of prophylactic allopurinol, adequate hydration, and/or urinary alkalinization should be considered.

Manifestations of fludarabine-induced tumor lysis syndrome may include hyperkalemia, hyperphosphatemia, hyperuricemia, hypocalcemia, metabolic acidosis, hematuria, urate crystalluria, and upper-quadrant and/or flank pain; renal dysfunction and/or failure may occur secondarily. Flank pain and/or hematuria often are the initial manifestations of the syndrome. If the syndrome develops, treatment with allopurinol, analgesics, IV fluids, and urinary alkalinization and correction of acid-base imbalances should be instituted as necessary. Metabolic (lactic)acidosis also has been reported in patients receiving the drug at dosages higher than those recommended for chronic lymphocytic leukemia.

Hyperglycemia has been reported in 6% or less of patients receiving fludarabine for chronic lymphocytic leukemia.

■ **Dermatologic Effects** Adverse dermatologic effects have been reported in up to 18% of patients receiving fludarabine for chronic lymphocytic leukemia. Rash (e.g., maculopapular) has been reported in up to 15% and pruritus and seborrhea in less than 5% of treated patients. Dermatomal herpes zoster or oral herpes simplex infection also has been reported; however, viral and bacterial infections are common complications of chronic lymphocytic leukemia. (See Cautions: Infectious Complications.)

■ **Other Adverse Effects** Fever has been reported in up to 69%, diaphoresis in up to 13%, and myalgia in up to 16% of patients receiving fludarabine.

Rarely, transfusion-associated graft-versus-host disease has occurred following transfusion of nonirradiated blood products in patients requiring blood transfusions during fludarabine therapy.

Abnormal liver function test results, cholelithiasis, liver failure, anaphylaxis, osteoporosis, arthralgia, dehydration, and/or hemorrhage have been reported in 6% or less of treated patients. Reversible hepatotoxicity and pancreatitis also have been reported in patients receiving the drug.

■ **Precautions and Contraindications** Fludarabine is a highly toxic drug with a low therapeutic index, and a therapeutic response is not likely to occur without some evidence of toxicity. The drug must be used only under constant supervision by clinicians experienced in therapy with cytotoxic agents. Most, but not all, adverse effects of fludarabine are reversible if detected promptly. If severe adverse effects occur during fludarabine therapy, the drug should be discontinued or dosage reduced and appropriate measures instituted as necessary. Fludarabine therapy should be reinstituted with caution if at all (depending on the effect), with adequate consideration of further need for the drug, and with awareness of possible recurrence of toxicity.

Hematologic function must be monitored frequently and carefully during and after fludarabine therapy. Periodic (e.g., prior to each course or more often if clinically indicated) assessment of peripheral blood cell counts is recommended to detect the possible development of anemia, thrombocytopenia, and/or neutropenia. Because these complications are potentially fatal, patients receiving fludarabine should be instructed to notify their clinician if fever, sore throat, or unusual bleeding or bruising occurs. Since life-threatening and sometimes fatal autoimmune hemolytic anemia that recurred upon rechallenge has been reported after one or more courses of fludarabine therapy, patients receiving fludarabine should be evaluated and monitored closely for hemolysis. (See Cautions: Hematologic Effects.)

The use of irradiated blood products should be considered in patients requiring blood transfusions during fludarabine therapy. Transfusion-associated graft-versus-host disease has occurred rarely following transfusion of nonirradiated blood products in patients receiving fludarabine.

Patients also should be observed closely for signs of nonhematologic toxicity during fludarabine therapy. While severe and potentially irreversible or fatal neurotoxic effects have been associated principally with dosages higher than those currently recommended for the treatment of chronic lymphocytic leukemia, such effects also have occurred rarely at relatively low dosages, and even patients receiving dosages currently recommended for this leukemia should be monitored for the possible development of these effects. (See Cautions: Nervous System Effects.)

Patients with a large initial tumor burden may be at particular risk of developing tumor lysis syndrome following initiation of fludarabine therapy. Since the drug can induce a rapid cytolytic response as early as the first week of therapy, precautions should be taken in patients considered at risk of developing this complication. (See Cautions: Metabolic Effects.)

Dosage of fludarabine should be adjusted carefully in patients with impaired renal function since the clearance of fludarabine (2-fluoro-ara-A) has been shown to correlate directly with creatinine clearance, suggesting renal excretion as an important means of elimination of the compound. In addition, patients with impaired renal function may be at increased risk of developing fludarabine-induced toxicity. Reduction of fludarabine dosage is necessary in patients with moderate renal impairment, and use of the drug is not recommended in patients with severe renal impairment (see Dosage and Administration: Dosage in Renal Impairment). The manufacturer states that the possibility that certain other patient populations (e.g., those with preexisting bone marrow impairment, geriatric patients) may be at increased risk for developing fludarabine-induced toxicity should be considered. Any such patient should be monitored closely for excessive toxicity and dosage modified or the drug discontinued accordingly.

Because of an increased incidence of infections with opportunistic agents in patients receiving purine analogs in combination with corticosteroids, prednisone should be omitted from regimens containing fludarabine or other purine analogs.

Fludarabine is contraindicated in patients with known hypersensitivity to the drug and/or any ingredient in the formulation.

■ **Pediatric Precautions** Current evidence from clinical studies has not demonstrated efficacy of fludarabine for any cancer in pediatric patients. Fludarabine was evaluated in 62 pediatric patients (median age: 10 years; range: 1–21 years) with refractory acute leukemia (45 patients) or solid tumors (17 patients). Pediatric patients with acute lymphocytic leukemia received an IV loading dose of fludarabine 10.5 mg/m^2 daily followed by a continuous IV infusion of 30.5 mg/m^2 daily for 5 days. Dose-limiting myelosuppression was observed in 12 pediatric patients with solid tumors receiving a loading dose of fludarabine 8 mg/m^2 daily followed by a continuous infusion of 23.5 mg/m^2 daily for 5 days. The maximum tolerated dose of fludarabine was a loading dose of 7 mg/m^2 daily followed by a continuous infusion of 20 mg/m^2 daily for 5 days.

Fludarabine-induced toxicity in children included bone marrow suppression, particularly thrombocytopenia. Other adverse effects reported in pediatric patients receiving fludarabine included fever, chills, asthenia, rash, nausea, vomiting, diarrhea, and infection. Peripheral neuropathy or pulmonary hypersensitivity reaction was not reported in this age group.

■ **Geriatric Precautions** Safety and efficacy of fludarabine in geriatric patients have not been studied specifically to date; however, chronic lymphocytic leukemia, for which safety and efficacy have been established, occurs principally in patients older than 50 years of age. Because geriatric patients may have decreased renal function and because patients with renal impairment may be at increased risk of fludarabine-induced toxicity, the manufacturer states that patients in this age group should be monitored closely and dosage adjusted accordingly. In addition, experience from at least one clinical study suggested that geriatric patients with advanced Rai stage chronic lymphocytic leukemia should be monitored particularly closely, and the possible need for substantial dosage reduction should be considered.

■ **Mutagenicity and Carcinogenicity** There was no evidence of mutagenicity when fludarabine was tested in bacteria (Ames test) or in a mammalian cell system (HGRPT assay in Chinese hamster ovary cells) with or without metabolic activation. However, fludarabine has been shown to be clastogenic; chromosomal aberrations were observed in vitro in Chinese hamster ovary cells exposed to the drug with metabolic activation. Fludarabine with or without metabolic activation also increased the rate of sister chromatid exchanges in this cell system. In addition, fludarabine was clastogenic in vivo (micronucleus test in mice), but was not mutagenic to germ cells (dominant lethal test in male mice).

Studies in animals to evaluate the carcinogenicity of fludarabine have not been performed.

■ **Pregnancy, Fertility, and Lactation** Fludarabine can cause fetal harm when administered to pregnant women, but potential benefits from use of the drug may be acceptable in certain conditions despite the possible risks to the fetus. Teratogenicity studies in animals have demonstrated that the drug induces skeletal malformations and external deformities at dosages similar to or less than the usual human dosage (on a mg/kg basis). There are no adequate and controlled studies in pregnant women. Women of childbearing potential should be advised to avoid becoming pregnant while receiving fludarabine, and the drug should be used during pregnancy only in life-threatening situations or severe disease for which safer drugs cannot be used or are ineffective. If fludarabine is administered during pregnancy or if the patient becomes pregnant while taking the drug, the patient should be informed of the potential hazard to the fetus.

Preclinical toxicology studies in animals have demonstrated dose-related effects on the male reproductive system, such as a decrease in mean testicular weight and degeneration and necrosis of spermatogenic epithelium. The possible effects of fludarabine on fertility in humans have not been evaluated adequately to date.

It is not known whether fludarabine is distributed into milk. Because of the potential for serious adverse reactions to fludarabine in nursing infants if the drug were distributed into milk, a decision should be made whether to discontinue nursing or the drug, taking into account the importance of the drug to the woman.

Drug Interactions

■ **Pentostatin** Concomitant therapy with fludarabine (principally 10 mg/m^2 daily for 4 days at 28-day intervals) and pentostatin (4 mg/m^{2}every 2 weeks) may be associated with severe and/or fatal pulmonary toxicity (e.g., pneumonitis). In one study, 4 of 6 patients receiving the drugs concomitantly for the treatment of refractory chronic lymphocytic leukemia reportedly developed such toxicity. While the mechanism of this possible increased toxicity currently is not known, concomitant therapy with these drugs is *not* recommended.

■ **Cytarabine** Cytarabine has been shown to decrease substantially the metabolism of subsequently administered fludarabine (2-fluoro-ara-A) to its pharmacologically active triphosphate (fludarabine triphosphate, 2-fluoro-ara-ATP) in vitro and in vivo. In addition, administration of cytarabine prior to a dose of fludarabine phosphate appeared to inhibit the antineoplastic effect of fludarabine in several patients with leukemia. It appears that cytarabine competes for deoxycytidine kinase, the rate-limiting enzyme required for intracellular conversion of both drugs to their active triphosphate. In contrast, pretreatment with fludarabine does not appear to inhibit the metabolic activation of cytarabine, but actually may stimulate such activation. The clinical importance of these findings requires further elucidation.

Chronic Toxicity

■ **Manifestations** During early studies of fludarabine using relatively high dosages (e.g., up to 96–150 mg/m² daily for 5–7 days or approximately 4–6 times the currently recommended dosage for chronic lymphocytic leukemia), severe, delayed, potentially irreversible or fatal nervous system toxicity was observed in up to 36% of patients receiving such dosages. Manifestations of this toxicity generally appeared 21–60 days following initial administration of the drug and included altered mental status (e.g., confusion, dementia), incontinence, generalized seizure, flaccid or spastic paralysis and/or quadriparesis, blurred vision, blindness (amaurosis), and/or coma.

Some patients with this fludarabine-induced neurotoxicity evidenced little to no abnormality in spinal fluid, EEG, or computed tomographic brain scans; however, autopsy findings have revealed focal or diffuse progressive CNS demyelination, particularly in the occipital lobe and spinal cord. (See Cautions: Nervous System Effects.) Leukoencephalopathy involving the subcortical white matter, optic nerves, and optical tract has been observed. The mechanism by which fludarabine produces this neurologic toxicity remains to be elucidated, and no predisposing factors other than dosage have been clearly identified. Manifestations of severe neurologic toxicity have been reported rarely in patients receiving the drug at relatively low dosages (e.g., equivalent to those currently recommended for chronic lymphocytic leukemia).

Other manifestations that are extensions of common adverse effects of fludarabine, such as myelosuppression, also may occur with overdosage.

The potential for developing long-term cumulative toxicity, particularly neurotoxic effects, with chronic fludarabine therapy at the currently recommended relatively low dosages is unknown. (See Cautions: Nervous System Effects.)

The contribution, if any, of 2-fluoroadenine to the toxic effects of fludarabine in humans remains to be established. While fludarabine is not metabolized to 2-fluoroadenine by mammalian purine nucleoside phosphorylase, the drug can be metabolized to this toxic metabolite by bacterial purine nucleoside phosphorylase. Despite the inability of the mammalian enzyme to catalyze the production of 2-fluoroadenine, this metabolite has been identified in plasma, urine, and CSF of animals receiving fludarabine. It has been suggested that systemic appearance of 2-fluoroadenine in mammals may result from biliary excretion of fludarabine and subsequent bacterial (e.g., by *Escherichia coli*) metabolism in the GI tract to, and enterohepatic circulation of, this toxic metabolite.

■ **Treatment** There is no known specific antidote for fludarabine overdosage. Management consists of discontinuance of the drug and initiation of supportive and symptomatic treatment. Transfusion with blood or blood components may be necessary for the management of substantial myelosuppression.

Pharmacology

Fludarabine phosphate is dephosphorylated in serum to fludarabine (2-fluoro-ara-adenine, 2-fluoro-ara-A), which is transported intracellularly via a carrier-mediated process and then is converted by deoxycytidine kinase to the nucleotide, fludarabine triphosphate (FATP, 2-fluoroarabinofuranosyladenine triphosphate, 2-fluoro-ara-ATP). 2-Fluoro-ara-ATP is thought to be the form required for the drug's cytotoxic effect. In sensitive malignant cells, the rate-limiting step in this process is the conversion of 2-fluoro-ara-A to 2-fluoro-ara-ATP by deoxycytidine kinase; in healthy cells, the importance of the intracellular transport mechanism as potentially rate limiting is increased relative to that in malignant cells. However, some evidence from patients with indolent but advanced lymphoproliferative malignancy indicates that response may not depend on intrinsic deoxycytidine kinase activity in tumor cells. Intracellular transport of fludarabine occurs preferentially into sensitive malignant cells compared with healthy cells.

While the exact mechanism(s) of action of fludarabine has not been elucidated fully and may be multifaceted, fludarabine triphosphate appears to inhibit α-DNA polymerase, ribonucleotide reductase, and DNA primase by competing with the physiologic substrate, deoxyadenosine triphosphate, resulting in inhibition of DNA synthesis. There also is evidence that the active phosphorylated form of the drug can be incorporated into growing DNA chains as a false nucleotide, thus interfering with chain elongation (prematurely terminating DNA synthesis), and/or may interfere with RNA and protein synthesis by decreasing the incorporation of uridine and leucine into RNA and protein, respectively. However, inhibition of RNA and protein synthesis appears to require drug concentrations higher than those required for inhibition of DNA synthesis.

Although both in vitro and in vivo studies have shown that T cells are more sensitive than B cells to the cytotoxic effects of fludarabine, the drug is highly active against B-cell lymphoproliferative disorders, including chronic lymphocytic leukemia. In addition, the cytolytic effect of the drug appears to be relatively rapid even in neoplasms such as chronic lymphocytic leukemia that are characterized by a slow proliferative rate.

A correlation appears to exist between intracellular accumulation of 2-fluoro-ara-ATP at 1 hour following infusion and the concentration of 2-fluoro-ara-A incorporated into nucleic acids. The ability of blast cells to synthesize DNA at 12–24 hours following administration of the drug was shown to be related inversely to the concentration of 2-fluoro-ara-ATP.

Although fludarabine has exhibited antiviral activity in vitro (e.g., against herpes simplex virus [HSV]types 1 and 2), it is *unlikely* that any clinically important antiviral activity could be achieved at less than toxic dosages of the drug in humans. In one study, the concentration of drug required for 99% inhibition of viral replication of HSV-1 and -2 was 100 times that required for 50% inhibition of growth of HeLa cells.

Pharmacokinetics

Pharmacokinetic data for fludarabine phosphate (2-fluoro-ara-AMP) are limited since the drug is dephosphorylated rapidly to fludarabine (2-fluoro-ara-A) following IV administration. Pharmacokinetic studies of the drug focus principally on fludarabine and fludarabine triphosphate (2-fluoro-ara-ATP), the active intracellular form. Therefore, while the drug is administered as, and dosages are expressed in terms of, the monophosphate salt, pharmacokinetic parameters generally are expressed in terms of fludarabine (2-fluoro-ara-A) and fludarabine triphosphate. A concentration of 1 μg of fludarabine or fludarabine phosphate per mL is approximately equivalent to 3.51 or 2.74 μmol/L, respectively.

■ **Absorption** Following IV administration, fludarabine phosphate is rapidly and apparently completely dephosphorylated to fludarabine (2-fluoro-ara-A). In plasma, the monophosphate is undetectable or becomes undetectable within several minutes after completion of IV administration. Following rapid IV injection over 2–5 minutes of a 260-mg/m² dose in one study, plasma concentrations of unchanged fludarabine phosphate were undetectable within 2–4 minutes after injection. Similar, rapid dephosphorylation of the drug also has been observed following IV administration in animals.

Following IV infusion over 30 minutes of daily 25-mg/m² doses in several adult patients, moderate accumulation of the drug was observed, with trough plasma concentrations increasing about twofold over the 5-day treatment period. In a limited number of pediatric patients, administration of 5–10 mg/m² of fludarabine phosphate as an IV loading dose followed by continuous IV infusion of 13–30 mg/m² daily over 5 days resulted in steady-state plasma fludarabine concentrations of 0.17–2.85 μg/mL. Peak concentrations of fludarabine triphosphate were achieved approximately 2 hours following completion of the infusion.

Areas under the concentration-time curve (AUCs) for fludarabine in plasma and fludarabine triphosphate in blast cells appear to be dose related, and a direct correlation reportedly exists between the quantity of fludarabine incorporated into nucleic acids and intracellular accumulation of fludarabine triphosphate. In nonleukemic patients, suppression of leukocyte counts appears to correlate with plasma fludarabine concentration and dose.

Fludarabine phosphate has been administered intraperitoneally in a few patients with solid peritoneal tumors. Following intraperitoneal infusion of 4, 8, or 12 mg/m² of fludarabine phosphate daily for 5 consecutive days, accumulation of fludarabine in peritoneal fluid exceeded that in plasma by a factor of approximately 8–13 based on mean peritoneal and plasma AUCs. Peak peritoneal fluid fludarabine concentrations averaged 4.1 or 3 μg/mL following a 4- or 8-mg/m² dose, respectively.

An oral preparation of fludarabine phosphate currently is not commercially available in the US, but the drug has been shown to be well absorbed from the GI tract following oral administration in animals. Following oral fludarabine phosphate doses of 86.7 or 260 mg/m² in dogs, peak fludarabine concentrations were achieved within 19–107.7 or 49.1–91.7 minutes, respectively; mean bioavailability was approximately 100 or 80%, respectively. Oral pharmacokinetic studies of the drug currently are under way in humans.

■ **Distribution** Limited data in animals and humans suggest that fludarabine (2-fluoro-ara-A) is widely distributed. In a few patients receiving the currently recommended dosage of 25 mg/m² of fludarabine phosphate IV daily for 5 days, the volume of distribution at steady state (V_{ss}) reportedly averaged 96–98 L/m². Following IV injection of fludarabine phosphate over 2–5 minutes in high doses (80–260 mg/m²), V_{ss} in a limited number of patients with advanced cancer averaged approximately 44 L/m². Tissue distribution studies in animals indicate that the highest concentrations of the drug are in liver, kidney, and spleen.

Although the extent to which fludarabine and/or metabolites of the drug distribute into the CNS in humans has not been determined to date, severe neurologic toxicity (e.g., blindness, coma) has been reported in patients receiving the drug, particularly in high dosages. (See Cautions: Nervous System Effects.) There is evidence from animal studies that fludarabine distributes into the CNS and that a toxic metabolite (2-fluoroadenine, possibly formed by bacteria in the GI tract), can be absorbed systematically via enterohepatic circulation and distributed into CSF. (See Chronic Toxicity: Manifestations.)

According to in vitro data, about 19–29% of fludarabine is bound to plasma proteins.

■ **Elimination** Fludarabine phosphate is dephosphorylated rapidly to fludarabine (2-fluoro-ara-A) following IV administration. (See the introductory discussion in Pharmacokinetics.) Plasma concentrations of fludarabine reportedly decline in a linear, dose-independent manner following IV administration of the drug. The elimination profile of fludarabine also has been reported to be either biphasic or triphasic, possibly because of differences in initial sampling times after IV administration and/or assay methods; however, reported terminal elimination half-lives have been similar. In a few patients receiving 18 or 25 mg/m^2 of fludarabine phosphate daily for 5 days, plasma fludarabine concentrations declined in a biphasic manner, with $t_{1/2\alpha}$ and $t_{1/2\beta}$ averaging approximately 36 minutes and 9.3 hours, respectively. In patients receiving high doses (80–260 mg/m^2) of fludarabine phosphate by rapid IV injection (over 2–5 minutes), elimination reportedly was triphasic, with the half-lives of the first, second, and third phases averaging approximately 5–7 minutes, 1.4–1.7 hours, and approximately 10 hours, respectively; however, using more sensitive sampling techniques, recent data describe a terminal elimination phase of 30 hours.

Fludarabine monophosphate initially is dephosphorylated, with subsequent transport of fludarabine into cells and intracellular phosphorylation to the triphosphate. (See Pharmacology.) Following administration of fludarabine phosphate 20–125 mg/m^2 as a 30-minute IV infusion daily for 5 days, the terminal elimination half-lives of fludarabine and fludarabine triphosphate were approximately 8–10 and 15 hours, respectively. An estimated terminal half-life of fludarabine (2-fluoro-ara-A) of about 20 hours was reported in cancer patients receiving fludarabine 25 mg/m^2 as a 30-minute IV infusion daily for 5 days.

In a limited number of pediatric patients, the plasma concentration profile of fludarabine exhibited both monoexponential and biexponential decay, with a mean $t_{1/2\alpha}$ of 10.5 hours in patients with monoexponential elimination and a $t_{1/2\alpha}$ and $t_{1/2\beta}$ of 1.2–1.4 and 12.4–19 hours, respectively, in patients with biexponential elimination.

Total body clearance of fludarabine appears to be directly correlated with creatinine clearance, suggesting renal excretion as an important means of elimination of the compound. Renal clearance accounts for about 40% of the total body clearance. Renal elimination appears to become more important at high dosages of the drug. In patients receiving 18–25 mg/m^2 of fludarabine phosphate IV daily for 5 days, approximately 24% of the dose was excreted in urine as fludarabine within 24 hours. In contrast, urinary excretion averaged 41–60% at IV doses of 80–260 mg/m^2.

Patients with moderate renal impairment (creatinine clearance 17–41 mL/minute per 1.73 m^2) receiving a reduced dose of fludarabine (20% less than the recommended dose) had a similar area under the plasma concentration-time curve (AUC) as patients with normal renal function receiving the usual recommended dose. Total body clearance averaged 172 mL/minute in patients with normal renal function and 124 mL/minute in patients with moderate renal impairment.

Unlike vidarabine, fludarabine is resistant to deamination by adenosine deaminase. However, arabinosyl-2-fluorohypoxanthine has been identified in urine of animals receiving fludarabine phosphate. It has been suggested that other metabolic pathways (e.g., deamination via adenosine monophosphate deaminase) may be responsible, but additional study is needed.

Chemistry and Stability

■ **Chemistry** Fludarabine phosphate, a synthetic purine nucleoside, is an antineoplastic agent. Fludarabine differs from the physiologic nucleosides, adenosine or deoxyadenosine, in that the sugar moiety is arabinose instead of ribose or deoxyribose, respectively, and by the addition of a fluorine atom to the purine base adenine. The drug is a purine antagonist antimetabolite. Fludarabine also is structurally related to vidarabine (9-β-D-arabinofuranosyladenine, ara-A), differing only by the presence of a fluorine atom at position 2 of the purine moiety and a phosphate group at position 5 of the arabinose moiety. Compared with vidarabine, these structural differences result in increased aqueous solubility and resistance to enzymatic degradation by adenosine deaminase.

Fludarabine (2-fluoro-ara-A) is commercially available as the monophosphate salt (2-fluoro-ara-AMP). Potency is expressed in terms of the salt. Monophosphorylation of fludarabine increases the drug's aqueous solubility while maintaining pharmacologic activity; the monophosphate undergoes rapid dephosphorylation in vivo. (See Pharmacokinetics.) Commercially available fludarabine phosphate powder for injection occurs as a white, lyophilized solid cake. During manufacture of the powder for injection, sodium hydroxide is added to adjust final pH. Following reconstitution of the drug with sterile water for injection to a concentration of 25 mg/mL, the solution has a pH of approximately 7.7 (range: 7.2–8.2). Fludarabine phosphate has solubilities of approximately 9 mg/mL in water and 28 or 57 mg/mL in aqueous buffers with a pH of 4 or 9, respectively.

Fludarabine phosphate also is commercially available as an aqueous injection containing 25 mg of the drug per mL. The injection also contains mannitol 25 mg/mL and sodium hydroxide to adjust pH to 6.8 (range: 6–7.1).

■ **Stability** Commercially available fludarabine phosphate powder for injection should be stored at 2–8°C. When stored as directed, the powder for injection is stable for at least 18 months after the date of manufacture. While early stability studies reported that the powder for injection was stable for at least 36 months when stored at 22–25°C, more recent studies employing assays with increased sensitivity have shown that the drug is less stable than this; therefore, the manufacturer currently recommends that fludarabine phosphate powder for injection *not*be stored at room temperature.

Fludarabine phosphate is relatively stable in aqueous solutions, with optimal stability occurring at an approximately neutral pH. When reconstituted to a final concentration of 25 mg/mL, aqueous solutions of the drug are stable for at least 16 days at room temperature and normal light conditions. Fludarabine phosphate is compatible with 5% dextrose or 0.9% sodium chloride injection. When diluted to a final concentration of 1 mg/mL, the drug is compatible in these diluents for at least 16 days at room temperature and normal light conditions. However, because such reconstituted and diluted fludarabine phosphate solutions contain no preservatives, the manufacturer recommends that they be used within 8 hours after preparation.

Commercially available fludarabine phosphate injection containing 25 mg/mL should be refrigerated at 2–8°C. The injection does not contain a preservative; ; unused portions should be discarded within 8 hours of initial vial entry. The injection is compatible with 5% dextrose or 0.9% sodium chloride injection.

Fludarabine phosphate has been reported to be physically incompatible with some drugs, including acyclovir sodium, amphotericin B, chlorpromazine hydrochloride, daunorubicin hydrochloride, ganciclovir sodium, hydroxyzine hydrochloride, miconazole (systemic form no longer commercially available in the US), or prochlorperazine edisylate, but the compatibility may depend on several factors (e.g., concentrations of the drugs, specific diluents used, resulting pH, temperature). Specialized references should be consulted for specific compatibility information.

Fludarabine phosphate is dephosphorylated in vitro by phosphatases present in heparinized whole blood samples. The addition of edetic acid (EDTA) to blood or plasma samples can inhibit this dephosphorylation. The monophosphate of fludarabine has been shown to be stable in blood containing 1 mg/mL of EDTA for at least 1 hour at 37°C and in plasma containing EDTA for at least 72 hours when refrigerated or for at least 2 weeks when frozen at −20°C. However, because the drug is rapidly dephosphorylated in vivo following IV administration, the addition of EDTA to blood specimens generally is not necessary unless pharmacokinetic characterization of the monophosphate during the first several minutes after injection is to be attempted.

For further information on the handling of antineoplastic agents, see the ASHP Guidelines on Handling Hazardous Drugs at http://www.ahfsdruginformation.com.

Preparations

Excipients in commercially available drug preparations may have clinically important effects in some individuals; consult specific product labeling for details.

Fludarabine Phosphate

Parenteral

For injection, for IV use only	50 mg	**Fludarabine Phosphate for Injection** **Fludara®, Berlex**
Injection, for IV use only	25 mg/mL*	**Fludarabine Phosphate Injection**

*available from one or more manufacturer, distributor, and/or repackager by generic (nonproprietary) name

†Use is not currently included in the labeling approved by the US Food and Drug Administration

Selected Revisions January 2009, © Copyright, May 1992, American Society of Health-System Pharmacists, Inc.

Fluorouracil

5-Fluorouracil, 5-FU

■ Fluorouracil, a pyrimidine antagonist, is an antimetabolite antineoplastic agent.

Uses

Fluorouracil is used for the palliative treatment of carcinoma of the colon, rectum, breast, stomach, and pancreas that is not amenable to surgery or irradiation. The drug also is used as an adjunct to surgery for the treatment of various solid tumors (e.g., adenocarcinoma of the colon, rectal carcinoma, breast cancer).

■ **GI Cancers** ***Combination Therapies for Colorectal Cancer*** Leucovorin calcium and levoleucovorin calcium are used to potentiate the antineoplastic activity of, and thus improve response to, fluorouracil in the palliative treatment of advanced colorectal carcinoma. Fluorouracil is designated an orphan drug by the US Food and Drug Administration (FDA) for use in combination with leucovorin for the treatment of metastatic adenocarcinoma of the colon and rectum. Such combined therapy is employed in an attempt to prolong survival relative to fluorouracil alone in patients with advanced disease. In vitro studies and clinical evidence have shown that the cytotoxicity of fluorouracil may be enhanced by reduced folates (e.g., leucovorin, levoleucovorin); it appears that elevated intracellular concentrations of reduced folates may stabilize the covalent ternary complex formed by fluorodeoxyuridylic acid, 5,10-methylenetetrahydrofolate, and thymidylate synthase, enhancing inhibition of this enzyme and thereby increasing the efficacy of fluorouracil.

Combination regimens including fluorouracil and either leucovorin or levoleucovorin, administered weekly or approximately monthly, have been evaluated in patients with advanced colorectal cancer in the adjuvant and metastatic setting.

The approximately monthly regimens studied in the North Central Cancer Treatment Group (Mayo/NCCTG) adjuvant study included 5-day courses of

IV fluorouracil 370 mg/m² plus IV leucovorin 200 mg/m² daily or fluorouracil 425 mg/m² plus leucovorin 20 mg/m² daily; both regimens were repeated at 4- to 5-week intervals. A commonly used regimen that is administered on a weekly schedule (often referred to as the high-dose leucovorin or Roswell Park regimen), consists of fluorouracil 500 mg/m² and leucovorin 500 mg/m² both given IV once weekly for 6 consecutive weeks. Results from the Intergroup 0089 study have demonstrated equal efficacy between the low-dose (monthly or Mayo Clinic schedule) and the high-dose (weekly or Roswell Park schedule) leucovorin regimens; however, because of ease of use and less toxicity, the high-dose regimen is considered a preferred regimen in the adjuvant setting.

A combination regimen of fluorouracil and leucovorin also has been evaluated as adjuvant treatment of colorectal cancer as a bimonthly continuous IV infusion (i.e., the LV5FU2 or deGramont regimen)†. The use of this regimen has been shown to be safer compared with the use of a direct IV injection ("bolus") regimen of fluorouracil and leucovorin. A simplified version of the LV5FU2 regimen also has been evaluated.

In the metastatic setting (i.e., patients with stage IV disease), the use of fluorouracil combined with leucovorin has not been shown to be any more efficacious than fluorouracil alone based on the results of a Southwestern Oncology Group (SWOG) study. However, the results of a more recent meta-analysis demonstrated improved responses and a small, but statistically significant improvement in overall survival with the fluorouracil/leucovorin combination regimens compared with fluorouracil alone.

Fluorouracil also has been used in combination with IV levoleucovorin given at one-half the usual dosage of leucovorin. Results from a comparative study demonstrated no substantial differences in response or tolerability between levoleucovorin and leucovorin when used in conjunction with fluorouracil for the palliative treatment of advanced colorectal cancer.

IV fluorouracil also has been used in combination with orally administered leucovorin in a limited number of patients with advanced colorectal carcinoma.

In addition to possible therapeutic potentiation, leucovorin and levoleucovorin may potentiate the risk of fluorouracil-induced toxicity (especially GI toxicity, including diarrhea, nausea, stomatitis, and vomiting, and, to a lesser degree, myelosuppression). (See Cautions: GI Effects.)

Monotherapy of Colorectal Cancer Fluorouracil has been administered as monotherapy of advanced colorectal cancer in various disease regimens. However, these regimens have been replaced by the use of fluorouracil and leucovorin combination regimens in the adjuvant setting for patients with stage III disease.

Hepatic Metastases Fluorouracil also has been studied as a form of regional adjuvant therapy (e.g., portal vein or hepatic artery infusion) of liver metastases associated with colon cancer†; however, the potential role of this drug in this setting remains to be more fully elucidated.

■ **Breast Cancer** Outcome may be improved when fluorouracil is used as an adjunct to surgery in certain women with breast cancer. Combination chemotherapy used as an adjunct to surgery has been shown to increase both disease-free (i.e., decreased recurrence) and overall survival in premenopausal and postmenopausal women with node-negative or -positive early (TNM stage I or II) breast cancer. Adjuvant combination chemotherapy that includes cyclophosphamide, methotrexate, and fluorouracil has been used most extensively and is considered a regimen of choice. Although adjuvant hormonal therapy with tamoxifen (with or without combination chemotherapy) generally is used for node-positive, estrogen-receptor-positive postmenopausal women, adjuvant combination chemotherapy (with or without tamoxifen) also can be used in such patients, but differences in toxicity profiles may influence the choice of regimen. For node-positive premenopausal women, adjuvant combination chemotherapy (with or without tamoxifen) generally is used. Adjuvant therapy with combination chemotherapy and/or tamoxifen has been used in women with node-negative disease.

Fluorouracil has been used as a component of combination chemotherapy as an adjunct to surgery in the treatment of early (TNM stage I or II) breast cancer in women with negative axillary lymph nodes and estrogen-receptor-negative tumors. Adjuvant therapy with such combination chemotherapy in both premenopausal and postmenopausal women has been associated with prolongation of disease-free survival and reduction of local, regional, and distant metastases, with tolerable adverse effects. Controversy currently exists regarding which patients with node-negative and estrogen-receptor-negative breast cancer are most likely to benefit from such adjuvant therapy following surgery. While some clinicians advocate the use of such adjuvant therapy in most or all patients with node-negative breast cancer, many clinicians suggest that such therapy should be offered selectively since the toxicities, costs, and/or other quality-of-life considerations outweigh the currently defined benefits in many patients with node-negative breast cancer. Patients with node-negative cancer and poor prognosis (e.g., presence of poor nuclear differentiation, tumor necrosis, tumor size exceeding 2 cm [some clinicians recommend tumor size exceeding 1 cm]) may be suitable candidates for adjuvant chemotherapy. Other women with node-negative breast cancer also may be candidates for adjuvant combination chemotherapy, and pooled analysis of a large number of randomized studies and other evidence have shown that effective adjuvant combination chemotherapy can increase both disease-free and overall survival in patients with node-negative disease, albeit less markedly than in those with node-positive disease.

Although all patients with node-negative breast cancer are at some risk for recurrence, women with small tumors (e.g., smaller than 1 cm) have an excellent prognosis, and the role of adjuvant combination chemotherapy in providing substantial benefit in such women or in other women with good prognostic indicators (e.g., favorable histologic type, diploid tumors with less than a 6–10% fraction of cells in the S phase) remains to be more fully elucidated. An expert panel convened by the National Institutes of Health has stated that most patients with node-negative breast cancer are cured by total or segmental (partial mastectomy, lumpectomy, breast conservation) mastectomy and axillary dissection, and suggests that the use of adjuvant therapy with combination chemotherapy in such patients be individualized based on consideration of the risk of recurrent disease without such adjuvant therapy, the expected reduction in risk and improvement in the quality of life with such adjuvant therapy, and the potential adverse effects of such therapy. The role of such adjuvant therapy in improving the quality of life in patients with node-negative breast cancer remains to be fully determined. The comparative efficacy and tolerability of adjuvant chemotherapy versus adjuvant hormonal (tamoxifen) therapy in women with node-negative disease also remains to be established, but tamoxifen has demonstrated efficacy in postmenopausal women with estrogen-receptor-positive and possibly also in receptor-negative disease, and by indirect analysis it has been suggested that tamoxifen may have an additive effect with combination chemotherapy in postmenopausal women.

Fluorouracil also has been used in conjunction with combination chemotherapy as adjuvant therapy following surgery in premenopausal and postmenopausal women with early breast cancer and positive nodes (stage II). In patients with node-positive early breast cancer, an effective regimen of adjuvant combination chemotherapy (e.g., cyclophosphamide, methotrexate, and fluorouracil; cyclophosphamide, doxorubicin, and fluorouracil; cyclophosphamide and doxorubicin with or without tamoxifen) is used to reduce the rate of recurrence and improve survival in both premenopausal and postmenopausal patients once treatment to control local disease (surgery, with or without radiation therapy) has been undertaken. These combinations have been tested and established as providing therapeutic benefit, and are superior to single-agent therapy with conventional agents; numerous other combination regimens providing apparently similar outcomes also have been used but are less common or have been studied less extensively. Although long-term (e.g., 6 months or longer) chemotherapy with adjuvant regimens is clinically superior to short-term (e.g., preoperative and perioperative) adjuvant regimens, clinical superiority between 6- versus 12-month regimens has not been demonstrated. There is some evidence that the addition of doxorubicin to a regimen of cyclophosphamide, methotrexate, and fluorouracil can improve outcome further in patients with more than 3 positive axillary lymph nodes, and that sequential (i.e., administering several courses of doxorubicin first) regimens are more effective than alternating regimens in such patients; in patients with fewer positive nodes, no additional benefit from doxorubicin has been demonstrated. The addition of doxorubicin to an adjuvant regimen of melphalan and fluorouracil improved outcome in women younger than 50 years of age with hormone-receptor-negative disease and in those 50–59 years of age with progestin-receptor-negative disease. The dose intensity of adjuvant combination chemotherapy also appears to be an important factor influencing clinical outcome in patients with early node-positive breast cancer, with response increasing with increasing dose intensity; therefore, arbitrary reductions in dose intensity should be avoided. In women with stage II disease and more than 10 positive lymph nodes, high-dose chemotherapy and autologous bone marrow transplant is an option currently being evaluated.

Fluorouracil also is used in the treatment of more advanced forms of breast cancer, including inoperable cancer. In stage III (locally advanced) breast cancer, combination chemotherapy (with or without hormonal therapy) is used sequentially following surgery and radiation therapy for operable disease and following biopsy and radiation therapy for inoperable disease; commonly employed effective regimens include cyclophosphamide, methotrexate, and fluorouracil; cyclophosphamide, doxorubicin, and fluorouracil; and cyclophosphamide, methotrexate, fluorouracil, and prednisone. These and other regimens also have been used in the treatment or more advanced (stage IV) and recurrent disease.

Fluorouracil alone has been reported to cause temporary objective remissions in patients with metastatic breast cancer; approximately 10–35% of patients respond. Response is improved in patients with metastatic disease when fluorouracil is used in combination with other antineoplastic agents. While continuous maintenance combination chemotherapy that included fluorouracil has been shown to delay disease progression after initial response or stabilization with induction therapy in women with metastatic disease and may improve quality of life, continuous maintenance therapy has not been shown to prolong overall survival compared with intermittent reinduction therapy that is initiated at the time of progression.

■ **Esophageal Cancer** Fluorouracil has been used alone and in combination therapy for the treatment of localized or advanced esophageal cancer†.

For the treatment of localized esophageal cancer, combined modality treatment consisting of combination chemotherapy with fluorouracil and cisplatin and concurrent radiation therapy may be used prior to surgery (as neoadjuvant therapy) or as an alternative to surgery (i.e., in patients who are not considered suitable surgical candidates or in an attempt to avoid perioperative mortality [less than 10%] and to relieve dysphagia). Combined modality therapy consisting of combination chemotherapy with fluorouracil and cisplatin and concurrent radiation therapy is more effective than radiation therapy alone in patients with localized esophageal carcinoma. Although the comparative benefit of combined chemotherapy and radiation versus surgery has not been established, some experts recommend combined modality treatment with combination chemotherapy (e.g., fluorouracil and cisplatin) and concurrent radiation therapy with or without surgery as primary treatment for localized, resectable esophageal cancer. (See Uses: Esophageal Cancer, in Cisplatin 10:00.)

For the palliative treatment of metastatic (local or distant) disease or recurrent or locally advanced esophageal disease that is not amenable to surgery or radiation therapy, fluorouracil is used in combination chemotherapy with cisplatin, and such combined therapy is considered a regimen of choice.

■ **Head and Neck Cancer** Fluorouracil is used in combination chemotherapy for the treatment of metastatic or recurrent squamous cell carcinoma of the head and neck†. Fluorouracil alone produces poor response rates (13–15%) in patients with advanced head or neck cancer; however, fluorouracil has a synergistic antitumor effect when used in combination with cisplatin. Combination chemotherapy with fluorouracil and cisplatin is commonly used for the palliative treatment of recurrent or metastatic head and neck cancer. (See Uses: Head and Neck Cancer in Cisplatin 10:00.)

Chemotherapy also has been administered in combination with radiation therapy for the palliative treatment of head and neck cancer in patients with locally advanced disease that is unresectable. Combination chemotherapy with fluorouracil and cisplatin administered in rapidly alternating sequence with radiation therapy has been shown to prevent local recurrence of tumor and prolong survival compared with radiation therapy alone in patients with unresectable locally advanced head and neck cancer. The use of chemotherapy combined with radiation therapy also is being investigated for larynx preservation; in 2 large randomized trials, patients receiving induction chemotherapy with fluorouracil and cisplatin followed by radiation therapy had similar survival rates as patients receiving laryngectomy and radiation therapy for locally advanced laryngeal or hypopharyngeal cancer. Induction chemotherapy with fluorouracil, cisplatin, and docetaxel also has been used prior to radiotherapy or chemoradiotherapy for the treatment of locally advanced squamous cell carcinoma of the head and neck. (See Uses: Head and Neck Cancer, in Docetaxel 10:00.)

■ **Cervical Cancer** Fluorouracil in combination with cisplatin is used concurrently with radiation therapy for the treatment of invasive cervical cancer†. Fluorouracil also is used in the treatment of metastatic or recurrent cervical cancer†. (See Uses: Cervical Cancer in Cisplatin 10:00 for an overview of therapy for cervical cancer.)

Concurrent Chemotherapy and Radiation Therapy for Invasive Cervical Cancer Fluorouracil is used in combination with cisplatin for concurrent chemotherapy and radiation therapy in patients with invasive cervical cancer (FIGO stages IB2 through IVA cervical cancer or FIGO stage IA2, IB, or IIA cervical cancer with poor prognostic factors, such as metastatic disease in pelvic lymph nodes, parametrial disease, or positive surgical margins, identified at the time of primary surgery), but randomized controlled studies are needed to determine if this combination regimen is superior to cisplatin alone. Results from one randomized trial suggest that cisplatin alone is as effective but less toxic than cisplatin-containing combination regimens for concomitant use with radiation therapy for the treatment of locally advanced cervical cancer.

Chemotherapy for Metastatic or Recurrent Cervical Cancer Response rates of about 10–20% have been reported with the use of fluorouracil alone or with leucovorin in advanced cervical cancer†. An overall response rate of 14% was observed in a small uncontrolled phase II study of patients receiving fluorouracil and leucovorin for recurrent adenocarcinoma of the cervix. The benefit of combination therapy with fluorouracil and cisplatin compared with cisplatin alone for metastatic or recurrent cervical cancer has not been established. Fluorouracil also has been used concurrently with radiation therapy for the treatment of recurrent pelvic disease following radical surgery for invasive cervical cancer. Further study is needed to define the role of fluorouracil in the treatment of advanced cervical cancer.

■ **Renal Cell Carcinoma** Fluorouracil has been used alone or in combination regimens for the treatment of metastatic renal cell carcinoma†. Fluorouracil alone has minimal activity in the treatment of metastatic renal cell carcinoma with response rates of about 5–7% in phase II studies. Fluorouracil also has been used in combination with aldesleukin and/or interferon alfa for the treatment of metastatic renal cell carcinoma. Because of variable efficacy and/or greater toxicity reported with such regimens, further study is required to establish the role of fluorouracil in combination therapy for the treatment of metastatic renal cell carcinoma. (See discussion of fluorouracil in combination regimens in Uses: Renal Cell Carcinoma in Aldesleukin 10:00 and Interferon Alfa 10:00.)

■ **Other Uses** Fluorouracil has been used as second-line therapy in the treatment of ovarian epithelial cancer†, including platinum-refractory disease. Fluorouracil also is used in the treatment of carcinoid tumors† and cancers of the liver† and biliary tract†. The optimal effectiveness and sequence of combination therapy of fluorouracil with other antineoplastic agents or with irradiation requires further investigation, and it should be kept in mind that any form of therapy that adds to the stress of the patient, interferes with nutrition, or depresses bone marrow function will increase fluorouracil toxicity.

For the use of fluorouracil in the treatment of actinic keratosis, see 84:92.

Dosage and Administration

■ **Administration** Fluorouracil is administered IV. Care should be taken to avoid extravasation of the drug. The usual injection formulation need not be further diluted. The 2.5- or 5-g pharmacy bulk package of fluorouracil is intended for preparation of individual doses of the drug and is *not* for direct IV infusion; after the vial has been entered, any unused portion should be discarded within 1 hour. The drug may be administered through a 25-gauge needle at any convenient rate. Fluorouracil also has been infused regionally into the venous or arterial blood supply of a tumor† (e.g., portal vein or hepatic artery infusions for liver metastases). For topical administration of fluorouracil, see 84:92.

■ **Dosage** ***General Dosage*** Dosage of fluorouracil is based on the patient's actual weight unless the patient is obese or has fluid retention. In these latter instances, dosage is based on ideal weight. Dosage also can be calculated according to body surface area.

Various dosage schedules for fluorouracil therapy have appeared in the literature. Dosage must be based on the clinical and hematologic response and tolerance of the patient in order to obtain optimum therapeutic results with minimum adverse effects. Clinicians should consult published protocols for the dosage of fluorouracil and other chemotherapeutic agents and the method and sequence of administration.

The initial course of fluorouracil therapy currently recommended by the manufacturers is as follows: a dose of 12 mg/kg is given once daily for 4 consecutive days; the manufacturers warn that the daily dose should not exceed 800 mg in this regimen. If further therapy is not precluded by toxic manifestations, a dose of 6 mg/kg is given on the sixth, eighth, tenth, and twelfth days, unless a toxic reaction occurs before then. Therapy is discontinued on the twelfth day. In patients considered poor risks and in patients not in an adequate nutritional state, the manufacturers suggest an initial dosage of 6 mg/kg daily for 3 days. If further therapy is not precluded by toxicity, 3 mg/kg may be given on the fifth, seventh, and ninth days, unless toxicity occurs before then. In poor-risk patients, dosage should not exceed 400 mg daily.

For patients in whom toxicity has not been a problem, the manufacturers state that therapy should be repeated at intervals of 30 days after the last dose of the previous course. Alternatively, when toxicity from the initial course of therapy has subsided, a single weekly maintenance dose of 10–15 mg/kg may be administered; weekly maintenance dosage should not exceed 1 g. The dosage schedule to be used in repeated courses depends on the patient's reaction to the previous course and should be adjusted accordingly.

Advanced Colorectal Carcinoma **Monthly Direct IV Injection ("Bolus") Schedule (Mayo Clinic Regimen).** A commonly used regimen, administered by IV injection ("bolus") on a monthly schedule, is leucovorin 20 mg/m^2 IV *or* an equivalent dose of levoleucovorin (10 mg/m^2 IV) followed by IV fluorouracil 425 mg/m^2; fluorouracil and either leucovorin or levoleucovorin are administered daily for 5 consecutive days. The regimen is repeated at 4-week intervals for 2 additional courses; thereafter, the regimen may be repeated at intervals of 4–5 weeks provided toxicity from the previous course has resolved completely. This regimen is frequently administered for a total of 6 cycles in the adjuvant setting.

Alternatively, leucovorin 200 mg/m^2 *or* an equivalent dose of levoleucovorin (100 mg/m^2) may be administered by slow IV injection (over a minimum of 3 minutes) and followed by IV fluorouracil 370 mg/m^2; fluorouracil and either leucovorin or levoleucovorin are administered daily for 5 consecutive days. The regimen is repeated at 4-week intervals for 2 additional courses; thereafter, the regimen may be repeated at intervals of 4–5 weeks provided toxicity from the previous course has resolved completely.

Weekly IV Infusion Schedule (Roswell Park Regimen). A commonly used regimen, administered by IV infusion on a weekly schedule, is leucovorin 500 mg/m^2 as a 2-hour IV infusion followed by fluorouracil 500 mg/m^2 as a slow IV injection administered 1 hour after the start of the leucovorin infusion†. Both drugs are administered weekly for 6 consecutive weeks followed by a 2-week rest; cycles are repeated every 8 weeks for a total of 4 courses in the adjuvant setting.

Dosage Modification for Mayo Clinic and Roswell Park Regimens. Dosage of fluorouracil in subsequent courses of therapy should be adjusted according to patient tolerance of the prior treatment course; dosage of leucovorin or levoleucovorin in subsequent courses is not adjusted because of toxicity. Daily fluorouracil dosage generally is reduced by 20% in patients who experienced moderate hematologic or GI toxicity in the prior course and by 30% in those patients who experienced severe toxicity. For patients who experienced no toxicity in the prior course of therapy, the dosage of fluorouracil may be increased by 10%. Other combination dosage regimens also have been used. (See Uses: Combination Therapies for GI Cancers.)

Bimonthly Infusion Schedule (Modified deGramont Regimen). A simplified version of the LV5FU2 regimen (deGramont regimen) consists of leucovorin 400 mg/m^2 as a 2-hour IV infusion on day 1 followed by fluorouracil 400 mg/m^2 as an IV injection on day 1; then fluorouracil 1500 mg/m^2 as a continuous IV infusion over 23 hours on days 1 and 2 (i.e., a total of 3000 mg/m^2 by continuous IV infusion over 46 hours); cycles are repeated every 2 weeks.

Breast Cancer Various fluorouracil-containing combination chemotherapy regimens have been used in the treatment of breast cancer, and published protocols should be consulted for dosages and the method and sequence of administration. The dose intensity of adjuvant combination chemotherapy appears to be an important factor influencing clinical outcome in patients with early node-positive breast cancer, with response increasing with increasing dose intensity; therefore, *arbitrary* reductions in dose intensity should be avoided.

One commonly employed regimen for the treatment of early breast cancer includes a fluorouracil dosage of 600 mg/m^2 IV on days 1 and 8 of each cycle combined with cyclophosphamide 100 mg/m^2 orally on days 1 through 14 of each cycle and methotrexate 40 mg/m^2 IV on days 1 and 8 of each cycle. In patients older than 60 years of age, the initial fluorouracil dosage was reduced to 400 mg/m^2 IV and the initial methotrexate dosage was reduced to 30 mg/m^2 IV. Dosage also was reduced if myelosuppression developed. Cycles generally were repeated monthly (i.e., allowing a 2-week rest period between cycles) for a total of 6–12 cycles (i.e., 6–12 months of therapy). Clinical superiority between 6- versus 12-month regimens has not been demonstrated.

There is some evidence that the addition of doxorubicin to a regimen of cyclophosphamide, methotrexate, and fluorouracil can improve outcome further in patients with early breast cancer and more than 3 positive axillary lymph nodes, and that sequential (i.e., administering several courses of doxorubicin first) regimens are more effective than alternating regimens in such patients; in patients with fewer positive nodes, no additional benefit from doxorubicin has been demonstrated. In the sequential regimen, 4 doses of doxorubicin hydrochloride 75 mg/m^2 IV were administered initially at 3-week intervals followed by 8 cycles of fluorouracil 600 mg/m^2 IV, cyclophosphamide 600 mg/m^2 IV, and methotrexate 40 mg/m^2 IV at 3-week intervals for a total of approximately 9 months of therapy. If myelosuppression developed with this sequential regimen, the subsequent cycle generally was delayed rather than reducing dosage.

Cautions

The major toxic effects of fluorouracil are on the normal, rapidly proliferating tissues particularly of the bone marrow and lining of the GI tract.

■ **GI Effects** Anorexia and nausea are common adverse effects of fluorouracil, and vomiting occurs frequently. These reactions generally occur during the first week of therapy, can often be alleviated by antiemetics, and generally subside within 2 or 3 days following therapy. Stomatitis is one of the most common and often the earliest sign of specific toxicity, appearing as early as the fourth day but more commonly on the fifth to eighth day of therapy. Diarrhea, which also occurs frequently, usually appears slightly later than stomatitis, but may occur concurrently or even in the absence of stomatitis. Esophagitis, proctitis, and GI ulceration and bleeding have been reported, and paralytic ileus occurred in two patients who received excessive dosage. Patients must be closely monitored for adverse GI effects. (See Cautions: Precautions and Contraindications.)

GI toxicities (particularly stomatitis and diarrhea) occur more frequently and may be more severe or prolonged in patients receiving leucovorin or levoleucovorin concomitantly with fluorouracil. A GI syndrome characterized by progression from mild GI symptoms to potentially fatal enterocolitis has been reported in several studies in patients with advanced colorectal carcinoma receiving combined therapy with the drugs; in these studies, adverse GI effects (e.g., severe diarrhea) were the dose-limiting toxicity. In one comparative study, severe (grade 3 or 4) diarrhea or stomatitis occurred in 18.9 or 8.6%, respectively, of patients receiving IV levoleucovorin (100 mg/m^2), 15.7 and 11.2%, respectively, of those receiving oral leucovorin (500 mg/m^2 in 4 divided doses), and 17.6 and 14.2%, respectively, of those receiving IV leucovorin (200 mg/m^2) concomitantly with fluorouracil. In one study, severe or exacerbated diarrhea occurred in 25 or 13% of patients receiving fluorouracil combined with high- (500-mg/m^2 doses) or low- (25-mg/m^2 doses) dose leucovorin, respectively. In another study, diarrhea required dose reduction in 50% of patients receiving fluorouracil and high-dose leucovorin. Death occurred in several geriatric patients who developed severe diarrhea, with or without nausea and vomiting, and subsequent dehydration during combined therapy. Limited data suggest that once-weekly administration of fluorouracil plus leucovorin may be associated with a higher risk of developing serious adverse GI effects than 5-day regimens administered at approximately monthly intervals. Severe diarrhea appears to be the dose-limiting toxicity associated with once-weekly administration of the combination, while diarrhea and/or mucositis appear to be the dose-limiting toxicities associated with the 5-day regimens. GI bleeding also has been associated with such fatal toxicity in some patients, and neutropenia, fever, sepsis (possibly related to disruption of the GI mucosa), and acute renal failure also were present in some but not all of the patients who died. Autopsy findings in 2 patients revealed evidence of enterocolitis, including hemorrhagic enterocolitis in one, as well as erosions of the gastric mucosa. In a patient who developed hypotension and abdominal pain and tenderness during combined fluorouracil and leucovorin therapy, there was histologic evidence of ileitis, duodenitis, and esophageal ulceration; the patient responded to hydration, parenteral nutrition, transfusions, and anti-infective therapy.

Combined therapy with fluorouracil and a reduced folate (leucovorin or levoleucovorin) should *not* be initiated or continued in patients with symptomatic GI toxicity until such symptoms have completely resolved. Fluorouracil dosage reduction may be necessary in patients who develop adverse GI effects, particularly in geriatric patients. Close monitoring is particularly important in patients who develop diarrhea with such combined therapy since rapid clinical deterioration and death can occur.

■ **Hematologic Effects** Leukopenia, predominantly of the granulocytopenic type, thrombocytopenia, and anemia occur commonly with fluorouracil therapy; leukopenia usually occurs after an adequate course of fluorouracil therapy. Pancytopenia and agranulocytosis also have occurred. The patient's hematologic status must be carefully monitored. (See Cautions: Precautions and Contraindications.) The nadir of the white blood cell count usually occurs from the ninth to the fourteenth day after therapy is initiated but may occur as late as the 25th day after the first dose of fluorouracil. Maximum thrombocytopenia has been reported to occur from the seventh to seventeenth day of therapy. Hematopoietic recovery is usually rapid and by the thirtieth day, blood cell counts have usually reached the normal range.

■ **Dermatologic and Sensitivity Reactions** Hair loss occurs frequently with fluorouracil therapy, and cosmetically significant alopecia has occurred in a substantial number of patients. Regrowth of hair has been reported even in patients receiving repeated courses of the drug. Partial loss of nails has occurred rarely, and diffuse melanosis of the nails has been reported. The most common type of dermatologic toxicity is a pruritic maculopapular rash which usually appears on the extremities and less frequently on the trunk. This rash is generally reversible and usually responsive to symptomatic treatment.

An erythematous, desquamative rash involving the hands and feet has been reported in patients receiving fluorouracil (in some cases, prolonged infusions of high dosages of the drug were administered). The rash may be accompanied by tingling or painful hands and feet, swollen palms and soles, and phalangeal tenderness. These adverse effects, referred to as palmar-plantar erythrodysesthesia or hand-foot syndrome, may gradually disappear over 5–7 days after discontinuance of fluorouracil therapy. Palmar-plantar dysesthesia syndrome may be treated with oral pyridoxine therapy; however, the safety and efficacy of pyridoxine in this condition have not been fully established.

Other dermatologic manifestations of fluorouracil toxicity have included dry skin and fissuring, diffuse erythema, and scaling. Exposure to strong sunlight may intensify skin reactions to the drug. Seborrheic dermatitis has been reported in a few patients, but could not always be definitely attributed to fluorouracil.

Photosensitivity manifested by erythema or increased pigmentation can occur with fluorouracil therapy. Rarely, anaphylaxis and generalized allergic reactions have occurred in patients receiving fluorouracil.

■ **Nervous System Effects** Disorientation, confusion, euphoria, ataxia, nystagmus, headache, and acute cerebellar syndrome (which may persist after therapy is discontinued) have occurred in patients receiving fluorouracil.

■ **Ocular Effects** Lacrimation, dacryostenosis, visual changes, and photophobia have been reported in patients receiving fluorouracil.

■ **Cardiovascular Effects** Myocardial ischemia and angina (including Prinzmetal variant angina) have occurred rarely in patients receiving fluorouracil. The exact mechanism(s) is not known, but the drug may cause these effects by inducing coronary artery vasospasm.

■ **Other Adverse Effects** Fever that occurred during the end of the second week following the first dose of fluorouracil, and which usually was not accompanied by demonstrable infection, has been reported. Epistaxis, thrombophlebitis, and vein pigmentation also have been reported.

■ **Precautions and Contraindications** Fluorouracil is a highly toxic drug with a very low therapeutic index. The drug can produce severe hematologic toxicity, GI hemorrhage, and even death. Fluorouracil should be given only by, or under the supervision of, a clinician who is experienced in cancer chemotherapy and in the use of antimetabolites. Patients should be hospitalized at least during the initial course of therapy and should be informed of the expected toxic effects, especially oral manifestations.

If intractable vomiting occurs, fluorouracil should be immediately discontinued. Patients should be questioned and the mouth examined daily for early evidence of stomatitis. Appearance of stomatitis, as evidenced by either oral mucosal erythema or ulceration at the inner margin of the lips, or of esophagopharyngitis as evidenced by a sore throat or dysphagia, necessitates cessation of therapy. Diarrhea necessitates immediate discontinuance of the drug. GI ulceration or bleeding, or hemorrhage at any site, also requires prompt cessation of treatment.

Since leucovorin calcium and levoleucovorin calcium enhance the toxicity of fluorouracil, combined therapy with fluorouracil and either leucovorin or levoleucovorin should be used with extreme caution in geriatric or debilitated patients since such patients are more likely to develop serious toxicity from fluorouracil.

Leukocyte counts with differential should be made before each dose of fluorouracil is given and if the leukocyte count falls to below 3500/mm^3 or decreases rapidly, or if there is a fall in the platelet count to below 100,000/mm^3, the drug should be discontinued. If the leukocyte count drops to less than 2000/mm^3, the patient should be placed in protective isolation and appropriate measures taken for the prevention of infection.

Toxicity of fluorouracil is enhanced when the drug is combined with therapy that interferes with nutrition, causes bone marrow suppression, or subjects the patient to stress. Patients in poor nutritional state, or whose bone marrow is depressed by previous therapy or by infiltration of malignant cells, are more likely to develop serious toxicity from fluorouracil than are patients in relatively good condition. Fluorouracil should be used with extreme caution in patients who have previously received high-dose pelvic irradiation therapy or alkylating agents and in patients with impaired liver or kidney function. The drug should also be used with extreme caution in patients with widespread metastatic involvement of the bone marrow. Rarely, severe and unexpected toxic reactions (including stomatitis, diarrhea, neutropenia, and neurotoxicity) have been reported in association with fluorouracil. These reactions have been attributed to deficiency of dipyrimidine dehydrogenase activity, which appears to cause prolonged clearance of fluorouracil. Recurrent, progressive toxicity and increased morbidity have resulted when rechallenge with fluorouracil (at a reduced dosage) was attempted in a small number of patients.

Fluorouracil is contraindicated in patients who are in a poor nutritional state and those who have depressed bone marrow function, potentially serious infections, or known hypersensitivity to fluorouracil.

■ **Pediatric Precautions** Safety and efficacy of fluorouracil in children have not been established.

■ **Mutagenicity and Carcinogenicity** Fluorouracil has been shown to be mutagenic in some but not all strains of *Salmonella typhimurium* and in *Saccharomyces cerevisiae*. In addition, the drug was mutagenic in the micronucleus test on mouse bone marrow cells and, at very high concentrations, produced chromosomal breaks in hamster fibroblasts in vitro. Although the risk of mutagenesis in patients receiving fluorouracil has not been evaluated, the possibility must be considered.

Long-term studies in animals to determine the carcinogenic potential of fluorouracil have not been performed; however, no evidence of carcinogenicity was observed in several animal studies following oral or IV administration of the drug for up to 1 year. In vitro, the drug has induced oncogenic transformation of fibroblasts from mouse embryo. The carcinogenic risk in humans is not known.

■ **Pregnancy, Fertility, and Lactation** Fluorouracil may cause fetal harm when administered to pregnant women. The drug has been shown to be teratogenic in animals at dosages 1–3 times the maximum recommended human therapeutic dosage. Fetal malformations included cleft palate, skeletal defects, and deformed appendages, paws, and tails. The drug has not been studied in animals for potential effects on perinatal and postnatal development; however, it does cross the placenta in rats and has caused increased resorptions and embryolethality in rats. In monkeys, doses greater than 40 mg/kg resulted in abortion of all embryos exposed to the drug. Although there is no evidence to date of teratogenicity caused by fluorouracil in humans, other drugs that inhibit DNA synthesis (e.g., methotrexate) have been reported to be teratogenic in humans. In addition, drugs that inhibit DNA, RNA, and protein synthesis like fluorouracil might be expected to have adverse effects on perinatal and postnatal development. There are no adequate and controlled studies using fluorouracil in pregnant women, and the drug should be used during pregnancy only in life-threatening situations or severe disease for which safer drugs cannot be used or are ineffective. Women of childbearing potential should be advised to avoid becoming pregnant during fluorouracil therapy. If the drug is used during pregnancy or if the patient becomes pregnant while receiving the drug, the patient should be informed of the potential hazard to the fetus.

Fluorouracil has not been adequately studied in animals to determine its effects on fertility and general reproductive performance. Following intraperitoneal administration of 125 or 250 mg/kg in rats, chromosomal aberrations and changes in chromosomal organization of spermatogonia were induced; spermatogonial differentiation was also inhibited, resulting in transient infertility. In a strain of mouse that is sensitive to the induction of sperm head abnormalities after exposure to a number of chemical mutagens and carcinogens, no abnormalities were produced at oral dosages of up to 80 mg/kg daily. Following intraperitoneal administration at weekly doses of 25 or 50 mg/kg weekly for 3 weeks during the preovulatory phases of oogenesis in female rats, the incidence of fertile matings was substantially reduced, development of preimplantation and postimplantation embryos was delayed, and the incidence of preimplantation lethality and chromosomal anomalies in the embryos was increased. In a limited study in rabbits, a single 25-mg/kg dose or daily doses of 5 mg/kg for 5 days had no effect on ovulation, appeared not to affect implantation, and had only a limited effect in producing zygote destruction. Drugs that inhibit DNA, RNA, and protein synthesis like fluorouracil might be expected to have adverse effects on gametogenesis.

It is not known whether fluorouracil is distributed into milk. Because fluorouracil inhibits DNA, RNA, and protein synthesis, it is recommended that women not nurse an infant while receiving the drug.

Pharmacology

Although the precise mechanisms of action of fluorouracil have not been fully elucidated, the main mechanism is thought to be the binding of the deoxyribonucleotide of the drug (FdUMP) and the folate cofactor, N^{5-10}-methylenetetrahydrofolate, to thymidylate synthase (TS) to form a covalently bound ternary complex, which inhibits the formation of thymidylate from uracil, thereby interfering with DNA synthesis. In addition, FUTP can be incorporated into RNA in place of uridine triphosphate (UTP), producing a fraudulent RNA and interfering with RNA processing and protein synthesis.

Pharmacokinetics

■ **Absorption** Following IV administration of fluorouracil, no intact drug is detected in plasma after 3 hours.

■ **Distribution** Fluorouracil is distributed into tumors, intestinal mucosa, bone marrow, liver, and other tissues. Despite its limited lipid solubility, the drug readily crosses the blood-brain barrier and distributes into CSF and brain tissue. Distribution studies in humans and animals have usually shown a higher concentration of the drug or its metabolites in the tumor than in surrounding tissue or in corresponding normal tissue. It has also been shown that there is a longer persistence of fluorouracil in some tumors than in the normal tissues of the host, perhaps due to impaired uracil catabolism. From these data, it has been suggested that the drug may possibly have some specificity against certain tumors in comparison with normal tissues.

Fluorouracil crosses the placenta in rats. It is not known whether the drug is distributed into human milk.

■ **Elimination** Following IV administration, the plasma elimination half-life averages about 16 minutes (range: 8–20 minutes) and is dose dependent.

A small portion of fluorouracil is anabolized in the tissues to 5-fluoro-2′-deoxyuridine and then to 5-fluoro-2′-deoxyuridine-5′-monophosphate, the active metabolite of the drug. The major portion of the drug is degraded in the liver. The metabolites are excreted as respiratory carbon dioxide and as urea, α-fluoro-β-alanine, α-fluoro-β-guanidopropionic acid, and α-fluoro-β-ureidopropionic acid in urine. Following a single IV dose of fluorouracil, approximately 15% of the dose is excreted in urine as intact drug within 6 hours; over 90% of this is excreted in the first hour.

Chemistry and Stability

■ **Chemistry** Fluorouracil is a fluorinated pyrimidine antagonist. The drug occurs as a white to practically white, practically odorless, crystalline powder and is sparingly soluble in water and slightly soluble in alcohol. The pH of the commercially available injection has been adjusted to approximately 9.2 with sodium hydroxide if needed.

■ **Stability** Fluorouracil injection should be stored at 15–30°C; freezing and exposure to light should be avoided. Slight discoloration of fluorouracil injection occurring during storage does not adversely affect potency or safety, but any precipitate formed during storage at low temperature must be dissolved by heating to 60°C and shaking vigorously; the solution should be cooled to body temperature before using. Precipitation of fluorouracil in the injection occurs commonly, particularly following exposure to low temperatures. The frequency of precipitation may increase during cold weather (e.g., winter months), and efforts should be taken to ensure storage in adequately heated areas during these periods to minimize such risk. The ease with which the precipitate will dissolve may depend on the size and location of the precipitated crystals; crystals that become lodged between the stopper and glass container may be more difficult to dissolve. In some cases, attempts to dissolve the precipitate with heat and agitation may be unsuccessful.

For further information on the handling of antineoplastic agents, see the ASHP Guidelines on Handling Hazardous Drugs at http://www.ahfsdruginformation.com.

Preparations

Excipients in commercially available drug preparations may have clinically important effects in some individuals; consult specific product labeling for details.

Fluorouracil

Parenteral

Injection, for IV use	50 mg/mL*	**Adrucil®**, Teva **Fluorouracil Injection**
	50 mg/mL (2.5 or 5 g) pharmacy bulk package*	**Adrucil®**, Teva **Fluorouracil Injection**

*available from one or more manufacturer, distributor, and/or repackager by generic (nonproprietary) name

†Use is not currently included in the labeling approved by the US Food and Drug Administration

Gemcitabine Hydrochloride

■ Gemcitabine hydrochloride, a synthetic pyrimidine nucleoside, is an antimetabolite antineoplastic agent.

Uses

■ **Ovarian Cancer** Gemcitabine is used in combination with carboplatin for the treatment of advanced ovarian epithelial cancer in patients whose disease has relapsed at least 6 months following completion of platinum-based therapy (i.e., platinum-sensitive recurrent ovarian cancer).

The current indication for use of gemcitabine in the treatment of ovarian cancer is based principally on the results of an open-label, randomized, phase 3 study in 356 patients with advanced ovarian cancer whose disease had relapsed at least 6 months following completion of first-line, platinum-based therapy. Patients were randomized to receive either combination therapy with gemcitabine (1 g/m² on days 1 and 8) and carboplatin (administered after gemcitabine on day 1 at the dose required to obtain an area under the plasma concentration-time curve [AUC] of 4 mg/mL per minute) or carboplatin alone (administered on day 1 at the dose required to obtain an AUC of 5 mg/mL per minute) on a 21-day cycle; 6 cycles of therapy were administered in the absence of progressive disease or unacceptable toxicity, with up to 10 cycles administered to those who derived benefit from therapy. Patients who received combination therapy with gemcitabine and carboplatin had prolonged median progression-free survival (8.6 versus 5.8 months) and a higher overall response rate (47.2 versus 30.9%) than patients who received carboplatin alone; median overall survival and median duration of response were similar for both groups. Grade 3 or 4 hematologic toxicity occurred more frequently in patients receiving combination therapy with gemcitabine and carboplatin than in those receiving carboplatin alone; neutropenia was the predominant toxicity. A greater proportion of patients receiving the gemcitabine and carboplatin regimen received red blood cell (27 versus 6.7%) and platelet transfusions (8 versus 3%) compared with those who received carboplatin alone. Although use of hematopoietic growth factors was higher in the group receiving gemcitabine and carboplatin (23.6%) than in the group receiving carboplatin alone (10.1%), the incidence of febrile neutropenia was low and similar in both groups.

■ **Breast Cancer** Gemcitabine is used in combination with paclitaxel for initial treatment of metastatic breast cancer following failure of adjuvant therapy with an anthracycline-containing regimen, unless such therapy was clinically contraindicated.

The current indication for use of gemcitabine in the treatment of breast cancer is based principally on the results of an open-label, randomized, phase 3 study in 529 patients with locally recurrent or metastatic breast cancer following failure of prior adjuvant or neoadjuvant therapy with an anthracycline-containing regimen, unless such therapy was clinically contraindicated. Patients were randomized to receive either combination therapy with gemcitabine (1.25 g/m^2 administered by IV infusion over 30–60 minutes on days 1 and 8) and paclitaxel (175 mg/m^2 administered by IV infusion over 3 hours before gemcitabine on day 1) or paclitaxel alone (175 mg/m^2 administered by IV infusion over 3 hours on day 1) in 21-day cycles; treatment was continued until disease progression, intolerable toxicity, or patient withdrawal occurred. Patients who received combination therapy with gemcitabine and paclitaxel had longer median overall survival (18.6 versus 15.8 months), median time to disease progression (6.14 versus 3.98 months), and median progression-free survival (5.9 versus 3.9 months), and a higher overall response rate (41.4 versus 26.2%) than patients who received paclitaxel alone; median duration of response was similar for both groups. Hematologic toxicity, particularly grade 3/4 neutropenia (47.9 versus 11.5%), was observed more frequently in patients receiving combination therapy with gemcitabine and paclitaxel than in those receiving paclitaxel alone. Febrile neutropenia occurred in 5% of patients who received combination therapy with gemcitabine and paclitaxel and in 1.2% of those who received paclitaxel alone.

■ **Pancreatic Cancer** Gemcitabine is used for the palliative treatment of locally advanced (nonresectable stage II or III) or metastatic (stage IV) adenocarcinoma of the pancreas. The drug can be used either as first-line therapy or as second-line therapy in patients previously treated with fluorouracil. Pancreatic cancer rarely is curable, and response to conventional chemotherapy, radiation therapy, and/or surgery generally is poor regardless of the stage of the cancer. Therefore, the principal goal of therapy for pancreatic cancer generally has been to provide palliation of associated symptoms (e.g., pain) and improvement in the quality of life.

The current indication for use of gemcitabine in the treatment of pancreatic cancer is based on limited data from a multicenter randomized study comparing the drug with fluorouracil in patients with locally advanced or metastatic pancreatic cancer who had not received previous chemotherapy, and from a multicenter open-label study in patients with advanced pancreatic cancer who previously had received fluorouracil alone or as a component of a chemotherapeutic regimen. In both clinical trials, gemcitabine was administered in an initial cycle of 1 g/m^2 IV over 30 minutes once weekly for up to 7 weeks (as tolerated) followed by a treatment-free week, and in subsequent cycles of once-weekly doses (adjusted according to hematologic tolerance) for 3 consecutive weeks each month. The primary efficacy parameter in these studies involved palliative effects grouped as "clinical benefit response." A clinical benefit response was defined as a reduction in pain intensity or analgesic consumption of at least 50% or an improvement in performance status of at least 20 points (on the Karnofsky scale) for a period of at least 4 consecutive weeks, without sustained worsening in any other parameter, or as a stabilization of these parameters combined with a marked, sustained weight gain (of at least 7% maintained for at least 4 weeks) that was not attributable to fluid accumulation.

In the comparative study, gemcitabine therapy was associated with statistically significant increases in clinical benefit response (occurring in 23.8 versus 4.8% of patients receiving gemcitabine or fluorouracil, respectively), survival (median of 5.65 versus 4.41 months with gemcitabine or fluorouracil therapy, respectively), and time to disease progression (9 versus 4 weeks, respectively) compared with fluorouracil therapy (administered IV over 30 minutes at a weekly dosage of 600 mg/m^2). However, there was no confirmed objective evidence of tumor response nor of weight gain with either therapy in this study. One-year survival probability based on Kaplan-Meier estimates was 18 or 2% for those receiving gemcitabine or fluorouracil, respectively.

In the open-label study, 27% of patients receiving gemcitabine as second-line therapy after previous fluorouracil-containing regimens exhibited a clinical benefit response. The median duration of clinical benefit response was 14 weeks (range: 4–69 weeks), and median survival in this study was 3.9 months.

■ **Non-small Cell Lung Cancer** ***Combination Therapy*** Gemcitabine is used in combination with cisplatin for the initial treatment of inoperable, locally advanced (stage IIIA or IIIB) or metastatic (stage IV) non-small cell lung cancer.

A small survival benefit has been demonstrated for the use of platinum-based (cisplatin) chemotherapy in selected patients with unresectable, locally advanced or metastatic non-small cell lung cancer who have a good performance status. Platinum-based chemotherapy regimens currently are preferred for the treatment of non-small cell lung cancer. (See Uses: Non-small Cell Lung Cancer in Cisplatin 10:00 for comprehensive discussion.) Use of chemotherapy for the treatment of advanced non-small cell lung cancer generally is advised only in patients with good performance status (ECOG performance status of 0 or 1, and 2 in selected patients) and evaluable lesions so that treatment can be discontinued if the disease does not respond. The decision to use chemotherapy must be individualized according to several factors, including patient preference, toxicity, survival benefit, quality of life, and cost of treatment.

In a large randomized trial comparing 4 chemotherapy regimens for advanced non-small cell lung cancer, median survival (8.1 versus 7.8 months) and response rate (22 versus 21%) were similar for patients receiving gemcitabine and cisplatin versus paclitaxel and cisplatin. Although median time to progression of disease was longer in patients receiving gemcitabine and cisplatin (4.2 months) compared with paclitaxel and cisplatin (3.4 months), patients receiving the gemcitabine-containing regimen were more likely to experience hematologic toxicity (thrombocytopenia or anemia) or renal toxicity. A higher percentage of patients receiving gemcitabine and cisplatin withdrew from the study because of complications of therapy compared with those receiving paclitaxel and cisplatin (27 versus 15%).

The current indication for gemcitabine in combination with cisplatin for the treatment of advanced non-small cell lung cancer is based principally on data from 2 randomized clinical studies involving a total of 657 patients. In a multicenter study, 522 patients with previously untreated, inoperable stage IIIA, IIIB, or IV non-small cell lung cancer were randomized to receive gemcitabine (1 g/m^2 IV on days 1, 8, and 15) and cisplatin (100 mg/m^2 IV on day 1) or cisplatin alone (100 mg/m^2 IV on day 1) on a 28-day cycle. Characteristics of the patients on the 2 study arms were similar except for tumor histology, with more patients receiving cisplatin alone having adenocarcinoma (48 versus 37%). Patients receiving combination therapy with gemcitabine and cisplatin had a longer median survival time (9 versus 7.6 months), a longer median time to disease progression (5.2 versus 3.7 months), and a higher objective response rate (26 versus 10%) than patients receiving cisplatin alone. Duration of response and quality of life (assessed using the FACT-L, a scale incorporating physical, social, emotional, and functional well-being as well as lung cancer symptoms) were similar for the 2 study groups. Combined therapy with gemcitabine and cisplatin was associated with greater toxicity, particularly myelosuppression, compared with cisplatin monotherapy, and dose adjustments were required in 90% of patients receiving gemcitabine and cisplatin compared with 16% of patients receiving cisplatin alone.

In a second multicenter, randomized study in 135 patients with stage IIIB or IV non-small cell lung cancer, patients were treated on 21-day cycles with cisplatin (100 mg/m^2 IV on day 1) and either gemcitabine (1.25 g/m^2 IV on days 1 and 8) or etoposide (100 mg/m^2 IV on days 1, 2, and 3). Median survival (8.7 versus 7 months) and quality of life (using the EORTC QLQ-C30 and LC13, which evaluate physical and psychologic functioning and symptoms related to lung cancer and its treatment) were similar in patients receiving gemcitabine/cisplatin or etoposide/cisplatin, respectively. A longer median time to disease progression (5 versus 4.1 months) and a higher objective response rate (33 versus 14%) were observed in patients receiving gemcitabine and cisplatin compared with those receiving etoposide and cisplatin. Thrombocytopenia (grade 3 or 4) was more frequent in patients receiving the gemcitabine-containing regimen than in those receiving the etoposide-containing regimen; although the incidence of grade 4 neutropenia was lower in patients receiving gemcitabine with cisplatin versus etoposide with cisplatin, the need for dose reductions or omission of scheduled doses for gemcitabine in twice as many patients as needed for etoposide may have contributed to this difference.

The use of gemcitabine in combination with other antineoplastic agents† for the treatment of non-small cell lung cancer is being investigated. In a randomized trial, patients with stage IIIB or IV non-small cell lung cancer receiving gemcitabine and docetaxel had similar response rates, median survival, and 1- or 2-year survival rates compared with those receiving cisplatin and docetaxel. Further study is needed to evaluate the role of platinum- and non-platinum-containing chemotherapy in the treatment of advanced non-small cell lung cancer.

Monotherapy Gemcitabine is an active agent in non-small cell lung cancer. In nonrandomized phase 2 studies of patients with advanced non-small cell lung cancer who had not received prior chemotherapy, objective response rates of approximately 20% (0–3% complete responses, 17–20% partial responses) have been observed with gemcitabine alone. In these studies, median duration of response ranged from 3.6–12.7 months, and median survival ranged from 7–9 months. Responses to gemcitabine also have been observed in patients with relapsed or refractory advanced non-small cell lung cancer who previously were treated with platinum-containing chemotherapy regimens. Gemcitabine therapy is well tolerated; because of the lower incidence of myelosuppression associated with its use compared with other agents used in the treatment of non-small cell lung cancer, the drug is particularly suited for use in combination chemotherapy regimens. Response rates do not appear to be significantly affected by age; there appears to be similar efficacy and no difference in adverse effects in patients 70 years of age or older versus younger patients receiving gemcitabine alone for advanced non-small cell lung cancer. Noncomparative studies suggest that patients with advanced non-small cell lung cancer receiving gemcitabine experience relief of symptoms (including cough, hemoptysis, chest pain, dyspnea, and anorexia) and improvement in performance status.

In 2 randomized phase 2 studies in patients with inoperable, locally advanced or metastatic non-small cell lung cancer that was previously untreated with chemotherapy, similar efficacy but less toxicity (leukopenia, nausea and vomiting, alopecia) was observed in those receiving gemcitabine alone versus combination therapy with cisplatin and etoposide.

Dosage and Other Considerations Although optimum dosage regimens have not been established, gemcitabine dosages of 1 or 1.25 g/m^2 administered by 30-minute IV infusion once weekly for 3 weeks followed by 1 week of rest have been used most commonly in patients receiving gemcitabine as monotherapy for advanced non-small cell lung cancer. Various dosage schedules have been studied for the combination of gemcitabine with cisplatin for the treatment of advanced non-small cell lung cancer; gemcitabine dosages of 1 g/m^2 administered once weekly for 3 weeks on a 4-week cycle or 1.25 g/m^2 administered once weekly for 2 weeks on a 3-week cycle have been used in large randomized trials (see Dosage and Administration: Dosage); gemcitabine doses of 1–1.5 g/m^2 have been used in combination with cisplatin in phase 2 studies. Other dosage schedules for gemcitabine (e.g., higher doses, lower doses administered over longer infusion periods) are being investigated in patients with advanced non-small cell lung cancer.

Further study is needed to define the role of gemcitabine used alone or in combination therapy for the treatment of advanced non-small cell lung cancer. No single chemotherapy regimen currently can be recommended as superior in the treatment of non-small cell lung cancer. Various chemotherapy regimens used alone or in combination with other treatment modalities, such as radiation therapy, are continually being evaluated for the treatment of advanced non-small cell lung cancer. Because current treatment is not satisfactory for almost all patients with non-small cell lung cancer except selected patients with early-stage, resectable disease, all patients may be considered for enrollment in clinical trials at the time of diagnosis.

■ **Bladder Cancer** Gemcitabine is an active agent that is used alone or in combination therapy for the treatment of advanced or metastatic bladder cancer†. Objective responses to gemcitabine have been observed in patients with metastatic bladder cancer that did not respond to previous treatment with cisplatin-based regimens, including some patients with hepatic metastases.

Gemcitabine is used in combination with cisplatin as an alternative to M-VAC (i.e., cisplatin, methotrexate, and vinblastine with doxorubicin) for the treatment of advanced or metastatic bladder cancer. In a large randomized trial of patients receiving either gemcitabine (1 g/m^2 over 30–60 minutes on days 1, 8, and 15) and cisplatin (70 mg/m^2 on day 2) or M-VAC for the treatment of advanced or metastatic bladder cancer, overall median survival (13.8 versus 14.8 months, respectively), median time to progressive disease (7.4 months for each regimen), and response rates (44 versus 38%, respectively, using intent-to-treat analysis) were similar. Prophylactic hematopoietic agents (growth factors) were not administered to either group; grade 3 or 4 anemia or grade 3 or 4 thrombocytopenia were observed more often in patients receiving gemcitabine and cisplatin whereas grade 3 or 4 neutropenia, neutropenic sepsis, grade 3 or 4 mucositis, and alopecia occurred more frequently in patients receiving M-VAC.

Gemcitabine also is used as a single agent for the treatment of advanced or metastatic bladder cancer. In a phase 2 study, gemcitabine 1.25 g/m^2 was administered IV once weekly for 3 weeks every 4 weeks in patients with advanced bladder cancer that did not respond to previous treatment with cisplatin-based chemotherapy. Among 25 evaluable patients, an overall response rate of 28% (12% complete responses, 16% partial responses) was reported, and symptomatic improvements in hematuria, dysuria, cystitis, and polyuria were observed. In two other phase 2 studies, IV gemcitabine 1.2 g/m^2 was administered once weekly for 3 weeks every 4 weeks in previously untreated patients with advanced or metastatic bladder cancer. Among 76 evaluable patients, overall response rates of 24–29% (8–11% complete responses, 16–18% partial responses) were observed. Gemcitabine appears to be well-tolerated in most patients with only mild toxicity.

Further study is needed to define the precise role of gemcitabine in the treatment of advanced or metastatic bladder cancer, particularly in combination regimens.

■ **Biliary Tract Cancer** Gemcitabine has been used in combination with cisplatin for the treatment of unresectable locally advanced or metastatic biliary tract cancer† (intrahepatic or extrahepatic cholangiocarcinoma, gallbladder cancer, or ampullary cancer), including unresectable recurrent disease following surgical resection.

Evidence concerning efficacy of chemotherapy regimens in the treatment of advanced biliary tract cancer is derived largely from small, nonrandomized, clinical studies and retrospective analyses; few large, randomized, controlled clinical trials have been conducted. Experts state that, in patients with biliary tract adenocarcinoma (the most common type of biliary tract cancer), chemotherapy can be recommended in individuals with unresectable locally advanced or metastatic disease and in those with recurrent disease following surgical resection, since there is some evidence from a randomized study in patients with unresectable pancreatic or biliary tract cancer indicating that use of chemotherapy for the treatment of unresectable biliary tract cancer is associated with prolonged survival and improved quality of life. Chemotherapy is recommended in such individuals with good performance status (ECOG performance status of 0 or 1). However, in patients with poor performance status (ECOG performance status of 2 or 3) or insufficient biliary decompression, the benefits of chemotherapy are limited and use of alternative therapy for palliation of associated symptoms (e.g., pain) and improvement in quality of life is recommended. In one retrospective analysis comparing chemotherapy with best supportive care in patients with advanced gallbladder cancer, a survival benefit was observed in patients with good performance status but not in those with poor performance status.

In a multicenter, randomized, phase 3 trial (Advanced Biliary Cancer [ABC]-02), 410 patients with unresectable locally advanced or metastatic biliary tract carcinoma, including unresectable recurrent disease following surgical resection, were randomized to receive either combination therapy with gemcitabine (1 g/m^2 administered by IV infusion over 30 minutes on days 1 and 8) and cisplatin (25 mg/m^2 administered by IV infusion over 1 hour on days 1 and 8) on a 21-day cycle or gemcitabine alone (1 g/m^2 administered by IV infusion over 30 minutes on days 1, 8, and 15) on a 28-day cycle. Patients without evidence of disease progression at 12 weeks could continue to receive their assigned regimen for an additional 12 weeks. Patients enrolled in the study generally had good baseline performance status (ECOG score of 0 or 1 in 88% of patients, score of 2 in 12%). Patients who had received prior systemic chemotherapy for locally advanced or metastatic biliary tract carcinoma (other than low-dose radiosensitizing chemotherapy given in conjunction with radiotherapy) were excluded from the study. At a median follow-up of 8.2 months, patients who received combination therapy with gemcitabine and cisplatin had longer median overall (11.7 versus 8.1 months) and progression-free (8 versus 5 months) survival, a higher 6-month progression-free survival rate (59.3 versus 42.5%), and higher rates of tumor control (complete or partial responses or stable disease) (81.4 versus 71.8%) compared with patients who received gemcitabine alone. Only one patient in each treatment group achieved a complete response. Grade 3 or 4 hematologic toxicity (most commonly neutropenia [25.3 versus 16.6%]) occurred more frequently in patients receiving combination therapy with gemcitabine and cisplatin, whereas grade 3 or 4 abnormalities in liver function (27.1 versus 16.7%), including elevations in serum ALT (SGPT) concentrations, occurred more frequently in patients receiving gemcitabine alone. Grade 3 or 4 infection occurred with similar frequency in both groups. Based on current evidence, combination therapy with gemcitabine and cisplatin is recommended (accepted) for use in the treatment of unresectable locally advanced or metastatic biliary tract cancer (intrahepatic or extrahepatic cholangiocarcinoma, gallbladder cancer, or ampullary cancer), including unresectable recurrent disease following surgical resection, in patients with good performance status (ECOG performance status of 0 or 1).

Dosage and Administration

■ **Reconstitution and Administration** Gemcitabine hydrochloride is administered by IV infusion. The manufacturer states that the drug is for IV use only.

Vials labeled as containing 200 mg or 1 g of gemcitabine should be reconstituted by adding 5 or 25 mL, respectively, of 0.9% sodium chloride injection without preservatives and shaking to dissolve. The resultant solutions have a gemcitabine concentration of 38 mg/mL, which accounts for the displacement volume of lyophilized powder (0.26 or 1.3 mL for vials labeled as containing 200 mg or 1 g, respectively). Smaller volumes should not be used for reconstitution since gemcitabine concentrations greater than 38 mg/mL may exceed the solubility of the drug and result in incomplete dissolution. The total volume upon reconstitution for vials labeled as containing 200 mg or 1 g is about 5.26 or 26.3 mL, respectively, and complete withdrawal of contents of the vials will provide 200 mg or 1 g, respectively. The reconstituted solutions can be infused IV without further dilution or as solutions that have been further diluted in 0.9% sodium chloride injection to gemcitabine concentrations as low as 0.1 mg/mL.

Reconstituted and diluted solutions of gemcitabine hydrochloride generally are infused IV over a period of 30 minutes; any unused portion after preparation of the appropriate dose should be discarded. Increased toxicity, including clinically important myelosuppression, was observed in clinical trials when gemcitabine was infused over periods exceeding 60 minutes. In a phase 1 study designed to assess maximally tolerated infusion rates, the risk of clinically important myelosuppression was particularly great with infusion periods of 4.5 hours (270 minutes) or longer. Because prolonged IV infusion of gemcitabine hydrochloride is associated with a prolonged half-life and increased toxicity, the manufacturer warns that the infusion time for the drug should *not* exceed 60 minutes. (See Description.)

Prior to administration, reconstituted and diluted solutions of gemcitabine hydrochloride should be inspected visually whenever solution and container permit. If discoloration or particulate matter is present, the solution should be discarded. When reconstituted and/or diluted as directed, gemcitabine hydrochloride solutions are stable for 24 hours at controlled room temperatures of 20–25°C. The solutions should *not* be refrigerated since crystallization may occur.

■ **Dosage** Dosage of gemcitabine hydrochloride is expressed in terms of gemcitabine and must be individualized based on body surface area and patient tolerance and response.

The manufacturer warns that gemcitabine should not be administered more frequently than once weekly since the risk of toxicity is increased with such dosing. In a phase 1 trial designed to assess the maximum tolerated dose on a schedule of 5 consecutive daily doses, patients developed intolerable hypotension and flu-like symptoms at gemcitabine dosages exceeding 10 mg/m^2 daily; the incidence and severity of these effects were dose related. In other dose-ranging phase 1 trials using twice-weekly schedules, maximum tolerated gemcitabine doses were 65 mg/m^2 when the drug was infused over 30 minutes and 150 mg/m^2 when the drug was injected over 5 minutes; in these trials, dose-limiting toxicities included thrombocytopenia and flu-like symptoms, particularly asthenia.

Ovarian Cancer For the treatment of advanced ovarian cancer in women whose disease has relapsed at least 6 months following completion of platinum-based therapy, the manufacturer recommends a regimen of gemcitabine 1 g/m^2 administered by 30-minute IV infusion on days 1 and 8 of a 21-day cycle; carboplatin (at a dose required to obtain an area under the plasma concentration-time curve [AUC] of 4 mg/mL per minute) should be administered IV on day 1 after gemcitabine administration.

Patients should have an absolute granulocyte count of at least 1500/mm^3 and a platelet count of at least 100,000/mm^3 prior to each cycle. If necessary, dosage of gemcitabine should be reduced or withheld according to the degree of hematologic toxicity. (See Hematologic Toxicity under Dosage: Dosage Modification for Toxicity and Contraindications for Continued Therapy, in Dosage and Administration.) For adjustment of carboplatin dosage according to the degree of hematologic toxicity, see Dosage and Administration: Dosage, in Carboplatin 10:00; the manufacturer's prescribing information also should be consulted. In case of severe (i.e., grade 3 or 4) nonhematologic toxicity other than nausea and vomiting, gemcitabine doses should be withheld or reduced. (See Nonhematologic Toxicity under Dosage: Dosage Modification for Toxicity and Contraindications for Continued Therapy, in Dosage and Administration.)

Breast Cancer For initial treatment of metastatic breast cancer in adults following failure of anthracycline-containing adjuvant chemotherapy or in whom such chemotherapy was contraindicated, the manufacturer recommends a regimen of gemcitabine 1.25 g/m^2 administered by 30-minute IV infusion on days 1 and 8 of a 21-day cycle; paclitaxel 175 mg/m^2 should be administered as a 3-hour IV infusion on day 1 before administration of gemcitabine.

Patients should have an absolute granulocyte count of at least 1500/mm^3 and a platelet count of at least 100,000/mm^3 prior to each cycle. If necessary, dosage of gemcitabine should be reduced or withheld according to the degree of hematologic toxicity. In case of severe (i.e., grade 3 or 4) nonhematologic toxicity other than alopecia or nausea and vomiting, gemcitabine doses should be withheld or reduced. (See Dosage Modification for Toxicity and Contraindications for Continued Therapy under Dosage and Administration: Dosage.) For adjustment of paclitaxel dosage according to the degree of hematologic or nonhematologic toxicity, see Dosage Modification for Toxicity and Contraindications for Continued Therapy under Dosage and Administration: Dosage, in Paclitaxel 10:00; the manufacturer's prescribing information also should be consulted.

Pancreatic Cancer The usual dosage of gemcitabine currently recommended by the manufacturer for the treatment of locally advanced or metastatic pancreatic carcinoma, either as first-line therapy in chemotherapy-naive patients or as second-line therapy in those previously treated with fluorouracil, is 1 g/m^2 once weekly. For the initial cycle, this dosage is repeated at weekly intervals as tolerated for up to 7 weeks, followed by a week of rest from treatment. If necessary during the course of the initial cycle, dosage should be reduced or withheld according to the degree of hematologic toxicity. (See Hematologic Toxicity under Dosage: Dosage Modification for Toxicity and Contraindications for Continued Therapy, in Dosage and Administration.) Subsequent cycles consist of once-weekly administration for 3 consecutive weeks of the usual or escalated dosage (see Dosage Escalation under Dosage: Pancreatic Cancer, in Dosage and Administration), if tolerated, or at dosages reduced according to the degree of hematologic toxicity, followed by a week of rest from treatment. In clinical trials, patients with pancreatic cancer reportedly received an average of 3 cycles of gemcitabine therapy. Because clearance of gemcitabine is reduced in women and geriatric patients, dosage reductions, including withholding of doses in some cases, may be more likely in these populations; however, there currently is no evidence that unusual dosage adjustments (i.e., other than those recommended in general for hematologic toxicity) would be required. In clinical trials, women tolerated the drug more poorly than men, were less likely to progress to subsequent cycles, and were more likely to experience hematologic toxicity (i.e., neutropenia and thrombocytopenia).

Dosage Escalation. Dosage escalation can be considered for patients with pancreatic cancer who successfully complete the initial 7-week or subsequent 3-week cycle of gemcitabine therapy at the full weekly dosage of 1 g/m^2, provided nadirs of the absolute granulocyte and platelet counts exceed 1500 and 100,000/mm^3, respectively, and nonhematologic toxicity exceeding a World Health Organization (WHO) grade of 1 is not present. In such patients, the dosage can be increased to 1.25 g/m^2 weekly. If a complete 3-week course at a dosage of 1.25 g/m^2 is tolerated (i.e., these hematologic parameters are met and there is no evidence of WHO grade 1 nonhematologic toxicity), dosage can be escalated further to 1.5 g/m^2 weekly given in 3-week cycles.

Non-small Cell Lung Cancer The optimum dosage regimen for gemcitabine when used in combination with cisplatin for the treatment of advanced non-small cell lung cancer has not been established. For the initial treatment of patients with inoperable, locally advanced (stage IIIA or IIIB) or metastatic (stage IV) non-small cell lung cancer, gemcitabine used in combination with cisplatin may be administered on either a 4-week schedule or a 3-week schedule with doses specific to the selected dosage schedule. For patients receiving combination therapy with gemcitabine and cisplatin on the *4-week schedule*, the manufacturer recommends a regimen of gemcitabine 1 g/m^2 administered by 30-minute IV infusion on days 1, 8, and 15 of each 28-day cycle; cisplatin 100 mg/m^2 should be administered IV on day 1 following completion of the gemcitabine infusion. For patients receiving combination therapy with gemcitabine and cisplatin on the *3-week schedule*, the manufacturer recommends a regimen of gemcitabine 1.25 g/m^2 administered by 30-minute IV infusion on days 1 and 8 of each 21-day cycle; cisplatin 100 mg/m^2 should be administered IV on day 1 following completion of the gemcitabine infusion.

If necessary, dosage of gemcitabine should be reduced or withheld according to the degree of hematologic toxicity. (See Hematologic Toxicity under Dosage: Dosage Modification for Toxicity and Contraindications for Continued Therapy, in Dosage and Administration.) For adjustment of cisplatin dosage according to the degree of hematologic toxicity, see Cautions: Precautions and Contraindications, in Cisplatin 10:00; the manufacturer's prescribing information also should be consulted. In case of severe (i.e., grade 3 or 4) nonhematologic toxicity other than alopecia or nausea and vomiting, gemcitabine and cisplatin doses should be withheld or reduced. (See Nonhematologic Toxicity under Dosage: Dosage Modification for Toxicity and Contraindications for Continued Therapy, in Dosage and Administration.) The manufacturer also recommends careful monitoring of serum concentrations of creatinine, potassium, calcium, and magnesium in patients receiving gemcitabine in combination with cisplatin. Appropriate administration, hydration, and dosage adjustment guidelines for cisplatin should be followed. (See Cisplatin 10:00.)

Biliary Tract Cancer When gemcitabine has been used in combination with cisplatin for the treatment of unresectable locally advanced or metastatic biliary tract cancer† in adults, including treatment of unresectable recurrent disease following surgical resection, gemcitabine 1 g/m^2 has been administered by 30-minute IV infusion on days 1 and 8 of each 21-day cycle, and cisplatin 25 mg/m^2 has been administered by 1-hour IV infusion on days 1 and 8 prior to gemcitabine administration. Treatment has been continued for 24 weeks (8 cycles of therapy) in the absence of disease progression or unacceptable toxicity.

Dosage Modification for Toxicity and Contraindications for Continued Therapy **Hematologic Toxicity.** A complete blood cell count (CBC), including differential and platelets, should be performed prior to each dose of gemcitabine. If myelosuppression is detected, therapy should be modified or temporarily withheld according to the degree of hematologic toxicity.

In patients receiving gemcitabine for the treatment of *advanced ovarian cancer*, the dosage of gemcitabine within a cycle of treatment should be adjusted according to the granulocyte and platelet counts obtained on day 8 of therapy. For patients with absolute granulocyte counts of at least 1500/mm^3 and platelet counts of at least 100,000/mm^3, no adjustment in dosage is necessary. For those with absolute granulocyte counts of 1000–1499/mm^3 *and/or* platelet counts of 75,000–99,999/mm^3, 50% of the full dose should be given. If the absolute granulocyte count is less than 1000/mm^3 *and/or* the platelet count is less than 75,000/mm^3, the dose should be withheld. The dosage of gemcitabine in combination with carboplatin for subsequent cycles should be adjusted according to observed toxicity. The dosage of gemcitabine in subsequent cycles should be reduced to 800 mg/m^2 on days 1 and 8 if any of the following hematologic toxicities occur: absolute granulocyte counts of less than 500/mm^3 for more than 5 days or less than 100/mm^3 for more than 3 days, febrile neutropenia, platelet counts of less than 25,000/mm^3, or cycle delay of more than one week due to toxicity. If any of these toxicities recur after the initial dosage reduction, gemcitabine should be administered on day 1 *only* at a dose of 800 mg/m^2 for the subsequent cycle.

In patients receiving gemcitabine for the treatment of *metastatic breast cancer*, the dosage of gemcitabine should be adjusted according to the granulocyte and platelet counts obtained on day 8 of therapy. For patients with absolute granulocyte counts of at least 1200/mm^3 and platelet counts exceeding 75,000/mm^3, no adjustment in dosage is necessary. For those with absolute granulocyte counts of 1000–1199/mm^3 *or* platelet counts of 50,000–75,000/mm^3, 75% of the full dose should be given. For those with absolute granulocyte counts of 700–999/mm^3 *and* platelet counts of at least 50,000/mm^3, 50% of the full dose should be given. If the absolute granulocyte count is less than 700/mm^3 *or* the platelet count is less than 50,000/mm^3, the dose should be withheld.

In patients receiving gemcitabine for the treatment of *locally advanced or metastatic pancreatic carcinoma* or *advanced non-small cell lung cancer* with absolute granulocyte counts of at least 1000/mm^3 and platelet counts of at least 100,000/mm^3, no adjustment in dosage is necessary. For those with absolute granulocyte counts of 500–999/mm^3 *or* platelet counts of 50,000–99,999/mm^3, 75% of the full dose should be given weekly. If the absolute granulocyte count is less than 500/mm^3 *or* the platelet count is less than 50,000/mm^3, the weekly dose should be withheld until the counts exceed these levels.

Nonhematologic Toxicity. The diagnosis of hemolytic-uremic syndrome should be considered and gemcitabine should be discontinued immediately in patients who develop anemia with evidence of microangiopathic hemolysis, elevation of serum bilirubin or LDH, reticulocytosis, and/or severe thrombocytopenia with or without evidence of renal failure (e.g., elevation of serum creatinine or BUN).

Gemcitabine should be discontinued immediately and appropriate supportive care (e.g., diuretics, corticosteroids) provided promptly in patients who develop severe adverse pulmonary effects.

In patients receiving gemcitabine for the treatment of *advanced ovarian cancer* who develop grade 3 or 4 nonhematologic toxicity other than nausea and vomiting, gemcitabine doses should be withheld or reduced by 50%.

In patients receiving gemcitabine for the treatment of *metastatic breast cancer* who develop grade 3 or 4 nonhematologic toxicity other than alopecia or nausea and vomiting, gemcitabine doses should be withheld or reduced by 50%.

In patients receiving gemcitabine in combination with cisplatin for the treatment of *advanced non-small cell lung cancer* who develop grade 3 or 4 nonhematologic toxicity other than alopecia or nausea and vomiting, gemcitabine and cisplatin doses should be withheld or reduced by 50%.

■ **Special Populations** The manufacturer states that there are insufficient data to recommend a dosage of gemcitabine in patients with renal or hepatic impairment. (See Adequate Patient Evaluation and Monitoring under Warnings/Precautions: General Precautions, in Cautions and see Hepatic Impairment and also see Renal Impairment under Warnings/Precautions: Specific Populations, in Cautions.)

Cautions

■ **Contraindications** Known hypersensitivity to gemcitabine or any ingredient in the formulation.

■ **Warnings/Precautions** ***Warnings*** **IV Administration.** Prolonged IV infusion of gemcitabine (i.e., over periods exceeding 60 minutes) and administration more frequent than once weekly may be associated with increased toxicity (e.g., myelosuppression). (See Dosage and Administration: Reconstitution and Administration.)

Hematologic Effects. The dose-limiting toxicity of gemcitabine is myelosuppression, including leukopenia, anemia, and thrombocytopenia. Patients receiving the drug may require red blood cell transfusions or, less frequently, platelet transfusions. Patients should be monitored for myelosuppression during therapy. A complete blood cell count (CBC), including differential and platelets, should be performed prior to each dose; dosage should be modified accordingly. (See Hematologic Toxicity under Dosage: Dosage Modification for Toxicity and Contraindications for Continued Therapy, in Dosage and Administration.)

Pulmonary Effects. Severe and sometimes fatal adverse pulmonary effects, including pulmonary edema, interstitial pneumonitis, pulmonary fibrosis, and adult respiratory distress syndrome (ARDS), have been reported in patients receiving one or more doses of gemcitabine; the drug should be discontinued immediately and appropriate supportive care (e.g., diuretics, corticosteroids) provided promptly in patients developing such effects. Onset of pulmonary symptoms has occurred up to 2 weeks following administration of the last dose of gemcitabine, and in rare instances, respiratory failure and death have occurred despite discontinuance of gemcitabine therapy. Dyspnea, unrelated to underlying disease and occasionally accompanied by bronchospasm, has been reported in patients receiving gemcitabine. Dose-limiting pulmonary toxicity, including esophagitis, pulmonary fibrosis, and pneumonitis, occurred in patients receiving gemcitabine and concurrent thoracic radiation therapy for non-small cell lung cancer. In addition, fatal pulmonary veno-occlusive disease has been reported in a patient who developed progressive dyspnea during gemcitabine therapy.

Renal Effects. Hemolytic-uremic syndrome and/or renal failure have been reported in patients receiving one or more doses of gemcitabine. In rare cases, renal failure leading to death or requiring dialysis has occurred despite discontinuance of gemcitabine therapy. Cases of renal failure leading to death typically were caused by hemolytic-uremic syndrome. The diagnosis of hemolytic-uremic syndrome should be considered and gemcitabine should be discontinued immediately in patients who develop anemia with evidence of microangiopathic hemolysis, elevation of serum bilirubin or LDH, reticulocytosis, severe thrombocytopenia and/or evidence of renal failure (e.g., elevation of serum creatinine or BUN).

Hepatic Effects. Serious hepatotoxicity, including hepatic failure and death, has been reported rarely in patients receiving gemcitabine alone or in combination with other potentially hepatotoxic drugs. In clinical studies, gemcitabine was associated with transient elevations in serum transaminases; however, there was no evidence of increasing hepatotoxicity with either longer duration of exposure to gemcitabine or with greater total cumulative dose. Elevated liver function test results, including increased concentrations of AST, ALT, γ-glutamyltransferase (GGT, γ-glutamyltranspeptidase, GGTP), alkaline phosphatase, and bilirubin, have been reported rarely during postmarketing surveillance.

Fetal/Neonatal Morbidity and Mortality. Gemcitabine may cause fetal harm; teratogenicity and embryolethality have been demonstrated in animals. There are no studies to date in humans. If gemcitabine is used during pregnancy or the patient becomes pregnant while receiving the drug, the patient should be apprised of the potential fetal hazard.

Sensitivity Reactions **Hypersensitivity Reactions.** Anaphylactoid reactions have been reported rarely during postmarketing surveillance in patients receiving gemcitabine.

General Precautions **Adequate Patient Evaluation and Monitoring.** Gemcitabine should be used under the supervision of a qualified clinician experienced in therapy with antineoplastic agents. Most adverse effects of the drug are reversible and do not require discontinuance of gemcitabine therapy, although withholding doses or reducing dosage may be necessary. (See Dosage Modification for Toxicity and Contraindications for Continued Therapy under Dosage and Administration: Dosage.)

Renal and hepatic function should be assessed prior to and periodically during gemcitabine therapy. A complete blood cell count, including differential and platelets, should be performed prior to each dose.

Cardiovascular Effects. Cardiovascular toxicity, including congestive heart failure, myocardial infarction, and arrhythmias (mainly supraventricular), has been reported rarely during postmarketing surveillance in patients receiving gemcitabine. Vasculitis and gangrene also have been reported rarely in patients receiving the drug.

Specific Populations **Pregnancy.** Category D. (See Fetal/Neonatal Morbidity and Mortality under Warnings/Precautions: Warnings, in Cautions.) (See Users Guide.)

Lactation. It is not known whether gemcitabine is distributed into milk. The manufacturer states that a decision should be made whether to discontinue nursing or the drug, taking into account the importance of the drug to the woman and the potential risk to nursing infants..

Pediatric Use. Efficacy of gemcitabine has not been established in children younger than 18 years of age. In a phase 1 study in pediatric patients with refractory leukemia†, the maximum tolerated dosage of gemcitabine was 10 mg/m^2 per minute for 6 hours (360 minutes) 3 times weekly, followed by 1 week of rest. When gemcitabine was administered at this dosage in a phase 2 study in patients with relapsed acute lymphoblastic leukemia† or acute myelogenous leukemia†, no clinically important activity was observed. Adverse effects reported in these studies were similar to those reported in adults and included bone marrow suppression, febrile neutropenia, increased serum transaminases, nausea, and rash/desquamation.

Geriatric Use. Because gemcitabine clearance is reduced and half-life is increased in geriatric patients, dosage reductions, including withholding of doses in some cases, may be more likely in this population; however, there currently is no evidence that unusual dosage adjustments (i.e., other than those recommended in general for hematologic and nonhematologic toxicity) would be required. Information derived from the safety database for gemcitabine monotherapy indicates that the frequency of adverse effects in patients older than 65 years of age is similar to that in younger adults; however, severe (grade 3/4) thrombocytopenia has occurred more frequently in geriatric patients. In the clinical study of gemcitabine given in combination with carboplatin for recurrent ovarian cancer, no overall differences in efficacy or safety were observed between geriatric and younger patients; however, grade 3/4 neutropenia occurred more frequently in geriatric patients 65 years of age or older.

Hepatic Impairment. Gemcitabine should be used with caution in patients with hepatic impairment. The effects of substantial hepatic insufficiency on the disposition of the drug have not been established. Use of gemcitabine in patients with current liver metastases or a history of hepatitis, alcoholism, or cirrhosis may lead to exacerbation of the underlying hepatic insufficiency. (See Dosage and Administration: Special Populations and see Adequate Patient Evaluation and Monitoring under Warnings/Precautions: General Precautions, in Cautions.)

Renal Impairment. Gemcitabine should be used with caution in patients with renal impairment. The effects of substantial renal insufficiency on the disposition of the drug have not been established. (See Dosage and Administration: Special Populations and see Adequate Patient Evaluation and Monitoring under Warnings/Precautions: General Precautions, in Cautions.)

Women. Because gemcitabine clearance is reduced and half-life is increased in women, dosage reductions, including withholding of doses in some cases, may be more likely in this population; however, there currently is no evidence that unusual dosage adjustments (i.e., other than those recommended in general for hematologic and nonhematologic toxicity) would be required. In clinical studies with gemcitabine therapy, women, especially older women, were more likely not to proceed to the next cycle and more likely to experience World Health Organization (WHO) grade 3/4 neutropenia and thrombocytopenia.

■ **Common Adverse Effects** Adverse effects reported in 10% or more of patients receiving gemcitabine monotherapy include myelosuppression (i.e., anemia, leukopenia, neutropenia, thrombocytopenia), proteinuria, hematuria, increased BUN, nausea, vomiting, pain, fever, rash, pruritus, dyspnea, constipation, diarrhea, hemorrhage, peripheral edema, edema, flu-like symptoms, infection, alopecia, stomatitis, somnolence, paresthesias, and increased serum AST, ALT, alkaline phosphatase, and bilirubin concentrations.

Drug Interactions

No formal drug interaction studies have been performed to date.

■ **Antineoplastic Agents** Based on data from patients with metastatic breast cancer, concomitant use of gemcitabine and paclitaxel appears to have minimal or no effect on the pharmacokinetics (i.e., clearance, half-life) of either drug.

Based on data from patients with non-small cell lung cancer, concomitant use of gemcitabine and carboplatin does not appear to alter the pharmacokinetics of either drug compared with use of each drug alone.

■ **Radiation Therapy** A pattern of tissue injury usually associated with radiation toxicity has been reported in association with concurrent and nonconcurrent use of gemcitabine and radiation therapy. Radiosensitizing activity of gemcitabine was observed in preclinical and clinical studies when the drug was administered with or within 7 days of radiation therapy (i.e., concurrent therapy). Gemcitabine has been associated with radiation recall reactions, but administration more than 7 days before or after radiation therapy (i.e., nonconcurrent therapy) does not otherwise appear to enhance toxicity. Available data suggest that gemcitabine therapy may be initiated once the acute effects of radiation therapy have resolved, or at least one week following radiation therapy.

Toxicity in patients receiving combined modality treatment is dependent on many factors, including doses of gemcitabine and radiation, frequency of gemcitabine administration, radiotherapy planning technique, and target tissue and volume. In one study in patients with non-small cell lung cancer who received gemcitabine therapy (dose of 1 g/m^2) and therapeutic thoracic radiation concurrently for up to 6 consecutive weeks, substantial toxicity (manifested as severe and potentially life-threatening mucositis, especially esophagitis and pneumonitis) was observed, particularly in those receiving large volumes of radiotherapy. Subsequent studies have suggested that toxicity is predictable and less severe when lower doses of gemcitabine are administered concurrently with radiation therapy; however, the optimal regimen for safe administration of gemcitabine with therapeutic dosages of radiation has not been established for all tumor types.

Description

Gemcitabine hydrochloride, a synthetic pyrimidine nucleoside, is an antineoplastic agent. The nucleoside analog consists of the pyrimidine base difluorocytidine, and the sugar moiety deoxyribose.

Like most antimetabolite antineoplastic agents, gemcitabine is cell-cycle specific, acting principally in the S phase of the cell cycle; the drug also may cause cellular arrest at the G_1—S border. The cytotoxic activity of gemcitabine (2′-deoxy-2′,2′-difluorocytidine) depends on intracellular conversion to its 5′-diphosphate and -triphosphate metabolites; thus, deoxydifluorocytidine-5′-diphosphate (dFdCDP, gemcitabine diphosphate) and -triphosphate (dFdCTP, gemcitabine triphosphate) and not unchanged gemcitabine are the pharmacologically active forms of the drug. Gemcitabine is phosphorylated by deoxycytidine kinase to gemcitabine monophosphate, which subsequently is phosphorylated to the corresponding diphosphate and triphosphate nucleosides, presumably by deoxycytidylate kinase and nucleoside diphosphate kinase, respectively. The cytotoxic effect of gemcitabine is attributed to the combined actions of its diphosphate and triphosphate nucleosides, which lead to inhibition of DNA synthesis.

Gemcitabine diphosphate inhibits ribonucleotide reductase, which is responsible for catalyzing the formation of deoxynucleoside triphosphates needed in DNA synthesis. By inhibiting this reductase, gemcitabine diphosphate interferes with subsequent *de novo* nucleotide production. Gemcitabine triphosphate inhibits DNA synthesis by competing with the physiologic substrate, deoxycytidine triphosphate, for DNA polymerase and incorporation into DNA. The reduction in intracellular concentrations of deoxycytidine triphosphate induced by gemcitabine diphosphate actually enhances the incorporation of gemcitabine triphosphate into DNA, a mechanism referred to as "self-potentiation." Following incorporation of gemcitabine triphosphate into the DNA chain, a single additional nucleotide, a normal base pair, is added and DNA synthesis is terminated, resulting in apoptosis (programmed cell death). DNA polymerase ε is unable to recognize the abnormal (gemcitabine) nucleotide and repair the DNA strand as a result of masking by the terminal normal base pair nucleotide (masked chain termination). This inability to recognize and excise the abnormal nucleotide results in a prolonged intracellular half-life of gemcitabine compared with other nucleoside analogs such as cytarabine and is thought to contribute to gemcitabine's expanded spectrum of antineoplastic activity relative to such agents. In CEM T lymphoblastoid cells, gemcitabine induces internucleosomal DNA fragmentation, which is characteristic of programmed cell death.

Following infusion of a single 1-g/m^2 dose over 30 minutes, gemcitabine is excreted principally in urine as unchanged drug (less than 10%) and as the inactive metabolite, 2′-deoxy-2′,2′-difluorouridine (dFdU). The inactive metabolite, dFdU, does not appear to accumulate with weekly dosing; however, it is excreted by the kidneys and may accumulate in patients with decreased renal function. The inactive metabolite also is found in plasma. The active metabolite, deoxydifluorocytidine-5′-triphosphate (dFdCTP, gemcitabine triphosphate), can be extracted from peripheral blood mononuclear cells. Volume of distribution and half-life of gemcitabine increase with longer infusion times. The half-life of gemcitabine ranges from 42–94 minutes and 4.1–10.6 hours following short and long infusions, respectively, depending on the patient's age and gender. Clearance is reduced and half-life increased in women and geriatric patients. Following a short (less than 70 minutes) infusion, the half-life of gemcitabine is approximately 42, 48, 61, and 79 minutes for men 29, 45, 65, and 79 years of age, respectively, and 49, 57, 73, and 94 minutes for women 29, 45, 65, and 79 years of age, respectively. The terminal phase half-life for the active metabolite, gemcitabine triphosphate, in mononuclear cells ranges from 1.7–19.4 hours.

For further information on the handling of antineoplastic agents, see the ASHP Guidelines on Handling Hazardous Drugs at http://www.ahfsdruginformation.com.

Advice to Patients

Risk of myelosuppression.

Importance of women informing clinicians if they are or plan to become pregnant or plan to breast-feed; necessity for clinicians to advise women to avoid pregnancy

Importance of informing clinicians of existing or contemplated concomitant therapy, including prescription and OTC drugs, as well as any concomitant illnesses.

Importance of informing patients of other important precautionary information. (See Cautions.)

Overview® (see Users Guide). For additional information on this drug until a more detailed monograph is developed and published, the manufacturer's labeling should be consulted. It is *essential* that the manufacturer's labeling be consulted for more detailed information on usual cautions, precautions, contraindications, potential drug interactions, laboratory test interferences, and acute toxicity.

Preparations

Excipients in commercially available drug preparations may have clinically important effects in some individuals; consult specific product labeling for details.

Gemcitabine Hydrochloride

Parenteral

For injection, for IV infusion	200 mg (of gemcitabine)	**Gemzar®**, Lilly
	1 g (of gemcitabine)	**Gemzar®**, Lilly

†Use is not currently included in the labeling approved by the US Food and Drug Administration

Gemtuzumab Ozogamicin GO

■ Gemtuzumab ozogamicin, a CD33-directed antibody-drug conjugate consisting of a recombinant humanized immunoglobulin G_4 (IgG_4) kappa monoclonal antibody (gemtuzumab) covalently linked to a cytotoxic calicheamicin derivative (*N*-acetyl-γ-calicheamicin), is an antineoplastic agent.

Uses

■ **Acute Myeloid Leukemia** Gemtuzumab ozogamicin is used as monotherapy or in combination with daunorubicin and cytarabine for the treatment of newly diagnosed CD33-positive acute myeloid leukemia (AML); the drug also is used as a single agent for the treatment of relapsed or refractory AML. Gemtuzumab ozogamicin has been designated an orphan drug by FDA for use in the treatment of AML.

Gemtuzumab ozogamicin was initially approved in May 2000 under the principles and procedures of the accelerated review policy of FDA for the treatment of CD33-positive AML in first relapse in patients 60 years of age or older who were not considered candidates for other cytotoxic chemotherapy; however, the manufacturer voluntarily withdrew the drug from the US market in October 2010 after a required postapproval study (Southwest Oncology Group [SWOG] S0106) failed to confirm clinical benefit and found that the drug was associated with an increased risk of fatal adverse events when used in combination with standard induction therapy. Subsequent review of exposure-response analyses suggested that use of lower or fractionated doses of gemtuzumab ozogamicin may reduce the drug's toxicity (e.g., hepatic veno-occlusive disease) without compromising efficacy (see Description), and following review of several clinical trials (ALFA-0701, AML-19, MyloFrance-1) that used lower dosages of gemtuzumab ozogamicin, FDA allowed the drug to be reintroduced in the US market.

Newly Diagnosed Acute Myeloid Leukemia **Combination Therapy.** Gemtuzumab ozogamicin is used in combination with daunorubicin and cytarabine for induction and consolidation therapy for newly diagnosed CD33-positive de novo AML. In adults with newly diagnosed CD33-positive de novo AML, the addition of gemtuzumab ozogamicin to standard induction and consolidation therapy with daunorubicin and cytarabine substantially prolonged event-free survival; however, subgroup analysis suggested an apparent lack of clinical benefit in patients with unfavorable cytogenetics. (See Decreased Efficacy in Patients with Unfavorable Cytogenetics under Warnings/Precautions: Other Warnings and Precautions, in Cautions.)

Efficacy of gemtuzumab ozogamicin in combination with daunorubicin and cytarabine for newly diagnosed CD33-positive AML is based principally on the results of an open-label, randomized phase 3 trial (ALFA-0701). In this trial, 271 patients 50–70 years of age with previously untreated de novo AML were randomized in a 1:1 ratio to receive therapy with gemtuzumab ozogamicin in combination with daunorubicin and cytarabine or standard therapy with daunorubicin and cytarabine alone. Patients in the standard therapy group received induction therapy with daunorubicin 60 mg/m^2 by IV infusion on days 1–3 and cytarabine 200 mg/m^2 by continuous IV infusion on days 1–7. Patients in the gemtuzumab ozogamicin group received the same dosages of daunorubicin and cytarabine in addition to gemtuzumab ozogamicin 3 mg/m^2 (up to a maximum of 4.5 mg) by IV infusion on days 1, 4, and 7. If complete remission (CR) was not achieved following the first induction cycle, a second induction cycle consisting of *only* daunorubicin and cytarabine was administered. If CR was achieved, consolidation therapy according to original treatment assignment was administered for 2 cycles. Consolidation therapy in the standard therapy group consisted of daunorubicin 60 mg/m² by IV infusion on day 1 and cytarabine 1 g/m² by IV infusion every 12 hours on days 1–4 of each consolidation cycle, with an additional dose of daunorubicin 60 mg/m² administered on day 2 of the second consolidation cycle. For consolidation therapy in the gemtuzumab ozogamicin group, the same dosages of daunorubicin and cytarabine as in the standard therapy group were administered with the addition of gemtuzumab ozogamicin 3 mg/m² (up to a maximum of 4.5 mg) on day 1 of each consolidation cycle. Allogeneic stem cell transplantation was permitted in patients who achieved CR; however, an interval of at least 2 months was recommended between the last dose of gemtuzumab ozogamicin and transplantation.

The primary measure of efficacy was event-free survival (defined as time to occurrence of any of the following events: failure to achieve CR or CR with incomplete platelet recovery [CRp] following induction therapy, relapse, or death from any cause). CR was defined as the presence of less than 5% blasts in bone marrow, absence of circulating blasts, full recovery of peripheral blood cell counts (platelet count exceeding 100,000/mm³, absolute neutrophil count [ANC] exceeding 1000/mm³, and hemoglobin concentration exceeding 9 g/dL) and transfusion independence. CRp was defined as the presence of less than 5% blasts in bone marrow, absence of circulating blasts, and incomplete recovery of platelet counts to greater than 100,000/mm³. Event dates for patients who failed to achieve protocol-specified CR or CRp were assigned as the date of bone marrow assessment following the last induction cycle.

The median age of patients in the ALFA-0701 study was 62 years, and 88% of the patients had an Eastern Cooperative Oncology Group (ECOG) performance status of 0–1. Baseline patient characteristics were generally balanced between the treatment groups; however, a larger proportion of gemtuzumab ozogamicin-treated patients were male compared with those receiving standard therapy (55 versus 44%). Overall, 59, 65, and 70% of patients had documented favorable/intermediate-risk cytogenetics and 33, 27, and 21% had poor/adverse-risk cytogenetics according to the National Comprehensive Cancer Network (NCCN), European LeukemiaNet (ELN), and cytogenetic risk classifications, respectively. Among patients with evaluable data on CD33 expression, 14% had low expression (defined as expression on less than 30% of blasts) and none had no expression of CD33 as detected by flow cytometry.

At the time of analysis, patients receiving gemtuzumab ozogamicin in combination with daunorubicin and cytarabine had a longer median event-free survival compared with those receiving standard therapy (17.3 versus 9.5 months; hazard ratio: 0.56). Because CR is the preferred end point in studies with patients with newly diagnosed AML, and CR and CRp are not considered to be equivalent measures of cytotoxic activity, an exploratory analysis limiting the definition of induction response to only CR and using the date of randomization as the event date was conducted by the FDA. In this exploratory analysis, median event-free survival also was prolonged in gemtuzumab ozogamicin-treated patients compared with standard therapy recipients (13.6 versus 8.8 months; hazard ratio: 0.68). Overall survival was not substantially different between the treatment groups. Results of a subgroup analysis based on relevant patient and disease characteristics suggested that the effect of gemtuzumab ozogamicin combined with daunorubicin and cytarabine on event-free survival and overall survival were consistent across most subgroups with the exception of patients with unfavorable cytogenetics, who did not appear to derive a benefit from the addition of gemtuzumab ozogamicin to standard therapy (hazard ratio: 1.11 for event-free survival and 1.55 for overall survival). (See Decreased Efficacy in Patients with Unfavorable Cytogenetics under Warnings/Precautions: Other Warnings and Precautions, in Cautions.)

Monotherapy. Gemtuzumab ozogamicin is used as a single agent for induction and continuation therapy for newly diagnosed CD33-positive AML. In adults with newly diagnosed CD33-positive AML, single-agent gemtuzumab ozogamicin therapy substantially prolonged overall survival compared with best supportive care.

Efficacy of gemtuzumab ozogamicin as single-agent therapy for newly diagnosed CD33-positive AML is based principally on the results of an open-label, randomized phase 3 study (AML-19) in adults with previously untreated AML (de novo or secondary to myelodysplasia). Patients were enrolled in this study if they were older than 75 years of age; however, patients 61–75 years of age who were unwilling to receive standard chemotherapy or had a World Health Organization (WHO) performance status of greater than 2 also were eligible for inclusion. A total of 237 adults were randomized (stratified by age, CD33 expression, baseline leukocyte count, WHO performance status, and treatment center) in a 1:1 ratio to receive gemtuzumab ozogamicin plus best supportive care or best supportive care alone. Patients in the gemtuzumab ozogamicin group received a single course of induction therapy with gemtuzumab ozogamicin 6 mg/m² by IV infusion on day 1 followed by 3 mg/m² by IV infusion on day 8. If patients were considered to be deriving clinical benefit (i.e., stable disease or better response) and were not experiencing substantial toxicity, gemtuzumab ozogamicin therapy was continued at a dosage of 2 mg/m² on day 1 of each 4-week cycle for up to 8 cycles until disease progression, relapse, or substantial toxicity occurred. The primary measure of efficacy was overall survival. The median age of patients in the study was 77 years (range: 62–88 years of age), and 65% of patients had a WHO performance status of 0 or 1. Baseline patient characteristics were generally balanced between the treatment groups; however, a larger proportion of gemtuzumab ozogamicin-treated patients were female (52 versus 39%) or had favorable/intermediate risk cytogenetics (50 versus 38%) compared with those receiving best supportive care. Among patients with evaluable data on CD33 expression, 10% had CD33 expression on less than 20% of blasts as detected by flow cytometry.

At the time of analysis, median overall survival was prolonged in gemtuzumab ozogamicin-treated patients compared with those who received best supportive care (4.9 versus 3.6 months; hazard ratio: 0.69). Results of a subgroup analysis based on relevant patient and disease characteristics suggested that the effect of gemtuzumab ozogamicin on overall survival was consistent across most subgroups; however, survival benefit for the drug versus best supportive care was not apparent in men (hazard ratio: 0.9) and those with CD33 expression on less than 20% of blasts (hazard ratio: 1.52).

Relapsed or Refractory Acute Myeloid Leukemia Gemtuzumab ozogamicin is used as a single agent for the treatment of relapsed or refractory CD33-positive AML in adults and pediatric patients 2 years of age or older. Use of gemtuzumab ozogamicin for this indication is based on CR rate and duration of response.

Efficacy of gemtuzumab ozogamicin as single-agent therapy for relapsed or refractory CD33-positive AML is based principally on the results of an open-label, noncomparative phase 2 trial (MyloFrance-1). In this trial, 57 patients with CD33-positive AML in first relapse received a single course of gemtuzumab ozogamicin 3 mg/m² by IV infusion on days 1, 4, and 7 followed by consolidation therapy with cytarabine (3 g/m² for patients younger than 55 years of age *or* 1 g/m² for patients 55 years of age or older and/or those with creatinine clearance less than 50 mL/minute) by IV infusion every 12 hours for 3 days. Hematopoietic stem cell transplantation (HSCT) was permitted following therapy with gemtuzumab ozogamicin; however, an interval of at least 90 days was recommended between gemtuzumab ozogamicin therapy and transplantation. The primary measures of efficacy were CR and duration of response. The median age of patients was 64 years (range: 22–80 years of age); 78% had intermediate-risk cytogenetics and 22% had poor-risk cytogenetics. The median duration of first remission following prior therapy was 10 months. This study excluded patients with therapy-related AML and those who had previously undergone autologous or allogeneic stem cell transplantation.

At the time of analysis, CR following a single course of gemtuzumab ozogamicin was achieved in 26% of the patients. Median relapse-free survival (defined as initial documentation of CR to date of relapse or death) was 11.6 months.

Dosage and Administration

■ General To minimize the risk of infusion-related reactions, a premedication regimen consisting of acetaminophen, an antihistamine (e.g., diphenhydramine), and a corticosteroid should be administered prior to administration of gemtuzumab ozogamicin. (See Infusion-related Effects under Warnings: Other Warnings and Precautions, in Cautions.) In *adults*, premedication with acetaminophen 650 mg and diphenhydramine hydrochloride 50 mg is recommended 1 hour prior to each gemtuzumab ozogamicin infusion, followed by methylprednisolone 1 mg/kg (or equivalent) within 30 minutes prior to infusion. In *pediatric patients*, premedication with acetaminophen 15 mg/kg (up to a maximum dose of 650 mg), diphenhydramine hydrochloride 1 mg/kg (up to a maximum dose of 50 mg), and methylprednisolone 1 mg/kg (or equivalent) is recommended 1 hour prior to each gemtuzumab ozogamicin infusion; additional doses of acetaminophen and diphenhydramine hydrochloride may be repeated at 4-hour intervals. If manifestations of an infusion-related reaction (e.g., pyrexia, chills, hypotension, dyspnea) occur during or within 4 hours of the infusion, methylprednisolone 1 mg/kg (or equivalent) may be administered.

Cytoreduction is recommended prior to administration of gemtuzumab ozogamicin in patients with hyperleukocytosis (leukocyte counts of 30,000/mm³ or greater).

Appropriate measures must be taken to prevent tumor lysis syndrome.

■ Reconstitution and Administration The usual precautions for handling and preparing solutions of cytotoxic drugs should be observed with gemtuzumab ozogamicin.

Gemtuzumab ozogamicin is administered by IV infusion over 2 hours using a 0.2-μm polyethersulfone inline filter. Prior to administration, commercially available gemtuzumab ozogamicin powder for injection must be reconstituted and diluted using proper aseptic technique.

Unopened vials of gemtuzumab ozogamicin powder for injection should be stored at 2–8°C until use; vials should not be frozen. The drug should be protected from light during storage and administration. During the infusion, only the infusion container (bag or syringe) must be protected from light.

Prior to reconstitution, gemtuzumab ozogamicin powder for injection should be brought to room temperature (approximately 5 minutes). The powder is reconstituted by adding 5 mL of sterile water for injection to a vial labeled as containing 4.5 mg of the drug to provide a solution containing 1 mg/mL. The vial should be gently swirled (not shaken) until the powder is dissolved, and the resulting solution should be inspected visually for particulate matter and discoloration. The reconstituted solution may contain small white to off-white, opaque to translucent, and amorphous to fiber-like particulates. If the reconstituted gemtuzumab ozogamicin solution is not diluted immediately, the solution may be stored under refrigeration at 2–8°C for up to 1 hour and should be protected from light; the solution should *not* be frozen.

To prepare the final diluted solution for infusion, the appropriate volume of reconstituted drug should be withdrawn and diluted with 0.9% sodium chloride injection to a final concentration of 0.075–0.234 mg/mL. The final diluted solution should be prepared in a syringe or IV bag depending on the dose. For doses of 3.9 mg or greater, the infusion solution may be prepared in either a syringe or infusion bag; for doses less than 3.9 mg, the infusion solution must be prepared in a syringe to minimize the potential for drug adsorption. The final diluted gemtuzumab ozogamicin solution for infusion should be mixed by gentle inversion and should *not* be shaken.

The manufacturer recommends immediate administration of diluted solutions of the drug. If immediate administration is not possible, the diluted solution may be stored under refrigeration (2–8°C) for up to 12 hours (including 1-hour storage of reconstituted solution in refrigerator, if needed, prior to dilution) and at room temperature for up to 6 hours (including 2-hour infusion time and an additional 1 hour, if needed, to allow refrigerated diluted solution to reach room temperature prior to administration). Diluted solutions of the drug should *not* be frozen and should be protected from light.

Gemtuzumab ozogamicin should *not* be admixed with or infused simultaneously through the same IV line with any other drug. Commercially available gemtuzumab ozogamicin powder for injection contains no preservatives and is intended for single use; any partially used vial should be discarded.

■ **Dosage** ***Acute Myeloid Leukemia*** **Combination Therapy for Newly Diagnosed CD33-positive Acute Myeloid Leukemia.** When used in combination with daunorubicin and cytarabine for induction therapy in patients with newly diagnosed CD33-positive de novo acute myeloid leukemia (AML), the recommended adult dosage of gemtuzumab ozogamicin is 3 mg/m^2 (up to a maximum dose of 4.5 mg) on days 1, 4, and 7. If complete remission is not achieved after the first induction cycle, a second cycle consisting of *only* daunorubicin and cytarabine may be administered.

Induction therapy should be followed by 2 cycles of consolidation therapy. Consolidation therapy should be administered 14 days after complete blood cell (CBC) counts have recovered following the prior cycle. For consolidation therapy, the recommended adult dosage of gemtuzumab ozogamicin is 3 mg/m^2 (up to a maximum dose of 4.5 mg) on day 1 in combination with daunorubicin and cytarabine.

If absolute neutrophil count (ANC) and platelet counts do not recover to greater than 500/mm^3 and greater than 100,000/mm^3, respectively, within 14 days after the planned start date of consolidation therapy, gemtuzumab ozogamicin should be omitted from the consolidation cycles.

Single-agent Therapy for Newly Diagnosed CD33-positive Acute Myeloid Leukemia. For induction therapy as a single agent in patients with newly diagnosed CD33-positive AML, the recommended adult dosage of gemtuzumab ozogamicin is 6 mg/m^2 on day 1 followed by 3 mg/m^2 on day 8 for one cycle. Induction therapy should be followed by up to 8 additional cycles of continuation therapy.

For continuation therapy, the recommended adult dosage of gemtuzumab ozogamicin is 2 mg/m^2 on day 1 of each 4-week cycle.

Single-agent Therapy for Relapsed or Refractory CD33-positive Acute Myeloid Leukemia. Gemtuzumab ozogamicin therapy for relapsed or refractory CD33-positive AML consists of a single course of treatment.

The recommended dosage of gemtuzumab ozogamicin in adults and pediatric patients 2 years of age or older with relapsed or refractory CD33-positive AML is 3 mg/m^2 (up to a maximum dose of 4.5 mg) on days 1, 4, and 7 for one cycle.

Dosage Modification for Toxicity If treatment-related toxicities occur, the manufacturer states that CBCs and blood chemistries should be monitored at least 3 times per week until resolution of the toxicity.

Hematologic Toxicity. If thrombocytopenia or neutropenia occurs in patients receiving gemtuzumab ozogamicin in combination with daunorubicin and cytarabine, discontinuance of gemtuzumab ozogamicin during consolidation therapy may be necessary. (See Combination Therapy for Newly Diagnosed CD33-positive Acute Myeloid Leukemia under Dosage: Acute Myeloid Leukemia, in Dosage and Administration.)

Hepatotoxicity. If serum aminotransferase (ALT and/or AST) elevations exceed 2.5 times the upper limit of normal (ULN) or total bilirubin concentrations exceed 2 times the ULN, therapy with gemtuzumab ozogamicin should be temporarily interrupted until ALT and AST recover to no more than 2.5 times the ULN and total bilirubin concentrations recover to no more than 2 times the ULN. If therapy is withheld for more than 2 days between sequential doses, the scheduled dose should be omitted.

If hepatic veno-occlusive disease occurs, gemtuzumab ozogamicin therapy should be discontinued.

Infusion-related Effects. If infusion-related reactions occur, gemtuzumab ozogamicin infusion should be interrupted and appropriate treatment (acetaminophen, diphenhydramine hydrochloride, and/or methylprednisolone) and supportive care should be provided. (See Dosage and Administration: General.)

Upon resolution of a mild or moderate infusion-related reaction, the infusion may be resumed but consideration should be given to reducing the rate of infusion by at least 50%. If the infusion-related reaction recurs, the infusion should be interrupted again and the same recommendations followed.

If severe or life-threatening infusion-related reactions (i.e., anaphylaxis, severe respiratory symptoms, clinically important hypotension) occur, therapy with gemtuzumab ozogamicin should be permanently discontinued.

Other Nonhematologic Toxicity. If other severe or life-threatening nonhematologic toxicity occurs, therapy with gemtuzumab ozogamicin should be temporarily interrupted until the toxicity has improved to no more than mild in severity. If therapy is withheld for more than 2 days between sequential doses, the scheduled dose should be omitted.

■ **Special Populations** The manufacturer makes no special dosage recommendations for patients with hepatic or renal impairment or for geriatric patients. (See Specific Populations under Cautions: Warnings/Precautions.)

Cautions

■ **Contraindications** Known hypersensitivity to gemtuzumab ozogamicin or any ingredient in the formulation.

■ **Warnings/Precautions** ***Warnings*** **Hepatotoxicity.** Hepatotoxicity, including severe and potentially fatal hepatic veno-occlusive disease (VOD; also known as sinusoidal obstruction syndrome), has been reported in patients receiving gemtuzumab ozogamicin therapy (either as monotherapy or as part of a combination chemotherapy regimen). Patients with underlying hepatic disease, those receiving higher dosages of gemtuzumab ozogamicin, and those receiving the drug before or after hematopoietic stem cell transplantation (HSCT) appear to be at greater risk of VOD. In the ALFA-0701 trial, VOD occurred in 6 of 131 gemtuzumab ozogamicin-treated patients (5%) during or following combination therapy with daunorubicin and cytarabine, or following subsequent HSCT; 3 of these cases were fatal. In this trial, the median time to onset of VOD following combination therapy with gemtuzumab ozogamicin, daunorubicin, and cytarabine was 9 days (range: 2–298 days); 1 patient developed VOD more than 28 days following the last dose of gemtuzumab ozogamicin, while the other 5 patients developed the condition within 28 days of receiving any dose of the drug. Hepatic VOD also was reported in 2 patients who received gemtuzumab ozogamicin for relapsed disease following therapy with daunorubicin and cytarabine during the randomized trial. In the Mylo-France-1 study, VOD was not observed during or following gemtuzumab ozogamicin monotherapy or following subsequent HSCT for relapsed or refractory acute myeloid leukemia (AML). In this study, none of the patients underwent HSCT within 3.5 months of gemtuzumab ozogamicin therapy. In a prospective observational study conducted to assess the safety of gemtuzumab ozogamicin during routine clinical practice, hepatic VOD was reported in 9.1% of the 482 patients who were evaluated.

In clinical trials, the risk of developing hepatic VOD was higher in adults receiving a higher dosage (9 mg/m^2 for 2 doses administered 14 days apart) of gemtuzumab ozogamicin monotherapy (see Description), those with preexisting moderate or severe hepatic impairment, and those receiving gemtuzumab ozogamicin before or after HSCT. The risk of developing VOD was increased by 8.7-fold in patients with preexisting moderate or severe hepatic impairment compared with those without such impairment. In addition, the risk was increased by 2.9-fold in patients who received gemtuzumab ozogamicin prior to HSCT and by 2.6-fold in those who received the drug after HSCT compared with those who received the drug but did not undergo HSCT. Although a relationship between development of hepatic VOD and timing of HSCT prior to or following higher dosages of gemtuzumab ozogamicin monotherapy has not been established, some clinicians recommend that patients wait at least 2–3.5 months after the last dose of gemtuzumab ozogamicin before undergoing HSCT because of evidence suggesting that intervals less than this time period may increase the risk of VOD.

Liver function test abnormalities, including elevations in serum aminotransferase (e.g., ALT and AST) and bilirubin concentrations, also have been reported in patients receiving gemtuzumab ozogamicin either in combination with daunorubicin and cytarabine or as monotherapy.

Patients receiving gemtuzumab ozogamicin should be closely monitored for signs and symptoms of hepatic VOD (e.g., elevated aminotransferase and/or total bilirubin concentrations, hepatomegaly [generally with pain], rapid weight gain, ascites). Liver function tests (i.e., ALT, AST, total bilirubin, alkaline phosphatase) should be assessed prior to each dose of gemtuzumab ozogamicin, and more frequently, as clinically indicated, during the post-HSCT period in patients proceeding to HSCT following therapy with gemtuzumab ozogamicin. If liver function test abnormalities occur, the manufacturer recommends more frequent monitoring of liver function tests and clinical manifestations of hepatotoxicity. Temporary interruption of therapy or drug discontinuance may be required if hepatotoxicity occurs. (See Hepatotoxicity under Dosage: Dosage Modification for Toxicity, in Dosage and Administration.) If hepatic VOD occurs, gemtuzumab ozogamicin therapy should be discontinued and patients should be treated according to standard practices.

Other Warnings and Precautions **Infusion-related Effects.** Life-threatening or fatal infusion-related reactions (e.g., pyrexia, chills, hypotension, tachycardia, hypoxia, respiratory failure) have been reported in patients receiving gemtuzumab ozogamicin therapy, generally during or within 24 hours following the infusion.

Premedication consisting of acetaminophen, an antihistamine (e.g., diphenhydramine), and a corticosteroid should be administered prior to each dose of gemtuzumab ozogamicin. Patients should be monitored during and for at least 1 hour following completion of each infusion. The manufacturer also recommends that vital signs be monitored frequently during infusions of the drug. If manifestations of an infusion-related reaction occur, especially dyspnea, bronchospasm, or hypotension, the gemtuzumab ozogamicin infusion should be immediately interrupted and the patient should be monitored until resolution of the reaction. All patients should receive appropriate treatment and supportive care; in addition, a reduction in infusion rate or permanent discontinuance of therapy may be required depending on the severity of the reaction. If severe or life-threatening infusion-related reactions (i.e., anaphylaxis, severe respiratory symptoms, clinically important hypotension) occur, gemtuzumab ozogamicin therapy should be permanently discontinued. (See Infusion-related Effects under Dosage: Dosage Modification for Toxicity, in Dosage and Administration.)

Hemorrhage. Serious or fatal hemorrhage associated with prolonged thrombocytopenia has been reported in patients receiving gemtuzumab ozogamicin therapy. In the ALFA-0701 trial, hemorrhage was reported in 90% of patients receiving gemtuzumab ozogamicin in combination with daunorubicin and cytarabine, and grade 3 or 4 hemorrhage was reported in 21% of patients. Fatal hemorrhagic events (i.e., cerebral, intracranial, and subdural hematoma) occurred in 3% of patients receiving gemtuzumab ozogamicin in combination with daunorubicin and cytarabine. In the ALFA-0701 trial, the risk of prolonged thrombocytopenia (platelet counts less than 50,000/mm^3 lasting longer than 42 days in the absence of active disease) increased following each treatment phase. Prolonged thrombocytopenia occurred in 19, 24, and 35% of patients following induction therapy, first consolidation cycle, and second consolidation cycle, respectively, with gemtuzumab ozogamicin in combination with daunorubicin and cytarabine compared with 7, 7, and 24%, respectively, of those receiving combination therapy with daunorubicin and cytarabine alone. Hemorrhage occurred at a lower incidence during consolidation therapy (5–6%) compared with induction therapy (18%). In the AML-19 study, hemorrhage was reported in 25% of patients receiving gemtuzumab ozogamicin monotherapy, and grade 3 or greater hemorrhage was reported in 13% of patients. Fatal hemorrhagic events occurred in 1% of patients receiving gemtuzumab monotherapy in this study. In the MyloFrance-1 trial, grade 3 or 4 hemorrhage was reported in 7 or 0%, respectively, of patients receiving gemtuzumab ozogamicin monotherapy.

Complete blood cell (CBC) counts should be assessed prior to each dose of gemtuzumab ozogamicin, and more frequently following treatment until resolution of cytopenias. Patients receiving gemtuzumab ozogamicin should be monitored for manifestations of bleeding during therapy. If hemorrhage or prolonged thrombocytopenia occurs, treatment delay or drug discontinuance may be required and supportive care should be instituted according to standard practice. (See Hematologic Toxicity under Dosage: Dosage Modification for Toxicity, in Dosage and Administration.)

Prolongation of QT Interval. Prolongation of the QT interval has been reported in patients receiving other antibody-drug conjugates containing calicheamicin.

ECG and serum electrolytes should be monitored prior to initiating gemtuzumab ozogamicin therapy and as clinically indicated in patients with a history of or predisposition to QT interval prolongation, including those with electrolyte abnormalities and those receiving concomitant drugs known to prolong the QT interval.

Decreased Efficacy in Patients with Unfavorable Cytogenetics. Results of a subgroup analysis in the ALFA-0701 trial suggested a lack of benefit for gemtuzumab ozogamicin in combination with daunorubicin and cytarabine compared with standard therapy alone in the subgroup of patients with unfavorable cytogenetics (hazard ratio: 1.11).

The manufacturer states that clinicians should consider the potential benefits and risks of continuing gemtuzumab ozogamicin in combination with daunorubicin and cytarabine in patients with newly diagnosed de novo AML following availability of cytogenetic test results. (See Combination Therapy under Acute Myeloid Leukemia: Newly Diagnosed Acute Myeloid Leukemia, in Uses.)

Fetal/Neonatal Morbidity and Mortality. There are no available data regarding the risk of gemtuzumab ozogamicin use in pregnant women; however, based on its mechanism of action and animal findings, the drug may cause fetal harm. Embryofetal toxicity (e.g., decreased fetal growth, embryofetal death) and teratogenicity (e.g., skeletal anomalies) have been demonstrated in rats receiving gemtuzumab ozogamicin at maternally toxic dosages that resulted in exposure levels approximately 0.4 times the human exposure at the maximum recommended dosage.

Pregnancy should be avoided during gemtuzumab ozogamicin therapy. The manufacturer recommends confirmation of pregnancy status prior to initiation of gemtuzumab ozogamicin, and women of childbearing potential should be advised to use effective contraceptive methods during and for at least 6 months after the last dose. In addition, men with female partners of childbearing potential should use effective methods of contraception during and for at least 3 months after the last dose. Patients should be apprised of the potential hazard to the fetus if gemtuzumab ozogamicin is used during pregnancy.

Impairment of Fertility. Results of animal studies suggest that gemtuzumab ozogamicin may impair male and female fertility. In one study, decreased numbers of implantation sites, corpora lutea, and viable embryos were observed in female rats receiving gemtuzumab ozogamicin at exposure levels approximately 0.4 times the human exposure at the maximum recommended dosage for 14 days prior to mating. In a fertility and general toxicology study, degeneration of reproductive tissues and adverse effects on sperm were observed in male animals receiving gemtuzumab ozogamicin at exposure levels approximately 1.2 times the human exposure at the maximum recommended dosage for 28 days followed by mating with untreated females either at the end of the dosing period or 9 weeks after the last dose. Adverse effects on male and female reproductive organs also have been observed in animals receiving other antibody-drug conjugates containing calicheamicin.

Immunogenicity. As with all therapeutic proteins, there is a potential for immunogenicity with gemtuzumab ozogamicin. Clinical trials did not evaluate the immunogenic potential of the drug at recommended dosages.

Specific Populations **Pregnancy.** Gemtuzumab ozogamicin may cause fetal harm if administered to pregnant women based on animal findings. (See Fetal/Neonatal Morbidity and Mortality under Warnings/Precautions: Other Warnings and Precautions, in Cautions.)

Lactation. It is not known whether gemtuzumab ozogamicin is distributed into human milk. Because of the potential for serious adverse reactions to gemtuzumab ozogamicin in nursing infants, women should be advised to discontinue nursing during therapy and for at least 1 month after discontinuance of therapy. The effects of the drug on nursing infants or on milk production are unknown.

Pediatric Use. Safety and efficacy of gemtuzumab ozogamicin alone or in combination with daunorubicin and cytarabine have not been established in pediatric patients with newly diagnosed AML.

Use of gemtuzumab ozogamicin monotherapy in pediatric patients 2 years of age or older with relapsed or refractory AML is supported by a noncomparative study that included 13 patients 2 years to less than 12 years of age and 15 patients 12–18 years of age; only 1 patient was younger than 2 years of age. No overall differences in safety and efficacy were observed by age.

Geriatric Use. In the ALFA-0701 trial evaluating gemtuzumab ozogamicin in combination with daunorubicin and cytarabine for newly diagnosed de novo AML, no overall differences in safety and efficacy were observed between geriatric patients 65 years of age or older and younger adults.

In the AML-19 study evaluating gemtuzumab ozogamicin monotherapy for newly diagnosed AML, all patients were 60 years of age or older and 65% were 75 years of age or older. No overall differences in safety and efficacy were observed by age.

In the MyloFrance-1 trial evaluating gemtuzumab ozogamicin monotherapy for relapsed or refractory AML, no overall differences in safety and efficacy were observed between geriatric patients 65 years of age or older and younger adults; however, pyrexia and infection of severe or greater severity occurred more frequently in geriatric patients compared with younger adults.

Hepatic Impairment. The pharmacokinetics of gemtuzumab ozogamicin do not appear to be substantially altered in patients with mild hepatic impairment. Data are not available in patients with moderate or severe hepatic impairment (total bilirubin concentration exceeding 1.5 times the upper limit of normal [ULN]).

Patients with moderate to severe hepatic impairment may have a higher risk of developing gemtuzumab ozogamicin-induced hepatic veno-occlusive disease. (See Hepatotoxicity under Warnings/Precautions: Warnings, in Cautions.)

Renal Impairment. The pharmacokinetics of gemtuzumab ozogamicin do not appear to be substantially altered in patients with mild or moderate renal impairment (creatinine clearance of 30–89 mL/minute). Data are not available in patients with severe renal impairment (creatinine clearance of 15–29 mL/minute).

■ **Common Adverse Effects** Adverse effects reported in at least 15% of adults receiving gemtuzumab ozogamicin in combination with daunorubicin and cytarabine for newly diagnosed de novo AML in the ALFA-0701 trial include hemorrhage, infection, prolonged thrombocytopenia (platelet counts less than 50,000/mm^3 lasting longer than 42 days in the absence of active disease), anemia, and neutropenia. Grade 3 or greater laboratory abnormalities reported in at least 10% of patients receiving gemtuzumab ozogamicin who had grade 2 or lesser severity of the laboratory abnormality at baseline include hypophosphatemia, hypokalemia, hyponatremia, elevated concentrations of alkaline phosphatase, and elevated concentrations of aminotransferases (ALT, AST).

Adverse effects reported in at least 15% of adults receiving gemtuzumab ozogamicin monotherapy for newly diagnosed AML in the AML-19 study include hepatotoxicity, fatigue, infection, cardiac effects, hemorrhage, febrile neutropenia, and metabolic abnormalities.

Adverse effects reported in at least 15% of patients receiving gemtuzumab ozogamicin monotherapy for relapsed or refractory AML include pyrexia, infection, elevated concentrations of ALT and/or AST, hemorrhage, nausea and vomiting, constipation, mucositis, headache, and rash. Grade 3 adverse effects reported in more than 30% of these patients include sepsis.

Drug Interactions

In vitro, gemtuzumab ozogamicin is unlikely to inhibit cytochrome P-450 (CYP) isoenzymes 1A2, 2A6, 2C8, 2C9, 2C19, 2D6, and 3A4/5 at clinically relevant concentrations. In vitro studies also indicate that the calicheamicin derivative of the antibody-drug conjugate is unlikely to inhibit CYP isoenzymes 1A2, 2B6, 2C8, 2C9, 2C19, 2D6, and 3A4/5 inhibit uridine diphosphate-glucuronosyltransferase (UGT) 1A1, 1A4, 1A6, 1A9, and 2B7, or induce CYP isoenzymes 1A2, 2B6, and 3A4 at clinically relevant concentrations.

The calicheamicin derivative of the antibody-drug conjugate also is unlikely to inhibit P-glycoprotein (P-gp), breast cancer resistance protein (BCRP), organic anion transporter (OAT) 1, OAT3, organic cation transporter (OCT) 2, organic anion transport protein (OATP) 1B1, and OATP1B3.

No formal drug interaction studies have been performed to date with gemtuzumab ozogamicin.

■ **Drugs that Prolong the QT Interval** ECG and electrolyte monitoring is recommended in patients receiving gemtuzumab ozogamicin concomitantly with other drugs known to prolong the QT interval. (See Prolongation of QT Interval under Warnings/Precautions: Other Warnings and Precautions, in Cautions.)

Description

Gemtuzumab ozogamicin, an anti-CD33 antibody-drug conjugate, is an antineoplastic agent. The anti-CD33 antibody, a recombinant humanized IgG_4 kappa immunoglobulin, is covalently linked to the cytotoxic antitumor antibiotic *N*-acetyl-γ-calicheamicin; the cytotoxic moiety is a derivative of calicheamicin, a natural product isolated from the microorganism *Micromonospora echinospora* subsp. *calichensis*. The formulation of gemtuzumab ozogamicin consists of both conjugated and unconjugated antibody; on average, approximately 2–3 moles of the calicheamicin derivative are attached to each mole of antibody. The antibody portion of gemtuzumab ozogamicin binds specifically to antigen CD33, a transmembrane glycoprotein that is expressed on the surface of leukemic blasts in more than 80% of patients with acute myeloid leukemia (AML). Following binding of the antibody portion of gemtuzumab ozogamicin to antigen CD33, the resultant complex is internalized by the myeloid cell. The calicheamicin derivative of the antibody-drug conjugate is released via hydrolytic cleavage of the linker and binds to DNA in the minor groove causing double-strand breaks and subsequent cell cycle arrest and apoptosis.

Maximum delivery of calicheamicin to leukemic blast cells appears to be dependent on saturation of a high percentage of antigen CD33; in a pharmacodynamic analysis, near maximal saturation of antigen CD33 in peripheral blood was observed with gemtuzumab ozogamicin doses as low as 2 mg/m². Although formal pharmacokinetic analyses have not been conducted in patients receiving a gemtuzumab ozogamicin dosage of 3 mg/m² on days 1, 4, and 7 (fractionated regimen), simulations suggest that peak plasma concentrations and systemic exposure of the drug are reduced following the initial dose and full course of a fractionated regimen compared with peak plasma concentrations following dosing with an unfractionated regimen (gemtuzumab ozogamicin 9 mg/m² for 2 doses administered 14 days apart). Because increased peak plasma concentrations following the initial dose of gemtuzumab ozogamicin 9 mg/m² have been correlated with an increased risk of hepatic veno-occlusive disease (VOD), these data suggest that a lower-dose fractionated regimen may reduce the risk of hepatic VOD without compromising efficacy. (See Uses: Acute Myeloid Leukemia.)

In vitro studies indicate that the calicheamicin derivative of the antibody-drug conjugate is extensively metabolized, primarily by nonenzymatic reduction. In vitro, the calicheamicin derivative is approximately 97% bound to plasma proteins. The terminal half-life of unconjugated gemtuzumab is 62 and 90 hours following the first and second doses, respectively, of the antibody-drug conjugate.

Advice to Patients

Risk of hepatotoxicity, including severe, life-threatening, or fatal hepatic veno-occlusive disease (VOD). Importance of informing patients that the risk of developing hepatic VOD may be increased in patients who have previously undergone or plan to undergo hematopoietic stem cell transplantation (HSCT). Importance of regular monitoring for signs and symptoms of hepatotoxicity (e.g., rapid weight gain, right upper-quadrant abdominal pain or tenderness, hepatomegaly, ascites) during therapy.

Risk of thrombocytopenia and hemorrhage. Importance of informing clinicians if signs and symptoms of bleeding occur.

Risk of infusion-related reactions. Importance of reporting signs and symptoms of such reactions, including fever, chills, rash, or breathing difficulty.

Risk of fetal harm. Necessity of advising women of childbearing potential and men who are partners of such women that they should use an effective method of contraception while receiving the drug and for at least 6 and 3 months, respectively, after discontinuance of therapy. Importance of women informing clinicians if they are or plan to become pregnant. If pregnancy occurs, advise pregnant women of potential risk to the fetus.

Importance of advising women to discontinue nursing during therapy and for at least 1 month after discontinuance of the drug.

Importance of informing clinicians of existing or contemplated concomitant therapy, including prescription and OTC drugs and dietary or herbal supplements, as well as any concomitant illnesses.

Importance of informing patients of other important precautionary information. (See Cautions.)

Overview® (see Users Guide). For additional information on this drug until a more detailed monograph is developed and published, the manufacturer's labeling should be consulted. It is *essential* that the manufacturer's labeling be consulted for more detailed information on usual cautions, precautions, contraindications, potential drug interactions, laboratory test interferences, and acute toxicity. For further information on the handling of antineoplastic agents, see the ASHP Guidelines on Handling Hazardous Drugs at http://www.ahfsdruginformation.com.

Preparations

Excipients in commercially available drug preparations may have clinically important effects in some individuals; consult specific product labeling for details.

Gemtuzumab Ozogamicin

Parenteral

For injection, for IV infusion	4.5 mg	**Mylotarg®**, Wyeth

Gilteritinib Fumarate

■ Gilteritinib, an inhibitor of multiple receptor tyrosine kinases including fms-like tyrosine kinase-3 (Flt-3), is an antineoplastic agent.

Uses

■ **Acute Myeloid Leukemia** Gilteritinib fumarate is used for the treatment of relapsed or refractory acute myeloid leukemia (AML) harboring fms-like tyrosine kinase-3 (Flt-3) mutation. Gilteritinib has been designated an orphan drug by FDA for the treatment of this cancer. An FDA-approved companion diagnostic test (e.g., LeukoStrat® CDx Flt-3 mutation assay) is required to confirm the presence of the Flt-3 mutation (peripheral blood or bone marrow) prior to initiation of therapy. The current indication is based on complete remission (CR) or complete remission with partial hematologic recovery (CRh) and improvement of hematologic deficits (determined by rate of conversion from transfusion dependence to transfusion independence).

The current indication for gilteritinib in the treatment of AML is based principally on the results of a planned interim analysis that was conducted in 138 patients randomized to receive gilteritinib in the open-label, controlled phase 3 study (ADMIRAL) in adults with relapsed or refractory AML with an internal tandem duplication (ITD) or a point mutation in the tyrosine kinase domain (TKD) of Flt-3 kinase as detected by the LeukoStrat® CDx Flt-3 mutation assay. The primary measures of efficacy were CR and CRh, duration of response, and loss of transfusion dependence (red blood cells [RBCs] and/or platelets). CR was defined as the presence of less than 5% blasts in bone marrow without evidence of extramedullary disease or myeloid differentiation, full recovery of peripheral blood cell counts (absolute neutrophil count [ANC] of at least 1000/mm³, platelet count of at least 100,000/mm³), and transfusion independence. CRh was defined as the presence of less than 5% blasts in bone marrow without evidence of extramedullary disease and with incomplete recovery of peripheral blood cell counts (ANC of at least 500/mm³, platelet count of at least 50,000/mm³). The median age of patients randomized to receive gilteritinib was 60 years (range: 20–84 years); 56% were Caucasian, 38% were 65 years of age or older, 46% were male, 82% had an Eastern Cooperative Oncology Group (ECOG) performance status of 0 or 1, 59% had previously untreated relapsed AML, 41% had primary refractory AML, 77% were transfusion dependent at baseline, and 20% had previously undergone stem cell transplantation. Flt-3-ITD mutations were present in 88% of patients and Flt-3-TKD (D835 or I836) mutations were present in 9% of patients. In this study, 369 adults were randomized in a 2:1 ratio to receive either gilteritinib (initial dosage of 120 mg once daily; dosage escalations up to 200 mg once daily were permitted) or a preselected salvage chemotherapy regimen (cytarabine 20 mg IV or subcutaneously twice daily for 10 days; azacitidine 75 mg/m² IV or subcutaneously daily for 7 days; mitoxantrone 8 mg/m² IV daily for 5 days in combination with etoposide 100 mg/m² IV daily for 5 days and cytarabine 1g/m² IV daily for 5 days [MEC]; fludarabine phosphate 30 mg/m² IV daily for 5 days, cytarabine 2 g/m² IV daily for 5 days, and idarubicin hydrochloride 10 mg/m² IV daily for 3 days with granulocyte colony-stimulating factor [G-CSF] 300 mcg/m² IV daily for 5 days [FLAG-IDA]). Gilteritinib therapy was continued until disease progression or unacceptable toxicity occurred. Allogeneic stem cell transplantation was permitted in patients who achieved CR.

At a median follow-up of 4.6 months, CR or CRh was achieved in 21% of gilteritinib-treated patients with a median response duration of 4.6 months; 11.6% of patients achieved CR. The median time to initial CR or CRh in gilteritinib-treated patients was 3.6 months. Approximately one-third (31%) of gilteritinib-treated patients who were transfusion dependent at baseline became transfusion independent during any 56-day period during the study. The majority (53%) of gilteritinib-treated patients who were transfusion independent at baseline remained transfusion independent during any 56-day period during the study.

Dosage and Administration

■ **General** Presence of the fms-like tyrosine kinase-3 (Flt-3) mutation (peripheral blood or bone marrow) must be confirmed by an FDA-approved companion diagnostic test prior to initiation of therapy with gilteritinib in patients with acute myeloid leukemia (AML). (See Uses: Acute Myeloid Leukemia.)

Complete blood cell (CBC) counts and blood chemistries, including creatine kinase (CK, creatine phosphokinase, CPK), should be assessed prior to initiation of gilteritinib therapy and monitored at least weekly for the first month of therapy, every other week for the following month of therapy, and then monthly thereafter.

Because prolongation of the QT interval may occur, ECGs should be performed prior to initiation of gilteritinib, on days 8 and 15 of cycle 1, and prior to initiation of cycles 2 and 3. (See Prolongation of QT Interval under Dosage: Dosage Modification for Toxicity, in Dosage and Administration.)

Restricted Distribution Program Gilteritinib fumarate can only be obtained through designated specialty pharmacies and distributors. Clinicians may contact the manufacturer (Astellas) at 844-632-9272 or consult the Xospata® website (https://www.xospata.com) for specific ordering and availability information.

■ **Administration** Gilteritinib fumarate is administered orally once daily without regard to meals. The drug should be taken at approximately the same time each day. The tablets should be swallowed whole with a cup of water; they should *not* be chewed, crushed, or broken.

■ **Dosage** Dosage of gilteritinib fumarate is expressed in terms of gilteritinib.

Acute Myeloid Leukemia For the treatment of relapsed or refractory AML with Flt-3 mutation, the recommended initial adult dosage of gilteritinib is 120 mg once daily on days 1–28 of each 28-day cycle. Therapy should be continued for at least 6 months to allow time for response or until disease progression or unacceptable toxicity occurs.

Dosage Modification for Toxicity **Reversible Posterior Leukoencephalopathy Syndrome.** If reversible posterior leukoencephalopathy syndrome (RPLS) occurs, gilteritinib therapy should be discontinued.

Prolongation of QT Interval. If the corrected QT (QT_c) interval exceeds 500 msec, gilteritinib should be withheld. When the QT_c interval improves to 480 msec or less or no more than 30 msec from baseline, gilteritinib may be resumed at a reduced dosage of 80 mg daily.

If the QT_c interval increases by more than 30 msec from baseline on days 8 *and* 9 of cycle 1, dosage reduction of gilteritinib to 80 mg daily should be considered.

Pancreatitis. If pancreatitis occurs, gilteritinib therapy should be withheld. Upon resolution of pancreatitis, gilteritinib may be resumed at a reduced dosage of 80 mg daily.

Other Toxicity. If other grade 3 or 4 adverse reaction occurs, therapy with gilteritinib should be withheld. When the toxicity improves to grade 1 or less, gilteritinib may be resumed at a reduced dosage of 80 mg daily.

■ **Special Populations** The manufacturer makes no special population dosage recommendations at this time. (See Specific Populations under Cautions: Warnings/Precautions.)

Cautions

■ **Contraindications** Gilteritinib fumarate is contraindicated in patients with hypersensitivity to the drug or any ingredient in the formulation. (See Sensitivity Reactions under Cautions: Warnings/Precautions.)

■ **Warnings/Precautions** ***Sensitivity Reactions*** **Hypersensitivity.** Anaphylactic reactions have been observed in 1% of patients receiving gilteritinib in clinical trials.

Reversible Posterior Leukoencephalopathy Syndrome Reversible posterior leukoencephalopathy syndrome (RPLS) has been reported rarely in patients receiving gilteritinib. In clinical trials, RPLS occurred in 1% of patients receiving gilteritinib. Manifestations of RPLS include seizure and altered mental status, which may resolve upon discontinuance of the drug. Brain imaging, preferably magnetic resonance imaging (MRI), is used to confirm the diagnosis. Gilteritinib therapy should be discontinued in patients who develop RPLS.

Prolongation of QT Interval Prolongation of the corrected QT (QT_c) interval has been observed in patients receiving gilteritinib. In clinical trials, an increase in the QT_c interval exceeding 60 msec from baseline occurred in 7% of gilteritinib-treated patients, and QT_c intervals exceeding 500 msec occurred in 1.4% of gilteritinib-treated patients.

ECGs should be assessed prior to initiation of gilteritinib, on days 8 and 15 of cycle 1, and prior to initiation of cycles 2 and 3. In addition, serum electrolytes (e.g., potassium, magnesium) should be assessed prior to initiation of gilteritinib therapy and monitored at least weekly for the first month of therapy, every other week for the following month of therapy, and then monthly thereafter. Because of the increased risk of QT interval prolongation in patients with hypokalemia and hypomagnesemia, such electrolyte abnormalities should be corrected prior to initiation of and during gilteritinib therapy. Temporary interruption and/or dosage reduction may be necessary in patients who experience prolongation of the QT_c interval during therapy with the drug. (See Prolongation of QT Interval under Dosage: Dosage Modification for Toxicity, in Dosage and Administration.)

Pancreatitis Pancreatitis has been reported rarely in patients receiving gilteritinib in clinical trials. Patients presenting with manifestations of pancreatitis (e.g., severe and persistent abdominal pain, which may be accompanied by nausea or vomiting) should be evaluated. Temporary interruption followed by dosage reduction may be necessary in patients who develop pancreatitis. (See Pancreatitis under Dosage: Dosage Modification for Toxicity, in Dosage and Administration.)

Fetal/Neonatal Morbidity and Mortality Gilteritinib may cause fetal harm in humans based on its mechanism of action and animal findings; the drug has been shown to be embryotoxic, fetotoxic, and teratogenic in animals. There are no available data regarding the risk of gilteritinib use in pregnant women to date to inform a drug-associated risk of adverse developmental outcomes. In animal reproduction studies, embryofetal toxicity (i.e., postimplantation loss, decreases in fetal body and placental weight) and teratogenic effects (i.e., gross external, visceral, and skeletal anomalies) were observed in rats receiving gilteritinib at exposure levels approximately 0.4 times the human exposure at the recommended dosage.

Placental transfer of gilteritinib has been observed in rats. Following administration of a radiolabeled dose of gilteritinib on gestation day 14, radioactivity of the drug in the fetus was similar to radioactivity of the drug observed in maternal plasma.

Pregnancy should be avoided during gilteritinib therapy. The manufacturer recommends confirmation of pregnancy status within 7 days prior to initiation of gilteritinib in women of reproductive potential and states that such women should be advised to use effective contraceptive methods while receiving gilteritinib and for at least 6 months after discontinuance of the drug. In addition, men with such female partners should use effective methods of contraception while receiving gilteritinib and for at least 4 months after discontinuance of the drug. Patients should be apprised of the potential hazard to the fetus if gilteritinib is used during pregnancy.

Impairment of Fertility Based on animal studies, gilteritinib may impair male fertility. The effect of the drug on fertility in humans is not known. In male dogs, gilteritinib was associated with degeneration and necrosis of germ cells, formation of spermatid giant cells, and single cell necrosis of the epididymal duct epithelia of the epididymal head.

Specific Populations **Pregnancy.** Gilteritinib may cause fetal harm if administered to pregnant women based on its mechanism of action and animal findings. (See Fetal/Neonatal Morbidity and Mortality under Cautions: Warnings/Precautions.)

The manufacturer recommends confirmation of pregnancy status in women of reproductive potential prior to initiation of gilteritinib therapy.

Lactation. Gilteritinib and/or its metabolite(s) are distributed into milk in rats. It is not known whether the drug or its metabolites distribute into human milk or if the drug has any effect on milk production or the nursing infant. Low amounts of gilteritinib are expected to distribute into human milk since the drug is highly bound to plasma proteins; however, the drug has a long half-life of 113 hours. Because of the potential for serious adverse reactions to gilteritinib in nursing infants, women should be advised to discontinue nursing during gilteritinib therapy and for at least 2 months after discontinuance of therapy.

Pediatric Use. Safety and efficacy of gilteritinib have not been established in pediatric patients.

Geriatric Use. In clinical trials evaluating gilteritinib in patients with relapsed or refractory acute myeloid leukemia (AML), 41% of patients receiving gilteritinib were 65 years of age or older, while 13% were 75 years of age or older. No overall differences in safety and efficacy were observed between geriatric patients and younger adults.

Hepatic Impairment. In a hepatic impairment study, systemic exposure of unbound gilteritinib in noncancer patients with mild or moderate hepatic impairment (Child-Pugh class A or B) was similar to that in individuals with normal hepatic function. The effects of severe hepatic impairment (Child-Pugh class C) on the pharmacokinetics of gilteritinib have not been established.

Renal Impairment. Formal pharmacokinetic studies of gilteritinib have not been conducted in patients with renal impairment; however, gilteritinib undergoes minimal renal elimination.

In a population pharmacokinetic analysis, serum creatinine concentrations did not have a substantial effect on the systemic exposure of gilteritinib in patients with relapsed or refractory AML; therefore, mild or moderate renal impairment (creatinine clearance of 30–80 mL/minute) is not expected to have clinically important effects on the systemic exposure of gilteritinib. The effects of severe renal impairment (creatinine clearance of 29 mL/minute or less) on the pharmacokinetics of gilteritinib have not been established.

■ **Common Adverse Effects** Adverse effects occurring in 10% or more of patients with relapsed or refractory AML receiving gilteritinib include myalgia/arthralgia, fatigue/malaise, pyrexia, dyspnea, edema, diarrhea without infectious etiology, rash, pneumonia, constipation, nausea, stomatitis, cough, headache, hypotension, dizziness, vomiting, renal impairment, abdominal pain, decreased appetite, sepsis, insomnia, dysgeusia, elevated concentrations of bilirubin, and hypertension. Laboratory abnormalities reported in more than 20% of patients with relapsed or refractory AML receiving gilteritinib include elevated concentrations of serum creatinine, hyperglycemia, hypertriglyceridemia, elevated concentrations of alkaline phosphatase, hypocalcemia, hypoalbuminemia, elevated concentrations of creatine kinase (CK, creatine phosphokinase, CPK), hypophosphatemia, elevated concentrations of aminotransferase (ALT or AST), hypokalemia, and hyponatremia.

Drug Interactions

Gilteritinib is metabolized principally by cytochrome P-450 (CYP) isoenzyme 3A4. In vitro studies indicate that gilteritinib is a weak inhibitor of CYP3A4.

In vitro, gilteritinib is a substrate of P-glycoprotein (P-gp). In vitro studies indicate that gilteritinib is a potent inhibitor of multidrug and toxin extrusion (MATE) transporter 1 and organic cation transporter (OCT) 2 and has the potential to inhibit breast cancer resistance protein (BCRP) and organic cation transporter (OCT) 1.

■ Drugs Affecting Hepatic Microsomal Enzymes and/or Efflux Transport Systems ***Inhibitors of CYP3A*** Concomitant use of gilteritinib with potent inhibitors of CYP3A may result in increased systemic exposure to gilteritinib. When the potent CYP3A4 and P-gp inhibitor itraconazole (200 mg twice daily on day 1 followed by 200 mg once daily on days 2–28) was administered concomitantly with gilteritinib (single 10-mg dose on day 6) in healthy individuals, peak plasma concentrations and area under the serum concentration-time curve (AUC) of gilteritinib were increased by approximately 20 and 120%, respectively. When the moderate CYP3A4 inhibitor fluconazole (400 mg on day 1 followed by 200 mg once daily on days 2–28) was administered concomitantly with gilteritinib (single 10-mg dose on day 6) in healthy individuals, peak plasma concentrations and AUC of gilteritinib were increased by approximately 16 and 40%, respectively.

Concomitant use of gilteritinib with potent inhibitors of CYP3A (e.g., itraconazole) should be avoided, and selection of an alternative drug with less CYP3A inhibition potential should be considered. If concomitant use of a potent CYP3A inhibitor cannot be avoided, patients should be monitored more frequently for signs of gilteritinib toxicity. If serious or life-threatening toxicity occurs, temporary interruption of gilteritinib therapy followed by dosage reduction may be necessary. (See Dosage Modification for Toxicity under Dosage and Administration: Dosage.)

Inducers of CYP3A and Efflux Transport Systems Concomitant use of gilteritinib with drugs that are combined P-gp and potent CYP3A inducers may result in decreased systemic exposure to gilteritinib and reduced gilteritinib efficacy. When the P-gp and potent CYP3A4 inducer rifampin (600 mg once daily for 21 days) was administered concomitantly with gilteritinib (single 20-mg dose on day 8) in healthy individuals, peak plasma concentrations and AUC of gilteritinib were decreased by approximately 30 and 70%, respectively.

Concomitant use of gilteritinib with drugs that are combined P-gp and potent CYP3A inducers (e.g., rifampin) should be avoided.

■ Drugs Metabolized by Hepatic Microsomal Enzymes When gilteritinib was administered concomitantly with the CYP3A substrate midazolam (single 2-mg dose on day 15) in patients with relapsed or refractory acute myeloid leukemia (AML), peak plasma concentrations and AUC of midazolam were increased by approximately 10%.

■ Drugs Affected by Multidrug and Toxin Extrusion Transporter When gilteritinib (200 mg once daily) was administered concomitantly with the MATE1 substrate cephalexin (single 500-mg dose on day 15) in patients with relapsed or refractory AML, peak plasma concentrations and AUC of cephalexin were decreased by less than 10%.

■ Drugs that Interact with Serotonin Type 2B Receptor or Nonspecific σ-receptors In vitro, gilteritinib is an inhibitor of type 2B serotonergic receptors (5-HT$_{2B}$) and nonspecific σ-receptors. Concomitant use of gilteritinib with drugs that bind to 5-HT$_{2B}$ or nonspecific σ-receptors (e.g., escitalopram, fluoxetine, sertraline) may result in reduced efficacy of such drugs. Concomitant use of gilteritinib with drugs that bind to 5-HT$_{2B}$ or nonspecific σ-receptors should be avoided unless use of the drugs that interact with 5-HT$_{2B}$ or nonspecific σ-receptors is considered necessary.

Description

Gilteritinib, an inhibitor of multiple receptor tyrosine kinases including fms-like tyrosine kinase-3 (Flt-3), is an antineoplastic agent. Receptor tyrosine kinases are involved in the initiation of various cascades of intracellular signaling events that lead to cell proliferation and/or influence processes critical to cell survival and tumor progression (e.g., angiogenesis, metastasis, inhibition of apoptosis), based on the respective kinase. Gilteritinib has been shown to inhibit Flt-3 signaling resulting in inhibition of cell proliferation induced by Flt-3 mutations (i.e., internal tandem duplications [ITD] and/or tyrosine kinase domain [TKD] point mutations in codon D835Y). The drug also has demonstrated apoptosis in leukemic cells harboring Flt-3-ITD mutations in the presence or absence of Flt-3-TKD point mutations. In vitro, gilteritinib has demonstrated potent inhibitory activity against AXL, an oncogenic tyrosine kinase commonly overexpressed in patients with acute myeloid leukemia (AML). AXL promotes Flt-3 signaling and may contribute to the development of resistance to receptor tyrosine kinase inhibitors; therefore, inhibitory activity against AXL may counteract a mechanism of resistance to the drug. The drug also has demonstrated inhibition of wild-type Flt-3, anaplastic lymphoma kinase (ALK), leukocyte receptor tyrosine kinase (LTK), and stem cell factor receptor (c-Kit). In patients with relapsed or refractory AML receiving gilteritinib 120 mg daily, greater than 90% inhibition of Flt-3 phosphorylation occurred within 24 hours of the initial dose. Inhibition above 90% also has been demonstrated on day 8 of cycle 1 in patients with relapsed or refractory AML receiving a gilteritinib dosage of at least 80 mg daily.

Peak plasma concentrations and area under the serum concentration-time curve (AUC) of gilteritinib are dose proportional over the gilteritinib dosage range of 20–450 mg daily in patients with relapsed or refractory AML. Following oral administration in a fasted state, the median time to peak plasma concentrations of gilteritinib is 4–6 hours. Steady-state concentrations of gilteritinib are reached within 15 days of once-daily dosing and the accumulation ratio is approximately tenfold. Administration of a single 40-mg dose of gilteritinib with a high-fat, high-calorie meal (800–1000 calories with 500–600 calories from fat) decreased peak plasma concentrations and AUC of gilteritinib by 26 and less than 10%, respectively, compared with administration in the fasted state. Following oral administration with a high-fat meal, the median time to peak plasma concentrations of gilteritinib was delayed by 2 hours.

Gilteritinib is metabolized principally by cytochrome P-450 (CYP) isoenzyme 3A4, via *N*-dealkylation and oxidation to the metabolites M17, M16, and M10; however, pharmacologic activity of these metabolites has not been established. The metabolites M17, M16, and M10 account for 10% or less of the total drug exposure. Gilteritinib is extensively distributed to tissues. Gilteritinib is highly bound (approximately 94%) to plasma proteins in vivo. In vitro, the drug is primarily bound to albumin. The estimated half-life of gilteritinib is 113 hours. Following administration of a radiolabeled dose of gilteritinib, 64.5% of the recovered dose is excreted in feces and 16.4% is eliminated in urine (10% or less as unchanged drug).

The pharmacokinetics of gilteritinib do not appear to be affected by age (20–87 years), gender, or ethnicity (Japanese versus non-Japanese).

Advice to Patients

Importance of instructing patients to read the manufacturer's patient information.

Importance of advising patients to swallow gilteritinib tablets whole with a cup of water and *not* to break, crush, or chew the tablets.

If a dose of gilteritinib is missed by 12 hours or less, importance of administering the missed dose on the same day as soon as it is remembered and taking the next dose at the regularly scheduled time on the following day. If a dose of gilteritinib is missed by more than 12 hours, importance of administering the next dose at the regularly scheduled time; an additional dose should not be administered to replace the missed dose. Patients should be advised not to take 2 doses within a 12-hour period.

Risk of reversible posterior leukoencephalopathy syndrome (RPLS). Importance of informing clinician immediately if manifestations of RPLS (e.g., seizure; altered mental status; rapidly worsening headache, decreased alertness, confusion, or visual disturbances) occur.

Risk of QT interval prolongation. Importance of informing clinician immediately if an abnormal heartbeat, loss of consciousness, or feelings of dizziness, lightheadedness, or faintness occur. Importance of monitoring electrolytes in patients with a history of electrolyte abnormalities (i.e., hypokalemia, hypomagnesemia).

Risk of pancreatitis. Importance of informing clinician immediately if manifestations of pancreatitis (e.g., severe and persistent abdominal pain, with or without nausea and vomiting) occur.

Risk of fetal harm. Necessity of advising women of reproductive potential that they should use effective methods of contraception while receiving the drug and for at least 6 months after discontinuance of therapy; necessity of advising men who are partners of such women that they should use effective methods of contraception while receiving the drug and for at least 4 months after discontinuance of therapy. Importance of women informing clinicians if they are or plan to become pregnant. If pregnancy occurs, advise pregnant women of potential risk to the fetus.

Importance of advising women to avoid breast-feeding while receiving the drug and for at least 2 months after discontinuance of therapy.

Importance of informing clinicians of existing or contemplated concomitant therapy, including prescription and OTC drugs and dietary or herbal supplements, as well as any concomitant illnesses (e.g., hypokalemia, hypomagnesemia).

Importance of informing patients of other important precautionary information. (See Cautions.)

Overview® (see Users Guide). For additional information on this drug until a more detailed monograph is developed and published, the manufacturer's labeling should be consulted. It is *essential* that the manufacturer's labeling be consulted for more detailed information on usual cautions, precautions, contraindications, potential drug interactions, laboratory test interferences, and acute toxicity. For further information on the handling of antineoplastic agents, see the ASHP Guidelines on Handling Hazardous Drugs at http://www.ahfsdruginformation.com.

Preparations

Gilteritinib fumarate can only be obtained through designated specialty pharmacies and distributors. (See Restricted Distribution Program under Dosage and Administration: General.)

Excipients in commercially available drug preparations may have clinically important effects in some individuals; consult specific product labeling for details.

Gilteritinib Fumarate

Oral

Tablets, film-coated	40 mg (of gilteritinib)	**Xospata®**, Astellas

Ibritumomab Tiuxetan

■ Ibritumomab, a murine anti-human antigen CD20 monoclonal antibody conjugated with the chelating agent tiuxetan, readily chelates the radioisotopes indium 111 and yttrium 90 and is used as a radioimmunotherapeutic agent.

Uses

■ **Non-Hodgkin's Lymphoma** ***Relapsed or Refractory Low-grade or Follicular Non-Hodgkin's Lymphoma*** Ibritumomab tiuxetan, as part of a specific therapeutic regimen (ibritumomab tiuxetan therapeutic regimen), is used for the treatment of relapsed or refractory low-grade or follicular B-cell non-Hodgkin's lymphoma (NHL); ibritumomab tiuxetan is designated an orphan drug by the US Food and Drug Administration (FDA) for this use.

Safety and efficacy of the ibritumomab tiuxetan therapeutic regimen in the treatment of relapsed or refractory low-grade or follicular B-cell NHL have been established in 3 studies in 214 patients with relapsed or refractory low-grade or follicular B-cell NHL, including follicular NHL that was refractory to rituximab therapy. Patients in these studies received an ibritumomab tiuxetan therapeutic regimen that consisted of 2 low doses (250 mg/m^2) of rituximab, an imaging dose (5 mCi) of ibritumomab tiuxetan labeled with indium 111 (indium In 111 ibritumomab tiuxetan) coupled with 2 or 3 whole body scans, and a standard (0.4 mCi/kg) or modified therapeutic dose (0.3 mCi/kg) of ibritumomab tiuxetan labeled with yttrium 90 (yttrium Y 90 ibritumomab tiuxetan).

The first study was a single-arm study in 54 patients with relapsed follicular NHL that was refractory to rituximab therapy. Patients had a World Health Organization (WHO) performance status of 0–2, less than 25% involvement of the bone marrow by lymphoma, no prior bone marrow transplantation, and acceptable hematologic, renal, and hepatic function. In this study, patients received the standard ibritumomab tiuxetan regimen and had an overall response rate (primary efficacy end point) of 74% (15% complete responses, 59% partial responses). The median duration of response was 6.4 months (range: 0.5 to longer than 49.9 months), and the median time to disease progression was 6.8 months (range: 1.1 to longer than 50.9 months). Long-term responses (duration of response at least 12 months) were observed in 19% of the patients in this study.

The second study was a randomized, open-label, comparative study in 130 patients with relapsed or refractory low-grade or follicular B-cell NHL. Patients received no prior rituximab therapy and had a WHO performance status of 0–2, less than 25% involvement of the bone marrow by lymphoma, no prior bone marrow transplantation, and acceptable hematologic function. In this study, patients were randomized to receive either the standard ibritumomab tiuxetan therapeutic regimen or IV rituximab (375 mg/m^2 once weekly for 4 weeks). The overall response rate (primary efficacy end point) was higher in patients receiving the ibritumomab tiuxetan therapeutic regimen (83% [38% confirmed complete responses]) than in those receiving rituximab (55% [18% confirmed complete responses]). Similarly, among patients with bulky or chemotherapy-resistant disease, the overall response rate was higher in patients who received the ibritumomab tiuxetan therapeutic regimen (70 or 73%, respectively) than in those who received rituximab (55 or 42%, respectively). However, the median duration of response and time to disease progression were similar between patients receiving the ibritumomab tiuxetan therapeutic regimen (14.3 and 12.1 months, respectively) and those receiving rituximab (11.5 and 10.1 months, respectively). Long-term responses (duration of response at least 12 months) were observed in 42% of the patients in this study.

The third study was a single-arm study in 30 patients with relapsed or refractory low-grade, follicular B-cell NHL who had a platelet count of 100,000–149,000/ mm^3. Patients with 25% or greater involvement of the bone marrow by lymphoma, prior myeloablative therapy with stem cell support, prior external beam radiation to greater than 25% of active marrow, or neutrophil count less than 1,500/mm^3 were excluded from the study. In this study, administration of yttrium Y 90 ibritumomab tiuxetan at a lower dosage (0.3 mCi/kg) resulted in an overall response rate of 89% and a median duration of response of 11.6 months; however, the incidence of adverse hematologic events was higher in this study than in previous studies. (See Hematologic Effects under Warnings/Precautions: Warnings, in Cautions.) Long-term responses (duration of response at least 12 months) were observed in 47% of the patients in this study.

Newly Diagnosed Follicular Non-Hodgkin's Lymphoma The ibritumomab tiuxetan therapeutic regimen is used for consolidation treatment of newly diagnosed follicular NHL in patients who have achieved partial or complete response to first-line induction chemotherapy.

Safety and efficacy of the ibritumomab tiuxetan therapeutic regimen as consolidation therapy for newly diagnosed follicular NHL have been established in a randomized, phase 3, open-label study in 414 patients who achieved partial or complete response to first-line induction chemotherapy. Patients had histologically confirmed grade 1 or 2 follicular NHL, stage III or IV disease, less than 25% involvement of the bone marrow by lymphoma, no prior external beam radiation or myeloablative therapy, and a platelet count of 150,000/ mm^3 or greater. Approximately 9.5% of patients previously received single-agent chlorambucil, 5% received fludarabine or a fludarabine-containing regimen, 71% received cyclophosphamide-containing combination chemotherapy (i.e., CHOP, CHOP-like, CVP/COP), and 14% received rituximab-containing combination chemotherapy as first-line induction therapy. In this study, patients were randomized to receive either the ibritumomab tiuxetan therapeutic regimen (consisting of 2 low doses [250 mg/m^2] of rituximab administered one week apart, with the second dose immediately followed by yttrium Y 90 ibritumomab tiuxetan [0.4 mCi/kg]) or no further therapy; yttrium Y 90 ibritumomab tiuxetan was administered between 6–12 weeks following the last dose of chemotherapy. The primary efficacy end point was prolongation of progression-free survival. After a median observation of 3.5 years, patients receiving the ibritumomab tiuxetan therapeutic regimen had longer median progression-free survival (38 months) compared with those receiving no further treatment (18 months). The number of deaths was too small to permit a reliable comparison of survival between the two treatment groups. Among patients with newly diagnosed follicular NHL who had partial response to first-line induction chemotherapy, complete response was achieved in 77% of patients receiving consolidation therapy, compared with 17.5% of those receiving no further treatment; the final complete response rate was 87.4% following consolidation with the ibritumomab tiuxetan therapeutic regimen compared with 53.3% following no further treatment. Among patients who were *bcl-2* polymerase chain reaction (PCR) positive after first-line induction chemotherapy, conversion to *bcl-2* PCR-negative status was observed in 90% of patients receiving consolidation therapy, compared with 36% of those receiving no further treatment.

Dosage and Administration

■ **General** Yttrium Y 90 ibritumomab tiuxetan is a radiopharmaceutical and should be prepared and used only by qualified clinicians experienced in the safe use and handling of radionuclides.

Because the ibritumomab tiuxetan therapeutic regimen may be associated with severe, potentially fatal infusion-related reactions, premedication with acetaminophen (650 mg orally) and an antihistamine (e.g., diphenhydramine [50 mg orally]) should be administered prior to each infusion of rituximab.

When used as consolidation therapy in patients with newly diagnosed follicular non-Hodgkin's lymphoma (NHL), the ibritumomab tiuxetan therapeutic regimen should be initiated when platelet counts are 150,000/mm^3 or greater, between 6–12 weeks following the last dose of first-line induction chemotherapy.

■ **Reconstitution and Administration** Rituximab is administered by IV infusion. The drug must be diluted prior to IV infusion and should not be mixed or diluted with other drugs. The manufacturer's labeling should be consulted for additional information on the reconstitution and administration of rituximab.

The manufacturer's labeling should be consulted for detailed information on the preparation of yttrium Y 90 ibritumomab tiuxetan.

Yttrium Y 90 ibritumomab tiuxetan is administered by slow IV injection (over 10 minutes). Prior to the injection of yttrium Y 90 ibritumomab tiuxetan, a 0.22-μm low-protein-binding filter should be placed in-line between the syringe and the infusion port. Following injection of the drug, the line should be flushed with at least 10 mL of 0.9% sodium chloride solution. Standard precautions should be taken to avoid extravasation of yttrium Y 90 ibritumomab tiuxetan (e.g., establishing a free-flowing IV line, ensuring adequate blood return upon needle aspiration) prior to administration of the radioimmunotherapeutic agent. The infusion site should be closely monitored for signs of extravasation (e.g., swelling, pain, discomfort); should manifestations of extravasation appear, the infusion should immediately be stopped and restarted in another limb, and a radiation safety officer should be consulted. Specific treatment for yttrium Y 90 ibritumomab tiuxetan-induced extravasation reactions has not been fully determined; however, the manufacturer states that recommendations for treatment of extravasation of vesicant chemotherapeutic agents (e.g., heating affected area to increase blood flow and accelerate drug clearance, moving affected area repeatedly to increase blood flow, using saline to increase volume in which radionucleotide is distributed to reduce absorbed radiation dose, using dimethylsulfoxide [DMSO] or other free-radical scavengers, liposuction, surgical excision and grafting [particularly after evidence of necrosis]) also may apply to radiopharmaceuticals.

Yttrium Y 90 ibritumomab tiuxetan can be routinely administered on an outpatient basis. Because no penetrating γ waves are produced during therapy with yttrium Y 90 ibritumomab tiuxetan, the risk of exposure to radiation is presumed to be low in health-care professionals, family members, and the patient's other close personal contacts. Although standard precautions for reducing the risk of radiation exposure (i.e., minimizing duration of exposure, maximizing distance from original source, using shielding) in such individuals are not necessary, some clinicians recommend that universal precautions for minimizing exposure to blood and other body fluids (e.g., saliva, urine, stool) should be followed.

■ **Dosage** The ibritumomab tiuxetan therapeutic regimen is intended for use as a single course of treatment. The regimen consists of 2 low doses of rituximab (to deplete peripheral B lymphocytes and to improve distribution of ibritumomab tiuxetan) and a therapeutic dose of yttrium Y 90 ibritumomab tiuxetan. Biodistribution evaluation (administration of an imaging dose of indium In 111 ibritumomab tiuxetan followed by 2 or 3 whole body scans) previously was required after the first dose of rituximab; however, such evaluation is no longer required as part of the ibritumomab tiuxetan therapeutic regimen.

For the treatment of relapsed or refractory low-grade or follicular B-cell NHL, or for consolidation treatment of newly diagnosed follicular NHL in patients who have achieved partial or complete response to first-line induction chemotherapy, the ibritumomab tiuxetan therapeutic regimen is administered in 2 steps. Step 1 (administered on day 1) involves IV infusion of rituximab. Step 2 (administered on day 7, 8, or 9) consists of a second IV infusion of rituximab, followed within 4 hours by IV injection of yttrium Y 90 ibritumomab tiuxetan.

Step 1 (administered on day 1) begins with IV infusion of a single dose (250 mg/m^2) of rituximab, infused at an initial rate of 50 mg/hour. If infusion-related events do not occur, the infusion rate may be increased in increments of 50 mg/hour every 30 minutes to a maximum infusion rate of 400 mg/hour. If *severe* infusion-related events develop, rituximab infusion should be immediately stopped and the ibritumomab tiuxetan therapeutic regimen discontinued. If *less severe* infusion-related events develop, rituximab infusion should be temporarily slowed or interrupted; the infusion may be resumed at one-half the previous rate when symptoms improve.

Step 2 (administered on day 7, 8, or 9) begins with a second IV infusion of rituximab (250 mg/m^2), infused at an initial rate of 100 mg/hour; the infusion rate may be increased, as tolerated, in increments of 100 mg/hour every 30 minutes to a maximum infusion rate of 400 mg/hour. If infusion-related events developed during administration of the first dose of rituximab (on day 1), the second dose of rituximab should be infused at an initial rate of 50 mg/hour, and the infusion rate should be increased in increments of 50 mg/hour every 30 minutes to a maximum infusion rate of 400 mg/hour. The second rituximab dose should be followed within 4 hours by slow IV injection (over 10 minutes) of yttrium Y 90 ibritumomab tiuxetan at a therapeutic dose of 0.4 mCi/kg (for patients with relapsed or refractory NHL or newly diagnosed NHL who have platelet counts of 150,000/mm^3 or greater) or 0.3 mCi/kg (for patients with relapsed or refractory NHL who have platelet counts of 100,000–149,000/mm^3). The prescribed, measured, and administered dose of yttrium Y 90 ibritumomab tiuxetan must not exceed the absolute maximum allowable dose of 32 mCi, regardless of the patient's weight.

■ Special Populations The manufacturer recommends that patients with relapsed or refractory NHL who have platelet counts of 100,000–149,000/mm^3 receive a lower therapeutic dose of yttrium Y 90 ibritumomab tiuxetan (0.3 mCi/kg). (See Dosage and Administration: Dosage.)

The manufacturer makes no other special population (e.g., hepatic or renal impairment) dosage recommendations at this time.

Cautions

■ Contraindications The manufacturer states that there are no contraindications to the use of ibritumomab tiuxetan.

■ Warnings/Precautions ***Warnings*** Yttrium Y 90 ibritumomab tiuxetan is a radiopharmaceutical and should be used only by qualified clinicians experienced in the safe use and handling of radionuclides.

Because the ibritumomab tiuxetan therapeutic regimen includes the use of rituximab, the prescribing information for rituximab also should be consulted for detailed information on the usual cautions, precautions, and contraindications of this drug.

Infusion-related Effects. Severe infusion-related effects, sometimes fatal, have been reported in patients receiving rituximab infusion, an essential component of the ibritumomab tiuxetan therapeutic regimen. In some patients, death has occurred within 24 hours of rituximab infusion. These fatal reactions were associated with hypoxia, pulmonary infiltrates, acute respiratory distress syndrome (ARDS), myocardial infarction (MI), ventricular fibrillation, or cardiogenic shock. Approximately 80% of fatal infusion reactions occurred in association with the initial infusion of rituximab, with a usual time of onset of severe reactions between 30–120 minutes after starting the infusion. If *severe* infusion-related effects (e.g., urticaria, hypotension, angioedema, hypoxia, bronchospasm, pulmonary infiltrates, ARDS, MI, ventricular fibrillation, cardiogenic shock) develop, rituximab and yttrium Y 90 ibritumomab tiuxetan should be immediately discontinued. If *less severe* infusion-related events develop, rituximab infusion should be temporarily slowed or interrupted. (See Dosage and Administration: Dosage.)For detailed information on infusion-related effects, including their management, see Cautions: Infusion-related Effects, in Rituximab 10:00.

Hematologic Effects. Cytopenias with delayed onset and prolonged duration, some complicated by hemorrhage and severe infection, are the most common severe adverse effects associated with the ibritumomab tiuxetan therapeutic regimen. When used according to recommended dosages, the incidences of severe thrombocytopenia and neutropenia are higher in patients with mild thrombocytopenia at baseline (platelet counts of 100,000–149,000/mm^3) compared with those with normal baseline platelet counts (150,000/mm^3 or greater). Among patients with relapsed or refractory non-Hodgkin's lymphoma (NHL) receiving yttrium Y 90 ibritumomab tiuxetan, severe neutropenia (absolute neutrophil count [ANC] less than 1000/mm^3) or thrombocytopenia (platelet count less than 50,000/mm^3) occurred in 57 or 61%, respectively, of patients with normal baseline platelet counts compared with 74 or 78%, respectively, of those with mild thrombocytopenia at baseline. Among patients with newly diagnosed NHL who had normal baseline platelet counts, severe neutropenia or thrombocytopenia occurred in 65 or 61% of patients, respectively. Grade 3 or 4 anemia occurred in 17% of patients with relapsed or refractory NHL and in 5% of patients with newly diagnosed NHL receiving the ibritumomab tiuxetan therapeutic regimen. In all patients, the median time to nadir ANC, platelet count, or hemoglobin concentration was 61–62, 49–53, or 68–69 days, respectively, following administration of yttrium Y 90 ibritumomab tiuxetan; severe neutropenia or thrombocytopenia persisted for a median of 22–29 or 24–35 days, respectively, and the median time to ANC or platelet count recovery was 12–15 days, respectively. Neutropenia and thrombocytopenia were more severe and more prolonged in patients who received the ibritumomab tiuxetan therapeutic regimen after first-line therapy with fludarabine or a fludarabine-containing regimen; in these patients, severe neutropenia or thrombocytopenia persisted for a median of 37 or 56 days, respectively, and the median time to ANC or platelet count recovery was 20 or 35 days, respectively. Filgrastim or erythropoietin was administered in 13 or 8%, respectively, of patients with relapsed or refractory NHL; granulocyte colony-stimulating factors or erythropoiesis-stimulating agents were administered in 14 or 5%, respectively, of patients with newly diagnosed NHL. Platelet transfusions were required in approximately 22% of all patients receiving the ibritumomab tiuxetan therapeutic regimen. Red blood cell transfusions were required in 20% of patients with relapsed or refractory NHL and in 2% of patients with newly diagnosed NHL. Severe cytopenias persisting more than 12 weeks following administration of the ibritumomab tiuxetan therapeutic regimen can occur. Severe hematologic effects occur more frequently in patients receiving the ibritumomab tiuxetan therapeutic regimen than in those receiving rituximab.

Patients should be monitored for manifestations of cytopenias and their complications (e.g., febrile neutropenia, hemorrhage) for up to 3 months following completion of the ibritumomab tiuxetan therapeutic regimen. (See Hematologic Monitoring under Warnings/Precautions: Other Warnings and Precautions, in Cautions.)Use of drugs that interfere with platelet function or coagulation following the ibritumomab tiuxetan therapeutic regimen should be avoided. (See Drug Interactions: Anticoagulants and Drugs Affecting Platelet Function.)

The ibritumomab tiuxetan therapeutic regimen should *not* be used in patients with 25% or greater involvement of the bone marrow by lymphoma and/or impaired bone marrow reserve.

Severe Cutaneous and Mucocutaneous Reactions. Severe cutaneous and mucocutaneous reactions, sometimes fatal, have been reported during postmarketing surveillance. These reactions have included erythema multiforme, Stevens-Johnson syndrome, toxic epidermal necrolysis, bullous dermatitis, and exfoliative dermatitis. The time to onset of these reactions was variable, ranging from a few days to 4 months following completion of the ibritumomab tiuxetan therapeutic regimen. The ibritumomab tiuxetan therapeutic regimen should be discontinued in patients experiencing a severe cutaneous or mucocutaneous reaction.

Other Warnings and Precautions **Altered Biodistribution.** In a postmarketing registry designed to collect biodistribution images and other information in reported cases of altered biodistribution, 12 of 953 patients (1.3%) reportedly had altered biodistribution.

Myelodysplastic Syndrome and Secondary Leukemia. Myelodysplastic syndrome (MDS) and/or acute myelogenous leukemia (AML) have been reported in about 19 of 746 (2.6%) patients with relapsed or refractory NHL receiving ibritumomab tiuxetan therapy in clinical studies or in the expanded-access trial; the median time to diagnosis of MDS or AML was 1.9 years following completion of therapy. Among the 211 patients included in clinical studies, MDS/AML was reported in about 5.2% of those receiving ibritumomab tiuxetan after a median follow-up of 6.5 years; the median time to diagnosis of MDS or AML was 2.9 years following ibritumomab tiuxetan therapy. Among the 535 patients included in the expanded-access trial, MDS/AML was reported in about 1.5% of those receiving ibritumomab tiuxetan after a median follow-up of 4.4 years; the median time to diagnosis of MDS or AML was 1.5 years following ibritumomab tiuxetan therapy. The cumulative incidence of MDS/AML among patients receiving ibritumomab tiuxetan has been increasing with longer follow-up; among the 211 patients included in clinical studies, the cumulative estimated incidence of MDS/secondary leukemia was 2.2% at 2 years and 5.9% at 5 years. Multiple cytogenetic abnormalities have been reported, particularly involving chromosome 5 and/or 7. The risk of developing MDS/AML does not appear to be associated with the number of prior treatments (0–1 versus 2–10).

Among 204 patients with newly diagnosed NHL, 1% were diagnosed with AML within 3 years after receiving the ibritumomab tiuxetan therapeutic regimen as consolidation therapy.

Fetal/Neonatal Morbidity and Mortality. Yttrium Y 90 ibritumomab tiuxetan may cause fetal harm when administered to pregnant women. There are no adequate and well-controlled studies to date in humans. Pregnancy should be avoided during therapy and for at least 12 months following completion of therapy. (See Advice to Patients.) If yttrium Y 90 ibritumomab tiuxetan is used during pregnancy or if the patient becomes pregnant while receiving therapy, the patient should be apprised of the potential hazard to the fetus.

Extravasation. Patients should be monitored closely for manifestations of extravasation (e.g., swelling, pain, discomfort) during infusion of yttrium Y 90 ibritumomab tiuxetan. If manifestations of extravasation appear, the infusion should immediately be stopped and restarted in another limb, and a radiation safety officer should be consulted. (See Dosage and Administration: Reconstitution and Administration.)

Hematologic Monitoring. Following the ibritumomab tiuxetan therapeutic regimen, complete blood cell counts (CBCs) and platelet counts should be monitored weekly until levels return to normal or as clinically indicated. Patients should be monitored for manifestations of cytopenias and their complications (e.g., febrile neutropenia, hemorrhage) for up to 3 months following completion of the ibritumomab tiuxetan therapeutic regimen. More frequent laboratory monitoring for thrombocytopenia is recommended in patients receiving anticoagulants or drugs affecting platelet function. (See Drug Interactions: Anticoagulants and Drugs Affecting Platelet Function.)

Radionuclide Precautions. The contents of the ibritumomab tiuxetan kit are not radioactive. However, institutional good radiation safety practices and patient management procedures should be employed during and after radiolabeling of ibritumomab tiuxetan with yttrium 90 to minimize exposure of patients and medical personnel to radiation.

Creutzfeldt-Jakob Disease and Viral Diseases. Because the ibritumomab tiuxetan therapeutic regimen contains albumin human, the preparations carry an extremely remote risk for transmitting viral diseases or Creutzfeldt-Jakob disease. No cases of transmission of viral diseases or Creutzfeldt-Jakob disease have been reported with albumin human. (See Risk of Transmissible Agents in Plasma-derived Preparations: Risk of Creutzfeldt-Jakob Disease under Cautions: Precautions and Contraindications, in Albumin Human 16:00.)

Infectious Complications. Among patients with relapsed or refractory NHL, infection was reported in 29% of patients within the first 3 months following initiation of the ibritumomab tiuxetan therapeutic regimen; severe (e.g., urinary tract infection, febrile neutropenia, sepsis, pneumonia, cellulitis, colitis, diarrhea, osteomyelitis, upper respiratory tract infection) or life-threatening infections (e.g., sepsis, empyema, pneumonia, febrile neutropenia, fever, biliary stent-associated cholangitis) occurred in 3 or 2% of patients, respectively. Infection was reported in 6% of patients during a follow-up period of 3 months to 4 years; severe or life-threatening infections occurred in 2 or 1% of these patients, respectively.

Among patients with newly diagnosed NHL, grade 3–4 infection (e.g., neutropenic sepsis, bronchitis, catheter sepsis, diverticulitis, herpes zoster infection, influenza, lower respiratory tract infection, sinusitis, upper respiratory tract infection) was reported in 8% of those receiving the ibritumomab tiuxetan therapeutic regimen as consolidation therapy.

Immunologic Effects. Transiently positive human antimurine antibody (HAMA) or human antichimeric antibody (HACA) responses were detected in about 1.3% of patients (6/446) receiving the ibritumomab tiuxetan therapeutic regimen in clinical studies. HAMA or HACA concentrations reverted to negative within 2 weeks to 3 months after completion of therapy; no patients had increasing concentrations of HAMA or HACA at the end of the studies.

Specific Populations **Pregnancy.** Category D. (See Users Guide.) (See Fetal/Neonatal Morbidity and Mortality under Warnings/Precautions: Other Warnings and Precautions, in Cautions.)

Lactation. Category D. (See Users Guide.) (See Fetal/Neonatal Morbidity and Mortality under Warnings/Precautions: Other Warnings and Precautions, in Cautions.)

Because human immunoglobulin G (IgG) is distributed into milk, it is expected that ibritumomab tiuxetan would be present in milk. Because of the potential for adverse reactions to yttrium Y 90 ibritumomab tiuxetan in nursing infants, a decision should be made whether to discontinue nursing or not administer the ibritumomab tiuxetan therapeutic regimen, taking into account the importance of the regimen to the woman.

Pediatric Use. Safety and efficacy of the ibritumomab tiuxetan therapeutic regimen have not been established in children younger than 18 years of age.

Geriatric Use. Of the 349 patients with relapsed or refractory NHL receiving the ibritumomab tiuxetan therapeutic regimen in clinical studies, 38% were 65 years of age or older and 12% were 75 years of age or older. Of the 206 patients with newly diagnosed NHL receiving the ibritumomab tiuxetan therapeutic regimen as consolidation therapy in the controlled clinical study, 14% were 65 years of age or older and 2% were 75 years of age or older.

No overall differences were observed between geriatric and younger patients in clinical studies; however, the possibility that some older patients may exhibit increased sensitivity to the ibritumomab tiuxetan therapeutic regimen cannot be ruled out.

■ **Common Adverse Effects** Adverse effects occurring in 10% or more of patients receiving the ibritumomab tiuxetan therapeutic regimen include cytopenias (e.g., thrombocytopenia, neutropenia, anemia), fatigue, nasopharyngitis, nausea, abdominal pain, asthenia, cough, diarrhea, and pyrexia.

Because the ibritumomab tiuxetan therapeutic regimen includes the use of rituximab, the prescribing information for rituximab also should be consulted for detailed information on the safety profile of this drug.

Drug Interactions

No formal drug interaction studies of ibritumomab tiuxetan have been performed.

■ **Hematopoietic Agents** In clinical studies, the use of hematopoietic growth factor was prohibited for the 2 weeks preceding ibritumomab tiuxetan therapy; altered biodistribution of ibritumomab tiuxetan characterized by increased uptake in the bone marrow may occur in patients with increased marrow activity caused by recent administration of hematopoietic growth factors.

■ **Anticoagulants and Drugs Affecting Platelet Function** Potential pharmacologic interaction (increased risk of thrombocytopenia, bleeding, and hemorrhage). Use of anticoagulants or drugs affecting platelet function following administration of the ibritumomab tiuxetan therapeutic regimen should be avoided. If such use cannot be avoided, more frequent laboratory monitoring for thrombocytopenia is recommended.

■ **Vaccines** The safety of immunization with live virus vaccines following the ibritumomab tiuxetan therapeutic regimen has not been studied. Live virus vaccines should not be administered within 12 months after completion of the regimen. The ability of patients to generate an immune response to any vaccine following therapy with the ibritumomab tiuxetan therapeutic regimen also has not been studied.

Description

Ibritumomab, a murine anti-human antigen CD20 monoclonal antibody conjugated with the chelating agent tiuxetan, readily chelates the radioisotopes indium 111 and yttrium 90. Ibritumomab tiuxetan radiolabeled with yttrium 90 (yttrium Y 90 ibritumomab tiuxetan) is used for radioimmunotherapy.

The immunologic component of yttrium Y 90 ibritumomab tiuxetan (ibritumomab) is an IgG_1 kappa immunoglobulin containing murine light- and heavy-chain sequences; ibritumomab is the parent murine monoclonal antibody from which the chimeric human-murine anti-human antigen CD20 monoclonal antibody rituximab was developed. Like rituximab, ibritumomab binds specifically to antigen CD20 (human B-lymphocyte-restricted differentiation antigen, Bp35), a hydrophobic transmembrane protein located on normal pre-B and mature B lymphocytes; antigen CD20 also is expressed on greater than 90% of B-cell non-Hodgkin's lymphomas (NHL) but is not found on hematopoietic stem cells, early pre-B cells, normal plasma cells, or other normal tissues. Results of in vitro studies indicate that, following binding of the Fab domain of ibritumomab to antigen CD20, the Fc domain triggers apoptosis of normal and malignant B cells through complement-dependent cytotoxicity (CDC) and antibody-dependent cell-mediated cytotoxicity (ADCC). The radioactive component of yttrium Y 90 ibritumomab tiuxetan (yttrium 90) induces cellular damage by forming free radicals in the target and neighboring cells and is responsible for the primary cytotoxic effect of the radioimmunotherapeutic agent.

Following IV injection, binding of ibritumomab tiuxetan has been observed on lymphoid cells of the bone marrow, lymph node, thymus, red and white pulp of the spleen, lymphoid follicles of the tonsil, and lymphoid nodules of other organs (e.g., large and small intestines).

In patients receiving the ibritumomab tiuxetan therapeutic regimen, the mean effective half-life of yttrium 90 activity in blood is 30 hours, and the mean area under the fraction of injected activity-time curve in blood is 39 hours. Approximately 7.2% of the injected dose of yttrium Y 90 ibritumomab tiuxetan is excreted in urine within 7 days.

Rapid and sustained depletion of circulating B cells occurs as a result of the cellular damage of B cells induced by the ibritumomab tiuxetan therapeutic regimen. Following completion of therapy, recovery of B cells begins at approximately 3 months, and median levels of B cells return to normal by 9 months. Median serum concentrations of IgG and IgA remain within the normal range throughout the period of B-cell depletion; median serum IgM concentrations decline to below normal values but return to normal by 6 months following treatment.

Advice to Patients

Risk of rituximab-related infusion reactions. Importance of taking premedications as prescribed and informing a clinician if severe infusion reactions occur.

Risk of cytopenias (e.g., thrombocytopenia, neutropenia, anemia). Importance of reporting to a clinician any signs or symptoms of cytopenias (e.g., bleeding, easy bruising, petechiae or purpura, pallor, weakness, fatigue, infection, pyrexia).

Importance of avoiding drugs that interfere with platelet function, unless directed by a clinician.

Risk of severe cutaneous or mucocutaneous reaction. Importance of promptly seeking medical evaluation if diffuse rash, bullae, or desquamation of the skin or oral mucosa develops.

Importance of not receiving live viral vaccines for 12 months after completion of therapy.

Importance of women informing clinicians immediately if they are or plan to become pregnant or plan to breast-feed. Necessity of advising women to use an effective method of contraception while receiving the ibritumomab tiuxetan therapeutic regimen and for at least 12 months following completion of therapy. Necessity of advising pregnant women of risk to the fetus. Importance of discontinuing nursing during and after therapy.

Importance of advising family members and other close contacts to follow standard precautions for minimizing exposure to blood and other body fluids (e.g., saliva, urine, stool).

Importance of informing clinicians of existing or contemplated concomitant therapy, including prescription and OTC drugs (e.g., live viral vaccines, medications that interfere with platelet function or coagulation) and dietary or herbal supplements, as well as any concomitant diseases.

Importance of informing patients of other important precautionary information. (See Cautions.)

Overview® (see Users Guide). For additional information on this drug until a more detailed monograph is developed and published, the manufacturer's labeling should be consulted. It is *essential* that the manufacturer's labeling be consulted for more detailed information on usual cau-

tions, precautions, contraindications, potential drug interactions, laboratory test interferences, and acute toxicity. For further information on the handling of antineoplastic agents, see the ASHP Guidelines on Handling Hazardous Drugs at http://www.ahfsdruginformation.com.

Preparations

Distribution is restricted to qualified and appropriately licensed clinicians and facilities equipped to handle radionuclides (e.g., nuclear pharmacies); the regimen is not available through community pharmacies.

Ibritumomab tiuxetan is commercially available as a kit that contains all of the nonradioactive ingredients necessary to prepare a single dose of yttrium Y 90 ibritumomab tiuxetan. Yttrium 90 chloride sterile solution is shipped directly from the supplier when the yttrium Y 90 ibritumomab tiuxetan (Y-90 Zevalin®) kit is ordered. Rituximab must be ordered separately.

Excipients in commercially available drug preparations may have clinically important effects in some individuals; consult specific product labeling for details.

Ibritumomab Tiuxetan

Parenteral

Kit	1 Vial, 3.2 mg/2 mL, Injection, for preparation of radioactive pharmaceutical, Ibritumomab Tiuxetan (Zevalin®, preservative-free)	**Y-90 Zevalin®** (available with 4 identification labels), Spectrum
	1 Vial, 50 mM/2 mL (Sodium Acetate Injection)	
	1 Vial (Formulation Buffer Injection; with albumin)	
	1 Vial (Reaction Vial, sterile, and empty)	

Ibrutinib

■ Ibrutinib, a selective irreversible inhibitor of Bruton's tyrosine kinase (BTK), is an antineoplastic agent.

Uses

Ibrutinib is used for the treatment of certain B-cell malignancies (mantle cell lymphoma, chronic lymphocytic leukemia [CLL]/small lymphocytic leukemia [SLL] with or without 17p deletion, marginal-zone lymphoma, Waldenstrom macroglobulinemia) and for the treatment of chronic graft-versus-host disease (GVHD).

■ **Mantle Cell Lymphoma** Ibrutinib is used for the treatment of mantle cell lymphoma in patients who have received at least one prior therapy. The current indication is based on overall response rate; clinical benefit (e.g., improvement in disease-related symptoms, increased survival) has not been established. Continued FDA approval for this indication may be contingent on confirmation of clinical benefit in additional trials. Ibrutinib has been designated an orphan drug by FDA for the treatment of this cancer.

The current indication for ibrutinib in the treatment of mantle cell lymphoma is based principally on the favorable response (compared with historical responses) demonstrated in a phase 2, open-label study (Study 1104) in patients who had received at least one prior therapy. The primary end point was overall response rate (complete plus partial responses) based on the International Working Group (IWG) criteria for non-Hodgkin's lymphoma. In this study, the investigator-assessed overall response rate was 65.8%; 17.1% of patients receiving the drug achieved a complete response. At the time of data analysis, responses were ongoing with a median duration of response for all responders of at least 17.5 months. The median age of patients enrolled in the study was 68 (range: 40–84) years; most patients (89%) had a baseline ECOG (Eastern Cooperative Oncology Group) performance status of 0 or 1. Patients in the study had received a median of 3 (range: 1–5) prior therapies for their disease; 11% of patients had undergone a stem-cell transplant. In this study, 111 patients received ibrutinib 560 mg orally once daily until disease progression or unacceptable toxicity occurred.

Effects of ibrutinib on investigator-assessed overall response rate and independent review facility-assessed overall response rate were comparable. The median time to complete or partial response was 1.9 months. A preliminary median progression-free survival of 13.9 months was estimated, but median overall survival was not yet reached. Following initiation of ibrutinib therapy, lymphocytosis (i.e., absolute lymphocyte count exceeding 5000/mm^3 and an increase of at least 50% from baseline) occurred in 33% of patients, generally during the initial few weeks of therapy, with a peak lymphocyte count occurring at a median of 4 weeks; lymphocytosis resolved in a median of 8 weeks. (See Description.)

■ **Chronic Lymphocytic Leukemia/Small Lymphocytic Lymphoma** Ibrutinib is used alone or in combination with bendamustine and rituximab for the treatment of CLL and SLL, including those with CLL/SLL harboring the 17p13.1 deletion (17p deletion) chromosomal abnormality. Ibrutinib has been designated an orphan drug by FDA for the treatment of these conditions.

Evidence of safety and efficacy of ibrutinib in the treatment of CLL and SLL is based principally on favorable results of an uncontrolled, open-label, multicenter study (Study 1102) and 3 randomized, controlled phase 3 studies (RESONATE, RESONATE-2, HELIOS); patients in Study 1102, RESONATE, and HELIOS had received at least one prior therapy for their disease and patients in the RESONATE-2 study were treatment-naive. Following initiation of ibrutinib therapy in these studies, lymphocytosis (i.e., absolute lymphocyte count exceeding 5000/mm^3 and an increase of at least 50% from baseline) occurred in 66% of patients, generally during the initial month of therapy; lymphocytosis resolved in a median of 14 weeks. However, when ibrutinib therapy was administered in combination with bendamustine and rituximab, lymphocytosis occurred in 7% of patients. (See Description.)

In Study 1102, the median age of patients was 67 years; all patients in the study had a baseline ECOG performance status of 0 or 1. Patients enrolled in the study had received a median of 4 prior therapies for their disease. In this study, 48 patients received ibrutinib 420 mg orally once daily until disease progression or unacceptable toxicity occurred. The overall response rate (as assessed by an independent review committee) was 58.3%; none of the patients achieved a complete response. At the time of data analysis, median duration of response had not been reached.

In the RESONATE study, 391 patients with CLL or SLL who were at risk for a poor outcome were treated with ibrutinib or the anti-CD20 antibody ofatumumab. Ibrutinib 420 mg was given orally once daily until disease progression or unacceptable toxicity occurred; ofatumumab was given by IV infusion in an initial dose of 300 mg (dose 1), followed by 2 g weekly for 7 doses (doses 2–8), then 2 g every 4 weeks for 4 doses (doses 9–12). The primary efficacy end point was progression-free survival as assessed by an independent review committee. The median age of patients in the study was 67 years (range: 30–88 years); all patients had a baseline ECOG performance status of 0 or 1 and 32% of patients harbored the 17p deletion chromosomal abnormality. Patients enrolled in the study had received a median of 2 (range: 1–13) prior therapies for their disease. Progression-free survival and overall survival had not been reached at the time of data analysis; however, patients receiving ibrutinib had a median reduction of 78% (range: 68–85%) in the risk of death or disease progression and a median reduction of 57% (range: 21–76%) in the risk of death compared with those receiving ofatumumab. The overall response rates with ibrutinib and ofatumumab were 42.6 and 4.1%, respectively; there were no complete responses in either group. In patients with CLL harboring the 17p deletion chromosomal abnormality, a similar reduction in the risk of death or progression (75%) and a higher overall response rate compared with those receiving ofatumumab (47.6 versus 4.7%) were observed.

In the HELIOS study, 578 patients with previously treated CLL or SLL received ibrutinib or placebo until disease progression or unacceptable toxicity in addition to therapy with bendamustine and rituximab (bendamustine/rituximab) for a maximum of six 28-day cycles. Ibrutinib 420 mg was given orally once daily; bendamustine 70 mg/m^2 was given IV on days 2 and 3 of cycle 1 and on days 1 and 2 of cycles 2–6; and rituximab 375 mg/m^2 was given IV on day 1 of cycle 1 followed by 500 mg/m^2 on day 1 of cycles 2–6. The primary efficacy end point was progression-free survival as assessed by an independent review committee. The median age of patients in the study was 64 years (range: 31–86 years); all patients had a baseline ECOG performance status of 0 or 1, 56% of patients had at least one tumor 5 cm or greater in size, and 26% of patients harbored the 11q22.3 deletion chromosomal abnormality. In this study, patients with CLL or SLL harboring the 17p deletion chromosomal abnormality were excluded because of known poor responses of such patients to bendamustine/rituximab. Patients enrolled in the study had received a median of 2 (range 1–11) prior therapies for their disease. At a median follow-up of 17 months, progression-free survival had not been reached in patients receiving ibrutinib in combination with bendamustine/rituximab; these patients had a median reduction of 80% (range: 72–85%) in the risk of death or disease progression. The overall response rates with ibrutinib in combination with bendamustine/rituximab or placebo in combination with bendamustine/rituximab were 82.7 or 67.8%, respectively; 8.3% of patients receiving ibrutinib in combination with bendamustine/rituximab achieved a complete response.

In the RESONATE-2 study, 269 geriatric patients with treatment-naive CLL or SLL were treated with ibrutinib or chlorambucil. Ibrutinib 420 mg was given orally once daily until disease progression or unacceptable toxicity occurred; chlorambucil was given orally at an initial dosage of 0.5 mg/kg (dose escalation up to 0.8 mg/kg was permitted if tolerated) on days 1 and 15 of each 28-day cycle for a maximum of 12 cycles. The primary efficacy end point was progression-free survival as assessed by an independent review committee. The median age of patients in the study was 73 years (range: 65–90 years); 91% patients had a baseline ECOG performance status of 0 or 1, 45% had Rai stage III or IV disease, and 20% of patients harbored the 11q22.3 deletion chromosomal abnormality. At a median follow-up of 28.1 months, progression-free survival and overall survival had not been reached; however, patients receiving ibrutinib had a median reduction of 84% (range: 72–91%) in the composite risk of death or disease progression and a median reduction of 84% (range: 44–95%) in the risk of death compared with those receiving chlorambucil. The overall response rates with ibrutinib and chlorambucil were 82.4 and 35.3%, respectively; complete responses were achieved in 3.7 and 1.5% of patients receiving ibrutinib and chlorambucil, respectively. Approximately one-half of the patients (41%) randomized to chlorambucil had therapy switched to ibrutinib; however, based on intent-to-treat analysis, patients receiving ibrutinib had a median reduction of 56% (range: 8–79%) in the risk of death compared with those receiving chlorambucil and a higher rate of 2-year overall survival (94.7 versus 84.3%).

■ **Marginal-zone Lymphoma** Ibrutinib is used for the treatment of marginal-zone lymphoma in patients who have received at least one prior anti-CD20-based therapy. The current indication is based on overall response rate; clinical benefit has not been established. Continued FDA approval for this indication may be contingent on confirmation of clinical benefit in additional trials. Ibrutinib has been designated an orphan drug by FDA for the treatment of this cancer.

The current indication for ibrutinib in the treatment of marginal-zone lymphoma is based principally on the favorable response demonstrated in a phase 2, open-label study (Study 1121) in patients who had received at least one prior anti-CD20-based therapy. The median age of patients enrolled in the study was 66 (range: 30–92) years; most patients (92%) had a baseline ECOG performance status of 0 or 1, 51% had mucosa-associated lymphoid tissue (MALT) lymphoma, 27% had nodal marginal-zone lymphoma, and 22% had splenic marginal-zone lymphoma. Patients in the study had received a median of 2 (range: 1–9) prior therapies for their disease. In this study, 63 patients received ibrutinib 560 mg orally once daily until disease progression or unacceptable toxicity occurred. The primary end point was overall response rate (complete plus partial responses) based on the 2007 IWG criteria for malignant lymphoma as assessed by an independent review committee. In this study, the overall response rate was 46%; 3.2% of patients receiving ibrutinib achieved a complete response. Results of a subgroup analysis based on disease subtype (i.e., MALT, nodal, or splenic marginal-zone lymphoma) suggested that the effect of ibrutinib on overall response rate was consistent across these subtypes. At the time of analysis, the median duration of response had not been reached. The median time to response was 4.5 (range: 2.3–16.4) months.

At a median follow-up of 19.4 months, the median progression-free survival was 14.2 months, but median overall survival was not yet reached. Median progression-free survival was 13.8, 19.4, or 8.3 months in patients with MALT lymphoma, splenic marginal-zone lymphoma, or nodal marginal-zone lymphoma, respectively. Following initiation of ibrutinib therapy, lymphocytosis (i.e., absolute lymphocyte count exceeding 5000/mm^3 and an increase of at least 50% from baseline) occurred in 11% of patients, with a peak lymphocyte count occurring at a median of 1 week; lymphocytosis resolved in a median of 11 weeks. (See Description.)

■ **Waldenstrom Macroglobulinemia** Ibrutinib is used for the treatment of Waldenstrom macroglobulinemia; the drug has been designated an orphan drug by FDA for the treatment of this condition.

Evidence of safety and efficacy of ibrutinib in the treatment of Waldenstrom macroglobulinemia is based principally on the results of an open-label, multicenter study (Study 1118) in patients who had received prior therapy for this disease. The median age of patients enrolled in the study was 63 years (range: 44–86 years); all patients had a baseline ECOG performance status of 0 or 1. Patients in the study had received a median of 2 (range: 1–11) prior therapies for their disease. In this study, 63 patients received ibrutinib 420 mg orally once daily until disease progression or unacceptable toxicity occurred. Response to ibrutinib treatment was assessed by investigators and an independent review committee (IRC) based on criteria from the International Workshop on Waldenstrom's Macroglobulinemia.

The IRC-assessed response rate, consisting of complete plus very good partial plus partial responses, was 61.9%; there were no complete responses. At the time of data analysis, responses were ongoing. The median time to response was 1.2 (range: 0.7–13.4) months. Substantial reductions from baseline in serum IgM concentration and bone marrow involvement and increases in hemoglobin concentration occurred with ibrutinib treatment, and overall toxicity (e.g., neutropenia, thrombocytopenia, bleeding, infection) was reported to be moderate.

■ **Chronic Graft-versus-host Disease** Ibrutinib is used for the treatment of chronic GVHD following failure of at least one prior systemic therapy; the drug has been designated an orphan drug by FDA for the treatment of this condition.

The current indication for ibrutinib in the treatment of chronic GVHD is based principally on the results of an open-label, multicenter study (Study 1129) in patients who required additional therapy following failure of first-line corticosteroid therapy. The median age of patients enrolled in the study was 56 (range: 19–74) years; 88% of patients had at least 2 organs involved at baseline and 60% of patients had a baseline Karnofsky performance status of 80 or less. The most common underlying malignancies resulting in stem cell transplantation were acute lymphocytic leukemia (ALL), acute myeloid leukemia (AML), and CLL. Patients in the study had received a median of 2 (range: 1–3) prior therapies for chronic GVHD. Approximately 50% of patients were receiving immunosuppressants and systemic corticosteroids (median daily prednisone [or equivalent] dosage was 0.3 mg/kg) at baseline. In this study, 42 patients received ibrutinib 420 mg orally once daily. Response to ibrutinib treatment was assessed by investigators based on criteria from the National Institutes of Health (NIH) Consensus Panel.

In this study, the overall response rate was 67%; 21% of patients receiving the drug achieved a complete response. At the time of data analysis, 48% of patients had sustained responses of 20 weeks or more. Responses in all organs affected by chronic GVHD (i.e., skin, mouth, GI tract, liver) were observed. The median time to response was 12.3 (range: 4.1–42.1) weeks. Exploratory analysis of patient-reported symptoms based on the Lee Symptom Scale showed at least a 7-point decrease in overall summary score in 24% of patients on at least 2 consecutive assessments (visits).

Dosage and Administration

■ **Administration** Ibrutinib is administered orally once daily at approximately the same time each day. The dose should be taken orally with water; capsules should *not* be opened, broken, or chewed, and tablets should not be cut, crushed, or chewed.

Ibrutinib capsules and tablets should be stored in the original packaging at 20–25°C, but may be exposed to temperatures ranging from 15–30°C.

■ **Dosage** ***Mantle Cell Lymphoma*** For the treatment of mantle cell lymphoma in patients who have received at least one prior therapy, the recommended dosage of ibrutinib is 560 mg once daily. Therapy should be continued until disease progression or unacceptable toxicity occurs.

Chronic Lymphocytic Leukemia/Small Lymphocytic Lymphoma For the treatment of chronic lymphocytic leukemia (CLL) or small lymphocytic lymphoma (SLL), including 17p deletion CLL/SLL, the recommended dosage of ibrutinib (as a single agent or in combination with bendamustine and rituximab) is 420 mg once daily. Therapy should be continued until disease progression or unacceptable toxicity occurs.

In the HELIOS study, patients received ibrutinib (420 mg once daily) continuously, bendamustine (70 mg/m^2 by IV infusion) on days 2 and 3 of cycle 1 and on days 1 and 2 of cycles 2–6, and rituximab 375 mg/m^2 by IV infusion on day 1 of cycle 1 followed by 500 mg/m^2 on day 1 of cycles 2–6. Ibrutinib therapy was continued until disease progression or unacceptable toxicity occurred. Treatment cycles were repeated every 28 days.

Marginal-zone Lymphoma For the treatment of marginal-zone lymphoma in patients who have received at least one prior anti-CD20-based therapy, the recommended dosage of ibrutinib is 560 mg once daily. Therapy should be continued until disease progression or unacceptable toxicity occurs.

Waldenstrom Macroglobulinemia For the treatment of Waldenstrom macroglobulinemia, the recommended dosage of ibrutinib is 420 mg once daily. Therapy should be continued until disease progression or unacceptable toxicity occurs.

Dosage adjustment is not necessary in patients undergoing plasmapheresis.

Chronic Graft-versus-host Disease For the treatment of chronic graft-versus-host disease (GVHD) following failure of at least one prior systemic therapy, the recommended dosage of ibrutinib is 420 mg once daily. Therapy should be continued until progression of chronic GVHD, recurrence of the underlying malignancy, or unacceptable toxicity. Ibrutinib should be discontinued when treatment for chronic GVHD is no longer necessary.

Dosage Modification for Toxicity Ibrutinib therapy should be withheld for the occurrence of grade 3 or higher nonhematologic toxicity, grade 3 or higher neutropenia with infection or fever, or grade 4 hematologic toxicity. Upon resolution or improvement of the toxicity (i.e., return to baseline or resolution to grade 1), ibrutinib therapy may be resumed (or discontinued) as described in Table 1.

Table 1: Dosage Modifications for Ibrutinib Toxicity

	Dosage Modification after Recovery from Toxicity	
Toxicity Occurrence	Mantle Cell Lymphoma or Marginal-zone Lymphoma (Starting Dosage = 560 mg daily)	CLL/SLL, Waldenstrom Macroglobulinemia, or Chronic GVHD (Starting Dosage = 420 mg daily)
First	Restart at 560 mg daily	Restart at 420 mg daily
Second	Restart at 420 mg daily	Restart at 280 mg daily
Third	Restart at 280 mg daily	Restart at 140 mg daily
Fourth	Discontinue ibrutinib	Discontinue ibrutinib

Dosage Modification with Concomitant Drugs or Foods Affecting Hepatic Microsomal Enzymes **B-Cell Malignancies (Mantle Cell Lymphoma, Marginal-zone Lymphoma, CLL/SLL, or Waldenstrom Macroglobulinemia).** Concomitant use of ibrutinib with *potent* CYP3A inhibitors should be avoided; however, if short-term (7 days or less) therapy with potent CYP3A inhibitors is necessary, ibrutinib therapy should be temporarily withheld during such therapy. If concomitant use with posaconazole oral suspension 100 mg once or twice daily or 200 mg twice daily or voriconazole 200 mg twice daily is required, the manufacturer recommends reducing the dosage of ibrutinib to 140 mg once daily. If concomitant use with posaconazole oral suspension 200 mg three times daily or 400 mg twice daily, posaconazole IV 300 mg once daily, or posaconazole delayed-release tablets 300 mg once daily is required, the manufacturer recommends reducing the dosage of ibrutinib to 70 mg once daily. If concomitant use of posaconazole or voriconazole is discontinued, the ibrutinib dosage should be returned to the dosage used prior to initiation of the antifungal agent. (See Drug Interactions: Drugs and Foods Affecting Hepatic Microsomal Enzymes.)

If concomitant use of ibrutinib and a *moderate* CYP3A inhibitor is necessary, the manufacturer recommends reducing the dosage of ibrutinib to 140 mg once daily. If concomitant use of the moderate CYP3A inhibitor is discontinued, the ibrutinib dosage should be returned to the dosage used prior to initiation of the moderate CYP3A inhibitor.

Patients receiving ibrutinib concomitantly with posaconazole, voriconazole, or a moderate inhibitor of CYP3A should be monitored for signs of ibrutinib toxicity, and therapy should be interrupted as appropriate. (See Dosage Modification for Toxicity under Dosage and Administration: Dosage.)

Chronic GVHD. Concomitant use of ibrutinib with *potent* CYP3A inhibitors should be avoided; however, if short-term (7 days or less) therapy with potent CYP3A inhibitors are necessary, ibrutinib therapy should be temporarily withheld during such therapy. If concomitant use with posaconazole oral suspension 100 mg once or twice daily or 200 mg twice daily or voriconazole 200 mg twice daily is required, the manufacturer recommends reducing the dosage of ibrutinib to 280 mg once daily. If concomitant use with posaconazole oral suspension 200 mg three times daily or 400 mg twice daily, posaconazole IV 300 mg once daily, or posaconazole delayed-release tablets 300 mg once daily is required, the manufacturer recommends reducing the dosage of ibrutinib to 140 mg once daily. If concomitant use of posaconazole or voriconazole is discontinued, the ibrutinib dosage used prior to initiation of the antifungals should be resumed. (See Drug Interactions: Drugs and Foods Affecting Hepatic Microsomal Enzymes.)

If concomitant use of ibrutinib and a *moderate* CYP3A inhibitor is necessary, the manufacturer recommends reducing the dosage of ibrutinib to 420 mg once daily. If concomitant use of the moderate CYP3A inhibitor is discontinued, the ibrutinib dosage should be returned to the dosage used prior to initiation of the moderate CYP3A inhibitor.

Patients receiving ibrutinib concomitantly with posaconazole, voriconazole, or a moderate inhibitor of CYP3A should be monitored for ibrutinib toxicity, and the dosage should be interrupted or adjusted as appropriate. (See Dosage Modification for Toxicity under Dosage and Administration: Dosage.)

■ **Special Populations** For patients with mild hepatic impairment (Child-Pugh class A), the manufacturer recommends an ibrutinib dosage of 140 mg once daily. For patients with moderate hepatic impairment (Child-Pugh class B), the manufacturer recommends an ibrutinib dosage of 70 mg once daily. Patients with hepatic impairment should be closely monitored for signs of toxicity. Use of ibrutinib in patients with severe hepatic impairment (Child-Pugh class C) should be avoided. (See Hepatic Impairment under Warnings/Precautions: Specific Populations, in Cautions.)

The manufacturer makes no specific dosage recommendations for geriatric patients or patients with renal impairment. (See Geriatric Use and also see Renal Impairment under Warnings/Precautions: Specific Populations, in Cautions.)

Cautions

■ **Contraindications** The manufacturer states that there are no known contraindications to the use of ibrutinib.

■ **Warnings/Precautions** ***Hemorrhage*** Hemorrhage, sometimes fatal, has been reported in patients receiving ibrutinib. Grade 3 or higher bleeding events (i.e., intracranial hemorrhage, subdural hematoma, GI bleeding, hematuria, postprocedural hemorrhage) occurred in up to 6% of patients treated with ibrutinib in clinical trials. Overall, hemorrhagic events, including bruising and petechiae, of any grade of severity occurred in approximately 50% of patients receiving ibrutinib in clinical trials. The mechanism of bleeding with ibrutinib therapy is unclear; there did not appear to be a correlation between thrombocytopenia and these events.

Concomitant use of ibrutinib with antiplatelet or anticoagulant therapies may increase the risk of hemorrhagic events; therefore, patients receiving concomitant antiplatelet or anticoagulant therapy should be monitored for manifestations of bleeding.

Because of the risk of bleeding, the potential benefits and risks of withholding ibrutinib therapy for at least 3–7 days prior to and following surgery (based on the type of surgery and bleeding risk) should be considered.

Infectious Complications Serious infections (bacterial, viral, or fungal), sometimes fatal, have been reported in patients receiving ibrutinib. Grade 3 or higher infections occurred in 14–29% of patients receiving ibrutinib in clinical trials. Progressive multifocal leukoencephalopathy (PML) and *Pneumocystis jirovecii* (formerly *P. carinii*) pneumonia also have been reported.

Patients should be monitored for signs and symptoms of infection and appropriate anti-infective treatment should be initiated as clinically indicated. Prophylaxis should be considered according to current standards of care in patients who are at increased risk for opportunistic infections.

Myelosuppression Cytopenias, including thrombocytopenia, anemia, and neutropenia, have been reported in patients receiving ibrutinib. Grade 3 or 4 neutropenia, thrombocytopenia, or anemia was reported in 13–29, 5–17, or 0–13%, respectively, of patients with B-cell malignancies receiving single-agent ibrutinib in clinical trials.

Complete blood cell (CBC) counts should be monitored monthly. Temporary interruption of ibrutinib therapy or dosage reduction may be necessary if myelosuppression occurs. (See Dosage Modification for Toxicity under Dosage and Administration: Dosage.)

Cardiac Effects Serious arrhythmias, sometimes fatal, have been reported in patients receiving ibrutinib, particularly those with cardiac risk factors, hypertension, acute infections, or a history of arrhythmias. Grade 3 or higher ventricular tachyarrhythmias or atrial fibrillation and atrial flutter occurred in 0–1% or 0–6%, respectively, of patients receiving ibrutinib in clinical trials. Patients receiving ibrutinib should be monitored periodically for arrhythmias. Patients should be managed as clinically indicated and ECG monitoring should be performed if symptoms of arrhythmia (e.g., palpitations, lightheadedness, syncope, angina) or new-onset dyspnea occur. If arrhythmia persists, dosage reduction should be considered and the potential benefit of the drug against the risks of continued therapy to the patient should be carefully weighed.

Hypertension has been reported in 6–17% of patients receiving ibrutinib in clinical trials. The median time to occurrence of hypertension was 4.6 months (range: 0.03–22 months). Patients should be monitored for the development of new-onset hypertension or hypertension that is not adequately controlled with medical management. If hypertension occurs, antihypertensive therapy should be initiated or adjusted as needed.

Development of Second Primary Malignancy Other malignancies, including non-skin carcinomas, have been reported in 3–16% of ibrutinib-treated patients in clinical trials. Non-melanoma skin cancer was the most frequent second primary malignancy, occurring in 2–13% of ibrutinib-treated patients.

Tumor Lysis Syndrome Tumor lysis syndrome has been reported infrequently in patients receiving ibrutinib. Potential for developing tumor lysis syndrome (e.g., large tumor burden) should be assessed at baseline and appropriate precautions taken. Patients should be monitored closely and treated as clinically indicated.

Fetal/Neonatal Morbidity and Mortality Based on findings in animals, ibrutinib may cause fetal harm if administered to pregnant women; the drug has been shown to be teratogenic, embryotoxic, and fetotoxic in animals. There are no available data regarding the risk of ibrutinib use in pregnant women to inform the drug-associated risk. Embryofetal toxicity (i.e., increased fetal resorption, postimplantation loss) and teratogenicity (i.e., visceral and skeletal anomalies) have been demonstrated in animals receiving ibrutinib at exposure levels 2–20 times the human exposure at the maximum recommended dosage (i.e., 420 or 560 mg daily).

Pregnancy should be avoided during ibrutinib therapy. Women of childbearing potential should be advised to use effective contraceptive methods during and for 1 month after discontinuance of the drug. In addition, men should avoid fathering a child during and for 1 month after discontinuance of the drug. If ibrutinib is used during pregnancy or if the patient becomes pregnant while receiving the drug, the patient should be apprised of the potential hazard to the fetus.

Specific Populations **Pregnancy.** Although there are no available data in pregnant women, ibrutinib may cause fetal harm based on animal findings. (See Fetal/Neonatal Morbidity and Mortality under Cautions: Warnings/Precautions.) If ibrutinib is used during pregnancy or if the patient becomes pregnant while receiving the drug, the patient should be apprised of the potential fetal hazard. (See Advice to Patients.)

In women of childbearing potential, the manufacturer recommends a pregnancy test prior to initiating ibrutinib therapy.

Lactation. It is not known whether ibrutinib or its metabolites are distributed into human milk or if the drug has any effect on milk production or the nursing infant. The benefits of breast-feeding and the importance of ibrutinib to the woman should be considered along with the potential adverse effects on the breast-fed child from the drug or from the underlying maternal condition.

Pediatric Use. Safety and efficacy of ibrutinib have not been established in pediatric patients.

Geriatric Use. In clinical trials, 62% of patients were 65 years of age or older and 21% were 75 years of age or older. No overall differences in efficacy were observed between geriatric and younger patients, but some adverse effects (i.e., anemia, grade 3 or higher pneumonia) occurred more frequently in geriatric patients.

Hepatic Impairment. Safety of ibrutinib has not been established in patients with hepatic impairment. In a single-dose study, systemic exposure of ibrutinib was increased 2.7-, 8.2-, or 9.8-fold in patients with mild (Child-Pugh class A), moderate (Child-Pugh class B), or severe (Child-Pugh class C) hepatic impairment, respectively, compared with that in individuals with normal hepatic function. In addition, peak plasma concentration of ibrutinib was increased 5.2-, 8.8-, or 7-fold in patients with mild, moderate, or severe hepatic impairment, respectively, compared with that in individuals with normal hepatic function.

Patients with hepatic impairment should be closely monitored for signs of toxicity during ibrutinib therapy, and the dosage should be adjusted as appropriate. (See Dosage Modification for Toxicity under Dosage and Administration: Dosage and also see Dosage and Administration: Special Populations.) Use of ibrutinib in patients with moderate or severe hepatic impairment should be avoided.

Renal Impairment. Systemic exposure of ibrutinib does not appear to be altered in patients with creatinine clearance exceeding 25 mL/minute. The manufacturer states that there is no experience with ibrutinib in patients with severe renal impairment (creatinine clearance less than 25 mL/minute) or in patients undergoing dialysis. (See Dosage and Administration: Special Populations.)

■ **Common Adverse Effects** Adverse effects reported in at least 20% of patients receiving ibrutinib for the treatment of previously treated mantle cell lymphoma in the principal clinical trial include thrombocytopenia, diarrhea, neutropenia, anemia, fatigue, musculoskeletal pain, peripheral edema, upper respiratory tract infection, nausea, bruising, dyspnea, constipation, rash, abdominal pain, vomiting, and decreased appetite.

Adverse effects reported in at least 20% of patients receiving ibrutinib for the treatment of CLL or SLL in the 4 principal clinical trials include thrombocytopenia, neutropenia, diarrhea, anemia, fatigue, musculoskeletal pain, upper respiratory tract infection, rash, nausea, bruising, pyrexia, hemorrhage, and cough.

Adverse effects reported in at least 20% of patients receiving ibrutinib for the treatment of previously treated marginal-zone lymphoma in the principal clinical trial include thrombocytopenia, fatigue, anemia, diarrhea, bruising, musculoskeletal pain, hemorrhage, rash, nausea, arthralgia, peripheral edema, cough, neutropenia, dyspnea, and upper respiratory tract infection.

Adverse effects reported in at least 20% of patients receiving ibrutinib for the treatment of previously treated Waldenstrom macroglobulinemia in the principal clinical trial include neutropenia, thrombocytopenia, diarrhea, rash, nausea, muscle spasms, and fatigue.

Adverse effects reported in at least 20% of patients receiving ibrutinib for the treatment of chronic GVHD following failure of at least one prior systemic therapy in the principal clinical trial include fatigue, bruising, diarrhea, thrombocytopenia, muscle spasms, stomatitis, hemorrhage, nausea, anemia, and pneumonia.

Other clinically important adverse effects include diarrhea and visual disturbances (i.e., blurry vision, decreased visual acuity). Diarrhea has been reported in 43% of patients receiving ibrutinib in clinical trials with a median time to onset of 10 days (range: 0–1.7 years). Blurry vision and decreased visual acuity have been reported in 10% of patients receiving ibrutinib in clinical trials with a median time to onset of 85 days (range: 1–414 days). Complete resolution of diarrhea or visual disturbances occurred in 82 or 61% of patients, respectively.

Drug Interactions

Metabolism of ibrutinib to an active dihydrodiol metabolite (PCI-45227) is mediated principally by cytochrome P-450 (CYP) isoenzyme 3A and, to a lesser extent, by CYP2D6.

In vitro studies indicate that ibrutinib and PCI-45227 are not expected to inhibit CYP isoenzymes 1A2, 2B6, 2C8, 2C9, 2C19, 2D6, or 3A or induce CYP isoenzymes 1A2, 2B6, or 3A at clinically relevant concentrations. In vitro studies indicate that ibrutinib may inhibit P-glycoprotein (P-gp) and breast cancer resistance protein (BCRP) transport at clinically relevant concentrations.

■ Drugs and Foods Affecting Hepatic Microsomal Enzymes

Inhibitors of CYP3A Concomitant use of ibrutinib with potent or moderate inhibitors of CYP3A may result in increased peak plasma concentrations and systemic exposure (area under the concentration-time curve [AUC]) of ibrutinib and an increased incidence of drug toxicity. When the potent CYP3A inhibitor ketoconazole (400 mg daily) was administered concomitantly with ibrutinib (single 40-mg dose), the peak plasma concentration and AUC of ibrutinib was increased by 29- and 24-fold, respectively. With multiple dosing of the potent CYP3A inhibitor voriconazole concomitantly with ibrutinib, the peak plasma concentration and AUC of ibrutinib was increased by 6.7- and 5.7-fold, respectively. Simulations using physiologically based pharmacokinetic models suggest that the potent CYP3A inhibitor posaconazole may increase the AUC of ibrutinib by threefold to tenfold under fed conditions. When the moderate CYP3A inhibitor erythromycin was administered concomitantly with ibrutinib, the peak plasma concentration and AUC of ibrutinib were increased by 3.4- and 3-fold, respectively.

Concomitant use of ibrutinib with *potent* CYP3A inhibitors should be avoided; however, if short-term (7 days or less) therapy with a potent CYP3A inhibitor (e.g., an anti-infective agent) is required, the manufacturer recommends withholding ibrutinib therapy during administration of the potent CYP3A inhibitor. If concomitant use of the potent CYP3A inhibitor posaconazole or voriconazole or a moderate CYP3A inhibitor is required, the manufacturer recommends reducing the daily dosage of ibrutinib. (See Concomitant Use with Drugs or Foods Affecting Hepatic Microsomal Enzymes under Dosage and Administration: Dosage.)

The manufacturer states that grapefruit products and Seville oranges are known to contain potent or moderate inhibitors of CYP3A and should be *avoided* during ibrutinib therapy.

Inducers of CYP3A Concomitant use of ibrutinib with potent or moderate inducers of CYP3A may result in decreased peak plasma concentrations and AUC of ibrutinib. Using a physiologically based pharmacokinetic model, administration of the potent CYP3A inducer rifampin (600 mg daily) concomitantly with ibrutinib (single 560-mg dose) reduced the peak plasma concentration and AUC of ibrutinib by approximately 13- and 10-fold, respectively. Other simulations using physiologically based pharmacokinetic models suggest that moderate inducers of CYP3A (e.g., efavirenz) may decrease the AUC of ibrutinib by up to threefold. Concomitant use of ibrutinib with potent CYP3A inducers (e.g., carbamazepine) should be avoided.

■ Substrates of Efflux Transport Systems

Concomitant use of ibrutinib with oral drugs that are substrates of P-gp or BCRP and have a narrow therapeutic index (e.g., digoxin, methotrexate) may result in increased concentrations of the substrate drug.

■ Anticoagulants and Antiplatelet Agents

Increased risk of hemorrhagic events. Patients should be monitored for bleeding manifestations.

Description

Ibrutinib is a selective, irreversible inhibitor of Bruton's tyrosine kinase (BTK); the drug is an antineoplastic agent. BTK, a member of the tyrosine protein kinase (Tec) family of kinases, is positioned early within the B-cell antigen receptor (BCR) signaling pathway. BCR is involved in the initiation of various cascades of intracellular signaling events, including activation of BTK, which leads to cell proliferation, differentiation, apoptosis, and cell migration essential for the development and survival of normal and malignant B-cells. Ibrutinib binds covalently to the active site of the tyrosine kinase BTK and irreversibly inhibits phosphorylation of tyrosine kinase, resulting in inhibition of downstream effector activity within the BCR signaling pathway.

In vitro kinase assays also have shown that ibrutinib inhibits (with up to tenfold less activity) the activity of several other receptor tyrosine kinases, including Bmx/Etk, epidermal growth factor receptor (EGFR), and members of the Src family of tyrosine kinases (e.g., Hck, Yes). In vivo, ibrutinib inhibits the proliferation and survival of malignant B-cells. The drug also has demonstrated cell migration and substrate adhesion of CLL cells and mantle cell lymphoma cells in vitro; the mobilization of cells from tissues to peripheral blood results in a transient increase in absolute lymphocyte count (lymphocytosis) in the peripheral blood. (See Uses.) In vitro and in vivo, ibrutinib has demonstrated substantial activity in activated B-cell-like diffuse large B-cell non-Hodgkin's lymphoma (ABC-DLBCL) cells expressing wild-type caspase recruitment domain-containing protein-11 (wild-type CARD-11), a nuclear factor-kappa B (NF-kB) signaling adaptor essential for the survival of ABC-DLBCL.

When given in a single dose of 1680 mg (3 times the maximum recommended daily dosage), ibrutinib did not prolong the QT interval to any clinically relevant extent. (See Cardiac Effects under Cautions: Warnings/Precautions.)

Following oral administration of ibrutinib in healthy, fasting individuals, the absolute bioavailability of the drug was 2.9%. Systemic exposure of ibrutinib increases with doses up to 840 mg in patients with B-cell malignancies. Following repeated doses of ibrutinib 420 or 560 mg daily, steady-state concentrations of the drug were achieved in 1 week and the accumulation ratio for the drug was 1–1.6. Administration of ibrutinib with a high-fat, high-calorie meal (800–1000 calories with fat accounting for approximately 50% of caloric content) resulted in an approximately twofold to fourfold increase in peak plasma concentrations and an approximately twofold increase in systemic exposure, compared with administration following overnight fasting. Ibrutinib is metabolized to several metabolites by the cytochrome P-450 (CYP) microsomal enzyme system, principally by the isoenzyme 3A. The active metabolite, PCI-45227 (a dihydrodiol metabolite), has demonstrated BTK inhibition approximately 15 times less than that of ibrutinib. In vitro, ibrutinib is 97.3% bound to plasma proteins. Ibrutinib is extensively distributed into tissue with an apparent volume of distribution at steady state of 10,000 L. Following administration of a single radiolabeled dose of ibrutinib, 80% of the dose was recovered in feces and less than 10% was recovered in urine; unchanged drug accounted for approximately 1% of the dose recovered in feces. The elimination half-life of ibrutinib is 4–6 hours. The clearance of ibrutinib does not appear to be affected by age or gender.

In vitro, the 50% inhibitory concentration of ibrutinib for collagen-induced platelet aggregation is 2026 ng/mL in blood samples from healthy donors, 1321 ng/mL in those with severe renal dysfunction, and 352 ng/mL in those taking warfarin. (See Hemorrhage under Cautions: Warnings/Precautions.) Clinically meaningful inhibition of adenosine diphosphate (ADP), arachidonic acid, ristocetin, and thrombin receptor agonist peptide-6 (TRAP-6) by ibrutinib have not been demonstrated.

Advice to Patients

Importance of advising patients to take ibrutinib as directed by their clinician and at approximately the same time each day. If a dose is missed, importance of administering the missed dose on the same day as soon as it is remembered. Patients should be advised not to take 2 doses on the same day to make up for a missed dose.

Importance of advising patients to take ibrutinib capsules or tablets orally with a glass of water; capsules should not be opened, broken, or chewed and tablets should not be cut, crushed, or chewed.

Risk of bleeding. Importance of promptly informing clinician of any episodes of unusual bleeding (e.g., severe headache, blood in stool or urine, prolonged or uncontrolled bleeding). Importance of notifying clinician before any planned surgeries, including dental procedures.

Risk of serious infection. Importance of reporting signs or symptoms of possible infection (e.g., chills, fever).

Risk of arrhythmia. Importance of informing clinician if palpitations, lightheadedness, dizziness, fainting, shortness of breath, or chest discomfort occurs.

Risk of hypertension; may require antihypertensive therapy.

Possible risk of developing a second primary malignancy (e.g., skin cancer).

Risk of tumor lysis syndrome. Importance of reporting signs or symptoms of tumor lysis syndrome (e.g., arrhythmia, seizure).

Risk of fetal harm. Apprise patient of potential hazard to the fetus if ibrutinib used during pregnancy. Women of childbearing potential should avoid becoming pregnant during therapy and for at least 1 month after discontinuance of therapy; men should also avoid fathering a child during therapy and for at least 1 month after discontinuance of therapy.

Risk of diarrhea. Importance of advising patients to maintain adequate hydration during ibrutinib therapy. Importance of informing clinician if diarrhea persists.

Importance of informing clinicians of existing or contemplated concomitant therapy, including prescription and OTC drugs and dietary or herbal supplements (e.g., St. John's wort), as well as any concomitant illnesses. Patients should be advised to avoid consuming grapefruit or Seville oranges.

Importance of informing patients of other important precautionary information. (See Cautions.)

Overview® (see Users Guide). For additional information on this drug until a more detailed monograph is developed and published, the manufacturer's labeling should be consulted. It is *essential* that the manufacturer's labeling be consulted for more detailed information on usual cautions, precautions, contraindications, potential drug interactions, laboratory test interferences, and acute toxicity. For further information on the handling of antineoplastic agents, see the ASHP Guidelines on Handling Hazardous Drugs at http://www.ahfsdruginformation.com.

Preparations

Excipients in commercially available drug preparations may have clinically important effects in some individuals; consult specific product labeling for details.

Ibrutinib

Oral		
Capsules	70 mg	**Imbruvica®**, Pharmacyclics (comarketed by Janssen Biotech)
	140 mg	**Imbruvica®**, Pharmacyclics (comarketed by Janssen Biotech)
Tablets	140 mg	**Imbruvica®**, Pharmacyclics (comarketed by Janssen Biotech)
	280 mg	**Imbruvica®**, Pharmacyclics (comarketed by Janssen Biotech)
	420 mg	**Imbruvica®**, Pharmacyclics (comarketed by Janssen Biotech)
	560 mg	**Imbruvica®**, Pharmacyclics (comarketed by Janssen Biotech)

IDArubicin Hydrochloride

■ Idarubicin hydrochloride, a semisynthetic anthracycline, is an antineoplastic agent.

Uses

■ **Acute Myeloid Leukemia** Idarubicin is used in combination with other antineoplastic agents for the treatment of acute myeloid (myelogenous, nonlymphocytic) leukemia (AML, ANLL), including French-American-British classifications M1 through M7, in adults, particularly younger adults. Cytarabine with either daunorubicin or idarubicin is a regimen of choice for remission induction in acute myeloid leukemia. Induction regimens are used to rapidly reduce the tumor burden in order to achieve complete remission, which generally is defined as less than 5% leukemic blast cells in the bone marrow, normalization of peripheral blood counts, and absence of any evidence of extramedullary disease. Optimal postremission therapy has not been established, but current approaches include consolidation chemotherapy with cytarabine-based regimens similar to standard induction regimens, consolidation chemotherapy with high-dose cytarabine-based regimens (for younger adults), high-dose chemotherapy or chemoradiotherapy with bone marrow infusion, or high-dose marrow-ablative therapy with stem cell transplantation. There is no evidence of benefit from prolonged administration of chemotherapy in the treatment of most types of AML, and most current treatment regimens in the US no longer employ maintenance therapy. An exception is type M3 AML (acute promyelocytic leukemia), for which improvement in overall survival and/or disease-free survival has been demonstrated with the use of maintenance therapy.

The current indication for idarubicin is based principally on the results of 4 randomized trials, 3 US studies (studies 1 through 3) and an Italian study (study 4), showing that combined therapy with idarubicin and cytarabine is at least as effective as with daunorubicin and cytarabine for induction therapy in patients with previously untreated AML. Patients with prior myelodysplastic syndrome, an indicator of poor prognosis, were excluded in study 1, but eligible for enrollment in studies 2–4. Both a higher rate of complete remission and prolonged overall survival in patients receiving idarubicin were reported in only one of the studies (study 1). Higher rates of complete remission (studies 1 and 2) and longer median survival (studies 1 and 3) associated with the idarubicin regimen each were reported in 2 of the 3 US studies. Long-term follow-up shows that, at 5 years, longer median survival in patients receiving idarubicin was maintained for only one of these 2 studies (study 1). Some clinicians have questioned the equivalence of the doses of daunorubicin and idarubicin used in these randomized trials, suggesting that the doses used may have contributed to any differences in patient outcome. No randomized trials comparing idarubicin versus higher dosages of daunorubicin in induction regimens for AML have been conducted to date, and the optimal dosage for daunorubicin in AML has not been established.

Analysis of pooled data for individual patients from 5 randomized studies (including the 4 randomized trials described in this discussion) indicates higher rates of complete remission (62 versus 53%) and survival at 5 years (13 versus 9%) in patients receiving idarubicin compared with those receiving daunorubicin. However, the difference in the rate of complete remission between idarubicin and daunorubicin appears to decrease with increasing age. Subgroup analysis of the data suggests a tendency toward a higher rate of early death (during the first 40 days of induction therapy) in patients aged 60 years and older receiving idarubicin compared with patients in the same age group receiving daunorubicin. Although the rate of later death (after 40 days of induction therapy) is lower for patients in all age groups receiving idarubicin compared with those receiving daunorubicin, there is a trend toward a lesser reduction in older patients compared with younger patients. The combined effect of these trends results in a difference in the rate of complete remission among older and younger patients receiving idarubicin. In addition, interim analysis of a phase 3 trial involving 363 patients aged 55 years and older with previously untreated AML shows no difference in response rate for patients receiving cytarabine, with idarubicin, daunorubicin, or mitoxantrone.

In study 1, a total of 130 patients 16–60 years of age (median age: approximately 40 years) with previously untreated AML received either idarubicin 12 mg/m^2 or daunorubicin 50 mg/m^2 IV daily for 3 days; both groups received cytarabine 25 mg/m^2 by rapid IV ("bolus") infusion followed by cytarabine 200 mg/m^2 continuous IV infusion daily for 5 days. Patients with a complete remission following 1 or 2 courses of induction therapy received 2 courses of consolidation therapy using the same doses as used in the induction regimen but for shorter periods (anthracycline for 2 days and cytarabine rapid IV loading dose followed by continuous IV infusion for 4 days). A rest period of 4–6 weeks is recommended before initiation of consolidation therapy and between the courses. Patients receiving idarubicin and cytarabine had a higher rate of complete remissions (78 versus 58%) and longer median survival (508 versus 435 days at a median follow-up of 2.5 years) than those receiving daunorubicin and cytarabine. Long-term follow-up shows that median survival at 5 years was longer in patients receiving the idarubicin regimen.

In study 2, a total of 230 patients aged 15 years to 60 years or older (median age about 60 years) with previously untreated AML received either idarubicin 12 mg/m^2 or daunorubicin 45 mg/m^2 IV daily for 3 days; both groups received cytarabine 100 mg/m^2 daily for 7 days by continuous IV infusion. Patients with complete remission following 1 or 2 courses of induction therapy received 3 courses of consolidation therapy at 21-day intervals or upon hematologic recovery using the same anthracycline (idarubicin 15 mg/m^2 or daunorubicin 50 mg/m^2), cytarabine 100 mg/m^2 by rapid IV infusion every 12 hours for 10 doses, and thioguanine 100 mg/m^2 orally every 12 hours for 10 doses. If severe myelosuppression occurred, treatment was delayed then resumed upon hematologic recovery, and subsequent courses were given with a 25% reduction in the dosage of all drugs. The study plan also included 4 courses of maintenance therapy to be given at 13-week intervals (2 days of the same anthracycline as used in induction and 5 days of cytarabine); however, this practice was discontinued following substantial toxicity, including 6 deaths from aplasia, among the first 47 patients enrolled in the trial. In this study, patients receiving idarubicin and cytarabine had a higher rate of complete remissions (69 versus 55%) than those receiving daunorubicin and cytarabine; similar median survival (328 versus 277 days) was observed between the groups.

In study 3, a total of 214 patients aged 18 years to 60 years or older (median age about 55 years) with previously untreated AML received either idarubicin 13 mg/m^2 or daunorubicin 45 mg/m^2 IV daily for 3 days; both groups received cytarabine 100 mg/m^2 daily for 7 days by continuous IV infusion. Patients with a complete remission following 1 or 2 courses of induction therapy received 2 courses of consolidation therapy using the same doses as used in the induction regimen but for shorter periods (anthracycline for 2 days and cytarabine for 5 days). Patients receiving idarubicin and cytarabine had a similar rate of complete remissions (67 versus 58%) but longer median survival (393 versus 281 days) than those receiving daunorubicin and cytarabine. However, an update of the study data shows no difference in survival at 5 years.

Patients with AML who have complete remission of disease following induction therapy generally receive consolidation chemotherapy. The optimal regimen has not been established, but consolidation chemotherapy typically consists of a cytarabine-based regimen similar to that used in induction therapy administered over a short-term period. In the 3 US studies comparing cytarabine regimens using either idarubicin or daunorubicin for AML, patients with complete remission of disease following 1 or 2 courses of induction therapy received consolidation chemotherapy including the same anthracycline. Maintenance therapy for AML generally is *not* recommended. In study 2, substantial hematologic toxicity, including 6 deaths from aplasia (5 of which were in those receiving idarubicin), occurred in patients receiving maintenance therapy; as for other anthracyclines, intensive maintenance therapy with idarubicin for AML is *not* recommended.

In addition to the 3 US studies, a multicenter, randomized study similar in design was conducted in Italy. In study 4, a total of 255 patients aged 55–78 years (median age about 62 years) with previously untreated AML received either idarubicin 12 mg/m^2 or daunorubicin 45 mg/m^2 IV daily for 3 days; both groups received cytarabine 100 mg/m^2 daily for 7 days by continuous IV infusion. Patients with a complete remission following 1 or 2 courses of induction therapy received consolidation therapy using the same dose of anthracycline as used in the induction regimen, cytarabine, and thioguanine; consolidation therapy was followed by a maintenance regimen with cytarabine and thioguanine. No difference was found in the rate of complete remissions (40 versus 39%) or median survival (87 versus 169 days) for patients receiving the idarubicin regimen compared with those receiving the daunorubicin regimen. A higher death rate during induction therapy was observed in patients receiving the idarubicin regimen; because this finding was not observed in patients of a similar age in the US studies, a difference in the level of supportive care has been suggested as a possible cause.

Idarubicin has been used in combination with cytarabine for the treatment of recurrent or refractory AML. Various agents are continually being evaluated for the treatment of recurrent AML.

■ **Other Uses** Idarubicin is being investigated as a component of combination regimens for the treatment of acute lymphocytic leukemia†.

Dosage and Administration

■ **Administration** Idarubicin is administered by IV injection. The drug is extremely irritating to tissues and, therefore, must *not* be given IM or subcutaneously. *Care should be taken to avoid extravasation of the drug.*

Idarubicin should be administered slowly (i.e., over 10–15 minutes) into a freely flowing IV infusion of 0.9% sodium chloride or 5% dextrose injection. The tubing for the IV infusion should be attached to a butterfly needle or other suitable device and preferably inserted into a large vein.

Although a stinging or burning sensation may be a symptom of extravasation during IV administration of idarubicin, extravasation may occur without these symptoms and even when blood returns well during initial aspiration of the infusion needle. If signs or symptoms of extravasation occur, administration of the drug should be discontinued immediately and the infusion restarted in another vein. In cases of known or suspected subcutaneous extravasation, intermittent ice packs (immediately for 30 minutes, then 30 minutes 4 times daily for 3 days) should be applied over the affected area and the involved extremity should be elevated. The involved extremity should be examined frequently, and plastic surgery consultation should be obtained promptly upon any sign of a local reaction (i.e., pain, erythema, edema, or vesication). In case of ulceration or severe persistent pain at the site of extravasation, early wide excision of the affected area should be considered.

Caution should be exercised in handling and preparing solutions of idarubicin. Because skin reactions may occur with accidental exposure to the drug, the manufacturer recommends the use of goggles, gloves, and protective gowns during preparation and administration of idarubicin. Skin accidentally exposed to the drug should be washed thoroughly with soap and water, and standard irrigation techniques should be used immediately in the event of eye involvement.

Parenteral idarubicin solutions should be inspected visually for particulate matter and discoloration prior to administration whenever solution and container permit. The manufacturer states that idarubicin should not be mixed with other drugs (unless specific compatibility data are available). Precipitation occurs when the drug is mixed with heparin, and prolonged contact with any alkaline solution will cause degradation of idarubicin.

■ **Dosage** ***Acute Myeloid Leukemia*** For remission induction therapy in patients with acute myeloid leukemia (AML), the recommended dosage of idarubicin is 12 mg/m^2 daily for 3 days by slow IV injection (over 10–15 minutes) in combination with cytarabine. Cytarabine may be administered as 100 mg/m^2 daily by continuous IV infusion for 7 days; this is the cytarabine schedule used in 3 of the 4 randomized trials on which the current indication is based. Cytarabine also has been administered as a 25-mg/m^2 IV loading dose followed by 200 mg/m^2 daily by continuous IV infusion for 5 days. A second induction course may be administered in the event of an incomplete antileukemic response after the first course.

Consolidation chemotherapy was administered to patients in the 3 US studies and the Italian study comparing the use of idarubicin and daunorubicin in the treatment of AML. (See Uses: Acute Myeloid Leukemia.)

Dosage Modification for Toxicity **GI Toxicity.** In patients who experience severe mucositis with the first course of induction therapy with idarubicin, administration of a second course should be delayed until the mucositis resolves, and the dosage of idarubicin should be reduced by 25%.

■ **Dosage in Renal and Hepatic Impairment** Hepatic or renal impairment may affect the disposition of idarubicin. The patient's hepatic and renal function should be evaluated prior to administration of idarubicin, and a dosage reduction should be considered if serum bilirubin and/or creatinine concentrations exceed the normal range. In several phase 3 clinical trials, idarubicin therapy was withheld in patients with serum bilirubin or creatinine concentrations exceeding 2 mg/dL. In one trial, patients with serum bilirubin concentrations of 2.6–5 mg/dL received idarubicin with a 50% reduction in dose. Idarubicin should not be given to patients who have a serum bilirubin concentration exceeding 5 mg/dL.

Cautions

Unless otherwise stated, the incidence of adverse effects reported is derived from data for 110 patients receiving the drug in combination with cytarabine during induction therapy for AML in one randomized clinical trial; these data are representative of the observations in other studies. Because patients receiving induction therapy for AML are seriously ill and are receiving multiple transfusions and concomitant medications, including potentially toxic anti-infective agents, it is difficult to determine the contribution of the study drug to adverse effects. Unless otherwise noted, these adverse effects occurred at a similar rate in patients receiving the daunorubicin regimen as induction therapy for AML.

During induction therapy in 3 US studies, hematologic toxicity, including duration of aplasia, and nonhematologic toxicity, including cardiac toxicity, were similar for the idarubicin and daunorubicin regimens in all 3 studies except for an increase in mucositis in patients receiving idarubicin in one study. During consolidation therapy, a longer duration of aplasia (in all 3 studies) and a higher incidence of mucositis (in 2 studies) were reported in patients receiving the idarubicin regimen. In addition, patients receiving the idarubicin regimen required more transfusions (in 2 studies reporting such data) and a greater number of days of IV anti-infective treatment (in study 3, which used a higher dose of idarubicin).

■ **Hematologic Effects and Infectious Complications** The major dose-limiting adverse effect of idarubicin, bone marrow suppression, occurs in all patients receiving therapeutic doses of the drug for the treatment of AML; myelosuppression also represents the therapeutic effect of the drug that is necessary to eradicate the leukemic clone. Deaths secondary to infection and/or bleeding have occurred in patients receiving idarubicin. Hemorrhage occurred in 63% of patients receiving idarubicin. In all 3 US studies comparing the idarubicin and daunorubicin regimens for AML, a longer duration of aplasia was reported during consolidation therapy in patients receiving idarubicin.

Infections occurred in 95% of patients receiving idarubicin. During consolidation therapy, the incidence and severity of infection was greater in patients receiving idarubicin compared with daunorubicin.

■ **Cardiac Effects** The incidence of adverse cardiac effects did not differ significantly for patients receiving idarubicin versus daunorubicin. Adverse cardiac effects were reported in 16% of patients receiving idarubicin versus 24% of patients receiving daunorubicin as a component of induction therapy for AML; such clinical myocardial toxicity was severe or life-threatening in 11% of those receiving idarubicin and in 21% of those receiving daunorubicin. Although data from animal studies suggest that idarubicin has reduced cardiotoxicity compared with daunorubicin and doxorubicin, no difference in cardiotoxicity was observed between idarubicin and daunorubicin during induction therapy for AML in the 3 US studies.

Myocardial toxicity associated with idarubicin was manifested by potentially fatal congestive heart failure (often attributed to fluid overload), acute life-threatening arrhythmias including atrial fibrillation, myocardial infarction, chest pain, asymptomatic decreases in left ventricular ejection fraction, or other cardiomyopathies. Cardiac insufficiency and arrhythmias generally were reversible and usually occurred in the setting of sepsis, anemia, and aggressive IV fluid administration. Adverse cardiac effects occurred more frequently in patients older than 60 years and in those with preexisting cardiac disease. Appropriate therapeutic measures for the management of congestive heart failure and/or arrhythmias should be used as clinically indicated. As with other anthracyclines, cardiac function should be monitored carefully in patients receiving idarubicin, particularly those at increased risk for myocardial toxicity.

For information on risk factors and monitoring for cardiotoxicity associated with idarubicin, see Precautions and Contraindications: Cardiac Toxicity. For additional information on the cardiotoxicity of anthracyclines, see Cautions: Cardiac Effects in Doxorubicin Hydrochloride 10:00.

■ **GI Effects** Adverse GI effects, including nausea and/or vomiting (82%), abdominal pain and/or diarrhea (73%), and mucositis (50%), have been reported frequently but were severe (equivalent to WHO grade 4 toxicity) in less than 5% of patients receiving idarubicin. The incidence of mucositis was higher in patients receiving the idarubicin regimen than in those receiving the daunorubicin regimen, especially during the consolidation treatment phase, in some US controlled trials.

Severe enterocolitis with perforation has been reported rarely in patients receiving the drug. (See Precautions and Contraindications: Other Precautions and Contraindications.).

■ **Dermatologic Effects** Alopecia occurs in about 77% of patients receiving idarubicin. Skin reactions, including generalized rash, urticaria, and a bullous erythematous rash of the palms and soles, occur in 46% of patients receiving the drug. Dermatologic reactions occurring in patients receiving idarubicin usually have been attributed to concomitant anti-infective therapy. Radiation recall reactions at the site of prior radiation therapy also have been reported in patients receiving idarubicin.

■ **Hepatic Effects** Changes in liver function test results have been reported in patients treated with idarubicin; these changes usually were transient and tended to occur in patients with sepsis who were receiving potentially hepatotoxic anti-infective agents. Severe changes in hepatic function (equivalent to WHO grade 4 toxicity) occurred in less than 5% of patients receiving idarubicin.

■ **Renal Effects** Alterations in renal function test results have been reported in patients treated with idarubicin; these changes usually were transient and tended to occur in patients with sepsis who were receiving potentially nephrotoxic anti-infective agents. Severe changes in renal function (equivalent to WHO grade 4 toxicity) occurred in 1% or less of patients receiving idarubicin.

■ **Local Effects** Extravasation of idarubicin can cause severe tissue necrosis. Other adverse local effects, including urticaria, hives, and erythematous streaking, also have been reported with idarubicin. For information on the management of extravasation of idarubicin, see Dosage and Administration: Administration.

■ **Nervous System Effects** Mental status changes, headache, peripheral neuropathy, seizures, and cerebellar abnormalities were reported in 41, 20, 7, 4, and 4%, respectively, of patients receiving idarubicin.

■ **Respiratory Effects** Adverse pulmonary effects have been reported in 39% of patients receiving idarubicin. Allergy-related pulmonary symptoms occurred in 2% of patients.

■ **Other Adverse Effects** Fever (not classified elsewhere) was reported in 26% of patients receiving idarubicin.

■ **Precautions and Contraindications** Idarubicin is a toxic drug with a low therapeutic index, and a therapeutic response is not likely to occur without evidence of toxicity. The drug must be used only under the supervision of clinicians experienced in the use of cytotoxic agents for leukemia therapy and only when the potential benefits of idarubicin therapy are thought to outweigh the possible risks. Close observation of the patient and careful laboratory monitoring are required; in addition, appropriate diagnostic and treatment facilities must be readily available in case the patient develops severe hemorrhagic conditions, infection, or other drug toxicity.

Hematologic Toxicity Idarubicin causes severe and sometimes fatal hematologic toxicity and generally should not be used in patients with preexisting bone marrow suppression caused by previous drug or radiation therapy unless the potential benefit outweighs the risk. Because idarubicin therapy causes severe myelosuppression which can lead to potentially fatal infection and/or bleeding (see Cautions: Hematologic Effects and Infectious Complications), complete blood cell counts should be monitored regularly during idarubicin therapy.

Cardiac Toxicity The potential benefit of idarubicin therapy must be weighed carefully against the risk of anthracycline-associated cardiotoxicity. The risk of idarubicin-induced cardiovascular toxicity is greater in patients who are older than 60 years of age, who have preexisting cardiac disease, or who have received prior therapy with anthracyclines or other cardiotoxic agents; the risk of cardiac toxicity also may be increased in patients with concomitant or previous radiation therapy to the mediastinal-pericardial area or in patients with anemia, bone marrow suppression, infections, or leukemic pericarditis and/or myocarditis.

The risk of anthracycline-induced cardiotoxicity increases with increasing dose; a cumulative dose of idarubicin beyond which the incidence of cardiotoxicity rapidly increases has not been determined. However, retrospective analysis of data from 115 evaluable patients (median age: 40 years, range: 13–82 years) receiving a median cumulative dose of idarubicin 96 mg/m^2 with a median follow-up of 225 days following the last dose of idarubicin suggests that the risk of congestive heart failure is low for cumulative idarubicin doses up to 150 mg/m^2 in patients with no risk factors for cardiac toxicity.

Cardiac function should be monitored carefully during idarubicin therapy. While there are no reliable methods for predicting which patients will develop congestive heart failure, anthracyline-induced cardiomyopathy usually is associated with a decrease in left ventricular ejection fraction from pretreatment baseline values.

For additional information on the cardiotoxicity of anthracyclines, see Cardiac Effects and also Precautions and Contraindications, under Cautions in Doxorubicin Hydrochloride 10.00.

Other Precautions and Contraindications Appropriate measures should be taken to prevent the occurrence of hyperuricemia related to the rapid lysis of leukemic cells. Any systemic infections should be treated before the initiation of idarubicin therapy.

Instrumental intervention may increase the risk of perforation in patients experiencing severe enterocolitis associated with idarubicin, and patients developing severe abdominal pain should be evaluated for the possibility of perforation.

Because hepatic or renal impairment may affect the disposition of idarubicin, hepatic and renal function should be evaluated before initiation of idarubicin therapy, and a dosage reduction should be considered if serum bilirubin and/or creatinine concentrations are elevated. Idarubicin is contraindicated in patients who have a serum bilirubin concentration exceeding 5 mg/dL; in some clinical trials, idarubicin therapy was not initiated if serum bilirubin and/or creatinine concentration exceeded 2 mg/dL. Changes in renal and hepatic function test results have been observed in patients receiving idarubicin, and frequent monitoring of these tests is recommended.

■ **Pediatric Precautions** Safety and efficacy of idarubicin in children have not been established. Although the drug has been used in induction therapy for children with acute myeloid leukemia, the efficacy and safety of idarubicin compared with the commonly used anthracycline daunorubicin have not been established.

■ **Geriatric Precautions** The risk of cardiovascular toxicity associated with idarubicin is greater in geriatric patients. Patients 60 years of age or older receiving induction therapy containing idarubicin experienced adverse cardiac effects, including congestive heart failure, serious arrhythmias, chest pain, myocardial infarction, and asymptomatic declines in left ventricular ejection fraction, more frequently than younger patients.

The difference in the rate of complete remission between idarubicin and daunorubicin appears to decrease with increasing age. (See Uses: Acute Myeloid Leukemia.)

■ **Mutagenicity and Carcinogenicity** Formal long-term studies to evaluate the carcinogenicity of idarubicin have not been performed to date. Mutagenic and carcinogenic properties of idarubicin and related compounds have been demonstrated in tests conducted in experimental models (including bacterial systems, mammalian cells in culture, and rats).

■ **Pregnancy, Fertility, and Lactation** Idarubicin can cause fetal toxicity when administered to pregnant women, but potential benefits may be acceptable in certain conditions despite possible risks to the fetus. A case of a human fetal death following maternal exposure to idarubicin during the second trimester of pregnancy has been reported. When administered to rats at a dosage of 1.2 mg/m^2 daily (equivalent to one-tenth the recommended human dosage), the drug was embryotoxic and teratogenic; this dosage was not toxic to dams. The drug was embryotoxic but not teratogenic in rabbits receiving 2.4 mg/m^2 daily (equivalent to one-fifth the recommended human dosage), a dosage which was toxic to dams.

Adequate, well-controlled studies in pregnant women have not been conducted. Idarubicin should be used during pregnancy only in life-threatening situations or severe disease for which safer drugs cannot be used or are ineffective. When the drug is administered during pregnancy or if the patient becomes pregnant while receiving the drug, the patient should be informed of the potential hazard to the fetus. Women of childbearing potential who are treated with idarubicin should be advised to avoid pregnancy. Men receiving idarubicin should be advised to use barrier contraception.

Studies have not been conducted to date to determine whether idarubicin affects fertility in males or females. When administered in male dogs at a dosage of 1.8 mg/m^2 daily 3 times per week (approximately one-seventh the recommended human dosage on a mg/m^2 basis) for 13 weeks (3 times the total human dose), idarubicin caused testicular atrophy and inhibition of spermatogenesis and sperm maturation resulting in few or no mature sperm; these effects were not readily reversible following an 8-week recovery period.

It is not known whether idarubicin or its metabolites are distributed into milk. Because of the potential for serious adverse reactions to idarubicin in nursing infants, nursing should be discontinued prior to idarubicin therapy.

Drug Interactions

Formal studies of drug interactions with idarubicin have not been performed to date.

Acute Toxicity

Two cases of fatal overdosage of idarubicin have been reported to date in patients receiving idarubicin 135 mg/m^2 over 3 days, or idarubicin 45 mg/m^2 and daunorubicin 90 mg/m^2 over 3 days. Manifestations of idarubicin overdosage may include severe, prolonged myelosuppression, acute cardiac toxicity or delayed cardiac failure, and possibly increased severity of GI toxicity. Severe arrhythmia was reported in one of the cases of fatal idarubicin overdose. In case of idarubicin overdose, appropriate supportive care, including platelet tranfusions, anti-infectives, and symptomatic treatment of mucositis, should be instituted. There is no known antidote to idarubicin, and it is considered unlikely that the drug is removed by conventional peritoneal dialysis or hemodialysis.

Pharmacology

Although the exact mechanism(s) of action has not been fully elucidated, idarubicin is a DNA-reactive agent. Idarubicin is thought to cause cytotoxicity by intercalation of the drug into DNA and/or inhibition of the enzyme topoisomerase II, resulting in disruption of nucleic acid synthesis.

Pharmacokinetics

■ **Absorption** Although an oral dosage form is not commercially available, idarubicin is known to be rapidly absorbed from the GI tract following oral administration; in contrast, other anthracyclines (i.e., doxorubicin, daunorubicin) are not absorbed to any appreciable extent following oral administration. Bioavailability varies widely in patients receiving oral idarubicin.

■ **Distribution** When administered by IV injection, idarubicin hydrochloride is rapidly and widely distributed in tissues and has a large volume of distribution. Measurement of idarubicin concentrations in nucleated blood and bone marrow cells in patients with leukemia has demonstrated that peak cellular idarubicin concentrations occur within a few minutes following IV injection. Concentrations of idarubicin and idarubicinol (the principal active metabolite of idarubicin) in nucleated blood and bone marrow cells exceed plasma concentrations by more than 100 times. The rate of disappearance of idarubicin was similar in plasma and cells, with a terminal half-life of approximately 15 hours. The terminal half-life of idarubicinol in cells was about 72 hours. The expected extent of drug and metabolite accumulation on days 2 and 3 of dosing is 1.7- and 2.3-fold, respectively, and no change is expected in the disposition of idarubicin during a 3-day dosing regimen.

At concentrations similar to the maximum plasma concentrations measured in pharmacokinetic studies, the extent of protein binding averaged 97 and 94% for idarubicin and idarubicinol, respectively. Protein binding of idarubicin and idarubicinol is not concentration dependent.

The distribution of idarubicin and idarubicinol into CSF has been studied in pediatric patients with leukemia receiving idarubicin on a schedule of once weekly for 3 weeks or once daily for 3 days every 3 weeks. Idarubicin (concentration 0.14 and 1.57 ng/mL) was detected in 2 of 21 CSF samples and idarubicinol (mean concentration 0.51 ng/mL; range, 0.22–1.05 ng/mL) was detected in 20 of the 21 samples; the clinical importance of these findings is unclear.

It is not known whether idarubicin or its metabolites are distributed into milk.

■ **Elimination** The pharmacokinetics of idarubicin have been evaluated in adult patients with leukemia and normal renal and hepatic function following IV administration of 10–12 mg/m² idarubicin daily for 3–4 days alone or in combination with cytarabine. The decline in plasma concentrations of idarubicin is best described by a 2- or 3-compartment open pharmacokinetic model. Elimination of idarubicin is slow, with an estimated mean terminal half-life of 22 hours (range: 4–48 hours) when given as a single agent and 20 hours (range: 7–38 hours) when administered in combination with cytarabine.

Idarubicin is metabolized by the enzyme aldoketoreductase to idarubicinol, the principal active metabolite, which has in vitro antitumor activity similar to idarubicin. The plasma clearance of idarubicin is about twice the expected hepatic blood flow, indicating extensive extrahepatic metabolism. Idarubicinol is eliminated more slowly than the parent drug, with an estimated mean elimination half-life exceeding 45 hours. Detectable plasma concentrations of idarubicinol are present for more than 8 days following IV administration of idarubicin. Idarubicin is excreted principally in bile; renal excretion (mostly as the metabolite idarubicinol) also plays a role.

The pharmacokinetics of idarubicin have been studied in pediatric patients with leukemia and appear to be linear. When idarubicin was administered IV at doses of 4.2–13.3 mg/m² per day, no difference in half-life was observed between daily and weekly administration (with 3 repeated doses for both regimens).

The pharmacokinetics of idarubicin in patients with hepatic and/or renal impairment have not been fully evaluated. The metabolism of idarubicin may be impaired in patients with moderate or severe hepatic dysfunction. Renal impairment also may affect the disposition of idarubicin.

Chemistry and Stability

■ **Chemistry** Idarubicin hydrochloride, a semisynthetic anthracycline, is an antineoplastic agent. The drug is structurally and pharmacologically related to the anthracycline daunorubicin. Idarubicin differs from daunorubicin in that idarubicin contains a hydrogen atom instead of a methoxy group at the 4-position of the D ring of the aglycone. Idarubicin has greater lipophilicity and consequently undergoes more rapid cellular uptake compared with other anthracyclines; these properties may result from the absence of the methoxy group.

Commercially available idarubicin hydrochloride injection occurs as a sterile, red-orange, isotonic, preservative-free solution. Hydrochloric acid is used to adjust the pH to 3.5.

■ **Stability** Idarubicin hydrochloride injection should be refrigerated at 2–8°C and protected from light. Vials of the injection should remain in the original package until immediately prior to use.

The manufacturer recommends that idarubicin generally *not* be mixed with other drugs; specialized references should be consulted for specific compatibility information. Precipitation occurs when the drug is mixed with heparin, and prolonged contact with any alkaline solution will cause degradation of the drug.

For further information on the handling of antineoplastic agents, see the ASHP Guidelines on Handling Hazardous Drugs at http://www.ahfsdruginformation.com.

Preparations

Excipients in commercially available drug preparations may have clinically important effects in some individuals; consult specific product labeling for details.

IDArubicin Hydrochloride

Parenteral

Injection, for IV infusion	1 mg/mL*	**Idamycin PFS®**, Pfizer **Idarubicin Hydrochloride Injection**

*available from one or more manufacturer, distributor, and/or repackager by generic (nonproprietary) name

†Use is not currently included in the labeling approved by the US Food and Drug Administration

Idelalisib

■ Idelalisib, an inhibitor of phosphoinositide 3-kinase isoform delta (PI3Kδ), is an antineoplastic agent.

REMS

FDA approved a REMS for idelalisib to ensure that the benefits outweigh the risks. The REMS may apply to one or more preparations of idelalisib and consists of the following: communication plan. See the FDA REMS page (https://www.accessdata.fda.gov/scripts/cder/rems/index.cfm).

Uses

■ **Chronic Lymphocytic Leukemia** Idelalisib is used in combination with rituximab for the treatment of relapsed chronic lymphocytic leukemia (CLL) in patients in whom monotherapy with rituximab would be considered appropriate therapy due to other comorbidities; idelalisib is designated an orphan drug by the US Food and Drug Administration (FDA) for the treatment of this cancer.

The current indication for idelalisib in the treatment of relapsed CLL is based principally on the results of a randomized, double-blind, placebo-controlled phase 3 study in adults with relapsed CLL who were unable to tolerate standard chemotherapy because of coexisting medical conditions, impaired renal function (creatinine clearance less than 60 mL/minute), and/or severe myelosuppression (grade 3 or higher neutropenia or thrombocytopenia) resulting from prior therapy with cytotoxic agents. In this study, 220 patients were randomized in a 1:1 ratio to receive either idelalisib (150 mg orally twice daily) in combination with rituximab (375 mg/m² administered by IV infusion initially, followed by 500 mg/m² by IV infusion every 2 weeks for 4 doses and then every 4 weeks for an additional 3 doses, for a total of 8 doses) or placebo in combination with rituximab. Patients received idelalisib until disease progression or unacceptable toxicity occurred. The primary end point of this study was progression-free survival as assessed by an independent review committee; secondary end points included overall survival, overall response rate, and lymph node response. The median age of patients was 71 years. Patients enrolled in the study had received a median of 3 prior therapies; the majority (96%) of patients had received previous treatment with an anti-CD20 monoclonal antibody. Approximately 45% of patients had previously received rituximab in combination with bendamustine, 34% received rituximab in combination with fludarabine and cyclophosphamide, 31% received single-agent rituximab, 17% received rituximab in combination with fludarabine, and 16% received chlorambucil.

This study was terminated prematurely at the request of the Independent Data Monitoring Committee because of improved progression-free survival observed during the first pre-specified interim analysis in patients receiving idelalisib in combination with rituximab. At the time of the second interim analysis, the progression-free survival benefit observed in patients receiving idelalisib in combination with rituximab remained statistically significant, although the median duration of progression-free survival had not yet been reached; the median progression-free survival in patients receiving placebo in combination with rituximab was 5.5 months. The overall response rate was 81% for patients receiving idelalisib in combination with rituximab and 13% for those receiving placebo in combination with rituximab; there were no complete responses in either group. Median overall survival had not been reached at the time of the interim analysis.

■ **Follicular B-cell Non-Hodgkin's Lymphoma** Idelalisib is used for the treatment of relapsed follicular B-cell non-Hodgkin's lymphoma (NHL) in patients who previously received at least 2 systemic therapies; idelalisib is designated an orphan drug by FDA for the treatment of this cancer. Labeling for use of idelalisib for the treatment of relapsed follicular B-cell NHL was approved under the principles and procedures of FDA's accelerated review process that allows approval based on analysis of surrogate markers of response. As a result of the accelerated review, labeling of idelalisib for the treatment of relapsed follicular B-cell NHL was based on improvement in objective response rate; clinical benefit (e.g., improvement in survival, amelioration of disease-related symptoms) has not been established. Continued approval for this indication may be contingent on verification of clinical benefit in confirmatory studies.

The current indication for idelalisib in the treatment of relapsed follicular B-cell NHL is based principally on the results of a multicenter, single-arm study in 72 adults with follicular B-cell NHL who previously received at least 2 systemic therapies and whose disease had relapsed within 6 months following therapy with rituximab and an alkylating agent. In this study, all patients received idelalisib 150 mg orally twice daily until disease progression or unacceptable toxicity occurred. The primary end point was overall response rate as assessed by an independent review committee. The median age of patients was 62 years; 92% of patients had a baseline ECOG performance status of 0 or 1. Patients enrolled in the study had received a median of 4 prior therapies. Approximately 49% of patients had previously received rituximab in combination with cyclophosphamide, doxorubicin, vincristine, and prednisone (CHOP); 50% received rituximab in combination with bendamustine; and 28% received rituximab in combination with cyclophosphamide, vincristine, and prednisone (CVP). Approximately 33% of patients had extranodal involvement, and 26% had bone marrow involvement. At the time of data analysis, the overall response rate was 54% (8% complete and 46% partial responses). The median duration of response was not evaluable; however, median time to response was 1.9 months.

■ **Small Lymphocytic Lymphoma** Idelalisib is used for the treatment of relapsed small lymphocytic lymphoma (SLL) in patients who previously received at least 2 systemic therapies; idelalisib is designated an orphan drug by FDA for the treatment of this cancer. Labeling for use of idelalisib for the treatment of relapsed SLL was approved under the principles and procedures of FDA's accelerated review process that allows approval based on analysis of surrogate markers of response. As a result of the accelerated review, labeling of idelalisib for the treatment of relapsed SLL was based on improvement in objective response rate; clinical benefit (e.g., improvement in survival, amelioration of disease-related symptoms) has not been established. Continued approval for this indication may be contingent on verification of clinical benefit in confirmatory studies.

The current indication for idelalisib in the treatment of relapsed SLL is based principally on the results of a multicenter, single-arm study in 26 adults with SLL who previously received at least 2 systemic therapies and whose disease had relapsed within 6 months of therapy with rituximab and an alkylating agent. In this study, all patients received idelalisib 150 mg orally twice daily until disease progression or unacceptable toxicity occurred. The primary end point was overall response rate as assessed by an independent review committee. The median age of patients was 65 years; 96% of patients had a baseline ECOG performance status of 0 or 1. Patients enrolled in the study had received a median of 4 prior therapies for their disease. Approximately 81% of patients had previously received rituximab in combination with bendamustine; 62% received rituximab with fludarabine and cyclophosphamide; and 35% received rituximab in combination with cyclophosphamide, doxorubicin, vincristine, and prednisone (CHOP). Approximately 27% of patients had extranodal involvement. At the time of data analysis, the overall response rate was 58%; there were no complete responses. The estimated median duration of response of 11.9 months, and median time to response was 1.9 months.

Dosage and Administration

■ **General** Liver function tests should be monitored prior to initiation of idelalisib, every 2 weeks during the first 3 months of therapy, every 4 weeks during the next 3 months, and then every 1–3 months thereafter. More frequent monitoring is recommended in patients who develop elevated serum aminotransferase or bilirubin concentrations during therapy. (See Hepatotoxicity under Dosage and Administration: Dosage Modification for Toxicity.)

Complete blood cell counts (CBC) should be monitored at least every 2 weeks during the first 3 months of therapy. More frequent monitoring is recommended in patients who develop myelosuppression during therapy. (See Myelosuppression under Dosage and Administration: Dosage Modification for Toxicity.)

Because idelalisib may cause hepatotoxicity or severe diarrhea, the manufacturer states that concomitant use of idelalisib with drugs that may cause hepatotoxicity or diarrhea should be avoided. (See Hepatotoxicity and also Diarrhea or Colitis under Warnings/Precautions: Warnings, in Cautions.)

■ **Administration** Idelalisib is administered orally without regard to meals. Idelalisib tablets should be swallowed whole.

■ **Dosage** *Chronic Lymphocytic Leukemia* For the treatment of relapsed chronic lymphocytic leukemia (CLL) in patients in whom monotherapy with rituximab would be considered appropriate therapy due to other comorbidities, the recommended maximum initial dosage of idelalisib in adults is 150 mg twice daily in combination with rituximab. Therapy should be continued until disease progression or unacceptable toxicity occurs. The manufacturer states that safety and efficacy of idelalisib beyond several months of therapy have not been established; in the phase 3 study in patients with relapsed CLL, the median duration of exposure to idelalisib was 5 months.

Follicular B-cell Non-Hodgkin's Lymphoma For the treatment of relapsed follicular B-cell non-Hodgkin's lymphoma (NHL) in patients who previously received at least 2 systemic therapies, the recommended maximum initial dosage of idelalisib in adults is 150 mg twice daily. Therapy should be continued until disease progression or unacceptable toxicity occurs. The manufacturer states that safety and efficacy of idelalisib beyond several months of therapy have not been established; in the single-arm study in patients with follicular B-cell NHL, the median duration of exposure to idelalisib was 6.1 months.

Small Lymphocytic Lymphoma For the treatment of relapsed small lymphocytic lymphoma (SLL) in patients who previously received at least 2 systemic therapies, the recommended maximum initial dosage of idelalisib in adults is 150 mg twice daily. Therapy should be continued until disease progression or unacceptable toxicity occurs. The manufacturer states that safety and efficacy of idelalisib beyond several months of therapy have not been established.

■ **Dosage Modification for Toxicity** Temporary interruption of therapy, dosage reduction, and/or permanent discontinuance of idelalisib may be necessary in patients who develop severe hepatotoxicity, diarrhea, or myelosuppression.

In patients experiencing other severe or life-threatening toxicities, therapy with idelalisib should be withheld until the toxicity has resolved. If clinically appropriate, idelalisib therapy may be resumed at a reduced dosage of 100 mg twice daily. If severe or life-threatening toxicities recur at a dosage of 100 mg twice daily, treatment with idelalisib should be permanently discontinued.

Hepatotoxicity In patients who exhibit increases in serum aminotransferase (ALT and/or AST) concentrations exceeding 3 up to 5 times the upper limit of normal (ULN) or bilirubin concentrations exceeding 1.5 up to 3 times the ULN, idelalisib therapy may be continued at the same dosage. Liver function tests should be monitored at least weekly until ALT, AST, and bilirubin concentrations return to within normal limits.

In patients who exhibit increases in ALT and/or AST concentrations exceeding 5 up to 20 times the ULN or bilirubin concentrations exceeding 3 up to 10 times the ULN, therapy with idelalisib should be withheld, and liver function tests should be monitored at least weekly. When ALT, AST, and bilirubin concentrations return to within normal limits, idelalisib therapy may be resumed at a reduced dosage of 100 mg twice daily.

In patients who exhibit increases in ALT and/or AST concentrations exceeding 20 times the ULN or bilirubin concentrations exceeding 10 times the ULN, therapy with idelalisib should be permanently discontinued.

Diarrhea In patients with moderate diarrhea (4–6 stools per day over baseline), idelalisib therapy may be continued at the same dosage; patients should be monitored at least weekly until diarrhea resolves.

In patients with severe diarrhea (7 or more stools per day over baseline) or diarrhea requiring hospitalization, therapy with idelalisib should be withheld, and patients should be monitored at least weekly. When diarrhea resolves, idelalisib therapy may be resumed at a reduced dosage of 100 mg twice daily.

In patients with life-threatening diarrhea, therapy with idelalisib should be permanently discontinued.

Myelosuppression In patients with absolute neutrophil counts (ANC) of 1000/mm^3 to less than 1500/mm^3 or platelet counts of 50,000/mm^3 to less than 75,000/mm^3, idelalisib therapy may be continued at the same dosage.

In patients with ANC of 500/mm^3 to less than 1000/mm^3 or platelet counts of 25,000/mm^3 to less than 50,000/mm^3, therapy with idelalisib may be continued at the same dosage; ANC and platelet counts should be monitored at least weekly.

In patients with ANC less than 500/mm^3 or platelet counts less than 25,000/mm^3, therapy with idelalisib should be withheld, and ANC and platelet counts should be monitored at least weekly. When ANC reaches or exceeds 500/mm^3 or platelet counts reach or exceed 25,000/mm^3, idelalisib may be resumed at a reduced dosage of 100 mg twice daily.

■ **Special Populations** The manufacturer makes no specific dosage recommendations for patients with preexisting hepatic impairment; however, such patients should be monitored for signs of toxicity, and dosage of idelalisib should be adjusted as appropriate. (See Hepatotoxicity under Dosage and Administration: Dosage Modifications for Toxicity and also see Hepatic Impairment under Warnings/Precautions: Specific Populations, in Cautions.)

No dosage adjustment is necessary in patients with creatinine clearance of 15 mL/minute or greater. (See Renal Impairment under Warnings/Precautions: Specific Populations, in Cautions.)

The manufacturer makes no specific dosage recommendations for geriatric patients. (See Geriatric Use under Warnings/Precautions: Specific Populations, in Cautions.)

Cautions

■ **Contraindications** Idelalisib is contraindicated in patients with a history of serious hypersensitivity reactions, including anaphylaxis and toxic epidermal necrolysis.

■ **Warnings/Precautions** *Warnings* **Hepatotoxicity.** Serious and/or fatal hepatotoxicity has been reported in 14% of patients receiving idelalisib. Elevations in aminotransferase (ALT or AST) concentrations exceeding 5 times the upper limit of normal (ULN) have occurred in patients receiving idelalisib. These elevations generally occurred during the initial 12 weeks of therapy; in the phase 3 study evaluating safety and efficacy of idelalisib in combination with rituximab in patients with relapsed chronic lymphocytic leukemia (CLL), elevations in ALT or AST concentrations occurred at a median of 93 or 92 days, respectively. Elevations in ALT or AST concentrations were reversible following temporary interruption of idelalisib therapy; however following resumption of therapy at a reduced dosage, recurrence of ALT and AST elevations was reported in 26% of patients.

Serum ALT and AST concentrations should be evaluated prior to initiation of therapy, every 2 weeks during the first 3 months of therapy, every 4 weeks during the next 3 months, and then every 1–3 months thereafter. If hepatotoxicity occurs, liver function tests should be monitored more frequently until levels return to within normal limits. Temporary interruption of therapy, dosage reduction, and/or permanent discontinuance of idelalisib may be necessary depending on the severity of hepatotoxicity. (See Hepatotoxicity under Dosage and Administration: Dosage Modification for Toxicity.) If ALT and/or AST concentrations increase to >20 times the ULN or bilirubin concentrations increase to >10 times the ULN, idelalisib therapy should be permanently discontinued. Idelalisib therapy also should be discontinued if hepatotoxicity recurs.

Concomitant use of idelalisib with drugs that may cause hepatotoxicity should be avoided.

Diarrhea or Colitis. Severe (grade 3 or greater) diarrhea or colitis has been reported in 14% of patients receiving idelalisib in clinical studies. Diarrhea can occur at any time and responds poorly to antimotility agents. Diarrhea resolves within a median of 1 week to 1 month following temporary interruption of idelalisib therapy and, in some instances, use of corticosteroids.

Patients receiving idelalisib should be monitored for the development of severe diarrhea or colitis. If moderate or severe diarrhea occurs, patients should be monitored at least weekly until diarrhea resolves. Temporary interruption of therapy, dosage reduction, and/or permanent discontinuance of idelalisib may be necessary depending on the severity of diarrhea. (See Diarrhea under Dosage and Administration: Dosage Modification for Toxicity.) If life-threatening diarrhea occurs, therapy with idelalisib should be permanently discontinued.

Concomitant use of idelalisib with drugs that may cause diarrhea should be avoided.

Intestinal Perforation. Severe or fatal intestinal perforation has been reported in patients receiving idelalisib. At the time of perforation, some patients had moderate to severe diarrhea. Idelalisib should be permanently discontinued if intestinal perforation occurs. (See Advice to Patients.)

Pneumonitis. Serious or fatal pneumonitis has been reported in patients receiving idelalisib.

Patients receiving idelalisib who present with pulmonary manifestations (e.g., cough, dyspnea, hypoxia, interstitial infiltrates on radiologic exam, a greater than 5% decrease in oxygen saturation) should be evaluated for pneumonitis. If pneumonitis is suspected, idelalisib therapy should be interrupted until the etiology of the pulmonary symptoms has been determined. Treatment for idelalisib-induced pneumonitis has included discontinuance of idelalisib and administration of corticosteroids.

Sensitivity Reactions Serious hypersensitivity reactions, including anaphylaxis, have been reported in patients receiving idelalisib. Idelalisib should be permanently discontinued, and supportive treatment instituted, in patients who experience a severe hypersensitivity reaction.

Other Warnings and Precautions **Dermatologic Effects.** Severe (grade 3 or greater) or life-threatening dermatologic reactions, including exfoliative dermatitis, rash (i.e., erythematous, generalized, macular, maculopapular, papular, pruritic, and exfoliative rash), and toxic skin reactions have been reported in patients receiving idelalisib. Toxic epidermal necrolysis has been reported in at least one patient receiving idelalisib in combination with rituximab and bendamustine in a clinical trial. Patients receiving idelalisib should be monitored for development of severe dermatologic reactions. If severe dermatologic reactions occur, idelalisib should be discontinued.

Neutropenia. Severe (grade 3 or 4) neutropenia has been reported in 31% of patients receiving idelalisib in clinical studies. Complete blood cell counts (CBC) should be monitored at least every 2 weeks during the first 3 months of therapy. If absolute neutrophil count (ANC) decreases to less than 1000/mm^3, CBCs should be monitored more frequently. Temporary interruption of idelalisib therapy followed by dosage reduction may be necessary depending on the severity of neutropenia. (See Myelosuppression under Dosage and Administration: Dosage Modification for Toxicity.)

Fetal/Neonatal Morbidity and Mortality. Idelalisib may cause fetal harm if administered to pregnant women; teratogenicity and embryofetal toxicity have been demonstrated in animals receiving idelalisib at dosages equivalent to 12–30 times the human exposure at the recommended dosage. Pregnancy should be avoided during therapy and for at least 1 month after drug discontinuance. (See Advice to Patients.) If idelalisib is used during pregnancy or if the patient becomes pregnant while receiving the drug, the patient should be apprised of the potential fetal hazard.

Specific Populations **Pregnancy.** Category D. (See Users Guide and see Fetal/Neonatal Morbidity and Mortality under Warnings/Precautions: Other Warnings and Precautions, in Cautions.)

Lactation. It is not known whether idelalisib is distributed into milk in humans. Because of the potential for serious adverse reactions to idelalisib in nursing infants, a decision should be made whether to discontinue nursing or the drug, taking into account the importance of the drug to the woman.

Pediatric Use. Safety and efficacy of idelalisib have not been established in pediatric patients younger than 18 years of age.

Geriatric Use. In clinical studies evaluating idelalisib in patients with relapsed CLL, follicular B-cell non-Hodgkin's lymphoma (NHL), and small lymphocytic lymphoma (SLL), 63% of patients were 65 years of age or older. No differences in efficacy were observed between geriatric patients and younger adults. However, patients 65 years of age or older with CLL or NHL had higher incidences of serious adverse reactions, death, or discontinuance of idelalisib due to adverse reactions compared with younger adults. (See Dosage and Administration: Special Populations.)

Hepatic Impairment. Systemic exposure of idelalisib is increased up to 1.7-fold in individuals with ALT, AST, or bilirubin concentrations above the ULN compared with individuals with normal hepatic function. Patients with preexisting hepatic impairment should be monitored for signs of toxicity during idelalisib therapy. (See Dosage and Administration: Special Populations.)

Safety and efficacy of idelalisib have not been established in patients with baseline ALT or AST concentrations exceeding 2.5 times the ULN or bilirubin concentrations exceeding 1.5 times the ULN because these patients were excluded from clinical studies of the drug.

Renal Impairment. Systemic exposure of idelalisib was unaffected following administration of a single 150-mg dose of idelalisib in patients with severe renal impairment (creatinine clearance of 15–29 mL/minute). (See Dosage and Administration: Special Populations.)

■ **Common Adverse Effects** Adverse effects reported in 5% or more of patients with relapsed chronic lymphocytic leukemia (CLL) receiving idelalisib in combination with rituximab and occurring at an incidence that is at least 2% higher than that reported with placebo in combination with rituximab include pyrexia, nausea, pneumonia, diarrhea, chills, rash, vomiting, decreased appetite, night sweats, headache, sepsis, sinusitis, pain, arthralgia, gastroesophageal reflux disease (GERD), stomatitis, bronchitis, nasal congestion, and urinary tract infection. Laboratory abnormalities reported in 10% or more of patients with relapsed CLL receiving idelalisib in combination with rituximab and at an incidence that is at least 5% higher than that reported with placebo in combination with rituximab include neutropenia, hypertriglyceridemia, hyperglycemia, elevated aminotransferase (ALT or AST) and γ-glutamyltransferase ([gamma]-glutamyltranspeptidase, GGT, GGTP) concentrations, decreased or increased lymphocyte count, hyponatremia, and hypoglycemia.

Adverse effects reported in 10% or more of patients receiving idelalisib alone for the treatment of indolent non-Hodgkin's lymphoma (NHL) include diarrhea, fatigue, nausea, cough, pyrexia, abdominal pain, pneumonia, rash, dyspnea, decreased appetite, vomiting, asthenia, upper respiratory tract infection, night sweats, insomnia, headache, and peripheral edema. Laboratory abnormalities reported in more than 20% of patients receiving idelalisib alone for the treatment of indolent NHL include neutropenia, elevated aminotransferase (ALT or AST) concentrations, decreased hemoglobin concentrations, and thrombocytopenia.

Drug Interactions

Idelalisib is metabolized by aldehyde oxidase, cytochrome P-450 (CYP) isoenzyme 3A, and, to a lesser extent, uridine diphosphate-glucuronosyl transferase (UGT) 1A4.

In vitro, idelalisib is a substrate of CYP3A, aldehyde oxidase, and UGT1A4. Idelalisib inhibits CYP isoenzymes 2C8, 2C19 and 3A, and its major metabolite (GS-563117) inhibits CYP isoenzymes 2C8, 2C9, 2C19, and 3A. Idelalisib and GS-563117 inhibit UGT1A1. Idelalisib and GS-563117 are not expected to inhibit CYP isoenzymes 1A, 2B6, and 2D6. In vitro studies show that idelalisib induces CYP isoenzymes 2B6 and 3A4 but does not induce CYP1A2; GS-563117 does not induce these enzymes.

In vitro, idelalisib is a substrate of efflux transporter P-glycoprotein (P-gp) and breast cancer resistance protein (BCRP); the drug is not a substrate of organic anion transport protein (OATP) 1B1, OATP1B3, renal organic anion transporter (OAT) 1, OAT3, or organic cation transporter (OCT) 2. GS-563117 is a substrate of P-gp and BCRP but not OATP1B1 or OATP1B3.

In vitro studies indicate that idelalisib inhibits P-gp, OATP1B1, and OATP1B3; the drug is not expected to inhibit BCRP, OCT2, OAT1, or OAT3. GS-563117 inhibits OATP1B1 and OATP1B3; the metabolite is not expected to inhibit P-gp, BCRP, OCT2, OAT1, or OAT3.

■ **Drugs Affecting Hepatic Microsomal Enzymes** ***Inhibitors of CYP3A Isoenzymes*** Concomitant use of idelalisib with potent inhibitors of CYP3A may result in increased systemic exposure to idelalisib. When the potent CYP3A and P-gp inhibitor ketoconazole (400 mg once daily for 4 days) was administered concomitantly with idelalisib (single 400-mg dose) in healthy individuals, area under the plasma concentration-time curve (AUC) of idelalisib increased by 1.8-fold; however, peak plasma concentrations of idelalisib were not affected. Patients receiving idelalisib concomitantly with CYP3A inhibitors should be monitored for signs of idelalisib toxicity. If severe adverse effects occur, temporary interruption of idelalisib therapy followed by dosage reduction may be necessary. (See Dosage and Administration: Dosage Modification for Toxicity.)

Inducers of CYP3A Isoenzymes Concomitant use of idelalisib with potent inducers of CYP3A may result in decreased systemic exposure to idelalisib. When the potent CYP3A and P-gp inducer rifampin (600 mg once daily for 8 days) was administered concomitantly with idelalisib (single 150-mg dose) in healthy individuals, AUC and peak plasma concentrations of idelalisib decreased by 75 and 58%, respectively. Concomitant use of idelalisib with potent CYP3A inducers (e.g., carbamazepine, phenytoin, rifampin, St. John's wort [*Hypericum perforatum*]) should be avoided.

■ **Drugs Metabolized by Hepatic Microsomal Enzymes** ***Substrates of CYP3A Isoenzymes*** Idelalisib is a potent inhibitor of CYP3A and may increase systemic exposure of other drugs metabolized by CYP3A. When the CYP3A substrate midazolam (single 5-mg oral dose) was administered concomitantly with idelalisib (150 mg twice daily for 15 doses) in healthy individuals, peak plasma concentration and AUC of midazolam were increased 2.4- and 5.4-fold, respectively. Concomitant use of idelalisib with CYP3A substrates should be avoided.

■ **Drugs Affecting the P-glycoprotein Transport System** When the potent CYP3A and P-gp inhibitor ketoconazole was administered concomitantly with idelalisib, systemic exposure to idelalisib was increased. (See Inhibitors of CYP3A Isoenzymes under Drug Interactions: Drugs Affecting Hepatic Microsomal Enzymes.)

Concomitant use of idelalisib with an inducer of P-gp may result in decreased systemic exposure to idelalisib. When the potent CYP3A and P-gp inducer rifampin was administered concomitantly with idelalisib, systemic exposure to idelalisib was decreased. (See Inducers of CYP3A Isoenzymes under Drug Interactions: Drugs Affecting Hepatic Microsomal Enzymes.) Concomitant use of idelalisib with potent P-gp inducers (e.g., rifampin) should be avoided.

■ **Substrates of P-glycoprotein or OATP Transport Systems** When the OATP1B1 and OATP1B3 substrate rosuvastatin (single 10-mg dose) was administered concomitantly with idelalisib (150 mg twice daily for 12 doses) in healthy individuals, systemic exposure to rosuvastatin was not affected.

When the P-gp substrate digoxin (single 0.5-mg dose) was administered concomitantly with idelalisib (150 mg twice daily for 19 doses) in healthy individuals, systemic exposure to digoxin was not affected.

Description

Idelalisib, a selective inhibitor of phosphoinositide 3-kinase isoform delta (PI3Kδ), is an antineoplastic agent. Phosphoinositide 3-kinases (PI3Ks) are lipid kinases consisting of a catalytic subunit that exists in 4 different isoforms (α, β, γ, δ). The delta isoform of PI3K (PI3Kδ) is highly expressed in hematopoietic cells and mediates B-cell receptor (BCR) signaling critical for B-cell homeostasis and function. Oversignaling of PI3K, particularly the delta isoform, has been implicated in the development of lymphoid malignancies. Idelalisib blocks constitutive PI3K/Akt signaling which results in apoptosis. The drug also has demonstrated inhibition of several cell signaling pathways, including BCR, CXCR4, and CXCR5, which are involved in the migration of B-cells to lymph nodes and bone marrow. Idelalisib induced apoptosis and inhibited proliferation in cell lines derived from malignant B-cells and in primary tumor cells. Treatment of lymphoma cells with idelalisib resulted in inhibition of chemotaxis and adhesion, and reduced cell viability.

Systemic exposure to idelalisib increases in a less than dose-proportional manner over a dosage range of 50–350 mg twice daily in the fasted state. Systemic exposure of idelalisib was increased by 1.4-fold following administration of a single dose of the drug with a high-fat meal compared with administration in the fasted state. Idelalisib is more than 84% bound to plasma proteins. Idelalisib is metabolized to its major metabolite, GS-563117, principally by cytochrome P-450 (CYP) isoenzyme 3A and aldehyde oxidase; the drug is metabolized only to a minor extent by uridine diphosphate-glucuronosyl transferase (UGT) 1A4. GS-563117 is inactive against PI3Kδ in vitro. The mean terminal half-life of idelalisib is 8.2 hours. Following oral administration of a single 150-mg dose of radiolabeled idelalisib, 78% of the dose was recovered in feces and 14% was recovered in urine; GS-563117 accounted for 44% of the dose recovered in feces and 49% of the dose recovered in urine.

Advice to Patients

Importance of instructing patients to read the manufacturer's patient information before starting idelalisib therapy and each time their prescription is refilled.

Importance of advising patients to take idelalisib exactly as prescribed and of not altering the dosage or discontinuing therapy unless advised to do so by their clinician. Importance of advising patients to swallow idelalisib tablets whole.

If a dose is missed, importance of advising patients to take it as soon as they remember unless the dose was missed by more than 6 hours, in which case they should not take the missed dose.

Risk of hepatotoxicity; importance of regular liver function test monitoring. Importance of advising patients to immediately report possible symptoms of hepatotoxicity (e.g., abdominal pain [especially right upper quadrant pain], jaundice, dark urine, bruising, bleeding diathesis) to their clinician.

Risk of severe diarrhea or colitis. Importance of immediately informing clinician if frequency of bowel movements increases by 6 or more a day.

Risk of intestinal perforation. Importance of immediately informing clinician if new or worsening abdominal pain, chills, fever, nausea, or vomiting occurs.

Risk of pneumonitis. Importance of immediately informing clinician if new or worsening respiratory symptoms (e.g., cough, dyspnea, wheezing) occur.

Risk of anaphylaxis or severe dermatologic reactions. Importance of immediately informing clinician if anaphylaxis or severe dermatologic reactions occur.

Risk of neutropenia. Importance of periodically monitoring blood cell counts during idelalisib therapy. Importance of immediately informing clinician if signs of infection (e.g., fever) occur.

Risk of fetal harm. Necessity of advising women of childbearing potential to avoid pregnancy and to consider using effective contraceptive methods while receiving idelalisib and for at least 1 month following discontinuance of therapy. Importance of women informing clinicians immediately if they become pregnant during therapy or think they may be pregnant. If pregnancy occurs, advise pregnant women of potential risk to the fetus.

Importance of advising women to avoid breast-feeding while receiving idelalisib therapy.

Importance of informing clinicians of existing or contemplated concomitant therapy, including prescription and OTC drugs and dietary or herbal supplements, as well as any concomitant illnesses (e.g., hepatic impairment).

Importance of informing patients of other important precautionary information. (See Cautions.)

Overview® (see Users Guide). For additional information on this drug until a more detailed monograph is developed and published, the manufacturer's labeling should be consulted. It is *essential* that the manufacturer's labeling be consulted for more detailed information on usual cautions, precautions, contraindications, potential drug interactions, laboratory test interferences, and acute toxicity. For further information on the handling of antineoplastic agents, see the ASHP Guidelines on Handling Hazardous Drugs at http://www.ahfsdruginformation.com.

Preparations

Excipients in commercially available drug preparations may have clinically important effects in some individuals; consult specific product labeling for details.

Idelalisib

Oral

Tablets, film-coated	100 mg	**Zydelig®**, Gilead Sciences
	150 mg	**Zydelig®**, Gilead Sciences

Ifosfamide

Isophosphamide

■ Ifosfamide, an alkylating agent structurally related to cyclophosphamide, is an antineoplastic agent.

Uses

Ifosfamide is used in conjunction with other antineoplastic agents for salvage therapy in the treatment of germ cell testicular neoplasms, and has been designated an orphan drug by the US Food and Drug Administration (FDA) for this use. The drug also has been designated an orphan drug by FDA for use in the treatment of various bone and soft tissue sarcomas, and usually is included as a component of various regimens for initial chemotherapy in these sarcomas. In addition, ifosfamide is used for initial or second- or third-line therapy in the treatment of various other malignancies including lung cancer†, cervical cancer†, and ovarian cancer†. Mesna, a uroprotective sulfhydryl (thiol) compound, is administered concomitantly with ifosfamide to minimize urotoxicity.

■ **Testicular Neoplasms** Ifosfamide is used as a component of various chemotherapeutic regimens for salvage therapy in patients with recurrent or refractory germ cell testicular cancer. Although the manufacturer states that such therapy is considered third-line, a regimen of ifosfamide, cisplatin, and either vinblastine sulfate or etoposide has induced complete responses in 20–45% of patients who previously received other cisplatin-based chemotherapy regimens, and is considered by most clinicians to be the standard initial salvage (i.e., second-line) regimen in patients with recurrent testicular cancer. Patients with minimal or moderate disease have a more favorable outcome with this salvage regimen than those with extensive disease. In a clinical study in patients with recurrent germ cell tumors (who had previously received at least 2 cisplatin-based chemotherapy regimens and were considered to have cisplatin-responsive disease), a regimen of ifosfamide, cisplatin, and either vinblastine sulfate or etoposide resulted in disease-free status in 36% of patients (with or without surgery) and median duration of disease control ranged from 3 to more than 42 weeks, median survival was 53 weeks, and 20% of patients had survival of 2 years or longer. In patients with refractory disease, high-dose chemotherapy (e.g., carboplatin and etoposide with or without ifosfamide) with autologous bone marrow transplant (ABMT) or peripheral stem cell rescue may produce durable complete remissions in some patients. Patients with progressive tumors during initial or salvage therapy and those with refractory mediastinal germ cell tumors generally appear to benefit less from high-dose chemotherapy and ABMT or peripheral stem cell rescue than those whose disease relapses after a response. Salvage surgery also may be considered for certain highly selected patients (e.g., those with chemorefractory disease confined to a single site).

The role of ifosfamide in the *initial* management of patients with advanced testicular cancer remains to be more fully elucidated. However, there is some evidence that response rate and survival in patients with previously untreated, advanced germ cell testicular cancer are similar and hematologic toxicity less pronounced with a regimen of ifosfamide, cisplatin, and etoposide compared with a regimen of cisplatin, etoposide, and bleomycin.

■ **Bone and Soft Tissue Sarcomas** Ifosfamide is used as a component of various chemotherapeutic regimens in conjunction with surgery and/or radiation therapy in the treatment of various bone and soft tissue sarcomas† in adults and children†. Regimens that include ifosfamide have been used for initial or second-line chemotherapy in these sarcomas.

Ifosfamide has been used in conjunction with other drugs (e.g., etoposide) and occasionally alone in the treatment of localized, metastatic, and recurrent osteosarcoma† in adults and children†. When used for initial therapy ofosteosarcoma†, ifosfamide has been included as a component of various chemotherapeutic regimens both preoperatively (as a neoadjunct) and postoperatively (as an adjunct) in conjunction with surgical resection of the tumor. Although ifosfamide is considered one of the more active drugs that can be used in the management of osteosarcoma, various regimens have been used in combination therapy for the disease and comparative efficacy is continually being evaluated. In addition, although chemotherapy is being used preoperatively in an attempt to increase the likelihood of a limb-sparing procedure (rather than amputation) as well as to evaluate the potential response to specific chemotherapy regimens, the role of preoperative therapy in affecting the extent of surgery required for complete ablation of the primary tumor and the prognostic value of response to such chemotherapy regarding possible disease recurrence remain to be more fully elucidated.

Ifosfamide also is used as a component of intensive combination chemotherapy for the management of metastatic and unresectable osteosarcoma. For metastatic disease, chemotherapy usually is used after, or where possible, before and after, surgical ablation of the primary tumor and, where possible, metastases; multiple thoracotomies may be required to remove recurrent pulmonary metastases. Even if the primary tumor and metastases are not resectable, intensive chemotherapy is indicated. For patients with recurrent or progressive metastatic disease confined to the lungs, combination chemotherapy may be used as an adjunct to aggressive surgical resection. The choice of further therapy depends on many factors including the site of recurrence and prior treatment (e.g., chemotherapy used for primary therapy) as well as patient-specific considerations. Ifosfamide used alone or in conjunction with etoposide has shown activity in up to one-third of patients with recurrent osteosarcoma.

Ifosfamide has been used alone or as a component of various chemotherapeutic regimens in the palliative treatment of advanced or recurrent adult soft tissue sarcomas†. In adults with advanced or metastatic soft tissue sarcoma, regimens that include doxorubicin with or without other agents (e.g., ifosfamide or cyclophosphamide, dacarbazine, vincristine) have been associated with response rates of 15–30% but with little or no impact on survival. Results from clinical studies in patients with advanced soft tissue sarcomas indicate that treatment with doxorubicin as a single agent is as effective as and has a more favorable adverse effect profile than combination regimens; however, a regimen of ifosfamide and doxorubicin may be useful in patients in whom substantial tumor-volume reduction is an important therapeutic end point. Additional studies, including studies using high-dose ifosfamide, are under way in an attempt to improve the prognosis in patients with advanced soft tissue sarcoma.

Although the manufacturer states that safe use of ifosfamide in children has not been definitely established, ifosfamide is used in conjunction with other antineoplastic agents for the treatment of Ewing's sarcoma†. Use of multiple-drug chemotherapy regimens in addition to radiation therapy and/or surgery has been shown to improve the rate of local control and the duration of survival in children with Ewing's sarcoma. While a regimen of vincristine, doxorubicin, and cyclophosphamide (with or without dactinomycin) has been widely used in the treatment of children with Ewing's sarcoma, the combination of ifosfamide and etoposide also has shown activity in the disease, and results from a large randomized study indicate that outcome may be improved in these children when ifosfamide and etoposide are given in alternating courses with vincristine, doxorubicin (or dactinomycin), and cyclophosphamide. A regimen employing alternating courses of chemotherapy that include ifosfamide and etoposide is considered by some clinicians to be the standard initial regimen in children with Ewing's sarcoma. Alternating courses of vincristine, doxorubicin, and cyclophosphamide with ifosfamide and etoposide may be used in patients with metastatic Ewing's sarcoma. There is some evidence that a regimen of ifosfamide and etoposide also may be effective for the treatment of recurrent Ewing's sarcoma in children who previously received other regimens.

Ifosfamide also has been used in various combination regimens for the treatment of rhabdomyosarcoma† in children. Although not considered standard initial therapy for the treatment of rhabdomyosarcoma by some clinicians, ifosfamide in conjunction with vincristine and etoposide or dactinomycin has been used successfully in a limited number of children with rhabdomyosarcoma and is considered by other clinicians as one of several alternative regimens that can be used initially (i.e., as first-line therapy). Regimens that have been most extensively evaluated to date include vincristine and dactinomycin for group I tumors and vincristine, dactinomycin, and cyclophosphamide for group II tumors; the addition of doxorubicin to this latter regimen does not appear to improve response. Substitution of ifosfamide for cyclophosphamide in this 3-drug regimen and combined therapy with vincristine, ifosfamide, and etoposide also have shown significant activity in this cancer. Rhabdomyosarcoma is curable in most children when optimal therapy is used, with more than 60% surviving 5 years after diagnosis. Ifosfamide also has been used in conjunction with etoposide in the treatment of recurrent rhabdomyosarcoma in children who have not previously received these drugs. Although such patients occasionally achieve a complete remission with second-line therapy, long-term prognosis generally is poor.

Ifosfamide also has shown activity in the management of Wilms' tumor, and has been used in conjunction with etoposide for second-line or salvage therapy in a limited number of children with recurrent Wilms' tumor†. Initial chemotherapy for Wilms' tumor usually includes vincristine and dactinomycin (with the addition of doxorubicin for more advanced stages), with regimens that include various combinations with drugs such as ifosfamide, etoposide, carboplatin, and cisplatin generally reserved for patients with relatively poor prognosis such as those with recurrent tumors of unfavorable histology, abdominal recurrence after radiation therapy, or recurrence within 6 months of nephrectomy or after initial 3-drug combination chemotherapy (e.g., vincristine, dactinomycin, and doxorubicin). Although Wilms' tumor is curable in most children, with more than 90% surviving 4 years after diagnosis, prognosis in patients with recurrence is variable, with the above patients having a relatively poor prognosis, and it remains to be established whether such second-line or salvage therapy (including regimens with autologous bone marrow transplant) can improve prognosis substantially in patients in whom it is relatively poor.

■ **Bladder Cancer** Ifosfamide is an active agent in the treatment of advanced or metastatic bladder cancer†. Concomitant mesna is used to prevent the urotoxicity associated with ifosfamide therapy. Ifosfamide has been used alone and in combination with other antineoplastic agents for the treatment of advanced urothelial carcinoma. Objective responses to ifosfamide have been observed in patients with advanced bladder cancer that did not respond to previous treatment with cisplatin-based regimens. However, the use of ifosfamide has been associated with substantial toxicity, including myelosuppression, nephrotoxicity, and encephalopathy, particularly in geriatric patients and patients who have received previous treatment with cisplatin-based regimens.

In a phase II trial of ifosfamide in 56 patients with advanced urothelial cancer who had received one prior chemotherapy regimen, typically consisting of cisplatin, methotrexate, and vinblastine with or without doxorubicin (abbreviated as M-VAC or CMV, respectively), objective responses occurred in 20% (9% complete responses, 11% partial responses) of patients. Dosage reduction was required for all patients because of excessive renal and CNS toxicity associated with the planned treatment schedule.

Combination therapy with ifosfamide, vinblastine, and gallium nitrate (abbreviated as VIG) produces response rates that appear to be comparable to those observed with M-VAC in patients with advanced or metastatic bladder cancer; however, because of the excessive toxicity (particularly hematologic and cardiac toxicity), sometimes fatal, associated with this regimen, no further clinical trials are planned for VIG in patients with transitional cell bladder carcinoma.

The role of ifosfamide in the treatment of advanced or metastatic bladder cancer has not been established. The use of ifosfamide in combination therapy with other antineoplastic agents (e.g., paclitaxel, cisplatin) as first-line or salvage therapy for advanced urothelial carcinoma is being investigated.

■ **Lung Cancer** Ifosfamide is used as a component of combination chemotherapy for the treatment of small cell lung cancer†. Combination chemotherapy regimens are superior to single-agent therapy for the treatment of small cell lung cancer and moderately intensive drug doses are superior to doses that produce minimal toxicity. Various regimens have been used in combination therapy and many 2- to 4-drug combination regimens have produced similar response rates. Ifosfamide is used in conjunction with etoposide and either carboplatin or cisplatin for the treatment of small cell lung cancer. In clinical studies that used regimens that included ifosfamide, an objective response occurred in 75–95% of patients who had limited disease and in 44–100% of patients who had extensive disease. The median duration of disease control with these ifosfamide regimens ranged from 5–45 weeks, and median duration of survival was 9–14 months. In at least one study, the addition of ifosfamide to a regimen of cisplatin and etoposide improved progression-free and overall survival but was associated with an increased incidence of myelosuppression.

Although optimum duration of chemotherapy has not been clearly defined, improvement in survival has not been observed when the duration of drug administration exceeds 3–6 or 6 months in patients with limited-stage or extensive-stage small cell lung cancer, respectively. While efficacy of the various available regimens is continually being evaluated, a combination chemotherapy regimen containing ifosfamide, a platinum-containing agent (carboplatin or cisplatin), and etoposide is one of several preferred or alternative regimens for the treatment of extensive-stage small cell lung carcinoma. Because the current prognosis for small cell lung carcinoma is unsatisfactory regardless of stage and despite considerable diagnostic and therapeutic advances, all patients with this cancer are candidates for inclusion in clinical trials at the time of diagnosis.

Ifosfamide has been used as a component of combination regimens with cisplatin (e.g., ifosfamide with mesna, cisplatin, and mitomycin) in the treatment of non-small cell lung carcinoma†; however, other platinum-containing regimens currently are preferred for the treatment of advanced non-small cell lung cancer. The addition of ifosfamide to cisplatin or carboplatin was associated with higher response rates but had no effect on survival and increased the frequency and severity of toxicity (e.g., leukopenia, thrombocytopenia, alopecia, vomiting) in patients with advanced non-small cell lung cancer.

■ **Cervical Cancer** Ifosfamide is an active agent in the treatment of metastatic or recurrent cervical cancer†. Response rates of 16–33% have been reported with use of ifosfamide as a single agent in advanced squamous cell carcinoma of the cervix. An overall response rate of 15% was observed in a small uncontrolled phase II study of patients receiving ifosfamide and mesna for recurrent or advanced adenocarcinoma, adenosquamous, or other nonsquamous carcinoma of the cervix.

Ifosfamide has been used in various combination regimens (e.g., cisplatin and ifosfamide with or without bleomycin) for the treatment of metastatic or recurrent cervical cancer. In a large randomized trial, higher response rates and increased duration of progression-free survival but greater toxicity and no difference in overall survival were observed for the combination of ifosfamide (with mesna) and cisplatin compared with cisplatin alone in patients with metastatic or recurrent squamous cell carcinoma of the cervix. Although high objective response rates have been observed with the combination regimen of ifosfamide, bleomycin, and cisplatin in women with metastatic or recurrent cervical cancer, toxicity is greater and survival is not improved in women receiving the combination regimen rather than cisplatin alone. The benefit of combination cisplatin-based chemotherapy regimens, such as cisplatin and ifosfamide, versus cisplatin alone has not been fully established, and further study is needed to define the role of ifosfamide in the treatment of advanced cervical cancer. (See Uses: Cervical Cancer in Cisplatin 10:00 for overview of treatment for cervical cancer.)

■ **Ovarian Cancer** Ifosfamide has been used alone or in conjunction with other antineoplastic agents for second-line (salvage) therapy in patients with advanced or recurrent ovarian carcinoma†. In patients with platinum-responsive disease (no disease progression within 5–12 months of discontinuing a platinum-based combination regimen), an objective response has been produced in 25–56% of patients treated with a salvage regimen of ifosfamide and carboplatin. In patients with platinum-refractory advanced ovarian carcinoma (i.e., disease that has progressed while treated with a platinum-based regimen or that has recurred shortly after completion of a platinum-based regimen), other drugs (e.g., paclitaxel) generally are preferred for initial second-line therapy. However, ifosfamide is one of several drugs that can be considered for salvage therapy in platinum-resistant disease, and partial or complete response has been observed in 12–20% of patients receiving salvage therapy with ifosfamide alone.

■ **Other Uses** Although ifosfamide has shown some activity when used in conjunction with other antineoplastic agents in the treatment of recurrent or advanced lymphomas† and is recommended by some clinicians as one of several alternatives that can be used for the treatment of advanced small noncleaved cell lymphoma (Burkitt's and non-Burkitt's) in children, regimens containing other antineoplastic agents generally are preferred for first-line treatment of lymphomas.

Ifosfamide has shown some activity when used as single-agent therapy in a limited number of patients for the management of advanced or recurrent uterine sarcoma†. Ifosfamide therapy has resulted in partial or complete responses in 32% of patients with mixed mesodermal sarcomas and partial responses in 17% of patients with leiomyosarcomas. There currently is no established standard therapy for recurrent uterine sarcoma, and further study is needed to determine the role of ifosfamide when used alone or in combination (e.g., with cisplatin) regimens for the treatment of these tumors.

Dosage and Administration

■ **Reconstitution and Administration** Ifosfamide is administered by IV infusion. IV infusions of ifosfamide should be administered over a period of at least 30 minutes; the drug also has been administered by continuous IV infusion.

To minimize urotoxicity, patients should be adequately hydrated prior to and during ifosfamide therapy (e.g., 2 liters of oral or IV fluid daily). In addition, a uroprotective agent such mesna should be administered during ifosfamide therapy to decrease the incidence of ifosfamide-induced bladder toxicity (e.g., hemorrhagic cystitis, hematuria); adequate uroprotection is particularly important at relatively high dosages.

Because of the carcinogenic potential of ifosfamide (see Cautions: Mutagenicity and Carcinogenicity), the usual precautions for handling and preparing solutions of cytotoxic drugs should be observed. The manufacturer recommends use of protective gloves when handling ifosfamide since accidental exposure may be associated with skin reactions. If ifosfamide solution comes in contact with skin or mucosa, affected skin areas should be washed immediately and thoroughly with soap and water and affected mucosa should be thoroughly rinsed with copious amounts of water.

Ifosfamide sterile powder is reconstituted by adding 20 or 60 mL of sterile water for injection or of sterile bacteriostatic water for injection containing benzyl alcohol or parabens to a vial labeled as containing 1 or 3 g of the drug, respectively, to provide solutions containing 50 mg/mL. These reconstituted solutions may be infused directly or further diluted to a concentration of 0.6–20 mg/mL with a compatible IV solution (see Chemistry and Stability: Stability).

Alternatively, commercially available aqueous isosfamide injection labeled as containing 100 mg/mL may be infused directly or diluted to 20 mg/mL in a compatible IV solution. (See Chemistry and Stability: Stability.) Dilution of each mL of the commercially available injection in 4 mL of IV solution will yield a final concentration of 20 mg/mL.

Ifosfamide solutions should be inspected visually for discoloration and particulate matter prior to administration.

■ **Dosage** Dosage of ifosfamide must be based on the clinical and hematologic response and tolerance of the patient in order to obtain optimum therapeutic response with minimal adverse effects. Although higher total doses of ifosfamide can be given by continuous infusion compared with short IV infusion with similar toxicity, the most effective dosage schedule has not been established. In patients who experience myelosuppression following a dose of ifosfamide, a subsequent course of the drug should not be administered until the patient's hematologic functions are within acceptable limits. (See Cautions: Precautions and Contraindications)

To minimize the risk of urotoxic effects, each dose of isosfamide must be accompanied by a mesna regimen. (See Dosage and Administration: Dosage, in Mesna 92:56)

Testicular Neoplasms For the treatment of recurrent germ cell testicular cancer in adults, the usual dosage of ifosfamide in combination chemotherapy regimens is 1.2 g/m^2 IV daily for 5 consecutive days every 3 weeks. In the study used to establish efficacy for this indication, ifosfamide-containing combination chemotherapy was given for a total of 4 courses.

Other Neoplasms For the treatment of other malignant neoplasms†, various dosage schedules and regimens of ifosfamide, alone or in conjunction with other antineoplastic agents, have been used. Clinicians should consult published protocols for dosages and the method and sequence of administration. While the dosage of ifosfamide used in the treatment of other malignant neoplasms generally has been similar to that used in the treatment of germ cell testicular cancer, dosage has varied. For the management of malignant neoplasms (i.e., sarcomas†, small cell lung cancer†, cervical cancer†, ovarian cancer†, uterine cancer†), ifosfamide has been given IV in a dosage of 1.2–2.5 g/m^2 daily for 3–5 days, with cycles of therapy repeated as necessary depending on the patient's response and dosage reduced as necessary depending on the patient's tolerance. Although higher doses have been used, they may be associated with substantially increased risk of toxicity (e.g., myelosuppression, neurotoxicity, nephrotoxicity).

■ **Dosage in Renal and Hepatic Impairment** Although ifosfamide has been used in a limited number of patients with renal and/or hepatic impairment, the manufacturer states that studies to determine the optimum dosage in such patients have not been conducted.

Cautions

The major adverse effects of ifosfamide are myelosuppression (leukopenia, thrombocytopenia), urinary tract and renal toxicity (bladder toxicity, nephrotoxicity, electrolyte effects), and neurotoxicity. The incidence and severity of bladder toxicity (e.g., hemorrhagic cystitis, hematuria) is reduced substantially when ifosfamide is administered in fractionated dosage schedules and given in conjunction with conventional uroprophylaxis (e.g., high fluid intake, frequent urination) and when mesna is used prophylactically as a uroprotective agent.

■ **Hematologic Effects** Hematologic toxicity is a major and dose-limiting adverse effect of ifosfamide. Myelosuppression, which is dose related, is manifested mainly by leukopenia and, to a lesser extent, thrombocytopenia. Leukopenia (leukocyte count less than 3000/mm^3) has been reported in 50% and thrombocytopenia (platelet count less than 100,000/mm$_3$) in 20% of patients receiving the usual dosage of ifosfamide (i.e., 1.2 g/m^2 IV daily for 5 days). At higher dosages, leukopenia occurs in almost all patients, and severe leukopenia (leukocyte count less than 1000/mm$_3$) occurs in 50% and platelet counts less than 50,000/mm^3 in 8% of patients receiving IV ifosfamide regimens totaling 10–12 g/m^2 per cycle. Severe myelosuppression occurs frequently when ifosfamide is used in conjunction with other antineoplastic agents. (See Drug Interactions: Myelosuppressive Therapy.)

Ifosfamide-induced myelosuppression generally is reversible. Leukocyte nadirs usually occur within 7–14 days after administration of ifosfamide, and leukocyte recovery generally occurs by the third week after administration of the drug.

Anemia has been reported in patients receiving ifosfamide.

■ **Genitourinary, Renal, and Electrolyte Effects** ***Bladder Toxicity*** Ifosfamide is toxic to the urothelium, producing effects that range in severity from microscopic to gross urinary bleeding. Prior to the introduction of the uroprotective agent, mesna, urotoxicity was a major dose-limiting adverse effect of ifosfamide despite vigorous hydration. Urotoxic effects attributed to ifosfamide include hemorrhagic cystitis, hematuria, dysuria, urinary frequency, and other manifestations of bladder irritation. Hematuria has been reported in 6–92% of patients receiving ifosfamide. When ifosfamide is administered in a dosage of 1.2 g/m^2 IV daily for 5 days without uroprotection (i.e., mesna), microscopic hematuria occurs in about 50% and gross hematuria in about 8% of patients.

Ifosfamide-induced bladder toxicity is attributed to chemical irritation of the epithelium of the bladder resulting from ifosfamide metabolites (e.g., acrolein) that accumulate in concentrated urine, and the incidence and severity of bladder toxicity can be reduced by conventional uroprophylaxis (e.g., high fluid intake, frequent urination), use of a fractionated ifosfamide dosage schedule, and concurrent administration of mesna. While most cells contain naturally occurring sulfhydryl (thiol) compounds (e.g., glutathione) and are able to inactivate such toxic metabolites, the concentration of thiols in urine is low. Studies in animals indicate that the initial urotoxic effect is disruption of the cell plasma membrane and cytoplasmic matrix. Various sulfhydryl (thiol) compounds (e.g., acetylcysteine, mesna) that can react with the toxic metabolites of ifosfamide have been studied for uroprotective activity. Oral acetylcysteine was one of the first agents tested for uroprotection, but acceptance was limited because of undesirable pharmacokinetic characteristics and resultant need for high dosages, and the poor patient tolerance (e.g., nausea, vomiting, bad taste) of such dosages. Mesna, 2-mercaptoethanesulfonate, acts specifically as a regional urologic detoxificant, and currently is preferred because of favorable pharmacodynamic properties (e.g., poor lipid solubility and distribution, extensive renal clearance) and documented lack of effect on the antitumor activity of concomitantly administered antineoplastic agents. Mesna substantially decreases the incidence and severity of ifosfamide-induced bladder toxicity. (See Drug Interactions: Mesna.)

Nephrotoxicity and Electrolyte Effects Potentially serious nephrotoxicity may occur in patients receiving ifosfamide. In clinical studies employing ifosfamide as single-agent therapy at the usual recommended dosage, nephrotoxicity was reported in 6% of patients. In a limited number of patients receiving high ifosfamide dosage (2–2.5 g/m^2 daily for 4 days), metabolic acidosis occurred in 31% of patients. Ifosfamide-induced nephrotoxicity may be evidenced by biochemical signs of renal dysfunction (e.g., aminoaciduria, glycosuria, proteinuria, cells or casts in the urine, increase in serum creatinine or BUN, decrease in creatinine clearance), glomerular impairment (e.g., acute or chronic renal failure), and/or renal tubular impairment (e.g., Fanconi's syndrome, renal tubular acidosis, nephrogenic diabetes insipidus). Although ifosfamide-induced renal toxicity may involve each of the 3 segments of the nephron, toxicity generally has been associated with proximal tubule dysfunction. Rarely, renal tubular acidosis has progressed to chronic renal failure.

Potentially irreversible Fanconi's syndrome, characterized by aminoaciduria, glycosuria, phosphaturia, bicarbonaturia, and kaliuresis, has been reported in children and adults and usually occurs after several courses of ifosfamide. Rarely, ifosfamide-induced phosphaturia may lead to hypophosphatemia and rickets. (See Cautions: Pediatric Precautions.) If electrolyte abnormalities develop in patients receiving ifosfamide, appropriate therapy to correct any electrolyte imbalance(s) should be instituted.

Nephrotoxicity may develop during ifosfamide therapy or following discontinuance of the drug. While the exact mechanism(s) is not known, renal toxicity may be caused by depletion of renal tubular glutathione by ifosfamide metabolites (e.g., acrolein, chloroacetaldehyde) or by alteration in amino acid, glucose, and/or phosphate renal cell transport by ifosfamide metabolites (e.g., 4-hydroxyifosfamide, chloroacetaldehyde). Ifosfamide-induced nephrotoxicity can be reversible; however, the long-term effects of the drug on renal function are not fully known. Although not clearly established, the risk of ifosfamide-induced nephrotoxicity appears to be increased in patients who have received previous or concurrent cisplatin therapy and in patients with preexisting renal impairment, infiltrating renal tumor, or prior nephrectomy. In addition, patients who are 5 years of age or younger or have received high cumulative doses of ifosfamide (e.g., 50 g/m^2) appear to be at increased risk for renal toxicity. (See Cautions: Pediatric Precautions.)Various ifosfamide regimens including direct IV injection, short infusion, or continuous infusion have been used in an attempt to decrease the incidence of nephrotoxicity; however, there are reports of serious renal toxicity with all schedules and a relative therapeutic advantage has not been established. While concomitant administration of mesna decreases the incidence of ifosfamide-induced bladder toxicity (e.g., hemorrhagic cystitis, hematuria), mesna does not prevent ifosfamide-induced nephrotoxicity.

■ **Nervous System Toxicity** Adverse nervous system effects occur in about 10–20% of patients receiving ifosfamide, and range in severity from mild somnolence and confusion to severe encephalopathy and coma. Ifosfamide-induced neurotoxicity usually is characterized by confusion, mutism, auditory and/or visual hallucinations, stupor, and coma. In addition, seizures, dizziness, disorientation, agitation, and cranial nerve dysfunction occur less frequently. Fatigue, malaise, polyneuropathy, extrapyramidal manifestations, and peripheral neuropathy have been reported in less than 1% of patients receiving ifosfamide.

If one or more signs of serious neurotoxicity (i.e., somnolence, confusion, hallucinations, and/or coma) occur during ifosfamide therapy, the drug should be discontinued and appropriate measures for supportive therapy instituted. If neurotoxicity is promptly detected and the drug discontinued, the effects generally are reversible and resolve within 2–4 days. Manifestations of emotional instability, impairment of short-term memory, and flattened affect may persist for 4–10 weeks in some patients. Rarely, neurotoxicity is irreversible, and fatal encephalopathy has been reported. Methylene blue has been used in the management of ifosfamide-induced encephalopathy and has been beneficial in some patients. (See Methylene Blue 92:12.)

While the exact mechanism(s) is not known, CNS toxicity may be caused by ifosfamide metabolites (e.g., chloroacetaldehyde), and it has been suggested that differences in the neurotoxic potentials of ifosfamide and cyclophosphamide may result from metabolic difference of the drugs. Patients with renal impairment, poor performance status, or previous exposure to cisplatin appear to be at increased risk of ifosfamide-related neurotoxicity. It is unclear whether neurotoxicity is dose related.

■ **GI Effects** Nausea and/or vomiting, which generally are moderate in severity, have been reported in 56–81% of patients receiving ifosfamide. The incidence and severity of nausea and vomiting are dose related, occurring in virtually all patients receiving high-dose ifosfamide. These GI effects generally begin within a few hours after administration of ifosfamide, last an average of 3 days, and respond to treatment with antiemetics. Anorexia, increased salivation, diarrhea, constipation, and stomatitis have been reported in less than 1% of patients receiving the drug.

■ **Dermatologic and Local Effects** Alopecia occurs in 74–83% of patients who receive ifosfamide alone, but may occur in up to 100% of patients who receive the drug in conjunction with other antineoplastic agents. Patients should be forewarned of the possibility of alopecia. Nonspecific dermatitis and hyperpigmentation have been reported in a limited number of patients receiving ifosfamide. Although ifosfamide-induced skin pigmentation generally is localized on dorsal and plantar surfaces of the hands and feet, genitalia, or areas occluded by bandages, it may cover large areas of the trunk. Hyperpigmentation appears more rapidly in dark- than in light-skinned individuals and may fade despite continued ifosfamide therapy or persist for several months after therapy with the drug has been completed.

Extravasation of ifosfamide can produce local pain, inflammation, and induration. Phlebitis has been reported in 1% of patients receiving the drug.

■ **Pulmonary Effects** Pulmonary symptoms have been reported in less than 1% of patients receiving ifosfamide. Rarely, potentially fatal interstitial pneumonitis has been reported in patients who received high ifosfamide dosage (2–4.5 g/m^2 IV daily for 4 days).

■ **Cardiac Effects** Cardiotoxicity has occurred in less than 1% of patients receiving ifosfamide. Rarely, severe, reversible cardiac dysfunction has occurred in patients who received high ifosfamide dosage (2.5–4.5 g/m^2 IV daily for 4 days) in conjunction with other antineoplastic agents. Myocardial depression occurred 6–23 days after initiation of ifosfamide therapy and resulted in a rapidly progressive syndrome of congestive heart failure and cardiopulmonary decompensation which, in most patients, was responsive to cardiac support therapy.

■ **Other Adverse Effects** Abnormalities in liver function test results (e.g., increases in serum concentration of liver enzymes and/or serum bilirubin) have occurred in 3% of patients receiving ifosfamide. Infection has occurred in 8% and fever of unknown origin in 1% of patients receiving the drug. Other adverse effects reported in less than 1% of patients include allergic reactions, coagulation disorders, hypertension, and hypotension. Acute pancreatitis has been reported rarely.

Although the clinical importance is unclear, the manufacturer states that ifosfamide therapy may interfere with normal wound healing.

■ **Precautions and Contraindications** Ifosfamide is a highly toxic drug with a low therapeutic index, and a therapeutic response is not likely to occur without some evidence of toxicity. The drug must be used only under constant supervision by clinicians experienced in therapy with cytotoxic agents.

To decrease the incidence and severity of bladder toxicity (e.g., hemorrhagic cystitis, hematuria) in patients receiving ifosfamide, most experts recommend use of conventional uroprophylaxis (e.g., adequate hydration, frequent urination) and administration of mesna, a uroprotective agent. These measures do not prevent hemorrhagic cystitis in all patients receiving ifosfamide and the urine of patients receiving the drug should be examined regularly for the presence of erythrocytes, which may precede hemorrhagic cystitis. A morning urine specimen should be examined for the presence of erythrocytes before each scheduled dose of ifosfamide. In patients who develop microscopic hematuria (more than 10 erythrocytes per high power field [HPF]), ifosfamide therapy should be discontinued until the hematuria resolves, and vigorous oral or parenteral hydration as well as mesna should be used in these patients for subsequent courses of ifosfamide. Because hemorrhagic cystitis can be severe and may be fatal, ifosfamide therapy should be discontinued or dosage of the drug reduced in patients who develop hematuria (more than 50 erythrocytes/HPF) while receiving usual dosages of ifosfamide in conjunction with mesna.

Ifosfamide should be used with caution in patients with impaired renal function. Because electrolyte abnormalities and/or acidosis, which rarely have been fatal, may occur in patients receiving ifosfamide, serum and urine chemistries, including phosphorus, potassium, alkaline phosphatase, and other appropriate laboratory studies should be monitored closely. If electrolyte abnormalities develop in patients receiving the drug, appropriate therapy to correct any imbalance(s) should be instituted.

Because patients who receive myelosuppressive drugs experience an increased frequency of infection and/or bleeding, hematologic status must be monitored carefully during ifosfamide therapy to determine the degree of hematopoietic suppression. The manufacturer states that ifosfamide is contraindicated in patients with severely depressed bone marrow function. Ifosfamide should be used with caution in patients with compromised bone marrow reserve as indicated by leukopenia, granulocytopenia, extensive bone marrow metastases, prior radiation therapy, or prior therapy with other cytotoxic agents. The manufacturer recommends that leukocyte counts, platelet counts, and hemoglobin concentrations be assessed prior to and at appropriate intervals during ifosfamide therapy. In patients who experience myelosuppression following a course of ifosfamide, subsequent courses generally should be withheld until leukocyte counts have recovered to greater than 4000/mm^3 and platelet counts exceed 100,000/mm^3. Unless ifosfamide therapy is considered clinically essential, the manufacturer states that the drug should not be administered to patients with leukocyte counts less than 2000/mm^3 and/or platelet counts less than 50,000/mm^3.

If serious neurotoxicity manifested as somnolence, confusion, hallucinations, and/or coma occurs during ifosfamide therapy, the drug should be discontinued and appropriate measures instituted. Most neurotoxic manifestations of ifosfamide are reversible if detected promptly.

Ifosfamide is contraindicated in patients with known hypersensitivity to the drug.

■ **Pediatric Precautions** Safety and efficacy of ifosfamide in children have not been established. Ifosfamide has been used in children 15 days to 17 years of age for the treatment of certain malignancies (e.g., Ewing's sarcoma, rhabdomyosarcoma, Wilms' tumor), and adverse effects of the drug reported in these children appear to be similar to those reported in adults. However, further study is needed to evaluate the safety of ifosfamide in children, especially those 5 years of age or younger who may be more susceptible to ifosfamide-induced renal toxicity than older children or adults. Severe nephrotoxicity leading to Fanconi's syndrome, which may be irreversible, has been reported in young children who received ifosfamide alone or in conjunction with other antineoplastic agents. Progressive tubular damage resulting in potentially debilitating hypophosphatemia and rickets has been reported rarely. Follow-up assessment of bone mineralization in a limited number of children who had received ifosfamide revealed essentially normal bone marrow density. Neurotoxicity and conjunctivitis and blurring of vision have been reported rarely in children receiving ifosfamide. A 4-year old child who received ifosfamide in conjunction with mesna developed severe, irreversible, encephalopathy that was fatal. In addition, encephalopathy, loss of developmental milestones, progressive brain atrophy, and cessation of brain growth was reported in one infant who received ifosfamide.

Although small differences in pharmacokinetic values have been reported in children, changes in these parameters are unlikely to be clinically relevant given the extensive interindividual variation in ifosfamide metabolism. If ifosfamide is used in children, the potential benefits of the drug should be weighed carefully against the drug's potentially serious adverse effects. Appropriate laboratory tests should be performed during, as well as after, ifosfamide therapy to monitor renal and bone biochemistries (e.g., urine glucose, urine protein, serum electrolytes) and appropriate supplementation initiated if renal tubular abnormalities are detected. Some clinicians recommend that the drug not be used in children with infiltrating renal tumors, prior nephrectomy, or any evidence of renal impairment.

■ **Geriatric Precautions** Ifosfamide has not been evaluated systematically in geriatric patients to date. In general, dosage of ifosfamide must be based on the clinical, renal, hematologic response and tolerance of the patient; the greater frequency of reduced drug clearance as well as decreased hepatic, renal, and hematopoietic function observed in the elderly should be considered. Although small differences in pharmacokinetic values have been reported in older individuals, changes in these parameters are unlikely to be clinically relevant given the extensive interindividual variation in ifosfamide metabolism.

■ **Mutagenicity and Carcinogenicity** Ifosfamide has been shown to be mutagenic in vitro in bacterial systems. In vivo, the drug increased dominant lethal mutations in male mice and recessive sex-linked lethal mutations in *Drosophila melanogaster* germ cells.

Ifosfamide has been shown to be carcinogenic in rats, and has been associated with an increased incidence of leiomyosarcomas and mammary fibroadenomas in female rats. Cyclophosphamide has been shown to cause urinary bladder tumors in mice, and acrolein, a toxic metabolite of both cyclophosphamide and ifosfamide, is the carcinogenic compound implicated in the development of these tumors. It has been suggested that concomitant use of mesna, by neutralizing the toxic effects of acrolein, may reduce the risk of bladder carcinoma induced by these oxazaphosphorine agents.

■ **Pregnancy, Fertility, and Lactation** Ifosfamide can cause fetal harm when administered to a pregnant woman, but potential benefits from use of the drug may be acceptable in certain conditions despite possible risk to the fetus. Ifosfamide has been shown to be teratogenic and embryotoxic in mice, rats, and rabbits in doses 0.05–0.075 times the human dose. There are no adequate or controlled studies to date using ifosfamide in pregnant women. Ifosfamide should be used during pregnancy only in life-threatening situations or for disease for which safer drugs cannot be used or are ineffective. If the drug is administered during pregnancy or if the patient becomes pregnant while receiving ifosfamide, the patient should be informed of the potential hazard to the fetus. Women of childbearing potential should be advised to avoid becoming pregnant during ifosfamide therapy.

The effects of ifosfamide on fertility have not been fully determined.

Ifosfamide is distributed into milk. Because of the potential for serious adverse reactions to ifosfamide in nursing infants, a decision should be made whether to discontinue nursing or the drug, taking into account the importance of the drug to the woman.

Drug Interactions

Although ifosfamide has been used concurrently with other drugs, including other cytotoxic agents, without unusual adverse effects, the possibility of adverse drug interactions cannot be excluded.

■ **Mesna** Concomitant administration of mesna substantially decreases the incidence and severity of ifosfamide-induced bladder toxicity (e.g., hemorrhagic cystitis, hematuria). Mesna is a synthetic sulfhydryl (thiol) compound. In urine, mesna interacts chemically with urotoxic ifosfamide metabolites (e.g., binding with double-bonds of acrolein) and precursors (e.g., binding with 4-hydroxyifosfamide to form 4-sulfethylthioifosfamide) resulting in detoxification of these metabolites. Although the incidence of ifosfamide-induced bladder toxicity (e.g., hemorrhagic cystitis, hematuria) is substantially lower in patients receiving concomitant mesna compared with that reported in patients receiving ifosfamide alone, mesna does not prevent ifosfamide-induced nephrotoxicity and does not prevent or decrease the incidence of nonrenal toxicities associated with the drug (i.e., myelosuppression, neurotoxicity, alopecia). Although mesna can undergo alkylation and presumably could reduce the cytotoxic effectiveness of ifosfamide by interfering with the mechanism of action, mesna and dimesna are hydrophilic and do not enter most cells, including tumor cells. There is no evidence from in vitro and in vivo tumor models that concomitant mesna interferes with the antitumor activity of ifosfamide.

Concomitant administration of mesna dosages up to 60 mg/kg reportedly does not exacerbate adverse GI effects associated with ifosfamide.

■ **Myelosuppressive Therapy** Concomitant use of ifosfamide and other myelosuppressive agents or radiation therapy may potentiate the hematologic toxicity of the other agents and vice versa. Severe myelosuppression occurs frequently when ifosfamide is used in conjunction with other antineoplastic agents. Patients receiving ifosfamide concomitantly with other myelosuppressive agents should be monitored carefully and dosage of the drugs and time of administration should be managed to minimize additive effects.

■ **Drugs Affecting Hepatic Microsomal Enzymes** Although specific studies have not been done and the clinical importance has not been determined, concomitant administration of drugs that affect cytochrome P-450 hepatic microsomal enzymes could alter the metabolism of ifosfamide resulting in increased or decreased conversion to active metabolites and theoretically could increase the toxicity or decrease the activity of the drug, respectively. In one study in mice, pretreatment with chlordiazepoxide, diazepam, or oxazepam resulted in increased plasma concentrations of active ifosfamide and potentiated the toxicity of the drug.

Acute Toxicity

■ **Manifestations** Limited information is available on the acute toxicity of ifosfamide. Overdosage of the drug would be expected to produce effects that are mainly extensions of common adverse reactions.

■ **Treatment** There is no known specific antidote for ifosfamide overdosage. While mesna is effective in preventing urotoxic effects of ifosfamide when administered prophylactically, the drug is not an antidote for systemic toxicity of the drug. Management of ifosfamide overdosage consists of discontinuance of the drug and initiation of supportive measures appropriate for the type of toxicity observed. Methylene blue has been used in the management of ifosfamide-induced encephalopathy. (See Cautions: Nervous System Toxicity.)

Pharmacology

The exact mechanism(s) of action of ifosfamide has not been conclusively determined, but it appears to be similar to that of other alkylating agents. Ifosfamide, like cyclophosphamide, requires biotransformation in the liver by mixed-function oxidases (cytochrome P-450 system) before it can exert its cytotoxic effects. Following conversion to active metabolites, ifosfamide functions as an alkylating agent, interfering with DNA replication and transcription of RNA, and ultimately resulting in disruption of nucleic acid function. Like other alkylating agents, ifosfamide is cycle-phase nonspecific.

Although the clinical importance is unclear, results of several in vitro and in vivo studies indicate that the cytotoxic activity of ifosfamide may be equal to or moderately greater than that of cyclophosphamide against some animal tumor models (e.g., murine leukemia L1210, Yoshida ascites sarcoma in rats, Lewis lung carcinoma in mice, C3H mammary tumor, Ridgeway osteogenic sarcoma, DS-carcinosarcoma, and TA-nephroblastoma in rats). Ifosfamide was less active than cyclophosphamide against intraperitoneal B16 melanoma and subcutaneous CD8 fl mammary cancer. In human tumor models, the spectrum of activity of ifosfamide resembled that of cyclophosphamide; however, ifosfamide produced higher response rates and less toxicity than cyclophosphamide. In vivo on a weight basis, cyclophosphamide may have greater antineoplastic activity than ifosfamide since a greater percentage of the ifosfamide dose is converted irreversibly to inactive metabolites.

Further study is needed to determine the extent of cross-resistance between ifosfamide, cyclophosphamide, and other alkylating agents. Although cross-resistance has been shown in certain cancer cell lines, cross-resistance with other nitrogen mustard alkylating agents does not appear to be complete.

Like cyclophosphamide and other alkylating agents, ifosfamide is immunosuppressive.

Pharmacokinetics

Ifosfamide is a prodrug and requires biotransformation before it can exert its antineoplastic effects. In vivo, ifosfamide is metabolized to a variety of both active and inactive metabolites and the pharmacokinetics of the drug and its metabolites are complex and have not been fully elucidated. Investigation of the pharmacokinetics of ifosfamide has been difficult, partly because many initial studies used assay methods that were not specific and could not reliably differentiate between ifosfamide and its various metabolites. In addition, identification and quantitation of some ifosfamide metabolites has been difficult because they are highly unstable and present only in very low concentrations. Most recently published pharmacokinetic studies have used improved analytical methods capable of measuring both ifosfamide and its most important metabolites.

■ **Absorption** Plasma concentrations of ifosfamide and its metabolites exhibit marked interindividual variation. Following IV administration of ifosfamide in a dosage of 1 or 2 g/m^2 daily given by continuous IV infusion over 24 hours, plasma drug concentrations after 3 days range from 10–18 or 15–36 mcg/mL, respectively. Peak plasma concentrations of ifosfamide mustard (isoforamide mustard), the principal alkylating metabolite, are reached within 20–30 minutes following IV administration of a single ifosfamide dose and average about 1% of concurrent ifosfamide concentrations on a molar basis. The area under the plasma concentration-time curve (AUC) of ifosfamide increases linearly over the dosage range of 1–5 g/m^2.

Although ifosfamide usually is given IV, the drug appears to be well absorbed following oral or subcutaneous administration, with reported bioavailabilities of 90–100%.

■ **Distribution** Ifosfamide and its metabolites appear to be distributed throughout the body, including the brain and CSF. Ifosfamide is distributed into milk.

The apparent volume of distribution of ifosfamide has been reported to be approximately 33 L, with slightly higher values reported in obese individuals and individuals older than 60 years of age.

■ **Elimination** Ifosfamide is metabolized to both active and inactive metabolites. Initial metabolism of ifosfamide occurs by 2 competing pathways, ring oxidation at the 4-carbon position and oxidation of one of the chloroethyl groups.

Ifosfamide is partially metabolized by mixed-function oxidases (cytochrome P-450 system) in the liver and, to a lesser extent, in the lung to 4-hydroxyifosfamide, which is in equilibrium with aldoifosfamide, the acyclic tautomer. Aldoifosfamide spontaneously splits into ifosfamide mustard, the primary alkylating metabolite, and to acrolein. Production of ifosfamide mustard appears to be catalyzed by phosphodiesterase I (5′-exonuclease) and/or spleen exonuclease (3′-exonuclease), found in serum, lymphocytes, and lymphatic tissue. Because 3′,5′-exonucleases linked to DNA-polymerases seem to be more active in catalyzing this reaction than unlinked exonuclease, production of ifosfamide mustard occurs predominately within cells. In addition, 4-hydroxyifosfamide may be enzymatically metabolized to 4-ketoifosfamide and aldoifosfamide may be enzymatically metabolized to carboxyifosfamide. 4-Hydroxyifosfamide also undergoes reversible reactions with sulfhydryl groups of proteins or amino acids to produce 4-thioifosfamide. The second metabolic pathway in the initial metabolism of ifosfamide involves side-chain oxidation and results in formation of chloroacetaldehyde, 2-dechloroethylifosfamide, and 3-dechloroethylifosfamide.

Plasma concentrations of ifosfamide reportedly decline in a linear, dose-independent manner following IV administration of up to about 4–5 g/m^2 of the drug. Plasma concentrations of ifosfamide mustard and chloroacetaldehyde reportedly decline in a manner similar to that of the parent drug. Administration of ifosfamide doses up to 5 g/m^2 has not been associated with saturation of the cytochrome P-450 system In adults with normal renal and hepatic function who receive a single ifosfamide dose by IV injection or short infusion, the terminal elimination half-life of ifosfamide ranges from 4–8 hours. Limited data indicate that the elimination half-life increases with age, averaging 2.1 hours in children 1–17 years of age and 6 hours in individuals older than 60 years of age; the elimination half-life also may be increased in obese individuals. An elimination half-life of 15 hours has been reported in adults with normal renal and hepatic function by one investigator; however, the assay method used in the study has been questioned and other investigators consistently have reported shorter half-lives. Following administration of ifosfamide over 3–5 days, the terminal elimination half-life decreases in a time-dependent manner, suggesting that ifosfamide induces its own hepatic metabolism. Because the ratio of ifosfamide metabolites remains unchanged, increases in metabolism presumably occur in both of the initial metabolic pathways. The elimination half-life of ifosfamide mustard is about 5–9 hours.

Ifosfamide and its metabolites are excreted principally in urine; about 14–34%, 10–14%, 4–7%, and 1–3% of a dose is excreted as unchanged drug, 3-dechloroethylifosfamide, 2-dechloroethylifosfamide, and carboxyifosfamide, respectively. Other metabolites (e.g., 4-hydroxyifosfamide, 4-ketoifosfamide) also appear to be excreted in the urine in very small amounts (less than 1% of the ifosfamide dose).

Chemistry and Stability

■ **Chemistry** Ifosfamide, an oxazaphosphorine derivative, is an alkylating agent structurally related to cyclophosphamide. Ifosfamide differs structurally from cyclophosphamide in that it contains one 2-chloroethyl group attached to the exocyclic nitrogen and a second 2-chloroethyl group attached to the cyclic nitrogen of the oxazaphosphorine ring, whereas both 2-chloroethyl groups contained in cyclophosphamide are attached to the exocyclic nitrogen. This structural difference in the spatial separation of the 2-chloroethyl groups results in ifosfamide having greater aqueous solubility, slower rate of activation, different alkylating metabolites, and a more effective DNA cross-linking distance than cyclophosphamide and appears to be responsible for the differences in antineoplastic activity and toxicity profiles associated with the drugs.

Ifosfamide occurs as an off-white to white, crystalline powder and is soluble in water. Following reconstitution of the commercially available sterile powder with sterile water for injection, ifosfamide solutions containing 50 mg/mL have a pH of 6.

Commercially available ifosfamide injection is an aqueous solution containing 100 mg/mL.

■ **Stability** Ifosfamide sterile powder for injection should be stored at 20–25°C. The powder should be protected from temperatures higher than 30°C, since ifosfamide reportedly liquefies at temperatures exceeding 35°C. Commercially available ifosfamide injection (100 mg/mL) should be refrigerated at 2–8°C.

Following reconstitution of ifosfamide sterile powder with sterile water for injection or with sterile bacteriostatic water for injection containing benzyl alcohol or parabens, solutions containing 50 mg of ifosfamide per mL are stable for up to 24 hours when kept refrigerated. Reconstituted ifosfamide solutions are compatible with 5% dextrose, 0.9% sodium chloride, lactated Ringer's, and sterile water for injection. Reconstituted solutions that have been further diluted to 0.6–20 mg/mL in one of these compatible IV fluids are physically and chemically stable in glass, polyvinyl chloride (PVC), or polyolefin containers for up to 24 hours when kept refrigerated. Intermediate concentrations and mixtures of these diluents (e.g., 2.5% dextrose, 0.45% sodium chloride, 5% dextrose and 0.9% sodium chloride) also may be used.

Following dilution of commercially available ifosfamide injection (100 mg/mL), solutions containing a final concentration of 20 mg/mL are physically and chemically compatible for 24 hours at 25°C in 5% dextrose, 5% dextrose and 0.2% sodium chloride, 5% dextrose and 0.33% sodium chloride, 5% dextrose and 0.45% sodium chloride, 5% dextrose and 0.9% sodium chloride, 0.9% sodium chloride, or lactated Ringer's injection.

Ifosfamide is physically and chemically compatible with mesna, and admixtures of the drugs reportedly are stable for at least 24 hours in 5% dextrose injection or lactated Ringer's injection.

For further information on the handling of antineoplastic agents, see the ASHP Guidelines on Handling Hazardous Drugs at http://www.ahfsdruginformation.com.

Preparations

Excipients in commercially available drug preparations may have clinically important effects in some individuals; consult specific product labeling for details.

Ifosfamide

Parenteral		
Kit	1 g, For injection, for IV infusion, Ifosfamide (Ifex® Kit) 100 mg/mL (1 g), Injection, Mesna (Mesnex®) (with benzyl alcohol)	**Ifex®/Mesnex® Kit,** Bristol-Myers Squibb
	100 mg/mL (1 g), Injection, Ifosfamide 100 mg/mL (1 g) Injection, Mesna (with benzyl alcohol)	**Ifosfamide Injection/Mesna Injection Kit**
	3 g, For injection, for IV infusion, Ifosfamide (Ifex®) 100 mg/mL (1 g), Injection, Mesna (Mesnex®) (with benzyl alcohol)	**Ifex®/Mesnex® Kit,** Bristol-Myers Squibb
	100 mg/mL (3 g), Injection, Ifosfamide 100 mg/mL (1 g) Injection, Mesna (with benzyl alcohol)	**Ifosfamide Injection/Mesna Injection Kit**

†Use is not currently included in the labeling approved by the US Food and Drug Administration

Imatinib Mesylate

■ Imatinib mesylate, an inhibitor of Bcr-Abl tyrosine kinase, is an antineoplastic agent.

Uses

■ **Chronic Myelogenous Leukemia** Imatinib is used for the treatment of Philadelphia chromosome-positive (Ph$^+$) chronic myelogenous leukemia (CML) in adult and pediatric patients.

Adult Patients **First-line Therapy for Chronic Phase CML.** Imatinib is used for the first-line treatment of Ph$^+$ CML in chronic phase in adult patients. The duration of follow-up for patients receiving imatinib for this use is limited.

The indication for this use is based on the results of an open-label, multicenter, randomized phase III trial in 1,106 patients receiving either imatinib or combination therapy with interferon alfa and cytarabine for newly diagnosed chronic phase Ph$^+$ CML. Single-agent therapy consisted of imatinib at an initial dose of 400 mg daily with dose escalations to 600 mg daily and then 800 mg daily as tolerated. Combination therapy consisted of interferon alfa 5 million units/m^2 given subcutaneously daily with cytarabine 20 mg/m^2 given subcutaneously daily for 10 days every month. Crossover therapy was allowed for treatment failure or unacceptable toxicity. The patients were mostly Caucasian (59% males and 41% females) with a median age of 51 years.

At the time of follow-up, 79% of patients initially receiving imatinib continued the assigned treatment; 7% of patients initially receiving interferon alfa and cytarabine continued the assigned treatment and the remainder either discontinued first-line therapy or crossed over to treatment with imatinib. The primary efficacy endpoint was progression-free survival, and progression was defined as death, progression to accelerated phase or blast phase CML, loss of complete hematologic response, loss of major cytogenetic response, or increasing white blood cell count in a patient with disease that did not achieve a complete hematologic response. According to intention-to-treat analysis, the estimated rate of progression-free survival at 30 months was higher in patients receiving imatinib (88%) than in those receiving interferon alfa and cytarabine (68%). The estimated rate of patients free of progression to accelerated phase

CML or blast crisis at 30 months was higher in patients receiving imatinib (95%) than in those receiving interferon alfa and cytarabine (90%).

The probability of remaining free of disease progression at 30 months was associated with molecular response to treatment achieved at 12 months: 100% probability of remaining free of disease progression for patients with complete cytogenetic response and major molecular response (a reduction of at least 3 logarithms in the amount of Bcr-Abl transcripts measured by real-time quantitative reverse transcriptase polymerase chain reaction), 93% for those with complete cytogenetic response but not major molecular response, and 82% for those without complete cytogenetic response. Secondary endpoints, including complete hematologic response and major cytogenetic response, were higher in patients receiving imatinib than in those receiving interferon alfa and cytarabine. Fluid retention (including superficial edema), muscle cramps, and rash occurred more frequently in patients receiving imatinib; fatigue, pyrexia, myalgia, and depression occurred more frequently in patients receiving interferon alfa and cytarabine.

Second-line Therapy for CML. Imatinib mesylate is used for the treatment of Ph$^+$ CML in patients who are in blast crisis, in the accelerated phase, or in the chronic phase of the disease after failure of interferon alfa therapy.

The current indication of imatinib is based principally on the results of 3 international, open-label, single-arm studies in more than 1000 patients with Ph$^+$ CML. The first study enrolled patients in the chronic phase of CML who failed interferon alfa therapy (i.e., inadequate hematologic response following 6 months of treatment, inadequate cytogenetic response following 1 year of treatment, hematologic or cytogenetic relapse, or intolerance to interferon). The second study enrolled patients who were in the accelerated phase of CML, while the third study enrolled patients in myeloid blast crisis. Patients in the chronic phase of CML received an initial imatinib dose of 400 mg daily (increased to 600 mg daily as necessary), while those in the accelerated phase or blast crisis received either 400 or 600 mg of the drug daily. The median duration of therapy with imatinib in patients with chronic phase, accelerated phase, or blast crisis was 29, 18, or 4 months, respectively.

Hematologic response (i.e., complete hematologic response, and, in patients in the accelerated phase or blast crisis, no evidence of leukemia or return to chronic phase of CML) occurred in 95, 71, or 31% of patients in the chronic phase, accelerated phase, or blast crisis, respectively. Complete hematologic response was achieved in approximately 95, 38, or 7% of these patients, respectively. Major cytogenetic response (i.e., complete or partial suppression of Ph$^+$ cells) occurred in 60, 21, or 7% of patients in the chronic phase, accelerated phase, or blast crisis, respectively, while complete cytogenetic response (i.e., no Ph$^+$ cells in metaphase) was achieved in 39, 16, or 2% of these patients, respectively. The rates of hematologic response and major cytogenetic response were higher in patients with accelerated phase CML or blast crisis who received an initial dosage of 600 mg of imatinib daily than in those who received an initial dosage of 400 mg daily.

Median time to hematologic response in patients receiving imatinib was 1 month; median duration of hematologic response is 10 months in patients in blast crisis and 29 months in those with accelerated phase CML receiving an initial dosage of imatinib 600 mg daily. About 88% of patients with late chronic phase CML, and 64% of patients with accelerated phase CML, who achieved an initial major cytogenetic response to imatinib therapy maintained that response for 2 years. About 27% of patients with blast crisis who achieved an initial hematologic response to imatinib therapy maintained that response for 2 years. In patients with late chronic phase CML receiving 2 years of imatinib therapy, estimated overall survival is 91%. In patients with accelerated CML, median survival was 21 months in patients receiving an initial imatinib dosage of 400 mg daily; median survival has not been reached in those receiving an initial imatinib dosage of 600 mg daily. In patients with blast crisis, median survival was 7 months.

Resistance to imatinib, particularly in patients with advanced-stage CML, has developed during therapy with the drug. In patients with myeloid blast crisis, development of imatinib resistance was observed as early as 42 days following initiation of therapy. Resistance to imatinib has not been evaluated in all patient groups; however, limited data from several open-label studies indicate a relapse rate of 4 or 43–80% in patients in chronic phase or blast crisis, respectively, who received the drug. Although the mechanism(s) of resistance to imatinib has not been fully determined to date, mutation and/or amplification (resulting in increased expression of Bcr-Abl tyrosine kinase) of the Bcr-Abl gene may be associated with decreased efficacy of the drug.

Pediatric Patients **First-line Therapy for Chronic Phase CML.** Imatinib is used for the first-line treatment of Ph$^+$ CML in chronic phase in pediatric patients. The duration of follow-up for patients receiving imatinib for this use is limited.

The indication for this use is based on the results of an open-label, uncontrolled phase II trial in 51 pediatric patients receiving imatinib 340 mg/m^2 daily for newly diagnosed chronic phase Ph$^+$ CML. After 8 weeks of imatinib therapy, complete hematologic response was observed in 78% of patients. The complete cytogenetic response rate (typically achieved between months 3 and 10) was 65%, which is comparable to the rate observed in adult patients.

Second-line Therapy for CML. Imatinib is used for the second-line treatment of Ph$^+$ CML in chronic phase in pediatric patients with disease that has recurred following stem cell transplantation or is resistant to interferon alfa therapy.

The indication for this use is based on the results of 2 small uncontrolled studies in pediatric patients receiving imatinib as second-line therapy for chronic phase CML. In the first study, which involved 14 pediatric patients ranging in age from 3 to 20 years of age, a complete cytogenetic response was observed in 7 patients. In the second study, which involved 3 patients, a complete cytogenetic response was observed in 2 patients.

■ **Gastrointestinal Stromal Tumors** Imatinib is used for the treatment of malignant gastrointestinal stromal tumors (GIST) in patients with unresectable tumor or metastatic disease that is Kit (CD117) positive. This indication is based on objective response rate; there currently are no controlled trials demonstrating a clinical benefit (e.g., lessening of disease-related symptoms, increased survival).

The indication for this use is based on the results of an open-label, multinational study in 147 patients receiving either imatinib 400 mg daily or imatinib 600 mg daily for up to 36 months for unresectable or metastatic malignant GIST. The objective response rate was 67% with a complete response in one patient and partial responses in 98 patients. The median time to response was 12 weeks. The study was not designed with adequate power to detect a statistically significant difference in response rates between the dose groups.

■ **Other Uses** Imatinib is used as a single agent for the treatment of relapsed or refractory Ph$^+$ acute lymphocytic leukemia (ALL), myelodysplastic syndrome (MDS) or myeloproliferative disease (MPD) associated with gene rearrangements of platelet-derived growth factor receptor (PDGFR), aggressive systemic mastocytosis (ASM), hypereosinophilic syndrome (HES) or chronic eosinophilic leukemia (CEL), and dermatofibrosarcoma protuberans (DFSP).

Dosage and Administration

■ **General** Imatinib mesylate should be used under the supervision of a qualified clinician experienced in the treatment of hematologic malignancies or malignant sarcomas as indicated.

In patients with elevated eosinophil concentrations, consider concomitant administration of prophylactic therapy with systemic corticosteroids (1–2 mg/kg) for 1–2 weeks upon initiation of imatinib therapy to reduce the risk of hypereosinophilic cardiac toxicity. (See Major Toxicities: Adverse Cardiovascular Effects and see General Precautions: Cardiovascular Toxicity.)

Imatinib mesylate is administered orally. In adults, imatinib doses of 400 or 600 mg should be administered once daily; an imatinib dosage of 800 mg daily should be administered as 400 mg twice daily using the 400-mg tablet to reduce exposure to iron. In children or adolescents, imatinib may be given as a once-daily dose or, alternatively, the daily dose may be divided equally in the morning and the evening.

Imatinib mesylate should be given with a meal and a large glass (240 mL) of water to minimize gastric irritation. Alternatively, for patients unable to swallow the tablets, the film-coated tablets may be dispersed in a glass of water or apple juice. The required number of tablets should be dispersed in 50 mL of beverage for each 100-mg tablet or 200 mL of beverage for each 400-mg tablet. The suspension should be administered immediately after complete disintegration of the tablet(s).

The manufacturer states that imatinib therapy may be continued as indicated in the absence of progressive disease or unacceptable toxicity.

Dosage of imatinib mesylate is expressed in terms of imatinib.

Chronic Myelogenous Leukemia **Adult Patients.** The recommended initial adult dosage of imatinib for the first-line treatment of Ph$^+$ chronic phase CML is 400 mg daily. Dose escalations to 600 mg daily, and then to 800 mg daily (administered as 400 mg twice daily), were permitted in patients receiving imatinib in the randomized trial.

The recommended adult dosage of imatinib for the second-line treatment of Ph$^+$ chronic phase CML is 400 mg daily; the recommended adult dosage for the second-line treatment of patients in accelerated phase or blast crisis is 600 mg daily. If there is inadequate hematologic response after at least 3 months of therapy, failure to achieve a cytogenetic response after 6–12 months of therapy, loss of a previously achieved hematologic or cytogenetic response, or evidence of disease progression, the manufacturer states that, in the absence of severe adverse drug or hematologic effects, adult dosage of imatinib may be increased to 600 mg daily in adults with chronic phase CML or to 800 mg daily (administered as 400 mg twice daily) in those with accelerated phase CML or blast crisis.

Pediatric Patients. The recommended pediatric dosage of imatinib for the first-line treatment of Ph$^+$ chronic phase CML is 340 mg/m^2 daily, and the daily dose should not exceed 600 mg.

The recommended pediatric dosage of imatinib for the second-line treatment of Ph$^+$ chronic phase CML that has recurred following stem cell transplantation or is resistant to interferon alfa therapy is 260 mg/m^2 daily.

Acute Lymphocytic Leukemia For the treatment of relapsed or refractory Ph$^+$ ALL, the recommended adult dosage of imatinib is 600 mg daily.

Myelodysplastic Syndrome/Myeloproliferative Diseases For the treatment of myelodysplastic syndrome or myeloproliferative disease associated with gene rearrangements of PDGFR, the recommended adult dosage of imatinib is 400 mg daily.

Aggressive Systemic Mastocytosis For the treatment of aggressive systemic mastocytosis (ASM) without the D816V c-Kit mutation, the recommended adult dosage of imatinib is 400 mg daily. For ASM with unknown status of the D816V c-Kit mutation that is not responding satisfactorily to other therapies, treatment with an adult imatinib dosage of 400 mg daily may be considered. For ASM without the D816V c-Kit mutation or of unknown D816V c-Kit mutational status that is associated with eosinophilia (a clonal hematologic disease related to the FIP1L1-PDGFRα fusion kinase), the recommended initial adult dosage of imatinib is 100 mg daily; if therapeutic response is insufficient, dose escalation from 100 mg to 400 mg may be attempted as tolerated. For ASM with the D816V c-Kit mutation, imatinib is ineffective and other therapy is indicated.

Hypereosinophilic Syndrome/Chronic Eosinophilic Leukemia For the treatment of hypereosinophilic syndrome (HES) or chronic eosinophilic leukemia (CEL) in patients without FIP1L1-PDGFRα fusion kinase expression or in patients in whom expression of FIP1L1-PDGFRα fusion kinase is unknown, the recommended adult dosage of imatinib is 400 mg daily. For HES or CEL with FIP1L1-PDGFRα fusion kinase expression, the recommended initial adult dosage of imatinib is 100 mg daily; if therapeutic response is insufficient, dose escalation from 100 to 400 mg may be attempted as tolerated.

Dermatofibrosarcoma Protuberans For unresectable, recurrent, and/or metastatic dermatofibrosarcoma protuberans, the recommended adult dosage of imatinib is 800 mg daily.

Gastrointestinal Stromal Tumors For the treatment of unresectable and/or metastatic malignant GIST, the recommended adult dosage of imatinib is 400 or 600 mg daily.

Dosage Modification for Toxicity **Dermatologic Toxicity.** Imatinib therapy should be discontinued in patients experiencing severe dermatologic toxicity, such as bullous skin reactions. (See Dermatologic Effects in Cautions: Major Toxicities.) In some patients, imatinib therapy was reinitiated at a lower dosage following resolution or lessening of the bullous skin reaction.

Fluid Retention/Edema. Management of edema may include diuretics, other supportive measures, and/or reduction of imatinib dosage. If severe fluid retention or edema develops, imatinib therapy should be interrupted until complete resolution occurs.

Hepatic Toxicity. In patients who exhibit substantial increases in bilirubin (more than 3 times the upper limit of normal) or hepatic transaminase concentrations (more than 5 times the upper limit of normal), the manufacturer recommends that therapy with imatinib be withheld until bilirubin concentrations decrease to less than 1.5 times the upper limit of normal or transaminase concentrations decrease to less than 2.5 times the upper limit of normal. Imatinib therapy may then be resumed at a reduced daily dosage (e.g., in adults, 400 mg to 300 mg, 600 mg to 400 mg, or 800 mg to 600 mg). In pediatric patients showing hepatic toxicity, daily imatinib doses can be reduced from 340 to 260 mg/m^2 daily or from 260 to 200 mg/m^2 daily.

Hematologic Toxicity. In *adult* patients with *chronic phase Ph$^+$ CML, myelodysplastic syndrome/myeloproliferative disease, aggressive systemic mastocytosis, or hypereosinophilic syndrome/chronic eosinophilic leukemia* receiving an initial imatinib dosage of 400 mg daily who experience a *first* occurrence of neutropenia (i.e., absolute neutrophil counts [ANC] less than 1000/mm^3) or thrombocytopenia (i.e., platelet counts less than 50,000/mm^3), the manufacturer recommends that subsequent doses of the drug be withheld until ANC reaches or exceeds 1500/mm^3 and platelet counts reach or exceed 75,000/mm^3. Imatinib therapy may then be resumed at the original starting dosage (400 mg daily). Following a *recurrence* of neutropenia or thrombocytopenia, imatinib therapy should be withheld until neutrophil and platelet counts return to acceptable levels (ANC of 1500/mm^3 or greater and platelet count of 75,000/mm^3 or greater), then reinitiated at a reduced dosage of 300 mg daily.

In *adult* patients with *aggressive systemic mastocytosis associated with eosinophilia, or hypereosinophilic syndrome/chronic eosinophilic leukemia with FIP1L1-PDGFRα fusion kinase expression* receiving an initial imatinib dosage of 100 mg daily who experience neutropenia (i.e., ANC less than 1000/mm^3) or thrombocytopenia (i.e., platelet counts less than 50,000/mm^3), the manufacturer recommends that subsequent doses of the drug be withheld until ANC reaches or exceeds 1500/mm^3 and platelet counts reach or exceed 75,000/mm^3. Imatinib therapy may then be resumed at the same dosage.

In *adult* patients with *accelerated phase or blast crisis Ph$^+$ CML or Ph$^+$ ALL* receiving an initial imatinib dosage of 600 mg daily who experience severe neutropenia (i.e., ANC less than 500/mm^3) or thrombocytopenia (i.e., platelet counts less than 10,000/mm^3) that is unrelated to the disease, the manufacturer recommends that dosage of imatinib be reduced to 400 mg daily. If cytopenia persists for 2 weeks, the dosage of imatinib should be reduced further to 300 mg daily. If cytopenia persists for 4 weeks, the manufacturer recommends that subsequent doses of the drug be withheld until ANC reaches or exceeds 1000/mm^3 and platelet counts reach or exceed 20,000/mm^3; imatinib therapy may then be reinitiated at a reduced dosage of 300 mg daily.

In *pediatric* patients with *newly diagnosed chronic phase Ph$^+$ CML* receiving an initial imatinib dosage of 340 mg/m^2 daily who experience a *first* occurrence of neutropenia (i.e., ANC less than 1000/mm^3) or thrombocytopenia (i.e., platelet counts less than 50,000/mm^3), the manufacturer recommends that subsequent doses of the drug be withheld until ANC reaches or exceeds 1500/mm^3 and platelet counts reach or exceed 75,000/mm^3. Imatinib therapy may then be resumed at the same dosage. Following a *recurrence* of neutropenia or thrombocytopenia, imatinib therapy should be withheld until neutrophil and platelet counts return to acceptable levels (ANC of 1500/mm^3 or greater and platelet count of 75,000/mm^3 or greater), then reinitiated at a reduced dosage of 260 mg/m^2 daily.

In *pediatric* patients with *recurrent or resistant chronic phase Ph$^+$ CML* receiving an initial imatinib dosage of 260 mg/m^2 daily who experience a *first* occurrence of neutropenia (i.e., ANC less than 1000/mm^3) or thrombocytopenia (i.e., platelet counts less than 50,000/mm^3), the manufacturer recommends that subsequent doses of the drug be withheld until ANC reaches or exceeds 1500/mm^3 and platelet counts reach or exceed 75,000/mm^3. Imatinib therapy may then be resumed at the same dosage. Following a *recurrence* of neutropenia or thrombocytopenia, imatinib therapy should be withheld until neutrophil and platelet counts return to acceptable levels (ANC of 1500/mm^3 or greater and platelet count of 75,000/mm^3 or greater), then reinitiated at a reduced dosage of 200 mg/m^2 daily.

In *adult* patients with *dermatofibrosarcoma protuberans* receiving an initial imatinib dosage of 800 mg daily who experience a *first* occurrence of neutropenia (i.e., ANC less than 1000/mm^3) or thrombocytopenia (i.e., platelet counts less than 50,000/mm^3), the manufacturer recommends that subsequent doses of the drug be withheld until ANC reaches or exceeds 1500/mm^3 and platelet counts reach or exceed 75,000/mm^3. Imatinib therapy may then be reinitiated at a reduced dosage of 600 mg daily. Following a *recurrence* of neutropenia or thrombocytopenia, imatinib therapy should be withheld until neutrophil and platelet counts return to acceptable levels (ANC of 1500/mm^3 or greater and platelet count of 75,000/mm^3 or greater), then reinitiated at a reduced dosage of 400 mg daily.

In *adult* patients with *GIST* receiving an initial imatinib dosage of 400 or 600 mg daily who experience a *first* occurrence of neutropenia (i.e., ANC less than 1000/mm^3) or thrombocytopenia (i.e., platelet counts less than 50,000/mm^3), the manufacturer recommends that subsequent doses of the drug be withheld until ANC reaches or exceeds 1500/mm^3 and platelet counts reach or exceed 75,000/mm^3. Imatinib therapy may then be resumed at the original starting dosage (400 or 600 mg daily). Following a *recurrence* of neutropenia or thrombocytopenia, imatinib therapy should be withheld until neutrophil and platelet counts return to acceptable levels (ANC of 1500/mm^3 or greater and platelet count of 75,000/mm^3 or greater), then reinitiated at a reduced dosage: 300 mg daily if the starting dose was 400 mg, or 400 mg daily if the starting dose was 600 mg.

■ **Special Populations** ***Hepatic Impairment*** Patients with mild to moderate hepatic impairment should receive an initial imatinib dosage of 400 mg daily. In patients with conditions normally requiring initial dosages less than 400 mg daily (e.g., pediatric patients with small body frame, adults with ASM or HES/CEL with FIP1L1-PDGFRα fusion kinase expression), therapy should be initiated at the recommended initial dosage, regardless of hepatic function.

Patients with severe hepatic impairment should receive an initial imatinib dosage of 300 mg daily. In patients with conditions normally requiring initial dosages less than 300 mg daily (e.g., pediatric patients with small body frame, adults with ASM or HES/CEL with FIP1L1-PDGFRα fusion kinase expression), therapy should be initiated at the recommended initial dosage, regardless of hepatic function. In patients with ASM or HES/CEL with FIP1L1-PDGFRα fusion kinase expression *and* severe hepatic impairment who require dosage escalation, dosage may be initially increased from 100 mg daily to 300 mg daily (rather than to 400 mg daily as usually recommended); liver function should be monitored carefully. If therapeutic response is insufficient in such patients, increasing the dosage to 400 mg daily as tolerated may be considered.

Cautions

■ **Contraindications** Known hypersensitivity to imatinib or any ingredient in the formulation.

■ **Warnings/Precautions** ***Warnings*** **Fetal/Neonatal Morbidity and Mortality.** May cause fetal harm; teratogenicity and embryolethality demonstrated in animals. No adequate and well-controlled studies to date in humans. Pregnancy should be avoided during therapy. If used during pregnancy, apprise of potential fetal hazard.

Major Toxicities **Cardiovascular Effects.** Severe congestive heart failure and left ventricular dysfunction have been reported during imatinib therapy, mostly in geriatric patients or patients with a history of cardiac disease. Monitor such patients carefully; evaluate and treat any patient with manifestations of cardiac failure.

In patients with hypereosinophilic syndrome and cardiac involvement, cardiogenic shock and left ventricular dysfunction has been associated with the initiation of imatinib therapy. In patients with this condition, withhold imatinib therapy and administer systemic corticosteroid therapy and supportive measures.

Dermatologic Effects. Bullous skin reactions, including erythema multiforme and Stevens-Johnson syndrome, have been reported in patients receiving imatinib. If dermatologic toxicity occurs, discontinue imatinib therapy. (See Dosage Modification for Toxicity, in Dosage and Administration.) Following resolution or lessening of the bullous skin reaction, imatinib therapy was reinitiated in some patients at a reduced dosage with or without concomitant administration of corticosteroids or antihistamines.

Fluid Retention/Edema. Fluid retention/edema occurred in about 60–80% of patients receiving imatinib for CML or GIST. Severe fluid retention (i.e., pleural effusion, pericardial effusion, pulmonary edema, ascites) or severe superficial edema (i.e., rapid weight gain, anasarca), occurred in 1–12% of patients receiving imatinib for CML or GIST in clinical studies. Other types of fluid retention and edema events, sometimes fatal, have occurred in patients receiving imatinib, including cardiac tamponade, cerebral edema, increased intracranial pressure, and papilledema. At least one patient with blast crisis who received imatinib in clinical studies died as a result of pleural effusion, congestive heart failure, and renal failure. In patients with CML, the incidence of these adverse effects appears to be increased in patients in blast crisis, in those receiving higher dosages (i.e., 600 mg daily), and in geriatric patients. Monitor signs (e.g., body weight) and symptoms of fluid retention regularly during imatinib therapy. If severe fluid retention develops, withhold imatinib therapy and provide appropriate treatment until complete resolution occurs.

Hematologic Effects. Cytopenias, including neutropenia, thrombocytopenia, and anemia, occurred in patients receiving imatinib for CML or GIST. For patients with CML, the frequency of cytopenias was dependent on the stage of disease. Cytopenias were less frequent in patients with newly diagnosed CML; the frequency of grade 3 or 4 neutropenia and thrombocytopenia was between 2-fold and 3-fold higher in patients with blast crisis or accelerated phase CML than in those with chronic phase CML. In pediatric patients receiving imatinib for CML, grade 3 or 4 cytopenias (neutropenia, thrombocytopenia, and anemia) occurred, usually within the first several months of therapy. Monitor complete blood cell counts (CBCs) weekly during the first month of therapy, every other week during the second month, and periodically (e.g., every 2–3 months) thereafter as clinically indicated. If hematologic toxicity occurs, withhold imatinib. (See Dosage Modification for Toxicity, in Dosage and Administration.)

Hepatic Effects. In patients receiving imatinib as first-line therapy for CML, grade 3 or 4 hyperbilirubinemia occurred in about 1%, and grade 3 or 4 elevations in ALT or AST in about 3–4%, of patients. In patients receiving imatinib as second-line therapy for CML, grade 3 or 4 hyperbilirubinemia occurred in up to 4% of patients, and elevations in alkaline phosphatase, ALT, and AST (grade 3 or 4 severity) occurred in up to 5% of patients. Fatal hepatic failure occurred in at least one patient who received imatinib concomitantly with acetaminophen. (See Drug Interactions: Acetaminophen.) In patients receiving imatinib for GIST, grade 3 or 4 elevations in ALT, AST, and bilirubin occurred in about 7, 5, and 3% of patients, respectively. Monitor liver function tests (i.e., transaminases, bilirubin, alkaline phosphatase) prior to initiation of therapy and monthly thereafter or as clinically indicated. If liver function test results are elevated, withhold imatinib. (See Dosage Modification for Toxicity, in Dosage and Administration.)

GI Effects. Nausea, vomiting, and diarrhea occur frequently in patients receiving imatinib. Gastrointestinal perforation, sometimes fatal, has occurred rarely in patients receiving imatinib.

Hemorrhage. Grade 3 or 4 hemorrhage has occurred in about 1% of patients receiving imatinib for first-line treatment of CML and 5% of those receiving the drug for GIST. In patients with GIST, hemorrhagic events included GI bleeds, intratumoral bleeds, or both; GI tumor sites may have been the source of GI bleeds.

Metabolic Effects. Hypophosphatemia associated with altered bone and mineral metabolism has been reported in patients receiving imatinib for CML or GIST.

General Precautions **Cardiovascular Toxicity.** Patients with cardiac disease or increased risk for cardiac failure should be monitored carefully for manifestations of cardiac failure during imatinib therapy.

Patients with elevated eosinophil concentrations are at increased risk for hypereosinophilic cardiac toxicity associated with imatinib. Patients with myelodysplastic syndrome (MDS)/myeloproliferative disease (MPD) or aggressive systemic mastocytosis (ASM) should be tested for elevated eosinophil concentrations. Perform an echocardiogram and measure serum troponin concentrations in patients with elevated eosinophil concentrations, including patients with hypereosinophilic syndrome/chronic eosinophilic leukemia or patients with MDS/MPD or ASM associated with high eosinophil concentrations. If the results of the echocardiogram or serum troponin concentrations are abnormal, consider the use of prophylactic therapy with systemic corticosteroids upon initiation of imatinib therapy. (See Dosage and Administration: General.)

GI Toxicity. Administer with food and a large glass of water to minimize GI irritation.

Long-term Therapy. Long-term safety data not available in humans. Severe hepatic and renal toxicity observed in animals receiving imatinib for as little as 2 weeks. Immunosuppression also reported in animals receiving imatinib for up to 39 weeks.

Specific Populations **Pregnancy.** Category D. (See Warnings: Fetal/Neonatal Morbidity and Mortality.)

Lactation. Imatinib and/or its metabolites are distributed into milk in rats; discontinue nursing because of potential risk in nursing infants.

Pediatric Use. Safety and efficacy of imatinib in children younger than 2 years of age have not been established. Imatinib has been used in a small number of pediatric patients for first-line or second-line treatment of CML. The duration of follow-up for patients receiving imatinib for newly diagnosed chronic phase CML is limited. Studies to date suggest that the safety and efficacy of imatinib are similar in children and adults, except musculoskeletal pain was less frequent and peripheral edema was not reported. Nausea and vomiting and myalgias were the most frequent adverse effects in children receiving imatinib.

Geriatric Use. With the exception of a higher incidence of edema (see Major Toxicities: Fluid Retention/Edema under Warnings/Precautions, in Cautions), no substantial differences in safety and efficacy relative to younger adults were observed.

Hepatic Impairment. Imatinib is metabolized extensively in the liver, and increased exposure to the drug and its major active metabolite is observed in patients with severe hepatic impairment. Close monitoring is recommended in these patients. (See Major Toxicities: Hepatic Effects, under Warnings/Precautions in Cautions.)

Renal Impairment. Safety and efficacy not established; use with caution.

■ **Common Adverse Effects** The most common adverse effects associated with imatinib therapy are fluid retention/edema, nausea and vomiting, muscle cramps, musculoskeletal pain, diarrhea, and rash. Other adverse effects occurring in 10% or more of patients receiving imatinib for CML or GIST include fatigue, asthenia, headache, dizziness, insomnia, depression, anxiety, joint pain, arthralgia, myalgia, back pain, abdominal pain, flatulence, dyspepsia, loose stools, anorexia, constipation, taste disturbance, nasopharyngitis, cough, pharyngolaryngeal pain, pharyngitis, sinusitis, upper respiratory tract infection, pneumonia, influenza, dyspnea, hemorrhage (including GI and CNS hemorrhage), pyrexia, increased weight, night sweats, rigors, hepatic toxicity, hypokalemia, pruritus, chest pain, and increased lacrimation.

Drug Interactions

■ **Drugs Affecting Hepatic Microsomal Enzymes** Cytochrome P-450 (CYP) isoenzyme 3A4 (CYP3A4) inhibitors (e.g., clarithromycin, erythromycin, itraconazole, ketoconazole): Potential pharmacokinetic interaction causing increased serum imatinib concentrations.

CYP3A4 inducers (e.g., carbamazepine, dexamethasone, phenobarbital, phenytoin, rifampin, St. John's wort): Potential pharmacokinetic interaction causing substantially decreased serum imatinib concentrations; alternative agents with less enzyme induction potential should be considered. For patients receiving a potent CYP3A4 inducer, such as rifampin or phenytoin, imatinib dosage should be increased by at least 50%, and clinical response should be monitored carefully.

■ **CYP3A4 Substrates** Imatinib appears to inhibit CYP3A4. Potential pharmacokinetic interaction (increased plasma CYP3A4-substrate concentrations) when imatinib is used with CYP3A4 substrates (e.g., cyclosporine, pimozide, triazolo-benzodiazepines, dihydropyridine calcium-channel blockers, certain HMG-CoA reductase inhibitors).

■ **Warfarin** Imatinib appears to inhibit CYP2C9 and CYP3A4. Potential pharmacokinetic and pharmacologic interaction (enhanced anticoagulant effect). Patients requiring anticoagulation therapy should receive heparin or low molecular weight heparin.

■ **CYP2D6 Substrates** Imatinib appears to inhibit CYP2D6. Potential pharmacokinetic interaction (increased CYP2D6 substrate plasma concentrations).

■ **Acetaminophen** Potential pharmacokinetic interaction (increased serum acetaminophen concentrations); caution is recommended. (See Major Toxicities: Hepatic Effects.)

Description

Imatinib mesylate, an inhibitor of Bcr-Abl tyrosine kinase, is an antineoplastic agent that is structurally and pharmacologically distinct from other currently available antineoplastic agents.

The Philadelphia chromosome, characteristic of chronic myelogenous leukemia (CML), is created by a reciprocal translocation between chromosomes 9 and 22. Translocation between these chromosomes results in production of an abnormal protein (Bcr-Abl tyrosine kinase) that exhibits enhanced tyrosine kinase activity (i.e., increased phosphorylation of tyrosine residues); phosphorylation of tyrosine residues on growth factor receptors is thought to be important in stimulating cell proliferation and inhibiting cell death (apoptosis). Imatinib competitively inhibits Bcr-Abl tyrosine kinase, thereby inhibiting tyrosine phosphorylation of proteins involved in Bcr-Abl signal transduction. The drug has been shown to inhibit proliferation and induce apoptosis of Bcr-Abl-positive cells as well as fresh leukemic cells from Philadelphia chromosome-positive CML.

Imatinib also appears to inhibit receptor tyrosine kinases for platelet-derived growth factor (PDGF) and stem cell factor (SCF), c-Kit, and PDGF-mediated and SCF-mediated cellular events. Data from in vitro studies shows that imatinib inhibits proliferation and induces apoptosis in gastrointestinal stromal tumor (GIST) cells, which express an activating c-kit mutation.

Imatinib is metabolized by the cytochrome P-450 (CYP) microsomal enzyme system, principally by the isoenzyme 3A4 (CYP3A4) and, to a lesser extent, by CYP1A2, CYP2D6, CYP2C9, and CYP2C19. The active metabolite, an *N*-demethylated piperazine derivative, formed principally by CYP3A4, accounts for approximately 15% of total plasma concentrations of the drug. Approximately 68 and 13% of an oral dose of imatinib is excreted in feces and urine, respectively, as active and inactive metabolites within 7 days.

Advice to Patients

Risks of severe fluid retention, cytopenia, and hepatotoxicity. Importance of women informing clinicians if they are or plan to become pregnant or to breast-feed; necessity of advising women to avoid pregnancy and nursing during therapy. Advise pregnant women of risk to the fetus.

Importance of informing clinicians of existing or contemplated concomitant therapy, including prescription and OTC drugs, as well as concomitant illnesses.

Overview (see Users Guide). For additional information until a more detailed monograph is developed and published, the manufacturer's labeling should be consulted. It is *essential* that the manufacturer's labeling be consulted for more detailed information on usual cautions, precautions, contraindications, potential drug interactions, laboratory test interferences, and acute toxicity. For further information on the handling of antineoplastic agents, see the ASHP Guidelines on Handling Hazardous Drugs at http://www.ahfsdruginformation.com.

Preparations

Excipients in commercially available drug preparations may have clinically important effects in some individuals; consult specific product labeling for details.

Imatinib Mesylate

Oral		
Tablets, film-coated	100 mg (of imatinib)	**Gleevec®**, Novartis
	400 mg (of imatinib)	**Gleevec®**, Novartis

Inotuzumab Ozogamicin

■ Inotuzumab ozogamicin, a CD22-directed antibody-drug conjugate consisting of a recombinant humanized immunoglobulin G_4 (IgG_4) kappa monoclonal antibody (inotuzumab) covalently linked to a cytotoxic calicheamicin derivative (*N*-acetyl-γ-calicheamicin), is an antineoplastic agent.

Uses

■ **B-cell Precursor Acute Lymphoblastic Leukemia** Inotuzumab ozogamicin is used for the treatment of relapsed or refractory B-cell precursor acute lymphoblastic leukemia (pre-B-ALL). The drug has been designated an orphan drug by FDA for use in treatment of pre-B-ALL.

The current indication for inotuzumab ozogamicin is based principally on the results of a randomized, open-label, international, multicenter phase 3 study (INO-VATE ALL) in 326 adults with relapsed or refractory pre-B-ALL that progressed following treatment with 1 or 2 induction chemotherapy regimens. Patients enrolled in the study were required to have at least 5% blast cells in their bone marrow. Patients were enrolled regardless of Philadelphia chromosome (Ph) status; however, patients with Ph-positive (Ph^+) disease must have failed prior therapy with at least one tyrosine kinase inhibitor and standard chemotherapy. Patients were randomized (stratified by duration of first remission, number of salvage therapies, and age) in a 1:1 ratio to receive inotuzumab ozogamicin or investigator's choice of chemotherapy. Patients randomized to inotuzumab ozogamicin received 0.8 mg/m² by IV infusion on day 1 followed by 0.5 mg/m² on days 8 and 15 of cycle 1 (21-day duration) and each subsequent 28-day cycle. Once complete remission (CR) or complete remission with incomplete hematologic recovery (CRi) was achieved, the dosage of inotuzumab ozogamicin was reduced to 0.5 mg/m² on days 1, 8, and 15 of each 28-day cycle. Inotuzumab ozogamicin was continued for up to 6 cycles. Patients randomized to the control group received combination therapy with fludarabine, cytarabine, and a granulocyte colony-stimulating factor (G-CSF); cytarabine in combination with mitoxantrone; or high-dose cytarabine.

The primary measures of efficacy in the INO-VATE ALL study were CR and CRi (as evaluated by a blinded independent central review committee), duration of remission, and proportion of patients who achieved complete remission who had results below the threshold for negative minimal residual disease (MRD-negative). CR was defined as the presence of less than 5% blasts in bone marrow without evidence of disease (absence of circulating blasts and resolution of extramedullary disease) and with full recovery of peripheral blood cell counts (platelet count of at least 100,000/mm³ and absolute neutrophil count [ANC] of at least 1000/mm³), CRi was defined as the presence of less than 5% blasts in bone marrow without evidence of disease and with incomplete recovery of peripheral blood cell counts (platelet count less than 100,000/mm³ and ANC less than 1000/mm³), and MRD-negativity was defined as the presence of less than 0.01% blasts using flow cytometry.

The median age of enrolled patients was 47 years (range: 18–79 years); 85% had Ph-negative (Ph^-) disease, 66% had received one prior treatment regimen for their disease, 33% had received 2 prior treatment regimens for their disease, 17% had undergone hematopoietic stem cell transplantation (HSCT) prior to study entry, and 63% were in first remission for less than 12 months. The primary efficacy population consisted of the initial 218 patients randomized in the study; all of these patients had CD22-positive pre-B-ALL with the majority (at least 90%) expressing CD22 on at least 70% of blast cells.

In the primary efficacy population of the INO-VATE ALL study, CR/CRi was reported in 80.7 or 29.4% of patients receiving inotuzumab ozogamicin or investigator's choice of chemotherapy, respectively; CR/CRi was achieved within the first 2 treatment cycles in 97% of patients receiving inotuzumab ozogamicin and 94% of patients receiving investigator's choice of chemotherapy. The majority of patients receiving inotuzumab ozogamicin (73%) or investigator's choice of chemotherapy (91%) achieved a response within the first treatment cycle. At the time of analysis, the median duration of response for patients achieving CR/CRi was 5.4 or 3.5 months in patients receiving inotuzumab ozogamicin or investigator's choice of chemotherapy, respectively; the median duration of response was more prolonged in inotuzumab ozogamicin-treated patients achieving CR (8 versus 4.9 months) and CRi (4.6 versus 2.9 months) compared with investigator's choice of chemotherapy-treated patients. Complete remission with partial hematologic recovery (CRh; defined as the presence of less than 5% blasts in bone marrow with partial recovery of peripheral blood cell counts [platelet count exceeding 50,000/mm³ and ANC exceeding 500/mm³]) was achieved in 29% of inotuzumab ozogamicin-treated patients and 6% of investigator's choice of chemotherapy-treated patients. MRD-negativity was reported in 89.7 or 69.4% of inotuzumab ozogamicin-treated patients who achieved CR or CRi, respectively, and in 31.6 or 23.1% of chemotherapy-treated patients who achieved CR or CRi, respectively. Effects of inotuzumab ozogamicin on CR, duration of response, and proportion of MRD-negative CR were comparable between the primary efficacy population and overall study population. Approximately one-half (48%) or 22% of inotuzumab ozogamicin-treated or chemotherapy-treated patients, respectively, in the overall study population underwent HSCT. Overall survival did not reach the prespecified level of statistical significance. Results of a subgroup analysis based on relevant patient and disease characteristics suggested that the effect of inotuzumab ozogamicin on CR and CRi generally was consistent across all subgroups; however, clinical benefit for the drug compared with chemotherapy was not apparent in the subgroups of patients with baseline Ph^+ disease and those bearing the t(4;11) chromosomal abnormality.

Dosage and Administration

■ **General** Because of the risk of infusion-related reactions, the manufacturer recommends a premedication regimen (i.e., corticosteroid, antipyretic, and antihistamine) prior to each inotuzumab ozogamicin infusion. Patients should be observed for symptoms of infusion-related reactions during and for at least 1 hour after the end of each infusion. (See Infusion-related Reactions under Warnings/Precautions: Other Warnings and Precautions, in Cautions.)

In patients with circulating lymphoblasts, cytoreduction with a combination of hydroxyurea, a corticosteroid, and/or vincristine until peripheral blast counts decrease to 10,000/mm³ or less is recommended prior to administration of the first dose of inotuzumab ozogamicin.

Restricted Distribution Inotuzumab ozogamicin is available only through a specialty pharmacy and specialty distributors. Clinicians may contact Pfizer Oncology Together at 877-744-5675 or consult the Pfizer Oncology Together website for specific availability information (https://www.pfizertogether.com/hcp/besponsa/reimbursement-information).

■ **Reconstitution and Administration** The usual precautions for handling and preparing solutions of cytotoxic drugs should be observed with inotuzumab ozogamicin.

Inotuzumab ozogamicin is administered by IV infusion at a rate of 50 mL/hour for 1 hour at room temperature. The manufacturer recommends administering final diluted solutions of the drug through polyvinyl chloride (PVC; diethylhexylphthalate [DEHP] or non-DEHP PVC), polyolefin (polypropylene and/or polyethylene), or polybutadiene administration sets with or without a filter. When a filter is used, a polyethersulfone (PES)-, polyvinylidene fluoride (PVDF)-, or hydrophilic polysulfone (HPS)-based filter is recommended; nylon or mixed cellulose ester (MCE) filters should *not* be used.

Unreconstituted inotuzumab ozogamicin powder for injection should be stored at 2–8°C. Unopened vials should be retained in the original package for protection from light; freezing of the vials should be avoided.

Prior to administration, commercially available inotuzumab ozogamicin powder for injection must be reconstituted and diluted. The powder for injection is reconstituted by adding 4 mL of sterile water for injection to each vial labeled as containing 0.9 mg of the drug to provide a solution containing 0.25 mg/mL. The vial should be gently swirled and inspected visually for particulate matter and discoloration prior to dilution and administration. The resulting solution should *not* be shaken. The reconstituted inotuzumab ozogamicin solution should be clear to opalescent, colorless to slightly yellow, and essentially free of visible particulates. The reconstituted solution may be diluted immediately, stored at 20–25°C for dilution within 4 hours, or stored at 2–8°C for dilution within 3 hours, and should be protected from light. The reconstituted solution should *not* be frozen.

For preparation of the final diluted inotuzumab ozogamicin solution for infusion, the required amount of reconstituted inotuzumab ozogamicin solution should be withdrawn from the vial using a syringe and injected into a PVC (DEHP or non-DEHP), polyolefin (polypropylene and/or polyethylene), or ethylene vinyl acetate (EVA) infusion bag containing 0.9% sodium chloride injection to achieve a total volume of 50 mL. Any unused reconstituted solution left in the vial should be discarded. The final diluted inotuzumab ozogamicin solution for infusion should be mixed by gentle inversion and should *not* be shaken.

If immediate administration of diluted inotuzumab ozogamicin solution for infusion is not possible, diluted solutions of the drug are stable for up to 4 hours after dilution when stored at room temperature or for up to 3 hours after dilution when stored under refrigeration (2–8°C); refrigerated diluted solutions of the drug should be brought to room temperature for approximately 1 hour prior to administration. Diluted solutions of the drug must be administered within 8 hours (including infusion time) of reconstitution and there should be no more than 4 hours between reconstitution and dilution of the solution. Diluted solutions of the drug should also be protected from light.

■ Dosage *B-cell Precursor Acute Lymphoblastic Leukemia*

For the treatment of relapsed or refractory B-cell precursor acute lymphoblastic leukemia (pre-B-ALL) in adults, the recommended dosage of inotuzumab ozogamicin during cycle 1 is 0.8 mg/m^2 on day 1, followed by 0.5 mg/m^2 on days 8 and 15 during a *3-week cycle*.

During subsequent cycles in patients who have *achieved complete remission (CR) or complete remission with incomplete hematologic recovery (CRi)*, the recommended dosage of inotuzumab ozogamicin is 0.5 mg/m^2 on days 1, 8, and 15 during each *4-week cycle*.

During subsequent cycles in patients who have *not achieved CR or CRi*, the recommended dosage of inotuzumab ozogamicin is 0.8 mg/m^2 on day 1, followed by 0.5 mg/m^2 on days 8 and 15 during each *4-week cycle*. However, if CR or CRi is not achieved within 3 cycles, treatment with the drug should be discontinued.

The recommended duration of inotuzumab ozogamicin therapy is 2 cycles in adults undergoing hematopoietic stem cell transplantation (HSCT) following inotuzumab ozogamicin treatment for pre-B-ALL. A third cycle may be considered in patients who do not achieve CR or CRi and minimal residual disease (MRD) negativity after 2 cycles (cycles 1–2). For patients not proceeding to HSCT, additional cycles of treatment, up to a maximum of 6 cycles, may be administered. (See Hepatotoxicity, including Hepatic Veno-occlusive Disease, under Warnings/Precautions: Warnings, in Cautions.)

Dosage Modification for Toxicity In patients who have required dosage reduction for toxicity, the dosage of inotuzumab ozogamicin must *not* be re-escalated in subsequent cycles.

Hematologic Toxicity. Dose delays may be required if absolute neutrophil count (ANC) and platelet counts have not recovered to recommended values prior to initiation of a new treatment cycle; interruption of inotuzumab ozogamicin therapy *within* treatment cycles (i.e., days 8 and/or 15) for hematologic toxicity is not necessary.

If ANC decreases to less than 1000/mm^3 in patients who had a baseline ANC of at least 1000/mm^3, initiation of the next cycle should be delayed until ANC reaches or exceeds 1000/mm^3. If prolonged neutropenia (i.e., lasting more than 28 days) occurs and is suspected to be related to inotuzumab ozogamicin, therapy with the drug should be discontinued.

If platelet count decreases to less than 50,000/mm^3 in patients who had a baseline platelet count of at least 50,000/mm^3, initiation of the next cycle should be delayed until platelet count reaches or exceeds 50,000/mm^3. If prolonged thrombocytopenia (i.e., lasting more than 28 days) occurs and is suspected to be related to inotuzumab ozogamicin, therapy with the drug should be discontinued.

If neutropenia or thrombocytopenia occurs in patients who had a baseline ANC of less than 1000/mm^3 and/or a platelet count of less than 50,000/mm^3, initiation of the next cycle should be delayed until one of the following occurs: ANC and platelet count return to at least baseline values for the prior cycle, ANC reaches or exceeds 1000/mm^3 and platelet count reaches or exceeds 50,000/mm^3, or most recent assessment of bone marrow reveals stable or improved disease and the neutropenia and thrombocytopenia are considered to be caused by the underlying disease and not toxicity to inotuzumab ozogamicin.

Hepatotoxicity. If hepatic veno-occlusive disease or other severe hepatotoxicity occurs, inotuzumab ozogamicin therapy should be permanently discontinued. (See Hepatotoxicity, including Hepatic Veno-occlusive Disease, under Warnings/Precautions: Warnings, in Cautions.)

In patients who exhibit increases in serum aminotransferase (ALT and/or AST) concentrations exceeding 2.5 times the upper limit of normal (ULN) or total bilirubin concentrations exceeding 1.5 times the ULN (except in patients with Gilbert's syndrome or hemolysis), therapy with inotuzumab ozogamicin should be temporarily interrupted until ALT and AST elevations decline to no more than 2.5 times the ULN and total bilirubin concentrations decline to no more than 1.5 times the ULN. Dosage reduction, dose omission, and/or permanent discontinuance of inotuzumab ozogamicin also may be necessary depending on the duration of the dosing interruption.

If therapy is withheld for less than 7 days (within a treatment cycle), the next dose may be administered upon resolution of toxicity; however, the schedule of administration should be adjusted to maintain a minimum of 6 days between doses. If therapy is withheld for 7 days or more but less than 14 days, the next dose within the treatment cycle should be omitted. If therapy is withheld for 14 days or more and adequate recovery has been achieved, the total dosage of inotuzumab ozogamicin should be reduced by 25% in the subsequent cycle. If further dosage reduction is necessary, the frequency of inotuzumab ozogamicin administration may be reduced from 3 to 2 doses per cycle in subsequent cycles. If dosage modification (dosage reduction then reduced frequency) of inotuzumab ozogamicin is not tolerated or elevated ALT, AST, and/or total bilirubin concentrations persist for more than 28 days despite interruption of therapy, the drug should be permanently discontinued.

Infusion-related Reactions. If infusion-related reactions occur, the inotuzumab ozogamicin infusion should be interrupted or permanently discontinued and appropriate treatment and supportive care should be provided. Depending on the severity of the reaction (except for severe or life-threatening reactions), discontinuance of the infusion or administration of corticosteroids and antihistamines should be considered.

If severe or life-threatening infusion-related reactions occur, inotuzumab ozogamicin should be permanently discontinued. (See Dosage and Administration: General and see also Infusion-related Reactions under Warnings/Precautions: Other Warnings and Precautions, in Cautions.)

Other Nonhematologic Toxicity. If other nonhematologic toxicity of grade 2 or greater severity occurs during inotuzumab ozogamicin therapy, therapy with the drug should be temporarily interrupted. Once the nonhematologic toxicity has returned to baseline or improved to grade 1, therapy with the drug may be resumed. Dosage reduction, dose omission, and/or permanent discontinuance of inotuzumab ozogamicin also may be necessary depending on the duration of the dosing interruption.

If therapy is withheld for less than 7 days (within a treatment cycle), the next dose may be administered upon resolution of toxicity; however, the schedule of administration should be adjusted to maintain a minimum of 6 days between doses. If therapy is withheld for 7 days or more but less than 14 days, the next dose within the treatment cycle should be omitted. If therapy is withheld for 14 days or more and adequate recovery has been achieved, the total dosage of inotuzumab ozogamicin should be reduced by 25% in the subsequent cycle. If further dosage reduction is necessary, the frequency of inotuzumab ozogamicin administration may be reduced from 3 to 2 doses per cycle in subsequent cycles. If dosage modification (dosage reduction then reduced frequency) of inotuzumab ozogamicin is not tolerated or the nonhematologic toxicity persists for more than 28 days despite interruption of therapy, the drug should be permanently discontinued.

■ Special Populations

The manufacturer states that no adjustment to the initial dosage of inotuzumab ozogamicin is necessary in patients with baseline serum ALT/AST concentrations 2.5 times the ULN or less and total bilirubin concentrations 1.5 times the ULN or less. There are limited data in patients with serum ALT/AST concentrations exceeding 2.5 times the ULN and/or total bilirubin concentrations exceeding 1.5 times the ULN; the manufacturer does not provide any specific dosage recommendations for such patients. (See Hepatic Impairment under Warnings/Precautions: Specific Populations, in Cautions.)

The manufacturer makes no specific dosage recommendations for patients with renal impairment. Inotuzumab ozogamicin has not been studied in patients with end-stage renal disease, including those receiving dialysis. (See Renal Impairment under Warnings/Precautions: Specific Populations, in Cautions.)

The manufacturer states that adjustment of the initial dosage of inotuzumab ozogamicin is not necessary in geriatric patients. (See Geriatric Use under Warnings/Precautions: Specific Populations, in Cautions.)

Cautions

■ Contraindications

The manufacturer states that there are no known contraindications to the use of inotuzumab ozogamicin.

■ Warnings/Precautions *Warnings*

Hepatotoxicity, including Hepatic Veno-occlusive Disease. Hepatotoxicity, including severe, life-threatening, and sometimes fatal hepatic veno-occlusive disease (VOD; also known as sinusoidal obstruction syndrome) and liver function test abnormalities, have been reported in patients receiving inotuzumab ozogamicin therapy. In the INO-VATE ALL study, hepatic VOD occurred during or following inotuzumab ozogamicin therapy in 5 of 164 patients (3%) without intervening hematopoietic stem cell transplantation (HSCT) and in 18 of 79 patients (23%) who underwent HSCT following therapy with the drug. A higher incidence of hepatic VOD was reported in inotuzumab ozogamicin-treated patients enrolled in Europe and Asia than in North America. Most cases were grade 3 or worse, and some cases resulted in death. The median time to onset of hepatic VOD in patients who underwent HSCT was 15 days (range: 3–57 days). Among patients who did not undergo HSCT, hepatic VOD was reported up to 56 days following the last dose of inotuzumab ozogamicin or during follow-up. In the INO-VATE ALL study, grade 3 or 4 elevations in serum ALT, AST, or total bilirubin concentrations occurred in 4, 4, or 5%, respectively, of patients receiving inotuzumab ozogamicin.

The risk of hepatic VOD is greater in patients who undergo HSCT following therapy with inotuzumab ozogamicin, those who receive a conditioning regimen containing 2 alkylating agents (e.g., busulfan in combination with other alkylating agents), and those whose most recent total bilirubin concentration is at or above the upper limit of normal (ULN) prior to HSCT. Other risk factors for developing hepatic VOD include ongoing or prior hepatic disease, history of HSCT, older age, heavily pretreated disease (i.e., later salvage line of therapy), and increased number of treatment cycles with inotuzumab ozogamicin. Patients who have experienced prior VOD or who have serious ongoing hepatic disease (e.g., cirrhosis, nodular regenerative hyperplasia, active hepatitis) also are at an increased risk of worsening hepatic disease, including developing VOD, following therapy with inotuzumab ozogamicin.

Because of the increased risk of hepatic VOD in patients undergoing HSCT, the manufacturer and some experts recommend reducing the inotuzumab ozogamicin treatment duration to 2 cycles in such patients; a third treatment cycle may be considered if complete remission (CR) or complete remission with incomplete hematologic recovery (CRi) and minimal residual disease (MRD) negativity are not achieved after 2 cycles.

Patients receiving inotuzumab ozogamicin should be closely monitored for signs and symptoms of hepatic VOD (e.g., elevated total bilirubin concentrations, hepatomegaly [which may be painful], rapid weight gain, ascites, edema, jaundice). Liver function tests (i.e., ALT, AST, total bilirubin, alkaline phosphatase) should be assessed prior to and following each dose of inotuzumab ozogamicin; however, because of the increased risk of hepatic VOD in patients who undergo HSCT, liver function tests should be closely monitored for the first month following HSCT and then less frequently thereafter, according to standard clinical practice. Some experts recommend preventing development of hepatic VOD in patients receiving inotuzumab ozogamicin with concurrent administration of drugs such as ursodiol. Dosage reduction, treatment delay, or drug discontinuance may be required if liver function test abnormalities occur during therapy with the drug. (See Hepatotoxicity under Dosage: Dosage Modification for Toxicity, in Dosage and Administration.)

If hepatic VOD occurs, inotuzumab ozogamicin therapy should be permanently discontinued. Supportive care, including maintaining an adequate fluid balance, is recommended by some experts in patients who develop hepatic VOD; continued administration of ursodiol also is recommended. Defibrotide sodium may be used in the treatment of patients with hepatic VOD with renal or pulmonary compromise. (For more information on hepatic VOD, including risk factors, clinical manifestations, and management, see Defibrotide Sodium 20:12.92.)

Increased Risk of Post-transplant Non-relapse Mortality. In the INO-VATE ALL study, inotuzumab ozogamicin was associated with a higher mortality rate at day 100 post-HSCT in patients who underwent HSCT following therapy with the drug compared with the investigator's choice of chemotherapy. The post-HSCT non-relapse mortality rate was 31 of 79 inotuzumab ozogamicin-treated patients (39%) and 8 of 35 chemotherapy-treated patients (23%). The most common causes of post-HSCT non-relapse mortality in patients receiving the drug were hepatic VOD and infectious complications. Among inotuzumab ozogamicin-treated patients, hepatic VOD occurred in 18 patients post-HSCT and resulted in 5 fatalities. Multiorgan failure or infection resulting in death occurred in 6 inotuzumab ozogamicin-treated patients with ongoing hepatic VOD at the time of death.

Patients receiving inotuzumab ozogamicin should be closely monitored for post-HSCT complications, including signs and symptoms of infection and hepatic VOD. (See Hepatotoxicity, including Hepatic Veno-occlusive Disease, under Warnings/Precautions: Warnings, in Cautions.)

Other Warnings and Precautions **Myelosuppression.** Neutropenia and thrombocytopenia resulting in severe, life-threatening, and sometimes fatal complications have been reported in patients receiving inotuzumab ozogamicin therapy. In the INO-VATE ALL study, thrombocytopenia and neutropenia were reported in 51 and 49%, respectively, of patients treated with the drug. Platelet counts recovered to greater than 50,000/mm^3 more than 45 days after the last dose of inotuzumab ozogamicin or chemotherapy in 9 or 2% of patients, respectively, who achieved CR or CRi at the end of therapy. Grade 4 thrombocytopenia or neutropenia occurred in 28 or 27%, respectively, of patients receiving the drug. Febrile neutropenia, which may be life-threatening, occurred in 26% of patients receiving inotuzumab ozogamicin. Infectious complications, sometimes serious, life-threatening or fatal, associated with neutropenia occurred in approximately one-half (48%) of patients receiving the drug. Fatal infection (i.e., pneumonia, neutropenic sepsis, sepsis, septic shock, pseudomonal sepsis) occurred in 8 of 164 patients (5%) receiving inotuzumab ozogamicin. Hemorrhage occurred in 33% of patients receiving the drug. Grade 3 or 4 hemorrhage was reported in 8 of 164 patients (5%) receiving inotuzumab ozogamicin. Fatal intra-abdominal hemorrhage occurred in one patient receiving the drug. The most common hemorrhagic event reported in the study was epistaxis.

Complete blood cell (CBC) counts should be monitored prior to each dose of inotuzumab ozogamicin. Prophylactic anti-infective therapy should be administered when appropriate and surveillance testing should be employed when appropriate during and following inotuzumab ozogamicin therapy. Patients should be monitored for signs and symptoms of complications associated with myelosuppression (e.g., infection, bleeding or hemorrhage). In patients who develop neutropenia, thrombocytopenia, or other complications associated with myelosuppression, temporary interruption of therapy, dosage reduction, or drug discontinuance may be required. (See Hematologic Toxicity under Dosage: Dosage Modification for Toxicity, in Dosage and Administration.)

Infusion-related Reactions. Infusion-related reactions have been reported in patients receiving inotuzumab ozogamicin therapy, generally during the first treatment cycle shortly after completion of the infusion. In the INO-VATE ALL study, infusion-related reactions occurred in 4 of 164 patients (2%) receiving inotuzumab ozogamicin; all infusion-related reactions were grade 2 severity. Infusion-related reactions resolved either spontaneously or following medical intervention.

The manufacturer states that premedication with a corticosteroid, antipyretic, and antihistamine should be administered prior to each dose of inotuzumab ozogamicin. Patients should also be closely monitored during and for at least 1 hour following infusions of the drug for the potential onset of infusion-related reactions, including symptoms such as fever, chills, rash, or breathing difficulty.

If an infusion-related reaction occurs, the infusion should be temporarily interrupted and, depending on the severity of the reaction, discontinuance of the infusion or administration of corticosteroids and antihistamines should be considered. Permanent discontinuance of inotuzumab ozogamicin is necessary in patients who experience severe or life-threatening infusion-related reactions. (See Infusion-related Reactions under Dosage: Dosage Modification for Toxicity, in Dosage and Administration.)

Prolongation of QT Interval. Prolongation of the QT interval has been reported in patients receiving inotuzumab ozogamicin therapy. In the INO-VATE ALL study, a QT_c interval (corrected for heart rate using Fridericia's formula [QT_cF]) exceeding 500 msec was not reported in any inotuzumab ozogamicin-treated patients; however, 3% of inotuzumab ozogamicin-treated patients had an increase in the QT_cF interval of 60 msec or more from baseline. Grade 2 prolongation of the QT interval occurred in 1% of patients receiving inotuzumab ozogamicin. In the INO-VATE ALL study, grade 3 or greater prolongation of the QT interval or torsades de pointes was not reported in any inotuzumab ozogamicin-treated patient. Analysis of central tendency showed a peak mean QT_cF interval change from baseline of 15.3 msec during day 1 of cycle 4.

Inotuzumab ozogamicin should be used with caution in patients with a history of or predisposition for prolongation of the QT_c interval, patients concurrently receiving other drugs known to prolong the QT interval, and in patients with electrolyte abnormalities. (See Drug Interactions: Drugs that Prolong the QT Interval.) The manufacturer recommends monitoring ECGs and serum electrolytes prior to initiation of inotuzumab ozogamicin therapy, following initiation of any drug known to prolong the QT_c interval, and periodically during therapy as clinically indicated.

Fetal/Neonatal Morbidity and Mortality. There are no available data on inotuzumab ozogamicin use in pregnant women; however, based on its mechanism of action and animal findings, inotuzumab ozogamicin may cause fetal harm. Embryofetal toxicity (e.g., increased resorption, fetal growth retardation) has been demonstrated in rats receiving inotuzumab ozogamicin at exposure levels approximately 0.4–2 times the human exposure at the maximum recommended dosage.

Pregnancy should be avoided during inotuzumab ozogamicin therapy. The manufacturer states that pregnancy status should be verified prior to initiation of inotuzumab ozogamicin therapy in women of childbearing potential and that such women should be advised to use effective contraceptive methods during therapy and for at least 8 months after discontinuance of the drug. In addition, men with female partners of childbearing potential should use effective methods of contraception during therapy and for at least 5 months after discontinuance of the drug. Patients should be apprised of the potential hazard to the fetus if inotuzumab ozogamicin is used during pregnancy or if the patient becomes pregnant while receiving the drug.

Impairment of Fertility. Results of animal studies suggest that inotuzumab ozogamicin may impair male and female fertility.

In a reproductive study, increased resorptions and decreased number of viable embryos and gravid uterine weights were observed following administration of inotuzumab ozogamicin daily for 2 weeks prior to mating through day 7 of gestation (at exposure levels approximately 2 times the human exposure at the maximum recommended dosage) in female animals. In toxicology studies, decreased ovarian and uterine weights and ovarian and uterine atrophy were observed followed administration of inotuzumab ozogamicin to female animals for 26 weeks.

In toxicology studies, decreased testicular weight, testicular atrophy, hypospermia, and prostatic and seminal vesicle atrophy were observed following administration of inotuzumab ozogamicin to male animals for 26 weeks; testicular degeneration and hypospermia were irreversible following discontinuance of the drug for 4 weeks.

Immunogenicity. There is a potential for immunogenicity with inotuzumab ozogamicin therapy. In clinical studies, anti-inotuzumab ozogamicin antibody formation occurred in 3% of patients receiving the drug; neutralizing antibodies were not detected in any of these patients. Clearance of inotuzumab ozogamicin was not affected by the presence of anti-inotuzumab ozogamicin antibodies.

Specific Populations **Pregnancy.** Inotuzumab ozogamicin may cause fetal harm if administered to pregnant women based on its mechanism of action and animal findings. (See Fetal/Neonatal Morbidity and Mortality under Warnings/Precautions: Other Warnings and Precautions, in Cautions.)

Pregnancy status should be verified in women of childbearing potential prior to initiation of inotuzumab ozogamicin therapy.

Lactation. It is not known whether inotuzumab ozogamicin or its metabolites are distributed into human milk or if the drug has any effect on milk production or the nursing infant. Because of the potential for adverse reactions to inotuzumab ozogamicin in nursing infants, women should be advised not to breast-feed while receiving the drug and for at least 2 months after discontinuance of therapy.

Pediatric Use. Safety and efficacy of inotuzumab ozogamicin have not been established in pediatric patients.

Geriatric Use. In the INO-VATE ALL study, 18% of patients were 65 years of age or older. No differences in efficacy or safety were observed between geriatric patients and younger adults in this study; however, thrombocytopenia, febrile neutropenia, and elevated concentrations of γ-glutamyltransferase (γ-glutamyltranspeptidase, GGT, GGTP) occurred more frequently in geriatric patients compared with younger adults.

Older age is associated with an increased risk for developing hepatic VOD in inotuzumab ozogamicin-treated patients. (See Hepatotoxicity, including Hepatic Veno-occlusive Disease, under Warnings/Precautions: Warnings, in Cautions)

Among patients 18–92 years of age, age did not appear to substantially affect the pharmacokinetics of inotuzumab ozogamicin. Initial dosage adjustment of the drug in geriatric patients is therefore not necessary.

Hepatic Impairment. Analysis of population pharmacokinetic data indicates that clearance of inotuzumab ozogamicin is not altered in patients with preexisting mild hepatic impairment (total bilirubin concentration not exceeding the ULN *with* AST concentration exceeding the ULN, or total bilirubin concentration exceeding the ULN but not more than 1.5 times the ULN *with* any AST concentration).

Although clearance of inotuzumab ozogamicin did not appear to be reduced in 4 patients with either moderate or severe hepatic impairment (total bilirubin concentration exceeding 1.5 times the ULN *with* any AST concentration), only limited data are available in such patients.

Renal Impairment. Analysis of population pharmacokinetic data indicates that clearance of inotuzumab ozogamicin is not altered in patients with renal impairment (creatinine clearance 15–89 mL/minute). Efficacy and safety of the drug in patients with end-stage renal disease with or without hemodialysis currently are unknown.

■ **Common Adverse Effects** Adverse effects reported in 20% or more of patients with relapsed or refractory acute lymphoblastic leukemia receiving inotuzumab ozogamicin as a single agent in the INO-VATE ALL study include thrombocytopenia, neutropenia, infection, anemia, leukopenia, fatigue, hemorrhage, pyrexia, nausea, headache, febrile neutropenia, elevated concentrations of aminotransferases (ALT, AST), abdominal pain, elevated concentrations of γ-glutamyltransferase (γ-glutamyltranspeptidase, GGT, GGTP), and hyperbilirubinemia.

Drug Interactions

In vitro studies indicate that *N*-acetyl-γ-calicheamicin dimethylhydrazide is primarily metabolized by nonenzymatic reduction. In vitro, *N*-acetyl-γ-calicheamicin dimethylhydrazide is unlikely to substantially inhibit cytochrome P-450 (CYP) isoenzymes 1A2, 2B6, 2C8, 2C9, 2C19, 2D6, and 3A4/5 or uridine diphosphate-glucuronosyltransferase (UGT) isoenzymes 1A1, 1A4, 1A6, 1A9, and 2B7 at clinically relevant concentrations. In vitro studies also indicate that *N*-acetyl-γ-calicheamicin dimethylhydrazide is unlikely to substantially induce CYP isoenzymes 1A2, 2B6, and 3A4 at clinically relevant concentrations. *N*-acetyl-γ-calicheamicin dimethylhydrazide is a substrate of P-glycoprotein (P-gp). *N*-acetyl-γ-calicheamicin dimethylhydrazide is unlikely to inhibit P-gp, breast cancer resistance protein (BCRP), organic anion transporter (OAT) 1 and OAT3, organic cation transporter (OCT) 2, and organic anion transport protein (OATP) 1B1 and OATP1B3.

In vitro studies indicate that inotuzumab ozogamicin is unlikely to substantially inhibit CYP isoenzymes 1A2, 2A6, 2B6, 2C8, 2C9, 2C19, 2D6, and 3A4/5 or induce CYP isoenzymes 1A2, 2B6, and 3A4 at clinically relevant concentrations.

■ **Drugs that Prolong the QT Interval** Concomitant use of inotuzumab ozogamicin and drugs known to prolong the QT interval or cause torsades de pointes may increase the risk of clinically important corrected QT (QT_c)-interval prolongation. The manufacturer recommends discontinuance of such drugs or concomitant use of alternative drugs not known to prolong the QT/QT_c interval while patients are receiving inotuzumab ozogamicin therapy. If concomitant use of other drugs known to prolong the QT/QT_c interval cannot be avoided, the manufacturer recommends more frequent monitoring of ECGs and serum electrolyte concentrations (i.e., prior to initiation of inotuzumab ozogamicin therapy, after initiation of any drug known to prolong the QT_c interval, and periodically during therapy as clinically indicated). (See Prolongation of QT Interval under Warnings/Precautions: Other Warnings and Precautions, in Cautions.)

■ **Antineoplastic Agents** ***Alkylating Agents*** Because the risk of developing hepatic veno-occlusive disease (VOD) is significantly higher in patients with relapsed or refractory acute lymphoblastic leukemia who undergo hematopoietic stem cell transplantation (HSCT) following inotuzumab ozogamicin therapy, including those who received conditioning regimens containing 2 alkylating agents (e.g., busulfan, melphalan, thiotepa), use of such conditioning regimens should be avoided in patients who received inotuzumab ozogamicin therapy prior to HSCT. (See Hepatotoxicity, including Hepatic Veno-occlusive Disease, under Warnings/Precautions: Warnings, in Cautions.)

■ **Hepatotoxic Drugs** Because hepatic VOD and liver function test abnormalities are associated with inotuzumab ozogamicin therapy, some experts recommend avoiding concomitant therapy with other drugs known to cause hepatotoxicity (e.g., azole antifungals) in patients receiving inotuzumab ozogamicin and high-dose conditioning regimens with alkylating agents, if possible. (See Hepatotoxicity, including Hepatic Veno-occlusive Disease, under Warnings/Precautions: Warnings, in Cautions.)

■ **Antifungal Agents** Because hepatic VOD and liver function test abnormalities are associated with inotuzumab ozogamicin therapy, some experts recommend avoiding concomitant therapy with other drugs known to cause hepatotoxicity such as azole antifungals. (See Hepatotoxicity, including Hepatic Veno-occlusive Disease, under Warnings/Precautions: Warnings, in Cautions.)

Description

Inotuzumab ozogamicin, a CD22-directed antibody-drug conjugate, is an antineoplastic agent. The antibody-drug conjugate consists of 3 components: a recombinant humanized immunoglobulin G_4 (IgG_4) kappa monoclonal antibody (inotuzumab), which is specific for human CD22; *N*-acetyl-γ-calicheamicin, a cytotoxic calicheamicin derivative that causes double-stranded DNA breaks; and an acid-cleavable linker (known as dimethylhydrazide), which covalently attaches *N*-acetyl-γ-calicheamicin to inotuzumab. *N*-acetyl-γ-calicheamicin is a semisynthetic derivative of the microorganism *Micromonospora echinospora* subsp. *calichensis*. On average, approximately 6 molecules of *N*-acetyl-γ-calicheamicin are attached to each inotuzumab molecule (range: 2–8).

The anticancer activity of inotuzumab ozogamicin appears to be produced by the binding of the antibody-drug conjugate to CD22-expressing tumor cells. The antibody portion of inotuzumab ozogamicin recognizes and binds specifically to human CD22, a transmembrane glycoprotein specific to B cells that is expressed on the surface of malignant cells in greater than 90% of B-cell acute lymphoblastic leukemia (ALL) cases, including B-cell precursor ALL. Following binding of the antibody-drug conjugate to CD22-expressing tumor cells, the resultant complex is internalized by the cell. *N*-acetyl-γ-calicheamicin is then released via hydrolytic cleavage of the linker and binds to DNA in the minor groove causing double-strand DNA breaks and subsequent cell cycle arrest and apoptosis.

The pharmacokinetics of inotuzumab ozogamicin following IV administration are characterized by a 2-compartment model with linear and time-dependent clearance components. Following repeated doses of inotuzumab ozogamicin in patients with ALL, mean peak plasma concentrations of the antibody-drug conjugate increased with subsequent cycles. Plasma concentrations of unconjugated *N*-acetyl-γ-calicheamicin are below the lower limit of quantification. Following repeated doses of inotuzumab ozogamicin, steady-state concentrations are reached by the fourth cycle of therapy; estimated systemic accumulation of the antibody-drug conjugate is 5.3-fold. In vitro studies indicate that *N*-acetyl-γ-calicheamicin is metabolized by nonenzymatic reduction. In vitro, *N*-acetyl-γ-calicheamicin dimethylhydrazide is approximately 97% bound to plasma proteins. The terminal elimination half-life of the antibody-drug conjugate is 12.3 days.

Population pharmacokinetic analyses indicate that age (range of 18–92 years), gender, and race (Asian versus non-Asian) do not have clinically important effects on the pharmacokinetics of the antibody-drug conjugate. Dosage of inotuzumab ozogamicin is based on body surface area (BSA) because disposition of the antibody-drug conjugate is significantly affected by BSA.

Advice to Patients

Risk of hepatotoxicity, including hepatic veno-occlusive disease (VOD) and elevated serum aminotransferase (ALT and/or AST) concentrations, during inotuzumab ozogamicin therapy. Importance of informing patients of the signs and symptoms of hepatic VOD (e.g., elevated serum bilirubin concentrations, rapid weight gain, abdominal swelling [which may be painful]) and advising them to seek immediate medical advice if such symptoms occur. Importance of informing patients to carefully consider the potential benefits and risks of inotuzumab ozogamicin treatment if they have a history of hepatic VOD or serious ongoing hepatic disease.

Risk of treatment-related mortality following hematopoietic stem cell transplantation (HSCT); most common causes are infectious complications or hepatic VOD. Importance of informing clinicians if signs and symptoms of infection occur.

Risk of myelosuppression. Importance of reporting signs and symptoms of myelosuppression (e.g., infection, bleeding/hemorrhage).

Risk of infusion-related reactions. Importance of advising patients to inform their clinician if symptoms of such reactions, including fever, chills, rash, or breathing difficulty, occur during infusion of inotuzumab ozogamicin.

Risk of QT-interval prolongation. Importance of informing clinicians if syncope or feelings of dizziness or faintness occur.

Risk of fetal harm. Necessity of advising women of childbearing potential and men who are partners of such women that they should use effective contraception while receiving the drug and for at least 8 and 5 months, respectively, after discontinuance of therapy. Importance of women informing clinicians if they are or plan to become pregnant. If pregnancy occurs, advise pregnant women of potential risk to the fetus.

Importance of advising women to avoid nursing during therapy and for at least 2 months after discontinuance of the drug.

Importance of informing clinicians of existing or contemplated concomitant therapy, including prescription and OTC drugs and dietary or herbal supplements, as well as any concomitant illnesses (e.g., hepatic impairment, cardiovascular disease).

Importance of informing patients of other important precautionary information. (See Cautions.)

Overview® (see Users Guide). For additional information on this drug until a more detailed monograph is developed and published, the manufacturer's labeling should be consulted. It is *essential* that the manufacturer's labeling be consulted for more detailed information on usual cautions, precautions, contraindications, potential drug interactions, laboratory test interferences, and acute toxicity. For further information on the handling of antineoplastic agents, see the ASHP Guidelines on Handling Hazardous Drugs at http://www.ahfsdruginformation.com.

Preparations

Distribution of inotuzumab ozogamicin is restricted. (See Restricted Distribution under Dosage and Administration: General.)

Excipients in commercially available drug preparations may have clinically important effects in some individuals; consult specific product labeling for details.

Inotuzumab Ozogamicin

Parenteral		
For injection, for IV infusion only	0.9 mg	**Besponsa®**, Wyeth

Interferon Alfa IFN

■ Interferon alfa is a family of proteins and glycoproteins with antiviral, antineoplastic, and immunomodulating activities. Interferon alfa is available in the US as interferon alfa-2b and interferon alfa-n3. For information on interferon alfa-n3, see Interferon Alfa 8:18.20. Interferon alfa also is available covalently bound to monomethoxy polyethylene glycol (PEG) (i.e., peginterferon alfa). For information on peginterferon alfa, see Peginterferon Alfa 8:18.20 and Peginterferon Alfa 10:00.

Uses

Interferon alfa is used in the treatment of various cancers, including hairy cell leukemia, AIDS-related Kaposi's sarcoma, follicular non-Hodgkin's lymphoma, and melanoma.

For information on use of interferon alfa in the treatment of various viral infections, see Interferon Alfa 8:18.20.

■ **Hairy Cell Leukemia** Interferon alfa (alfa-2a [no longer commercially available in the US], alfa-2b) is used for the treatment of hairy cell leukemia (leukemic reticuloendotheliosis). Results from a limited number of studies in which comparative efficacy was not a specific objective suggest that both interferon subtypes have similar efficacy in patients with this disease.

Therapy with interferon alfa produces complete response in 10% and clinically important tumor regression or disease stabilization (complete or partial responses; overall response) in approximately 80% of patients with hairy cell leukemia, including in previously untreated patients (i.e., those who have not undergone splenectomy) as well as in those with progressive disease in whom splenectomy has been performed. The drug does not appear to be curative. Because of their apparent greater efficacy (i.e., higher complete response rate), cladribine or pentostatin is preferred for most patients with hairy cell leukemia who require treatment. (See Cladribine 10:00 and also see Pentostatin 10:00.) Because of the availability of effective drug therapies, splenectomy is becoming less important as a therapeutic option in patients with hairy cell leukemia. Additional studies and long-term follow-up are needed to elucidate optimal therapy for hairy cell leukemia.

Reductions in splenomegaly and in the number of leukemic cells in peripheral blood generally are the initial signs of response to interferon alfa therapy in patients with hairy cell leukemia. Interferon alfa also may decrease bone marrow hypercellularity and hairy cell infiltrates and result in substantial and sustained improvements in granulocyte and platelet counts in peripheral blood and hemoglobin concentrations. Most patients with hairy cell leukemia have at least one abnormality in their hematologic profile prior to interferon therapy, and response to the drug is characterized by complete or partial normalization of hematologic values, including hemoglobin concentration and granulocyte and platelet counts in peripheral blood and bone marrow. Patients who respond to interferon alfa therapy have an increased performance status, a decreased number of infections as granulocyte counts improve, and substantially reduced requirements for red blood cell and platelet transfusions. Clinical improvement in patients treated with interferon alfa may be apparent within the first month of therapy and usually is apparent within 6 months; however, up to 9–12 months or more of therapy may be required for clinical response.

Clinical response to interferon alfa therapy in hairy cell leukemia generally is similar whether or not the patient has undergone splenectomy, although limited data suggest that response may occur more rapidly in splenectomized patients. In addition, some studies indicate that the incidence of complete remission may be greater in previously untreated patients than in splenectomized patients. Because of the availability of more effective agents such as cladribine and pentostatin, splenectomy is a less important therapeutic option in patients with hairy cell leukemia. Some clinicians suggest that splenectomy may be considered in patients who do not respond to therapy with cladribine, pentostatin, or interferon alfa or when massive splenomegaly or splenic rupture with pain and infection are present. Although interferon alfa generally appears equally effective in patients with mild or severe disease, differences in response rate observed in these studies may have been related to initiation of interferon alfa therapy at an earlier clinical stage of the disease in previously untreated patients. In most patients with substantial splenomegaly, interferon alfa therapy reduces the spleen to normal or near-normal size and produces a reversal of the hematologic abnormalities in peripheral blood that result from hypersplenism. In some of these patients, interferon therapy may reverse hypersplenism which, if not reversed, could have necessitated splenectomy. In those patients who exhibit persistent splenomegaly despite interferon alfa therapy, splenectomy may be required. Limited evidence also suggests that the addition of interferon alfa to antimicrobial therapy in patients with hairy cell leukemia and unresponsive mycobacterial or fungal infections may result in microbiologic and/or clinical cure of the infection, apparently through restoration by interferon alfa of impaired immune function; therefore, some clinicians suggest that interferon may be particularly beneficial and preferable therapy in patients with hairy cell leukemia who have recurrent opportunistic infections.

During the initial 1–3 months of interferon alfa therapy, marked depression in hematopoiesis may occur, as evidenced by a substantial decrease in the monocyte, granulocyte, and polymorphonuclear leukocyte counts in peripheral blood; however, peripheral blood counts generally improve with continued therapy. It has not been established whether the initial transient decrease in circulating granulocytes observed in many patients may increase their risk of infection; however, individuals with hairy cell leukemia have required red blood cell and platelet transfusions during this period of transient myelosuppression. (See Cautions: Precautions and Contraindications.) Interferon alfa therapy does not appear to adversely affect hemoglobin concentration and platelet count in patients with normal pretreatment values of these parameters. Following this initial interferon-induced depression in hematopoiesis, peripheral hematologic parameters generally return to normal over several (e.g., 2–6) months, with platelet count usually returning first, followed by hemoglobin concentration and granulocyte and monocyte counts, and these parameters may continue to improve throughout the initial 9–12 months of therapy.

In addition to restoring peripheral blood counts to normal or near-normal values, interferon alfa produces substantial decreases in the leukemic cell index (the product of the percentages of bone marrow cellularity and leukemic cell infiltrates in the marrow). While return of peripheral blood hematologic values to normal usually occurs after only 2–6 months of therapy, evidence suggests that prolonged (at least 9–12 months) therapy with interferon alfa generally is necessary to decrease leukemic cell infiltration in bone marrow; several patients categorized as having minor responses to interferon therapy reportedly have had a greater than 50% decrease in or complete clearing of leukemic cells in bone marrow despite persistence of neutropenia. Limited evidence suggests that interferon therapy produces a decrease in leukocyte counts in most patients who have leukocytosis prior to therapy.

Interferon alfa may reverse the clinical and laboratory manifestations (e.g., splenomegaly, anemia and other cytopenias, leukemic infiltration) of hairy cell leukemia and has induced objective remissions that may persist for 2 years or longer (range: 0.5 months to longer than 2 years). During the first 3 months following discontinuance of interferon alfa therapy in patients with hairy cell leukemia, an increase in the percentage of leukemic infiltrates in bone marrow frequently is evident. However, this change represents a relative rather than an absolute increase in bone marrow leukemic cells related to the rapid exit of normal myeloid and erythroid precursors from the bone marrow following discontinuance of interferon alfa therapy. Although patients usually are not refractory to a second course of interferon alfa therapy, such therapy generally is not required unless the progressive increase in leukemic infiltrates in bone marrow is accompanied by one or more peripheral blood cytopenias. Deterioration in peripheral blood cell counts does not occur rapidly after discontinuance of interferon alfa therapy; however, within 7–12 months after completion of therapy, peripheral blood platelet and granulocyte counts may decrease to 60% of those achieved at the end of an initial course of therapy. A second course of interferon alfa therapy may be required 2–19 months after completion of the initial course because of this reduction in platelet and granulocyte counts, suggesting that maintenance therapy with interferon alfa may be necessary for prolonged remission in patients with hairy cell leukemia.

Limited evidence suggests that response to interferon alfa therapy during long-term treatment of hairy cell leukemia may be dose related, although conflicting data have been reported. In one study, most patients who received 1 million units/m^2 of interferon alfa achieved normalization of hematologic values and a reduction in leukemic bone marrow infiltration but had delayed increases in granulocyte count relative to individuals treated with 2 or 4 million units/m^2; a few patients achieved only partial responses despite prolonged therapy (i.e., for approximately 1 year). In another study, there was a relatively high incidence of disease progression in patients with hairy cell leukemia who were treated with very low (200,000 units/m^2) dosages of interferon alfa, which is unusual in patients treated with standard dosages (e.g., 2 million units/m^2) of the drug. Most patients whose disease progressed on this low-dose regimen demonstrated a hematologic response within 3 months of increasing the interferon alfa dosage to that of a standard regimen. While low-dose regimens of interferon alfa are *not* recommended for initial therapy or for relapse of hairy cell leukemia because of the risk of disease progression and associated neutropenia and thrombocytopenia, low-dose therapy with the drug may prove to be useful for maintenance in patients whose disease is in remission, but additional study and experience are needed.

Response to interferon alfa therapy may be monitored periodically (e.g., monthly) by determining peripheral blood hemoglobin concentration and platelet, granulocyte, and leukemic cell counts in peripheral blood and bone marrow and comparing these with baseline values. Although the manufacturer and some clinicians state that therapy should be discontinued if the patient does not respond within 6 months, other clinicians suggest that therapy be continued for at least 12 months unless there is evidence of disease progression; onset of response has been noted as late as 9–12 months following initiation of treatment in some patients, and limited evidence suggests that prolonged therapy (e.g., 12–18 months or longer) may improve the possibility of a response, including complete remission. However, it has not been established whether achieving complete remission offers any advantage in terms of performance status or survival. In addition, the possible advantage of prolonged maintenance therapy compared with more aggressive induction regimens requires further study.

The optimum duration of interferon alfa therapy for hairy cell leukemia has not been clearly established, although it appears that therapy should continue for at least 6 months. Extending interferon alfa therapy up to a total duration of 18–24 months can maintain therapeutic response during treatment, but does not appear to influence the clinical course of the disease once interferon has been discontinued. Optimum duration of therapy cannot be defined until the biochemical and pharmacologic factors that predict prolonged survival have been identified. Bone marrow histology does not completely normalize in most patients following treatment with interferon alfa, and many (e.g., 20–50%) patients who respond to initial therapy relapse within 6–12 months after discontinuance of the drug. Although limited evidence suggests that early disease relapse following completion of treatment may be more common in patients with severe neutropenia or hyperleukocytosis at the time of diagnosis, other studies have not confirmed a correlation between these baseline hematologic findings and duration of remission. Limited data suggest that the best indicators of relapse following interferon alfa therapy in patients with hairy cell leukemia may be the neutrophil (leukocyte) alkaline phosphatase (NAP or LAP) score and the percentage of hairy cells in bone marrow. In one study, patients whose NAP score was less than 30 had the best prognosis (as measured by time from discontinuance of interferon therapy until further antileukemic therapy was needed); patients with greater than 30% leukemic cells in bone marrow had a poor prognosis, while an NAP score of 30 or greater and 30% or less leukemic cells in bone marrow was associated with an intermediate prognosis. Further studies are needed to determine which clinical and/or laboratory indices are most useful in predicting relapse and the need for subsequent maintenance therapy following interferon therapy or splenectomy.

Limited data are available on long-term survival in patients with hairy cell leukemia treated with interferon alfa. The survival rate at 24–48 months for patients who respond to the drug ranges from approximately 87–94%, while the corresponding survival rate for comparable controls treated with standard therapies, including antineoplastic agents (principally chlorambucil) or supportive care (e.g., transfusions), has ranged from approximately 35–75% at 14–40 months.

■ AIDS-related Kaposi's Sarcoma Interferon alfa (alfa-2a [no longer commercially available in the US], alfa-2b) is used for the palliative treatment of AIDS-related Kaposi's sarcoma in selected adults, and is designated an orphan drug by the US Food and Drug Administration (FDA) for the treatment of this disease. The likelihood of response to interferon alfa treatment is greater in patients without systemic symptoms who have limited lymphadenopathy and relatively intact immune systems as indicated by CD4$^+$ T-cell counts. Patients who have constitutional ("B") symptoms (e.g., fever, night sweats, weight loss) and/or who have a history of opportunistic infection at the time of diagnosis of Kaposi's sarcoma generally respond poorly to interferon. For advanced AIDS-related Kaposi's sarcoma, a liposomal anthracycline (doxorubicin or daunorubicin) or paclitaxel are recommended as drugs of choice (see Uses: AIDS-related Kaposi's Sarcoma in Doxorubicin 10:00, Daunorubicin 10:00, and Paclitaxel 10:00).

In contrast to the usual protracted, indolent course of the classic (e.g., Mediterranean) form of Kaposi's sarcoma, Kaposi's sarcoma in patients with human immunodeficiency virus (HIV) infection often is rapidly progressive. AIDS-related Kaposi's sarcoma may progress to multifocal, widespread lesions that involve the skin, oral mucosa, and lymph nodes as well as visceral organs such as the GI tract, lung, liver, and spleen; such lesions often are numerous and may be cosmetically unattractive or disfiguring and accompanied by lymphedema. All patients with AIDS-related Kaposi's sarcoma should be receiving highly active antiretroviral therapy; in some patients, initiation of antiretroviral therapy alone may result in tumor regression and resolution of lesions.

Interferon alfa should *not* be used in patients with visceral AIDS-related Kaposi's sarcoma associated with rapidly progressive or life-threatening disease since such patients require rapid cytoreduction, while the response to interferon generally is slow and poor. It has been suggested that disease progression theoretically could occur in such patients secondary to interferon's immunosuppressive properties.

Although response rates are variable, interferon alfa therapy is associated with clinically important tumor regression or disease stabilization in a substantial proportion of patients with AIDS-related Kaposi's sarcoma who do not have a history of opportunistic infections or "B" symptoms; major (complete plus partial) responses occur in approximately 20–50% of such patients receiving high-dose (36–54 million units daily) therapy with the drug. The variability in overall response rates may be explained in part by the relative severity of AIDS in patients in different studies, and response rates exceeding 50% may occur in patients with a relatively good prognosis.

Antiretroviral effects of interferon alfa have been demonstrated in vitro and in vivo, and some studies have reported an apparent correlation between these effects (e.g., as evidenced by decreased viral shedding and p24 antigenemia) and clinical response to interferon therapy in patients with AIDS-related Kaposi's sarcoma. The antiviral effects of interferon alfa have been most prominent in patients with the most competent (in terms of baseline CD4$^+$ T-cell counts) immune systems. However, the effects of interferon alfa on immune function are not clearly defined or consistent, since substantial improvement in immunologic status (as measured in vitro) has not been observed when the drug was used alone and progression of immunodeficiency has occurred in some patients during interferon alfa therapy. In responding patients with early AIDS and Kaposi's sarcoma, interferon alfa reportedly improved quality of life by inducing substantial tumor regression, and such patients also had a lower incidence of opportunistic infection than those not responding to such therapy. Interferon alfa has produced improvement at all disease sites (although not always concomitantly), including skin, lymph nodes, and GI tract, and Kaposi's lesions generally begin to regress within 4–8 weeks following initiation of therapy.

Response to interferon alfa therapy appears to be related to multiple factors, including pretreatment immune status of the patient, presence of disease symptoms, and interferon dosage. Patients with AIDS-related Kaposi's sarcoma who are most likely to respond to therapy with interferon alfa are those who have had no prior opportunistic infections and those with relatively normal CD4$^+$ T-cell counts, limited lymphadenopathy, and no systemic manifestations (e.g., weight loss, fever, night sweats). Evidence suggests that relative preservation of immune function may be required for interferon alfa to be active as an antitumor agent, and the severity of clinical manifestations in patients with AIDS-related Kaposi's sarcoma appears to be associated with the degree of immunologic impairment in these patients. Pretreatment determinations of immune function (as assessed by total lymphocyte count, CD4$^+$ T-cell counts, and the ratio of CD8$^+$ T-cells) frequently have been associated with clinical outcome and response to therapy. Patients with CD4$^+$ T-cell counts exceeding 400/ mm^3 appear to have the highest response rates (approximately 40–50%) to interferon alfa therapy; in some studies in which pretreatment levels of CD4$^+$ T cells were not substantially higher in responding than in nonresponding patients, therapy with interferon alfa was associated with a marked increase in the number of these T cells.

Response of AIDS-related Kaposi's sarcoma to interferon alfa therapy also appears to be related to interferon dosage, although some evidence that did not show a clear dose effect also has been reported; dosages of 20 million or more units/m^2 daily appear to be associated with better and more rapid responses than low dosages (e.g., 1–3 million units/m^2 daily). Initial therapy with high dosages (e.g., 30–50 million units daily) of interferon alfa has produced major responses in approximately 40–45% of patients with less-advanced AIDS (e.g., patients with CD4$^+$ T-cell counts exceeding 400/ mm^3 who have not experienced severe opportunistic infections); comparable response rates with a somewhat reduced incidence of adverse effects have been achieved when interferon alfa therapy was initiated at a low dosage (e.g., 3 million units daily) and dosage was increased over several days to 36 million units daily. Interferon alfa dosages of less than 3 million units daily generally are not as effective as higher dosages in inducing tumor regression, while dosages exceeding 36 million units (up to a maximum of 54 million units) daily generally have been associated with an unacceptable degree of adverse effects. In one study, patients who responded to therapy with 36 million units of interferon alfa daily during the first month of treatment reportedly developed new lesions when the dosing frequency was decreased to 3 times weekly.

Patients without detectable acid-labile, endogenous interferon activity in serum prior to treatment generally are more likely to respond to therapy with exogenously administered interferon alfa. Initial response to interferon alfa therapy, but not the duration of response or survival, generally has been independent of the stage of Kaposi's sarcoma (as determined by the location and extent of tumor involvement). Some evidence indicates that the presence of visceral disease or extensive dissemination of the tumor is not necessarily an indicator of poor prognosis to therapy; however, not all sites respond equally (e.g., pulmonary disease may respond relatively poorly). Limited data also suggest that response of cutaneous lesions to interferon alfa therapy in patients with AIDS-related Kaposi's sarcoma may depend on the cytologic and/or histochemical characteristics of the lesions. Papular and nodular lesions, which are composed principally of endothelial cells, usually undergo partial or complete regression with interferon alfa therapy, while flat hemorrhagic lesions consisting of pericytial cells generally remain unchanged.

The optimum duration of therapy with interferon alfa in patients with AIDS-related Kaposi's sarcoma has not been determined. The median duration of response for patients receiving therapy with the drug has been approximately 7 months; however, complete and partial responses have persisted for longer than 3 years in some patients who received maintenance therapy for variable periods. Patients who were asymptomatic prior to treatment or who achieved a complete response with therapy generally had more rapid responses and longer durations of remission than symptomatic patients or those who achieved partial responses. Some clinicians suggest that unless an opportunistic infection or severe interferon-associated adverse effects occurs, consideration should be given to continuing interferon alfa therapy indefinitely, with appropriate dosage adjustment, provided a response or disease stabilization is observed; however, the effect of such a regimen on duration of response has not been fully elucidated. In one study, patients who received 6 months of maintenance therapy with interferon alfa after attaining complete responses (i.e., complete gross and histologic clearing of lesions) while on the drug were still disease free 5 months after cessation of maintenance therapy. Further long-term follow-up is needed to determine an optimum duration of interferon alfa therapy for patients with AIDS-related Kaposi's sarcoma.

No treatment, including interferon alfa, has been shown conclusively to alter the natural history of AIDS-related Kaposi's sarcoma, although responders generally survive longer than nonresponders and thus the drug appears to affect disease progression. In one clinical study, patients who achieved a major (complete plus partial) response with high-dose (36–54 million units daily) interferon alfa therapy had a median survival exceeding 28 months, while nonresponders had a median survival of only 14 months. In another study in patients receiving an interferon alfa-2b dosage of 30 million units/m^2 three times weekly, the median survival in responders and nonresponders reportedly was 22.6 and 9.7 months, respectively. Responding patients with a pretreatment CD4$^+$ T-cell count exceeding 200 cells/ mm^3 reportedly survived longer than responders who had lower baseline CD4$^+$ T-cell counts and longer than nonresponders, regardless of their baseline CD4$^+$ T-cell counts; median survival was approximately 31 months in patients who had CD4$^+$ T-cell counts exceeding 200/ mm^3 and only about 9 months in those who had CD4$^+$ T-cell counts less than or equal to 200/ mm^3. Some limited long-term follow-up data from patients with AIDS-related Kaposi's sarcoma treated with interferon alfa suggest that patients whose tumors regressed with interferon therapy had a substantial reduction in opportunistic infections and longer survival compared with nonresponders. However, whether these differences in response are attributable to interferon or are part of the natural history of AIDS-related Kaposi's sarcoma has not been determined. Limited placebo-controlled studies have not shown any effect of interferon alfa on survival in patients with AIDS-related Kaposi's sarcoma who have had at least one opportunistic infection, although therapy with the drug in such patients has not been extensively evaluated. Some clinicians suggest that cytotoxic antineoplastic therapy may be preferable to interferon alfa treatment in patients with a poor prognosis because antineoplastic therapy is possibly more effective and response more rapid, and there is no evidence that such therapy predisposes these patients to infection or that interferon alfa therapy is superior; in patients with a favorable prognosis, the efficacy of antineoplastic therapy appears to be comparable to that of interferon. Controlled, comparative studies, in which clinical endpoints for survival and time to first opportunistic infection are well defined, and long-term follow-up of patients with early HIV infection and Kaposi's sarcoma are needed to determine whether interferon alfa or other therapies can produce meaningful improvements in survival and/or quality of life.

Interferon alfa also has been used for the treatment of classic Mediterranean Kaposi's sarcoma†. In at least one patient with laryngeal involvement, the drug produced complete regression of these lesions. However, there is a paucity of information regarding the efficacy of such therapy, and the advanced age of patients with this form of Kaposi's may limit their tolerance of the drug's adverse effects. In addition, radiation therapy and/or conventional antineoplastic therapy generally are preferred when treatment is indicated in this form of Kaposi's.

■ Non-Hodgkin's and Cutaneous T-cell Lymphomas Interferon alfa (alfa-2b) is labeled by the FDA for use in conjunction with anthracycline-containing combination chemotherapy for the treatment of clinically aggressive follicular non-Hodgkin's lymphoma in adults. Interferon alfa also has been used for the treatment of low-grade adult non-Hodgkin's lymphomas† and for the treatment of cutaneous T-cell lymphomas†.

Although other agents generally are preferred, the safety and efficacy of interferon alfa-2b in conjunction with a combination chemotherapy regimen has been evaluated for initial treatment in patients with clinically aggressive, large-tumor-burden, stage III/IV follicular non-Hodgkin's lymphoma. In a randomized, controlled trial, 130 patients received CHVP chemotherapy alone and 135 patients received CHVP therapy and interferon alfa-2b (5 million units subcutaneously 3 times weekly) for 18 months. CHVP chemotherapy consisted of cyclophosphamide 600 mg/m^2, doxorubicin 25 mg/m^2, and teniposide 60 mg/m^2 administered IV on day 1 with oral prednisone (40 mg/m^2 daily on days 1–5). Treatment consisted of 6 CHVP cycles administered monthly, followed by an additional 6 cycles administered every 2 months for 1 year. Patients in both treatment groups received a total of 12 CHVP cycles over 18 months. The group receiving CHVP and interferon alfa-2b had longer progression-free survival than those receiving CHVP alone (2.9 years versus 1.5 years). After a median follow-up of 6.1 years, the median survival for patients treated with CHVP alone was 5.5 years while median survival for patients treated with CHVP and interferon alfa-2b had not been reached. In 3 other randomized, controlled studies, use of interferon alfa in conjunction with anthracycline-containing combination chemotherapy regimens was associated with prolonged progression-free survival. Differences in overall survival were not consistently observed.

The manufacturer states that efficacy of interferon alfa-2b in the treatment of low-grade, low-tumor-burden follicular non-Hodgkin's lymphoma has not been determined. Interferon alfa given alone has produced objective clinical responses in approximately 40–60% of patients with low-grade lymphocytic adult non-Hodgkin's lymphomas†. However, these diseases typically have a long, indolent course, and improved survival with available therapies, including interferon alfa, in low-grade adult lymphocytic lymphomas has not been documented. Interferon alfa generally appears to have little therapeutic value in intermediate- or high-grade adult non-Hodgkin's lymphomas†, although occasional responses have been reported with high dosages of the drug. Features of B- and T-cell types that might predict response to interferon alfa in non-Hodgkin's lymphomas have not been identified, and further study is warranted to determine which, if any, subpopulation of patients with higher-grade lymphomas is most likely to benefit from interferon alfa therapy.

Responses to interferon alfa therapy in low-grade lymphocytic adult non-Hodgkin's lymphomas generally have been noted in patients with advanced disease who have received extensive prior treatment with regimens containing either anthracycline-derivative antineoplastic agents (e.g., doxorubicin) or radiation therapy; objective responses have been noted in approximately 40–50% of patients with advanced low-grade lymphocytic lymphoma refractory to standard treatment regimens, with complete responses occurring in approximately 6–15% of patients. Whether interferon alfa can produce comparable responses in patients with early-stage, low-grade lymphocytic lymphoma who have not received prior therapy has not been established to date; studies are ongoing. Evidence suggests that relatively low doses of interferon alfa (e.g., 2–3 million units/m^2) may be as effective as but less toxic than the high doses (e.g., 50 million units/m^2) initially used in the treatment of lymphocytic adult non-Hodgkin's lymphomas†; however, limited data suggest that patients who experience disease relapse while receiving low doses of interferon alfa may not respond to subsequent therapy with higher doses of the drug.

Systemic therapy with interferon alfa has produced response rates of approximately 40–75% in patients with cutaneous T-cell lymphomas† (CTCL; e.g., mycosis fungoides, Sézary syndrome). Such responses have been reported in patients who have failed to respond to topical or systemic therapy with other drugs as well as in previously untreated patients; many clinicians consider interferon alfa the most effective single-agent therapy for patients whose disease is refractory to standard treatment (topical mechlorethamine, psoralen plus UVA light, total electron-beam irradiation, antineoplastic agents) for these neoplasms. In one study in a limited number of patients with advanced, refractory CTCL, objective responses lasting 3 to more than 36 months (median duration approximately 5 months) were noted in 45% of patients receiving interferon alfa in an initial dosage of 50 million units/m^2 IM 3 times weekly. However, as with other non-Hodgkin's lymphomas, the optimum therapeutic regimen for interferon alfa in patients with CTCL has not been determined, and the effects of the drug on survival when given to patients with earlier stages of the disease and/or in combination with antineoplastic or other therapies are being evaluated. Large cutaneous lesions in patients with CTCL have undergone a substantial decrease in size during interferon alfa therapy, and extracutaneous responses (e.g., reductions in the size of palpable lymph nodes and in the number of circulating malignant cells) have also occurred.

Prognosis for patients with CTCL† depends on stage of the disease, type of skin lesion, and presence or absence of peripheral blood, lymph node, or visceral involvement; however, responses to interferon alfa appear to be unrelated to disease stage and/or prior therapy. Limited data suggest that response to interferon alfa may depend on dosage and scheduling of the drug. Highest response rates reportedly occur with doses ranging from 6–50 million units. Among patients with CTCL, those with mycosis fungoides appear most responsive to interferon therapy. Complete remissions with interferon alfa therapy have been reported in approximately 10–27% of patients with CTCL, generally in patients receiving high doses (e.g., 50 million units/m^2).

Preliminary evidence suggests that the combination of interferon alfa and phototherapy (psoralen plus UVA light irradiation) is effective and generally well tolerated in patients with CTCL†, although individuals with the more aggressive large-cell variant of the disease may be less likely to respond to this regimen. In one study, intralesional administration† of low doses of interferon alfa appeared to be more effective than a fivefold higher dose administered IM in patients with plaque-phase mycosis fungoides, suggesting that intralesional concentrations of the drug may be an important determinant of therapeutic response.

■ Melanoma ***Adjuvant Therapy*** Interferon alfa (alfa-2a [no longer commercially available in the US], alfa-2b) is used as an adjunct to surgery (within 56 days of surgery) in adults with malignant melanoma who are disease free but at high risk for systemic recurrence. Use of adjuvant therapy with interferon alfa following surgical resection prolongs disease-free but not overall survival in patients at high risk for recurrence of disease, particularly among patients with node-positive melanoma.

In a large randomized trial, patients receiving adjuvant therapy with interferon alfa-2b within 56 days of surgery for deep primary (T4) or regionally metastatic (N1) melanoma had prolonged disease-free and overall survival but experienced substantial toxicity compared with patients receiving surgery alone. Patients with Breslow's classification greater than 4 mm, and those with any Breslow's classification with primary or recurrent lymph node involvement, were included in the study. Adjuvant therapy consisted of IV interferon alfa-2b 20 million units/m^2 5 days per week for 4 weeks followed by maintenance therapy with 10 million units/m^2 subcutaneously 3 days per week for 48 weeks. Median overall survival of 3.82 or 2.78 years, respectively, was observed in patients receiving adjuvant interferon alfa therapy or undergoing surgery alone while median time to relapse was 1.72 or 0.98 years, respectively, with such treatment. The estimated 5-year overall survival rate was 46 or 37% in patients receiving adjuvant therapy or undergoing surgery alone, respectively. Although interpretation of the data is limited because stratification was performed to ensure balance rather than to make comparisons between the patient groups, subgroup analysis demonstrated benefit of adjuvant therapy with interferon alfa-2b only among patients with node-positive disease; the small number of patients with node-negative disease enrolled in the trial does not allow any meaningful conclusions regarding efficacy of adjuvant therapy with interferon alfa in this group. Toxicity was substantial with 67% of patients experiencing severe (grade 3) toxicity at some point during the year of treatment; depending on the individual patient and the relative value placed on time spent with toxicity and survival time with relapsed disease, the quality-of-life-adjusted gain in survival time may or may not be significant in patients receiving adjuvant therapy with interferon alfa.

In a subsequent 3-arm randomized trial comparing adjuvant therapy with high-dose IV interferon alfa-2b (followed by maintenance therapy with subcutaneous interferon alfa-2b), adjuvant therapy with low-dose subcutaneous interferon alfa-2b, or observation following surgical resection of deep primary (T4) or primary or recurrent regionally metastatic (N1) melanoma, disease-free survival was prolonged in patients receiving high-dose interferon alfa versus observation; however, overall survival did not differ among the groups. Results from another large trial in patients randomized to receive observation or adjuvant therapy with high-dose IM interferon alfa-2a (no longer commercially available in the US) 3 days a week for 12 weeks following surgery for primary melanomas greater than 1.69 mm in thickness with or without nodal involvement did not detect a difference in recurrence or survival rates, but subset analysis suggested a trend toward increased rate and duration of disease-free survival in patients with node-positive disease receiving adjuvant interferon alfa. Use of adjuvant therapy with interferon alfa may be a reasonable option in selected patients (e.g., those with deep primary tumors or node-positive disease), but further study is needed to establish the role of adjuvant therapy with interferon alfa in patients with high-risk, localized melanoma.

Metastatic Melanoma Interferon alfa has been used alone for the treatment of metastatic melanoma† in selected patients. Response rates averaging about 16% (with approximately 4% complete responses) have been reported in patients with metastatic melanoma receiving interferon alfa as a single agent administered daily or 3 times per week.

Monotherapy with IM interferon alfa dosages ranging from 10–20 million units/m^2 3 times weekly has been used in patients with metastatic melanoma. However, therapy with interferon alfa alone in tolerable dosages appears unlikely to alter survival in patients with this metastatic disease. The median duration of response following therapy with interferon alfa alone in patients with metastatic melanoma has been reported to be 5 months, but some patients have achieved complete responses lasting longer than 2–3 years. A relatively prolonged course of interferon alfa therapy (i.e., approximately 3 months) may be required to produce responses in patients with metastatic melanoma.

Prognostic factors that reliably identify patients with metastatic melanoma who are likely to respond favorably to interferon alfa therapy have not been identified to date. Most responses to interferon alfa monotherapy have occurred in patients with subcutaneous and small-volume disease. However, long-term responses have been observed in patients with visceral- and nonvisceral-dominant disease, in previously treated and untreated patients, and in those treated with monotherapy or combination drug therapy. Limited data suggest that intralesional therapy with interferon alfa has clinical activity in patients with melanoma, but efficacy of the drug given by this route has not been compared with that of systemic interferon therapy.

Interferon alfa also has been used in combination therapy for the treatment of metastatic melanoma. Results from a small randomized trial suggested that the combination of interferon alfa and dacarbazine was superior to dacarbazine alone, but other studies did not confirm these findings. The addition of interferon alfa did not increase response rate or prolong survival in patients receiving high-dose IV aldesleukin or continuous IV infusion aldesleukin and IV cisplatin for the treatment of metastatic melanoma. The use of interferon alfa and aldesleukin in combination with conventional chemotherapeutic agents (e.g., cisplatin, dacarbazine) is being investigated for the treatment of metastatic melanoma. A large randomized trial is under way to investigate the comparative efficacy and toxicity of concurrent biochemotherapy with interferon alfa-2b, aldesleukin, cisplatin, vinblastine, and dacarbazine versus combination chemotherapy with cisplatin, vinblastine, and dacarbazine.

■ **Basal Cell and Squamous Cell Skin Cancers** Interferon alfa has been used effectively by intralesional injection in the treatment of basal cell carcinoma†. The response of these lesions to interferon alfa therapy appears to be related to the dose and duration of therapy with the drug, increasing with increasing total dose and duration. While response was poor in patients treated with intralesional injection of 0.9 million units 3 times weekly for 3 weeks in one study and in those treated with a single 10 million-unit dose of a long-acting (protamine zinc) interferon alfa injection in another study, a good response was observed in other studies employing larger total doses and/or more prolonged therapy. In a large, multicenter study, a histologic cure rate exceeding 80% was observed at 1 year in patients receiving intralesional therapy with 1.5 million units of interferon alfa 3 times weekly for 3 weeks. A similar histologic cure rate was observed after 4 months in another study in which patients received intralesional interferon alfa therapy with a long-acting injection at a dosage of 10 million units once weekly for 3 weeks; however, the risk of adverse effects appears to be increased with this regimen compared with the lower-dose, more frequently administered regimen employing the immediate-release injection. As with other (e.g., surgical) therapy, patients treated with intralesional interferon alfa therapy for basal cell carcinoma should be followed closely for evidence of residual cancer. In addition, some clinicians caution that, pending further accumulation of data, the possibility that the lesions occasionally may be transformed into epidermoid cysts by interferon alfa therapy should be considered, since there may be some attendant risk of carcinoma reversion. Although intralesional interferon alfa appears to be safe and effective in the treatment of basal cell carcinoma, and offers the potential for improved cosmetic results and patient acceptance compared with surgical management of this cancer, the role of interferon therapy compared with other therapies (e.g., surgery, cryosurgery, curettage and electrodessication) remains to be more fully elucidated.

Limited evidence also suggests that intralesional therapy with interferon alfa can produce clinical and/or histologic responses in patients with squamous cell carcinoma† or keratoacanthoma†. Clinical improvement also has been reported in a limited number of patients with actinic (solar) keratosis†, which either disappeared or showed histologic improvement with intralesional interferon alfa therapy. However, experience with interferon alfa in the treatment of these skin disorders is less extensive than in the treatment of basal cell carcinoma, and further study is needed to determine the potential role of the drug in the treatment of these disorders.

■ **Chronic Myelogenous Leukemia** Interferon alfa (alfa-2a [no longer commercially available in the US], alfa-2b†) is used for the treatment of adult-type (Philadelphia chromosome-positive) chronic myelogenous (myelocytic, myeloid) leukemia (CML) in patients who are in the chronic phase of the disease and who have been minimally pretreated (within 1 year of diagnosis). In patients with CML, interferon alfa can produce complete or partial hematologic remissions and cytogenetic responses. Although the cytogenetic responses may be prolonged in some patients, further study and follow-up are needed to determine whether the drug can improve long-term survival in patients with this disease. Limited data suggest that pediatric patients with adult-type CML (i.e., Philadelphia-positive disease) also may exhibit a good therapeutic response to interferon alfa similar to that achieved in adults; however, children with juvenile-type CML† (i.e., Philadelphia-negative disease) generally are unresponsive to chemotherapy or interferon alfa. (See Pediatric Precautions.)

Complete hematologic remission, generally characterized by relative normalization of leukocyte and platelet counts, reduction in leukocyte alkaline phosphatase concentrations, marked reduction of splenomegaly, and decreased bone marrow cellularity, has been achieved in approximately 22–80% of patients receiving 2–5 million units/m^2 of interferon alfa daily or 3 times weekly for prolonged periods (e.g., 1–3 years). A cytogenetic response (i.e., suppression of Philadelphia chromosome-positive cells) generally occurs in at least 10–70% of patients achieving complete hematologic remission with interferon alfa therapy. Unlike the transient suppression of the Philadelphia chromosome generally observed with intensive cytotoxic antineoplastic therapy, interferon alfa has produced complete suppression of this chromosome for about 2–8 years or longer in some patients. However, interferon-induced decreases in bone marrow cellularity and suppression of Philadelphia chromosome-positive cells are delayed compared with hematologic improvement, with median times to complete hematologic and cytogenetic remission reported in early studies as 3.4 and 9 months, respectively, but in more recent studies as 5–6.7 and greater than 18 months, respectively. In addition, while the ability of interferon alfa to suppress the malignant Philadelphia chromosome-positive clone and favor reemergence of a normal clone of marrow cells suggests that the drug is potentially curative, only intensive chemotherapy, alone or combined with radiation therapy, followed by bone marrow transplantation has been shown to be curative to date.

Hematologic and cytogenetic responses to interferon alfa therapy appear to be greatest in newly diagnosed, previously untreated patients with low- to intermediate-risk disease (i.e., low to moderately high leukocytosis, splenomegaly, and presence of the Philadelphia chromosome) who have early chronic-phase CML (i.e., those who are treated within 12 months of diagnosis); response rates are approximately fourfold to sixfold higher in the early chronic phase compared with the accelerated and blast phases of the disease. In addition, limited data indicate that response rates to interferon alfa are increased in patients who are white and younger than 60 years of age. Interferon alfa reportedly can control the thrombocytosis that may occur during the initial and/or accelerated phase of CML, but the drug generally has little or no long-term therapeutic effect in the accelerated or blast phase of the disease. However, some evidence indicates that interferon alfa-treated patients with CML who enter blast crisis frequently have a lymphoid blast phenotype, which in a subset of patients appears to be associated with greater response to subsequent antineoplastic therapy, rather than the more typical myeloid blast transformation. There is some evidence to suggest that response to interferon alfa in patients with CML also may be dose related, as evidenced in one study by a higher response rate in patients receiving 5 million versus 2 million units/m^2 three times weekly; some clinicians suggest an interferon alfa dosage of 5 million units/m^2 given daily. However, additional study is needed to determine the optimum dosage of interferon alfa in the treatment of CML.

Results of a randomized, multicenter, controlled study in newly diagnosed or minimally treated patients (those who received less than 100 mg of busulfan or less than 50 g of hydroxyurea) with CML demonstrate a longer median survival in patients receiving interferon alfa (44% of patients receiving interferon alfa also received intermittent single-drug chemotherapy) versus those receiving conventional therapy with antineoplastic agents (e.g., hydroxyurea, busulfan). Median survival of 69–72 or 52–55 months, respectively, was reportedly observed in patients receiving interferon alfa or conventional chemotherapy while overall hematologic response rate was 60% (40% had complete response) or 70% (30% had complete response) in patients receiving interferon alfa or conventional chemotherapy, respectively. Usually, cytogenetic responses were only observed in patients who had complete hematologic remissions, and longer survival was observed in patients with cytogenetic response. In addition, the time of disease progression from chronic to blastic phase was

69–72 or 45–46 months in patients receiving interferon alfa or conventional chemotherapy, respectively.

Concomitant administration of interferon alfa-2b† with cytarabine has been associated with increased survival in patients with CML. Results of a randomized controlled study in previously untreated patients with CML demonstrate a longer survival in patients receiving interferon alfa-2b (5 million units/m^2 given subcutaneously daily) in combination with cytarabine (20 mg/m^2 daily for 10 days given subcutaneously 2 weeks after initiation of interferon alfa-2b therapy and monthly thereafter) versus those receiving interferon alfa-2b without cytarabine; patients from both groups also received hydroxyurea 50 mg/kg daily until a complete hematologic remission was achieved. After 3 years, median survival rate of about 86 or 79%, respectively, reportedly was observed in patients receiving combined interferon alfa-2b therapy with cytarabine or interferon alfa-2b without cytarabine while overall hematologic response rate was 66 or 55% in patients receiving combined interferon alfa-2b therapy with cytarabine or interferon alfa-2b without cytarabine, respectively. Major cytogenetic response rate after 12 months was 41 or 24% in patients receiving combined interferon alfa-2b therapy with cytarabine or interferon alfa-2b without cytarabine, respectively. Longer survival was observed in patients with cytogenetic response. Some patients underwent allogeneic or autologous bone marrow transplantation, and the 2-year survival rate after allogeneic bone marrow transplantation was 56 or 59% in patients receiving combined interferon alfa-2b therapy with cytarabine or interferon alfa-2b without cytarabine, respectively, while 2-year survival rate after autologous bone marrow transplantation was 61 or 68% in patients receiving combined interferon alfa-2b therapy with cytarabine or interferon alfa-2b without cytarabine, respectively. Patients who did not have complete hematologic or major cytogenetic responses within 6 or 12 months, respectively, were allowed to cross over to combined treatment with interferon alfa-2b and cytarabine. Among patients who received initial therapy with interferon alfa-2b without cytarabine, but then crossed over to receive combined treatment with interferon alfa-2b and cytarabine, complete and partial responses of 2 and 6%, respectively, were observed.

Further studies and follow-up of previously untreated patients receiving interferon alfa for CML are needed to determine whether the drug alters the natural course of the disease. However, results of several studies indicate that patients with CML who achieve a complete hematologic and cytogenetic response to interferon alfa therapy have a substantially longer survival rate than those who have partial or no response; complete elimination of malignant cells in peripheral blood and bone marrow (as determined by Southern blot and polymerase chain reaction analyses) has been reported following prolonged therapy with the drug. Longer survival usually is associated with slower progression to the blastic phase.

■ **Renal Cell Carcinoma** ***Overview*** Interferon alfa, alone or in combination therapy, is used for the treatment of metastatic renal cell carcinoma† in selected patients. There is no generally accepted standard drug therapy for metastatic renal cell carcinoma. Because of the poor response to systemic therapy, surgical resection often is included in the management of metastatic renal cell carcinoma. (See Uses: Renal Cell Carcinoma in Aldesleukin 10:00 for an overview of therapy for metastatic renal cell carcinoma.)

Various forms of systemic drug therapy, including cytotoxic agents, hormonal agents, and biologic agents (e.g., interferon alfa, aldesleukin, antiangiogenic and other targeted therapy), have been studied in patients with metastatic renal cell carcinoma. Response rates with cytotoxic chemotherapy generally have been poor (10% or less) for any regimen that has been studied in adequate numbers of patients with metastatic renal cell carcinoma. Evidence suggests that the incidence of tumor regression associated with interferon alfa therapy is similar to or possibly greater than that associated with conventional hormonal or antineoplastic drug therapy for this disease, and that adverse effects associated with interferon therapy may be less debilitating than those associated with these therapies. Results of studies with hormonal therapy (e.g., medroxyprogesterone acetate, tamoxifen) has been studied in the treatment of metastatic renal cell carcinoma, results have been disappointing, and these agents are no longer used.

Immunotherapy with interferon alfa or aldesleukin is used for the systemic treatment of metastatic renal cell carcinoma despite low response rates. Interferon alfa produces objective responses in only 5–30% (overall about 10–15%) of patients with metastatic disease†, and complete responses are uncommon (about 1%). The overall response rates associated with either interferon alfa or aldesleukin monotherapy appear to be similar (10–15 versus 15%, respectively), but evidence suggests that the incidence of complete or durable response is lesser with interferon alfa than with aldesleukin (1 versus 5%). In addition, a survival benefit has been associated with interferon-alfa-containing regimens in patients with metastatic renal cell carcinoma whereas such data are lacking for aldesleukin. Results of large randomized trials and analysis of pooled data from several randomized studies indicate that interferon alfa, used alone or in combination, modestly increases response rates and prolongs survival in patients with metastatic renal cell carcinoma compared with conventional antineoplastic or hormonal agents.

Whether higher response rates or more durable responses are observed in patients with metastatic renal cell carcinoma receiving immunotherapy with cytokines, such as interferon alfa, than in those receiving supportive care only has not been fully established. Results from a randomized, placebo-controlled trial showed no benefit in overall response rate, rate of durable complete response, time to disease progression, or duration of survival with use of the cytokine interferon gamma-1b for metastatic renal cell carcinoma. Most of the evidence for the use of interferon alfa in the treatment of metastatic renal cell carcinoma is based on results from noncomparative, phase II studies; interferon alfa has not been studied in placebo-controlled trials, and evidence from randomized trials comparing interferon alfa monotherapy or interferon alfa-containing regimens with other agents is limited.

Because the prognosis for patients with metastatic renal cell carcinoma is poor and conventional cytokine therapy has minimal activity with substantial toxicity, all patients with this cancer should be considered for inclusion in clinical trials at the time of diagnosis. Supportive care (e.g., adequate analgesia for pain management, surgery for solitary brain metastasis or spinal cord compression, radiation therapy for palliation of metastases, particularly painful bone metastases) remains a mainstay of therapy for patients with metastatic renal cell cancer.

The use of interferon alfa as adjuvant therapy for completely resected, locally advanced renal cell carcinoma did not improve survival or reduce the risk of relapse. No systemic therapy has been shown to reduce the risk of relapse or prolong survival in patients with localized renal cell carcinoma at high risk of recurrence; preliminary results from a small randomized trial suggest that adjuvant therapy with ex vivo activated T cells (ALT) and high-dose cimetidine delays disease recurrence.

Monotherapy for Metastatic Renal Cell Carcinoma Most evidence for the use of interferon alfa as a single agent for the treatment of metastatic renal cell carcinoma is based on uncontrolled phase II studies. Evidence from controlled, comparative studies evaluating the efficacy of interferon alfa as a single agent versus other agents in the treatment of metastatic renal cell carcinoma is limited.

Although evidence suggests that the incidence of complete or durable response is lesser with interferon alfa (1 versus 5%), the overall response rates associated with either interferon alfa or aldesleukin monotherapy appear to be similar (10–15 versus 15%, respectively). In addition, interferon alfa therapy is less toxic than high-dose aldesleukin therapy, and 2 large randomized trials have demonstrated a survival benefit for interferon-alfa-containing regimens in patients with metastatic renal cell carcinoma

Combination Therapy for Metastatic Renal Cell Carcinoma Interferon alfa has been used in various combination regimens with other agents including biologic response modifiers (e.g., aldesleukin), and/or conventional chemotherapeutic agents (e.g., fluorouracil, vinblastine) for the treatment of metastatic renal cell carcinoma. According to analysis of pooled data from several randomized studies, higher overall response rate (14 versus 8%) and prolonged survival were observed for regimens containing interferon alfa compared with antineoplastic or hormonal regimens for the treatment of metastatic renal cell carcinoma.

Interferon alfa has been used in combination with aldesleukin for the treatment of metastatic renal cell carcinoma. A collective response rate of about 20% (5% complete responses, 15% partial responses), similar to the overall response rate of 15% observed with aldesleukin monotherapy has been observed in patients with metastatic renal cell carcinoma receiving interferon alfa in combination with aldesleukin.

A retrospective analysis indicates that similar efficacy and less toxicity are observed in patients receiving subcutaneous interferon alfa and subcutaneous aldesleukin compared with continuous IV infusion of aldesleukin alone for advanced renal cell carcinoma. In a large, randomized trial, patients with metastatic renal cell carcinoma receiving subcutaneous interferon alfa-2a (no longer commercially available in the US) combined with continuous IV infusion of aldesleukin had a higher response rate and higher rate of event-free survival at 1 year but no difference in overall survival compared with those receiving either agent alone; less toxicity was observed in patients receiving interferon alfa than in those receiving aldesleukin, either alone or in combination therapy. The low response rates observed for monotherapy with interferon alfa or aldesleukin in this trial may have contributed to the differences observed in comparison with the combination therapy.

Limited evidence from a randomized, phase II trial suggests that the addition of interferon alfa-2b to a high-dose, intermittent IV infusion regimen of aldesleukin did not improve response rate, and incidence of complete response and duration of response appeared to be more favorable for patients receiving high-dose aldesleukin monotherapy for advanced renal cell carcinoma. At a median follow-up of 72 months in another randomized phase II trial, median duration of response was longer (53 versus 14 months) and the rate of progression-free survival at 3 years was higher (13 versus 3%) for patients receiving high-dose IV aldesleukin alone compared with those receiving IV interferon alfa-2b and high-dose IV aldesleukin. Another phase II randomized trial indicates that toxicity is greater but overall survival is not improved when subcutaneous interferon alfa is added to a regimen of subcutaneous aldesleukin. In a randomized trial, no survival difference was observed in patients receiving subcutaneous interferon alfa, subcutaneous aldesleukin, and oral tamoxifen versus oral tamoxifen alone.

Interferon alfa, with or without aldesleukin, also has been used in combination with conventional chemotherapeutic agents (e.g., fluorouracil, vinblastine) for the treatment of metastatic renal cell carcinoma.

In a phase III randomized trial, median survival was prolonged (16.9 versus 9.4 months) and response rate was higher (16.5 versus 2.5%) but grade 4 toxicity was more frequent (18 versus 2%) in patients receiving subcutaneous interferon alfa-2a (no longer commercially available in the US) and IV vinblastine than in those receiving IV vinblastine alone. The role of vinblastine in combination with interferon alfa remains to be established. Variable results have been reported for the benefit versus toxicity of combination regimens with interferon alfa and conventional antineoplastic agents compared with interferon alfa monotherapy.Response rates in patients with advanced renal cell carcinoma are similar or increased when vinblastine is added to interferon alfa therapy, but no difference in survival has been observed; in some studies, increased toxicity has been reported with the addition of vinblastine. No differences in overall response rates, progression-free survival, or overall survival were observed in a large randomized trial of interferon alfa-2a (no longer commercially available in the US) and 13-cis-retinoic acid (isotretinoin) versus interferon alfa-2a alone.

Interferon alfa also has been used in combination with aldesleukin and fluorouracil for the treatment of metastatic renal cell carcinoma. Although early reports from small uncontrolled studies suggested that interferon alfa used in combination with aldesleukin and fluorouracil produced favorable response rates, longer follow-up and subsequent phase II studies did not confirm higher response rates or comparable durability of responses, and some variations of the 3-drug regimen showed substantial toxicity. Results from one randomized trial indicate that the addition of fluorouracil does not improve response rate in patients receiving a regimen of subcutaneous interferon alfa and subcutaneous aldesleukin. In another randomized trial, patients receiving combination therapy with subcutaneous interferon alfa-2a (no longer commercially available in the US), subcutaneous aldesleukin, and IV fluorouracil had higher response rates and prolonged overall and progression-free survival compared with those receiving oral tamoxifen alone. Further study is required to establish the comparative efficacy and toxicity of combination therapy with interferon alfa, aldesleukin, and fluorouracil. In small, uncontrolled studies, the addition of fluorouracil did not appear to improve response rates compared with interferon alfa alone but added toxicities associated with fluorouracil.

Evidence from a randomized trial indicates that the addition of coumarin and cimetidine, potential immunomodulating agents, did not improve response rates or survival duration in patients receiving interferon alfa for metastatic renal cell carcinoma. The addition of aspirin did not enhance or interfere with the efficacy of interferon alfa therapy for metastatic renal cell carcinoma, nor did it lessen overall treatment-associated toxicity. Concomitant treatment with prednisone (10–20 mg daily) reportedly may improve the subjective tolerability of therapy by reducing flu-like symptoms without reducing response rates in patients with renal cell carcinoma receiving interferon alfa at dosages of 18 million units or more 3 times weekly; however, prednisone had little effect on the hepatic toxicity associated with high-dose interferon alfa therapy.

Other Considerations The optimum dosage and duration of interferon alfa therapy for patients with metastatic renal cell carcinoma have not been established, but limited data suggest that response to the drug may be dose dependent; dosages of interferon alfa ranging from 5–20 million units daily or 3 times weekly appear to be required to achieve optimum response with manageable toxicity. The period from initiation of treatment to occurrence of an objective response averages 3–4 months, and responses to interferon alfa rarely last longer than 2 years.

Although median duration of survival generally appears to be greater in patients with renal cell carcinoma who respond to interferon alfa than in those who do not, it is unclear whether therapy with the drug actually results in a prolonged survival or merely selects out patients with a better initial prognosis. Factors associated with higher rates of response to interferon alfa therapy include a low tumor burden with lung-predominant metastases (including mediastinum, pleural, and mediastinal node metastases), good performance status, prior nephrectomy, prolonged disease-free interval between nephrectomy and disease recurrence, relatively low nadir granulocyte counts, and perhaps in vitro sensitivity of the tumor to interferon alfa, as determined by clonogenic assay. Although reliable criteria for selecting patients most likely to benefit from cytokine therapy have not been established, prognostic factors have been identified that are associated with poor outcome despite treatment with interferon alfa and/or aldesleukin (e.g., multiple sites of metastasis, metastasis to the liver, metastasis within 1 year following diagnosis of primary tumor.

Except in rare cases, interferon alfa has not exhibited antitumor activity against unresected renal cell carcinoma or retroperitoneal, brain, or hepatic metastases. Patient selection appears to have considerable influence on outcome of therapy, and no single prognostic factor appears to correlate strongly with therapeutic response. Many patients with renal cell carcinoma who respond to interferon alfa therapy develop anti-interferon antibodies which, in some but not all studies, appear to have been associated with loss of response to therapy. However, many factors influence the frequency, magnitude, and importance of this antibody response, and further studies are needed to determine whether such antibody development affects outcome of therapy with interferon alfa in patients with renal cell carcinoma. (See Dermatologic, Local, Sensitivity, and Immunologic Reactions: Antibody Formation, in Cautions.)

■ Bladder Cancer Intravesical therapy† with interferon alfa has been used in the prophylaxis or treatment of superficial bladder cancer†. Although intravesicular BCG generally is preferred for superficial bladder cancer, responses to intravesical interferon alfa have been noted in patients with disease that failed to respond to or is refractory to other intravesical agents (e.g., BCG).

Interferon alfa administered intravesically has been used alone or in combination therapy as adjuvant or prophylactic therapy to prevent the recurrence of superficial bladder cancer following transurethral resection (TUR). Interferon alfa used alone as an intravesical agent generally appears to be less effective but less toxic than intravesical therapy with BCG or chemotherapeutic agents for the *prophylaxis* of superficial bladder cancer. At a mean follow-up of 43 months, relapse rates were similar in patients with stage T1, grade 2 or 3 or relapsed grade 1, bladder cancer receiving TUR with or without adjuvant intravesical therapy with interferon alfa-2b 60 million units once weekly for 12 weeks and then once monthly for up to 1 year of treatment. In a comparative study, intravesical interferon alfa-2b was inferior to intravesical mitomycin for preventing tumor recurrence in patients with papillary bladder tumors. In a small randomized trial, interferon alfa-2a (no longer commercially available in the US) was inferior to BCG as intravesical therapy for recurrent stage T1, grade 1 to 3, superficial bladder cancer. In a large randomized trial using a single intravesical instillation immediately following TUR, interferon alfa-2b was inferior to epirubicin for preventing recurrence of stage Ta or T1 superficial bladder cancer.

Interferon alfa also has been used in combination therapy for the prophylaxis of superficial bladder cancer. In a few randomized studies with small numbers of patients, combination therapy with interferon alfa and epirubicin administered intravesically did not appear to be more effective than either agent alone in preventing or delaying the recurrence of superficial bladder cancer at low risk of recurrence. Further study is needed to evaluate the additive or synergistic effects of interferon alfa used in combination therapy with other intravesical agents (e.g., BCG) for the prophylaxis of superficial bladder cancer.

Limited evidence suggests that interferon alfa administered intravesically is an active agent in the *treatment* of superficial bladder cancer, both as primary therapy and as secondary therapy after intravesical administration of other agents has failed. The drug has produced objective response rates ranging from 30–60% when administered intravesically for the treatment of superficial cancer of the bladder. Complete responses to intravesical interferon alfa have been observed in some patients with noninvasive papillary tumors and/or carcinoma in situ, including patients with recurrent disease or disease refractory to intravesical therapy with BCG live or cytotoxic agents. Limited data suggest that high intravesical doses (e.g., 100 million units) of interferon alfa may be more effective, with minimal toxicity, than lower doses (e.g., 10 million units) in achieving complete responses in patients with carcinoma *in situ*.

Responses have been reported in small numbers of patients receiving intralesional administration (into the base of the tumor or surrounding tissue) of interferon alfa for papillary tumors of the bladder. In limited numbers of patients, little or no efficacy has been demonstrated for the use of interferon alfa administered IM for the prophylaxis or treatment of superficial bladder cancer. Continuous intra-arterial administration† of interferon alfa showed no efficacy and considerable toxicity in 5 patients with advanced bladder cancer.

Intravesical administration of interferon has been associated with minimal toxicity; local symptoms rarely have been observed, and the most commonly observed systemic toxicity has consisted of mild to moderate flu-like symptoms. Comparative studies in larger numbers of patients are needed to determine the role of interferon alfa therapy in the prophylaxis and treatment of superficial bladder cancer.

■ Ovarian Cancer Agents other than interferon alfa are preferred for the treatment of ovarian cancer. Interferon alfa has been administered intraperitoneally† for the treatment of minimal residual epithelial ovarian cancer† in a limited number of patients. Interferon alfa appears to be an active agent in ovarian cancer when administered intraperitoneally, particularly in patients with small-volume, platinum-sensitive disease. Further studies are needed to establish the role of interferon alfa administered intraperitoneally as a single agent or in combination with conventional antineoplastic agents to patients with minimal or no evidence of residual ovarian carcinoma.

Objective responses (mostly partial responses) have been reported in less than 20% of a small number of patients with advanced ovarian cancer receiving IV or IM administration of interferon alfa.

■ Multiple Myeloma Interferon alfa has been used for the palliative treatment of multiple myeloma† in patients whose disease has relapsed or become refractory to conventional antineoplastic therapy (e.g., melphalan plus prednisone); the drug also has been used as induction therapy in a limited number of patients with the disease. Although therapy with interferon alfa alone appears to produce objective responses in only 10–30% of patients with relapsed or refractory disease, limited data suggest that some of these patients may respond to reinstitution of antineoplastic therapy following treatment with interferon alfa. Responses to interferon alfa therapy may be more common in patients who have relapsed from previous therapy than in individuals with initially refractory disease. Limited data indicate that interferon alfa may prolong duration of response and survival when given as maintenance therapy to patients following successful induction therapy with antineoplastic agents. In one study in patients who achieved an objective response following multiple courses of induction chemotherapy (a regimen of melphalan and prednisone or a regimen of vincristine, melphalan, cyclophosphamide, and prednisone [VMCP] alternating with vincristine, carmustine, doxorubicin, and prednisone [VBAP]), the median duration of response for those who subsequently received interferon alfa maintenance therapy (3 million units/m^2 subcutaneously 3 times weekly) compared with those who did not was 26 versus 14 months and the median duration of survival was 52 versus 39 months; differences in survival between interferon alfa maintenance and no maintenance were particularly evident in the subset of patients who had achieved a substantial objective response to induction chemotherapy; Previously *untreated* patients receiving interferon alfa in a combined regimen with conventional antineoplastic therapy (i.e., melphalan and prednisone) may have at best a marginally improved response rate compared with those receiving antineoplastic therapy alone, although no substantial difference in overall survival was observed.

When used for induction of remission in a limited number of previously untreated patients with multiple myeloma, therapy with interferon alfa has been associated with response rates of up to 50–75%. Evidence suggests that patients most likely to benefit from interferon therapy are those who have received limited or no prior treatment, those with early-stage disease, and those who have a small tumor burden. Patients responding to interferon alfa therapy may have subjective improvement in bone pain, recalcification of osteolytic lesions, decreases in bone marrow plasma cells, decreased concentrations of monoclonal (M-component) immunoglobulins (e.g., myeloma or Bence-Jones proteins) in serum and/or urine, and an increase in performance status. IgM synthesis and decreased serum concentrations of IgG, IgA, and IgM reportedly normalize in patients who respond to interferon, which suggests that interferon alfa stimulates the recovery of normal immune function in these individuals; this restoration to normal of immunoglobulin concentrations is uncommon in patients who respond to therapy with antineoplastic agents alone.Preliminary results of studies in which multiple-drug regimens of antineoplastic agents (e.g., vincristine, carmustine, melphalan, cyclophosphamide, and prednisone) have been alternated with courses of interferon alfa suggest that such alternating therapy may increase the rate of response and duration of survival in patients with multiple myeloma, although combined therapy also may increase toxicity (e.g., neutropenia). Further long-term follow-up, and randomized studies comparing such alternating regimens with antineoplastic therapy alone, are needed to confirm these results.

■ **Other Uses** Interferon alfa has been used for the management of various angiomatous (angiogenic) disorders† in a limited number of patients. Although experience to date is limited, interferon alfa has been used with encouraging results in some such conditions that previously were fatal in most cases (e.g, pulmonary hemangiomatosis†). Initiation of interferon alfa therapy in a 12-year-old boy with pulmonary hemangiomatosis resulted in substantial improvement in pulmonary function, pulmonary angiograms, exercise tolerance, and other manifestations (e.g., digital clubbing) of this disorder; the condition has remained in remission for at least 30 months with long-term interferon alfa maintenance therapy. Encouraging results also have been observed following initiation of interferon alfa therapy in several other patients with pulmonary hemangiomatosis or other angiomatous disorders, and in at least 2 infants with progressive hemangioendotheliomas†. It has been suggested that interferons may inhibit angiogenesis in part by inhibiting proliferation of endothelial cells, smooth muscle cells, and fibroblasts that have been stimulated by fibroblast growth factor (FGF); decreasing collagen production; and increasing endothelial prostacyclin production. Other mechanisms also may be involved. Additional study and experience are needed to establish the role of interferon alfa in the management of these disorders and to determine the optimum dosage and duration of therapy. Some clinicians recommend that, pending further accumulation of data, interferon alfa therapy be reserved for consistently life-threatening or fatal angiomatous conditions for which effective alternative treatment is not available (e.g., pulmonary hemangiomatosis), patients with life-threatening complications of angiomatous disease that fail to respond adequately to conventional therapy or in whom such therapy is not tolerated (e.g., those developing excessive corticosteroid toxicity during the management of Kasabach-Merritt [hemangioma-thrombocytopenia] syndrome†), conditions that seriously compromise vital organs or structures, and conditions that result in disfigurement, disability, or potential amputation.

Interferon alfa also has been used in the treatment of metastatic small intestinal carcinoid tumors†. The drug has reduced the frequency and/or severity of symptoms associated with the carcinoid syndrome and has produced substantial reductions in urinary 5-hydroxyindoleacetic acid concentrations, serum human chorionic gonadotropin concentrations, and serum pancreatic peptide tumor markers.

Dosage and Administration

■ **Reconstitution and Administration** Interferon alfa-2b is administered by IM, subcutaneous, or intralesional injection or by IV infusion.

Interferon alfa-2b may be *self-administered* if the clinician determines that the patient and/or their caregiver are competent to reconstitute and safely administered the drug after appropriate training and with medical follow-up as necessary. Patients and/or their caregivers who administer interferon alfa in a home setting should be cautioned against reuse of syringes and needles, supplied with a puncture-resistant container for the safe disposal of such equipment after use, and instructed on the proper disposal of full disposal containers.

Interferon alfa-2b is available in various strengths in single-dose vials containing a powder for injection that requires reconstitution prior to injection and in multiple-dose vials containing solution for injection. Not all dosage forms and strengths are appropriate for all indications.

Interferon alfa solutions should be inspected visually for discoloration and particulate matter prior to administration whenever solution and container permit.

Patients should be well hydrated during interferon alfa therapy, especially during initial stages of treatment.

Some adverse effects associated with interferon alfa therapy (e.g., flu-like syndrome) may be prevented or ameliorated by administering the drug in the evening or at bedtime. In addition, the incidence of adverse effects may be reduced by administration of acetaminophen or other nonopiate analgesic at the time the interferon alfa dose is given.

IV Administration **Melanoma.** For use as an adjunct to surgery in the treatment of malignant melanoma, interferon alfa-2b is given initially by IV infusion (induction therapy) and then by subcutaneous injection (maintenance therapy). (See Melanoma under Reconstitution and Administration: Subcutaneous Injection, in Dosage and Administration.)

IV solutions should be prepared using single-dose vials of interferon alfa-2b powder for injection containing 10, 18, or 50 million units of the drug. Solutions of the drug commercially available in multiple-dose vials should not be used for IV administration.

Single-dose vials of interferon alfa-2b containing 10, 18, or 50 million units of the drug should be reconstituted by adding 1 mL of the sterile water for injection diluent provided by the manufacturer and gently swirling the vial; the resultant solution contains 10, 18, or 50 million units/mL, respectively.

The appropriate dose of reconstituted solution should be withdrawn from the vial and added to 100 mL of 0.9% sodium chloride injection. The final concentration of the IV solution should not be less than 10 million units/100 mL (100,000 units/mL).

IV solutions of interferon alfa-2b should be given by IV infusion over 20 minutes.

IM Injection IM injections of interferon alfa-2b should be made into the anterolateral thigh, upper arm, or outer area of the buttocks.

Hairy Cell Leukemia. For IM injection for the treatment of hairy cell leukemia, single-dose vials of interferon alfa-2b powder for injection containing 10 million units of the drug should be reconstituted with 1 mL of the sterile water for injection diluent provided by the manufacturer and the vial gently swirled; the resultant solution contains 10 million units/mL. The appropriate dose of reconstituted solution should be administered IM undiluted.

Alternatively, the appropriate dose of interferon alfa-2b solution for injection from a multiple-dose vial containing 6 or 10 million units/mL can be administered IM undiluted.

Interferon alfa-2b should not be administered IM in patients with hairy cell leukemia and platelet counts less than 50,000/mm^3.

AIDS-related Kaposi's Sarcoma. For IM injection for the treatment of AIDS-related Kaposi's sarcoma, single-dose vials of interferon alfa-2b powder for injection containing 50 million units should be reconstituted with 1 mL of the sterile water for injection diluent provided by the manufacturer and the vial gently swirled; the resultant solution contains 50 million units/mL. The appropriate dose of reconstituted solution should be administered IM undiluted.

Multiple-dose vials containing interferon alfa-2b solution for injection should not be used for treatment of AIDS-related Kaposi's sarcoma.

Subcutaneous Injection Subcutaneous injections of interferon alfa-2b should be made into the anterolateral thigh, upper arm, or abdomen (avoiding the navel). Subcutaneous injections should not be made into an area where the skin is irritated, red, bruised, infected, or has scars, stretch marks, or lumps.

Hairy Cell Leukemia. For subcutaneous injection for the treatment of hairy cell leukemia, single-dose vials of interferon alfa-2b powder for injection containing 10 million units of the drug should be reconstituted with 1 mL of the sterile water for injection provided by the manufacturer and the vial gently swirled; the resultant solution contains 10 million units/mL. The appropriate dose of reconstituted solution should be administered subcutaneously undiluted.

Alternatively, the appropriate dose of interferon alfa-2b solution for injection from a multiple-dose vial containing 6 or 10 million units/mL can be administered subcutaneously undiluted.

AIDS-related Kaposi's Sarcoma. For subcutaneous injection for the treatment of AIDS-related Kaposi's sarcoma, single-dose vials of interferon alfa-2b powder for injection containing 50 million units should be reconstituted with 1 mL of the sterile water for injection diluent provided by the manufacturer and the vial gently swirled; the resultant solution contains 50 million units/mL. The appropriate dose of reconstituted solution should be administered subcutaneously undiluted.

Multiple-dose vials containing interferon alfa-2b solution for injection should not be used for treatment of AIDS-related Kaposi's sarcoma.

Follicular non-Hodgkin's Lymphoma. For subcutaneous injection for the treatment of follicular non-Hodgkin's lymphoma, single-dose vials of interferon alfa-2b powder for injection containing 10 million units should be reconstituted with 1 mL of the sterile water for injection diluent provided by the manufacturer and the vial gently swirled; the resultant solution contains 10 million units/mL. The appropriate dose of reconstituted solution should be administered subcutaneously undiluted.

Alternatively, the appropriate dose of interferon alfa-2b solution for injection from a multiple-dose vial containing 6 or 10 million units/mL can be administered subcutaneously undiluted.

Melanoma. For use as an adjunct to surgery in the treatment of malignant melanoma, interferon alfa-2b is given initially by IV infusion (induction therapy) and then by subcutaneous injection (maintenance therapy). (See Melanoma under Reconstitution and Administration: IV Administration, in Dosage and Administration.)

For subcutaneous injection for maintenance therapy, single-dose vials of interferon alfa-2b powder for injection containing 10 or 18 million units of the drug should be reconstituted with 1 mL of the sterile water for injection diluent provided by the manufacturer and the vial gently swirled; the resultant solution contains 10 or 18 million units/mL, respectively. The appropriate dose of reconstituted solution should be administered subcutaneously undiluted.

Alternatively, the appropriate dose of interferon alfa-2b solution for injection from a multiple-dose vial containing 6 or 10 million units/mL can be administered subcutaneously undiluted.

■ **Dosage** ***Hairy Cell Leukemia*** The usual adult dosage of interferon alfa-2b for induction of remission in hairy cell leukemia is 2 million units/m^2 given by IM or subcutaneous injection 3 times weekly. The drug should be administered subcutaneously (not IM) in patients with platelet counts less than 50,000/mm^3.

Improvement in one or more hematologic variables generally occurs within 2 months after initiation of interferon alfa therapy in patients with hairy cell leukemia; however, improvement in granulocyte and platelet counts may require up to 6 months or longer of interferon alfa therapy. The manufacturer states that interferon alfa-2b therapy should be continued for up to 6 months; patients who are responding may benefit from continued treatment, but the drug should be discontinued if disease progresses or fails to respond after 6 months of treatment. Some clinicians suggest that therapy with interferon alfa be continued for at least 12 months before discontinuance for nonresponse is considered, unless there is evidence of disease progression. The minimum effective dosage and optimum duration of therapy with interferon alfa for hairy cell leukemia have not been clearly established.

If severe adverse effects occur during interferon alfa-2b therapy, dosage should be decreased by 50% or the drug should be temporarily discontinued. If adverse effects abate, interferon alfa-2b therapy may be resumed using reduced dosage (1 million units/m^2 3 times weekly). The drug should be permanently discontinued if severe adverse effects persist or if they recur when reduced dosage is used.

AIDS-Related Kaposi's Sarcoma For the treatment of AIDS-related Kaposi's sarcoma, the manufacturer recommends that adults receive interferon alfa-2b in a dosage of 30 million units/m^2 3 times weekly given by IM or subcutaneous injection. The manufacturer states that interferon alfa-2b should be continued until disease progression or maximal response has been achieved after 16 weeks of treatment. Response to interferon alfa is slow, and the maximum effect occurs after 6 or more months of treatment.

If severe adverse effects occur during interferon alfa-2b therapy, dosage should be decreased by 50% or the drug should be temporarily discontinued. If adverse effects abate, interferon alfa-2b therapy may be resumed using reduced dosage. The drug should be permanently discontinued if severe adverse effects persist or if they recur when reduced dosage is used.

Follicular non-Hodgkin's Lymphoma If interferon alfa-2b is used in conjunction with anthracycline-containing chemotherapy for the treatment of follicular lymphoma, the manufacturer recommends that adults receive interferon alfa-2b in a dosage of 5 million units given by subcutaneous injection 3 times weekly for up to 18 months.

When interferon alfa-2b is added to the chemotherapy regimen, myelosuppressive drug dosage has been reduced by 25% from full dose and the cycle length increased by 33% (e.g., from 21 to 28 days). The chemotherapy cycle should be delayed if neutrophil counts are less than 1500/mm^3 or platelet counts are less than 75,000/mm^3.

Interferon alfa-2b therapy should be withheld if neutrophil counts are less than 1000/mm^3 or platelet counts are less than 50,000/mm^3. Dosage of interferon alfa-2b should be decreased by 50% (2.5 million units 3 times weekly) if neutrophil counts are greater than 1000/mm^3 but less than 1500/mm^3. If hematologic toxicity resolves (absolute neutrophil count greater than 1500/mm^3), interferon alfa-2b dosage may be reescalated to the initial starting dosage (5 million units 3 times weekly). Interferon alfa-2b therapy should be permanently discontinued if serum AST concentrations exceed 5 times the upper limit of normal or if serum creatinine concentrations exceed 2 mg/dL.

Melanoma For use as an adjunct to surgery in the treatment malignant melanoma, interferon alfa-2b is given in 2 phases (induction therapy and maintenance therapy).

For induction therapy, the recommended adult dosage of interferon alfa-2b is 20 million units/m^2 daily given by IV infusion 5 consecutive days per week for 4 weeks. For maintenance therapy, the recommended adult dosage of interferon alfa-2b is 10 million units/m^2 given by subcutaneous injection 3 times weekly for 48 weeks.

If severe adverse effects occur during interferon alfa-2b therapy (e.g., granulocyte counts greater than 250/mm^3 but less than 500/mm^3, serum ALT and/or AST concentrations greater than 5–10 times the upper limit of normal), the drug should be withheld until adverse effects abate. Interferon alfa-2b therapy may then be resumed at 50% of the previous dosage. If toxicity does not abate when the drug is withheld, serious adverse effects recur with reduced dosage, or granulocyte counts decrease to less than 250/mm^3 or serum ALT and/or AST concentrations increase to more than 10 times the upper limit of normal, interferon alfa-2b therapy should be permanently discontinued.

Cautions

Almost all patients experience adverse effects at some time during the course of interferon alfa therapy. However, evaluation of some adverse effects and establishment of a causal relationship to interferon alfa have been difficult since the drug has been used principally in patients with serious underlying diseases, such as acquired immunodeficiency syndrome (AIDS), various cancers, and/or viral hepatitis.

The incidence and severity of many adverse effects associated with interferon alfa therapy may be related to the underlying disease, type and dosage (including duration of therapy) of interferon alfa administered, route of administration (e.g., systemic versus local injection), and age and/or performance status of the patient. Patients receiving relatively low dosages and local administration of interferon alfa (e.g., in the management of exophytic genital warts) generally appear to have a lower incidence of adverse effects compared with patients receiving relatively high systemic dosages (e.g., in the management of AIDS-related Kaposi's sarcoma), although most types of adverse effects reported with systemic administration of the drug also have been reported with local administration. When administered 2–3 times weekly, interferon alfa doses of 1–9 million units generally are well tolerated while doses of 18 million units or more usually produce moderate to severe adverse effects and those of 36 million units or more usually produce severe adverse effects. Intermittent doses of 50 million units or more rarely are tolerated for periods exceeding 8 weeks, and intermittent or daily doses of 100 million units or more rarely are tolerated for periods exceeding 4–8 or 1–2 weeks, respectively.

The most common adverse effect associated with interferon alfa therapy is a flu-like syndrome, which generally occurs within the first several hours to days and has been reported in up to 98% of patients receiving the drug.

Most of the adverse effects associated with interferon alfa therapy are mild to moderate in degree of severity and diminish in intensity and frequency with continued therapy. However, adverse effects may be severe enough to require discontinuance of the drug in about 3–11% of patients; the likelihood that intolerance will require dosage reduction and/or discontinuance increases with increasing doses. Noncompliance secondary to adverse effects also may increase with increasing doses. Some interferon alfa-induced adverse effects may be alleviated by dosage reduction or may subside despite continued therapy at the same dosage.

For information on adverse effects, cautions, and precautions related to use of interferon alfa for the treatment of viral infections, see Cautions in Interferon Alfa 8:18.20.

■ **Flu-like Syndrome** A flu-like syndrome develops to some degree in almost all patients receiving 1 million units or more of interferon alfa but its severity appears to be dose related. The syndrome is characterized by the development of fever (in about 40–98% of patients), fatigue/malaise (in about 50–95% of patients), myalgia (in about 30–75% of patients), chills (in about 40–65% of patients), headache (in about 20–70% of patients), arthralgia (in about 5–24% of patients), rigors, tachycardia, anorexia, dry mouth, dysgeusia, back pain, sweating, and dizziness. Abdominal cramps and diarrhea also may be associated with the syndrome.

Fever frequently reaches 38–40°C within 6 hours of administration of interferon alfa, generally persists for 2–12 hours if untreated, and usually is preceded by chills, which can be severe. Pretreatment with a nonsteroidal anti-inflammatory agent (NSAIA) or acetaminophen may minimize the risk of developing fever and/or its severity. Such pretreatment also may attenuate some other effects (e.g., myalgia) associated with interferon alfa-induced flu-like syndrome. However, fever usually becomes self-limiting after the first several weeks of therapy, manifesting as a low-grade fever that does not require specific treatment. Therefore, subsequent development of high fever during prolonged interferon alfa therapy should prompt consideration of other possible causes (e.g., infection). The pyrogenic response to interferon alfa therapy may be mediated by a drug-induced increase of hypothalamic prostaglandin (PGE_2) production and/or release rather than by an increase in interleukin-1. This response does not appear to be secondary to an exogenous pyrogenic contaminant in interferon alfa preparations. Patients receiving high doses of interferon alfa (e.g., 50–120 million units) may experience a sharp febrile response accompanied by severe rigors and occasionally may develop peripheral cyanosis, vasoconstriction, nausea, vomiting, severe myalgias, intense headaches, and exhaustion. Transient hypotension and syncope also may occur in these patients, especially when the drug is administered IV.

There is considerable interindividual variation in the development of tolerance to interferon alfa-induced flu-like effects; however, tolerance of such effects appears to be optimized by employing relatively low (e.g., 10 million units or less 3–7 times weekly) dosages of interferon alfa, and such dosages usually permit continuous treatment for prolonged periods. In patients receiving daily interferon alfa therapy, fever and other flu-like symptoms usually diminish within a few days to weeks; malaise often recurs with each dose for the first few weeks of therapy. In patients receiving less frequent, intermittent therapy with the drug, flu-like symptoms may recur with each dose, particularly when the interval between doses exceeds 3 days or therapy is temporarily withheld and subsequently reinstituted.

A persistent and pervasive fatigue, which usually is preceded by fever and is characterized by weakness or tiredness, also can occur as a component of an interferon alfa-induced chronic flu-like syndrome; such patients frequently report a feeling of lassitude and/or lack of motivation to participate in normal activities (e.g., job absenteeism, social withdrawal), thus exhibiting decreased performance status. Fatigue/malaise may be the most prominent adverse effect associated with continued interferon alfa therapy and may include an increased need for sleep, anorexia and weight loss, myalgias, backache, headache, difficulty concentrating, chilliness, and low-grade fever. Although manifestations of this fatigue usually are intermittent, they can be severe enough to substantially impair physical activity and require interruption of therapy. Fatigue may be an important dose-limiting effect of interferon alfa therapy in patients receiving high dosages of the drug; dosage reduction or interruption of therapy with the drug usually is required in such patients but may only ameliorate rather than eliminate such symptoms. Tolerance to fatigue may be enhanced with intermittent dosing schedules, and some patients may better tolerate the drug when it is administered in the evening rather than in the morning. However, persistent and pervasive fatigue also has been reported in patients receiving relatively low dosages (e.g., 2–10 million units/m^2 three times weekly) of the drug.

It has been postulated that interferon alfa-induced fatigue may result from a neurotoxic effect of the drug preferentially manifesting as a frontal lobe or more generalized encephalopathy. Therefore, some clinicians have suggested that a distinct (from the flu-like syndrome), reversible neurasthenia syndrome may exist. However, the possibility that such manifestations may be secondary to the patient's underlying condition cannot be excluded, and additional study is necessary. This neurasthenia syndrome has been described as a constant, pervasive, nonspecific symptom complex, manifested characteristically as a psychomotor retardation (i.e., sudden adynamic state with loss of cognitive, verbal, and motor spontaneity, incentive, and interest). While intellectual activity may be disturbed, formal intellect appears to be preserved (i.e., drive rather than ability is impaired). For additional information on these and other adverse nervous system effects, see Cautions: Nervous System Effects.

■ **Musculoskeletal Effects** Myalgia and arthralgia, often associated with a flu-like syndrome, are the most frequent adverse musculoskeletal effects of interferon alfa, occurring in up to 70 and 24% of patients, respectively.These effects generally are transient, mild, and self-limiting. More severe myalgias, generally involving the lower extremities and associated with limitation of movement, have been observed in patients with chronic myelogenous leukemia receiving the drug. Such myalgias frequently require 1–2 weeks of bed rest and corticosteroid and/or analgesic (e.g., opiate) therapy for relief. These severe myalgias generally were not associated with an increase in serum muscle enzymes, and electromyograms have failed to reveal evidence of myositis. Skeletal pain, which frequently is one of the first adverse effects associated with interferon alfa therapy, has been reported in some patients with multiple myeloma who were receiving the drug; however, arthralgias were not observed in patients with metastatic osseous lesions associated with renal cell carcinoma or other malignancies.

Muscle (e.g., leg cramps) and bone disorders have been reported in less than 5% of patients receiving interferon alfa. Back pain, muscle pain, and stiffness of the shoulders have been reported in 1–4% of patients. Muscle weakness, arthrosis, polyarticular arthropathies, and arthritis have been reported in less than 1% of patients receiving the drug. Interferon alfa-associated arthropathies may be autoimmune in nature in some patients.

■ **GI Effects** Anorexia has been reported in about 19–65% of patients with hairy cell leukemia or AIDS-related Kaposi's sarcoma receiving interferon alfa. Anorexia and associated weight loss also are common in other patients during continued therapy with the drug. Anorexia, which usually occurs after continued dosing of the drug, also may be accompanied by flu-like symptoms and may require dosage reduction. Occasionally, associated weight loss may be striking and dose limiting, especially in patients who were underweight prior to initiating therapy with the drug.

Nausea, vomiting, diarrhea, dysgeusia (metallic or salty taste), and abdominal pain have been reported in about 17–50, 6–50, 20–45, 13–25, and 5–20% of patients, respectively, receiving interferon alfa therapy. Dysgeusia may be particularly likely during initiation of therapy and, at high dosages, may be accompanied by saburral (foulness resulting from accumulation of epithelial matter and debris) tongue and/or halitosis. Hypogeusia (especially for meat) also has been reported, and alterations in taste may be accompanied by alterations in smell. Diarrhea, which can be severe at high doses, generally is watery and usually is not accompanied by abdominal cramps or blood, mucus, or fat in the stools. Nausea rarely may require antiemetic therapy.

Dry mouth or gingivitis has been reported in up to 28 or 14% of patients, respectively, receiving interferon alfa. Stomatitis and eructation has been reported in up to 6% of patients. Dyspepsia, hypersalivation, thirst, GI hemorrhage melena, esophagitis, hyperesthesia of the tongue, discoloration of the GI mucosa, gastric ulcer, oral pain, bleeding gums, and hyperplasia of the gums have been reported rarely.

■ **Nervous System Effects** Although interferon alfa distributes poorly into the CNS, adverse nervous system effects have been reported in patients receiving the drug and have ranged from mild mental disturbances (e.g., anxiety, irritability), fatigue, and headache to more severe delirium and global dysfunction with mental obtundation and stupor. In some cases, the patient's underlying condition may have contributed to or caused the observed effect. Patients, especially geriatric patients, receiving relatively high systemic dosages of the drug and those with underlying CNS impairment appear to be particularly likely to develop adverse nervous system effects. However, nervous system effects also have been reported in patients receiving relatively low dosages (e.g., 2–10 million units/m^2 three times weekly) of the drug. Most adverse nervous system effects are mild and rapidly (e.g., within a few days) reversible following dosage reduction or interruption of interferon alfa therapy, although several (e.g., 2–4) weeks may be required for resolution, especially in severe cases.

Depression, suicidal behavior (e.g., suicidal ideation, suicide attempts), and suicides have been reported in association with the use of interferon alfa. If severe depression occurs, discontinuance of interferon alfa therapy generally is required.

The most common adverse nervous system effects associated with interferon alfa therapy are fatigue (usually as a component of a flu-like or neurasthenia syndrome) (see Cautions: Flu-like Syndrome), headache, malaise, and dizziness, which have been reported in up to 95, 10–50, 20–70, and 9–40% of patients, respectively. Headache also may be a component of a flu-like syndrome and, in some cases, was described as migraine. Depression (including exacerbation of underlying depression, which can be debilitating), circumoral and/or peripheral paresthesias (e.g., tingling of the extremities), unspecified pain, altered mental status, amnesia, and confusion have been reported in up to 28, up to 21, up to 17, up to 17, up to 14, and up to 12% of patients, respectively, receiving interferon alfa therapy. In some patients, especially geriatric patients, with malignancy receiving relatively high systemic dosages of the drug, alterations in mental status have been severe, manifesting as substantial mental obtundation and coma. In addition, paresthesia may be severe in some patients and may be more likely in patients previously exposed to vinca alkaloid therapy. (See Antineoplastic Agents: Vinca Alkaloids, in Drug Interactions.)

Somnolence, sleep disturbances (e.g., hypersomnia, insomnia), anxiety, hypoesthesia, nervousness, emotional lability, and vertigo have been reported in 5% or less of patients receiving interferon alfa. Lethargy, tremor, hallucinations, abnormal thinking, psychomotor retardation, stupor, coma, stroke, and transient ischemic attacks have been reported in less than 1% of patients receiving interferon alfa. Impaired coordination, extrapyramidal reactions, paralysis, bradykinesia, hypertonia, dysphasia, and aphasia also have been reported in less than 1% of patients receiving the drug.

Patients receiving interferon alfa also have developed decreased tendon reflexes, hyporeflexia, mild to marked motor loss, and slowing of motor and sensory conduction velocities. Such changes were suggestive of a mild sensory motor neuropathy; in some patients with preexisting neurologic dysfunction and/or receiving high dosages of the drug, severe neurotoxicity (e.g., polyradiculopathy) and neurogenic muscle atrophy (e.g., neuralgic amyotrophy) were reported. Exacerbation of neurologic manifestations also has been reported in some patients with multiple sclerosis following initiation of interferon alfa therapy. (See Cautions: Precautions and Contraindications.)

Reversible EEG abnormalities, which may be severe, have been reported in patients receiving interferon alfa and were characterized by progressive slowing of background activity, with a dominant slowing of alpha rhythm and appearance of diffuse slow waves (e.g., theta and delta), and mainly involved the frontal and temporal lobes. Other EEG abnormalities (e.g., paroxysmal bursts of moderate- to high-voltage frontal rhythmic delta waves) also have been reported. Seizures have been reported occasionally in patients receiving the drug. The risk of EEG abnormalities does not appear to correlate with serum interferon alfa concentrations, and the drug generally was undetectable in the CSF of these patients. However, the risk of such abnormalities may be increased with increasing dosages, and some patients may tolerate reduced interferon alfa dosages.

EEG abnormalities reported in patients receiving interferon alfa often have been associated with profound but selective CNS dysfunction (e.g., psychomotor retardation, marked somnolence, fatigue, confusion, disorientation, social withdrawal, general mental slowing, expressive dysphagia) that was characteristic of a frontal lobe neurasthenia syndrome. However, other clinicians have described the syndrome as a more complex and generalized encephalopathy. The syndrome also may mimic viral encephalitis. Patients with manifestations of this syndrome most notably exhibit a sudden adynamic state (psychomotor retardation) that includes loss of higher mental function such as cognitive, verbal, and motor spontaneity, incentive, expressions, gestures, and interest; such patients may exhibit moderate to severe behavioral changes. Loss of libido also may occur. The mechanism(s) for this possible neurotoxic reaction has not been elucidated, although alterations in central neurotransmitters may contribute, at least in part, since metoclopramide or methylphenidate occasionally have reversed neuropsychiatric effects associated with interferon alfa therapy.

Other neuropsychiatric effects associated with interferon alfa therapy have included phobias, obsessional thoughts and rituals, tearfulness, delirium (which may include clouding of consciousness, agitation, paranoia, and suicidal ideation), disruption of interpersonal relationships, irritability, and psychosis. In some cases, the patient's underlying condition may have contributed to the observed effects. Difficulty in concentration, mental clouding, disorientation to time and space, visuospatial disorientation, numbness, and speech disorders also have been reported. Delirium appears to be the most severe adverse neuropsychiatric effect associated with interferon alfa therapy and appears to be a continuum of such effects since patients developing delirium usually are irritable, depressed, withdrawn, and agitated and occasionally suicidal, paranoid, and anxious. In patients receiving relatively low doses of the drug, delirium appears to occur only rarely and probably only in patients with underlying CNS dysfunction (e.g., those with a history of CNS insult or injury). Tearfulness that develops in some patients receiving interferon alfa usually is labile, often unpredictable and uncontrollable (e.g., characterized by excessive sentimentality), and out of proportion to the precipitating situation (e.g., gestures of kindness, viewing television news).

Patients with a history of brain injury, severe substance abuse, or brain dysfunction such as mild organic brain syndrome associated with early hepatic failure may be at increased risk of developing delirium. In addition, the risk of adverse neuropsychiatric effects appears to be increased with increasing dosages. However, even during long-term interferon alfa therapy at relatively low dosages, neuropsychiatric effects reportedly occur in up to 20% of patients, and they are some of the most frequent reasons for dosage reduction or discontinuance of the drug during prolonged therapy. Patients with a history of alcohol or substance abuse may be vulnerable to interferon alfa-induced neuropsychiatric effects during prolonged therapy, developing craving, fear of recidivism to abuse, or actual relapse; therefore, such patients should be advised of the possibility of this effect and offered counseling if necessary.

Because the goal of interferon alfa therapy generally is to continue therapy if possible until the optimum benefit is achieved, efforts aimed at detecting and managing adverse psychiatric effects often become important during prolonged therapy. It is important that patients and their partners and family members be apprised of the potential for such effects and encouraged to aid clinicians in early detection. They should be advised that the onset of these effects often is insidious, and they initially may manifest as irritability and resultant problems at work or with interpersonal relationships. Tolerance of interferon alfa-induced adverse neuropsychiatric effects can be increased by providing encouragement, counseling, and reassurance that the effects are drug related and generally resolve once therapy is complete; dosage adjustment and symptomatic management may be required. Simple reassurance that irritability and associated effects are caused by interferon alfa and will decrease with dosage adjustment often is sufficient to relieve anxiety and make the effects tolerable. When irritability and associated symptoms are severe, reassurance may be insufficient to enable the patient to function socially or control their mood and behavior; dosage reduction (e.g., by one half) in such cases may improve neuropsychiatric manifestations within a few days.There is limited evidence that methylphenidate or metoclopramide may provide relief in some patients, but controlled studies are needed to confirm this finding. Rarely, discontinuance of interferon alfa therapy may be necessary. If delirium or severe depression occurs, dosage reduction or interruption of interferon alfa therapy generally is required. Limited data suggest that fluoxetine may be useful in treating depression associated with interferon alfa therapy. Because of the potential severity of delirium, discontinuance of interferon alfa and close observation (e.g., in a hospital setting) has been recommended for patients who develop this effect.

■ **Hematologic Effects** Adverse hematologic effects occur frequently in patients receiving interferon alfa but, unlike the marked myelosuppression that frequently occurs with conventional antineoplastic (cytotoxic) agents, interferon alfa generally is mildly myelosuppressive and produces hematologic toxicity that generally is well tolerated and transient. Hematologic toxicity occasionally may be apparent within a few hours of interferon alfa administration and may not be cumulative. The incidence of adverse hematologic effects appears to be decreased in patients with exophytic genital warts receiving local, low-dose therapy compared with patients with AIDS-related Kaposi's sarcoma or other malignancies.

The predominant manifestations of interferon alfa-induced hematologic toxicity include leukopenia (mainly neutropenia), anemia, and thrombocytopenia, which occur in about 3–69, 5–69, and 3–42% of patients, respectively. Thrombocytopenia and anemia generally are well tolerated, although thrombocytopenia occasionally may be severe enough to require discontinuance of interferon alfa. Marked decreases in erythrocytes can occur in patients with preexisting anemia. Leukopenia (e.g., granulocytopenia) also occasionally may be severe enough to require discontinuance of the drug. Reductions in interferon alfa dosage can ameliorate decreased blood cell counts. Following discontinuance of interferon alfa therapy, recovery from leukopenia and/or thrombocytopenia generally are rapid (e.g., within a few days), while recovery from anemia generally is slow (e.g., within weeks to a few months). Despite these adverse hematologic effects associated with interferon alfa therapy, patients generally do not experience abnormal blood loss, evidence of hemolysis, or bleeding diathesis. However, transient myelosuppression occasionally may be severe enough to require red blood cell and/or platelet transfusions.

Leukopenia, which may occur within a few hours of administration of interferon alfa, usually is asymptomatic and dose-related, may be dose-limiting, and may result both from granulocytopenia and lymphocytopenia. Leukopenia may improve following conversion to intermittent (e.g., every 3 or more days) administration or interruption of interferon alfa therapy. Interferon alfa-induced leukopenia appears to result from reversibly impaired bone marrow release of mature cells and/or from depletion or sequestration of circulating leukocytes rather than from direct myelotoxicity (e.g., maturation arrest). However, there is in vitro evidence that interferons may inhibit myeloid and erythroid progenitor cells. In patients with normal pretreatment blood cell counts, the risk of infection may not be increased substantially by interferon alfa-induced leukopenia since the leukocytic response to infection does not appear to be impaired by the drug in such patients. However, leukopenia may be more frequent and severe in patients with multiple myeloma or lymphoma, and these and other patients with preexisting leukopenia may be at increased risk of infection during interferon therapy.

Decreased hemoglobin concentration have occurred in patients, receiving chronic interferon alfa therapy. Prolonged administration of the drug occasionally may result in a normochromic, normocytic anemia; recovery from anemia generally requires weeks to months following discontinuance of interferon alfa, suggesting that some interference with erythropoiesis may be involved. Positive direct antiglobulin (Coombs') test results occasionally have been observed in patients receiving interferon alfa. Rarely, immunologically mediated hemolytic anemia has occurred, which generally improved following discontinuance of the drug and administration of corticosteroids; anemia recurred in several patients who were rechallenged with the drug.

Interferon alfa-induced thrombocytopenia usually is mild and asymptomatic and generally develops slowly over several weeks, and its incidence appears to be related to the patient's underlying condition. Patients with chronic lymphocytic leukemia or multiple myeloma appear to be at increased risk of developing thrombocytopenia during therapy with drug compared with patients with solid tumors. Platelet counts usually reach a nadir within 2–4 weeks. In some patients (e.g., those with malignant erythrocytosis or thrombocytosis associated with renal cell carcinoma or chronic myelocytic leukemia), the anemic and thrombocytopenic effects of interferon alfa may be therapeutically beneficial. Immunologically mediated thrombocytopenia (e.g., as reflected by platelet-associated immunoglobulin) has been reported rarely and disappeared following discontinuance of the drug and administration of corticosteroids. In several patients, thrombocytopenia has recurred following rechallenge with interferon alfa, and in at least one such patient, the drug subsequently was tolerated following splenectomy. Occasionally, immunologically mediated thrombocytopenia may be severe and result in bleeding complications. In a patient with preexisting thrombocytopenic purpura, rapid deterioration of the purpura, which became unresponsive to corticosteroid and IV immune globulin therapy, occurred following initiation of interferon alfa therapy; the patient died several weeks later from intracerebral hemorrhage. Purpura and cyanosis have been reported in less than 1% of patients receiving interferon alfa therapy. Petechiae have been reported rarely, but a causal relationship to interferon alfa has not been established. In some patients with leukemia who were receiving interferon alfa therapy, prolongation of prothrombin and partial thromboplastin times occurred.

■ **Hepatic Effects** Increased serum concentrations of AST (SGOT) and ALT (SGPT) have been reported in about 10–50% of patients receiving interferon alfa therapy, although such increases appear to be dose-related and have been reported in up to 80% of patients receiving relatively high dosages of the drug. In addition, increases in these enzymes generally are more marked in patients with preexisting elevations. Increased serum concentrations of LDH, alkaline phosphatase, and bilirubin also have been reported frequently in patients receiving the drug, although less commonly than increased aminotransferase (transaminase) concentrations. Changes in LDH and alkaline phosphatase concentrations occur principally in patients with preexisting abnormalities and do not necessarily correlate with aminotransferase changes. Increases in hepatic enzymes generally are mild to moderate and transient. (See Cautions: Precautions and Contraindications.) However, substantial increases occasionally may occur in patients receiving relatively high dosages of interferon alfa; such increases generally are reversible following dosage reduction or discontinuance of the drug. Elevations of serum aminotransferase concentrations generally return to normal within several days to a week following discontinuance of interferon alfa.

■ **Respiratory Effects** Dyspnea, cough (which may be nonproductive), pharyngitis, sinusitis, and drying of the oropharynx have been reported in up to 34% of patients receiving interferon alfa and may be severe. Nasal congestion, rhinitis, and rhinorrhea have been reported in up to 2–10% of patients. Antihistamines reportedly may alleviate some of these symptoms. Pulmonary infiltrates, pneumonitis, and pneumonia have been reported rarely in patients treated with interferon alfa; fatalities reportedly have occurred. Such effects have been reported most frequently in patients with chronic hepatitis C virus (HCV) infection receiving interferon alfa, but they also have occurred in patients receiving the drug for oncologic diseases. The etiology of these adverse effects has not been established. Epistaxis, drainage of sinus secretions, throat tightness, wheezing, and bronchospasm have been reported less frequently. Pneumonia or respiratory disorder was reported in at least one patient receiving the drug. While a causal relationship has not been established, some clinicians suggest that immunomodulating effects of interferons could predispose to the development of pulmonary sarcoidosis during prolonged therapy.

■ **Dermatologic, Sensitivity, and Immunologic Reactions** ***Dermatologic Reactions*** The most common adverse dermatologic effects of interferon alfa are rash and transient alopecia or thinning of the hair, which occur in about 25% or less of patients.

Interferon alfa-induced rash, which may be maculopapular, papular, macular, or urticarial, generally is intermittent or transient, does not require dosage reduction, and does not progress to more serious manifestations. Rash occurs most frequently on the extremities and trunk and, occasionally, on the neck and may be accompanied by pruritus and erythema. In several patients with rash, skin testing failed to show evidence of a true hypersensitivity reaction, and limited evidence suggests that some local erythematous reactions may result in part from a direct interferon alfa-induced vasodilation. In at least one patient with repeated flare-ups of rash, skin biopsy revealed evidence of mild vasculitis. While it previously was believed that many adverse dermatologic effects associated with interferon alfa therapy resulted from impurities in early preparations of the drug rather than from the drug itself, experience with currently available purified preparations suggests otherwise.

Interferon alfa-induced alopecia usually has been associated with prolonged (e.g., 3 months or longer) therapy and is manifested as thinning and slight to mild hair loss, which occasionally becomes more marked when therapy with the drug is interrupted. Hair loss generally is reversible but often persists for 1–3 months after discontinuance of interferon alfa; occasionally, an irreversible androgenetic (male-pattern) alopecia has developed in patients receiving prolonged therapy. It has been suggested that alopecia and hair thinning may result from the cytotoxic activity of interferon alfa. In addition, hair loss in some patients may be a manifestation of hypothyroidism associated with interferon alfa therapy. (See Cautions: Endocrine Effects.) Excessive growth of eyelashes also has been reported, and abnormal hair texture has been reported rarely.

Dry skin and dermatitis have been reported in approximately 8–13% of patients receiving interferon alfa. Excessive sweating or night sweats have been reported in 2–8% of patients. Acne, nail disorder, epidermal necrolysis, photosensitivity, skin discoloration, and exfoliative dermatitis have been reported less frequently.

In some patients with psoriasis, interferon alfa exacerbated the disease within 2–4 weeks of initiation of therapy with the drug for other conditions. Endogenous interferons (e.g., gamma and possibly alfa) have been detected in psoriatic blister fluid from patients with the disease, suggesting that local production of interferons may contribute in part to the pathogenesis of this skin condition.

Cutaneous vascular lesions with punctate telangiectasis have developed in patients with malignant melanoma who were receiving interferon alfa. The lesions developed principally on the trunk and extremities, but not at the sites of injection, after 4–8 months of therapy and showed histologic evidence of increased production of epidermis and proliferation of mature dermal blood vessels; it was suggested that these effects may have resulted indirectly secondary to interferon alfa-induced effects on interleukin-1 and/or epidermal thymocyte activating factor.

Sensitivity Reactions and Autoimmune Disorders Severe, acute hypersensitivity reactions, characterized by urticaria, angioedema, bronchoconstriction, or anaphylaxis, have been reported rarely with interferon alfa. If a severe hypersensitivity reaction occurs during interferon alfa therapy, the drug should be discontinued and the patient given appropriate therapy. Sensitivity to allergens, which may be severe, has been reported occasionally in patients receiving interferon alfa, and anaphylactic reactions have been reported rarely. Autoimmune diseases, which rarely were fatal, including thrombocytopenia, vasculitis, Raynaud's phenomenon, rheumatoid arthritis, lupus erythematosus, and rhabdomyolysis, have occurred in patients receiving interferon alfa. The mechanism(s) of these effects has not been determined, and a direct causal relationship to interferon alfa has not been established. Patients who develop an autoimmune disease while receiving interferon alfa therapy should be monitored closely and the drug discontinued if necessary. In addition, a systemic lupus erythematous (SLE)-like syndrome, manifested as myalgia, low-grade arthritis, leukopenia, and a high titer of antinuclear (ANA) and anti-double-stranded DNA antibodies, was observed in at least one patient receiving interferon alfa and resolved following administration of a corticosteroid and discontinuance of the drug; the syndrome recurred following interferon alfa rechallenge. Antinuclear antibodies also have been reported in other patients receiving the drug, some of whom had positive titers prior to therapy. There is some evidence to suggest that interferons (particularly alfa) may be involved, at least in part, in the pathogenesis of SLE. Parotitis and epididymitis, which were described as allergic or autoimmune reactions and subsequently progressed to unilateral scrotal and bilateral facial parotid swelling, also have been reported in at least one patient receiving the drug; resolution occurred 1 week after discontinuance of interferon alfa therapy but manifestations returned following rechallenge. Other possibly autoimmune sequelae of interferon alfa therapy have included hemolytic anemia, thyroid abnormalities, and hepatitis.

Antibody Formation Numerous studies have confirmed that interferon neutralizing antibodies, probably of the IgG class, develop occasionally in patients receiving natural, partially purified interferons as well as in those receiving highly purified recombinant interferons, but their clinical importance has not been fully established. Such antibodies also can be present in patients with no history of exposure to exogenous interferon preparations. The prevalence of interferon neutralizing antibodies has not been clearly elucidated, in part because of differences in detection methods, sampling times, and interest in monitoring. In studies in which antibodies were monitored, the reported prevalence of their development showed considerable variability, ranging from 0–30% in patients receiving interferon alfa--2b. There is some evidence to suggest that patients with renal cell carcinoma or Kaposi's sarcoma may be at increased risk of developing neutralizing antibodies to interferon alfa. The reason for the increased risk of developing antibodies in these patients is not known, but it has been suggested that exogenously administered interferon alfa may induce phenotypic changes in these tumor cells and that newly exposed antigens may cross react with the interferon alfa molecule. Some, but not all, evidence suggests that the risk of developing neutralizing antibodies increases with increasing duration of interferon alfa therapy. In addition, other factors such as type of interferon preparation, dose, dosing regimen, and route of administration have been suggested to affect the risk of antibody development, but carefully designed, comparative studies using standardized assay techniques are needed to more fully elucidate the relative risk associated with various interferon preparations and regimens.

The presence of interferon alfa neutralizing antibodies does not appear to alter the spectrum, incidence, or severity of interferon alfa-associated adverse effects, and dosage adjustment or interruption of therapy usually is not necessary; however, some evidence suggests that certain adverse effects occasionally may abate once such antibodies develop. Patients with detectable levels of interferon alfa neutralizing antibodies do not appear to be at increased risk of developing adverse effects that might be attributable to immune complex formation (e.g., renal, lung, or articular disorders or collagen vascular disease), and no correlation appears to exist between the development of interferon alfa neutralizing antibodies and the development of interferon alfa-associated autoimmune factors (e.g., antinuclear or antithyroid antibodies, rheumatoid factor) or disorders.

While many patients who develop interferon neutralizing antibodies continue to respond to interferon alfa therapy, other patients, some of whom had previously responded to therapy with the drug, exhibit evidence of disease progression and decreased serum interferon concentrations as neutralizing antibodies develop. In patients who continue to respond to interferon alfa therapy despite the development of antibodies, data are conflicting regarding the effect of such antibodies on the duration of response; some evidence suggests that the duration of response may be adversely affected (i.e., shortened), while other evidence suggests that the time to onset and the duration of response, including survival rates, are not affected.

Anti-interferon antibodies elicited by recombinant DNA-derived preparations usually do not neutralize the natural, partially purified, multispecies human interferon alfa obtained from leukocytes but instead neutralize a restricted range of recombinant DNA-derived interferon alfa species. Preliminary evidence suggests that patients who develop anti-interferon antibodies and show evidence of disease progression while receiving recombinant interferon alfa therapy may respond to treatment with a preparation of natural interferon alfa (e.g., a purified preparation of natural leukocyte interferon). There also is evidence that antibodies to recombinant interferon alfa-2a (no longer commercially available in the US) or interferon alfa-2b can cross-react with some naturally occurring interferon alfa subtypes. In addition, limited evidence suggests that some neutralizing antibodies to interferon alfa-2a also can neutralize interferon alfa-2b. Therefore, substituting one recombinant interferon alfa preparation for another may not provide effective second-line therapy in patients who develop anti-interferon antibodies to a given interferon preparation and show evidence of disease progression.

■ **Renal, Electrolyte, Fluid, and Genitourinary Effects** Proteinuria is the most common adverse renal effect associated with interferon alfa therapy and occurs in about 15–20% of patients. Proteinuria generally is mild, rarely exceeds 1 g daily, is not associated with a decrease in serum protein, and has not been clearly related to prior renal impairment or to dose of interferon alfa. Urinary excretion of leukocytes and erythrocytes have been reported in about 5–14% of patients. Increased BUN and serum creatinine concentrations have been reported in up to 10% of patients. The possibility that the patient's underlying condition (e.g., multiple myeloma) may have contributed to the development of renal dysfunction should be considered. However, in some patients with multiple myeloma and preexisting light-chain proteinuria, interferon alfa was well tolerated and did not produce worsening of renal function.

Acute renal failure and nephrotic syndrome accompanied by interstitial nephritis and minimal change nephropathy have been reported rarely in patients receiving interferon alfa; manifestations in such patients have included peripheral edema, marked nonselective proteinuria, and decreased creatinine clearance. Renal function improved following discontinuance of interferon alfa, but adverse renal effects recurred upon rechallenge with the drug. Nephrotic syndrome, secondary to membranoproliferative glomerulonephritis and associated with hypertension and proteinuria, has been reported in at least one patient receiving long-term interferon alfa therapy. Although measurements of urinary albumin and β_2-microglobulin in a limited number of patients receiving short-term (up to 28 days) interferon alfa therapy did not reveal glomerular or tubular lesions, glomerulonephritis has been reported in animals receiving high doses of the drug, and the drug has produced nephrotoxic effects at the proximal renal tubule cell membrane (e.g., inhibition of glucose and alanine uptake) in animals similar to those produced by other low-molecular-weight proteins.

Dehydration has been reported in less than 1% of patients receiving interferon alfa, and may be secondary to fever, loss of appetite, and/or other factors. Some patients receiving high dosages of the drug have developed hyperkalemia and hypercalcemia. Hyponatremia, probably secondary to a syndrome of inappropriate secretion of antidiuretic hormone (SIADH), and hypocalcemia also have been reported in some patients receiving high dosages.

Transient impotence has been reported in up to 6% of patients receiving interferon alfa. Micturition disorders, nocturia, dysuria, and polyuria occurred in 1% or less of patients receiving the drug. Menstrual irregularities also have been reported.

■ **Ocular and Otic Effects** Visual disturbances have been reported in up to 7% of patients receiving interferon alfa. Ocular pain, including that associated with ocular rotation, blurred vision, and stye (hordeolum) formation have been reported in 1–6% of patients receiving the drug. Conjunctivitis, lacrimal gland disorder, photophobia, and abnormal vision have been reported in less than 1% of patients, and periorbital edema has been reported in at least one patient. Retinal hemorrhages, cotton-wool spots, and retinal artery or vein obstruction have been observed rarely in patients receiving interferon alfa, but the mechanism of these adverse effects has not been determined. Although most cases of interferon alfa-associated visual loss have been mild and nonprogressive, at least one patient receiving interferon alfa-2b as adjuvant therapy (following surgical resection of melanoma at high risk of recurrence) experienced permanent and irreversible loss of visual function. Adverse retinal effects develop most commonly after several months of therapy with the drug; however, such effects occasionally have developed in patients receiving interferon alfa for shorter periods. Therefore, patients who experience ocular disturbances or changes in visual acuity or in visual fields during interferon alfa therapy should have an ophthalmologic examination. Baseline ophthalmologic examinations are recommended prior to initiation of interferon alfa therapy. (See Cautions: Precautions and Contraindications.)

Hearing disorders have been reported in less than 5% of patients and earache and tinnitus in less than 1% of patients receiving interferon alfa therapy.

■ Endocrine and Metabolic Effects Thyroid dysfunction (hypothyroidism or hyperthyroidism) has been reported occasionally in patients receiving interferon alfa and, in some patients, may not resolve spontaneously following discontinuance of the drug. Most such cases reported to date were in patients receiving the drug for the treatment of breast cancer, carcinoid tumors, or chronic HCV infection. However, the possibility that any patient receiving interferon alfa could develop thyroid abnormalities should be considered. In some patients, clinical manifestations as well as laboratory evidence of thyroid dysfunction were observed, and thyroidal therapy (thyroid replacement for hyperthyroidism, antithyroid agents for hyperthyroidism) was required. Although the mechanism by which interferon alfa may alter thyroid function has not been established, antibodies to thyroid microsomal antigen, thyroid receptors, and thyroglobulin have been observed in interferon-treated patients with thyroid dysfunction, suggesting an autoimmune mechanism (e.g., Graves' disease, thyroiditis). While a causal relationship to interferon alfa has not been clearly established, and some evidence suggests that interferon gamma present as a contaminant in interferon alfa preparations may in part be responsible, thyroid dysfunction has been reported in patients receiving highly purified interferon alfa preparations and a temporal relationship has been observed.If manifestations of possible thyroid dysfunction develop in a patient receiving interferon alfa, the patient's thyroid function should be evaluated and appropriate therapy instituted if needed. Interferon alfa therapy should be discontinued in patients whose serum thyrotropin concentrations cannot be maintained in the normal range with antithyroid therapy or hormone replacement therapy, depending on the thyroid dysfunction. However, thyroid dysfunction is not always reversible by discontinuance of the drug.

Increased concentrations of follicle-stimulating hormone (FSH, follitropin) and low concentrations of testosterone have been reported occasionally in patients receiving interferon alfa. Serum estradiol and progesterone concentrations were decreased in certain women and in at least one man receiving the drug. Inconsistent fluctuations of prolactin, somatotropin (growth hormone), thyrotropin (TSH), and insulin also were observed in some of these women. Gynecomastia and loss of libido have been reported in less than 5% and virilization in less than 1% of patients receiving interferon alfa. Increased serum concentrations of 11-hydroxycorticosteroids also have been reported.

Weight loss, which often is associated with anorexia (see Cautions: GI Effects) and may be severe, has been reported in up to 25% of patients receiving interferon alfa therapy. Cachexia has been reported in less than 1% of patients receiving interferon alfa. Interferon alfa has produced glycosuria in healthy adults.

Hypertriglyceridemia, which has been severe (e.g., serum triglyceride concentration exceeding 1000 mg/dL) in some cases but reversible upon drug discontinuance, has been reported in patients receiving interferon alfa. (See Cautions: Precautions and Contraindications.) Serum total and/or HDL-cholesterol concentrations have decreased or increased in patients and healthy individuals receiving the drug.

■ Cardiovascular Effects The most common adverse cardiovascular effects of interferon alfa therapy include edema (e.g., facial, peripheral) and hypotension, which occur in up to 9% of patients. Certain adverse cardiovascular effects (e.g., tachycardia, vasoconstriction, distal cyanosis, hypotension) may be related to the febrile reaction that occurs frequently during initial therapy with interferon alfa, and substantial hemodynamic changes may occur in some patients. Hypotension may occur during administration of interferon alfa or up to 2 days after therapy and may be severe, requiring dosage reduction and/or supportive therapy such as fluid replacement to maintain intravascular volume; however, hypotension that develops gradually during interferon alfa therapy may not respond to volume repletion. The risk of hypotension appears to increase with age and increasing dosages. Chest pain, which may be severe, and vasodilation have been reported in less than 5% of patients receiving interferon alfa. Flushing also has been reported in less than 5% of patients receiving the drug, and vasovagal reactions, heat intolerance, and hot sensation at the bottom of the foot have been reported in 2% or less of patients.

Cardiac arrhythmias, which were mainly supraventricular (e.g., paroxysmal atrial tachycardia, sinus tachycardia, atrial fibrillation), have been reported in less than 3% of patients receiving interferon alfa therapy, although ventricular arrhythmias (e.g., ventricular premature complexes) also have been reported. Most individuals in whom cardiac arrhythmias occurred were geriatric patients and some had preexisting heart disease, a history of arrhythmias, or received a potentially cardiotoxic drug (e.g., doxorubicin). Rarely, arrhythmias associated with interferon alfa therapy may be life-threatening. Hypertension and palpitationshave been reported in less than 3% of patients receiving interferon alfa.

Cardiomyopathy, which generally is reversible, has been reported in up to 2% of patients receiving interferon alfa. Cardiomyopathy has been reported in some patients without a history of heart disease. Frank manifestations of congestive heart failure (e.g., cardiomegaly, pulmonary congestion, pleural effusions, T-wave flattening, fluid retention, shortness of breath, dyspnea) can occur in these patients, and it has been suggested that patients with limited cardiac reserve may be at risk of developing congestive heart failure secondary to acute cardiovascular changes associated with severe febrile reactions induced by interferon alfa. A causal relationship to the drug has not been established, but a temporal relationship was observed in several case reports. In several patients with AIDS-related Kaposi's sarcoma who developed cardiomyopathy during prolonged, high-dose therapy with the drug, it was suggested that a synergistic interaction between the HIV infection and interferon alfa may have been responsible in part for the observed myocardial depression. However, other mechanisms (e.g., interferon alfa-induced impairment of myocyte metabolic processes) also appear to be involved. The incidence of hypotension, arrhythmias, and cardiomyopathy in patients with preexisting heart disease is not known. These adverse cardiovascular effects may require dosage reduction, discontinuance of interferon alfa, or supportive therapy. In patients without preexisting cardiac dysfunction, return to normal function can occur following discontinuance of the drug.

Raynaud's phenomenon, bradycardia, cardiac failure, peripheral ischemia, and syncope have been reported in less than 1% of patients receiving interferon alfa therapy. Sudden death and/or myocardial infarction also have been reported rarely (in less than 1% of patients); these adverse effects usually occurred in individuals with a prior history of heart disease, including previous myocardial infarction and ischemic heart disease (e.g., angina), and a causal relationship to interferon alfa has not been established. However, myocardial infarction also has been reported in some patients without a history of heart disease. Nonmalignant pericardial effusion has been reported in at least one patient with renal cell carcinoma who received interferon alfa, suggesting the possibility of an interferon-induced perimyocarditis.

■ Local Reactions Adverse local effects associated with parenteral administration of interferon alfa generally have been mild to moderate and were reported in up to 12–20% of patients. Burning, pruritus, pain, edema, erythema, rash, and vesiculation may occur at the injection site. Aseptic skin necrosis was reported in a few patients after inadvertent intra-arterial injection of interferon alfa.

■ Infectious Complications Infectious complications have been reported in patients receiving interferon alfa, possibly secondary in part to neutropenia induced by the drug. Patients with preexisting cirrhosis (hepatic decompensation) and those with multiple myeloma, lymphoma, or other preexisting leukopenia may be at increased risk of developing such complications during therapy with the drug. Serious bacterial infections (e.g., cellulitis, septicemia, peritonitis, pneumonia, lung abscess, brain abscess) appear to be particularly likely during interferon alfa therapy for viral hepatitis in patients with cirrhosis, being reported in 5 of 7 such patients in one study. Candidiasis (moniliasis) has been reported in up to 18% of patients with AIDS-related Kaposi's sarcoma receiving relatively high doses of the drug; the infection has been reported less frequently in other patients receiving lower dosages. Exacerbation or reactivation of herpes simplex (e.g., herpes labialis) has been reported in 1–8% of patients receiving the drug. Abscess formation, furunculosis, viral or fungal infections, nonherpetic cold sores, and sepsis occurred in less than 1% of patients receiving the drug. Swollen lymph nodes and lymphadenopathy have been reported in 1% of patients, and mucositis has been reported in at least one patient.

■ Precautions and Contraindications Interferon alfa-2b is contraindicated in patients with known hypersensitivity to interferon alfa or any ingredient in the preparation. If a severe hypersensitivity reaction occurs during interferon alfa therapy, the drug should be discontinued and the patient given appropriate therapy.

Interferon alfa-2b is contraindicated in patients with autoimmune hepatitis or decompensated liver disease.

Interferon alfa may cause or aggravate fatal or life-threatening neuropsychiatric, autoimmune, ischemic, and infectious disorders. Patients should be closely monitored with periodic clinical and laboratory evaluations and the drug discontinued in those with persistently severe or worsening signs or symptoms of these disorders. In many, but not all cases, these disorders resolve after interferon alfa is discontinued.

The potential benefit to the patient must be carefully weighed against the possible risks involved, and the patient should be apprised of these risks. Patients should be instructed about the proper use of interferon alfa and should read the patient information and medication guide provided by the manufacturer.

Interferon alfa should be used with caution in patients with a history of preexisting psychiatric disorders, especially those with a history of depression. All patients receiving interferon alfa should be informed that depression and suicidal ideation may be adverse effects of treatment and should be advised to immediately report these effects to a clinician if they occur. All patients should be closely monitored for evidence of depression and other psychiatric symptoms. Patients who develop such symptoms should be carefully monitored during therapy and for 6 months after discontinuing therapy. If symptoms persist or worsen, or suicidal ideation or aggressive behavior toward others is identified, interferon alfa should be discontinued and the patient followed with appropriate psychiatric intervention. If severe depression and/or other psychiatric condition develops, interferon alfa therapy should be discontinued immediately and appropriate psychiatric intervention provided.

Use of interferons may be associated with exacerbation of psychiatric symptoms in patients with concomitant psychiatric and substance use disorders. When initiating treatment in patients with a history of psychiatric conditions or substance use disorders, clinicians should consider the need for drug screening and periodic clinical evaluation, including psychiatric symptom monitoring.

Re-emergence or development of neuropsychiatric symptoms or substance use should prompt early intervention.

Because interferon therapy has been associated with fever and flu-like symptoms (see Cautions: Flu-like Syndrome), the drug should be used with caution in patients with debilitating diseases such as cardiac disease (e.g., unstable angina, uncontrolled congestive heart failure), pulmonary disease (chronic obstructive pulmonary disease), or diabetes mellitus (who may be prone to ketoacidosis). The acute and generally self-limiting manifestations associated with the flu-like syndrome may exacerbate these preexisting conditions. In addition, the drug also should be used with caution in patients with cardiac disease or a history of any cardiac condition since hypotension, arrhythmias, myocardial infarction, sudden death, and cardiomyopathy have been reported occasionally in patients receiving the drug. (See Cautions: Cardiovascular Effects.) Patients with a history of cardiac disease must be monitored carefully when receiving interferon alfa therapy. Electrocardiographic monitoring should be performed prior to initiating and periodically during interferon alfa therapy in patients with preexisting cardiac disease and/or advanced stages of cancer. Certain adverse cardiovascular effects, (e.g., tachycardia, vasoconstriction, distal cyanosis, hypotension) may be related to the febrile reaction that occurs frequently during initial therapy with interferon alfa, and the drug should be used with caution in individuals with limited cardiac reserve. Because patients with underlying massive hemangiomas also may be at increased risk of developing substantial hemodynamic changes during initiation of interferon alfa therapy, the hemodynamic status of such patients should be monitored closely when therapy with the drug is started and for several days thereafter; if such changes occur, dosage should be reduced or the drug discontinued, and supportive and symptomatic care should be initiated as necessary.

Pulmonary infiltrates, pneumonitis, and pneumonia have been reported rarely in patients treated with interferon alfa; fatalities have occurred. Baseline chest radiographs are suggested before interferon alfa therapy is initiated, and should be performed when clinically indicated in patients who develop fever, cough, dyspnea, or other respiratory symptoms. If there is evidence of pulmonary infiltrates or pulmonary function impairment, the patient should be closely monitored and, if appropriate, interferon alfa should be discontinued. Recurrence of respiratory failure has occurred with interferon rechallenge.

Although fever frequently occurs during initiation of interferon alfa therapy, any change in pattern of fever should be regarded as a possible sign of some underlying condition (e.g., infection) rather than assumed to be induced by the drug. In addition, the subsequent development of high fever during prolonged interferon alfa therapy should prompt consideration of such other possible causes. The possibility that patients with viral hepatitis and cirrhosis and those with multiple myeloma, lymphoma, or other preexisting leukopenia may be at increased risk of infection during interferon alfa therapy should be considered. (See Cautions: Hematologic Effects and Cautions: Infectious Complications.)

Increased serum concentrations of AST and/or ALT have been reported in patients receiving interferon alfa. (See Cautions: Hepatic Effects.) Therefore, the drug should be used with caution in patients with hepatic disease, and liver function tests should be performed prior to initiating interferon alfa therapy and periodically thereafter. In patients with melanoma, liver function tests should be monitored weekly during the induction phase and monthly during the maintenance phase of interferon alfa therapy.

Adverse renal effects and fluid and electrolyte abnormalities (e.g., dehydration) have been reported occasionally in patients receiving interferon alfa. (See Cautions: Renal, Electrolyte, Fluid, and Genitourinary Effects.) In addition, all patients should be well hydrated during interferon alfa therapy, especially during initial stages of therapy. Electrolytes should be evaluated prior to initiation of therapy with the drug and monitored periodically thereafter. Because of the risk of acute rejection episodes, interferon alfa should be used with caution in renal transplant recipients, particularly when relatively high doses are considered. (See Cautions: Renal, Electrolyte, Fluid, and Genitourinary Effects.)

Because of the risk of potential adverse nervous system effects associated with interferon alfa therapy (see Cautions: Nervous System Effects), the drug should be used with caution in patients with seizure disorders, brain metastases, and/or compromised CNS; the drug should only be used in these patients if the possible benefits of therapy outweigh the potential risks. Because of the risk for adverse CNS effects and possible symptomatic exacerbation of previously asymptomatic brain lesions, some clinicians state that consideration should be given to performing computerized tomography scans prior to initiation of interferon alfa therapy in patients with malignancies that have a high incidence of brain metastasis; if brain metastases are detected, the drug should be used with caution and high doses probably should be avoided. In addition, all patients receiving interferon alfa should be monitored periodically for the possible development of drug-related neuropsychiatric effects; efforts at early detection and intervention are important, since a possible association to interferon alfa therapy may be overlooked by the patient until their life has been severely affected. (See Cautions: Nervous System Effects.) Because partners or family members may be the first to observe such changes, they should be advised that the drug can induce changes in mood and personality that potentially can affect interpersonal relationships. Patients should be warned that interferon alfa may impair their ability to perform hazardous activities requiring mental alertness (e.g., operating machinery, driving a motor vehicle), especially at high doses, and that CNS depressants (e.g., opiates, sedatives) should be used concomitantly with caution. In addition, because the drug can cause mental clouding and impair concentration ability, especially at high doses, patients whose job or life-style requires unimpaired intellectual function should be advised that their mental abilities may be impaired during interferon alfa therapy.

Baseline ophthalmologic examinations should be performed in all patients prior to initiation of interferon alfa therapy. Patients with preexisting ophthalmologic disorders (e.g., diabetic or hypertensive retinopathy) should receive ophthalmologic examinations periodically during therapy. A prompt and complete ophthalmologic examination should be performed in any patient who develops ocular symptoms; the drug should be discontinued in patients who develop new or worsening ophthalmologic disorders .

Serum TSH concentrations should be determined prior to initiation of interferon alfa therapy since thyroid dysfunction (hypothyroidism or hyperthyroidism) has been reported occasionally in patients receiving interferon alfa. Patients with preexisting thyroid dysfunction whose serum thyrotropin concentrations cannot be maintained in the normal range with antithyroid therapy or hormone replacement therapy should not receive interferon alfa therapy. In addition, if manifestations of possible thyroid dysfunction develop in a patient receiving interferon alfa, the patient's thyroid function should be evaluated and appropriate therapy instituted if needed. (See Cautions: Endocrine and Metabolic Effects.)

Patients with preexisting diabetes mellitus and those who develop diabetes mellitus during interferon alfa therapy may continue to receive interferon alfa as long as their diabetes can be controlled with drug therapy. Patients with diabetes that cannot be controlled with drug therapy should discontinue interferon alfa therapy.

The possibility that interferon alfa may precipitate or exacerbate manifestations of autoimmune disorders (e.g., arthropathies, systemic lupus erythematosus, psoriasis, hemolytic anemia, thrombocytopenia, hepatitis, sarcoidosis) should be considered in patients receiving the drug. (See Cautions: Hepatic Effects.) In addition, since potentially fatal autoimmune diseases have occurred in patients receiving interferon alfa (see Cautions: Sensitivity Reactions and Autoimmune Disorders), patients who develop an autoimmune disease while receiving interferon alfa therapy should be monitored closely and the drug discontinued if necessary.

Interferon alfa should be used with caution in patients with myelosuppression and in those receiving drugs that may be myelosuppressive. Complete blood cell counts, platelet counts, and appropriate blood chemistry tests should be performed before initiating interferon alfa therapy and periodically thereafter. In patients with melanoma, differential leukocyte counts should be monitored weekly during the induction phase and monthly during the maintenance phase of interferon alfa therapy. Interferon alfa should be used with caution in patients with coagulation disorders (e.g., thrombophlebitis, pulmonary embolism, hemophilia), preexisting leukopenia, or increased risk of infection.

Because substantial increases in serum triglyceride concentrations have been reported with interferon alfa therapy, some clinicians suggest that serum triglyceride concentrations be monitored during interferon alfa therapy. (See Cautions: Endocrine and Metabolic Effects.) Since hypertriglyceridemia may result in pancreatitis, discontinuance of interferon alfa therapy should be considered in patients with persistently elevated triglycerides (e.g., serum triglyceride concentration exceeding 1000 mg/dL) associated with symptoms of potential pancreatitis (e.g., abdominal pain, nausea, vomiting).

Pancreatitis, sometimes fatal, has occurred in patients receiving interferon. Interferon alfa should be suspended in patients with signs and symptoms of pancreatitis (e.g., abdominal pain, nausea, vomiting); the drug should be discontinued if a diagnosis of pancreatitis is established.

■ **Pediatric Precautions** Safety and efficacy of interferon alfa-2b have not been established in pediatric patients for any indications other than treatment of chronic hepatitis B virus (HBV) and chronic HCV infection. (See Interferon Alfa 8:18.20.)

In general, adverse effects (e.g., fever, chills, GI effects, nervous system effects, hematologic effects, hepatic effects, local effects at the injection site) observed in adolescents and younger children appear to be dose related, generally reversible, and similar to those observed in adults, although children may be more likely than adults to develop alopecia or thinning of the hair during prolonged therapy. In addition, delay in weight and height increases compared with baseline have been reported in pediatric patients receiving interferon alfa for the treatment of chronic HBV or HCV infection.

■ **Geriatric Precautions** Clinical studies of interferon alfa have not included sufficient numbers of patients 65 years of age and older to determine whether geriatric patients respond differently than younger adults. In studies evaluating use of interferon alfa in conjunction with oral ribavirin, geriatric patients had a higher frequency of anemia (67%) than younger patients (28%). There also is some evidence that adverse cardiovascular effects and confusion are reported more frequently in geriatric patients than in younger adults. Alterations in mental status associated with interferon alfa therapy can be severe in geriatric patients; mental obtundation and coma have been reported. (See Cautions: Cardiovascular Effects and Cautions: Nervous System Effects.)

Interferon alfa should be used with caution in geriatric patients because of age-related decreases in hepatic, renal, bone marrow, and/or cardiac function and concomitant disease and drug therapy. Dosage reduction or interruption of interferon alfa therapy and/or initiation of appropriate supportive measures may be necessary.

■ **Mutagenicity and Carcinogenicity** Studies using interferon alfa-2b (Intron® A) have not shown evidence of mutagenicity. Studies to determine the carcinogenic potential of interferon alfa-2b have not been performed to date.

■ Pregnancy, Fertility, and Lactation Interferon alfa should be used during pregnancy only when potential benefits justify possible risks to the fetus. Women of childbearing potential should use an effective method of contraception during therapy with the drug.

Although there are no adequate and controlled studies to date in humans, interferon alfa-2b has exhibited abortifacient activity in rhesus monkeys when given in dosages of 15 and 30 million units/kg daily (estimated human equivalent of 5 and 10 million units/kg, respectively, based on body surface area adjusted for a 60-kg adult).

Interferon alfa may impair fertility. Menstrual cycle abnormalities have been observed in nonhuman primates and menstrual cycle irregularities and decreased serum estrogen and progesterone concentrations have been reported in humans receiving interferon alfa. Impaired spermatogenesis and transient impotence have been reported occasionally. Interferon alfa-2b should be used with caution in fertile males.

It is not known whether interferon alfa is distributed into milk, but murine interferons distribute into milk in mice. Because of the potential for serious adverse effects to interferon alfa in nursing infants if the drug were distributed into milk, a decision should be made whether to discontinue nursing or the drug, taking into account the importance of the drug to the woman.

Drug Interactions

■ Antineoplastic Agents Interferon alfa should be used with caution in patients receiving drugs that are potentially myelosuppressive.

The antineoplastic activity of interferon alfa and certain cytotoxic agents (e.g., cisplatin, cyclophosphamide, doxorubicin, eflornithine [difluoromethylornithine, DFMO], fluorouracil, mechlorethamine, melphalan, methotrexate, mitomycin, nitrosoureas, vinblastine, vincristine) may be additive or synergistic in vitro and in vivo against some tumors. However, animal and in vitro studies may not accurately predict human response, and results of preliminary clinical studies using various combinations of interferon alfa and conventional antineoplastic agents generally have been disappointing. The mechanism(s) of potential synergistic activity has not been fully elucidated, but it appears to be complex. In addition, the resultant activity appears to depend not only on the specific cytotoxic drug that is combined with interferon alfa, but also on the concentrations, relative amounts, and duration and sequence of exposure of the drugs. Further studies are needed to determine the potential interactions between interferon alfa and antineoplastic agents, and to establish the optimum regimens, including dosages and sequencing.

There is some evidence to suggest that combined therapy with interferon alfa and vinblastine or etoposide may produce greater systemic toxicity without enhanced therapeutic benefits in patients with AIDS-related Kaposi's sarcoma. (See the discussions on Vinca Alkaloids and on Etoposide that follow.)

Interferon alfa combined with carmustine or eflornithine has produced additive or synergistic antineoplastic activity in vitro and in animal models. While the clinical importance of these experimental data remains to be determined, limited evidence from clinical trials suggests that combined therapy with interferon alfa and carmustine, dacarbazine, or eflornithine does not appear to produce unacceptable toxicity but may be beneficial in some advanced cancers. Further long-term, controlled studies are needed to establish the potential therapeutic benefits of these combinations.

Vinca Alkaloids Limited data indicate that the antineoplastic activity of interferon alfa and vinblastine does not appear to be additive against renal cell carcinoma† or AIDS-related Kaposi's sarcoma. However, vinblastine may potentiate the toxicity of interferon alfa when these drugs are used concomitantly. In patients with metastatic renal cell carcinoma, increased incidence and/or severity of hepatic toxicity and hematologic toxicity were reported with the addition of vinblastine to interferon alfa. In a limited number of patients with AIDS-related Kaposi's sarcoma, the incidence of nausea, vomiting, thrombocytopenia, hepatic dysfunction, and fever usually was comparable to that observed with interferon alfa alone, but granulocytopenia, neurotoxicity, and malaise occurred at a higher incidence and with a greater degree of severity in patients receiving vinblastine concomitantly with interferon alfa; 70% of the patients with AIDS-related Kaposi's sarcoma experienced severe fatigue, chills, and asthenia.

Neurotoxicity (e.g., paresthesia, peripheral neuropathy) in patients receiving interferon alfa usually occurs more frequently in those who have previously received or are concomitantly receiving vinca alkaloids (e.g., vinblastine, vincristine). The mechanism of this additive neurotoxic effect is not known; however, mild sensorimotor neuropathy was observed in patients who underwent neurologic evaluation. Some clinicians suggest that high doses of interferon alfa may produce severe neuronal lesions and neurogenic muscle atrophy.

Etoposide Response rates in patients with AIDS-related Kaposi's sarcoma receiving combination chemotherapy with interferon alfa and etoposide suggest that the combination has no synergistic antineoplastic activity against this malignancy, and the incidence of toxicity (e.g., hematologic effects) is higher with the combination than with either drug alone.

■ Antiviral Agents ***Antiretroviral Agents*** Concomitant use of interferon alfa and zidovudine can increase the risk of hematologic (e.g., neutropenia, thrombocytopenia) and hepatic toxicity. The increased risk of such toxicity may be synergistic, although the mechanism of such potential synergy is not known. In a study in patients with AIDS-related Kaposi's sarcoma in which tolerance to varying subcutaneous interferon alfa dosages of 5–35 million units daily and oral zidovudine dosages of 50–250 mg every 4 hours daily were evaluated, the incidence of neutropenia, thrombocytopenia, and hepatic toxicity was higher than expected (based on experience with either drug alone) in patients receiving a 100- or 250-mg regimen of zidovudine combined with interferon alfa. In addition, interferon alfa dosages of 15 units or more daily were not tolerated in any patient receiving the 100- or 250-mg zidovudine regimen. Life-threatening toxicity, consisting of acute respiratory decompensation that possibly was caused by intrapulmonary hemorrhage associated with severe thrombocytopenia, developed 5 days after initiation of interferon therapy and resolved in at least one patient within a week after discontinuance of therapy.

Potentially fatal hepatic decompensation has been reported in HIV-infected patients coinfected with hepatitis C virus (HCV) who received antiretroviral therapy concomitantly with interferon alfa with or without ribavirin. Patients receiving zidovudine with interferon alfa with or without ribavirin should be closely monitored for toxicities (e.g., hepatic decompensation, neutropenia, anemia). Discontinuance of zidovudine should be considered as medically appropriate. Dosage reduction or discontinuance of interferon alfa and/or ribavirin also should be considered if worsening clinical toxicities, including hepatic decompensation (e.g., Child-Pugh score exceeding 6), occur.

Although no major alterations in the pharmacokinetics of zidovudine or interferon alfa were apparent in HIV-infected patients with Kaposi's sarcoma receiving both drugs, a trend for increased area under the plasma concentration-time curve (AUC) and decreased clearance of zidovudine after 3 weeks of administration of interferon alfa was observed in some other patients.

HCV Antivirals In vitro, interferon alfa-2b and boceprevir have had additive effects against HCV without evidence of antagonism.

In vitro, interferon alfa and simeprevir have had synergistic effects against HCV; there is no in vitro evidence of antagonism.

There is no in vitro evidence of antagonistic anti-HCV effects between interferon alfa and sofosbuvir or telaprevir.

Telbivudine Peripheral neuropathy has been reported when alfa interferons were used concomitantly with telbivudine. In one study, increased risk and severity of peripheral neuropathy were observed in patients receiving conjugated interferon alfa (peginterferon alfa-2a) concomitantly with telbivudine compared with those receiving telbivudine alone. The safety and efficacy of concomitant use of telbivudine with any interferon for treatment of chronic hepatitis B virus (HBV) infection have not been established.

■ Biologic Response Modifiers ***Aldesleukin*** Hypersensitivity reactions, consisting of erythema, pruritus, and hypotension, have been reported in patients receiving combination regimens that included sequential administration of high-dose aldesleukin and antineoplastic agents, specifically, interferon alfa, dacarbazine, cisplatin, and tamoxifen. These hypersensitivity reactions occurred within hours of administration of chemotherapy, and medical intervention was required in some patients.

Interferon alfa used in combination with aldesleukin has been associated with the development or exacerbation of autoimmune disease and inflammatory disorders. Exacerbation or presentation of thyroiditis, inflammatory arthritis, oculo-bulbar myasthenia gravis, crescentic IgA glomerulonephritis, Stevens-Johnson syndrome, or bullous pemphigoid has been reported following concurrent use of interferon alfa and aldesleukin. In one patient who developed rapidly progressive renal failure following combination therapy with interferon alfa and aldesleukin for metastatic renal cell carcinoma, renal biopsy revealed crescentic glomerulonephritis.

The incidence of myocardial injury, including myocardial infarction, myocarditis, ventricular hypokinesia, and severe rhabdomyolysis, appears to be increased in patients receiving concurrent interferon alfa and aldesleukin.

■ Effects on Hepatic Clearance of Drugs Interferon alfa has been shown to inhibit the metabolism of theophylline, possibly via the hepatic cytochrome P-450 (microsomal) enzyme system. (See Pharmacology: Effects on Cytochrome P-450 System.) It is not known whether interferon alfa itself interacts with the cytochrome P-450 enzyme system or the drug exerts this effect through an interaction with the immune system. Concomitant use of interferon alfa with theophylline in healthy adults or in patients with chronic active hepatitis B has prolonged the terminal elimination half-life and increased areas under the plasma concentration-time curves (AUCs) of theophylline by reducing hepatic clearance of the drug. Concomitant use of interferon alfa and theophylline has resulted in a 100% increase in serum theophylline concentrations. It appears that the reduction of hepatic clearance of theophylline was greatest in individuals who were the fast metabolizer phenotype.

Interferon alfa also may inhibit metabolism of barbiturates. Initiation of interferon alfa in a patient stabilized on phenobarbital resulted in increased serum phenobarbital concentrations and manifestations of toxicity (e.g., lethargy, fatigue). Although these adverse effects can be induced by interferon alone, associated serum phenobarbital concentrations of 54 mcg/mL suggested that they were manifestations of barbiturate toxicity. While the mechanism of this potential interaction was not determined, it was suggested that inhibition of barbiturate metabolism may have resulted from inhibition of the hepatic cytochrome P-450 enzyme system.

Further studies and experience are needed to establish the clinical importance of this potential drug interaction and to determine whether interferon alfa interacts with other drugs that are metabolized by the hepatic cytochrome P-

450 (microsomal) enzyme system. It has been reported that interferon alfa also inhibits the metabolism of antipyrine.

■ **Radiation Therapy** Interferon has been used as an adjunct to radiation therapy in patients with various neoplasms; however, severe toxicity has been reported in some patients receiving such combined therapy. Severe oral mucositis, manifested by ulceration, bleeding, soreness, or edema of the lips, tongue, oral mucosa, oropharynx, or esophagus, has been reported in a limited number of patients with AIDS-related Kaposi's sarcoma receiving concomitant administration of interferon alfa and radiation therapy. Severe mucositis, accompanied by airway obstruction, respiratory distress, life-threatening hemorrhage, or oropharyngeal edema, also has been reported in some patients with chronic myelogenous leukemia receiving interferon alfa and total body irradiation prior to bone marrow transplantation. In some patients with small cell lung cancer, interferon alfa appeared to potentiate the effects of radiation therapy; an increased incidence of severe radiation pneumonitis and esophagitis has been observed in these patients. Interferons may have either radioprotective or radiosensitizing properties, depending on the tumor cell type and/or type of interferon; however, some other evidence suggests that the drugs may not affect cellular sensitivity to radiation.

Patients receiving interferon alfa with radiation therapy should be closely monitored. Further studies are needed to evaluate the exact nature of interaction between radiation and interferon alfa therapy and to determine the safety and efficacy of the concomitant administration of these therapies.

Acute Toxicity

Studies in mice, rats, and cynomolgus monkeys receiving parenteral recombinant interferon alfa-2b 0.1 or 1 million units daily; 4, 20, or 100 million units/kg daily; and 1.1 million units/kg daily or 0.25, 0.75, or 2.5 million units/kg daily, respectively, for up to 9 days, 3 months, and 1 month, respectively, have revealed no evidence of toxicity. However, in cynomolgus monkeys receiving parenteral recombinant interferon alfa-2b 4, 20, or 100 million units/kg daily for 3 months, toxicity was observed at the mid- and high doses and mortality was observed at the high dose. Because interferon alfa-induced effects generally are species specific, animal toxicity studies may not be predictive of human response.

Pharmacology

■ **Mechanism of Action** Interferon alfa exists as at least 23 proteins and, occasionally, glycoproteins that possess complex antiviral, antineoplastic, and immunomodulating activities. Interferons, including interferon alfa, are biologic response modifiers. Endogenous interferon alpha is produced and secreted in response principally to viral (especially double-stranded RNA viruses) infection mainly by peripheral blood leukocytes (e.g., monocytes; macrophages; non-B, non-T lymphocytes, natural killer [NK] cells) and interferon beta by fibroblasts and epithelial cells, although certain other synthetic and biologic substances (e.g., certain bacteria and other microorganisms capable of intracellular growth, endotoxins, surface glycoproteins, lipopolysaccharides, polynucleotides) also can induce their production. In addition, other cells may produce and secrete these interferons. Interferons are produced endogenously according to information encoded by species of interferon genes, and exert virus-nonspecific antiviral activity, at least in homologous cells, through cellular metabolic processes involving synthesis of RNA and proteins.

The precise mechanisms of action of interferons have not been fully elucidated but appear to be complex, and the resultant activities appear to be substantially interrelated. Unlike classic antiviral and cytotoxic agents, the antiviral and antineoplastic properties of interferons appear to result from a complex cascade of biologic modulation and pharmacologic effects rather than from direct virucidal or cytocidal effects. The drugs affect many cell functions producing restoration, augmentation, and/or modulation of the host's immune system; direct antiproliferative and antineoplastic activities; modulation of cell differentiation; and modulation of cellular transcription and translation, including a reduction in oncogene expression. Some or all of these effects may be interrelated and ultimately responsible for the antiviral and antineoplastic activity of interferons.

Interferons must bind to specific cell surface receptors in order to exert biologic and pharmacologic effects (e.g., antiviral activity); such binding appears to involve high-affinity sites. In addition, some evidence suggests that the principal effects of interferons result not from direct intracellular actions but rather from ligand-receptor complexes at the cell surface that can mediate and induce intracellular events. The biologic and pharmacologic effects of interferons are relatively species specific, and such specificity may reside at the receptor level. In addition, there is some evidence that while interferon alfa and interferon beta bind to and compete for the same receptors, interferon gamma appears to bind to other receptors and therefore potentially acts via different cellular pathways; synergistic antiviral and antineoplastic activities may result from combined use of interferon gamma with interferon alfa or beta.

The mechanism(s) by which interferons ultimately elicit various intracellular effects has not been fully elucidated, but binding at the cell surface appears to induce differential gene transcription and translation of cellular mRNA; this selective increase in gene expression results in modulation of RNA and protein synthesis. Interferons can either enhance or suppress transcription and translation, with resultant alteration in the synthesis of numerous cellular proteins. However, it is not clear whether intact interferon, interferon degradation products, interferon receptors, or receptor-ligand complexes must be incorporated within the cell to elicit cellular responses, or whether interferon-receptor complexes at the cell surface are capable of generating intracellular signals that mediate interferon modulation of gene expression. Likewise, the importance of a second messenger or other mediators (e.g., cyclic adenosine monophosphate [cAMP], cyclic guanosine monophosphate [cGMP], diacylglycerol, prostaglandins) in eliciting intracellular effects of interferons has not been determined. While changes in intracellular concentrations of cAMP and cGMP occur soon after interferons bind to cell surface receptors, the biologic and pharmacologic importance of these changes is uncertain since the antiviral and antineoplastic effects of interferons do not appear to depend on changes in intracellular concentrations of cyclic nucleotides. Receptor binding of interferons does not activate a protein kinase with tyrosine phosphorylating activity nor does interferon binding inhibit the epidermal growth factor (EGF)-induced increase in protein kinase activity. Inhibition of viral replication is merely one of the multiple biologic effects mediated by interferons that involve selective gene activation and the synthesis of newly induced mRNAs and proteins. The antiviral and antiproliferative effects of interferons depend both on de novo RNA and protein synthesis; however, there is no convincing evidence to suggest that the clinical antineoplastic effects of interferon are linked to the antiviral properties of the drug in humans. The antiviral activity of interferon alfa generally is evident at lower doses than are the antiproliferative effects of the drug.

Antiviral Effects The antiviral effects of interferons are complex. In addition, the potential therapeutic effect of interferons against viral infections also is complex and appears to depend on the immunomodulating as well as antiviral effects of the drug. Interferons generally can prevent but not cure certain viral infections, although progression of the infection may occur in some cases secondary to adverse immunologic effects of the drugs. Administration of interferons does not directly improve signs and symptoms of viral infections; in fact, endogenous interferons have been implicated as mediating some of the manifestations (e.g., fever, malaise, myalgia) associated with such infections.

Interferon alfa exhibits a broad spectrum of antiviral activity against numerous viruses including human immunodeficiency virus (HIV), human papillomaviruses (HPV), hepatitis B virus (HBV), hepatitis C virus (HCV), hepatitis D virus (HDV), herpes simplex virus (HSV) types 1 and 2, cytomegalovirus (CMV), varicella-zoster virus (VZV), poliovirus, vaccinia virus, rhinoviruses, coronaviruses, adenoviruses, encephalomyocarditis virus (a cardiovirus), and vesicular stomatitis virus (a vesiculovirus). The antiviral activity of interferons against a given virus appears to depend in part on the host cell and the ability of the interferon to induce an antiviral mechanism within that cell, the inoculum size, and the interferon type and subtype employed.

Interferons exhibit virus-nonspecific antiviral activity through cellular metabolic processes involving synthesis of RNA and proteins. Interferon-induced inhibition of viral replication appears to involve several mechanisms, and different mechanisms may apply to various types of viruses. The degree of viral inhibition may be determined in part by the replicative characteristics of the virus as well as the dose of interferon. Inhibition of viral replication involves several processes, and the replicative properties of the individual virus and the host cell-virus interaction may determine which steps of viral proliferation are affected by interferons. For most viruses, however, inhibition of viral protein synthesis appears to be the principal process involved.

The antiviral properties of interferons generally are only evident when cells are exposed to the drugs before viral exposure. Although interferons may inhibit viral penetration, the drugs generally do not prevent the virion or viral nucleic acid from entering the cell and do not directly produce cellular resistance to viral infection, but rather mediate transcription of mRNA with resultant formation of potent antiviral proteins; such changes in gene expression occur rapidly (e.g., within several hours) after exposure to the drugs. These proteins can inhibit viral replication by inhibiting viral protein synthesis or enhancing the degradation of viral nucleic acid. Interferon-mediated inhibition of mRNA methylation and the drug's effects on viral uncoating, assembly, and release also may contribute to the antiviral activity.

The antiviral activity of interferons appears to depend in part on two enzymes, a 2′-5′-oligoadenylate synthetase (polymerase) and a protein kinase; synthesis of these enzymes is induced when cells are exposed to the drugs. The activity of these enzyme systems depends on the presence of double-stranded RNA (dsRNA) formed during viral replication, and it has been suggested that interferons may have an effect on dsRNA that contributes to their antiviral activity. Interferon-induced degradation of mRNA and resultant inhibition of protein synthesis, inactivation of transfer RNA (tRNA), and inhibition of post-transcriptional modifications of mRNA are mediated principally by the actions of 2′-5′-oligoadenylate synthetase, protein kinase, and a 2′-phosphodiesterase.

Interferons induce an endonuclease system that can cleave single-stranded RNA regions of the RNA-replicative intermediate of RNA viruses and host-cell single-stranded RNA. Induction of 2′-5′-oligoadenylate synthetase, a nucleotide polymerase and the first enzyme in this system, by interferons converts ATP to several 2′-5′-linked oligonucleotides (polyadenylic acids). In the presence of dsRNA, certain 2′-5′-linked oligonucleotides can activate a latent ribonuclease (endoribonuclease RNase L, RNase F) that cleaves the replicative intermediate of RNA viruses and host single-stranded RNA. The oligonucleotides (polyadenylic acids) also are potent inhibitors of mRNA-dependent protein synthesis and can enhance the degradation of mRNA. Activation of the ribonuclease by the oligonucleotides is reversible. While these effects appear to be involved in the antiviral activity of interferons against RNA viruses, it remains to be elucidated whether the action of interferons on these enzymes also is involved in antiviral activity against DNA viruses.

The presence of the 2′-5′-phosphodiester linkage in these oligoadenylates makes them resistant to most cellular nucleases; however, a 2′-5′-phosphodiesterase that can degrade the oligonucleotides has been detected in murine and human cells. This enzyme, which has greater affinity for 2′-5′- phosphodiester bonds than for 3′-5′ bonds present in DNA and RNA, can rapidly hydrolyze the oligoadenylates to ATP and AMP, can reportedly cleave the cytosine-cytosine-adenine (CCA) terminus from tRNA, and may be responsible for the reversible tRNA inhibition of translation in interferon-treated cells.

In addition to effects of the drugs on gene transcription, interferons reportedly decrease the extent of methylation of cap structures on mRNA transcripts. 5′-Terminal cap structures are present on most eukaryotic cellular and viral mRNA, and the extent of methylation on the cap may influence its stability and the efficacy of translation of proteins, including viral proteins.

Interferons also induce the synthesis of a protein kinase, which, when activated by dsRNA in the presence of ATP, phosphorylates and inactivates one of the proteins (eIF-2) necessary for initiation of elongation (protein synthesis), a ribosome-associated protein P-1, and possibly the enzyme itself. The inactive eIF-2 cannot participate in the initial stage of protein synthesis. The resultant inhibition of protein synthesis can prevent the formation of the viral coat protein and thereby inhibit the formation of viral progeny. While the protein kinase also is capable of phosphorylating other substrates, such as histones, in interferon-treated cells, it is not known whether such substrates are physiologic substrates for the enzyme. The action of the protein kinase can be antagonized by the presence of a phosphoprotein phosphatase that dephosphorylates the phosphorylated P-1 and the eIF-2.

Although the precise role of protein kinase in the antiviral activity of interferons remains to be more fully elucidated, the increase in protein kinase activity induced by interferons correlates well with the establishment of antiviral activity, at least in some virus cell systems, and is a function of the duration of drug exposure and the concentration of interferon. In murine cells, for example, the rate and extent of antiviral activity induced by the drugs have been shown to be correlated with their ability to induce the P-1/eIF-2 protein kinase, suggesting that induction of the enzyme and phosphorylation of eIF-2 may contribute substantially to the antiviral effects of interferons, at least in this cell line. Likewise, declines in antiviral and protein kinase activities have been shown to be correlated, and such activities can be reinduced with subsequent reexposure to interferons. Continuous exposure to interferons prevents the decline in protein kinase activity and prolongs the antiviral activity induced by the drugs. In other virus-cell systems, however, other mechanisms may be principally responsible for the antiviral activity of interferons.

The extent to which the oligoadenylate synthetase and protein kinase systems contribute to the antiviral activity of interferons remains to be more fully elucidated, but other mechanisms also appear to be involved. Viral replication probably can be inhibited at more than one stage of the viral replicative cycle presumably secondary to different mediators of interferon actions, and not all pathways may be functioning in a given interferon-exposed cell. Thus, even within the same cell line, interferons may inhibit the replication of certain viruses but not others.

The biochemical basis for the selectivity of interferons against virus-infected rather than uninfected host cells has not been established. The oligoadenylate synthetase system cannot adequately explain the selectivity of the drugs for viral replication since endoribonuclease RNase L cleaves viral and host mRNA nonselectively in vitro; in some in vivo systems, however, viral protein synthesis is inhibited preferentially with respect to host protein synthesis. It has been suggested that the dsRNA-induced RNase system works at a subcellular level, and that the close proximity of ribosomes, ribosomal RNA, ds-RNA, 2′-5′-oligonucleotide synthetase, polyadenylate, and 2′-phosphodiesterase to each other may contribute to interferon selectivity for virally infected cells. The protein kinase-mediated inhibition of protein synthesis that inhibits binding of tRNA to the ribosome may discriminate between cellular and viral RNA, and may exhibit some selectivity for viral nucleic acid.

Interferons also may inhibit viral replication by augmenting the response of immune effector cells involved in the recognition and killing of virally infected cells. However, interferon-induced inhibition of viral replication does not eliminate the infection; instead, the antiviral effect of the drugs minimizes the viral burden to the host's immune system. Thus, the antiviral efficacy of interferons depends on the host's immunologic status.

For information on antiviral uses of interferon alfa, see Interferon Alfa 8:18.20.

Antiproliferative Effects Interferons exhibit antiproliferative (growth inhibitory) activity against normal and malignant cells with resultant antineoplastic effects in vitro and in vivo, and can alter both the structure and behavior of these cells. In addition, the drugs can inhibit the growth of primary tumors as well as metastatic foci. The mechanism(s) of this antiproliferative activity has not been fully elucidated but appears to be complex. The ability of interferons to inhibit or enhance the synthesis of specific proteins, to modify expression of cell surface antigens, and/or to induce modulation of the immune system may be involved. Although some evidence suggests that the antiviral and antiproliferative activities of interferons may share some common biochemical and physiologic pathways, the possible roles of the 2′-5′-oligoadenylate synthetase and protein kinase systems (see Mechanism of Action: Antiviral Effects, in Pharmacology) in mediating the antiproliferative effects of interferons have not been clearly established. It has been suggested that the oligoadenylate synthetase system may be involved in the regulation of cellular proliferation and may contribute to the antiproliferative effects of interferons, since levels of this enzyme decrease substantially in rapidly proliferating cells and increase when cell growth is inhibited. Other evidence also indicates that the oligoadenylate synthetase system may contribute to the antiproliferative effects of interferon. However, there also is evidence to suggest that no correlation exists between the antiproliferative activity of interferons and induction of these enzyme systems by the drugs, and, in some studies, the relative antiproliferative activity of various interferons actually was the reverse of the relative antiviral activity.

The antineoplastic activity of interferons may result from a direct antiproliferative effect on the tumor cell and/or the ability of the drugs to induce a host response to the tumor. However, the drugs generally do not appear to be directly cytocidal to tumor cells; instead, the cytostatic effects of interferons may decrease the rate of cell proliferation to a level incompatible with cell survival. Interferons also may alter the host-tumor relationship by affecting host humoral factors (e.g., growth factors) or by modulating the response of immune effector cells (e.g., natural killer [NK] cells, T and B cells). However, evidence from studies in immunocompromised mice suggests that inhibition of tumor growth by interferons can occur independently of certain cellular immunologic mechanisms of the host. The ability of the drugs to modify cell surface morphology and function may result in altered transport of substances necessary for cell survival and thus contribute to their antiproliferative activity. The biologic effects of interferons on the host also may contribute to their antineoplastic properties since interferon-induced inhibition of tumor growth has been observed with some malignant cell lines despite resistance of the cells to the antiproliferative properties of the drugs. In addition, interferons have exhibited antineoplastic activity against tumors that lacked receptors for the drug, suggesting that an indirect effect may have been responsible for the observed activity against some cells.

Inhibition of Cell Division. Interferon-induced prolongation of the cell cycle appears to be principally responsible for the antiproliferative effects of the drugs. Interferons inhibit or reduce the synthesis of RNA and protein during the G_1 (first "gap," post-mitotic, or presynthesis) phase of the cell cycle that is required for cells to enter the S (DNA synthetic) phase of the cell cycle. Interferons also inhibit ornithine decarboxylase, the rate-limiting enzyme in the synthesis of polyamines, which are necessary for the assembly of DNA. Interferons prolong all phases of the cell cycle, induce cells to enter the nonproliferative G_0 (resting) phase, and delay cells at the G_0/G_1 border from entering the cell cycle; the antiproliferative effects of the drugs may be more pronounced in this latter subpopulation of cells. These antiproliferative effects are dose dependent and reversible, with normal growth rate being restored within 24–72 hours after removal from exposure to the drug. Continued treatment with interferons in vitro and in vivo results in a more prolonged inhibition of cell proliferation. The antiproliferative effects of interferons on normal hematopoietic stem and progenitor cells may be responsible for the reversible myelosuppression that may occur secondary to therapy with the drugs.

The cytostatic property of interferons is not differentially selective for transformed or malignant cell populations, and thus can affect normal cells. Optimum antiproliferative activity generally is attained when interferons are administered repeatedly and are in direct contact with the cells or tumor. Human cell lines reported to be sensitive to the drugs include a lymphoblastoid cell line, osteosarcoma, myeloid leukemia, colon carcinoma, , hepatoma, neuroblastoma, and normal, hyperplastic, and malignant breast tissue. Interferon alfa also inhibits colony formation of transplantable murine tumors and fresh biopsies of human tumors including melanoma, lung cancer, myeloma, ovarian carcinoma, sarcoma, adenocarcinoma of unknown primary origin, acute leukemia, and renal cell carcinoma.

Effect on Cell Phenotype and Oncogene Expression. Interferons can decrease the transcription and expression of several oncogenes (e.g., c-*myc*, c-*mos*, c-*abl*, c-Ha-*ras*, c-*sis*, c-*src*) and in growth factor receptors, and can inhibit the expression of a protein induced by platelet-derived growth factor (the formation of this factor depends on the c-*sis* oncogene). In some transformed cell lines, this decrease in transcription and expression of the oncogene product has been correlated with inhibition of tumor cell proliferation. Long-term exposure of some transformed cell lines to interferons can lead to a reversion of the cells to a more normal phenotype, characterized by more normal growth characteristics and cellular morphology. This phenotypic reversion has been associated with a specific decrease in oncogene expression and loss of tumorigenicity and oncogenic potential of the cells. The interferon-induced reduction in c-Ha-*ras* and c-*myc* RNA appears to be selective for the oncogene transcripts; however, despite this selective decrease in the levels of the oncogene mRNA and the expression of their gene products, interferons do not alter the quantity or distribution of the transfected DNA present in the cell. Interferons principally may act at the level of gene transcription and subsequent mRNA translation; however, some evidence suggests that this effect on oncogene expression may be mediated in part by interferon-induced decreases in the number of copies of viral genome.

It has been suggested that expression of the c-*myc* gene plays a major role in the malignant transformation of some cells. Therefore, although a causal relationship between modulation of oncogene expression by interferons and growth inhibition has not been established, it has been proposed that the decrease in expression of this and other oncogenes by the drugs may contribute to their antiproliferative activity. Interferon-mediated decreases in the expression of c-*myc* gene in a Burkitt's lymphoma cell line has been proposed as a model for interferon-induced cellular differentiation. Decreased c-*myc* oncogene expression occurs relatively early during interferon exposure and does not appear to be mediated by the accumulation of cells at the $_0$/G_1 border of the cell cycle. Interferons disrupt DNA replication in these cells in several ways, including inhibiting the synthesis of Okazaki fragments (short segments of base pairs that are formed and subsequently joined during DNA replication) and decreasing the stability of these newly synthesized replicons. A cell line resistant to the antiproliferative effects of an interferon does not exhibit this drug-induced decrease in oncogene expression. Similar observations regarding changes in the expression of c-*myc*, c-*mos*, and c-*ras* genes generally have been noted in patients with hairy cell leukemia who have received interferon alfa therapy, and the gradual reduction in the percentage of cells in bone marrow expressing the Philadelphia chromosome associated with interferon alfa therapy in patients with chronic myelogenous leukemia also may reflect the tendency of the leukemic cells to progress from a malignant phenotype and genotype toward a more normal nonmalignant state.

Limited evidence suggests that oncogenes present in transformed cell lines may modulate cellular sensitivity to different types of interferons, resulting in some cell types that are resistant to the effects of one interferon type (e.g., gamma) while sensitive to another interferon type (e.g., alfa). Interferons can inhibit the growth of numerous cell lines, without altering the level of the c-*myc* mRNA transcript or distribution of cells in the cell cycle, and can block the platelet-derived growth factor (PGDF)-induced stimulation of cell proliferation without affecting the increased expression of c-*myc* that precedes this stimulation. However, other evidence indicates that the importance of modulation of oncogene expression and alterations in phenotypic expression and differentiation of malignant cells in the antineoplastic activity of interferons remains to be established.

Effect on Cell Differentiation. Interferons generally enhance cellular differentiation, but can inhibit the functional and morphologic differentiation of some cells (e.g., fibroblasts).Interferons can alter the phenotypic expression of prenatural killer (NK) cells and lymphocytes (e.g., T cells) and can augment the expression of Fc receptors on the cell surface of immune effector cells that require these receptors for immunologic reactivity. These changes in phenotypic expression, interferon-mediated increases in phagocytosis by macrophages or monocytes, augmentation of antibody-dependent cell-mediated cytotoxicity by killer (K) cells, and enhancement of histamine release by basophils presumably are related to the ability of interferons to modulate cellular differentiation. Interferons also can enhance or inhibit the maturation of normal monocyte and macrophage precursors, activate monocytes and macrophages, and enhance the differentiation of a human leukemic cell line to macrophages and/or granulocytes. Evidence from studies in which interferons stimulated their own immunologic neutralization by augmenting the expression of certain cell surface antigens also indicates that the drugs enhance cell differentiation.

Other Antiproliferative Mechanisms. There is limited evidence that some of the biologic and pharmacologic effects, including antiproliferative effects, of interferons may be mediated in part by prostaglandins. Prostaglandins can modulate cell proliferation and function as immunomodulators, and interferons have been shown to stimulate prostaglandin biosynthesis. In addition, the absence of cyclooxygenase in some cells may explain the resistance of these cells to the antiviral and antiproliferative effects of interferons. However, prostaglandins also produce effects on the immune system that can oppose those induced by interferons. In addition, cyclooxygenase inhibitors and exogenous prostaglandins have complex effects on the biologic activity of interferons, and interferons do not appear to affect phospholipase or cyclooxygenase activities. Further study is needed to establish the role, if any, of the cyclooxygenase system and prostaglandins in the biologic effects mediated by interferons.

It also has been suggested that the biologic and pharmacologic effects of interferons may be related partly to their ability to alter intracellular concentrations of cyclic nucleotides (e.g., cAMP, cGMP). Cells exposed to cyclic nucleotide derivatives or agents that increase the intracellular concentration of cyclic nucleotides exhibit increased sensitivity to the antiviral and antiproliferative properties of interferons. Interferon-induced elevations in the concentration of cAMP and cGMP occur prior to or concomitantly with the development of the antiproliferative and antiviral effects of the drugs and do not occur in cells resistant to the effects of interferons. However, such increases in cAMP and cGMP apparently are not essential to the antiviral and antiproliferative actions of interferons, since blocking these increases does not reduce the activity of the drugs. In addition, because of the complex role of cyclic nucleotides in the regulation of cell proliferation, it remains to be determined whether these second messengers have an established role in mediating these effects of interferons.

Effects on Cell Plasma Membrane. Agents (e.g., amphotericin B, colchicine, vinblastine) that alter plasma membrane and cytoskeletal components can inhibit the antiviral effects of interferons, whereas agents (e.g., sodium butyrate) that increase synthesis of microfilaments and the number of cellular desmosomes may enhance the action of interferons. Interferons can alter the cell surface expression of gangliosides and other membrane components and can decrease the unsaturated fatty acid content of major phospholipids, which may lead to a more rigid lipid bilayer in the plasma membrane and a decrease in cell motility. The overall cellular net charge becomes more negative, as does the intramembranous charge.

Interferons can alter the ion flux across plasma membranes and can increase neuronal excitability, decrease the release of plasminogen activator from the plasma membrane, increase the size and number of actin filaments, alter the cell surface distribution of fibronectin, and increase cell volume and surface area. These changes in cell size and degree of arrangement, polymerization, and amount of actin generally correlate with a decrease in the rate of cell proliferation.

Interferons also can alter nucleoside transport and cell surface antigen and immunoglobulin expression and can produce a relative increase in histocompatibility antigens on lymphocytes. Expression of membrane receptors for Fc fragments of IgG and IgM can be increased and decreased, respectively, by interferons alfa or beta.

Immune System Effects Interferons are cytokines that exhibit complex and variable immunologic activity, including both immunomodulating and immunosuppressive effects. The immunomodulating activity of interferons may have important effects on the immunologic relationship between tumors and the host. However, despite the wide range of regulatory actions of interferons on the immune system and the possibility that these actions may contribute at least in part to the antineoplastic activity of the drugs, there currently is little direct evidence to support the theory that the antineoplastic activity of interferons *depends* on their effects on the immune system. While interferons generally exhibit similar pharmacologic actions, including many actions involving the immune system, differences between interferon types appear to be greatest for immunologic effects, with interferon gamma appearing to be the most distinct, particularly in its macrophage (phagocyte)-activating properties.

Interferons can influence the proliferation of immune effector cells, such as those that are cytotoxic to tumor cells, and can also modulate antibody production and the release of other lymphokines (e.g., interleukin-2 [IL-2], MIF, LIF), which may be important in the host's immune response to tumors. Interferons also may alter host response to tumors and other cells by modulating the expression of cell surface antigens, including major histocompatibility antigens (e.g., interferon alfa increases class I histocompatibility molecules on lymphocytes and interferon gamma increases both class I and II molecules) and tumor-associated antigens, which may alter the immunogenicity of tumor and other cells. Interferons also can enhance natural killer (NK) cell activity and macrophage activity, although there currently is no direct evidence that such enhancement of the cytotoxicity of immune effector cells is responsible for the therapeutic effects of interferons. While some evidence also suggests that the effect of interferons on the host immune system may be an important determinant of the antiproliferative activity of the drugs and that the antineoplastic activity of interferons may be mediated in part by their effects on the host's immune system, other evidence suggests that the effects of the drugs on host response may be mediated by nonimmune mechanisms, such as depletion of growth factors and inhibition of angiogenesis and stroma development.

Interferons, principally interferon gamma but also interferon alfa, can modulate cellular and humoral immune responses and can enhance the cytotoxicity of immune effector cells and the phagocytic activity of macrophages. In addition, the secretion of interferons alfa and beta is increased in activated macrophages, and mature B cells express receptors for interferons that probably contribute as governing signals to the complex immune responses of these cells. Interferon gamma appears to be a particularly important macrophage-activating cytokine (lymphokine); this interferon type, but not alfa or beta, exhibits clinically important effects on the production of intracellular, superoxide radicals that are capable of mediating killing activity against certain microorganisms. There also is limited evidence that interferons can stimulate lymphocytic infiltration. Although interferons can enhance antibody production, the effect of the drugs on the production of antibody to tumor-associated antigens has not been clearly established.

Interferons also may augment cytotoxicity of cytotoxic T cells (CTL, killer T cells) and lymphokine-activated killer (LAK) cells by potentiating interleukin-2 (IL-2) release. While it has been suggested that interferon-mediated stimulation of LAK production may increase the host's response against tumor cells, some in vitro evidence indicates that interferons can inhibit the proliferation of interleukin-2-stimulated lymphocytes and can inhibit the induction of LAK activity.

Effects on Natural Killer Cell and Killer Cell Activity. Interferons, including interferon alfa, augment natural killer (NK) cell activity, but there reportedly is substantial variation in the ability of the numerous subtypes of interferon alfa to enhance NK-cell activity. NK cells possess some surface characteristics of both the myeloid and lymphoid lineage, and are defined in part by their ability to lyse certain types of tumor cells and normal targets. In animal models, NK cells can inhibit the formation of metastatic foci in the host, and interferons reportedly can augment this antimetastatic effect of these immune effector cells. Interferons augment NK-cell cytotoxicity directly and do not require the presence of an accessory cell population. In vitro, human NK-cell activity may increase 16-fold in the presence of interferon alfa, although substantial individual variation exists in response to interferon enhancement of NK-cell activity.

Interferons enhance NK-cell activity by increasing the proportion of NK cells that become cytotoxic and by decreasing both their cell cycle time and the time required for the cells to lyse their targets. An acceleration in lytic kinetics results, and the increased recyclability of NK cells allows the same effector cell to lyse more than one target. Interferons also can recruit cytotoxic cells from a non-cytotoxic pre-NK cell population that is capable of binding but not lysing target cells and can enhance NK-cell binding to less sensitive targets. Limited data suggest that the recruitment of pre-NK cells may be the principal mechanism by which interferons enhance NK-cell activity. Interferons are only capable of activating pre-NK cells and NK cells when present before these effector cells bind their target cells, and NK cells are activated only while in the presence of interferon. The drugs can enhance NK-cell activity against fresh or freshly frozen tumor cells of diverse origin; however, they consistently have failed to enhance the activity of the same effector cells against autologous tumor cells.

Interferons also may have effects on NK-cell activity that could negatively affect host responses. For example, interferons are capable of protecting malignant cells from NK cell-mediated lysis. Interferons also can inhibit the host's immune response by decreasing NK-cell activity and by inducing increased resistance to NK cell-mediated lysis. This inhibition of NK cell activity may serve to protect from NK cell-mediated lysis any target cell population that expresses interferon receptors. Some evidence suggests that this protection of target cells from NK cell-mediated lysis may provide a mechanism whereby interferons could activate NK cells to lyse tumor cells preferentially while ensuring that normal cells were protected; however, other evidence indicates that certain malignant cells that possess interferon receptors also can be protected from NK cell-mediated cytotoxicity by preexposure to an interferon. This interferon-induced target cell protection from NK-cell lysis requires de novo RNA and protein synthesis, is specific for NK cell-mediated lysis, and is not accompanied by a decrease in antibody-dependent cellular cytotoxicity. It has been suggested that interferon-induced protection from NK cell-mediated cytolysis actually may result in a slight enhancement of immune-mediated target-cell killing secondary to increased expression of histocompatibility antigens and a stimulation of the alloimmune response from cytotoxic T cells (CTL, killer T cells).

The dose, schedule, and route of interferon administration can have profound effects on NK-cell activity. The optimum dose of interferons required for immune stimulation has not been established, but for interferon alfa, some evidence suggests that lower doses achieve higher NK-cell activity when the drug is administered for sustained periods and that NK-cell activity actually is depressed with continued administration of the drug. Other studies, however, have shown either consistent increases or decreases in NK-cell activity, or have shown individual variation and no consistent changes in such activity. Therefore, it has been suggested that a threshold dose of interferon exists, above which there is a negative influence on NK cells. The long-term effects of interferon alfa on NK-cell activity also have varied, with reports of increases or decreases in such activity. In one study, low-dose interferon alfa produced an increase in NK-cell activity within 48 hours, but this increase was not sustained despite repeated administration of the drug. High-dose interferon alfa gave a more sustained increase of NK-cell activity but did not produce the same initial increase observed with the low dose. In a study in which interferon alfa was administered on an intermittent schedule, the drug produced a dose-related decrease in NK-cell activity over a 6-week period, following an initial stimulatory effect. In addition, the route and schedule of administration appear to influence the effect of interferons on NK-cell activity. In general, no clearly defined relationship exists between stimulation of NK-cell activity by interferons and the clinical antineoplastic activity of these drugs.

Interferons generally enhance antibody-dependent cell-mediated cytotoxicity (ADCC) against a variety of antibody-coated target cells. While the mechanism of this enhancement in ADCC is not known, killer (K) cells, the subpopulation of lymphocytes that mediates ADCC, may be involved since these cells have Fc receptors to IgG, and interferons are known to enhance expression of these receptors.

Effects on Macrophage and Monocyte Activity. Interferon-induced activation of macrophages and monocytes results in morphologic changes in these cells, increased phagocytic activity, and nonspecific cytotoxicity against tumor cells and other target cells. Interferons enhance the number of phagocytic cells and the degree of phagocytosis of individual cells. Interferons also enhance Fc receptor-mediated phagocytosis. Activated macrophages can recognize cell-surface properties characteristic of transformed cells and can selectively destroy these malignant cells.

Interferon-mediated enhancement in macrophage phagocytosis can be neutralized by anti-interferon globulin. In addition, such enhancement of macrophage killing of leukemic cells can be suppressed when these effector cells are incubated with PGE_1, PGE_2, or hydrocortisone after interferon treatment, although the prostaglandins have no effect on unstimulated macrophages. This effect of prostaglandins may be mediated by increased intracellular concentrations of cAMP. (See Other Antiproliferative Mechanisms, under Mechanism of Action: Antiproliferative Effects, in Pharmacology.)

Effects on T Cells. Interferons have varied effects on T cells, a cell population that may influence tumor growth in several ways. T cells may interact directly with tumor cells or indirectly through regulatory influences on other immune effector cell types. The effects of the drugs on T cells most likely reflect the diverse functional activities of various T-cell subsets. While there is some in vitro and in vivo evidence that the drug either has no effect on or actually decreases (secondary to the drug's antiproliferative activity) CTL-mediated killing, other evidence indicates that interferon alfa can enhance killing by CTL cells despite decreases in T-Cell proliferation. Therefore, interferon alfa may produce a selective increase in a specific population of cytotoxic T cells.

Interferon alfa also can affect delayed-type hypersensitivity responses, but the nature of the drug's effect depends on the timing of interferon administration. Interferon alfa inhibits delayed hypersensitivity reactions when the drug is administered prior to sensitization or secondary challenge with antigen but enhances the response when it is administered a few hours after sensitization.Antigen-specific leukocyte-induced inhibition of granulocyte migration and leukocyte migration inhibition reactions resulting from exposure of lymphocytes to phytohemagglutin can be partially or totally suppressed by interferon alfa. Interferons also can modulate lymphokine release from mitogen-stimulated lymphocytes. Relatively low concentrations of interferon alfa reportedly can decrease or increase production by mitogen (concanavalin A)-stimulated lymphocytes of the lymphokines—leukocyte inhibitory factor (LIF) and macrophage inhibitory factor (MIF, migration inhibiting factor), while higher concentrations of the drug reportedly inhibit production of these migration inhibitory factors.

Limited data suggest that interferons may augment suppressor T-cell activity. Antigen-specific suppressor T cells may play a particularly crucial role in suppressing the host's immune response to tumors; however, it has not been established how interferons may affect this subset of suppressor T cells.

Interferon alfa can modulate the expression of cell surface receptors on T cells (see Pharmacology: Effect on Cell Surface Antigens) and can increase the expression of IgG Fc receptors. Interferon alfa's effect on CTL-cell activity in mixed lymphocyte culture (MLC) appears to depend on the duration of exposure of the lymphocytes to interferon.

Effects on B Cells. Interferons can either enhance or suppress B-cell responses depending on dose and sequence of administration relative to antigenic stimulation. Low or high doses of interferon alfa followed by antigen stimulation can increase or decrease antibody production, respectively. Interferons enhance the B-cell responses when added during late stages (48–72 hours after antigen) of the response, presumably secondary to a modulatory effect on T cells. Exposure to interferon prior to or immediately after exposure to antigen generally suppresses antibody response. In animal studies, B-cell antibody production and the proper functioning of memory cells generally was inhibited by interferons when the drugs were given prior to antigen exposure. More generally, in vivo administration of interferons 48–72 hours after antigen results in a twofold to sixfold enhancement of the antibody response.

Interferon-induced suppression of antibody responses affects both IgM and IgG antibodies. Interferon alfa also can modulate IgE production and action, and the drug has depressed the ability of spleen cells to elicit an anaphylactic response, probably by inhibiting IgE synthesis or release. However, exogenous addition of antibody enhances interferon alfa-mediated histamine release from human basophils in vitro via a mechanism that requires de novo RNA synthesis.

Effect on Cell Surface Antigens. Interferons also may affect immune responses by modulating cell surface antigen expression and by enhancing expression of transplantation antigens and alloantigens. In addition, interferon alfa has enhanced the expression of a major histocompatibility complex (MHC) class I antigen on hepatocytes infected with hepatitis B virus, thereby resulting in a more efficient induction of cytotoxic T-cell (CTL, killer T-cell) activity against viral antigens, and elimination of the infected cells from the liver. A similar immune-mediated mechanism has been suggested for tumor cells, since interferons are known to increase the expression of MHC antigens and tumor associated antigens on melanoma and other tumor cells.

■ **Effect on Hepatic Cytochrome P-450 System** Interferons, including interferon alfa, and various agents that induce their production and/or secretion (e.g., viruses, quinacrine, tilorone, polyribonucleotides, endotoxin) have been shown to depress to varying degrees the hepatic cytochrome P-450 (microsomal) enzyme system, and the ability of interferon-inducing agents to depress this oxidative (monooxygenase) enzyme system may be mediated by interferons rather than by a direct effect of the agents. Depression of the cytochrome P-450 system has been manifested as reductions in the amount of hepatic microsomal protein, including the cytochrome P-450 and b_5 hemoproteins, and in the activities of several cytochrome P-450-dependent enzymes.

It remains to be established whether interferon-induced depression of the cytochrome P-450 enzyme system results from increased degradation, suppressed synthesis, or inhibition of cytochrome P-450. Evidence mainly from studies with interferon inducers suggests that increased degradation of hepatic hemoproteins rather than suppressed synthesis may be principally involved; however, other evidence from such studies suggests that decreased synthesis of the apoprotein of cytochrome P-450, probably secondary to disturbances in heme turnover, is an important mechanism. A second mediator (e.g., interleukin-1), in addition to interferons, also has been suggested. The importance of the effects of interferons on the cytochrome P-450 enzyme system remains to be established, but interferon alfa can inhibit the metabolism of certain drugs (e.g., theophylline) (see Drug Interactions: Effects on Hepatic Clearance of Drugs), possibly secondary to depression of this enzyme system. In addition, the extent of effect on the cytochrome P-450 system depends in part on the type and subtype of interferon employed.

■ **Other Effects** Interferons appear to be intrinsically pyrogenic. The pyrogenic response associated with administration of interferon alfa may be mediated by a drug-induced increase in the production and/or release of prostaglandin (PGE_2) in the hypothalamus rather than by an increase in interleukin-1. The response does not appear to be secondary to an exogenous pyrogenic contaminant in interferon alfa preparations.

Resistance

Cells that are sensitive to the antiviral and antiproliferative effects of interferon alfa possess specific high-affinity saturable interferon receptor sites on their cell surface; however, the presence of such receptors is not necessarily a sufficient criterion for ensuring cellular sensitivity to the drug. Tumor cells may be resistant to the antiproliferative effects of interferon alfa despite the presence of functional, specific high-affinity interferon receptors on their cell surface. Resistance to the antiproliferative effects of interferon alfa usually occurs at the cellular level; however, the precise mechanism responsible for resistance to the drugs may differ among cell populations.

An association has been observed between the presence of neutralizing anti-interferon antibody and clinical resistance to interferon alfa in some patients with hairy cell leukemia, suggesting that resistance to the drug may not always arise at the intracellular level. However, a causal relationship between the presence of antibodies and disease progression and/or resistance to interferon alfa therapy was not established, and some patients who developed neutralizing antibodies to interferon continued to respond to the drug. Therefore, the development of antibodies should not necessarily be interpreted as indicating resistance to the drug. For a more complete discussion of anti- interferon antibodies, see Dermatologic, Local, Sensitivity, and Immunologic Reactions: Antibody Formation, in Cautions.

Pharmacokinetics

Few, if any, studies in humans are available that directly compare the pharmacokinetics of recombinant DNA-derived (e.g., interferon alfa-2a [no longer commercially available in the US], interferon alfa-2b) and mixtures of naturally occurring human interferons. Some data suggest that the overall disposition of these preparations is similar and that these interferons produce comparable serum concentration-time profiles in humans and several species of animals following IM administration. Although substantial interindividual variability in serum interferon concentrations has been observed after administration of recombinant interferon alfa-2a in healthy individuals and patients with disseminated cancer, the overall disposition of the drug was similar following IM or IV dosing in these individuals and in patients with amyotrophic lateral sclerosis (ALS), except for the possibility of a higher clearance in patients with ALS. Observed differences in interferon pharmacokinetics among patient populations may be related to differences in disease states, dosing schedules, or inherent interindividual variability.

In most studies of the pharmacokinetics of recombinant and mixtures of naturally occurring human interferons, interferon concentration or activity in serum, urine, or CSF was determined using hemadsorption inhibition tests with ^{51}Cr-labeled erythrocytes, bioassays, radioimmunoassays, or enzyme-linked immunosorbent assays (ELISA). In patients with normal renal function, both ELISA and a bioassay based on inhibition of viral cytopathic effect give comparable results for serum concentrations of interferon alfa-2a; bioassay results with interferon alfa-2b reportedly also correlate well with those of radioimmunoassay.

■ **Absorption** For systemic effects, interferon alfa is administered parenterally because the drug is susceptible to degradation by proteolytic enzymes in the GI tract. Interferon alfa is well absorbed following IM or subcutaneous injection; the apparent fraction of the dose absorbed after IM or subcutaneous injection exceeds 80%. Peak serum interferon alfa concentrations following IV administration of the drug generally occur within 15–60 minutes and are substantially greater than those attained after IM or subcutaneous administration. However, serum interferon alfa concentrations following IM or subcutaneous administration generally are maintained for longer periods of time than those produced by rapid IV injection or rapid (e.g., 40 minutes or less) IV infusion. Following a 36 million-unit dose of interferon alfa administered by IV infusion or by IM or subcutaneous injection, peak serum interferon alfa concentrations averaged approximately 2320, 340, or 290 units/mL, respectively; 24 hours after administration, concentrations of interferon alfa administered by all of these routes were less than 17 units/mL. Depending on the administered dose, serum interferon concentrations generally are detectable for approximately 4–8 hours after rapid IV injection or infusion or for approximately 16–30 hours after IM or subcutaneous injection.

Following IM administration of interferon alfa in doses of 1 million to 198 million units, peak serum interferon alfa concentrations ranged from 18–1000 units/mL 1–8 hours (range: 2–12 hours) after the injection. Dose-proportional increases in serum interferon alfa concentration were observed following IM doses of up to 198 million units; AUC also increased with increasing doses of interferon alfa, although route of administration did not have a consistent effect on this value. Limited data suggest that the time required to achieve peak serum drug concentrations following IM administration of interferon alfa may increase slightly with increasing doses up to 72 million units; however, this has not been a consistent finding. Following IM administration of recombinant interferon alfa-2a (no longer commercially available in the US) in patients with various solid and hematologic malignancies, serum interferon alfa concentrations achieved at 3, 4, and 8 hours were 14, 12, and 16 units/mL after 3-million-unit doses; 37, 38, and 46 units/mL with 9-million-unit doses; or 62, 108, and 182 units/mL with 18-million-unit doses. In patients with chronic lymphocytic leukemia or advanced non-Hodgkin's lymphoma, peak serum interferon alfa concentrations 4–8 hours after IM administration of 5 million or 50 million units of recombinant interferon alfa-2a ranged from 91–542 or from 1009–3725 units/mL, respectively.

The serum concentration-time profile of interferon alfa following subcutaneous administration appears to be comparable to that following IM administration, although peak serum drug concentrations after subcutaneous injection are attained somewhat later. Following subcutaneous injection of recombinant interferon alfa-2a (no longer commercially available in the US) or alfa-2b in doses ranging from 1 million to 36 million units, mean peak serum interferon alfa concentrations ranged from 18–346 units/mL and were generally achieved in 6–8 hours (range: 3–12 hours).

Following intralesional injection of interferon alfa-n3 into anogenital warts, systemic plasma concentrations of the drug were undetectable (detection limit of 3 units/mL); however, some systemic absorption apparently occurs since adverse systemic effects have been reported in patients receiving intralesional therapy. Following intralesional injection of 3 million units of interferon alfa-2b weekly per wart for 4 weeks, serum concentrations of the drug ranged from 5–40 units/mL. The drug also was absorbed systemically following intralesional injection of interferon alfa-2b or a mixture of naturally occurring human interferon alfa at dosages of 18–30 million units weekly in patients with malignant melanoma; peak serum concentrations of the drug occurred 6 hours after injection, achieving a median of 95 units/mL. Some percutaneous absorption of interferon alfa also appears to occur following topical application of the drug, since adverse systemic effects have been reported rarely.

Interferon alfa can achieve high and sustained CSF concentrations following intrathecal† or intraventricular† administration. (See Pharmacokinetics: Distribution.) Following intraperitoneal† administration, interferon alfa reportedly is absorbed systemically, resulting in high, sustained serum concentrations after several weeks of therapy; interferon alfa was still detectable in serum 5 days following intraperitoneal administration, but intraperitoneal concentrations were 30–1000 times those achieved in serum.

Following topical application to the eye (into the lower conjunctival sac) of 0.25, 0.75, 2.5, or 5 million units of a buffered solution of interferon alfa, concentrations of the drug in the nasal cavity at 1 hour were 602, 1461, 1197, or 4360 units/mL, respectively; detectable concentrations were present for at least 8 hours following administration. The extent of intraocular penetration of interferon alfa following topical application of the eye currently is not known.

■ **Distribution** Limited data on the tissue distribution of interferon in animals suggest that mixtures of naturally occurring human or animal interferons are widely and rapidly distributed into body tissues after parenteral administration, with the highest concentrations occurring in spleen, kidney, liver, and lung. Limited evidence also indicates interferon uptake and/or binding by other types of tissue or tumors. Although a similar pattern of tissue distribution was noted in animals given certain recombinant DNA-derived interferons (human interferon alfa-2c), animal studies in which recombinant interferon alfa-2a (no longer commercially available in the US) or alfa-2b were used suggest that the these interferons are not concentrated in any organ or that only the kidney, which appears to be the principal site of interferon metabolism, demonstrates substantial uptake of the drugs. (See Pharmacokinetics: Elimination.) Studies with radiolabeled recombinant interferon alfa-2a in patients with osteosarcoma indicate uptake of the drug by the liver and by tumor tissue; differences in peak plasma concentrations following administration of human leukocyte interferon suggest that interferon alfa binds to a greater degree to tumors of the lymph nodes and bone marrow than to breast tumors. Following IM or subcutaneous injection of human recombinant interferon alfa-2a into the shank muscle of animals, interferon alfa readily distributes into lymph tissue.

Differences in volume of distribution and in other pharmacokinetic values among various recombinant interferons have been demonstrated in a few studies; however, the overall disposition of recombinant interferon alfa-2a in mice, dogs, monkeys, and humans appears to be similar (i.e., species independent). The volume of distribution of interferon alfa in humans reportedly approximates 20–60% of body weight; in healthy individuals who received 36 million units of recombinant interferon alfa-2a IV over 40 minutes, the volume of distribution at steady state (V_{ss}) ranged from 0.23–0.75 L/kg (mean: 0.4 L/kg).

Interferon alfa does not readily distribute into CSF following systemic administration of mixtures of naturally occurring human or recombinant interferons in animals or humans, although low concentrations have been detected in CSF following administration of large systemic doses. Following IM injection of a mixture of naturally occurring human leukocyte interferon, no interferon activity was detectable (i.e., concentration less than 20 units/mL) in CSF at 4 hours after a dose of 3 million units in an infant or at 6 and 8 hours after a dose of 30 million units in a 12-year-old boy. Using a radioimmunoassay (detection limit 2.5 units/mL), CSF interferon alfa concentrations of 3.1–3.8 units/mL were noted from 0.5–8 hours following a dose of recombinant interferon alfa-2b in a woman with disseminated breast cancer receiving 27 million units daily as a 30-minute IV infusion for 5 successive days every 3 weeks; corresponding serum interferon alfa concentrations ranged from 22–3065 units/mL. In a limited number of patients with amyotrophic lateral sclerosis, interferon alfa concentrations in CSF were undetectable (i.e., less than 2.6 units/mL) following IV infusion of a single 18-million units dose of recombinant interferon alfa-2a but ranged from 2.9–11.9 units/mL (550- to 1100-fold less than corresponding serum concentrations) following a dose of 50 million units; CSF concentrations were detectable after 1 hour and, in 2 patients, for at least 24 hours after the dose. In both animals and man, higher CSF concentrations of interferon alfa can be achieved by intrathecal† or intraventricular† administration. Distribution of interferon alfa into serum following injection into CSF occurs slowly; a stable serum concentration was maintained for 12–24 hours following intrathecal injection of 10 million units of human leukocyte interferon in monkeys. Intrathecal administration of interferon alfa in animals produced CSF interferon concentrations that were approximately 16- to 30-fold greater than corresponding serum concentrations. In a neonate who received 600,000 units of a mixture of naturally occurring human interferon alfa intrathecally once or twice daily for disseminated herpes simplex infection, CSF interferon alfa concentrations measured 12 or 24 hours after the dose ranged from 800–8000 units/mL. The presence of interferon alfa in CSF does not ensure penetration of the drug into parenchymal brain tissue; virus has been recovered postmortem from the brain tissue of a patient with disseminated herpes simplex infection in whom relatively high CSF concentrations of interferon alfa were attained following intrathecal injection of the drug. However, survival was substantially greater in monkeys infected with rabies virus and treated with intrathecally administered human leukocyte interferon than in those not treated, suggesting that interferon does reach grey and white matter of the brain.

It is not known whether interferon crosses the placenta in humans. Studies in mice indicate that murine interferon is distributed into milk; it is not known whether interferon is distributed into human milk.

■ Elimination Interferon alfa is rapidly cleared from plasma following rapid IV injection or IV infusion in animals or humans, while more prolonged concentrations are observed following IM or subcutaneous administration. In healthy individuals and patients with normal renal function, plasma concentrations of interferon alfa appear to decline in a biphasic manner. Limited data from studies in humans receiving recombinant interferon alfa-2a (no longer commercially available in the US) or recombinant interferon alfa-2b suggest that variability in the reported elimination half-life of interferon alfa may be related to route or method of administration, interindividual variability in drug disposition, and/or presence of disease. However, the serum concentrations and clearance of partially purified human leukocyte interferon or recombinant interferon alfa-2a was not appreciably altered in several patients with chronic renal failure.

Following a brief IV infusion, the terminal elimination half-life of recombinant interferon alfa-2a averaged 5.1 hours (range 3.7–8.5 hours) in healthy individuals and ranged from approximately 0.75–2 hours in a limited number of patients with disseminated cancer. Elimination half-life of recombinant interferon alfa-2a was more prolonged following continuous IV infusion for 14 days in a few patients with leukemia, ranging from 4.6–9.8 hours. In healthy individuals who received a 30-minute IV infusion of recombinant interferon alfa-2b, elimination half-life averaged approximately 2 hours (range: 0.5–2.9 hours). Elimination half-life of recombinant interferon alfa-2a or alfa-2b averaged approximately 2–3.5 hours following IM or subcutaneous administration in healthy individuals and approximately 2.6–11.5 hours following IM administration in patients with disseminated cancer.

In a study using isolated, perfused rabbit kidneys, the plasma disappearance rate of recombinant interferon alfa was greater than that of a mixture of naturally occurring interferon alfa. Following a single, rapid IV injection or a 14-day continuous IV infusion of interferon alfa-2a, total body clearance of the drug from plasma was 1.9–3.6 or 0.6–1.4 mL/minute per kg, respectively. Although conflicting data have been reported, accumulation of interferon alfa appears to occur with multiple IM dosing.

The metabolism of recombinant interferon alfa appears to be similar to that of mixtures of naturally occurring human interferon alfa in general. Interferon alfa appears to be metabolized principally in the kidney. Interferon alfa generally is undetectable or present only in trace quantities in urine, and the drug reappears in systemic circulation in negligible concentrations following its passage through the kidney; studies in which interferons have been detected in urine reported no correlation between urine and serum concentrations of the drug. In animals and humans, the total body clearance of recombinant interferon alfa exceeds the creatinine clearance, which also suggests that renal tubular secretion, extrarenal elimination, and/or renal and/or extrarenal catabolism contribute to elimination of the drug. Studies in isolated, perfused kidney preparations demonstrate that interferon alfa is freely filtered through the glomeruli. Approximately 90–96% of the drug is absorbed by the renal tubule, where it undergoes rapid proteolytic degradation at the brush border or in the lysosomes of the tubular epithelium. Studies of human leukocyte or recombinant interferons in isolated liver perfusate systems suggest that hepatic metabolism and subsequent biliary excretion is a minor pathway of elimination for interferon alfa.

In a limited number of patients with chronic renal failure who received single, low doses (i.e., 3 million units) of partially purified or recombinant interferon alfa, the serum concentrations and clearance of the drugs were not substantially altered; however, it has been suggested that interferon alfa may accumulate in body fluids of patients with markedly depressed glomerular filtration rate (GFR) and creatinine clearance. Limited evidence in patients receiving recombinant interferon alfa-2a suggests that hemodialysis is not effective in removing interferon alfa from the body.

Chemistry and Stability

■ Chemistry Interferon alfa is a family of highly homologous, species-specific proteins and, occasionally, glycoproteins that possess complex antiviral, antineoplastic, and immunomodulating activities. Because of the relative species-specific activity of interferons, interferons intended for human use are of human origin (e.g., prepared using donor-provided human cells such as leukocytes, using cultured human cell lines such as lymphoblastoid cells, or using recombinant techniques that employ human genes). At least 23 structurally similar subtypes of human interferon alfa (e.g., interferon alfa-2a, interferon alfa-2b) have been identified.

Interferon alfa is commercially available in the US as interferon alfa-2b and interferon alfa-n3. Interferon alfa-2b is of recombinant DNA origin and interferon alfa-n3 is derived from human leukocytes. For additional information on interferon alfa-2b and interferon alfa-n3, see Interferon Alfa 8:18.20.

Interferons are produced and secreted principally by peripheral blood leukocytes, fibroblasts, and epithelial cells in response to viral infection or certain other synthetic and biologic inducers (e.g., double-stranded RNA, certain bacteria and other microorganisms, endotoxin, surface glycoproteins). By definition, interferons exist as proteins or glycoproteins, are produced endogenously according to information encoded by species of interferon genes, and exert virus-nonspecific antiviral activity, at least in homologous cells, through cellular metabolic processes involving synthesis of RNA and proteins. In addition to interferon alfa, interferon beta and interferon gamma have been identified and are classified according to antigenic specificity and/or biologic properties. Interferon alfa and interferon beta have been referred to as type I interferons in part because of their general acid stability, and interferon gamma has been referred to as a type II interferon in part because of its general acid lability; however, some subtypes may not possess the acid stability profile indicated by this classification. Although interferon alfa, interferon beta, and interferon gamma also have been referred to as leukocyte or lymphoblastoid interferon, fibroblast interferon, and lymphocyte or immune interferon, respectively, these descriptions are considered misnomers since interferons alfa and beta can both be produced by leukocytes and fibroblasts, and production of interferon gamma can be induced by mitogen-stimulated mechanisms.

Human interferon alfa proteins generally contain 165 or 166 amino acids and have molecular weights ranging from 16,000–28,000 daltons, with most subtypes containing 166 amino acids and having molecular weights of 18,000–20,000. While the precise subtype composition of interferon alfa-n3 (α-interferons, leukocyte interferon, HuIFN-α (Le)) currently is not known, interferon alfa proteins present in the mixture consist of approximately 166 amino acids each and have molecular weights ranging from 16,000–27,000 daltons. The precise subtype composition of interferon alfa-n1 (α-interferons, lymphoblastoid interferon, HuIFN-α (Ly); not commercially available in the US), which is a mixture of at least 8 interferon alfa proteins but is derived from lymphoblastoid cells rather than from leukocytes, also currently is not known. Interferon alfa-2a (HuIFN-αA, Ro 22-8181; no longer commercially available in the US) and interferon alfa-2b (Sch 38500) are biosynthetic (recombinant DNA origin) forms of interferon alfa (rHuIFN-α) that consist of 165 amino acids. Interferons alfa-2a and alfa-2b have molecular weights of approximately 19,000 daltons and differ at position 23 in the amino acid sequence, with alfa-2a possessing a lysine group and alfa-2b an arginine group at this position. The importance, if any, of this single amino acid difference has not been established, and it remains to be elucidated whether clinically important differences in therapeutic and/or toxicologic profiles exist. Compared with other interferon alfa subtypes, interferon alfa-2a and interferon alfa-2b both have a deletion at position 44 in the amino acid sequence. In addition, although 2 large molecular segments are identical in various interferon alfa subtypes, the amino acid sequences of the subtypes differ from one another by several amino acids and are 70–90% homologous. Interferon alfa-2c (not commercially available in the US) differs structurally from interferon alfa-2b by the presence of an arginine group rather than a histidine group at position 34 in the amino acid sequence. The structure-activity relationships for interferons have not been clearly established. While both the amino and carboxy terminal regions of the molecules may be involved in eliciting antiviral activity, studies to determine which region(s) of the molecules confers various degrees of activity have yielded conflicting results. In addition, some evidence indicates that different regions may be involved in eliciting various activities of the drug.

Interferon Alfa-2b Interferon alfa-2b is prepared from cultures of genetically modified *Escherichia coli* using recombinant DNA technology. The bacteria is modified by the addition of a plasmid that incorporates an interferon alfa-2b gene from human leukocytes for human interferon alfa synthesis. Because a single gene is used for the preparation, single molecular species (i.e., 2b) rather than a mixture of interferon alfa subtypes is present in commercially available preparations of interferon alfa-2b. Trace amounts of residual *E. coli* protein may be produced during fermentation. Although tetracycline hydrochloride is included in the nutrient medium used during the fermentation process, it is undetectable in the final preparation of interferon alfa-2b.

Potency of interferon alfa-2b is expressed in International Units (IU) as tested against the activity of specific international reference preparations of interferons established by the World Health Organization (WHO). Interferon alfa-2b (recombinant DNA origin) commercially available in the US has a specific activity that is approximately 2.6 million units/mg of protein as measured by high performance liquid chromatography (HPLC) assay.

Interferon alfa-2b is commercially available in the US as a sterile powder for injection in single-dose vials or as a sterile solution in multiple-dose vials. The powder for injection occurs as a white to cream-colored lyophilized powder and contains dibasic and monobasic sodium phosphate as a buffer, glycine, and albumin human. Following reconstitution with the sterile water for injection diluent provided by the manufacturer, the injection occurs as a clear and colorless to light yellow solution. Commercially available solutions of interferon alfa-2b are clear and colorless and contain dibasic and monobasic sodium phosphate, edetate disodium, and polysorbate 80; *m*-cresol is added as a preservative.

■ **Stability** Commercially available interferon alfa-2b powder for injection in single-dose vials should be stored in a refrigerator at 2–8°C. Following reconstitution of the powder for injection with the sterile water for injection diluent provided by the manufacturer, the solution should be used immediately, but may be stored at 2–8°C for up to 24 hours.

Commercially available interferon alfa-2b solution for injection in multiple-dose vials should be stored at 2–8°C and should not be frozen or exposed to heat. After the initial dose is administered, any solution remaining in the vial should be discarded after 1 month.

For further information on the handling of antineoplastic agents, see the ASHP Guidelines on Handling Hazardous Drugs at http://www.ahfsdruginformation.com

Preparations

Excipients in commercially available drug preparations may have clinically important effects in some individuals; consult specific product labeling for details.

Interferon Alfa-2b (Recombinant DNA Origin)

Parenteral		
For injection	10 million units	**Intron® A** (available as single-dose vials with sterile water for injection diluent), Schering
	18 million units	**Intron® A** (available as single-dose vials with sterile water for injection diluent), Schering
	50 million units	**Intron® A** (available as single-dose vials with sterile water for injection diluent), Schering
Injection	6 million units/mL (18 million units)	**Intron® A** (available as multiple-dose vials), Schering
	10 million units/mL (25 million units)	**Intron® A** (available as multiple-dose vials), Schering

†Use is not currently included in the labeling approved by the US Food and Drug Administration

Selected Revisions April 2016, © Copyright, December 1990, American Society of Health-System Pharmacists, Inc.

Ipilimumab

■ Ipilimumab, a recombinant, fully human monoclonal antibody that binds to cytotoxic T-lymphocyte-associated antigen 4 (CTLA-4), is an antineoplastic agent.

REMS

FDA approved a REMS for ipilimumab to ensure that the benefits outweigh the risk. However, FDA later rescinded REMS requirements. See the FDA REMS page (https://www.accessdata.fda.gov/scripts/cder/rems/index.cfm).

Uses

■ **Melanoma** Ipilimumab is used for the treatment of unresectable or metastatic melanoma. Ipilimumab is designated an orphan drug by the US Food and Drug Administration (FDA) for the treatment of this cancer.

Efficacy of ipilimumab is based principally on observed survival benefits from a randomized, phase 3, double-blind, controlled study in 676 adults with previously treated (e.g., aldesleukin [23% of patients], dacarbazine, temozolomide, fotemustine [not commercially available in the US], carboplatin) unresectable or metastatic melanoma. Eligible patients (59% male, median 57 years of age, 71% with TNM metastasis stage M1c, 98% with Eastern Cooperative Oncology Group [ECOG] performance status of 0 or 1, positive for human leukocyte antigen [HLA]-A2*0201 allele) were randomized (3:1:1) to receive ipilimumab with glycoprotein 100 (gp100) melanoma peptide vaccine (an investigational vaccine), ipilimumab monotherapy, or gp100 vaccine monotherapy. Patients received induction regimens of ipilimumab (or placebo, as assigned) as a 90-minute IV infusion of 3 mg/kg followed by gp100 vaccine (or placebo, as assigned) as 2 separate 1-mg subcutaneous injections every 3 weeks for 4 doses. This study excluded patients with autoimmune disease, primary ocular melanoma or untreated active CNS metastasis, and those receiving immunosuppressive agents (including long-term corticosteroids). Assessment of tumor response occurred at 12 and 24 weeks and every 3 months thereafter. Median survival in patients receiving ipilimumab (with or without gp100 vaccine) was 10 months versus 6 months in patients receiving gp100 vaccine monotherapy. After a median follow-up of 28 months, rates of overall survival at 12, 18, and 24 months in patients receiving ipilimumab monotherapy were 45.6, 33.2, and 23.5%, respectively, compared with 25.3, 16.3, and 13.7%, respectively, in patients receiving gp100 vaccine monotherapy. Based on investigator assessment, best overall response rate was 10.9 or 1.5% in those receiving ipilimumab monotherapy or gp100 vaccine monotherapy, respectively.

Another phase 3 study evaluated ipilimumab as part of a combination chemotherapy regimen with dacarbazine in 502 adults with previously untreated, unresectable or metastatic melanoma. Patients were randomized to receive either ipilimumab and dacarbazine or dacarbazine and placebo. Treatment consisted of ipilimumab at higher than recommended doses (i.e., 10 mg/kg) and dacarbazine at doses of 850 mg/m². Patients received induction regimens of ipilimumab and dacarbazine or dacarbazine and placebo IV at 1, 4, 7, and 10 weeks followed by dacarbazine alone every 3 weeks for 22 weeks. Patients with stable disease or an objective response during induction therapy were eligible to receive a maintenance regimen of ipilimumab or placebo every 12 weeks until disease progression, development of adverse effects, or study completion. This study excluded patients receiving any prior treatment for metastatic disease or concomitant therapy with immunosuppressive agents (including long-term corticosteroids), or those with brain metastasis, primary ocular or mucosal melanoma, or autoimmune disease. Patients receiving ipilimumab and dacarbazine had increased median overall survival (11.2 months) compared with those receiving dacarbazine and placebo (9.1 months) with higher 1-year (47.3 versus 36.3%), 2-year (28.5 versus 17.9%), and 3-year (20.8 versus 12.2%) survival rates, respectively.

Ipilimumab therapy has shown variable patterns of clinical response that differ from the patterns observed with conventional chemotherapeutic agents. While disease regression shortly after initiation of ipilimumab therapy has been reported in some patients, durable stable disease (potentially with small decreases in total tumor burden over a long period of time), response after apparent disease progression, and reduced total tumor burden despite development of new lesions also have been observed. These variable response patterns to ipilimumab have all been associated with improved survival. Utilization of conventional response criteria for measurement of disease progression (e.g., Response Evaluation Criteria in Solid Tumors [RECIST], modified World Health Organization [WHO] criteria) may identify progressive disease before the full benefits of immunotherapy have been realized and may not detect all clinical responses to ipilimumab. Response criteria specific for immunotherapeutic agents that account for total tumor burden and uniquely define progressive disease have been proposed, but have not been prospectively validated. While there is some evidence that development of immune-mediated adverse events correlates with antitumor response to ipilimumab, the occurrence of high-grade immune-mediated adverse events is not required for a clinical response to ipilimumab, nor does this type of adverse reaction ensure a clinical response to the drug. Definitive criteria (e.g., biomarkers, genetic polymorphisms, preexisting antitumor immune response) to reliably identify patients who are likely to respond favorably to ipilimumab have not been established to date.

Dosage and Administration

■ **Administration** Ipilimumab is administered by IV infusion.

Ipilimumab is available as a 5-mg/mL, preservative-free, injection concentrate in single-use vials containing 50 or 200 mg of the drug.

Ipilimumab injection concentrate should be protected from light, stored at 2–8°C, and should not be frozen.

Ipilimumab injection concentrate must be diluted prior to administration. Prior to dilution, the appropriate number of vials containing ipilimumab injection concentrate should stand at room temperature for approximately 5 minutes. For IV infusion, the appropriate dose should be withdrawn from the vial(s) and injected into an IV bag. The injection concentrate should then be diluted with 0.9% sodium chloride or 5% dextrose injection to achieve a final ipilimumab concentration of 1–2 mg/mL. This diluted solution should be mixed by gentle inversion. Vials containing ipilimumab injection concentrate and diluted solutions of the drug should not be shaken. The diluted solution may be refrigerated or stored at controlled room temperature for no more than 24 hours. Any partially used vials, including unused diluted solution, should be discarded.

Ipilimumab injection concentrate should not be admixed or infused with other drugs. Final diluted ipilimumab solutions should be infused IV over 90 minutes using an in-line, sterile, nonpyrogenic, low-protein-binding filter. The IV line should be flushed with 0.9% sodium chloride or 5% dextrose injection after each dose.

■ **Dosage** The recommended adult dosage of ipilimumab for the treatment of unresectable or metastatic melanoma is 3 mg/kg given by IV infusion once every 3 weeks for a total of 4 doses.

Dosage Modification for Toxicity Ipilimumab therapy should be permanently discontinued in patients experiencing any severe or life-threatening immune-mediated adverse reactions. (See Warnings under Cautions: Warnings/Precautions.)

Ipilimumab therapy should be temporarily withheld in patients experiencing any moderate immune-mediated adverse reactions or symptomatic endocrinopathy. (See Warnings under Cautions: Warnings/Precautions.) If the adverse reaction completely or partially resolves to grade 0 or 1 and the patient is receiving 7.5 mg or less of prednisone per day (or equivalent), ipilimumab may be resumed at a dosage of 3 mg/kg every 3 weeks until all 4 planned doses have been administered or 16 weeks have elapsed since the first dose, whichever occurs first.

Ipilimumab therapy should be permanently discontinued in patients experiencing persistent moderate immune-mediated adverse reactions and in those unable to reduce corticosteroid dosage to 7.5 mg or less of prednisone per day (or equivalent).

Ipilimumab therapy should be permanently discontinued in patients unable to complete the full treatment course within 16 weeks after receiving the first dose.

■ **Special Populations** No special population dosage recommendations at this time.

Cautions

■ **Contraindications** The manufacturer states that there are no known contraindications to the use of ipilimumab.

■ **Warnings/Precautions** *Warnings* Severe, sometimes fatal, immune-mediated adverse reactions have occurred with ipilimumab treatment. These reactions are a result of T-cell activation and proliferation, and may involve any organ system. The most common, severe immune-mediated adverse reactions are enterocolitis, hepatitis, dermatitis (including toxic epidermal necrolysis), neuropathy, and endocrinopathy. These reactions have usually manifested during ipilimumab treatment, but also have occurred weeks or months after discontinuing the drug.

Patients should be evaluated for manifestations of enterocolitis, dermatitis, neuropathy, and endocrinopathy using appropriate laboratory tests (e.g., liver function and thyroid function tests) prior to each dose of ipilimumab. If severe immune-mediated adverse reactions occur, the drug should be discontinued and high-dose systemic corticosteroid therapy should be initiated. (See REMS and also see Dosage Modification for Toxicity under Dosage and Administration: Dosage.)

Immune-mediated GI Effects. Immune-mediated enterocolitis, sometimes fatal, has occurred with ipilimumab therapy. Among patients receiving ipilimumab for unresectable or metastatic melanoma in a phase 3 clinical trial, severe or life-threatening (grade 3–5) immune-mediated enterocolitis (i.e., diarrhea [7 or more stools per day above baseline], fever, ileus, peritoneal signs) occurred in 7% of patients. Moderate (grade 2) immune-mediated enterocolitis (i.e., diarrhea [up to 6 stools per day above baseline], abdominal pain, mucus or blood in stool) occurred in 5% of patients. In addition, intestinal perforation occurred in 1% and fatal immune-mediated enterocolitis occurred in 0.8% of patients receiving ipilimumab. The incidence and severity of enterocolitis appear to be dose dependent.

The majority of patients experiencing severe, life-threatening, or fatal (grade 3–5) enterocolitis required hospitalization and the median time to onset was 7.4 weeks (range 1.6–13.4 weeks) after initiation of ipilimumab. Treatment with high-dose corticosteroids (40 mg or more of prednisone per day [or equivalent]) was used in 85% of these patients (median daily dosage of 80 mg of prednisone [or equivalent], median duration of 2.3 weeks [up to 13.9 weeks] followed by tapering of the corticosteroid dosage). Infliximab was administered to 8% of patients experiencing moderate, severe, or life-threatening immune-mediated enterocolitis following an inadequate response to corticosteroid therapy. The majority (74%) of patients experiencing grade 3–5 enterocolitis had complete resolution, while 3% improved to grade 2 enterocolitis, and 24% did not report improvement.

Among the 5% of patients experiencing moderate (grade 2) enterocolitis, the median time to onset was 6.3 weeks (range 0.3–18.9 weeks) after initiation of ipilimumab; 54% of such patients were treated with corticosteroids. High-dose corticosteroid therapy (40 mg or more of prednisone per day [or equivalent], median duration of 10 days) was administered in 25% of patients followed by tapering of the corticosteroid dosage, while 29% were treated with less than 40 mg of prednisone per day [or equivalent] for a median duration of 5.1 weeks. The majority (79%) of patients experiencing grade 2 enterocolitis had complete resolution, while 11% reported improvement, and 11% did not report improvement.

Patients should be monitored for manifestations of enterocolitis, including diarrhea, abdominal pain, and mucus or blood in the stool with or without fever, and for manifestations of bowel perforation, including peritoneal signs and ileus. Infectious etiologies should be ruled out in symptomatic patients; for severe or persistent symptoms, endoscopic evaluation should be considered.

Ipilimumab should be permanently discontinued in patients experiencing severe or life-threatening adverse GI reactions, including colitis with abdominal pain, fever, ileus, or peritoneal signs; an increase in stool frequency of 7 or more per day above baseline; stool incontinence; a need for IV hydration exceeding 24 hours; or GI hemorrhage or perforation. Once bowel perforation has been ruled out, systemic corticosteroid therapy should be initiated at a dosage of 1–2 mg/kg per day of prednisone (or equivalent). Once symptoms have resolved or severity of symptoms is reduced, corticosteroid dosage should be tapered over at least 1 month. Dosage tapering schedules less than 1 month in duration have resulted in recurrence or worsening of enterocolitis in some patients. If symptoms persist, patients should continue to be monitored for GI perforation or peritonitis. Repeating the endoscopic evaluation and initiating alternative immunosuppressive therapy (e.g., infliximab) may be considered.

In cases of moderate enterocolitis, ipilimumab should be temporarily withheld and antidiarrheal therapy initiated. If symptoms persist for longer than 1 week, systemic corticosteroid therapy should be initiated at a dosage of 0.5 mg/kg per day of prednisone (or equivalent). Therapy with ipilimumab may be resumed once symptoms have resolved or improved to mild severity and daily prednisone dosage is 7.5 mg or less (or equivalent). Ipilimumab should be permanently discontinued in patients unable to reduce corticosteroid dosage to 7.5 mg or less of prednisone per day (or equivalent) or in those unable to complete the full ipilimumab treatment course within 16 weeks after receiving the first dose. (See Dosage Modification for Toxicity under Dosage and Administration: Dosage.)

Symptomatic treatment with antidiarrheal agents (e.g., diphenoxylate and atropine, loperamide) is used by some clinicians for grade 1 or 2 diarrhea associated with ipilimumab therapy. Treatment guidelines from some experts recommend the use of budesonide for treatment of grade 2 diarrhea and high-dose corticosteroid therapy for treatment of grade 3 or 4 diarrhea. Prophylactic use of budesonide also has been investigated to reduce the frequency of grade 2 or greater diarrhea associated with ipilimumab. However, in one randomized, double-blind study, prophylactic therapy with budesonide during ipilimumab therapy did *not* result in a decreased frequency of grade 2 or greater diarrhea.

Immune-mediated Hepatic Effects. Severe, sometimes fatal, hepatotoxicity, including immune-mediated hepatitis, has occurred with ipilimumab therapy. Among patients receiving ipilimumab for unresectable or metastatic melanoma in a phase 3 clinical trial, severe, life-threatening, or fatal (grade 3–5) hepatotoxicity (i.e., serum AST or ALT concentrations exceeding 5 times the upper limit of normal [ULN] or total bilirubin concentrations exceeding 3 times the ULN) occurred in 2% of patients. In addition, moderate (grade 2) hepatotoxicity (i.e., serum AST or ALT concentrations 2.5–5 times the ULN or total bilirubin concentrations 1.5–3 times the ULN) occurred in 2.5% of patients. Of patients receiving ipilimumab during clinical trials, 0.4% of patients required hospitalization for hepatotoxicity and 0.2% experienced fatal hepatotoxicity. Mycophenolate therapy has been used in patients with persistent, severe hepatitis despite treatment with high-dose corticosteroids. The incidence and severity of hepatitis appear to be dose dependent.

Patients should be assessed for manifestations of hepatotoxicity using appropriate laboratory tests (e.g., AST, ALT, and bilirubin concentrations) prior to each dose of ipilimumab. Infectious and malignant etiologies should be ruled out and liver function tests should be evaluated more frequently in patients experiencing hepatotoxicity until resolution of the toxicity.

Ipilimumab should be permanently discontinued in patients experiencing severe or life-threatening hepatotoxicity. In such patients, systemic corticosteroid therapy should be initiated at a dosage of 1–2 mg/kg per day of prednisone (or equivalent). Once liver function tests indicate a sustained improvement or have returned to baseline levels, corticosteroid therapy should be tapered over at least 1 month. If severe or life-threatening hepatotoxicity persists, alternative immunosuppressive therapy may be considered.

In cases of moderate (grade 2) hepatotoxicity, ipilimumab therapy should be temporarily withheld. Ipilimumab may be resumed once serum ALT and AST concentrations are less than 2.5 times the ULN and total bilirubin is less than 1.5 times the ULN or these values have returned to baseline. (See Dosage Modification for Toxicity under Dosage and Administration: Dosage.)

Ipilimumab should be permanently discontinued if the patient is unable to complete the full treatment course within 16 weeks after receiving the first dose.

Immune-mediated Dermatologic Effects. Immune-mediated dermatitis, sometimes fatal, has occurred with ipilimumab therapy. Among patients receiving ipilimumab for unresectable or metastatic melanoma in a phase 3 clinical trial, severe, life-threatening, or fatal (grade 3–5) immune-mediated dermatitis (e.g., Stevens-Johnson syndrome; toxic epidermal necrolysis; rash complicated by full thickness dermal ulceration; or necrotic, bullous, or hemorrhagic manifestations) occurred in 2.5% of patients. One patient required hospitalization for severe dermatitis, and one death occurred as a result of toxic epidermal necrolysis. In addition, moderate (grade 2) immune-mediated dermatitis occurred in 12% of patients. Among patients experiencing moderate, severe, or life-threatening immune-mediated dermatitis, the median onset was 3.1 weeks (up to 17.3 weeks) following initiation of ipilimumab therapy.

Treatment of severe dermatitis with high-dose corticosteroids was utilized in 54% of these patients (median daily dosage of 60 mg of prednisone [or equivalent], duration up to 14.9 weeks followed by tapering of the corticosteroid dosage). The majority (86%) of these patients had complete resolution occurring in up to 15.6 weeks.

Among patients experiencing moderate dermatitis during ipilimumab treatment in the clinical study, 40% were treated with systemic corticosteroids (median daily dosage of 60 mg of prednisone [or equivalent], median duration of 2.1 weeks), 11% were treated with topical corticosteroids, and 49% did not receive treatment with either systemic or topical corticosteroids. The majority (70%) of patients experiencing moderate dermatitis had complete resolution, while 11% reported improvement, and 19% did not report improvement.

Patients should be monitored for manifestations of dermatitis, (e.g., rash, pruritus). Dermatitis should be considered immune mediated unless another etiology can be identified.

Ipilimumab should be permanently discontinued in patients experiencing severe or life-threatening dermatitis. In such patients, systemic corticosteroid therapy should be initiated at a dosage of 1–2 mg/kg per day of prednisone (or equivalent). Once dermatitis is controlled, corticosteroid dosage should be tapered over at least 1 month.

Ipilimumab should be withheld for moderate (diffuse, 50% or less of skin surface) signs and symptoms of dermatitis. Topical or systemic corticosteroids should be administered if there is no symptomatic improvement within 1 week. Ipilimumab may be resumed once dermatitis is resolved or severity is reduced (i.e., localized rash) and daily prednisone dosage is 7.5 mg or less (or equivalent).

For mild dermatitis (including localized rash and pruritus), the patient should be treated symptomatically. Topical or systemic corticosteroid therapy should be administered if there is no symptomatic improvement within 1 week. (See Dosage Modification for Toxicity under Dosage and Administration: Dosage.)

Immune-mediated Neurologic Effects. Severe or fatal immune-mediated neurologic reactions, including sensory neuropathy, motor neuropathy, Guillain-Barré syndrome, and myasthenia gravis, have occurred with ipilimumab therapy. Among patients receiving ipilimumab for unresectable or metastatic melanoma in a phase 3 clinical trial, one death attributed to Guillain-Barré syndrome and one case of severe (grade 3) peripheral motor neuropathy were reported. Additional cases of Guillain-Barré syndrome and myasthenia gravis have been reported in other clinical studies with the drug.

Patients should be monitored for symptoms of motor or sensory neuropathy (e.g., unilateral or bilateral weakness, sensory alterations, paresthesia). Unless an alternative etiology is identified, such symptoms should be considered immune mediated.

Ipilimumab should be permanently discontinued in patients experiencing severe neurologic reactions, including new or worsening severe neuropathy (interfering with daily activities), Guillain-Barré syndrome, or myasthenia gravis. Severe neuropathy should be appropriately managed and consideration given to initiating systemic corticosteroids at a dosage of 1–2 mg/kg per day of prednisone (or equivalent).

Ipilimumab should be withheld in patients experiencing moderate neuropathy that does not interfere with daily activities and appropriate medical intervention should be initiated. Therapy with ipilimumab may be resumed once symptoms have resolved or returned to baseline. Ipilimumab should be permanently discontinued in patients unable to complete the full treatment course within 16 weeks after receiving the first dose. (See Dosage Modification for Toxicity under Dosage and Administration: Dosage.)

Immune-mediated Endocrine Effects. Immune-mediated endocrinopathies have occurred with ipilimumab therapy and were most frequently manifested as hypopituitarism, adrenal insufficiency, adrenal crisis, hyperthyroidism, or hypothyroidism. Among patients receiving ipilimumab for unresectable or metastatic melanoma in a phase 3 clinical trial, severe or life-threatening (grade 3–4) immune-mediated endocrinopathies (i.e., requiring hospitalization and/or urgent medical intervention, interfering with activities of daily living) occurred in 1.8% of patients. While all of these patients developed hypopituitarism, some developed other concomitant endocrinopathies that included adrenal insufficiency, hypogonadism, and hypothyroidism; 66% of these patients required hospitalization. In addition, moderate (grade 2) immune-mediated endocrinopathies (requiring hormone replacement or medical intervention) occurred in 2.3% of patients and included hypothyroidism, adrenal insufficiency, hypopituitarism, hyperthyroidism, and Cushing's syndrome. In patients experiencing moderate to severe immune-mediated endocrinopathies, the median onset was 11 weeks (up to 19.3 weeks) after the initiation of ipilimumab. Long-term hormone replacement therapy (including adrenal or thyroid hormones) was necessary in 81% of these patients experiencing moderate or severe endocrinopathies associated with ipilimumab therapy.

Patients should be monitored for manifestations of hypophysitis, adrenal insufficiency, adrenal crisis, hyperthyroidism, and hypothyroidism. Clinical presentation may consist of fatigue, headache, mental status change, abdominal pain, unusual bowel habits, hypotension, or nonspecific symptoms that may resemble other causes (including brain metastasis, underlying disease). Such signs and symptoms of endocrinopathy should be considered immune mediated unless another etiology can be identified. Thyroid function tests and clinical chemistry values should be evaluated prior to the first dose of ipilimumab and each subsequent dose of the drug, and as clinically indicated throughout treatment. In a limited number of patients, imaging studies that revealed enlargement of the pituitary gland were used to diagnose hypophysitis.

Ipilimumab therapy should be withheld in patients with symptoms of endocrinopathy. In such patients, systemic corticosteroid therapy should be initiated at a dosage of 1–2 mg/kg per day of prednisone (or equivalent) in conjunction with appropriate hormone replacement therapy. Ipilimumab may be resumed once symptoms have resolved or returned to baseline, the patient is stable on hormone replacement therapy (if indicated), and corticosteroid dosage does not exceed 7.5 mg of prednisone daily (or equivalent). (See Dosage Modification for Toxicity under Dosage and Administration: Dosage.) Ipilimumab should be permanently discontinued in patients unable to reduce corticosteroid dosage to 7.5 mg or less of prednisone daily (or equivalent) or in those unable to complete the full ipilimumab treatment course within 16 weeks after receiving the first dose of drug.

Other Warnings/Precautions **Other Immune-mediated Effects.** Other immune-mediated adverse reactions, including nephritis, pneumonitis, meningitis, pericarditis, uveitis, iritis, and hemolytic anemia have occurred with ipilimumab therapy. Among patients receiving ipilimumab for unresectable or metastatic melanoma in a phase 3 clinical trial, such immune-mediated reactions were observed in less than 1% of patients. In addition, immune-mediated reactions such as myocarditis, angiopathy, temporal arteritis, vasculitis, polymyalgia rheumatica, conjunctivitis, blepharitis, episcleritis, scleritis, leukocytoclastic vasculitis, erythema multiforme, psoriasis, pancreatitis, arthritis, and autoimmune thyroiditis were reported in less than 1% of patients in clinical trials of the drug.

Ipilimumab should be permanently discontinued in patients experiencing clinically important or severe immune-mediated adverse reactions. In patients experiencing severe immune-mediated reactions, systemic corticosteroid therapy should be initiated at a dosage of 1–2 mg/kg per day of prednisone (or equivalent). Ipilimumab should be permanently discontinued in patients unable to reduce corticosteroid dosage to 7.5 mg or less of prednisone daily (or equivalent) or in those unable to complete the full ipilimumab treatment course within 16 weeks after receiving the first dose of drug.

In patients experiencing uveitis, iritis, or episcleritis, therapy with an ophthalmic corticosteroid preparation should be administered. Ipilimumab should be permanently discontinued in patients experiencing immune-mediated ocular disease unresponsive to topical corticosteroid therapy.

Immunogenicity. There is a potential for immunogenicity with ipilimumab therapy. Development of binding antibodies to ipilimumab were detected by electrochemiluminescence (ECL) in 1.1% of patients receiving the drug during clinical trials. Among these patients, infusion-related reactions consistent with hypersensitivity or anaphylaxis were not observed. Neutralizing antibodies to ipilimumab also were not detected in these patients. The ability of the ECL assay to detect anti-ipilimumab antibodies is limited by the presence of circulating drug. In a cohort of patients with the lowest trough concentrations of ipilimumab after receiving 0.3 mg/kg of drug, 6.9% tested positive for ipilimumab-binding antibodies.

Because the observed incidence of antibody positivity may be influenced by several factors including assay methodology, sample handling, timing of sample collection, concomitant drug therapy, and underlying disease, comparison of the incidence of antibodies to ipilimumab to that of other drugs may be misleading.

Specific Populations **Pregnancy.** Category C. (See Users Guide.)

Lactation. It is not known whether ipilimumab is distributed into milk. A decision should be made whether to discontinue nursing or the drug, taking into account the importance of the drug to the woman.

Pediatric Use. Safety and efficacy of ipilimumab have not been established in pediatric patients younger than 18 years of age.

Geriatric Use. No substantial difference in safety and efficacy relative to younger adults have been observed.

Hepatic Impairment. Ipilimumab has not been studied in patients with hepatic impairment.

Renal Impairment. Ipilimumab has not been studied in patients with renal impairment.

■ **Common Adverse Effects** Adverse effects reported in 5% or more of patients receiving ipilimumab include fatigue, diarrhea, pruritus, rash, and colitis.

Drug Interactions

No formal drug interaction studies have been performed to date.

Description

Ipilimumab, a recombinant, fully human monoclonal antibody that binds to cytotoxic T-lymphocyte-associated antigen 4 (CTLA-4), is an antineoplastic agent. The drug is an IgG_1 kappa immunoglobulin that is produced in mammalian (Chinese hamster ovary) cell culture.

Ipilimumab has high affinity and specificity for CTLA-4, an inducible receptor expressed on the surface of T-cells after activation. CTLA-4 competes with CD28, a costimulatory T-cell receptor, for the ligands CD80 (B7-1) and CD86 (B7-2) on antigen-presenting cells. The interaction between CTLA-4 and CD80 or CD86 results in inhibition of T-cell activation and proliferation. Anti-CTLA-4 antibodies block the interaction with CD80 and CD86, and allow for prolonged T-cell activation and enhanced immune response. The antineoplastic effects of the drug are indirect and appear to result from augmented T-cell-mediated antitumor immune response. An initial increase in total tumor burden (e.g., enlargement of baseline lesions, development of new lesions) observed in the absence of substantial clinical deterioration during ipilimumab therapy may not indicate treatment failure, but may be a result of lymphocytic infiltration of the lesions or tumor growth prior to complete immune system activation.

The pharmacokinetics of ipilimumab following IV administration is characterized by a 2-compartment model with first-order elimination and dose-dependent clinical effects. Plasma concentrations and area under the serum concentration-time curve (AUC) reportedly are dose proportional in the ipilimumab dosage range of 0.3–10 mg/kg with minimal systemic accumulation when administered every 3 weeks. Steady-state concentrations are reached by the third infusion dose and terminal half-life is approximately 14.7 days. Systemic clearance of ipilimumab increases with increasing body weight, but this is not considered clinically important when the drug is dosed based on body weight. Clearance of the drug is not affected by age, gender, anti-ipilimumab antibody status, previous antineoplastic therapy, baseline lactate dehydrogenase concentrations, human leukocyte antigen (HLA)-A2*0201 allele status, performance status, or concomitant use of budesonide. Renal impairment (i.e., baseline creatinine clearance of 29 mL/min or greater) did not have a clinically important effect on the pharmacokinetics of ipilimumab. In patients with various degrees of hepatic impairment, baseline serum ALT, AST, and total bilirubin concentrations also did not have a clinically important effect on the pharmacokinetics of the drug.

Advice to Patients

Risk of severe, and potentially fatal, immune-mediated adverse reactions, including enterocolitis, hepatitis, dermatitis, neuropathy, and endocrinopathy. (See REMS.)

Importance of promptly contacting clinician if signs or symptoms of immune-mediated reactions (e.g., changes in bowel movements or diarrhea, rash or pruritus, weakness or paresthesia, fatigue, headache, mental status changes, abdominal pain, hypotension) occur.

Importance of advising patient to read the manufacturer's medication guide before beginning treatment and each time the drug is administered.

Importance of women informing clinicians if they are or plan to become pregnant or plan to breast-feed. Ipilimumab may cause fetal harm. Importance of advising nursing women not to breast-feed during therapy with the drug.

Importance of informing clinicians of existing or contemplated concomitant therapy, including prescription and OTC drugs, as well as any concomitant illnesses, including autoimmune disease, history of organ transplantation, or liver damage.

Importance of informing patients of other important precautionary information. (See Cautions.)

Overview® (see Users Guide). For additional information on this drug until a more detailed monograph is developed and published, the manufacturer's labeling should be consulted. It is *essential* that the manufacturer's labeling be consulted for more detailed information on usual cautions, precautions, contraindications, potential drug interactions, laboratory test interferences, and acute toxicity.

Preparations

Excipients in commercially available drug preparations may have clinically important effects in some individuals; consult specific product labeling for details.

Ipilimumab (recombinant)

Parenteral		
Injection concentrate, for IV infusion only	5 mg/mL (50 or 200 mg)	Yervoy®, Bristol-Myers Squibb

Irinotecan Hydrochloride

■ Irinotecan, a type I DNA topoisomerase inhibitor, is an antineoplastic agent.

Uses

Irinotecan is commercially available in 2 types of formulations: conventional (nonencapsulated) and liposomal irinotecan hydrochloride. The efficacy and safety of irinotecan for each indication is based on research and clinical experience using a specific formulation.

■ **GI Cancers** ***Combination Therapy for Colorectal Cancer*** Conventional irinotecan hydrochloride is used as a component of first-line therapy in combination with fluorouracil and leucovorin for the treatment of metastatic carcinoma of the colon or rectum.

The current indication for use of conventional irinotecan in combination therapy for advanced colorectal cancer is based principally on data from 2 phase 3, multinational, randomized, controlled trials evaluating the combination of conventional irinotecan with fluorouracil and leucovorin compared with fluorouracil and leucovorin alone. In both studies, the addition of irinotecan to fluorouracil and leucovorin prolonged survival and increased objective response rate and time to tumor progression.

In a randomized trial involving 3 treatment arms, combination therapy with conventional irinotecan and rapid IV ("bolus") fluorouracil/leucovorin weekly for 4 weeks every 6 weeks was compared with a standard regimen of rapid IV ("bolus") fluorouracil/leucovorin daily for 5 consecutive days every 4 weeks and with conventional irinotecan alone weekly for 4 weeks every 6 weeks. Higher confirmed objective response rate (39 vs 21%), longer median time to disease progression (7 vs 4.3 months), and prolonged median survival (14.8 vs 12.6 months) were observed in patients receiving combination therapy with irinotecan and fluorouracil/leucovorin compared with fluorouracil/leucovorin alone. This difference in survival with the triple-drug regimen was noted even though 56% of the patients receiving fluorouracil/leucovorin received an irinotecan-based regimen after the conclusion of the study. Outcome was similar for patients receiving irinotecan alone compared with fluorouracil/leucovorin. Grade 3 diarrhea and grade 3 or 4 vomiting occurred more frequently in patients receiving the irinotecan-containing combination regimen, whereas grade 3 or 4 mucositis, grade 4 neutropenia, and neutropenic fever were more common in patients receiving fluorouracil/leucovorin. No difference between the irinotecan-combination and fluorouracil/leucovorin treatment groups was observed in a quality-of-life analysis, and the incidence of treatment-related mortality was approximately 1% in each of the 3 groups.

In another randomized trial, the addition of conventional irinotecan to infusional fluorouracil/leucovorin increased objective response rate (35 vs 22%), median time to disease progression (6.7 vs 4.4 months) and median survival (17.4 vs 14.1 months). Diarrhea, neutropenia, leukopenia, and asthenia occurred with greater frequency and severity in patients receiving irinotecan-based combination chemotherapy compared with those receiving fluorouracil/leucovorin alone.

Higher rates of hospitalization, neutropenic fever, thromboembolism, treatment discontinuance during the first cycle, and early deaths were associated with a baseline performance status of 2 (vs 0 or 1) regardless of treatment regimen. Diarrhea and neutropenia occurred frequently and were often severe in patients receiving irinotecan-based combination therapy or fluorouracil/leucovorin alone; comparison of data from the randomized trial including a group of patients receiving irinotecan alone reveals that nausea, vomiting, and alopecia each occurs at a higher incidence or with greater severity in patients receiving irinotecan, whereas neutropenic fever and mucositis are more commonly associated with fluorouracil/leucovorin.

The optimal dosage regimen for conventional irinotecan-based combination therapy has not been established. An unexpectedly high rate of death associated with use of the conventional irinotecan and rapid IV ("bolus") fluorouracil/leucovorin regimen (3 times the rate of death in the comparative regimens) resulted in the suspension of enrollment in 2 randomized trials (one for metastatic colon cancer and one for adjuvant treatment of resectable colon cancer). Most of the deaths occurred during or immediately after the first 6-week cycle of treatment, particularly during the first 3–4 weeks, and were attributed to the combined effect of several moderate or severe toxicities described either as a GI syndrome or as a vascular syndrome. (See GI Toxicity and Cardiovascular Toxicity under Dosage: Dosage Modification for Toxicity and Contraindications for Continued Therapy, in Dosage and Administration.) A direct comparison of the safety and efficacy of the 2 regimens has not been performed; however, lower rates of treatment-related mortality have been reported when fluorouracil was administered by IV infusion.

Monotherapy for Colorectal Cancer Conventional irinotecan hydrochloride is used as a single agent for the treatment of metastatic carcinoma of the colon or rectum in patients whose disease has recurred or progressed following initial therapy with fluorouracil-based antineoplastic regimens. The drug originally became commercially available in the US under the principles and procedures of the FDA's accelerated review policy that allows approval based on effects on a clinical endpoint (e.g., tumor shrinkage) other than survival, irreversible morbidity, or quality of life pending completion of studies to establish and define the degree of clinical benefit. Conventional irinotecan received full approval following the completion of randomized trials demonstrating prolonged survival in patients receiving the drug for this use.

Evidence of clinical benefit of conventional irinotecan is based principally on data from 2 randomized trials in which conventional irinotecan 300–350 mg/m² was administered once every 3 weeks and in 3 phase 2 trials in which conventional irinotecan 125 mg/m² was administered once weekly for 4 weeks followed by a 2-week rest period. In 2 randomized trials involving a total of 535 patients with metastatic carcinoma of the colon or rectum that recurred or progressed following fluorouracil-containing chemotherapy, survival was prolonged in those receiving conventional irinotecan compared with those receiving fluorouracil or supportive care.

In a randomized trial of patients with metastatic colorectal cancer that progressed within 6 months following treatment with fluorouracil, patients receiving conventional irinotecan 300–350 mg/m² as a single 90-minute infusion once every 3 weeks and supportive care had longer median survival (9.2 vs 6.5 months) than those receiving supportive care alone. Patients receiving irinotecan had longer time to development of pain (6.9 vs 2 months), longer time to deterioration of performance status (5.7 vs 3.3 months), and longer time to weight loss of 5% or greater (6.4 vs 4.2 months) compared with those receiving supportive care alone; although patients receiving irinotecan had a higher rate of diarrhea than those receiving supportive care alone, other quality-of-life measures were comparable or better for patients receiving the drug. In addition, patients with a baseline performance status of 1 or 2 receiving irinotecan and supportive care or supportive care alone showed an improvement in performance status of 33.3 or 11.3%, respectively. Supportive care included the use of anti-infectives, analgesics, corticosteroids, transfusions, psychotherapy, or any other symptomatic therapy as clinically indicated, including palliative radiation therapy. Approximately 21% of patients treated with irinotecan and supportive care also received other chemotherapy regimens, and 31% of patients treated with supportive care also received various chemotherapy regimens.

In another randomized trial, patients with recurrent or refractory metastatic colorectal cancer receiving conventional irinotecan 300–350 mg/m² as a single 90-minute IV infusion once every 3 weeks had longer median survival (10.8 vs 8.5 months) than those receiving fluorouracil by continuous IV infusion. The rate of survival at 1 year was higher in patients receiving irinotecan compared with those receiving fluorouracil (45 vs 32%); the quality of life as assessed by the European Organization of Research and Treatment of Cancer

Quality of Life Questionnaire (EORTC QLQ-C30) was similar and both treatments were equally well tolerated.

In an open-label, single-agent, multicenter study involving 132 patients with metastatic cancer of the colon or rectum that recurred or progressed following therapy with fluorouracil-containing regimens, the intent-to-treat response rate was 12% in patients receiving conventional irinotecan at a starting dose of 350 mg/m^2 administered by 30-minute IV infusion once every 3 weeks. In 3 phase 2 clinical trials, 304 patients with metastatic colorectal cancer who previously had been treated with a fluorouracil-containing antineoplastic regimen received conventional irinotecan 125 mg/m^2 once weekly. These open-label, single-agent trials evaluated the surrogate endpoint of tumor response rate and did *not* provide information on actual clinical benefit (e.g., decrease in disease-related symptoms, increase in survival) of irinotecan therapy. Patients received irinotecan in repeated 6-week cycles, each cycle consisting of once-weekly, 90-minute IV infusions of irinotecan for 4 weeks followed by a 2-week drug-free period. In one trial, an initial weekly irinotecan hydrochloride dose of 150 mg/m^2 was administered to a few patients; however, these patients developed unacceptably high rates of severe diarrhea, dehydration, and febrile neutropenia, and subsequent patients in the trial received an initial dose of 125 mg/m^2. In another trial, the initial dose of irinotecan hydrochloride was reduced from 125 to 100 mg/m^2 to evaluate the therapeutic ratio of this initial dose. In these trials, 34, 63, or 3% of patients received initial irinotecan hydrochloride doses of 100, 125, or 150 mg/m^2, respectively.

Intent-to-treat analysis of the pooled data from the 3 trials revealed an overall response rate of 15% (2 complete and 27 partial responses) among patients who received the recommended initial conventional irinotecan hydrochloride dose of 125 mg/m^2; however, the response rate was only 7.8% among patients who received an initial dose of 100 mg/m^2. More than 50% of patients responding to irinotecan in these trials had failed to respond to previous fluorouracil-based regimens administered for colorectal cancer with metastases. The median response duration for patients receiving an initial irinotecan hydrochloride dose of 125 mg/m^2 was 5.8 months (range: 2.6–15.1 months). Among patients with disease responding to irinotecan, all but 2 patients achieved responses by the second 6-week cycle of irinotecan therapy; one response was observed by the fourth and one after the eighth cycle of therapy.

Among patients receiving irinotecan on a weekly dosage schedule in phase 2 trials, response rates were similar regardless of gender, age (greater than or less than 65 years), primary cancer site (colon or rectum), history of previous pelvic radiation therapy, or number of metastatic lesions (single or multiple). The response rate among patients with a performance status of zero (i.e., fully active; able to perform all predisease activities without restriction) was 18.5%, while the response rate among those with a performance status of 1 (i.e., restricted in physically strenuous activity but ambulatory and able to perform work of a light or sedentary nature [e.g., light housework, office work]) or 2 (i.e., ambulatory and capable of all self-care but unable to carry out any work activities; up and about more than 50% of waking hours) was 8.2%. Patients with a performance status of 3 or 4 have not been studied.

■ Pancreatic Cancer Liposomal irinotecan hydrochloride is used in combination with fluorouracil and leucovorin for the treatment of metastatic adenocarcinoma of the pancreas in patients whose disease has progressed following gemcitabine-based chemotherapy; liposomal irinotecan is designated an orphan drug by FDA for the treatment of this cancer.

The current indication for use of liposomal irinotecan in combination therapy with fluorouracil and leucovorin for the treatment of metastatic adenocarcinoma of the pancreas in patients whose disease has progressed following gemcitabine-based chemotherapy is based principally on data from a randomized, controlled, open-label phase 3 study (NAPOLI-1). In patients with previously treated metastatic adenocarcinoma of the pancreas, liposomal irinotecan has been shown to prolong overall survival compared with fluorouracil and leucovorin alone.

In this study, 417 patients were randomized in a 1:1:1 ratio to receive liposomal irinotecan (70 mg/m^2 by IV infusion over 90 minutes) in combination with fluorouracil and leucovorin (leucovorin 400 mg/m^2 by IV infusion over 30 minutes followed by fluorouracil 2.4 g/m^2 by IV infusion over 46 hours) administered every 2 weeks, liposomal irinotecan (100 mg/m^2 by IV infusion over 90 minutes) administered every 3 weeks, *or* fluorouracil and leucovorin (leucovorin 200 mg/m^2 by IV infusion over 30 minutes followed by fluorouracil 2 g/m^2 by IV infusion over 24 hours) administered on days 1, 8, 15, and 22 of each 6-week cycle. The initial dosage of liposomal irinotecan was reduced by 20 mg/m^2 in patients who were homozygous for the UGT1A1*28 allele; however, the dose was increased to the full dosage following the first cycle if adverse events did not occur. Treatment was continued until disease progression or unacceptable toxicity occurred. The primary measure of efficacy was overall survival. The median age of patients was 63 years; 53% had a baseline Karnofsky performance status of 90–100, 67% had liver metastasis, and 31% had lung metastasis. All patients enrolled in the study had received prior therapy with gemcitabine; 54% had received prior therapy with gemcitabine in combination with another agent, and 13% had received prior therapy with gemcitabine in combination with albumin-bound paclitaxel.

In this study, patients randomized to receive liposomal irinotecan in combination with fluorouracil and leucovorin had longer median overall survival (6.1 versus 4.2 months) and progression-free survival (3.1 versus 1.5 months) compared with patients receiving fluorouracil and leucovorin alone; however, improvement in overall survival was not demonstrated in patients receiving liposomal irinotecan alone compared with those receiving fluorouracil and leucovorin (4.9 versus 4.2 months, respectively). In addition, patients receiving liposomal irinotecan in combination with fluorouracil and leucovorin had a higher overall response rate compared with those receiving fluorouracil and leucovorin alone (7.7 versus 0.8%, respectively). Results of a subgroup analysis (based on age, disease stage, Karnofsky performance status, baseline albumin concentration, previous lines of therapy for metastatic disease, prior exposure to radiation therapy or surgery, prior exposure to fluorouracil-, irinotecan-, or platinum-based chemotherapy) suggested that the drug's effect on overall survival was consistent across most subgroups.

■ Small Cell Lung Cancer Conventional irinotecan is used in combination with cisplatin for the initial treatment of extensive small cell lung cancer†.

A phase 3, randomized trial was terminated early when interim analysis of the data showed that median overall survival was prolonged (12.8 versus 9.4 months) and the rate of survival at 2 years was higher (19.5 versus 5.2%) in patients receiving irinotecan and cisplatin versus etoposide and cisplatin for extensive small cell lung cancer. Patients received a regimen of conventional irinotecan 60 mg/m^2 on days 1, 8, and 15 and cisplatin 60 mg/m^2 on day 1 during a 4-week cycle for 4 cycles; or a regimen of etoposide 100 mg/m^2 on days 1, 2, and 3 and cisplatin 80 mg/m^2 on day 1 during a 3-week cycle for 4 cycles. Severe or life-threatening diarrhea occurred more frequently in patients receiving irinotecan and cisplatin, whereas severe or life-threatening myelosuppression occurred more frequently in those receiving etoposide and cisplatin. Interim analysis of another randomized trial using a modified irinotecan-containing regimen suggests that overall survival is similar in patients receiving a regimen of either irinotecan and cisplatin or etoposide and cisplatin.

In phase 2 studies, objective response rates of 16–47% have been observed in patients receiving conventional irinotecan alone, typically at initial doses of 100–125 mg/m^2 infused IV over a period of 90 minutes once weekly, for refractory or relapsed small cell lung cancer. Higher doses of irinotecan are associated with increased frequency and severity of adverse effects, particularly neutropenia.

Because the current prognosis for small cell lung cancer is unsatisfactory regardless of stage and despite considerable diagnostic and therapeutic advances, all patients with this cancer are candidates for inclusion in clinical trials at the time of diagnosis.

■ Cervical Cancer Conventional irinotecan is being investigated as an active agent in the treatment of metastatic or recurrent cervical cancer†. Objective response rates of 13–21% have been reported with use of irinotecan as a single agent for advanced squamous cell carcinoma of the cervix. Although no responses to irinotecan were observed in one small uncontrolled phase 2 study of patients with platinum-resistant advanced squamous cell carcinoma of the cervix, responses to the drug have been reported in similar patients in another phase 2 study. The benefit of combination chemotherapy regimens vs single-agent therapy (e.g., cisplatin alone) has not been fully established, and further study is needed to determine the role of irinotecan in the treatment of advanced cervical cancer. (See Uses: Cervical Cancer in Cisplatin 10:00 for an overview of therapy for cervical cancer.)

Dosage and Administration

Irinotecan is commercially available in 2 types of formulations: conventional (nonencapsulated) and liposomal irinotecan hydrochloride. The properties of irinotecan may differ according to formulation, and the dosage and reconstitution instructions for irinotecan are specific to formulation. Liposomal irinotecan hydrochloride may *not* be substituted for other formulations of irinotecan hydrochloride.

Dosage of liposomal irinotecan hydrochloride is expressed in terms of anhydrous irinotecan, whereas dosage of conventional irinotecan hydrochloride is expressed in terms of the hydrated salt.

In addition to GI and hematologic toxicity, other severe adverse effects have occurred in patients receiving conventional or liposomal irinotecan. Hypersensitivity reactions, including severe anaphylactic or anaphylactoid reactions, have been reported. Renal impairment and acute renal failure have occurred, usually in patients who became volume-depleted from severe vomiting and/or diarrhea. Cardiovascular and thromboembolic events also have been reported in patients receiving conventional irinotecan. (See Cardiovascular Toxicity under Dosage: Dosage Modification for Toxicity and Contraindications for Continued Therapy, in Dosage and Administration.)

The manufacturer of conventional irinotecan recommends close monitoring in patients older than 65 years of age because of increased risk of treatment-related toxicity, such as early and late diarrhea, during therapy with conventional irinotecan. Patients receiving conventional irinotecan/fluorouracil/leucovorin therapy should be monitored closely (e.g., weekly assessment), particularly during the first cycle of treatment, since most of the treatment-related toxicities leading to early death occurred within the first 3–4 weeks. Changes in serum electrolytes and/or acid-base balance, including hyponatremia or hypernatremia, hypokalemia, and/or metabolic acidosis, may be an early indication of treatment-related toxicity; patients with abnormalities in serum sodium, potassium, and/or bicarbonate concentrations, with or without concomitant elevations in BUN or serum creatinine concentrations, should be evaluated carefully for dehydration and receive aggressive medical management, including fluid and electrolyte replacement.

Liposomal irinotecan hydrochloride can only be obtained through select specialty distributors. Clinicians may consult the Onivyde® website for specific availability information (https://www.onivyde.com).

■ **Administration** Conventional or liposomal irinotecan hydrochloride is administered by IV infusion. Care should be taken to avoid extravasation of conventional irinotecan, and the infusion site should be monitored for signs of inflammation. Should manifestations of extravasation appear, the infusion should immediately be stopped and restarted in another vein. The manufacturer of conventional irinotecan recommends that extravasation of the drug be treated by flushing the infusion site promptly with sterile water and applying an ice pack.

Procedures for proper handling and disposal of antineoplastic drugs (e.g., use of protective clothing and gloves) should be used to avoid exposure to conventional or liposomal irinotecan during preparation of IV solutions. If conventional irinotecan hydrochloride for injection concentrate or a solution of the drug comes in contact with the skin or mucous membranes, the skin should be washed immediately and thoroughly with soap and water or the mucosa should be flushed with copious amounts of water.

Conventional Irinotecan Hydrochloride *Commercially available conventional irinotecan hydrochloride for injection concentrate must be diluted prior to IV administration.* For IV infusion, the manufacturer recommends diluting the drug in 5% dextrose injection to a final irinotecan hydrochloride concentration of 0.12–2.8 mg/mL. In most clinical trials, the dose of conventional irinotecan hydrochloride was diluted in 250–500 mL of 5% dextrose injection. The manufacturer states that although 5% dextrose injection is the preferred diluent, 0.9% sodium chloride injection also may be used for dilution of conventional irinotecan. The diluted solution of conventional irinotecan should be infused over a period of 90 minutes; more rapid infusion rates may increase the likelihood of cholinergic symptoms (e.g., early diarrhea, diaphoresis, flushing, abdominal cramping, rhinitis, increased salivation, miosis, lacrimation).

Solutions of conventional irinotecan hydrochloride prepared in 5% dextrose injection are physically and chemically stable for up to 24 hours when stored at room temperature (approximately 25°C) under ambient fluorescent lighting or for up to 48 hours when protected from light and refrigerated at 2–8°C. For conventional irinotecan hydrochloride solutions prepared in 5% dextrose injection, the manufacturer recommends administration of such drug solutions within 24 hours if refrigerated or within 4 hours if maintained at room temperature because of the potential for microbial contamination during preparation of the admixtures; however, if dilution is performed under strict aseptic conditions (e.g., under laminar airflow conditions), administration of solutions prepared in 5% dextrose injection and stored at room temperature should be completed within 12 hours. Solutions of conventional irinotecan hydrochloride prepared in 0.9% sodium chloride are stable for up to 24 hours when stored at room temperature (approximately 25°C) under ambient fluorescent lighting. The manufacturer states that solutions of conventional irinotecan hydrochloride prepared in 0.9% sodium chloride may occasionally develop visible particulates when refrigerated at 2–8°C; therefore, solutions prepared in sodium chloride injection should *not* be refrigerated but should be stored at room temperature and used within 4 hours. However, if dilution is performed under strict aseptic conditions (e.g., under laminar airflow conditions), administration of solutions prepared in 0.9% sodium chloride injection and stored at room temperature should be completed within 12 hours. Freezing of commercially available conventional irinotecan hydrochloride for injection concentrate or IV admixtures of the drug may result in formation of a precipitate and should be avoided.

Conventional irinotecan hydrochloride for injection concentrate should be inspected visually for particulate matter in the vial and again in the syringe when transferring the drug solution to prepare admixtures of the drug. The manufacturer states that other drugs should not be added to IV solutions of conventional irinotecan hydrochloride.

Liposomal Irinotecan Hydrochloride *Liposomal irinotecan hydrochloride for injection concentrate must be diluted prior to IV infusion.* The concentrate should be diluted in 500 mL of 5% dextrose injection or 0.9% sodium chloride injection. The diluted solution of liposomal irinotecan should be infused over a period of 90 minutes. The manufacturer states that in-line filters should *not* be used during administration of liposomal irinotecan hydrochloride. Any unused solution should be discarded.

Solutions of liposomal irinotecan hydrochloride should be administered within 24 hours of preparation when stored under refrigeration at 2–8°C or within 4 hours when stored at room temperature. The diluted drug should be protected from light and should *not* be frozen. Prior to administration, the diluted solution should be allowed to come to room temperature.

■ **Dosage** Because irinotecan often causes neutropenia, leukopenia, and anemia, which can be severe, the drug should *not* be used in patients with severe bone marrow failure. In addition, concurrent radiation therapy has not been adequately studied and is not recommended. Because conventional irinotecan hydrochloride for injection concentrate contains sorbitol, the drug should *not* be given to patients with hereditary fructose intolerance. Treatment with conventional or liposomal irinotecan should *not* be initiated until resolution of bowel obstruction.

Irinotecan is considered an antineoplastic agent of *moderate emetic risk* (i.e., incidence of emesis without antiemetics exceeds 30% but does not exceed 90%). Because nausea and/or vomiting occur frequently in patients receiving irinotecan therapy and may be severe, effective antiemetic therapy (e.g., dexamethasone 8 mg and a 5-HT_3 serotonin receptor antagonist such as palonosetron) should be administered orally or IV at least 30 minutes prior to irinotecan therapy. Additional oral antiemetic therapy also should be considered for subsequent home use by the patient as needed. Unless clinically contraindicated, clinicians should consider prophylactic or therapeutic administration of antimuscarinic therapy (e.g., 0.25–1 mg of atropine sulfate by IV or subcutaneous injection) for patients experiencing rhinitis, increased salivation, miosis, lacrimation, diaphoresis, flushing, bradycardia, abdominal cramping, or early diarrhea (i.e., diarrhea with an onset during or shortly after [within 24 hours of] administration of irinotecan); such symptoms are expected to occur more frequently in patients receiving higher doses of irinotecan.

Dosage adjustment may be required according to the patient's status for activity of UGT1A1, a uridine diphosphate-glucuronosyltransferase (UGT) enzyme involved in the metabolism of SN-38, an active metabolite of irinotecan. In patients who are homozygous for the UGT1A1*28 allele, UGT1A1 activity is reduced, and the risk of irinotecan-induced neutropenia is increased; reduction in the initial dosage of conventional irinotecan by at least one dose level should be considered in such patients. The optimal dosage reduction for conventional irinotecan has not been established, and subsequent dosage adjustment may be necessary according to patient tolerance. The recommended initial dose of liposomal irinotecan in patients with metastatic adenocarcinoma of the pancreas who are homozygous for the UGT1A1*28 allele is 50 mg/m^2; the dose may be increased to 70 mg/m^2 as tolerated during subsequent cycles. In patients who are heterozygous for the UGT1A1*28 allele, UGT1A1 activity is intermediate, and the risk of irinotecan-induced neutropenia may be increased. Clinical results have been variable with conventional irinotecan.

Inadvertent overdosage of conventional irinotecan has occurred in several patients, including at least one fatal case, because the manufacturer's label on the vial was misread. Therefore, particular care should be taken to ensure that the correct dose of the drug is administered, including careful attention to the concentration of conventional irinotecan for injection concentrate present in the vial and the appropriate volume needed to provide the prescribed dose.

Patients should be instructed to contact their clinician if any of the following occur during irinotecan therapy: diarrhea for the first time during treatment; black or bloody stools; symptoms of dehydration, such as lightheadedness, dizziness, or faintness; inability to take fluids by mouth because of nausea or vomiting; inability to control diarrhea within 24 hours; new-onset cough or dyspnea; manifestations of severe hypersensitivity reactions; or fever or evidence of infection. Patients should be warned about the potential for dizziness or visual disturbances that may occur within 24 hours following the administration of conventional irinotecan and be advised not to drive or operate machinery if these symptoms occur. Patients also should be alerted to the possibility of alopecia during conventional or liposomal irinotecan therapy.

Colorectal Cancer **Combination Therapy.** For use in a combination regimen as first-line therapy for metastatic carcinoma of the colon or rectum, conventional irinotecan is administered with leucovorin and fluorouracil. For all regimens, the dose of leucovorin should be administered immediately following conventional irinotecan, and then followed immediately by administration of fluorouracil. The optimal dosage regimen for conventional irinotecan-based combination therapy has not been established; an unexpectedly high rate of death has been reported in 2 clinical trials using irinotecan with fluorouracil given by rapid IV injection ("bolus"), and some clinicians prefer administration of fluorouracil by IV infusion in this regimen. (See Combination Therapy for Colorectal Cancer in Uses: GI Cancers.)

In regimen 1, the initial dose of conventional irinotecan hydrochloride is 125 mg/m^2 infused IV over a period of 90 minutes followed by leucovorin 20 mg/m^2 given by rapid IV injection and then fluorouracil 500 mg/m^2 given by rapid IV injection ("bolus"). Treatment is given weekly for 4 weeks on days 1, 8, 15, and 22 during a 6-week cycle; the next cycle begins on day 43.

In regimen 2, the initial dose of conventional irinotecan hydrochloride is 180 mg/m^2 infused IV over a period of 90 minutes followed by leucovorin 200 mg/m^2 infused IV over 2 hours, then fluorouracil 400 mg/m^2 by rapid IV injection ("bolus"), and then fluorouracil 600 mg/m^2 infused IV over 22 hours. Treatment is given during a 6-week cycle with administration of conventional irinotecan on days 1, 15, and 29, and administration of the leucovorin and fluorouracil (rapid IV injection ["bolus"] and infusional) component of the regimen on days 1, 2, 15, 16, 29, and 30, with the next cycle beginning on day 43.

Patients who have received prior pelvic or abdominal radiation therapy, who have a performance status of 2, or who have modestly elevated baseline total serum bilirubin concentrations (i.e., 1–2 mg/dL) are at increased risk for irinotecan-induced toxicity such as grade 3 or 4 neutropenia; the manufacturer states that reduction of the initial dose of conventional irinotecan hydrochloride by one dose level (e.g., to 100 mg/m^2 for regimen 1 or to 150 mg/m^2 for regimen 2) should be considered in such patients. The manufacturer states that specific dosage recommendations for conventional irinotecan for patients with baseline total serum bilirubin concentrations exceeding 2 mg/dL currently are not available.

During a cycle of therapy or when initiating a subsequent cycle of therapy, the dose level should be reduced as necessary based on modification for toxicity. (See Table 1 and Table 2.) Further reductions in dose level in decrements of 20% may be warranted in patients who continue to experience toxicity. Unless intolerable toxicity develops, treatment with additional cycles may be administered every 6 weeks in patients who continue to experience clinical benefit.

Table 1. Dosage Regimens and Dosage Modifications for Conventional Irinotecan-based Combination Therapy for Metastatic Colon or Rectal Cancer

Regimen/Agent	Initial Dosage and Dosage Modifications for Combination Therapy (mg/m²)		
	Initial Dosage	Reduced Dosage Level 1	Reduced Dosage Level 2
Regimen 1 [a]			
Irinotecan hydrochloride	125	100	75
Leucovorin	20	20	20
Fluorouracil	500	400	300
Regimen 2 [b]			
Irinotecan hydrochloride	180	150	120
Leucovorin	200	200	200
Fluorouracil bolus	400	320	240
Fluorouracil infusion	600	480	360

[a] Treatment on days 1, 8, 15, and 22.

[b] Administration of irinotecan on days 1, 15, and 29, and administration of leucovorin, bolus fluorouracil, and infusional fluorouracil on days 1, 2, 15, 16, 29, and 30.

Outside of a well-designed clinical trial, irinotecan should not be used in combination with the "Mayo clinic" regimen of rapid IV injection ("bolus") fluorouracil/leucovorin (i.e., administration for 4–5 consecutive days every 4 weeks) because of increased toxicity, including deaths.

Monotherapy. For the treatment of metastatic carcinoma of the colon or rectum in patients whose disease has recurred or progressed following fluorouracil-based antineoplastic therapy, conventional irinotecan may be administered on a weekly dosage schedule or once every 3 weeks with doses specific to the selected dosage schedule.

The recommended initial dose of conventional irinotecan hydrochloride as a single agent for the treatment of metastatic carcinoma of the colon or rectum in patients receiving the drug on a *weekly dosage schedule* is 125 mg/m² infused IV over a period of 90 minutes. The dose of conventional irinotecan is administered once weekly for 4 weeks followed by a 2-week rest period. Additional cycles (i.e., weekly doses for 4 weeks followed by a 2-week rest period) may be administered every 6 weeks in patients who attain a response or whose disease remains stable, provided intolerable toxicity does not develop.

The recommended initial dose of conventional irinotecan hydrochloride for the treatment of metastatic carcinoma of the colon or rectum in patients receiving the drug *once every 3 weeks* is 350 mg/m² infused IV over a period of 90 minutes. The dose of conventional irinotecan is administered once every 3 weeks for as long as intolerable toxicity does not occur and the patient continues to experience clinical benefit.

Patients who have received prior pelvic or abdominal radiation therapy, who have a performance status of 2, or who have modestly elevated baseline total serum bilirubin concentrations (i.e., 1–2 mg/dL) are at increased risk for irinotecan-induced toxicity such as grade 3 or 4 neutropenia; the manufacturer states that reduction of the initial dose of conventional irinotecan hydrochloride by one dose level (e.g., to 100 mg/m² for the weekly dosage schedule or to 300 mg/m² for the once-every-3-weeks dosage schedule) should be considered in such patients. A reduced initial dose of 300 mg/m² also is recommended for patients 70 years of age or older who are receiving the once-every-3-weeks dosage schedule of conventional irinotecan hydrochloride; however, the manufacturer states that geriatric patients receiving the weekly dosage schedule of conventional irinotecan may receive the usual initial dose of the drug. Reduction in the initial dose of conventional irinotecan may be considered in patients with baseline total serum bilirubin concentrations exceeding 2 mg/dL; the manufacturer states that specific dosage recommendations for conventional irinotecan for such patients currently are not available.

Pancreatic Cancer For use in a combination regimen for metastatic adenocarcinoma of the pancreas that has progressed following gemcitabine-based therapy, liposomal irinotecan is administered with leucovorin and fluorouracil. Liposomal irinotecan is *not* indicated as a single agent for the treatment of metastatic adenocarcinoma of the pancreas.

The recommended initial dose of liposomal irinotecan is 70 mg/m² infused IV over a period of 90 minutes followed by leucovorin 400 mg/m² infused IV over 30 minutes and then fluorouracil 2.4 g/m² infused IV over 46 hours. Treatment is repeated every 2 weeks.

The manufacturer makes no specific dosage recommendations for liposomal irinotecan for patients with total serum bilirubin concentrations exceeding the upper limit of normal (ULN).

Dosage Modification for Toxicity and Contraindications for Continued Therapy Dosage of conventional or liposomal irinotecan should be modified as necessary based on individual patient tolerance; the patient should be monitored carefully to obtain optimum therapeutic response with minimum adverse effects. Among those receiving conventional or liposomal irinotecan-based combination therapy, doses of fluorouracil also should be modified as necessary based on individual patient tolerance.

The manufacturer states that a new cycle of conventional irinotecan therapy should not be undertaken until the granulocyte count has recovered to at least 1500/mm³, the platelet count has recovered to at least 100,000/mm³, and treatment-related diarrhea has fully resolved. If the patient experiences multiple toxicities, adjustment of conventional irinotecan hydrochloride dose within a cycle of therapy and prior to starting a new cycle of therapy should be based on the preceding toxicity requiring the largest dose reduction. Treatment should be delayed for 1–2 weeks to allow for recovery from treatment-related toxicities. If the patient experiences an irinotecan-induced toxicity that does not resolve after delaying drug administration for 2 weeks, discontinuance of the drug should be considered.

Among patients receiving conventional irinotecan as a single agent, initial doses of conventional irinotecan hydrochloride are based on body surface area alone, but subsequent doses within a cycle of therapy or for a new cycle of therapy in patients receiving the drug on a *weekly dosage schedule* should be adjusted in increments of 25–50 mg/m² to a dose within the range of 50–150 mg/m² based on the worst toxicity encountered with the previous dose of conventional irinotecan; subsequent doses for a new cycle of therapy in patients receiving the drug *once every 3 weeks* should be decreased in increments of 50 mg/m² to a dose as low as 200 mg/m² based on the worst toxicity encountered with the previous dose of conventional irinotecan. If the patient experiences no toxicity within a cycle of therapy using the once-every-3-weeks dosage schedule, the current conventional irinotecan hydrochloride dose should be maintained for the subsequent cycle of therapy. If the patient experiences no toxicity during an entire 6-week cycle of therapy using the weekly dosage schedule, the dose of conventional irinotecan hydrochloride may be increased by 25 mg/m² at the start of the next cycle; however, the dose should not exceed 150 mg/m².

The Recommended Dosage Modifications tables (Tables 2–4) describe recommended modifications in conventional irinotecan hydrochloride dose based on commonly observed toxicities of the drug for patients receiving combination or single-agent therapy with the drug. The dose-limiting toxicities of conventional irinotecan are diarrhea and neutropenia.

Recommended dosage modifications for liposomal irinotecan based on observed toxicities of the drug are described in the following sections on specific types and severities of toxicity.

For a more complete discussion of dosage modifications, cautions, and precautions associated with conventional or liposomal irinotecan therapy, the respective manufacturer's labeling should be consulted.

GI Toxicity. Conventional or liposomal irinotecan may induce both early and late forms of diarrhea, both of which may be severe. Early diarrhea (occurring during or within 24 hours of administration of conventional or liposomal irinotecan) is cholinergic in nature and generally is transient; diarrhea may be accompanied by diaphoresis, flushing, rhinitis, increased salivation, miosis, lacrimation, bradycardia, and abdominal cramping and may be prevented or ameliorated by administration of atropine sulfate (e.g., 0.25–1 mg by IV or subcutaneous injection) unless administration of the drug is clinically contraindicated. Late diarrhea (occurring more than 24 hours after administration of conventional or liposomal irinotecan) can be life-threatening since it may be prolonged and may lead to dehydration, electrolyte imbalance, or sepsis.

Patients receiving conventional irinotecan in combination with rapid IV ("bolus") fluorouracil/leucovorin have experienced early death induced or exacerbated by treatment-related GI toxicity, typically during or immediately following the first cycle of treatment. This GI syndrome is manifested by diarrhea, nausea, vomiting, anorexia, and abdominal cramping, and is often associated with severe dehydration, neutropenia, fever, and electrolyte abnormalities. Radiographic findings include dilated bowel, air-fluid levels without anatomic obstruction, and thickened bowel wall. An independent panel of clinicians that reviewed the causes of these early deaths has recommended close monitoring and prompt, aggressive treatment of toxicity in conjunction with treatment discontinuance in patients experiencing unresolved drug-related toxicity.

Late diarrhea, as an isolated event or as part of the GI syndrome, should be treated promptly with intensive oral loperamide hydrochloride therapy (e.g., 4 mg at the onset of diarrhea, then 2 mg every 2 hours until the patient is diarrhea-free for 12 hours). Use of loperamide at these doses should not exceed 48 consecutive hours because of the risk of paralytic ileus. The efficacy of other antiperistaltic agents in the management of irinotecan-induced diarrhea is unclear. During the night, the patient may take loperamide hydrochloride 4 mg every 4 hours. Baseline bowel patterns should be documented prior to initiation of irinotecan therapy, and any increase in the frequency of bowel movements or change in stool consistency should prompt initiation of loperamide therapy. Premedication with loperamide is not recommended. If diarrhea persists for more than 24 hours despite loperamide therapy, or if diarrhea occurs with fever, some clinicians recommend a 7-day course of oral fluoroquinolone therapy. If diarrhea persists for longer than 48 hours, some clinicians advise discontinuance of loperamide and hospitalization of the patient for parenteral hydration. Prophylactic treatment with an oral fluoroquinolone also should be initiated in patients with an absolute neutrophil count below 500/mm³, even in the absence of fever or diarrhea.

Cases of late diarrhea complicated by colitis, ulceration, bleeding, ileus, and infection have occurred in patients receiving conventional irinotecan; megacolon and intestinal perforation also have been reported. Anti-infective therapy should be initiated promptly in patients who develop ileus.

Patients with bowel obstruction should *not* receive conventional or liposomal irinotecan.

Patients with diarrhea should be monitored carefully and given fluid and electrolyte replacement if they become dehydrated or anti-infective therapy if they develop ileus, fever, or severe neutropenia. Some clinicians recommend appropriate anti-infective therapy in any patient with prolonged diarrhea, regardless of neutrophil count, with treatment continued until resolution. Delayed initiation of anti-infective therapy, premature discontinuance of anti-infective therapy, or selection of inappropriate anti-infectives probably contributed to early deaths among patients receiving conventional irinotecan with rapid IV ("bolus") fluorouracil/leucovorin. Patients experiencing severe diarrhea that does not resolve to baseline bowel function for at least 24 hours without the use of antidiarrheal medications or anti-infectives should *not* receive further treatment with the conventional irinotecan/fluorouracil/leucovorin regimen.

Following the first treatment with conventional irinotecan-based 3-drug combination therapy, subsequent weekly chemotherapy treatments should be delayed until pretreatment bowel function has been restored for at least 24 hours without the need for antidiarrhea medication. If NCI grade 2, 3, or 4 late diarrhea occurs, administration of conventional irinotecan should be interrupted until the patient recovers, and subsequent doses of the drug should be reduced within the current treatment cycle. An independent panel of clinicians that reviewed the causes of early deaths in patients receiving the 3-drug regimen has recommended that the same guidelines for dosage modification be followed for abdominal cramping; if grade 2 or higher abdominal cramping occurs, treatment should be interrupted until the cramping has fully resolved, and subsequent doses of the drug should be reduced within the current treatment cycle. Among patients receiving conventional irinotecan as a single agent, subsequent doses within the treatment cycle should be reduced in those experiencing grade 2 diarrhea. If severe (NCI grade 3 or 4) diarrhea occurs, administration of conventional irinotecan should be interrupted until the patient recovers, and subsequent doses of the drug should be reduced.

If grade 2–4 diarrhea occurs in patients receiving liposomal irinotecan, therapy with the drug should be withheld until diarrhea resolves to grade 1 or less. Liposomal irinotecan therapy may then be resumed at a reduced dosage (i.e., 70 mg/m^2 reduced to 50 mg/m^2 or 50 mg/m^2 reduced to 43 mg/m^2). If grade 2–4 diarrhea recurs following dosage reduction, therapy should be withheld again until diarrhea resolves to grade 1 or less; therapy may then be resumed at a further reduced dosage (i.e., 50 mg/m^2 reduced to 43 mg/m^2 or 43 mg/m^2 reduced to 35 mg/m^2). If grade 2–4 diarrhea recurs at this reduced dosage, treatment with liposomal irinotecan should be discontinued.

Hematologic Toxicity. Conventional or liposomal irinotecan can induce severe myelosuppression, particularly neutropenia, and deaths caused by sepsis have been reported in patients treated with the drug. In studies using the weekly dosage schedule for conventional irinotecan monotherapy, patients with even modestly elevated (i.e., 1–2 mg/dL) total serum bilirubin concentrations and those who had received prior pelvic or abdominal radiation therapy were at increased risk of grade 3 or 4 neutropenia associated with the drug. The risk of myelosuppression also may be greater in patients with deficient glucuronidation of bilirubin (e.g., Gilbert's syndrome) who are receiving conventional irinotecan. Complications of neutropenia should be managed promptly with anti-infective therapy.

Therapy with conventional irinotecan should be interrupted during a treatment cycle if neutropenic fever occurs or if the absolute neutrophil count (ANC) drops below 1000/mm^3. Following recovery to an ANC of at least 1000/mm^3, subsequent doses of conventional irinotecan should be reduced according to the level of neutropenia observed (see the Recommended Dosage Modifications tables [Tables 2–4]). Blood tests should be obtained no sooner than 48 hours before scheduled treatment and trends in the ANC as well as absolute values should be considered; in patients with a rapidly falling ANC, conventional irinotecan therapy should be interrupted even if the current ANC is considered adequate to permit treatment.

The manufacturer of liposomal irinotecan recommends that complete blood cell (CBC) counts be obtained on days 1 and 8 of each cycle and more frequently if clinically indicated. Therapy with liposomal irinotecan should be interrupted if neutropenic fever occurs or if the ANC drops below 1500/mm^3. Following recovery to an ANC of at least 1500/mm^3, subsequent doses of liposomal irinotecan should be reduced if grade 3 or 4 neutropenia or neutropenic fever was observed.

Cardiovascular Toxicity. Patients receiving conventional irinotecan in combination with rapid IV ("bolus") fluorouracil/leucovorin have experienced early death induced or exacerbated by treatment-related cardiovascular toxicity, typically during or immediately following the first cycle of treatment. This vascular syndrome is characterized by an acute, fatal myocardial infarction, pulmonary embolus, or cerebrovascular accident that occurs during or shortly after receiving chemotherapy. An underlying cardiovascular or thromboembolic condition, if present, was considered stable or well-compensated at the time of treatment. Vascular syndrome may occur as an isolated event or in association with GI or other toxicities of conventional irinotecan-based therapy. Cardiovascular and thromboembolic events also have been reported in patients receiving conventional irinotecan with fluorouracil administered as an IV infusion.

Pulmonary Toxicity. Interstitial lung disease (ILD), sometimes fatal, has been reported in patients receiving conventional irinotecan-based therapy. Patients who have preexisting lung disease or those who have received pneumotoxic drugs, radiation therapy, or hematopoietic agents (i.e., granulocyte or granulocyte-macrophage colony-stimulating factors [G-CSF, GM-CSF]) may be at greater risk for ILD. Patients at risk for developing ILD should be closely monitored for respiratory symptoms before and during irinotecan-based therapy. If manifestations of ILD (i.e., new or progressive dyspnea, cough, or fever) occur, therapy with conventional or liposomal irinotecan should be withheld pending results of clinical investigation. Conventional or liposomal irinotecan should be discontinued in patients who are diagnosed with treatment-related ILD.

Hypersensitivity Reactions. If severe hypersensitivity reactions, including anaphylaxis, occur, therapy with conventional or liposomal irinotecan should be permanently discontinued.

Grade 3 or 4 Toxicity. If grade 3 or 4 adverse events occur in patients receiving liposomal irinotecan, therapy with the drug should be withheld until the toxicity resolves to grade 1 or less. Liposomal irinotecan therapy may then be resumed at a reduced dosage (i.e., 70 mg/m^2 reduced to 50 mg/m^2 or 50 mg/m^2 reduced to 43 mg/m^2). If grade 3 or 4 adverse events recur following dosage reduction, therapy should be withheld again until the toxicity resolves to grade 1 or less; therapy may then be resumed at a further reduced dosage (i.e., 50 mg/m^2 reduced to 43 mg/m^2 or 43 mg/m^2 reduced to 35 mg/m^2). If grade 3 or 4 adverse events recur at this reduced dosage, treatment with liposomal irinotecan should be discontinued.

Table 2. Recommended Dosage Modifications for Conventional Irinotecan in Combination Therapy with Fluorouracil and Leucovorin

The administration of chemotherapy treatments should be delayed until pretreatment bowel function has been restored for at least 24 hours without the need for antidiarrhea medication. A new cycle of conventional irinotecan-based combination therapy should not begin until the granulocyte count has recovered to ≥1500/mm^3, the platelet count has recovered to ≥100,000/mm^3, and treatment-related diarrhea is fully resolved. Treatment should be delayed 1–2 weeks to allow for recovery from treatment-related toxicities. If the patient has not recovered after a 2-week delay, consideration should be given to discontinuing conventional irinotecan.

Toxicity – NCI Grade (Value)[a]	During a Cycle of Therapy[b]	At the Start of Subsequent Cycles of Therapy[b]
No toxicity	Maintain dose level	Maintain dose level
Neutropenia		
1 (1500 to 1999/mm^3)	Maintain dose level	Maintain dose level
2 (1000 to 1499/mm^3)	Decrease by 1 dose level	Maintain dose level
3 (500 to 999/mm^3)	Omit dose until resolved to ≤ grade 2, then decrease by 1 dose level	Decrease by 1 dose level
4 (<500/mm^3)	Omit dose until resolved to ≤ grade 2, then decrease by 2 dose levels	Decrease by 2 dose levels
Neutropenic fever	Omit dose until resolved, then decrease by 2 dose levels	
Other hematologic toxicities	Dose modifications for leukopenia or thrombocytopenia during a cycle of therapy and at the start of subsequent cycles of therapy are also based on NCI toxicity criteria and are the same as recommended for neutropenia above	
Diarrhea		
1 (2–3 stools/day > pretreatment)	Delay dose until resolved to baseline, then resume the same dose	Maintain dose level
2 (4–6 stools/day > pretreatment)	Omit dose until resolved to baseline, then decrease by 1 dose level	Maintain dose level
3 (7–9 stools/day > pretreatment)	Omit dose until resolved to baseline, then decrease by 1 dose level	Decrease by 1 dose level
4 (≥10 stools/day > pretreatment)	Omit dose until resolved to baseline, then decrease by 2 dose levels	Decrease by 2 dose levels
Other nonhematologic toxicities[c]		
1	Maintain dose level	Maintain dose level
2	Omit dose until resolved to ≤ grade 1, then decrease by 1 dose level	Maintain dose level
3	Omit dose until resolved to ≤ grade 2, then decrease by 1 dose level	Decrease by 1 dose level
4	Omit dose until resolved to ≤ grade 2, then decrease by 2 dose levels	Decrease by 2 dose levels
	Note: For mucositis/stomatitis, decrease only fluorouracil, not conventional irinotecan	*Note*: For mucositis/stomatitis, decrease only fluorouracil, not conventional irinotecan

[a] National Cancer Institute Common Toxicity Criteria (version 1.0).

[b] All dose modifications should be based on the worst preceding toxicity.

[c] Excluding alopecia, anorexia, asthenia.

Table 3. Recommended Dosage Modifications for Single-Agent *Weekly* Dosage Schedule of Conventional Irinotecan[a]

A new cycle of conventional irinotecan therapy should not begin until the granulocyte count has recovered to ≥1500/mm³, the platelet count has recovered to ≥100,000/mm³, and treatment-related diarrhea is fully resolved. Treatment should be delayed 1–2 weeks to allow for recovery from treatment-related toxicities. If the patient has not recovered after a 2-week delay, consideration should be given to discontinuing conventional irinotecan.

Toxicity – NCI Grade[b]	During a Cycle of Therapy[a]	At the Start of the Next Cycle of Therapy[a]
No toxicity	Maintain dose level	Increase dose by 25 mg/m² up to a maximum dose of 150 mg/m²
Neutropenia		
1 (1500 to 1999/mm³)	Maintain dose level	Maintain dose level
2 (1000 to 1499/mm³)	Decrease dose by 25 mg/m²	Maintain dose level
3 (500 to 999/mm³)	Omit dose until resolved to ≤ grade 2, then decrease dose by 25 mg/m²	Decrease dose by 25 mg/m²
4 (<500/mm³)	Omit dose until resolved to ≤ grade 2, then decrease dose by 50 mg/m²	Decrease dose by 50 mg/m²
Neutropenic fever	Omit dose until resolved, then decrease dose by 50 mg/m²	Decrease dose by 50 mg/m²
Other hematologic toxicities	Dose modifications for leukopenia, thrombocytopenia, and anemia during a cycle of therapy are also based on NCI toxicity criteria and are the same as recommended for neutropenia above	Dose modifications for leukopenia, thrombocytopenia, and anemia at the start of subsequent cycles of therapy are also based on NCI toxicity criteria and are the same as recommended for neutropenia above
Diarrhea		
1 (2–3 stools/day > pretreatment)	Maintain dose level	Maintain dose level
2 (4–6 stools/day > pretreatment)	Decrease dose by 25 mg/m²	Maintain dose level
3 (7–9 stools/day > pretreatment)	Omit dose until resolved to ≤ grade 2, then decrease dose by 25 mg/m²	Decrease dose by 25 mg/m²
4 (≥10 stools/day > pretreatment)	Omit dose until resolved to ≤ grade 2, then decrease dose by 50 mg/m²	Decrease dose by 50 mg/m²
Other nonhematologic toxicities[c]		
1	Maintain dose level	Maintain dose level
2	Decrease dose by 25 mg/m²	Decrease dose by 25 mg/m²
3	Omit dose until resolved to ≤ grade 2, then decrease dose by 25 mg/m²	Decrease dose by 25 mg/m²
4	Omit dose until resolved to ≤ grade 2, then decrease dose by 50 mg/m²	Decrease dose by 50 mg/m²

[a] All dose modifications should be based on the worst preceding toxicity.

[b] National Cancer Institute Common Toxicity Criteria (version 1.0).

[c] Excluding alopecia, anorexia, asthenia.

Table 4. Recommended Dosage Modifications for Single-Agent *Once-Every-3-Weeks* Schedule of Conventional Irinotecan[a]

A new cycle of conventional irinotecan therapy should not begin until the granulocyte count has recovered to ≥1500/ mm³, the platelet count has recovered to ≥100,000/ mm³, and treatment-related diarrhea is fully resolved. Treatment should be delayed 1–2 weeks to allow for recovery from treatment-related toxicities. If the patient has not recovered after a 2-week delay, consideration should be given to discontinuing conventional irinotecan.

Toxicity – NCI Grade[b]	At the Start of the Next Cycle of Therapy[a]
No toxicity	Maintain dose level
Neutropenia	
1 (1500 to 1999/mm³)	Maintain dose level
2 (1000 to 1499/mm³)	Maintain dose level
3 (500 to 999/mm³)	Decrease dose by 50 mg/m²
4 (<500/mm³)	Decrease dose by 50 mg/m²
Neutropenic fever	Decrease dose by 50 mg/m²
Other hematologic toxicities	Dose modifications for leukopenia, thrombocytopenia, and anemia at the start of subsequent cycles of therapy are also based on NCI toxicity criteria and are the same as recommended for neutropenia above
Diarrhea	
1 (2–3 stools/day > pretreatment)	Maintain dose level
2 (4–6 stools/day > pretreatment)	Maintain dose level
3 (7–9 stools/day > pretreatment)	Decrease dose by 50 mg/m²
4 (≥10 stools/day > pretreatment)	Decrease dose by 50 mg/m²
Other nonhematologic toxicities[c]	
1	Maintain dose level
2	Decrease dose by 50 mg/m²
3	Decrease dose by 50 mg/m²
4	Decrease dose by 50 mg/m²

[a] All dose modifications should be based on the worst preceding toxicity.

[b] National Cancer Institute Common Toxicity Criteria (version 1.0).

[c] Excluding alopecia, anorexia, asthenia.

■ **Dosage in Renal and Hepatic Impairment** ***Conventional Irinotecan Hydrochloride*** Safety and efficacy of conventional irinotecan hydrochloride have not been evaluated systematically in patients with renal impairment. The manufacturer makes no specific recommendations regarding dosage adjustment in patients with renal impairment, but states that use of conventional irinotecan in patients requiring dialysis is not recommended.

In patients with hepatic impairment, clearance of conventional irinotecan is decreased and exposure to the SN-38 active metabolite is increased. In clinical trials for GI cancer using either dosage schedule, conventional irinotecan was not administered to patients with serum bilirubin concentrations exceeding 2 mg/dL; specific dosage recommendations are not available for such patients. The drug also was *not* administered to patients who had serum aminotransferase concentrations exceeding 3 times the ULN in the absence of hepatic metastases or to those with hepatic metastases who had serum aminotransferase concentrations exceeding 5 times the ULN. The manufacturer states that reduction of the initial dose of conventional irinotecan hydrochloride by one dose level (e.g., to 100 mg/m² for regimen 1 or to 150 mg/m² for regimen 2 as first-line combination therapy; to 100 mg/m² for the weekly dosage schedule or to 300 mg/m² for the once-every-3-weeks dosage schedule as monotherapy) should be considered for patients with modestly elevated serum bilirubin concentrations (i.e., 1–2 mg/dL). (See Colorectal Cancer under Dosage and Administration: Dosage.)

Liposomal Irinotecan Hydrochloride In a population pharmacokinetic analysis of liposomal irinotecan hydrochloride, systemic exposure to the SN-38 active metabolite in patients with mild (creatinine clearance of 60–89 mL/minute) or moderate (creatinine clearance of 30–59 mL/minute) renal impairment was similar to that in patients with normal renal function. Pharmacokinetic data in patients with severe renal impairment (creatinine clearance less than 30 mL/minute) are limited. The manufacturer makes no specific dosage recommendations for patients with renal impairment.

Formal pharmacokinetic studies with liposomal irinotecan hydrochloride have not been conducted in patients with hepatic impairment. Data from a population pharmacokinetic analysis indicate that average steady-state concentrations of total SN-38 are increased by 37% in patients with baseline serum bilirubin concentrations of 1–2 mg/dL compared with patients with baseline serum bilirubin concentrations of less than 1 mg/dL; however, elevated concentrations of serum aminotransferases (ALT or AST) did not affect total SN-38 concentrations. The drug has not been studied in patients with serum bilirubin concentrations exceeding 2 mg/dL, and patients with bilirubin concentrations exceeding the ULN were not included in the pivotal clinical trial evaluating liposomal irinotecan therapy for metastatic pancreatic cancer. The manufacturer makes no specific recommendations regarding dosage adjustment in patients with hepatic impairment.

Description

Irinotecan (CPT-11), a semisynthetic derivative of camptothecin, is an antineoplastic agent. Camptothecins are alkaloids with antitumor activity that are extracted from plants such as *Camptotheca acuminata*. Conventional and liposomal preparations of irinotecan hydrochloride are commercially available as the trihydrate. Each mL of conventional irinotecan hydrochloride for injection concentrate contains 20 mg of the drug in terms of the hydrated salt. Each mL of liposomal irinotecan hydrochloride for injection concentrate contains 4.3 mg of the drug in terms of the anhydrous base.

Irinotecan is a type I DNA topoisomerase inhibitor. DNA topoisomerases (i.e., types I and II) are enzymes in the cell nucleus that regulate DNA topology (3-dimensional conformation) and facilitate nuclear processes such as DNA replication, recombination, and repair. During these processes, type I DNA topoisomerase creates transient (reversible) single-stranded breaks in double-stranded DNA, allowing intact single DNA strands to pass through the break and relieve the topologic constraints (e.g., torsional strain) inherent in supercoiled DNA. The 3′-DNA terminus of the broken DNA strands bind covalently with the topoisomerase enzyme to form a catalytic intermediate, termed a cleavable complex. After the DNA is sufficiently relaxed and the strand passage reaction is complete, DNA topoisomerase reattaches the broken DNA strands to form the chemically unaltered topoisomers that allow transcription to proceed. Irinotecan is a water-soluble precursor to the lipophilic active metabolite SN-38 (7-ethyl-10-hydroxycamptothecin), which is 1000 times as potent as irinotecan in vitro as an inhibitor of type I DNA topoisomerase. However, the precise contribution of SN-38 to the pharmacologic activity of administered irinotecan is unknown because of the variable in vitro cytotoxic potency reported for SN-38 relative to the parent drug and differences in the area under the plasma concentration-time curve and plasma protein binding of SN-38 compared with irinotecan.

Irinotecan, its active metabolite SN-38, and other type I topoisomerase inhibitors are believed to exert their cytotoxic effects during the S-phase of DNA synthesis through an interaction with the DNA–DNA topoisomerase cleavable complex. The cleavable complex is bound and stabilized by irinotecan and/or SN-38, preventing the topoisomerase from religating the single-strand breaks. The ternary complex of irinotecan/SN-38, DNA, and DNA topoisomerase interferes with the moving replication fork, inducing replication arrest and lethal double-stranded breaks in DNA. This DNA damage is not efficiently repaired and apparently leads to apoptosis (programmed cell death).

SumMon® (see Users Guide). For additional information on this drug until a more detailed monograph is developed and published, the manufacturer's labeling should be consulted. It is *essential* that the labeling be consulted for detailed information on the usual cautions, precautions, and contraindications. For further information on the handling of antineoplastic agents, see the ASHP Guidelines on Handling Hazardous Drugs at http://www.ahfsdruginformation.com.

Preparations

Distribution of liposomal irinotecan hydrochloride is restricted. (See Dosage and Administration.)

Excipients in commercially available drug preparations may have clinically important effects in some individuals; consult specific product labeling for details.

Irinotecan Hydrochloride (Trihydrate)

Parenteral

Concentrate, for injection, for IV infusion only	20 mg/mL (40 and 100 mg)*	**Camptosar®**, Pfizer

*available from one or more manufacturer, distributor, and/or repackager by generic (nonproprietary) name

Irinotecan Hydrochloride Liposomal (Trihydrate)

Parenteral

Concentrate, for injection, for IV infusion only	4.3 mg (of irinotecan) per mL (43 mg)	**Onivyde®**, Merrimack

†Use is not currently included in the labeling approved by the US Food and Drug Administration

Ivosidenib

■ Ivosidenib, a potent and selective inhibitor of isocitrate dehydrogenase-1 (IDH1), is an antineoplastic agent.

Uses

■ **Acute Myeloid Leukemia** ***Newly Diagnosed Acute Myeloid Leukemia*** Ivosidenib is used for the treatment of newly diagnosed acute myeloid leukemia (AML) with susceptible isocitrate dehydrogenase-1 (IDH1) mutation in patients who are 75 years of age or older or who are not candidates for intensive induction chemotherapy. Susceptible IDH1 mutations are defined as those resulting in increased 2-hydroxyglutarate levels in the leukemic cells and where efficacy of ivosidenib is predicted by clinically meaningful remissions at the recommended dosage of the drug and/or inhibition of IDH1 mutation activity is expected at ivosidenib concentrations sustainable at the recommended dosage. Ivosidenib has been designated an orphan drug by FDA for the treatment of this cancer. An FDA-approved diagnostic test (e.g., Abbott RealTi*me*® IDH1 assay) is required to confirm the presence of IDH1 mutation (peripheral blood or bone marrow) prior to initiation of therapy. The current indication is based on complete remission (CR) or complete remission with partial hematologic recovery (CRh), duration of response, and improvement of hematologic deficits (determined by the proportion of transfusion-dependent patients achieving transfusion independence). CR was defined as the presence of less than 5% blasts in bone marrow without evidence of disease and with full recovery of peripheral blood cell counts (platelet count exceeding 100,000/mm^3 and absolute neutrophil count [ANC] exceeding 1000/mm^3). CRh was defined as the presence of less than 5% blasts in bone marrow without evidence of disease and with partial recovery of peripheral blood cell counts (platelet count exceeding 50,000/mm^3 and ANC exceeding 500/mm^3).

The current indication for ivosidenib in the treatment of newly diagnosed AML with IDH1 mutation is based principally on the results for a cohort of patients with newly diagnosed AML with IDH1 mutation who received ivosidenib in an open-label, multicenter, noncomparative, phase 1, dose-escalation and dose-expansion study (AG120-C-001) in adults with advanced hematologic malignancies harboring IDH1 mutation (as detected by the Abbott RealTi*me*® IDH1 mutation test). This cohort of patients included 28 adults with newly diagnosed AML who were 75 years of age or older or who were not candidates for intensive induction chemotherapy. Patients were not candidates for intensive induction chemotherapy if they met at least one of the following criteria: baseline Eastern Cooperative Oncology Group (ECOG) performance status of 2 or greater, severe cardiac or pulmonary disease, hepatic impairment (bilirubin concentration exceeding 1.5 times the upper limit of normal [ULN]), or creatinine clearance less than 45 mL/minute.

The median age of patients enrolled in the newly diagnosed AML cohort of this phase 1 study was 77 years (range: 64–87 years); 86% were white, 68% were 75 years of age or older, 54% were male, 78% had an ECOG performance status of 0 or 1, 68% had adverse-risk cytogenetics, 32% had intermediate-risk cytogenetics, 61% were transfusion dependent at baseline, 68% had AML with myelodysplasia-related changes (AML-MRC), 21% had de novo AML, and 11% had therapy-related AML (t-AML; secondary AML). Approximately one-half (46%) of patients enrolled in the cohort had received prior therapy with a hypomethylating agent for an antecedent hematologic disorder. IDH1 mutations at codon R132C, R132G, R132H, R132L, or R132S were present in 86, 4, 7, 4, or 0%, respectively, of patients enrolled in the newly diagnosed AML cohort. Patients received an initial ivosidenib dosage of 500 mg orally once daily. Therapy was continued until disease progression or unacceptable toxicity occurred or stem cell transplantation was required. Following ivosidenib therapy, 7% of patients with newly diagnosed AML underwent stem cell transplantation. The median duration of ivosidenib therapy was 4.3 months.

At a median follow-up of 8.1 months, CR or CRh was achieved in 42.9% of patients receiving ivosidenib for newly diagnosed AML; 28.6% of patients achieved CR. The median duration of best response (CR or CRh) had not been reached at the time of the analysis. The median time to best response was 2.8 months; the majority (92%) of these patients achieved an initial best response within 6 months of initiating ivosidenib therapy. Among patients who were transfusion dependent at baseline, 41.2% became transfusion independent during any 56-day period during the study. The majority (54.5%) of patients who were transfusion independent at baseline remained transfusion independent during any 56-day period during the study.

Relapsed or Refractory Acute Myeloid Leukemia Ivosidenib is used for the treatment of relapsed or refractory AML with susceptible IDH1 mutation. Susceptible IDH1 mutations are defined as those resulting in increased 2-hydroxyglutarate levels in the leukemic cells and where efficacy of ivosidenib is predicted by clinically meaningful remissions at the recommended dosage of the drug and/or inhibition of IDH1 mutation activity is expected at ivosidenib concentrations sustainable at the recommended dosage. Ivosidenib has been designated an orphan drug by FDA for the treatment of this cancer. An FDA-approved diagnostic test (e.g., Abbott RealTi*me*® IDH1 assay) is required to confirm the presence of IDH1 mutation (peripheral blood or bone marrow) prior to initiation of therapy. The current indication is based on CR or CRh, duration of response, and improvement of hematologic deficits (determined by the proportion of transfusion-dependent patients achieving transfusion independence). CR was defined as the presence of less than 5% blasts in bone marrow without evidence of disease and with full recovery of peripheral blood cell counts (platelet count exceeding 100,000/mm^3 and ANC exceeding 1000/mm^3). CRh was defined as the presence of less than 5% blasts in bone marrow without evidence of disease and with partial recovery of peripheral blood cell counts (platelet count exceeding 50,000/mm^3 and ANC exceeding 500/mm^3).

The current indication for ivosidenib in the treatment of relapsed or refractory AML with IDH1 mutation is based principally on the results for a cohort of patients with relapsed or refractory AML with IDH1 mutation who received ivosidenib in an open-label, multicenter, noncomparative, phase 1, dose-escalation and dose-expansion study (AG120-C-001) in adults with advanced hematologic malignancies harboring IDH1 mutation (as detected by the Abbott RealTi*me*® IDH1 mutation test). This cohort of patients included 174 adults with relapsed or refractory AML.

The median age of patients enrolled in the relapsed or refractory AML cohort of this phase 1 study was 67 years (range: 18–87 years); 62% were white, 64% were 65 years of age or older, 51% were male, 77% had an ECOG performance status of 0 or 1, 37% had previously untreated relapsed AML, 26% had refractory AML, 37% had primary refractory AML, 60% had intermediate-risk cytogenetics, 27% had poor-risk cytogenetics, 63% were transfusion dependent at baseline, and 23% had previously undergone stem cell transplantation. Patients enrolled in the cohort had received a median of 2 prior therapies. IDH1 mutations at codon R132C, R132H, R132G, R132S, or R132L were present in 59, 25, 7, 6, or 4%, respectively, of patients enrolled in the relapsed or refractory AML cohort. Patients received an initial ivosidenib dosage of 500 mg orally once daily. Therapy was continued until disease progression or unacceptable toxicity occurred or stem cell transplantation was required. Following ivosidenib therapy, 12% of patients underwent stem cell transplantation. The median duration of ivosidenib therapy was 4.1 months.

At a median follow-up of 8.3 months, CR or CRh was achieved in 32.8% of patients receiving ivosidenib for relapsed or refractory AML with a median response duration of 8.2 months; 24.7% of patients achieved CR. The median time to best response (CR or CRh) was 2 months; all of these patients achieved an initial best response within 6 months of initiating ivosidenib therapy. Approximately one-third (37.3%) of patients who were transfusion dependent at baseline became transfusion independent during any 56-day period during the study. The majority (59.4%) of patients who were transfusion independent at baseline remained transfusion independent during any 56-day period during the study.

Dosage and Administration

■ **General** Presence of the isocitrate dehydrogenase-1 (IDH1) mutation (peripheral blood or bone marrow) must be confirmed prior to initiation of therapy with ivosidenib. Because IDH1 mutation may emerge during treatment, patients without this mutation at diagnosis of acute myeloid leukemia (AML) should be retested at the time of relapse.

Because differentiation syndrome or leukocytosis may occur, complete blood cell (CBC) counts and blood chemistries should be monitored at baseline, at least once weekly for the initial month of therapy, every other week for the next month, and then once monthly thereafter. Laboratory abnormalities should be managed promptly. (See Dosage: Dosage Modification for Toxicity.)

Because elevations in serum creatine kinase (CK, creatine phosphokinase, CPK) concentrations were observed in healthy volunteers, serum CK concentrations should be monitored once weekly for the first month of therapy. In clinical trials, no cases of rhabdomyolysis were reported; however, the actual frequency of this adverse effect is unknown because serum CK concentrations were not routinely monitored.

Because prolongation of the QT interval may occur, electrocardiograms (ECGs) should be monitored at least once weekly for the first 3 weeks of therapy and then at least once monthly thereafter. More frequent monitoring may be required in patients who have risk factors for developing QT interval prolongation. (See Prolongation of QT Interval under Warnings/Precautions: Other Warnings and Precautions, in Cautions.)

Restricted Distribution Ivosidenib can only be obtained through designated specialty pharmacies and distributors. Clinicians may contact the manufacturer (Agios Pharmaceuticals) at 844-409-1141 or consult the Tibsovo® website (https://www.tibsovopro.com) for specific ordering and availability information.

■ **Administration** Ivosidenib is administered orally at approximately the same time each day without regard to meals; however, administration with a high-fat meal should be avoided because of increased systemic exposure of the drug. (See Description.) The tablets should be swallowed whole; they should *not* be chewed, crushed, or split.

■ **Dosage** ***Acute Myeloid Leukemia*** **Newly Diagnosed Acute Myeloid Leukemia.** For the treatment of newly diagnosed AML with IDH1 mutation in patients who are 75 years of age or older or who are not candidates for intensive induction chemotherapy, the recommended adult dosage of ivosidenib is 500 mg once daily. Therapy should be continued until disease progression or unacceptable toxicity occurs. In the principal efficacy study (AG120-C-001), most patients with newly diagnosed AML achieved best response within 6 months of initiating ivosidenib; therefore, the manufacturer states that therapy should be continued for at least 6 months to allow time for response.

In patients who present with leukocytosis (leukocyte count exceeding 25,000/mm³ or increase in total leukocyte count of more than 15,000/mm³ from baseline) in the absence of infection, hydroxyurea therapy should be initiated according to standard practices and leukapheresis should be performed as needed. If leukocytosis persists, temporary interruption of ivosidenib therapy may be necessary. (See Leukocytosis under Dosage: Dosage Modification for Toxicity, in Dosage and Administration.)

Relapsed or Refractory Acute Myeloid Leukemia. For the treatment of relapsed or refractory AML with IDH1 mutation, the recommended adult dosage of ivosidenib is 500 mg once daily. Therapy should be continued until disease progression or unacceptable toxicity occurs. In the principal efficacy study (AG120-C-001), most patients with relapsed or refractory AML achieved best response within 6 months of initiating ivosidenib; therefore, the manufacturer states that therapy should be continued for at least 6 months to allow time for response.

In patients who present with leukocytosis (leukocyte count exceeding 25,000/mm³ or increase in total leukocyte count of more than 15,000/mm³ from baseline) in the absence of infection, hydroxyurea therapy should be initiated according to standard practices and leukapheresis should be performed as needed. If leukocytosis persists, temporary interruption of ivosidenib therapy may be necessary. (See Leukocytosis under Dosage: Dosage Modification for Toxicity, in Dosage and Administration.)

Dosage Modification for Toxicity **Differentiation Syndrome.** If severe signs or symptoms (e.g., pyrexia, acute respiratory distress, pulmonary infiltrates, pleural or pericardial effusion, hypotension, peripheral edema, rapid weight gain, hepatic or renal impairment, multiorgan dysfunction) persist for more than 48 hours despite systemic corticosteroid therapy, ivosidenib therapy should be withheld until the toxicity improves to grade 2 or less. (See Differentiation Syndrome under Warnings/Precautions: Warnings, in Cautions.)

Leukocytosis. If leukocytosis persists despite hydroxyurea therapy, ivosidenib therapy should be withheld. Upon resolution of leukocytosis, ivosidenib may be resumed at the initial dosage (500 mg daily). (See Acute Myeloid Leukemia under Dosage and Administration: Dosage.)

Prolongation of QT Interval. For corrected QT (QT_c) interval of 480–500 msec, ivosidenib therapy should be withheld. When the QT_c interval improves to 480 msec or less, ivosidenib may be resumed at a dosage of 500 mg daily.

If the QT_c interval exceeds 500 msec, ivosidenib therapy should be withheld. When the QT_c interval improves to 480 msec or less or no more than 30 msec from baseline, ivosidenib may be resumed at a reduced dosage of 250 mg daily. If an alternate etiology for QT_c interval prolongation is confirmed, the dosage of ivosidenib may be re-escalated to 500 mg daily.

If symptomatic QT_c interval prolongation (e.g., life-threatening arrhythmias) occurs, ivosidenib therapy should be permanently discontinued.

Guillain-Barré Syndrome. If Guillain-Barré syndrome occurs, ivosidenib therapy should be permanently discontinued.

Other Toxicity. If a grade 3 or greater adverse reaction occurs, ivosidenib therapy should be withheld. When the toxicity improves to grade 2 or less, ivosidenib therapy may be resumed at a reduced dosage of 250 mg daily; the dosage of ivosidenib may be re-escalated to 500 mg daily when the toxicity improves to grade 1 or less.

If a grade 3 or greater adverse reaction recurs, ivosidenib therapy should be discontinued.

Concomitant Use with Drugs Affecting Hepatic Microsomal Enzymes Concomitant use of ivosidenib with drugs that are potent inhibitors of cytochrome P-450 (CYP) isoenzyme 3A4 should be avoided, and selection of an alternative drug with less CYP3A4 inhibition potential is recommended. If concomitant use with a potent CYP3A4 inhibitor cannot be avoided, the manufacturer recommends reducing the dosage of ivosidenib from 500 mg once daily to 250 mg once daily. When concomitant use of the potent CYP3A4 inhibitor is discontinued, the ivosidenib dosage should be returned (after at least 5 elimination half-lives of the potent CYP3A4 inhibitor) to 500 mg once daily. (See Inhibitors of CYP3A4 under Drug Interactions: Drugs Affecting Hepatic Microsomal Enzymes.)

■ **Special Populations** No initial dosage adjustment is necessary in patients with mild or moderate preexisting hepatic impairment (Child-Pugh class A or B). Ivosidenib has not been studied in patients with preexisting severe hepatic impairment (Child-Pugh class C); the manufacturer states that clinicians should consider potential risks and benefits of the drug prior to initiating therapy in such patients. (See Hepatic Impairment under Warnings/Precautions: Specific Populations, in Cautions.)

No initial dosage adjustment is necessary in patients with mild or moderate preexisting renal impairment (estimated glomerular filtration rate [eGFR] 30 to less than 90 mL/minute per 1.73 m²). Ivosidenib has not been studied in patients with preexisting severe renal impairment (eGFR less than 30 mL/minute per 1.73 m²) or in those requiring dialysis; the manufacturer states that clinicians should consider potential risks and benefits of the drug prior to initiating therapy in such patients. (See Renal Impairment under Warnings/Precautions: Specific Populations, in Cautions.)

The manufacturer makes no special dosage recommendations for geriatric patients. (See Geriatric Use under Warnings/Precautions: Specific Populations, in Cautions.)

Cautions

■ **Contraindications** The manufacturer states that there are no known contraindications to the use of ivosidenib.

■ **Warnings/Precautions** ***Warnings*** **Differentiation Syndrome.** Differentiation syndrome, which may be life-threatening or fatal, occurred in 25% of ivosidenib-treated patients with newly diagnosed acute myeloid leukemia (AML) and 19% of ivosidenib-treated patients with relapsed or refractory AML in the AG120-C-001 study. Differentiation syndrome resolved following completion of therapy or temporary interruption of therapy in 86% of patients with newly diagnosed AML experiencing differentiation syndrome and 79% of those with relapsed or refractory AML experiencing differentiation syndrome. Differentiation syndrome following therapy with an isocitrate dehydrogenase-1 (IDH1) inhibitor, including ivosidenib, is associated with rapid proliferation and differentiation of myeloid cells. In patients receiving ivosidenib, differentiation syndrome has been characterized by acute respiratory distress (dyspnea and/or hypoxia), pulmonary infiltrates, renal impairment, multiorgan dysfunction, pyrexia, pulmonary or peripheral edema, rapid weight gain, rash, hypotension, tumor lysis syndrome, leukocytosis without infectious etiology, and pleural or pericardial effusions. Differentiation syndrome has been observed with or without concomitant leukocytosis as early as 1 day or up to 3 months after initiation of ivosidenib.

Manifestations of differentiation syndrome may be clinically indistinguishable from manifestations of disease progression or other acute comorbidities; therefore, differentiation syndrome should be suspected if there is no clear alternate etiology. If signs or symptoms suggestive of differentiation syndrome occur, IV or oral corticosteroid therapy (e.g., 10 mg of dexamethasone IV every 12 hours [or equivalent]) should be initiated for at least 3 days and hemodynamic parameters should be monitored until symptoms improve. If concomitant leukocytosis occurs in the absence of infection, hydroxyurea therapy should be initiated according to standard practices and leukapheresis should be performed as needed. Signs or symptoms of differentiation syndrome may recur if systemic corticosteroid and/or hydroxyurea therapy is discontinued prematurely; therefore, corticosteroid and hydroxyurea therapy should be continued until symptoms resolve, followed by tapering of the corticosteroid and/or hydroxyurea dosage. If severe signs or symptoms of differentiation syndrome persist for more than 48 hours despite corticosteroid therapy, ivosidenib should be temporarily interrupted until symptoms improve to grade 2 or less. (See Differentiation Syndrome under Dosage: Dosage Modification for Toxicity, in Dosage and Administration.)

Other Warnings and Precautions **Prolongation of QT Interval.** Prolongation of the corrected QT (QT_c) interval and ventricular arrhythmias have been observed in patients receiving ivosidenib. The prolongation appears to occur in a plasma concentration-dependent manner. Following administration of ivosidenib 500 mg daily, a QT_c interval change from baseline of approximately 17.2 msec has been observed at steady-state peak plasma concentrations. In the AG120-C-001 study, 14% of ivosidenib-treated patients with hematologic malignancies had an increase in the QT_c interval exceeding 60 msec from baseline and 9% had a QT_c interval exceeding 500 msec. In addition, ventricular fibrillation was reported in one patient. Patients were excluded from the study if they had a baseline QT_c interval of 450 msec or greater (except those with preexisting bundle branch block), history of long QT syndrome, or uncontrolled or clinically important cardiovascular disease.

Patients with congenital long QT syndrome, congestive heart failure (CHF), or electrolyte abnormalities, and those receiving cytochrome P-450 (CYP) isoenzyme 3A4 inhibitors or drugs known to prolong the QT_c interval (e.g., antiarrhythmic agents, fluoroquinolone anti-infectives, azole antifungals, type 3 serotonin [5-HT_3] receptor antagonists) may be at increased risk for QT interval prolongation during ivosidenib therapy; therefore, more frequent monitoring (i.e., electrocardiograms [ECGs], serum electrolytes) may be necessary. (See Drug Interactions: Drugs that Prolong QT Interval and also see Inhibitors of CYP3A4 under Drug Interactions: Drugs Affecting Hepatic Microsomal Enzymes.)

ECGs should be monitored at least once weekly for the first 3 weeks of ivosidenib therapy and then at least once monthly thereafter. Blood chemistries also should be monitored at baseline, at least once weekly for the initial month of therapy, every other week for the next month, and then once monthly thereafter. Any electrolyte abnormalities that occur prior to initiation of ivosidenib therapy or during therapy should be corrected as clinically indicated. If QT interval prolongation occurs, temporary interruption, dosage reduction, or discontinuance of ivosidenib may be necessary (See Prolongation of QT Interval under Dosage: Dosage Modification for Toxicity, in Dosage and Administration), and ECGs should be monitored at least once weekly until 2 weeks following resolution of the toxicity.

Guillain-Barré Syndrome. Guillain-Barré syndrome occurred in 2 of 258 patients (less than 1%) receiving ivosidenib in the AG120-C-001 study.

Patients receiving ivosidenib therapy should be monitored for signs or symptoms of motor and/or sensory neuropathy (e.g., unilateral or bilateral weakness, sensory alterations, paresthesias, difficulty breathing). Ivosidenib therapy should be discontinued in patients who develop Guillain-Barré syndrome.

Specific Populations **Pregnancy.** Ivosidenib may cause fetal harm in humans based on animal findings. There are no available data regarding use of ivosidenib in pregnant women to inform a drug-associated risk of adverse developmental outcomes. In animal reproduction studies, embryofetal toxicity (e.g., decreased fetal weight, abortion) and teratogenicity (e.g., skeletal and visceral anomalies) were observed in rats and rabbits receiving ivosidenib at exposures levels approximately 2 times the human exposure at the recommended dosage.

Pregnancy should be avoided during ivosidenib therapy. Patients should use adequate methods of contraception while receiving therapy with ivosidenib. (See Drug Interactions: Hormonal Contraceptives.) Patients should be apprised of the potential hazard to the fetus if ivosidenib is used during pregnancy.

Lactation. It is not known whether ivosidenib or its metabolites are distributed into human milk. Because of the potential for serious adverse reactions to ivosidenib in nursing infants, women should be advised to discontinue nursing during ivosidenib therapy and for at least 1 month after the last dose. The effects of the drug on nursing infants or on the production of milk are unknown.

Pediatric Use. Safety and efficacy of ivosidenib have not been established in pediatric patients.

Geriatric Use. In the AG120-C-001 study, 97% of ivosidenib-treated patients with newly diagnosed AML were 65 years of age or older and 56% were 75 years of age or older.

In the AG120-C-001 study, 63% of ivosidenib-treated patients with relapsed or refractory AML were 65 years of age or older and 22% were 75 years of age or older; no overall differences in safety and efficacy were observed between geriatric patients in this cohort and younger adults.

Hepatic Impairment. Following administration of a single 500-mg dose of ivosidenib, systemic exposure of ivosidenib in individuals with mild or moderate hepatic impairment (Child-Pugh class A or B) increased by 85 or 71%, respectively, compared with individuals with normal hepatic function. The pharmacokinetic profile of ivosidenib has not been established in patients with severe hepatic impairment (Child-Pugh class C).

Renal Impairment. In a population pharmacokinetic analysis, mild or moderate renal impairment (estimated glomerular filtration rate [eGFR] 30 to less than 90 mL/minute per 1.73 m^2) did not have clinically important effects on systemic exposure to ivosidenib. The pharmacokinetic profile of ivosidenib has not been established in patients with severe renal impairment (eGFR less than 30 mL/minute per 1.73 m^2) and those requiring dialysis.

■ **Common Adverse Effects** Adverse effects reported in 10% or more of patients receiving ivosidenib for the treatment of newly diagnosed AML in the AG120-C-001 study include diarrhea, fatigue, edema, decreased appetite, leukocytosis, nausea, arthralgia, abdominal pain, dyspnea, differentiation syndrome, myalgia, constipation, dizziness, mucositis, vomiting, QT interval prolongation, cough, neuropathy, pruritus, rash, decreased weight, dyspepsia, and headache. Laboratory abnormalities reported in 10% or more of patients receiving ivosidenib for the treatment of newly diagnosed AML include decreased hemoglobin concentrations, elevated concentrations of alkaline phosphatase, decreased potassium concentrations, decreased sodium concentrations, elevated concentrations of uric acid, elevated concentrations of aminotransferases (i.e., ALT, AST), elevated concentrations of serum creatinine, decreased magnesium concentrations, decreased calcium concentrations, and decreased phosphate concentrations.

Adverse effects reported in 10% or more of patients receiving ivosidenib for the treatment of relapsed or refractory AML in the AG120-C-001 study include fatigue, leukocytosis, arthralgia, diarrhea, dyspnea, edema, nausea, mucositis, rash, QT interval prolongation, pyrexia, cough, constipation, differentiation syndrome, decreased appetite, myalgia, vomiting, abdominal pain, chest pain, headache, pleural effusion, hypotension, and neuropathy. Laboratory abnormalities reported in 10% or more of patients receiving ivosidenib for the treatment of relapsed or refractory AML include decreased hemoglobin concentrations, decreased sodium concentrations, decreased magnesium concentrations, increased uric acid concentrations, decreased potassium concentrations, elevated concentrations of alkaline phosphatase, elevated concentrations of aminotransferases (i.e., ALT, AST), decreased phosphate concentrations, elevated concentrations of serum creatinine, and elevated concentrations of bilirubin.

Drug Interactions

Ivosidenib is metabolized principally by cytochrome P-450 (CYP) isoenzyme 3A4 and, to a lesser extent, by *N*-dealkylation and hydrolysis.

In vitro studies indicate that ivosidenib is an inducer of CYP3A4 resulting in induction of its own metabolism. In vitro, the drug also has the potential to induce CYP isoenzymes 2B6, 2C8, and 2C9.

In vitro, ivosidenib is an inhibitor of P-glycoprotein (P-gp) and organic anion transporter (OAT) 3, but does not inhibit breast cancer resistance protein (BCRP), organic anion transport protein (OATP) 1B1, OATP1B3, organic anion transporter (OAT) 1, and organic cation transporter (OCT) 2 at clinically relevant concentrations. In vitro, the drug is a substrate for P-gp, but is not a substrate for BCRP, OATP1B1, or OATP1B3.

■ **Drugs Affecting Hepatic Microsomal Enzymes** ***Inhibitors of CYP3A4*** Concomitant use of ivosidenib with moderate or potent inhibitors of CYP3A4 may increase systemic exposure to ivosidenib and increase the risk of toxicity (e.g., prolongation of QT interval). When the potent CYP3A4 inhibitor itraconazole (200 mg once daily for 18 days) was administered concomitantly with ivosidenib (single 250-mg dose) in healthy individuals, area under the serum concentration-time curve (AUC) of ivosidenib was increased by 169% and peak plasma concentrations were unchanged. Simulations suggest that concomitant use of ivosidenib (single 500-mg dose) and the moderate CYP3A4 inhibitor fluconazole (400 mg on day 1, then 200 mg once daily for 29 days) would result in a 73% increase in AUC of ivosidenib and unchanged peak plasma concentrations; however, concomitant use of ivosidenib (500 mg once daily for 15 days) and fluconazole (400 mg on day 1, then 200 mg once daily for 14 days) may increase AUC and peak plasma concentration of ivosidenib by 90 and 52%, respectively, at steady state.

Because of the potential for moderate (e.g., fluconazole) and potent (e.g., itraconazole) CYP3A4 inhibitors to increase exposure to ivosidenib, selection of an alternative drug with less CYP3A4 inhibition potential should be considered. If concomitant use of a potent CYP3A4 inhibitor cannot be avoided, the manufacturer recommends reducing the dosage of ivosidenib from 500 mg once daily to 250 mg once daily. When concomitant use of the potent CYP3A4 inhibitor is discontinued, the ivosidenib dosage should be returned (after at least 5 elimination half-lives of the potent CYP3A4 inhibitor) to 500 mg once daily. Patients receiving ivosidenib concomitantly with moderate or potent CYP3A4 inhibitors should be monitored for signs of ivosidenib toxicity (i.e., QT interval prolongation). (See Prolongation of QT Interval under Warnings/Precautions: Other Warnings and Precautions, in Cautions.)

Inducers of CYP3A4 Concomitant use of ivosidenib with potent inducers of CYP3A4 may decrease ivosidenib plasma concentrations. Simulations suggest that concomitant use of ivosidenib (500 mg once daily) and the potent CYP3A4 inducer rifampin (600 mg once daily for 15 days) may decrease AUC and peak plasma concentration of ivosidenib by 33 and 19%, respectively.

Concomitant use of ivosidenib with potent CYP3A4 inducers (e.g., rifampin) should be avoided.

■ **Drugs Metabolized by Hepatic Microsomal Enzymes** ***Substrates of CYP3A4*** Concomitant use of ivosidenib with sensitive CYP3A4 substrates may decrease plasma concentrations of the substrate drug and decrease therapeutic efficacy of the drug. Simulations suggest that concomitant use of ivosidenib (500 mg once daily) and the sensitive CYP3A substrate midazolam (single 5-mg dose) may decrease AUC and peak plasma concentration of midazolam by 83 and 74%, respectively. Simulations also suggest that concomitant use of ivosidenib and CYP3A4 substrates such as itraconazole may result in a clinically important decrease of systemic exposure to itraconazole at steady state.

Concomitant use of ivosidenib with sensitive substrates of CYP3A4 should be avoided, and selection of an alternative drug should be considered. If concomitant use with sensitive substrates of CYP3A4 cannot be avoided, patients should be monitored for loss of efficacy of the substrate drug. Because concomitant use of ivosidenib with itraconazole or ketoconazole (CYP3A4 substrates) may decrease antifungal efficacy of itraconazole or ketoconazole, the manufacturer states that concomitant use of ivosidenib with itraconazole or ketoconazole is not recommended.

Substrates of CYP2C9 Ivosidenib has the potential to induce CYP2C9 and may decrease plasma concentrations of drugs that are sensitive substrates of CYP2C9 (e.g., warfarin).

Concomitant use of ivosidenib with sensitive substrates of CYP2C9 should be avoided, and selection of an alternative drug should be considered. If concomitant use with sensitive substrates of CYP2C9 cannot be avoided, patients should be monitored for loss of efficacy of the substrate drug.

■ **Drugs that Prolong QT Interval** Because ivosidenib has been associated with QT interval prolongation, concomitant use of ivosidenib with other drugs known to prolong the QT interval (e.g., antiarrhythmic agents, fluoroquinolone anti-infectives, azole antifungals, type 3 serotonin [5-HT_3] receptor antagonists) should be avoided, and selection of an alternative drug should be considered. If concomitant use of drugs known to prolong the QT interval cannot be avoided, ECGs and serum electrolytes should be monitored more frequently. (See Prolongation of QT Interval under Warnings/Precautions: Other Warnings and Precautions, in Cautions.)

■ **Hormonal Contraceptives** Concomitant use of ivosidenib with hormonal contraceptives may result in decreased plasma concentrations of the hormonal contraceptive and decreased contraceptive efficacy. The manufacturer states that an alternative nonhormonal contraceptive should be considered during ivosidenib therapy.

■ **Drugs Affecting Gastric Acidity** Concomitant administration of ivosidenib and drugs that increase the pH of the upper GI tract (e.g., antacids, histamine H_2-receptor antagonists, proton-pump inhibitors) does not affect the pharmacokinetics of ivosidenib.

Description

Ivosidenib, a potent and selective inhibitor of isocitrate dehydrogenase-1 (IDH1), is an antineoplastic agent. Isocitrate dehydrogenases (IDH) are metabolic enzymes in the citric acid cycle responsible for the oxidative decarboxylation of isocitrate to α-ketoglutarate, which is essential for normal cellular processes. Approximately 6–16% of acute myeloid leukemia (AML) cases carry IDH1 mutations. IDH1 mutations cause a reduction of α-ketoglutarate to the oncometabolite 2-hydroxyglutarate, which competitively inhibits α-ketoglutarate-dependent dioxygenases resulting in epigenetic dysregulation and subsequent histone and DNA hypermethylation and differentiation arrest of hematopoietic stem cells.

Susceptible IDH1 mutations are defined as those resulting in increased 2-hydroxyglutarate levels in the leukemic cells and where efficacy of ivosidenib is predicted by clinically meaningful remissions at the recommended dosage of ivosidenib and/or inhibition of IDH1 mutation activity is expected at ivosidenib concentrations sustainable at the recommended dosage. The most common ivosidenib-susceptible IDH1 mutations are R132C and R132H substitution mutations. In vitro studies indicate that ivosidenib inhibits IDH1 with R132C, R132H, R132G, R132L, or R132S mutation at much lower concentrations than IDH1 wild-type enzymes.

Ivosidenib has demonstrated decreased 2-hydroxyglutarate levels and induction of myeloid cell differentiation in vitro and in mice bearing tumor xenografts that expressed IDH1 mutation. Ivosidenib also has demonstrated decreased 2-hydroxyglutarate levels, reduced blast cell counts, and increased percentages of mature myeloid cells in patients with AML that expressed IDH1 mutation. The clinical importance of persistent IDH1 mutations in patients who achieve complete remission has not been established; however, persistent IDH1 mutations may indicate continued differentiation of abnormal myeloblast cells into mature granulocytes.

Peak plasma concentrations and area under the serum concentration-time curve (AUC) of ivosidenib are less than dose proportional over the ivosidenib dosage range of 200–1200 mg daily. Following oral administration of a single dose, median time to peak plasma concentrations of ivosidenib is approximately 3 hours. Following repeated administration of ivosidenib, steady-state concentrations of the drug are achieved in 14 days and accumulation of the drug is observed (approximately 1.9- and 1.5-fold increases in AUC and peak plasma concentrations, respectively). Pharmacokinetics of ivosidenib at steady state in patients with newly diagnosed AML and those with relapsed or refractory disease are similar. Administration of ivosidenib (single 500-mg dose) with a high-fat meal (approximately 900–1000 calories with 500–600 calories from fat) increased peak plasma concentrations and AUC of ivosidenib by 98 and approximately 25%, respectively, in healthy individuals compared with administration in the fasted state; administration of ivosidenib with a high-fat meal should be avoided. (See Dosage and Administration: Administration.)

Ivosidenib is metabolized principally by cytochrome P-450 (CYP) isoenzyme 3A4 and, to a lesser extent, by *N*-dealkylation and hydrolysis. Following oral administration of a radiolabeled dose of the drug, unchanged ivosidenib accounted for greater than 92% of plasma total radioactivity. In vitro, ivosidenib is highly bound (92–96%) to plasma proteins. The terminal half-life of ivosidenib is 93 hours. Following administration of a radiolabeled dose of ivosidenib, 77% of the radioactivity was recovered in feces (67% of the dose as unchanged drug) and 17% was recovered in urine (10% of the dose as unchanged drug).

Clearance of ivosidenib does not appear to be affected substantially by age (18–89 years), sex, race, body weight (38–150 kg), or Eastern Cooperative Oncology Group (ECOG) performance status.

Advice to Patients

Importance of instructing patients to read the manufacturer's patient information (medication guide).

Importance of advising patients to swallow ivosidenib tablets whole and to *not* chew, crush, or split the tablets. Importance of avoiding high-fat meals while taking the drug.

Importance of advising patients to take ivosidenib as directed by their clinician at approximately the same time each day. If a dose is missed by 12 hours or less, importance of administering the missed dose on the same day as soon as it is remembered and taking the next dose at the regularly scheduled time on the following day. If a dose is vomited, importance of administering the next dose at the regularly scheduled time; an additional dose should not be administered to replace the vomited dose. Patients should be advised not to take 2 doses within a 12-hour period.

Risk of developing differentiation syndrome. Importance of informing clinician immediately if manifestations of differentiation syndrome (e.g., pyrexia, cough, difficulty breathing, rash, decreased urination, hypotension, rapid weight gain, peripheral edema) occur.

Risk of tumor lysis syndrome. Importance of monitoring blood chemistry and maintaining adequate hydration during ivosidenib therapy.

Risk of QT interval prolongation. Importance of informing clinician if manifestations of QT interval prolongation (e.g., feelings of dizziness, lightheadedness, faintness) occur. Importance of informing patients that electrocardiograms (ECGs) and serum electrolytes must be monitored during ivosidenib therapy.

Risk of Guillain-Barré syndrome. Importance of informing clinician if manifestations of Guillain-Barré syndrome (e.g., weakness or tingling sensation in legs, arms, or upper body; unilateral or bilateral numbness and pain; altered sensory function; burning or prickling sensation; difficulty breathing) occur.

Risk of adverse GI effects. Importance of informing clinician if diarrhea, nausea, vomiting, mucositis, constipation, decreased appetite, or abdominal pain occurs.

Importance of women informing clinicians if they are or plan to become pregnant or plan to breast-feed. Apprise patient of potential hazard to the fetus if used during pregnancy.

Importance of advising women to avoid breast-feeding while receiving the drug for at least 1 month after the last dose.

Importance of informing clinicians of existing or contemplated concomitant therapy, including prescription and OTC drugs and dietary or herbal supplements, as well as any concomitant illnesses.

Importance of informing patients of other important precautionary information. (See Cautions.)

Overview® (see Users Guide). For additional information on this drug until a more detailed monograph is developed and published, the manufacturer's labeling should be consulted. It is *essential* that the manufacturer's labeling be consulted for more detailed information on usual cautions, precautions, contraindications, potential drug interactions, laboratory test interferences, and acute toxicity. For further information on the handling of antineoplastic agents, see the ASHP Guidelines on Handling Hazardous Drugs at http://www.ahfsdruginformation.com.

Preparations

Ivosidenib can only be obtained through designated specialty pharmacies and distributors. (See Restricted Distribution under Dosage and Administration: General.)

Excipients in commercially available drug preparations may have clinically important effects in some individuals; consult specific product labeling for details.

Ivosidenib

Oral

Tablets, film-coated	250 mg	**Tibsovo®**, Agios

Ixabepilone

Azaepothilone B

■ Ixabepilone, a microtubule inhibitor that is a semisynthetic derivative of epothilone B, is an epothilone antineoplastic agent.

Uses

■ **Breast Cancer** ***Combination Therapy*** Ixabepilone is used in combination with oral capecitabine for the treatment of metastatic or locally advanced breast cancer in patients whose disease is resistant to treatment with an anthracycline and a taxane or in patients whose cancer is taxane-resistant and for whom further anthracycline therapy is contraindicated. Anthracycline resistance is defined as progression during therapy or within 6 months in the adjuvant setting or 3 months in the metastatic setting. Taxane resistance is defined as progression during therapy or within 12 months in the adjuvant setting or 4 months in the metastatic setting.

The current indication for ixabepilone and capecitabine combination therapy is based mainly on the results of an open-label, multicenter, multinational, randomized, phase 3 trial comparing the efficacy and safety of ixabepilone in combination with capecitabine and capecitabine given as monotherapy in patients with metastatic or locally advanced breast cancer. In this trial, 752 patients received ixabepilone (40 mg/m^2 IV every 3 weeks) in combination with capecitabine (1000 mg/m^2 orally given twice daily for 2 weeks followed by a 1-week rest period) or capecitabine monotherapy (1250 mg/m^2 orally given twice daily for 2 weeks followed by a 1-week rest period). All patients were previously treated with and demonstrated tumor progression or resistance to anthracyclines and taxanes. Patients who had received a minimum cumulative dose of 240 mg/m^2 of doxorubicin or 360 mg/m^2 of epirubicin were also eligible. Patients in the combination treatment group received a median of 5 cycles of treatment and patients in the capecitabine monotherapy treatment group received a median of 4 cycles of treatment.

Patients receiving combination therapy with ixabepilone and capecitabine in this study demonstrated a longer progression-free survival (5.7 versus 4.1 months, respectively) and a higher objective tumor response rate (approximately 35 versus 14%, respectively) compared with patients receiving capecitabine monotherapy. No difference in overall survival (12.9 versus 11.1 months, respectively) between patients receiving combination therapy with ixabepilone and capecitabine and patients receiving capecitabine monotherapy was observed.

A second open-label, multicenter, multinational, randomized, phase 3 trial compared the efficacy and safety of ixabepilone in combination with capecitabine and capecitabine given as monotherapy in patients with metastatic or locally advanced breast cancer. In this trial, 1221 patients received ixabepilone (40 mg/m^2 IV every 3 weeks) in combination with capecitabine (1000 mg/m^2 orally given twice daily for 2 weeks followed by a 1-week rest period) or capecitabine monotherapy (1250 mg/m^2 orally given twice daily for 2 weeks followed by a 1-week rest period). All patients were previously treated with, but not necessarily resistant to, anthracyclines and taxanes. In the 79% of patients with measurable disease, patients receiving combination therapy with ixabepilone and capecitabine in this study demonstrated longer progression-free survival (6.2 versus 4.4 months, respectively) and a higher objective tumor response rate (approximately 43 versus 29%, respectively) compared with patients receiving capecitabine monotherapy. No significant difference in overall survival (16.4 versus 15.6 months, respectively) between patients receiving combination therapy with ixabepilone and capecitabine and patients receiving capecitabine monotherapy was observed.

Monotherapy Ixabepilone is used as monotherapy for the treatment of metastatic or locally advanced breast cancer in patients whose tumors are resistant or refractory to anthracyclines, taxanes, and capecitabine.

The current indication for use of ixabepilone as a single agent is based primarily on the results of a multicenter, single-arm study involving 126 women with metastatic or locally advanced breast cancer. The study enrolled patients whose tumors had recurred or progressed following 2 or more chemotherapy regimens including an anthracycline, a taxane, and capecitabine; patients who had received a minimum cumulative dose of 240 mg/m^2 of doxorubicin or 360 mg/m^2 of epirubicin were also eligible. The patients in this study were heavily pretreated (88% had previously received 2 or more chemotherapy regimens for metastatic disease) and 86% had liver and/or lung metastases. Ixabepilone 40 mg/m^2 was given as a 3-hour IV infusion every 3 weeks; patients received a median of 4 cycles (range: 1–18 cycles) of therapy with the drug. The objective tumor response rates based on independent radiologic review and investigator assessments were approximately 12% (with all partial responses) and 18%, respectively. The median time to response was approximately 6 weeks, median duration of response was approximately 6 months, and median progression-free survival was approximately 3 months.

The possible role of ixabepilone in the initial therapy of advanced breast cancer† also is being studied.

Dosage and Administration

■ **General** To minimize risk of hypersensitivity reactions, the manufacturer states that all patients should be premedicated with diphenhydramine hydrochloride 50 mg orally (or similar antihistamine) and a histamine H_2-receptor antagonist (e.g., ranitidine 150–300 mg orally) approximately 1 hour before beginning the ixabepilone infusion. Patients who experienced a prior hypersensitivity reaction to the drug must also be premedicated with corticosteroids (e.g., dexamethasone 20 mg, given either IV 30 minutes prior to infusion or orally 60 minutes prior to infusion).

■ **Reconstitution and Administration** Ixabepilone is administered by IV infusion only over 3 hours.

Ixabepilone is commercially available as the Ixempra® kit, which contains 2 single-use vials: one of the vials contains ixabepilone powder for injection and the other vial contains diluent. Ixabepilone powder for injection must be reconstituted and diluted prior to administration. The kit should be removed from the refrigerator and allowed to stand at room temperature for approximately 30 minutes prior to reconstitution. A white precipitate may be observed in the diluent vial when first removed from the refrigerator, but this precipitate will dissolve to form a clear solution once the diluent warms to room temperature.

Procedures for proper handling and disposal of antineoplastic drugs should be followed. To minimize risk of dermal exposure, impervious gloves should be worn when handling vials containing ixabepilone, regardless of the setting, including unpacking and inspection, transport within a facility, and dose preparation and administration. For additional information on proper procedures for handling antineoplastic agents, see the ASHP Guidelines on Handling Hazardous Drugs at http://www.ahfsdruginformation.com.

Ixabepilone powder for injection is reconstituted by adding 8 mL of the supplied diluent to the vial labeled as containing 15 mg of ixabepilone or 23.5 mL of the supplied diluent to the vial labeled as containing 45 mg of ixabepilone to provide a solution containing 2 mg/mL; only the supplied diluent should be used when reconstituting the powder. The vial should be gently swirled and inverted until the powder completely dissolves. Following reconstitution, the solution should be diluted with an appropriate infusion fluid as soon as possible, but may be stored in the vial for up to one hour at room temperature and room light. The appropriate dose should then be withdrawn and diluted in the appropriate volume of infusion fluid supplied in diethylhexylphthalate (DEHP)-free bags. Acceptable infusion fluids for dilution of reconstituted ixabepilone solution include lactated Ringer's injection, Plasma-Lyte A Injection pH 7.4®, or 0.9% sodium chloride injection with 2 mEq sodium bicarbonate injection (i.e., 2 mL of 8.4% w/v sodium bicarbonate solution or 4 mL of 4.2% w/v sodium bicarbonate solution) added to adjust the pH to between 6 and 9. For most doses, a 250-mL bag of infusion fluid is sufficient; however, it is necessary to check the final infusion concentration of each dose based on the volume of infusion fluid to be used; the final infusion concentration must be between 0.2–0.6 mg/mL. The infusion bag should be mixed thoroughly by manual rotation. Once diluted, the solution is stable at room temperature and room light for up to 6 hours; administration of diluted ixabepilone must be completed within this 6-hour period. Diluents other than those specified by the manufacturer should not be used.

The drug should be administered through an appropriate 0.2- to 1.2-μm inline filter. Only DEHP-free infusion containers and administration sets should be used.

■ **Dosage** For the management of breast cancer in adults, 40 mg/m^2 of ixabepilone is administered IV over 3 hours every 3 weeks, either as monotherapy or in combination with capecitabine. Dosages for patients with a body surface area greater than 2.2 m^2 should be calculated based on 2.2 m^2.

The use of potent inhibitors of cytochrome P-450 isoenzyme 3A4 (CYP3A4), including amprenavir (no longer commercially available in the US), atazanavir, clarithromycin, delavirdine, indinavir, itraconazole, ketoconazole, nefazodone, nelfinavir, ritonavir, saquinavir, telithromycin, and voriconazole, should be avoided during ixabepilone therapy. If concomitant administration of a potent CYP3A4 inhibitor is necessary during ixabepilone therapy, a dosage reduction to 20 mg/m^2 should be considered. Upon discontinuance of the CYP3A4 inhibitor, approximately 1 week should elapse before adjusting the ixabepilone dosage back to the usual recommended dosage of 40 mg/m^2. (See Drug Interactions.)

The use of potent inducers of CYP3A4, including carbamazepine, dexamethasone, phenobarbital, phenytoin, rifabutin, and rifampin, should be avoided during ixabepilone therapy. The use of an alterative concomitant medication with no or minimal enzyme induction potential should be considered. If concomitant administration of a potent CYP3A4 inducer is necessary during ixabepilone therapy, dosage may be gradually increased from 40 mg/m^2 to 60 mg/m^2, based on individual tolerance. If the dosage is increased, ixabepilone should be administered as a 4-hour IV infusion. Upon discontinuance of the CYP3A4 inducer, the ixabepilone dosage should be returned to the dosage used prior to initiation of the inducer. (See Drug Interactions.)

■ **Dosage Modification for Toxicity** Patients receiving ixabepilone should be evaluated during treatment by periodic clinical observation and laboratory tests, including complete blood cell counts. If toxicities are present, treatment should be delayed to allow recovery. Dosage adjustment guidelines for monotherapy and combination therapy with ixabepilone are shown in Table 1. If toxicities recur, an additional 20% dosage reduction should be made.

Table 1. Dosage Adjustment Guidelines for Nonhematologic and Hematologic Toxicities

Ixabepilone (Monotherapy or Combination Therapy)	Ixabepilone Dosage Modification
Nonhematologic:	
Grade 2 neuropathy (moderate) lasting ≥7 days	Decrease dosage by 20%
Grade 3 neuropathy (severe) lasting <7 days	Decrease dosage by 20%
Grade 3 neuropathy (severe) lasting ≥7 days or disabling neuropathy	Discontinue treatment
Any grade 3 toxicity (severe) other than neuropathy	Decrease dosage by 20%
Transient grade 3 arthralgia/myalgia or fatigue	No change in ixabepilone dosage
Grade 3 hand-foot syndrome (palmar-plantar erythrodysesthesia)	No change in ixabepilone dosage
Any grade 4 toxicity (disabling)	Discontinue treatment
Hematologic:	
Neutrophils <500/mm³ for ≥7 days	Decrease dosage by 20%
Febrile neutropenia	Decrease dosage by 20%
Platelets <25,000/mm³ or platelets <50,000/mm³ with bleeding	Decrease dosage by 20%
Capecitabine (when used in combination with ixabepilone)	**Capecitabine Dosage Modification**
Nonhematologic:	
All types and grades of nonhematologic toxicities	Consult the full prescribing information for capecitabine
Hematologic:	
Platelets <25,000/mm³ or <50,000/mm³ with bleeding	Hold for concurrent diarrhea or stomatitis until platelet count >50,000/mm³, then continue at same dosage
Neutrophils <500/mm³ for ≥7 days or febrile neutropenia	Hold for concurrent diarrhea or stomatitis until neutrophil count >1000/mm³, then continue at same dosage

Dosage adjustments at the start of a cycle should be based on nonhematologic toxicity or blood counts from the preceding cycle following the guidelines in Table 1. Patients should not begin a new cycle of treatment unless the neutrophil count is at least 1500/mm³, platelet count is at least 100,000/mm³, and nonhematologic toxicities have improved to grade 1 (mild) or resolved.

■ Special Populations

Table 2. Dosage Adjustments for Ixabepilone Monotherapy in Patients with Hepatic Impairment

Severity	Transaminase and Bilirubin Concentrations[a]	Ixabepilone Dosage[b]
Mild	AST and ALT ≤2.5 × ULN and bilirubin ≤1 × ULN	40 mg/m²
	AST and ALT ≤10 × ULN and bilirubin ≤1.5 × ULN	32 mg/m²
Moderate	AST and ALT ≤10 × ULN and bilirubin >1.5 × ULN to ≤3 × ULN	20–30 mg/m²

[a] Excluding patients whose total bilirubin is elevated due to Gilbert's disease.

[b] Dosage recommendations are for first course of therapy; further dosage decreases in subsequent courses should be made based on individual tolerance.

Ixabepilone in combination with capecitabine is contraindicated in patients with serum AST or ALT concentrations exceeding 2.5 times the upper limit of normal (ULN) or serum bilirubin concentrations elevated above the upper limit of normal (i.e., exceeding 1 times the upper limit of normal). Patients receiving combination treatment who have serum AST and ALT concentrations not exceeding 2.5 times the upper limit of normal and serum bilirubin concentrations not exceeding the upper limit of normal may receive the usual dosage of ixabepilone (40 mg/m²).

For ixabepilone monotherapy, patients with hepatic impairment should be dosed based on the guidelines in Table 2. In patients with moderate hepatic impairment, the manufacturer recommends an initial ixabepilone dosage of 20 mg/m², which may then be increased up to a maximum dosage of 30 mg/m² in subsequent cycles, if tolerated. Ixabepilone monotherapy in patients with serum AST or ALT concentrations exceeding 10 times the upper limit of normal or serum bilirubin concentrations exceeding 3 times the upper limit of normal is not recommended. Limited data are available for patients with baseline AST or ALT concentrations exceeding 5 times the upper limit of normal; the drug should be used with caution in such patients.

Cautions

■ Contraindications

History of severe (grade 3 or 4) hypersensitivity reaction to agents containing polyoxyl 35 castor oil (Cremophor® EL, polyoxyethylated castor oil).

Neutrophil count less than 1500/mm³ or platelet count less than 100,000/mm³.

Ixabepilone in combination with capecitabine is contraindicated in patients with serum AST or ALT concentrations exceeding 2.5 times the upper limit of normal or serum bilirubin concentrations elevated above the upper limit of normal (i.e., exceeding 1 times the upper limit of normal).

■ Warnings/Precautions

Warnings

Toxicity in Hepatic Impairment. Patients with baseline serum AST or ALT concentrations exceeding 2.5 times the upper limit of normal or serum bilirubin concentrations exceeding 1.5 times the upper limit of normal experienced greater toxicity than patients with baseline AST or ALT concentrations not exceeding 2.5 times the upper limit of normal or serum bilirubin concentrations not exceeding 1.5 times the upper limit of normal when treated with ixabepilone 40 mg/m² in combination with capecitabine or as monotherapy in breast cancer clinical studies. In patients with hepatic impairment receiving combined ixabepilone and capecitabine, the overall frequency of grade 3 or 4 adverse effects, febrile neutropenia, serious adverse effects, and toxicity-related deaths was greater. In patients with hepatic impairment receiving ixabepilone monotherapy, grade 4 neutropenia, febrile neutropenia, and serious adverse effects were more frequent. Safety and pharmacokinetics of ixabepilone monotherapy were evaluated in patients with varying degrees of hepatic impairment, and exposure was found to be increased in patients with elevated serum AST or bilirubin concentrations.

Ixabepilone in combination with capecitabine is contraindicated in patients with baseline serum AST or ALT concentrations exceeding 2.5 times the upper limit of normal or serum bilirubin concentrations elevated above the upper limit of normal (i.e., exceeding 1 times the upper limit of normal). Patients with hepatic impairment who are treated with ixabepilone monotherapy should receive a reduced dosage depending on the degree of hepatic impairment (see Table 2 under Dosage and Administration: Special Populations). Ixabepilone monotherapy in patients with serum AST or ALT concentrations exceeding 10 times the upper limit of normal or serum bilirubin concentrations exceeding 3 times the upper limit of normal is not recommended. Limited data are available for patients with serum AST or ALT concentrations exceeding 5 times the upper limit of normal; caution should be used when treating these patients.

Other Warnings and Precautions

Peripheral Neuropathy. Peripheral neuropathy, mostly sensory in nature but also motor neuropathy, occurs commonly in ixabepilone-treated patients and was reported in over 60% of patients receiving the drug in controlled studies. Although generally mild to moderate in severity, grade 3 or 4 neuropathy was reported in 14 and 23% of patients receiving ixabepilone monotherapy and ixabepilone combined with capecitabine, respectively, in controlled trials. Neuropathy generally develops early during treatment, with approximately 75% of new-onset or worsening neuropathy occurring during the first 3 cycles. Peripheral neuropathy was often characterized as paresthesia or dysesthesia and manifested as a symmetrical, stocking-and-glove distribution with more pronounced effects in the lower extremities.

All patients receiving ixabepilone should therefore be monitored for symptoms of neuropathy, including burning sensation, hyperesthesia or hypoesthesia, paresthesia, discomfort, and neuropathic pain. In clinical trials, peripheral neuropathy was managed through dosage reductions, treatment delays, and treatment discontinuance. Patients experiencing new or worsening neuropathic symptoms may require a dosage reduction and/or treatment delay. (See Dosage and Administration: Dosage Modification for Toxicity.) Neuropathy was the most frequent cause of treatment discontinuance due to drug toxicity, but generally was reversible. In clinical studies involving ixabepilone monotherapy or combined ixabepilone and capecitabine therapy, peripheral neuropathy improved or did not worsen in at least 80% of patients following dosage reduction. In patients with grade 3 or 4 neuropathy, documented improvement to baseline or grade 1 neuropathy was reported in 76–79% of patients 12 weeks after onset of the neuropathy.

Patients with diabetes mellitus or preexisting peripheral neuropathy may be at increased risk of developing severe neuropathy. The manufacturer states that prior therapy with neurotoxic chemotherapeutic agents did not predict the development of neuropathy. However, some evidence suggests that previous exposure to other neurotoxic drugs (including taxanes) may increase the risk of ixabepilone-associated neuropathy. The manufacturer states that ixabepilone should be used with caution in patients with diabetes mellitus or preexisting peripheral neuropathy.

Hematologic Effects. Myelosuppression is one of the major and dose-limiting adverse effects of ixabepilone and is primarily manifested as neutropenia. In clinical studies, grade 4 neutropenia (less than 500 cells/mm³) occurred in 36% of patients treated with ixabepilone plus capecitabine and 23% of patients treated with ixabepilone monotherapy. Febrile neutropenia and infection with neutropenia were reported in 5 and 6%, respectively, of patients treated with ixabepilone plus capecitabine, and 3 and 5%, respectively, of patients treated with ixabepilone monotherapy. Neutropenia-related death occurred in 1.9% of patients with normal hepatic function or mild hepatic impairment treated with ixabepilone plus capecitabine. The incidence of neutropenia-related death was higher (29%) in patients with serum AST or ALT concentrations exceeding 2.5 times the upper limit of normal or serum bilirubin concentrations exceeding 1.5 times the upper limit of normal. Neutropenia-related death occurred in 0.4% of patients receiving ixabepilone monotherapy. No neutropenia-related deaths were reported in patients with serum AST or ALT concentrations exceeding 2.5 times the upper limit of normal or serum bilirubin concentrations exceeding 1.5 times the upper limit of normal treated with ixabepilone monotherapy.

Ixabepilone should not be administered to patients with a neutrophil count less than 1500/mm³. Frequent determinations of peripheral blood cell counts are recommended for all patients receiving the drug to monitor for myelosuppression. Patients who experience severe neutropenia or thrombocytopenia should have their dosage reduced. (See Dosage and Administration: Dosage Modification for Toxicity.)

Hypersensitivity Reactions. Patients with a history of severe hypersensitivity reaction to agents containing polyoxyl 35 castor oil (Cremophor® EL, polyoxyethylated castor oil), such as paclitaxel, should *not* be treated with ixabepilone. All patients receiving ixabepilone should be premedicated with an antihistamine and a histamine H_2-receptor antagonist approximately 1 hour before beginning the ixabepilone infusion and should also be observed for hypersensitivity reactions (e.g., flushing, rash, dyspnea, bronchospasm). (See Dosage and Administration: General.) If a severe hypersensitivity reaction develops, the infusion of ixabepilone should be stopped and aggressive supportive treatment (e.g., epinephrine, corticosteroids) instituted. Severe hypersensitivity reactions (including anaphylaxis) have occurred in 9 out of 1323 (approximately 1%) of patients receiving the drug in clinical trials; 3 out of 9 of these were able to be retreated. The manufacturer states that patients who experience a hypersensitivity reaction in one cycle of ixabepilone treatment must be premedicated in subsequent cycles with a corticosteroid in addition to the antihistamine and a histamine H_2-receptor antagonist, and extension of the infusion time should be considered. (For more information on hypersensitivity reactions associated with the polyoxyl 35 castor oil vehicle, see Cautions: Sensitivity Reactions, in Cyclosporine 92:44.)

Cardiovascular Effects. The incidence of adverse cardiovascular effects (myocardial ischemia and ventricular dysfunction) was higher in patients receiving combined ixabepilone and capecitabine therapy (1.9%) than in those receiving capecitabine alone (0.3%). Supraventricular arrhythmias were observed in patients receiving combination treatment (0.5%) but not those receiving capecitabine alone. The manufacturer recommends that ixabepilone be used with caution in patients with a history of cardiac disease. Discontinuance of the drug should be considered in patients who develop cardiac ischemia or impaired cardiac function.

Potential for Cognitive Impairment from Excipient. Since the diluent in the commercially available Ixempra® kit contains dehydrated alcohol, the possibility of adverse CNS effects, including cognitive impairment, and other effects of alcohol should be considered. (See Advice to Patients.)

Radiation Recall. Radiation recall has been reported in patients receiving ixabepilone.

Specific Populations **Pregnancy.** Category D. (See Users Guide.)

Lactation. Not known whether ixabepilone is distributed into human milk; however, in lactating rats given radiolabeled ixabepilone, concentrations of radioactivity in milk were comparable to those in plasma and declined in parallel with plasma concentrations of the drug. Discontinue nursing or the drug, taking into account the importance of the drug to the woman.

Pediatric Use. Safety and efficacy not established in pediatric patients younger than 18 years of age.

Geriatric Use. Clinical studies of ixabepilone did not include sufficient numbers of patients 65 years of age and older to determine whether geriatric patients respond differently than younger patients. In clinical studies, 45 out of 431 breast cancer patients receiving ixabepilone and capecitabine in combination were 65 years of age or older and 3 patients were 75 years of age or older. Overall, the incidence of grade 3 or 4 adverse reactions was higher in geriatric patients 65 years of age and older compared with younger patients (82 and 68%, respectively); these reactions included stomatitis, diarrhea, palmar-plantar erythrodysesthesia syndrome, peripheral neuropathy, febrile neutropenia, fatigue, and asthenia. Toxicity-related deaths occurred in 2 out of 43 (4.7%) patients 65 years of age or older with normal baseline hepatic function or mild hepatic impairment. In clinical studies, 32 out of 240 breast cancer patients receiving ixabepilone as monotherapy were 65 years of age or older and 6 patients were 75 years of age or older. No overall differences in safety were observed in these patients compared with those younger than 65 years of age.

Hepatic Impairment. Patients with baseline serum AST or ALT concentrations exceeding 2.5 times the upper limit of normal or serum bilirubin concentrations exceeding 1.5 times the upper limit of normal experienced greater toxicity than patients with baseline AST or ALT concentrations not exceeding 2.5 times the upper limit of normal or serum bilirubin concentrations not exceeding 1.5 times the upper limit of normal when treated with ixabepilone 40 mg/m² in combination with capecitabine or as monotherapy in breast cancer clinical studies. Ixabepilone and capecitabine combination therapy is contraindicated in patients with serum AST or ALT concentrations exceeding 2.5 times the upper limit of normal or serum bilirubin concentrations elevated above the upper limit of normal (i.e., exceeding 1 times the upper limit of normal). (See Toxicity in Hepatic Impairment under Warnings/Precautions: Warnings, in Cautions.)

Dosage reduction depending on the degree of hepatic impairment is recommended if ixabepilone is used as monotherapy in patients with hepatic impairment. Because there is a need for dosage adjustment based on hepatic function, assessment of hepatic function is recommended before initiation of ixabepilone and periodically thereafter. (See Dosage and Administration: Special Populations.) Caution is also advised if ixabepilone monotherapy is used in patients with hepatic impairment.

Renal Impairment. Ixabepilone is minimally excreted via the kidneys. No controlled pharmacokinetic studies have been conducted with the drug in patients with renal impairment. In addition, ixabepilone and capecitabine combination therapy has not been evaluated in patients with a calculated creatinine clearance of less than 50 mL/minute. Ixabepilone given as monotherapy has not been evaluated in patients with serum creatinine concentrations exceeding 1.5 times the upper limit of normal. In a population pharmacokinetic analysis of ixabepilone monotherapy, there was no meaningful effect of mild and moderate renal insufficiency (creatinine clearance exceeding 30 mL/minute) on the pharmacokinetics of the drug. The manufacturer does not make specific dosage adjustment recommendations for ixabepilone in renal impairment.

■ **Common Adverse Effects** Adverse effects reported in 20% or more of patients receiving ixabepilone included peripheral sensory neuropathy, fatigue/asthenia, myalgia/arthralgia, alopecia, nausea, vomiting, stomatitis/mucositis, diarrhea, and musculoskeletal pain. Incidence of adverse effects was generally higher in patients receiving both ixabepilone and capecitabine than in those receiving ixabepilone alone. Adverse effects reported in 20% or more of patients receiving ixabepilone in combination with capecitabine included palmar-plantar erythrodysesthesia (hand-foot syndrome), anorexia, abdominal pain, nail disorder, and constipation. Adverse hematologic effects reported in 40% or more of patients include neutropenia, leukopenia, anemia, and thrombocytopenia.

Drug Interactions

■ **Drugs Affecting or Metabolized by Hepatic Microsomal Enzymes** ***Inhibitors of Cytochrome P-450 (CYP) 3A4 Isoenzyme*** Pharmacokinetic interaction (increased plasma ixabepilone concentrations) may occur during concomitant administration of potent CYP3A4 inhibitors (e.g., amprenavir [no longer commercially available in the US], atazanavir, clarithromycin, delavirdine, indinavir, itraconazole, ketoconazole, nefazodone, nelfinavir, ritonavir, saquinavir, telithromycin, voriconazole); concomitant use of ixabepilone with these drugs should be avoided. Concurrent administration of ixabepilone with ketoconazole increased the area under the plasma concentration-time curve (AUC) of ixabepilone by 79% compared with ixabepilone treatment alone. Close monitoring for toxicity and reduction of ixabepilone dosage to 20 mg/m² should be considered if concomitant therapy with a potent CYP3A4 inhibitor and ixabepilone is needed. Upon discontinuance of the CYP3A4 inhibitor, approximately 1 week should elapse before adjusting the ixabepilone dosage back to the usual recommended dosage of 40 mg/m².

Because the effect of mild or moderate CYP3A4 inhibitors (e.g., erythromycin, fluconazole, verapamil) on exposure to ixabepilone has not been studied, caution should be used during concomitant administration of these drugs and use of alternative therapeutic agents that do not inhibit CYP3A4 should be considered. Patients receiving CYP3A4 inhibitors during ixabepilone therapy should be closely monitored for acute toxicity (e.g., frequent monitoring of peripheral blood counts between cycles of ixabepilone).

Inducers of CYP3A4 Pharmacokinetic interaction (decreased and possibly subtherapeutic plasma ixabepilone concentrations) may occur during concomitant use with potent CYP3A4 inducers (e.g., carbamazepine, dexamethasone, phenobarbital, phenytoin, rifabutin, rifampin); concomitant use of ixabepilone with these drugs should be avoided. Concurrent administration of ixabepilone with rifampin decreased the AUC of ixabepilone by 43% compared with ixabepilone treatment alone. If concurrent administration of other drugs is indicated during ixabepilone therapy, drugs with no or minimal enzyme induction potential should be considered. If concomitant administration of a potent CYP3A4 inducer is necessary during ixabepilone therapy, dosage may be gradually increased from 40 mg/m² to 60 mg/m², and patients should be monitored carefully for toxicity. (See Dosage and Administration: Dosage.) A dosage of 60 mg/m² over 4 hours is predicted to result in an AUC of ixabepilone in the range observed at the usual recommended dosage without concomitant enzyme inducers. Upon discontinuance of the CYP3A4 inducer, the ixabepilone dosage should be returned to the dosage used prior to initiation of the inducer.

Since St. John's wort (*Hypericum perforatum*) may cause unpredictable decreases in plasma ixabepilone concentrations, such concomitant use should be avoided.

Substrates of CYP3A4 and other CYP Isoenzymes At clinically relevant plasma concentrations, ixabepilone does not inhibit CYP isoenzymes 3A4, 1A2, 2A6, 2B6, 2C8, 2C9, 2C19, or 2D6 and does not induce CYP isoenzymes 3A4, 1A2, 2B6, or 2C9; pharmacokinetic interaction is unlikely when ixabepilone is used with substrates of these isoenzymes.

■ **Drugs Affecting the P-glycoprotein Transport System** In vitro studies indicate that ixabepilone is a weak inhibitor and a substrate for the P-glycoprotein transport system.

■ **Capecitabine** Concomitant administration of ixabepilone with capecitabine has decreased peak ixabepilone and capecitabine concentrations by 19 and 27%, respectively, and increased fluorouracil AUC by 14% compared with separate administration of these drugs. This pharmacokinetic interaction is unlikely to be clinically important and effectiveness of combination therapy with these drugs has been demonstrated in clinical trials.

■ **Grapefruit** Grapefruit juice and other grapefruit products should be avoided because of the potential for increased plasma ixabepilone concentrations.

Description

Ixabepilone is a microtubule inhibitor belonging to the epothilone class of antineoplastic agents. Epothilones are naturally occurring products of fermentation from the myxobacterium *Sorangium cellulosum.* Ixabepilone is a semisynthetic derivative of epothilone B, a 16-membered polyketide macrolide, with a chemically modified lactam substitution for the naturally existing lactone. Ixabepilone binds to β-tubulin subunits on microtubules and stabilizes and suppresses microtubule activity resulting in mitotic arrest and apoptosis. Although ixabepilone appears to share a similar antimicrotubule mechanism of action with taxanes, the drug differs structurally from taxanes and does not appear to be affected by common mechanisms of taxane resistance.

Ixabepilone is active in xenografts that are resistant to multiple antineoplastic agents, including taxanes, anthracyclines, and vinca alkaloids. The drug has also demonstrated synergistic antitumor activity in combination with capecitabine in vivo. In addition to direct antitumor activity, ixabepilone possesses antiangiogenic activity.

Ixabepilone is extensively metabolized in the liver, principally by oxidative metabolism via the cytochrome P-450 (CYP) isoenzyme 3A4. The drug is eliminated primarily as metabolized drug, with more than 30 inactive metabolites eliminated in urine and feces. No single metabolite accounted for more than 6% of the administered dose. Following IV administration of a single dose of radiolabeled drug, approximately 86% of the dose was eliminated within 7 days, 65% in feces and 21% in urine. Unchanged ixabepilone accounted for less than 2 and 6% of the dose in feces and urine, respectively. The drug has a terminal elimination half-life of approximately 52 hours (range: 20–72 hours). No accumulation in plasma is expected when the drug is administered once every 3 weeks.

Advice to Patients

Importance of reading the patient information provided by the manufacturer.

Risk of neuropathy. Importance of patients notifying clinicians if they develop any numbness, tingling, or burning of the hands or feet.

Importance of patients notifying clinicians if they develop a fever of 100.5°F or higher or other signs and symptoms of potential infection (e.g., chills, cough, burning or pain upon urination).

Importance of patients notifying clinicians if they experience urticaria, pruritus, rash, flushing, swelling, dyspnea, chest tightness, and/or other hypersensitivity-related symptoms following IV infusion of ixabepilone.

Importance of patients notifying clinicians if they notice chest pain, difficulty breathing, palpitations, or unusual weight gain.

Importance of patients informing clinicians if they are allergic to a drug such as paclitaxel that contains polyoxyl 35 castor oil (Cremophor® EL, polyethoxylated castor oil).

Importance of patients informing clinicians if they have hepatic impairment. Importance of undergoing blood tests to determine liver function before and during ixabepilone therapy. Importance of not taking ixabepilone in combination with capecitabine if hepatic impairment is present.

Importance of not drinking grapefruit juice while receiving ixabepilone therapy.

Importance of informing patients that Ixempra® contains alcohol and may cause drowsiness or dizziness. Importance of avoiding certain activities (e.g., operating machinery, driving a motor vehicle) if patient feels drowsy or dizzy.

Importance of informing clinicians of existing or contemplated concomitant therapy, including prescription and OTC drugs and dietary or herbal supplements (e.g., St. John's wort), as well as any concomitant illnesses (e.g., diabetes mellitus, liver disease).

Importance of women informing clinicians if they are or plan to become pregnant or plan to breast-feed. Apprise patient of potential hazard to the fetus if used during pregnancy; women of childbearing potential should avoid becoming pregnant.

Importance of informing patients of other important precautionary information. (See Cautions.)

Overview® (see Users Guide). For additional information on this drug until a more detailed monograph is developed and published, the manufacturer's labeling should be consulted. It is *essential* that the manufacturer's labeling be consulted for more detailed information on usual cautions, precautions, contraindications, potential drug interactions, laboratory test interferences, and acute toxicity. For further information on the handling of antineoplastic agents, see the ASHP Guidelines on Handling Hazardous Drugs at http://www.ahfsdruginformation.com.

Preparations

Excipients in commercially available drug preparations may have clinically important effects in some individuals; consult specific product labeling for details.

Ixabepilone

Parenteral		
For injection, for IV infusion only	15 mg	**Ixempra®**, Bristol-Myers Squibb
	45 mg	**Ixempra®**, Bristol-Myers Squibb

†Use is not currently included in the labeling approved by the US Food and Drug Administration

Ixazomib Citrate

■ Ixazomib, an inhibitor of the 20S proteasome, is an antineoplastic agent.

Uses

■ **Multiple Myeloma** Ixazomib is used in combination with lenalidomide and dexamethasone for the treatment of multiple myeloma in patients who have received at least one prior therapy. Ixazomib is designated an orphan drug by FDA for this use.

The current indication for ixazomib in combination with lenalidomide and dexamethasone in patients with relapsed and/or refractory multiple myeloma who have received at least one prior therapy is based principally on the results of a randomized, double-blind, placebo-controlled study in 722 patients (age range: 30–91 years, median age 66 years). Patients refractory to lenalidomide or proteasome inhibitors were not included in the study.

In this study, patients were randomized in a 1:1 ratio to receive either the combination of ixazomib, lenalidomide, and dexamethasone or the combination of placebo, lenalidomide, and dexamethasone until disease progression or unacceptable toxicity occurred. Randomization was stratified based on the number of previous lines of therapy (1 versus 2 or 3), myeloma International Staging System (stage I or II versus III), and prior therapy with a proteasome inhibitor (exposed or naive). Most patients in the study were Caucasian (85%), had relapsed multiple myeloma (77%), were in stage I or II of multiple myeloma (88%), and had received one prior line of therapy (61%). Light chain disease was reported in 23% of patients, while 12% of patients had free light chain-measurable only disease. Patients received oral ixazomib 4 mg or placebo on days 1, 8, and 15 plus oral lenalidomide 25 mg on days 1 through 21; all patients also received oral dexamethasone 40 mg on days 1, 8, 15, and 22 of each 28-day cycle. Patients with renal impairment received an initial dose of lenalidomide according to the manufacturer's labeling for the drug. Thromboprophylaxis also was recommended for all patients in both treatment groups according to the manufacturer's labeling for lenalidomide. At the clinician's discretion, antiemetics were administered in 19 or 12% of patients assigned to the ixazomib or placebo regimen, respectively; antivirals in 64 or 60%, respectively; and antihistamines in 27 or 19%, respectively, for prophylaxis and/or management of symptoms. The primary end point of the study was progression-free survival defined as the time from randomization to time of first documentation of disease progression, according to the 2011 International Myeloma Working Group Consensus Uniform Response Criteria as assessed by a blinded independent review committee based on central laboratory results. Response was assessed every 4 weeks until disease progression occurred.

Improvement in progression-free survival was demonstrated in patients receiving the ixazomib regimen compared with those receiving the placebo regimen. Progressive disease or death was reported in 36% of patients randomly assigned to the ixazomib treatment group compared with 43% of those assigned to the placebo group (hazard ratio 0.74). Median times to response were 1.1 months in the ixazomib treatment group and 1.9 months in the placebo group, and median duration of response was 20.5 or 15 months for the ixazomib or placebo groups, respectively, in the evaluable population. Furthermore, the overall response rates were 78 and 72% in patients receiving the ixazomib and placebo regimens, respectively. A non-inferential progression-free survival analysis was conducted at a median follow-up of 23 months with 372 progression-free survival events; the hazard ratio of progression-free survival was 0.82 for patients receiving the ixazomib regimen compared with the placebo regimen. Estimated median progression-free survival was 20 months in patients receiving the ixazomib regimen and 15.9 months in those receiving the placebo regimen. A planned interim analysis measuring overall survival also was conducted simultaneously, with 35% of the required number of deaths for final overall analysis. Deaths were reported in 81 or 90 patients receiving the ixazomib or placebo regimen, respectively, and an overall survival benefit was not demonstrated.

Dosage and Administration

■ **General** Before a new cycle of ixazomib therapy is initiated, absolute neutrophil count (ANC) should be at least 1000/mm³; platelet count should be at least 75,000/mm³; and at clinician's discretion, nonhematologic toxicities generally should be returned to grade 1 or less or to baseline.

Clinicians should consult the respective manufacturers' labeling for additional information regarding lenalidomide and dexamethasone used in combination regimens.

If capsule breakage occurs, direct contact of the contents of ixazomib capsules with the skin or eyes should be avoided. If contact with the skin or eyes occurs, the skin should be washed thoroughly with soap and water, and the eyes should be flushed thoroughly with water.

■ **Administration** Ixazomib is administered once weekly on the same day and at approximately the same time for the first 3 weeks of each 4-week cycle.

Ixazomib is administered orally at least 1 hour before or at least 2 hours after food.

Ixazomib and dexamethasone should not be administered simultaneously on days that patients receive both medications, because dexamethasone is given with food, while ixazomib is given on an empty stomach.

Ixazomib capsules should be swallowed whole with water and should *not* be crushed, chewed, or opened.

If vomiting occurs after a dose of ixazomib is administered, the dose should not be repeated. Instead, the next dose should be administered at the regularly scheduled time.

If a dose of ixazomib is delayed or missed, the dose should be administered only if there are at least 72 hours until the next scheduled dose. A missed dose should *not* be administered within 72 hours of the next scheduled dose, and the dose should *not* be doubled to make up for the missed dose.

■ **Dosage** Dosage of ixazomib citrate is expressed in terms of ixazomib.

Multiple Myeloma For use in combination with lenalidomide and dexamethasone in the treatment of multiple myeloma in patients who have received at least one prior therapy, the recommended initial dosages in each 28-day cycle are ixazomib 4 mg administered orally once weekly on days 1, 8, and 15; lenalidomide 25 mg administered orally once daily on days 1–21; and dexamethasone 40 mg administered orally on days 1, 8, 15, and 22. Treatment should be continued until disease progression or unacceptable toxicity occurs.

Dosage Modification for Toxicity Management of some adverse effects may require temporary interruption of therapy, dosage reduction, and/or permanent discontinuance of ixazomib therapy. Up to 2 dosage reductions for toxicity may be made. If dosage modification from 4 mg is necessary, an initial dosage reduction to 3 mg once weekly is recommended. If further dosage reduction is necessary, the dosage should be reduced to 2.3 mg once weekly. Dosages less than 2.3 mg once weekly are not recommended.

Dosage Modification for Hematologic Toxicity. If ANC is less than 500/mm^3, ixazomib and lenalidomide should be withheld until ANC is at least 500/mm^3. The addition of granulocyte colony-stimulating factors also should be considered based on clinical guidelines. When ANC returns to at least 500/mm^3, lenalidomide should be reduced by 1 dose level according to the manufacturer's labeling, and ixazomib should be resumed at the previous dosage (i.e., 4, 3, or 2.3 mg). If ANC less than 500/mm^3 recurs, ixazomib and lenalidomide should be withheld until ANC is at least 500/mm^3; the ixazomib dose should then be reduced by 1 dose level (i.e., a dose of 4 mg reduced to 3 mg or a dose of 3 mg reduced to 2.3 mg), and lenalidomide should be resumed at the previous dosage following resolution of toxicity. For additional occurrences of neutropenia, dosage modifications of ixazomib and lenalidomide should be alternated. Following a second dosage reduction of ixazomib, the treatment regimen should be discontinued if ANC below 500/mm^3 recurs.

If the platelet count is less than 30,000/mm^3, ixazomib and lenalidomide should be withheld until platelet count is at least 30,000/mm^3. When the platelet count returns to at least 30,000/mm^3, ixazomib may be continued at the previous dosage (i.e., 4, 3, or 2.3 mg), and lenalidomide should be reduced by 1 dose level according to the manufacturer's labeling. If platelet count less than 30,000/mm^3 recurs, ixazomib and lenalidomide should be withheld until platelet count is at least 30,000/mm^3. Following return of platelet count to at least 30,000/mm^3, ixazomib should be resumed at 1 dose level lower than the previous dosage (i.e., a dose of 4 mg reduced to 3 mg or a dose of 3 mg reduced to 2.3 mg), and lenalidomide should be resumed at the previous dosage. For additional occurrences of thrombocytopenia, dosage modifications of ixazomib and lenalidomide should be alternated. Following a second dosage reduction of ixazomib, the treatment regimen should be discontinued if platelet count below 30,000/mm^3 recurs.

Dosage Modification for Peripheral Neuropathy. If grade 1 *with pain* or grade 2 peripheral neuropathy occurs, ixazomib should be withheld until peripheral neuropathy resolves to grade 1 or less *without pain* or returns to baseline. Following resolution, ixazomib should be resumed at the previous dosage (i.e., 4, 3, or 2.3 mg). The treatment regimen should be discontinued if grade 1 *with pain* or grade 2 peripheral neuropathy occurs following a second dosage reduction of ixazomib.

If grade 2 *with pain* or grade 3 peripheral neuropathy occurs, ixazomib should be withheld and, at the clinician's discretion, generally should resolve to grade 1 or less or to baseline prior to resuming ixazomib. Following resolution, ixazomib should be resumed at 1 dose level lower than the previous dosage (i.e., a dose of 4 mg reduced to 3 mg or a dose of 3 mg reduced to 2.3 mg). The treatment regimen should be discontinued if grade 2 *with pain* or grade 3 peripheral neuropathy occurs following a second dosage reduction of ixazomib.

If any grade 4 peripheral neuropathy occurs, the treatment regimen should be discontinued.

Dosage Modification for Dermatologic Toxicity. If grade 2 or 3 rash occurs, lenalidomide should be withheld until rash resolves to grade 1 or less. Following resolution, lenalidomide should be resumed at 1 dose level lower than the previous dosage according to the manufacturer's labeling. If grade 2 or 3 rash recurs, ixazomib and lenalidomide should be withheld until rash resolves to grade 1 or less. Following resolution, ixazomib should be resumed at 1 dose level lower than the previous dosage (i.e., a dose of 4 mg reduced to 3 mg or a dose of 3 mg reduced to 2.3 mg), and lenalidomide should be resumed at the previous dosage. For additional occurrences of rash, dosage modifications of ixazomib and lenalidomide should be alternated. The treatment regimen should be discontinued if grade 2 or 3 rash occurs following a second dosage reduction of ixazomib.

If any grade 4 rash occurs, the treatment regimen should be discontinued.

Dosage Modification for Other Nonhematologic Toxicity. If other grade 3 or 4 nonhematologic toxicity occurs, ixazomib should be withheld and, at the clinician's discretion, generally should resolve to patient's condition at baseline or to grade 1 or less prior to resuming ixazomib. If the nonhematologic toxicity is attributable to ixazomib, then ixazomib should be resumed at 1 dose level lower than the previous dosage (i.e., a dose of 4 mg reduced to 3 mg or a dose of 3 mg reduced to 2.3 mg) following resolution of toxicity. The treatment regimen should be discontinued if grade 3 or 4 nonhematologic toxicity occurs following a second dosage reduction of ixazomib.

■ **Special Populations** The initial dosage of ixazomib should be reduced to 3 mg weekly in patients with moderate (total bilirubin exceeding 1.5 to 3 times the upper limit of normal [ULN]) or severe (total bilirubin exceeding 3 times the ULN) hepatic impairment.

The initial dosage of ixazomib should be reduced to 3 mg weekly in patients with severe renal impairment (creatinine clearance less than 30 mL/minute) or in those with end-stage renal disease (ESRD) requiring dialysis. Ixazomib is not dialyzable; therefore, the drug can be administered without regard to the timing of dialysis.

Clinicians should consult the manufacturer's labeling for lenalidomide for specific dosage recommendations of the drug in patients with hepatic or renal impairment.

Cautions

■ **Contraindications** The manufacturer states there are no known contraindications to the use of ixazomib.

■ **Warnings/Precautions** ***Thrombocytopenia*** Thrombocytopenia has been reported frequently in patients receiving ixazomib with platelet nadirs usually occurring on days 14–21 of each 28-day cycle and resolving to baseline by the beginning of the next cycle. Platelet count was 10,000/mm^3 or less during treatment in 3 or 1% of patients receiving the ixazomib or placebo regimen, respectively. Less than 1% of patients receiving either regimen had a platelet count of 5000/mm^3 or less during treatment. Treatment was discontinued because of thrombocytopenia at similar rates in the 2 treatment groups. Platelet transfusions were required in 6 or 5% of patients receiving the ixazomib or placebo regimen, respectively. Platelet counts should be monitored at least monthly in patients receiving ixazomib. However, more frequent monitoring should be considered during the first 3 treatment cycles. Thrombocytopenia should be managed with dosage modifications and platelet transfusions according to the standard of care. (See Dosage Modification for Hematologic Toxicity under Dosage: Dosage Modification for Toxicity, in Dosage and Administration.)

GI Toxicity Diarrhea was reported in 42 or 36% of patients receiving the ixazomib or placebo regimen, respectively; constipation in 34 or 25%, respectively; nausea in 26 or 21%, respectively; and vomiting in 22 or 11%, respectively. Use of antidiarrheal or antiemetic drugs and/or supportive care was required occasionally. In the principal efficacy study, 1% of patients receiving the ixazomib regimen discontinued 1 or more of the 3 drugs as a result of diarrhea, compared with less than 1% of patients in the placebo group. Dosage modifications should be made for patients who experience grade 3 or 4 adverse GI effects. (See Dosage Modification for Other Nonhematologic Toxicity under Dosage: Dosage Modification for Toxicity, in Dosage and Administration.)

Peripheral Neuropathy Peripheral neuropathy has been reported in patients receiving ixazomib. Most cases were grade 1 (18 or 14% of patients receiving the ixazomib or placebo regimen, respectively) or grade 2 (8 or 5% of patients receiving the ixazomib or placebo regimen, respectively). Grade 3 peripheral neuropathy was reported in 2% of patients receiving either treatment regimen; no cases of grade 4 or serious peripheral neuropathy were reported. Peripheral sensory neuropathy was reported in 19 or 14% of patients receiving the ixazomib or placebo regimen, respectively; peripheral motor neuropathy was not commonly reported in those receiving either treatment regimen. Peripheral neuropathy resulted in discontinuance of 1 or more of the 3 drugs in 1% of patients receiving either treatment regimen. Patients should be monitored for symptoms of peripheral neuropathy, and dosage modifications may be required in those experiencing new or worsening symptoms. (See Dosage Modification for Peripheral Neuropathy under Dosage: Dosage Modification for Toxicity, in Dosage and Administration.)

Peripheral Edema Peripheral edema was reported in 25 or 18% of patients receiving the ixazomib or placebo regimen, respectively. Most cases were grade 1 (16% of patients receiving the ixazomib treatment regimen compared with 13% of patients receiving the placebo regimen) or grade 2 (7% of patients receiving the ixazomib treatment regimen compared with 4% of patients receiving the placebo regimen). Grade 3 peripheral edema was also reported in 2 or 1% of patients receiving the ixazomib or placebo regimen, respectively. No cases of grade 4 peripheral edema were reported, and no patients required discontinuance of treatment because of peripheral edema. If peripheral edema occurs, patients should be assessed for underlying causes and supportive care should be provided, as warranted. Dosing of dexamethasone should be modified based on the manufacturer's labeling for the drug; dosage of ixazomib should be adjusted for grade 3 or 4 symptoms. (See Dosage Modification for Other Nonhematologic Toxicity under Dosage: Dosage Modification for Toxicity, in Dosage and Administration.)

Dermatologic Reactions Rash was reported in 19 or 11% of patients receiving the ixazomib or placebo regimen, respectively. Most adverse dermatologic reactions were grade 1 (10% in the ixazomib treatment group compared with 7% in the placebo group) or grade 2 (6% in the ixazomib treatment group compared with 3% in the placebo group). Grade 3 rash was reported in 3% of patients receiving the ixazomib regimen and 1% of patients receiving the placebo regimen. No cases of grade 4 or serious rash were reported. The most common types of rash reported in patients receiving either regimen included maculopapular and macular rash. Rash resulted in discontinuance of 1 or more of the 3 drugs in less than 1% of patients receiving either treatment regimen. Rash should be managed with supportive care or with dosage modification if grade 2 or higher rash occurs. (See Dosage Modification for Dermatologic Toxicity under Dosage: Dosage Modification for Toxicity, in Dosage and Administration.)

Hepatotoxicity Hepatotoxicity, including drug-induced hepatic injury, hepatocellular injury, hepatic steatosis, cholestatic hepatitis, and hepatotoxicity, has been reported in less than 1% of patients receiving ixazomib. Hepatic impairment also has been reported (6% in the ixazomib group compared with 5% in the placebo group). Hepatic enzymes should be monitored regularly, and dosage modifications should be made in patients experiencing grade 3 or 4 symptoms. (See Dosage Modification for Other Nonhematologic Toxicity under Dosage: Dosage Modification for Toxicity, in Dosage and Administration.)

Fetal/Neonatal Morbidity and Mortality Ixazomib can cause fetal harm based on its mechanism of action and animal findings. There are no adequate and well-controlled studies in pregnant women. Ixazomib caused embryofetal toxicity (e.g., skeletal variations/abnormalities, decreased fetal weight, trend toward decreased fetal viability, increased postimplantation loss) in pregnant rats and rabbits receiving the drug at dosages resulting in exposures slightly higher than those observed in patients receiving the recommended dosage. Women of childbearing potential should be advised to avoid becoming pregnant while receiving ixazomib. If ixazomib is used during pregnancy, or if the patient becomes pregnant while receiving ixazomib, the patient should be apprised of the potential hazard to the fetus. Women of childbearing potential and men who are partners of such women must use effective contraception during ixazomib treatment and for 90 days following the last dose of the drug.

Specific Populations **Pregnancy.** Based on its mechanism of action and animal findings, ixazomib can cause fetal harm if administered to pregnant women. (See Fetal/Neonatal Morbidity and Mortality under Cautions: Warnings/Precautions.)

Lactation. It is not known whether ixazomib or its metabolites are distributed into milk. Because of the potential for serious adverse effects to ixazomib in nursing infants, women should discontinue nursing during ixazomib therapy.

Pediatric Use. Safety and efficacy of ixazomib have not been established in pediatric patients.

Geriatric Use. Of the total number of patients in clinical studies evaluating ixazomib, 55% were 65 years of age or older and 17% were 75 years of age or older. No overall differences in safety or efficacy were observed between geriatric patients and younger adults, and other clinical experience has not demonstrated differences in responses between the geriatric and younger patients. However, greater sensitivity of some older patients cannot be ruled out.

Hepatic Impairment. The pharmacokinetics of ixazomib were similar in patients with normal hepatic function and in those with mild hepatic impairment (total bilirubin less than or equal to the upper limit of normal [ULN] and aspartate aminotransferase (AST) concentrations exceeding the ULN, or total bilirubin exceeding 1 to 1.5 times the ULN and any AST concentration) based on a population pharmacokinetic analysis. The pharmacokinetics of ixazomib were characterized in patients with normal hepatic function receiving 4 mg, in those with moderate hepatic impairment (total bilirubin exceeding 1.5 to 3 times the ULN) receiving 2.3 mg, and in those with severe hepatic impairment (total bilirubin exceeding 3 times the ULN) receiving 1.5 mg. Dose-normalized mean area under the concentration-time curve (AUC) increased by 20% in those with moderate or severe hepatic impairment compared with patients with normal hepatic function. In patients with moderate or severe hepatic impairment, the initial dosage of ixazomib should be reduced. (See Dosage and Administration: Special Populations.)

Renal Impairment. The pharmacokinetics of ixazomib were similar in patients with normal renal function and in those with mild (creatinine clearance 60–89 mL/minute) or moderate (creatinine clearance 30–59 mL/minute) renal impairment based on a population pharmacokinetic analysis. Pre- and post-dialyzer concentrations of ixazomib measured during hemodialysis were also similar, suggesting that ixazomib is not dialyzable. The pharmacokinetics of ixazomib were characterized at a dose of 3 mg in patients with normal renal function (creatinine clearance 90 mL/minute or greater), severe renal impairment (creatinine clearance less than 30 mL/minute), or end-stage renal disease (ESRD) requiring dialysis. Mean AUC was increased by 39% in patients with severe renal impairment or ESRD requiring dialysis compared with those with normal renal function. The initial dosage of ixazomib should be reduced in patients with severe renal impairment or ESRD requiring dialysis. (See Dosage and Administration: Special Populations.)

■ **Common Adverse Effects** Nonhematologic adverse effects reported in 5% or more of patients receiving ixazomib in combination with lenalidomide and dexamethasone, and at an incidence at least 5% higher than that reported with placebo given in combination with lenalidomide and dexamethasone, include rash, upper respiratory tract infection, back pain, vomiting, peripheral edema, nausea, peripheral neuropathy, constipation, and diarrhea.

Thrombocytopenia was reported in 20% or more of patients receiving the ixazomib regimen and at a frequency greater than that observed with the placebo regimen.

Drug Interactions

Ixazomib is a low-affinity substrate of P-glycoprotein (P-gp); the drug is not a substrate of breast cancer resistance protein (BCRP), multidrug resistance protein (MRP) 2, or hepatic organic anion transport protein (OATP).

Ixazomib is not a reversible or time-dependent inhibitor of cytochrome (CYP) P-450 isoenzymes 1A2, 2B6, 2C8, 2C9, 2C19, 2D6, or 3A4/5. Ixazomib also is not an inhibitor of P-gp, BCRP, MRP2, OATP 1B1 or 1B3, organic cation transporter (OCT) 2, organic anion transporter (OAT) 1 or 3, or multidrug and toxin extrusion (MATE) 1 or MATE2K transporters.

Ixazomib does not induce CYP isoenzymes 1A2, 2B6, or 3A4/5 or corresponding immunoreactive protein concentrations and is not expected to produce pharmacokinetic interactions via CYP inhibition or induction. Additionally, ixazomib is not expected to cause transporter-mediated pharmacokinetic interactions.

■ **Drugs Affecting or Affected by Hepatic Microsomal Enzymes** Concomitant administration of ixazomib with potent CYP1A2 inhibitors did not result in a clinically important change in the systemic exposure of ixazomib based on a population pharmacokinetic analysis.

Concomitant use of ixazomib and potent CYP3A inducers (e.g., carbamazepine, phenytoin, rifampin, and St. John's wort) can potentially decrease the systemic exposure of ixazomib. Concomitant use of ixazomib and potent CYP3A inducers should be avoided.

■ **Carbamazepine** Concomitant administration of ixazomib with carbamazepine, a potent CYP3A inducer, can potentially decrease the systemic exposure of ixazomib. Concomitant use of ixazomib and carbamazepine should be avoided.

■ **Clarithromycin** Concomitant administration of ixazomib and clarithromycin, a potent CYP3A inhibitor, did not result in a clinically important change in the systemic exposure of ixazomib.

■ **Phenytoin** Concomitant administration of ixazomib with phenytoin, a potent CYP3A inducer, can potentially decrease the systemic exposure of ixazomib. Concomitant use of ixazomib and phenytoin should be avoided.

■ **Rifampin** Concomitant administration of ixazomib with rifampin, a potent CYP3A inducer, decreased the peak plasma concentration and area under the concentration-time curve (AUC) of ixazomib by 54 and 74%, respectively. Concomitant use of ixazomib and rifampin should be avoided.

■ **St. John's Wort** Concomitant administration of ixazomib with St. John's wort (*Hypericum perforatum*), a potent CYP3A inducer, can potentially decrease the systemic exposure of ixazomib. Concomitant use of ixazomib and St. John's wort should be avoided.

Description

Ixazomib citrate is a prodrug of ixazomib, a boron-containing selective inhibitor of the 20S proteasome; ixazomib is an antineoplastic agent. Ixazomib citrate is rapidly hydrolyzed to its active form (ixazomib). Ixazomib reversibly binds the $\beta5$ subunit of the 20S proteasome and inhibits its chymotrypsin-like activity. In vitro, ixazomib induces caspase-mediated apoptosis of multiple myeloma cell lines and has demonstrated cytotoxicity against myeloma cells obtained from patients who had relapsed following previous therapies, including bortezomib, lenalidomide, and dexamethasone. Concomitant use of ixazomib and lenalidomide has demonstrated synergistic cytotoxic effects in multiple myeloma cell lines, and ixazomib has demonstrated antitumor activity in a mouse multiple myeloma tumor xenograft model in vivo.

Mean absolute oral bioavailability of ixazomib is 58% based on a population pharmacokinetic analysis. Following oral administration, the median time to peak plasma concentration is 1 hour. The terminal half-life of ixazomib is 9.5 days. Systemic exposure of the drug increases in a dose-proportional manner over a dosage range of 0.2–10.6 mg, and following weekly oral dosing, the accumulation is twofold. A high-fat meal decreases the area under the concentration-time curve (AUC) and peak plasma concentration of ixazomib by 28 and 69%, respectively. Metabolism by multiple cytochrome P-450 (CYP) isoenzymes and through non-CYP-dependent pathways is expected to be the primary clearance mechanism of ixazomib. Age, gender, body surface area, or race do not demonstrate a clinically important effect on the clearance of ixazomib based on a population pharmacokinetic analysis.

Advice to Patients

Importance of instructing patients to read the manufacturer's patient information carefully before starting ixazomib therapy and before each treatment.

Importance of instructing patients to take ixazomib exactly as prescribed at least 1 hour before or 2 hours after food. Advise patients that capsules should be swallowed whole with water and that capsules should *not* be crushed, chewed, or opened.

Importance of advising patients that ixazomib should be administered once weekly on the same day and at approximately the same time for the first 3 weeks of each 4-week cycle.

Importance of advising patients that ixazomib and dexamethasone should not be administered simultaneously, because dexamethasone should be administered with food, while ixazomib should be given on an empty stomach.

Importance of informing patients that if a dose is missed, the dose should be taken as soon as possible if there are at least 72 hours until the next scheduled dose. Patients should be advised not to take a missed dose if it is within 72 hours of the next scheduled dose.

If vomiting occurs following administration of ixazomib, a replacement dose should *not* be administered. Patients should be advised to resume dosing at time of the next scheduled dose.

Advise patients that direct contact with the contents of ixazomib capsules should be avoided. If capsule breakage occurs, direct contact with the skin or eyes should be avoided. If contact occurs, the skin should be washed thoroughly with soap and water, and the eyes should be flushed thoroughly with water.

Importance of advising patients to store capsules in original carton until time of use.

Risk of thrombocytopenia. Importance of advising patients of the signs or symptoms of thrombocytopenia (e.g., bleeding, easy bruising).

Risk of GI toxicity. Importance of advising patients to report diarrhea, constipation, nausea, and vomiting to their clinician if adverse GI effects persist.

Risk of peripheral neuropathy. Importance of advising patients to report new or worsening symptoms of peripheral neuropathy (e.g., tingling, numbness, pain, burning sensation in feet or hands, weakness in arms or legs) to their clinician.

Risk of peripheral edema. Importance of advising patients to report unusual swelling of their extremities or weight gain from swelling to their clinician.

Risk of cutaneous reactions. Importance of advising patients to report new or worsening rash to their clinician.

Risk of hepatotoxicity. Importance of advising patients to report jaundice or right upper quadrant abdominal pain to their clinician.

Risk of fetal harm. Importance of advising women of childbearing potential and men who are partners of such women to use effective contraception during treatment and for 90 days following discontinuance of the drug. Importance of immediately informing clinician if the patient or their partner becomes pregnant during treatment or within 90 days of the last dose.

Importance of advising patients to discontinue nursing while receiving ixazomib.

Importance of informing clinicians of existing or contemplated concomitant therapy, including prescription and OTC drugs and herbal supplements, as well as any concomitant illnesses.

Importance of informing patients of other precautionary information. (See Cautions.)

Overview® (see Users Guide). For additional information on this drug until a more detailed monograph is developed and published, the manufacturer's labeling should be consulted. It is *essential* that the manufacturer's labeling be consulted for more detailed information on usual cautions, precautions, contraindications, potential drug interactions, laboratory test interferences, and acute toxicity. For further information on the handling of antineoplastic agents, see the ASHP Guidelines on Handling Hazardous Drugs at http://www.ahfsdruginformation.com.

Preparations

Excipients in commercially available drug preparations may have clinically important effects in some individuals; consult specific product labeling for details.

Ixazomib Citrate

Oral

Capsules	2.3 mg (of ixazomib)	**Ninlaro®**, Takeda
	3 mg (of ixazomib)	**Ninlaro®**, Takeda
	4 mg (of ixazomib)	**Ninlaro®**, Takeda

Lapatinib Ditosylate

■ Lapatinib, an inhibitor of human epidermal growth factor receptor type 2 (HER2/ERBB2) and epidermal growth factor receptor (HER1/EGFR/ERBB1) tyrosine kinases, is an antineoplastic agent.

Uses

■ **Breast Cancer** ***Advanced or Metastatic Breast Cancer*** Lapatinib ditosylate is used in combination with letrozole (an aromatase inhibitor) for the treatment of hormone receptor-positive metastatic breast cancer that overexpresses the HER2 protein in postmenopausal women who are candidates for hormonal therapy. Lapatinib ditosylate also is used in combination with capecitabine for the treatment of advanced or metastatic breast cancer that overexpresses the HER2 protein in patients who have received prior therapy including an anthracycline, a taxane, and trastuzumab.

Combination Therapy with Lapatinib and Letrozole. Lapatinib ditosylate is used in combination with letrozole for the treatment of hormone receptor-positive metastatic breast cancer that overexpresses the HER2 protein in postmenopausal women who are candidates for hormonal therapy. Use of lapatinib ditosylate in combination with an aromatase inhibitor has not been compared with a trastuzumab-containing chemotherapy regimen for the treatment of metastatic breast cancer.

Safety and efficacy of lapatinib in combination with letrozole for this indication have been evaluated in a phase 3, randomized, double-blind, controlled clinical study in postmenopausal women with hormone receptor-positive (estrogen- and/or progesterone-positive) metastatic breast cancer; 17% of patients enrolled in this study had HER2-overexpressing tumors. Patients were randomized to receive lapatinib (1.5 g once daily) and letrozole (2.5 mg once daily) or letrozole (2.5 mg once daily) and placebo. Patients who had received prior therapy for advanced or metastatic disease were excluded from the study. However, prior adjuvant or neoadjuvant chemotherapy, radiation therapy, or antiestrogen therapy was allowed; adjuvant use of aromatase inhibitors and trastuzumab was allowed if such treatment was completed at least one year prior to study entry. Approximately one-half of the 219 patients with HER2-overexpressing tumors had previously received antiestrogens and/or chemotherapy, approximately one-third had received adjuvant antiestrogen therapy within 6 months of study entry, and less than 1% had received prior trastuzumab therapy.

In the subgroup of patients with HER2-overexpressing tumors, those receiving combined therapy with lapatinib and letrozole had longer median progression-free survival (35.4 versus 13 weeks) and a higher objective response rate (28 versus 15%) compared with those receiving letrozole alone. However, in the subgroup of patients with HER2-negative tumors, combined therapy with lapatinib and letrozole did not improve progression-free survival or response rate over that observed with letrozole alone.

Combination Therapy with Lapatinib and Capecitabine. Lapatinib ditosylate is used in combination with capecitabine for the treatment of advanced or metastatic breast cancer that overexpresses the HER2 protein in patients who have received prior therapy including an anthracycline, a taxane, and trastuzumab.

Safety and efficacy of lapatinib (in combination with capecitabine) in the treatment of HER2-overexpressing advanced or metastatic breast cancer have been evaluated in a phase 3, open-label, randomized, controlled clinical study. The study enrolled patients with locally advanced or metastatic breast cancer that had progressed following treatment with regimens that included an anthracycline, a taxane, and trastuzumab. Patients were randomized to receive lapatinib (1.25 g once daily, continuously) in conjunction with capecitabine (2 g/m^2 daily on days 1–14 every 21 days) or capecitabine monotherapy (2.5 g/m^2 daily on days 1–14 every 21 days).

Enrollment in this study was terminated early when a planned interim analysis indicated that patients receiving lapatinib in combination with capecitabine had a longer median time to progression (8.4 versus 4.4 months) and longer median progression-free survival (8.4 versus 4.1 months) than did those receiving capecitabine alone. At the time of the interim analysis, overall survival and overall response rates did not differ substantially between the 2 treatment groups. The mortality rate was 22% in both groups; overall response rates were 22% for patients receiving lapatinib in combination with capecitabine and 14% for those receiving capecitabine monotherapy. Two efficacy analyses performed 4 months later (one an independent assessment and the other an investigator assessment that incorporated updated tumor assessment data) indicated that response rates were higher in patients receiving lapatinib in combination with capecitabine than in those receiving capecitabine alone (23.7 versus 13.9%, respectively [independent analysis]); 31.8 versus 17.4%, respectively [investigator analysis]). These analyses, like the interim analysis, indicated that median time to progression was longer in patients receiving lapatinib in combination with capecitabine than in those receiving capecitabine alone (27.1 versus 18.6 weeks, respectively [independent analysis]; 23.9 versus 18.3 weeks, respectively [investigator analysis]). Based on these results, the study was unblinded and combination therapy with lapatinib and capecitabine was offered to all patients who had been receiving capecitabine alone. Early termination of the study and patient crossover resulted in insufficient power to detect a survival benefit with the combination regimen; at 2 years after the independent and investigator analyses, median overall survival was 75 weeks for patients receiving lapatinib in combination with capecitabine compared with 65.9 weeks for those receiving capecitabine alone.

Dosage and Administration

■ **Administration** Lapatinib ditosylate is administered orally once daily. The manufacturer states that the drug should be administered at least one hour before or one hour after meals. The daily dosage should not be divided because administration of the same total daily dosage in divided doses results in greater systemic exposure (approximately twofold) to the drug. Patients should be advised not to double the next dose if a dose is missed.

■ **Dosage** Dosage of lapatinib ditosylate monohydrate is expressed in terms of lapatinib.

For use in combination with letrozole for the treatment of hormone receptor-positive, HER2-overexpressing metastatic breast cancer in postmenopausal women, the recommended dosage of lapatinib is 1.5 g orally once daily, given continuously in combination with letrozole 2.5 mg once daily. In a clinical trial evaluating this regimen, treatment was continued until disease progression occurred or the patient withdrew from the study.

For use in combination with capecitabine for the treatment of HER2-overexpressing advanced or metastatic breast cancer in patients who have received prior therapy including an anthracycline, a taxane, and trastuzumab, the recommended adult dosage of lapatinib is 1.25 g orally once daily on days 1–21 in combination with capecitabine 2 g/m^2 daily (administered orally in 2 divided doses approximately 12 hours apart) on days 1–14 of each 21-day cycle. Treatment should be continued until disease progression or unacceptable toxicity occurs.

■ **Dosage Modification** ***Decreased Left Ventricular Ejection Fraction*** Lapatinib should be discontinued in patients with decreased left ventricular ejection fraction (LVEF) of National Cancer Institute (NCI) Common Terminology Criteria for Adverse Events (CTCAE) grade 2 or greater and in patients with an LVEF that drops below the institution's lower limit of normal. Lapatinib may be restarted at a reduced dosage after a minimum of 2 weeks if the LVEF returns to normal and the patient is asymptomatic. Lapatinib should be restarted at a reduced dosage of 1.25 g once daily when given in combination with letrozole for the treatment of hormone receptor-positive, HER2-overexpressing metastatic breast cancer and at a reduced dosage of 1 g once daily when given in combination with capecitabine for the treatment of HER2-overexpressing, advanced or metastatic breast cancer. (See Decreased Left Ventricular Ejection Fraction under Cautions: Warnings/Precautions.)

Hepatic Toxicity If severe changes in liver function occur, lapatinib therapy should be discontinued permanently. Lapatinib therapy should *not* be reinitiated in patients who have experienced severe changes in liver function. (See Hepatic Toxicity under Cautions: Warnings/Precautions.)

GI Toxicity If severe diarrhea occurs, interruption or discontinuance of lapatinib therapy may be required.

Pulmonary Toxicity If manifestations of grade 3 or higher interstitial lung disease or pneumonitis develop, lapatinib therapy should be discontinued.

Other Toxicity Interruption or discontinuance of lapatinib therapy may be considered in patients experiencing toxicity (other than decreased LVEF) of NCI grade 2 or greater. For patients receiving lapatinib in combination with letrozole for the treatment of hormone receptor-positive, HER2-overexpressing metastatic breast cancer, the manufacturer states that lapatinib can be restarted at a reduced dosage of 1.25 g daily once the toxicity improves to grade 1 or less; if the toxicity recurs, lapatinib can be restarted at a dosage of 1.25 g daily (i.e., restarted without further dosage reduction). For patients receiving lapatinib in combination with capecitabine for the treatment of HER2-overexpressing, advanced or metastatic breast cancer, the manufacturer states that lapatinib can be restarted at the same dosage (1.25 g daily) once the toxicity improves to grade 1 or less; however, if the toxicity recurs, lapatinib should be restarted at a lower dosage (1 g daily).

Concomitant Use with Drugs Affecting Hepatic Microsomal Enzymes Concomitant use of lapatinib with potent *inhibitors* of cytochrome P-450 (CYP) isoenzyme 3A4 should be avoided. (See Drug Interactions: Drugs Affecting or Metabolized by Hepatic Microsomal Enzymes.) If concomitant use of lapatinib with a potent CYP3A4 inhibitor cannot be avoided, reduction of lapatinib dosage (to 500 mg daily) should be considered based on pharmacokinetic considerations; however, no clinical data on this dosage adjustment in this patient population are available. If the potent CYP3A4 inhibitor is discontinued, a period of approximately 1 week should elapse before lapatinib dosage is increased to the usual recommended dosage.

Concomitant use of lapatinib with potent CYP3A4 *inducers* should be avoided. (See Drug Interactions: Drugs Affecting or Metabolized by Hepatic Microsomal Enzymes.) If concomitant use of lapatinib with a potent CYP3A4 inducer cannot be avoided, a gradual increase in lapatinib dosage should be considered based on pharmacokinetic considerations. Lapatinib dosage should be increased gradually as tolerated from a dosage of 1.5 g daily up to 5.5 g daily when given in combination with letrozole for the treatment of hormone receptor-positive, HER2-overexpressing metastatic breast cancer and from a dosage of 1.25 g daily up to 4.5 g daily when given in combination with capecitabine for the treatment of HER2-overexpressing, advanced or metastatic breast cancer. However, no clinical data on these dosage adjustments in these patient populations are available. If the potent CYP3A4 inducer is discontinued, lapatinib dosage should be reduced to the usual recommended dosage.

■ **Special Populations** In patients with severe hepatic impairment (Child-Pugh class C), a reduced lapatinib dosage should be considered based on pharmacokinetic considerations. A reduced dosage of 1 g once daily should be considered when lapatinib is given in combination with letrozole for the treatment of hormone receptor-positive, HER2-overexpressing metastatic breast cancer; a reduced dosage of 750 mg once daily should be considered when lapatinib is given in combination with capecitabine for the treatment of HER2-overexpressing, advanced or metastatic breast cancer. However, no clinical data on these dosage adjustments in these patient populations are available. (See Hepatic Impairment under Warnings/Precautions: Specific Populations, in Cautions.)

Cautions

■ **Contraindications** Lapatinib is contraindicated in patients with known hypersensitivity (e.g., anaphylaxis) to the drug or any ingredient in the formulation.

■ **Warnings/Precautions** ***Decreased Left Ventricular Ejection Fraction*** Lapatinib has been reported to cause decreased left ventricular ejection fraction (LVEF). Clinical studies indicate that the majority (more than 57%) of decreases in LVEF associated with the drug occur within the first 12 weeks of lapatinib treatment. Data on long-term exposure are limited. However, LVEF decreases are rare, generally reversible, and nonprogressive. Caution should be exercised if lapatinib is administered to patients with conditions that could impair LVEF. The manufacturer recommends evaluating LVEF in patients prior to the initiation of lapatinib and periodically during treatment.

Lapatinib should be discontinued in patients with decreased LVEF of NCI-CTCAE grade 2 or greater and in patients with an LVEF that drops below the institution's lower limit of normal. (See Decreased Left Ventricular Ejection Fraction under Dosage and Administration: Dosage Modification.)

Hepatic Toxicity Hepatic toxicity, which may be severe, and deaths have been reported in patients receiving lapatinib. The cause of the deaths is uncertain.

Hepatic toxicity manifested by abnormal liver function test results, including serum concentrations of ALT (SGPT) or AST (SGOT) greater than 3 times the upper limit of normal and serum concentrations of total bilirubin greater than 2 times the upper limit of normal, have been observed in less than 1% of patients receiving lapatinib in clinical trials. Hepatic toxicity may occur within days to several months following initiation of lapatinib therapy.

Liver function tests (serum concentrations of transaminases, bilirubin, and alkaline phosphatase), should be monitored before initiation of lapatinib therapy, every 4–6 weeks during therapy, and as clinically indicated. If severe changes in liver function occur, lapatinib therapy should be discontinued permanently.

Diarrhea Diarrhea, including severe diarrhea, has been reported in patients receiving lapatinib. In clinical trials, diarrhea occurred in 64–65% of patients receiving lapatinib in combination with letrozole or capecitabine. Grade 3 or 4 diarrhea occurred in 9 or less than 1%, respectively, of patients receiving lapatinib in combination with letrozole and in 13 or 1%, respectively, of those receiving lapatinib in combination with capecitabine.

Diarrhea should be proactively managed with antidiarrheal agents. Management of severe diarrhea may include oral or IV electrolytes and fluids, and interruption or discontinuance of lapatinib therapy.

Interstitial Lung Disease/Pneumonitis Lapatinib therapy (alone or in combination with other antineoplastics) has been associated with interstitial lung disease and pneumonitis. Patients should be monitored for pulmonary symptoms, and the drug should be discontinued if symptoms suggestive of grade 3 or higher interstitial lung disease or pneumonitis develop.

Prolongation of QT Interval QT interval prolongation has been reported in patients receiving lapatinib; the drug should be administered with caution to patients who have or may develop prolongation of the corrected QT (QT_c) interval (e.g., patients with hypokalemia, hypomagnesemia, or congenital long QT syndrome; those receiving concomitant drugs that may prolong the QT_c interval). Hypokalemia or hypomagnesemia should be corrected prior to lapatinib administration. Monitoring of the electrocardiogram (ECG) and electrolytes should be considered.

Fetal/Neonatal Morbidity and Mortality Lapatinib may cause fetal harm; fetal anomalies, abortion, and death of offspring within days after birth have been demonstrated in animals. Pregnancy should be avoided during therapy. (See Advice to Patients.) If lapatinib is used during pregnancy or if the patient becomes pregnant while receiving the drug, the patient should be apprised of the potential hazard to the fetus.

Therapy Monitoring Liver function tests, including serum concentrations of transaminases, bilirubin, and alkaline phosphatase, should be monitored before initiation of lapatinib therapy, every 4–6 weeks during therapy, and as clinically indicated.

Specific Populations **Pregnancy.** Category D. (See Fetal/Neonatal Morbidity and Mortality under Cautions: Warnings/Precautions.)

Lactation. It is not known whether lapatinib is distributed into human milk. A decision should be made whether to discontinue nursing or the drug, taking into account the importance of the drug to the woman.

Pediatric Use. Safety and efficacy have not been established in children.

Geriatric Use. No substantial differences in safety or efficacy have been observed in geriatric patients relative to younger adults, but increased sensitivity cannot be ruled out.

Hepatic Impairment. Lapatinib should be used with caution in patients with severe hepatic impairment (Child-Pugh class C); systemic exposure to the drug may be increased. Dosage reduction should be considered in patients with severe hepatic impairment. (See Dosage and Administration: Special Populations.)

Renal Impairment. Safety and efficacy have not been established in patients with renal impairment or in patients undergoing hemodialysis. However, renal impairment is unlikely to affect lapatinib pharmacokinetics since less than 2% of the drug and its metabolites are eliminated by the kidneys.

■ **Common Adverse Effects** Adverse effects reported in 10% or more of patients receiving lapatinib in combination with either letrozole or capecitabine include diarrhea, nausea, vomiting, rash, dry skin, fatigue, and liver function test (AST, ALT, total bilirubin) abnormalities. Anorexia, alopecia, pruritus, nail disorder, asthenia, headache, and epistaxis also were reported in

10% or more of patients receiving lapatinib in combination with letrozole, and stomatitis, dyspepsia, palmar-plantar erythrodysesthesia (hand-foot syndrome), mucosal inflammation, pain, dyspnea, insomnia, and hematologic (hemoglobin, platelets, neutrophils) abnormalities also were reported in 10% or more of patients receiving lapatinib in combination with capecitabine.

Drug Interactions

■ **Drugs Affecting or Metabolized by Hepatic Microsomal Enzymes** Potent inhibitors of cytochrome P-450 (CYP) isoenzyme 3A4 (CYP3A4): Concomitant use of lapatinib with potent inhibitors of CYP3A4 (e.g., atazanavir, clarithromycin, indinavir, itraconazole, ketoconazole, nefazodone, nelfinavir, ritonavir, saquinavir, telithromycin, voriconazole) should be avoided. In drug interaction studies with ketoconazole (200 mg twice daily for 7 days), systemic lapatinib exposure increased approximately 3.6-fold, and lapatinib half-life increased 1.7-fold. If concomitant use of lapatinib with a potent CYP3A4 inhibitor cannot be avoided, reduction of lapatinib dosage should be considered. (See Concomitant Use with Drugs Affecting Hepatic Microsomal Enzymes under Dosage and Administration: Dosage Modification.)

Potent inducers of CYP3A4: Concomitant use of lapatinib with potent CYP3A4 inducers (e.g., carbamazepine, dexamethasone, phenobarbital, phenytoin, rifabutin, rifampin, rifapentine, St. John's wort [*Hypericum perforatum*]) should be avoided. In drug interaction studies, carbamazepine (100 mg twice daily for 3 days and 200 mg twice daily for 17 days) decreased systemic lapatinib exposure approximately 72%. If concomitant use of lapatinib with a potent CYP3A4 inducer cannot be avoided, lapatinib dosage should be adjusted. (See Concomitant Use with Drugs Affecting Hepatic Microsomal Enzymes under Dosage and Administration: Dosage Modification.)

Substrates of CYP isoenzymes: Lapatinib inhibits CYP2C8 in vitro at clinically relevant concentrations and is a weak inhibitor of CYP3A4 in vivo, but does not appear to substantially inhibit CYP isoenzymes 1A2, 2C9, 2C19, and 2D6, or UGT enzymes in vitro. Concomitant administration of lapatinib with oral or IV midazolam (a CYP3A4 substrate) increased midazolam exposure (as measured by area under the concentration-time curve [AUC] over 24 hours) by 45 or 22%, respectively. The manufacturer states that caution should be exercised and that a dosage reduction of the substrate drug should be considered when lapatinib is administered concomitantly with a CYP2C8 or CYP3A4 substrate with a narrow therapeutic index.

■ **Drugs that are Substrates or Inhibitors of P-glycoprotein Transport System** Lapatinib is both a substrate and an inhibitor of the efflux transporter P-glycoprotein (P-gp, ABCB1). Caution should be exercised if lapatinib is administered with drugs that are substrates or inhibitors of P-gp; increased plasma concentrations of the substrate drug or lapatinib are likely. When lapatinib is used concomitantly with a P-gp substrate with a narrow therapeutic index, consideration should be given to reducing the dosage of the P-gp substrate drug.

■ **Drugs that Prolong the QT Interval** Because lapatinib may cause prolongation of the QT interval, lapatinib should be used with caution in patients receiving concomitant therapy with other drugs (e.g., antiarrhythmic agents) known to prolong the QT interval.

■ **Capecitabine** Concomitant administration of lapatinib with capecitabine did not substantially alter the pharmacokinetics of either drug or the metabolites of capecitabine.

■ **Digoxin** Concomitant administration of lapatinib and oral digoxin (a P-gp substrate) increased systemic exposure (AUC) of digoxin by approximately 2.8-fold. In patients receiving digoxin, serum digoxin concentrations should be measured prior to initiation of lapatinib therapy and monitored throughout concomitant therapy. If serum digoxin concentrations exceed 1.2 ng/mL, digoxin dosage should be reduced by 50%.

■ **Paclitaxel** In patients receiving lapatinib and paclitaxel (a CYP2C8 and P-gp substrate) concomitantly, systemic exposure (AUC over 24 hours) of paclitaxel was increased by 23%. However, the manufacturer states that because of limitations of the study design, these data may underestimate the potential increase in paclitaxel exposure during concomitant use.

■ **Grapefruit** Grapefruit products should be avoided because of the potential for increased plasma lapatinib concentrations.

Description

Lapatinib, a tyrosine kinase inhibitor, is an antineoplastic agent. The drug inhibits the intracellular tyrosine kinase domains of both epidermal growth factor receptor (HER1/EGFR/ERBB1) and human epidermal growth factor receptor type 2 (HER2/ERBB2). Lapatinib has been shown to inhibit ERBB-driven tumor cell growth in vitro and in various animal models. The drug also has exhibited additive antineoplastic activity with fluorouracil (the active metabolite of capecitabine) in vitro. Lapatinib has been shown in vitro to retain significant antineoplastic activity against breast cancer cell lines selected for long-term growth in trastuzumab-containing medium, suggesting a lack of cross-resistance between lapatinib and trastuzumab.

Hormone receptor-positive breast cancer cells that overexpress EGFR and HER2 tend to be resistant to endocrine (antiestrogen) therapies. Similarly, hormone receptor-positive breast cancer cells that initially lack EGFR or HER2 may upregulate these receptor pathways as the tumor becomes resistant to endocrine therapy. In vitro data indicate that complex interactions between pathways involving the estrogen receptor and epidermal growth factor receptors (e.g., EGFR, HER2) may result in enhanced signal transduction and eventually lead to sustained tumor growth. Therefore, combined use of endocrine therapy (e.g., letrozole) and therapy targeting EGFR/HER2 (e.g., lapatinib) in women with hormone receptor-positive, HER2-overexpressing breast cancer may delay or prevent the emergence of acquired endocrine resistance resulting from increased EGFR and HER2 signaling.

Lapatinib is metabolized by the cytochrome P-450 (CYP) enzyme system, principally by isoenzymes 3A4 and 3A5, and is a substrate of P-glycoprotein. In vitro studies using human liver microsomes indicate that lapatinib does not significantly inhibit CYP isoenzymes 1A2, 2C9, 2C19, and 2D6, but studies suggest that lapatinib does inhibit CYP isoenzymes 3A4 and 2C8 as well as human P-glycoprotein. Steady-state concentrations of the drug are reached in approximately 6–7 days, indicating an effective half-life of 24 hours. Systemic exposure of lapatinib is increased threefold to fourfold when the drug is administered with a meal and is increased approximately twofold when the total daily dose is administered in divided doses instead of once daily.

Advice to Patients

Importance of women informing clinicians if they are or plan to become pregnant or plan to breast-feed.

Importance of taking lapatinib once daily; dividing the total daily dose is not recommended. Importance of taking the drug at least one hour before or after a meal. If a dose of lapatinib is missed, the next dose should be taken at the regularly scheduled time; the dose should not be doubled.

Importance of informing patients that decreased left ventricular ejection fraction (LVEF) has been reported; importance of informing clinicians if symptoms such as shortness of breath, palpitation, or fatigue occur.

Risk of diarrhea associated with lapatinib use; importance of advising patient about appropriate countermeasures to prevent and/or manage diarrhea. Importance of advising patient to inform clinician if severe diarrhea occurs.

Importance of informing clinicians of existing or contemplated concomitant therapy, including prescription and OTC drugs and herbal supplements, as well as any concomitant illnesses. Importance of not consuming grapefruit products during lapatinib therapy.

Importance of informing patients of other important precautionary information. (See Cautions.)

Overview® (see Users Guide). For additional information on this drug until a more detailed monograph is developed and published, the manufacturer's labeling should be consulted. It is *essential* that the manufacturer's labeling be consulted for more detailed information on usual cautions, precautions, contraindications, potential drug interactions, laboratory test interferences, and acute toxicity.

Preparations

Excipients in commercially available drug preparations may have clinically important effects in some individuals; consult specific product labeling for details.

Lapatinib Ditosylate

Oral

Tablets, film-coated	250 mg (of lapatinib)	**Tykerb®**, GlaxoSmithKline

Larotrectinib Sulfate

■ Larotrectinib, a potent and selective inhibitor of tropomyosin receptor kinase (Trk) A, TrkB, and TrkC, is an antineoplastic agent.

Uses

■ **Solid Tumors with Neurotrophic Receptor Tyrosine Kinase Gene Fusion** Larotrectinib sulfate is used for the treatment of solid tumors harboring a neurotrophic receptor tyrosine kinase (*NTRK*) gene fusion (without a known acquired mutation for resistance) in patients who have metastatic disease or may experience severe morbidity following surgical resection and whose disease progressed following prior therapy or those who are not candidates for other treatment options. The presence of *NTRK* fusion should be confirmed prior to initiation of therapy. An FDA-approved diagnostic test for detection of *NTRK* fusion is not currently available; however, in clinical studies, presence of *NTRK* fusion was determined by fluorescence in situ hybridization (FISH), reverse transcription-polymerase chain reaction (RT-PCR), or next-generation sequencing (NGS). Larotrectinib has been designated an orphan drug by FDA for the treatment of these cancers. The accelerated approval of larotrectinib for this indication is based on overall response rate and duration of response. Continued approval for this indication may be contingent on verification and description of clinical benefit of larotrectinib in confirmatory studies.

The incidence of solid tumors harboring activating *NTRK* fusions has not been fully characterized; however, 1500–5000 cases are estimated per year in the US. Although a relatively small subset (less than 1%) of patients with common solid tumors (e.g., lung, colon, or prostate cancer) harbor *NTRK* fusions, such fusions have been frequently reported in certain rare cancers (i.e., 91–100% of mammary analogue secretory carcinomas, secretory breast carcinomas, or infantile fibrosarcomas; 61% of congenital mesoblastic nephromas; 12–15% of papillary thyroid cancers).

The current indication for larotrectinib in the treatment of solid tumors harboring *NTRK* fusion is based principally on data from 3 open-label noncomparative studies (LOXO-TRK-14001, SCOUT, and NAVIGATE) evaluating larotrectinib in patients with unresectable or metastatic solid tumors harboring *NTRK* fusion. The primary efficacy population consisted of the initial 55 adult and pediatric patients enrolled in the LOXO-TRK-14001, SCOUT, and NAVIGATE studies with solid tumors harboring an *NTRK* fusion. Patients were eligible for these studies if they experienced disease progression following prior systemic therapy, if available, or if severe morbidity following surgical resection for locally advanced disease was expected. In these studies, adult patients received larotrectinib 100 mg orally twice daily and pediatric patients (18 years of age or younger) received larotrectinib 100 mg/m² (maximum dose of 100 mg) orally twice daily. Therapy was continued until the occurrence of unacceptable toxicity or disease progression. The primary efficacy end points were overall response rate and duration of response (as evaluated by a blinded independent review committee) according to Response Evaluation Criteria in Solid Tumors (RECIST). In the primary efficacy population, the median age of patients was 45 years (range: 4 months to 76 years); 78% of patients were 18 years of age or older, 22% were younger than 18 years of age, 93% had an Eastern Cooperative Oncology Group (ECOG) performance status of 0 or 1, 67% were white, 7% were Hispanic or Latino, 4% were Asian, and 4% were black. Most patients (82%) had metastatic disease and 18% had unresectable locally advanced disease. The majority (98%) of patients in the primary efficacy population had received prior surgery, radiation therapy, or systemic therapy for their disease; 82% of these patients had received a median of 2 prior systemic therapies and 35% had received at least 3 prior systemic therapies. The most common cancers in the primary efficacy population were salivary gland tumors (22%), soft tissue sarcoma (20%), infantile fibrosarcoma (13%), and thyroid cancer (9%).

At the time of data analysis, the overall response rate in the primary efficacy population was 75%; complete response was achieved in 22% of patients. The median duration of response had not been reached at the time of the analysis; however, 73, 63, or 39% of patients had durable responses of 6, 9, or 12 months or longer, respectively. The overall response rate in patients with infantile fibrosarcoma, thyroid carcinoma, gastrointestinal stromal tumor (GIST), soft tissue sarcoma, salivary gland cancer, lung cancer, melanoma, or colon cancer was 100, 100, 100, 91, 83, 75, 50, or 25%, respectively. Stable disease was reported in patients with cholangiocarcinoma, appendix cancer, or pancreatic cancer while progressive disease was reported in one patient with breast cancer. The most common *NTRK* fusion was *ETV6-NTRK3*; however, *NTRK* fusions were inferred in 3 patients with infantile fibrosarcoma with documented *ETV6* translocation as detected by FISH. The overall response rate in patients with tumors harboring inferred *ETV6-NTRK3*, *IRF2BP2-NTRK1*, *SQSTM1-NTRK1*, documented *ETV6-NTRK3*, *TPM3-NTRK1*, or *LMNA-NTRK1* fusion was 100, 100, 100, 84, 56, or 40%, respectively. Although *PDE4DIP-NTRK1*, *PPL-NTRK1*, *STRN-NTRK2*, *TPM4-NTRK3*, *TPR-NTRK1*, and *TRIM63-NTRK1* fusions were detected in one patient each, patients with tumors harboring these *NTRK* fusions achieved complete or partial responses.

Dosage and Administration

■ **General** Presence of a neurotrophic receptor tyrosine kinase (*NTRK*) gene fusion must be confirmed prior to initiation of therapy with larotrectinib. (See Uses: Solid Tumors with Neurotrophic Receptor Tyrosine Kinase Gene Fusion.)

Restricted Distribution Larotrectinib sulfate can only be obtained through designated specialty pharmacies and distributors. Clinicians may contact the manufacturer (Bayer) at 844-634-8725 or consult the Vitrakvi® website (https://www.vitrakvi.com) for specific ordering and availability information.

■ **Administration** Larotrectinib is administered orally (as capsules or oral solution) twice daily without regard to meals. The capsules should be swallowed whole with water; they should *not* be chewed or crushed. The oral solution should be administered using an oral dosing syringe according to the manufacturer's directions.

Larotrectinib capsules should be stored at room temperature of 20–25°C, but may be exposed to 15–30°C.

Larotrectinib oral solution should be stored in a refrigerator at 2–8°C; the oral solution should not be frozen. Unused portions of larotrectinib oral solution should be discarded after 90 days of opening the bottle.

■ **Dosage** Dosage of larotrectinib sulfate is expressed in terms of larotrectinib.

The oral solution and capsules may be interchanged at equal doses.

Solid Tumors with Neurotrophic Receptor Tyrosine Kinase Gene Fusion For the treatment of solid tumors harboring *NTRK* fusion (without a known acquired mutation for resistance) in patients who have metastatic disease or may experience severe morbidity following surgical resection and whose disease progressed following prior therapy or those who are not candidates for other treatment options, the recommended dosage of larotrectinib in *adult and pediatric patients with a body surface area (BSA) of at least 1 m²* is 100 mg twice daily. In *pediatric patients with a BSA less than 1 m²*, the recommended dosage of larotrectinib is 100 mg/m² twice daily.

Larotrectinib therapy should be continued until disease progression or unacceptable toxicity occurs.

Dosage Modification for Toxicity If a grade 3 or 4 adverse reaction occurs, larotrectinib therapy should be withheld. If the grade 3 or 4 adverse reaction resolves to grade 1 or baseline within 4 weeks of withholding larotrectinib, the drug should be resumed at a reduced dosage (or discontinued) as described in Table 1. If the grade 3 or 4 adverse reaction does not resolve within 4 weeks of withholding larotrectinib, the drug should be permanently discontinued.

Table 1. Dosage Modifications for Larotrectinib Toxicity.

	Dosage Modification after Recovery from Toxicity	
Toxicity Occurrence	Adult and Pediatric Patients with BSA of 1 m² or More (Starting Dosage = 100 mg twice daily)	Pediatric Patients with BSA Less than 1 m² (Starting Dosage = 100 mg/m² twice daily)
First	Restart at 75 mg twice daily	Restart at 75 mg/m² twice daily
Second	Restart at 50 mg twice daily	Restart at 50 mg/m² twice daily
Third	Restart at 100 mg once daily	Restart at 25 mg/m² twice daily
Fourth	Permanently discontinue larotrectinib	Permanently discontinue larotrectinib

Concomitant Use with CYP3A4 Inhibitors or Inducers Concomitant use of larotrectinib with *potent inhibitors of cytochrome P-450 (CYP) isoenzyme 3A4* should be avoided; however, if such concomitant use cannot be avoided, the manufacturer recommends reducing the dosage of larotrectinib by 50% (e.g., dosage of 100 mg twice daily reduced to 50 mg twice daily; dosage of 100 mg/m² twice daily reduced to 50 mg/m² twice daily). When concomitant use of the potent CYP3A4 inhibitor is discontinued, the larotrectinib dosage should be returned (after at least 3–5 elimination half-lives of the CYP3A4 inhibitor) to the dosage used prior to initiation of the potent CYP3A4 inhibitor. (See Inhibitors of CYP3A4 under Drug Interactions: Drugs and Foods Affecting Hepatic Microsomal Enzymes.)

Concomitant use of larotrectinib with *potent inducers of CYP3A4* should be avoided; however, if such concomitant use cannot be avoided, the manufacturer recommends doubling the dosage of larotrectinib (e.g., dosage of 100 mg twice daily increased to 200 mg twice daily; dosage of 100 mg/m² twice daily increased to 200 mg/m² twice daily). When concomitant use of the potent CYP3A4 inducer is discontinued, the larotrectinib dosage should be returned (after at least 3–5 elimination half-lives of the CYP3A4 inducer) to the dosage used prior to initiation of the potent CYP3A4 inducer. (See Inducers of CYP3A4 under Drug Interactions: Drugs and Foods Affecting Hepatic Microsomal Enzymes.)

■ **Special Populations** For patients with moderate or severe hepatic impairment (Child-Pugh class B or C), the manufacturer recommends reducing the initial dosage of larotrectinib by 50% (e.g., dosage of 100 mg twice daily reduced to 50 mg twice daily; dosage of 100 mg/m² twice daily reduced to 50 mg/m² twice daily). No initial dosage adjustment is necessary in patients with mild hepatic impairment (Child-Pugh class A). (See Hepatic Impairment under Warnings/Precautions: Specific Populations, in Cautions.)

The manufacturer states that no adjustment to the dosage of larotrectinib is necessary in patients with renal impairment. (See Renal Impairment under Warnings/Precautions: Specific Populations, in Cautions.)

The manufacturer makes no specific dosage recommendations for geriatric patients. (See Geriatric Use under Warnings/Precautions: Specific Populations, in Cautions.)

Cautions

■ **Contraindications** The manufacturer states that there are no known contraindications to the use of larotrectinib sulfate.

■ **Warnings/Precautions** ***Neurologic Effects*** Larotrectinib can cause a variety of adverse neurologic effects including delirium, dysarthria, dizziness, gait disturbance, paresthesia, memory impairment, and tremor. In the principal efficacy studies of larotrectinib in patients with unresectable or metastatic solid tumors, neurologic events occurred in 53% of 176 patients receiving the drug and were grade 3 or 4 in 6 or 0.6%, respectively, of patients. Most patients (65%) experienced neurologic events within 3 months of initiation of larotrectinib therapy; however, neurologic events have occurred as early as 1 day or as late as 2.2 years following initiation of the drug. Grade 4 encephalopathy also was reported in 1 of 176 patients (0.6%) receiving larotrectinib. Temporary interruption or dosage reduction of larotrectinib was necessary because of dizziness, gait disturbance, delirium, memory impairment, or tremor in 3, 1, 1, 1, or 1%, respectively, of patients receiving the drug.

Temporary interruption of larotrectinib therapy followed by dosage reduction or permanent discontinuance of therapy may be necessary in patients experiencing neurologic events during therapy with the drug, and such patients should be advised not to drive or operate machinery. (See Dosage Modification for Toxicity under Dosage and Administration: Dosage.)

Hepatotoxicity Elevations in aminotransferase (ALT and/or AST) concentrations have been reported in patients receiving larotrectinib. In the principal efficacy studies of larotrectinib in patients with unresectable or metastatic solid tumors, elevations in serum concentrations of ALT or AST occurred in 45% of 176 patients receiving the drug and were grade 3 or 4 in 6 or 0.6%, respectively, of patients. The median time to occurrence of elevated ALT or AST concentration was 2 months (range: 1 month to 2.6 years). Temporary interruption or dosage reduction of larotrectinib was necessary because of elevated AST or ALT concentrations in 4 or 6%, respectively, of patients receiving the drug. Therapy was discontinued because of elevations in ALT or AST concentrations in 2% of patients receiving the drug.

Liver function tests, including ALT and AST concentrations, should be monitored every 2 weeks for the first month of therapy and then monthly thereafter or more frequently as clinically indicated. Temporary interruption of larotrectinib therapy followed by dosage reduction or permanent discontinuance of therapy may be necessary if hepatotoxicity occurs. (See Dosage Modification for Toxicity under Dosage and Administration: Dosage.)

Fetal/Neonatal Morbidity and Mortality Larotrectinib may cause fetal harm in humans based on its mechanism of action and animal findings; embryofetal toxicity and teratogenicity have been demonstrated in animals. There are no available data regarding use of larotrectinib in pregnant women. Larotrectinib has been shown to cross the placenta in animals. In animal reproduction studies, fetal anasarca and omphalocele were observed in rats and rabbits receiving larotrectinib at exposure levels approximately 11 and 0.7 times the human exposure, respectively, at the recommended dosage. Literature reports in individuals with congenital mutations in the tropomyosin receptor kinase (Trk) pathway suggest an association between decreased Trk-mediated signaling and obesity, developmental delays, cognitive impairment, insensitivity to pain, and anhidrosis.

Pregnancy should be avoided during larotrectinib therapy. The manufacturer recommends confirmation of pregnancy status prior to initiation of larotrectinib in women of reproductive potential and states that such women should be advised to use effective contraceptive methods while receiving larotrectinib and for at least 1 week after discontinuance of the drug. In addition, men with such female partners should use effective methods of contraception while receiving larotrectinib and for at least 1 week after discontinuance of the drug. Patients should be apprised of the potential hazard to the fetus if larotrectinib is used during pregnancy.

Impairment of Fertility Based on animal studies, larotrectinib may impair female fertility. The effect of the drug on fertility in humans is not known. In a repeat-dose toxicity study, decreased uterine weight, uterine atrophy, decreased corpora lutea, and increased incidence of anestrus were observed in female rats receiving larotrectinib at exposure levels approximately 10–45 times the human exposure at the recommended dosage.

Specific Populations **Pregnancy.** Larotrectinib may cause fetal harm if administered to pregnant women based on its mechanism of action and animal findings. (See Fetal/Neonatal Morbidity and Mortality under Cautions: Warnings/Precautions.)

Lactation. It is not known whether larotrectinib or its metabolites are distributed into human milk. Because of the potential for serious adverse reactions to larotrectinib in breast-fed infants, women should be advised not to breast-feed while receiving the drug and for 1 week after the last dose. The effects of the drug on breast-fed infants or on the production of milk are unknown.

Pediatric Use. Safety and efficacy of larotrectinib have not been established in pediatric patients younger than 28 days. Efficacy of larotrectinib in pediatric patients with solid tumors harboring a neurotrophic receptor tyrosine kinase (*NTRK*) gene fusion has been established in 3 noncomparative studies that included 12 pediatric patients 28 days of age or older. Based on limited safety data in 44 pediatric patients receiving larotrectinib, some grade 3 or 4 adverse effects and laboratory abnormalities (i.e., weight gain, neutropenia) occurred more frequently in pediatric patients compared with adults; however, because the studies were uncontrolled, it is unclear whether this effect was related to larotrectinib or to other confounding factors (e.g., differences in susceptibility to infection). No differences in pharmacokinetics were observed between pediatric patients and adults.

Geriatric Use. In clinical trials evaluating larotrectinib in patients with unresectable or metastatic solid tumors, 22% of patients receiving larotrectinib were 65 years of age or older, while 5% were 75 years of age or older. There is insufficient experience in patients 65 years of age or older to determine whether geriatric patients respond differently than younger patients.

Hepatic Impairment. Following administration of a single 100-mg dose of larotrectinib, the area under the plasma concentration-time curve (AUC) in individuals with mild, moderate, or severe hepatic impairment (Child-Pugh class A, B, or C) was increased by 1.3-, 2-, or 3.2-fold, respectively, compared with individuals with normal hepatic function; peak plasma concentrations were increased by 1.5-fold in individuals with severe hepatic impairment compared with individuals with normal hepatic function. Initial dosage adjustment is required in patients with moderate or severe hepatic impairment. (See Dosage and Administration: Special Populations.)

Renal Impairment. Following administration of a single 100-mg dose of larotrectinib to individuals with end-stage renal disease requiring dialysis, AUC and peak plasma concentrations were increased by 1.5- and 1.3-fold, respectively, compared with individuals with normal renal function (creatinine clearance of 90 mL/minute or greater). Larotrectinib has not been studied in patients with moderate or severe renal impairment (creatinine clearance of 60 mL/minute or less).

■ **Common Adverse Effects** Adverse effects reported in at least 10% of patients receiving larotrectinib include fatigue, nausea, dizziness, cough, vomiting, constipation, diarrhea, dyspnea, pyrexia, peripheral edema, weight gain, myalgia/arthralgia, headache, abdominal pain, decreased appetite, muscular weakness, back or extremity pain, hypertension, fall, and nasal congestion. Laboratory abnormalities reported in at least 5% of patients receiving larotrectinib include elevated concentrations of aminotransferases (i.e., ALT, AST), anemia, hypoalbuminemia, elevated concentrations of alkaline phosphatase, and neutropenia.

Drug Interactions

Larotrectinib is metabolized principally by cytochrome P-450 (CYP) isoenzyme 3A4.

In vitro studies indicate that larotrectinib is an inhibitor of CYP3A4. In vitro, larotrectinib does not inhibit or induce CYP isoenzymes 1A2, 2B6, 2C8, 2C9, 2C19, or 2D6 at clinically relevant concentrations.

In vitro, larotrectinib is a substrate of the efflux transporters P-glycoprotein (P-gp) and breast cancer resistance protein (BCRP), but is not a substrate for organic anion transporter (OAT) 1, OAT3, organic cation transporter (OCT) 1, OCT2, organic anion transport protein (OATP) 1B1, or OATP1B3. In vitro studies indicate that larotrectinib does not inhibit P-gp, BCRP, OAT1, OAT3, OCT1, OCT2, OATP1B1, OATP1B3, bile salt export pump (BSEP), multidrug and toxin extrusion (MATE) transporter 1, and MATE2K at clinically relevant concentrations.

■ **Drugs and Foods Affecting Hepatic Microsomal Enzymes** ***Inhibitors of CYP3A4*** Concomitant use of larotrectinib with potent inhibitors of CYP3A4 may increase systemic exposure to larotrectinib and possible toxicity. When the potent CYP3A inhibitor itraconazole (200 mg once daily for 7 days) was administered concomitantly with larotrectinib (single 100-mg dose), peak plasma concentration and area under the plasma concentration-time curve (AUC) of larotrectinib were increased by 2.8- and 4.3-fold, respectively. The potential for moderate or weak CYP3A inhibitors to alter larotrectinib pharmacokinetics has not been established.

Concomitant use of larotrectinib with potent inhibitors of CYP3A4 (e.g., itraconazole, grapefruit juice) should be avoided. If concomitant use of a potent CYP3A4 inhibitor cannot be avoided, the manufacturer recommends reducing the dosage of larotrectinib by 50% (e.g., dosage of 100 mg twice daily reduced to 50 mg twice daily; dosage of 100 mg/m^2 twice daily reduced to 50 mg/m^2 twice daily). When concomitant use of the potent CYP3A4 inhibitor is discontinued, the larotrectinib dosage should be returned (after at least 3–5 elimination half-lives of the CYP3A4 inhibitor) to the dosage used prior to initiation of the potent CYP3A4 inhibitor.

Inducers of CYP3A4 Concomitant use of larotrectinib with potent inducers of CYP3A4 may decrease systemic exposure to larotrectinib and reduce larotrectinib efficacy. When the potent CYP3A inducer rifampin (600 mg once daily for 11 days) was administered concomitantly with larotrectinib (single 100-mg dose), peak plasma concentration and AUC of larotrectinib were decreased by 71 and 81%, respectively. The potential for moderate or weak CYP3A inducers to alter larotrectinib pharmacokinetics has not been established.

Concomitant use of larotrectinib with potent inducers of CYP3A4 (e.g., rifampin, St. John's wort [*Hypericum perforatum*]) should be avoided. If concomitant use of a potent CYP3A4 inducer cannot be avoided, the manufacturer recommends doubling the dosage of larotrectinib (e.g., dosage of 100 mg twice daily increased to 200 mg twice daily; dosage of 100 mg/m^2 twice daily increased to 200 mg/m^2 twice daily). When concomitant use of the potent CYP3A4 inducer is discontinued, the larotrectinib dosage should be returned (after at least 3–5 elimination half-lives of the CYP3A4 inducer) to the dosage used prior to initiation of the potent CYP3A4 inducer.

■ **Drugs Metabolized by Hepatic Microsomal Enzymes** ***Substrates of CYP3A4*** Larotrectinib may increase systemic exposure and risk of adverse effects of other drugs metabolized by CYP3A4. When the sensitive CYP3A4 substrate midazolam (single 2-mg dose) was administered concomitantly with larotrectinib (100 mg twice daily for 10 days) in healthy individuals, peak plasma concentration and AUC of midazolam were both increased by 1.7-fold; peak plasma concentration and AUC of the major metabolite of midazolam (1-hydroxymidazolam) were both increased by 1.4-fold. Concomitant use with sensitive substrates of CYP3A4 (e.g., midazolam) should be avoided. If concomitant use of a sensitive CYP3A4 substrate cannot be avoided, the patient should be monitored for CYP3A4 substrate-related toxicity.

■ **Drugs Affecting the P-glycoprotein Transport System** When the P-gp inhibitor rifampin (single 600-mg dose) was administered concomitantly with larotrectinib (single 100-mg dose) in healthy individuals, peak plasma concentration and AUC of larotrectinib were increased by 1.8- and 1.7-fold, respectively. (See Drug Interactions: Drugs and Foods Affecting Hepatic Microsomal Enzymes.)

Description

Larotrectinib, a potent and selective inhibitor of tropomyosin receptor kinase (Trk) A, TrkB, and TrkC, is an antineoplastic agent. The Trk family of tyrosine kinases (encoded by the neurotrophic receptor tyrosine kinase genes *NTRK1*, *NTRK2*, and *NTRK3*) are involved in the initiation of various cascades of intracellular signaling events (i.e., Ras/MAPK/ERK, PI3K/Akt, and PLCγ1/Pkc signal transduction pathways), which leads to cell proliferation, differentiation, apoptosis, and regulation of processes critical to neuron survival in the central and peripheral nervous systems. Chromosomal rearrangements of the *NTRK1*, *NTRK2*, and *NTRK3* genes result in fusions with an unrelated gene. These *NTRK* gene fusions encode a constitutively active chimeric Trk oncogenic fusion protein resulting in dysregulation of Trk signaling and subsequent tumorigenesis. In vitro biochemical assays have shown that larotrectinib inhibits the activity of wild-type TrkA, TrkB, and TrkC. In vitro and in vivo, larotrectinib has demonstrated antitumor activity in cell lines with Trk expression from constitutive activation, deletion of a protein regulatory domain, or overexpression of wild-type Trk. Larotrectinib also has demonstrated inhibition of tyrosine kinase nonreceptor 2 (TNK2).

Clinical resistance to larotrectinib has been attributed to secondary point mutations of the NTRK kinase domain in 90% of cases. Larotrectinib has shown minimal activity in cell lines with point mutations in the TrkA kinase domain, including the acquired resistance mutation G595R. Acquired resistance to larotrectinib also has been identified in cell lines with G623R, G696A, or F617L point mutations in the TrkC kinase domain.

Following oral administration of larotrectinib capsules, systemic exposure to larotrectinib increases in a dose-proportional manner over a dose range of 100–400 mg and increases in a slightly more than dose-proportional manner over a dose range of 600–900 mg. Following oral administration of larotrectinib capsules at a dosage of 100 mg twice daily, peak plasma concentrations of the drug were achieved in approximately 1 hour and steady-state concentrations were achieved within 3 days. The mean absolute oral bioavailability of larotrectinib capsules was 34%. The area under the plasma-concentration time curve (AUC) for larotrectinib oral solution was similar to the AUC for larotrectinib capsules; peak plasma concentrations were 36% higher for larotrectinib oral solution compared with larotrectinib capsules. Administration of larotrectinib capsules (single 100-mg dose) with a high-fat meal decreased peak plasma concentrations by 35% and delayed the time to peak plasma concentrations by 2 hours compared with administration in the fasted state, but did not substantially affect the extent of absorption. Larotrectinib is metabolized principally by cytochrome P-450 (CYP) isoenzyme 3A4. Larotrectinib is 70% bound to plasma proteins, and binding is independent of larotrectinib concentration. Following oral administration of a single 100-mg radiolabeled dose of larotrectinib, 58% of the dose was recovered in feces (5% as unchanged drug) and 39% was recovered in urine (20% as unchanged drug). The terminal half-life of larotrectinib is 2.9 hours.

The pharmacokinetics of larotrectinib do not appear to be affected by age (range of 28 days to 82 years), sex, or body weight (range of 3.8–179 kg).

Advice to Patients

Importance of instructing patients to read the manufacturer's patient information.

Importance of advising patients to take larotrectinib exactly as prescribed and to not alter the dosage or discontinue therapy unless advised to do so by their clinician. Importance of advising patients to swallow larotrectinib capsules whole and to not chew or crush the capsules.

Importance of advising patients to take a missed dose as soon as it is remembered unless the dose was missed by more than 6 hours, in which case they should not take the missed dose. If a dose is vomited, importance of administering the next dose at the regularly scheduled time.

Risk of adverse neurologic effects. Importance of informing clinician if new or worsening manifestations of neurologic events (e.g., confusion; speech difficulties; dizziness; coordination difficulties; tingling, numbness, or burning sensation in hands and feet) occur. Necessity of advising patients to avoid driving or operating hazardous machinery if they experience neurologic events.

Risk of hepatotoxicity; importance of regular liver function test monitoring. Importance of immediately informing clinician if signs or symptoms of hepatotoxicity (e.g., loss of appetite, nausea, vomiting, abdominal pain [especially right upper quadrant pain]) occur.

Risk of fetal harm. Necessity of advising women of reproductive potential to avoid pregnancy and to use effective contraceptive methods while receiving larotrectinib and for at least 1 week following discontinuance of therapy. Importance of advising men who are partners of such women that they should use effective methods of contraception while receiving the drug and for at least 1 week after the drug is discontinued. Importance of women informing clinicians if they become pregnant during therapy or think they may be pregnant. Advise men and women of reproductive potential of potential risk to the fetus.

Importance of advising women to avoid breast-feeding while receiving larotrectinib and for 1 week after discontinuance of therapy.

Risk of impaired female fertility.

Importance of informing clinicians of existing or contemplated concomitant therapy, including prescription and OTC drugs and dietary or herbal supplements (e.g., St. John's wort [*Hypericum perforatum*], grapefruit, grapefruit juice), as well as any concomitant illnesses (e.g., hepatic impairment).

Importance of informing patients of other important precautionary information. (See Cautions.)

Overview® (see Users Guide). For additional information on this drug until a more detailed monograph is developed and published, the manufacturer's labeling should be consulted. It is *essential* that the manufacturer's labeling be consulted for more detailed information on usual cautions, precautions, contraindications, potential drug interactions, laboratory test interferences, and acute toxicity. For further information on the handling of antineoplastic agents, see the ASHP Guidelines on Handling Hazardous Drugs at http://www.ahfsdruginformation.com.

Preparations

Larotrectinib sulfate can only be obtained through designated specialty pharmacies and distributors. (See Restricted Distribution under Dosage and Administration: General.)

Excipients in commercially available drug preparations may have clinically important effects in some individuals; consult specific product labeling for details.

Larotrectinib Sulfate

Oral		
Capsules	25 mg (of larotrectinib)	**Vitrakvi®**, Loxo Oncology
	100 mg (of larotrectinib)	**Vitrakvi®**, Loxo Oncology
Solution	20 mg (of larotrectinib) per mL	**Vitrakvi®**, Loxo Oncology

Lenalidomide

■ Lenalidomide, a thalidomide analog, is an immunomodulatory agent with antineoplastic and antiangiogenic activity.

REMS

FDA approved a REMS for lenalidomide to ensure that the benefits outweigh the risks. The REMS may apply to one or more preparations of lenalidomide and consists of the following: elements to assure safe use and implementation system. See the FDA REMS page (https://www.accessdata.fda.gov/scripts/cder/rems/index.cfm).

Uses

■ **Myelodysplastic Syndromes** Lenalidomide is used in the management of red blood cell transfusion-dependent anemia associated with low-risk or intermediate-1-risk myelodysplastic syndromes (MDS) in individuals with a cytogenetic deletion abnormality involving the long arm of chromosome 5 (a deletion 5q abnormality), with or without additional cytogenetic abnormalities. Lenalidomide is designated an orphan drug by the US Food and Drug Administration (FDA) for use in MDS.

The current indication for lenalidomide is based principally on results from an uncontrolled, open-label, multicenter trial (MDS-003) in 148 patients with transfusion-dependent anemia (i.e., requiring at least 2 units of red blood cells within 8 weeks prior to study treatment) secondary to MDS; all patients enrolled in the trial had a cytogenetic abnormality involving a deletion between bands 31 and 33 of the long (q) arm of chromosome 5, designated as del(5)(q31-33), either in isolation or in association with additional cytogenetic abnormalities. Most (81%) of the patients in this trial had low-risk or intermediate-1-risk MDS, as determined by the International Prognosis Scoring System (IPSS), a method for evaluating MDS prognosis (i.e., survival and risk of transformation to acute myeloid leukemia [AML]) based on the karyotype, percentage of blast cells in the bone marrow, and number of cytopenias. Patients received lenalidomide at a dosage of either 10 mg once daily or 10 mg once daily for 21 days of each 28-day period. Sequential dosage reductions (to 5 mg daily or 5 mg every other day) as well as interruptions in the dosage regimen were allowed for management of toxicity. Transfusion independence, defined as the absence of red blood cell transfusions during any period of 56 consecutive days (8 weeks) during therapy, was achieved in 67% of patients; the transfusion-free period was sustained for a median of 44 weeks (range: 0 to more than 67 weeks) following the end of this 56-day period of transfusion independence. Response to lenalidomide was rapid; the median time to response was 4.6 weeks, and 90% of patients who achieved a transfusion benefit with therapy did so within 3 months.

Lenalidomide also has been studied for the management of transfusion-dependent low-risk or intermediate-1-risk MDS in patients *without* the deletion 5q (del[5q]) chromosomal abnormality (non-del[5q])†. In a multicenter, phase 2, noncomparative clinical trial (MDS-002), 214 patients with transfusion-dependent anemia (i.e., requiring at least 2 units of red blood cells within 8 weeks prior to study treatment) secondary to low-risk or intermediate-1-risk MDS without the deletion 5q chromosomal abnormality received lenalidomide 10 mg once daily on days 1–21 of a 28-day cycle or 10 mg once daily continuously. Treatment was administered cyclically upon initiation of the study, but the schedule was amended when data from a prior study in MDS suggested a faster onset of response to lenalidomide, with no apparent increase in toxicity, with continuous administration; patients were permitted to switch from cyclic to continuous treatment. Sustained (for at least 8 weeks) hematologic improvement involving the erythroid cell line was reported in 43% of patients in this study, with 26% of patients achieving transfusion independence accompanied by an increase in hemoglobin concentration of at least 1 g/dL after a median of 4.8 weeks of treatment; the median duration of transfusion independence was 41 weeks. An additional 17% of patients had a 50% or greater reduction in transfusions. When the study data were analyzed to exclude minor responses and to use a more stringent definition of baseline transfusion dependence (transfusion of 4 or more units of red blood cells in response to a hemoglobin concentration of 9 g/dL or less within 8 weeks prior to study treatment), 62% of patients had baseline transfusion dependence and 30% of those patients achieved a reduction in transfusion requirements equaling 4 or more units during any 8-week period during therapy. In the subset of patients without baseline transfusion dependence, 37% achieved a sustained (for at least 8 weeks) increase in hemoglobin concentration of at least 1.5 g/dL during therapy. Overall, 17 or 33% of patients achieved sustained (for at least 8 weeks) transfusion independence or hematologic improvement involving the erythroid cell line. Grade 3/4 neutropenia and thrombocytopenia occurred in 30 and 25% of patients, respectively. There were no apparent differences in response and few differences in adverse effects between those who initiated therapy with cyclic administration and those who received only continuous daily dosing. Efficacy of lenalidomide is being evaluated in a phase 3, placebo-controlled, clinical trial (MDS-005) in patients with low-risk or intermediate-1-risk MDS without the deletion 5q chromosomal abnormality who have transfusion-dependent anemia and are unresponsive to therapy with erythropoiesis-stimulating agents or have endogenous erythropoietin concentrations exceeding 500 mU/mL.

A post-hoc analysis of the MDS-002 and MDS-003 clinical trials demonstrated a correlation between treatment-related cytopenias and likelihood of achieving transfusion independence in patients with the deletion 5q chromosomal abnormality; however, no relationship between the development of treatment-related cytopenias and response could be established for lower-risk MDS patients without the deletion 5q abnormality.

Use of lenalidomide for the treatment of transfusion-dependent low-risk or intermediate-1-risk MDS without the deletion 5q chromosomal abnormality is a reasonable choice (accepted, with possible conditions). However, randomized controlled studies in adequate numbers of patients are lacking; additional data are needed to further elucidate clinical benefit (i.e., hematologic improvement-erythroid response) and to assess the relevance of prognostic factors (e.g., transfusion requirement, baseline platelet count, duration of MDS, serum lactate dehydrogenase concentration) to lenalidomide response.

■ **Multiple Myeloma** Lenalidomide is used in combination with dexamethasone for the treatment of multiple myeloma in patients who have received at least one prior therapy for this condition. Lenalidomide is designated an orphan drug by the US Food and Drug Administration (FDA) for use in multiple myeloma.

The current indication for lenalidomide is based principally on results from 2 randomized, double-blind, placebo-controlled, multicenter studies (MM-009 and MM-010) involving a total of 692 patients with multiple myeloma who had received at least one prior therapy. Patients were randomized to receive lenalidomide and placebo (25 mg once daily on days 1–21 of a 28-day cycle and placebo once daily on days 22–28 of each 28-day cycle) or placebo (on days 1–28 of each 28-day cycle); all patients also received oral dexamethasone 40 mg once daily on days 1–4, 9–12, and 17–20 of each 28-day cycle for the first 4 cycles of therapy, followed by dexamethasone 40 mg once daily on days 1–4 of each subsequent 28-day cycle. Sequential dosage reductions (i.e., to 15 mg daily, 10 mg daily, and 5 mg daily) and dosage interruptions of lenalidomide were allowed for management of toxicity . In both studies, treatment was to continue until disease progression. Time to progression was substantially longer in patients receiving lenalidomide and dexamethasone compared with those receiving dexamethasone and placebo (about 37 versus about 20 weeks, respectively). Patients receiving lenalidomide also experienced substantially higher overall (51–53 versus 16–19%), complete (8 versus 1%), and partial (43–44 versus 16–19%) response rates compared with those receiving dexamethasone and placebo, respectively. The median duration of follow-up in these 2 studies was 20.1 and 22.3 weeks.

Longer-term follow-up data from these 2 studies demonstrated an improved overall response rate (60.6 versus 21.9%), higher complete response rate (15 versus 2%), more prolonged duration of response (median of 15.8 versus 7 months), and a more prolonged time to progression (median of 13.4 versus 4.6 months) in patients receiving lenalidomide and dexamethasone compared with patients receiving dexamethasone and placebo, respectively. At a median follow-up of 48 months for surviving patients, a substantial benefit in overall survival (median of 38 versus 31.6 months) also was demonstrated.

A pooled subgroup analysis of data from the MM-009 and MM-010 studies in patients with relapsed or refractory multiple myeloma treated with lenalidomide and dexamethasone and who had received prior thalidomide therapy revealed a substantially lower complete response rate, a shorter median time to progression, and a shorter progression-free survival compared with patients who were thalidomide-naive; however, the median overall survival among patients who had or had not received prior thalidomide therapy was found to be similar (36.1 and 33.3 months, respectively).

Dosage and Administration

■ **Administration** Lenalidomide capsules should be administered orally with water once daily. The capsules should be swallowed intact and should not be broken, chewed, or opened. No more than a 28-day supply of lenalidomide should be dispensed at one time. Food does not appear to alter extent of absorption, but may reduce peak plasma concentrations of the drug; however, the manufacturer makes no specific recommendation regarding administration of lenalidomide capsules with food.

■ **Dosage** *Myelodysplastic Syndromes* For the management of transfusion-dependent anemia associated with low-risk or intermediate-1-risk myelodysplastic syndromes (MDS) in individuals with a cytogenetic deletion abnormality involving the long arm of chromosome 5 (a deletion 5q abnormality), with or without additional cytogenetic abnormalities, the recommended initial dosage in adults is 10 mg once daily.

When used in adults for the treatment of transfusion-dependent low-risk or intermediate-1-risk MDS without the deletion 5q chromosomal abnormality†, lenalidomide has been administered at a dosage of 10 mg once daily.

Dosage Modification for Toxicity in Patients with Myelodysplastic Syndromes. Because lenalidomide is associated with substantial thrombocytopenia and neutropenia in patients with this condition, complete blood cell counts (CBCs) should be monitored weekly for the first 8 weeks of therapy and at least monthly thereafter. Therapy should be interrupted or dosage reduced accordingly (see tables 1-6).

Table 1. Dosage Adjustment for Thrombocytopenia Occurring Within 4 Weeks After Initiation of Therapy with Lenalidomide 10 mg Daily

Platelet Count	Lenalidomide Dosage Adjustment
If baseline platelet count is ≥100,000/mm³ and:	
Count decreases to <50,000/mm³	Interrupt therapy
If count returns to ≥50,000/mm³ following interruption in therapy	Resume at 5 mg daily
If baseline count is <100,000/mm³ and:	
Count decreases to 50% of baseline	Interrupt therapy
If baseline count was ≥60,000/mm³ and count returns to ≥50,000/mm³ following interruption in therapy	Resume at 5 mg daily
If baseline count was <60,000/mm³ and count returns to ≥30,000/mm³ following interruption in therapy	Resume at 5 mg daily

Table 2. Dosage Adjustment for Thrombocytopenia Occurring More Than 4 Weeks After Initiation of Therapy with Lenalidomide 10 mg Daily

Platelet Count	Lenalidomide Dosage Adjustment
If count decreases to <30,000/mm³ or decreases to <50,000/mm³ with platelet infusions	Interrupt therapy
If count returns to ≥30,000/mm³ (without hemostatic failure) following interruption in therapy	Resume at 5 mg daily

Table 3. Dosage Adjustment for Thrombocytopenia Occurring During Therapy with Lenalidomide 5 mg Daily

Platelet Count	Lenalidomide Dosage Adjustment
If count decreases to <30,000/mm³ or decreases to <50,000/mm³ with platelet infusions	Interrupt therapy
If count returns to ≥30,000/mm³ (without hemostatic failure) following interruption in therapy	Resume at 5 mg every other day

Table 4. Dosage Adjustment for Neutropenia Occurring Within 4 Weeks After Initiation of Therapy with Lenalidomide 10 mg Daily

Absolute Neutrophil Count (ANC)	Lenalidomide Dosage Adjustment
If baseline ANC is ≥1000/mm³ and:	
Count decreases to <750/mm³	Interrupt therapy
If count returns to ≥1000/mm³ following interruption in therapy	Resume at 5 mg daily
If baseline ANC is <1000/mm³ and:	
Count decreases to <500/mm³	Interrupt therapy
If count returns to ≥500/mm³ following interruption in therapy	Resume at 5 mg daily

Table 5. Dosage Adjustment for Neutropenia Occurring More Than 4 Weeks After Initiation of Therapy with Lenalidomide 10 mg Daily

ANC	Lenalidomide Dosage Adjustment
If count decreases to <500/mm³ for ≥7 days or decreases to <500/mm³ associated with fever (>38.5°C)	Interrupt therapy
If count returns to ≥500/mm³ following interruption in therapy	Resume at 5 mg daily

Table 6. Dosage Adjustment for Neutropenia Occurring During Therapy with Lenalidomide 5 mg Daily

ANC	Lenalidomide Dosage Adjustment
If count decreases to <500/mm³ for ≥7 days or decreases to <500/mm³ associated with fever (≥38.5°C)	Interrupt therapy
If count returns to ≥500/mm³ following interruption in therapy	Resume at 5 mg every other day

Multiple Myeloma For the management of multiple myeloma in adults who have received at least one prior therapy, the recommended initial dosage of lenalidomide is 25 mg once daily (as a single 25-mg capsule) on days 1–21 of repeated 28-day cycles. The effect of substituting lower-strength capsules to achieve a 25-mg dose is not known. Patients should also receive an oral 40-mg dexamethasone dose once daily on days 1–4, 9–12, and 17–20 of each 28-day cycle for the first 4 cycles of therapy, followed by an oral 40-mg dexamethasone dose once daily on days 1–4 of each subsequent 28-day cycle.

Dosage Modification for Toxicity in Patients with Multiple Myeloma. Because lenalidomide is associated with thrombocytopenia and neutropenia in patients with this condition, complete blood cell counts (CBCs) should be monitored every 2 weeks for the first 3 months of therapy and at least monthly thereafter. Therapy should be interrupted or dosage reduced accordingly (see tables). For grade 3 or 4 toxicities other than neutropenia and thrombocytopenia that are considered related to lenalidomide therapy, interrupt treatment and resume at next lower dosage level (see tables 7 and 8) when toxicity resolves or decreases in severity to grade 2 or lower.

Table 7. Dosage Adjustment for Thrombocytopenia Occurring During Therapy with Lenalidomide 25 mg Daily

Platelet Count	Lenalidomide Dosage Adjustment
If count decreases to <30,000/mm³	Interrupt therapy and follow CBCs weekly
If count returns to ≥30,000/mm³ following interruption in therapy	Resume at 15 mg daily
For each subsequent decrease to <30,000/mm³	Interrupt therapy
If count returns to ≥30,000/mm³ following interruption in therapy for subsequent decreases to <30,000/mm³	Resume at a dosage of 5 mg less than previous dosage (minimum dosage of 5 mg daily); do not administer dosages lower than 5 mg daily

Table 8. Dosage Adjustment for Neutropenia Occurring During Therapy with Lenalidomide 25 mg Daily

ANC	Lenalidomide Dosage Adjustment
If count decreases to <1000/mm³	Interrupt therapy, add a granulocyte colony-stimulating factor (G-CSF), and monitor CBCs weekly
If count returns to ≥1000/mm³ following interruption in therapy and no other toxicity is present	Resume at 25 mg daily
If count returns to ≥1000/mm³ following interruption in therapy and if other toxicity is present	Resume at 15 mg daily
For each subsequent decrease to <1000/mm³	Interrupt therapy
If count returns to ≥1000/mm³ following interruption in therapy for subsequent decreases to <1000/mm³	Resume at a dosage of 5 mg less than previous dosage (minimum dosage of 5 mg daily); do not administer dosages lower than 5 mg daily

■ Special Populations

Table 9. Initial Recommended Dosage in Patients with Myelodysplastic Syndromes and Renal Impairment

Creatinine clearance in mL/min	Dose	Interval
Mild Impairment: At least 60	10 mg	Once daily
Moderate Impairment: 30–less than 60	5 mg	Once daily
Severe Impairment: Less than 30 (not requiring dialysis)	5 mg	Every 48 hours
End-stage Renal Disease: Less than 30 (requiring dialysis)	5 mg	3 times a week (following each dialysis)

Table 10. Initial Recommended Dosage in Patients with Multiple Myeloma and Renal Impairment

Creatinine clearance in mL/min	Dose	Interval
Mild Impairment: At least 60	25 mg	Once daily
Moderate Impairment: 30–less than 60	10 mg	Once daily
Severe Impairment: Less than 30 (not requiring dialysis)	15 mg	Every 48 hours
End-stage Renal Disease: Less than 30 (requiring dialysis)	5 mg	Once daily; on dialysis days, administer dose after dialysis

Because lenalidomide is eliminated primarily by the kidneys, adjustments to the initial dosage are recommended to provide appropriate drug exposure in patients with moderate or severe renal impairment as well as in patients on hemodialysis. Based on a pharmacokinetic study in patients with renal impairment due to nonmalignant conditions, adjustment to the initial lenalidomide dosage is recommended for patients with creatinine clearances of less than 60 mL/minute (see tables 9 and 10). Nondialysis patients with creatinine clearances of less than 11 mL/minute and hemodialysis patients with creatinine clearances less than 7 mL/minute have not been studied.

After initiation of lenalidomide therapy in renally impaired patients, subsequent dosage adjustments should be based on individual patient tolerance. (See Dosage and Administration: Dosage.)

In patients on hemodialysis, lenalidomide should be given *after* the completion of the dialysis session on days when hemodialysis is scheduled to ensure adequate therapeutic plasma concentrations and avoid the need for a supplemental dose of the drug.

Because lenalidomide is excreted substantially by the kidneys and geriatric patients are more likely to have decreased renal function, careful dosage selection and monitoring of renal function are advised in such patients.

■ Restricted Distribution Program

Because lenalidomide is an analog of thalidomide (a known human teratogen that can cause severe, life-threatening birth defects if administered during pregnancy), commercially available lenalidomide must be obtained through a restricted distribution program, the RevAssist® program, designed to help ensure that fetal exposure to the drug does not occur. Clinicians, pharmacists, and patients must be registered in the RevAssist® program before they can prescribe, dispense, and receive lenalidomide, and compliance with all terms outlined in the program is mandatory. The RevAssist® program controls access to lenalidomide; educates RevAssist® participants (clinicians, pharmacists, patients) about the risks associated with lenalidomide and the procedural requirements for safe use of the drug; and monitors compliance with the registration, education, and safety requirements of the program. For information regarding the RevAssist® program, Celgene should be contacted by phone (888-423-5436) or by the Internet (http://www.revlimid.com).

Cautions

■ Contraindications

Lenalidomide is contraindicated in women who are pregnant and in females of childbearing potential. The drug should be used in women of childbearing potential only when alternative therapies are not available and adequate precautions are taken to avoid pregnancy. (See Dosage and Administration: Restricted Distribution Program and also see Fetal/Neonatal Morbidity and Mortality under Warnings/Precautions: Warnings, in Cautions.)

Lenalidomide is contraindicated in patients with known hypersensitivity to the drug or any ingredient in the formulation.

■ Warnings/Precautions

Warnings **Fetal/Neonatal Morbidity and Mortality.** May cause fetal toxicity. No studies to date in humans. There is insufficient information regarding the teratogenic potential of lenalidomide; because of structural similarity to thalidomide, lenalidomide is contraindicated in women who are or may become pregnant. All female patients of childbearing potential and all sexually mature males receiving lenalidomide must use effective contraceptive measures (which may include abstinence) to help ensure that fetal exposure to lenalidomide does not occur. Contraceptive measures are indicated even in females with a history of infertility. The only females who do not need to observe mandatory contraceptive measures are those who have undergone hysterectomy, bilateral oophorectomy, or who are postmenopausal and have had no menses for at least 24 consecutive months. All female patients of childbearing potential must use 2 reliable forms of contraception simultaneously (unless the patient chooses to remain continuously abstinent from engaging in heterosexual sexual contact) during lenalidomide therapy or interruptions of therapy, and continue such contraception until 4 weeks after lenalidomide therapy is discontinued. The patient must use at least 2 birth control methods; preferably one should be a highly effective birth control method (intrauterine device [IUD], hormonal contraceptives, tubal ligation, vasectomized partner) and one additional effective barrier method (latex condom, diaphragm, cervical cap). Sexually mature males (including those who have successfully undergone vasectomy) receiving lenalidomide must completely avoid unprotected sexual contact with women of childbearing potential because it is not known whether lenalidomide is present in semen. While receiving lenalidomide and for at least 4 weeks after discontinuing the drug, sexually mature males must use a latex condom each time they have sexual contact with a woman of childbearing potential. All females of childbearing potential must be tested for pregnancy within 10–14 days prior and again within the 24 hours immediately prior to the first dose of lenalidomide using a reliable serum pregnancy test with the sensitivity to detect human serum or urine chorionic gonadotropin (HCG) concentrations of at least 50 mIU/mL.

The prescribing clinician should not provide the woman with a prescription for lenalidomide until a written report of the pregnancy test is available indicating that results are negative. Pregnancy tests must then be repeated at regular intervals during lenalidomide therapy (i.e., weekly during the first month, then every 2 or 4 weeks in women with irregular or regular menstrual cycles, respectively). Pregnancy tests and counseling also should be performed if a patient misses her period or if there is any abnormality in menstrual bleeding. The drug should be discontinued during the evaluation period. If lenalidomide is inadvertently administered during pregnancy or if the patient becomes pregnant while receiving the drug, lenalidomide should be immediately discontinued and the patient informed of the potential hazard to the fetus; the patient should be referred to an obstetrician/gynecologist experienced in reproductive toxicity, and the clinician should notify Celgene (888-423-5436) and the FDA via the MedWatch program (800-FDA-1088). (See Dosage and Administration: Restricted Distribution Program and also see Cautions: Contraindications.)

Hematologic Effects. Lenalidomide is associated with substantial neutropenia and thrombocytopenia. In a clinical trial, grade 3 or 4 hematologic toxicity was reported in 80% of patients with myelodysplastic syndromes (MDS; involving a cytogenetic deletion abnormality on the long arm of chromosome 5 [a deletion 5q abnormality]) receiving lenalidomide. Dosage delay or reduction secondary to neutropenia and/or thrombocytopenia was required in 80% of such patients, and a second dosage delay or reduction was required in 34% of patients. Median time to onset of grade 3 or 4 neutropenia (occurring in 48% of patients) was 42 days (range: 14–411 days), and median time to documented recovery was 17 days (range: 2–170 days) while median time to onset of grade 3 or 4 thrombocytopenia (occurring in 54% of patients) was 28 days (range: 8–290 days) and median time to documented recovery was 22 days (range: 5–224 days). Complete blood counts (CBCs) should be monitored weekly for the first 8 weeks of therapy and at least monthly thereafter. If hematologic toxicity occurs, dosage interruption and/or reduction may be required (see Dosage and Administration: Dosage Modification for Toxicity in Patients with Myelodysplastic Syndromes). Supportive therapy (including blood products) and/or a granulocyte colony-stimulating factor (G-CSF) also may be required.

Pooled analyses of clinical studies in patients with multiple myeloma receiving lenalidomide and dexamethasone indicate that grade 3 or 4 hematologic toxicity occurred more frequently in patients receiving lenalidomide and dexamethasone than in those receiving placebo and dexamethasone. CBCs should be monitored every 2 weeks for the first 12 weeks of therapy and at least monthly thereafter. If hematologic toxicity occurs, dosage interruption and/or reduction may be required (see Dosage and Administration: Dosage Modification for Toxicity in Patients with Multiple Myeloma).

Deep Venous Thrombosis and Pulmonary Embolism. Lenalidomide substantially increases the risk of deep venous thrombosis and pulmonary embolism in patients with multiple myeloma receiving combination therapy that includes lenalidomide. Venous thromboembolic events also have occurred in patients with MDS or mantle cell lymphoma who were receiving lenalidomide monotherapy. Although the risk of venous thromboembolism in MDS patients receiving lenalidomide is not well characterized and the background risk in untreated patients is unknown, a low incidence of venous thromboembolism (0.53%) has been reported during the first 3 years of exposure to the drug in the US. Patients and clinicians should be observant for signs and symptoms of thromboembolism. In addition, patients should be advised to seek medical care if they develop shortness of breath, chest pain, or swelling of the arms or legs. It is not known whether prophylactic therapy with anticoagulants or antiplatelet agents reduces the risk of thromboembolism associated with lenalidomide.

The manufacturer and some experts state that decisions regarding use of thromboprophylaxis and selection of an appropriate thromboprophylaxis regimen (e.g., aspirin, anticoagulant) should be based on careful assessment of the patient's risk factors for thromboembolism. The International Myeloma Working Group (IMWG) currently recommends thromboprophylaxis with aspirin for multiple myeloma patients receiving lenalidomide with one or no underlying individual and/or myeloma-related risk factors for venous thromboembolism and thromboprophylaxis with a low molecular weight heparin for those with 2 or more individual and/or myeloma-related risk factors. The IMWG also recommends that thromboprophylaxis with a low molecular weight heparin be considered in lenalidomide-treated patients receiving high-dose dexamethasone, doxorubicin, or multiple antineoplastic agents, independent of additional risk factors. The IMWG states that although full-dose warfarin (international normalized ratio [INR] 2–3) is an alternative to low molecular weight heparin, there is limited clinical experience with this approach. The American Society of Clinical Oncology (ASCO) currently recommends pharmacologic thromboprophylaxis for multiple myeloma patients receiving lenalidomide in conjunction with dexamethasone or antineoplastic agents, and states that those at lower risk for thromboembolism may receive either aspirin or a low molecular weight heparin, while those at higher risk should receive a low molecular weight heparin.

Sensitivity Reactions **Angioedema, Stevens-Johnson Syndrome, and Toxic Epidermal Necrolysis.** Angioedema and serious dermatologic reactions, including Stevens-Johnson syndrome and toxic epidermal necrolysis, have been reported in lenalidomide-treated patients. These reactions can be fatal. Patients who have experienced a grade 4 rash associated with thalidomide therapy should *not* receive lenalidomide. Discontinuance or interruption of lenalidomide therapy should be considered in patients who experience a grade 2 or 3 rash. Lenalidomide must be discontinued if angioedema, a grade 4 skin rash, or an exfoliative or bullous rash occurs or if Stevens-Johnson syndrome or toxic epidermal necrolysis is suspected, and the drug should not be resumed following discontinuance for these reactions.

General Precautions **Tumor Lysis Syndrome.** Lenalidomide has antineoplastic activity and therefore the complications of tumor lysis syndrome may occur. Patients at risk of tumor lysis syndrome are those with a high tumor burden prior to treatment. Such patients should be monitored closely and appropriate precautions taken.

Specific Populations **Pregnancy.** Category X. (See Dosage and Administration: Restricted Distribution Program and also see Fetal/Neonatal Morbidity and Mortality under Warnings/Precautions: Warnings, in Cautions.)

Lactation. Not known whether lenalidomide is distributed into human milk; discontinue nursing or the drug, taking into account the importance of the drug to the woman.

Pediatric Use. Safety and efficacy not established in patients younger than 18 years of age.

Geriatric Use. No substantial differences in efficacy or overall frequency of adverse effects relative to younger adults; however, an increased incidence of serious adverse events has been reported in patients older than 65 years of age compared with younger patients.

Because lenalidomide is excreted substantially by the kidneys and geriatric patients are more likely to have decreased renal function, careful dosage selection and monitoring of renal function are advised in such patients.

Renal Impairment. In a single-dose (25-mg) pharmacokinetic study, the elimination half-life of lenalidomide increased and clearance of the drug decreased as creatinine clearance decreased from mild to severe renal impairment. Patients with moderate and severe renal impairment had a threefold increase in half-life and a 66–75% decrease in drug clearance compared with healthy individuals. In patients on hemodialysis, an approximate 4.5-fold increase in elimination half-life and an 80% decrease in clearance have been observed following single-dose administration of lenalidomide compared with healthy individuals. Approximately 30% of an administered dose of the drug was removed during a single hemodialysis session. In multiple myeloma patients, patients with mild renal impairment had 56% higher AUC values compared with those with normal renal function.

Because lenalidomide is excreted substantially by the kidneys, adjustment to the initial dosage is recommended to provide appropriate drug exposure in patients with moderate or severe renal impairment (creatinine clearance less than 60 mL/minute) and in patients on hemodialysis. Lenalidomide is partially removed by hemodialysis. On days when hemodialysis is scheduled, lenalidomide should be given *after* the completion of the dialysis session. (See Dosage and Administration: Special Populations.)

Safety and efficacy of lenalidomide have not been studied in nondialysis patients with creatinine clearances less than 11 mL/minute or in end-stage renal disease patients on hemodialysis with creatinine clearances less than 7 mL/minute. (See Dosage and Administration: Special Populations.)

■ **Common Adverse Effects** Adverse effects reported in 10% or more of patients receiving lenalidomide for the treatment of transfusion-dependent anemia secondary to MDS include thrombocytopenia, neutropenia, diarrhea, pruritus, rash, fatigue, constipation, nausea, nasopharyngitis, arthralgia, back pain, fever, peripheral edema, cough, dizziness, headache, muscle cramps, dyspnea, pharyngitis, asthenia, epistaxis, upper respiratory tract infection, dry skin, abdominal pain, anemia, pneumonia, hypokalemia, limb pain, urinary tract infection, anorexia, edema, insomnia, and vomiting.

Adverse effects reported in 10% or more of patients receiving lenalidomide in combination with dexamethasone for the management of previously treated multiple myeloma include constipation, fatigue, insomnia, muscle cramps, diarrhea, neutropenia, anemia, asthenia, fever, nausea, headache, peripheral edema, dizziness, dyspnea, tremor, weight loss, thrombocytopenia, rash, back pain, hyperglycemia, muscle weakness, blurred vision, cough, dyspepsia, anorexia, upper respiratory tract infection, dysgeusia, paresthesia, hypokalemia, pneumonia, arthralgia, and vomiting.

Drug Interactions

■ **Drugs Affecting or Metabolized by Hepatic Microsomal Enzymes** Drug interactions with lenalidomide unlikely.

■ **Digoxin** Potential pharmacokinetic interaction (increased peak plasma digoxin concentrations). Manufacturer recommends periodic monitoring of plasma digoxin concentrations in patients receiving lenalidomide and digoxin concurrently.

■ **Warfarin** Drug interaction with lenalidomide unlikely.

Description

Lenalidomide, a thalidomide analog, is an immunomodulatory agent with antineoplastic and antiangiogenic activity. Lenalidomide appears to have a positive effect on erythropoiesis in transfusion-dependent patients with low-risk or intermediate-1-risk myelodysplastic syndromes (MDS) occurring in association with certain cytogenetic abnormalities (i.e., deletions between bands 31 and 33 of the long [q] arm of chromosome 5, with or without other cytogenetic abnormalities). However, the mechanism of action of lenalidomide in the management of transfusion-dependent anemia in such patients has not been fully elucidated. Lenalidomide affects ligand-induced responses (angiogenesis, inflammation, cell adhesion, immune response), and these actions may be integral to its activity in MDS. The drug has been shown to inhibit production of proinflammatory cytokines (e.g., tumor necrosis factor [TNF; TNF-α]), increase production of interleukin-2 and interferon gamma, and increase cytolytic T-cell and natural killer (NK) cell responses. Lenalidomide also has been shown to inhibit the growth of multiple myeloma cells from patients with multiple myeloma and of human multiple myeloma cell line by inducing cell cycle arrest and apoptosis.

Lenalidomide is principally eliminated by the kidneys via glomerular filtration and active tubular secretion; approximately 66% of the drug is excreted in urine as unchanged drug. In vitro studies indicate that lenalidomide is neither metabolized by nor inhibits or induces cytochrome P-450 enzymes.

Advice to Patients

Importance of educating patients regarding the RevAssist® restricted distribution program for obtaining lenalidomide. (See Dosage and Administration: Restricted Distribution Program.)

Importance of advising patients to swallow capsules intact and not to break, chew, or open capsules.

Necessity of monitoring blood cell counts for low white blood cells (neutropenia) and low platelets (thrombocytopenia) during lenalidomide therapy.

Risk of deep venous thrombosis and pulmonary embolism; importance of advising patients to seek medical care if they develop symptoms of shortness of breath, chest pain, or swelling of the arms or legs.

Importance of advising women of risk of teratogenicity secondary to structural similarity with thalidomide. Importance of advising women to take precautions to avoid fetal exposure to lenalidomide (see Fetal/Neonatal Morbidity and Mortality under Warnings/Precautions: Warnings, in Cautions) and to avoid breast-feeding while undergoing lenalidomide therapy. Importance of women informing a clinician immediately if they are or plan to become pregnant or plan to breast-feed. Importance of advising men to use a latex condom during any sexual contact with females of childbearing potential.

Importance of advising patients that they cannot donate blood while taking lenalidomide.

Importance of informing clinicians of existing or contemplated concomitant therapy, including prescription and OTC drugs, as well as any concomitant illnesses.

Importance of informing patients of other important precautionary information. (See Cautions.)

Overview® (see Users Guide). For additional information on this drug until a more detailed monograph is developed and published, the manufacturer's labeling should be consulted. It is *essential* that the manufacturer's labeling be consulted for more detailed information on usual cautions, precautions, contraindications, potential drug interactions, laboratory test interferences, and acute toxicity.

Preparations

Because lenalidomide is an analog of thalidomide (a known human teratogen that can cause severe, life-threatening birth defects if administered during pregnancy), commercially available lenalidomide must be obtained through a restricted distribution program (RevAssist®), designed to help ensure that fetal exposure to the drug does not occur. See Dosage and Administration: Restricted Distribution Program.

Excipients in commercially available drug preparations may have clinically important effects in some individuals; consult specific product labeling for details.

Lenalidomide

Oral		
Capsules	5 mg	Revlimid®, Celgene
	10 mg	Revlimid®, Celgene
	15 mg	Revlimid®, Celgene
	25 mg	Revlimid®, Celgene

†Use is not currently included in the labeling approved by the US Food and Drug Administration

Lenvatinib Mesylate

■ Lenvatinib, an inhibitor of multiple receptor tyrosine kinases, is an antineoplastic agent.

Uses

■ **Differentiated Thyroid Cancer** Lenvatinib mesylate is used for the treatment of locally recurrent or metastatic, progressive, radioactive iodine (iodine-131)-refractory differentiated thyroid cancer (DTC). The drug has been designated an orphan drug by the FDA for the treatment of this cancer. Currently available evidence indicates that lenvatinib therapy is associated with significantly prolonged progression-free survival and improved response rates compared with placebo in patients with locally recurrent or metastatic, radioactive iodine-refractory differentiated thyroid cancer.

Differentiated thyroid cancer, including papillary and follicular (including Hürthle cell) thyroid cancer, is the most common type of thyroid cancer. Differentiated thyroid cancer is usually treated with surgery and radioactive iodine therapy.

The current indication for lenvatinib is based principally on the results of a randomized, multicenter, double-blind, placebo-controlled, phase 3 study (the SELECT study) conducted in patients with locally recurrent or metastatic, radioactive iodine-refractory differentiated thyroid cancer and radiographic evidence of progressive disease within 12 months prior to randomization. Patients in the study were considered refractory to radioactive iodine if at least one of the following occurred: uptake of radioactive iodine did not occur in at least 1 measurable lesion on any iodine-131 scan, progression of at least 1 measurable lesion with iodine uptake within 12 months of radioactive iodine therapy, or cumulative iodine-131 activity exceeding 600 mCi with the last dose administered at least 6 months prior to study entry. In this study, 392 patients were randomized in a 2:1 ratio to receive either lenvatinib (24 mg) or placebo orally once daily in 28-day cycles until disease progression or intolerable toxicity occurred. The primary efficacy end point of this study was progression-free survival (as evaluated by a blinded independent review committee) according to Response Evaluation Criteria in Solid Tumors (RECIST); secondary endpoints included objective response rate and overall survival.

The median age of patients enrolled in the SELECT study was 63 years; 24% of the patients had received one prior therapy with a vascular endothelial growth factor (VEGF) or vascular endothelial growth factor receptor (VEGFR) inhibitor. Most patients (66%) had papillary thyroid cancer and 34% had follicular thyroid cancer; of the patients with follicular histology, 44 and 11% had Hürthle and clear cell subtypes, respectively. Most patients (67%) in the lenvatinib treatment arm did not demonstrate uptake of radioactive iodine on any scan and 59% of the patients in the lenvatinib treatment arm had progressed within 12 months of prior radioactive iodine therapy. The median cumulative radioactive iodine activity administered prior to study entry was 350 mCi.

The median progression-free survival was substantially longer in patients receiving lenvatinib (18.3 months) compared with those receiving placebo (3.6 months) in the SELECT study. Improved progression-free survival was observed in the lenvatinib-treated patients regardless of gender, age, ethnicity, previous therapy with a tyrosine kinase inhibitor, geographic region, histologic findings, and baseline thyrotropin concentrations. The objective response rate was 65% for patients receiving lenvatinib and 2% for those receiving placebo; partial response was achieved in 63% and complete response was achieved in 2% of the lenvatinib-treated patients. Median overall survival had not been reached at the time of the analysis. Upon radiographic confirmation of progression, 83% of patients previously randomized to receive placebo crossed over to receive open-label lenvatinib treatment; the median progression-free survival among evaluable patients entering the open-label phase was 10.1 months and the objective response rate was 52.3%.

Dosage and Administration

■ **General** ***Restricted Distribution Program*** Lenvatinib mesylate can only be obtained through designated specialty pharmacies. Clinicians may contact the manufacturer (Eisai) at 855-347-2448 or consult the Lenvima® website for specific ordering and availability information (http://www.lenvima.com).

■ **Administration** Lenvatinib mesylate is administered orally without regard to meals. (See Description.) The drug should be taken at the same time each day.

If a dose of lenvatinib mesylate is missed and cannot be taken within 12 hours, the missed dose should be skipped and the next dose should be taken at the regularly scheduled time.

If lenvatinib is used following sorafenib or other antineoplastic agents, there is a potential risk for additive toxicities unless there is an adequate washout period between treatments. In clinical trials, the minimum washout period was 4 weeks.

■ **Dosage** Dosage of lenvatinib mesylate is expressed in terms of lenvatinib.

Differentiated Thyroid Cancer The recommended adult dosage of lenvatinib for the treatment of locally recurrent or metastatic, progressive, radioactive iodine-refractory differentiated thyroid cancer is 24 mg (two 10-mg capsules and one 4-mg capsule) once daily. Therapy should be continued until disease progression or unacceptable toxicity occurs.

Dosage Modification for Toxicity Dosing interruption and/or dosage reduction or discontinuance of lenvatinib therapy may be necessary based on severity and persistence of an adverse effect. If dosage reduction from 24 mg once daily is necessary, the dosage should be reduced to 20 mg (two 10-mg capsules) once daily. If the toxicity recurs on a dosage of 20 mg once daily, the dosage should be reduced to 14 mg (one 10-mg capsule and one 4-mg capsule) once daily. If the toxicity recurs on a dosage of 14 mg once daily, the dosage should be reduced to 10 mg (one 10-mg capsule) once daily. The manufacturer provides no specific recommendations for further dosage reductions.

Grade 2 or 3 Toxicity or Grade 4 Laboratory Abnormalities. For a first occurrence of a persistent and intolerable grade 2 or 3 adverse reaction or grade 4 laboratory abnormality, lenvatinib should be withheld until the toxicity or laboratory abnormality resolves or improves to grade 1 or less or to baseline. Lenvatinib therapy may then be resumed at a reduced dosage of 20 mg (two 10-mg capsules) once daily.

If the toxicity recurs or another persistent and intolerable grade 2 or 3 adverse reaction or grade 4 laboratory abnormality occurs on a dosage of 20 mg once daily, lenvatinib should be withheld until the toxicity resolves or improves to grade 1 or less or to baseline. Lenvatinib therapy may then be resumed at a reduced dosage of 14 mg (one 10-mg capsule and one 4-mg capsule) once daily.

If the toxicity recurs or another persistent and intolerable grade 2 or 3 adverse reaction or grade 4 laboratory abnormality occurs on a dosage of 14 mg once daily, lenvatinib should be withheld until the toxicity resolves or improves to grade 1 or less or to baseline. Lenvatinib therapy may then be resumed at a reduced dosage of 10 mg (one 10-mg capsule) once daily. The manufacturer provides no specific recommendations for further dosage reductions.

The safety of resumption of lenvatinib therapy after resolution of grade 4 adverse reactions has not been studied; the manufacturer provides no specific dosage recommendations for such patients.

Cardiovascular Toxicity. If grade 3 hypertension persists despite optimal antihypertensive therapy, lenvatinib should be withheld until the hypertension improves to grade 2 or less. The drug may then be resumed at a reduced dosage. Lenvatinib therapy should be discontinued if life-threatening hypertension occurs. (See Hypertension under Cautions: Warnings/Precautions.)

If grade 3 cardiac dysfunction (i.e., decreased ventricular function, cardiac failure, or pulmonary edema) occurs, lenvatinib should be withheld until the cardiac dysfunction improves to grade 1 or less or to baseline. The drug may then be resumed at a reduced dosage or discontinued, depending on the severity and persistence of the cardiac dysfunction. If grade 4 cardiac dysfunction occurs, lenvatinib therapy should be discontinued. (See Cardiac Dysfunction under Cautions: Warnings/Precautions.)

If grade 3 or greater QT-interval prolongation occurs, lenvatinib should be withheld until the toxicity improves to grade 1 or less or to baseline. Lenvatinib therapy may then be resumed at a reduced dosage. (See Prolongation of QT Interval under Cautions: Warnings/Precautions.)

Arterial Thromboembolism. If an arterial thromboembolic event occurs, lenvatinib therapy should be discontinued. (See Arterial Thromboembolic Events under Cautions: Warnings/Precautions.)

Hemorrhage. If grade 3 hemorrhage occurs, lenvatinib should be withheld until the toxicity improves to grade 1 or less or to baseline. Lenvatinib therapy may then be resumed at a reduced dosage or discontinued, depending on the severity and persistence of the hemorrhage.

If grade 4 hemorrhage occurs, lenvatinib therapy should be discontinued. (See Hemorrhage under Cautions: Warnings/Precautions.)

Nephrotoxicity. If grade 3 or 4 renal impairment or renal failure occurs, lenvatinib should be withheld until the toxicity improves to grade 1 or less or to baseline. Lenvatinib therapy may then be resumed at a reduced dosage or discontinued, depending on the severity and persistence of the nephrotoxicity. (See Renal Failure and Impairment under Cautions: Warnings/Precautions.)

Hepatotoxicity. If grade 3 or 4 hepatotoxicity occurs, lenvatinib should be withheld until the toxicity improves to grade 1 or less or to baseline. The drug may then be resumed at a reduced dosage or discontinued, depending on the severity and persistence of the hepatotoxicity. If hepatic failure occurs, lenvatinib therapy should be discontinued. (See Hepatic Toxicity under Cautions: Warnings/Precautions.)

Proteinuria. Lenvatinib therapy should be interrupted for proteinuria of 2 g or more per 24 hours and resumed at a reduced dosage when proteinuria declines below this level.

If nephrotic syndrome occurs, treatment with lenvatinib should be discontinued. (See Proteinuria under Cautions: Warnings/Precautions.)

GI Toxicity. Because nausea, vomiting, and diarrhea occur frequently in patients receiving lenvatinib, initiation of therapy for these adverse GI effects (e.g., with antiemetic and/or antidiarrheal agents) is recommended prior to interruption of therapy or dosage modification.

If GI perforation or a life-threatening fistula occurs, lenvatinib therapy should be discontinued. (See GI Perforation and Fistula Formation under Cautions: Warnings/Precautions.)

Reversible Posterior Leukoencephalopathy Syndrome. If reversible posterior leukoencephalopathy syndrome (RPLS) occurs, lenvatinib should be withheld until the RPLS has fully resolved. Lenvatinib therapy may then be resumed at a reduced dosage or discontinued, depending on the severity and persistence of neurologic symptoms. (See Reversible Posterior Leukoencephalopathy Syndrome under Cautions: Warnings/Precautions.)

■ Special Populations

For patients with severe hepatic impairment (Child-Pugh class C), the manufacturer recommends a reduced lenvatinib dosage of 14 mg (one 10-mg capsule and one 4-mg capsule) once daily. Dosage adjustment is not necessary in patients with mild or moderate hepatic impairment (Child-Pugh class A or B). (See Hepatic Impairment under Warnings/Precautions: Specific Populations, in Cautions.)

For patients with severe renal impairment (creatinine clearance less than 30 mL/minute), the manufacturer recommends a reduced lenvatinib dosage of 14 mg (one 10-mg capsule and one 4-mg capsule) once daily. Dosage adjustment is not necessary in patients with mild (creatinine clearance of 60–89 mL/minute) or moderate (creatinine clearance of 30–59 mL/minute) renal impairment. Use of lenvatinib in patients with end-stage renal disease has not been studied, and the manufacturer provides no specific dosage recommendations for such patients. (See Renal Impairment under Warnings/Precautions: Specific Populations, in Cautions.)

The manufacturer makes no specific dosage recommendations for geriatric patients. (See Geriatric Use under Warnings/Precautions: Specific Populations, in Cautions.)

Cautions

■ Contraindications

The manufacturer states that there are no known contraindications to the use of lenvatinib mesylate.

■ Warnings/Precautions

Hypertension In the SELECT study, hypertension occurred in 73% of patients receiving lenvatinib compared with 16% of those receiving placebo. Grade 3 hypertension was reported in 44% of lenvatinib-treated patients compared with 4% of those receiving placebo, and grade 4 hypertension was reported in less than 1% of the lenvatinib-treated patients and in none of those receiving placebo. Hypertension usually developed early during lenvatinib therapy; the median time to onset of new or worsening hypertension was 16 days after initiating the drug. Hypertension necessitated discontinuance of therapy in approximately 1% of lenvatinib-treated patients.

Blood pressure should be assessed and controlled, if necessary, prior to initiating lenvatinib therapy. Blood pressure should be monitored following 1 week of therapy, every 2 weeks for the first 2 months of therapy, and then at least monthly thereafter. If hypertension occurs, patients should be managed medically (i.e., with antihypertensive therapy) as needed to control blood pressure during therapy. Interruption of lenvatinib therapy followed by dosage reduction is necessary when grade 3 hypertension occurs despite optimal antihypertensive therapy. Lenvatinib therapy should be discontinued if life-threatening hypertension occurs. (See Cardiovascular Toxicity under Dosage: Dosage Modification for Toxicity, in Dosage and Administration.)

Cardiac Dysfunction In the SELECT study, cardiac dysfunction (defined as decreased left or right ventricular function, cardiac failure, or pulmonary edema) was reported in 7% of patients receiving lenvatinib (grade 3 or greater in 2%) and in 2% of those receiving placebo (no cases of grade 3 or greater). Decreased ejection fraction was the most commonly reported finding (as assessed by echocardiography) in these cases. Decreases in ejection fraction exceeding 20% were reported in 2% of patients receiving lenvatinib compared with none of those receiving placebo.

Patients receiving lenvatinib should be monitored for manifestations of cardiac decompensation. Dosing interruption followed by dosage reduction or discontinuance of the drug is necessary when grade 3 cardiac dysfunction occurs. Lenvatinib therapy should be discontinued if grade 4 cardiac dysfunction occurs. (See Cardiovascular Toxicity under Dosage: Dosage Modification for Toxicity, in Dosage and Administration.)

Arterial Thromboembolic Events In the SELECT study, arterial thromboembolic events (e.g., cerebrovascular accident, transient ischemic attack, myocardial infarction) were reported in 5% of patients receiving lenvatinib (grade 3 or greater in 3%) and in 2% of patients receiving placebo (grade 3 or greater in 1%).

Lenvatinib therapy should be discontinued if an arterial thromboembolic event occurs. The safety of resuming lenvatinib therapy following such an event has not been established, and the drug has not been evaluated in patients who have had an arterial thromboembolic event within the previous 6 months.

Hepatic Toxicity Elevations in aminotransferase (ALT or AST) concentrations, acute hepatitis, and hepatic failure have been reported in patients receiving lenvatinib. In the SELECT study, grade 3 or greater elevations in ALT or AST concentrations occurred in 4 or 5%, respectively, of patients receiving lenvatinib. Among 1108 patients treated with lenvatinib in clinical studies, hepatic failure (including fatal cases) and acute hepatitis occurred in 3 patients and 1 patient, respectively.

Liver function tests should be evaluated prior to initiation of therapy and monitored every 2 weeks for the first 2 months of therapy and then at least monthly thereafter during therapy. Interruption of therapy followed by dosage reduction or discontinuance of lenvatinib is necessary when grade 3 or greater hepatic toxicity occurs. Lenvatinib therapy should be discontinued if hepatic failure occurs. (See Hepatotoxicity under Dosage: Dosage Modification for Toxicity, in Dosage and Administration.)

Proteinuria In the SELECT study, proteinuria was reported in 34% of patients receiving lenvatinib compared with 3% of those receiving placebo. Grade 3 proteinuria was reported in 11% of lenvatinib-treated patients compared with none of those receiving placebo. Proteinuria usually occurred early during therapy.

Patients should be monitored for proteinuria prior to initiation of lenvatinib and periodically during treatment with the drug. In patients with a 2+ or greater urine dipstick reading for proteinuria, a 24-hour urine protein measurement should be obtained. If proteinuria of 2 g or more per 24 hours is present, lenvatinib therapy should be interrupted and later resumed at a reduced dosage when proteinuria declines to below 2 g per 24 hours. Lenvatinib therapy should be discontinued if nephrotic syndrome occurs. (See Proteinuria under Dosage: Dosage Modification for Toxicity, in Dosage and Administration.)

Renal Failure and Impairment Renal impairment and renal failure have been reported in patients receiving lenvatinib. In the SELECT study, renal impairment was reported in 14% of patients receiving lenvatinib compared with 2% of those receiving placebo. Grade 3 or greater renal impairment or failure occurred in 3% of lenvatinib-treated patients compared with 1% of those receiving placebo. Dehydration and hypovolemia caused by diarrhea and vomiting was the main risk factor for developing severe renal impairment.

Dosing interruption followed by dosage reduction or discontinuance of lenvatinib is necessary when grade 3 or 4 renal toxicity or renal failure occurs. (See Nephrotoxicity under Dosage: Dosage Modification for Toxicity, in Dosage and Administration.)

GI Perforation and Fistula Formation GI perforation and fistula formation have been reported in patients receiving lenvatinib or other tyrosine kinase inhibitors. In most cases, GI perforation and fistulae occurred in patients with risk factors (e.g., prior surgery, recent sigmoidoscopy or colonoscopy, radiotherapy, underlying tumor, diverticulitis, bowel obstruction). In the SELECT study, GI perforation or fistula formation was reported in 2% of lenvatinib-treated patients and in 0.8% of those receiving placebo.

Lenvatinib should be discontinued in patients who develop GI perforation or a life-threatening fistula. (See GI Toxicity under Dosage: Dosage Modification for Toxicity, in Dosage and Administration.)

Prolongation of QT Interval Prolongation of the QT interval has been reported in patients receiving lenvatinib. In the SELECT study, prolongation of the QT interval or the corrected QT (QT_c) interval was reported in 9% of lenvatinib-treated patients and in 2% of those receiving placebo. Grade 3 or 4 prolongation of the QT interval was reported in 2% of lenvatinib-treated patients compared with none of those receiving placebo.

ECGs should be monitored during lenvatinib therapy in patients with congenital long QT syndrome, congestive heart failure, bradyarrhythmias, and/or in those concurrently receiving other drugs known to prolong the QT interval (see Drug Interactions: Drugs that Prolong the QT Interval). In addition, serum electrolyte concentrations (i.e., potassium, magnesium, calcium) should be monitored in all patients receiving the drug. Any electrolyte abnormalities that occur during lenvatinib therapy should be corrected. Interruption of therapy followed by dosage reduction upon improvement to grade 1 or less or to baseline is necessary when grade 3 or greater QT-interval prolongation occurs in patients receiving the drug. (See Cardiovascular Toxicity under Dosage: Dosage Modification for Toxicity, in Dosage and Administration.)

Hypocalcemia In the SELECT study, grade 3 or 4 hypocalcemia was reported in 9% of patients receiving lenvatinib compared with 2% of those receiving placebo. In most patients, lenvatinib-associated hypocalcemia responded to calcium replacement and temporary interruption of therapy followed by dosage reduction.

Blood calcium concentrations should be monitored at least monthly during lenvatinib therapy. If hypocalcemia occurs, calcium replacement therapy should be administered as necessary. Temporary interruption of lenvatinib therapy followed by dosage reduction may be necessary, depending on the presence of ECG changes and the severity and persistence of the hypocalcemia. (See Dosage Modification for Toxicity under Dosage and Administration: Dosage.)

Reversible Posterior Leukoencephalopathy Syndrome Reversible posterior leukoencephalopathy syndrome (RPLS) occurred rarely (3 cases; less than 1%) in patients treated with lenvatinib in clinical studies. RPLS is a neurologic disorder that may manifest with severe headache, seizures, weakness, confusion, blindness, or other visual disturbances; hypertension also may be present. Magnetic resonance imaging (MRI) is necessary to confirm the diagnosis of RPLS.

Interruption of lenvatinib therapy until the RPLS is fully resolved is necessary. Upon resolution, the drug may be resumed at a reduced dosage or discontinued, depending on the severity and persistence of the neurologic manifestations. (See Reversible Posterior Leukoencephalopathy Syndrome under Dosage: Dosage Modification for Toxicity, in Dosage and Administration.)

Hemorrhage In the SELECT study, hemorrhagic events occurred in 35% of patients receiving lenvatinib compared with 18% of those receiving placebo. The incidence of grade 3–5 hemorrhage was similar between the 2 groups (2 and 3% in patients receiving lenvatinib or placebo, respectively). The most common hemorrhagic event in the study was epistaxis. Fatal intracranial hemorrhage occurred in 1 of 16 lenvatinib-treated patients who had CNS metastases at baseline. Hemorrhagic events necessitated discontinuance of therapy in 1% of the lenvatinib-treated patients.

Interruption of lenvatinib therapy followed by dosage reduction or discontinuance of the drug is necessary when grade 3 hemorrhage occurs. (See Hemorrhage under Dosage: Dosage Modification for Toxicity, in Dosage and Administration.) If grade 4 hemorrhage occurs, lenvatinib therapy should be discontinued.

Impairment of Thyroid-stimulating Hormone Suppression Lenvatinib impairs exogenous thyroid suppression. Among patients with a normal thyroid-stimulating hormone (TSH) concentration at baseline in the SELECT study, elevated TSH concentrations (exceeding 5 microunits/mL) were observed in 57% of patients treated with lenvatinib.

TSH concentrations should be monitored monthly during lenvatinib therapy, and thyroid replacement therapy should be adjusted as necessary in patients with differentiated thyroid cancer receiving the drug.

Fetal/Neonatal Morbidity and Mortality Lenvatinib may cause fetal harm in humans based on its mechanism of action and animal findings; the drug has been shown to be teratogenic, embryotoxic, and fetotoxic in animals. There are no available data regarding the risk of lenvatinib use in pregnant women to date. In animal reproduction studies, dose-related decreases in mean fetal body weight; delayed fetal ossifications; and dose-related increases in fetal external, visceral, and skeletal anomalies were observed in rats at dosages below the recommended human dosage. Postimplantation loss was observed in more than 80% of pregnant rats at a lenvatinib dosage of 1 mg/kg per day (approximately 0.5 times the recommended human dosage based on body surface area). Fetal external, visceral, and skeletal anomalies and postimplantation loss (including one fetal death) also were observed in rabbits receiving dosages below the recommended human dosage; the drug also was abortifacient.

Pregnancy should be avoided during lenvatinib therapy. Women of childbearing potential should be advised to use an effective method of contraception while receiving lenvatinib and for at least 2 weeks after discontinuance of therapy. If lenvatinib is used during pregnancy or if the patient becomes pregnant while receiving the drug, the patient should be apprised of the potential fetal hazard. (See Advice to Patients.)

Impairment of Fertility Results of animal studies suggest that lenvatinib may impair male and female fertility. The effect of the drug on fertility in humans is not known.

Specific Populations **Pregnancy.** Lenvatinib may cause fetal harm if administered to pregnant women based on its mechanism of action and animal findings. (See Fetal/Neonatal Morbidity and Mortality under Cautions: Warnings/Precautions.)

Lactation. Lenvatinib and its metabolites are distributed into milk in rats at concentrations higher than maternal plasma; it is not known whether the drug is distributed into milk in humans. Because of the potential for serious adverse reactions to lenvatinib in nursing infants, women should be advised to discontinue nursing during lenvatinib therapy.

Pediatric Use. Safety and efficacy of lenvatinib have not been established in pediatric patients.

Growth retardation (decreased weight gain, food consumption, and femur and tibia width and/or length), secondary delays in physical development, and reproductive organ immaturity have been observed in juvenile rats receiving daily oral administration of lenvatinib for 8 weeks.

Geriatric Use. In the SELECT study, 45% of patients receiving lenvatinib were 65 years of age or older and 11% were 75 years of age or older. No overall differences in safety and efficacy were observed between these geriatric patients and younger adults.

In a pharmacokinetic population analysis, age did not have a substantial effect on the clearance of lenvatinib.

Hepatic Impairment. Following administration of a single 10-mg dose of lenvatinib, dose-adjusted total exposure to the drug in individuals with mild or moderate hepatic impairment (Child-Pugh class A or B) was 119 or 107% higher, respectively, compared with individuals with normal hepatic function; no dosage adjustment is required in patients with mild or moderate hepatic impairment.

Following administration of a single 5-mg dose of lenvatinib, dose-adjusted total exposure to the drug was 180% in individuals with severe hepatic impairment (Child-Pugh class C) compared with that in individuals with normal hepatic function; therefore, dosage adjustment is necessary in patients with severe hepatic impairment. (See Dosage and Administration: Special Populations.)

Renal Impairment. Following administration of a single 24-mg dose of lenvatinib, total exposure to lenvatinib in individuals with mild (creatinine clearance 60–89 mL/minute) and moderate (creatinine clearance 30–59 mL/minute) renal impairment was similar compared with individuals with normal renal function and was approximately 20% higher in those with severe renal impairment (creatinine clearance less than 30 mL/minute). The manufacturer recommends dosage adjustment in patients with severe renal impairment, who may be at increased risk for renal and other toxicity with the drug. Lenvatinib has not been studied in patients with end-stage renal disease. (See Dosage and Administration: Special Populations and also see Proteinuria and Renal Failure and Impairment under Cautions: Warnings/Precautions.)

■ **Common Adverse Effects** Adverse effects reported in 20% or more of patients receiving lenvatinib for differentiated thyroid cancer and at an incidence that is at least 5% higher than that reported with placebo include hypertension, diarrhea, fatigue, arthralgia/myalgia, decreased appetite, weight loss, nausea, stomatitis, headache, vomiting, proteinuria, palmar-plantar erythrodysesthesia (hand-foot syndrome), abdominal pain, dysphonia, constipation, oral pain, cough, rash, and peripheral edema.

Grade 3 or 4 laboratory abnormalities reported in 2% or more of patients receiving lenvatinib for differentiated thyroid cancer and at an incidence that is at least 2% higher than that reported with placebo include hypocalcemia, hypokalemia, elevated concentrations of hepatic aminotransferase enzymes (i.e., ALT, AST), lipase, or serum creatinine, and thrombocytopenia. Laboratory abnormalities (all grades) that occurred in more than 5% of lenvatinib-treated patients and at an incidence that is twofold or higher than that reported with placebo include hypoalbuminemia, elevated concentrations of alkaline phosphatase, hypomagnesemia, hypoglycemia, hyperbilirubinemia, hypercalcemia, hypercholesterolemia, increased concentrations of amylase, and hyperkalemia.

Drug Interactions

Lenvatinib is metabolized principally by cytochrome P-450 (CYP) isoenzyme 3A4. In vitro studies indicate that lenvatinib inhibits CYP isoenzymes 2C8, 1A2, 2B6, 2C9, 2C19, 2D6, and 3A, and also uridine diphosphate-glucuronosyl transferases (UGT) 1A1 and 1A4, but does not inhibit CYP isoenzymes 2A6 or 2E1. The drug shows little to no inhibition of UGT 1A6, 1A9, or 2B7 or aldehyde oxidase. Lenvatinib also induces CYP3A, but does not induce CYP isoenzymes 1A1, 1A2, 2B6, or 2C9, and UGT 1A1, 1A4, 1A6, 1A9, or 2B7.

In vitro, lenvatinib is an inhibitor of organic anion transporter (OAT) 1, OAT3, organic cation transporter (OCT) 1, OCT2, organic anion transport protein (OATP) 1B1, and bile salt export pump (BSEP), and shows little to no inhibition of OATP1B3; the clinical relevance of these findings is not known. In vitro, the drug is a substrate for P-glycoprotein (P-gp) and breast cancer resistance protein (BCRP), but is not a substrate for OAT1, OAT3, OCT1, OCT2, OATP1B1, OATP1B3, or BSEP.

■ **Drugs Affecting Hepatic Microsomal Enzymes and/or Efflux Transport Systems** ***Inhibitors of CYP3A and Efflux Transport Systems*** When ketoconazole (a CYP3A4, P-gp, and BCRP inhibitor) 400 mg was administered once daily for 18 days with a single 5-mg dose of lenvatinib on day 5, peak plasma concentrations and systemic exposure of lenvatinib were increased by 19 and 15%, respectively. The manufacturer states that dosage adjustment is not necessary when lenvatinib is used concomitantly with CYP3A, P-gp, and BCRP inhibitors.

When the P-gp inhibitor, rifampin (single 600-mg dose), was administered concomitantly with lenvatinib (single 24-mg dose), peak plasma concentrations and systemic exposure of lenvatinib were increased by 33 and 31%, respectively.

Inducers of CYP3A and Efflux Transport Systems When rifampin (a CYP3A and P-gp inducer) 600 mg was administered once daily for 21 days with a single 24-mg dose of lenvatinib on day 15, systemic exposure of lenvatinib was decreased by 18% and peak plasma concentrations were unchanged. The manufacturer states that dosage adjustment is not necessary when lenvatinib is used concomitantly with CYP3A and P-gp inducers.

■ **Drugs Metabolized by Hepatic Microsomal Enzymes** ***Substrates of CYP3A4*** Clinically important pharmacokinetic interactions between drugs that are substrates of CYP3A4 (e.g., midazolam) and lenvatinib are not expected during concurrent use.

Substrates of CYP2C8 Clinically important pharmacokinetic interactions between drugs that are substrates of CYP2C8 (e.g., repaglinide) and lenvatinib are not expected during concurrent use.

Other CYP Substrates In vitro studies indicate that clinically important effects are not expected with concurrent use of lenvatinib and drugs metabolized by CYP1A2, 2B6, 2C9, 2C19, or 2D6.

■ **Drugs that Prolong the QT Interval** Because lenvatinib has been associated with QT-interval prolongation, the manufacturer recommends ECG monitoring in lenvatinib-treated patients concurrently receiving other drugs known to prolong the QT interval, including class IA antiarrhythmics (e.g., quinidine, procainamide) and class III antiarrhythmics (e.g., amiodarone, sotalol). In addition, electrolyte monitoring and correction of any electrolyte abnormalities is recommended in all patients receiving lenvatinib. (See Prolongation of QT Interval under Cautions: Warnings/Precautions.)

Description

Lenvatinib, an inhibitor of multiple receptor tyrosine kinases, is an antineoplastic agent. Receptor tyrosine kinases (RTKs) are involved in the initiation of various cascades of intracellular signaling events that lead to cell proliferation and/or influence processes critical to cell survival and tumor progression (e.g., angiogenesis, metastasis, inhibition of apoptosis), based on the respective kinase. Lenvatinib inhibits the kinase activities of vascular endothelial growth factor (VEGF) receptors VEGFR-1, VEGFR-2, and VEGFR-3. The drug also inhibits other RTKs involved in pathogenic angiogenesis, tumor growth, and cancer progression, including fibroblast growth factor (FGF) receptors (FGFR1, FGFR2, FGFR3, and FGFR4), the platelet-derived growth factor receptor (PDGFR), stem cell factor receptor (c-Kit), and ret proto-oncogene (RET).

Following oral administration, lenvatinib is rapidly absorbed with peak plasma concentrations usually occurring within 1–4 hours. Peak plasma concentrations and systemic exposure to lenvatinib are proportional to dose following single or repeated administration of the drug over the dosage range of 3.2–32 mg once daily. Administration of lenvatinib with food delayed the rate of absorption (time to reach peak concentrations delayed by 2 hours), but did not affect the extent of absorption. Lenvatinib is metabolized in the liver principally by cytochrome P-450 (CYP) 3A4, aldehyde oxidase, and nonenzymatic processes. Lenvatinib is highly bound (98–99%) to plasma proteins. The elimination half-life of the drug is approximately 28 hours. Following oral administration of a single radiolabeled dose of lenvatinib, approximately 64% of the dose is recovered in the feces and approximately 25% of the dose is recovered in urine within 10 days.

Advice to Patients

Importance of instructing patients to read the manufacturer's patient information before starting lenvatinib therapy and each time their prescription is refilled.

If a dose is missed by more than 12 hours, importance of advising patients to skip that dose and take the next dose at the regularly scheduled time.

Risk of hypertension developing or worsening during therapy. Importance of regular monitoring of blood pressure during treatment. Importance of informing clinician if hypertension occurs.

Risk of cardiac dysfunction. Importance of immediately informing clinician if symptoms of cardiac dysfunction (e.g., shortness of breath, peripheral edema) occur.

Risk of arterial thromboembolic events. Importance of advising patients to seek immediate medical attention for new onset chest pain or acute neurologic symptoms consistent with myocardial infarction or stroke (e.g., severe chest pain or pressure, shortness of breath, unilateral numbness or weakness, difficulty talking, severe headache, vision changes, arm, back, neck, or jaw pain).

Risk of hepatotoxicity. Importance of liver function test monitoring before and during lenvatinib therapy. Importance of immediately reporting any possible manifestations of hepatotoxicity (e.g., jaundice, dark or "tea-colored" urine, light-colored stools).

Risk of proteinuria and renal impairment or failure. Importance of advising patients that they will be monitored regularly for renal function and proteinuria during lenvatinib therapy.

Increased risk of GI perforation or fistula formation. Importance of seeking immediate medical attention if severe abdominal pain occurs.

Increased risk of hemorrhagic events. Importance of advising patients to contact their clinician if bleeding or symptoms of severe bleeding occur.

Risk of QT-interval prolongation. Importance of informing patients that ECGs and/or serum electrolytes may be monitored during lenvatinib therapy.

Risk of hypocalcemia. Importance of monitoring calcium concentrations during therapy.

Risk of reversible posterior leukoencephalopathy syndrome (RPLS). Importance of contacting clinician promptly if severe headache, seizures, weakness, confusion, or visual disturbances occur during therapy.

Risk of impairment of exogenous thyroid suppression. Importance of monitoring thyroid-stimulating hormone (TSH) during therapy.

Risk of fetal harm. Necessity of advising women of childbearing potential to avoid pregnancy and to use an effective method of contraception during therapy and for at least 2 weeks after discontinuance of lenvatinib. Importance of women informing their clinicians if they are or plan to become pregnant. If pregnancy occurs, advise pregnant women of potential risk to the fetus.

Importance of advising women to avoid breast-feeding during lenvatinib therapy.

Importance of informing clinicians of existing or contemplated concomitant therapy, including prescription and OTC drugs, as well as any concomitant illnesses (e.g., cardiovascular disease [including congenital long QT syndrome]).

Importance of informing patients of other important precautionary information. (See Cautions.)

Overview® (see Users Guide). For additional information on this drug until a more detailed monograph is developed and published, the manufacturer's labeling should be consulted. It is *essential* that the manufacturer's labeling be consulted for more detailed information on usual cautions, precautions, contraindications, potential drug interactions, laboratory test interferences, and acute toxicity. For further information on the handling of antineoplastic agents, see the ASHP Guidelines on Handling Hazardous Drugs at http://www.ahfsdruginformation.com.

Preparations

Distribution of lenvatinib mesylate is restricted. (See Restricted Distribution Program under Dosage and Administration: General.)

Excipients in commercially available drug preparations may have clinically important effects in some individuals; consult specific product labeling for details.

Lenvatinib Mesylate

Oral		
Capsules	4 mg (of lenvatinib)	**Lenvima®**, Eisai
	10 mg (of lenvatinib)	**Lenvima®**, Eisai
Kits	10 Capsules, Lenvatinib mesylate 10 mg (of lenvatinib) (Lenvima®) 5 Capsules, Lenvatinib mesylate 4 mg (of lenvatinib) (Lenvima®)	**Lenvima® 24 mg Daily Dose** (available in a package containing 6 blister cards), Eisai
	10 Capsules, Lenvatinib mesylate 10 mg (of lenvatinib) (Lenvima®)	**Lenvima® 20 mg Daily Dose** (available in a package containing 6 blister cards), Eisai
	5 Capsules, Lenvatinib mesylate 10 mg (of lenvatinib) (Lenvima®) 5 Capsules, Lenvatinib mesylate 4 mg (of lenvatinib) (Lenvima®)	**Lenvima® 14 mg Daily Dose** (available in a package containing 6 blister cards), Eisai
	5 Capsules, Lenvatinib mesylate 10 mg (of lenvatinib) (Lenvima®)	**Lenvima® 10 mg Daily Dose** (available in a package containing 6 blister cards), Eisai

Lorlatinib

■ Lorlatinib, an inhibitor of multiple receptor tyrosine kinases including anaplastic lymphoma kinase (ALK) and c-ros oncogene-1 (ROS-1), is an antineoplastic agent.

Uses

■ **Non-small Cell Lung Cancer** Lorlatinib is used for the treatment of anaplastic lymphoma kinase (ALK)-positive metastatic non-small cell lung cancer (NSCLC) in patients whose disease has progressed on crizotinib and at least one other ALK inhibitor for metastatic disease, or progressed on alectinib as the initial ALK inhibitor for metastatic disease, or progressed on ceritinib as the initial ALK inhibitor for metastatic disease. The accelerated approval of lorlatinib for this indication is based on tumor response rate and duration of response; continued approval for this indication may be contingent on verification and description of clinical benefit in a confirmatory study. The drug has been designated an orphan drug by the FDA for the treatment of ALK-positive or c-ros oncogene-1 (ROS-1)-positive NSCLC.

A relatively small subset of patients with NSCLC (approximately 3–7%) have ALK-positive disease, which indicates potential responsiveness to ALK inhibitor therapy (e.g., alectinib, brigatinib, ceritinib, crizotinib). Patients with this form of lung cancer typically are nonsmokers or have a history of light smoking, and are younger in age and often have adenocarcinoma histology. Although crizotinib is highly active in patients with ALK-positive NSCLC, most patients treated with the drug eventually experience disease progression, limiting the drug's long-term therapeutic potential. Disease progression in patients receiving ALK inhibitors (e.g., alectinib, ceritinib, crizotinib) can result from acquired resistance mutations in ALK, amplification of gene expression, activation of alternate signaling pathways, and/or progression of brain metastases (e.g., because of poor distribution of crizotinib into the CSF). (See Description.)

The current indication for lorlatinib is based principally on the results of a multicenter, nonrandomized, open-label, phase 2 study that enrolled a total of 215 adults with metastatic ALK-positive NSCLC who had experienced disease progression while receiving therapy with crizotinib or other ALK inhibitors (e.g., alectinib, ceritinib, brigatinib) with or without prior chemotherapy. The study also included treatment-naive patients with ALK-positive NSCLC and patients with ROS1-positive NSCLC who were not included in the efficacy analysis of lorlatinib for this indication. Patients received lorlatinib 100 mg orally once daily until disease progression, unacceptable toxicity, death, or study withdrawal occurred. The primary efficacy end points were overall response rate and intracranial overall response rate according to the Response Evaluation Criteria in Solid Tumors (RECIST 1.1) as evaluated by a central independent review committee (IRC); additional outcome measures included duration of response and intracranial duration of response. The median age of patients included in the study analysis was 53 years (range: 29–85 years), 51% of patients were white and 34% were Asian, and 59% were female. All patients had metastatic disease and 95% had adenocarcinoma histology. Approximately 30% of patients evaluated had disease progression during crizotinib therapy, and 13, 35, or 22% had disease progression during prior therapy with 1 (non-crizotinib), 2, or 3 ALK inhibitors, respectively. CNS metastases were present in 69% of patients and 60% of such patients had previously received radiation to the brain. The IRC-assessed overall response rate with lorlatinib was 48%; partial responses were achieved in 44% of patients and 4% had a complete response. The median duration of response was 12.5 months. In the subgroup of 89 patients with measurable brain metastases at baseline, the IRC-assessed intracranial overall response rate was 60% (38% partial responses and 21% complete responses) and the median duration of intracranial response was 19.5 months.

A phase 3 controlled trial comparing lorlatinib with crizotinib as first-line, single-agent therapy in treatment-naive patients with ALK-positive NSCLC† (the CROWN trial) is under way. Lorlatinib currently is not FDA-labeled for use in patients with treatment-naive ALK-positive NSCLC.

Dosage and Administration

■ **General** Because lorlatinib can cause hyperlipidemia, serum cholesterol and triglyceride concentrations should be assessed prior to initiating therapy, 1 and 2 months after initiating therapy, and then periodically thereafter. (See Hyperlipidemia under Dosage: Dosage Modification for Toxicity, in Dosage and Administration.)

Because lorlatinib can cause atrioventricular (AV) block, ECG monitoring is recommended prior to initiating therapy and periodically thereafter. (See Atrioventricular Block under Dosage: Dosage Modification for Toxicity, in Dosage and Administration.)

Restricted Distribution Lorlatinib is available only through specialty pharmacies. Clinicians may consult the Lorbrena® website (https://www.lorbrena.com) for specific information regarding distribution of the drug.

■ **Administration** Lorlatinib is administered orally once daily at the same time each day without regard to food. (See Description.) The tablets should be swallowed whole and should *not* be crushed, chewed, or split. The manufacturer states that lorlatinib tablets should not be taken if they are broken, cracked, or otherwise not intact.

If a dose of lorlatinib is missed, the dose should be taken as soon as it is remembered unless the next dose is due within 4 hours. Two doses should not be taken at the same time. If vomiting occurs after taking a dose, the next dose should be taken at the regularly scheduled time; an additional dose should not be taken.

■ **Dosage** ***Non-small Cell Lung Cancer*** For the treatment of anaplastic lymphoma kinase (ALK)-positive metastatic non-small cell lung cancer (NSCLC) that has progressed on crizotinib and at least one other ALK inhibitor or progressed on initial therapy with alectinib or ceritinib, the recommended adult dosage of lorlatinib is 100 mg once daily. Therapy with the drug should be continued until disease progression or unacceptable toxicity occurs.

Dosage Modification for Toxicity Dosing interruption and/or dosage reduction of lorlatinib may be necessary based on individual safety and tolerability.

In the principal efficacy study, interruption of therapy or dosage reduction because of adverse reactions was necessary in approximately 48 or 24%, respectively, of patients receiving lorlatinib at the recommended dosage (most commonly for edema, peripheral neuropathy, cognitive effects, or mood effects).

If dosage reduction is necessary, an initial dosage reduction to 75 mg once daily is recommended. If further dosage reduction is necessary, the dosage should be reduced to 50 mg once daily. If a dosage of 50 mg once daily is not tolerated, lorlatinib should be permanently discontinued.

CNS Effects. If grade 1 adverse CNS effects occur, lorlatinib therapy may be continued at the same dosage or therapy may be interrupted until recovery to baseline. Therapy may then be resumed at the same dosage or at the next lower dosage.

If grade 2 or 3 adverse CNS effects occur, lorlatinib therapy should be interrupted until recovery to grade 0 or 1. Therapy may then be resumed at the next lower dosage.

If grade 4 adverse CNS effects occur, lorlatinib therapy should be permanently discontinued. (See CNS Effects under Cautions: Warnings/Precautions.)

Hyperlipidemia. If grade 4 hypercholesterolemia (serum cholesterol concentration exceeding 500 mg/dL) and/or grade 4 hypertriglyceridemia (serum triglyceride concentration exceeding 1000 mg/dL) occurs, lorlatinib therapy should be interrupted and appropriate antilipemic therapy should be initiated, the dosage of existing antilipemic therapy should be increased, or the existing antilipemic regimen should be changed to a new lipid-lowering therapy. Lorlatinib therapy may be resumed at the same dosage upon recovery of hypercholesterolemia and/or hypertriglyceridemia to grade 2 or less.

If severe hypercholesterolemia and/or hypertriglyceridemia *recurs* despite optimal antilipemic therapy, therapy should then be resumed at the next lower dosage of lorlatinib. (See Hyperlipidemia under Cautions: Warnings/Precautions.)

Atrioventricular Block. If second-degree atrioventricular (AV) block occurs, lorlatinib therapy should be interrupted until the PR interval is less than 200 msec. Lorlatinib should then be resumed at the next lower dosage.

If complete AV block occurs, lorlatinib therapy should be interrupted until a pacemaker is placed *or* the PR interval is less than 200 msec. If a pacemaker is placed, lorlatinib therapy may be resumed at the same dosage. If a pacemaker is *not* placed, lorlatinib therapy should be resumed at the next lower dosage.

If complete AV block *recurs*, a pacemaker should be placed or lorlatinib therapy should be permanently discontinued.

Interstitial Lung Disease/Pneumonitis. If treatment-related interstitial lung disease/pneumonitis of any grade occurs, lorlatinib therapy should be permanently discontinued. (See Interstitial Lung Disease/Pneumonitis under Cautions: Warnings/Precautions.)

Other Toxicity. If any other grade 1 or 2 adverse reaction occurs, lorlatinib therapy may be continued at the same dosage or reduced to the next lower dosage.

If any other grade 3 or 4 adverse reaction occurs, lorlatinib therapy should be interrupted until recovery to grade 2 or less, or to baseline. Lorlatinib therapy may then be resumed at the next lower dosage.

Concomitant Use of Drugs Affecting Hepatic Microsomal Enzymes Concomitant use of lorlatinib with *potent* inducers of cytochrome P-450 (CYP) isoenzyme 3A is contraindicated. Potent CYP3A inducers should be discontinued for 3 plasma half-lives of the potent CYP3A inducer prior to initiating lorlatinib therapy. Concomitant use of lorlatinib with *moderate* CYP3A inducers should be avoided. (See Serious Hepatotoxicity with Concurrent Use of Potent CYP3A Inducers under Cautions: Warnings/Precautions.)

Concomitant use of lorlatinib with *potent* CYP3A inhibitors should be avoided. If concomitant use of a potent CYP3A inhibitor cannot be avoided, the initial dosage of lorlatinib should be reduced from 100 mg once daily to 75 mg once daily. In patients who have had a dosage reduction to 75 mg once daily because of adverse reactions, the dosage of lorlatinib should be reduced to 50 mg once daily during concomitant use of a potent CYP3A inhibitor. If concomitant use of the potent CYP3A inhibitor is discontinued, the lorlatinib dosage should be increased (after 3 plasma half-lives of the CYP3A inhibitor) back to the dosage that was used prior to initiation of the potent CYP3A inhibitor. (See Inhibitors of CYP3A under Drug Interactions: Drugs Affecting Hepatic Microsomal Enzymes.)

■ **Special Populations** No dosage adjustment is necessary in patients with mild hepatic impairment (total bilirubin concentrations not exceeding the upper limit of normal [ULN] with AST concentrations exceeding the ULN, or total bilirubin concentrations exceeding 1 but not exceeding 1.5 times the ULN with any AST concentration). The recommended dosage of lorlatinib has not been established in patients with moderate or severe hepatic impairment. (See Hepatic Impairment under Warnings/Precautions: Specific Populations, in Cautions.)

No dosage adjustment is necessary in patients with mild or moderate renal impairment (creatinine clearance of 30–89 mL/minute). The recommended dosage of lorlatinib has not been established in patients with severe renal impairment (creatinine clearance less than 30 mL/minute). (See Renal Impairment under Warnings/Precautions: Specific Populations, in Cautions.)

The manufacturer makes no specific dosage recommendations for geriatric patients. (See Geriatric Use under Warnings/Precautions: Specific Populations, in Cautions.)

Cautions

■ **Contraindications** Lorlatinib is contraindicated in patients receiving potent cytochrome P-450 (CYP) isoenzyme 3A inducers because of the potential for serious hepatotoxicity. (See Serious Hepatotoxicity with Concurrent Use of Potent CYP3A Inducers under Cautions: Warnings/Precautions.)

■ **Warnings/Precautions** ***Serious Hepatotoxicity with Concurrent Use of Potent CYP3A Inducers*** Severe hepatotoxicity occurred in 10 of 12 healthy individuals receiving a single dose of lorlatinib with multiple daily doses of rifampin (a potent CYP3A inducer) during a drug interaction study. Grade 3 or 4 elevations in ALT or AST concentrations occurred in 83% and grade 2 elevations occurred in 8% of individuals who received the drugs concomitantly during the study. ALT or AST elevations occurred within 3 days of concomitant administration and returned to within normal limits after a median of 15 days (range: 7–34 days). The median time to recovery was 18 days following grade 3 or 4 elevations in ALT or AST concentrations and 7 days following grade 2 elevations. Concomitant use of lorlatinib with drugs that are *potent* CYP3A inducers is contraindicated. Potent CYP3A inducers should be discontinued for 3 plasma half-lives of the potent CYP3A inducer prior to initiating lorlatinib therapy.

Concomitant use of lorlatinib with drugs that are *moderate* CYP3A inducers should be avoided. If concomitant use cannot be avoided, AST, ALT, and bilirubin concentrations should be monitored 48 hours after initiation of lorlatinib and at least 3 times during the first week of concomitant therapy. If grade 2 or higher hepatotoxicity persists during concomitant use, either lorlatinib or the moderate CYP3A inducer should be discontinued, depending on the relative importance of each drug to the patient. (See Inducers of CYP3A under Drug Interactions: Drugs Affecting Hepatic Microsomal Enzymes.)

CNS Effects Lorlatinib can cause a wide variety of adverse CNS effects, including seizures, hallucinations, and changes in cognitive function (including memory impairment, cognitive disorder, and amnesia), mood (including suicidal ideation/suicidality, irritability, anxiety, depression, and labile affect), speech, mental status, and sleep. Although adverse CNS effects associated with lorlatinib therapy generally are mild in severity and intermittent and improve or resolve upon dosage modification, treatment interruption, dosage reduction, or drug discontinuance may be required depending on their severity. (See CNS Effects under Dosage: Dosage Modification for Toxicity, in Dosage and Administration.)

In the principal efficacy study of metastatic non-small cell lung cancer (NSCLC), adverse CNS effects were reported in 54% of patients receiving lorlatinib in dosages ranging from 10–200 mg daily given in single or divided doses. Cognitive, mood, or speech effects occurred in 29, 24, or 14% of lorlatinib-treated patients, respectively, and severe effects (i.e., grade 3 or 4) occurred in 2.1, 1.8, or 0.3% of these patients, respectively. Hallucinations or mental status changes occurred in 7 or 2.1% of patients, respectively, and were severe in 0.6 or 1.8% of patients, respectively. Seizures occurred in 3% of lorlatinib-treated patients, sometimes in conjunction with other neurologic findings. Effects on sleep occurred in 10% of patients receiving the drug. The median time to first onset of any adverse CNS effect was 1.2 months (range: 1 day to 1.7 years). Overall, treatment interruption, dosage reduction, or permanent discontinuance of lorlatinib because of adverse CNS effects was required in 9, 8, or 1.5%, respectively, of patients in the study.

Hyperlipidemia Increases in serum cholesterol and triglyceride concentrations may occur in patients receiving lorlatinib. Hypercholesterolemia or hypertriglyceridemia occurred in 90% or more of patients receiving the recommended dosage of lorlatinib in the principal efficacy study and 80% of patients receiving lorlatinib required initiation of antilipemic therapy. Grade 3 or 4 elevations in serum total cholesterol or triglyceride concentrations occurred in 17% of patients treated with lorlatinib. Treatment interruption or dosage reduction of lorlatinib was required in approximately 7 or 3% of patients, respectively, due to hypercholesterolemia or hypertriglyceridemia. The median time to onset of hypercholesterolemia or hypertriglyceridemia was 15 days; the median time to initiation of antilipemic therapy was 21 days.

Serum cholesterol and triglycerides should be assessed prior to initiating lorlatinib therapy, 1 and 2 months after initiating therapy, and periodically thereafter. Antilipemic therapy should be initiated or the dosage of existing antilipemic therapy should be increased in patients with hyperlipidemia. Temporary interruption followed by resumption of lorlatinib therapy at the same dosage or at a reduced dosage may be necessary, depending on the severity of the hyperlipidemia. (See Hyperlipidemia under Dosage: Dosage Modification for Toxicity, in Dosage and Administration.)

Atrioventricular Block PR-interval prolongation and atrioventricular (AV) block may occur in patients receiving lorlatinib. In the principal efficacy study, AV block occurred in 1% of patients who received lorlatinib at the recommended dosage and had a baseline ECG; 0.3% of these patients experienced grade 3 AV block and underwent pacemaker placement. ECG monitoring is recommended prior to initiating lorlatinib and periodically during therapy. If AV block occurs, lorlatinib therapy should be interrupted; dosage reduction may be necessary unless a pacemaker is placed. If complete AV block recurs in patients without a pacemaker, lorlatinib should be permanently discontinued. (See Atrioventricular Block under Dosage: Dosage Modification for Toxicity, in Dosage and Administration.)

Interstitial Lung Disease/Pneumonitis Severe or life-threatening adverse pulmonary reactions consistent with interstitial lung disease (ILD)/pneumonitis may occur in patients receiving lorlatinib. In the principal efficacy study, ILD or pneumonitis occurred in 1.5% of patients receiving lorlatinib at any dosage, and grade 3 or 4 ILD or pneumonitis occurred in 1.2% of patients receiving the drug. One patient (0.3%) discontinued the drug because of ILD/pneumonitis.

Patients receiving lorlatinib who present with worsening of respiratory symptoms indicative of ILD or pneumonitis (e.g., dyspnea, cough, fever) should be promptly evaluated. (See Advice to Patients.) Lorlatinib therapy should be immediately interrupted in patients with suspected ILD/pneumonitis. The drug should be permanently discontinued in patients with treatment-related ILD or pneumonitis of any severity. (See Interstitial Lung Disease/Pneumonitis under Dosage: Dosage Modification for Toxicity, in Dosage and Administration.)

Fetal/Neonatal Morbidity and Mortality Lorlatinib may cause fetal harm if administered to pregnant women based on its mechanism of action and animal findings. There are no clinical data on the use of lorlatinib in pregnant women. Malformations, increased post-implantation loss, and abortion were observed when the drug was administered to pregnant animals during the period of organogenesis at maternal exposures that were equal to or less than human exposure at the recommended dosage of 100 mg once daily based on area under the concentration-time curve (AUC).

Pregnancy should be avoided during lorlatinib therapy. The manufacturer recommends confirmation of pregnancy status prior to initiation of lorlatinib in women of childbearing potential; such women should use effective nonhormonal contraception during lorlatinib therapy and for at least 6 months after the drug is discontinued. In addition, men with female partners of childbearing potential should use effective methods of contraception while receiving lorlatinib and for at least 3 months after the drug is discontinued. Pregnant women and women of reproductive potential should be apprised of the potential fetal hazard. (See Drug Interactions: Hormonal Contraceptives and see also Advice to Patients.)

Impairment of Fertility Based on findings in male reproductive organs in animal studies, lorlatinib may transiently impair male fertility.

Specific Populations **Pregnancy.** Although there are no clinical data in pregnant women to date, animal studies and its mechanism of action suggest that lorlatinib may cause fetal harm. (See Fetal/Neonatal Morbidity and Mortality under Cautions: Warnings/Precautions.)

Lactation. It is not known whether lorlatinib or its metabolites are distributed into either human or animal milk or if the drug has any effect on milk production or the nursing infant. Because of the potential for adverse reactions to lorlatinib in nursing infants, women should be advised not to breast-feed while receiving the drug and for 7 days after the drug is discontinued.

Pediatric Use. Safety and efficacy of lorlatinib have not been established in pediatric patients.

Geriatric Use. In the principal efficacy study evaluating lorlatinib in patients with NSCLC, approximately 18% of patients receiving lorlatinib at the recommended dosage were 65 years of age or older. Although data are limited, no clinically important differences in safety or efficacy were observed between geriatric patients and younger adults in this study.

Age (19–85 years) does not appear to have clinically important effects on the pharmacokinetics of lorlatinib.

Hepatic Impairment. Mild hepatic impairment (total bilirubin concentrations not exceeding the upper limit of normal [ULN] with AST concentrations exceeding the ULN, or total bilirubin concentrations exceeding 1 but not exceeding 1.5 times the ULN with any AST concentration) did not have clinically important effects on the pharmacokinetics of lorlatinib; dosage adjustment in patients with mild hepatic impairment is therefore not necessary.

Pharmacokinetics of lorlatinib have not been studied to date in patients with moderate or severe hepatic impairment.

Renal Impairment. Mild to moderate renal impairment (creatinine clearance of 30–89 mL/minute) did not have clinically important effects on the pharmacokinetics of lorlatinib; dosage adjustment in patients with mild or moderate renal impairment is therefore not necessary.

Pharmacokinetics of lorlatinib have not been studied to date in patients with severe renal impairment.

■ **Common Adverse Effects** Adverse effects reported in 20% or more of patients receiving the recommended dosage of lorlatinib in the principal efficacy study include edema (including generalized and localized edema, swelling, and peripheral, eyelid, facial, or periorbital edema), peripheral neuropathy, cognitive effects (including memory impairment, cognitive disorder, and amnesia), dyspnea, fatigue/asthenia, weight gain, arthralgia, mood effects, and diarrhea.

Laboratory abnormalities reported in 20% or more of patients receiving the recommended dosage of lorlatinib in the principal efficacy study include hypercholesterolemia, hypertriglyceridemia, hyperglycemia, increased AST or ALT concentrations, hypoalbuminemia, anemia, thrombocytopenia, lymphopenia, increased lipase or amylase concentrations, increased alkaline phosphatase concentrations, hypophosphatemia, hyperkalemia, and hypomagnesemia.

Drug Interactions

Lorlatinib is metabolized principally by cytochrome P-450 (CYP) isoenzyme 3A4 and uridine diphosphate-glucuronosyltransferase (UGT) 1A4, with minor contributions by CYP isoenzymes 2C8, 2C19, and 3A5 and UGT1A3. In vitro studies indicate that lorlatinib inhibits P-glycoprotein (P-gp), organic cation transporter (OCT) 1, organic anion transporter (OAT) 3, multidrug and toxin extrusion (MATE) 1, and intestinal breast cancer resistance protein (BCRP).

In vitro studies indicate that lorlatinib is a time-dependent inhibitor as well as an inducer of CYP3A and that it activates the pregnane X receptor (PXR); the net effect in vivo is induction. Lorlatinib induces CYP2B6 and activates the human constitutive androstane receptor (CAR). Lorlatinib and its major metabolite M8 do not inhibit CYP isoenzymes 1A2, 2B6, 2C8, 2C9, 2C19, or 2D6 nor UGT isoenzymes 1A1, 1A4, 1A6, 1A9, 2B7, or 2B15. M8 does not inhibit CYP3A nor induce CYP isoenzymes 1A2, 2B6, and CYP3A.

Lorlatinib does not inhibit organic anion transporting polypeptide (OATP) 1B1, OATP1B3, OAT1, OCT2, MATE2K, and systemic BCRP. M8 does not inhibit P-gp, BCRP, OATP1B1, OATP1B3, OAT1, OAT3, OCT1, OCT2, MATE1, and MATE2K.

■ **Drugs Affecting Hepatic Microsomal Enzymes** ***Inducers of CYP3A*** Concomitant use of lorlatinib with *potent* CYP3A inducers may result in severe hepatotoxicity. Grade 3 or 4 elevations in serum ALT or AST concentrations occurred in 83% and grade 2 elevations occurred in 8% of healthy individuals who received the potent CYP3A inducer rifampin (600 mg daily on days 1–8) and lorlatinib (single 100-mg dose on day 8) in a drug interaction study. Elevations in hepatic enzymes occurred within 3 days of concomitant administration. In addition, peak plasma concentrations and area under the concentration-time curve (AUC) of lorlatinib were decreased by 76 and 85%, respectively. The mechanism of hepatotoxicity is thought to be through activation of the PXR by lorlatinib and rifampin, which are both PXR agonists.

Concomitant use of lorlatinib with *potent* CYP3A inducers is contraindicated. Potent CYP3A inducers must be discontinued and 3 plasma half-lives of the potent CYP3A inducer must elapse prior to initiation of lorlatinib therapy. (See Serious Hepatotoxicity with Concurrent Use of Potent CYP3A Inducers under Cautions: Warnings/Precautions.)

The effect of concomitant use of lorlatinib and *moderate* CYP3A inducers on the risk of hepatotoxicity and the pharmacokinetics of lorlatinib is not known.

Concomitant use of lorlatinib with drugs that are *moderate* CYP3A inducers should be avoided. If concomitant use cannot be avoided, ALT, AST, and bilirubin concentrations should be assessed 48 hours after initiation of lorlatinib and at least 3 times during the first week of concomitant therapy. If grade 2 or higher hepatotoxicity persists during concomitant therapy, lorlatinib or the moderate CYP3A inducer should be discontinued, taking into account the relative importance of each drug to the patient. (See Concomitant Use of Drugs Affecting Hepatic Microsomal Enzymes under Dosage and Administration: Dosage.)

Inhibitors of CYP3A Concomitant use of lorlatinib with potent inhibitors of CYP3A may increase plasma concentrations of lorlatinib, which may increase the incidence and severity of adverse effects. Concurrent administration of itraconazole (200 mg daily) and lorlatinib (single 100-mg dose) in healthy individuals increased peak plasma concentrations and AUC of lorlatinib by 24 and 42%, respectively.

Concomitant use of lorlatinib with potent CYP3A inhibitors should be avoided. If concomitant use cannot be avoided, the initial lorlatinib dosage should be reduced from 100 mg daily to 75 mg daily. In patients who have had a dosage reduction to 75 mg daily, the dosage of lorlatinib should be reduced to 50 mg daily during concomitant use with a potent CYP3A inhibitor. If concomitant use of the potent CYP3A inhibitor is discontinued, the lorlatinib dosage should be increased back to the dosage that was tolerated prior to initiation of the potent CYP3A inhibitor after 3 plasma half-lives of the potent CYP3A inhibitor have elapsed.

■ **Drugs Metabolized by Hepatic Microsomal Enzymes** Concomitant use of lorlatinib and drugs metabolized by CYP3A may result in decreased concentrations and reduced efficacy of the CYP3A substrate. When lorlatinib (150 mg daily for 15 days) was administered concurrently with midazolam (single 2-mg oral dose), peak plasma concentrations and AUC of midazolam decreased by 50 and 64%, respectively.

Concomitant use of lorlatinib and CYP3A substrates where minimal concentration changes may result in serious therapeutic failure should be avoided. If concomitant use cannot be avoided, dosage adjustment of the CYP3A substrate may be required; specific product labeling for the CYP3A substrate should be consulted.

■ **Drugs Affecting Gastric pH** Concomitant administration of lorlatinib and the proton-pump inhibitor rabeprazole did not have a clinically important effect on the pharmacokinetics of lorlatinib.

■ **Hormonal Contraceptives** Concomitant use of lorlatinib and hormonal contraceptives may result in reduced efficacy of the hormonal contraceptive. Women of childbearing potential should therefore use effective nonhormonal contraception during lorlatinib therapy and for at least 6 months after the drug is discontinued. (See Fetal/Neonatal Morbidity and Mortality under Cautions: Warnings/Precautions.)

Description

Lorlatinib, an inhibitor of multiple tyrosine kinases, including anaplastic lymphoma kinase (ALK) and c-ros oncogene-1 (ROS1) as well as TYK1, FER, FPS, TRKA, TRKB, TRKC, FAK, FAK2, and ACK, is an antineoplastic agent. The drug inhibits phosphorylation of ALK and ALK-mediated signal transduction, specifically STAT3, AKT, ERK, and S6.

Activating mutations or translocations of the ALK gene have been identified in several malignancies and can result in the expression of oncogenic fusion proteins (e.g., echinoderm microtubule-associated protein-like 4 [EML4]-ALK). Such ALK gene rearrangements have been identified in approximately 3–7% of patients with non-small cell lung cancer (NSCLC). Formation of ALK fusion proteins such as EML4-ALK results in activation and dysregulation of the gene's expression and signaling, which can contribute to increased cell proliferation and survival in tumors expressing these proteins.

Although the ALK inhibitor crizotinib has demonstrated improved outcomes in patients with NSCLC harboring ALK mutations, secondary resistance to crizotinib eventually develops, generally within the first 1–2 years of treatment. Clinical resistance to crizotinib has been attributed to several possible mechanisms, including acquired resistance mutations of ALK, amplification of gene expression, and activation of alternate signaling pathways. More potent ALK inhibitors (e.g., alectinib, ceritinib) were developed to overcome resistance to crizotinib; however, resistance to these drugs also develops over time. Secondary mutations of ALK are responsible for about 30% of cases of acquired crizotinib resistance while about 50% of cases of acquired resistance to other ALK inhibitors are attributed to ALK mutations, with G1202R predominating. The CNS is a common site of disease progression in crizotinib-treated patients because of poor distribution of the drug into CSF; development and/or progression of brain metastases occurs in approximately one-third to one-half of patients during crizotinib treatment.

In vitro, lorlatinib demonstrates greater potency than alectinib, ceritinib, and crizotinib in its activity against wild-type ALK and is active against cell lines expressing ALK mutations that confer resistance to crizotinib, including G1202R (which also confers resistance to alectinib and ceritinib), G1269A, and L1196M. Lorlatinib also demonstrated dose-dependent antitumor activity in mice bearing NSCLC tumor xenografts that expressed EML4-ALK fusions with either ALK variant 1 or ALK mutations, including G1202R and I1171T mutations that were detected in tumors of patients at the time of disease progression in patients receiving therapy with other ALK inhibitors. Lorlatinib also demonstrated antitumor activity and prolonged survival in mice bearing intracranial EML4-ALK-positive tumor xenografts and antitumor activity in patients with CNS metastases who had received prior treatment with other ALK inhibitors (e.g., alectinib, ceritinib, crizotinib).

Peak plasma concentration of lorlatinib is dose proportional and systemic exposure to lorlatinib is slightly less than dose proportional at steady state over the oral dosage range of 10–200 mg once daily. Following oral administration, peak plasma concentrations of lorlatinib are achieved at a median of 1.2 hours. The mean absolute bioavailability of lorlatinib is 81%. Administration of lorlatinib with a high-fat, high-calorie meal has no clinically important effect on the pharmacokinetics of lorlatinib. Lorlatinib is 66% bound to plasma proteins in vitro and is distributed into CSF at a CSF-to-plasma ratio of 0.75. Lorlatinib is metabolized principally by cytochrome P-450 (CYP) isoenzyme 3A4 and uridine diphosphate-glucuronosyltransferase (UGT) 1A4, with minor contributions by CYP isoenzymes 2C8, 2C19, and 3A5, and UGT1A3. The major metabolite, M8, is pharmacologically inactive. Following oral administration of a single dose of radiolabeled lorlatinib, 48% of the dose is eliminated in urine (less than 1% as unchanged drug) and 41% of the dose is eliminated in feces (about 9% as unchanged drug). Oral clearance of lorlatinib is higher at steady state than following a single dose, suggesting that autoinduction occurs. The mean plasma half-life of lorlatinib is 24 hours. Age (19–85 years), sex, race/ethnicity, body weight, and CYP3A5 or CYP2C19 metabolizer phenotypes do not have clinically important effects on the pharmacokinetics of lorlatinib.

Advice to Patients

Importance of instructing patients to read the manufacturer's patient information.

Importance of advising patients to take lorlatinib exactly as prescribed and of not altering the dosage or discontinuing therapy unless advised to do so by their clinician. Importance of advising patients to swallow lorlatinib tablets whole without regard to food and not to crush, chew, or split the tablets. If a dose of lorlatinib is missed, the missed dose should be taken as soon as possible unless it is within 4 hours of the next dose, in which case the missed dose should not be taken. Patients should be informed to not take 2 doses at the same time to make up for a missed dose. If vomiting occurs after taking a dose, the next dose should be taken at the regularly scheduled time; an additional dose should not be taken.

Risk of severe hepatotoxicity when used concomitantly with potent cytochrome P-450 (CYP) isoenzyme 3A inducers.

Importance of informing clinicians of existing or contemplated concomitant therapy, including prescription and OTC drugs (e.g., antilipemic agents, rifampin, oral contraceptives) and dietary or herbal supplements (e.g., St. John's wort), as well as any concomitant illnesses (e.g., history of depression or other mood disorders, hyperlipidemia, cardiac arrhythmias, pulmonary disease).

Risk of adverse CNS effects. Importance of advising patients to notify their clinician if they experience new or worsening CNS symptoms such as changes in cognitive function or mood, suicidal ideation, hallucinations, or seizures.

Risk of hyperlipidemia. Importance of informing patients about the need for monitoring serum cholesterol and triglyceride concentrations during lorlatinib therapy. Patients should be advised that initiation of antilipemic therapy or an increase in the dosage of existing antilipemic agents may be required.

Risk of atrioventricular (AV) block. Importance of patients immediately contacting their clinician if they experience new or worsening cardiac symptoms such as dizziness, faintness, or arrhythmia during therapy.

Risk of severe or life-threatening interstitial lung disease/pneumonitis. Importance of advising patients that symptoms may be similar to those of lung cancer and to contact their clinician immediately if they experience any new or worsening respiratory symptoms (e.g., dyspnea or shortness of breath, cough, fever).

Risk of fetal harm. Necessity of advising women of childbearing potential that they should use effective, nonhormonal methods of contraception while receiving lorlatinib and for at least 6 months after discontinuance of therapy and of also advising such women that oral contraceptives and other hormonal forms of contraception may not be effective during lorlatinib therapy. Importance of advising men with female partners of childbearing potential to use effective methods of contraception while receiving the drug and for at least 3 months after the drug is discontinued. Importance of also advising men of reproductive potential that lorlatinib may transiently impair fertility and to discuss any concerns about fertility with their clinician.

Importance of women informing their clinicians if they are or plan to become pregnant. If pregnancy occurs, the patient should be advised of the potential risk to the fetus.

Importance of advising women to avoid breast-feeding while receiving lorlatinib and for 7 days after discontinuance of therapy.

Importance of informing patients of other important precautionary information. (See Cautions.)

Overview® (see Users Guide). For additional information on this drug until a more detailed monograph is developed and published, the manufacturer's labeling should be consulted. It is *essential* that the manufacturer's labeling be consulted for more detailed information on usual cautions, precautions, contraindications, potential drug interactions, laboratory test interferences, and acute toxicity. For further information on the handling of antineoplastic agents, see the ASHP Guidelines on Handling Hazardous Drugs at http://www.ahfsdruginformation.com.

Preparations

Distribution of lorlatinib is restricted. (See Restricted Distribution under Dosage and Administration: General.)

Excipients in commercially available drug preparations may have clinically important effects in some individuals; consult specific product labeling for details.

Lorlatinib

Oral		
Tablets, film-coated	25 mg	**Lorbrena®**, Pfizer
	100 mg	**Lorbrena®**, Pfizer

†Use is not currently included in the labeling approved by the US Food and Drug Administration

Lutetium Lu 177 Dotatate

Lutetium 177Lu Oxodotreotide, 177Lu-DOTA-Tyr3-octreotate, 177Lu-DOTA-octreotate, 177Lu-dotatate

■ Lutetium Lu 177 dotatate, a lutetium 177 radiolabeled tetraazacyclododecane-tetra-acetic acid (DOTA)-somatostatin analog conjugate consisting of the somatostatin analog octreotide linked to a chelator (DOTA), is a peptide receptor radionuclide agent.

Uses

■ Neuroendocrine Tumors of Gastroenteropancreatic Origin

Lutetium Lu 177 dotatate is used for the treatment of somatostatin receptor-positive neuroendocrine tumors of gastroenteropancreatic origin (GEP-NET), including foregut, midgut, and hindgut neuroendocrine tumors. Lutetium Lu 177 dotatate has been designated an orphan drug by FDA for use in this condition.

The current indication for lutetium Lu 177 dotatate is based principally on the results of a randomized, multicenter, open-label phase 3 study (Neuroendocrine Tumors Therapy [NETTER-1]) in patients with progressive, well-differentiated, somatostatin receptor-positive, unresectable, locally advanced or metastatic midgut neuroendocrine tumors, with supporting data from an open-label, noncomparative, retrospective phase ½ study (ERASMUS) in a cohort of patients with GEP-NETs of the foregut, midgut, and hindgut.

In the NETTER-1 study, 229 patients were randomized (stratified by somatostatin receptor expression and duration of octreotide) in a 1:1 ratio to receive either lutetium Lu 177 dotatate (7.4 GBq administered as an IV infusion every 8 weeks for up to 4 doses [maximum cumulative dose of 29.6 GBq] or until disease progression or unacceptable toxicity occurred or the patient withdrew from the study) plus best supportive care (long-acting [extended-release] octreotide 30 mg administered as an IM injection 4–24 hours following each dose of lutetium Lu 177 dotatate and then every 4 weeks until disease progression or week 76 of study enrollment) or high-dose long-acting octreotide (60 mg administered as an IM injection every 4 weeks) alone. All patients were permitted to receive rescue therapy with short-acting octreotide; however, administration of short-acting octreotide was not permitted within 24 hours prior to administration of lutetium Lu 177 dotatate. The primary measure of efficacy was progression-free survival (as evaluated by a blinded independent review committee according to Response Evaluation Criteria in Solid Tumors [RECIST]); additional outcome measures were objective response rate, duration of response, and overall survival.

The median age of patients enrolled in the NETTER-1 study was 64 years; 90% were Caucasian, 51% were male, 96% had liver metastases, 77% had serum chromogranin A (CgA) concentrations exceeding 2 times the upper limit of normal (ULN), 74% had received a stable dosage of octreotide for more than 6 months, 69% had low-grade primary tumors (defined as Ki67 expression in 2% or less of tumor cells as detected by immunohistochemistry assay), 65% had serum 5-hydroxyindoleacetic acid (5-HIAA) concentrations exceeding 2 times the ULN, 65% had alkaline phosphatase concentrations not more than the ULN, and 12% had received prior therapy with everolimus. The most common primary tumor site was the ileum (74%), and the median Karnofsky performance score of patients enrolled in the study was 90. Eligible patients also were required to have well-differentiated primary tumors (defined as Ki67 expression in 20% or less of tumor cells), Karnofsky performance status of at least 60, confirmed presence of somatostatin receptors on all lesions, and creatinine clearance of at least 50 mL/minute. This study excluded patients who received prior peptide receptor radionuclide therapy (PRRT) or external beam radiation therapy to more than 25% of the bone marrow.

At a median follow-up of 10.5 months in the NETTER-1 study, median progression-free survival had not been reached in patients receiving lutetium Lu 177 dotatate in combination with long-acting octreotide; however, the risk of disease progression or death in patients receiving lutetium Lu 177 dotatate in combination with long-acting octreotide was reduced by 79% compared with those receiving high-dose long-acting octreotide. At the time of the primary analysis, lutetium Lu 177 dotatate in combination with long-acting octreotide reduced the risk of death by 48% compared with high-dose long-acting octreotide; however, the prespecified level of statistical significance was not achieved. In addition, patients receiving lutetium Lu 177 dotatate in combination with long-acting octreotide had higher objective response rates compared with those receiving high-dose long-acting octreotide (13 versus 4%); complete responses were achieved in 1% of patients receiving lutetium Lu 177 dotatate in combination with long-acting octreotide and none of those receiving high-dose long-acting octreotide. At the time of the analysis, the median duration of response had not been reached in patients receiving lutetium Lu 177 dotatate in combination with long-acting octreotide and was 1.9 months in those receiving high-dose long-acting octreotide. Results of a subgroup analysis (based on age, gender, tumor grade, baseline CgA concentrations, baseline 5-HIAA concentrations, grade of somatostatin receptor expression, baseline alkaline phosphatase concentration, and presence of extrahepatic metastases) suggested that the effect of lutetium Lu 177 dotatate on progression-free survival was consistent across all subgroups.

In the ERASMUS study, lutetium Lu 177 dotatate was initially provided under a PRRT expanded access program without a formal clinical protocol or prespecified statistical analysis plan; however, a protocol specific for lutetium Lu 177 dotatate was generated several years following initiation of the program and allowed for retrospective analysis. In this study, 360 patients with GEP-NETs of the foregut, midgut, or hindgut received lutetium Lu 177 dotatate (7.4 GBq) administered as an IV infusion every 6–13 weeks for up to 4 doses; patients enrolled in the study received a median dose of 29.6 GBq and approximately one-half of patients (55%) received concomitant therapy with a somatostatin analog. Patients also received an amino acid solution containing *l*-lysine and *l*-arginine administered as an IV infusion over 4 hours beginning 30 minutes prior to administration of lutetium Lu 177 dotatate. The primary measure of efficacy was objective response rate as assessed by the investigator according to RECIST. The median age of patients enrolled in the cohort of patients with GEP-NETs of the foregut, midgut, or hindgut was 61 years; 61% had a baseline Karnofsky performance status of at least 90, 60% had disease progression within 12 months of study enrollment, 52% were male, and 15% had received prior chemotherapy. Baseline tumor assessments were obtained in 39% of patients. In the cohort of patients with GEP-NET of the foregut, midgut, or hindgut, the objective response rate was 16% with a median duration of response of 35 months; complete response was achieved in less than 1% of patients.

Dosage and Administration

■ **General** Lutetium Lu 177 dotatate is a radiopharmaceutical and should be prepared and used only by a qualified clinician (i.e., authorized by an appropriate regulatory agency) experienced in the safe use and handling of radionuclides. Procedures for proper handling (e.g., use of waterproof gloves, shields, tongs) and disposal of radionuclides should be followed when preparing and administering lutetium Lu 177 dotatate.

To minimize the risk of nephrotoxicity associated with lutetium Lu 177 dotatate, an amino acid solution containing *l*-lysine and *l*-arginine should be administered by IV infusion 30 minutes prior to each lutetium Lu 177 dotatate infusion and continued during and for at least 3 hours after the lutetium Lu 177 dotatate infusion. The amino acid solution may be administered through the same IV line (equipped with a 3-way valve) with lutetium Lu 177 dotatate or through a separate IV line in the opposite arm. The amino acid solution should be administered as a 1.5–2.2 L solution containing 18–24 g of *l*-lysine and 18–24 g of *l*-arginine with an osmolarity of less than 1050 mOsm/L. (See Renal Effects under Cautions: Warnings/Precautions.) To minimize the risk of nausea associated with the amino acid infusion, the manufacturer recommends premedication with an antiemetic (e.g., granisetron, ondansetron) 30 minutes prior to each amino acid infusion. The manufacturer states that no dosage adjustment of the amino acid solution is necessary when the dosage of lutetium Lu 177 dotatate is reduced.

Patients should be adequately hydrated (e.g., one glass of water every hour) during and after administration of lutetium Lu 177 dotatate to ensure good urinary output. (See Renal Effects under Cautions: Warnings/Precautions.)

■ **Administration** Lutetium Lu 177 dotatate is administered by IV infusion. *The radiopharmaceutical should not be administered by rapid IV injection, such as IV push or bolus.* The IV line should be flushed with 25 mL of 0.9% sodium chloride injection after IV administration of lutetium Lu 177 dotatate.

Lutetium Lu 177 dotatate should *not* be injected directly into any IV solution. Precautions for reducing the risk of radiation exposure (i.e., use of waterproof gloves, shielding, tongs) should be followed.

Lutetium Lu 177 dotatate vials must be stored below 25°C in the lead shielded container provided by the manufacturer; the shelf-life of lutetium Lu 177 dotatate is 72 hours.

Prior to administration, lutetium Lu 177 dotatate injection should be inspected visually for particulate matter and discoloration. The solution should be clear and colorless to slightly yellow; the solution should not be used if it is discolored or if particulate matter is present. The level of radioactivity of lutetium Lu 177 dotatate in the vial should be confirmed with a calibrated radioactivity measurement system (e.g., Geiger counter).

For IV infusion, a short (2.5 cm in length) 20-gauge needle should be inserted into a vial containing 370 MBq/mL (equivalent to 10 mCi/mL) of lutetium Lu 177 dotatate and then connected to a primed administration set and infusion bag containing 500 mL of 0.9% sodium chloride injection; the short 20-gauge needle must remain *above* the lutetium Lu 177 dotatate solution. Lutetium Lu 177 dotatate should *not* be injected directly into the 0.9% sodium chloride solution. The administration set connected to the short needle should be clamped to prevent flow of 0.9% sodium chloride solution into the lutetium Lu 177 dotatate vial during preparation of the infusion. A longer (9 cm in length) 18-gauge needle should be inserted into the same vial containing 370 MBq/mL (equivalent to 10 mCi/mL) of lutetium Lu 177 dotatate. The tip of the long needle should be securely positioned at the bottom of the lutetium Lu 177 dotatate vial for the duration of the infusion. The long needle should be connected to a dedicated IV line, primed with 0.9% sodium chloride solution, for infusion of lutetium Lu 177 dotatate to the patient.

During the infusion, the flow of 0.9% sodium chloride injection into the vial increases pressure in the vial, which facilitates flow of lutetium Lu 177 dotatate from the vial to the patient. The 0.9% sodium chloride solution should flow (regulated by clamp) into the lutetium Lu 177 dotatate vial via the short needle. Alternatively, an infusion pump may be used to control the flow rate of 0.9% sodium chloride solution. If an infusion pump is used, the 0.9% sodium chloride solution should be set at an initial rate of 50–100 mL/hour for 5–10 minutes followed by an increase to 200–300 mL/hour for 25–30 minutes for a total infusion time of 30–40 minutes.

To ensure complete administration of the radiopharmaceutical, the level of solution in the vial containing lutetium Lu 177 dotatate should remain constant during the entire infusion. Once the radioactivity emission in the vial stabilizes for at least 5 minutes, the lutetium Lu 177 dotatate infusion may be completed by removing the long needle from the vial and clamping the administration set connected to the 0.9% sodium chloride solution.

Any unused portion in the vial or administration set should be discarded according to local and federal regulations.

■ **Dosage** ***Neuroendocrine Tumors of Gastroenteropancreatic Origin*** For the treatment of somatostatin receptor-positive neuroendocrine tumors of gastroenteropancreatic origin (GEP-NET), including foregut, midgut, and hindgut neuroendocrine tumors, the recommended adult dosage of lutetium Lu 177 dotatate is 7.4 GBq (equivalent to 200 mCi) administered by IV infusion over 30–40 minutes every 8 weeks for a total of 4 doses.

In the NETTER-1 study, lutetium Lu 177 dotatate was used in combination with long-acting (extended-release) octreotide; rescue therapy with short-acting (immediate-release) octreotide also was permitted. When lutetium Lu 177 dotatate is used in combination with short- or long-acting octreotide, the manufacturer states that short- or long-acting octreotide should *not* be administered within 24 hours or 4 weeks, respectively, prior to each dose of lutetium Lu 177 dotatate. (See Drug Interactions: Octreotide.)

When lutetium Lu 177 dotatate is used in combination with long-acting octreotide, the manufacturer states that a single 30-mg dose of long-acting octreotide acetate may be administered by IM injection between 4–24 hours following each dose of lutetium Lu 177 dotatate and should *not* be administered within 4 weeks prior to administration of lutetium Lu 177 dotatate. Following discontinuance of lutetium Lu 177 dotatate therapy, long-acting octreotide acetate (30 mg administered by IM injection every 4 weeks) may be continued until disease progression or for a treatment duration of up to 18 months.

Dosage Modification for Toxicity If adverse reactions occur, interruption of therapy, dosage reduction, and/or permanent discontinuance of lutetium Lu 177 dotatate may be necessary based on severity of the adverse effect.

Dosage adjustment of amino acids is not necessary when the dosage of lutetium Lu 177 dotatate is reduced.

Hematologic Toxicity. If grade 2–4 thrombocytopenia occurs, lutetium Lu 177 dotatate therapy should be withheld until thrombocytopenia improves to grade 1 or less. Lutetium Lu 177 dotatate may then be resumed at a reduced dosage of 3.7 GBq (equivalent to 100 mCi); if grade 2–4 thrombocytopenia does not recur, the dosage of lutetium Lu 177 dotatate may be re-escalated to 7.4 GBq (equivalent to 200 mCi). If grade 2–4 thrombocytopenia recurs or does not improve within 16 weeks of withholding therapy, lutetium Lu 177 dotatate should be permanently discontinued. (See Hematologic Effects under Cautions: Warnings/Precautions.)

If grade 3 or 4 neutropenia or anemia occurs, lutetium Lu 177 dotatate therapy should be withheld until the toxicity improves to grade 2 or less. Lutetium Lu 177 dotatate may then be resumed at a reduced dosage of 3.7 GBq (equivalent to 100 mCi); if grade 3 or 4 neutropenia or anemia does not recur, the dosage of lutetium Lu 177 dotatate may be re-escalated to 7.4 GBq (equivalent to 200 mCi). If grade 3 or 4 neutropenia or anemia recurs or does not improve within 16 weeks of withholding therapy, lutetium Lu 177 dotatate should be permanently discontinued.

Renal Toxicity. If nephrotoxicity (i.e., increase in serum creatinine concentration from baseline of 40% or more; creatinine clearance less than 40 mL/minute; decrease in creatinine clearance from baseline of 40% or more) occurs, lutetium Lu 177 dotatate therapy should be withheld until the toxicity completely resolves. Lutetium Lu 177 dotatate may then be resumed at a reduced dosage of 3.7 GBq (equivalent to 100 mCi); if the toxicity does not recur, the dosage of lutetium Lu 177 dotatate may be re-escalated to 7.4 GBq (equivalent to 200 mCi). If nephrotoxicity recurs or does not improve within 16 weeks of withholding therapy, the drug should be permanently discontinued. (See Renal Effects under Cautions: Warnings/Precautions.)

Hepatotoxicity. If hepatotoxicity (i.e., elevations in bilirubin concentration exceeding 3 times the upper limit of normal [ULN]; serum albumin less than 3 g/dL with prothrombin ratio less than 70%) occurs, lutetium Lu 177 dotatate therapy should be withheld until the toxicity completely resolves. Lutetium Lu 177 dotatate may then be resumed at a reduced dosage of 3.7 GBq (equivalent to 100 mCi); if the toxicity does not recur, the dosage of lutetium Lu 177 dotatate may be re-escalated to 7.4 GBq (equivalent to 200 mCi). If hepatotoxicity recurs or does not improve within 16 weeks of withholding therapy, lutetium Lu 177 dotatate should be permanently discontinued. (See Hepatic Toxicity under Cautions: Warnings/Precautions.)

Other Toxicity. If grade 3 or 4 nonhematologic toxicity occurs, lutetium Lu 177 dotatate therapy should be withheld until the toxicity improves to grade 2 or less. Lutetium Lu 177 dotatate may then be resumed at a reduced dosage of 3.7 GBq (equivalent to 100 mCi); if the toxicity does not recur, the dosage of lutetium Lu 177 dotatate may be re-escalated to 7.4 GBq (equivalent to 200 mCi). If grade 3 or 4 nonhematologic toxicity recurs or does not improve within 16 weeks of withholding therapy, lutetium Lu 177 dotatate should be permanently discontinued.

■ **Special Populations** The manufacturer states that no adjustment to the initial dosage of lutetium Lu 177 dotatate is necessary in patients with mild or moderate hepatic impairment. Lutetium Lu 177 dotatate has not been studied in patients with severe hepatic impairment (total bilirubin concentration exceeding 3 times the upper limit of normal [ULN] with any AST concentration), and the manufacturer provides no specific dosage recommendations for such patients. (See Hepatic Impairment under Warnings/Precautions: Specific Populations, in Cautions.)

The manufacturer states that no adjustment to the initial dosage of lutetium Lu 177 dotatate is necessary in patients with mild to moderate renal impairment (creatinine clearance of 30 mL/minute or greater). Lutetium Lu 177 dotatate has not been studied in patients with severe renal impairment (creatinine clearance of less than 30 mL/minute) or end-stage renal disease, and the manufacturer provides no specific dosage recommendations for such patients. (See Renal Impairment under Warnings/Precautions: Specific Populations, in Cautions.)

The manufacturer makes no specific dosage recommendations for geriatric patients. (See Geriatric Use under Warnings/Precautions: Specific Populations, in Cautions.)

Cautions

■ **Contraindications** The manufacturer states that there are no known contraindications to the use of lutetium Lu 177 dotatate.

■ **Warnings/Precautions** ***Radiation Exposure*** The radioactive component of lutetium Lu 177 dotatate (lutetium 177) contributes to a patient's lifetime cumulative radiation exposure, and development of new malignancies is a known risk of long-term radiation exposure. (See Myelodysplastic Syndrome and Acute Leukemia under Cautions: Warnings/Precautions.)

Because radioactivity can be detected in urine for up to 30 days following administration of lutetium Lu 177 dotatate, institutional good radiation safety practices and patient management procedures should be employed during and after administration of lutetium Lu 177 dotatate to minimize exposure of patients, medical personnel, and household contacts to radiation.

Hematologic Effects Adverse hematologic effects (e.g., anemia, neutropenia, thrombocytopenia) occur frequently in patients receiving lutetium Lu 177 dotatate in combination with long-acting (extended-release) octreotide. In the Neuroendocrine Tumors Therapy (NETTER-1) study, anemia, thrombocytopenia, and neutropenia occurred in 81, 53, and 26%, respectively, of patients receiving lutetium Lu 177 dotatate in combination with long-acting octreotide, compared with 54, 17, and 11%, respectively, of patients receiving high-dose long-acting octreotide. Following the initial dose of lutetium Lu 177 dotatate, nadir platelet counts occurred in a median of 5.1 weeks. Thrombocytopenia resolved in 68% of patients in a median of 2 months and improved to grade 3 or less in an additional 25% of patients.

Some data suggest that preexisting renal impairment, leukocyte count below 4000/mm^3, advanced age (i.e., older than 70 years of age), extensive tumor mass, and high tumor uptake on octreotide scintigraphy (i.e., OctreoScan®) may result in increased potential for developing grade 3 or 4 hematologic toxicity.

Complete blood cell (CBC) counts should be monitored prior to and periodically during lutetium Lu 177 dotatate therapy. Temporary interruption followed by dosage reduction or discontinuance of lutetium Lu 177 dotatate may be necessary if hematologic toxicity occurs during therapy with lutetium Lu 177 dotatate. (See Hematologic Toxicity under Dosage: Dosage Modification for Toxicity, in Dosage and Administration.)

Myelodysplastic Syndrome and Acute Leukemia In the NETTER-1 study, myelodysplastic syndrome (MDS) was reported in 2.7% of patients receiving lutetium Lu 177 dotatate in combination with long-acting octreotide compared with none of those receiving high-dose long-acting octreotide. In the ERASMUS study, MDS or acute leukemia was reported in 1.8 or 0.5%, respectively, of patients receiving lutetium Lu 177 dotatate; the median time to occurrence was 28 months (range: 9–41 months) or 55 months (range: 32–155 months), respectively, following initiation of therapy.

Renal Effects Because peptide analogs such as octreotide are extensively reabsorbed in the renal proximal tubules, accumulation of the radioactive component of lutetium Lu 177 dotatate (lutetium 177) in renal interstitium results in inflammation and fibrosis and subsequent acute or chronic renal damage. In the ERASMUS study, renal failure was reported in 8 patients (less than 1%) receiving lutetium Lu 177 dotatate at 3–36 months following initiation of therapy; 2 of these patients had preexisting renal impairment or risk factors for renal failure (e.g., diabetes mellitus, hypertension) and required dialysis. Available data have suggested that advanced age (i.e., older than 60 years of age), poorly controlled diabetes mellitus, hypertension, prior platinum-containing therapy, and preexisting renal impairment may be risk factors for developing nephrotoxicity associated with peptide receptor radionuclide therapy (PRRT).

Coadministration of positively charged amino acids (e.g., *l*-lysine, *l*-arginine) with PRRT has been shown to minimize the risk of nephrotoxicity by reducing reabsorption of peptide receptor radionuclides, such as lutetium Lu 177 dotatate, in the proximal tubules which subsequently reduces the dose of radiation to the kidneys. In the ERASMUS study, coadministration of the amino acids *l*-lysine and *l*-arginine reduced the median radiation dose to the kidneys by 47% and increased the mean beta-phase plasma clearance of lutetium Lu 177 dotatate by 36%. The manufacturer states that an amino acid solution containing *l*-lysine and *l*-arginine should be administered 30 minutes prior to each lutetium Lu 177 dotatate infusion and continued during and for at least 3 hours after the lutetium Lu 177 dotatate infusion. (See Dosage and Administration: General.) Patients also should be adequately hydrated (e.g., one glass of water every hour) during and after administration of lutetium Lu 177 dotatate to ensure good urinary output.

Renal function (i.e., serum creatinine) should be monitored prior to and periodically during lutetium Lu 177 dotatate therapy; monitoring should be more frequent in those with mild or moderate renal impairment. If nephrotoxicity occurs, temporary interruption of therapy followed by dosage reduction or discontinuance of lutetium Lu 177 dotatate may be necessary. (See Renal Toxicity under Dosage: Dosage Modification for Toxicity, in Dosage and Administration.)

Hepatic Toxicity In the ERASMUS study, hepatic tumor hemorrhage, edema, or necrosis was reported in 2 patients receiving lutetium Lu 177 dotatate, with one patient also experiencing intrahepatic congestion and cholestasis. The risk of developing hepatic toxicity is increased in patients with hepatic metastasis.

Liver function tests (i.e., serum aminotransferase, bilirubin, serum albumin) should be monitored prior to and periodically during lutetium Lu 177 dotatate therapy. If hepatotoxicity occurs, temporary interruption of therapy followed by dosage reduction or discontinuance of lutetium Lu 177 dotatate may be necessary. (See Hepatotoxicity under Dosage: Dosage Modification for Toxicity, in Dosage and Administration.)

Carcinoid Hormonal Crisis In the ERASMUS study, carcinoid hormonal crisis (also known as neuroendocrine hormonal crisis), which may manifest as flushing, diarrhea, bronchospasm, or hypotension, was reported in 1% of patients, generally during or within 24 hours of the initial dose of lutetium Lu 177 dotatate. Hypercalcemia also was reported in 2 patients.

Patients receiving lutetium Lu 177 dotatate should be monitored for manifestations of carcinoid hormonal crisis and should be managed (e.g., IV somatostatin analog, hydration, corticosteroids, electrolytes) as clinically indicated if such crises occur.

Fetal/Neonatal Morbidity and Mortality Based on its mechanism of action, lutetium Lu 177 dotatate may cause fetal harm. There are no available data regarding the risk of lutetium Lu 177 dotatate use in pregnant women or animals to date.

Pregnancy should be avoided during lutetium Lu 177 dotatate therapy. Pregnancy status should be verified prior to initiation of lutetium Lu 177 dotatate, and women of reproductive potential should be advised to use effective contraceptive methods while receiving the radiopharmaceutical and for 7 months after the final dose. In addition, men with female partners of reproductive potential should use effective methods of contraception while receiving the radiopharmaceutical and for 4 months after the final dose. If lutetium Lu 177 dotatate is used during pregnancy or if the patient becomes pregnant while receiving the radiopharmaceutical, the patient should be apprised of the potential fetal hazard. (See Advice to Patients.)

Impairment of Fertility Lutetium Lu 177 dotatate may impair male and female fertility. The cumulative radiation exposure following the recommended course of lutetium Lu 177 dotatate (29.6 GBq) results in an absorbed radiation dose in the testis and ovaries that is comparable to the dose at which external beam radiotherapy causes reversible or permanent infertility.

Specific Populations **Pregnancy.** Lutetium Lu 177 dotatate may cause fetal harm if administered to pregnant women based on its mechanism of action. (See Fetal/Neonatal Morbidity and Mortality under Cautions: Warnings/Precautions.)

Lactation. It is not known whether lutetium Lu 177 dotatate distributes into milk in human or animals or whether the radiopharmaceutical has any effects on nursing infants and on milk production. Because of the potential for serious adverse reactions to lutetium Lu 177 dotatate in nursing infants, women should be advised to discontinue nursing during lutetium Lu 177 dotatate therapy and for 2.5 months after the last dose.

Pediatric Use. Safety and efficacy of lutetium Lu 177 dotatate have not been established in pediatric patients.

Geriatric Use. In clinical trials, 33% of patients receiving lutetium Lu 77 dotatate were 65 years of age or older. No differences in serious adverse effects or response rate were observed between geriatric patients and younger adults; however, some data suggest that advanced age may increase the risk for developing nephrotoxicity or grade 3 or 4 hematologic toxicity. (See Hematologic Effects and also see Renal Effects under Cautions: Warnings/Precautions.)

Hepatic Impairment. A dedicated hepatic impairment trial for lutetium Lu 177 dotatate has not been conducted to date; however, lutetium Lu 177 dotatate does not undergo hepatic elimination. (See Dosage and Administration: Special Populations.)

Safety of lutetium Lu 177 dotatate has not been established in patients with severe hepatic impairment (total bilirubin concentration exceeding 3 times the upper limit of normal [ULN] with any AST concentration).

Renal Impairment. In the NETTER-1 study, an association between creatinine clearance and adverse hematologic effects was not observed in patients receiving lutetium Lu 177 dotatate. However, since lutetium Lu 177 dotatate is eliminated mainly by the kidneys, mild to moderate renal impairment may result in an increased potential for adverse reactions. (See Hematologic Effects and also see Renal Effects under Cautions: Warnings/Precautions.) Renal function should be monitored more frequently in patients with mild to moderate renal impairment. Safety of lutetium Lu 177 dotatate has not been established in patients with severe renal impairment (creatinine clearance of less than 30 mL/minute) or end-stage renal disease. (See Dosage and Administration: Special Populations.)

■ **Common Adverse Effects** Adverse effects reported in at least 10% of patients receiving lutetium Lu 177 dotatate in combination with long-acting octreotide in the NETTER-1 study include nausea, vomiting, fatigue, musculoskeletal pain, abdominal pain, diarrhea, decreased appetite, dizziness, headache, peripheral edema, flushing, alopecia, distension, anxiety, hypertension, renal failure, cough, and constipation. Laboratory abnormalities reported in at least 10% of patients receiving lutetium Lu 177 dotatate in combination with long-acting octreotide include lymphopenia, elevated concentrations of serum creatinine, hyperglycemia, anemia, elevated concentrations of γ-glutamyltransferase (γ-glutamyltranspeptidase, GGT, GGTP), elevated concentrations of alkaline phosphatase, leukopenia, thrombocytopenia, elevated concentrations of aminotransferases (i.e., AST, ALT), hyperuricemia, hypocalcemia, elevated concentrations of bilirubin, hypokalemia, neutropenia, hyperkalemia, hypernatremia, and hypoglycemia.

In a retrospective analysis of data from the ERASMUS study for a subset of 811 patients with somatostatin receptor-positive tumors (neuroendocrine or other primary tumor sites), serious adverse reactions following a median follow-up exceeding 4 years included MDS, acute leukemia, renal failure, hypotension, cardiac failure, myocardial infarction, and carcinoid crisis. Most (81%) of these patients received a cumulative lutetium Lu 177 dotatate dose of 22.2 GBq or more.

Drug Interactions

In vitro studies indicate that nonradioactive lutetium dotatate (lutetium Lu 175 dotatate) is not an inhibitor or inducer of cytochrome P-450 (CYP) isoenzyme 1A2, 2B6, 2C9, 2C19, or 2D6.

In vitro, nonradioactive lutetium dotatate is not an inhibitor of P-glycoprotein (P-gp), breast cancer resistance protein (BCRP), organic anion transporter (OAT) 1, OAT3, organic anion transport protein (OATP) 1B1, OATP1B3, organic cation transporter (OCT) 1, or OCT2.

■ **Corticosteroids** The prescribing information for lutetium Lu 177 dotatate in the US does not provide information concerning the concurrent use of corticosteroids during therapy. However, the manufacturer in the European Union recommends avoiding concomitant use of lutetium Lu 177 dotatate and long-term use of high-dose corticosteroids because some evidence suggests that corticosteroids may induce down-regulation of somatostatin receptor type 2 (SSRT2). Patients receiving corticosteroid therapy for chronic conditions should be carefully evaluated for sufficient somatostatin receptor expression. The manufacturer in the European Union also states that intermittent use of corticosteroids should be avoided because of insufficient data; however, if concomitant use cannot be avoided, a single dose of a corticosteroid may be administered at least 1 hour following completion of the lutetium Lu 177 dotatate infusion.

■ **Octreotide** Because somatostatin analogs such as octreotide are competitive inhibitors with lutetium Lu 177 dotatate in binding to somatostatin receptors, concomitant use of lutetium Lu 177 dotatate with somatostatin analogs (e.g., octreotide) may reduce lutetium Lu 177 dotatate efficacy.

When lutetium Lu 177 dotatate is used in combination with short-acting (immediate-release) or long-acting (extended-release) octreotide, the manufacturer states that short- or long-acting octreotide should *not* be administered within 24 hours or 4 weeks, respectively, prior to each dose of lutetium Lu 177 dotatate.

When lutetium Lu 177 dotatate is used in combination with long-acting octreotide, the manufacturer states that a single 30-mg dose of long-acting octreotide acetate may be administered by IM injection between 4–24 hours after each dose of lutetium Lu 177 dotatate and should *not* be administered within 4 weeks prior to administration of lutetium Lu 177 dotatate. Following discontinuance of lutetium Lu 177 dotatate therapy, long-acting octreotide acetate (30 mg administered by IM injection every 4 weeks) may be continued until disease progression or for a treatment duration of up to 18 months.

Description

Lutetium Lu 177 dotatate, a lutetium 177 radiolabeled tetraazacyclododecane-tetra-acetic acid (DOTA)-somatostatin analog conjugate consisting of the somatostatin analog octreotide linked to a chelator (DOTA), is a peptide receptor radionuclide agent. The peptide portion of lutetium Lu 177 dotatate binds specifically to somatostatin receptors, with the highest affinity for somatostatin receptor type 2 (SSRT2). Following binding of the somatostatin analog component of lutetium Lu 177 dotatate to somatostatin receptors, the resultant complex is internalized by the cell. The radioactive component of lutetium Lu 177 dotatate (lutetium 177) induces cellular damage by forming free radicals in target and neighboring cells and is responsible for the primary cytotoxic effect of the peptide receptor radionuclide agent.

Following IV administration, lutetium Lu 177 dotatate rapidly distributes into kidneys, tumor lesions, liver, spleen, and, sometimes, pituitary gland and thyroid within 4 hours. In patients receiving lutetium Lu 177 dotatate at the recommended dosage, the mean effective half-life of lutetium Lu 177 dotatate in the blood is 3.5 hours. Coadministration of the amino acids *l*-lysine and *l*-arginine reduces the median radiation dose to the kidneys by 47% and increases the mean β-phase plasma clearance of lutetium Lu 177 dotatate by 36%. Lutetium Lu 177 dotatate does not undergo hepatic metabolism. Lutetium Lu 177 dotatate is eliminated by the kidneys; 44, 58, or 65% of the dose is recovered in urine within 5, 24, or 48 hours, respectively. Following IV administration of lutetium Lu 177 dotatate, more than 99% of the dose is expected to be eliminated within 14 days. In vivo, nonradioactive lutetium dotatate (lutetium Lu 175 dotatate) is 43% bound to plasma proteins. The mean effective and terminal half-lives of lutetium Lu 177 dotatate are 3.5 and 71 hours, respectively.

Advice to Patients

Importance of advising patients to follow standard precautions for minimizing radiation exposure to household contacts.

Risk of myelosuppression (e.g., thrombocytopenia, neutropenia, anemia). Importance of monitoring complete blood cell (CBC) counts prior to and periodically during lutetium Lu 177 dotatate therapy. Importance of informing clinician if any signs or symptoms of myelosuppression or infection (e.g., fever, chills, dizziness, shortness of breath, bleeding, easy bruising) occur.

Risk of myelodysplastic syndrome (MDS) and acute leukemia.

Risk of renal toxicity. Importance of monitoring renal function prior to and periodically during lutetium Lu 177 dotatate therapy. Importance of advising patients to maintain adequate hydration during and after administration of lutetium Lu 177 dotatate to ensure good urinary output.

Risk of hepatotoxicity. Importance of liver function test monitoring prior to and periodically during lutetium Lu 177 dotatate therapy.

Risk of carcinoid hormonal crisis. Importance of informing clinician if manifestations of carcinoid hormonal crisis (e.g., severe flushing, diarrhea, bronchospasm, hypotension) occur.

Risk of fetal harm. Necessity of advising women of reproductive potential that they should use effective methods of contraception while receiving lutetium Lu 177 dotatate and for 7 months after the final dose. Necessity of advising male patients with female partners of reproductive potential that they should use effective methods of contraception while receiving lutetium Lu 177 dotatate and for 4 months after the final dose. Importance of women informing clinicians if they are or plan to become pregnant. Apprise patient of potential fetal hazard if used during pregnancy.

Importance of advising women to avoid breast-feeding while receiving lutetium Lu 177 dotatate and for 2.5 months after the last dose.

Risk of impaired male and female fertility.

Importance of informing clinicians of existing or contemplated concomitant therapy, including prescription and OTC drugs and dietary or herbal supplements, as well as any concomitant diseases.

Importance of informing patients of other important precautionary information. (See Cautions.)

Overview® (see Users Guide). For additional information on this drug until a more detailed monograph is developed and published, the manufacturer's labeling should be consulted. It is *essential* that the manufacturer's labeling be consulted for more detailed information on usual cautions, precautions, contraindications, potential drug interactions, laboratory test interferences, and acute toxicity. For further information on the handling of antineoplastic agents, see the ASHP Guidelines on Handling Hazardous Drugs at http://www.ahfsdruginformation.com.

Preparations

Excipients in commercially available drug preparations may have clinically important effects in some individuals; consult specific product labeling for details.

Lutetium Lu 177 Dotatate

Parenteral		
Injection, for IV infusion only	370 MBq/mL (equivalent to 10 mCi/mL)	**Lutathera®** (available in a lead-shielded container), Advanced Accelerator Applications

Melphalan

Phenylalanine Mustard

■ Melphalan, a nitrogen mustard-derivative alkylating agent, is an antineoplastic agent.

Uses

■ **Multiple Myeloma** Melphalan is used alone and as a component of various chemotherapeutic regimens in the treatment of multiple myeloma. The drug usually is used orally; however, melphalan hydrochloride also can be used IV in the palliative treatment of multiple myeloma in patients in whom oral therapy is not feasible, and melphalan injection is designated an orphan drug by the US Food and Drug Administration (FDA) for use in this condition. Comparative studies have shown the efficacy of IV melphalan hydrochloride in combination with prednisone in the treatment of multiple myeloma to be equivalent to that of orally administered melphalan in combination with prednisone.

Although not curative, melphalan can prolong the survival of patients with multiple myeloma. Although melphalan is used mainly in combination chemotherapy, about one-third of patients who receive the drug alone have an objective response, which may be characterized by a decrease in the amount of abnormal proteins present in urine or serum, a decrease in the number of myeloma cells in the bone marrow, an increase in hemoglobin, improved renal function, a decreased frequency of infection due in part to an increased concentration of normal immunoglobulins, normalization of serum calcium, and/or lack of progression and, rarely, recalcification of bone lesions. Subjective response, which occurs in most patients who receive melphalan alone, is characterized by relief of pain and increased mobility and performance status. Response to melphalan may occur gradually over several months; therefore, it is important that repeated courses or continuous therapy be administered in order that maximum benefit from the drug may be obtained. Many clinicians believe that 3–12 months of therapy with melphalan may be necessary to evaluate the response to the drug.

Comparative studies have shown the effectiveness of melphalan in the treatment of multiple myeloma to be equivalent to that of cyclophosphamide, and most experts consider melphalan or cyclophosphamide to be the drug of choice for the treatment of multiple myeloma. Some experts prefer cyclophosphamide to melphalan in patients with severe thrombocytopenia because of the relative platelet-sparing effect of cyclophosphamide. In some patients resistant to melphalan, cyclophosphamide in high doses may be useful. Controlled trials of intermittent regimens of melphalan with prednisone have shown this combination to be superior in most patients to the use of intermittent or daily regimens of melphalan alone for remission induction; the median duration of survival is apparently increased compared to that produced by melphalan alone. In patients who achieve a remission, continued maintenance therapy after the first year of treatment does not appear to prolong the duration of remission or survival; however, some clinicians continue therapy because most patients relapse and some of these patients may become unresponsive to further chemotherapy. Melphalan also has been used in other combination regimens with agents such as carmustine, cyclophosphamide, fluoxymesterone, lomustine, procarbazine hydrochloride, testosterone, and vincristine sulfate, but the best combination or sequential therapy to achieve the maximum response and duration of survival has not been established.

■ **Ovarian Cancer** Melphalan may be used in the palliative treatment of nonresectable epithelial carcinoma of the ovary. An objective response occurs in 30–50% of patients who receive melphalan alone. Response rates, including complete response rates, are higher for cisplatin-based combination therapy; however, the best combination or sequential therapy in the treatment of advanced ovarian tumors has not been established, and the comparative safety and efficacy of various regimens are continually being evaluated. Tumor regression has occurred in some patients receiving intraperitoneal† administration of melphalan for the treatment of advanced ovarian cancer confined to the peritoneal cavity and/or associated with malignant ascites.

■ **Breast Cancer** Melphalan has been used alone or with other antineoplastic agents as an adjunct to surgery in the treatment of breast cancer†. Melphalan appears to increase disease-free survival principally in patients younger than 50 years of age with 1–3 involved axillary lymph nodes; however, combination therapy containing melphalan and/or other agents appears to be more effective in these and other subgroups of patients. Some clinicians have recommended that melphalan no longer be used *alone* as adjunctive therapy.

Combination chemotherapy used as an adjunct to surgery has been shown to increase both disease-free (i.e., decreased recurrence) and overall survival in premenopausal and postmenopausal women with node-negative or -positive early (TNM stage I or II) breast cancer. Adjuvant combination chemotherapy has produced overall reductions in the annual rates of recurrence and death of 28 and 16%, respectively, with overall 5-year disease-free survival rates of 58.8 versus 49.6% for patients with early breast cancer receiving combination chemotherapy versus those who did not. Although adjuvant combination chemotherapy that includes cyclophosphamide, methotrexate, and fluorouracil has been used most extensively and is considered a regimen of choice, several melphalan-containing regimens appear to produce similar outcomes in early breast cancer but have been used less commonly and/or studied less extensively. Melphalan has been used for adjunctive treatment of early breast cancer in combination with fluorouracil for premenopausal women and in combination with fluorouracil and tamoxifen for postmenopausal women with estrogen-receptor-positive/progestin-receptor-positive tumors. Melphalan also has been used in combination with doxorubicin and fluorouracil, since the addition of doxorubicin to an adjuvant regimen of melphalan and fluorouracil (without tamoxifen) has been shown to improve outcome in women younger than 50 years of age with hormone-receptor-negative disease and in those 50–59 years of age with progestin-receptor-negative disease. Melphalan also has been used as a component of these and other regimens for the treatment of locally advanced (stage III) disease.

■ **Melanoma** Melphalan is used in isolated limb perfusion† for palliative treatment of locally recurrent or unresectable in-transit metastatic melanoma† of the extremities. Use of melphalan in combination regimens (e.g., melphalan, tumor necrosis factor, and interferon gamma) for perfusion therapy of limb melanoma is being investigated. No survival benefit has been shown for use of isolated limb perfusion with melphalan as adjuvant therapy for melanoma of the extremities.

■ **Other Uses** Melphalan has been used in the treatment of polycythemia vera†; its effect is reportedly about equivalent to that of chlorambucil, but faster in onset.

Melphalan has been used with prednisone in the treatment of amyloidosis†. In a randomized study in patients with primary amyloidosis, combined therapy with melphalan and prednisone produced an objective response (as measured by disappearance or a reduction of at least 50% in serum or urinary monoclonal protein concentration) in about 29% of patients compared with 28% of patients receiving combined therapy with melphalan, prednisone, and colchicine and 3% of patients receiving colchicine alone. A median survival duration of 18 months was reported in patients receiving melphalan with prednisone compared with 17 months in those receiving melphalan, prednisone, and colchicine and 8.5 months in those receiving colchicine monotherapy. Objective response has been observed within 1 year following initiation of chemotherapy in about 70% of those who responded, while 21% of patients who responded required an additional year of chemotherapy. Patients with cardiac amyloidosis had a much shorter survival (about 5 months) after randomization than those with amyloidosis associated with nephrotic syndrome (16 months), or peripheral neuropathy (about 34 months). In addition, at 12 months following initiation of chemotherapy, patients who showed an objective response had a median overall survival of about 50 months compared with 36 months for those without an objective response. Additional studies are needed to evaluate the efficacy of high-dose melphalan therapy and other agents in the management of primary amyloidosis.

Melphalan has also been used in the treatment of scleromyxedema†, chronic myelogenous leukemia†, osteogenic sarcoma†, advanced prostatic carcinoma†, and testicular seminoma†.

Melphalan also has been administered by regional isolation perfusion† in the treatment of certain sarcomas†.

Dosage and Administration

■ **Reconstitution and Administration** Melphalan is administered orally, and melphalan hydrochloride is administered by IV injection. Melphalan hydrochloride also has been administered intra-arterially†, intraperitoneally†, and by regional isolation perfusion† (e.g., for melanoma).

Melphalan hydrochloride powder for injection is reconstituted by adding 10 mL of the diluent provided by the manufacturer to a vial labeled as containing 50 mg of melphalan using a 20-gauge or larger needle to provide a solution containing 5 mg/mL. The diluent should be added rapidly and the vial should be shaken vigorously until a clear solution is obtained. Reconstituted solutions of melphalan hydrochloride should be inspected visually for particulate matter and discoloration prior to administration whenever solution and container permit. The reconstituted solution should not be refrigerated, since a precipitate may form at 5°C. The reconstituted solution of melphalan hydrochloride should be diluted further with 0.9% sodium chloride injection to provide a solution with a concentration not exceeding 0.45 mg/mL. Dilution of reconstituted solutions of the drug should be performed immediately because a citrate derivative of melphalan has been detected in the solution within 30 minutes of reconstitution of melphalan hydrochloride for injection. Because approximately 1% of the labeled strength of melphalan hydrolyzes every 10 minutes following dilution with 0.9% sodium chloride, the solution of melphalan hydrochloride should be administered soon after dilution. Melphalan is administered by IV infusion, usually over 15–20 minutes. Administration of melphalan hydrochloride should be completed within 60 minutes of reconstitution.

The manufacturer recommends that procedures for proper handling and disposal of antineoplastic drugs (e.g., use of gloves) be used, since adverse dermatologic effects associated with exposure to the drug may occur. If melphalan solution comes in contact with the skin or mucous membranes, the affected area should be washed thoroughly with soap and water. For further information on the handling of cytotoxic drugs, see the guidelines at the end of Antineoplastic Agents 10:00 and consult special references on the handling and disposal of cytotoxic drugs.

■ **Dosage** Dosage of melphalan must be adjusted carefully according to the clinical and hematologic response and tolerance of the patient in order to obtain optimum therapeutic results with minimum adverse effects. It is usually necessary to maintain some degree of myelosuppression. The leukocyte count generally serves as a guide to dosage adjustments and is usually maintained between 3000–4000/mm^3. Dosage adjustments based on the blood cell nadir and blood counts taken on the day of melphalan therapy should be considered.

Dosage of melphalan hydrochloride is expressed in terms of melphalan.

Multiple Myeloma For the treatment of multiple myeloma, various dosage schedules for oral melphalan or IV melphalan hydrochloride have been used. The drug may be administered continually or intermittently. The clinician should consult published protocols for the dosage of melphalan and other chemotherapeutic agents and the method and sequence of administration.

Oral Dosage. The manufacturer recommends a usual initial oral dosage of melphalan of 6 mg given as a single daily dose. Subsequent dosage should be adjusted as required based on blood counts performed approximately weekly. After 2–3 weeks, the drug should be discontinued for up to 4 weeks until the leukocyte and platelet counts increase, at which time an oral maintenance dosage of 2 mg daily may be instituted. Alternatively, most clinicians recommend an intermittent oral melphalan dosage schedule of 0.15 mg/kg daily for 7 successive days or 0.25 mg/kg daily for 4 successive days, administered at intervals of 4–6 weeks, usually with prednisone.

Other clinicians have used oral melphalan dosages of 10 mg daily for 7–10 days. In these patients, maximum suppression of leukocyte and platelet counts occurred within 3–5 weeks while recovery reportedly occurred within 4–8 weeks. When platelet and leukocyte counts exceeded 100,000 and 4000, respectively, a continuous maintenance therapy of 2 mg daily was initiated; dosage was adjusted at 1–3 mg daily depending on hematologic response. The manufacturer states that it is desirable to maintain a substantial degree of bone marrow depression in order to keep the leukocyte count at 3000–3500.

IV Dosage. The manufacturer states that an exact dosage conversion from oral to parenteral melphalan cannot be made. Clinicians should consult published protocols for specific information on parenteral dosage regimens using IV melphalan hydrochloride for specific diseases.

The manufacturer states that the usual IV dosage of melphalan is 16 mg/m^2 given by IV infusion once at 2-week intervals for 4 doses; then, after satisfactory recovery from toxicity, the same dose should be repeated at 4-week intervals. In some controlled clinical studies in patients with multiple myeloma, dosage reductions of 25% were employed when platelet counts were 75,000–99,999 or leukocyte counts were 3000–3999 and dosage reductions of 50%

were used when platelet counts were 50,000–74,999 or leukocyte counts were 2000–2999; IV melphalan was discontinued when platelet or leukocyte counts fell below these values.

Ovarian Cancer For the treatment of ovarian carcinoma, the usual dosage of melphalan is 0.2 mg/kg daily for 5 successive days, administered at intervals of 4–5 weeks.

■ **Dosage in Renal Impairment** Dosage reduction should be considered in patients with renal impairment who are receiving IV melphalan hydrochloride therapy, since increased bone marrow suppression was observed in patients with BUN concentrations of 30 mg/dL or more. When dosage of IV melphalan hydrochloride is reduced by 50% in these patients, the risk of severe leukopenia and drug-related death may be reduced from about 50 to 11% and 10 to 3% of patients, respectively.

Cautions

Adverse systemic effects reported with IV melphalan hydrochloride usually are similar to those reported with oral melphalan; however, results of controlled clinical studies indicate that the incidence of severe myelosuppression was higher in patients receiving the drug IV compared with those receiving the drug orally.

■ **Hematologic Effects** Hematologic toxicity is the major and dose-limiting adverse effect of both oral and IV melphalan and is manifested principally by leukopenia and thrombocytopenia. Anemia, hemolytic anemia, pancytopenia, and agranulocytosis may also occur. Myelosuppression usually occurs after 2–3 weeks of melphalan therapy, but leukopenia may occur after 5 days in a few patients. Leukocyte and platelet counts usually return to normal levels during the fifth week, but leukopenia or thrombocytopenia may persist for 6 weeks or longer after the drug is discontinued. However, irreversible bone marrow depression has been reported in some patients receiving the drug. The patient's hematologic status must be carefully monitored. (See Cautions: Precautions and Contraindications.) Melphalan has reportedly caused positive direct Coombs' test results and concurrent hemolytic anemia. Severe leukopenia may occur in patients with renal impairment receiving IV melphalan hydrochloride therapy; dosage reduction (i.e., by 50%) should be considered in these patients. (See Dosage and Administration: Dosage in Renal Impairment.)

■ **Cardiovascular Effects** Arterial or venous thrombosis, or pulmonary embolism, sometimes fatal, has been reported in patients receiving melphalan administered by regional isolation perfusion.

■ **Nervous System Effects** Adverse neurologic effects, including transient paralysis, limb pain, nerve injury, and peripheral neuritis, have been associated with administration of melphalan by regional isolation perfusion.

■ **Local Effects** Phlebitis and extravasation have been reported in patients receiving IV melphalan hydrochloride.

Administration of melphalan by regional isolation perfusion may cause erythema and/or edema of the perfused area, thrombophlebitis, necrotizing fasciitis, and varying degrees of vesiculation and tissue necrosis; amputation sometimes has been necessary.

■ **GI Effects** Mild nausea and vomiting occur infrequently after usual doses but may be common after large doses of melphalan. Occasional diarrhea, stomatitis, and oral ulceration also have been reported.

■ **Dermatologic and Hypersensitivity Reactions** Dermatologic reactions including maculopapular and urticarial rashes, dermatitis, skin hypersensitivity, allergic reactions, pruritus, and, rarely, alopecia have been reported in patients receiving melphalan. Anaphylaxis has also been reported. Hypersensitivity reactions including urticaria, pruritus, exanthema, rash, edema, tachycardia, bronchospasm, dyspnea, hypotension, and anaphylaxis have been reported in about 2% of patients receiving the drug IV; in several patients, rechallenge with oral melphalan produced rash, pruritus, and chest pain. Hypersensitivity reactions occur most commonly after several courses of IV therapy with the drug. If a hypersensitivity reaction to IV melphalan hydrochloride occurs, the drug should be discontinued and appropriate symptomatic treatment initiated (e.g., plasma volume expanders, vasopressors, corticosteroids, antihistamines) at the discretion of the clinician.

Skin ulceration at the injection site and skin necrosis (rarely requiring skin grafting) have been reported in patients receiving IV melphalan therapy.

■ **Other Adverse Effects** Vasculitis, pulmonary fibrosis, and interstitial pneumonitis have been reported in patients receiving melphalan. Hepatotoxicity (e.g., hepatic veno-occlusive disease) has been reported in patients receiving IV melphalan hydrochloride. Hepatotoxicity also has been reported in patients receiving oral melphalan. Rarely, menstrual irregularities and bronchopulmonary dysplasia have occurred following prolonged melphalan therapy.

■ **Precautions and Contraindications** Melphalan is a highly toxic drug with a low therapeutic index, and a therapeutic response is not likely to occur without some evidence of toxicity. The drug must be used only under constant supervision by physicians experienced in therapy with cytotoxic agents. Melphalan should be used only when the possible benefits outweigh the possible risks. Patients should be advised that the major toxicities associated with melphalan are bone marrow depression, hypersensitivity reactions, infertility, nonlymphocytic leukemia, myeloproliferative syndrome, and GI and pulmonary toxicities. Patients who receive myelosuppressive drugs experience an increased frequency of infections as well as possible hemorrhagic complications. Because these complications are potentially fatal, the patient should be instructed to notify the physician if fever, sore throat, persistent cough, or unusual bleeding or bruising occurs. The patient's hematologic status must be carefully monitored and blood counts performed approximately weekly in patients receiving oral melphalan therapy. The manufacturer states that complete blood counts (leukocyte count with differential, platelet count, hemoglobin) should be performed prior to initiation of IV melphalan hydrochloride therapy and before each subsequent IV dose. Therapy should be discontinued temporarily or dosage decreased at the first sign of abnormal bone marrow depression (specifically, if the leukocyte count falls below 3000/mm^3 or the platelet count falls below 100,000/mm^3); when blood counts have returned to acceptable levels, therapy may be resumed if indicated. Treatment of severe hematologic toxicity may consist of supportive therapy, antibiotics for complicating infections, and transfusions with blood components. Melphalan should be used with extreme caution in patients whose bone marrow reserve may have been compromised by prior irradiation or chemotherapy, or whose bone marrow function is recovering from previous cytotoxic therapy. Patients also should be instructed to notify the physician if rash, signs or symptoms of vasculitis, nausea, vomiting, amenorrhea, weight loss, or unusual lumps/masses occur.

The manufacturer states that there may be cross-sensitivity between melphalan and chlorambucil manifested by rash.

Melphalan is contraindicated in patients with known hypersensitivity to the drug or in patients whose disease was resistant to prior therapy with the drug. It has not been clearly determined whether dosage of oral melphalan should routinely be reduced in patients with impaired renal function; the manufacturer states that patients with azotemia should be closely monitored in order to make dosage reductions, if necessary, at the earliest possible time. The manufacturer states that although renal elimination of melphalan appears to be low dosage reduction should be considered in patients with renal impairment who are receiving melphalan hydrochloride IV, since increased bone marrow suppression was observed in patients with BUN concentrations of 30 mg/dL or more. A 50% reduction in IV melphalan dosage was associated with a decreased risk of leukopenia and drug-related death. (See Dosage and Administration: Dosage in Renal Impairment.)

■ **Pediatric Precautions** Safety and efficacy of melphalan in pediatric patients have not been established.

■ **Geriatric Precautions** In clinical studies, the responses to melphalan in geriatric patients did not differ substantially from those observed in younger patients. However, dosage of melphalan should be selected carefully in geriatric patients and the greater frequency of decreased hepatic, renal, and/or cardiac function and of concomitant disease and drug therapy observed in the elderly also should be considered.

■ **Mutagenicity and Carcinogenicity** Melphalan is potentially mutagenic. The drug has caused chromatid or chromosome damage in humans. Structural chromosomal and chromatid aberrations also have been observed in bone marrow cells of Wistar rats receiving IM doses of 6 and 60 mg/m^2. Melphalan is potentially carcinogenic and has been associated with the development of acute myelogenous (nonlymphocytic) leukemia, myeloproliferative syndrome, and carcinoma in patients with multiple myeloma, ovarian carcinoma, or breast cancer, especially with prolonged continuous dosing of the drug. Evidence from clinical studies suggests that the estimated 10-year cumulative risk of developing acute leukemia or myeloproliferative syndrome following melphalan therapy is 19.5 or less than 2% in patients receiving cumulative doses of 730–9652 or less than 600 mg of the drug, respectively. However, a cumulative dose below which there is no risk of melphalan-induced secondary malignancy has not been established to date. Although the benefits of melphalan therapy in the palliative treatment of multiple myeloma and ovarian carcinoma are generally believed to outweigh the potential risks, the possibility of development of a secondary malignancy must be considered. There are no adequate and controlled carcinogenicity studies in animals; however, intraperitoneal administration of melphalan dosages of 5.4–10.8 mg/m^2 in rats and 2.25–4.5 mg/m^2 in mice 3 times a week for 6 months were associated with peritoneal sarcomas and lung tumors, respectively.

■ **Pregnancy, Fertility, and Lactation** Melphalan can cause fetal harm when administered to pregnant women. Although there are no adequate and controlled studies to date using melphalan in pregnant women, the drug has been shown to be teratogenic and embryotoxic in rats. In rats given oral melphalan dosages of 6–18 mg/m^2 daily for 10 days or intraperitoneal dosages of 18 mg/m^2, teratogenic effects, including anomalies of the brain (e.g., meningocele, encephalocele, deformation, underdevelopment) and eyes (e.g., anophthalmia, microphthalmia), hepatocele (exomphalos), and reduction in size of mandibles and tails occurred. If melphalan is administered during pregnancy or if the patient becomes pregnant while receiving the drug, the patient should be informed of the potential hazard to the fetus. Women of childbearing potential should be advised to avoid becoming pregnant while receiving melphalan.

Ovarian suppression and amenorrhea may occur during melphalan therapy in premenopausal women. Reversible and irreversible suppression of testicular function also have been reported in patients receiving the drug.

It is not known whether melphalan is distributed into milk. Because of the potential for serious adverse reactions to melphalan in nursing infants if the drug were distributed into milk, a decision should be made whether to discontinue nursing or the drug, taking into account the importance of the drug to the woman. The manufacturer states that IV melphalan should not be administered to nursing women.

Drug Interactions

■ **Food** Food appears to decrease the bioavailability of melphalan. Following oral administration of melphalan, bioavailability of the drug was about 85–93 and 49–58% in the fasted and nonfasted state, respectively. Some clinicians state that oral melphalan should not be administered with food.

■ **Cyclosporine** Melphalan may increase cyclosporine-induced nephrotoxicity. Severe renal failure has been reported in patients receiving a single dose of IV melphalan followed by usual dosages of cyclosporine. Renal function should be monitored carefully in patients receiving cyclosporine and melphalan concomitantly; dosage reduction of cyclosporine may be necessary in patients receiving high-dose melphalan therapy.

■ **Other Drugs** Plasma elimination of melphalan may be enhanced by interferon alfa-induced fever, resulting in a decreased area under the plasma concentration-time curve (AUC) of melphalan. The clinical importance of this interaction remains to be determined.

Concomitant administration of cisplatin may affect pharmacokinetics of melphalan secondary to cisplatin-induced renal impairment, which may result in decreased clearance of melphalan. IV melphalan may reduce the threshold for carmustine-induced pulmonary toxicity. Concomitant nalidixic acid and melphalan use in children may result in an increased incidence of severe hemorrhagic necrotic enterocolitis.

Cimetidine appears to inhibit GI absorption of melphalan resulting in reduced serum concentrations of melphalan; patients receiving cimetidine and melphalan concomitantly should be monitored for decreased melphalan activity.

Acute Toxicity

■ **Pathogenesis** The oral LD_{50} of melphalan is 21 mg/kg in mice.

■ **Manifestations** Overdosage with melphalan doses up to 290 mg/m² was associated with severe nausea, vomiting, ulceration of the mouth, decreased consciousness, seizures, muscular paralysis, and cholinomimetic effects. In addition, overdosage with melphalan dosages up to 50 mg daily for 16 days may be associated with vomiting, ulceration of the mouth, diarrhea, and hemorrhage of the GI tract. Several fatalities following melphalan overdosage have been reported to date. One child who received standard supportive care survived a single melphalan dose of 254 mg/m². In patients receiving high doses of melphalan (i.e., greater than 100 mg/m²), severe mucositis, stomatitis, colitis, diarrhea, and GI bleeding have been reported. Elevations in liver enzymes, hepatic veno-occlusive disease, nephrotoxicity, and adult respiratory distress syndrome have occurred rarely. In some patients, severe hyponatremia caused by inappropriate antidiuretic hormone secretion (SIADH) has been reported. The principal toxic effect of melphalan is bone marrow suppression. The patient's hematologic status should be monitored carefully for 3–6 weeks following melphalan overdosage.

■ **Treatment** Treatment of severe hematologic toxicity may consist of supportive therapy, anti-infectives for complicating infections, and blood product transfusions, at the discretion of the clinician. Results of an uncontrolled study suggest that administration of autogenous (autologous) bone marrow or a biosynthetic hematopoietic agent (e.g., filgrastim, sargramostim) may shorten the period of melphalan-induced pancytopenia. Melphalan is not removed by hemodialysis or hemoperfusion.

Pharmacology

Melphalan, as an alkylating agent, interferes with DNA replication and transcription of RNA, and ultimately results in the disruption of nucleic acid function. Melphalan also possesses some immunosuppressive activity.

Pharmacokinetics

The pharmacokinetics of orally administered melphalan have been studied extensively in adults.

■ **Absorption** Absorption of melphalan from the GI tract is incomplete and extremely variable. In a crossover study of single 0.6 mg/kg IV and oral doses of melphalan, the areas under the plasma concentration-time curves (AUCs) following oral administration were 25–89% of those following IV administration. In one study in fasting patients given a single oral melphalan dose of 0.6 mg/kg, average peak plasma melphalan concentrations of 280 ng/mL were reached within 2 hours. In adult patients with myeloma who received single IV melphalan doses of 10 or 20 mg/m², mean peak plasma concentrations of the drug were 1.2 or 2.8 ng/mL, respectively. Monohydroxy and dihydroxy derivatives of melphalan are present in plasma within 30 minutes after oral administration of the drug.

■ **Distribution** Melphalan is rapidly distributed throughout total body water. Melphalan distributes into CSF in low concentrations. The volume of distribution of melphalan at steady state (V_{ss}) has been reported to be approximately 0.5 L/kg. The drug reportedly is 60–90% bound to plasma proteins, mainly albumin and to a lesser extent (about 20%) to α_1-acid glycoprotein (α_1-AGP). About 30% of melphalan is irreversibly bound to plasma proteins. Interactions of melphalan with immunoglobulins have been found to be negligible. Experimental evidence indicates that melphalan may alkylate plasma proteins. It is not known whether melphalan crosses the placenta. It is also not known whether melphalan or its metabolites are distributed into milk.

■ **Elimination** Following a single oral dose in one study, the terminal plasma half-life of melphalan was 1.5 hours. Monohydroxy and dihydroxy derivatives of melphalan have apparent terminal plasma half-lives 2–3 times longer than unchanged melphalan. Plasma concentrations of melphalan appear to decline in a biphasic manner following IV administration of the drug. Following IV administration of melphalan hydrochloride in adult patients, the half-life of melphalan is about 10 minutes in the initial distribution phase ($t_{1/2\alpha}$) and about 75 minutes in the terminal elimination phase ($t_{1/2\beta}$).

Melphalan is apparently eliminated from plasma mainly by spontaneous hydrolysis, forming the monohydroxy and dihydroxy derivatives of the drug; no other metabolites have been identified in humans. In vitro in human plasma, melphalan undergoes first-order hydrolysis. Following IV administration of melphalan hydrochloride, total body clearance of the drug averages 7–9 mL/minute per kg in adult patients, although considerable interindividual variation in body clearance exists. In adult patients, total body clearance of melphalan may be decreased following multiple IV doses (e.g., 0.5 mg/kg every 6 weeks). Total body clearance decreased from 8.1 mL/minute per kg after the first course of therapy to 5.5 mL/minute per kg after the third course of therapy; body clearance did not decrease appreciably after the third course of therapy with melphalan. About 20–35% of an oral dose is excreted in urine as the drug and its metabolites within 24 hours. Approximately 10% of a single oral dose of melphalan is excreted in urine unchanged within 24 hours. Although renal elimination of melphalan appears to be low, results of one pharmacokinetic study indicate that there may be a direct correlation between renal function and elimination rate constant of the drug, while a negative correlation may exist between the area under the plasma concentration-time curve (AUC) of the drug and renal function. In one study using orally administered melphalan C 14, 20–50% of the dose was excreted in feces within 6 days.

Chemistry and Stability

■ **Chemistry** Melphalan, a nitrogen mustard derivative, is a bifunctional alkylating agent. The drug is the L-isomer of the phenylalanine derivative of mechlorethamine. Melphalan occurs as an off-white to buff powder that has a faint odor and is practically insoluble in water and slightly soluble in alcohol. Melphalan hydrochloride for injection is commercially available as a sterile, nonpyrogenic, lyophilized powder. The powder for injection also contains povidone. A sterile diluent containing water for injection, sodium citrate, propylene glycol, and alcohol is provided by the manufacturer for reconstitution. The reconstituted injection has a pH of about 7; the pK_a of melphalan is approximately 2.5.

■ **Stability** Melphalan tablets should be stored in well-closed, light-resistant, glass containers at a temperature less than 40°C, preferably between 15–30°C. Following reconstitution with sterile diluent, melphalan hydrochloride solution containing 5 mg of melphalan per mL is stable for up to 90 minutes at room temperature; this reconstituted solution should not be refrigerated since a precipitate may form at 5°C. The reconstituted solution should be diluted further with 0.9% sodium chloride injection to provide a solution with a concentration not exceeding 0.45 mg/mL. This diluted solution is stable for 60 minutes at room temperature.

For further information on the handling of antineoplastic agents, see the ASHP Guidelines on Handling Hazardous Drugs at http://www.ahfsdruginformation.com.

Preparations

Excipients in commercially available drug preparations may have clinically important effects in some individuals; consult specific product labeling for details.

Melphalan

Oral

Tablets, film-coated	2 mg	**Alkeran®**, GlaxoSmithKline

Melphalan Hydrochloride

Parenteral

For injection	50 mg (of melphalan)	**Alkeran®**, GlaxoSmithKline

†Use is not currently included in the labeling approved by the US Food and Drug Administration

Selected Revisions January 2009, © Copyright, August 1981, American Society of Health-System Pharmacists, Inc.

Mercaptopurine

6-Mercaptopurine, 6-MP

■ Mercaptopurine, a purine antagonist, is an antineoplastic agent and immunosuppressant.

Uses

■ **Acute Lymphocytic Leukemia** Mercaptopurine is used as first-line therapy in conjunction with methotrexate for maintenance of drug-induced remissions in adults and pediatric patients with acute lymphocytic leukemia (ALL). Maintenance therapy is considered essential once a complete hematologic remission is obtained.

■ **Inflammatory Bowel Disease** Mercaptopurine has been used in the management of moderately to severely or chronically active Crohn's disease† to maintain clinical remission in corticosteroid-dependent patients and to provide benefit in patients with fistulizing Crohn's disease†. Mercaptopurine (e.g., 1.5 mg/kg daily) has been used in conjunction with corticosteroids to induce remission in patients with mildly to severely active refractory Crohn's disease; however, onset of action of mercaptopurine is slow and usually several months (at least 3 months) are required to achieve clinical response. Therefore, the role, if any, of mercaptopurine in the management of acute disease activity is uncertain. Mercaptopurine is used in patients with chronically active steroid-dependent Crohn's disease.

Limited data indicate that mercaptopurine may be effective in maintaining remission in patients with corticosteroid-induced clinical remissions and in allowing reduction of oral corticosteroid therapy in steroid-dependent patients. In several studies, clinical response associated with mercaptopurine has been substantially higher than that associated with placebo. Results of long-term follow-up studies indicate that treatment with mercaptopurine may be effective for up to 4 years, although in some studies clinical benefits have persisted longer. Limited data indicate that relapse rates after 4 years of immunosuppressive therapy may be similar whether therapy has been maintained or discontinued; however, further larger studies are needed to confirm such data.

Mercaptopurine also has been effective in the management of fistulizing Crohn's disease†. Current clinical practice concerning use of mercaptopurine is based on a meta-analysis of 5 controlled trials in which fistula closure was considered a secondary end point and in several uncontrolled case studies. Data from these studies indicate that long-term (several years) therapy with mercaptopurine may be effective in the management of fistulizing Crohn's disease. However, because there currently are no controlled studies employing fistula closing as a primary end point, additional study is needed to more clearly establish efficacy.

Mercaptopurine has been used effectively in pediatric patients with intractable Crohn's disease† who have been refractory to corticosteroids, sulfasalazine, and/or anti-infectives, usually for several years. While mercaptopurine (1.5 mg/kg daily; maximum daily dosage of 75 mg), administered conjunctively with existing drug regimens, decreased disease activity (including frequency of perianal lesions) during the first 6 months of therapy, continued improvement was evident 7–12 months after initiation of such therapy. In addition, during mercaptopurine therapy, corticosteroid requirements were reduced substantially and in several patients, corticosteroids were discontinued.

For more information on the management of Crohn's disease, see Uses; Crohn's Disease, in Mesalamine 56:36.

Mercaptopurine also has been used for the treatment of ulcerative colitis†.

Risks and benefits of mercaptopurine therapy should be carefully considered in patients with inflammatory bowel disease†, especially in adolescents and young adults with the disease. Cases of hepatosplenic T-cell lymphoma have been reported in patients receiving mercaptopurine for the management of inflammatory bowel disease. (See Cautions: Malignancies and Lymphoproliferative Disorders.)

■ **Other Uses** Mercaptopurine has been included in combination regimens used as maintenance therapy for lymphoblastic lymphoma†, an aggressive form of non-Hodgkin's lymphoma.

Dosage and Administration

■ **Administration** Mercaptopurine is administered orally. An evening schedule is recommended for the administration of mercaptopurine and methotrexate as maintenance therapy for ALL in children.

■ **Dosage** Dosage of mercaptopurine must be individualized based on clinical and hematologic response and tolerance of the patient in order to obtain optimum therapeutic results with minimum adverse effects. Clinicians should consult published protocols for the dosage of mercaptopurine and other chemotherapeutic agents and the method and sequence of administration.

Acute Lymphocytic Leukemia For use in maintenance therapy for acute lymphocytic leukemia (ALL) after remission is attained, maintenance dosage of mercaptopurine varies from one patient to another, but the usual dosage is 1.5–2.5 mg/kg daily administered once daily. Mercaptopurine is used in conjunction with methotrexate as a standard maintenance regimen for childhood ALL.

Crohn's Disease For the management of Crohn's disease†, adults usually have received an initial mercaptopurine dosage of 1–1.5 mg/kg daily, which has been increased in some patients to 125 mg daily.

Pediatric patients with Crohn's disease have received a mercaptopurine dosage of 1–1.5 mg/kg daily up to a maximum of 75 mg daily.

Dosage Adjustment for TPMT Deficiency Patients with inherited deficiency of thiopurine *S*-methyl transferase (TPMT) activity are at increased risk of life-threatening myelotoxicity; substantial dosage reduction may be required in these individuals when initiating mercaptopurine therapy. (See Cautions: Precautions and Contraindications.)

For patients with homozygous TPMT deficiency (i.e., little or no TPMT activity), substantial reduction of mercaptopurine dosage is required to avoid severe toxicity. The optimal initial dosage of mercaptopurine in these patients has not been established. Some clinicians have recommended that for patients with TPMT deficiency the initial dosage of mercaptopurine be reduced to one-tenth of the usual dosage with further dosage adjustments based on the occurrence of myelotoxicity.

For patients with heterozygous TPMT deficiency (i.e., low or intermediate TPMT activity), most will tolerate usual dosages of mercaptopurine, but some will require dosage reduction.

Dosage Adjustment for Concomitant Use of Allopurinol Patients who receive allopurinol and mercaptopurine concomitantly should have the dosage of mercaptopurine reduced to 25–33% of the usual dose to avoid severe toxicity. (See Drug Interactions: Allopurinol.)

Dosage Modification for Toxicity and Contraindications for Continued Therapy **Hematologic Toxicity.** Because mercaptopurine may have a delayed hematologic effect, therapy should be discontinued temporarily at the first sign of an unexpected abnormally large or rapid decrease in any of the formed elements of the blood that is not attributable to the disease process or another drug. If the bone marrow status is uncertain, bone marrow examination (aspiration and/or biopsy) may be helpful in distinguishing between progression of leukemia, resistance to therapy, and marrow hypoplasia induced by mercaptopurine. The decision to increase or decrease mercaptopurine dosage or to continue or discontinue mercaptopurine therapy depends on the severity and rapidity with which hematologic effects occur.

In patients with clinical or laboratory evidence of severe bone marrow toxicity, particularly myelosuppression, TPMT testing should be considered. (For information on dosage adjustment according to TPMT activity, see Dosage Adjustment for TPMT Deficiency under Dosage and Administration: Dosage. For information on genetic polymorphism and variability in the metabolism of mercaptopurine, see Cautions: Precautions and Contraindications.) For patients who experience excessive myelosuppression, it may be possible to reduce the dosage of mercaptopurine and administer the usual dosage of other myelosuppressive chemotherapy needed for treatment. Substantial reduction of mercaptopurine dosage to about 10% of the usual dosage typically is required in patients who are homozygous-deficient for TPMT.

Hepatic Toxicity. If deterioration of liver function tests, jaundice, hepatomegaly, anorexia with tenderness in the right hypochondrion, or other evidence of toxic hepatitis or biliary stasis occurs, mercaptopurine should be discontinued until the exact etiology can be determined.

Pancreatic Toxicity. Pancreatitis has occurred in patients receiving mercaptopurine for the treatment of inflammatory bowel disease. If manifestations of pancreatitis, such as epigastric pain, back pain, fever, nausea, and elevated serum amylase concentration, occur, mercaptopurine therapy should be discontinued permanently. Reinitiation of mercaptopurine therapy in such patients causes recurrent pancreatitis and is *not* recommended.

■ **Dosage in Renal Impairment** Lower doses of mercaptopurine should be used to initiate therapy in patients with impaired renal function to avoid accumulation of the drug and its metabolites and increased risk of toxicity.

■ **Dosage in Hepatic Impairment** In patients with impaired hepatic function, consideration should be given to administering reduced dosages of mercaptopurine.

Cautions

The principal effects of mercaptopurine are bone marrow depression and hepatotoxicity.

■ **Malignancies and Lymphoproliferative Disorders** Mercaptopurine is mutagenic in animals and humans, is carcinogenic in animals, and may increase the risk of neoplasia in patients. Cases of hepatosplenic T-cell lymphoma have been reported in patients receiving mercaptopurine for the management of inflammatory bowel disease.

Hepatosplenic T-cell lymphoma, a rare, aggressive, usually fatal type of T-cell lymphoma, has been reported during postmarketing experience mainly in adolescents and young adults with Crohn's disease or ulcerative colitis who received treatment with thiopurine analogs (mercaptopurine or azathioprine) and/or tumor necrosis factor (TNF) blocking agents. Although most of the reported cases occurred in patients who had received a combination of immunosuppressive agents, including TNF blocking agents and thiopurine analogs (mercaptopurine or azathioprine), cases have been reported in patients receiving mercaptopurine or azathioprine alone. As of December 31, 2010, the US Food and Drug Administration (FDA) had identified 3 cases of hepatosplenic T-cell lymphoma in patients with Crohn's disease who had received mercaptopurine without concomitant or sequential immunosuppressive therapy. The 3 cases of hepatosplenic T-cell lymphoma were fatal and occurred in men 18–33 years of age (mean age: 24 years) following 3–8 years of mercaptopurine therapy. In addition, FDA identified 25 cases of hepatosplenic T-cell lymphoma in patients with Crohn's disease or ulcerative colitis who had received a TNF blocking agent (infliximab or both infliximab and adalimumab); in 22 of these cases, a thiopurine analog (mercaptopurine or azathioprine) was used concomitantly. In some cases, potential confounding factors could not be excluded because complete medical histories were not available. Since patients with certain conditions (e.g., Crohn's disease) may be at increased risk for lymphoma, it may be difficult to measure the added risk of treatment with TNF blocking agents, azathioprine, and/or mercaptopurine. (See Cautions: Precautions and Contraindications.)

■ **Hematologic Effects** The most consistent dose-dependent toxicity of mercaptopurine is myelosuppression manifested by anemia, leukopenia, thrombocytopenia, or any combination of these effects. These findings also may reflect progression of disease. Life-threatening infection and bleeding have occurred in patients with mercaptopurine-induced granulocytopenia and thrombocytopenia, respectively.

In many patients with severe depression of the formed elements of the blood caused by mercaptopurine, bone marrow examined by aspiration and/or biopsy may appear hypoplastic; however, in some patients it may appear normocellular. The qualitative changes in erythroid elements of the blood (toward the megaloblastic series) that are characteristic of treatment with folic acid antagonists and some other antimetabolites are not observed with mercaptopurine therapy.

Individuals who are homozygous deficient (2 nonfunctional alleles) for an inherited defect in the TPMT (thiopurine *S*-methyltransferase) gene are unusually sensitive to the myelosuppressive effects of mercaptopurine and are prone to the development of rapid bone marrow suppression following initiation of therapy. Substantial dosage reductions generally are required in such patients to avoid the development of life-threatening bone marrow suppression. Tolerance of mercaptopurine may vary in individuals who are heterozygous deficient (one nonfunctional allele) for the defect in the TPMT gene. Although some of these patients may experience greater toxicity, most will tolerate usual doses of mercaptopurine. (See Dosage Adjustment for TPMT Deficiency under Dosage and Administration: Dosage.)

Concomitant use of allopurinol may exacerbate the myelotoxicity associated with mercaptopurine therapy. Reduction of mercaptopurine dosage is required. (See Drug Interactions: Allopurinol and Dosage Adjustment for Concomitant Use of Allopurinol under Dosage and Administration: Dosage.) Patients receiving drugs that inhibit TPMT activity (e.g., olsalazine, mesalamine, sulfasalazine) also may be at greater risk for bone marrow toxicity. (See Drug Interactions: 5-Aminosalicylates.)

Hematologic status must be carefully monitored in patients receiving the drug. (See Cautions: Precautions and Contraindications.) Dosage adjustment may be required in patients experiencing hematologic toxicity. (See Hematologic Toxicity under Dosage: Dosage Modification for Toxicity and Contraindications for Continued Therapy, in Dosage and Administration.)

■ **Hepatic Effects** Hepatotoxicity manifested by rapid onset of jaundice, cholestasis, ascites, hepatic encephalopathy, and/or elevated hepatic enzyme concentrations, usually associated with hepatic necrosis and severe fibrosis, may occur in patients receiving mercaptopurine; deaths from hepatic necrosis have occurred. In some cases, hepatotoxicity has been associated with anorexia and diarrhea. Hepatic function must be carefully monitored in patients receiving mercaptopurine. (See Cautions: Precautions and Contraindications.) Although hepatic injury can occur at any dosage, the incidence appears to increase when dosage exceeds 2.5 mg/kg daily. The histologic pattern of mercaptopurine-induced hepatotoxicity usually includes features of both intrahepatic cholestasis and parenchymal cell necrosis; features of either form of hepatic injury may predominate. The precise mechanism of hepatic injury is not clear, and the relative contribution to this injury of a direct toxic effect of the drug and/or a hypersensitivity reaction is not known. Clinical studies with mercaptopurine have given varying incidences of hepatotoxicity induced by the drug. In a large number of patients with various neoplastic diseases receiving mercaptopurine dosages of 2.5–5 mg/kg daily, definitive clinical evidence of drug-induced hepatotoxicity was absent, although biochemical evidence of hepatitis occasionally occurred in previously transfused patients. In several other studies in adults and pediatric patients with leukemia, the incidence of hepatotoxicity during mercaptopurine therapy generally ranged from 0–6%, although jaundice was reported in 40% of patients receiving the drug in one study, particularly when dosage exceeded 2.5 mg/kg daily. Clinically detectable jaundice usually occurs at 1–2 months, but has been reported as early as 1 week and as late as 8 years after initiation of mercaptopurine therapy. In some patients, jaundice has cleared following discontinuance of the drug and reappeared when therapy was reinstituted.

Dosage adjustment may be required in patients experiencing hepatic toxicity. (See Hepatic Toxicity under Dosage: Dosage Modification for Toxicity and Contraindications for Continued Therapy, in Dosage and Administration.)

■ **GI Effects** Adverse GI effects, which occur less frequently in pediatric patients than in adults, have been reported occasionally. Nausea, vomiting, and anorexia are uncommon during initial therapy with mercaptopurine but may occur more frequently with continued administration of the drug. Intestinal ulceration has occurred in patients receiving mercaptopurine. Mild diarrhea and sprue-like syndrome have been observed occasionally but a causal relationship to mercaptopurine has not been established. Other adverse GI effects include epigastric distress, abdominal pain, and mucositis. Rarely, oral lesions resembling candidiasis rather than characteristic folic acid antagonist ulcerations have been reported in patients receiving mercaptopurine.

■ **Renal Effects** As a result of extensive purine catabolism accompanying rapid cellular destruction, hyperuricemia and/or hyperuricosuria may occur in patients receiving mercaptopurine for leukemia. In some patients, oliguria and, rarely, renal insufficiency may result. Hematuria, crystalluria, and accompanying flank pain have also been reported. These effects may be minimized by adequate hydration, alkalinization of the urine, and/or administration of allopurinol. Reduction of mercaptopurine dosage is required for concomitant use of allopurinol. (See Dosage Adjustment for Concomitant Use of Allopurinol under Dosage and Administration: Dosage.)

■ **Metabolic Effects** Tumor lysis syndrome with hyperuricemia and/or hyperuricosuria may occur as a result of rapid cell lysis in patients receiving mercaptopurine as antineoplastic therapy. Prophylactic use of a xanthine oxidase inhibitor such as allopurinol may be used to minimize these adverse effects, but reduction of mercaptopurine dosage is required. (See Cautions: Renal Effects.)

■ **Pancreatic Effects** An increased risk of pancreatitis has been associated with mercaptopurine in patients receiving the drug for the management of inflammatory bowel disease. Manifestations of pancreatitis included epigastric pain, back pain, fever, nausea, and elevated serum amylase concentration. Mercaptopurine therapy should be discontinued permanently in patients experiencing pancreatitis. (See Pancreatic Toxicity under Dosage: Dosage Modification for Toxicity and Contraindications for Continued Therapy, in Dosage and Administration.)

■ **Dermatologic Effects** Rashes, hyperpigmentation, and alopecia have occurred in patients receiving mercaptopurine.

■ **Other Adverse Effects** Drug fever rarely has been reported in patients receiving mercaptopurine. Other causes of pyrexia, such as sepsis, should be ruled out before attributing the effect to the drug in patients with acute leukemia. Other infrequently occurring adverse effects of mercaptopurine include fever, headache, and excessive weakness. Oligospermia has been reported.

■ **Precautions and Contraindications** Mercaptopurine is a highly toxic drug with a low therapeutic index, and a therapeutic response is not likely to occur without some evidence of toxicity. The drug must be used only under constant supervision by clinicians experienced in therapy with cytotoxic agents.

Patients who have received mercaptopurine therapy should be monitored for the occurrence of malignancies. Because therapy with thiopurine analogs (mercaptopurine or azathioprine) and/or TNF blocking agents may increase the risk of malignancies, including hepatosplenic T-cell lymphoma, the risks and benefits of these agents should be carefully considered, especially in adolescents and young adults with Crohn's disease or ulcerative colitis. Patients and caregivers should be informed of the potential increased risk of hepatosplenic T-cell lymphoma, especially in adolescents and young adults with inflammatory bowel disease who receive treatment with thiopurine analogs (mercaptopurine or azathioprine) and/or TNF blocking agents, and should be advised of the relative risks and benefits of these and other immunosuppressive agents. Patients and caregivers should be informed of the signs and symptoms of malignancies such as hepatosplenic T-cell lymphoma (e.g., splenomegaly, hepatomegaly, abdominal pain, persistent fever, night sweats, weight loss), and advised to contact a clinician if such signs or symptoms occur. Patients should be advised not to discontinue therapy without consulting a clinician. (See Cautions: Malignancies and Lymphoproliferative Disorders.)

Patients with inherited deficiency of thiopurine *S*-methyl transferase (TPMT) activity are at increased risk of life-threatening myelotoxicity; substantial dosage reduction may be required in these individuals when initiating mercaptopurine therapy. Prior to initiation of mercaptopurine therapy, TPMT genotype in genomic DNA or phenotype of TPMT activity in red blood cells should be determined to identify patients who are either homozygous or heterozygous for the nonfunctional allele of the TPMT gene. Among Caucasians and African Americans, about 10% of patients will have one nonfunctional allele of the TPMT gene (heterozygous deficient) causing low or intermediate TPMT activity. In these patients, higher concentrations of thioguanine nucleotides will accumulate, and mercaptopurine toxicity is more likely. About 0.3% (approximately 1 in 300 patients) will have two nonfunctional alleles of the TMPT gene (homozygous deficient) causing little or no detectable TPMT activity. Substantial reduction of mercaptopurine dosage is required in these patients to avoid excessive cellular accumulation of thioguanine nucleotides and resulting toxicity. (See Dosage Adjustment for TPMT Deficiency under Dosage and Administration: Dosage.)

The TPMT status of a patient may be determined by genotypic or phenotypic testing. Genotypic testing reveals the allelic pattern for the TPMT gene. For about 95% of individuals with reduced activity of the TPMT gene, 3 alleles have been identified: TPMT*2, TPMT*3A, and TPMT*3C. Individuals who are homozygous for any of these alleles are TPMT deficient and those who are heterozygous for these alleles have low or intermediate TPMT activity. Phenotypic testing assesses the level of thiopurine nucleotides or TPMT activity in erythrocytes. Concomitant use of some drugs or recent blood transfusions can cause inaccurate measurements of TPMT activity, so caution is advised in interpreting the results of phenotypic testing.

Patients should be informed that the major toxicities of mercaptopurine are myelosuppression and liver and GI toxicity. Patients who receive myelosuppressive drugs experience an increased frequency of infections as well as possible hemorrhagic complications. Because these complications are potentially fatal, the patient should be instructed to notify the clinician if fever, sore throat, signs of infection, bleeding from any site, or symptoms of anemia occur. Patients also should be instructed to notify the clinician if they experience jaundice, nausea, or vomiting.

The patient's hematologic status must be carefully monitored and hematologic studies (hemoglobin or hematocrit, total leukocyte count, differential cell count, and quantitative platelet count) performed at least once a week during mercaptopurine therapy. Bone marrow examination also may be useful for the evaluation of marrow status. Adjustment of mercaptopurine dosage for hematologic toxicity may be required. (See Dosage and Administration: Dosage: Dosage Modification for Toxicity and Contraindications for Continued Therapy: Hematologic Toxicity.)

Serum transaminase, alkaline phosphatase, and bilirubin concentrations should be determined at weekly intervals during initiation of mercaptopurine therapy and at monthly intervals thereafter. More frequent testing may be advisable in patients with preexisting liver disease or in those receiving other hepatotoxic drugs; concomitant administration of mercaptopurine and other hepatotoxic agents requires particular caution. (See Drug Interactions: Hepatotoxic Drugs.)

Concomitant use with allopurinol or drugs that inhibit TPMT (e.g., olsalazine, mesalamine, sulfasalazine) may exacerbate mercaptopurine toxicity. If allopurinol and mercaptopurine are used concomitantly, the dosage of mercaptopurine should be reduced to 25–33% of the usual dosage. (See Drug Interactions: Allopurinol.)

Patients receiving mercaptopurine may exhibit decreased cellular hypersensitivities and impaired allograft rejection. Induction of immunity to infectious agents or vaccines will be subnormal in these patients. These effects must be considered with regard to intercurrent infections and risk of subsequent neoplasia.

Mercaptopurine is contraindicated in patients whose disease was resistant to prior therapy with the drug. Mercaptopurine is contraindicated in individuals who are hypersensitive to the drug or any component in the formulation.

■ **Pediatric Precautions** Acute lymphocytic leukemia is a common cancer in children and mercaptopurine used in conjunction with methotrexate is an established regimen for maintenance therapy.

Cases of hepatosplenic T-cell lymphoma have been reported in adolescents receiving mercaptopurine for the management of inflammatory bowel disease. (See Cautions: Malignancies and Lymphoproliferative Disorders.)

■ **Geriatric Precautions** Clinical studies of mercaptopurine did not include sufficient numbers of patients 65 years of age and older to determine whether geriatric patients respond differently than younger patients. While other clinical experience has not revealed age-related differences in response or tolerance, drug dosage generally should be titrated carefully in geriatric patients, usually initiating therapy at the low end of the dosage range. The greater frequency of decreased hepatic, renal, and/or cardiac function and of concomitant disease and drug therapy observed in the elderly also should be considered.

■ **Mutagenicity and Carcinogenicity** Mercaptopurine causes chromosomal aberrations in animals and humans and induces dominant-lethal mutations in male mice. The drug is potentially carcinogenic in humans, but the extent of risk is not known. Mercaptopurine may increase the risk of neoplasia in patients; cases of hepatosplenic T-cell lymphoma have been reported in patients receiving mercaptopurine for the management of inflammatory bowel disease. (See Cautions: Malignancies and Lymphoproliferative Disorders.)

■ **Pregnancy, Fertility, and Lactation** Mercaptopurine is potentially teratogenic. The drug can cause fetal toxicity when administered to pregnant women, but potential benefits from use of the drug may be acceptable in certain conditions despite possible risks to the fetus. Women who receive mercaptopurine during the first trimester of pregnancy have an increased incidence of abortion; the risk of malformation in offspring surviving first trimester exposure to the drug is not known. In one series of 28 women who received mercaptopurine after the first trimester of pregnancy, one aborted, one delivered a stillborn child, and three women died without delivering; no macroscopically abnormal fetuses were observed.

There are no adequate and well-controlled studies to date using mercaptopurine in pregnant women. Mercaptopurine should be used during pregnancy only in life-threatening situations or severe disease for which safer drugs cannot be used or are ineffective, and the drug should be used with particular caution during the first trimester of pregnancy. Women of childbearing potential should be advised to avoid becoming pregnant during mercaptopurine therapy. When the drug is administered during pregnancy or if the patient becomes pregnant while receiving the drug, the patient should be informed of the potential hazard to the fetus.

The effect of mercaptopurine on fertility in humans is not known. In mice, the surviving female offspring of mothers who received chronic low doses of mercaptopurine during pregnancy were either were sterile or had pregnancies with smaller litters and more dead fetuses than control animals.

It is not known whether mercaptopurine is distributed into milk. Because of the potential for serious adverse reactions to mercaptopurine in nursing infants, a decision should be made whether to discontinue nursing or the drug, taking into account the importance of the drug to the woman.

Drug Interactions

■ **Allopurinol** In dosages of 300–600 mg daily, allopurinol inhibits the oxidative metabolism of mercaptopurine by xanthine oxidase, thus increasing the possibility of toxic effects of mercaptopurine, particularly bone marrow depression. If allopurinol and mercaptopurine are administered concomitantly, the dosage of mercaptopurine should be reduced to 25–33% of the usual dosage, and subsequent dosage adjusted according to the patient response and toxic effects.

■ **Hepatotoxic Drugs** Because of possible increased risk of liver toxicity, caution should be exercised and hepatic function should be closely monitored in patients receiving mercaptopurine and other hepatotoxic agents. In one study, a high incidence of hepatotoxicity was reported in patients receiving mercaptopurine and doxorubicin, which is not believed to be hepatotoxic.

■ **5-Aminosalicylates** In vitro evidence indicates that aminosalicylate derivatives inhibit TPMT (thiopurine *S*-methyltransferase). Concomitant use with these drugs (e.g., olsalazine, mesalamine, sulfasalazine) may exacerbate the myelotoxicity associated with mercaptopurine therapy and caution is advised.

■ **Myelosuppressive Drugs** The dosage of mercaptopurine may need to be reduced when the drug is used concomitantly with other drugs that cause myelosuppression. Exacerbation of myelosuppression associated with mercaptopurine has been observed in patients receiving trimethoprim-sulfamethoxazole.

■ **Warfarin** Mercaptopurine has been reported to inhibit the anticoagulant activity of warfarin.

Laboratory Test Interferences

Mercaptopurine may interfere with SMA (sequential multiple analyzer) 12/60 determinations, giving falsely elevated serum glucose and uric acid values.

Acute Toxicity

The oral LD_{50} of mercaptopurine is 480 mg/kg in mice and 425 mg/kg in rats.

Manifestations of mercaptopurine overdosage reflect common adverse effects of the drug that may be immediate (e.g., anorexia, nausea, vomiting, diarrhea) or delayed (e.g., myelosuppression, hepatic dysfunction, gastroenteritis).

There is no known antidote for mercaptopurine overdosage. Management of unintended toxicity consists primarily of discontinuance of the drug. Induction of emesis may be helpful immediately following accidental overdosage. Because of rapid intracellular incorporation of mercaptopurine into longlasting active metabolites, hemodialysis is thought to be ineffective in clearing the drug.

Pharmacology

Mercaptopurine is converted intracellularly to a ribonucleotide, which functions as a purine antagonist. Ultimately, the synthesis of RNA and DNA is inhibited. There usually is complete cross-resistance between mercaptopurine and thioguanine.

Mercaptopurine is also a powerful immunosuppressant that strongly inhibits the primary immune response, selectively suppressing humoral immunity; some inhibition of the cellular immune response also occurs.

Pharmacokinetics

■ **Absorption** Absorption of mercaptopurine from the GI tract is variable and incomplete, but about 50% of a dose is usually absorbed. The absolute bioavailability of oral mercaptopurine appears to be lower and extremely variable. However, factors influencing absorption of mercaptopurine are not known. In one study in patients with acute lymphocytic leukemia given oral and IV mercaptopurine doses of 75 mg/m^2, the absolute bioavailability of oral mercaptopurine averaged 16% (range 5–37%); it was suggested that the drug undergoes metabolism in the GI mucosa during absorption and/or on first pass through the liver. After a single oral dose, maximum serum concentrations are reached within 2 hours, and the drug is not detectable in the serum after 8 hours. Because purine antagonists rapidly enter into anabolic and catabolic pathways of purines, blood concentration measurements actually represent several compounds and the interpretation of blood concentrations is difficult.

■ **Distribution** Mercaptopurine and its metabolites are distributed throughout total body water. The volume of distribution of mercaptopurine usually exceeds total body water content. Although the drug reportedly crosses the blood-brain barrier, CSF concentrations are not sufficient for the treatment of meningeal leukemia. It is not known whether mercaptopurine is distributed into milk.

■ **Elimination** Following IV administration of mercaptopurine (an IV preparation of the drug currently is not commercially available in the US), the elimination half-life of the drug is reportedly 21 minutes in pediatric patients and 47 minutes in adults.

Mercaptopurine is metabolized via 2 major pathways. Mercaptopurine is rapidly and extensively oxidized to 6-thiouric acid in the liver by the enzyme xanthine oxidase. Because xanthine oxidase is inhibited by allopurinol, concomitant use of this drug decreases the metabolism of mercaptopurine and its active metabolites and leads to toxicity. If allopurinol and mercaptopurine are used concomitantly, the dosage of mercaptopurine must be reduced to avoid toxicity. (See Dosage Adjustment for Concomitant Use of Allopurinol under Dosage and Administration: Dosage.)

Another major catabolic pathway is thiol methylation of mercaptopurine to form the inactive metabolite methyl-6-MP. This reaction is catalyzed by the enzyme thiopurine *S*-methyltransferase (TPMT). Variability in TPMT activity in patients because of a genetic polymorphism in the TPMT gene causes interindividual differences in the metabolism of mercaptopurine and resulting systemic exposure to the drug and its active metabolites. (For information on dosage adjustment according to TPMT activity, see Dosage Adjustment for TPMT Deficiency under Dosage and Administration: Dosage. For information on genetic polymorphism and variability in the metabolism of mercaptopurine, see Cautions: Precautions and Contraindications.) Dethiolation can also occur, with large portions of the sulfur being excreted as inorganic sulfate.

Mercaptopurine is excreted in urine as unchanged drug and metabolites. In one study in adults with normal renal function, about 11% of an oral dose was recovered in the urine within 6 hours.

Chemistry and Stability

■ **Chemistry** Mercaptopurine is a chemical analog of the physiologic purines, adenine and hypoxanthine. Mercaptopurine, like azathioprine and thioguanine, is a purine antagonist antimetabolite. Mercaptopurine occurs as an odorless or nearly odorless, slightly yellow crystalline powder, is insoluble in water and soluble in hot alcohol, and has a pK_a of 7.6.

■ **Stability** Mercaptopurine tablets should be stored in well-closed containers at a temperature between 15–25°C.

An oral suspension of mercaptopurine containing 50 mg/mL has been prepared extemporaneously from the commercially available tablets. The tablets were crushed, mixed with a volume of suspending agent (Cologel®) equal to one-third the final volume, and then the suspension was brought to the final volume with a 2:1 mixture of simple syrup and wild cherry syrup. The resulting suspension was stable for at least 14 days when stored in an amber glass bottle at room temperature.

For further information on the handling of antineoplastic agents, see the ASHP Guidelines on Handling Hazardous Drugs at http://www.ahfsdruginformation.com.

Preparations

Excipients in commercially available drug preparations may have clinically important effects in some individuals; consult specific product labeling for details.

Mercaptopurine

Oral		
Tablets	50 mg*	**Mercaptopurine Tablets**
		Purinethol® (scored), Teva

*available from one or more manufacturer, distributor, and/or repackager by generic (nonproprietary) name

†Use is not currently included in the labeling approved by the US Food and Drug Administration

Methotrexate
Methotrexate Sodium

Amethopterin, MTX

■ Methotrexate, a folic acid antagonist, is an antineoplastic agent and immunosuppressant.

Uses

■ **Trophoblastic Neoplasms** Methotrexate is used in the treatment of trophoblastic neoplasms (choriocarcinoma, chorioadenoma destruens, and hydatidiform mole) in women except in those with impaired renal or hepatic function or who have failed to respond to previous therapy with methotrexate. These latter patients may be treated with dactinomycin. Methotrexate therapy is most effective in patients who have had the disease for only a short period prior to initiation of chemotherapy, who have low initial gonadotropin concentrations, and who do not have metastases. Complete remissions have been attained in about 75% of patients with metastases and in a higher percentage of patients without metastases. Methotrexate has also been used prophylactically against malignant trophoblastic disease in patients with hydatidiform mole.

In contrast to uterine choriocarcinoma, testicular choriocarcinomas are usually resistant to methotrexate alone. In patients with metastatic tumors of the testes, combination therapy utilizing methotrexate, dactinomycin, and chlorambucil has produced objective responses, as evidenced by decrease in size of metastases and tumor masses and/or lowered urinary chorionic gonadotropin concentrations in approximately 33–50% or more of patients treated. Following initial treatment, repeated courses of therapy at 1- to 3-month intervals for several years appear to be necessary in order to suppress tumor growth. In a few patients there has been an apparently permanent remission but control of tumor growth is often of only short duration.

■ **Leukemias** Methotrexate also is used as a component of various chemotherapeutic regimens in the palliative treatment of acute leukemias. Present regimens are most effective in the treatment of acute lymphocytic (lymphoblastic) leukemia and have been reported to produce remissions in 90% of patients treated. Methotrexate has been used with corticosteroids to induce remissions, but the drug is now most frequently used alone or in combination with other antineoplastic agents for maintenance therapy following induction of remission with vincristine sulfate and prednisone. Combination chemotherapy usually produces longer remissions than use of a single drug. Methotrexate alone rarely is effective in the treatment of acute myeloblastic leukemia; remissions are short with relapses common and resistance develops rapidly. Methotrexate, however, may produce remissions in adults who have responded initially to mercaptopurine and who have become resistant to this drug. In addition, methotrexate has been used in combination regimens in induction of remissions of acute myeloblastic leukemia.

Leukemic infiltration into the meninges and CSF has been relieved temporarily by intrathecal administration of methotrexate. The drug may be effective in patients whose systemic disease has become resistant to methotrexate since leukemic cells in the CNS usually retain their original degree of sensitivity to methotrexate; however, poor responses generally occur in patients with initial methotrexate resistance. Focal leukemic involvement of the CNS may not respond to intrathecal methotrexate and usually responds best to radiation therapy. Methotrexate is also used prophylactically against meningeal leukemia.

■ **Osteosarcoma** High-dose methotrexate, followed by rescue therapy with either leucovorin or levoleucovorin, is used in combination chemotherapy regimens as an adjunct to surgical resection or amputation of the primary tumor in patients with nonmetastatic osteosarcoma. These regimens appear to prolong the relapse-free survival in such patients. Methotrexate is designated an orphan drug by the US Food and Drug Administration (FDA) for use in osteogenic sarcoma.

■ **Breast Cancer** Methotrexate has been used alone or, more commonly, in combination chemotherapy for the treatment of breast cancer.

Combination chemotherapy used as an adjunct to surgery has been shown to increase both disease-free (i.e., decreased recurrence) and overall survival in premenopausal and postmenopausal women with node-negative or -positive early (TNM stage I or II) breast cancer. Adjuvant combination chemotherapy in early breast cancer has produced overall reductions in the annual rates of recurrence and death of 28 and 16%, respectively, with overall 5-year disease-free survival rates of 58.8 versus 49.6% for patients receiving combination chemotherapy versus those who did not. Adjuvant combination chemotherapy that includes methotrexate, cyclophosphamide, and fluorouracil has been used most extensively and is considered a regimen of choice. Although adjuvant hormonal therapy with tamoxifen (with or without combination chemotherapy) generally is used for node-positive, estrogen-receptor-positive postmenopausal women, adjuvant combination chemotherapy (with or without tamoxifen) also can be used in such patients, but differences in toxicity profiles may influence the choice of regimen. For node-positive premenopausal women, adjuvant combination chemotherapy (with or without tamoxifen) generally is used. Adjuvant therapy with combination chemotherapy and/or tamoxifen has been used in women with node-negative disease.

Controversy currently exists regarding which patients with node-negative and estrogen-receptor-negative breast cancer are most likely to benefit from such adjuvant therapy following surgery (see Uses: Breast Cancer, in Fluorouracil 10:00), but such patients with poor prognosis are reasonable candidates for adjuvant chemotherapy with an effective regimen (e.g., 6–12 months of methotrexate, cyclophosphamide, and fluorouracil initiated within 6 weeks of surgery); other node-negative patients also may be suitable candidates, but toxicities, costs, and other quality-of-life considerations should be weighed in assessing potential benefit. All patients with node-negative breast cancer are at some risk of recurrence, and effective adjuvant combination chemotherapy can increase both disease-free and overall survival, albeit less markedly than in patients with node-positive disease.

In patients with node-positive early breast cancer (i.e., stage II), an effective regimen of adjuvant combination chemotherapy (e.g., methotrexate, cyclophosphamide, and fluorouracil; cyclophosphamide, doxorubicin, and fluorouracil; cyclophosphamide and doxorubicin with or without tamoxifen) is used to reduce the rate of recurrence and improve survival in both premenopausal and postmenopausal patients once treatment to control local disease (surgery, with or without radiation therapy) has been undertaken. These combinations have been tested and established as providing therapeutic benefit, and are superior to single-agent therapy with conventional agents; numerous other combination regimens providing apparently similar outcomes also have been used but are less common or have been studied less extensively. Although long-term (e.g., 6 months or longer) chemotherapy with adjuvant regimens is clinically superior to short-term (e.g., preoperative and perioperative) adjuvant regimens, clinical superiority between 6- versus 12-month regimens has not been demonstrated. There is some evidence that the addition of doxorubicin to a regimen of methotrexate, cyclophosphamide, and fluorouracil can improve outcome further in patients with more than 3 positive axillary lymph nodes, and that sequential (i.e., administering several courses of doxorubicin first) regimens are more effective than alternating regimens in such patients; in patients with fewer positive nodes, no additional benefit from doxorubicin has been demonstrated. The dose intensity of adjuvant combination chemotherapy also appears to be an important factor influencing clinical outcome in patients with early node-positive breast cancer, with response increasing with increasing dose intensity; therefore, arbitrary reductions in dose intensity should be avoided. In women with stage II disease and more than 10 positive lymph nodes, high-dose chemotherapy and autologous bone marrow transplant is an option currently being evaluated.

In stage III (locally advanced) breast cancer, combination chemotherapy (with or without hormonal therapy) is used sequentially following surgery and radiation therapy for operable disease and following biopsy and radiation therapy for inoperable disease; commonly employed effective regimens include methotrexate, cyclophosphamide, and fluorouracil; cyclophosphamide, doxorubicin, and fluorouracil; and methotrexate, cyclophosphamide, fluorouracil, and prednisone. These and other regimens also have been used in the treatment or more advanced (stage IV) and recurrent disease.

■ **Lymphoma** Methotrexate may also be useful in the treatment of Burkitt's lymphoma, advanced stages (III and IV, Peters' Staging System) of lymphosarcoma, especially in children when used with other drugs, and in advanced cases of mycosis fungoides (cutaneous T-cell lymphoma). Although radiation therapy is generally used for treatment of localized histiocytic lymphoma, lymphosarcoma, and mycosis fungoides, chemotherapy may be useful in the treatment of generalized stages of these diseases. Hodgkin's disease responds poorly to methotrexate therapy.

■ **Psoriasis** Methotrexate is used in carefully selected patients in the symptomatic control of severe, recalcitrant, disabling psoriasis that is not adequately responsive to other forms of therapy; however, the drug is not curative. Methotrexate should be used in the treatment of psoriasis only after the diagnosis has been definitely established, as by biopsy and/or after dermatologic consultation. Although methotrexate has been reported to produce beneficial effects in up to 75% of patients with psoriasis, there has been only one brief controlled study and the long-term effects of the drug and optimal dosage have not been established. Prior to initiation of methotrexate therapy, patients should be carefully screened to exclude pregnant women and patients with renal, hepatic or hematopoietic disease, or infections. The potential benefit to the patient must be carefully weighed against the possible risks involved and patients should be informed of potential toxicity.

Methotrexate has also been used topically in the treatment of psoriasis; however, results of one study indicated that the drug had little visible effect on the psoriatic lesions and another reported that the usefulness of topical methotrexate was limited by adverse effects on the surrounding skin.

■ **Rheumatoid Arthritis** Methotrexate is used for the management of rheumatoid arthritis in adults whose symptoms progress despite an adequate regimen of nonsteroidal anti-inflammatory agents (NSAIAs). Methotrexate is one of several disease-modifying antirheumatic drugs (DMARDs) that can be used when DMARD therapy is appropriate.

Pharmacologic therapy for rheumatoid arthritis usually consists of combinations of nonsteroidal anti-inflammatory agents (NSAIAs), DMARDs, and/or corticosteroids. The ultimate goal in managing rheumatoid arthritis is to prevent or control joint damage, prevent loss of function, and decrease pain. Although NSAIAs may be useful for initial symptomatic treatment of rheumatoid arthritis, these drugs do not alter the course of the disease or prevent joint destruction. DMARDs have the potential to reduce or prevent joint damage, preserve joint integrity and function, and reduce total health care costs, and all patients with rheumatoid arthritis are candidates for DMARD therapy. DMARDs should be initiated early in the disease course and should not be delayed beyond 3 months in patients with active disease (i.e., ongoing joint pain, substantial morning stiffness, fatigue, active synovitis, persistent elevation of erythrocyte sedimentation rate [ESR] or C-reactive protein [CRP], radiographic evidence of joint damage) despite an adequate regimen of NSAIAs. DMARDs commonly used in the treatment of rheumatoid arthritis include methotrexate, etanercept, hydroxychloroquine, infliximab, leflunomide, and sulfasalazine. Less frequently used DMARDs include azathioprine, cyclosporine, minocycline, penicillamine, and/or oral or injectable gold compounds. The role of anakinra, a recombinant human interleukin-1 (IL-1) receptor antagonist, in the management of rheumatoid arthritis remains to be established.

While many factors influence the choice of a DMARD, methotrexate has substantially greater long-term efficacy than other DMARDs and is used as the initial or anchor DMARD in many patients with rheumatoid arthritis. Because residual inflammation generally persists in patients receiving maximum dosages of a single DMARD, many rheumatoid arthritis patients are candidates for combination therapy to achieve optimum control. Although the most effective combination regimen of DMARDs has not been determined, regimens that have been found efficacious in clinical studies include combinations of methotrexate and cyclosporine, etanercept, hydroxychloroquine, infliximab, leflunomide, or sulfasalazine.

Low-dose oral corticosteroids and local injection of corticosteroids are effective in relieving symptoms in patients with active rheumatoid arthritis. In addition, limited evidence indicates that low-dose corticosteroids slow the rate of joint damage.

Several international groups of rheumatologists have issued consensus reports that address the role of tumor necrosis factor (TNF) blocking agents (e.g., etanercept, infliximab) in the management of rheumatoid arthritis. These groups state that use of TNF blocking agents is most appropriate in patients with active disease (5 swollen joints and elevated acute-phase response [ESR of 28 mm/hour or greater, or CRP level of 2 mg/dL or greater]) despite adequate exposure to methotrexate or other effective DMARD. A course of methotrexate in a dosage of at least 20 mg weekly (or lower dosage if toxicity develops) for 3 months is considered an adequate course of DMARD therapy, and failure with such a course should prompt consideration of modification of the therapeutic regimen (e.g., initiation of a TNF blocking agent). Other factors to consider when deciding whether to use a TNF blocking agent in the treatment of rheumatoid arthritis are differences in the aggressiveness of the disease, extent of structural damage, effects of the disease on quality of life, and toxicity of previously used DMARDs.

Once therapy with a TNF blocking agent has been started, patients should be assessed for therapeutic response (e.g., a 20% reduction in swollen joint count with a 20% reduction in acute-phase response). While therapy should be continued indefinitely in those who have responded to therapy and are not experiencing substantial adverse effects, therapy with the TNF blocking agent should be discontinued in patients who have not responded after 12 weeks.

Administration of methotrexate alone is not a complete treatment for rheumatoid arthritis, and the drug should be used only as part of a comprehensive treatment program, including nondrug therapies such as rest and physical therapy. Most patients with active rheumatoid arthritis will show some benefit from methotrexate therapy, although improvement often plateaus during the first 6 months of therapy with the drug (occasionally being maintained for 2 years or longer) and may wane during continued use. There is no substantial evidence that methotrexate permanently arrests or reverses the underlying disease process, although the drug slows its progression in some patients. NSAIA and/or low-dose corticosteroid therapy may be continued when methotrexate therapy is initiated; however, the possible increased risk of toxicity with concomitant use of methotrexate and NSAIAs should be considered. (See Drug Interactions: Protein Bound Drugs and Weak Organic Acids, and also Nonsteroidal Anti-inflammatory Agents.) Depending on the patient's response to methotrexate, corticosteroid dosage may be gradually reduced. The manufacturer of methotrexate states that combined use of methotrexate and gold compounds, penicillamine, hydroxychloroquine, sulfasalazine, or other antirheumatic cytotoxic or immunosuppressive agents has not been adequately studied to date and may increase the risk of adverse effects.

■ **Head and Neck Cancer** Methotrexate is used alone and in combination therapy for the palliative treatment of recurrent or metastatic head and neck carcinoma. When used alone, at a dosage of 40–60 mg/m² once weekly, methotrexate produces an average objective response rate of 30%. Duration of response is short at an average of 4 months.

In a randomized study, patients with recurrent or metastatic squamous cell carcinoma of the head and neck who received cisplatin and fluorouracil, carboplatin and fluorouracil, or methotrexate alone had objective response rates of 32, 21, or 10%, respectively. Although the objective response rate achieved with cisplatin and fluorouracil was greater than that observed with methotrexate alone, combination chemotherapy was associated with increased toxicity and no difference in survival was observed. In patients with recurrent or metastatic head and neck cancer who cannot tolerate combination therapy with cisplatin and fluorouracil, weekly low-dose methotrexate may be used.

Methotrexate frequently is used in combination regimens with other antineoplastic agents (e.g., bleomycin, fluorouracil, vincristine). Combination therapy with cisplatin, methotrexate, bleomycin, and vincristine has been used for the treatment of recurrent or metastatic squamous cell carcinoma of the head and neck. Further study is needed to establish the comparative benefit of methotrexate-containing regimens in the treatment of advanced head and neck cancer.

■ **Crohn's Disease** Methotrexate has been used for its anti-inflammatory effects in the management of Crohn's disease†. Results of several open-label, and double-blind, placebo-controlled studies in adults indicate that use of methotrexate can result in clinical response (including clinical remission) in patients with chronically active Crohn's disease who have not responded to prior therapies (e.g., corticosteroids, other immunosuppressants), although efficacy of orally administered methotrexate has not been consistently reported in placebo-controlled clinical studies.

Safety and efficacy of parenteral methotrexate in the management of active Crohn's disease was evaluated in a double-blind placebo-controlled multicenter 16-week study that included 141 adults with chronically active Crohn's disease who had inadequate response to a corticosteroid (i.e. , prednisone). To be included in the study, patients had to have a chronically active disease unresponsive to a minimum of 3-months of therapy with prednisone (12.5 mg daily) with at least one attempt to discontinue the corticosteroid. At baseline, patients had a median Crohn's Disease Activity Index (CDAI) of 181–190. The CDAI score is based on subjective observations by the patient (e.g., the daily number of liquid or very soft stools, severity of abdominal pain, general well-being) and objective evidence (e.g., number of extraintestinal manifestations, presence of an abdominal mass, use or nonuse of antidiarrheal drugs, the hematocrit, body weight). Patients were randomized to receive IM methotrexate (94 patients; 25 mg once weekly) or placebo (47 patients). Patients continued to receive prednisone, which was tapered over 10 weeks (starting 2 weeks after randomization), unless their condition worsened; however, no other drugs used for management of Crohn's disease (e.g., oral or topical derivatives of 5-aminosalicylic acid, budesonide, other immunosuppressive agents, topical corticosteroids) were allowed. The primary outcome was clinical remission (defined as a CDAI index of 150 points or less and discontinuance of prednisone) at the end of the trial (16 weeks). Clinical remission at the end of the study was reported in 39 or 19% of patients receiving methotrexate or placebo, respectively. In addition, patients receiving methotrexate used less prednisone overall and had a lower mean average CDAI score than those receiving placebo (170 points for methotrexate versus 193 points for placebo). Many patients in this study who entered remission after 16–24 weeks of treatment with IM methotrexate (25 mg weekly) were enrolled in a new trial which evaluated the safety and efficacy of parenteral methotrexate for maintenance therapy of Crohn's disease. In this multicenter, double-blind, placebo-controlled trial, 76 patients with chronically active Crohn's disease in remission were randomized to receive 15 mg of IM methotrexate once weekly (40 patients) or placebo (36 patients) for 40 weeks; no other treatment for Crohn's disease was allowed. After 40 weeks, a greater proportion of patients receiving methotrexate were free of relapse (defined as an increase of baseline CDAI of 100 points or more, or the need to initiate therapy for active disease) than those receiving placebo (65% for methotrexate versus 39% for placebo); in addition, a smaller proportion of patients receiving methotrexate required prednisone therapy for relapse when compared with those receiving placebo (28% for methotrexate versus 58% for placebo).

Safety and efficacy of oral methotrexate in the management of chronically active Crohn's disease was evaluated in 2 other randomized double-blind, placebo-controlled trials in 59 corticosteroid-dependent adults. Patients received a weekly oral methotrexate dosage of 12.5 mg for 9 months in one trial and 15–22.5 mg for up to 1 year in the other. Efficacy (measured by reduction of dosage of corticosteroids, reduction in CDAI, or reduction in Harvey Bradshaw index) of oral methotrexate was similar to that of oral mercaptopurine (50 mg daily) in one of the studies and to placebo in both studies.

Some clinicians state that pediatric patients† with corticosteroid-dependent or corticosteroid-resistant, moderately to severely active Crohn's disease† who had an inadequate response to or were intolerant of azathioprine or mercaptopurine, may receive methotrexate (10–15 mg/m² weekly) for the management of such disease. (See Cautions: Pediatric Precautions.)

For further information on the management of Crohn's disease, see Uses: Crohn's Disease, in Mesalamine 56:36.

■ Other Uses Methotrexate is used in combination regimens with cisplatin and vinblastine, with or without doxorubicin, for the treatment of invasive and advanced bladder cancer. (See Uses: Bladder Cancer, in Cisplatin 10:00.) Because methotrexate is absorbed through the ileum, placement of a Foley catheter or frequent emptying of the reservoir is advised in patients with long ileal loops or internal reservoirs during administration of methotrexate-containing regimens for the treatment of advanced or metastatic bladder cancer. Because elimination of methotrexate may be impaired and risk of toxicity increased in patients with renal dysfunction, edema, pleural fluid collections, or ascites, use of leucovorin rescue or deletion of methotrexate is advised if methotrexate-containing regimens are being considered for the treatment of advanced or metastatic bladder cancer in such patients.

Methotrexate has been used in second-line therapy for the treatment of recurrent small cell lung cancer. Although methotrexate is labeled for use in the treatment of the squamous cell type of non-small cell lung cancer, other agents are preferred for the treatment of this neoplasm.

Methotrexate has been used in treating a variety of solid tumors†. In some studies, the drug has been administered by intra-arterial infusion alone or in conjunction with IM leucovorin calcium in the palliative management of carcinomas capable of being infused via a single artery. Low-dose oral methotrexate has been used in patients with chronic progressive multiple sclerosis†. Results of several clinical studies indicate that low-dose methotrexate (7.5 mg weekly for up to 2 years) reduces both disease activity (as assessed by magnetic resonance imaging [MRI]) and sustained progression of disability (as assessed by the Expanded Disability Status Scale, the Ambulation Index, and standardized tests of upper extremity function). Patients with secondary progressive multiple sclerosis benefited the most from methotrexate therapy.

Methotrexate has been used for its immunosuppressive and/or anti-inflammatory effects in the treatment of psoriatic arthritis†, systemic lupus erythematosus†, vasculitis†, dermatomyositis†, polymyositis†, Wegener's granulomatosis†, and a variety of dermatologic and chronic refractory ocular diseases†. Controlled studies have shown that oral or parenteral methotrexate therapy is effective in the short-term management of psoriatic arthritis; however, because of its potential toxicities, methotrexate is generally used in the management of this condition only in patients whose disease is severe and/or unresponsive to conventional therapy.

Dosage and Administration

■ Reconstitution and Administration Methotrexate is administered orally. Methotrexate sodium is administered by IM, IV, or intrathecal injection; the drug may also be administered intra-arterially.

Methotrexate sodium injection and powder for injection should be reconstituted according to the manufacturers' directions.

For the treatment of meningeal leukemia, methotrexate must be administered intrathecally since passage of the drug from the blood to CSF is minimal. Prior to intrathecal administration of methotrexate, a volume of CSF approximately equivalent to the volume of methotrexate solution to be injected (e.g., 5–15 mL) is usually removed. If a lumbar puncture is traumatic, methotrexate should not be administered intrathecally. Two days should elapse before again attempting the injection. Methotrexate should be injected intrathecally only if there is easy flow of blood-free spinal fluid. Some clinicians recommend that the entire volume of methotrexate injection be injected intrathecally in 15–30 seconds. Aspiration should not be performed. *For intrathecal injection, preservative-free methotrexate solutions containing 1 mg/mL are used*; solutions may be prepared using preservative-free 0.9% sodium chloride injection as a diluent. *Methotrexate formulations or diluents containing preservatives must not be used for intrathecal administration or high-dose methotrexate therapy.*

Methotrexate sodium solutions should be inspected visually for particulate matter and discoloration whenever solution and container permit.

■ Dosage Methotrexate should only be used under the supervision of a clinician who is experienced in cancer chemotherapy and in the use of antimetabolites. (See Cautions: Precautions and Contraindications.) Dosage of methotrexate sodium is expressed in terms of methotrexate. Various dosage schedules for methotrexate therapy alone and in combination with other antineoplastic agents and/or radiation therapy have appeared in the literature; dosage, route of administration, and duration of therapy must be individualized according to the disease being treated, other therapy being employed, and the condition, response, and tolerance of the patient. In patients in whom discontinuance of methotrexate has been required, therapy should be reinstituted with caution, giving complete consideration to further need for the drug and the possibility of recurrence of toxicity. Clinicians should consult published protocols for additional dosages of methotrexate and other chemotherapeutic agents and the method and sequence of administration.

Careful review of the intended use for methotrexate should be undertaken to ensure that inadvertent overdosage (e.g., administering antineoplastic rather than anti-inflammatory dosages) does not occur. Dosages used in rheumatic conditions (e.g., rheumatoid arthritis, psoriasis) and certain inflammatory GI conditions (e.g., Crohn's disease†) are substantially lower than those used to treat cancer, and intermittent dosing rather than daily dosing is used for such inflammatory conditions. It is essential that any order for daily dosing of the drug be reviewed carefully to ensure that the intended use is an antineoplastic one. Inadvertent daily administration of the drug for non-cancer uses can prove fatal. Regimens for rheumatic conditions and certain inflammatory GI conditions employ intermittent dosing, usually once weekly as a single dose or once weekly as 3-divided doses at 12-hour intervals. Clinicians also should ensure that printed materials (e.g., discharge instructions) patients and/or their caregivers receive describe the correct dosing regimen for their condition, and they should be instructed carefully about their prescribed regimen, paying particular attention to the frequency of administration.

Trophoblastic Neoplasms For the treatment of trophoblastic neoplasms, the usual dosage of methotrexate is 15–30 mg daily, administered orally or IM for 5 days. A repeat course may be given after a period of one or more weeks provided all signs of residual toxicity have disappeared. Three to five courses of therapy are usually employed. Therapy is usually evaluated by 24-hour quantitative analysis of urinary chorionic gonadotropin which should return to normal or less than 50 IU/24 hours, usually after the third or fourth course. Complete resolution of measurable lesions usually occurs 4–6 weeks later. One or two courses of methotrexate therapy are usually given after normalization of urinary chorionic gonadotropin hormone concentrations is achieved. In the treatment of trophoblastic disease in women, regimens alternating courses of methotrexate therapy and dactinomycin therapy or combining administration of methotrexate and mercaptopurine or methotrexate, dactinomycin, and chlorambucil have also been used. In the treatment of trophoblastic disease in women, 10–15 mg of methotrexate daily has also been administered via the hypogastric artery† until toxicity or therapeutic response occurred. Combination chemotherapy with methotrexate, chlorambucil, and dactinomycin has been used in the treatment of metastatic testicular tumors in men.

Leukemia Although methotrexate is not generally a drug of choice for induction of remission of lymphoblastic leukemia, oral methotrexate dosage of 3.3 mg/m² daily and prednisone 60 mg/m² daily for 4–6 weeks have been used. After a remission is attained, maintenance therapy with methotrexate is administered twice weekly, orally or by IM injection, for a total weekly dose of 30 mg/m². Administration of the drug in twice-weekly doses appears to be more effective than daily drug administration. Alternatively, 2.5 mg/kg has been administered IV every 14 days.

For the treatment of meningeal leukemia, an intrathecal methotrexate dosage of 12 mg/m² or an empiric dose of 15 mg, administered at 2- to 5-day intervals until CSF cell counts return to normal, has been suggested; this is then followed by one additional dose of the drug. Alternatively, 12 mg/m² has been administered once weekly for 2 weeks and then once monthly thereafter. For prophylaxis against meningeal leukemia, a methotrexate dose of 12 mg/m² or 15 mg has been used; the intervals for administration differ from the regimen used in the treatment of meningeal leukemia, and specialized references and the medical literature should be consulted for specific recommendations. However, because the volume of CSF is related to age and not body surface area, dosage regimens based on body surface area may result in inadequate CSF concentrations in children and high, potentially neurotoxic CSF concentrations in adults; therefore, some clinicians recommend that intrathecal dosage be based on the patient's age. Clinical studies indicate that intrathecal methotrexate dosage regimens based on age may be more effective and less neurotoxic than dosage regimens based on body surface area. The suggested intrathecal doses based on age are 6 mg for children younger than 1 year of age, 8 mg for children 1 year of age, 10 mg for children 2 years of age, and 12 mg for children 3 years of age or older and for adults; geriatric patients may require reduced doses because of reduced CSF turnover and decreasing brain volume. *Regardless of the method used to determine intrathecal methotrexate dosage, the dose should be carefully checked prior to administration to minimize the risk of inadvertent intrathecal overdosage.* Because methotrexate appears in systemic circulation following intrathecal administration, systemic administration of the drug should be appropriately adjusted, reduced, or discontinued. Systemic administration of leucovorin calcium simultaneously with intrathecal methotrexate may prevent systemic toxicity without abolishing the activity of the antimetabolite in the CNS. The manufacturers state that focal leukemic involvement of the CNS may not respond to intrathecal methotrexate therapy and may be best treated with radiation therapy.

Osteosarcoma The recommended initial dose for high-dose methotrexate treatment of nonmetastatic osteosarcoma is 12 g/m² administered by IV infusion over 4 hours (followed by leucovorin or levoleucovorin rescue) on postoperative weeks 4, 5, 6, 7, 11, 12, 15, 16, 29, 30, 44, and 45, on a schedule in combination with other chemotherapy agents (e.g., doxorubicin, cisplatin, the combination of bleomycin, cyclophosphamide, and dactinomycin [BCD regimen]). If the initial dosage is not sufficient to produce peak serum methotrexate concentrations of 454 mcg/mL (1000 μM [10^{-3} mol/L]) at the end of the infusion, the dose may be increased to 15 g/m² in subsequent treatments.

Leucovorin and levoleucovorin are used as rescue therapy following a high-dose methotrexate regimen to prevent acute toxicity. Leucovorin is administered orally, IM, or by IV injection starting 24 hours after the beginning of the methotrexate infusion. If the patient experiences GI toxicity (e.g., nausea, vomiting), leucovorin should be administered parenterally. The usual dosage of leucovorin is 15 mg (approximately 10 mg/m²) orally, IM, or by IV injection every 6 hours for a total of 60 hours or a total of 10 doses. (See Leucovorin Calcium 92:12.)

Levoleucovorin is administered as an IV infusion at a rate no faster than 160 mg of levoleucovorin per minute every 6 hours for a total of 60 hours or a total of 10 doses, starting 24 hours after the beginning of the methotrexate infusion. (See Levoleucovorin Calcium 92:12.)

Patients receiving high-dose methotrexate regimens must be well hydrated and carefully monitored. (See Cautions: Precautions and Contraindications.) For specific information on dosage modifications, cautions, and precautions associated with high-dose methotrexate therapy, the manufacturer's prescribing information should be consulted.

Breast Cancer Various methotrexate-containing combination chemotherapy regimens have been used in the treatment of breast cancer, and published protocols should be consulted for dosages and the method and sequence of administration. The dose intensity of adjuvant combination chemotherapy appears to be an important factor influencing clinical outcome in patients with early node-positive breast cancer, with response increasing with increasing dose intensity; therefore, *arbitrary* reductions in dose intensity should be avoided.

One commonly employed regimen for the treatment of early breast cancer includes a methotrexate dosage of 40 mg/m² (administered IV) on days 1 and 8 of each cycle combined with cyclophosphamide 100 mg/m² on days 1 through 14 of each cycle and fluorouracil 600 mg/m² on days 1 and 8 of each cycle. In patients older than 60 years of age, the initial methotrexate dosage was reduced to 30 mg/m² and the initial fluorouracil dosage was reduced to 400 mg/m². Dosage also was reduced if myelosuppression developed. Cycles generally were repeated monthly (i.e., allowing a 2-week rest period between cycles) for a total of 6–12 cycles (i.e., 6–12 months of therapy). Clinical superiority between 6- versus 12-month regimens has not been demonstrated.

There is some evidence that the addition of doxorubicin to a regimen of cyclophosphamide, methotrexate, and fluorouracil can improve outcome further in patients with early breast cancer and more than 3 positive axillary lymph nodes, and that sequential (i.e., administering several courses of doxorubicin first) regimens are more effective than alternating regimens in such patients; in patients with fewer positive nodes, no additional benefit from doxorubicin has been demonstrated. In the sequential regimen, 4 doses of doxorubicin hydrochloride 75 mg/m² were administered initially at 3-week intervals followed by 8 cycles of methotrexate 40 mg/m², cyclophosphamide 600 mg/m², and fluorouracil 600 mg/m² at 3-week intervals for a total of approximately 9 months of therapy. If myelosuppression developed with this sequential regimen, the subsequent cycle generally was delayed rather than reducing dosage.

Burkitt's Lymphoma and Lymphosarcoma The usual dosage of methotrexate for the treatment of stages I or II of Burkitt's lymphoma is 10–25 mg/day orally for 4–8 days. Methotrexate is commonly given concomitantly with other antineoplastic agents in the treatment of stage III Burkitt's lymphoma and lymphosarcomas. In all stages, several courses of drug therapy are usually administered interposed with 7- to 10-day rest periods. Stage III lymphosarcomas may respond to combined drug therapy with methotrexate given in doses of 0.625–2.5 mg/kg daily.

Mycosis Fungoides Clinical response occurs in up to 50% of patients receiving single-agent therapy with methotrexate for mycosis fungoides (cutaneous T-cell lymphoma). In early stages of the disease, the usual dosage is 5–50 mg orally once weekly. The need for dosage reduction or discontinuance of therapy is determined by response to therapy and hematologic monitoring. Methotrexate also has been administered twice weekly in doses of 15–37.5 mg in patients with disease that has responded poorly to once-weekly dosing. In patients with advanced stages of mycosis fungoides, combination chemotherapy regimens that include IV methotrexate in higher doses followed by leucovorin rescue have been used.

Psoriasis For the management of psoriasis, a single 5- to 10-mg dose of methotrexate should be given 1 week prior to initiation of methotrexate therapy to detect idiosyncratic reactions. Optimum dosage has not been established and dosage must be based on individual requirements and response. Dosage must be constantly supervised by a physician who is experienced in the use of antineoplastic agents.

There are 2 dosage schedules suggested by the manufacturers. To avoid potentially lethal overdosage, patients should be instructed carefully about their dosage regimen, paying particular attention to the frequency of administration.

The divided oral dosage schedule, which is based on cellular kinetic studies, consists of 2.5 mg of methotrexate administered orally at 12-hour intervals for 3 doses each week; in this regimen, dosage may be increased gradually by 2.5 mg/week, but weekly dosage should usually not exceed 25 mg and should *not* exceed 30 mg.

In the weekly single-dosage schedule, the manufacturers suggest that 10–25 mg may be administered orally, IM, or IV as a single dose once weekly. The usual oral dose in the weekly single-dosage schedule is 7.5–25 mg, with an occasional patient requiring up to 37.5 mg; dosage may be increased gradually by 2.5–5 mg/week. The usual IM or rapid IV dose in the weekly single-dosage schedule is 7.5–50 mg, with an occasional patient requiring up to 100 mg; dosage may be increased gradually. The manufacturers state that the oral, IM, or IV dose in the weekly single-dosage schedule should usually not exceed 50 mg.

In most patients, substantial improvement usually occurs within 4 weeks and optimum results occur in 2–3 months. Cessation of methotrexate usually results in a recurrence of symptoms in 2 weeks to 6 months. After optimal response is achieved, each schedule should be reduced to the lowest possible dose with the longest possible rest period. Conventional topical therapy should be resumed as soon as possible.

Psoriatic Arthritis The optimum dosage of methotrexate in the management of psoriatic arthritis† has not been clearly established, although oral and parenteral dosage regimens similar to those used in the management of psoriasis have been employed. Clinicians should consult specialized references for detailed information on specific dosage regimens.

Rheumatoid Arthritis For the management of rheumatoid arthritis, a single test dose of methotrexate may be given prior to initiation of therapy to detect possible sensitivity to adverse effects associated with the drug. Optimum dosage has not been fully established and dosage must be based on individual requirements and response. Patients receiving methotrexate therapy for rheumatoid arthritis must be constantly supervised by a physician who is experienced in the use of antineoplastic agents. The mnemonic dispensing packages (Rheumatrex® Dose Pack) may be used for initial methotrexate therapy and are suitable for maintenance therapy in patients receiving weekly methotrexate doses of 5–20 mg; however, use of these dispensing packages is *not* recommended for titration to weekly doses higher than 20 mg. To avoid potentially lethal overdosage, patients should be instructed carefully about their dosage regimen, paying particular attention to the frequency of administration.

For the management of rheumatoid arthritis, methotrexate is administered in low-dose, intermittent (i.e., weekly rather than daily) regimens. The usual initial dosage in adults is 7.5 mg orally once weekly. This dosage may be administered either in a single-dosage schedule consisting of a single 7. 5-mg oral dose once weekly or in a divided-dosage schedule consisting of 2.5 mg of methotrexate administered orally at 12-hour intervals for 3 doses each week. Dosage in either the single- or divided-dosage schedule may be gradually increased until an optimum therapeutic response is achieved. However, dosage usually should not exceed 20 mg weekly, since higher dosages have been associated with a substantially increased incidence and severity of serious adverse reactions (e.g., bone marrow suppression). After an optimum response to the drug is achieved, the weekly dosage should be reduced to the lowest possible effective level. Therapeutic response in patients with rheumatoid arthritis usually is apparent within 3–6 weeks, but optimum response may not be achieved for another 3 or more months of therapy. The optimum duration of therapy is unknown; however, limited data from long-term clinical studies indicate that initial clinical improvement may be maintained for prolonged periods (e.g., 2 years or longer) with continued methotrexate therapy. Following discontinuance of the drug, rheumatoid arthritis usually worsens within 3–6 weeks.

Parenteral methotrexate regimens in the management of rheumatoid arthritis are variable, but have often consisted of 7.5–15 mg given IM once weekly in adults†.

Crohn's Disease For the management of Crohn's disease†, methotrexate has been administered in low-dose, intermittent (i.e., weekly rather than daily) regimens. For the management of chronically active, refractory Crohn's disease, methotrexate has been administered once weekly either IM in a dosage of 25 mg for 16 weeks or orally in a dosage of 12.5–22.5 mg for up to 1 year. For maintenance therapy of Crohn's disease, an IM methotrexate dosage of 15 mg weekly has been used.

Cautions

The major toxic effects of methotrexate are on normal, rapidly proliferating tissues, particularly of the bone marrow and lining of the GI tract. These adverse effects generally are dose related and are reversible if detected early. Ulcerations of the oral mucosa are usually the earliest signs of toxicity, but in some patients bone marrow depression coincides with or precedes the appearance of mouth lesions.

■ **Hematologic Effects** Leukopenia, thrombocytopenia, anemia, and hemorrhage from various sites may result from methotrexate therapy and may develop rapidly. In one study using single IV doses of methotrexate, the nadir of hemoglobin concentrations occurred in 6–13 days and was followed by recovery; reticulocytes reached their nadir in 2–7 days followed by recovery with rebound between 9 and 19 days. Leukocytes generally had two periods of depression; the first occurred in 4–7 days with recovery in 7–13 days and the second in 12–21 days with recovery in 15–29 days. Platelets reached their minimum in 5–12 days and recovered in number in 15–27 days.

Thrombocytopenia has been reported in approximately 5%, leukopenia and pancytopenia in approximately 1.5%, and decreased hematocrit and epistaxis in less than 1% of patients receiving 12–18 weeks of methotrexate for the management of rheumatoid arthritis.

■ **GI Effects** Toxic effects of methotrexate on oral and GI mucosa are manifested by gingivitis, glossitis, pharyngitis, stomatitis, enteritis, ulcerations and bleeding of the mucous membranes of the mouth or other portions of the GI tract, abdominal distress, anorexia, nausea, vomiting, hematemesis, diarrhea, and melena. If ulcerative stomatitis or diarrhea occurs, methotrexate therapy must be interrupted in order to prevent hemorrhagic enteritis and death from intestinal perforation.

Pancreatitis also has been reported in patients receiving methotrexate.

■ **Hepatic Effects** Methotrexate therapy has been associated with both acute and chronic hepatotoxicity. Acutely, elevations in serum aminotransferase (transaminase) concentrations frequently occur 1–3 days after a dose of the drug. Such elevations generally are transient, asymptomatic, and do not appear to be predictive of subsequent hepatic damage. Elevated liver function test results reportedly occurred in approximately 15% of patients receiving 12–18 weeks of methotrexate for the management of rheumatoid arthritis.

Hepatotoxicity manifested as hepatic fibrosis or cirrhosis or other histologic changes in the liver has occurred during long-term methotrexate therapy; such hepatotoxicity may require hepatic allotransplantation and can be fatal. In patients with psoriasis, when such changes occur, they often may *not* be preceded by symptoms of hepatotoxicity or abnormal liver function test results; in patients with rheumatoid arthritis, prolonged, substantial abnormalities in liver function test results may precede appearance of hepatic fibrosis or cirrhosis. Chronic hepatotoxicity generally has been associated with prolonged (2 years or longer) methotrexate therapy and cumulative doses of 1.5 g or more. Although accurate estimates of the incidence of chronic hepatotoxicity currently are not available, the incidence appears to be greater in patients receiving frequent (e.g., daily), small doses of the drug (such as the daily-dosage regimen used for psoriasis) than in those receiving intermittent regimens (such as those used for neoplastic disease and possibly rheumatoid arthritis). The risk of developing chronic hepatotoxicity in patients receiving methotrexate therapy for the management of psoriasis appears to be related to the cumulative dose of the drug, and presence of concurrent conditions such as alcoholism, obesity, or diabetes as well as advanced age appear to contribute to this risk. Although clinical experience is limited, these risk factors also may apply to patients receiving methotrexate therapy for the management of rheumatoid arthritis. In one retrospective analysis in a limited number of patients with rheumatoid arthritis who underwent periodic percutaneous liver biopsy as routine monitoring for potential hepatotoxicity while receiving intermittent methotrexate regimens for an average of 32 months, progressive hepatic changes, principally progression to mild to moderate fatty infiltration with portal inflammation, occurred in about 20% of these patients; alterations in liver function test results were not predictive of such changes. In this study, fibrosis that developed in patients with rheumatoid arthritis was considered mild and no patient with rheumatoid arthritis developed cirrhosis; however, the drug was discontinued in most patients when fibrosis was evident and additional study and experience are necessary to better elucidate the potential risk of hepatotoxicity associated with methotrexate therapy for arthritis.

Although various pathologic hepatic changes including atrophy, necrosis, fatty changes, fibrosis, and cirrhosis have been observed in patients with methotrexate-induced hepatotoxicity, no specific pathologic finding appears to be characteristic of methotrexate hepatotoxicity. The rate of progression of hepatic lesions with continued therapy and the potential reversibility of such lesions following discontinuance of the drug currently are not known. (See Cautions: Precautions and Contraindications.)

■ **Respiratory Effects** Pulmonary toxicity, which can progress rapidly and is potentially fatal, has been associated with methotrexate therapy. Adverse pulmonary effects, including pulmonary fibrosis and acute or chronic interstitial pneumonitis, appear to occur at any time during therapy at any dosage of the drug, including low dosages. Although the clinical presentation of methotrexate-induced pulmonary toxicity is variable, manifestations commonly include fever, cough (especially one that is dry and nonproductive), dyspnea, chest pain, hypoxemia (which can be severe), and/or radiographic evidence of pulmonary infiltrates (usually diffuse and/or alveolar). Lung biopsies have revealed variable degrees of interstitial inflammation, granulomatous inflammation, and/or fibrosis. Because patients with rheumatoid arthritis may have underlying interstitial pulmonary changes associated with their disease, it may be difficult to differentiate such changes from potential methotrexate-induced changes; however, rheumatoid changes generally progress more slowly. In addition, a potential association between preexisting rheumatoid pulmonary changes and susceptibility to methotrexate-induced pulmonary toxicity has been suggested but requires further elucidation.

The possibility of methotrexate-induced pulmonary toxicity should be considered in any patient who develops pulmonary manifestations (e.g., dry, nonproductive cough; dyspnea) while receiving the drug. If such manifestations occur, methotrexate should be discontinued and careful clinical evaluation of the patient performed, including exclusion of possible infectious causes. Management of methotrexate-induced pulmonary toxicity mainly is supportive and may include mechanical ventilation; limited evidence suggests that administration of relatively high dosages of corticosteroids may provide some benefit, but additional experience is necessary. In addition, pulmonary toxicity induced by the drug may not be fully reversible and fatalities have been reported.

■ **Dermatologic and Sensitivity Reactions** Severe, occasionally fatal cutaneous or sensitivity reactions (e.g., toxic epidermic necrolysis, Stevens-Johnson syndrome, exfoliative dermatitis, skin necrosis, erythema multiforme) have been reported in pediatric and adult patients within days of receiving single or multiple oral, IM, IV, or intrathecal doses of methotrexate. These reactions occurred following high-, intermediate-, or low-dose methotrexate therapy in patients with neoplastic or non-neoplastic diseases. Recovery has been reported after discontinuance of the drug. Other adverse dermatologic effects of methotrexate include erythematous rashes, pruritus, dermatitis, urticaria, folliculitis, photosensitivity, depigmentation, hyperpigmentation, petechiae, ecchymoses, telangiectasia, acne, and furunculosis. Alopecia occasionally occurs. Regrowth of hair usually occurs after methotrexate is discontinued but may require several months. Burning and erythema may occur in psoriatic areas for 1–2 days following each dose of the drug and psoriatic lesions may be aggravated by concomitant exposure to ultraviolet radiation. In addition, painful plaque erosions rarely have been reported in patients receiving methotrexate for the treatment of psoriasis.

■ **Effects following Intrathecal Administration** Following intrathecal administration of methotrexate, acute chemical arachnoiditis manifested by headache, back pain, nuchal rigidity, and/or fever; subacute myelopathy manifested by paraparesis/paraplegia involving one or more spinal nerve roots; chronic leukoencephalopathy (which may be progressive and even fatal) manifested by confusion, irritability, somnolence, ataxia, dementia, and occasionally seizures and coma; and increased CSF pressure have occurred. Systemic toxicity also may occur following intrathecal and intra-arterial administration. Leukoencephalopathy, manifested by mental confusion, tremors, ataxia, irritability, somnolence, and seizures, and rarely progressing to coma and death, has been reported in patients receiving simultaneous oral and intrathecal methotrexate therapy. Leukoencephalopathy also has occurred following IV administration of methotrexate to patients who had received craniospinal irradiation. In addition, chronic leukoencephalopathy also has been reported in patients receiving repeated high doses of methotrexate with leucovorin rescue, but without cranial irradiation. Discontinuance of methotrexate may not be associated with complete recovery.

Inadvertent intrathecal overdosage of methotrexate has occurred rarely. In cases in which the inadvertent intrathecal dose was less than 100 mg and the error was usually rapidly recognized and appropriate therapy promptly instituted, the patients experienced no or only mild neurotoxicity. In cases in which the dose exceeded 100 mg, severe neurotoxicity occurred, manifested as prompt burning or numbness in the lower extremities, stupor, agitation, seizures, and/or respiratory insufficiency∞ some cases, brain damage or fatal necrotizing leukoencephalopathy resulted despite prompt treatment, but complete recovery following prompt and aggressive therapy has been reported.

Inadvertent intrathecal overdosage of methotrexate constitutes a medical emergency, requiring prompt treatment and management. Although data are limited, management may be guided by the dose administered, time elapsed since administration, and anticipated severity of neurotoxicity. Regardless of the dose administered, as soon as the overdose is recognized, a repeat lumbar puncture should be performed immediately and CSF allowed to drain to gravity.

The efficacy of CSF drainage alone as a means for removing the drug is a function of the dose administered and time elapsed since administration, and decreases as these factors increase. If the dose exceeds 100 mg, prompt neurosurgical intervention with ventriculolumbar perfusion following immediate CSF drainage should be considered; continuous CSF drainage or multiple CSF exchanges may also be considered but are not likely to be as effective.

Other treatment measures may include high-dose parenteral leucovorin calcium therapy to minimize systemic toxicity, corticosteroids to minimize CNS inflammatory reactions, and other supportive therapy as necessary. Efficacy of carboxypeptidase G2 (glucarpidase) has not been established in the management of severe overdoses of intrathecal methotrexate; however, successful use of the drug in this setting has been reported. Successful treatment with intrathecal glucarpidase in a 6-year-old patient who received a 600-mg dose of methotrexate intrathecally has been reported; the patient also was treated with CSF drainage, ventriculolumbar perfusion, IV dexamethasone, IV leucovorin calcium, and hydration and alkalinization. While the addition of leucovorin to the ventriculolumbar perfusion fluid has been suggested and employed, its value is not known and the possibility that it may be epileptogenic via this route of administration should be considered. Intrathecal administration of leucovorin is contraindicated, and the drug has contributed to at least one death when administered by this route. The possible benefits of prophylactic anticonvulsant therapy are probably outweighed by the potential for obscuring acute neurologic symptoms and causing additional adverse effects.

■ **Cardiovascular Effects** Pericarditis, pericardial effusion, hypotension, and thromboembolic complications (e.g., thrombophlebitis; pulmonary embolism; arterial, cerebral, deep vein, or retinal vein thrombosis) have been reported in patients receiving methotrexate therapy.

■ **Other Adverse Effects** Headaches, drowsiness, blurred vision, eye discomfort, conjunctivitis, severe visual changes of unknown etiology, tinnitus, malaise, undue fatigue, and dizziness may occur in patients receiving methotrexate. A transient acute neurologic syndrome manifested by confusion, hemiparesis, seizures, and coma has been reported in patients receiving high-dose methotrexate therapy. The exact cause of this stroke-like encephalopathy is not known; however, it has been suggested that the syndrome may have been related to hemorrhage or complications from intra-arterial catheterization. Other reported complications from intra-arterial infusion techniques include arterial spasm, thrombosis, hemorrhage, infection at the catheter site, and thrombophlebitis. Transient subtle cognitive dysfunction, mood alteration, unusual cranial sensations, leukoencephalopathy, or encephalopathy have been reported in some patients receiving low-dose methotrexate therapy.

Other reported adverse effects of methotrexate include chills and fever, sweating, arthralgia, myalgia, decreased resistance to infection, septicemia, upper respiratory infection, osteoporosis including aseptic necrosis of the femoral head, hypogammaglobulinemia, cystitis, dysuria, vaginal discharge, gynecomastia, loss of libido, impotence, diabetes, abnormal tissue cell changes, and even sudden death.

Severe nephropathy manifested by azotemia, hematuria, and renal failure may occur in patients receiving methotrexate; fatalities have been reported. In one study, postmortem examination revealed extensive necrosis of the epithelium of the convoluted tubules. In patients with renal impairment, methotrexate accumulation and increased toxicity or additional renal damage may occur.

Soft tissue necrosis and osteonecrosis have been reported rarely in patients receiving methotrexate. The risk of soft tissue necrosis and osteonecrosis associated with methotrexate may be elevated in patients receiving concomitant radiotherapy.

Elevations in serum uric acid concentrations may occur in patients receiving methotrexate as a result of cell destruction and hepatic and renal damage. In some patients, uric acid nephropathy and acute renal failure may result. Tumor lysis syndrome associated with other cytotoxic drugs (e.g., fludarabine, cladribine), also has been reported in patients with rapidly growing tumors who were receiving methotrexate. Pharmacologic and appropriate supportive treatment may prevent or alleviate this complication. Methotrexate also was reported to precipitate acute gouty arthritis in two patients being treated for psoriasis. Administration of large volumes of fluids, alkalinization of the urine, and/or administration of allopurinol may be useful in preventing acute attacks of hyperuricemia and uric acid nephropathy.

Nodulosis, vasculitis, and reversible lymphomas (see Precautions and Contraindications) have been reported rarely in patients receiving methotrexate. Sometimes fatal opportunistic infections have been reported in patients receiving methotrexate for neoplastic or non-neoplastic diseases. The most frequent infection was *Pneumocystis carinii* pneumonia; however, other infections (e.g., nocardiosis, histoplasmosis, cryptococcosis, herpes zoster, herpes simplex hepatitis, disseminated herpes simplex) also were reported.

■ **Precautions and Contraindications** Methotrexate is a highly toxic drug with a very low therapeutic index and a therapeutic response is not likely to occur without some evidence of toxicity. The drug can produce hepatotoxicity, severe hematologic toxicity, and GI hemorrhage; severe infection and even death may result. When methotrexate is used in combination with other antineoplastic agents and/or radiation therapy, toxic reactions may be more severe than would occur with methotrexate therapy alone. Concomitant use of methotrexate and radiation therapy may result in an increased risk of soft tissue necrosis and osteonecrosis (see Cautions: Other Adverse Effects). Although doses of methotrexate used in the management of psoriasis and rheumatoid arthritis are usually lower than those used in antineoplastic chemotherapy, severe toxicity may occur in any patient receiving the drug and deaths have been reported with the use of methotrexate in the management of malignancy, psoriasis, and rheumatoid arthritis.

Since methotrexate may produce severe toxicity, which may be fatal, the manufacturer states that the drug should *only* be used in patients with life-threatening neoplastic diseases or in those with severe, recalcitrant, disabling psoriasis or rheumatoid arthritis that is not adequately responsive to other forms of therapy.

The use of high-dose methotrexate regimens employed in the adjunctive treatment of osteosarcoma requires a meticulous understanding of the risks associated with such therapy and of leucovorin rescue. Particular attention to leukocyte counts, serum bilirubin and ALT (SGPT) concentrations, presence of mucositis or persistent pleural effusions, renal function, hydration, urinary alkalinization, fluid and electrolyte balance, and pharmacokinetic monitoring must be ensured when such regimens are used. The manufacturer's labeling and published protocols should be consulted for specific recommendations, including dosage guidelines based on these findings.

Methotrexate must be used only under constant supervision by a clinician who is experienced in the use of antimetabolites. Patients should be fully informed of the risks involved and should be instructed to report promptly any symptoms of toxicity. Because methotrexate is a highly toxic drug, the manufacturers recommend that patients be given no more than a 7-day supply of the drug at one time or, if an intermittent regimen is used (i.e., weekly rather than daily doses), no more than a 1-month supply (e.g., using a mnemonic dispensing package); refills should be only by direct order (i.e., written or oral) of the prescribing clinician. In addition, patients receiving intermittent regimens consisting of weekly rather than daily doses of the drug for the management of rheumatic conditions (e.g., rheumatoid arthritis, psoriasis) and certain inflammatory GI conditions (e.g., Crohn's disease†) should be carefully instructed about their regimen and the frequency of methotrexate administration since mistaken daily use of the drug has resulted in fatalities; patients should be provided with and encouraged to read a copy of the patient instructions supplied by the manufacturer.

Patients receiving methotrexate should be closely monitored for hematologic, renal, hepatic, and pulmonary toxicities, with complete hematologic studies, urinalysis, renal function tests, liver function tests, and chest radiographs. Liver biopsy and bone marrow aspiration studies may be advisable, especially in patients receiving high-dose or prolonged methotrexate therapy. Particular attention to close monitoring is recommended for patients with renal impairment or with pleural effusions or other third-space compartments (e.g., ascites) since elimination of the drug may be impaired. In addition, consideration should be given to evacuating accumulated fluid if possible in patients with substantial compartmental third-spacing prior to methotrexate therapy; monitoring serum concentrations of the drug, reducing drug dosage, or, occasionally, discontinuance of methotrexate also is recommended. Dehydrated patients also are at risk of increased serum methotrexate concentrations. The patient's bleeding time, coagulation time, blood group, and blood type should be on record in case the need for transfusion or surgery arises. If toxic effects or adverse reactions occur, dosage should be reduced or the drug discontinued and appropriate corrective measures taken; however, it should be considered that serious toxic reactions may occur in the absence of abnormal laboratory test results. Severe, occasionally fatal cutaneous reactions have been reported in patients receiving single or multiple oral, IM, IV, or intrathecal doses of methotrexate. These reactions usually occur within days of administration of the drug and recovery has been reported after discontinuance of methotrexate. (See Cautions: Dermatologic and Sensitivity Reactions.)

Hematologic studies must be performed prior to and at frequent intervals during methotrexate therapy. Complete blood cell counts, including differential and platelet counts, generally should be determined at least once weekly in patients receiving the drug for the treatment of neoplastic disease, and at least once monthly in patients receiving the drug for psoriasis or rheumatoid arthritis. If a profound drop in blood cell count occurs, the drug must be immediately discontinued and appropriate alternative therapy instituted. If profound leukopenia and fever occur, the patient should be closely observed and antibiotic therapy should be initiated if there are signs of infection. Blood or platelet transfusions may be necessary in patients with severe bone marrow depression.

There is poor correlation between liver function test results and chronic hepatotoxicity in patients receiving methotrexate, and liver scans are of minimal value in detecting methotrexate hepatotoxicity; liver biopsy is currently the only reliable measure of hepatotoxicity. Nonetheless, hepatic function must be determined prior to initiation of methotrexate and liver function tests, including serum albumin concentrations, should be repeated periodically throughout therapy (at 1- to 2-month intervals in patients treated for psoriasis or rheumatoid arthritis). In patients being treated for psoriasis, liver biopsy should be performed before instituting methotrexate or shortly thereafter (i.e., 2–4 months after). Repeat liver biopsies are recommended after a total cumulative dose of 1.5 g and after additional cumulative doses of 1–1.5 g. In patients with psoriasis, a relationship between abnormal liver function test results and hepatic fibrosis or cirrhosis has not been established, and prolonged, substantial abnormalities in liver function test results may *not* precede appearance of hepatic fibrosis or cirrhosis in such patients. When a pre-methotrexate liver biopsy is not feasible, a liver scan might be useful to detect occult liver disease. Because some patients may discontinue methotrexate after 2–4 months of therapy (due to adverse effects or lack of efficacy), pre-methotrexate liver biopsy might be postponed in patients with psoriasis until this initial period is completed; if long-term methotrexate therapy is anticipated, liver biopsy should then be performed. Abnormal liver function test results frequently occur 1–2 days following a dose of methotrexate, and it is recommended that liver function tests be performed at least 1 week after the last dose of the drug. Because these tests generally return to normal within a few days, repeat tests should be done before performing a liver biopsy. If substantial abnormal liver function test results develop and persist, methotrexate therapy should be withheld for 1–2 weeks and liver function tests repeated. Liver function test results should generally return to normal within 1–2 weeks following discontinuance of the drug; however, if substantial abnormal liver function test results persist, a liver biopsy is recommended.

The decision to perform liver biopsies during methotrexate therapy for rheumatoid arthritis must be carefully individualized. Age at first use of methotrexate and duration of therapy reportedly are risk factors for methotrexate-induced hepatotoxicity. Although unconfirmed to date, it is not known if other risk factors similar to those observed in patients with psoriasis also are present in patients with rheumatoid arthritis. In patients with a history of excessive alcohol consumption, those with prolonged, substantial abnormal liver function test results, or those with chronic hepatitis B or C, liver biopsy should be performed before instituting methotrexate therapy. In patients with rheumatoid arthritis, prolonged, substantial abnormal liver function test results may precede appearance of fibrosis or cirrhosis. In patients with normal liver function, history and physical examination, and no other risk factors (obesity, diabetes mellitus, impaired renal function, history of liver disease, history of IV drug abuse, family history of inheritable liver disease, history of significant exposure to known hepatotoxic drugs), a liver biopsy is recommended after a cumulative methotrexate dosage of approximately 1.5 g. In addition, a liver biopsy should be performed during therapy in patients with prolonged, substantial abnormal liver function test results or with serum albumin concentration below normal values (but whose rheumatoid arthritis is under control). If pre-methotrexate and the first post-methotrexate therapy biopsies show no serious abnormalities and the patient has no risk factors, repeat liver biopsies are recommended every 2–3 years or after additional cumulative dosages of 1–1.5 g. Patients with grade I, II, or IIIA pathologic changes may continue to receive methotrexate therapy, but some clinicians state that those with grade IIIA changes should have a repeat liver biopsy after approximately 6 months of continuous methotrexate therapy. Patients with prolonged, substantial abnormal liver function test results who refuse liver biopsy or those with grade IIIB or IV pathologic changes should not receive further methotrexate therapy; however, occasional patients may require additional therapy with careful follow-up liver biopsies. Concomitant administration of methotrexate and other drugs with hepatotoxic potential including alcohol should be avoided.

Renal function tests should be performed prior to and periodically during methotrexate therapy (at 1- to 2-month intervals in patients with psoriasis or rheumatoid arthritis; more frequent monitoring usually is necessary in patients receiving methotrexate for the treatment of neoplastic disease). If renal impairment develops during methotrexate therapy, dosage should be reduced or the drug discontinued until renal function is improved or restored. In addition, tumor lysis syndrome associated with other cytotoxic drugs (e.g., fludarabine, cladribine) also has been reported in patients with rapidly growing tumors who were receiving methotrexate. Pharmacologic and appropriate supportive treatment may prevent or alleviate this complication.

Malignant lymphomas may occur in patients receiving low-dose methotrexate therapy; such lymphomas may regress following withdrawal of the drug and therefore may not require cytotoxic therapy. However, if lymphomas do not regress following discontinuance of methotrexate, appropriate therapy should be instituted. The manufacturers state that the potential benefits of methotrexate therapy (alone or in combination with other drugs) should be weighed against these potential risks, especially in children or young adults.

Since potentially fatal opportunistic infections (e.g., *Pneumocystis carinii* pneumonia) have been reported in patients receiving methotrexate therapy, the possibility of *P. carinii* pneumonia should be considered in patients who develop pulmonary symptoms. In addition, pulmonary function tests may be useful if methotrexate-induced pulmonary toxicity is suspected, particularly if baseline values are available. For other precautions associated with the potential toxic effects of the drug on the lungs, see Cautions: Pulmonary Effects.

The immunosuppressive action of methotrexate must be considered when evaluating use of the drug in patients in whom immune responses may be important or essential. In patients at high risk for acquired immunodeficiency syndrome (AIDS), an HIV antibody determination should be considered because of the potential for additive immunosuppression and increased risk of opportunistic infections. Two psoriatic patients developed tuberculosis while receiving methotrexate and it has been suggested that, in addition to a chest radiograph, a tuberculin skin test should be performed prior to initiation of methotrexate therapy. If the initial tuberculin test is positive, isoniazid preventive therapy (see 8:16.04) should be initiated concomitantly with methotrexate therapy. Since an accurate evaluation of the tuberculin test is not possible in patients receiving methotrexate, chest radiographs should be repeated every 6 months during therapy in these patients.

Methotrexate should be used with extreme caution in patients with infection, peptic ulcer, ulcerative colitis, or debility, and in very young or geriatric patients. Methotrexate should be used with extreme caution, if at all, in patients with malignant disease who have preexisting liver damage or impaired hepatic function, preexisting bone marrow depression, aplasia, leukopenia, thrombocytopenia, or anemia; the drug is usually contraindicated in patients with impaired renal function. In the management of psoriasis or rheumatoid arthritis, methotrexate is contraindicated in patients with preexisting blood dyscrasias such as bone marrow hypoplasia, leukopenia, thrombocytopenia, or clinically important anemia; those with overt or laboratory evidence of immunodeficiency syndromes; and those with excessive alcohol consumption, alcoholic liver disease, or chronic liver disease.

■ Pediatric Precautions The manufacturer states that safety and efficacy of methotrexate in pediatric patients for the management of any conditions other than cancer chemotherapy or polyarticular-course juvenile rheumatoid arthritis have not been established. Severe neurotoxic effects, manifested mainly by focal or generalized seizures, have been reported with increased frequency in pediatric patients with acute lymphoblastic leukemia who were receiving intermediate-dose IV methotrexate (1 g/m^2). Leukoencephalopathy and/or microangiopathic calcifications usually were observed in diagnostic imaging procedures of symptomatic patients.

■ Mutagenicity and Carcinogenicity Methotrexate has been reported to cause chromosome damage. Although patients who had previously received methotrexate have conceived and borne normal children, both men and women should be advised to avoid conception during and immediately following methotrexate therapy so that normal production of germinal cells may be reestablished. (See Cautions: Pregnancy, Fertility, and Lactation.) It has been suggested that methotrexate may be carcinogenic; however, extensive epidemiologic studies are required before its carcinogenicity can be confirmed or refuted. Malignant lymphomas (e.g., non-Hodgkin's lymphoma) may occur in patients receiving low-dose oral methotrexate therapy; such lymphomas may regress following withdrawal of the drug and, therefore, may not require cytotoxic therapy. However, if lymphomas do not regress following discontinuance of methotrexate, appropriate therapy should be instituted. Therefore, the manufacturers state that the potential benefits of methotrexate therapy (alone or in combination with other drugs) should be weighed against these potential risks, especially in children or young adults.

■ Pregnancy, Fertility, and Lactation Abortion, fetal death, and/or congenital anomalies have occurred in pregnant women receiving methotrexate, especially during the first trimester of pregnancy. Methotrexate is contraindicated in the management of psoriasis or rheumatoid arthritis in pregnant women. Women of childbearing potential should not receive methotrexate until pregnancy is excluded. For the management of psoriasis or rheumatoid arthritis, methotrexate therapy in women should be started immediately following a menstrual period and appropriate measures should be taken in men or women to avoid conception during and for at least 12 weeks following methotrexate therapy. Both men and women receiving methotrexate should be informed of the potential risk of adverse effects on reproduction. Women of childbearing potential should be fully informed of the potential hazard to the fetus should they become pregnant during methotrexate therapy. In cancer chemotherapy, methotrexate should not be used in pregnant women or women of childbearing potential who might become pregnant unless the potential benefits to the mother outweigh the possible risks to the fetus.

Defective oogenesis or spermatogenesis, transient oligospermia, menstrual dysfunction, and infertility have been reported in patients receiving methotrexate.

Methotrexate is distributed into breast milk. Because of the potential for serious adverse reactions to methotrexate in nursing infants, the drug is contraindicated in nursing women.

Drug Interactions

■ Protein-bound Drugs and Weak Organic Acids Because methotrexate is partly bound to serum proteins, its toxicity may be increased as a result of displacement by certain drugs such as salicylates, sulfonamides, sulfonylureas, phenytoin, phenylbutazone, tetracyclines, chloramphenicol, and aminobenzoic acid. Until the clinical importance of these findings is established, these drugs should be given cautiously in patients receiving methotrexate. In addition, the possibility that weak organic acids, including salicylates, may delay renal excretion of methotrexate and increase accumulation should be considered.

■ Nonsteroidal Anti-inflammatory Agents Severe, sometimes fatal, toxicity (including hematologic and GI toxicity) has occurred following administration of a NSAIA (e.g., indomethacin, ketoprofen) concomitantly with methotrexate (particularly with high-dose therapy) in patients with various malignant neoplasms, psoriasis, or rheumatoid arthritis. The toxicity was associated with elevated and prolonged serum concentrations of methotrexate. The exact mechanism of the interaction remains to be established, but it has been suggested that NSAIAs may inhibit renal elimination of methotrexate, possibly by decreasing renal perfusion via inhibition of renal prostaglandin synthesis or by competing for renal elimination.

NSAIAs should be avoided in patients receiving relatively high dosages of methotrexate (e.g., those used in the treatment of neoplastic disease). The risk of concomitant low-dose, intermittent (e.g., 5–15 mg weekly) methotrexate therapy and NSAIAs has not been fully elucidated, but the drugs have been used concomitantly in many patients receiving methotrexate for the management of rheumatoid arthritis. However, in clinical studies in which the drugs were used concomitantly, the patients often were monitored closely and were receiving relatively stable dosages of NSAIAs; in addition, those with conditions that might predispose to methotrexate toxicity generally were excluded from the studies. NSAIAs should be used with caution in patients receiving low-dose methotrexate regimens such as those employed in the management of rheumatoid arthritis, and the possibility of increased and prolonged serum methotrexate concentrations and resultant toxicity should be considered. Although intermittent regimens also are used in the management of psoriasis, methotrexate dosages in such regimens usually are higher than those used in the management of rheumatoid arthritis and therefore are more likely to result in toxicity during concomitant NSAIA therapy; serious toxicity, including at least one death, has been reported in several patients with psoriasis receiving combined therapy with the drugs. Further study is needed to evaluate the interaction between NSAIAs and methotrexate.

■ Penicillins Concomitant use of penicillins (e.g., amoxicillin, carbenicillin) may decrease renal clearance of methotrexate, presumably by inhibiting renal tubular secretion of the drug. Increased serum concentrations of methotrexate, resulting in GI or hematologic toxicity, have been reported in patients receiving low- or high-dose methotrexate therapy concomitantly with penicillins, and patients receiving the drugs concomitantly should be carefully monitored.

■ Proton-Pump Inhibitors Although no formal drug interaction studies have been conducted with methotrexate and proton-pump inhibitors, data from case reports, population pharmacokinetic studies, and retrospective analyses suggest that concomitant use of methotrexate (particularly at high dosages) with proton-pump inhibitors (e.g., esomeprazole, omeprazole, pantoprazole) may decrease methotrexate clearance, resulting in elevated and prolonged serum concentrations of methotrexate and/or its metabolite hydroxymethotrexate and possibly leading to methotrexate toxicities. Increased concentrations of methotrexate and/or hydroxymethotrexate with or without associated adverse effects (e.g., renal toxicity, adverse hematologic effects, severe mucositis, myalgia) have been reported when methotrexate dosages ranging from 300 mg/m^2 to 12 g/m^2 were administered concomitantly with proton-pump inhibitors. Although the majority of reported cases occurred in patients receiving high dosages of methotrexate, methotrexate toxicity also has been reported following concomitant administration of *low* dosages of methotrexate (15 mg per week) with a proton-pump inhibitor. Therefore, the manufacturers of proton-pump inhibitors state that temporary discontinuance of proton-pump inhibitor therapy may be considered in some patients receiving high-dose methotrexate. Some clinicians specifically recommend withholding proton-pump inhibitor therapy for several days before, during, and for several days after methotrexate administration; in patients in whom acid suppression is clinically indicated during methotrexate therapy, substitution of a histamine H_2-receptor antagonist (e.g., ranitidine) for the proton-pump inhibitor may be considered. Pending further evaluation, some clinicians state that these recommendations should extend to patients receiving low-dose methotrexate.

■ **Other Drugs** Drugs with similar pharmacologic activity such as pyrimethamine should not be given to patients receiving methotrexate.

Concomitant use of other potentially hepatotoxic drugs (e.g., retinoids, azathioprine, sulfasalazine) and methotrexate may increase the risk of hepatotoxicity; patients receiving concomitant therapy with these drugs should be closely monitored.

Although concomitant use of methotrexate with cisplatin exhibits possible synergistic antineoplastic effects, cisplatin may alter renal elimination of methotrexate. Caution is advised if high-dose methotrexate is administered in conjunction with cisplatin for the treatment of osteosarcoma.

Co-trimoxazole should be used with caution in patients receiving methotrexate, since sulfonamides can displace methotrexate from plasma protein-binding sites resulting in increased free methotrexate concentrations.

It has been suggested that folic acid preparations including vitamin products may decrease the effectiveness of methotrexate therapy and should not be given to patients receiving methotrexate; however, there have been no clinical studies to support or refute this hypothesis.

Methotrexate increases plasma mercaptopurine concentrations; dosage adjustment may be necessary.

Probenecid diminishes renal tubular transport of methotrexate; patients should be carefully monitored during concomitant use of these agents.

Methotrexate may decrease clearance of theophylline; serum theophylline concentrations should be monitored in patients receiving theophylline concomitantly with methotrexate.

Vaccination with live virus vaccines generally should not be performed in patients receiving methotrexate. Disseminated vaccinia infection has been reported following smallpox vaccination in at least one patient receiving methotrexate. Although the antibody response to killed virus vaccines is not normal, partial or complete protection may still be attained and these vaccines may be used if necessary in patients receiving methotrexate.

Acute Toxicity

■ **Treatment** Treatment of toxicity resulting from impaired elimination or an inadvertent overdosage of methotrexate consists of administration of a folic acid antidote (i.e., leucovorin, levoleucovorin) with or without a carboxypeptidase G2 (i.e., glucarpidase); however, glucarpidase is indicated only for the treatment of toxic plasma methotrexate concentrations (exceeding 0.454 mcg/mL [1 *μM*]) in patients with delayed methotrexate clearance due to renal impairment. Because of the potential for subtherapeutic concentrations of methotrexate, glucarpidase should not be used in patients who exhibit the expected clearance of methotrexate or in those with normal or mildly impaired renal function.

In cases of inadvertent overdosage of methotrexate, leucovorin or levoleucovorin should be administered as soon as possible. In patients with impaired elimination of methotrexate, leucovorin or levoleucovorin should be administered within 24 hours of methotrexate administration when there is delayed methotrexate excretion. Leucovorin or levoleucovorin should *not* be administered intrathecally. As the time interval between methotrexate administration and rescue therapy with leucovorin or levoleucovorin increases, the effectiveness of either drug in counteracting methotrexate toxicity may decrease. Serum creatinine and methotrexate concentrations should be determined at 24-hour intervals. The optimal dose of leucovorin or levoleucovorin should be determined based on serum methotrexate concentrations. (See Leucovorin Calcium 92:12 and Levoleucovorin Calcium 92:12.)

If glucarpidase is used, rescue therapy with leucovorin or levoleucovorin should be continued following administration of the drug; however, because leucovorin is a substrate for glucarpidase (and the pharmacokinetics of levoleucovorin and leucovorin are comparable), leucovorin and levoleucovorin should not be administered within 2 hours before or after a dose of glucarpidase. During the first 48 hours following administration of glucarpidase, leucovorin or levoleucovorin should be administered at the dose utilized prior to administration of glucarpidase. After 48 hours, the dose of leucovorin or levoleucovorin should be determined based on plasma methotrexate concentrations. (See Glucarpidase 92:12.)

For specific information on dosage modifications, cautions, and precautions associated with impaired methotrexate elimination or an inadvertent overdosage, the manufacturer's prescribing information should be consulted.

If accidental overdosage of intrathecal methotrexate occurs, intensive systemic supportive therapy (e.g., administration of high-dose leucovorin calcium, alkaline diuresis, rapid CSF drainage, ventriculolumbar perfusion) may be required (see Cautions: Effects following Intrathecal Administration).

In case of severe overdosage of methotrexate, hydration and urinary alkalinization may be needed to prevent precipitation of the drug and/or its metabolites in the renal tubules. Hemodialysis and peritoneal dialysis generally have been ineffective in improving the elimination of methotrexate. However, effective clearance of methotrexate has been reported with the use of acute, intermittent hemodialysis with a high-flux polysulfone dialyzer (the F-80B Fresenius Dialyzer) in a small number of patients with acute renal failure secondary to methotrexate or with end-stage renal disease unrelated to methotrexate therapy.

For additional information on the treatment of intrathecal methotrexate overdosage, see Cautions: Effects following Intrathecal Administration.

Pharmacology

Methotrexate and its polyglutamate metabolites reversibly inhibit dihydrofolate reductase, the enzyme that reduces folic acid to tetrahydrofolic acid. Inhibition of tetrahydrofolate formation limits the availability of one-carbon fragments necessary for synthesis of purines and the conversion of deoxyuridylate to thymidylate in the synthesis of DNA and cell reproduction. The affinity of dihydrofolate reductase for methotrexate is far greater than its affinity for folic acid or dihydrofolic acid and, therefore, even very large doses of folic acid given simultaneously will not reverse the effects of methotrexate. Leucovorin calcium, a derivative of tetrahydrofolic acid, may block the effects of methotrexate if given shortly after the antineoplastic agent. Results of one study indicate that methotrexate also causes an increase in intracellular deoxyadenosine triphosphate, which is thought to inhibit ribonucleotide reduction, and polynucleotide ligase, an enzyme concerned in DNA synthesis and repair. Tissues with high rates of cellular proliferation such as neoplasms, psoriatic epidermis, bone marrow, the lining of the GI tract, hair matrix, and fetal cells are most sensitive to the effects of methotrexate.

Resistance to methotrexate may develop and has been associated with decreased cellular uptake of the drug, increased dihydrofolate reductase activity (associated with increased synthesis of the enzyme), decreased binding of methotrexate to dihydrofolate reductase (because of mutated dihydrofolate reductase protein), and decreased intracellular concentrations of polyglutamylated metabolites of methotrexate; however, the precise mechanism of this resistance development has not been established.

Methotrexate also has immunosuppressive activity, in part possibly as a result of inhibition of lymphocyte multiplication. The mechanism(s) of action in the management of rheumatoid arthritis of the drug is not known, although suggested mechanisms have included immunosuppressive and/or anti-inflammatory effects.

Pharmacokinetics

■ **Absorption** Oral absorption of methotrexate appears to be highly variable and dose dependent. While older studies demonstrated good absorption from the GI tract with relatively low oral doses of methotrexate, more recent studies indicate that the oral bioavailability of the drug may be below 50% even at relatively low doses (i.e., 15 mg/m² or lower). The bioavailability of methotrexate decreases with increasing oral doses (suggesting the presence of a saturable absorption process) and absorption is substantially reduced at doses exceeding 80 mg/m². Studies investigating the use of divided doses of methotrexate in an attempt to improve the oral bioavailability of the drug have shown conflicting results. It has been suggested that poor bioavailability should be assumed with oral methotrexate doses of 100 mg/m² or greater, regardless of the dosage schedule used. Food delays absorption and decreases peak serum concentrations of the drug. Peak serum concentrations of methotrexate generally are achieved in 1–2 hours following oral administration in adults.

Oral administration of methotrexate in pediatric patients with leukemia reportedly results in wide variability in the rate and extent of oral absorption. Oral bioavailability of 23–95%, with a 20-fold difference between the highest and lowest peak serum concentration measurements (range: 0.11–2.3 *μM*), has been reported in pediatric patients receiving oral methotrexate 20 mg/m² for the treatment of leukemia. Substantial variability in the time to peak serum concentration also has been observed; in patients receiving methotrexate at an oral dose of 15 mg/m², the time to peak serum concentration ranged from 0.67–4 hours.

Methotrexate appears to be completely absorbed following IM administration at doses of up to at least 100 mg. Peak serum concentrations are achieved 30–60 minutes after IM administration of the drug. Serum concentrations following intra-arterial administration are similar to those achieved following IV administration.

■ **Distribution** Methotrexate is actively transported across cell membranes. At serum methotrexate concentrations exceeding 0.1 μmol/mL, passive diffusion becomes a major means of intracellular transport of the drug. The drug is widely distributed into body tissues with highest concentrations in the kidneys, gallbladder, spleen, liver, and skin. Following systemic administration of a single dose of methotrexate, the drug inhibits DNA synthesis in psoriatic epidermis for 12–16 hours. Following oral or IV administration of the drug to animals, synovial fluid methotrexate concentrations are higher in inflamed than in uninflamed joints; concurrent administration of salicylates did not affect distribution of methotrexate into joints, but pretreatment with prednisone reduced the amount of drug distributed into inflamed joints relative to that into normal joints. In patients receiving long-term, oral methotrexate therapy for rheumatoid arthritis, the ratio of synovial fluid to serum concentrations of methotrexate ranged from 0.9–1.2. Methotrexate distributes into third space fluids, and the presence of pleural effusions or ascites can substantially alter the disposition of the drug (see Pharmacokinetics: Elimination). Slow release of methotrexate from third space accumulations may prolong the terminal half-life and may increase the risk of drug toxicity with high doses (i.e., exceeding 250 mg/m²).

Methotrexate is retained for several weeks in the kidneys and for months in the liver. Sustained serum concentrations and tissue accumulation of methotrexate may result from repeated daily doses. Following IV administration, an initial volume of distribution of approximately 0.18 L/kg and a steady-state volume of distribution of approximately 0.4–0.8 L/kg have been reported. According to the manufacturer, the drug does not reach therapeutic concentrations in the CSF when given orally or parenterally. However, high-dose systemic methotrexate therapy can result in peak CSF concentrations above the therapeutic threshold of 0.001 μmol/mL and has been used to prevent meningeal leukemia and lymphoma. Following IV administration of methotrexate, CSF drug concentrations are dose related; a CSF concentration of 0.0001 μmol/mL was reported after a dose of 500 mg/m²y 24-hour IV infusion, and CSF concentrations exceeding 0.01 μmol/mL were observed following an IV bolus dose of 7500 mg/m². Intrathecal administration of methotrexate may result in potentially cytotoxic serum drug concentrations that can persist for 24–48 hours.

Methotrexate crosses the placental barrier. Methotrexate is distributed into breast milk; the highest reported breast milk plasma concentration ratio, which occurred 10 hours after administration of a 22.5-mg oral dose, was 0.08:1. (See Cautions: Pregnancy, Fertility, and Lactation.)

At serum concentrations of 0.001–0.1 μmol/mL, about 50% of the drug is bound to plasma proteins (primarily albumin).

■ **Elimination** In patients receiving methotrexate for the treatment of psoriasis or rheumatoid arthritis, or as low-dose antineoplastic therapy (i.e., less than 30 mg/m²), a terminal half-life of about 3–10 hours has been reported. Higher doses of methotrexate have been associated with a longer elimination half-life of about 8–15 hours.

Plasma concentrations of methotrexate following high-dose IV infusion appear to decline in a biphasic manner. The half-life of the initial phase ($t_{1/2\alpha}$) averages 1.5–3.5 hours in patients with normal total body clearance and the half-life in the terminal phase ($t_{1/2\beta}$) is about 8–15 hours.

After absorption, methotrexate undergoes hepatic and intracellular metabolism to form methotrexate polyglutamates, metabolites which by hydrolysis may be converted back to methotrexate. Methotrexate polyglutamates inhibit dihydrofolate reductase and thymidylate synthetase. Small amounts of these polyglutamate metabolites may remain in tissues for extended periods; the retention and prolonged action of these active metabolites vary among different cells, tissues, and tumors. In addition, small amounts of methotrexate polyglutamates may be converted to 7-hydroxymethotrexate; accumulation of this metabolite may become substantial following administration of high doses of methotrexate, since the aqueous solubility of 7-hydroxymethotrexate is threefold to fivefold lower than that of the parent compound. Following oral administration of methotrexate, the drug also is partially metabolized by the intestinal flora.

The drug is excreted primarily by the kidneys via glomerular filtration and active transport. Small amounts are excreted in the feces, probably via the bile. Methotrexate has a biphasic excretion pattern. Up to 92% of a single dose is excreted within 24 hours following IV administration followed by excretion of 1–2% of the retained dose daily. In one study, 58–92% of an IV methotrexate dose of 0.1–10 mg/kg was excreted in the urine within 24 hours. Only slightly less urinary excretion occurred following oral administration of 0.1 mg/kg. Following oral administration of 10 mg/kg, however, only 15% of the dose was excreted in the urine within 24 hours and 48% within 5 days. About 39% of the larger oral dose was recovered in the feces as compared to 7–9% following 0.1 mg/kg administered orally and 2–5% of 0.1–10 mg/kg administered IV. Enterohepatic recirculation of methotrexate may occur. Methotrexate excretion is impaired and accumulation occurs more rapidly in patients with impaired renal function, pleural effusions, or those with other third-space compartments (e.g., ascites). In addition, simultaneous administration of other weak organic acids such as salicylates may suppress methotrexate clearance.

Chemistry and Stability

■ **Chemistry** Methotrexate is a mixture containing at least 85% 4-amino-10-methylfolic acid, calculated on the anhydrous basis, and small amounts of related compounds. Methotrexate is a folic acid antagonist. Structurally, the primary constituent of methotrexate differs from folic acid in the substitution of an amino group for a hydroxyl group in the pteridine nucleus and in the addition of a methyl group on the amino nitrogen between the pteroyl and benzoyl groups. Methotrexate is a weak acid that occurs as an orange-brown, crystalline powder and is practically insoluble in water and in alcohol. Great care should be taken to prevent inhaling particles of the chemical and exposing the skin to it. Methotrexate sodium occurs as a yellow powder and is soluble in water. Methotrexate sodium injection has a pH of 7.5–9. Commercially available injections of methotrexate sodium are available with benzyl alcohol as a preservative or without a preservative.

■ **Stability** Methotrexate sodium tablets should be protected from light and stored in well-closed containers at 20–25°C. Methotrexate sodium injection and powder for injection should be protected from light and stored at 20–25°C. Stability and compatibility of methotrexate sodium solutions depend on several factors including the formulation of methotrexate sodium used, presence of preservatives, concentration of drug(s), specific diluents used, resulting pH, and temperature; the manufacturers' labeling and specialized references should be consulted for specific information.

For further information on the handling of antineoplastic agents, see the ASHP Guidelines on Handling Hazardous Drugs at http://www.ahfsdruginformation.com.

Preparations

Excipients in commercially available drug preparations may have clinically important effects in some individuals; consult specific product labeling for details.

Methotrexate Sodium

Oral		
Tablets	2.5 mg (of methotrexate)*	**Methotrexate Sodium Tablets** (scored)
		Rheumatrex® Dose Pack (scored), Dava
Tablets, film coated	5 mg (of methotrexate)	**Trexall®** (scored), Duramed
	7.5 mg (of methotrexate)	**Trexall®** (scored), Duramed
	10 mg (of methotrexate)	**Trexall®** (scored), Duramed
	15 mg (of methotrexate)	**Trexall®** (scored), Duramed
Parenteral		
For injection	1 g (of methotrexate)*	**Methotrexate Sodium for Injection**
Injection	10 mg (of methotrexate) per mL*	**Methotrexate Sodium Injection Isotonic**
	25 mg (of methotrexate) per mL*	**Methotrexate Sodium Injection Isotonic**

*available from one or more manufacturer, distributor, and/or repackager by generic (nonproprietary) name

†Use is not currently included in the labeling approved by the US Food and Drug Administration

Midostaurin

■ Midostaurin, an inhibitor of multiple receptor tyrosine kinases including fms-like tyrosine kinase-3 (Flt-3), is an antineoplastic agent.

Uses

■ **Acute Myeloid Leukemia** Midostaurin is used in combination with cytarabine and daunorubicin as a component of induction therapy followed by use in combination with high-dose cytarabine as a component of consolidation therapy for newly diagnosed acute myeloid leukemia (AML) harboring fms-like tyrosine kinase-3 (Flt-3) mutation. Midostaurin has been designated an orphan drug by FDA for the treatment of this cancer. An FDA-approved companion diagnostic test (e.g., LeukoStrat® CDx Flt-3 mutation assay) is required to confirm the presence of the Flt-3 mutation prior to initiation of therapy. In patients with newly diagnosed AML harboring Flt-3 mutation, the addition of midostaurin to cytarabine-based induction and consolidation therapy substantially prolonged survival. Flt-3 mutation is detectable in approximately 30% of patients with newly diagnosed AML.

The current indication for midostaurin in the treatment of AML is based principally on the results of a randomized, double-blind, placebo-controlled, phase 3 study (RATIFY) in adults with newly diagnosed AML harboring an internal tandem duplication (ITD) mutation or a point mutation in the tyrosine kinase domain (TKD) of the Flt-3 kinase.

In this study, 717 adults were randomized in a 1:1 ratio to receive either midostaurin or placebo in combination with standard cytarabine-based induction and consolidation therapy. Midostaurin (50 mg twice daily) or placebo was administered on days 8–21 of each cycle of induction therapy and each 28-day cycle of consolidation therapy. Induction therapy consisted of daunorubicin 60 mg/m² daily by short IV infusion on days 1–3 and cytarabine 200 mg/m² daily by continuous IV infusion on days 1–7 of each cycle for up to 2 cycles; a second cycle of induction therapy with the same drug combination was administered if definitive evidence of clinically important residual leukemia was present in the bone marrow on day 21. Patients who achieved complete remission (defined as less than 5% leukemic blast cells in the bone marrow, absence of leukemic blast cells in peripheral blood, absolute neutrophil count [ANC] exceeding 1000/mm³, platelet count exceeding 100,000/mm³, and absence of extramedullary disease) following induction therapy received consolidation therapy. Consolidation therapy consisted of high-dose cytarabine (3 g/m² by IV infusion over 3 hours every 12 hours) on days 1, 3, and 5 of each 28-day cycle for up to 4 cycles. Patients who remained in complete remission received post-consolidation therapy with midostaurin (50 mg twice daily continuously) or placebo, according to the original treatment assignment, in 28-day cycles for up to 12 cycles (maintenance phase).

Patients in this study were stratified according to subtype of Flt-3 mutation (TKD or ITD); patients with ITD mutations were further stratified based on mutant-to-wild-type Flt-3 allelic ratio (high ITD was defined as an allelic ratio of 0.7 or greater, and low ITD was defined as an allelic ratio of less than 0.7). Patients who proceeded to stem cell transplantation were included in the efficacy analysis, but study treatment was discontinued. The primary measure of efficacy was overall survival. In this study, 25% of patients received a second cycle of induction therapy, 62% received at least one cycle of consolidation therapy, and 29% received maintenance therapy. Among the patients who received maintenance therapy with midostaurin, 58% of these patients completed 12 cycles of therapy. Following initial complete remission, induction failure, or salvage therapy after relapse, 59% of midostaurin-treated patients and 55% of placebo recipients underwent stem cell transplantation.

The median age of patients enrolled in the RATIFY study was 47 years (range: 18–60 years); 44% were male, 88% had an Eastern Cooperative Oncology Group (ECOG) performance status of 0 or 1, and 95% had de novo AML. Approximately one-half of patients had a low Flt-3-ITD allelic ratio, 30% had a high Flt-3-ITD allelic ratio, and 23% had Flt-3-TKD mutations. In addition, nucleophosmin 1 (NPM1) mutation was present in 58% of 563 patients evaluated for this mutation. Baseline characteristics were generally balanced between treatment groups; however, a larger proportion of patients receiving placebo were female (59 versus 52%) or had NPM1 mutation (60 versus 55%) compared with those receiving midostaurin.

After a minimum follow-up of approximately 3.5 years, midostaurin in combination with cytarabine-based induction and consolidation therapy reduced the risk of death by 23% compared with placebo in combination with cytarabine-based induction and consolidation therapy. Because overall survival curves (based on Kaplan-Meier estimates) for both treatment groups reached a plateau after approximately 36 months, median overall survival could not be reliably estimated; however, at a follow-up of 6 years, the mean survival time in midostaurin-treated patients was 44 months compared with 38.6 months in placebo recipients. Median event-free survival (events defined as failure to obtain a complete remission within 60 days of initiation of therapy, relapse, or death from any cause) was prolonged in midostaurin-treated patients compared with placebo recipients (8.2 versus 3 months; hazard ratio: 0.78); however, many patients were classified as having an early event because of failure to achieve protocol-specified complete remission, and event dates for these patients were assigned as the date of last adequate response assessment prior to day 60. Therefore, because of the potential for bias in the estimated effect size, an exploratory analysis of event-free survival in which events were defined as failure to obtain complete remission at any time during induction therapy (assigned as an event beginning on study day 1), relapse, or death from any cause was conducted. In this exploratory analysis, median event-free survival also was prolonged in midostaurin-treated patients compared with placebo recipients (10.6 versus 5.6 months; hazard ratio: 0.72). Median disease-free survival also was prolonged in midostaurin-treated patients compared with placebo recipients (26.7 versus 15.5 months). Subgroup analysis according to Flt-3 mutation subtype suggested that the favorable overall survival benefit of midostaurin in combination with chemotherapy was consistent across these subgroups; however, overall survival did not differ significantly between midostaurin-treated patients and placebo recipients within these subgroups.

Midostaurin is not indicated for use as single-agent induction therapy in patients with AML.

■ **Systemic Mastocytosis** Midostaurin is used for the treatment of aggressive systemic mastocytosis (ASM), systemic mastocytosis with associated hematologic neoplasm (SM-AHN; also known as systemic mastocytosis with an associated hematologic non-mast-cell-lineage disease [SM-AHNMD]), and mast cell leukemia; midostaurin has been designated an orphan drug by FDA for the treatment of these conditions. Systemic mastocytosis is characterized by multifocal infiltrates of neoplastic mast cells in various internal organs, including the bone marrow, spleen, liver, and GI tract; symptoms are related to release of vasoactive mediators and to organ damage resulting from neoplastic mast cell infiltration. In 2 open-label, noncomparative, phase 2 studies in patients with advanced systemic mastocytosis, overall responses (major plus partial responses) were observed in 52–60% of evaluable patients.

The first study enrolled 116 adults with advanced systemic mastocytosis whose disease had relapsed or progressed following 0–2 prior therapies for systemic mastocytosis; 89 of these patients had at least one measurable clinical finding (C-finding) related to organ damage caused by infiltrating neoplastic mast cells (i.e., transfusion-independent and transfusion-dependent anemia or thrombocytopenia, hypoalbuminemia, neutropenia, liver function test abnormalities, weight loss) and were evaluable for response in the primary efficacy analysis. Patients enrolled in the study were required to have adequate renal and hepatic function (i.e., serum creatinine concentrations not exceeding 2 mg/dL; total bilirubin concentrations not exceeding 1.5 times the upper limit of normal [ULN] or 3 times the ULN if disease related and aminotransferase concentrations not exceeding 2.5 times the ULN or 5 times the ULN if disease related). This study excluded patients with corrected QT (QT_c) intervals exceeding 450 msec, cardiovascular disease (e.g., left ventricular ejection fraction less than 50%, recent myocardial infarction, poorly controlled hypertension), or evidence of pulmonary infiltrates, and those with acute-stage or life-threatening SM-AHN. All patients received midostaurin 100 mg orally twice daily in continuous 28-day cycles until disease progression, death, or unacceptable toxicity occurred or treatment was discontinued for other reasons. The median duration of treatment was 11 months; however, 17% of patients were still receiving midostaurin therapy at the time of analysis.

In this study, the primary measure of efficacy was overall response rate (major plus partial responses) occurring within the first 6 treatment cycles and lasting at least 8 weeks as assessed by the study steering committee using modified Valent response criteria; major response was defined as complete resolution of at least one C-finding, and partial response was defined as improvement of at least one C-finding by greater than 20%. Subtypes of major response included complete remission (absence of mast cell organ infiltration and organomegaly and a reduction in serum tryptase concentrations, an indicator of disease burden, to less than 20 ng/mL), incomplete remission (greater than 50% reduction in mast cell organ infiltration and/or organomegaly and/or serum tryptase concentrations), and pure clinical response (no more than 50% reduction in serum tryptase concentrations but no substantial change in mast cell organ infiltration and organomegaly). Patients receiving concomitant high-dose corticosteroid therapy were excluded from the primary efficacy analysis. The median age of response-evaluable patients was 64 years; 97% of these patients were Caucasian, 64% of patients were male, 36% had received prior therapy for systemic mastocytosis, and 82% of the patients had D816V c-Kit mutation at baseline.

The overall response rate in this study was 60% in the primary efficacy population and 46% in the intent-to-treat population. In the primary efficacy population, major response was achieved in 45% of patients, generally within the first 3 months of therapy. The complete plus incomplete remission rate was 21% in the primary efficacy population, with incomplete remission reported in 38, 16, or 25% of patients with ASM, SM-AHN, or mast cell leukemia, respectively; there were no complete remissions. The median time to incomplete remission was 0.5 months. At the time of analysis, responses were ongoing, with a median response duration of at least 24.1 months in the primary efficacy population. In the primary efficacy population, median progression-free survival was 17 months and the preliminary estimate of median overall survival was 26.8 months. In a post-hoc analysis, median overall survival was substantially prolonged in patients who achieved a response compared with those who did not achieve a response (44.4 versus 15.4 months). Results of a subgroup analysis (based on age, gender, exposure to prior therapy, and presence of D816V c-Kit mutation) suggested that the effects of midostaurin on response rates were consistent across all subgroups.

A post-hoc analysis of this study using the more-stringent International Working Group-Myeloproliferative Neoplasms Research and Treatment and European Competence Network on Mastocytosis (IWG-MRT-ECNM) consensus response criteria was conducted in 115 evaluable patients. In this post-hoc analysis, overall responses lasting at least 12 weeks were achieved in 17% of patients; complete remission was achieved in 2% of patients. Among patients with ASM, SM-AHN, or mast cell leukemia, overall response rates were 31, 11, or 19%, respectively. Overall response rates were 17% in patients with D816V c-Kit mutation at baseline as well as in those who had received prior therapy for systemic mastocytosis. Although the overall response rate and depth of response were lower using the IWG-MRT-ECNM response criteria, responses were durable, lasting at least 6 months.

In a second similarly designed trial, 26 patients with previously treated or untreated advanced systemic mastocytosis received midostaurin (100 mg orally twice daily after meals) in 28-day cycles for up to 12 cycles; however, 3 patients were not evaluable for response because the subtype of systemic mastocytosis was not confirmed. An overall response (as assessed by the investigators using Valent response criteria) that occurred within the first 2 cycles and lasted for at least 8 weeks was achieved in 52% of evaluable patients, including 10 of 17 patients with SM-AHN and 2 of 6 patients with mast cell leukemia; however, patients receiving concomitant corticosteroid therapy were included in the response assessment. At the time of analysis, responses were ongoing, with a median response duration of at least 29.3 months.

Dosage and Administration

■ **General** Presence of the fms-like tyrosine kinase-3 (Flt-3) mutation must be confirmed by an FDA-approved companion diagnostic test prior to initiation of therapy with midostaurin in patients with acute myeloid leukemia (AML). (See Uses: Acute Myeloid Leukemia.)

Because nausea and vomiting occur frequently in patients receiving midostaurin, premedication with an antiemetic agent should be administered prior to midostaurin therapy. In the principal efficacy studies evaluating midostaurin in patients with advanced systemic mastocytosis, antiemetic agents (e.g., serotonin type 3 [5-HT_3] receptor antagonists) were administered 1–2 hours prior to each dose of midostaurin, with additional antiemetic agents administered as required following midostaurin administration.

Clinicians should consult the respective manufacturers' labelings or published protocols for information on the dosage, method of administration, and administration sequence of other antineoplastic agents used in combination regimens for the treatment of AML.

■ **Administration** Midostaurin is administered orally twice daily, at intervals of approximately 12 hours, with food. The capsules should be swallowed whole and should *not* be opened or crushed.

■ **Dosage** ***Acute Myeloid Leukemia*** For use in conjunction with cytarabine and daunorubicin as a component of induction therapy followed by use in conjunction with high-dose cytarabine as a component of consolidation therapy for newly diagnosed AML with Flt-3 mutation, the recommended adult dosage of midostaurin is 50 mg twice daily on days 8–21 of each cycle.

In the RATIFY study, patients who received midostaurin as a component of induction and consolidation therapy also received post-consolidation therapy† with midostaurin (50 mg twice daily continuously) for up to 12 additional 28-day cycles. (See Uses: Acute Myeloid Leukemia.)

Systemic Mastocytosis For the treatment of aggressive systemic mastocytosis (ASM), systemic mastocytosis with an associated hematologic neoplasm (SM-AHN), or mast cell leukemia, the recommended adult dosage of midostaurin is 100 mg twice daily. Therapy should be continued until disease progression or unacceptable toxicity occurs.

Dosage Adjustment of Midostaurin for Systemic Mastocytosis In the principal efficacy studies evaluating midostaurin in patients with advanced systemic mastocytosis, adverse effects resulting in dosage modifications occurred, generally within the initial 5 months of therapy, in 56% of patients receiving midostaurin. The median time to first dosage modification for toxicity was 1.6 months.

Patients should be monitored for adverse effects at least weekly for the first 4 weeks of therapy, every other week for the following 8 weeks of therapy, and then monthly thereafter.

Hematologic Toxicity. If absolute neutrophil count (ANC) decreases to less than 1000/mm³ in patients with systemic mastocytosis (except in patients with mast cell leukemia) or ANC decreases to less than 500/mm³ in patients who have a baseline ANC of 500–1500/mm³, midostaurin therapy should be withheld. When ANC reaches or exceeds 1000/mm³, midostaurin may be resumed at a reduced dosage of 50 mg twice daily. If a reduced dosage of 50 mg twice daily is tolerated, the midostaurin dosage may be returned to 100 mg twice daily.

If platelet count decreases to less than 50,000/mm³ in patients with systemic mastocytosis (except in patients with mast cell leukemia) or platelet count decreases to less than 25,000/mm³ in patients who have a baseline platelet count of 25,000–75,000/mm³, midostaurin therapy should be withheld. When platelet count reaches or exceeds 50,000/mm³, midostaurin may be resumed at a reduced dosage of 50 mg twice daily. If a reduced dosage of 50 mg twice daily is tolerated, the midostaurin dosage may be returned to 100 mg twice daily.

If hemoglobin concentration decreases to less than 8 g/dL in patients with systemic mastocytosis (except in patients with mast cell leukemia) or life-threatening anemia occurs in patients who have a baseline hemoglobin concentration of 8–10 g/dL, midostaurin therapy should be withheld. When hemoglobin concentration reaches or exceeds 8 g/dL, midostaurin may be resumed at a reduced dosage of 50 mg twice daily. If a reduced dosage of 50 mg twice daily is tolerated, the midostaurin dosage may be returned to 100 mg twice daily.

If prolonged treatment-related neutropenia, thrombocytopenia, or anemia (i.e., lasting more than 21 days) occurs, midostaurin therapy should be discontinued.

GI Effects. If grade 3 or 4 nausea and/or vomiting occurs in patients with systemic mastocytosis despite optimal antiemetic therapy, midostaurin therapy should be withheld for 3 days (6 doses). Upon resumption of therapy, the dosage of midostaurin should be reduced to 50 mg twice daily. If a reduced dosage of 50 mg twice daily is tolerated, the midostaurin dosage may be returned to 100 mg twice daily.

Other Nonhematologic Effects. If other grade 3 or 4 nonhematologic toxicity occurs in patients with systemic mastocytosis, midostaurin therapy should be withheld until the toxicity resolves to grade 2 or less. Upon resumption of therapy, the dosage of midostaurin should be reduced to 50 mg twice daily. If a reduced dosage of 50 mg twice daily is tolerated, the midostaurin dosage may be returned to 100 mg twice daily.

■ **Special Populations** The manufacturer makes no special population dosage recommendations at this time. (See Specific Populations under Cautions: Warnings/Precautions.)

Cautions

■ **Contraindications** Midostaurin is contraindicated in patients with known hypersensitivity to the drug or any ingredient in the formulation. (See Sensitivity Reactions under Cautions: Warnings/Precautions.)

■ **Warnings/Precautions** *Sensitivity Reactions* **Hypersensitivity.** Hypersensitivity reactions, characterized by dyspnea, flushing, chest pain, or angioedema, have been reported. In the principal efficacy studies evaluating midostaurin in patients with systemic mastocytosis, 1 of 142 patients receiving midostaurin experienced anaphylactic shock.

Fetal/Neonatal Morbidity and Mortality There are no adequate and well-controlled studies of midostaurin in pregnant women; however, based on its mechanism of action and animal findings, midostaurin may cause fetal harm. Embryofetal toxicity (i.e., decreased fetal weight, fetal growth retardation, abortion) have been demonstrated in animals receiving midostaurin at exposure levels of approximately 0.01 times the human exposure at the recommended dosage. Late embryofetal death also has been demonstrated in animals receiving midostaurin at exposure levels of approximately 0.004 times the human exposure at the recommended dosage.

Pregnancy should be avoided during midostaurin therapy. The manufacturer states that confirmation of pregnancy status must be obtained no more than 7 days prior to initiation of midostaurin therapy, and women of childbearing potential and men who are partners of such women should be advised to use effective contraceptive methods during and for at least 4 months after discontinuance of the drug. Patients should be apprised of the potential hazard to the fetus if midostaurin is used during pregnancy.

Interstitial Lung Disease/Pneumonitis Interstitial lung disease (ILD) and pneumonitis, sometimes fatal, have occurred in patients receiving midostaurin as monotherapy or in combination with chemotherapy.

Patients receiving midostaurin should be monitored for pulmonary symptoms suggestive of ILD or pneumonitis. (See Advice to Patients.) Midostaurin should be discontinued in patients who experience manifestations of ILD or pneumonitis without an infectious etiology.

Prolongation of QT Interval In a placebo- and active-controlled study of the effects of midostaurin on the QT interval, clinically important QT-interval prolongation was not observed when midostaurin was administered at a dosage of 75 mg twice daily for 3 days, and no relationship between change in QT interval and plasma concentrations of the drug and its active metabolites was observed. However, the duration of the study was not adequate to determine whether the active metabolite CGP-52421 prolongs the QT interval at steady-state exposures. In clinical studies evaluating use of midostaurin in patients with advanced systemic mastocytosis, prolongation of the QT interval (corrected for heart rate using Fridericia's formula [QT_cF]) by more than 60 msec from baseline occurred in 6.3% of midostaurin-treated patients and the QT_cF interval exceeded 480 or 500 msec in 4.7 or 0%, respectively, of midostaurin-treated patients. In a randomized study evaluating use of midostaurin in patients with acute myeloid leukemia (AML), prolongation of the QT_cF interval by more than 60 msec from baseline occurred in 18.4% of patients receiving midostaurin compared with 10.7% of those receiving placebo, and the QT_cF interval exceeded 480 or 500 msec in 10.1 or 6.2%, respectively, of midostaurin-treated patients compared with 5.7 or 2.6%, respectively, of patients receiving placebo.

The manufacturer states that periodic monitoring of ECGs should be considered in patients receiving midostaurin concomitantly with other drugs that are known to prolong the QT interval. (See Drug Interactions: Drugs that Prolong the QT Interval.)

Impairment of Fertility Results of animal studies suggest that midostaurin may impair male and female fertility. It is not known whether these effects are reversible.

Specific Populations **Pregnancy.** Midostaurin may cause fetal harm if administered to pregnant women based on its mechanism of action and animal findings. (See Fetal/Neonatal Morbidity and Mortality under Cautions: Warnings/Precautions.)

Confirmation of pregnancy status must be obtained no more than 7 days prior to initiation of midostaurin therapy.

Lactation. Midostaurin and its metabolites are distributed into milk in rats; it is not known whether the drug or its metabolites are distributed into milk in humans. Because of the potential for serious adverse reactions to midostaurin in nursing infants, women should be advised to discontinue nursing during midostaurin therapy. Women may begin nursing 4 months after discontinuance of therapy. The effects of the drug on nursing infants or on milk production are unknown.

Pediatric Use. Safety and efficacy of midostaurin have not been established in pediatric patients.

Geriatric Use. In phase 3 clinical trials evaluating midostaurin in patients with advanced systemic mastocytosis, 45% of patients were 65 years of age or older, while 11% were 75 years of age or older. No overall differences in safety and efficacy were observed between geriatric patients and younger adults, but greater sensitivity in some older patients cannot be ruled out.

Clinical studies evaluating midostaurin in patients with AML did not include sufficient numbers of patients 65 years of age and older to determine whether geriatric patients respond differently than younger adults.

The manufacturer states that midostaurin should be used with caution in geriatric patients, considering the patient's eligibility for concomitant chemotherapy and the greater frequency of concomitant disease and drug therapy observed in this age group.

Hepatic Impairment. Analysis of population pharmacokinetic data indicates that the pharmacokinetics of midostaurin and its metabolites are not influenced by mild (total bilirubin concentration between 1–1.5 times the upper limit of normal [ULN] or AST concentration exceeding the ULN) or moderate (total bilirubin concentration between 1.5–3 times the ULN with any AST concentration) hepatic impairment. The effects of severe hepatic impairment (total bilirubin concentration exceeding 3 times the ULN with any AST concentration) on the pharmacokinetics of midostaurin have not been established.

Renal Impairment. Analysis of population pharmacokinetic data indicates that the pharmacokinetics of midostaurin and its metabolites are not influenced by mild to moderate renal impairment (creatinine clearance of 30 mL/minute or greater). The effects of severe renal impairment (creatinine clearance 15–29 mL/minute) on the pharmacokinetics of midostaurin have not been established.

■ **Common Adverse Effects** Adverse effects reported in 10% or more of patients with previously untreated AML receiving midostaurin in combination with chemotherapy and occurring at an incidence at least 2% higher than that reported with placebo in combination with chemotherapy include febrile neutropenia, nausea, mucositis, vomiting, headache, petechiae, musculoskeletal pain, epistaxis, device-related infection, hyperglycemia, upper respiratory tract infection, hemorrhoids, arthralgia, hyperhidrosis, prolonged activated partial thromboplastin time (aPTT), insomnia, and renal impairment; however, grade 1 or 2 adverse effects were not reported in all clinical sites enrolled in the study. Laboratory abnormalities reported in 10% or more of patients with previously untreated AML receiving midostaurin in combination with chemotherapy and at an incidence at least 2% higher than that reported with placebo in combination with chemotherapy include hypocalcemia, elevated ALT concentrations, and hypernatremia.

Adverse effects reported in 10% or more of patients with advanced systemic mastocytosis receiving midostaurin alone include nausea, vomiting, diarrhea, edema, musculoskeletal pain, abdominal pain, fatigue, upper respiratory tract infection, constipation, pyrexia, headache, dyspnea, arthralgia, cough, urinary tract infection, GI hemorrhage, rash, dizziness, pleural effusion, epistaxis, insomnia, prolonged QT interval, renal impairment, herpes simplex virus infection, and pneumonia. Laboratory abnormalities reported in 20% or more of patients with advanced systemic mastocytosis receiving midostaurin alone include hyperglycemia, lymphopenia, leukopenia, anemia, thrombocytopenia, neutropenia, elevated alkaline phosphatase concentrations, hypocalcemia, elevated concentrations of pancreatic enzymes (e.g., amylase, lipase), hyperuricemia, elevated aminotransferase (ALT or AST) and γ-glutamyltransferase (γ-glutamyltranspeptidase, GGT, GGTP) concentrations, hyponatremia, hyperbilirubinemia, hypoalbuminemia, hypokalemia, elevated concentrations of serum creatinine, hyperkalemia, hypophosphatemia, and hypomagnesemia.

Drug Interactions

Midostaurin and its active metabolites (CGP-52421 and CGP-62221) are metabolized principally by cytochrome P-450 (CYP) isoenzyme 3A4. In vitro studies indicate that midostaurin, CGP-52421, and CGP-62221 are inhibitors of CYP isoenzymes 1A2, 2C8, 2C9, 2C19, 2D6, and 2E1 and inducers of CYP isoenzymes 1A2, 2B6, 2C8, 2C9, 2C19, and 3A.

In vitro, midostaurin, CGP-52421, and CGP-62221 are inhibitors of organic anion transport protein (OATP) 1A1 and inducers of multidrug resistance protein (MRP) 2 at clinically relevant concentrations. In vitro studies suggest that midostaurin is not a substrate of P-glycoprotein (P-gp) or MRP2.

■ Drugs and Foods Affecting Hepatic Microsomal Enzymes

Inhibitors of CYP3A Concomitant use of midostaurin with potent inhibitors of CYP3A may result in increased systemic exposure to midostaurin and its active metabolites (CGP-52421 and CGP-62221) and an increased incidence of adverse effects. The extent of the pharmacokinetic interaction appears to be dependent on the duration of midostaurin dosing, such that the increase in midostaurin concentrations may be larger and the potential for adverse effects greater when potent CYP3A inhibitors are administered during the first week of midostaurin therapy. (See Description.) In healthy individuals, the potent CYP3A4 inhibitor ketoconazole (400 mg daily for 10 days) increased the area under the concentration-time curve (AUC) and peak plasma concentrations of midostaurin (single 50-mg dose) by 10.4- and 1.8-fold, respectively, and prolonged the elimination half-life of midostaurin from 23.3 hours to 90.6 hours. In addition, the AUCs of CGP-62221 and CGP-52421 were increased by 3.5- and 1.2-fold, respectively; however, peak plasma concentrations of these active metabolites were decreased by twofold. When itraconazole (100 mg twice daily on days 22–28) was administered concomitantly with midostaurin (100 mg twice daily on days 1–2 followed by 50 mg twice daily on days 3–28) in patients with acute myeloid leukemia (AML), trough plasma concentrations of midostaurin, CGP-62221, and CGP-52421 were increased by 2.1-, 1.2-, and 1.3-fold, respectively, on day 28.

Because of the potential for potent CYP3A inhibitors (e.g., clarithromycin; cobicistat; conivaptan; diltiazem; *ritonavir-boosted* elvitegravir; grapefruit products; idelalisib; *ritonavir-boosted* indinavir; itraconazole; ketoconazole; the fixed combination of lopinavir and ritonavir [lopinavir/ritonavir]; nefazodone; nelfinavir; the fixed combination of ombitasvir, paritaprevir, and ritonavir [with or without dasabuvir]; posaconazole; ritonavir; *ritonavir-boosted* saquinavir; *ritonavir-boosted* tipranavir; voriconazole) to increase exposure to midostaurin and its active metabolites, selection of an alternative drug with less CYP3A inhibition potential should be considered. (See Drug Interactions: Grapefruit.) Alternatively, patients should be monitored for adverse effects, especially during the first week of midostaurin therapy (including the first week of midostaurin therapy in each cycle when used in combination with chemotherapy).

Inducers of CYP3A Concomitant use of midostaurin with potent inducers of CYP3A may result in decreased systemic exposure to midostaurin, CGP-52421, and CGP-62221, and reduced midostaurin efficacy. When the potent CYP3A4 inducer rifampin (600 mg daily for 14 days) was administered concomitantly with midostaurin (single 50-mg dose) in healthy individuals, the AUCs of midostaurin, CGP-52421, and CGP-62221 were decreased by 96, 59, and 92%, respectively.

Concomitant use with potent CYP3A4 inducers (e.g., carbamazepine, enzalutamide, mitotane, phenytoin, rifampin) should be avoided. Although the CYP3A4 induction potential of St. John's wort [*Hypericum perforatum*] varies among preparations, St. John's wort is generally considered a potent CYP3A4 inducer and concomitant use should be avoided. Some clinicians also recommend avoiding concomitant use with moderate CYP3A4 inducers.

■ Drugs Metabolized by Hepatic Microsomal Enzymes

When midostaurin (100 mg on day 3 followed by 50 mg twice daily on days 4–6) was administered concomitantly with the sensitive CYP3A substrate midazolam (4 mg on days 1, 3, and 8) in healthy individuals, the AUCs of midazolam and its active metabolite, 1-hydroxymethylmidazolam, were not appreciably affected; however, because the extent of enzyme induction after only 4 days of midostaurin administration may not fully reflect the enzyme induction potential at steady state, the findings are not considered to be conclusive. (See Description.)

■ Drugs that Prolong the QT Interval

Although a controlled study of the effects of midostaurin on the QT interval did not reveal clinically important effects, some patients receiving the drug during clinical trials have experienced QT-interval prolongation. Therefore, the manufacturer states that periodic monitoring of ECGs should be considered in patients receiving midostaurin concomitantly with other drugs that are known to prolong the QT interval. (See Prolongation of QT Interval under Cautions: Warnings/Precautions.)

■ Grapefruit

Although the CYP3A inhibition potential of grapefruit juice may be influenced by the concentration, dose, and specific preparation, grapefruit juice is generally considered to be a potent CYP3A inhibitor. Patients receiving midostaurin should be advised to avoid consuming grapefruit products.

Description

Midostaurin, an inhibitor of multiple receptor tyrosine kinases including fms-like tyrosine kinase 3 (Flt-3), is an antineoplastic agent. Receptor tyrosine kinases are involved in the initiation of various cascades of intracellular signaling events that lead to cell proliferation and/or influence processes critical to cell survival and tumor progression (e.g., angiogenesis, metastasis, inhibition of apoptosis), based on the respective kinase. Midostaurin has been shown to inhibit Flt-3 signaling resulting in inhibition of Flt-3-induced cell proliferation. The drug also induced apoptosis in leukemic cells expressing Flt-3 mutations (i.e., internal tandem duplications [ITD], tyrosine kinase domain [TKD] point mutations) or overexpressing wild-type Flt-3 and platelet-derived growth factor receptors (PDGFR). In vitro, midostaurin or its active metabolites (CGP-62221 and CGP-52421) exhibit inhibitory activity against wild-type Flt-3, mutant Flt-3, vascular endothelial growth factor receptor 2 (VEGFR-2), PDGFR-α, PDGFR-β, and members of the protein kinase C (PKC) family of tyrosine kinases. The drug also has demonstrated inhibition of stem cell factor receptor (c-Kit) signaling resulting in apoptosis in mast cells and inhibition of c-Kit-induced cell proliferation and histamine release.

Following repeated administration of midostaurin, trough concentrations of midostaurin and its metabolites (CGP-62221 and CGP-52421) exhibit time-dependent pharmacokinetics and there is a lack of proportionality between dosage and systemic exposure, possibly because of autoinduction of its own metabolism. Maximum trough concentrations of both midostaurin and CGP-62221 are achieved in 8 days and then decline substantially (by about 50–60%) to steady-state values by day 28; however, plasma concentrations of CGP-52421 continue to increase until day 28. Maximum trough and steady-state concentrations of midostaurin, CGP-62221, and CGP-52421 achieved at a midostaurin dosage of 50 mg twice daily (given with food) are similar to those achieved at a dosage of 100 mg twice daily (also given with food).

Following oral administration in a fasted state, midostaurin is rapidly absorbed with peak plasma concentrations occurring within 1–3 hours. Administration of a single 50-mg dose of midostaurin with a high-fat, high-calorie meal (900–1000 calories with 50% of calories from fat) increased the area under the concentration-time curve (AUC) of midostaurin by 1.6-fold and decreased peak plasma concentrations of the drug by 27% compared with administration in the fasted state. When the drug was administered with a standard meal (450 calories with 25% of calories from fat), the AUC of midostaurin was increased by 1.2-fold and peak plasma concentrations were decreased by 20% compared with administration in the fasted state. Following oral administration with a standard or high-fat meal, the median time to peak plasma concentrations of midostaurin ranged from 2.5–3 hours. (See Dosage and Administration: Administration.)

Midostaurin and its metabolites are highly bound (greater than 99.8%) to plasma proteins (mainly to α_1-acid glycoprotein) in vitro.

Midostaurin is metabolized principally by cytochrome P-450 (CYP) isoenzyme 3A4. Major metabolites of the drug include active hydroxyl (CGP-52421) and *O*-demethylated (CGP-62221) derivatives. CGP-52421 and CGP-62221 also are metabolized by CYP3A4 and account for approximately 38 and 28%, respectively, of total plasma concentrations of the drug. The terminal half-lives of midostaurin, CGP-62221, and CGP-52421 are 21, 32, and 482 hours, respectively. Following oral administration of midostaurin, 95% of the recovered dose is excreted in feces (4% as unchanged drug and 91% as metabolites) and 5% is eliminated in urine.

Data from a population pharmacokinetic analysis indicate that age (20–94 years), gender, and race do not have clinically important effects on the pharmacokinetics of midostaurin.

Advice to Patients

Importance of instructing patients to read the manufacturer's patient information before initiating midostaurin therapy.

If a dose is missed or vomited, importance of administering the next dose at the regularly scheduled time; an additional dose should *not* be administered to make up for a missed dose.

Risk of interstitial lung disease or pneumonitis. Importance of informing clinician immediately if new or worsening cough, chest pain, or shortness of breath occurs.

Risk of diarrhea, nausea, or vomiting. Importance of informing clinician if any of these symptoms occur or persist despite optimal supportive therapy.

Risk of impaired fertility in men and women.

Risk of fetal harm. Necessity of advising women of child-bearing potential and men who are partners of such women that they should use an effective method of contraception while receiving the drug and for at least 4 months after discontinuance of therapy. Importance of women informing clinicians if they are or plan to become pregnant. If pregnancy occurs, advise pregnant women of potential risk to the fetus.

Importance of advising women to avoid breast-feeding while receiving the drug and for at least 4 months after discontinuance of therapy.

Importance of informing clinicians of existing or contemplated concomitant therapy, including prescription and OTC drugs, as well as any concomitant illnesses.

Importance of informing patients of other important precautionary information. (See Cautions.)

Overview® (see Users Guide). For additional information on this drug until a more detailed monograph is developed and published, the manufacturer's labeling should be consulted. It is *essential* that the manufacturer's labeling be consulted for more detailed information on usual cautions, precautions, contraindications, potential drug interactions, laboratory test interferences, and acute toxicity. For further information on the handling of antineoplastic agents, see the ASHP Guidelines on Handling Hazardous Drugs at http://www.ahfsdruginformation.com.

Preparations

Excipients in commercially available drug preparations may have clinically important effects in some individuals; consult specific product labeling for details.

Midostaurin

Oral		
Capsules	25 mg	**Rydapt®**, Novartis

†Use is not currently included in the labeling approved by the US Food and Drug Administration

Necitumumab

■ Necitumumab, a recombinant, fully human IgG_1 kappa monoclonal antibody that binds to human epidermal growth factor receptor (EGFR), is an antineoplastic agent.

Uses

■ **Non-small Cell Lung Cancer** Necitumumab is used in combination with gemcitabine and cisplatin for the first-line treatment of metastatic squamous non-small cell lung cancer (NSCLC). Necitumumab is designated an orphan drug by FDA for the treatment of this cancer.

The current indication for necitumumab in the treatment of metastatic squamous NSCLC is based principally on the results of a randomized, multinational, open-label, controlled phase 3 study (SQUIRE) in adults with chemotherapy-naive metastatic (stage IV) squamous NSCLC. In this study, 1093 patients were randomized (stratified by ECOG performance status and race) in a 1:1 ratio to receive either necitumumab (800 mg by IV infusion on days 1 and 8) in combination with gemcitabine (1.25 g/m² by IV infusion on days 1 and 8) and cisplatin (75 mg/m² by IV infusion on day 1) or gemcitabine in combination with cisplatin every 3 weeks for a maximum of 6 cycles in the absence of disease progression or unacceptable toxicity. Patients demonstrating at least stable disease while receiving necitumumab, gemcitabine, and cisplatin continued to receive necitumumab as single-agent therapy until disease progression or unacceptable toxicity occurred. The primary measure of efficacy was overall survival; secondary end points included overall response rate and investigator-assessed progression-free survival. The median age of patients was 62 years (range: 32–86 years), 83% were male, 84% were Caucasian, and most were smokers (91%). Baseline ECOG performance status was 0 or 1 for 91% of the patients and 2 for the remaining 9% of the patients; 91% of the patients had metastatic disease in 2 or more sites. The median duration of follow-up was approximately 25 months. Patients receiving necitumumab in combination with gemcitabine and cisplatin had a substantially longer median overall survival (11.5 versus 9.9 months) and investigator-assessed progression-free survival (5.7 versus 5.5 months) compared with patients receiving gemcitabine and cisplatin alone. No significant difference in overall response rate was observed between the 2 treatment groups in this study (31 versus 29%, respectively).

In a randomized, open-label, multicenter phase 3 study (INSPIRE) in adults with chemotherapy-naive metastatic *nonsquamous* NSCLC, patients were randomized to receive either necitumumab in combination with pemetrexed and cisplatin or pemetrexed and cisplatin alone every 3 weeks. This study was terminated prematurely because an increased incidence of death due to any cause and of thromboembolic events was observed in the group of patients treated with necitumumab, pemetrexed, and cisplatin. At the time of study termination, 633 patients had been enrolled; the median age of patients was 61 years and 89% had adenocarcinoma histology. The median duration of follow-up for the necitumumab plus pemetrexed and cisplatin and the pemetrexed and cisplatin alone groups was 24.5 and 25.6 months, respectively. The addition of necitumumab to pemetrexed and cisplatin was not found to improve overall survival (the primary measure of efficacy), progression-free survival, or overall response rate in this study.

The manufacturer states that necitumumab is *not* indicated for the treatment of *nonsquamous* NSCLC†. (See Increased Toxicity and Mortality in Nonsquamous NSCLC under Warnings/Precautions: Other Warnings and Precautions, in Cautions.)

Dosage and Administration

■ **General** To minimize the risk of infusion-related reactions in patients who have previously experienced a grade 1 or 2 infusion-related reaction to necitumumab, premedication with an antihistamine (e.g., diphenhydramine or equivalent) is recommended prior to all subsequent infusions of the drug. Patients who have experienced a second occurrence of a grade 1 or 2 infusion-related reaction should receive an antihistamine (diphenhydramine or equivalent), acetaminophen (or equivalent), and dexamethasone (or equivalent) prior to each subsequent necitumumab infusion. (See Infusion-related Reactions under Dosage: Dosage Modification for Toxicity, in Dosage and Administration and also under Warnings/Precautions: Other Warnings and Precautions, in Cautions.)

Serum electrolyte concentrations, including magnesium, potassium, and calcium, should be monitored closely and electrolyte abnormalities corrected aggressively, as clinically appropriate, prior to each infusion of necitumumab and for at least 8 weeks following the last dose of the drug. (See Electrolyte Abnormalities under Dosage: Dosage Modification for Toxicity, in Dosage and Administration.)

■ **Administration** Necitumumab is administered by IV infusion over 60 minutes; the infusion solution should be administered using an infusion pump. Diluted necitumumab infusion solution should *not* be administered in the same IV line with any other drug or electrolytes. The IV line should be flushed with 0.9% sodium chloride injection at the end of the infusion.

Necitumumab injection concentrate must be diluted prior to administration. Prior to dilution, the injection concentrate should be inspected visually for particulate matter and discoloration. The injection concentrate should be clear to slightly opalescent and colorless to slightly yellow and should *not* be used if particulate matter or discoloration is present.

Necitumumab is diluted by adding the appropriate volume of necitumumab injection concentrate (containing 16 mg/mL) to an infusion container containing the appropriate volume of 0.9% sodium chloride injection to yield a final volume of 250 mL. Necitumumab injection concentrate should *not* be diluted with solutions containing dextrose or other solutions. Necitumumab also should *not* be admixed with any other drug or electrolytes. The diluted necitumumab infusion solution should be mixed by gentle inversion and should *not* be shaken. Diluted necitumumab infusion solution may be stored at room temperature (up to 25°C) for up to 4 hours or under refrigeration (2–8°C) for up to 24 hours; the diluted infusion solution should *not* be frozen.

Diluted necitumumab infusion solution should be inspected visually for particulate matter and discoloration prior to administration; if particulate matter or discoloration is evident, the diluted solution should be discarded.

Any unused portion left in the vial should be discarded since necitumumab injection concentrate contains no preservative.

Unopened vials of necitumumab injection concentrate should be protected from light and stored in the original carton at 2–8°C, and should *not* be frozen or shaken.

■ **Dosage** ***Non-small Cell Lung Cancer*** For the first-line treatment of metastatic squamous non-small cell lung cancer (NSCLC), the recommended adult dosage of necitumumab is 800 mg administered as a 60-minute IV infusion on days 1 and 8 of each 3-week cycle. The drug is given in combination with gemcitabine and cisplatin.

Necitumumab should be administered by IV infusion prior to IV infusion of gemcitabine and cisplatin.

Treatment with necitumumab should be continued until disease progression or unacceptable toxicity occurs.

Dosage Modification for Toxicity **Infusion-related Reactions.** If a grade 1 infusion-related reaction occurs, the infusion rate should be reduced by 50% for the duration of the infusion.

If a grade 2 infusion-related reaction occurs, the infusion should be interrupted until resolution to grade 1 or less; the infusion should then be resumed at a 50% reduced infusion rate for all subsequent infusions.

If grade 3 or 4 infusion-related reactions occur, necitumumab should be *permanently* discontinued. (See Infusion-related Reactions under Warnings/Precautions: Other Warnings and Precautions, in Cautions.)

Dermatologic Toxicity. If grade 3 rash or acneiform rash develops, necitumumab therapy should be withheld. If toxicity improves to grade 2 or less, the drug should be resumed at a reduced dosage of 400 mg for at least 1 treatment cycle. If symptoms do not worsen, the dosage may be increased to 600 mg and then to 800 mg in subsequent cycles. If dermatologic toxicity worsens or becomes intolerable at a dosage of 400 mg, necitumumab therapy should be *permanently* discontinued. If grade 3 rash or acneiform rash does *not* improve to grade 2 or less within 6 weeks of withholding necitumumab, therapy should be *permanently* discontinued.

If grade 3 skin induration/fibrosis or grade 4 dermatologic toxicity occurs, necitumumab therapy should be *permanently* discontinued. (See Dermatologic Toxicity under Warnings/Precautions: Other Warnings and Precautions, in Cautions.)

Electrolyte Abnormalities. If grade 3 or 4 electrolyte abnormalities occur, necitumumab therapy should be withheld until resolution to grade 2 or less; treatment may be resumed at the previous dosage upon improvement of hypomagnesemia and related electrolyte abnormalities to grade 2 or less. (See Cardiopulmonary Arrest and also see Hypomagnesemia under Warnings/Precautions: Warnings, in Cautions.)

■ **Special Populations** The manufacturer provides no specific dosage recommendations for geriatric patients or for patients with hepatic or renal impairment. (See Specific Populations under Cautions: Warnings/Precautions.)

No dosage adjustment is necessary based on body weight, race, or gender.

Cautions

■ **Contraindications** The manufacturer states there are no contraindications to the use of necitumumab.

■ **Warnings/Precautions** ***Warnings*** **Cardiopulmonary Arrest.** Cardiopulmonary arrest and/or sudden death occurred in 15 (3%) of 538 patients receiving necitumumab in combination with gemcitabine and cisplatin compared with 3 (0.6%) of 541 patients receiving gemcitabine and cisplatin alone for metastatic squamous non-small cell lung cancer (NSCLC) in the primary efficacy study. Twelve of the 15 patients died within 30 days of the last dose of necitumumab and had comorbid conditions (including 3 patients with a history of coronary artery disease, 4 with hypomagnesemia, 7 with chronic obstructive pulmonary disease, and 5 with hypertension); 11 of the 12 patients had an unwitnessed death. Patients with substantial coronary artery disease, myocardial infarction within 6 months, uncontrolled hypertension, and uncontrolled congestive heart failure were excluded from this study. The incremental risk of cardiopulmonary arrest or sudden death with necitumumab therapy in patients with a history of coronary artery disease, congestive heart failure, or arrhythmias compared with those without these cardiovascular conditions is not known.

Serum electrolyte concentrations, including magnesium, potassium, and calcium, should be closely monitored prior to each necitumumab infusion and for at least 8 weeks following the last dose of the drug. Necitumumab therapy should be withheld for grade 3 or 4 electrolyte abnormalities. (See Electrolyte Abnormalities under Dosage: Dosage Modification for Toxicity, in Dosage and Administration.) Electrolyte abnormalities should be aggressively corrected, as clinically appropriate.

Hypomagnesemia. Hypomagnesemia occurred in 83% of patients receiving necitumumab in combination with gemcitabine and cisplatin compared with 70% of patients receiving gemcitabine and cisplatin alone in the primary efficacy study, and severe (grade 3 or 4) hypomagnesemia occurred in 20% of patients receiving necitumumab with gemcitabine and cisplatin compared with 7% of patients receiving gemcitabine and cisplatin alone. The median time to development of hypomagnesemia and accompanying electrolyte abnormalities was 6 weeks, and about half of the cases developed within 4–9 weeks following initiation of necitumumab therapy.

Serum electrolyte concentrations, including magnesium, potassium, and calcium, should be monitored prior to each necitumumab infusion during therapy and for at least 8 weeks following completion of therapy. If electrolyte abnormalities occur, they should be corrected, as clinically appropriate. Necitumumab therapy should be withheld for grade 3 or 4 electrolyte abnormalities. (See Electrolyte Abnormalities under Dosage: Dosage Modification for Toxicity, in Dosage and Administration.)

Other Warnings and Precautions **Thromboembolic Events.** Venous and arterial thromboembolic events, including some fatal events, have been reported in patients receiving necitumumab in combination with gemcitabine and cisplatin. The most common venous thromboembolic events were pulmonary embolism and deep-vein thrombosis and the most common arterial thromboembolic events were stroke/cerebral ischemia and myocardial infarction. In the primary efficacy study, venous thromboembolism (VTE) was reported in 9 or 5% of patients and was grade 3 or higher in 5 or 3% of patients receiving necitumumab with chemotherapy or chemotherapy alone, respectively. The incidence of fatal events was similar between treatment groups. Arterial thromboembolism was reported in 5 or 4% of patients and was grade 3 or higher in 4 or 2% of patients receiving necitumumab with chemotherapy or chemotherapy alone, respectively. The relative risk of venous or arterial thromboembolic events was approximately threefold higher in patients with a history of thromboembolic events than in patients without such a history.

Necitumumab should be *permanently* discontinued in patients who develop a serious or life-threatening venous or arterial thromboembolic event.

Dermatologic Toxicity. Dermatologic toxicity, including rash, acneiform dermatitis, acne, dry skin, pruritus, generalized rash, skin fissures, maculopapular rash, and erythema, was reported in 79% of patients receiving necitumumab in combination with gemcitabine and cisplatin in the primary efficacy study. Severe dermatologic toxicity occurred in 8% of patients receiving this regimen. Dermatologic toxicity usually developed within the first 2 weeks of therapy and resolved within 17 weeks after onset.

Sun exposure should be limited during necitumumab therapy. (See Advice to Patients.)

Reduction in dosage or discontinuance of therapy may be required in patients who develop dermatologic toxicity. (See Dermatologic Toxicity under Dosage: Dosage Modification for Toxicity, in Dosage and Administration.)

Infusion-related Reactions. Infusion-related reactions of any severity occurred in 1.5% and grade 3 reactions occurred in 0.4% of necitumumab-treated patients in the primary efficacy study. Most infusion-related reactions occurred after the first or second infusion of the drug. None of the patients received premedication for infusion-related reactions for the first dose of necitumumab in this study.

Patients should be monitored for manifestations of infusion-related reactions during and following infusions of necitumumab. If infusion-related reactions occur, premedication should be given for all subsequent infusions. (See General under Dosage and Administration.) Reduction in the infusion rate, temporary interruption of therapy, or permanent discontinuance of necitumumab may be necessary depending on the severity of the reaction. (See Infusion-related Reactions under Dosage: Dosage Modification for Toxicity, in Dosage and Administration.)

Increased Toxicity and Mortality in Nonsquamous NSCLC. In the INSPIRE study in patients with *nonsquamous* NSCLC, necitumumab in combination with pemetrexed and cisplatin was associated with an increased incidence of serious toxicity and mortality compared with pemetrexed and cisplatin alone. In this study, more patients receiving necitumumab in combination with pemetrexed and cisplatin compared with those receiving pemetrexed and cisplatin alone experienced serious toxicity (51 versus 41%, respectively), fatal toxicity (16 versus 10%), and cardiopulmonary arrest and/or sudden death (3.3 versus 1.3%). (See Uses: Non-small Cell Lung Cancer.)

The manufacturer states that necitumumab is *not* indicated for the treatment of *nonsquamous* NSCLC†.

Fetal/Neonatal Morbidity and Mortality. Based on animal studies and its mechanism of action, necitumumab may cause fetal harm if administered to pregnant women. Disruption or depletion of epidermal growth factor receptor (EGFR) in animal models has been shown to impair embryofetal development (including effects on placental, lung, cardiac, skin, and neural development). The absence of EGFR signaling has resulted in embryolethality and postnatal deaths in animals. Women of childbearing potential should use effective contraception while receiving necitumumab and for 3 months after the final dose of the drug. If necitumumab is used during pregnancy or if the patient becomes pregnant while receiving the drug, the patient should be apprised of the potential fetal hazard.

Specific Populations **Pregnancy.** Based on animal studies and its mechanism of action, necitumumab may cause fetal harm if administered to pregnant women. (See Fetal/Neonatal Morbidity and Mortality under Warnings/Precautions: Other Warnings and Precautions, in Cautions.)

Lactation. It is not known whether necitumumab is distributed into human milk. The effects of the drug on nursing infants and on milk production also are unknown. Because of the potential for serious adverse reactions to necitumumab in nursing infants, women should be advised not to breast-feed while receiving the drug and for 3 months after the last dose.

Pediatric Use. Safety and efficacy of necitumumab have not been established in pediatric patients.

Geriatric Use. In the principal efficacy study evaluating necitumumab in patients with metastatic squamous NSCLC, 39% of patients were 65 years of age or older and 20% were 70 years of age or older. In a subgroup analysis of this study, an overall survival benefit was not observed in patients 70 years of age or older receiving necitumumab in combination with gemcitabine and cisplatin. Although the overall safety of necitumumab was generally similar for subgroups of patients younger than 70 years of age and those 70 years of age or older, a higher incidence of venous thromboembolic events, including pulmonary embolism, was observed in patients 70 years of age or older receiving necitumumab with gemcitabine plus cisplatin compared with younger patients in this study.

In a population pharmacokinetic analysis, patient age (range: 19–84 years) did not substantially affect systemic exposure of necitumumab.

Hepatic Impairment. Formal studies evaluating the effect of hepatic impairment on the pharmacokinetics of necitumumab have not been conducted to date. In a population pharmacokinetic analysis, systemic exposure to necitumumab was unaffected in patients with mild to moderate hepatic impairment. The manufacturer states that no patients with severe hepatic impairment were enrolled in clinical trials with the drug.

Renal Impairment. Formal studies evaluating the effect of renal impairment on the pharmacokinetics of necitumumab have not been conducted to date. However, a population pharmacokinetic analysis indicates that renal function (as assessed by estimated creatinine clearance in a range of 11–250 mL/minute) does not affect systemic exposure of the drug.

■ **Common Adverse Effects** Adverse effects reported in at least 15% of patients receiving necitumumab in combination with gemcitabine and cisplatin in the primary efficacy study and at an incidence more than 2% higher than that reported with gemcitabine and cisplatin alone include rash, vomiting, diarrhea, and acneiform dermatitis.

Laboratory abnormalities reported in more than 10% of patients receiving necitumumab in combination with gemcitabine and cisplatin in the primary efficacy study and at an incidence more than 2% higher than that reported with gemcitabine and cisplatin alone include hypomagnesemia, hypokalemia, hypocalcemia, and hypophosphatemia.

Drug Interactions

■ **Antineoplastic Agents** Concomitant use of necitumumab with gemcitabine and cisplatin in patients with advanced solid tumors increased peak plasma concentration and systemic exposure of gemcitabine by 63 and 22%, respectively, compared with administration of gemcitabine and cisplatin alone; systemic exposure to cisplatin was unchanged.

Concomitant use of necitumumab with gemcitabine and cisplatin did not substantially affect systemic exposure of necitumumab.

Description

Necitumumab, a recombinant, fully human IgG_1 kappa monoclonal antibody that binds to human epidermal growth factor receptor (EGFR), is an antineoplastic agent.

Necitumumab binds with high affinity and specificity to the extracellular domain of the epidermal growth factor (EGF) binding site of human EGFR and competitively inhibits the interaction of EGFR with its ligands. The mechanism by which necitumumab inhibits EGFR appears to be similar to that of cetuximab, a recombinant chimeric (human-murine) monoclonal antibody used in the treatment of colorectal cancer and squamous cell carcinoma of the head and neck; cetuximab also has been used in the treatment of non-small cell lung cancer (NSCLC)†. While EGFR-activating mutations are rare in squamous-cell histologic type cancers, overexpression of EGFR has been observed in the majority (60–80%) of these tumors. Blockade of EGFR results in inhibition of ligand-induced phosphorylation and downstream signaling pathways, which play an important role in cell proliferation, invasion, metastasis, angiogenesis, and inhibition of apoptosis (programmed cell death). Binding of necitumumab induces EGFR internalization and degradation in vitro; in addition, in vitro binding leads to antibody-dependent cell-mediated cytotoxicity (ADCC) in EGFR-expressing cells.

In mice bearing xenografts of human cancers, including NSCLC, necitumumab in combination with gemcitabine and cisplatin demonstrated increased antitumor activity compared with gemcitabine and cisplatin alone.

In contrast to cetuximab, which has been associated with hypersensitivity reactions in about 20% of patients when used for NSCLC†, necitumumab is a fully human antibody and is therefore potentially less immunogenic. In the primary efficacy study of necitumumab in patients with metastatic squamous cell NSCLC, hypersensitivity/infusion-related reactions were reported in 1.5% of patients receiving the drug.

Based on a population pharmacokinetic analysis, steady-state necitumumab concentrations are predicted to be reached in approximately 100 days following IV infusion of necitumumab 800 mg on days 1 and 8 of each 21-day cycle. The elimination half-life of necitumumab in patients receiving the recommended dosage regimen is approximately 14 days.

Advice to Patients

Risk of electrolyte abnormalities, including hypomagnesemia, hypokalemia, and hypocalcemia. Importance of advising patients to take electrolyte replacement therapy exactly as advised by their clinician.

Risk of venous and arterial thromboembolic events.

Risk of skin reactions. Importance of advising patients to minimize sun exposure with protective clothing and use of sunscreen during necitumumab therapy.

Risk of infusion-related reactions. Importance of informing patients to report signs and symptoms of infusion reactions (e.g., fever, chills, breathing problems) to a healthcare professional.

Risk of fetal harm. Necessity of advising women of childbearing potential to use effective methods of contraception while receiving necitumumab and for 3 months after the last dose of the drug. If a patient becomes pregnant during therapy, apprise patient of potential hazard to the fetus.

Importance of advising women to avoid breast-feeding while receiving necitumumab therapy and for 3 months following the last dose of the drug.

Importance of informing patients of other important precautionary information. (See Cautions.)

Overview® (see Users Guide). For additional information on this drug until a more detailed monograph is developed and published, the manufacturer's labeling should be consulted. It is *essential* that the manufacturer's labeling be consulted for more detailed information on usual cautions, precautions, contraindications, potential drug interactions, laboratory test interferences, and acute toxicity. For further information on the handling of antineoplastic agents, see the ASHP Guidelines on Handling Hazardous Drugs at http://www.ahfsdruginformation.com.

Preparations

Excipients in commercially available drug preparations may have clinically important effects in some individuals; consult specific product labeling for details.

Necitumumab (Recombinant)

Parenteral

Concentrate, for injection, for IV infusion only	16 mg/mL (800 mg)	**Portrazza®, Lilly**

†Use is not currently included in the labeling approved by the US Food and Drug Administration

Nelarabine

Nelzarabine

■ Nelarabine, a prodrug of the deoxyguanosine analog 9-β-D-arabinofuranosylguanine (ara-G), is an antimetabolite antineoplastic agent.

Uses

■ **Acute Lymphocytic Leukemia** *Acute T-cell Leukemia* Nelarabine is used for the treatment of acute T-cell lymphocytic (lymphoblastic) leukemia (ALL) and T-cell lymphoblastic lymphoma in patients whose disease is refractory to or has relapsed after at least 2 prior chemotherapy regimens. Nelarabine is designated an orphan drug by the US Food and Drug Administration (FDA) for use in these conditions. Nelarabine became commercially available in the US under the principles and procedures of the accelerated review policy of the FDA, which allows approval based on analysis of surrogate markers of response rather than clinical end points. The current indication for nelarabine is based on induction of complete responses; randomized clinical trials showing increased survival or other clinical benefits have not been conducted to date.

Safety and efficacy of nelarabine were evaluated in an open-label, single-arm, multicenter trial in 39 adults with relapsed or refractory T-cell ALL or T-cell lymphoblastic lymphoma.

Among the 28 trial patients (mean age: 34 years, range: 16–65 years; 82% male; 61% white) with disease that was refractory to or had relapsed after at least 2 prior induction regimens, nelarabine (1500 mg/m² IV over 2 hours on days 1, 3, and 5, with treatment cycles repeated every 21 days) resulted in a complete response rate of 18%, a rate of complete response without full hematologic recovery of 4%, a duration of response (complete or complete without full hematologic recovery) of 4 to longer than 195 weeks, and a median overall survival of about 21 weeks.

Pediatric Patients. Safety and efficacy of nelarabine also were evaluated in an open-label, single-arm, multicenter trial in 84 children and young adults 21 years of age and younger (mean age: about 12 years) with relapsed or refractory T-cell ALL or T-cell lymphoblastic lymphoma. Among the 39 trial patients with disease that was refractory to or had relapsed after at least 2 prior induction regimens, nelarabine (650 mg/m² IV over 1 hour daily for 5 consecutive days and repeated every 21 days) resulted in a complete response rate of 13%, a rate of complete response without full hematologic recovery of 10%, a duration of response (complete or complete without full hematologic recovery) of about 3–9 weeks, and a median overall survival of about 13 weeks.

Dosage and Administration

■ **Administration** Nelarabine is administered by IV infusion over 2 hours in adults and over 1 hour in children. Nelarabine injection should *not* be diluted prior to administration. The appropriate dose of nelarabine should be withdrawn from the required number of vials and transferred into empty polyvinylchloride (PVC) infusion bags or glass containers prior to administration. The drug should be inspected visually for particulate matter and discoloration prior to administration.

Appropriate measures (e.g., administration of IV fluids, allopurinol, and alkalinization of urine) should be taken to prevent hyperuricemia of tumor lysis syndrome. (See Tumor Lysis Syndrome under Warnings/Precautions: Warnings, in Cautions.)

The usual precautions for handling and preparing solutions of cytotoxic drugs should be observed when preparing or administering nelarabine.

■ **Dosage** The optimal duration of treatment in adult or pediatric patients has not been clearly established. In clinical trials, treatment generally was continued until evidence of disease progression, unacceptable toxicity, bone marrow transplantation, or lack of clinical benefit was observed or until patients became candidates for bone marrow transplantation.

Nelarabine should be discontinued in patients experiencing neurotoxicity of NCI Common Toxicity Criteria grade 2 or greater. (See Neurotoxicity under Warnings/Precautions: Warnings, in Cautions.) Dosage may be delayed for other toxicity (e.g., hematologic toxicity).

Acute Lymphocytic Leukemia The recommended adult dosage of nelarabine for the treatment of relapsed or refractory T-cell ALL or T-cell lymphoblastic lymphoma is 1500 mg/m² given by IV infusion over 2 hours on days 1, 3, and 5 and then every 21 days thereafter.

The recommended pediatric dosage of nelarabine for the treatment of relapsed or refractory T-cell ALL or T-cell lymphoblastic lymphoma is 650 mg/m² IV over 1 hour daily for 5 consecutive days and then every 21 days thereafter.

■ **Special Populations** Dosage adjustment is not necessary in patients with mild renal impairment (creatinine clearance of 50 mL/minute or greater). Insufficient data are available to support a dosage recommendation for patients with moderate to severe renal impairment (creatinine clearance of less than 50 mL/minute) or hepatic impairment.

Cautions

■ **Contraindications** Known hypersensitivity to nelarabine or any ingredient in the formulation.

■ **Warnings/Precautions** *Warnings* Nelarabine should be used under the supervision of a qualified clinician experienced in therapy with antineoplastic agents.

Neurotoxicity. Neurotoxicity, usually manifested by somnolence, confusion, seizures, peripheral neuropathy (ranging from numbness and paresthesias to motor weakness and paralysis), ataxia, and hypoesthesia (which may be severe and irreversible), is the dose-limiting toxicity of nelarabine.

Severe neurotoxic effects also have included coma, status epilepticus, craniospinal demyelination, and ascending peripheral neuropathy (similar in presentation to Guillain-Barré syndrome).

Patients who have received prior or concomitant intrathecal chemotherapy or prior craniospinal irradiation may be at increased risk for nelarabine-induced neurotoxicity. Patients should be closely monitored for neurologic toxicity, and the drug should be discontinued in patients experiencing neurologic events of NCI Common Toxicity Criteria grade 2 or greater.

Fetal/Neonatal Morbidity and Mortality. May cause fetal harm; teratogenicity demonstrated in animals. No studies to date in humans. Pregnancy should be avoided during therapy. If used during pregnancy or the patient becomes pregnant while receiving nelarabine, apprise of potential fetal hazard.

General Precautions **Hematologic Toxicity.** The principal manifestations of hematologic toxicity include leukopenia, thrombocytopenia, anemia, and neutropenia.

Tumor Lysis Syndrome. Appropriate measures (e.g., hydration, urinary alkalinization, allopurinol) to prevent hyperuricemia should be used in patients at risk for tumor lysis syndrome.

Immunization. The manufacturer recommends that live virus vaccines be avoided during therapy with the drug.

Adequate Patient Monitoring. Complete blood cell counts, including platelet count, should be performed at regular intervals in all patients receiving nelarabine. Patients receiving nelarabine should be closely monitored for adverse neurologic effects; the drug should be discontinued in patients experiencing neurotoxic events of NCI Common Toxicity grade 2 or greater.

Specific Populations **Pregnancy.** Category D. (See Users Guide.) (See Fetal/Neonatal Morbidity and Mortality under Warnings/Precautions: Warnings, in Cautions.)

Lactation. Not known whether nelarabine or ara-G is distributed into human milk; discontinue nursing during nelarabine therapy.

Pediatric Use. Safety and efficacy for treatment of relapsed or refractory T-cell ALL and T-cell lymphoblastic lymphoma have been established in patients 2.5–21 years of age. (See Pediatric Patients under Acute Lymphocytic Leukemia: Acute T-cell Leukemia, in Uses.)

Geriatric Use. Experience in those 65 years of age and older insufficient to determine whether they respond differently from younger adults. Incidence of adverse neurologic effects appears to increase with increasing age, especially in those 65 years of age and older. Renal impairment, which occurs more commonly in geriatric patients, may result in reduced clearance of ara-G.

Hepatic Impairment. Nelarabine has not been studied in patients with hepatic impairment. Because of the possibility of an increased risk of adverse reactions, closely monitor patients with severe hepatic impairment (serum bilirubin greater than 3 mg/dL).

Renal Impairment. Clearance of ara-G is reduced in patients with decreased renal function. Because of the possibility of an increased risk of adverse reactions, closely monitor patients with severe renal impairment (creatinine clearance of less than 30 mL/minute).

■ **Common Adverse Effects** Adverse effects reported in 5% or more of adults receiving nelarabine include anemia, thrombocytopenia, neutropenia, febrile neutropenia, somnolence, dizziness, peripheral neurologic disorders, peripheral neuropathy, peripheral motor neuropathy, peripheral sensory neuropathy, hypoesthesia, headache, paresthesia, ataxia, depressed level of consciousness, tremor, fatigue, pyrexia, asthenia, confusion, insomnia, depression, muscular weakness, myalgia, arthralgia, back pain, extremity pain, abnormal gait, nausea, diarrhea, vomiting, constipation, abdominal pain, anorexia, stomatitis, abdominal distension, sinus tachycardia, peripheral edema, edema, pain, rigors, chest pain, noncardiac chest pain, infection, pneumonia, sinusitis, increased serum AST concentrations, dehydration, hyperglycemia, cough, dyspnea, pleural effusion, epistaxis, exertional dyspnea, wheezing, petechiae, and hypotension.

Adverse effects reported in 5% or more of pediatric patients receiving nelarabine include anemia, neutropenia, thrombocytopenia, leukopenia, headache, peripheral neurologic disorders, peripheral neuropathy, peripheral sensory neuropathy, somnolence, hypoesthesia, seizures, increased serum transaminase concentrations, hyperbilirubinemia, hypoalbuminemia, hypokalemia, hypocalcemia, increased serum creatinine concentrations, hypoglycemia, hypomagnesemia, vomiting, asthenia, and infection.

Drug Interactions

■ **Drugs Affecting or Metabolized by Hepatic Microsomal Enzymes** Nelarabine does not appear to substantially inhibit any of the cytochrome P-450 (CYP) isoenzymes, including 1A2, 2A6, 2B6, 2C8, 2C9, 2C19, 2D6, or 3A4 in vitro (at concentrations up to 100 μM).

■ **Fludarabine** In a limited number of patients with refractory leukemia, fludarabine did not affect the pharmacokinetics of nelarabine, ara-G, or ara-GTP.

Description

Nelarabine, a prodrug of the deoxyguanosine analog ara-G, is an antimetabolite antineoplastic agent. Nelarabine is demethylated by adenosine deaminase (ADA) to ara-G, monophosphorylated by deoxyguanosine kinase and deoxycytidine kinase, and subsequently converted to the active 5′-triphosphate, ara-GTP. Ara-GTP accumulates in leukemic blasts and is incorporated into DNA, inducing fragmentation and apoptosis. Other mechanisms may contribute to the pharmacologic and toxicologic effects of the drug.

Nelarabine and ara-G are extensively distributed throughout the body and are not substantially bound to human plasma proteins (less than 25%). Following IV administration of nelarabine in adult patients with refractory leukemia or lymphoma, nelarabine and ara-G are rapidly eliminated from the plasma with a half-life of about 30 minutes and 3 hours, respectively. Mean clearance of nelarabine is about 30% higher in pediatric patients than in adult patients, while clearance of ara-G is similar in the two groups. Nelarabine and ara-G are partially (5–10 and 20–30%, respectively, of the administered dose) excreted by the kidneys.

Advice to Patients

Risk of somnolence; avoid driving or operating machinery.

Importance of patients notifying clinicians if they develop new or worsening symptoms of peripheral neuropathy (e.g., tingling or numbness in fingers, hands, toes, or feet; difficulty with fine motor coordination tasks such as buttoning clothing; unsteadiness while walking; weakness arising from a low chair or climbing stairs; increased tripping over uneven surfaces).

Importance of patients notifying clinicians immediately if they develop seizures.

Importance of patients notifying clinicians if fever or other symptom of infection, unusual bleeding or bruising, breathing difficulty, excessive fatigue, pallor, GI effects (e.g., nausea, vomiting, diarrhea, constipation), headache, drowsiness, or blurred vision occurs.

Importance of advising women to use an effective method of contraception and to avoid breast-feeding while undergoing nelarabine therapy. Importance of women informing a clinician immediately if they are or plan to become pregnant or plan to breast-feed.

Importance of informing clinicians of existing or contemplated concomitant therapy, including prescription and OTC drugs, as well as any concomitant illnesses.

Importance of informing patients of other important precautionary information. (See Cautions.)

Overview® (see Users Guide). For additional information on this drug until a more detailed monograph is developed and published, the manufacturer's labeling should be consulted. It is *essential* that the manufacturer's labeling be consulted for more detailed information on usual cautions, precautions, contraindications, potential drug interactions, laboratory test interferences, and acute toxicity.

Preparations

Excipients in commercially available drug preparations may have clinically important effects in some individuals; consult specific product labeling for details.

Nelarabine

Parenteral

Injection, for IV use	5 mg/mL (250 mg)	**Arranon®**, GlaxoSmithKline

Neratinib Maleate

■ Neratinib, a potent, selective, and irreversible inhibitor of human epidermal growth factor receptor type 2 (HER2), HER4, and epidermal growth factor receptor (EGFR) tyrosine kinases, is an antineoplastic agent.

Uses

■ **Breast Cancer** ***Extended Adjuvant Therapy for Early-stage Breast Cancer*** Neratinib is used as extended adjuvant therapy in patients with human epidermal growth factor receptor type 2 (HER2)-positive, early-stage breast cancer who have received adjuvant trastuzumab therapy.

The current indication for neratinib is based principally on the results of a randomized, double-blind, placebo-controlled phase 3 study (ExteNET) in women with HER2-positive early-stage breast cancer who completed neoadjuvant and adjuvant trastuzumab therapy within 2 years of randomization. In this study, 2840 patients were randomized (stratified by hormone receptor status, nodal status, and adjuvant trastuzumab regimen) to receive either neratinib (240 mg orally once daily) or placebo. Treatment was continued for 12 months unless disease progression, new breast cancer, or unacceptable toxicity occurred, or treatment was discontinued for other reasons. The primary measure of efficacy was invasive disease-free survival. The median age of patients enrolled in the study was 52 years; 81% of the patients were white, 99.7% had an ECOG (Eastern Cooperative Oncology Group) performance status of 0 or

1, 57% had hormone receptor-positive disease, and 30% had 4 or more positive nodes. Most patients (81%) were enrolled within 1 year of completion of adjuvant trastuzumab therapy; the median time from completion of adjuvant trastuzumab therapy to randomization was 4.4 or 4.6 months in patients randomized to neratinib or placebo, respectively.

At a follow-up of 2 years and 28 days, neratinib reduced the risk of disease recurrence or death by 34% compared with placebo; estimated 2-year invasive disease-free survival rates were 94.2 or 91.9% in patients receiving neratinib or placebo, respectively. Results of an exploratory analysis in approximately 75% of the intent-to-treat population suggested that the treatment effect of neratinib on invasive disease-free survival was maintained at 5 years (hazard ratio: 0.73). Subgroup analysis suggested that neratinib had a greater effect on invasive disease-free survival relative to placebo in patients with hormone receptor-positive disease than in those with hormone receptor-negative disease (hazard ratio: 0.49 and 0.93, respectively), in those who received sequential adjuvant trastuzumab therapy than in those who received adjuvant trastuzumab concurrently with chemotherapy (hazard ratio: 0.46 and 0.80, respectively), and in those who completed adjuvant trastuzumab therapy within 1 year of randomization than in those who completed adjuvant trastuzumab therapy 1–2 years prior to randomization (hazard ratio: 0.63 and 0.92, respectively). Median overall survival had not been reached at the time of the efficacy analysis.

Dosage and Administration

■ **General** To minimize the incidence and severity of treatment-related diarrhea, antidiarrheal prophylaxis with loperamide during the initial 2 cycles of neratinib is recommended. The manufacturer recommends loperamide hydrochloride 4 mg 3 times daily during weeks 1–2 (days 1–14), followed by administration twice daily during weeks 3–8 (days 15–56), and then as needed; however, the daily dosage of loperamide hydrochloride should not exceed 16 mg. The dosage of loperamide should be adjusted until the patient reaches a stool frequency of 1–2 per day. (See Diarrhea under Cautions: Warnings/Precautions.)

Restricted Distribution Program Neratinib maleate can only be obtained through designated specialty pharmacies. Clinicians may consult the Nerlynx® website (https://nerlynx.com/hcp/access-and-support/how-to-get-nerlynx) for specific ordering and availability information.

■ **Administration** Neratinib maleate is administered orally with food. (See Description.) The drug should be taken at approximately the same time each day.

Neratinib tablets should be swallowed whole; tablets should *not* be chewed, crushed, or split.

■ **Dosage** Dosage of neratinib maleate is expressed in terms of neratinib.

Breast Cancer The recommended adult dosage of neratinib for the extended adjuvant treatment of human epidermal growth factor receptor type 2 (HER2)-positive early-stage breast cancer following adjuvant trastuzumab-based therapy is 240 mg once daily given continuously for one year.

Dosage Modification for Toxicity Dosage interruption and/or reduction or discontinuance of neratinib therapy may be necessary based on severity of adverse reactions. Dosage adjustment of neratinib is recommended based on individual safety and tolerability. If dosage reduction from 240 mg once daily is necessary, the dosage should be reduced to 200 mg once daily. If the toxicity recurs at a dosage of 200 mg once daily, the dosage should be reduced to 160 mg once daily. If the toxicity recurs at a dosage of 160 mg once daily, the dosage should be reduced to 120 mg once daily. If the toxicity recurs at a dosage of 120 mg once daily, neratinib therapy should be discontinued.

Neratinib should be discontinued in patients experiencing persistent grade 2 or greater adverse effects that do not recover to grade 0 or 1 or any toxicity that requires a treatment delay of greater than 3 weeks.

Grade 3 or 4 Toxicity. If grade 3 toxicity occurs, neratinib should be withheld until the toxicity improves to grade 1 or less or to baseline within 3 weeks. The drug may then be resumed at a reduced dosage.

If grade 4 toxicity occurs, neratinib therapy should be permanently discontinued.

GI Toxicity. If diarrhea of any severity occurs in association with dehydration, pyrexia, hypotension, renal failure, or grade 3 or 4 neutropenia, neratinib therapy should be temporarily interrupted. Patients experiencing diarrhea should modify their diet and maintain fluid intake of approximately 2 L per day to avoid dehydration. If diarrhea improves to grade 1 or less or to baseline within 1 week of withholding the drug, neratinib therapy may then be resumed at the same dosage. If greater than 1 week is required for improvement to grade 1 or less or to baseline, neratinib therapy should be resumed at a reduced dosage. Once diarrhea improves to grade 1 or less or to baseline, patients should receive loperamide hydrochloride 4 mg with each subsequent dose of neratinib. If diarrhea recurs to grade 2 or greater severity at a reduced dosage of 120 mg once daily, neratinib should be permanently discontinued.

If grade 1 diarrhea (less than 4 stools per day over baseline) occurs, antidiarrheal therapy should be adjusted and patients should modify their diet and maintain fluid intake of approximately 2 L per day to avoid dehydration. Once diarrhea improves or returns to baseline, patients should receive loperamide hydrochloride 4 mg with each subsequent dose of neratinib.

If grade 2 diarrhea (4–6 stools per day over baseline) lasting 5 days or longer or grade 3 diarrhea (7 or more stools per day over baseline, fecal incontinence, requiring hospitalization, limiting self-care activities of daily living) lasting longer than 2 days occurs, neratinib should be temporarily interrupted. Patients experiencing grade 2 or 3 diarrhea also should modify their diet and maintain fluid intake of approximately 2 L per day to avoid dehydration. If diarrhea improves to grade 1 or less or to baseline within 1 week of withholding the drug, neratinib therapy may then be resumed at the same dosage. If greater than 1 week is required for improvement to grade 1 or less or to baseline, neratinib therapy should be resumed at a reduced dosage. Loperamide hydrochloride 4 mg should be administered with subsequent doses of neratinib. If diarrhea recurs to grade 2 or greater severity at a reduced dosage of 120 mg once daily, neratinib should be permanently discontinued.

If grade 2 diarrhea lasting less than 5 days or grade 3 diarrhea lasting less than 2 days occurs, antidiarrheal therapy should be adjusted and patients should modify their diet and maintain fluid intake of approximately 2 L per day to avoid dehydration. Once diarrhea improves to grade 1 or less or to baseline, patients should receive loperamide hydrochloride 4 mg with each subsequent dose of neratinib.

If grade 4 diarrhea associated with life-threatening consequences or requiring urgent intervention occurs, neratinib should be permanently discontinued. (See Diarrhea under Cautions: Warnings/Precautions.)

Hepatotoxicity. For grade 3 elevations of serum ALT (i.e., exceeding 5 but not exceeding 20 times the upper limit of normal [ULN]) or bilirubin concentrations (i.e., exceeding 3 but not exceeding 10 times the ULN), neratinib should be withheld. If hepatotoxicity improves to grade 1 or less within 3 weeks, the drug may then be resumed at a reduced dosage. If grade 3 elevations of serum ALT or bilirubin concentrations recur despite one dose reduction, neratinib should be permanently discontinued.

For grade 4 elevations of serum ALT (i.e., exceeding 20 times the ULN) or bilirubin concentrations (i.e., exceeding 10 times the ULN), neratinib should be permanently discontinued. (See Hepatic Toxicity under Cautions: Warnings/Precautions.)

■ **Special Populations** For patients with severe preexisting hepatic impairment (Child-Pugh class C), the manufacturer recommends an initial neratinib dosage of 80 mg once daily. No dosage adjustment is necessary in patients with mild or moderate hepatic impairment (Child-Pugh class A or B). (See Hepatic Impairment under Warnings/Precautions: Specific Populations, in Cautions.)

No dosage adjustment is necessary in patients with renal impairment. (See Renal Impairment under Warnings/Precautions: Specific Populations, in Cautions.)

There are currently no specific dosage recommendations for geriatric patients. (See Geriatric Use under Warnings/Precautions: Specific Populations, in Cautions.)

Cautions

■ **Contraindications** The manufacturer states that there are no known contraindications to the use of neratinib.

■ **Warnings/Precautions** ***Diarrhea*** Severe diarrhea associated with dehydration, hypotension, and renal impairment has been reported in patients receiving neratinib. In the ExteNET study in patients with human epidermal growth factor receptor type 2 (HER2)-positive early-stage breast cancer, diarrhea was reported in 95% of patients receiving neratinib and was grade 3 in severity in 40% of patients. The majority (93%) of patients experienced diarrhea during the first month of therapy; the median time to onset of grade 3 or greater diarrhea was 8 days. The median cumulative duration of grade 3 or greater diarrhea was 5 days. In a small study, the incidence and time to onset of grade 1 or greater diarrhea was not ameliorated by administering the total daily dosage of neratinib in 2 divided doses (120 mg twice daily) instead of the recommended 240 mg once daily.

The manufacturer recommends antidiarrheal prophylaxis with loperamide during the initial 2 cycles of neratinib. (See Dosage and Administration: General.) Patients receiving neratinib should be monitored for development of diarrhea and treated as necessary with appropriate therapy (e.g., antidiarrheal agents, fluid replacement). Additional antidiarrheal agents may be necessary for the management of loperamide-refractory diarrhea. Stool cultures should be performed as clinically indicated to exclude infectious causes in patients experiencing grade 3 or 4 diarrhea or diarrhea of any severity associated with dehydration, pyrexia, or neutropenia. Liver function tests also should be evaluated in patients experiencing grade 3 or greater diarrhea. (See Hepatic Toxicity under Cautions: Warnings/Precautions.) Temporary interruption followed by dosage reduction or discontinuance of neratinib may be necessary depending on the severity of the diarrhea. (See GI Toxicity under Dosage: Dosage Modification for Toxicity, in Dosage and Administration.)

Hepatic Toxicity Elevations in aminotransferase (ALT or AST) concentrations have been reported in patients receiving neratinib. In the ExteNET study, elevations in ALT or AST concentrations 2 times the upper limit of normal (ULN) or more occurred in 9.7 or 5.1% of patients receiving neratinib, respectively; severe (grade 3 or greater) elevations occurred in 1.7% of patients. Hepatotoxicity or elevations in ALT or AST concentrations led to discontinuance of neratinib in 1.7% of patients.

Liver function tests (i.e., serum ALT, AST, total bilirubin, alkaline phosphatase concentrations) should be evaluated prior to initiation of therapy, monthly for the first 3 months of therapy, every 3 months thereafter during therapy, and as clinically indicated. Serum ALT, AST, total and fractionated bilirubin, and alkaline phosphatase concentrations as well as prothrombin time should be evaluated in patients experiencing grade 3 or greater diarrhea requiring IV fluid replacement and in those experiencing signs or symptoms of hepatotoxicity (e.g., worsening fatigue, nausea, vomiting, right upper quadrant pain or tenderness, pyrexia, rash, eosinophilia). (See Diarrhea under Cautions: Warnings/Precautions.) If grade 3 or 4 serum ALT or bilirubin elevations occur, temporary interruption followed by dosage reduction or discontinuance of neratinib may be necessary; alternate causes of hepatotoxicity also should be considered. (See Hepatotoxicity under Dosage: Dosage Modification for Toxicity, in Dosage and Administration.)

Fetal/Neonatal Morbidity and Mortality There are no adequate and well-controlled studies of neratinib in pregnant women; however, based on its mechanism of action and animal findings, neratinib may cause fetal harm. Embryofetal toxicity (i.e., increased fetal resorption, abortion) and teratogenicity (i.e., external, visceral, and skeletal anomalies) have been demonstrated in animals receiving neratinib at exposure levels approximately 0.2 times the human exposure at the maximum recommended dosage. Effects on long-term memory have been observed in male pups when pregnant rats received the drug from day 7 of gestation through day 20 of lactation at a dosage approximately 0.2 times the maximum recommended human dosage based on body surface area.

Pregnancy should be avoided during neratinib therapy. Women of childbearing potential should be advised to use effective contraceptive methods while receiving neratinib and for at least 1 month after discontinuance of the drug. In addition, men with such female partners should use effective methods of contraception while receiving neratinib and for 3 months after discontinuance of the drug. Patients should be apprised of the potential hazard to the fetus if neratinib is used during pregnancy.

Specific Populations **Pregnancy.** Neratinib may cause fetal harm if administered to pregnant women based on its mechanism of action and animal findings. (See Fetal/Neonatal Morbidity and Mortality under Cautions: Warnings/Precautions.)

Lactation. It is not known whether neratinib or its metabolites are distributed into milk. Because of the potential for serious adverse reactions to neratinib in nursing infants, women should be advised to discontinue nursing while receiving neratinib and for at least 1 month after the drug is discontinued. The effects of the drug or its metabolites on nursing infants or on the production of milk are unknown.

Pediatric Use. Safety and efficacy of neratinib have not been established in pediatric patients.

Geriatric Use. In the ExteNET study, 12% of patients receiving neratinib in the safety population were 65 years of age or older and 1.8% were 75 years of age or older. Patients 65 years of age or older had higher incidences of serious adverse reactions (e.g., vomiting, diarrhea, renal failure, dehydration) or discontinuance of neratinib due to adverse reactions compared with younger adults.

Hepatic Impairment. Following administration of a single 120-mg dose of neratinib, peak plasma concentrations and systemic exposure of neratinib in individuals with mild or moderate hepatic impairment (Child-Pugh class A or B) were similar to those in individuals with normal hepatic function but were increased by 273 and 281%, respectively, in those with severe hepatic impairment (Child-Pugh class C); therefore, dosage adjustment is necessary in patients with severe hepatic impairment. (See Dosage and Administration: Special Populations.)

Renal Impairment. The effects of renal impairment on the pharmacokinetics of neratinib have not been established; however, the drug is not extensively eliminated in urine. No dosage adjustment is necessary in such patients.

■ **Common Adverse Effects** Adverse effects reported in 10% or more of patients receiving neratinib for the extended adjuvant treatment of HER2-positive early-stage breast cancer include diarrhea, nausea, abdominal pain, fatigue, vomiting, headache, rash, stomatitis, decreased appetite, muscle spasms, dizziness, and dyspepsia.

Drug Interactions

Neratinib is primarily metabolized by cytochrome P-450 (CYP) isoenzyme 3A4 and, to a lesser extent, by flavin-containing monooxygenase (FMO).

■ Drugs and Foods Affecting Hepatic Microsomal Enzymes

Inhibitors of CYP3A4 Concomitant use of neratinib with potent or moderate inhibitors of CYP3A4 may result in increased systemic exposure to neratinib and an increased incidence of adverse effects. Concomitant administration of the potent CYP3A4 inhibitor ketoconazole (400 mg daily for 5 days) with neratinib (single 240-mg dose) in healthy individuals increased the peak plasma concentration and area under the plasma concentration-time curve (AUC) of neratinib by 321 and 481%, respectively. Although moderate CYP3A4 inhibitors have not been specifically studied in drug interaction studies to date, the potential for clinically important pharmacokinetic interactions between neratinib and moderate CYP3A4 inhibitors should be considered.

Concomitant use of neratinib with potent (e.g., clarithromycin; cobicistat; conivaptan; diltiazem; *ritonavir-boosted* elvitegravir; grapefruit products; idelalisib; *ritonavir-boosted* indinavir; itraconazole; ketoconazole; the fixed combination of lopinavir and ritonavir [lopinavir/ritonavir]; nefazodone; nelfinavir; the fixed combination of ombitasvir, paritaprevir, and ritonavir [with or without dasabuvir]; posaconazole; ritonavir; *ritonavir-boosted* saquinavir; *ritonavir-boosted* tipranavir; voriconazole) or moderate (e.g., aprepitant, cimetidine, ciprofloxacin, clotrimazole, crizotinib, cyclosporine, dronedarone, erythromycin, fluconazole, fluvoxamine, imatinib, verapamil) inhibitors of CYP3A4 should be avoided.

Inducers of CYP3A4 Concomitant use of neratinib with potent or moderate inducers of CYP3A4 may result in decreased systemic exposure to neratinib and its active *N*-desmethyl (M6) and dimethylamine *N*-oxide (M7) metabolites and reduced neratinib efficacy. When the potent CYP3A4 inducer rifampin was administered concomitantly with neratinib (single 240-mg dose) in healthy individuals, the AUCs of neratinib and its active metabolites (M6 and M7) were decreased by 87 and 37–49%, respectively, and the peak plasma concentration of neratinib was decreased by 76%. Although moderate CYP3A4 inducers have not been specifically studied in drug interaction studies to date, the potential for clinically important pharmacokinetic interactions between neratinib and moderate CYP3A4 inducers should be considered.

Concomitant use with potent (e.g., carbamazepine, enzalutamide, mitotane, phenytoin, rifampin, St. John's wort [*Hypericum perforatum*]) or moderate (e.g., bosentan, efavirenz, etravirine, modafinil) CYP3A4 inducers should be avoided.

■ **Drugs Affecting Gastric Acidity** Concomitant use of neratinib with drugs affecting gastric acidity may decrease the solubility of neratinib and subsequently reduce its bioavailability and efficacy. Concomitant administration of the proton-pump inhibitor lansoprazole (30 mg daily for 7 days) with neratinib (single 240-mg dose) in healthy individuals decreased the peak plasma concentration and AUC of neratinib by 71 and 65%, respectively. Although other drugs affecting gastric acidity (e.g., antacids, histamine H_2-receptor antagonists) have not been specifically studied in drug interaction studies to date, clinically important pharmacokinetic interactions between neratinib and these drugs appear likely.

Concomitant use with proton-pump inhibitors and histamine H_2-receptor antagonists should be avoided; however, antacids may be administered 3 hours prior to administration of neratinib.

■ **Substrates of P-Glycoprotein Transport Systems** Concomitant use of neratinib with P-glycoprotein (P-gp) substrates (e.g., digoxin, dabigatran, fexofenadine) may result in increased systemic exposure of the substrate drug. When the P-gp substrate digoxin (single 0.5-mg dose) was administered concomitantly with neratinib (240 mg once daily) in healthy individuals, peak plasma concentrations and AUC of digoxin increased by 54 and 32%, respectively.

Caution should be exercised and a dosage reduction for substrates with a narrow therapeutic index (e.g., digoxin) should be considered.

Description

Neratinib, a potent, selective, and irreversible inhibitor of human epidermal growth factor receptor type 2 (HER2), HER4, and epidermal growth factor receptor (EGFR) tyrosine kinases, is an antineoplastic agent. In vitro, neratinib and its active metabolites (M3, M6, M7, M11) exhibit inhibitory activity against EGFR, HER2, and HER4. In vitro, the drug has been shown to reduce phosphorylation of EGFR and HER2 resulting in inhibition of downstream signaling of the mitogen-activated protein kinase (MAPK) and phosphoinositide 3-kinase (PI3K/Akt) pathways. Neratinib has demonstrated antitumor activity in mice bearing tumor xenografts that expressed EGFR and HER2.

Neratinib exhibits nonlinear pharmacokinetics. Peak plasma concentrations and areas under the serum concentration-time curve (AUCs) of neratinib are less than dose proportional over the dosage range of 40–400 mg once daily. Peak plasma concentrations of neratinib and its major active metabolites (M3, M6, and M7) are achieved about 2–8 hours following oral administration of the drug. Following repeated doses of neratinib 240 mg once daily, the mean accumulation ratio for the drug was 1.14. Oral administration of neratinib with a high-fat meal or standard breakfast increased peak plasma concentrations by 1.7- or 1.2-fold, respectively, and increased AUC by 2.2- or 1.1-fold, respectively, compared with administration in the fasting state. In vitro, neratinib is highly bound (greater than 99%) to plasma proteins (mainly to albumin and α_1-acid glycoprotein), independent of concentration. Neratinib is metabolized principally by cytochrome P-450 (CYP) isoenzyme 3A4 and, to a lesser extent, by flavin-containing monooxygenase (FMO). Major metabolites of the drug include active pyridine *N*-oxide (M3), *N*-desmethyl (M6), dimethylamine *N*-oxide (M7), and bis-*N*-oxide (M11) derivatives which account for 15, 33, 22, and 4%, respectively, of total plasma concentrations of the drug. Following repeated administration of neratinib, the mean elimination half-lives of neratinib, M3, M6, and M7 are 14.6, 21.6, 13.8, and 10.4 hours, respectively. Following oral administration of a single radiolabeled dose of neratinib, approximately 97.1% of the recovered dose is excreted in feces and 1.13% is eliminated in urine.

Data from a population pharmacokinetic analysis indicate that age, gender, and race do not have clinically important effects on the pharmacokinetics of neratinib.

Advice to Patients

Importance of reading the manufacturer's patient information.

If a dose is missed, importance of administering the next dose at the regularly scheduled time; an additional dose should *not* be administered to make up for a missed dose.

Risk of diarrhea. Importance of informing patients how to manage diarrhea (e.g., dietary modification, antidiarrheal agents) to maintain 1–2 bowel movements per day. Importance of informing clinician if severe diarrhea or diarrhea associated with weakness, dizziness, or fever occurs.

Risk of hepatotoxicity. Importance of advising patients to immediately report possible signs and symptoms of hepatotoxicity (e.g., worsening fatigue, nausea, vomiting, right upper quadrant pain, jaundice, fever, rash, pruritus) to their clinician.

Risk of fetal harm. Necessity of advising women of childbearing potential to use effective methods of contraception while receiving neratinib and for at least 1 month after the drug is discontinued. Importance of advising men who are partners of such women to use effective methods of contraception while receiving the drug and for 3 months after discontinuance of therapy. Importance of women informing clinicians if they are or plan to become pregnant. If pregnancy occurs, advise pregnant women of potential risk to the fetus.

Importance of advising women to avoid breast-feeding while receiving the drug and for at least 1 month after discontinuance of therapy.

Importance of informing clinicians of existing or contemplated concomitant therapy, including prescription and OTC drugs, as well as any concomitant illnesses.

Importance of informing patients of other important precautionary information. (See Cautions.)

Overview® (see Users Guide). For additional information on this drug until a more detailed monograph is developed and published, the manufacturer's labeling should be consulted. It is *essential* that the manufacturer's labeling be consulted for more detailed information on usual cautions, precautions, contraindications, potential drug interactions, laboratory test interferences, and acute toxicity. For further information on the handling of antineoplastic agents, see the ASHP Guidelines on Handling Hazardous Drugs at http://www.ahfsdruginformation.com.

Preparations

Distribution of neratinib maleate is restricted. (See Restricted Distribution Program under Dosage and Administration: General.)

Excipients in commercially available drug preparations may have clinically important effects in some individuals; consult specific product labeling for details.

Neratinib Maleate

Oral

Tablets, film-coated	40 mg (of neratinib)	**Nerlynx®**, Puma Biotechnology

Nilotinib

■ Nilotinib, an inhibitor of Bcr-Abl tyrosine kinase, is an antineoplastic agent.

Uses

■ **Chronic Myelogenous Leukemia** Nilotinib is used for the treatment of newly diagnosed Philadelphia chromosome-positive (Ph^+) chronic myelogenous leukemia (CML) in adults who are in the chronic phase of the disease. Nilotinib also is used for the treatment of Ph^+ CML in adults who are in the chronic or accelerated phase of the disease after failure (secondary to resistance or intolerance) of prior therapy that included imatinib. Nilotinib is designated an orphan drug by the US Food and Drug Administration (FDA) for use in the treatment of CML.

Treatment of Newly Diagnosed Chronic Phase CML Nilotinib is used for the treatment of newly diagnosed Ph^+ CML in adults who are in the chronic phase of the disease. The indication for this use is based on major molecular and cytogenetic response rates obtained at 12 months from an ongoing open-label, multicenter, randomized, phase 3 study (Evaluating Nilotinib Efficacy and Safety in Clinical Trials—Newly Diagnosed Patients [ENESTnd]) in patients with newly diagnosed, chronic phase Ph^+ CML. Additional follow-up data are need to establish long-term efficacy of nilotinib for this use.

In this study, 846 patients who had been diagnosed with chronic phase Ph^+ CML within the previous 6 months and who had received no prior tyrosine kinase inhibitor therapy (except imatinib administered for 2 weeks or less) and no other therapies for CML (except hydroxyurea or anagrelide) for periods longer than 2 weeks were randomized to receive nilotinib 300 mg twice daily, nilotinib 400 mg twice daily, or imatinib 400 mg once daily (with the option to increase imatinib dosage to 400 mg twice daily in patients with suboptimal response or treatment failure). The primary analysis in this study was performed when all patients had completed 12 months of therapy (or had discontinued treatment prior to that date). At the data cutoff date, patients in all 3 groups had received a median of 18.6 months of treatment.

Major molecular response (defined as a Bcr-Abl transcript level of 0.1% or less in peripheral blood) at 12 months of treatment was achieved in 44 or 43% of patients receiving nilotinib 300 or 400 mg twice daily, respectively, compared with 22% of patients receiving imatinib. Complete cytogenetic response (defined as complete eradication of Ph^+ metaphases in cells obtained from a bone marrow sample) was achieved at 12 months in 80 or 78% of patients receiving nilotinib 300 or 400 mg twice daily, respectively, compared with 65% of patients receiving imatinib. The Kaplan-Meier estimate of the median time to achieve a major molecular response was 8.6 or 11 months for patients receiving nilotinib 300 or 400 mg twice daily, respectively; at the data cutoff point, the median time to achieve a major molecular response with imatinib had not yet been determined. Disease progression (i.e., transformation from chronic phase to accelerated or blast phase of CML) occurred by the data cutoff date in less than 1% of patients receiving nilotinib and in 4% of patients receiving imatinib.

Among patients with a poor prognosis (based on high Sokal risk score, a CML-specific prognostic indicator based on age, spleen size, platelet count, and peripheral blast count), major molecular response at 12 months of treatment was achieved in 41 or 32% of those receiving nilotinib 300 or 400 mg twice daily, respectively, compared with 17% of those receiving imatinib. Complete cytogenetic response was achieved in 74 or 63% of poor-risk patients receiving nilotinib 300 or 400 mg twice daily, respectively, compared with 49% of poor-risk patients receiving imatinib.

Adverse dermatologic effects (i.e., rash, pruritus, alopecia), headache, and elevated transaminase and bilirubin concentrations occurred more commonly in patients receiving nilotinib, whereas adverse GI effects (i.e., nausea, diarrhea, vomiting), muscle spasm, edema, and grade 3/4 neutropenia occurred more commonly in patients receiving imatinib.

Treatment of Chronic or Accelerated Phase CML Following Prior Treatment Failure Nilotinib is used for the treatment of Ph^+ CML in adults who are in the chronic or accelerated phase of the disease after failure (secondary to resistance or intolerance) of prior therapy that included imatinib. The indication for this use is based on overall hematologic and cytogenetic response rates.

Safety and efficacy of nilotinib for this indication have been evaluated in one open-label, multicenter, phase 2 trial in adults with CML in the chronic or accelerated phase; patients were intolerant of or had disease that was resistant to imatinib. In 321 patients in the chronic phase of CML, treatment with nilotinib (400 mg twice daily) resulted in a major cytogenetic response (defined as elimination or substantial reduction [to 35% or less] of Ph^+ hematopoietic cells) in 51% of patients; 37% achieved a complete cytogenetic response, while 15% achieved a partial response. The median time to major cytogenetic response was 2.8 months (range: 1–28 months), and the duration of major cytogenetic response exceeded 18 months in 62% of those who responded. The estimated 24-month overall survival rate was 87%. In 137 patients in the accelerated phase of CML, treatment with nilotinib (400 mg twice daily) resulted in confirmed hematologic response in 39% of patients; 30% achieved a complete hematologic response, while 9% had no evidence of leukemia. The median time to first hematologic response was 1 month (range: 1–14 months), and the duration of hematologic response exceeded 18 months in 44% of those who responded. At the time of data analysis, all patients in the trial had been followed for at least 24 months or had discontinued therapy early; the median duration of nilotinib treatment was 18.4 months for patients with CML in the chronic phase and 8.7 months for those with CML in the accelerated phase. At the time of data analysis, median durations of response had not been reached.

Among patients in this study who were tested for Bcr-Abl mutations following imatinib treatment failure, 24 different Bcr-Abl mutations were detected in 42 or 54% of those with chronic or accelerated phase CML, respectively.

Dosage and Administration

■ **Administration** Nilotinib is administered orally twice daily (approximately 12 hours apart in the morning and evening). Because food increases the bioavailability of nilotinib, the manufacturer states that the drug should be administered at least 1 hour before or 2 hours after any food. The manufacturer states that nilotinib capsules should be swallowed whole with water. Alternatively, for patients who are unable to swallow capsules, nilotinib capsules may be opened and the contents of each capsule dispersed in one teaspoonful of applesauce; the mixture should be swallowed immediately (within 15 minutes) and not stored for later use. The manufacturer states that foods other than applesauce should not be used and that no more than one teaspoonful of applesauce should be mixed with the contents of each capsule.

Nilotinib may be administered in conjunction with hematopoietic growth factors (e.g., erythropoietin, filgrastim, sargramostim), if clinically indicated. The drug also may be administered concomitantly with hydroxyurea or anagrelide, if clinically indicated.

■ **Dosage** ***Chronic Myelogenous Leukemia*** The recommended adult oral dosage of nilotinib for the treatment of newly diagnosed Philadelphia chromosome-positive (Ph^+) CML in the chronic phase is 300 mg twice daily. In one phase 3 clinical trial, nilotinib was administered for a median of 18.6 months.

The recommended adult oral dosage of nilotinib for the treatment of Ph^+ CML in the chronic or accelerated phase after failure of prior therapy that included imatinib is 400 mg twice daily. In one phase 2 clinical trial, nilotinib was administered for a median of 18.4 or 8.7 months in patients with CML in the chronic or accelerated phase, respectively.

■ **Dosage Modification** ***Concomitant Use with Drugs Affecting or Metabolized by Hepatic Microsomal Enzymes*** Because concomitant use of nilotinib with potent inhibitors of cytochrome P-450 (CYP) isoenzyme 3A4 may result in increased plasma concentrations of nilotinib, concomitant therapy with such drugs should be avoided. (See Inhibitors of CYP3A4 under Drug Interactions: Drugs Affecting or Metabolized by Hepatic Microsomal Enzymes.) If treatment with a potent CYP3A4 inhibitor is required, the manufacturer of nilotinib recommends that therapy with nilotinib be interrupted. However, if such concomitant use cannot be avoided, reduction of nilotinib dosage to 200 mg once daily in patients receiving nilotinib as first-line therapy for CML or 300 mg once daily in those receiving nilotinib following failure of prior therapy that included imatinib should be considered. The manufacturer states that these dosage recommendations are based on pharmacokinetic studies of nilotinib and that there is no clinical experience with use of these dosages in patients concomitantly receiving the drug with a potent CYP3A4 inhibitor. In addition, patients receiving such concomitant therapy should be closely monitored for prolongation of the QT interval. If the potent inhibitor is later discontinued, the nilotinib dosage may be adjusted upward to the usual indicated dosage after a suitable washout period.

Because concomitant use of nilotinib with potent CYP3A4 inducers may result in decreased plasma concentrations of nilotinib, concomitant therapy with such drugs should be avoided. (See Inducers of CYP3A4 under Drug Interactions: Drugs Affecting or Metabolized by Hepatic Microsomal Enzymes.) Because of the drug's nonlinear pharmacokinetic profile (see Description), the use of higher nilotinib dosages is unlikely to compensate for the reduction in nilotinib exposure.

Prolongation of QT Interval Nilotinib is associated with plasma concentration-dependent prolongation of the QT interval. (See Prolongation of QT Interval under Warnings/Precautions: Warnings, in Cautions.) Hypomagnesemia or hypokalemia should be treated before the drug is initiated. ECGs should be obtained to monitor the QT interval at baseline and 7 days after initiation of nilotinib; ECGs should be repeated approximately 7 days after any dosage adjustments.

Nilotinib therapy should be withheld if the QT interval corrected for rate (QT_c) exceeds 480 msec. The patient's serum potassium and magnesium concentrations should be determined; if serum concentrations are below the lower limits of normal, supplements should be administered. The patient's concomitant drug usage should be reviewed; other drugs that prolong the QT interval should be avoided. (See Drug Interactions: Drugs that Prolong the QT Interval.) Treatment may be resumed within 2 weeks at the prior dosage (300 mg twice daily in patients receiving nilotinib as first-line therapy for CML or 400 mg twice daily in those receiving nilotinib following failure of prior therapy that included imatinib) if the QT interval corrected for heart rate using Fridericia's formula (QT_cF) returns to less than 450 msec and to within 20 msec of baseline. If QT_cF is between 450 msec and 480 msec after nilotinib has been withheld for 2 weeks, therapy with the drug may be resumed at a reduced dosage of 400 mg once daily. If QT_cF exceeds 480 msec following this dosage reduction, nilotinib should be discontinued.

Myelosuppression Temporary interruption or dosage reduction of nilotinib therapy is indicated in patients who develop neutropenia or thrombocytopenia that is not related to the underlying CML. Nilotinib therapy should be withheld if absolute neutrophil counts (ANC) decrease to less than 1000/mm^3 and/or platelet counts decrease to less than 50,000/mm^3. Treatment may be resumed within 2 weeks at the prior dosage (300 mg twice daily in patients receiving nilotinib as first-line therapy for CML or 400 mg twice daily in those receiving nilotinib following failure of prior therapy that included imatinib) when ANC exceeds 1000/mm^3 and platelet counts exceed 50,000/mm^3. If blood counts remain low for more than 2 weeks, nilotinib dosage should be reduced to 400 mg once daily.

Increased Serum Concentrations of Lipase, Amylase, Bilirubin, and/or Hepatic Transaminases Nilotinib therapy should be withheld in patients who experience elevated lipase, amylase, bilirubin, and/or hepatic transaminase concentrations of grade 3 or higher (as defined by the National Cancer Institute [NCI] Common Terminology Criteria for Adverse Events [CTCAE]). Treatment may be resumed at a reduced dosage of 400 mg once daily (in patients receiving nilotinib either as first-line therapy for CML or following failure of prior therapy that included imatinib) if the toxicity decreases in intensity to grade 1 or less.

Other Nonhematologic Effects Nilotinib therapy should be withheld in patients experiencing other clinically important moderate or severe nonhematologic adverse effects; once the adverse effect has resolved, treatment may be resumed at a reduced dosage of 400 mg once daily. If clinically appropriate, escalation of the dosage back to 300 mg twice daily (in patients receiving nilotinib as first-line therapy for CML) or 400 mg twice daily (in those receiving nilotinib following failure of prior therapy that included imatinib) should be considered.

■ **Special Populations** If use of nilotinib is required in patients with hepatic impairment, reduction of the initial dosage is recommended. The manufacturer states that, if possible, alternative therapy should be considered. (See Hepatic Impairment under Warnings/Precautions: Specific Populations, in Cautions.)

When nilotinib is used for the treatment of newly diagnosed, chronic phase Ph$^+$ CML in patients with mild, moderate, or severe hepatic impairment (Child-Pugh class A, B, or C, respectively), an initial dosage of 200 mg twice daily, followed by dosage escalation to 300 mg twice daily as tolerated, is recommended.

When nilotinib is used for the treatment of chronic or accelerated phase Ph$^+$ CML after failure of prior therapy that included imatinib, an initial dosage of 300 mg twice daily, followed by dosage escalation to 400 mg twice daily as tolerated, is recommended for patients with mild or moderate hepatic impairment (Child-Pugh class A or B, respectively). When nilotinib is used for this indication in patients with severe hepatic impairment (Child-Pugh class C), an initial dosage of 200 mg twice daily, followed by dosage escalation as tolerated to 300 mg twice daily and then to 400 mg twice daily, is recommended.

The manufacturer makes no specific dosage recommendations for geriatric patients or patients with renal impairment. (See Geriatric Use and also Renal Impairment under Warnings/Precautions: Specific Populations, in Cautions.)

Cautions

■ **Contraindications** Hypokalemia, hypomagnesemia, or long QT syndrome.

■ **Warnings/Precautions** ***Warnings*** **Prolongation of QT Interval.** Nilotinib is associated with plasma concentration-dependent prolongation of the QT interval. In the clinical trial in patients with newly diagnosed chronic phase CML, an increase in the QT interval (corrected for heart rate using Fridericia's formula [QT_cF]) of more than 60 msec from baseline was observed in one patient (0.4%) receiving nilotinib 300 mg twice daily; QT_cF did not exceed 500 msec in any patient. In the clinical trial in patients with chronic or accelerated phase CML who received nilotinib (400 mg twice daily) after failure of prior treatment, increases in QT_cF of more than 60 msec from baseline were observed in 4.1% of patients, and QT_cF exceeded 500 msec in less than 1% of patients (4 patients). Prolongation of the QT interval can result in torsades de pointes, leading to syncope, seizure, and/or sudden death. (See Sudden Death under Warnings/Precautions: Warnings, in Cautions.)

Nilotinib should not be used in patients with hypokalemia, hypomagnesemia, or long QT syndrome. Because hypokalemia and hypomagnesemia may further prolong the QT interval, these electrolyte abnormalities should be corrected prior to administration of nilotinib, and these electrolytes should be monitored periodically during therapy.

Substantial prolongation of the QT interval may occur when nilotinib is administered inappropriately with food or used concomitantly with potent CYP3A4 inhibitors or with drugs known to prolong the QT interval; therefore, concurrent use of such agents and administration with food should be avoided (see Dosage and Administration: Administration and see Drug Interactions).

ECGs should be obtained to monitor the QT interval at baseline and 7 days after initiation of the drug, and should be repeated periodically thereafter, as well as approximately 7 days after any dosage adjustments. (See Prolongation of QT Interval under Dosage and Administration: Dosage Modification.)

Sudden Death. Sudden death has been reported in 0.3% of patients with CML who received nilotinib in clinical trials. The early occurrence of some of these deaths relative to the initiation of nilotinib suggests the possibility that ventricular repolarization abnormalities may have contributed to their occurrence. (See Prolongation of QT Interval under Warnings/Precautions: Warnings, in Cautions.)

■ **Other Warnings and Precautions** ***Myelosuppression*** In the clinical trial evaluating nilotinib 400 mg twice daily after failure of prior therapy, grade 3/4 neutropenia, thrombocytopenia, and anemia occurred in 31, 30, and 11%, respectively, of patients in the chronic phase of CML and in 42, 42, and 27%, respectively, of patients in the accelerated phase of CML. In the clinical trial in patients with newly diagnosed chronic phase CML, grade 3/4 neutropenia, thrombocytopenia, and anemia occurred in 12, 10, and 4%, respectively, of patients receiving nilotinib 300 mg twice daily. The manufacturer states that myelosuppression generally was reversible and usually was managed by withholding nilotinib or reducing the dosage. Complete blood cell counts should be monitored every 2 weeks during the first 2 months of therapy and monthly (or as clinically indicated) thereafter. If hematologic toxicity occurs, interruption of nilotinib therapy and/or dosage reduction may be necessary. (See Myelosuppression under Dosage and Administration: Dosage Modification.)

Elevated Serum Lipase In clinical trials, grade 3/4 elevations in serum lipase occurred in 7% of patients with newly diagnosed chronic phase CML who received nilotinib 300 mg twice daily and in 18% of those with chronic or accelerated phase CML who received nilotinib 400 mg twice daily after failure of prior therapy. Caution is recommended in patients with a previous history of pancreatitis. Serum lipase should be monitored monthly or as clinically indicated, and interruption of therapy and/or dosage reduction may be necessary in some patients. If lipase elevations are accompanied by abdominal symptoms, nilotinib therapy should be interrupted and diagnostic testing to exclude pancreatitis considered. (See Increased Serum Concentrations of Lipase, Amylase, Bilirubin, and/or Hepatic Transaminases under Dosage and Administration: Dosage Modification.)

Hepatic Effects In clinical trials, grade 3/4 elevations in hepatic enzymes (AST/ALT and/or alkaline phosphatase) and/or bilirubin occurred in up to 4% of patients with newly diagnosed chronic phase CML who received nilotinib 300 mg twice daily and in up to 9% of those with chronic or accelerated phase CML who received nilotinib 400 mg twice daily after failure of prior therapy. Hepatic function tests should be monitored monthly or as clinically indicated, and interruption of therapy and/or dosage reduction may be necessary in some patients. (See Increased Serum Concentrations of Lipase, Amylase, Bilirubin, and/or Hepatic Transaminases under Dosage and Administration: Dosage Modification.)

A pharmacogenetic analysis of 97 patients that evaluated the polymorphisms of uridine diphosphate-glucuronosyltransferase (UGT) 1A1 and its potential association with hyperbilirubinemia during nilotinib treatment found that the (TA)7/(TA)7 genotype was associated with an increase in the risk of hyperbilirubinemia relative to the (TA)6/(TA)6 and (TA)6/(TA)7 genotypes. The largest increases in bilirubin were observed in patients with the (TA)7/(TA)7 genotype (UGT1A1*28).

Electrolyte Abnormalities Electrolyte abnormalities (hypophosphatemia, hypokalemia, hyperkalemia, hypocalcemia, and hyponatremia) of grade 3 or 4 in severity occurred in up to 5% of patients with newly diagnosed chronic phase CML who received nilotinib 300 mg twice daily and in up to 17% of those with chronic or accelerated phase CML who received nilotinib 400 mg twice daily after failure of prior therapy. Electrolyte abnormalities must be corrected prior to initiation of nilotinib therapy, and these electrolytes should be monitored periodically during therapy.

Total Gastrectomy Because median steady-state trough concentrations of nilotinib are reduced by 53% in patients who have undergone total gastrectomy, more frequent follow-up of these patients should be considered. If necessary, increased dosage of nilotinib or institution of alternative therapy may be considered.

Lactose-Intolerant Patients Since nilotinib capsules contain lactose, use of the drug in patients with rare hereditary problems of galactose intolerance, severe lactase deficiency with severe intolerance to lactose-containing products, or glucose-galactose malabsorption is not recommended.

Fetal/Neonatal Morbidity and Mortality Nilotinib may cause fetal harm; maternal and embryofetal toxicity have been demonstrated in animals. No adequate and well-controlled studies have been conducted to date in humans. Pregnancy should be avoided during therapy. If used during pregnancy or if the patient becomes pregnant while receiving nilotinib, the patient should be apprised of the potential fetal hazard.

Specific Populations **Pregnancy.** Category D. (See Fetal/Neonatal Morbidity and Mortality under Warnings/Precautions: Other Warnings and Precautions, in Cautions.)

Lactation. Nilotinib is distributed into milk in rats. It is not known whether the drug is distributed into milk in humans. Because of the potential for serious adverse effects from nilotinib in nursing infants, the manufacturer states that a decision should be made whether to discontinue nursing or the drug, taking into account the importance of the drug to the woman.

Pediatric Use. Safety and efficacy not established in pediatric patients.

Geriatric Use. In the clinical trial evaluating nilotinib in patients with newly diagnosed, chronic phase Ph$^+$ CML, approximately 12% of patients were 65 years of age or older. No differences in major molecular response rates were observed between geriatric patients 65 years of age or older and younger adults.

In the clinical trial evaluating nilotinib in patients with chronic or accelerated phase CML after failure of prior therapy that included imatinib, approximately 30% of patients were 65 years of age or older. In patients in the chronic phase of CML, no difference was found in major cytogenetic response rates in patients 65 years of age and older relative to younger adults. In patients in the accelerated phase of CML, the hematologic response rate was 29% in those 65 years of age and older compared with 44% in those younger than 65 years of age.

No major differences in safety were observed in patients 65 years of age and older compared with younger adults.

Cardiac Disorders. Clinical trials of nilotinib excluded patients with a history of uncontrolled or clinically important cardiovascular disease, including recent myocardial infarction, congestive heart failure, unstable angina, and clinically important bradycardia. Caution is advised in patients with such cardiac disorders. (See Prolongation of QT Interval under Warnings/Precautions: Warnings, in Cautions.)

Hepatic Impairment. Nilotinib exposure is increased in patients with hepatic impairment. Following administration of a single 200-mg dose of the drug in individuals with mild to moderate (Child-Pugh class A or B) or severe (Child-Pugh class C) hepatic impairment, area under the concentration-time curve (AUC) was increased by 35 or 56%, respectively, compared with values observed in individuals with normal hepatic function. The manufacturer recommends that alternative therapy be considered, if possible, in patients with hepatic impairment. If nilotinib therapy is required in patients with hepatic impairment, reduction of the initial dosage and close monitoring of the QT interval are recommended. (See Dosage and Administration: Special Populations.)

Renal Impairment. Nilotinib has not been studied in patients with renal impairment; however, since nilotinib and its metabolites are not renally excreted, a decrease in total body clearance is not anticipated in patients with renal impairment.

■ **Common Adverse Effects** Adverse nonhematologic effects reported in 10% or more of patients receiving nilotinib include rash, pruritus, headache, nausea, fatigue, myalgia, nasopharyngitis, constipation, diarrhea, abdominal pain, vomiting, arthralgia, pyrexia, upper respiratory infection, back pain, cough, and asthenia. Common grade 3 or 4 adverse hematologic effects include thrombocytopenia, neutropenia, and anemia, which appear to occur more commonly in patients with chronic or accelerated phase CML who are receiving nilotinib (400 mg twice daily) after failure of prior therapy than in patients receiving the drug (300 mg twice daily) for treatment of newly diagnosed chronic phase CML.

Drug Interactions

■ **Drugs Affecting or Metabolized by Hepatic Microsomal Enzymes** ***Drugs Metabolized by Hepatic Microsomal Enzymes*** In vitro studies indicate that nilotinib is a competitive inhibitor of cytochrome P-450 (CYP) isoenzymes 3A4, 2C8, 2C9, and 2D6 and has the potential to increase concentrations of drugs metabolized by these enzymes. In a single-dose study, concomitant administration of nilotinib with midazolam (a CYP3A4 substrate) to healthy individuals increased midazolam exposure by 30%. In another study in healthy individuals, administration of a single dose of nilotinib did not alter the pharmacokinetics or pharmacodynamics of warfarin (a CYP2C9 substrate). Caution should be exercised if nilotinib is used concomitantly with substrates of these enzymes that have a narrow therapeutic index.

In vitro studies also suggest that nilotinib may induce CYP isoenzymes 2B6, 2C8, and 2C9, and thereby has the potential to decrease concentrations of drugs that are metabolized by these enzymes.

Inhibitors of CYP3A4 Nilotinib plasma concentration may be increased during concomitant use with potent CYP3A4 inhibitors (e.g., atazanavir, clarithromycin, indinavir, itraconazole, ketoconazole, nefazodone, nelfinavir, ritonavir, saquinavir, telithromycin, voriconazole); concomitant use of nilotinib with these drugs should be avoided. In healthy individuals receiving ketoconazole (400 mg once daily for 6 days), systemic exposure (as measured by the area under the concentration-time curve [AUC]) to nilotinib was increased approximately threefold. If therapy with any of these drugs is required, therapy with nilotinib should be interrupted. If concomitant use of nilotinib with a potent CYP3A4 inhibitor cannot be avoided, reduction of nilotinib dosage should be considered. (See Concomitant Use with Drugs Affecting or Metabolized by Hepatic Microsomal Enzymes under Dosage and Administration: Dosage Modification.) In addition, patients should be closely monitored for prolongation of the QT interval.

Inducers of CYP3A4 Decreased nilotinib plasma concentrations may occur during concomitant use with potent CYP3A4 inducers (e.g., dexamethasone, carbamazepine, phenobarbital, phenytoin, rifabutin, rifampin, rifapentine, St. John's wort [*Hypericum perforatum*]). In healthy individuals receiving rifampin (600 mg once daily for 12 days), a CYP3A4 inducer, systemic exposure (as measured by AUC) to nilotinib was decreased approximately 80%. Concomitant use of nilotinib with potent CYP3A4 inducers should be avoided since adjustment of nilotinib dosage is considered unlikely to compensate for the reduction in nilotinib exposure; alternative drugs with less potential for CYP3A4 induction should be selected. (See Concomitant Use with Drugs Affecting or Metabolized by Hepatic Microsomal Enzymes under Dosage and Administration: Dosage Modification.)

■ **Drugs Affecting Gastric Acidity** Drugs that increase the pH of the upper GI tract may decrease the solubility of nilotinib and reduce its bioavailability. In healthy individuals, concomitant oral administration of the proton-pump inhibitor esomeprazole (40 mg once daily for 6 days) with nilotinib (a single 400-mg dose given concomitantly with the sixth dose of esomeprazole) resulted in a 34% reduction in the AUC of nilotinib. Increasing the dose level of nilotinib is not likely to compensate for the loss of exposure, and separation of doses may not eliminate the interaction because proton-pump inhibitors have an extended effect on the pH of the upper GI tract. The manufacturer states that nilotinib and proton-pump inhibitors should be used concomitantly with caution.

The effects of histamine H_2-receptor antagonists and antacids on the pharmacokinetics of nilotinib have not been established to date. If use of a histamine H_2-receptor antagonist or antacid is necessary, the manufacturer recommends that doses of the acid-lowering drug and doses of nilotinib be separated by at least several hours.

■ **Drugs Metabolized by Uridine Diphosphate-glucuronosyltransferase** In vitro studies indicate that nilotinib is a competitive inhibitor of uridine diphosphate-glucuronosyltransferase (UGT) 1A1, potentially increasing the concentrations of drugs metabolized by this enzyme. Caution should be exercised when nilotinib is used concomitantly with drugs metabolized by UGT1A1 that have a narrow therapeutic index.

■ **Substrates or Inhibitors of P-Glycoprotein Transport Systems** Nilotinib inhibits the efflux transporter P-glycoprotein (Pgp, ABCB1). If nilotinib is administered with drugs that are substrates of Pgp, increased concentrations of the substrate drug are likely, and caution should be exercised.

Nilotinib also is a Pgp substrate. If nilotinib is administered with drugs that inhibit Pgp, increased concentrations of nilotinib are likely, and caution should be exercised.

■ **Drugs that Prolong the QT Interval** The administration of nilotinib with antiarrhythmics (e.g., amiodarone, disopyramide, procainamide, quinidine, sotalol) or other drugs that prolong the QT interval (e.g., chloroquine, clarithromycin, haloperidol, methadone, moxifloxacin, pimozide) should be avoided. (See Prolongation of QT Interval under Warnings/Precautions:

Warnings, in Cautions.) If therapy with any of these drugs is required, therapy with nilotinib should be interrupted. If interruption of treatment with nilotinib is not possible, patients who require treatment with a drug that prolongs the QT interval should be closely monitored for prolongation of the QT interval. (See Prolongation of QT Interval under Dosage and Administration: Dosage Modification.)

■ **Grapefruit** Grapefruit products and other foods that are known to inhibit CYP3A4 should be avoided.

■ **Imatinib** In a phase 1 clinical trial, administration of nilotinib (400 mg twice daily) in conjunction with imatinib (400 mg once or twice daily) resulted in a 30–50% increase in nilotinib AUC and an increase of approximately 20% in imatinib AUC.

Description

Nilotinib, an inhibitor of Bcr-Abl tyrosine kinase, is an antineoplastic agent. Chronic myelogenous leukemia (CML) is a clonal myeloproliferative disorder characterized by the expansion of hematopoietic cells carrying the Philadelphia chromosome (Ph), resulting from a reciprocal translocation of the long arms of chromosomes 9 and 22. A novel fusion gene is formed, Bcr-Abl, which encodes a constitutively active, cytoplasmic form of protein tyrosine kinase. The unregulated activity of the Abl tyrosine kinase in Bcr-Abl is the cause of CML. Nilotinib is an orally active aminopyrimidine-derivative tyrosine kinase inhibitor that functions through competitive inhibition at the ATP-binding site of Bcr-Abl, leading to the inhibition of tyrosine phosphorylation of proteins that are involved in the intracellular signal transduction that Bcr-Abl mediates.

Clinical resistance to imatinib in CML has been attributed to several mechanisms, but point mutations in the Bcr-Abl kinase domain appear to the most common, occurring in 30–90% of patients who develop resistance. The ability of nilotinib to overcome imatinib resistance resulting from Bcr-Abl kinase domain mutations has been demonstrated in vitro. In preclinical studies in cell-line models, nilotinib inhibited most (32 of 33) imatinib-resistant Bcr-Abl kinase domain mutant forms.

Nilotinib is extensively metabolized by the cytochrome P-450 (CYP) microsomal enzyme system, principally by the isoenzyme 3A4. Nilotinib is the principal circulating component in the serum, and none of the metabolites substantially contribute to the pharmacologic activity of the drug. Following oral administration of a single radiolabeled dose of nilotinib, 93% of the radioactivity was recovered in feces within 7 days; unchanged drug accounted for 69% of the dose recovered in feces. Food increases the bioavailability of nilotinib. When the drug was administered 30 minutes after a high-fat meal, systemic exposure (as measured by the area under the concentration-time curve [AUC]) was increased by 82% relative to administration in the fasted state. However, single-dose administration of two intact 200-mg nilotinib capsules was bioequivalent to single-dose administration of two 200-mg capsules when the contents of each capsule were dispersed in a teaspoonful of applesauce and ingested within 15 minutes following dispersal. (See Dosage and Administration: Administration.) Steady-state exposure of nilotinib is dose dependent; at dosages exceeding 400 mg once daily, the increase in exposure is less than proportional to the increase in dose. Steady-state exposure at a dosage of 400 mg twice daily is 13% higher than exposure at a dosage of 300 mg twice daily.

In vitro studies indicate that nilotinib inhibits CYP isoenzymes 3A4, 2C8, 2C9, and 2D6; the drug also inhibits uridine diphosphate-glucuronosyltransferase (UGT) 1A1 and P-glycoprotein. In addition, in vitro studies suggest that nilotinib induces CYP isoenzymes 2B6, 2C8, and 2C9. (See Drug Interactions.)

Advice to Patients

A copy of the manufacturer's patient information (medication guide) for nilotinib should be provided to all patients with each prescription of the drug. Importance of patients reading the medication guide prior to initiation of therapy and each time the prescription is refilled.

Risk of QT-interval prolongation. Importance of informing clinicians immediately if feelings of lightheadedness or faintness or an irregular heartbeat occurs.

Importance of advising patients to swallow nilotinib capsules whole with water. Alternatively, patients who cannot swallow capsules may be instructed to open nilotinib capsules, sprinkle the contents of each capsule on one teaspoonful of applesauce, and swallow the mixture immediately (within 15 minutes). Advise patients that foods other than applesauce should not be used and that no more than one teaspoonful of applesauce should be mixed with the contents of each capsule.

Importance of advising patients that nilotinib is a long-term therapy. Importance of not altering the dosage or discontinuing nilotinib therapy without first consulting clinician.

Importance of advising patients that if a dose of nilotinib is missed, the next dose should be taken at the regularly scheduled time; the dose should not be doubled.

Importance of advising patients to take nilotinib at least 2 hours after eating any food, and to wait at least 1 hour before eating any food. Advise patients receiving nilotinib twice daily to take the doses approximately 12 hours apart.

Importance of advising patients to avoid any grapefruit products or any other foods known to inhibit cytochrome P-450 (CYP) isoenzyme 3A4 while taking nilotinib. Advise patients to separate doses of nilotinib and doses of antacids or H_2-receptor antagonists by at least several hours.

Importance of informing clinicians if patient is lactose intolerant.

Importance of advising women of childbearing potential to use an effective method of contraception and to avoid breast-feeding while undergoing nilotinib therapy. Importance of women informing a clinician immediately if they are or plan to become pregnant or plan to breast-feed. If pregnancy occurs, advise patient of risk to the fetus.

Importance of informing clinicians of existing or contemplated concomitant therapy, including prescription and OTC drugs and herbal products (e.g., St. John's wort), as well as any concomitant illnesses (e.g., long QT syndrome).

Importance of informing patients of other important precautionary information. (See Cautions.)

Overview® (see Users Guide). For additional information on this drug until a more detailed monograph is developed and published, the manufacturer's labeling should be consulted. It is *essential* that the manufacturer's labeling be consulted for more detailed information on usual cautions, precautions, contraindications, potential drug interactions, laboratory test interferences, and acute toxicity.

Preparations

Excipients in commercially available drug preparations may have clinically important effects in some individuals; consult specific product labeling for details.

Nilotinib

Oral		
Capsules	150 mg	**Tasigna®**, Novartis
	200 mg	**Tasigna®**, Novartis

Niraparib Tosylate

■ Niraparib tosylate, an inhibitor of poly(adenosine diphosphate [ADP]-ribose) polymerase (PARP), is an antineoplastic agent.

Uses

■ **Ovarian, Fallopian Tube, and Primary Peritoneal Cancer** Niraparib is used as maintenance therapy for the treatment of recurrent epithelial ovarian, fallopian tube, or primary peritoneal cancer in patients in complete or partial response following platinum-based chemotherapy. The drug has been designated an orphan drug by the FDA for the treatment of this cancer. In patients with platinum-sensitive epithelial ovarian, fallopian tube, or primary peritoneal cancer, maintenance therapy with niraparib has been shown to prolong progression-free survival compared with placebo, regardless of BRCA mutation status.

The current indication for niraparib maintenance therapy is based principally on the results of a randomized, double-blind, placebo-controlled phase 3 study (NOVA) in adults with platinum-sensitive epithelial ovarian, fallopian tube, or primary peritoneal cancer. Patients in the NOVA study were enrolled into 1 of 2 cohorts based on BRCA mutation status (confirmed or suspected deleterious); those with germline BRCA mutations were assigned to the germline BRCA-mutated (gBRCA-mutation) cohort and those without germline BRCA mutations were assigned to the non-gBRCA-mutation cohort (including those with wild-type gBRCA using the BRACAnalysis CDx diagnostic test). The non-gBRCA-mutation cohort in this study included patients with homologous recombination deficiency (HRD)-positive tumors, including those with somatic BRCA mutations and other defects, as well as patients with HRD-negative tumors.

In the NOVA study, 553 patients were randomized in a 2:1 ratio to receive either niraparib (300 mg once daily) or placebo within 8 weeks following the last dose of platinum-based chemotherapy. Treatment was continued until disease progression or unacceptable toxicity occurred or the patient withdrew from the study. Patients randomized to receive placebo were not permitted to cross over to niraparib therapy upon disease progression. Patients were stratified according to time to progression following the penultimate platinum-based regimen, concomitant use of bevacizumab with the penultimate or last platinum-based regimen, and best response following the most recent platinum-based regimen.

The primary end point of the NOVA study was progression-free survival as assessed by a blinded independent central review committee according to Response Evaluation Criteria in Solid Tumors (RECIST) and, in some cases, additional criteria (e.g., increasing serum cancer antigen-125 [CA-125] concentrations, clinical signs and symptoms) were considered. The median age of patients ranged from 57–64 years in those receiving niraparib and 58–67 years in those receiving placebo; 86% of all patients were white and 67 and 69% of patients in the niraparib and placebo groups, respectively, had a baseline ECOG performance status of 0. All enrolled patients had previously received at least 2 platinum-based regimens; approximately 40% of all patients had received 3 or more previous lines of therapy, 26% of the niraparib-treated patients had previously received bevacizumab therapy, 51% of all patients were in complete response following platinum-based chemotherapy, and 6–12 months had elapsed since penultimate platinum-based chemotherapy in 39% of patients in both the niraparib and placebo groups. Patients receiving niraparib had a substantially longer median progression-free survival than those receiving placebo in both the gBRCA-mutation (21 versus 5.5 months; hazard ratio: 0.26) and non-gBRCA-mutation cohorts (9.3 versus 3.9 months; hazard ratio: 0.45). Median progression-free survival also was significantly longer in niraparib-treated patients with HRD-positive epithelial ovarian, fallopian tube, or primary peritoneal cancer in the non-gBRCA-mutation cohort compared with those receiving placebo (12.9 versus 3.8 months; hazard ratio: 0.38). At the time of the progression-free survival analysis, limited overall survival data were available; deaths were reported in 17% of patients across the 2 cohorts. Niraparib therapy was associated with moderate bone marrow toxicity in this study. (See Hematologic Effects under Cautions: Warnings/Precautions.)

Dosage and Administration

■ **General** Because myelosuppression and cases of myelodysplastic syndrome (MDS) and acute myeloid leukemia (AML) have been reported in patients receiving niraparib, the manufacturer states that complete blood cell (CBC) counts should be monitored weekly for the first month of therapy, monthly for the next 11 months of therapy, and then periodically thereafter. (See Myelodysplastic Syndrome/Acute Myeloid Leukemia and also see Hematologic Effects under Cautions: Warnings/Precautions.)

■ **Administration** Niraparib tosylate is administered orally without regard to meals at approximately the same time each day. (See Description.) The manufacturer states that bedtime administration may help relieve nausea.

The capsules should be swallowed whole.

■ **Dosage** Dosage of niraparib tosylate monohydrate is expressed in terms of niraparib.

Ovarian, Fallopian Tube, and Primary Peritoneal Cancer The recommended adult dosage of niraparib for maintenance therapy of recurrent epithelial ovarian, fallopian tube, or primary peritoneal cancer in patients who are in complete or partial response to platinum-containing chemotherapy is 300 mg (three 100-mg capsules) once daily.

Niraparib therapy should be initiated no later than 8 weeks following the most recent platinum-based chemotherapy regimen. Therapy should be continued until disease progression or unacceptable toxicity occurs.

If a dose of niraparib is missed or vomited, patients should *not* take an extra dose. The next dose should be taken at the regularly scheduled time.

Dosage Modification for Toxicity Dosing interruption and/or dosage reduction or discontinuance of niraparib therapy may be necessary based on severity and persistence of an adverse effect. If dosage reduction from 300 mg once daily is necessary, the dosage should be reduced to 200 mg once daily. If the toxicity recurs on a dosage of 200 mg once daily, the dosage should be reduced to 100 mg once daily. If the toxicity recurs on a dosage of 100 mg once daily, niraparib therapy should be discontinued.

Hematologic Toxicity. For platelet counts less than 100,000/mm^3, niraparib therapy should be withheld for no more than 28 days and CBCs should be monitored weekly until platelet counts reach or exceed 100,000/mm^3. For the first occurrence of a platelet count less than 100,000/mm^3, niraparib therapy may then be resumed at the same dosage or a reduced dosage of 200 mg once daily. For subsequent occurrences of a platelet count less than 100,000/mm^3, the daily dosage of niraparib should be reduced in decrements of 100 mg; however, if a dosage of 100 mg once daily requires further reduction or platelet counts do not return to acceptable levels within 28 days of withholding the drug, niraparib should be discontinued. (See Myelodysplastic Syndrome/Acute Myeloid Leukemia and also see Hematologic Effects under Cautions: Warnings/Precautions.)

For platelet counts less than 75,000/mm^3, niraparib therapy should be withheld for no more than 28 days and CBCs should be monitored weekly until platelet counts reach or exceed 100,000/mm^3. Upon resumption of therapy, the daily dosage of niraparib should be reduced in decrements of 100 mg. If platelet counts do not return to acceptable levels within 28 days of withholding the drug or a platelet count less than 75,000/mm^3 recurs on a reduced dosage of 100 mg once daily, niraparib therapy should be discontinued.

For platelet counts of 10,000/mm^3 or less, niraparib therapy should be withheld for no more than 28 days and platelet transfusion should be considered; however, the manufacturer states that if there are other risk factors such as concomitant use of anticoagulants or antiplatelet agents, withholding these drugs and/or a platelet transfusion may be considered at a higher platelet count. Upon completion of platelet transfusion, CBCs should be monitored weekly for 1 month. Niraparib therapy may be resumed at a reduced dosage once platelet counts reach or exceed 100,000/mm^3 and 7 or more days have elapsed since platelet transfusion. Upon resumption of therapy, CBCs should be monitored weekly for an additional month to ensure the platelet count is stable.

For neutropenia (absolute neutrophil count [ANC] less than 1,000/mm^3) or anemia (hemoglobin concentration less than 8 g/dL), niraparib therapy should be withheld for no more than 28 days and CBCs should be monitored weekly. Niraparib therapy may be resumed when ANC reaches or exceeds 1,500/mm^3 or hemoglobin concentrations reach or exceed 9 g/dL. Upon resumption of therapy, the daily dosage of niraparib should be reduced in 100-mg decrements. If ANC and/or hemoglobin concentrations do not return to acceptable levels within 28 days of withholding the drug or if the dosage has already been reduced to 100 mg once daily, niraparib therapy should be discontinued.

If MDS/AML is confirmed, niraparib therapy should be discontinued.

Nonhematologic Toxicity. For grade 3 or greater nonhematologic toxicity in situations in which prophylaxis is not considered feasible or if the adverse reaction persists despite treatment, niraparib therapy should be withheld until the toxicity resolves, but for no longer than 28 days. Upon resumption of therapy, the daily dosage of niraparib should be reduced in decrements of 100 mg; however, if a dosage of 100 mg once daily requires further reduction, the drug should be discontinued.

If prolonged grade 3 or greater nonhematologic toxicity (lasting more than 28 days) occurs on a dosage of 100 mg once daily, niraparib should be discontinued.

■ **Special Populations** No initial dosage adjustment of niraparib is necessary in patients with mild hepatic impairment. There are limited data in patients with moderate to severe hepatic impairment; the manufacturer currently provides no specific dosage recommendations for such patients. (See Hepatic Impairment under Warnings/Precautions: Specific Populations, in Cautions.)

No initial dosage adjustment of niraparib is necessary in patients with mild (creatinine clearance 60–89 mL/minute) or moderate (creatinine clearance 30–59 mL/minute) renal impairment. Niraparib has not been studied in patients with severe renal impairment (creatinine clearance less than 30 mL/minute) or end-stage renal disease requiring hemodialysis, and the manufacturer provides no specific dosage recommendations for such patients. (See Renal Impairment under Warnings/Precautions: Specific Populations, in Cautions.)

The manufacturer makes no specific dosage recommendations for geriatric patients. (See Geriatric Use under Warnings/Precautions: Specific Populations, in Cautions.)

Cautions

■ **Contraindications** The manufacturer states that there are no known contraindications to the use of niraparib.

■ **Warnings/Precautions** ***Myelodysplastic Syndrome/Acute Myeloid Leukemia*** Myelodysplastic syndrome (MDS) and acute myeloid leukemia (AML), including fatal cases, have been reported in niraparib-treated patients. Overall, MDS/AML have been reported in 7 of 751 patients (0.9%) receiving niraparib in clinical studies. In the principal efficacy study, MDS/AML occurred in 5 of 367 patients (1.4%) receiving niraparib and in 2 of 179 patients (1.1%) receiving placebo. All of these patients had received previous chemotherapy with platinum-containing agents, and some also had received other DNA-damaging antineoplastic agents and radiotherapy. The duration of niraparib therapy in patients who developed MDS/AML varied from less than 1 month to 2 years.

Complete blood cell (CBC) counts should be monitored in patients receiving niraparib. (See Hematologic Effects under Cautions: Warnings/Precautions.) If MDS/AML is confirmed, niraparib should be discontinued.

Hematologic Effects Adverse hematologic effects (e.g., thrombocytopenia, anemia, neutropenia) are often reported in patients receiving niraparib therapy. In the principal efficacy study, grade 3 or greater thrombocytopenia, anemia, and neutropenia occurred in 29, 25, and 20%, respectively, of patients receiving niraparib. Discontinuance of therapy was necessary in 3, 1, and 2% of patients experiencing thrombocytopenia, anemia, and neutropenia, respectively.

Niraparib therapy should not be initiated until patients have recovered from hematologic toxicity caused by previous chemotherapy (to grade 1 or less). CBC counts should be monitored weekly for the first month of therapy, monthly for the next 11 months, and then periodically thereafter. (See Hematologic Toxicity under Dosage: Dosage Modification for Toxicity, in Dosage and Administration.) If clinically important hematologic toxicity develops and persists for more than 4 weeks following interruption of niraparib therapy, patients should be referred to a hematologist for further evaluation, including bone marrow analysis and cytogenetic testing of a blood sample. (See Myelodysplastic Syndrome/Acute Myeloid Leukemia under Cautions: Warnings/Precautions.)

Cardiovascular Effects Hypertension and hypertensive crisis have been reported in niraparib-treated patients. Tachycardia and other cardiac arrhythmias, palpitations, and angina also have occurred in patients receiving the drug. In the principal efficacy study, grade 3 or greater hypertension occurred in 9% of niraparib-treated patients compared with 2% of those receiving placebo; discontinuance of therapy was necessary in less than 1% of patients receiving niraparib or placebo. Maximum mean increases from baseline in pulse rate, systolic blood pressure, and diastolic blood pressure were 24.1 beats per minute, 24.5 mm Hg, and 16.5 mm Hg, respectively, in patients receiving niraparib compared with 15.8 beats per minute, 18.3 mm Hg, and 11.6 mm Hg, respectively, in those receiving placebo.

In a randomized, placebo-controlled study in patients with cancer, substantial changes in the mean QT interval corrected for rate (QT_c) (i.e., greater than 20 msec) were not observed when niraparib 300 mg was administered once daily.

Blood pressure and heart rate should be monitored monthly for the first year of niraparib therapy and then periodically thereafter. Patients with cardiovascular disorders, particularly those with coronary insufficiency, cardiac arrhythmias, and/or hypertension, should be closely monitored. Hypertension should be managed with antihypertensive therapy and adjustment of the niraparib dosage, if necessary. (See Nonhematologic Toxicity under Dosage: Dosage Modification for Toxicity, in Dosage and Administration.)

Fetal/Neonatal Morbidity and Mortality Based on its mechanism of action, niraparib may cause fetal harm (e.g., teratogenicity, embryofetal death) in humans. There are no data regarding use of niraparib in pregnant women to inform the drug-associated risk. Niraparib has the potential to cause teratogenicity and/or embryofetal death since the drug is genotoxic and targets actively dividing cells in animals and patients (e.g., bone marrow). Due to the potential risk to the fetus based on its mechanism of action, animal developmental and reproductive toxicology studies have not been conducted with niraparib.

Pregnancy should be avoided during niraparib therapy. Women of childbearing potential should be advised to use effective contraceptive methods while receiving niraparib and for at least 6 months after discontinuance of therapy. If niraparib is used during pregnancy or if the patient becomes pregnant while receiving the drug, the patient should be apprised of the potential risk to the fetus and the potential risk for loss of the pregnancy.

Impairment of Fertility Results of animal studies suggest that niraparib may impair male fertility. The effect of the drug on fertility in humans is not known.

Fertility studies have not been conducted with niraparib in animals. In a general toxicity study, reduced sperm, spermatids, and germ cells in epididymides and testes were observed in male animals receiving niraparib at exposure levels approximately 0.3 and 0.012 times the human exposure at the recommended dosage. A trend toward reversibility of these findings 4 weeks after discontinuance of therapy was observed.

Specific Populations **Pregnancy.** Although there are no available data in pregnant women, niraparib may cause fetal harm based on its mechanism of action. (See Fetal/Neonatal Morbidity and Mortality under Cautions: Warnings/Precautions.) If niraparib is used during pregnancy or if the patient becomes pregnant while receiving the drug, the patient should be apprised of the potential fetal hazard and potential for loss of the pregnancy. (See Advice to Patients.)

In women of childbearing potential, the manufacturer recommends a pregnancy test prior to initiating niraparib therapy.

Lactation. It is not known whether niraparib or its metabolites are distributed into human milk or if the drug has any effect on milk production or the nursing infant. Because of the potential for serious adverse reactions to niraparib in nursing infants, women should be advised to discontinue nursing while receiving the drug and for 1 month after the drug is discontinued.

Pediatric Use. Safety and efficacy of niraparib have not been established in pediatric patients.

Geriatric Use. In the principal efficacy study evaluating niraparib in patients with ovarian, fallopian tube, or primary peritoneal cancer, 35% of patients were 65 years of age or older and 8% were 75 years of age or older. No overall differences in safety and efficacy were observed between geriatric patients and younger adults. However, the possibility of increased sensitivity to the drug in some geriatric patients cannot be ruled out.

Hepatic Impairment. Population pharmacokinetic analyses indicate that systemic exposure to niraparib in patients with mild hepatic impairment is similar to that in patients with normal hepatic function; therefore, no initial dosage adjustment of niraparib is necessary in such patients.

Pharmacokinetics and safety of niraparib in patients with moderate to severe hepatic impairment have not been evaluated to date. (See Dosage and Administration: Special Populations.)

Renal Impairment. Population pharmacokinetic analyses indicate that the pharmacokinetics of niraparib in patients with mild or moderate renal impairment (creatinine clearance 30–89 mL/minute) are similar to those in patients with normal renal function; therefore, no initial dosage adjustment of the drug is necessary in such patients.

Pharmacokinetics and safety of niraparib in patients with severe renal impairment (creatinine clearance less than 30 mL/minute) or end-stage renal disease requiring hemodialysis have not been established to date. (See Dosage and Administration: Special Populations.)

■ **Common Adverse Effects** Adverse effects reported in 10% or more of patients receiving niraparib monotherapy for ovarian, fallopian tube, or primary peritoneal cancer in the principal efficacy study include nausea, fatigue/asthenia, constipation, vomiting, abdominal pain and/or distension, insomnia, headache, decreased appetite, nasopharyngitis, rash, diarrhea, dyspnea, hypertension, mucositis/stomatitis, myalgia, back pain, dizziness, dyspepsia, cough, arthralgia, urinary tract infection, anxiety, dry mouth, dysgeusia, and palpitations.

Laboratory abnormalities reported in 25% or more of patients receiving niraparib include anemia or decreased hemoglobin concentrations, thrombocytopenia or decreased platelet count, leukopenia or decreased leukocyte count, neutropenia or decreased absolute neutrophil count (ANC), and elevated concentrations of aminotransferases (e.g., AST, ALT).

Drug Interactions

Niraparib is principally metabolized by carboxylesterases to form a major inactive metabolite, M1, which subsequently undergoes glucuronidation by uridine diphosphate-glucuronosyltransferases (UGT) to form the M10 metabolite. In vivo, niraparib is a substrate of carboxylesterases and UGT.

In vitro studies indicate that neither niraparib nor its major metabolite (M1) are inhibitors of cytochrome P-450 (CYP) isoenzymes 1A2, 2B6, 2C8, 2C9, 2C19, 2D6, and 3A4 or inducers of CYP3A4. The drug is a weak inducer of CYP1A2 in vitro.

In vitro studies indicate that niraparib is a substrate, but not an inhibitor, of P-glycoprotein (P-gp). Niraparib is also a substrate and a weak inhibitor of breast cancer resistance protein (BCRP). In vitro, neither niraparib nor M1 is a substrate or inhibitor of bile salt export pump (BSEP), organic anion transport protein (OATP) 1B1, OATP1B3, organic cation transporter (OCT) 1, OCT2, organic anion transporter (OAT) 1, and OAT3. In vitro studies also show that M1 is not a substrate or inhibitor of P-gp and BCRP.

■ **Drugs Affecting Gastric Acidity** Although not specifically studied in drug interaction studies to date, clinically important pharmacokinetic interactions between niraparib and drugs affecting gastric acidity (e.g., histamine H_2-receptor antagonists, proton-pump inhibitors) appear unlikely based on the drug's solubility in an acidic pH range.

■ **Anticoagulants and Antiplatelet Agents** There is a potential for increased risk of adverse hematologic effects and hemorrhagic events in patients concurrently receiving niraparib and anticoagulants or antiplatelet agents. (See Hematologic Toxicity under Dosage: Dosage Modification for Toxicity, in Dosage and Administration and see also Hematologic Effects under Cautions: Warnings/Precautions.)

Description

Niraparib, an inhibitor of mammalian poly(adenosine diphosphate [ADP]-ribose) polymerase (PARP) enzymes PARP-1 and PARP-2, is an antineoplastic agent. The drug is a highly selective inhibitor of PARP-1 and PARP-2, which are involved in detection of DNA damage and its repair. In vitro studies have demonstrated that niraparib-induced cytotoxicity may involve inhibition of PARP enzymatic activity and increased formation of PARP-DNA complexes, which result in DNA damage, apoptosis, and cell death. In vitro, niraparib exhibits cytotoxic activity in tumor cell lines with or without deficiencies in BRCA1/2. In addition, niraparib reduced tumor growth in xenograft models of human cancer cell lines with BRCA1/2 deficiencies in mice and in patient-derived xenograft tumor models with homologous recombination deficiency expressing either mutated or wild-type BRCA1/2.

Following oral administration, the absolute bioavailability of niraparib is approximately 73%. Peak plasma concentrations and areas under the serum concentration-time curve (AUCs) of niraparib are proportional to dose following repeated administration of the drug over the dosage range of 30–400 mg once daily. Following oral administration, niraparib is rapidly absorbed with peak plasma concentrations occurring within 3 hours. Repeated administration of niraparib 30–400 mg daily resulted in a twofold niraparib accumulation ratio. Oral administration of niraparib with a high-fat meal (800–1000 calories with fat accounting for approximately 50% of the caloric content) resulted in a decrease in peak plasma concentrations of approximately 22% and an increase in AUC of approximately 7%; however, these effects were not considered clinically important. The drug is 83% bound to plasma proteins. Following oral administration of multiple doses of niraparib (300 mg once daily), the mean terminal half-life of niraparib was 36 hours. Niraparib is metabolized to inactive metabolites principally by amide hydrolysis followed by glucuronidation. Following oral administration of a single radiolabeled dose of niraparib, 47.5% of the radioactivity was recovered in urine (11% of the dose as unchanged drug) and 38.8% was recovered in feces (19% of the dose as unchanged drug). Population pharmacokinetic analyses indicate that age (18–65 years), gender, and race/ethnicity do not have clinically important effects on the pharmacokinetics of niraparib.

Advice to Patients

Importance of instructing patients to read the manufacturer's patient information.

Importance of advising patients to take niraparib capsules once daily at approximately the same time each day, either with or without food, and to swallow the capsules whole. Importance of advising patients that administration of the drug at bedtime may help alleviate any nausea symptoms.

If a dose is missed or vomited, importance of advising patients not to take an extra dose and to take the next normal dose at the regularly scheduled time.

Risk of myelodysplastic syndrome and acute myeloid leukemia. Importance of informing clinician if fatigue/asthenia, fever, weight loss, frequent infections, bruising, unusual bleeding (including hematuria or bloody stool), or shortness of breath occurs.

Risk of bone marrow suppression. Importance of periodic hematologic monitoring during niraparib therapy. Importance of informing clinician if new onset of bleeding, fever, or symptoms of infection occur.

Risk of adverse cardiovascular effects, including hypertension and increased heart rate. Importance of advising patients to undergo monthly blood pressure and heart rate monitoring during the first year of treatment and periodically thereafter and to contact their clinician if elevated blood pressure occurs.

Risk of fetal harm and pregnancy loss. Necessity of advising women of childbearing potential to avoid pregnancy and to use effective contraception while receiving niraparib and for at least 6 months following discontinuance of therapy. Importance of women informing clinicians immediately if they become pregnant during therapy or think they may be pregnant. If pregnancy occurs, advise pregnant women of potential risk to the fetus.

Importance of advising women to avoid breast-feeding while receiving niraparib and for 1 month following discontinuance of therapy.

Importance of informing clinicians of existing or contemplated concomitant therapy, including prescription and OTC drugs and dietary or herbal supplements, as well as any concomitant illnesses (e.g., cardiovascular disease, including hypertension, coronary insufficiency, or cardiac arrhythmias).

Importance of informing patients of other important precautionary information. (See Cautions.)

Overview® (see Users Guide). For additional information on this drug until a more detailed monograph is developed and published, the manufacturer's labeling should be consulted. It is *essential* that the manufacturer's labeling be consulted for more detailed information on usual cautions, precautions, contraindications, potential drug interactions, laboratory test interferences, and acute toxicity. For further information on the handling of antineoplastic agents, see the ASHP Guidelines on Handling Hazardous Drugs at http://www.ahfsdruginformation.com.

Preparations

Excipients in commercially available drug preparations may have clinically important effects in some individuals; consult specific product labeling for details.

Niraparib Tosylate

Oral

Capsules	100 mg (of niraparib)	**Zejula®**, Tesaro

Nivolumab

■ Nivolumab, a fully human anti-programmed-death receptor-1 (anti-PD-1) monoclonal antibody, is an antineoplastic agent. The drug is an IgG_4 kappa immunoglobulin.

Uses

■ **Melanoma** ***Unresectable or Metastatic Melanoma*** Nivolumab is used as monotherapy or in combination with ipilimumab for the treatment of unresectable or metastatic melanoma; nivolumab is designated an orphan drug by FDA for the treatment of this cancer.

The current indications for nivolumab as monotherapy or in combination with ipilimumab for the treatment of unresectable or metastatic melanoma are based principally on the results of an open-label, multicenter, randomized phase 3 study (CheckMate-037) and results of 2 multicenter, double-blind, randomized phase 3 studies (CheckMate-066 and CheckMate-067).

The CheckMate-037 study included 405 adults with unresectable or metastatic melanoma that had progressed during or following therapy with ipilimumab and, in those with tumors bearing the b-Raf serine-threonine kinase (BRAF) V600 mutation, therapy with a BRAF inhibitor. Patients were randomized (stratified by programmed-death ligand-1 [PD-L1] expression status, BRAF mutation status, and response to prior ipilimumab therapy) in a 2:1 ratio to receive either nivolumab (3 mg/kg administered by IV infusion every 2 weeks) or investigator's choice of chemotherapy (either dacarbazine 1 g/m^2 every 3 weeks or carboplatin at the dose required to obtain an area under the plasma concentration-time curve [AUC] of 6 mg/mL per minute in combination with paclitaxel 175 mg/m^2 every 3 weeks) until disease progression or unacceptable toxicity occurred. However, clinically stable patients with disease progression could continue treatment if they were considered to be deriving clinical benefit. In a planned noncomparative interim analysis, efficacy in the initial 120 patients randomized to receive nivolumab was evaluated based on overall response rate (as evaluated by a blinded independent central review committee) and duration of response. The median age of patients in the initial nivolumab-treated cohort was 58 years; all patients in this cohort had an Eastern Cooperative Oncology Group (ECOG) performance status of 0 or 1. Most patients (76%) in this cohort had TNM metastasis stage M1c disease, 68% had received 2 or more prior systemic therapies for their disease, 56% had elevated LDH concentrations, 22% had tumors bearing the BRAF V600 mutation, and 18% had a history of brain metastasis. Demographic characteristics of the entire study population were similar to those of the initial nivolumab-treated cohort. This study excluded patients receiving immunosuppressive agents and those with autoimmune disease, ocular melanoma, active brain metastasis, or a history of immune-mediated adverse effects with prior ipilimumab therapy (i.e., any grade 4 immune-mediated adverse effect [except for endocrinopathies] or grade 3 immune-mediated adverse effect that persisted for more than 12 weeks).

After a minimum follow-up of 6 months in the CheckMate-037 study, the overall response rate in the initial cohort of nivolumab-treated patients was 32%; complete response was achieved in 4 patients. At the time of analysis, the median duration of response had not been reached; most (87%) of the patients who responded to nivolumab had ongoing responses. Exploratory analysis suggested higher objective response rates for nivolumab compared with investigator's choice of chemotherapy regardless of BRAF mutation status or prior ipilimumab benefit; although a response benefit was observed for nivolumab compared with chemotherapy in patients with negative PD-L1 expression, the benefit of nivolumab relative to that of chemotherapy appeared to be greater in those with positive PD-L1 expression (defined as PD-L1 expression of any intensity on at least 5% of tumor cells as detected by immunohistochemistry assay). In the entire study population, median overall survival was 15.7 or 14.4 months in patients receiving nivolumab or investigator's choice of chemotherapy, respectively.

In the CheckMate-066 study, 418 patients with previously untreated unresectable or metastatic BRAF wild-type melanoma were randomized (stratified by PD-L1 expression status and stage of metastasis) to receive either nivolumab (3 mg/kg administered by IV infusion every 2 weeks) or dacarbazine (1 g/m^2 every 3 weeks) until disease progression or unacceptable toxicity occurred. However, patients with disease progression could continue receiving treatment if they were considered to be deriving clinical benefit. The primary measure of efficacy was overall survival; additional outcome measures were progression-free survival and overall response rate. The median age of patients was 65 years; 99.5% were Caucasian and 59% were male. Most patients (99%) enrolled in the study had an ECOG performance status of 0 or 1; however, a larger proportion of patients receiving nivolumab had an ECOG performance status of 0 compared with those receiving dacarbazine (71 versus 58%). Most patients (61%) had TNM metastasis stage M1c disease, 74% had cutaneous melanoma, 11% had mucosal melanoma, 37% had elevated LDH concentrations, 35% had positive PD-L1 expression (defined as PD-L1 expression of any intensity on at least 5% of tumor cells as detected by immunohistochemistry assay), and 4% had a history of brain metastasis. Patients with a history of serious autoimmune disease, ocular/uveal melanoma, or active brain or leptomeningeal metastasis were excluded from the study.

In the CheckMate-066 study, median overall survival in patients receiving nivolumab had not been reached at the time of the interim analysis; however, nivolumab reduced the risk of death by 58% compared with dacarbazine. At the time of the initial interim analysis, patients receiving nivolumab had a higher overall response rate (34 versus 9%) and longer median progression-free survival (5.1 versus 2.2 months) compared with patients receiving dacarbazine. After a minimum follow-up of 38.4 or 38.5 months in patients receiving nivolumab or dacarbazine, respectively, median overall survival was 37.5 months in patients receiving nivolumab compared with 11.2 months in those receiving dacarbazine. Progression-free survival for nivolumab- and dacarbazine-treated patients at the time of the updated analysis remained similar to the initial interim results. At the time of the updated analysis, overall response rates in nivolumab- and dacarbazine-treated patients were 42.9 and 14.4%, respectively; complete responses were achieved in 19 and 1.4% of nivolumab- and dacarbazine-treated patients, respectively. Median duration of response had not been reached in those receiving nivolumab and was 6 months in those receiving dacarbazine. The median time to complete or partial response was 2.1 months in nivolumab-treated patients and 2.9 or 2.2 months, respectively, in dacarbazine-treated patients. A planned subgroup analysis indicated that the effect of nivolumab on progression-free survival and overall survival was consistent regardless of PD-L1 expression (less than 5% versus 5% or more of tumor cells).

In the CheckMate-067 study, 945 patients with previously untreated unresectable or metastatic melanoma were randomized (stratified by PD-L1 expression status, BRAF V600 mutation status, and stage of metastasis) to receive one of 3 regimens: nivolumab (1 mg/kg by IV infusion) in combination with ipilimumab (3 mg/kg by IV infusion) every 3 weeks for 4 doses, followed by nivolumab monotherapy (3 mg/kg by IV infusion every 2 weeks); nivolumab (3 mg/kg by IV infusion every 2 weeks) and placebo; or ipilimumab (3 mg/kg by IV infusion every 3 weeks for 4 doses) and placebo. Treatment was continued until disease progression or unacceptable toxicity occurred; however, patients with disease progression could continue receiving treatment if they were considered to be deriving clinical benefit. The primary measures of efficacy were progression-free survival and overall survival; additional outcome measures were overall response rate and duration of response. In this study, the median age of patients was 61 years; 97% were Caucasian, 65% were male, 46% had positive PD-L1 expression (defined as PD-L1 expression of any intensity on at least 5% of tumor cells as detected by immunohistochemistry assay), 36% had elevated LDH concentrations, 32% had BRAF V600 mutation-positive melanoma, 22% had received prior adjuvant therapy, and 4% had a history of brain metastasis. All patients enrolled in the study had an ECOG performance status of 0 or 1. Most patients (93%) had metastatic disease; 58% of patients had TNM metastasis stage M1c disease. Patients with autoimmune disease, conditions requiring therapy with immunosuppressive agents, ocular melanoma, or active brain metastasis were excluded from the study.

After a minimum follow-up of 28 months in the CheckMate-067 study, overall survival rate was higher in patients receiving nivolumab in combination with ipilimumab and in those receiving nivolumab compared with those receiving ipilimumab (59 and 55%, respectively, versus 37%). Progression-free survival also was prolonged in patients receiving nivolumab in combination with ipilimumab and in those receiving nivolumab compared with those receiving ipilimumab (11.7 and 6.9 months, respectively, versus 2.9 months). In addition, patients receiving nivolumab in combination with ipilimumab and those receiving nivolumab had higher overall response rates compared with those receiving ipilimumab (50 and 40%, respectively, versus 14%); complete responses were achieved in 8.9, 8.5, or 1.9% of patients receiving combination therapy with nivolumab and ipilimumab, nivolumab, or ipilimumab, respectively. After a minimum follow-up of 28 months, 55, 56, or 39% of patients receiving these respective treatments had durable responses of 24 months or more. After a minimum follow-up of 48 months, median overall survival was 36.9 or 19.9 months in patients receiving nivolumab or ipilimumab, respectively, but had not been reached in those receiving nivolumab in combination with ipilimumab. Progression-free survival at a minimum follow-up of 48 months in patients receiving combination therapy with nivolumab and ipilimumab, nivolumab, or ipilimumab remained similar to the initial interim results. The study was not designed to assess whether combination therapy with nivolumab and ipilimumab results in improved survival relative to nivolumab alone. Results of a subgroup analysis (based on age, geographic region, ECOG performance status, PD-L1 expression status, BRAF V600 mutation status, stage of metastasis, tumor burden, and number of lesions) suggested that the progression-free survival and overall survival benefit of nivolumab or nivolumab in combination with ipilimumab versus ipilimumab was consistent across all subgroups.

Adjuvant Therapy for Locally Advanced or Metastatic Melanoma Nivolumab is used as adjuvant therapy of locally advanced or metastatic melanoma following complete resection.

The current indication for nivolumab as adjuvant therapy for locally advanced or metastatic melanoma is based principally on the results of a randomized, double-blind phase 3 study (CheckMate-238) in patients with completely resected stage IIIB, IIIC, or IV melanoma. In this study, 906 patients were randomized (stratified by disease stage and PD-L1 expression status) to receive either nivolumab (3 mg/kg administered by IV infusion every 2 weeks) or ipilimumab (10 mg/kg by IV infusion every 3 weeks for 4 doses then every 12 weeks beginning at week 24) for up to 1 year or until disease recurrence or unacceptable toxicity occurred. The primary measure of efficacy was recurrence-free survival. The median age of patients enrolled in the study was 55 years; 95% were Caucasian, 90% had a baseline ECOG performance status of 0, 58% were male, 81% had stage IIIB or IIIC disease, 42% had BRAF V600 mutation-positive melanoma, 48% had macroscopic lymph node involvement, 34% had positive PD-L1 expression (defined as PD-L1 expression of any intensity on at least 5% of tumor cells as detected by a clinical trial assay), 32% had tumor ulceration, and 8% had elevated LDH concentrations. Patients were eligible for enrollment in the study following complete resection of melanoma within 12 weeks prior to randomization. The study excluded patients with a history of autoimmune disease, ocular/uveal melanoma, or any condition requiring therapy with systemic corticosteroids or immunosuppressive agents; those who had received prior therapy for melanoma other than surgery; those who had received adjuvant radiation therapy following neurosurgical resection; and those who had received adjuvant therapy with interferon alfa 6 months or more prior to randomization.

After a minimum follow-up of 18 months, median recurrence-free survival had not been reached in either group; however, nivolumab reduced the risk of recurrence or death by 35% compared with ipilimumab. At 18 months, the recurrence-free survival rate was 66.4 or 52.7% in patients receiving nivolumab or ipilimumab, respectively. Results of a subgroup analysis (based on age, gender, disease stage, PD-L1 status, BRAF mutation status, presence of tumor ulceration, lymph node involvement, and disease subtype) suggested that the effect of nivolumab on recurrence-free survival was consistent across most subgroups; however, a recurrence-free survival benefit for nivolumab versus ipilimumab was not apparent in patients with stage IV M1c disease, those with microscopic lymph node involvement and ulceration of the primary tumor, or those with a mucosal subtype.

■ **Non-small Cell Lung Cancer** Nivolumab is used for the treatment of metastatic non-small cell lung cancer (NSCLC) that has progressed during or following therapy with platinum-based chemotherapy and, in those with epidermal growth factor receptor (EGFR) mutation- or anaplastic lymphoma kinase (ALK)-positive tumors, therapy with an EGFR or ALK inhibitor. The current indication for use of nivolumab for the treatment of previously treated metastatic NSCLC is based principally on the results of 2 randomized open-label studies (CheckMate-017 and CheckMate-057) and a supportive multicenter, noncomparative phase 2 study (CheckMate-063).

In the CheckMate-017 study, 272 patients with metastatic squamous NSCLC that had progressed during or following therapy with one platinum-containing, 2-drug combination regimen were randomized to receive either nivolumab (3 mg/kg administered by IV infusion every 2 weeks) or docetaxel (75 mg/m^2 administered by IV infusion every 3 weeks). The primary measure of efficacy was overall survival. The median age of patients enrolled in the study was 63 years; all patients enrolled in the study had an ECOG performance status of 0 or 1. Patients were eligible for enrollment in the study regardless of tumor expression of PD-L1. This study excluded patients with autoimmune disease, any condition requiring therapy with immunosuppressive agents, symptomatic interstitial lung disease, or untreated brain metastasis.

At the time of data analysis in the CheckMate-017 study, median overall survival (9.2 versus 6 months) and progression-free survival (3.5 versus 2.8 months) were prolonged and overall response rates (20 versus 9%) were higher in patients receiving nivolumab compared with those receiving docetaxel; complete response was achieved in 1 patient receiving nivolumab and none of those receiving docetaxel. Median overall survival, median progression-free survival, and overall response rates remained similar at the time of a 24-month analysis. Among patients with evaluable PD-L1 expression, there were no clear differences in overall survival based on PD-L1 expression.

In the CheckMate-057 study, 582 patients with metastatic nonsquamous NSCLC that had progressed during or following therapy with one platinum-containing, 2-drug combination regimen were randomized to receive either nivolumab (3 mg/kg administered by IV infusion every 2 weeks) or docetaxel (75 mg/m^2 administered by IV infusion every 3 weeks) until disease progression or unacceptable toxicity occurred. The primary measure of efficacy was overall survival; additional outcome measures were overall response rate and progression-free survival. The median age of patients enrolled in the study was 62 years; all patients enrolled in the study had an ECOG performance status of 0 or 1, 93% had adenocarcinoma histology, 14% had EGFR mutation-positive disease, 3.6% had ALK-positive disease, and 40% had received maintenance therapy as part of their first-line regimen. This study excluded patients with autoimmune disease, symptomatic interstitial lung disease, untreated brain metastasis, or any condition requiring therapy with immunosuppressive agents.

At the time of the interim analysis in the CheckMate-057 study, patients receiving nivolumab had longer median overall survival compared with those receiving docetaxel (12.2 versus 9.4 months). Although not statistically significant, progression-free survival appeared to be shorter in patients receiving nivolumab compared with those receiving docetaxel (2.3 versus 4.2 months). Patients receiving nivolumab had a higher overall response rate compared with those receiving docetaxel (19 versus 12%); complete responses were achieved in 1.4 or 0.3% of patients receiving nivolumab or docetaxel, respectively. At the time of analysis, the median duration of response was 17 months in patients receiving nivolumab and 6 months in those receiving docetaxel; however, responses were ongoing in nivolumab-treated patients. Median overall survival, median progression-free survival, and overall response rates remained similar at the time of a 24-month analysis. Subgroup analysis based on relevant patient characteristics (prior maintenance therapy, line of therapy, age, gender, ECOG performance status, smoking status, EGFR mutation status, KRAS mutation status) suggested that nivolumab had a greater effect on overall survival relative to docetaxel in most patient subgroups; however, a survival benefit for nivolumab versus docetaxel was not apparent for patients receiving the drug as third-line therapy, those who had never smoked, and those with EGFR mutation-positive disease. Subgroup analysis also indicated that increasing levels of PD-L1 expression were associated with overall survival and progression-free survival benefits for nivolumab compared with docetaxel.

In the CheckMate-063 study, 117 patients with advanced squamous NSCLC that had progressed following therapy with a platinum-based regimen and at least one additional systemic therapy received nivolumab 3 mg/kg administered by IV infusion every 2 weeks. The primary measure of efficacy was overall response rate (as evaluated by an independent central review committee); an additional outcome measure was duration of response. The median age of patients enrolled in the study was 65 years; all patients enrolled in the study had an ECOG performance status of 0 or 1. Patients were eligible for enrollment in the study regardless of their PD-L1 status. This study excluded patients with autoimmune disease, symptomatic interstitial lung disease, or untreated brain metastasis. After a minimum follow-up of 10 months, the overall response rate was 15%; there were no complete responses. At the time of analysis, 76% of the responders had ongoing responses; 59% of these patients had durable responses of 6 months or more.

■ **Small Cell Lung Cancer** Nivolumab is used for the treatment of metastatic small cell lung cancer (SCLC) that has progressed following therapy with platinum-based chemotherapy and at least one other line of therapy; nivolumab has been designated an orphan drug by FDA for the treatment of this cancer. The accelerated approval of nivolumab for the treatment of metastatic SCLC that has progressed following therapy with platinum-based chemotherapy and at least one other line of therapy is based on objective response rate and duration of response; continued approval for this indication may be contingent on verification and description of clinical benefit of nivolumab in confirmatory studies.

The current indication for nivolumab in the treatment of previously treated metastatic SCLC is based principally on the results for a cohort of patients with metastatic SCLC who received nivolumab monotherapy in an ongoing, multicenter, open-label phase ½ study (CheckMate-032). This cohort of patients included 109 adults with metastatic SCLC that had progressed following therapy with platinum-based chemotherapy and at least one other line of therapy who received nivolumab (3 mg/kg administered by IV infusion over 60 minutes every 2 weeks). The primary measure of efficacy was objective response rate (as evaluated by a blinded independent central review committee according to RECIST). The median age of patients enrolled in this SCLC cohort was 64 years (6% of patients were 75 years of age or older); 99% had a baseline ECOG performance status of 0 or 1, 94% were Caucasian, 93% were former or current smokers, 56% were male, and 7% had brain metastases. Approximately 65% had platinum-sensitive disease (defined as disease progression 90 days or more following the last dose of platinum-containing therapy). All patients enrolled in the cohort had received 2 or more prior lines of therapy; 94% had received 2 or 3 lines of therapy and 6% had received 4 or 5 lines of therapy. Patients were eligible for enrollment in the study regardless of tumor expression of PD-L1. This study excluded patients with autoimmune disease, any condition requiring therapy with immunosuppressive agents, symptomatic interstitial lung disease, or untreated brain metastasis.

The overall response rate in the CheckMate-032 study for patients receiving nivolumab monotherapy for treatment of metastatic SCLC that had progressed following treatment with platinum-based chemotherapy and at least one other line of therapy was 12%; complete responses were achieved in 0.9% of patients.

At the time of analysis, 77, 62, or 39% of the responders had durable responses of at least 6, 12, or 18 months, respectively.

■ **Renal Cell Carcinoma** ***Previously Treated Advanced Renal Cell Carcinoma*** Nivolumab is used as monotherapy for the treatment of advanced renal cell carcinoma previously treated with antiangiogenic therapy. In patients with advanced renal cell carcinoma, nivolumab therapy has been shown to prolong overall survival and increase response rate compared with everolimus.

The current indication for nivolumab as monotherapy in the treatment of advanced renal cell carcinoma is based principally on the results of a randomized, open-label phase 3 study (CheckMate-025) in adults with advanced renal cell carcinoma that had progressed during or following treatment with 1 or 2 prior antiangiogenic therapies. In this study, 821 patients were randomized (stratified by geographic region, Memorial Sloan-Kettering Cancer Center [MSKCC] risk category, number of prior therapies including an antiangiogenic agent) to receive either nivolumab (3 mg/kg administered by IV infusion every 2 weeks) or everolimus (10 mg orally once daily). The primary measure of efficacy was overall survival. The median age of patients enrolled in the study was 62 years (9% of patients were 75 years of age or older); 88% were Caucasian, 75% were male, 81% had MSKCC favorable- or intermediate-risk disease, and 77% had received one prior antiangiogenic therapy. All patients enrolled in the study had a baseline Karnofsky performance status of 70 or greater. Patients were eligible for enrollment in the study regardless of tumor expression of PD-L1. This study excluded patients with active autoimmune disease, any history of or active brain metastasis, or any condition requiring therapy with immunosuppressive agents, and those previously treated with a mammalian target of rapamycin (mTOR) inhibitor.

After a minimum follow-up of 14 months, patients receiving nivolumab had longer median overall survival compared with those receiving everolimus (25 versus 19.6 months). Results of a subgroup analysis suggested that the effect of nivolumab on overall survival was consistent regardless of MSKCC risk category, number of prior therapies including an antiangiogenic agent, and geographic region; however, an overall survival benefit for nivolumab versus everolimus was not apparent in the small group of patients 75 years of age or older. Patients receiving nivolumab also had higher objective response rates (21.5 versus 3.9%), with a median response duration of 23 months for those receiving nivolumab and 13.7 months for those receiving everolimus. The median time to response was 3 months (range: 1.4–13 months) for nivolumab-treated patients. This study was terminated prematurely at the request of the independent data monitoring committee because of improved overall survival observed during the prespecified interim analysis in patients receiving nivolumab.

First-line Therapy for Advanced Renal Cell Carcinoma Nivolumab is used in combination with ipilimumab for the treatment of intermediate- or poor-risk, previously untreated, advanced renal cell carcinoma. In patients with intermediate- or poor-risk, previously untreated, advanced renal cell carcinoma, nivolumab in combination with ipilimumab has been shown to prolong overall survival and increase response rate compared with sunitinib. Efficacy of nivolumab in combination with ipilimumab in patients with favorable-risk†, previously untreated, advanced renal cell carcinoma has not been established.

The current indication for nivolumab in combination with ipilimumab in the treatment of intermediate- or poor-risk, previously untreated, advanced renal cell carcinoma is based principally on the results of a randomized, open-label phase 3 study (CheckMate-214) in adults with previously untreated advanced renal cell carcinoma. In this study, 1082 patients were randomized (stratified by geographic region and International Metastatic Renal Cell Carcinoma Database Consortium [IMDC] risk score) to receive either nivolumab (3 mg/kg by IV infusion) in combination with ipilimumab (1 mg/kg by IV infusion) every 3 weeks for 4 doses, followed by nivolumab monotherapy (3 mg/kg by IV infusion every 2 weeks), or sunitinib (50 mg orally once daily for 4 consecutive weeks of each 6-week cycle). Treatment was continued until disease progression or unacceptable toxicity occurred. The primary measures of efficacy were overall survival, progression-free survival (as evaluated by an independent review committee according to RECIST), and objective response rate (as evaluated by an independent review committee according to RECIST) in patients with intermediate- or poor-risk disease (defined as patients with at least one prognostic risk factor according to IMDC criteria). The median age of patients enrolled in the study was 61 years (8% of patients were 75 years of age or older); 87% were Caucasian and 73% were male. All patients enrolled in the study had a baseline Karnofsky performance status of 70 or greater. Patients were eligible for enrollment in the study regardless of tumor expression of PD-L1. This study excluded patients with active autoimmune disease, any history of or active brain metastasis, or any condition requiring therapy with immunosuppressive agents.

At a median follow-up of 25.2 months, median overall survival for patients with intermediate- or poor-risk disease receiving nivolumab in combination with ipilimumab had not been reached; however, nivolumab in combination with ipilimumab reduced the risk of death by 37% compared with sunitinib. Progression-free survival was 11.6 months in patients receiving nivolumab in combination with ipilimumab and 8.4 months in those receiving sunitinib; however, the difference was not statistically significant. Patients with intermediate- or poor-risk disease receiving nivolumab in combination with ipilimumab also had higher objective response rates (41.6 versus 26.5%); complete response was achieved in 9.4% of patients receiving nivolumab in combination with ipilimumab and 1.2% of those receiving sunitinib. At the time of analysis, the median duration of response had not been reached in patients receiving nivolumab in combination with ipilimumab and was 18.2 months in those receiving sunitinib. Results of a subgroup analysis (based on age, gender, geographic region, IMDC risk category, prior nephrectomy, baseline level of PD-L1 expression, and site of metastases) in patients with intermediate- or poor-risk disease suggested a survival benefit for nivolumab in combination with ipilimumab relative to sunitinib across subgroups. In an exploratory analysis, an overall survival benefit for the nivolumab-ipilimumab combination regimen compared with sunitinib was not apparent in the subgroup of patients who had favorable-risk disease (hazard ratio: 1.45).

■ **Hodgkin Lymphoma** Nivolumab is used for the treatment of classical Hodgkin lymphoma (cHL) that has relapsed or progressed following autologous stem cell transplantation and subsequent therapy with brentuximab vedotin or following failure of at least 3 systemic therapies (including autologous stem cell transplantation); nivolumab has been designated an orphan drug by FDA for the treatment of this cancer. The accelerated approval of nivolumab for this indication is based on objective response rate. Continued approval for this indication may be contingent on verification and description of clinical benefit of nivolumab in confirmatory studies.

The current indication for nivolumab in the treatment of cHL is based principally on analysis of combined data from a cohort of patients in an open-label, multicenter, noncomparative phase 2 study (CheckMate-205) and an open-label, multicenter phase 1 dose-escalation study (CheckMate-039); 95 patients with cHL that had relapsed or progressed following autologous stem cell transplantation and subsequent therapy with brentuximab vedotin and 258 patients with cHL that had relapsed or progressed following autologous stem cell transplantation were included in the pooled analysis. The primary measure of efficacy was objective response rate as assessed by an independent review committee; an additional outcome measure was duration of response. Patients in both studies received nivolumab 3 mg/kg administered by IV infusion every 2 weeks. Treatment was continued until disease progression, maximum clinical benefit, or unacceptable toxicity occurred. Patients were eligible for enrollment in these studies regardless of tumor expression of PD-L1. The studies excluded patients with an ECOG performance status of 2 or greater, autoimmune disease, or symptomatic interstitial lung disease; those who had received an allogeneic stem cell transplant; those who had received radiation therapy to the chest area within 24 weeks prior to enrollment; and those with a history of pulmonary toxicity who had an adjusted diffusion lung capacity for carbon monoxide (DLCO) of 60% or less.

In the cohort of patients who had relapsed or had experienced disease progression following autologous stem cell transplantation and subsequent therapy with brentuximab vedotin, the median age of patients was 37 years; 87% were Caucasian and 64% were male. The median number of previous systemic therapies for patients in this cohort was 5 (range: 2–15). The overall response rate for patients in this cohort was 66%; complete response was achieved in 6% of patients in this cohort. At a median follow-up of 9.9 months, the estimated median duration of response was 13.1 months for patients in this cohort. The median time to response was 2 months (range: 0.7–11.1 months).

In the cohort of patients who had relapsed or had experienced disease progression following autologous stem cell transplantation, the median age of patients was 34 years; 86% were Caucasian and 59% were male. Most patients (85%) in this cohort had received at least 3 prior therapies; the median number of previous therapies was 4 (range: 2–15). Most patients (76%) in this cohort had received prior therapy with brentuximab vedotin; 78% of patients received brentuximab vedotin following stem cell transplantation, 17% received the drug prior to stem cell transplantation, and 5% received the drug prior to and following stem cell transplantation. The overall response rate for patients in this cohort was 69%; complete response was achieved in 14% of patients in this cohort. At a median follow-up of 6.7 months, the median duration of response had not been reached. The median time to response was 2 months (range: 0.7–11.1 months).

■ **Head and Neck Cancer** Nivolumab is used for the treatment of metastatic or recurrent squamous cell carcinoma of the head and neck that has progressed during or following therapy with platinum-based chemotherapy. In patients with metastatic or recurrent squamous cell carcinoma of the head and neck, nivolumab therapy has been shown to prolong overall survival compared with standard chemotherapy.

The current indication for nivolumab in the treatment of metastatic or recurrent squamous cell carcinoma of the head and neck is based principally on the results of a randomized, open-label phase 3 study (CheckMate-141) in adults with metastatic or recurrent squamous cell carcinoma of the head and neck that had progressed during or within 6 months following platinum-based chemotherapy in the neoadjuvant, adjuvant, primary (unresectable locally advanced), or metastatic setting. In this study, 361 patients were randomized (stratified by prior cetuximab use) to receive either nivolumab (3 mg/kg administered by IV infusion every 2 weeks) or investigator's choice of standard chemotherapy (cetuximab 400 mg/m^2 by IV infusion followed by cetuximab 250 mg/m^2 by IV infusion weekly; methotrexate 40–60 mg/m^2 by IV infusion weekly; or docetaxel 30–40 mg/m^2 by IV infusion weekly) until disease progression or unacceptable toxicity occurred. However, nivolumab therapy could be continued in patients with disease progression if they were considered to be deriving clinical benefit. The primary measure of efficacy was overall survival; additional outcome measures were overall response rate and progression-free survival. The median age of patients enrolled in the study was 60 years; most patients (98%) had an ECOG performance status of 0 or 1, 90% had metastatic disease, 83% were Caucasian, 83% were male, 76% were former or current smokers, 55% had received at least 2 prior therapies, 51% had unknown human papillomavirus (HPV) status, and 25% had HPV-positive disease (as assessed by p16 immunohistochemistry assay). This study excluded patients with autoimmune disease, untreated brain metastasis, conditions requiring therapy with immunosuppressive agents, human immunodeficiency virus (HIV) infection, hepatitis B virus (HBV) or hepatitis C virus (HCV) infection, recurrent or metastatic carcinoma of the nasopharynx, squamous cell carcinoma of unknown primary histology, or salivary gland or nonsquamous histology (e.g., mucosal melanoma).

A planned interim analysis indicated that patients receiving nivolumab had longer overall survival compared with patients receiving standard chemotherapy (7.5 versus 5.1 months). The median follow-up at the time of the interim analysis was 5.1 months. Results of the interim analysis suggested a numerical, but not statistically significant, increase in overall response rate with nivolumab compared with standard chemotherapy; progression-free survival was similar in both groups. Results of a subgroup analysis (based on age, ECOG performance status, prior cetuximab therapy, lines of prior therapy, investigator's choice of standard chemotherapy, site of primary tumor, and platinum-refractory disease in the primary setting) suggested that the effect of nivolumab on overall survival was consistent across all subgroups. A planned exploratory analysis indicated a survival benefit for nivolumab compared with standard chemotherapy regardless of PD-L1 expression or p16 tumor status; although the survival benefit appeared to be more pronounced in patients with PD-L1 expression on 1% or more of tumor cells compared with those with PD-L1 expression levels of less than 1% (hazard ratios: 0.55 and 0.89, respectively) and in patients with p16-positive tumors compared with those with p16-negative tumors (hazard ratios: 0.56 and 0.73, respectively), these interactions were not statistically significant.

■ Urothelial Carcinoma Nivolumab is used for the treatment of locally advanced or metastatic urothelial carcinoma that has progressed during or following platinum-containing therapy or within 12 months of platinum-containing therapy in the neoadjuvant or adjuvant setting. The accelerated approval of nivolumab for this indication is based on objective response rate and duration of response. Continued approval for this indication may be contingent on verification and description of clinical benefit of nivolumab in confirmatory studies.

The current indication for nivolumab in the treatment of locally advanced or metastatic urothelial carcinoma is based principally on the results of a multicenter, noncomparative phase 2 study (CheckMate-275) in adults with locally advanced or metastatic urothelial carcinoma that had progressed during or following platinum-containing therapy for metastatic disease or within 12 months of platinum-containing therapy in the neoadjuvant or adjuvant setting. The primary measure of efficacy was objective response rate as assessed by a blinded independent review committee according to Response Evaluation Criteria in Solid Tumors (RECIST 1.1). In this study, the median age of patients was 66 years; 86% were Caucasian, 84% had visceral metastases, 78% were male, and 27% had nonbladder urothelial carcinoma. All patients enrolled in the study had an ECOG performance status of 0 or 1. Approximately one-third (29%) of patients had received at least 2 prior therapies for metastatic disease and 34% had disease progression following platinum-containing therapy in the neoadjuvant or adjuvant setting; 36, 23, or 7% of patients had received prior treatment with cisplatin-, carboplatin-, or both cisplatin- and carboplatin-based regimens, respectively, for metastatic disease. Patients received nivolumab 3 mg/kg administered by IV infusion every 2 weeks until disease progression or unacceptable toxicity occurred; however, patients with disease progression could continue treatment if they were considered to be deriving clinical benefit. Patients with active brain or leptomeningeal metastases, autoimmune disease, or any condition requiring therapy with immunosuppressive agents were excluded from the study. Patients were eligible for enrollment in the study regardless of their PD-L1 status.

At a minimum follow-up of 6 months, the objective response rate was 19.6%; complete responses were achieved in 2.6% of patients. Among patients who had received prior therapy only in the neoadjuvant and adjuvant setting, the objective response rate was 23.4%. At the time of analysis, the estimated median duration of response was 10.3 months; however, 77% of the patients who responded to nivolumab had ongoing responses. The median time to response was 1.9 months (range: 1.6–7.2 months). In the planned subgroup analysis based on PD-L1 expression (as detected by an immunohistochemistry assay [Dako PD-L1 IHC 28-8 pharmDx]), the objective response rate with nivolumab therapy was 15.1% in patients with PD-L1 expression on less than 1% of tumor cells and 25% in those with PD-L1 expression on 1% or more of tumor cells; complete responses were achieved in 0.7 or 4.8% of patients in these respective subgroups. The median progression-free survival as assessed by the blinded independent review committee was 2 months. At a median follow-up of 7 months, median overall survival was 8.7 months in the overall population, 11.3 months in those with PD-L1 expression of 1% or more, and 6 months in those with PD-L1 expression of less than 1%. Results of a subgroup analysis (based on site of metastasis, ECOG performance status, Bellmunt risk factors, baseline hemoglobin concentration, baseline creatinine clearance, site of primary tumor, and prior therapy for advanced or metastatic disease) suggested that the drug's effect on tumor response was consistent across most subgroups; however, the effect on tumor response appeared to be reduced in patients with increasing number of Bellmunt risk factors.

■ Colorectal Cancer Nivolumab is used as monotherapy or in combination with ipilimumab for the treatment of metastatic colorectal cancer with high microsatellite instability (MSI-H) or mismatch repair deficiency (dMMR) that has progressed following fluoropyrimidine-, oxaliplatin-, and irinotecan-containing therapy. The accelerated approval of nivolumab as a single agent or in combination with ipilimumab for this indication is based on objective response rate and duration of response. Continued approval for this indication may be contingent on verification and description of clinical benefit of nivolumab in confirmatory studies.

Although some solid tumors, such as colorectal cancer, are generally unresponsive to anti-PD-1 therapy, a subpopulation of patients with solid tumors with MSI-H or dMMR has been shown to be particularly responsive to anti-PD-1 therapy. Deficiencies in the DNA mismatch repair pathway as a result of germline or somatic mutations in mismatch repair genes subsequently result in elevated levels of DNA instability in regions of short tandem repeat sequences (microsatellites) that are prone to replication errors (MSI-H). It has been postulated that the increased mutational burden in tumors with microsatellite instability produces tumor-specific neoantigens responsible for elevated levels of tumor-infiltrating lymphocytes and upregulation of immune checkpoint proteins such as PD-1 and PD-L1, suggesting that patients with solid tumors with MSI-H or dMMR are good candidates for immune checkpoint therapy. Clinical studies have demonstrated increased response rates in patients with solid tumors, particularly colorectal cancer, with MSI-H or dMMR receiving anti-PD-1 therapy. In a phase 2 study evaluating pembrolizumab, an anti-PD-1 antibody, in patients with solid tumors with dMMR or proficient mismatch repair (pMMR), the objective response rate (40 versus 0%) and progression-free survival rate (78 versus 11%) were substantially higher in patients with colorectal cancer with dMMR compared with those with pMMR colorectal cancer; response rates in patients with noncolorectal cancers with dMMR were similar to those in patients with colorectal cancer with dMMR.

The current indication for nivolumab as a single agent or in combination with ipilimumab is based principally on the results of an open-label, multicenter, noncomparative phase 2 study (CheckMate-142) in adults with MSI-H or dMMR metastatic colorectal cancer who had experienced disease progression during or following at least one prior therapy, including fluoropyrimidine- and oxaliplatin- or irinotecan-containing therapy, or who had not tolerated such therapies. Objective response rate was assessed by a blinded independent review committee according to RECIST 1.1. In this study, patients assigned to the monotherapy cohort received nivolumab 3 mg/kg administered as an IV infusion every 2 weeks until disease progression or unacceptable toxicity occurred, and patients assigned to the combination therapy cohort received nivolumab 3 mg/kg administered as an IV infusion and ipilimumab 1 mg/kg administered as an IV infusion on day 1 of each 21-day cycle for 4 doses, followed by single-agent nivolumab therapy (3 mg/kg administered as an IV infusion every 2 weeks) until disease progression or unacceptable toxicity occurred; however, patients in both cohorts could continue single-agent nivolumab beyond initial disease progression if they were considered to be deriving clinical benefit. Patients with active autoimmune disease, active brain metastasis, any condition requiring therapy with immunosuppressive agents, history of HIV infection, or HBV or HCV infection were excluded from the study.

In the cohort of 74 patients who received single-agent nivolumab, the median age of patients was 53 years; 98% had an ECOG performance status of 0 or 1, 88% were Caucasian, 59% were male, and 36% had a history of Lynch syndrome. Most patients (72%) had previously received fluoropyrimidine-, oxaliplatin-, and irinotecan-containing therapy and 42% of patients had previously received anti-EGFR therapy; 30, 28, 19, or 16% of patients had received 1, 2, 3, or 4 or more prior lines of therapy for metastatic disease, respectively. At a median follow-up of 12 months, the objective response rate was 32%; complete responses were achieved in 2.7% of patients. At the time of analysis, 63 or 38% of patients had durable responses of at least 6 or 12 months, respectively. Among patients previously treated with fluoropyrimidine-, oxaliplatin-, and irinotecan-containing therapy, the objective response rate was 28%; complete responses were achieved in 1.9% of patients who had received such prior therapy; and 67 or 40% of the responders had durable responses of at least 6 or 12 months, respectively. Objective responses were observed regardless of PD-L1 expression (on tumor cells or tumor-infiltrating immune cells), presence of mutated or wild-type BRAF or KRAS, or history of Lynch syndrome.

In the cohort of 119 patients who received nivolumab in combination with ipilimumab, the median age of patients was 58 years; 92% were Caucasian, 59% were male, and 29% had a history of Lynch syndrome. All patients enrolled in the combination therapy cohort had a baseline ECOG performance status of 0 or 1. Most patients (69%) had previously received fluoropyrimidine-, oxaliplatin-, and irinotecan-containing therapy and 29% of patients had previously received anti-EGFR therapy; 10, 40, 24, or 15% of patients had received 1, 2, 3, or 4 or more prior lines of therapy for metastatic disease, respectively. At a median follow-up of 13.4 months, the objective response rate was 49%; complete responses were achieved in 4.2% of patients. At the time of analysis, 83 or 19% of patients had durable responses of at least 6 or 12 months, respectively. Among patients previously treated with fluoropyrimidine-, oxaliplatin-, and irinotecan-containing therapy, the objective response rate was 46%; complete responses were achieved in 3.7% of patients who had received such prior therapy; and 89 or 21% of the responders had durable responses of at least 6 or 12 months, respectively.

■ **Hepatocellular Carcinoma** Nivolumab is used for the treatment of hepatocellular carcinoma previously treated with sorafenib; nivolumab has been designated an orphan drug by FDA for the treatment of this cancer. The accelerated approval of nivolumab for this indication is based on objective response rate and duration of response. Continued approval for this indication may be contingent on verification and description of clinical benefit of nivolumab in confirmatory studies.

The current indication for nivolumab in the treatment of previously treated hepatocellular carcinoma is based principally on the results for a cohort of patients with hepatocellular carcinoma in an open-label, multicenter, noncomparative, phase ½ study (CheckMate-040); the cohort included 154 adults with advanced hepatocellular carcinoma who had experienced disease progression during sorafenib therapy or who had not tolerated such therapy. The primary measure of efficacy was objective response rate according to RECIST 1.1 and modified RECIST for hepatocellular carcinoma as assessed by a blinded independent review committee. The median age of patients in the hepatocellular carcinoma cohort was 63 years; 99% had Child-Pugh class A hepatic impairment, 77% were male, 71% had extrahepatic spread, 46% were Caucasian, 31% had active HBV infection, 37% had α-fetoprotein concentrations of 0.4 mg/L or more, 29% had macrovascular invasion, 21% had active HCV infection, and 19% had received at least 2 prior systemic therapies. All patients enrolled in the hepatocellular carcinoma cohort had an ECOG performance status of 0 or 1 and previously had received sorafenib therapy; sorafenib was discontinued because of intolerable toxicity in 23% of patients. Alcohol consumption or nonalcoholic liver disease was the cause of hepatocellular carcinoma in 18 or 6.5% of patients, respectively. Prior therapies included surgical resection, locoregional therapy, and radiation therapy in 66, 58, and 24% of patients, respectively. Patients received nivolumab 3 mg/kg administered as an IV infusion every 2 weeks until disease progression or unacceptable toxicity occurred. The study excluded patients with autoimmune disease, brain metastasis, a history of hepatic encephalopathy, current or prior episodes of clinically important ascites, HIV infection, active HBV and HCV coinfection, or active HBV and hepatitis D virus (HDV) coinfection.

At the time of analysis, the objective response rate according to RECIST 1.1 or modified RECIST for patients in the hepatocellular carcinoma cohort of this study was 14.3 or 18.2%, respectively; according to these response criteria, complete response was achieved in 1.9 or 3.2%, respectively, of patients. The median duration of response had not been reached; however, 91% of patients who responded to the drug had durable responses of 6 months or more and 55% had durable responses of 12 months or more.

Dosage and Administration

■ **Administration** Nivolumab is administered by IV infusion over 30 minutes. *The drug should not be administered by rapid IV injection, such as IV push or bolus.* Following nivolumab administration, the IV administration line should be flushed with 0.9% sodium chloride injection or 5% dextrose injection.

For IV infusion over 30 minutes, the appropriate dose of nivolumab injection (containing 10 mg/mL) should be diluted with an appropriate volume of 0.9% sodium chloride or 5% dextrose injection to a final concentration of 1–10 mg/mL. The total volume of the infusion solution must not exceed 160 mL; for adults and pediatric patients weighing less than 40 kg, the total volume of the infusion solution must not exceed 4 mL per kg of body weight. Prior to dilution, the injection should be inspected visually for particulate matter and discoloration. The solution should be clear to opalescent and colorless to pale yellow; the solution should not be used if it is cloudy or discolored or if foreign particles other than translucent to white proteinaceous particles are present. The diluted solution should be mixed by gentle inversion and should *not* be shaken. Nivolumab should be administered through a sterile, nonpyrogenic, low-protein-binding 0.2- to 1.2-μm inline filter.

Diluted solutions of the drug are stable for up to 8 hours after dilution (including infusion time) when stored at room temperature or up to 24 hours after dilution when stored under refrigeration (2–8°C); diluted solutions of the drug should *not* be frozen.

Any unused portion in the vial or infusion bag should be discarded since nivolumab injection contains no preservative.

Nivolumab should *not* be administered simultaneously through the same IV line with any other drug or admixed with ipilimumab in the same infusion bag. When nivolumab is used in combination with ipilimumab, separate inline filters should be used for each infusion.

■ **Dosage** Clinicians should consult published protocols for information on the dosage, method of administration, and administration sequence of other antineoplastic agents used in combination regimens with nivolumab.

Melanoma **Monotherapy for Unresectable or Metastatic Melanoma.** When used as monotherapy for the treatment of unresectable or metastatic melanoma, the recommended adult dosage of nivolumab is 240 mg administered every 2 weeks or 480 mg administered every 4 weeks as a 30-minute IV infusion. Therapy should be continued until disease progression or unacceptable toxicity occurs.

Combination Therapy for Unresectable or Metastatic Melanoma. When used in combination with ipilimumab for the treatment of unresectable or metastatic melanoma, the recommended adult dosage of nivolumab is 1 mg/kg administered as a 30-minute IV infusion in combination with ipilimumab 3 mg/kg administered as a 90-minute IV infusion every 3 weeks for up to 4 doses or until unacceptable toxicity occurs, followed by single-agent nivolumab therapy at a dosage of 240 mg administered every 2 weeks or 480 mg administered every 4 weeks as a 30-minute IV infusion until disease progression or unacceptable toxicity occurs. Nivolumab should be administered before ipilimumab.

If nivolumab therapy is temporarily interrupted for toxicity, ipilimumab should also be withheld.

Adjuvant Therapy for Locally Advanced or Metastatic Melanoma. For the adjuvant therapy of completely resected locally advanced or metastatic melanoma, the recommended adult dosage of nivolumab is 240 mg administered every 2 weeks or 480 mg administered every 4 weeks as a 30-minute IV infusion. Therapy should be continued for up to 1 year or until disease recurrence or unacceptable toxicity occurs.

Non-small Cell Lung Cancer For the treatment of metastatic non-small cell lung cancer (NSCLC) that has progressed during or following therapy with platinum-based chemotherapy and, in those with epidermal growth factor receptor (EGFR) mutation- or anaplastic lymphoma kinase (ALK)-positive tumors, therapy with an FDA-labeled EGFR or ALK inhibitor, the recommended adult dosage of nivolumab is 240 mg administered every 2 weeks or 480 mg administered every 4 weeks as a 30-minute IV infusion. Therapy should be continued until disease progression or unacceptable toxicity occurs.

Small Cell Lung Cancer For the treatment of metastatic small cell lung cancer (SCLC) that has progressed following therapy with platinum-based chemotherapy and at least one other line of therapy, the recommended adult dosage of nivolumab is 240 mg administered every 2 weeks as a 30-minute IV infusion. Therapy should be continued until disease progression or unacceptable toxicity occurs.

Renal Cell Carcinoma **Monotherapy for Advanced Renal Cell Carcinoma.** When used as monotherapy for the treatment of advanced renal cell carcinoma previously treated with antiangiogenic therapy, the recommended adult dosage of nivolumab is 240 mg administered every 2 weeks or 480 mg administered every 4 weeks as a 30-minute IV infusion. Therapy should be continued until disease progression or unacceptable toxicity occurs.

Combination Therapy for Advanced Renal Cell Carcinoma. When used in combination with ipilimumab for the treatment of intermediate- or poor-risk, previously untreated, advanced renal cell carcinoma, the recommended adult dosage of nivolumab is 3 mg/kg administered as a 30-minute IV infusion in combination with ipilimumab 1 mg/kg administered as a 30-minute IV infusion every 3 weeks for 4 doses, followed by single-agent nivolumab therapy at a dosage of 240 mg administered every 2 weeks or 480 mg administered every 4 weeks as a 30-minute IV infusion until disease progression or unacceptable toxicity occurs. Nivolumab should be administered before ipilimumab.

If nivolumab therapy is temporarily interrupted for toxicity, ipilimumab should also be withheld.

Hodgkin Lymphoma For the treatment of classical Hodgkin lymphoma (cHL) that has relapsed or progressed following autologous stem cell transplantation and subsequent therapy with brentuximab vedotin or following failure of at least 3 systemic therapies (including autologous stem cell transplantation), the recommended adult dosage of nivolumab is 240 mg administered every 2 weeks or 480 mg administered every 4 weeks as a 30-minute IV infusion. Therapy should be continued until disease progression or unacceptable toxicity occurs.

Head and Neck Cancer For the treatment of metastatic or recurrent squamous cell carcinoma of the head and neck that has progressed during or following therapy with platinum-based chemotherapy, the recommended adult dosage of nivolumab is 240 mg administered every 2 weeks or 480 mg administered every 4 weeks as a 30-minute IV infusion. Therapy should be continued until disease progression or unacceptable toxicity occurs.

Urothelial Carcinoma For the treatment of locally advanced or metastatic urothelial carcinoma that has progressed during or following platinum-containing therapy or within 12 months of platinum-containing therapy in the neoadjuvant or adjuvant setting, the recommended adult dosage of nivolumab is 240 mg administered every 2 weeks or 480 mg administered every 4 weeks as a 30-minute IV infusion. Therapy should be continued until disease progression or unacceptable toxicity occurs.

Colorectal Cancer **Monotherapy for Metastatic Colorectal Cancer.** When used as monotherapy for the treatment of metastatic colorectal cancer with high microsatellite instability (MSI-H) or mismatch repair deficiency (dMMR) that has progressed following fluoropyrimidine-, oxaliplatin-, and irinotecan-containing therapy in adults and adolescents (12 years of age and older), the recommended dosage of nivolumab is 240 mg administered as a 30-minute IV infusion every 2 weeks. Therapy should be continued until disease progression or unacceptable toxicity occurs.

Combination Therapy for Metastatic Colorectal Cancer. When used in combination with ipilimumab for the treatment of metastatic colorectal cancer with MSI-H or dMMR that has progressed following fluoropyrimidine-, oxaliplatin-, and irinotecan-containing therapy in adults and adolescents (12 years of age and older), the recommended dosage of nivolumab is 3 mg/kg administered as a 30-minute IV infusion in combination with ipilimumab 1 mg/kg administered as a 30-minute IV infusion every 3 weeks for 4 doses, followed by single-agent nivolumab therapy at a dosage of 240 mg administered every 2 weeks as a 30-minute IV infusion until disease progression or unacceptable toxicity occurs. Nivolumab should be administered before ipilimumab.

If nivolumab therapy is temporarily interrupted for toxicity, ipilimumab should also be withheld.

Hepatocellular Carcinoma For the treatment of hepatocellular carcinoma previously treated with sorafenib, the recommended adult dosage of nivolumab is 240 mg administered every 2 weeks or 480 mg administered every 4 weeks as a 30-minute IV infusion. Therapy should be continued until disease progression or unacceptable toxicity occurs.

Therapy Interruption for Toxicity If immune-mediated adverse effects occur, temporary or permanent discontinuance of nivolumab may be required based on severity of the reaction.

Nivolumab should be permanently discontinued in patients experiencing persistent grade 2 or 3 immune-mediated adverse effects lasting 12 weeks or longer and in those requiring a corticosteroid dosage of 10 mg or more of prednisone daily (or equivalent) for more than 12 weeks. (See Cautions: Warnings/Precautions.)

Nivolumab should be permanently discontinued in patients experiencing any life-threatening or grade 4 immune-mediated adverse effect. Therapy with the drug also should be permanently discontinued if grade 3 immune-mediated adverse effects recur.

Immune-mediated Pneumonitis. If grade 2 immune-mediated pneumonitis occurs, nivolumab therapy should be interrupted until the toxicity resolves to grade 0 or 1. (See Immune-mediated Pneumonitis under Cautions: Warnings/Precautions.)

If grade 3 or 4 immune-mediated pneumonitis occurs, nivolumab therapy should be permanently discontinued.

Immune-mediated GI Effects. If grade 2 or 3 immune-mediated colitis or diarrhea occurs, nivolumab therapy should be interrupted until the toxicity resolves to grade 0 or 1; however, if grade 3 immune-mediated colitis or diarrhea occurs in patients receiving nivolumab in combination with ipilimumab, nivolumab therapy should be permanently discontinued. If colitis recurs upon reinitiation of therapy, nivolumab therapy should be permanently discontinued. (See Immune-mediated GI Effects under Cautions: Warnings/Precautions.)

If grade 4 immune-mediated colitis or diarrhea occurs, nivolumab therapy should be permanently discontinued.

Immune-mediated Hepatic Effects. For serum aminotransferase (ALT or AST) elevations exceeding 3 times but not more than 5 times the upper limit of normal (ULN) or total bilirubin concentrations exceeding 1.5 times but not more than 3 times the ULN (i.e., grade 2) in patients *without* hepatocellular carcinoma, nivolumab therapy should be interrupted until the toxicity resolves to grade 0 or 1. (See Immune-mediated Hepatic Effects under Cautions: Warnings/Precautions.)

For ALT or AST elevations exceeding 5 times the ULN or total bilirubin concentrations exceeding 3 times the ULN (i.e., grade 3 or greater) in patients *without* hepatocellular carcinoma, nivolumab therapy should be permanently discontinued.

For ALT or AST elevations exceeding 3 times but not more than 5 times the ULN in patients *with* hepatocellular carcinoma and baseline ALT and AST concentrations within normal limits, nivolumab therapy should be interrupted until the toxicity resolves to baseline.

For ALT or AST elevations exceeding 5 times but not more than 10 times the ULN in patients *with* hepatocellular carcinoma and baseline ALT or AST concentrations exceeding the ULN but not more than 3 times the ULN, nivolumab therapy should be interrupted until the toxicity resolves to baseline.

For ALT or AST elevations exceeding 8 times but not more than 10 times the ULN in patients *with* hepatocellular carcinoma and baseline ALT or AST concentrations exceeding 3 times but not more than 5 times the ULN, nivolumab therapy should be interrupted until the toxicity resolves to baseline.

For ALT or AST elevations exceeding 10 times the ULN or total bilirubin concentrations exceeding 3 times the ULN in patients *with* hepatocellular carcinoma, nivolumab therapy should be permanently discontinued.

Immune-mediated Endocrine Effects. If grade 2 or 3 immune-mediated hypophysitis, grade 2 immune-mediated adrenal insufficiency, or grade 3 immune-mediated hyperglycemia occurs, nivolumab therapy should be interrupted until the toxicity resolves to grade 0 or 1. (See Immune-mediated Endocrine Effects under Cautions: Warnings/Precautions.)

If grade 4 immune-mediated hypophysitis, grade 3 or 4 immune-mediated adrenal insufficiency, or grade 4 immune-mediated hyperglycemia occurs, nivolumab therapy should be permanently discontinued.

The manufacturer states that there are no recommended dosage modifications of nivolumab for patients with immune-mediated hypothyroidism or hyperthyroidism.

Immune-mediated Renal Effects. For serum creatinine elevations exceeding 1.5 times but not more than 6 times the ULN or exceeding 1.5 times baseline values (i.e., grade 2 or 3), nivolumab therapy should be interrupted until the toxicity resolves to grade 0 or 1. (See Immune-mediated Renal Effects under Cautions: Warnings/Precautions.)

For elevated serum creatinine concentrations exceeding 6 times the ULN (i.e., grade 4), nivolumab therapy should be permanently discontinued.

Immune-mediated Dermatologic Effects. If grade 3 immune-mediated rash occurs or Stevens-Johnson syndrome or toxic epidermal necrolysis is suspected, nivolumab therapy should be interrupted until the toxicity resolves to grade 0 or 1. (See Immune-mediated Dermatologic Effects under Cautions: Warnings/Precautions.)

If grade 4 immune-mediated rash occurs or Stevens-Johnson syndrome or toxic epidermal necrolysis is confirmed, nivolumab therapy should be permanently discontinued.

Immune-mediated CNS Effects. If new-onset moderate or severe neurologic signs or symptoms occur, nivolumab therapy should be interrupted until the toxicity resolves to grade 0 or 1. (See Immune-mediated CNS Effects under Cautions: Warnings/Precautions.)

If immune-mediated encephalitis occurs, nivolumab therapy should be permanently discontinued.

Other Immune-mediated Adverse Effects. If grade 3 immune-mediated myocarditis occurs, nivolumab therapy should be permanently discontinued.

If any other grade 3 immune-mediated adverse effects occur, nivolumab therapy should be interrupted until the toxicity resolves to grade 0 or 1. If the grade 3 adverse effect recurs, nivolumab therapy should be permanently discontinued. (See Other Immune-mediated Effects under Cautions: Warnings/Precautions.)

Infusion-related Reactions. If mild or moderate infusion-related reactions occur, the infusion should be interrupted or the infusion rate should be reduced. (See Infusion-related Effects under Cautions: Warnings/Precautions.)

If severe or life-threatening infusion-related reactions occur, nivolumab therapy should be permanently discontinued.

■ **Special Populations** No dosage adjustment is necessary in patients with mild or moderate preexisting hepatic impairment. Nivolumab has not been studied in patients with severe preexisting hepatic impairment, and the manufacturer provides no specific dosage recommendations for such patients. (See Hepatic Impairment under Warnings/Precautions: Specific Populations, in Cautions.)

No dosage adjustment is necessary in patients with mild, moderate, or severe preexisting renal impairment. (See Renal Impairment under Warnings/Precautions: Specific Populations, in Cautions.)

The manufacturer makes no special dosage recommendations for geriatric patients. (See Geriatric Use under Warnings/Precautions: Specific Populations, in Cautions.)

Cautions

■ **Contraindications** The manufacturer states there are no known contraindications to the use of nivolumab.

■ **Warnings/Precautions** ***Immune-mediated Pneumonitis*** Immune-mediated pneumonitis (defined as pneumonitis of no clear alternate etiology requiring corticosteroid therapy), sometimes fatal, has occurred in patients receiving nivolumab therapy.

In clinical studies evaluating single-agent nivolumab, immune-mediated pneumonitis occurred in 3.1% of patients receiving nivolumab; the median time to onset of immune-mediated pneumonitis was 3.5 months (range: 1 day to 22.3 months). Nivolumab was temporarily interrupted or permanently discontinued because of immune-mediated pneumonitis in 1.3 or 1.1%, respectively, of patients receiving the drug. Most patients (89%) experiencing immune-mediated pneumonitis received high-dose corticosteroid therapy (40 mg or more of prednisone daily [or equivalent]) for a median duration of 26 days (range: 1 day to 6 months). Following tapering of the corticosteroid dosage, complete resolution of immune-mediated pneumonitis occurred in 67% of patients. Following reinitiation of nivolumab therapy, immune-mediated pneumonitis recurred in approximately 8% of patients.

In clinical studies evaluating nivolumab 1 mg/kg in combination with ipilimumab 3 mg/kg, immune-mediated pneumonitis occurred in 6% of patients with melanoma receiving combination therapy; the median time to onset of immune-mediated pneumonitis was 1.6 months (range: 24 days to 10.1 months). Combination therapy with nivolumab 1 mg/kg and ipilimumab 3 mg/kg was temporarily interrupted or permanently discontinued because of immune-mediated pneumonitis in 3.7 or 2.2%, respectively, of patients receiving the drug combination. Most patients (84%) experiencing immune-mediated pneumonitis received high-dose corticosteroid therapy (40 mg or more of prednisone daily [or equivalent]) for a median duration of 30 days (range: 5 days to 11.8 months). Complete resolution of immune-mediated pneumonitis occurred in 68% of patients. Following reinitiation of combination therapy with nivolumab 1 mg/kg and ipilimumab 3 mg/kg, immune-mediated pneumonitis recurred in approximately 13% of patients.

In clinical studies evaluating nivolumab 3 mg/kg in combination with ipilimumab 1 mg/kg, immune-mediated pneumonitis occurred in 4.4 or 1.7% of patients with renal cell carcinoma or colorectal cancer, respectively, receiving combination therapy; the median time to onset of immune-mediated pneumonitis was 2.6 months (range: 8 days to 9.2 months) in patients with renal cell carcinoma and 1.9 months (range: 27 days to 3 months) in patients with colorectal cancer. Combination therapy with nivolumab 3 mg/kg and ipilimumab 1 mg/kg was temporarily interrupted or permanently discontinued because of immune-mediated pneumonitis in 1.7 or 1.8%, respectively, of patients receiving the drug combination. All patients experiencing immune-mediated pneumonitis received systemic corticosteroid therapy. The majority (92%) of patients experiencing immune-mediated pneumonitis received high-dose corticosteroid therapy (40 mg or more of prednisone daily [or equivalent]) for a median duration of 19 days (range: 4 days to 3.2 months); however, adjunctive therapy with infliximab was required in approximately 8% of patients. Complete resolution of immune-mediated pneumonitis occurred in 81% of patients. Following reinitiation of combination therapy with nivolumab 3 mg/kg and ipilimumab 1 mg/kg, immune-mediated pneumonitis recurred in one patient with colorectal cancer.

Patients receiving nivolumab should be monitored clinically and by radiographic imaging for manifestations of pneumonitis. In patients who develop grade 2 or greater immune-mediated pneumonitis, systemic corticosteroid therapy should be initiated at a dosage of 1–2 mg/kg of prednisone daily (or equivalent) followed by tapering of the corticosteroid dosage. Temporary interruption or discontinuance of nivolumab may be necessary if immune-mediated pneumonitis occurs during therapy with the drug. (See Therapy Interruption for Toxicity under Dosage and Administration: Dosage.)

Immune-mediated GI Effects Immune-mediated colitis (defined as colitis of no clear alternate etiology requiring corticosteroid therapy), sometimes fatal, has occurred in patients receiving nivolumab therapy.

In clinical studies evaluating single-agent nivolumab, immune-mediated colitis occurred in 2.9% of patients receiving nivolumab; the median time to onset of immune-mediated colitis was 5.3 months (range: 2 days to 20.9 months). Nivolumab was temporarily interrupted or permanently discontinued because of immune-mediated colitis in 1 or 0.7%, respectively, of patients receiving the drug. Most (approximately 91%) of the 58 patients experiencing immune-mediated colitis received high-dose corticosteroid therapy (40 mg or more of prednisone daily [or equivalent]) for a median duration of 23 days (range: 1 day to 9.3 months); however, adjunctive therapy with infliximab was required in 4 patients. Complete resolution of immune-mediated colitis occurred in 74% of patients. Following reinitiation of nivolumab therapy, immune-mediated colitis recurred in approximately 16% of patients.

In clinical studies evaluating nivolumab 1 mg/kg in combination with ipilimumab 3 mg/kg, immune-mediated colitis occurred in 26% of patients with melanoma receiving combination therapy and was fatal in 3 patients; the median time to onset of immune-mediated colitis was 1.6 months (range: 3 days to 15.2 months). Combination therapy with nivolumab 1 mg/kg and ipilimumab 3 mg/kg was temporarily interrupted or permanently discontinued because of immune-mediated colitis in 7 or 16%, respectively, of patients receiving the drug combination. Most patients (96%) experiencing immune-mediated colitis received high-dose corticosteroid therapy (40 mg or more of prednisone daily [or equivalent]) for a median duration of 1.1 months (range: 1 day to 12 months); however, adjunctive therapy with infliximab was required in approximately 23% of patients. Complete resolution of immune-mediated colitis occurred in 75% of patients. Following reinitiation of combination therapy with nivolumab 1 mg/kg and ipilimumab 3 mg/kg, immune-mediated colitis recurred in approximately 28% of patients.

In clinical studies evaluating nivolumab 3 mg/kg in combination with ipilimumab 1 mg/kg, immune-mediated colitis occurred in 10 or 7% of patients with renal cell carcinoma or colorectal cancer, respectively, receiving combination therapy; the median time to onset of immune-mediated colitis was 1.7 months (range: 2 days to 19.2 months) in patients with renal cell carcinoma and 2.4 months (range: 22 days to 5.2 months) in patients with colorectal cancer. Combination therapy with nivolumab 3 mg/kg and ipilimumab 1 mg/kg was temporarily interrupted or permanently discontinued because of immune-mediated colitis in 3.9 or 3.2%, respectively, of patients receiving the drug combination. All patients experiencing immune-mediated colitis received systemic corticosteroid therapy. Most patients (80%) experiencing immune-mediated colitis received high-dose corticosteroid therapy (40 mg or more of prednisone daily [or equivalent]) for a median duration of 21 days (range: 1 day to 27 months); however, adjunctive therapy with infliximab was required in approximately 23% of patients with immune-mediated colitis. Complete resolution of immune-mediated colitis occurred in 88% of patients. Following reinitiation of combination therapy with nivolumab 3 mg/kg and ipilimumab 1 mg/kg, immune-mediated colitis recurred in 2 patients with renal cell carcinoma.

Patients receiving nivolumab should be monitored for manifestations of colitis. In patients who develop grade 3 or 4 immune-mediated colitis, systemic corticosteroid therapy should be initiated at a dosage of 1–2 mg/kg of prednisone daily (or equivalent) followed by tapering of the corticosteroid dosage. In patients who experience grade 2 immune-mediated colitis for more than 5 days, systemic corticosteroid therapy should be initiated at a dosage of 0.5–1 mg/kg of prednisone daily (or equivalent) followed by tapering of the corticosteroid dosage; if immune-mediated colitis worsens or fails to improve, the systemic corticosteroid dosage should be increased to 1–2 mg/kg of prednisone daily (or equivalent). Temporary interruption or discontinuance of nivolumab may be necessary if immune-mediated colitis occurs during therapy with the drug. (See Therapy Interruption for Toxicity under Dosage and Administration: Dosage.)

Immune-mediated Hepatic Effects Immune-mediated hepatitis (defined as hepatitis of no clear alternate etiology requiring corticosteroid therapy) has occurred in patients receiving nivolumab therapy.

In clinical studies evaluating single-agent nivolumab, immune-mediated hepatitis occurred in 1.8% of patients receiving nivolumab; the median time to onset of immune-mediated hepatitis was 3.3 months (range: 6 days to 9 months). Nivolumab was temporarily interrupted or permanently discontinued because of immune-mediated hepatitis in 1 or 0.7%, respectively, of patients receiving the drug. All 35 patients experiencing immune-mediated hepatitis received high-dose corticosteroid therapy (40 mg or more of prednisone daily [or equivalent]) for a median duration of 23 days (range: 1 day to 2 months); however, adjunctive therapy with mycophenolic acid was required in 2 patients. Complete resolution of immune-mediated hepatitis occurred in 74% of patients. Following reinitiation of nivolumab therapy, immune-mediated hepatitis recurred in approximately 29% of patients.

In clinical studies evaluating nivolumab 1 mg/kg in combination with ipilimumab 3 mg/kg, immune-mediated hepatitis occurred in 13% of patients with melanoma receiving combination therapy; the median time to onset of immune-mediated hepatitis was 2.1 months (range: 15 days to 11 months). Combination therapy with nivolumab 1 mg/kg and ipilimumab 3 mg/kg was temporarily interrupted or permanently discontinued because of immune-mediated hepatitis in 5 or 6%, respectively, of patients receiving the drug combination. Most patients (92%) experiencing immune-mediated hepatitis received high-dose corticosteroid therapy (40 mg or more of prednisone daily [or equivalent]) for a median duration of 1.1 months (range: 1 day to 13.2 months). Complete resolution of immune-mediated hepatitis occurred in 75% of patients. Following reinitiation of combination therapy with nivolumab 1 mg/kg and ipilimumab 3 mg/kg, immune-mediated hepatitis recurred in approximately 11% of patients.

In clinical studies evaluating nivolumab 3 mg/kg in combination with ipilimumab 1 mg/kg, immune-mediated hepatitis occurred in 7 or 8% of patients with renal cell carcinoma or colorectal cancer, respectively, receiving combination therapy; the median time to onset of immune-mediated hepatitis was 2 months (range: 14 days to 26.8 months) in patients with renal cell carcinoma and 2.2 months (range: 22 days to 10.5 months) in patients with colorectal cancer. Combination therapy with nivolumab 3 mg/kg and ipilimumab 1 mg/kg was temporarily interrupted or permanently discontinued because of immune-mediated hepatitis in 3.5 or 3.6%, respectively, of patients receiving the drug combination. All patients experiencing immune-mediated hepatitis received systemic corticosteroid therapy. The majority (94%) of patients experiencing immune-mediated hepatitis received high-dose corticosteroid therapy (40 mg or more of prednisone daily [or equivalent]) for a median duration of 1 month (range: 1 day to 7 months); however, adjunctive therapy with mycophenolate was required in approximately 19% of patients with immune-mediated hepatitis. Complete resolution of immune-mediated hepatitis occurred in 83% of patients; upon resumption of combination therapy with nivolumab 3 mg/kg and ipilimumab 1 mg/kg, no patients had recurrence of immune-mediated hepatitis.

Liver function tests should be performed prior to initiation of nivolumab therapy and periodically during therapy. If grade 3 or 4 elevations of serum ALT or AST concentrations (with or without concomitant elevations of total bilirubin concentrations) occur in patients *without* hepatocellular carcinoma, systemic corticosteroid therapy should be initiated at a dosage of 1–2 mg/kg of prednisone daily (or equivalent) followed by tapering of the corticosteroid dosage. If grade 2 elevations of serum ALT or AST concentrations occur in patients *without* hepatocellular carcinoma, systemic corticosteroid therapy should be initiated at a dosage of 0.5–1 mg/kg of prednisone daily (or equivalent). In patients who develop immune-mediated hepatitis, temporary interruption of therapy or drug discontinuance may be required. (See Therapy Interruption for Toxicity under Dosage and Administration: Dosage.) Whenever nivolumab therapy is temporarily interrupted or discontinued because of immune-mediated hepatitis in patients *with* hepatocellular carcinoma, systemic corticosteroid therapy should be initiated at a dosage of 1–2 mg/kg of prednisone daily (or equivalent) followed by tapering of the corticosteroid dosage.

Immune-mediated Endocrine Effects Immune-mediated endocrinopathies, such as hypophysitis, thyroid dysfunction (i.e., hypothyroidism, hyperthyroidism), adrenal insufficiency, and diabetes mellitus (including diabetic ketoacidosis), have occurred in patients receiving nivolumab therapy.

Hypophysitis. In clinical studies evaluating single-agent nivolumab, immune-mediated hypophysitis occurred in 0.6% of patients receiving nivolumab; the median time to occurrence was 4.9 months (range: 1.4–11 months). Nivolumab was temporarily interrupted or permanently discontinued because of immune-mediated hypophysitis in 0.2 or 0.1%, respectively, of patients receiving the drug. Approximately 67% of patients experiencing immune-mediated hypophysitis received hormone replacement therapy and 33% received high-dose corticosteroid therapy (40 mg or more of prednisone daily [or equivalent]) for a median duration of 14 days (range: 5–26 days).

In clinical studies evaluating nivolumab 1 mg/kg in combination with ipilimumab 3 mg/kg, immune-mediated hypophysitis occurred in 9% of patients with melanoma receiving combination therapy; the median time to occurrence was 2.7 months (range: 27 days to 5.5 months). Combination therapy with nivolumab 1 mg/kg and ipilimumab 3 mg/kg was temporarily interrupted or permanently discontinued because of immune-mediated hypophysitis in 3.9 or 1%, respectively, of patients receiving the drug combination. Approximately 75% of patients experiencing immune-mediated hypophysitis received hormone replacement therapy and 56% received high-dose corticosteroid therapy (40 mg or more of prednisone daily [or equivalent]) for a median duration of 19 days (range: 1 day to 2 months).

In clinical studies evaluating nivolumab 3 mg/kg in combination with ipilimumab 1 mg/kg, immune-mediated hypophysitis occurred in 4.6 or 3.4% of patients with renal cell carcinoma or colorectal cancer, respectively, receiving combination therapy; the median time to onset of immune-mediated hypophysitis was 2.8 months (range: 1.3–7.3 months) in patients with renal cell carcinoma and 3.7 months (range: 2.8–5.5 months) in patients with colorectal cancer. Combination therapy with nivolumab 3 mg/kg and ipilimumab 1 mg/kg was temporarily interrupted or permanently discontinued because of immune-mediated hypophysitis in 2.6 or 1.2%, respectively, of patients receiving the drug combination. Approximately 72% of patients experiencing immune-mediated hypophysitis received hormone replacement therapy and 55% received high-dose corticosteroid therapy (40 mg or more of prednisone daily [or equivalent]) for a median duration of 13 days (range: 1 day to 1.6 months).

Patients receiving nivolumab should be monitored for manifestations of hypophysitis. If grade 2 or greater hypophysitis occurs, hormone replacement therapy should be administered as clinically indicated and systemic corticosteroid therapy should be initiated at a dosage of 1 mg/kg of prednisone daily (or equivalent) followed by tapering of the corticosteroid dosage. If immune-mediated hypophysitis occurs, temporary interruption or discontinuance of nivolumab may be necessary. (See Therapy Interruption for Toxicity under Dosage and Administration: Dosage.)

Adrenal Insufficiency. In clinical studies evaluating single-agent nivolumab, immune-mediated adrenal insufficiency occurred in 1% of patients receiving nivolumab; the median time to occurrence was 4.3 months (range: 15 days to 21 months). Nivolumab was temporarily interrupted or permanently discontinued because of immune-mediated adrenal insufficiency in 0.5 or 0.1%, respectively, of patients receiving the drug. Most patients (85%) experiencing immune-mediated adrenal insufficiency received hormone replacement therapy and 25% received high-dose corticosteroid therapy (40 mg or more of prednisone daily [or equivalent]) for a median duration of 11 days (range: 1 day to 1 month).

In clinical studies evaluating nivolumab 1 mg/kg in combination with ipilimumab 3 mg/kg, immune-mediated adrenal insufficiency occurred in 5% of patients with melanoma receiving combination therapy; the median time to occurrence was 3 months (range: 21 days to 9.4 months). Combination therapy with nivolumab 1 mg/kg and ipilimumab 3 mg/kg was temporarily interrupted or permanently discontinued because of immune-mediated adrenal insufficiency in 1.7 or 0.5%, respectively, of patients receiving the drug combination. Approximately one-half (57%) of patients experiencing immune-mediated adrenal insufficiency received hormone replacement therapy and 33% received high-dose corticosteroid therapy (40 mg or more of prednisone daily [or equivalent]) for a median duration of 9 days (range: 1 day to 2.7 months).

In clinical studies evaluating nivolumab 3 mg/kg in combination with ipilimumab 1 mg/kg, immune-mediated adrenal insufficiency occurred in 7 or 5.9% of patients with renal cell carcinoma or colorectal cancer, respectively, receiving combination therapy; the median time to onset of immune-mediated adrenal insufficiency was 3.4 months (range: 2–22.3 months) in patients with renal cell carcinoma and 3.7 months (range: 2.5–13.4 months) in patients with colorectal cancer. Combination therapy with nivolumab 3 mg/kg and ipilimumab 1 mg/kg was temporarily interrupted or permanently discontinued because of immune-mediated adrenal insufficiency in 2.6 or 1.2%, respectively, of patients receiving the drug combination. Approximately 94% of patients experiencing immune-mediated adrenal insufficiency received hormone replacement therapy and 27% received high-dose corticosteroid therapy (40 mg or more of prednisone daily [or equivalent]) for a median duration of 12 days (range: 2 days to 5.6 months).

Patients receiving nivolumab should be monitored for manifestations of adrenal insufficiency. If grade 3 or 4 adrenal insufficiency occurs, systemic corticosteroid therapy should be initiated at a dosage of 1–2 mg/kg of prednisone daily (or equivalent) followed by tapering of the corticosteroid dosage. If immune-mediated adrenal insufficiency occurs, temporary interruption or discontinuance of nivolumab may be necessary. (See Therapy Interruption for Toxicity under Dosage and Administration: Dosage.)

Thyroid Dysfunction. In clinical studies evaluating single-agent nivolumab, immune-mediated hypothyroidism or thyroiditis-associated hypothyroidism occurred in 9% of patients receiving nivolumab; the median time to occurrence was 2.9 months (range: 1 day to 16.6 months). Most patients (79%) experiencing immune-mediated hypothyroidism received thyroid hormone replacement therapy with levothyroxine and 4% also required therapy with corticosteroids. Resolution of immune-mediated hypothyroidism or thyroiditis-associated hypothyroidism occurred in 35% of patients. In addition, immune-mediated hyperthyroidism has been reported in 2.7% of patients receiving single-agent nivolumab in clinical studies; the median time to occurrence was 1.5 months (range: 1 day to 14.2 months). Approximately one-half of patients (48%) experiencing immune-mediated hyperthyroidism received therapy with antithyroid agents or corticosteroids; 26, 9, 4 or 9% of patients received methimazole, carbimazole (not commercially available in the US), propylthiouracil, or corticosteroids, respectively. Resolution of immune-mediated hyperthyroidism occurred in 76% of patients.

In clinical studies evaluating nivolumab 1 mg/kg in combination with ipilimumab 3 mg/kg, immune-mediated hypothyroidism or thyroiditis-associated hypothyroidism occurred in 22% of patients with melanoma receiving combination therapy; the median time to occurrence was 2.1 months (range: 1 day to 10.1 months). Most patients (73%) experiencing immune-mediated hypothyroidism received thyroid hormone replacement therapy with levothyroxine. Resolution of immune-mediated hypothyroidism or thyroiditis-associated hypothyroidism occurred in 45% of patients. In addition, immune-mediated hyperthyroidism has been reported in 8% of patients receiving nivolumab 1 mg/kg in combination with ipilimumab 3 mg/kg in clinical studies; the median time to occurrence was 23 days (range: 3 days to 3.7 months). Approximately one-half of patients (53%) experiencing immune-mediated hyperthyroidism received therapy with antithyroid agents; 29% of patients received methimazole and 24% received carbimazole. Resolution of immune-mediated hyperthyroidism occurred in 94% of patients.

In clinical studies evaluating nivolumab 3 mg/kg in combination with ipilimumab 1 mg/kg, immune-mediated hypothyroidism or thyroiditis-associated hypothyroidism occurred in 22 or 15% of patients with renal cell carcinoma or colorectal cancer, respectively, receiving combination therapy; the median time to occurrence was 2.2 months (range: 1 day to 21.4 months) in patients with renal cell carcinoma and 2.3 months (range: 22 days to 9.8 months) in patients with colorectal cancer. Approximately 81 or 78% of patients with renal cell carcinoma or colorectal cancer, respectively, who were experiencing immune-mediated hypothyroidism received thyroid hormone replacement therapy with levothyroxine. In addition, immune-mediated hyperthyroidism has been reported in 12% of patients with renal cell carcinoma or colorectal cancer who were receiving nivolumab 3 mg/kg in combination with ipilimumab 1 mg/kg; the median time to occurrence was 1.4 months (range: 6 days to 14.2 months) in patients with renal cell carcinoma and 1.1 months (range: 21 days to 5.4 months) in patients with colorectal cancer. Approximately 15% of patients experiencing immune-mediated hyperthyroidism received therapy with methimazole and 2% received carbimazole.

Thyroid function should be evaluated prior to initiation of nivolumab therapy and periodically during therapy. In patients who develop immune-mediated hypothyroidism, thyroid hormone replacement therapy should be initiated. If immune-mediated hyperthyroidism occurs, appropriate medical therapy should be initiated.

Diabetes Mellitus. Immune-mediated type 1 diabetes mellitus and diabetic ketoacidosis have occurred in patients receiving nivolumab therapy.

In clinical studies evaluating single-agent nivolumab, immune-mediated type 1 diabetes mellitus occurred in 0.9% of patients receiving nivolumab; the median time to occurrence was 4.4 months (range: 15 days to 22 months). Two of 17 patients with immune-mediated type 1 diabetes mellitus experienced diabetic ketoacidosis.

In clinical studies evaluating nivolumab 1 mg/kg in combination with ipilimumab 3 mg/kg, immune-mediated type 1 diabetes mellitus occurred in 1.5% of patients with melanoma receiving combination therapy; the median time to occurrence was 2.5 months (range: 1.3–4.4 months). Combination therapy with nivolumab 1 mg/kg and ipilimumab 3 mg/kg was temporarily interrupted or permanently discontinued in 2 of the 6 patients with immune-mediated type 1 diabetes mellitus.

In clinical studies evaluating nivolumab 3 mg/kg in combination with ipilimumab 1 mg/kg, immune-mediated type 1 diabetes mellitus occurred in 2.7% of patients with renal cell carcinoma receiving combination therapy; the median time to occurrence was 3.2 months (range: 19 days to 16.8 months). Combination therapy with nivolumab 3 mg/kg and ipilimumab 1 mg/kg was temporarily interrupted or permanently discontinued in 33 or 20%, respectively, of patients with immune-mediated type 1 diabetes mellitus.

Patients receiving nivolumab should be monitored for hyperglycemia. If grade 3 immune-mediated hyperglycemia occurs, nivolumab therapy should be temporarily interrupted until blood glucose concentrations have stabilized. If grade 4 immune-mediated hyperglycemia occurs, nivolumab therapy should be permanently discontinued. (See Therapy Interruption for Toxicity under Dosage and Administration: Dosage.)

Immune-mediated Renal Effects Immune-mediated nephritis (defined as renal dysfunction or grade 2 or greater elevations in serum creatinine concentrations with no clear alternate etiology and requiring corticosteroid therapy) has occurred in patients receiving nivolumab therapy.

In clinical studies evaluating single-agent nivolumab, immune-mediated nephritis and renal dysfunction occurred in 1.2% of patients receiving nivolumab; the median time to onset of immune-mediated nephritis and renal dysfunction was 4.6 months (range: 23 days to 12.3 months). Nivolumab was temporarily interrupted or permanently discontinued because of immune-mediated nephritis and renal dysfunction in 0.8 or 0.3%, respectively, of patients receiving the drug. All patients experiencing immune-mediated nephritis and renal dysfunction received high-dose corticosteroid therapy (40 mg or more of prednisone daily [or equivalent]) for a median duration of 21 days (range: 1 day to 15.4 months). Complete resolution of immune-mediated nephritis and renal dysfunction occurred in 48% of patients; upon resumption of nivolumab, no patients had recurrence of immune-mediated nephritis or renal dysfunction.

In clinical studies evaluating nivolumab 1 mg/kg in combination with ipilimumab 3 mg/kg, immune-mediated nephritis and renal dysfunction occurred in 2.2% of patients with melanoma receiving combination therapy; the median time to onset of immune-mediated nephritis and renal dysfunction was 2.7 months (range: 9 days to 7.9 months). Combination therapy with nivolumab 1 mg/kg and ipilimumab 3 mg/kg was temporarily interrupted or permanently discontinued because of immune-mediated nephritis and renal dysfunction in 0.5 or 0.7%, respectively, of patients receiving the drug combination. Approximately 67% of patients experiencing immune-mediated nephritis and renal dysfunction received high-dose corticosteroid therapy (40 mg or more of prednisone daily [or equivalent]) for a median duration of 13.5 days (range: 1 day to 1.1 months). Complete resolution of immune-mediated nephritis and renal dysfunction occurred in all patients. Following reinitiation of combination therapy with nivolumab 1 mg/kg and ipilimumab 3 mg/kg in 2 patients, neither patient had recurrence of immune-mediated nephritis or renal dysfunction.

In clinical studies evaluating nivolumab 3 mg/kg in combination with ipilimumab 1 mg/kg, immune-mediated nephritis and renal dysfunction occurred in 4.6 or 1.7% of patients with renal cell carcinoma or colorectal cancer, respectively, receiving combination therapy; the median time to onset of immune-mediated nephritis and renal dysfunction was 3 months (range: 1 day to 13.2 months) in these patients. Combination therapy with nivolumab 3 mg/kg and ipilimumab 1 mg/kg was temporarily interrupted or permanently discontinued because of immune-mediated nephritis and renal dysfunction in 2.3 or 1.2%, respectively, of patients receiving the drug combination. Most patients (78%) experiencing immune-mediated nephritis and renal dysfunction received high-dose corticosteroid therapy (40 mg or more of prednisone daily [or equivalent]) for a median duration of 17 days (range: 1 day to 6 months). Complete resolution of immune-mediated nephritis and renal dysfunction occurred in 63% of patients. Following reinitiation of combination therapy with nivolumab 3 mg/kg and ipilimumab 1 mg/kg, immune-mediated nephritis and renal dysfunction recurred in one patient with renal cell carcinoma.

Renal function should be evaluated prior to initiation of nivolumab therapy and periodically during therapy. In patients who develop grade 4 elevations in serum creatinine concentrations, systemic corticosteroid therapy should be initiated at a dosage of 1–2 mg/kg of prednisone daily (or equivalent) followed by tapering of the corticosteroid dosage. In patients who develop grade 2 or 3 elevations in serum creatinine concentrations, systemic corticosteroid therapy should be initiated at a dosage of 0.5–1 mg/kg of prednisone daily (or equivalent); if renal function worsens or fails to improve, the systemic corticosteroid dosage should be increased to 1–2 mg/kg of prednisone daily (or equivalent). Temporary interruption or discontinuance of nivolumab may be necessary if elevations in serum creatinine concentrations occur during therapy with the drug. (See Therapy Interruption for Toxicity under Dosage and Administration: Dosage.)

Immune-mediated Dermatologic Effects Immune-mediated rash has occurred in patients receiving nivolumab therapy. Severe, sometimes fatal, skin reactions (including Stevens-Johnson syndrome and toxic epidermal necrolysis) have been reported with the drug.

In clinical studies evaluating single-agent nivolumab, immune-mediated rash occurred in 9% of patients receiving nivolumab; the median time to onset of immune-mediated rash was 2.8 months (range: less than 1 day to 25.8 months). Nivolumab was temporarily interrupted or permanently discontinued because of immune-mediated rash in 0.8 or 0.3%, respectively, of patients receiving the drug. Most patients (85%) experiencing immune-mediated rash received topical corticosteroid therapy and approximately 16% of patients received high-dose corticosteroid therapy (40 mg or more of prednisone daily [or equivalent]) for a median duration of 12 days (range: 1 day to 8.9 months). Complete resolution of immune-mediated rash occurred in 48% of patients. Following reinitiation of nivolumab therapy, immune-mediated rash recurred in approximately 1.4% of patients.

In clinical studies evaluating nivolumab 1 mg/kg in combination with ipilimumab 3 mg/kg, immune-mediated rash occurred in 22.6% of patients with melanoma receiving combination therapy; the median time to onset of immune-mediated rash was 18 days (range: 1 day to 9.7 months). Combination therapy with nivolumab 1 mg/kg and ipilimumab 3 mg/kg was temporarily interrupted or permanently discontinued because of immune-mediated rash in 3.9 or 0.5%, respectively, of patients receiving the drug combination. Approximately 17% of patients experiencing immune-mediated rash received high-dose corticosteroid therapy (40 mg or more of prednisone daily [or equivalent]) for a median duration of 14 days (range: 2 days to 4.7 months). Complete resolution of immune-mediated rash occurred in 47% of patients. Following reinitiation of combination therapy with nivolumab 1 mg/kg and ipilimumab 3 mg/kg, immune-mediated rash recurred in approximately 6% of patients.

In clinical studies evaluating nivolumab 3 mg/kg in combination with ipilimumab 1 mg/kg, immune-mediated rash occurred in 16 or 14% of patients with renal cell carcinoma or colorectal cancer, respectively, receiving combination therapy; the median time to onset of immune-mediated rash was 1.5 months (range: 1 day to 20.9 months) in patients with renal cell carcinoma and 26 days (range: 5 days to 9.8 months) in patients with colorectal cancer. Combination therapy with nivolumab 3 mg/kg and ipilimumab 1 mg/kg was temporarily interrupted or permanently discontinued because of immune-mediated rash in 2.6 or 0.5%, respectively, of patients receiving the drug combination. All patients experiencing immune-mediated rash received systemic corticosteroid therapy; 19% of patients received high-dose corticosteroid therapy (40 mg or more of prednisone daily [or equivalent]) for a median duration of 22 days (range: 1 day to 23 months). Complete resolution of immune-mediated rash occurred in 66% of patients. Following reinitiation of combination therapy with nivolumab 3 mg/kg and ipilimumab 1 mg/kg, immune-mediated rash recurred in approximately 3% of patients.

In patients who develop grade 3 or 4 immune-mediated rash, systemic corticosteroid therapy should be initiated at a dosage of 1–2 mg/kg of prednisone daily (or equivalent) followed by tapering of the corticosteroid dosage. Temporary interruption or discontinuance of nivolumab may be necessary if immune-mediated rash occurs during therapy with the drug. (See Therapy Interruption for Toxicity under Dosage and Administration: Dosage.) If Stevens-Johnson syndrome or toxic epidermal necrolysis is suspected, nivolumab therapy should be temporarily interrupted and the patient should be referred for evaluation and treatment by a specialist. If Stevens-Johnson syndrome or toxic epidermal necrolysis is confirmed, nivolumab should be permanently discontinued.

Immune-mediated CNS Effects Immune-mediated encephalitis of no clear alternate etiology, sometimes fatal, has occurred in patients receiving nivolumab therapy.

In clinical studies evaluating single-agent nivolumab, immune-mediated encephalitis occurred in 0.2% of patients receiving nivolumab. Following 7.2 months of nivolumab therapy, fatal limbic encephalitis occurred in one patient despite discontinuance of nivolumab therapy and administration of systemic corticosteroid therapy. Immune-mediated encephalitis occurred following allogeneic stem cell transplantation in 2 patients.

In clinical studies evaluating nivolumab 1 mg/kg in combination with ipilimumab 3 mg/kg, immune-mediated encephalitis occurred in one patient with melanoma receiving the drug combination after 1.7 months of exposure.

In clinical studies evaluating nivolumab 3 mg/kg in combination with ipilimumab 1 mg/kg, immune-mediated encephalitis occurred in one patient with renal cell carcinoma receiving the drug combination after approximately 4 months of exposure and one patient with colorectal cancer receiving the drug combination after 15 days of exposure. One patient received high-dose corticosteroid therapy (40 mg or more of prednisone daily [or equivalent]) and adjunctive therapy with infliximab.

In patients with new moderate to severe neurologic manifestations suggestive of encephalitis (e.g., headache, pyrexia, confusion, memory loss, hallucinations, fatigue/asthenia, somnolence, drowsiness, seizures, stiff neck), nivolumab should be withheld and adequate evaluation (e.g., consultation with a neurologist, brain magnetic resonance imaging [MRI] scan, lumbar puncture) should be performed to exclude other causes (e.g., infection). If immune-mediated encephalitis is confirmed, nivolumab should be permanently discontinued and systemic corticosteroid therapy should be initiated at a dosage of 1–2 mg/kg of prednisone daily (or equivalent) followed by tapering of the corticosteroid dosage.

Other Immune-mediated Effects Other immune-mediated adverse effects, including myocarditis, rhabdomyolysis, myositis, uveitis, iritis, pancreatitis, facial and abducens nerve paresis, demyelination, polymyalgia rheumatica, autoimmune neuropathy, Guillain-Barré syndrome, hypopituitarism, systemic inflammatory response syndrome, gastritis, duodenitis, sarcoidosis, histiocytic necrotizing lymphadenitis (Kikuchi lymphadenitis), motor dysfunction, vasculitis, aplastic anemia, pericarditis, and myasthenic syndrome, have occurred rarely in patients receiving nivolumab as a single agent or in combination with ipilimumab. Some cases have resulted in death. Immune-mediated adverse effects may occur following discontinuance of nivolumab therapy.

If an immune-mediated adverse effect is suspected, adequate evaluation should be performed to exclude other causes. Depending on the severity of the immune-mediated adverse effect, nivolumab therapy should be interrupted or permanently discontinued and high-dose corticosteroid therapy and, if indicated, hormone replacement therapy should be initiated. Once the toxicity has resolved to grade 0 or 1, the corticosteroid dosage should be tapered over at least 1 month. If clinically appropriate, nivolumab may be restarted following completion of the corticosteroid taper. (See Therapy Interruption for Toxicity under Dosage and Administration: Dosage.)

If uveitis occurs in conjunction with other immune-mediated adverse effects, a Vogt-Koyanagi-Harada-like syndrome (which has been observed in patients receiving nivolumab as a single agent or in combination with ipilimumab) should be considered. Systemic corticosteroid therapy may be required to reduce the risk of permanent vision loss.

Infusion-related Effects Infusion-related reactions have occurred in patients receiving nivolumab therapy. Severe infusion-related reactions have been reported rarely in patients receiving nivolumab in clinical studies.

In clinical studies evaluating single-agent nivolumab, infusion-related reactions occurred in 6.4% of patients receiving nivolumab as a 60-minute IV infusion.

In clinical studies evaluating nivolumab 1 mg/kg in combination with ipilimumab 3 mg/kg, infusion-related reactions occurred in 2.5% of patients with melanoma receiving combination therapy.

In clinical studies evaluating nivolumab 3 mg/kg in combination with ipilimumab 1 mg/kg, infusion-related reactions occurred in 5.1 or 4.2% of patients with renal cell carcinoma or colorectal cancer, respectively, receiving combination therapy.

In a pharmacokinetic and safety comparison of 30- and 60-minute IV nivolumab infusions, infusion-related reactions occurred in 2.7 or 2.2% of patients receiving the drug over 30 or 60 minutes, respectively, and resulted in dose delay, temporary interruption of therapy, or permanent drug discontinuance in 1.4 or 0.5%, respectively, of patients.

In patients experiencing mild or moderate infusion-related reactions, interruption of the infusion or a reduction in the infusion rate may be necessary. For patients experiencing severe or life-threatening infusion-related reactions, nivolumab therapy should be permanently discontinued.

Allogeneic Stem Cell Transplantation-related Complications Patients who undergo allogeneic stem cell transplantation either before or after receiving therapy with an anti-programmed-death receptor-1 (anti-PD-1) monoclonal antibody, including nivolumab, may experience serious or fatal transplant-related complications, including hyperacute, acute, or chronic graft-versus-host disease (GVHD); hepatic veno-occlusive disease following allogeneic stem cell transplantation with a reduced-intensity conditioning regimen; and corticosteroid-requiring febrile syndrome with no identified infectious cause. These complications may occur despite other intervening therapy between administration of the anti-PD-1 monoclonal antibody and transplantation.

In clinical studies evaluating nivolumab in patients with classical Hodgkin lymphoma (cHL), 17 patients underwent allogeneic stem cell transplantation following discontinuance of nivolumab. Fatal transplant-related complications occurred in 6 of the 17 patients (35%); 5 of the fatal cases occurred in the setting of severe or refractory GVHD. Hyperacute GVHD occurred in 2 patients (12%), and grade 3 or greater GVHD occurred in 5 patients (29%). Hepatic veno-occlusive disease occurred in one patient following allogeneic stem cell transplantation with a reduced-intensity conditioning regimen; death occurred following development of GVHD and multiorgan failure.

Potential benefits and risks of anti-PD-1 monoclonal antibody therapy administered either before or after allogeneic stem cell transplantation should be considered. Patients who receive nivolumab should be monitored closely for early manifestations of stem cell transplantation-related complications and such conditions should be managed promptly if they occur.

Fetal/Neonatal Morbidity and Mortality Nivolumab may cause fetal harm if administered to pregnant women. Blockade of signaling of the programmed death 1 (PD-1) and ligand 1 (PD-L1) pathway in animals has been shown to disrupt maternal immune tolerance to the fetus and has been associated with increased fetal loss and immune-mediated disorders. Therefore, inhibition of this pathway by nivolumab may increase the risk of fetal loss (e.g., abortion, stillbirth) or neonatal death. In cynomolgus monkeys receiving nivolumab (at exposure levels of 9 and 42 times the human exposure at a dose of 3 mg/kg), the incidence of fetal loss during the first and third trimesters was higher compared with concurrent or historical controls. Human immunoglobulin G_4 (IgG_4) has been shown to cross the placenta; therefore, fetal exposure to nivolumab may occur. The effects of nivolumab may be greater during the second and third trimesters of pregnancy.

Pregnancy should be avoided during nivolumab therapy. Women of childbearing potential should be advised to use an effective method of contraception while receiving nivolumab and for at least 5 months after the last dose of the drug. If nivolumab is used during pregnancy or if the patient becomes pregnant while receiving the drug, the patient should be apprised of the potential fetal hazard.

Treatment-related Mortality Increased mortality has been reported in clinical trials in patients with multiple myeloma who received an anti-PD-1 monoclonal antibody, including nivolumab, in combination with an immunomodulatory agent (i.e., lenalidomide, pomalidomide) and dexamethasone; nivolumab is *not* currently FDA-labeled for use in patients with multiple myeloma. The manufacturer of nivolumab states that use of an anti-PD-1 or anti-PD-L1 antibody in combination with a thalidomide analog and dexamethasone in patients with multiple myeloma is *not* recommended outside of a controlled clinical trial.

Immunogenicity There is a potential for immunogenicity with nivolumab therapy. Development of anti-nivolumab antibodies was detected by electrochemiluminescence (ECL) in 11.2, 37.8, or 23.8–26% of patients receiving nivolumab monotherapy, nivolumab 1 mg/kg in combination with ipilimumab 3 mg/kg, or nivolumab 3 mg/kg in combination with ipilimumab 1 mg/kg, respectively. Neutralizing antibodies to nivolumab were detected in 0.7, 4.6, or 0.5–1.9% of patients receiving these respective treatments. No effects on safety (including infusion-related reactions) or efficacy were observed in the presence of anti-nivolumab antibodies. No effects on nivolumab pharmacokinetics were observed in patients receiving single-agent nivolumab; however, clearance of nivolumab increased by 20% in the presence of anti-nivolumab antibodies in patients receiving nivolumab in combination with ipilimumab.

Specific Populations **Pregnancy.** Nivolumab may cause fetal harm if administered to pregnant women based on its mechanism of action and animal findings. The effects of nivolumab may be greater during the second and third trimesters of pregnancy. (See Fetal/Neonatal Morbidity and Mortality under Cautions: Warnings/Precautions.)

Lactation. It is not known whether nivolumab is distributed into human milk. Because many drugs are distributed into human milk and because of the potential for serious adverse reactions to nivolumab in nursing infants, women should be advised to discontinue nursing during nivolumab therapy.

Pediatric Use. Safety and efficacy of nivolumab for the treatment of melanoma, non-small cell lung cancer (NSCLC), small cell lung cancer (SCLC), renal cell carcinoma, cHL, squamous cell carcinoma of the head and neck, urothelial carcinoma, and hepatocellular carcinoma have not been established in pediatric patients younger than 18 years of age.

Safety and efficacy of nivolumab as monotherapy or in combination with ipilimumab for the management of metastatic colorectal cancer with high microsatellite instability (MSI-H) or mismatch repair deficiency (dMMR) have not been established in pediatric patients younger than 12 years of age. Because the clinical course of MSI-H or dMMR metastatic colorectal cancer is similar in adults and pediatric patients, safety and efficacy of nivolumab as monotherapy or in combination with ipilimumab for the treatment of MSI-H or dMMR metastatic colorectal cancer in adolescents 12 years of age or older are supported by extrapolation of data from clinical studies evaluating nivolumab in adults, population pharmacokinetic analyses indicating that age and body weight do not have clinically important effects on systemic exposure to the drug, and evidence that exposure to monoclonal antibodies generally is similar in adults and adolescents.

Geriatric Use. Some clinical studies of nivolumab monotherapy in patients with melanoma (CheckMate-037), cHL (CheckMate-205 and CheckMate-039), squamous cell carcinoma of the head and neck (CheckMate-141), MSI-H or dMMR metastatic colorectal cancer (CheckMate-142), hepatocellular carcinoma (CheckMate-040), or SCLC (CheckMate-032) did not include sufficient numbers of patients 65 years of age and older to determine whether geriatric patients respond differently than younger adults; however, no clinically important differences in safety or efficacy were observed between patients 65 years of age and older and younger adults in other clinical studies in patients with melanoma (CheckMate-066, CheckMate-067, and CheckMate-238), NSCLC (CheckMate-017 and CheckMate-057), renal cell carcinoma (CheckMate-025), or urothelial carcinoma (CheckMate-275).

In the CheckMate-067 study, 41% of patients with unresectable or metastatic melanoma receiving nivolumab 1 mg/kg in combination with ipilimumab 3 mg/kg were 65 years of age or older, and 11% were 75 years of age or older. No overall differences in safety and efficacy were observed between geriatric patients and younger adults.

In the CheckMate-214 study, 38% of patients with advanced renal cell carcinoma receiving nivolumab 3 mg/kg in combination with ipilimumab 1 mg/kg were 65 years of age or older, and 8% were 75 years of age or older. No overall difference in safety was observed between geriatric patients and younger adults. In addition, no overall difference in efficacy was observed between geriatric patients with intermediate- or poor-risk disease and younger adults.

Hepatic Impairment. Analysis of population pharmacokinetic data indicates that nivolumab clearance in patients with hepatocellular carcinoma or other malignancies and mild hepatic impairment (total bilirubin concentration not exceeding the ULN *with* AST concentration exceeding the ULN, or total bilirubin concentration more than 1 times but no more than 1.5 times the ULN *with* any AST concentration) and those with hepatocellular carcinoma and moderate hepatic impairment (total bilirubin concentration more than 1.5 times but not more than 3 times the ULN *with* any AST concentration) is similar to that in patients with normal hepatic function. Data are not available for patients with severe hepatic impairment (total bilirubin concentration exceeding 3 times the ULN *with* any AST concentration).

Renal Impairment. Analysis of population pharmacokinetic data indicates that nivolumab clearance in patients with mild, moderate, or severe renal impairment (estimated glomerular filtration rate [GFR] 15–89 mL/minute per 1.73 m^2) is similar to that in patients with normal renal function.

■ Common Adverse Effects

Adverse effects reported in 10% or more of patients receiving nivolumab as a single agent for the treatment of unresectable or metastatic melanoma and at an incidence that is at least 5% higher than that reported with the comparator chemotherapy regimen(s) in either the CheckMate-037 or CheckMate-066 study include fatigue, musculoskeletal pain, rash, pruritus, cough, upper respiratory infection, edema, vitiligo, and erythema. Laboratory abnormalities reported in 10% or more of patients receiving nivolumab for the treatment of unresectable or metastatic melanoma and at an incidence that is at least 5% higher than that reported with chemotherapy include elevated concentrations of hepatic aminotransferase enzymes (i.e., ALT, AST), hyponatremia, elevated concentrations of alkaline phosphatase,hyperkalemia, and elevated concentrations of bilirubin.

Adverse effects reported in 10% or more of patients receiving nivolumab as a single agent for the treatment of unresectable or metastatic melanoma and at an incidence that is at least 5% higher than that reported with ipilimumab in the CheckMate-067 study include fatigue, musculoskeletal pain, cough, upper respiratory infection, arthralgia, hypothyroidism, and vitiligo. Laboratory abnormalities reported in 20% or more of patients receiving nivolumab as a single agent for the treatment of unresectable or metastatic melanoma and at an incidence that is at least 5% higher than that reported with ipilimumab include hyperglycemia, lymphopenia and elevated concentrations of lipase.

Adverse effects reported in 10% or more of patients receiving nivolumab in combination with ipilimumab for the treatment of unresectable or metastatic melanoma and at an incidence that is at least 5% higher than that reported with ipilimumab in the CheckMate-067 study include fatigue, diarrhea, rash, nausea, pyrexia, vomiting, decreased appetite, cough, dyspnea, upper respiratory infection, arthralgia, hypothyroidism, weight loss, and hyperthyroidism. Laboratory abnormalities reported in 20% or more of patients receiving nivolumab in combination with ipilimumab for the treatment of unresectable or metastatic melanoma and at an incidence that is at least 5% higher than that reported with ipilimumab include elevated concentrations of hepatic aminotransferase enzymes (i.e., ALT, AST), hyperglycemia, anemia, hyponatremia, elevated concentrations of pancreatic enzymes (i.e., lipase, amylase), elevated concentrations of alkaline phosphatase, lymphopenia, hypocalcemia, and elevated concentrations of serum creatinine.

Adverse effects reported in 10% or more of patients receiving nivolumab for the adjuvant therapy of locally advanced or metastatic melanoma following complete resection and at an incidence that is at least 5% higher than that reported with ipilimumab in the CheckMate-238 study include musculoskeletal pain, upper respiratory infection, and arthralgia. Laboratory abnormalities reported in 10% or more of patients receiving nivolumab for the adjuvant therapy of locally advanced or metastatic melanoma following complete resection and at an incidence that is at least 5% higher than that reported with ipilimumab include lymphopenia, leukopenia, and neutropenia.

Adverse effects reported in 10% or more of patients receiving nivolumab as a single agent for the treatment of metastatic NSCLC and at an incidence that is at least 5% higher than that reported with docetaxel in the CheckMate-017 and CheckMate-057 studies combined include cough, decreased appetite, and pruritus. Laboratory abnormalities reported in 10% or more of patients receiving nivolumab for the treatment of metastatic NSCLC and at an incidence that is at least 5% higher than that reported with docetaxel include elevated concentrations of hepatic aminotransferase enzymes (i.e., ALT, AST), alkaline phosphatase, serum creatinine, and thyroid-stimulating hormone (TSH).

Adverse effects reported in patients receiving nivolumab as a single agent for the treatment of metastatic SCLC in the CheckMate-032 study were generally similar to those observed in patients with other malignancies. Adverse effects reported in 20% or more of patients receiving nivolumab as a single agent for the treatment of metastatic SCLC include fatigue, decreased appetite, musculoskeletal pain, dyspnea, nausea, diarrhea, constipation, and cough.

Adverse effects reported in more than 15% of patients receiving nivolumab as a single agent for the treatment of advanced renal cell carcinoma previously treated with antiangiogenic therapy and at an incidence that is at least 5% higher than that reported with everolimus in the CheckMate-025 study include constipation, back pain, arthralgia, pruritus, and upper respiratory infection. Laboratory abnormalities reported in more than 15% of patients receiving nivolumab for the treatment of advanced renal cell carcinoma and at an incidence that is at least 5% higher than that reported with everolimus include hyponatremia, hyperkalemia, and hypercalcemia.

Adverse effects reported in more than 15% of patients receiving nivolumab in combination with ipilimumab for the treatment of intermediate- or poor-risk, previously untreated, advanced renal cell carcinoma and at an incidence that is at least 5% higher than that reported with sunitinib in the CheckMate-214 study include rash, pruritus, and pyrexia. Laboratory abnormalities reported in more than 15% of patients receiving nivolumab in combination with ipilimumab for the treatment of intermediate- or poor-risk, previously untreated, advanced renal cell carcinoma and at an incidence that is at least 5% higher than that reported with sunitinib include elevated concentrations of amylase.

Adverse effects reported in 10% or more of patients receiving nivolumab as a single agent for the treatment of cHL in the CheckMate-205 and CheckMate-039 studies combined include upper respiratory infection, fatigue, cough, diarrhea, pyrexia, musculoskeletal pain, rash, nausea, pruritus, vomiting, headache, abdominal pain, arthralgia, dyspnea, constipation, infusion-related reactions, pneumonia, hypothyroidism/thyroiditis, peripheral neuropathy, and nasal congestion. Laboratory abnormalities reported in 10% or more of patients receiving nivolumab for the treatment of cHL include leukopenia, neutropenia, thrombocytopenia, elevated concentrations of hepatic aminotransferase enzymes (i.e., ALT, AST), lymphopenia, anemia, elevated concentrations of pancreatic enzymes (i.e., lipase, amylase), elevated concentrations of alkaline phosphatase, hyponatremia, hypokalemia, elevated concentrations of serum creatinine, hypocalcemia, hyperkalemia, hypomagnesemia, and elevated concentrations of bilirubin.

Adverse effects reported in 10% or more of patients receiving nivolumab as a single agent for the treatment of recurrent or metastatic squamous cell carcinoma of the head and neck and at an incidence higher than that reported with the comparator chemotherapy regimens in the CheckMate-141 study include cough and dyspnea. Laboratory abnormalities reported in 10% or more of patients receiving nivolumab for the treatment of recurrent or metastatic squamous cell carcinoma of the head and neck and at an incidence higher than that reported with chemotherapy include elevated concentrations of alkaline phosphatase, elevated concentrations of amylase, hypercalcemia, hyperkalemia, and elevated concentrations of TSH.

Adverse effects reported in 10% or more of patients receiving nivolumab as a single agent for the treatment of locally advanced or metastatic urothelial carcinoma in the CheckMate-275 study include asthenia/fatigue/malaise, musculoskeletal pain, decreased appetite, nausea, cough, diarrhea, pyrexia, urinary tract infection, constipation, rash, thyroid disorders, dyspnea, abdominal pain, edema, pruritus, vomiting, and arthralgia. Laboratory abnormalities reported in 10% or more of patients receiving nivolumab for the treatment of locally advanced or metastatic urothelial carcinoma include hyperglycemia, lymphopenia, hyponatremia, anemia, elevated concentrations of serum creatinine, elevated concentrations of alkaline phosphatase, hypocalcemia, elevated concentrations of hepatic aminotransferase enzymes (i.e., ALT, AST), elevated concentrations of pancreatic enzymes (i.e., lipase, amylase), hyperkalemia, hypomagnesemia, thrombocytopenia, and leukopenia.

Adverse effects reported in 10% or more of patients receiving nivolumab as a single agent for the treatment of metastatic colorectal cancer with MSI-H or dMMR in the CheckMate-142 study include fatigue, diarrhea, abdominal pain, nausea, musculoskeletal pain, vomiting, cough, pyrexia, rash, constipation, upper respiratory infection, arthralgia, hyperglycemia, pruritus, headache, decreased appetite, dizziness, and edema. Laboratory abnormalities reported in 10% or more of patients receiving nivolumab as a single agent for the treatment of metastatic colorectal cancer with MSI-H or dMMR include anemia, elevated concentrations of alkaline phosphatase, lymphopenia, elevated concentrations of hepatic aminotransferase enzymes (i.e., ALT, AST), elevated concentrations of pancreatic enzymes (i.e., lipase, amylase), hyponatremia, neutropenia, hypocalcemia, hypomagnesemia, thrombocytopenia, elevated concentrations of bilirubin, hypokalemia, elevated concentrations of serum creatinine, and hyperkalemia.

Adverse effects reported in 10% or more of patients receiving nivolumab in combination with ipilimumab for the treatment of metastatic colorectal cancer with MSI-H or dMMR in the CheckMate-142 study include fatigue, diarrhea, musculoskeletal pain, pyrexia, abdominal pain, pruritus, nausea, rash, decreased appetite, vomiting, cough, headache, constipation, arthralgia, hypothyroidism, dyspnea, insomnia, hyperthyroidism, dizziness, dry skin, and decreased weight. Laboratory abnormalities reported in 10% or more of patients receiving nivolumab in combination with ipilimumab for the treatment of metastatic colorectal cancer with MSI-H or dMMR include anemia, elevated concentrations of hepatic aminotransferase enzymes (i.e., ALT, AST), elevated concentrations of pancreatic enzymes (i.e., lipase, amylase), elevated concentrations of alkaline phosphatase, hyponatremia, thrombocytopenia, elevated concentrations of serum creatinine, lymphopenia, hyperkalemia, elevated concentrations of bilirubin, hypomagnesemia, neutropenia, hypocalcemia, and hypokalemia.

Adverse effects reported in patients receiving nivolumab as a single agent for the treatment of advanced hepatocellular carcinoma in the CheckMate-040 study were generally similar to those observed in patients with other malignancies; however, a higher incidence of elevated concentrations of hepatic aminotransferase enzymes (i.e., ALT, AST) and bilirubin were reported in these patients.

Drug Interactions

No formal drug interaction studies have been performed to date.

■ **Ipilimumab** Concomitant administration of nivolumab 1 mg/kg and ipilimumab 3 mg/kg increased nivolumab clearance by 29% but did not alter clearance of ipilimumab; however, concomitant administration of nivolumab 3 mg/kg and ipilimumab 1 mg/kg did not alter clearance of either drug.

Description

Nivolumab, a fully human anti-programmed-death receptor-1 (anti-PD-1) monoclonal antibody, is an antineoplastic agent. The drug is an IgG_4 kappa immunoglobulin.

Nivolumab is selective for PD-1, an immune-checkpoint receptor expressed on activated T cells, monocytes, B cells, natural killer (NK) T cells, and dendritic cells. Overexpression of PD-1 ligands on the surface of tumor cells results in activation of PD-1 and suppression of cytotoxic T-cell activity. Nivolumab blocks the interaction between PD-1 and its ligands, resulting in enhanced immune response, including enhanced antitumor immune response. The drug also has been shown to reduce tumor growth in syngeneic mouse tumor models. The combination of nivolumab and an anti-cytotoxic T-lymphocyte-associated antigen 4 (anti-CTLA-4) antibody (i.e., ipilimumab) also has demonstrated enhanced T-cell function, including enhanced antitumor immune response, compared with either drug alone. Combined blockade of PD-1 and CTLA-4 also has been shown to enhance antitumor activity in syngeneic mouse tumor models.

Systemic exposure to nivolumab is proportional to dose over the dosage range of 0.1–10 mg/kg every 2 weeks. Following repeated 3-mg/kg doses of nivolumab every 2 weeks, steady-state concentrations are reached by 12 weeks; systemic accumulation of the drug is 3.7-fold. Based on dose-exposure relationships, no clinically important differences in safety and efficacy have been observed between nivolumab 240 mg every 2 weeks and nivolumab 3 mg/kg every 2 weeks in patients with melanoma, non-small cell lung cancer (NSCLC), renal cell carcinoma, urothelial carcinoma, metastatic colorectal cancer with high microsatellite instability (MSI-H), or hepatocellular carcinoma. In addition, the predicted exposure to nivolumab administered as a 30-minute IV infusion is comparable to that observed following administration as a 60-minute IV infusion. Although nivolumab clearance decreases over time (by about 25% from baseline to steady state) in patients with metastatic tumors, the decrease in clearance is not considered clinically important. Nivolumab clearance does not decrease over time in patients with completely resected melanoma; clearance in this patient population is 24% lower than that observed at steady state in patients with metastatic melanoma. The mean terminal half-life of nivolumab is approximately 25 days.

Clearance of nivolumab does not appear to be affected by age (range of 29–87 years), body weight (35–160 kg), gender, race, baseline LDH concentration, programmed death ligand 1 (PD-L1) expression, solid tumor type, tumor burden, renal impairment, or mild hepatic impairment.

Advice to Patients

Importance of advising patients to read the manufacturer's medication guide before beginning treatment and each time nivolumab is administered.

Risk of immune-mediated pneumonitis. Importance of informing clinician immediately if new or worsening cough, chest pain, or shortness of breath occurs.

Risk of immune-mediated colitis. Importance of informing clinician immediately if diarrhea, severe abdominal pain, or changes in stool occur.

Risk of immune-mediated hepatitis. Importance of informing clinician immediately if signs and symptoms of liver damage (e.g., jaundice, severe nausea or vomiting, abdominal pain [particularly in the right upper quadrant], lethargy, easy bruising or bleeding, lack of appetite, dark urine, drowsiness) occur.

Risk of immune-mediated endocrine effects. Importance of informing clinician immediately if manifestations of hypophysitis, hyperthyroidism, hypothyroidism, adrenal insufficiency, or diabetes mellitus occur.

Risk of immune-mediated nephritis or renal dysfunction. Importance of informing clinician immediately if signs and symptoms of nephritis (e.g., decreased urine output, hematuria, peripheral edema, lack of appetite) occur.

Risk of immune-mediated rash. Importance of informing clinician immediately if a rash develops.

Risk of immune-mediated encephalitis. Importance of informing clinician immediately if signs and symptoms of encephalitis (e.g., headache, fever, confusion, memory loss, hallucinations, fatigue, asthenia, somnolence, drowsiness, seizures, stiff neck) occur.

Risk of infusion-related reactions. Importance of informing clinician immediately if signs and symptoms of such reactions, including dizziness, chills, fever, breathing difficulty, pruritus, flushing, and feeling of faintness, occur.

Risk of allogeneic stem cell transplantation-related complications.

Risk of fetal harm. Necessity of advising women of childbearing potential that they should use an effective method of contraception while receiving nivolumab and for at least 5 months after the last dose of the drug. Importance of women informing clinicians if they are or plan to become pregnant. If pregnancy occurs, advise pregnant women of potential risk to the fetus.

Importance of advising women to avoid breast-feeding while receiving nivolumab therapy.

Importance of informing clinicians of existing or contemplated concomitant therapy, including prescription and OTC drugs, as well as any concomitant illnesses (e.g., autoimmune disorders, history of organ transplantation, liver damage, pulmonary disorders).

Importance of informing patients of other important precautionary information. (See Cautions.)

Overview® (see Users Guide). For additional information on this drug until a more detailed monograph is developed and published, the manufacturer's labeling should be consulted. It is *essential* that the manufacturer's labeling be consulted for more detailed information on usual cautions, precautions, contraindications, potential drug interactions, laboratory test interferences, and acute toxicity. For further information on the handling of antineoplastic agents, see the ASHP Guidelines on Handling Hazardous Drugs at http://www.ahfsdruginformation.com.

Preparations

Excipients in commercially available drug preparations may have clinically important effects in some individuals; consult specific product labeling for details.

Nivolumab

Parenteral

Injection, for IV infusion only	10 mg/mL (40, 100, and 240 mg)	**Opdivo®**, Bristol-Myers Squibb

†Use is not currently included in the labeling approved by the US Food and Drug Administration

Obinutuzumab

■ Obinutuzumab, a recombinant humanized anti-CD20 monoclonal antibody, is an antineoplastic agent; the drug also is referred to as a type II anti-CD20 monoclonal antibody.

Uses

■ **Chronic Lymphocytic Leukemia** Obinutuzumab is used in combination with chlorambucil for the treatment of previously untreated chronic lymphocytic leukemia (CLL); obinutuzumab is designated an orphan drug by the US Food and Drug Administration (FDA) for the treatment of this cancer.

The current indication for obinutuzumab is based principally on results of an open-label, randomized, active-controlled, multicenter study in 781 patients with previously untreated CD20-positive CLL. Patients were randomized in a 2:2:1 ratio to receive obinutuzumab in combination with chlorambucil, rituximab in combination with chlorambucil, or chlorambucil alone. After 118 patients had been assigned to the chlorambucil monotherapy group, randomization to this group was closed and randomization to the 2 combination regimens continued in a 1:1 ratio. The primary measure of efficacy was progression-free survival as assessed by the investigator; secondary end points included overall survival, progression-free survival as assessed by an independent review facility (IRF), and overall response rate. The median age of patients was 73 years; 22, 42, or 36% of the patients had Binet stage A, B, or C disease, respectively. Most patients had more than 3 coexisting medical conditions (82%) or a creatinine clearance of less than 70 mL/minute (65%). Therapy was administered in 4-week cycles for a total of 6 cycles. Dosages of the drugs were obinutuzumab 1 g by IV infusion once weekly for 3 doses during cycle 1, followed by 1 g by IV infusion every 4 weeks for an additional 5 cycles; chlorambucil 0.5 mg/kg on days 1 and 15 of each cycle; and rituximab 375 mg/m^2 on day 1 of cycle 1, followed by 500 mg/m^2 every 4 weeks for an additional 5 cycles. Because of a high rate of infusion-related reactions in patients receiving obinutuzumab 1 g once weekly for 3 doses during cycle 1, the study protocol was amended to divide the initial 1-g dose of obinutuzumab on day 1 of cycle 1 into 2 infusions (100 mg on day 1 and 900 mg on day 2 of cycle 1). (See Infusion-related Effects under Warnings/Precautions: Other Warnings and Precautions, in Cautions.)

In patients receiving obinutuzumab in combination with chlorambucil, median IRF-assessed progression-free survival was prolonged compared with that in patients receiving chlorambucil alone (23 versus 11.1 months, respectively). Effects of obinutuzumab on investigator-assessed progression-free survival and IRF-assessed progression-free survival were comparable. Patients receiving obinutuzumab in combination with chlorambucil appeared to have a higher overall response rate (75.9 versus 32.1%, respectively) and a longer median duration of response (15.2 versus 3.5 months, respectively) compared with those receiving chlorambucil alone; 27.8% of patients receiving obinutuzumab in combination with chlorambucil achieved a complete response compared with 0.9% of those receiving chlorambucil alone. At the time of the primary analysis for comparison of obinutuzumab in combination with chlorambucil versus rituximab in combination with chlorambucil, obinutuzumab-treated patients appeared to have a higher overall response rate (78.4 versus 65.1%) and longer progression-free survival (26.7 versus 15.2 months) than rituximab-treated patients. Effects on overall survival remain to be established; however, a planned interim analysis suggested a trend toward a survival benefit in patients receiving obinutuzumab in combination with chlorambucil compared with those receiving chlorambucil alone, but no difference in overall survival between obinutuzumab- or rituximab-treated patients. Infusion-related reactions and grade 3 or 4 neutropenia occurred more frequently in patients receiving obinutuzumab.

Dosage and Administration

■ **General** Patients at high risk of tumor lysis syndrome (i.e., patients with a high number of circulating malignant cells [lymphocyte count of 25,000/mm^3 or greater] or a large tumor burden) should receive adequate hydration and prophylaxis with an antihyperuricemic agent (e.g., allopurinol) beginning 12–24 hours prior to the first dose of obinutuzumab. (See Tumor Lysis Syndrome under Warnings/Precautions: Other Warnings and Precautions, in Cautions.)

Obinutuzumab should be administered only in settings where adequate monitoring can be performed and appropriate medical support is available for management of potential infusion-related reactions. (See Infusion-related Effects under Warnings/Precautions: Other Warnings and Precautions, in Cautions.)

To minimize the risk of infusion-related events associated with obinutuzumab, the manufacturer recommends a premedication regimen (e.g., a corticosteroid, an antihistamine, and acetaminophen) prior to obinutuzumab infusions. Hydrocortisone has not been effective in reducing the rate of infusion-related events associated with obinutuzumab and is not recommended as premedication. Acetaminophen 650 mg to 1 g should be administered at least 30 minutes prior to *each* obinutuzumab infusion. On days 1 and 2 of cycle 1, an antihistamine (e.g., diphenhydramine hydrochloride 50 mg) and IV corticosteroid (dexamethasone 20 mg or methylprednisolone 80 mg) also should be administered at least 30 minutes and 1 hour, respectively, prior to infusion of obinutuzumab. Recommendations for antihistamine and/or corticosteroid premedication prior to subsequent doses of obinutuzumab (days 8 and 15 of cycle 1 and day 1 of cycles 2–6) are based on the patient's tolerance of the previous infusion. Patients who have experienced a grade 1 or 2 infusion-related reaction should receive an antihistamine prior to subsequent doses, while those who have experienced a grade 3 infusion-related reaction should receive both an antihistamine and a corticosteroid prior to subsequent doses. In addition, corticosteroid premedication is recommended for patients with a high circulating lymphocyte count (exceeding 25,000/mm^3) prior to the next dose of obinutuzumab. Recommended dosages of antihistamines and corticosteroids are the same as those used prior to the initial infusion. (See Infusion-related Effects under Warnings/Precautions: Other Warnings and Precautions, in Cautions.)

Because hypotension may occur during administration of obinutuzumab, consideration should be given to withholding antihypertensive therapy for 12 hours prior to, during, and for 1 hour following each obinutuzumab infusion until blood pressure has stabilized; however, the potential risks and benefits of withholding antihypertensive therapy should be considered in patients at increased risk of hypertensive crisis. (See Infusion-related Effects under Warnings/Precautions: Other Warnings and Precautions, in Cautions.)

Anti-infective prophylaxis is strongly recommended during therapy with obinutuzumab in patients with neutropenia; antiviral and antifungal prophylaxis should be considered. (See Infectious Complications under Warnings/Precautions: Other Warnings and Precautions, in Cautions.)

■ **Administration** Obinutuzumab is administered by IV infusion. *The drug should not be administered by rapid IV injection, such as IV push or bolus.*

Unopened vials of obinutuzumab injection concentrate should be protected from light, stored at 2–8°C, and should not be frozen or shaken.

Dilution Prior to administration, obinutuzumab injection concentrate must be diluted using proper aseptic technique. The manufacturer states that obinutuzumab may be administered following dilution to a final concentration of 0.4–4 mg/mL.

Obinutuzumab injection concentrate should be inspected visually for particulate matter and discoloration. Solutions of the drug should be clear and colorless to slightly brown.

Diluted solutions of obinutuzumab for administration on day 1 (100 mg) and day 2 (900 mg) of cycle 1 may be prepared on the same day. For simultaneous preparation of both doses, 40 mL of obinutuzumab injection concentrate should be withdrawn from a vial labeled as containing 1 g in 40 mL. For the 100-mg dose, 4 mL of the injection concentrate is added to a PVC or non-PVC polyolefin infusion bag containing 100 mL of 0.9% sodium chloride to yield a final concentration of approximately 1 mg/mL. The diluted solution of the drug for day 1 of cycle 1 should be administered immediately. For the 900-mg dose, the remaining 36 mL of obinutuzumab injection concentrate is added to a PVC or non-PVC polyolefin infusion bag containing 250 mL of 0.9%

sodium chloride to yield a final concentration of approximately 3.1 mg/mL. The diluted solution of the drug for day 2 of cycle 1 should be stored at 2–8°C for up to 24 hours; the solution should be brought to room temperature and then administered immediately.

For a 1-g dose of obinutuzumab, 40 mL of obinutuzumab injection concentrate should be withdrawn from a vial labeled as containing 1 g in 40 mL and added to an infusion bag containing 250 mL of 0.9% sodium chloride to yield a final concentration of approximately 3.4 mg/mL. The manufacturer recommends immediate administration of diluted solutions of the drug. If immediate administration is not possible, diluted solutions of the drug may be stored at 2–8°C for up to 24 hours; the solution should be brought to room temperature and then administered immediately.

Diluted obinutuzumab solutions should be mixed by gentle inversion and should *not* be shaken. Obinutuzumab injection concentrate should *not* be diluted in 5% dextrose injection. Obinutuzumab should *not* be admixed with any other drug. Commercially available obinutuzumab injection concentrate contains no preservatives and is intended for single use; any partially used vials should be discarded.

Rate of Administration The initial obinutuzumab dose (100 mg; day 1 of cycle 1) should be infused IV at a rate of 25 mg/hour over 4 hours. The second dose of obinutuzumab (900 mg; day 2 of cycle 1) should be infused at an initial rate of 50 mg/hour; if infusion-related reactions do not occur, the infusion rate may be increased in increments of 50 mg/hour every 30 minutes to a maximum rate of 400 mg/hour. Subsequent doses of obinutuzumab (1 g each; days 8 and 15 of cycle 1 and day 1 of cycles 2–6) should be infused at an initial rate of 100 mg/hour; if infusion-related events do not occur, the infusion rate may be increased in increments of 100 mg/hour every 30 minutes to a maximum rate of 400 mg/hour.

If infusion-related reactions occur, the infusion rate should be reduced or obinutuzumab therapy should be interrupted depending on the severity of the reaction. If the infusion-related reaction is grade 4 in severity, therapy with obinutuzumab should be permanently discontinued. If the infusion-related reaction is grade 3, the obinutuzumab infusion should be interrupted; once the reaction has resolved, the infusion may be resumed but the rate of infusion should be reduced by at least 50%. If no further infusion-related reactions occur, the infusion rate may be increased in increments and intervals appropriate for the treatment cycle dose. If a grade 3 infusion-related reaction recurs, treatment with obinutuzumab should be permanently discontinued. For grade 1 and 2 infusion-related reactions, the infusion rate should be reduced or the infusion should be interrupted until the reaction has resolved; if infusion-related reactions do not occur upon resumption or continuation at a reduced rate, the infusion rate may be increased in increments and intervals appropriate for the treatment cycle dose. (See Infusion-related Effects under Warnings/Precautions: Other Warnings and Precautions, in Cautions.)

■ **Dosage** For the treatment of previously untreated chronic lymphocytic leukemia (CLL) in adults, obinutuzumab is administered in combination with chlorambucil in 4-week cycles for a maximum of 6 cycles. During cycle 1, the recommended dosage of obinutuzumab is 100 mg on day 1, followed by 900 mg on day 2, and then 1 g once weekly for 2 doses (days 8 and 15). During cycles 2–6, the recommended dosage of obinutuzumab is 1 g every 4 weeks (day 1 of each cycle). Patients who do not complete the day 1 dose in cycle 1 may proceed to receive the day 2 dose if continued therapy with the drug is appropriate.

If a dose is missed, the missed dose should be administered as soon as possible; waiting until the next scheduled dose is not recommended. The schedule of administration should be adjusted to maintain the recommended 4-week interval between doses.

Although volume of distribution and steady-state clearance of obinutuzumab increase with increasing body weight, the manufacturer states that dosage adjustment based on body weight is not necessary.

Therapy Interruption for Toxicity **Infusion-related Effects.** If infusion-related reactions occur, the infusion rate should be reduced or obinutuzumab therapy should be interrupted depending on the severity of the reaction, and appropriate symptomatic and supportive therapy should be provided. (See Rate of Administration under Dosage and Administration: Administration.) If a grade 4 infusion-related reaction occurs, obinutuzumab therapy should be permanently discontinued.

Hematologic Toxicity. If grade 3 or 4 cytopenia occurs, temporary interruption of obinutuzumab therapy should be considered.

Infectious Complications. If infection occurs, temporary interruption of obinutuzumab therapy should be considered.

Other Nonhematologic Toxicity. If grade 2 or greater nonhematologic toxicity occurs, temporary interruption of obinutuzumab therapy should be considered.

■ **Special Populations** There are no special population dosage recommendations at this time. Obinutuzumab has not been studied in patients with hepatic impairment or in patients with renal impairment with a creatinine clearance of less than 30 mL/minute. The recommended adult dosage for treatment of CLL is based on clinical trial experience mainly in geriatric patients. (See Specific Populations under Cautions: Warnings/Precautions.)

Cautions

■ **Contraindications** The manufacturer states there are no known contraindications to the use of obinutuzumab.

■ **Warnings/Precautions** ***Warnings*** **Patients Infected with Hepatitis B Virus.** Reactivation of hepatitis B virus (HBV) infection has been reported in patients receiving anti-CD20 monoclonal antibodies, such as obinutuzumab, and has resulted in fulminant hepatitis, hepatic failure, and death. HBV reactivation has been reported in patients who are hepatitis B surface antigen-positive [HBsAg-positive]; HBsAg-negative and hepatitis B core antibody-positive [anti-HBc-positive]; or HBsAg-negative, anti-HBc-positive, and hepatitis B surface antibody-positive [anti-HBs-positive].

Following review of the Adverse Event Reporting System (AERS) database, the US Food and Drug Administration (FDA) identified 106 cases of fatal HBV-related acute liver injury in patients receiving rituximab (between November 1997 and August 2012) and 3 such cases in patients receiving ofatumumab (between October 2009 and August 2012); 32 of these case reports contained sufficient data to meet the criteria for HBV reactivation. In this review, acute liver injury was attributed to HBV reactivation if seroconversion of HBsAg from negative to positive occurred in those with either anti-HBc or a history of HBV, or if an increase in serum HBV DNA level occurred in those who were HBsAg-positive prior to therapy with an anti-CD20 monoclonal antibody (i.e., rituximab, ofatumumab). HBV reactivation was diagnosed by seroconversion of HBsAg in most (69%) cases. In this review, the duration of rituximab or ofatumumab therapy prior to diagnosis of HBV reactivation was highly variable, ranging from 63 days after initiation of the drug to 12 months following the last dose; however, delayed onset of HBV reactivation (up to 24 months following completion of rituximab therapy) has been reported. Among patients with HBV reactivation, 10% had received HBV antiviral prophylaxis and 28% had received antiviral treatment for HBV reactivation. All of the patients experiencing HBV reactivation had received recent or concomitant therapy with other immunosuppressive agents.

All patients should be screened for HBV infection by measuring HBsAg and anti-HBc before initiating treatment with obinutuzumab. Hepatitis experts should be consulted regarding monitoring and use of antiviral therapy in those with evidence of HBV infection (HBsAg-positive with any antibody status or HBsAg-negative and anti-HBc-positive); although data are limited, treatment guidelines from some experts recommend the use of prophylactic antiviral therapy in patients who are chronic carriers of HBV. Patients with evidence of current or prior HBV infection should be monitored for clinical and laboratory evidence of hepatitis or HBV reactivation during obinutuzumab therapy and for several months thereafter, since reactivation has occurred more than 12 months following completion of anti-CD20 monoclonal antibody therapy. Obinutuzumab and any concomitant chemotherapy should be discontinued immediately if HBV reactivation occurs, and appropriate treatment for HBV infection should be initiated. Experts in the management of HBV infection should be consulted regarding resumption of obinutuzumab therapy once control of the reactivated HBV infection has been achieved. It has not been established whether obinutuzumab can be safely readministered in patients who develop HBV reactivation.

Progressive Multifocal Leukoencephalopathy. JC virus infection causing progressive multifocal leukoencephalopathy (PML), which can be fatal, has been reported in patients receiving obinutuzumab. The possible diagnosis of PML should be considered in any patient receiving obinutuzumab who experiences new onset or worsening of neurologic manifestations suggestive of PML (e.g., confusion, vision changes, changes in speech or walking, dizziness or vertigo). If PML is suspected, the drug should be withheld and diagnostic evaluation, including consultation with a neurologist, brain magnetic resonance imaging (MRI) scan, and lumbar puncture, should be considered. If PML is confirmed, obinutuzumab should be permanently discontinued; dosage reduction or discontinuance of concomitant immunosuppressive therapy should be considered.

Other Warnings and Precautions **Infusion-related Effects.** Infusion-related reactions, sometimes severe or life-threatening, have been reported in patients receiving obinutuzumab. Infusion-related reactions generally occur more frequently during the first 2 infusions (total dose of 1 g) than during subsequent infusions of the drug; infusion-related reactions have occurred within 24 hours of administration. Infusion-related effects may include bronchospasm, larynx and throat irritation, wheezing, dyspnea, laryngeal edema, flushing, hypertension, hypotension, tachycardia, nausea, vomiting, diarrhea, pyrexia, headache, and chills.

In the phase 3 clinical trial evaluating obinutuzumab in patients with chronic lymphocytic leukemia (CLL), infusion-related reactions occurred in most (89%) of the first 53 patients who received the drug; during cycle 1 of therapy, these patients received obinutuzumab 1 g at weekly intervals for 3 doses. Subsequent study protocol amendments resulted in the initial 1-g dose of obinutuzumab being divided and administered as 2 infusions (100 mg on day 1 and 900 mg on day 2 of cycle 1) and also led to changes in premedication requirements. In a subgroup of 45 patients who received the drug following these protocol amendments, 47% experienced infusion-related reactions following the first 2 infusions (total dose of 1 g), and less than 2% experienced infusion-related reactions during subsequent infusions. Among patients receiving the drug either before or after the protocol modifications, infusion-related reactions occurred in approximately two-thirds of patients after administration of the first 1 g of obinutuzumab and were severe or life-threatening (grade 3 or 4) in approximately 21% of patients; infusion-related reactions (all less than grade 3) occurred in 3% of patients after administration of the second 1-g dose of obinutuzumab (day 8 of cycle 1) and in less than 1% of patients after subsequent doses.

To minimize the risk of infusion-related reactions, patients receiving obinutuzumab should be premedicated with acetaminophen, an antihistamine, and a corticosteroid prior to administration of the drug. (See Dosage and Administration: General.) Patients should be monitored closely during infusions of the drug for manifestations of infusion-related reactions. Patients with preexisting cardiac or pulmonary conditions may be at greater risk for severe infusion-related reactions; more frequent monitoring during and following an infusion is indicated in these patients. Because hypotension may occur during administration of obinutuzumab, withholding antihypertensive therapy should be considered. (See Dosage and Administration: General.)

In patients experiencing infusion-related reactions, interruption of the infusion or a reduction in the infusion rate may be necessary. (See Rate of Administration under Dosage and Administration: Administration.) For patients experiencing a grade 4 infusion-related reaction (e.g., anaphylaxis, acute life-threatening respiratory symptoms, other life-threatening infusion-related reaction), the manufacturer recommends permanent discontinuance. Appropriate treatment and supportive care (e.g., corticosteroid, epinephrine, bronchodilator, oxygen) should be provided as clinically indicated for infusion-related reactions.

Tumor Lysis Syndrome. Tumor lysis syndrome consisting of rapid reduction in tumor volume followed by acute renal failure, hyperkalemia, hypocalcemia, hyperuricemia, and/or hyperphosphatemia, may occur within 12–24 hours of completion of the initial infusion of obinutuzumab. In the phase 3 clinical trial evaluating obinutuzumab combined with chlorambucil in patients with previously untreated CLL, grade 3 or 4 tumor lysis syndrome was reported in 2% of obinutuzumab-treated patients compared with none of those receiving chlorambucil alone. The risk of tumor lysis syndrome is increased in patients with a high number of circulating malignant cells (lymphocyte count of 25,000/mm^3 or greater) or a large tumor burden. Appropriate measures (e.g., prophylactic antihyperuricemic therapy and adequate hydration beginning 12–24 hours prior to obinutuzumab infusion) should be used in patients at high risk for tumor lysis syndrome. If tumor lysis syndrome develops, patients should receive appropriate medical treatment, including correction of electrolyte abnormalities, monitoring of renal function and fluid balance, and supportive care (e.g., dialysis) as clinically indicated.

Infectious Complications. Serious bacterial, new or reactivated viral, or fungal infections may occur during and following completion of obinutuzumab therapy. In the phase 3 clinical trial evaluating obinutuzumab combined with chlorambucil in patients with previously untreated CLL, the incidence of infection was similar between obinutuzumab-treated patients and those receiving chlorambucil alone; infection was reported in 38% of obinutuzumab-treated patients and was grade 3 or 4 in severity in 9% of patients. The manufacturer states that obinutuzumab should not be used in patients with active infections. The risk of infection may be increased in patients with a history of recurring or chronic infections.

Hematologic Effects. Grade 3 or 4 neutropenia and thrombocytopenia have been reported in patients receiving obinutuzumab in combination with chlorambucil. In the phase 3 clinical trial evaluating obinutuzumab combined with chlorambucil in patients with previously untreated CLL, delayed-onset neutropenia (occurring 28 days or more after completion of therapy) was reported in 16% of obinutuzumab-treated patients compared with 12% of those receiving chlorambucil alone. Prolonged neutropenia (lasting longer than 28 days) also may occur. Acute-onset thrombocytopenia (occurring within 24 hours after completion of therapy) occurred in 5% of obinutuzumab-treated patients.

Complete blood cell counts (CBCs) and platelet counts should be monitored at regular intervals during obinutuzumab therapy; if grade 3 or 4 neutropenia or thrombocytopenia occurs, the manufacturer recommends more frequent hematologic monitoring until resolution. If neutropenia occurs, the manufacturer strongly recommends anti-infective prophylaxis during therapy with obinutuzumab; antiviral and antifungal prophylaxis should be considered. Clinicians should monitor for signs or symptoms of infection; if infection develops, appropriate treatment should be instituted. Transfusion of blood products (i.e., platelets) may be necessary.

Immunization. The safety and efficacy of immunization with live or attenuated viral vaccines during or following obinutuzumab therapy have not been established. The manufacturer recommends that live viral vaccines be avoided during obinutuzumab therapy and until B-cell counts have recovered.

Immunogenicity. Antibodies to obinutuzumab have been detected in patients receiving the drug; the clinical relevance of such antibodies is not known. Anti-obinutuzumab antibodies were detected in approximately 13% of obinutuzumab-treated patients at 1 or more time points during a 12-month follow-up period. Neutralizing antibodies have not been assessed.

Specific Populations **Pregnancy.** Category C. (See Users Guide.)

Although obinutuzumab did not produce teratogenic effects when administered to pregnant cynomolgus monkeys from early gestation until parturition, the presence of the drug was detected and B-cell depletion was observed in the offspring on day 28 postpartum; B-cell count and immune function returned to normal within 6 months of birth. Women of childbearing potential should use effective contraceptive methods during treatment and for 12 months following obinutuzumab therapy.

Lactation. It is not known whether obinutuzumab is distributed into human milk. Because human immunoglobulin G (IgG) is distributed into milk in humans, and because of the potential for serious adverse reactions to obinutuzumab in nursing infants, a decision should be made whether to discontinue nursing or the drug, taking into account the importance of the drug to the woman.

Pediatric Use. Safety and efficacy of obinutuzumab have not been established in pediatric patients.

Geriatric Use. In the phase 3 clinical trial evaluating obinutuzumab in combination with chlorambucil for the treatment of previously untreated CLL, 82% of patients were 65 years of age or older and 45% were 75 years of age or older. Although no overall differences in efficacy were observed between geriatric and younger patients, the incidences of serious adverse events (45 versus 30%, respectively) and fatal adverse events (5 versus 2%, respectively) were higher among patients 75 years of age or older compared with younger patients. Age does not appear to affect the pharmacokinetics of obinutuzumab.

Hepatic Impairment. Obinutuzumab has not been studied in patients with hepatic impairment.

Renal Impairment. A population pharmacokinetic analysis indicated that the pharmacokinetics of obinutuzumab are not influenced by baseline creatinine clearance exceeding 30 mL/minute. Obinutuzumab has not been studied in patients with baseline creatinine clearance less than 30 mL/minute.

■ **Common Adverse Effects** Adverse effects reported in 5% or more of patients receiving obinutuzumab in combination with chlorambucil and at an incidence that is at least 2% higher than that reported with chlorambucil alone include infusion-related reactions, pyrexia, cough, and musculoskeletal disorders.

Laboratory abnormalities reported in 5% or more of patients receiving obinutuzumab in combination with chlorambucil and at an incidence that is at least 2% higher than that reported with chlorambucil alone include neutropenia, lymphopenia, leukopenia, thrombocytopenia, hypocalcemia, hyperkalemia, hyponatremia, elevated aminotransferase (i.e., AST, ALT) concentrations, elevated serum creatinine concentration, hypoalbuminemia, elevated serum alkaline phosphatase concentration, and hypokalemia.

Drug Interactions

No formal drug interaction studies have been performed to date.

Description

Obinutuzumab, a recombinant humanized anti-CD20 monoclonal antibody, is an antineoplastic agent; the drug also is referred to as a type II anti-CD20 monoclonal antibody. The drug is an IgG_1 kappa immunoglobulin produced by recombinant DNA technology in mammalian cell (Chinese hamster ovary) culture. Obinutuzumab binds specifically to the class II epitope of antigen CD20, a glycoprotein expressed on the surface of normal and malignant B-lymphocytes, including B-cell chronic lymphocytic leukemia (B-CLL) cells. Following binding of obinutuzumab to antigen CD20, the Fc domain triggers host immune responses (i.e., antibody-dependent cell-mediated cytotoxicity [ADCC], antibody-dependent cellular phagocytosis [ADCP], complement-dependent cytotoxicity [CDC]) causing lysis of the B-cells.

Unlike rituximab (a type I anti-CD20 monoclonal antibody), obinutuzumab (a type II anti-CD20 monoclonal antibody) is relatively ineffective in inducing CDC activity, but elicits more potent homotypic adhesion and direct induction of programmed cell death. Obinutuzumab is an anti-CD20 monoclonal antibody with a nonfucosylated Fc domain engineered to enhance the binding affinity of the drug for Fcγ receptors, activating Fc receptors expressed by immune effectors (e.g., natural killer [NK] cells, macrophages), which results in enhanced ADCC against malignant B cells relative to rituximab. In addition, modification of elbow hinge sequences within the antibody may account for enhanced type II antibody properties of the drug, such as increased direct induction of programmed cell death. Obinutuzumab was tenfold to 25-fold more potent than rituximab at depleting B-cells in blood obtained from healthy individuals and also was more effective than rituximab in depleting B-cells in blood obtained from an individual with chronic lymphocytic leukemia (CLL).

In patients with CLL, obinutuzumab caused circulating $CD19^+$ B-cell depletion (defined as a $CD19^+$ B-cell count less than 70 cells/mm^3). Initial B-cell recovery occurred approximately 9 months following completion of obinutuzumab therapy in some patients; however, in other patients, B-cell depletion persisted at 18 months. Depletion of B-cells has not been shown to be directly correlated to clinical response. Obinutuzumab exhibits linear and time-dependent nonlinear clearance. Following repeated administration of obinutuzumab during a treatment course, clearance by the nonlinear pathway diminishes. The terminal half-life of obinutuzumab is approximately 28–30 days in patients with CLL.

Advice to Patients

Risk of infusion-related reactions; importance of reporting signs and symptoms of such reactions, including dizziness, nausea, chills, fever, vomiting, diarrhea, breathing difficulty, or chest pain.

Risk of tumor lysis syndrome; importance of reporting symptoms of tumor lysis syndrome (e.g., nausea, vomiting, diarrhea, lethargy).

Risk of infection; importance of reporting signs or symptoms of infection (e.g., cough, fever).

Risk of progressive multifocal leukoencephalopathy; importance of reporting new or worsening neurologic symptoms (e.g., confusion, dizziness or loss of balance, difficulty speaking or walking, changes in vision).

Risk of reactivation of hepatitis B virus (HBV) infection; importance of reporting worsening fatigue or icteric changes. Importance of informing clinician of presence of HBV carrier state or of any history of HBV infection.

Advise patients that they should not receive a live viral vaccine if they have recently received obinutuzumab.

Importance of routine monitoring of blood cell counts.

Necessity of advising women to avoid pregnancy and breast-feeding while receiving therapy. Necessity of advising women receiving obinutuzumab to use an effective method of contraception during therapy and for 12 months after the last dose of obinutuzumab.

Importance of informing clinicians of existing or contemplated concomitant therapy, including prescription and OTC drugs, as well as any concomitant illnesses.

Importance of informing patients of other important precautionary information. (See Cautions.)

Overview® (see Users Guide). For additional information on this drug until a more detailed monograph is developed and published, the manufacturer's labeling should be consulted. It is *essential* that the manufacturer's labeling be consulted for more detailed information on usual cautions, precautions, contraindications, potential drug interactions, laboratory test interferences, and acute toxicity. For further information on the handling of antineoplastic agents, see the ASHP Guidelines on Handling Hazardous Drugs at http://www.ahfsdruginformation.com.

Preparations

Excipients in commercially available drug preparations may have clinically important effects in some individuals; consult specific product labeling for details.

Obinutuzumab

Parenteral

Injection, for IV infusion only	25 mg/mL (1 g)	**Gazyva®**, Genentech

Ofatumumab

HuMax-CD20, 2F2

■ Ofatumumab, a recombinant fully human anti-CD20 monoclonal antibody, is an antineoplastic agent.

Uses

■ **Chronic Lymphocytic Leukemia** Ofatumumab is used for the treatment of B-cell chronic lymphocytic leukemia (B-CLL) that is refractory to both fludarabine and alemtuzumab. Efficacy was determined based on durable objective response rate; clinical benefit (e.g., decrease in disease-related symptoms, increase in survival) has not been established. Ofatumumab is designated an orphan drug by the US Food and Drug Administration (FDA) for the treatment of this cancer.

The current indication for ofatumumab is based principally on interim results for a subset of 59 patients with fludarabine- and alemtuzumab-refractory B-CLL who were enrolled in a phase 2, open-label, noncomparative study (Hx-CD20-406) involving 154 patients with refractory or relapsed B-CLL; the study also included a subset of 79 patients with fludarabine-refractory B-CLL who were not considered candidates for alemtuzumab therapy because of the presence of bulky lymphadenopathy. In this study, drug refractoriness was defined as failure to achieve at least a partial response to fludarabine or alemtuzumab or disease progression within 6 months following completion of such therapy. The primary measure of efficacy was overall response rate evaluated over 24 weeks of treatment using the 1996 National Cancer Institute-sponsored Working Group Guidelines for CLL. The median age of patients with fludarabine- and alemtuzumab-refractory B-CLL was 64 years; these patients had received a median of 5 prior therapies for their disease, including fludarabine (100% of patients), alemtuzumab (100%), alkylating agents (93%), and rituximab (59%). Patients received an initial dose of ofatumumab 300 mg (dose 1) with a subsequent increase to 2 g administered weekly for 7 doses (doses 2–8), followed by 2 g administered monthly for 4 doses (doses 9–12); all doses were administered by IV infusion. Prior to each ofatumumab infusion, patients received acetaminophen, an antihistamine, and a corticosteroid as prophylaxis for infusion-related reactions. The investigator-determined overall response rate in patients with fludarabine- and alemtuzumab-refractory B-CLL was 42% with a median response duration of 6.5 months; there were no complete responses. Antitumor activity of ofatumumab also was observed in other patients with relapsed or refractory B-CLL enrolled in this study or in an open-label dose-escalation study.

Dosage and Administration

■ **General** Ofatumumab should be administered only in settings where adequate monitoring can be performed and appropriate medical support is available for management of potential infusion-related reactions. (See Infusion-related Effects under Warnings/Precautions: Other Warnings and Precautions, in Cautions.)

To minimize the risk of infusion-related events associated with ofatumumab, the manufacturer recommends premedication with oral acetaminophen 1 g (or equivalent agent), an oral or IV antihistamine (cetirizine hydrochloride 10 mg or equivalent), and an IV corticosteroid (prednisolone 100 mg [IV formulation not commercially available in the US] or equivalent [e.g., methylprednisolone 80 mg]) administered 30 minutes to 2 hours prior to *each* ofatumumab infusion. Depending on individual patient tolerance of ofatumumab infusions, reduction of the corticosteroid dose administered prior to ofatumumab doses 3–8 and 10–12 may be feasible; however, the dose of corticosteroid administered prior to ofatumumab doses 1, 2, and 9 should *not* be reduced. Over the course of doses 3–8, the corticosteroid dose may be gradually reduced with successive infusions if the previous infusion did not result in an infusion reaction of grade 3 or greater. If dose 9 of ofatumumab does not result in an infusion reaction of grade 3 or greater, a prednisolone dose of 50–100 mg (or equivalent) may be administered prior to doses 10–12.

■ **Administration** Ofatumumab is administered by IV infusion. *The drug should not be administered by rapid IV injection, such as IV push or bolus.* After dilution, ofatumumab infusion solution should be administered using an administration set and the inline filter provided by the manufacturer. Solutions of the drug should be administered via an infusion pump. Other IV solutions or drugs should not be administered simultaneously through the same IV line with ofatumumab infusion. The infusion line should be flushed with 0.9% sodium chloride injection before and after IV ofatumumab administration.

The manufacturer states that no incompatibilities between ofatumumab and PVC or polyolefin bags and administration sets have been observed.

Dilution Commercially available ofatumumab injection concentrate must be diluted prior to IV administration.

Ofatumumab injection concentrate and diluted solutions of the drug should be inspected visually for particulate matter and discoloration prior to administration. Solutions of the drug should be clear to opalescent and colorless but may contain a small amount of visible translucent-to-white, amorphous ofatumumab particulates; the drug should be discarded if the solution is discolored or cloudy or if foreign particulate matter is present. The vials should *not* be shaken.

For a 300-mg dose of ofatumumab (dose 1 in the 12-dose regimen), the injection concentrate is prepared for infusion by first withdrawing and discarding 15 mL of solution from an infusion bag containing 1 L of 0.9% sodium chloride injection; a total of 15 mL of ofatumumab injection concentrate is then withdrawn from 3 single-use vials (each labeled as containing 100 mg in 5 mL) of the drug and added to the infusion bag to yield a final concentration of 0.3 mg/mL.

For a 2-g dose of ofatumumab (doses 2–12 in the 12-dose regimen), the injection concentrate is prepared for infusion by first withdrawing and discarding 100 mL of solution from an infusion bag containing 1 L of 0.9% sodium chloride injection; a total of 100 mL of ofatumumab injection concentrate is then withdrawn from 2 single-use vials (each labeled as containing 1 g in 50 mL) of the drug and added to the infusion bag to yield a final concentration of 2 mg/mL.

Following addition of the injection concentrate to the infusion fluid, the IV bag should be gently inverted to mix the solution. The diluted drug may be stored at 2–8°C for up to 24 hours; infusion of diluted ofatumumab solutions should begin within 12 hours of preparation. Ofatumumab should not be admixed with any other drug.

Rate of Administration The initial ofatumumab dose (300 mg; dose 1) should be infused IV as a 0.3-mg/mL solution at an initial rate of 3.6 mg/hour (12 mL/hour); if infusion-related events do not occur, the infusion rate may be doubled (from 12 mL/hour to 25, 50, 100, and then 200 mL/hour) every 30 minutes to a maximum rate of 60 mg/hour (200 mL/hour). The second dose of ofatumumab (2 g; dose 2) should be infused as a 2-mg/mL solution at an initial rate of 24 mg/hour (12 mL/hour); if infusion-related events do not occur, the infusion rate may be doubled (from 12 mL/hour to 25, 50, 100, and then 200 mL/hour) every 30 minutes to a maximum rate of 400 mg/hour (200 mL/hour). Subsequent doses of ofatumumab (2 g each; doses 3–12) should be infused as a 2-mg/mL solution at an initial rate of 50 mg/hour (25 mL/hour); if infusion-related events do not occur, the infusion rate may be doubled (from 25 mL/hour to 50, 100, 200, and then 400 mL/hour) every 30 minutes to a maximum rate of 800 mg/hour (400 mL/hour).

In patients experiencing infusion-related reactions of *any* severity, the manufacturer recommends interruption of the infusion. If the reaction is grade 4 in severity, the infusion should not be resumed. If the reaction is grade 1–3, the infusion may be restarted once the reaction has resolved completely or if it remains grade 2 or less in severity. For grade 1 and 2 reactions, the infusion should be resumed at one-half the previous infusion rate. For grade 3 reactions, the infusion should be resumed at 12 mL/hour. After the infusion has been resumed, the infusion rate may be increased as tolerated by doubling the rate (as described in the previous paragraph) every 30 minutes. (See Infusion-related Effects under Warnings/Precautions: Other Warnings and Precautions, in Cautions.)

■ **Dosage** The recommended adult dosage of ofatumumab for the treatment of B-cell chronic lymphocytic leukemia (B-CLL) that is refractory to fludarabine and alemtuzumab is an initial dose of 300 mg (dose 1) followed one week later by 2 g administered weekly for 7 doses (doses 2–8), then followed 4 weeks later by 2 g administered every 4 weeks for 4 doses (doses 9–12).

■ **Special Populations** No special population dosage recommendations at this time.

Cautions

■ **Contraindications** The manufacturer states there are no known contraindications to the use of ofatumumab.

■ **Warnings/Precautions** ***Warnings*** **Patients Infected with Hepatitis B Virus.** Reactivation of hepatitis B virus (HBV) infection has been reported in patients receiving anti-CD20 monoclonal antibodies, including ofatumumab, and has resulted in fulminant hepatitis, hepatic failure, and death. HBV reactivation has been reported in patients who are hepatitis B surface antigen-positive [HBsAg-positive]; HBsAg-negative and hepatitis B core antibody-positive [anti-HBc-positive]; or HBsAg-negative, anti-HBc-positive, and hepatitis B surface antibody-positive [anti-HBs-positive].

Following review of the Adverse Event Reporting System (AERS) database, the US Food and Drug Administration (FDA) identified 106 cases of fatal HBV-related acute liver injury in patients receiving rituximab (between November 1997 and August 2012) and 3 such cases in patients receiving ofatumumab (between October 2009 and August 2012); 32 of these case reports contained sufficient data to meet the criteria for HBV reactivation. In this review, acute liver injury was attributed to HBV reactivation if seroconversion of HBsAg from negative to positive occurred in those with either anti-HBc or a history of HBV, or if an increase in serum HBV DNA level occurred in those who were HBsAg-positive prior to therapy with an anti-CD20 monoclonal antibody (i.e., rituximab, ofatumumab). HBV reactivation was diagnosed by seroconversion of HBsAg in most (69%) cases. In this review, the duration of rituximab or ofatumumab therapy prior to diagnosis of HBV reactivation was highly variable, ranging from 63 days after initiation of the drug to 12 months following the last dose; however, delayed onset of HBV reactivation (up to 24 months following completion of rituximab therapy) has been reported. All of the patients experiencing HBV reactivation had received recent or concomitant therapy with other immunosuppressive agents. Among patients with HBV reactivation, 10% received HBV antiviral prophylaxis and 28% received antiviral treatment for HBV reactivation.

To decrease the risk of HBV reactivation, all patients should be screened for HBV infection by measuring HBsAg and anti-HBc before initiating treatment with ofatumumab. Hepatitis experts should be consulted regarding monitoring and use of antiviral therapy in those with evidence of HBV infection (HBsAg-positive with any antibody status or HBsAg-negative and anti-HBc-positive); although data are limited, treatment guidelines from some experts recommend the use of prophylactic antiviral therapy in patients who are chronic carriers of HBV. Patients with evidence of current or prior HBV infection should be monitored for clinical and laboratory evidence of hepatitis or HBV reactivation during ofatumumab therapy and for several months thereafter, since reactivation has occurred more than 12 months following completion of anti-CD20 monoclonal antibody therapy. Ofatumumab and any concomitant chemotherapy should be discontinued immediately if HBV reactivation occurs, and appropriate treatment for HBV infection should be initiated. Concomitant chemotherapy should be discontinued until the HBV infection has been controlled or has resolved. Clinicians with expertise in managing HBV infection should be consulted regarding resumption of ofatumumab therapy once control of the reactivated HBV infection has been achieved. It has not been established whether ofatumumab can be safely readministered in patients who develop HBV reactivation.

Progressive Multifocal Leukoencephalopathy. Progressive multifocal leukoencephalopathy (PML), which may be fatal, has been reported in patients receiving anti-CD20 monoclonal antibodies, including ofatumumab. The possible diagnosis of PML should be considered in any patient receiving ofatumumab who experiences new onset or worsening of neurologic manifestations. If PML is suspected, the drug should be discontinued and diagnostic evaluation, including consultation with a neurologist, should be considered as clinically indicated.

Other Warnings and Precautions **Infusion-related Effects.** In patients experiencing infusion-related reactions of *any* severity, the ofatumumab infusion should be interrupted. For patients experiencing a grade 4 reaction, the manufacturer recommends that the infusion not be resumed. For patients experiencing a grade 1–3 reaction, the infusion may be restarted at a slower infusion rate (see Rate of Administration under Dosage and Administration: Administration) once the reaction has completely resolved or if it remains at grade 2 or less in severity. Appropriate treatment and supportive care should be provided for severe infusion reactions including angina or any other manifestation of myocardial ischemia.

In a clinical trial in patients with moderate to severe chronic obstructive pulmonary disease, grade 3 bronchospasm occurred in 2 of 5 patients during ofatumumab infusions.

Tumor Lysis Syndrome. Tumor lysis syndrome has been reported in patients receiving anti-CD20 monoclonal antibodies, including ofatumumab. Appropriate measures (e.g., aggressive IV hydration, antihyperuricemic therapy, correction of blood chemistries, monitoring of renal function) should be employed as clinically indicated.

Hematologic Effects. Severe, prolonged (lasting 1 week or longer) neutropenia and anemia have been reported; thrombocytopenia may occur. In patients with relapsed or refractory B-CLL (Hx-CD20-406 study), grade 3 or 4 neutropenia occurred in 24 or 18%, respectively, of patients with a normal baseline neutrophil count. In the subset of patients with fludarabine- and alemtuzumab-refractory B-CLL, the incidences of grade 3–4 neutropenia and anemia were 12 and 8%, respectively.

Complete blood cell counts (CBCs) and platelet counts should be monitored at regular intervals during ofatumumab therapy; if a grade 3 or 4 cytopenia occurs, the manufacturer recommends more frequent hematologic monitoring.

Hepatitis B Virus Infection. Fatal HBV infection has been reported in patients who were not previously infected with the virus. Patients should be monitored for clinical and laboratory evidence of hepatitis.

Intestinal Obstruction. Small bowel obstruction has been reported in patients receiving ofatumumab. A diagnostic evaluation should be performed in patients who present with symptoms suggestive of intestinal obstruction (e.g., abdominal pain, repeated vomiting).

Immunization. The safety of immunization with live viral vaccines during or following ofatumumab therapy has not been established. The manufacturer recommends that live viral vaccines be avoided in patients who have recently received ofatumumab therapy. The ability of patients who have received ofatumumab therapy to generate a primary or anamnestic humoral response to any vaccine also has not been studied.

Therapy Monitoring. CBCs and platelet counts should be monitored at regular intervals during ofatumumab therapy; the manufacturer recommends more frequent monitoring if a grade 3 or 4 cytopenia occurs.

Infectious Complications. Bacterial, viral, or fungal infections were reported in 70% of patients with relapsed or refractory B-CLL (Hx-CD20-406 study) receiving ofatumumab; serious (grade 3 or 4) or fatal infections occurred in 29 or 12%, respectively, of patients receiving the drug. In the subset of patients with fludarabine- and alemtuzumab-refractory B-CLL, the incidence of fatal infections was 17%.

Immunogenicity. There is potential for immunogenicity with the use of therapeutic proteins such as ofatumumab. In one study, tests for antibodies to ofatumumab yielded negative results in 33 and 39% of patients tested after the eighth and twelfth doses, respectively, of the drug; test results were inconclusive in the remainder of patients because of interference by high concentrations of circulating ofatumumab with the enzyme-linked immunosorbent assay (ELISA).

Specific Populations **Pregnancy.** Category C. (See Users Guide.)

Lactation. It is not known whether ofatumumab is distributed into milk in humans. Human immunoglobulin G (IgG) is distributed into milk, although systemic absorption of these maternal antibodies in breast-fed infants does not appear to be substantial. Because the effects of local GI and limited systemic exposure to ofatumumab are unknown, the drug should be used with caution in nursing women.

Pediatric Use. Safety and efficacy have not been established in children.

Geriatric Use. Clinical studies of ofatumumab in patients with refractory CLL did not include sufficient numbers of patients 65 years of age and older to determine whether geriatric patients respond differently than younger patients. Among patients 21–86 years of age, age did not appear to substantially affect the pharmacokinetics of the drug.

Hepatic Impairment. Safety and efficacy have not been established.

Renal Impairment. Safety and efficacy have not been established. Among patients with baseline creatinine clearances within the range of 33–287 mL/minute, creatinine clearance did not appear to substantially affect the pharmacokinetics of ofatumumab.

■ **Common Adverse Effects** Adverse events reported in 10% or more of patients receiving ofatumumab include neutropenia, pneumonia, pyrexia, cough, diarrhea, anemia, fatigue, dyspnea, rash, nausea, bronchitis, and upper respiratory infection.

Drug Interactions

No formal drug interactions studies have been performed to date.

Description

Ofatumumab, a recombinant fully human anti-CD20 monoclonal antibody, is an antineoplastic agent. The drug is an IgG_1 kappa immunoglobulin that was generated using transgenic mice and hybridoma technology and is produced in a recombinant murine cell line. Ofatumumab binds specifically to antigen CD20, a glycoprotein expressed on the surface of normal and malignant B-lymphocytes, including B-cell chronic lymphocytic leukemia (B-CLL) cells. Following binding of the Fab domain of ofatumumab to antigen CD20, the Fc domain triggers a host immune response causing lysis of the B-cell; the exact mechanism of cell lysis has not been fully elucidated but is thought to involve complement-dependent cytotoxicity (CDC) and antibody-dependent cell-mediated cytotoxicity (ADCC).

Whereas rituximab (a chimeric human-murine anti-CD20 monoclonal antibody) recognizes the large-loop epitope on antigen CD20 to elicit a CDC response, ofatumumab recognizes an epitope that also includes the small loop, which is located in closer proximity to the cell membrane. Compared with rituximab, ofatumumab exhibits higher affinity for antigen CD20 in vitro (as manifested by slower dissociation from the CD20 binding site) and appears to display more potent CDC activity against B-cell lines in vitro (due to enhanced cytotoxicity against both rituximab-resistant and low-CD20-expressing B-CLL cells). In addition, because ofatumumab recognizes an epitope of the antigen binding site that is located in closer proximity to the cell membrane, ofatumumab may be more efficient than rituximab in binding complement proteins (C1q), which may explain the greater complement-mediated lysis of CD20-expressing B-cells observed with ofatumumab in nonclinical models. The clinical importance of these differences remains to be established.

In patients with fludarabine- and alemtuzumab-refractory B-CLL, the median decrease in circulating CD19+ B-cells after doses 8 and 12 in the 12-dose ofatumumab regimen was 91 and 85%, respectively. The time required for lymphocytes, including CD19+ B-cells, to recover to normal levels following treatment with ofatumumab has not been fully determined.

Ofatumumab is eliminated through both an antigen CD20-independent route and a B-cell-mediated route. Clearance is dose dependent over the dose range of 100 mg to 2 g; after sequential doses of the drug, clearance is decreased substantially because of B-cell depletion. In one study, the mean half-life determined between the fourth and twelfth doses was approximately 14 days (range 2.3–61.5 days).

Advice to Patients

Risk of infusion-related reactions; importance of reporting signs and symptoms of such reactions, including fever, chills, rash, or breathing difficulty, that occur within 24 hours of an infusion of the drug.

Risk of cytopenias; importance of reporting bleeding, easy bruising, petechiae, pallor, worsening weakness, or fatigue.

Risk of infection; importance of reporting signs or symptoms of infection (e.g., cough, fever).

Risk of progressive multifocal leukoencephalopathy; importance of reporting new or worsening neurologic symptoms (e.g., confusion, dizziness or loss of balance, difficulty speaking or walking, changes in vision).

Risk of reactivation of hepatitis B virus (HBV) infection; importance of reporting worsening fatigue or icteric changes. Importance of informing clinician of presence of HBV carrier state or of any history of HBV infection.

Risk of small bowel obstruction; importance of reporting new or worsening abdominal pain or nausea or a marked increase in feeling unwell.

Importance of routine monitoring of blood cell counts.

Advise patients that they should not receive a live viral vaccine if they have recently received ofatumumab.

Importance of women informing clinicians if they are or plan to become pregnant or plan to breast-feed.

Importance of informing clinicians of existing or contemplated concomitant therapy, including prescription and OTC drugs, as well as any concomitant illnesses.

Importance of informing patients of other important precautionary information. (See Cautions.)

Overview® (see Users Guide). For additional information on this drug until a more detailed monograph is developed and published, the manufacturer's labeling should be consulted. It is *essential* that the manufacturer's labeling be consulted for more detailed information on usual cautions, precautions, contraindications, potential drug interactions, laboratory test interferences, and acute toxicity. For further information on the handling of antineoplastic agents, see the ASHP Guidelines on Handling Hazardous Drugs at http://www.ahfsdruginformation.com.

Preparations

Excipients in commercially available drug preparations may have clinically important effects in some individuals; consult specific product labeling for details.

Ofatumumab (recombinant)

Parenteral		
For injection concentrate, for IV infusion	20 mg/mL	Arzerra®, GlaxoSmithKline

Olaparib

■ Olaparib, an inhibitor of poly(adenosine diphosphate [ADP]-ribose) polymerase (PARP), is an antineoplastic agent.

Uses

■ **Ovarian Cancer** Olaparib is used as single-agent therapy for the treatment of adults with confirmed or suspected deleterious germline BRCA-mutated (gBRCA-mutated) advanced ovarian cancer previously treated with 3 or more chemotherapy regimens. The drug has been designated an orphan drug by the FDA for the treatment of this cancer. An FDA-approved companion diagnostic test (BRACAnalysis CDx) is required to confirm the presence of mutations in the BRCA genes (BRCA1 and BRCA2) prior to initiation of olaparib therapy. Women with mutations that result in defective BRCA genes are more likely to develop ovarian cancer. It is estimated that approximately 10–15% of all cases of ovarian cancer are associated with these hereditary BRCA mutations.

Olaparib received FDA approval for the treatment of gBRCA-mutated advanced ovarian cancer in December 2014 under the agency's accelerated review program, which allows approval of a drug to treat a serious or life-threatening disease based on clinical data demonstrating that the drug has an effect on a surrogate endpoint that is likely to predict clinical benefit to patients (e.g., prolongation of overall survival, amelioration of disease-related symptoms). Olaparib's accelerated approval for this indication was based on the drug's effect on objective response rate and duration of response; continued approval may be contingent on verification and description of clinical benefit of olaparib in confirmatory trials (e.g., SOLO-2 study).

In June 2014, the FDA Oncologic Drugs Advisory Committee (ODAC) initially reviewed olaparib for potential use as maintenance therapy in patients with platinum-sensitive relapsed ovarian cancer with germline BRCA mutation. The committee reviewed data from a multicenter, double-blind, placebo-controlled, phase 2 study of olaparib (study 19), which included a preplanned retrospective analysis of outcomes by BRCA status and concluded that, despite a 7-month median improvement in progression-free survival, the results of the analysis did not support accelerated approval of olaparib as maintenance therapy in patients with platinum-sensitive ovarian cancer harboring deleterious BRCA1 or BRCA2 mutations. ODAC recommended postponing consideration of accelerated approval of olaparib for the treatment of deleterious BRCA1- or BRCA2-mutated advanced ovarian cancer until results of the confirmatory study, SOLO-2, became available. Following ODAC's initial decision, the manufacturer submitted additional information supporting olaparib's approval for a different indication: use in patients with germline BRCA-mutated advanced ovarian cancer who have received 3 or more chemotherapy regimens. FDA's subsequent accelerated approval for this indication was based principally on efficacy data from a multicenter, open-label, noncomparative, phase 2 study of olaparib (study 1; also called study 42) as well as safety data from several other clinical studies, including a placebo-controlled study.

In the principal efficacy study (study 1), 137 adult patients with confirmed or suspected deleterious BRCA-mutated ovarian cancer previously treated with 3 or more chemotherapy regimens received olaparib monotherapy (400 mg twice daily) until disease progression or unacceptable toxicity occurred. The median age of patients enrolled in the study was 58 years. Most of the patients had an ECOG performance status of 0–1 (93%) and confirmed or suspected deleterious BRCA1 or BRCA2 mutation was verified retrospectively in 97% of the patients for whom blood samples were available by the companion diagnostic test, BRACAnalysis CDx, which is FDA-labeled for selection of patients for olaparib therapy. Patients enrolled in the study received a median of 5 prior chemotherapy regimens. The primary efficacy end points were overall response rate and duration of response. The overall response rate in this study was 34%, with a complete response reported in 2% and a partial response reported in 32% of the patients. At the time of the analysis, the median duration of response was 7.9 months.

Dosage and Administration

■ **General** Because myelodysplastic syndrome (MDS) and acute myelogenous leukemia (AML) have been reported in patients receiving olaparib, the manufacturer states that complete blood cell (CBC) counts should be obtained prior to initiation of olaparib and monthly during therapy with the drug. (See Myelodysplastic Syndrome/Acute Myeloid Leukemia under Cautions: Warnings/Precautions.)

Restricted Distribution Program Olaparib can only be obtained through a specialty pharmacy. Clinicians may contact the specialty pharmacy at 844-275-2360 or consult the Lynparza® website for specific ordering and availability information (http://www.lynparza.com/assets/pdf/how-to-order-lynparza.pdf).

■ **Administration** Olaparib is administered orally twice daily. The prescribing information for olaparib in the US does not provide specific instructions concerning administration with regard to food; in the European Union, the manufacturer recommends taking olaparib at least one hour after meals and preferably up to 2 hours before the next meal since food can delay absorption of the drug. (See Description.) The capsules should be swallowed whole and should *not* be chewed, dissolved, or opened.

Olaparib capsules should be stored at 25°C but may be exposed to temperatures ranging from 15–30°C; exposure to temperatures greater than 40°C should be avoided. The capsules should not be taken if they are suspected of having been exposed to temperatures exceeding 40°C or if the capsules appear deformed or show evidence of leakage.

■ **Dosage** ***Ovarian Cancer*** The recommended adult dosage of olaparib for the treatment of confirmed or suspected deleterious germline BRCA-mutated (as detected by an FDA-approved companion diagnostic test) advanced ovarian cancer is 400 mg (eight 50-mg capsules) twice daily (total daily dosage of 800 mg). Therapy should be continued until disease progression or unacceptable toxicity occurs.

If a dose of olaparib is missed, patients should *not* take an extra dose. The next dose should be taken at the regularly scheduled time.

Dosage Modification for Toxicity If adverse reactions occur, interruption of therapy or dosage reduction of olaparib should be considered. The recommended initial dosage reduction is to 200 mg (four 50-mg capsules) twice daily (total daily dosage of 400 mg). If further dosage reduction is necessary, the dosage should be reduced to 100 mg (two 50-mg capsules) twice daily (total daily dosage of 200 mg). Dosages less than 100 mg twice daily are not recommended.

Concomitant Use of Drugs Affecting Hepatic Microsomal Enzymes Concomitant use of olaparib with drugs that are moderate or potent inhibitors of cytochrome P-450 (CYP) isoenzyme 3A should be avoided. If concomitant use of a *potent* CYP3A inhibitor cannot be avoided, the manufacturer recommends reducing the dosage of olaparib to 150 mg (three 50-mg capsules) twice daily. If concomitant use of a *moderate* CYP3A inhibitor cannot be avoided, the manufacturer recommends reducing the dosage of olaparib to 200 mg (four 50-mg capsules) twice daily. (See Inhibitors of CYP3A under Drug Interactions: Drugs Affecting Hepatic Microsomal Enzymes.)

■ **Special Populations** The manufacturer makes no specific dosage recommendations for patients with hepatic impairment. (See Hepatic Impairment under Warnings/Precautions: Specific Populations, in Cautions.)

The manufacturer states that no adjustment to the initial dosage of olaparib is necessary in patients with mild renal impairment; however, such patients should be closely monitored for possible toxicity during therapy. Olaparib has not been studied in patients with moderate or severe renal impairment, including in those receiving dialysis, and the manufacturer provides no specific dosage recommendations for such patients. (See Renal Impairment under Warnings/Precautions: Specific Populations, in Cautions.)

The manufacturer makes no specific dosage recommendations for geriatric patients. (See Geriatric Use under Warnings/Precautions: Specific Populations, in Cautions.)

Cautions

■ **Contraindications** The manufacturer states that there are no known contraindications to the use of olaparib.

■ **Warnings/Precautions** ***Myelodysplastic Syndrome/Acute Myeloid Leukemia*** In clinical studies, myelodysplastic syndrome (MDS) and acute myeloid leukemia (AML) were reported in less than 1% of olaparib-treated patients; all of these patients had received previous chemotherapy with platinum-containing agents and/or other DNA-damaging antineoplastic agents. Most of the MDS/AML cases (77%) were fatal. The duration of olaparib therapy in patients who developed secondary MDS/cancer therapy-related AML varied from less than 6 months to over 2 years.

Complete blood cell (CBC) counts should be monitored at baseline and then monthly in patients receiving olaparib. In addition, olaparib therapy should not be initiated until patients have recovered from hematologic toxicity caused by previous chemotherapy (to grade 1 or less). If prolonged hematologic toxicity occurs during therapy, olaparib should be withheld and CBC counts should be monitored weekly until recovery to grade 1 or less. If hematologic toxicity persists for more than 4 weeks following interruption of therapy, patients should be referred to a hematologist for further evaluation, including bone marrow analysis and cytogenetic testing of a blood sample. If MDS/AML is confirmed, olaparib should be discontinued.

Pneumonitis Pneumonitis, which was fatal in some cases, has been reported in less than 1% of patients receiving olaparib therapy. The cases of pneumonitis reported to date had no consistent clinical pattern and were confounded by predisposing factors (including cancer and/or metastases in lungs, preexisting pulmonary disease, history of smoking, and previous chemotherapy and/or radiotherapy).

Olaparib therapy should be interrupted and prompt diagnostic evaluation should occur in patients who have new or worsening pulmonary symptoms (see Advice to Patients) or if a radiologic abnormality occurs. If pneumonitis is confirmed, olaparib should be discontinued and the patient treated appropriately.

Fetal/Neonatal Morbidity and Mortality Based on its mechanism of action and animal findings, olaparib may cause fetal harm in humans; the drug has been shown to be teratogenic, embryotoxic and fetotoxic, and embryolethal in animals. Pregnancy should be avoided during olaparib therapy. If contraceptive methods are being considered, women of childbearing potential should be advised to use highly effective contraception while receiving olaparib and for at least 1 month after discontinuance of therapy. If olaparib is used during pregnancy or if the patient becomes pregnant while receiving the drug, the patient should be apprised of the potential risk to the fetus and the potential risk for loss of the pregnancy. (See Advice to Patients.)

Specific Populations **Pregnancy.** Category D. (See Users Guide and see Fetal/Neonatal Morbidity and Mortality under Cautions: Warnings/Precautions.)

Lactation. It is not known whether olaparib is distributed into human milk. Because many drugs are distributed into human milk and because of the potential for serious adverse reactions to olaparib in nursing infants, a decision should be made whether to discontinue nursing or the drug, taking into account the importance of the drug to the woman.

Pediatric Use. Safety and efficacy of olaparib have not been established in pediatric patients. In addition, pharmacokinetic studies of olaparib in pediatric patients have not been conducted to date.

Geriatric Use. In clinical studies evaluating olaparib in patients with advanced solid tumors (the majority [69%] of whom had ovarian cancer), 20% of patients were 65 years of age or older. The safety profile of olaparib was similar regardless of patient age in these studies, except that grade 3 or greater adverse reactions occurred more frequently in patients 65 years of age or older compared with younger patients (approximately 53 versus 43%, respectively). (See Dosage and Administration: Special Populations.)

Hepatic Impairment. The safety, efficacy, and pharmacokinetics of olaparib have not been studied in patients with hepatic impairment. Patients with serum bilirubin concentrations exceeding 1.5 times the upper limit of normal (ULN) and ALT and/or AST concentrations 2.5 or more times the ULN in the absence of liver metastases or ALT and/or AST concentrations exceeding 5 times the ULN in the presence of liver metastases were excluded from clinical studies of the drug. (See Dosage and Administration: Special Populations.)

Renal Impairment. Mean peak plasma concentrations and systemic exposure of olaparib were increased by 1.2- and 1.5-fold, respectively, in patients with mild renal impairment (creatinine clearance 50–80 mL/minute) compared with individuals with normal renal function. The manufacturer recommends that patients with mild renal impairment be closely monitored for possible olaparib toxicity. (See Dosage and Administration: Special Populations.)

The pharmacokinetics of olaparib have not been studied in patients with moderate or severe renal impairment (creatinine clearance less than 50 mL/minute) or in those receiving dialysis.

■ **Common Adverse Effects** Adverse effects reported in 20% or more of patients receiving olaparib monotherapy for ovarian cancer in clinical trials include fatigue (including asthenia), nausea, abdominal pain or discomfort, vomiting, diarrhea, nasopharyngitis or pharyngitis, dyspepsia, back pain, headache, dermatitis or rash, decreased appetite, myalgia, arthralgia or musculoskeletal pain, cough, and dysgeusia.

Laboratory abnormalities reported in 20% or more of patients receiving olaparib include anemia, elevated mean corpuscular volume (MCV), lymphopenia, thrombocytopenia, elevated serum creatinine, and neutropenia.

Drug Interactions

Olaparib is metabolized principally by cytochrome P-450 (CYP) isoenzyme 3A4. In vitro, olaparib is a substrate of CYP3A4 and P-glycoprotein (P-gp). In vitro studies also indicate that olaparib inhibits CYP3A4 and induces CYP2B6 at higher concentrations than are achieved clinically.

In vitro, olaparib is an inhibitor of breast cancer resistance protein (BCRP), organic anion transport protein (OATP) 1B1, organic cation transporter (OCT) 1 and OCT2, organic anion transporter (OAT) 3, and multidrug and toxic compound extrusion (MATE) 1 and MATE2K; the clinical relevance of these findings is not known.

■ **Drugs Affecting Hepatic Microsomal Enzymes** ***Inhibitors of CYP3A*** Concomitant use of olaparib with moderate or potent inhibitors of CYP3A may result in increased plasma concentrations of olaparib. When the potent CYP3A inhibitor itraconazole was administered concomitantly with olaparib, peak plasma concentrations and systemic exposure of olaparib were increased by 1.4- and 2.7-fold, respectively. Simulations using physiologically-based pharmacokinetic models suggest that concomitant administration of fluconazole, a moderate CYP3A inhibitor, and olaparib may increase peak plasma concentrations and systemic exposure of olaparib by 1.1-fold and two-fold, respectively.

Concomitant use of olaparib with moderate (e.g., amprenavir [no longer commercially available in the US], aprepitant, atazanavir, ciprofloxacin, crizotinib, diltiazem, erythromycin, fluconazole, fosamprenavir, imatinib, *ritonavir-boosted* darunavir, verapamil) or potent inhibitors of CYP3A (e.g., boceprevir, clarithromycin, indinavir, itraconazole, ketoconazole, *ritonavir-boosted* lopinavir, nefazodone, nelfinavir, posaconazole, ritonavir, saquinavir, telaprevir [no longer commercially available in the US], telithromycin, voriconazole) should be avoided, and selection of an alternative drug with less CYP3A inhibition potential should be considered. If concomitant use of the moderate or potent CYP3A inhibitor cannot be avoided, the manufacturer recommends reducing the dosage of olaparib to 150 mg twice daily during concomitant administration of a potent CYP3A inhibitor and to 200 mg twice daily during concomitant administration of a moderate CYP3A inhibitor. (See Concomitant Use of Drugs Affecting Hepatic Microsomal Enzymes under Dosage and Administration: Dosage.)

Inducers of CYP3A Concomitant use of olaparib with moderate or potent inducers of CYP3A may result in decreased plasma concentrations of olaparib. When the potent CYP3A inducer rifampin was administered concomitantly with olaparib, peak plasma concentrations and systemic exposure of olaparib were decreased by 71 and 87%, respectively. Simulations using physiologically-based pharmacokinetic models suggest that concomitant administration of the moderate CYP3A inducer efavirenz and olaparib may decrease peak plasma concentrations and systemic exposure of olaparib by 20–30 and 50–60%, respectively.

Concomitant use of olaparib with moderate (e.g., bosentan, efavirenz, etravirine, modafinil, nafcillin) or potent inducers of CYP3A (e.g., carbamazepine, phenytoin, rifampin, St. John's wort [*Hypericum perforatum*]) should be avoided. If concomitant use of a moderate CYP3A inducer cannot be avoided, the potential for reduced efficacy of olaparib should be considered.

■ **Antineoplastic Agents** Myelosuppression may be potentiated or prolonged when olaparib is used concomitantly with other antineoplastic agents known to cause myelosuppression. (See Myelodysplastic Syndrome/Acute Myeloid Leukemia under Cautions: Warnings/Precautions.)

■ **Grapefruit and Seville Oranges** The manufacturer states that grapefruit products and Seville oranges are known to inhibit CYP3A and should be avoided because of the potential for increased plasma olaparib concentrations during concurrent use.

Description

Olaparib, an inhibitor of mammalian poly(adenosine diphosphate [ADP]-ribose) polymerase (PARP) enzymes, including PARP-1, PARP-2, and PARP-3, is an antineoplastic agent. PARP enzymes are involved in normal cellular homeostasis, including DNA transcription, cell cycle regulation, and DNA repair. In vitro studies have demonstrated that olaparib-induced cytotoxicity may involve inhibition of PARP enzymatic activity and increased formation of PARP-DNA complex, which result in disruption of cellular homeostasis and apoptosis. PARP inhibitors such as olaparib appear to be selective for tumor cells that harbor certain homologous recombination deficiencies, including those harboring BRCA1 and BRCA2 mutations. In vitro, olaparib inhibited growth of select tumor cell lines. In addition, olaparib reduced tumor growth of xenograft models of human cancer in mice both as a single agent or following platinum-based chemotherapy. Increased cytotoxicity and anti-tumor activity were observed following olaparib treatment in BRCA-deficient cell lines and mouse tumor models.

Following oral administration, olaparib is rapidly absorbed with peak plasma concentrations usually occurring within 1–3 hours. Following repeated doses of olaparib, systemic accumulation of the drug was not observed. Steady-state concentrations are reached within 3–4 days. Administration of olaparib with a high-fat meal delayed the rate of absorption (time to peak concentrations delayed by 2 hours), but did not substantially affect the extent of absorption (mean area under the serum concentration-time curve [AUC] increased by approximately 20%). Limited data suggest that systemic exposure of olaparib increases less than proportionally with dose over the dose range of 100–400 mg; however, data were variable across the studies. Olaparib is primarily metabolized by the cytochrome P-450 (CYP) isoenzyme 3A4. Following oral administration of a single radiolabeled dose of olaparib, 44% of the radioactivity was recovered in urine and 42% was recovered in feces; the majority of the dose was excreted as metabolites. Olaparib is approximately 82% bound to plasma proteins when given at the recommended dosage. The mean terminal plasma half-life of the drug is 11.9 hours.

Advice to Patients

Importance of providing a copy of written patient information (medication guide) each time olaparib is dispensed. Importance of advising patients to read the patient information before taking olaparib and each time the prescription is refilled.

Importance of advising patients to swallow olaparib capsules whole and not to chew, dissolve, or open the capsules. Importance of also advising patients to avoid grapefruit, grapefruit juice, and Seville oranges while taking the drug.

If a dose is missed, importance of advising patients not to take an extra dose and to take the next normal dose at the regularly scheduled time.

Importance of informing patients that olaparib capsules should be stored at room temperature (20–25°C) and that exposure to temperatures greater than 40°C should be avoided. Importance of advising patients that olaparib capsules should not be taken if they are suspected of having been exposed to temperatures exceeding 40°C or if they appear deformed or show evidence of leakage.

Risk of MDS/AML. Importance of informing clinician if fatigue/asthenia, fever, weight loss, frequent infections, bruising, unusual bleeding (including hematuria or bloody stool), or shortness of breath occurs.

Importance of hematologic monitoring during olaparib therapy.

Risk of pneumonitis. Importance of informing clinician if new or worsening respiratory symptoms, including shortness of breath, fever, cough, or wheezing, occur.

Importance of advising patients that mild or moderate nausea and/or vomiting commonly occurs with olaparib therapy; patients experiencing these symptoms should contact their clinician for advice on available antiemetic treatment options.

Risk of fetal harm and pregnancy loss. Necessity of advising women of childbearing potential to avoid pregnancy and to use a highly effective method of contraception while receiving olaparib and for at least 1 month following discontinuance of therapy. Importance of women informing clinicians immediately if they become pregnant during therapy or think they may be pregnant. If pregnancy occurs, advise pregnant women of potential risk to the fetus.

Importance of advising women to avoid breast-feeding while receiving olaparib therapy.

Importance of informing clinicians of existing or contemplated concomitant therapy, including prescription and OTC drugs and dietary or herbal supplements (e.g., St. John's wort), as well as any concomitant illnesses (e.g., respiratory disorders, liver or kidney damage).

Importance of informing patients of other important precautionary information. (See Cautions.)

Overview® (see Users Guide). For additional information on this drug until a more detailed monograph is developed and published, the manufacturer's labeling should be consulted. It is *essential* that the manufacturer's labeling be consulted for more detailed information on usual cautions, precautions, contraindications, potential drug interactions, laboratory test interferences, and acute toxicity. For further information on the handling of antineoplastic agents, see the ASHP Guidelines on Handling Hazardous Drugs at http://www.ahfsdruginformation.com.

Preparations

Distribution of olaparib is restricted. (See Restricted Distribution Program under Dosage and Administration: General.)

Excipients in commercially available drug preparations may have clinically important effects in some individuals; consult specific product labeling for details.

Olaparib

Oral

Capsules	50 mg	**Lynparza®**, AstraZeneca

Olaratumab

■ Olaratumab, a recombinant human IgG_1 monoclonal antibody that specifically binds to platelet-derived growth factor receptor alpha (PDGFR-α), is an antineoplastic agent.

Uses

■ **Soft Tissue Sarcoma** Olaratumab is used in combination with doxorubicin for the treatment of soft tissue sarcoma that is not amenable to curative treatment with surgery or radiation therapy; patients must have a histologic subtype for which an anthracycline-containing regimen is appropriate. The accelerated approval of olaratumab for this indication is based on progression-free and overall survival. Continued approval for this indication may be contingent on verification and description of clinical benefit of olaratumab in confirmatory studies. Olaratumab has been designated an orphan drug by FDA for the treatment of this cancer.

The current indication for olaratumab is based principally on the results of an open-label, randomized, phase 1b/phase 2 study in adults with locally advanced or metastatic soft tissue sarcoma (excluding Kaposi's sarcoma) that was not amenable to curative treatment with surgery or radiation therapy. Patients with a histologic subtype that may be treated with an anthracycline-containing regimen were enrolled; however, prior use of an anthracycline was not permitted. In the phase 2 portion of this study, 133 adults were randomized in a 1:1 ratio to receive either olaratumab (15 mg/kg by IV infusion on days 1 and 8 of each 21-day cycle) in combination with doxorubicin hydrochloride (75 mg/m^2 by IV infusion on day 1 of each 21-day cycle for a maximum of 8 cycles) or doxorubicin alone; patients were permitted to receive dexrazoxane prior to doxorubicin during cycles 5–8. Olaratumab was continued until disease progression or unacceptable toxicity occurred. The primary end point of this study was progression-free survival as assessed by independent blinded review according to Response Evaluation Criteria in Solid Tumors (RECIST); secondary end points included overall survival and overall response rate. The median age of patients enrolled in the phase 2 portion of this study was 58 years (range: 22–86 years); 86% of patients were white, 95% had an ECOG (Eastern Cooperative Oncology Group) performance status of 0 or 1, 38% had leiomyosarcoma histology, and 1.5% had synovial sarcoma histology. Most patients (65%) had not received chemotherapy for metastatic disease. About one-half of the patients randomized to doxorubicin alone received single-agent olaratumab following disease progression.

At the time of analysis, patients receiving olaratumab and doxorubicin had longer median progression-free survival compared with patients receiving doxorubicin alone (8.2 versus 4.4 months, respectively). A planned analysis of overall survival indicated that patients receiving olaratumab and doxorubicin had longer median overall survival compared with patients receiving doxorubicin alone (26.5 versus 14.7 months, respectively). In addition, patients receiving combined therapy with olaratumab and doxorubicin appeared to have a higher overall response rate (18.2 versus 7.5%, respectively) compared with those receiving doxorubicin alone. A subset analysis of overall survival based on clinically relevant baseline patient and disease characteristics consistently showed treatment benefit with combined therapy with olaratumab and doxorubicin compared with doxorubicin alone. However, given the small size of the study and the heterogeneity of the study population, confirmation of clinical benefit is necessary.

Dosage and Administration

■ **General** Clinicians should consult the respective manufacturers' labelings for information on the dosage and method of administration of other antineoplastic agents used in combination regimens.

Because of the risk of infusion-related reactions associated with olaratumab, the manufacturer recommends premedication with diphenhydramine hydrochloride 25–50 mg and dexamethasone phosphate 10–20 mg administered IV prior to olaratumab on day 1 of cycle 1. Severe infusion-related reactions can occur despite premedication. Olaratumab should be administered in a setting where resuscitation equipment is readily available. (See Infusion-related Effects under Cautions: Warnings/Precautions.)

Restricted Distribution Program Olaratumab can only be obtained through specialty distributors and pharmacies. Clinicians may consult the Lartruvo® website for specific availability information (https://www.lartruvo.com/hcp/resources).

■ **Administration** Olaratumab is administered by IV infusion over 60 minutes. *The drug should not be administered by rapid IV injection, such as IV push or bolus.* Olaratumab should *not* be administered simultaneously through the same IV line with any other drug or electrolytes. The infusion line should be flushed with 0.9% sodium chloride injection after olaratumab administration.

Dilution Prior to administration, olaratumab injection concentrate must be diluted.

Olaratumab injection concentrate and diluted solutions of the drug should be inspected visually for particulate matter and discoloration; the drug should be discarded if the solution is discolored or if particulate matter is present. Olaratumab injection concentrate should be clear to slightly opalescent and colorless to slightly yellow. The vials should *not* be shaken or frozen.

Olaratumab is diluted by withdrawing the appropriate dose (15 mg/kg) of olaratumab injection concentrate from a vial labeled as containing 10 mg/mL and diluting it in 0.9% sodium chloride injection to yield a final volume of 250 mL. The diluted olaratumab solution for infusion should be mixed by gentle inversion and should *not* be shaken. Olaratumab injection concentrate should *not* be diluted in dextrose-containing solutions or any other solutions. Commercially available olaratumab injection concentrate contains no preservatives and is intended for single use; any partially used vials should be discarded.

Diluted olaratumab solution may be stored under refrigeration (2–8°C) for up to 24 hours followed by an additional 4 hours (including infusion time) at room temperature (below 25°C); the diluted solution should be brought to room temperature prior to administration.

■ **Dosage** ***Soft Tissue Sarcoma*** For the treatment of soft tissue sarcoma that is not amenable to curative treatment with surgery or radiation therapy, but for which an anthracycline-containing regimen is appropriate, the recommended dosage of olaratumab is 15 mg/kg administered by IV infusion over 60 minutes on days 1 and 8 of each 21-day cycle until disease progression or unacceptable toxicity occurs. For cycles 1–8, doxorubicin also is administered.

Dosage Modification for Toxicity **Infusion-related Effects.** If grade 1 or 2 infusion-related reactions occur, the olaratumab infusion should be interrupted; upon resolution of the infusion-related reaction, the infusion may be resumed but the rate of infusion should be reduced by 50%. If grade 3 or 4 infusion-related reactions occur, olaratumab should be permanently discontinued. (See Infusion-related Effects under Cautions: Warnings/Precautions.)

Neutropenia. If febrile neutropenia, neutropenic infection, or prolonged grade 4 neutropenia (lasting longer than 1 week) occurs, olaratumab therapy should be withheld until the absolute neutrophil count (ANC) reaches or exceeds 1000/mm^3; therapy may then be resumed at a *permanently* reduced dosage of 12 mg/kg.

■ **Special Populations** The manufacturer makes no specific dosage recommendations for geriatric patients or patients with hepatic or renal impairment. (See Specific Populations under Cautions: Warnings/Precautions.)

Cautions

■ **Contraindications** The manufacturer states there are no known contraindications to the use of olaratumab.

■ **Warnings/Precautions** ***Infusion-related Effects*** Infusion-related reactions, sometimes fatal, have been reported in patients receiving olaratumab. In clinical studies, infusion-related reactions occurred in 14% of patients receiving the drug, with the first occurrence generally reported during the first 2 cycles. The frequency of infusion-related reactions was similar regardless of administration of premedication. Infusion-related reactions may include flushing, dyspnea, bronchospasm, fever/chills, severe hypotension, anaphylactic shock, or cardiac arrest. In clinical studies, infusion-related reactions requiring interruption of the infusion or permanent discontinuance of olaratumab therapy occurred in 10 or 2.3% of patients, respectively. Olaratumab therapy was resumed in all patients experiencing grade 1 or 2 infusion-related reactions; however, grade 1 or 2 infusion-related reactions recurred in 12 of 59 patients (20%) following resumption of the infusion.

The manufacturer states that premedication with IV diphenhydramine hydrochloride and IV dexamethasone phosphate should be administered prior to the first dose of olaratumab during cycle 1. (See Dosage and Administration: General.) Patients should be monitored during and following infusions of the drug for manifestations of infusion-related reactions. If infusion-related reactions occur, temporary interruption of the infusion followed by reduction in the infusion rate or permanent discontinuance of olaratumab may be required. (See Infusion-related Effects under Dosage: Dosage Modification for Toxicity, in Dosage and Administration.)

Combination Therapy When olaratumab in used in combination with doxorubicin, the usual cautions, precautions, and contraindications associated with doxorubicin must be considered in addition to those associated with olaratumab. For further information regarding warnings and precautions associated with doxorubicin, see Cautions in Doxorubicin Hydrochloride 10:00.

Fetal/Neonatal Morbidity and Mortality There are no adequate and well-controlled studies of olaratumab in pregnant women; however, based on its mechanism of action and animal findings, olaratumab can cause fetal harm. In animal models, disruption of platelet-derived growth factor receptor alpha (PDGFR-α) signaling has been associated with teratogenicity (i.e., cleft face, spina bifida) and embryofetal lethality. Teratogenicity (i.e., abnormal eyelid development, skeletal malformations) was observed in pregnant mice receiving 50 or 150 mg/kg of an antimurine PDGFR-α antibody IV every 3 days (exposure levels less than the human exposure at the recommended olaratumab dosage); however, embryotoxicity (i.e., postimplantation loss) occurred at a dose as low as 5 mg/kg.

Pregnancy should be avoided during olaratumab therapy. Women of childbearing potential should be advised to use an effective method of contraception while receiving olaratumab and for 3 months after discontinuance of therapy. If olaratumab is used during pregnancy or if the patient becomes pregnant while receiving the drug, the patient should be apprised of the potential fetal hazard.

Immunogenicity There is potential for immunogenicity with the use of therapeutic proteins such as olaratumab. Anti-olaratumab antibodies were detected by enzyme-linked immunosorbent assay (ELISA) in 13 of 370 patients (3.5%) treated with olaratumab in clinical studies; neutralizing antibodies were detected in all of these patients. The clinical importance of anti-olaratumab antibodies has not been established.

Impairment of Fertility In animal models, loss of PDGFR-α signaling resulted in decreased testicular size, Leydig cell loss, and spermatogenic arrest, suggesting that olaratumab may impair male fertility. The effect of olaratumab on fertility in humans is not known.

Specific Populations **Pregnancy.** Olaratumab can cause fetal harm if administered to pregnant women based on its mechanism of action and animal findings. (See Fetal/Neonatal Morbidity and Mortality under Cautions: Warnings/Precautions.)

Lactation. It is not known whether olaratumab is distributed into milk. Because of the potential for serious adverse reactions to olaratumab in nursing infants, women should be advised to discontinue nursing during olaratumab therapy. Women may begin nursing 3 months after discontinuance of therapy. The effects of the drug on nursing infants or on milk production are unknown.

Pediatric Use. Safety and efficacy of olaratumab have not been established in pediatric patients.

Geriatric Use. Clinical studies of olaratumab did not include sufficient numbers of patients 65 years of age and older to determine whether geriatric patients respond differently than younger patients. Among patients 22–85 years of age, age did not appear to substantially affect the pharmacokinetics of the drug.

Hepatic Impairment. Mild (total bilirubin concentration not exceeding the upper limit of normal [ULN] with AST concentration exceeding the ULN, or total bilirubin concentration more than 1 times but not more than 1.5 times the ULN with any AST concentration) to moderate (total bilirubin concentration more than 1.5 times but not more than 3 times the ULN with any AST concentration) hepatic impairment did not appear to substantially affect the pharmacokinetics of olaratumab. Olaratumab has not been studied in patients with severe hepatic impairment (total bilirubin concentration exceeding 3 times the ULN with any AST concentration).

Renal Impairment. Mild to moderate renal impairment (creatinine clearance of 30–89 mL/minute) did not appear to substantially affect the pharmacokinetics of olaratumab. Olaratumab has not been studied in patients with severe renal impairment (creatinine clearance of 15–29 mL/minute).

■ **Common Adverse Effects** Adverse effects reported in 10% or more of patients receiving olaratumab in combination with doxorubicin and at an incidence that is at least 5% higher than that reported with doxorubicin alone include nausea, fatigue, musculoskeletal pain, mucositis, alopecia, vomiting, diarrhea, decreased appetite, abdominal pain, pyrexia, neuropathy, headache, peripheral edema, infusion-related reactions (including hypersensitivity and angioedema), anxiety, and dry eyes. Laboratory abnormalities reported in more than 10% of patients receiving olaratumab in combination with doxorubicin and at an incidence that is at least 5% higher than that reported with doxorubicin alone include lymphopenia, neutropenia, thrombocytopenia, hyperglycemia, leukopenia, increased activated partial thromboplastin time (aPTT), hypokalemia, hypophosphatemia, increased alkaline phosphatase concentrations, and hypomagnesemia.

Drug Interactions

■ **Antineoplastic Agents** ***Doxorubicin*** Concomitant administration of olaratumab (15 mg/kg) with doxorubicin (75 mg/m^2) in patients with solid tumors did not substantially alter systemic exposure to olaratumab or doxorubicin.

Description

Olaratumab, a recombinant human IgG_1 monoclonal antibody that specifically binds to platelet-derived growth factor receptor alpha (PDGFR-α), is an antineoplastic agent. PDGFR-α, a receptor tyrosine kinase (RTK) expressed on cells of mesenchymal origin, is involved in intracellular signaling events that lead to cell proliferation, differentiation, and migration essential for the development and survival of mesenchymal cells. Overactivity of PDGFR-α signaling can influence processes critical for tumor progression (e.g., oncogenesis, metastasis, maintenance of the tumor microenvironment). Olaratumab binds specifically to PDGFR-α and blocks the interaction of PDGFR-α with its ligands

(PDGF-AA and PDGF-BB) and PDGFR-α activation by PDGF-AA, PDGF-BB, and PDGF-CC, resulting in inhibition of downstream signaling. In vitro and in vivo, olaratumab with or without doxorubicin has demonstrated antitumor activity against selected sarcoma cell lines; the drug also has been shown to disrupt PDGFR-α signaling in tumor implant models.

Steady-state concentrations are reached during cycle 3 following administration of olaratumab 15 mg/kg IV on days 1 and 8 along with doxorubicin hydrochloride 75 mg/m^2 IV on day 1 of each 21-day cycle. The estimated elimination half-life of olaratumab is approximately 11 days.

The pharmacokinetics of olaratumab do not appear to be affected substantially by age (22–85 years), gender, race, mild to moderate renal impairment, and mild to moderate hepatic impairment. Clearance of the drug increases with increasing body weight.

Advice to Patients

Risk of infusion-related reactions; importance of reporting signs and symptoms of such reactions, including flushing, dyspnea, bronchospasm, and fever/chills.

Risk of fetal harm. Necessity of advising women of childbearing potential that they should use an effective method of contraception while receiving the drug and for 3 months after discontinuance of therapy. Importance of women informing clinicians if they are pregnant. If pregnancy occurs, advise pregnant women of potential risk to the fetus.

Necessity of advising women to avoid breast-feeding during therapy and for 3 months after discontinuance of therapy.

Importance of informing clinicians of existing or contemplated concomitant therapy, including prescription and OTC drugs, as well as any concomitant illnesses.

Importance of informing patients of other important precautionary information. (See Cautions.)

Overview® (see Users Guide). For additional information on this drug until a more detailed monograph is developed and published, the manufacturer's labeling should be consulted. It is *essential* that the manufacturer's labeling be consulted for more detailed information on usual cautions, precautions, contraindications, potential drug interactions, laboratory test interferences, and acute toxicity. For further information on the handling of antineoplastic agents, see the ASHP Guidelines on Handling Hazardous Drugs at http://www.ahfsdruginformation.com.

Preparations

Distribution of olaratumab is restricted. (See Restricted Distribution Program under Dosage and Administration: General.)

Excipients in commercially available drug preparations may have clinically important effects in some individuals; consult specific product labeling for details.

Olaratumab

Parenteral

For injection concentrate, for IV infusion	10 mg/mL (190 and 500 mg)	**Lartruvo®**, Lilly

Omacetaxine Mepesuccinate

Homoharringtonine, HHT

■ Omacetaxine mepesuccinate, a protein synthesis inhibitor, is an antineoplastic agent.

Uses

■ **Chronic Myelogenous Leukemia.** Omacetaxine mepesuccinate is used for the treatment of chronic myelogenous leukemia (CML) in adults who are in the chronic or accelerated phase of the disease after failure (secondary to resistance and/or intolerance) of prior therapy with 2 or more tyrosine kinase inhibitors. The drug has been designated an orphan drug by the US Food and Drug Administration (FDA) for use in this condition. The current indication for omacetaxine mepesuccinate is based on hematologic and cytogenetic response rates; there currently are no controlled trials demonstrating a clinical benefit (e.g., improvement in disease-related symptoms, increased survival) with the drug.

The current indication for omacetaxine mepesuccinate is based principally on data from 2 open-label, noncomparative, multicenter trials in adults with CML following failure of prior tyrosine kinase inhibitor therapy; the inclusion criteria for one of the trials also required that patients have the T315I Bcr-Abl mutation (see Description). Efficacy of the drug was evaluated using a combined cohort of patients from these trials who had received at least 2 tyrosine kinase inhibitors (imatinib, dasatinib, or nilotinib) and had, at a minimum, documented evidence of resistance or intolerance to dasatinib and/or nilotinib. Resistance was defined as a lack of or loss of complete hematologic response by 12 weeks, cytogenetic response by 24 weeks, or major cytogenetic response by 52 weeks or as progressive leukocytosis. Intolerance to tyrosine kinase inhibitors was defined as grade 3 or 4 nonhematologic toxicity that did not resolve with adequate intervention, grade 4 hematologic toxicity lasting more than 7 days, or any toxicity of grade 2 or worse that was unacceptable to the patient. In these trials, omacetaxine mepesuccinate was administered at an induction dosage of 1.25 mg/m^2 subcutaneously twice daily for 14 days of a 28-day treatment cycle; once a response was achieved, dosage was reduced to 1.25 mg/m^2 twice daily for 7 days every 28 days for maintenance therapy. Patients were eligible to receive up to 24 months of maintenance treatment.

The efficacy analysis included a total of 76 patients with chronic phase CML and 35 patients with accelerated phase CML. These patients were heavily pretreated; about 47% of patients with chronic phase CML and 63% of those with accelerated phase CML had a history of treatment failure following 3 tyrosine kinase inhibitors (imatinib, dasatinib, and nilotinib), and most also had received other therapies for CML (e.g., hydroxyurea, interferon, cytarabine). In patients with chronic phase CML, treatment with omacetaxine mepesuccinate resulted in a major cytogenetic response (defined as elimination or substantial reduction [to 35% or less] of Philadelphia chromosome-positive [Ph$^+$] hematopoietic cells) in 18% of the patients; the mean time to major cytogenetic response was 3.5 months and the median duration of such response was 12.5 months. The complete cytogenetic response rate in patients with chronic phase CML was 8%. Among patients with accelerated phase CML, 14% achieved a major hematologic response (defined as complete hematologic response or no evidence of leukemia); the mean time to major hematologic response was 2.3 months and the median duration of such response was 4.7 months. None of the patients with accelerated phase CML achieved a major cytogenetic response.

Dosage and Administration

■ **General** Because omacetaxine mepesuccinate may cause myelosuppression, complete blood cell counts (CBCs) should be monitored routinely (i.e., weekly during induction and initial maintenance cycles, then every 2 weeks thereafter or as clinically indicated).

■ **Reconstitution and Administration** Omacetaxine mepesuccinate is administered by subcutaneous injection.

Although the drug has been self-administered in clinical trials, the manufacturer states that omacetaxine mepesuccinate should be prepared and administered by a healthcare professional; procedures for proper handling (e.g., use of gloves or protective clothing) and disposal of antineoplastic agents should be followed. If omacetaxine mepesuccinate comes in contact with the skin, the affected area should be washed immediately and thoroughly with soap and water.

Omacetaxine mepesuccinate powder for injection should be stored at 20–25°C until use and retained in the original carton for protection from light. Prior to administration, the lyophilized powder should be reconstituted by adding 1 mL of 0.9% sodium chloride injection to a vial labeled as containing 3.5 mg of the drug to provide a solution containing 3.5 mg/mL. Following addition of the diluent, the vial should be gently swirled until a clear solution is obtained; complete dissolution of the powder usually occurs in less than 1 minute. If not used immediately, reconstituted solutions of omacetaxine mepesuccinate may be stored at room temperature and administered within 12 hours of reconstitution or stored at 2–8°C and administered within 24 hours of reconstitution; the solution should be protected from light during storage.

■ **Dosage** The recommended induction dosage of omacetaxine mepesuccinate for adults with chronic or accelerated phase chronic myelogenous leukemia (CML) following failure of prior therapy with 2 or more tyrosine kinase inhibitors is 1.25 mg/m^2 twice daily for 14 consecutive days of a 28-day cycle. Cycles should be repeated every 28 days until a hematologic response is achieved. Patients should then receive a maintenance dosage of 1.25 mg/m^2 twice daily for 7 consecutive days of a 28-day treatment cycle.

The optimal duration of omacetaxine mepesuccinate therapy has not been established; the manufacturer recommends that treatment be continued as long as the patient is deriving clinical benefit. In clinical trials, the median duration of therapy was 7.4 months (median of 6 treatment cycles) in patients with chronic phase CML and 1.9 months (median of 2 treatment cycles) in those with accelerated phase CML.

Dosage Modification for Toxicity **Hematologic Toxicity.** Treatment cycles should be delayed and/or the number of dosing days per cycle reduced in patients who experience hematologic toxicities (e.g., neutropenia, thrombocytopenia). If grade 4 neutropenia (absolute neutrophil count [ANC] less than 500/mm^3) or grade 3 thrombocytopenia (platelet count less than 50,000/mm^3) occurs, the subsequent treatment cycle should be delayed until the ANC is at least 1000/mm^3 and the platelet count is at least 50,000/mm^3. In addition, the number of consecutive dosing days in the subsequent treatment cycle should be reduced by 2 (e.g., to 12 days in patients receiving an induction dosage or to 5 days in those receiving a maintenance dosage).

Nonhematologic Toxicity. Clinically important nonhematologic toxicities (e.g., diarrhea, hyperglycemia) should be managed symptomatically; in addition, therapy with omacetaxine mepesuccinate should be interrupted and/or delayed until such toxicities have resolved.

■ **Special Populations** The manufacturer makes no special population dosage recommendations at this time. Because omacetaxine mepesuccinate is not substantially eliminated renally (i.e., less than 15% of a dose is recovered as unchanged drug in urine), some clinicians suggest that dosage adjustments may not be required in patients with renal impairment.

Cautions

■ **Contraindications** The manufacturer states that there are no contraindications to the use of omacetaxine mepesuccinate.

■ **Warnings/Precautions** ***Hematologic Effects*** Myelosuppression is the major dose-limiting toxicity associated with omacetaxine mepesuccinate therapy. In an analysis of pooled data from 3 trials involving 163 patients with chronic or accelerated phase chronic myelogenous leukemia (CML), grade 3 or 4 thrombocytopenia was reported in 85–88% of patients, grade 3 or 4 neutropenia was reported in 71–81% of patients, and grade 3 or 4 anemia was reported in 62–80% of patients receiving omacetaxine mepesuccinate. Myelosuppression generally was reversible and was managed with treatment delays and/or a reduction in the number of dosing days per treatment cycle; however, some patients developed serious infections, febrile neutropenia, or major bleeding as a complication of myelosuppression. Fatalities related to severe myelosuppression were reported in approximately 3% of patients in the 3 clinical trials combined.

Complete blood cell counts (CBCs) should be performed routinely during omacetaxine mepesuccinate therapy. The manufacturer and other experts recommend that CBCs be monitored weekly during induction and initial maintenance cycles, then every 2 weeks or as clinically indicated thereafter. Dosage modifications may be required if severe hematologic toxicities occur. (See Hematologic Toxicity under Dosage: Dosage Modification for Toxicity, in Dosage and Administration.) In clinical trials, administration of hematopoietic agents (e.g., filgrastim, epoetin alfa, darbepoetin alfa) was required in some patients who developed myelosuppression. Patients with neutropenia should be monitored frequently for symptoms of infection and fever because of an increased risk of infections. (See Advice to Patients.)

Bleeding Omacetaxine mepesuccinate causes severe thrombocytopenia, which can increase the risk of bleeding. (See Hematologic Effects, under Cautions: Warnings/Precautions.) Severe bleeding events, including at least 4 cases of fatal cerebral hemorrhage and 3 cases of severe, but nonfatal GI hemorrhage, have been reported in patients with CML receiving omacetaxine mepesuccinate in clinical trials. Most of these bleeding events were associated with severe thrombocytopenia.

Platelet counts should be monitored routinely during omacetaxine mepesuccinate therapy as part of the recommended CBC monitoring schedule. (See Advice to Patients and also see Drug Interactions: Drugs Affecting Hemostasis.)

Hyperglycemia Omacetaxine mepesuccinate may cause glucose intolerance and hyperglycemia. In clinical trials in patients receiving the drug for treatment of chronic or accelerated phase CML, hyperglycemia was reported in about 66% of patients; about 11% of the patients had grade 3 or 4 hyperglycemia, which included at least 1 case of hyperosmolar nonketotic hyperglycemia.

Blood glucose concentrations should be monitored frequently during omacetaxine mepesuccinate therapy, particularly in patients with preexisting diabetes mellitus or risk factors for diabetes mellitus. Patients with poorly controlled diabetes mellitus should not receive omacetaxine mepesuccinate until good glycemic control has been established.

Fetal /Neonatal Morbidity and Mortality Omacetaxine mepesuccinate may cause fetal harm; fetotoxic effects, including delayed fetal development (e.g., incomplete or reduced ossification, decreased fetal body weight), and embryolethality have been demonstrated in animals. There are no adequate and well-controlled studies in pregnant women.

Women of childbearing potential should be advised to avoid pregnancy during omacetaxine mepesuccinate therapy. If the drug is used during pregnancy or if the patient becomes pregnant while receiving the drug, the patient should be apprised of the potential fetal hazard.

Specific Populations **Pregnancy.** Category D. (See Users Guide.) (See Fetal/Neonatal Morbidity and Mortality, under Cautions: Warnings/Precautions.)

Lactation. It is not known whether omacetaxine mepesuccinate is distributed into milk. Because many drugs are distributed into milk and because of the potential for serious adverse effects of omacetaxine mepesuccinate in nursing infants, a decision should be made whether to discontinue nursing or the drug, taking into account the importance of the drug to the woman.

Pediatric Use. Safety and efficacy of omacetaxine mepesuccinate have not been established in pediatric patients. The drug has been used in a limited number of acutely ill children with refractory or recurrent leukemia; however, long-term effects of the drug on growth and development are not known.

Geriatric Use. In the cohort of patients in whom efficacy of omacetaxine mepesuccinate as third-line or subsequent therapy for CML was evaluated, approximately 30% of patients with chronic phase CML and 46% of those with accelerated phase CML were 65 years of age or older. Differences in response rates were observed between these patients and younger adults; older patients with accelerated phase CML had higher rates of major hematologic response compared with younger adults (31 versus 0%), while older patients with chronic phase CML had lower rates of major cytogenetic response than younger adults (9 versus 23%). Age-related differences in safety also were observed, with geriatric patients 65 years of age or older experiencing a higher incidence of toxicity, particularly hematologic toxicity.

Hepatic Impairment. Formal studies evaluating the effects of hepatic impairment on the disposition of omacetaxine mepesuccinate have not been conducted. In a population pharmacokinetic analysis, mild hepatic impairment (total bilirubin concentration not exceeding 1.5 times the upper limit of normal [ULN] and AST greater than the ULN) did not appear to affect the pharmacokinetics of the drug.

Renal Impairment. Formal studies evaluating the effects of renal impairment on the disposition of omacetaxine mepesuccinate have not been conducted. In a population pharmacokinetic analysis, creatinine clearances of 50–80 or less than 50 mL/minute did not appear to affect the pharmacokinetics of the drug.

■ **Common Adverse Effects** Adverse effects reported in 10% or more of patients with chronic phase or accelerated phase CML receiving omacetaxine mepesuccinate following failure of therapy with 2 or more tyrosine kinase inhibitors include thrombocytopenia, anemia, neutropenia, leukopenia, bone marrow failure, febrile neutropenia, lymphopenia, diarrhea, nausea, vomiting, constipation, abdominal pain, fatigue, asthenia, anorexia, extremity pain, back pain, headache, insomnia, arthralgia, peripheral edema, injection site reaction, pyrexia, infection, chills, cough, dyspnea, epistaxis, alopecia, rash, and increased serum concentrations of glucose, uric acid, and creatinine.

Drug Interactions

Clinical drug interaction studies have not been conducted to date with omacetaxine mepesuccinate. In vitro studies indicate that the drug is not a substrate of cytochrome P-450 (CYP) isoenzymes and does not inhibit major CYP isoenzymes at clinically relevant concentrations; the potential for omacetaxine mepesuccinate to induce CYP isoenzymes has not been determined.

In vitro studies indicate that omacetaxine mepesuccinate is a substrate of P-glycoprotein (P-gp), but does not appear to inhibit P-gp at clinically relevant concentrations.

■ **Drugs Affecting Hemostasis** Since omacetaxine mepesuccinate can cause severe thrombocytopenia, which can increase the risk of bleeding, the manufacturer states that concomitant use of the drug with aspirin, anticoagulants, or nonsteroidal anti-inflammatory agents (NSAIAs) should be avoided in patients with platelet counts less than 50,000/mm^3.

Description

Omacetaxine mepesuccinate, a protein synthesis inhibitor, is an antineoplastic agent. The drug is a semisynthetic form of a natural cephalotaxine alkaloid found in the leaves of various members of the *Cephalotaxus* genus of evergreen trees native to Asia. Although the exact mechanism of action of omacetaxine mepesuccinate has not been fully elucidated, the drug is known to inhibit protein synthesis at the point of early protein translation by binding to the A-site cleft in the peptidyl-transferase center of the large ribosomal subunit, thereby interfering with peptide elongation. Preliminary data suggest that omacetaxine mepesuccinate induces apoptosis by causing a rapid loss of short-lived proteins, such as the antiapoptotic protein myeloid cell leukemia-1 (Mcl-1), that are upregulated in leukemic cells and act to regulate proliferation and survival of these cells. The drug has been shown in vitro to reduce levels of Mcl-1 as well as levels of Bcr-Abl tyrosine kinase, an abnormal protein that is associated with the development of chronic myelogenous leukemia (CML). Unlike tyrosine kinase inhibitors, omacetaxine mepesuccinate exerts its antileukemic effects independent of direct Bcr-Abl binding.

Clinical resistance to tyrosine kinase inhibitors in CML has been attributed to several mechanisms, but point mutations in the Bcr-Abl kinase domain appear to be the most common, occurring in up to 40–60% of patients who develop resistance. One of these mutations is the T315I Bcr-Abl mutation, which confers resistance to the tyrosine kinase inhibitors bosutinib, dasatinib, imatinib, and nilotinib. Omacetaxine mepesuccinate has exhibited antileukemic activity against CML in the presence of the Bcr-Abl T315I mutation in vivo in murine models and in early clinical studies. In vitro, the drug has exhibited additive or synergistic activity with imatinib when the drugs were used sequentially against imatinib-resistant cell lines.

Omacetaxine mepesuccinate is rapidly absorbed following subcutaneous administration; peak plasma concentrations of the drug are achieved in approximately 30 minutes. Omacetaxine mepesuccinate is primarily hydrolyzed by plasma esterases to an inactive 4'-desmethyl derivative; the drug undergoes minimal hepatic microsomal oxidation and/or esterase-mediated metabolism in vitro. The major route of elimination of omacetaxine mepesuccinate is not known; following subcutaneous administration, approximately 12–15% of a dose is excreted unchanged in urine and the mean elimination half-life is approximately 6–7 hours.

Advice to Patients

Importance of advising patients that omacetaxine mepesuccinate can decrease blood cell counts and that routine monitoring of blood cell counts is necessary. Importance of patients informing a clinician immediately if they experience fever or other symptoms of infection, shortness of breath, substantial fatigue, or any unusual bleeding or bruising; confusion, slurred speech, or altered vision also may be symptoms suggestive of bleeding.

Importance of advising patients with diabetes mellitus about the increased risk of hyperglycemia and the need for careful blood glucose monitoring during therapy.

Importance of advising patients of the possibility of adverse GI effects, including nausea, diarrhea, abdominal pain, constipation, and vomiting, and to notify a clinician if such manifestations persist.

Importance of advising patients to avoid driving or operating machinery if fatigue occurs.

Importance of advising patients that omacetaxine mepesuccinate may cause rash or hair loss and to immediately report a severe or worsening rash or itching.

Importance of informing clinicians of existing or contemplated concomitant therapy, including prescription and OTC drugs, as well as any concomitant illnesses.

Importance of women informing clinicians if they are or plan to become pregnant or plan to breast-feed. Importance of advising women of childbearing age about the potential for fetotoxic effects, and to avoid pregnancy and nursing while receiving the drug.

Importance of informing patients of other important precautionary information. (See Cautions.)

Overview® (see Users Guide). For additional information on this drug until a more detailed monograph is developed and published, the manufacturer's labeling should be consulted. It is *essential* that the manufacturer's labeling be consulted for more detailed information on usual cautions, precautions, contraindications, potential drug interactions, laboratory test interferences, and acute toxicity. For further information on the handling of antineoplastic agents, see the ASHP Guidelines on Handling Hazardous Drugs at http://www.ahfsdruginformation.com.

Preparations

Excipients in commercially available drug preparations may have clinically important effects in some individuals; consult specific product labeling for details.

Omacetaxine Mepesuccinate

Parenteral		
For Injection, for subcutaneous use	3.5 mg	**Synribo®**, Teva

Osimertinib Mesylate

■ Osimertinib mesylate, a third-generation inhibitor of receptor tyrosine kinases, is an antineoplastic agent.

Uses

■ **Non-small Cell Lung Cancer** ***First-line Therapy for Metastatic Non-small Cell Lung Cancer*** Osimertinib mesylate is used for the first-line treatment of metastatic non-small cell lung cancer (NSCLC) in patients whose tumors harbor epidermal growth factor receptor (EGFR) exon 19 deletions (del19) or exon 21 (L858R) substitution mutations as detected by an FDA-approved diagnostic test (e.g., cobas® EGFR Mutation Test). Information on FDA-approved companion diagnostic tests for the detection of EGFR mutations in NSCLC is available at http://www.fda.gov/CompanionDiagnostics. Osimertinib has been designated an orphan drug by FDA for the treatment of EGFR mutation-positive NSCLC. A progression-free survival benefit has been observed in adults with previously untreated EGFR mutation-positive metastatic NSCLC receiving osimertinib compared with patients receiving erlotinib or gefitinib.

EGFR-activating mutations are present in approximately 15–22% of NSCLC cases in North America and Europe and are present in up to 30–50% of cases in patients of East Asian descent. The majority of EGFR mutations are exon 19 deletions and an L858R substitution in exon 21, which together account for about 90% of EGFR mutations in patients with NSCLC. (See Description.)

The current indication for osimertinib in the first-line treatment of metastatic NSCLC is based principally on the results of a randomized, multicenter, double-blind phase 3 study (FLAURA) in adults with previously untreated locally advanced or metastatic NSCLC. In this study, 556 patients were randomized (stratified by race and EGFR mutation) in a 1:1 ratio to receive either osimeritinib (80 mg orally once daily) or investigator's choice of gefitinib (250 mg orally once daily) or erlotinib (150 mg orally once daily) until disease progression or unacceptable toxicity occurred. The primary measure of efficacy was progression-free survival (as evaluated by the investigator). Patients with CNS metastases not requiring corticosteroid therapy and whose condition was neurologically stable for at least 2 weeks following completion of surgery or radiation therapy were eligible for this study. The median age of patients was 64 years (range: 26–93 years); most patients (95%) had metastatic disease, 64% had never smoked, 63% were female, 62% were of Asian ancestry, and 7% had received prior adjuvant or neoadjuvant chemotherapy. All enrolled patients had a World Health Organization (WHO) performance status of 0 or 1 and were required to have evidence of an EGFR mutation (confirmed by the cobas® EGFR Mutation Test or a clinical trial assay); 63% of patients had exon 19 deletions, 37% had exon 21 (L858R) substitution mutations, and less than 1% also had T790M mutations. Approximately 20% of the patients randomized to investigator's choice of erlotinib or gefitinib received osimertinib therapy following disease progression.

At a median follow-up of 15 or 9.7 months in patients receiving osimertinib or investigator's choice of erlotinib or gefitinib, respectively, patients receiving osimertinib had a longer median progression-free survival than those receiving erlotinib or gefitinib (18.9 versus 10.2 months; hazard ratio of 0.46). Effects of osimertinib on investigator-assessed progression-free survival and progression-free survival as assessed by a blinded independent central review committee (BICR) were comparable. The objective response rate in osimertinib-treated patients was 77% compared with 69% in those receiving erlotinib or gefitinib; complete responses were achieved in 2 or 1% of patients, respectively. Patients receiving osimertinib had a longer median duration of response (17.6 versus 9.6 months) compared with those receiving erlotinib or gefitinib. At the time of the progression-free survival analysis, median overall survival had not been reached. Results of subgroup analyses (based on age, gender, WHO performance status, race, smoking status, EGFR mutation, or presence of brain metastases) suggested that the effect of osimertinib on progression-free survival was consistent across all subgroups. In the subgroup of 41 patients with baseline measurable CNS metastases, BICR-assessed CNS objective response rates were 77 or 63% in the osimertinib or investigator's choice of EGFR tyrosine kinase inhibitor groups, respectively, with durable responses of 6 months or more in 47 or 33% of patients, respectively, or 12 months or more in 47 or 33% of patients, respectively; complete responses were achieved in 18% of patients receiving osimertinib and none of those receiving erlotinib or gefitinib.

Previously Treated Metastatic Non-small Cell Lung Cancer Osimertinib mesylate is used for the treatment of metastatic NSCLC in patients with the EGFR T790M mutation (as detected by an FDA-approved diagnostic test) who experienced disease progression during or following EGFR tyrosine kinase inhibitor therapy. Osimertinib is designated an orphan drug by FDA for the treatment of EGFR mutation-positive NSCLC.

The current indication for osimertinib in the treatment of metastatic NSCLC following failure of prior EGFR tyrosine kinase inhibitor therapy is based principally on the results of a randomized, multicenter, open-label, active-controlled study (AURA3) in 419 adults with metastatic EGFR T790M mutation-positive NSCLC (confirmed by the cobas® EGFR Mutation Test) whose disease had progressed while receiving prior systemic therapy, including a first-line EGFR tyrosine kinase inhibitor (e.g., gefitinib, erlotinib, afatinib). Patients were randomized in a 2:1 ratio to receive osimertinib (80 mg orally once daily) or platinum-based chemotherapy (pemetrexed 500 mg/m^2 in combination with either cisplatin 75 mg/m^2 or carboplatin dosed to a target area under the plasma concentration-time curve [AUC] of 5 mg/mL per minute by IV infusion once every 3 weeks for a maximum of 6 cycles); patients receiving platinum-based chemotherapy whose disease had not progressed after 4 cycles were permitted to receive maintenance pemetrexed therapy. Treatment was continued until disease progression, unacceptable toxicity, or study withdrawal occurred. The primary efficacy end point of the study was progression-free survival as assessed by the investigator according to Response Evaluation Criteria in Solid Tumors (RECIST 1.1); secondary end points included objective response rate, duration of response, and overall survival. The median age of patients was 62 years; the majority of patients were female (64%), of Asian ancestry (65%), had never smoked (68%), and had adenocarcinoma histology (84%). Thirty-four percent of the patients had CNS metastases at baseline, among which 11% had measurable disease.

At a median follow-up of 8.3 months, patients receiving osimertinib in the AURA3 study had a longer median investigator-assessed progression-free survival compared with patients receiving platinum-based chemotherapy (10.1 versus 4.4 months). Analysis of progression-free survival according to BICR resulted in similar findings as the investigator assessment. Patients receiving osimertinib also had a higher objective response rate (65 versus 29%) and a longer median duration of response (11 versus 4.2 months) compared with those receiving platinum-based chemotherapy. Complete response was achieved in 1% of patients in both treatment groups. At the time of analysis, overall survival data were not available. In the subgroup of patients with baseline measurable CNS metastases, BICR-assessed CNS objective response rates were 57 or 25% in the osimertinib or platinum-based chemotherapy groups, respectively, with durable responses of 6 months or more in 47 or 0% of patients receiving these respective treatments, or 9 months or more in 12 or 0% of patients receiving these respective treatments; complete responses were achieved in 7% of patients receiving osimertinib and none of those receiving platinum-based chemotherapy.

Dosage and Administration

■ **General** Confirmation of the presence of epidermal growth factor receptor (EGFR) exon 19 deletions (del19) or exon 21 (L858R) substitution mutations in tumor or plasma specimens by an FDA-approved diagnostic test (e.g., cobas® EGFR Mutation Test) is necessary prior to initiating therapy with osimertinib for the first-line treatment of metastatic non-small cell lung cancer (NSCLC). Patients with a negative plasma del19 or L858R mutation result should be reevaluated for the feasibility of a tumor biopsy.

Confirmation of the presence of EGFR T790M mutation in tumor or plasma specimens by an FDA-approved diagnostic test (e.g., cobas® EGFR Mutation Test) is necessary prior to initiating therapy with osimertinib for the treatment of previously treated metastatic NSCLC. Because of the high rate of false-negative results, plasma testing is recommended only when a tumor biopsy cannot be obtained; patients with a negative plasma T790M result should be reevaluated for the feasibility of a tumor biopsy.

Restricted Distribution Osimertinib can only be obtained through a limited network of specialty pharmacies. Clinicians may consult the Tagrisso® website (https://www.tagrissohcp.com) for specific information regarding distribution of the drug.

■ **Administration** Osimertinib is administered orally once daily without regard to meals. The tablets should be swallowed whole and should *not* be crushed.

For patients unable to swallow solids, osimertinib tablets may be dispersed in a container with 60 mL (2 ounces) of noncarbonated water and immediately swallowed; no other liquids should be used. When preparing the drug dispersion, the water should be stirred (without crushing, heating, or ultrasonicating) until the tablet is dispersed (the tablet will not completely dissolve). Following administration, the container should be rinsed with an additional 120–240 mL (4–8 ounces) of water and the contents swallowed immediately to ensure that the full dose is given.

Alternatively, if administration through a nasogastric tube is required, the tablet should be dispersed in a container with 15 mL of noncarbonated water and drawn into a syringe; the container should then be rinsed with an additional 15 mL of water to transfer any residue to the syringe. The resulting 30-mL drug dispersion should be administered through the nasogastric tube, and the tube should be flushed with appropriate volumes of water (approximately 30 mL).

If a dose of osimertinib is missed, the next dose should be taken at the regularly scheduled time; the missed dose should not be taken.

■ **Dosage** Dosage of osimertinib mesylate is expressed in terms of osimertinib.

Non-small Cell Lung Cancer The recommended adult dosage of osimertinib for the initial treatment of EGFR del19 or L858R mutation-positive metastatic NSCLC is 80 mg once daily. Osimertinib therapy should be continued until disease progression or unacceptable toxicity occurs.

The recommended adult dosage of osimertinib for the treatment of EGFR T790M mutation-positive metastatic NSCLC following failure of prior EGFR tyrosine kinase inhibitor therapy is 80 mg once daily. Osimertinib therapy should be continued until disease progression or unacceptable toxicity occurs.

Dosage Modification for Toxicity or Drug Interactions **Dosage Modification for Pulmonary Effects.** If interstitial lung disease or pneumonitis occurs, osimertinib therapy should be permanently discontinued. (See Interstitial Lung Disease/Pneumonitis under Cautions: Warnings/Precautions.)

Dosage Modification for Cardiac Effects. If corrected QT (QT_c) interval exceeds 500 msec on at least 2 separate ECGs, osimertinib therapy should be withheld until the QT_c interval is less than 481 msec or returns to baseline (if baseline QT_c interval is 481 msec or more). Osimertinib therapy may then be resumed at a reduced dosage of 40 mg daily. If QT_c-interval prolongation is accompanied by signs and/or symptoms of life-threatening arrhythmia, the drug should be permanently discontinued. (See Prolongation of QT Interval under Cautions: Warnings/Precautions.)

If symptomatic congestive heart failure occurs, osimertinib should be permanently discontinued. (See Cardiomyopathy under Cautions: Warnings/Precautions.)

Dosage Modification for Other Toxicity. If any other grade 3 or higher adverse reaction occurs, osimertinib therapy should be interrupted for up to 3 weeks. If the adverse reaction improves to grade 2 or less within this time period, the drug may be resumed at the original dosage or at a reduced dosage of 40 mg daily. If there is no improvement within 3 weeks of withholding osimertinib, the drug should be permanently discontinued.

Concomitant Use with CYP3A Inducers. If osimertinib is used concomitantly with a potent inducer of cytochrome P-450 (CYP) isoenzyme 3A, osimertinib dosage should be increased to 160 mg daily. The usual dosage of 80 mg daily should be resumed 3 weeks after the potent CYP3A inducer is discontinued. No dosage adjustment is required when osimertinib is used concomitantly with moderate and/or weak CYP3A inducers. (See Drug Interactions: Drugs Affecting Hepatic Microsomal Enzymes.)

■ **Special Populations** The manufacturer makes no specific dosage recommendations for geriatric patients. (See Geriatric Use under Warnings/Precautions: Specific Populations, in Cautions.)

No dosage adjustment is necessary in patients with mild to severe renal impairment (creatinine clearance 15–89 mL/minute). Insufficient data are available to provide dosage recommendations for patients with end-stage renal disease (creatinine clearance less than 15 mL/minute). (See Renal Impairment under Warnings/Precautions: Specific Populations, in Cautions.)

No dosage adjustment is necessary in patients with mild to moderate hepatic impairment (Child-Pugh class A or B; total bilirubin concentration not exceeding the upper limit of normal [ULN] with AST concentration exceeding the ULN; or total bilirubin concentration 1–3 times the ULN with any AST concentration). Insufficient data are available to provide dosage recommendations for patients with severe hepatic impairment. (See Hepatic Impairment under Warnings/Precautions: Specific Populations, in Cautions.)

Cautions

■ **Contraindications** The manufacturer states that there are no known contraindications to the use of osimertinib mesylate.

■ **Warnings/Precautions** ***Interstitial Lung Disease/Pneumonitis*** Severe or fatal interstitial lung disease/pneumonitis may occur in patients receiving osimertinib. Across all clinical studies, interstitial lung disease or pneumonitis occurred in 3.9% of 1142 osimertinib-treated patients and was fatal in 0.4% of patients receiving the drug.

Osimertinib therapy should be withheld in patients who experience any respiratory manifestations suggestive of interstitial lung disease (e.g., dyspnea, cough, fever). (See Advice to Patients.) If a diagnosis of interstitial lung disease is confirmed, the drug should be permanently discontinued.

Prolongation of QT Interval Prolongation of the corrected QT (QT_c) interval has been reported in patients receiving osimertinib. The prolongation appears to occur in a concentration-dependent manner. Across all clinical studies, QT_c-interval prolongation exceeding 500 msec or an increase from baseline QT_c interval of greater than 60 msec occurred in 0.9 or 3.6%, respectively, of 1142 osimertinib-treated patients. Patients with baseline QT_c interval exceeding 470 msec were excluded from these studies.

The manufacturer recommends periodic monitoring of ECG and serum electrolytes during osimertinib therapy in patients at risk for QT-interval prolongation, including those with congenital long QT syndrome, congestive heart failure, or electrolyte abnormalities, and in those receiving concomitant drugs known to prolong the QT interval with known risk of torsades de pointes. (See Drug Interactions: Drugs that Prolong the QT Interval.) If QT-interval prolongation occurs, dosage reduction, temporary interruption, or permanent discontinuance of therapy may be necessary. (See Dosage Modification for Cardiac Effects under Dosage: Dosage Modification for Toxicity or Drug Interactions, in Dosage and Administration.) If QT_c-interval prolongation is accompanied by signs and/or symptoms of life-threatening arrhythmia, osimertinib therapy should be permanently discontinued.

Cardiomyopathy Cardiomyopathy has been reported in patients receiving osimertinib. Across all clinical studies, cardiomyopathy (defined as acute or chronic cardiac failure, congestive heart failure, pulmonary edema, or decreased ejection fraction) was reported in 2.6% of 1142 osimertinib-treated patients; fatal cardiomyopathy occurred in 0.1% of patients receiving the drug. Across all clinical studies, decreases in left ventricular ejection fraction (LVEF) to less than 50% with a decline of more than 10% from baseline was reported in 3.9% of 908 osimertinib-treated patients who had baseline and follow-up LVEF assessments.

In patients with cardiac risk factors, cardiac function (including LVEF) should be assessed prior to initiating osimertinib and periodically during therapy; LVEF should be assessed in any patient who develops cardiac complications during osimertinib therapy. Osimertinib should be permanently discontinued in patients who develop symptomatic congestive heart failure.

Keratitis Keratitis has been reported in 0.7% of 1142 patients receiving osimertinib in clinical studies. Patients who develop manifestations suggestive of keratitis (e.g., eye inflamation, lacrimation, photosensitivity, blurred vision, eye pain, red eye) should be referred promptly to an ophthalmologist for evaluation.

Fetal/Neonatal Morbidity and Mortality Osimertinib may cause fetal harm if administered to pregnant women based on its mechanism of action and animal findings. Embryofetal toxicity (e.g., postimplantation loss and early embryonic death, decreased fetal weight) has been demonstrated in animals at dose exposures of approximately 1.5 times those observed in humans at the recommended dosage. There are no adequate and well-controlled studies in pregnant women.

Pregnancy should be avoided during therapy. The manufacturer states that pregnancy status should be confirmed prior to initiation of osimertinib therapy in women of childbearing potential and that such women should be advised to use effective contraception during osimertinib therapy and for 6 weeks after the drug is discontinued. In addition, men with female partners of childbearing potential should use effective methods of contraception while receiving the drug and for 4 months after the drug is discontinued.

Impairment of Fertility Results of animal studies suggest that osimertinib may impair female and male fertility. In female rats, administration of osimertinib at a dosage of 20 mg/kg daily (producing peak plasma osimertinib concentrations approximately 1.5 times those observed with the recommended human dosage) from 2 weeks before mating to pregnancy day 8 had no effect on estrus cycles or pregnancy rates, but caused early embryonic deaths; the effects of osimertinib on fertility appeared to be reversible when female rats were mated 1 month after discontinuance of the drug.

Increased preimplantation embryonic loss was observed in untreated female rats mated to osimertinib-treated male rats; it is not known whether these effects are reversible.

Specific Populations **Pregnancy.** Although there are no available data in pregnant women, animal studies suggest that osimertinib may cause fetal harm. (See Fetal/Neonatal Morbidity and Mortality under Cautions: Warnings/Precautions.) If osimertinib is used during pregnancy or if the patient becomes pregnant while receiving the drug, the patient should be apprised of the potential fetal hazard. (See Advice to Patients.)

Lactation. It is not known whether osimertinib is distributed into human milk or if the drug has any effect on milk production or the nursing infant. Adverse effects (e.g., reduced growth rates, neonatal deaths) have been observed in the offspring of rats administered osimertinib during gestation and early lactation. Because of the potential for serious adverse reactions to osimertinib in nursing infants, women should be advised to discontinue nursing while receiving the drug and for 2 weeks after the drug is discontinued.

Pediatric Use. Safety and efficacy of osimertinib have not been established in pediatric patients.

Geriatric Use. In clinical studies of osimertinib, 43% of patients were 65 years of age or older. No overall differences in efficacy were observed based on age; however, an exploratory analysis suggests a higher incidence of grade 3 or 4 adverse reactions and more frequent dosage modifications for adverse reactions in geriatric patients compared with younger adults.

Hepatic Impairment. Population pharmacokinetic analysis suggests that the pharmacokinetics of osimertinib are not substantially altered in patients with mild to moderate hepatic impairment (Child-Pugh class A or B; total bilirubin concentration not exceeding the upper limit of normal [ULN] with AST concentration exceeding the ULN; or total bilirubin concentration 1–3 times the ULN with any AST concentration). The drug has not been studied in patients with severe (total bilirubin concentration 3–10 times the ULN with any AST concentration) hepatic impairment.

Renal Impairment. Population pharmacokinetic analysis suggests that the pharmacokinetics of osimertinib are not substantially altered in patients with mild to severe renal impairment (creatinine clearance of 15–89 mL/minute). The drug has not been studied in patients with end-stage renal disease (creatinine clearance less than 15 mL/minute).

■ **Common Adverse Effects** Adverse effects reported in more than 20% of patients receiving osimertinib for the initial treatment of non-small cell lung cancer (NSCLC) harboring epidermal growth factor receptor (EGFR) exon 19 deletions (del19) or exon 21 (L858R) substitution mutations in the FLAURA study include diarrhea, rash, dry skin, nail toxicity, stomatitis, and fatigue. Laboratory abnormalities reported in at least 20% of patients receiving osimertinib for the initial treatment of EGFR del19 or L858R mutation-positive metastatic NSCLC include lymphopenia, anemia, thrombocytopenia, neutropenia, hyperglycemia, hypermagnesemia, hyponatremia, and elevated concentrations of aminotransferases (i.e., AST, ALT).

Adverse effects reported in more than 20% of patients receiving osimertinib for the treatment of previously treated EGFR T790M mutation-positive metastatic NSCLC in the AURA3 study include diarrhea, rash, dry skin, nail toxicity, and fatigue. Laboratory abnormalities reported in at least 20% of patients receiving osimertinib for the treatment of previously treated EGFR T790M mutation-positive metastatic NSCLC include lymphopenia, thrombocytopenia, anemia, hypermagnesemia, neutropenia, hyponatremia, hyperglycemia, and hypokalemia.

Drug Interactions

Osimertinib mesylate is metabolized principally by cytochrome P-450 (CYP) isoenzyme 3A. In vitro studies indicate that osimertinib induces CYP1A2; the drug does not inhibit CYP1A2, 2A6, 2B6, 2C8, 2C9, 2C19, 2D6, or 2E1.

Osimertinib is a substrate of P-glycoprotein (P-gp) and breast cancer resistance protein (BCRP), but not a substrate of organic anion transport protein (OATP) 1B1 or OATP1B3. Osimertinib inhibits BCRP but does not inhibit organic anion transporter (OAT) 1, OAT3, OATP1B1, OATP1B3, multidrug and toxin extrusion transporter (MATE) 1, MATE2K, or organic cation transporter (OCT) 2.

■ **Drugs Affecting Hepatic Microsomal Enzymes** When the potent CYP3A4 inhibitor itraconazole (200 mg twice daily) was administered concomitantly with osimertinib, peak plasma concentrations of osimertinib decreased by 20% and area under the plasma concentration-time curve (AUC) increased by 24%; however, these changes were not considered to be clinically important.

Concomitant use of osimertinib with potent inducers of CYP3A may decrease plasma concentrations of osimertinib. When the potent CYP3A4 inducer rifampin (600 mg daily for 21 days) was administered concomitantly with osimertinib (80 mg once daily) in patients with epidermal growth factor receptor (EGFR) mutation-positive non-small cell lung cancer (NSCLC), peak plasma concentrations and AUC of osimertinib decreased by 73 and 78%, respectively. Because of the potential for reduced efficacy of osimertinib, concomitant administration of osimertinib and potent CYP3A inducers (e.g., rifampin) should be avoided. If concomitant use cannot be avoided, dosage of osimertinib should be increased. (See Concomitant Use with CYP3A Inducers under Dosage: Dosage Modification for Toxicity or Drug Interactions, in Dosage and Administration.)

■ **Drugs Metabolized by Hepatic Microsomal Enzymes** When the CYP3A4 substrate simvastatin (single 40-mg dose) was administered concomitantly with osimertinib (80 mg daily) in patients with EGFR mutation-positive NSCLC, peak plasma concentrations and (AUC) of simvastatin were not substantially affected.

■ **Drugs Transported by Breast Cancer Resistance Protein** Concomitant use of osimertinib and drugs that are substrates of BCRP (e.g., rosuvastatin) may increase exposure and toxicity of the BCRP substrate. When the BCRP substrate rosuvastatin (single 20-mg dose) was administered concomitantly with osimertinib (80 mg daily) in patients with EGFR mutation-positive NSCLC, peak plasma concentrations and AUC of rosuvastatin were increased by 72 and 35%, respectively. Patients receiving BCRP substrates concomitantly with osimertinib should be monitored for adverse effects of the substrate drug, unless otherwise specified in the manufacturer's labeling for the substrate.

■ **Drugs Affected by the P-glycoprotein Transport System** Concomitant use of osimertinib and drugs that are substrates of P-gp (e.g., fexofenadine) may increase exposure and toxicity of the P-gp substrate. When the P-gp substrate fexofenadine was administered concomitantly with osimertinib, peak plasma concentrations and AUC of fexofenadine were increased by 76 and 56%, respectively, following a single dose, and by 25 and 27%, respectively, at steady state. Patients receiving P-gp substrates concomitantly with osimertinib should be monitored for adverse effects of the substrate drug, unless otherwise specified in the manufacturer's labeling for the substrate drug.

■ **Drugs that Prolong the QT Interval** Concomitant use of osimertinib and drugs that prolong the QT interval may result in additive effects on QT-interval prolongation. Concomitant use of drugs known to prolong the QT interval with known risk of torsades de pointes should be avoided when possible. If concomitant use of drugs known to prolong the QT interval with known risk of torsades de pointes cannot be avoided, the manufacturer recommends periodic monitoring of ECG and electrolytes. (See Prolongation of QT Interval under Cautions: Warnings/Precautions.)

■ **Drugs Affecting Gastric Acidity** Concomitant administration of a single 80-mg dose of osimertinib with omeprazole (40 mg daily for 5 days) did not affect systemic exposure to osimertinib.

Description

Osimertinib mesylate, a third-generation inhibitor of receptor tyrosine kinases, is an antineoplastic agent. The drug binds irreversibly and selectively to certain mutant forms of the epidermal growth factor receptor (EGFR), including EGFR-sensitizing mutations (e.g., exon 19 deletion [del19], exon 21 substitution [L858R]) and the secondary T790M mutation.

Although first- and second-generation EGFR tyrosine kinase inhibitors (e.g., afatinib, erlotinib, gefitinib) have demonstrated improved outcomes in patients with non-small cell lung cancer (NSCLC) harboring EGFR mutations (e.g., del19, L858R), secondary resistance eventually develops following approximately 9–13 months of treatment. Clinical resistance to EGFR tyrosine kinase inhibitors has been attributed to the development of a secondary mutation, EGFR T790M, in approximately 50–60% of cases; this mutation results in production of a bulky methionine side chain in the receptor kinase domain of EGFR that is thought to sterically hinder the binding of first-generation (reversible) EGFR tyrosine kinase inhibitors to EGFR. Second-generation (irreversible) EGFR tyrosine kinase inhibitors (e.g., afatinib, dacomitinib) were developed to overcome this resistance; however, their clinical use has been limited by dose-limiting toxicities (e.g., skin rash, GI toxicity) possibly due to activity against wild-type EGFR. Osimertinib, a third-generation EGFR tyrosine kinase inhibitor, exhibits approximately ninefold greater affinity for mutant forms of EGFR than wild-type EGFR. In vitro studies and studies in animal tumor xenograft models indicate that the drug has antitumor activity against NSCLC cell lines expressing EGFR mutations L858R/T790M, L858R, T790M/del19, and del19 and, to a lesser extent, wild-type EGFR. Osimertinib also inhibits the activity of HER2/ErbB2, HER3/ErbB3, HER4/ErbB4, ACK1, and BLK at clinically relevant concentrations in vitro.

Following oral administration, median time to peak plasma osimertinib concentrations is approximately 6 hours (range 3–24 hours) with steady-state concentrations achieved within approximately 15 days. Dose-proportional increases in area under the plasma concentration-time curve (AUC) and peak plasma concentration of osimertinib are observed over a dose range of 20–240 mg. Administration of osimertinib with a high-fat meal slightly increased the AUC and peak plasma concentration of the drug by 19 and 14%, respectively, compared with the fasted state. (See Dosage and Administration: Administration.) Limited data in animals suggest that osimertinib distributes into the brain. Osimertinib is predominantly metabolized by the cytochrome P-450 (CYP) isoenzyme 3A. Two active metabolites (AZ7550 and AZ5104) have been identified, each accounting for approximately 10% of total drug exposure; AZ7550 has a similar potency to osimertinib, but AZ5104 exhibits higher potency against mutant EGFR and wild-type EGFR. Osimertinib is 95% bound to plasma proteins. Osimertinib is principally eliminated in feces (68%) and to a lesser extent in urine (14%); approximately 2% of an administered dose is eliminated as unchanged drug. The mean elimination half-life of osimertinib is 48 hours.

The pharmacokinetics of osimertinib do not appear to be affected by age, gender, or race (Asian versus non-Asian), body weight, baseline albumin concentration, line of therapy, or smoking status.

Advice to Patients

Importance of instructing patients to read the manufacturer's patient information.

Risk of severe or fatal interstitial lung disease/pneumonitis. Importance of immediately informing clinician if new or worsening respiratory symptoms (e.g., difficulty breathing, shortness of breath, cough, fever) occur.

Risk of QT_c-interval prolongation. Importance of immediately informing clinician if any possible symptoms of QT-interval prolongation (e.g., dizziness, lightheadedness, syncope) occur.

Risk of cardiomyopathy. Importance of immediately informing clinician if manifestations of heart failure (e.g., palpitations, shortness of breath, edema) occur.

Risk of keratitis. Importance of informing clinician if manifestations of keratitis (e.g., eye inflammation, lacrimation, photosensitivity, eye pain, red eye, changes in vision) occur.

Risk of fetal harm. Necessity of advising women of childbearing potential to use effective methods of contraception while receiving osimertinib and for 6 weeks after the drug is discontinued. Necessity of advising men with female partners of childbearing potential to use effective methods of contraception while receiving the drug and for 4 months after the drug is discontinued. Importance of women informing their clinician if they are pregnant or think they may be pregnant. If pregnancy occurs, the patient should be advised of the potential risk to the fetus.

Importance of advising women to avoid breast-feeding while receiving osimertinib therapy and for 2 weeks after the drug is discontinued.

Importance of informing clinicians of existing or contemplated concomitant therapy, including prescription and OTC drugs and dietary or herbal supplements, as well as any concomitant illnesses.

Importance of informing patients of other important precautionary information. (See Cautions.)

Overview® (see Users Guide). For additional information on this drug until a more detailed monograph is developed and published, the manufacturer's labeling should be consulted. It is *essential* that the manufacturer's labeling be consulted for more detailed information on usual cautions, precautions, contraindications, potential drug interactions, laboratory test interferences, and acute toxicity. For further information on the handling of antineoplastic agents, see the ASHP Guidelines on Handling Hazardous Drugs at http://www.ahfsdruginformation.com.

Preparations

Osimertinib mesylate can only be obtained through select specialty distributors. (See Restricted Distribution under Dosage and Administration: General.)

Excipients in commercially available drug preparations may have clinically important effects in some individuals; consult specific product labeling for details.

Osimertinib Mesylate

Oral		
Tablets, film-coated	40 mg (of osimertinib)	**Tagrisso®**, AstraZeneca
	80 mg (of osimertinib)	**Tagrisso®**, AstraZeneca

Oxaliplatin

■ Oxaliplatin is a platinum-containing antineoplastic agent.

Uses

■ **Colorectal Cancer** Oxaliplatin, in combination with fluorouracil and leucovorin, is used as adjuvant therapy for stage III cancer of the colon in patients who have undergone complete resection of the primary tumor. Oxaliplatin also is used in combination with fluorouracil and leucovorin in the treatment of advanced cancer of the colon and rectum.

Oxaliplatin also has been used in combination with capecitabine† (a prodrug of fluorouracil) as adjuvant therapy following the complete resection of the primary tumor in patients with stage III colon cancer.

Adjuvant Therapy for Stage III Colon Cancer **Oxaliplatin in Combination with Fluorouracil and Leucovorin.** Oxaliplatin, in combination with fluorouracil and leucovorin, is used as adjuvant therapy for stage III cancer of the colon in patients who have undergone complete resection of the primary tumor. This indication is based on survival benefit observed with the combination of oxaliplatin, fluorouracil, and leucovorin compared with the combination of fluorouracil and leucovorin.

Use of oxaliplatin, in combination with fluorouracil and leucovorin, as adjuvant therapy for stage III colon cancer is based principally on evidence of improved disease-free and overall survival from a multicenter, open-label, randomized study (Multicenter International Study of Oxaliplatin/5-Fluorouracil/Leucovorin in the Adjuvant Treatment of Colon Cancer [MOSAIC]) in 2246 patients with stage II or III colon cancer who had undergone complete resection of the primary tumor. Eligible patients were randomized to receive a 2-day combination regimen of oxaliplatin, fluorouracil, and leucovorin (leucovorin 200 mg/m² administered by IV infusion over 2 hours, followed by fluorouracil 400 mg/m² administered by IV injection and fluorouracil 600 mg/m² administered by IV infusion over 22 hours, administered for 2 consecutive days; oxaliplatin 85 mg/m² was administered by IV infusion over 2 hours concurrently with leucovorin on the first day only) or a 2-day combination regimen of fluorouracil and leucovorin (leucovorin 200 mg/m² administered by IV infusion over 2 hours, followed by fluorouracil 400 mg/m² administered by IV injection and fluorouracil 600 mg/m² administered by IV infusion over 22 hours). Treatment with both regimens was repeated at intervals of 2 weeks for a total of 12 cycles.

Among patients with stage III colon cancer, treatment with the oxaliplatin/fluorouracil/leucovorin regimen was associated with higher rates of disease-free survival at 5 years and overall survival at 6 years (66 and 73%, respectively) compared with the fluorouracil/leucovorin regimen (59 and 69%, respectively). At a median follow-up of 9.5 years, the disease-free and overall survival benefit of oxaliplatin/fluorouracil/leucovorin in patients with stage III colon cancer was maintained (10-year disease-free and overall survival rates of 62 and 67%, respectively, with oxaliplatin/fluorouracil/leucovorin compared with 54 and 59%, respectively, with fluorouracil/leucovorin). Among patients with stage II disease, 5-year disease-free survival rates and 6-year overall survival rates with the 2 regimens were similar. Likewise, 10-year disease-free and overall survival rates failed to show a benefit for oxaliplatin/fluorouracil/leucovorin compared with fluorouracil/leucovorin in patients with stage II disease. Grade 3 and 4 hematologic toxicity (neutropenia, thrombocytopenia, anemia) occurred more commonly with oxaliplatin/fluorouracil/leucovorin than with fluorouracil/leucovorin, although the incidence of febrile neutropenia was low with both regimens. Grade 3 and 4 GI toxicity (nausea, vomiting, diarrhea) also occurred more commonly with oxaliplatin/fluorouracil/leucovorin. Peripheral sensory neuropathy was reported in 92% of patients receiving oxaliplatin/fluorouracil/leucovorin compared with 16% of those receiving fluorouracil/leucovorin (see Neuropathy under Warnings/Precautions: Other Warnings and Precautions, in Cautions).

Oxaliplatin and Capecitabine. Efficacy and safety of oxaliplatin in combination with capecitabine† as adjuvant therapy in patients with stage III colon cancer have been evaluated in an open-label, randomized phase 3 study (NO16968; XELOXA). In this study, 1886 patients were randomized to receive either combination therapy with oxaliplatin (130 mg/m² administered by IV infusion over 2 hours on day 1) and capecitabine (1 g/m² administered orally twice daily on days 1–14) on a 3-week cycle for 8 cycles or combination therapy with IV fluorouracil and leucovorin (Mayo Clinic or Roswell Park regimen). The Mayo Clinic regimen consisted of fluorouracil 425 mg/m² administered by rapid IV injection ("bolus") and leucovorin 20 mg/m² administered by rapid IV infusion on days 1–5 of each 4-week cycle for a total of 6 cycles (24 weeks), and the Roswell Park regimen consisted of fluorouracil 500 mg/m² administered by rapid IV injection ("bolus") and leucovorin 500 mg/m² administered as a 2-hour IV infusion on day 1 of weeks 1–6 of each 8-week cycle for a total of 4 cycles (32 weeks). Patients were enrolled no more than 8 weeks following surgery with curative intent, by which time full recovery from surgery was required. The median age of patients was 61–62 years. Most patients (99%) enrolled in the study had a baseline ECOG performance status of 0 or 1. The primary measure of efficacy was disease-free survival.

At a median follow-up of 74 months, patients who received oxaliplatin in combination with capecitabine had higher disease-free (66.1 versus 59.8%; hazard ratio: 0.8) and relapse-free (69.3 versus 62.2%; hazard ratio: 0.78) survival rates compared with patients who received fluorouracil and leucovorin. At a median follow-up of 83 months, patients who received oxaliplatin in combination with capecitabine also had a higher overall survival rate (74.4 versus 69.6%; hazard ratio: 0.83) compared with those who received fluorouracil and leucovorin. Subgroup analysis based on prognostic factors (e.g., age, regional lymph node involvement, baseline carcinoembryonic antigen [CEA] concentration) suggested that the effect of capecitabine in combination with oxaliplatin on disease-free and overall survival was consistent across the subgroups, including those 70 years of age or older; however, the effect size appeared to be reduced in patients 70 years of age or older compared with younger patients. Neurosensory toxicity (any grade: 78 versus 8%; grade 3 or 4: 11 versus less than 1%), grade 3 or 4 hand-foot syndrome (5 versus less than 1%), and grade 3 or 4 thrombocytopenia (5% versus less than 1%) occurred more frequently in patients receiving oxaliplatin in combination with capecitabine, while grade 3 or 4 neutropenia (9 versus 16%), febrile neutropenia (less than 1 versus 4%), and stomatitis (less than 1 versus 9%) occurred more frequently in those receiving fluorouracil and leucovorin.

Use of combination therapy with oxaliplatin and capecitabine also was investigated in a randomized, multicenter, phase 3 study in patients with high-risk stage II or stage III colorectal cancer who had undergone complete resection of the primary tumor; however, interpretation of the results is limited by the failure to meet the planned accrual of 800 patients in the study to demonstrate superiority. In this study, 408 patients were randomized to receive either combination therapy with oxaliplatin (130 mg/m² on day 1) and capecitabine (1 g/m² twice daily on days 1–14) on a 3-week cycle for 8 cycles or combination therapy with an oxaliplatin, fluorouracil, and leucovorin (modified FOLFOX6) regimen on a 2-week cycle for 12 cycles. At a median follow-up of 74.7 months, median disease-free and overall survival had not been reached; however, 3-year disease-free and overall survival rates were similar between patients receiving capecitabine in combination with oxaliplatin (79.5 and 86.9%, respectively) compared with patients receiving modified FOLFOX6 (79.8 and 87.2%, respectively).

Based on current evidence, combination therapy with oxaliplatin and capecitabine is a reasonable choice (accepted, treatment option) for use as adjuvant therapy in patients with stage III colon cancer who have undergone complete resection of the primary tumor.

Treatment of Advanced Colorectal Cancer Oxaliplatin, in combination with fluorouracil and leucovorin, is used in the treatment of advanced cancer of the colon and rectum. The combination regimen has been studied as first-line therapy for unresectable cancer of the colon or rectum and also as second-line therapy in patients whose disease has recurred or progressed during or within 6 months following first-line therapy with the combination of fluorouracil, leucovorin, and irinotecan.

First-line Therapy for Advanced Colorectal Cancer. Use of oxaliplatin, in combination with fluorouracil and leucovorin, as first-line therapy for advanced colorectal cancer is based principally on evidence of improved response and survival from a multicenter, open-label, randomized study conducted by the North Central Cancer Treatment Group (NCCTG N9741) in patients with previously untreated unresectable colorectal cancer. The oxaliplatin/fluorouracil/leucovorin regimen was compared with 2 other regimens (oxaliplatin plus irinotecan and the combination of irinotecan, fluorouracil, and leucovorin) in 795 concurrently randomized patients with previously untreated unresectable colorectal cancer.

In this study, the oxaliplatin/fluorouracil/leucovorin combination was administered as a 2-day regimen (leucovorin 200 mg/m^2 administered by IV infusion over 2 hours, followed by fluorouracil 400 mg/m^2 administered by IV injection and fluorouracil 600 mg/m^2 administered by IV infusion over 22 hours, administered for 2 consecutive days; oxaliplatin 85 mg/m^2 was administered by IV infusion over 2 hours concurrently with leucovorin on the first day only); therapy was repeated at intervals of 2 weeks. The irinotecan/oxaliplatin regimen consisted of oxaliplatin 85 mg/m^2 and irinotecan 200 mg/m^2, both administered by IV infusion on day 1 and repeated at 3-week intervals. The irinotecan/fluorouracil/leucovorin regimen consisted of irinotecan 125 mg/m^2 administered by IV infusion, fluorouracil 500 mg/m^2 administered by IV injection, and leucovorin 20 mg/m^2 administered by IV injection on days 1, 8, 15, and 22 and repeated at 6-week intervals.

Overall response rates were higher with oxaliplatin/fluorouracil/leucovorin therapy (45%) compared with irinotecan/fluorouracil/leucovorin (31%) or irinotecan/oxaliplatin (35%) therapy. The median time to disease progression was similar with the irinotecan/oxaliplatin (6.5 months) and irinotecan/fluorouracil/leucovorin (6.9 months) regimens, but was longer (8.7 months) with the oxaliplatin/fluorouracil/leucovorin regimen. Median overall survival of patients receiving oxaliplatin/fluorouracil/leucovorin therapy (19.5 months) was longer than that of patients receiving irinotecan/fluorouracil/leucovorin therapy (15 months) but did not differ from that of patients receiving irinotecan/oxaliplatin (17.4 months). Grade 3 and 4 GI toxicity (nausea, vomiting, diarrhea) and febrile neutropenia were more commonly associated with the irinotecan-containing regimens, whereas grade 3 and 4 paresthesias were more commonly associated with the oxaliplatin/fluorouracil/leucovorin regimen.

Second-line Therapy for Advanced Colorectal Cancer. Use of oxaliplatin, in combination with fluorouracil and leucovorin, as second-line therapy for advanced colorectal cancer is based principally on response rate and an interim analysis showing improved time to radiographic progression of the disease in a multicenter, randomized, open-label, controlled study in over 450 patients (of more than 800 patients enrolled) with advanced colorectal cancer that had recurred or progressed during or within 6 months following first-line therapy with the combination of fluorouracil, leucovorin, and irinotecan. There currently are no data demonstrating a clinical benefit (e.g., improvement in disease-related symptoms, increased survival).

In this study, eligible patients with unresectable, measurable, and histologically proven disease were randomized to receive oxaliplatin alone (85 mg/m^2 administered by IV infusion over 2 hours), a 2-day combination regimen of fluorouracil and leucovorin (leucovorin 200 mg/m^2 administered by IV infusion over 2 hours, followed by fluorouracil 400 mg/m^2 administered by IV injection and fluorouracil 600 mg/m^2 administered by IV infusion over 22 hours), or a 2-day combination regimen of oxaliplatin, fluorouracil, and leucovorin (leucovorin 200 mg/m^2 administered by IV infusion over 2 hours, followed by fluorouracil 400 mg/m^2 administered by IV injection and fluorouracil 600 mg/m^2 administered by IV infusion over 22 hours, administered for 2 consecutive days; oxaliplatin 85 mg/m^2 was administered by IV infusion over 2 hours concurrently with leucovorin on the first day only). Therapy was repeated at intervals of 2 weeks until radiographic progression, toxicity, or 13 months since the first dose had elapsed, whichever occurred first. Patients randomized to receive oxaliplatin monotherapy or fluorouracil/leucovorin received a median of 3 cycles, while those randomized to receive oxaliplatin/fluorouracil/leucovorin received a median of 6 cycles.

Partial response rates were higher in patients receiving oxaliplatin/fluorouracil/leucovorin (9%) than in those who received oxaliplatin monotherapy (1%) or fluorouracil/leucovorin (0%). There were no complete responses in any group. In addition, the median time to radiographic disease progression was longer in patients receiving oxaliplatin/fluorouracil/leucovorin (4.6 months) than in those who received oxaliplatin alone (1.6 months) or fluorouracil/leucovorin (2.7 months).

Dosage and Administration

■ Reconstitution and Administration

Oxaliplatin is administered by IV infusion over 2 hours. Commercially available oxaliplatin powder for injection must be reconstituted and diluted prior to administration; the commercially available concentrate for injection must be diluted prior to administration. Reconstitution or final dilution of the drug must *never* be performed with a sodium chloride solution or other chloride-containing solutions. Because aluminum has been reported to cause degradation of platinum compounds (see Chemistry and Stability, in Cisplatin 10:00), the manufacturer states that needles or IV administration sets containing aluminum parts should not be used for the reconstitution or dilution of oxaliplatin.

Oxaliplatin sterile powder for injection is reconstituted by adding 10 mL (to the vial labeled as containing 50 mg of oxaliplatin) or 20 mL (to the vial labeled as containing 100 mg of oxaliplatin) of water for injection or 5% dextrose injection to provide a solution containing 5 mg/mL; the reconstituted drug may be stored in the vial under refrigeration for up to 24 hours. Alternatively, the commercially available concentrate for injection containing oxaliplatin 5 mg/mL can be used. The appropriate dose should be withdrawn and diluted in 250–500 mL of 5% dextrose injection prior to administration; the diluted drug may be stored under refrigeration for up to 24 hours or at room temperature for up to 6 hours. Oxaliplatin solutions should be inspected visually for particulate matter and/or discoloration prior to administration and should be discarded if either is present. The commercially available concentrate for injection must be protected from light and freezing; following dilution, protection from light is not required. The manufacturer states that oxaliplatin powder for injection is not sensitive to light.

The manufacturer states that oxaliplatin solutions must not be mixed or administered simultaneously through the same IV line with alkaline drugs or media (e.g., basic solutions of fluorouracil). The infusion line should be flushed with 5% dextrose injection prior to administration of oxaliplatin or any concomitant drug.

Leucovorin is administered by IV infusion over 2 hours concurrently with oxaliplatin but in a separate container using a Y-type administration set. The dose of fluorouracil then is administered by direct IV injection over 2–4 minutes, followed by the maintenance dose administered by IV infusion over 22 hours. The respective manufacturer's prescribing information should be consulted for additional information on the reconstitution and administration of fluorouracil and leucovorin.

The manufacturer of oxaliplatin recommends that procedures for proper handling and disposal of antineoplastic drugs (e.g., use of gloves) be used to avoid exposure to oxaliplatin during preparation of IV solutions. If oxaliplatin solution comes in contact with the skin or mucous membranes, the skin should be washed immediately and thoroughly with soap and water or the mucosa should be flushed with copious amounts of water. Since oxaliplatin is an antineoplastic agent, the manufacturer states that consideration should be given to handling and disposal according to guidelines issued for cytotoxic drugs, although there is no general agreement that all of the procedures recommended in such guidelines are necessary or appropriate. For further information on the handling of antineoplastic agents, see the ASHP Guidelines on Handling Hazardous Drugs at http://www.ahfsdruginformation.com.

■ General Dosage

For the management of advanced cancer of the colon or rectum, or for adjuvant therapy of stage III cancer of the colon following complete resection of the primary tumor, an oxaliplatin dosage of 85 mg/m^2 is administered by IV infusion on day 1 as part of a 2-day combination regimen that includes fluorouracil and leucovorin. The 2-day regimen may be repeated at intervals of 2 weeks. Because this regimen may be associated with an increased incidence of grade 3 or 4 nausea and vomiting compared with the combination regimen containing only fluorouracil and leucovorin, the manufacturer of oxaliplatin states that premedication with antiemetics, including selective inhibitors of type 3 serotonergic (5-HT_3) receptors (e.g., dolasetron, granisetron, ondansetron) with or without dexamethasone, should be considered prior to each 2-day cycle. (See GI Effects under Warnings/Precautions: Other Warnings and Precautions, in Cautions.) According to the manufacturer, hydration prior to administration of oxaliplatin is not necessary.

The combination regimen of oxaliplatin, fluorouracil, and leucovorin (FOLFOX4) is administered over 2 consecutive days. On day 1, oxaliplatin 85 mg/m^2 and leucovorin 200 mg/m^2 (diluted with 5% dextrose injection) are administered concurrently (in separate containers using a Y-type administration set) by IV infusion over 2 hours. Fluorouracil 400 mg/m^2 then is administered by IV injection over 2–4 minutes followed by fluorouracil 600 mg/m^2 (diluted with 500 mL of 5% dextrose injection) administered as an IV infusion over 22 hours. On day 2, leucovorin 200 mg/m^2 is administered by IV infusion over 2 hours, followed by fluorouracil 400 mg/m^2 administered by IV injection over 2–4 minutes and fluorouracil 600 mg/m^2 administered as an IV infusion over 22 hours. When this regimen is used as adjuvant therapy for stage III colon cancer, a total of 12 cycles (6 months) of therapy is recommended. In patients with advanced colorectal cancer, treatment with the regimen is recommended until evidence of disease progression or unacceptable toxicity occurs.

An alternative regimen of oxaliplatin, fluorouracil, and leucovorin (i.e., modified FOLFOX6) also has been used for treatment of advanced colorectal cancer and for adjuvant therapy of colon cancer, and is one of several regimens recommended by the National Comprehensive Cancer Network (NCCN) for the treatment of advanced or metastatic colon cancer and for adjuvant therapy of colon cancer. The modified FOLFOX6 regimen is administered over 2 consecutive days. Oxaliplatin 85 mg/m^2 and leucovorin 400 mg/m^2 (or, alternatively, leucovorin 350 mg) (diluted with 5% dextrose injection) are administered concurrently (in separate containers using a Y-type administration set) by IV infusion over 2 hours. Fluorouracil 400 mg/m^2 then is administered by IV injection over 5 minutes followed by fluorouracil 1200 mg/m^2 administered as an IV infusion daily for 2 days (i.e., 2400 mg/m^2 administered as an IV infusion over 46–48 hours [total fluorouracil dosage of 2800 mg/m² per cycle]). Clinicians should consult individual protocols for specific dosage information.

When oxaliplatin has been used in combination with capecitabine† (CapeOx) as adjuvant therapy following the complete resection of the primary tumor in patients with stage III colon cancer, oxaliplatin 130 mg/m² has been administered by IV infusion over 2 hours on day 1 and capecitabine 1 g/m² has been administered orally twice daily on days 1–14 of each 3-week cycle. Treatment has been continued for 8 cycles of therapy.

■ Dose Modification for Toxicity The management of certain adverse effects (e.g., neurosensory effects, GI or hematologic toxicity) may require modification of oxaliplatin dosage or duration of infusion. Increasing the duration of oxaliplatin infusion from 2 to 6 hours may minimize acute toxicities; adjustment of infusion duration for fluorouracil or leucovorin is not necessary.

Adjuvant Therapy for Stage III Colon Cancer In patients treated for stage III colon cancer (adjuvant setting) who experience persistent grade 2 adverse neurosensory effects that do not resolve, reduction of oxaliplatin dosage to 75 mg/m² should be considered; in those with persistent grade 3 neurosensory effects, discontinuance of oxaliplatin should be considered. Dosage modification for fluorouracil or leucovorin is not necessary in these patients.

In patients treated for stage III colon cancer (adjuvant setting) who have recovered from grade 3 or 4 GI toxicity (that occurred despite prophylactic treatment), grade 4 neutropenia, or grade 3 or 4 thrombocytopenia, the manufacturer of oxaliplatin recommends reducing the dosage of oxaliplatin to 75 mg/m² and that of fluorouracil by 20% (i.e., 300 mg/m² by IV injection over 2–4 minutes and 500 mg/m² by IV infusion over 22 hours). Administration of the next dose should be delayed until neutrophil counts are at least 1500/mm³ and platelet counts are at least 75,000/mm³.

Therapy for Advanced Colorectal Cancer In patients with advanced colorectal cancer who experience persistent grade 2 adverse neurosensory effects that do not resolve, reduction of oxaliplatin dosage to 65 mg/m² should be considered; in those with persistent grade 3 neurosensory effects, discontinuance of oxaliplatin should be considered. Dosage modification for fluorouracil or leucovorin is not necessary in these patients.

In patients with advanced colorectal cancer who have recovered from grade 3 or 4 GI toxicity (that occurred despite prophylactic treatment), grade 4 neutropenia, or grade 3 or 4 thrombocytopenia, the manufacturer of oxaliplatin recommends reducing the dosage of oxaliplatin to 65 mg/m² and that of fluorouracil by 20% (i.e., 300 mg/m² by IV injection over 2–4 minutes and 500 mg/m² by IV infusion over 22 hours). Administration of the next dose should be delayed until neutrophil counts are at least 1500/mm³ and platelet counts are at least 75,000/mm³.

■ Special Populations No special population dosage recommendations at this time. However, safety and efficacy have not been established in patients with renal impairment and caution should be exercised. (See Renal Impairment under Warnings/Precautions: Specific Populations, in Cautions.) No adjustment of initial dosage was necessary in geriatric patients (65 years of age or older) receiving oxaliplatin in combination with fluorouracil and leucovorin as second-line therapy for advanced colorectal cancer.

Cautions

■ Contraindications Known hypersensitivity to oxaliplatin, any ingredient in the formulation, or other platinum-containing compounds.

■ Warnings/Precautions ***Warnings*** **Anaphylaxis.** Anaphylactic/anaphylactoid and other hypersensitivity reactions (grade 3 or 4) have been reported in 2–3% of patients with colorectal cancer receiving oxaliplatin. These allergic reactions (e.g., rash, urticaria, erythema, pruritus, bronchospasm, hypotension), which rarely may be fatal, are similar in nature and severity to those associated with other platinum-containing antineoplastic agents. Other manifestations may include facial flushing, infusion-associated diarrhea, shortness of breath, diaphoresis, chest pain, disorientation, and syncope. Allergic reactions may occur within minutes following administration of oxaliplatin and during any cycle of treatment and should be managed with appropriate supportive therapy; epinephrine, corticosteroids, and antihistamines may be used to alleviate manifestations. Discontinuance of therapy may be required.

Other Warnings and Precautions Oxaliplatin should be used under the supervision of a qualified clinician experienced in therapy with antineoplastic agents.

Because the oxaliplatin therapeutic regimen includes the use of fluorouracil and leucovorin, the usual cautions, precautions, and contraindications of these drugs also should be considered.

Neuropathy. Treatment with oxaliplatin is consistently associated with acute or persistent neuropathy, both of which are principally peripheral neuropathies. The duration and severity of peripheral neuropathy appear to increase with increasing cumulative dosage of oxaliplatin. Peripheral sensory neuropathy occurred in 92% of patients receiving the combination of oxaliplatin, fluorouracil, and leucovorin as adjuvant therapy for colon cancer; grade 3 events occurred in 12% of patients. In patients with advanced colorectal cancer, peripheral sensory neuropathy occurred in 82 or 74% of patients receiving the oxaliplatin/fluorouracil/leucovorinregimen as first- or second-line therapy, respectively; grade 3 or 4 events occurred in 19% of those receiving the regimen as first-line therapy and 7% of those receiving the regimen as second-line therapy. The median onset of grade 3 peripheral sensory neuropathy was cycle 9 of adjuvant therapy and cycle 6 of second-line therapy.

Acute, reversible sensory neuropathy that is principally peripheral has been reported in 56% of patients receiving oxaliplatin/fluorouracil/leucovorin therapy; acute neurotoxicity has been reported in approximately 30% of patients during an individual treatment cycle. Grade 3 or 4 acute neuropathy occurred in 2% of patients receiving the oxaliplatin/fluorouracil/leucovorin regimen as second-line therapy for advanced colorectal cancer. In the adjuvant setting, 12% of patients experienced grade 3 peripheral neuropathy during treatment. Differences among studies in the reporting of oxaliplatin-associated neuropathy reflect the use of different grading scales. In studies in patients with advanced colorectal cancer, neuropathy was graded using a study-specific scale (range of 1–4) for characterizing paresthesias and dysesthesias; in the study of adjuvant therapy, the National Cancer Institute Common Toxicity Criteria (NCI-CTC Version 2.0) scale for grading neuropathy (applicable range of 0–3) was used.

Manifestations of acute peripheral neuropathy include transient paresthesia, dysesthesia, and hypoesthesia in the hands, feet, perioral area, or throat; jaw spasm, abnormal tongue sensation, dysarthria, ocular pain, and a feeling of chest pressure also have been observed. These symptoms may occur within hours or 1–2 days following administration of oxaliplatin, resolve within 14 days, and frequently recur with further administration of the drug. Because symptoms of acute sensory neuropathy may be precipitated or exacerbated by exposure to cold temperature or cold objects,patients should be advised to refrain from ingesting cold beverages or food, to avoid exposure to cold temperatures, and to use gloves when handling cold or frozen objects; the manufacturer states that ice (e.g., for mucositis prophylaxis) should be avoided during infusion of oxaliplatin. (See Advice to Patients.)

An acute syndrome of pharyngolaryngeal dysesthesia (grade 3 or 4), characterized by subjective sensations of dysphagia or dyspnea without laryngospasm or bronchospasm (i.e., no stridor or wheezing), has been reported in 1–2% of patients with advanced colorectal cancer receiving oxaliplatin in clinical studies; symptoms usually resolve within hours of onset. Some evidence indicates that prolonging the duration of oxaliplatin infusion may reduce the incidence of laryngopharyngeal dysesthesia.

Persistent sensory neuropathy that is principally peripheral has been reported in 48% of patients receiving oxaliplatin/fluorouracil/leucovorin therapy. Symptoms of persistent neuropathy usually include paresthesias, dysesthesias, and hypoesthesias; however, impaired proprioception, which can interfere with daily activities (e.g., writing, buttoning clothing, swallowing, walking), also has been observed. Persistent neuropathy can occur without any prior acute neuropathic event and typically persists for more than 14 days following administration of oxaliplatin. Approximately 80% of patients who developed grade 3 persistent neuropathy during clinical studies had progressed from prior grade 1 or 2 neuropathic events. Symptoms of persistent neuropathy may improve in some patients upon discontinuance of oxaliplatin. Long-term follow-up of patients receiving adjuvant therapy with the oxaliplatin/fluorouracil/leucovorin regimen indicated that the incidence of peripheral sensory neuropathy after completion of such therapy was 39% at 6 months with a decline to 21% at 18 months; the incidence of grade 3 neurotoxicity was 1% at 6 and 18 months and 0.7% at 48 months. Persistent grade 3 or 4 neuropathy occurred in 6% of patients receiving the oxaliplatin/fluorouracil/leucovorin regimen as second-line therapy for advanced colorectal cancer.

Preventive strategies, including the use of intermittent oxaliplatin regimens (i.e., "stop and go" schedule) and other potential neuromodulatory regimens (e.g., amifostine, carbamazepine, gabapentin, glutathione), have been evaluated to reduce the incidence and severity of oxaliplatin-induced neurotoxicity; however, due to the lack of adequate data from well-conducted clinical trials, there is insufficient evidence to support the use of any preventive therapy. In a retrospective cohort study in patients with advanced colorectal cancer, the incidence of grade 3 distal paresthesias was lower in those who received IV infusions of calcium gluconate and magnesium sulfate (immediately before and after infusions of oxaliplatin) compared with those who did not receive such infusions (7 versus 26%). Calcium gluconate and magnesium sulfate infusions are being evaluated in randomized, double-blind, placebo-controlled studies in patients receiving oxaliplatin/fluorouracil/leucovorin-based regimens for colorectal cancer. Preliminary data from one of these studies suggest a reduction in neurotoxicity in patients receiving prophylactic calcium and magnesium therapy; however, data from another study suggested that addition of calcium and magnesium to the chemotherapy regimen had a negative effect on clinical response and antitumor activity. Additional data are needed to define the role of prophylactic calcium and magnesium therapy in reducing the severity and duration of acute and chronic oxaliplatin-induced neurotoxicity and to confirm the effects, if any, of such therapy on clinical response to oxaliplatin-based regimens used in the treatment of colorectal cancer.

Pulmonary Toxicity. Pulmonary fibrosis, which may be fatal, occurred in less than 1% of patients receiving oxaliplatin in clinical trials. In patients receiving the oxaliplatin/fluorouracil/leucovorin regimen as adjuvant therapy, the combined incidence of grade 3 cough and dyspnea was less than 1% (with no reports of grade 4 pulmonary toxicity); grade 3 or 4 pulmonary toxicity (cough, dyspnea, hypoxia) was reported in 7% of patients receiving first-line oxaliplatin/fluorouracil/leucovorin therapy for advanced colorectal cancer. In the study of adjuvant oxaliplatin/fluorouracil/leucovorin therapy, one death secondary to eosinophilic pneumonia was reported. If unexplained respiratory manifestations (e.g., nonproductive cough, dyspnea, crackles, radiographic evidence of pulmonary infiltrates) develop, the manufacturer states that oxaliplatin should be discontinued temporarily until further pulmonary investigation excludes interstitial lung disease or pulmonary fibrosis.

Hepatic Effects. Increased concentrations of transaminases (ALT [SGPT], AST [SGOT]) and alkaline phosphatase occurred in 57 and 42%, respectively, of patients receiving oxaliplatin/fluorouracil/leucovorin as adjuvant therapy compared with 34 and 20%, respectively, of patients receiving fluorouracil/leucovorin; the incidence of hyperbilirubinemia was similar in both treatment groups. Liver biopsy specimens from patients receiving oxaliplatin/fluorouracil/leucovorin therapy have revealed evidence of hepatic vascular conditions (e.g., peliosis hepatis, nodular regenerative hyperplasia or sinusoidal changes, perisinusoidal fibrosis, veno-occlusive lesions). In patients with abnormal liver function test results or portal hypertension that cannot be explained by metastases to the liver, hepatic vascular toxicity should be considered and, if appropriate, investigated.

The manufacturer recommends that hepatic function tests (e.g., transaminases, bilirubin) be performed prior to each cycle of oxaliplatin.

Fetal/Neonatal Morbidity and Mortality. Oxaliplatin may cause fetal harm; teratogenicity and embryolethality demonstrated in animals. No adequate and well-controlled studies to date in humans. Pregnancy should be avoided during therapy. (See Advice to Patients.) If oxaliplatin is used during pregnancy or if the patient becomes pregnant while receiving the drug, apprise of the potential hazard to the fetus.

GI Effects. The incidence of grade 3 or 4 nausea and vomiting in patients with colon cancer was higher with adjuvant oxaliplatin/fluorouracil/leucovorin therapy compared with adjuvant fluorouracil/leucovorin therapy; in addition, the incidence of grade 3 or 4 GI toxicity (nausea, vomiting, diarrhea, mucositis/stomatitis) was higher with oxaliplatin/fluorouracil/leucovorin than with fluorouracil/leucovorin given as second-line therapy for advanced colorectal cancer. In patients receiving first-line therapy for advanced colorectal cancer, the incidence of grade 3 or 4 vomiting and diarrhea was lower with oxaliplatin/fluorouracil/leucovorin than with irinotecan/fluorouracil/leucovorin. In patients with advanced colorectal cancer, the incidence of adverse GI effects appeared to be similar across cycles of treatment. Certain adverse GI effects (e.g., diarrhea, mucositis) may be exacerbated by addition of oxaliplatin to fluorouracil/leucovorin therapy and should be managed with appropriate supportive therapy. The manufacturer states that ice (e.g., for mucositis prophylaxis) should be avoided during and following IV infusion of oxaliplatin to prevent precipitation or exacerbation of acute neurologic symptoms. (See Neuropathy under Warnings/Precautions: Other Warnings and Precautions, in Cautions.)

Thrombocytopenia and Bleeding. In clinical trials, thrombocytopenia and hemorrhage occurred more frequently in patients receiving oxaliplatin/fluorouracil/leucovorin therapy than in those receiving fluorouracil/leucovorin. Grade 3 or 4 thrombocytopenia was reported in 2% of patients receiving adjuvant oxaliplatin/fluorouracil/leucovorin therapy; in patients with advanced colorectal cancer, the incidence was 3–5%. Grade 3 or 4 GI bleeding was reported in 0.2% of patients receiving adjuvant oxaliplatin/fluorouracil/leucovorin therapy. Epistaxis was reported in 10% of patients receiving oxaliplatin/fluorouracil/leucovorin compared with 2% of patients receiving irinotecan/fluorouracil/leucovorin and 1% of those receiving irinotecan/oxaliplatin as first-line therapy for advanced colorectal cancer. The manufacturer recommends that platelet counts be performed prior to administration of each cycle of oxaliplatin.

Prolongation of the prothrombin time and international normalized ratio (INR), occasionally associated with hemorrhage, has been reported in patients receiving oxaliplatin/fluorouracil/leucovorin therapy concomitantly with anticoagulant therapy. Careful monitoring is recommended for patients receiving oxaliplatin/fluorouracil/leucovorin therapy concomitantly with oral anticoagulants (e.g., warfarin).

Neutropenia and Infectious Complications. Grade 3 or 4 neutropenia occurred in 29 or 12%, respectively, of patients receiving oxaliplatin/fluorouracil/leucovorin as adjuvant therapy and in 35 or 18%, respectively, of those receiving oxaliplatin/fluorouracil/leucovorin therapy for advanced colorectal cancer. Febrile neutropenia or documented infection with severe neutropenia occurred in 1.8% of patients receiving this adjuvant regimen. Among patients with advanced colorectal cancer, febrile neutropenia occurred in 4 or 6% of those receiving oxaliplatin/fluorouracil/leucovorin as first- or second-line therapy, respectively, and neutropenia with infection occurred in 8% of those receiving first-line oxaliplatin/fluorouracil/leucovorin therapy.

The manufacturer recommends that a leukocyte count with differential be performed prior to each cycle of oxaplatin.

Thromboembolism. Thromboembolic events occurred in 6% of patients receiving adjuvant or first-line therapy with the oxaliplatin/fluorouracil/leucovorin regimen and in 9% of patients receiving this regimen as second-line therapy.

Renal Effects. Increased serum creatinine concentrations were reported in approximately 5–10% of patients receiving oxaliplatin/fluorouracil/leucovorin therapy for advanced colorectal cancer; grade 3 or 4 elevation in serum creatinine concentrations was reported in approximately 1% of patients receiving this regimen as second-line therapy.

The manufacturer recommends that renal function tests (e.g., serum creatinine) be performed prior to administration of each cycle of oxaliplatin.

Dermatologic Effects. Injection site reactions, including erythema, swelling, and pain, have been reported in clinical studies. Extravasation may result in local pain and inflammation, which may be severe and lead to complications (e.g., necrosis).

The incidence of alopecia in patients receiving oxaliplatin/fluorouracil/leucovorin therapy appears to be similar to that in patients receiving fluorouracil/leucovorin therapy. The incidence of palmar-plantar erythrodysesthesia (hand-foot syndrome) was similar in patients receiving either oxaliplatin/fluorouracil/leucovorin or fluorouracil/leucovorin as second-line therapy for advanced colorectal cancer; however, among patients receiving these regimens as first-line therapy, the incidence was higher with oxaliplatin/fluorouracil/leucovorin (7%) than with fluorouracil/leucovorin (2%).

Ocular Effects. Adverse ocular effects, including conjunctivitis, abnormal lacrimation, and abnormal visual disturbances, have been reported with oxaliplatin administered in combination with fluorouracil and leucovorin in clinical trials. Cases of decreased visual acuity, visual field disturbances (including tunnel vision), optic neuritis, ocular pain, and transient vision loss have been reported, sometimes on the day of or within several days following an oxaliplatin infusion; all events were reversible.

Laboratory Monitoring. Blood cell counts (e.g., leukocyte count with differential, platelet count), hemoglobin, and blood chemistry tests (including ALT, AST, bilirubin, and creatinine) should be performed prior to administration of each cycle of oxaliplatin. Patients receiving the combination of oxaliplatin, fluorouracil, and leucovorin concomitantly with oral anticoagulants may require closer monitoring of prothrombin time and INR (see Drug Interactions: Anticoagulants).

Specific Populations **Pregnancy.** Category D. (See Fetal/Neonatal Morbidity and Mortality under Warnings/Precautions: Other Warnings and Precautions, in Cautions.)

Lactation. It is not known whether oxaliplatin or its metabolites are distributed into milk. Discontinue nursing or the drug, taking into account the importance of the drug to the woman.

Pediatric Use. Efficacy of oxaliplatin has not been established in children younger than 18 years of age. No substantial antitumor activity has been reported in phase 1 and 2 clinical trials in patients 7 months to 22 years of age with solid tumors.

Geriatric Use. No differences in clearance of ultrafilterable platinum were observed between geriatric (65 years of age and older) and younger patients in clinical studies; however, the incidence of certain adverse effects (i.e., granulocytopenia, leukopenia, diarrhea, dehydration, hypokalemia, fatigue, syncope) was higher in geriatric patients than in younger adults. In the study of adjuvant therapy for colon cancer, a descriptive subset analysis indicated that the effect on disease-free survival of the oxaliplatin/fluorouracil/leucovorin regimen compared with that of fluorouracil/leucovorin in patients 65 years of age or older was inconclusive. In patients receiving the oxaliplatin/fluorouracil/leucovorin regimen as first-line therapy for advanced colorectal cancer, no differences in efficacy were observed in patients 65 years of age or older compared with the overall study population.

Renal Impairment. Safety and efficacy of the combination regimen of oxaliplatin, fluorouracil, and leucovorin in patients with renal impairment have not been evaluated. However, clearance of the platinum ultrafiltrate appears to decrease with decreasing renal function. Limited data indicate that the area under the plasma concentration-time curve (AUC) of platinum increases by about 60, 140, or 190% in patients with mild (creatinine clearance of 50–80 mL/minute), moderate (creatinine clearance of 30 to less than 50 mL/minute), or severe renal impairment (creatinine clearance of less than 30 mL/minute), respectively, compared with that in patients with normal renal function. Therefore, the manufacturer states that the oxaliplatin/fluorouracil/leucovorin regimen should be used with caution in patients with renal impairment. However, the pharmacodynamic relationship between platinum ultrafiltrate concentrations and safety or efficacy of oxaliplatin has not been established.

■ **Common Adverse Effects** The most common adverse effects of the oxaliplatin/fluorouracil/leucovorin regimen administered as adjuvant therapy are adverse neurologic (i.e., peripheral sensory neuropathy), GI (nausea, vomiting, diarrhea, and mucositis), and hematologic (anemia, neutropenia, and thrombocytopenia) effects; fatigue; and increases in serum transaminase and alkaline phosphatase concentrations. Other adverse effects reported in 15% or more of patients receiving adjuvant oxaliplatin/fluorouracil/leucovorin therapy include skin disorder, alopecia, fever, infection, constipation, bilirubinemia, abdominal pain, and epistaxis.

In patients with advanced colorectal cancer receiving the oxaliplatin/fluorouracil/leucovorin regimen as first- or second-line therapy, the most common adverse effects are adverse neurologic (i.e., neuropathy, including paresthesia and acute or persistent neuropathy), hematologic (anemia, neutropenia, leukopenia, and thrombocytopenia), and GI (nausea, vomiting, and diarrhea) effects and fatigue. Other adverse effects reported in 15% or more of patients receiving oxaliplatin/fluorouracil/leucovorin as first- or second-line therapy include increase in serum transaminase concentrations, mucositis, alopecia, pharyngolaryngeal dysesthesia, anorexia, cough, abdominal pain, constipation, fever, increase in alkaline phosphatase concentration, dyspnea, back pain, headache, edema, rhinitis, and pain.

Drug Interactions

■ **Anticoagulants** Prolongation of prothrombin time and international normalized ratio (INR), occasionally associated with hemorrhage, has been reported in patients receiving oxaliplatin/fluorouracil/leucovorin therapy concomitantly with anticoagulant therapy. Careful monitoring is recommended for patients receiving oxaliplatin/fluorouracil/leucovorin therapy concomitantly with oral anticoagulants (e.g., warfarin).

■ **Fluorouracil** Pharmacokinetic interaction unlikely when recommended dosages and administration schedule (see Dosage and Administration) are used. Potential pharmacokinetic interaction (20% increase in plasma fluorouracil concentrations) during concomitant use of fluorouracil and 130 mg/m² of oxaliplatin at intervals of 3 weeks.

■ **Other Antineoplastic Agents** Pharmacokinetic interaction with irinotecan or topotecan unlikely.

■ **Nephrotoxic Drugs** Potential pharmacokinetic interaction (decreased clearance of platinum-containing compounds); however, this interaction has not been specifically studied.

■ **Protein-bound Drugs** In vitro data indicate that erythromycin, granisetron, paclitaxel, salicylates, and valproate sodium are unlikely to displace platinum from plasma proteins.

■ **Drugs Affecting Hepatic Microsomal Enzymes** Pharmacokinetic interaction with drugs metabolized by cytochrome P-450 (CYP) isoenzymes or those that induce or inhibit these isoenzymes unlikely. However, no studies have been conducted.

Description

Oxaliplatin is a platinum-containing antineoplastic agent. The drug is an organoplatinum complex, consisting of a platinum atom complexed with 1,2-diaminocyclohexane (DACH) and a labile oxalate ligand. Oxaliplatin must undergo nonenzymatic activation before antineoplastic activity occurs. In physiologic solutions, the labile oxalate ligand of oxaliplatin presumably is displaced, forming several transient reactive complexes (e.g., monoaquo DACH platinum, diaquo DACH platinum) that covalently bind to specific DNA base sequences, producing intrastrand and interstrand DNA cross-links. Cross-links between specific DNA base sequences (i.e., adjacent guanine residues, adjacent adenine and guanine residues, guanine residues separated by an intervening nucleotide) produced by transient reactive intermediates of oxaliplatin are thought to inhibit DNA replication and transcription. Some evidence indicates that the presence of the bulky DACH carrier ligand of oxaliplatin may contribute to a greater degree of inhibition of DNA synthesis and cytotoxicity compared with that observed with cisplatin and may result in the lack of cross-resistance between oxaliplatin and cisplatin. Oxaliplatin is cycle-phase nonspecific.

Oxaliplatin has been shown to exhibit antitumor activity against colon carcinoma in vivo. Synergistic antiproliferative activity of oxaliplatin and fluorouracil has been demonstrated in vitro and in vivo in several tumor models (i.e., HT29 [colon], GR [mammary], L1210 [leukemia]).

Because oxaliplatin undergoes rapid and extensive nonenzymatic biotransformation to numerous platinum-containing transient reactive intermediates, pharmacokinetic parameters of the drug generally are expressed in terms of platinum-containing complexes rather than the parent compound. Following a 2-hour IV infusion of oxaliplatin, approximately 15% of the administered platinum is present in the systemic circulation while the remaining 85% is rapidly distributed into tissues or eliminated in urine. A fraction of the platinum-containing complexes distributed into peripheral tissues is irreversibly bound to and accumulates (approximately twofold) in erythrocytes, where the complexes appear to have no relevant activity. Approximately 90% of the platinum in the systemic circulation is irreversibly bound to plasma proteins, principally albumin and gamma globulins. It is thought that antineoplastic activity of oxaliplatin resides only in platinum-containing species present in the ultrafilterable plasma fraction (biotransformed, nonprotein-bound species); however, the pharmacodynamic relationship between platinum ultrafiltrate concentrations and safety or efficacy of oxaliplatin has not been established. There is no evidence that platinum accumulates in plasma following administration of 85 mg/m² dosages of oxaliplatin once every 2 weeks; however, a progressive accumulation of platinum in erythrocytes has been reported.

Oxaliplatin undergoes rapid and extensive nonenzymatic biotransformation; there is no evidence of cytochrome P-450 (CYP)-mediated metabolism in vitro. As many as 17 platinum-containing derivatives, including several cytotoxic species (e.g., monochloro DACH platinum, dichloro DACH platinum, monoaquo DACH platinum, diaquo DACH platinum) and various noncytotoxic species, have been isolated from plasma ultrafiltrate samples from patients receiving oxaliplatin. Distribution of platinum-containing derivatives appears to be triphasic, with the half-lives of the first, second, and third phases averaging approximately 0.43, 16.8, and 391 hours, respectively. Platinum-containing derivatives are eliminated principally by renal excretion; renal clearance of ultrafilterable platinum appears to be directly proportional to glomerular filtration rate (GFR). Following administration of a single 2-hour IV infusion of oxaliplatin, approximately 54 or 2% of platinum-containing derivatives is excreted in urine and feces, respectively, within 5 days.

Advice to Patients

Risk of neuropathy. Importance of understanding that symptoms of acute sensory neuropathy may be precipitated or exacerbated by exposure to cold temperature or cold objects; importance of avoiding cold drinks or use of ice and of covering exposed skin prior to exposure to cold temperature or cold objects. Importance of reading manufacturer's patient information for further instructions to minimize exposure to cold temperature or cold objects.

Risk of anemia, leukopenia, neutropenia, and thrombocytopenia; importance of informing a clinician immediately if fever, particularly if associated with persistent diarrhea, or evidence of infection develops.

Risk of dizziness, nausea, vomiting, visual abnormalities (e.g., transient vision loss), and other neurologic symptoms that may affect gait and balance; such effects may affect ability to drive or operate machinery.

Importance of understanding other potential risks associated with therapy. (See Cautions: Warnings/Precautions.) Importance of *immediately* seeking medical attention if symptoms of anaphylactic/anaphylactoid reactions (e.g., swelling of the throat, difficulty breathing) occur. Importance of informing a clinician of persistent vomiting, diarrhea, signs of dehydration, cough or shortness of breath, or other signs of allergic reactions (e.g., rash).

Importance of women informing clinicians immediately if they are or plan to become pregnant or plan to breast-feed; necessity of advising women to avoid pregnancy during therapy. Advise pregnant women of risk to the fetus.

Importance of informing clinicians of existing or contemplated concomitant therapy, including prescription and OTC drugs, as well as concomitant illness. Importance of informing patients of other important precautionary information (see Cautions).

Overview® (see Users Guide). For additional information on this drug until a more detailed monograph is developed and published, the manufacturer's labeling should be consulted. It is *essential* that the manufacturer's labeling be consulted for more detailed information on usual cautions, precautions, contraindications, potential drug interactions, laboratory test interferences, and acute toxicity. For further information on the handling of antineoplastic agents, see the ASHP Guidelines on Handling Hazardous Drugs at http://www.ahfsdruginformation.com.

Preparations

Excipients in commercially available drug preparations may have clinically important effects in some individuals; consult specific product labeling for details.

Oxaliplatin

Parenteral

For injection, for IV infusion	50 mg	**Eloxatin**®, Sanofi-Aventis
	100 mg	**Eloxatin**®, Sanofi-Aventis
For injection concentrate, for IV infusion	5 mg/mL (50, 100, and 200 mg)	**Eloxatin**®, Sanofi-Aventis

†Use is not currently included in the labeling approved by the US Food and Drug Administration

PACLitaxel

Taxol

■ Paclitaxel is a natural or semisynthetic diterpene antineoplastic agent extracted from the bark of the Western (Pacific) yew (*Taxus brevifolia*) or the needles and twigs of *Taxus baccata*.

Uses

Paclitaxel is commercially available in 2 types of formulations: conventional paclitaxel (in a nonaqueous solution) and albumin-bound paclitaxel. The efficacy and safety of paclitaxel for each indication is based on research and clinical experience using a specific formulation. Albumin-bound paclitaxel currently is labeled for use only in the second-line therapy of metastatic breast cancer, first-line therapy of non-small cell lung cancer in combination with carboplatin, and first-line therapy of metastatic adenocarcinoma of the pancreas in combination with gemcitabine. The functional properties of paclitaxel may differ substantially according to formulation; therefore, albumin-bound paclitaxel may *not* be substituted for or used in combination with other formulations of paclitaxel.

■ **Ovarian Cancer** Paclitaxel is used alone or in combination therapy for the treatment of ovarian cancer.

Adjuvant Therapy for Early-stage Ovarian Epithelial Cancer The use of platinum-based therapy, such as carboplatin and paclitaxel, is being investigated for adjuvant treatment following surgery in poor-prognosis early-stage ovarian epithelial cancer†. (See Uses: Ovarian Cancer: Adjuvant Therapy for Early-stage Ovarian Epithelial Cancer in Carboplatin 10:00.)

First-line Therapy for Advanced Ovarian Epithelial Cancer A platinum-containing agent in combination with paclitaxel is a preferred regimen for the initial treatment of advanced ovarian epithelial cancer.

Carboplatin Versus Cisplatin. Randomized trials have demonstrated that carboplatin is as effective as but less toxic than cisplatin when used in combination with paclitaxel for the initial treatment of advanced ovarian cancer. Carboplatin in combination with paclitaxel† currently is a preferred regimen for the initial treatment of advanced ovarian epithelial cancer. (See Uses: Ovarian Cancer: First-line Therapy for Advanced Ovarian Epithelial Cancer in Carboplatin 10:00.)

Platinum-containing Agent With Paclitaxel Versus Platinum-containing Agent With Cyclophosphamide. Evidence from randomized trials indicates that combined paclitaxel and cisplatin therapy is superior to combined cyclophosphamide and cisplatin therapy for the initial treatment of advanced epithelial ovarian cancer.

The current indication for the use of paclitaxel in combination with cisplatin for the initial treatment of advanced ovarian epithelial cancer is based principally on a comparative study in which 410 patients (386 evaluable patients) with suboptimally debulked (greater than 1 cm residual tumor mass) stage III or IV ovarian cancer who had no prior chemotherapy were randomized to receive paclitaxel 135 mg/m² (administered by 24-hour IV infusion) with cisplatin 75 mg/m² versus cyclophosphamide 750 mg/m² with cisplatin 75 mg/m². Among 216 evaluable patients with measurable disease, those receiving paclitaxel and cisplatin had an overall objective response of 73% (51% complete responses, 22% partial responses) compared with 60% (31% complete responses, 29% partial responses) for those receiving cisplatin and cyclophosphamide; the higher response rate for the combination of paclitaxel and cisplatin was maintained according to intention-to-treat analysis of 240 women with measurable disease (62 versus 48%). Patients receiving paclitaxel and cisplatin also had a longer median time to progression (evaluable patients: 18 versus 13 months; intention-to-treat analysis: 16.6 versus 13 months) and increased median overall survival (evaluable patients: 38 versus 24 months; intention-to-treat analysis: 35.5 versus 24.2 months) than those receiving cyclophosphamide and cisplatin. Higher frequencies of severe neutropenia (81 versus 58%), alopecia (55 versus 37%), asthenia (17 versus 10%), diarrhea (16 versus 8%), febrile neutropenia (15 versus 4%), myalgia/arthralgia (9 versus 2%), and hypersensitivity reactions (8 versus 1%) were observed in patients receiving paclitaxel and cisplatin compared with those receiving cyclophosphamide and cisplatin.

In a confirmatory randomized trial involving 680 patients with advanced ovarian cancer, longer median survival (35.6 versus 25.9 months), longer median time to progression (15.3 versus 11.5 months), and higher response rates (59 versus 45%) were observed for combination therapy with paclitaxel (175 mg/m² administered as a 3-hour IV infusion) and cisplatin versus cyclophosphamide and cisplatin. Limited evidence from subset analysis suggests that the same patterns were observed in patients with non-optimally debulked disease. Higher frequencies of neurotoxicity (87 versus 52%, severe in 21 versus 2%), myalgia/arthralgia (60 versus 27%), and diarrhea (37 versus 29%) were observed in patients receiving paclitaxel and cisplatin compared with those receiving cyclophosphamide and cisplatin.

At a follow-up of 6.5 years, the survival benefit associated with the paclitaxel and cisplatin regimen in both randomized trials has been maintained.

Combination therapy with paclitaxel and cisplatin is preferable to either high-dose cisplatin or paclitaxel alone for the initial treatment of advanced ovarian cancer.

Intraperitoneal Cisplatin and Paclitaxel. Combined IV and intraperitoneal therapy with IV paclitaxel, intraperitoneal cisplatin, and intraperitoneal paclitaxel† has been used for the treatment of optimally debulked stage III epithelial ovarian cancer.

The National Cancer Institute (NCI) recommends use of a combined IV and intraperitoneal regimen for eligible patients with advanced epithelial ovarian cancer because of a substantial survival benefit. Based on clinical trials, NCI recommends that use of a regimen containing intraperitoneal cisplatin (100 mg/m²) and a taxane (either IV only or IV plus intraperitoneal) should be strongly considered following primary surgery in patients with optimally debulked stage III epithelial ovarian cancer. Although an optimal intraperitoneal chemotherapy regimen has not been established, favorable results were observed following sequential administration of IV paclitaxel, intraperitoneal cisplatin, and intraperitoneal paclitaxel in the Gynecologic Oncology Group (GOG)-172 study.

In this randomized, phase 3 trial (GOG-172), 429 patients with previously untreated stage III epithelial ovarian cancer or primary peritoneal cancer, with no residual mass exceeding 1 cm in diameter following surgery, received either combined IV and intraperitoneal therapy or IV therapy. All patients enrolled in this study had good baseline GOG performance status (0–2) and adequate bone marrow, renal, and hepatic function. Most patients (88%) had ovarian cancer, and serous adenocarcinoma was the most common histologic type (79% of patients). The primary end points of the study were progression-free survival and overall survival. Combined IV and intraperitoneal therapy consisted of IV paclitaxel 135 mg/m² by 24-hour infusion on day 1, followed by intraperitoneal cisplatin 100 mg/m² on day 2 and intraperitoneal paclitaxel 60 mg/m² on day 8. IV therapy consisted of IV paclitaxel 135 mg/m² by 24-hour infusion on day 1 followed by IV cisplatin 75 mg/m² on day 2. Both regimens were repeated every 21 days for up to 6 cycles. Patients who received combined IV and intraperitoneal therapy had longer median progression-free (23.8 versus 18.3 months) and overall (65.6 versus 49.7 months) survival compared with patients who received IV therapy.

Most (83%) of the patients receiving IV therapy completed 6 cycles of their assigned chemotherapy regimen; however, only 42% of patients receiving combined IV and intraperitoneal therapy completed 6 cycles of assigned chemotherapy; patients who could not complete the intraperitoneal regimen received IV therapy for the remaining treatment cycles. The most common reason for discontinuance of intraperitoneal therapy was catheter-related complications. Grade 3 or 4 leukopenia (76 versus 64%), GI effects (46 versus 24%), metabolic effects (27 versus 7%), fatigue (18 versus 4%), neurologic effects (19 versus 9%), infection (16 versus 6%), thrombocytopenia (12 versus 4%), and pain (11 versus 1%) occurred more frequently in patients receiving combined IV and intraperitoneal therapy than in those receiving IV therapy. Although patients receiving combined IV and intraperitoneal therapy reported less improvement in abdominal discomfort before cycle 4, improvement in abdominal discomfort was similar in both treatment groups 1 year after completion of therapy. Among patients who received combined IV and intraperitoneal therapy, quality of life was worse during and shortly after completion of therapy (before cycle 4 and at 3–6 weeks following therapy) compared with those who received IV therapy. Quality of life scores were similar for the groups at 1 year after completion of treatment, except for greater persistence of moderate paresthesias in patients receiving combined IV and intraperitoneal therapy.

Retrospective review of baseline data (patient and disease characteristics) from two phase 3 clinical trials (including GOG-172) for patients receiving intraperitoneal therapy for optimally debulked stage III epithelial ovarian cancer suggested that extent of residual tumor mass, histology, and age were important predictors of survival in such patients. Patients with clear cell histology appeared to derive less benefit from intraperitoneal therapy compared with those with serous histology (hazard ratio for progression-free and overall survival of 2.66 and 3.88, respectively). In addition, each additional year of age was associated with a 1% increase in the risk of death. Although patients enrolled in the studies had optimally debulked (1 cm or less residual tumor mass) disease, survival was greater in patients with only microscopic residual disease.

Retrospective analysis of data from patients receiving a modified IV and intraperitoneal regimen suggests that a reduced dosage of intraperitoneal cisplatin administered in conjunction with a shortened IV paclitaxel infusion time may result in less toxicity and produce a survival benefit similar to that reported in the GOG-172 study (67 months versus 65.6 months reported in GOG-172). The modified IV and intraperitoneal regimen consisted of IV paclitaxel 135 mg/m² by 3-hour infusion on day 1, followed by intraperitoneal cisplatin 75 mg/m² on day 2 and intraperitoneal paclitaxel 60 mg/m² on day 8 of each 21-day cycle. Most patients (80%) completed 4 or more cycles of therapy and 55% completed 6 cycles. The frequency of grade 3 or 4 neutropenia (12%), GI effects (8%), metabolic effects (5%), neurologic effects (6%), infection (2%), fatigue (2%), and thrombocytopenia (0%) in this series of patients receiving the modified IV and intraperitoneal regimen appeared to be lower than toxicity rates reported in the GOG-172 study. By shortening the infusion time for IV paclitaxel to 3 hours, the modified regimen also may provide an outpatient alternative to inpatient administration over 24 hours. However, randomized controlled trials are needed to establish comparative safety and efficacy of this modified regimen. The modified IV and intraperitoneal schedule containing the lower intraperitoneal cisplatin dosage and the 3-hour IV paclitaxel infusion also has been studied in conjunction with a third cytotoxic drug, but with evidence of excessive toxicity.

Based on current evidence, combined IV and intraperitoneal therapy with IV paclitaxel, intraperitoneal cisplatin, and intraperitoneal paclitaxel is recommended (accepted) for use as initial adjuvant treatment of optimally debulked stage III epithelial ovarian cancer in patients with good performance status (GOG performance status of 0–2).

Second-line Therapy for Advanced Ovarian Epithelial Cancer

Paclitaxel is used alone or in combination therapy as second-line or subsequent therapy in patients with advanced ovarian epithelial cancer.

Paclitaxel is used alone as second-line or subsequent therapy in patients with advanced ovarian epithelial cancer. In the treatment of advanced ovarian cancer refractory to prior chemotherapy, paclitaxel alone produces an objective response in about 35% (range: 16–48%) of patients. Patients whose cancer is resistant to platinum-containing therapy (defined as tumor progression while on platinum-containing therapy or tumor relapse within 6 months after completion of a platinum-containing regimen) who then receive paclitaxel therapy reportedly have had response rates of 14–35%.

The current indication of paclitaxel monotherapy for recurrent or refractory ovarian cancer was initially based on data from 5 phase I and II clinical studies involving 189 patients, a multicenter randomized phase III study involving 407 patients, and interim analysis of experience from an additional 300 patients who received the drug under a treatment IND protocol. According to the manufacturer, patients in 2 of the phase II clinical studies receiving an initial dose of paclitaxel of 135–170 mg/m² administered by 24-hour IV infusion had objective response rates (complete or partial responses) of 22% and 30%. The median duration of overall response in these 2 studies was about 7 months, and the median survival was 8.1 and 15.9 months. Similar responses were observed in other clinical studies using higher initial doses of paclitaxel or concomitant administration of paclitaxel and filgrastim, a recombinant human granulocyte colony-stimulating factor (G-CSF).

The response rates observed in these phase II studies were confirmed in a large case series in which 1000 patients with platinum-refractory ovarian cancer who received paclitaxel 135 mg/m² administered by 24-hour IV infusion had an overall objective response rate of 22%. According to the manufacturer, patients in a phase III study with a bifactorial design receiving paclitaxel 135 or 175 mg/m² as a 3- or 24-hour IV infusion had an overall objective response rate of 16.2% with 6 complete responses and 60 partial responses. The duration of response measured from the first day of treatment was 8.3 months (range: 3.2–21.6 months). Median time to disease progression was 3.7 months (range: 0.1 to longer than 25 months), and median survival was 11.5 months (range: 0.2 to longer than 26 months).

Response rates did not differ significantly according to dose or infusion schedule. Patients receiving a paclitaxel dose of either 175 or 135 mg/m² had objective (partial or complete) response rates of 20 or 15%, respectively. Patients receiving paclitaxel doses by either 3- or 24-hour IV infusion had objective (partial or complete) response rates of 16 or 19%, respectively. Median time to disease progression was longer in patients receiving 175 mg/m^2 than in those receiving 135 mg/m^2 (4.2 versus 3.1 months) and similar in patients receiving paclitaxel by 3-hour IV infusion or 24-hour IV infusion (4 versus 3.7 months). No difference in survival was observed according to dose or infusion schedule. Median survival was 11.6 or 11 months in patients receiving paclitaxel 175 or 135 mg/m^2, respectively, and 11.7 or 11.2 months in patients receiving paclitaxel by 3- or 24-hour infusion, respectively. Although severity of myelosuppression was affected by dose, the most important factor was duration of infusion; the same paclitaxel doses administered by 24-hour IV infusion were more myelotoxic than those administered by 3-hour IV infusion. The results of this randomized study support the use of paclitaxel doses of 135 or 175 mg/m^2 administered by 3-hour IV infusion, but the power of the study was inadequate to determine whether a particular dosage schedule for paclitaxel produced superior efficacy.

Paclitaxel also has been used in combination therapy with a platinum agent (carboplatin or cisplatin) as second-line or subsequent therapy† for advanced ovarian epithelial cancer. Analysis of combined data for 802 patients involved in parallel randomized, multicenter trials indicates that median survival and median progression-free survival are prolonged in patients receiving combination therapy with paclitaxel and a platinum agent (a regimen of paclitaxel and carboplatin in 80% of patients) rather than platinum-based therapy alone (a regimen of carboplatin alone in 71% of patients) for the treatment of relapsed platinum-sensitive ovarian cancer.

Dosage and Other Considerations Response rates for paclitaxel therapy vary with tumor histology, volume of residual tumor, and development of resistance to previous platinum-based chemotherapy.

Current evidence suggests that increased dose intensity (amount of paclitaxel per unit time) may affect response to paclitaxel but that paclitaxel doses exceeding 175 mg/m^2 are more toxic and do not improve survival in patients with advanced ovarian cancer. In addition to dose effect, the effect of duration of infusion of paclitaxel has been studied in patients with ovarian cancer. Efficacy was similar but toxicity, particularly myelosuppression, was greater when paclitaxel alone was administered by 24-hour versus 3-hour infusion for the subsequent therapy of advanced ovarian cancer. Limited evidence suggests that subsequent therapy with prolonged infusion of paclitaxel (96-hour IV infusion) does not produce response in patients with advanced ovarian cancer that was resistant to previous therapy with the drug administered by 3-hour or 24-hour IV infusion.

The effect of duration of infusion on the efficacy and toxicity of paclitaxel administered as a component of combination therapy also has not been fully established. Increased incidence and severity of neurotoxicity is associated with administration of paclitaxel by 3-hour IV infusion in combination therapy with cisplatin in patients with gynecologic cancers. In a large randomized trial, patients with advanced ovarian cancer receiving paclitaxel (175 mg/m^2 administered as a 3-hour IV infusion) and cisplatin had an increased incidence of severe neurosensory toxicity compared with those receiving cyclophosphamide and cisplatin. Prolonged paclitaxel infusions do not appear to offer benefit in the treatment of ovarian cancer. In a randomized trial comparing 96-hour infusion of paclitaxel 120 mg/m^2 with 24-hour infusion of paclitaxel 135 mg/m^2 (each in a combination regimen of paclitaxel and cisplatin) for suboptimal stage III or IV ovarian epithelial cancer, median survival rates were similar between the groups but the relative death rate was approximately 5% greater among patients receiving the prolonged infusion of paclitaxel.

Maintenance therapy with paclitaxel for advanced ovarian cancer† is being investigated. In a randomized trial, patients receiving 12 months of single-agent paclitaxel therapy following complete response to induction therapy with platinum/paclitaxel therapy for advanced ovarian cancer experienced longer progression-free survival but greater neurotoxicity than those receiving 3 months of such therapy. Because the trial was terminated according to study design following a planned interim analysis that detected the difference in progression-free survival, and cross-over treatment was allowed, overall survival data may be unavailable. Whether maintenance therapy with paclitaxel is superior to treatment upon progression of disease is unclear, and a confirmatory randomized trial is needed. Until further evidence is available, clinicians should discuss maintenance paclitaxel therapy and offer it as an option for patients with advanced ovarian cancer that has a complete response to induction therapy.

■ Breast Cancer

Adjuvant Therapy for Breast Cancer **Adjuvant Therapy for Node-positive Breast Cancer.** Paclitaxel is administered sequentially to standard doxorubicin-containing combination chemotherapy as adjuvant therapy for node-positive breast cancer, particularly in patients with hormone receptor-negative disease.

The current indication for paclitaxel as adjuvant therapy is based on data from a multicenter, randomized trial involving 3170 patients with node-positive breast cancer. Following completion of 4 courses of doxorubicin and cyclophosphamide (AC), patients received paclitaxel (175 mg/m^2 as a 3-hour IV infusion once every 3 weeks for 4 courses) or no additional chemotherapy. Patients with hormone receptor-positive disease were assigned to receive tamoxifen, and patients who had received segmental mastectomies were assigned to receive radiation therapy following recovery from treatment-related toxicity. At a median follow-up of 30.1 months, patients receiving AC followed by adjuvant therapy with paclitaxel had a 22% reduction in the risk of disease recurrence and a 26% reduction in the risk of death compared with patients receiving AC alone. Subset analysis according to number of positive nodes, tumor size, menopausal status, and hormone receptor status suggests a similar effect of adjuvant paclitaxel on disease-free or overall survival in all of the larger subsets except for patients with hormone receptor-positive tumors, who experienced a smaller reduction in risk for disease recurrence or death.

The study was also designed to assess the efficacy and toxicity of 3 dose levels of doxorubicin (60, 75, or 90 mg/m^2). No effect on disease-free or overall survival was observed for doxorubicin doses exceeding 60 mg/m^2; higher incidences of severe hematologic toxicities (including severe thrombocytopenia and platelet transfusions), infections, mucositis, and cardiovascular events were observed for higher doses of doxorubicin. Higher frequencies of severe (grade 3 or 4) toxicity, including neurosensory toxicity, myalgia/arthralgia, neurologic pain (5 versus 1%), flu-like symptoms (5 versus 3%), and hyperglycemia (3 versus 1%), were observed in patients receiving AC followed by paclitaxel compared with those receiving AC alone. Two deaths (0.1%) were attributed to treatment with adjuvant paclitaxel.

In another randomized trial, involving 3060 patients with node-positive breast cancer, disease-free survival was longer in patients receiving paclitaxel (versus no additional therapy) following postoperative chemotherapy with doxorubicin and cyclophosphamide.

Differing dosage schedules are being investigated for the use of paclitaxel as adjuvant therapy for node-positive breast cancer (e.g., increased dose density, concurrent versus sequential administration of doxorubicin and cyclophosphamide with paclitaxel). In a randomized trial, increased dose density of the doxorubicin, cyclophosphamide, and paclitaxel regimen with treatment every 2 weeks rather than every 3 weeks was associated with prolonged disease-free and overall survival, but no effect was observed for concurrent administration (doxorubicin/cyclophosphamide followed by paclitaxel) versus sequential administration (doxorubicin followed by paclitaxel and then cyclophosphamide). Further follow-up of this study and a confirmatory trial are needed to establish the effect of dose densification for this regimen.

Adjuvant Therapy for Early-stage HER2-positive Breast Cancer. Paclitaxel-containing adjuvant therapy is used in conjunction with trastuzumab for the treatment of operable HER2-positive breast cancer†. In several large randomized trials, the addition of trastuzumab to standard adjuvant chemotherapy in patients with operable HER2-positive breast cancer reduced the risk of death and/or prolonged disease-free survival. See Adjuvant Therapy for Early-stage Breast Cancer under Uses: Breast Cancer, in Trastuzumab 10:00.

First-line Therapy for Advanced Breast Cancer **Paclitaxel and Gemcitabine.** Paclitaxel is used in combination with gemcitabine for the initial treatment of metastatic breast cancer following failure of adjuvant chemotherapy; prior therapy in such patients should have included an anthracycline antineoplastic agent (e.g., doxorubicin) unless clinically contraindicated.

The current indication for combination therapy with paclitaxel and gemcitabine for the first-line treatment of metastatic breast cancer is based on data from a randomized, multinational, phase III trial involving 529 patients who had prior adjuvant or neoadjuvant anthracycline therapy unless clinically contraindicated. Patients were randomized to receive either combination therapy with paclitaxel and gemcitabine (paclitaxel 175 mg/m^2 by 3-hour IV infusion followed by gemcitabine 1250 mg/m^2 by 30-minute IV infusion on day 1 and then the same dosage of gemcitabine on day 8) or paclitaxel alone (paclitaxel 175 mg/m^2 by 3-hour IV infusion on day 1) in 21-day cycles. Longer median time to disease progression (5.2 versus 2.9 months) and higher response rates (40.8 versus 22.1%) were observed in patients receiving paclitaxel and gemcitabine compared with those receiving paclitaxel monotherapy. In an interim analysis, a trend toward prolonged survival was noted among patients receiving combination therapy with paclitaxel and gemcitabine. Greater toxicity was reported in patients receiving combination therapy with paclitaxel and gemcitabine than in those receiving paclitaxel alone, including neutropenia (all: 69 versus 31%, severe: 48 versus 11%), anemia (69 versus 51%), thrombocytopenia (26 versus 7%), elevated serum ALT (SGPT) concentrations (18 versus 6%), and elevated serum AST (SGOT) concentrations (16 versus 5%).

Paclitaxel With or Without Doxorubicin. Paclitaxel has been used alone or in combination with doxorubicin as first-line chemotherapy for metastatic breast cancer†.

In a randomized trial with crossover, patients with metastatic breast cancer who had no previous chemotherapy with anthracyclines or taxanes received paclitaxel 200 mg/m^{2}administered by 3-hour IV infusion or doxorubicin IV 75 mg/m^2 for 7 courses or until disease progression or unacceptable toxicity were observed; patients with disease progression were crossed over to therapy with the alternative agent. Although overall survival did not differ, lower response rates and shorter median progression-free survival were observed among patients receiving initial therapy with paclitaxel versus doxorubicin; arthralgia/myalgia and sensory neurotoxicity were associated with paclitaxel whereas mucositis, gastrointestinal toxicity, grade 4 neutropenia, febrile neutropenia, and cardiotoxicity were more frequently observed with doxorubicin.

In a randomized, phase III, multicenter trial, patients with metastatic breast cancer receiving first-line therapy with doxorubicin and paclitaxel had higher response rates, longer median time to progression, and longer median survival than those receiving cyclophosphamide, doxorubicin, and fluorouracil (CAF). Neutropenia (including grade 3 or 4 neutropenia), arthralgia/myalgia, peripheral neuropathy, and diarrhea occurred more frequently in patients receiving doxorubicin and paclitaxel, whereas nausea and vomiting was more common in those receiving CAF. In another randomized trial, similar response rates, median progression-free survival, and median survival were observed for patients receiving doxorubicin and paclitaxel versus doxorubicin and cyclophosphamide as first-line therapy for metastatic breast cancer.

Results from a phase III trial comparing a combination of paclitaxel and doxorubicin to either agent alone (with subsequent crossover to the alternative agent) as first-line therapy for metastatic breast cancer showed a higher overall response rate and longer time to treatment failure with the combination regimen; however, overall survival and quality of life were similar for combination therapy compared with either agent alone. Results from a randomized study comparing paclitaxel monotherapy to a standard combination chemotherapy regimen (CMFP [cyclophosphamide, methotrexate, fluorouracil, and prednisolone]) showed a similar objective response rate, time to progression, and overall survival duration with the 2 regimens.

The choice of single-agent or combination chemotherapy as first-line therapy for metastatic breast cancer may depend on the rate of disease progression, the presence of comorbid conditions, and clinician and patient preferences.

Paclitaxel and Trastuzumab for HER2-positive Metastatic Breast Cancer. Paclitaxel is used in combination with trastuzumab (Herceptin®, Genentech), a humanized anti-HER2 antibody, for the initial treatment of metastatic breast cancer in patients with tumors that overexpress the HER2 protein. (See First-line Therapy for Advanced Breast Cancer under Uses: Breast Cancer, in Trastuzumab 10:00.)

The current indication for combination therapy with paclitaxel and trastuzumab for the initial treatment of metastatic breast cancer is based on data from a randomized, controlled, multicenter trial involving 469 patients with 2+ or 3+ HER2-overexpressing breast tumors (based on a 0–3+ scale). Patients were randomized to receive chemotherapy alone or chemotherapy combined with trastuzumab (4 mg/kg IV loading dose followed by once-weekly doses of 2 mg/kg IV). Chemotherapy consisted of an anthracycline and cyclophosphamide unless patients had received prior adjuvant chemotherapy with an anthracycline, in which case chemotherapy consisted of paclitaxel 175 mg/m^2 administered by 3-hour IV infusion every 21 days for at least 6 cycles. Longer median time to disease progression (6.7 versus 2.5 months), higher overall response rate (38 versus 15%), and longer median duration of response (8.3 versus 4.3 months) were reported for combination therapy with paclitaxel and trastuzumab compared with paclitaxel alone in patients with metastatic breast cancer characterized by excess production of the HER2 protein.

Second-line Therapy for Advanced Breast Cancer **Conventional Paclitaxel.** Paclitaxel is used as monotherapy for the treatment of breast cancer in patients who have metastatic disease refractory to conventional combination chemotherapy or who have experienced relapse within 6 months of adjuvant chemotherapy; prior therapy in such patients should have included an anthracycline antineoplastic agent (e.g., doxorubicin) unless clinically contraindicated.

The current indication for use of paclitaxel as a single agent in advanced breast cancer is based principally on data from a multicenter, randomized study involving 471 patients who were treated previously with 1 or 2 regimens of chemotherapy. For 454 evaluable patients in the study, overall response rate was 26%, median time to disease progression was 3.5 months, and median survival was 11.7 months. The median duration of response was 8.1 months. Patients receiving a paclitaxel dose of either 175 or 135 mg/m^2 administered as a 3-hour infusion had similar rates of objective (partial or complete) response of 28 or 22%, respectively. Median time to progression of disease was longer (4.2 versus 3 months) but median survival was similar (11.7 versus 10.5 months) for patients receiving paclitaxel doses of 175 or 135 mg/m^2, respectively.

In this randomized study, 60% of patients had symptomatic disease with impaired performance status at study entry and 73% had visceral metastases. Overall, 30% of these patients had disease that progressed following adjuvant chemotherapy, 39% had metastatic disease refractory to conventional chemotherapy, and 31% of patients had disease that progressed or failed to respond in both settings. Of the patients in this study, 67% had received an anthracycline antineoplastic agent and 23% had disease considered resistant to this class of agents.

Two uncontrolled phase II studies of paclitaxel therapy were conducted in a total of 53 patients with metastatic breast cancer who had been treated previously with a maximum of one regimen of antineoplastic therapy (including some patients who had received no prior chemotherapy). Treatment consisted of paclitaxel as a 24-hour IV infusion at initial doses of 250 mg/m^2 (with G-CSF support) or 200 mg/m^2, and overall objective response rates of 57 and 52% were observed. Dose reductions were required in patients who experienced severe hematologic (e.g., neutropenia) or nonhematologic (e.g., infection, neurotoxicity) toxicity; therefore, the median dose of paclitaxel per course was 203 mg/m^2 for both studies. Overall, response rates were not influenced by initial dose or dose intensity of paclitaxel or by concomitant administration of filgrastim.

In another phase II study of patients whose disease was refractory to at least 2 regimens of antineoplastic therapy, including anthracycline therapy, an overall response rate of 30% (partial responses only) was observed with a paclitaxel dose of 200 mg/m^2 given as a 24-hour infusion with concomitant administration of filgrastim. In phase II studies that evaluated the use of a 3-hour infusion schedule, patients with metastatic breast cancer that was refractory to previous chemotherapy, including anthracyclines, who received paclitaxel doses of 175–225 mg/m^2 had overall response rates (partial or complete) of 18–38%.

The optimal dosage regimen of paclitaxel when used as single-agent therapy in patients with metastatic breast cancer has not been established. The effect of dose on the efficacy and toxicity of paclitaxel has been studied in patients with metastatic breast cancer. In patients with metastatic breast cancer receiving paclitaxel administered as a 3-hour IV infusion, paclitaxel doses exceeding 175 mg/m^2 are associated with greater toxicity, particularly hematologic and neurosensory toxicity, but do not appear to increase response rate or prolong survival. The use of a weekly schedule of paclitaxel to increase dose density is being investigated. In a phase II study, an overall response rate of 53% was observed in patients with metastatic breast cancer receiving paclitaxel 100 mg/m^2 administered once weekly until disease progression (median of 14 infusions per patient); this regimen was notable for lack of myelosuppression although peripheral neuropathy prohibited dose escalation above paclitaxel 100 mg/m^2.

The effect of duration of infusion on the efficacy and toxicity of paclitaxel has been studied in patients with metastatic breast cancer. Evidence from a randomized trial indicates that response rate is higher in patients with advanced breast cancer receiving high-dose paclitaxel (250 mg/m^2) by 24- versus 3-hour IV infusion but event-free survival and survival are similar; hematologic toxicity, including febrile neutropenia, occurs more frequently with the 24-hour infusion of paclitaxel whereas severe neurotoxicity is more common with the 3-hour infusion. No difference in response rate, duration of response, or survival was observed in patients with metastatic breast cancer receiving paclitaxel 140 mg/m^2 by 96-hour IV infusion or paclitaxel 250 mg/m^2 by 3-hour IV infusion.

Albumin-bound Paclitaxel. Albumin-bound paclitaxel is used as monotherapy for the treatment of breast cancer in patients who have metastatic disease refractory to conventional combination chemotherapy or who have experienced relapse within 6 months of adjuvant chemotherapy; prior therapy in such patients should have included an anthracycline antineoplastic agent (e.g., doxorubicin) unless clinically contraindicated.

The current indication for use of albumin-bound paclitaxel as a single agent in advanced breast cancer is based principally on data from 2 single-arm open-label studies and a randomized trial.

In a randomized trial involving 460 patients with metastatic breast cancer, patients received either albumin-bound paclitaxel 260 mg/m^2 by 30-minute IV infusion or paclitaxel 175 mg/m^2 by 3-hour IV infusion. Most patients in the study had visceral metastases, had received prior chemotherapy in the adjuvant and/or metastatic setting, and had received therapy with anthracyclines. Patients with metastatic breast cancer receiving albumin-bound paclitaxel had a higher rate of reconciled target lesion response (21.5%) than those receiving conventional paclitaxel (11.1%). The reconciled target lesion response rate was based on independent radiologic assessment of tumor response reconciled with the investigator assessment of response for the first 6 cycles of therapy. Compared with conventional paclitaxel, albumin-bound paclitaxel was associated with a lower incidence of grade 4 neutropenia (9 versus 22%) and hypersensitivity reactions (all: 4 versus 12%, severe: 0 versus 2%), but a higher frequency of sensory neuropathy (all: 71 versus 56%, severe: 10 versus 2%), asthenia (47 versus 39%), nausea (30 versus 22%), diarrhea (27 versus 15%), and vomiting (18 versus 10%).

Objective responses to albumin-bound paclitaxel were observed in 2 phase II studies in patients with metastatic breast cancer. In one study, patients received albumin-bound paclitaxel 300 mg/m^2 by 30-minute IV infusion once every 3 weeks. In the other study, patients received albumin-bound paclitaxel 175 mg/m^2 by 30-minute IV infusion once every 3 weeks.

■ **Non-small Cell Lung Cancer** ***Adjuvant Therapy*** Platinum-containing therapy, such as paclitaxel and carboplatin, is used in selected patients for the adjuvant treatment of completely resected non-small cell lung cancer†. In a randomized trial, patients receiving 4 cycles of paclitaxel and carboplatin therapy following surgery for stage IB non-small cell lung cancer had a higher overall survival rate at 4 years (71%) than those in an observation group (59%). Analysis of pooled data abstracted from randomized trials suggests that adjuvant chemotherapy prolongs survival in patients with resected non-small cell lung cancer.

Therapy for Advanced Disease Currently preferred regimens for the initial treatment of advanced non-small cell lung cancer in patients with good performance status include a platinum-containing agent in combination with another cytotoxic agent such as paclitaxel, docetaxel, gemcitabine, pemetrexed, or vinorelbine.

Although the primary objective of treatment in patients with advanced non-small cell lung carcinoma is palliation, small improvements in survival have been demonstrated with the use of platinum-based chemotherapy.

Conventional Paclitaxel and Carboplatin. Paclitaxel and carboplatin is used in the treatment of advanced non-small cell lung cancer†. Similar response rates and median survival were observed in a randomized trial in which patients received paclitaxel and carboplatin versus regimens of cisplatin in combination with paclitaxel, gemcitabine, or docetaxel for advanced non-small cell lung cancer. Paclitaxel and carboplatin (paclitaxel 225 mg/m^2 by 3-hour IV infusion on day 1 followed on the same day by carboplatin at the dose required to obtain an AUC of 6 mg/mL per minute) was less toxic than the other regimens and was selected as a reference regimen for further studies. However, another randomized trial showed a survival benefit in patients receiving cisplatin/paclitaxel rather than carboplatin/paclitaxel for advanced non-small cell lung cancer. In this study, paclitaxel 200 mg/m^2 by 3-hour IV infusion was administered with either cisplatin 80 mg/m² or carboplatin at the dose required to obtain an AUC of 6 mg/mL per minute. In another randomized trial, response rates, median survival, and 1- and 2-year survival rates were similar in patients receiving either paclitaxel/carboplatin or vinorelbine/cisplatin for advanced non-small cell lung cancer; grade 3 peripheral neuropathy occurred more frequently in patients receiving paclitaxel and carboplatin whereas grade 3 or 4 leukopenia and grade 3 nausea and vomiting were more frequent in patients receiving vinorelbine and cisplatin. Further study is needed to clarify the comparative efficacy of carboplatin and cisplatin in the treatment of non-small cell lung cancer.

Weekly schedules of paclitaxel and carboplatin for the treatment of advanced non-small cell lung cancer are being investigated.

Conventional Paclitaxel and Cisplatin. Paclitaxel and cisplatin is used in the treatment of advanced non-small cell lung cancer. Combination chemotherapy with paclitaxel and cisplatin is associated with higher response rates and similar survival compared with other cisplatin-containing regimens (e.g., cisplatin with etoposide, cisplatin with teniposide).

The current indication for the use of paclitaxel in combination with cisplatin for the initial treatment of advanced non-small cell lung cancer is based on a comparative study in which 599 patients with stage IIIB or IV non-small cell lung cancer who had not received previous chemotherapy were randomized to receive paclitaxel at a dose of 135 or 250 mg/m² administered by 24-hour IV infusion followed by IV cisplatin 75 mg/m² versus IV cisplatin 75/mg/m² with IV etoposide 100 mg/m². Patients receiving the higher dose of paclitaxel received concomitant administration of granulocyte colony-stimulating factor [G-CSF]). Patients receiving paclitaxel (135 or 250 mg/m²) combined with cisplatin had higher response rates (25 or 23%, respectively, versus 12%) but similar median survival (9.3 or 10 months, respectively, versus 7.4 months) compared with those receiving combination therapy with etoposide and cisplatin. Longer time to progression of disease was observed in patients receiving the higher dose of paclitaxel combined with cisplatin compared with etoposide and cisplatin (4.9 versus 2.7 months). Quality of life assessed by the Functional Assessment of Cancer Therapy-Lung (FACT-L) questionnaire showed a more favorable score in the Lung Cancer Specific Symptoms subscale for patients receiving the lower dose of paclitaxel combined with cisplatin compared with etoposide and cisplatin.

Similar response rates and median survival were observed in patients receiving paclitaxel doses of either 250 or 135 mg/m², but greater toxicity occurred in patients receiving the higher dose, including arthralgia/myalgia (42 versus 21%), severe neurosensory toxicity (28 versus 13%), and severe hypersensitivity reactions (4 versus 1%). Although patients received concomitant administration of G-CSF with the higher dose of paclitaxel, severe neutropenia was common in patients receiving paclitaxel 250 or 135 mg/m² with cisplatin (65 or 74%, respectively) and occurred more frequently than in patients receiving etoposide with cisplatin (55%). Other adverse effects that occurred more frequently in patients receiving paclitaxel 250 or 135 mg/m² by 24-hour IV infusion followed by cisplatin than in those receiving etoposide with cisplatin included arthralgia/myalgia (42 or 21%, respectively, versus 9%) and severe neurosensory toxicity (28 or 13%, respectively, versus 8%).

Conventional Paclitaxel and Gemcitabine. Paclitaxel also is used in non-platinum-based combination regimens for the treatment of advanced non-small cell lung cancer†. In a phase III randomized trial, efficacy and toxicity were similar in patients with advanced non-small cell lung cancer receiving initial treatment with paclitaxel/gemcitabine or paclitaxel/carboplatin. Treatment consisted of paclitaxel 200 mg/m² as a 3-hour IV infusion on day 1 followed by either gemcitabine (1000 mg/m² as a 30-minute IV infusion on days 1 and 8) or carboplatin (at the dose required to obtain an AUC of 6 mg/mL per minute as a 1-hour IV infusion on day 1) with treatment cycles repeated every 3 weeks for up to 6 cycles. Treatment-related toxicity was mild in both groups.

Albumin-bound Paclitaxel and Carboplatin. Albumin-bound paclitaxel in combination with carboplatin is used for the initial treatment of advanced non-small cell lung cancer in patients who are not candidates for curative surgery or radiation therapy. Combination chemotherapy with albumin-bound paclitaxel and carboplatin is associated with higher response rates and similar survival compared with conventional paclitaxel and carboplatin.

The current indication for albumin-bound paclitaxel in combination with carboplatin is based principally on the results of a randomized, multicenter, open-label trial in patients with previously untreated advanced non-small cell lung cancer. In this study, 1052 patients with stage IIIB or IV non-small cell lung cancer were randomized to receive either albumin-bound paclitaxel (100 mg/m² by 30-minute IV infusion) on days 1, 8, and 15 followed by IV carboplatin (at the dose required to obtain an AUC of 6 mg/mL per minute) on day 1 of each 21-day cycle or conventional paclitaxel (200 mg/m² by 3-hour IV infusion) followed by IV carboplatin (at the dose required to obtain an AUC of 6 mg/mL per minute) on day 1 of each 21-day cycle. Treatment was continued until disease progression or unacceptable toxicity occurred. Patients receiving albumin-bound paclitaxel combined with carboplatin had higher overall response rates (33 versus 25%) but similar median overall survival (12.1 versus 11.2 months) and progression-free survival (6.3 versus 5.8 months) compared with those receiving conventional paclitaxel combined with carboplatin. Albumin-bound paclitaxel therapy was associated with higher overall response rates (41 versus 24%) compared with conventional paclitaxel therapy in patients with squamous cell histology and was as effective as conventional paclitaxel in patients with nonsquamous cell histology (response rate of 26 versus 25% in patients with nonsquamous cell histology receiving therapy with albumin-bound paclitaxel or conventional paclitaxel, respectively). Grade 3 or greater thrombocytopenia (18 versus 9%) and anemia (27 versus 7%) occurred more frequently in patients receiving albumin-bound paclitaxel, whereas grade 3 or greater neutropenia (58 versus 47%) and sensory neuropathy (12 versus 3%) occurred more frequently in those receiving conventional paclitaxel.

Conventional Paclitaxel. Paclitaxel appears to be one of the most active single agents in patients with non-small cell lung carcinoma who have not received prior chemotherapy. In phase II studies of patients with advanced non-small cell lung carcinoma who had not received prior chemotherapy, objective response rates of 21–24% (0–4% complete responses, 20–21% partial responses) and 1-year survival rates of approximately 40% have been observed with paclitaxel alone at doses of 200–250 mg/m² administered by 24-hour infusion every 3 weeks. Response rates of 10–26% have been observed in additional phase II studies of patients who had not received previous chemotherapy for advanced disease with paclitaxel doses of 135–225 mg/m² administered over shorter periods of infusion (i.e., 1 or 3 hours). Limited evidence suggests that paclitaxel is not active against disease refractory to platinum-containing chemotherapy.

Intrapleural injections of paclitaxel have been used for the treatment of malignant pleural effusions† in a limited number of patients with non-small cell lung cancer.

■ AIDS-related Kaposi's Sarcoma

Paclitaxel alone is used for the palliative treatment of advanced or refractory AIDS-related (epidemic) Kaposi's sarcoma. Use of a liposomal anthracycline (doxorubicin or daunorubicin) is a first-line therapy of choice for advanced AIDS-related Kaposi's sarcoma (see Uses: AIDS-related Kaposi's Sarcoma in Doxorubicin 10:00 or Daunorubicin 10:00).

Although the comparative efficacy of paclitaxel versus other treatments for advanced AIDS-related Kaposi's sarcoma (e.g., liposomal doxorubicin; liposomal daunorubicin; combination therapy with conventional doxorubicin, bleomycin, and a vinca alkaloid [vinblastine or vincristine]) has not been established, paclitaxel has shown substantial activity in patients with advanced disease (e.g., extensive mucocutaneous disease, lymphedema, symptomatic visceral disease). Objective responses to paclitaxel therapy have been reported in patients with poor prognostic factors, including low baseline helper/inducer ($CD4^+$, $T4^+$) T-cell counts (less than 200/mm³), visceral involvement (e.g., pulmonary disease), or history of opportunistic infection, as well as in patients who have received prior systemic chemotherapy. However, the depressed immunologic status of the patient limits the therapeutic benefit of systemic chemotherapy, and there currently are no data showing unequivocal evidence of improved survival with any treatment for AIDS-related Kaposi's sarcoma; new therapies are continually being evaluated.

The current indication for use of paclitaxel in advanced AIDS-related Kaposi's sarcoma is based on limited data from 2 uncontrolled phase II studies involving 59 patients who previously had received systemic therapy, including interferon alfa (32%), liposomal daunorubicin (31%), liposomal doxorubicin (2%), and/or conventional doxorubicin-containing chemotherapy (42%); 64% of the patients had received previous chemotherapy with anthracycline agents. Most of these patients experienced progression of disease during, or could not tolerate, previous systemic therapy for AIDS-related Kaposi's sarcoma. According to the manufacturer, the overall objective response rate was 59% (3% complete responses, 56% partial responses). A cutaneous (i.e., objective) response was defined principally as flattening of the size of all previously raised lesions by at least 50%. The median duration of response measured from the first day of treatment was 10.4 months (range: 7–11 months). Median time to disease progression was 6.2 months (range: 4.6–8.7 months).

Retrospective analysis of the data showed that some patients receiving paclitaxel as second-line therapy for AIDS-related Kaposi's sarcoma experienced additional clinical benefits, including improvement of pulmonary function in those with pulmonary involvement, increased ambulation, resolution of ulcers, decreased analgesic requirements for pain caused by foot lesions, and resolution of facial lesions. Rapid, substantial improvement in tumor-associated lymphedema also has been observed in patients receiving paclitaxel for advanced AIDS-related Kaposi's sarcoma.

The optimum dosage regimen for paclitaxel in the treatment of AIDS-related Kaposi's sarcoma has not been established. In the first phase II study, paclitaxel was administered IV over 3 hours at an initial dosage of 135 mg/m² once every 3 weeks. The paclitaxel dose was to be increased by 20 mg/m² for each subsequent cycle of therapy to a maximum dose of 175 mg/m²; however, at least 12 of 29 patients required dose reduction to less than 135 mg/m² because of dose-limiting toxicity, particularly neutropenia. Patients in this study initially did not receive concomitant therapy with granulocyte colony-stimulating factor (i.e., filgrastim), but the study protocol was later modified to allow concomitant administration of filgrastim to reduce the severity of paclitaxel-associated myelosuppression. In the second phase II study, paclitaxel was administered IV over 3 hours at a dosage of 100 mg/m² once every 2 weeks. Concomitant administration of a granulocyte colony-stimulating factor (G-CSF) was initiated as clinically indicated, and most of the patients in this study were already receiving G-CSF prior to the initiation of paclitaxel therapy. The dose intensity of paclitaxel per week was 38–39 mg/m² for both studies.

Although direct comparison of data from these uncontrolled phase II studies is not possible, a higher incidence of hematologic toxicity was reported in patients receiving paclitaxel 135 mg/m² compared with that reported in patients receiving paclitaxel 100 mg/m², including severe neutropenia (76 versus 35%), febrile neutropenia (55 versus 9%), and opportunistic infections (76 versus 54%). The higher incidence of hematologic toxicity in patients receiving paclitaxel 135 mg/m² may have been at least partially secondary to the delayed administration of G-CSF in these patients. The manufacturer recommends concomitant administration of a granulocyte colony-stimulating factor (e.g., filgrastim) as clinically indicated in patients with AIDS-related Kaposi's sarcoma to reduce the severity of myelosuppression associated with paclitaxel therapy.

The incidence of nonhematologic toxicity also appears to be higher in patients receiving higher doses of paclitaxel. Certain adverse effects occurred more frequently in patients receiving the higher dose of paclitaxel (135 versus 100 mg/m²) for AIDS-related Kaposi's sarcoma, including arthralgia and/or myalgia (93 versus 48%), peripheral neuropathy (79 versus 46%), and hypersensitivity reaction (14 versus 9%).

Other schedules of paclitaxel therapy have been investigated in patients with AIDS-related Kaposi's sarcoma. Some responses have been reported in patients with advanced AIDS-related Kaposi's sarcoma receiving paclitaxel administered by continuous 96-hour infusion (initial dosage of 105 mg/m² with or without filgrastim) following progression of disease or absence of response with administration of the drug by 3-hour infusion. Further study is needed to determine the optimal dosage and schedule of paclitaxel for the treatment of advanced AIDS-related Kaposi's sarcoma.

Optimal therapy for the treatment of advanced AIDS-related Kaposi's sarcoma has not been established. The potential effects of systemic chemotherapy on the patient's immune and hematologic status must be considered in the management of AIDS-related Kaposi's sarcoma.

■ **Pancreatic Cancer** Albumin-bound paclitaxel in combination with gemcitabine is used as first-line therapy in patients with metastatic adenocarcinoma of the pancreas. Combination chemotherapy with albumin-bound paclitaxel and gemcitabine is associated with higher response rates and prolonged overall and progression-free survival compared with gemcitabine monotherapy.

The current indication for albumin-bound paclitaxel in combination with gemcitabine is based principally on the results of a randomized, multicenter, open-label trial in patients with previously untreated metastatic adenocarcinoma of the pancreas. In this study, 861 patients with metastatic adenocarcinoma of the pancreas were randomized (stratified according to performance status, presence of liver metastases, and geographic region) to receive either albumin-bound paclitaxel (125 mg/m² administered IV over 30–40 minutes) followed by gemcitabine (1 g/m² administered IV over 30–40 minutes) on days 1, 8, and 15 of each 28-day cycle or gemcitabine (1 g/m² IV over 30–40 minutes) alone once weekly for 7 weeks followed by a treatment-free week, and then once weekly for 3 consecutive weeks (days 1, 8, and 15) of each subsequent 28-day cycle. Median overall survival was prolonged in patients receiving albumin-bound paclitaxel combined with gemcitabine compared with those receiving gemcitabine alone (8.5 versus 6.7 months); 1-year survival was reported in 35% of patients receiving combined therapy and 22% of those receiving gemcitabine alone. Median progression-free survival also was prolonged in patients receiving albumin-bound paclitaxel combined with gemcitabine compared with those receiving gemcitabine alone (5.5 versus 3.7 months). The median time to treatment failure was 5.1 months in patients receiving combined therapy and 3.6 months in those receiving gemcitabine monotherapy. Patients receiving albumin-bound paclitaxel combined with gemcitabine had higher overall response rates (23 versus 7%); one patient receiving combined therapy achieved a complete response compared with none of those receiving gemcitabine alone. Subgroup analysis suggested that combined therapy consistently had a greater effect than gemcitabine monotherapy on overall and progression-free survival in patients with more advanced disease (i.e., those with poor performance status, presence of liver metastasis, more than 3 sites of metastatic disease, or carbohydrate antigen [CA] 19-9 level of 59 or more times the upper limit of normal). Compared with gemcitabine monotherapy, combined therapy was associated with a higher incidence of grade 3 or greater neutropenia (38 versus 27%), leukopenia (31 versus 16%), thrombocytopenia (13 versus 9%), febrile neutropenia (3 versus 1%), fatigue (17 versus 7%), peripheral neuropathy (17 versus 1%), and diarrhea (6 versus 1%).

■ **Small Cell Lung Cancer** Paclitaxel is an active agent in the treatment of small cell lung cancer†.

In phase II studies of patients with previously untreated extensive-stage small cell lung cancer, objective response rates of 35–41% (mostly partial responses) have been observed with paclitaxel alone (using a regimen of paclitaxel 250 mg/m² by 24-hour IV infusion every 3 weeks). Responses to paclitaxel (175 mg/m² by 3-hour IV infusion every 3 weeks) used alone or in combination therapy have been reported in patients with advanced small cell lung cancer that has relapsed following one or more previous chemotherapy regimens. In phase I and II studies, combination therapy with paclitaxel (e.g., cisplatin, etoposide, and paclitaxel; carboplatin, etoposide, and paclitaxel) has produced high response rates in patients with limited- or extensive-stage small cell lung cancer; however, randomized studies to date have not demonstrated a survival benefit from adding paclitaxel to standard combination regimens.

In a randomized trial, response rates and median survival were similar but toxicity was greater when paclitaxel was added to etoposide and cisplatin for previously untreated extensive-stage small cell lung cancer. Another randomized trial was terminated early because excessive toxicity and toxicity-related mortality occurred when paclitaxel was added to etoposide/cisplatin for the initial treatment of limited-stage or extensive-stage small cell lung cancer. Based on experience in these randomized trials, the addition of paclitaxel to standard regimens for the treatment of small-cell lung cancer is *not* recommended.

Concomitant administration of granulocyte colony-stimulating factor (G-CSF) has been used in some patients with small cell lung cancer to reduce the severity of myelosuppression associated with paclitaxel therapy; however, use of G-CSF generally is not required when paclitaxel is administered by short IV infusion (e.g., 1 or 3 hours).

Because the current prognosis for patients with small cell lung cancer is unsatisfactory regardless of stage and despite considerable diagnostic and therapeutic advances, all patients with this cancer are candidates for inclusion in clinical trials at the time of diagnosis.

■ **Esophageal Cancer** Paclitaxel has been used alone or in combination therapy for the treatment of esophageal cancer†. Like cisplatin, paclitaxel is active against both histologic types of esophageal cancer (i.e., squamous cell carcinoma and adenocarcinoma).

In a phase II study of patients with advanced esophageal cancer who had not received prior chemotherapy, an objective response rate of 32% (2% complete responses, 30% partial responses) has been observed with paclitaxel alone using an initial paclitaxel dosage of 250 mg/m² administered as a 24-hour IV infusion every 3 weeks. Response rates did not differ significantly according to histologic type; patients with adenocarcinoma and squamous cell carcinoma of the esophagus had objective response rates of 34 and 28%, respectively. Concomitant administration of granulocyte colony-stimulating factor was used to reduce the severity of myelosuppression associated with paclitaxel therapy, particularly with longer infusion schedules and higher doses of the drug.

The use of paclitaxel in combination with other antineoplastic agents (e.g., cisplatin, fluorouracil) for the treatment of advanced esophageal cancer is being investigated. The use of paclitaxel-containing regimens (with or without radiation therapy) prior to surgical resection is being investigated for the treatment of esophageal cancer. Optimal therapy for esophageal cancer has not been established, and new therapies are continually being evaluated. Because the prognosis for most patients with esophageal cancer remains poor, all newly diagnosed patients should be considered for enrollment in clinical trials comparing various treatment modalities.

■ **Bladder Cancer** Paclitaxel is an active agent in the treatment of transitional cell bladder cancer†. Paclitaxel has been used alone and in combination therapy for the treatment of advanced or metastatic bladder cancer.

In a phase II study of 26 patients with advanced transitional cell bladder cancer who had not received prior chemotherapy, objective responses occurred in 42% (27% complete responses, 15% partial responses) of patients receiving paclitaxel 250 mg/m² by 24-hour IV infusion every 21 days. Concomitant administration of granulocyte colony-stimulating factor (i.e., filgrastim) was used to reduce the severity of myelosuppression associated with paclitaxel therapy. Only partial responses have been reported in a small number of patients receiving paclitaxel alone or in combination with other antineoplastic agents for advanced or metastatic bladder cancer refractory to previous chemotherapy and/or radiation therapy. A low response rate (10%, partial responses only) was observed in patients receiving paclitaxel 80 mg/m² by 1-hour IV infusion once weekly for 4 weeks for previously treated advanced urothelial cancer.

Because paclitaxel is eliminated principally via hepatic metabolism, it may be a reasonable alternative in patients with advanced transitional cell urothelial cancer who have renal impairment and cannot tolerate the renal toxicity associated with cisplatin-based regimens. Paclitaxel also may be a useful alternative for the treatment of advanced or metastatic bladder cancer in patients with poor performance status who cannot tolerate standard platinum-based regimens.

Combination therapy with paclitaxel followed by carboplatin has been investigated as an active regimen in patients with advanced bladder cancer. Although high response rates were observed in earlier phase II studies of paclitaxel and carboplatin for previously untreated advanced bladder cancer, lower response rates were reported for this combination in a later phase II study and another phase II study involving patients with cisplatin-treated disease. Limited evidence from a small randomized trial that did reach full enrollment suggests that response rates and survival are similar but toxicity is lesser in patients receiving paclitaxel/carboplatin versus cisplatin, methotrexate, vinblastine, and doxorubicin (M-VAC). In this study, paclitaxel 225 mg/m² by 3-hour IV infusion was administered on day 1 followed by carboplatin at the dose required to obtain an AUC of 6 mg/mL per minute administered over 30 minutes; this cycle was administered every 3 weeks for a maximum of 6 cycles. Combination therapy with paclitaxel and carboplatin may be a reasonable option for the treatment of advanced bladder cancer in patients with renal dysfunction. The use of weekly dosing schedules of paclitaxel and carboplatin for patients with advanced bladder cancer is being investigated.

The use of paclitaxel in combination therapy with other antineoplastic agents (e.g., cisplatin, ifosfamide, gemcitabine) is being evaluated for the palliative treatment of advanced or metastatic bladder cancer. New chemotherapy regimens are continually being evaluated for the treatment of bladder cancer.

■ **Head and Neck Cancer** Paclitaxel is an active agent in the treatment of head and neck cancer†.

Paclitaxel is used in combination with cisplatin for the palliative treatment of advanced head and neck cancer. In a randomized trial involving patients with locally advanced, recurrent, or metastatic head and neck cancer, similar response rates and survival were observed in those receiving cisplatin and paclitaxel (paclitaxel 175 mg/m² by 3-hour IV infusion on day 1 followed by cisplatin 75 mg/m² IV on day 1) versus those receiving cisplatin and fluorouracil (cisplatin 100 mg/m² on day 1 and fluorouracil 1000 mg/m² per 24 hours by continuous IV infusion day 1 through 4). Hematologic toxicities and stomatitis were more common in the patients receiving cisplatin and fluorouracil, but the frequency of neurotoxicity was similar between the groups. The use of paclitaxel in combination with other antineoplastic agents is being investigated.

Paclitaxel has been used alone for the treatment of advanced head and neck cancer. In phase II studies of patients with advanced or unresectable locally advanced squamous cell carcinoma of the head and neck, objective response rates of 36–40% (7–12% complete responses, 24–33% partial responses) have been observed with paclitaxel alone using a regimen of paclitaxel 250 mg/m² as a 24-hour IV infusion administered every 3 weeks. Long-term follow-up for one of these studies indicates a median survival of 9.2 months with paclitaxel monotherapy in patients with advanced head and neck cancer.

The effect of dose on the efficacy and toxicity of paclitaxel has been studied in patients with advanced head and neck cancer. Results of a randomized clinical trial indicate that response rates and duration of survival are similar when paclitaxel doses of 200 mg/m² (with granulocyte colony-stimulating factor [G-CSF]) or 135 mg/m²(without G-CSF) are administered by 24-hour infusion followed by cisplatin 75 mg/m² with treatment cycles administered every 3 weeks; however, unacceptably high rates of hematologic toxicity occurred and neither regimen is recommended for use in the treatment of advanced head and neck cancer. Concomitant administration of granulocyte colony-stimulating factor has been used in patients with squamous cell carcinoma of the head and neck to reduce the severity of myelosuppression associated with paclitaxel therapy, particularly with high doses of the drug.

Paclitaxel also has been administered by IV infusion over shorter periods (e.g., 1 or 3 hours) in patients with head and neck cancer. The effect of duration of infusion on the efficacy and toxicity of paclitaxel has been studied in patients with advanced head and neck cancer. Interim analysis from a randomized study shows that toxicity is greater in patients with recurrent or metastatic squamous cell carcinoma of the head and neck receiving paclitaxel 175 mg/m² administered by 24-hour IV infusion versus 3-hour IV infusion. Paclitaxel has been administered by IV infusion over longer periods in patients with head and neck cancer; low response rates were observed for a regimen of paclitaxel 120 or 140 mg/m² by 96-hour IV infusion in patients with advanced squamous cell carcinoma of the head and neck.

In addition to its antitumor activity, in vitro studies indicate that paclitaxel is a radiosensitizer, and the use of paclitaxel in combination with radiation therapy is being investigated in patients with advanced head and neck cancer. Paclitaxel-containing therapy has been used with concurrent radiation therapy in the treatment of advanced head or neck cancer. Paclitaxel-containing therapy is being investigated as induction therapy preceding surgery and/or radiation therapy, or concurrent chemotherapy and radiation therapy, in the treatment of locally advanced squamous cell carcinoma of the head and neck. The prognosis for patients with advanced head and neck cancer generally is poor; the optimal timing and regimens of chemotherapy used alone or in the combined modality treatment of advanced head and neck cancer have not been established, and new therapies are continually being evaluated.

■ **Cervical Cancer** Paclitaxel is an active agent in the treatment of cervical cancer†. (See Uses: Cervical Cancer in Cisplatin 10:00 for an overview of therapy for cervical cancer.)

Paclitaxel and Radiation Therapy for Locally Advanced Cervical Cancer The use of paclitaxel as a radiation sensitizer is being investigated in patients with locally advanced cervical cancer†. Additional comparative studies are needed to determine the optimum chemotherapy regimens and schedules to be used concurrently with radiation therapy for the treatment of locally advanced cervical cancer.

Paclitaxel for Advanced Cervical Cancer Paclitaxel is an active agent in the treatment of metastatic or recurrent cervical cancer†. Objective response rates of 17–25% have been observed in patients receiving paclitaxel as a single agent for advanced squamous cell carcinoma of the cervix. An objective response rate of 31% was reported in patients receiving paclitaxel alone for advanced nonsquamous cervical cancer.

Paclitaxel and Cisplatin for Advanced Cervical Cancer Paclitaxel and cisplatin is used in the treatment of advanced cervical cancer. Objective responses of 40–45% for combination therapy with cisplatin and paclitaxel have been reported in patients who previously had not received chemotherapy for advanced or recurrent cervical cancer. In a randomized trial involving patients with advanced squamous cell cervical cancer, response rate was higher (36 versus 19%) and progression-free survival was longer (4.8 versus 2.8 months) in those receiving paclitaxel and cisplatin than in those receiving cisplatin alone; overall survival was similar between the groups (9.7 versus 8.8 months). In this study, patients received either paclitaxel and cisplatin (paclitaxel 135 mg/m² by 24-hour IV infusion followed immediately by IV cisplatin 50 mg/m²) or single-agent cisplatin (same dosage of cisplatin used for combination therapy) every 3 weeks.

■ **Endometrial Cancer** Paclitaxel is used in the treatment of endometrial cancer†.

Paclitaxel is an active agent that has been used in the treatment of advanced or recurrent endometrial cancer. Paclitaxel and carboplatin, with or without radiation therapy, is used in the palliative treatment of advanced or recurrent endometrial cancer. In a randomized trial, similar response rates, progression-free survival, and overall survival were observed for patients receiving doxorubicin and cisplatin versus doxorubicin and paclitaxel (with filgrastim) for advanced endometrial cancer. In another randomized trial, higher response rate and prolonged progression-free and overall survival but greater neurotoxicity was observed with the addition of paclitaxel to doxorubicin and cisplatin for advanced endometrial cancer. A phase III randomized trial comparing doxorubicin, cisplatin, paclitaxel and filgrastim (G-CSF) versus carboplatin and paclitaxel for advanced endometrial cancer is under way.

The use of adjuvant radiation therapy and chemotherapy with cisplatin and paclitaxel following surgery for high-risk endometrial cancer confined to the uterus is being investigated.

■ **Other Uses** Paclitaxel is used in the treatment of gastric cancer†. Paclitaxel is used in the treatment of relapsed or refractory testicular cancer†.

Dosage and Administration

■ **Reconstitution and Administration** Paclitaxel is administered by IV infusion. Paclitaxel also has been administered intraperitoneally†.

Paclitaxel is commercially available in 2 types of formulations: conventional paclitaxel (in a nonaqueous solution) and albumin-bound paclitaxel. The properties of paclitaxel may differ according to formulation, and the dosage and reconstitution instructions for paclitaxel are specific to formulation. Albumin-bound paclitaxel may *not* be substituted for or used in combination with other formulations of paclitaxel.

Caution should be exercised in handling and preparing solutions of conventional or albumin-bound paclitaxel. Because dermatologic reactions (e.g., tingling, burning, erythema) may occur with accidental exposure to the drug, the manufacturers recommend the use of protective gloves during preparation and administration of paclitaxel. Skin accidentally exposed to the drug should be washed immediately and thoroughly with soap and water. If the drug comes into contact with mucous membranes, thorough flushing with water should be used immediately. Dyspnea, chest pain, ocular burning, sore throat, and nausea have been reported upon inhalation, and inadvertent inhalation should be avoided during preparation and administration of paclitaxel solutions.

Paclitaxel for injection concentrate, diluted solutions of conventional paclitaxel, and reconstituted suspensions of albumin-bound paclitaxel should be inspected visually for particulate matter and discoloration whenever solution and container permit.

Medication errors have occurred that involved confusion between paclitaxel (Taxol®) and docetaxel (Taxotere®). To avoid medication errors, the prescriber should print both the brand and generic names for paclitaxel on the prescription order form. If a handwritten prescription is difficult to read, the pharmacist should confirm the drug name with the prescriber. If the prescription is confirmed verbally, the drug names should be spelled out. Pharmacy labels and preprinted order forms should list both the generic and brand names using upper- and lower-case fonts (i.e., PACLItaxel and TaxOL). Two pharmacists should provide independent confirmation that the correct drug is being administered before chemotherapy is dispensed, and two nurses should confirm that the correct drug has been dispensed for the correct patient before administering the medication.

IV Administration Adverse local effects have occurred following extravasation of paclitaxel during administration, and the injection site should be monitored closely during infusion of conventional or albumin-bound paclitaxel for possible infiltration of the drug. (See Cautions: Local Effects.)

Conventional Paclitaxel. *Paclitaxel for injection concentrate must be diluted prior to IV infusion.* For IV infusion, the manufacturer recommends diluting the concentrate in 0.9% sodium chloride injection, 5% dextrose injection, 5% dextrose and 0.9% sodium chloride injection, or 5% dextrose in Ringer's injection to a final paclitaxel concentration of 0.3–1.2 mg/mL.

Undiluted paclitaxel for injection concentrate should not be placed in plasticized polyvinyl chloride (PVC) equipment or devices used to prepare solutions for infusion. To minimize exposure of the patient to leached DEHP, *diluted* paclitaxel solutions preferably should be stored in glass or polypropylene bottles or in plastic (polypropylene or polyolefin) bags and administered through polyethylene-lined administration sets. Leaching of unacceptable amounts of DEHP has been reported with some administration sets labeled as not containing PVC (probably because of pumping segments made of heavily plasticized PVC); therefore, compatibility of administration sets with paclitaxel solutions should be verified prior to their use. (See Chemistry and Stability: Stability.)

Because a small number of fibers (within acceptable USP limits) have been detected in paclitaxel solutions prepared from the commercially available for injection concentrate, a hydrophilic, microporous inline filter with a pore size not exceeding 0.22 μm is necessary during administration of paclitaxel solutions. The manufacturer reports that use of filter devices such as IVEX-2® filters, which incorporate short inlet and outlet PVC-coated tubing, has not resulted in significant leaching of DEHP. (See Chemistry and Stability: Stability.) The Chemo Dispensing Pin® device or similar devices with spikes should *not* be used with vials of paclitaxel; this type of device can cause the stopper to collapse and contaminate the paclitaxel solution.

Albumin-bound Paclitaxel. Albumin-bound paclitaxel in the form of lyophilized powder must be reconstituted to an injectable suspension prior to IV infusion. Using aseptic technique, 20 mL of 0.9% sodium chloride injection should be injected slowly (over a minimum period of 1 minute) into the vial containing the lyophilized paclitaxel. The flow from the sterile syringe should be injected onto the inside wall of the vial; injection of 0.9% sodium chloride injection directly onto the lyophilized cake should be avoided because it causes foaming. Once injection of the 20 mL of 0.9% sodium chloride injection into the vial is complete, the vial should be allowed to sit for a minimum of 5 minutes to ensure thorough wetting of the lyophilized cake/powder. The vial then should be swirled and/or inverted gently for at least 2 minutes until the cake/powder is completely dissolved; foaming should be avoided. If foaming or clumping occurs, the reconstituted paclitaxel suspension should be allowed to stand for at least 15 minutes until foam subsides.

The reconstituted suspension has a final paclitaxel concentration of 5 mg/mL. The exact dosing volume of the injectable suspension should be calculated using the following formula: dosing volume in mL equals total dose in mg divided by 5 mg/mL. Before the dosing volume is withdrawn from the vial, the suspension should be inspected. The reconstituted paclitaxel suspension should appear milky and homogeneous with no visible particulates. If particulates are visible or settling has occurred, the vial should be inverted *gently* to ensure complete resuspension of the particles in solution. Then the appropriate dosing volume of paclitaxel suspension should be withdrawn from the vial and injected into an empty sterile PVC IV bag. Unlike conventional paclitaxel, DEHP-free containers or administration sets are not required for the preparation or administration of albumin-bound paclitaxel suspension. Unlike conventional paclitaxel, the use of an inline filter is *not* recommended for the IV infusion of albumin-bound paclitaxel suspension.

The injection site should be monitored closely during the infusion for possible infiltration of the drug. According to the manufacturer, limiting the infusion of albumin-bound paclitaxel to 30 minutes as directed reduces the likelihood of infusion-related reactions.

Intraperitoneal Instillation **Conventional Paclitaxel.** For intraperitoneal† administration in the Gynecologic Oncology Group (GOG)-172 study in patients with advanced epithelial ovarian cancer, the paclitaxel dose was diluted in 1 L of 0.9% sodium chloride solution that was warmed to 37°C and infused through a surgically implanted peritoneal catheter, followed by intraperitoneal infusion of an additional liter of warmed saline solution. Following peritoneal infusion, the patient was asked to roll into a different position every 15 minutes for the next 2 hours to disperse the drug throughout the peritoneal cavity.

Various implanted access ports and connecting catheters have been used for intraperitoneal administration of chemotherapeutic agents. The intraperitoneal catheter may be placed at the time of primary (cytoreductive) surgery as long as contamination of the peritoneal cavity has not occurred. Timing of placement of the intraperitoneal catheter (at the time of primary surgery versus delayed insertion) does not appear to affect tolerance of intraperitoneal therapy or treatment completion rates. The intraperitoneal catheter should be removed as soon as intraperitoneal therapy is completed to avoid catheter-related complications. Further study is needed to optimize techniques for intraperitoneal therapy to minimize the risk of complications (e.g., infection, catheter obstruction, catheter retraction, bowel perforation, pain, leakage, port access problems). Specialized sources should be consulted for guidance on how to administer intraperitoneal therapy.

Supportive therapy should include premedication to prevent hypersensitivity reactions to paclitaxel.

■ **Dosage** Paclitaxel is commercially available in 2 types of formulations: conventional paclitaxel (in a nonaqueous solution) and albumin-bound paclitaxel. The functional properties of paclitaxel may differ according to formulation, and the dosage instructions for paclitaxel are specific to formulation. Albumin-bound paclitaxel may *not* be substituted for or used in combination with other formulations of paclitaxel. Clinicians should consult the respective manufacturer's labeling and published protocols for formulation-specific regimens and specific dosages, methods of administration, and administration sequence of other antineoplastic agents used in combination regimens.

Dosage of albumin-bound paclitaxel is expressed in terms of paclitaxel.

Conventional or albumin-bound paclitaxel should not be administered to patients with baseline neutrophil counts less than 1500/mm³. In patients with HIV infection, conventional paclitaxel should not be administered if baseline neutrophil counts are less than 1000/mm³. To monitor the occurrence of paclitaxel-induced bone marrow suppression, mainly neutropenia, which may be severe and result in infection, it is recommended that frequent peripheral blood cell counts be performed in all patients receiving paclitaxel.

Conventional Paclitaxel All patients should be premedicated before administration of conventional paclitaxel to prevent severe hypersensitivity reactions.

For patients receiving paclitaxel for the treatment of solid tumors, the manufacturer recommends the following premedication regimen: oral dexamethasone 20 mg administered approximately 12 and 6 hours before paclitaxel; IV diphenhydramine hydrochloride (or similar antihistamine) 50 mg administered 30–60 minutes before paclitaxel; and either IV cimetidine hydrochloride (300 mg of cimetidine) or ranitidine hydrochloride (50 mg of ranitidine) administered 30–60 minutes before paclitaxel.

For patients with HIV infection who are receiving conventional paclitaxel for the treatment of AIDS-related Kaposi's sarcoma, the manufacturer recommends the following premedication regimen: oral dexamethasone 10 mg administered approximately 12 and 6 hours before paclitaxel; IV diphenhydramine hydrochloride (or similar antihistamine) 50 mg administered 30–60 minutes before paclitaxel; and either IV cimetidine hydrochloride (300 mg of cimetidine) or ranitidine hydrochloride (50 mg of ranitidine) administered 30–60 minutes before paclitaxel. This is the same premedication regimen as for other patients receiving paclitaxel with the exception of a reduced dose of oral dexamethasone (10 mg).

Concomitant administration of filgrastim is used to reduce the severity of myelosuppression in patients receiving paclitaxel therapy, particularly those who are at high risk for febrile neutropenia. Because of immunosuppression in patients with advanced HIV disease, the manufacturer recommends concomitant administration of a granulocyte colony-stimulating factor (e.g., filgrastim) as clinically indicated to reduce the severity of myelosuppression associated with paclitaxel in patients with AIDS-related Kaposi's sarcoma.

Albumin-bound Paclitaxel Unlike conventional paclitaxel, which requires premedication prior to administration to prevent severe hypersensitivity reactions, premedication generally is *not* required prior to administration of albumin-bound paclitaxel. However, premedication may be necessary in patients who experienced a hypersensitivity reaction during a previous course of therapy with the drug.

Ovarian Cancer **Conventional Paclitaxel as First-line Therapy for Advanced Ovarian Epithelial Cancer.** When used in combination therapy with cisplatin for the initial treatment of advanced ovarian cancer, there are 2 recommended paclitaxel-containing regimens. Differences in toxicity should be considered when selecting the appropriate regimen for a patient. One recommended regimen is conventional paclitaxel 175 mg/m² administered by 3-hour IV infusion followed by cisplatin 75 mg/m² IV with cycles repeated every 3 weeks. Another recommended regimen is conventional paclitaxel 135 mg/m² administered by 24-hour IV infusion followed by cisplatin 75 mg/m² IV with cycles repeated every 3 weeks.

Intraperitoneal Conventional Paclitaxel and Cisplatin as First-line Therapy for Advanced Ovarian Epithelial Cancer. When combined therapy with IV and intraperitoneal conventional paclitaxel and intraperitoneal cisplatin† has been used for the initial adjuvant treatment of optimally debulked stage III epithelial ovarian cancer, IV paclitaxel 135 mg/m² by 24-hour infusion on day 1, followed by intraperitoneal cisplatin 100 mg/m² on day 2 and intraperitoneal paclitaxel 60 mg/m² on day 8, has been administered every 21 days for up to 6 cycles. Modified IV and intraperitoneal regimens are being investigated. (See Uses: Ovarian Cancer.)

Conventional Paclitaxel as Second-line or Subsequent Therapy for Advanced Ovarian Epithelial Cancer. When used as monotherapy in patients with metastatic carcinoma of the ovary that failed to respond to first-line or subsequent chemotherapy, the recommended regimen is conventional paclitaxel 135 or 175 mg/m² infused IV over 3 hours and repeated every 3 weeks as tolerated. Optimal dosage of paclitaxel has not been established in this patient population.

Breast Cancer **Conventional Paclitaxel as Adjuvant Therapy for Node-positive Breast Cancer.** For the adjuvant therapy of node-positive breast cancer, conventional paclitaxel 175 mg/m² is administered as a 3-hour IV infusion once every 3 weeks for 4 courses following the completion of doxorubicin-containing combination chemotherapy. In a large randomized trial on which this indication is based, patients received 4 courses of doxorubicin and cyclophosphamide followed by adjuvant therapy with paclitaxel.

Conventional or Albumin-bound Paclitaxel as Second-line Therapy for Advanced Breast Cancer. For metastatic breast cancer that is refractory to initial chemotherapy or breast cancer that has relapsed within 6 months of adjuvant therapy, *conventional* paclitaxel 175 mg/m² is administered as a 3-hour IV infusion once every 3 weeks.

For metastatic breast cancer that is refractory to combination chemotherapy or breast cancer that has relapsed within 6 months of adjuvant therapy, *albumin-bound* paclitaxel 260 mg/m² is administered as a 30-minute IV infusion once every 3 weeks.

Non-small Cell Lung Cancer **Conventional Paclitaxel and Cisplatin.** When used in combination therapy with cisplatin for the initial treatment of advanced non-small cell lung cancer in patients who are not candidates for potentially curative surgery and/or radiation therapy, the recommended regimen is conventional paclitaxel 135 mg/m² administered by 24-hour IV infusion followed by cisplatin 75 mg/m² IV with cycles repeated every 3 weeks. A regimen of conventional paclitaxel 175 mg/m² administered by 3-hour IV infusion followed by cisplatin 80 mg/m² IV with cycles repeated every 3 weeks also has been used in patients with advanced non-small cell lung cancer.

Albumin-bound Paclitaxel and Carboplatin. When used in combination therapy with carboplatin for the initial treatment of advanced non-small cell lung cancer in patients who are not candidates for potentially curative surgery and/or radiation therapy, the recommended regimen is albumin-bound paclitaxel 100 mg/m² administered by 30-minute IV infusion on days 1, 8, and 15 and IV carboplatin at the dose required to obtain an area under the concentration-time curve (AUC) of 6 mg/mL per minute on day 1 of each 21-day cycle.

AIDS-related Kaposi's Sarcoma **Conventional Paclitaxel.** For patients with advanced HIV infection, paclitaxel therapy should be initiated only if the neutrophil count is at least 1000/mm³.

For patients with AIDS-related Kaposi's sarcoma that has failed to respond to first-line or subsequent chemotherapy, there are 2 recommended paclitaxel regimens. One recommended regimen is conventional paclitaxel 135 mg/m² administered by 3-hour IV infusion once every 3 weeks. Another recommended regimen is conventional paclitaxel 100 mg/m² administered by 3-hour IV infusion once every 2 weeks. Both of these regimens achieve a dose intensity of 45–50 mg/m² per week. In phase II studies, greater toxicity was observed with the higher-dose schedule, and patients with poor performance status were treated with paclitaxel 100 mg/m² once every 2 weeks.

Pancreatic Cancer **Albumin-bound Paclitaxel and Gemcitabine.** When used in combination therapy with gemcitabine for the initial treatment of metastatic adenocarcinoma of the pancreas, the recommended regimen is albumin-bound paclitaxel 125 mg/m² administered IV over 30–40 minutes followed by gemcitabine 1 g/m² administered IV over 30–40 minutes on days 1, 8, and 15 of each 28-day cycle.

Dosage Modification for Toxicity and Contraindications for Continued Therapy with Conventional Paclitaxel **Hematologic Toxicity.** For patients receiving conventional paclitaxel, repeat cycles of the drug should be withheld until platelet counts exceed 100,000/mm³ *and* neutrophil counts are at least 1500/mm³ in patients with solid tumors or are at least 1000/mm³ in patients with advanced AIDS-related Kaposi's sarcoma.

For patients receiving conventional paclitaxel who experience severe neutropenia (neutrophil count less than 500/mm³ for at least 7 days), a 20% reduction in the dose of conventional paclitaxel is recommended for subsequent courses of therapy.

The incidence and severity of hematologic toxicity (i.e., neutropenia) have been shown to increase with dose and duration of infusion for conventional paclitaxel. The use of supportive therapy, such as G-CSF, with administration of conventional paclitaxel is recommended for patients who have experienced severe neutropenia.

Sensitivity Reactions. Mild symptoms (e.g., flushing, skin reactions, dyspnea, hypotension, tachycardia) do not require interruption of therapy. If signs or symptoms of a severe reaction (e.g., hypotension requiring treatment, dyspnea requiring bronchodilators, angioedema, generalized urticaria) occur during administration of paclitaxel, the infusion should be discontinued immediately and aggressive symptomatic therapy instituted as necessary. Such therapy may include epinephrine, IV fluids, and additional doses of antihistamine (e.g., diphenhydramine) and corticosteroid as clinically indicated.

Further therapy with conventional paclitaxel should *not* be undertaken in any patient who experienced a severe hypersensitivity reaction during a previous course of therapy with the drug. It is not known whether patients who have exhibited hypersensitivity to conventional paclitaxel can tolerate subsequent therapy with albumin-bound paclitaxel.

Hepatic Toxicity. In patients with preexisting hepatic impairment, dose reduction is recommended depending on the degree of hepatic impairment for the first course of therapy with conventional paclitaxel. Further dose reduction may be required during subsequent courses of paclitaxel therapy based on hepatic toxicity. (See Dosage of Conventional Paclitaxel in Hepatic Impairment under Dosage and Administration: Dosage in Renal and Hepatic Impairment.)

Cardiovascular Toxicity. If a patient develops substantial conduction abnormalities during administration of paclitaxel, appropriate therapy should be initiated and continuous cardiac monitoring should be performed during subsequent therapy with the drug. Paclitaxel infusions occasionally must be interrupted or discontinued because of initial or recurrent hypertension.

Neurologic Toxicity. For patients who experience severe peripheral neuropathy while receiving conventional paclitaxel, the manufacturer recommends a 20% reduction in the dose for subsequent courses of therapy. The incidence and severity of neurotoxicity increase with paclitaxel dose.

Dosage Modification for Toxicity and Contraindications for Continued Therapy with Albumin-bound Paclitaxel for Breast Cancer
Hematologic Toxicity. For patients receiving albumin-bound paclitaxel, repeat cycles of the drug should be withheld until neutrophil counts exceed 1500/mm³ and platelet counts exceed 100,000/mm³.

For patients who experience severe neutropenia (neutrophil count less than 500/mm³ for at least 7 days) while receiving albumin-bound paclitaxel for breast cancer, the manufacturer recommends a reduction in dose to albumin-bound paclitaxel 220 mg/m² for subsequent courses of therapy. For patients who experience recurrence of severe neutropenia, further reduction in dose to albumin-bound paclitaxel 180 mg/m² is recommended.

Sensitivity Reactions. Further therapy with paclitaxel should *not* be undertaken in any patient who experienced a severe hypersensitivity reaction during a previous course of therapy with the drug. It is not known whether patients who have exhibited hypersensitivity to conventional paclitaxel can tolerate subsequent therapy with albumin-bound paclitaxel.

Hepatic Toxicity. In patients with preexisting hepatic impairment, dose reduction is recommended depending on the degree of hepatic impairment for the first course of therapy with albumin-bound paclitaxel. Further dose reduction may be required during subsequent courses of albumin-bound paclitaxel therapy based on hepatic toxicity. (See Dosage of Albumin-bound Paclitaxel in Hepatic Impairment under Dosage and Administration: Dosage in Renal and Hepatic Impairment.)

Neurologic Toxicity. Sensory neuropathy associated with albumin-bound paclitaxel is dose and schedule dependent. In patients with breast cancer, the incidence and severity of sensory neuropathy associated with albumin-bound paclitaxel increased with cumulative dose of the drug.

For patients who experience grade 1 or 2 sensory neuropathy while receiving albumin-bound paclitaxel, dosage modification generally is not required.

For patients with breast cancer who experience severe sensory neuropathy while receiving albumin-bound paclitaxel, treatment should be withheld until resolution to grade 1 or 2 severity followed by reduction in dose to albumin-bound paclitaxel 220 mg/m² for subsequent courses of therapy. For patients who experience recurrence of severe sensory neuropathy, treatment should be withheld until resolution to grade 1 or 2 severity followed by further reduction in dose to albumin-bound paclitaxel 180 mg/m² for subsequent courses of therapy.

Dosage Modification for Toxicity and Contraindications for Continued Therapy with Albumin-bound Paclitaxel for Non-small Cell Lung Cancer **Hematologic Toxicity.** For patients receiving albumin-bound paclitaxel, repeat cycles of the drug should be withheld until neutrophil counts are at least 1500/mm³ and platelet counts are at least 100,000/mm³.

For patients who experience severe neutropenia (neutrophil count less than 500/mm³ for at least 7 days) or thrombocytopenia (platelet count less than 50,000/mm³) while receiving albumin-bound paclitaxel for non-small cell lung cancer, the manufacturer recommends dose reduction upon resumption of therapy.

For patients with non-small cell lung cancer who experience severe neutropenia or febrile neutropenia (neutrophil count less than 500/mm³ with fever exceeding 38°C) while receiving albumin-bound paclitaxel and carboplatin, treatment should be delayed until neutrophil counts are at least 1500/mm³ on day 1 or at least 500/mm³ on day 8 or 15 of the cycle; treatment may then be resumed at a permanently reduced dose of albumin-bound paclitaxel 75 mg/m² and a target carboplatin AUC of 4.5 mg/mL per minute. Following a second episode of severe neutropenia or febrile neutropenia, treatment should again be delayed; treatment may be resumed at a permanently reduced dose of albumin-bound paclitaxel 50 mg/m² and a target carboplatin AUC of 3 mg/mL per minute. Albumin-bound paclitaxel and carboplatin should be discontinued following a third episode of severe neutropenia or febrile neutropenia.

If initiation of a repeat cycle of therapy for non-small cell lung cancer is delayed by more than 7 days because the patient's neutrophil count is less than 1500/mm³, permanent dose reduction of albumin-bound paclitaxel to 75 mg/m² and a target carboplatin AUC of 4.5 mg/mL per minute is recommended. Following a second such treatment delay, permanent dose reduction of albumin-bound paclitaxel to 50 mg/m² and a target carboplatin AUC of 3 mg/mL per minute is recommended. Albumin-bound paclitaxel and carboplatin should be discontinued following a third such delay.

For patients with non-small cell lung cancer who experience severe thrombocytopenia while receiving albumin-bound paclitaxel and carboplatin, treatment should be delayed until platelet counts are at least 100,000/mm³ on day 1 or at least 50,000/mm³ on day 8 or 15 of the cycle; treatment may then be resumed at a permanently reduced dose of albumin-bound paclitaxel 75 mg/m² and a target carboplatin AUC of 4.5 mg/mL per minute. Albumin-bound paclitaxel and carboplatin should be discontinued following a second episode of severe thrombocytopenia.

Sensitivity Reactions. Further therapy with paclitaxel should *not* be undertaken in any patient who experienced a severe hypersensitivity reaction during a previous course of therapy with the drug. It is not known whether patients who have exhibited hypersensitivity to conventional paclitaxel can tolerate subsequent therapy with albumin-bound paclitaxel.

Hepatic Toxicity. In patients with preexisting hepatic impairment, dose reduction is recommended depending on the degree of hepatic impairment for the first course of therapy with albumin-bound paclitaxel. Further dose reduction may be required during subsequent courses of albumin-bound paclitaxel therapy based on hepatic toxicity. (See Dosage of Albumin-bound Paclitaxel in Hepatic Impairment under Dosage and Administration: Dosage in Renal and Hepatic Impairment.)

Neurologic Toxicity. Sensory neuropathy associated with albumin-bound paclitaxel is dose and schedule dependent.

For patients who experience grade 1 or 2 peripheral neuropathy while receiving albumin-bound paclitaxel, dosage modification generally is not required.

For patients with non-small cell lung cancer who experience grade 3 or 4 peripheral neuropathy while receiving albumin-bound paclitaxel and carboplatin, treatment should be withheld until resolution to grade 1 or less followed by a permanent reduction in dose to albumin-bound paclitaxel 75 mg/m² and a target carboplatin AUC of 4.5 mg/mL per minute. Following a second episode of grade 3 or 4 peripheral neuropathy, treatment should again be withheld until resolution to grade 1 or less; treatment may then be resumed at a permanently reduced dose of albumin-bound paclitaxel 50 mg/m² and a target carboplatin AUC of 3 mg/mL per minute. Albumin-bound paclitaxel and carboplatin should be discontinued following a third episode of grade 3 or 4 peripheral neuropathy.

Dosage Modification for Toxicity and Contraindications for Continued Therapy with Albumin-bound Paclitaxel for Pancreatic Cancer When dosage modification is necessary for patients receiving albumin-bound paclitaxel and gemcitabine for pancreatic cancer, dosage of albumin-bound paclitaxel should be reduced in decrements of 25 mg/m² (i.e., 1 dose level) and dosage of gemcitabine should be reduced in decrements of 200 mg/m² (i.e., 1 dose level); however, if a dose of albumin-bound paclitaxel 75 mg/m² or gemcitabine 600 mg/m² requires further reduction, both drugs should be discontinued.

Hematologic Toxicity. For patients receiving albumin-bound paclitaxel, repeat cycles of the drug should be withheld until neutrophil counts are at least

1500/mm^3 and platelet counts are at least 100,000/mm^3. See Table 1 for recommended dosage modifications for hematologic toxicity occurring either within a cycle or at the start of a repeat cycle of albumin-bound paclitaxel and gemcitabine therapy in patients with pancreatic cancer.

Table 1. Recommended Dosage Modifications for Hematologic Toxicity During or at the Start of a Cycle of Albumin-bound Paclitaxel and Gemcitabine for Pancreatic Cancer

Cycle Day and Cell Counts (cells/mm^3)	Albumin-bound Paclitaxel and Gemcitabine Dosage Modification
Day 1:	
Neutrophil count <1500 or platelet count <100,000	Delay start of cycle until recovery
Day 8:	
Neutrophil count 500 to <1000 or platelet count 50,000 to <75,000	Reduce dose of both drugs by 1 dose level
Neutrophil count <500 or platelet count <50,000	Withhold day 8 dose of both drugs
Day 15 (when day 8 doses were reduced or given without modification):	
Neutrophil count 500 to <1000 or platelet count 50,000 to <75,000	Reduce dose of both drugs by 1 dose level from day 8
Neutrophil count <500 or platelet count <50,000	Withhold day 15 dose of both drugs
Day 15 (when day 8 doses were withheld):	
Neutrophil count ≥1000 or platelet count ≥75,000	Reduce dose of both drugs by 1 dose level from day 1
Neutrophil count 500 to <1000 or platelet count 50,000 to <75,000	Reduce dose of both drugs by 2 dose levels from day 1
Neutrophil count <500 or platelet count <50,000	Withhold day 15 dose of both drugs

For patients with pancreatic cancer who experience grade 3 or 4 febrile neutropenia while receiving albumin-bound paclitaxel and gemcitabine, therapy should be withheld until fever resolves and neutrophil count reaches or exceeds 1500/mm^3; albumin-bound paclitaxel and gemcitabine may then be resumed at 1 dose level lower than the previous dosage.

Sensitivity Reactions. Further therapy with paclitaxel should *not* be undertaken in any patient who experienced a severe hypersensitivity reaction during a previous course of therapy with the drug. It is not known whether patients who have exhibited hypersensitivity to conventional paclitaxel can tolerate subsequent therapy with albumin-bound paclitaxel.

Hepatic Toxicity. In patients with preexisting hepatic impairment, dose reduction is recommended depending on the degree of hepatic impairment for the first course of therapy with albumin-bound paclitaxel. Further dose reduction may be required during subsequent courses of albumin-bound paclitaxel therapy based on hepatic toxicity. (See Dosage of Albumin-bound Paclitaxel in Hepatic Impairment under Dosage and Administration: Dosage in Renal and Hepatic Impairment.)

Neurologic Toxicity. Sensory neuropathy associated with albumin-bound paclitaxel is dose and schedule dependent.

For patients who experience grade 1 or 2 peripheral neuropathy while receiving albumin-bound paclitaxel, dosage modification generally is not required.

For patients with pancreatic cancer who experience grade 3 or 4 peripheral neuropathy while receiving albumin-bound paclitaxel and gemcitabine, treatment with albumin-bound paclitaxel should be withheld until resolution to grade 1 or less; the drug may then be resumed at 1 dose level lower than the previous dosage. No modification of gemcitabine dosage is required.

Dermatologic Toxicity. For patients with pancreatic cancer who experience grade 2 or 3 cutaneous toxicity while receiving albumin-bound paclitaxel and gemcitabine, the dose of albumin-bound paclitaxel and gemcitabine should be reduced by 1 dose level. If cutaneous toxicity persists, treatment should be discontinued.

GI Toxicity. For patients with pancreatic cancer who experience grade 3 mucositis or diarrhea while receiving albumin-bound paclitaxel and gemcitabine, treatment should be withheld until resolution to grade 1 or less; albumin-bound paclitaxel and gemcitabine may then be resumed at 1 dose level lower than the previous dosage.

Pulmonary Toxicity. For patients with pancreatic cancer who develop signs and symptoms of pneumonitis while receiving albumin-bound paclitaxel and gemcitabine, therapy should be interrupted during evaluation of suspected pneumonitis. Albumin-bound paclitaxel and gemcitabine should be permanently discontinued in patients diagnosed with pneumonitis.

■ Dosage in Renal and Hepatic Impairment

The effect of renal impairment on the disposition of paclitaxel has not been fully established. Reduction of paclitaxel dosage in patients with impaired renal function does not appear to be necessary.

Paclitaxel is metabolized mainly in the liver, and increased toxicity may occur in patients with hepatic impairment.

Dosage of Conventional Paclitaxel in Hepatic Impairment

Toxicity associated with paclitaxel, particularly grade 3 or 4 myelosuppression, may be exacerbated in patients with serum total bilirubin concentrations greater than 2 times the upper limit of normal. Paclitaxel should be used with extreme caution in patients with hepatic impairment, and dosage reduction is recommended depending on the degree of hepatic impairment. Such patients should be monitored closely for the development of profound myelosuppression.

For patients receiving conventional paclitaxel as a 24-hour IV infusion for ovarian or non-small cell lung cancer, the usual dose of 135 mg/m^2 may be administered for the first course of therapy in those who have serum transaminase concentrations less than 2 times the upper limit of normal and serum bilirubin concentrations up to 1.5 mg/dL; for patients with elevated serum transaminase concentrations less than 10 times the upper limit of normal and serum bilirubin concentrations up to 1.5 mg/dL, a reduced dose of paclitaxel 100 mg/m^2 is recommended; for patients with elevated serum transaminase concentrations less than 10 times the upper limit of normal and serum bilirubin concentrations of 1.6–7.5 mg/dL, a reduced dose of paclitaxel 50 mg/m^2 is recommended. For patients with elevated serum transaminase concentrations at least 10 times the upper limit of normal or serum bilirubin concentrations exceeding 7.5 mg/dL, paclitaxel therapy is *not* recommended.

For patients receiving conventional paclitaxel as a 3-hour IV infusion for ovarian or breast cancer, the usual dose of 175 mg/m^2 may be administered for the first course of therapy in those who have serum transaminase concentrations less than 10 times the upper limit of normal and serum bilirubin concentrations up to 1.25 times the upper limit of normal; for patients with serum transaminase concentrations less than 10 times the upper limit of normal and serum bilirubin concentrations of 1.26–2 times the upper limit of normal, a reduced dose of paclitaxel 135 mg/m^2 is recommended; for patients with serum transaminase concentrations less than 10 times the upper limit of normal and serum bilirubin concentrations of 2.01–5 times the upper limit of normal, a reduced dose of paclitaxel 90 mg/m^2 is recommended. For patients with elevated serum transaminase concentrations at least 10 times the upper limit of normal or serum bilirubin concentrations exceeding 5 times the upper limit of normal, paclitaxel therapy is *not* recommended.

Further reduction of paclitaxel dosage for subsequent courses of therapy should be based on patient tolerance.

Dosage of Albumin-bound Paclitaxel in Hepatic Impairment

Patients should be monitored closely since toxicity associated with paclitaxel may be exacerbated in patients with hepatic impairment. Paclitaxel should be used with caution in patients with hepatic impairment, and dosage reduction is recommended depending on the degree of hepatic impairment. No adjustment of the initial dosage is required in patients with mild hepatic impairment.

Breast Cancer. For patients receiving albumin-bound paclitaxel for breast cancer, the usual dose of 260 mg/m^2 may be administered for the first course of therapy in those who have mild hepatic impairment (AST concentrations less than 10 times the upper limit of normal and elevated serum bilirubin concentrations up to 1.25 times the upper limit of normal).

For patients with moderate hepatic impairment (AST concentrations less than 10 times the upper limit of normal and serum bilirubin concentrations of 1.26–2 times the upper limit of normal), a reduced initial dose of albumin-bound paclitaxel 200 mg/m^2 is recommended. For patients with severe hepatic impairment (AST concentrations less than 10 times the upper limit of normal and serum bilirubin concentrations of 2.01–5 times the upper limit of normal), a reduced initial dose of albumin-bound paclitaxel 130 mg/m^2 is recommended. If the 130-mg/m^2 dose of albumin-bound paclitaxel is tolerated, the dose may be increased to 200 mg/m^2 in subsequent cycles. For patients with serum AST concentrations exceeding 10 times the upper limit of normal or serum bilirubin concentrations exceeding 5 times the upper limit of normal, albumin-bound paclitaxel therapy is *not* recommended. Further reduction of albumin-bound paclitaxel dosage for subsequent courses of therapy should be based on patient tolerance.

Non-small Cell Lung Cancer. For patients receiving albumin-bound paclitaxel for non-small cell lung cancer, the usual dose of 100 mg/m^2 may be administered for the first course of therapy in those who have mild hepatic impairment (AST concentrations less than 10 times the upper limit of normal and elevated serum bilirubin concentrations up to 1.25 times the upper limit of normal).

For patients with moderate hepatic impairment (AST concentrations less than 10 times the upper limit of normal and serum bilirubin concentrations of 1.26–2 times the upper limit of normal), a reduced initial dose of albumin-bound paclitaxel 75 mg/m^2 is recommended. For patients with severe hepatic impairment (AST concentrations less than 10 times the upper limit of normal and serum bilirubin concentrations of 2.01–5 times the upper limit of normal), a reduced initial dose of albumin-bound paclitaxel 50 mg/m^2 is recommended. If the 50-mg/m^2 dose of albumin-bound paclitaxel is tolerated, the dose may be increased to 75 mg/m^2 in subsequent cycles. For patients with serum AST concentrations exceeding 10 times the upper limit of normal or serum bilirubin concentrations exceeding 5 times the upper limit of normal, albumin-bound paclitaxel therapy is *not* recommended. Patients with serum bilirubin concentrations exceeding the upper limit of normal were excluded from clinical studies evaluating use of the drug in non-small cell lung cancer. Further reduction of albumin-bound paclitaxel dosage for subsequent courses of therapy should be based on patient tolerance.

Pancreatic Cancer. For patients receiving albumin-bound paclitaxel for pancreatic cancer, the usual dose of 125 mg/m^2 may be administered for the first course of therapy in those who have mild hepatic impairment (AST concentrations less than 10 times the upper limit of normal and elevated serum bilirubin concentrations up to 1.25 times the upper limit of normal). For patients with AST concentrations less than 10 times the upper limit of normal and serum bilirubin concentrations of 1.26–5 times the upper limit of normal, AST concentrations exceeding 10 times the upper limit of normal, or serum bilirubin concentrations exceeding 5 times the upper limit of normal, albumin-bound paclitaxel therapy is *not* recommended. Patients with serum bilirubin concentrations exceeding the upper limit of normal were excluded from clinical studies evaluating use of the drug in pancreatic cancer. Further reduction of albumin-bound paclitaxel dosage for subsequent courses of therapy should be based on patient tolerance.

Cautions

■ Hematologic Effects and Infectious Complications The major and dose-limiting adverse effect of paclitaxel is bone marrow suppression, manifested by neutropenia, leukopenia, thrombocytopenia, and anemia. The frequency and severity of hematologic toxicity increase with higher dose, especially at conventional paclitaxel doses exceeding 190 mg/m^2. Paclitaxel-induced neutropenia does not appear to increase with cumulative exposure and does not appear to be more frequent or more severe in patients who have received prior radiation therapy. In clinical studies, myelosuppression was more profound when paclitaxel was given after cisplatin rather than with the alternative sequence (i.e., paclitaxel before cisplatin), apparently because plasma clearance of paclitaxel was decreased by approximately 33% when the drugs were administered in this sequence.

Neutropenia and Leukopenia Paclitaxel-induced neutropenia, which is dose and schedule dependent, generally is rapidly reversible.

Conventional Paclitaxel. Neutropenia (neutrophil count less than 2000/mm^3) occurred in 90% of patients with ovarian or breast cancer and in 95–100% of patients with AIDS-related Kaposi's sarcoma receiving paclitaxel as a single agent in clinical trials. Severe neutropenia (neutrophil count less than 500/mm^3) occurred in 52% of patients during paclitaxel monotherapy for ovarian or breast cancer. In a phase III clinical trial of patients with metastatic ovarian cancer receiving subsequent therapy with paclitaxel alone at a dose of 135 or 175 mg/m^2 administered as an infusion over 3 hours, severe neutropenia occurred in 14 or 27%, respectively. In patients with AIDS-related Kaposi's sarcoma receiving paclitaxel 100 or 135 mg/m^2 by 3-hour IV infusion, severe neutropenia occurred in 35 or 76%, respectively.

In a randomized trial in patients receiving initial treatment for advanced ovarian cancer, grade 4 neutropenia occurred in 81%, and febrile neutropenia occurred in 15%, of patients receiving paclitaxel 135 mg/m^2 by 24-hour IV infusion followed by cisplatin; episodes of fever associated with grade 4 neutropenia were reported in approximately 3% of courses. In another randomized trial in patients receiving initial treatment for advanced ovarian cancer, grade 4 neutropenia occurred in 33%, and febrile neutropenia occurred in 4%, of patients receiving paclitaxel 175 mg/m^2 by 3-hour IV infusion followed by cisplatin. In patients with node-positive breast cancer receiving cyclophosphamide and doxorubicin followed by paclitaxel, grade 4 neutropenia was reported in 76% of patients but it occurred during the period of paclitaxel therapy in only 15% of patients. In patients with non-small cell lung cancer receiving initial treatment with paclitaxel 135 mg/m^2 by 24-hour IV infusion followed by cisplatin, neutropenia occurred in 89% of patients and was severe in 74% of patients.

The onset of neutropenia usually occurs by 8–10 days and neutrophil nadirs generally occur at a median of 10–12 days following paclitaxel administration; neutrophil counts commonly recover by 15–21 days after administration. Subsequent paclitaxel courses of therapy generally do not result in lower neutrophil nadirs than the initial course, suggesting that the drug may not be irreversibly toxic to stem cells. Some data suggest that the addition of filgrastim to paclitaxel therapy may reduce the duration and severity of neutropenia and/or allow dose intensification. There also is some evidence that shorter paclitaxel infusion times (e.g., 3 hours) may result in a lower frequency and severity of neutropenia. In a phase III trial of subsequent therapy for patients with metastatic ovarian cancer, neutropenia, including severe neutropenia, occurred more frequently in patients receiving paclitaxel doses by 24-hour infusion than in those receiving the drug by 3-hour infusion; duration of infusion had a greater effect on paclitaxel-induced myelosuppression than did the amount of dose (135 versus 175 mg/m^2).

Leukopenia (less than 4000/mm^3) occurred in 90% of patients with ovarian or breast cancer receiving paclitaxel as a single agent in clinical trials and was severe (less than 1000/mm^3) in 17% of patients.

Albumin-bound Paclitaxel. Neutropenia (neutrophil count less than 2000/mm^3) occurred in 80%, severe neutropenia (neutrophil count less than 500/mm^3) occurred in 9%, and febrile neutropenia occurred in 2% of patients receiving albumin-bound paclitaxel for metastatic breast cancer. In a phase III clinical trial of patients with advanced non-small cell lung cancer receiving therapy with albumin-bound paclitaxel 100 mg/m^2 by 30-minute IV infusion in combination with carboplatin, grade 3 or 4 neutropenia occurred in 47% of patients. In patients with metastatic pancreatic cancer receiving albumin-bound paclitaxel 125 mg/m^2 by 30- to 40-minute IV infusion in combination with gemcitabine, grade 3 or 4 neutropenia occurred in 38% of patients.

Infectious Complications **Conventional Paclitaxel.** Fever was associated with 12% of all paclitaxel treatment courses in patients with solid tumors receiving the drug as a single agent. Among patients receiving paclitaxel monotherapy for ovarian or breast cancer, at least one episode of infection was reported in 30% of patients, and 9% of all treatment courses were associated with an infectious episode. These infectious episodes, including sepsis, pneumonia, and peritonitis, were fatal in 1% of all patients. In a phase III trial of paclitaxel as subsequent therapy for patients with metastatic ovarian cancer, infectious episodes occurred in 20 or 26% of patients receiving paclitaxel 135 or 175 mg/m^2, respectively, by 3-hour infusion. Urinary and respiratory tract infections were the most frequently reported infectious complications.

In patients with node-positive breast cancer receiving cyclophosphamide and doxorubicin followed by paclitaxel, severe infection was reported in 14% of patients. In patients with non-small cell lung cancer receiving initial treatment with paclitaxel 135 mg/m^2 by 24-hour IV infusion followed by cisplatin, infections occurred in 38% of patients.

Among patients receiving paclitaxel for AIDS-related Kaposi's sarcoma, at least one episode of opportunistic infection was reported in 61% of patients. In patients with AIDS-related Kaposi's sarcoma, febrile neutropenia (neutrophil count less than 500/mm^3 with fever exceeding 38°C and IV anti-infectives and/or hospitalization required) occurred in 55% of patients receiving paclitaxel 135 mg/m^2 and in 9% of those receiving paclitaxel 100 mg/m^2.

Albumin-bound Paclitaxel. Infection was reported in 24% of patients receiving albumin-bound paclitaxel for metastatic breast cancer. Oral candidiasis, respiratory tract infections, and pneumonia were the most frequently reported infectious complications. In patients with metastatic breast cancer, febrile neutropenia occurred in 2% of patients receiving albumin-bound paclitaxel as a single agent.

Among patients receiving albumin-bound paclitaxel combined with gemcitabine for pancreatic cancer, pyrexia was reported in 41% of patients and urinary tract infections were reported in 11% of patients. Other infections reported in less than 10% of patients were oral candidiasis and pneumonia. In patients with pancreatic cancer, sepsis (irrespective of neutrophil count) occurred in 5% of patients receiving albumin-bound paclitaxel combined with gemcitabine; biliary obstruction or the presence of a biliary stent appear to be risk factors for sepsis.

Thrombocytopenia **Conventional Paclitaxel.** Thrombocytopenia (platelet count less than 100,000/mm^3) developed less frequently than neutropenia, with at least one episode occurring in 20% of patients with ovarian or breast cancer receiving paclitaxel alone as subsequent therapy in clinical trials, and was severe (platelet count less than 50,000/mm^3) in 7% of patients. In patients with AIDS-related Kaposi's sarcoma receiving paclitaxel 135 or 100 mg/m^2, thrombocytopenia occurred in 52 or 27% of patients, and was severe in 17 or 5%, respectively.

In randomized trials for the initial treatment of advanced ovarian cancer, thrombocytopenia (platelet count less than 130,000/mm^3) was reported in 21% of patients receiving paclitaxel 175 mg/m^2 by 3-hour IV infusion followed by cisplatin, and thrombocytopenia (platelet count less than 100,000/mm^3) was reported in 26% of patients receiving paclitaxel 135 mg/m^2 by 24-hour IV infusion followed by cisplatin. In patients with node-positive breast cancer receiving cyclophosphamide and doxorubicin followed by paclitaxel, severe thrombocytopenia (platelet count less than 50,000/mm^3) was reported in 25% of patients. In patients with non-small cell lung cancer receiving initial treatment with paclitaxel 135 mg/m^2 by 24-hour IV infusion followed by cisplatin, thrombocytopenia occurred in 48% of patients and was severe (platelet count less than 50,000/mm^3) in 6% of patients.

Platelet nadirs usually occur 8 or 9 days after administration of the drug. Bleeding episodes occurred in 14% of patients with ovarian or breast cancer receiving paclitaxel alone as subsequent therapy and in 4% of all treatment courses, but most episodes were localized, and the frequency of such events was unrelated to paclitaxel dose or schedule; 2% of patients received platelet transfusions. In a phase III clinical trial of subsequent therapy for metastatic ovarian carcinoma, bleeding episodes were reported in 10% of patients receiving paclitaxel (135 or 175 mg/m^2) by 3-hour infusion; none of the patients who were treated with the 3-hour infusion received platelet transfusions.

Albumin-bound Paclitaxel. Thrombocytopenia (platelet count less than 100,000/mm^3) occurred in 2%, and was severe (platelet count less than 50,000/mm^3) in less than 1%, of patients receiving albumin-bound paclitaxel for metastatic breast cancer. Bleeding was reported in 2% of patients. In a phase III clinical trial of patients with advanced non-small cell lung cancer receiving therapy with albumin-bound paclitaxel 100 mg/m^2 by 30-minute IV infusion in combination with carboplatin, grade 3 or 4 thrombocytopenia occurred in 18% of patients; epistaxis occurred in 7% of patients. In patients with metastatic pancreatic cancer receiving albumin-bound paclitaxel 125 mg/m^2 by 30- to 40-minute IV infusion in combination with gemcitabine, grade 3 or 4 thrombocytopenia occurred in 13% of patients; epistaxis occurred in 15% of patients.

Anemia **Conventional Paclitaxel.** Anemia (hemoglobin less than 11 g/dL) occurred in 78% of patients with ovarian or breast cancer receiving paclitaxel monotherapy in clinical trials and was severe (less than 8 g/dL) in 16% of patients. No consistent relationship between paclitaxel dose or schedule and the frequency of anemia was observed. Anemia occurred in 69% of patients with a baseline hemoglobin of 11 g/dL or higher at study entry, and 7% had severe anemia. Among patients receiving paclitaxel alone as subsequent therapy for ovarian or breast cancer, packed red blood cell transfusions were administered to 25% of all patients and to 12% of patients with a baseline hemoglobin of 11 g/dL or higher. In patients with AIDS-related Kaposi's sarcoma receiving paclitaxel 135 or 100 mg/m^2, anemia occurred in 86 or 73% of patients, and was severe in 34 or 25%, respectively.

In randomized trials for the initial treatment of advanced ovarian cancer, anemia (hemoglobin less than 12 g/dL) was reported in 96% of patients receiving paclitaxel 175 mg/m^2 by 3-hour IV infusion followed by cisplatin, and anemia (hemoglobin less than 11 g/dL) was reported in 88% of patients receiving paclitaxel 135 mg/m^2 by 24-hour IV infusion followed by cisplatin. In patients with node-positive breast cancer receiving cyclophosphamide and doxorubicin followed by paclitaxel, severe anemia (hemoglobin less than 8 g/dL) was reported in 21% of patients. In patients receiving paclitaxel 135 mg/m^2 by 24-hour IV infusion followed by cisplatin for the initial treatment of advanced non-small cell lung cancer, anemia occurred in 94% of patients and was severe (hemoglobin less than 8 g/dL) in 22% of patients.

Albumin-bound Paclitaxel. Anemia (hemoglobin less than 11 g/dL) occurred in 33%, and was severe (hemoglobin less than 8 g/dL) in 1%, of patients receiving albumin-bound paclitaxel for metastatic breast cancer.

Anemia of grade 3 or 4 severity occurred in 28% of patients receiving albumin-bound paclitaxel combined with carboplatin for non-small cell lung cancer.

Eosinophilia Eosinophilia was reported in 40% of patients receiving a paclitaxel dose of 135 mg/m^2 for AIDS-related Kaposi's sarcoma.

■ **Sensitivity Reactions** ***Conventional Paclitaxel*** Anaphylaxis and severe hypersensitivity reactions have occurred in 2–4% of patients receiving conventional paclitaxel in clinical trials. Paclitaxel frequently causes hypersensitivity reactions, and all patients receiving the conventional formulation of the drug should be premedicated to prevent severe reactions. (See Dosage and Administration: Dosage.) Fatal hypersensitivity reactions have occurred in patients receiving conventional paclitaxel despite premedication.

In clinical trials involving use of paclitaxel alone as subsequent therapy for ovarian or breast cancer, 20% of all courses of paclitaxel therapy were associated with hypersensitivity reactions; reactions occurred in 41% of patients despite premedication and were severe in 2%. The frequency and severity of hypersensitivity reactions were not affected by the dose or schedule of paclitaxel administration in patients receiving the drug alone as subsequent therapy for ovarian cancer. The frequency and severity of hypersensitivity reactions were not affected by dose in patients receiving the drug alone as subsequent therapy for breast cancer. In patients with AIDS-related Kaposi's sarcoma receiving paclitaxel 135 or 100 mg/m^2, hypersensitivity reactions occurred in 14 or 9% of patients, respectively.

In randomized trials for the initial treatment of advanced ovarian cancer, hypersensitivity reactions were reported in 11% of patients receiving paclitaxel 175 mg/m^2 by 3-hour IV infusion followed by cisplatin and in 8% of patients receiving paclitaxel 135 mg/m^2 by 24-hour IV infusion followed by cisplatin. In patients with node-positive breast cancer receiving cyclophosphamide and doxorubicin followed by paclitaxel, severe hypersensitivity reactions were reported in 4% of patients; all patients were designated to receive premedication. In patients with non-small cell lung cancer receiving initial treatment with paclitaxel 135 mg/m^2 by 24-hour IV infusion followed by cisplatin, hypersensitivity reactions occurred in 16% of patients and were severe in 1%.

The most frequent manifestations of minor hypersensitivity reactions were flushing (28%), rash (12%), hypotension (4%), dyspnea (2%), tachycardia (2%), and hypertension (1%), as observed in patients receiving paclitaxel alone as subsequent therapy for ovarian or breast cancer. Rarely, chills and back pain have been reported in association with hypersensitivity reactions in patients receiving paclitaxel. The frequency of hypersensitivity reactions remained relatively stable during the entire treatment period.

Severe reactions, which generally occur within the first hour of paclitaxel infusion, are characterized by dyspnea and hypotension requiring treatment, flushing, chest pains, tachycardia, angioedema, and generalized urticaria, and are probably histamine mediated. Delayed onset of urticarial rash, 7–10 days following completion of a course of therapy, has been observed in patients receiving paclitaxel for AIDS-related Kaposi's sarcoma. Discontinuance of paclitaxel therapy and aggressive management of symptoms are required in patients experiencing severe hypersensitivity reactions. (See Dosage Modification for Toxicity and Contraindications for Continued Therapy: Sensitivity Reactions in Dosage and Administration: Dosage.)

The exact cause of the hypersensitivity reactions is not known, but they may result from the polyoxyl 35 castor oil (Cremophor® EL, polyethoxylated castor oil) in the paclitaxel for injection concentrate or from paclitaxel itself. (For information on hypersensitivity reactions associated with this vehicle, see Cautions: Sensitivity Reactions, in Cyclosporine 92:44.)

Other cutaneous reactions associated with hypersensitivity to paclitaxel, including acral erythema, generalized pustular dermatosis, and bullous fixed drug eruption, have been reported.

Albumin-bound Paclitaxel Hypersensitivity reactions occurred in 4% of patients receiving albumin-bound paclitaxel for metastatic breast cancer; no severe hypersensitivity reactions were reported. Hypersensitivity reactions, which were grade 1 or 2 in severity, occurred on the day that albumin-bound paclitaxel was administered and consisted of dyspnea in 1%, and flushing, hypotension, chest pain, or arrhythmia, each in less than 1% of patients. However, severe and sometimes fatal hypersensitivity reactions have been reported during postmarketing experience in patients receiving albumin-bound paclitaxel. The use of albumin-bound paclitaxel in patients who have experienced hypersensitivity reactions to conventional paclitaxel has not been studied.

■ **Nervous System Effects** The frequency and severity of adverse neurologic effects were dose dependent in patients receiving therapy with conventional or albumin-bound paclitaxel. The frequency and severity of neurologic toxicity in patients receiving paclitaxel were influenced by prior and/or concomitant therapy with neurotoxic agents.

Peripheral Neuropathy **Conventional Paclitaxel.** Peripheral neuropathy was reported in 60% of all patients receiving paclitaxel alone as subsequent therapy for ovarian or breast cancer in clinical trials, and in 52% of patients without preexisting neuropathy. Among patients receiving paclitaxel alone as subsequent therapy for ovarian or breast cancer, paclitaxel-induced neuropathy was severe in 3% of patients (2% of patients without preexisting neuropathy) and required discontinuance of the drug in 1% of patients. The frequency and severity of peripheral neuropathy increased with the higher dose but did not appear to be affected by the schedule of paclitaxel administration in patients receiving the drug alone as subsequent therapy for ovarian cancer. The frequency and severity of peripheral neuropathy increased with the higher dose in patients receiving the drug alone as subsequent therapy for breast cancer. In patients with AIDS-related Kaposi's sarcoma receiving paclitaxel 135 or 100 mg/m^2, peripheral neuropathy occurred in 79 or 46% of patients, and was severe in 10 or 2%, respectively.

Comparison across studies in patients with ovarian cancer suggests that higher incidences of neurotoxicity and severe neurotoxicity occur when paclitaxel 175 mg/m^2 by 3-hour IV infusion is followed by cisplatin. In randomized trials for the initial treatment of advanced ovarian cancer, neuromotor or neurosensory toxicity was reported in 87% (severe in 21%) of patients receiving paclitaxel 175 mg/m^2 by 3-hour IV infusion followed by cisplatin, and peripheral neuropathy was reported in 25% (severe in 3%) of patients receiving paclitaxel 135 mg/m^2 by 24-hour IV infusion followed by cisplatin. In patients with node-positive breast cancer receiving cyclophosphamide and doxorubicin followed by paclitaxel, grade 2 or 3 neurosensory toxicity occurred during the period of paclitaxel therapy in 15% of patients. In patients with advanced non-small cell lung cancer receiving initial treatment with paclitaxel 135 mg/m^2 by 24-hour IV infusion followed by cisplatin, neuromotor toxicity occurred in 37% of patients and was severe in 6%; neurosensory toxicity occurred in 48% of patients and was severe in 13%. This incidence of severe neurotoxicity in patients with non-small cell lung cancer receiving paclitaxel followed by cisplatin is higher than the incidence (severe peripheral neuropathy in 3%) reported in patients with ovarian or breast cancer receiving paclitaxel alone.

The neuropathy usually is sensory in nature and is characterized by paresthesia with numbness and tingling in a stocking-and-glove distribution. Perioral numbness also has been reported, and many patients experience burning pain (often associated with hyperesthesia), particularly in the feet. The onset may be rapid, occurring within a few days. Pruritus preceding the onset of peripheral neuropathy has been reported in patients receiving high doses of paclitaxel by 3-hour IV infusion; paclitaxel-induced pruritus was relieved by treatment with tricyclic antidepressant therapy. One patient experienced a "recall" reaction of severe peripheral neuropathy following extravasation of paclitaxel.

The frequency and severity of peripheral neuropathy are dose dependent and increase with cumulative dose; toxicity may be dose limiting or require dose modification.

The frequency and severity of paclitaxel-induced neurotoxicity increase with dose, especially at doses exceeding 190 mg/m^2. Among patients receiving paclitaxel alone as subsequent therapy for ovarian or breast cancer, neurologic manifestations were apparent in 27% of patients following the initial course of therapy and in 34–51% of patients receiving 2–10 courses of therapy; such manifestations tended to worsen with increasing exposure to the drug. Sensory manifestations usually improve or resolve within several months after discontinuance of paclitaxel. Infrequently, motor neuron toxicity also has occurred in patients receiving the drug.

Preexisting neuropathies resulting from previous therapies are not a contraindication to paclitaxel therapy; however, the incidence of paclitaxel-related neurotoxicity appears to be increased in patients with preexisting neuropathy or other risk factors for neuropathy.

Albumin-bound Paclitaxel. Sensory neuropathy occurred in 71%, and was severe in 10 %, of patients receiving albumin-bound paclitaxel for metastatic breast cancer. The frequency of sensory neuropathy increased with the cumulative dose of albumin-bound paclitaxel. In the randomized trial comparing albumin-bound paclitaxel with conventional paclitaxel for metastatic breast cancer, 24 (10%) of 229 patients receiving albumin-bound paclitaxel developed grade 3 peripheral neuropathy, and none developed grade 4 peripheral neuropathy. Of these 24 patients, amelioration of symptoms at a median of 22 days was documented in 14 patients; 10 patients resumed treatment at a reduced dose of albumin-bound paclitaxel, and 2 patients discontinued therapy with the drug. Improvement was not documented in the other 10 patients, and 4 of these patients discontinued therapy with albumin-bound paclitaxel.

Peripheral neuropathy occurred in 48%, and was severe in 3%, of patients receiving albumin-bound paclitaxel combined with carboplatin for non-small cell lung cancer. In the randomized trial comparing albumin-bound paclitaxel combined with carboplatin with conventional paclitaxel combined with carboplatin for non-small cell lung cancer, 3% of patients receiving albumin-bound paclitaxel combined with carboplatin developed grade 3 peripheral neuropathy and none developed grade 4 peripheral neuropathy. Grade 3 peripheral neuropathy improved to grade 1 or resolved in 59% of these patients following interruption or discontinuance of albumin-bound paclitaxel therapy. In comparison, severe (grade 3 or 4) peripheral neuropathy occurred in 12% of patients receiving conventional paclitaxel combined with carboplatin.

Peripheral neuropathy occurred in 54%, and was severe in 17%, of patients receiving albumin-bound paclitaxel combined with gemcitabine for metastatic pancreatic cancer. In the randomized trial comparing albumin-bound paclitaxel combined with gemcitabine with gemcitabine monotherapy for pancreatic cancer, 17% of patients receiving albumin-bound paclitaxel developed grade 3 peripheral neuropathy, and none developed grade 4 peripheral neuropathy. The median time to onset of grade 3 peripheral neuropathy was 140 days following albumin-bound paclitaxel administration. Amelioration of grade 3 peripheral neuropathy to grade 1 severity or less at a median of 29 days following discontinuance of the drug was reported. Albumin-bound paclitaxel was resumed at a reduced dosage in 44% of patients with grade 3 peripheral neuropathy.

Other Nervous System Effects **Conventional Paclitaxel.** Rarely, seizures (including tonoclonic seizures), syncope, ataxia, and neuroencephalopathy have occurred during or immediately following administration of paclitaxel. Autonomic neuropathy resulting in paralytic ileus has been reported rarely in patients receiving paclitaxel. A case of acute and temporary worsening of parkinsonian syndrome following paclitaxel infusion has been reported in a geriatric patient with Parkinson's disease.

The formulation of conventional paclitaxel contains ethyl alcohol, and some adverse neurologic effects of paclitaxel appear to be related to the effects of alcohol, particularly when high doses of conventional paclitaxel are administered over short infusion periods (e.g., 3 hours). CNS toxicity, rarely fatal, has been reported in pediatric patients receiving high doses of conventional paclitaxel by 3-hour IV infusion. (See Cautions: Pediatric Precautions.) Ethanol intoxication has been reported in a patient receiving high doses of conventional paclitaxel (348 mg/m^2) by 3-hour IV infusion.

Albumin-bound Paclitaxel. In patients receiving albumin-bound paclitaxel combined with gemcitabine for pancreatic cancer, depression occurred in 12%, and was severe in less than 1%, of patients. Headache occurred in 14%, and was severe in less than 1%, of patients receiving albumin-bound paclitaxel combined with gemcitabine for pancreatic cancer.

Cranial nerve palsies, vocal cord paresis, and autonomic neuropathy resulting in paralytic ileus have been reported in patients receiving albumin-bound paclitaxel.

■ Cardiovascular Effects

Hypotension and Bradycardia **Conventional Paclitaxel.** Hypotension and bradycardia are the most common adverse cardiovascular effects of paclitaxel. During the first 3 hours of paclitaxel IV infusion in clinical trials of paclitaxel used alone as subsequent therapy for ovarian or breast cancer, hypotension occurred in 12% of all patients and 3% of all treatment courses, and bradycardia occurred in 3% of all patients and 1% of all treatment courses. In a phase III trial of patients receiving paclitaxel alone as subsequent therapy for metastatic ovarian cancer, the frequency of hypotension or bradycardia did not appear to be influenced by paclitaxel dose or schedule. The frequency of hypotension or bradycardia did not appear to be influenced by prior anthracycline therapy. In a phase II study in patients receiving paclitaxel 135 mg/m^2 by 3-hour IV infusion for AIDS-related Kaposi's sarcoma, hypotension and bradycardia occurred in 17 and 3% of all patients, respectively. Hypotension was reported in 9% of patients receiving paclitaxel 100 mg/m^2 by 3-hour IV infusion for AIDS-related Kaposi's sarcoma.

In patients with advanced non-small cell lung cancer receiving initial treatment with paclitaxel 135 mg/m^2 by 24-hour IV infusion followed by cisplatin, adverse cardiovascular effects occurred in 33% of patients and were severe in 13%.

Most episodes of bradycardia and hypotension associated with paclitaxel were asymptomatic and did not require further treatment or discontinuance of the drug, although hypotension associated with severe hypersensitivity reactions to the drug may require intervention. Chest pain is a frequent manifestation of a severe hypersensitivity reaction. (See Cautions: Sensitivity Reactions.) Atypical chest pain also has been reported during paclitaxel infusion and may be another manifestation of a hypersensitivity reaction.

Albumin-bound Paclitaxel. During the 30-minute IV infusion, hypotension occurred in 5%, and bradycardia occurred in less than 1%, of patients receiving albumin-bound paclitaxel for metastatic breast cancer. Most episodes of hypotension or bradycardia were asymptomatic and did not require treatment or discontinuance of the paclitaxel infusion.

Hypertension Hypertension, often associated with a hypersensitivity reaction, has been observed in patients during administration of conventional paclitaxel. Hypertension also has been reported in patients receiving albumin-bound paclitaxel.

ECG Abnormalities ECG abnormalities in patients receiving conventional or albumin-bound paclitaxel generally were asymptomatic, were not dose limiting, and did not require therapeutic intervention.

Conventional Paclitaxel. ECG abnormalities were present in 23% of all paclitaxel-treated patients during clinical trials of the drug as a single agent for the subsequent therapy of ovarian or breast cancer, developing in 14% of patients with normal baseline ECGs during therapy with the drug. The most frequent ECG abnormalities included nonspecific repolarization, sinus bradycardia, sinus tachycardia, and premature beats. Among patients with normal baseline ECGs, prior therapy with anthracyclines did not influence the frequency of ECG abnormalities.

Albumin-bound Paclitaxel. ECG abnormalities were observed in 60% of all patients receiving albumin-bound paclitaxel for metastatic breast cancer and developed in 35% of patients with normal baseline ECGs. The most frequent ECG abnormalities included nonspecific repolarization, sinus bradycardia, and sinus tachycardia.

Arrhythmias, Conduction Abnormalities, and Other Severe Cardiovascular Effects **Conventional Paclitaxel.** Severe adverse cardiovascular effects occurred in about 1% of all patients receiving paclitaxel alone as subsequent therapy for ovarian or breast cancer in clinical trials. These effects included arrhythmias (e.g., asymptomatic ventricular tachycardia, bigeminy, syncope, hypertension, and venous thrombosis. In one patient treated with paclitaxel 175 mg/m^2 over 24 hours, syncope was accompanied by progressive hypotension and resulted in death. Severe conduction abnormalities, such as complete atrioventricular (AV) block requiring pacemaker insertion, have occurred in less than 1% of patients receiving paclitaxel. Atrial fibrillation and supraventricular tachycardia have been reported rarely in patients receiving paclitaxel. Junctional tachycardia has been reported in patients receiving paclitaxel. A higher incidence of severe adverse cardiovascular effects (12–13%) was reported in patients with advanced non-small cell lung cancer receiving paclitaxel in combination with cisplatin; difference in the cardiovascular risk factors in this patient population may have contributed to this increase.

Rarely, vascular toxicity, including myocardial infarction, has been reported in patients receiving paclitaxel. In one case, fatal myocardial infarction not preceded by an arrhythmia occurred during paclitaxel infusion in a patient with atherosclerotic cardiovascular disease. A patient with no history of cardiac disease experienced acute myocardial infarction while receiving paclitaxel therapy for metastatic breast cancer and subsequently died; previous radiation therapy to the left breast may have increased the risk of myocardial infarction in this patient. In another patient, sudden death occurred 7 days following completion of paclitaxel infusion; the immediate cause of death was determined to be acute pulmonary edema, which was probably caused by acute heart failure. Cerebrovascular infarction occurred 36 hours following completion of paclitaxel infusion in a patient with metastatic ovarian cancer; although the mechanism is not clear, it has been suggested that administration of paclitaxel precipitated thrombus formation in a patient predisposed to thromboembolic disorder by underlying disease.

Albumin-bound Paclitaxel. Severe adverse cardiovascular effects occurred in about 3% of patients receiving albumin-bound paclitaxel for metastatic breast cancer. These effects included chest pain, cardiac arrest, cardiac ischemia, myocardial infarction, supraventricular tachycardia, edema, thrombosis, pulmonary thromboembolism, pulmonary embolism, and hypertension. Cerebrovascular events (strokes) and transient ischemic attacks also have been reported in patients receiving albumin-bound paclitaxel for metastatic breast cancer. Other adverse cardiovascular effects reported in patients receiving albumin-bound paclitaxel include tachycardia and AV block.

Congestive Heart Failure and Cardiomyopathy **Conventional Paclitaxel.** Congestive heart failure, with progressive deterioration and death in at least one patient, has been reported in patients receiving paclitaxel who had also received previous chemotherapy, including anthracyclines. Although congestive heart failure has been associated with anthracycline therapy, suspected paclitaxel-induced myocardial damage detected by electron microscopy has been reported. Cardiomyopathy associated with acute renal failure has been reported in a patient receiving paclitaxel for AIDS-related Kaposi's sarcoma; although this may have been a complication of the underlying disease, a causal relationship with the administration of paclitaxel could not be ruled out.

Albumin-bound Paclitaxel. Congestive heart failure and left ventricular dysfunction have been reported in patients receiving albumin-bound paclitaxel, generally in those who previously received cardiotoxic drugs such as anthracyclines or had a history of cardiac disease.

Edema **Conventional Paclitaxel.** In clinical trials of paclitaxel as a single agent for the subsequent therapy of ovarian or breast cancer, edema occurred in 21% of all patients receiving paclitaxel, 17% of patients without baseline edema, and 5% of treatment courses in patients without baseline edema. Severe edema occurred in 1% of patients receiving subsequent therapy with paclitaxel alone for ovarian or breast cancer, and none of these patients required discontinuance of the drug. Edema in patients receiving paclitaxel commonly was focal and disease related; frequency of edema did not increase with length of time spent in the study.

Albumin-bound Paclitaxel. Edema occurred in 10% of patients receiving albumin-bound paclitaxel for metastatic breast cancer, and none had severe edema. Peripheral edema occurred in 10% of patients receiving albumin-bound paclitaxel combined with carboplatin for non-small cell lung cancer, and none had severe edema. In patients receiving albumin-bound paclitaxel combined with gemcitabine for pancreatic cancer, peripheral edema occurred in 46%, and was severe in 3%, of patients.

■ GI Effects

The most common GI toxicities associated with paclitaxel therapy are nausea and vomiting, diarrhea, and mucositis; these adverse effects usually are mild to moderate in severity. Intestinal obstruction, intestinal perforation, pancreatitis, ischemic colitis, and dehydration have occurred in patients receiving paclitaxel. Neutropenic enterocolitis (typhlitis) has been reported rarely in patients receiving conventional paclitaxel (alone or in combination therapy) despite concomitant administration of granulocyte colony-stimulating factor.

Conventional Paclitaxel Nausea and vomiting occurred in 52% of patients with ovarian or breast cancer and in 69% of patients with AIDS-related Kaposi's sarcoma receiving paclitaxel monotherapy in clinical trials. Higher incidences of nausea and vomiting are reported in clinical trials of combination therapy with paclitaxel and cisplatin for the initial treatment of advanced ovarian cancer (65 and 88%) or non-small cell lung cancer (85 and 87%). In patients with node-positive breast cancer receiving cyclophosphamide and doxorubicin followed by paclitaxel, severe nausea and vomiting was reported in 18% of patients.

Diarrhea and mucositis occurred in 38 and 31%, respectively, of patients receiving paclitaxel alone as subsequent therapy for ovarian or breast cancer. In patients with AIDS-related Kaposi's sarcoma receiving paclitaxel, diarrhea and mucositis occurred in 79 and 28% of patients, respectively; one-third of patients with AIDS-related Kaposi's sarcoma reported diarrhea before initiation of paclitaxel therapy. In randomized trials for the initial treatment of advanced ovarian cancer, diarrhea was reported in 37% of patients receiving paclitaxel 175 mg/m^2 by 3-hour IV infusion followed by cisplatin and in 16% of patients receiving paclitaxel 135 mg/m^2 by 24-hour IV infusion followed by cisplatin. In patients with node-positive breast cancer receiving cyclophosphamide and doxorubicin followed by paclitaxel, severe mucositis was reported in 4% of patients. In patients with non-small cell lung cancer receiving initial treatment with paclitaxel 135 mg/m^2 by 24-hour IV infusion followed by cisplatin, mucositis occurred in 18% of patients and was severe in 1%.

Paclitaxel-induced mucositis is characterized by diffuse ulceration of the lips, oral cavity, and pharynx; dysphagia and pain reflecting esophageal involvement may occur. In clinical trials of paclitaxel as a single agent for the subsequent therapy for ovarian or breast cancer, mucositis was schedule dependent and occurred more frequently in patients receiving paclitaxel by 24-hour infusion than in those receiving the drug by 3-hour infusion.

Anorexia and taste perversion have been reported with use of paclitaxel.

Albumin-bound Paclitaxel Nausea occurred in 30% and was severe in 3%, diarrhea occurred in 26% and was severe in less than 1%, and vomiting occurred in 18% and was severe in 4% of patients receiving albumin-bound paclitaxel for metastatic breast cancer. Mucositis was reported in 7% of patients receiving albumin-bound paclitaxel for metastatic breast cancer and was severe in less than 1%.

In the randomized trial comparing albumin-bound paclitaxel combined with gemcitabine with gemcitabine monotherapy for pancreatic cancer, nausea occurred in 54% and was severe in 6%, diarrhea occurred in 44% and was severe in 6%, and vomiting occurred in 36% and was severe in 6% of patients receiving albumin-bound paclitaxel. Mucositis was reported in 10% of patients receiving albumin-bound paclitaxel combined with gemcitabine for pancreatic cancer and was severe in 1%. Decreased appetite, dehydration, and dysgeusia were reported in 36, 21, and 16%, respectively, of patients receiving albumin-bound paclitaxel combined with gemcitabine.

■ **Dermatologic Effects** ***Conventional Paclitaxel*** Alopecia occurred in 87% of patients receiving paclitaxel alone as subsequent therapy for ovarian or breast cancer in clinical trials. In randomized trials for the initial treatment of advanced ovarian cancer, alopecia was reported in 96% of patients receiving paclitaxel 175 mg/m^2 by 3-hour IV infusion followed by cisplatin and in 55% of patients receiving paclitaxel 135 mg/m^2 by 24-hour IV infusion followed by cisplatin. In patients with node-positive breast cancer receiving cyclophosphamide and doxorubicin followed by paclitaxel, alopecia occurred during the period of paclitaxel therapy in 46% of patients.

Alopecia, which usually is complete, generally occurs 14–21 days after administration of paclitaxel with a sudden onset, often occurring in a single day. In addition, patients often experience a loss of all body hair including axillary, pubic, and extremity hair and eyelashes and eyebrows. Paclitaxel-induced alopecia is reversible, usually within 6–8 weeks after treatment, and patients receiving multiple courses of therapy often experience hair regrowth after 5–7 cycles.

Transient skin changes have been observed in patients with paclitaxel-induced hypersensitivity reactions. (See Cautions: Sensitivity Reactions.) Nail changes (changes in pigmentation, discoloration of nail bed) occurred in 2% of patients receiving paclitaxel monotherapy for ovarian or breast cancer. Severe nail changes, including dark discoloration of hands and/or feet followed by nail raising and paronychia with exudation and subungual hemorrhage, partial or complete loss of nails, or pain in the nail beds, have been reported in patients receiving paclitaxel on a weekly schedule for metastatic breast cancer. Radiation recall dermatitis associated with paclitaxel, resulting in extensive desquamation and necrosis in one patient with metastatic breast cancer, has been reported in several patients. Maculopapular rash, pruritus, Stevens-Johnson syndrome, and toxic epidermal necrolysis have been reported rarely in patients receiving paclitaxel.

Albumin-bound Paclitaxel Alopecia occurred in 90% of patients receiving albumin-bound paclitaxel for metastatic breast cancer. Nail changes, such as changes in pigmentation or discoloration of the nail bed, were uncommon in patients receiving albumin-bound paclitaxel.

In a randomized trial comparing albumin-bound paclitaxel combined with gemcitabine with gemcitabine monotherapy for pancreatic cancer, alopecia occurred in 50% of patients receiving albumin-bound paclitaxel. Rash was reported in 30% of patients receiving albumin-bound paclitaxel combined with gemcitabine for pancreatic cancer and was severe in 2%.

Skin abnormalities related to radiation recall, generalized or maculopapular rash, erythema, pruritus, photosensitivity reactions, Stevens-Johnson syndrome, and toxic epidermal necrolysis also have been reported in patients receiving albumin-bound paclitaxel.

■ **Local Effects** Specific treatment for paclitaxel-induced extravasation reactions currently is unknown, and the injection site should be monitored closely for possible infiltration of the drug during infusion of conventional or albumin-bound paclitaxel.

Conventional Paclitaxel Injection site reactions occurred in 13% of patients receiving paclitaxel alone as subsequent therapy for ovarian or breast cancer in clinical studies. Injection site reactions, including reactions secondary to extravasation, usually were mild and were characterized by erythema, tenderness, skin discoloration, or swelling at the injection site. Such reactions have been observed more frequently in patients receiving paclitaxel by 24-hour infusion than in those receiving the drug by 3-hour infusion. Recurrence of skin reactions at a previous site of extravasation (i.e., "recall" reactions) following administration of paclitaxel at a different injection site has been reported rarely.

Rarely, severe local effects of paclitaxel, such as phlebitis, cellulitis, induration, skin exfoliation, necrosis, and fibrosis have been reported. In some patients, the onset of injection site reaction occurred during prolonged infusion of paclitaxel; delayed onset of injection site reactions, 3–13 days following completion of paclitaxel infusion, also has been reported.

Albumin-bound Paclitaxel Injection site reactions occurred in less than 1% of patients receiving albumin-bound paclitaxel for metastatic breast cancer.

■ **Musculoskeletal Effects** Arthralgia and/or myalgia usually were transient, occurred 2 or 3 days after administration of conventional or albumin-bound paclitaxel, and resolved within a few days.

Conventional Paclitaxel Arthralgia and/or myalgia occurred in 60% of patients receiving paclitaxel alone as subsequent therapy for ovarian or breast cancer in clinical trials and was severe in 8% of patients. In patients with AIDS-related Kaposi's sarcoma receiving paclitaxel 135 or 100 mg/m^2, arthralgia and/or myalgia occurred in 93 or 48% of patients, and was severe in 14 or 16%, respectively.

In randomized trials for the initial treatment of advanced ovarian cancer, myalgia or arthralgia was reported in 60% of patients receiving paclitaxel 175 mg/m^2 by 3-hour IV infusion followed by cisplatin and in 9% of patients receiving paclitaxel 135 mg/m^2 by 24-hour IV infusion followed by cisplatin. In patients with node-positive breast cancer receiving cyclophosphamide and doxorubicin followed by paclitaxel, grade 2 or 3 myalgias occurred during the period of paclitaxel therapy in 23% of patients. In patients with advanced non-small cell lung cancer receiving initial treatment with paclitaxel 135 mg/m^2 by 24-hour IV infusion followed by cisplatin, arthralgia/myalgia occurred in 21% of patients and was severe in 3%.

In clinical trials of patients with ovarian or breast cancer, the frequency and severity of arthralgia and/or myalgia did not appear to be dose or schedule dependent and did not vary throughout the treatment period.

Albumin-bound Paclitaxel Myalgia and/or arthralgia occurred in 44%, and was severe in 8%, of patients receiving albumin-bound paclitaxel for metastatic breast cancer. In a phase III clinical trial of patients with advanced non-small cell lung cancer receiving therapy with albumin-bound paclitaxel 100 mg/m^2 by 30-minute IV infusion in combination with carboplatin, arthralgia or myalgia occurred in 13 or 10% of patients, respectively, and was severe in less than 1% of patients. In patients with advanced pancreatic cancer receiving albumin-bound paclitaxel 125 mg/m^2 by 30- to 40-minute IV infusion in combination with gemcitabine, arthralgia, myalgia, or extremity pain occurred in 11, 10, or 11% of patients, respectively, and was severe in 1% of patients.

■ **Hepatic Effects** Hepatic necrosis and hepatic encephalopathy resulting in death have occurred rarely in patients receiving conventional paclitaxel and may occur in patients receiving albumin-bound paclitaxel. Fatal hepatic coma occurred following administration of conventional paclitaxel in a patient with breast cancer and hepatic metastases.

Conventional Paclitaxel Abnormalities in liver function test results have occurred in patients receiving paclitaxel for ovarian or breast cancer but do not appear to be dose or schedule related. In patients with normal baseline hepatic function, increased serum alkaline phosphatase concentrations occurred in 22%, increased serum AST (SGOT) concentrations occurred in 19%, and increased serum bilirubin concentrations occurred in 7% of patients receiving paclitaxel monotherapy for ovarian or breast cancer. Prolonged exposure to paclitaxel has not been associated with cumulative hepatic toxicity.

Albumin-bound Paclitaxel Among patients with normal baseline hepatic function, increased serum AST (SGOT) concentrations occurred in 39%, increased serum alkaline phosphatase concentrations occurred in 36%, and increased serum bilirubin concentrations occurred in 7%, of patients receiving albumin-bound paclitaxel for metastatic breast cancer in a randomized trial. Elevations in serum GGT concentrations (grade 3 or 4) occurred in 14% of patients receiving albumin-bound paclitaxel.

■ **Renal Effects** ***Conventional Paclitaxel*** Renal toxicity, including acute renal failure, has been reported in patients with HIV infection receiving paclitaxel. In patients with AIDS-related Kaposi's sarcoma receiving paclitaxel 135 or 100 mg/m^2 by 3-hour IV infusion, elevation of serum creatinine occurred in 34 or 18% of patients, and was severe in 7 or 5%, respectively.

Elevations of serum creatinine generally were reversible; however, discontinuance of paclitaxel therapy was required in one patient suspected of having severe HIV nephropathy.

Albumin-bound Paclitaxel Elevations of serum creatinine occurred in 11%, and were severe in 1%, of patients receiving albumin-bound paclitaxel for metastatic breast cancer. No interruptions, delay, or reductions in dose of albumin-bound paclitaxel were required for renal toxicity.

■ **Respiratory Effects** Lung fibrosis has been reported rarely in patients receiving conventional paclitaxel and may occur in patients receiving albumin-bound paclitaxel.

Conventional Paclitaxel Radiation pneumonitis and interstitial pneumonia have been reported in patients receiving paclitaxel and concurrent radiation therapy. Possible radiation recall pneumonitis has been reported in a patient who received paclitaxel 12 days following completion of radiation therapy for metastatic adenocarcinoma of the lung. Adverse respiratory effects associated with hypersensitivity to paclitaxel, including pneumonitis and transient pulmonary infiltrates, also have been reported. Pulmonary embolism has been reported rarely in patients receiving paclitaxel.

Albumin-bound Paclitaxel Dyspnea was reported in 12%, and cough in 7%, of patients receiving albumin-bound paclitaxel for metastatic breast cancer. Pneumothorax has been reported in less than 1% of patients following treatment with albumin-bound paclitaxel for metastatic breast cancer. Cough was reported in 17% of patients receiving albumin-bound paclitaxel combined with gemcitabine for pancreatic cancer.

Pneumonitis, interstitial pneumonia, pulmonary embolism, and radiation pneumonitis have been reported in patients receiving albumin-bound paclitaxel. Pneumonitis was reported in 4% of patients, and was fatal in 2 of 17 patients, following treatment with albumin-bound paclitaxel combined with gemcitabine for pancreatic cancer.

■ **Ocular Effects** ***Conventional Paclitaxel*** Optic nerve disturbances and visual disturbances have been reported following administration of paclitaxel, particularly in patients receiving high doses. Rare reports of abnormalities in visual evoked potentials suggest persistent damage of the optic nerve related to paclitaxel. Other visual disturbances reported in association with paclitaxel infusion (e.g., scintillating scotomata, photopsia) generally appear to be reversible. Conjunctivitis and increased lacrimation have been reported rarely in patients receiving paclitaxel.

Albumin-bound Paclitaxel Ocular or visual disturbances occurred in 13% of 366 patients receiving albumin-bound paclitaxel for metastatic breast cancer in single-arm studies or a randomized trial. Severe ocular or visual disturbances occurred in 1% of patients and consisted of keratitis and blurred vision in patients receiving high doses (300 or 375 mg/m^2) of albumin-bound paclitaxel. These adverse ocular effects generally have been reversible; however, rare reports of abnormal visual evoked potentials in patients receiving conventional paclitaxel suggest that persistent damage of the optic nerve may occur. Reduced visual acuity due to cystoid macular edema has been reported in patients receiving albumin-bound paclitaxel or other taxanes; following discontinuance of therapy, cystoid macular edema improves and visual acuity may return to baseline. Conjunctivitis and increased lacrimation have been reported rarely in patients receiving conventional paclitaxel and may occur in patients receiving albumin-bound paclitaxel.

■ **Otic Effects** Ototoxicity, including hearing loss and tinnitus, has been reported in patients receiving paclitaxel.

■ **Other Adverse Effects** ***Conventional Paclitaxel*** Asthenia and malaise have been reported in patients receiving paclitaxel. In a randomized trial for the initial treatment of advanced ovarian cancer, asthenia was reported in 17% of patients receiving paclitaxel 135 mg/m^2 by 24-hour IV infusion followed by cisplatin.

Albumin-bound Paclitaxel Asthenia was reported in 47%, and was severe in 8%, of patients receiving albumin-bound paclitaxel for metastatic breast cancer. Fatigue and asthenia were reported in 59 and 19%, respectively, of patients receiving albumin-bound paclitaxel combined with gemcitabine for pancreatic cancer, and were severe in 18 or 7%, respectively, of patients. In addition, hypokalemia was reported in 12%, and was severe in 4%, of patients receiving albumin-bound paclitaxel combined with gemcitabine for pancreatic cancer.

■ **Precautions and Contraindications** Paclitaxel is a toxic drug with a low therapeutic index, and a therapeutic response is not likely to occur without evidence of toxicity. The drug must be used only under constant supervision by clinicians experienced in therapy with cytotoxic agents and only when the potential benefits of paclitaxel therapy are thought to outweigh the possible risks. In addition, appropriate diagnostic and treatment facilities must be readily available in case the patient develops any severe hypersensitivity reactions to paclitaxel therapy (e.g., hypotension, dyspnea requiring bronchodilators, angioedema, generalized urticaria).

Paclitaxel (conventional or albumin-bound paclitaxel) should *not* be used in patients with known severe hypersensitivity to the drug. In addition, paclitaxel for injection concentrate should *not* be used in patients with known severe hypersensitivity to the polyoxyl 35 castor oil vehicle. (See Cautions: Sensitivity Reactions.) To prevent severe hypersensitivity reactions, patients should be pretreated with corticosteroids (e.g., dexamethasone), diphenhydramine, and H_2-receptor antagonists (e.g., cimetidine, ranitidine) before receiving conventional paclitaxel. Premedication generally is not required in patients receiving albumin-bound paclitaxel. (See Dosage and Administration: Dosage.)

At least one commercially available formulation of paclitaxel injection contains metabisulfite, a sulfite that may cause serious allergic-type reactions in certain susceptible individuals. The overall incidence of sulfite sensitivity in the general population is probably low, but in susceptible individuals, exposure to sulfites can result in acute bronchospasm or, less frequently, life-threatening anaphylaxis. The paclitaxel formulation containing metabisulfite should be used with caution in atopic, nonasthmatic individuals.

Paclitaxel therapy (with conventional or albumin-bound paclitaxel) should not be administered to patients with baseline neutrophil counts less than 1500/mm^3. In patients with HIV infection, paclitaxel therapy should not be administered if baseline neutrophil counts are less than 1000/mm^3. To monitor the occurrence of paclitaxel-induced bone marrow suppression, mainly neutropenia, which may be severe and result in infection, it is recommended that frequent peripheral blood cell counts, including blood cell counts prior to each dose of the drug, be performed in all patients. (See Dosage and Administration: Dosage.) Because sepsis has been reported in patients receiving albumin-bound paclitaxel, administration of a broad-spectrum anti-infective should be initiated if the patient becomes febrile (regardless of neutrophil count).

Reduction in dosage of paclitaxel and close monitoring are required in patients with hepatic impairment. (See Dosage and Administration: Dosage in Renal and Hepatic Impairment.)

Because paclitaxel may cause adverse cardiovascular effects, including hypotension, bradycardia, and hypertension, frequent monitoring of vital signs is recommended, particularly during the first hour of the drug infusion; however, continuous cardiac monitoring is not required except in patients with preexisting serious conduction abnormalities.

Because albumin-bound paclitaxel may cause life-threatening pneumonitis, monitoring for manifestations of pneumonitis is recommended.

Patients should be warned that the alcohol contained in conventional paclitaxel may impair their ability to perform hazardous activities requiring mental alertness (e.g., operating machinery, driving a motor vehicle) following paclitaxel infusion, particularly when high doses of the drug are administered over short infusion periods (e.g., 3 hours), and that CNS depressants (e.g., opiates, sedatives) should be used concomitantly with caution.

Because albumin-bound paclitaxel contains albumin, a derivative of human blood, there is a remote risk of transmission of disease, such as viral disease or Creutzfeldt-Jakob disease, associated with its use. To date, no cases of transmission of bloodborne illness have been associated with use of albumin.

■ **Pediatric Precautions** Safety and efficacy of conventional or albumin-bound paclitaxel in children have not been established.

The manufacturer reports that CNS toxicity, rarely fatal, has been observed in pediatric patients receiving high doses of conventional paclitaxel (350–420 mg/m^2) by 3-hour IV infusion in a clinical trial. Because paclitaxel injection contains dehydrated alcohol, toxicity may have resulted from IV administration of large amounts of alcohol over a short period of time. The use of concomitant antihistamine as a component of the premedication regimen may intensify the toxic effect of the alcohol. However, the possibility of a direct toxic effect of paclitaxel itself cannot be ruled out.

■ **Geriatric Precautions** When the total number of patients studied in clinical trials of conventional paclitaxel for advanced ovarian, breast, or non-small cell lung cancer and in the study for the adjuvant treatment of breast cancer is considered, 17% were 65 years of age or older, and 1% were 75 years of age or older. Clinical studies of conventional paclitaxel did not include sufficient numbers of patients 65 years of age and older to determine whether geriatric patients respond differently than younger patients. In a study of paclitaxel for the first-line treatment of advanced ovarian cancer, median survival was lower in geriatric patients than in younger patients. Geriatric patients are at increased risk for certain adverse effects of paclitaxel, including severe myelosuppression and severe neuropathy. In 2 clinical studies of conventional paclitaxel for non-small cell lung cancer, geriatric patients had a higher incidence of cardiovascular toxicity than younger patients.

In a randomized trial evaluating albumin-bound paclitaxel for the treatment of metastatic breast cancer, 13% of patients receiving albumin-bound paclitaxel were 65 years of age or older, and less than 2% were 75 years of age or older. No difference in toxicity of albumin-bound paclitaxel was observed between geriatric and younger patients.

In a randomized trial evaluating albumin-bound paclitaxel combined with carboplatin for the treatment of advanced non-small cell lung cancer, 31% of patients receiving albumin-bound paclitaxel combined with carboplatin were 65 years of age or older, and less than 3.5% were 75 years of age or older. Although no overall differences in efficacy were observed between geriatric and younger patients, toxicity (i.e., myelosuppression, peripheral neuropathy, arthralgia) occurred more frequently in patients 65 years of age or older.

In a clinical trial evaluating albumin-bound paclitaxel combined with gemcitabine for the treatment of metastatic pancreatic cancer, 41% of patients receiving albumin-bound paclitaxel combined with gemcitabine were 65 years of age or older, and less than 10% were 75 years of age or older. Although no overall differences in efficacy were observed between geriatric and younger patients, toxicity (i.e., diarrhea, decreased appetite, dehydration, epistaxis) occurred more frequently in patients 65 years of age or older. The clinical trial did not include sufficient numbers of patients older than 75 years of age to determine whether these patients respond differently than younger patients.

■ **Mutagenicity and Carcinogenicity** Paclitaxel has been shown to induce chromosome aberrations in human lymphocytes in vitro, and the drug was mutagenic in the micronucleus test in mice in vivo; however, paclitaxel was not mutagenic in the Ames test or the CHO/HGPRT gene mutation assay.

Studies to determine the carcinogenic potential of paclitaxel have not been performed to date.

■ **Pregnancy, Fertility, and Lactation** Paclitaxel can cause fetal toxicity when administered to pregnant women, but potential benefits may be acceptable in certain conditions despite the possible risks to the fetus.

Reproduction studies in rabbits receiving IV conventional paclitaxel doses of 3 mg/kg daily (approximately 0.2 times the maximum recommended human dose on a mg/m^2 basis) during organogenesis revealed evidence of maternal toxicity, embryotoxicity, and fetotoxicity. The drug caused intrauterine mortality, increased resorptions, and increased fetal deaths. Reproduction studies in rats receiving IV paclitaxel doses of 1 mg/kg daily (approximately 0.04 times the maximum recommended human dose on a mg/m^2 basis) during organogenesis resulted in embryotoxicity and fetotoxicity. No teratogenic effects were observed in the offspring of rats receiving daily IV paclitaxel doses of 1 mg/kg; however, the teratogenic potential of higher paclitaxel doses could not be assessed because of extensive fetal mortality.

Reproduction studies in rats receiving albumin-bound paclitaxel at IV doses of 6 mg/m^2 (approximately 2% of the maximum recommended human dose on a mg/m^2 basis) on gestation days 7 to 17 resulted in embryotoxicity and fetotoxicity. The drug caused intrauterine mortality, increased resorptions, reduced numbers of litters, increased fetal deaths, reduction in fetal body weight, and increased fetal anomalies including soft tissue and skeletal malformations, such as eye bulge, folded retina, microphthalmia, and dilation of brain ventricles. Fetal anomalies also occurred in the offspring of rats receiving lower doses of albumin-bound paclitaxel (IV doses of 3 mg/m^2 or approximately 1% of the maximum recommended human dose on a mg/m^2 basis).

There are no adequate and well-controlled studies to date using paclitaxel in pregnant women. Paclitaxel should be used during pregnancy only in life-threatening situations or for severe disease for which safer drugs cannot be used or are ineffective. When paclitaxel is used during pregnancy or if the patient becomes pregnant while receiving the drug, the patient should be informed of the potential hazard to the fetus. Women of childbearing potential should be advised to avoid becoming pregnant during therapy with paclitaxel. Men receiving albumin-bound paclitaxel should be advised to avoid fathering a child.

At an IV dose of 1 mg/kg daily, conventional paclitaxel reduced fertility in rats.

Reduced fertility with decreased pregnancy rates and increased loss of embryos in mated females occurred in male rats given albumin-bound paclitaxel at a dose of 42 mg/m^2 weekly (approximately 16% of the daily maximum recommended human dose on a mg/m^2 basis) for 11 weeks prior to mating with untreated female rats. Fetal anomalies, including soft tissue and skeletal malformations, occurred in the offspring of male rats receiving lower doses of albumin-bound paclitaxel (IV doses of 3 and 12 mg/m^2 or approximately 1–5% of the maximum recommended human dose on a mg/m^2 basis). Testicular atrophy/degeneration has been observed with the administration of a single dose of albumin-bound paclitaxel in rats receiving 54 mg/m^2 and dogs receiving 175 mg/m^2.

It is not known whether paclitaxel is distributed into human milk. However, in lactating rats given radiolabeled paclitaxel, concentrations of radioactivity in milk were higher than those in plasma and declined in parallel with plasma concentrations of the drug. Because of the potential for serious adverse reactions to paclitaxel in nursing infants, a decision should be made whether to discontinue nursing or the drug, taking into account the importance of the drug to the woman.

Drug Interactions

■ **CNS Depressants** Concomitant administration of CNS depressants such as antihistamines or opiates with paclitaxel should be undertaken with caution as these drugs may cause potentiation of CNS depression caused by the alcohol contained in the paclitaxel formulation.

■ **Drugs Affecting Hepatic Microsomal Enzymes** Although specific studies have not been performed and the clinical importance has not been determined, concomitant administration of drugs that affect cytochrome P-450 (CYP) hepatic microsomal enzymes could alter the metabolism of paclitaxel. Metabolism of paclitaxel is mediated by CYP2C8 and CYP3A4, and the possibility exists that drugs that induce these isoenzymes may reduce plasma paclitaxel concentrations. Conversely, concomitant administration of paclitaxel with drugs that inhibit CYP2C8 and/or CYP3A4 may increase plasma paclitaxel concentrations. In addition, concomitant administration of paclitaxel with other drugs that are metabolized by CYP2C8 and/or CYP3A4 may result in decreased metabolism of the drug(s) because of competition for the enzyme. Caution should be exercised when paclitaxel is used concomitantly with drugs that are substrates, inhibitors, or inducers of CYP2C8 and/or CYP3A4.

Lower steady-state or peak plasma concentrations of paclitaxel, increased rates of clearance, and reduced toxicity have been reported in patients receiving anticonvulsants known to induce CYP enzymes (e.g., phenobarbital, phenytoin). Histamine H_2-receptor antagonists are a component of the premedication regimen used to prevent severe hypersensitivity reactions in patients receiving conventional paclitaxel; no pharmacokinetic, toxicologic, or pharmacologic differences were observed in a prospective, crossover trial in which patients received either cimetidine or famotidine despite the variable effects of these drugs on cytochrome P-450 enzyme activity. In addition, no difference in paclitaxel steady-state concentrations was observed between cycles in a small number of patients who received standard-dose (i.e., 300 mg) versus high-dose (i.e., 2400 mg) cimetidine during subsequent cycles of paclitaxel therapy. The potential interaction between paclitaxel and protease inhibitors (e.g., indinavir, nelfinavir, ritonavir, saquinavir), which are substrates and/or inhibitors of the CYP3A4 isoenzyme, has not been studied in clinical trials.

Results of in vitro studies show that the metabolism of paclitaxel to its principal metabolite, 6α-hydroxypaclitaxel, was inhibited by ketoconazole, verapamil, diazepam, quinidine, dexamethasone, cyclosporine, teniposide, etoposide, or vincristine; however, the concentrations of drugs used in these studies exceeded the plasma concentrations found in vivo following typical therapeutic doses. Other agents that inhibited the metabolism of paclitaxel in vitro include testosterone, 17α-ethinyl estradiol, retinoic acid, or quercetin (a specific inhibitor of CYP2C8).

■ **Antineoplastic Agents** Sequence-dependent drug interactions have been reported to occur when paclitaxel is administered with other antineoplastic agents, including cisplatin, doxorubicin, and cyclophosphamide. In a phase I trial using escalating doses of IV conventional paclitaxel 110–200 mg/m^2 sequentially administered with IV cisplatin 50 or 75 mg/m^2, increased severity of myelosuppression was observed when paclitaxel was administered following cisplatin compared with the alternative sequence (paclitaxel administered preceding cisplatin). Pharmacokinetic studies show that administration of cisplatin followed by conventional paclitaxel decreases paclitaxel clearance by approximately 25–33%. When cisplatin and paclitaxel must be administered sequentially, the sequence of paclitaxel followed by cisplatin is recommended. Increased severity of neutropenia and thrombocytopenia have been reported when paclitaxel is administered (by 24-hour IV infusion) followed by cyclophosphamide.

Use of paclitaxel in combination therapy with doxorubicin may result in increased plasma concentrations of doxorubicin and its active metabolite doxorubicinol; this interaction may contribute to the antitumor efficacy as well as the increased incidence of cardiac toxicity when paclitaxel is used in conjunction with doxorubicin. Synergistic cytotoxicity with paclitaxel followed by doxorubicin has been observed in *in vitro* studies and may result from a paclitaxel-induced increase in activity of DNA topoisomerase II, one of the intracellular targets involved in doxorubicin cytotoxicity.

Administration of conventional paclitaxel followed by carboplatin was associated with similar rates of neutropenia but less severe thrombocytopenia compared with carboplatin alone; a pharmacodynamic mechanism for the interaction between the drugs has been postulated since the pharmacokinetics of the agents were unchanged. When administration of albumin-bound paclitaxel was followed immediately by carboplatin, no clinically important changes in paclitaxel exposure occurred; although mean exposure to free carboplatin was about 23% higher than the targeted exposure (6 mg/mL per minute), mean half-life and clearance of carboplatin were consistent with values reported for carboplatin alone.

The potential for pharmacokinetic interactions between paclitaxel and gemcitabine has not been elucidated.

■ **Protein-bound Drugs** In vitro data indicate that paclitaxel is highly bound (89–98%) to plasma proteins; however, the presence of cimetidine, ranitidine, dexamethasone, or diphenhydramine did not displace paclitaxel from plasma proteins.

Acute Toxicity

■ **Manifestations** Limited information is available on acute overdosage of paclitaxel. Overdosage with paclitaxel would be expected to produce effects such as myelosuppression, peripheral or sensory neurotoxicity, and mucositis.

Overdosage of conventional paclitaxel in pediatric patients may be associated with acute ethanol toxicity because of the presence of dehydrated alcohol in the formulation. (See Cautions: Pediatric Precautions.)

■ **Treatment** There is no known specific antidote for paclitaxel overdosage. Management of paclitaxel overdosage consists of discontinuance of the drug and initiation of supportive measures appropriate for the type of toxicity observed. Paclitaxel appears to be minimally removed by hemodialysis.

Pharmacology

Paclitaxel is an antimicrotubule antineoplastic agent. Unlike some other common antimicrotubule agents (e.g., vinca alkaloids, colchicine, podophyllotoxin), which inhibit microtubule assembly, paclitaxel and docetaxel (a semisynthetic taxoid) promote microtubule assembly.

Microtubules are organelles that exist in a state of dynamic equilibrium with their components, tubulin dimers. They are an essential part of the mitotic spindle and also are involved in maintenance of cell shape and motility, and transport between organelles within the cell.

By binding in a reversible, concentration-dependent manner to the β-subunit of tubulin at the *N*-terminal domain, paclitaxel enhances the polymerization of tubulin, the protein subunit of the spindle microtubules, even in the absence of factors that are normally required for microtubule assembly (e.g., guanosine triphosphate [GTP]), and induces the formation of stable, nonfunctional microtubules. Paclitaxel promotes microtubule stability even under conditions that typically cause depolymerization in vitro (e.g., cold temperature, the addition of calcium, the presence of antimitotic drugs). While the precise mechanism of action of the drug is not understood fully, paclitaxel disrupts the dynamic equilibrium within the microtubule system and blocks cells in the late G_2 phase and M phase of the cell cycle, inhibiting cell replication.

Evidence suggests that paclitaxel also may induce cell death by triggering apoptosis. In addition, paclitaxel and docetaxel enhance the effects of ionizing radiation, possibly by blocking cells in the G_2 phase, the phase of the cell cycle in which cells are most radiosensitive. Preclinical evidence suggests that cross-resistance between paclitaxel and docetaxel is incomplete.

Pharmacokinetics

Conventional paclitaxel exhibits nonlinear, dose-dependent pharmacokinetics, particularly when the drug is administered over shorter periods of infusion (e.g., 3 hours). Both saturable distribution and elimination contribute to the nonlinear disposition of conventional paclitaxel. Although the relevance of these findings in humans is unknown, a study in mice comparing the pharmacokinetic profiles of differing formulations of paclitaxel suggests that the nonlinear distribution of conventional paclitaxel may be related to the formulation vehicle, polyoxyl 35 castor oil (Cremophor® EL, polyoxyethylated castor oil). Because of the nonlinearity of pharmacokinetics for conventional paclitaxel, relatively small changes in dose may lead to large changes in peak plasma concentrations and total drug exposure. The pharmacokinetics of conventional paclitaxel in patients with AIDS-related Kaposi's sarcoma have not been evaluated. In addition, the disposition of conventional paclitaxel and its metabolites has not been evaluated in geriatric patients.

■ **Absorption** ***Conventional Paclitaxel*** Peak plasma concentrations and areas under the plasma concentration-time curve (AUCs) following IV administration of paclitaxel exhibit marked interindividual variation. Plasma concentrations of paclitaxel increase during continuous IV administration of the drug and decline immediately following completion of the infusion. Following 24-hour IV infusion of paclitaxel at doses of 135 or 175 mg/m² in patients with advanced ovarian cancer, peak plasma concentrations averaged 195 or 365 ng/mL, respectively; the increase in dose (30%) was associated with a disproportionately greater increase in peak plasma concentration (87%), but the increase in AUC was proportional. When paclitaxel was administered by continuous IV infusion over 3 hours at doses of 135 or 175 mg/m² in patients with advanced ovarian cancer, peak plasma concentrations averaged 2.17 or 3.65 mcg/mL, respectively; the increase in dose (30%) was associated with disproportionately greater increases in peak plasma concentration (68%) and AUC (89%).

Albumin-bound Paclitaxel For the dose range 80–375 mg/m², increase in dose of albumin-bound paclitaxel was associated with a proportional increase in AUC. The duration of infusion did not affect the pharmacokinetic disposition of albumin-bound paclitaxel. Following 30-minute or 3-hour IV infusion of albumin-bound paclitaxel 260 mg/m² in patients with metastatic breast cancer, the peak plasma concentration averaged 18,741 ng/mL.

■ **Distribution** At plasma concentrations ranging from 0.1–50 mcg/mL, 88–98% of paclitaxel is bound to plasma proteins.

Conventional Paclitaxel Following IV administration, paclitaxel is widely distributed into body fluids and tissues. Paclitaxel has a large volume of distribution that appears to be affected by dose and duration of infusion. Following administration of paclitaxel doses of 135 or 175 mg/m² by IV infusion over 24 hours in patients with advanced ovarian cancer, the mean apparent volume of distribution at steady state ranged from 227–688 L/m². The steady-state volume of distribution ranged from 18.9–260 L/m² in children with solid tumors or refractory leukemia receiving paclitaxel 200–500 mg/m²by 24-hour IV infusion.

Paclitaxel does not appear to readily penetrate the CNS, but paclitaxel has been detected in ascitic fluid following IV infusion of the drug. It is not known whether paclitaxel is distributed into human milk, but in lactating rats given radiolabeled paclitaxel, concentrations of radioactivity in milk were higher than those in plasma and declined in parallel with plasma concentrations of the drug.

Albumin-bound Paclitaxel Paclitaxel bound to nanoparticles of the serum protein albumin is delivered via endothelial transport mediated by albumin receptors, and the resulting concentration of paclitaxel in tumor cells is increased compared with that achieved using an equivalent dose of conventional paclitaxel.

Like conventional paclitaxel, albumin-bound paclitaxel has a large volume of distribution. Following 30-minute or 3-hour IV infusion of 80–375 mg/m² albumin-bound paclitaxel, the volume of distribution averaged 632 L/m². The volume of distribution of albumin-bound paclitaxel 260 mg/m² by 30-minute IV infusion was 53% larger than the volume of distribution of conventional paclitaxel 175 mg/m² by 3-hour IV infusion.

■ **Elimination** Paclitaxel is extensively metabolized in the liver. Metabolism of paclitaxel to its major metabolite, 6α-hydroxypaclitaxel, is mediated by cytochrome P-450 isoenzyme CYP2C8, while metabolism to 2 of its minor metabolites, 3′-*p*-hydroxypaclitaxel and 6α,3′-*p*-dihydroxypaclitaxel, is catalyzed by CYP3A4.

Conventional Paclitaxel Following IV infusion of paclitaxel over periods ranging from 6–24 hours in adults with malignancy, plasma concentrations of paclitaxel appeared to decline in a biphasic manner in some studies, with an average distribution half-life ($t_{1/2\alpha}$) of 0.34 hours and an average elimination half-life ($t_{1/2\beta}$) of 5.8 hours. However, additional studies, particularly those in which paclitaxel is administered over shorter periods of infusion, show that the drug exhibits nonlinear pharmacokinetic behavior. In patients receiving paclitaxel 175 mg/m²administered by 3-hour IV infusion, the distribution half-life ($t_{1/2\alpha}$) averages 0.27 hours and the elimination half-life ($t_{1/2\beta}$) averages 2.33 hours.

The plasma clearance of paclitaxel was studied in patients with ovarian cancer; the total body clearance averaged 12.2 L/hour per m² in those receiving paclitaxel 175 mg/m² by 3-hour IV infusion, 17.7 L/hour per m² in those receiving paclitaxel 135 mg/m² by 3-hour IV infusion, and 21.7 L/hour per m² in those receiving paclitaxel 135 mg/m² by 24-hour IV infusion.

Paclitaxel and its metabolites are excreted principally in the feces via biliary elimination. Urinary excretion of paclitaxel is minimal, with unchanged drug in urine typically accounting for less than 10% of an administered dose. Following IV administration of paclitaxel over 1, 6, or 24 hours, 1.3–12.6% of the dose was excreted as unchanged drug in the urine. In patients receiving 3-hour IV infusions of radiolabeled paclitaxel, a mean of 71% of the radioactivity (about 5% of which was unchanged drug) was excreted in the feces in 120 hours and 14% was recovered in urine.

Administration of cisplatin followed by paclitaxel decreases paclitaxel clearance by approximately 25–33%. When cisplatin and paclitaxel must be administered sequentially, the sequence of paclitaxel followed by cisplatin is recommended. (See Drug Interaction: Antineoplastic Agents.)

The effect of renal impairment on the elimination of conventional paclitaxel has not been fully established. Paclitaxel is metabolized mainly in the liver, and limited data indicate that clearance of conventional paclitaxel is reduced in patients with hepatic impairment. The frequency and severity of myelotoxicity associated with paclitaxel may be increased in patients with elevated serum total bilirubin concentrations, and dosage reduction is advised. (See Dosage in Renal and Hepatic Impairment.)

Paclitaxel appears to be minimally removed by hemodialysis. In a patient undergoing hemodialysis approximately 24 hours following administration of paclitaxel 135 mg/m² by 3-hour IV infusion, paclitaxel was not detected in the dialysate; AUC and clearance of paclitaxel were within the range of values reported for patients not undergoing dialysis.

Albumin-bound Paclitaxel Following 30-minute or 3-hour IV infusion of 80–375 mg/m² albumin-bound paclitaxel, plasma concentrations of paclitaxel declined in a biphasic manner with initial rapid distribution to the peripheral compartment and then a slower phase of elimination; the terminal half-life of albumin-bound paclitaxel was about 27 hours. The total body clearance of albumin-bound paclitaxel averaged 15 L/hour per m². The plasma clearance of albumin-bound paclitaxel 260 mg/m² by 30-minute IV infusion was 43% higher than the plasma clearance of conventional paclitaxel 175 mg/m² by 3-hour IV infusion.

Urinary excretion of albumin-bound paclitaxel is minimal. Following 30-minute IV infusion of albumin-bound paclitaxel 260 mg/m², about 4% of the dose was excreted in the urine as unchanged drug and less than 1% was excreted as metabolites. Approximately 20% of the dose was excreted in feces.

Following 30-minute IV infusion of albumin-bound paclitaxel 260 or 200 mg/m² in patients with mild or moderate hepatic impairment, respectively, systemic exposure to the drug was similar to values previously reported for patients with normal hepatic function. In patients with severe hepatic impairment, systemic exposure following 30-minute IV infusion of albumin-bound paclitaxel 130 mg/m² was lower than reported exposure levels for patients with normal hepatic function. In addition, mean nadir neutrophil counts in cycle 1 were higher in patients with severe hepatic impairment compared with patients with mild or moderate hepatic impairment. Doses of 200 mg/m² have not been evaluated in patients with severe hepatic impairment but are predicted to result in systemic exposure levels similar to those reported for patients with normal hepatic function. Pharmacokinetics of albumin-bound paclitaxel have not been elucidated in patients with AST concentrations exceeding 10 times the upper limit of normal or bilirubin concentrations of 5 or more times the upper limit of normal.

The effect of renal impairment on the elimination of albumin-bound paclitaxel has not been established.

Chemistry and Stability

■ **Chemistry** Paclitaxel, a natural product extracted from the bark of the Western (Pacific) yew (*Taxus brevifolia*) or produced from the needles and twigs of a more prevalent yew (*Taxus baccata*) using a semisynthetic process, is an antineoplastic agent. Paclitaxel also is obtained from *Taxus media*. The taxanes (paclitaxel and docetaxel) differ structurally from other currently available antineoplastic agents. Because of paclitaxel's complex, unusual chemistry, supplies initially were limited to drug extracted from the slow-growing Western (Pacific) yew. An alternative method allowing preparation of the drug in larger yields (i.e., a semisynthetic method using a precursor extracted from needles and twigs of a more prevalent yew) has been developed; semisynthetic paclitaxel is bioequivalent to the natural drug. Additional sources of the drug (e.g., production of paclitaxel by *Taxomyces andreanae*, an endophytic fungus associated with Pacific yew) continue to be explored.

Paclitaxel is a complex diterpene with a taxane ring system and a four-membered oxetane ring. An ester side chain at position 13 of the taxane ring is essential for the drug's cytotoxic activity. In addition, presence of an accessible hydroxyl group at position 2′ of this ester side chain enhances the drug's activity. Paclitaxel differs structurally from docetaxel by the presence of an acetyl group rather than a hydroxyl group on position 10 of the baccatin III ring and by a benzamide phenyl group instead of a trimethylmethoxy moiety on the 3′ position of the side chain at position 13 of the taxane ring.

Paclitaxel occurs as a white to off-white crystalline powder. Paclitaxel is highly lipophilic and insoluble in water.

Conventional Paclitaxel Because paclitaxel is extremely hydrophobic, the commercially available injection concentrate is a sterile, nonaqueous solution of the drug in polyoxyl 35 castor oil (Cremophor® EL, polyoxyethylated castor oil) and dehydrated alcohol. Commercially available paclitaxel for injection concentrate is a clear, colorless to slightly yellow, viscous solution. Following dilution of paclitaxel for injection concentrate with 5% dextrose and 0.9% sodium chloride injection or 5% dextrose and Ringer's injection, solutions containing 0.6 or 1.2 mg of paclitaxel per mL maintain a pH of 4.4–5.6 for up to 27 hours.

Albumin-bound Paclitaxel Paclitaxel is commercially available as protein-bound particles consisting of paclitaxel bound to albumin; the mean particle size of albumin-bound paclitaxel is about 130 nm. Albumin-bound paclitaxel is a sterile, white to yellow lyophilized powder that must be reconstituted for use as an injectable suspension; there are no solvents. Each single-use vial contains 100 mg of paclitaxel and approximately 900 mg of human albumin.

■ **Stability** ***Conventional Paclitaxel*** Commercially available paclitaxel for injection concentrate should be stored in unopened vials at 20–25°C and retained in the original package for protection from light. Neither freezing nor refrigeration adversely affects paclitaxel for injection concentrate. Refrigeration may result in precipitation of the drug or formulation vehicle; however, the precipitate typically will dissolve at room temperature without loss of potency. If freezing occurs, paclitaxel for injection concentrate may be thawed at room temperature until precipitate dissolves; the manufacturer states that the chemical or physical stability of the injection is not affected. If the solution remains cloudy or if an insoluble precipitate remains at room temperature, the vial should be discarded. When stored under recommended conditions, unopened vials of commercially available paclitaxel for injection concentrate are stable until the date indicated on the package.

The manufacturer states that, when diluted as directed, paclitaxel solutions are stable for up to 27 hours when stored at approximately 25°C under ambient lighting conditions.

Contact of undiluted paclitaxel for injection concentrate with plasticized polyvinyl chloride (PVC) equipment or devices used to prepare solutions for infusion is *not* recommended. Polyoxyl 35 castor oil can cause leaching of diethylhexylphthalate (DEHP) from PVC containers and, following dilution of paclitaxel for injection concentrate in PVC containers, substantial leaching of DEHP occurs in a time- and concentration-dependent manner. To minimize exposure of the patient to leached DEHP, diluted paclitaxel solutions preferably should be stored in glass or polypropylene bottles or in plastic (polypropylene or polyolefin) bags and administered through polyethylene-lined administration sets. Leaching of unacceptable amounts of DEHP has been reported with some administration sets labeled as not containing PVC (probably because of pumping segments made of heavily plasticized PVC); therefore, compatibility of administration sets with paclitaxel solutions should be verified prior to their use.

Solutions of paclitaxel prepared with 5% dextrose injection or 0.9% sodium chloride injection at concentrations of 0.3–1.2 mg/mL reportedly were chemically and physically stable for up to 48 hours when prepared and stored in polyolefin containers at ambient temperature (20–23°C) under normal fluorescent light; however, in this study, physical stability was determined only by the absence of gross precipitation. In another study, paclitaxel solutions of 0.1 and 1 mg/mL in 5% dextrose injection or 0.9% sodium chloride injection were stable for up to 3 days when prepared and stored in polyolefin bags at 4, 22, or 32°C. Extemporaneously compounded admixtures of paclitaxel 1 mg/mL in 5% dextrose solution with addition of dehydrated alcohol injection to achieve a final ethanol concentration of 20 or 25% were chemically and physically stable for up to 7 days when prepared and stored in polyolefin containers at 4, 22, or 32°C.

Solutions of paclitaxel have been reported to be physically incompatible with various drugs, including amphotericin B, chlorpromazine hydrochloride, hydroxyzine hydrochloride, methylprednisolone sodium succinate, and mitoxantrone hydrochloride. The physical and/or chemical compatibility of paclitaxel with other drugs depends on several factors (e.g., concentrations of the drugs, specific diluents used, resulting pH, temperature); studies evaluating the stability of paclitaxel with other drugs, particularly other antineoplastic agents, are ongoing. Specialized references should be consulted for specific information.

Because a small number of fibers (within acceptable USP limits) have been detected in paclitaxel solutions prepared from the commercially available for injection concentrate, a hydrophilic, microporous inline filter with a pore size not exceeding 0.22 μm is necessary during administration of paclitaxel solutions. The manufacturer reports that use of filter devices such as IVEX-2® filters, which incorporate short inlet and outlet PVC-coated tubing, has not resulted in significant leaching of DEHP.

Diluted solutions of paclitaxel may appear hazy. When such solutions are passed through a 0.22-μm filter, no clinically important loss of potency is observed, suggesting that the haze is caused by the formulation vehicle rather than precipitation of the drug.

Albumin-bound Paclitaxel Commercially available albumin-bound paclitaxel for injectable suspension should be stored in unopened vials at 20–25°C and retained in the original package for protection from bright light. Neither freezing nor refrigeration adversely affects albumin-bound paclitaxel for injectable suspension. When stored under recommended conditions, unopened vials of commercially available albumin-bound paclitaxel for injectable suspension are stable until the date indicated on the package.

Reconstituted suspensions of albumin-bound paclitaxel should be used immediately; if immediate use is not possible, vials of reconstituted albumin-bound paclitaxel suspension may be placed in the original carton to protect them from bright light and refrigerated at 2–8°C for up to 8 hours. After 8 hours, any unused portion of the reconstituted albumin-bound paclitaxel suspension should be discarded.

Before the dosing volume is withdrawn from the vial, the suspension should be inspected. Settling of the reconstituted albumin-bound paclitaxel suspension may occur. Mild agitation of the vial should ensure complete resuspension of the albumin-bound paclitaxel. If particulates are visible after mild agitation of the vial, the suspension should be discarded and another reconstituted albumin-bound paclitaxel suspension should be prepared. When reconstituted as directed, albumin-bound paclitaxel suspension is stable in the IV infusion bag for up to 4 hours when stored at approximately 25°C under ambient lighting conditions.

For further information on the handling of antineoplastic agents, see the ASHP Guidelines on Handling Hazardous Drugs at http://www.ahfsdruginformation.com.

Preparations

Excipients in commercially available drug preparations may have clinically important effects in some individuals; consult specific product labeling for details.

PACLitaxel

Parenteral

For injection, concentrate, for IV infusion	6 mg/mL*	**Onxol®**, Teva **Paclitaxel Injection**

*available from one or more manufacturer, distributor, and/or repackager by generic (nonproprietary) name

PACLitaxel (albumin-bound)

Parenteral

For injectable suspension, for IV infusion	100 mg (of paclitaxel)	**Abraxane®**, Celgene

†Use is not currently included in the labeling approved by the US Food and Drug Administration

Palbociclib

■ Palbociclib, a reversible and selective inhibitor of cyclin-dependent kinase (CDK) 4 and 6, is an antineoplastic agent.

Uses

■ **Breast Cancer** Palbociclib is used in combination with letrozole or fulvestrant for the treatment of hormone receptor-positive, human epidermal growth factor receptor type 2 (HER2)-negative advanced or metastatic breast cancer.

Initial Therapy for Advanced Breast Cancer Palbociclib is used in combination with letrozole for the initial treatment of hormone receptor-positive, HER2-negative advanced or metastatic breast cancer in postmenopausal women. The accelerated approval of palbociclib for this indication is based on progression-free survival. Continued approval for this indication may be contingent on verification and description of clinical benefit of palbociclib in confirmatory studies.

The current indication for palbociclib is based principally on the results of a randomized, multicenter, open-label phase 2 study (PALOMA-1/TRIO-18) in postmenopausal women with previously untreated estrogen receptor-positive, HER2-negative metastatic breast cancer. The primary measure of efficacy was progression-free survival as assessed by the investigator according to Response Evaluation Criteria in Solid Tumors (RECIST). The median age of patients was 63 years; 43% of the patients had received prior chemotherapy, 33% had received neoadjuvant or adjuvant endocrine therapy prior to diagnosis of advanced breast cancer, and 49% of the patients had not received prior systemic therapy in the neoadjuvant or adjuvant setting. All patients enrolled in the study had a baseline ECOG performance status of 0 or 1. The majority of patients (98%) had metastatic disease and 48 or 19% of patients had visceral or bone-only disease, respectively. In this study, 165 patients were randomized (stratified according to disease site and disease-free interval following adjuvant treatment or de novo metastatic disease) in a 1:1 ratio to receive either palbociclib (125 mg orally once daily for 3 consecutive weeks of each 4-week cycle) in combination with letrozole (2.5 mg orally once daily continuously) or letrozole alone. Patients were treated until disease progression, unacceptable toxicity, death, or withdrawal of patient consent occurred.

In this study, patients receiving palbociclib in combination with letrozole had a longer median progression-free survival (20.2 versus 10.2 months based on intent-to-treat analysis) compared with patients receiving letrozole alone. Patients receiving palbociclib in combination with letrozole also had higher overall response rates compared with those receiving letrozole alone (55.4 versus 39.4%) with a median response duration of 20.3 months for those receiving palbociclib in combination with letrozole and 11.1 months for those receiving letrozole alone; complete responses were achieved in 2% of patients in the palbociclib treatment group. A subset analysis of progression-free survival based on clinically relevant baseline patient and disease characteristics consistently showed treatment benefit with palbociclib and letrozole combination therapy compared with letrozole alone. Median overall survival had not been reached at the time of the final efficacy analysis.

Previously Treated Advanced Breast Cancer Palbociclib is used in combination with fulvestrant for the treatment of hormone receptor-positive, HER2-negative advanced or metastatic breast cancer in women with disease progression following endocrine therapy.

The current indication for palbociclib is based principally on the results of a randomized, double-blind, placebo-controlled phase 3 study (PALOMA-3) in women with hormone receptor-positive, HER2-negative metastatic breast cancer. The primary measure of efficacy was progression-free survival as assessed by the investigator according to RECIST. The median age of patients was 57 years. All patients enrolled in the study had a baseline ECOG performance status of 0 or 1. The majority of patients (80%) were postmenopausal and 60 or 23% of patients had visceral or bone-only disease, respectively. All patients enrolled in the study had received prior systemic therapy, 75% of patients had received prior chemotherapy, and 25% of patients had not received prior therapy for metastatic disease. Patients who had received prior therapy with a cyclin-dependent kinase (CDK) inhibitor, fulvestrant, everolimus, or a phosphoinositide 3-kinase (PI3K)/mammalian target of rapamycin (mTOR) inhibitor were excluded from the study. In this study, 521 patients were randomized (stratified according to sensitivity to endocrine therapy, menopausal status, and presence of visceral metastases) in a 2:1 ratio to receive either palbociclib (125 mg orally once daily for 3 consecutive weeks of each 4-week cycle) in combination with fulvestrant (500 mg IM on days 1 and 15 during cycle 1 and then on day 1 of each 4-week cycle thereafter) or placebo in combination with fulvestrant. Patients were treated until disease progression, symptomatic deterioration, unacceptable toxicity, death, or withdrawal of patient consent occurred. Premenopausal or perimenopausal patients received goserelin acetate for at least 4 weeks prior to and during the study.

In this study, patients receiving palbociclib in combination with fulvestrant had a longer median progression-free survival (9.5 versus 4.6 months) compared with patients receiving placebo in combination with fulvestrant. Patients receiving palbociclib in combination with fulvestrant also had higher overall response rates compared with those receiving placebo in combination with fulvestrant (24.6 versus 10.9%) with a response duration of 9.3 months for those receiving palbociclib in combination with fulvestrant and 7.6 months for those receiving placebo in combination with fulvestrant. A subset analysis of progression-free survival based on clinically relevant baseline patient and disease characteristics consistently showed treatment benefit with palbociclib and fulvestrant combination therapy compared with placebo and fulvestrant therapy. Median overall survival had not been reached at the time of the final efficacy analysis.

Dosage and Administration

■ **General** Complete blood cell counts (CBCs) should be monitored at baseline, prior to initiation of each cycle, and as clinically indicated; additional monitoring of CBCs should be obtained on day 14 of cycles 1 and 2. More frequent monitoring may be required in patients who develop hematologic toxicity during therapy. (See Hematologic Toxicity under Dosage and Administration: Dosage Modification for Toxicity.)

Clinicians should consult the respective manufacturers' labelings for information on dosage adjustments, adverse effects, and contraindications of other antineoplastic agents used in combination regimens.

Restricted Distribution Palbociclib can only be obtained through a limited network of specialty pharmacies. Specific information regarding distribution of palbociclib is available from the manufacturer at https://www.ibrance.com/getting-ibrance.

■ **Administration** Palbociclib is administered orally with food at approximately the same time each day. (See Description.) Palbociclib capsules should be swallowed intact and should *not* be chewed, crushed, or opened.

If a dose of palbociclib is missed or vomited, patients should *not* double the dose or take extra doses. The next dose should be taken at the regularly scheduled time.

■ **Dosage** ***Breast Cancer*** **Initial Therapy for Advanced Breast Cancer.** For the initial treatment of hormone receptor-positive, HER2-negative advanced or metastatic breast cancer in postmenopausal women, the recommended dosage of palbociclib is 125 mg once daily on days 1–21 of each 28-day cycle in combination with letrozole 2.5 mg once daily given continuously throughout the 28-day cycle. In the PALOMA-1/TRIO-18 study, therapy was continued until disease progression or unacceptable toxicity occurred.

Previously Treated Advanced Breast Cancer. For the treatment of hormone receptor-positive, HER2-negative advanced or metastatic breast cancer in women with disease progression following endocrine therapy, the recommended dosage of palbociclib is 125 mg once daily on days 1–21 of each 28-day cycle in combination with fulvestrant 500 mg IM on days 1 and 15 during cycle 1, and then on day 1 of each 28-day cycle thereafter. In the PALOMA-3 study, therapy was continued until disease progression or unacceptable toxicity occurred.

Premenopausal or perimenopausal patients receiving combination therapy with palbociclib and fulvestrant should be treated with a luteinizing hormone-releasing hormone (LHRH) agonist (e.g., goserelin) according to current standards of care.

Dosage Modification for Toxicity Management of some adverse effects may require temporary interruption of therapy, dosage reduction, and/or permanent discontinuance of palbociclib therapy. Dosage adjustment of palbociclib is recommended based on individual safety and tolerability. Up to 2 dosage reductions for toxicity may be made. If dosage modification is necessary, an initial dosage reduction to 100 mg once daily is recommended. If further dosage reduction is necessary, the dosage should be reduced to 75 mg once daily. Dosages less than 75 mg once daily are not recommended.

Hematologic Toxicity. For grade 3 febrile neutropenia (absolute neutrophil count [ANC] 500 to less than 1000/mm^3 associated with fever of 38.5°C or more and/or infection), palbociclib therapy should be interrupted. The next cycle should be delayed until ANC reaches or exceeds 1000/mm^3. Upon resumption of therapy, the dosage of palbociclib should be reduced. (See Neutropenia under Cautions: Warnings/Precautions.)

If grade 3 hematologic toxicity is reported after CBC monitoring on day 1 of any cycle, therapy with palbociclib should be interrupted; monitoring of CBCs should be repeated within 1 week. The next cycle should be delayed until the toxicity resolves to grade 2 or less; therapy with palbociclib may be continued at the same dosage.

If grade 3 hematologic toxicity is reported after CBC monitoring on day 14 of cycle 1 or 2, palbociclib may be continued at the same dosage; monitoring of CBCs should be repeated on day 21.

If prolonged grade 3 neutropenia (i.e., lasting longer than 7 days) occurs or grade 3 neutropenia recurs in subsequent cycles, resumption of therapy at a reduced dosage may then be considered.

For grade 4 hematologic toxicity, therapy with palbociclib should be interrupted. The next cycle should be delayed until the toxicity resolves to grade 2 or less. Upon resumption of therapy, the dosage of palbociclib should be reduced.

An exception is made for patients with grade 3 or 4 lymphopenia presenting without an associated clinical event such as an opportunistic infection; no dosage modification is required in such patients.

Nonhematologic Toxicity. If persistent grade 3 or greater nonhematologic toxicity occurs despite appropriate medical management, palbociclib therapy should be withheld until the toxicity resolves to grade 1 or less, or to grade 2 or less if the toxicity is not considered a safety risk for the patient. Upon resumption of therapy, the palbociclib dosage should be reduced.

Concomitant Use with Drugs or Foods Affecting Hepatic Microsomal Enzymes Concomitant use of palbociclib with drugs that are potent inhibitors of cytochrome P-450 (CYP) isoenzyme 3A should be avoided; an alternative drug with no or minimal CYP3A inhibition potential should be considered. If concomitant use of a potent CYP3A inhibitor cannot be avoided, the manufacturer recommends reducing the dosage of palbociclib to 75 mg once daily. If concomitant use of the potent CYP3A inhibitor is discontinued, the palbociclib dosage should be returned (after 3–5 terminal half-lives of the CYP3A inhibitor) to the dosage used prior to initiation of the potent CYP3A inhibitor. (See Drugs Affecting Hepatic Microsomal Enzymes under Drug Interactions.)

■ **Special Populations** The manufacturer makes no specific dosage recommendations for geriatric patients or patients with hepatic or renal impairment. (See Specific Populations under Cautions: Warnings/Precautions.)

Cautions

■ **Contraindications** The manufacturer states that there are no known contraindications to the use of palbociclib.

■ **Warnings/Precautions** ***Neutropenia*** Neutropenia commonly occurs in patients receiving palbociclib. In the principal efficacy studies, grade 3 or greater neutropenia occurred in 62 or 66% of patients receiving palbociclib in combination with letrozole or those receiving palbociclib in combination with fulvestrant, respectively. The median time to occurrence of neutropenia was 15 days (range: 13–117 days). The median duration of grade 3 or greater neutropenia was 7 days. Febrile neutropenia has been observed in 1% of patients receiving palbociclib. In the PALOMA-3 study, fatal neutropenic sepsis occurred in one patient.

Complete blood cell (CBC) counts should be monitored at baseline, prior to initiation of each cycle, and as clinically indicated; additional monitoring of CBCs should be obtained on day 14 of cycles 1 and 2. More frequent monitoring may be necessary in patients who develop hematologic toxicity during therapy. Temporary interruption, dosage reduction, or treatment delay may be necessary if neutropenia occurs during therapy with the drug. (See Hematologic

Toxicity under Dosage: Dosage Modification for Toxicity, in Dosage and Administration.)

Pulmonary Embolism Pulmonary embolism has occurred during palbociclib therapy. In the principal efficacy studies, pulmonary embolism occurred in 5 or 1% of patients receiving palbociclib in combination with letrozole or those receiving palbociclib in combination with fulvestrant, respectively, compared with none of those receiving letrozole alone or fulvestrant in combination with placebo.

Patients should be monitored for signs and symptoms of pulmonary embolism. Appropriate treatment should be provided if pulmonary embolism occurs.

Fetal/Neonatal Morbidity and Mortality There are no adequate and well-controlled studies of palbociclib in pregnant women; however, based on its mechanism of action and animal findings, palbociclib may cause fetal harm. Embryofetal toxicity (i.e., decreased fetal weight) and teratogenicity (i.e., skeletal alterations) have been demonstrated in rats and rabbits receiving palbociclib at exposure levels of approximately 4 and 9 times the human exposure at the recommended dosage, respectively; however, embryofetal toxicity was not observed in the offspring of female rats receiving the drug from 15 days prior to breeding through day 7 of gestation at exposure levels of approximately 4 times the human exposure at the recommended dosage.

Pregnancy should be avoided during palbociclib therapy. Women of childbearing potential should be advised to use an effective method of contraception while receiving palbociclib and for at least 3 weeks after discontinuance of therapy. Male patients should be advised to use an effective method of contraception while receiving palbociclib and for 3 months after discontinuance of therapy each time they have sexual contact with women of childbearing potential. Patients should be apprised of the potential hazard to the fetus if used during pregnancy.

Impairment of Male Fertility Results of animal studies suggest that palbociclib may impair male fertility. Adverse effects on male reproductive organs and sperm (i.e., decreased organ weight, atrophy or degeneration, intratubular cellular debris, hypospermia, low sperm motility and density, decreased secretion) were observed in rats and dogs receiving palbociclib at exposure levels of approximately 10 or more and 0.1 times the human exposure at the recommended dosage, respectively, in a repeat-dose toxicity study; effects on male reproductive organs were partially reversible following a 4- and 12-week nondosing period in rats and dogs, respectively. Decreased fertility also was observed in male rats receiving palbociclib at exposure levels 20 times the human exposure at the recommended dosage.

Specific Populations **Pregnancy.** Palbociclib may cause fetal harm if administered to pregnant women based on its mechanism of action and animal findings. (See Fetal/Neonatal Morbidity and Mortality under Cautions: Warnings/Precautions.)

Lactation. It is not known whether palbociclib is distributed into milk. Because many drugs are distributed into human milk and because of the potential for serious adverse reactions to palbociclib in nursing infants, women should be advised to discontinue nursing during therapy and for 3 weeks after discontinuance of the drug. The effects of the drug on nursing infants or on milk production are unknown.

Pediatric Use. Safety and efficacy of palbociclib have not been established in pediatric patients younger than 18 years of age.

Geriatric Use. In the PALOMA-1/TRIO-18 study, 44% of palbociclib-treated patients were 65 years of age or older and 10% were 75 years of age or older. In the PALOMA-3 study, 25% of palbociclib-treated patients were 65 years of age or older. No overall differences in safety and efficacy were observed between geriatric and younger patients. (See Dosage and Administration: Special Populations.)

Hepatic Impairment. In a population pharmacokinetic analysis, no clinically important differences in systemic exposure of palbociclib were observed between patients with mild hepatic impairment (total bilirubin concentration not exceeding the upper limit of normal [ULN] with AST concentration exceeding the ULN, or total bilirubin concentration exceeding 1 to 1.5 times the ULN with any AST concentration) and those with normal hepatic function. Formal pharmacokinetic studies have not been conducted in patients with moderate or severe hepatic impairment (total bilirubin concentration exceeding 1.5 times the ULN with any AST concentration). (See Dosage and Administration: Special Populations.)

Renal Impairment. In a population pharmacokinetic analysis, no clinically important differences in systemic exposure of palbociclib were observed between patients with mild (creatinine clearance of 60 to less than 90 mL/minute) or moderate renal impairment (creatinine clearance of 30 to less than 60 mL/minute) and those with normal renal function. Formal pharmacokinetic studies have not been conducted in patients with severe renal impairment. (See Dosage and Administration: Special Populations.)

■ **Common Adverse Effects** Adverse effects reported in 10% or more of patients with advanced or metastatic breast cancer receiving palbociclib in combination with letrozole in the PALOMA-1/TRIO-18 study include neutropenia, leukopenia, fatigue, anemia, upper respiratory infection (including influenza, laryngitis, nasopharyngitis, pharyngitis, rhinitis, sinusitis), nausea, stomatitis (including oropharyngeal pain), alopecia, diarrhea, hot flush, arthralgia, thrombocytopenia, decreased appetite, vomiting, dyspnea, back pain, headache, asthenia, peripheral neuropathy, bone pain, constipation, cough, epistaxis, musculoskeletal pain, dizziness, and extremity pain.

Adverse effects reported in 10% or more of patients with advanced or metastatic breast cancer receiving palbociclib in combination with fulvestrant in the PALOMA-3 study include neutropenia, leukopenia, infections, fatigue, nausea, anemia, stomatitis, headache, diarrhea, thrombocytopenia, constipation, vomiting, alopecia, rash, decreased appetite, hot flush, arthralgia, cough, pyrexia, back pain, dizziness, and dyspnea.

Drug Interactions

Palbociclib is metabolized principally by cytochrome P-450 (CYP) isoenzyme 3A and sulfotransferase (SULT) 2A1. In vitro studies indicate that palbociclib does not inhibit CYP isoenzymes 1A2, 2A6, 2B6, 2C8, 2C9, 2C19, and 2D6 or induce CYP isoenzymes 1A2, 2B6, 2C8, and 3A4 at clinically relevant concentrations; however, in vivo studies indicate that the drug is a weak time-dependent inhibitor of CYP3A.

In vitro studies indicate that palbociclib has a low potential for inhibition of P-glycoprotein (P-gp), breast cancer resistance protein (BCRP), organic cation transporter (OCT) 2, organic anion transporter (OAT) 1, OAT 3, organic anion transport protein (OATP) 1B1 and OATP1B3 at clinically relevant concentrations.

■ **Drugs Affecting Hepatic Microsomal Enzymes** ***Inhibitors of CYP3A*** Concomitant use of palbociclib with potent inhibitors of CYP3A may result in increased peak plasma concentrations and systemic exposure (area under the concentration-time curve [AUC]) of palbociclib. When the potent CYP3A inhibitor itraconzole (200 mg daily) was administered concomitantly with palbociclib (single 125-mg dose) in healthy individuals, the peak plasma concentrations and AUC of palbociclib were increased by 34 and 87%, respectively.

Concomitant use of palbociclib with potent inhibitors of CYP3A (e.g., clarithromycin, indinavir, itraconazole, ketoconazole, *ritonavir-boosted* lopinavir, nefazodone, nelfinavir, posaconazole, ritonavir, saquinavir, telithromycin, verapamil, voriconazole) should be avoided, and selection of an alternative drug with no or minimal CYP3A inhibition potential should be considered. If concomitant use of a potent CYP3A inhibitor cannot be avoided, the manufacturer recommends dosage reduction of palbociclib to 75 mg once daily. If concomitant use of the potent CYP3A inhibitor is discontinued, the palbociclib dosage should be returned (after 3–5 terminal half-lives of the CYP3A inhibitor) to the dosage used prior to initiation of the potent CYP3A4 inhibitor.

Inducers of CYP3A Concomitant use of palbociclib with potent or moderate inducers of CYP3A may result in decreased peak plasma concentrations and AUC of palbociclib. When the potent CYP3A inducer rifampin (600 mg daily) was administered concomitantly with palbociclib (single 125-mg dose) in healthy individuals, the peak plasma concentrations and AUC of palbociclib were decreased by 70 and 85%, respectively. When the moderate CYP3A inducer modafinil (400 mg daily) was administered concomitantly with palbociclib (single 125-mg dose) in healthy individuals, peak plasma concentrations and AUC of palbociclib were decreased by 11 and 32%, respectively.

Concomitant use of palbociclib with moderate (e.g., bosentan, efavirenz, etravirine, modafinil, nafcillin) or potent inducers of CYP3A (e.g., carbamazepine, phenytoin, rifampin, St. John's wort [*Hypericum perforatum*]) should be avoided.

■ **Drugs Metabolized by Hepatic Microsomal Enzymes** ***Substrates of CYP3A*** When the CYP3A substrate midazolam was administered concomitantly with palbociclib in healthy individuals, peak plasma concentrations and AUC of midazolam were increased by 37 and 61%, respectively. If concomitant use of palbociclib with CYP3A substrates with a narrow therapeutic index (e.g., alfentanil, cyclosporine, dihydroergotamine, ergotamine, everolimus, fentanyl, pimozide, quinidine, sirolimus, tacrolimus) cannot be avoided, a dosage reduction of the CYP3A substrate should be considered.

■ **Drugs Affecting Gastric Acidity** When multiple doses of the proton-pump inhibitor rabeprazole were administered concomitantly with palbociclib (single 125-mg dose) in healthy individuals, peak plasma concentrations and AUC of palbociclib were decreased by 41 and 13%, respectively, under fed conditions and by 80 and 62%, respectively, under fasting conditions. Because effects on gastric pH are less marked with histamine H_2-receptor antagonists or antacids compared with proton-pump inhibitors, decreases in palbociclib exposure are expected to be minimal when H_2-receptor antagonists or antacids are used concomitantly with palbociclib under fed conditions. Clinically important effects on palbociclib exposure were not observed when antacids, histamine H_2-receptor antagonists, or proton-pump inhibitors were used concomitantly with palbociclib under fed conditions.

■ **Fulvestrant** Concomitant administration of palbociclib and fulvestrant did not affect the pharmacokinetics of either drug.

■ **Goserelin** Concomitant administration of palbociclib and goserelin did not affect the pharmacokinetics of either drug.

■ **Grapefruit** Grapefruit products are CYP3A inhibitors and should be avoided because of the potential for increased plasma palbociclib concentrations during concurrent use.

■ **Letrozole** Concomitant administration of palbociclib and letrozole did not affect the pharmacokinetics of either drug.

Description

Palbociclib, a reversible and selective inhibitor of cyclin-dependent kinase (CDK) 4 and 6, is an antineoplastic agent. Several mechanisms contribute to the dysregulation of the cell cycle during the G1 into S phase, including amplification or overexpression of the cyclin D oncogene or the loss of intrinsic CDK inhibitors (i.e., p16, p15, p18, p19, p21, p27, p57) in breast cancer. Palbociclib specifically inhibits CDK4 and 6 and blocks the interaction of CDK4 and 6 with cyclin D, resulting in inhibition of phosphorylation of the tumor suppressor protein retinoblastoma and inhibition of progression of the cell cycle from the G1 into S phase. In vitro, palbociclib has demonstrated reduced cellular proliferation of estrogen receptor-positive breast cancer cell lines by inhibiting the G1 into S phase of the cell cycle. Decreased phosphorylation of retinoblastoma protein resulting in reduced E2F expression and signaling and increased cell growth arrest have been reported in breast cancer cell lines treated with palbociclib and antiestrogens compared with either drug alone. In vitro, the combination of palbociclib with antiestrogens increased cell senescence for up to 6 days following discontinuance of therapy in estrogen receptor-positive breast cancer cell lines. The combination of palbociclib and letrozole also has demonstrated increased inhibition of retinoblastoma protein phosphorylation, downstream signaling, and tumor growth compared with either drug alone in patient-derived estrogen receptor-positive breast tumor xenografts.

Following oral administration, the mean absolute bioavailability of palbociclib is 46%. Area under the serum concentration-time curve (AUC) and peak plasma concentrations of palbociclib are dose proportional over a dosage range of 25–225 mg. Peak plasma concentrations of palbociclib are achieved about 6–12 hours following oral administration of the drug. Following repeated doses of palbociclib administered once daily, steady-state concentrations of the drug were achieved in 8 days and the median accumulation ratio for the drug was 2.4.

Absorption and systemic exposure to palbociclib were decreased in approximately 13% of individuals receiving the drug in a fasting state; systemic exposure to palbociclib increased when the drug was administered with food in these individuals, but administration with food did not alter systemic exposure to a clinically important extent in other individuals. Administration of palbociclib with food reduces the interindividual variability in systemic exposure to palbociclib. Oral administration of palbociclib with a low-fat, low-calorie (approximately 400–500 calories) or high-fat, high-calorie meal (approximately 800–1000 calories) resulted in increases in systemic exposure of 12 or 21%, respectively, and increases in peak plasma concentrations of 27 or 38%, respectively, compared with administration in the fasting state. When an oral dose of palbociclib was administered between 2 moderate-fat, standard-calorie meals (approximately 500–700 calories per meal) (i.e., single dose administered 1 hour after the first meal and 2 hours before the second meal), systemic exposure and peak plasma concentrations of the drug were increased by 13 and 24%, respectively, compared with administration in the fasting state.

Palbociclib is metabolized in the liver principally by cytochrome P-450 (CYP) isoenzyme 3A and sulfotransferase (SULT) 2A1. In vitro, palbociclib is approximately 85% bound to plasma proteins. Following oral administration of a single radiolabeled dose of palbociclib, 74.1% of the radioactivity was recovered in feces and 17.5% was recovered in urine; the majority of the dose was excreted as metabolites. The mean plasma elimination half-life of the drug is 29 hours.

Population pharmacokinetic analyses indicate that age (22–89 years), gender, and body weight do not have clinically important effects on the exposure of palbociclib.

Advice to Patients

Importance of taking palbociclib with food. Avoid grapefruit and grapefruit juice while taking the drug.

Importance of advising patients to swallow palbociclib capsules whole and not to chew, crush, or open the capsules.

If a dose is missed or vomited, importance of administering the next dose at the regularly scheduled time; an additional dose should not be administered to make up for a missed dose.

Risk of myelosuppression or infection. Importance of informing clinician immediately if signs or symptoms of myelosuppression or infection (e.g., fever, chills, dizziness, shortness of breath, weakness, increased tendency to bleed and/or bruise) occur.

Risk of pulmonary embolism. Importance of informing clinician immediately if signs or symptoms of pulmonary embolism (e.g., shortness of breath, chest pain, tachypnea, tachycardia) occur.

Risk of fetal harm. Necessity of advising women of childbearing potential and men who are partners of such women that they should use an effective method of contraception during treatment and for at least 3 weeks in women or 3 months in men after discontinuance of therapy. Importance of women informing clinicians if they are or plan to become pregnant. If pregnancy occurs, advise patient of potential risk to the fetus.

Risk of serious adverse reactions in nursing infants. Importance of advising women to discontinue nursing during therapy and for 3 weeks after discontinuance of the drug.

Importance of informing clinicians of existing or contemplated concomitant therapy, including prescription and OTC drugs and dietary or herbal supplements (e.g., St. John's wort), as well as any concomitant illnesses.

Importance of informing patients of other important precautionary information. (See Cautions.)

Overview® (see Users Guide). For additional information on this drug until a more detailed monograph is developed and published, the manufacturer's labeling should be consulted. It is *essential* that the manufacturer's labeling be consulted for more detailed information on usual cautions, precautions, contraindications, potential drug interactions, laboratory test interferences, and acute toxicity. For further information on the handling of antineoplastic agents, see the ASHP Guidelines on Handling Hazardous Drugs at http://www.ahfsdruginformation.com.

Preparations

Distribution of palbociclib is restricted. (See Restricted Distribution under Dosage and Administration: General.)

Excipients in commercially available drug preparations may have clinically important effects in some individuals; consult specific product labeling for details.

Palbociclib

Oral		
Capsules	75 mg	**Ibrance®**, Pfizer
	100 mg	**Ibrance®**, Pfizer
	125 mg	**Ibrance®**, Pfizer

Panitumumab

■ Panitumumab, a recombinant human IgG_2 kappa monoclonal antibody that binds to the human epidermal growth factor receptor (EGFR; also called an epidermal growth factor receptor [EGFR] inhibitor), is an antineoplastic agent.

Uses

■ **Colorectal Cancer** Panitumumab is used as a single agent for the treatment of metastatic colorectal cancer that is refractory to fluoropyrimidine-, oxaliplatin-, and irinotecan-containing chemotherapy regimens in adult patients with tumors that express the epidermal growth factor receptor (EGFR). The current indication for panitumumab monotherapy in the treatment of EGFR-expressing metastatic colorectal cancer is based on progression-free survival; there currently are no data available demonstrating an improvement in disease-related symptoms or increased survival with the drug.

Because retrospective stratified analyses of metastatic colorectal cancer trials have not shown a treatment benefit for panitumumab in patients whose tumors had *KRAS* mutations in codon 12 or 13, use of the drug is *not* recommended for the treatment of colorectal cancer with such mutations.

Safety and efficacy of panitumumab in the management of metastatic colorectal cancer have principally been evaluated in an open-label, multinational, randomized, controlled trial (designated study 1 by the manufacturer). Patients enrolled in this trial were required to have immunohistochemical evidence of EGFR expression (using the DAKO EGFR pharmDx® test kit). In this trial, 463 patients with metastatic colorectal cancer whose disease had progressed during or following treatment with a regimen containing a fluoropyrimidine, oxaliplatin, and irinotecan were randomized to receive panitumumab 6 mg/kg administered by IV infusion once every 2 weeks plus best supportive care or best supportive care alone until disease progression occurred or unacceptable toxicity developed. Patients randomized to best supportive care alone were eligible to cross over to panitumumab therapy upon disease progression.

In this study, mean progression-free survival was longer in patients receiving panitumumab combined with best supportive care (96 days) compared with those receiving best supportive care alone (60 days). The panitumumab-treated patients also had a 46% lower relative progression rate compared with those receiving best supportive care alone. About 75% of the patients randomized to best supportive care alone crossed over to panitumumab therapy following disease progression; the median time to crossover was 8.4 weeks. Partial response was reported in 19 patients in this study for an overall response rate of 8% in patients receiving panitumumab combined with best supportive care; no patient receiving best supportive care alone had an objective response. The median duration of response in patients demonstrating partial response was 17 weeks. No difference in overall survival was observed between the 2 treatment groups in this study.

The presence of mutations in the *KRAS* (also called *K-ras*) gene in codon 12 or 13 in colorectal cancer tumor tissue has been associated with a lack of benefit from therapy with anti-EGFR monoclonal antibodies (e.g., cetuximab, panitumumab); such mutations appear to be present in approximately 30–50% of primary colorectal tumors. Retrospective subset analyses from 7 randomized clinical studies evaluating cetuximab or panitumumab either as monotherapy or in combination with chemotherapy in metastatic colorectal cancer suggest that these anti-EGFR monoclonal antibodies are not effective for the treatment of patients with colorectal cancer containing *KRAS* mutations in codon 12 or 13. The analyses also demonstrated improved tumor response, progression-free survival, and overall survival in patients receiving these anti-EGFR monoclonal antibodies whose tumors did not contain mutations in codon 12 or 13 (wild type) compared with abnormal (mutated) *KRAS* tumors in most of these studies. In the principal clinical study evaluating panitumumab monotherapy for colorectal cancer (study 1), *KRAS* status was determined in 427 out of 463 patients, with *KRAS* mutations found in 43% of patients. Clinical efficacy of panitumumab in this study was found to be limited to patients with wild-type (nonmutated) *KRAS*, with response rates of 17 and 0% for the wild-type and mutated groups, respectively; patients with wild-type *KRAS* also had a longer overall survival. The American Society of Clinical Oncology (ASCO) and some clinicians recommend that all patients with metastatic colorectal cancer who are potential candidates for EGFR inhibitor therapy (e.g., panitumumab, cetuximab) have their tumor tested for *KRAS* mutations in a Clinical Laboratory Improvement Amendments (CLIA)-accredited laboratory. If *KRAS* mutation in codon 12 or 13 is detected, the use of panitumumab is *not* recommended.

Panitumumab is *not* approved for use in combination with chemotherapy for the treatment of metastatic colorectal cancer. (See Use in Combination with other Chemotherapeutic Regimens under Warnings/Precautions: Other Warnings and Precautions, in Cautions.)

Dosage and Administration

■ **General** Premedication to minimize the risk of infusion-related reactions does not appear to be necessary; however, the manufacturer states that appropriate medical resources for the treatment of severe reactions should be available during panitumumab infusions.

■ **Administration** Panitumumab is administered by IV infusion. *The drug should not be administered by rapid IV injection, such as IV push or bolus.* Doses of panitumumab of 1 g or less should be infused over 60 minutes; doses exceeding 1 g should be infused over 90 minutes.

Panitumumab injection should be inspected visually for particulate matter and discoloration prior to administration. Solutions of the drug should be colorless but may contain a small amount of visible, translucent-to-white, amorphous, proteinaceous panitumumab particulates; the solution should *not* be administered if discoloration is observed. The vials should *not* be shaken.

For IV infusion, the appropriate dose (6 mg/kg) of panitumumab injection (containing 20 mg/mL) should be withdrawn into a syringe and diluted in 0.9% sodium chloride injection to a total volume of 100 mL using aseptic technique; doses exceeding 1 g should be diluted in 0.9% sodium chloride injection to a total volume of 150 mL. The final concentration should not exceed 10 mg of panitumumab per mL. The diluted solution should be mixed by gentle inversion, should *not* be shaken, and should *not* be mixed or diluted with other drugs or infusion solutions. The diluted infusion solution may be stored at room temperature for up to 6 hours or at 2–8°C for up to 24 hours; freezing should be avoided.

After dilution, panitumumab infusion solution should be administered IV through an appropriate 0.2- or 0.22-μm inline filter. Solutions of the drug should be administered using an infusion pump and infused through a peripheral IV line or indwelling IV catheter; the infusion line should be flushed with 0.9% sodium chloride injection before and after IV panitumumab administration.

Panitumumab injection should be protected from direct sunlight and stored at 2–8°C; freezing should be avoided.

Any unused portion left in the vial should be discarded since the injection contains no preservative.

■ **Dosage** For the management of previously treated, EGFR-expressing metastatic colorectal cancer as monotherapy in adults, the recommended dosage of panitumumab is 6 mg/kg administered as a single IV infusion over 60 minutes every 14 days. Doses exceeding 1 g should be infused over 90 minutes. In the randomized controlled trial evaluating panitumumab monotherapy for metastatic colorectal cancer, a median of 5 doses was administered.

■ **Dosage Modification for Toxicity** ***Infusion-related Reactions*** In patients who develop mild or moderate (grade 1 or 2) infusion-related reactions, the infusion rate should be reduced by 50% for the duration of that infusion. In patients who develop severe (grade 3 or 4) infusion-related reactions, panitumumab therapy should be immediately and *permanently* discontinued.

Dermatologic Toxicity In patients who experience severe (grade 3 or 4) or intolerable dermatologic toxicity, panitumumab therapy should be withheld. If toxicity does not improve to grade 2 or less within 1 month, therapy should be *permanently* discontinued. If dermatologic toxicity improves to grade 2 or less and the patient is symptomatically improved after withholding no more than 2 doses, treatment may be resumed at 50% of the original dosage. The dosage may then be increased in increments of 25% of the original dosage up to the recommended dosage of 6 mg/kg if toxicity does not recur. If toxicity recurs, therapy should be *permanently* discontinued.

■ **Special Populations** There are no special population dosage recommendations at this time.

Cautions

■ **Contraindications** The manufacturer states that there are no known contraindications to the use of panitumumab.

■ **Warnings/Precautions** ***Warnings*** **Dermatologic, Mucosal, and Ocular Toxicity.** Dermatologic toxicity was reported in approximately 90% of patients and was severe (grade 3 or 4) in 16% of patients in a large, controlled trial. Such toxicity may be manifested as dermatitis acneiform, pruritus, erythema, rash, skin exfoliation, paronychia, dry skin, and/or skin fissures. Severe dermatologic toxicity may result in infectious complications, including sepsis, septic death, and abscesses requiring incision and drainage. Mucosal toxicity, including oral mucositis and stomatitis, was reported in 6–7% of patients receiving panitumumab therapy; one case of grade 3 mucosal inflammation was reported. Ocular toxicity, including conjunctivitis, ocular hyperemia, increased lacrimation, and eye/eyelid irritation, was reported in 15% of patients. Paronychia was reported in 25% of patients receiving panitumumab, with severe cases (grade 3 or 4) reported in 2%; other nail disorders were reported in 9% of patients. Median time to development of dermatologic, nail, or ocular toxicity was 14 days and median time to most severe toxicity was 15 days after the first dose of panitumumab; the median time to resolution after the last dose of panitumumab was 84 days. Severe toxicity necessitated dose interruption in 11% of panitumumab-treated patients.

Panitumumab should be withheld for severe or life-threatening dermatologic toxicity. If severe adverse dermatologic effects occur, patients should be monitored for possible inflammatory or infectious complications and appropriate therapy should be initiated. Prevention and treatment should be carefully individualized and may require specialized care; topical and/or systemic antibiotics, topical emollients, topical corticosteroids, and/or systemic antihistamines may be helpful in some cases. Dosage modifications, including possible discontinuance of therapy, may be required. (See Dermatologic Toxicity under Dosage and Administration: Dosage Modification for Toxicity.)

Infusion-related Reactions. Infusion-related reactions occurred in 4% and severe reactions (grade 3 or 4) occurred in approximately 1% of patients taking panitumumab in the monotherapy clinical trial (Study 1). In all clinical studies, severe infusion reactions occurred in approximately 1% of the panitumumab-treated patients. Serious infusion reactions included anaphylactic reactions, bronchospasm, and hypotension. No fatalities were reported; however, fatalities have occurred with other monoclonal antibody products. A reduction in infusion rate or discontinuance of therapy may be necessary depending on the severity of the reaction. (See Infusion-related Reactions under Dosage and Administration: Dosage Modification for Toxicity.)

Other Warnings and Precautions **Use in Combination with other Chemotherapeutic Regimens.** Panitumumab is *not* indicated for use in combination with chemotherapy.

In an interim analysis of a randomized, open-label, multicenter trial (designated study 2 by the manufacturer), addition of panitumumab to a bevacizumab plus chemotherapy regimen (containing either oxaliplatin or irinotecan and fluorouracil) in the first-line treatment of metastatic colorectal cancer resulted in poorer outcomes (i.e., decreased overall survival time) and increased toxicity (i.e., higher incidence of grade 3–5 adverse reactions). Grade 3/4 adverse reactions occurred more frequently in panitumumab-treated patients compared with those in non-panitumumab-containing treatment arms and included dermatologic toxicity (e.g., rash, acneiform dermatitis), diarrhea, dehydration (mainly in patients with diarrhea), hypokalemia, stomatitis or mucositis, and hypomagnesemia. Grade 3–5 pulmonary embolism also occurred more frequently in panitumumab-treated patients compared with non-panitumumab-containing treatment arms (7 and 4%, respectively). Because of the toxicities experienced, patients randomized to panitumumab, bevacizumab, and chemotherapy received a lower mean relative dose intensity of each agent (oxaliplatin, irinotecan, direct IV injection ["bolus"] fluorouracil, and/or infusional fluorouracil) over the first 24 weeks compared with those receiving bevacizumab plus chemotherapy.

In another clinical study, addition of panitumumab to irinotecan, bolus fluorouracil, and leucovorin (the IFL regimen) resulted in an increased incidence and severity of chemotherapy-induced diarrhea (58% incidence of grade 3/4 diarrhea; one case of grade 5 diarrhea). Grade 3 diarrhea was reported in 25% of patients receiving panitumumab plus irinotecan, continuous fluorouracil infusion, and leucovorin (FOLFIRI regimen).

Severe diarrhea and dehydration, which may lead to acute renal failure and other complications, have been observed in patients receiving panitumumab in combination with chemotherapy. (See Drug Interactions.)

Pulmonary Effects. Pulmonary fibrosis (including 2 fatalities; 1 case occurred in a patient with preexisting idiopathic pulmonary fibrosis) reported in less than 1% of patients receiving panitumumab. Caution should be used in patients with preexisting lung disease; such patients were excluded from clinical trials. Panitumumab should be *permanently* discontinued in patients who develop interstitial lung disease, pneumonitis, or lung infiltrates during therapy.

Electrolyte Effects. Electrolyte abnormalities, including decreased serum magnesium concentrations, reported; grade 3 or 4 hypomagnesemia requiring oral or IV electrolyte repletion occurred in approximately 2% of patients in one study. In some patients, both hypomagnesemia and hypocalcemia have occurred. Hypomagnesemia usually developed 6 weeks or longer following initiation of panitumumab therapy.

Serum electrolytes (including magnesium and calcium) should be monitored periodically during and for 8 weeks following completion of panitumumab therapy.

Appropriate treatment (e.g., oral or IV electrolyte repletion) should be instituted if necessary.

Photosensitivity. Exposure to sunlight can exacerbate dermatologic toxicity; the manufacturer recommends that patients apply sunscreen, wear hats, and limit sun exposure during therapy and for 2 months following the last dose of the drug.

Fetal/Neonatal Morbidity and Mortality. Panitumumab may cause fetal harm; embryolethality and abortifacient effects have been demonstrated in animals. No studies to date in pregnant women. Pregnancy should be avoided during therapy and for 6 months after the last dose. If panitumumab is used during pregnancy or if the patient becomes pregnant while receiving the drug, apprise of the potential fetal hazard and/or risk for loss of the pregnancy. (See Advice to Patients.)

EGFR Testing. The manufacturer states that pretreatment assessment for EGFR expression is necessary for selecting patients appropriate for panitumumab therapy. However, panitumumab has demonstrated antitumor activity in patients with low or negative EGFR levels. Some authorities state that routine EGFR expression testing is not recommended and that patients should not be included or excluded from panitumumab therapy based solely on EGFR test results.

If testing is conducted, EGFR expression should be assessed by laboratories with demonstrated proficiency in the specific technology being utilized. Improper assay performance may lead to unreliable results.

Immunologic Effects. Panitumumab appears to have a relatively low immunogenic potential. Anti-panitumumab antibodies were detected in the sera of less than 1% and in 4.6% of panitumumab-treated patients using the acid dissociation ELISA and Biacore® screening immunoassays, respectively. In patients whose sera tested positive in screening bioassays, neutralizing antibodies were detected in 1.6 and 0.8% of post-dose samples and follow-up samples, respectively, using an in vitro biological assay. There appears to be no relationship between the appearance of antibodies to panitumumab using screening immunoassays and the pharmacokinetic and tolerability profile of the drug.

Specific Populations **Pregnancy.** Category C. (See Users Guide.) (See Fetal/Neonatal Morbidity and Mortality under Warnings/Precautions: Other Warnings and Precautions, in Cautions.) Amgen's Pregnancy Surveillance Program may be contacted at 800-772-6436.

Lactation. It is not known whether panitumumab is distributed into milk; however, human immunoglobulin G (IgG) is distributed into human milk. Published data suggest that breast milk antibodies do not enter the neonatal and infant circulation in substantial amounts. Because many drugs are excreted into human milk and because of the potential for serious adverse reactions in nursing infants from panitumumab, a decision should be made whether to discontinue nursing or the drug, taking into account the importance of the drug to the mother. If nursing is interrupted, based on the mean half-life of panitumumab, nursing should not be resumed earlier than 2 months following the last dose of panitumumab.

Pediatric Use. Safety and efficacy not established in pediatric patients younger than 18 years of age.

Geriatric Use. In the randomized, controlled study, 42% of the patients with metastatic colorectal cancer who received panitumumab were 65 years of age and older. Although the clinical study of panitumumab did not include a sufficient number of geriatric patients to determine whether they respond differently than younger patients, no apparent differences in safety and efficacy relative to younger adults were reported.

■ **Common Adverse Effects** The most common adverse effects in patients receiving panitumumab monotherapy in metastatic colorectal cancer include dermatologic toxicity, including erythema (65%), acne (13%) or acneiform dermatitis (57%), pruritus (57%), skin exfoliation (25%), skin rash (22%), skin fissures (20%), and dry skin (10%); hypomagnesemia (38%); paronychia (25%); fatigue (26%); GI toxicity, including abdominal pain (25%), nausea (23%), diarrhea (21%), including diarrhea resulting in dehydration, constipation (21%), and vomiting (19%); ocular toxicity, including conjunctivitis, increased lacrimation, ocular hyperemia, and eye/eyelid irritation (15%); cough (14%); peripheral edema (12%); dehydration; and general deterioration (11%).

Drug Interactions

No formal drug interaction studies of panitumumab have been performed.

■ **Bevacizumab** Increased toxicity (pulmonary embolism, dermatologic toxicity, diarrhea, dehydration, hypomagnesemia) may result during concurrent therapy with bevacizumab and panitumumab. The manufacturer states that use of panitumumab in combination chemotherapy regimens is not approved. (See Use in Combination with other Chemotherapeutic Regimens under Warnings/Precautions: Other Warnings and Precautions, in Cautions.)

■ **Fluoropyrimidines (e.g., Fluorouracil)** Pharmacokinetic interaction is unlikely. However, the manufacturer states that use of panitumumab in combination chemotherapy regimens is not approved.

■ **Irinotecan** Pharmacokinetic interaction is unlikely.

Increased incidence and severity of chemotherapy-induced diarrhea reported following addition of panitumumab to irinotecan, direct IV injection ("bolus") fluorouracil, and leucovorin (the IFL regimen) in a clinical study. The manufacturer states that use of panitumumab in combination chemotherapy regimens is not approved. (See Use in Combination with other Chemotherapeutic Regimens under Warnings/Precautions: Other Warnings and Precautions, in Cautions.)

■ **Paclitaxel** Pharmacokinetic interaction is unlikely. However, the manufacturer states that use of panitumumab in combination chemotherapy regimens is not approved.

■ **Radiation Therapy** Potential pharmacologic interaction (increased risk of dermatological toxicity). Although experience with concurrent panitumumab and radiation therapy is limited to date, combined use of cetuximab (another EGFR inhibitor) and radiation therapy has been associated with an increased risk of high-grade radiation dermatitis, rash, and mucositis.

Description

Panitumumab, a recombinant human IgG_2 kappa monoclonal antibody that specifically binds to the human epidermal growth factor receptor (EGFR, HER1, c-erbB-1), is an antineoplastic agent. The drug is an immunoglobulin containing a fully human framework.

Human epidermal growth factor receptor (EGFR, HER1, c-erbB-1) is a transmembrane glycoprotein that belongs to the subfamily of type I receptor tyrosine kinases, which includes EGFR (HER1, c-erbB-1), HER2/*neu*, HER3, and HER4. While EGFR is expressed in many normal epithelial tissues (e.g., skin, hair follicle), overexpression of the glycoprotein is detected in human carcinomas (e.g., colon, rectum). Interaction of EGFR with its normal ligands (e.g., EGF, transforming growth factor [TGF]-α) results in phosphorylation and activation of a series of intracellular proteins that, in turn, regulate transcription of genes involved with cellular growth and survival, motility, and proliferation. Signal transduction through EGFR leads to activation of the wild-type (nonmutated) *KRAS* gene. However, the presence of an activating somatic mutation of the *KRAS* gene (mutated *KRAS*) in a cancer cell can lead to dysregulation of signaling pathways and resistance to EGFR inhibitor therapy (e.g., cetuximab and panitumumab).

Panitumumab binds specifically and with high affinity to the extracellular domain of EGFR on both normal and tumor cells and competitively blocks the cellular action of EGF and other ligands (e.g., TGF-α). In nonclinical studies, binding of panitumumab to EGFR blocks phosphorylation and activation of receptor-associated kinases resulting in inhibition of cell growth, induction of apoptosis (programmed cell death), decreased proinflammatory cytokine and vascular endothelial growth factor production, and internalization of the EGFR. In vitro tests and in vivo animal studies have demonstrated that panitumumab inhibits the growth and survival of selected human tumor cell lines that overexpress EGFR, while such antitumor effects were not observed in human cancer xenografts that lacked EGFR expression.

Following administration of the recommended regimen of panitumumab (6 mg/kg by IV infusion every 2 weeks), steady-state panitumumab concentrations are achieved by the third infusion. The mean elimination half-life of panitumumab following multiple dosing is approximately 7.5 days.

Advice to Patients

Risk of severe skin reactions (such as pimples, itching, red colored skin, rash, peeling skin, dry skin, and cracks in the skin); these reactions also may happen to the stomach and intestine lining, eyes, and nails. Importance of informing patients to report skin and ocular or visual changes to a healthcare professional.

Risk of severe infusion reactions during IV infusion. Importance of informing patients to report sudden symptoms (such as trouble breathing, shortness of breath, fever, chills, and low blood pressure) to a healthcare professional.

Risk of a severe lung problem called pulmonary fibrosis; importance of informing patients to report persistent or recurrent coughing, wheezing, dyspnea, or new onset facial swelling to a healthcare professional.

Importance of informing patients to report diarrhea and dehydration to a healthcare professional.

Importance of informing patients to use sunscreen and hats and limit sun exposure during therapy and for 2 months following the last dose of the drug to avoid exacerbation of adverse dermatologic effects.

Importance of advising patients that periodic monitoring of serum electrolytes (including magnesium and calcium) is required.

Risk of potential embryofetal lethality. Necessity of advising women and men to use an effective method of contraception during panitumumab therapy and for 6 months following the last dose of the drug; women should avoid breast-feeding during therapy and for 2 months following discontinuance of the drug. Importance of women informing clinicians if they are or plan to become pregnant or plan to breast-feed; panitumumab may affect ability of women to become pregnant. If pregnancy occurs, advise patient of risk to the fetus and/or the potential risk for loss of the pregnancy.

Importance of informing clinicians of existing or contemplated concomitant therapy, including prescription and OTC drugs and dietary or herbal supplements, as well as any concomitant illnesses, particularly pulmonary disease.

Importance of informing patients of other important precautionary information. (See Cautions.)

Overview® (see Users Guide). For additional information on this drug until a more detailed monograph is developed and published, the manufacturer's labeling should be consulted. It is *essential* that the manufacturer's labeling be consulted for more detailed information on usual cautions, precautions, contraindications, potential drug interactions, laboratory test interferences, and acute toxicity. For further information on the handling of antineoplastic agents, see the ASHP Guidelines on Handling Hazardous Drugs at http://www.ahfsdruginformation.com.

Preparations

Excipients in commercially available drug preparations may have clinically important effects in some individuals; consult specific product labeling for details.

Panitumumab (Recombinant)

Parenteral	
Injection, for IV infusion only	20 mg/mL (100, 200, and 400 mg) **Vectibix**®, Amgen

Selected Revisions August 2014, © Copyright, January 2008, American Society of Health-System Pharmacists, Inc.

Panobinostat Lactate

■ Panobinostat lactate, a histone deacetylase (HDAC) inhibitor, is an antineoplastic agent.

REMS

FDA approved a REMS for panobinostat to ensure that the benefits outweigh the risks. The REMS may apply to one or more preparations of panobinostat and consists of the following: communication plan. See the FDA REMS page (https://www.accessdata.fda.gov/scripts/cder/rems/index.cfm).

Uses

■ **Multiple Myeloma** Panobinostat lactate is used in combination with bortezomib and dexamethasone for the treatment of multiple myeloma in patients who have received at least 2 prior therapies, including bortezomib and an immunomodulatory agent. Panobinostat has been designated an orphan drug by the US Food and Drug Administration (FDA) for use in this condition. The accelerated approval of panobinostat for this indication is based on progression-free survival; continued FDA approval for this indication may be contingent on verification and description of clinical benefit of panobinostat in confirmatory studies.

Approval of panobinostat for the labeled indication is based principally on data for a subset of patients who were enrolled in PANORAMA1, a randomized, double-blind, placebo-controlled, phase 3, multicenter study evaluating the efficacy of panobinostat in combination with bortezomib and dexamethasone in 768 patients with relapsed multiple myeloma who had received 1–3 prior therapies. Patients with primary refractory or bortezomib-refractory disease and those who had received prior treatment with a deacetylase inhibitor were excluded from the study. The median number of prior therapies was 1; 48% of patients enrolled in the study had received 2 or 3 prior therapies, and 57% of patients had undergone prior stem cell transplantation. The most common agents used in prior antineoplastic regimens were corticosteroids (90%), melphalan (80%), thalidomide (53%), cyclophosphamide (47%), bortezomib (44%), and lenalidomide (19%). The median age of patients in the study was 63 years (range 28–84); 53% of patients were male; 65, 30, and 3% were Caucasian, Asian, and black, respectively; and 93% had an Eastern Cooperative Oncology Group (ECOG) performance status of 0 or 1. Treatment consisted of either the combination of panobinostat, bortezomib, and dexamethasone or the combination of placebo, bortezomib, and dexamethasone administered in 21-day cycles; randomization to these regimens was stratified by prior use of bortezomib and the number of prior therapies. Patients received either oral panobinostat (20 mg) or placebo 3 times weekly during weeks 1 and 2 (days 1, 3, 5, 8, 10, and 12) of each 21-day cycle. IV bortezomib (1.3 mg/m^2) was administered twice weekly during weeks 1 and 2 (days 1, 4, 8, and 11) of cycles 1–8 and once weekly during weeks 1 and 2 (days 1 and 8) of cycles 9–16. Oral dexamethasone (20 mg) was administered on the day of and the day after bortezomib administration. Treatment was administered for a maximum of 16 cycles (48 weeks).

In PANORAMA1, the primary end point was progression-free survival, as assessed by investigators using modified European Group for Blood and Marrow Transplantation (EBMT) criteria; median duration of follow-up was 29 months in both treatment groups. Median progression-free survival was 12 months in those who received the combination of panobinostat, bortezomib, and dexamethasone and 8.1 months in those who received the combination of placebo, bortezomib, and dexamethasone; overall response rates were 61 and 55%, respectively. Overall survival was not significantly different between treatment groups at the time of interim analysis. Serious adverse effects (60 versus 42%) and grade 3 or 4 adverse effects (96 versus 82%) occurred more frequently in patients receiving panobinostat, bortezomib, and dexamethasone compared with those receiving placebo, bortezomib, and dexamethasone; grade 3 or 4 diarrhea (25 versus 8%), asthenia or fatigue (24 versus 12%), peripheral neuropathy (18 versus 15%), thrombocytopenia (67 versus 31%), lymphopenia (53 versus 40%), and neutropenia (34 versus 11%) were reported more frequently with the combination of panobinostat, bortezomib, and dexamethasone than with the combination of placebo, bortezomib, and dexamethasone.

The benefit-to-risk assessment appeared to be more favorable in patients with more heavily pretreated disease. In the subgroup of 193 patients who had received prior treatment with both bortezomib and an immunomodulatory agent and had received a median of 2 prior therapies (76% had received 2 or more prior therapies), median progression-free survival was 10.6 months in those receiving panobinostat, bortezomib, and dexamethasone compared with 5.8 months in those receiving placebo, bortezomib, and dexamethasone. In this subgroup of patients, the overall response rate (complete, near complete, and partial responses) was 59% in patients receiving panobinostat, bortezomib, and dexamethasone compared with 41% in those receiving placebo, bortezomib, and dexamethasone.

Dosage and Administration

■ **General** Because of the risk of cardiac toxicity, an ECG should be performed prior to initiation of panobinostat therapy to confirm that the QT interval (corrected for heart rate using Fridericia's formula; QT_cF) is less than 450 msec. In addition, serum concentrations of electrolytes, including potassium and magnesium, should be determined prior to therapy and any abnormalities corrected. (See Cardiac Effects under Warnings/Precautions: Warnings, in Cautions.)

Because of the risk of myelotoxicity, the complete blood cell count (CBC) should be determined prior to initiation of therapy to verify that baseline platelet and absolute neutrophil counts (ANCs) are within acceptable limits (at least 100,000/mm^3 and 1500/mm^3, respectively). (See Hematologic Effects under Warnings/Precautions: Other Warnings and Precautions, in Cautions.)

Procedures for proper handling and disposal of antineoplastic agents should be followed. Exposure to the contents of panobinostat capsules, including exposure to crushed or broken capsules, should be avoided. If such contact with the skin or mucous membranes occurs, the affected areas should be washed thoroughly.

Restricted Distribution Program Panobinostat can only be obtained through a limited network of specialty pharmacies. Clinicians may contact the manufacturer at 888-669-6682 or http://www.farydak.com for specific availability information.

■ **Administration** Panobinostat lactate is administered orally once daily on each scheduled day at approximately the same time. The drug may be administered without regard to food.

The manufacturer states that panobinostat lactate capsules should be swallowed whole with a cup of water, and the capsules should not be opened, crushed, or chewed.

■ **Dosage** Dosage of panobinostat lactate is expressed in terms of panobinostat.

When used in combination with bortezomib and dexamethasone for the treatment of multiple myeloma in adults who have received at least 2 prior therapies, including bortezomib and an immunomodulatory agent, the recommended initial oral dosage of panobinostat is 20 mg given 3 times weekly during weeks 1 and 2 (days 1, 3, 5, 8, 10, and 12) of each 21-day cycle for up to 8 cycles. During cycles 1–8, the recommended dosage of IV bortezomib is 1.3 mg/m^2 given twice weekly during weeks 1 and 2 (days 1, 4, 8, and 11) of each cycle, and the recommended dosage of oral dexamethasone is 20 mg given 4 times weekly during weeks 1 and 2 (days 1, 2, 4, 5, 8, 9, 11, and 12) of each cycle. Continuation of treatment for an additional 8 cycles (cycles 9–16) should be considered for patients who derive clinical benefit from the regimen and do not experience unresolved severe or clinically important toxicity. For cycles 9–16, the recommended dosage of panobinostat is the same as in cycles 1–8 (i.e., 20 mg 3 times weekly during weeks 1 and 2 [days 1, 3, 5, 8, 10, and 12] of each 21-day cycle). However, during cycles 9–16, the recommended dosage of IV bortezomib is reduced to 1.3 mg/m^2 once weekly during weeks 1 and 2 (days 1 and 8) of each cycle, and the recommended dosage of oral dexamethasone is reduced to 20 mg twice weekly during weeks 1 and 2 (days 1, 2, 8, and 9) of each cycle. The total duration of treatment may be up to 16 cycles (48 weeks).

The initial dose of panobinostat should be reduced to 10 mg in patients receiving a potent cytochrome P-450 (CYP) 3A inhibitor (e.g., clarithromycin, conivaptan, indinavir, itraconazole, ketoconazole, lopinavir/ritonavir). (See Drug Interactions: Drugs Affecting or Metabolized by Hepatic Microsomal Enzymes.)

Dosage Modification for Toxicity Therapy with panobinostat and bortezomib may be temporarily interrupted and subsequent dosage reductions may be required in patients who experience adverse effects. If dosage modification of panobinostat is necessary, the dose should be reduced in decrements of 5 mg while maintaining the 3-week treatment cycle. If a reduction in dosage to less than 10 mg 3 times weekly is necessary, panobinostat should be discontinued.

Dosage Modification for GI Toxicity. If grade 2 diarrhea (increase of 4–6 stools per day over baseline) occurs, panobinostat therapy should be interrupted; interruption of bortezomib therapy also should be considered. Once diarrhea has resolved, therapy with both drugs may be resumed at the previous dosages. If grade 3 diarrhea (increase of 7 or more stools per day over baseline) occurs, or if IV fluids or hospitalization is required, therapy with both panobinostat and bortezomib should be interrupted; once diarrhea has resolved, therapy with both drugs may be resumed at reduced dosages. If grade 4 (life-threatening) diarrhea occurs, both drugs should be permanently discontinued. (See GI Effects under Warnings/Precautions: Warnings, in Cautions.)

If grade 3 or 4 nausea or vomiting occurs, panobinostat therapy should be interrupted; once nausea and vomiting have resolved, panobinostat therapy may be resumed at a reduced dosage.

Dosage Modification for Cardiac Toxicity. If the QT interval (corrected for heart rate using Fridericia's formula; QT_cF) increases to 480 msec or greater, panobinostat therapy should be interrupted and any electrolyte abnormalities corrected. If QT interval prolongation does not resolve, panobinostat should be permanently discontinued.

Dosage Modification for Hematologic Toxicity. Treatment interruption or dosage reduction of panobinostat is required in patients who experience thrombocytopenia, neutropenia, or anemia. Platelet transfusions should be considered in patients with severe thrombocytopenia; if thrombocytopenia does not improve despite the recommended treatment modifications or despite repeated platelet transfusions, panobinostat should be discontinued. If grade 3 or 4 neutropenia occurs, dosage reduction and/or use of granulocyte colony-stimulating factors (G-CSFs) should be considered. If neutropenia does not improve despite these measures or if severe infection occurs, panobinostat should be discontinued.

If grade 3 thrombocytopenia (platelet count of 25,000 to less than 50,000/mm^3) occurs, panobinostat and bortezomib may be continued at the current dosages, with monitoring of platelet counts performed at least weekly. If grade 3 thrombocytopenia is accompanied by bleeding or if grade 4 thrombocytopenia (platelet count less than 25,000/mm^3) occurs, therapy with panobinostat and bortezomib should be interrupted and platelet counts monitored at least weekly. Once the platelet count has recovered to 50,000/mm^3 or greater, panobinostat therapy may be resumed at a reduced dosage. Once the platelet count has recovered to 75,000/mm^3 or greater, bortezomib therapy may be resumed at the previous dosage if only 1 dose was omitted prior to recovery or at a reduced dosage if 2 or more consecutive doses or 2 or more doses within the same cycle were omitted.

For grade 3 neutropenia with an ANC of 750–1000/mm^3, therapy with panobinostat and bortezomib may be continued at the current dosages. Following 2 or more occurrences of grade 3 neutropenia with an ANC of 500–750/mm^3, bortezomib may be continued at the current dosage but panobinostat therapy should be interrupted; once ANC has recovered to 1000/mm^3 or greater, therapy with panobinostat may be resumed at the previous dosage.

For grade 3 neutropenia that is accompanied by febrile neutropenia of any grade, therapy with both panobinostat and bortezomib should be interrupted. Once febrile neutropenia has resolved and ANC has recovered to 1000/mm^3 or greater, therapy with panobinostat may be resumed at a reduced dosage, and bortezomib therapy may be resumed at the previous dosage if only 1 dose was omitted prior to recovery or at a reduced dosage if 2 or more consecutive doses or 2 or more doses within the same cycle were omitted.

For grade 4 neutropenia (ANC less than 500/mm^3), therapy with both panobinostat and bortezomib should be interrupted. Once ANC has recovered to 1000/mm^3 or greater, therapy with panobinostat may be resumed at a reduced dosage, and bortezomib therapy may be resumed at the previous dosage if only 1 dose was omitted prior to recovery or at a reduced dosage if 2 or more consecutive doses or 2 or more doses within the same cycle were omitted.

If grade 3 anemia (hemoglobin concentration less than 8 g/dL) occurs, panobinostat therapy should be interrupted. Once hemoglobin concentration increases to 10 g/dL or higher, panobinostat therapy may be resumed at a reduced dosage.

Dosage Modification for Other Toxicity. In patients who experience grade 3 or 4 adverse effects other than thrombocytopenia, neutropenia, or GI toxicity, dosage modification of panobinostat is required. For grade 3 or 4 toxicity or for a grade 2 recurrence of such toxicity, panobinostat therapy should be interrupted until the toxicity resolves to grade 1 or less; panobinostat may then be resumed at a reduced dosage. In those who experience a grade 3 or 4 toxicity recurrence, further reduction in dosage may be considered once the toxicity has resolved to grade 1 or less.

■ **Special Populations** The initial dose of panobinostat should be reduced to 15 mg in patients with mild hepatic impairment and 10 mg in patients with moderate hepatic impairment. Use of panobinostat should be avoided in patients with severe hepatic impairment. Patients should be monitored frequently for adverse effects and dosage should be adjusted as needed for toxicity. (See Hepatic Impairment under Warnings/Precautions: Specific Populations, in Cautions.)

Cautions

■ **Contraindications** The manufacturer states there are no known contraindications to the use of panobinostat.

■ **Warnings/Precautions** ***Warnings*** **GI Effects.** GI toxicity is common in patients receiving panobinostat. In the PANORAMA1 study in patients with relapsed multiple myeloma, severe diarrhea occurred in 25% of patients receiving panobinostat in combination with bortezomib and dexamethasone. Diarrhea of any grade occurred in 68% of patients receiving the panobinostat-containing regimen, compared with 42% of patients receiving bortezomib and dexamethasone alone. Diarrhea can occur at any time in patients receiving panobinostat. Thus, the patient's fluid and electrolyte status, including serum concentrations of potassium, magnesium, and phosphate, should be monitored prior to initiation of panobinostat therapy and then weekly (or more frequently as clinically indicated) during treatment; any abnormalities should be corrected to prevent dehydration and electrolyte disturbances. Patients who experience diarrhea, nausea, or vomiting may require treatment interruption or dosage reduction. (See Dosage Modification for Toxicity under Dosage and Administration: Dosage.) Antidiarrheal therapy (e.g., loperamide) should be initiated at the first sign of abdominal cramping, loose stools, or onset of diarrhea. Patients initiating panobinostat therapy should have antidiarrheal agents on hand. Prophylactic use of antiemetics should be considered as clinically indicated.

Cardiac Effects. Severe or fatal cardiac ischemic events, severe arrhythmias, and ECG changes have occurred in patients receiving panobinostat.

In the PANORAMA1 study in patients with relapsed multiple myeloma, arrhythmias and cardiac ischemic events occurred in 12 and 4%, respectively, of patients receiving panobinostat in combination with bortezomib and dexamethasone, compared with 5 and 1%, respectively, of patients receiving bortezomib and dexamethasone alone. Panobinostat should not be initiated in patients with a history of recent myocardial infarction or unstable angina.

ECG abnormalities such as ST-segment depression and T-wave abnormalities also occurred more frequently in patients receiving panobinostat in combination with bortezomib and dexamethasone (22 and 40%, respectively) compared with those receiving bortezomib and dexamethasone alone (4 and 18%, respectively). Panobinostat may prolong the QT interval. In the PANORAMA1 study, prolongation of the QT interval (corrected for heart rate using Fridericia's formula; QT_cF) to 451–480 or 481–500 msec occurred in 10.8 or 1.3%, respectively, of patients receiving panobinostat in combination with bortezomib and dexamethasone; no episodes in which the QT_cF interval exceeded 500 msec were observed. In this study, the maximum increase in the QT_cF interval from baseline was 31–60 msec or more than 60 msec in 14.5 or 0.8%, respectively, of patients. Pooled clinical data from more than 500 patients who received panobinostat as a single agent for various indications and at various dosages indicated that the QT_cF interval exceeded 500 msec in approximately 1% of patients overall and in 5% or more of those receiving a panobinostat dose of 60 mg or higher.

ECGs should be performed prior to initiation of panobinostat therapy and periodically during treatment as clinically indicated. Because arrhythmias may be exacerbated by electrolyte disturbances, serum concentrations of electrolytes, including potassium and magnesium, also should be monitored prior to and during treatment, and any abnormalities should be corrected. During the PANORAMA1 study in patients with relapsed multiple myeloma, ECGs were performed at baseline and prior to initiation of each treatment cycle for the first 8 cycles and serum electrolytes were monitored prior to the beginning of each cycle, at day 11 of cycles 1–8, and at the start of each cycle for cycles 9–16. Panobinostat should not be initiated in patients with a QT_cF interval exceeding 450 msec or clinically important ST-segment or T-wave abnormalities. If the QT_cF interval increases to 480 msec or greater during treatment, panobinostat therapy should be interrupted and any electrolyte abnormalities corrected. Panobinostat should be permanently discontinued if QT interval prolongation does not resolve.

Other Warnings and Precautions **Hemorrhagic Events.** Serious, sometimes fatal, hemorrhage has been reported in patients receiving panobinostat. In the PANORAMA1 study in patients with relapsed multiple myeloma, 5 patients receiving panobinostat in combination with bortezomib and dexamethasone died from a hemorrhagic event, compared with 1 patient receiving bortezomib and dexamethasone alone. All 5 panobinostat-treated patients had grade 3 or greater thrombocytopenia at the time of the event. Grade 3 or 4 hemorrhage was reported in 4% of patients receiving panobinostat in combination with bortezomib and dexamethasone and 2% of patients receiving bortezomib and dexamethasone alone.

Hematologic Effects. Panobinostat may cause severe thrombocytopenia, neutropenia, and anemia. In the PANORAMA1 study in patients with relapsed multiple myeloma, grade 3 or 4 thrombocytopenia occurred in 67% of patients receiving panobinostat in combination with bortezomib and dexamethasone, compared with 31% of patients receiving bortezomib and dexamethasone alone. Patients receiving panobinostat in combination with bortezomib and dexamethasone were more likely to receive a platelet transfusion (33 versus 10%) or to require treatment interruption and/or dosage modification because of thrombocytopenia (31 versus 11%) compared with those receiving bortezomib and dexamethasone alone.

Severe neutropenia occurred in 34% of patients receiving panobinostat in combination with bortezomib and dexamethasone, compared with 11% of patients receiving bortezomib and dexamethasone alone. Neutropenia resulted in treatment interruption and/or dosage modification in 10% of patients receiving the panobinostat-containing regimen. Patients receiving panobinostat in combination with bortezomib and dexamethasone were more likely to receive a granulocyte colony-stimulating factor (13 versus 4%) compared with those receiving bortezomib and dexamethasone alone.

Complete blood cell counts (CBCs) should be monitored prior to initiation of therapy and then weekly (or more frequently as clinically indicated) during treatment. CBCs should be monitored more frequently in patients older than 65 years of age because an increased frequency of myelosuppression has been observed in these patients. Treatment interruptions or dosage reductions may be necessary. (See Dosage Modification for Toxicity under Dosage and Administration: Dosage.)

Infectious Complications. Local and systemic infections, including pneumonia, bacterial infections, invasive fungal infections, and viral infections, have been reported in patients receiving panobinostat. Severe infections occurred in 31% of patients receiving panobinostat in combination with bortezomib and dexamethasone compared with 24% of patients receiving bortezomib and dexamethasone alone; infections were fatal in 10 patients who received the panobinostat-containing regimen and 6 patients who received bortezomib and dexamethasone alone. Infections of all grades occurred at similar frequencies in both treatment groups. Panobinostat therapy should not be initiated in patients with active infections. Patients should be monitored for signs and symptoms of infection during treatment. If infection develops, appropriate anti-infective treatment should be initiated promptly and interruption or discontinuance of panobinostat considered.

Hepatotoxicity. Hepatic dysfunction, principally elevations in aminotransferase and total bilirubin concentrations, has occurred in patients receiving panobinostat. Hepatic function should be monitored prior to and regularly during treatment. If liver function test abnormalities are observed, dosage modifications may be considered (see Dosage and Administration: Special Populations), and the patient should be monitored until concentrations return to normal or pretreatment values.

Fetal/Neonatal Morbidity and Mortality. Panobinostat may cause fetal harm; teratogenicity has been demonstrated in animals.

Pregnancy should be avoided during panobinostat therapy. A pregnancy test should be performed in women of childbearing potential prior to initiation of therapy and periodically during treatment. Women of childbearing potential who are sexually active should be advised to use effective contraception while receiving panobinostat and for at least 1 month following the last dose of the drug. Men who are sexually active should use condoms while receiving panobinostat and for 3 months following the last dose. If panobinostat is used during pregnancy or if the patient becomes pregnant while receiving the drug, the patient should be apprised of the potential fetal hazard.

Specific Populations **Pregnancy.** Panobinostat may cause fetal harm; teratogenicity has been demonstrated in animals. (See Fetal/Neonatal Morbidity and Mortality under Warnings/Precautions: Other Warnings and Precautions, in Cautions.)

Lactation. It is not known whether panobinostat is distributed into human milk. A decision should be made whether to discontinue nursing or the drug, taking into account the importance of the drug to the woman.

Pediatric Use. Safety and efficacy of panobinostat have not been established in pediatric patients.

Geriatric Use. In clinical trials evaluating panobinostat in patients with relapsed multiple myeloma, 42% of patients were 65 years of age or older. Although no overall differences in efficacy were observed between geriatric patients and younger adults, patients 65 years of age or older had a higher frequency of selected adverse effects, were more likely to discontinue treatment because of adverse effects (45 versus 30%), and had a higher rate of death not related to disease progression (9 versus 5%) compared with younger adults. Monitoring for potential toxicity (especially GI toxicity, myelosuppression, and cardiac toxicity) should be performed more frequently in patients older than 65 years of age.

Hepatic Impairment. Safety and efficacy of panobinostat have not been established in patients with hepatic impairment. In a pharmacokinetic study in patients with advanced cancer, the area under the concentration-time curve (AUC) of panobinostat was increased by 43% in patients with mild hepatic impairment (bilirubin concentration at or below the upper limit of normal [ULN] and AST concentration exceeding the ULN, or bilirubin concentration more than 1 times but not more than 1.5 times the ULN and any AST concentration) and by 105% in those with moderate hepatic impairment (bilirubin concentration exceeding 1.5 times but not more than 3 times the ULN and any AST concentration). Use of panobinostat should be avoided in patients with severe hepatic impairment. Patients with mild or moderate hepatic impairment should receive a reduced initial dosage of the drug and should be monitored frequently for adverse effects. (See Dosage and Administration: Special Populations.)

Renal Impairment. In a pharmacokinetic study in patients with advanced cancer and various degrees of renal function, systemic exposure to panobinostat was not substantially altered by mild to severe renal impairment. Panobinostat has not been studied in patients with end-stage renal disease or patients undergoing dialysis, and it is not known if panobinostat is dialyzable.

■ **Common Adverse Effects** Adverse effects reported in 10% or more of patients receiving panobinostat in combination with bortezomib and dexamethasone, and at an incidence that is at least 5% higher than that reported with bortezomib and dexamethasone alone, include decreased appetite, arrhythmia, diarrhea, fatigue, nausea, peripheral edema, pyrexia, vomiting, and weight loss.

Laboratory abnormalities reported in 10% or more of patients receiving panobinostat in combination with bortezomib and dexamethasone, and at an incidence that is at least 5% higher than that reported with bortezomib and dexamethasone alone, include anemia, hyperbilirubinemia, hypermagnesemia, hyperphosphatemia, hypoalbuminemia, hypocalcemia, hypokalemia, hyponatremia, hypophosphatemia, increased serum creatinine concentrations, leukopenia, lymphopenia, neutropenia, and thrombocytopenia.

Drug Interactions

Panobinostat is a substrate of cytochrome P-450 (CYP) isoenzyme 3A and, in vitro, has been shown to inhibit CYP isoenzymes 2D6, 2C19, and 3A4 (in a time-dependent manner). Panobinostat also is a substrate of P-glycoprotein (P-gp).

In vitro studies indicate that panobinostat does not inhibit CYP isoenzymes 1A2, 2C8, 2C9, or 2E, nor does it induce CYP isoenzymes 1A1/2, 2B6, 2C8/9/19, or 3A or uridine diphosphate-glucuronosyl transferase (UGT) 1A1.

In vitro, panobinostat inhibits organic anion transporter (OAT) 3, organic anion transporter protein (OATP) 1B1 and 1B3, and organic cation transporter (OCT) 1 and 2; panobinostat does not inhibit P-gp, breast cancer resistance protein (BCRP), or OAT1. Panobinostat does not induce P-gp or multidrug resistance protein (MRP) 2 transporters.

■ **Drugs Affecting or Metabolized by Hepatic Microsomal Enzymes** ***Inhibitors of CYP3A*** In patients with advanced cancer, concomitant administration of panobinostat (single 20-mg dose) with the potent CYP3A inhibitor ketoconazole (400 mg daily) increased peak plasma concentration and area under the plasma concentration-time curve (AUC) of panobinostat by 62 and 73%, respectively, compared with administration of panobinostat alone. Time to peak plasma concentration was unchanged. Dose of panobinostat should be reduced to 10 mg when panobinostat is used concomitantly with a potent CYP3A inhibitor (e.g., clarithromycin, conivaptan, indinavir, itraconazole, ketoconazole, lopinavir/ritonavir, nefazodone, nelfinavir, posaconazole, ritonavir, saquinavir, telithromycin, voriconazole). Star fruit, pomegranate or pomegranate juice, and grapefruit or grapefruit juice should be avoided, as these foods are known to inhibit CYP3A isoenzymes.

Inducers of CYP3A A decrease in panobinostat exposure is likely if panobinostat is used concomitantly with potent inducers of CYP3A. Simulations using a physiologically based pharmacokinetic model suggest that systemic exposure of panobinostat may be decreased by approximately 70% in the presence of a potent CYP3A inducer (e.g., rifampin). Concomitant use of panobinostat and potent inducers of CYP3A should be avoided.

Substrates of CYP2D6 In patients with advanced cancer, panobinostat increased the median peak plasma concentration and AUC of the CYP2D6 substrate dextromethorphan by approximately 80 and 60%, respectively, but the extent of change in dextromethorphan exposure was highly variable. Concomitant use of panobinostat with sensitive CYP2D6 substrates (e.g., atomoxetine, desipramine, dextromethorphan, metoprolol, nebivolol, perphenazine, tolterodine, venlafaxine) or CYP2D6 substrates with a narrow therapeutic index (e.g., thioridazine, pimozide) should be avoided. If concomitant use of panobinostat and CYP2D6 substrates cannot be avoided, patients should be monitored frequently for adverse reactions.

Substrates of CYP3A Simulations using a physiologically based pharmacokinetic model suggest that panobinostat may increase exposure of the CYP3A substrate midazolam by less than 10%; the clinical relevance of this finding is unknown.

■ **Drugs that Prolong QT Interval** Concomitant use of antiarrhythmic agents (e.g., amiodarone, disopyramide, procainamide, quinidine, sotalol) or other drugs known to prolong the QT interval (e.g., chloroquine, clarithromycin, methadone, moxifloxacin, pimozide) with panobinostat is not recommended. The manufacturer states that antiemetic agents that are known to prolong the QT interval (e.g., dolasetron, ondansetron, tropisetron) may be used concomitantly with frequent ECG monitoring.

■ **Drugs that Affect Gastric pH** Although aqueous solubility of panobinostat is pH dependent, with higher pH resulting in lower solubility, simulations using a physiologically based pharmacokinetic model suggest that changes in gastric pH will not substantially alter oral absorption of panobinostat.

Description

Panobinostat, a histone deacetylase (HDAC) inhibitor, is an antineoplastic agent. HDAC enzymes catalyze the removal of acetyl groups from the lysine residues of proteins, including histones and transcription factors. Overexpression of HDAC enzymes or aberrant recruitment of HDAC enzymes to oncogenic transcription factors causing hypoacetylation of core nucleosomal histones has been observed in some cancer cells. Hypoacetylation of histones is associated with a condensed chromatin structure and repression of gene transcription. Inhibition of HDAC activity allows for the accumulation of acetyl groups on histone lysine residues, resulting in an open chromatin structure and transcriptional activation. Panobinostat inhibits the enzymatic activity of HDAC isoforms in classes I, II, and IV at low nanomolar concentrations. In vitro, panobinostat causes the accumulation of acetylated histones and other proteins and induces cell cycle arrest and/or apoptosis of some transformed cells. Increased levels of acetylated histones have been observed in xenografts from mice treated with panobinostat.

Panobinostat is extensively metabolized via reduction, hydrolysis, oxidation, and glucuronidation. Metabolism by cytochrome P-450 (CYP) isoenzyme 3A accounts for approximately 40% of the total hepatic panobinostat elimination; minor contributions from CYP 2D6 and 2C19 have been observed in vitro. In vitro, uridine diphosphate-glucuronosyl transferase (UGT) 1A1, 1A3, 1A7, 1A8, 1A9, and 2B4 contribute to the glucuronidation of the drug. Panobinostat is excreted in feces (44–77%) and urine (29–51%), mainly as metabolites; only a small portion of a dose is excreted as unchanged drug (less than 3.5% in feces and less than 2.5% in urine). The terminal elimination half-life of panobinostat in patients with advanced cancer is approximately 37 hours.

Advice to Patients

Importance of instructing patients to read the manufacturer's medication guide carefully before starting panobinostat therapy and each time the prescription is refilled.

Importance of advising patients to take panobinostat exactly as prescribed and not to alter the dose or discontinue the drug without first consulting their clinician.

Importance of advising patients that a missed dose should be taken as soon as possible, up to 12 hours after the scheduled administration time. If a dose is vomited, the dose should not be repeated; instead, the next dose should be taken at the regularly scheduled time.

Importance of swallowing the capsules whole and of not opening, crushing, or chewing capsules. If powder from the capsules accidentally contacts the skin or eyes, importance of washing the skin with soap and water or flushing the eyes with water.

Risk of cardiac toxicity and ECG changes; importance of advising patients to report chest pain or discomfort, changes in heart rate, palpitations, lightheadedness, fainting, dizziness, blue discoloration of lips, shortness of breath, and swelling of lower limbs or skin.

Risk of thrombocytopenia and bleeding. Importance of advising patients to immediately contact their clinician if they experience any episodes or observe any signs or symptoms of bleeding; importance of informing patients that it might take longer than usual for bleeding to stop.

Importance of advising patients that regular blood tests will be performed to monitor blood cell counts and chemistries.

Risk of neutropenia and potentially severe and life-threatening infections. Importance of advising patients to contact their clinician immediately if they develop a fever or any other signs or symptoms of infection.

Risk of severe nausea, vomiting, and diarrhea, which may require treatment. Importance of advising patients to contact their clinician at the onset of diarrhea, if persistent vomiting occurs, or if signs of dehydration are present, and to consult with their clinician prior to taking medications with laxative properties.

Risk of fetal harm. Importance of advising women of childbearing potential to avoid pregnancy while receiving panobinostat. Sexually active women should be advised to use effective contraception while receiving the drug and for at least 1 month after the last dose. Sexually active men should be advised to use condoms while receiving panobinostat and for at least 3 months after the last dose.

Importance of advising women not to breast-feed while taking panobinostat.

Importance of informing clinicians of existing or contemplated concomitant therapy, including prescription and OTC drugs and herbal supplements, as well as any concomitant illnesses. Importance of avoiding star fruit and pomegranate or grapefruit products.

Importance of informing patients of other precautionary information. (See Cautions.)

Overview® (see Users Guide). For additional information on this drug until a more detailed monograph is developed and published, the manufacturer's labeling should be consulted. It is *essential* that the manufacturer's labeling be consulted for more detailed information on usual cautions, precautions, contraindications, potential drug interactions, laboratory test interferences, and acute toxicity. For further information on the handling of antineoplastic agents, see the ASHP Guidelines on Handling Hazardous Drugs at http://www.ahfsdruginformation.com.

Preparations

Distribution of panobinostat is restricted. (See Restricted Distribution under Dosage and Administration: General.)

Excipients in commercially available drug preparations may have clinically important effects in some individuals; consult specific product labeling for details.

Panobinostat Lactate

Oral		
Capsules	10 mg (of panobinostat)	Farydak®, Novartis
	15 mg (of panobinostat)	Farydak®, Novartis
	20 mg (of panobinostat)	Farydak®, Novartis

PAZOPanib Hydrochloride

■ Pazopanib hydrochloride, an inhibitor of multiple receptor tyrosine kinases, is an antineoplastic agent.

Uses

■ **Renal Cell Carcinoma** Pazopanib hydrochloride is used for the treatment of advanced renal cell carcinoma.

The current indication for pazopanib hydrochloride is based principally on the results of a randomized, double-blind, placebo-controlled, multicenter, phase 3 study (VEG105192) in 435 patients 18 years of age and older (median age: 59 years) with locally advanced and/or metastatic clear-cell (or predominantly clear-cell) renal cell carcinoma. This study initially enrolled patients whose disease had progressed following one prior cytokine-based regimen (i.e., aldesleukin, interferon alfa); the study protocol was subsequently amended (after enrollment of 7 patients) to include patients who had received no prior therapy (treatment-naive patients). Because other drugs (e.g., sorafenib, sunitinib) had been approved in the US for treatment of renal cell carcinoma, the US Food and Drug Administration (FDA) expressed concerns about the use of a placebo control, and agreement was not reached on the study design. The VEG105192 study, thus, was conducted outside of the US in countries where patients did not have access to established therapies (e.g., aldesleukin, interferon alfa, sorafenib, sunitinib) or where cytokines were not recognized as standard treatment for renal cell carcinoma.

In this study, 435 patients (233 treatment-naive and 202 cytokine-pretreated patients) were randomized in a 2:1 ratio to receive either pazopanib (800 mg daily) or placebo along with best supportive care. Treatment in both groups was continued until disease progression, unacceptable toxicity, death, or discontinuance of therapy for other reasons occurred; upon disease progression, patients previously randomized to receive placebo were permitted to cross over to open-label pazopanib. The median duration of treatment was 7.4 or 3.8 months in patients randomized to receive pazopanib or placebo, respectively. Enrolled patients had clear cell histology (90%) or predominantly clear cell histology (10%); 88–89% had undergone nephrectomy, and approximately 50% had metastatic disease involving 3 or more organs. Radiographic assessment of efficacy was performed every 6 weeks during the first 24 weeks of therapy and then every 8 weeks thereafter. The primary measure of efficacy was progression-free survival; the secondary end points included overall survival, overall response rate, and duration of response.

The median progression-free survival in the overall population was 9.2 months in patients receiving pazopanib compared with 4.2 months in those receiving placebo; the effect size appeared to be larger in the treatment-naive subgroup (11.1 versus 2.8 months) but also was clinically important in the cytokine-pretreated subgroup (7.4 versus 4.2 months). Improved progression-free survival was observed in patients receiving pazopanib regardless of Memorial Sloan-Kettering Cancer Center (MSKCC) risk category, gender, age, or ECOG performance status. The overall response rate for all patients receiving pazopanib was 30%, and the median duration of response was 58.7 weeks. Response rates were similar among treatment-naive (32%) and cytokine-pretreated (29%) subgroups of patients who received pazopanib. The median time to response was 11.9 weeks. At the time of data analysis, patients had not been followed for a sufficient time too establish the effects of the drug on overall survival; despite an observed favorable (albeit not statistically significant) trend in improved overall survival, some clinicians anticipate that crossover from placebo to pazopanib therapy at the time of disease progression, along with improved access to other therapies (e.g., vascular endothelial growth factor receptor [VEGFR] inhibitors, mammalian target of rapamycin [mTOR] inhibitors), will confound the data, making analysis of overall survival difficult.

A randomized study comparing pazopanib with sunitinib as first-line treatment for advanced and/or metastatic renal cell carcinoma is under way.

Dosage and Administration

■ **Administration** Pazopanib hydrochloride is administered orally once daily. The drug should be administered without food (i.e., at least 1 hour before or 2 hours after a meal). Pazopanib hydrochloride tablets should be swallowed whole and should not be crushed; crushing the tablets has been shown to increase the rate of absorption and systemic exposure to the drug. (See Description.)

■ **Dosage** Dosage of pazopanib hydrochloride is expressed in terms of pazopanib.

The recommended adult dosage of pazopanib for the treatment of advanced renal cell carcinoma is 800 mg once daily. The dosage should not exceed 800 mg daily. Therapy should be continued for as long as the patient derives clinical benefit from the drug or until unacceptable toxicity occurs. In the VEG105192 study, patients received pazopanib hydrochloride for a median duration of 7.4 months.

Dosage adjustments should be considered if hepatotoxicity occurs or when pazopanib is used in conjunction with potent inhibitors of cytochrome P-450 (CYP) isoenzyme 3A4. (See Dosage Modification under Dosage and Administration: Dosage.)

Dosage Modification When dosage modification is necessary, dosage of pazopanib generally should be reduced by 400 mg daily initially; subsequent dosage adjustments should be made in increments or decrements of 200 mg daily, depending on individual patient tolerability.

Hepatotoxicity. Liver function tests should be performed prior to initiation of pazopanib, at least once every 4 weeks for at least the first 4 months of therapy or as clinically indicated, and periodically thereafter. If hepatotoxicity occurs, pazopanib dosage should be reduced, or therapy should be interrupted or permanently discontinued. (See Table 1.)

Table 1. Recommended Dosage Modifications for Hepatotoxicity

ALT (SGPT) and/or Bilirubin Concentrations	Recommended Action
Serum ALT concentration 3–8 times the upper limit of normal (ULN)	Continue pazopanib; monitor liver function weekly until serum ALT concentration returns to grade 1 or baseline
Serum ALT concentration >8 times the ULN	Interrupt pazopanib therapy until serum ALT concentration returns to grade 1 or baseline; if benefit outweighs risk, reinitiate pazopanib at a reduced dosage of 400 mg or less once daily; following reinitiation, monitor liver function weekly for 8 weeks; if serum ALT concentration rises to >3 times the ULN, discontinue pazopanib *permanently*
Serum ALT concentration >3 times the ULN *and* mild, indirect (unconjugated) hyperbilirubinemia in patients with known Gilbert's syndrome	Manage per recommendations for patients with isolated serum ALT elevations
Serum ALT concentration >3 times the ULN *and* serum bilirubin concentration >2 times the ULN	Discontinue pazopanib *permanently*; monitor liver function until hepatotoxicity resolves

Concomitant Use with Drugs Affecting Hepatic Microsomal Enzymes. Concomitant use of pazopanib with potent inhibitors of CYP3A4 may result in increased plasma concentrations of pazopanib and should be *avoided*. (See Drug Interactions: Drugs and Foods Affecting Hepatic Microsomal Enzymes.) If concomitant use with a potent CYP3A4 inhibitor cannot be avoided, the manufacturer recommends reducing the dosage of pazopanib to 400 mg daily. This dosage is predicted to adjust the area under the plasma concentration-time curve (AUC) of pazopanib to the range observed in the absence of CYP3A4 inhibitors; however, there are no clinical data with use of this dosage in patients concomitantly receiving potent CYP3A4 inhibitors. The manufacturer states that further reductions in pazopanib dosage may be required if adverse effects occur during therapy.

Concomitant use of pazopanib with potent inducers of CYP3A4 may result in decreased plasma concentrations of pazopanib and should be *avoided*. (See Drug Interactions: Drugs and Foods Affecting Hepatic Microsomal Enzymes.)

■ **Special Populations** No dosage adjustment is necessary in patients with mild hepatic impairment (total serum bilirubin concentration not exceeding 1.5 times the ULN with any level of ALT). The manufacturer recommends that dosage of pazopanib be reduced to 200 mg once daily in patients with moderate hepatic impairment (total serum bilirubin concentration exceeding 1.5 times, but not more than 3 times, the ULN with any level of ALT). Safety of pazopanib has not been established in patients with severe hepatic impairment (total serum bilirubin concentration exceeding 3 times the ULN with any level of ALT); therefore, the manufacturer recommends that the drug *not* be used in such patients.

Renal impairment is not expected to influence pazopanib exposure; therefore, the manufacturer states that dosage adjustment is not necessary in patients with renal impairment.

Cautions

■ **Contraindications** The manufacturer states there are no known contraindications to the use of pazopanib.

■ **Warnings/Precautions** ***Warnings*** **Hepatic Effects.** Severe or fatal hepatotoxicity, manifested as increases in serum concentrations of aminotransferases (ALT [SGPT], AST [SGOT]) and bilirubin, has been reported in patients receiving pazopanib. Most (92.5%) cases of aminotransferase elevations (of any grade) occurred during the first 18 weeks of therapy. In the randomized, placebo-controlled study (VEG105192) in patients with renal cell carcinoma, increases in ALT concentrations exceeding 3 or 10 times the upper limit of normal (ULN) were reported in approximately 18 or 4%, respectively, of patients receiving pazopanib. Concurrent increases in concentrations of ALT (exceeding 3 times the ULN) *and* bilirubin (exceeding twice the ULN) in the absence of substantial (exceeding 3 times the ULN) increases in alkaline phosphatase concentrations were reported in approximately 2% of patients receiving pazopanib. In an analysis of data from 11 studies involving 977 patients who received pazopanib as a single agent for a variety of tumor types (including 586 patients with renal cell carcinoma), death (resulting from disease progression and hepatic failure) occurred in approximately 0.2% of patients receiving pazopanib.

Because pazopanib inhibits uridine diphosphate-glucuronosyltransferase (UGT) 1A1 (an enzyme that catalyzes the glucuronidation of bilirubin for elimination), mild elevations in indirect (unconjugated) bilirubin may occur in patients with deficient glucuronidation of bilirubin (i.e., Gilbert's syndrome). (See Description.)

Liver function tests should be performed prior to initiation of pazopanib, at least once every 4 weeks for at least the first 4 months of therapy or as clinically indicated, and periodically thereafter. If hepatotoxicity occurs, pazopanib dosage should be reduced, or therapy should be interrupted or permanently discontinued. (See Hepatotoxicity under Dosage: Dosage Modification, in Dosage and Administration.)

Other Warnings and Precautions **Prolongation of QT Interval and Torsades de Pointes.** Prolongation of the QT interval and torsades de pointes have been reported in patients receiving pazopanib. In the VEG105192 study, prolongation of the QT interval (500–549 msec) was reported in approximately 1 or 0% of patients receiving pazopanib or placebo, respectively. In an analysis of pooled data from 3 studies involving 558 patients with renal cell carcinoma, prolongation of the QT interval (500 msec or greater) or torsades de pointes was reported in approximately 2% or less than 1%, respectively, of patients receiving pazopanib.

Pazopanib should be used with caution in patients with a history of prolongation of the QT interval, in patients receiving antiarrhythmic agents or other drugs that cause prolongation of the QT interval, and in patients with relevant preexisting cardiac disease. ECG should be monitored prior to initiation of pazopanib and periodically during treatment; serum electrolytes (e.g., calcium, magnesium, potassium) should be maintained within the normal range.

Hemorrhage. Hemorrhage, sometimes severe or fatal, has been reported in patients receiving pazopanib. In the VEG105192 study, hemorrhage was reported in approximately 13 or 5% of patients receiving pazopanib or placebo, respectively. The most common hemorrhagic events reported with pazopanib in this study included hematuria, epistaxis, hemoptysis, and rectal hemorrhage; severe hemorrhagic events included pulmonary, GI, and genitourinary hemorrhage. Fatal hemorrhage was reported in approximately 1 or 0% of patients receiving pazopanib or placebo, respectively. In an analysis of pooled data from 3 studies involving 586 patients with renal cell carcinoma, hemorrhage (all grades) or grade 3–5 hemorrhage was reported in approximately 16 or 2%, respectively, of patients receiving pazopanib; cerebral/intracranial hemorrhage or fatal hemorrhage was reported in less than 1% or approximately 1%, respectively, of patients receiving pazopanib.

Pazopanib has not been evaluated in patients with a history of hemoptysis or patients with cerebral or clinically important GI hemorrhage within the past 6 months; therefore, the manufacturer recommends that pazopanib be *avoided* in such patients.

Thromboembolism. Arterial thromboembolic events, sometimes severe or fatal, have been reported in patients receiving pazopanib. In the VEG105192 study, myocardial infarction/ischemia, cerebrovascular accident, or transient ischemic attack (TIA) was reported in approximately 2, less than 1, or 1%, respectively, of patients receiving pazopanib, compared with 0% of patients receiving placebo. In an analysis of pooled data from 3 studies involving 586 patients with renal cell carcinoma, thromboembolic events (i.e., myocardial infarction, angina, ischemic stroke, transient ischemic attacks) (all grades) or grade 3–5 events were reported in approximately 3 or 2%, respectively, of patients receiving pazopanib; fatal arterial thromboembolism was reported in approximately 0.3% of patients receiving pazopanib.

Pazopanib should be used with caution in patients who are at increased risk or who have a history of arterial thromboembolic events. Pazopanib has not been evaluated in patients who had experienced an arterial thromboembolic event within the past 6 months; therefore, the manufacturer recommends that pazopanib be *avoided* in such patients.

GI Effects. GI perforation or fistula, sometimes fatal, has been reported in patients receiving pazopanib. In an analysis of pooled data from 3 studies involving 586 patients with renal cell carcinoma, GI perforation or fistula was reported in approximately 0.9% of patients receiving pazopanib; fatal perforation was reported in approximately 0.3% of patients receiving pazopanib.

Pazopanib should be used with caution in patients at increased risk for GI perforation or fistula formation. Patients receiving pazopanib should be monitored for manifestations of GI perforation or fistula formation.

Hypertension. Hypertension (systolic blood pressure of 150 mm Hg or greater or diastolic blood pressure of 100 mm Hg or greater) has been reported in patients receiving pazopanib. Most (88%) cases occurred during the first 18 weeks of therapy. In the VEG105192 study, hypertension was reported in approximately 40 or 10% of patients receiving pazopanib or placebo, respectively; grade 3 hypertension was reported in approximately 4 or less than 1% of patients receiving pazopanib or placebo, respectively. In an analysis of pooled data from 3 studies involving 586 patients with renal cell carcinoma, hypertension was reported in approximately 47% of patients, and hypertensive crisis was reported in at least one patient receiving pazopanib. The majority of hypertension cases were managed with antihypertensive therapy or by reduction in pazopanib dosage.

Blood pressure should be adequately controlled prior to initiation of pazopanib. Patients receiving pazopanib should be monitored for hypertension and treated with antihypertensive therapy as needed. If hypertension persists despite use of antihypertensive therapy, dosage of pazopanib may be reduced (i.e., by 400 mg daily initially, then by 200 mg daily, depending on individual patient tolerability). If hypertension is severe or persistent despite use of antihypertensive therapy *and* reduction of pazopanib dosage, pazopanib should be discontinued.

Wound-healing Complications. The effect of pazopanib on wound healing has not been established. Because inhibitors of vascular endothelial growth factor receptor (VEGFR), including pazopanib, may impair wound healing, pazopanib should be discontinued at least 7 days prior to scheduled surgery; the decision to resume pazopanib therapy postoperatively should be based on clinical assessment of the adequacy of wound healing. If wound dehiscence occurs, pazopanib should be discontinued.

Hypothyroidism. Hypothyroidism has been reported in patients receiving pazopanib. In the VEG105192 study, increases in thyroid-stimulating hormone (TSH) concentrations were reported in 27 or 5% of patients receiving pazopanib or placebo, respectively; hypothyroidism was reported in 7 or 0% of patients receiving pazopanib or placebo, respectively. In an analysis of pooled data from 3 studies involving 586 patients with renal cell carcinoma, hypothyroidism was reported in 4% of patients receiving pazopanib.

Proactive monitoring of thyroid function tests is recommended.

Proteinuria. Proteinuria has been reported in patients receiving pazopanib. In the VEG105192 study, proteinuria was reported in 9% of patients receiving pazopanib. In an analysis of pooled data from 3 studies involving 586 patients with renal cell carcinoma, proteinuria (all grades) was reported in approximately 8% of patients, and grade 3 or grade 4 proteinuria each was reported in less than 1% of patients.

Urinalysis should be performed prior to initiation of pazopanib and periodically during therapy. If grade 4 proteinuria occurs, pazopanib should be discontinued.

Fetal/Neonatal Morbidity and Mortality. Pazopanib may cause fetal harm; the drug has been shown to be teratogenic, embryotoxic, fetotoxic, and abortifacient in animals. There are no adequate and well-controlled studies in pregnant women. Pregnancy should be avoided during therapy. If used during pregnancy or if the patient becomes pregnant while receiving pazopanib, the patient should be apprised of the potential fetal hazard.

Adequate Patient Evaluation and Monitoring. Liver function tests, ECG, electrolytes, blood pressure, and urinalysis should be monitored prior to initiation of pazopanib and periodically during therapy. Proactive monitoring of thyroid function tests is recommended.

Specific Populations **Pregnancy.** Category D. (See Fetal/Neonatal Morbidity and Mortality under Warnings/Precautions: Other Warnings and Precautions, in Cautions , and also see Users Guide.)

Lactation. It is not known whether pazopanib is distributed into human milk. Because many drugs are distributed into human milk and because of the potential for serious adverse reactions to pazopanib in nursing infants, a decision should be made whether to discontinue nursing or the drug, taking into account the importance of the drug to the woman.

Pediatric Use. Safety and efficacy have not been established in pediatric patients younger than 18 years of age.

Geriatric Use. In an analysis of pooled data from 3 studies involving 586 patients with renal cell carcinoma, 33% of patients were 65 years of age and older, and 6% were older than 75 years of age. Although no overall differences in safety or efficacy were observed in geriatric patients, patients older than 60 years of age may be at greater risk of hepatotoxicity (i.e., serum ALT concentration exceeding 3 times the ULN). Other reported clinical experience has not identified differences in responses between geriatric and younger patients, but greater sensitivity in some older patients cannot be ruled out.

Hepatic Impairment. The safety and pharmacokinetic profile of pazopanib have not been fully established in patients with hepatic impairment. In clinical studies with pazopanib, only patients with bilirubin concentrations not exceeding 1.5 times the ULN *and* aminotransferase (ALT, AST) concentrations not exceeding twice the ULN were included. An analysis of pharmacokinetic data indicated that pazopanib clearance in patients with mild hepatic impairment (total serum bilirubin concentration not exceeding 1.5 times the ULN with any level of ALT) was similar to that in patients with normal hepatic function. Pazopanib clearance was decreased by 50% in patients with moderate hepatic impairment (total serum bilirubin concentration exceeding 1.5 times, but not more than 3 times, the ULN with any level of ALT) compared with that in patients with normal hepatic function, and the maximum tolerated dosage in such patients was 200 mg daily; therefore, dosage adjustment is necessary in patients with moderate hepatic impairment. (See Dosage and Administration: Special Populations.) The safety and pharmacokinetics of pazopanib in patients with severe hepatic impairment have not been established; therefore, the manufacturer recommends that pazopanib *not* be used this patient population.

Renal Impairment. In a population pharmacokinetic analysis involving patients with various cancers, creatinine clearances of 30–150 mL/minute did not substantially affect clearance of pazopanib. The safety, efficacy, and pharmacokinetic profile of pazopanib have not been established in patients with severe renal impairment (creatinine clearance less than 30 mL/minute) or in patients undergoing peritoneal dialysis or hemodialysis. Because renal impairment is unlikely to affect the pharmacokinetics (e.g., exposure) of pazopanib (i.e., less than 4% of a radiolabeled oral dose of pazopanib is recovered in urine), the manufacturer states that no dosage adjustment is necessary in patients with renal impairment.

■ **Common Adverse Effects** Adverse effects reported in 10% or more of patients receiving pazopanib in the VEG105192 study include diarrhea, hypertension, hair color changes (depigmentation), nausea, anorexia, vomiting, fatigue, asthenia, abdominal pain, and headache.

Laboratory abnormalities reported in more than 10% of patients receiving pazopanib in the VEG105192 study that occurred more frequently (5% or more) than with placebo include increased aminotransferase (ALT, AST) concentrations, increased glucose concentrations, leukopenia, increased bilirubin concentrations, neutropenia, decreased phosphorus concentrations, thrombocytopenia, lymphocytopenia, decreased sodium concentrations, decreased magnesium concentrations, and decreased glucose concentrations.

Drug Interactions

Pazopanib is metabolized principally by cytochrome P-450 (CYP) isoenzyme 3A4 and, to a lesser extent, by CYP isoenzymes 1A2 and 2C8. Results of drug interaction studies in cancer patients suggest that pazopanib is a weak inhibitor of CYP isoenzymes 3A4, 2C8, and 2D6 but has no effect on CYP isoenzymes 1A2, 2C9, or 2C19. In vitro studies indicate that pazopanib also may induce CYP3A4.

In vitro studies indicate that pazopanib inhibits uridine diphosphate-glucuronosyltransferase (UGT) 1A1 and organic anion transport protein (OATP) 1B1; the drug appears to be a substrate of P-glycoprotein (Pgp) and breast cancer resistant protein (BCRP).

■ **Drugs and Foods Affecting Hepatic Microsomal Enzymes** Inhibitors of CYP3A4: Pharmacokinetic interaction (increased peak plasma concentrations and area under the plasma concentration-time curve [AUC] of pazopanib) observed during concomitant use of pazopanib ophthalmic solution with ketoconazole (a potent inhibitor of CYP3A4 and an inhibitor of Pgp) or during concomitant use of pazopanib oral tablets with lapatinib (a substrate and weak inhibitor of CYP3A4, Pgp, and BCRP). Concomitant use of pazopanib with a *potent* CYP3A4 inhibitor (e.g., clarithromycin, ketoconazole, ritonavir) should be *avoided*; if concomitant use cannot be avoided, pazopanib dosage should be reduced. (See Concomitant Use with Drugs Affecting Hepatic Microsomal Enzymes under Dosage: Dosage Modification, in Dosage and Administration.) The manufacturer states that concomitant use with grapefruit or grapefruit juice also should be *avoided*.

Inducers of CYP3A4: Potential pharmacokinetic interaction (decreased plasma concentrations of pazopanib). Concomitant use of pazopanib with a potent inducer of CYP3A4 (e.g., rifampin) should be *avoided*, and selection of an alternative agent with minimal or no enzyme induction potential should be considered. If long-term use of a potent CYP3A4 inducer is required, pazopanib should not be initiated.

■ **Drugs Metabolized by Hepatic Microsomal Enzymes** Substrates of CYP isoenzymes 3A4, 2D6, or 2C8: Pharmacokinetic interaction (increased exposure to substrate) observed during concomitant use with midazolam (a CYP3A4 substrate), dextromethorphan (a CYP2D6 substrate), or paclitaxel (a CYP3A4 and CYP2C8 substrate). Concomitant use with substrates of CYP isoenzymes 3A4, 2D6, or 2C8 that have a narrow therapeutic index is not recommended.

Substrates of CYP isoenzymes 1A2, 2C9, or 2C19: No clinically relevant pharmacokinetic interaction with caffeine (a CYP1A2 substrate), warfarin (a CYP2C9 substrate), or omeprazole (a CYP2C19 substrate).

■ **Drugs Transported by Organic Anion Transport Protein (OATP)** Potential pharmacokinetic interaction (increased plasma concentration of drugs transported by OATP1B1).

■ **Drugs Metabolized by Uridine Diphosphate-glucuronosyltransferase (UGT)** Potential pharmacokinetic interaction (increased plasma concentration of drugs metabolized by UGT1A1).

■ **Drugs that Prolong the QT Interval** Risk of prolonged QT interval and torsades de pointes. Pazopanib should be used with caution in patients receiving antiarrhythmic agents or other drugs that cause prolongation of the QT interval. (See Prolongation of QT Interval and Torsades de Pointes under Warnings/Precautions: Other Warnings and Precautions, in Cautions.)

Description

Pazopanib hydrochloride, an inhibitor of multiple receptor tyrosine kinases, is an antineoplastic agent. Receptor tyrosine kinases (RTKs) are involved in the initiation of various cascades of intracellular signaling events that lead to cell proliferation and/or influence processes critical to cell survival and tumor progression (e.g., angiogenesis, metastasis, inhibition of apoptosis), based on the respective kinase. Pazopanib inhibits signal transduction pathways involving multiple receptor tyrosine kinases, principally vascular endothelial growth factor receptors (i.e., VEGFR-1, VEGFR-2, VEGFR-3), platelet-derived growth factor receptors (i.e., PDGFR-α, PDGFR-β), and stem cell factor receptor (i.e., c-Kit); the drug has modest inhibitory effects on fibroblast growth factor receptors (i.e., FGFR1, FGFR3), transmembrane glycoprotein receptor tyrosine kinase (c-Fms), leukocyte-specific protein tyrosine kinase (Lck), and interleukin-2 receptor inducible T-cell kinase (Itk). In vitro, pazopanib has been shown to inhibit ligand-induced autophosphorylation of VEGFR-2, PDGFR-β, and c-Kit. In vivo, pazopanib inhibited VEGF-induced VEGFR-2 phosphorylation in mouse lungs and in human umbilical vein endothelial cells (HUVEC), angiogenesis in a mouse model, and the growth of some human tumor xenografts in mice.

Pazopanib appears to be as potent as sorafenib and sunitinib against VEGFR (i.e., VEGFR-1, VEGFR-2, VEGFR-3) and less potent than sunitinib against fms-like tyrosine kinase 3 (Flt-3). Differences in potencies against non-VEGF receptors may account for variabilities in non-VEGFR-related ("off-target") adverse effects observed with pazopanib (e.g., hepatotoxicity, lower incidence of palmar-plantar erythrodysesthesia [hand-foot syndrome] and rash compared with sorafenib or sunitinib [based on indirect cross-study comparison], lower incidence of and less severe myelosuppression compared with sunitinib [based on indirect cross-study comparison]). The relatively lower incidence of and less severe myelosuppressive effects reported with pazopanib may be explained, in part, by the drug's lower potency against Flt-3 (a regulator of hematopoiesis).

Pazopanib is incompletely absorbed from the GI tract, with reported bioavailabilities of 14–39%. Following oral administration, peak plasma concentrations of pazopanib occurred at a median of 2–4 hours. Administration of a single 400-mg crushed tablet increased the peak plasma concentrations and area under the plasma concentration-time curve (AUC) by approximately twofold and 46%, respectively, and decreased the time to peak plasma concentrations by approximately 2 hours, compared with administration of the whole tablet. Administration of pazopanib with food (i.e., low-fat or high-fat meal) resulted in an approximately twofold increase in peak plasma concentrations and AUC of the drug. Pazopanib is more than 99% bound to plasma proteins; in vitro studies suggest that pazopanib is a substrate of P-glycoprotein (Pgp) and breast cancer resistant protein (BCRP). Pazopanib is metabolized by the cytochrome P-450 (CYP) microsomal enzyme system, principally by the isoenzyme 3A4 (CYP3A4) and, to a lesser extent, by CYP1A2 and CYP2C8 (see Drug Interactions); in plasma, pazopanib metabolites accounted for less than 10% of the administered dose. The mean half-life of pazopanib is approximately 30.9 hours. Approximately 82% of a radiolabeled dose of pazopanib is excreted in feces (67% of which is unchanged drug), and less than 4% is eliminated in urine. Hemodialysis is not expected to enhance elimination of pazopanib because the drug is highly bound to plasma proteins and is not substantially excreted renally.

Pazopanib inhibits uridine diphosphate-glucuronosyltransferase (UGT) 1A1, an enzyme that catalyzes the glucuronidation of bilirubin for elimination. Patients who are homozygous for the UGT1A1*28 allele (characterized by a mutation in the promoter region of the UGT1A1 gene) have reduced expression of UGT1A1, which may manifest as mild hyperbilirubinemia (i.e., Gilbert's syndrome). Mild elevations of indirect (unconjugated) bilirubin concentrations may occur in patients with Gilbert's syndrome receiving pazopanib. A pooled pharmacogenetic analysis of 236 Caucasian patients that evaluated the polymorphisms of UGT1A1 and its potential association with hyperbilirubinemia during pazopanib treatment found that the (TA)7/(TA)7 genotype (UGT1A1*28/*28, underlying genetic susceptibility to Gilbert's syndrome) was associated with an increase in the risk of hyperbilirubinemia relative to the (TA)6/(TA)6 and (TA)6/(TA)7 genotypes.

Advice to Patients

Pazopanib medication guide should be provided to the patient each time the drug is dispensed; importance of patient reading the medication guide prior to initiating pazopanib therapy and each time the prescription is refilled.

Importance of taking pazopanib hydrochloride tablets without food (i.e., at least 1 hour before or 2 hours after a meal). Importance of swallowing the tablets whole and not crushing the tablets. Avoid grapefruit or grapefruit juice while taking the drug.

If a dose of pazopanib is missed by less than 12 hours, the dose should be taken as soon as it is remembered, and the next dose should be taken at the regularly scheduled time. Do not take more than one dose at a time.

Risk of adverse hepatic effects. Importance of immediately reporting any manifestations of hepatotoxicity (e.g., jaundice, unusual fatigue, unusual darkening of urine, nausea, vomiting, loss of appetite, right-upper quadrant pain, easy bruising).

Risk of adverse cardiovascular effects. Importance of monitoring blood pressure regularly during therapy. Importance of immediately reporting irregular or fast heart beat, fainting, or manifestations of a heart attack or stroke (e.g., chest pain or pressure; pain in arms, back, neck, or jaw; shortness of breath; numbness or weakness on one side of body; trouble talking; headache; dizziness).

Risk of bleeding. Importance of promptly informing clinicians of any unusual bleeding, bruising, or wounds that do not heal.

Risk of adverse GI effects (e.g., diarrhea, nausea, vomiting, GI perforation). Importance of understanding measures to manage mild diarrhea and notifying clinician if moderate or severe diarrhea occurs. Importance of immediately reporting any manifestations of GI perforation (e.g., abdominal pain or swelling, vomiting blood, black sticky stools).

Risk of depigmentation of hair and skin.

Importance of women informing clinicians if they are or plan to become pregnant or plan to breast-feed. Apprise patient of potential hazard to the fetus if used during pregnancy; women of childbearing potential should avoid becoming pregnant.

Importance of informing clinicians of existing or contemplated concomitant therapy, including prescription and OTC drugs and dietary or herbal supplements, as well as any concomitant illnesses (e.g., cardiovascular disease, hepatic impairment).

Importance of informing patients of other important precautionary information. (See Cautions.)

Overview® (see Users Guide). For additional information on this drug until a more detailed monograph is developed and published, the manufacturer's labeling should be consulted. It is *essential* that the manufacturer's labeling be consulted for more detailed information on usual cautions, precautions, contraindications, potential drug interactions, laboratory test interferences, and acute toxicity.

Preparations

Excipients in commercially available drug preparations may have clinically important effects in some individuals; consult specific product labeling for details.

PAZOPanib Hydrochloride

Oral

Tablets, film-coated	200 mg (of pazopanib)	**Votrient®**, GlaxoSmithKline

Pegaspargase

PEG-L-asparaginase

■ Pegaspargase, an *Escherichia coli*-derived asparaginase enzyme that is conjugated with polyethylene glycol (PEG), is an antineoplastic agent.

Uses

■ **Acute Lymphocytic Leukemia** ***First-line Therapy for Acute Lymphocytic Leukemia*** Pegaspargase is used as a component of combination chemotherapy for the first-line treatment of childhood and adult acute lymphocytic (lymphoblastic) leukemia (ALL). Pegaspargase is used as a component of induction therapy; the drug also is used as a component of intensification (consolidation) treatment regimens administered following achievement of remission and prior to initiation of maintenance therapy.

Various drugs have been used for combination chemotherapy of childhood and adult ALL, and comparative efficacy of these regimens is continually being evaluated. Treatment of ALL typically includes remission induction therapy, followed by intensification (consolidation) therapy, and then 2–3 years of maintenance therapy (e.g., methotrexate and mercaptopurine with or without pulses of vincristine and prednisone). The intensity of both induction and postinduction therapies is based on assessment of the patient's risk of relapse. Additional therapy (e.g., intrathecal administration of methotrexate with or without intrathecal cytarabine and hydrocortisone, with or without systemic methotrexate and leucovorin rescue in children; intrathecal methotrexate given alone or in conjunction with cranial radiation or systemic methotrexate and leucovorin rescue in adults) is needed for prophylaxis of CNS involvement (meningeal leukemia) in patients with ALL. Other regimens are preferred in certain subsets of patients with ALL (e.g., B-cell ALL, T-cell ALL, Philadelphia chromosome-positive ALL). Certain patients with a poor prognosis or with a poor response to initial treatment may be candidates for hematopoietic stem cell transplantation. Specialized references and experts should be consulted for additional information.

An asparaginase preparation is used in combination with a corticosteroid (dexamethasone or prednisone) and vincristine as an induction regimen for non-high-risk childhood ALL. The use of intensive induction regimens with 4 or more drugs, including an asparaginase preparation, a corticosteroid (e.g., prednisone), vincristine, and an anthracycline (e.g., daunorubicin), with or without cyclophosphamide, may improve the rate of event-free survival but is associated with greater toxicity. An induction regimen containing 4 or more drugs does not appear to be necessary to achieve favorable outcomes in patients at low or standard risk of treatment failure provided adequate intensification therapy is provided following achievement of remission. Therefore, some clinicians reserve such regimens for patients with high-risk childhood ALL. However, other clinicians have elected to use a 4- or 5-drug induction regimen for all patients with childhood ALL regardless of presenting features. Multiple-drug induction regimens produce a complete remission in more than 95% of children with ALL.

Either pegaspargase or asparaginase (Escherichia coli) may be used as the asparaginase component in first-line combination chemotherapeutic regimens for childhood ALL; however, because pegaspargase has similar efficacy and toxicity as asparaginase (Escherichia coli) but requires less frequent administration, many clinicians prefer pegaspargase for use during both induction and postinduction phases of treatment in pediatric patients with newly diagnosed ALL. (Asparaginase [Escherichia coli] no longer is commercially available in the US.) Asparaginase (Erwinia chrysanthemi) may be used in patients who are hypersensitive to *E. coli*-derived asparaginase (asparaginase [Escherichia coli] or pegaspargase). (See Asparaginase [Erwinia chrysanthemi] 10:00.)

Induction regimens for adult ALL typically include prednisone, vincristine, and an anthracycline; some regimens also add other drugs, such as an asparaginase preparation (see Asparaginase [Erwinia chrysanthemi] 10:00) or cyclophosphamide. Such induction regimens produce a complete remission in about 85% of adults with ALL.

The current indication for pegaspargase in the first-line treatment of ALL is based on an open-label, randomized, active-controlled, multicenter study involving 118 pediatric patients 1–9 years of age with previously untreated standard-risk ALL. Patients received either pegaspargase or native asparaginase (Escherichia coli) as a component of combination chemotherapy. The dosage schedule for pegaspargase was 2500 units/m² IM on day 3 of the 4-week induction phase and on day 3 of each of the two 8-week delayed intensification treatment phases. The dosage schedule for native asparaginase (Escherichia coli) was 6000 units/m² IM 3 times weekly for a total of 9 doses during the induction phase and for a total of 6 doses during each delayed intensification treatment phase.

At specified time points during all phases of treatment, the proportion of patients with the target level of asparagine depletion (serum asparagine concentration of 1 μM or less) was similar among patients receiving pegaspargase-containing therapy or asparaginase (Escherichia coli) containing therapy. For both groups, serum asparagine concentrations typically decreased within 4 days following the first dose of drug and remained low for approximately 3 weeks. Similar magnitude and duration of reduction in CSF asparagine concentrations were observed for the 2 groups. Similar toxicity was observed between the groups. Pharmacokinetic analysis during induction therapy showed that pegaspargase has a longer elimination half-life (5.5 days) than native asparaginase (Escherichia coli) (1.1 days).

Binding or neutralizing antibodies to pegaspargase were detected in 2% of patients during induction therapy, in 10% of patients during the first phase of delayed intensification therapy, and in 11% of patients during the second phase of delayed intensification therapy. The effect of the development of binding antibodies on the pharmacokinetic disposition, antileukemic efficacy, or risk of clinical allergic reactions associated with pegaspargase therapy has not been fully established. Reduced activity of pegylated asparaginase has been demonstrated in sera that tested positive for antibodies to the drug in samples collected from pediatric patients receiving pegaspargase for ALL.

Pegaspargase also is used as a component of combination chemotherapy for first-line treatment of adult ALL. In one study (Cancer and Leukemia Group B [CALGB] study 9511) in 102 adults with previously untreated ALL or acute undifferentiated leukemia, treatment with a combination chemotherapy regimen that included pegaspargase resulted in complete responses in 77% of patients. The pegaspargase dosage schedule for the first 21 patients was 2000 units/m^2 (maximum dose of 3750 units) given by subcutaneous injection† on day 5 of the 4-week induction phase and on day 15 of the 8-week early intensification treatment phase; subsequent patients received pegaspargase 2000 units/m^2 (maximum dose of 3750 units) by subcutaneous injection† on days 5 and 22 of the induction phase and on days 15 and 43 of the early intensification treatment phase. Patients who achieved asparagine depletion (defined as asparaginase concentrations exceeding 0.03 units/mL for 14 consecutive days following at least one pegaspargase dose) had prolonged disease-free and overall survival (median: 25 and 31 months, respectively) compared with those who did not achieve asparagine depletion (median: 12 and 13 months, respectively), although the differences were not statistically significant following adjustment for other patient characteristics. Complete response rates and relapse rates did not differ between patients who achieved asparagine depletion and those who did not achieve asparagine depletion. Larger studies are needed to more fully evaluate these findings.

Acute Lymphocytic Leukemia and Hypersensitivity to Native Asparaginase Pegaspargase is used as a component of combination chemotherapy for the treatment of ALL in patients who are hypersensitive to native (nonconjugated) forms of asparaginase. In several open-label studies in patients with multiply-relapsed acute leukemia (principally lymphocytic) and hypersensitivity to asparaginase, remission was reinduced in 50% of patients (36% complete and 14% partial) when pegaspargase was used as a component of combination chemotherapy. This response rate is comparable to that reported for reinduction of relapsed acute leukemia when native asparaginase (Escherichia coli) (no longer commercially available in the US) was used as a component of a combination regimen. Although pegaspargase is less immunogenic than native (nonconjugated) asparaginase, hypersensitivity reactions to the PEG-conjugated enzyme (i.e., pegaspargase) can occur.

Dosage and Administration

■ **Administration** Pegaspargase is administered by IM injection or IV infusion. Pegaspargase also may be administered by subcutaneous† injection.

Parenteral pegaspargase solutions should be inspected visually for particulate matter, cloudiness, and discoloration prior to administration whenever solution and container permit. The drug should be discarded if the solution is discolored or cloudy or if particulate matter is present. No more than one dose should be used from each single-use vial; any unused portion should be discarded since the drug contains no preservative. Because freezing inactivates the enzyme, pegaspargase injection or diluted solutions should *not* be used if there is any possibility that freezing may have occurred, even if there is no change in the appearance of the solution. Pegaspargase injection or diluted solutions that have been shaken or vigorously agitated should not be used. In addition, pegaspargase injection that has been stored at room temperature for more than 48 hours should not be used.

For IM injection, commercially available pegaspargase injection is administered undiluted. The manufacturer recommends that not more than 2 mL be administered at any one injection site; IM doses exceeding 2 mL should be divided and administered at separate sites.

For IV infusion, pegaspargase injection should be diluted in 100 mL of sodium chloride injection or 5% dextrose injection and administered over a period of 1–2 hours through an infusion that is already running. After the drug has been diluted for IV infusion, pegaspargase solutions should be used immediately. If immediate use is not possible, pegaspargase diluted solutions should be stored at 2–8°C. Storage after dilution of the drug should not exceed 48 hours from the time of preparation to completion of administration. The diluted solution should be protected from direct sunlight.

Procedures for proper handling and disposal of antineoplastic drugs should be followed when preparing or administering asparaginase preparations.

■ **Dosage** Dosage of pegaspargase is expressed in international units (IU, units) and must be individualized according to body surface area. Following administration of pegaspargase, patients should be monitored for 1 hour for anaphylaxis or serious allergic reactions. (See Cautions: Precautions and Contraindications.)

Acute Lymphocytic Leukemia For induction therapy of acute lymphocytic leukemia (ALL), pegaspargase usually is initiated as part of a multiple-drug regimen that includes vincristine and a corticosteroid and may include an anthracycline (e.g., daunorubicin, doxorubicin). Clinicians should consult published protocols for the dosage of pegaspargase and other chemotherapeutic agents and the method and sequence of administration. For the induction of remission of ALL, the usual dosage of pegaspargase is 2500 units/m^2 administered IM or IV as a single dose no more frequently than every 14 days. While the optimum duration of the induction remission regimen remains to be established, a 28-day, 1- or 2-dose regimen has been evaluated. When patients are in remission, pegaspargase may be used as part of an intensification treatment regimen prior to initiation of maintenance therapy. When pegaspargase has been administered IM or IV as a component of intensification therapy, a dose of 2500 units/m^2 has been given at various dosing intervals. Doses of pegaspargase should be administered no more frequently than every 14 days.

For first-line treatment of adult ALL, pegaspargase has been administered as a component of combination chemotherapy at a dosage of 2000 units/m^2 (maximum dose of 3750 units) given by subcutaneous† injection on days 5 and 22 of a 4-week induction phase and on days 15 and 43 of an 8-week early intensification treatment phase.

Contraindications for Continued Therapy **Anaphylaxis and Allergic Reactions.** Pegaspargase therapy should be discontinued in patients with anaphylaxis or serious allergic reactions.

Thrombosis. Pegaspargase therapy should be discontinued in patients experiencing serious thrombotic reactions.

Pancreatitis. Pegaspargase therapy should be discontinued in patients with pancreatitis.

Cautions

Serious adverse effects associated with pegaspargase therapy include anaphylaxis and serious allergic reactions, serious thrombosis, pancreatitis, glucose intolerance, and coagulopathy. Among patients receiving pegaspargase as a component of combination therapy in first-line treatment for ALL, the most common adverse effects are allergic reactions (including anaphylaxis), hyperglycemia, pancreatitis, CNS thrombosis, coagulopathy, hyperbilirubinemia, and elevated serum transaminase concentrations. Like other asparaginase preparations, pegaspargase rarely causes severe bone marrow depression, and usually does not significantly affect GI or oral mucosa or hair follicles. In general, except for hypersensitivity reactions, adults receiving pegaspargase have a somewhat higher incidence of known asparaginase toxicities than children. There does not appear to be a substantial difference in adverse effects following IV versus IM administration of the drug.

Although pegaspargase is less immunogenic than native (nonconjugated) asparaginase, the most frequent adverse effects remain hypersensitivity reactions, including life-threatening anaphylaxis. Most other adverse effects of pegaspargase are similar to those of native asparaginase and may be attributed to asparagine and glutamine depletion and, therefore, decreased protein synthesis in tissues with high rates of protein synthesis (e.g., liver [including clotting factors], kidneys, pancreas, CNS) or to increased blood concentrations of ammonia as a product of the breakdown of asparagine.

■ **Sensitivity Reactions** The most frequent adverse effects of pegaspargase are hypersensitivity or allergic reactions, which may include acute anaphylaxis, bronchospasm, hypotension, laryngeal edema, urticaria, chills, systemic rash, and local erythema or swelling. Pegaspargase is less immunogenic than native forms of asparaginase derived from *Escherichia coli* or *Erwinia chrysanthemi* (formerly *Erwinia carotovora*; also known as *Pectobacterium chrysanthemi*) ; however, in patients with known hypersensitivity to these forms of asparaginase, hypersensitivity reactions to pegaspargase, including life-threatening anaphylaxis, can occur.

Among patients in a randomized trial receiving pegaspargase in combination chemotherapy as first-line therapy for ALL, grade 3 or 4 clinical allergic reactions occurred in 2% of patients.

In clinical trials for relapsed ALL, the incidence of clinical allergic reactions to pegaspargase was 32% in patients with hypersensitivity to native asparaginase and 10% in asparaginase-nonhypersensitive patients. Grade 3 or 4 clinical allergic reactions occurred in 8% of patients with hypersensitivity to native asparaginase and 2% of asparaginase-nonhypersensitive patients. About 56% of the hypersensitive patients in clinical trials for relapsed ALL were previously hypersensitive to asparaginase (Escherichia coli) and 44% were previously hypersensitive to both asparaginase (Escherichia coli) and asparaginase (Erwinia chrysanthemi). Therapy-limiting (i.e., requiring discontinuance of the respective drug) hypersensitivity reactions to pegaspargase occurred in 14% of patients in clinical trials who were previously hypersensitive to asparaginase (Escherichia coli) and in 26% of patients who were previously hypersensitive to both asparaginase (Escherichia coli) and asparaginase (Erwinia chrysanthemi). The incidence of therapy-limiting hypersensitivity reactions to pegaspargase in clinical trials was 9% overall (19% in asparaginase-hypersensitive patients and 3% in asparaginase-nonhypersensitive patients). Therapy-limiting anaphylactic reactions occurred in 1% of patients. The probability of a previously hypersensitive or nonhypersensitive patient completing 8 doses of pegaspargase therapy without developing a therapy-limiting hypersensitivity reaction was 77 and 95%, respectively.

■ **Hematologic Effects** Thrombosis, including superficial and deep-vein thrombosis, sagittal sinus thrombosis, thrombosis involving a central venous catheter, and stroke, is one of the most common adverse effects of pegaspargase and may be severe. Thrombosis occurred in 4% of patients receiving the drug for relapsed ALL in clinical trials.

Coagulopathy, sometimes severe, is a common adverse effect of pegaspargase. Among patients in a randomized trial receiving pegaspargase in combination chemotherapy as first-line therapy for ALL, grade 3 or 4 coagulopathy (prolonged prothrombin time, prolonged partial thromboplastin time, or hypofibrinogenemia) occurred in 2% of patients. Interim data from a multifactorial design study in which 2770 patients received pegaspargase in combination chemotherapy as first-line therapy for ALL shows a higher rate of grade 3 or 4 coagulopathy (7%). Decreased antithrombin III concentrations also have been reported in patients receiving pegaspargase.

Disseminated intravascular coagulation, clinical hemorrhage (which may be fatal), and decreases in plasma concentrations of protein C and protein S also have been reported.

Coagulation tests should be performed at baseline and periodically during and following pegaspargase therapy. Treatment with fresh frozen plasma to replace coagulation factors should be initiated in patients with severe or symptomatic coagulopathy.

■ **Pancreatic Effects** Impairment of pancreatic function occurs frequently in patients receiving pegaspargase and may be caused by decreased insulin synthesis or necrosis and inflammation of the cells of the pancreas. Among patients in a randomized trial receiving pegaspargase in combination chemotherapy as first-line therapy for ALL, grade 3 or 4 pancreatitis occurred in 2% of patients.

Pancreatitis, which sometimes may be fulminant and fatal, occurred in 1% of patients receiving pegaspargase for relapsed ALL in clinical trials. An increased incidence of pancreatitis has been observed in some clinical trials in nonhypersensitive patients who received pegaspargase as part of combination chemotherapy regimens that resulted in prolonged asparagine depletion and included repeated intermediate-dose methotrexate or high-dose cytarabine. Increased serum amylase concentrations have occurred in patients receiving pegaspargase.

■ **Metabolic Effects** Glucose intolerance, sometimes irreversible, is a serious adverse effect of pegaspargase. Among patients in a randomized trial receiving pegaspargase in combination chemotherapy as first-line therapy for ALL, grade 3 or 4 hyperglycemia occurred in 5% of patients.

Mild to severe hyperglycemia may occur in patients receiving pegaspargase. Hyperglycemia requiring insulin therapy occurred in 3% of patients receiving the drug for relapsed ALL in clinical trials. Hypoproteinemia and hypoalbuminemia also have been reported.

■ **Hepatic Effects** Hyperbilirubinemia and elevated serum aminotransferase (ALT, AST) concentrations are among the most common adverse effects of pegaspargase. Among patients in a randomized trial receiving pegaspargase in combination chemotherapy as first-line therapy for ALL, grade 3 or 4 increased serum aminotransferase (AST or ALT) concentrations occurred in 3% and grade 3 or 4 hyperbilirubinemia occurred in 2% of patients. Interim data from a multifactorial design study in which 2770 patients received pegaspargase in combination chemotherapy as first-line therapy for ALL shows a higher rate of grade 3 or 4 increased serum aminotransferase concentrations (11%).

Jaundice, abnormal liver function test results, increased serum concentrations of bilirubin (direct and indirect), and hypoalbuminemia, which may be associated with peripheral edema, also have occurred in patients receiving pegaspargase.

■ **GI Effects** Nausea, vomiting, abdominal pain, diarrhea, and constipation have occurred in patients receiving pegaspargase. Patients who experience abdominal pain should be evaluated for evidence of pancreatitis.

■ **Nervous System Effects** CNS thrombosis (e.g., sagittal sinus thrombosis, stroke) is one of the most common adverse effects of pegaspargase. Among patients in a randomized trial receiving pegaspargase in combination chemotherapy as first-line therapy for ALL, grade 3 or 4 CNS thrombosis occurred in 3% of patients. Interim data from a multifactorial design study in which 2770 patients received pegaspargase in combination chemotherapy as first-line therapy for ALL showed a 2% rate of grade 3 or 4 CNS thrombosis/hemorrhage.

Peripheral neuritis, neuropathy, neurologic disorder, and dizziness also have been reported in patients receiving pegaspargase.

■ **Cardiovascular Effects** Hypotension (which may be severe) occurred in patients receiving pegaspargase in clinical trials.

■ **Immunologic Effects** Antibody formation has been detected in patients receiving pegaspargase. In one clinical trial, antibodies to the drug were detected in 2% of patients during induction therapy, in 10% of patients during the first phase of delayed intensification therapy, and in 11% of patients during the second phase of delayed intensification therapy. The effect of the development of binding antibodies on the pharmacokinetic disposition or antileukemic efficacy of pegaspargase or on the risk of clinical allergic reactions associated with such therapy has not been fully established.

■ **Other Effects** Fever, increased BUN, fatigue, pain in the extremities (which may be local or diffuse), injection site reactions (including pain, swelling, or erythema), and facial edema have occurred in patients receiving pegaspargase.

■ **Precautions and Contraindications** Because pegaspargase may cause severe or, rarely, even fatal adverse effects, the potential benefit of the drug to the patient must be weighed carefully against the possible risks involved, and the patient should be apprised of these risks.

Serious clinical allergic reactions to pegaspargase, including life-threatening anaphylaxis, may occur during therapy with the drug, particularly in patients with known hypersensitivity to other forms of asparaginase. Patients receiving pegaspargase should be informed of the possibility of serious allergic reactions, including life-threatening anaphylaxis, and should be monitored for 1 hour after administration of the drug. Appropriate agents for maintenance of an adequate airway and treatment of a hypersensitivity reaction, such as an antihistamine, epinephrine, oxygen, and IV corticosteroid, should be readily available whenever pegaspargase is administered.

Because of the risk of coagulopathy associated with pegaspargase therapy, coagulation tests (including fibrinogen levels, prothrombin time, and partial thromboplastin time) should be performed at baseline and periodically during and following pegaspargase therapy.

Patients should be informed to report immediately any possible manifestations of serious adverse effects, such as swellings or difficulty breathing (possibly serious allergic reactions); severe headache, arm or leg swelling, sudden shortness of breath, or chest pain (possibly thrombosis); severe abdominal pain (possibly pancreatitis); or excessive thirst or increase in the volume or frequency of urination (possibly glucose intolerance). Pegaspargase should be discontinued if pancreatitis, a serious thrombotic event, or anaphylaxis or other serious allergic reaction occurs.

Pegaspargase is contraindicated in patients with a history of serious thrombosis associated with prior asparaginase therapy. Pegaspargase is contraindicated in patients with a history of pancreatitis associated with prior asparaginase therapy. The drug also is contraindicated in patients who have had clinically important hemorrhagic events associated with prior asparaginase therapy. Pegaspargase also is contraindicated in patients who have had previous serious allergic reactions to the drug such as urticaria, systemic rash, bronchospasm, laryngeal edema, local erythema or swelling, or hypotension.

■ **Pediatric Precautions** The safety and efficacy of pegaspargase have been evaluated in a randomized trial involving children 1–9 years of age receiving the drug as first-line therapy for standard-risk ALL. The safety and efficacy of pegaspargase also have been evaluated in children with ALL and hypersensitivity to asparaginase.

■ **Geriatric Precautions** Clinical studies of pegaspargase did not include sufficient numbers of patients 65 years of age and older to determine whether geriatric patients respond differently than younger patients.

■ **Mutagenicity and Carcinogenicity** Pegaspargase did not exhibit mutagenic activity when tested against *Salmonella typhimurium* strains in the Ames assay. Studies to determine the carcinogenic potential of pegaspargase have not been performed to date.

■ **Pregnancy, Fertility, and Lactation** Animal reproduction studies have not been performed with pegaspargase, and it is not known whether the drug can cause fetal harm when administered to pregnant women. Pegaspargase should be used during pregnancy only when clearly needed.

Studies to determine the effects of pegaspargase on fertility have not been performed to date, and it is not known whether the drug can affect reproductive capacity.

It is not known whether pegaspargase is distributed into human milk. Because of the potential for serious adverse effects in nursing infants if pegaspargase were distributed into milk, a decision should be made whether to discontinue nursing or the drug, taking into account the importance of the drug to the woman.

Drug Interactions

No formal studies of interactions between pegaspargase and other drugs have been conducted.

During the period of its inhibition of protein synthesis and cell replication, pegaspargase may interfere with the action of other antineoplastic agents that require cell replication for their cytotoxic effects (e.g., methotrexate).

Acute Toxicity

Limited information is available on the acute toxicity of pegaspargase. Among 3 patients who received an overdosage of pegaspargase 10,000 units/m² as an IV infusion, 2 patients experienced adverse effects. The infusion rate was slowed and an antihistamine was administered when one patient developed a rash 10 minutes after the initiation of the pegaspargase infusion. Another patient experienced a slight increase in serum concentrations of liver enzymes.

Pharmacology

Pegaspargase selectively kills leukemic cells by depleting them of plasma asparagine, an amino acid that is needed for synthesis of protein, RNA, and DNA. Because of a lack of asparagine synthase, some leukemic cells cannot synthesize asparagine and depend on an exogenous source for survival. Treatment with the enzyme L-asparaginase or pegylated asparaginase breaks down extracellular asparagine into aspartic acid and ammonia, causing depletion of asparagine and killing the leukemic cells. Because of their ability to synthesize asparagine, normal cells are less affected by the depletion of asparagine.

Pegaspargase is a modified form of *Escherichia coli*-derived asparaginase that is less immunogenic than the native enzyme and also has an increased plasma half-life.

Pharmacokinetics

Pharmacokinetic assessments of pegaspargase are based on an enzymatic assay that measures asparaginase activity.

■ **Absorption** In 34 pediatric patients receiving pegaspargase 2500 units/m^2 IM as first-line therapy for standard-risk ALL, pegaspargase plasma concentrations exceeded 0.1 unit/mL in more than 90% of samples for approximately 20 days in those receiving the drug during induction therapy and both phases of delayed intensification therapy.

In 25 adults receiving a single dose of pegaspargase 2000 units/m^2 IV as part of a standard induction regimen of first-line therapy for ALL, the peak serum concentration of asparaginase enzymatic activity averaged 1 unit/mL.

In 3 pharmacokinetic studies involving a total of 37 patients receiving pegaspargase 2500 units/m^2 IM every 2 weeks for relapsed ALL, the area under the concentration-time curve was 9.5±4 units/mL per day in patients who were previously hypersensitive to native asparaginase (Escherichia coli) and 9.8±6 units/mL per day in patients who were not hypersensitive to asparaginase (Escherichia coli).

■ **Distribution** In 25 adults receiving a single dose of pegaspargase 2000 units/m^2 IV as part of a standard induction regimen of first-line therapy for ALL, the volume of distribution was 2.43 L/m^2 (equivalent to plasma volume).

Distribution of pegaspargase into the CSF is reflected by the decrease in CSF asparagine concentrations, which reportedly is similar to that achieved with asparaginase (Escherichia coli) (no longer commercially available in the US). It is not known whether pegaspargase is distributed into milk.

■ **Elimination** In 34 pediatric patients receiving pegaspargase 2500 units/m^2 IM as first-line therapy for standard-risk ALL, the elimination half-life of pegaspargase was about 5.8 days during the induction phase; the elimination half-life was similar for phases 1 and 2 of delayed intensification therapy.

In 25 adults receiving a single dose of pegaspargase 2000 units/m^2 IV as part of a standard induction regimen of first-line therapy for ALL, the elimination half-life was 7 days.

In 3 pharmacokinetic studies involving a total of 37 patients receiving pegaspargase 2500 units/m^2 IM every 2 weeks for relapsed ALL, the plasma half-life of pegaspargase was 3.2±1.8 days in 9 patients who were previously hypersensitive to native asparaginase (Escherichia coli) and 5.7±3.2 days in 28 patients who were not hypersensitive to asparaginase (Escherichia coli).

Chemistry and Stability

■ **Chemistry** Pegaspargase is an antineoplastic agent. The drug is prepared by conjugating covalently polyethylene glycol (PEG) monomethyl ether to *Escherichia coli*-derived asparaginase, resulting in the formation of monomethoxypolyethylene glycol succinimidyl asparaginase (pegaspargase). The asparaginase component is a tetrameric enzyme that is produced endogenously by *E. coli* and consists of identical 34.5 kilodalton subunits. Approximately 69–82 molecules of PEG are linked to the enzyme; the molecular weight of each PEG molecule is about 5 kilodaltons. By modifying the nonconjugated (native) enzyme with PEG, resultant pegaspargase has a reduced immunogenic potential and increased plasma half-life compared with native *E. coli*-derived asparaginase.

Pegaspargase is commercially available as a clear, colorless, isotonic sterile solution that is preservative-free. Phosphate-buffered saline solution is added to adjust the pH to 7.3.

The activity of pegaspargase is expressed in International Units (IU; units); 1 unit of L-asparaginase is the amount of enzyme required to generate 1 μmol of ammonia per minute at pH 7.3 and 37°C. The preparation has a specific activity of at least 85 units per milligram of protein. Each 5-mL vial of the drug contains pegaspargase 3750 units.

■ **Stability** Pegaspargase injection should be stored at 2–8°C and protected from light. Pegaspargase injection should not be administered if the drug has been stored at room temperature (15–25°C) for more than 48 hours. Because pegaspargase injection contains no preservative, any unused portion should be discarded.

Pegaspargase diluted solutions should be used immediately after the drug has been diluted for IV infusion. If immediate use is not possible, pegaspargase diluted solutions should be stored at 2–8°C. Storage after dilution of the drug should not exceed 48 hours from the time of preparation to completion of administration. The diluted solution should be protected from direct sunlight.

Pegaspargase injection or diluted solution should not be administered if the drug has been frozen. Pegaspargase injection or diluted solution should not be shaken or agitated vigorously, and if this happens, the drug should be discarded. If pegaspargase injection or diluted solution appears cloudy or discolored, or if particulate matter is present, the drug should be discarded.

For further information on the handling of antineoplastic agents, see the ASHP Guidelines on Handling Hazardous Drugs.

Preparations

Excipients in commercially available drug preparations may have clinically important effects in some individuals; consult specific product labeling for details.

Pegaspargase

Parenteral

Injection	750 units/mL	**Oncaspar®**, Sigma-Tau

†Use is not currently included in the labeling approved by the US Food and Drug Administration

Peginterferon Alfa

■ Peginterferon alfa contains interferon alfa (recombinant DNA origin) covalently bound to monomethoxy polyethylene glycol (PEG). Peginterferon alfa-2b is used as an antineoplastic agent. Peginterferon alfa-2a and peginterferon alfa-2b are used as antiviral agents (see Peginterferon Alfa 8:18.20). For information on nonconjugated interferon alfa, see Interferon Alfa 8:18.20 and Interferon Alfa 10:00.

Uses

■ **Melanoma** Peginterferon alfa-2b (Sylatron®) is used as an adjuvant to surgery for the treatment of melanoma in adults with microscopic or gross nodal involvement who have undergone definitive surgical resection including complete lymphadenectomy. Adjuvant treatment with peginterferon alfa-2b should be initiated in such patients within 84 days of surgery.

Efficacy and safety of peginterferon alfa-2b for the adjuvant treatment of melanoma were evaluated in a phase 3, open-label, randomized controlled study (EORTC 18991). Adults with surgically resected stage 3 melanoma were randomized (within 84 days of regional lymph node dissection) to observation alone or treatment with peginterferon alfa-2b (Sylatron®; 6 mcg/kg subcutaneously once weekly for 8 weeks [induction], then 3 mcg/kg subcutaneously once weekly for up to 5 years [maintenance]). Demographics and baseline characteristics were similar between groups (median age 50 years, 42% female, 54% with 1 pathologically positive lymph node, 34% with 2–4 positive nodes, 12% with 5 or more positive nodes). Patients randomized to the peginterferon alfa-2b group received the induction dosage of 6 mcg/kg once weekly for a median of 8 weeks; during this time, 36% of patients required dosage reductions, 29% required dosage delays (average delay 1.2 weeks), and 16% did not continue on to the maintenance dosage. Of the patients who continued to the maintenance dosage of 3 mcg/kg once weekly, the median duration of treatment was 14.3 months; during this time, 52% of patients required dosage reductions and 70% required dosage delays (average delay 2.2 weeks). The median relapse-free survival was 34.8 months in the peginterferon alfa-2b group and 25.5 months in the observation group. There was no statistically significant difference in survival between the peginterferon alfa-2b group and the observation group.

Dosage and Administration

■ **General** Several peginterferon alfa subtypes (alfa-2a, alfa-2b), dosage forms, and strengths are commercially available, and care should be taken to ensure that the correct preparation is used.

Of the commercially available peginterferon alfa preparations, only peginterferon alfa-2b (Sylatron®) should be used for adjuvant treatment of melanoma. Patients should be cautioned *not* to change brands of peginterferon alfa without consulting their clinician.

■ **Reconstitution and Administration** Peginterferon alfa-2b is administered by subcutaneous injection once weekly.

Subcutaneous injections of peginterferon alfa-2b should be made into the thigh, outer surface of the upper arm, or abdomen (avoiding areas of the navel and waistline). Injection sites should be rotated.

Peginterferon alfa-2b may be *self-administered* if the clinician determines that the patient and/or their caregiver are competent to safely administer the drug after appropriate training and with medical follow-up as necessary. Patients and/or their caregivers who administer peginterferon alfa-2b in a home setting should be carefully instructed in the proper administration of the drug, including aseptic technique. They should be cautioned against reuse of syringes and needles and should be given instruction regarding the proper, safe disposal of such equipment after use.

Administration of peginterferon alfa-2b (Sylatron®) with an antipyretic at bedtime may minimize adverse flu-like effects. The manufacturer recommends administration of acetaminophen 0.5–1 g orally 30 minutes prior to the first dose of peginterferon alfa-2b and as needed for subsequent doses.

Single-dose vials containing lyophilized peginterferon alfa-2b should be stored at 25°C, but may be exposed to temperatures ranging from 15–30°C; the drug should not be frozen or exposed to heat.

Peginterferon alfa-2b lyophilized powder for injection must be reconstituted prior to administration using *only* sterile water for injection. Prior to reconstitution, peginterferon alfa-2b should appear as a white to off-white powder. Single-dose vials labeled as containing 200, 300, or 600 mcg of peginterferon alfa-2b per 0.5 mL contain 296, 444, or 888 mcg of lyophilized drug, respectively.

Peginterferon alfa-2b in single-dose vials should be reconstituted by adding 0.7 mL of the sterile water diluent provided by the manufacturer and gently swirling the vial; the vial should not be shaken.

Reconstituted peginterferon alfa-2b should be inspected visually for particulate matter and discoloration prior to administration; the solution should be clear and colorless and should not be used if discolored or cloudy or if particulates are present.

If the reconstituted solution is not used immediately, it may be stored for up to 24 hours at 2–8°C; the solution should not be frozen.

No more than 0.5 mL of reconstituted solution should be withdrawn from each vial. Peginterferon alfa-2b vials are for single-use only; any unused portions should be discarded.

■ Dosage

Dosage modification may be necessary if adverse effects occur. (See Dosage and Administration: Dosage Modification for Toxicity.)

Melanoma When peginterferon alfa-2b (Sylatron®) is used as an adjuvant to surgery for treatment of melanoma in adults with microscopic or gross nodal involvement who have undergone definitive surgical resection including lymphadenectomy, the recommended dosage is 6 mcg/kg subcutaneously once weekly for 8 doses (induction), followed by 3 mcg/kg subcutaneously once weekly for up to 5 years (maintenance). Peginterferon alfa-2b should be initiated within 84 days of surgery.

■ Dosage Modification for Toxicity

Peginterferon alfa-2b (Sylatron®) should be permanently discontinued if the patient experiences persistent or worsening severe neuropsychiatric disorders, develops grade 4 nonhematologic toxicity, is unable to tolerate a dosage of 1 mcg/kg once weekly, or develops new or worsening retinopathy.

Peginterferon alfa-2b should be withheld if the patient has an absolute neutrophil count (ANC) less than 500/mm^3, platelet count less than 50,000/mm^3, Eastern Cooperative Oncology Group (ECOG) performance status of 2 or greater, or grade 3 or higher nonhematologic toxicity. Peginterferon alfa-2b may be resumed using a reduced dosage when the patient exhibits all of the following: ANC 500/mm^3 or greater, platelet count 50,000/mm^3 or greater, ECOG performance status 0 or 1, *and* nonhematologic toxicity that has completely resolved or improved to grade 1.

If dosage modification of peginterferon alfa-2b is required during weeks 1–8 of treatment (induction) because of adverse reactions, a 3-step decrease from the original dosage of 6 mcg/kg once weekly is recommended (i.e., dosage should be decreased to 3 mcg/kg once weekly; if needed, decrease to 2 mcg/kg once weekly; then, if needed, further decrease to 1 mcg/kg once weekly). If the patient is unable to tolerate peginterferon alfa-2b at a dosage of 1 mcg/kg once weekly, the drug should be permanently discontinued.

If dosage modification of peginterferon alfa-2b is required during weeks 9–260 of treatment (maintenance) because of adverse reactions, a 2-step decrease from the original dosage of 3 mcg/kg once weekly is recommended (i.e., dosage should be decreased to 2 mcg/kg once weekly; if needed, decrease to 1 mcg/kg once weekly). If the patient is unable to tolerate peginterferon alfa-2b at a dosage of 1 mcg/kg once weekly, the drug should be permanently discontinued.

■ Special Populations

Hepatic Impairment Peginterferon alfa-2b (Sylatron®) has not been studied in patients with melanoma who have hepatic impairment. The drug is contraindicated in those with hepatic decompensation (Child-Pugh score greater than 6, class B and C).

Renal Impairment When peginterferon alfa-2b (Sylatron®) is used as an adjuvant to surgery for treatment of melanoma in adults with moderate renal impairment (creatinine clearance 30–50 mL/minute per 1.73 m^2), dosage should be reduced to 4.5 mcg/kg subcutaneously once weekly for 8 doses (induction), followed by 2.25 mcg/kg subcutaneously once weekly for up to 5 years (maintenance). In adults with severe renal impairment (creatinine clearance less than 30 mL/minute per 1.73 m^2) and adults with end-stage renal disease requiring dialysis, dosage of peginterferon alfa-2b should be reduced to 3 mcg/kg subcutaneously once weekly for 8 doses (induction), followed by 1.5 mcg/kg subcutaneously once weekly for up to 5 years (maintenance). (See Renal Impairment under Warnings/Precautions: Specific Populations, in Cautions.)

Dosage adjustments of peginterferon alfa-2b (Sylatron®) are not needed in adults with creatinine clearance exceeding 50 mL/minute per 1.73 m^2.

Cautions

■ Contraindications

Peginterferon alfa-2b (Sylatron®) is contraindicated in patients with a history of anaphylaxis to peginterferon alfa-2b or interferon alfa-2b and in those with autoimmune hepatitis or hepatic decompensation (Child-Pugh score greater than 6, class B and C).

■ Warnings/Precautions

Warnings **Neuropsychiatric Effects.** Peginterferon alfa-2b (Sylatron®) can cause life-threatening or fatal neuropsychiatric reactions. The risk of serious depression, with suicidal ideation and completed suicides, and other serious neuropsychiatric disorders (e.g., homicidal ideation, increased risk of relapse in recovering drug addicts) are increased with alpha interferons, including peginterferon alfa-2b.

In a clinical study of peginterferon alfa-2b in patients with melanoma, depression occurred in 59 or 24% of patients in the peginterferon alfa-2b or observation group, respectively; severe or life-threatening depression occurred in 7 or less than 1% of patients, respectively. In postmarketing experience, adverse neuropsychiatric reactions have been reported up to 6 months after discontinuance of peginterferon alfa-2b. Aggressive behavior, psychoses, hallucinations, bipolar disorders, mania, and encephalopathy also have been reported with peginterferon alfa-2b and interferon alfa-2b.

Patients and their caregivers should be advised to immediately contact a clinician if the patient experiences symptoms of depression or suicidal ideation. Patients should be monitored and evaluated for signs and symptoms of depression and other psychiatric symptoms every 3 weeks during the first 8 weeks of treatment and every 6 months thereafter; monitoring should be continued for at least 6 months after the last dose of peginterferon alfa-2b.

Peginterferon alfa-2b should be permanently discontinued if the patient develops persistent severe or worsening psychiatric symptoms or behaviors, and the patient should be referred for psychiatric evaluation. These disorders may not resolve after peginterferon alfa-2b is discontinued.

Other Warnings/Precautions **Cardiovascular Effects.** Adverse cardiac effects (e.g., myocardial infarction, bundle-branch block, ventricular tachycardia, supraventricular arrhythmia) occurred in 4% of patients receiving peginterferon alfa-2b in a clinical study compared with 2% of patients in the observation group. In postmarketing experience, hypotension, cardiomyopathy, and angina pectoris have occurred in patients receiving peginterferon alfa-2b.

Peginterferon alfa-2b should be permanently discontinued if new onset of ventricular arrhythmia or cardiovascular decompensation occurs.

Ocular Effects. Peginterferon alfa-2b can cause decreased visual acuity or blindness due to retinopathy. Certain retinal or ocular changes may be induced or aggravated by treatment with peginterferon alfa-2b or other alpha interferons (e.g., macular edema, retinal artery or vein thrombosis, retinal hemorrhages and cotton wool spots, optic neuritis, papilledema, serous retinal detachment). In a clinical study in patients with melanoma, 2 patients receiving peginterferon alfa-2b developed partial loss of vision due to retinal thrombosis or retinopathy. The overall incidence of serious retinal disorders, visual disturbances, blurred vision, and reduction in visual acuity was less than 1% in both the peginterferon alfa-2b and observation groups.

An eye examination, including assessment of visual acuity and indirect ophthalmoscopy or fundus photography, should be performed at baseline in patients with preexisting retinopathy and at any time vision changes occur during peginterferon alfa-2b treatment.

Peginterferon alfa-2b should be permanently discontinued in patients who develop new or worsening retinopathy.

Hepatic Effects. Peginterferon alfa-2b increases the risk of hepatic decompensation and death in patients with cirrhosis. Hepatic function (i.e., serum bilirubin, ALT, AST, alkaline phosphatase, LDH) should be assessed at 2 weeks, 8 weeks, 2 months, and 3 months following initiation of peginterferon alfa-2b and every 6 months thereafter during treatment.

Peginterferon alfa-2b should be permanently discontinued if the patient exhibits evidence of severe (grade 3) hepatic injury or hepatic decompensation (Child-Pugh score greater than 6, class B and C).

Endocrine Effects. Peginterferon alfa-2b can cause new onset or worsening hypothyroidism, hyperthyroidism, or diabetes mellitus. In a clinical study in patients with melanoma, 1% of patients developed hypothyroidism. The overall incidence of endocrine disorders was 2% in patients receiving peginterferon alfa-2b compared with less than 1% for patients in the observation group.

Thyroid-stimulating hormone (TSH) levels should be assessed within the 4 weeks preceding initiation of peginterferon alfa-2b, at 3 and 6 months following initiation of the drug, and every 6 months thereafter during treatment.

Peginterferon alfa-2b should be permanently discontinued in patients who develop hypothyroidism, hyperthyroidism, or diabetes mellitus that cannot be effectively managed.

Antibody Formation. In a clinical study evaluating peginterferon alfa in patients with melanoma, the overall incidence of binding antibodies to peginterferon alfa-2b was approximately 35% (50/144); one patient developed neutralizing antibodies. Antibody development occurred in more patients receiving peginterferon alfa-2b than the observation group (52 and 18%, respectively). The effects of antibody formation on pharmacokinetics, safety, and efficacy of peginterferon alfa-2b have not been fully elucidated.

The percentage of individuals who test positive for antibody formation is highly dependent on the sensitivity and specificity of the assay used. The observed incidence of antibody positivity in an assay may be influenced by several factors (e.g., assay methodology, sample handling, timing of sample collection, concomitant medications, underlying disease). Therefore, comparison of the incidence of antibodies to peginterferon alfa-2b (Sylatron®) with the incidence of antibodies to other peginterferon or interferon preparations may be misleading.

Specific Populations **Pregnancy.** Category C. (See Users Guide.)

Lactation. It is not known whether peginterferon alfa-2b is distributed into human milk. Studies in mice indicate that mouse interferons are distributed into milk. Because of the potential for adverse reactions to peginterferon alfa-2b in nursing infants, a decision should be made whether to discontinue nursing or the drug, taking into account the importance of the drug to the mother.

Pediatric Use. Safety and efficacy of peginterferon alfa-2b (Sylatron®) have not been established in children younger than 18 years of age.

Geriatric Use. There are insufficient data to determine whether patients older than 65 years of age respond differently to peginterferon alfa-2b than younger adults.

Hepatic Impairment. Safety and efficacy of peginterferon alfa-2b have not been studied in patients with melanoma who have hepatic impairment. The drug is contraindicated in patients with hepatic decompensation (Child-Pugh score greater than 6, class B and C) and should be discontinued if hepatic decompensation occurs during treatment.

Renal Impairment. Because the mean exposure (area under the concentration-time curve [AUC]) of peginterferon alfa-2b is increased 1.4-fold in individuals with moderate renal impairment and increased 2.1-fold in individuals with severe renal impairment and in those with end-stage renal disease requiring dialysis when compared with the AUC in individuals with normal renal function, dosage of the drug should be decreased 25% in adults with moderate renal impairment and decreased 50% in adults with severe renal impairment and in those with end-stage renal impairment requiring dialysis. (See Renal Impairment under Dosage and Administration: Special Populations.)

■ **Common Adverse Effects** In a clinical trial evaluating peginterferon alfa-2b for adjuvant treatment of melanoma, essentially all patients receiving the drug experienced adverse effects at some time during the course of treatment; the drug was discontinued in 33% because of adverse effects. The most common adverse effects (occurring in greater than 50% of patients) are flu-like symptoms (fatigue, headache, myalgia, pyrexia, chills), anorexia, arthralgia, injection site reaction, depression, nausea, and elevated AST and ALT concentrations.

Drug Interactions

■ **Drugs Metabolized by Hepatic Microsomal Enzymes** The following information on possible interactions with drugs metabolized by cytochrome P-450 (CYP) enzymes is based on studies using peginterferon alfa-2b in a dosage of 1 mcg/kg once weekly. The effects of peginterferon alfa-2b given in dosages recommended for adjuvant treatment of melanoma (6 mcg/kg once weekly and 3 mcg/kg once weekly) on the pharmacokinetics of drugs metabolized by CYP enzymes have not been studied.

In healthy individuals who received *multiple doses* of peginterferon alfa-2b (1 mcg/kg subcutaneously once weekly for 4 weeks) and received probe drugs of metabolic enzymes (e.g., caffeine, tolbutamide, dextromethorphan, midazolam) before the first and after the fourth dose of peginterferon alfa-2b, CYP2C9 activity increased to 125% of baseline and CYP2D6 activity decreased to 51% of baseline; there was no clinically important effect on activity of CYP1A2 or CYP3A4.

In a 2-way crossover trial in healthy individuals who received probe drugs of metabolic enzymes (e.g., caffeine, tolbutamide, dextromethorphan, midazolam, dapsone) with or without a *single dose* of peginterferon alfa-2b (1 mcg/kg subcutaneously), there was no effect on the activity of CYP1A2, CYP2C9, CYP2D6, CYP3A4, or *N*-acetyltransferase (NAT) enzymes.

If peginterferon alfa-2b dosages used for adjuvant treatment of melanoma are used concomitantly with drugs metabolized by CYP2C9 or CYP2D6, the therapeutic effects of these drugs may be altered.

Description

Peginterferon alfa-2b is used as an antineoplastic agent. The mechanism by which peginterferon alfa-2b exerts therapeutic effects in the adjuvant treatment of melanoma is unknown; the drug is a pleiotropic cytokine. Peginterferon alfa-2b contains interferon alfa-2b (recombinant DNA origin) covalently bound to monomethoxy polyethylene glycol (PEG). As a result of conjugation with PEG, the apparent clearance of peginterferon alfa-2b is lower and mean half-life of the drug is greater than that reported for nonconjugated interferon alfa-2b. Consequently, peginterferon alfa-2b can be administered less frequently than nonconjugated preparations.

Pharmacokinetics of peginterferon alfa-2b were studied in adults receiving the drug for adjuvant treatment of melanoma. Initial treatment in these patients using a dosage of 6 mcg/kg subcutaneously once weekly for 8 doses (induction) resulted in mean peak serum concentrations of 4.4 ng/mL at week 8; the mean terminal half-life was approximately 51 hours and the mean accumulation from week 1 to week 8 was 1.7. After dosage was decreased to 3 mcg/kg subcutaneously once weekly (maintenance), peak serum concentrations at week 4 of the lower dosage were 2.5 ng/mL and the mean terminal half–life was 43 hours. Renal clearance accounts for approximately 30% of total peginterferon alfa-2b clearance. Following a single 4.5-mg subcutaneous dose of peginterferon alfa-2b, the mean exposure (area under the concentration-time curve [AUC]) of the drug was increased 1.4-fold in individuals with moderate renal impairment (creatinine clearance 30–50 mL/minute per 1.73 m^2) and was increased 2.1-fold in those with severe renal impairment (creatinine clearance less than 30 mL/minute per 1.73 m^2) or end-stage renal disease requiring dialysis when compared with the AUC in individuals with normal renal function (creatinine clearance exceeding 80 mL/minute per 1.73 m^2).

Advice to Patients

Advise patients of the importance of reading the manufacturer's patient information and medication guide.

Advise patients receiving peginterferon alfa-2b (Sylatron®) that administration with an antipyretic at bedtime may minimize common flu-like symptoms (e.g., chills, fever, muscle aches, joint pain, headaches, tiredness).

Advise patients to maintain hydration if they experience flu-like symptoms.

Importance of not reusing or sharing syringes or needles. Importance of proper disposal of vials, syringes, and needles.

Importance of informing clinicians of existing or previous treatment for mental illness, including depression, suicidal thoughts, or suicide attempts. Importance of reporting any sign or symptom of depression or suicidal ideation to clinician during treatment and up to 6 months after the last dose. Advise patients that immediate discontinuance of the drug may be necessary in severe cases.

Importance of informing clinicians of existing or contemplated concomitant therapy, including herbal supplements, prescription and OTC drugs, as well as concomitant illnesses.

Importance of women informing clinicians if they are or plan to become pregnant or plan to breast-feed. Importance of using peginterferon alfa-2b during pregnancy only if potential benefits justify potential risks to the fetus.

Importance of advising patients of other important precautionary information. (See Cautions.)

Overview® (see Users Guide). For additional information on this drug until a more detailed monograph is developed and published, the manufacturer's labeling should be consulted. It is *essential* that the manufacturer's labeling be consulted for more detailed information on usual cautions, precautions, contraindications, potential drug interactions, laboratory test interferences, and acute toxicity.

Preparations

Excipients in commercially available drug preparations may have clinically important effects in some individuals; consult specific product labeling for details.

Peginterferon Alfa-2b

Parenteral

For injection, for subcutaneous use	200 mcg/0.5 mL	**Sylatron®** (available as single-dose vials with 1.25 mL vial sterile water for injection diluent, Safety-Lok® syringes with safety sleeve, and alcohol swabs), Schering
	300 mcg/0.5 mL	**Sylatron®** (available as single-dose vials with 1.25 mL vial sterile water for injection diluent, Safety-Lok® syringes with safety sleeve, and alcohol swabs), Schering
	600 mcg/0.5 mL	**Sylatron®** (available as single-dose vials with 1.25 mL vial sterile water for injection diluent, Safety-Lok® syringes with safety sleeve, and alcohol swabs), Schering

Pembrolizumab

Lambrolizumab

■ Pembrolizumab, a humanized anti-programmed-death receptor-1 (anti-PD-1) monoclonal antibody, is an antineoplastic agent.

Uses

■ **Melanoma** ***Unresectable or Metastatic Melanoma*** Pembrolizumab is used for the treatment of unresectable or metastatic melanoma; pembrolizumab has been designated an orphan drug by FDA for the treatment of this cancer.

The current indication for pembrolizumab in the treatment of unresectable or metastatic melanoma is based principally on the results of an open-label, randomized phase 3 study (KEYNOTE-006) and a randomized phase 2 study (KEYNOTE-002).

In the KEYNOTE-006 study, 834 patients with ipilimumab-naive unresectable or metastatic melanoma who had received no more than one prior systemic therapy for metastatic disease were randomized (stratified by number of prior therapies, Eastern Cooperative Oncology Group [ECOG] performance status, and programmed-death ligand-1 [PD-L1] expression) in a 1:1:1 ratio to receive pembrolizumab 10 mg/kg administered as a 30-minute IV infusion every 2 or 3 weeks for up to 24 months or ipilimumab 3 mg/kg every 3 weeks administered as a 90-minute IV infusion for a maximum of 4 cycles. Treatment was continued for the specified duration or until the occurrence of unacceptable toxicity or disease progression that was symptomatic, rapidly progressive, associated with a decline in performance status, requiring urgent intervention, or confirmed in 4–6 weeks by repeat radiographic studies. The primary measures of efficacy were overall survival and progression-free survival (as evaluated by a blinded independent central review committee according to Response Evaluation Criteria in Solid Tumors [RECIST] modified to follow no more than 10 target lesions and no more than 5 target lesions per organ); additional outcome measures were objective response rate and duration of response.

The median age of patients enrolled in the KEYNOTE-006 study was 62 years; 98% were Caucasian and 60% were male. All patients enrolled in the study had an ECOG performance status of 0 or 1. Most patients (80%) had positive PD-L1 expression (defined as PD-L1 expression of any intensity on at least 1% of tumor cells as detected by an investigational assay), 65% had stage M1c disease, 66% had not received prior systemic therapies for metastatic disease, 68% had LDH concentrations within normal limits, 36% had tumors bearing the b-Raf serine-threonine kinase (BRAF) mutation, and 9% had a history of brain metastases. Approximately one-half of patients (46%) with BRAF mutation-positive disease had received prior therapy with a BRAF inhibitor. This study excluded patients with ocular melanoma, active brain metastases, autoimmune disease, conditions requiring therapy with immunosuppressive agents, human immunodeficiency virus (HIV) infection, or hepatitis B virus (HBV) or hepatitis C virus (HCV) infection.

In the KEYNOTE-006 study, a planned interim analysis indicated prolonged median progression-free survival in patients receiving pembrolizumab every 3 or 2 weeks compared with those receiving ipilimumab (4.1 or 5.5 months, respectively, versus 2.8 months; hazard ratio for both dosages: 0.58). The median follow-up period at the time of interim analysis was 7.9 months. After a minimum follow-up of 12 months, the risk of death in patients receiving pembrolizumab every 3 or 2 weeks was reduced by 31 or 37%, respectively, compared with those receiving ipilimumab. Patients receiving pembrolizumab every 3 or 2 weeks also had a higher objective response rate compared with those receiving ipilimumab (33 or 34%, respectively, versus 12%); complete responses were achieved in 5–6% of patients treated with pembrolizumab compared with 1% of those treated with ipilimumab. At the time of interim analysis, the median duration of response had not been reached in any group; however, responses were ongoing in 97, 89, or 88% of patients receiving pembrolizumab every 3 weeks, pembrolizumab every 2 weeks, or ipilimumab, respectively. Because of the survival benefit observed at the interim analysis, this study was terminated prematurely at the request of the independent data monitoring committee and patients previously randomized to receive ipilimumab were permitted to cross over to open-label pembrolizumab therapy. Overall survival, progression-free survival, and objective response rates for pembrolizumab- and ipilimumab-treated patients at the time of final analysis (at a median follow-up of 22.9 months) remained similar to the interim results; in the final analysis, no substantial differences in efficacy were observed between the 2 pembrolizumab dosage regimens. Results of a subgroup analysis (based on age, sex, ECOG performance status, serum LDH concentration, BRAF mutation status, number of prior therapies, PD-L1 status, and baseline tumor size) suggested that the effect of pembrolizumab on overall survival was consistent across all subgroups.

In the KEYNOTE-002 study, 540 patients with unresectable or metastatic melanoma were randomized (stratified by ECOG performance status, serum LDH concentrations, and BRAF mutation status) in a 1:1:1 ratio to receive pembrolizumab 2 or 10 mg/kg by IV infusion every 3 weeks or investigator's choice of chemotherapy (dacarbazine 1 g/m^2 IV every 3 weeks; temozolomide 200 mg/m^2 orally once daily for 5 days every 28 days; carboplatin at the dose required to obtain an area under the plasma concentration-time curve [AUC] of 6 mg/mL per minute in combination with paclitaxel 225 mg/m^2 IV every 3 weeks for 4 cycles followed by carboplatin at the dose required to obtain an AUC of 5 mg/mL per minute and paclitaxel 175 mg/m^2 IV every 3 weeks; paclitaxel 175 mg/m^2 IV every 3 weeks; or carboplatin at the dose required to obtain an AUC of 5 or 6 mg/mL per minute IV every 3 weeks). Treatment with pembrolizumab was continued until the occurrence of unacceptable toxicity or disease progression that was symptomatic, rapidly progressive, associated with a decline in performance status, requiring urgent intervention, or confirmed in 4–6 weeks by repeat radiographic studies. Patients randomized to receive chemotherapy were permitted to cross over to pembrolizumab therapy following disease progression.

Patients were enrolled in the KEYNOTE-002 study if their disease had progressed within 24 weeks of ipilimumab therapy and was refractory following at least 2 doses of ipilimumab (at a dose of at least 3 mg/kg) and, in those with tumors bearing the BRAF V600 mutation, refractory to therapy with a BRAF or mitogen-activated extracellular signal-regulated kinase (MEK) inhibitor. The primary measures of efficacy were progression-free survival (as evaluated by a blinded independent central review committee according to RECIST modified to follow no more than 10 target lesions and no more than 5 target lesions per organ) and overall survival; additional outcome measures were objective response rate (as evaluated by a blinded independent central review committee according to RECIST modified to follow no more than 10 target lesions and no more than 5 target lesions per organ) and duration of response. The median age of patients enrolled in the study was 62 years; 98% were Caucasian, 61% were male, 40% had elevated LDH concentrations at baseline, and 23% had tumors bearing the BRAF mutation. All patients enrolled in the study had an ECOG performance status of 0 or 1. Most patients (82%) had stage M1c disease and 73% had received at least 2 prior therapies for advanced or metastatic disease. This study excluded patients with uveal melanoma, active brain metastases or carcinomatous meningitis, autoimmune disease, active infection requiring systemic therapy, a history of HIV infection, or active HBV or HCV infection.

In the KEYNOTE-002 study, a planned interim analysis for progression-free survival indicated a 43 or 50% reduction in the risk of disease progression or death in patients receiving pembrolizumab 2 or 10 mg/kg, respectively, compared with those receiving chemotherapy. The median follow-up period at the time of interim analysis was 10 months. Patients receiving pembrolizumab at either dosage also had a higher objective response rate compared with those receiving chemotherapy (21–25% versus 4%); complete responses were achieved in 2–3% of patients treated with pembrolizumab compared with none of those treated with chemotherapy. At the final analysis (at a median follow-up of 28 months), median overall survival was prolonged in patients receiving pembrolizumab 2 or 10 mg/kg compared with those receiving chemotherapy (13.4 or 14.7 months, respectively, versus 11 months). Pembrolizumab 2 or 10 mg/kg reduced the risk of death by 14 or 26%, respectively, compared with chemotherapy; however, the prespecified level of statistical significance was not achieved. At the time of final analysis, the median duration of response was 22.8 months in patients receiving pembrolizumab 2 mg/kg, had not been reached in those receiving pembrolizumab 10 mg/kg, and was 6.8 months in those receiving chemotherapy. Progression-free survival and objective response rates for pembrolizumab- and chemotherapy-treated patients at the time of final analysis remained similar to the interim results; no substantial differences in efficacy were observed between the 2 pembrolizumab dosage regimens. Results of a subgroup analysis (based on ECOG performance status, baseline serum LDH concentration, BRAF mutation status, number of prior therapies, PD-L1 status, baseline tumor size, prior chemotherapy regimen, best response to ipilimumab, and disease stage) suggested that the effect of pembrolizumab on overall survival was consistent across all subgroups.

Adjuvant Therapy for Locally Advanced Melanoma Pembrolizumab is used as adjuvant therapy of melanoma with lymph node involvement following complete resection.

The current indication for use of pembrolizumab as adjuvant therapy of melanoma with lymph node involvement following complete resection is based principally on the results of a phase 3 randomized, double-blind, placebo-controlled study (KEYNOTE-054). In this study, 1019 adults with completely resected stage III melanoma were randomized (stratified by disease stage and geographic region) in a 1:1 ratio to receive either pembrolizumab (200 mg by IV infusion every 3 weeks) or placebo for up to 18 doses (approximately one year) or until disease progression or unacceptable toxicity occurred. Upon disease recurrence, patients could cross over to pembrolizumab therapy or receive repeat treatment with the drug. Patients were eligible for enrollment in the study following complete regional lymphadenectomy and, if indicated, radiation therapy within 13 weeks prior to initiation of study treatment. The primary measure of efficacy was recurrence-free survival in the entire study population and in the subset of patients with PD-L1-positive tumors (defined as a PD-L1 expression combined positive score of at least 1%, as measured by a clinical trial immunohistochemistry assay).

The median age of patients enrolled in the KEYNOTE-054 study was 54 years; 62% were male, 84% had positive PD-L1 expression, and 50% had tumors bearing the BRAF V600 mutation. Approximately one-half of patients (46%) had stage IIIB melanoma, 20% had stage IIIC disease with 4 or more positive lymph nodes, 18% had stage IIIC disease with 1–3 positive lymph nodes, and 16% had stage IIIA disease. All patients had an ECOG performance status of 0 or 1. The study excluded patients who had received prior systemic therapy for melanoma and those with autoimmune disease, uncontrolled infection, or any condition requiring use of systemic glucocorticoids.

At a median follow-up of 15 months in the KEYNOTE-054 study, median recurrence-free survival had not been reached in patients receiving pembrolizumab; however, pembrolizumab reduced the risk of recurrence or death by 43% compared with placebo. A recurrence-free survival benefit was observed for pembrolizumab regardless of tumor PD-L1 expression. For patients with PD-L1 positive tumors, pembrolizumab reduced the risk of recurrence or death by 46% compared with placebo. Results of an exploratory analysis (based on age, sex, disease stage, number of positive lymph nodes, microscopic versus macroscopic lymph node involvement, presence of tumor ulceration, and BRAF mutation status) suggested that the effect of pembrolizumab on recurrence-free survival was consistent across subgroups.

■ **Non-small Cell Lung Cancer** ***First-line Therapy for Metastatic Non-small Cell Lung Cancer*** **Monotherapy.** Pembrolizumab is used as a single agent for the initial treatment of metastatic non-small cell lung cancer (NSCLC) with high PD-L1 expression (defined as PD-L1 expression of any intensity on at least 50% of tumor cells [i.e., tumor proportion score of at least 50%]) and without epidermal growth factor receptor (EGFR) or anaplastic lymphoma kinase (ALK) genomic aberrations. An FDA-approved diagnostic test is required to confirm the presence of high PD-L1 expression prior to initiation of therapy.

The current indication for use of pembrolizumab as a single agent for the initial treatment of metastatic NSCLC in patients with high PD-L1 expression is based principally on the results of an open-label, randomized phase 3 study (KEYNOTE-024). In this study, 305 patients with previously untreated metastatic NSCLC with high PD-L1 expression (tumor proportion score of at least 50%) were randomized (stratified by ECOG performance status, histology, and geographic region) in a 1:1 ratio to receive either pembrolizumab (200 mg by IV infusion every 3 weeks for up to 24 months) or investigator's choice of platinum-based chemotherapy (pemetrexed 500 mg/m^2 IV and carboplatin at the dose required to obtain an AUC of 5–6 mg/mL per minute on day 1 of each 3-week cycle for 4–6 cycles, followed by an option to continue pemetrexed maintenance therapy; pemetrexed 500 mg/m^2 IV and cisplatin 75 mg/m^2 on day 1 of each 3-week cycle for 4–6 cycles, followed by an option to continue pemetrexed maintenance therapy; gemcitabine 1.25 g/m^2 on days 1 and 8 and cisplatin 75 mg/m^2 on day 1 of each 3-week cycle for 4–6 cycles; gemcitabine 1.25 g/m^2 on days 1 and 8 and carboplatin at the dose required to obtain an AUC of 5–6 mg/mL per minute on day 1 of each 3-week cycle for 4–6 cycles; paclitaxel 200 mg/m^2 and carboplatin at the dose required to obtain an AUC of 5–6 mg/mL per minute on day 1 of each 3-week cycle for 4–6 cycles, followed by an option to continue pemetrexed maintenance therapy). Treatment was continued for the specified duration or until disease progression or unacceptable toxicity occurred; however, clinically stable patients with disease progression could continue treatment if they were considered to be deriving clinical benefit. In addition, patients randomized to receive platinum-based chemotherapy were permitted to cross over to pembrolizumab therapy upon disease progression. Approximately 44% of the patients randomized to platinum-based chemotherapy crossed over to pembrolizumab therapy following disease progression. The primary measure of efficacy was progression-free survival (as evaluated by a blinded independent central review committee according to RECIST modified to follow no more than 10 target lesions and no more than 5 target lesions per organ); additional outcome measures were overall survival and objective response rate (as evaluated by a blinded independent central review committee according to RECIST modified to follow no more than 10 target lesions and no more than 5 target lesions per organ).

The median age of patients enrolled in the KEYNOTE-024 study was 65 years; 82% were Caucasian, 82% had nonsquamous histology, 61% were male, 18% had squamous histology, 15% were of Asian ancestry, and 9% had a history of brain metastases. With one exception, all patients had a baseline ECOG performance status of 0 or 1. This study excluded patients with EGFR or ALK genomic aberrations, untreated brain metastases, active autoimmune disease that required systemic therapy within 2 years of randomization, conditions requiring therapy with systemic corticosteroids or immunosuppressive agents, active interstitial lung disease or a history of pneumonitis requiring glucocorticoid therapy, or irradiation of the thoracic region at a dose exceeding 30 Gy within 26 weeks of enrollment.

In the KEYNOTE-024 study, patients receiving pembrolizumab had a longer median progression-free survival (10.3 versus 6 months based on intent-to-treat analysis; hazard ratio: 0.5) and overall survival (30 versus 14.2 months; hazard ratio: 0.6) compared with patients receiving platinum-based chemotherapy. Patients receiving pembrolizumab also had higher objective response rates compared with those receiving platinum-based chemotherapy (45 versus 28%); complete responses were achieved in 4 or 1% of patients receiving pembrolizumab or platinum-based chemotherapy, respectively. At the second interim analysis (at a median follow-up of 11.2 months), the median duration of response had not been reached in patients receiving pembrolizumab. The median time to response was similar in both treatment groups (2.2 months). Results of a subgroup analysis (based on age, sex, geographic region, ECOG performance status, histology, smoking status, presence of brain metastases, and prior use of pemetrexed in combination with platinum-based chemotherapy) suggested that the effect of pembrolizumab on progression-free survival was evident across all subgroups.

Combination Therapy for Metastatic Nonsquamous NSCLC. Pembrolizumab is used in combination with pemetrexed and a platinum-containing antineoplastic agent (carboplatin or cisplatin) for the initial treatment of metastatic nonsquamous NSCLC without EGFR or ALK genomic aberrations.

Efficacy of pembrolizumab in combination with pemetrexed and a platinum-containing antineoplastic agent (carboplatin or cisplatin) for the initial treatment of metastatic nonsquamous NSCLC is based principally on the results of a randomized, double-blind, phase 3 study (KEYNOTE-189). In this study, 616 adults with previously untreated metastatic NSCLC with nonsquamous histology were randomized (stratified by PD-L1 expression, platinum-containing antineoplastic agent, and smoking status) in a 2:1 ratio to receive either pembrolizumab in combination with pemetrexed and investigator's choice of a platinum-containing antineoplastic agent (carboplatin or cisplatin) or placebo in combination with pemetrexed and investigator's choice of a platinum-containing antineoplastic agent; 72% of patients enrolled in the study received carboplatin. Those randomized to the pembrolizumab combination regimen received pembrolizumab (200 mg by IV infusion) in combination with pemetrexed (500 mg/m^2 by IV infusion) and either carboplatin (at the dose required to obtain an AUC of 5 mg/mL per minute by IV infusion) or cisplatin (75 mg/m^2 by IV infusion) on day 1 of each 21-day cycle for 4 cycles followed by pembrolizumab (200 mg by IV infusion) in combination with pemetrexed (500 mg/m^2 by IV infusion) every 3 weeks. Those randomized to the placebo combination regimen received placebo in combination with pemetrexed and either carboplatin or cisplatin at the same dosages for 4 cycles followed by placebo in combination with pemetrexed (500 mg/m^2 by IV infusion) every 3 weeks. Treatment was continued for up to 24 months or until disease progression or unacceptable toxicity occurred; however, clinically stable patients with disease progression could continue treatment if they were considered to be deriving clinical benefit. In addition, patients randomized to receive placebo in combination with pemetrexed and a platinum-containing antineoplastic agent were permitted to cross over to single-agent pembrolizumab upon disease progression. Approximately 41% of patients randomized to receive the placebo combination regimen crossed over to therapy with an anti-programmed-death receptor-1 (PD-1) or anti-programmed-death ligand-1 (PD-L1) antibody following disease progression.

The primary measures of efficacy in the KEYNOTE-189 study were overall survival and progression-free survival (as evaluated by a blinded independent central review committee according to RECIST modified to follow no more than 10 target lesions and no more than 5 target lesions per organ); additional outcome measures were objective response rate (as evaluated by a blinded independent central review committee according to RECIST modified to follow no more than 10 target lesions and no more than 5 target lesions per organ) and duration of response.

The median age of patients enrolled in the KEYNOTE-189 study was 64 years; 94% were Caucasian, 59% were male, 56% had a baseline ECOG performance status of 1, 31% had a PD-L1 expression tumor proportion score of less than 1%, 18% had a history of brain metastases, 12% had never smoked, and 3% were of Asian ancestry. This study excluded patients with EGFR or ALK genomic aberrations, conditions requiring therapy with systemic corticosteroids or immunosuppressive agents, active autoimmune disease requiring systemic therapy within the previous 2 years, symptomatic brain metastases, history of pneumonitis requiring therapy with glucocorticoids, or irradiation of the thoracic region at a dose exceeding 30 Gy within 26 weeks of enrollment.

At a median follow-up of 10.5 months in the KEYNOTE-189 study, patients receiving the pembrolizumab combination regimen had a longer median progression-free survival compared with patients receiving the placebo combination regimen (8.8 versus 4.9 months; hazard ratio: 0.52). Although median overall survival for patients receiving the pembrolizumab combination regimen had not been reached at the time of analysis, median overall survival appeared to be prolonged in patients receiving pembrolizumab in combination with pemetrexed and a platinum-containing antineoplastic agent compared with those receiving placebo in combination with pemetrexed and a platinum-containing antineoplastic agent (hazard ratio: 0.49). Patients receiving the pembrolizumab combination regimen also had higher objective response rates compared with those receiving the placebo combination regimen (48 versus 19%); complete responses were achieved in 0.5% of patients in both treatment groups. At the time of analysis, the median duration of response was 11.2 and 7.8 months in patients receiving the pembrolizumab combination regimen and those receiving the placebo combination regimen, respectively.

Results of a subgroup analysis (based on age, sex, ECOG performance status, smoking status, presence of brain metastases, level of PD-L1 expression, and platinum-containing antineoplastic agent) suggested that the effect of pembrolizumab on overall survival and progression-free survival was evident across all subgroups. Subgroup analysis also indicated that the effect of pembrolizumab on objective response rate was evident regardless of level of PD-L1 expression, but objective response rates were substantially greater in patients with PD-L1 expression of any intensity on at least 50% of tumor cells (i.e., tumor proportion score of at least 50%) who received the pembrolizumab combination regimen compared with those who received the placebo combination regimen (61.4 versus 22.9%).

Combination Therapy for Metastatic Squamous NSCLC. Pembrolizumab is used in combination with carboplatin and paclitaxel (conventional or albumin-bound) for the initial treatment of metastatic squamous NSCLC.

Efficacy of pembrolizumab in combination with carboplatin and paclitaxel (conventional or albumin-bound) for the initial treatment of metastatic squamous NSCLC is based principally on the results of a randomized, double-blind phase 3 study (KEYNOTE-407). In this study, 559 adults with previously untreated metastatic NSCLC with squamous histology were randomized (stratified by PD-L1 expression, geographic region, and paclitaxel formulation) in a 1:1 ratio to receive either pembrolizumab in combination with carboplatin and investigator's choice of paclitaxel formulation (conventional or albumin-bound paclitaxel) or placebo in combination with carboplatin and investigator's choice of paclitaxel formulation; 60% of patients enrolled in the study received conventional paclitaxel. Those randomized to the pembrolizumab-carboplatin-paclitaxel regimen received pembrolizumab (200 mg by IV infusion) in combination with carboplatin (at the dose required to obtain an AUC of 6 mg/mL per minute by IV infusion) on day 1 of each 21-day cycle for 4 cycles and either conventional paclitaxel (200 mg/m^2) on day 1 of each 21-day cycle or albumin-bound paclitaxel (100 mg/m^2) on days 1, 8, and 15 of each 21-day cycle for 4 cycles followed by pembrolizumab (200 mg by IV infusion) every 3 weeks. Those randomized to the placebo-carboplatin-paclitaxel regimen received placebo in combination with carboplatin and either conventional or albumin-bound paclitaxel at the same dosages for 4 cycles followed by placebo every 3 weeks. Therapy was continued for up to 24 months or until disease progression or unacceptable toxicity occurred; however, clinically stable patients with disease progression could continue receiving pembrolizumab if they were considered to be deriving clinical benefit. In addition, patients randomized to receive placebo-carboplatin-paclitaxel were permitted to cross over to single-agent pembrolizumab upon disease progression. Approximately 32% of patients randomized to receive placebo-carboplatin-paclitaxel crossed over to therapy with an anti-PD-1 or anti-PD-L1 antibody following disease progression.

The primary measures of efficacy in the KEYNOTE-407 study were progression-free survival and objective response rate (as evaluated by a blinded independent central review committee according to RECIST modified to follow no more than 10 target lesions and no more than 5 target lesions per organ) and overall survival; an additional outcome measure was duration of response (as evaluated by a blinded independent central review committee according to RECIST modified to follow no more than 10 target lesions and no more than 5 target lesions per organ).

The median age of patients enrolled in the KEYNOTE-407 study was 65 years; 81% were male, 77% were Caucasian, 71% had a baseline ECOG performance status of 1, 35% had a PD-L1 expression tumor proportion score of less than 1%, 19% were of East Asian ancestry, and 8% had a history of brain metastases. This study excluded patients with conditions requiring therapy with immunosuppressive agents, active autoimmune disease requiring systemic therapy within the previous 2 years, symptomatic brain metastases, history of pneumonitis requiring therapy with glucocorticoids, or irradiation of the thoracic region at a dose exceeding 30 Gy within 26 weeks of enrollment.

At a median follow-up of 7.8 months in the KEYNOTE-407 study, patients receiving pembrolizumab-carboplatin-paclitaxel had a longer median overall survival (15.9 versus 11.3 months based on intent-to-treat analysis; hazard ratio: 0.64) and progression-free survival (6.4 versus 4.8 months based on intent-to-treat analysis; hazard ratio: 0.56) compared with patients receiving placebo-carboplatin-paclitaxel. In the primary efficacy population (consisting of the initial 204 patients enrolled in the study), patients receiving pembrolizumab-carboplatin-paclitaxel had higher objective response rates compared with those receiving placebo-carboplatin-paclitaxel (58 versus 35%); the median duration of response was 7.2 and 4.9 months in patients receiving these respective treatments.

Results of a subgroup analysis (based on age, sex, ECOG performance status, level of PD-L1 expression, and paclitaxel formulation) suggested that the effect of pembrolizumab on overall survival and progression-free survival was evident across all subgroups. Subgroup analysis also indicated that the effect of pembrolizumab on objective response rate was evident regardless of level of PD-L1 expression, but objective response rates were substantially greater in patients with PD-L1 expression of any intensity on at least 50% of tumor cells (i.e., tumor proportion score of at least 50%) who received pembrolizumab-carboplatin-paclitaxel compared with those who received placebo-carboplatin-paclitaxel (60.3 versus 32.9%).

Previously Treated Metastatic Non-small Cell Lung Cancer Pembrolizumab is used as a single agent for the treatment of PD-L1-positive (defined as PD-L1 expression of any intensity on at least 1% of tumor cells [i.e., tumor proportion score of at least 1%]) metastatic NSCLC that has progressed during or following platinum-based chemotherapy, and, if the tumor is EGFR- or ALK-positive, during or following an FDA-labeled anti-EGFR or anti-ALK therapy. An FDA-approved diagnostic test is required to confirm the presence of PD-L1 expression prior to initiation of therapy.

The current indication for use of pembrolizumab as a single agent for the treatment of metastatic NSCLC in patients with disease progression during or following platinum-based chemotherapy is based principally on the results of an open-label, randomized phase 2/3 study (KEYNOTE-010). Patients were enrolled in the study if PD-L1 expression of any intensity on at least 1% of tumor cells was detected by immunohistochemistry assay (PD-L1 IHC 22C3 pharmDx). In this study, 1033 patients were randomized (stratified by level of PD-L1 expression, ECOG performance status, and geographic region) in a 1:1:1 ratio to receive pembrolizumab 2 or 10 mg/kg by IV infusion every 3 weeks or docetaxel 75 mg/m^2 by IV infusion every 3 weeks. Treatment was continued for up to 24 months or until the occurrence of unacceptable toxicity or disease progression that was symptomatic, rapidly progressive, associated with a decline in performance status, requiring urgent intervention, or confirmed in 4–6 weeks by repeat radiographic studies. The primary measures of efficacy were overall survival and progression-free survival (as evaluated by a blinded independent central review committee according to RECIST modified to follow no more than 10 target lesions and no more than 5 target lesions per organ) in the total population and in patients with high PD-L1 expression (defined as PD-L1 expression of any intensity on at least 50% of tumor cells); additional outcome measures were objective response rate and duration of response.

The median age of patients enrolled in the KEYNOTE-010 study was 63 years; 72% were Caucasian, 70% had nonsquamous histology, 66% had an ECOG performance status of 1, 61% were male, 43% had high PD-L1 expression, 21% were of Asian ancestry, 21% had squamous histology, 15% had a history of brain metastases, 8% had EGFR genomic aberrations, and 1% had ALK genomic aberrations. Most of the patients (91%) had metastatic disease; all patients enrolled in the study had received prior therapy with a platinum-containing, 2-drug combination regimen and 29% had received at least 2 prior therapies for metastatic disease. This study excluded patients with active autoimmune disease requiring systemic corticosteroids, conditions requiring therapy with immunosuppressive agents, active brain metastases or carcinomatous meningitis; interstitial lung disease or a history of pneumonitis requiring corticosteroid therapy, or irradiation of the thoracic region at a dose exceeding 30 Gy within 26 weeks of enrollment.

In the total patient population of the KEYNOTE-010 study, median overall survival was prolonged in patients receiving pembrolizumab 2 or 10 mg/kg compared with those receiving docetaxel (10.4 or 12.7 months, respectively, versus 8.5 months; hazard ratio: 0.71 or 0.61, respectively). Among patients with high PD-L1 expression, median overall survival also was prolonged in patients receiving pembrolizumab 2 or 10 mg/kg compared with those receiving docetaxel (14.9 or 17.3 months, respectively, versus 8.2 months; hazard ratio: 0.54 or 0.5, respectively). In the total patient population, no difference in median progression-free survival was observed between patients receiving pembrolizumab 2 or 10 mg/kg and those receiving docetaxel; however, among those with high PD-L1 expression, median progression-free survival was prolonged in patients receiving pembrolizumab at either dosage compared with those receiving docetaxel (5.2 versus 4.1 months; hazard ratio: 0.58–0.59). Patients receiving pembrolizumab at either dosage also had higher objective response rates compared with those receiving docetaxel in the total patient population (18–19 versus 9%) and in the cohort of patients with high PD-L1 expression (29–30% versus 8%). Complete responses were not achieved in any treatment group. At a median follow-up of 13.1 months, the median duration of response had not been reached in patients receiving pembrolizumab. The median time to response in the cohort of patients with high PD-L1 expression was similar in each treatment group (9 weeks). Results of a subgroup analysis (based on age, sex, ECOG performance status, PD-L1 expression, new or archival tumor sample, EGFR mutation status, and histology) suggested that the effect of pembrolizumab on overall survival was consistent across all subgroups.

■ **Head and Neck Cancer** Pembrolizumab is used for the treatment of recurrent or metastatic head and neck squamous cell carcinoma that has progressed during or following platinum-containing therapy. The accelerated approval of pembrolizumab for this indication is based on objective response rate and duration of response. Continued approval for this indication may be contingent on verification and description of clinical benefit of pembrolizumab in confirmatory studies.

The current indication for pembrolizumab in the treatment of recurrent or metastatic head and neck squamous cell carcinoma is based principally on the results for a cohort of patients with head and neck squamous cell carcinoma in an open-label, multicenter, nonrandomized, phase 1b study (KEYNOTE-012); the cohort of patients with head and neck squamous cell carcinoma included 174 adults with head and neck squamous cell carcinoma that had progressed during or following platinum-containing therapy for recurrent or metastatic disease or following platinum-containing therapy as part of induction, concurrent, or adjuvant therapy. Patients were enrolled in the study if PD-L1 expression of any intensity on at least 1% of tumor cells was detected by immunohistochemistry assay. Patients were eligible for enrollment in the study regardless of their human papillomavirus (HPV) status. Patients received pembrolizumab 10 mg/kg administered as an IV infusion every 2 weeks or 200 mg administered as an IV infusion every 3 weeks for up to 24 months or until the occurrence of unacceptable toxicity or disease progression that was symptomatic, rapidly progressive, associated with a decline in performance status, requiring urgent intervention, or confirmed after at least 4 weeks by repeat radiographic studies. Reinitiation of pembrolizumab was permitted for subsequent disease progression for up to one additional year.

The median age of patients enrolled in the head and neck squamous cell carcinoma cohort of the KEYNOTE-012 study was 60 years; 87% had metastatic disease, 82% were male, 75% were Caucasian, 63% previously had received cetuximab therapy, 33% had HPV-positive tumors, 16% were of Asian ancestry, and 6% were black. All patients enrolled in the study had an ECOG performance status of 0 or 1. In the cohort of patients with head and neck squamous cell carcinoma, the median number of prior therapies was 2. This study excluded patients with active autoimmune disease, conditions requiring therapy with immunosuppressive agents, interstitial lung disease, brain metastases, infections requiring systemic therapy, HIV infection, or HBV or HCV infection.

At a median follow-up of 8.9 months, the objective response rate for patients in the head and neck squamous cell carcinoma cohort of the KEYNOTE-012 study was 16%; complete response was achieved in 5% of patients. At the time of analysis, the median duration of response had not been reached; however, 82% of patients who responded to pembrolizumab had durable responses of 6 months or more. Objective response rates and duration of response were similar in both dosage groups and those with HPV-negative or HPV-positive disease. Objective response rate was similar in an expansion cohort of patients who received a fixed dosage of pembrolizumab (200 mg administered by IV infusion every 3 weeks). Adverse effects were similar between both dosage regimens.

■ **Hodgkin Lymphoma** Pembrolizumab is used for the treatment of refractory classical Hodgkin lymphoma (cHL) and cHL that has relapsed following at least 3 prior therapies; pembrolizumab has been designated an orphan drug by FDA for the treatment of this cancer. The accelerated approval of pembrolizumab for this indication is based on objective response rate and duration of response. Continued approval for this indication may be contingent on verification and description of clinical benefit of pembrolizumab in confirmatory studies.

The current indication for use of pembrolizumab for the treatment of relapsed or refractory cHL is based principally on the results of an open-label, multicenter, noncomparative phase 2 study (KEYNOTE-087). Patients were enrolled in 3 cohorts: those with disease progression following autologous stem cell transplantation and subsequent therapy with brentuximab vedotin, those with disease progression following salvage chemotherapy and brentuximab vedotin, and those with disease progression following autologous transplantation only. In this study, 210 patients received pembrolizumab 200 mg by IV infusion every 3 weeks for up to 24 months or until disease progression or unacceptable toxicity occurred; however, clinically stable patients were permitted to continue pembrolizumab therapy despite disease progression at the time of the initial assessment. The primary measure of efficacy was objective response rate (as evaluated by a blinded independent central review committee according to revised International Working Group [IWG] criteria).

The median age of patients enrolled in the KEYNOTE-087 study was 35 years; 88% were Caucasian and 9% were 65 years of age or older. With one exception, all patients had a baseline ECOG performance status of 0 or 1. Patients in this study had received a median of 4 prior therapies for cHL; 58% of patients were refractory to their most recent therapy (35% of these patients had primary refractory disease and 14% were refractory to all prior therapies), 61% had undergone prior autologous stem cell transplantation, 83% previously had received brentuximab vedotin, and 36% had received prior radiation therapy. This study excluded patients with active noninfectious pneumonitis; those who had received an allogeneic stem cell transplant within the past 5 years; those who had received an allogeneic stem cell transplant and experienced symptoms of graft-versus-host disease (GVHD); and those with CNS involvement, active autoimmune disease that required systemic therapy in the past 2 years, conditions requiring therapy with immunosuppressive agents, active infection requiring systemic therapy, HIV infection, or active HBV or HCV infection.

At a median follow-up of 9.4 months, the objective response rate was 69% with a median response duration of 11.1 months; complete response was achieved in 22% of patients. Objective response rates were similar in each cohort.

■ Primary Mediastinal Large B-cell Lymphoma Pembrolizumab is used for the treatment of refractory primary mediastinal large B-cell lymphoma (PMBL) and PMBL that has relapsed following at least 2 prior therapies; pembrolizumab has been designated an orphan drug by FDA for the treatment of this cancer. The accelerated approval of pembrolizumab for this indication is based on objective response rate and duration of response. Continued approval for this indication may be contingent on verification and description of clinical benefit of pembrolizumab in confirmatory studies.

The current indication for use of pembrolizumab for the treatment of relapsed or refractory PMBL is based principally on the results of an open-label, multicenter, noncomparative phase 2 study (KEYNOTE-170). In this study, 53 patients received pembrolizumab 200 mg by IV infusion every 3 weeks for up to 24 months or until disease progression or unacceptable toxicity occurred. The primary measures of efficacy were objective response rate (as evaluated by a blinded independent central review committee according to revised IWG criteria) and duration of response.

The median age of patients enrolled in the KEYNOTE-170 study was 33 years; 92% were Caucasian and 43% were male. All patients had a baseline ECOG performance status of 0 or 1. Patients in this study had received a median of 3 prior therapies for PMBL; 49% of patients had relapsed disease refractory to their most recent therapy, 36% had primary refractory disease, 32% had received prior radiation therapy, 26% had undergone prior autologous stem cell transplantation, and 15% had untreated relapsed disease. All patients had received prior therapy with rituximab. This study excluded patients with active noninfectious pneumonitis; those who had received an allogeneic stem cell transplant within the past 5 years; those who had received an allogeneic stem cell transplant and experienced symptoms of graft-versus-host disease (GVHD); those with active autoimmune disease; and those with conditions requiring therapy with immunosuppressive agents or active infection requiring systemic therapy.

At a median follow-up of 9.7 months, the objective response rate was 45% with a median time to response of 2.8 months; complete response was achieved in 11% of patients. At the time of analysis, median duration of response had not been reached.

Pembrolizumab is not recommended for the treatment of PMBL in patients who require urgent cytoreduction.

■ Urothelial Carcinoma Pembrolizumab is used for the treatment of locally advanced or metastatic urothelial carcinoma that has progressed during or following platinum-containing therapy or within 12 months of platinum-containing therapy in the neoadjuvant or adjuvant setting. Pembrolizumab also is used for the treatment of locally advanced or metastatic urothelial carcinoma in patients with high PD-L1 expression (defined as a PD-L1 expression combined positive score of at least 10%) who are not candidates for cisplatin-containing therapy and those who are not candidates for platinum-containing chemotherapy regardless of PD-L1 expression. An FDA-approved diagnostic test is required to confirm the presence of high PD-L1 expression prior to initiation of pembrolizumab therapy in patients who are not candidates for cisplatin. The accelerated approval of pembrolizumab for the treatment of locally advanced or metastatic urothelial carcinoma in patients who are not candidates for cisplatin or platinum-containing therapy is based on objective response rate and duration of response. Continued approval for use of pembrolizumab for this indication may be contingent on verification and description of clinical benefit of pembrolizumab in confirmatory studies.

The current indication for pembrolizumab in the treatment of locally advanced or metastatic urothelial carcinoma that has progressed during or following platinum-containing therapy or within 12 months of platinum-containing therapy in the neoadjuvant or adjuvant setting is based principally on the results of an open-label, multicenter, randomized, phase 3 study (KEYNOTE-045). In this study, 542 patients with locally advanced or metastatic urothelial carcinoma that had progressed following platinum-containing therapy or within 12 months following platinum-containing therapy in the neoadjuvant or adjuvant setting were randomized (stratified by ECOG performance status, presence of liver metastases, baseline hemoglobin concentration, and time elapsed since last dose of chemotherapy) in a 1:1 ratio to receive either pembrolizumab (200 mg by IV infusion) or investigator's choice of chemotherapy (paclitaxel 175 mg/m^2 IV, docetaxel 75 mg/m^2 IV, or vinflunine 320 mg/m^2 IV [not commercially available in the US]) every 3 weeks. Treatment was continued for up to 24 months or until the occurrence of unacceptable toxicity or disease progression that was symptomatic, rapidly progressive, associated with a decline in performance status, requiring urgent intervention, or confirmed by repeat radiographic studies. The primary measures of efficacy were overall survival and progression-free survival (as evaluated by a blinded independent central review committee according to RECIST modified to follow no more than 10 target lesions and no more than 5 target lesions per organ); additional outcome measures were objective response rate (as evaluated by a blinded independent central review committee according to RECIST modified to follow no more than 10 target lesions and no more than 5 target lesions per organ) and duration of response.

The median age of patients enrolled in the KEYNOTE-045 study was 66 years; 98% had an ECOG performance status of 0 or 1, 96% had metastatic disease, 87% had visceral metastases (including 34% with metastases to the liver), 74% were male, 72% were Caucasian, 23% were of Asian ancestry, and 21% had received at least 2 prior systemic therapies for metastatic disease. The lower or upper urinary tract was the primary site of the tumor in 86 or 14% of patients, respectively. Most patients (76%) had received prior therapy with cisplatin, 23% had received carboplatin, and 1% had received therapy containing other platinum agents; 15% of patients had disease progression following platinum-containing therapy in the neoadjuvant or adjuvant setting. Patients with active brain metastases or carcinomatous meningitis, autoimmune disease, interstitial lung disease, conditions requiring therapy with immunosuppressive agents, active infection requiring systemic therapy, a history of HIV infection, active HBV or HCV infection, or at least one poor prognostic factor for second-line therapy (i.e., hemoglobin concentration less than 10 g/dL, liver metastases, last dose of chemotherapy less than 3 months prior to enrollment) were excluded from the study.

In the KEYNOTE-045 study, median overall survival was prolonged in patients receiving pembrolizumab compared with those receiving chemotherapy (10.3 versus 7.4 months; hazard ratio: 0.73); however, a difference in median progression-free survival was not observed between the treatment groups. Patients receiving pembrolizumab also had higher objective response rates compared with those receiving chemotherapy (21 versus 11%); complete responses were achieved in 7 or 3% of patients receiving pembrolizumab or chemotherapy, respectively. Median duration of response had not been reached in patients receiving pembrolizumab. The median follow-up period at the time of the analysis was 9 months. Results of a subgroup analysis (based on age, sex, ECOG performance status, smoking status, histology, PD-L1 expression, site of primary tumor, site of metastases, presence of liver metastases, baseline hemoglobin concentration, number of risk factors, setting of most recent therapy, time elapsed since most recent therapy, previous platinum therapy, and investigator's choice of chemotherapy) suggested that the effect of pembrolizumab on overall survival was consistent across all subgroups; however, an overall survival benefit for the drug compared with chemotherapy was not apparent in the subgroup of patients who had never smoked (hazard ratio: 1.06).

The current indication for pembrolizumab in the treatment of locally advanced or metastatic urothelial carcinoma in patients who are not candidates for cisplatin-containing therapy is based principally on the results of an open-label, multicenter, noncomparative, phase 2 study (KEYNOTE-052). In this study, 370 patients with locally advanced or metastatic urothelial carcinoma who were not candidates for cisplatin-containing therapy received pembrolizumab 200 mg by IV infusion every 3 weeks. Treatment was continued for up to 24 months or until the occurrence of unacceptable toxicity or disease progression that was symptomatic, rapidly progressive, associated with a decline in performance status, requiring urgent intervention, or confirmed by repeat radiographic studies. The primary measure of efficacy was objective response rate (as evaluated by an independent central review committee according to RECIST modified to follow no more than 10 target lesions and no more than 5 target lesions per organ) and duration of response.

The median age of patients enrolled in the KEYNOTE-052 study was 74 years; 89% were Caucasian, 87% had metastatic disease, 85% had visceral metastases (including 21% with metastases to the liver), and 77% were male. The lower or upper urinary tract was the primary site of the tumor in 81 or 19% of patients, respectively. Most patients (90%) were treatment-naive and 10% had received platinum-containing therapy in the neoadjuvant or adjuvant setting. Approximately one-third (30%) of patients had high expression of PD-L1 (defined as a combined positive score of at least 10% as detected by an immunohistochemistry assay); the median age of these patients was 73 years, 87% were Caucasian, 68% were male, 82% had metastatic disease, 81% had a primary tumor in the lower urinary tract, 18% had a primary tumor in the upper urinary tract, 76% had visceral metastases (including 11% with metastases to the liver), 90% were treatment-naive, and 10% had received platinum-containing therapy in the neoadjuvant or adjuvant setting. Reasons for cisplatin ineligibility included baseline renal impairment (creatinine clearance less than 60 mL/minute), poor performance status (ECOG performance status of 2), poor performance status and baseline renal impairment, or other reasons (i.e., New York Heart Association [NYHA] class III heart failure, peripheral neuropathy or hearing loss of grade 2 or greater severity) in 50, 32, 9, or 9%, respectively, of patients in the total patient population and 45, 37, 10, or 8%, respectively, of patients in the subset of patients with high PD-L1 expression. Patients with active brain metastases and/or carcinomatous meningitis, autoimmune disease, interstitial lung disease, conditions requiring therapy with immunosuppressive agents, active infection requiring systemic therapy, a history of HIV infection, or active HBV or HCV infection were excluded from the study.

In the KEYNOTE-052 study, the objective response rate was 29%; complete response was achieved in 7% of patients. Among patients with high PD-L1 expression, the objective response rate was 47%; complete response was achieved in 15% of patients. At a median follow-up of 7.8 months, median duration of response had not been reached.

Decreased survival with pembrolizumab monotherapy compared with platinum-based therapy has been reported in an ongoing clinical trial (KEYNOTE-361) in patients with previously untreated metastatic urothelial carcinoma with low PD-L1 expression; pembrolizumab monotherapy is *not* currently FDA-labeled for use in such patients. In this trial, patients with previously untreated metastatic urothelial carcinoma who were eligible for platinum-containing therapy were randomized to receive pembrolizumab monotherapy, pembrolizumab in combination with platinum-based therapy (cisplatin or carboplatin in combination with gemcitabine), or platinum-based therapy alone. A preliminary data analysis showed decreased survival of patients with low PD-L1 expression who were receiving pembrolizumab monotherapy compared with those receiving platinum-based therapy. Therefore, at the request of the independent data monitoring committee, enrollment in the pembrolizumab monotherapy group was halted for patients with low expression of PD-L1 (defined as a PD-L1 expression combined positive score of less than 10%).

■ Solid Tumors with High Microsatellite Instability or Mismatch Repair Deficiency Pembrolizumab is used for the treatment of unresectable or metastatic solid tumors with high microsatellite instability (MSI-H) or mismatch repair deficiency (dMMR) that have progressed following prior therapy in patients who are not candidates for other treatment options; in the treatment of unresectable or metastatic MSI-H or dMMR colorectal cancer, pembrolizumab is used in patients who have experienced disease progression following therapy with a fluoropyrimidine, oxaliplatin, and irinotecan. The accelerated approval of pembrolizumab for this indication is based on objective response rate and duration of response. Continued approval for this indication may be contingent on verification and description of clinical benefit of pembrolizumab in confirmatory studies.

Although some solid tumors, such as colorectal cancer, are generally unresponsive to anti-PD-1 therapy, a subpopulation of patients with solid tumors with MSI-H or dMMR has been shown to be particularly responsive to anti-PD-1 therapy. Deficiencies in the DNA mismatch repair pathway as a result of germline or somatic mutations in mismatch repair genes subsequently result in elevated levels of DNA instability in regions of short tandem repeat sequences (microsatellites) that are prone to replication errors (MSI-H). It has been postulated that the increased mutational burden in tumors with microsatellite instability produces tumor-specific neoantigens responsible for elevated levels of tumor-infiltrating lymphocytes and upregulation of immune checkpoint proteins such as PD-1 and PD-L1, suggesting that patients with solid tumors with MSI-H or dMMR are good candidates for immune checkpoint therapy. Clinical studies have demonstrated increased response rates in patients with solid tumors, particularly colorectal cancer, with MSI-H or dMMR receiving anti-PD-1 therapy. In a phase 2 study evaluating pembrolizumab in patients with solid tumors with dMMR or proficient mismatch repair (pMMR), the objective response rate (40 versus 0%) and progression-free survival rate (78 versus 11%) were substantially higher in patients with colorectal cancer with dMMR compared with those with pMMR colorectal cancer; response rates in patients with noncolorectal cancers with dMMR were similar to those in patients with colorectal cancer with dMMR.

The current indication for pembrolizumab in the treatment of unresectable or metastatic MSI-H or dMMR solid tumors, including colorectal cancer, is based principally on pooled results for 149 patients with MSI-H or dMMR solid tumors across 5 open-label, multicenter, noncomparative trials (KEYNOTE-016, KEYNOTE-164, KEYNOTE-012, KEYNOTE-028, KEYNOTE-158). In these trials, patients received either pembrolizumab 200 mg IV every 3 weeks or pembrolizumab 10 mg/kg IV every 2 weeks for up to 24 months or until the occurrence of unacceptable toxicity or disease progression that was symptomatic, rapidly progressive, associated with a decline in performance status, or requiring urgent intervention. The primary measures of efficacy were objective response rate (as evaluated by a blinded independent central review committee according to RECIST modified to follow no more than 10 target lesions and no more than 5 target lesions per organ) and duration of response.

The median age of patients included in the pooled analysis was 55 years; 98% had metastatic disease, 77% were Caucasian, 19% were of Asian ancestry, and 2% were black. Most patients with metastatic colorectal cancer (84%) and 53% of those with other solid tumors had received at least 2 prior therapies. Patients evaluated in the pooled analysis had received a median of 2 prior therapies for metastatic or unresectable disease. Patients with active autoimmune disease or conditions requiring therapy with immunosuppressive agents were excluded from these trials.

In the pooled cohort of patients with MSI-H or dMMR solid tumors, the objective response rate was 39.6%; complete response was achieved in 7.4% of patients. At the time of analysis, the median duration of response had not been reached; however, 78% of the patients who responded to pembrolizumab had durable responses of 6 months or more. Among patients with colorectal cancer or other solid tumors, the objective response rate was 36 or 46%, respectively.

The safety and efficacy of pembrolizumab in pediatric patients with MSI-H CNS malignancies have not been established; use of pembrolizumab is *not* indicated for use in these patients.

■ Gastric Cancer Pembrolizumab is used for the treatment of recurrent, locally advanced or metastatic, PD-L1-positive (defined as a combined positive score of at least 1%, reflecting the proportion of PD-L1-staining tumor cells, macrophages, and lymphocytes relative to tumor cells in the tumor microenvironment) gastric adenocarcinoma, including adenocarcinoma of the gastroesophageal junction, that has progressed during or following at least 2 prior therapies, including fluoropyrimidine- and platinum-containing chemotherapy, and, if the tumor overexpresses the human epidermal growth factor receptor type 2 (HER2) protein, during or following therapy with an anti-HER2 agent. An FDA-approved diagnostic test is required to confirm the presence of PD-L1 expression prior to initiation of therapy. The accelerated approval of pembrolizumab for this indication is based on objective response rate and duration of response. Continued approval for this indication may be contingent on verification and description of clinical benefit of pembrolizumab in confirmatory studies.

The current indication for pembrolizumab in the treatment of gastric cancer is based principally on the results of an open-label phase 2 trial (KEYNOTE-059) in a cohort of 143 patients with gastric adenocarcinoma, including adenocarcinoma of the gastroesophageal junction, that had progressed during or following at least 2 prior therapies; with a PD-L1-expression combined positive score of at least 1%, as detected by an immunohistochemistry assay (PD-L1 IHC 22C3 pharmDx); and with either microsatellite stable disease or unknown microsatellite instability (MSI) or mismatch repair (MMR) status. Patients enrolled in the study must have received a platinum- and fluoropyrimidine-containing regimen and, in those with tumors overexpressing the HER2 protein, therapy with an anti-HER2 agent. In this study, patients received pembrolizumab 200 mg by IV infusion every 3 weeks. Treatment was continued for up to 24 months or until the occurrence of unacceptable toxicity or disease progression that was symptomatic, rapidly progressive, associated with a decline in performance status, requiring urgent intervention, or confirmed after at least 4 weeks by repeat radiographic studies. The primary measures of efficacy were objective response rate (as evaluated by a blinded independent central review committee according to RECIST modified to follow no more than 10 target lesions and no more than 5 target lesions per organ) and duration of response.

The median age of patients enrolled in the KEYNOTE-059 trial was 64 years; 82% were Caucasian, 77% were male, and 11% were of Asian ancestry. Most patients (85%) had metastatic disease; 51 or 49% had received at least 2 or 3 prior therapies, respectively, for recurrent or metastatic disease. All enrolled patients had a baseline ECOG performance status of 0 or 1. Patients with active autoimmune disease, conditions requiring therapy with immunosuppressive agents, or clinical evidence of ascites were excluded from the trial.

In the KEYNOTE-059 trial, the objective response rate was 13.3%; complete response was achieved in 1.4% of patients. At the time of analysis, the median duration of response had not been reached; however, 58% of the patients who responded to pembrolizumab had durable responses of at least 6 months and 26% had durable responses of at least 12 months. Among 7 patients with MSI-H tumors, 4 patients achieved an objective response, including 1 patient with a complete response; median duration of response had not been reached.

■ Cervical Cancer Pembrolizumab is used for the treatment of recurrent or metastatic, PD-L1-positive (defined as a combined positive score of at least 1%) cervical cancer that has progressed during or following chemotherapy. An FDA-approved diagnostic test is required to confirm the presence of PD-L1 expression prior to initiation of therapy. The accelerated approval of pembrolizumab for this indication is based on objective response rate and duration of response. Continued approval for this indication may be contingent on verification and description of clinical benefit of pembrolizumab in confirmatory studies.

The current indication for pembrolizumab in the treatment of recurrent or metastatic cervical cancer is based principally on the results for a subset of 77 patients with PD-L1-positive cervical cancer (part of a cohort of 98 patients with cervical cancer) in an open-label, multicenter, nonrandomized, phase 2 study (KEYNOTE-158). These 77 patients had a PD-L1 combined positive score of at least 1% as detected by an immunohistochemistry assay (PD-L1 IHC 22C3 pharmDx) and had received at least one prior chemotherapy regimen in the metastatic setting. Patients received pembrolizumab 200 mg administered as an IV infusion every 3 weeks. Treatment was continued for up to 24 months or until unacceptable toxicity or disease progression occurred; however, patients with disease progression could receive additional doses of the drug until disease progression was confirmed, unless disease progression was symptomatic, rapidly progressive, associated with a decline in performance status, or requiring urgent intervention.

The median age of the 77 patients in the KEYNOTE-158 study with PD-L1-positive cervical cancer was 45 years; 81% were Caucasian, 14% were of Asian ancestry, 3% were black, 92% had squamous cell carcinoma, 6% had adenocarcinoma, and 1% had adenosquamous histology. Of these 77 patients, 95% had metastatic disease and 65% had received at least 2 prior therapies for recurrent or metastatic disease. All of the patients had an ECOG performance status of 0 or 1. The study excluded patients with autoimmune disease or conditions requiring therapy with immunosuppressive agents.

At a median follow-up of 11.7 months, the objective response rate in the KEYNOTE-158 study for patients with PD-L1-positive cervical cancer who had received at least one prior chemotherapy regimen for metastatic disease was 14.3%; complete response was achieved in 2.6% of patients. At the time of analysis, the median duration of response had not been reached; however, 91% of patients who responded to pembrolizumab had durable responses of 6 months or more. Objective responses were not observed in patients with a PD-L1 combined positive score of less than 1%.

■ Hepatocellular Carcinoma Pembrolizumab is used for the treatment of hepatocellular carcinoma previously treated with sorafenib; pembrolizumab has been designated an orphan drug by FDA for the treatment of this cancer. The accelerated approval of pembrolizumab for this indication is based on objective response rate and duration of response. Continued approval for this indication may be contingent on verification and description of clinical benefit of pembrolizumab in confirmatory studies.

The current indication for pembrolizumab in the treatment of previously treated hepatocellular carcinoma is based principally on the results of a phase 2, nonrandomized, noncomparative study (KEYNOTE-224) in 104 adults with hepatocellular carcinoma who had experienced disease progression during or following sorafenib therapy or who had not tolerated such therapy. Patients received pembrolizumab 200 mg administered as an IV infusion every 3 weeks for up to 24 months or until unacceptable toxicity or disease progression occurred; however, clinically stable patients with disease progression could continue treatment if they were considered to be deriving clinical benefit. The primary measures of efficacy were objective response rate (as evaluated by a blinded independent central review committee according to RECIST modified to follow no more than 10 target lesions and no more than 5 target lesions per organ) and duration of response. The study excluded patients with active autoimmune disease, any condition requiring immunosuppressive therapy, more than one etiology of hepatitis, brain metastasis, clinical evidence of ascites, hepatic encephalopathy, or esophageal or gastric variceal bleeding within the prior 6 months. The study also excluded patients who had received any prior systemic therapy other than sorafenib for advanced hepatocellular carcinoma; sorafenib was discontinued because of intolerable toxicity in 20% of patients.

The median age of patients enrolled in the KEYNOTE-224 study was 68 years; 83% were male, 81% were Caucasian, and 14% were of Asian ancestry. All patients had an ECOG performance status of 0 or 1. Most patients (94%) had Child-Pugh class A hepatic impairment, 64% had extrahepatic disease, 17% had vascular invasion, 9% had both extrahepatic disease and vascular invasion, 38% had α-fetoprotein concentrations of 0.4 mg/L or more, 21% were seropositive for HBV, 25% were seropositive for HCV, and 9% were seropositive for both HBV and HCV. At a median duration of follow-up of 12.3 months, the objective response rate was 17%; complete response was achieved in 1% of patients. The median duration of response had not been reached at the time of analysis; however, 89% of patients who responded to the drug had durable responses of 6 months or more and 56% had durable responses of 12 months or more. Results of a subgroup analysis (based on age, sex, geographic region, performance status, etiology, disease stage, α-fetoprotein concentration, presence of extrahepatic disease, presence of macrovascular invasion, reason for sorafenib discontinuance) suggested that objective response rates were generally similar across subgroups.

■ **Merkel Cell Carcinoma** Pembrolizumab is used for the treatment of recurrent, locally advanced or metastatic Merkel cell carcinoma; pembrolizumab has been designated an orphan drug by FDA for the treatment of this cancer. The accelerated approval of pembrolizumab for this indication is based on objective response rate and duration of response. Continued approval for this indication may be contingent on verification and description of clinical benefit of pembrolizumab in confirmatory studies.

The current indication for pembrolizumab in the treatment of recurrent, locally advanced or metastatic Merkel cell carcinoma is based principally on the results of a phase 2, noncomparative, nonrandomized study (KEYNOTE-017) in 50 adults with recurrent locally advanced or metastatic Merkel cell carcinoma who had not received prior systemic therapy for advanced disease. Patients received pembrolizumab 2 mg/kg administered as an IV infusion every 3 weeks for up to 24 months or until the occurrence of unacceptable toxicity or disease progression that was symptomatic, rapidly progressive, associated with a decline in performance status, requiring urgent intervention, or confirmed in at least 4 weeks with repeat radiographic studies. The primary measures of efficacy were objective response rate (as evaluated by a blinded independent central review committee according to RECIST) and duration of response. The study excluded patients with active autoimmune disease or any condition requiring immunosuppressive therapy. The median age of patients enrolled in the KEYNOTE-017 study was 71 years (80% were 65 years of age or older); 68% were male and 90% were Caucasian. All patients had an ECOG performance status of 0 or 1. Most patients (86%) had stage IV disease; 14% had stage IIIB disease. Prior therapies included surgery or radiation therapy in 84 or 70% of patients, respectively. At a median follow-up of 14.9 months, the objective response rate was 56%; complete response was achieved in 24% of patients. The median duration of response had not been reached at the time of analysis; however, 96% of patients who responded to the drug had durable responses of 6 months or more and 54% had durable responses of 12 months or more.

Dosage and Administration

■ **Reconstitution and Administration** Pembrolizumab is administered by IV infusion over 30 minutes.

Pembrolizumab is commercially available as an injection concentrate and as a lyophilized powder. The lyophilized powder must be reconstituted and then diluted to prepare a final pembrolizumab infusion solution. Pembrolizumab injection concentrate must be diluted prior to IV administration.

Prior to administration, commercially available pembrolizumab powder for injection must be reconstituted and diluted using proper aseptic technique. The powder is reconstituted by adding 2.3 mL of sterile water for injection to a vial labeled as containing 50 mg of the drug to provide a solution containing 25 mg/mL. The diluent should be directed toward the wall of the vial and not directly at the pembrolizumab powder. The vial should be gently swirled and allowed to stand for up to 5 minutes to let the bubbles dissipate; the vial should not be shaken.

The reconstituted pembrolizumab solution or commercially available injection concentrate should be inspected visually for particulate matter and discoloration prior to dilution and administration. The solution should be clear to slightly opalescent and colorless to slightly yellow, and should not be used if visible particles are present.

For preparation of the final diluted pembrolizumab solution for infusion, the required amount of reconstituted pembrolizumab solution or commercially available injection concentrate should be injected into an infusion bag containing a sufficient volume of 0.9% sodium chloride injection or 5% dextrose injection to yield a final solution with a pembrolizumab concentration of 1–10 mg/mL. The final diluted pembrolizumab solution for infusion should be mixed by gentle inversion. Reconstituted and diluted solutions of the drug are stable for up to 6 hours (including infusion time) after reconstitution of the lyophilized powder or dilution of the injection concentrate when stored at room temperature or up to 24 hours when stored under refrigeration (2–8°C); diluted solutions of the drug should be brought to room temperature prior to administration. Reconstituted and diluted solutions of the drug should not be frozen. Pembrolizumab should be administered through a sterile, nonpyrogenic, low-protein-binding 0.2- to 5-μm inline or add-on filter.

Pembrolizumab should *not* be administered simultaneously through the same IV line with any other drug. Commercially available pembrolizumab for injection and pembrolizumab injection concentrate contain no preservatives and are intended for single use only; any unused portions should be discarded.

■ **Dosage** Clinicians should consult published protocols for information on the dosage, method of administration, and administration sequence of other antineoplastic agents used in combination regimens with pembrolizumab.

Melanoma **Unresectable or Metastatic Melanoma.** For the treatment of unresectable or metastatic melanoma, the recommended adult dosage of pembrolizumab is 200 mg administered as a 30-minute IV infusion every 3 weeks. Therapy should be continued until disease progression or unacceptable toxicity occurs.

Adjuvant Therapy for Locally Advanced Melanoma. For the adjuvant therapy of completely resected advanced melanoma with regional nodal involvement, the recommended adult dosage of pembrolizumab is 200 mg administered as a 30-minute IV infusion every 3 weeks. Therapy should be continued for up to 12 months or until disease recurrence or unacceptable toxicity occurs.

Non-small Cell Lung Cancer **Monotherapy for Metastatic Non-small Cell Lung Cancer (NSCLC).** For the initial treatment of metastatic NSCLC in patients with epidermal growth factor receptor (EGFR)- and anaplastic lymphoma kinase (ALK)-negative tumors with high levels of programmed-death ligand-1 (PD-L1) expression (defined as PD-L1 expression of any intensity on at least 50% of tumor cells), the recommended adult dosage of pembrolizumab is 200 mg administered as a 30-minute IV infusion every 3 weeks. Therapy should be continued for up to 24 months or until disease progression or unacceptable toxicity occurs.

For the treatment of PD-L1-positive (defined as PD-L1 expression of any intensity on at least 1% of tumor cells) metastatic NSCLC that has progressed during or following platinum-based chemotherapy and, if the tumor is EGFR- or ALK-positive, during or following therapy with an FDA-labeled anti-EGFR or anti-ALK agent, the recommended adult dosage of pembrolizumab is 200 mg administered as a 30-minute IV infusion every 3 weeks. Therapy should be continued for up to 24 months or until disease progression or unacceptable toxicity occurs.

Selection of single-agent pembrolizumab for the treatment of metastatic NSCLC should be based on the presence of PD-L1 expression. (See Uses: Non-small Cell Lung Cancer.)

Combination Therapy for Metastatic NSCLC. For the initial treatment of metastatic nonsquamous NSCLC without EGFR or ALK genomic aberrations, the recommended adult dosage of pembrolizumab is 200 mg administered as a 30-minute IV infusion every 3 weeks in combination with pemetrexed and a platinum-containing antineoplastic agent (carboplatin, cisplatin). Pembrolizumab should be administered before pemetrexed and the platinum-containing antineoplastic agent. Therapy should be continued for up to 24 months or until disease progression or unacceptable toxicity occurs.

For the initial treatment of metastatic squamous NSCLC, the recommended adult dosage of pembrolizumab is 200 mg administered as a 30-minute IV infusion every 3 weeks in combination with carboplatin and paclitaxel (conventional or albumin-bound). Pembrolizumab should be administered before carboplatin and paclitaxel. Therapy should be continued for up to 24 months or until disease progression or unacceptable toxicity occurs.

Head and Neck Cancer For the treatment of recurrent or metastatic head and neck squamous cell carcinoma that has progressed during or following platinum-containing therapy, the recommended adult dosage of pembrolizumab is 200 mg administered as a 30-minute IV infusion every 3 weeks. Therapy should be continued for up to 24 months or until disease progression or unacceptable toxicity occurs.

Hodgkin Lymphoma For the treatment of refractory classical Hodgkin lymphoma (cHL) and cHL that has relapsed following at least 3 prior therapies, the recommended *adult* dosage of pembrolizumab is 200 mg administered as a 30-minute IV infusion every 3 weeks. The recommended *pediatric* dosage of pembrolizumab for this indication is 2 mg/kg (up to a maximum of 200 mg) administered as a 30-minute IV infusion every 3 weeks. Therapy should be continued for up to 24 months or until disease progression or unacceptable toxicity occurs.

Primary Mediastinal Large B-cell Lymphoma For the treatment of refractory primary mediastinal large B-cell lymphoma (PMBL) or PMBL that has relapsed following at least 2 prior therapies, the recommended *adult* dosage of pembrolizumab is 200 mg administered as a 30-minute IV infusion every 3 weeks. The recommended *pediatric* dosage of pembrolizumab for this indication is 2 mg/kg (up to 200 mg) administered as a 30-minute IV infusion every 3 weeks. Therapy should be continued for up to 24 months or until disease progression or unacceptable toxicity occurs.

Pembrolizumab is not recommended for the treatment of PMBL in patients who require urgent cytoreduction.

Urothelial Carcinoma For the treatment of locally advanced or metastatic urothelial carcinoma that has progressed during or following platinum-containing therapy or within 12 months of platinum-containing therapy in the neoadjuvant or adjuvant setting, locally advanced or metastatic urothelial carcinoma in patients with high levels of PD-L1 expression (defined as PD-L1 expression combined positive score of at least 10%) who are not candidates for cisplatin-containing therapy, or locally advanced or metastatic urothelial carcinoma in patients who are not candidates for platinum-containing chemotherapy regardless of PD-L1 expression, the recommended adult dosage of pembrolizumab is 200 mg administered as a 30-minute IV infusion every 3 weeks. Therapy should be continued for up to 24 months or until disease progression or unacceptable toxicity occurs.

Selection of pembrolizumab therapy for the treatment of locally advanced or metastatic urothelial carcinoma in patients who are not candidates for cisplatin-containing therapy should be based on the presence of PD-L1 expression. (See Uses: Urothelial Carcinoma.)

Solid Tumors with High Microsatellite Instability or Mismatch Repair Deficiency For the treatment of unresectable or metastatic solid tumors with high microsatellite instability (MSI-H) or mismatch repair deficiency (dMMR) that have progressed following prior therapy in patients who are not candidates for other treatment options or for the treatment of unresectable or metastatic MSI-H or dMMR colorectal cancer that has progressed following therapy with a fluoropyrimidine, oxaliplatin, and irinotecan, the recommended *adult* dosage of pembrolizumab is 200 mg administered as a 30-minute IV infusion every 3 weeks. The recommended *pediatric* dosage of pembrolizumab for this indication is 2 mg/kg (up to a maximum of 200 mg) administered as a 30-minute IV infusion every 3 weeks. Therapy should be continued for up to 24 months or until disease progression or unacceptable toxicity occurs.

Gastric Cancer For the treatment of recurrent, locally advanced or metastatic, PD-L1-positive (defined as a PD-L1 expression combined positive score of at least 1%) gastric adenocarcinoma, including adenocarcinoma of the gastroesophageal junction, that has progressed during or following at least 2 prior therapies, including fluoropyrimidine- and platinum-containing chemotherapy, and, if the tumor overexpresses the human epidermal growth factor receptor type 2 (HER2) protein, during or following therapy with an anti-HER2 agent, the recommended adult dosage of pembrolizumab is 200 mg administered as a 30-minute IV infusion every 3 weeks. Therapy should be continued for up to 24 months or until disease progression or unacceptable toxicity occurs.

Initiation of pembrolizumab therapy should be based on the presence of PD-L1 expression; if PD-L1 expression is not detected in an archival tumor specimen, the feasibility of obtaining a new tumor specimen should be considered. (See Uses: Gastric Cancer.)

Cervical Cancer For the treatment of recurrent or metastatic, PD-L1-positive (defined as a PD-L1 expression combined positive score of at least 1%) cervical cancer that has progressed during or following chemotherapy, the recommended adult dosage of pembrolizumab is 200 mg administered as a 30-minute IV infusion every 3 weeks. Therapy should be continued for up to 24 months or until disease progression or unacceptable toxicity occurs.

Initiation of pembrolizumab therapy should be based on the presence of PD-L1 expression. (See Uses: Cervical Cancer.)

Hepatocellular Carcinoma For the treatment of hepatocellular carcinoma previously treated with sorafenib, the recommended adult dosage of pembrolizumab is 200 mg administered as a 30-minute IV infusion every 3 weeks. Therapy should be continued for up to 24 months or until disease progression or unacceptable toxicity occurs.

Merkel Cell Carcinoma For the treatment of recurrent, locally advanced or metastatic Merkel cell carcinoma, the recommended *adult* dosage of pembrolizumab is 200 mg administered as a 30-minute IV infusion every 3 weeks. The recommended *pediatric* dosage of pembrolizumab for this indication is 2 mg/kg (up to a maximum of 200 mg) administered as a 30-minute IV infusion every 3 weeks. Therapy should be continued for up to 24 months or until disease progression or unacceptable toxicity occurs.

Therapy Interruption for Toxicity If immune-mediated adverse effects occur, temporary or permanent discontinuance of pembrolizumab may be required based on severity of the reaction.

Pembrolizumab should be permanently discontinued in patients experiencing persistent grade 2 or 3 immune-mediated adverse effects (except for endocrinopathies) that do not recover to grade 0 or 1 within 12 weeks of the last dose of pembrolizumab. Therapy with the drug also should be permanently discontinued in patients unable to reduce corticosteroid dosage to less than 10 mg of prednisone daily (or equivalent) within 12 weeks.

Pembrolizumab should be permanently discontinued in patients experiencing any life-threatening immune-mediated adverse effect (except for endocrinopathies or hematologic toxicity in patients with cHL or PMBL). Therapy with the drug also should be permanently discontinued if grade 3 or 4 immune-mediated adverse effects recur.

Hematologic Toxicity. If grade 4 hematologic toxicity occurs in patients with cHL or PMBL, pembrolizumab therapy should be interrupted until the toxicity resolves to grade 0 or 1.

Immune-mediated Pneumonitis. If grade 2 immune-mediated pneumonitis occurs, pembrolizumab therapy should be interrupted until the toxicity resolves to grade 0 or 1 *and* the corticosteroid dosage has been tapered. (See Immune-mediated Pneumonitis under Cautions: Warnings/Precautions.)

If grade 3 or 4 immune-mediated pneumonitis occurs or grade 2 immune-mediated pneumonitis recurs, pembrolizumab therapy should be permanently discontinued.

Immune-mediated GI Effects. If grade 2 or 3 immune-mediated colitis occurs, pembrolizumab therapy should be interrupted until the toxicity resolves to grade 0 or 1 *and* the corticosteroid dosage has been tapered. (See Immune-mediated GI Effects under Cautions: Warnings/Precautions.)

If grade 4 immune-mediated colitis occurs, pembrolizumab therapy should be permanently discontinued.

Immune-mediated Hepatic Effects. For serum aminotransferase (ALT or AST) elevations exceeding 3 times but not more than 5 times the upper limit of normal (ULN) or total bilirubin concentrations exceeding 1.5 times but not more than 3 times the ULN in patients *without* hepatocellular carcinoma, pembrolizumab therapy should be interrupted until the toxicity resolves to grade 0 or 1 *and* the corticosteroid dosage has been tapered. (See Immune-mediated Hepatic Effects under Cautions: Warnings/Precautions.)

For ALT or AST elevations exceeding 5 times the ULN or total bilirubin concentrations exceeding 3 times the ULN in patients *without* hepatocellular carcinoma, pembrolizumab therapy should be permanently discontinued. In addition, in patients with liver metastasis with baseline grade 2 serum aminotransferase elevations, pembrolizumab therapy should be permanently discontinued if ALT or AST concentrations increase by 50% or more from baseline for at least 1 week.

For ALT or AST concentrations that are 5 or more times the ULN in patients *with* hepatocellular carcinoma and baseline ALT and AST concentrations less than 2 times the ULN, pembrolizumab therapy should be interrupted until the toxicity resolves to grade 0 or 1 or the AST and ALT concentrations return to baseline.

For ALT or AST concentrations exceeding 3 times the baseline concentrations in patients *with* hepatocellular carcinoma and baseline ALT or AST concentrations of 2 or more times the ULN, pembrolizumab therapy should be interrupted until the toxicity resolves to grade 0 or 1 or the AST and ALT concentrations return to baseline.

For total bilirubin concentrations exceeding 2 mg/dL in patients *with* hepatocellular carcinoma and baseline total bilirubin concentrations of less than 1.5 mg/dL, pembrolizumab therapy should be interrupted until the toxicity resolves to grade 0 or 1 or the bilirubin concentrations return to baseline.

For total bilirubin concentrations exceeding 3 mg/dL (regardless of the baseline concentration) in patients *with* hepatocellular carcinoma, pembrolizumab therapy should be interrupted until the toxicity resolves to grade 0 or 1 or the bilirubin concentrations return to baseline.

For ALT or AST concentrations exceeding 10 times the ULN in patients *with* hepatocellular carcinoma, pembrolizumab therapy should be permanently discontinued.

For Child-Pugh score of 9 or more in patients *with* hepatocellular carcinoma, pembrolizumab therapy should be permanently discontinued.

If GI bleeding suggestive of portal hypertension, new onset of clinically detectable ascites, or encephalopathy occurs in patients *with* hepatocellular carcinoma, pembrolizumab therapy should be permanently discontinued.

Immune-mediated Endocrine Effects. If grade 2 immune-mediated hypophysitis or severe hyperglycemia occurs, pembrolizumab therapy should be interrupted. (See Immune-mediated Endocrine Effects under Cautions: Warnings/Precautions.)

If grade 3 or 4 immune-mediated endocrinopathies, including hypophysitis and hyperthyroidism, occur, pembrolizumab therapy should be interrupted until the patient is clinically stable or the drug should be discontinued.

Immune-mediated Renal Effects. If grade 2 immune-mediated nephritis occurs, pembrolizumab therapy should be interrupted until the toxicity resolves to grade 0 or 1 *and* the corticosteroid dosage has been tapered. (See Immune-mediated Renal Effects under Cautions: Warnings/Precautions.)

If grade 3 or 4 immune-mediated nephritis occurs, pembrolizumab therapy should be permanently discontinued.

Immune-mediated Dermatologic Effects. If a grade 3 immune-mediated skin reaction occurs or Stevens-Johnson syndrome or toxic epidermal necrolysis is suspected, pembrolizumab therapy should be interrupted until the toxicity resolves to grade 0 or 1. (See Immune-mediated Dermatologic Effects under Cautions: Warnings/Precautions.)

If a grade 4 immune-mediated skin reaction occurs or Stevens-Johnson syndrome or toxic epidermal necrolysis is confirmed, pembrolizumab therapy should be permanently discontinued.

Other Immune-mediated Adverse Effects. If any other grade 2 immune-mediated adverse effects occur, pembrolizumab therapy should be interrupted until the toxicity resolves to grade 0 or 1 *and* the corticosteroid dosage has been tapered. (See Other Immune-mediated Effects under Cautions: Warnings/Precautions.)

If any other grade 3 immune-mediated adverse effects occur, pembrolizumab therapy should be interrupted until the toxicity resolves to grade 0 or 1 *and* the corticosteroid dosage has been tapered, or the drug should be permanently discontinued (depending on the severity and type of reaction).

If any other grade 4 immune-mediated adverse effects occur, pembrolizumab therapy should be permanently discontinued.

Infusion-related Reactions. If grade 1 or 2 infusion-related reactions occur, the infusion should be interrupted or the infusion rate should be slowed.

If grade 3 or 4 infusion-related reactions occur, pembrolizumab therapy should be permanently discontinued.

■ **Special Populations** The manufacturer makes no special dosage recommendations for patients with preexisting hepatic or renal impairment or for geriatric patients. (See Specific Populations under Cautions: Warnings/Precautions.)

Cautions

■ **Contraindications** The manufacturer states there are no known contraindications to the use of pembrolizumab.

■ **Warnings/Precautions** ***Immune-mediated Pneumonitis*** Immune-mediated pneumonitis, sometimes fatal, has occurred in patients receiving pembrolizumab therapy.

In clinical studies evaluating single-agent pembrolizumab, immune-mediated pneumonitis occurred in 3.4% of patients and was grade 3 or greater in approximately 1.3% of patients receiving the drug. The median time to onset of immune-mediated pneumonitis was 3.3 months and the median duration was 1.5 months. Most patients (67%) experiencing immune-mediated pneumonitis received systemic corticosteroid therapy; 79% of these patients received high-dose corticosteroid therapy for a median duration of 8 days followed by tapering of the corticosteroid dosage. Immune-mediated pneumonitis occurred more frequently in patients who had received prior thoracic irradiation compared with those who had not received thoracic irradiation (6.9 versus 2.9%). Pembrolizumab was discontinued because of immune-mediated pneumonitis in 1.3% of patients receiving the drug. Immune-mediated pneumonitis resolved in 59% of patients.

Patients receiving pembrolizumab should be monitored for pulmonary symptoms indicative of pneumonitis. If pneumonitis is suspected, patients should be evaluated for pneumonitis using radiographic imaging. In patients who develop grade 2 or greater pneumonitis, systemic corticosteroid therapy should be initiated (1–2 mg/kg of prednisone daily [or equivalent]) followed by tapering of the corticosteroid dosage. Temporary interruption or discontinuance of pembrolizumab may be necessary if immune-mediated pneumonitis occurs during therapy with the drug. (See Therapy Interruption for Toxicity under Dosage and Administration: Dosage.)

Immune-mediated GI Effects Immune-mediated colitis has occurred in patients receiving pembrolizumab therapy.

In clinical studies evaluating single-agent pembrolizumab, immune-mediated colitis occurred in 1.7% of patients and was grade 3 or 4 in approximately 1.2% of patients receiving the drug. The median time to onset of immune-mediated colitis was 3.5 months and the median duration was 1.3 months. Most patients (69%) experiencing immune-mediated colitis received systemic corticosteroid therapy; 82% of these patients received high-dose corticosteroid therapy for a median duration of 7 days followed by tapering of the corticosteroid dosage. Pembrolizumab was discontinued because of immune-mediated colitis in 0.5% of patients receiving the drug. Immune-mediated colitis resolved in 85% of patients.

Patients receiving pembrolizumab should be monitored for manifestations of colitis. In patients who develop grade 2 or greater colitis, systemic corticosteroid therapy should be initiated (1–2 mg/kg of prednisone daily [or equivalent]) followed by tapering of the corticosteroid dosage. Temporary interruption or discontinuance of pembrolizumab may be necessary if immune-mediated colitis occurs during therapy with the drug. (See Therapy Interruption for Toxicity under Dosage and Administration: Dosage.)

Immune-mediated Hepatic Effects Immune-mediated hepatitis has occurred in patients receiving pembrolizumab therapy.

In clinical studies evaluating single-agent pembrolizumab, immune-mediated hepatitis occurred in 0.7% of patients and was grade 3 or 4 in approximately 0.5% of patients receiving the drug. The median time to onset of immune-mediated hepatitis was 1.3 months and the median duration was 1.8 months. Most patients (68%) experiencing immune-mediated hepatitis received systemic corticosteroid therapy; 92% of these patients received high-dose corticosteroid therapy for a median duration of 5 days followed by tapering of the corticosteroid dosage. Pembrolizumab was discontinued because of immune-mediated hepatitis in 0.2% of patients receiving the drug. Immune-mediated hepatitis resolved in 79% of patients.

Patients receiving pembrolizumab should be assessed for changes in liver function. If grade 2 hepatitis occurs, systemic corticosteroid therapy should be initiated at a dosage of 0.5–1 mg/kg of prednisone daily (or equivalent) followed by tapering of the corticosteroid dosage. In patients who develop grade 3 or greater hepatitis, systemic corticosteroid therapy should be initiated at a dosage of 1–2 mg/kg of prednisone daily (or equivalent) followed by tapering of the corticosteroid dosage. In patients who develop elevations of serum aminotransferase or bilirubin concentrations, temporary interruption of therapy or drug discontinuance may be required. (See Therapy Interruption for Toxicity under Dosage and Administration: Dosage.)

Immune-mediated Endocrine Effects Immune-mediated endocrinopathies, including hypophysitis, thyroid dysfunction (i.e., hyperthyroidism, hypothyroidism, thyroiditis), and diabetes mellitus, have occurred in patients receiving pembrolizumab therapy.

Hypophysitis. In clinical studies evaluating single-agent pembrolizumab, immune-mediated hypophysitis occurred in 0.6% of patients and was grade 3 or 4 in approximately 0.4% of patients receiving pembrolizumab. The median time to onset of immune-mediated hypophysitis was 3.7 months and the median duration was 4.7 months. Most patients (94%) experiencing immune-mediated hypophysitis received systemic corticosteroid therapy; 38% of these patients received high-dose corticosteroid therapy. Pembrolizumab was discontinued because of immune-mediated hypophysitis in 0.1% of patients receiving the drug. Immune-mediated hypophysitis resolved in 41% of patients.

Patients should be monitored for manifestations of hypophysitis (including hypopituitarism and adrenal insufficiency) during pembrolizumab therapy. If hypophysitis occurs, systemic corticosteroid therapy and hormone replacement therapy should be administered as clinically indicated. In patients who develop hypophysitis, temporary interruption or discontinuance of pembrolizumab may be required. (See Therapy Interruption for Toxicity under Dosage and Administration: Dosage.)

Thyroid Dysfunction. In clinical studies evaluating single-agent pembrolizumab, immune-mediated hyperthyroidism occurred in 3.4% of patients and was grade 2 or 3 in 0.9% of patients receiving pembrolizumab. The median time to onset of immune-mediated hyperthyroidism was 1.4 months and the median duration was 2.1 months. Pembrolizumab was discontinued because of immune-mediated hyperthyroidism in less than 0.1% of patients receiving the drug. Immune-mediated hyperthyroidism resolved in 74% of patients.

In clinical studies evaluating single-agent pembrolizumab, immune-mediated hypothyroidism occurred in 8.5% of patients and was grade 2 or 3 in 6.3% of patients receiving pembrolizumab. The median time to onset of immune-mediated hypothyroidism was 3.5 months and the median duration was not reached but ranged from 2 days to more than 27 months. Pembrolizumab was discontinued because of immune-mediated hypothyroidism in less than 0.1% of patients receiving the drug. Immune-mediated hypothyroidism resolved in 20% of patients. In clinical studies evaluating pembrolizumab in patients with squamous cell carcinoma of the head and neck, new-onset or worsening immune-mediated hypothyroidism occurred in 15% of patients and was grade 3 in 0.5% of patients receiving the drug; 54% of patients with immune-mediated hypothyroidism had no history of hypothyroidism.

In clinical studies evaluating single-agent pembrolizumab, immune-mediated thyroiditis occurred in 0.6% of patients and was grade 2 in 0.3% of patients receiving pembrolizumab. The median time to onset of immune-mediated thyroiditis was 1.2 months.

Thyroid function should be evaluated prior to initiation of therapy, periodically during therapy, and as clinically indicated. Patients should be monitored for manifestations of hyperthyroidism, hypothyroidism, or thyroiditis during pembrolizumab therapy. In patients who develop hypothyroidism, thyroid hormone replacement therapy should be initiated as clinically indicated. If hyperthyroidism occurs, antithyroid agents and β-adrenergic blocking agents (β-blockers) should be initiated as clinically indicated. In patients who develop hyperthyroidism, temporary interruption or discontinuance of pembrolizumab may be required. (See Therapy Interruption for Toxicity under Dosage and Administration: Dosage.)

Diabetes Mellitus. In clinical studies evaluating single-agent pembrolizumab, immune-mediated type 1 diabetes mellitus and diabetic ketoacidosis occurred in 0.2% of patients receiving pembrolizumab.

Patients receiving pembrolizumab should be monitored for manifestations of diabetes mellitus (e.g., hyperglycemia). If type 1 diabetes mellitus occurs, insulin should be initiated. If severe hyperglycemia occurs, pembrolizumab therapy should be temporarily interrupted and antidiabetic agents should be initiated. (See Therapy Interruption for Toxicity under Dosage and Administration: Dosage.)

Immune-mediated Renal Effects Immune-mediated nephritis has occurred in patients receiving pembrolizumab therapy.

In clinical studies evaluating single-agent pembrolizumab, immune-mediated nephritis occurred in 0.3% of patients and was grade 3 or 4 in approximately 0.2% of patients receiving the drug. The median time to onset of immune-mediated nephritis was 5.1 months and the median duration was 3.3 months. Most patients (89%) experiencing immune-mediated nephritis received systemic corticosteroid therapy; 88% of these patients received high-dose corticosteroid therapy for a median duration of 15 days followed by tapering of the corticosteroid dosage. Pembrolizumab was discontinued because of immune-mediated nephritis in 0.1% of patients receiving the drug. Immune-mediated nephritis resolved in 56% of patients.

In clinical studies evaluating pembrolizumab in combination with pemetrexed and a platinum-containing antineoplastic agent, immune-mediated nephritis occurred in 1.7% of patients receiving combination therapy and was grade 3 or 4 in 1.5% of patients receiving combination therapy. The median time to onset of immune-mediated nephritis was 3.2 months and the duration ranged from 1.6–16.8 months or more. Most patients (86%) experiencing immune-mediated nephritis received systemic corticosteroid therapy; all of these patients received high-dose corticosteroid therapy for a median duration of 3 days followed by tapering of the corticosteroid dosage. Pembrolizumab was discontinued because of immune-mediated nephritis in 1.2% of patients receiving pembrolizumab in combination with pemetrexed and a platinum-containing agent. Immune-mediated nephritis resolved in 29% of patients.

Patients receiving pembrolizumab should be monitored for changes in renal function. In patients who develop nephritis, temporary interruption of therapy or drug discontinuance may be required. (See Therapy Interruption for Toxicity under Dosage and Administration: Dosage.) If grade 2 or greater nephritis occurs, systemic corticosteroid therapy should be initiated (1–2 mg/kg of prednisone daily [or equivalent]) followed by tapering of the corticosteroid dosage.

Immune-mediated Dermatologic Effects Immune-mediated rash, including Stevens-Johnson syndrome, toxic epidermal necrolysis (sometimes fatal), exfoliative dermatitis, and bullous pemphigoid, may occur in patients receiving pembrolizumab therapy.

Patients receiving pembrolizumab should be monitored for severe skin reactions. If an immune-mediated skin reaction is suspected, adequate evaluation should be performed to exclude other causes. Temporary interruption or discontinuance of pembrolizumab may be necessary if immune-mediated rash occurs during therapy with the drug; systemic corticosteroid therapy also should be initiated. (See Therapy Interruption for Toxicity under Dosage and Administration: Dosage.) If Stevens-Johnson syndrome or toxic epidermal necrolysis is suspected, pembrolizumab therapy should be temporarily interrupted and the patient referred for evaluation and treatment by a specialist. If Stevens-Johnson syndrome or toxic epidermal necrolysis is confirmed, pembrolizumab should be permanently discontinued.

Other Immune-mediated Effects Other immune-mediated adverse effects, which may be severe or fatal and may affect any organ system or tissue, have occurred in patients receiving pembrolizumab therapy.

In clinical studies evaluating single-agent pembrolizumab, uveitis, myositis, pancreatitis, arthritis, hemolytic anemia, sarcoidosis, encephalitis, Guillain-Barré syndrome, myasthenia gravis, and vasculitis have occurred in patients receiving the drug. In these clinical studies, such immune-mediated adverse effects were observed in less than 1% of patients; however, arthritis occurred in 1.5% of patients. In addition, immune-mediated adverse effects such as myelitis and myocarditis have been reported in other clinical trials of the drug and during postmarketing experience. Immune-mediated rejection of solid organ transplants also has been reported during postmarketing experience in patients who received pembrolizumab. Immune-mediated adverse effects generally occur during therapy with an anti-programmed-death receptor-1 (anti-PD-1) or anti-programmed-death ligand-1 (anti-PD-L1) antibody, but also may occur following discontinuance of the drug.

If an immune-mediated adverse effect is suspected, adequate evaluation should be performed to exclude other causes. Depending on the type and severity of the immune-mediated adverse effect, pembrolizumab therapy should be interrupted until the toxicity resolves to grade 0 or 1 or the drug should be discontinued, and systemic corticosteroid therapy should be initiated. (See Therapy Interruption for Toxicity under Dosage and Administration: Dosage.) Once the toxicity has resolved to grade 0 or 1, the corticosteroid dosage should be tapered over at least 1 month. Based on limited data, systemic immunosuppressive therapy may be considered in patients experiencing immune-mediated adverse effects inadequately controlled with systemic corticosteroid therapy. Because pembrolizumab may increase the risk of rejection in solid organ transplant recipients, the risk of possible organ rejection should be weighed against potential benefits of the drug.

Infusion-related Effects Severe or life-threatening infusion-related reactions, including hypersensitivity reactions and anaphylaxis, have occurred in 0.2% of patients receiving single-agent pembrolizumab.

Patients receiving pembrolizumab should be monitored for signs and symptoms of infusion-related reactions. In patients experiencing grade 3 or 4 infusion-related reactions, the pembrolizumab infusion should be stopped and the drug permanently discontinued.

Allogeneic Stem Cell Transplantation-related Immune-mediated Complications Immune-mediated complications, including graft-versus-host disease (GVHD) and hepatic veno-occlusive disease, have occurred in patients who underwent allogeneic stem cell transplantation prior to or following therapy with pembrolizumab. Some cases have resulted in death. Immune-mediated complications following allogeneic stem cell transplantation may occur despite other intervening therapy between pembrolizumab administration and transplantation.

In clinical trials evaluating pembrolizumab in patients with classical Hodgkin lymphoma (cHL), 6 of 23 patients (26%) who underwent allogeneic stem cell transplantation following therapy with pembrolizumab developed GVHD; one case resulted in death. Severe hepatic veno-occlusive disease following reduced-intensity conditioning occurred in 2 patients, which resulted in one fatality. Hyperacute GVHD resulting in death also has been reported in patients with lymphoma who received an anti-PD-1 antibody prior to allogeneic stem cell transplantation. In patients with a history of allogeneic stem cell transplantation, acute GVHD (including fatal acute GVHD) has occurred following pembrolizumab therapy. Patients with a history of GVHD following allogeneic stem cell transplantation may be at increased risk for developing GVHD following therapy with pembrolizumab.

In patients who previously underwent allogeneic stem cell transplantation, the potential benefit of pembrolizumab therapy should be weighed against the risks of developing GVHD. Patients who receive pembrolizumab should be monitored closely for early manifestations of stem cell transplantation-related immune-mediated complications (e.g., hyperacute GVHD, grade 3 or 4 acute GVHD, corticosteroid-requiring febrile syndrome, hepatic veno-occlusive disease) and such conditions should be managed promptly if they occur.

Treatment-related Mortality Increased mortality has been reported in clinical trials in patients with multiple myeloma receiving pembrolizumab in combination with an immunomodulatory agent (i.e., lenalidomide, pomalidomide); pembrolizumab is *not* currently FDA-labeled for use in patients with multiple myeloma. In 2 randomized, controlled phase 3 trials (KEYNOTE-183 and KEYNOTE-185) enrolling 550 patients with multiple myeloma, interim analyses indicated that the risk of death was increased by 61 or 106%, respectively, in patients receiving pembrolizumab in combination with an immunomodulatory agent (pomalidomide or lenalidomide, respectively) and low-dose dexamethasone compared with those receiving the immunomodulatory agent and low-dose dexamethasone. Because of these findings, these trials were terminated at FDA's request.

The manufacturer of pembrolizumab states that an anti-PD-1 or anti-PD-L1 antibody should *not* be used in combination with an immunomodulatory agent and dexamethasone in patients with multiple myeloma outside of a controlled clinical trial. FDA recommends that ongoing clinical trials evaluating an anti-PD-1 or anti-PD-L1 agent in combination with an immunomodulatory agent or in combination with other drugs for use in hematologic malignancies be evaluated for permanent discontinuance or protocol amendments.

Fetal/Neonatal Morbidity and Mortality Pembrolizumab may cause fetal harm if administered to pregnant women. Blockade of signaling of the PD-1 and PD-L1 pathway in animals has been shown to disrupt maternal immune tolerance to the fetus and has been associated with increased fetal loss and immune-mediated disorders. Therefore, inhibition of this pathway by pembrolizumab may increase the risk of fetal loss (e.g., abortion, stillbirth). Human immunoglobulin G_4 (IgG_4) has been shown to cross the placenta; therefore, fetal exposure to pembrolizumab may occur and increase the risk of immune-mediated disorders or alter normal immune response of the developing fetus.

Pregnancy should be avoided during pembrolizumab therapy. The manufacturer states that pregnancy status should be verified prior to initiation of pembrolizumab therapy in women of childbearing potential and such women should be advised to use a highly effective method of contraception while receiving pembrolizumab and for at least 4 months after the last dose. If pembrolizumab is used during pregnancy or if the patient becomes pregnant while receiving the drug, the patient should be apprised of the potential fetal hazard.

Immunogenicity There is a potential for immunogenicity with pembrolizumab therapy. The ability of the electrochemiluminescence (ECL) assay to detect anti-pembrolizumab antibodies is limited by the presence of circulating drug. Development of anti-pembrolizumab antibodies was detected in 2.1% of patients receiving pembrolizumab 2 mg/kg every 3 weeks, 200 mg every 3 weeks, or 10 mg/kg every 2 or 3 weeks; neutralizing antibodies to pembrolizumab were detected in 0.5% of patients receiving the drug at these dosages. No effects of antibody formation on pharmacokinetics or safety (i.e., infusion-related reactions) of the drug were observed.

Specific Populations **Pregnancy.** Pembrolizumab may cause fetal harm if administered to pregnant women based on its mechanism of action. (See Fetal/Neonatal Morbidity and Mortality under Cautions: Warnings/Precautions.)

Pregnancy status should be verified in women of childbearing potential prior to initiation of pembrolizumab therapy.

Lactation. It is not known whether pembrolizumab is distributed into human milk. The effects of pembrolizumab on nursing infants or on milk production also are unknown. Because of the potential for serious adverse reactions to pembrolizumab in nursing infants, women should be advised to discontinue nursing during pembrolizumab therapy and for 4 months after the last dose.

Pediatric Use. Efficacy of pembrolizumab has not been established in pediatric patients with melanoma, non-small cell lung cancer (NSCLC), squamous cell carcinoma of the head and neck, urothelial carcinoma, gastric cancer, cervical cancer, or hepatocellular carcinoma.

Safety and efficacy of pembrolizumab for the treatment of solid tumors with high microsatellite instability (MSI-H), cHL, or primary mediastinal large B-cell lymphoma (PMBL) in pediatric patients is supported by extrapolation of data from clinical studies evaluating pembrolizumab in adults, safety data in pediatric patients, pharmacokinetic analysis indicating that age (range of 15–94 years) does not have clinically important effects on clearance of the drug, and limited data indicating that exposure to pembrolizumab in pediatric patients is similar to that in adults.

Based on limited data in pediatric patients (range: 2–18 years of age) receiving a median of 3 doses of pembrolizumab (2 mg/kg every 3 weeks), plasma concentrations of pembrolizumab in pediatric patients were similar to those observed in adults receiving the same dosage of the drug. The safety profile of pembrolizumab was generally similar between pediatric patients and adults, but some adverse effects (i.e., fatigue, vomiting, abdominal pain, elevated serum aminotransferase concentrations, hyponatremia) occurred more frequently in pediatric patients.

Geriatric Use. In clinical trials evaluating pembrolizumab for melanoma, NSCLC, squamous cell carcinoma of the head and neck, cHL, and urothelial carcinoma, 46% of patients were 65 years of age or older and 16% were 75 years of age or older. No overall differences in safety and efficacy were observed between geriatric patients and younger adults.

Hepatic Impairment. Analysis of population pharmacokinetic data indicates that clearance of pembrolizumab is not altered in patients with mild hepatic impairment (total bilirubin concentration not exceeding the ULN *with* AST concentration exceeding the ULN, or total bilirubin concentration more than 1 times but not more than 1.5 times the ULN *with* any AST concentration). Insufficient data are available for patients with moderate or severe hepatic impairment.

Renal Impairment. Analysis of population pharmacokinetic data indicates that clearance of pembrolizumab is not altered in patients with renal impairment (estimated glomerular filtration rate [GFR] of 15 mL/minute per 1.73 m^2 or greater).

■ **Common Adverse Effects** Adverse effects reported in 10% or more of patients receiving pembrolizumab for the treatment of unresectable or metastatic melanoma and at an incidence that is at least 2% higher than that reported with ipilimumab or chemotherapy in the KEYNOTE-006 or KEYNOTE-002 studies include pruritus, rash, constipation, fatigue, arthralgia, cough, decreased appetite, pyrexia, abdominal pain, vitiligo, back pain, dyspnea, asthenia, hypothyroidism, and nausea. Laboratory abnormalities reported in 20% or more of patients receiving pembrolizumab for the treatment of unresectable or metastatic melanoma and at an incidence that is at least 2% higher than that reported with ipilimumab or chemotherapy include hyperglycemia, hypertriglyceridemia, hypoalbuminemia, hyponatremia, anemia, lymphopenia, elevated concentrations of aminotransferases (i.e., ALT, AST), elevated concentrations of alkaline phosphatase, decreased concentrations of bicarbonate, hypocalcemia, and hypercholesterolemia.

Adverse effects reported in 10% or more of patients receiving pembrolizumab as adjuvant therapy for completely resected advanced melanoma with regional lymph node involvement in the KEYNOTE-054 study include diarrhea, pruritus, nausea, arthralgia, hypothyroidism, cough, rash, asthenia, influenza-like illness, weight loss, and hyperthyroidism. Laboratory abnormalities reported in 20% or more of patients receiving pembrolizumab as adjuvant therapy include elevated concentrations of aminotransferases (i.e., ALT, AST) and lymphopenia.

Adverse effects reported in 20% or more of patients receiving pembrolizumab in combination with pemetrexed and a platinum-containing antineoplastic agent (carboplatin or cisplatin) for the initial treatment of metastatic nonsquamous NSCLC and at an incidence that is at least 2% higher than that reported with placebo plus pemetrexed and a platinum-containing agent in the KEYNOTE-189 study include nausea, fatigue, constipation, diarrhea, rash, and pyrexia. Laboratory abnormalities reported in 20% or more of patients receiving pembrolizumab in combination with pemetrexed and a platinum-containing agent (i.e., carboplatin, cisplatin) for the initial treatment of metastatic nonsquamous NSCLC and at an incidence that is at least 2% higher than that reported with placebo plus pemetrexed and a platinum-containing agent include anemia, hyperglycemia, neutropenia, elevated concentrations of aminotransferases (i.e., ALT, AST), elevated concentrations of serum creatinine, hyponatremia, hypophosphatemia, hypocalcemia, and hyperkalemia.

Adverse effects reported in patients receiving pembrolizumab in combination with carboplatin and paclitaxel (conventional or albumin-bound) for the initial treatment of metastatic squamous NSCLC in the KEYNOTE-407 study were similar to those reported in patients receiving the drug in combination with pemetrexed and a platinum-containing antineoplastic agent (carboplatin, cisplatin) for the initial treatment of metastatic nonsquamous NSCLC in the KEYNOTE-189 study; however, higher incidences of alopecia and peripheral neuropathy were reported in patients receiving pembrolizumab in combination with carboplatin and paclitaxel compared with placebo plus carboplatin and paclitaxel.

Adverse effects reported in 10% or more of patients receiving pembrolizumab as a single agent for the treatment of previously treated, PD-L1-positive metastatic NSCLC and at an incidence that is at least 2% higher than that reported with docetaxel in the KEYNOTE-010 study include decreased appetite, dyspnea, nausea, cough, rash, constipation, vomiting, arthralgia, back pain, and pruritus. Laboratory abnormalities reported in 20% or more of patients receiving pembrolizumab for the treatment of previously treated, PD-L1-positive metastatic NSCLC and at an incidence that is at least 2% higher than that reported with docetaxel include hyponatremia, elevated concentrations of alkaline phosphatase, and elevated concentrations of aminotransferases (i.e., ALT, AST).

Adverse effects reported in 20% or more of patients receiving pembrolizumab for the treatment of recurrent metastatic head and neck squamous cell carcinoma in the KEYNOTE-012 study include fatigue, decreased appetite, and dyspnea. Adverse effects in patients receiving pembrolizumab for the treatment of head and neck squamous cell carcinoma were similar to those reported in patients receiving the drug for the treatment of melanoma or NSCLC; however, a higher incidence of facial edema and new or worsening hypothyroidism were reported in patients with head and neck squamous cell carcinoma.

Adverse effects reported in 10% or more of patients receiving pembrolizumab for the treatment of relapsed or refractory cHL in the KEYNOTE-087 study include fatigue, cough, pyrexia, musculoskeletal pain, diarrhea, rash, vomiting, hypothyroidism, nausea, upper respiratory tract infection, dyspnea, headache, pruritus, arthralgia, and peripheral neuropathy. Laboratory abnormalities reported in 20% or more of patients receiving pembrolizumab for the treatment of relapsed or refractory cHL include elevated concentrations of aminotransferases (i.e., ALT, AST), anemia, thrombocytopenia, and neutropenia.

Adverse effects reported in 10% or more of patients receiving pembrolizumab for the treatment of relapsed or refractory PMBL in the KEYNOTE-170 study include musculoskeletal pain, upper respiratory tract infection, pyrexia, cough, fatigue, dyspnea, abdominal pain, diarrhea, arrhythmia, headache, and nausea. Laboratory abnormalities reported in 15% or more of patients receiving pembrolizumab for the treatment of relapsed or refractory PMBL include anemia, hyperglycemia, leukopenia, lymphopenia, neutropenia, hypophosphatemia, elevated concentrations of aminotransferases (i.e., ALT, AST), hypoglycemia, elevated concentrations of alkaline phosphatase, elevated concentrations of serum creatinine, hypocalcemia, and hypokalemia.

Adverse effects reported in 10% or more of cisplatin-ineligible patients receiving pembrolizumab for the treatment of locally advanced or metastatic urothelial carcinoma in the KEYNOTE-052 study include fatigue, musculoskeletal pain, decreased appetite, constipation, rash, diarrhea, pruritus, urinary tract infection, abdominal pain, nausea, cough, peripheral edema, hematuria, vomiting, dyspnea, pyrexia, arthralgia, and weight loss. Laboratory abnormalities reported in 10% or more of cisplatin-ineligible patients receiving pembrolizumab for the treatment of locally advanced or metastatic urothelial carcinoma include anemia, elevated concentrations of aminotransferases (i.e., ALT, AST), elevated concentrations of serum creatinine, and hyponatremia.

Adverse effects reported in 10% or more of patients receiving pembrolizumab for the treatment of previously treated locally advanced or metastatic urothelial carcinoma and at an incidence that is at least 2% higher than that reported with chemotherapy in the KEYNOTE-045 study include musculoskeletal pain, pruritus, rash, cough, vomiting, dyspnea, and hematuria. Laboratory abnormalities reported in 20% or more of patients receiving pembrolizumab for the treatment of previously treated locally advanced or metastatic urothelial carcinoma and at an incidence that is at least 2% higher than that reported with chemotherapy include elevated concentrations of alkaline phosphatase, serum creatinine, and AST.

Adverse effects reported in the KEYNOTE-059 study in patients receiving pembrolizumab for the treatment of gastric cancer were similar to those reported in other studies in patients receiving the drug for the treatment of melanoma or NSCLC.

Adverse effects reported in 10% or more of patients receiving pembrolizumab for the treatment of recurrent or metastatic cervical cancer in the KEYNOTE-158 study include fatigue, musculoskeletal pain, diarrhea, abdominal pain, pain, decreased appetite, hemorrhage, nausea, pyrexia, vomiting, infection (including urinary tract infection), rash, peripheral edema, constipation, headache, hypothyroidism, and dyspnea. Laboratory abnormalities reported in 20% or more of patients receiving pembrolizumab for the treatment of recurrent or metastatic cervical cancer include anemia, lymphopenia, hypoalbuminemia, elevated concentrations of alkaline phosphatase, hyperglycemia, hyponatremia, elevated concentrations of aminotransferases (i.e., ALT, AST), elevated concentrations of serum creatinine, hypocalcemia, and hypokalemia.

Adverse effects reported in the KEYNOTE-224 study in patients receiving pembrolizumab for the treatment of hepatocellular carcinoma generally were similar to those reported in other studies in patients receiving the drug for the treatment of melanoma or NSCLC; however, higher incidences of ascites, immune-mediated hepatitis, elevated concentrations of aminotransferases (i.e., ALT, AST), and hyperbilirubinemia were reported in patients with hepatocellular carcinoma.

Adverse effects reported in the KEYNOTE-017 study in patients receiving pembrolizumab for the treatment of Merkel cell carcinoma were similar to those reported in other studies in patients receiving the drug for the treatment of melanoma or NSCLC; however, higher incidences of hyperglycemia and elevated AST concentrations were reported in patients with Merkel cell carcinoma.

Drug Interactions

No formal drug interaction studies have been performed to date.

Description

Pembrolizumab, a humanized anti-programmed-death receptor-1 (anti-PD-1) monoclonal antibody, is an antineoplastic agent. The drug is an IgG_4 kappa immunoglobulin.

Pembrolizumab is highly selective for PD-1, an immune-checkpoint receptor expressed on activated T-cells, monocytes, B-cells, natural killer (NK) T-cells, and dendritic cells. Overexpression of PD-1 ligands on the surface of tumor cells results in activation of PD-1 and suppression of cytotoxic T-cell activity. Pembrolizumab blocks the interaction between PD-1 and its ligands, resulting in enhanced immune response, including enhanced antitumor immune response. The drug also has been shown to reduce tumor growth in syngeneic mouse tumor models.

Area under the serum concentration-time curve (AUC), peak plasma concentration, and trough concentration of pembrolizumab are proportional to dose over the dosage range of 2–10 mg/kg every 3 weeks. Following repeated doses of pembrolizumab every 3 weeks, steady-state concentrations are reached by 16 weeks; systemic accumulation of the drug is 2.1-fold. Based on dose-exposure safety and efficacy relationships, the manufacturer states that there are no clinically important differences in safety and efficacy between pembrolizumab 200 mg every 3 weeks and pembrolizumab 2 mg/kg every 3 weeks in patients with melanoma or non-small cell lung cancer (NSCLC). Clearance of pembrolizumab is approximately 23% lower at steady state than following the initial dose; however, this difference is not considered clinically important. The mean terminal half-life of pembrolizumab is 22 days.

The pharmacokinetics of pembrolizumab do not appear to be affected by age (range of 15–94 years), gender, race (89% Caucasian), renal impairment, mild hepatic impairment, or tumor burden.

Advice to Patients

Importance of advising patient to read the manufacturer's medication guide before beginning treatment and each time the drug is administered.

Risk of immune-mediated pneumonitis. Importance of informing clinician immediately if new or worsening cough, chest pain, or shortness of breath occurs.

Risk of immune-mediated colitis. Importance of informing clinician immediately if diarrhea, severe abdominal pain, or changes in stool occur.

Risk of immune-mediated hepatitis. Importance of informing clinician immediately if signs and symptoms of liver damage (e.g., jaundice, nausea, vomiting, dark urine, abdominal pain [particularly in the right upper quadrant], easy bruising or bleeding, lack of appetite) occur.

Risk of immune-mediated hypophysitis. Importance of informing clinician immediately if persistent or unusual headache, extreme weakness, dizziness or fainting, or vision changes occur.

Risk of immune-mediated nephritis. Importance of informing clinician immediately if signs and symptoms of renal damage (e.g., decreased urine output, change in color of urine) occur.

Risk of immune-mediated hyperthyroidism or hypothyroidism. Importance of informing clinician immediately if symptoms of abnormal thyroid function occur.

Risk of immune-mediated type 1 diabetes mellitus. Importance of informing clinician immediately if signs and symptoms of diabetes mellitus occur.

Risk of immune-mediated severe skin reactions. Importance of informing clinician immediately if severe skin reactions or signs and symptoms of Stevens-Johnson syndrome or toxic epidermal necrolysis develop.

Risk of other immune-mediated adverse effects. Importance of informing clinician immediately if manifestations of other potential immune-mediated adverse effects occur.

Risk of infusion-related reactions. Importance of informing clinician immediately if signs and symptoms of such reactions (e.g., dizziness, chills, fever, difficulty breathing, pruritus, flushing, feeling of faintness) occur.

Risk of immune-mediated rejection of a solid organ transplant. Importance of informing clinician immediately if signs and symptoms of solid organ transplant rejection occur.

Risk of immune-mediated complications following allogeneic stem cell transplantation.

Importance of laboratory monitoring during pembrolizumab therapy.

Risk of fetal harm. Necessity of advising women of childbearing potential that they should use a highly effective method of contraception while receiving the drug and for 4 months after the last dose. Importance of women informing clinicians if they are or plan to become pregnant. If pregnancy occurs, advise pregnant women of potential risk to the fetus.

Importance of advising women to avoid breast-feeding while receiving pembrolizumab therapy and for 4 months after the last dose.

Importance of informing clinicians of existing or contemplated concomitant therapy, including prescription and OTC drugs, as well as any concomitant illnesses (e.g., autoimmune disorders, history of organ transplantation, liver damage).

Importance of informing patients of other important precautionary information. (See Cautions.)

Overview® (see Users Guide). For additional information on this drug until a more detailed monograph is developed and published, the manufacturer's labeling should be consulted. It is *essential* that the manufacturer's labeling be consulted for more detailed information on usual cautions, precautions, contraindications, potential drug interactions, laboratory test interferences, and acute toxicity. For further information on the handling of antineoplastic agents, see the ASHP Guidelines on Handling Hazardous Drugs at http://www.ahfsdruginformation.com.

Preparations

Excipients in commercially available drug preparations may have clinically important effects in some individuals; consult specific product labeling for details.

Pembrolizumab

Parenteral

For injection, for IV use	50 mg	**Keytruda®**, Merck
Concentrate, for injection, for IV use	25 mg/mL (100 mg)	**Keytruda®**, Merck

PEMEtrexed Disodium

■ Pemetrexed, a folic acid antagonist, is an antineoplastic agent.

Uses

■ **Malignant Pleural Mesothelioma** Pemetrexed is used in combination with cisplatin for the treatment of malignant pleural mesothelioma in adults whose disease is unresectable or who otherwise are not candidates for potentially curative surgery. This malignancy occurs infrequently, is linked to asbestos exposure, and previously was considered unresponsive to chemotherapy, with a median survival of 6–8 months following diagnosis. Pemetrexed is designated an orphan drug by the US Food and Drug Administration (FDA) for use in this condition.

Efficacy of pemetrexed and cisplatin in the treatment of malignant pleural mesothelioma was established in a randomized, phase III, comparative, multicenter study in 448 adults who had not received previous chemotherapy. Patients were randomized to receive pemetrexed (500 mg/m^2) in combination with cisplatin (75 mg/m^2) on day 1 or cisplatin (75 mg/m^2) on day 1; both regimens were administered every 21 days. Patients studied were predominantly older (median age: 61 years) white males; approximately 68% of patients had tumors of epithelial histology, and 78% had stage III or IV disease. After 117 patients were treated, the study protocol was changed and patients started receiving folic acid and vitamin B_{12}supplementation because of hematologic and GI toxicity. The primary outcome measure was survival. Patients receiving the combination regimen had a longer median survival (12.1 versus 9.3 months), a longer time to progression (5.7 versus 3.9 months), a higher overall response rate (41.3 versus 16.7%), and improvement in lung function compared with patients receiving cisplatin alone. Addition of folic acid and vitamin B_{12} supplementation reduced toxicity and did not adversely affect survival.

■ **Non-small Cell Lung Cancer** Pemetrexed is used alone for the treatment of locally advanced or metastatic non-small cell lung cancer in adults who have received prior chemotherapy. This indication is based on the surrogate end point of tumor response rate; there are no controlled clinical studies to date demonstrating improvement in disease-related symptoms or increased survival with pemetrexed therapy.

Pemetrexed has been evaluated in a randomized, phase III, multicenter study in adults with stage III or IV (25 or 75% of patients, respectively) non-small cell lung cancer not amenable to potentially curative therapy. All patients in this study had received prior chemotherapy for advanced disease. Patients were randomized to receive pemetrexed (500 mg/m^2) or docetaxel (75 mg/m^2) on day 1; the regimens were administered every 21 days. Patients receiving pemetrexed also received folic acid and vitamin B_{12} supplementation. Response rates and clinical benefit (complete or partial response or stable disease) rates were similar in patients receiving pemetrexed or docetaxel. Overall response rates were 9.1 or 8.8% in patients receiving pemetrexed or docetaxel, respectively. Median survival (the primary end point of the study) was 8.3 or 7.9 months in those receiving pemetrexed or docetaxel, respectively; however, efficacy of pemetrexed in terms of survival could not be established, since a reliable and consistent effect of docetaxel on survival could not be estimated from historical study data, and crossover between treatments at the time of disease progression may have confounded interpretation of the survival data. Median progression-free survival was 2.9 months and 1-year survival rate was 29.7% in both treatment groups.

Dosage and Administration

■ **Reconstitution and Administration** Pemetrexed is administered by IV infusion over 10 minutes.

The usual precautions for handling and preparing solutions of cytotoxic drugs should be observed with pemetrexed. The manufacturer recommends use of protective gloves when handling the drug. If pemetrexed comes in contact with skin or mucosa, affected skin areas should be washed immediately and thoroughly with soap and water and affected mucosa should be thoroughly rinsed with copious amounts of water.

Pemetrexed is not a vesicant. Extravasation should be managed according to local standard of practice; there is no specific antidote for extravasation of pemetrexed.

Vials labeled as containing 500 mg of pemetrexed should be reconstituted by adding 20 mL of 0.9% sodium chloride injection without preservatives to provide a solution containing 25 mg/mL. The vial should be gently swirled until the powder is completely dissolved. The appropriate volume of reconstituted solution must be further diluted with 0.9% sodium chloride injection without preservatives to a volume of 100 mL prior to administration. Pemetrexed is incompatible with diluents containing calcium (e.g., lactated Ringer's injection, Ringer's injection); pemetrexed should not be diluted with these solutions, diluents other than 0.9% sodium chloride injection without preservatives, or other drugs. Because reconstituted and/or diluted pemetrexed solutions contain no preservatives, any unused portions of these solutions should be discarded. When reconstituted and/or diluted as directed, pemetrexed solutions are stable for 24 hours at controlled room temperature under ambient lighting.

■ **General Dosage** Dosage of pemetrexed disodium heptahydrate is expressed in terms of anhydrous pemetrexed.

All patients should be premedicated with a corticosteroid before pemetrexed administration to reduce the incidence and severity of cutaneous reactions. A regimen of oral dexamethasone 4 mg twice daily for 3 days, starting 1 day prior to pemetrexed administration, has been used in clinical studies.

All patients should be instructed to take a low-dose oral folic acid preparation or a multivitamin preparation containing folic acid daily to reduce toxicity. At least 5 daily doses of folic acid must be taken during the 7-day period preceding the first dose of pemetrexed; dosing should continue during the full course of therapy and for 21 days after the last dose of pemetrexed. Folic acid dosages ranged from 0.35–1 mg daily in clinical studies; the most commonly used dosage was 0.4 mg daily. Patients also must receive one IM injection of vitamin B_{12} during the week preceding the first dose of pemetrexed and every 3 cycles thereafter; injections administered subsequent to the initial dose may be given the same day as pemetrexed. A dose of 1 mg of vitamin B_{12} was used in clinical studies.

Malignant Pleural Mesothelioma The recommended adult dosage of pemetrexed is 500 mg/m² infused IV over 10 minutes in conjunction with cisplatin 75 mg/m² infused IV over 2 hours beginning approximately 30 minutes after completion of the pemetrexed infusion on day 1 of a 21-day cycle. Patients should be adequately hydrated before and after administration of cisplatin; clinicians should consult published protocols for information related to specific regimens.

Chemotherapy in subsequent cycles should be delayed until absolute neutrophil counts (ANCs) are at least 1500/mm³, platelet counts are at least 100,000/mm³, and creatinine clearances are at least 45 mL/minute.

Non-small Cell Lung Cancer The recommended adult dosage of pemetrexed is 500 mg/m² infused IV over 10 minutes on day 1 of a 21-day cycle.

Chemotherapy in subsequent cycles should be delayed until ANCs are at least 1500/mm³, platelet counts are at least 100,000/mm³, and creatinine clearances are at least 45 mL/minute.

Dosage Modification for Toxicity After the first treatment cycle, subsequent doses of pemetrexed as a single agent or in combination with cisplatin should be adjusted based on nadir hematologic counts (i.e., ANCs, platelet counts) and maximum nonhematologic toxicity.

Treatment may be delayed to allow sufficient time for recovery from hematologic toxicity; if pemetrexed therapy is resumed following such toxicity, subsequent doses should be reduced according to the nadir ANCs and platelet counts observed (see Table 1). Therapy should be discontinued if the patient experiences grade 3 or 4 hematologic toxicity after 2 dose reductions.

Table 1. Recommended Dosage Modification for Hematologic Toxicity of Pemetrexed Monotherapy or Pemetrexed and Cisplatin Combination Therapy

Toxicity	Dose of Pemetrexed	Dose of Cisplatin
Nadir ANC <500/mm³ and nadir platelets ≥50,000/mm³	75% of previous dose	75% of previous dose
Nadir platelets <50,000/mm³, regardless of nadir ANC	50% of previous dose	50% of previous dose

If the patient experiences grade 3 or 4 nonhematologic toxicity (except neurotoxicity), therapy should be interrupted until the toxicity resolves or decreases in intensity to at least pretreatment values. If pemetrexed therapy is then resumed, subsequent doses should be reduced according to the type and severity of the toxicity (see Table 2). Therapy should be discontinued if the patient experiences grade 3 or 4 nonhematologic toxicity (except neurotoxicity) after 2 dose reductions. These recommendations for dosage modifications for grade 3 or 4 nonhematologic toxicity apply to grade 4 but not to grade 3 elevations in serum transaminase values; dosage modification is not required for grade 3 elevations in serum transaminase values.

Table 2. Recommended Dosage Modification for Nonhematologic Toxicity (Except Neurotoxicity) of Pemetrexed Monotherapy or Pemetrexed and Cisplatin Combination Therapy

Toxicity and National Cancer Institute (NCI) Common Toxicity Criteria Grade	Dose of Pemetrexed	Dose of Cisplatin
Any grade 3 or 4 nonhematologic toxicity (except neurotoxicity), excluding grade 3 or 4 mucositis or grade 3 elevation in serum transaminase values	75% of previous dose	75% of previous dose
Any diarrhea requiring hospitalization (regardless of grade) or grade 3 or 4 diarrhea	75% of previous dose	75% of previous dose
Grade 3 or 4 mucositis	50% of previous dose	100% of previous dose

If the patient experiences grade 2 neurotoxicity, the pemetrexed dose may be maintained at the current level but subsequent doses of cisplatin should be reduced (see Table 3). Therapy should be discontinued immediately if grade 3 or 4 neurotoxicity occurs.

Table 3. Recommended Dosage Modifications for Neurotoxicity of Pemetrexed Monotherapy or Pemetrexed and Cisplatin Combination Therapy

NCI Common Toxicity Criteria Grade	Dose of Pemetrexed	Dose of Cisplatin
0–1	100% of previous dose	100% of previous dose
2	100% of previous dose	50% of previous dose

■ **Special Populations** In clinical trials, patients with creatinine clearances of 45 mL/minute and greater did not require dosage reductions other than those recommended for all patients. Information concerning patients with creatinine clearances less than 45 mL/minute is insufficient to date to make dosage recommendations for these patients, and use in such patients currently is *not* recommended.

Dosage reductions other than those recommended for all patients are not needed in geriatric patients 65 years of age or older.

Cautions

■ **Contraindications** Known hypersensitivity to pemetrexed or any ingredient in the formulation.

■ **Warnings/Precautions** ***Warnings*** **Hematologic Toxicity.** The principal manifestations of hematologic toxicity include neutropenia, thrombocytopenia, and/or anemia; myelosuppression is the most common dose-limiting toxicity. Absolute neutrophil count (ANC) reaches nadir at day 8–10 and returns to baseline approximately 4–8 days after nadir.

Folate and Vitamin B_{12} Supplementation. Patients must receive folic acid and vitamin B_{12} to prevent treatment-related hematologic and GI toxicity. Patients receiving supplemental folic acid and vitamin B_{12} in clinical studies had a reduction in grade 3/4 hematologic and nonhematologic toxicities (i.e., neutropenia, febrile neutropenia, infection with grade 3/4 neutropenia) and an overall reduction in toxicity.

Sensitivity Reactions **Dermatologic Effects.** Rash reported. Premedication with a corticosteroid reduces the incidence and severity of cutaneous reactions.

General Precautions **Adequate Patient Evaluation and Monitoring.** Pemetrexed should be administered only under the supervision of qualified clinicians experienced in the use of cytotoxic therapy.

Complete blood cell counts, including platelet counts, should be performed in all patients receiving pemetrexed. Patients should be monitored for nadir and recovery; blood cell counts were monitored before each dose and on days 8 and 15 of each treatment cycle in clinical studies.

Renal and hepatic function should be monitored periodically.

Other Considerations. Not known whether pemetrexed accumulates in fluid collections such as pleural effusions or ascites; such accumulations could increase toxicity. Some clinicians suggest that large effusions be drained before pemetrexed therapy.

Specific Populations **Pregnancy.** Category D. (See Users Guide.)

Lactation. Not known whether pemetrexed or its metabolites are distributed into human milk. Because of the potential for serious adverse reactions to pemetrexed in nursing infants, nursing should be discontinued prior to therapy.

Pediatric Use. Safety and efficacy not established in children.

Geriatric Use. Age-related differences in the pharmacokinetics of pemetrexed were not observed in adults 26–80 years of age.

Age-based dosage adjustments are not necessary in geriatric patients 65 years of age or older.

Hepatic Impairment. Pemetrexed has not been studied in patients with hepatic impairment. Patients with serum bilirubin concentrations exceeding 1.5 times the upper limit of normal were excluded from clinical studies. Patients with serum transaminase concentrations exceeding 3 times the upper limit of normal who had no evidence of hepatic metastases were excluded from clinical studies; patients with serum transaminase concentrations 3–5 times the upper limit of normal who had hepatic metastases were included in clinical studies.

Pemetrexed is not appreciably metabolized by the liver. Elevated serum transaminase or total bilirubin concentrations do not affect pharmacokinetics of pemetrexed.

Renal Impairment. Pemetrexed is eliminated principally unchanged by renal excretion; renal impairment is associated with reduced clearance of and increased systemic exposure to pemetrexed.

Dosage adjustment is not needed in patients with creatinine clearance of 45 mL/minute or greater. Information concerning patients with creatinine clearance less than 45 mL/minute is insufficient to date to make dosage recommendations for these patients; use of the drug in these patients currently is *not* recommended. Repeat cycles of pemetrexed should be withheld until creatinine clearances are at least 45 mL/minute.

Concomitant use of pemetrexed with cisplatin has not been evaluated in patients with moderate renal impairment.

Caution is advised if nonsteroidal anti-inflammatory agents (NSAIAs) are used concomitantly with pemetrexed in patients with renal impairment. (See Drug Interactions: Nonsteroidal Anti-inflammatory Agents.)

■ **Common Adverse Effects** Common adverse effects include hematologic effects, fever and infection, stomatitis/pharyngitis, rash/desquamation, nausea, fatigue, dyspnea, vomiting, constipation, chest pain, and anorexia.

Drug Interactions

■ **Drugs Metabolized by Hepatic Microsomal Enzymes** Pharmacokinetic interaction unlikely with drugs metabolized by cytochrome P-450 (CYP) isoenzymes 1A2, 2C9, 2D6, or 3A.

■ **Cisplatin** Pharmacokinetic interaction unlikely.

■ **Nonsteroidal Anti-inflammatory Agents** Pharmacokinetic interaction (decreased clearance of pemetrexed; increased pemetrexed AUC) with ibuprofen. The manufacturer states that ibuprofen (up to 400 mg 4 times daily) may be used concomitantly with pemetrexed in patients with normal renal function (creatinine clearance of 80 mL/minute or greater); however, caution is advised if ibuprofen is used concomitantly with pemetrexed in patients with mild to moderate renal impairment (creatinine clearance of 45–79 mL/minute). Patients with mild to moderate renal impairment should not receive nonsteroidal anti-inflammatory agents (NSAIAs) having short half-lives (e.g., ibuprofen) for 2 days before, the day of, and for 2 days after administration of pemetrexed.

Data are not available to date regarding possible interactions with NSAIAs having longer half-lives, and the manufacturer states that all patients receiving such NSAIAs should interrupt therapy with the NSAIA for at least 5 days before, the day of, and for 2 days after administration of pemetrexed. If concomitant use of a NSAIA is necessary, the patient should be closely monitored for toxicity, particularly myelosuppression and renal and GI toxicity.

Pharmacokinetic interaction unlikely with low to moderate aspirin dosage (325 mg every 6 hours). Effect of higher aspirin dosage on pemetrexed pharmacokinetics not known.

■ **Nephrotoxic Drugs** Possible pharmacokinetic interaction (delayed clearance of pemetrexed).

■ **Probenecid** Possible pharmacokinetic interaction (delayed clearance of pemetrexed). Pharmacokinetic interaction also possible with other substances secreted at the renal tubule.

■ **Vitamins** Pharmacokinetic interaction unlikely with oral folic acid and vitamin B_{12} given IM.

Description

Pemetrexed, a folic acid antagonist, exerts its antineoplastic activity by disrupting folate-dependent metabolic processes that are essential for cell replication. Pemetrexed inhibits the folate-dependent enzymes thymidylate synthase, dihydrofolate reductase, and phosphoribosylglycinamide formyltransferase (glycinamide ribonucleotide formyltransferase), enzymes involved in *de novo* biosynthesis of thymidine and purine nucleotides. Pemetrexed enters cells through the reduced folate carrier and membrane folate binding protein transport systems and undergoes extensive intracellular polyglutamation by tetrahydrofolylpolyglutamate synthase (folylpolyglutamate synthase). The polyglutamate forms are retained for long periods in the cells and are inhibitors of thymidylate synthase and phosphoribosylglycinamide formyltransferase. Polyglutamation is a time- and concentration-dependent process that occurs in tumor cells and, to a lesser extent, in normal tissues.

Preclinical studies have shown that pemetrexed inhibits the in vitro growth of mesothelioma cell lines (MSTO-211H, NCI-H2052). Synergistic inhibitory effects have been observed in the MSTO-211H mesothelioma cell line when pemetrexed was combined with cisplatin.

Advice to Patients

Importance of taking folic acid and vitamin B_{12} to reduce the risk of adverse effects. Importance of taking a corticosteroid for 3 days during each treatment cycle to reduce the risk of a skin reaction.

Importance of recognizing and reporting adverse effects of pemetrexed, including myelosuppressive effects, infectious complications, and GI symptoms (i.e., diarrhea, mucositis). Necessity of monitoring blood cell counts and serum creatinine. Necessity of dosage adjustment or delay in treatment if toxicity occurs.

Importance of women informing clinicians if they are or plan to become pregnant or to breast-feed. Apprise patient of potential hazard to the fetus if used during pregnancy; women of childbearing potential should avoid becoming pregnant.

Importance of informing clinicians of existing or contemplated concomitant therapy, including prescription and OTC drugs, especially nonsteroidal anti-inflammatory agents.

Overview® (see Users Guide). For additional information on this drug until a more detailed monograph is developed and published, the manufacturer's labeling should be consulted. It is *essential* that the manufacturer's labeling be consulted for more detailed information on usual cautions, precautions, contraindications, potential drug interactions, laboratory test interferences, and acute toxicity.

Preparations

Excipients in commercially available drug preparations may have clinically important effects in some individuals; consult specific product labeling for details.

PEMEtrexed Disodium

Parenteral

For injection, for IV infusion only	500 mg (of pemetrexed)	**Alimta®**, Lilly

Pertuzumab

■ Pertuzumab, a recombinant humanized anti-human epidermal growth factor receptor type 2 (anti-*HER2*/*ERBB2*) monoclonal antibody, is an antineoplastic agent.

Uses

■ **Breast Cancer** Pertuzumab is used in combination with trastuzumab and docetaxel for the treatment of metastatic breast cancer in patients whose tumors overexpress the human epidermal growth factor receptor type 2 (*HER2*) protein and who have not received prior anti-*HER2* therapy or chemotherapy for metastatic disease.

The current indication for pertuzumab is based principally on the results of a randomized, double-blind, placebo-controlled, phase 3 study (CLEOPATRA) in adults with *HER2*-overexpressing metastatic breast cancer. Patients were eligible for enrollment in the study if they had disease demonstrating an immunohistochemistry (IHC) assay score of 3+ or a fluorescent *in situ* hybridization (FISH) amplification ratio of 2 or higher. In addition, patients with prior adjuvant or neoadjuvant chemotherapy were required to have a disease-free interval of more than 12 months before diagnosis of metastatic breast cancer and enrollment into the study; patients may have received one prior hormonal treatment for metastatic disease before study enrollment.

In this study, 808 patients were randomized (stratified according to prior treatment and geographic region) in a 1:1 ratio to receive either pertuzumab (840 mg by IV infusion initially, followed by 420 mg by IV infusion every 3 weeks thereafter) in combination with trastuzumab (8 mg/kg by IV infusion initially, followed by 6 mg/kg by IV infusion every 3 weeks thereafter) and docetaxel (75 mg/m^2 by IV infusion initially, followed by 75 or 100 mg/m^2 every 3 weeks thereafter) *or* placebo in combination with trastuzumab and docetaxel. Patients received pertuzumab and trastuzumab until disease progression, withdrawal of patient consent, or unacceptable toxicity occurred; docetaxel was continued for at least 6 cycles. The primary measure of efficacy was progression-free survival as assessed by an independent review facility (IRF-assessed progression-free survival); secondary end points included overall survival, progression-free survival as assessed by the investigator (investigator-assessed progression-free survival), objective response rate, and duration of response. The median age of patients enrolled in the study was 54 years (range: 22–89 years). Approximately half of the patients had received prior adjuvant or neoadjuvant chemotherapy, including regimens consisting of an anthracycline (39%), taxane (23%), trastuzumab (11%), or hormonal therapy (25%); approximately 11% of patients with hormone receptor-positive tumors had received hormonal therapy for metastatic disease. All except 2 of the enrolled patients were women. Approximately 89% of patients had an IHC score of 3+, and approximately 95% of patients had FISH-positive tumors.

Patients randomized to receive pertuzumab in combination with trastuzumab and docetaxel had a longer median IRF-assessed progression-free survival compared with patients receiving placebo in combination with trastuzumab and docetaxel (18.5 versus 12.4 months, respectively). Effects of pertuzumab on investigator-assessed progression-free survival and IRF-assessed progression-free survival were comparable. Prolonged progression-free survival was observed in pertuzumab-treated patients regardless of age, race, geographic region, or prior adjuvant or neoadjuvant therapy. In addition, patients receiving pertuzumab in combination with trastuzumab and docetaxel appeared to have a higher objective response rate (80.2 versus 69.3%, respectively) and a longer median duration of response (20.2 versus 12.5 months, respectively) compared with those receiving placebo in combination with trastuzumab and docetaxel. Effects on overall survival remain to be established; however, a planned interim analysis suggested a trend toward a survival benefit in the pertuzumab group compared with the control group. The median follow-up period at the time of interim analysis was 19.3 months in both treatment arms; the median duration of treatment was estimated to be 18.1 months for pertuzumab-treated patients and 11.8 months for placebo-treated patients. At the time of interim analysis, pertuzumab- or placebo-treated patients had received a mean of 19.9 or 16.2 treatment cycles, respectively; both groups received a median of 8 docetaxel cycles.

Dosage and Administration

■ **General** Because infusion or hypersensitivity reactions may occur, patients should be closely observed for 60 minutes after the first infusion of pertuzumab and for 30 minutes after subsequent infusions of the drug. (See Infusion or Hypersensitivity Reactions under Warnings/Precautions: Sensitivity Reactions, in Cautions.)

Restricted Distribution Pertuzumab can only be obtained through select specialty distributors. Specific information regarding distribution of pertuzumab is available from the manufacturer at 800-551-2231 or http://www.perjeta.com.

■ **Administration** Pertuzumab is administered by IV infusion. The initial dose of pertuzumab should be administered by IV infusion over 60 minutes; subsequent doses may be administered by IV infusion over 30–60 minutes. (See General under Dosage and Administration.) *Pertuzumab solutions should not be administered by rapid IV injection, such as IV push or bolus.*

Prior to administration, pertuzumab injection must be diluted using proper aseptic technique. Pertuzumab injection is diluted by adding the appropriate volume of pertuzumab 30 mg/mL solution to a polyvinyl chloride (PVC) or non-PVC polyolefin infusion bag containing 250 mL of 0.9% sodium chloride injection; the bag should be inverted gently to mix the solution and should *not* be shaken. Pertuzumab injection should *not* be diluted in 5% dextrose injection. Any unused portion left in the vial should be discarded since the injection contains no preservative. Pertuzumab solutions should be inspected visually for particulate matter and discoloration prior to dilution and administration. Following dilution, pertuzumab infusion solution may be administered immediately or stored at 2–8°C for up to 24 hours. Diluted pertuzumab solution should not be admixed with any other drug.

Unopened vials of pertuzumab injection should be protected from light and stored in the original carton at 2–8°C until use; vials should *not* be frozen or shaken.

Procedures for proper handling (e.g., use of gloves) and disposal of antineoplastic drugs should be followed when preparing or administering pertuzumab.

■ **Dosage** ***Breast Cancer*** For the treatment of metastatic breast cancer that overexpresses the human epidermal growth factor receptor type 2 (*HER2*) protein, the recommended initial dose of pertuzumab is 840 mg (administered by IV infusion over 60 minutes) in combination with trastuzumab 8 mg/kg (administered by IV infusion over 90 minutes) and docetaxel 75 mg/m^2 (administered by IV infusion). The initial regimen is followed every 3 weeks thereafter by pertuzumab 420 mg (administered by IV infusion over 30–60 minutes) in combination with trastuzumab 6 mg/kg (administered by IV infusion over 30–90 minutes) and docetaxel 75 or 100 mg/m^2.

In the CLEOPATRA study, pertuzumab and trastuzumab were continued for a mean of 19.9 cycles, and docetaxel was continued for a median of 8 cycles.

If a dose is missed or delayed, and the time between 2 sequential infusions is less than 6 weeks, a pertuzumab dose of 420 mg should be administered; waiting until the next scheduled dose is not recommended. If the time between 2 sequential infusions is 6 weeks or longer, the initial pertuzumab dose of 840 mg should be re-administered, followed by a pertuzumab dosage of 420 mg every 3 weeks thereafter.

Dosage Modification for Toxicity and Contraindications for Continued Therapy Dosage reductions are not recommended for pertuzumab. If toxicities occur, reduction in infusion rate or temporary or permanent discontinuance of pertuzumab should be considered based on causality.

Infusion or Hypersensitivity Reactions. If clinically important infusion reactions occur, the infusion rate should be reduced or pertuzumab therapy interrupted, and appropriate medical therapy should be initiated. If severe infusion or hypersensitivity reactions occur, pertuzumab infusion should be immediately discontinued, and permanent discontinuance of pertuzumab therapy should be considered. Patients should be monitored carefully until signs and symptoms have completely resolved. (See Infusion or Hypersensitivity Reactions under Warnings/Precautions: Sensitivity Reactions, in Cautions.)

Left Ventricular Dysfunction. If left ventricular ejection fraction (LVEF) decreases to less than 40% *or* to 40–45% with an absolute decrease from baseline of 10% or more, pertuzumab and trastuzumab should be withheld for at least 3 weeks. (See Left Ventricular Dysfunction under Warnings/Precautions: Other Warnings and Precautions, in Cautions.)

LVEF should be reassessed within approximately 3 weeks. If LVEF has recovered to greater than 45% *or* to 40–45% with an absolute decrease from baseline of less than 10%, pertuzumab therapy may be resumed. If LVEF has not improved or has declined further, discontinuance of pertuzumab and trastuzumab should be strongly considered, unless the benefits for the individual patient outweigh the risks.

The prescribing information for docetaxel should be consulted for detailed information on dosage modifications for this drug.

Pertuzumab should be withheld or discontinued if trastuzumab is withheld or discontinued; however, if docetaxel is discontinued, therapy with pertuzumab and trastuzumab may be continued.

■ **Special Populations** Dosage adjustment is not necessary based on body weight or baseline albumin concentration. (See Description.)

No dosage adjustment is necessary in patients with mild (creatinine clearance of 60–90 mL/minute) or moderate (creatinine clearance of 30–60 mL/minute) renal impairment. The manufacturer makes no specific dosage recommendations for patients with severe renal impairment (creatinine clearance less than 30 mL/minute) because data are limited in this population. (See Renal Impairment under Warnings/Precautions: Specific Populations, in Cautions.)

The manufacturer makes no specific dosage recommendations for geriatric patients. (See Geriatric Use under Warnings/Precautions: Specific Populations, in Cautions.)

Cautions

■ **Contraindications** The manufacturer states that there are no known contraindications to the use of pertuzumab.

■ **Warnings/Precautions** ***Warnings*** **Fetal/Neonatal Morbidity and Mortality.** Pertuzumab may cause fetal harm if administered to pregnant women; the drug has been shown to be embryotoxic and fetotoxic in animals. In pregnant cynomolgus monkeys, exposure to pertuzumab at concentrations 2.5–20 times that of human clinical exposure (based on peak plasma concentrations) resulted in oligohydramnios, delayed fetal kidney development, and embryo-fetal death.

There are no adequate and well-controlled studies to date in pregnant women; however, based on findings from animal studies, the manufacturer states that the embryotoxic and fetotoxic effects of pertuzumab are likely to be present during all trimesters of pregnancy. Therefore, pregnancy status should be verified prior to initiation of pertuzumab, and women of childbearing potential should be advised to use effective contraceptive methods during and for 6 months after discontinuance of the drug.

If pertuzumab is used during pregnancy or if the patient becomes pregnant while receiving the drug, the patient should be apprised of the potential fetal hazard. (See Pregnancy under Warnings/Precautions: Specific Populations, in Cautions.) Patients who become pregnant during pertuzumab therapy should be monitored for development of oligohydramnios; if oligohydramnios occurs, appropriate fetal testing within the standards of care should be performed. Efficacy of IV hydration in the management of oligohydramnios secondary to pertuzumab exposure is unknown.

Sensitivity Reactions **Infusion or Hypersensitivity Reactions.** Infusion reactions, including hypersensitivity and anaphylaxis, have been reported in patients receiving pertuzumab. In the CLEOPATRA study in which the initial dose of pertuzumab was administered one day before trastuzumab and docetaxel during the first cycle (to allow for evaluation of pertuzumab-related infusion reactions), infusion reactions were reported in 13% of patients receiving pertuzumab compared with 9.8% of those receiving placebo; the most common infusion reactions were pyrexia, chills, fatigue, headache, asthenia, hypersensitivity, and vomiting. During the second cycle when pertuzumab, trastuzumab, and docetaxel were administered on the same day, the most common infusion reactions included fatigue, dysgeusia, hypersensitivity, myalgia, and vomiting.

In the CLEOPATRA study, hypersensitivity or anaphylactic reactions occurred in 10.8 or 9.1% of patients receiving pertuzumab or placebo, respectively; grade 3–4 hypersensitivity or anaphylactic reactions occurred in 2 or 2.5% of patients, respectively. Anaphylaxis occurred in 4 patients receiving pertuzumab and 2 patients receiving placebo.

Patients should be observed closely for 60 minutes after the first infusion of pertuzumab and for 30 minutes after subsequent infusions of the drug. If infusion or hypersensitivity reactions occur, reduction in infusion rate or temporary or permanent discontinuance of pertuzumab may be required. (See Infusion or Hypersensitivity Reactions under Dosage: Dosage Modification for Toxicity and Contraindications for Continued Therapy, under Dosage and Administration.)

Other Warnings and Precautions **Left Ventricular Dysfunction.** Decreases in left ventricular ejection fraction (LVEF) have been reported with inhibitors of human epidermal growth factor receptor type 2 (*HER2*), including pertuzumab. In the CLEOPATRA study, pertuzumab in combination with trastuzumab and docetaxel was not associated with an increased incidence of symptomatic left ventricular systolic dysfunction (LVSD) or decreases in LVEF compared with placebo in combination with trastuzumab and docetaxel. LVSD occurred in 4.4% of pertuzumab-treated patients and in 8.3% of placebo-treated patients; symptomatic LVSD (congestive heart failure) occurred in 1 and 1.8% of patients, respectively. Pooled analysis of data from several studies evaluating use of pertuzumab as a single agent or in combination with either chemotherapy or targeted therapy for the treatment of various malignancies demonstrated that the median time to development of LVSD and symptomatic heart failure was around cycle 4, with 87% of the events occurring between cycles 1 and 7. In this pooled analysis, no substantial increases in cardiac dysfunction were observed following use of pertuzumab in combination with trastuzumab or non-anthracycline-based chemotherapy.

Pertuzumab has not been studied in patients with a baseline LVEF of 50% or lower, prior history of congestive heart failure, decreases in LVEF to less than 50% during prior trastuzumab therapy, or conditions that could impair left ventricular function (e.g., uncontrolled hypertension, recent myocardial infarction, serious cardiac arrhythmia requiring treatment, cumulative prior anthracycline exposure greater than 360 mg/m^2 of doxorubicin or its equivalent). However, patients who have received prior anthracycline therapy or who have had prior radiation therapy to the chest area may be at greater risk for development of LVSD.

LVEF should be assessed prior to initiation of pertuzumab and at regular intervals (e.g., every 3 months) during treatment. If substantial decreases in LVEF occur, temporary or permanent discontinuance of pertuzumab may be required. (See Left Ventricular Dysfunction under Dosage: Dosage Modification for Toxicity and Contraindications for Continued Therapy, in Dosage and Administration.)

Evaluation of *HER2*. Detection of *HER2* overexpression is necessary prior to initiating therapy because safety and efficacy of pertuzumab have been established only in patients with *HER2*-overexpressing tumors. In clinical practice and clinical research studies, the methods of *HER2* evaluation most commonly used are immunohistochemistry (IHC) assays, which directly measure overexpression of the *HER2* protein, and fluorescent *in situ* hybridization (FISH), which measures amplification of the *HER2* oncogene. (See Evaluation of *HER2/neu* in Breast Cancer under Uses: Breast Cancer, in Trastuzumab 10:00.) In the CLEOPATRA study, patients with breast cancer were required to have disease demonstrating an IHC score of 3+ (as determined by the Dako Herceptest®) or a FISH amplification ratio of 2 or higher (as determined by the

Dako *HER2* FISH PharmDx® test kit). Limited data are available for patients whose breast tumors are FISH-positive but lack *HER2* overexpression.

Assessment of *HER2* status should be performed by laboratories with demonstrated proficiency in the specific technology being used. Improper assay performance, including use of suboptimally fixed tissue, failure to use specified reagents, deviation from specific assay instructions, and failure to include appropriate controls for assay validation, can lead to unreliable results.

Immunogenicity. As with all therapeutic proteins, there is a potential for immunogenicity. In the CLEOPATRA study, anti-pertuzumab antibodies were detected in 11 of 386 patients (2.8%) receiving pertuzumab in combination with trastuzumab and docetaxel and in 23 of 372 patients (6.2%) receiving placebo in combination with trastuzumab and docetaxel. Anaphylactic or hypersensitivity reactions related to the presence of anti-pertuzumab antibodies were not observed in these patients.

The presence of pertuzumab in the serum sample may interfere with assays used to measure antibodies to the drug. In addition, the assay may be detecting antibodies to trastuzumab. Therefore, data may not accurately reflect the true incidence of anti-pertuzumab antibody formation.

Prolongation of QT Interval. In a subset of 20 patients enrolled in the CLEOPATRA study, no large (i.e., more than 20 msec) increases in the corrected QT (QT_c) interval were observed in patients receiving pertuzumab in combination with trastuzumab and docetaxel. However, smaller increases (i.e., less than 10 msec) in QT_c interval cannot be excluded because of study limitations.

Specific Populations **Pregnancy.** Category D. (See Fetal/Neonatal Morbidity and Mortality under Warnings/Precautions: Warnings, in Cautions.)

If pertuzumab is used during pregnancy or if the patient becomes pregnant while receiving the drug, the patient should be apprised of the potential fetal hazard; the patient should be encouraged to enroll in the MotHER Pregnancy Registry (800-690-6720), and clinicians should immediately notify the Genentech Adverse Event Line (888-835-2555).

Lactation. It is not known whether pertuzumab is distributed into milk; however, human immunoglobulin G (IgG) is distributed into milk. (See Description.) Because of the potential for serious adverse reactions to pertuzumab in nursing infants, a decision should be made whether to discontinue nursing or the drug, taking into account the long elimination half-life of the drug and the importance of the drug to the woman.

Pediatric Use. Safety and efficacy of pertuzumab have not been established in children younger than 18 years of age.

Geriatric Use. In the CLEOPATRA study, 15% of patients were 65 years of age or older, and 1% were 75 years of age or older. No overall differences in safety and efficacy were observed between geriatric and younger patients. In a population pharmacokinetic analysis, no substantial differences in pharmacokinetics were observed between geriatric and younger adults.

Hepatic Impairment. The pharmacokinetics of pertuzumab have not been studied in patients with hepatic impairment.

Renal Impairment. In a population pharmacokinetic analysis, systemic exposure to pertuzumab was similar between patients with mild (creatinine clearance of 60–90 mL/minute) or moderate (creatinine clearance of 30–60 mL/minute) renal impairment and those with normal renal function. Pharmacokinetic data in patients with severe renal impairment (creatinine clearance less than 30 mL/minute) are limited. (See Dosage and Administration: Special Populations.)

■ **Common Adverse Effects** The most common adverse effects occurring in more than 30% of patients receiving pertuzumab in combination with trastuzumab and docetaxel include diarrhea, alopecia, neutropenia, nausea, fatigue, rash, and peripheral neuropathy. The most common grade 3 or 4 adverse effects reported in more than 2% of patients receiving pertuzumab in combination with trastuzumab and docetaxel include neutropenia, febrile neutropenia, leukopenia, diarrhea, peripheral neuropathy, anemia, asthenia, and fatigue.

Drug Interactions

■ **Antineoplastic Agents** No drug-drug interactions between pertuzumab and trastuzumab, or between pertuzumab and docetaxel, were observed in a substudy of 37 patients enrolled in the CLEOPATRA study.

Description

Pertuzumab, a recombinant humanized anti-human epidermal growth factor receptor type 2 (anti-*HER2/ERBB2*) monoclonal antibody, is an antineoplastic agent. The drug is an IgG_1 kappa immunoglobulin produced by recombinant DNA technology in mammalian cell (Chinese hamster ovary) culture. Pertuzumab also is referred to as a *HER2/neu* receptor antagonist.

Pertuzumab binds specifically to the extracellular dimerization domain (subdomain II) of the *HER2* protein, blocking heterodimerization of *HER2* with other ligand-bound members of the *HER/ERBB* family (i.e., epidermal growth factor receptor [*HER1*/EGFR/*ERBB1*], *HER3/ERBB3*, *HER4/ERBB4*). Blockade of *HER2* heterodimerization (particularly with *HER3*) by pertuzumab results in inhibition of ligand-activated intracellular signaling through 2 major signal pathways, mitogen-activated protein kinase (MAPK) and phosphoinositide 3-kinase (PI3K/Akt), potentially causing cell growth arrest and apoptosis, respectively. Similar to trastuzumab, pertuzumab also mediates antibody-dependent cell-mediated cytotoxicity (ADCC).

Pertuzumab binds to a different *HER2* domain than trastuzumab and exhibits complementary mechanisms of action with trastuzumab; the combined use of these agents, therefore, may result in more comprehensive inhibition of *HER2* signaling. Pertuzumab alone inhibits proliferation of human tumor cells, while the combination of pertuzumab and trastuzumab has been shown to substantially augment antitumor activity in *HER2*-overexpressing xenograft models.

The pharmacokinetics of pertuzumab are linear over a dose range of 2–25 mg/kg. Following administration of an initial dose of 840 mg followed by a maintenance dosage of 420 mg every 3 weeks thereafter, steady-state concentrations of pertuzumab were reached after the first maintenance dose. The median half-life of pertuzumab is 18 days.

The pharmacokinetics of pertuzumab do not appear to be affected by age, gender, or ethnicity (Japanese versus non-Japanese). Baseline serum albumin concentration and lean body weight had a minor influence on pharmacokinetic parameters; therefore, the manufacturer states that dosage adjustment based on body weight or baseline albumin concentration is not necessary.

Advice to Patients

Risk of fetal harm (e.g., embryo-fetal death, birth defects). Necessity of advising women of childbearing potential to use effective contraceptive methods during and for 6 months after discontinuance of pertuzumab. Encourage women who have been exposed to pertuzumab during pregnancy to enroll in the MotHER Pregnancy Registry by contacting 800-690-6720. (See Fetal/Neonatal Morbidity and Mortality under Warnings/Precautions: Warnings, in Cautions.)

Importance of discontinuing breast-feeding during therapy.

Risk of infusion or hypersensitivity reactions.

Risk of decreased left ventricular ejection fraction (LVEF).

Importance of informing clinicians of existing or contemplated concomitant therapy, including prescription and OTC drugs, as well as any concomitant illnesses.

Importance of informing patients of other important precautionary information. (See Cautions.)

Overview® (see Users Guide). For additional information on this drug until a more detailed monograph is developed and published, the manufacturer's labeling should be consulted. It is *essential* that the manufacturer's labeling be consulted for more detailed information on usual cautions, precautions, contraindications, potential drug interactions, laboratory test interferences, and acute toxicity. For further information on the handling of antineoplastic agents, see the ASHP Guidelines on Handling Hazardous Drugs at http://www.ahfsdruginformation.com.

Preparations

Pertuzumab can only be obtained through select specialty distributors. Specific information regarding distribution of pertuzumab is available from the manufacturer at 800-551-2231 or http://www.perjeta.com.

Excipients in commercially available drug preparations may have clinically important effects in some individuals; consult specific product labeling for details.

Pertuzumab

Parenteral

Injection, for IV infusion	30 mg/mL (420 mg)	**Perjeta®**, Genentech

Pomalidomide

■ Pomalidomide, a thalidomide analog, is an immunomodulatory agent with antineoplastic and antiangiogenic activity.

REMS

FDA approved a REMS for pomalidomide to ensure that the benefits outweigh the risk. The REMS may apply to one or more preparations of pomalidomide and consists of the following: elements to assure safe use and implementation system. See the FDA REMS page (https://www.accessdata.fda.gov/scripts/cder/rems/index.cfm).

Uses

■ **Multiple Myeloma** Pomalidomide is used for the treatment of multiple myeloma in patients who have received at least 2 prior therapies including lenalidomide and bortezomib and have demonstrated disease progression during or within 60 days following completion of their last therapy. Pomalidomide has been designated an orphan drug by the US Food and Drug Administration (FDA) for use in multiple myeloma. The current indication is based on overall response rate; there currently are no clinical trials demonstrating a clinical benefit (e.g., improvement in disease-related symptoms, increased survival).

The current indication for pomalidomide is based principally on the results of a randomized, open-label, multicenter, phase 2 trial (MM-002) in adults with relapsed multiple myeloma who had received lenalidomide and bortezomib. Patients were enrolled if their disease was refractory to their most recent therapy (i.e., disease progression during or within 60 days following completion of their most recent therapy). In this trial, 221 patients were randomized in a 1:1 ratio to receive pomalidomide (4 mg once daily on days 1–21 of a 28-day cycle) alone or in combination with low-dose dexamethasone (40 mg once daily on days 1, 8, 15, and 22 of a 28-day cycle; patients older than 75 years of age received reduced doses [i.e., 20 mg] of dexamethasone); treatment was continued until disease progression or unacceptable toxicity occurred or treatment was discontinued for other reasons. Patients who received pomalidomide alone could add low-dose dexamethasone to their treatment regimen upon disease progression. All enrolled patients were required to receive thromboprophylaxis (i.e., aspirin 81–100 mg once daily or other antithrombotic therapy if aspirin was contraindicated). The primary end point of this study was progression-free survival; secondary end points included objective response rate, duration of response, time to response, and overall survival. The median age of enrolled patients was 63 years, and patients had received a median of 5 prior therapies for multiple myeloma. Most of the patients (approximately 75%) had undergone stem cell transplantation and approximately 60% of patients had disease that was refractory to both bortezomib and lenalidomide. A planned interim analysis indicated that patients receiving pomalidomide in combination with low-dose dexamethasone had a higher overall response rate than patients receiving pomalidomide alone (29.2 versus 7.4%), with a median response duration of 7.4 months; one patient receiving pomalidomide in combination with low-dose dexamethasone achieved a complete response compared with none of those receiving pomalidomide alone. The median follow-up at the time of the interim analysis was 9.6 weeks.

Use of pomalidomide in combination with dexamethasone also was investigated in an open-label, multicenter, phase 3 trial (MM-003) in patients with relapsed or refractory multiple myeloma. In this trial, 455 patients were randomized in a 2:1 ratio to receive pomalidomide (4 mg once daily on days 1–21 of a 28-day cycle) in combination with low-dose dexamethasone (40 mg once daily on days 1, 8, 15, and 22 of a 28-day cycle) or high-dose dexamethasone alone (40 mg daily on days 1–4, 9–12, and 17–20 of a 28-day cycle); patients older than 75 years of age received reduced doses (i.e., 20 mg) of dexamethasone. Patients enrolled in the trial had received a median of 5 prior therapies. Most patients (72%) in this trial had disease that was refractory to both lenalidomide and bortezomib. At a median follow-up of 18 weeks, patients receiving pomalidomide in combination with low-dose dexamethasone had longer median progression-free survival compared with those receiving high-dose dexamethasone alone (15.7 versus 8 weeks; hazard ratio: 0.45). Although median overall survival for patients receiving the combination regimen had not been reached at the time of analysis, overall survival appeared to be prolonged in patients receiving pomalidomide in combination with low-dose dexamethasone compared with those receiving high-dose dexamethasone alone.

Dosage and Administration

■ **General** ***Restricted Distribution Program*** *Because pomalidomide is an analog of thalidomide (a known human teratogen that can cause severe, life-threatening birth defects), commercially available pomalidomide must be obtained through a restricted distribution program, the Pomalyst Risk Evaluation and Mitigation Strategy (REMS)® program, designed to help ensure that fetal exposure to the drug does not occur.* Clinicians, pharmacists, and patients must be registered in the Pomalyst REMS® program before they can prescribe, dispense, and receive pomalidomide, and compliance with all terms outlined in the program is mandatory. The Pomalyst REMS® program controls access to pomalidomide; educates program participants (clinicians, pharmacists, patients) about the risks associated with pomalidomide and the procedural requirements for safe use of the drug; and monitors compliance with the registration, education, and safety requirements of the program. Clinicians may contact 888-423-5436 or visit http://www.celgeneriskmanagement.com for additional information and to enroll in the program. (See Fetal/Neonatal Morbidity and Mortality under Warnings/Precautions: Warnings, in Cautions.)

■ **Administration** Pomalidomide capsules should be administered orally with water once daily. The drug should be administered without food (i.e., at least 2 hours before or 2 hours after a meal). The capsules should be swallowed intact and should not be broken, chewed, or opened. No more than a 28-day supply of pomalidomide should be prescribed and dispensed at one time.

Exposure to the contents of the capsules should be avoided. If such contact with the skin or mucous membranes occurs, affected areas of skin should be washed thoroughly with soap and water and affected mucosa should be rinsed thoroughly with water.

Procedures for proper handling and disposal of antineoplastic drugs should be followed when administering pomalidomide.

■ **Dosage** ***Multiple Myeloma*** For the treatment of multiple myeloma in adults who have received at least 2 prior therapies including lenalidomide and bortezomib, the recommended initial dosage of pomalidomide is 4 mg once daily on days 1–21 of repeated 28-day cycles. The drug may be used in combination with low-dose dexamethasone. (See Uses: Multiple Myeloma.) In clinical studies, therapy was continued for as long as the patient derived clinical benefit from the drug or until unacceptable toxicity occurred. New cycles of therapy should *not* be undertaken until neutrophil counts reach or exceed 500/mm³ and platelet counts reach or exceed 50,000/mm³.

Dosage Modification for Toxicity Dosage of pomalidomide should be adjusted in 1-mg decrements if toxicities requiring dosage modification occur; if a dosage of 1 mg daily is not tolerated, pomalidomide should be discontinued.

Hematologic Toxicity. For the first occurrence of neutropenia (absolute neutrophil count [ANC] less than 500/mm³), febrile neutropenia (temperature of 38.5°C or higher *and* ANC less than 1000/mm³), or thrombocytopenia (platelet count less than 25,000/mm³), pomalidomide therapy should be withheld and complete blood cell counts (CBCs) should be monitored weekly; therapy may be resumed at a reduced dosage of 3 mg daily when ANC reaches or exceeds 500/mm³ and platelet counts exceed 50,000/mm³. (See Hematologic Effects under Warnings/Precautions: Other Warnings and Precautions, in Cautions.)

For subsequent occurrences of neutropenia (ANC less than 500/mm³) or thrombocytopenia (platelet count less than 25,000/mm³), therapy should be withheld again until ANC reaches or exceeds 500/mm³ and platelet counts reach or exceed 50,000/mm³ and then may be resumed at a dosage further reduced by 1 mg daily.

Grade 3 or 4 Toxicity. If grade 3 or 4 toxicities other than neutropenia or thrombocytopenia occur, pomalidomide therapy should be interrupted; following resolution of the toxicity or improvement to grade 2 or less, pomalidomide therapy may be resumed at a reduced dosage of 1 mg daily less than the previous dosage.

■ **Special Populations** No dosage adjustment is necessary in geriatric patients.

Use of pomalidomide should be avoided in patients with serum aminotransferase (ALT and AST) concentrations exceeding 3 times the upper limit of normal (ULN) and bilirubin concentrations exceeding 2 mg/dL. Use of pomalidomide also should be avoided in patients with serum creatinine concentrations exceeding 3 mg/dL. Safety and efficacy have not been established in these patients.

Cautions

■ **Contraindications** Pomalidomide is contraindicated in women who are pregnant. (See Restricted Distribution Program under Dosage and Administration: Generaland also see Fetal/Neonatal Morbidity and Mortality under Warnings/Precautions: Warnings, in Cautions.)

■ **Warnings/Precautions** ***Warnings*** **Fetal/Neonatal Morbidity and Mortality.** Pomalidomide may cause fetal toxicity; pomalidomide is a structural analog of thalidomide, a known human teratogen, and teratogenic and other fetotoxic effects of pomalidomide (e.g., musculoskeletal anomalies and deformities; absence of internal organs, including bladder and thyroid; defects of internal organ systems, including cardiovascular, respiratory, renal, hepatic, and CNS abnormalities; increased fetal resorptions) have been demonstrated in animals. Therefore, pomalidomide is contraindicated in women who are pregnant.

All female patients of childbearing potential and all sexually mature males receiving pomalidomide must use effective contraceptive measures (which may include abstinence) to help ensure that fetal exposure to the drug does not occur. Contraceptive measures are indicated even in females with a history of infertility. The only females who do not need to observe mandatory contraceptive measures are those who have undergone hysterectomy or bilateral oophorectomy and those who are postmenopausal and have had no menses for 24 or more consecutive months. All female patients of childbearing potential must use 2 reliable forms of contraception simultaneously (unless the patient chooses to remain continuously abstinent from engaging in heterosexual sexual contact) beginning 4 weeks prior to initiation of therapy, during therapy and treatment interruptions, and then for 4 weeks following discontinuance of pomalidomide therapy. At least one contraceptive method should be a highly effective method (intrauterine device [IUD], hormonal contraceptives, tubal ligation, vasectomized partner); the other may be an effective barrier method (latex or synthetic condom, diaphragm, cervical cap). Sexually mature males receiving pomalidomide must completely avoid unprotected sexual contact with women of childbearing potential and must *not* donate semen while receiving pomalidomide and for 4 weeks after discontinuing the drug. (See Description.) While receiving pomalidomide and for up to 28 days after discontinuing the drug, sexually mature males (including those who have successfully undergone vasectomy) must use a latex or synthetic condom each time they have sexual contact with a woman of childbearing potential.

Because pomalidomide may cause fetal harm and because of the possibility that the drug may be present in blood and be transfused into a woman who is pregnant, patients receiving pomalidomide must *not* donate blood during therapy and for at least 1 month following discontinuance of the drug.

All females of childbearing potential must be tested for pregnancy within 10–14 days and again within 24 hours immediately prior to initiation of pomalidomide therapy. The prescribing clinician should *not* provide the patient with a prescription for pomalidomide until reports of the pregnancy tests are available indicating that the results are negative. Pregnancy tests must then be repeated at regular intervals during pomalidomide therapy (i.e., weekly during the first month, then every 2 or 4 weeks in women with irregular or regular menstrual cycles, respectively). Pregnancy tests and counseling also should be performed if a patient misses her period or if there is any abnormality in menstrual bleeding. The drug should be discontinued during the evaluation period. If the drug is used during pregnancy or if the patient becomes pregnant while receiving the drug, pomalidomide should be immediately discontinued and the patient informed of the potential hazard to the fetus; the patient should be referred to an obstetrician/gynecologist experienced in reproductive toxicity, and the clinician should notify Celgene (888-423-5436) and the US Food and Drug Administration (FDA) via the MedWatch program (800-332-1088). (See Restricted Distribution Program under Dosage and Administration: General.)

Venous Thromboembolic Events. Serious venous thromboembolic events have been reported in patients receiving pomalidomide. In the pivotal multiple myeloma trial, deep-vein thrombosis or pulmonary embolism occurred in 3% of patients receiving pomalidomide alone or in combination with low-dose dexamethasone. In this trial, all patients were required to receive an antithrombotic agent for prevention of venous thromboembolism; antithrombotic agents used for prophylaxis or treatment included aspirin (81% of patients), heparin (21%), warfarin (16%), and clopidogrel (3%). The manufacturer and some experts state that decisions regarding use of thromboprophylaxis and selection of an appropriate thromboprophylaxis regimen (e.g., aspirin, anticoagulant) should be based on careful assessment of the patient's risk factors for thromboembolism. (See Cautions: Thromboembolic Events, in Thalidomide 92:20.)

Sensitivity Reactions **Hypersensitivity Reactions.** Patients who have had serious hypersensitivity reactions to thalidomide or lenalidomide may be at increased risk for hypersensitivity reactions to pomalidomide; such patients were excluded from the pivotal multiple myeloma trial.

Other Warnings and Precautions **Hematologic Effects.** In the pivotal multiple myeloma trial, grade 3 or 4 neutropenia, anemia, or thrombocytopenia was reported in 43, 21, or 21%, respectively, of patients receiving pomalidomide alone or in combination with low-dose dexamethasone; febrile neutropenia was reported in 3% of patients.

Complete blood cell counts (CBCs) should be monitored weekly for the first 8 weeks of therapy and monthly thereafter. If hematologic toxicity occurs, dosage interruption and/or reduction may be required. (See Hematologic Toxicity under Dosage: Dosage Modification for Toxicity, in Dosage and Administration.)

Nervous System Effects. In the pivotal multiple myeloma trial, dizziness or confusion occurred in 18 or 12%, respectively, of patients receiving pomalidomide alone or in combination with dexamethasone; grade 3 or 4 dizziness occurred in 1% of patients, and grade 3 or 4 confusion occurred in 3% of patients. (See Advice to Patients.) Neuropathy was reported in 18% of patients, and peripheral neuropathy was reported in 9% of patients.

Development of Second Primary Malignancy. Acute myelogenous leukemia (AML) has been reported in patients receiving pomalidomide as investigational therapy for uses other than multiple myeloma.

Specific Populations **Pregnancy.** Category X. (See Restricted Distribution Program under Dosage and Administration: General and also see Fetal/Neonatal Morbidity and Mortality under Warnings/Precautions: Warnings, in Cautions.)

Lactation. Pomalidomide is distributed into milk in rats; it is not known whether pomalidomide is distributed into milk in humans. Because of the potential for serious adverse reactions to pomalidomide in nursing infants, a decision should be made whether to discontinue nursing or the drug, taking into account the importance of the drug to the woman.

Pediatric Use. Safety and efficacy of pomalidomide have not been established in pediatric patients younger than 18 years of age.

Geriatric Use. In clinical trials evaluating pomalidomide in patients with multiple myeloma, 41% of patients were 65 years of age or older and 12% were 75 years of age or older. Although no overall differences in efficacy were observed between geriatric and younger patients, pneumonia occurred more frequently in patients 65 years of age or older compared with younger patients. (See Dosage and Administration: Special Populations.)

Hepatic Impairment. Pomalidomide has not been studied in patients with hepatic impairment; however, the drug is extensively metabolized in the liver. (See Dosage and Administration: Special Populations.)

Renal Impairment. Pomalidomide has not been studied in patients with renal impairment; however, about 73% of a radiolabeled dose of the drug is excreted by the kidneys, mainly as metabolites. (See Dosage and Administration: Special Populations.)

■ Common Adverse Effects Adverse effects occurring in more than 20% of patients receiving pomalidomide with or without low-dose dexamethasone include fatigue, asthenia, pyrexia, peripheral edema, neutropenia, anemia, thrombocytopenia, constipation, diarrhea, nausea, pneumonia, upper respiratory tract infection, back pain, musculoskeletal chest pain, dyspnea, cough, decreased appetite, hypercalcemia, rash, and dizziness.

Drug Interactions

No formal drug interaction studies have been performed to date.

■ Drugs Affecting or Metabolized by Hepatic Microsomal Enzymes Metabolism of pomalidomide is mediated primarily by cytochrome P-450 (CYP) isoenzymes 1A2 and 3A4. Concomitant use of pomalidomide with potent inhibitors of CYP1A2 or CYP3A (e.g., ketoconazole) may increase exposure to pomalidomide and should be avoided. Conversely, concomitant use of pomalidomide with potent inducers of CYP1A2 (e.g., cigarette smoking) or CYP3A (e.g., rifampin) may decrease exposure to pomalidomide and also should be avoided. When the weak CYP3A inducer dexamethasone (20–40 mg once daily) was administered concomitantly with pomalidomide (4 mg once daily) in patients with multiple myeloma, pharmacokinetics of pomalidomide were unchanged.

Pomalidomide does not inhibit or induce CYP isoenzymes in vitro.

■ Drugs Affecting Efflux Transport Systems Pomalidomide is a substrate of the efflux transporter P-glycoprotein (P-gp); potent inhibitors or inducers of this transport protein may potentially alter pomalidomide exposure. Concomitant use of pomalidomide with potent inhibitors or inducers of P-gp should be avoided.

Pomalidomide does not inhibit or induce transporters in vitro.

Description

Pomalidomide, a thalidomide analog, is an immunomodulatory agent with antineoplastic and antiangiogenic activity. The drug has been shown to inhibit production of proinflammatory cytokines (e.g., tumor necrosis factor [TNF; TNF-α], interleukin-6) and increase cytolytic T-cell and natural killer (NK) cell responses. Pomalidomide has been shown to inhibit the growth of hematopoietic tumor cells, including lenalidomide-resistant multiple myeloma cell lines, by inducing apoptosis. The drug has shown synergistic antitumor effects when combined with dexamethasone in lenalidomide-sensitive and lenalidomide-resistant cell lines. Pomalidomide has been shown to inhibit angiogenesis in vitro and in mice bearing tumor xenografts.

Pomalidomide is extensively metabolized in the liver, principally by cytochrome P-450 (CYP) isoenzymes 1A2 and 3A4, with minor contributions from CYP isoenzymes 2C19 and 2D6. Following multiple-dose oral administration (2 mg once daily for 4 days) in healthy men, pomalidomide concentrations in semen were approximately 67% of plasma concentrations at 4 hours after a dose (near-peak plasma concentrations). (See Fetal/Neonatal Morbidity and Mortality under Warnings/Precautions: Warnings, in Cautions.) The median terminal half-life of pomalidomide in patients with multiple myeloma is 7.5 hours. Following oral administration of a single 2-mg dose of radiolabeled pomalidomide, approximately 73% of the dose was recovered in urine and 15% was recovered in feces; unchanged drug accounted for only 2% of the dose recovered in urine and 8% of the dose recovered in feces.

Advice to Patients

Importance of educating patients regarding the Pomalyst Risk Evaluation and Mitigation Strategy (REMS)® restricted distribution program for obtaining pomalidomide. (See REMS and also see Restricted Distribution Program under Dosage and Administration: General.)

Importance of advising patients to swallow capsules intact and not to break, chew, or open capsules.

Importance of advising patients that a missed dose may be taken up to 12 hours after the scheduled administration time; if more than 12 hours have elapsed, the missed dose should be omitted and the regular dosing schedule resumed the following day. Importance of not taking 2 doses at the same time to make up for a missed dose.

Risk of fetal harm. Necessity of advising women of childbearing potential to use effective methods of contraception beginning 4 weeks prior to initiation of therapy, throughout therapy, during dosage interruptions, and for at least 4 weeks after discontinuance of therapy (see Fetal/Neonatal Morbidity and Mortality under Warnings/Precautions: Warnings, in Cautions); importance of obtaining pregnancy tests at appropriate intervals during therapy and of immediately discontinuing therapy and contacting their clinician if pregnancy is suspected. Necessity of advising men (including those who have successfully undergone vasectomy) to use a latex or synthetic condom during sexual encounters with women of childbearing potential; these contraceptive measures are required during and for at least 28 days after discontinuance of pomalidomide therapy. Availability of information on emergency contraception at 888-668-2528.

Importance of advising women to avoid breast-feeding while receiving pomalidomide therapy.

Importance of advising men to avoid donating semen while receiving pomalidomide and for 4 weeks after discontinuing therapy with the drug.

Importance of advising patients to avoid donating blood while receiving pomalidomide and for 1 month after discontinuing therapy with the drug.

Risk of neutropenia, thrombocytopenia, and anemia. Importance of regular monitoring of blood cell counts during pomalidomide therapy. Importance of informing clinician if signs and symptoms of neutropenia, thrombocytopenia, or anemia occur.

Risk of severe hypersensitivity reactions in patients who have had hypersensitivity reactions to thalidomide or lenalidomide.

Risk of venous thromboembolic events; importance of advising patients to seek medical care if shortness of breath, chest pain, or swelling of the arms or legs occurs.

Risk of dizziness or confusion; importance of avoiding activities where dizziness or confusion could cause serious harm to self or others. Importance of not taking other drugs that may cause dizziness or confusion without consulting their clinician.

Risk of neuropathy. Importance of informing clinician if signs and symptoms of neuropathy occur.

Possible risk of developing a second primary malignancy (i.e., acute myelogenous leukemia [AML]).

Importance of not smoking during pomalidomide therapy, since smoking may reduce the drug's efficacy.

Importance of informing clinicians of existing or contemplated concomitant therapy, including prescription and OTC drugs and dietary or herbal supplements, as well as any concomitant illnesses.

Importance of informing patients of other important precautionary information. (See Cautions.)

Overview® (see Users Guide). For additional information on this drug until a more detailed monograph is developed and published, the manufacturer's labeling should be consulted. It is *essential* that the manufacturer's labeling be consulted for more detailed information on usual cautions, precautions, contraindications, potential drug interactions, laboratory test interferences, and acute toxicity. For further information on the handling of antineoplastic agents, see the ASHP Guidelines on Handling Hazardous Drugs at http://www.ahfsdruginformation.com.

Preparations

Because pomalidomide is an analog of thalidomide (a known human teratogen that can cause severe, life-threatening birth defects), distribution of pomalidomide is restricted. (See REMS and also see Restricted Distribution Program under Dosage and Administration: General.)

Excipients in commercially available drug preparations may have clinically important effects in some individuals; consult specific product labeling for details.

Pomalidomide

Oral		
Capsules	1 mg	**Pomalyst®**, Celgene
	2 mg	**Pomalyst®**, Celgene
	3 mg	**Pomalyst®**, Celgene
	4 mg	**Pomalyst®**, Celgene

Selected Revisions April 2016,

PRALAtrexate PDX

■ Pralatrexate, a folic acid antagonist, is an antineoplastic agent.

Uses

■ **Peripheral T-cell Lymphoma** Pralatrexate is used for the treatment of relapsed or refractory peripheral T-cell lymphoma (PTCL) and is designated an orphan drug by the US Food and Drug Administration (FDA) for use in this condition. The current indication for pralatrexate is based on overall response rate; clinical benefit (e.g., improvement in progression-free or overall survival) has not been established.

The current indication for pralatrexate is based principally on the results of a phase 2, open-label, single-arm, multicenter study (PROPEL) in 109 evaluable patients 21–85 years of age (median age: 59 years) with relapsed or refractory peripheral T-cell lymphoma who had received at least one prior treatment. Patients enrolled in this study had received a median of 3 prior treatments; 63% of patients did not have evidence of response to their most recent treatment prior to study entry, and 24% of patients did not have evidence of response to any previous treatments. In this study, patients received pralatrexate (30 mg/m² administered by rapid IV injection over 3–5 minutes) once weekly for 6 weeks, followed by one week of rest; this 7-week cycle was continued until disease progression or unacceptable toxicity occurred. Response and disease progression, assessed at the end of cycle 1 and then every 14 weeks thereafter, were evaluated by independent central review using the International Workshop Criteria (IWC). Treatment with pralatrexate resulted in an overall response rate (complete and partial responses) of 27%. Approximately 66% of responses occurred during the first cycle of treatment; the median time to first response was 45 days. The median duration of response reportedly was 9.4 months; however, this estimate for duration of response may not be accurate since the long interval (14 weeks) between efficacy assessments and the lack of subsequent assessments in some patients make it difficult to determine the actual time when a response or progression occurred. Because of these study limitations, durable response (response lasting at least 14 weeks and confirmed by subsequent assessments) was considered by some clinicians to be a preferred efficacy parameter over duration of response; durable response was achieved in 12% of patients receiving pralatrexate.

Dosage and Administration

■ **General** Pralatrexate should be administered under the supervision of a qualified clinician experienced in the use of antineoplastic agents. In addition, adequate diagnostic and treatment facilities must be readily available for appropriate management of complications.

All patients should be instructed to take a low dose (1–1.25 mg) of oral folic acid daily to reduce toxicity. Folic acid should be initiated 10 days prior to the first dose of pralatrexate; folic acid should be continued during the full course of therapy and for 30 days after the last dose of pralatrexate. Patients also should receive an IM injection of vitamin B_{12} (1 mg) no more than 10 weeks prior to the first dose of pralatrexate and every 8–10 weeks thereafter; injections administered subsequent to the initial dose may be given on the same day as pralatrexate.

Complete blood cell counts (CBCs) and severity of mucositis and other treatment-related toxicities (e.g., hepatotoxicity) should be assessed weekly during therapy (i.e., just prior to each dose). Prior to administering any dose of pralatrexate, mucositis should be grade 1 or lower, platelet counts should be at least 100,000/mm³ (prior to the first dose) or at least 50,000/mm³ (prior to subsequent doses), and absolute neutrophil counts (ANCs) should be at least 1000/mm³. Serum chemistry tests, including hepatic and renal function tests, should be performed before administration of the first and fourth pralatrexate doses of each treatment cycle. (See Dosage Modification for Toxicity under Dosage and Administration: Dosage.)

■ **Administration** Pralatrexate is administered undiluted by rapid IV injection over 3–5 minutes into the side port of a free-flowing IV infusion of 0.9% sodium chloride injection.

The usual precautions for handling, preparing, and administering solutions of cytotoxic drugs should be observed with pralatrexate. The manufacturer recommends use of gloves and other protective clothing when handling the drug. If pralatrexate comes in contact with skin or mucosa, affected skin areas should be washed immediately and thoroughly with soap and water and affected mucosa should be thoroughly flushed with water.

The appropriate volume of pralatrexate 20-mg/mL injection should be aseptically withdrawn into a syringe for immediate use. Pralatrexate injection should *not* be diluted. Because pralatrexate injection contains no preservatives, any unused portions should be discarded.

Pralatrexate injection should be stored in the original carton at 2–8°C and protected from light until use. When stored in the original carton at room temperature, unopened vials of pralatrexate injection are stable for 72 hours; any vials left at room temperature for longer than 72 hours should be discarded.

■ **Dosage** ***Peripheral T-cell Lymphoma*** The recommended adult dosage of pralatrexate for the treatment of relapsed or refractory peripheral T-cell lymphoma is 30 mg/m² (administered by rapid IV injection over 3–5 minutes) once weekly for 6 weeks, followed by one week of rest; this 7-week cycle should be continued until disease progression or toxicity occurs. In the phase 2, open-label, single-arm, multicenter study (PROPEL), pralatrexate was administered for a median of 70 days.

CBCs and severity of mucositis and other treatment-related toxicities (e.g., hepatotoxicity) should be assessed weekly during therapy (i.e., just prior to each dose). Prior to administering any subsequent doses of pralatrexate, mucositis should be grade 1 or lower, platelet counts should be at least 50,000/mm³, and ANCs should be at least 1000/mm³. (See Dosage Modification for Toxicity under Dosage and Administration: Dosage.)

Dosage Modification for Toxicity After the initial dose, subsequent doses of pralatrexate should be adjusted based on severity of mucositis, hematologic counts (i.e., ANCs, platelet counts), and/or presence of other treatment-related toxicities (e.g., hepatotoxicity) determined on the day of treatment. Depending on the severity of the toxicity, subsequent doses of pralatrexate may be omitted and/or reduced, or pralatrexate therapy may be discontinued permanently. (See Tables 1, 2, and 3.) The manufacturer states that omitted doses should *not* be made up at the end of the treatment cycle; in addition, dosages reduced following drug-related adverse effects should *not* be re-escalated.

Table 1. Recommended Dosage Modification for Mucositis

Mucositis Grade[a] on Day of Treatment	Recommended Action
Grade 2	Omit dose; when mucositis improves (to grade 1 or lower), resume pralatrexate at prior dose
Grade 2 recurrence	Omit dose; when mucositis improves (to grade 1 or lower), resume pralatrexate at a reduced dose of 20 mg/m²
Grade 3	Omit dose; when mucositis improves (to grade 1 or lower), resume pralatrexate at a reduced dose of 20 mg/m²
Grade 4	Discontinue pralatrexate permanently

[a] Per National Cancer Institute (NCI) Common Terminology Criteria for Adverse Events (NCI CTCAE version 3.0).

Table 2. Recommended Dosage Modification for Hematologic Toxicity

Blood Count on Day of Treatment	Duration of Toxicity	Recommended Action
Platelet count <50,000/mm³	1 week	Omit dose; when platelet count ≥50,000/mm³, resume pralatrexate at prior dose
	2 weeks	Omit dose; when platelet count ≥50,000/mm³, resume pralatrexate at a reduced dose of 20 mg/m²
	3 weeks	Discontinue pralatrexate permanently

ANC of 500–1000/mm³ without fever	1 week	Omit dose; when ANC ≥1000/mm³, resume pralatrexate at prior dose
ANC of 500–1000/mm³ with fever or ANC <500/mm³	1 week	Omit dose; initiate growth factor (e.g., filgrastim, sargramostim) support; when ANC ≥1000/mm³, resume pralatrexate at prior dose and continue growth factor support
	2 weeks or recurrence	Omit dose; initiate growth factor (e.g., filgrastim, sargramostim) support; when ANC ≥1000/mm³, resume treatment at a reduced dose of 20 mg/m² and continue growth factor support
	3 weeks or second recurrence	Discontinue pralatrexate permanently

Table 3. Recommended Dosage Modification for Other Treatment-related Toxicities (e.g., Hepatotoxicity)

Toxicity Grade[b] on Day of Treatment	Recommended Action
Grade 3	Omit dose; when toxicity improves (to grade 2 or lower), resume pralatrexate at a reduced dose of 20 mg/m²
Grade 4	Discontinue pralatrexate permanently

[b] Per National Cancer Institute (NCI) Common Terminology Criteria for Adverse Events (NCI CTCAE version 3.0).

■ **Special Populations** Dosage reductions other than those recommended for all patients are not needed in geriatric patients (65 years of age and older) who have normal renal function.

Cautions

■ **Contraindications** The manufacturer states that there are no known contraindications to the use of pralatrexate.

■ **Warnings/Precautions** ***Hematologic Toxicity*** The principal manifestations of hematologic toxicity include thrombocytopenia, anemia, and neutropenia. In the phase 2, open-label, single-arm, multicenter study (PROPEL), thrombocytopenia, anemia, and neutropenia were reported in 41, 34, and 24%, respectively, of patients receiving pralatrexate. Dosage of pralatrexate should be adjusted based on the absolute neutrophil count (ANC) and platelet count just prior to each dose (i.e., determined on day of treatment). (See Dosage Modification for Toxicity under Dosage and Administration: Dosage.)

Mucositis Mucositis (i.e., stomatitis or mucosal inflammation of the GI and genitourinary tracts) was reported in 70% of patients receiving pralatrexate in the PROPEL study. Mucositis typically occurs within 2–5 days after initiation of pralatrexate. In the PROPEL study, grade 3 or 4 mucositis occurred in 17 or 4% of patients, respectively, with a median time to onset of 15 days and a median duration of 13 days.

In several analyses of patients receiving pralatrexate, the severity of mucositis appeared to be related to higher baseline concentrations of methylmalonic acid (MMA, a marker of vitamin B deficiency) or higher systemic exposure (i.e., area under the plasma concentration-time curve [AUC]) to pralatrexate. Mucositis also appeared to occur somewhat more frequently in geriatric patients (65 years of age and older) than in younger adults.

To reduce pralatrexate-induced mucositis, the manufacturer recommends supplementation with folic acid and vitamin B_{12} before and during therapy with pralatrexate. (See Dosage and Administration: General.) The manufacturer and the National Comprehensive Cancer Network (NCCN) also recommend other strategies to prevent oral mucositis, including maintaining fluid and protein intake, establishing an effective oral hygiene protocol, using topical therapies (e.g., oral cryotherapy when feasible), and avoiding irritants (e.g., alcohol or alcohol-containing medications, tobacco, specific foods).

If mucositis occurs during pralatrexate therapy, pain may be relieved by altering eating and drinking habits, using topical anesthetics (e.g., "magic mouthwash"), and/or using systemic (e.g., opiate) analgesics. The manufacturer's labeling and/or published guidelines should be consulted for specific recommendations on the management of mucositis. If mucositis is grade 2 or higher, subsequent doses of pralatrexate should be omitted and/or reduced, or pralatrexate therapy discontinued permanently. (See Dosage Modification for Toxicity under Dosage and Administration: Dosage.)

Folate and Vitamin B_{12} Supplementation Patients must receive folic acid and vitamin B_{12} to prevent treatment-related hematologic and GI toxicity (i.e., mucositis). (See Dosage and Administration: General.) Administration of supplemental folic acid and vitamin B_{12} has been shown to normalize MMA concentrations and reduce the severity of GI toxicity.

Fetal/Neonatal Morbidity and Mortality Pralatrexate may cause fetal harm; embryotoxicity, fetotoxicity, and fetal lethality have been demonstrated in animals. Pregnancy should be avoided during therapy. If used during pregnancy or if the patient becomes pregnant while receiving pralatrexate, the patient should be apprised of the potential fetal hazard.

Hepatotoxicity Elevations in serum aminotransferase (transaminase) concentrations (i.e., AST [SGOT], ALT [SGPT]) have been reported with pralatrexate. Persistent abnormalities in liver function test results may indicate hepatotoxicity. Liver function tests should be performed before administration of the first and fourth pralatrexate doses of each treatment cycle. If hepatotoxicity is grade 3 or higher, subsequent doses of pralatrexate should be omitted and/or reduced, or pralatrexate therapy discontinued permanently. (See Table 3.)

Adequate Patient Evaluation and Monitoring Pralatrexate should be administered under the supervision of qualified clinicians experienced in the use of cytotoxic therapy.

Complete blood cell counts (CBCs), including platelet counts and ANCs, should be obtained prior to initiation of pralatrexate therapy and monitored weekly during therapy (i.e., just prior to each dose). Severity of mucositis should be assessed prior to each scheduled dose of pralatrexate. In addition, serum chemistry tests, including hepatic and renal function tests, should be performed before administration of the first and fourth pralatrexate doses of each treatment cycle.

Specific Populations **Pregnancy.** Category D. (See Users Guide.) (See Fetal/Neonatal Morbidity and Mortality under Cautions: Warnings/Precautions.)

Lactation. It is not known whether pralatrexate is distributed into human milk. Because of the potential for serious adverse reactions to pralatrexate in nursing infants, a decision should be made whether to discontinue nursing or the drug, taking into account the importance of the drug to the woman.

Pediatric Use. Safety and efficacy of pralatrexate have not been established in pediatric patients.

Geriatric Use. In the PROPEL study, 36% of patients were 65 years of age and older. Although no overall differences in safety and efficacy were observed in geriatric patients, some data indicate that geriatric patients (65 years of age and older) may be at increased risk of developing mucositis compared with younger adults. (See Mucositis under Cautions: Warnings/Precautions.) While the manufacturer states that no dosage adjustment is required in geriatric patients with normal renal function, it should be noted that age-related decline in renal function may result in reduced clearance of and increased exposure to pralatrexate.

Hepatic Impairment. Safety and efficacy of pralatrexate have not been established in patients with hepatic impairment. Patients were excluded from the pralatrexate lymphoma clinical trials if their total bilirubin concentrations exceeded 1.5 mg/dL and their AST (SGOT) or ALT (SGPT) concentrations were more than 2.5 times the upper limit of normal (or more than 5 times the upper limit of normal if there was documented hepatic involvement with the lymphoma).

Renal Impairment. Safety and efficacy of pralatrexate have not been established in patients with renal impairment; however, data from a population pharmacokinetic analysis indicate that drug clearance decreases with declining creatinine clearance. Pralatrexate should be used with caution in patients with moderate or severe renal impairment.

■ **Common Adverse Effects** The most common adverse effects of pralatrexate include mucositis, thrombocytopenia, nausea, and fatigue. Other common adverse effects reported in more than 20% of patients include anemia, constipation, pyrexia, edema, cough, epistaxis, vomiting, neutropenia, and diarrhea. The most common *serious* adverse effects of pralatrexate include pyrexia, mucositis, sepsis, febrile neutropenia, dehydration, dyspnea, and thrombocytopenia.

Drug Interactions

No formal drug interaction studies have been performed to date.

In vitro studies indicate that pralatrexate is not a substrate, inhibitor, or inducer of cytochrome P-450 (CYP) isoenzymes. Pralatrexate also is not a substrate or inhibitor of the P-glycoprotein transport system.

■ **Drugs Affecting or Metabolized by Hepatic Microsomal Enzymes** Pharmacokinetic interaction unlikely with drugs affecting or metabolized by CYP isoenzymes.

■ **Drugs Eliminated by Renal Excretion** Possible pharmacokinetic interaction (delayed clearance of pralatrexate) with drugs that undergo substantial renal excretion (e.g., co-trimoxazole, nonsteroidal anti-inflammatory agents [NSAIAs]).

■ **Probenecid** Pharmacokinetic interaction (delayed clearance of and increased exposure to pralatrexate).

Description

Pralatrexate, a 10-deazaaminopterin analog of methotrexate, is an antineoplastic agent. Pralatrexate differs structurally from methotrexate in that pralatrexate contains a carbon with a propargyl side chain instead of a nitrogen with a methyl side chain in the 10-position. This structural modification allows pralatrexate to selectively and efficiently enter cells expressing reduced-folate carrier type 1 (RFC-1), a protein that is overexpressed on fetal and certain cancer cell types (including some T-cell lymphomas). In addition, the modified structure also allows pralatrexate to undergo enhanced intracellular polyglutamylation by the enzyme folylpolyglutamate synthetase (FPGS), resulting in enhanced retention and accumulation of the drug inside the cells; polyglutamylation is a time- and concentration-dependent process that occurs in tumor cells and, to a lesser extent, in normal tissues. Like methotrexate, polyglutamylated pralatrexate exerts its antineoplastic activity by disrupting folate-dependent metabolic processes that are essential for cell replication. Specifically, pralatrexate inhibits dihydrofolate reductase (DHFR), an enzyme involved in the synthesis of deoxythymidine and purine nucleotides. Reduction in the pool of available nucleotides, primarily thymine and to a lesser extent adenine and guanine, interrupts DNA synthesis and induces S-phase arrest, resulting in cytostasis and apoptosis (programmed cell death).

In preclinical studies, pralatrexate demonstrated greater affinity for RFC-1 (resulting in enhanced intracellular transport), enhanced polyglutamylation (resulting in increased intracellular drug retention and accumulation), and improved cytotoxicity compared with other folic acid antagonists (e.g., methotrexate, pemetrexed). Down-regulation and/or inhibition of effective RFC-1 transport and/or polyglutamylation have been proposed as possible mechanisms of resistance to methotrexate and other folic acid antagonists.

Following rapid IV injection of pralatrexate (30 mg/m^2 over 3–5 minutes) once weekly for 6 weeks in 7-week cycles, peak plasma concentration and area under the plasma concentration-time curve (AUC) of the drug increased proportionally with dose. In vitro studies indicate that pralatrexate is approximately 67% bound to plasma proteins. Following multiple treatment cycles, no accumulation of pralatrexate was observed. Pralatrexate is not substantially metabolized by phase I hepatic cytochrome P-450 (CYP) isoenzymes or phase II hepatic glucuronidases; the drug has low potential to induce or inhibit the activity of CYP isoenzymes. In vitro studies indicate that pralatrexate is not a substrate or inhibitor of the P-glycoprotein transport system. The terminal elimination half-life of pralatrexate is 12–18 hours. Following a single rapid IV injection of pralatrexate (30 mg/m^2 over 3–5 minutes), approximately 34% of pralatrexate is excreted unchanged in urine. Because of the contribution of renal excretion to overall clearance of pralatrexate, age-related decline in renal function may lead to a reduction in clearance of and corresponding increase in plasma exposure to the drug. In a population pharmacokinetic analysis, drug clearance decreased with decreasing creatinine clearance. There was no substantial effect of gender on pharmacokinetics of pralatrexate.

Advice to Patients

Importance of taking folic acid and vitamin B_{12} to reduce the risk of adverse effects.

Risk of mucositis. Importance of immediately informing clinicians of redness and/or soreness in the mucous membranes, including the mouth, lips, throat, and other areas along the GI tract and genital areas. Importance of understanding measures to prevent mucositis and to minimize discomfort should it occur. (See Mucositis under Cautions: Warnings/Precautions.)

Risk of thrombocytopenia, anemia, and neutropenia. Importance of reporting any unusual bleeding (e.g., nosebleed), bruising, weakness, fatigue, pallor, shortness of breath, or fever or other manifestations of infection (e.g., chills, cough, pain or burning upon urination).

Necessity of obtaining complete blood cell counts (CBCs) as well as renal and liver function tests periodically.

Importance of women informing clinicians if they are or plan to become pregnant or plan to breast-feed. Apprise patient of potential hazard to the fetus if used during pregnancy; women of childbearing potential should avoid becoming pregnant.

Importance of informing clinicians of existing or contemplated concomitant therapy, including prescription (e.g., co-trimoxazole, probenecid) and OTC drugs (e.g., nonsteroidal anti-inflammatory agents [NSAIAs]), as well as any concomitant illnesses.

Importance of informing patients of other important precautionary information. (See Cautions.)

Overview® (see Users Guide). For additional information on this drug until a more detailed monograph is developed and published, the manufacturer's labeling should be consulted. It is *essential* that the manufacturer's labeling be consulted for more detailed information on usual cautions, precautions, contraindications, potential drug interactions, laboratory test interferences, and acute toxicity.

Preparations

Excipients in commercially available drug preparations may have clinically important effects in some individuals; consult specific product labeling for details.

PRALAtrexate

Parenteral

Injection, for IV use only	20 mg/mL	**Folotyn®** (available in single-dose vials), Allos

Ramucirumab

■ Ramucirumab, a recombinant human IgG_1 monoclonal antibody, is a vascular endothelial growth factor receptor (VEGFR)-2 antagonist.

Uses

■ **Gastric Cancer** Ramucirumab is used alone or in combination with paclitaxel for the treatment of advanced or metastatic gastric adenocarcinoma, including adenocarcinoma of the gastroesophageal junction, that has progressed during or following fluoropyrimidine- or platinum-based chemotherapy; ramucirumab is designated an orphan drug by FDA for the treatment of this cancer.

The current indication for ramucirumab in the treatment of gastric cancer is based principally on the results of 2 randomized, double-blind, placebo-controlled phase 3 studies (REGARD and RAINBOW) in patients with locally advanced or metastatic gastric adenocarcinoma, including adenocarcinoma of the gastroesophageal junction, who had received platinum- and/or fluoropyrimidine-containing regimens. In both studies, the primary measure of efficacy was overall survival.

In the REGARD study, 355 patients were randomized in a 2:1 ratio to receive either ramucirumab (8 mg/kg by IV infusion) or placebo every 2 weeks; all patients received best supportive care. Treatment was continued until disease progression, unacceptable toxicity, or death occurred. The median age of patients was 60 years; all except one of the enrolled patients had a baseline ECOG performance status of 0 or 1. Most patients (81%) enrolled in the study had received prior combined chemotherapy with a platinum compound and a fluoropyrimidine; 15% of patients had received fluoropyrimidine-containing regimens without a platinum compound, and 4% had received platinum-containing regimens without a fluoropyrimidine. At the time of the primary analysis, patients receiving ramucirumab had longer median overall survival (5.2 versus 3.8 months) and progression-free survival (2.1 versus 1.3 months) compared with patients receiving placebo. Results of an exploratory subgroup analysis (based on age, gender, race, and geographic region) suggested a lack of an overall survival benefit in women; patients in North America, Europe, Australia, and New Zealand; and patients categorized as "other" race.

In the RAINBOW study, 665 patients were randomized in a 1:1 ratio to receive either ramucirumab (8 mg/kg by IV infusion over 1 hour on days 1 and 15 of each 28-day cycle) in combination with paclitaxel (80 mg/m^2 by IV infusion over 1 hour on days 1, 8, and 15 of each 28-day cycle) or placebo in combination with paclitaxel. The median age of patients was 61 years; all patients enrolled in the study had a baseline ECOG performance status of 0 or 1. Most patients (81%) enrolled in the study had received prior combined chemotherapy with a platinum compound and a fluoropyrimidine; 15% of patients had received fluoropyrimidine-containing chemotherapy without a platinum compound, and 4% had received platinum-containing regimens without a fluoropyrimidine. Final analysis of overall survival, using derived data, indicated that patients receiving ramucirumab in combination with paclitaxel had longer median overall survival (9.6 versus 7.4 months) and median progression-free survival (4.4 versus 2.9 months) compared with patients receiving placebo in combination with paclitaxel. The objective response rate (complete and partial responses) was 28% for patients receiving ramucirumab in combination with paclitaxel compared with 16% for those receiving placebo in combination with paclitaxel. Data from this study indicate that effects of ramucirumab on survival were consistent across various patient subgroups (including women and patients in Europe, North America, and Australia) and support the hypothesis that results of the exploratory subgroup analysis of the REGARD study were likely limited by small sample size and random effects.

■ **Non-small Cell Lung Cancer** Ramucirumab is used in combination with docetaxel for the treatment of metastatic non-small cell lung cancer (NSCLC) that has progressed during or following platinum-based chemotherapy. Patients with epidermal growth factor receptor (EGFR)- or anaplastic lymphoma kinase (ALK)-positive tumors also should have documented disease progression during or following an FDA-labeled anti-EGFR or anti-ALK therapy prior to initiating therapy with ramucirumab.

The current indication for ramucirumab in the treatment of metastatic NSCLC is based principally on the results of a randomized, double-blind, placebo-controlled phase 3 study (REVEL) in patients with locally advanced or metastatic NSCLC that had progressed during or following platinum-based chemotherapy. The primary measure of efficacy was overall survival. In this study, 1253 patients were randomized in a 1:1 ratio to receive either ramucirumab (10 mg/kg by IV infusion on day 1 of each 21-day cycle) in combination with docetaxel (75 mg/m^2 by IV infusion on day 1 of each 21-day cycle) or placebo in combination with docetaxel; because an increased incidence of neutropenia and febrile neutropenia was noted in patients in East Asia, these patients received a reduced docetaxel dosage (60 mg/m^2 every 21 days). Treatment was continued until disease progression, death, or unacceptable toxicity occurred, or treatment was discontinued for other reasons. The median duration of treatment was 3.5 months for patients receiving ramucirumab in combination with docetaxel. The median age of patients was 62 years. All patients enrolled in the study had a baseline ECOG performance status of 0 or 1, and 73% had nonsquamous histology. The majority (99%) of patients had received previous platinum-based chemotherapy. In addition to platinum-based chemotherapy,

38% of patients also had received pemetrexed; 25% had received gemcitabine; 24% had received a taxane; and 14% had received bevacizumab.

Patients randomized to receive ramucirumab in combination with docetaxel had a longer median overall survival (10.5 versus 9.1 months) and progression-free survival (4.5 versus 3 months) compared with patients receiving placebo in combination with docetaxel. In addition, patients receiving ramucirumab in combination with docetaxel appeared to have a higher investigator-assessed objective response rate (complete and partial responses) (23 versus 14%) and higher disease control rate (64 versus 53%) compared with those receiving placebo in combination with docetaxel.

■ **Colorectal Cancer** Ramucirumab is used in combination with fluorouracil, leucovorin (folinic acid), and irinotecan (the combination of fluorouracil, leucovorin, and irinotecan is hereafter referred to as FOLFIRI in this monograph) for the treatment of metastatic colorectal cancer that has progressed during or following combination therapy with oxaliplatin, bevacizumab, and a fluoropyrimidine. Results of a randomized, placebo-controlled study (RAISE) demonstrated improved overall and progression-free survival with such second-line ramucirumab therapy; an increase in the frequency of certain adverse effects with ramucirumab therapy generally was manageable with appropriate dosage adjustments and supportive therapy.

In the RAISE study, 1072 patients were randomly assigned to receive either ramucirumab 8 mg/kg by IV infusion over 1 hour or placebo in combination with FOLFIRI. The FOLFIRI regimen consisted of irinotecan 180 mg/m^2 by IV infusion over 90 minutes concurrent with (or followed by) leucovorin 400 mg/m^2 by IV infusion over 2 hours, followed by fluorouracil 400 mg/m^2 by IV injection over 2–4 minutes, then fluorouracil 2.4 g/m^2 by IV infusion over 46–48 hours. Treatment was repeated every 2 weeks and continued until radiographically confirmed disease progression or unacceptable toxicity occurred; if one or more components of treatment were discontinued for toxicity, patients were permitted to continue therapy with the remaining treatment component(s) until disease progression or unacceptable toxicity occurred. The median duration of treatment was 4.4 months for patients receiving ramucirumab in combination with FOLFIRI. The median age of patients was 62 years; 76% of patients were white, 49% had a baseline ECOG performance status of 0, 49% had *KRAS* mutations, and 24% had experienced disease progression within less than 6 months after beginning first-line therapy.

Patients receiving the ramucirumab-FOLFIRI regimen had a longer median overall survival (13.3 versus 11.7 months) and a longer progression-free survival (5.7 versus 4.5 months) than patients receiving the placebo-FOLFIRI regimen. In addition, results of a subgroup analysis (based on age, disease stage, ECOG performance status, *KRAS* mutation status, time to disease progression, number of metastatic sites, presence of metastasis only in the liver, site of primary tumor, and baseline carcinoembryonic antigen [CEA] concentration) suggested that the drug's effect on overall and progression-free survival was consistent across all subgroups. Ramucirumab therapy was associated with a higher incidence of grade 3 or worse treatment-emergent adverse effects (e.g., neutropenia, hypertension). (See Cautions.)

Dosage and Administration

■ **General** Ramucirumab should be administered only in settings where adequate monitoring can be performed and appropriate medical support is available for management of potential infusion-related reactions. (See Infusion-related Effects under Warnings/Precautions: Other Warnings and Precautions, in Cautions.)

To minimize the risk of infusion-related reactions associated with ramucirumab, premedication with an antihistamine (e.g., IV diphenhydramine hydrochloride) is recommended prior to each infusion. Patients who have experienced a grade 1 or 2 infusion-related reaction also should receive dexamethasone (or equivalent) and acetaminophen prior to subsequent infusions.

Ramucirumab can only be obtained through a limited network of specialty pharmacies. Clinicians may contact the manufacturer (Eli Lilly) by telephone at 800-545-5979 or consult the Cyramza® website for specific ordering and availability information (http://www.cyramzahcp.com).

■ **Administration** Ramucirumab is administered by IV infusion over 1 hour. *The drug should not be administered by rapid IV injection, such as IV "push" or "bolus."*

Ramucirumab injection concentrate *must* be diluted prior to administration.

Diluted ramucirumab solution should be inspected visually for particulate matter and discoloration prior to administration; if particulate matter or discoloration is evident, the diluted solution should be discarded.

Diluted ramucirumab solution should be administered using an infusion pump. The manufacturer recommends administering the drug through a low-protein-binding 0.22-μm inline filter. Diluted ramucirumab solution should *not* be administered in the same IV line with any other drug or electrolyte solution. The IV line should be flushed with 0.9% sodium chloride injection at the end of the infusion.

Unopened vials of ramucirumab injection concentrate should be protected from light, stored at 2–8°C, and should not be frozen or shaken.

Dilution Prior to dilution, ramucirumab injection concentrate should be inspected visually for particulate matter and discoloration; if particulate matter or discoloration is evident, the solution should be discarded.

Ramucirumab is diluted by withdrawing the appropriate dose (8 mg/kg) of ramucirumab injection concentrate from the vial labeled as containing 10 mg/mL and diluting in 0.9% sodium chloride injection to yield a final volume of 250 mL. The diluted ramucirumab solution for infusion should be mixed by gentle inversion and should *not* be shaken. Ramucirumab injection concentrate should *not* be diluted in diluents containing dextrose. Ramucirumab should *not* be admixed with any other drug or electrolytes. Commercially available ramucirumab injection concentrate contains no preservatives and is intended for single use; any partially used vials should be discarded.

Diluted ramucirumab solution may be stored at room temperature (below 25°C) for up to 4 hours or under refrigeration (2–8°C) for up to 24 hours; the diluted solution should not be frozen.

■ **Dosage** ***Gastric Cancer*** For the treatment of advanced or metastatic gastric adenocarcinoma, including adenocarcinoma of the gastroesophageal junction, that has progressed during or following fluoropyrimidine- or platinum-based chemotherapy, the recommended adult dosage of ramucirumab (as a single agent or in combination with paclitaxel) is 8 mg/kg administered by IV infusion every 2 weeks.

When used in combination with paclitaxel, ramucirumab should be administered before administration of paclitaxel. In the RAINBOW study, patients received ramucirumab (8 mg/kg by IV infusion over 1 hour) on days 1 and 15 of each 28-day cycle and paclitaxel (80 mg/m^2 by IV infusion over 1 hour) on days 1, 8, and 15 of each 28-day cycle.

Treatment with ramucirumab should be continued until disease progression or unacceptable toxicity occurs. In the REGARD study in which ramucirumab was used as a single agent, patients received a median of 4 doses of ramucirumab. In the RAINBOW study in which ramucirumab was used in combination with paclitaxel, patients received a median of 9 doses of ramucirumab.

Non-small Cell Lung Cancer For the treatment of metastatic non-small cell lung cancer (NSCLC) that has progressed during or following platinum-based chemotherapy, the recommended adult dosage of ramucirumab is 10 mg/kg administered by IV infusion every 3 weeks in combination with docetaxel.

Ramucirumab should be administered before administration of docetaxel.

Treatment with ramucirumab should be continued until disease progression or unacceptable toxicity occurs. In the REVEL study, patients received a median of 4.5 doses of ramucirumab.

Colorectal Cancer For the treatment of metastatic colorectal cancer that has progressed during or following combination therapy with oxaliplatin, bevacizumab, and a fluoropyrimidine, the recommended dosage of ramucirumab in adults is 8 mg/kg administered by IV infusion every 2 weeks in combination with FOLFIRI (i.e., fluorouracil, leucovorin [folinic acid], and irinotecan).

Ramucirumab should be administered before FOLFIRI.

Treatment with ramucirumab should be continued until disease progression or unacceptable toxicity occurs. In the RAISE study, patients received a median of 8 doses of ramucirumab over a median of 4.4 months.

Dosage Modification for Toxicity If toxicities occur, temporary or permanent discontinuance of ramucirumab may be required based on causality.

Ramucirumab should be *permanently discontinued* in patients who develop severe (grade 3 or 4) bleeding, arterial thromboembolic events, clinically important hypertension that is not controlled with antihypertensive therapy, hypertensive crisis, hypertensive encephalopathy, grade 3 or 4 infusion-related effects, GI perforation, nephrotic syndrome, proteinuria exceeding 3 g per 24 hours, or reversible posterior leukoencephalopathy syndrome (RPLS). (See Cautions: Warnings/Precautions.)

Ramucirumab therapy should be *temporarily suspended* prior to surgery or if wound healing complications develop during therapy. Therapy also should be temporarily interrupted in patients who develop severe hypertension or proteinuria. (See Hypertension and also Proteinuria under Dosage: Dosage Modification for Toxicity, in Dosage and Administration.)

Infusion-related Effects. If grade 1 or 2 infusion-related reactions occur, the infusion rate should be reduced by 50%. If grade 3 or 4 infusion-related reactions occur, ramucirumab should be permanently discontinued. (See Infusion-related Effects under Warnings/Precautions: Other Warnings and Precautions, in Cautions.)

Hypertension. If severe hypertension occurs, ramucirumab therapy should be interrupted until hypertension is controlled. Ramucirumab should be permanently discontinued in patients with clinically important hypertension that is not controlled with antihypertensive therapy or in patients who develop hypertensive crisis or hypertensive encephalopathy. (See Hypertension under Warnings/Precautions: Other Warnings and Precautions, in Cautions.)

Proteinuria. Ramucirumab therapy should be interrupted for proteinuria of 2 g or more per 24 hours; when proteinuria declines below this level, ramucirumab may be resumed at a reduced dosage of 6 mg/kg every 2 weeks (in patients receiving ramucirumab for advanced or metastatic gastric adenocarcinoma or metastatic colorectal cancer) or 8 mg/kg every 3 weeks (in patients receiving ramucirumab for metastatic NSCLC). If proteinuria recurs, therapy should be withheld again; when proteinuria declines below 2 g per 24 hours, ramucirumab may then be resumed at a reduced dosage of 5 mg/kg every 2 weeks (in patients receiving ramucirumab for advanced or metastatic gastric adenocarcinoma or metastatic colorectal cancer) or 6 mg/kg every 3 weeks (in patients receiving ramucirumab for metastatic NSCLC). If nephrotic syndrome or proteinuria exceeding 3 g per 24 hours occurs, treatment with ramucirumab should be permanently discontinued. (See Proteinuria under Warnings/Precautions: Other Warnings and Precautions, in Cautions.)

■ **Special Populations** No dosage adjustment is necessary in patients with mild hepatic impairment (total bilirubin concentration within the upper limit of normal [ULN] and AST concentration exceeding the ULN, or total bilirubin concentration ranging from more than 1 to 1.5 times the ULN and any AST concentration). (See Hepatic Impairment under Warnings/Precautions: Specific Populations, in Cautions.)

No dosage adjustment is necessary in patients with renal impairment. (See Renal Impairment under Warnings/Precautions: Specific Populations, in Cautions.)

The manufacturer makes no specific dosage recommendations for geriatric patients. (See Geriatric Use under Warnings/Precautions: Specific Populations, in Cautions.)

Cautions

■ **Contraindications** The manufacturer states there are no known contraindications to the use of ramucirumab.

■ **Warnings/Precautions** ***Warnings*** **Hemorrhage.** Ramucirumab is associated with an increased risk of hemorrhage and GI hemorrhage, including severe and sometimes fatal hemorrhage.

In the REGARD study, severe bleeding was reported in 3.4% of patients receiving ramucirumab compared with 2.6% of those receiving placebo, and red blood cell transfusions were required in 11% of patients receiving ramucirumab compared with 8.7% of those receiving placebo. In the RAINBOW study, severe bleeding was reported in 4.3% of patients receiving ramucirumab in combination with paclitaxel compared with 2.4% of those receiving placebo plus paclitaxel. Patients with gastric cancer receiving nonsteroidal anti-inflammatory agents (NSAIAs) were excluded from the REGARD and RAINBOW studies; therefore, the risk of gastric hemorrhage associated with ramucirumab is unknown in such patients.

In the REVEL study, severe bleeding was reported in 2.4% of patients with metastatic non-small cell lung cancer (NSCLC) receiving ramucirumab in combination with docetaxel compared with 2.3% of those receiving placebo plus docetaxel. Pulmonary hemorrhage was reported in 7% of patients with nonsquamous histology receiving ramucirumab in combination with docetaxel compared with 6% of those receiving placebo plus docetaxel; among patients with squamous histology, pulmonary hemorrhage was reported in 10% of patients receiving ramucirumab in combination with docetaxel compared with 12% of those receiving placebo plus docetaxel. Patients with NSCLC receiving therapeutic anticoagulation, long-term therapy with NSAIAs, or antiplatelet therapy other than once-daily aspirin, and those with radiographic evidence of major airway or blood vessel invasion or intratumor cavitation, were excluded from the REVEL study; therefore, the risk of pulmonary hemorrhage associated with ramucirumab is unknown in such patients.

In the RAISE study, severe bleeding was reported in 2.5% of patients with metastatic colorectal cancer receiving ramucirumab in combination with FOLFIRI (i.e., fluorouracil, leucovorin [folinic acid], and irinotecan) compared with 1.7% of those receiving placebo plus FOLFIRI.

Ramucirumab should be permanently discontinued if severe (grade 3 or 4) hemorrhage occurs during therapy with the drug.

GI Perforation. GI perforation, potentially fatal, has been reported with antiangiogenic agents that are inhibitors of vascular endothelial growth factor receptor (VEGFR), including ramucirumab. In clinical trials, GI perforation was reported in 4 of 570 patients (0.7%) receiving ramucirumab as a single agent. In the RAINBOW study, GI perforation was reported in 1.2% of patients receiving ramucirumab in combination with paclitaxel compared with 0.3% of patients receiving placebo plus paclitaxel. In the REVEL study, GI perforation was reported in 1% of patients receiving ramucirumab in combination with docetaxel compared with 0.3% of patients receiving placebo plus docetaxel. In the RAISE study, GI perforation was reported in 1.7% of patients receiving ramucirumab in combination with FOLFIRI compared with 0.6% of those receiving placebo plus FOLFIRI.

Ramucirumab should be permanently discontinued in patients who develop GI perforation.

Impaired Wound Healing. Data are lacking on the effects of ramucirumab in patients with serious or non-healing wounds; however, inhibitors of VEGFR may impair wound healing. Ramucirumab should be discontinued in patients with impaired wound healing.

The manufacturer recommends that ramucirumab be discontinued prior to scheduled surgery. The decision to resume therapy postoperatively should be based on clinical assessment of the adequacy of wound healing. If wound healing complications develop during ramucirumab therapy, the drug should be discontinued until the wound is fully healed.

Other Warnings and Precautions **Arterial Thromboembolic Events.** Severe, sometimes fatal, arterial thromboembolic events (including myocardial infarction, cardiac arrest, cerebrovascular accident, and cerebral ischemia) have been reported in patients receiving ramucirumab. In the REGARD study, arterial thromboembolic events were reported in 1.7% of patients receiving ramucirumab compared with none of those receiving placebo.

Ramucirumab should be permanently discontinued if a severe arterial thromboembolic event occurs during therapy with the drug.

Hypertension. Ramucirumab is associated with an increased risk of severe hypertension. In the REGARD study, grade 3 or 4 hypertension was reported in 8% of patients receiving ramucirumab compared with 3% of those receiving placebo. In the RAINBOW study, grade 3 or greater hypertension was reported in 15% of patients receiving ramucirumab in combination with paclitaxel compared with 3% of those receiving placebo plus paclitaxel. In the REVEL study, grade 3 or greater hypertension was reported in 6% of patients receiving ramucirumab in combination with docetaxel compared with 2% of those receiving placebo plus docetaxel. In the RAISE study, grade 3 or greater hypertension was reported in 11% of patients receiving ramucirumab in combination with FOLFIRI compared with 3% of those receiving placebo plus FOLFIRI.

Hypertension should be controlled prior to initiating therapy with ramucirumab. Blood pressure should be monitored every 2 weeks or more frequently as clinically indicated during therapy with the drug. If severe hypertension occurs, ramucirumab therapy should be interrupted until hypertension is controlled. Ramucirumab should be permanently discontinued in patients with clinically important hypertension that is not controlled with antihypertensive therapy or in patients who develop hypertensive crisis or hypertensive encephalopathy.

Infusion-related Effects. Infusion-related reactions, sometimes severe, have been reported in patients receiving ramucirumab. In clinical studies, infusion-related reactions occurred in 16% of patients receiving ramucirumab without premedication. Infusion-related reactions generally occurred more frequently during or following the first 2 infusions. Infusion-related reactions may include bronchospasm, supraventricular tachycardia, hypotension, rigors/tremors, back pain/spasms, chest pain and/or tightness, chills, flushing, dyspnea, wheezing, hypoxia, and paresthesia.

Premedication with an antihistamine (e.g., IV diphenhydramine hydrochloride) should be administered prior to each infusion of ramucirumab. (See Dosage and Administration: General.) Patients should be monitored during infusions of the drug for manifestations of infusion-related reactions. If infusion-related reactions occur, reduction in the infusion rate or permanent discontinuance of ramucirumab may be required. (See Infusion-related Effects under Dosage: Dosage Modification for Toxicity, under Dosage and Administration.)

Hepatic Effects. New-onset or worsening encephalopathy, ascites, or hepatorenal syndrome has been reported in patients with preexisting Child-Pugh class B or C cirrhosis receiving ramucirumab as a single agent.

Reversible Posterior Leukoencephalopathy Syndrome. Reversible posterior leukoencephalopathy syndrome (RPLS) has been reported in less than 0.1% of patients receiving ramucirumab in clinical studies.

If signs or symptoms of RPLS develop, diagnosis of RPLS should be confirmed by magnetic resonance imaging (MRI), and ramucirumab therapy should be discontinued. Symptoms of RPLS may resolve or improve within days, but some patients can experience ongoing neurologic sequelae or death.

Proteinuria. Proteinuria has been reported in patients receiving ramucirumab. In the RAINBOW study, proteinuria of any grade occurred in 17% of patients receiving ramucirumab in combination with paclitaxel compared with 6% of those receiving placebo plus paclitaxel. In the RAISE study, grade 3 or greater proteinuria occurred in 3% of patients receiving ramucirumab in combination with FOLFIRI compared with 0.2% of those receiving placebo plus FOLFIRI; among these patients, nephrotic syndrome occurred in 0.6% of patients receiving ramucirumab in combination with FOLFIRI versus none of those receiving placebo plus FOLFIRI.

Urine dipstick proteinuria and/or urinary protein-to-creatinine ratio should be monitored for development or worsening of proteinuria during therapy.

Ramucirumab therapy should be interrupted in patients with urine protein levels of 2 g or more per 24 hours and resumed at a reduced dosage when proteinuria declines below this level. If urine protein levels exceed 3 g per 24 hours or if nephrotic syndrome occurs, treatment with ramucirumab should be permanently discontinued. (See Proteinuria under Dosage: Dosage Modification for Toxicity, in Dosage and Administration.)

Thyroid Dysfunction. Hypothyroidism has been reported in patients receiving ramucirumab in combination with FOLFIRI. In the RAISE study, hypothyroidism occurred in 2.6% of patients receiving ramucirumab in combination with FOLFIRI compared with 0.9% of those receiving placebo plus FOLFIRI. Among patients with normal baseline thyroid-stimulating hormone (TSH) concentrations, increases in TSH concentrations were reported in 46% of patients receiving ramucirumab in combination with FOLFIRI compared with 4% of those receiving placebo plus FOLFIRI.

Thyroid function should be monitored during ramucirumab therapy.

Fetal/Neonatal Morbidity and Mortality. There are no adequate and well-controlled studies of ramucirumab in pregnant women; however, based on its mechanism of action, ramucirumab can cause fetal harm. In animals, angiogenesis, vascular endothelial growth factors (VEGF), and vascular endothelial growth factor receptor 2 (VEGFR-2) have a critical role in female reproduction, embryofetal development, and postnatal development. Teratogenicity (i.e., poor development of cranial region, forelimbs, forebrain, heart, blood vessels) has been observed in animals following disruption of VEGF signaling.

Pregnancy should be avoided during ramucirumab therapy. Women of childbearing potential should be advised to use an effective method of contraception while receiving ramucirumab and for at least 3 months after discontinuance of therapy. Patients should be apprised of the potential hazard to the fetus if the drug is used during pregnancy.

Immunogenicity. Antibodies to ramucirumab have been detected in patients receiving the drug. In clinical studies, anti-ramucirumab antibodies were detected in 86 of 2890 patients (3%) receiving ramucirumab. Neutralizing antibodies were detected in 14 of the 86 patients who tested positive for anti-ramucirumab antibodies.

Impairment of Fertility. Results of animal studies suggest that inhibitors of VEGFR, such as ramucirumab, may impair female fertility or ability to maintain pregnancy.

Specific Populations **Pregnancy.** Based on its mechanism of action, ramucirumab may cause fetal harm if administered to pregnant women. (See Fetal/Neonatal Morbidity and Mortality under Cautions: Warnings/Precautions.)

Lactation. It is not known whether ramucirumab is distributed into human milk. Human immunoglobulin G (IgG) is distributed into milk; however, published data suggest that antibodies contained in breast milk do not enter the neonatal and infant circulation in substantial amounts. Nevertheless, because of the potential for serious adverse reactions to ramucirumab in nursing infants, the manufacturer states that nursing during ramucirumab therapy is not recommended. Data are lacking on the effects of the drug in nursing infants or on the production of milk.

Pediatric Use. Safety and efficacy of ramucirumab have not been established in pediatric patients younger than 18 years of age.

In animals, exposure to ramucirumab at concentrations 0.2 times that of human clinical exposure resulted in toxicities in bone (i.e., thickening of epiphyseal growth plates, osteochondropathy).

Geriatric Use. In the REGARD and RAINBOW studies, 36% of patients with advanced or metastatic gastric adenocarcinoma receiving ramucirumab were 65 years of age or older, and 7% were 75 years of age or older. No overall differences in safety or efficacy were observed between geriatric and younger adults.

In the REVEL study, 36% of patients with metastatic NSCLC receiving ramucirumab in combination with docetaxel were 65 years of age or older, and 7% were 75 years of age or older. In an exploratory subgroup analysis, survival benefit was not observed in patients 65 years of age or older receiving ramucirumab in combination with docetaxel (hazard ratio 1.10).

In the RAISE study, 40% of patients with metastatic colorectal cancer receiving ramucirumab in combination with FOLFIRI were 65 years of age or older, and 10% were 75 years of age or older. No overall differences in safety or efficacy were observed between geriatric and younger adults in this study.

Hepatic Impairment. In a population pharmacokinetic analysis, no clinically meaningful differences in the average steady-state concentrations of ramucirumab were observed between patients with mild (total bilirubin concentration within the upper limit of normal [ULN] and AST concentration exceeding the ULN, or total bilirubin concentration ranging from more than 1 to 1.5 times the ULN and any AST concentration) or moderate (total bilirubin concentration ranging from 1.5 to 3 times the ULN and any AST concentration) hepatic impairment and those with normal hepatic function. Formal pharmacokinetic studies have not been conducted in patients with severe (total bilirubin concentration exceeding 3 times the ULN and any AST concentration) hepatic impairment. (See Dosage and Administration: Special Populations.)

New-onset or worsening encephalopathy, ascites, or hepatorenal syndrome has been reported in patients with preexisting Child-Pugh class B or C cirrhosis receiving ramucirumab as a single agent. Ramucirumab should be used in patients with Child-Pugh class B or C cirrhosis only if the potential benefit outweighs the risk of clinical deterioration.

Renal Impairment. In a population pharmacokinetic analysis, no clinically meaningful differences in the average steady-state concentrations of ramucirumab were observed between patients with mild (creatinine clearance of 60–89 mL/minute), moderate (creatinine clearance of 30–59 mL/minute), or severe (creatinine clearance of 15–29 mL/minute) renal impairment and those with normal renal function. (See Dosage and Administration: Special Populations.)

■ **Common Adverse Effects** Adverse effects reported in 5% or more of patients with advanced or metastatic gastric adenocarcinoma receiving ramucirumab as a single agent in the REGARD study and occurring at an incidence at least 2% higher than that reported with placebo include hypertension, diarrhea, bleeding or hemorrhage, headache, proteinuria, and hyponatremia. Clinically important adverse effects reported in less than 5% of patients receiving ramucirumab as a single agent in the REGARD study include neutropenia, epistaxis, rash, anemia, intestinal obstruction, arterial thromboembolic events, GI perforation, and infusion-related reactions.

Adverse effects reported in 5% or more of patients with advanced or metastatic gastric adenocarcinoma receiving ramucirumab in combination with paclitaxel in the RAINBOW study and occurring at an incidence at least 2% higher than that reported with placebo plus paclitaxel include fatigue or asthenia, neutropenia, diarrhea, epistaxis, peripheral edema, hypertension, stomatitis, proteinuria, thrombocytopenia, hypoalbuminemia, and GI hemorrhage. Clinically important adverse effects reported in less than 5% of patients receiving ramucirumab in combination with paclitaxel in the RAINBOW study include sepsis and GI perforation.

Adverse effects reported in 5% or more of patients with metastatic NSCLC receiving ramucirumab in combination with docetaxel in the REVEL study and occurring at an incidence at least 2% higher than that reported with placebo plus docetaxel include neutropenia, fatigue or asthenia, stomatitis or mucosal inflammation, epistaxis, febrile neutropenia, peripheral edema, thrombocytopenia, increased lacrimation, hypertension, diarrhea, decreased appetite, neuropathy, leukopenia, pyrexia, myalgia, arthralgia, back pain, dysgeusia, and insomnia. Clinically important adverse effects reported in less than 5% of patients receiving ramucirumab in combination with docetaxel in the REVEL study include hyponatremia and proteinuria.

Adverse effects reported in the RAISE study in 5% or more of patients with metastatic colorectal cancer receiving ramucirumab in combination with FOLFIRI and at an incidence at least 2% higher than that reported with placebo plus FOLFIRI include diarrhea, neutropenia, fatigue, hemorrhage, decreased appetite, epistaxis, stomatitis, vomiting, constipation, abdominal pain, thrombocytopenia, hypertension, peripheral edema, mucosal inflammation, proteinuria, pyrexia, headache, decreased weight, cough, liver injury or liver failure, palmar-plantar erythrodysesthesia (hand-foot syndrome), GI hemorrhage, venous thromboembolic event, hypoalbuminemia, and infusion-related reactions. Clinically important adverse effects reported in less than 5% of patients receiving ramucirumab in combination with FOLFIRI include GI perforation.

Drug Interactions

■ **Antineoplastic Agents** ***Docetaxel*** Concomitant administration of ramucirumab (10 mg/kg) with docetaxel (75 mg/m^2) in patients with solid tumors did not substantially alter systemic exposure to ramucirumab or docetaxel.

Irinotecan Concomitant administration of ramucirumab with irinotecan in patients with solid tumors did not substantially alter systemic exposure to ramucirumab or irinotecan (including its active metabolite SN-38).

Paclitaxel Concomitant administration of ramucirumab (8 mg/kg) with paclitaxel (80 mg/m^2) in patients with solid tumors did not substantially alter systemic exposure to ramucirumab or paclitaxel.

Description

Ramucirumab, a recombinant human IgG_1 monoclonal antibody, is a vascular endothelial growth factor receptor (VEGFR)-2 antagonist. Ramucirumab binds specifically to VEGFR-2 and blocks the interaction of VEGFR-2 with its ligands (VEGF-A, VEGF-C, and VEGF-D), resulting in inhibition of VEGF-stimulated activation of both VEGFR-2 and downstream signaling pathways. The VEGFR signaling pathway plays an important role in the pathogenesis and progression of several types of tumors since it is a pivotal mediator of tumor angiogenesis; the pathway also regulates tumor growth and metastatic spread. In vitro assays have shown that binding of ramucirumab to VEGFR-2 blocks ligand-induced phosphorylation and activation of the receptor. Ramucirumab has been shown to inhibit VEGF-induced endothelial cell proliferation and migration in vitro. Ramucirumab also has been shown to inhibit angiogenesis in vivo.

Following administration of 8 mg/kg every 2 weeks in patients with advanced or metastatic gastric adenocarcinoma, the mean elimination half-life of ramucirumab was 15 days. Following administration of 10 mg/kg every 21 days in patients with metastatic non-small cell lung cancer [NSCLC]), the mean elimination half-life of ramucirumab was 23 days. Data from a population pharmacokinetic analysis indicate that age, gender, and race do not have clinically important effects on the pharmacokinetics of ramucirumab.

Advice to Patients

Risk of severe bleeding. Importance of informing clinician of any episodes or symptoms of bleeding (e.g., lightheadedness).

Risk of arterial thromboembolic events.

Risk of hypertension. Importance of receiving routine monitoring of blood pressure and informing clinician if blood pressure is elevated or if manifestations of hypertension (e.g., severe headache, lightheadedness, neurologic symptoms) occur.

Importance of informing clinician if severe diarrhea, vomiting, or severe abdominal pain occurs.

Risk of wound healing complications. Importance of informing clinician of any scheduled surgery.

Risk of fetal or neonatal toxicity and miscarriage. Necessity of advising women receiving ramucirumab to use an effective method of contraception during and for at least 3 months after the last dose of ramucirumab. Importance of immediately informing clinician if the patient becomes pregnant during therapy. If pregnancy occurs, apprise patient of potential hazard to the fetus.

Importance of discontinuing nursing while receiving ramucirumab therapy.

Importance of informing clinicians of existing or contemplated concomitant therapy, including prescription and OTC drugs and dietary or herbal supplements (e.g., nonsteroidal anti-inflammatory agents [NSAIAs]), as well as any concomitant illnesses (e.g., hypertension, hepatic disease).

Importance of informing patients of other important precautionary information. (See Cautions.)

Overview® (see Users Guide). For additional information on this drug until a more detailed monograph is developed and published, the manufacturer's labeling should be consulted. It is *essential* that the manufacturer's labeling be consulted for more detailed information on usual cautions, precautions, contraindications, potential drug interactions, laboratory test interferences, and acute toxicity. For further information on the handling of antineoplastic agents, see the ASHP Guidelines on Handling Hazardous Drugs at http://www.ahfsdruginformation.com.

Preparations

Excipients in commercially available drug preparations may have clinically important effects in some individuals; consult specific product labeling for details.

Ramucirumab (Recombinant)

Parenteral

Concentrate for injection, for IV infusion only	10 mg/mL (100 and 500 mg)	**Cyramza®**, Eli Lilly

Selected Revisions August 2017, © Copyright, April 2015, American Society of Health-System Pharmacists, Inc.

Regorafenib

■ Regorafenib, an inhibitor of multiple receptor tyrosine kinases, is an antineoplastic agent.

Uses

■ **Colorectal Cancer** Regorafenib is used for the treatment of metastatic colorectal cancer in patients who have received fluoropyrimidine-, oxaliplatin-, and irinotecan-containing regimens; a vascular endothelial growth factor inhibitor (anti-VEGF therapy); and, in those with tumors bearing the wild-type (nonmutated) *KRAS* gene, an epidermal growth factor receptor inhibitor (anti-EGFR therapy).

The current indication for regorafenib in the treatment of metastatic colorectal cancer is based principally on the results of a randomized, double-blind, placebo-controlled phase 3 study (CORRECT) in patients with previously treated metastatic colorectal cancer. The primary measure of efficacy was overall survival. The median age of patients was 61 years. Patients enrolled in the study had received a median of 3 prior therapies for their disease; all patients had received previous treatment with bevacizumab and with fluoropyrimidine-, oxaliplatin-, and irinotecan-containing regimens. With one exception, all patients with tumors bearing the wild-type *KRAS* gene had previously received panitumumab or cetuximab therapy. In this study, 760 patients were randomized in a 2:1 ratio to receive either regorafenib (160 mg orally once daily) or placebo for 3 consecutive weeks of each 4-week cycle; all patients received best supportive care. Treatment was continued until disease progression, death, or unacceptable toxicity occurred or treatment was discontinued for other reasons. The median duration of treatment was 1.7 months for patients receiving regorafenib. Results of a planned interim analysis indicated that patients receiving regorafenib had a longer median overall survival (6.4 versus 5 months; hazard ratio for death: 0.77) and longer median progression-free survival (2 versus 1.7 months) than those receiving placebo. Overall response rates were low (1 versus 0.4%, respectively) and were not substantially different between regorafenib-treated patients and placebo-treated patients, suggesting that the drug's main effect in this patient population was disease stabilization; none of the patients achieved a complete response. Subgroup analysis according to primary site of disease suggested that regorafenib had a greater effect on overall survival relative to placebo in patients with colon cancer than in those with rectal cancer (hazard ratio: 0.7 and 0.95, respectively); an overall survival benefit for the drug versus placebo was not apparent in the small subgroup of patients with primary disease involving both the colon and rectum (hazard ratio: 1.09). Subgroup analysis suggested that the drug's effect on progression-free survival was uniform across all 3 subgroups.

■ **GI Stromal Tumor** Regorafenib is used for the treatment of locally advanced, unresectable, or metastatic GI stromal tumor (GIST) in patients who previously received imatinib and sunitinib therapy; regorafenib has been designated an orphan drug by FDA for the treatment of this cancer.

The current indication for regorafenib in the treatment of GIST is based principally on the results of a randomized, double-blind, placebo-controlled phase 3 study (GRID) in patients with locally advanced, unresectable, or metastatic GIST following failure of both imatinib and sunitinib therapy. The primary measure of efficacy was progression-free survival based on radiographic evidence. The median age of patients was 60 years; all patients enrolled in the study had a baseline ECOG performance status of 0 or 1. In this study, 199 patients were randomized in a 2:1 ratio to receive either regorafenib (160 mg orally once daily) or placebo for 3 consecutive weeks of each 4-week cycle; all patients received best supportive care. Treatment cycles were continued until disease progression or unacceptable toxicity occurred or treatment was discontinued for other reasons; upon radiographic progression, patients previously randomized to receive placebo were permitted to cross over to open-label regorafenib treatment. The median duration of treatment was 5.7 months for patients receiving regorafenib. A planned interim analysis indicated that patients receiving regorafenib had longer median progression-free survival (4.8 months) compared with those receiving placebo (0.9 months). The overall response rate was 4.5% for patients receiving regorafenib and 1.5% for those receiving placebo; none of the patients achieved a complete response. Median overall survival had not been reached at the time of the interim analysis; however, no significant difference in overall survival was observed between the treatment groups.

■ **Hepatocellular Carcinoma** Regorafenib is used for the treatment of hepatocellular carcinoma in patients who previously received sorafenib therapy; regorafenib has been designated an orphan drug by FDA for the treatment of this cancer.

The current indication for regorafenib in the treatment of hepatocellular carcinoma is based principally on the results of a randomized, double-blind, placebo-controlled phase 3 study (RESORCE) in patients with Barcelona Clinic Liver Cancer (BCLC) stage B or C hepatocellular carcinoma following failure of sorafenib therapy. Patients were enrolled in the study if they were not eligible for surgical or locoregional therapies; 81% of patients enrolled in the study had macroscopic vascular invasion and/or extrahepatic disease. Patients who permanently discontinued prior therapy with sorafenib because of toxicity or who were unable to tolerate a sorafenib dosage of 400 mg once daily were excluded from the study. The median age of patients was 63 years; 98% had mild (Child-Pugh class A) hepatic impairment, 88% were male, 87% had BCLC stage C disease, 61% had received prior locoregional therapies, and 41% were Asian. All patients enrolled in the study had a baseline ECOG performance status of 0 or 1. Chronic hepatitis B virus (HBV) infection, alcohol consumption, chronic hepatitis C virus (HCV) infection, or nonalcoholic steatohepatitis were risk factors for underlying cirrhosis in 38, 25, 21, or 7% of patients, respectively. The median duration of prior sorafenib treatment was 7.8 months. The primary measure of efficacy was overall survival.

In this study, 573 patients were randomized in a 2:1 ratio to receive either regorafenib (160 mg orally once daily) or placebo for 3 consecutive weeks of each 4-week cycle; all patients received best supportive care. Treatment cycles were continued until disease progression or unacceptable toxicity occurred or treatment was discontinued for other reasons; placebo recipients were permitted to cross over to open-label regorafenib treatment after the primary analysis. The median duration of treatment was 3.5 months for patients receiving regorafenib. Median overall survival was 10.6 months in patients receiving regorafenib compared with 7.8 months in those receiving placebo. In addition, patients receiving regorafenib had prolonged progression-free survival (3.1 versus 1.5 months) and higher objective response rates (11 versus 4%) according to modified Response Evaluation Criteria in Solid Tumors (RECIST) assessment for hepatocellular carcinoma (mRECIST) compared with those receiving placebo; complete responses were achieved in 0.5% of regorafenib-treated patients. Use of either mRECIST or RECIST version 1.1 to assess progression-free survival and objective response rates resulted in comparable findings. Subgroup analysis according to disease etiology (HCV infection, HBV infection, alcohol consumption), tumor burden (presence or absence of macroscopic vascular invasion and/or extrahepatic disease), ECOG performance status (0 or 1), Child-Pugh score (A5 or A6), α-fetoprotein (AFP) concentration, age, gender, and geographic region suggested that regorafenib consistently improved median overall and progression-free survival and time to progression across all subgroups.

Dosage and Administration

■ **Administration** Regorafenib is administered orally with water following a low-fat meal containing less than 600 calories and less than 30% fat (see Description) at the same time each day. The tablets should be swallowed whole.

■ **Dosage** Dosage of regorafenib, which is commercially available as the monohydrate, is expressed in terms of anhydrous regorafenib.

Colorectal Cancer For the treatment of metastatic colorectal cancer in patients who previously received fluoropyrimidine-, oxaliplatin-, and irinotecan-containing regimens, anti-vascular endothelial growth factor (anti-VEGF) therapy, and, in those with tumors bearing the wild-type (nonmutated) *KRAS* gene, anti-epidermal growth factor receptor (anti-EGFR) therapy, the recommended dosage of regorafenib is 160 mg once daily for 21 days followed by a 7-day rest period; courses of therapy are given in 28-day cycles. Therapy should be continued until disease progression or unacceptable toxicity occurs.

GI Stromal Tumor For the treatment of locally advanced, unresectable, or metastatic GI stromal tumor (GIST) in patients who previously received imatinib and sunitinib therapy, the recommended dosage of regorafenib is 160 mg once daily for 21 days followed by a 7-day rest period; courses of therapy are given in 28-day cycles. Therapy should be continued until disease progression or unacceptable toxicity occurs.

Hepatocellular Carcinoma For the treatment of hepatocellular carcinoma in patients who previously received sorafenib therapy, the recommended dosage of regorafenib is 160 mg once daily for 21 days followed by a 7-day rest period; courses of therapy are given in 28-day cycles. Therapy should be continued until disease progression or unacceptable toxicity occurs.

Dosage Modification for Toxicity When dosage modification is necessary, the daily dosage of regorafenib should be reduced in decrements of 40 mg; however, if a dosage of 80 mg daily is not tolerated, regorafenib should be permanently discontinued.

Grade 3 or 4 Toxicity. If grade 3 or 4 toxicity occurs, regorafenib therapy should be interrupted. If the toxicity is grade 4, the manufacturer states that therapy should be permanently discontinued; the manufacturer states that therapy may be resumed following recovery from grade 4 toxicity *only* if the potential benefits of resuming therapy outweigh the risks. When therapy is resumed following recovery from the first episode of grade 3 or 4 toxicity (except hepatotoxicity or infection), regorafenib should be administered at a reduced dosage of 120 mg daily; if grade 3 or 4 toxicity (except hepatotoxicity or infection) occurs at a dosage of 120 mg daily, therapy should be withheld again until recovery occurs and then may be resumed at a further reduced dosage of 80 mg daily. (See Hepatotoxicity and also see Infectious Complications under Dosage: Dosage Modification for Toxicity, in Dosage and Administration.) If the patient does not tolerate a dosage of 80 mg daily, regorafenib therapy should be permanently discontinued.

Dermatologic Toxicity. For the first episode of grade 2 palmar-plantar erythrodysesthesia (hand-foot syndrome) of any duration, dosage of regorafenib should be reduced to 120 mg daily. If grade 2 palmar-plantar erythrodysesthesia does not improve within 7 days of dosage reduction or if it recurs at a dosage of 120 mg daily, therapy should be withheld; when therapy is resumed, the dosage should be further reduced to 80 mg daily. If the patient does not tolerate a dosage of 80 mg daily, regorafenib therapy should be permanently discontinued. (See Dermatologic Effects under Warnings/Precautions: Other Warnings and Precautions, in Cautions.)

If grade 3 palmar-plantar erythrodysesthesia occurs, regorafenib therapy should be withheld for at least 7 days; following recovery, therapy may be resumed at a reduced dosage of 120 mg daily. If grade 3 palmar-plantar erythrodysesthesia recurs at a dosage of 120 mg daily, therapy should be withheld again for at least 7 days; following recovery, therapy may be resumed at a further reduced dosage of 80 mg daily. If the patient does not tolerate a dosage of 80 mg daily, regorafenib therapy should be permanently discontinued.

For recommended dosage modifications in patients experiencing grade 4 palmar-plantar erythrodysesthesia, see Grade 3 or 4 Toxicity under Dosage: Dosage Modification for Toxicity, in Dosage and Administration.

Hepatotoxicity. In patients who exhibit grade 3 serum aminotransferase (ALT and/or AST) elevations (i.e., exceeding 5 times the upper limit of normal [ULN], but not more than 20 times the ULN), regorafenib therapy should be interrupted; following recovery, therapy may be resumed at a reduced dosage of 120 mg daily *only* if the potential benefits of resuming therapy outweigh the risk of hepatotoxicity. If grade 3 elevations in ALT or AST recur at a dosage of 120 mg daily, treatment with regorafenib should be permanently discontinued. (See Hepatic Toxicity under Warnings/Precautions: Warnings, in Cautions.)

Following any occurrence of grade 4 ALT and/or AST elevations (i.e., exceeding 20 times the ULN), regorafenib therapy should be permanently discontinued.

Following any occurrence of grade 2 or higher AST and/or ALT elevations (i.e., exceeding 3 times the ULN) *and* bilirubin concentrations exceeding twice the ULN, regorafenib therapy should be permanently discontinued.

Hypertension. If symptomatic grade 2 hypertension occurs, regorafenib therapy should be interrupted. (See Cardiovascular Effects under Warnings/Precautions: Other Warnings and Precautions, in Cautions.) For recommended dosage modifications in patients with grade 3 or 4 hypertension, see Grade 3 or 4 Toxicity under Dosage: Dosage Modification for Toxicity, in Dosage and Administration.

Infectious Complications. If grade 3 or 4 infection develops or worsening infection of any grade occurs, regorafenib therapy should be interrupted; following resolution of the infection, therapy may be resumed at the same dosage. (See Infectious Complications under Warnings/Precautions: Other Warnings and Precautions, in Cautions.)

■ Special Populations

The manufacturer makes no specific dosage recommendations for geriatric patients.

No dosage adjustment is necessary in patients with mild (total bilirubin concentration not exceeding the ULN with AST concentration exceeding the ULN *or* total bilirubin concentration exceeding the ULN, but no more than 1.5 times the ULN) or moderate (total bilirubin concentration exceeding 1.5 times, but not more than 3 times the ULN with any AST concentration) preexisting hepatic impairment; however, patients with hepatic impairment should be closely monitored for adverse effects. Use of regorafenib in patients with severe preexisting hepatic impairment (total bilirubin concentration exceeding 3 times the ULN) is *not* recommended because safety and efficacy have not been established in these patients.

No dosage adjustment is necessary in patients with mild to severe renal impairment. The pharmacokinetics of regorafenib have not been studied in patients with end-stage renal disease requiring dialysis; therefore, the manufacturer states that an appropriate dosage for these patients has not been established.

Although hepatotoxicity and palmar-plantar erythrodysesthesia occur more frequently in Asian patients, the manufacturer states that no initial dosage adjustment is necessary in this population.

Cautions

■ Contraindications

The manufacturer states there are no known contraindications to the use of regorafenib.

■ Warnings/Precautions

Warnings

Hepatic Toxicity. Severe and sometimes fatal hepatotoxicity has been reported in patients receiving regorafenib, generally during the initial 2 months of therapy; hepatic toxicity is usually characterized by a hepatocellular pattern of injury. In the CORRECT study, fatal hepatic failure was reported more frequently in patients with metastatic colorectal cancer receiving regorafenib compared with those receiving placebo (1.6 versus 0.4%). Among patients receiving regorafenib for GI stromal tumor (GIST) in the GRID study, fatal hepatic failure occurred in 0.8% of patients. In the RESORCE study, the incidence of fatal hepatic failure was not increased in patients with hepatocellular carcinoma receiving regorafenib compared with those receiving placebo. In an analysis of pooled data from 3 trials involving patients with metastatic colorectal cancer, GIST, or hepatocellular carcinoma, liver function test abnormalities were reported more frequently in Asian patients receiving regorafenib compared with Caucasian patients.

Serum aminotransferase (ALT and AST) and bilirubin concentrations should be evaluated prior to initiation of therapy, at least every 2 weeks for the first 2 months of therapy, and then monthly thereafter or more frequently as clinically indicated. If aminotransferase and/or bilirubin concentrations rise above pretreatment levels, liver function tests should be monitored weekly until the elevated concentrations have returned to baseline values or have decreased to less than 3 times the upper limit of normal (ULN). Temporary interruption of therapy followed by dosage reduction or permanent drug discontinuance may be necessary depending on the severity and persistence of the toxicity (i.e., elevated liver function test results or hepatocellular necrosis). (See Hepatotoxicity under Dosage: Dosage Modification for Toxicity, in Dosage and Administration.)

Other Warnings and Precautions

Infectious Complications. Infections, sometimes fatal, have been reported in patients receiving regorafenib. In clinical studies, infection was reported in 32% (grade 3 or greater in 9%) of patients receiving regorafenib compared with 17% of those receiving placebo. Urinary tract infections, nasopharyngitis, mucocutaneous and systemic fungal infections, and pneumonia were the most common infections, occurring in 5.7, 4, 3.3, and 2.6% of patients, respectively. Fatal infections, most commonly respiratory infections, occurred in 1% of regorafenib-treated patients compared with 0.3% of those receiving placebo.

Temporary interruption of therapy may be necessary depending on the severity of the infection. (See Infectious Complications under Dosage: Dosage Modification for Toxicity, in Dosage and Administration.)

Hemorrhage. Hemorrhage, sometimes fatal, has been reported in patients receiving regorafenib. In clinical studies, hemorrhage was reported more frequently in regorafenib-treated patients compared with patients receiving placebo (18.2 versus 9.5%); grade 3 or greater hemorrhage occurred in 3% of regorafenib-treated patients. Fatal hemorrhage (CNS bleeding or respiratory, GI, or genitourinary tract bleeding) was reported in 0.7% of patients receiving regorafenib.

If severe or life-threatening hemorrhage occurs, regorafenib should be permanently discontinued. If regorafenib is used in patients receiving a coumarin-derivative anticoagulant (e.g., warfarin), the international normalized ratio (INR) should be monitored more frequently. (See Drug Interactions: Warfarin.)

GI Perforation and Fistula Formation. GI perforation occurred in 0.6% of 4518 patients receiving regorafenib in clinical trials; 8 deaths were reported. In placebo-controlled trials, GI fistula formation was reported in 0.8 or 0.2% of patients receiving regorafenib or placebo, respectively.

Regorafenib should be permanently discontinued in patients with GI perforation or fistula formation.

Dermatologic Effects. In clinical studies, skin reactions, including palmar-plantar erythrodysesthesia (hand-foot syndrome) and severe rash requiring dosage modification, occurred in 71.9% of patients receiving regorafenib and 25.5% of those receiving placebo. Palmar-plantar erythrodysesthesia was reported in 53% of patients receiving regorafenib and 8% of those receiving placebo; the onset generally occurred during the first cycle of therapy. Grade 3 palmar-plantar erythrodysesthesia, grade 3 rash, severe erythema multiforme, and severe Stevens-Johnson syndrome were reported more frequently in patients receiving regorafenib compared with those receiving placebo. Toxic epidermal necrolysis also occurred in patients receiving regorafenib in clinical trials. In an analysis of pooled data from 3 trials involving patients with metastatic colorectal cancer, GIST, or hepatocellular carcinoma, palmar-plantar erythrodysesthesia was reported more frequently in Asian patients receiving regorafenib compared with Caucasian patients.

Dosage reduction, temporary interruption of therapy, or permanent drug discontinuance may be necessary depending on the severity and persistence of the toxicity; other symptomatic and supportive measures also should be employed. (See Dermatologic Toxicity under Dosage: Dosage Modification for Toxicity, in Dosage and Administration.)

Cardiovascular Effects. In the CORRECT study, hypertension was reported more frequently in patients with metastatic colorectal cancer receiving regorafenib compared with those receiving placebo (30 versus 8%). In the GRID study, hypertension occurred in 59% of patients with GIST receiving regorafenib compared with 27% of those receiving placebo. In the RESORCE study, hypertension occurred in 31% of patients with hepatocellular carcinoma receiving regorafenib compared with 6% of those receiving placebo. Hypertensive crisis has been reported. Onset of hypertension generally occurred during the first cycle of therapy. Blood pressure should be controlled before regorafenib therapy is initiated. Blood pressure should be monitored weekly during the first 6 weeks of regorafenib therapy and thereafter should be monitored every cycle, or more frequently, as clinically indicated. If hypertension is severe or uncontrolled, temporary or permanent discontinuance of therapy is recommended. (See Hypertension under Dosage: Dosage Modification for Toxicity, in Dosage and Administration.)

In clinical studies, cardiac ischemia or infarction occurred more frequently in patients receiving regorafenib than in those receiving placebo (0.9 versus

0.2%). Therapy should be interrupted in patients who develop new or acute-onset cardiac ischemia or cardiac infarction. Upon resolution of acute cardiac ischemic events, therapy may be resumed if the potential benefits outweigh the risk of further cardiac ischemia.

Reversible Posterior Leukoencephalopathy Syndrome. Reversible posterior leukoencephalopathy syndrome (RPLS) has occurred in patients receiving regorafenib. This complication occurred in one of 4800 patients treated with regorafenib in clinical trials. RPLS is a syndrome of subcortical vasogenic edema that may manifest with headache, seizures, visual disturbances, confusion, or altered mental function. Magnetic resonance imaging (MRI) is necessary to confirm the diagnosis of RPLS.

The possible diagnosis of RPLS should be considered in any patient receiving regorafenib who presents with neurologic manifestations suggestive of RPLS. Regorafenib should be discontinued in patients who develop RPLS.

Wound Healing Complications. The effect of regorafenib on wound healing has not been specifically studied to date; however, inhibitors of vascular endothelial growth factor receptor (VEGFR) may impair wound healing.

The manufacturer recommends that regorafenib be discontinued at least 2 weeks prior to scheduled surgery. The decision to resume therapy postoperatively should be based on clinical assessment of the adequacy of wound healing. Regorafenib should be discontinued in patients with wound dehiscence.

Fetal/Neonatal Morbidity and Mortality. Regorafenib may cause fetal harm if administered to pregnant women; embryolethality and teratogenicity have been demonstrated in animals. Regorafenib produced developmental toxicity, including cardiovascular, genitourinary, and skeletal abnormalities, when administered to pregnant animals in dosages associated with exposure levels lower than those associated with the recommended human dosage. Pregnancy should be avoided during therapy and for 2 months after drug discontinuance. If regorafenib is used during pregnancy or if the patient becomes pregnant while receiving the drug, the patient should be apprised of the potential fetal hazard. (See Advice to Patients.)

Impairment of Fertility. Results of animal studies suggest that regorafenib may impair male and female fertility. The effect of regorafenib on fertility in humans is not known.

Specific Populations **Pregnancy.** Regorafenib may cause fetal harm if administered to pregnant women based on its mechanism of action and animal findings. (See Fetal/Neonatal Morbidity and Mortality under Warnings/Precautions: Other Warnings and Precautions, in Cautions.)

Lactation. Regorafenib and its metabolites are distributed into milk in rats; it is not known whether the drug is distributed into milk in humans. Because of the potential for serious adverse reactions to regorafenib in nursing infants, women should be advised to discontinue nursing during regorafenib therapy. The effects of the drug on nursing infants or on milk production are unknown. Women may begin nursing 2 weeks after discontinuance of therapy.

Pediatric Use. Safety and efficacy of regorafenib have not been established in pediatric patients younger than 18 years of age.

Persistent growth and thickening of the femoral epiphyseal growth plate, as well as dose-dependent angiectasis and dentin alteration, have been observed in animals receiving repeated doses of regorafenib at exposure levels lower than those associated with the recommended human dosage.

Geriatric Use. In clinical studies, 40% of patients were 65 years of age or older and 10% were 75 years of age or older. No overall differences in safety and efficacy were observed between geriatric patients and younger adults, but grade 3 or 4 hypertension occurred more frequently in geriatric patients.

Hepatic Impairment. In a population pharmacokinetic analysis, no clinically meaningful differences in the mean systemic exposure to regorafenib and its active *N*-oxide (M-2) and *N*-oxide and *N*-desmethyl (M-5) metabolites were observed in patients with hepatocellular carcinoma and mild (total bilirubin concentration not exceeding the ULN with AST concentration exceeding the ULN *or* total bilirubin concentration exceeding the ULN, but no more than 1.5 times the ULN) or moderate (total bilirubin concentration exceeding 1.5 times, but not more than 3 times, the ULN with any AST concentration) hepatic impairment compared with patients with normal hepatic function; no dosage adjustment is required in patients with mild or moderate hepatic impairment. However, patients with mild or moderate hepatic impairment should be monitored closely for adverse effects. Regorafenib has not been studied in patients with severe hepatic impairment (total bilirubin concentration exceeding 3 times the ULN); therefore, use of the drug is not recommended in these patients.

Renal Impairment. Following administration of regorafenib (160 mg daily for 21 days), systemic exposure to regorafenib and its active M-2 and M-5 metabolites in patients with severe renal impairment (creatinine clearance 15–29 mL/minute) was similar to that in patients with normal renal function; no dosage adjustment is recommended in patients with mild to severe renal impairment. However, regorafenib has not been studied in patients with end-stage renal disease requiring dialysis, and an appropriate dosage for these patients has not been established.

■ **Common Adverse Effects** Adverse effects reported in 10% or more of patients receiving regorafenib for the treatment of metastatic colorectal cancer following failure of prior therapy include asthenia/fatigue, pain, decreased appetite, palmar-plantar erythrodysesthesia (hand-foot syndrome), diarrhea, mucositis, weight loss, infection, dysphonia, hypertension, fever, rash, hemorrhage, headache, and nausea. Laboratory abnormalities reported in 20% or more of patients receiving regorafenib for the treatment of metastatic colorectal cancer include proteinuria, anemia, elevated concentrations of hepatic enzymes (e.g., AST, ALT), hypocalcemia, hypophosphatemia, lymphopenia, elevated concentrations of pancreatic enzymes (e.g., amylase, lipase), hyperbilirubinemia, thrombocytopenia, hyponatremia, hypokalemia, and increased international normalized ratio (INR).

Adverse effects reported in 10% or more of patients receiving regorafenib for the treatment of locally advanced, unresectable, or metastatic GIST following failure of prior therapy include palmar-plantar erythrodysesthesia, pain, hypertension, asthenia/fatigue, diarrhea, mucositis, dysphonia, infection, decreased appetite, rash, alopecia, fever, nausea, hypothyroidism, vomiting, headache, muscle spasms, weight loss, hemorrhage, myalgia, constipation, and hoarseness. Laboratory abnormalities reported in 20% or more of patients receiving regorafenib for the treatment of locally advanced, unresectable, or metastatic GIST include proteinuria, elevated concentrations of hepatic enzymes (e.g., AST, ALT), hypophosphatemia, hyperbilirubinemia, lymphopenia, and hypokalemia.

Adverse effects reported in 10% or more of patients receiving regorafenib for the treatment of hepatocellular carcinoma following failure of prior therapy include pain, palmar-plantar erythrodysesthesia, asthenia/fatigue, diarrhea, decreased appetite, hypertension, infection, fever, dysphonia, hemorrhage, nausea, mucositis, weight loss, vomiting, and muscle spasms. Laboratory abnormalities reported in 20% or more of patients receiving regorafenib for the treatment of previously treated hepatocellular carcinoma include elevated concentrations of hepatic enzymes (e.g., AST, ALT), hyperbilirubinemia, hypophosphatemia, lymphopenia, thrombocytopenia, proteinuria, increased INR, elevated concentrations of pancreatic enzymes (e.g., amylase, lipase), hypokalemia, and hypocalcemia.

Drug Interactions

■ **Drugs and Foods Affecting Hepatic Microsomal Enzymes** Metabolism of regorafenib to M-2 (an active *N*-oxide metabolite) is mediated by cytochrome P-450 isoenzyme 3A4 (CYP3A4); the enzyme responsible for conversion of M-2 to M-5 (an active *N*-oxide and *N*-desmethyl metabolite) has not been established to date. Therefore, concomitant use of regorafenib with potent inhibitors of CYP3A4 may result in increased systemic exposure to the parent drug, decreased systemic exposure to M-2 and M-5, and an increased incidence of adverse effects. In healthy individuals, the potent CYP3A4 inhibitor ketoconazole (400 mg daily for 18 days) increased the area under the concentration-time curve (AUC) of regorafenib (single 160-mg dose administered 5 days after initiation of ketoconazole) by 33% and decreased the AUCs of both M-2 and M-5 by approximately 93%. Concomitant use of regorafenib with potent inhibitors of CYP3A4 (e.g., clarithromycin, grapefruit juice, itraconazole, ketoconazole, nefazodone, posaconazole, telithromycin, voriconazole) should be avoided.

Concomitant use of regorafenib with potent inducers of CYP3A4 may result in decreased systemic exposure to the parent drug, increased systemic exposure to M-5, and reduced regorafenib efficacy. In healthy individuals, the potent CYP3A4 inducer rifampin (600 mg daily for 9 days) decreased the AUC of regorafenib (single 160-mg dose administered 7 days after initiation of rifampin) by 50% and increased the AUC of M-5 by 264%; the AUC of M-2 was not substantially altered. Concomitant use of regorafenib with potent inducers of CYP3A4 (e.g., carbamazepine, phenobarbital, phenytoin, rifampin, St. John's wort [*Hypericum perforatum*]) should be avoided.

■ **Drugs Metabolized by Hepatic Microsomal Enzymes** In vitro studies have suggested that regorafenib inhibits CYP isoenzymes 2B6, 2C8, 2C9, 2C19, and 3A4; that the active M-2 metabolite inhibits CYP isoenzymes 2C8, 2C9, 2D6, and 3A4; and that the active M-5 metabolite inhibits CYP2C8. In vitro studies also have suggested that regorafenib does not induce CYP isoenzymes 1A2, 2B6, 2C19, or 3A4. However, when patients with advanced solid tumors received a single dose of midazolam (2 mg; a CYP3A4 substrate), rosiglitazone (4 mg; a CYP2C8 substrate), warfarin sodium (10 mg; a CYP2C9 substrate), or omeprazole (40 mg; a CYP2C19 substrate) following 2 weeks of regorafenib administration (160 mg once daily), the AUCs of midazolam and rosiglitazone were not substantially altered, the AUC of warfarin was increased by 25%, and plasma concentrations of omeprazole measured 6 hours after administration were not substantially altered.

■ **Drugs Affected by Transport Systems** In vitro data indicate that regorafenib is an inhibitor of the efflux transporter breast cancer resistance protein (BCRP). Therefore, concomitant use of regorafenib with drugs that are substrates of BCRP may result in increased systemic exposure to the substrate drug. When regorafenib (160 mg once daily for 14 days) was administered prior to the BCRP substrate rosuvastatin (single 5-mg dose), peak plasma concentration and AUC of rosuvastatin were increased 4.6- and 3.8-fold, respectively. Patients receiving regorafenib concomitantly with BCRP substrates (e.g., atorvastatin, fluvastatin, methotrexate) should be closely monitored for signs of toxicity associated with the substrate drug.

Although in vitro data also indicate that regorafenib is an inhibitor of the efflux transporter P-glycoprotein (P-gp), clinical data indicate that regorafenib does not alter the pharmacokinetics of digoxin (a P-gp substrate). No clinically meaningful interactions between regorafenib and P-gp substrates are expected.

■ **Drugs Affecting Transport Systems** In vitro studies indicate that the active M-2 and M-5 metabolites of regorafenib are substrates of P-gp and BCRP. Inhibitors or inducers of these efflux transporters may alter M-2 and

M-5 exposure; however, the clinical importance of these in vitro findings is not known.

■ **Drugs Metabolized by Uridine Diphosphate-glucuronosyltransferase (UGT)** In vitro studies indicate that regorafenib and its active metabolites competitively inhibit UGT1A1 and UGT1A9 at clinically relevant concentrations. In patients receiving an irinotecan-containing regimen concomitantly with regorafenib, the AUCs of irinotecan and its active metabolite SN-38 (a UGT1A1 substrate) were increased by 28 and 44%, respectively, when a dose of irinotecan hydrochloride (180 mg/m² as a 1.5-hour IV infusion) was given 5 days after completion of a series of 7 doses of regorafenib (160 mg orally once daily).

■ **Antibiotics** When regorafenib (single 160-mg dose) was administered concomitantly with neomycin sulfate (1 g orally 3 times daily for 5 days) in healthy individuals, the AUC of regorafenib was not substantially altered; however, the AUCs of M-2 and M-5 were decreased by 76 and 86%, respectively. The effect of other antibiotics on systemic exposure of regorafenib and its active metabolites has not been established.

■ **Antineoplastic Agents** ***Fluorouracil*** In patients receiving a fluorouracil-containing regimen concomitantly with regorafenib, the pharmacokinetics of fluorouracil were not substantially altered when fluorouracil (400 mg/m² by IV injection, followed by continuous IV infusion of 2400 mg/m² over 46 hours) was given 5 days after completion of a series of 7 doses of regorafenib (160 mg orally once daily).

Irinotecan In patients receiving an irinotecan-containing regimen concomitantly with regorafenib, the AUCs of irinotecan and its active metabolite SN-38 were increased by 28 and 44%, respectively. (See Drug Interactions: Drugs Metabolized by Uridine Diphosphate-glucuronosyltransferase [UGT].)

Oxaliplatin In patients receiving an oxaliplatin-containing regimen concomitantly with regorafenib, the AUCs of total and unbound platinum were increased by 39 and 17%, respectively, when oxaliplatin (85 mg/m² as a 2-hour IV infusion) was given 5 days after completion of a series of 7 doses of regorafenib (160 mg orally once daily).

■ **Warfarin** When regorafenib is used in patients receiving a coumarin-derivative anticoagulant (e.g., warfarin), international normalized ratio (INR) should be monitored more frequently. (See Hemorrhage under Warnings/Precautions: Other Warnings and Precautions, in Cautions.) When a single dose of warfarin sodium (10 mg; a CYP2C9 substrate) was administered following 2 weeks of therapy with regorafenib (160 mg once daily), the AUC of warfarin was increased by 25%.

Description

Regorafenib, an inhibitor of multiple receptor tyrosine kinases (RTKs), is an antineoplastic agent. Receptor tyrosine kinases are involved in the initiation of various cascades of intracellular signaling events that lead to cell proliferation and/or influence processes critical to cell survival and tumor progression (e.g., angiogenesis, metastasis, inhibition of apoptosis), based on the respective kinase. In vitro, regorafenib or its active metabolites (M-2 and M-5) exhibit inhibitory activity against vascular endothelial growth factor receptors (i.e., VEGFR-1, VEGFR-2, VEGFR-3), platelet-derived growth factor receptors (i.e., PDGFR-α, PDGFR-β), fibroblast growth factor receptors (i.e., FGFR1, FGFR2), and tyrosine kinase with immunoglobulin and epidermal growth factor homology (i.e., TIE-2) at clinically relevant concentrations; the drug also has a broad spectrum of inhibitory effects on other receptor kinases involved in normal cellular functions and pathologic processes (e.g., RET, c-Kit, DDR2, TrkA, EphA-2, Raf-1, b-Raf, mutant b-Raf, SAPK2, Ptk5, Bcr-Abl, CSF-1R). Regorafenib has been shown to inhibit tumor angiogenesis in vivo. The drug also has demonstrated inhibition of tumor growth in mice bearing tumor xenografts, including human colorectal carcinoma, GI stromal tumor (GIST), and hepatocellular carcinoma. In addition, regorafenib has demonstrated inhibition of tumor metastasis in xenograft models of human colorectal carcinoma in mice.

When regorafenib is administered in dosages exceeding 60 mg daily, steady-state exposure to the drug, as measured by area under the serum concentration-time curve (AUC), increases in a less than dose-proportional manner. Regorafenib is metabolized principally by cytochrome P-450 (CYP) isoenzyme 3A4 and uridine diphosphate-glucuronosyl transferase (UGT) 1A9. The main circulating metabolites, M-2 (an *N*-oxide metabolite) and M-5 (an *N*-oxide and *N*-desmethyl metabolite), have been shown to be equipotent to regorafenib in biochemical and cellular assays. Regorafenib and its active metabolites are highly bound (more than 99%) to plasma proteins. Regorafenib undergoes enterohepatic circulation. Following oral administration of a single 160-mg dose of regorafenib, the terminal half-life of regorafenib and M-2 were similar (28 and 25 hours, respectively); however, elimination of M-5 was slower, with a terminal half-life of approximately 51 hours. Following oral administration of 120 mg of radiolabeled regorafenib (as an oral solution), approximately 71% of the dose was recovered in feces (47% of the dose as unchanged drug and 24% as metabolites) and 19% was recovered in urine within 12 days.

Bioavailability of regorafenib and its active metabolites is affected by the presence of food and the fat content of the meal. Administration of a single 160-mg dose of regorafenib with a high-fat meal (945 calories and 54.6 g of fat) increased the AUC of regorafenib by 48% and decreased the AUCs of M-2 and M-5 by 20 and 51%, respectively, compared with administration in the fasted state. When the drug was administered with a low-fat meal (319 calories and 8.2 g of fat), the AUCs of regorafenib, M-2, and M-5 were increased by 36, 40, and 23%, respectively, compared with administration in the fasted state. (See Dosage and Administration: Administration.) In clinical trials establishing safety and efficacy, regorafenib was administered with a low-fat meal.

Age, gender, ethnicity, and body weight do not have clinically important effects on the pharmacokinetics of regorafenib.

Advice to Patients

Importance of taking regorafenib with water at the same time each day following a low-fat meal (containing less than 600 calories and less than 30% fat). If a dose is missed, importance of administering the missed dose on the same day as soon as it is remembered. Patients should be informed to not take 2 doses on the same day to make up for a missed dose. Importance of avoiding grapefruit juice while taking the drug.

Risk of severe or life-threatening hepatotoxicity and importance of liver function test monitoring. Importance of promptly informing clinician of signs and symptoms of severe liver damage (e.g., jaundice, nausea, vomiting, dark urine, changes in sleep pattern).

Risk of infection. Importance of promptly informing clinician of signs and symptoms of infection (e.g., fever, severe cough or sore throat, shortness of breath, burning or pain upon urination, unusual vaginal discharge or irritation).

Risk of severe bleeding. Importance of informing clinician of signs and symptoms of unusual bleeding (e.g., bruising, lightheadedness).

Risk of palmar-plantar erythrodysesthesia (hand-foot syndrome) or rash. Importance of informing clinician of skin changes (e.g., redness, pain, blisters, bleeding, swelling).

Risk of hypertension developing or worsening during therapy. Importance of regular monitoring of blood pressure during treatment. Importance of informing clinician of signs and symptoms of hypertension (e.g., severe headache, lightheadedness, neurologic symptoms).

Risk of myocardial ischemia and infarction. Importance of seeking immediate medical attention if chest pain, shortness of breath, or feelings of dizziness or faintness occur during regorafenib therapy.

Risk of reversible posterior leukoencephalopathy syndrome (RPLS). Importance of immediately informing clinician if severe headache, seizure, confusion, or visual and neurologic disturbances occur during regorafenib therapy.

Risk of GI perforation. Importance of promptly informing clinician if severe abdominal pain, persistent abdominal swelling, chills, nausea, vomiting, dehydration, or high fever occurs.

Risk of wound healing complications. Importance of informing clinician of any recent or scheduled surgery.

Risk of fetal harm. Necessity of advising women of childbearing potential and men who are partners of such women that they should use effective methods of contraception while receiving the drug and for 2 months after discontinuance of therapy. Importance of patients informing their clinicians if they or their partners are pregnant or think they may be pregnant.

Importance of advising women to avoid breast-feeding while receiving regorafenib therapy and for 2 weeks after the final dose.

Importance of informing clinicians of existing or contemplated concomitant therapy, including prescription and OTC drugs and dietary or herbal supplements (e.g., St. John's wort), as well as any concomitant illnesses (e.g., hypertension or other cardiovascular disease, hepatic disease, bleeding disorders).

Importance of storing regorafenib tablets in the original container, tightly closed; importance of not removing the desiccant from the bottle or placing the tablets in daily or weekly pill boxes. Any unused tablets should be discarded 7 weeks after the container is first opened.

Importance of informing patients of other important precautionary information. (See Cautions.)

Overview® (see Users Guide). For additional information on this drug until a more detailed monograph is developed and published, the manufacturer's labeling should be consulted. It is *essential* that the manufacturer's labeling be consulted for more detailed information on usual cautions, precautions, contraindications, potential drug interactions, laboratory test interferences, and acute toxicity. For further information on the handling of antineoplastic agents, see the ASHP Guidelines on Handling Hazardous Drugs at http://www.ahfsdruginformation.com.

Preparations

Excipients in commercially available drug preparations may have clinically important effects in some individuals; consult specific product labeling for details.

Regorafenib

Oral		
Tablets, film-coated	40 mg	**Stivarga®**, Bayer

Ribociclib Succinate

■ Ribociclib, a selective inhibitor of cyclin-dependent kinases 4 (CDK4) and 6 (CDK6), is an antineoplastic agent.

Uses

■ **Breast Cancer** ***Initial Therapy for Advanced Breast Cancer*** Ribociclib is used in combination with an aromatase inhibitor for the initial treatment of hormone receptor-positive, human epidermal growth factor receptor type 2 (HER2)-negative advanced or metastatic breast cancer in postmenopausal women. A statistically significant progression-free survival benefit has been observed in postmenopausal women with previously untreated, hormone receptor-positive, HER2-negative advanced or metastatic breast cancer receiving combined therapy with ribociclib and letrozole compared with patients receiving placebo in combination with letrozole.

The current indication for ribociclib is based principally on the results of a randomized, double-blind, placebo-controlled phase 3 study (MONALEESA-2) in postmenopausal women with previously untreated hormone receptor-positive, HER2-negative advanced breast cancer. In this study, 668 patients were randomized (stratified by site of metastases) to receive either ribociclib (600 mg orally once daily for 21 days followed by a 7-day rest period) in combination with letrozole (2.5 mg orally once daily continuously) or placebo in combination with letrozole (2.5 mg orally once daily continuously). Treatment was continued until disease progression, death, or unacceptable toxicity occurred or treatment was discontinued for other reasons. Patients randomized to receive placebo were not permitted to cross over to open-label ribociclib therapy upon disease progression. The primary measure of efficacy was progression-free survival as assessed by the investigator according to Response Evaluation Criteria in Solid Tumors (RECIST). The median age of patients was 62 years; 82% of the patients were white; 34% had de novo metastatic disease, 21% had bone-only disease, and 59% had visceral involvement; 47% had received prior chemotherapy, and 51% had received neoadjuvant or adjuvant endocrine therapy prior to diagnosis of advanced breast cancer. All patients enrolled in the study had a baseline ECOG performance status of 0 or 1.

At the time of a planned interim analysis of MONALEESA-2 results, the progression-free survival benefit observed in patients receiving ribociclib in combination with letrozole was statistically significant, although the median duration of progression-free survival had not yet been reached; the median progression-free survival in patients receiving placebo in combination with letrozole was 14.7 months. The results of the progression-free survival analysis based on an independent, blinded, central radiologic assessment were consistent with the investigator assessment. Ribociclib and letrozole combination therapy was associated with higher rates of progression-free survival at 12 and 18 months (72.8 and 63%, respectively) compared with those receiving placebo in combination with letrozole (60.9 and 42.2%, respectively). Among patients with measurable disease, patients receiving ribociclib in combination with letrozole had higher overall response rates compared with those receiving placebo in combination with letrozole (52.7 versus 37.1%). A subset analysis of progression-free survival based on clinically relevant baseline patient and disease characteristics consistently showed treatment benefit with ribociclib and letrozole combination therapy compared with placebo in combination with letrozole. Median overall survival had not been reached at the time of the interim efficacy analysis.

Dosage and Administration

■ **General** Ribociclib succinate is commercially available alone (Kisqali®) and copackaged with letrozole (Kisqali® Femara® Co-Pack).

Because ribociclib may cause neutropenia and hepatotoxicity, the manufacturer states that complete blood cell (CBC) counts and liver function tests should be monitored at baseline, every 2 weeks for cycles 1–2, prior to initiation of cycles 3–6, and then as clinically indicated. (See Hematologic Toxicity and also see Hepatic Toxicity under Dosage: Dosage Modification, in Dosage and Administration.)

Because ribociclib may prolong the QT interval, ribociclib therapy should only be initiated in patients with corrected QT (QT_c) intervals less than 450 msec. Electrolyte abnormalities should be corrected prior to administration of the drug.

Clinicians should consult the respective manufacturers' labelings for information on dosage and administration (including dosage adjustments), adverse effects, and contraindications of other antineoplastic agents used in combination regimens.

■ **Administration** Ribociclib is administered orally without regard to food at approximately the same time each day, preferably in the morning. The tablets should be swallowed intact and should *not* be broken, chewed, crushed, or split.

If a dose of ribociclib is missed or vomited, patients should *not* take an extra dose. The next dose should be taken at the regularly scheduled time.

■ **Dosage** Dosage of ribociclib succinate is expressed in terms of ribociclib.

Breast Cancer **Initial Therapy for Advanced Breast Cancer.** For the initial treatment of hormone receptor-positive, human epidermal growth factor receptor type 2 (HER2)-negative advanced or metastatic breast cancer in postmenopausal women, the recommended dosage of ribociclib is 600 mg once daily on days 1–21 of each 28-day cycle in combination with letrozole 2.5 mg once daily given continuously throughout the 28-day cycle. In the MONALEESA-2 study, therapy was continued until disease progression or unacceptable toxicity occurred.

Dosage Modification Dosage interruption and/or reduction, or discontinuance of ribociclib therapy, may be necessary based on severity of adverse reactions. Dosage adjustment of ribociclib is recommended based on individual safety and tolerability. If dosage reduction from 600 mg once daily is necessary, the dosage should be reduced to 400 mg once daily. If the toxicity recurs at a dosage of 400 mg once daily, the dosage should be reduced to 200 mg once daily. If the toxicity recurs at a dosage of 200 mg once daily, ribociclib therapy should be discontinued.

Hematologic Toxicity. For grade 4 neutropenia (i.e., absolute neutrophil count [ANC] less than 500/mm³), ribociclib therapy should be interrupted until neutropenia improves to grade 2 or less. Upon resumption of therapy, the dosage of ribociclib should be reduced. (See Neutropenia under Cautions: Warnings/Precautions.)

For grade 3 febrile neutropenia (i.e., ANC 500 to less than 1000/mm³ associated with a single episode of fever of 38.5°C or more *or* fever exceeding 38°C for more than 1 hour *and/or* infection), ribociclib therapy should be interrupted until neutropenia improves to grade 2 or less. Upon resumption of therapy, the dosage of ribociclib should be reduced.

For the first occurrence of grade 3 neutropenia (i.e., ANC 500 to less than 1000/mm³), ribociclib therapy should be interrupted; therapy may be resumed at the same dosage when neutropenia improves to grade 2 or less. For subsequent occurrences of grade 3 neutropenia, ribociclib therapy should be withheld again; therapy may then be resumed at a reduced dosage when neutropenia improves to grade 2 or less.

For grade 1 or 2 neutropenia (i.e., ANC 1000/mm³ to less than the lower limit of normal [LLN]), ribociclib therapy may be continued at the same dosage.

Hepatic Toxicity. For grade 4 serum aminotransferase (ALT and/or AST) elevations (i.e., exceeding 20 times the upper limit of normal [ULN]) with total bilirubin concentrations no more than 2 times the ULN, ribociclib therapy should be discontinued. (See Hepatic Toxicity under Cautions: Warnings/Precautions.)

For the first occurrence of grade 3 serum ALT and/or AST elevations (i.e., exceeding 5 times the ULN, but no more than 20 times the ULN) with total bilirubin concentrations no more than 2 times the ULN, ribociclib therapy should be interrupted; therapy may be resumed at a reduced dosage when the toxicity improves to baseline or better grade. If grade 3 hepatotoxicity recurs at a reduced dosage, ribociclib therapy should be discontinued.

For the first occurrence of grade 2 serum ALT and/or AST elevations (i.e., exceeding 3 times the ULN, but no more than 5 times the ULN) with total bilirubin concentrations no more than 2 times the ULN *in patients with preexisting ALT and/or AST concentrations no more than 3 times the ULN*, ribociclib therapy should be interrupted; therapy may be resumed at the same dosage when the toxicity improves to baseline or better grade. For subsequent occurrences, ribociclib therapy should be withheld again; therapy may then be resumed at a reduced dosage when the toxicity improves to baseline or better grade.

If grade 2 serum ALT and/or AST elevations with total bilirubin concentrations no more than 2 times the ULN persist *in patients with preexisting ALT and/or AST concentrations exceeding 3 times the ULN, but no more than 5 times the ULN*, ribociclib therapy may be continued without interruption.

If grade 1 serum ALT and/or AST elevations (i.e., exceeding the ULN, but no more than 3 times the ULN) with total bilirubin concentrations no more than 2 times the ULN occur, ribociclib therapy may be continued without dosage adjustment.

For serum ALT and/or AST elevations exceeding 3 times the ULN with concomitant total bilirubin concentrations exceeding 2 times the ULN (irrespective of baseline hepatic function) in the absence of cholestasis, ribociclib therapy should be discontinued.

Cardiovascular Toxicity. If the QT_c interval exceeds 480 msec, ribociclib therapy should be interrupted; therapy may be resumed at the same dosage when the QT_c interval improves to less than 481 msec. If QT_c-interval prolongation (i.e., 481 msec or greater) recurs, therapy should be withheld again; therapy may then be resumed at a reduced dosage when the QT_c interval improves to less than 481 msec.

If the QT_c interval exceeds 500 msec on at least 2 separate ECGs during a single visit, ribociclib therapy should be interrupted; therapy may be resumed at a reduced dosage when the QT_c-interval improves to less than 481 msec.

When QT_c-interval prolongation (exceeding 500 msec or increase of more than 60 msec from baseline) occurs concurrently with torsades de pointes, polymorphic ventricular tachycardia, unexplained syncope, or signs and/or symptoms of serious arrhythmia, ribociclib therapy should be permanently discontinued.

Other Toxicity. For grade 4 adverse reactions, ribociclib therapy should be discontinued.

For grade 3 adverse reactions, ribociclib therapy should be interrupted; therapy may be resumed at the same dosage when the toxicity improves to grade 1 or less. For subsequent occurrences of grade 3 adverse reactions, ribociclib therapy should be withheld again; therapy may then be resumed at a reduced dosage when the toxicity improves to grade 1 or less.

For grade 1 or 2 adverse reactions, ribociclib therapy may be continued at the same dosage; however, patients should receive appropriate medical therapy and additional monitoring as clinically indicated.

Concomitant Use with Drugs and Foods Affecting Hepatic Microsomal Enzymes. Concomitant use of ribociclib with drugs that are potent inhibitors of cytochrome P-450 (CYP) isoenzyme 3A should be avoided, and selection of an alternative drug with less CYP3A inhibition potential is recommended. If concomitant use of a potent CYP3A inhibitor cannot be avoided, the manufacturer recommends reducing the dosage of ribociclib from 600 mg once daily to 400 mg once daily. When concomitant use of the potent CYP3A inhibitor is discontinued, the ribociclib dosage should be returned (after at least 5 elimination half-lives of the CYP3A inhibitor) to the dosage used prior to initiation of the potent CYP3A inhibitor. (See Inhibitors of CYP3A under Drug Interactions: Drugs and Foods Affecting Hepatic Microsomal Enzymes.)

■ **Special Populations** For patients with moderate or severe preexisting hepatic impairment (Child-Pugh class B or C), the manufacturer recommends an initial ribociclib dosage of 400 mg once daily. No dosage adjustment is necessary in patients with mild hepatic impairment (Child-Pugh class A). The manufacturer provides no specific dosage recommendations in patients with baseline grade 3 or greater serum ALT and/or AST elevations. (See Hepatic Impairment under Warnings/Precautions: Specific Populations, in Cautions.)

There are currently no special dosage recommendations for geriatric patients or patients with renal impairment. (See Geriatric Use and also see Renal Impairment under Warnings/Precautions: Specific Populations, in Cautions.)

Cautions

■ **Contraindications** The manufacturer states that there are no known contraindications to the use of ribociclib.

■ **Warnings/Precautions** ***Prolongation of QT Interval*** Prolongation of the corrected QT (QT_c) interval has been observed in ribociclib-treated patients. The prolongation appears to occur in a plasma concentration-dependent manner. Following administration of ribociclib 600 mg once daily, an estimated mean increase in QT_c interval exceeding 20 msec is expected at mean steady-state peak plasma concentrations. In a pharmacokinetic/pharmacodynamic study evaluating potential effects of ribociclib on the QT_c interval, the mean QT_c interval increase from baseline was 22.9 msec (range: 21.6–24.1 msec) at clinically relevant concentrations. In the MONALEESA-2 study, an increase in the QT_c interval exceeding 60 msec from baseline occurred in 3% of ribociclib-treated patients, and QT_c intervals exceeding 500 msec occurred in 0.3% of ribociclib-treated patients. Prolongation of the QT_c interval usually occurred within the first 4 weeks of treatment and was reversible upon dosage interruption. In addition, syncope was reported in 2.7% of patients receiving combined therapy with ribociclib and letrozole compared with 0.9% of patients receiving placebo and letrozole. In this study, sudden death occurred in one patient with grade 3 hypokalemia and grade 2 prolongation of the QT interval. Torsades de pointes was not observed in the MONALEESA-2 study in patients receiving combined therapy with ribociclib and letrozole.

Ribociclib should be avoided in patients with congenital long QT syndrome, uncontrolled or clinically important cardiac disease (e.g., myocardial infarction, congestive heart failure, unstable angina, bradyarrhythmias), electrolyte abnormalities, or other risk factors for developing prolongation of the QT interval.

Prolongation of the QT interval may occur when ribociclib is used concomitantly with potent CYP3A inhibitors or with drugs known to prolong the QT_c interval; therefore, concurrent use of such agents should be avoided. (See Concomitant Use with Drugs and Foods Affecting Hepatic Microsomal Enzymes under Dosage: Dosage Modification, in Dosage and Administration and also see Drug Interactions.)

ECGs should be monitored at baseline, around day 14 of cycle 1, prior to initiation of cycle 2, and then as clinically indicated. More frequent ECG monitoring is recommended in patients who develop QT_c-interval prolongation during therapy. In addition, serum electrolytes (i.e., potassium, calcium, phosphorus, magnesium) should be monitored at baseline, prior to initiation of cycles 1–6, and then as clinically indicated. Ribociclib therapy should only be initiated in patients with QT_c intervals less than 450 msec. Electrolyte abnormalities should be corrected prior to administration of the drug. Temporary interruption, dosage reduction, or discontinuance of ribociclib may be necessary if QT_c-interval prolongation occurs during therapy with the drug. (See Cardiovascular Toxicity under Dosage: Dosage Modification, in Dosage and Administration.)

Hepatic Toxicity Drug-induced hepatotoxicity has occurred in patients receiving ribociclib. In the MONALEESA-2 study, grade 3 or 4 elevations in serum ALT concentrations were reported in 10% of patients receiving combined therapy with ribociclib and letrozole compared with 1% of those receiving placebo and letrozole; grade 3 or 4 elevations in serum AST concentrations were reported in 7 and 2% of patients receiving these respective treatments. The median time to onset of grade 3 or greater elevations in ALT/AST concentrations was 57 days; these elevations in ALT/AST resolved to grade 2 or less in approximately 24 days. Serum aminotransferase elevations exceeding 3 times the upper limit of normal (ULN) with concurrent elevations in total bilirubin concentrations exceeding 2 times the ULN, normal alkaline phosphatase concentrations, and absence of cholestasis were reported in 1% of patients; these adverse hepatic effects were reversible upon discontinuance of ribociclib therapy.

Liver function tests should be monitored at baseline, every 2 weeks during cycles 1 and 2, prior to initiation of cycles 3–6, and then as clinically indicated. More frequent monitoring is recommended if elevations in serum aminotransferase concentrations occur. Temporary interruption, dosage reduction, or discontinuance of ribociclib may be necessary if hepatotoxicity occurs during therapy with the drug.

Neutropenia Neutropenia commonly occurs in patients receiving ribociclib. In the MONALEESA-2 study, grade 3 or 4 neutropenia occurred in 60 or 1% of patients receiving ribociclib in combination with letrozole or those receiving placebo in combination with letrozole, respectively. The median time to occurrence of grade 2 or greater neutropenia was 16 days. The median duration of grade 3 or greater neutropenia was 15 days. Febrile neutropenia has been observed in 1.5% of patients receiving ribociclib in combination with letrozole. Discontinuance of ribociclib due to neutropenia occurred in 0.9% of ribociclib-treated patients.

Complete blood cell (CBC) counts should be monitored at baseline, every 2 weeks during cycles 1 and 2, prior to initiation of cycles 3–6, and then as clinically indicated. Temporary interruption, dosage reduction, or discontinuance of ribociclib may be necessary if neutropenia occurs during therapy with the drug.

Fetal/Neonatal Morbidity and Mortality There are no adequate and well-controlled studies of ribociclib in pregnant women; however, based on its mechanism of action and animal findings, ribociclib may cause fetal harm. Embryofetal toxicity (e.g., decreased fetal weight) and teratogenicity (e.g., external, visceral, and skeletal abnormalities) have been demonstrated in rats and rabbits receiving ribociclib at exposure levels of approximately 0.6 and 1.5 times, respectively, the human exposure at the recommended dosage. Maternal toxicity, abortion, and embryolethality were not observed in rabbits receiving ribociclib at exposure levels approximately 1.5 times the human exposure at the recommended dosage; however, reduced maternal body weight gain was observed in rats receiving ribociclib at exposure levels approximately 0.6 times the human exposure at the recommended dosage.

Pregnancy should be avoided during ribociclib therapy. The manufacturer recommends confirmation of pregnancy status prior to initiation of ribociclib, and women of childbearing potential should be advised to use effective contraceptive methods during and for at least 3 weeks after discontinuance of the drug. Patients should be apprised of the potential hazard to the fetus if ribociclib is used during pregnancy.

Impairment of Fertility Results of animal studies suggest that ribociclib may impair male fertility.

In a general toxicology study, testicular atrophy was observed following administration of ribociclib daily (at exposure levels as low as 0.03 times the human exposure at the recommended dosage) for 3 weeks of each 4-week cycle to male animals for 26–39 weeks.

Specific Populations **Pregnancy.** Ribociclib may cause fetal harm if administered to pregnant women based on its mechanism of action and animal findings. (See Fetal/Neonatal Morbidity and Mortality under Cautions: Warnings/Precautions.)

Confirmation of pregnancy status prior to initiation of ribociclib therapy is recommended.

Lactation. Ribociclib and its metabolites are distributed into milk in rats; it is not known whether the drug is distributed into milk in humans. Because of the potential for serious adverse reactions to ribociclib in nursing infants, women should be advised to discontinue nursing during and for at least 3 weeks after discontinuance of ribociclib therapy. The effects of the drug or its metabolites on nursing infants or on milk production are unknown.

Pediatric Use. Safety and efficacy of ribociclib have not been established in pediatric patients.

In a phase 1 dose-escalation study, 32 patients 1–21 years of age with relapsed or refractory neuroblastoma, malignant rhabdoid tumors, or other tumors with documented cyclin D–cyclin-dependent kinase (CDK) 4/6–inhibitor of CDK4 (INK4)–retinoblastoma (Rb) pathway (cyclin D-CDK4/6-INK4-Rb pathway) abnormalities received ribociclib in dosages ranging from 280–470 mg/m² orally once daily for 21 days followed by a 7-day rest period. Grade 3 fatigue and grade 4 thrombocytopenia were dose-limiting toxicities associated with ribociclib therapy. Hematologic dose-limiting toxicities were not observed in patients receiving ribociclib 350 mg/m².

Based on the results of this dose-escalation study, a ribociclib dosage of 350 mg/m² orally once daily for 21 days followed by a 7-day rest period has been recommended for phase 2 studies in pediatric patients.

Geriatric Use. In the MONALEESA-2 study, 45% of patients were 65 years of age or older and 11% were 75 years of age or older. No overall differences in safety and efficacy were observed between geriatric patients and younger adults.

Among patients 23–84 years of age, age did not appear to substantially affect systemic exposure to ribociclib.

Hepatic Impairment. Mean systemic exposure of ribociclib is increased less than twofold in individuals with preexisting moderate (Child-Pugh class B) or severe (Child-Pugh class C) hepatic impairment compared with individuals with normal hepatic function; however, systemic exposure of ribociclib was unaffected in individuals with preexisting mild (Child-Pugh class A) hepatic impairment. Population pharmacokinetic analysis also indicated that systemic exposure to ribociclib in patients with mild hepatic impairment was similar to that in patients with normal hepatic function. Dosage adjustment is required in patients with preexisting moderate or severe hepatic impairment. (See Dosage and Administration: Special Populations.)

Renal Impairment. Population pharmacokinetic analysis indicated that systemic exposure to ribociclib in patients with mild or moderate renal impairment (estimated glomerular filtration rate [GFR] 30 to less than 90 mL/minute per 1.73 m^2) was similar to that in patients with normal renal function.

Pharmacokinetics of ribociclib have not been established in patients with severe renal impairment (estimated GFR less than 30 mL/minute per 1.73 m^2). (See Dosage and Administration: Special Populations.)

■ **Common Adverse Effects** Adverse effects reported in 10% or more of patients with advanced breast cancer receiving ribociclib in combination with letrozole and at an incidence that is at least 2% higher than that reported with placebo in combination with letrozole in the MONALEESA-2 study include neutropenia, nausea, infection (most commonly urinary tract and upper respiratory tract infections), fatigue, diarrhea, alopecia, leukopenia, vomiting, constipation, headache, hot flush, back pain, decreased appetite, anemia, elevated concentrations of aminotransferases (i.e., AST, ALT), rash, pruritus, pyrexia, dyspnea, insomnia, peripheral edema, stomatitis, abdominal pain, and lymphopenia.

Laboratory abnormalities reported in 10% or more of patients receiving ribociclib in combination with letrozole include decreased leukocyte count, decreased neutrophil count, decreased hemoglobin concentrations, decreased lymphocyte count, decreased platelet count, elevated concentrations of serum creatinine, and decreased concentrations of serum phosphorus or potassium.

Drug Interactions

Ribociclib is metabolized mainly in the liver via oxidation by cytochrome P-450 (CYP) isoenzyme 3A4. In vitro studies indicate that ribociclib is a reversible inhibitor of CYP isoenzymes 1A2, 2E1, and 3A4/5 at clinically relevant concentrations; the drug demonstrates time-dependent inhibition of CYP3A4/5. In vitro studies indicate that ribociclib does not inhibit CYP isoenzymes 2A6, 2B6, 2C8, 2C9, 2C19, and 2D6 at clinically relevant concentrations. In vitro, ribociclib does not exhibit time-dependent inhibition of CYP isoenzymes 1A2, 2C9, and 2D6 or induce CYP isoenzymes 1A2, 2B6, 2C9, and 3A4 at clinically relevant concentrations.

In vitro studies indicate that ribociclib may inhibit breast cancer resistance protein (BCRP), organic cation transporter (OCT) 2, multidrug and toxic compound extrusion protein (MATE) 1, and bile salt export pump (BSEP), but has a low potential for inhibition of P-glycoprotein (P-gp), MATE2K, OCT1, organic anion transport protein (OATP) 1B1, and OATP1B3 at clinically relevant concentrations.

■ **Drugs and Foods Affecting Hepatic Microsomal Enzymes** ***Inhibitors of CYP3A*** Concomitant use of ribociclib with potent inhibitors of CYP3A may result in increased peak plasma concentrations and systemic exposure (area under the concentration-time curve [AUC]) of ribociclib. When the potent CYP3A inhibitor ritonavir (100 mg twice daily for 14 days) was administered concomitantly with ribociclib (single 400-mg dose) in healthy individuals, the peak plasma concentrations and AUC of ribociclib were increased by 1.7- and 3.2-fold, respectively. In addition, peak plasma concentrations and AUC of a major metabolite of ribociclib (LEQ803) were decreased by 96 and 98%, respectively. Simulations using physiologically based pharmacokinetic models suggest that moderate inhibitors of CYP3A4 (e.g., erythromycin) may increase the peak plasma concentrations and AUC of ribociclib by 1.3- and 1.9-fold, respectively.

Concomitant use of ribociclib with potent inhibitors of CYP3A (e.g., clarithromycin, conivaptan, indinavir, itraconazole, ketoconazole, lopinavir/ritonavir, nefazodone, nelfinavir, posaconazole, ritonavir, saquinavir, voriconazole) should be avoided, and selection of an alternative drug with less CYP3A inhibition potential should be considered. If concomitant use of a potent CYP3A inhibitor cannot be avoided, the manufacturer recommends dosage reduction of ribociclib to 400 mg once daily. If concomitant use of the potent CYP3A inhibitor is discontinued, the ribociclib dosage should be returned (after at least 5 terminal half-lives of the CYP3A inhibitor) to the dosage used prior to initiation of the potent CYP3A4 inhibitor.

Concomitant use of ribociclib with grapefruit or pomegranate products may increase systemic exposure of ribociclib. Grapefruit and pomegranate are known to inhibit CYP3A. Therefore, grapefruit or pomegranate products should be avoided during ribociclib therapy.

Inducers of CYP3A Concomitant use of ribociclib with potent inducers of CYP3A may result in decreased peak plasma concentrations and AUC of ribociclib. When the potent CYP3A4 inducer rifampin (600 mg twice daily for 14 days) was administered concomitantly with ribociclib (single 600-mg dose) in healthy individuals, the peak plasma concentrations and AUC of ribociclib were decreased by 81 and 89%, respectively. In addition, peak plasma concentrations of LEQ803 increased by 1.7-fold and AUC decreased by 27%. Simulations using physiologically based pharmacokinetic models suggest that moderate inducers of CYP3A (e.g., efavirenz) may decrease the peak plasma concentrations and AUC of ribociclib by 37 and 60%, respectively.

Concomitant use of ribociclib with potent inducers of CYP3A (e.g., carbamazepine, phenytoin, rifampin, St. John's wort [*Hypericum perforatum*]) should be avoided, and selection of an alternative drug with no or minimal CYP3A induction potential should be considered.

■ **Drugs Metabolized by Hepatic Microsomal Enzymes** ***Substrates of CYP3A*** Ribociclib inhibits CYP3A4/5 in vitro and potentially can increase plasma concentrations of other drugs metabolized by CYP3A. When the CYP3A4 substrate midazolam (single 5-mg dose on day 8) was administered concomitantly with ribociclib (400 mg once daily for 8 days), peak plasma concentrations and AUC of midazolam were increased by 2.1- and 3.8-fold, respectively. Simulations using physiologically based pharmacokinetic models suggest that concomitant use of ribociclib 600 mg once daily with midazolam may increase the peak plasma concentrations and AUC of midazolam by 2.4- and 5.2-fold, respectively. The manufacturer states that caution should be exercised and that a dosage reduction of the substrate drug should be considered when ribociclib is administered concomitantly with CYP3A substrates that have a narrow therapeutic index (e.g., alfentanil, cyclosporine, dihydroergotamine, ergotamine, everolimus, fentanyl, sirolimus, tacrolimus).

Substrates of CYP1A2 Ribociclib is a weak inhibitor of CYP1A2 at clinically relevant concentrations. When the CYP1A2 substrate caffeine (single 100-mg dose on day 8) was administered concomitantly with ribociclib (400 mg once daily for 8 days), peak plasma concentrations of caffeine decreased by 10% and AUC increased by 20%.

■ **Drugs Affecting Gastric Acidity** In a population pharmacokinetic analysis, concomitant administration of ribociclib and drugs that increase gastric pH (e.g., proton-pump inhibitors) did not appear to affect the absorption of ribociclib. Simulations using physiologically based pharmacokinetic models suggest that drugs affecting gastric acidity are not expected to affect the pharmacokinetics of ribociclib.

■ **Drugs that Prolong the QT Interval** Concomitant use of ribociclib with antiarrhythmic agents (e.g., amiodarone, disopyramide, procainamide, quinidine, sotalol) or other drugs that prolong the QT interval (e.g., bepridil [no longer commercially available in the US], chloroquine, clarithromycin, haloperidol, methadone, moxifloxacin, IV ondansetron, pimozide) should be avoided. (See Prolongation of QT Interval under Cautions: Warnings/Precautions.)

■ **Anastrozole** Concomitant administration of ribociclib and anastrozole did not affect the pharmacokinetics of either drug.

■ **Exemestane** Concomitant administration of ribociclib and exemestane did not affect the pharmacokinetics of either drug.

■ **Letrozole** Concomitant administration of ribociclib and letrozole did not affect the pharmacokinetics of either drug.

Description

Ribociclib, a selective inhibitor of cyclin-dependent kinases 4 (CDK4) and 6 (CDK6), is an antineoplastic agent. Several mechanisms contribute to the dysregulation of the cell cycle during the G1 into S phase, including amplification or overexpression of the cyclin D oncogene or the loss of intrinsic CDK inhibitors (i.e., p16, p15, p18, p19, p21, p27, p57) in breast cancer. Ribociclib specifically inhibits CDK4 and CDK6 and blocks the interaction of CDK4 and CDK6 with cyclin D, resulting in inhibition of phosphorylation of the tumor suppressor protein retinoblastoma and inhibition of progression of the cell cycle from the G1 into S phase. In vitro, ribociclib has demonstrated decreased phosphorylation of retinoblastoma protein and reduced cellular proliferation of breast cancer cell lines by inhibiting the G1 into S phase of the cell cycle. In addition, ribociclib reduced tumor volume, which correlated with inhibition of retinoblastoma protein phosphorylation, in xenograft models of human cancer. The combination of ribociclib and an antiestrogen agent (e.g., letrozole) also has demonstrated increased inhibition of tumor growth compared with either drug alone in patient-derived estrogen receptor-positive breast tumor xenografts.

Area under the serum concentration-time curve (AUC) and peak plasma concentrations of ribociclib are more than dose proportional over a dosage range of 50–1200 mg. Peak plasma concentrations of ribociclib are achieved about 1–4 hours following oral administration of the drug. Following repeated doses of ribociclib 600 mg once daily, steady-state concentrations of the drug were achieved in 8 days and the mean accumulation ratio for the drug was 2.5. Oral administration of ribociclib with a high-fat, high-calorie meal (approximately 800–1000 calories with fat accounting for approximately 50% of the caloric content) did not affect the rate or extent of absorption of the drug. Ribociclib is approximately 70% bound to plasma proteins. Ribociclib is metabolized mainly in the liver via oxidation by cytochrome P-450 (CYP) isoenzyme 3A4. Clinical activity from the main circulating metabolites (CCI284, LEQ803, and a secondary glucuronide) is negligible, and these metabolites account for 18–22% of total plasma concentrations of the drug. Following oral administration of a single radiolabeled dose of ribociclib, 69% of the radioactivity was recovered in feces and 23% was recovered in urine. The mean plasma elimination half-life of the drug is 29.7–54.7 hours.

Population pharmacokinetic analysis indicated that age (23–84 years), gender, race, and body weight do not have clinically important effects on the exposure of ribociclib.

Advice to Patients

Importance of advising patients to swallow ribociclib succinate tablets whole and *not* to break, chew, crush, or split the tablets.

If a dose is missed or vomited, importance of administering the next dose at the regularly scheduled time; an additional dose should not be administered to make up for a missed dose.

Risk of QT-interval prolongation. Importance of informing clinicians immediately if an abnormal heartbeat or feelings of dizziness or faintness occur.

Risk of hepatotoxicity. Importance of advising patients to immediately report possible symptoms of hepatotoxicity (e.g., fatigue, anorexia, right upper quadrant pain, jaundice, dark urine, bleeding diathesis) to their clinician.

Risk of neutropenia. Importance of informing clinician immediately if signs or symptoms of neutropenia or infection (e.g., fever, chills) occur.

Risk of fetal harm. Necessity of advising women of childbearing potential to use an effective method of contraception during treatment and for at least 3 weeks after discontinuance of therapy. Importance of women informing clinicians if they are or plan to become pregnant. Apprise patient of potential fetal hazard if used during pregnancy.

Importance of advising women to discontinue nursing during therapy and for at least 3 weeks after discontinuance of the drug.

Importance of informing clinicians of existing or contemplated concomitant therapy, including prescription and OTC drugs and dietary or herbal supplements (e.g., St. John's wort), as well as any concomitant illnesses (e.g., hepatic impairment, cardiovascular disease [including congenital long QT syndrome]).

Importance of informing patients of other important precautionary information. (See Cautions.)

Overview® (see Users Guide). For additional information on this drug until a more detailed monograph is developed and published, the manufacturer's labeling should be consulted. It is *essential* that the manufacturer's labeling be consulted for more detailed information on usual cautions, precautions, contraindications, potential drug interactions, laboratory test interferences, and acute toxicity. For further information on the handling of antineoplastic agents, see the ASHP Guidelines on Handling Hazardous Drugs at http://www.ahfsdruginformation.com.

Preparations

Excipients in commercially available drug preparations may have clinically important effects in some individuals; consult specific product labeling for details.

Ribociclib Succinate

Oral

Tablets, film-coated	200 mg (of ribociclib)	**Kisqali®**, Novartis

Ribociclib Succinate Combinations

Oral

Kit	Ribociclib succinate 200 mg (of ribociclib) (21, 42, or 63 film-coated tablets)	**Kisqali® Femara® Co-Pack,** Novartis
	Letrozole 2.5 mg (28 film-coated tablets)	

riTUXimab

■ Rituximab, a chimeric human-murine anti-human antigen CD20 monoclonal antibody, is an antineoplastic agent.

Uses

■ **Non-Hodgkin's Lymphoma** Rituximab is used alone or in combination with other chemotherapy regimens for the treatment of B-cell non-Hodgkin's lymphoma (NHL) and is designated an orphan drug by the US Food and Drug Administration (FDA) for the treatment of this cancer.

Relapsed or Refractory Low-grade or Follicular Non-Hodgkin's Lymphoma **Immunotherapy with Rituximab.** Rituximab is used as a single agent for the treatment of relapsed or refractory low-grade or follicular, antigen CD20-positive, B-cell NHL. Treatment of advanced-stage or relapsed low-grade NHL generally is palliative, and many therapeutic options have been employed, including single-agent chemotherapy, combination chemotherapy and/or radiation therapy, and aggressive management with combination chemotherapy and bone marrow or peripheral stem cell transplantation. Although most patients with relapse of low-grade or follicular NHL initially achieve an objective clinical response to treatment, further relapse eventually occurs, and subsequent therapy is associated with lower response rates and shorter durations of remission. The optimal management of indolent recurrent NHL has not been established, and new therapies are continually being evaluated.

The current indication for use of rituximab in the treatment of relapsed or refractory low-grade or follicular NHL is based on data from noncomparative studies. The use of rituximab for the treatment of relapsed or refractory low-grade or follicular B-cell NHL has been investigated in clinical studies including a total of 296 patients receiving rituximab regimens of 4 or 8 once-weekly doses administered as initial treatment, initial treatment of bulky disease, or retreatment.

In a multicenter, open-label, single-arm study, 166 patients with relapsed or refractory low-grade or follicular B-cell NHL who received rituximab 375 mg/m^2 as an IV infusion once weekly for 4 weeks had an overall response rate of 48% (6% complete responses, 42% partial responses). Patients with bulky disease (tumor masses greater than 10 cm) or with greater than 5000 lymphocytes/mm^3 in the peripheral blood were excluded from the study. The median time to onset of response was 50 days, and the median duration of response was 11.2 months (range: 1.9–42.1 or more months). Resolution of disease-related signs and symptoms was reported in 64% (25/39) of patients with such manifestations (including B symptoms) at the time of study entry. According to multivariate analysis, overall response rate was higher in patients with International Working Formulation (IWF) histologic lymphoma subtypes B, C, or D than in those with subtype A (58 versus 12%). In addition, overall response rate was higher in patients whose largest lesion was less than 5 cm versus greater than 7 cm (maximum, 21 cm) in greatest diameter (53 versus 38%), and in patients with chemosensitive versus chemoresistant relapse (defined as duration of response of less than 3 months) (53 versus 36%). Response rates did not differ according to age, presence of extranodal disease or bone marrow involvement, or history of prior anthracycline therapy. The overall response rate in patients receiving rituximab who had been treated previously with autologous bone marrow transplantation was 78%.

Rituximab also has been administered once weekly in an 8-week regimen. In a multicenter, single-arm study, 37 patients with relapsed or refractory low-grade NHL who received rituximab 375 mg/m^2 as an IV infusion once weekly for 8 weeks had an overall response rate of 57% (14% complete responses, 43% partial responses). The projected median duration of response was 13.4 months (range: 2.5–36.5 or more months). Treatment with 8 weekly doses of rituximab was associated with a higher overall incidence of grade 3 and 4 adverse effects compared with a regimen of 4 weekly doses (70 versus 57%).

Rituximab appears to have activity in patients with relapsed or refractory low-grade NHL who have bulky disease (single lesion exceeding 10 cm in diameter) but is associated with an increased incidence of clinically important adverse events, including neutropenia, anemia, dyspnea, hypotension, and abdominal pain, in such patients. In pooled data from multiple studies, 39 patients with relapsed or refractory, bulky disease, low-grade NHL who received rituximab 375 mg/m^2 as an IV infusion once weekly for 4 weeks had an overall response rate of 36% (3% complete responses, 33% partial responses) and a median duration of response of 6.9 months (range: 2.8–25 or more months).

Responses also have been observed in patients with NHL receiving additional courses of rituximab for refractory disease or for relapse of disease that initially responded to the drug. In a multicenter, single-arm study, an overall response rate of 38% (10% complete responses, 28% partial responses) and a projected median duration of response of 15 months (range: 3–25.1 or more months) were reported in 60 patients receiving retreatment with rituximab 375 mg/m^2 once weekly for 4 weeks for relapsed or refractory, low-grade or follicular B-cell NHL following an objective clinical response to one or more prior courses of rituximab at a median of 14.5 months prior to retreatment. Among the 60 patients, 55 patients received their second course of rituximab, 3 patients received their third course, and 2 patients received both their second and third course of rituximab in the study. The incidence of grade 3 or 4 adverse effects was similar in patients retreated with rituximab and patients receiving initial treatment with rituximab (58 and 57%, respectively).

Maintenance therapy with rituximab following induction chemotherapy (with or without rituximab) has been shown to offer benefit in patients with relapsed or refractory indolent NHL. In a phase 3 randomized trial, progression-free survival was prolonged in patients receiving 2 years of maintenance therapy with rituximab following chemotherapy with cyclophosphamide, vincristine, and prednisone (CVP) for advanced indolent NHL compared with those receiving CVP alone. In another randomized trial, duration of response was prolonged in patients receiving maintenance therapy with rituximab following salvage chemotherapy (with or without rituximab) for recurring or refractory follicular or mantle cell lymphoma compared with those receiving induction chemotherapy alone. In a phase 3 randomized trial, median progression-free survival and median overall survival were prolonged in patients receiving maintenance therapy with rituximab following chemotherapy with either cyclophosphamide, doxorubicin, vincristine, and prednisone (CHOP) or rituximab-CHOP for relapsed or resistant follicular NHL compared with those receiving induction chemotherapy alone.

Radioimmunotherapy with Rituximab and Ibritumomab. Rituximab is used as a required component of a therapeutic regimen with ibritumomab tiuxetan (ibritumomab tiuxetan therapeutic regimen) for the treatment of relapsed or refractory low-grade or follicular B-cell NHL, including follicular NHL that is refractory to rituximab therapy. Limited evidence indicates that the overall response rate is higher in such patients receiving the ibritumomab tiuxetan therapeutic regimen compared with standard rituximab immunotherapy; comparative effects on survival have not been established. The regimen consists of an initial rituximab dose (administered on day 1) and a second rituximab dose (administered on day 7, 8, or 9) followed within 4 hours by a therapeutic dose of yttrium Y 90 ibritumomab tiuxetan. For additional information on the use of rituximab as part of the ibritumomab tiuxetan therapeutic regimen for NHL, see Ibritumomab Tiuxetan 10:00.

Rituximab in Combination with Bendamustine. Efficacy and safety of rituximab in combination with bendamustine† for the treatment of relapsed or refractory indolent NHL or relapsed or refractory mantle cell lymphoma† in patients who had received up to 3 prior treatment regimens has been studied in 2 open-label, phase 2 studies.

In both studies, patients received rituximab 375 mg/m² IV on day 1, followed by bendamustine hydrochloride 90 mg/m² daily as an IV infusion on days 2 and 3, administered on a 28-day cycle for a total of 4 cycles. An additional dose of rituximab was administered one week prior to the first rituximab-bendamustine treatment cycle and repeated at 28 days following the last rituximab-bendamustine treatment cycle. Patients achieving a response between the second and fourth treatment cycles were permitted to receive an additional 2 cycles of rituximab-bendamustine treatment in the second study. Overall response rates in the 2 studies were similar (90–92%), with 41–60% of patients exhibiting complete responses. Overall and complete response rates were higher in patients with no prior exposure to rituximab (100 and 48%, respectively) than in those with prior rituximab exposure (86 and 35%, respectively). Median progression-free survival was similar in both studies (24 and 23 months). At the time of the data analysis, median duration of survival had not been reached in the first study; however, the actuarial 48-month survival rate was 55%.

Small numbers of patients in each study (16 and 12, respectively) had relapsed or refractory mantle cell lymphoma. Overall and complete response rates for these patients were 75–92 and 42–50%, respectively. Median progression-free survival was 18 months in the first study; median response duration was 19 months in the second study.

Based on current evidence and because of the favorable toxicity profile, combination therapy with rituximab and bendamustine is recommended (accepted) for use in the treatment of relapsed or refractory indolent NHL or mantle cell lymphoma.

For further information on the use of combination therapy with rituximab and bendamustine for the treatment of relapsed or refractory indolent NHL or mantle cell lymphoma, see Relapsed or Refractory Non-Hodgkin's Lymphoma or Mantle Cell Lymphoma under Uses: Non-Hodgkin's Lymphoma, in Bendamustine 10:00.

Previously Untreated Follicular Non-Hodgkin's Lymphoma

Immunotherapy with Rituximab. Rituximab is used in combination with chemotherapy for the treatment of previously untreated follicular, antigen CD20-positive, B-cell NHL.

In an open-label, multicenter, randomized trial, 322 patients with previously untreated follicular B-cell NHL received either rituximab with cyclophosphamide, vincristine, and prednisone (CVP) or CVP alone. CVP was administered in eight 3-week cycles; in the combined modality regimen, rituximab 375 mg/m² was administered on day 1 of each cycle of CVP. Among patients receiving rituximab, 85% received the maximum dosage (a total of 8 doses). The median age of the patients was 52 years, and 26% of the patients were 60 years of age or older. Most of the patients had stage III or IV disease, 50% had an International Prognostic Index score of at least 2, and the diagnosis of follicular NHL was centrally confirmed in 95% of the patients.

Median progression-free survival was prolonged in patients with advanced follicular NHL receiving rituximab with CVP (2.4 years) compared with those receiving CVP alone (1.4 years). The risk of disease progression, relapse, or death was reduced (hazard ratio: 0.44, range: 0.29–0.65) in patients receiving the rituximab-containing regimen. Patients receiving rituximab and CVP experienced higher incidences of neutropenia (8 versus 3%) and infusion-related toxicity, including rash (17 versus 5%), cough (15 versus 6%), flushing (14 versus 3%), rigors (10 versus 2%), pruritus (10 versus 1%), and chest tightness (7 versus 1%) than those receiving CVP alone.

Radioimmunotherapy with Rituximab and Ibritumomab. Rituximab is used as a required component of a therapeutic regimen with ibritumomab tiuxetan (ibritumomab tiuxetan therapeutic regimen) for consolidation treatment of newly diagnosed follicular NHL in patients who have achieved partial or complete response to first-line induction chemotherapy. Data from a phase 3, open-label study indicate that median progression-free survival is longer in such patients receiving consolidation therapy with the ibritumomab tiuxetan therapeutic regimen compared with those receiving no further treatment; comparative effects on survival have not been established. The regimen consists of an initial rituximab dose (administered on day 1) and a second rituximab dose (administered on day 7, 8, or 9) followed within 4 hours by a therapeutic dose of yttrium Y 90 ibritumomab tiuxetan. For additional information on the use of rituximab as part of the ibritumomab tiuxetan therapeutic regimen for NHL, see Ibritumomab Tiuxetan 10:00.

Previously Untreated Indolent Non-Hodgkin's Lymphoma or Mantle Cell Lymphoma Efficacy and safety of rituximab in combination with bendamustine† for the treatment of previously untreated advanced-stage indolent NHL or previously untreated advanced-stage mantle cell lymphoma† have been studied in two phase 3 studies (Study Group Indolent Lymphomas [StiL] NHL 1-2003 and BRIGHT).

In the StiL NHL 1-2003 study in 514 patients with previously untreated mantle cell lymphoma or CD20-positive indolent NHL, rituximab in combination with bendamustine was noninferior to rituximab in combination with cyclophosphamide, doxorubicin, vincristine, and prednisone (R-CHOP) in terms of progression-free survival; median progression-free survival was 69.5 and 31.2 months in patients receiving rituximab in combination with bendamustine and those receiving R-CHOP, respectively. Overall response rates were similar in patients receiving rituximab in combination with bendamustine and those receiving R-CHOP (93 versus 91%, respectively); however, the complete response rate was higher in the rituximab-bendamustine group (40 versus 30%). Although median overall survival had not been reached in either group at the time of analysis, substantial differences were not observed between the treatment groups.

In the BRIGHT study in 447 patients with previously untreated mantle cell lymphoma or CD20-positive indolent NHL, rituximab in combination with bendamustine was noninferior to standard combination chemotherapy (R-CHOP or rituximab in combination with cyclophosphamide, vincristine, and prednisone [R-CVP]) for attainment of complete response; complete response was achieved in 31% of patients receiving rituximab in combination with bendamustine and 25% of those receiving R-CHOP or R-CVP. Although complete response rates in patients with indolent NHL (mainly follicular lymphoma) tended to favor the rituximab-bendamustine regimen over R-CHOP or R-CVP, subset analysis failed to establish noninferiority of the rituximab-bendamustine regimen in patients with indolent NHL or follicular lymphoma. In the subset of patients with mantle cell lymphoma, complete response rates were higher in patients receiving rituximab in combination with bendamustine compared with those receiving R-CHOP or R-CVP. Overall response rates were higher in patients receiving rituximab in combination with bendamustine compared with those receiving R-CHOP or R-CVP (97 versus 91%).

Based on current evidence, use of rituximab in combination with bendamustine may be considered a reasonable choice (accepted, with possible conditions) for the treatment of previously untreated advanced-stage indolent NHL or mantle cell lymphoma; however, the histologic subtype of NHL should be considered when selecting a combination chemotherapy regimen.

For further information on the use of combination therapy with rituximab and bendamustine for the treatment of previously untreated advanced-stage indolent NHL or mantle cell lymphoma, see Previously Untreated, Indolent Non-Hodgkin's Lymphoma or Mantle Cell Lymphoma under Uses: Non-Hodgkin's Lymphoma, in Bendamustine 10:00.

Nonprogressing Low-grade Non-Hodgkin's Lymphoma Rituximab is used as a single agent for the treatment of nonprogressing (including stable disease) low-grade, antigen CD20-positive, B-cell NHL following first-line combination chemotherapy with cyclophosphamide, vincristine, and prednisone (CVP). This indication is based on data from an open-label, multicenter, randomized trial in which 322 patients with previously untreated low-grade B-cell NHL (IWF histologic subtype A, B, or C) received 6 or 8 cycles of CVP followed by rituximab or no further treatment.

In the combined modality regimen, patients received rituximab 375 mg/m² once weekly for 4 weeks (4 doses total) every 6 months for up to 16 doses total; 59% of the patients received the maximum dosage of rituximab. The median age of patients receiving rituximab was 58 years; 37% of the patients in the study were 60 years of age or older. Most of the patients had stage III or IV disease, 63% had an International Prognostic Index score of at least 2, and the diagnosis of low-grade NHL was centrally confirmed in 62% of the patients.

The risk of disease progression, relapse, or death was reduced (estimated hazard ratio: 0.36–0.49) in patients receiving the rituximab-containing regimen. Patients receiving rituximab following CVP experienced higher incidences of grade 3 or 4 neutropenia (4 versus 1%) than those receiving no further treatment; other adverse effects that occurred more frequently in patients receiving rituximab included fatigue (39 versus 14%), anemia (35 versus 20%), peripheral sensory neuropathy (30 versus 18%), infection (19 versus 9%), pulmonary toxicity (18 versus 10%), hepatobiliary toxicity (17 versus 7%), rash and/or pruritus (17 versus 5%), arthralgia (12 versus 3%), and weight gain (11 versus 4%).

Previously Untreated Diffuse Large B-cell Non-Hodgkin's Lymphoma Rituximab is used in combination with cyclophosphamide, doxorubicin, vincristine, and prednisone (CHOP) or other anthracycline-based regimens for the treatment of previously untreated diffuse large B-cell, antigen CD20-positive, NHL. This indication is based on data from 3 open-label, multicenter, randomized trials involving a total of 1854 patients who received rituximab with combination chemotherapy (CHOP or other anthracycline-based regimen) or combination chemotherapy alone for previously untreated diffuse large B-cell NHL. The addition of rituximab to chemotherapy was shown to offer benefit in older patients with advanced-stage disease as well as younger patients with early-stage disease.

In the first randomized trial (the NCI-sponsored E4494 trial), 632 patients (60 years of age or older) with diffuse large B-cell NHL (IWF histologic subtype F, G, or H B-cell NHL or diffuse large B-cell NHL including primary mediastinal B-cell lymphoma according to the Revised European-American Lymphoma [REAL] classification) received 6 or 8 cycles of CHOP with or without rituximab 375 mg/m² (2 doses preceding the first 21-day cycle of chemotherapy and then 1 dose preceding cycles 3, 5, and 7 for a total of 4 or 5 doses). Most of the patients (73%) had stage III or IV disease, 30% had extranodal disease in at least 2 sites, 56% had an International Prognostic Index score of at least 2, 86% had an ECOG performance status less than 2, and the diagnosis of diffuse large B-cell NHL was centrally confirmed in 62% of the patients. Median progression-free survival was prolonged in patients with diffuse large B-cell NHL receiving rituximab and CHOP (3.1 years) compared with those receiving CHOP alone (1.6 years). The risk of disease progression, relapse, or death was reduced (hazard ratio: 0.69) in patients receiving the rituximab-containing regimen. Patients with disease that responded to treatment with rituximab and CHOP then received either additional rituximab therapy or no further therapy. The statistical evaluation of the data for induction therapy with rituximab was designed to exclude the effect of additional rituximab therapy; additional rituximab therapy did not affect survival.

In the second randomized trial (the Groupe d'Etude des Lymphomes de l'Adulte trial), 399 patients (60 years of age or older, median age: 69 years) with diffuse large B-cell NHL received up to 8 cycles of CHOP with or without rituximab 375 mg/m^2 on day 1 of each 21-day cycle. Most of the patients (80%) had stage III or IV disease, 52% had extranodal disease in at least 2 sites, 60% had an age-adjusted International Prognostic Index score of at least 2, and 80% had an ECOG performance status less than 2. Median event-free survival was prolonged in patients with diffuse large B-cell NHL receiving rituximab and CHOP (2.9 years) compared with those receiving CHOP alone (1.1 years). The risk of disease progression, relapse, change in therapy, or death from any cause was reduced (hazard ratio: 0.60) in patients receiving the rituximab-containing regimen. Estimated overall survival at 5 years was 58% for patients receiving rituximab-CHOP versus 46% for patients receiving CHOP alone.

In the third randomized trial (the MabThera International Trial M39045), 823 patients (18–60 years of age) with diffuse large B-cell NHL received an anthracycline-containing chemotherapy regimen with or without rituximab. Among all patients, 28% had stage III or IV disease, 49% had bulky disease, and 34% had extranodal disease; 100% had an International Prognostic Index score of 1 or less, and 99% had an ECOG performance status less than 2. The main end point of the study was time to treatment failure. The risk of disease progression, failure to achieve a complete response, relapse, or death was reduced (hazard ratio: 0.45) in patients receiving the rituximab-containing regimen.

Patients with diffuse large B-cell NHL receiving rituximab and CHOP in clinical trials experienced a higher incidence of certain adverse effects. Grade 3 or 4 thrombocytopenia (9 versus 7%) and grade 3 or 4 lung disorder (6 versus 3%) occurred more frequently in patients receiving rituximab-CHOP than in those receiving CHOP alone. Other adverse effects that occurred more frequently in patients 60 years of age or older who received rituximab and CHOP included pyrexia (56 versus 46%), lung disorder (31 versus 24%), cardiac disorder (29 versus 21%), and chills (13 versus 4%). In the second randomized trial, the higher incidence of cardiac disorders in patients receiving rituximab and CHOP was caused mainly by increased frequency of supraventricular arrhythmias or tachycardia (4.5 versus 1%). Other severe adverse effects that occurred more frequently in patients receiving rituximab and CHOP than in those receiving CHOP alone (in one or more studies) were viral infection, neutropenia, and anemia.

Responses to rituximab therapy have been observed in patients with recurrent aggressive antigen CD20-positive NHL†.

■ **Chronic Lymphocytic Leukemia** Rituximab is used in combination with fludarabine and cyclophosphamide (R-FC) for the treatment of previously untreated and previously treated antigen CD20-positive chronic lymphocytic leukemia (CLL). Rituximab is designated an orphan drug by FDA for the treatment of this cancer.

Previously Untreated Chronic Lymphocytic Leukemia Rituximab is used in combination with fludarabine and cyclophosphamide (R-FC) for the treatment of previously untreated antigen CD20-positive chronic lymphocytic leukemia (CLL). This indication is based principally on the results of a multicenter, open-label, randomized study (CLL8) in which 817 adult patients with previously untreated CLL were randomized to receive 6 cycles of either FC (fludarabine 25 mg/m^2 and cyclophosphamide 250 mg/m^2, administered IV on days 1–3 of each 28-day cycle) or FC in combination with rituximab (rituximab 375 mg/m^2 administered by IV infusion on day 0 during the first FC cycle, followed by rituximab 500 mg/m^2 IV on day 1 during subsequent FC cycles). The median age of patients in this study was 61 years, and 30% of the patients were 65 years of age or older. Approximately 5, 64, or 31% of patients in this study had Binet stage A, stage B, or stage C disease, respectively. More than 99% of patients had an ECOG performance status of 0–1.

At a median follow-up of 37.7 months, patients receiving R-FC experienced prolonged median progression-free survival (51.8 versus 32.8 months), a higher overall response rate (95 versus 88%), a higher complete response rate (44 versus 22%), and a higher overall survival rate (84 versus 79%, although median survival has not been reached) compared with patients receiving FC. In patients receiving R-FC, the largest benefit on progression-free survival, overall response, and complete response was observed in those with Binet stage A or stage B CLL; in addition, only patients with Binet stage A or stage B CLL experienced an improved benefit in overall survival. Based on results of an exploratory analysis (stratified by age), the addition of rituximab to FC resulted in no additional benefit in progression-free survival in patients 70 years of age or older.

Patients receiving R-FC experienced higher incidences of adverse hematologic effects (i.e., neutropenia, leukopenia, febrile neutropenia, pancytopenia) compared with those receiving FC; however, this was not associated with an increase in infection rate. Patients receiving R-FC also experienced a higher incidence of infusion-related effects. The treatment-related mortality rate was similar (2%) in patients receiving R-FC compared with those receiving FC.

Previously Treated Chronic Lymphocytic Leukemia Rituximab is used in combination with fludarabine and cyclophosphamide (R-FC) for the treatment of previously treated antigen CD20-positive chronic lymphocytic leukemia (CLL). This indication is based principally on the results of a multicenter, open-label, randomized study (REACH) in which 552 adult patients with previously treated CLL were randomized to receive 6 cycles of either FC (fludarabine 25 mg/m^2 and cyclophosphamide 250 mg/m^2, administered IV on days 1–3 of each 28-day cycle) or FC in combination with rituximab (rituximab 375 mg/m^2 administered by IV infusion on day 0 during the first FC cycle, followed by 500 mg/m^2 IV on day 1 during subsequent FC cycles). The median age in this study was 63 years, and 44% of the patients were 65 years of age or older. Approximately 9, 60, or 31% of patients in this study had Binet stage A, stage B, or stage C disease, respectively. Most patients (82%) had received previous treatment with an alkylating agent (27% alkylator refractory, 55% alkylator sensitive), and 17% had previously received (and demonstrated response to) fludarabine; fludarabine-refractory patients or patients who had received previous treatment with interferon, rituximab, other monoclonal antibodies, or stem-cell transplantation were excluded from the study. All patients had an ECOG performance status of 0–1.

At a median follow-up of 25 months, patients receiving R-FC experienced prolonged median progression-free survival (27 versus 21.9 months), a higher overall response rate (61 versus 49%), and a higher complete response rate (9 versus 3%) compared with patients receiving FC. Among patients receiving R-FC, improved progression-free survival was observed in patients across all Binet stages as well as in patients with high lymphocyte counts, poor renal function, or poor prognostic factors (e.g., del11q, unmutated IgVH, positive ZAP-70). Based on results of an exploratory analysis (stratified by age), the addition of rituximab to FC resulted in no additional benefit in progression-free survival in patients 65 years or older. No difference in overall survival has been observed with the R-FC regimen compared with the FC regimen.

Patients receiving R-FC experienced higher incidences of grade 3 or 4 neutropenia; however, this was not associated with an increase in the overall incidence of infections or grade 3 or 4 infections. Hepatitis B (primary infection and reactivation) was reported in 3% of patients receiving R-FC and in less than 1% of those receiving FC.

■ **Rheumatoid Arthritis** Rituximab in combination with methotrexate is used for the treatment of moderately to severely active rheumatoid arthritis (RA) in adults with disease that has shown an inadequate response to therapy with at least one tumor necrosis factor (TNF; TNF-α) antagonist. This indication is based mainly on data from 2 randomized, double-blind, placebo-controlled studies in patients at least 18 years of age who had a diagnosis of RA according to American College of Rheumatology (ACR) criteria and had active disease (at least 8 swollen joints and 8 tender joints).

In the first randomized study, patients received an IV infusion of either rituximab 1 g or placebo on days 1 and 15 (for a total of 2 doses) in combination with continued therapy with oral or parenteral methotrexate 10–25 mg weekly for 24 weeks. Patients were permitted to receive additional courses of rituximab (given as 2 separate doses of 1 g each) in combination with methotrexate in an open-label extension study at intervals determined by clinical evaluation, but no sooner than 16 weeks after the previous dose of rituximab. IV glucocorticoid was administered prior to each rituximab infusion, and oral glucocorticoid was administered on a tapering schedule from baseline through day 14. At 24 weeks, the number of patients achieving a response measured as a percentage improvement (20%, 50%, or 70%) in disease symptoms according to ACR criteria was higher for those receiving rituximab and methotrexate compared with those receiving placebo and methotrexate (ACR 20: 51 versus 18%, ACR 50: 27 versus 5%, ACR 70: 12 versus 1%). Favorable responses were noted for all components of the ACR response including reduced counts for swollen and tender joints, improvement according to physician and patient global assessments, reduced pain, reduced disability, and reduced serum C-reactive protein (CRP) concentrations. Although all patients experienced similar benefits at week 4 following a brief course of IV and oral glucocorticoids, the number of patients experiencing ACR responses (at all levels) from week 8 through week 24 was higher among those receiving rituximab and methotrexate. Results of the open-label extension study indicate that the combination of rituximab and methotrexate is more effective than methotrexate alone in delaying radiographic progression of structural damage (defined as changes in the Genant-modified total Sharp score [TSS], erosion score [ES], and joint space narrowing [JSN] score) after one year of therapy; progression of structural damage was further delayed following 2 years of therapy. Approximately 57% of patients receiving rituximab in combination with methotrexate had no progression of structural damage after 2 years of therapy.

In the second randomized study, all patients received the first course of rituximab (2 separate doses of 1 g each) in combination with methotrexate. Patients who experienced ongoing disease activity were randomized to receive either a second course of rituximab (2 separate doses of 1 g each) in combination with methotrexate or placebo in combination with methotrexate, generally between weeks 24–28. At week 48, 54, 29, or 14% of patients receiving rituximab in combination with methotrexate achieved ACR 20, ACR 50, or ACR 70, respectively, compared with 45, 26, or 13%, respectively, of those receiving methotrexate alone.

Efficacy of rituximab has been established in 4 controlled studies in patients with RA who had an inadequate response to nonbiologic disease-modifying antirheumatic drugs (DMARDs) and in one controlled study in methotrexate-naive patients; however, a favorable risk-benefit ratio has not been established for the use of rituximab in these patient populations. In one of the 4 controlled studies, 342 adult patients with moderately to severely active RA who had an inadequate response to methotrexate were randomized to receive methotrexate in combination with either rituximab 1 g (given as 2 separate does of 500 mg each), rituximab 2 g (given as 2 separate does of 1 g each), or placebo. At 24 weeks, more patients receiving methotrexate in combination with rituximab 2 g had clinically meaningful improvement in physical function, as reflected by improvement in the Health Assessment Questionnaire Disability Index (HAQ-DI) score, than patients receiving methotrexate with placebo (58 versus 48%). In addition, patients receiving methotrexate in combination with rituximab experienced greater improvement from baseline in HAQ-DI score at 24 weeks than did patients receiving methotrexate with placebo. These improvements were maintained at 48 weeks. Improvements in HAQ-DI score observed with the 2 rituximab dosages (1 g or 2 g) were similar; however, radiographic responses were not assessed. In another randomized study, 161 patients with active RA despite treatment with methotrexate received one of the following regimens: oral methotrexate (at least 10 mg weekly), rituximab (1 g IV on days 1 and 15), rituximab (same dosage) and cyclophosphamide (750 mg IV on days 3 and 17), or rituximab (same dosage) and methotrexate (at least 10 mg weekly). At week 24, the proportion of patients achieving an ACR 50 response was greater in those receiving rituximab-methotrexate (43%) or rituximab-cyclophosphamide (41%) than in those receiving methotrexate alone (13%). Responses at all levels of improvement (i.e., ACR 20, 50, and 70 responses) were maintained at week 48 in the rituximab-methotrexate group.

Efficacy of rituximab also has been established in one randomized, double-blind, placebo-controlled study in methotrexate-naive patients. In this study, patients with moderately to severely active RA were randomized to receive methotrexate (7.5 mg weekly initially, then titrated up to 20 mg weekly by week 8) in combination with either rituximab 1 g (500 mg IV on days 1 and 15), rituximab 2 g (1 g IV on days 1 and 15), or placebo. After a minimum of 24 weeks, patients with ongoing disease activity were permitted to receive retreatment with additional courses of their assigned treatment. Following one year of therapy, the proportion of patients achieving ACR 20, ACR 50, or ACR 70 was similar among those receiving methotrexate with either dose of rituximab, which was higher than the proportion of patients receiving methotrexate with placebo. However, only the combination of methotrexate with high dose rituximab (2 g) was shown to be more effective than methotrexate alone in delaying radiographic progression of structural damage (as assessed by TSS). Despite the demonstrated efficacy in patients who had an inadequate response to DMARDs and in methotrexate-naive patients, a favorable risk-benefit ratio has not been established for the use of rituximab in these patient populations; therefore, the use of rituximab for RA in patients with disease that has no prior inadequate response to one or more TNF antagonists currently is *not* recommended.

Adverse effects during the 24-hour period following the first infusion, such as acute infusion reactions, occurred more frequently in patients receiving rituximab-methotrexate than in those receiving placebo-methotrexate (overall adverse effects: 32 versus 23%, acute infusion reactions: 27 versus 19%).

■ **Other Uses** Rituximab has been used in the treatment of other forms of NHL, including lymphoplasmacytic lymphoma (Waldenstrom's macroglobulinemia)†. Rituximab also has been used in the treatment of relapsed or refractory hairy cell leukemia†.

Rituximab has been used for the treatment of idiopathic thrombocytopenic purpura (ITP; also known as immune thrombocytopenic purpura)† in adult patients. Results of a meta-analysis indicated an overall response (platelet counts exceeding 50,000/mm³) or complete response (platelet counts exceeding 150,000/mm³) rate of approximately 63 or 46%, respectively; however, because of the lack of controlled randomized studies, efficacy of rituximab compared with standard treatments for ITP cannot be determined, and indiscriminate use of rituximab for the treatment of ITP in adult patients should be *avoided.* Rituximab also has been used in children with severe chronic ITP refractory to standard therapy†. However, because of the low response rate (30–60%) and potentially serious adverse effects (including progressive multifocal leukoencephalopathy [PML]), some experts recommend that rituximab be reserved for pediatric patients with chronic ITP who have failed splenectomy.

Rituximab and immune globulin IV has been used in the treatment of refractory pemphigus vulgaris†.

Dosage and Administration

■ **Reconstitution and Administration** Rituximab is administered by IV infusion. Rituximab solutions should *not* be administered undiluted nor by rapid IV injection.

Rituximab for injection concentrate *must* be diluted prior to IV infusion. For IV infusion, the appropriate dose of rituximab for injection concentrate should be withdrawn and diluted in the appropriate volume of 0.9% sodium chloride or 5% dextrose injection to yield a final rituximab concentration of 1–4 mg/mL. Aseptic technique should be used, and the IV bag should be gently inverted to mix the solution. Any unused solution remaining in the vial should be discarded. No other drug should be added to or administered in the same IV line with rituximab infusion. Prior to administration, rituximab solutions should be inspected visually for particulate matter and discoloration. If particulate matter or discoloration is evident, the solution should not be used.

The initial rituximab dose should be infused at an initial rate of 50 mg/hour; if infusion-related events do not occur, the infusion rate may be increased in increments of 50 mg/hour every 30 minutes to a maximum infusion rate of 400 mg/hour. In patients who tolerate the first infusion well, subsequent rituximab infusions may be administered at an initial infusion rate of 100 mg/hour; the rate of infusion may be increased in increments of 100 mg/hour every 30 minutes as tolerated to a maximum infusion rate of 400 mg/hour.

Patients with previously untreated follicular non-Hodgkin's lymphoma (NHL) or previously untreated diffuse large B-cell NHL who are receiving rituximab in combination with a glucocorticoid-containing chemotherapy regimen may receive the second rituximab dose at an accelerated infusion rate if they tolerate the first dose (administered at the standard rate) without experiencing grade 3 or 4 infusion-related events. In such patients, the second rituximab infusion may be administered over a total infusion time of 90 minutes, with 20% of the total dose administered over the first 30 minutes and the remaining 80% of the total dose administered over the next 60 minutes. Those who tolerate this 90-minute infusion may receive subsequent rituximab doses (through cycle 6 or 8) at the same 90-minute infusion rate. Patients should receive the glucocorticoid component of the chemotherapy regimen prior to each rituximab infusion to reduce the incidence and severity of infusion reactions. Patients with clinically important cardiovascular disease (i.e., uncontrolled hypertension, myocardial infarction [MI], unstable angina, New York Heart Association [NYHA] functional class II or greater congestive heart failure [CHF], ventricular arrhythmia requiring medication within the past year, NYHA class II or greater peripheral vascular disease) or with a high circulating lymphocyte count (5000/mm³ or greater) before cycle 2 should *not* receive rituximab over 90 minutes, as these patients were excluded from the phase 3 noncomparative trial (RATE) evaluating this infusion rate.

■ **Dosage** To minimize the risk of infusion-related events (see Cautions: Infusion-Related Effects) associated with rituximab, premedication with acetaminophen and an antihistamine is recommended before each infusion of the drug. Because transient hypotension may occur during administration of rituximab, it may be appropriate to withhold antihypertensive therapy during the 12-hour period preceding each rituximab infusion.

Non-Hodgkin's Lymphoma **Immunotherapy for Relapsed or Refractory Low-grade or Follicular Non-Hodgkin's Lymphoma.** For the treatment of relapsed or refractory low-grade or follicular, antigen CD20-positive, B-cell NHL, the recommended dosage of rituximab is 375 mg/m² administered by IV infusion once weekly for 4 weeks or 8 weeks. Patients who subsequently develop progressive disease following response to previous rituximab therapy may receive an additional course of rituximab 375 mg/m² by IV infusion once weekly for 4 weeks.

Radiotherapy for Relapsed or Refractory Low-grade or Follicular Non-Hodgkin's Lymphoma. When used in conjunction with ibritumomab as a component of a radioimmunotherapeutic regimen for relapsed or refractory low-grade or follicular B-cell NHL, rituximab 250 mg/m² should be infused on day 1 and then again on day 7, 8, or 9; the second dose of rituximab should be followed within 4 hours by a therapeutic dose of yttrium Y 90 ibritumomab tiuxetan. For additional dosage information regarding the use of rituximab as part of the ibritumomab tiuxetan therapeutic regimen, see Ibritumomab Tiuxetan 10:00.

Combination Therapy for Relapsed or Refractory Indolent Non-Hodgkin's Lymphoma or Mantle Cell Lymphoma. When rituximab has been used in combination with bendamustine† in adults with relapsed or refractory indolent NHL or relapsed or refractory mantle cell lymphoma†, rituximab 375 mg/m² has been administered by IV infusion on day 1, followed by IV infusion (over 30–60 minutes) of bendamustine hydrochloride 90 mg/m² on days 2 and 3. The bendamustine-rituximab regimen has been administered on a 28-day cycle for a total of 4–6 cycles. An additional dose of rituximab has been administered one week prior to the first bendamustine-rituximab treatment cycle and repeated at 28 days following the last bendamustine-rituximab treatment cycle.

Previously Untreated Follicular Non-Hodgkin's Lymphoma. For the treatment of previously untreated follicular, antigen CD20-positive, B-cell NHL, the recommended dosage of rituximab is 375 mg/m² administered by IV infusion on day 1 of each cycle of chemotherapy for up to 8 doses.

When used in conjunction with ibritumomab as a component of a radioimmunotherapeutic regimen for consolidation treatment of follicular NHL in patients who have achieved partial or complete response to first-line induction chemotherapy, rituximab 250 mg/m² should be infused on day 1 and then again on day 7, 8, or 9; the second dose of rituximab should be followed within 4 hours by a therapeutic dose of yttrium Y 90 ibritumomab tiuxetan. For additional dosage information regarding the use of rituximab as part of the ibritumomab tiuxetan therapeutic regimen, see Ibritumomab Tiuxetan 10:00.

Combination Therapy for Previously Untreated Indolent Non-Hodgkin's Lymphoma or Mantle Cell Lymphoma. When rituximab has been used in combination with bendamustine† in adults with previously untreated advanced-stage indolent NHL or previously untreated advanced-stage mantle cell lymphoma†, rituximab 375 mg/m² has been administered by IV infusion on day 1, followed by IV infusion (over 30–60 minutes) of bendamustine hydrochloride 90 mg/m² on days 1 and 2. The bendamustine-rituximab regimen has been administered on a 28-day cycle for up to 8 cycles.

Nonprogressing, Low-grade Non-Hodgkin's Lymphoma. For the treatment of nonprogressing (including stable disease), low-grade, antigen CD20-positive, B-cell NHL following first-line therapy with 6–8 cycles of chemotherapy with cyclophosphamide, vincristine, and prednisone (CVP), the recommended dosage of rituximab is 375 mg/m² administered by IV infusion once weekly for 4 doses every 6 months for up to 16 doses total.

Previously Untreated Diffuse Large B-cell Non-Hodgkin's Lymphoma. For the treatment of previously untreated diffuse large B-cell NHL, the recommended dosage of rituximab is 375 mg/m^2 administered by IV infusion on day 1 of each cycle of chemotherapy (such as cyclophosphamide, doxorubicin, vincristine, and prednisone [CHOP]) for up to 8 doses total.

Chronic Lymphocytic Leukemia For patients receiving rituximab in combination with fludarabine and cyclophosphamide for chronic lymphocytic leukemia, prophylaxis against *Pneumocystis jiroveci* (formerly *Pneumocystis carinii*) pneumonia (PCP) (i.e., co-trimoxazole) and herpes virus infection (i.e., acyclovir/valacyclovir) is recommended during treatment and for up to 12 months following discontinuance of therapy.

Previously Untreated Chronic Lymphocytic Leukemia. For the treatment of previously untreated antigen CD20-positive chronic lymphocytic leukemia, the recommended dosage of rituximab is 375 mg/m^2 administered by IV infusion on day 0 of the *first* cycle of chemotherapy with fludarabine and cyclophosphamide (FC, administered on days 1–3 of each 28-day cycle), followed by 500 mg/m^2 administered by IV infusion on day 1 of *subsequent* FC cycles (cycles 2–6, administered every 28 days), for up to 6 doses total.

Previously Treated Chronic Lymphocytic Leukemia. For the treatment of previously treated antigen CD20-positive chronic lymphocytic leukemia, the recommended dosage of rituximab is 375 mg/m^2 administered by IV infusion on day 0 of the *first* cycle of chemotherapy with fludarabine and cyclophosphamide (FC, administered on days 1–3 of each 28-day cycle), followed by 500 mg/m^2 administered by IV infusion on day 1 of *subsequent* FC cycles (cycles 2–6, administered every 28 days), for up to 6 doses total.

Rheumatoid Arthritis For patients receiving rituximab for rheumatoid arthritis, glucocorticoid (methylprednisolone 100 mg IV or its equivalent) should be administered 30 minutes prior to each infusion to reduce the incidence and severity of infusion reactions.

When used in combination with methotrexate to reduce the signs and symptoms of moderately to severely active rheumatoid arthritis (RA) in adults with disease that has shown an inadequate response to therapy with at least one tumor necrosis factor (TNF; TNF-α) antagonist, rituximab 1 g is administered as an IV infusion on days 1 and 15 (for a total of 2 doses per course). Subsequent courses of rituximab and methotrexate may be administered every 24 weeks or based on clinical evaluation, but not sooner than every 16 weeks.

Dosage Modification for Toxicity and Contraindications for Continued Therapy Depending on the severity of the symptoms, the manufacturer recommends temporary or permanent discontinuance of rituximab when severe adverse effects occur; slower infusion rates should be employed when rituximab therapy is reinitiated following interruption of the infusion because of severe drug-related reactions (e.g., infusion-related effects).

Infusion-related Effects. In patients experiencing signs and symptoms of a severe infusion reaction (e.g., urticaria, hypotension, angioedema, hypoxia, bronchospasm, pulmonary infiltrates, acute respiratory distress syndrome, myocardial infarction, ventricular fibrillation, cardiogenic shock, anaphylactoid events), appropriate medications and supportive care (e.g., epinephrine, glucocorticoids, oxygen, bronchodilators) should be provided as clinically indicated. Depending on the severity of the infusion reaction and the required interventions, rituximab infusion should be temporarily or permanently discontinued. Once manifestations of infusion reactions have resolved, the infusion may be resumed but the rate of infusion should be reduced by at least 50%.

Mucocutaneous Effects. In the event of a severe mucocutaneous reaction, rituximab should be discontinued, and the patient should undergo prompt medical evaluation. (See Cautions: Mucocutaneous and Dermatologic Effects and also see Mucocutaneous and Dermatologic Effects under Cautions: Precautions and Contraindications.) Skin biopsy may be useful to diagnose the mucocutaneous reaction and guide treatment. The safety of readministration of rituximab in patients who have experienced a severe mucocutaneous reaction to the drug has not been determined.

Progressive Multifocal Leukoencephalopathy. In patients who develop progressive multifocal leukoencephalopathy (PML), rituximab therapy should be discontinued and reductions or discontinuance of any concomitant chemotherapy or immunosuppressive therapy should be considered. (See Cautions: Progressive Multifocal Leukoencephalopathy and also see Nervous System Effects under Cautions: Precautions and Contraindications.)

Hepatitis B Virus Reactivation. In patients with reactivation of hepatitis B virus (HBV) infection, rituximab therapy and any concomitant chemotherapy should be discontinued, and appropriate treatment, including antiviral therapy, should be initiated. It has not been established whether rituximab can be safely readministered in patients who develop HBV reactivation. Clinicians with expertise in managing HBV infection should be consulted regarding resumption of rituximab therapy once control of the reactivated infection has been achieved. (See Cautions: Hepatitis B Virus Reactivation and also see Hepatic Effects under Cautions: Precautions and Contraindications.)

Infectious Complications. In patients who develop severe infections, rituximab therapy should be discontinued, and appropriate anti-infective therapy should be initiated. (See Cautions: Infectious Complications and also see Infectious Complications under Cautions: Precautions and Contraindications.)

Cardiovascular Effects. Rituximab infusion should be discontinued in the event of clinically important adverse cardiac events or serious or life-threatening cardiac arrhythmias. In patients who develop serious arrhythmias during rituximab therapy, or who have a history of arrhythmia or angina, cardiac monitoring should be instituted during and following all infusions of rituximab. (See Cautions: Cardiovascular Effects and also see Cardiovascular Effects under Cautions: Precautions and Contraindications.)

Renal Effects. Rituximab therapy should be discontinued in patients who experience oliguria or increases in serum creatinine concentrations. (See Cautions: Renal Effects.)

Respiratory Effects. Some clinicians recommend discontinuance of rituximab if interstitial lung disease is suspected. The manufacturer states the safety of continuing or reinitiating rituximab therapy in patients who have experienced pneumonitis or bronchiolitis obliterans has not been established. (See Cautions: Respiratory Effects and also see Respiratory Effects under Cautions: Precautions and Contraindications.)

Cautions

Serious adverse effects, sometimes fatal, have occurred in patients receiving rituximab. Severe or fatal infusion-related reactions; tumor lysis syndrome associated with fatal renal failure; severe or fatal mucocutaneous reactions; progressive multifocal leukoencephalopathy causing death; hepatitis B reactivation with fulminant hepatitis, hepatic failure, and death; other severe or fatal, bacterial, fungal, and viral infections; serious or life-threatening cardiac arrhythmias; severe or fatal renal toxicity; and fatal bowel obstruction and perforation have occurred in patients receiving rituximab.

Adverse effects, including serious adverse effects, commonly occur with rituximab therapy. In clinical studies of rituximab in patients with relapsed or refractory low-grade or follicular non-Hodgkin's lymphoma (NHL), adverse effects were reported in 99% of patients, and grade 3 or 4 adverse effects were reported in 57% of patients. The most common adverse effects reported in 25% or more of patients in clinical studies are infusion-related reactions, fever, lymphopenia, chills, infection, and asthenia.

The incidence of adverse effects in patients with NHL is based on data collected from clinical trials involving 1606 patients receiving rituximab alone or in combination with chemotherapy, including data collected from 356 patients (median age: 57 years) with relapsed or refractory, low-grade NHL during a 12-month observation period following use of rituximab as a single agent in nonrandomized, single-arm clinical studies. Most patients with NHL received rituximab 375 mg/m^2 IV, given as a single agent weekly for up to 8 doses, in combination with chemotherapy for up to 8 doses, or following chemotherapy for up to 16 doses. Unless otherwise specified for a particular adverse effect in the following discussion, incidence rates for adverse effects in patients with NHL are based mainly on the data for patients receiving single-agent rituximab for relapsed or refractory low-grade or follicular NHL. Many adverse effects of rituximab in patients with NHL generally were mild or moderate in severity; the incidence of grade 3 or 4 adverse effects often was 1% or less with the exception of a smaller subset of certain adverse effects that occurred more frequently with greater severity (e.g., grade 3 or 4 lymphopenia in 40%, grade 3 or 4 neutropenia in 6%).

The incidence of adverse effects in patients with chronic lymphocytic leukemia (CLL) is based on data from clinical trials involving 676 patients receiving rituximab in combination with chemotherapy. The most common adverse effects reported in 25% or more of patients are infusion-related reactions and neutropenia.

Incidence rates for adverse effects in patients with rheumatoid arthritis (RA) are based mainly on data from 2578 patients receiving methotrexate with either rituximab or placebo in phase 2 and 3 studies. The most common adverse effects reported in 10% or more of patients are upper respiratory tract infection, nasopharyngitis, urinary tract infection, and bronchitis; other important adverse effects include infusion-related effects, serious infections, and cardiovascular events.

■ **Infusion-related Effects** Severe infusion-related effects, sometimes fatal, have been reported in patients receiving rituximab. Severe reactions typically occurred during the first infusion, with time to onset of 30–120 minutes. Fatal reactions have occurred within 24 hours of infusion, approximately 80% of which was associated with the first infusion. Manifestations and sequelae of an infusion-related reaction include urticaria, hypotension, angioedema, hypoxia, bronchospasm, pulmonary infiltrates, acute respiratory distress syndrome, myocardial infarction, ventricular fibrillation, cardiogenic shock, anaphylactoid events, or death. (See Infusion-related Effects under Dosage: Dosage Modification for Toxicity and Contraindications for Continued Therapy, in Dosage and Administration and also see Infusion-related Effects under Cautions: Precautions and Contraindications.) Acute infusion-related reactions observed with rituximab result from the release and/or activation of cytokines during B-cell depletion, often referred to as cytokine-release syndrome. Reported risk factors for cytokine-release syndrome and subsequent infusion-related reactions induced by rituximab include older age, high tumor burden, elevated cytokine or complement levels, and B-lymphocyte aggregation or tumor cell agglutination at baseline.

The manufacturer reports that approximately 70 cases of serious infusion-related events, 8 of which were fatal, have been reported out of an estimated 12,000–14,000 patients worldwide who received rituximab therapy between November 1997 and December 1998. In 7 of the 8 fatal cases, manifestations developed during the initial infusion of rituximab, and death in most cases was preceded by severe bronchospasm, dyspnea, hypotension, and/or angioedema. Severe respiratory events, including hypoxia, pulmonary infiltrates, and adult respiratory distress syndrome, contributed to 6 of the 8 deaths. In some cases, manifestations worsened over time, while in others, initial improvement was followed by clinical deterioration. Therefore, patients experiencing any severe infusion-related manifestation should be monitored closely until complete resolution occurs. (See Infusion-related Effects under Dosage: Dosage Modification for Toxicity and Contraindications for Continued Therapy, in Dosage and Administration and also see Infusion-related Effects under Cautions: Precautions and Contraindications.)

Among patients receiving rituximab for NHL, the incidence of infusion reactions was 77% during the first infusion and decreased with each subsequent infusion. Manifestations of infusion-related reactions in these patients included fever, chills/rigors, nausea, pruritus, angioedema, hypotension, headache, bronchospasm, urticaria, rash, vomiting, myalgia, dizziness, and hypertension. These reactions generally occurred within 30–120 minutes of starting the first rituximab infusion and usually resolved with slowing or interruption of the infusion and administration of supportive care, including diphenhydramine, acetaminophen, and IV sodium chloride injection.

Among patients with previously untreated follicular NHL or previously untreated diffuse large B-cell NHL who did not experience a grade 3 or 4 infusion-related reaction to rituximab during the first treatment cycle and who received rituximab as a 90-minute infusion during subsequent treatment cycles, the incidence of grade 3 or 4 infusion-related reactions was 1.1% during cycle 2 and 2.8% during cycles 2–8. During cycle 2, the incidence of grade 3 or 4 infusion-related reactions was 3.5% among patients with follicular NHL receiving rituximab in combination with cyclophosphamide, vincristine, and prednisone (CVP) and 0% among patients with diffuse large B-cell NHL receiving rituximab in combination with cyclophosphamide, doxorubicin, vincristine, and prednisone (CHOP).

Among patients receiving rituximab in combination with fludarabine and cyclophosphamide (FC) for CLL, grade 3 and 4 infusion reactions (defined as nausea, pyrexia, chills, hypotension, vomiting, or dyspnea occurring during or within 24 hours after initiation of rituximab infusion) occurred in 9 or 7% of previously untreated or previously treated patients, respectively.

Among patients receiving rituximab and methotrexate for RA, adverse effects occurred during the 24-hour period following the infusion in 32% of patients following the first infusion and in 11% of patients following the second infusion. Acute infusion reactions (manifested by fever, chills, rigors, pruritus, urticaria, rash, angioedema, sneezing, throat irritation, cough, and/or bronchospasm, with or without associated hypotension or hypertension) occurred in 27% of patients following the first infusion and in 9% of patients following the second infusion. Serious acute infusion reactions occurred in less than 1% of patients. Dosage modification of rituximab (stopping, slowing, or interrupting the infusion) for infusion-related toxicity was required after the first course of therapy in 10% of patients receiving rituximab and methotrexate. The percentage of patients experiencing acute infusion reactions decreased with subsequent courses of rituximab. Although the administration of IV glucocorticoids prior to rituximab infusions reduced the incidence and severity of acute infusion reactions, the administration of oral glucocorticoids provided no clear benefit in preventing such reactions. Antihistamines and acetaminophen also were administered prior to rituximab infusions to prevent infusion-related effects.

■ Tumor Lysis Syndrome Tumor lysis syndrome, consisting of rapid reduction in tumor volume followed by acute renal failure, hyperkalemia, hypocalcemia, hyperuricemia, or hyperphosphatemia, occurring within 12–24 hours of completion of the initial infusion of rituximab, has been reported in patients with NHL and sometimes has been fatal. The risk of tumor lysis syndrome is increased in patients with a high number of circulating malignant cells (25,000/mm^3 or greater) or a large tumor burden. (See Tumor Lysis Syndrome under Cautions: Precautions and Contraindications.)

■ Mucocutaneous and Dermatologic Effects Severe mucocutaneous reactions, sometimes fatal, have been reported in patients receiving rituximab. Severe mucocutaneous reactions associated with rituximab therapy include paraneoplastic pemphigus (an uncommon disorder which is a manifestation of the underlying malignancy), Stevens-Johnson syndrome, lichenoid dermatitis, vesiculobullous dermatitis, and toxic epidermal necrolysis. The onset of severe mucocutaneous reactions is variable but has occurred as early as the first day of rituximab administration. (See Mucocutaneous Effects under Dosage: Dosage Modification for Toxicity and Contraindications for Continued Therapy, in Dosage and Administration and also see Mucocutaneous and Dermatologic Effects under Cautions: Precautions and Contraindications.)

Adverse effects involving the skin or appendages were reported in 44% of patients receiving single-agent rituximab for NHL in clinical studies and were grade 3 or 4 in severity in 2% of patients. Rash, night sweats, pruritus, and urticaria were reported in 15, 15, 14, and 8% of patients, respectively.

Among patients receiving rituximab and methotrexate for RA, pruritus occurred in 5%, and urticaria in 2%, of patients.

■ Progressive Multifocal Leukoencephalopathy Progressive multifocal leukoencephalopathy (PML) secondary to JC infection, sometimes fatal, has been reported in patients receiving rituximab for hematologic malignancies or autoimmune diseases (e.g., RA, systemic lupus erythematosus [SLE]†). Most patients with hematologic malignancies who were diagnosed with PML had received rituximab in combination with chemotherapy or as part of a hematopoietic stem cell transplantation. Patients with autoimmune diseases who developed PML had received prior or concurrent immunosuppressive therapy. Most cases of PML were diagnosed within 12 months of the last infusion of rituximab. PML usually causes death or severe disability, and no therapy is known to prevent, treat, or cure this condition.

In a report from the Research on Adverse Drug Events and Reports (RADAR) project, 52 cases of PML were identified in patients with B-cell lymphoid malignancy (e.g., CLL, NHL); all of these patients had received prior therapies that affect immune function (e.g., alkylating agents, purine analogs, corticosteroids, drugs that prevent allogeneic stem cell or solid organ graft rejection). Reported manifestations of PML, which progressed over weeks to months, included confusion, mental status changes, focal motor weakness, hemiparesis, loss of motor coordination, and speech and vision changes. According to the report, a median of 6 rituximab doses was administered prior to diagnosis of PML, and the median time to diagnosis of PML was 5.5 months following the last dose of rituximab. The case-fatality rate of PML derived from this report was 90%, with a median time to death of 2 months after diagnosis of PML.

Two fatal cases of PML have been reported in patients with RA receiving rituximab; these patients had possible risk factors for PML (e.g., prior chemotherapy and radiation therapy, long-standing lymphopenia). In addition, at least one case of PML has been reported in a patient with RA receiving rituximab who had *not* received prior therapy with a tumor necrosis factor (TNF) antagonist. The manufacturer states that the reported incidence of PML is rare (3 out of 100,000 patients); however, data suggest that patients with RA who receive rituximab are at increased risk of developing PML. (See Progressive Multifocal Leukoencephalopathy under Dosage: Dosage Modification for Toxicity and Contraindications for Continued Therapy, in Dosage and Administration and also see Nervous System Effects under Cautions: Precautions and Contraindications.)

■ Hepatitis B Virus Reactivation Reactivation of hepatitis B virus (HBV) infection has been reported in patients receiving anti-CD20 monoclonal antibodies, including rituximab, and has resulted in fulminant hepatitis, hepatic failure, and death. HBV reactivation has been reported in patients who are hepatitis B surface antigen-positive [HBsAg-positive]; HBsAg-negative and hepatitis B core antibody-positive [anti-HBc-positive]; or HBsAg-negative, anti-HBc-positive, and hepatitis B surface antibody-positive [anti-HBs-positive].

Following review of the Adverse Event Reporting System (AERS) database, the US Food and Drug Administration (FDA) identified 106 cases of fatal HBV-related acute liver injury in patients receiving rituximab (between November 1997 and August 2012) and 3 such cases in patients receiving ofatumumab (between October 2009 and August 2012); 32 of these case reports contained sufficient data to meet the criteria for HBV reactivation. In this review, acute liver injury was attributed to HBV reactivation if seroconversion of HBsAg from negative to positive occurred in those with either anti-HBc or a history of HBV, or if an increase in serum HBV DNA level occurred in those who were HBsAg-positive prior to therapy with an anti-CD20 monoclonal antibody (i.e., rituximab, ofatumumab). HBV reactivation was diagnosed by seroconversion of HBsAg in most (69%) cases. In this review, the duration of rituximab or ofatumumab therapy prior to diagnosis of HBV reactivation was highly variable, ranging from 63 days after initiation of the drug to 12 months following the last dose; however, delayed onset of HBV reactivation (up to 24 months following completion of rituximab therapy) has been reported. All of the patients experiencing HBV reactivation had received recent or concomitant therapy with other immunosuppressive agents. Among patients with HBV reactivation, 10% received HBV antiviral prophylaxis and 28% received antiviral treatment for HBV reactivation. (See Hepatitis B Virus Reactivation under Dosage: Dosage Modification for Toxicity and Contraindications for Continued Therapy, in Dosage and Administration and also see Hepatic Effects under Cautions: Precautions and Contraindications.)

■ Infectious Complications Serious, including fatal, bacterial, fungal, and new or reactivated viral infections, have been reported during and following completion of rituximab-based therapy. Infections have been reported in some patients with prolonged hypogammaglobulinemia (i.e., hypogammaglobulinemia lasting longer than 11 months following rituximab therapy). New or reactivated viral infections include cytomegalovirus, herpes simplex virus, parvovirus B19, varicella zoster virus, West Nile virus, and hepatitis B and C. (See Infectious Complications under Dosage: Dosage Modification for Toxicity and Contraindications for Continued Therapy, in Dosage and Administration and also see Infectious Complications under Cautions: Precautions and Contraindications.) An increased incidence of fatal infections has been observed in patients receiving rituximab for HIV-associated lymphoma†.

Infection was reported in 31% of patients receiving rituximab for NHL in clinical studies; severe (grade 3 or 4) infections, including sepsis, occurred in 4% of patients. The incidence of bacterial, viral, and fungal infections was 19, 10, and 1%, respectively; 6% of patients had infections of unknown etiology. In patients with NHL receiving rituximab monotherapy, B-cell depletion occurred in 70–80% of patients with NHL, and reduction in serum concentrations of IgG and IgM occurred in 14% of patients.

Among patients receiving rituximab and methotrexate for RA in clinical studies, 39% of patients experienced an infection; the most common infections were nasopharyngitis, upper respiratory tract infection, urinary tract infection, bronchitis, and sinusitis. Serious infection was reported in approximately 2% of patients with RA receiving rituximab; the most common serious infections were pneumonia, lower respiratory tract infection, cellulitis, and urinary tract infection. Fatal serious infections included pneumonia, sepsis, and colitis. The incidence of serious infection remained stable in patients receiving subsequent courses of rituximab. In 185 patients with active RA receiving rituximab, subsequent treatment with a biologic disease-modifying antirheumatic drug (DMARD) did not appear to increase the incidence of serious infection.

JC virus infection causing progressive multifocal leukoencephalopathy (PML), sometimes fatal, has been reported in patients receiving rituximab. (See Cautions: Progressive Multifocal Leukoencephalopathy.)

■ Cardiovascular Effects Myocardial infarction, ventricular fibrillation, cardiogenic shock, and/or hypotension have occurred as severe manifestations and sequelae of infusion-related reactions and sometimes led to death in patients receiving rituximab. (See Cautions: Infusion-related Effects.) Other severe adverse cardiac effects, including rare instances of fatal cardiac failure with onset of manifestations weeks after rituximab therapy, have been reported. Cardiac arrhythmias and angina also have been reported. (See Cardiovascular Effects under Dosage: Dosage Modification for Toxicity and Contraindications for Continued Therapy, in Dosage and Administration and also see Cardiovascular Effects under Cautions: Precautions and Contraindications.)

Adverse cardiovascular effects were reported in about 25% of patients receiving single-agent rituximab for NHL in clinical studies and were grade 3 or 4 in severity in 3% of patients. Hypotension, peripheral edema, and hypertension were reported in 10, 8, and 6% of patients, respectively.

Among patients receiving rituximab and methotrexate for RA, serious adverse cardiovascular effects, sometimes fatal, occurred in about 2% of patients; hypertension was reported in 8% of patients.

■ Renal Effects Severe, including fatal, renal toxicity can occur after rituximab administration in patients with NHL. Acute renal failure requiring dialysis and sometimes resulting in death, has occurred in patients who experience tumor lysis syndrome. (See Cautions: Tumor Lysis Syndrome, and see Renal Effects under Dosage: Dosage Modification for Toxicity and Contraindications for Continued Therapy, in Dosage and Administration, and also see Tumor Lysis Syndrome under Cautions: Precautions and Contraindications.)

Renal toxicity associated with rituximab also has occurred in patients with NHL receiving concomitant cisplatin therapy† during clinical studies. Combined therapy with rituximab and cisplatin currently is not approved by the US Food and Drug Administration (FDA).

■ GI Effects Abdominal pain, bowel obstruction, and bowel perforation, sometimes fatal, can occur in patients receiving rituximab in combination with chemotherapy. In postmarketing reports in patients with NHL, the mean time to documented GI perforation was 6 days (range: 1–77 days).

Adverse GI effects were reported in about 37% of patients receiving single-agent rituximab for NHL in clinical studies and were grade 3 or 4 in severity in 2% of patients. Nausea and vomiting occurred in 23 and 10% of patients, respectively. Abdominal pain and diarrhea occurred in 14 and 10% of patients, respectively.

Among patients receiving rituximab and methotrexate for RA, nausea occurred in 8%, dyspepsia in 3%, and upper abdominal pain in 2% of patients.

Patients receiving rituximab who have complaints suggestive of bowel obstruction, such as abdominal pain or repeated vomiting, should receive a diagnostic evaluation.

■ Respiratory Effects Adverse respiratory effects, including acute respiratory distress syndrome, bronchospasm, dyspnea, hypoxia, and pulmonary infiltrates, have occurred as severe manifestations and sequelae of infusion-related reactions to rituximab and sometimes have been fatal. Patients with preexisting pulmonary conditions should be closely monitored for possible infusion-related toxicity. (See Cautions: Infusion-related Effects and also see Infusion-related Effects under Cautions: Precautions and Contraindications.)

Delayed pulmonary toxicity (e.g., bronchiolitis obliterans [presenting during and up to 6 months following rituximab infusion], pneumonitis [including interstitial pneumonitis]), sometimes fatal, has been reported in patients receiving rituximab alone or in combination with other chemotherapeutic agents. In several reports evaluating cases of interstitial lung disease (i.e., interstitial pneumonitis), the most common manifestations observed included dyspnea, fever, and cough. In these reports, if interstitial lung disease was suspected, immediate discontinuance of rituximab was required, and patients were managed with corticosteroid therapy (e.g., methylprednisolone, prednisolone, prednisone) and other clinically appropriate measures (e.g., antibiotics). The manufacturer states the safety of continuing or reinitiating rituximab therapy in patients experiencing pneumonitis or bronchiolitis obliterans has not been established. Interstitial pneumonitis reportedly recurred in a limited number of patients following rechallenge with rituximab. (See Respiratory Effects under Dosage: Dosage Modification for Toxicity and Contraindications for Continued Therapy, in Dosage and Administration and also see Respiratory Effects under Cautions: Precautions and Contraindications.)

Adverse respiratory effects were reported in about 38% of patients receiving single-agent rituximab for NHL in clinical studies and were grade 3 or 4 in severity in 4% of patients. Increased cough, bronchospasm, and dyspnea were reported in 13, 8, and 7% of patients, respectively. Rhinitis, throat irritation, and sinusitis occurred in 12, 9, and 6% of patients, respectively.

Among patients receiving rituximab and methotrexate for RA, rhinitis occurred in 3%, and throat irritation in 2%, of patients.

■ Metabolic and Electrolyte Effects Among patients receiving single-agent rituximab for NHL, hyperglycemia and increases in LDH were reported in 9 and 7% of patients, respectively.

Among patients receiving rituximab and methotrexate for RA in controlled clinical studies, hypophosphatemia and hyperuricemia were reported in 12 and 1.5% of patients, respectively. The majority of cases of hypophosphatemia occurred during the rituximab infusion and was considered transient; hypophosphatemia reportedly occurred more frequently in patients who received glucocorticoids.

■ Hematologic Effects Adverse hematologic effects, mainly manifested by lymphopenia, occur frequently in patients receiving rituximab. Adverse hematologic or lymphatic system effects were reported in 67% of patients receiving single-agent rituximab for NHL in clinical studies and were grade 3 or 4 in severity in 48% of patients. Lymphopenia was reported in 48% of patients and was grade 3 or 4 in severity in 40% of patients; the median duration of lymphopenia was 14 days (range: 1–588 days).

Grade 3 and 4 cytopenias occurred in 48% of patients receiving single-agent rituximab for NHL in clinical studies. Neutropenia and leukopenia each were reported in 14% of patients and were grade 3 or 4 in severity in 6 and 4% of patients, respectively. The median duration of neutropenia was 13 days (range: 2–116 days). Thrombocytopenia occurred in 12% of patients and was grade 3 or 4 in severity in 2% of patients. Agranulocytosis has been reported in patients receiving rituximab.

Anemia was reported in 8% of patients receiving single-agent rituximab for NHL and was grade 3 or 4 in severity in 3% of patients. At least one case of transient aplastic anemia (pure red cell aplasia) and two cases of hemolytic anemia have been reported in patients receiving rituximab therapy for NHL.

Prolonged pancytopenia, marrow hypoplasia, late onset neutropenia, and hyperviscosity syndrome in lymphoplasmacytic lymphoma (Waldenstrom's macroglobulinemia) have been reported in patients with hematologic malignancies receiving rituximab.

Complete blood cell counts (CBC) and platelet counts should be monitored regularly during rituximab therapy with more frequent monitoring in patients who develop cytopenias. (See Hematologic Effects under Cautions: Precautions and Contraindications.) Cytopenias associated with rituximab may persist for an extended duration (i.e., months) following discontinuance of the drug.

■ Immunologic Effects Administration of rituximab is associated with rapid and sustained depletion of B cells from the peripheral blood and tissues. (See Pharmacology.)

In patients with NHL, sustained and clinically important reductions in serum IgM and IgG concentrations were observed from 5 through 11 months following rituximab therapy; serum IgM and/or IgG concentrations below the normal range were observed in 14% of patients. In clinical studies of patients receiving rituximab for rheumatoid arthritis, total and individual serum immunoglobulin concentrations were reduced at 6 months with the greatest change observed in IgM concentrations. Following 24 weeks of therapy with rituximab, decreases in serum IgM, IgG, or IgA concentrations to below the lower limit of normal were observed in 10, 2.8, or 0.8% of patients, respectively; following repeated courses of rituximab, decreases in serum IgM, IgG, or IgA concentrations to below the lower limit of normal were observed in 23.3, 5.5, or 0.5% of patients, respectively. The clinical importance of decreased immunoglobulin concentrations in patients receiving rituximab for rheumatoid arthritis is uncertain.

Adverse immunologic and/or autoimmune effects reported in patients receiving rituximab include uveitis, optic neuritis, systemic vasculitis, pleuritis, lupus-like syndrome, serum sickness, polyarticular arthritis, and vasculitis with rash.

Among 356 patients with low-grade or follicular NHL receiving single-agent rituximab in clinical studies, positive human antichimeric antibody (HACA) responses were detected in 4 patients (1.1%), 3 of whom achieved an objective clinical response.

Among 2578 patients with RA receiving rituximab, positive HACA responses were detected in 273 patients (11%). Positive HACA responses typically were detected at any time after administration of rituximab and were not associated with increased infusion reactions or other adverse effects. Upon retreatment, the incidence of infusion reactions was similar between HACA-positive and HACA-negative patients; most infusion reactions were mild to moderate. Four HACA-positive patients with RA experienced serious infusion reactions; however, the temporal relationship between HACA positivity and infusion reaction was variable among these patients. The clinical importance of HACA formation in patients receiving rituximab is unclear.

The immune response to various antigens have been evaluated in a randomized, controlled study in patients with RA receiving either rituximab in combination with methotrexate or methotrexate alone. The proportion of patients demonstrating an immune response to pneumococcal vaccine (i.e., measured as an increase in antibody titers to at least 6 of 12 serotypes) was lower in patients receiving rituximab in combination with methotrexate (19%) than in patients receiving methotrexate alone (61%). In addition, a smaller proportion of patients receiving rituximab in combination methotrexate developed detectable concentrations of anti-keyhole limpet hemocyanin (KLH) antibodies after vaccination compared with patients receiving methotrexate alone (47 versus 93%). The immune response to tetanus toxoid (a recall antigen) and delayed-type hypersensitivity (DTH) response to a candida skin test, however, were similar in patients receiving rituximab in combination with methotrexate compared with patients receiving methotrexate alone. Most patients receiving rituximab in combination with methotrexate had B-cell counts below the lower limit of normal at the time of immunization; the clinical implications of these findings are not known.

■ Nervous System Effects Adverse nervous system effects were reported in about one-third of patients receiving single-agent rituximab for NHL in clinical studies. Headache, dizziness, and anxiety were reported in 19, 10, and 5% of patients, respectively.

Among patients receiving rituximab and methotrexate for RA, anxiety, migraine, and paresthesia each occurred in 2% of patients.

PML secondary to JC infection, sometimes fatal, has been reported in patients receiving rituximab for hematologic malignancies or autoimmune diseases (e.g., RA, systemic lupus erythematosus [SLE]†). (See Cautions: Progressive Multifocal Leukoencephalopathy.)

■ **Musculoskeletal Effects** Adverse musculoskeletal effects were reported in about 26% of patients receiving single-agent rituximab for NHL in clinical studies and were grade 3 or 4 in severity in 3% of patients. Back pain, myalgia, and arthralgia, each was reported in 10% of patients.

Among patients receiving rituximab and methotrexate for RA, arthralgia occurred in 6% of patients.

■ **Other Adverse Effects** Fever occurred in 53% of patients receiving rituximab monotherapy for NHL. Chills were reported in 33% of patients with NHL and were grade 3 or 4 in severity in 3% of patients. Other adverse effects in patients receiving single-agent rituximab for NHL included asthenia in 26%, pain in 12%, angioedema in 11%, and flushing in 5% of patients.

Among patients receiving rituximab and methotrexate for RA, pyrexia occurred in 5%, chills in 3%, and asthenia in 2% of patients.

The incidences and types of adverse effects reported in patients with RA were similar following a single course versus repeated courses of rituximab. In a clinical study in which patients received an initial course of methotrexate in combination with rituximab, followed by a second course of methotrexate in combination with either rituximab or placebo, the safety profile reported in patients receiving methotrexate plus rituximab was similar to that reported in patients receiving methotrexate plus placebo.

■ **Precautions and Contraindications** The use of rituximab is *not* recommended in patients with severe, active infections.

Serious adverse effects, including infusion-related reactions, tumor lysis syndrome, mucocutaneous reactions, progressive multifocal leukoencephalopathy, hepatitis B reactivation with fulminant hepatitis, bacterial/fungal/viral infections, cardiac arrhythmias, renal toxicity, and bowel obstruction and perforation, have occurred in patients receiving rituximab and have sometimes been fatal. (See Cautions for further discussion of adverse effects.)

Interruption or discontinuance of rituximab therapy is required in patients experiencing severe or life-threatening adverse reactions. Reinitiation at a slower infusion rate (minimum of 50% reduction in rate) is required if rituximab therapy is resumed following complete resolution of symptoms. (See Dosage Modification for Toxicity and Contraindications for Continued Therapy under Dosage and Administration: Dosage.)

Rituximab may be administered in an outpatient setting; however, appropriate diagnostic and treatment facilities, including medications for the treatment of severe adverse reactions, such as infusion-related reactions, hypersensitivity reactions, and cardiac arrhythmias, must be readily available.

Infusion-related Effects To minimize the risk of infusion-related effects associated with rituximab, premedication is recommended before each infusion of the drug. (See Dosage and Administration.) Patients (particularly those with preexisting cardiac or pulmonary conditions, those with a high number of circulating malignant B-cells [i.e., 25,000/mm^3 or greater], and patients with a history of a cardiopulmonary reaction to rituximab) should be carefully monitored during rituximab infusions. If an infusion reaction occurs, the rituximab infusion should be interrupted and appropriate medications and supportive care provided as clinically indicated. (See Infusion-related Effects under Dosage and Administration: Dosage Modification for Toxicity and Contraindications for Continued Therapy, in Dosage and Administration.)

Because infusion reactions may occur during or within 24 hours after rituximab infusion, patients should be instructed to notify a clinician if they experience any of the following symptoms during or following rituximab infusion: hives (red itchy welts) or rash; itching; swelling of the lips, tongue, throat, or face; sudden cough; shortness of breath, difficulty breathing, or wheezing; weakness; dizziness or feeling faint; palpitations; or chest pain.

Tumor Lysis Syndrome Patients receiving rituximab should be closely monitored for development of tumor lysis syndrome, including manifestations of renal failure. The manufacturer states that patients at high risk of tumor lysis syndrome (i.e., patients with a high number of circulating malignant cells [25,000/mm^3 or greater] or a high tumor burden) should receive aggressive IV hydration and anti-hyperuricemic therapy. If tumor lysis syndrome develops, patients should receive appropriate medical treatment, including correction of electrolyte abnormalities, monitoring of renal function and fluid balance, and any necessary supportive care (e.g., dialysis) as clinically indicated.

Mucocutaneous and Dermatologic Effects Severe mucocutaneous reactions, sometimes fatal, have been reported in patients receiving rituximab. Patients should be instructed to notify a clinician or to immediately seek medical attention if they experience any of the following symptoms at any time during rituximab therapy: painful sores or ulcers on the skin, lips, or in the mouth; blisters; peeling skin; rash; or pustules. (See Mucocutaneous Effects under Dosage: Dosage Modification for Toxicity and Contraindications for Continued Therapy, in Dosage and Administration and also see Cautions: Mucocutaneous and Dermatologic Effects.)

Nervous System Effects Neurologic function should be monitored during rituximab therapy. The possible diagnosis of PML should be considered in any patient receiving rituximab who experiences new onset of neurologic manifestations. Diagnostic evaluation, including consultation with a neurologist, brain magnetic resonance imaging (MRI) scan, and lumbar puncture, should be considered as clinically indicated.

Patients receiving rituximab should be advised to immediately inform a clinician if they experience any of the following symptoms: confusion, trouble thinking, loss of balance, change in walking or talking, decreased strength or weakness on one side of the body, or blurred or loss of vision.

Hepatic Effects To decrease the risk of HBV reactivation, all patients should be screened for HBV infection by measuring HBsAg and anti-HBc before initiating treatment with rituximab. Hepatitis experts should be consulted regarding monitoring and use of antiviral therapy in those with evidence of HBV infection (HBsAg-positive with any antibody status or HBsAg-negative and anti-HBc-positive); although data are limited, treatment guidelines from some experts recommend the use of prophylactic antiviral therapy in patients who are chronic carriers of HBV. Patients with evidence of current or prior HBV infection should be monitored for clinical and laboratory evidence of hepatitis or HBV reactivation during rituximab therapy and for several months thereafter, since reactivation has occurred more than 12 months following completion of therapy. Rituximab and any concomitant chemotherapy should be discontinued immediately if HBV reactivation occurs, and appropriate treatment for HBV infection should be initiated. Concomitant chemotherapy should be discontinued until the HBV infection has been controlled or has resolved. Clinicians with expertise in managing HBV infection should be consulted regarding resumption of rituximab therapy once control of the reactivated HBV infection has been achieved. It has not been established whether rituximab can be safely readministered in patients who develop HBV reactivation. (See Hepatitis B Virus Reactivation under Dosage: Dosage Modification for Toxicity and Contraindications for Continued Therapy, in Dosage and Administration.)

Infectious Complications Serious, sometimes fatal, infections, have been reported with rituximab therapy. (See Cautions: Infectious Complications.) The manufacturer states that rituximab should *not* be used in patients with severe, active infections.

Patients receiving rituximab in combination with fludarabine and cyclophosphamide for treatment of CLL should receive prophylaxis against *Pneumocystis jiroveci* (formerly *Pneumocystis carinii*) pneumonia (PCP) (i.e., co-trimoxazole) and herpes virus infection (e.g., acyclovir or valacyclovir) during treatment and for up to 12 months following discontinuance of therapy.

Patients should be advised to inform a clinician before initiating rituximab therapy if they have an infection, a weakened immune system, or a history of severe infections (e.g., hepatitis B or C virus, cytomegalovirus, herpes simplex virus, parvovirus B19, varicella zoster virus [chickenpox or shingles], West Nile virus). Patients also should be advised to immediately inform a clinician if they experience any of the following symptoms: fever; persistent runny nose or sore throat; cough; tiredness; body aches; earache; headache; pain during urination; white patches in the mouth or throat; or cuts, scrapes, or incisions that are red, warm, swollen, or painful. (See Infectious Complications under Dosage: Dosage Modification for Toxicity and Contraindications for Continued Therapy, in Dosage and Administration.)

Cardiovascular Effects Cardiac monitoring should be performed during and after all infusions of rituximab in patients who develop clinically important arrhythmias or who have a history of arrhythmia or angina. Because patients with RA are at increased risk for cardiovascular toxicity compared with the general population, such patients should be monitored carefully throughout the rituximab infusion. (See Cautions: Cardiovascular Effects and also see Cardiovascular Effects under Dosage: Dosage Modification for Toxicity and Contraindications for Continued Therapy, in Dosage and Administration.)

Patients receiving rituximab should be advised to inform a clinician if they experience chest pain or irregular heart beats.

Vaccination Status The manufacturer makes no specific recommendations regarding vaccination in patients with NHL receiving rituximab; however, the US Centers for Disease Control and Prevention (CDC) and US Public Health Service Advisory Committee on Immunization Practices (ACIP) have established guidelines on the use of vaccines in individuals with altered immunocompetence.

Prior to administering rituximab therapy for RA, the manufacturer states that clinicians should follow CDC guidelines and administer *non-live* (i.e., inactivated) vaccines at least 4 weeks prior to a course of rituximab. Some experts state that appropriate vaccination (e.g., to prevent influenza) may be given during rituximab therapy when clinically indicated; however, immune responses have been shown to be submaximal.

The manufacturer states that administration of vaccines containing *live* virus is *not* recommended prior to or during rituximab therapy. However, some experts state that live, attenuated vaccines may be administered in patients with RA, but only *before* initiation of rituximab therapy.

Prior to initiation of rituximab therapy, patients should be advised to inform their clinician if they recently received or are scheduled to receive any vaccines. Patients also should be advised to inform their clinician if any household contacts are scheduled to receive vaccines.

Hematologic Effects In patients with lymphoid malignancies receiving rituximab as a single agent, CBCs and platelet counts should be obtained prior to each rituximab course. In those receiving rituximab in combination with chemotherapy, CBCs and platelet counts should be obtained at weekly to monthly intervals; more frequent monitoring is recommended in patients who develop cytopenias.

In patients with RA receiving rituximab, CBCs and platelet counts should be obtained every 2–4 months during treatment.

Cytopenias associated with rituximab may persist for an extended duration (i.e., months) following discontinuance of the drug.

Respiratory Effects Patients with preexisting pulmonary conditions should be closely monitored for possible infusion-related toxicity.

Patients presenting with manifestations of delayed pulmonary toxicity (e.g., dyspnea, fever, cough) that are *not* associated with an acute infusion-related reaction should undergo prompt medical evaluation (i.e., pulse oximetry or blood gases, chest CT, pulmonary function tests documenting a restrictive pattern and decreased pulmonary diffusion capacity for carbon monoxide [DL_{CO}], other evaluations to rule out an infectious etiology or interstitial fibrosis) for possible interstitial lung disease. If interstitial lung disease is suspected, some clinicians recommend that rituximab be discontinued and corticosteroid (i.e., glucocorticoid) therapy, along with other clinically appropriate measures (e.g., antibiotics), initiated. (See Cautions: Respiratory Effects.)

Other Precautions and Contraindications Prior to each treatment session, the patient should be given a copy of the manufacturer's patient information (medication guide) and an opportunity to discuss any questions.

The manufacturer states there are no known contraindications to the use of rituximab.

■ **Pediatric Precautions** Safety and efficacy of rituximab in children have not been established. The pharmacokinetics of rituximab have not been studied in children or adolescents.

■ **Geriatric Precautions** Clinical studies of rituximab in low-grade or follicular, antigen CD20-positive, B-cell NHL did not include sufficient numbers of patients 65 years of age and older to determine whether geriatric patients respond differently than younger patients. Among patients with diffuse large B-cell NHL in 3 randomized trials, 927 patients received rituximab in combination with chemotherapy; of these, 396 (43%) were 65 years of age or older and 123 (13%) were 75 years of age or older. Although no overall difference in efficacy was observed between geriatric and younger patients, geriatric patients were more likely to experience certain adverse effects, such as supraventricular arrhythmias and severe respiratory effects, including pneumonia and pneumonitis.

Among the 676 patients with previously untreated or previously treated chronic lymphocytic leukemia (CLL) receiving rituximab in 2 randomized studies (CLL8 and REACH studies), 243 (36%) were 65 years of age or older and 100 (15%) were 70 years of age or older. Based on results of an exploratory analysis (stratified by age), the addition of rituximab to fludarabine and cyclophosphamide (FC) resulted in no additional benefit in previously untreated patients 70 years of age or older or in previously treated patients 65 years of age or older. (See Uses: Chronic Lymphocytic Leukemia.) Previously untreated geriatric patients received lower dosages of fludarabine and cyclophosphamide compared with younger patients, while previously treated geriatric patients received lower dosages of fludarabine, cyclophosphamide, *and* rituximab. Compared with younger patients, patients 70 years of age or older experienced higher incidences of grade 3 or 4 adverse effects, including neutropenia, febrile neutropenia, anemia, and pancytopenia (among patients with previously untreated CLL), and neutropenia, anemia, thrombocytopenia, pancytopenia, and infections (among patients with previously treated CLL).

Among the 2578 patients with RA enrolled in studies worldwide, 12% were 65–75 years of age and 2% were 75 years of age or older. In one clinical trial among patients receiving rituximab and methotrexate for RA, ACR 20 response rates were similar (53 versus 51%) in geriatric (65 years of age or older) and younger patients, respectively. The incidences of adverse effects were similar in older and younger patients; however, the rates of serious adverse effects, including serious infections, malignancies, and cardiovascular events, were higher in older patients.

■ **Mutagenicity and Carcinogenicity** Long-term animal studies to determine the mutagenic or carcinogenic potential of rituximab have not been performed to date.

■ **Pregnancy, Fertility, and Lactation** Although rituximab has been shown to cross the monkey placenta, results of an embryofetal developmental toxicity study in which IV rituximab was administered to pregnant cynomolgus monkeys during early gestation did not indicate teratogenicity. However, a decrease in levels of lymphoid tissue B cells was observed in the offspring of treated dams. In another developmental toxicity study in cynomolgus monkeys receiving rituximab during prenatal and postnatal periods, decreased levels of B cells and immunosuppression were observed in the offspring; levels of B cells and immune function returned to normal within 6 months of birth. There are no adequate and well-controlled studies in pregnant women. Postmarketing data indicate that B-cell lymphocytopenia generally lasting less than 6 months can occur in infants exposed to rituximab in utero. Rituximab was detected postnatally in the serum of infants exposed to the drug in utero. The manufacturer states that rituximab should be used during pregnancy only if the potential benefit justifies the potential risk to the fetus. Individuals of childbearing potential should use effective contraception during treatment and for up to 12 months following rituximab therapy.

Studies have not been conducted to date to determine whether rituximab affects fertility in males or females.

Rituximab is distributed into milk in lactating cynomolgus monkeys. It is not known whether rituximab is distributed into milk in humans. IgG is distributed into human milk; however, published data suggest that antibodies in breast milk do not enter the neonatal and infant circulations in substantial amounts. The unknown risks to the infant from oral ingestion of rituximab should be weighed against the known benefits of breastfeeding.

Drug Interactions

Formal drug interaction studies of rituximab have not been conducted.

■ **Antirheumatic Agents** The safety of concomitant use of rituximab with biologic agents or nonbiologic disease-modifying antirheumatic drugs (DMARDs) other than methotrexate in patients with rheumatoid arthritis (RA) exhibiting peripheral B cell depletion following treatment with rituximab has not been established. Such patients should be monitored closely for signs of infection if biologic agents and/or DMARDs are used concomitantly. In clinical trials, concomitant administration of methotrexate or cyclophosphamide did not alter the pharmacokinetic disposition of rituximab in patients with RA.

■ **Cisplatin** Renal toxicity has been reported in patients receiving cisplatin in combination with rituximab for NHL in clinical studies. If rituximab is administered concomitantly with cisplatin (e.g., in the clinical trial setting), *extreme caution* should be used, and patients should be monitored closely for signs of renal toxicity.

■ **Cyclophosphamide** Concomitant administration of rituximab with cyclophosphamide in patients with chronic lymphocytic leukemia (CLL) did not alter systemic exposure to cyclophosphamide.

■ **Fludarabine** Concomitant administration of rituximab with fludarabine in patients with CLL did not alter systemic exposure to fludarabine.

■ **Live Vaccines** The safety of immunization with live viral vaccines following rituximab therapy has not been established. The manufacturer states that use of vaccines containing live virus is *not* recommended prior to or during rituximab therapy. (See Cautions: Immunologic Effects and also see Vaccination Status under Cautions: Precautions and Contraindications.)

Acute Toxicity

Limited information is available on the acute toxicity of rituximab. Overdosage has not been reported in clinical studies with patients receiving rituximab in single doses of up to 500 mg/m^2.

Pharmacology

Rituximab is an antineoplastic agent that binds specifically to antigen CD20 (human B-lymphocyte-restricted differentiation antigen, Bp35), a hydrophobic transmembrane protein located on pre-B and mature B lymphocytes. Antigen CD20 also is expressed on greater than 90% of B-cell non-Hodgkin's lymphomas (NHL) but is not found on hematopoietic stem cells, early pre-B cells, normal plasma cells, or other normal tissues. Antigen CD20 is involved in the regulation of cell cycle initiation and differentiation and also may function as a calcium ion channel.

Following binding of the Fab domain of rituximab to antigen CD20 on B lymphocytes, the Fc domain triggers a host immune response causing lysis of normal and malignant B cells; the exact mechanism of cell lysis has not been fully elucidated but is thought to involve complement-dependent cytotoxicity (CDC) and antibody-dependent cell-mediated cytotoxicity (ADCC). Rapid and sustained depletion of circulating and tissue-based B cells occurs as a result of the lysis of B cells induced by rituximab. Depletion of circulating B cells lasted for up to 6–9 months in 83% of patients receiving rituximab for NHL in a clinical study.Antigen CD20 is not shed from the cell surface and does not internalize following antibody binding. Circulation of free CD20 antigen does not occur. Following completion of rituximab therapy, recovery of B cells begins at approximately 6 months, and median levels of B cells return to normal by 12 months.

Inhibition of cellular proliferation and induction of apoptosis by rituximab have been demonstrated in some NHL cell lines. Rituximab also has been shown to increase the in vitro sensitivity of certain chemoresistant human lymphoma cell lines to some cytotoxic agents, including doxorubicin.

B cells may contribute to the pathogenesis of rheumatoid arthritis and associated chronic synovitis by involvement in the production of rheumatoid factor and other autoantibodies, presentation of antigen, activation of T cells, and/or production of inflammatory cytokines. By binding and causing lysis of B cells, rituximab interferes with the autoimmune and inflammatory processes in rheumatoid arthritis. In patients with rheumatoid arthritis, nearly complete depletion of peripheral B lymphocytes (CD19 counts below the lower limit of quantification [20/μL]) occurred within 2 weeks following the first dose of rituximab. In most patients, depletion of circulating B cells lasted for at least 6 months. A small number of patients (approximately 4%) experienced prolonged peripheral B-cell depletion (more than 3 years) after a single course of treatment. Rituximab therapy also was associated with the reduction of certain biologic markers of inflammation, including interleukin-6, C-reactive protein, serum amyloid protein, S100 A8/S100 A9 heterodimer complex, anti-citrullinated peptide, and rheumatoid factor.

Pharmacokinetics

The pharmacokinetic disposition of rituximab when administered in conjunction with 6 cycles of combination chemotherapy with CHOP (i.e., cyclophosphamide, doxorubicin, vincristine, and prednisone) is similar to that observed with rituximab alone.

The pharmacokinetics of rituximab have not been studied in children or adolescents. The effects of renal or hepatic impairment on the pharmacokinetic disposition of rituximab have not been formally studied.

■ Absorption In a study of 203 patients with non-Hodgkin's lymphoma (NHL) receiving rituximab 375 mg/m² by IV infusion once weekly for 4 weeks, rituximab was detected in the serum of patients 3–6 months after completion of treatment.

In patients with rheumatoid arthritis (RA) receiving rituximab, the peak serum concentration averaged 183 mcg/mL following two 500-mg doses and 381 mcg/mL following two 1-g doses.

■ Distribution Following IV infusion, binding of rituximab has been observed on lymphoid cells in the thymus, the white pulp of the spleen, and a majority of B lymphocytes in peripheral blood and lymph nodes. Little or no binding has been observed upon examination of non-lymphoid tissues.

Based on a population pharmacokinetic analysis of data in 2005 patients with RA, the volume of distribution of rituximab was 3.1 L.

It is not known whether rituximab crosses the placenta or distributes into milk in humans; however, IgG distributes into milk in humans. (See Cautions: Pregnancy, Fertility, and Lactation.)

■ Elimination Based on a population pharmacokinetic analysis of data in 298 patients with NHL receiving rituximab once weekly or once every 3 weeks, the estimated median terminal elimination half-life was 22 days (range: 6–52 days). Patients with higher CD19-positive cell count or larger measurable tumor lesions at pretreatment had a higher rate of clearance. Age and gender had no effect on the pharmacokinetics of rituximab in patients with NHL.

In 21 patients with chronic lymphocytic leukemia (CLL) receiving rituximab 375 mg/m² approximately every 28 days, the estimated median terminal half-life was 32 days (range: 14–62 days).

Based on a population pharmacokinetic analysis of data in 2005 patients with RA, the estimated clearance of rituximab was 0.335 L/day (approximately 0.014 L/hour), and the mean terminal elimination half-life was 18 days (range: 5–78 days). Age, weight, and gender had no effect on the pharmacokinetics of rituximab in patients with RA.

Chemistry and Stability

■ Chemistry Rituximab, a chimeric human-murine anti-human antigen CD20 monoclonal antibody, is an antineoplastic agent.

The rituximab antibody is an IgG_1 kappa immunoglobulin containing murine light-chain and heavy-chain variable region sequences and human constant region sequences. Because of the presence of human constant region sequences, the chimeric antibody is characterized by lower immunogenicity, longer half-life, and more effective lysis of tumor cells compared with murine monoclonal antibodies.

Rituximab binds specifically to antigen CD20, a hydrophobic transmembrane protein located on pre-B and mature B lymphocytes.

Commercially available rituximab concentrate for injection occurs as a sterile, clear, colorless, preservative-free solution. The product is formulated for IV administration in 9 mg/mL sodium chloride, 7.35 mg/mL sodium citrate dihydrate, 0.7 mg/mL polysorbate 80, and water for injection and has been adjusted to a pH of 6.5.

■ Stability Vials of rituximab should be stored at 2–8°C and should not be frozen or shaken; when stored under recommended conditions, commercially available rituximab liquid concentrate for injection should be stable up to the date of expiration marked on the vial. Vials of rituximab should be protected from direct sunlight.

Following dilution of rituximab as recommended, solutions of the drug may be stored for 24 hours at 2–8°C. Rituximab solutions for infusion have been shown to be stable for an additional 24 hours at room temperature; however, since rituximab solutions do not contain a preservative, diluted solutions should be stored at 2–8°C. No incompatibilities between rituximab and polyvinylchloride or polyethylene bags have been observed.

For further information on the handling of antineoplastic agents, see the ASHP Guidelines on Handling Hazardous Drugs at http://www.ahfsdruginformation.com.

Preparations

Excipients in commercially available drug preparations may have clinically important effects in some individuals; consult specific product labeling for details.

riTUXimab

Parenteral

For injection concentrate, for IV infusion	10 mg/mL (100 and 500 mg)	**Rituxan®**, Biogen Idec (also promoted by Genentech)

†Use is not currently included in the labeling approved by the US Food and Drug Administration

Rucaparib Camsylate

■ Rucaparib, an inhibitor of poly(adenosine diphosphate [ADP]-ribose) polymerase (PARP), is an antineoplastic agent.

Uses

■ Ovarian Cancer Rucaparib is used as single-agent therapy for the treatment of deleterious germline and/or somatic BRCA-mutated advanced ovarian cancer previously treated with 2 or more chemotherapy regimens. The accelerated approval of rucaparib for this indication is based on overall response rate and duration of response. Continued approval for this indication may be contingent on verification and description of clinical benefit of rucaparib in confirmatory studies. The drug has been designated an orphan drug by FDA for the treatment of this cancer. An FDA-approved companion diagnostic test (FoundationFocus® CDx BRCA) is required to confirm the presence of mutations in the BRCA genes (BRCA1 and/or BRCA2) prior to initiation of rucaparib therapy. Women with mutations that result in defective BRCA genes are more likely to develop ovarian cancer. It is estimated that approximately 10–15% of all cases of ovarian cancer are associated with these hereditary BRCA mutations.

The current indication for rucaparib as single-agent therapy is based on response rates obtained in 2 multicenter, single-arm, open-label phase 2 or 1/2 studies (ARIEL2 parts 1 and 2, CO-338-010 part 2A) for a group of 106 patients with deleterious germline and/or somatic BRCA-mutated advanced ovarian cancer, including primary peritoneal and fallopian tube cancer, that had progressed following treatment with 2 or more chemotherapy regimens, including at least 2 platinum-based regimens. Patients in both studies received rucaparib 600 mg orally twice daily until disease progression or unacceptable toxicity occurred. The median age of patients enrolled in both studies was 59 years. Most of the patients were Caucasian (78%) and all of the enrolled patients had an ECOG performance status of 0 or 1. About one-half of patients had received 3 or more prior chemotherapy regimens. Confirmed deleterious BRCA mutations were detected in tumor tissue samples but not in blood specimens in 18 of 106 patients enrolled in both studies. Results of the clinical trial assay used to detect BRCA mutation were verified retrospectively by the FoundationFocus® CDx BRCA test in 64 of 67 patients for whom tumor tissue samples were available. The primary efficacy end point in both studies was overall response rate as assessed by the investigator according to Response Evaluation Criteria in Solid Tumors (RECIST); duration of response was also evaluated.

In these studies, the combined overall response rate was 54%, with a complete response reported in 9% and a partial response reported in 45% of the patients. At the time of the analysis, the median duration of response was 9.2 months (range: 6.6–11.6 months). An independent review committee assessed overall response rate as 42% with a median duration of response of 6.7 months (range: 5.5–11.1 months). Subgroup analysis according to previous therapy suggested that rucaparib had a higher overall response rate in patients with platinum-sensitive disease than in those with platinum-resistant disease (66 versus 25%); responses were observed in none of the 7 patients with platinum-refractory disease.

Approximately 50% of patients with high-grade serous ovarian cancers have aberrations in the homologous recombination repair pathway that result in subsequent loss or duplication of chromosomal regions (also known as genomic loss of heterozygosity [LOH]); BRCA mutations or aberrations in other homologous recombination genes account for approximately 21 or 20%, respectively, of such cancers with homologous recombination deficiency. Poly (adenosine diphosphate [ADP]-ribose) polymerase (PARP) inhibitors appear to be selective for tumor cells that harbor homologous recombination deficiencies, and prolonged progression-free survival has been observed with PARP inhibitor therapy in patients with or without BRCA mutation. Although an optimal method for identifying homologous recombination deficiency in cancers with wild-type BRCA is unknown, measurement of genomic instability based on loss of heterozygosity has been used.

In part 1 of the ARIEL2 study, patients with platinum-sensitive, high-grade ovarian cancer that had progressed following treatment with at least 1 platinum-based regimen were classified into predefined homologous recombination deficiency subgroups based on BRCA mutation status (germline and/or somatic BRCA mutation, wild-type BRCA with high LOH, and wild-type BRCA with low LOH). Pretreatment tumor tissue samples with 14% or more of genomic LOH were considered high LOH. The primary efficacy end point in part 1 of the ARIEL2 study was progression-free survival. Patients with BRCA mutations and those with wild-type BRCA expression with high LOH had longer progression-free survival, higher overall response rates, and longer times to progression compared with those with wild-type BRCA expression with low LOH. Results of an exploratory analysis suggested that among patients with BRCA wild-type tumors, analysis of genomic LOH may be a predictor of response to rucaparib in patients with platinum-sensitive disease with mutations in a homologous recombination gene other than BRCA1 or BRCA2; however, larger randomized studies are needed to confirm the predictive ability of the biomarker.

Dosage and Administration

■ General Confirmation of the diagnosis of deleterious germline and/or somatic BRCA-mutated advanced ovarian cancer by an FDA-approved companion diagnostic test is necessary for selecting patients for rucaparib therapy.

Because myelodysplastic syndrome (MDS) and acute myelogenous leukemia (AML) have been reported in patients receiving rucaparib, the manufacturer states that complete blood cell (CBC) counts should be obtained prior to initiation of rucaparib and monthly during therapy with the drug. (See Myelodysplastic Syndrome/Acute Myeloid Leukemia under Cautions: Warnings/Precautions.)

Restricted Distribution Program Rucaparib camsylate can only be obtained through select specialty distributors. Clinicians may contact the manufacturer (Clovis Oncology) by telephone at 844-779-7707 or consult the Rubraca® Connections website for specific availability information (http://www.rubracaconnections.com/pages/hcp_home.html).

■ **Administration** Rucaparib camsylate is administered orally twice daily. The drug may be given without regard to meals.

■ **Dosage** Dosage of rucaparib camsylate is expressed in terms of rucaparib.

Ovarian Cancer The recommended adult dosage of rucaparib as monotherapy for the treatment of previously treated deleterious germline and/or somatic BRCA-mutated advanced ovarian cancer is 600 mg (two 300-mg tablets) twice daily. Therapy should be continued until disease progression or unacceptable toxicity occurs.

Dosage Modification for Toxicity If adverse reactions occur, interruption of therapy or dosage reduction of rucaparib should be considered. If dosage reduction from 600 mg twice daily is necessary, the recommended dosage is 500 mg twice daily. If dosage reduction from 500 mg twice daily is necessary, the recommended dosage is 400 mg twice daily. If further dosage reduction is necessary, the dosage should be reduced to 300 mg twice daily.

■ **Special Populations** The manufacturer states that no adjustment to the initial dosage of rucaparib is necessary in patients with mild hepatic impairment (total bilirubin concentration not exceeding the upper limit of normal [ULN] with AST concentration exceeding the ULN *or* total bilirubin concentration exceeding the ULN, but not more than 1.5 times the ULN, with any AST concentration). There are limited data in patients with moderate hepatic impairment and no data in patients with severe hepatic impairment; the manufacturer provides no specific dosage recommendations for such patients. (See Hepatic Impairment under Warnings/Precautions: Specific Populations, in Cautions.)

The manufacturer states that no adjustment to the initial dosage of rucaparib is necessary in patients with mild or moderate renal impairment (creatinine clearance 30–89 mL/minute). Rucaparib has not been studied in patients with severe renal impairment (creatinine clearance less than 30 mL/minute), including in those receiving dialysis, and the manufacturer provides no specific dosage recommendations for such patients. (See Renal Impairment under Warnings/Precautions: Specific Populations, in Cautions.)

The manufacturer makes no specific dosage recommendations for geriatric patients. (See Geriatric Use under Warnings/Precautions: Specific Populations, in Cautions.)

Cautions

■ **Contraindications** The manufacturer states that there are no known contraindications to the use of rucaparib.

■ **Warnings/Precautions** ***Myelodysplastic Syndrome/Acute Myeloid Leukemia*** In clinical studies evaluating rucaparib in patients with ovarian cancer, myelodysplastic syndrome (MDS) and acute myeloid leukemia (AML) were reported in 2 of 377 patients (0.5%) receiving rucaparib at 57 or 539 days following initiation of therapy. In another clinical study evaluating rucaparib in patients with ovarian cancer, AML was reported in 2 patients (less than 1%) receiving rucaparib at 107 or 427 days following initiation of therapy; AML was fatal in one patient. All of these patients had received previous chemotherapy with platinum-containing agents and/or other DNA-damaging antineoplastic agents.

Complete blood cell (CBC) counts should be monitored at baseline and then monthly in patients receiving rucaparib. In addition, rucaparib therapy should not be initiated until hematologic toxicity caused by previous chemotherapy has resolved to grade 1 or less. If prolonged hematologic toxicity occurs during therapy, rucaparib should be withheld and CBC counts should be monitored weekly until recovery to grade 1 or less occurs. If hematologic toxicity persists for more than 4 weeks following interruption of therapy, patients should be referred to a hematologist for further evaluation, including bone marrow analysis and cytogenetic testing of a blood sample. If MDS/AML is confirmed, rucaparib should be discontinued.

Fetal/Neonatal Morbidity and Mortality Based on its mechanism of action and animal findings, rucaparib may cause fetal harm. Embryotoxicity (i.e., postimplantation loss) was observed in pregnant rats receiving rucaparib at exposure levels equivalent to approximately 0.04 times the human exposure at the recommended rucaparib dosage. The manufacturer recommends confirmation of pregnancy status prior to initiation of rucaparib, and women of childbearing potential should be advised to use effective contraceptive methods during rucaparib therapy and for 6 months after discontinuance of the drug. If rucaparib is used during pregnancy or if the patient becomes pregnant while receiving the drug, the patient should be apprised of the potential risk to the fetus and the potential risk for loss of the pregnancy.

Prolongation of QT Interval In an open-label, noncomparative study evaluating potential effects of rucaparib on the QT interval, a significant relationship between the increase from baseline in QT interval (corrected for heart rate using Fridericia's formula [QT_cF]) and systemic exposure to rucaparib (administered at dosages ranging from 40 mg once daily to 840 mg twice daily) was observed. At the estimated 95th percentile for steady-state peak plasma concentrations attained with a rucaparib dosage of 600 mg twice daily, the mean increase from baseline in the QT_cF interval was 14.9 msec (range: 11.1–18.7 msec).

Specific Populations **Pregnancy.** Rucaparib may cause fetal harm if administered to pregnant women based on its mechanism of action and animal findings. (See Fetal/Neonatal Morbidity and Mortality under Cautions: Warnings/Precautions.)

Confirmation of pregnancy status prior to initiation of rucaparib therapy is recommended.

Lactation. It is not known whether rucaparib is distributed into milk. Because of the potential for serious adverse reactions to rucaparib in nursing infants, women should be advised to discontinue nursing during rucaparib therapy. Women may begin nursing 2 weeks after discontinuance of therapy. The effects of the drug on nursing infants or on milk production are unknown.

Pediatric Use. Safety and efficacy of rucaparib have not been established in pediatric patients.

Geriatric Use. In clinical studies evaluating rucaparib in women with ovarian cancer, 42% of patients were 65 years of age or older. No overall differences in safety were observed between geriatric patients and younger adults. However, the possibility of increased sensitivity to the drug in some geriatric patients cannot be ruled out. Clinical experience with rucaparib in patients 65 years of age or older with BRCA-mutated ovarian cancer is insufficient to determine whether geriatric patients respond differently than younger adults.

In pharmacokinetic population analyses, age did not have a clinically important effect on systemic exposure to rucaparib.

Hepatic Impairment. In population pharmacokinetic analyses, the pharmacokinetics of rucaparib were similar in patients with mild hepatic impairment (total bilirubin concentration not exceeding the upper limit of normal [ULN] with AST concentration exceeding the ULN *or* total bilirubin concentration exceeding the ULN, but not more than 1.5 times the ULN, with any AST concentration) and those with normal hepatic function. (See Dosage and Administration: Special Populations.)

The pharmacokinetic profile of rucaparib has not been established in patients with moderate or severe hepatic impairment (total bilirubin concentration exceeding 1.5 times the ULN).

Renal Impairment. Systemic exposure to rucaparib was increased by approximately 15 or 32% in patients with mild (creatinine clearance 60–89 mL/minute) or moderate (creatinine clearance 30–59 mL/minute) renal impairment, respectively, compared with individuals with normal renal function. (See Dosage and Administration: Special Populations.)

The pharmacokinetics of rucaparib have not been established in patients with severe renal impairment (creatinine clearance less than 30 mL/minute) or in those receiving dialysis.

■ **Common Adverse Effects** Adverse effects reported in 20% or more of patients receiving rucaparib include asthenia/fatigue, nausea, vomiting, anemia, constipation, decreased appetite, dysgeusia, diarrhea, abdominal pain, dyspnea, abdominal distention, and thrombocytopenia. Laboratory abnormalities reported in 35% or more of patients receiving rucaparib include elevated serum creatinine concentrations, elevated concentrations of aminotransferases (i.e., AST, ALT), decreased hemoglobin concentrations, decreased lymphocyte concentrations, decreased absolute neutrophil count (ANC), and elevated cholesterol concentrations.

Drug Interactions

Rucaparib is metabolized principally by cytochrome P-450 (CYP) isoenzyme 2D6 and, to a lesser extent, by CYP isoenzymes 1A2 and 3A4. In vitro studies also indicate that rucaparib is a reversible inhibitor of CYP isoenzymes 1A2, 2C19, 2C9, and 3A and, to a lesser extent, CYP isoenzymes 2C8 and 2D6 and uridine diphosphate-glucuronosyltransferase (UGT) 1A1. In vitro, rucaparib induces CYP1A2 and downregulates CYP isoenzymes 2B6 and 3A4 at clinically relevant concentrations.

Rucaparib is a potent inhibitor of multidrug and toxic compound extrusion (MATE) 1 and MATE2K, and a moderate inhibitor of organic cation transporter (OCT) 1. Rucaparib also is a weak inhibitor of multidrug resistance protein (MRP) 4, organic anion transport protein (OATP) 1B1, OATP1B3, organic anion transporter (OAT) 1, and OAT3, but does not inhibit MRP2, MRP3, or bile salt export pump (BSEP) at ultratherapeutic concentrations (300 micromolar [$3 \times 10^{-4}M$]). In vitro, the 50% inhibitory concentrations of rucaparib for breast cancer resistance protein (BCRP) and P-glycoprotein (P-gp) are 55 micromolar ($5.5 \times 10^{-5}M$) and 283 micromolar ($2.83 \times 10^{-4}M$), respectively.

In vitro studies indicate that rucaparib is a substrate of the efflux transporters P-gp and BCRP, but is not a substrate for OAT1, OAT3, OCT2, OATP1B1, or OATP1B3.

■ **Proton-pump Inhibitors** In population pharmacokinetic analyses, concomitant administration of rucaparib with proton-pump inhibitors did not have a clinically meaningful effect on systemic exposure to rucaparib.

Description

Rucaparib camsylate, an inhibitor of mammalian poly(adenosine diphosphate [ADP]-ribose) polymerase (PARP) enzymes, including PARP-1, PARP-2, and PARP-3, is an antineoplastic agent. PARP enzymes are involved in normal cellular homeostasis, including DNA transcription, cell cycle regulation, and DNA repair.

In vitro studies have demonstrated that rucaparib-induced cytotoxicity may involve inhibition of PARP enzymatic activity and increased formation of PARP-DNA complexes, which result in disruption of cellular homeostasis and apoptosis. PARP inhibitors, such as rucaparib, appear to be selective for tumor cells that harbor certain homologous recombination deficiencies, including those harboring BRCA1 and BRCA2 mutations. (See Uses: Ovarian Cancer.) Rucaparib reduced tumor growth of xenograft models of human cancer (with or without deficiencies in BRCA) in mice.

Following oral administration, the mean absolute bioavailability of rucaparib is 36% (range: 30–45%). Rucaparib exhibits linear, time-independent, dose-proportional pharmacokinetics over the dosage range of 240–840 mg twice daily. Following oral administration at the recommended dosage, the median time to peak plasma concentrations of rucaparib is 1.9 hours. Repeated twice-daily administration of rucaparib resulted in 3.5- to 6.2-fold mean rucaparib accumulation (based on area under the concentration-time curve [AUC]). Administration of rucaparib (single 600-mg dose) with a high-fat meal in patients with solid tumors decreased the rate but only modestly increased the extent of absorption; time to peak plasma concentration was delayed by 2.5 hours, and peak plasma concentration and AUC were increased by 20 and 38%, respectively, relative to fasted conditions. Rucaparib is metabolized principally by cytochrome P-450 (CYP) isoenzyme 2D6 and, to a lesser extent, by CYP isoenzymes 1A2 and 3A4. Genetic polymorphisms of CYP2D6 (i.e., poor, intermediate, or ultrarapid metabolizer) or CYP1A2 (i.e., hyperinducers) do not substantially affect systemic exposure to rucaparib at steady state. In vitro, rucaparib is 70% bound to plasma proteins at therapeutic concentrations. The mean terminal half-life of the drug is 17–19 hours.

Data from population pharmacokinetic analyses indicate that age, race, and body weight do not have clinically important effects on systemic exposure to rucaparib.

Advice to Patients

Importance of reading the manufacturer's patient information.

If a dose is missed or vomited, importance of administering the next dose at the regularly scheduled time; an additional dose should not be administered to make up for a missed dose.

Risk of myelodysplastic syndrome (MDS) and acute myeloid leukemia (AML). Importance of informing clinician if fatigue/asthenia, fever, weight loss, frequent infections, bruising, unusual bleeding (including hematuria or bloody stool), shortness of breath, abnormal complete blood cell (CBC) counts, or requirement for blood product transfusions occurs.

Importance of hematologic monitoring during rucaparib therapy.

Risk of photosensitivity reactions. Importance of limiting exposure to sunlight during rucaparib therapy and of wearing protective clothing and using sunscreen when exposure cannot be avoided.

Risk of fetal harm and pregnancy loss. Necessity of advising women of childbearing potential to avoid pregnancy and to use an effective method of contraception while receiving rucaparib and for 6 months following discontinuance of therapy. Importance of women informing clinicians immediately if they are pregnant or become pregnant during therapy. If pregnancy occurs, advise pregnant women of potential risk to the fetus.

Importance of advising women to avoid breast-feeding while receiving rucaparib and for 2 weeks following discontinuance of therapy.

Importance of informing clinicians of existing or contemplated concomitant therapy, including prescription and OTC drugs and dietary or herbal supplements, as well as any concomitant illnesses.

Importance of informing patients of other important precautionary information. (See Cautions.)

Overview® (see Users Guide). For additional information on this drug until a more detailed monograph is developed and published, the manufacturer's labeling should be consulted. It is *essential* that the manufacturer's labeling be consulted for more detailed information on usual cautions, precautions, contraindications, potential drug interactions, laboratory test interferences, and acute toxicity. For further information on the handling of antineoplastic agents, see the ASHP Guidelines on Handling Hazardous Drugs at http://www.ahfsdruginformation.com.

Preparations

Distribution of rucaparib is restricted. (See Restricted Distribution Program under Dosage and Administration: General.)

Excipients in commercially available drug preparations may have clinically important effects in some individuals; consult specific product labeling for details.

Rucaparib Camsylate

Oral		
Tablets, film-coated	200 mg (of rucaparib)	**Rubraca®**, Clovis Oncology
	250 mg (of rucaparib)	**Rubraca®**, Clovis Oncology
	300 mg (of rucaparib)	**Rubraca®**, Clovis Oncology

Ruxolitinib Phosphate

■ Ruxolitinib phosphate, a selective inhibitor of Janus kinase (JAK) 1 and 2, is an antineoplastic agent.

Uses

■ **Intermediate- or High-Risk Myelofibrosis** Ruxolitinib phosphate is used for the treatment of intermediate- or high-risk myelofibrosis, including primary myelofibrosis, post-polycythemia vera myelofibrosis, and post-essential thrombocythemia myelofibrosis. Ruxolitinib is designated an orphan drug by the US Food and Drug Administration (FDA) for use in the treatment of these conditions.

Efficacy and safety of ruxolitinib were established in 2 randomized phase 3 studies (Controlled Myelofibrosis Study with Oral JAK Inhibitor Treatment I and II [COMFORT-I and COMFORT-II]) in patients with myelofibrosis (primary myelofibrosis, post-polycythemia vera myelofibrosis, or post-essential thrombocythemia myelofibrosis). In these studies, patients had palpable splenomegaly at least 5 cm below the costal margin and a risk category of intermediate-2 (2 prognostic factors) or high risk (3 or more prognostic factors) based on the International Working Group (IWG) consensus criteria. The International Prognostic Scoring System (IPSS) includes 5 risk factors for estimating survival from time of diagnosis, including age greater than 65 years, hemoglobin level less than 10 g/dL, leukocyte count greater than 25,000/mm^3, circulating myeloblasts of 1% or greater, and presence of constitutional symptoms. The presence of 0, 1, 2, or 3 or more risk factors indicate low, intermediate-1, intermediate-2, or high risk, respectively.

In both clinical studies, ruxolitinib starting dosage was based on platelet count; for initial treatment, patients with platelet counts of 100,000–200,000/mm^3 received an initial ruxolitinib dosage of 15 mg twice daily and patients with platelet counts exceeding 200,000/mm^3 received ruxolitinib 20 mg twice daily. Dosages were then individualized based on tolerability, efficacy, and platelet counts; patients with platelet counts exceeding 100,000 but not exceeding 125,000/mm^3 received a maximum dosage of 20 mg twice daily, patients with platelet counts exceeding 75,000 but not exceeding 100,000/mm^3 received a maximum dosage of 10 mg twice daily, and those with platelet counts exceeding 50,000 but not exceeding 75,000/mm^3 received a maximum dosage of 5 mg twice daily.

COMFORT-I was a double-blind, randomized, placebo-controlled study in 309 patients with myelofibrosis who were refractory to or not candidates for available therapy. The median age was 68 years, and median spleen volume (as measured by magnetic resonance imaging [MRI] or computed tomography [CT]) was 2595 cm^3 (upper limit of normal 300 cm^3). The primary end point of this study was the proportion of patients achieving a 35% or greater reduction from baseline in spleen volume (measured by MRI or CT) at 24 weeks. A 35% or greater reduction in spleen volume from baseline was achieved in a substantially larger proportion of patients receiving ruxolitinib compared with those receiving placebo (41.9 versus 0.7%).

COMFORT-II was an open label, randomized study in 219 patients with myelofibrosis randomized in a 2:1 ratio to receive either ruxolitinib or best available therapy (selected by the investigator on a patient-by-patient basis). The median age of patients enrolled in the study was 66 years and median spleen volume (as measured by MRI or CT) was 2381 cm^3. Among patients receiving best available therapy, the most commonly used drugs were hydroxyurea (47% of patients) and glucocorticoids (16% of patients); 33% of patients in this treatment arm received no therapy. The primary efficacy end point was the proportion of patients achieving 35% or greater reduction from baseline in spleen volume (measured by MRI or CT) at 48 weeks. A 35% or greater reduction in spleen volume from baseline was achieved in a substantially larger proportion of patients receiving ruxolitinib compared with those receiving best available therapy (28.5 versus 0%).

Dosage and Administration

■ **General** A complete blood cell count (CBC), including platelet count, must be performed prior to initiating therapy, every 2–4 weeks until dosage is stabilized, and then as clinically indicated.

Restricted Distribution Program Patients must obtain ruxolitinib through the Incyte Connecting to Access, Reimbursement, Education, and Support (IncyteCARES) program. The clinician and patient must jointly complete a prescription and reimbursement application. Following verification of prescription information and review of healthcare benefits, an authorized specialty pharmacy ships ruxolitinib directly to the patient. To enroll in this program, the patient should call 855-452-5234 or visit http://www.jakafi.com.

■ **Administration** Ruxolitinib is administered orally and can be taken with or without food. If a dose is missed, the patient should not take an additional dose, but should take the next scheduled dose.

For patients unable to swallow tablets, ruxolitinib can be dispersed in a glass of water containing approximately 40 mL and administered through a nasogastric tube (8 French or larger). The water should be stirred for approximately 10 minutes; once the tablet has dispersed, the suspension should be administered within 6 hours through a nasogastric tube using an appropriate syringe. Following administration, the tube should be rinsed with approximately 75 mL of water.

■ **Dosage** Dosage of ruxolitinib phosphate is expressed in terms of ruxolitinib.

Intermediate- or High-Risk Myelofibrosis The recommended initial dosage of ruxolitinib is based on platelet count. In patients with platelet counts exceeding 200,000/mm³, the recommended initial adult dosage of ruxolitinib for the treatment of intermediate- or high-risk myelofibrosis is 20 mg twice daily. In patients with platelet counts of 100,000–200,000/mm³, the recommended initial adult dosage is 15 mg twice daily. Dosage should be titrated based on efficacy and safety up to a maximum recommended dosage of 25 mg twice daily. (See Dosage Modification for Thrombocytopenia and also Dosage Modification for Insufficient Clinical Response under Dosage and Administration: Dosage.)

Dosage of ruxolitinib should be tapered gradually (e.g., by 5 mg twice daily on a weekly basis) when the drug is discontinued for reasons other than thrombocytopenia.

Dosage Modification for Thrombocytopenia Treatment with ruxolitinib should be interrupted in patients with platelet counts less than 50,000/mm³. Therapy may be restarted or dosage increased following recovery of platelet counts to acceptable levels. When restarting therapy, dosages at least 5 mg twice daily below the original dosage should be used. For maximum dosages that may be used when restarting ruxolitinib after therapy interruption for thrombocytopenia, see Table 1.

Table 1. Maximum Dosages for Restarting Ruxolitinib Following Interruption for Thrombocytopenia

Current Platelet Count (per mm³)	Maximum Dosage for Restarting Therapy
≥125,000	20 mg twice daily
100,000 to <125,000	15 mg twice daily
75,000 to <100,000	10 mg twice daily for at least 2 weeks; if stable, may increase to 15 mg twice daily
50,000 to <75,000	5 mg twice daily for at least 2 weeks; if stable, may increase to 10 mg twice daily
<50,000	Continue to withhold therapy

To avoid therapy interruption as a result of thrombocytopenia, patients receiving ruxolitinib should be monitored for declining platelet counts and dosage reductions should be considered (see Table 2).

Table 2. Recommended Dosage Modifications to Avoid Ruxolitinib Therapy Interruption for Thrombocytopenia

	Ruxolitinib Dosage at Time of Platelet Decline				
Current Platelet Count (per mm³)	25 mg twice daily	20 mg twice daily	15 mg twice daily	10 mg twice daily	5 mg twice daily
	Modified Ruxolitinib Dosage				
100,000 to <125,000	20 mg twice daily	15 mg twice daily	Maintain dosage level	Maintain dosage level	Maintain dosage level
75,000 to <100,000	10 mg twice daily	10 mg twice daily	10 mg twice daily	Maintain dosage level	Maintain dosage level
50,000 to <75,000	5 mg twice daily	5 mg twice daily	5 mg twice daily	5 mg twice daily	Maintain dosage level
<50,000	Withhold therapy	Withhold therapy	Withhold therapy	Withhold therapy	Withhold therapy

Dosage Modification for Insufficient Clinical Response If clinical response is considered insufficient and platelet and neutrophil counts are adequate, dosage may be increased in increments of 5 mg twice daily (e.g., from 15 mg twice daily to 20 mg twice daily) to a maximum of 25 mg twice daily. Dosage increases should be considered in patients who meet all of the following conditions: failure to achieve a reduction from pretreatment baseline spleen size of either 50% in palpable length or 35% in volume as measured by CT or MRI; platelet counts exceeding 125,000/mm³ at 4 weeks with no counts less than 100,000/mm³; absolute neutrophil counts (ANCs) exceeding 750/mm³.

Dosage should not be increased during the first 4 weeks of therapy or more frequently than every 2 weeks.

If there is no spleen size reduction or symptomatic improvement after 6 months of therapy with ruxolitinib, the drug should be discontinued.

Limited clinical data indicate that long-term maintenance dosages of 5 mg twice daily have not been associated with adequate responses, and continued use at this dosage should be limited to patients in whom benefits outweigh the potential risks.

Dosage Modification for Concomitant Use with Drugs and Food Affecting Hepatic Microsomal Enzymes Because concomitant use of ruxolitinib with potent inhibitors of cytochrome P-450 (CYP) isoenzyme 3A4 may result in increased plasma concentrations of ruxolitinib, the recommended initial dosage is 10 mg twice daily in patients with platelet counts of 100,000/mm³ or greater receiving such concomitant therapy. Additional dosage modifications should be made after careful monitoring of safety and efficacy. Concomitant use of ruxolitinib and potent CYP3A4 inhibitors should be avoided in patients with platelet counts less than 100,000/mm³. No dosage adjustment is recommended in patients receiving concomitant therapy with ruxolitinib and weak or moderate CYP3A4 inhibitors. (See Drug Interactions: Drugs and Food Affecting Hepatic Microsomal Enzymes.)

■ **Special Populations** In patients with mild to severe hepatic impairment and platelet counts of 100,000–150,000/mm³, the recommended initial dosage of ruxolitinib is 10 mg twice daily. Subsequent dosage modifications should be made based on careful monitoring of safety and efficacy. Ruxolitinib should be avoided in patients with hepatic impairment and platelet counts less than 100,000/mm³.

In patients with platelet counts of 100,000–150,000/mm³ and moderate or severe renal impairment (creatinine clearance of 15–59 mL/minute), the recommended initial dosage of ruxolitinib is 10 mg twice daily.

In patients with end-stage renal disease (ESRD) (i.e., creatinine clearance of less than 15 mL/minute) receiving dialysis, the recommended initial dosage of ruxolitinib is 15 mg in patients with platelet counts of 100,000–200,000/mm³ and 20 mg in patients with platelet counts exceeding 200,000/mm³; the 15- or 20-mg dose should be administered *following completion* of each dialysis session only on days when hemodialysis is scheduled. Subsequent dosage modifications should be made based on careful monitoring of safety and efficacy. Ruxolitinib should be avoided in patients with ESRD who are not receiving dialysis and in patients with moderate or severe renal impairment with platelet counts less than 100,000/mm³.

The manufacturer makes no specific dosage recommendations for geriatric patients. (See Geriatric Use under Warnings/Precautions: Specific Populations, in Cautions.)

Cautions

■ **Contraindications** The manufacturer states that there are no known contraindications to the use of ruxolitinib phosphate.

■ **Warnings/Precautions** ***Thrombocytopenia, Anemia, and Neutropenia*** Ruxolitinib can cause adverse hematologic reactions, including thrombocytopenia, anemia, and neutropenia. A complete blood cell count (CBC) must be performed before initiating therapy with ruxolitinib. Grade 3 or 4 thrombocytopenia occurred in 12.9% of patients receiving ruxolitinib compared with 1.3% of patients receiving placebo in the Controlled Myelofibrosis Study with Oral JAK Inhibitor Treatment I (COMFORT-I). The median time to onset of grade 3 or 4 thrombocytopenia was approximately 8 weeks. Patients with platelet counts of 100,000–200,000/mm³ prior to initiation of ruxolitinib had a higher incidence of grade 3 or 4 thrombocytopenia compared with patients with platelet counts exceeding 200,000/mm³ (16.5 versus 7.2%).

Thrombocytopenia generally was reversible and usually was managed by reducing the dosage or temporarily withholding ruxolitinib. If clinically indicated, platelet transfusions may be administered.

Grade 3 or 4 anemia occurred in 45.2% of patients receiving ruxolitinib compared with 19.2% of patients receiving placebo in COMFORT-I. Patients who develop anemia may require blood transfusions; dosage modification of ruxolitinib also may be considered in such patients.

In COMFORT-I , grade 3 or 4 neutropenia occurred in 7.1% of patients receiving ruxolitinib compared with 2% of patients receiving placebo. Neutropenia (absolute neutrophil count [ANC] less than 500/mm³) generally was reversible and managed by temporarily withholding ruxolitinib.

CBCs should be monitored as clinically indicated and dosing adjusted as required.

Infectious Complications Patients should be assessed for the risk of developing serious bacterial, mycobacterial, fungal, and viral infections. Active serious infections should have resolved prior to initiating therapy with ruxolitinib. Clinicians should carefully observe patients receiving ruxolitinib for signs and symptoms of infection and should promptly initiate appropriate treatment.

Herpes zoster infection occurred in 1.9% of patients receiving ruxolitinib in a clinical study. Clinicians should inform patients about the early signs and symptoms of herpes zoster and advise patients to seek treatment as soon as possible for this condition.

Withdrawal of Therapy Following interruption or discontinuance of ruxolitinib therapy, symptoms of myelofibrosis generally return to pretreatment levels within approximately 1 week. In isolated cases, patients with myelofibrosis who discontinued ruxolitinib during an acute concomitant illness experienced worsening of the clinical course of their disease. However, it has not been established whether discontinuance of therapy contributed to the clinical deterioration in these patients. Gradual tapering of the dosage should be considered when ruxolitinib is discontinued for reasons other than thrombocytopenia. (See Dosage and Administration: General.)

Withdrawal manifestations, characterized by acute relapse of disease symptoms, accelerated splenomegaly, worsening of cytopenias, and occasional hemodynamic decompensation (including septic shock-like syndrome with severe hypoxia, hypotension, fever, and confusion), have been reported in some patients following discontinuance of ruxolitinib. Some experts recommend that ruxolitinib dosage should be tapered gradually over a 2-week period under close medical supervision.

Specific Populations **Pregnancy.** Category C. (See Users Guide.)

Lactation. Ruxolitinib and/or its metabolites are distributed into milk in rats; it is not known whether ruxolitinib is distributed into human milk. Because of the potential for serious adverse reactions to ruxolitinib in nursing infants, a decision should be made whether to discontinue nursing or the drug, taking into account the importance of the drug to the woman.

Pediatric Use. Safety and efficacy of ruxolitinib in children have not been established.

Geriatric Use. In clinical studies of ruxolitinib, approximately 52% of patients with myelofibrosis were 65 years of age or older. No overall differences in safety or efficacy relative to younger adults were observed.

Hepatic Impairment. Following a single 25-mg dose of ruxolitinib, mean area under the plasma concentration-time curve (AUC) for the drug was increased by 87, 28, or 65% in patients with mild (Child-Pugh class A), moderate (Child-Pugh class B), or severe (Child-Pugh class C) hepatic impairment, respectively, compared with patients with normal hepatic function. Terminal elimination half-life was prolonged in patients with hepatic impairment (4.1–5 hours) compared with healthy individuals (2.8 hours). Dosage reduction of ruxolitinib is recommended in patients with any degree of hepatic impairment and platelet counts of 100,000–150,000/mm^3. (See Dosage and Administration: Special Populations.)

Renal Impairment. The pharmacokinetic profile of ruxolitinib in patients with various degrees of renal impairment was similar to that in individuals with normal renal function. However, exposure to ruxolitinib metabolites increased with increasing severity of renal impairment. Dosage reduction of ruxolitinib is recommended in patients with end-stage renal disease requiring dialysis and in patients with moderate or severe renal impairment (creatinine clearance of 15–59 mL/minute) and platelet counts of 100,000–150,000/mm^3. (See Dosage and Administration: Special Populations.)

■ **Common Adverse Effects** Adverse effects reported in more than 10% of patients receiving ruxolitinib include thrombocytopenia, anemia, neutropenia, bruising, dizziness, and headache.

Drug Interactions

Ruxolitinib is metabolized mainly by cytochrome P-450 (CYP) isoenzyme 3A4.

In vitro data indicate that neither ruxolitinib nor its M18 metabolite is an inhibitor of P-glycoprotein (P-gp), breast cancer resistance protein (BCRP), organic anion-transporting polypeptides (OATP) 1B1 and 1B3, organic cation transporters (OCT) 1 and 2, and organic anion transporters (OAT) 1 and 3 at clinically relevant concentrations. Ruxolitinib also is not a substrate for P-gp.

■ **Drugs and Food Affecting Hepatic Microsomal Enzymes** Because ruxolitinib is mainly metabolized by CYP3A4, potent inhibitors or inducers of this isoenzyme are expected to alter the drug's pharmacokinetics. Ruxolitinib and its M18 metabolite do not inhibit CYP1A2, 2B6, 2C8, 2C9, 2C19, 2D6, or 3A4 in vitro. Ruxolitinib also does not induce CYP1A2, 2B6, or 3A4 at clinically relevant concentrations.

Concomitant use of ruxolitinib with potent inhibitors of CYP3A4 (e.g., boceprevir, clarithromycin, conivaptan, grapefruit juice, indinavir, itraconazole, ketoconazole, lopinavir/ritonavir, mibefradil [no longer commercially available in the US], nefazodone, nelfinavir, posaconazole, ritonavir, saquinavir, telaprevir, telithromycin, voriconazole) has resulted in increased peak plasma concentrations and area under the serum concentration-time curve (AUC) of ruxolitinib. Dosage reduction of ruxolitinib is recommended when the drug is used concomitantly with potent CYP3A4 inhibitors. Patients should be monitored closely during concomitant therapy and dosage should be titrated based on safety and efficacy. (See Dosage Modification for Concomitant Use with Drugs and Food Affecting Hepatic Microsomal Enzymes under Dosage and Administration: Dosage and also see Drug Interactions: Ketoconazole.)

Concomitant use of ruxolitinib with weak or moderate CYP3A4 inhibitors (e.g., erythromycin) also has resulted in increased peak plasma concentrations and AUC of ruxolitinib, but does not appear to be a clinically important interaction. Dosage adjustment of ruxolitinib is not recommended when used concomitantly with weak or moderate CYP3A4 inhibitors.

Concomitant use of ruxolitinib with CYP3A4 inducers (e.g., rifampin) has resulted in decreased peak plasma concentrations and AUC of ruxolitinib. However, no dosage adjustment is recommended when the drug is used concomitantly with CYP3A4 inducers. The manufacturer states that patients should be monitored closely during concomitant therapy and dosage should be titrated based on safety and efficacy.

■ **Ketoconazole** Concomitant administration of ruxolitinib (single 10-mg dose) with ketoconazole (200 mg twice daily for 4 days) increased peak plasma concentrations and AUC of ruxolitinib by 33 and 91%, respectively. Half-life of ruxolitinib also was prolonged from 3.7 to 6 hours with concomitant use of ketoconazole. Dosage reduction is recommended when ruxolitinib is administered with potent CYP3A4 inhibitors (e.g., ketoconazole). (See Dosage Modification for Concomitant Use with Drugs and Food Affecting Hepatic Microsomal Enzymes under Dosage and Administration: Dosage.) Patients should be closely monitored and the dosage titrated based on safety and efficacy.

■ **Erythromycin** Concomitant administration of ruxolitinib (single 10-mg dose) with erythromycin (500 mg twice daily for 4 days) increased ruxolitinib peak plasma concentrations and AUC by 8 and 27%, respectively. No dosage adjustment is recommended when ruxolitinib is administered with weak or moderate CYP3A4 inhibitors (e.g., erythromycin). In patients receiving a stable dosage of ruxolitinib, clinicians should use caution when initiating treatment with a moderate CYP3A4 inhibitor, especially in patients with low platelet counts.

■ **Rifampin** Concomitant administration of ruxolitinib (single 50-mg dose) with rifampin (600 mg once daily for 10 days) decreased ruxolitinib peak plasma concentrations and AUC by 32 and 61%, respectively. No dosage adjustment is recommended when ruxolitinib is administered with a CYP3A4 inducer. Patients should be closely monitored and the dosage titrated based on safety and efficacy.

Description

Ruxolitinib phosphate, a selective inhibitor of Janus kinase (JAK) 1 and 2, is an antineoplastic agent. JAK1 and 2 mediate the signaling of cytokines and growth factors that are important for hematopoiesis and immune function. JAK signaling involves recruitment of signal transducers and activators of transcription (STAT) to cytokine receptors, activation, and subsequent localization of STATs to the nucleus leading to modulation of gene expression. Myelofibrosis is a myeloproliferative neoplasm known to be associated with dysregulated JAK1 and 2 signaling. Ruxolitinib demonstrated dose- and time-dependent inhibition of cytokine-induced phosphorylated STAT3 with maximal inhibition occurring 1–2 hours after single-dose administration (ranging from 5–200 mg) in healthy individuals at all dosage levels.

Following oral administration, absorption of ruxolitinib is approximately 95%, and mean systemic bioavailability is estimated to be about 80%. Following oral administration of ruxolitinib, peak plasma concentrations are achieved within 1–2 hours. The mean half-life of ruxolitinib following a single oral dose is approximately 3 hours, and the mean half-life of ruxolitinib and its metabolites is approximately 5.8 hours. Cytochrome P-450 (CYP) isoenzyme 3A4 is the major enzyme responsible for metabolism of ruxolitinib. Two major active metabolites were identified in the plasma of healthy individuals; all active metabolites contribute 18% of the overall pharmacodynamic activity of ruxolitinib. Following administration of a single oral dose of radiolabeled ruxolitinib in healthy individuals, elimination was predominantly through metabolism with 74 and 22% of radioactivity excreted in urine and feces, respectively. Unchanged drug accounted for less than 1% of the excreted total radioactivity.

Advice to Patients

Importance of informing patients that ruxolitinib is associated with thrombocytopenia, anemia, and neutropenia, and to have complete blood cell counts (CBCs) monitored before and during treatment. Patients should be advised to contact their clinicians if unusual bleeding, bruising, fatigue, shortness of breath, or fever occurs.

Patients should be advised to notify a clinician immediately if signs and/or symptoms of infection (e.g., chills, aches, fever, nausea, vomiting, weakness) occur.

Importance of informing patients about early signs and symptoms of herpes zoster (e.g., painful skin rash or blisters) and advising patients to seek treatment as soon as possible.

Importance of informing patients with end-stage renal disease receiving dialysis to take their dose of ruxolitinib *following completion* of the dialysis session only on days when hemodialysis is scheduled.

Inform patients of importance of adherence to the dosing schedule; patients should not change their dosage or stop taking ruxolitinib without consulting their clinician. Patients should be aware that after treatment discontinuance, myelofibrosis signs and symptoms are expected to return.

Importance of not drinking grapefruit juice while receiving ruxolitinib therapy.

Importance of not doubling the next dose if a dose is missed; the next dose should be taken at the regularly scheduled time.

Importance of women informing clinicians if they are or plan to become pregnant or plan to breast-feed. Importance of advising women not to breast-feed during therapy with the drug.

Importance of informing clinicians of existing or contemplated concomitant therapy, including prescription and OTC drugs, as well as any concomitant illnesses (e.g., fungal, bacterial, or human immunodeficiency virus [HIV] infections).

Importance of informing patients of other important precautionary information. (See Cautions.)

Overview® (see Users Guide). For additional information on this drug until a more detailed monograph is developed and published, the manufacturer's labeling should be consulted. It is *essential* that the manufacturer's labeling be consulted for more detailed information on usual cautions, precautions, contraindications, potential drug interactions, laboratory test interferences, and acute toxicity.

Preparations

Distribution of ruxolitinib is restricted. (See Restricted Distribution Program under Dosage and Administration: General.)

Excipients in commercially available drug preparations may have clinically important effects in some individuals; consult specific product labeling for details.

Ruxolitinib Phosphate

Oral

Tablets	5 mg (of ruxolitinib)	**Jakafi®**, Incyte Corporation
	10 mg (of ruxolitinib)	**Jakafi®**, Incyte Corporation
	15 mg (of ruxolitinib)	**Jakafi®**, Incyte Corporation
	20 mg (of ruxolitinib)	**Jakafi®**, Incyte Corporation
	25 mg (of ruxolitinib)	**Jakafi®**, Incyte Corporation

Siltuximab

■ Siltuximab, a recombinant chimeric (human-murine) monoclonal antibody and interleukin-6 (IL-6) antagonist, is an antineoplastic agent.

Uses

■ Multicentric Castleman's Disease Siltuximab is used for the treatment of multicentric Castleman's disease (MCD) in patients who are human immunodeficiency virus (HIV)-negative and human herpes virus type 8 (HHV-8)-negative; siltuximab is designated an orphan drug by the FDA for the treatment of this disease.

MCD is a rare lymphoproliferative disorder that is associated with excessive release of interleukin-6 (IL-6) and other proinflammatory cytokines. The disease usually affects adults. Although the pathogenesis of MCD is not fully understood, excessive production and dysregulation of IL-6 appear to play a prominent role in the multicentric form of the disease, and lead to stimulation of the production of acute phase reactants in the liver. As a result, patients with MCD often experience systemic manifestations such as fever, night sweats, anorexia, weight loss, weakness and fatigue, edema, effusions, pruritus, pain, and/or dyspnea. Laboratory abnormalities, such as anemia, elevated concentrations of inflammatory markers (e.g., C-reactive protein), hypergammaglobulinemia, and hypoalbuminemia, also may be present. (See Description.)

The current indication for siltuximab is based principally on the results of a randomized, double-blind, placebo-controlled, multinational phase 2 study in adults with MCD who were HIV-negative and HHV-8-negative. A total of 79 patients with symptomatic MCD were randomized (2:1) to receive siltuximab plus best supportive care or to placebo plus best supportive care in this study. Best supportive care included management of effusions; use of antipyretic, antipruritic, antihistamine, and analgesic medications; management of infections; transfusions; and standard treatment of infusion-related reactions. Siltuximab was given in a dosage of 11 mg/kg by IV infusion every 3 weeks until treatment failure (defined as disease progression based on increased symptoms, radiologic progression, or deterioration in performance status) or unacceptable toxicity. The primary measure of efficacy was durable tumor and symptomatic response, which was defined as tumor response assessed by independent review and complete resolution or stabilization of disease-related symptoms for at least 18 weeks without treatment failure. Upon treatment failure, patients previously randomized to receive placebo were permitted to cross over to open-label siltuximab treatment. The median patient age in the study was 48 years (range: 20–78 years); the histologic subtype of MCD was similar in both treatment arms, with 33% hyaline vascular subtype, 23% plasmacytic subtype, and 44% mixed subtype. At baseline, 55 and 65% of the patients in the siltuximab and placebo arms, respectively, had received prior systemic therapies for their disease and 25 and 35% of the patients in the siltuximab and placebo arms, respectively, were concurrently receiving corticosteroid therapy. Durable tumor and symptomatic response was observed in 34% of patients receiving siltuximab compared with none of those receiving placebo. Tumor response rates also were substantially higher in patients receiving siltuximab compared with those receiving placebo (38 versus 4%). At the time of analysis, median time to treatment failure had not been reached in patients receiving siltuximab; however, the median time to treatment failure was 134 days in patients receiving placebo. In addition, in patients who were anemic when entering the study, hemoglobin concentrations increased by at least 1.5 g/dL following 13 weeks of therapy in 61% of siltuximab-treated patients compared with none of those receiving placebo.

In a separate analysis of patient-reported outcomes (e.g., patient perception of symptoms, functional status, and well being) from this study, the siltuximab-treated patients reported substantial and durable improvements in fatigue compared with those receiving placebo. Fatigue was improved at the end of the first cycle of therapy and continued to improve throughout the study. In addition, patients receiving siltuximab experienced significant improvement from baseline in most of the domains assessed by the Short Form-36 (SF-36) Health Survey (physical, role emotional, vitality, bodily pain, and mental health domains).

In an interim analysis of a long-term extension study of siltuximab therapy in 19 patients with MCD, patients who had received in total a median of 81 doses of the drug over a median follow-up period of 5.1 years were all alive and control of their disease was maintained. Chronic siltuximab therapy was well tolerated, and there was no evidence of new or cumulative toxicity.

The manufacturer states that siltuximab was not studied in HIV- and HHV-8-positive patients with MCD† because the drug did not bind to virally produced IL-6 in a nonclinical study. (See Description.) However, it has been suggested by some clinicians that anti-IL6 therapy may still help to decrease the activity of human IL-6, which is elevated in most patients with HIV-associated MCD, and thereby help to control the disease. There currently is very little experience treating HIV- and HHV-8-associated MCD with anti-IL-6 therapy. Clinical trials are needed to determine whether siltuximab is effective in this population.

Dosage and Administration

■ General Because of the risk of infusion-related reactions and hypersensitivity, siltuximab should be administered in a setting in which resuscitation equipment, medications, and personnel trained to provide resuscitation are available. (See Infusion-related Reactions and Hypersensitivity under Cautions: Warnings/Precautions.)

Complete blood cell (CBC) counts should be obtained prior to each dose of siltuximab for the first 12 months of therapy and then every 3 cycles thereafter. Clinicians should be aware that siltuximab therapy may increase hemoglobin concentrations in patients with multicentric Castleman's disease (MCD). (See Hematologic Toxicity under Dosage: Therapy Interruption for Toxicity, in Dosage and Administration.)

Siltuximab should not be administered to patients with severe infections until the infection resolves. (See Concurrent Active Severe Infections under Cautions: Warnings/Precautions.)

■ Administration Siltuximab is administered by IV infusion over 60 minutes.

Unopened vials of siltuximab lyophilized powder for injection should be protected from light and stored at 2–8°C.

Prior to administration, commercially available siltuximab lyophilized powder for injection must be reconstituted and diluted using proper aseptic technique. Based on the indicated dosage of siltuximab, the appropriate number of vials of the drug should be reconstituted. The vials containing siltuximab lyophilized powder should be removed from the refrigerator and allowed to come to room temperature (15–25°C) over approximately 30 minutes prior to reconstitution; the drug should remain at room temperature for the duration of the preparation. A 21-gauge, 1.5-inch needle is recommended by the manufacturer for preparation. The lyophilized powder is reconstituted by adding 5.2 mL of sterile water for injection to a vial labeled as containing 100 mg of siltuximab or by adding 20 mL of sterile water for injection to a vial labeled as containing 400 mg of siltuximab to provide a solution containing 20 mg/mL. The vials should then be gently swirled to facilitate dissolution of the lyophilized powder, which should dissolve in less than 1 hour. The vials should *not* be shaken or swirled vigorously. The contents of the reconstituted vials should not be removed until all of the solids have completely dissolved. The reconstituted solution should be inspected visually for particulate matter and discoloration prior to dilution and should not be used if particles are present or if the solution appears discolored or visibly opaque. The reconstituted siltuximab solution should be kept at room temperature for no more than 2 hours prior to addition into the infusion bag.

Reconstituted siltuximab solution should then be diluted in 5% dextrose injection to provide a total volume of 250 mL (i.e., if a 250-mL bag of 5% dextrose injection is used, a volume of the diluent equal to the total required volume of reconstituted siltuximab solution should be removed from the bag prior to addition of the reconstituted siltuximab solution). The total required volume of reconstituted siltuximab solution should then be added slowly to the diluent in a diethylhexyl phthalate (DEHP)-plasticized polyvinylchloride (PVC) or non-PVC (polyolefin) infusion bag. The diluted solution should then be mixed by gentle inversion. Diluted infusion solutions of the drug are stable for up to 4 hours after dilution of the reconstituted solution (including infusion time) when stored at room temperature. Siltuximab infusion solution should be administered by IV infusion through a 0.2-μm inline polyethersulfone filter. The diluted infusion solution should be administered through PVC- or polyurethane-lined administration sets.

Siltuximab should *not* be administered simultaneously through the same IV line with any other drug. Commercially available vials of siltuximab for injection contain no preservatives and are intended for single use only; any unused portions of the reconstituted or diluted solutions should be discarded. Procedures for proper disposal should be followed.

■ Dosage ***Multicentric Castleman's Disease*** For the treatment of MCD in adults who are human immunodeficiency virus (HIV)-negative and human herpes virus type 8 (HHV-8)-negative, the recommended dosage of siltuximab is 11 mg/kg administered as a 60-minute infusion every 3 weeks. Therapy should be continued until treatment failure (i.e., disease progression based on increased symptoms, radiologic progression, or deterioration in performance status) occurs.

Therapy Interruption for Toxicity **Hematologic Toxicity.** A delay in administration of the *first* dose of siltuximab should be considered in patients with an absolute neutrophil count (ANC) of less than 1000/mm^3, platelet count of less than 75,000/mm^3, and/or hemoglobin concentration of 17 g/dL or more. The dosage of siltuximab should *not* be reduced in such cases.

For *subsequent* doses, the manufacturer recommends that a delay in therapy be considered if the ANC is less than 1000/mm^3, the platelet count is less than 50,000/mm^3, and/or the hemoglobin concentration is 17 g/dL or more. The dosage of siltuximab should *not* be reduced in such cases.

Infusion-related Reactions and Hypersensitivity. If mild to moderate infusion-related reactions occur, the siltuximab infusion should be temporarily interrupted. If the reaction resolves, the infusion may be resumed at a slower infusion rate. Treatment with antihistamines, acetaminophen, and/or corticosteroids should be considered in such cases. Siltuximab should be discontinued if the patient is unable to tolerate the infusion following these interventions.

If severe infusion-related reactions or cytokine release syndromes occur, therapy with the drug should be *permanently* discontinued.

Siltuximab should be immediately and *permanently* discontinued in patients who experience anaphylaxis. (See Cautions: Contraindications and also see Infusion-related Reactions and Hypersensitivity under Cautions: Warnings/Precautions.)

■ **Special Populations** No initial dosage adjustment is necessary in patients with mild or moderate hepatic impairment (Child-Pugh class A or B). The manufacturer currently does not provide dosage recommendations for patients with severe hepatic impairment. (See Hepatic Impairment under Warnings/Precautions: Specific Populations, in Cautions.)

In patients with renal impairment, no initial dosage adjustment is necessary in patients with a creatinine clearance of 15 mL/minute or greater. The manufacturer currently does not provide dosage recommendations for patients with a creatinine clearance of less than 15 mL/minute and for patients with end-stage renal disease. (See Renal Impairment under Warnings/Precautions: Specific Populations, in Cautions.)

The manufacturer makes no specific dosage recommendations for geriatric patients. (See Geriatric Use under Warnings/Precautions: Specific Populations, in Cautions.)

Cautions

■ **Contraindications** Severe hypersensitivity reaction to siltuximab or any ingredient in the formulation. (See Infusion-related Reactions and Hypersensitivity under Cautions: Warnings/Precautions.)

■ **Warnings/Precautions** ***Concurrent Active Severe Infections*** Siltuximab may mask signs and symptoms of acute inflammation (i.e., suppression of fever and acute phase reactants such as C-reactive protein [CRP]).

Siltuximab should not be used in patients with severe infections until the infection has resolved.

Patients receiving siltuximab should be closely monitored for possible infections. If an infection develops, anti-infective therapy should be initiated promptly and siltuximab therapy should be withheld until the infection resolves.

Immunization Because inhibition of interleukin-6 (IL-6) may interfere with the normal immune response to new antigens, live vaccines should not be administered to patients receiving siltuximab. (See Advice to Patients.)

Infusion-related Reactions and Hypersensitivity Anaphylactic reaction occurred in 1 of 750 siltuximab-treated patients. If signs of anaphylaxis or other severe allergic reactions occur, the infusion of siltuximab should be discontinued and no further therapy with the drug should be given. (See Contraindications under Cautions.)

Infusion-related reactions were reported in 4.8% of patients receiving siltuximab monotherapy. Manifestations include back pain, chest pain or discomfort, nausea and vomiting, flushing, erythema, and palpitations.

In patients experiencing mild or moderate infusion-related reactions, temporary interruption of the siltuximab infusion is recommended. If the reaction resolves, the infusion may be resumed at a slower infusion rate. Treatment with antihistamines, acetaminophen, and corticosteroids should be considered in such cases. Siltuximab should be discontinued if the patient is unable to tolerate the infusion following these interventions.

If severe infusion-related reactions or cytokine release syndromes occur, siltuximab therapy should be permanently discontinued.

GI Perforation GI perforation has occurred in patients receiving siltuximab in clinical trials; however, no cases were reported in multicentric Castleman's disease (MCD) trials of the drug.

Siltuximab should be used with caution in patients who may be at increased risk for GI perforation (e.g., those with diverticulitis or ulcers). Patients should be evaluated promptly if symptoms associated with or suggestive of GI perforation occur (e.g., stomach pain, nausea, change in bowel habits, fever).

Immunogenicity There is a potential for immunogenicity with siltuximab therapy. Anti-siltuximab antibodies were detected by enzyme immunoassay (EIA) and electrochemiluminescence-based immunoassay (ECLIA) methods in 1 of 411 patients (0.2%) treated with siltuximab in clinical studies. Further analyses of the single positive sample indicated a low titer of anti-siltuximab antibodies with non-neutralizing capabilities. No evidence of altered toxicity of the drug was observed in the patient who developed the antibodies.

Specific Populations **Pregnancy.** There are no adequate and well-controlled studies in pregnant women. Maternal and fetal toxicity was not observed when siltuximab was administered to pregnant animals; however, siltuximab crossed the placenta and fetal serum concentrations were similar to maternal concentrations. Administration of a human antibody to IL-6 to pregnant animals caused decreased globulin concentrations in pregnant animals and offspring.

Infants born to pregnant women treated with siltuximab may be at an increased risk of infection; therefore, caution is advised in the administration of live vaccines in these infants. Pregnancy should be avoided during siltuximab therapy. The drug should be used during pregnancy only if the potential benefit justifies the potential risk to the fetus. Women of childbearing potential should use contraception during siltuximab treatment and for 3 months following discontinuance of the drug.

Lactation. It is not known whether siltuximab is distributed into human milk or absorbed systemically after ingestion. Because many drugs and immunoglobulins are distributed into human milk and because of the potential for adverse reactions to siltuximab in nursing infants, a decision should be made whether to discontinue nursing or the drug, taking into account the importance of the drug to the woman.

Pediatric Use. MCD usually affects adults. Safety and efficacy of siltuximab have not been established in pediatric patients younger than 18 years of age.

Geriatric Use. In clinical trials evaluating siltuximab as single-agent therapy, 35% of patients were 65 years of age or older. Although no overall differences in safety were observed between geriatric patients and younger adults in these clinical trials and in other clinical experience, the possibility of increased sensitivity to the drug in some geriatric patients cannot be ruled out. Clinical studies evaluating siltuximab for the treatment of MCD did not include sufficient numbers of patients 65 years of age and older to determine the effect of age on the drug's efficacy for this condition.

In a population pharmacokinetic analysis, age (range: 18–85 years) did not affect exposure of siltuximab.

Hepatic Impairment. A population pharmacokinetic analysis of data from 377 patients enrolled in siltuximab clinical trials indicates that clearance of the drug is similar in patients with preexisting mild or moderate hepatic impairment (Child-Pugh class A or B) and those with normal hepatic function. Patients with severe hepatic impairment (Child-Pugh class C) were excluded from clinical studies of the drug.

Renal Impairment. Analysis of population pharmacokinetic data from 377 patients enrolled in siltuximab clinical trials indicates that clearance of the drug is similar in patients with preexisting mild, moderate, or severe renal impairment (creatinine clearance 15–89 mL/minute) and those with normal renal function. The potential effect of end-stage renal disease on siltuximab pharmacokinetics is not known since clinical and pharmacokinetic data are very limited. (See Dosage and Administration: Special Populations.)

■ **Common Adverse Effects** Adverse effects reported in more than 10% of patients receiving siltuximab for the treatment of MCD and at an incidence that is at least 10% higher than that reported with placebo include rash (e.g., maculopapular, papular, generalized, pruritic), pruritus, upper respiratory tract infection, weight gain, localized edema, abdominal pain, thrombocytopenia, nasopharyngitis, and hyperuricemia.

Drug Interactions

Formal drug interaction studies have not been conducted to date with siltuximab.

■ **Drugs Metabolized by Hepatic Microsomal Enzymes** Possible increased metabolism of drugs that are metabolized by cytochrome P-450 (CYP) isoenzymes. Because cytokines such as interleukin-6 (IL-6) may down-regulate CYP enzymes, inhibition of IL-6 by siltuximab may restore CYP enzyme activity to higher levels. Effects of siltuximab on CYP enzyme activity may persist for several weeks after the drug is discontinued.

Following initiation or discontinuance of siltuximab therapy, patients receiving certain drugs metabolized by CYP isoenzymes (i.e., those with a low therapeutic index that require individualized dosing [e.g., cyclosporine, theophylline, warfarin]) should be monitored for therapeutic effect and/or changes in serum concentrations, and dosages of these drugs should be adjusted as needed. Caution also is advised when siltuximab is used concomitantly with CYP3A4 substrates (e.g., oral contraceptives, atorvastatin, lovastatin) for which a reduction in efficacy would be undesirable.

■ **Vaccines** Live vaccines should not be administered to patients receiving siltuximab. (See Immunization under Cautions: Warnings/Precautions.)

Description

Siltuximab is a recombinant chimeric (human-murine) monoclonal antibody specific for human interleukin-6 (IL-6) that is produced in Chinese hamster ovary cells. The drug is an IgG_1 kappa immunoglobulin that binds human IL-6 and thereby prevents its binding to both soluble and membrane-bound IL-6 receptors. IL-6 is known to be involved in a variety of normal physiologic processes including induction of immunoglobulin secretion, initiation of hepatic acute phase protein synthesis, and cell proliferation and differentiation.

Overproduction of IL-6 appears to play a critical role in the disease process of multicentric Castleman's disease (MCD), resulting in plasma cell proliferation and a variety of systemic manifestations (e.g., lymphadenopathy, hepatosplenomegaly, ascites, pleural effusion, edema, fever, fatigue, night sweats, anorexia, cachexia, anemia, pain, pruritus, sensory neuropathy). Although the cause of MCD in patients who are *not* infected with human immunodeficiency virus (HIV) and human herpes virus type 8 (HHV-8) has not been fully elucidated, HHV-8 is a well established cause of hypercytokinemia in HIV-infected and in some HIV-negative patients with MCD. Siltuximab did not bind to virally produced IL-6 in a nonclinical study. (See Uses: Multicentric Castleman's Disease.)

Pharmacokinetics of siltuximab are approximately proportional to dose over the dosage range of 2.8–11 mg/kg given by IV infusion every 3 weeks. When given as an IV infusion once every 3 weeks, steady-state concentrations of siltuximab are achieved by the sixth infusion (within 18 weeks); systemic accumulation of the drug is approximately 1.7-fold higher at steady state when compared with single-dose administration. The dosage of siltuximab is based on body weight because body weight was the only significant covariate for clearance of the drug in a population pharmacokinetic analysis. The mean terminal half-life of siltuximab following the first IV infusion is 20.6 days.

Advice to Patients

Importance of advising patients about potential benefits and risks of siltuximab. Importance of patients reading the manufacturer's patient information prior to initiation of therapy and each time they receive an infusion of the drug.

Risk of increased susceptibility to infection. Importance of instructing patients to immediately contact their clinician if they develop symptoms suggesting an infection in order to ensure rapid evaluation and appropriate treatment.

Importance of advising patients that they should not receive live vaccines during siltuximab therapy. Importance of informing clinician of recent or scheduled vaccinations and of discussing recommended vaccinations with their clinician prior to beginning siltuximab therapy.

Risk of infusion-related and allergic reactions. Importance of immediately reporting signs and symptoms of such reactions, including dizziness, lightheadedness, wheezing, swelling of the lips, rash, breathing difficulty, or chest pain or tightness.

Importance of advising patients to report any new or worsening medical conditions to their clinician.

Importance of women informing clinicians if they are or plan to become pregnant or plan to breast-feed. Importance of advising women not to breast-feed during therapy. Necessity of advising women of childbearing potential to use effective contraception while receiving siltuximab and for 3 months after the drug is discontinued.

Importance of informing clinicians of existing or contemplated concomitant therapy, including prescription and OTC drugs, as well as any concomitant illnesses (e.g., infections, GI disease).

Importance of informing patients of other important precautionary information. (See Cautions.)

Overview® (see Users Guide). For additional information on this drug until a more detailed monograph is developed and published, the manufacturer's labeling should be consulted. It is *essential* that the manufacturer's labeling be consulted for more detailed information on usual cautions, precautions, contraindications, potential drug interactions, laboratory test interferences, and acute toxicity. For further information on the handling of antineoplastic agents, see the ASHP Guidelines on Handling Hazardous Drugs at http://www.ahfsdruginformation.com.

Preparations

Excipients in commercially available drug preparations may have clinically important effects in some individuals; consult specific product labeling for details.

Siltuximab

Parenteral		
For injection, for IV infusion	100 mg	**Sylvant®**, Janssen Biotech
	400 mg	**Sylvant®**, Janssen Biotech

†Use is not currently included in the labeling approved by the US Food and Drug Administration

Sonidegib

■ Sonidegib, a hedgehog signaling pathway inhibitor, is an antineoplastic agent.

Uses

■ **Basal Cell Carcinoma** Sonidegib is used for the treatment of locally advanced basal cell carcinoma in adults whose disease recurred following surgery or radiation therapy, and in those who are not candidates for surgery or radiation therapy.

The current indication for sonidegib in the treatment of locally advanced basal cell carcinoma is based principally on the results of a randomized, double-blind, noncomparative phase 2 study (BOLT) in patients with locally advanced or metastatic basal cell carcinoma. The primary measure of efficacy was objective response rate (as evaluated by a blinded independent central review committee). Tumor response was evaluated in patients with locally advanced disease using a modification of the Response Evaluation Criteria in Solid Tumors (RECIST) version 1.1 in addition to radiographic assessment of target lesions, digital clinical photography, and tumor biopsy. Complete response in locally advanced disease was defined as the absence of tumor in all modalities used for assessment. Response by digital clinical photography was evaluated using World Health Organization (WHO) adapted criteria; partial response was defined as a 50% or greater reduction in lesion size (i.e., sum of the product of perpendicular diameters of lesions) and complete response was defined as disappearance of all lesions.

In this study, the median age of patients was 67 years (range: 25–92 years); 3 patients had a diagnosis of nevoid basal cell carcinoma syndrome (also known as Gorlin syndrome). Most of the patients (76%) had received prior therapy for basal cell carcinoma, including surgery (73%), radiation therapy (18%), and topical or photodynamic therapy (21%). Approximately half of the patients had aggressive histology (micronodular, infiltrative, multifocal, basosquamous, or sclerosing basal cell carcinoma). In this study, 66 patients with locally advanced basal cell carcinoma received sonidegib 200 mg orally once daily. Treatment was continued until disease progression, death, or unacceptable toxicity occurred or treatment was discontinued for other reasons. Patients enrolled in the study with locally advanced basal cell carcinoma were required to have lesions for which radiation therapy was contraindicated or inappropriate (e.g., diagnosis of nevoid basal cell carcinoma syndrome or limitations due to location of tumor), had disease recurrence following surgery or radiation therapy, or had unresectable disease.

Among patients with locally advanced basal cell carcinoma receiving sonidegib 200 mg once daily, 38 of 66 patients (58%) achieved an objective response; 5% of patients receiving the 200-mg dosage achieved a complete response. At the time of analysis, 31 of 38 responders (82%) had ongoing responses; 4 of 7 patients who experienced disease progression maintained a response for 6 months or longer. Objective response rates were similar between patients with locally advanced basal cell carcinoma receiving sonidegib 200 or 800 mg once daily. Results of a subgroup analysis (based on histology and geographic region) suggested that the drug's effect on objective response was consistent among these subgroups.

Dosage and Administration

■ **General** Because sonidegib may cause fetal harm, women of childbearing potential must be tested for pregnancy prior to initiation of the drug. (See Fetal/Neonatal Morbidity and Mortality under Warnings/Precautions: Warnings, in Cautions.)

Because sonidegib may cause adverse musculoskeletal effects, the manufacturer states that serum creatine kinase (CK, creatine phosphokinase, CPK) and creatinine concentrations should be evaluated at baseline, periodically during therapy, and as clinically indicated. More frequent monitoring may be necessary if toxicity occurs. (See Musculoskeletal Effects under Warnings/Precautions: Other Warnings and Precautions, in Cautions.)

■ **Administration** Sonidegib is administered orally once daily on an empty stomach, at least 1 hour before or 2 hours after a meal. (See Description and also see Advice to Patients.)

■ **Dosage** ***Basal Cell Carcinoma*** For the treatment of locally advanced basal cell carcinoma following failure of prior surgery or radiation therapy, the recommended dosage of sonidegib in adults is 200 mg once daily. Therapy should be continued until disease progression or unacceptable toxicity occurs.

Dosage Modification for Toxicity **Musculoskeletal Effects.** For the first occurrence of elevations in serum CK concentrations of 2.5–10 times the upper limit of normal (ULN) or first occurrence of severe or intolerable adverse musculoskeletal effects, sonidegib therapy should be withheld until the toxicity has resolved. Sonidegib may then be resumed at a dosage of 200 mg once daily.

If recurrent elevations in serum CK concentrations of 2.5–5 times the ULN occur, sonidegib therapy should be withheld until the toxicity has resolved. Sonidegib may then be resumed at a dosage of 200 mg once daily.

If elevations in serum CK concentrations exceeding 2.5 times the ULN with worsening renal function or exceeding 10 times the ULN occur, sonidegib therapy should be permanently discontinued.

For recurrent elevations in serum CK concentrations exceeding 5 times the ULN or for recurrent severe intolerable adverse musculoskeletal effects, sonidegib therapy should be permanently discontinued.

■ **Special Populations** No dosage adjustment is recommended based on age, body weight, gender, or ethnicity.

No dosage adjustment is necessary in patients with mild hepatic impairment (i.e., total bilirubin concentrations not exceeding the ULN with AST concentrations exceeding the ULN, or total bilirubin concentrations exceeding the ULN, but no more than 1.5 times the ULN). Sonidegib has not been studied in patients with moderate or severe hepatic impairment. (See Hepatic Impairment under Warnings/Precautions: Specific Populations, in Cautions.)

No dosage adjustment is necessary in patients with renal impairment. (See Renal Impairment under Warnings/Precautions: Specific Populations, in Cautions.)

The manufacturer makes no specific dosage recommendations for geriatric patients. (See Geriatric Use under Warnings/Precautions: Specific Populations, in Cautions.)

Cautions

■ **Contraindications** The manufacturer states that there are no known contraindications to the use of sonidegib.

■ **Warnings/Precautions** ***Warnings*** **Fetal/Neonatal Morbidity and Mortality.** There are no adequate and well-controlled studies of sonidegib in pregnant women; however, based on its mechanism of action and animal findings, sonidegib may cause fetal harm. The drug has been shown to cause embryofetal toxicity (i.e., abortion, fetal resorption) and teratogenic effects (i.e., severe midline defects, absent digits, severe craniofacial anomalies, other irreversible malformations) in rabbits receiving sonidegib at exposure levels of approximately 0.05 times the human exposure at the recommended dosage.

Pregnancy should be avoided during sonidegib therapy. Women of childbearing potential should be advised to use an effective method of contraception while receiving sonidegib and for at least 20 months after discontinuance of therapy. Patients should be apprised of the potential hazard to the fetus if the drug is used during pregnancy. While receiving sonidegib and for at least 8 months after discontinuing the drug, sexually mature males (including those who have successfully undergone vasectomy) must use a condom each time they have sexual contact with a pregnant woman or woman of childbearing potential and must *not* donate semen while receiving sonidegib and for at least 8 months after discontinuing the drug.

Because sonidegib may cause fetal harm and because of the possibility that the drug may be present in blood and be transfused into a woman who is pregnant, patients receiving sonidegib must *not* donate blood or blood products during therapy and for at least 20 months following discontinuance of the drug.

All females of childbearing potential must be tested for pregnancy prior to initiation of sonidegib therapy. If a female patient or female partner of a male patient receiving sonidegib therapy becomes pregnant during therapy or within 20 or 8 months, respectively, after discontinuance of the drug, the clinician should notify the manufacturer (Novartis) at 888-669-6682.

Other Warnings and Precautions **Musculoskeletal Effects.** Musculoskeletal effects, possibly accompanied by elevations of serum creatine kinase (CK, creatine phosphokinase, CPK) concentrations, commonly occur during treatment with inhibitors of the hedgehog pathway, including sonidegib. In clinical studies evaluating sonidegib (dosage range of 100 mg to 3 g) in 571 patients with advanced malignancies, rhabdomyolysis (defined as serum CK concentrations exceeding 10 times the baseline value and serum creatinine concentrations of 1.5 or more times the baseline value) occurred in 1 patient receiving sonidegib 800 mg. In the BOLT study, musculoskeletal effects or increased serum CK concentrations occurred in 68% (grade 3 or 4 in 9%) or 61% (grade 3 or 4 in 8%), respectively, of patients receiving sonidegib 200 mg daily. The most common musculoskeletal effects reported in this study included muscle spasms, musculoskeletal pain, and myalgia; musculoskeletal pain and myalgia usually preceded elevations in serum CK concentrations. The median time to occurrence of grade 2 or greater elevations in serum CK concentrations was 12.9 weeks (range: 2–39 weeks) and the median time for resolution of toxicity to grade 1 or less was 12 days (range: 8–14 days). Adverse musculoskeletal effects requiring medical intervention, including magnesium supplementation, muscle relaxants, and/or opiates or other analgesics, occurred in 29% of patients receiving sonidegib 200 mg daily; 5% of patients receiving this dosage of the drug required IV hydration or hospitalization.

Serum CK and creatinine concentrations should be evaluated at baseline, periodically during sonidegib therapy, and as clinically indicated; patients who develop musculoskeletal symptoms *and* elevations in CK concentrations exceeding 2.5 times the upper limit of normal (ULN) should be monitored at least weekly until the toxicity has resolved. Temporary interruption, dosage reduction, or discontinuance of sonidegib may be necessary depending on severity of musculoskeletal symptoms during therapy with the drug. (See Musculoskeletal Effects under Dosage: Dosage Modification for Toxicity, in Dosage and Administration.)

Impairment of Female Fertility. Results of animal studies suggest that sonidegib may impair female fertility. Infertility was observed in female rats receiving sonidegib at dosages of 20 mg/kg or more daily (dosages approximately 1.3 times the human exposure at the recommended dosage). A reduced incidence of pregnancy, increased number of early resorptions, and decreased incidence of viable fetuses also were observed in female rats receiving the drug at dosages approximately 0.12 times the human exposure at the recommended dosage. In a repeat-dose toxicity study, degeneration of reproductive organs (i.e., uterus, ovaries) was observed in female rats receiving sonidegib at exposure levels of approximately 2 or more times the human exposure at the recommended dosage.

Specific Populations **Pregnancy.** Sonidegib may cause fetal harm if administered to pregnant women based on its mechanism of action and animal findings. (See Fetal/Neonatal Morbidity and Mortality under Warnings/Precautions: Warnings, in Cautions.)

Lactation. It is not known whether sonidegib is distributed into milk. Because of the potential for serious adverse reactions to sonidegib in nursing infants, women should be advised to discontinue nursing while receiving sonidegib and for at least 20 months after discontinuance of therapy. The effects of the drug on nursing infants or on milk production are unknown.

Pediatric Use. Safety and efficacy of sonidegib have not been established in pediatric patients.

Data in animals suggest possible adverse effects on bone, teeth, reproductive tissues, and nerve fibers in juvenile rats receiving sonidegib at exposure levels of approximately 1.2 times the human exposure at the recommended dosage.

Geriatric Use. In the BOLT study, 54% of patients receiving sonidegib (200 or 800 mg once daily) were 65 years of age or older and 28% were 75 years of age or older. No overall differences in efficacy were observed between geriatric and younger adults; however, grade 3 or 4 adverse effects, serious adverse effects, or adverse effects requiring interruption or discontinuance of therapy occurred more frequently in patients 65 years of age or older compared with younger adults. (See Dosage and Administration: Special Populations.)

Hepatic Impairment. In a population pharmacokinetic analysis, no clinically important differences in systemic exposure of sonidegib were observed between patients with mild hepatic impairment and those with normal hepatic function. The effects of moderate or severe hepatic impairment on the pharmacokinetics of sonidegib have not been established. (See Dosage and Administration: Special Populations.)

Renal Impairment. In a population pharmacokinetic analysis, no clinically important differences in systemic exposure of sonidegib were observed between patients with mild (creatinine clearance of 60–89 mL/minute) or moderate (creatinine clearance of 30–59 mL/minute) renal impairment and those with normal renal function. (See Dosage and Administration: Special Populations.)

■ **Common Adverse Effects** Adverse effects reported in 10% or more of patients with advanced basal cell carcinoma receiving sonidegib in the principal efficacy study include muscle spasms, alopecia, dysgeusia, fatigue, nausea, diarrhea, musculoskeletal pain, weight loss, decreased appetite, myalgia, abdominal pain, headache, pain, vomiting, pruritus, and arthralgia.

Laboratory abnormalities reported in more than 15% of patients receiving sonidegib include elevated concentrations of serum creatinine, elevated concentrations of serum CK, hyperglycemia, elevated concentrations of lipase, anemia, lymphopenia, elevated concentrations of aminotransferases (i.e., AST, ALT), and elevated concentrations of amylase.

Amenorrhea lasting at least 18 months also has been reported in 2 of 14 premenopausal women receiving sonidegib (200 or 800 mg once daily).

Drug Interactions

Sonidegib is metabolized principally by cytochrome P-450 (CYP) isoenzyme 3A. In vitro studies indicate that sonidegib inhibits CYP isoenzymes 2B6 and 2C9, but does not induce CYP 1A2, 2B6, or 3A.

In vitro studies indicate that sonidegib inhibits breast cancer resistance protein (BCRP, ABCG2), but does not inhibit P-glycoprotein (P-gp, ABCB1), multidrug resistance protein 2 (MRP2, ABCC2), organic cation transporter (OCT) 1, OCT2, organic anion transporter (OAT) 1, OAT3, organic anion transport protein (OATP) 1B1, and OATP1B3. In vitro studies also indicate that the drug is not a substrate of P-gp, MRP2, or BCRP.

■ **Drugs Affecting Hepatic Microsomal Enzymes** ***Inhibitors of CYP3A*** Concomitant use of sonidegib with moderate or potent inhibitors of CYP3A may result in increased peak plasma concentrations and systemic exposure of sonidegib. When the potent CYP3A inhibitor ketoconazole (200 mg twice daily for 14 days) was administered concomitantly with sonidegib (single 800-mg dose) in healthy individuals, peak plasma concentrations and area under the plasma concentration-time curve (AUC) of sonidegib were increased by 1.5- and 2.2-fold, respectively. Simulations using physiologically based pharmacokinetic models suggest that a similar increase in AUC would occur in cancer patients receiving concomitant administration of sonidegib (200 mg once daily) and a potent CYP3A inhibitor for 14 days. Simulations using physiologically based pharmacokinetic models suggest that concomitant administration of erythromycin, a moderate CYP3A inhibitor, and sonidegib (200 mg once daily) for 14 days or 4 months may increase AUC of sonidegib by 1.8- or 2.8-fold, respectively.

Concomitant use of sonidegib with potent (e.g., itraconazole, ketoconazole, nefazodone, posaconazole, saquinavir, telithromycin, voriconazole) or moderate (e.g., atazanavir, diltiazem, fluconazole) inhibitors of CYP3A should be avoided. If concomitant short-term (less than 14 days) therapy with a moderate CYP3A inhibitor cannot be avoided, the manufacturer recommends monitoring for adverse musculoskeletal effects and other toxicities.

Inducers of CYP3A Concomitant use of sonidegib with moderate or potent inducers of CYP3A may result in decreased peak plasma concentrations and AUC of sonidegib. When the potent CYP3A inducer rifampin (600 mg daily for 14 days) was administered concomitantly with sonidegib (single 800-mg dose) in healthy individuals, the peak plasma concentrations and AUC of sonidegib were decreased by 54 and 72%, respectively. Simulations using physiologically based pharmacokinetic models suggest that concomitant administration of efavirenz, a moderate CYP3A inducer, and sonidegib (200 mg once daily) for 14 days or 4 months may decrease AUC of sonidegib by 56 or 69%, respectively, in cancer patients.

Concomitant use of sonidegib with moderate or potent inducers of CYP3A (e.g., carbamazepine, efavirenz, modafinil, phenobarbital, phenytoin, rifabutin, rifampin, St. John's wort [*Hypericum perforatum*]) should be avoided.

■ **Drugs Affecting Gastric Acidity** In a population pharmacokinetic analysis, concomitant administration of a proton-pump inhibitor or histamine H_2-receptor antagonist and sonidegib decreased systemic exposure of sonidegib by 30–34%.

Description

Sonidegib is an antineoplastic agent that inhibits the hedgehog pathway by binding to and selectively inhibiting smoothened, a transmembrane protein involved in hedgehog signal transduction. The hedgehog signaling pathway plays an important role during embryonic organ and tissue development and is a key regulator of bone development and maintenance of tissues and stem cells in adults and during postnatal development. However, genetic mutations that allow for aberrant activation of the hedgehog pathway have been implicated in the development of several malignancies such as basal cell carcinoma. Inhibition of smoothened by sonidegib results in inhibition of the hedgehog pathway.

Following oral administration, less than 10% of sonidegib is absorbed. Area under the serum concentration-time curve (AUC) and peak plasma concentrations of sonidegib are dose proportional over a dosage range of 100–400 mg. Peak plasma concentrations of sonidegib are achieved 2–4 hours following oral administration of a single dose of sonidegib (100 mg to 3 g) under fasting conditions in cancer patients. Following administration of sonidegib, steady-state concentrations of the drug are achieved in approximately 4 months and the estimated accumulation is 19-fold. Administration of sonidegib with a high-fat meal (approximately 1000 calories with 50% of calories from fat) increased systemic exposure (AUC and peak plasma concentrations) of sonidegib by 7.4- to 7.8-fold. In a population pharmacokinetic analysis, administration of sonidegib with a high-fat meal increased bioavailability of the drug fivefold. Sonidegib is metabolized in the liver principally by cytochrome P-450 (CYP) isoenzyme 3A. In vitro, sonidegib is more than 97% bound to plasma proteins.

Following oral administration of sonidegib, approximately 70% of the absorbed dose is recovered in feces and 30% is recovered in urine; unchanged drug is not excreted in urine. The estimated plasma elimination half-life of the drug is 28–29.6 days.

Population pharmacokinetic analyses indicate that age, gender, body weight, and ethnicity generally do not have clinically important effects on the exposure of sonidegib. A cross-study comparison indicates that systemic exposure following administration of sonidegib (single 200-mg dose) is increased by 1.7-fold in healthy Japanese individuals compared with individuals from Western countries.

Advice to Patients

Importance of advising patients to take sonidegib on an empty stomach, at least 1 hour before or 2 hours after a meal. If a dose of sonidegib is missed, patients should be instructed to take the next dose at the regularly scheduled time.

Risk of adverse musculoskeletal effects. Importance of monitoring serum creatine kinase (CK, creatine phosphokinase, CPK) and creatinine concentrations before and during sonidegib therapy. Importance of immediately reporting dark urine, decreased urine output, inability to urinate, or new or worsening unexplained muscle pain, tenderness, or weakness that occurs during therapy or persists following discontinuance of sonidegib.

Risk of fetal harm. Necessity of advising women of childbearing potential to use effective methods of contraception during sonidegib therapy and for at least 20 months after discontinuance of therapy (see Fetal/Neonatal Morbidity and Mortality under Warnings/Precautions: Warnings, in Cautions); importance of obtaining pregnancy tests prior to initiation of therapy. Female patients and female partners of men receiving sonidegib therapy should contact clinician if pregnancy is suspected or confirmed. Advise pregnant women potentially exposed to the drug of potential risk to the fetus.

Necessity of advising men (including those who have successfully undergone vasectomy) to use a condom during sexual encounters with women of childbearing potential; these contraceptive measures are required during and for at least 8 months after discontinuance of sonidegib therapy.

Risk of serious adverse reactions in nursing infants. Importance of advising women to avoid breast-feeding while receiving sonidegib therapy and for at least 20 months after discontinuance of therapy.

Importance of advising men to avoid donating semen while receiving sonidegib and for at least 8 months after discontinuing therapy with the drug.

Importance of advising patients to avoid donating blood or blood products while receiving sonidegib and for at least 20 months after discontinuing therapy with the drug.

Importance of informing clinicians of existing or contemplated concomitant therapy, including prescription and OTC drugs and dietary or herbal supplements (e.g., St. John's wort), as well as any concomitant illnesses.

Importance of informing patients of other important precautionary information. (See Cautions.)

Overview® (see Users Guide). For additional information on this drug until a more detailed monograph is developed and published, the manufacturer's labeling should be consulted. It is *essential* that the manufacturer's labeling be consulted for more detailed information on usual cautions, precautions, contraindications, potential drug interactions, laboratory test interferences, and acute toxicity. For further information on the handling of antineoplastic agents, see the ASHP Guidelines on Handling Hazardous Drugs at http://www.ahfsdruginformation.com.

Preparations

Excipients in commercially available drug preparations may have clinically important effects in some individuals; consult specific product labeling for details.

Sonidegib

Oral

Capsules	200 mg	**Odomzo®**, Novartis

SORAfenib Tosylate

■ Sorafenib tosylate, an inhibitor of several serine/threonine and receptor tyrosine kinases, is an antineoplastic agent.

Uses

■ **Hepatocellular Carcinoma** Sorafenib tosylate is used for the treatment of unresectable hepatocellular carcinoma and is designated an orphan drug by the US Food and Drug Administration (FDA) for the treatment of this cancer.

The current indication for sorafenib tosylate in the treatment of unresectable hepatocellular carcinoma is based principally on the results of a randomized, double-blind, placebo-controlled phase 3 study (Sorafenib Hepatocellular Carcinoma Assessment Randomized Protocol [SHARP] trial) in patients with previously untreated advanced hepatocellular carcinoma. In this study, 602 patients were randomized in a 1:1 ratio to receive either sorafenib (400 mg orally twice daily) or placebo. Treatment was continued until disease progression, death, or unacceptable toxicity occurred.

Patients were enrolled in the study if they were not eligible for or had disease progression after surgical or locoregional therapies; approximately 70% of patients enrolled in the study had macroscopic vascular invasion, extrahepatic spread, or both. The majority of enrolled patients had mild (Child-Pugh class A) hepatic impairment (97%) and a baseline ECOG performance status of 0 (54%) or 1 (38%). Chronic hepatitis C virus (HCV) infection, alcohol consumption, or chronic hepatitis B virus (HBV) infection was the cause of hepatocellular carcinoma in 28, 26, or 18% of patients, respectively. The median duration of treatment was 5.3 months for patients receiving sorafenib and 4.3 months for those receiving placebo.

The primary measure of efficacy was overall survival; secondary end points included time to progression (based on independent radiologic review) and disease control rate. A planned second interim analysis indicated that patients receiving sorafenib had a longer median overall survival than those receiving placebo (10.7 versus 7.9 months; hazard ratio for death: 0.69). Final analysis of the time to disease progression (which occurred at an earlier time point than the survival analysis) indicated that patients receiving sorafenib had a longer median time to progression compared with those receiving placebo (5.5 versus 2.8 months). Patients receiving sorafenib had higher disease control rates compared with those receiving placebo (43 versus 32%). The proportion of patients with disease stabilization was slightly higher among those receiving sorafenib compared with those receiving placebo (71 versus 67%, respectively); however, partial response rates were low (2 versus 1%, respectively) and none of the patients achieved a complete response. Subgroup analysis according to disease etiology (HCV, HBV, alcohol consumption), tumor burden (presence or absence of macroscopic vascular invasion and/or extrahepatic spread), ECOG performance status (0–2), tumor stage (Barcelona Clinic Liver Cancer [BCLC] stage), and prior therapy (resection/ablation or chemoembolization) suggested that sorafenib consistently improved median overall survival across all subgroups; an effect on time to progression was not apparent in the small subgroup of HBV-positive patients.

Efficacy of sorafenib also was demonstrated in a supportive phase 3 study conducted in the Asia-Pacific area (i.e., China, South Korea, Taiwan). In this study, 271 adults with previously untreated advanced hepatocellular carcinoma were randomized in a 2:1 ratio to receive either sorafenib (400 mg orally twice daily) or placebo. In contrast to the SHARP trial, most patients in this study were HBV-positive (73%) and had an ECOG performance status of 1 (69%). Although absolute overall survival, time to progression, and disease control were poorer in this study as compared to the SHARP trial, patients in this study who received sorafenib had a longer median overall survival (6.5 versus 4.2 months), longer median time to progression (2.8 versus 1.4 months), and higher disease control rate (35.3 versus 15.8%) than those who received placebo.

Additional studies are need to more fully evaluate the efficacy and safety of sorafenib for the treatment of hepatocellular carcinoma in patients with more severe (i.e., Child-Pugh class B) hepatic impairment. (See Hepatic Impairment under Warnings/Precautions: Specific Populations, in Cautions.)

■ **Renal Cell Carcinoma** Sorafenib tosylate is used for the treatment of advanced renal cell carcinoma and is designated an orphan drug by FDA for the treatment of this cancer. Safety and efficacy of sorafenib tosylate in the treatment of advanced renal cell carcinoma were established in 2 randomized, controlled clinical trials (one phase 2 and one phase 3).

In the phase 3 trial, patients with unresectable and/or metastatic clear cell renal carcinoma who had received one prior systemic (e.g., cytokine) therapy were randomized to receive sorafenib 400 mg twice daily or placebo. Patients receiving sorafenib had a longer median progression-free survival (167 versus 84 days), an increased rate of progression-free survival at 12 weeks (79 versus 50%), and a decreased risk of progression compared with those receiving placebo. Effects on overall survival remain to be established; 2 planned interim analyses suggested a numerical but not statistically significant increase in overall survival with sorafenib compared with placebo. At the time of the first interim survival analysis, partial response, stable disease, and progressive disease were observed in 10, 74, and 12%, respectively, of patients receiving sorafenib and in 2, 53, and 37%, respectively, of patients receiving placebo.

The phase 2 trial included patients with metastatic malignancies, including individuals with untreated or previously treated renal cell carcinoma. Following a 12-week run-in induction period during which all patients received sorafenib 400 mg twice daily, tumor response was assessed and those with stable disease (i.e., less than 25% change from baseline in bidimensional tumor measurements) were randomized to receive either sorafenib 400 mg twice daily or placebo for an additional 12 weeks, those with tumor shrinkage (at least 25% reduction from baseline) continued to receive sorafenib in an open-label arm of the study, and those with tumor growth (at least 25% increase from baseline) discontinued therapy with the drug. Of the 202 patients with renal cell carcinoma who were enrolled in the run-in induction phase, 65 were randomized to receive either sorafenib or placebo and 79 were assigned to receive open-label treatment with the drug. Patients in the placebo group who experienced disease progression were allowed to cross over to open-label sorafenib. In the subgroup of patients randomized to receive sorafenib or placebo, those receiving sorafenib had a higher rate of progression-free survival at 24 weeks (50 versus 18%) and a longer median progression-free survival (163 versus 41 days) than did those receiving placebo.

Dosage and Administration

■ **Administration** Because administration with a high-fat meal may decrease oral bioavailability of sorafenib, the manufacturer recommends that sorafenib tosylate be administered orally at least 1 hour before or 2 hours after a meal.

■ **Dosage** Dosage of sorafenib tosylate is expressed in terms of sorafenib.

Hepatocellular Carcinoma For the treatment of unresectable hepatocellular carcinoma, the recommended adult dosage of sorafenib is 400 mg twice daily. Therapy should be continued for as long as the patient derives clinical benefit from the drug or until unacceptable toxicity occurs.

Renal Cell Carcinoma For the treatment of advanced renal cell carcinoma, the recommended adult dosage of sorafenib is 400 mg twice daily. Therapy should be continued for as long as the patient derives clinical benefit from the drug or until unacceptable toxicity occurs.

Dosage Modification for Toxicity Dosage of sorafenib may be reduced or therapy temporarily interrupted in patients who develop suspected adverse effects, such as cutaneous toxicity (see Table 1). If dosage reduction is necessary, sorafenib dosage may be decreased to 400 mg once daily. If further dosage reduction is required, sorafenib dosage may be decreased to 400 mg every other day.

Table 1: Suggested Dosage Modification for Cutaneous Toxicity

Cutaneous Toxicity Grade	Occurrence	Suggested Dosage Modification
Grade 1: numbness, dysesthesia, paresthesia, tingling, painless swelling, erythema, or discomfort of the hands or feet that does not disrupt the patient's normal activities	Any occurrence	Continue therapy with sorafenib and consider topical therapy for symptomatic relief
Grade 2: painful erythema and swelling of the hands or feet and/or discomfort affecting the patient's normal activities	1st occurrence	Continue therapy with sorafenib and consider topical therapy for symptomatic relief If improvement is not evident within 7 days, see below
	No improvement within 7 days or 2nd or 3rd occurrence	Interrupt sorafenib therapy until toxicity resolves to grade 0 or 1 When resuming therapy, decrease sorafenib dosage by one dose level (e.g., to 400 mg once daily or 400 mg every other day)
	4th occurrence	Discontinue sorafenib therapy
Grade 3: moist desquamation, ulceration, blistering or severe pain of the hands or feet, or severe discomfort that causes the patient to be unable to work or perform activities of daily living	1st or 2nd occurrence	Interrupt sorafenib therapy until toxicity resolves to grade 0 or 1 When resuming therapy, decrease sorafenib dosage by one dose level (e.g., to 400 mg once daily or 400 mg every other day)
	3rd occurrence	Discontinue sorafenib therapy

■ **Special Populations** The manufacturer makes no specific dosage recommendations for geriatric patients.

No dosage adjustment is necessary in patients with mild (Child-Pugh class A) or moderate (Child-Pugh class B) hepatic impairment. Sorafenib has not been studied in patients with severe (Child-Pugh class C) hepatic impairment. (See Hepatic Impairment under Warnings/Precautions: Specific Populations, in Cautions.)

No dosage adjustment is necessary in patients with mild to severe renal impairment; however, the drug has not been studied in patients with renal impairment requiring dialysis. (See Renal Impairment under Warnings/Precautions: Specific Populations, in Cautions.)

Cautions

■ **Contraindications** Known hypersensitivity to sorafenib or any ingredient in the formulation.

In combination with carboplatin and paclitaxel in patients with squamous cell lung cancer. (See Increased Mortality in Squamous Cell Carcinoma of the Lung under Cautions: Warnings/Precautions.)

■ **Warnings/Precautions** *Cardiovascular Effects* In the phase 3 trial of sorafenib in patients with unresectable hepatocellular carcinoma, cardiac ischemia or infarction occurred in 2.7% of patients receiving sorafenib compared with 1.3% of those receiving placebo. In the phase 3 trial in patients with advanced renal cell carcinoma, cardiac ischemia or infarction occurred more frequently in patients receiving sorafenib than in those receiving placebo (2.9 versus 0.4%). Temporary or permanent discontinuance of sorafenib should be considered in patients who develop cardiac ischemia and/or infarction.

In the phase 3 trial of sorafenib in patients with unresectable hepatocellular carcinoma, hypertension occurred in approximately 9.4% of patients receiving sorafenib compared with 4.3% of those receiving placebo. In the phase 3 trial in patients with advanced renal cell carcinoma, hypertension was reported more frequently in patients receiving sorafenib compared with those receiving placebo (16.9 versus 1.8%). Hypertension usually was mild or moderate, occurred early in the course of treatment, and was managed with standard antihypertensive therapy. Blood pressure should be monitored weekly during the first 6 weeks of sorafenib therapy and thereafter should be monitored and treated, if required, in accordance with established medical practice. If hypertension is severe or persistent despite initiation of antihypertensive therapy, temporary or permanent discontinuance of sorafenib should be considered.

Sorafenib may prolong the QT interval, which may increase the risk of ventricular arrhythmias. In a small multicenter, open-label, nonrandomized trial evaluating the effects of sorafenib (400 mg twice daily) on the QT interval in patients with advanced cancer, no large (i.e., exceeding 20 msec) increases in the corrected QT (QT_c) interval were observed. Following the first 28-day treatment cycle (cycle 1), the maximum mean change in QT_c interval was 8.5 msec, which was observed at 6 hours following the first dose of cycle 2. Sorafenib should be avoided in patients with congenital long QT syndrome. ECGs and serum electrolytes (potassium, calcium, and magnesium) should be monitored in patients with congestive heart failure, bradyarrhythmias, or electrolyte abnormalities, and in those who are receiving drugs known to prolong the QT interval (e.g., class IA and III antiarrhythmic agents).

Hemorrhage Sorafenib may increase the risk of bleeding. However, in the phase 3 trial of sorafenib in patients with unresectable hepatocellular carcinoma, the incidence of bleeding from esophageal varices was lower in patients receiving sorafenib compared with those receiving placebo (2.4 versus 4%); similarly, fatal hemorrhage from any site occurred in 2.4% of patients receiving sorafenib and 4% of those receiving placebo. In the phase 3 trial in patients with advanced renal cell carcinoma, bleeding (regardless of causality) was reported in 15.3 or 8.2% of patients receiving sorafenib or placebo, respectively; grade 3 and 4 bleeding were reported in 2 and 0%, respectively, of patients receiving sorafenib compared with 1.3 and 0.2%, respectively, of patients receiving placebo. Fatal hemorrhage occurred in one patient in each treatment group in this study. Permanent discontinuance of sorafenib should be considered if any bleeding episode requires medical intervention.

Infrequent bleeding events or elevations in the international normalized ratio (INR) have been reported in some patients receiving concomitant therapy with warfarin and sorafenib. Patients receiving such concomitant therapy should be monitored regularly for changes in prothrombin time (PT) or INR and for clinical bleeding episodes. (See Drug Interactions: Warfarin.)

Dermatologic Effects Palmar-plantar erythrodysesthesia (commonly referred to as hand-foot syndrome) and rash are common adverse effects of sorafenib. In the phase 3 trial of sorafenib in patients with unresectable hepatocellular carcinoma, hand-foot syndrome and rash occurred in 21 and 19%, respectively, of patients receiving sorafenib compared with 3 and 14%, respectively, of patients receiving placebo. In the phase 3 trial in patients with advanced renal cell carcinoma, hand-foot syndrome and rash occurred in 30 and 40%, respectively, of patients receiving the drug compared with 7 and 16%, respectively, of patients receiving placebo. Rash and hand-foot syndrome usually are grade 1 or 2 and generally appear during the first 6 weeks of treatment with sorafenib. Management of dermatologic toxicities may include topical therapies for symptomatic relief, temporary interruption of therapy, and/or dosage modification of sorafenib; in severe or persistent cases, permanent discontinuance of sorafenib therapy may be necessary. (See Dosage Modification for Toxicity under Dosage and Administration: Dosage.)

Cases of severe and possibly life-threatening dermatologic toxicities, including Stevens-Johnson syndrome and toxic epidermal necrolysis, have been reported. If Stevens-Johnson syndrome or toxic epidermal necrolysis is suspected, sorafenib therapy should be discontinued.

GI Effects GI perforation, sometimes associated with apparent intra-abdominal tumor, has been reported rarely in patients receiving sorafenib. Sorafenib therapy should be discontinued if GI perforation occurs.

Wound-healing Complications The effect of sorafenib on wound healing has not been established. The manufacturer recommends that sorafenib therapy be temporarily interrupted in patients undergoing major surgery. There is limited clinical experience regarding the timing of reinitiation of sorafenib therapy following major surgery; therefore, the decision to resume sorafenib therapy should be based on clinical assessment of the adequacy of wound healing.

Increased Mortality in Squamous Cell Carcinoma of the Lung Subset analysis of data from 2 randomized controlled trials in patients with previously untreated advanced (stage IIIB or IV) non-small cell lung cancer revealed an increased risk of mortality in patients with squamous cell carcinoma receiving sorafenib in combination with carboplatin and paclitaxel (hazard ratio of 1.81) and in those receiving sorafenib in combination with gemcitabine and cisplatin (hazard ratio of 1.22) compared with those receiving the corresponding dual regimen (i.e., therapy with carboplatin and paclitaxel or with gemcitabine and cisplatin, respectively). Sorafenib in combination with carboplatin and paclitaxel is contraindicated in patients with squamous cell carcinoma of the lung. In addition, the manufacturer states that use of sorafenib in combination with gemcitabine and cisplatin is *not* recommended in patients with squamous cell carcinoma of the lung.

Safety and efficacy of sorafenib in patients with non-small cell lung cancer have not been established.

Hepatic Effects Serious or fatal drug-induced hepatitis characterized by a hepatocellular pattern of hepatic injury with substantially elevated serum aminotransferase concentrations may occur; increased serum concentrations of bilirubin and increased INR also may occur. The manufacturer states that liver function tests should be monitored regularly in patients receiving sorafenib. Sorafenib therapy should be discontinued if substantially elevated serum aminotransferase concentrations occur and other possible causes (i.e., viral hepatitis, malignancy progression) have been ruled out.

Fetal/Neonatal Morbidity and Mortality Sorafenib may cause fetal harm if administered to pregnant women; teratogenicity and embryolethality have been demonstrated in animals. Although there are no adequate and well-controlled studies in humans, sorafenib has been shown to have teratogenic and embryolethal effects (i.e., postimplantation loss, resorptions, skeletal retardation, retarded fetal weight) in rats and rabbits when given in dosages lower than the usual human dosage. Pregnancy should be avoided during therapy. (See Advice to Patients.) If sorafenib is used during pregnancy or if the patient becomes pregnant while receiving the drug, the patient should be apprised of the potential hazard to the fetus.

Women of childbearing potential and men receiving the drug should use an effective contraceptive method during sexual encounters during and for at least 2 weeks following discontinuance of sorafenib therapy.

Specific Populations **Pregnancy.** Category D. (See Fetal/Neonatal Morbidity and Mortality under Cautions: Warnings/Precautions.)

Lactation. Sorafenib is distributed into milk in rats; it is not known whether the drug is distributed into milk in humans. Because many drugs are distributed into human milk and because of the potential for serious adverse reactions to sorafenib in nursing infants, a decision should be made whether to discontinue nursing or the drug, taking into account the importance of the drug to the woman.

Pediatric Use. Safety and efficacy of sorafenib have not been established in children younger than 18 years of age.

Geriatric Use. In clinical trials evaluating sorafenib in patients with unresectable hepatocellular carcinoma or advanced renal cell carcinoma, 59 or 32%, respectively, of patients were 65 years of age or older, and 19 or 4%, respectively, were 75 years of age or older. No substantial differences in safety and efficacy relative to younger adults have been observed, but increased sensitivity to the drug cannot be ruled out.

Hepatic Impairment. Systemic exposure to sorafenib in patients with mild or moderate (Child-Pugh class A or B) hepatic impairment, including both patients with hepatocellular carcinoma and individuals without such disease, is similar to that observed in individuals with normal hepatic function. In patients with hepatocellular carcinoma, systemic exposure and peak plasma concentrations of the drug were slightly higher in those with moderate (Child-Pugh class B) hepatic impairment compared with those with mild (Child-Pugh class A) hepatic impairment; however, the differences were not clinically meaningful. (See Dosage and Administration: Special Populations.)

Limited safety and efficacy data are available for patients with hepatocellular carcinoma and moderate (Child-Pugh class B) hepatic impairment. In a phase 2 study in patients with hepatocellular carcinoma, median overall survival was shorter in patients with moderate (Child-Pugh class B) hepatic impairment than in those with mild (Child-Pugh class A) hepatic impairment (3.2 versus 9.5 months, respectively). Shorter median overall survival in patients with moderate hepatic impairment also has been reported from several prospective and retrospective studies of sorafenib use for hepatocellular carcinoma.

Safety and efficacy of sorafenib have not been established in patients with severe (Child-Pugh class C) hepatic impairment.

Renal Impairment. No relationship between renal function and systemic exposure to sorafenib was observed following administration of a single 400-mg dose of sorafenib in individuals with normal renal function or mild (creatinine clearance of 50–80 mL/minute), moderate (creatinine clearance of 30–49 mL/minute), or severe (creatinine clearance less than 30 mL/minute) renal impairment. Pharmacokinetic parameters of sorafenib have not been evaluated in patients with renal impairment requiring dialysis.

■ **Common Adverse Effects** Adverse effects reported in 10% or more of patients receiving sorafenib for the treatment of unresectable hepatocellular carcinoma and more frequently with the drug than with placebo include hypoalbuminemia, diarrhea, lymphopenia, fatigue, thrombocytopenia, increased INR, increased lipase concentrations, hypophosphatemia, increased amylase concentrations, abdominal pain, weight loss, anorexia, hypocalcemia, nausea, hand-foot syndrome, rash/desquamation, vomiting, alopecia, constipation, pruritus, hepatic impairment, dry skin, and hypertension.

Adverse effects reported in 10% or more of patients receiving sorafenib for the treatment of advanced renal cell carcinoma and more frequently with the drug than with placebo include hypophosphatemia, diarrhea, increased lipase concentrations, rash/desquamation, fatigue, hand-foot syndrome, increased amylase concentrations, alopecia, nausea, lymphopenia, pruritus, neutropenia, hypertension, anorexia, vomiting, constipation, hemorrhage, dyspnea, sensory neuropathy, hypocalcemia, thrombocytopenia, dry skin, pain (abdominal, joint, headache), and weight loss.

Drug Interactions

■ **Drugs Affecting Hepatic Microsomal Enzymes** Sorafenib is partially metabolized by cytochrome P-450 (CYP) isoenzyme 3A4; however, when the potent CYP3A4 inhibitor ketoconazole (400 mg daily for 7 days) was administered concomitantly with sorafenib (single 50-mg dose) in healthy individuals, mean systemic exposure to sorafenib was unchanged. These data suggest that clinically important interactions with drugs that inhibit CYP3A4 are unlikely.

Concomitant use of sorafenib with inducers of CYP3A4 may result in increased metabolism of and decreased systemic exposure to sorafenib. In healthy individuals, the potent CYP3A4 inducer rifampin (600 mg daily for 5 days) decreased systemic exposure to sorafenib (single 400-mg dose) by 37%. Concomitant use of sorafenib with potent inducers of CYP3A4 (e.g., carbamazepine, dexamethasone, phenobarbital, phenytoin, rifabutin, rifampin, St. John's wort [*Hypericum perforatum*]) should be avoided when possible.

■ **Drugs Metabolized by Hepatic Microsomal Enzymes** In vitro studies using human hepatic microsomes indicate that sorafenib competitively inhibits CYP isoenzymes 2B6, 2C8, 2C9, 2C19, 2D6, and 3A4. However, concomitant administration of sorafenib with cyclophosphamide (a CYP2B6 substrate) or paclitaxel (a CYP2C8 substrate) did not result in clinically important changes in enzyme inhibition, suggesting that sorafenib, when administered at the recommended dosage, may not result in clinically important inhibition of CYP2B6 or CYP2C8 (see Drug Interactions: Antineoplastic Agents). In addition, sorafenib does not appear to alter systemic exposure to dextromethorphan (a CYP2D6 substrate), midazolam (a CYP3A4 substrate), or omeprazole (a CYP2C19 substrate), suggesting that clinically important interactions with drugs that are metabolized by these isoenzymes also are unlikely. When warfarin (a CYP2C9 substrate) was administered concomitantly with sorafenib, mean changes from baseline in prothrombin time (PT)/international normalized ratio (INR) did not appear to be greater in patients receiving sorafenib as compared with placebo, suggesting that the risk for clinically important inhibition of CYP2D6 by sorafenib also may be low (See Drug Interactions: Warfarin).

The manufacturer states that sorafenib is unlikely to induce CYP isoenzymes 1A2 or 3A4.

■ **Drugs Metabolized by Uridine Diphosphate-glucuronosyltransferase** In vitro studies indicate that sorafenib inhibits glucuronidation by the uridine diphosphate-glucuronosyltransferase (UGT) 1A1 and 1A9 pathways; sorafenib may increase systemic exposure to UGT 1A1 or 1A9 substrates. Caution is advised when sorafenib is used concomitantly with drugs predominantly metabolized by the UGT 1A1 or 1A9 pathway (e.g., irinotecan, whose active metabolite SN-38 is metabolized by UGT 1A1). (See Drug Interactions: Antineoplastic Agents.)

■ **Drugs Affecting Gastric Acidity** Because the aqueous solubility of sorafenib is dependent on pH, drugs that increase the pH of the upper GI tract (e.g., proton-pump inhibitors) may potentially decrease the solubility of sorafenib. However, concomitant administration of the proton-pump inhibitor omeprazole (40 mg once daily for 5 days) with a single dose of sorafenib did not result in clinically important changes in systemic exposure to sorafenib. The manufacturer states that dosage adjustment of sorafenib is not necessary when sorafenib is administered concurrently with drugs affecting gastric acidity.

■ **Substrates of P-Glycoprotein Transport System** In vitro data indicate that sorafenib is an inhibitor of the efflux transporter P-glycoprotein (P-gp). Concomitant use of sorafenib with drugs that are substrates of P-gp (e.g., digoxin) may result in increased systemic exposure to the substrate drug.

■ **Antibiotics** In healthy individuals, neomycin (1 g 3 times daily for 5 days) decreased the mean systemic exposure to sorafenib (single 400-mg dose) by 54%. Bacterial glucuronidases in the GI tract may cleave sorafenib conjugates, allowing reabsorption of unconjugated drug; neomycin interferes with this enterohepatic circulation process, thereby reducing bioavailability of sorafenib. The effect of other antibiotics on the pharmacokinetics of sorafenib has not been established.

■ **Antineoplastic Agents** When docetaxel was administered concomitantly with sorafenib, systemic exposure and peak plasma concentration of docetaxel were increased by 36–80 and 16–32%, respectively. Caution is advised.

When irinotecan was administered concomitantly with sorafenib, systemic exposure to irinotecan and its active metabolite SN-38 was increased by 26–42 and 67–120%, respectively. Caution is advised. (See Drug Interactions: Drugs Metabolized by Uridine Diphosphate-glucuronosyltransferase.)

When doxorubicin was used concomitantly with sorafenib, systemic exposure to doxorubicin was increased by 21%.

Concomitant use of capecitabine with sorafenib did not substantially alter systemic exposure to sorafenib but increased systemic exposure to capecitabine and its active metabolite fluorouracil by 15–50 and 0–52%, respectively.

Concomitant use of paclitaxel and carboplatin with continuous sorafenib therapy increased systemic exposure to sorafenib and to paclitaxel and its major metabolite 6-hydroxypaclitaxel (a metabolite formed by CYP2C8) by 47, 29, and 50%, respectively, but did not alter the pharmacokinetics of carboplatin. (See Increased Mortality in Squamous Cell Carcinoma of the Lung under Cautions: Warnings/Precautions.)

Sorafenib does not appear to affect the pharmacokinetics of cisplatin, cyclophosphamide, gemcitabine, or oxaliplatin.

■ **Warfarin** When warfarin (a CYP2C9 substrate) was administered concomitantly with sorafenib, mean changes from baseline in PT/INR did not appear to be greater in patients receiving sorafenib as compared with placebo. However, infrequent bleeding events or elevations in INR have been reported in some patients receiving concomitant therapy with warfarin and sorafenib. (See Hemorrhage under Cautions: Warnings/Precautions.)

Description

Sorafenib tosylate, an inhibitor of several serine/threonine and receptor tyrosine kinases, is an antineoplastic agent. Serine/threonine and receptor tyrosine kinases are involved in various cascades of intracellular signaling events that lead to cell proliferation and/or influence processes critical to cell survival and tumor progression (e.g., angiogenesis, apoptosis, metastasis), based on the respective kinase. Although the exact mechanism of antineoplastic activity of sorafenib has not been fully elucidated, sorafenib appears to inhibit signal transduction pathways involving multiple intracellular (e.g., c-Raf, b-Raf, mutant b-Raf) and cell surface kinases (e.g., c-Kit, Flt-3, RET, vascular endothelial growth factor receptor [VEGFR]-1, VEGFR-2, VEGFR-3, platelet-derived growth factor receptor [PDGFR]-*β*) in vitro. In vivo, sorafenib inhibited angiogenesis and growth of human hepatocellular carcinoma, renal cell carcinoma, and several other human tumor xenografts in immunocompromised mice.

Sorafenib is metabolized mainly in the liver via oxidation by cytochrome P-450 (CYP) isoenzyme 3A4, as well as via glucuronidation by uridine diphosphate-glucuronosyltransferase (UGT) 1A9. At least 8 metabolites of sorafenib have been identified. The main circulating metabolite, a pyridine *N*-oxide derivative, is pharmacologically active and accounts for approximately 9–16% of total plasma concentrations of the drug. Approximately 77% of an oral dose of sorafenib is excreted in feces and 19% is eliminated in urine; unchanged sorafenib, which accounts for 51% of a dose, is recovered in feces but not in urine. The pharmacokinetics of sorafenib do not appear to be affected by age or gender; however, systemic exposure to the drug was 30% lower in Asians than in Caucasians.

Advice to Patients

If a dose is missed, importance of administering the next dose at the regularly scheduled time; a double dose should *not* be administered to make up for a missed dose.

Importance of women informing clinicians if they are or plan to become pregnant or plan to breast-feed. Necessity of advising women to avoid pregnancy during therapy and for at least 2 weeks following completion of sorafenib therapy, as well as advising women to discontinue nursing while receiving therapy. Necessity of advising women and men to use effective contraceptive methods during sorafenib therapy and for at least 2 weeks following completion of therapy. Advise women of the potential risk to the fetus (e.g., birth defects) and/or the potential risk for loss of the pregnancy.

Risk of hand-foot syndrome and rash; importance of advising patient about appropriate countermeasures.

Risk of hypertension, particularly during the first 6 weeks of sorafenib therapy. Importance of monitoring blood pressure regularly during therapy.

Risk of bleeding. Importance of patients promptly informing clinicians of any episodes of bleeding.

Risk of bleeding or elevation in international normalized ratio (INR) in patients receiving concomitant therapy with warfarin and sorafenib. Importance of monitoring INR regularly during therapy.

Risk of potential GI perforation. Importance of informing clinician immediately if high fever, nausea, vomiting, or severe stomach or abdominal pain occurs.

Risk of potential cardiac ischemia and/or infarction. Importance of patients immediately informing clinicians of any episodes of chest pain or other symptoms of cardiac ischemia.

Risk of wound healing complications. Importance of informing clinician of any scheduled surgery.

Risk of QT-interval prolongation. Importance of informing clinicians immediately if an abnormal heartbeat or feelings of dizziness or faintness occur.

Risk of hepatitis and importance of regular liver function test monitoring. Importance of advising patients to report signs and symptoms of hepatitis (e.g., jaundice, dark tea-colored urine, light-colored stool, worsening nausea or vomiting, abdominal pain).

Importance of informing clinicians of existing or contemplated concomitant therapy, including prescription and OTC drugs and herbal supplements (e.g., St. John's wort), as well as any concomitant illnesses (e.g., cardiovascular disease [including congenital long QT syndrome]).

Importance of informing patients of other important precautionary information. (See Cautions.)

Overview® (see Users Guide). For additional information on this drug until a more detailed monograph is developed and published, the manufacturer's labeling should be consulted. It is *essential* that the manufacturer's labeling be consulted for more detailed information on usual cautions, precautions, contraindications, potential drug interactions, laboratory test interferences, and acute toxicity.

Preparations

Excipients in commercially available drug preparations may have clinically important effects in some individuals; consult specific product labeling for details.

SORAfenib Tosylate

Oral		
Tablets, film-coated	200 mg (of sorafenib)	**NexAVAR®**, Bayer (comarketed by Onyx)

Selected Revisions August 2014, © Copyright, May 2006, American Society of Health-System Pharmacists, Inc.

SUNItinib Malate

■ Sunitinib malate, an inhibitor of multiple receptor tyrosine kinases, is an antineoplastic agent.

Uses

■ **Gastrointestinal Stromal Tumor** Sunitinib malate is used for the treatment of gastrointestinal stromal tumor (GIST) in adults who are intolerant of or whose disease has progressed during imatinib therapy.

The current indication for sunitinib malate is based principally on the results of 2 studies (one randomized, double-blind, placebo-controlled, phase 3 study and one open-label, single-arm, phase 1/2 dose-escalation study) in patients with GIST who were intolerant of or whose disease had progressed during imatinib therapy. In the phase 3 study, 312 patients were randomized in a 2:1 ratio to receive either sunitinib (50 mg) or placebo given once daily for 4 consecutive weeks followed by a 2-week period without treatment. Treatment cycles were repeated until disease progression or withdrawal from the study for other reasons occurred. A planned interim analysis indicated that patients receiving sunitinib had a longer median time to tumor progression (27.3 versus 6.4 weeks) and a longer median progression-free survival (24.1 versus 6 weeks) than those receiving placebo. Following these favorable results, the study was unblinded, and study investigators permitted patients previously randomized to receive placebo to cross over to open-label sunitinib; those previously randomized to receive sunitinib were permitted to continue therapy based on clinical judgment. After the study was unblinded, 94.3% of patients initially randomized to receive placebo crossed over to receive sunitinib therapy. Updated analysis confirmed that, following administration of a median of 5–6 treatment cycles, patients receiving sunitinib (i.e., those originally randomized to sunitinib and those who switched from placebo to sunitinib) had a longer median time to tumor progression (28.4 weeks) than those who received placebo (8.7 weeks); the time to tumor progression in patients who switched from placebo to sunitinib was not statistically different from that in patients originally randomized to sunitinib therapy. At the planned final analysis, median overall survival was 72.7 weeks in patients receiving sunitinib compared with 64.9 weeks in those receiving placebo.

In the open-label, single-arm, dose-escalation study, treatment with sunitinib given in 6-week cycles at a dosage of 50 mg once daily for 4 consecutive weeks followed by a 2-week drug-free period produced partial responses in 5 of 55 patients (9.1%).

■ **Renal Cell Carcinoma** Sunitinib malate is used for the treatment of advanced renal cell carcinoma.

The current indication for sunitinib malate is based principally on the results of a large randomized trial and 2 uncontrolled studies.

In a multicenter randomized trial, 750 patients received either sunitinib or interferon alfa as initial treatment for metastatic renal cell cancer. Treatment consisted of sunitinib 50 mg once daily for 4 consecutive weeks followed by a 2-week period without treatment, or interferon alfa 9 million units subcutaneously 3 times a week, until disease progression, intolerable toxicity, or withdrawal from the study occurred. Progression-free survival was prolonged (47.3 versus 22 weeks) and overall response rate was higher (27.5 versus 5.3%) in patients receiving sunitinib compared with those receiving interferon alfa. At the planned final analysis, median overall survival was 114.6 weeks in patients receiving sunitinib compared with 94.9 weeks in those receiving interferon alfa. The median overall survival for the interferon alfa-treated group included 6.7% of patients who crossed over to treatment with sunitinib and 32% of patients who received poststudy therapy with sunitinib.

Patients receiving sunitinib had a greater frequency of ventricular dysfunction, including left ventricular ejection fraction (LVEF) below the lower limit of normal (27 versus 15%) and decline in LVEF (7 versus 2%), than those receiving interferon alfa. Hypertension (34 versus 4%), including grade 3 hypertension (13 versus less than 1%), and bleeding events (37 versus 10%) occurred more frequently in patients receiving sunitinib than in those receiving interferon alfa.

The use of sunitinib also was investigated in 2 single-arm, phase 2 studies in 169 patients with metastatic renal cell carcinoma who were intolerant of cytokine-based therapy (e.g., aldesleukin, interferon alfa, combination of aldesleukin and interferon alfa) and/or whose disease had progressed during or following completion of such therapy. Approximately 95% of enrolled patients had at least some component of clear-cell histology, and 97% had undergone nephrectomy. Metastatic disease present at the time of study entry included lung (82%), liver (23%), and bone (35%) metastases; patients with known brain metastases or leptomeningeal disease were excluded from both studies. All patients in both studies received sunitinib (dosage schedule of 50 mg once daily for 4 consecutive weeks followed by a 2-week period without treatment) until disease progression, intolerable toxicity, or withdrawal from the study occurred. Data analysis from the first study revealed a partial response rate of 34% and a median progression-free survival of 8.3 months; the median overall survival had not been reached at the time of this analysis. Data analysis from the second study revealed a partial response rate of 36.5% and a median time to tumor progression of 8.7 months. In these studies, more than 90% of partial responses were observed during the first 4 cycles of sunitinib therapy, with the latest response observed during cycle 10.

■ **Neuroendocrine Tumors of Pancreatic Origin** Sunitinib malate is used for the treatment of progressive, well-differentiated neuroendocrine tumors of pancreatic origin (PNET) in patients with unresectable, locally advanced, or metastatic disease.

The current indication for sunitinib malate is based principally on the results of a randomized, double-blind, placebo-controlled, multicenter, phase 3 study in patients with unresectable, locally advanced, or metastatic well-differentiated PNET that had progressed within the previous 12 months. In this study, 171 patients were randomized in a 1:1 ratio to receive either sunitinib (37.5 mg) or placebo orally once daily; therapy was given continuously (i.e., without a scheduled off-treatment period). Approximately 27 or 29% of patients randomized to receive sunitinib or placebo, respectively, also received concomitant therapy with a somatostatin analog. Treatment with sunitinib or placebo was continued until disease progression, unacceptable toxicity, or death occurred; upon disease progression, patients previously randomized to receive placebo were permitted to cross over to open-label sunitinib therapy in an extension study. The primary end point of this study was progression-free survival; secondary end points included safety, overall response rate, time to tumor response, response duration, and overall survival. Median duration of treatment was approximately 4.6 months in patients receiving sunitinib and 3.7 months in those receiving placebo. This study was terminated prematurely (prior to the prespecified interim analysis) after an independent data monitoring committee found longer median progression-free survival among patients randomized to receive sunitinib and higher incidences of death and severe adverse effects among those randomized to receive placebo. Data analysis revealed a median progression-free survival of 10.2 months in patients receiving sunitinib compared with 5.4 months in patients receiving placebo, although the magnitude of effect on progression-free survival may have been overestimated by early termination of the study. Objective response was observed in 9.3% (25% complete and 75% partial responses) of patients receiving sunitinib compared with none of those receiving placebo. Overall survival had not been reached at the time of this analysis; however, death had occurred in 9 patients receiving sunitinib compared with 21 patients receiving placebo.

Dosage and Administration

■ **Administration** Sunitinib malate is administered orally without regard to meals.

■ **Dosage** Dosage of sunitinib malate is expressed in terms of sunitinib.

Gastrointestinal Stromal Tumor For the treatment of gastrointestinal stromal tumor (GIST) in adults who are intolerant of or whose disease has progressed during imatinib therapy, sunitinib is given in 6-week cycles at a recommended dosage of 50 mg once daily for 4 consecutive weeks followed by a 2-week period without the drug. In clinical studies, therapy was continued for as long as the patient derived clinical benefit from the drug or until unacceptable toxicity occurred.

Renal Cell Carcinoma For the treatment of advanced renal cell carcinoma in adults, sunitinib is given in 6-week cycles at a recommended dosage of 50 mg once daily for 4 consecutive weeks followed by a 2-week period without the drug. In clinical studies, therapy was continued for as long as the patient derived clinical benefit from the drug or until unacceptable toxicity occurred.

Neuroendocrine Tumors of Pancreatic Origin For the treatment of progressive, well-differentiated neuroendocrine tumors of pancreatic origin (PNET) in adults with unresectable, locally advanced, or metastatic disease, sunitinib is given continuously (i.e., without an off-treatment period) at a recommended dosage of 37.5 mg once daily. In the principal efficacy study, sunitinib was continued until disease progression, unacceptable toxicity, or death occurred.

Dosage Modification Dosage of sunitinib should be adjusted in increments or decrements of 12.5 mg daily (i.e., 1 dose level), depending on individual patient safety and tolerability; however, in the principal efficacy study in patients with progressive, well-differentiated PNET, the maximum dosage administered was 50 mg daily. In clinical studies in patients with GIST or advanced renal cell carcinoma, dosages reduced following drug-related adverse effects generally were not re-escalated, even in the absence of toxicity; however, re-escalation back to the previous dosage was permitted based on clinical judgment. Initiation of the *next* treatment cycle could be delayed if additional time (i.e., more than 2 weeks) was required to recover from toxicities that developed during the previous treatment cycle.

Cardiovascular Toxicity. If manifestations of congestive heart failure develop, the drug should be discontinued. In patients without clinical evidence of congestive heart failure but in whom left ventricular ejection fraction (LVEF) is less than 50% and is reduced from baseline by more than 20%, interruption of therapy and/or dosage reduction is recommended. In the event that severe hypertension occurs, temporary interruption of therapy is recommended until the blood pressure is controlled.

In clinical studies in patients with GIST or advanced renal cell carcinoma, sunitinib therapy was temporarily withheld in patients who developed certain grade 2 (i.e., asymptomatic decrease in LVEF from baseline by 20% and to a level below the lower limit of normal [LVEF of less than 50%], nonurgent ventricular paroxysmal dysrhythmia requiring intervention) or grade 3 cardiac toxicities. When manifestations resolved or decreased in intensity to grade 1 or less, patients who originally experienced grade 2 cardiac toxicity could resume sunitinib therapy at the same dosage (if the toxicity resolved within 1 week) or at 1 dose level lower than the previous dosage; patients who originally experienced grade 3 cardiac toxicity could resume therapy at 1 dose level lower than the previous dosage. Patients who developed grade 4 cardiac toxicity were required to *permanently* discontinue therapy.

In clinical trials, sunitinib therapy was interrupted or discontinued in patients experiencing venous thromboembolic events, such as pulmonary embolism or deep-vein thrombosis.

Hematologic Toxicity. In clinical studies in patients with GIST or advanced renal cell carcinoma, sunitinib therapy was temporarily withheld in patients who developed grade 3 or 4 hematologic toxicity (excluding lymphopenia). When manifestations resolved or decreased in intensity to grade 2 or less, patients who originally experienced grade 3 hematologic toxicity could resume sunitinib therapy at the same dosage; patients who originally experienced grade 4 hematologic toxicity could resume therapy at 1 dose level lower than the previous dosage. Patients who experienced grade 3 or 4 lymphopenia could continue therapy without interruption.

Proteinuria. Sunitinib therapy should be interrupted and dosage reduced for proteinuria of or exceeding 3 g per 24 hours. If nephrotic syndrome occurs or if proteinuria recurs despite dosage reduction, treatment with sunitinib should be discontinued. (See Proteinuria under Warnings/Precautions: Other Warnings and Precautions, in Cautions.)

Other Nonhematologic Toxicity. In clinical studies in patients with GIST or advanced renal cell carcinoma, sunitinib therapy was temporarily withheld in patients who developed grade 3 or 4 nonhematologic toxicity. When manifestations resolved or decreased in intensity to grade 1 or less, patients with GIST who originally experienced grade 3 nonhematologic toxicity could resume sunitinib therapy at the same dosage, while those with advanced renal cell carcinoma could resume therapy at the same dosage or at 1 dose level lower than the previous dosage; patients who originally experienced grade 4 nonhematologic toxicity could resume therapy at 1 dose level lower than the previous dosage or discontinue therapy based on clinical judgment.

Concomitant Use with Drugs Affecting Hepatic Microsomal Enzymes. Concomitant use of sunitinib with potent inhibitors or inducers of cytochrome P-450 (CYP) isoenzyme 3A4 may alter the combined plasma concentrations of sunitinib and its primary active metabolite. (See Drug Interactions: Drugs and Foods Affecting Hepatic Microsomal Enzymes.) If concomitant use of sunitinib with a potent CYP3A4 *inhibitor* cannot be avoided, reduction of sunitinib dosage to no less than 37.5 mg daily (in patients receiving sunitinib for GIST or advanced renal cell carcinoma) or no less than 25 mg daily (in patients receiving sunitinib for progressive, well-differentiated PNET) should be considered. If concomitant use with a CYP3A4 *inducer* cannot be avoided, an increase in sunitinib dosage up to a maximum of 87.5 mg daily (in patients receiving sunitinib for GIST or advanced renal cell carcinoma) or 62.5 mg daily (in patients receiving sunitinib for progressive, well-differentiated PNET) should be considered, and the patient should be monitored carefully for toxicity.

■ **Special Populations** The manufacturer states that initial dosage adjustment is not necessary in patients with mild or moderate hepatic impairment (Child-Pugh class A or B). (See Hepatic Impairment under Warnings/Precautions: Specific Populations, in Cautions.)

The manufacturer states that initial dosage adjustment is not necessary in patients with mild, moderate, or severe renal impairment; subsequent dosage modifications should be based on safety and tolerability. Initial dosage adjustment is not necessary in patients with end-stage renal disease receiving hemodialysis; however, subsequent dosages may be increased gradually up to twofold based on safety and tolerability. (See Renal Impairment under Warnings/Precautions: Specific Populations, in Cautions.)

Cautions

■ **Contraindications** The manufacturer states there are no known contraindications to the use of sunitinib.

■ **Warnings/Precautions** ***Warnings*** **Hepatotoxicity.** Severe hepatotoxicity, sometimes fatal, has been reported in patients receiving sunitinib. Hepatic failure has been reported in patients receiving sunitinib in clinical trials (0.3%) and during postmarketing surveillance. Manifestations of hepatic failure include jaundice, elevated aminotransferase concentrations and/or hyperbilirubinemia in conjunction with encephalopathy, coagulopathy, and/or renal failure.

Liver function tests (ALT, AST, and bilirubin concentrations) should be monitored prior to initiation of sunitinib, during therapy, and as clinically indicated. If grade 3 or 4 hepatotoxicity occurs, sunitinib therapy should be temporarily interrupted; if hepatotoxicity does not resolve, sunitinib should be discontinued. Sunitinib should not be restarted in patients who subsequently experience severe changes in liver function tests or exhibit other manifestations of hepatic failure.

Safety of sunitinib in patients with AST and/or ALT concentrations exceeding 2.5 times the upper limit of normal or, if caused by liver metastases, exceeding 5 times the upper limit of normal has not been established.

Other Warnings and Precautions **Fetal/Neonatal Morbidity and Mortality.** Sunitinib can cause fetal harm because of its inhibitory effects on angiogenesis. Teratogenicity, embryotoxicity, and fetotoxicity have been demonstrated in animals. Pregnancy should be avoided during therapy. If sunitinib is used during pregnancy or if the patient becomes pregnant while receiving the drug, the patient should be apprised of the potential fetal hazard.

Cardiovascular Effects. Cardiovascular events (including heart failure, myocardial disorders, and cardiomyopathy), sometimes fatal, have been reported in patients receiving sunitinib during postmarketing surveillance.

Decreases in left ventricular ejection fraction (LVEF) to below the lower limit of normal were reported in 11% of patients with gastrointestinal stromal tumor (GIST) receiving sunitinib in the randomized, controlled study. Of the 22 cases of LVEF reported in patients with GIST, 9 cases resolved without intervention, 5 resolved following intervention (e.g., dosage reduction, initiation of antihypertensive or diuretic therapy), and 6 did not resolve despite discontinuance of sunitinib therapy. Grade 3 reductions in left ventricular systolic function (i.e., LVEF less than 40%) were reported in 3 patients with GIST receiving sunitinib, 2 of whom died without receiving further sunitinib therapy. Fatal heart failure in one patient in each group and fatal cardiac arrest in two patients in each group were reported in patients with GIST receiving sunitinib or placebo in the randomized, controlled study.

Among patients receiving sunitinib for advanced renal cell carcinoma in the randomized trial, 27% had an LVEF below the lower limit of normal, and 7% experienced a decline in LVEF (to a value below 50% or as a reduction greater than 20% from the baseline value). Left ventricular dysfunction was reported in 1% and congestive heart failure in less than 1% of patients receiving sunitinib.

Among patients receiving sunitinib for progressive, well-differentiated neuroendocrine tumors of pancreatic origin (PNET) in the principal efficacy study, fatal cardiac failure was reported in 2% of patients compared with none of those receiving placebo.

Venous thromboembolic events, such as pulmonary embolism or deep-vein thrombosis, occurred in 3% of patients receiving sunitinib for GIST and 2% of patients receiving the drug for advanced renal cell carcinoma.

Because patients with a history of cardiovascular disease (e.g., myocardial infarction [MI], severe or unstable angina, coronary or peripheral artery bypass graft, symptomatic congestive heart failure, cerebrovascular accident or transient ischemic attack, pulmonary embolism) within 12 months prior to sunitinib administration were excluded from clinical studies, it is unknown whether patients with these concomitant conditions may be at a higher risk of developing drug-related left ventricular dysfunction. Clinicians should weigh this risk against potential benefits of the drug. These patients should be carefully monitored for clinical signs and symptoms of congestive heart failure during sunitinib therapy; baseline and periodic evaluations of LVEF also should be considered in such patients. In patients without cardiac risk factors, a baseline evaluation of ejection fraction should be considered.

If manifestations of congestive heart failure develop, sunitinib should be discontinued. In patients without clinical evidence of congestive heart failure but in whom LVEF is less than 50% and is reduced from baseline by more than 20%, interruption of therapy and/or dosage reduction is recommended. (See Cardiovascular Toxicity under Dosage: Dosage Modification, in Dosage and Administration.)

Prolongation of QT Interval and Torsades de Pointes. Sunitinib prolongs the QT interval in a dose-dependent manner, which may increase the risk of ventricular arrhythmias, including torsades de pointes. Torsades de pointes has been reported in less than 0.1% of patients receiving sunitinib.

Sunitinib should be used with caution in patients with a history of prolongation of the QT interval, those receiving antiarrhythmic agents, and those with relevant preexisting cardiac disease, bradycardia, or electrolyte disturbances. Periodic monitoring with on-treatment ECGs and serum magnesium and potassium concentrations should be considered. Caution and reduction of sunitinib dosage should be considered in patients concomitantly receiving potent CYP3A4 inhibitors. (See Concomitant Use with Drugs Affecting Hepatic Microsomal Enzymes under Dosage: Dosage Modification, in Dosage and Administration.)

Hypertension. Hypertension has been reported in 15% of patients with GIST receiving sunitinib in the randomized, controlled study compared with 11% of those receiving placebo. Grade 3 hypertension occurred in 4% of patients with GIST receiving sunitinib compared with none of those receiving placebo. Severe hypertension (systolic blood pressure exceeding 200 mm Hg or diastolic blood pressure exceeding 110 mm Hg) occurred in 4% of patients with GIST receiving sunitinib compared with 1% of those receiving placebo. None of the patients with GIST discontinued sunitinib because of hypertension.

Among patients receiving sunitinib for advanced renal cell carcinoma in the randomized trial, 34% of patients experienced hypertension, including 13% with grade 3 hypertension. Severe hypertension (systolic blood pressure exceeding 200 mm Hg or diastolic blood pressure exceeding 110 mm Hg) occurred in 9% of patients receiving sunitinib compared with 1% of those receiving interferon alfa for advanced renal cell carcinoma. Sunitinib dosage was reduced or therapy temporarily interrupted in 6% of patients. Four patients, including 1 patient with malignant hypertension, discontinued sunitinib therapy because of hypertension.

Among patients receiving sunitinib for progressive, well-differentiated PNET in the principal efficacy study, 27% of patients experienced hypertension, including 10% with grade 3 hypertension. Severe hypertension (systolic blood pressure exceeding 200 mm Hg or diastolic blood pressure exceeding 110 mm Hg) occurred in 10% of patients receiving sunitinib compared with 3% of those receiving placebo for progressive, well-differentiated PNET. Sunitinib dosage was reduced or therapy temporarily interrupted in 8% of patients. One patient discontinued sunitinib therapy because of hypertension.

Patients should be monitored for development of hypertension and treated as needed with standard antihypertensive therapy. If severe hypertension occurs, temporary interruption of therapy is recommended until the blood pressure is controlled.

Hemorrhage. Hemorrhagic events (including GI, respiratory, tumor, urinary tract, and brain hemorrhage), sometimes fatal, have been reported in patients receiving sunitinib during postmarketing surveillance. Less common bleeding events reported in patients receiving sunitinib include rectal, gingival, upper GI, genital, and wound bleeding.

Bleeding events have been reported in 18% of patients with GIST receiving sunitinib in the randomized, controlled study compared with 17% of those receiving placebo. The most common bleeding event reported was epistaxis. In the randomized, controlled study in patients with GIST, grade 3 or 4 bleeding events were reported in 7 or 9% of patients receiving sunitinib or placebo, respectively; fatal GI bleeding was reported in one patient receiving placebo.

Among patients receiving sunitinib for advanced renal cell carcinoma in the randomized trial, 37% had bleeding events. Most bleeding events were grade 1 or 2; a grade 5 bleeding event (i.e., gastric bleed) occurred in one treatment-naive patient.

Bleeding events (excluding epistaxis) have been reported in 22% of patients with progressive, well-differentiated PNET receiving sunitinib in the principal efficacy study compared with 10% of those receiving placebo. Epistaxis was reported in 20% of patients receiving sunitinib, and grade 3 epistaxis was reported in 1% of patients. Other grade 3 or 4 bleeding events were reported in 0% of patients receiving sunitinib compared with 4% of those receiving placebo.

Tumor-related hemorrhage has been reported in patients receiving sunitinib. These events may occur suddenly and, in the case of pulmonary tumors, may present as severe and life-threatening hemoptysis or pulmonary hemorrhage. Pulmonary hemorrhage, sometimes fatal, has been reported in clinical trials and during postmarketing surveillance in patients receiving sunitinib for GIST, advanced renal cell carcinoma, or metastatic lung cancer†. Grade 3 and 4 tumor hemorrhage occurred in 5 of 202 evaluable patients (3%) with GIST receiving sunitinib in the randomized, controlled study; tumor hemorrhages were observed as early as cycle 1 and as late as cycle 6. One of these 5 patients discontinued sunitinib; none of the other 4 patients postponed or discontinued therapy because of tumor hemorrhage. No patients with GIST receiving placebo experienced intratumoral hemorrhage. Patients receiving sunitinib should be monitored carefully with periodic clinical and laboratory evaluations (e.g., serial complete blood counts [CBCs], physical examinations) for development of tumor hemorrhage.

Serious, sometimes fatal GI complications, including GI perforation, have occurred rarely in patients with intra-abdominal malignancies treated with sunitinib.

Osteonecrosis of the Jaw. Osteonecrosis of the jaw (ONJ) has been reported in patients receiving sunitinib in clinical studies and during postmarketing surveillance. Symptoms may include jaw pain, numbness or feeling of heaviness in the jaw, loosening of a tooth, toothache, or swelling or sores inside the mouth. The risk of ONJ may be increased in patients with dental disease or in those receiving concomitant bisphosphonate therapy.

Prior to initiating sunitinib, a routine oral examination and appropriate preventive dentistry should be performed. If possible, invasive dental procedures should be avoided during sunitinib treatment, particularly in patients who previously received or currently are receiving bisphosphonate therapy. (See Advice to Patients.)

Tumor Lysis Syndrome. Tumor lysis syndrome, sometimes fatal, has been reported principally in patients with GIST or advanced renal cell carcinoma receiving sunitinib in clinical studies and during postmarketing surveillance. The risk of tumor lysis syndrome is increased in patients with a large tumor burden; such patients should be monitored closely and treated as clinically indicated.

Thyroid Dysfunction. Thyroid dysfunction has been reported in patients receiving sunitinib in clinical studies and during postmarketing surveillance.

In a prospective, observational cohort study, abnormal serum thyroid-stimulating hormone (TSH) concentrations occurred in 26 of 42 patients (62%) receiving sunitinib for a median of 37 weeks for GIST: 15 patients (36%) developed persistent, primary hypothyroidism, 4 patients (9.5%) developed isolated TSH suppression, and 7 patients (17%) had transient, mild TSH elevations. The risk of developing hypothyroidism increased with increasing duration of therapy. Among 73 patients receiving sunitinib for advanced renal cell carcinoma, the results of thyroid function tests were available for 66 patients; 56 of the 66 patients (85%) had at least one abnormality in thyroid function consistent with hypothyroidism, and 47 of the 56 patients with an abnormality in thyroid function (84%) had manifestations possibly related to hypothyroidism. Among 17 patients receiving thyroid hormone replacement therapy, 9 patients experienced an improvement in their condition.

Treatment-emergent acquired hypothyroidism occurred in 4% of patients receiving sunitinib for GIST in a clinical study. Among patients receiving sunitinib for advanced renal cell carcinoma in the randomized trial, hypothyroidism was reported in 16% of patients. Hypothyroidism has been reported in 7% of patients with progressive, well-differentiated PNET receiving sunitinib in the principal efficacy study.

Hyperthyroidism, sometimes followed by hypothyroidism, has been reported in clinical studies and during postmarketing surveillance.

Baseline thyroid function should be measured in all patients, and hypothyroidism or hyperthyroidism should be treated as clinically indicated before initiation of sunitinib therapy. All patients should be monitored closely for manifestations of thyroid dysfunction, including hypothyroidism, hyperthyroidism, and thyroiditis, during sunitinib therapy; if signs and/or symptoms suggestive of thyroid dysfunction occur, thyroid function tests should be performed and treatment instituted as clinically indicated.

Wound-healing Complications. Impaired wound healing has been reported during sunitinib therapy. The manufacturer recommends temporary interruption of sunitinib therapy prior to major surgical procedures. There is limited clinical experience regarding the timing of reinitiation of sunitinib therapy following major surgery; therefore, the decision to resume sunitinib therapy should be based on clinical assessment of the adequacy of wound healing.

Proteinuria. Proteinuria and nephrotic syndrome, sometimes resulting in renal failure or death, have occurred in patients receiving sunitinib therapy. Patients should be monitored for the development or worsening of proteinuria. Urinalysis should be performed prior to initiation of sunitinib and periodically during therapy; further assessment with a 24-hour urine collection should be performed as clinically indicated. Sunitinib therapy should be interrupted and dosage reduced for proteinuria of or exceeding 3 g per 24 hours. If nephrotic syndrome occurs or if proteinuria recurs despite dosage reduction, treatment with sunitinib should be discontinued. The safety of continued sunitinib therapy in patients with moderate to severe proteinuria has not been systematically evaluated.

Dermatologic Effects. Severe and sometimes fatal cutaneous reactions, including erythema multiforme, Stevens-Johnson syndrome, and toxic epidermal necrolysis, have been reported. Sunitinib should be discontinued if manifestations of erythema multiforme, Stevens-Johnson syndrome, or toxic epidermal necrolysis (e.g., worsening skin rash, often with blisters or mucosal lesions) occur. Sunitinib therapy must not be resumed if Stevens-Johnson syndrome or toxic epidermal necrolysis is suspected.

Cases of necrotizing fasciitis, including fatalities, also have been reported in patients receiving sunitinib. Necrotizing fasciitis has occurred secondary to fistula formation and has included sites such as the perineum. If necrotizing fasciitis occurs, therapy with sunitinib should be discontinued.

Endocrine Effects. Adrenal toxicity (characterized histologically by hemorrhage, necrosis, congestion, hypertrophy, and inflammation) has been reported in animals; however, no evidence of adrenal hemorrhage or necrosis has been demonstrated in humans. Abnormal response to rapid corticotropin (ACTH) stimulation tests (e.g., decreased plasma cortisol concentrations) has been observed in some patients; however, no clinical evidence of adrenal insufficiency has been observed. Patients who experience stress (e.g., surgery, trauma, severe infection) should be monitored for development of adrenal insufficiency.

Neurologic Effects. Seizures and radiologic evidence of reversible posterior leukoencephalopathy syndrome (RPLS), sometimes fatal, have been reported in less than 1% of patients receiving sunitinib. If seizures and manifestations of RPLS (e.g., hypertension, headache, decreased alertness, altered mental functioning, visual loss, cortical blindness) occur, sunitinib therapy should be temporarily interrupted and medical management (including control of hypertension) instituted. When manifestations resolve, sunitinib therapy may be resumed at the discretion of the clinician.

Pancreatitis. Pancreatitis has been reported in 1% of patients receiving sunitinib for advanced renal cell carcinoma or progressive, well-differentiated PNET. If manifestations of pancreatitis occur, sunitinib therapy should be discontinued.

Microangiopathic Hemolytic Anemia. Cases of microangiopathic hemolytic anemia have been reported in patients with solid tumors receiving bevacizumab in combination with sunitinib†. In a phase 1 study involving 25 patients receiving bevacizumab at a fixed dose and sunitinib at escalating dose levels, 5 of 12 patients receiving bevacizumab with the highest dose level of sunitinib had laboratory findings consistent with microangiopathic hemolytic anemia. Of these 5 patients, 2 patients had evidence of severe microangiopathic hemolytic anemia, including thrombocytopenia, anemia, reticulocytosis, reduced serum haptoglobin concentrations, schistocytes on peripheral smear, modest increases in serum creatinine concentrations, severe hypertension, RPLS, and proteinuria. These findings were reversed within 3 weeks following discontinuance of both drugs without other interventions.

Use of bevacizumab in combination with sunitinib is *not* recommended. Clinicians should report cases of microangiopathic hemolytic anemia associated with bevacizumab therapy to the manufacturer or the US Food and Drug Administration (FDA).

Clinical and Laboratory Monitoring. Complete blood cell (CBC) counts (including platelet count) and serum chemistry tests (including phosphate) should be obtained in all patients at the beginning of *each* treatment cycle.

Specific Populations **Pregnancy.** Category D. (See Users Guide and see Fetal/Neonatal Morbidity and Mortality under Warnings/Precautions: Other Warnings and Precautions, in Cautions.)

Lactation. Sunitinib and/or its metabolites are extensively distributed into milk in rats, with a milk-to-plasma ratio of up to 12:1. It is not known whether sunitinib or its primary active metabolite is distributed into human milk. Because of the potential for serious adverse reactions to sunitinib in nursing infants, a decision should be made whether to discontinue nursing or the drug, taking into account the importance of the drug to the woman.

Pediatric Use. Safety and efficacy of sunitinib have not been established in pediatric patients.

Geriatric Use. Of the 825 patients receiving sunitinib for GIST or advanced renal cell carcinoma in clinical studies, 34% were 65 years of age or older. In the principal efficacy study evaluating sunitinib in adults with progressive, well-differentiated PNET, 27% of patients receiving sunitinib were 65 years of age or older. No overall differences in safety and efficacy were observed relative to younger adults.

Hepatic Impairment. Following administration of a single dose of sunitinib, systemic exposure in patients with mild or moderate (Child-Pugh class A or B) hepatic impairment was similar to that in individuals with normal hepatic function; no initial dosage adjustment is required in patients with mild or moderate hepatic impairment. Safety and efficacy of sunitinib have not been established in patients with severe (Child-Pugh class C) hepatic impairment.

Clinical studies for cancer that were conducted excluded patients with AST or ALT concentrations exceeding 2.5 times the upper limit of normal or, if caused by liver metastases, exceeding 5 times the upper limit of normal.

Renal Impairment. Following administration of a single dose of sunitinib, systemic exposure in patients with severe renal impairment (creatinine clearance less than 30 mL/minute) was similar to that in individuals with normal renal function (creatinine clearance exceeding 80 mL/minute). In individuals with end-stage renal disease undergoing hemodialysis, systemic exposure to sunitinib was decreased by 47% compared with those with normal renal function. No initial dosage adjustment is required in patients with renal impairment or in those with end-stage renal disease undergoing hemodialysis; however, adjustments to subsequent dosages may be necessary. (See Dosage and Administration: Special Populations.)

■ Common Adverse Effects The most common adverse effects occurring in 20% or more of patients receiving sunitinib for GIST, advanced renal cell carcinoma, or progressive, well-differentiated PNET in randomized trials are fatigue, asthenia, fever, diarrhea, nausea, mucositis/stomatitis, vomiting, dyspepsia, abdominal pain, constipation, hypertension, peripheral edema, rash, hand-foot syndrome, skin discoloration, dry skin, changes in hair color, altered taste, headache, back pain, arthralgia, extremity pain, cough, dyspnea, anorexia, and bleeding.

Adverse effects reported in 10% or more of patients with GIST receiving sunitinib in the randomized, controlled study that occurred more frequently than with placebo include diarrhea, skin abnormalities (e.g., skin discoloration, rash, hand-foot syndrome), anorexia, mucositis/stomatitis, asthenia, altered taste, constipation, hypertension, and myalgia/limb pain. Laboratory abnormalities reported in 10% or more of patients with GIST receiving sunitinib that occurred more frequently than with placebo include neutropenia, lymphopenia, thrombocytopenia, anemia, elevated concentrations of hepatic enzymes (i.e., AST, ALT, alkaline phosphatase), elevated concentrations of bilirubin, elevated concentrations of pancreatic enzymes (i.e., amylase, lipase), elevated creatinine concentrations, hypokalemia, hypernatremia, and decreased LVEF.

Adverse effects reported in 10% or more of patients with advanced renal cell carcinoma receiving sunitinib include diarrhea, fatigue, nausea, anorexia, altered taste, mucositis/stomatitis, pain in extremity, vomiting, bleeding, hypertension, dyspepsia, abdominal pain, arthralgia, back pain, cough, asthenia, dyspnea, peripheral edema, constipation, headache, fever, skin abnormalities (e.g., skin discoloration, dry skin, rash, hand-foot syndrome), changes in hair color, weight loss, decreased ejection fraction, hypothyroidism, insomnia, chills, flatulence, oral pain, alopecia, nasopharyngitis, oropharyngeal pain, chest pain, dry mouth, gastroesophageal reflux disease (GERD), erythema, pruritus, glossodynia, dizziness, upper respiratory tract infection, depression, and hemorrhoids. Laboratory abnormalities reported in 10% or more of patients with advanced renal cell carcinoma receiving sunitinib include anemia, leukopenia, neutropenia, lymphopenia, thrombocytopenia, elevated creatinine concentrations, elevated concentrations of hepatic enzymes (i.e., AST, ALT, alkaline phosphatase), elevated concentrations of pancreatic enzymes (i.e., amylase, lipase), elevated serum creatine kinase, hyperuricemia, electrolyte abnormalities (i.e., hypocalcemia, hypokalemia, hyperkalemia, hypernatremia, hyponatremia, hypercalcemia, abnormal serum phosphorus), elevated concentrations of bilirubin, hyperglycemia, hypoglycemia, and abnormal serum albumin.

Adverse effects reported in 10% or more of patients with progressive, well-differentiated PNET receiving sunitinib that occurred more frequently than with placebo include diarrhea, stomatitis/oral syndromes, nausea, abdominal pain, asthenia, vomiting, fatigue, changes in hair color, hypertension, skin abnormalities (e.g., hand-foot syndrome, rash, dry skin), bleeding, dysgeusia, epistaxis, headache, insomnia, weight loss, dyspepsia, and arthralgia. Laboratory abnormalities reported in 10% or more of patients with progressive, well-differentiated PNET receiving sunitinib include neutropenia, lymphopenia, thrombocytopenia, anemia, elevated concentrations of hepatic enzymes (i.e., AST, ALT, alkaline phosphatase), elevated concentrations of bilirubin, elevated concentrations of pancreatic enzymes (i.e., amylase, lipase), elevated creatinine concentrations, electrolyte abnormalities (i.e., hypokalemia, hyperkalemia, hyponatremia, hypocalcemia, hypomagnesemia, hypophosphatemia), hyperglycemia, hypoglycemia, and hypoalbuminemia.

Drug Interactions

Sunitinib and its primary active metabolite are metabolized principally by cytochrome P-450 (CYP) isoenzyme 3A4. However, in vitro studies indicate that the drug does not inhibit or induce major CYP isoenzymes.

■ Drugs and Foods Affecting Hepatic Microsomal Enzymes Concomitant use of sunitinib with potent inhibitors of CYP3A4 (e.g., atazanavir, clarithromycin, indinavir, itraconazole, ketoconazole, nefazodone, nelfinavir, ritonavir, saquinavir, telithromycin, voriconazole, grapefruit) may result in increased plasma concentrations of sunitinib. When the potent CYP3A4 inhibitor ketoconazole was administered concomitantly with a single dose of sunitinib in healthy individuals, peak plasma concentrations and area under the plasma concentration-time curve (AUC) of sunitinib and its primary active metabolite increased by 49 and 51%, respectively. Selection of an alternative agent with minimal or no enzyme inhibition potential is recommended during sunitinib therapy. If concomitant use of sunitinib with a potent CYP3A4 inhibitor cannot be avoided, reduction of sunitinib dosage to no less than 37.5 mg daily (in patients receiving sunitinib for GIST or advanced renal cell carcinoma) or no less than 25 mg daily (in patients receiving sunitinib for progressive, well-differentiated PNET) should be considered.

Concomitant use of sunitinib with inducers of CYP3A4 (e.g., carbamazepine, dexamethasone, phenobarbital, phenytoin, rifabutin, rifampin, rifapentine, St. John's wort [*Hypericum perforatum*]) may result in decreased plasma concentrations of sunitinib. When the potent CYP3A4 inducer rifampin was administered concomitantly with a single dose of sunitinib in healthy individuals, peak plasma concentrations and AUC of sunitinib and its primary active metabolite decreased by 23 and 46%, respectively. Selection of an alternative agent with minimal or no enzyme induction potential is recommended during sunitinib therapy. If concomitant use of sunitinib with a CYP3A4 inducer cannot be avoided, an increase in sunitinib dosage up to a maximum of 87.5 mg daily (in patients receiving sunitinib for GIST or advanced renal cell carcinoma) or 62.5 mg daily (in patients receiving sunitinib for progressive, well-differentiated PNET) should be considered, and the patient should be monitored carefully for toxicity. St. John's wort may cause unpredictable decreases in plasma sunitinib concentrations and should be *avoided* during sunitinib therapy.

■ **Drugs Metabolized by Hepatic Microsomal Enzymes** In vitro studies indicate that sunitinib and its primary active metabolite are unlikely to have clinically relevant interactions with drugs metabolized by CYP isoenzymes 1A2, 2A6, 2B6, 2C8, 2C9, 2C19, 2D6, 2E1, 3A4/5, or 4A9/11.

■ **Antiarrhythmics** Sunitinib prolongs the QT interval, which may increase the risk of ventricular arrhythmias, including torsades de pointes. The drug should be used with caution in patients receiving antiarrhythmic agents. (See Prolongation of QT Interval and Torsades de Pointes under Warnings/Precautions: Other Warnings and Precautions, in Cautions.)

■ **Bisphosphonates** Concomitant use of sunitinib with bisphosphonates (e.g., alendronate, etidronate, ibandronate, pamidronate, risedronate, zoledronic acid) may increase the risk of developing osteonecrosis of the jaw (ONJ). (See Osteonecrosis of the Jaw under Warnings/Precautions: Other Warnings and Precautions, in Cautions.)

Description

Sunitinib malate, an inhibitor of multiple receptor tyrosine kinases, is an antineoplastic agent. Receptor tyrosine kinases (RTKs) are involved in the initiation of various cascades of intracellular signaling events that lead to cell proliferation and/or influence processes critical to cell survival and tumor progression (e.g., angiogenesis, metastasis, inhibition of apoptosis), based on the respective kinase. Although the exact mechanism of antineoplastic activity of sunitinib has not been fully elucidated, data from biochemical and cellular assays indicate that sunitinib may inhibit signal transduction pathways involving multiple receptor (i.e., cell surface) tyrosine kinases, including platelet-derived growth factor receptors (i.e., PDGFR-α, PDGFR-β), vascular endothelial growth factor receptors (i.e., VEGFR-1, VEGFR-2, VEGFR-3), stem cell factor receptor (i.e., c-Kit), fms-like tyrosine kinase 3 (Flt-3), colony stimulating factor receptor type 1 (CSF-1R), and the glial cell line-derived neurotrophic factor receptor (RET). Sunitinib-induced inhibition of signal transduction pathways involving PDGFR-β, VEGFR-2, and c-Kit has been confirmed in tumor xenografts expressing receptor tyrosine kinase targets in vivo. Sunitinib has been shown to inhibit growth of tumor cells expressing dysregulated target receptor tyrosine kinases (i.e., PDGFR, RET, c-Kit) in vitro; the drug also has been shown to inhibit PDGFR-β- and VEGFR-2-dependent tumor angiogenesis in vivo.

Following oral administration, peak plasma concentrations of sunitinib generally occur within 6–12 hours. Food has no effect on bioavailability of sunitinib. Sunitinib is metabolized principally by cytochrome P-450 (CYP) isoenzyme 3A4 to several metabolites. The main circulating metabolite, an *N*-desethyl derivative, has been shown to be equipotent to sunitinib in biochemical and cellular assays; this metabolite accounts for approximately 23–37% of total plasma concentrations of the drug and also is metabolized by CYP3A4. Steady-state concentrations of sunitinib and its primary active metabolite are achieved within 10–14 days. Sunitinib and its primary active metabolite are 95 and 90% bound to human plasma proteins in vitro, respectively. Following oral administration of a single dose in healthy volunteers, the terminal half-life of sunitinib or its primary active metabolite is approximately 40–60 or 80–110 hours, respectively. Approximately 61% of an oral dose of sunitinib is excreted in feces and 16% is eliminated in urine, mainly as sunitinib and the primary metabolite; minor metabolites are recovered in feces and urine but generally are not found in plasma.

Population pharmacokinetic analyses of demographic data indicate that the pharmacokinetics of sunitinib or its primary active metabolite are not substantially affected by age, body weight, creatinine clearance, race, gender, or ECOG performance status. The pharmacokinetics of sunitinib have not been evaluated in pediatric patients.

Advice to Patients

Importance of reading the manufacturer's patient information prior to beginning sunitinib therapy and rereading it each time the prescription is refilled.

Risk of hepatotoxicity. Importance of contacting clinician promptly if manifestations of hepatotoxicity (e.g., abdominal pain [particularly in the right upper quadrant], dark urine, generalized pruritus, jaundice) occur.

Risk of adverse GI effects (e.g., diarrhea, nausea, vomiting, dyspepsia, mouth pain/irritation/stomatitis, taste disturbance). Supportive care for adverse GI effects requiring treatment may include antiemetic or antidiarrheal therapy.

Risk of adverse dermatologic effects (e.g., skin discoloration resulting from the drug color [yellow]; hair or skin depigmentation; skin dryness, thickness, or cracking; blisters or rash on the hands and soles of the feet), including severe cutaneous reactions (e.g., Stevens-Johnson syndrome, toxic epidermal necrolysis). Importance of informing clinician immediately if severe dermatologic reactions occur.

Increased risk of bleeding. Importance of promptly informing clinician of any manifestations or episodes of bleeding (e.g., abdominal pain or swelling; hematemesis; black, sticky stools; hematuria; headache; change in mental status).

Risk of osteonecrosis of the jaw. Importance of advising patient that their clinician should examine their mouth before sunitinib therapy. Importance of informing dentist about sunitinib treatment prior to dental procedures.

Risk of thyroid dysfunction. Importance of informing clinician if symptoms of abnormal thyroid function (e.g., persistent or worsening fatigue, hair loss, weight gain or loss, irregular menstrual cycles, feeling hot or cold) occur.

Risk of fatigue, hypertension, and edema.

Importance of women informing clinicians if they are or plan to become pregnant or plan to breast-feed. Necessity of advising women to avoid pregnancy while receiving therapy. Advise pregnant women of risk to the fetus and/or the potential risk for loss of the pregnancy.

Importance of informing clinicians of existing or contemplated concomitant therapy, including prescription and OTC drugs and herbal supplements (e.g., St. John's wort), as well as any concomitant illnesses.

Importance of informing patients of other important precautionary information. (See Cautions.)

Overview® (see Users Guide). For additional information on this drug until a more detailed monograph is developed and published, the manufacturer's labeling should be consulted. It is *essential* that the manufacturer's labeling be consulted for more detailed information on usual cautions, precautions, contraindications, potential drug interactions, laboratory test interferences, and acute toxicity. For further information on the handling of antineoplastic agents, see the ASHP Guidelines on Handling Hazardous Drugs at http://www.ahfsdruginformation.com.

Preparations

Excipients in commercially available drug preparations may have clinically important effects in some individuals; consult specific product labeling for details.

SUNItinib Malate

Oral		
Capsules	12.5 mg (of sunitinib)	**Sutent®**, Pfizer
	25 mg (of sunitinib)	**Sutent®**, Pfizer
	37.5 mg (of sunitinib)	**Sutent®**, Pfizer
	50 mg (of sunitinib)	**Sutent®**, Pfizer

†Use is not currently included in the labeling approved by the US Food and Drug Administration

Talazoparib Tosylate

■ Talazoparib, a potent and selective inhibitor of poly(adenosine diphosphate [ADP]-ribose) polymerase (PARP), is an antineoplastic agent.

Uses

■ **Breast Cancer** Talazoparib tosylate is used as a single agent for the treatment of confirmed or suspected deleterious germline BRCA-mutated (gBRCA-mutated), human epidermal growth factor receptor type 2 (HER2)-negative locally advanced or metastatic breast cancer. An FDA-approved companion diagnostic test (BRACAnalysis CDx®) is required to confirm the presence of mutations in the BRCA genes (BRCA1 and/or BRCA2) prior to initiation of talazoparib therapy. Currently available evidence indicates that talazoparib therapy is associated with substantially prolonged progression-free survival and improved response rates compared with standard single-agent chemotherapy in adults with confirmed or suspected deleterious gBRCA-mutated, HER2-negative locally advanced or metastatic breast cancer.

The current indication for talazoparib is based principally on the results of a randomized, open-label phase 3 study (EMBRACA) in adults with confirmed or suspected deleterious gBRCA-mutated, HER2-negative locally advanced or metastatic breast cancer, with supporting data from an open-label, 2-cohort phase 2 study (ABRAZO).

In the EMBRACA study, 431 patients were randomized (stratified by number of prior therapies, hormone receptor status, presence of brain metastases) in a 2:1 ratio to receive either talazoparib (1 mg orally once daily continuously) or investigator's choice of single-agent chemotherapy (capecitabine 1.25 g/m^2 orally twice daily for 14 days of each 21-day cycle; eribulin mesylate 1.4 mg/m^2 IV on days 1 and 8 of each 21-day cycle; gemcitabine 1.25 g/m^2 IV on days 1 and 8 of each 21-day cycle; or vinorelbine 30 mg/m^2 IV on days 1 and 8 of each 21-day cycle). Treatment was continued until disease progression or unacceptable toxicity occurred or the patient withdrew from the study. All patients enrolled in the study were required to have received prior therapy with an anthracycline and/or a taxane in the neoadjuvant, adjuvant, locally advanced, or metastatic setting unless such therapy was contraindicated; however, patients with previously untreated locally advanced or metastatic breast cancer without a history of adjuvant chemotherapy could be enrolled if the patient was a candidate for the control arm. Patients whose disease progressed during platinum-based chemotherapy for advanced breast cancer and those who had received prior therapy with a poly(adenosine diphosphate [ADP]-ribose) polymerase (PARP) inhibitor were excluded from the study.

In the EMBRACA study, the median age of patients receiving talazoparib was 45 years; 67% were Caucasian, 11% were of Asian ancestry, 4% were black or African American, and 1% were male. The median age of patients receiving standard single-agent chemotherapy was 50 years; 75% were Caucasian, 11% were of Asian ancestry, 1% were black or African American, and 2% were male. Most of the patients enrolled in the study had an ECOG performance status of 0 or 1 (98%), and confirmed or suspected deleterious BRCA1 or BRCA2 mutation was verified by the companion diagnostic test BRACAnalysis CDx® in 82% of patients. Approximately one-half (56%) of all patients had estrogen receptor-positive and/or progesterone receptor-positive breast cancer and 44% were hormone receptor-negative. Patients enrolled in the study had received a median of one prior chemotherapy regimen for advanced disease; 38% of patients had previously untreated advanced or metastatic disease, 37% had received one prior chemotherapy regimen, 20% had received 2 prior chemotherapy regimens, and 5% had received 3 or more previous lines of chemotherapy. Among talazoparib-treated patients, 91, 85, or 16% of patients had previously received taxane-, anthracycline-, or platinum-containing chemotherapy, respectively. The primary measure of efficacy was progression-free survival (as evaluated by a blinded independent central review committee according to Response Evaluation Criteria in Solid Tumors [RECIST]).

In the EMBRACA study at a median follow-up of 11.2 months, median progression-free survival was 8.6 months in patients receiving talazoparib compared with 5.6 months in those receiving standard single-agent chemotherapy. The results of the progression-free survival analysis based on investigator assessment were consistent with the independent blinded central radiologic assessment. In addition, patients receiving talazoparib had higher objective response rates (50.2 versus 18.4%) compared with those receiving standard single-agent chemotherapy. The median duration of response in patients receiving talazoparib or standard single-agent chemotherapy was 6.4 or 3.9 months, respectively. Median overall survival had not been reached at the time of the analysis. Results of a subgroup analysis (based on number of prior therapies, hormone receptor status, history of brain metastases) suggested that the drug's effect on progression-free survival was consistent across all subgroups. Talazoparib substantially improved quality of life (using the European Organisation for Research and Treatment of Cancer Quality of Life Questionnaire Core 30 [EORTC QLQ-C30] and BR23) and delayed clinically meaningful deterioration in physical and psychologic functioning and symptoms related to breast cancer and associated treatment.

In the ABRAZO study, 84 patients were enrolled into 1 of 2 cohorts based on prior therapy; 49 patients with platinum-sensitive disease (defined as those who achieved a complete or partial response to platinum-containing chemotherapy for at least 8 weeks following the last dose of platinum therapy) were assigned to the platinum-sensitive cohort and 35 patients with heavily pretreated disease (defined as those who had received 3 or more chemotherapy regimens that did not contain a platinum agent) were assigned to the heavily pretreated cohort. Patients received talazoparib 1 mg orally once daily until disease progression or unacceptable toxicity occurred. The primary measure of efficacy was objective response rate as assessed by an independent central review committee according to RECIST. The median age of patients enrolled in the study was 50 years, and patients had received a median of 3 prior therapies for their disease. The majority (59%) of patients in the platinum-sensitive cohort had triple-negative breast cancer (estrogen receptor-negative, progesterone receptor-negative, and HER2-negative) compared with 17% of those in the heavily pretreated cohort. One-half of all patients had BRCA2 mutation-positive disease and 49% had BRCA1 mutation-positive disease. The objective response rate in patients with platinum-sensitive or heavily pretreated disease was 21 or 37%, respectively, with a median duration of response of 5.8 or 3.8 months, respectively; complete response was achieved in 4% of patients with platinum-sensitive disease and in none of those with heavily pretreated disease.

Dosage and Administration

■ **General** Confirmation of the diagnosis of deleterious germline BRCA-mutated locally advanced or metastatic breast cancer by an FDA-approved companion diagnostic test is necessary for selecting patients for talazoparib therapy.

Because myelodysplastic syndrome (MDS) and acute myeloid leukemia (AML) have been reported in patients receiving talazoparib, the manufacturer states that complete blood cell (CBC) counts should be obtained prior to initiation of talazoparib and monthly during therapy with the drug. (See Myelodysplastic Syndrome/Acute Myeloid Leukemia under Cautions: Warnings/Precautions.)

Restricted Distribution Talazoparib tosylate can only be obtained through select specialty pharmacies. Clinicians may contact the manufacturer (Pfizer) by telephone at 877-744-5675 or consult the Pfizer Oncology together® website for specific availability information (https://www.pfizeroncologytogether.com/hcp).

■ **Administration** Talazoparib tosylate is administered orally once daily. The drug may be given without regard to meals.

The capsules should be swallowed whole and should *not* be dissolved or opened.

■ **Dosage** Dosage of talazoparib tosylate is expressed in terms of talazoparib.

Breast Cancer The recommended adult dosage of talazoparib as monotherapy for the treatment of confirmed or suspected deleterious germline BRCA-mutated locally advanced or metastatic breast cancer is 1 mg once daily. Therapy should be continued until disease progression or unacceptable toxicity occurs.

Dosage Modification If adverse reactions occur, interruption of therapy or dosage reduction of talazoparib should be considered. If dosage reduction from 1 mg once daily is necessary, the recommended dosage is 0.75 mg once daily. If dosage reduction from 0.75 mg once daily is necessary, the recommended dosage is 0.5 mg once daily. If further dosage reduction is necessary, the dosage should be reduced to 0.25 mg once daily. If the toxicity recurs on a dosage of 0.25 mg once daily, talazoparib therapy should be discontinued.

Hematologic Toxicity. For hemoglobin concentrations less than 8 g/dL, talazoparib therapy should be withheld. When hemoglobin concentrations reach or exceed 9 g/dL, talazoparib may be resumed at a reduced dosage. (See Myelodysplastic Syndrome/Acute Myeloid Leukemia and also see Hematologic Effects under Cautions: Warnings/Precautions.)

For platelet counts less than 50,000/mm^3, talazoparib therapy should be withheld. When platelet count reaches or exceeds 75,000/mm^3, talazoparib may be resumed at a reduced dosage.

For absolute neutrophil count (ANC) less than 1000/mm^3, talazoparib therapy should be withheld. When ANC reaches or exceeds 1500/mm^3, talazoparib may be resumed at a reduced dosage.

If MDS/AML is confirmed, talazoparib therapy should be discontinued.

Nonhematologic Effects. If grade 3 or 4 nonhematologic toxicity occurs, talazoparib therapy should be withheld. When the nonhematologic toxicity resolves to grade 1 or less, dosage reduction of talazoparib or discontinuance of therapy may be considered.

Concomitant Use of Drugs Affecting the P-glycoprotein Transport System. Concomitant use of talazoparib with *potent* inhibitors of P-glycoprotein (P-gp) (i.e., amiodarone, carvedilol, clarithromycin, itraconazole, verapamil) should be avoided; if concomitant use of these P-gp inhibitors cannot be avoided, the manufacturer recommends reducing the dosage of talazoparib from 1 mg once daily to 0.75 mg once daily. If concomitant use of the P-gp inhibitor is discontinued, the talazoparib dosage should be returned (after 3–5 terminal half-lives of the P-gp inhibitor) to the dosage used prior to initiation of the P-gp inhibitor. (See Inhibitors of P-gp under Drug Interactions: Drugs Affecting Efflux Transport Systems.)

■ **Special Populations** The manufacturer states that no adjustment to the dosage of talazoparib is necessary in patients with mild hepatic impairment (total bilirubin concentration not exceeding the upper limit of normal [ULN] with AST concentration exceeding the ULN or total bilirubin concentration exceeding the ULN, but not more than 1.5 times the ULN, with any AST concentration). Talazoparib has not been studied in patients with moderate to severe hepatic impairment (total bilirubin concentration exceeding 1.5 times the ULN with any AST concentration), and the manufacturer provides no specific dosage recommendations for such patients. (See Hepatic Impairment under Warnings/Precautions: Specific Populations, in Cautions.)

For patients with moderate renal impairment (creatinine clearance 30–59 mL/minute), the manufacturer recommends a talazoparib dosage of 0.75 mg once daily. No dosage adjustment is necessary in patients with mild renal impairment (creatinine clearance 60–89 mL/minute). Talazoparib has not been studied in patients with severe renal impairment (creatinine clearance less than 30 mL/minute) or in those receiving dialysis, and the manufacturer provides no specific dosage recommendations for such patients. (See Renal Impairment under Warnings/Precautions: Specific Populations, in Cautions.)

The manufacturer makes no specific dosage recommendations for geriatric patients. (See Geriatric Use under Warnings/Precautions: Specific Populations, in Cautions.)

Cautions

■ **Contraindications** The manufacturer states that there are no known contraindications to the use of talazoparib.

■ **Warnings/Precautions** ***Myelodysplastic Syndrome/Acute Myeloid Leukemia*** In clinical studies evaluating talazoparib in patients with solid tumors, myelodysplastic syndrome (MDS) and acute myeloid leukemia (AML) were reported in 2 of 584 patients (0.3%) receiving talazoparib at 4 or 24 months following initiation of therapy. Both of these patients had received previous chemotherapy with platinum-containing agents and/or other DNA-damaging antineoplastic agents.

Complete blood cell (CBC) counts should be monitored at baseline and then monthly in patients receiving talazoparib. (See Hematologic Effects under Cautions: Warnings/Precautions.) In addition, talazoparib therapy should not be initiated until patients have adequately recovered from hematologic toxicity caused by previous chemotherapy. If prolonged hematologic toxicity occurs during therapy, talazoparib should be withheld and CBC counts should be monitored weekly until recovery occurs. If hematologic toxicity persists for more than 4 weeks following interruption of therapy, patients should be referred to a hematologist for further evaluation, including bone marrow analysis and cytogenetic testing of a blood sample. If MDS/AML is confirmed, talazoparib should be discontinued.

Hematologic Effects Adverse hematologic effects (e.g., anemia, neutropenia, thrombocytopenia) are frequently reported in patients receiving talazoparib therapy. In clinical trials, grade 3 or greater anemia, neutropenia, and thrombocytopenia occurred in 39, 21, and 15%, respectively, of patients receiving talazoparib. Therapy was discontinued because of anemia, neutropenia, or thrombocytopenia in 0.7, 0.3, or 0.3%, respectively, of patients receiving the drug.

Talazoparib therapy should not be initiated until patients have adequately recovered from hematologic toxicity caused by previous chemotherapy. CBC counts should be monitored at baseline and then monthly in patients receiving talazoparib. Temporary interruption, dosage reduction, or discontinuance of talazoparib may be necessary if hematologic toxicity occurs during therapy with the drug. (See Hematologic Toxicity under Dosage: Dosage Modification, in Dosage and Administration.) If hematologic toxicity develops and persists for more than 4 weeks following interruption of talazoparib therapy, patients should be referred to a hematologist for further evaluation, including bone marrow analysis and cytogenetic testing of a blood sample. (See Myelodysplastic Syndrome/ Acute Myeloid Leukemia under Cautions: Warnings/Precautions.)

Fetal/Neonatal Morbidity and Mortality Based on its mechanism of action and animal findings, talazoparib may cause fetal harm. Embryotoxicity (i.e., embryofetal death, decreased fetal weight) and teratogenicity were observed in pregnant rats receiving talazoparib at exposure levels equivalent to 0.24 times the human exposure at the recommended talazoparib dosage. The manufacturer recommends confirmation of pregnancy status prior to initiation of talazoparib, and women of reproductive potential should be advised to use effective contraceptive methods during talazoparib therapy and for at least 7 months after discontinuance of the drug. In addition, men who are partners of such women, including those who are pregnant, should use effective methods of contraception while receiving the drug and for at least 4 months after the drug is discontinued. Patients should be apprised of the potential fetal hazard if talazoparib is used during pregnancy.

Impairment of Fertility Results of animal studies suggest that talazoparib may impair male fertility. The effect of the drug on fertility in humans is not known.

Specific Populations **Pregnancy.** Talazoparib may cause fetal harm if administered to pregnant women based on its mechanism of action and animal findings. (See Fetal/Neonatal Morbidity and Mortality under Cautions: Warnings/Precautions.)

Confirmation of pregnancy status prior to initiation of talazoparib therapy is recommended.

Lactation. It is not known whether talazoparib is distributed into milk. Because of the potential for serious adverse reactions to talazoparib in nursing infants, women should be advised to discontinue nursing during talazoparib therapy and for at least 1 month after discontinuance of therapy. The effects of the drug on nursing infants or on milk production are unknown.

Pediatric Use. Safety and efficacy of talazoparib have not been established in pediatric patients.

The pharmacokinetic profile of talazoparib has not been established in patients younger than 18 years of age.

Geriatric Use. In clinical studies evaluating talazoparib in patients with advanced solid tumors, 17% of patients were 65 years of age or older and 4% were 75 years of age or older. No overall differences in safety were observed between geriatric patients and younger adults. However, the possibility of increased sensitivity to the drug in some geriatric patients cannot be ruled out.

Hepatic Impairment. Pharmacokinetics of talazoparib were unaffected following administration of the drug in individuals with mild hepatic impairment (total bilirubin concentration not exceeding the upper limit of normal [ULN] with AST concentration exceeding the ULN or total bilirubin concentration exceeding the ULN, but not more than 1.5 times the ULN, with any AST concentration). (See Dosage and Administration: Special Populations.)

The pharmacokinetics of talazoparib have not been established in patients with moderate to severe hepatic impairment (total bilirubin concentration exceeding 1.5 times the ULN with any AST concentration).

Renal Impairment. Clearance of talazoparib was decreased by 14.4 or 37.1% in patients with mild (creatinine clearance 60–89 mL/minute) or moderate (creatinine clearance 30–59 mL/minute) renal impairment, respectively, compared with individuals with normal renal function. (See Dosage and Administration: Special Populations.)

The pharmacokinetics of talazoparib have not been established in patients with severe renal impairment (creatinine clearance less than 30 mL/minute) or in those receiving dialysis.

■ **Common Adverse Effects** Adverse effects reported in 20% or more of patients receiving talazoparib include fatigue, anemia, nausea, neutropenia, headache, thrombocytopenia, alopecia, vomiting, diarrhea, and decreased appetite. Laboratory abnormalities reported in 25% or more of patients receiving talazoparib include decreased hemoglobin concentrations, decreased leukocyte count, decreased lymphocyte concentrations, decreased absolute neutrophil count (ANC), decreased platelet count, elevated glucose concentrations, elevated concentrations of aminotransferases (i.e., AST, ALT), elevated alkaline phosphatase concentrations, and decreased calcium concentrations.

Drug Interactions

In vitro studies indicate that talazoparib is not an inhibitor of cytochrome P-450 (CYP) isoenzymes 1A2, 2B6, 2C8, 2C9, 2C19, 2D6, and 3A4/5 or an inducer of CYP isoenzymes 1A2, 2B6, or 3A4.

In vitro, talazoparib is not an inhibitor of uridine diphosphate-glucuronosyltransferases (UGT) 1A1, 1A4, 1A6, 1A9, 2B7, and 2B15.

In vitro studies indicate that talazoparib is a substrate, but not an inhibitor, of P-glycoprotein (P-gp) and breast cancer resistance protein (BCRP). In vitro, talazoparib is not a substrate or inhibitor of organic anion transport protein (OATP) 1B1, OATP1B3, organic cation transporter (OCT) 1, OCT2, organic anion transporter (OAT) 1, OAT3, bile salt export pump (BSEP), and multidrug and toxic compound extrusion protein (MATE) 1 and MATE2K.

■ **Drugs Affecting or Metabolized by Hepatic Microsomal Enzymes** Talazoparib undergoes minimal hepatic metabolism; drug interactions are unlikely with inhibitors or inducers of CYP isoenzymes.

■ **Drugs Affecting Efflux Transport Systems** ***Inhibitors of P-gp*** Concomitant use of talazoparib with inhibitors of P-gp may result in increased systemic exposure of talazoparib. In a population pharmacokinetic analysis, concomitant administration of a *potent* P-gp inhibitor (i.e., amiodarone, carvedilol, clarithromycin, itraconazole, verapamil) with talazoparib increased the systemic exposure of talazoparib by approximately 45% and resulted in an increase in talazoparib dosage reductions. However, concomitant use of talazoparib with a *moderate* or *weak* P-gp inhibitor (i.e., azithromycin, atorvastatin, diltiazem, felodipine, fluvoxamine, quercetin) in clinical studies did not have a clinically meaningful effect on systemic exposure to talazoparib.

Concomitant use of talazoparib with *potent* P-gp inhibitors such as amiodarone, carvedilol, clarithromycin, itraconazole, or verapamil should be avoided; if concomitant use of these P-gp inhibitors cannot be avoided, the manufacturer recommends reducing the dosage of talazoparib from 1 mg once daily to 0.75 mg once daily. If concomitant use of the P-gp inhibitor is discontinued, the talazoparib dosage should be returned (after 3–5 terminal half-lives of the P-gp inhibitor) to the dosage used prior to initiation of the P-gp inhibitor. Patients receiving talazoparib concomitantly with a *moderate* or *weak* P-gp inhibitor should be monitored for signs of talazoparib toxicity. If adverse effects occur, temporary interruption of talazoparib therapy followed by dosage reduction may be necessary. (See Dosage and Administration: Dosage Modification.)

Inducers of P-gp The effect of inducers of P-gp on the pharmacokinetics of talazoparib have not been studied.

Inhibitors of BCRP Although not specifically studied in drug interaction studies to date, concomitant use of talazoparib with inhibitors of BCRP may result in increased systemic exposure of talazoparib.

Concomitant use of talazoparib with BCRP inhibitors should be avoided. If concomitant use cannot be avoided, patients should be monitored for signs of talazoparib toxicity.

■ **Drugs Affecting Gastric Acidity** Concomitant administration of talazoparib with drugs that reduce gastric acidity such as proton-pump inhibitors, antacids, and histamine H_2-receptor antagonists does not have a clinically meaningful effect on absorption of talazoparib.

Description

Talazoparib, a potent and selective inhibitor of mammalian poly(adenosine diphosphate [ADP]-ribose) polymerase (PARP) enzymes, including PARP-1 and PARP-2, is an antineoplastic agent. PARP enzymes are involved in normal cellular homeostasis, including DNA transcription, cell cycle regulation, and DNA repair. In vitro studies have demonstrated that talazoparib-induced cytotoxicity may involve inhibition of PARP enzymatic activity and increased formation of PARP-DNA complex, which result in DNA damage, decreased cell proliferation, and apoptosis. PARP inhibitors, such as talazoparib, appear to be selective for tumor cells that harbor certain homologous recombination deficiencies, including those harboring BRCA1 and BRCA2 mutations. In vitro, talazoparib is at least 18- or 37-fold more potent than rucaparib and olaparib in BRCA-deficient or phosphatase and tensin homolog (PTEN)-deficient tumor cells lines, respectively. In vitro, talazoparib is 922- and 231-fold more potent than rucaparib and olaparib in estrogen receptor-negative, progesterone receptor-negative, and human epidermal growth factor receptor type 2 (HER2)-negative breast tumor cell lines harboring BRCA1 mutation. In addition, talazoparib demonstrated antitumor activity in patient-derived xenograft tumor models harboring either mutated or wild-type BRCA1/2.

Talazoparib exhibits linear pharmacokinetics over the dosage range of 0.025–2 mg. Following oral administration, the median time to peak plasma concentrations of talazoparib is 1–2 hours. Following repeated oral administration of talazoparib at a dosage of 1 mg daily, the median accumulation ratio of talazoparib is 2.3–5.2. Steady-state concentrations are reached within 2–3 weeks. Administration of talazoparib (single 0.5-mg dose) with a high-fat, high-calorie meal (800–1000 calories with fat accounting for approximately 50–75% of the caloric content) decreased the rate of absorption (time to peak concentrations delayed by 3 hours) and the mean peak plasma concentrations (decreased by 46%), but did not substantially affect the extent of absorption. Talazoparib undergoes minimal hepatic metabolism. Talazoparib is metabolized by mono-oxidation, dehydrogenation, cysteine conjugation of mono-desfluorotalazoparib, and glucuronide conjugation. Following oral administration of a radiolabeled dose of talazoparib, approximately 68.7% of the radioactivity was recovered in urine (54.6% of the dose as unchanged drug) and 19.7% was recovered in feces (13.6% of the dose as unchanged drug). In vitro, talazoparib is 74% bound to plasma proteins, and binding is independent of talazoparib concentration. The mean terminal half-life of the drug is 90 hours.

The pharmacokinetics of talazoparib do not appear to be affected substantially by age (18–88 years), gender, race, or body weight (36–162 kg).

Advice to Patients

Importance of reading the manufacturer's patient information.

Importance of advising patients to take talazoparib capsules once daily without regard to meals. Importance of advising patients to swallow talazoparib capsules whole and not to dissolve or open the capsules.

If a dose is missed or vomited, importance of administering the next dose at the regularly scheduled time; an additional dose should not be administered to make up for a missed dose.

Risk of myelodysplastic syndrome (MDS) and acute myeloid leukemia (AML). Importance of informing clinician if fatigue/asthenia, fever, weight loss, frequent infections, bruising, unusual bleeding (including hematuria or bloody stool), shortness of breath, abnormal complete blood cell (CBC) counts, or requirement for blood product transfusions occurs.

Risk of bone marrow suppression. Importance of hematologic monitoring during talazoparib therapy.

Risk of fetal harm and pregnancy loss. Necessity of advising women of reproductive potential to use effective contraception during talazoparib therapy and for at least 7 months after the last dose of the drug. Necessity of advising men who are partners of such women, including those who are pregnant, that they should use effective contraception during talazoparib therapy and for at least 4 months after the last dose of the drug. Importance of women informing clinicians immediately if they are pregnant or become pregnant during therapy. If pregnancy occurs, advise pregnant women of potential risk to the fetus.

Importance of advising women to avoid breast-feeding while receiving talazoparib and for at least 1 month following discontinuance of therapy.

Importance of informing clinicians of existing or contemplated concomitant therapy, including prescription and OTC drugs and dietary or herbal supplements, as well as any concomitant illnesses.

Importance of informing patients of other important precautionary information. (See Cautions.)

Overview® (see Users Guide). For additional information on this drug until a more detailed monograph is developed and published, the manufacturer's labeling should be consulted. It is *essential* that the manufacturer's labeling be consulted for more detailed information on usual cautions, precautions, contraindications, potential drug interactions, laboratory test interferences, and acute toxicity. For further information on the handling of antineoplastic agents, see the ASHP Guidelines on Handling Hazardous Drugs at http://www.ahfsdruginformation.com.

Preparations

Talazoparib tosylate can only be obtained through designated specialty pharmacies. (See Restricted Distribution under Dosage and Administration: General.)

Excipients in commercially available drug preparations may have clinically important effects in some individuals; consult specific product labeling for details.

Talazoparib Tosylate

Oral		
Capsules	0.25 mg (of talazoparib)	**Talzenna®**, Pfizer

Selected Revisions July 2019, © Copyright, November 2018, American Society of Health-System Pharmacists, Inc.

Talimogene Laherparepvec

T-VEC, OncoVEX^{GM-CSF}

■ Talimogene laherparepvec, a live, attenuated herpes simplex virus type 1 (HSV-1)-derived oncolytic virus encoding granulocyte-macrophage colony-stimulating factor (GM-CSF), is an antineoplastic agent.

Uses

■ **Melanoma** Talimogene laherparepvec is used intralesionally for the local treatment of unresectable cutaneous, subcutaneous, and nodal lesions in patients with recurrent melanoma following initial surgery. The current indication is based on durable response rate; there currently are no controlled trials demonstrating a clinical benefit (e.g., increased survival) or an effect on visceral metastases.

The current indication for talimogene laherparepvec is based principally on the results of an open-label, randomized, phase 3 study (OPTiM) in 436 adults with unresectable stage IIIB, stage IIIC, or metastatic melanoma. The primary measure of efficacy was durable response rate (complete plus partial responses lasting at least 6 months). Because immunotherapeutic agents such as talimogene laherparepvec are associated with delayed therapeutic responses and pseudoprogression in which new lesions develop prior to tumor regression, tumor responses were assessed according to modified WHO response criteria to allow continued treatment despite disease progression (i.e., development of new lesions or progression of existing lesions). Patients were allowed to have received prior systemic therapy for melanoma. Patients with active cerebral metastases, bony metastases, extensive visceral disease, or primary ocular or mucosal melanoma; those with evidence of immunosuppression; and those receiving a systemic antiviral agent active against herpes simplex virus type 1 (HSV-1) (e.g., acyclovir) were excluded from the study. The mean age of patients was 63 years (range: 22–94 years), 98% of patients were white, 70% had an ECOG performance status of 0, 70% had metastatic disease, and 58% of patients were seropositive for wild-type HSV-1 at baseline. Approximately 50% of patients had received prior therapy for melanoma (other than or in addition to surgery, adjuvant therapy, or radiation therapy).

In this study, patients were randomized in a 2:1 ratio to receive either talimogene laherparepvec or sargramostim (granulocyte-macrophage colony-stimulating factor [GM-CSF]). Patients in the talimogene laherparepvec group received up to 4 mL of the drug by intralesional injection per treatment visit at a concentration of 1 million (1×10^6) plaque-forming units (PFU)/mL on day 1, followed by a concentration of 100 million (1×10^8) PFU/mL on day 21 and every 2 weeks thereafter. Patients in the sargramostim group received sargramostim 125 mcg/m^2 once daily administered by subcutaneous injection on days 1–14 of each 28-day cycle. Treatment was continued until no injectable lesions were present or for at least 6 months despite disease progression (i.e., an increase in size of one or more existing lesions and/or development of any new lesions) unless alternative therapy was clinically indicated or unacceptable toxicity occurred. After 6 months of therapy, treatment was continued until clinically relevant disease progression (i.e., progressive disease associated with reduced performance status and/or a clinical indication for alternative therapy) occurred, unacceptable toxicity occurred, patient consent was withdrawn, lack of response by 12 months was observed, complete remission occurred, or no injectable lesions were present (talimogene laherparepvec group only). After 12 months, patients with stable or responding disease could continue treatment for an additional 6 months, unless disease progression occurred or no injectable lesions were present.

At the time of the primary analysis, the durable response rate was 16.3% in patients receiving talimogene laherparepvec compared with 2.1% in those receiving sargramostim. The median time to response was 4.1 months (range: 1.2–16.7 months) in patients receiving talimogene laherparepvec. The median time to treatment failure was 8.2 months in patients receiving talimogene laherparepvec and 2.9 months in those receiving sargramostim. No difference in overall survival was observed between patients receiving talimogene laherparepvec and those receiving sargramostim (22.9 versus 19 months, respectively). Results of an exploratory subgroup analysis (based on disease stage, line of therapy, gender, performance status, and HSV-1 status) suggested greater clinical benefit (i.e., durable response rate, overall response rate, overall survival) in patients with previously untreated metastatic melanoma and in those with stage IIIB, IIIC, or IVM1a disease.

Dosage and Administration

■ **General** ***Restricted Distribution Program*** Talimogene laherparepvec can only be obtained through specialty distributors. Clinicians may consult the Imlygic® website for specific availability information (http://www.imlygic.com).

■ **Administration** Talimogene laherparepvec is administered by intralesional injection using a 22- to 26-gauge needle; syringes calibrated in small increments (e.g., 0.5-mL insulin syringes) are recommended for better injection control. The oncolytic virus should be injected into cutaneous, subcutaneous, and/or nodal lesions that are visible, palpable, or detectable by ultrasound guidance. *The oncolytic virus should not be administered by IV injection.*

During shipping and storage, talimogene laherparepvec should be kept frozen at a temperature of −90 to −70°C. Prior to administration, frozen suspensions of the oncolytic virus must be completely thawed at room temperature (20–25°C) for approximately 30 minutes in the original carton; the suspension should *not* be exposed to temperatures exceeding 25°C. The suspension may be mixed by gentle swirling and should *not* be shaken. After thawing, talimogene laherparepvec should be administered immediately. If immediate administration is not possible, suspensions containing talimogene laherparepvec 1 million (1×10^6) plaque-forming units (PFU)/mL or 100 million (1×10^8) PFU/mL may be refrigerated at 2–8°C in the original vial and carton (for protection from light) for 12 or 48 hours, respectively; vials refrigerated beyond the specified times should be discarded. Once thawed, the suspension should not be refrozen.

The manufacturer states that aseptic technique must be observed when preparing talimogene laherparepvec syringes since the suspension contains no preservative. The appropriate volume (up to 0.1–4 mL depending on lesion size) (see Dosage and Administration: Dosage) of talimogene laherparepvec suspension should be withdrawn from a vial labeled as containing 1 million (1×10^6) PFU/mL (initial dose) or 100 million (1×10^8) PFU/mL (subsequent doses) using a sterile syringe with an 18- to 26-gauge needle; the needle should be replaced with a 22- to 26-gauge needle for intralesional injection. Care should be taken to avoid aerosolization of the oncolytic virus. The manufacturer recommends preparing talimogene laherparepvec in a biologic safety cabinet. Talimogene laherparepvec should be administered immediately following preparation of the syringe.

The manufacturer's labeling should be consulted for detailed information on the administration of talimogene laherparepvec. Prior to administration, lesions and surrounding areas should be cleaned with alcohol and allowed to dry. Topical or local anesthetics may be administered prior to injection of talimogene laherparepvec; however, anesthetic agents should be injected around the periphery of the lesion and should *not* be injected directly into the lesion. Talimogene laherparepvec should be injected into a lesion using a single insertion point; however, multiple insertion points may be used if a lesion is larger than the radial reach of the needle. From the single insertion point, the needle should be pulled back without exiting the lesion and redirected along multiple tracks until the full dose has been evenly and completely dispersed within the lesion. Following administration, the needle should be withdrawn slowly from the lesion to avoid leakage of talimogene laherparepvec from the insertion point. The manufacturer states that a new needle should be used if a needle is completely withdrawn from a lesion and each time a different lesion is injected.

Following administration of talimogene laherparepvec, pressure should be applied to the injection site with sterile gauze for at least 30 seconds and the injection site and surrounding area should be cleaned with alcohol. Health-care personnel should change gloves and apply an absorbent pad and dry occlusive dressing over the injected lesion(s); the exterior of the dry occlusive dressing should be wiped with alcohol. (See Advice to Patients.)

Preparation and Administration Precautions Health-care personnel who are immunocompromised or pregnant should *not* handle talimogene laherparepvec or come into direct contact with injection sites, dressings, or body fluids of treated patients. (See Accidental Exposure under Cautions: Warnings/Precautions.)

Procedures for proper handling (e.g., use of gloves, protective clothing, and eyewear or face shield) and disposal of biohazard waste, including administration equipment (e.g., vial, syringe, needle, cotton gauze, gloves, masks, dressings), should be followed when preparing or administering talimogene laherparepvec. Health-care personnel should cover open wounds prior to handling talimogene laherparepvec suspension.

If accidental occupational exposure occurs (e.g., through a splash to the eyes or mucosa), the affected area should be flushed with water for at least 15 minutes. If talimogene laherparepvec suspension comes in contact with broken skin or a needlestick injury occurs, the affected area should be cleaned thoroughly with soap and water and/or a disinfectant.

If spillage of talimogene laherparepvec occurs, the affected area should be treated with a virucidal agent such as sodium hypochlorite 1% and absorbent materials should be used to blot the area.

■ Dosage

Dosage of talimogene laherparepvec is expressed in plaque-forming units (PFU).

Melanoma The recommended injection volume of talimogene laherparepvec for the treatment of unresectable cutaneous, subcutaneous, and nodal lesions in patients with recurrent melanoma following initial surgery is dependent on the size of the lesion (see Table 1); however, the total injection volume of talimogene laherparepvec for all injected lesions combined should *not* exceed 4 mL per treatment visit. If lesions are clustered together, the cluster should be injected as a single lesion according to the injection volumes in Table 1. Talimogene laherparepvec 1 million (1×10^6) PFU/mL should be used for the initial treatment visit, followed 3 weeks later by treatment with talimogene laherparepvec 100 million (1×10^8) PFU/mL; all subsequent doses of the oncolytic virus (including reinitiation of therapy) should be administered at 2-week intervals using talimogene laherparepvec 100 million PFU/mL.

Treatment of all lesions may not be possible in one treatment visit or even over the full course of treatment; the lesions treated at any given visit may include previously injected and/or uninjected lesions. Highest priority should be given to treating the largest lesion(s) at the initial treatment visit and any new lesions (i.e., lesions that developed after the previous treatment visit) at subsequent treatment visits; remaining lesions should be prioritized by lesion size until the maximum injection volume of talimogene laherparepvec has been reached or until all injectable lesions have been treated. Treatment should be continued for at least 6 months or until no injectable lesions are present. If new unresectable cutaneous, subcutaneous, or nodal lesions appear after a complete response was achieved, therapy with talimogene laherparepvec may be reinitiated.

Table 1. Injection Volume Based on Lesion Size

Lesion Size (longest dimension)	Injection Volume
>5 cm	Up to 4 mL
>2.5–5 cm	Up to 2 mL
>1.5–2.5 cm	Up to 1 mL
>0.5–1.5 cm	Up to 0.5 mL
≤0.5 cm	Up to 0.1 mL

■ Special Populations

The manufacturer makes no special population dosage recommendations at this time.

Cautions

■ Contraindications

Talimogene laherparepvec is contraindicated in immunosuppressed individuals (including those with a history of primary or acquired immunodeficiencies, acquired immunodeficiency syndrome [AIDS] or other clinical manifestations of human immunodeficiency virus [HIV] infection, leukemia, or lymphoma, and those receiving immunosuppressive therapy). (See Herpes Infection under Cautions: Warnings/Precautions.)

Talimogene laherparepvec is contraindicated in pregnant women. (See Pregnancy under Warnings/Precautions: Specific Populations, in Cautions.)

■ Warnings/Precautions

Fetal/Neonatal Morbidity and Mortality There are no adequate and well-controlled studies of talimogene laherparepvec in pregnant women. However, wild-type herpes simplex virus type 1 (HSV-1) may cross the placenta and transmission of the virus may occur during birth; fetal or neonatal infection with the wild-type virus can cause serious adverse effects (e.g., multiorgan failure, death). The potential exists for similar adverse effects to occur in a fetus or neonate exposed to the attenuated talimogene laherparepvec virus. Embryofetal toxicity was not observed when talimogene laherparepvec was administered IV (at dosages approximately 60 times, on a plaque-forming units [PFU] per kg basis, the maximum recommended human dose) to pregnant mice during the period of organogenesis; however, limitations of the study design limit applicability of these data to humans.

Pregnancy should be avoided during talimogene laherparepvec therapy. Women of childbearing potential should be advised to use an effective method of contraception while receiving talimogene laherparepvec. Patients should be apprised of the potential hazard to the fetus if the drug is used during pregnancy.

Accidental Exposure Accidental exposure may lead to transmission of talimogene laherparepvec and subsequent herpes infection. Accidental needlestick injury and exposure in or near the eyes (eye splash) have been reported by health-care personnel during preparation and administration of talimogene laherparepvec.

Health-care personnel, close contacts (e.g., household contacts, caregivers, sex partners, persons sharing the same bed), pregnant women, and neonates should not have direct contact with talimogene laherparepvec injection sites, dressings, or body fluids of treated patients. Health-care personnel who are immunocompromised or pregnant should *not* prepare or administer talimogene laherparepvec. Caregivers should wear protective gloves when applying or changing occlusive dressings and observe procedures for proper disposal of used dressings, gloves, and cleaning materials. (See Advice to Patients.)

If accidental exposure to talimogene laherparepvec occurs, the affected area should be cleaned thoroughly with soap and water and/or a disinfectant. Exposed individuals should be monitored for signs and symptoms of herpes infection and should receive appropriate treatment as clinically indicated. (See Herpes Infection under Cautions: Warnings/Precautions and also see Advice to Patients.)

Because touching or scratching injection sites or occlusive dressings may result in inadvertent transfer of talimogene laherparepvec to other areas of the body, patients should be advised to avoid touching or scratching injection sites or occlusive dressings. (See Description.)

Herpes Infection Herpes infections, including cold sores and herpetic keratitis, have been reported in patients receiving talimogene laherparepvec in clinical studies. Talimogene laherparepvec is a genetically modified preparation of live, attenuated HSV-1; therefore, life-threatening disseminated herpes infection may occur in immunosuppressed individuals. (See Cautions: Contraindications.)

If herpes-like lesions develop in patients or close contacts, standard hygienic practices should be followed to prevent virus transmission. Herpes-like lesions should be evaluated by a clinician and reported to the manufacturer by telephone at 855-465-9442; patients or close contacts may participate in follow-up testing for further characterization of the infection.

Antiviral agents active against HSV-1 (e.g., acyclovir) may affect the efficacy of talimogene laherparepvec. (See Drug Interactions: Antiviral Agents.) Clinicians should consider whether the potential benefit of treating herpes infections with antiviral therapy outweighs the risk in patients receiving talimogene laherparepvec.

Injection Site Complications Impaired healing at the injection site, cellulitis, and systemic bacterial infections have been reported in patients receiving talimogene laherparepvec in clinical studies. Necrosis or ulceration of tumor tissue also may occur. Talimogene laherparepvec may increase the risk of impaired healing at injection sites in patients with underlying risk factors (e.g., previous radiation at the injection site, lesions in poorly vascularized areas). Impaired healing at an injection site resulting in infection and subsequent amputation of a lower extremity occurred in one patient 6 months after talimogene laherparepvec administration; however, wound complications previously had occurred in the affected area following surgery and radiation therapy.

If injection site complications, particularly necrosis resulting in open wounds, occur, the manufacturer recommends careful wound care and infection precautions. If persistent infection or impaired healing of an injection site occurs, clinicians should consider whether the benefit of continuing talimogene laherparepvec therapy outweighs the risks.

Immune-mediated Events Immune-mediated events, including glomerulonephritis, vasculitis, pneumonitis, worsening psoriasis, and vitiligo, have been reported in patients receiving talimogene laherparepvec in clinical studies.

Before initiating talimogene laherparepvec therapy in patients with underlying autoimmune disease or continuing such therapy in patients who experience immune-mediated events, clinicians should consider whether the benefit of talimogene laherparepvec therapy outweighs the risks.

Plasmacytoma Plasmacytoma has been reported in proximity to the talimogene laherparepvec injection site in a patient with smoldering multiple myeloma.

Before initiating talimogene laherparepvec therapy in patients with multiple myeloma or continuing such therapy in patients who develop plasmacytoma, clinicians should consider whether the benefit of talimogene laherparepvec therapy outweighs the risks.

Specific Populations **Pregnancy.** Talimogene laherparepvec may cause serious adverse effects similar to those observed in a fetus or neonate exposed to wild-type HSV-1. (See Fetal/Neonatal Morbidity and Mortality under Cautions: Warnings/Precautions.)

Lactation. It is not known whether talimogene laherparepvec is distributed into milk. Because many drugs are distributed into milk, women should be advised to discontinue nursing or talimogene laherparepvec, taking into account the developmental and health benefits of breast-feeding and the importance of the therapy to the woman. The effects of talimogene laherparepvec on nursing infants or on milk production are unknown.

Pediatric Use. Safety and efficacy of talimogene laherparepvec have not been established in pediatric patients.

Geriatric Use. In the OPTiM study in patients with unresectable melanoma, 48% of talimogene laherparepvec-treated patients were 65 years of age or older. In clinical studies, no overall differences in safety and efficacy were observed between geriatric patients and younger adults.

Hepatic Impairment. The pharmacokinetic profile of talimogene laherparepvec has not been fully established in patients with hepatic impairment.

Renal Impairment. The pharmacokinetic profile of talimogene laherparepvec has not been fully established in patients with renal impairment.

■ **Common Adverse Effects** Adverse effects reported in 25% or more of patients receiving talimogene laherparepvec and at an incidence that is at least 5% higher than that reported with sargramostim include fatigue, chills, pyrexia, influenza-like illness, injection site pain, and nausea.

Drug Interactions

No formal drug interaction studies have been performed to date.

■ **Antiviral Agents** Antiviral agents may affect the efficacy of talimogene laherparepvec. Talimogene laherparepvec is a genetically modified preparation of live, attenuated herpes simplex virus type 1 (HSV-1) and is susceptible to acyclovir. (See Herpes Infection under Cautions: Warnings/Precautions.)

Description

Talimogene laherparepvec, a live, attenuated herpes simplex virus type 1 (HSV-1)-derived oncolytic virus encoding granulocyte-macrophage colony-stimulating factor (GM-CSF), is an antineoplastic agent. Oncolytic viruses are native or genetically modified virus strains that display a preferential tropism for neoplastic cells in which they replicate and cause cell death without damaging normal tissue. The viral genome may be modified to attenuate pathogenicity and enhance therapeutic activity (e.g., increase viral tropism for neoplastic cells, enhance tumor-selective viral replication and lytic capacity, include transgenes to induce host antitumor immunity). Talimogene laherparepvec is a preparation of live, attenuated HSV-1 with several modifications that confer oncolytic properties. Modifications to the talimogene laherparepvec virus include deletion of the ICP34.5 and ICP47 genes to provide decreased pathogenicity in normal tissues, selective replication in tumor cells, tumor cell lysis, and enhanced antitumor immune response. The talimogene laherparepvec virus also is encoded to express GM-CSF to recruit antigen-presenting cells to the tumor microenvironment, enhance dendritic cell function, and promote cytotoxic T-cell responses to tumor-associated antigens. The precise mechanism of action of talimogene laherparepvec is unknown.

Following repeated intratumoral administration of talimogene laherparepvec in mice, the highest concentrations of talimogene laherparepvec viral DNA were detected in the injected tumor; oncolytic viral DNA also was detected in blood, spleen, lymph nodes, liver, heart, and kidneys, but not in bone marrow, eyes, lachrymal glands, nasal mucosa, or feces. Talimogene laherparepvec viral DNA was detected in the treated tumor or in blood up to 84 or 14 days, respectively, following the last injection. Preliminary data from a phase 2 trial evaluating the distribution and viral shedding of talimogene laherparepvec after repeated intralesional administration indicated that talimogene laherparepvec viral DNA was detected in blood and urine in 85 and 20% of patients, respectively, with peak concentrations in urine detected on the same day as administration. Infectious talimogene laherparepvec virus was detected at the site of injection in 3 of 20 patients at a single time point within one week of the initial injection. Although infectious talimogene laherparepvec virus was not detected on the exterior of occlusive dressings, talimogene laherparepvec viral DNA was detected at this site in 14 of 20 patients; in 13 patients, measurable levels of talimogene laherparepvec viral DNA decreased over time with no measurable viral DNA on the exterior of occlusive dressings by the third treatment.

Advice to Patients

Importance of advising patients to read the manufacturer's medication guide before beginning treatment and each time talimogene laherparepvec is administered.

Risk of virus transmission. Close contacts should avoid direct contact with injection sites, dressings, or body fluids of treated patients.

Importance of keeping injection sites covered for at least one week following each treatment or longer if weeping or oozing occurs. Importance of replacing the dressing if it falls off.

Importance of advising patients to avoid touching or scratching injection sites or occlusive dressings to prevent inadvertent transfer of talimogene laherparepvec to other areas of the body.

Importance of informing patients and/or caregivers of the risks associated with accidental exposure. Importance of advising patients and/or caregivers to wear protective gloves when applying or changing occlusive dressings and to dispose of used dressings and cleaning materials in a sealed plastic bag in household waste.

If accidental exposure to talimogene laherparepvec occurs, importance of thoroughly cleaning the affected area with soap and water and/or a disinfectant. Importance of informing clinician if herpes-like lesions occur.

Importance of informing patients and/or caregivers that individuals who are pregnant or immunocompromised should not change dressings or clean injection sites.

Risk of fetal harm. Necessity of advising women of childbearing potential that they should use an effective method of contraception while receiving the oncolytic virus. If pregnancy occurs, importance of advising pregnant women of potential risk to the fetus.

Importance of advising women not to breast-feed during therapy.

Importance of informing clinicians of existing or contemplated concomitant therapy, including prescription and OTC drugs, as well as any concomitant illnesses.

Importance of informing patients of other important precautionary information. (See Cautions.)

Overview® (see Users Guide). For additional information on this drug until a more detailed monograph is developed and published, the manufacturer's labeling should be consulted. It is *essential* that the manufacturer's labeling be consulted for more detailed information on usual cautions, precautions, contraindications, potential drug interactions, laboratory test interferences, and acute toxicity. For further information on the handling of antineoplastic agents, see the ASHP Guidelines on Handling Hazardous Drugs at http://www.ahfsdruginformation.com.

Preparations

Distribution of talimogene laherparepvec is restricted. (See Restricted Distribution Program under Dosage and Administration: General.)

Excipients in commercially available drug preparations may have clinically important effects in some individuals; consult specific product labeling for details.

Talimogene Laherparepvec

Parenteral		
Injection, for intralesional use	1 million (1 × 10^6) PFU per mL	**Imlygic®**, Amgen
	100 million (1 × 10^8) PFU per mL	**Imlygic®**, Amgen

Temozolomide

■ Temozolomide, a prodrug that has little, if any, pharmacologic activity until hydrolyzed in vivo, is an alkylating antineoplastic agent.

Uses

■ **Brain Tumors** ***Glioblastoma Multiforme*** Temozolomide is used concomitantly with radiation therapy for the treatment of newly diagnosed glioblastoma multiforme in adults; temozolomide also is used as maintenance therapy for glioblastoma multiforme.

The current indication is based on a randomized trial involving 573 patients with newly diagnosed glioblastoma multiforme. Treatment consisted of temozolomide 75 mg/m² once daily with radiation therapy for 42 days (up to a maximum of 49 days) followed by a 4-week rest period and then maintenance therapy with up to 6 cycles of temozolomide (150 or 200 mg/m²) on days 1–5 of every 28-day cycle; or radiation therapy alone. Salvage therapy with temozolomide was administered upon disease progression to 22% of patients receiving initial therapy with temozolomide and radiation therapy and 57% of patients receiving initial therapy with radiation therapy alone.

Overall survival was prolonged (unadjusted hazard ratio for death: 0.63) and median survival was increased by 2.5 months (14.6 versus 12.1 months) in patients receiving concomitant temozolomide and radiation therapy followed by maintenance therapy with temozolomide compared with those receiving radiation therapy alone as initial therapy for glioblastoma multiforme. Nausea (36 versus 16%), vomiting (20 versus 6%), anorexia (19 versus 9%), constipation (18 versus 6%), and thrombocytopenia (4 versus 1%) occurred more frequently in patients receiving concomitant temozolomide and radiation therapy than in those receiving radiation therapy alone.

Anaplastic Astrocytoma Temozolomide is used in the treatment of refractory anaplastic astrocytoma in adults whose disease has progressed after initial therapy with a nitrosourea and procarbazine. The current indication is based on tumor response rates in this population from an uncontrolled phase 2 study. In a single-arm, multicenter study in 162 patients with relapsed anaplastic astrocytoma who had a baseline Karnofsky performance status of 70 or greater, efficacy in a subgroup of 54 patients with refractory disease (i.e., progression following treatment with a nitrosourea and procarbazine) was demonstrated by an overall (complete plus partial) tumor response rate of 22% and a complete response rate of 9%. Median durations of all responses and complete responses were 50 and 64 weeks, respectively. Progression-free survival at 6 and 12 months was 45 and 29%, respectively; median progression-free survival was 4.4 months; 12-month overall survival was 65%; and median overall survival was 15.9 months.

Dosage and Administration

■ **General** Temozolomide is administered orally or by IV infusion.

The recommended dosage of temozolomide by IV infusion over 90 minutes is the same as the dose for the oral capsule formulation. Bioequivalence of oral and IV doses of temozolomide has been established only when temozolomide for injection is administered by IV infusion over 90 minutes; infusion over a shorter or longer duration may result in suboptimal dosing or an increase in infusion-related adverse reactions.

Opportunistic infections, such as *Pneumocystis jiroveci* (formerly *P. carinii*) pneumonia (PCP), may occur in patients receiving temozolomide. The risk of PCP is higher when temozolomide is administered as a longer dosage regimen. Prophylaxis for PCP (e.g., inhaled pentamidine or oral co-trimoxazole) is required for all patients receiving concomitant temozolomide and radiation therapy for the 42-day regimen. For patients experiencing lymphocytopenia during the concomitant phase of therapy, PCP prophylaxis should be continued until recovery from lymphocytopenia occurs. Regardless of the regimen, all patients receiving temozolomide, particularly those receiving concomitant corticosteroids, should be monitored closely for the development of PCP.

■ **Reconstitution and Administration** When given orally, temozolomide is administered once daily and should be swallowed intact with a full glass of water. If capsules are accidentally opened or damaged, precautions should be taken to avoid inhalation of capsule contents or contact with the skin or mucous membranes. The manufacturer recommends use of gloves and safety glasses to avoid exposure in case of breakage of the capsules. Although the drug may be administered with food, administration on an empty stomach may reduce the incidence of nausea and vomiting. Because food may decrease the rate and extent of absorption of temozolomide, the drug should be administered in a consistent manner relative to food intake. (See Advice to Patients.) Bedtime administration may be advisable. Antiemetics may be administered prior to and/or following temozolomide administration.

Based on the dose prescribed, the number of each strength capsules needed (e.g., for a dose of 275 mg daily for 5 days, dispense five 250-mg capsules, five 20-mg capsules, and five 5-mg capsules) should be determined. Each strength of capsules should be dispensed in a separate container. Each container should be labeled with the strength per capsule and with the appropriate number of capsules to be taken each day. The patient should be instructed to take the appropriate number of capsules from each container to equal the total daily dose.

Temozolomide for injection should be stored at 2–8°C and must be reconstituted prior to administration. If vials are accidentally opened or damaged, precautions should be taken to avoid inhalation of vial contents or contact with the skin or mucous membranes. The manufacturer recommends use of gloves and safety glasses to avoid exposure in case of breakage of the vial. Prior to reconstitution, temozolomide for injection should be brought to room temperature. Temozolomide for injection should be reconstituted by adding 41 mL of sterile water for injection to a vial labeled as containing 100 mg of temozolomide to provide a solution containing 2.5 mg/mL of the drug; reconstituted vials should be gently swirled but not shaken. The reconstituted solution may be stored at room temperature (25°C) for up to 14 hours (including infusion time). Reconstituted temozolomide for injection should be inspected visually for particulate matter prior to administration; the drug should be discarded if the solution contains visible particulate matter. The reconstituted solution should not be further diluted prior to administration. Using aseptic technique, up to 40 mL from each vial of reconstituted solution needed to reach the calculated dosage should be transferred to an empty 250-mL polyvinylchloride (PVC) infusion bag; compatibility studies with non-PVC bags have not been conducted. Temozolomide for injection should be administered by IV infusion over 90 minutes using an infusion pump. IV lines should be flushed before and after each temozolomide infusion. The manufacturer states that other drugs should not be infused through the same IV line.

■ **Dosage** ***Glioblastoma Multiforme*** **Concomitant Phase.** During the concomitant phase of therapy, the initial oral or IV dosage of temozolomide for the treatment of newly diagnosed glioblastoma multiforme is 75 mg/m^2 daily. Temozolomide is to be administered daily for 42 days concomitantly with focal radiation therapy (60 Gy administered in 30 fractions). No dosage reductions for temozolomide are recommended during the concomitant phase of therapy, but interruptions or discontinuance may be required according to toxicity.

A complete blood cell count (CBC) should be obtained prior to treatment and weekly during treatment. Criteria for the continuance of temozolomide dosing are as follows: absolute neutrophil count (ANC) of at least 1500/mm^3, platelet count of at least 100,000/mm^3, and nonhematologic toxicities that are grade 1 or less in severity (except alopecia, nausea, and vomiting). If these criteria are met, the daily temozolomide dose should be continued throughout the 42-day concomitant phase of therapy (for up to 49 days) in the treatment period.

Temozolomide dosing should be *interrupted* for any of the following criteria: ANC of 500–1499/mm^3, platelet count of 10,000–99,000/mm^3, or any grade 2 nonhematologic toxicity (except alopecia, nausea, and vomiting). Temozolomide therapy may be resumed when all of the criteria for the continuance of temozolomide dosing are met.

Temozolomide dosing should be *discontinued* for any of the following criteria: ANC less than 500/mm^3, platelet count less than 10,000/mm^3, or any grade 3 or 4 nonhematologic toxicity (except alopecia, nausea, and vomiting). Patients experiencing any of these toxicities should not receive any further concomitant therapy with temozolomide and are not eligible for maintenance therapy.

Maintenance Phase. For patients who complete the concomitant phase of therapy, the maintenance phase of therapy is initiated after a 4-week rest period following completion of temozolomide and radiation therapy. The maintenance phase of therapy consists of up to 6 cycles of temozolomide therapy as tolerated.

During the maintenance phase of therapy, the temozolomide dose is administered once daily for 5 days followed by a 23-day rest period for a 28-day cycle. The initial oral or IV dosage of temozolomide (for cycle 1) is 150 mg/m^2 once daily for 5 days followed by a 23-day rest period. The dose level for subsequent cycles of therapy depends on toxicity.

A CBC should be obtained prior to treatment on day 1 and on day 22 (21 days following the first dose of temozolomide) or within 48 hours of that day and then weekly, and dosing should not resume until the dosing criteria for continuance of therapy are met. Criteria for the continuance of maintenance temozolomide dosing are as follows: ANC that exceeds 1500/mm^3, platelet count that exceeds 100,000/mm^3, and nonhematologic toxicities that are grade 2 or less in severity (except alopecia, nausea, and vomiting).

For patients who meet the dosing criteria following cycle 1, the dosage of temozolomide may be *increased* to 200 mg/m^2 once daily for 5 days for cycle 2 and maintained at this level for each subsequent cycle for which the dosing criteria are met. For patients who experience toxicity during cycle 1, the temozolomide dose should *not* be increased for cycle 2 or any subsequent cycle of therapy.

The temozolomide dose (administered once daily for 5 days) should be *reduced* by 50 mg/m^2 (for example, from 150 mg/m^2 to 100 mg/m^2, or from 200 mg/m^2 to 150 mg/m^2) for the subsequent cycle of therapy for any of the following criteria: ANC less than 1000/mm^3, platelet count less than 50,000/mm^3, or any grade 3 nonhematologic toxicity (except alopecia, nausea, and vomiting). Dose reductions for the next cycle of therapy should be based on the lowest blood count or the worst nonhematologic toxicity that occurred during the previous cycle of therapy.

Temozolomide dosing should be *discontinued* for any of the following criteria: the dose reduction for toxicity during a previous cycle would result in a dose lower than temozolomide 100 mg/m^2 for the subsequent cycle, recurrence of the same grade 3 nonhematologic toxicity (except alopecia, nausea, and vomiting) following dose reduction, or any grade 4 nonhematologic toxicity (except alopecia, nausea, and vomiting).

Anaplastic Astrocytoma The initial oral or IV dosage of temozolomide for the treatment of refractory anaplastic astrocytoma in adults is 150 mg/m^2 daily for 5 consecutive days of a 28-day treatment cycle.

Subsequent dosage is adjusted based on nadir platelet and ANC during the previous cycle and on ANC and platelet counts on day 29 (i.e., day 1 of the next cycle). A CBC should be obtained prior to treatment on day 1 and on day 22 (i.e., 21 days after the first dose) of the cycle or within 48 hours of that day and weekly until the ANC and platelet counts exceed 1500 and 100,000/mm^3, respectively. The next cycle should be withheld until these counts are exceeded. If both nadir and day-of-dosing ANC and platelet counts exceed 1500 and 100,000/mm^3, respectively, then temozolomide dosage may be increased to 200 mg/m^2 daily for 5 consecutive days of the next 28-day cycle. If either the ANC is between 1000–1500/mm^3 or the platelet count is between 50,000–100,000/mm^3 during any cycle, therapy should be postponed until the ANC and platelet counts exceed 1500 and 100,000/mm^3, respectively, at which time a dosage of 150 mg/m^2 daily for 5 consecutive days should be used. If either the ANC or platelet count declines to less than 1000 or 50,000/mm^3, respectively, during any cycle, dosage for the next cycle should be reduced *by* 50 mg/m^2 daily, but not to less than the lowest recommended dosage of 100 mg/m^2 daily.

Temozolomide therapy can be continued until disease progression occurs. Although therapy was continued for up to 2 years in the clinical study establishing efficacy, the optimum duration is not known.

■ **Special Populations** ***Renal and Hepatic Impairment*** Use with caution in patients with severe hepatic or renal impairment. Pharmacokinetics in patients with mild to moderate hepatic impairment is similar to those in patients with normal hepatic function. Drug clearance is not affected by renal function in patients with creatinine clearances of 36–130 mL/minute per m^2.

Geriatric and Female Patients Among patients receiving temozolomide for anaplastic astrocytoma, geriatric patients and women had a greater risk of developing myelosuppression, but the manufacturer makes no specific recommendations regarding dosage adjustment other than usual adjustment for ANC and platelet counts. (See Warnings: Hematologic Effects, in Cautions.)

Dosage should be selected with caution in geriatric patients because of age-related decreases in hepatic, renal, and/or cardiac function and concomitant disease and drug therapy.

Cautions

■ **Contraindications** Known hypersensitivity (e.g., urticaria, allergic reaction including anaphylaxis, toxic epidermal necrolysis, Stevens-Johnson syndrome) to temozolomide or any ingredient in the formulation. Known hypersensitivity to dacarbazine (DTIC), since both drugs are metabolized to 5-(3-methyltriazen-1-yl)-imidazole-4-carboxamide (MTIC).

■ **Warnings/Precautions** ***Warnings*** **Hematologic Effects.** Thrombocytopenia and neutropenia are dose-limiting toxicities for all patients receiving temozolomide. Prolonged pancytopenia, which may result in aplastic anemia and in some cases has been fatal, has been reported. In some cases, assessment has been complicated by exposure to concomitant medications (e.g., carbamazepine, phenytoin, co-trimoxazole) which may be associated with aplastic anemia.

Among patients receiving temozolomide for newly diagnosed glioblastoma multiforme, grade 3 or 4 platelet abnormalities including thrombocytopenia occurred in 14% and grade 3 or 4 neutrophil abnormalities including neutropenia occurred in 8%.

Among patients receiving temozolomide for anaplastic astrocytoma, greater incidence of grade 4 thrombocytopenia and/or neutropenia in women and geriatric patients. Occurs late in the treatment cycle; nadirs occur at a median of 26 days for platelets and 28 days for neutrophils. Usually develops during the first few cycles of temozolomide therapy, resolves within 14 days, and is not cumulative. Hospitalization, blood transfusion, or drug discontinuance for myelosuppression may be required. Pancytopenia, leukopenia, and anemia also reported. Periodic blood cell count monitoring and possible dosage adjustment, schedule interruption, or discontinuance of therapy required. (See Dosage and Administration: General.)

Carcinogenic Effects. Myelodysplastic syndrome and secondary malignancies, including myeloid leukemia, have been observed.

Pneumocystis jiroveci (Pneumocystis carinii) Pneumonia. Temozolomide may be associated with a risk of *Pneumocystis jiroveci* (formerly known as *Pneumocystis carinii*) pneumonia (PCP), particularly with longer dosage regimens. All patients (particularly those receiving corticosteroids) should be monitored closely for development of PCP (regardless of regimen). PCP prophylaxis is required for all patients receiving temozolomide in conjunction with radiation therapy for glioblastoma multiforme; prophylaxis in patients who develop lymphocytopenia should be continued until lymphocytopenia resolves (grade 1 or less). (See Dosage and Administration: General.)

Fetal/Neonatal Morbidity and Mortality. May cause fetal harm; teratogenicity and embryolethality demonstrated in animals. No adequate and well-controlled studies to date in humans. Pregnancy should be avoided during therapy. If used during pregnancy, apprise of potential fetal hazard.

Hepatic Effects. Reactivation of hepatitis B resulting in death has been reported in a patient receiving temozolomide for glioblastoma. Hepatitis screening and prophylactic therapy with antiviral agents as clinically indicated should be considered in patients receiving temozolomide.

Sensitivity Reactions Allergic reactions, including cases of anaphylaxis and erythema multiforme, have been reported.

General Precautions **Dispensing.** Patients may need to take combinations of temozolomide capsules of different strengths to receive the correct daily dose. (See Dosage and Administration: Reconstitution and Administration.) To minimize the risk of inappropriate dosing, the clinician or pharmacist should provide written instructions for the dosage schedule.

Specific Populations **Pregnancy.** Category D. See Users Guide. (See Warnings: Fetal/Neonatal Morbidity and Mortality, in Cautions.)

Lactation. Not known whether temozolomide is distributed in milk; discontinue nursing because of potential risk in nursing infants.

Pediatric Use. Safety and efficacy in pediatric patients have not been established. Efficacy was not demonstrated in open-label studies of children 3–18 years of age receiving temozolomide mostly for CNS tumors. Similar toxicity was observed in pediatric patients and adults.

Geriatric Use. Experience in those 65 years of age and older insufficient to determine whether they respond differently than younger adults. Caution is advised. (See Warnings: Hematologic Effects, in Cautions and also see Special Populations: Geriatric and Female Patients, in Dosage and Administration.)

An increased incidence of grade 4 thrombocytopenia and/or neutropenia has been reported in patients 70 years of age or older compared with younger patients receiving temozolomide for refractory anaplastic astrocytoma.

Similar toxicity in geriatric patients (65 years of age or older) and younger patients receiving temozolomide for newly diagnosed glioblastoma multiforme.

Severe Hepatic or Renal Impairment. Use with caution. (See Dosage and Administration: Special Populations.)

■ **Common Adverse Effects** Among patients receiving temozolomide for newly diagnosed glioblastoma multiforme, alopecia, fatigue, nausea, vomiting, anorexia, headache, and constipation were most frequent. About half (49%) of patients experienced at least one severe or life-threatening adverse effect, most commonly fatigue (13%), convulsions (6%), headache (5%), or thrombocytopenia (5%).

Among patients receiving temozolomide for anaplastic astrocytoma, nausea, vomiting, headache, and fatigue most frequent and clearly drug related. Adverse effects usually were mild to moderate in severity and self-limiting, with nausea and vomiting controllable with antiemetics. Nausea and vomiting were severe in 10 and 6%, respectively. Myelosuppression also clearly drug related. (See Warnings: Hematologic Effects, in Warnings/Precautions.)

Among patients receiving temozolomide by IV infusion, adverse reactions probably related to treatment that were not reported in patients receiving oral temozolomide include pain, irritation, pruritus, warmth, swelling, erythema at the injection site, petechiae, and hematoma.

Description

Temozolomide, an imidazotetrazine derivative, is an antineoplastic agent. Temozolomide is a prodrug and has little, if any, pharmacologic activity until hydrolyzed in vivo to 5-(3-methyltriazen-1-yl)imidazole-4-carboxamide (MTIC). Following administration of temozolomide, the drug undergoes rapid, nonenzymatic hydrolysis at physiologic pH to MTIC. MTIC is thought to exert its cytotoxic effects by acting as an alkylating agent at the O^6 and N^7 positions of guanine in DNA.

Cytochrome P-450 (CYP) isoenzymes play only a minor role in temozolomide and MTIC metabolism.

Advice to Patients

Importance of adherence to dosage and laboratory appointment schedules.

Importance of *Pneumocystis jiroveci* pneumonia (PCP) prophylaxis for patients with glioblastoma multiforme (see Warnings: Pneumocystis jiroveci Pneumonia, under Warnings/Precautions: Warnings, in Cautions). Importance of patients informing clinicians of signs and symptoms of PCP infection (e.g., shortness of breath, fever, chills, dry cough).

Importance of women informing clinicians immediately if they are or plan to become pregnant or plan to breast-feed; necessity of advising women and men to avoid pregnancy during therapy. Necessity of advising pregnant patient of the risk to the fetus.

Importance of informing clinicians of existing or contemplated concomitant therapy, including prescription and OTC drugs, as well as concomitant illnesses.

Importance of taking temozolomide in a consistent manner relative to food intake to ensure consistent bioavailability and clinical effect. Necessity of swallowing capsules whole, without chewing; need for precautions to avoid exposure to capsule contents (carcinogen potential) and for correct, safe storage and disposal (away from children and pets) of antineoplastic drugs.

Advise of risk of nausea and vomiting. Premedication with antiemetics and bedtime dosing recommended.

Advise of risk of low platelet counts and possible risk of bleeding. Importance of patients informing clinicians of any unusual bruising or bleeding.

Importance of providing a copy of manufacturer's patient information, including written, patient-specific instructions for how to take the medication. (See Dispensing under Warnings/Precautions: General Precautions, in Cautions.)

Overview (see Users Guide). For additional information until a more detailed monograph is developed and published, the manufacturer's labeling should be consulted. It is *essential* that the manufacturer's labeling be consulted for more detailed information on usual cautions, precautions, contraindications, potential drug interactions, laboratory test interferences, and acute toxicity. For further information on the handling of antineoplastic agents, see the ASHP Guidelines on Handling Hazardous Drugs.

Preparations

Excipients in commercially available drug preparations may have clinically important effects in some individuals; consult specific product labeling for details.

Temozolomide

Oral		
Capsules	5 mg	**Temodar®**, Schering
	20 mg	**Temodar®**, Schering
	100 mg	**Temodar®**, Schering
	140 mg	**Temodar®**, Schering
	180 mg	**Temodar®**, Schering
	250 mg	**Temodar®**, Schering
Parenteral		
For injection, for IV infusion	100 mg	**Temodar® for Injection**, Schering

Temsirolimus

■ Temsirolimus, an inhibitor of mammalian target of rapamycin (mTOR) kinase, is an antineoplastic agent.

Uses

■ **Renal Cell Carcinoma** Temsirolimus is used for the treatment of advanced renal cell carcinoma and is designated an orphan drug by the US Food and Drug Administration (FDA) for use in this condition. Some clinicians consider temsirolimus a first-line therapy in poor-risk patients.

The current indication for temsirolimus is based principally on the results of a randomized, open-label, multicenter phase 3 study in 626 patients with previously untreated, poor-prognosis, advanced renal cell carcinoma. In this study, patients were randomized to receive temsirolimus (25 mg IV weekly), interferon alfa (3 million units, increased to up to 18 million units, subcutaneously 3 times weekly), or combination therapy with temsirolimus (15 mg IV weekly) and interferon alfa (3 million units, increased to up to 6 million units, subcutaneously 3 times weekly). Approximately 80% of the patients had some component of clear-cell carcinoma histology, 67% had undergone nephrectomy, and approximately 80% had been diagnosed as having metastatic disease within 12 months prior to study entry. Median overall survival was prolonged in patients receiving temsirolimus alone (10.9 months) compared with those receiving interferon alfa alone (7.3 months.) However, the combination of temsirolimus and interferon alfa did not significantly improve overall survival (8.4 months) compared with interferon alfa alone. Median progression-free survival times, as determined by radiologic assessments performed at 8-week intervals, were 5.5, 3.1, or 4.7 months in patients receiving temsirolimus alone, interferon alfa alone, or the combination regimen, respectively.

Dosage and Administration

■ **General** To minimize risk of hypersensitivity reactions, the manufacturer states that premedication with IV diphenhydramine hydrochloride 25–50 mg (or a similar antihistamine) should be administered about 30 minutes before beginning temsirolimus infusion.

■ **Administration** ***IV Administration*** Temsirolimus is administered by IV infusion.

An infusion pump is used to administer the drug.

Temsirolimus for injection concentrate contains polysorbate 80, which can cause leaching of diethylhexylphthalate (DEHP) from polyvinyl chloride (PVC) infusion bags and administration sets. To minimize exposure of patients to leached DEHP, the final diluted solution of temsirolimus should be stored in glass or polypropylene bottles or in plastic (polypropylene or polyolefin) bags. An inline polyethersulfone filter with a pore size not exceeding 5 μm should be used, and polyethylene-lined administration sets also are recommended.

Temsirolimus for injection concentrate should be protected from light, stored at 2–8°C, and protected from excessive room light and sunlight during handling and preparation.

Dilution. *To avoid precipitation, temsirolimus for injection concentrate must be diluted in a 2-step process prior to administration.*

In the first dilution step, 1.8 mL of the nonaqueous diluent supplied by the manufacturer should be added to a vial labeled as containing 25 mg/mL of temsirolimus (initial total volume of 1.2 mL); the resultant solution contains approximately 10 mg/mL of the drug in a total volume of 3 mL. Contents of the vial should be mixed well by inversion, allowing sufficient time for air bubbles to subside. Temsirolimus solutions that have been diluted to 10 mg/mL (initial dilution) may be stored for up to 24 hours at controlled room temperature.

In the second dilution step, the appropriate dose of temsirolimus should be withdrawn from the vial, then rapidly diluted in 250 mL of 0.9% sodium chloride injection in a suitable container (polypropylene, polyolefin, polyethylene, or glass). The final diluted solution should be mixed by gently inverting the bag or bottle; shaking the container should be avoided to prevent excessive foaming of the solution. Precipitation will occur if *undiluted* temsirolimus for injection concentrate is added directly to an aqueous infusion solution (e.g., 0.9% sodium chloride injection). Administration of the final diluted solution of temsirolimus should be completed within 6 hours of the time that the diluted temsirolimus mixture is added to the sodium chloride injection.

Rate of Administration. Final diluted temsirolimus solutions should be infused IV over 30–60 minutes.

■ **Dosage** ***Renal Cell Carcinoma*** **General Dosage.** The recommended adult dosage of temsirolimus in the treatment of advanced renal cell carcinoma is 25 mg once weekly. Therapy should be continued for as long as the patient derives clinical benefit from the drug or until unacceptable toxicity occurs.

Dosage adjustments of temsirolimus should be considered when used in conjunction with potent inhibitors or inducers of cytochrome P-450 isoenzyme 3A4. (See Drug Interactions.)

Dosage Modification for Toxicity. Therapy should be temporarily interrupted if hematologic toxicities (e.g., absolute neutrophil count less than 1000/mm^3, platelet count less than 75,000/mm^3) or National Cancer Institute (NCI) Common Terminology Criteria for Adverse Events (CTCAE) grade 3 or greater toxicity occurs.

Following resolution of toxicity to grade 2 or less, consideration should be given to resuming temsirolimus at a reduced weekly dosage that is 5 mg less than the previous dosage, but not less than 15 mg weekly.

■ **Special Populations** Dosage reduction or discontinuance may be warranted in patients with hepatic impairment to reduce potential for toxicity, but no specific dosage recommendations at this time. No dosage adjustment is recommended in patients with renal impairment. Temsirolimus has not been studied in patients undergoing hemodialysis. The manufacturer makes no specific geriatric dosage recommendations at this time. (See Specific Populations under Cautions: Warnings/Precautions.)

Cautions

■ **Contraindications** The manufacturer states that there are no known contraindications to the use of temsirolimus.

■ **Warnings/Precautions** ***Sensitivity Reactions*** **Hypersensitivity Reactions.** Anaphylaxis, dyspnea, flushing, and chest pain have been reported.

Temsirolimus should be used with caution in patients with known hypersensitivity to the drug or its metabolites (e.g., sirolimus), polysorbate 80, or any other ingredient in the formulation.

Pretreatment with an antihistamine prior to each dose of temsirolimus is recommended to prevent hypersensitivity reactions. Temsirolimus should be used with caution in patients with known hypersensitivity to antihistamines or with conditions requiring avoidance of antihistamines.

If a hypersensitivity reaction develops, the infusion should be discontinued and the patient observed for at least 30–60 minutes. Treatment may be resumed with administration of a histamine H_1-receptor antagonist (e.g., diphenhydramine hydrochloride), if not previously used, and/or with a histamine H_2-receptor antagonist (e.g., famotidine 20 mg, ranitidine 50 mg) administered IV approximately 30 minutes before restarting the temsirolimus infusion. IV infusion may be resumed at a slower rate (infusion time of up to 60 minutes).

Hyperglycemia Hyperglycemia is likely to develop. Patients may require initiation or increased dosage of insulin and/or an oral hypoglycemic agent. Glucose concentrations should be monitored prior to and during therapy.

Immunosuppression Immunosuppression may occur. Patients should be carefully observed for infections, including opportunistic infections.

Use of live vaccines and close contact with those who have received live vaccines should be avoided during temsirolimus therapy.

Interstitial Lung Disease Interstitial lung disease, sometimes fatal, has occurred. Patients should be observed for signs and symptoms (e.g., dyspnea, cough, hypoxia, fever) and radiographic changes. If interstitial lung disease is suspected, temsirolimus should be discontinued and consideration should be given to use of corticosteroids and/or antibiotics.

Hyperlipemia Hyperlipemia with increased triglycerides and cholesterol is likely to develop. Initiation or increased dosage of a lipid-lowering agent may be required. Serum cholesterol and triglycerides should be monitored prior to and during therapy.

Bowel Perforation Bowel perforations, sometimes fatal, have been reported. Patients with metabolic acidosis, fever, abdominal pain, bloody stools, diarrhea, and/or acute abdomen should be promptly evaluated.

Acute Renal Failure Acute renal failure that is rapidly progressive and sometimes fatal has occurred, which was not clearly related to disease progression. Renal function should be monitored prior to and during therapy. Some patients do not respond to dialysis.

Wound Healing Complications Abnormal wound healing has been reported. The drug should be used with caution in patients during the perioperative period.

Intracerebral Hemorrhage Increased risk of intracerebral bleeding, sometimes fatal, has been reported in patients with primary CNS tumors or metastases and/or in those receiving anticoagulation therapy. (See Drug Interactions: Anticoagulants.)

Drug and Food Interactions Patients should avoid concomitant use of temsirolimus with certain drugs (e.g., potent inhibitors or inducers of cytochrome P-450 isoenzyme 3A4) or foods (e.g., grapefruit juice); if alternative treatment cannot be given, adjustment of temsirolimus dosage is recommended. (See Drug Interactions.)

Fetal/Neonatal Morbidity and Mortality Temsirolimus may cause fetal harm. Animal studies indicate adverse effects on embryofetal development.

Women should avoid becoming pregnant during and for 3 months after discontinuing temsirolimus therapy. If used during pregnancy or if patient becomes pregnant, apprise of potential fetal hazard.

Male patients with partners of childbearing potential also should use reliable contraception during temsirolimus treatment and for 3 months after the last dose.

Adequate Patient Evaluation and Monitoring Complete blood cell counts (CBCs) and chemistry panels should be monitored periodically in patients receiving temsirolimus. In clinical trials, CBC was assessed prior to and on a weekly basis during therapy; chemistry panels were assessed every 2 weeks. These tests may be monitored more or less frequently during temsirolimus therapy at the discretion of the clinician.

Glucose and lipid profiles and renal function tests also should be monitored periodically.

Specific Populations **Pregnancy.** Category D. (See Fetal/Neonatal Morbidity and Mortality under Cautions, and also see Users Guide.)

Lactation. Not known whether temsirolimus is distributed into milk; discontinue nursing or the drug, taking into account the importance of the drug to the woman.

Pediatric Use. Safety and efficacy not established in pediatric patients.

Geriatric Use. Insufficient experience in patients 65 years of age or older to determine whether geriatric patients respond differently than younger adults.

Hepatic Impairment. Safety and efficacy in patients with hepatic impairment not studied specifically to date; studies in this patient population are ongoing.

Renal Impairment. Safety and efficacy in patients with renal impairment not studied specifically to date. Renal impairment is not expected to substantially alter systemic exposure to the drug.

■ **Common Adverse Effects** Adverse reactions reported in 30% or more of patients receiving temsirolimus include rash, asthenia, mucositis/stomatitis, nausea, edema, anorexia, anemia, hyperglycemia, hyperlipemia, hypertriglyceridemia, lymphopenia, increased alkaline phosphatase, increased serum creatinine, hypophosphatemia, thrombocytopenia, increased AST (SGOT) levels, and leukopenia.

Drug Interactions

Both temsirolimus and its principal active metabolite, sirolimus, are metabolized by cytochrome P-450 (CYP) isoenzyme 3A4. In vitro studies using human liver microsomes indicate that temsirolimus inhibits CYP isoenzymes 2D6 and 3A4.

■ **Drugs Affecting Hepatic Microsomal Enzymes** CYP3A4 inhibitors: Potential pharmacokinetic interaction (increased plasma concentrations of the principal active metabolite sirolimus). Concomitant use with a potent CYP3A4 inhibitors should be avoided; if no alternative is available, consideration should be given to temsirolimus dosage adjustment.

CYP3A4 inducers: Potential pharmacokinetic interaction (decreased plasma concentrations of the principal active metabolite sirolimus). Concomitant use with potent CYP3A4 inducers should be avoided; if no alternative is available, consideration should be given to temsirolimus dosage adjustment.

For specific recommendations when temsirolimus is used concomitantly with a potent inhibitor or inducer of CYP3A4, see the following sections on interactions with specific drugs or drug classes.

■ **Drugs Metabolized by Hepatic Microsomal Enzymes** Substrates of CYP2D6 and CYP3A4: No evidence of clinically important effects in drug interaction studies with substrates of CYP2D6; no effect on substrates of CYP3A4 is anticipated.

■ **Angiotensin-converting Enzyme Inhibitors** Angioedema-type reactions observed during concomitant therapy with angiotensin-converting enzyme (ACE) inhibitors. Caution is advised.

■ **Anticoagulants** Increased risk of intracerebral bleeding in patients receiving concomitant therapy. Caution is advised.

■ **Anticonvulsants** Decreased plasma sirolimus concentrations may occur during concomitant therapy with anticonvulsants that are potent CYP3A4 inducers (e.g., carbamazepine, phenobarbital, phenytoin). Temsirolimus dosage should be increased from 25 mg weekly to 50 mg weekly; if the anticonvulsant is discontinued, temsirolimus dosage should be resumed at previous level.

■ **Azole Antifungals** Increased plasma sirolimus concentrations may occur during concomitant therapy with azole antifungals (e.g., itraconazole, ketoconazole, voriconazole). Temsirolimus dosage should be decreased from 25 mg weekly to 12.5 mg weekly; if the antifungal is discontinued, an interval of 1 week should be allowed before resuming previous level of temsirolimus dosage.

■ **Antimycobacterials** Decreased plasma sirolimus concentrations reported during concomitant therapy with rifamycin antimycobacterials (e.g., rifabutin, rifampin). Temsirolimus dosage should be increased from 25 mg weekly to 50 mg weekly; if the antimycobacterial is discontinued, temsirolimus dosage should be resumed at previous level.

■ **Dexamethasone** Decreased plasma sirolimus concentrations may occur during concomitant therapy with dexamethasone. Temsirolimus dosage should be increased from 25 mg weekly to 50 mg weekly; if dexamethasone is discontinued, temsirolimus dosage should be resumed at previous level.

■ **Grapefruit Juice** Increased plasma sirolimus concentrations may occur during concomitant use with grapefruit juice. Such concomitant use should be avoided.

■ **HIV Protease Inhibitors** Increased plasma sirolimus concentrations may occur during concomitant therapy with HIV protease inhibitors (e.g., atazanavir, indinavir, nelfinavir, ritonavir, saquinavir). Temsirolimus dosage should be decreased from 25 mg weekly to 12.5 mg weekly; if the HIV protease inhibitor is discontinued, an interval of 1 week should be allowed before resuming previous level of temsirolimus dosage.

■ **Macrolides** Increased plasma sirolimus concentrations may occur during concomitant therapy with macrolide anti-infectives (e.g., clarithromycin, telithromycin). Temsirolimus dosage should be decreased from 25 mg weekly to 12.5 mg weekly; if the macrolide is discontinued, an interval of 1 week should be allowed before resuming previous level of temsirolimus dosage.

■ **Nefazodone** Increased plasma sirolimus concentrations may occur during concomitant therapy with nefazodone. Temsirolimus dosage should be decreased from 25 mg weekly to 12.5 mg weekly; if nefazodone is discontinued, an interval of 1 week should be allowed before resuming previous level of temsirolimus dosage.

■ **St. John's Wort (*Hypericum perforatum*)** Unpredictable decreases in plasma temsirolimus concentrations reported with concomitant use. Concomitant use should be avoided.

■ **Sunitinib** Increased risk of dose-limiting toxicity requiring hospitalization (e.g., grade 3/4 erythematous maculopapular rash, gout/cellulitis) reported with concurrent use.

Description

Temsirolimus, an inhibitor of mammalian target of rapamycin (mTOR) kinase, is an antineoplastic agent. Receptor tyrosine kinases (RTKs) are involved in the initiation of various cascades of intracellular signaling events that lead to cell proliferation and/or influence processes critical to cell survival and tumor progression (e.g., angiogenesis, metastasis), inhibition of apoptosis. Although the exact mechanism of action has not been fully elucidated, temsirolimus binds with high affinity to the intracellular protein FK506 binding protein-12 in vitro, forming a drug-protein complex that inhibits the activation of mTOR, which regulates cell division. This disruption of mTOR signaling suppresses proteins that regulate cell-cycle progression, thereby blocking cells in the G_1 phase of the cell cycle. Inhibition of mTOR by temsirolimus also has been associated with reduced expression of hypoxia inducible factor 1α and 2α (HIF-1α and HIF-2α) in vitro, resulting in reduced expression of vascular endothelial growth factor (VEGF) and a potential antiangiogenic effect.

Temsirolimus inhibited T lymphocyte activity in mice, but the effects were reversible and T lymphocyte activity returned to normal within 24 hours of discontinuance. No consistent effect on lymphocyte population or activation was demonstrated in humans. However, infections may result from immunosuppression.

Temsirolimus is metabolized by hydrolysis to sirolimus, the principal active metabolite. Both temsirolimus and sirolimus also are metabolized by cytochrome P-450 (CYP) isoenzyme 3A4. Although temsirolimus is metabolized to sirolimus, temsirolimus itself exhibits antitumor activity and is not considered a prodrug. Following IV administration of a single radiolabeled dose of temsirolimus, approximately 78% of the total radioactivity is recovered in feces and 4.6% in urine within 14 days.

Advice to Patients

Risk of serious allergic reactions, including anaphylaxis; importance of immediately reporting any facial swelling or difficulty breathing.

Risk of increased blood glucose levels; importance of reporting excessive thirst or any increase in volume or frequency of urination.

Risk of increased triglyceride and/or cholesterol levels.

Risk of increased susceptibility to infection; risk of renal failure.

Risk of abnormal wound healing in the event that surgery is performed within a few weeks of therapy initiation or during therapy.

Risk of interstitial lung disease, which may be fatal; importance of reporting any new or worsening respiratory symptoms.

Risk of bowel perforation, which may be fatal; importance of reporting any new or worsening abdominal pain or blood in stools.

Importance of advising patients with CNS tumors and/or receiving anticoagulant therapy of the potential for increased risk of intracerebral bleeding, which may be fatal.

Risk of decreased efficacy of vaccination; importance of not receiving live vaccines and of avoiding close contact with those who have received live vaccines.

Importance of informing clinicians of existing or contemplated concomitant therapy, including prescription and OTC drugs, as well as any concomitant illnesses.

Importance of women informing clinicians if they are or plan to become pregnant or plan to breast-feed; necessity for clinicians to advise women of childbearing potential and men with partners of childbearing potential to avoid pregnancy and to use effective contraceptive methods during therapy and for 3 months following discontinuance of therapy.

Importance of informing patients of other important precautionary information. (See Cautions.)

Overview® (see Users Guide). For additional information on this drug until a more detailed monograph is developed and published, the manufacturer's labeling should be consulted. It is *essential* that the manufacturer's labeling be consulted for more detailed information on usual cautions, precautions, contraindications, potential drug interactions, laboratory test interferences, and acute toxicity.

Preparations

Excipients in commercially available drug preparations may have clinically important effects in some individuals; consult specific product labeling for details.

Temsirolimus

Parenteral		
For injection concentrate, for IV infusion only	25 mg/mL (30 mg)	**Torisel®**, Wyeth

Topotecan Hydrochloride

■ Topotecan, a semisynthetic derivative of camptothecin is an antineoplastic agent.

Uses

■ **Ovarian Cancer** Topotecan is used IV for the treatment of advanced ovarian cancer in patients with disease that has recurred or progressed following therapy with platinum-based (i.e., cisplatin, carboplatin) regimens. The current indication for use of IV topotecan is based principally on data from 2 clinical trials (including a multicenter, randomized study comparing topotecan with paclitaxel) in patients with advanced ovarian cancer. In these clinical trials, topotecan was administered at an initial dosage of 1.5 mg/m² IV over 30 minutes once daily for 5 days (as tolerated) followed by 16 treatment-free days (total of 21 days per treatment course); dosage of topotecan in subsequent cycles was adjusted according to hematologic tolerance.

In a randomized trial of patients receiving IV topotecan versus paclitaxel (175 mg/m² IV over 3 hours once every 21 days), respectively, the overall response rate (21 versus 14%), the median response duration (25.9 versus 21.6 weeks), and the median survival duration (63 versus 53 weeks) were similar. In patients receiving topotecan, the median time to response was longer (7.6 versus 6 weeks), but median time to disease progression was prolonged (18.9 versus 14.7 weeks), compared with patients receiving paclitaxel. Patients with disease that did not respond to, or progressed during, the initially assigned therapy were allowed to subsequently receive the alternative therapy. Among

61 patients receiving topotecan following initial therapy with paclitaxel, 8 patients (13%) had an objective response (all partial responses); among 49 patients receiving paclitaxel following initial therapy with topotecan, 5 patients (10%) had an objective response (2 complete responses, 3 partial responses). Hematologic toxicity, including grade 4 neutropenia, grade 4 thrombocytopenia, and grade 3 or 4 anemia, occurred more frequently during topotecan therapy. In a separate analysis of a subset of patients with disease resistant to platinum-containing therapy (defined as tumor progression during therapy or relapse within 6 months following completion of therapy), treatment with topotecan or paclitaxel was associated with an overall response rate of 12 or 7%, respectively; all responses were partial responses except for 1 complete response in a patient receiving topotecan.

In an open-label trial, responses were observed in 14% of patients receiving IV topotecan as second-line therapy for resistant or recurrent ovarian cancer following treatment with a platinum-containing regimen. The median duration of response in these patients was 22 weeks (range: 4.6–41.9 weeks), the median time to disease progression was 11.3 weeks (range: 0.7–72.1 weeks), and the median survival was 67.9 weeks (range: 1.4–112.9 weeks).

■ **Small Cell Lung Cancer** Topotecan is used orally and IV as second-line therapy for treatment-sensitive small cell lung cancer. The current indication for use of oral topotecan monotherapy is based principally on data from a randomized, open-label, multicenter phase 3 trial comparing oral topotecan and best supportive care with best supportive care alone in 141 patients with recurrent small cell lung cancer. Eligible patients included those who achieved a complete or partial response to first-line chemotherapy, those who were not considered suitable for further IV chemotherapy (i.e., those with resistant disease based on short disease-free interval, presence of comorbidities, or those who refused additional parenteral chemotherapy), and patients who had relapsed at least 45 days after the completion of a prior chemotherapy regimen (i.e., to ensure adequate bone marrow recovery). The median treatment-free interval after first-line therapy for patients randomized to oral topotecan and best supportive care or best supportive care alone was 84 or 90 days, respectively. Patients randomized to oral topotecan received a dosage of 2.3 mg/m^2 daily on days 1–5 of a 21-day cycle; patients received a median of 4 cycles (range: 1–10). Based on an intent-to-treat analysis, an improvement in median overall survival (i.e., all-cause mortality) was observed in patients receiving topotecan and best supportive care (25.9 weeks) compared with those receiving best supportive care alone (13.9 weeks); 6-month survival rates also improved in patients receiving oral topotecan (49%) compared with those receiving best supportive care alone (26%). An improvement in median survival also was reported in poor-risk patients receiving oral topotecan including those with chemoresistant disease (defined by a disease-free interval of 60 days or less) or with an Eastern Cooperative Oncology Group (ECOG) performance status of 2 or less. In the oral topotecan group, partial response and stabilization of disease were achieved in 7 and 44% of patients, respectively. Responses from patient questionnaires also indicated a slower decline in health-related quality of life measures (performed at 3-month intervals) in patients receiving oral topotecan; control of symptoms such as dyspnea, sleep interference, and fatigue was greater with use of oral topotecan and best supportive care compared with best supportive care alone.

In the group receiving oral topotecan, grade 3/4 cytopenias, including neutropenia, thrombocytopenia, and anemia, were reported in 61, 37, and 25% of patients, respectively. Severe (grade 3/4) diarrhea also was reported in 5% of patients receiving the drug.

Safety and efficacy of oral topotecan have been compared directly with IV topotecan as second-line therapy in a randomized, open-label, phase 3 study of 309 patients with recurrent, treatment-sensitive small cell lung cancer. Eligible patients included those with disease recurrence at least 90 days following completion of first-line chemotherapy. Patients were randomized to receive either oral topotecan (2.3 mg/m^2 daily) or IV topotecan (1.5 mg/m^2 over 30 minutes daily) on days 1–5 of a 21-day cycle; patients received a median of 4 cycles. Overall response was similar between the two treatment groups with rates of 18.3 and 21.9% reported for oral and IV topotecan, respectively. Similar improvement in median survival time also was reported for patients receiving oral topotecan (33 weeks) compared with IV topotecan (35 weeks). However, the trial was not adequately powered to demonstrate an improvement in survival outcome for one particular regimen.

In this study, the incidence of grade 3 neutropenia was similar in both treatment groups; however, grade 4 neutropenia was reported more frequently (64 versus 47%) in patients receiving IV compared with oral topotecan, respectively. Antibiotic usage also was slightly higher in patients receiving IV topotecan compared with those receiving oral therapy. In addition, granulocyte colony-stimulating factor (G-CSF, filgrastim) was used in a higher percentage (25 versus 16%) of patients receiving oral than IV topotecan, respectively. Diarrhea was a frequently reported adverse event with oral topotecan; grade 3/4 diarrhea occurred in 7.9 compared with 2.7% of patients receiving oral or IV topotecan, respectively. In patients reporting diarrhea with oral topotecan, the symptoms were characterized as self-limiting or manageable with standard antidiarrhea treatment (e.g., loperamide).

Some experts state that use of oral topotecan is a reasonable alternative for patients with recurrent small cell lung cancer who cannot tolerate the IV formulation of the drug.

In the clinical studies submitted to support the labeled indication of IV topotecan for use in small cell lung cancer, treatment-sensitive small cell lung cancer was defined as disease initially responding to first-line chemotherapy with subsequent relapse no sooner than 60–90 days following completion of first-line therapy.

The current indication for use of IV topotecan in recurrent small cell lung cancer is based principally on data from a randomized, multicenter, phase 3 trial and 3 uncontrolled, phase 2 studies. Results from a large randomized trial indicate that IV topotecan used as a single agent is as effective as combination chemotherapy with cyclophosphamide, doxorubicin, and vincristine (CAV) for the treatment of recurrent small cell lung cancer. In this trial, 211 patients with small cell lung cancer that relapsed at least 60 days following completion of first-line chemotherapy were randomized to receive either IV topotecan (1.5 mg/m^2 IV over 30 minutes daily on days 1–5) or combination chemotherapy with CAV (sequential administration of cyclophosphamide 1000 mg/m^2, doxorubicin 45 mg/m^2, and vincristine 2 mg on day 1) on a 21-day cycle; in patients experiencing an objective response, therapy was continued until disease progression or unacceptable toxicity occurred, or for at least 6 courses past the maximal response. About 80% of the patients receiving IV topotecan or CAV had received a platinum-containing agent and etoposide, with or without other agents, as initial treatment for small cell lung cancer. The overall response rate was similar in patients receiving IV topotecan (24.3%, all partial responses) or CAV (18.3%, 1% complete responses). Among patients receiving IV topotecan or CAV, respectively, the median time to progression (13.3 versus 12.3 weeks) and the median survival duration (25 versus 24.7 weeks) also were comparable. IV topotecan was more effective than CAV for palliation of symptoms, including dyspnea, anorexia, hoarseness, fatigue, and interference with daily activity.

Grade 4 neutropenia was reported in about 70% of patients receiving either IV topotecan or CAV but occurred more frequently in treatment courses with CAV (51.4%) versus IV topotecan (37.8%). IV topotecan was associated with a higher incidence of grade 4 thrombocytopenia (29 versus 5%) and grade 3 or 4 anemia (42 versus 20%) than combination chemotherapy with CAV. Cardiac toxicity with reduction in left ventricular ejection fraction occurred more frequently in patients receiving CAV than in those receiving IV topotecan (17.1 versus 7.7%, respectively).

In 3 uncontrolled phase 2 studies of IV topotecan for the treatment of recurrent or progressive small cell lung cancer, objective response rates ranged from 11–31% in patients with treatment-sensitive disease (defined as progression of disease at least 90 days following completion of therapy) and from 2–7% in patients with refractory disease (defined as progression of disease during, or within 90 days of completion of, first-line therapy).

■ **Cervical Cancer** Topotecan is used IV in combination with cisplatin for the treatment of stage IVB, recurrent or persistent cervical cancer that is not amenable to curative treatment with surgery and/or radiation therapy.

The current indication for use of IV topotecan in combination with cisplatin for advanced cervical cancer is based on the results of a randomized trial in which patients received cisplatin alone, topotecan and cisplatin, or methotrexate, vinblastine, doxorubicin, and cisplatin (MVAC). Following 4 deaths related to treatment, the MVAC arm of the trial was closed, and the data for these patients were excluded from this analysis. In the remaining arms, treatment consisted of combination therapy with topotecan 0.75 mg/m^2 IV over 30 minutes for 3 consecutive days starting on day 1 of a 21-day course plus cisplatin 50 mg/m^2 on day 1; or cisplatin alone (same cisplatin dosage as in combination regimen). About half (56%) of the patients in each arm had received previous treatment with cisplatin (alone or with other agents) as first-line therapy.

Among 293 patients receiving either IV topotecan and cisplatin or cisplatin alone for advanced cervical cancer, median survival was prolonged (9.4 versus 6.5 months, hazard ratio: 0.76) for patients receiving the combination regimen. Despite greater hematologic toxicity among patients receiving combination therapy, quality of life scores were similar in patients receiving topotecan and cisplatin or cisplatin alone. Adverse dermatologic effects, infection/febrile neutropenia, cardiovascular and hepatic toxicity, and stomatitis/pharyngitis were more frequent in patients receiving combination therapy with topotecan and cisplatin compared with cisplatin alone.

Dosage and Administration

■ **Reconstitution and Administration** Topotecan hydrochloride capsules are administered orally and may be taken with or without food. The capsules should be swallowed whole and should not be crushed, chewed, divided, or opened. If vomiting occurs following administration of oral topotecan, a replacement dose should *not* be administered.

Topotecan hydrochloride for injection concentrate is administered by IV infusion only. Care should be taken to avoid extravasation of the drug; inadvertent extravasation of topotecan has been associated with mild local reactions such as erythema and bruising.

Commercially available topotecan hydrochloride for injection concentrate must be diluted prior to IV administration. The drug is reconstituted by adding 4 mL of sterile water for injection to the vial labeled as containing 4 mg of topotecan in order to provide a solution containing 1 mg/mL of topotecan. The calculated daily dose of topotecan is then diluted in a suitable volume (e.g., 50–250 mL) of 5% dextrose or 0.9% sodium chloride injection and infused IV over a period of 30 minutes. The manufacturer states that solutions of topotecan hydrochloride should be prepared immediately before use since the lyophilized drug does not contain a preservative.

Topotecan hydrochloride for injection concentrate should be inspected visually for particulate matter in the vial and again in the syringe when transferring the drug solution to prepare admixtures of the drug. As with all parenteral products, diluted solutions of the drug should be inspected visually for particulate matter and discoloration prior to administration whenever solution and container permit.

The manufacturer recommends that procedures for proper handling and disposal of antineoplastic drugs (e.g., use of protective clothing and gloves, preparation of drug solutions under a vertical laminar flow hood) be used to avoid exposure to topotecan during preparation of IV solutions. If topotecan hydrochloride or a solution of the drug comes in contact with the skin or mucous membranes, the skin should be washed immediately and thoroughly with soap and water or the mucosa should be flushed with copious amounts of water.

■ **Dosage** Dosage of oral and IV topotecan hydrochloride is expressed in terms of topotecan. Dosage of the drug must be individualized based on body surface area and patient tolerance.

Ovarian Cancer For the treatment of metastatic cancer of the ovary in patients with disease that has recurred or progressed following therapy with platinum-based (i.e., cisplatin, carboplatin) regimens, the recommended initial dose of topotecan is 1.5 mg/m^2 infused IV over a period of 30 minutes; this dose is administered daily for 5 consecutive days followed by a 16-day rest period for a 21-day treatment course. In patients without progression of disease, the manufacturer recommends a minimum of 4 courses of topotecan therapy (provided that intolerable toxicity does not develop) because median time to response was 9–12 weeks in 3 clinical trials in patients with metastatic ovarian cancer, and response may not be achieved if therapy with the drug is discontinued prematurely.

Small Cell Lung Cancer **Oral.** When used orally for the treatment of recurrent small cell lung cancer following initial response to chemotherapy, the recommended initial dosage of topotecan is 2.3 mg/m^2 administered once daily for 5 consecutive days followed by a 16-day rest period for a 21-day treatment course. The calculated daily dosage should be rounded to the nearest 0.25 mg, and the minimum number of capsules containing 0.25 and 1 mg should be prescribed. The same number of 0. 25-mg and 1-mg capsules should be administered for each of the 5 dosing days. Although the manufacturer does not recommend a specific number of cycles for the treatment of small cell lung cancer, at least 4 treatment cycles of oral topotecan were used in a controlled clinical trial.

IV. When used IV for the treatment of recurrent small cell lung cancer following initial response to chemotherapy, the recommended initial dosage of topotecan is 1.5 mg/m^2 infused over a period of 30 minutes; this dosage is administered daily for 5 consecutive days followed by a 16-day rest period for a 21-day treatment course. In patients without progression of disease, the manufacturer recommends a minimum of 4 courses of IV topotecan therapy (provided that intolerable toxicity does not develop) because median time to response was 5–7 weeks in 4 small clinical trials in patients with small cell lung cancer, and response may not be achieved if therapy with the drug is discontinued prematurely.

Cervical Cancer For the treatment of stage IVB, recurrent or persistent cervical cancer that is not amenable to curative treatment with surgery and/or radiation therapy, the recommended dose of topotecan is 0.75 mg/m^2 infused IV over a period of 30 minutes; this dose is administered daily for 3 consecutive days (days 1–3) and on day 1 is followed by IV cisplatin 50 mg/m^2 for each 21-day course.

Dosage Modification for Toxicity The dose-limiting toxicity of topotecan therapy is myelosuppression. Because neutropenia occurs frequently during topotecan therapy and may be severe and potentially fatal, it is essential that bone marrow function be monitored through evaluation of peripheral blood cell counts before and during topotecan therapy.

Before the initial course of therapy with either oral or IV topotecan, patients must have a baseline neutrophil count of at least 1500/mm^3 and a platelet count of at least 100,000/mm^3. Bone marrow reserves should be evaluated frequently during topotecan therapy using peripheral blood cell counts, and subsequent courses of therapy should be withheld until the neutrophil count exceeds 1000/mm^3, platelet count exceeds 100,000/mm^3, and hemoglobin concentration is at least 9 g/dL (with transfusion if necessary).

Oral. If severe neutropenia (defined by National Cancer Institute [NCI] Common Toxicity Criteria as grade 4, (i.e., an absolute neutrophil count [ANC] less than 500/mm^3) occurs with any course of oral topotecan therapy for small cell lung cancer and is associated with fever or infection or has a duration of 7 days or longer, or if moderate neutropenia (i.e., ANC 500–1000/mm^3) persists beyond day 21 of a treatment course, the dosage of topotecan in subsequent courses should be reduced by 0.4 mg/m^2 daily (to 1.9 mg/m^2).

If the platelet count falls below 25,000/mm^3 during any course of oral topotecan therapy, the dosage of topotecan should be reduced by 0.4 mg/m^2 daily (to 1.9 mg/m^2) in subsequent courses.

If grade 3 or 4 diarrhea occurs during any course of oral topotecan therapy, the dosage of topotecan in subsequent courses should be reduced by 0.4 mg/m^2 daily (to 1.9 mg/m^2). The manufacturer states that the same dosage modification for oral topotecan also may be necessary in patients reporting mild diarrhea (grade 2) during therapy. (See Warnings: GI Effects.)

IV. If severe neutropenia (defined by NCI Common Toxicity Criteria as grade 4, (i.e., ANC less than 500/mm^3) occurs with any course of IV topotecan monotherapy of ovarian or small cell lung cancer, the dose of topotecan in subsequent courses should be reduced by 0.25 mg/m^2 (to 1.25 mg/m^2); alternatively, G-CSF (filgrastim) may be administered following the subsequent course. If severe neutropenia occurs in a treatment course and therapy with filgrastim is preferred to reduction of IV topotecan dosage in the subsequent course, filgrastim should be initiated 24 hours after the final dose of IV topotecan in the subsequent treatment course (i.e., beginning on day 6 of the 21-day treatment course) since concurrent therapy with filgrastim and IV topotecan can increase the severity and duration of neutropenia.

If the platelet count falls below 25,000/mm^3 with any course of IV topotecan monotherapy, the dose of topotecan in subsequent courses should be reduced by 0.25 mg/m^2 (to 1.25 mg/m^2).

Myelosuppression may be greater when IV topotecan is used in combination with other cytotoxic agents, and dose reduction may be necessary. (See Drug Interactions: Antineoplastic Agents.) If severe febrile neutropenia (i.e., ANC less than 1000/mm^3 with temperature of 38°C) occurs when IV topotecan is being used in combination with cisplatin for treatment of cervical cancer, the dose of topotecan should be reduced by 20% to 0.6 mg/m^2 for subsequent courses of therapy. Similarly, if the platelet count falls below 25,000/mm^3, the dose of IV topotecan should be reduced by 20% to 0.6 mg/m^2. If severe febrile neutropenia occurs in a treatment course and therapy with filgrastim is preferred to reduction of topotecan dosage in the subsequent course, filgrastim should be initiated 24 hours after the final dose of topotecan in the subsequent treatment course (i.e., beginning on day 4 of the 21-day treatment course). If febrile neutropenia occurs despite the use of filgrastim, the dose of IV topotecan should be further reduced by 20% to 0.45 mg/m^2 for subsequent courses of therapy. For administration and hydration guidelines for cisplatin and for recommendations for dosage reduction for cisplatin in the event of hematologic toxicity, see the manufacturer's labeling for cisplatin.

■ **Dosage in Renal and Hepatic Impairment** In patients with impaired renal function receiving oral or IV topotecan monotherapy, the dosage of topotecan must be modified in response to the degree of renal impairment.

For patients receiving oral topotecan for treatment of small cell lung cancer, dosage adjustment is *not*recommended for patients with creatinine clearance of 50–80 mL/minute; however, for patients with creatinine clearance of 30–49 mL/minute, the dosage of oral topotecan should be reduced to 1.8 mg/m^2 daily (rounded to the nearest 0.25 mg). The manufacturer states that insufficient data are available to provide a dosage recommendation for oral topotecan in patients with creatinine clearance less than 30 mL/minute.

For patients receiving IV topotecan, no dosage adjustment is recommended for patients with creatinine clearance of 40–60 mL/minute; however the dosage of IV topotecan should be reduced to 0.75 mg/m^2 in patients with creatinine clearance of 20–39 mL/minute. The manufacturer states that insufficient data are available to provide a dosage recommendation for IV topotecan in patients with creatinine clearance less than 19 mL/minute.

In patients with cervical cancer, therapy with IV topotecan and cisplatin should be initiated only in those with serum creatinine concentrations of 1.5 mg/dL or less. In the clinical trial, cisplatin therapy was discontinued in patients with a serum creatinine concentration exceeding 1.5 mg/dL. No data are available regarding the safety or efficacy of continued therapy with topotecan following discontinuance of cisplatin therapy in patients with cervical cancer.

In geriatric patients, no adjustments in either oral or IV topotecan dosage appear to be required other than those related to decreases in renal function with age. Because geriatric patients are more likely to have decreased renal function and because patients with renal impairment may be at increased risk of topotecan-induced toxicity, care should be taken in dosage selection for patients in this age group and renal function should be monitored.

Clinically important alterations in the pharmacokinetics of oral or IV topotecan in patients with impaired hepatic function (i.e., plasma bilirubin greater than 1.5 to less than 15 mg/dL) have not been observed to date, and the manufacturer makes no specific recommendations for dosage modification in such patients.

Cautions

The data on adverse effects are based on the experience of 682 patients with lung cancer (recurrent small cell lung cancer and non-small cell lung cancer) receiving at least one dose of oral topotecan in clinical studies. Among patients receiving oral topotecan for lung cancer, the treatment-related death rate was 5.7%. In addition, safety data are reported based on the experience of 879 patients receiving IV topotecan 1.5 mg/m^2 daily for 5 days for metastatic ovarian cancer (453 patients) or recurrent or progressive small cell lung cancer (426 patients) and 140 patients receiving IV topotecan 0.75 mg/m^2 daily for 3 consecutive days with cisplatin 50 mg/m^2 on day 1 for advanced cervical cancer. Among patients receiving IV topotecan for ovarian cancer, the treatment-related death rate was 1%. Among patients receiving IV topotecan for small cell lung cancer, the treatment-related death rate was 5%.

■ **Hematologic Effects and Infectious Complications** Hematologic toxicity generally occurs in all patients receiving oral or IV topotecan. Myelosuppression, mainly neutropenia, may be severe in patients receiving topotecan, and can result in infection and death. Topotecan-induced neutropenia is not cumulative over time. Pancytopenia also has been reported with topotecan.

Leukopenia is the dose-limiting toxicity of topotecan, and the white blood cell count decreases with increasing dosage or increasing area under the concentration-time curve (AUC) of topotecan. For orally administered topotecan, an association between topotecan AUC on day 1 and observed myelosuppression has been established. The AUC of the pharmacologically active form of the drug, topotecan lactone (i.e., over a treatment course), also may correlate with the level of hematologic toxicity (i.e., leukopenia). Among patients receiving oral topotecan for lung cancer (recurrent small cell lung cancer and non-small cell lung cancer), leukopenia (less than 3000 cells/mm^3) occurred in 86% of patients and grade 4 leukopenia (less than 1000 cells/mm^3) was reported in 15% of patients.

Among patients receiving IV topotecan for ovarian cancer or small cell lung cancer, leukopenia (less than 3000 cells/mm^3) occurred in 97% and grade 4 leukopenia (less than 1000 cells/mm^3) occurred in 32% of patients. Following the first cycle of topotecan 1.5 mg/m^2 IV for 5 days, an 80–90% decrease in white blood cell count typically is observed at nadir.

Among patients receiving oral topotecan for lung cancer (recurrent small cell lung cancer and non-small cell lung cancer), neutropenia occurred in 83% and grade 3 and 4 neutropenia (less than 500 cells/mm^3) occurred in 24 and 32% of patients, respectively. Grade 4 neutropenia was most common during the first course of therapy (20% of patients) and occurred for a median duration of 7 days. Febrile neutropenic episodes were reported in 4% of patients; fatal sepsis occurred in 1% of patients receiving oral topotecan in clinical trials.

Among patients receiving IV topotecan for ovarian cancer or small cell lung cancer, neutropenia (less than 1500 cells/mm^3) occurred in 97% and grade 4 neutropenia (less than 500 cells/mm^3) occurred in 78% of patients. Grade 4 neutropenia was common during the first course of therapy (60% of patients). Grade 4 neutropenia occurred in 39% of all treatment courses for a median duration of 7 days. The nadir neutrophil count was reached at a median of 12 days. Intravenous topotecan-induced sepsis or febrile neutropenia occurred in 23% of patients; fatal sepsis occurred in 1% of patients receiving IV topotecan in clinical trials. Among patients receiving IV topotecan and cisplatin for cervical cancer, neutropenia (less than 2000 cells/mm^3) occurred in 89%, grade 3 neutropenia (less than 1000 cells/mm^3 to 500 cells/mm^3) occurred in 26%, and grade 4 neutropenia (less than 500 cells/mm^3) occurred in 48% of patients. Infection or febrile neutropenia occurred in 28% of such patients and was grade 3 in 15% and grade 4 in 4% of patients.

Among patients receiving oral topotecan for lung cancer (recurrent small cell lung cancer and non-small cell lung cancer), thrombocytopenia occurred in 81%; grade 4 thrombocytopenia (less than 10,000 cells/mm^3) occurred in 6% of patients for a median duration of 3 days.

Among patients receiving IV topotecan for ovarian cancer or small cell lung cancer, thrombocytopenia (less than 75,000 cells/mm^3) occurred in 69% and grade 4 thrombocytopenia (less than 25,000 cells/mm^3) occurred in 27% of patients. Grade 4 thrombocytopenia occurred in 9% of all treatment courses for a median duration of 5 days. The nadir platelet count was reached at a median of 15 days. Platelet transfusions were administered to 15% of patients in 4% of treatment courses with IV topotecan. Among patients receiving IV topotecan and cisplatin for cervical cancer, thrombocytopenia (less than 130,000 cells/mm^3) occurred in 74%, grade 3 thrombocytopenia (less than 50,000 cells/mm^3 to 10,000 cells/mm^3) occurred in 26%, and grade 4 thrombocytopenia (less than 10,000 cells/mm^3) occurred in 7% of patients.

Among patients receiving oral topotecan for lung cancer (recurrent small cell lung cancer and non-small cell lung cancer), anemia occurred in 98% and grade 3 or 4 anemia (hemoglobin less than 8 g/dL) occurred in 25% of patients.

Among patients receiving IV topotecan for ovarian cancer or small cell lung cancer, anemia (hemoglobin less than 10 g/dL) occurred in 89% and grade 3 or 4 anemia (hemoglobin less than 8 g/dL) occurred in 37% of patients. Grade 3 or 4 anemia occurred in 14% of all treatment courses. The nadir erythrocyte count was reached at a median of 15 days. Red blood cell transfusions were administered to 52% of patients in 22% of treatment courses with topotecan. Among patients receiving IV topotecan and cisplatin for cervical cancer, anemia (hemoglobin less than 12 g/dL) occurred in 94%, grade 3 anemia (less than 8 g/dL to 6.5 g/dL) occurred in 34%, and grade 4 anemia (less than 6.5 g/dL) occurred in 6% of patients.

■ **Neutropenic Colitis** Neutropenic colitis (typhlitis), a sequela of drug-induced neutropenia, has been reported with oral and IV topotecan and can be fatal. Cases of neutropenic colitis have occurred in patients receiving IV topotecan as part of some combination chemotherapy regimens†, in patients with acute leukemia†, or in pediatric patients†.

The possibility of neutropenic colitis should be considered in patients who develop fever, neutropenia, and abdominal pain during topotecan therapy. (See Cautions: GI Effects.)

■ **GI Effects** Diarrhea (sometimes severe and requiring hospitalization) has been reported with oral topotecan. Topotecan-related diarrhea is associated with substantial morbidity and in some cases, may be life-threatening. Among patients with recurrent small cell lung cancer receiving oral topotecan in a controlled clinical trial, diarrhea occurred in 14% of patients with 5% of these patients reporting grade 3/4 diarrhea. The median time to onset for grade 2 diarrhea (or worse) in this study was 9 days. Data pooled from 4 lung cancer trials (in patients with small cell lung cancer or non-small cell lung cancer) demonstrated a 22% incidence of diarrhea with 4.4% of patients reporting grade 3/4 diarrhea. In these trials, the incidence of diarrhea was 28% in patients 65 years of age or older compared with 19% in patients younger than 65 years of age; grade 3/4 diarrhea also was reported more frequently in patients 65 years of age or older (8%) compared with those younger than 65 years of age (3%). In another study comparing oral and IV topotecan regimens, the incidence of diarrhea was higher (36 versus 20%) in patients receiving oral topotecan.

Diarrhea may occur at the same time as neutropenia and its sequelae. (See Cautions: Neutropenic Colitis.) Severe diarrhea was temporally associated with the onset of severe neutropenia (e.g., occurring within 5 days) in 5% of patients receiving oral topotecan in clinical trials.

Among patients receiving oral topotecan for small cell lung cancer in a clinical trial, nausea or vomiting occurred in 27 or 19% of patients, respectively.

Among patients receiving IV topotecan for ovarian cancer or small cell lung cancer, adverse GI effects included nausea (64%), vomiting (45%), diarrhea (32%), constipation (29%), abdominal pain (22%), and stomatitis (18%). Grade 3 or 4 abdominal pain occurred in 6% of patients receiving topotecan for ovarian cancer and in 2% of patients receiving the drug for small cell lung cancer. Anorexia was reported in 19% of patients. Grade 3 or 4 intestinal obstruction was reported in 5% of patients in a clinical trial receiving topotecan for advanced ovarian cancer.

Among patients receiving IV topotecan and cisplatin for cervical cancer, adverse GI effects included nausea in 55%, vomiting in 40%, and stomatitis/pharyngitis in 6% of patients. Unspecified other GI disorders were reported in 63% of patients.

■ **Respiratory Effects** Interstitial lung disease (sometimes fatal) has been reported during postmarketing experience with IV topotecan. Risk factors for developing interstitial lung disease include pulmonary fibrosis, lung cancer, exposure to thoracic radiation, use of drugs known to cause pulmonary toxicity, use of colony-stimulating factors (i.e., hematopoietic growth factors), and a history of interstitial lung disease. Patients should be monitored for symptoms suggestive of interstitial lung disease, including cough, fever, dyspnea, and/or hypoxia. If a new diagnosis of interstitial lung disease is confirmed, the manufacturer states that topotecan therapy should be discontinued.

Dyspnea was reported in 22% and coughing in 15% of patients receiving IV topotecan for ovarian cancer or small cell lung cancer. Grade 3 or 4 dyspnea occurred in 6% of patients receiving IV topotecan for ovarian cancer and in 9% of patients receiving the drug for small cell lung cancer. Grade 3 or 4 pneumonia was reported in 8% of patients receiving IV topotecan for recurrent or progressive small cell lung cancer in a clinical trial. Among patients receiving IV topotecan and cisplatin for cervical cancer, adverse respiratory effects occurred in 17% of patients.

■ **Dermatologic Effects** Among patients receiving oral topotecan for small cell lung cancer in a clinical trial, alopecia occurred in 10% of patients.

Among patients receiving IV topotecan for ovarian cancer or small cell lung cancer, adverse dermatologic effects such as alopecia (49%) and rash (16%), including pruritus, erythematous rash, urticaria, dermatitis, bullous eruption, and maculopapular rash have been reported. Total alopecia (grade 2) occurred in 31% of patients receiving IV topotecan for ovarian cancer or small cell lung cancer.

Among patients receiving IV topotecan and cisplatin for cervical cancer, adverse dermatologic effects occurred in 48% of patients.

Severe dermatitis or pruritus has occurred rarely in patients receiving IV topotecan.

■ **Nervous System Effects** Headache was reported in 18% of patients and paresthesia, generally mild, was reported in 7% of patients receiving IV topotecan for ovarian cancer or small cell lung cancer.

Among patients receiving IV topotecan and cisplatin for cervical cancer, adverse nervous system effects occurred in 38% of patients, including neuropathy in 3% of patients.

■ **Genitourinary Effects** Among patients receiving IV topotecan and cisplatin for cervical cancer, adverse genitourinary effects occurred in 36% of patients.

■ **Cardiovascular Effects** Among patients receiving IV topotecan and cisplatin for cervical cancer, adverse cardiovascular effects occurred in 25% of patients. Hemorrhage was reported in 15% and coagulation in 6% of such patients. Severe bleeding (associated with thrombocytopenia) has occurred rarely in patients receiving IV topotecan.

■ **Hepatic Effects** Transient elevations in serum aminotransferase concentrations (grade 1 in 8%, grade 3 or 4 in 4%) occurred in patients receiving IV topotecan for ovarian cancer or small cell lung cancer. Grade 3 or 4 elevations in serum bilirubin concentrations occurred in less than 2% of such patients.

Among patients receiving IV topotecan and cisplatin for cervical cancer, adverse hepatic effects occurred in 24% of patients.

■ **Musculoskeletal Effects** Grade 3 or 4 arthralgia was reported in 1% of patients receiving IV topotecan for advanced ovarian cancer in a clinical trial.

Among patients receiving IV topotecan and cisplatin for cervical cancer, adverse musculoskeletal effects occurred in 14% of patients.

■ **Sensitivity Reactions** Anaphylactoid reactions and angioedema have occurred rarely in patients receiving IV topotecan. Allergic manifestations have been reported.

■ **Local Effects** Erythema and bruising, generally mild, have occurred following inadvertent extravasation of IV topotecan.

■ **Other Adverse Effects** Among patients receiving oral topotecan for small cell lung cancer in a clinical trial, fatigue was reported in 11% and asthenia was reported in 3% of patients.

Among patients receiving IV topotecan for ovarian cancer or small cell lung cancer, other adverse effects included fatigue in 29%, pyrexia in 28%, asthenia in 25%, and pain (including body pain, back pain, and skeletal pain) in 23% of patients. Grade 3 or 4 chest pain and malaise each was reported in 2% of patients receiving IV topotecan for advanced ovarian cancer in a clinical trial.

Among patients receiving IV topotecan and cisplatin for cervical cancer, adverse constitutional effects, including fatigue, lethargy, malaise, asthenia, fever without neutropenia, rigors, chills, sweating, and weight change (gain or loss) occurred in 69%, pain in 59%, and adverse metabolic or laboratory effects in 39% of patients. Other adverse effects reported in patients receiving topotecan and cisplatin for cervical cancer were allergic/immunologic or endocrine effects in 6%, sexual/reproductive effects in 5%, and ocular effects in 5% of patients.

■ **Precautions and Contraindications** Topotecan should be used IV under the supervision of a qualified clinician experienced in therapy with antineoplastic agents. Appropriate management of complications is possible only when adequate diagnostic and treatment facilities are readily available.

Patients should be advised to use caution when driving or operating machinery if they experience symptoms of asthenia or fatigue, which can occur with the use of chemotherapeutic agents, including topotecan.

Myelosuppression, principally neutropenia, is the dose-limiting toxicity of topotecan, and use of the drug is contraindicated in patients with severe myelosuppression. Oral and IV topotecan therapy should *not* be initiated in patients with baseline neutrophil counts less than 1500/mm^3 or platelet counts less than 100,000/mm^3. Frequent monitoring of peripheral blood cell counts is required during topotecan therapy. Patients should be informed that topotecan may decrease blood cell counts and that frequent blood tests will be performed to monitor for the development of bone marrow suppression. Patients also should be advised to contact their clinician if fever, other signs of infection (e.g., chills, cough, burning pain on urination), or bleeding develops during therapy.

Patients should be advised of the risk of potentially severe diarrhea with oral topotecan. Patients also should be informed about diarrhea prevention and/or proactive management of early signs and symptoms of diarrhea and instructed to contact their clinician if severe diarrhea develops, including symptoms of diarrhea 3 or more times a day, with fever, and/or with abdominal pain or cramps. If diarrhea occurs, clinicians are advised to aggressively manage the condition in accordance with published clinical guidelines. Aggressive management of diarrhea may include the use of antidiarrhea agents and anti-infectives, changes in fluid intake and diet, and/or hospitalization.

Topotecan can cause fetal toxicity when administered to pregnant women. If the drug is administered during pregnancy or if the patient becomes pregnant while receiving the drug, the patient should be informed of the potential hazard to the fetus. The manufacturer states that use of oral topotecan is contraindicated in pregnant and nursing women. (See Cautions: Pregnancy and Lactation.)

Topotecan also is contraindicated in patients with a known history of hypersensitivity reactions to the drug or any component of the formulation.

■ **Pediatric Precautions** Safety and efficacy of topotecan in children have not been established.

■ **Geriatric Precautions** Because elimination of oral and IV topotecan may be prolonged in patients with renal impairment and geriatric patients may have decreased renal function, the risk of adverse effects may be greater in such patients. Careful dosage selection and monitoring of renal function are advised in geriatric patients receiving topotecan.

Among 682 patients receiving oral topotecan for thoracic cancer, 33% were 65 years of age or older and 5% were 75 years of age or older. In clinical trials, diarrhea was reported more frequently (28 versus 19%) with the use of oral topotecan in patients 65 years of age or older than in those younger than 65 years of age.

Among 879 patients receiving IV topotecan for metastatic ovarian cancer or recurrent or progressive small cell lung cancer, 32% were 65 years of age or older and 4% were 75 years of age or older. Among 140 patients receiving IV topotecan and cisplatin for cervical cancer, 6% were 65 years of age or older and 3% were 75 years of age or older. Although no overall differences in safety and efficacy were observed between geriatric and younger patients receiving IV topotecan, the possibility that some geriatric patients may exhibit increased sensitivity to IV topotecan cannot be ruled out.

■ **Mutagenicity** Topotecan is mutagenic. Topotecan exhibited mutagenic activity in L5178Y mouse lymphoma cells. Topotecan was clastogenic to cultured human lymphocytes (with and without metabolic activation) and mouse bone marrow. Topotecan did not demonstrate mutagenic activity in bacterial cells.

■ **Carcinogenicity** Although studies to determine the carcinogenic potential of topotecan have not been performed to date, the drug is known to be genotoxic to mammalian cells and is a probable carcinogen.

■ **Pregnancy and Lactation** ***Pregnancy*** Topotecan can cause fetal toxicity when administered to pregnant women. The manufacturer states that use of oral topotecan is contraindicated in pregnant women.

Reproduction studies in rabbits receiving an IV topotecan dosage of 0.1 mg/kg daily (approximately equivalent to the IV clinical dose in humans on a mg/m^2 basis) on gestation days 6–20 revealed evidence of maternal toxicity, embryolethality, and reduced fetal body weight. Reproduction studies in rats receiving an IV topotecan dosage of 0.23 mg/kg daily (approximately equivalent to the IV clinical dose in humans on a mg/m^2 basis) for 14 days before mating through gestation day 6 showed fetal resorption, microphthalmia, preimplant loss, and mild maternal toxicity. The offspring of rats receiving an IV topotecan dosage of 0.1 mg/kg daily (approximately equivalent to half the IV clinical dose in humans on a mg/m^2 basis) on gestation days 6–17 experienced an increase in postimplantation mortality and total fetal malformations. The most frequent malformations affected the eye (microphthalmia, anophthalmia, rosette formation of the retina, coloboma of the retina, ectopic orbit), brain (dilated lateral and third ventricles), skull, and vertebrae.

There are no adequate and well-controlled studies to date using topotecan in pregnant women. If topotecan is used during pregnancy or if the patient becomes pregnant while receiving the drug, the patient should be informed of the potential hazard to the fetus. Women of childbearing potential should be advised to use effective contraceptive measures to avoid becoming pregnant during therapy with topotecan.

Lactation In lactating rats receiving IV topotecan at a dosage of 4.72 mg/m^2, high concentrations of the drug (i.e., up to 48 times higher than plasma concentrations) were distributed into milk. It is not known whether topotecan is distributed into human milk. The manufacturer states that use of oral topotecan is contraindicated in nursing women. Because of the potential for serious adverse reactions to topotecan in nursing infants, nursing should be discontinued during therapy.

Drug Interactions

■ **Drugs Metabolized by Hepatic Microsomal Enzymes** In vitro drug interaction studies show no evidence that topotecan affects substrates of cytochrome P-450 (CYP) isoenzymes, including CYP1A2, CYP2A6, CYP2C8, CYP2C9, CYP2C19, CYP2D6, CYP2E, CYP3A, or CYP4A; however, in vivo drug interaction studies evaluating the effects of topotecan on CYP isoenzymes have not been performed to date. In vitro data also indicate that dihydropyrimidine dehydrogenase (DPD) enzyme activity is not affected by topotecan.

■ **Drugs that Inhibit Efflux Transport Systems** Topotecan is a substrate of the efflux transporters *P*-glycoprotein (Pgp, ABCB1) and ABCG2 (breast cancer resistance protein [BCRP]). Concomitant use of elacridar (not commercially available in the US), an inhibitor of both *P*-glycoprotein and ABCG2 transporters, with oral topotecan resulted in a 2.5-fold increase in the area under the plasma concentration-time curve (AUC) for both topotecan lactone, the pharmcologically active form of the drug, and total topotecan. Concomitant use of oral topotecan with inhibitors of *P*-glycoprotein (e.g., cyclosporine, ketoconazole, ritonavir, saquinavir) also resulted in substantial increases in topotecan exposure. In one study, concomitant use of cyclosporine administered within 4 hours of an oral dose of topotecan resulted in a 2- to 3-fold increase in the AUCs of both topotecan lactone and total topotecan. The manufacturer states that concomitant use of oral topotecan with Pgp inhibitors should be avoided. If topotecan is used concomitantly with a Pgp (ABCB1) and/or an ABCG2 inhibitor, careful monitoring for signs of toxicity should be performed.

■ **Hematopoietic Agents** Concurrent administration of granulocyte colony-stimulating factor (G-CSF) can prolong the duration of neutropenia associated with IV topotecan therapy. If G-CSF (filgrastim) is to be used concomitantly, therapy should be initiated 24 hours after the final dose of IV topotecan (i.e., beginning on day 6 of the 21-day treatment course for monotherapy or beginning on day 4 of the 21-day treatment course for combination therapy with IV topotecan and cisplatin).

■ **Antineoplastic Agents** The severity of drug-induced myelosuppression may be increased when IV topotecan is used in combination with other cytotoxic agents, and dosage reduction may be necessary. Severe myelotoxicity, in some cases resulting in fatalities from sepsis, has occurred during combined therapy with IV topotecan and other antineoplastic agents (e.g., cisplatin, paclitaxel). A sequence-dependent interaction has been reported when IV topotecan is administered concomitantly with cisplatin; lower doses of each drug were required with administration of cisplatin on day 1 of the topotecan dosing schedule compared with administration of cisplatin on day 5 of the topotecan dosing schedule.

■ **Ranitidine** Concurrent administration of ranitidine did not result in any change to the pharmacokinetics of oral topotecan.

Acute Toxicity

Limited information is available on the acute toxicity of topotecan. Overdosage of oral or IV topotecan would be expected to cause bone marrow suppression. A patient who erroneously received a single IV dose of 35 mg/m^2 rather than the intended dose of 17.5 mg/m^2 experienced severe neutropenia (nadir of 320/mm^3) 14 days later followed by recovery without incident. The LD_{10} of IV topotecan in mice is 75 mg/m^2. There is no known specific antidote for overdosage with topotecan. If acute overdosage occurs with oral or IV topotecan, patients should be observed closely for bone marrow suppression and supportive measures, including prophylactic use of granulocyte colony-stimulating factor (G-CSF) and/or antibiotic therapy should be considered.

Pharmacology

Topotecan, a semisynthetic derivative of camptothecin, is an antineoplastic agent. Topotecan is a type I DNA topoisomerase inhibitor. DNA topoisomerases (i.e., types I and II) are enzymes in the cell nucleus that regulate DNA topology (3-dimensional conformation) and facilitate nuclear processes such as DNA replication, recombination, and repair. During these processes, type I DNA topoisomerase creates transient (reversible) single-stranded breaks in double-stranded DNA, allowing intact single DNA strands to pass through the break and relieve the topologic constraints (e.g., torsional strain) inherent in supercoiled DNA. The 3′-DNA terminus of the broken DNA strand binds covalently with the topoisomerase enzyme to form a catalytic intermediate, termed a cleavable complex. After the DNA is sufficiently relaxed and the strand passage reaction is complete, DNA topoisomerase reattaches the broken DNA strands to form the chemically unaltered topoisomers that allow transcription to proceed.

Topotecan and other type I topoisomerase inhibitors are believed to exert their cytotoxic effects during the S-phase of DNA synthesis through an interaction with the DNA-DNA topoisomerase cleavable complex. The cleavable complex is bound and stabilized by topotecan, preventing the topoisomerase from religating the single-strand breaks. The ternary complex of topotecan, DNA, and DNA topoisomerase interferes with the moving replication fork, inducing replication arrest and lethal double-stranded breaks in DNA. This DNA damage is not efficiently repaired and apparently leads to apoptosis (programmed cell death).

Pharmacokinetics

■ **Absorption** Following oral administration, topotecan is rapidly absorbed with peak plasma concentrations occurring within 1–2 hours. Oral bioavailability of topotecan is approximately 40%. Administration of a high-fat meal with oral topotecan did not affect the extent of absorption, but delayed the time to achieve maximum serum concentrations for both total topotecan (from 3–4 hours) and topotecan lactone, its pharmacologically active form (from 1.5–3 hours). Oral topotecan may be given without regard to food.

Area under the plasma concentration-time curve (AUC) is approximately proportional to dose following oral or IV administration of topotecan. IV topotecan exhibits multiexponential pharmacokinetics.

■ **Distribution** Following oral or IV administration, about 35% of the drug is bound to plasma proteins. It is not known whether topotecan is distributed into human milk.

■ **Elimination** At a pH of 4 or less, the lactone moiety of topotecan undergoes hydrolysis to create the pharmacologically active form of the drug; this process is reversible and, at physiologic pH, the drug is present mostly in ring-opened hydroxy form. Topotecan is metabolized in the liver to *N*-desmethyl topotecan.

Following oral administration, about 57% of topotecan (administered daily for 5 days) is excreted in urine as unchanged drug (20%) and as the *N*-desmethyl metabolite (2%). Approximately 33% of the oral dose of topotecan was eliminated in feces as total topotecan and approximately 2% as *N*-desmethyl topotecan.

Following IV administration, about 74% of a topotecan dose is excreted, mostly unchanged in urine (51%) and feces (18%) within 9 days; excretion of *N*-desmethyl topotecan in urine is approximately 3% and in feces is approximately 2%. *O*-Glucuronide metabolites of topotecan and *N*-desmethyl topotecan also have been detected in urine following oral and IV (less than 2% of the administered IV dose) administration of the drug.

Topotecan has a terminal half-life of 3–6 hours following oral administration and 2–3 hours following IV administration of the drug.

No substantial gender-related differences in pharmacokinetics were reported in patients receiving oral topotecan. The average plasma clearance of IV topotecan was 24% higher in males than in females, mainly because of difference in body size.

Following oral administration, exposure to topotecan lactone was 10 or 20% higher in patients with mild (creatinine clearance of 50–80 mL/minute) or moderate renal impairment (creatinine clearance of 30–49 mL/minute), respectively, than in patients with normal renal function. The manufacturer states that no apparent differences in pharmacokinetics were observed in geriatric patients with creatinine clearance of 60 mL/minute or more receiving oral topotecan. Dosage adjustment of oral topotecan is not required for patients with mild renal impairment; however, in patients with moderate renal impairment, reduction to a level that is predicted to adjust the AUC to within the normal range is recommended. (See Dosage and Administration: Dosage in Renal and Hepatic Impairment.)

In patients with impaired renal function, the clearance of IV topotecan is reduced and half-life may be prolonged. In patients with creatinine clearance of 40–60 mL/minute, plasma clearance of IV topotecan was decreased by approximately 67% compared with patients having normal renal function. In patients with creatinine clearance of 20–39 mL/minute, plasma clearance was reduced to about 34% of control values and half-life was increased to approximately 5 hours. Dosage reduction is recommended in patients with impaired renal function according to the degree of renal impairment. (See Dosage and Administration: Dosage in Renal and Hepatic Impairment.)

Following oral administration, substantial differences in the pharmacokinetics of topotecan were not observed in patients based on measurement of hepatic function (e.g., serum bilirubin or transaminase concentrations). In patients with impaired hepatic function (i.e., serum bilirubin concentrations of 1.7–15 mg/dL), the clearance of IV topotecan was reduced by approximately 67% compared with patients having normal hepatic function, and half-life was slightly prolonged (from 2 to 2.5 hours). However, the usual recommended dosage of IV topotecan was tolerated in such patients with hepatic impairment.

Chemistry and Stability

■ **Chemistry** Topotecan, a semisynthetic derivative of camptothecin, is an antineoplastic agent. Camptothecins are alkaloids with antitumor activity that are extracted from plants such as *Camptotheca acuminata*. Topotecan is a type I DNA topoisomerase inhibitor. Topotecan is soluble in water.

Commercially available capsules contain topotecan hydrochloride equivalent to 0.25 or 1 mg of topotecan as free base.

Commercially available topotecan for injection concentrate is a sterile lyophilized, buffered, light yellow to greenish powder. Each single-dose vial contains topotecan hydrochloride equivalent to 4 mg of topotecan as free base. Hydrochloric acid and/or sodium hydroxide may be used to adjust the pH to 2.5–3.5.

Reconstituted solutions of IV topotecan are yellow to yellow-green.

■ **Stability** Commercially available topotecan capsules should be stored at 2–8°C. Bottles containing topotecan capsules should be stored in their original containers (i.e., outer cartons) and protected from light and heat.

Commercially available topotecan for injection concentrate should be stored in unopened vials at 20–25°C and retained in the original package for protection from light. When stored under recommended conditions, unopened vials of commercially available topotecan for injection concentrate are stable until the date indicated on the package.

Following reconstitution of vials of topotecan hydrochloride, solutions of the drug are stable for up to 24 hours when stored at controlled room temperature (approximately 20–25°C) in ambient light. When topotecan is further diluted to concentrations of 10 or 500 mcg/mL in Viaflex IV bags containing 5% dextrose or 0.9% sodium chloride injection, such solutions reportedly are stable for up to 4 days when stored at room temperature. However, the manufacturer states that diluted solutions of topotecan for IV infusion should be administered within 24 hours because of microbiologic considerations.

For further information on the handling of antineoplastic agents, see the ASHP Guidelines on Handling Hazardous Drugs at http://www.ahfsdruginformation.com.

Preparations

Excipients in commercially available drug preparations may have clinically important effects in some individuals; consult specific product labeling for details.

Topotecan Hydrochloride

Oral		
Capsules	0.25 mg (of topotecan)	**Hycamtin®**, GlaxoSmithKline
	1 mg (of topotecan)	**Hycamtin®**, GlaxoSmithKline
Parenteral		
For injection concentrate, for IV infusion only	4 mg (of topotecan)	**Hycamtin®**, GlaxoSmithKline

†Use is not currently included in the labeling approved by the US Food and Drug Administration

Trabectedin

■ Trabectedin, a synthetic alkaloid originally isolated from the marine ascidian *Ecteinascidia turbinata*, is an alkylating antineoplastic agent.

Uses

■ **Soft Tissue Sarcomas** Trabectedin is used for the treatment of unresectable or metastatic liposarcoma or leiomyosarcoma in patients who have received prior therapy with an anthracycline-containing regimen. Trabectedin has been designated an orphan drug by FDA for the treatment of soft tissue sarcoma. In patients with unresectable or metastatic leiomyosarcoma or liposarcoma following therapy with either an anthracycline- and ifosfamide-containing chemotherapy regimen or an anthracycline-containing chemotherapy regimen and an additional chemotherapy regimen, trabectedin has been shown to prolong progression-free survival.

The efficacy and safety of trabectedin were demonstrated in a randomized, open-label, active-controlled, multicenter, phase 3 study (study 1) conducted in patients 15 years of age and older with unresectable, locally advanced or metastatic leiomyosarcoma or liposarcoma following therapy with at least either an anthracycline- and ifosfamide-containing chemotherapy regimen or an anthracycline-containing chemotherapy regimen and one or more additional cytotoxic chemotherapy regimen(s). In this study, 518 patients were randomized (stratified by histologic subtype, ECOG performance status, and number of prior chemotherapy regimens) in a 2:1 ratio to receive trabectedin (initial dosage of 1.5 mg/m^2 by IV infusion over 24 hours) or dacarbazine (initial dosage of 1 g/m^2 by IV infusion over 20–120 minutes) on day 1 of each 21-day cycle. Patients assigned to receive trabectedin also received dexamethasone phosphate 20 mg IV prior to each infusion of the drug. Treatment was continued until disease progression or unacceptable toxicity occurred. Patients randomized to receive dacarbazine were not permitted to cross over to trabectedin therapy upon disease progression.

The efficacy end points of this study were progression-free survival as assessed by the investigator according to Response Evaluation Criteria in Solid Tumors (RECIST), objective response rate, overall survival, and duration of response. The median age of enrolled patients was 56 years (range: 17–81 years); 76% of patients were white, 12% were black, and 4% were Asian; 30% were male; 73% had leiomyosarcomas and 27% had liposarcomas; and 49% had a baseline ECOG performance status of 0. The majority (89%) of patients had received at least 2 prior chemotherapy regimens; 90, 81, 74, and 59% of patients had previously received doxorubicin, gemcitabine, docetaxel, and ifosfamide, respectively, and approximately 10% of patients had previously received pazopanib.

Final analysis of median progression-free survival in study 1 indicated that patients treated with trabectedin had a substantially longer median progression-free survival compared with patients treated with dacarbazine (4.2 versus 1.5 months). The progression-free survival benefit for trabectedin was confirmed by independent blinded review. The objective response rate was 7% in patients receiving trabectedin and 6% in those receiving dacarbazine; complete responses were not achieved in either treatment group. At the time of analysis, the median duration of response for all responders was 6.9 months in patients receiving trabectedin and 4.2 months in those receiving dacarbazine. No substantial difference in overall survival was observed between the 2 treatment groups in this study. Results of a subgroup analysis (based on age, gender, ethnicity, histologic subtype, ECOG performance status, number of prior chemotherapy regimens, and body mass index [BMI]) suggested that trabectedin's effect on progression-free survival was consistent across all subgroups.

Dosage and Administration

■ **General** To help prevent nausea and vomiting and reduce the risk of hepatotoxicity associated with trabectedin therapy, premedication with dexamethasone phosphate 20 mg should be administered IV 30 minutes prior to each infusion of trabectedin. Additional antiemetics may be administered as needed.

Because trabectedin may cause neutropenia and associated sepsis, the manufacturer states that the neutrophil count should be assessed prior to administration of each dose of the drug and periodically throughout the treatment cycle. (See Neutropenic Sepsis under Cautions: Warnings/Precautions.)

Because trabectedin may cause rhabdomyolysis, the manufacturer states that serum creatine kinase (CK, creatine phosphokinase, CPK) concentrations should be assessed prior to administration of each dose of the drug. (See Rhabdomyolysis under Cautions: Warnings/Precautions.)

Because hepatotoxicity may occur with trabectedin, liver function tests should be assessed prior to each infusion of the drug. (See Hepatic Toxicity under Cautions: Warnings/Precautions.)

Because cardiomyopathy may occur with trabectedin, the manufacturer states that left ventricular ejection fraction (LVEF) should be assessed by echocardiogram or multiple gated acquisition (MUGA) scan prior to initiation of trabectedin and at 2- to 3-month intervals thereafter. (See Cardiomyopathy under Cautions: Warnings/Precautions.)

Restricted Distribution Program Trabectedin can only be obtained through specialty distributors. Clinicians may consult the Yondelis® website for specific availability information (http://www.yondelis.com/ordering).

■ **Administration** Procedures for proper handling and disposal of antineoplastic agents should be followed.

Trabectedin is administered by continuous IV infusion over 24 hours via a central venous line using an infusion set with a 0.2-μm polyethersulfone inline filter.

Unreconstituted vials of trabectedin powder for injection should be stored at 2–8°C.

Prior to administration, commercially available trabectedin powder for injection must be reconstituted and diluted using proper aseptic technique. The lyophilized powder is reconstituted by adding 20 mL of sterile water for injection to a vial labeled as containing 1 mg of trabectedin to provide a solution containing 0.05 mg/mL of the drug. The vial should then be shaken until complete dissolution of the powder occurs and inspected visually for particulate matter and discoloration prior to dilution. The solution should be clear and colorless to pale brownish-yellow; the vial should be discarded if particulate matter or discoloration is present. The reconstituted trabectedin solution should be diluted immediately. Any partially used vials should be discarded.

For preparation of the final diluted trabectedin solution for infusion, the appropriate volume of reconstituted solution should be withdrawn from the vial and further diluted in 500 mL of 0.9% sodium chloride injection or 5% dextrose injection. Final diluted solutions of trabectedin are stable for 30 hours following reconstitution when stored at 2–8°C or room temperature in ambient light. Administration of the drug must be completed within 30 hours following reconstitution. Any unused portion of reconstituted solution or diluted infusion solution should be discarded. Trabectedin should not be admixed with any other drug.

Trabectedin may adsorb to certain infusion materials; however, the manufacturer states that diluted solutions of trabectedin are compatible with type I colorless glass vials; polyvinylchloride (PVC) and polyethylene bags and tubing; polyethylene and polypropylene mixture bags; polyethersulfone inline filters; titanium, platinum, or plastic ports; silicone and polyurethane catheters; and infusion pumps having contact surfaces made of PVC, polyethylene, or polyethylene/polypropylene.

■ **Dosage** ***Soft Tissue Sarcomas*** For the treatment of unresectable or metastatic liposarcoma or leiomyosarcoma in patients who have received prior therapy with an anthracycline-containing regimen, the recommended adult dosage of trabectedin is 1.5 mg/m² administered as a continuous IV infusion over 24 hours every 3 weeks. Treatment should be continued until disease progression or unacceptable toxicity occurs.

Dosage Modification for Toxicity If adverse reactions occur, interruption of therapy, dosage reduction, and/or permanent discontinuance of trabectedin should be considered. When dosage reduction is necessary, an initial dosage reduction to 1.2 mg/m² every 3 weeks is recommended. If further dosage reduction is necessary, the dosage should be reduced to 1 mg/m² every 3 weeks. If a dosage of 1 mg/m² every 3 weeks is not tolerated, trabectedin should be permanently discontinued.

Dosage of trabectedin should *not* be re-escalated following a dosage reduction.

Trabectedin should be permanently discontinued in patients experiencing persistent adverse reactions requiring a treatment delay of more than 3 weeks.

Hematologic Toxicity. For an absolute neutrophil count (ANC) less than 1500/mm³ or a platelet count less than 100,000/mm³, trabectedin therapy should be withheld for up to 3 weeks. Therapy may then be resumed at the same dosage.

If an ANC less than 1000/mm³ and signs or symptoms of infection (e.g., fever) occurred during the preceding cycle, the trabectedin dosage should be reduced.

If an ANC less than 500/mm³ occurred for more than 5 days during the preceding cycle, the trabectedin dosage should be reduced.

If platelet counts less than 25,000/mm³ occurred during the preceding cycle, the trabectedin dosage should be reduced.

If life-threatening or prolonged and severe neutropenia occurred during the preceding cycle, the trabectedin dosage should be permanently reduced. (See Neutropenic Sepsis under Cautions: Warnings/Precautions.)

Hepatic Toxicity. For elevations in total bilirubin concentrations exceeding the upper limit of normal (ULN) or serum aminotransferase (ALT or AST) or alkaline phosphatase concentrations exceeding 2.5 times the ULN, trabectedin therapy should be withheld for up to 3 weeks. Therapy may then be resumed at the same dosage.

If total bilirubin concentrations exceeded the ULN, AST or ALT concentrations exceeded 5 times the ULN, or alkaline phosphatase concentrations exceeded 2.5 times the ULN during the preceding cycle, the trabectedin dosage should be reduced.

If severe hepatic dysfunction (total bilirubin concentrations at least 2 times the ULN *and* AST or ALT concentrations at least 3 times the ULN with alkaline phosphatase concentrations less than 2 times the ULN) occurred during the preceding cycle, trabectedin therapy should be permanently discontinued. (See Hepatic Toxicity under Cautions: Warnings/Precautions.)

Creatine Kinase Elevation. For serum CK concentrations exceeding 2.5 times the ULN, trabectedin therapy should be withheld for up to 3 weeks. Therapy may then be resumed at the same dosage.

If serum CK concentrations exceeded 5 times the ULN during the preceding cycle, the trabectedin dosage should be reduced.

If rhabdomyolysis occurs, trabectedin should be permanently discontinued. (See Rhabdomyolysis under Cautions: Warnings/Precautions.)

Cardiovascular Toxicity. For left ventricular ejection fraction (LVEF) values less than the lower limit of normal (LLN) or evidence of cardiomyopathy, trabectedin therapy should be withheld for up to 3 weeks. Therapy may then be resumed at the same dosage.

If LVEF less than the LLN with an absolute decrease from baseline of 10% or more or clinical evidence of cardiomyopathy occurred during the preceding cycle, the trabectedin dosage should be reduced.

If symptomatic cardiomyopathy or prolonged left ventricular dysfunction (LVEF does not recover to LLN within 3 weeks) occurs, trabectedin therapy should be permanently discontinued. (See Cardiomyopathy under Cautions: Warnings/Precautions.)

Other Nonhematologic Toxicity. For any other grade 3 or 4 nonhematologic adverse effects, trabectedin therapy should be withheld for up to 3 weeks. Therapy may then be resumed at the same dosage.

If any other grade 3 or 4 nonhematologic adverse effects occurred during the preceding cycle, the trabectedin dosage should be reduced.

■ **Special Populations** Pending further study of the effect of hepatic impairment on trabectedin pharmacokinetics, the manufacturer states that dosage adjustment is not necessary in patients with normal serum bilirubin concentrations and serum ALT or AST concentrations up to 2.5 times the ULN or in those with liver metastases. Trabectedin should *not* be used in patients with serum bilirubin concentrations exceeding the ULN or serum aminotransferase (ALT or AST) concentrations exceeding 2.5 times the ULN. The manufacturer states that there is no recommended dosage of the drug in patients with serum bilirubin concentrations that are above the institutional ULN. (See Hepatic Impairment under Warnings/Precautions: Specific Populations, in Cautions.)

No dosage adjustment is necessary in patients with mild or moderate renal impairment (creatinine clearance of 30–89 mL/minute). Trabectedin has not been studied in patients with severe renal impairment or in those with end-stage renal disease and the manufacturer does not provide specific dosage recommendations for such patients. (See Renal Impairment under Warnings/Precautions: Specific Populations, in Cautions.)

The manufacturer makes no specific dosage recommendations for geriatric patients. (See Geriatric Use under Warnings/Precautions: Specific Populations, in Cautions.)

Cautions

■ **Contraindications** Trabectedin is contraindicated in patients with known severe hypersensitivity, including anaphylaxis, to the drug.

In the European Medicines Agency (EMEA) labeling, the manufacturer states that concurrent use of trabectedin with yellow fever vaccine is contraindicated. (See Live Vaccines under Drug Interactions.)

■ **Warnings/Precautions** ***Neutropenic Sepsis*** Neutropenic sepsis, sometimes fatal, has been reported in patients receiving trabectedin. In the principal efficacy study evaluating trabectedin in patients with liposarcoma or leiomyosarcoma, grade 3 or 4 neutropenia occurred in 43% of patients receiving the drug. The median time to first occurrence of grade 3 or 4 neutropenia was 16 days (range: 8 days to 9.7 months) and the median time to complete resolution of neutropenia was 13 days (range: 3 days to 2.3 months). Febrile neutropenia (defined as grade 3 or 4 neutropenia with fever of 38.5°C or higher) occurred in 5% of trabectedin-treated patients. Neutropenic sepsis occurred in 10 of 378 patients (2.6%) receiving trabectedin; 5 of these patients had febrile neutropenia, which was fatal in 4 patients (1.1%).

Absolute neutrophil count (ANC) should be monitored prior to each dose of trabectedin and periodically throughout the treatment cycle. Temporary interruption, dosage reduction, or discontinuance of trabectedin may be necessary if neutropenia occurs during therapy with the drug. (See Hematologic Toxicity under Dosage: Dosage Modification for Toxicity, in Dosage and Administration and see also Advice to Patients.)

Rhabdomyolysis Trabectedin can cause rhabdomyolysis and musculoskeletal toxicity. In the principal efficacy study, rhabdomyolysis resulting in death occurred in 3 of 378 patients (0.8%) receiving trabectedin. Elevations of serum creatine kinase (CK, creatine phosphokinase, CPK) were reported in 32% (grade 3 or 4 in 6%) of patients receiving trabectedin and in 9% (grade 3 in 0.6%) of patients receiving dacarbazine. Renal failure occurred in 11 of 24 patients experiencing grade 3 or 4 serum CK elevations during trabectedin therapy; rhabdomyolysis resulting in renal failure occurred in 4 of these patients. The median time to first occurrence of grade 3 or 4 CK elevations was 2 months (range: 1–11.5 months) and the median time to complete resolution was 14 days (range: 5 days to 1 month).

Serum CK concentrations should be evaluated prior to each dose of trabectedin. Temporary interruption, dosage reduction, or discontinuance of trabectedin may be necessary if elevated CK concentrations occur during therapy with the drug. (See Creatine Kinase Elevation under Dosage: Dosage Modification for Toxicity, in Dosage and Administration.) Trabectedin should be permanently discontinued if rhabdomyolysis occurs.

Hepatic Toxicity Hepatotoxicity, including hepatic failure, may occur with trabectedin. In the principal efficacy study, grade 3 or 4 elevations in liver function tests (i.e., ALT, AST, total bilirubin, or alkaline phosphatase) occurred in 35% of patients receiving trabectedin. Patients with serum bilirubin concentrations exceeding the upper limit of normal (ULN), serum aminotransferase concentrations exceeding 2.5 times the ULN, or significant chronic liver disease (e.g., cirrhosis, hepatitis) were excluded from this study. The median time to development of grade 3 or 4 elevations in serum aminotransferase (ALT or AST) concentrations was 29 days (range: 3 days to 11.5 months). The majority (85%) of patients experiencing grade 3 or 4 elevations in liver function tests had complete resolution; the median time to complete resolution was 13 days (range: 4 days to 4.4 months). Drug-induced hepatic injury (defined as concurrent elevations in ALT or AST concentrations exceeding 3 times the ULN, alkaline phosphatase concentrations less than 2 times the ULN, and total bilirubin concentrations at least 2 times the ULN) occurred in 1.3% of patients receiving trabectedin. Elevations in aminotransferase concentrations exceeding 8 times the ULN occurred in 18% of patients receiving the drug.

Liver function tests should be performed prior to administration of each dose of trabectedin. Temporary interruption, dosage reduction, or discontinuance of trabectedin based on the severity and duration of the elevation in the liver function test result may be necessary. (See Hepatic Toxicity under Dosage: Dosage Modification for Toxicity, in Dosage and Administration.)

Cardiomyopathy Cardiomyopathy (including heart failure, congestive heart failure, decreased left ventricular ejection fraction [LVEF], diastolic dysfunction, or right ventricular dysfunction) may occur with trabectedin therapy. In the principal efficacy study, cardiomyopathy occurred in 6% (grade 3 or 4 in 4%) of patients receiving trabectedin and in 2.3% (grade 3 or 4 in 1.2%) of those receiving dacarbazine; cardiomyopathy resulting in death occurred in one patient receiving trabectedin and in none of those receiving dacarbazine. Patients with New York Heart Association (NYHA) class II to IV heart failure, left ventricular dysfunction at baseline, or history of myocardial infarction within 6 months prior to therapy initiation were excluded from the principal efficacy study evaluating trabectedin in patients with liposarcoma or leiomyosarcoma. The median time to development of grade 3 or 4 cardiomyopathy in trabectedin-treated patients was 5.3 months (range: 26 days to 15.3 months).

LVEF should be assessed using echocardiogram or multiple gated acquisition (MUGA) scan prior to initiation of trabectedin and then every 2 to 3 months during treatment. Temporary interruption, dosage reduction, or discontinuance of trabectedin may be necessary if decreased LVEF occurs during therapy with the drug. (See Cardiovascular Toxicity under Dosage: Dosage Modification for Toxicity, in Dosage and Administration.)

Extravasation Resulting in Tissue Necrosis Extravasation of trabectedin may cause tissue necrosis requiring debridement. Tissue necrosis may develop more than 1 week following the extravasation. Severe local tissue inflammation and necrosis associated with extravasation of trabectedin from central venous access devices have been reported in 2 patients; both patients had full-thickness injuries that required surgical debridement, suggesting that trabectedin is a vesicant.

Specific treatment for extravasation of trabectedin has not been established. Because of the risk of extravasation and resulting tissue necrosis, the manufacturer states that a central venous line should be used to administer the drug. (See Dosage and Administration: Administration.)

Fetal/Neonatal Morbidity and Mortality Based on its mechanism of action, trabectedin may cause fetal harm if administered to pregnant women. There are no available data concerning the use of trabectedin during pregnancy. Animal reproductive and developmental studies at relevant dosages have not been conducted with trabectedin; however, the drug has been shown to cross the placenta in pregnant animals. Pregnancy should be avoided during therapy. Women of childbearing potential should use effective methods of contraception while receiving the drug and for at least 2 months after the last dose of the drug.

Trabectedin may damage spermatozoa, possibly resulting in genetic and fetal abnormalities. Men with female partners of childbearing potential should use effective methods of contraception during trabectedin therapy and for at least 5 months after the last dose of the drug.

Impairment of Fertility Trabectedin may result in decreased fertility in males and females. Fertility studies were not performed with trabectedin. In male animals, limited evidence of hemorrhage and degeneration in testes was observed with repeated administration of trabectedin at dosages approximately 0.2 times the recommended human dosage.

Specific Populations **Pregnancy.** Trabectedin may cause fetal harm if administered to pregnant women based on its mechanism of action. (See Fetal/Neonatal Morbidity and Mortality under Cautions: Warnings/Precautions.)

Lactation. It is not known whether trabectedin is distributed into milk. The effects of the drug on nursing infants and on milk production also are unknown. Because of the potential for serious adverse reactions to trabectedin in nursing infants, women should be advised to discontinue nursing while receiving the drug. In the European Union, the manufacturer also recommends discontinuing nursing for 3 months after discontinuance of the drug.

Pediatric Use. Safety and efficacy of trabectedin have not been established in pediatric patients with liposarcoma or leiomyosarcoma.

In a phase 2 study evaluating the pharmacokinetics of trabectedin 1.5 mg/m^2 by IV infusion over 24 hours in pediatric patients (12–21 years of age) weighing 15 kg or more with rhabdomyosarcoma, Ewing sarcoma, or nonrhabdomyosarcoma soft tissue sarcoma, pharmacokinetic parameters were generally similar to those observed in adults.

Geriatric Use. Clinical studies of trabectedin did not include sufficient numbers of patients 65 years of age and older to determine whether geriatric patients respond differently than younger adults. (See Dosage and Administration: Special Populations.)

Population pharmacokinetic analyses in adults indicate that age (19–83 years) does not have clinically important effects on the pharmacokinetics of trabectedin.

Hepatic Impairment. Because trabectedin is extensively metabolized in the liver, hepatic impairment is likely to affect the pharmacokinetics of the drug. A population pharmacokinetic analysis showed no relationship between serum aminotransferase or bilirubin concentrations and the clearance of trabectedin. In a phase 1 trial, the pharmacokinetics of trabectedin were not substantially affected in cancer patients with liver metastases (stratified by serum alkaline phosphatase concentrations) within a dosage range of 0.75–1.3 mg/m^2. However, the manufacturer states that the effect of any degree of hepatic impairment on trabectedin exposure is not known.

Pending further study of the drug in patients with hepatic impairment, the manufacturer states that trabectedin dosage adjustment is not necessary in patients with normal serum bilirubin concentrations and serum ALT or AST concentrations up to 2.5 times the ULN or in those with liver metastases.

Pharmacokinetic data for trabectedin in patients with moderate to severe hepatic impairment and those with total bilirubin concentrations exceeding the ULN are not yet available. In addition, trabectedin may cause hepatotoxicity. (See Hepatic Toxicity under Cautions: Warnings/Precautions.) The prescribing information indicates that trabectedin should not be used in patients with moderate to severe hepatic impairment and states that there is no recommended dosage of the drug in patients with serum bilirubin concentrations above the ULN.

Renal Impairment. In a population pharmacokinetic analysis, mild to moderate renal impairment did not have clinically important effects on the pharmacokinetics of trabectedin. The pharmacokinetics of trabectedin have not been systematically studied in patients with severe renal impairment or end-stage renal disease. However, hemodialysis is not expected to enhance elimination of trabectedin because the drug is highly bound to plasma proteins and is not substantially excreted renally.

Trabectedin dosage adjustment is not necessary in patients with mild (creatinine clearance 60–89 mL/minute) or moderate (creatinine clearance 30–59 mL/minute) renal impairment. The manufacturer does not provide specific dosage recommendations for patients with severe renal impairment or end-stage renal disease.

■ **Common Adverse Effects** Adverse effects reported in 10% or more of patients receiving trabectedin for the treatment of advanced leiomyosarcoma or liposarcoma and at an incidence that is at least 2% higher than that reported with dacarbazine include nausea, vomiting, constipation, decreased appetite, diarrhea, fatigue (includes asthenia and malaise), peripheral edema, dyspnea, headache, arthralgia, myalgia, and insomnia.

Laboratory abnormalities reported in more than 10% of patients receiving trabectedin for the treatment of advanced leiomyosarcoma or liposarcoma and at an incidence that is at least 2% higher than that reported with dacarbazine include anemia, increased concentrations of alkaline phosphatase, neutropenia, hypoalbuminemia, thrombocytopenia, increased concentrations of serum creatinine, increased concentrations of CK, increased concentrations of aminotransferases (i.e., ALT, AST), and hyperbilirubinemia.

Drug Interactions

Trabectedin is metabolized principally by cytochrome P-450 (CYP) isoenzyme 3A4; other CYP isoenzymes (e.g., 2C9, 2C19, 2D6, and 2E1) may contribute to the drug's metabolism to a minor extent. In vitro studies indicate that trabectedin has limited inhibition or induction potential of CYP isoenzymes 1A2, 2A6, 2B6, 2C9, 2C19, 2D6, 2E1, and 3A4 at clinically relevant concentrations.

In vitro studies indicate that trabectedin undergoes glucuronidation by uridine diphosphate-glucuronosyltransferase (UGT) 2B15.

Trabectedin is a substrate of P-glycoprotein (P-gp).

■ **Drugs and Foods Affecting Hepatic Microsomal Enzymes**

Inhibitors of CYP3A Concomitant use of trabectedin with potent inhibitors of CYP3A may result in increased peak plasma concentrations and systemic exposure of trabectedin. When the potent CYP3A inhibitor ketoconazole (200 mg twice daily for 7.5 days) was administered concomitantly with trabectedin (single 0.58 mg/m² dose on day 1), peak plasma concentrations and area under the plasma concentration-time curve (AUC) of trabectedin were increased by 22 and 66%, respectively, compared with a single 1.3 mg/m² dose of trabectedin.

Concomitant use of trabectedin with potent inhibitors of CYP3A (e.g., aprepitant, clarithromycin, conivaptan, indinavir, itraconazole, ketoconazole, *ritonavir-boosted* lopinavir, nefazodone, nelfinavir, posaconazole, ritonavir, saquinavir, telithromycin, voriconazole) should be avoided. If concomitant short-term (less than 14 days) therapy with a potent CYP3A inhibitor cannot be avoided, the manufacturer recommends administering the potent CYP3A inhibitor 1 week following completion of the trabectedin infusion and discontinuing the potent CYP3A inhibitor 1 day prior to the next trabectedin infusion.

Inducers of CYP3A Concomitant use of trabectedin with potent inducers of CYP3A may result in decreased peak plasma concentrations and systemic exposure of trabectedin. When the potent CYP3A inducer rifampin (600 mg daily for 6 days) was administered concomitantly with trabectedin (single dose of 1.3 mg/m² IV on day 6), peak plasma concentrations and AUC of trabectedin were decreased by 21 and 31%, respectively.

Concomitant use of trabectedin with potent CYP3A inducers (e.g., phenobarbital, rifampin, St. John's wort [*Hypericum perforatum*]) should be avoided.

Grapefruit Grapefruit products are potent CYP3A inhibitors and should be avoided in patients receiving trabectedin because of the potential for increased plasma concentrations of the drug during concurrent use.

■ **Drugs Affecting Efflux Transport Systems** Trabectedin is a substrate of the efflux transporter P-gp. Concomitant use of trabectedin with drugs that inhibit P-gp (e.g., cyclosporine, verapamil) may affect the pharmacokinetics (i.e., distribution and elimination) of trabectedin. The clinical relevance of this interaction is not known; therefore, P-gp inhibitors and trabectedin should be used concomitantly with caution.

■ **Antineoplastic Agents** Pharmacokinetic analyses indicate no clinically important pharmacokinetic interactions between trabectedin and doxorubicin or docetaxel.

Pharmacokinetics of trabectedin were not affected when gemcitabine, carboplatin, or paclitaxel was administered prior to trabectedin.

Concurrent administration of trabectedin and carboplatin, cisplatin, or paclitaxel did not alter the pharmacokinetics of carboplatin, cisplatin, or paclitaxel.

■ **Alcohol and Other Hepatotoxic Drugs** The prescribing information for trabectedin in the US does not provide information concerning the concurrent use of potentially hepatotoxic drugs and alcohol during therapy. However, the manufacturer in the European Union recommends caution during concomitant use of trabectedin and other drugs with hepatotoxic potential and states that alcohol should be avoided during trabectedin therapy. (See Hepatic Toxicity under Cautions: Warnings/Precautions.)

■ **Drugs Associated with Rhabdomyolysis** Drugs associated with rhabdomyolysis such as HMG CoA reductase inhibitors (statins; e.g., atorvastatin, fluvastatin, lovastatin, pravastatin, simvastatin) should be used with caution in patients receiving trabectedin because the risk of rhabdomyolysis may be increased in such patients. (See Rhabdomyolysis under Cautions: Warnings/Precautions.)

■ **Live Vaccines** The prescribing information for trabectedin in the US does not provide information concerning the use of live vaccines during therapy. In the European Union, the manufacturer states that concomitant use of live attenuated vaccines is not recommended during trabectedin therapy and that use of yellow fever vaccine with trabectedin is specifically contraindicated.

Description

Trabectedin, a synthetic tetrahydroisoquinoline alkaloid originally isolated from the marine ascidian *Ecteinascidia turbinata*, is an alkylating antineoplastic agent. Unlike conventional alkylating agents that bind to DNA in the major groove, trabectedin forms covalent adducts with guanine residues in the minor groove of DNA, which induces bending of the DNA helix toward the major groove. This adduct formation triggers a cascade of events that can alter the subsequent actions of DNA binding proteins, including transcription factors and DNA repair pathways, resulting in G_2/M phase arrest, inhibition of progression of cells from the S phase, and, subsequently, cell growth arrest and apoptosis. Trabectedin has demonstrated antiproliferative activity in vitro and in vivo against a range of human tumor cell lines and experimental tumors, including malignancies such as sarcoma, breast cancer, non-small cell lung cancer, ovarian cancer, and melanoma.

The pharmacokinetics of trabectedin appear to be biphasic with an initial rapid decline in plasma concentrations of the drug followed by a slower rate of disappearance. Pharmacokinetics of trabectedin are dose proportional over a dosage range of 0.024–1.8 mg/m². The drug exhibits time-independent exposure. Following repeated doses of trabectedin administered every 3 weeks, systemic accumulation of the drug was not observed. Trabectedin is extensively metabolized in the liver, principally by cytochrome P-450 (CYP) isoenzyme 3A4. The drug is approximately 97% bound to plasma proteins, and protein binding is independent of plasma drug concentration over the range of 0.01-0.1 mcg/mL. Trabectedin is principally excreted via biliary elimination. Following IV infusion of trabectedin over 3 or 24 hours, 58% of the administered dose is recovered in feces and 6% is recovered in urine within 24 days; a negligible amount of unchanged drug is excreted in feces and urine. The terminal half-life of trabectedin is approximately 7.3 days.

Advice to Patients

Importance of instructing patients to read the manufacturer's patient information.

Risk of myelosuppression. Importance of monitoring absolute neutrophil counts (ANC) prior to each dose of trabectedin and periodically throughout the treatment cycle. Importance of promptly informing clinician if fever, unusual bruising, bleeding, fatigue, or pallor occurs.

Risk of rhabdomyolysis. Importance of creatine kinase (CK, creatine phosphokinase, CPK) monitoring. Importance of advising patients to promptly inform clinician if they experience severe muscle pain or weakness.

Risk of hepatotoxicity. Importance of monitoring liver function tests prior to each dose of trabectedin. Importance of immediately contacting clinician if possible manifestations of hepatotoxicity (e.g., jaundice, abdominal pain [particularly in the right upper quadrant], severe nausea or vomiting, difficulty concentrating, disorientation, confusion) occur.

Risk of cardiomyopathy. Importance of cardiac monitoring before initiating trabectedin and periodically during therapy. Importance of immediately contacting clinician if new chest pain, shortness of breath, fatigue, lower extremity edema, or heart palpitations occur.

Risk of hypersensitivity reactions. Importance of advising patients to seek immediate medical attention if symptoms of an allergic reaction, including difficulty breathing, chest tightness, wheezing, severe dizziness or lightheadedness, swelling of the lips, or rash, occur.

Risk of extravasation. Importance of contacting a clinician if redness, swelling, pruritus, or discomfort or leakage at the injection site occurs.

Risk of fetal harm. Necessity of advising women of childbearing potential to use effective contraception during trabectedin therapy and for at least 2 months after the last dose of the drug. Necessity of advising men who are partners of such women that they should use effective contraception during trabectedin therapy and for at least 5 months after the last dose of the drug. If pregnancy occurs, advise patient of potential risk to the fetus.

Importance of advising women to avoid breast-feeding while receiving trabectedin. (See Lactation under Warnings/Precautions: Specific Populations, in Cautions.)

Importance of informing clinicians of existing or contemplated concomitant therapy, including prescription and OTC drugs and dietary or herbal supplements (e.g., St. John's wort), as well as any concomitant illnesses.

Importance of advising patients to avoid grapefruit during trabectedin therapy.

Importance of informing patients of other important precautionary information. (See Cautions.)

Overview® (see Users Guide). For additional information on this drug until a more detailed monograph is developed and published, the manu-

facturer's labeling should be consulted. It is *essential* that the manufacturer's labeling be consulted for more detailed information on usual cautions, precautions, contraindications, potential drug interactions, laboratory test interferences, and acute toxicity. For further information on the handling of antineoplastic agents, see the ASHP Guidelines on Handling Hazardous Drugs at http://www.ahfsdruginformation.com.

Preparations

Distribution of trabectedin is restricted. (See Restricted Distribution Program under Dosage and Administration: General.)

Excipients in commercially available drug preparations may have clinically important effects in some individuals; consult specific product labeling for details.

Trabectedin

Parenteral

For injection, for IV infusion	1 mg	**Yondelis®**, Janssen

Trametinib Dimethyl Sulfoxide

■ Trametinib, an inhibitor of mitogen-activated extracellular signal-regulated kinase (MEK) 1 and MEK2 in cells with b-Raf serine-threonine kinase (BRAF) V600E or V600K mutations, is an antineoplastic agent.

Uses

■ **Melanoma** Trametinib, alone or in combination therapy, is used for the treatment of unresectable or metastatic melanoma in selected patients; the drug also is used in combination therapy for the adjuvant treatment of melanoma in selected patients.

Trametinib is *not* indicated for use in patients with melanoma who have experienced disease progression following treatment with a BRAF inhibitor.

Adjuvant Therapy for Melanoma Trametinib is used in combination with dabrafenib as adjuvant therapy following complete resection of melanoma with b-Raf serine-threonine kinase (BRAF) V600E or V600K mutation and nodal involvement. An FDA-approved diagnostic test (e.g., THxID® BRAF kit) is required to confirm the presence of the BRAF V600E or V600K mutation prior to initiation of therapy.

The current indication for trametinib in combination with dabrafenib as adjuvant therapy following complete resection of melanoma with BRAF V600E or V600K mutation and nodal involvement is based principally on the results of a randomized, double-blind, placebo-controlled phase 3 study (COMBI-AD) in patients who had undergone complete resection of stage III melanoma with BRAF V600E or V600K mutation (as detected by the bioMerieux THxID® BRAF V600 mutation test) and involvement of regional lymph nodes. In this study, 870 patients were randomized (stratified by disease stage and BRAF mutation status) in a 1:1 ratio to receive trametinib 2 mg once daily with dabrafenib 150 mg twice daily or placebo for up to 12 months. Patients enrolled in this study must have had undergone complete resection of melanoma with complete lymphadenectomy within 12 weeks of randomization. The primary measure of efficacy was relapse-free survival. The median age of patients enrolled in the study was 51 years; 99% of patients were Caucasian, 55% were male, 91% had a baseline Eastern Cooperative Oncology Group (ECOG) performance status of 0, 65% had macroscopic lymph node involvement, 41% had tumor ulceration, 41% had stage IIIb disease, and 40% had stage IIIc disease. The majority (91%) of patients had BRAF V600E mutation and 9% had a V600K mutation. Patients who had mucosal or ocular melanoma, unresectable in-transit metastases, or distant metastatic disease and those who had previously received systemic therapy (including radiation therapy) were not eligible to enroll in the study.

After a median follow-up of 2.8 years, median relapse-free survival had not been reached in patients receiving trametinib in combination with dabrafenib and was 16.6 months in those receiving placebo; however, trametinib in combination with dabrafenib reduced the risk of relapse by 53% compared with placebo. In an updated analysis of this study at a median follow-up of 44 or 42 months for patients receiving trametinib in combination with dabrafenib or those receiving placebo, respectively, relapse-free survival remained similar to the primary results. Trametinib in combination with dabrafenib was associated with a numerically, but not significantly, higher estimated 3-year overall survival rate as compared with placebo. Results of a subgroup analysis (based on disease stage, lymph node involvement, presence of tumor ulceration) suggested that the effect of trametinib in combination with dabrafenib was consistent across all subgroups.

Unresectable or Metastatic Melanoma **Monotherapy.** Trametinib is used as monotherapy for the treatment of unresectable or metastatic melanoma with BRAF V600E or V600K mutations. Trametinib has been designated an orphan drug by the FDA as monotherapy for the treatment of this cancer. An FDA-approved diagnostic test (e.g., THxID® BRAF kit) is required to confirm the presence of the BRAF V600E or V600K mutation prior to initiation of therapy.

The current indication for trametinib monotherapy is based principally on the results of a randomized, open-label, phase 3 study (METRIC study) in patients with unresectable or metastatic melanoma positive for V600E or V600K BRAF mutations. Trametinib improved progression-free survival and overall survival when compared with conventional chemotherapy. This study randomized 322 adults (median 54 years of age, 54% male, more than 99% white, 36% with elevated LDH) in a 2:1 ratio to receive oral trametinib 2 mg daily or investigator's choice of chemotherapy (dacarbazine 1 g/m² or paclitaxel 175 mg/m²) every 3 weeks. In this study, 87% of patients with unresectable or metastatic melanoma had BRAF V600E mutations compared with 12% of enrolled patients with V600K mutations. The majority of patients (66%) had not received prior chemotherapy for advanced melanoma; prior use of MEK inhibitors, BRAF inhibitors, or ipilimumab was not allowed. Once disease progression had occurred, patients originally randomized to conventional chemotherapy were allowed to cross over to trametinib treatment. Median progression-free survival was 4.8 months in patients randomized to trametinib versus 1.5 months in patients randomized to conventional chemotherapy. The objective response rate was 22% among those randomized to trametinib and 8% among those randomized to conventional chemotherapy. Median duration of response was 5.5 months for patients randomized to trametinib and was not yet reached for those randomized to conventional chemotherapy.

Trametinib is *not* indicated for use in patients with melanoma who have experienced disease progression following treatment with a BRAF inhibitor. In an open-label, phase 2 study in patients with unresectable or metastatic melanoma with BRAF mutations, no confirmed objective responses were observed in the cohort of 40 patients who had previously received treatment with a BRAF inhibitor. The median progression-free survival among these patients was 1.8 months.

Combination Therapy. Trametinib is used in combination with dabrafenib for the treatment of unresectable or metastatic melanoma with BRAF V600E or V600K mutation. Trametinib has been designated an orphan drug by the FDA when used in combination with dabrafenib for the treatment of this cancer. An FDA-approved diagnostic test (e.g., THxID® BRAF kit) is required to confirm the presence of the BRAF V600E or V600K mutation prior to initiation of therapy.

The current indication for trametinib in combination with dabrafenib in the treatment of unresectable or metastatic melanoma with BRAF V600E or V600K mutation is based principally on the results of a randomized phase 3 study (COMBI-D) in patients with previously untreated stage IIIc or IV cutaneous melanoma with BRAF V600E or V600K mutation. The primary measure of efficacy was progression-free survival. In this study, 423 patients were randomized in a 1:1 ratio to receive either trametinib (2 mg once daily) in combination with dabrafenib (150 mg twice daily) or dabrafenib in combination with placebo. Treatment was continued until disease progression or unacceptable toxicity occurred or the patient withdrew from the study; however, patients with disease progression could continue receiving treatment if they met prespecified criteria for continuation. The median age of patients was 56 years; greater than 99% were Caucasian, 72% had an ECOG performance status of 0, 66% had stage M1c disease, 65% had normal LDH concentrations, and 2 patients had a history of brain metastases. Most patients (85%) had BRAF V600E mutation and 15% had a V600K mutation. At a median follow-up of 9 months, median progression-free survival or overall survival was 9.3 or 25.1 months, respectively, in patients receiving trametinib and dabrafenib compared with 8.8 or 18.7 months, respectively, in those receiving placebo and dabrafenib. An updated progression-free survival analysis confirmed prolonged median progression-free survival (11 versus 8.8 months; hazard ratio for death or disease progression: 0.67) in patients receiving trametinib in combination with dabrafenib compared with those receiving placebo and dabrafenib. A final analysis for overall survival estimated a prolonged median overall survival (25.1 versus 18.7 months) and a reduction in the risk of death (29%) in patients receiving trametinib in combination with dabrafenib. In addition, patients receiving trametinib and dabrafenib had higher overall response rates (66 versus 51%) compared with those receiving placebo and dabrafenib; complete responses were achieved in 10 or 8% of patients receiving trametinib in combination with dabrafenib or placebo in combination with dabrafenib, respectively. The median duration of response in patients receiving trametinib and dabrafenib or those receiving placebo and dabrafenib was 9.2 or 10.2 months, respectively. Results of a subgroup analysis (based on age, gender, disease stage, baseline ECOG performance status, baseline serum LDH concentration, visceral involvement, number of disease sites, and BRAF V600 mutation status) suggested that the effects of combination therapy with trametinib and dabrafenib on progression-free survival and overall survival were consistent across all subgroups.

■ **Non-small Cell Lung Cancer** Trametinib is used in combination with dabrafenib for the treatment of metastatic non-small cell lung cancer (NSCLC) with BRAF V600E mutation. Trametinib has been designated an orphan drug by the FDA when used in combination with dabrafenib for the treatment of this cancer. An FDA-approved diagnostic test (e.g., THxID® BRAF kit) is required to confirm the presence of the BRAF V600E mutation prior to initiation of therapy.

The current indication for trametinib in combination with dabrafenib in the treatment of metastatic NSCLC with BRAF V600E mutation is based principally on the results of an open-label, multicenter, nonrandomized, 3-cohort, phase 2 study (BRF113928). Patients in the BRF113928 study were enrolled into 2 cohorts: those previously treated with 1–3 systemic therapies with disease progression following at least one platinum-containing regimen and those with treatment-naive metastatic NSCLC. The cohort of patients with previously treated disease received either single-agent dabrafenib (150 mg twice daily) or trametinib (2 mg once daily) in combination with dabrafenib (150 mg twice daily). The cohort of patients with previously untreated disease received trametinib (2 mg once daily) in combination with dabrafenib (150 mg twice daily). Treatment was continued until disease progression or unacceptable toxicity occurred or the patient withdrew from the study. Patients with prior exposure to BRAF or mitogen-activated extracellular signal-regulated kinase (MEK) inhibitors were not eligible to enroll in the study; however, prior exposure to epidermal growth factor receptor (EGFR) or anaplastic lymphoma kinase (ALK) inhibitors was permitted in patients with EGFR- or ALK-positive tumors. The primary measure of efficacy was objective response rate as assessed by an independent review committee according to Response Evaluation Criteria in Solid Tumors (RECIST) and duration of response. The median age of patients was 66 years; 98% had squamous cell histology, 90% had an ECOG performance status of 0 or 1, 81% were Caucasian, 60% had a history of smoking, 48% were male, 32% were nonsmokers, 14% were Asian, 11% had received adjuvant chemotherapy, 8% were current smokers, 3% were black, and 2% were Hispanic. The majority (99%) of patients had metastatic disease; brain or liver metastases were present in 6 or 14% of these patients, respectively. Among the cohort of patients with previously treated disease, 58% had received only one prior systemic therapy for metastatic disease.

In the cohort of patients with previously treated disease, the objective response rate was 27 or 63% in patients receiving single-agent dabrafenib or combination therapy with trametinib and dabrafenib, respectively, and the median duration of response was 9.9 or 12.6 months, respectively. In the cohort of patients receiving trametinib in combination with dabrafenib for treatment-naive disease, the objective response rate was 61%. In the overall study population, 52 or 59–64% of the patients who responded to single-agent dabrafenib or trametinib and dabrafenib combination therapy, respectively, had durable responses of 6 months or more.

■ **Anaplastic Thyroid Cancer** Trametinib is used in combination with dabrafenib for the treatment of locally advanced or metastatic anaplastic thyroid cancer with BRAF V600E mutation when no satisfactory locoregional treatment options are available. Dabrafenib has been designated an orphan drug by the FDA when used in combination with trametinib for the treatment of this cancer. An FDA-approved diagnostic test (e.g., THxID® BRAF kit) is required to confirm the presence of the BRAF V600E mutation prior to initiation of therapy.

The current indication for trametinib in combination with dabrafenib in the treatment of anaplastic thyroid cancer with BRAF V600E mutation is based principally on the results of an activity-estimating, open-label, multicenter, nonrandomized, multicohort, phase 2 trial (BRF117019) in patients with rare BRAF V600E mutation-positive malignancies, including anaplastic thyroid cancer. In this trial, a cohort of 26 patients with locally advanced, unresectable, or metastatic anaplastic thyroid cancer received trametinib (2 mg once daily) in combination with dabrafenib (150 mg twice daily). Treatment was continued until disease progression or unacceptable toxicity occurred or the patient withdrew from the study. Patients with prior exposure to BRAF or MEK inhibitors, symptomatic or untreated CNS metastases, airway obstruction, or inability to swallow or retain oral drugs were not eligible to enroll in the study. The primary measure of efficacy was objective response rate as assessed by an independent review committee according to RECIST and duration of response. The median age of patients enrolled in the anaplastic thyroid cancer cohort was 70 years; 50% were male, 50% were Caucasian, 46% were Asian, and 54% had a history of differentiated thyroid cancer. All patients had an ECOG performance status of 0 or 1. The majority (92%) of patients had previously undergone surgery, 81% had received prior external beam radiation therapy, and 54% had received systemic therapy. The objective response rate in 23 evaluable patients in the anaplastic thyroid cancer cohort was 61%; complete response was achieved in 4% of the evaluable patients. Durable responses of 6 months or more were observed in 64% of responders.

Dosage and Administration

■ **General** An FDA-approved diagnostic test (e.g., THxID® BRAF kit) is required to confirm the presence of the b-Raf serine-threonine kinase (BRAF) V600E or V600K mutation prior to initiation of trametinib monotherapy for the treatment of unresectable or metastatic melanoma or combination therapy with trametinib and dabrafenib for the treatment of unresectable or metastatic melanoma or for the adjuvant treatment of melanoma; the presence of BRAF V600E mutation must be confirmed prior to initiation of combination therapy with trametinib and dabrafenib for the treatment of metastatic non-small cell lung cancer (NSCLC) or locally advanced or metastatic anaplastic thyroid cancer.

■ **Administration** Trametinib should be administered orally once daily, approximately every 24 hours, at least 1 hour before or 2 hours after a meal.

■ **Dosage** Dosage of trametinib dimethyl sulfoxide is expressed in terms of trametinib.

Melanoma **Adjuvant Therapy for Melanoma.** For use in combination with dabrafenib as adjuvant treatment following complete resection of melanoma with BRAF V600E or V600K mutation and nodal involvement, the recommended adult dosage of trametinib is 2 mg once daily. Therapy should be continued for up to 1 year or until disease progression or unacceptable toxicity occurs.

Unresectable or Metastatic Melanoma. For the treatment of unresectable or metastatic melanoma with BRAF V600E orV600K mutation, the recommended adult dosage of trametinib (as a single agent or in combination with dabrafenib) is 2 mg once daily. Therapy should be continued until disease progression or unacceptable toxicity occurs.

Non-small Cell Lung Cancer For use in combination with dabrafenib for the treatment of metastatic NSCLC with BRAF V600E mutation, the recommended adult dosage of trametinib is 2 mg once daily. Therapy should be continued until disease progression or unacceptable toxicity occurs.

Anaplastic Thyroid Cancer For use in combination with dabrafenib for the treatment of locally advanced or metastatic anaplastic thyroid cancer with BRAF V600E mutation when no satisfactory locoregional treatment options are available, the recommended adult dosage of trametinib is 2 mg once daily. Therapy should be continued until disease progression or unacceptable toxicity occurs.

Dosage Modification for Toxicity Dosage of trametinib may be reduced or therapy temporarily interrupted in patients who develop adverse effects. Up to 2 dosage reductions for toxicity may be made. If dosage modification of trametinib is necessary, an initial dosage reduction to 1.5 mg daily is recommended. If further dosage modification is necessary, dosage reduction to 1 mg daily may be considered. For patients unable to tolerate a dosage of trametinib 1 mg daily, the drug should be permanently discontinued.

For further information regarding dosage modification when trametinib is used in combination with dabrafenib, including information regarding dabrafenib dosage modification for toxicity, see Dosage and Administration: Dosage Modification for Toxicity, in Dabrafenib 10:00.

Dosage Modification for New Primary Cutaneous Malignancies. If new primary cutaneous malignancies occur, no dosage modification of trametinib is recommended.

Dosage Modification for New Primary Noncutaneous Malignancies. If new noncutaneous malignancies occur during combination therapy with trametinib and dabrafenib, no dosage modification of trametinib is required.

Dosage Modification for Febrile Drug Reactions. If fever (temperature exceeding 40°C) or fever complicated by rigors, hypotension, dehydration, or renal failure occurs, trametinib treatment should be interrupted until the adverse reaction resolves. Once fever has resolved, trametinib may be resumed at the same or a reduced dosage.

Dosage Modification for Dermatologic Effects. If grade 2 skin toxicity develops and is intolerable, trametinib should be withheld for up to 3 weeks. If grade 2 toxicity improves within 3 weeks of withholding trametinib, the drug should be resumed at a reduced dosage. If grade 2 skin toxicity does not improve within 3 weeks of withholding trametinib, the drug should be permanently discontinued.

If grade 3 or 4 skin toxicity occurs, trametinib should be withheld for up to 3 weeks. If grade 3 or 4 skin toxicity does not improve within 3 weeks of withholding trametinib, the drug should be permanently discontinued. If grade 3 or 4 skin toxicity improves within 3 weeks of withholding trametinib, the drug may be resumed at a reduced dosage.

Dosage Modification for Cardiac Effects. If an asymptomatic decrease in left ventricular ejection fraction (LVEF) from baseline of 10% or more and to a level below institution-specific lower limit of normal occurs, trametinib should be withheld for up to 4 weeks. If LVEF improves to normal values within 4 weeks of withholding trametinib, the drug may be resumed at a reduced dosage. If LVEF does not improve to normal values within 4 weeks of withholding trametinib, the drug should be permanently discontinued.

If symptomatic congestive heart failure (CHF) or a decrease in LVEF from baseline exceeding 20% and to a level below institution-specific lower limit of normal occurs, trametinib should be permanently discontinued.

Dosage Modification for Hemorrhage. If grade 3 hemorrhagic events occur, trametinib should be withheld. If improvement is observed, trametinib may be resumed at a lower dosage. If grade 3 hemorrhagic events do not improve, trametinib should be permanently discontinued.

If any grade 4 hemorrhagic events occur, trametinib should be permanently discontinued.

Dosage Modification for Venous Thromboembolism. If uncomplicated deep-vein thrombosis (DVT) or pulmonary embolism (PE) occurs, use of trametinib should be interrupted for up to 3 weeks. If improvement to grade 0 or 1 is observed within 3 weeks, trametinib may be resumed at a lower dosage. If no improvement is observed within 3 weeks, trametinib should be permanently discontinued.

If life-threatening PE occurs, trametinib should be permanently discontinued.

Dosage Modification for Ocular Effects. If retinal pigment epithelial detachment occurs, trametinib should be withheld for up to 3 weeks. If retinal pigment epithelial detachment improves within 3 weeks of withholding trametinib, the drug may be resumed at the same or a reduced dosage. If retinal pigment epithelial detachment does not improve within 3 weeks of withholding trametinib, the drug may be resumed at a reduced dosage or permanently discontinued.

If retinal vein occlusion occurs, trametinib should be permanently discontinued.

If uveitis occurs during combination therapy with trametinib and dabrafenib, no dosage modification of trametinib is necessary.

Dosage Modification for Pulmonary Effects. If interstitial lung disease or pneumonitis occurs, trametinib should be permanently discontinued.

Dosage Modification for Other Toxicity. If an intolerable grade 2 or any grade 3 adverse reaction occurs, trametinib should be withheld. If the grade 3 adverse reaction improves to grade 0 or 1, the drug should be resumed at a reduced dosage. If the grade 3 adverse reaction does not improve to grade 0 or 1, the drug should be permanently discontinued.

At the first occurrence of any grade 4 adverse reaction, trametinib should be withheld until the adverse reaction improves to grade 0 or 1 and then may be resumed at a reduced dosage. If the grade 4 adverse reaction does not improve to grade 0 or 1, trametinib should be permanently discontinued. If there is a recurrent grade 4 adverse reaction, trametinib also should be permanently discontinued.

■ **Special Populations** In patients with mild hepatic impairment (total bilirubin concentration not exceeding the ULN with AST concentration exceeding the ULN or total bilirubin concentration exceeding the ULN, but no more than 1.5 times the ULN, with any AST concentration), dosage adjustments are not necessary. However, appropriate dosage has not been established in patients with moderate to severe hepatic impairment.

In patients with mild or moderate renal impairment (glomerular filtration rate [GFR] 30–89 mL/minute per 1.73 m^2), dosage adjustments are not necessary. Appropriate dosage has not been established in patients with severe renal impairment.

The manufacturer does not make any specific dosage recommendations for geriatric patients.

Cautions

■ **Contraindications** The manufacturer states there are no known contraindications to the use of trametinib.

■ **Warnings/Precautions** ***Combination Therapy*** When combination therapy with trametinib includes the use of dabrafenib, the manufacturer's prescribing information for dabrafenib should be consulted for detailed information on the usual cautions, precautions, and contraindications of this drug. For further information regarding warnings and precautions associated with dabrafenib, also see Cautions: Warnings/Precautions, in Dabrafenib 10:00.

Development of New Primary Malignancies New primary cutaneous and noncutaneous malignancies are a known class effect of b-Raf serine-threonine kinase (BRAF) inhibitors (i.e., dabrafenib, encorafenib, vemurafenib).

In the COMBI-D study, basal cell carcinoma occurred in 3.3% of patients receiving trametinib in combination with dabrafenib compared with 6% of those receiving dabrafenib monotherapy. Additional occurrences of basal cell carcinoma were reported in 2 of the 7 patients who developed basal cell carcinoma following combination therapy with trametinib and dabrafenib. Cutaneous squamous cell carcinoma or new primary melanoma occurred in 3 or 0.5%, respectively, of patients receiving trametinib in combination with dabrafenib.

In the COMBI-AD study, cutaneous squamous cell carcinoma or new primary melanoma occurred in 1 or less than 1%, respectively, of patients receiving trametinib in combination with dabrafenib. In the BRF113928 study, cutaneous squamous cell carcinoma occurred in 3.2% of patients receiving trametinib in combination with dabrafenib.

In the COMBI-D, COMBI-AD, and BRF113928 studies, noncutaneous malignancies occurred in 1.4, 1, and 1.1%, respectively, of patients receiving trametinib in combination with dabrafenib.

Although the mechanism for development of cutaneous squamous cell carcinoma has not been fully determined, it has been suggested that paradoxical activation of mitogen-activated protein kinase (MAPK) signaling may lead to accelerated growth of such skin lesions as well as development of other primary malignancies. Some data suggest that mitogen-activated extracellular signal-regulated kinase (MEK) inhibitors (i.e., binimetinib, cobimetinib, trametinib) block the paradoxical activation of the MAPK pathway induced by BRAF inhibitors; therefore, combination therapy with a BRAF inhibitor and an MEK inhibitor may reduce the risk of developing cutaneous squamous cell carcinoma. Findings from a meta-analysis of randomized controlled studies that assessed the relative risk of development of cutaneous squamous cell carcinoma in cancer patients receiving a BRAF inhibitor indicate that the risk of cutaneous squamous cell carcinoma is higher in patients receiving a BRAF inhibitor than in patients receiving combination therapy with a BRAF inhibitor and an MEK inhibitor.

Dermatologic evaluations should be performed prior to initiation of combination therapy with trametinib and dabrafenib, every 2 months during therapy, and for up to 6 months following discontinuance of combination therapy. Close monitoring for signs and symptoms of new noncutaneous malignancies should be performed. In patients developing new primary cutaneous malignancies or noncutaneous malignancies during combination therapy, dosage modification of trametinib is not necessary.

Hemorrhage Hemorrhage, including major hemorrhagic events (i.e., symptomatic bleeding in a critical area or organ), has occurred when trametinib is used in combination with dabrafenib. In the COMBI-D study, hemorrhage occurred in 19% of patients receiving trametinib in combination with dabrafenib. Gastric hemorrhage or fatal intracranial hemorrhage occurred in 6 or 1.4%, respectively, of patients receiving trametinib in combination with dabrafenib. In the BRF113928 study, retroperitoneal and subarachnoid hemorrhage were fatal in 2.2% of patients receiving trametinib in combination with dabrafenib. In the COMBI-AD study, no fatal hemorrhagic events were observed in patients receiving combination therapy with trametinib and dabrafenib.

If hemorrhagic events occur, dosage modification and/or treatment discontinuance may be necessary. For grade 3 hemorrhagic events, use of trametinib should be interrupted. If improvement occurs, trametinib may be resumed at a lower dosage level. If improvement does not occur, trametinib should be permanently discontinued. For grade 4 hemorrhagic events, trametinib should be permanently discontinued.

Colitis and GI Perforation Colitis and GI perforation, sometimes fatal, have occurred in patients receiving trametinib as monotherapy or as combination therapy with dabrafenib. In clinical studies, colitis or GI perforation occurred in 0.6 or 0.3%, respectively, of patients receiving trametinib.

Patients should be monitored closely for manifestations of colitis and GI perforation.

Venous Thromboembolism Venous thromboembolism (VTE) has occurred when trametinib is used in combination with dabrafenib. In the COMBI-D, COMBI-AD, or BRF113928 studies, deep-vein thrombosis (DVT) and pulmonary embolism (PE) occurred in 2.8, 2, or 4.3%, respectively, of patients receiving trametinib in combination with dabrafenib.

Patients should be advised to immediately seek medical care if they develop symptoms of DVT or PE such as shortness of breath, chest pain, or arm or leg swelling. Dosage modification or treatment discontinuance may be necessary if DVT or PE occurs. (See Dosage Modification for Venous Thromboembolism under Dosage: Dosage Modification for Toxicity, in Dosage and Administration.)

Cardiac Effects Cardiomyopathy, including cardiac failure, has occurred in patients receiving trametinib monotherapy or combination therapy with dabrafenib.

In the METRIC study, 7% of patients receiving trametinib and no patients receiving conventional chemotherapy (IV dacarbazine or paclitaxel) experienced cardiomyopathy (defined as cardiac failure, left ventricular dysfunction, decreased left ventricular ejection fraction [LVEF]). Dosage modification and/or treatment discontinuance was necessary in 4% of trametinib-treated patients as a result of adverse cardiac effects. Cardiomyopathy resolved in most of these patients (71%). Across all clinical trials evaluating single-agent trametinib, 11% of patients receiving trametinib experienced an absolute decrease in LVEF from baseline of 10% or more and to a level below institution-specific lower limit of normal. An absolute decrease in LVEF from baseline of 20% or more and to a level below institution-specific lower limit of normal occurred in 5% of trametinib-treated patients.

In the COMBI-D study, 6% of patients receiving trametinib in combination with dabrafenib experienced an absolute decrease in LVEF from baseline of 10% or more and to a level below institution-specific lower limit of normal. Dosage interruption, dosage reduction, or discontinuance of trametinib was necessary in 4.4, 2.4, or 1.5%, respectively, of patients receiving trametinib in combination with dabrafenib. Cardiomyopathy resolved in most of these patients (83%).

In the COMBI-AD study, 3% of patients receiving trametinib in combination with dabrafenib experienced an absolute decrease in LVEF from baseline exceeding 10% and to a level below institution-specific lower limit of normal. Dosage interruption, dosage reduction, or discontinuance of trametinib was necessary in 2.1, 1.6, or 0.2%, respectively, of patients receiving combination therapy with trametinib and dabrafenib. Cardiomyopathy resolved in most of these patients (86%).

In the BRF113928 study, 9% of patients receiving trametinib in combination with dabrafenib experienced an absolute decrease in LVEF from baseline exceeding 10% and to a level below institution-specific lower limit of normal. Dosage interruption or discontinuance of trametinib therapy was necessary in 5 or 2.2%, respectively, of patients receiving combination therapy with trametinib and dabrafenib. Cardiomyopathy resolved in 50% of these patients.

Before initiation of trametinib therapy, LVEF should be assessed using echocardiogram or multigated radionuclide angiography (MUGA). LVEF should be assessed 1 month after initiation of trametinib and then every 2–3 months during treatment. Trametinib should be withheld in patients experiencing an absolute decrease in LVEF from baseline of 10% or more and to a level below institution-specific lower limit of normal. Trametinib should be permanently discontinued in patients experiencing symptomatic cardiomyopathy or persistent, asymptomatic left ventricular dysfunction (i.e., decrease in LVEF from baseline exceeding 20% and to a level below institution-specific lower limit of normal) that does not resolve within 4 weeks. (See Dosage Modification for Cardiac Effects under Dosage: Dosage Modification for Toxicity, in Dosage and Administration.)

Ocular Effects Retinal pigment epithelial detachment and retinal vein occlusion have occurred in patients receiving trametinib monotherapy or combination therapy with dabrafenib.

Retinal pigment epithelial detachment may be bilateral and multifocal, occurring in the macular region of the retina or other sites in the retina. Routine ophthalmologic examinations were not performed to detect asymptomatic retinal pigment epithelial detachment in clinical trials evaluating trametinib in patients with melanoma or non-small cell lung cancer (NSCLC); therefore, the true incidence of this adverse effect is unknown.

Retinal vein occlusion may lead to macular edema, decreased visual function, neovascularization, and glaucoma. Retinal vein occlusion occurred in 0.2% of patients receiving trametinib in clinical trials.

Ophthalmologic examinations should be performed periodically and as clinically indicated during trametinib therapy. If visual disturbances are reported, ophthalmologic evaluations should be performed urgently (within 24 hours).

If retinal pigment epithelial detachment is diagnosed, trametinib should be withheld. If repeat ophthalmologic evaluation confirms resolution of retinal pigment epithelial detachment within 3 weeks, trametinib may be resumed at the same or a reduced dosage. If no improvement is observed within 3 weeks, trametinib may be resumed at a reduced dosage or permanently discontinued. (See Dosage Modification for Ocular Effects under Dosage: Dosage Modification for Toxicity, in Dosage and Administration.)

If retinal vein occlusion is diagnosed, trametinib should be permanently discontinued.

If uveitis occurs in patients receiving combination therapy with trametinib and dabrafenib, no dosage modification of trametinib is required.

Pulmonary Effects Interstitial lung disease or pneumonitis has been reported in patients receiving trametinib monotherapy or combination therapy with dabrafenib. In clinical trials, interstitial lung disease or pneumonitis occurred in 2% of patients receiving trametinib monotherapy. In the METRIC study, 2.4% of patients developed interstitial lung disease or pneumonitis; all of those patients required hospitalization. In the COMBI-AD, COMBI-D, and BRF113928 studies, pneumonitis occurred in less than 1, 1, and 2.2%, respectively, of patients receiving trametinib in combination with dabrafenib.

In patients presenting with new or progressive pulmonary symptoms (including cough, dyspnea, hypoxia, pleural effusion, infiltrates), trametinib should be withheld pending results of clinical investigation. Trametinib should be permanently discontinued in patients diagnosed with treatment-related interstitial lung disease or pneumonitis. (See Dosage Modification for Pulmonary Effects under Dosage: Dosage Modification for Toxicity, in Dosage and Administration.)

Febrile Drug Reactions Serious febrile drug reactions (including fever accompanied by hypotension, rigors/chills, dehydration, or renal failure) have occurred in patients receiving combination therapy with trametinib and dabrafenib.

Across all clinical studies evaluating combination therapy with trametinib and dabrafenib in patients with unresectable or metastatic melanoma, the incidence of pyrexia was 57%; approximately 50% of these patients experienced at least 3 discrete episodes. In these studies, serious febrile reactions or fever of any severity complicated by hypotension, severe rigors/chills, dehydration, renal failure, or syncope occurred in 17% of patients receiving combination therapy with trametinib and dabrafenib. Fever was complicated by severe chills/rigors, dehydration, renal failure, or syncope in 0.4, 1.8, 0.5, or 0.7%, respectively, of patients receiving combination therapy with trametinib and dabrafenib.

If serious febrile reactions or fever accompanied by hypotension, rigors/chills, dehydration, or renal failure occurs, trametinib therapy should be interrupted and the patient evaluated for manifestations of infection. If severe pyrexia occurs, renal function should be monitored (e.g., serum creatinine) during and following severe pyrexia. Dosage modification or treatment discontinuance may be necessary. (See Dosage Modification for Febrile Drug Reactions under Dosage: Dosage Modification for Toxicity, in Dosage and Administration.) Prophylactic antipyretics should be administered in patients resuming trametinib following a serious febrile reaction or fever associated with complications. For second or subsequent occurrences of prolonged fever (lasting longer than 3 days) or fever associated with complications (e.g., dehydration, hypotension, renal failure, severe chills/rigors) without evidence of an active infection, corticosteroids (e.g., prednisone 10 mg daily) should be administered for at least 5 days.

Dermatologic Effects Dermatologic toxicity, including severe reactions (sometimes requiring hospitalization), has occurred in patients receiving trametinib monotherapy. In the METRIC study, adverse dermatologic reactions (including rash, dermatitis, acneiform rash, palmar-plantar erythrodysesthesia syndrome [hand-foot syndrome], and erythema) were reported in 87% of patients receiving trametinib. Severe dermatologic toxicity occurred in 12% of patients and 6% required hospitalization, most commonly for severe dermatologic toxicity or secondary skin infection requiring IV antibiotics. Dosage reduction or treatment discontinuance was required in 12 or 1%, respectively, of patients with dermatologic toxicity.

Serious dermatologic toxicity also has occurred in patients receiving trametinib in combination with dabrafenib. In the COMBI-D study, the incidence of any dermatologic toxicity was 55% in patients receiving trametinib in combination with dabrafenib; none of these cases were serious or severe. Patients in this study did not require permanent discontinuance of trametinib for dermatologic toxicity; however, dosage reduction was required in 5% of patients. Across clinical trials evaluating trametinib in combination with dabrafenib in patients with unresectable or metastatic melanoma, severe dermatologic toxicity occurred in 0.7% of patients receiving trametinib in combination with dabrafenib.

If dermatologic toxicity occurs, dosage modification or treatment discontinuance may be necessary. (See Dosage Modification for Dermatologic Effects under Dosage: Dosage Modification for Toxicity, in Dosage and Administration.)

Hyperglycemia Hyperglycemia has occurred in patients receiving combination therapy with trametinib and dabrafenib. In the COMBI-D study, grade 3 or 4 hyperglycemia occurred in 5 or 0.5%, respectively, of patients receiving dabrafenib in combination with trametinib. In this study, intensification of hypoglycemic therapy was required in 27% of patients with a history of diabetes mellitus receiving trametinib in combination with dabrafenib.

Serum glucose concentrations should be monitored prior to initiation of therapy and as clinically appropriate in patients with preexisting diabetes mellitus or hyperglycemia.

Fetal/Neonatal Morbidity and Mortality Trametinib may cause fetal harm in humans based on its mechanism of action and animal findings; the drug has been shown to be abortifacient and embryotoxic in rabbits at dosages resulting in exposures as low as 0.3 times the human exposure at recommended dosages.

Women with reproductive potential should use highly effective contraceptive methods while receiving trametinib and for 4 months following discontinuance of the drug. If pregnancy is confirmed or suspected during therapy, the patient should contact her clinician. If a woman is or becomes pregnant while taking trametinib, she should be informed of the risk to the fetus.

Impairment of Fertility Results of animal studies suggest that trametinib may reduce female fertility. In fertility studies, impairment of fertility (increased follicular cysts and reduced corpora lutea) was observed in female animals receiving trametinib at exposure levels equivalent to 0.3 times the human exposure at the recommended dosage.

Specific Populations **Pregnancy.** Trametinib may cause fetal harm if administered to pregnant women based on its mechanism of action and animal findings. (See Fetal/Neonatal Morbidity and Mortality under Cautions: Warnings/Precautions.)

Lactation. It is not known whether trametinib is distributed into human milk. Because of the potential for serious adverse reactions to trametinib in breast-fed infants, women should be advised not to breast-feed while receiving the drug and for 4 months after the last dose. The effects of the drug on breast-fed infants or on the production of milk are unknown.

Pediatric Use. Safety and efficacy of trametinib have not been established in pediatric patients.

Geriatric Use. Clinical experience with trametinib monotherapy in patients 65 years of age or older is insufficient to determine whether geriatric patients respond differently than younger adults.

In the COMBI-D, COMBI-V, and COMBI-AD studies evaluating trametinib in combination with dabrafenib in patients with melanoma, 21% of patients were 65 years of age or older and 5% were 75 years of age or older. No overall differences in efficacy were observed between geriatric patients and younger adults, but some adverse effects (i.e., peripheral edema, anorexia) occurred more frequently in geriatric patients with metastatic melanoma.

Clinical experience with trametinib in patients 65 years of age or older with NSCLC is insufficient to determine whether geriatric patients respond differently than younger adults.

Hepatic Impairment. In population pharmacokinetic analyses, systemic exposure of trametinib was not affected in patients with mild hepatic impairment (total bilirubin concentration not exceeding the ULN with AST concentration exceeding the ULN or total bilirubin concentration exceeding the ULN, but no more than 1.5 times the ULN, with any AST concentration). (See Dosage and Administration: Special Populations.)

The pharmacokinetic profile of trametinib has not been established in patients with moderate or severe hepatic impairment.

Renal Impairment. In population pharmacokinetic analyses, systemic exposure of trametinib was not affected in patients with mild to moderate renal impairment (glomerular filtration rate [GFR] 30–89 mL/minute per 1.73 m^2). (See Dosage and Administration: Special Populations.)

The pharmacokinetic profile of trametinib has not been established in patients with severe renal impairment.

■ Common Adverse Effects

Adverse effects reported in 20% or more of patients receiving trametinib monotherapy for the treatment of unresectable or metastatic melanoma with BRAF V600E or V600K mutation and at an incidence that is at least 5% higher than that reported with conventional chemotherapy in the METRIC study include rash, diarrhea, and lymphedema. Laboratory abnormalities reported in 20% or more of patients receiving trametinib monotherapy for the treatment of unresectable or metastatic melanoma with BRAF V600E or V600K mutation and at an incidence that is at least 5% higher than that reported with conventional chemotherapy include elevated concentrations of aminotransferases (i.e., AST, ALT), hypoalbuminemia, anemia, and elevated concentrations of alkaline phosphatase.

Adverse effects reported in 20% or more of patients receiving trametinib in combination with dabrafenib for the treatment of previously untreated unresectable or metastatic melanoma with BRAF V600E or V600K mutation in the COMBI-D and COMBI-V studies include pyrexia, diarrhea, fatigue, nausea, rash, chills, headache, vomiting, arthralgia, hypertension, and cough. Laboratory abnormalities reported in 20% or more of patients receiving trametinib in combination with dabrafenib for the treatment of previously untreated unresectable or metastatic melanoma with BRAF V600E or V600K mutation include hyperglycemia, elevated concentrations of alkaline phosphatase, hypophosphatemia, and hyponatremia.

Adverse effects reported in 20% or more of patients receiving trametinib in combination with dabrafenib for the adjuvant treatment of melanoma with BRAF V600E or V600K mutation in the COMBI-AD study include pyrexia, fatigue, nausea, headache, chills, rash, diarrhea, arthralgia, vomiting, and myalgia. Laboratory abnormalities reported in 20% or more of patients receiving trametinib in combination with dabrafenib for the adjuvant treatment of melanoma with BRAF V600E or V600K mutation include hyperglycemia, elevated concentrations of aminotransferases (i.e., AST, ALT), neutropenia, hypophosphatemia, elevated concentrations of alkaline phosphatase, lymphopenia, anemia, and hypoalbuminemia.

Adverse effects reported in 20% or more of patients receiving trametinib in combination with dabrafenib for the treatment of metastatic NSCLC with BRAF V600E mutation in the BRF113928 study include pyrexia, fatigue, nausea, vomiting, diarrhea, dry skin, decreased appetite, edema, rash, chills, hemorrhage, cough, and dyspnea. Laboratory abnormalities reported in 20% or more of patients receiving trametinib in combination with dabrafenib for the treatment of metastatic NSCLC with BRAF V600E mutation include hyperglycemia, elevated concentrations of alkaline phosphatase, elevated concentrations of aminotransferases (i.e., AST, ALT), hyponatremia, leukopenia, anemia, neutropenia, lymphopenia, hypophosphatemia, and elevated concentrations of serum creatinine.

Adverse effects reported in the BRF117019 study in patients receiving trametinib in combination with dabrafenib for the treatment of locally advanced or metastatic anaplastic thyroid cancer were similar to those reported in other studies in patients receiving combination therapy with trametinib and dabrafenib for the treatment of melanoma or NSCLC.

Drug Interactions

Formal drug interaction studies have not been conducted with trametinib.

In vitro studies have indicated that trametinib induces cytochrome P-450 (CYP) 3A; however, cross-study comparisons with a sensitive CYP3A4 substrate showed that trametinib had no clinically relevant effects on pharmacokinetics of the sensitive CYP3A4 substrate.

In vitro studies have indicated that trametinib is an inhibitor of CYP2C8.

Trametinib is a substrate of P-glycoprotein (P-gp) and bile salt export pump (BSEP). Pharmacokinetic interactions are unlikely with drugs that inhibit the P-gp transport system since trametinib exhibits high passive permeability and bioavailability.

Trametinib is not a substrate for CYP isoenzymes, breast cancer resistance protein (BCRP), organic anion transporter polypeptide (OATP) 1B1, OATP1B3, OATP2B1, organic cation transporter (OCT) 1, multidrug resistance-associated protein (MRP) 2, or multidrug and toxic compound extrusion 1 (MATE1). Trametinib is not an inhibitor of CYP 1A2, 2A6, 2B6, 2C9, 2C19, 2D6, or 3A4, and also is not an inhibitor of OATP1B1, OATP1B3, organic anion transporter (OAT) 1, OAT3, OCT2, P-gp, BCRP, BSEP, MRP2, or MATE1.

Concomitant administration of trametinib 2 mg once daily with dabrafenib 150 mg twice daily resulted in no change in area under the concentration-time curve (AUC) of trametinib compared with administration of trametinib alone.

Description

Trametinib, a selective inhibitor of mitogen-activated extracellular signal regulated kinase (MEK) 1 and MEK2 activation and kinase activity in cells with b-Raf serine-threonine kinase (BRAF) V600E or V600K mutations, is an antineoplastic agent. MEK proteins are upstream regulators of the extracellular signal-related kinase (ERK) pathway, which promotes cellular proliferation. Approximately 50% of cutaneous melanomas carry a BRAF mutation. The most common BRAF mutation is the substitution of glutamic acid for valine at codon 600 (BRAF V600E); a less frequently occurring BRAF mutation is the substitution of lysine for valine at codon 600 (BRAF V600K). BRAF V600 mutations result in activation of the BRAF pathway that includes MEK 1 and 2. The mutation of BRAF V600E activates the mitogen-activated protein kinase (MAPK) and extracellular signal-regulated kinase (ERK) signal transduction pathway, which enhances cell proliferation and tumor progression (e.g., metastasis). Trametinib inhibits BRAF V600 mutation-positive melanoma cell growth in vitro and in vivo by decreasing cell proliferation, causing cell cycle arrest, and inducing apoptosis.

Clinical resistance to monotherapy with a BRAF inhibitor, generally occurring 6–7 months following initiation of therapy, has been attributed to several possible resistance mechanisms mostly relying on reactivation of the MAPK/ERK pathway. Complete inhibition of the MAPK/ERK pathway resulting in durable responses may be achieved with the use of combination therapy with a BRAF inhibitor (i.e., dabrafenib, encorafenib, vemurafenib) and an MEK inhibitor (i.e., binimetinib, cobimetinib, trametinib). Use of trametinib and dabrafenib in combination resulted in greater growth inhibition of melanoma cell lines testing positive for BRAF V600 mutations in vitro. In addition, combination therapy was associated with prolonged inhibition of tumor growth in melanoma xenografts testing positive for BRAF V600 mutations compared with either drug alone.

Following oral administration, the absolute bioavailability of trametinib is 72%. Peak plasma concentrations of trametinib occur within 1.5 hours after oral administration. Following administration of a single trametinib dose within the dosage range of 0.125–10 mg, the drug exhibits dose-proportional increases in peak plasma concentrations and greater than proportional increases in area under the concentration-time curve (AUC). After repeated once-daily dosing of 0.125–4 mg, increases in peak plasma concentrations and AUC are dose proportional. Trametinib is 97.4% bound to plasma proteins. Administration of a single dose of trametinib with a high-fat, high-calorie meal (approximately 1000 calories) decreased peak plasma concentrations and AUC of the drug by 70 and 24%, respectively, and delayed the rate of absorption (time to reach peak concentrations delayed by 4 hours). (See Dosage and Administration: Administration.) Trametinib is principally metabolized by deacetylation with or without mono-oxygenation or in combination with glucuronidation in vitro. The estimated terminal half-life of trametinib is 3.9–4.8 days. Following oral administration of a radiolabeled dose of trametinib, more than 80% of the dose is recovered in feces and less than 20% is recovered in urine.

Advice to Patients

Importance of advising patient to read the manufacturer's patient information before beginning treatment and each time the prescription is refilled.

Importance of taking trametinib at least 1 hour before or 2 hours after a meal.

Importance of taking a missed dose as soon as it is remembered, but only if it can be taken at least 12 hours before the next scheduled dose.

Importance of proper storage of trametinib (e.g., storing the tablets in the manufacturer's original bottle at 2–8°C). Importance of not removing the desiccant from the bottle and not storing the tablets in pill boxes.

Risk of new primary cutaneous and noncutaneous malignancies with trametinib and dabrafenib combination therapy. Importance of contacting a clinician promptly if dermatologic changes (i.e., new lesions or changes to existing lesions) or signs and/or symptoms of other malignancies occur.

Risk of intracranial and GI hemorrhage with trametinib and dabrafenib combination therapy. Importance of contacting a clinician promptly if signs and/or symptoms of unusual bleeding or hemorrhage occur.

Risk of colitis or GI perforation. Importance of contacting a clinician promptly if unusual bleeding, diarrhea, abdominal pain or tenderness, fever, or nausea occurs.

Risk of deep-vein thrombosis and pulmonary embolism with trametinib and dabrafenib combination therapy. Importance of contacting a clinician promptly if sudden onset of breathing difficulty, leg pain, or swelling occurs.

Risk of cardiomyopathy. Importance of immediately contacting a clinician if manifestations of heart failure occur.

Risk of visual disturbances that may lead to blindness. Importance of contacting a clinician if changes in vision occur.

Risk of interstitial lung disease (or pneumonitis). Importance of immediately contacting a clinician if cough or dyspnea occurs.

Risk of serious febrile reactions with trametinib and dabrafenib combination therapy. Importance of contacting a clinician if fever develops.

Risk of skin toxicities (possibly requiring hospitalization). Importance of contacting a clinician if progressive or intolerable rash occurs.

Risk of hypertension. Importance of monitoring blood pressure regularly during therapy and of contacting a clinician if manifestations of hypertension occur.

Risk of diarrhea (sometimes severe). Importance of contacting a clinician if severe diarrhea occurs.

Risk of fetal harm if taken during pregnancy. Importance of female patients using highly effective contraception during trametinib treatment and for 4 months after discontinuance of the drug. Importance of contacting a clinician if pregnancy is suspected or confirmed during treatment.

Risk of serious adverse reactions in nursing infants of women receiving trametinib. Importance of discontinuing breast-feeding during therapy and for 4 months after the last dose.

Importance of advising women of reproductive potential that trametinib may reduce female fertility.

Importance of informing clinicians of existing or contemplated concomitant therapy, including prescription and OTC drugs and dietary or herbal supplements, as well as any concomitant illnesses (e.g., cardiovascular disease).

Importance of informing patients of other important precautionary information. (See Cautions.)

Overview® (see Users Guide). For additional information on this drug until a more detailed monograph is developed and published, the manufacturer's labeling should be consulted. It is *essential* that the manufacturer's labeling be consulted for more detailed information on usual cautions, precautions, contraindications, potential drug interactions, laboratory test interferences, and acute toxicity. For further information on the handling of antineoplastic agents, see the ASHP Guidelines on Handling Hazardous Drugs at http://www.ahfsdruginformation.com.

Preparations

Excipients in commercially available drug preparations may have clinically important effects in some individuals; consult specific product labeling for details.

Trametinib Dimethyl Sulfoxide

Oral		
Tablets	0.5 mg (of trametinib)	**Mekinist®**, Novartis
	2 mg (of trametinib)	**Mekinist®**, Novartis

Trastuzumab

Trastuzumab (Herceptin®) should not be confused with ado-trastuzumab emtansine (Kadcyla®). The latter agent is an anti-human epidermal growth factor receptor type 2 (anti-*HER2*) antibody-drug conjugate; the anti-*HER2* antibody trastuzumab, a humanized immunoglobulin (IgG_1), is conjugated with the microtubule inhibitor DM1 (derivative of maytansine) via the linker MCC (4-[N-maleimidomethyl] cyclohexane-1-carboxylate).

The original generic name for Kadcyla®, as established by the US Adopted Name (USAN) Council in 2009, was trastuzumab emtansine. Because of the similarity between the original generic name (trastuzumab emtansine) and the generic name for Herceptin® (trastuzumab), the US Food and Drug Administration (FDA) approved the addition of the prefix "ado" to the generic name for Kadcyla® (i.e., ado-trastuzumab emtansine); however, the potential exists for dispensing or prescribing errors involving these drugs. The manufacturer of ado-trastuzumab emtansine (Kadcyla®) states that this drug should *not* be substituted for or used with trastuzumab (Herceptin®). Therefore, extra care should be exercised to ensure the accuracy of prescriptions for trastuzumab (Herceptin®) or ado-trastuzumab emtansine (Kadcyla®).

To avoid medication errors, the Institute for Safe Medication Practices (ISMP), the FDA, and the manufacturer of ado-trastuzumab emtansine (Kadcyla®) recommend that prescribers communicate both the brand and generic names for ado-trastuzumab emtansine (Kadcyla®) on the prescription order form. (See Dispensing and Administration Precautions under Dosage and Administration: Reconstitution and Administration and also under Cautions: Precautions and Contraindications.)

■ Trastuzumab, a recombinant DNA-derived humanized anti-*HER2* monoclonal antibody, is an antineoplastic agent.

Uses

■ **Breast Cancer** ***Overview*** Trastuzumab is used as monotherapy for the treatment of metastatic breast cancer that has relapsed following prior chemotherapy in patients with tumors that overexpress the *HER2* protein. Trastuzumab also is used in combination with paclitaxel for the initial treatment of metastatic breast cancer in patients with tumors that overexpress the *HER2* protein. Trastuzumab is used in conjunction with standard adjuvant chemotherapy for the treatment of operable HER2-positive breast cancer. The benefit of combination therapy with trastuzumab and chemotherapy appears to be largely limited to patients with disease testing 3+ for HER2 overexpression. Trastuzumab, the second monoclonal antibody approved for the treatment of cancer and the first monoclonal antibody approved for the treatment of breast cancer, received fast-track and priority review from the US Food and Drug Administration (FDA).

Although the use of trastuzumab in combination with an anthracycline and cyclophosphamide for the initial treatment of *HER2*-overexpressing metastatic breast cancer has been investigated in a large, randomized clinical trial, the clinical benefit obtained with this regimen did not outweigh the increased risk of serious cardiac toxicity, and an indication for the use of trastuzumab with this combination regimen did *not* receive approval from the FDA.

Trastuzumab also is *not* indicated for the treatment of metastatic breast cancer in patients with tumors that do not overexpress the *HER2* protein.

Patients with metastatic breast tumors with 2+ or 3+ overexpression of *HER2* protein (based on a 0–3+ scale with 3+ being the highest degree of overexpression) as determined by an immunohistochemical assay using 4D5 and CB11 murine monoclonal anti-*HER2* antibodies (known as the Clinical Trial Assay [CTA]) were eligible for enrollment in clinical trials of trastuzumab. About 33% of women with metastatic breast cancer screened for eligibility for enrollment in clinical trials of trastuzumab were found to have 2+- or 3+-*HER2*-overexpressing tumors; among patients enrolled in the pivotal clinical trials, about 75% had 3+-overexpressing tumors and 25% had 2+-overexpressing tumors. Although these studies were not designed to include stratification by degree of *HER2* overexpression, and the small number of patients with 2+-overexpressing tumors limits interpretation of the data, retrospective analysis of the data from clinical trials suggests that benefit of trastuzumab (i.e., higher response rates, increased time to progression of disease) may be limited to patients with tumors that have 3+ overexpression of the *HER2* protein. Further study is needed to establish the benefit of trastuzumab in patients with 2+-overexpressing (weakly positive) breast tumors.

Evaluation of HER2/neu in Breast Cancer The methods of *HER2/neu* evaluation most commonly used in routine clinical practice and clinical research studies are immunohistochemistry (IHC) assays, which directly measure overexpression of the *HER2/neu* protein, and fluorescent *in situ* hybridization (FISH), which measures amplification of the *HER2/neu* oncogene. The presence of HER2 overexpression may be inferred when HER2 gene amplification is detected using the FISH assay. HercepTest® and PATHWAY® (IHC assays) and PathVysion®, INFORM®, and HER2 FISH pharmDx® (FISH assays) are examples of appropriate commercial assays that may be used to identify candidates for trastuzumab therapy.

Findings from small studies show conflicting results for the agreement of IHC and FISH testing, with some studies citing high levels of concordance, while others report levels as low as 49%. Some experts argue for use of a FISH assay as the primary screening tool because of greater accuracy whereas others argue for use of an IHC assay because of lesser time and cost requirements. In addition, overexpression of the *HER2* protein has been observed in the absence of detectable *HER2* gene amplification (i.e., FISH-negative). In a large quality control and quality assurance study in which both FISH and IHC test results were available for 2913 of 2963 breast cancer specimens, the concordance rate was 65% when IHC scores of 2+ and 3+ were grouped together; the concordance rate increased to 96% when results for the IHC 2+ specimens were excluded from the analysis. The FISH assay had a higher failure rate (5 versus 0.08%), higher cost, and longer testing and interpretation times than the IHC assay.

Because of limitations in the accuracy and precision of each of these types of assays, use of a single methodology for the evaluation of HER2 overexpression is not advised. Many experts currently recommend initial screening using an IHC assay followed by confirmation of positive results using a FISH assay, particularly for 2+ HER2-overexpressing tumors. The precision of *HER2/neu* evaluation may vary according to the type of assay and assay procedures used. Further study of these methods, particularly regarding their comparative efficacy in predicting disease prognosis and response to therapy, is needed to establish the optimum procedure for determining the *HER2/neu* status of breast cancer.

The reliability of HER2 testing is improved when performed in large-volume central laboratories compared with local laboratories. Assessment of *HER2* overexpression in breast tumors using IHC or FISH methodology should be performed by laboratories with demonstrated proficiency in the specific technology being used. Improper assay performance, including use of suboptimally fixed tissue, failure to use specified reagents, deviation from specific assay instructions, and failure to include appropriate controls for assay validation, can lead to unreliable results. For full instructions on assay performance, refer to the prescribing information for each assay kit.

Detection of HER2 Protein Overexpression. The IHC assay used to test breast tumors for *HER2* overexpression in the pivotal trials of trastuzumab is a research assay known as the Clinical Trial Assay (CTA). The DAKO HercepTest® is a commercially available immunohistochemical test that is used to measure *HER2* protein in tumors and to help identify patients who may be candidates for treatment with trastuzumab. In the randomized trial involving patients with metastatic breast cancer (study 3), data suggest that benefit of combination therapy with trastuzumab and chemotherapy was largely limited to patients with disease testing 3+ for HER2 overexpression on the CTA.

The HercepTest® has been assessed for concordance with the CTA. The low specificity reported for the HercepTest® when used according to manufacturer guidelines and the FDA-approved scoring system raises concerns about large numbers of false-positive specimens resulting in inappropriate use of trastuzumab. In one study using tissue specimens from 48 cases of invasive breast cancer, consideration of the level of staining of nonneoplastic epithelium in a specimen as an internal control helped compensate for variability in tissue fixation and processing and improved the specificity of the HercepTest® from 42% to 93%.

Detection of HER2 Gene Amplification. Measurement of the number of HER2 gene copies using the FISH assay to detect gene amplification may be used as a surrogate measurement of protein overexpression. PathVysion® is a commercially available FISH assay that is used to identify patients who may be candidates for trastuzumab therapy.

In a retrospective analysis of known CTA 2+ or 3+ tumor specimens from patients with metastatic breast cancer receiving trastuzumab and chemotherapy in a randomized trial (study 3), the data suggest that benefit of treatment was greater in patients with FISH-positive tumors than in those with FISH-negative tumors; however, time to progression of disease was prolonged in patients receiving combination therapy with trastuzumab and chemotherapy for CTA 2+ or 3+ tumors regardless of the FISH test status. This treatment effect was particularly strong among patients receiving trastuzumab and chemotherapy for CTA 3+ tumors even if the tumor was FISH-negative. There are insufficient data to determine whether the FISH assay can be used to identify a subgroup of patients with CTA 2+ tumors who would be unlikely to benefit from trastuzumab therapy.

Adjuvant Therapy for Early-stage Breast Cancer Trastuzumab is used in conjunction with standard adjuvant chemotherapy (doxorubicin and cyclophosphamide followed by paclitaxel) for the treatment of HER2-overexpressing, node-positive breast cancer.

In several large randomized trials, the addition of trastuzumab to standard adjuvant chemotherapy in patients with operable HER2-positive breast cancer reduced the risk of death and/or prolonged disease-free survival.

The current indication for trastuzumab as adjuvant therapy for HER2-overexpressing, node-positive breast cancer is based on 2 North American randomized clinical trials. In the National Surgical Adjuvant Breast and Bowel Project trial B-31 (study 1), 2043 women were randomly assigned to receive either doxorubicin and cyclophosphamide followed by paclitaxel or the same regimen with trastuzumab given concurrently with paclitaxel. In the North Central Cancer Treatment Group trial N9831 (study 2), 1633 of the 2766 patients enrolled were randomly assigned to receive either doxorubicin and cyclophosphamide followed by paclitaxel or the same regimen with trastuzumab given concurrently with paclitaxel.

A total of 3752 patients were randomly assigned to treatment in the 2 trials prior to a planned interim analysis. In a combined analysis of data from patient groups from the 2 trials at a median follow-up of 2 years, disease-free survival at 3 years was prolonged (hazard ratio: 0.48, absolute disease-free survival rate: 87 versus 75%) and the risk of death at 3 years was decreased (hazard ratio: 0.67, absolute survival rate: 94 versus 92%) in patients receiving trastuzumab in combination with standard adjuvant chemotherapy compared with those receiving standard adjuvant chemotherapy alone. Subgroup analysis of the data from study 2 exploring efficacy according to HER2 overexpression showed a strong effect on disease-free survival (hazard ratio: 0.42) for the addition of trastuzumab to adjuvant chemotherapy in patients with disease that was 3+ HER2-overexpressing and FISH-positive. Because of the small number of events in the other subgroups, it is not known whether adjuvant therapy including trastuzumab would benefit patients with breast tumors that are FISH-positive but lack 3+ HER2 overexpression.

Trastuzumab also was used as adjuvant therapy for operable HER2-positive breast cancer in an international multicenter randomized trial. In the Herceptin Adjuvant (HERA) trial, 5081 women received trastuzumab (1 or 2 years) or underwent observation following neoadjuvant and/or adjuvant chemotherapy for operable HER2-positive breast cancer. At a median follow-up of 1 year among 3387 patients receiving either 1 year of trastuzumab therapy or observation, the rate of disease-free survival was prolonged in patients receiving trastuzumab (hazard ratio for an event: 0.54, absolute difference in disease-free survival at 2 years of 8.4 percentage points). At a median follow-up of 2 years, prolonged survival has been observed in patients receiving 1 year of trastuzumab therapy compared with observation (hazard ratio for death: 0.66, absolute difference in death rate at 3 years of 2.7 percentage points).

Patients were eligible for enrollment in the randomized trials if they had operable breast cancer that was identified as HER2-positive with either 3+ HER2 overexpression according to the IHC assay or positive results for amplification of the HER2 gene according to the FISH assay. HER2 testing was performed at a reference laboratory (study 1) or HER2 test results were confirmed by a central laboratory prior to randomization (study 2). For 1153 tumor specimens in study 2 which tested as IHC 3+ using HercepTest® at a local laboratory, 85% were concordant and 15% were discordant when testing was confirmed by a central laboratory. For 414 tumor specimens in study 2 which tested as FISH-positive using PathVysion® at a local laboratory, 94% were concordant and 6% were discordant when testing was confirmed by a central laboratory.

In the 2 North American trials, most patients (91%) had node-positive disease. The median age of the patients was 49 years (range: 22–80 years), and most were Caucasian (84%). Most patients had intermediate-grade (27%) or high-grade (66%) breast tumors, and 53% had hormone receptor-positive disease. The benefit of trastuzumab appeared to be similar among patients with hormone receptor-positive or hormone receptor-negative breast tumors. Because of the lack of data in these trials, it is unknown whether the addition of trastuzumab to standard adjuvant chemotherapy would benefit patients with node-negative breast cancer. In the international trial, the median age of the patients was 49 years; about one-third of the patients had node-negative breast cancer, and 48% had hormone receptor-negative tumors. In this trial, the benefit of 1 year of trastuzumab therapy did not appear to differ according to nodal or estrogen receptor status.

In both North American trials, for the comparison groups receiving trastuzumab given concurrently with paclitaxel, an initial dose of trastuzumab 4 mg/kg was administered with the first dose of paclitaxel followed by trastuzumab 2 mg/kg once weekly for 51 weeks. The same regimen of adjuvant chemotherapy with doxorubicin and cyclophosphamide was used in both trials (four 21-day cycles of doxorubicin 60 mg/m^2 and cyclophosphamide 600 mg/m^2), but the regimens for paclitaxel differed: 80 mg/m^2 once weekly or 175 mg/m^2 once every 3 weeks for a total of 12 weeks in trial B-31 (study 1) and 80 mg/m^2 once weekly in trial N9831 (study 2). When administered, radiation therapy was initiated following the completion of chemotherapy. Patients with estrogen receptor-positive and/or progesterone receptor-positive tumors also received hormonal therapy.

In trial N9831 (study 2), a third group of patients received adjuvant chemotherapy with doxorubicin and cyclophosphamide, followed by paclitaxel therapy, and then trastuzumab therapy. Further follow-up is needed before the comparative efficacy of concurrent versus sequential paclitaxel and trastuzumab therapy can be assessed, but an interim analysis of the data from this trial suggests that concurrent therapy may be more effective.

In the international trial, differing regimens of neoadjuvant and/or adjuvant chemotherapy (including both anthracyclines and taxanes in about 26% of patients) were followed by an initial dose of trastuzumab 8 mg/kg and then trastuzumab 6 mg/kg once every 3 weeks.

Increased risk of cardiac toxicity was associated with trastuzumab therapy. Among patients receiving adjuvant therapy for breast cancer, those receiving trastuzumab and paclitaxel following completion of doxorubicin and cyclophosphamide therapy experienced a higher incidence of symptomatic, laboratory-confirmed cardiomyopathy compared with those receiving paclitaxel alone (2 versus 0.4%). The cumulative incidence of class III or IV congestive heart failure or death from cardiac causes at 3 years in patients receiving trastuzumab was 4.1% in trial B-31 (study 1) and 2.9% in trial N9831 (study 2). The incidence of class III or IV congestive heart failure in patients receiving trastuzumab was 0.5% at 1 year in the international trial.

Patients were eligible for enrollment in the North American randomized trials if they did not have previous or currently active cardiac disease based on symptoms or test findings (ECG, radiographs, and left ventricular ejection fraction [LVEF]) or uncontrolled hypertension (diastolic blood pressure exceeding 100 mm Hg or systolic blood pressure exceeding 200 mm Hg). Cardiac function was monitored at regular intervals, and trastuzumab therapy was not initiated or was discontinued if clinical manifestations or decline in LVEF indicated cardiac toxicity. Trastuzumab therapy was permanently discontinued in patients who developed congestive heart failure or persistent/recurrent LVEF decline. Similar eligibility criteria, cardiac monitoring, and stopping rules for cardiotoxicity were applied in the international trial. Further follow-up is needed to fully assess the risk of cardiotoxicity associated with trastuzumab as adjuvant therapy for operable HER2-positive breast cancer.

Increased risk of pulmonary toxicity also was associated with trastuzumab therapy. Among patients receiving adjuvant therapy for breast cancer in the 2 North American trials (studies 1 and 2), those receiving trastuzumab and paclitaxel following completion of doxorubicin and cyclophosphamide therapy experienced a higher incidence of dyspnea, the most common pulmonary toxicity, compared with those receiving paclitaxel alone (study 1: 12 versus 4%, study 2: 2.5 versus 0.1%). Pneumonitis/pulmonary infiltrates (0.7 versus 0.3%) and deaths from respiratory failure (3 deaths versus 1 death) also occurred more frequently in patients receiving trastuzumab compared with chemotherapy alone.

For patients with node-positive, HER2-positive operable breast cancer, trastuzumab should be added to standard adjuvant chemotherapy unless contraindicated. For patients with node-negative, HER2-positive operable breast cancer†, the use of trastuzumab in conjunction with standard adjuvant chemotherapy should be considered with careful weighing of possible benefit versus the risk of cardiac toxicity. Careful patient selection and monitoring of cardiac function is required in all patients receiving trastuzumab as adjuvant therapy. Further follow-up of these clinical trials and additional studies are needed to answer other questions, such as the optimal dosing schedule, timing of administration (concurrent versus sequential), and duration of therapy for trastuzumab, and to fully evaluate the nature and risk of cardiotoxicity associated with trastuzumab in this patient population.

A randomized trial is under way comparing the addition of trastuzumab to anthracycline-containing versus non-anthracycline-containing adjuvant chemotherapy to determine whether similar efficacy can be achieved with less cardiac toxicity for HER2-positive operable breast cancer. Other regimens and schedules for adjuvant trastuzumab therapy are being investigated. For a small subgroup of 232 patients with HER2-positive tumors among 1010 women receiving adjuvant chemotherapy for node-positive or high-risk node-negative early breast cancer in a randomized trial, the addition of trastuzumab to chemotherapy with either docetaxel or vinorelbine compared with chemotherapy alone (prior to treatment with an anthracycline-containing regimen) prolonged recurrence-free survival. This shortened schedule for trastuzumab (9 weekly infusions) preceding the use of an anthracycline was not associated with decreased left ventricular ejection fraction or cardiac failure.

First-line Therapy for Advanced Breast Cancer The current indication for use of trastuzumab in combination with paclitaxel for the initial treatment of metastatic breast cancer is based on data from a randomized, controlled, multicenter clinical trial involving 469 patients with 2+ or 3+ *HER2*-overexpressing metastatic breast cancer. Patients were randomized to receive combination therapy with trastuzumab (4-mg/kg IV initial dose followed by once-weekly doses of 2 mg/kg IV) and chemotherapy or chemotherapy alone. For patients who had received prior adjuvant therapy with an anthracycline, chemotherapy consisted of paclitaxel 175 mg/m^2 IV over 3 hours every 21 days for at least 6 cycles; for all other patients, chemotherapy consisted of an anthracycline (doxorubicin hydrochloride 60 mg/m^2 or epirubicin hydrochloride 75 mg/m^2 every 21 days) and cyclophosphamide (600 mg/m^2 every 21 days) for 6 cycles. Trastuzumab therapy was continued until disease progression or intolerable toxicity was observed. The median age of the patients was 52 years (range: 25–77 years) and most (89%) were Caucasian.

Longer time to disease progression (7.2 versus 4.5 months), higher overall response rate (45 versus 29%), longer median duration of response (8.3 versus 5.8 months), and longer median survival (25.1 versus 20.3 months) were reported in patients receiving trastuzumab in combination with chemotherapy compared with those receiving chemotherapy alone. With the exception of overall survival, the magnitude of benefit was greater with the addition of trastuzumab to paclitaxel versus an anthracycline and cyclophosphamide despite the poorer prognosis of patients in the paclitaxel subgroup; in addition, the incidence and severity of cardiac toxicity were greater in patients receiving trastuzumab combined with an anthracycline and cyclophosphamide.

The benefit of adding trastuzumab to conventional chemotherapy was greater in patients with 3+-*HER2*-overexpressing breast tumors than in those with 2+-*HER2*-overexpressing breast tumors. Although the study was not designed to include stratification by degree of *HER2* overexpression, and the small number of patients with 2+-overexpressing tumors limits interpretation of the data, retrospective analysis suggests that response to trastuzumab is limited to the patients with the highest level of *HER2* overexpression (3+). The relative risk for disease progression in patients receiving trastuzumab in combination with chemotherapy versus those receiving chemotherapy alone was lower among patients with 3+ versus 2+ *HER2*-overexpressing disease (relative risk 0.42 versus 0.76) using the CTA methodology; lower relative risk for disease progression represents longer time to disease progression.

Compared with patients receiving paclitaxel alone, those receiving trastuzumab and paclitaxel experienced a longer median time to disease progression (6.7 versus 2.5 months) and a higher overall response rate (38 versus 15%); median duration of response was 8 versus 4 months and median survival was 22 versus 18 months. Because of the difference in patient characteristics between the groups (i.e., poorer prognosis for patients in the paclitaxel subgroup), the results of this clinical trial cannot be used to compare the efficacy and safety of combination therapy with trastuzumab and paclitaxel versus standard first-line therapy of an anthracycline and cyclophosphamide for metastatic breast cancer.

Combination therapy with trastuzumab, paclitaxel, and carboplatin† is used in the treatment of HER2-overexpressing metastatic breast cancer. In a phase 3 randomized trial, the addition of carboplatin to trastuzumab and paclitaxel increased response rate and prolonged progression-free survival in patients with HER2-overexpressing metastatic breast cancer. Combination therapy with vinorelbine and trastuzumab† is being investigated as an active regimen for the treatment of HER2-overexpressing metastatic breast cancer. (See Uses: Breast Cancer in Vinorelbine 10:00.) Another ongoing study will compare the efficacy of trastuzumab in combination with paclitaxel for tumors with overexpression versus normal expression of *HER2* in patients with recurrent or metastatic breast cancer.

Second-line or Salvage Therapy for Advanced Breast Cancer The current indication for use of trastuzumab as monotherapy for metastatic breast cancer is based on data from a single-arm, open-label, multicenter clinical trial in 222 patients with 2+ or 3+ *HER2*-overexpressing metastatic breast cancer that relapsed following 1 or 2 previous chemotherapy regimens. Among patients enrolled in the study, 66% had received prior adjuvant chemotherapy, 68% had received 2 prior chemotherapy regimens for metastatic disease, and 25% had received prior myeloablative therapy with hematopoietic rescue. About 72% of the patients had visceral disease (i.e., lung or liver metastases), and patients with only bone metastases, a characteristic that generally is associated with an indolent course of disease, were ineligible for enrollment in the trial.

Patients received an initial dose of trastuzumab 4 mg/kg IV followed by once weekly doses of 2 mg/kg IV; the overall response rate was 14% (2% complete responses, 12% partial responses), the median duration of response was 9 months, and the median survival was 13 months. Trastuzumab therapy was continued until disease progression or intolerable toxicity was observed. Complete responses to trastuzumab were observed only in patients with metastatic breast disease limited to the skin and the lymph nodes.

Retrospective analysis suggests that response to trastuzumab is related to the degree of *HER2* overexpression with an overall response rate of 18% in patients with 3+ overexpressing tumors versus 6% in those with 2+ overexpressing tumors. According to retrospective analysis of the tumor specimens, the overall response rate was 20% in patients with FISH-positive tumors compared with no responses in those with FISH-negative tumors.

Among 352 patients (including 213 patients in the multicenter clinical trial) receiving trastuzumab as monotherapy for metastatic breast cancer, the median age of the patients was 50 years (range: 28–86 years), and most were Caucasian (86%).

Dosage and Administration

■ Reconstitution and Administration

Trastuzumab is administered by IV infusion. The initial dose of trastuzumab should be administered as an IV infusion over 90 minutes; if the first infusion is well tolerated, subsequent doses may be administered by IV infusion over 30 minutes. Trastuzumab solutions should *not* be administered by rapid IV injection, such as IV push or bolus. The usual precautions for handling and preparing cytotoxic drugs should be observed when reconstituting or administering trastuzumab.

Commercially available trastuzumab powder for injection must be reconstituted prior to administration. Trastuzumab is supplied with a diluent of bacteriostatic water for injection, which contains 1.1% benzyl alcohol; reconstitution using the 20 mL of supplied diluent results in a solution containing 21 mg/mL of trastuzumab. Alternatively, for patients sensitive to benzyl alcohol, 20 mL of sterile water for injection may be used for reconstitution.

Trastuzumab must be handled carefully during reconstitution; shaking the reconstituted solution of trastuzumab or causing excessive foaming during the addition of diluent may cause problems with dissolution and the amount of the drug that can be withdrawn from the vial. Using a sterile syringe, the 20 mL of supplied diluent should be injected slowly into the vial with the stream of diluent directed into the lyophilized cake of trastuzumab. The vial should be swirled gently to aid reconstitution; because trastuzumab may be sensitive to shear-induced stress (e.g., agitation, rapid expulsion from a syringe), the reconstituted solution of the drug should *not* be shaken. Slight foaming of the reconstituted trastuzumab solution is not unusual, and the vial should be allowed to stand undisturbed for 5 minutes following reconstitution. The reconstituted solution of trastuzumab should be clear to slightly opalescent, colorless to pale yellow, and free of visible particulate matter.

Immediately upon reconstitution with bacteriostatic water for injection, the vial containing trastuzumab solution must be labeled to indicate the date by which the contents should be used (i.e., 28 days from the date of reconstitution); unused portions should be discarded after 28 days. For administration in patients with known hypersensitivity to benzyl alcohol, trastuzumab should be reconstituted using sterile water for injection; the resulting solution must be used *immediately*, and any unused solution should be discarded.

Reconstituted solutions of trastuzumab should be further diluted prior to administration by adding an appropriate volume of trastuzumab 21 mg/mL solution to a polyvinyl chloride or polyethylene infusion bag containing 250 mL of 0.9% sodium chloride injection; the bag should be inverted gently to mix the solution. Trastuzumab solutions for infusion should *not* be diluted in or administered through an IV line containing 5% dextrose injection, and trastuzumab should not be mixed or diluted with other drugs. Prior to administration, trastuzumab solutions should be inspected visually for particulate matter and discoloration.

Dispensing and Administration Precautions Trastuzumab (Herceptin®) should not be confused with ado-trastuzumab emtansine (Kadcyla®). Because of the similarity between the original generic name of Kadcyla® (trastuzumab emtansine) and the generic name for Herceptin® (trastuzumab), the US Food and Drug Administration (FDA) approved the addition of the prefix "ado" to the generic name for Kadcyla® (i.e., ado-trastuzumab emtansine). However, the potential exists for dispensing or prescribing errors involving these drugs. Extra care should be exercised to ensure the accuracy of prescriptions for trastuzumab (Herceptin®) or ado-trastuzumab emtansine (Kadcyla®). To avoid medication errors, the Institute for Safe Medication Practices (ISMP), the FDA, and the manufacturer of ado-trastuzumab emtansine (Kadcyla®) recommend that prescribers communicate both the brand and generic names for ado-trastuzumab emtansine (Kadcyla®) on the prescription order form. (See Special Alerts.)

■ Dosage

Adjuvant Therapy for Early-stage Breast Cancer For the adjuvant treatment of HER2-overexpressing, node-positive breast cancer, trastuzumab is given concurrently with paclitaxel following adjuvant chemotherapy with doxorubicin and cyclophosphamide; an initial dose of trastuzumab 4 mg/kg is administered (given with the first dose of paclitaxel), followed by trastuzumab 2 mg/kg once weekly for 51 weeks. Trastuzumab should *not* be administered concurrently with doxorubicin and cyclophosphamide. Following the completion of therapy with doxorubicin and cyclophosphamide, trastuzumab is administered weekly for 52 weeks, concurrently with paclitaxel for the first 12 weeks, then as monotherapy.

Therapy for Advanced Breast Cancer When used for the treatment of metastatic breast cancer that overexpresses the *HER2* protein, either as monotherapy for treatment of disease that has relapsed following prior chemotherapy or in combination therapy with paclitaxel for initial treatment, the manufacturer recommends an initial trastuzumab dose of 4 mg/kg administered by IV infusion over 90 minutes, followed by once-weekly doses of 2 mg/kg IV.

Patients should be observed for fever and chills or other infusion-associated symptoms during trastuzumab infusion. (See Cautions: Infusion-related Effects.) If prior infusions were well tolerated, subsequent weekly doses of trastuzumab 2 mg/kg IV may be administered over 30 minutes. Trastuzumab therapy is administered until disease progression occurs. In clinical trials, once-weekly administration of trastuzumab was continued until disease progression or intolerable toxicity was observed.

Among patients receiving trastuzumab and chemotherapy as first-line therapy for metastatic breast cancer, 58% of patients received trastuzumab for at least 6 months and 9% received trastuzumab for at least 12 months. Among patients receiving trastuzumab monotherapy as second-line or salvage therapy for metastatic breast cancer, 31% of patients received trastuzumab for at least 6 months and 16% received trastuzumab for at least 12 months.

Dosage Modification for Toxicity and Contraindications for Continued Therapy **Respiratory Toxicity.** Infusion of trastuzumab should be interrupted in patients experiencing dyspnea, and discontinuance of trastuzumab therapy should be considered strongly in patients who develop pneumonitis or acute respiratory distress syndrome. (Also see Infusion-related Toxicity under Dosage: Dosage Modification for Toxicity and Contraindications for Continued Therapy, in Dosage and Administration.)

Infusion-related Toxicity. Discontinuance of trastuzumab should be strongly considered for infusion reactions manifesting as anaphylaxis, angioedema, pneumonitis, or acute respiratory distress syndrome.

Infusion of trastuzumab should be interrupted in all patients experiencing dyspnea or clinically important hypotension and appropriate medical therapy, which may include epinephrine, corticosteroids, diphenhydramine, bronchodilators, and oxygen, should be instituted. Patients should be evaluated and monitored carefully until signs and symptoms have resolved completely. Permanent discontinuance of trastuzumab therapy should be strongly considered in all patients experiencing severe or life-threatening infusion reactions. For mild or moderate infusion reactions, the rate of infusion of trastuzumab may be slowed.

According to the manufacturer, the most appropriate method for identifying patients who may safely receive additional infusions of trastuzumab following a severe infusion-related reaction to the drug has not been determined. Following complete recovery from a severe infusion-related reaction, some patients have tolerated subsequent infusions of the drug, typically accompanied by prophylactic treatment including antihistamines and/or corticosteroids, but others have experienced severe reactions to additional infusions of trastuzumab despite the use of premedication.

Mild to moderate infusion-related symptoms, such as chills or fever, have been treated with acetaminophen, diphenhydramine, and/or meperidine, and, in some patients, the rate of infusion of trastuzumab was reduced. Permanent discontinuance of the drug because of such infusion-related symptoms was required in less than 1% of patients.

Sensitivity Reactions. Discontinuance of trastuzumab should be strongly considered for infusion reactions manifesting as anaphylaxis or angioedema.

Infusion of trastuzumab should be interrupted in all patients experiencing dyspnea or clinically important hypotension and appropriate medical therapy should be instituted. See Infusion-related Toxicity under Dosage: Dosage Modification for Toxicity and Contraindications for Continued Therapy, in Dosage and Administration.

Cardiovascular Toxicity. Careful assessment of cardiac function and monitoring of clinical condition are required in patients receiving trastuzumab. For cardiac monitoring requirements, see Cardiovascular Effects under Cautions: Precautions and Contraindications. Trastuzumab-induced decline in left ventricular ejection fraction (LVEF) may be asymptomatic. If clinical manifestations of cardiotoxicity or a clinically important decrease in LVEF occurs, trastuzumab therapy should be interrupted or discontinued. Medical management of cardiac dysfunction may result in recovery of LVEF to at least 50% in some patients.

For patients receiving adjuvant therapy, left ventricular function should be assessed before initiation of trastuzumab and frequently during therapy. If LVEF decreases by 16 percentage points or more from the baseline value, or if LVEF decreases by 10 or more percentage points from the baseline value to a value that is below the lower limit of normal, trastuzumab therapy should be discontinued for 4 weeks. After 4 weeks, cardiac function should be reassessed; if there are no clinical manifestations of cardiotoxicity, LVEF returns to normal limits, and the absolute decrease in LVEF from baseline is 15 percentage points or less, trastuzumab therapy can be resumed. If LVEF decline is persistent (greater than 8 weeks) and 2 consecutive holds are placed on therapy, or if therapy has been interrupted on more than 3 occasions for cardiomyopathy, therapy with trastuzumab should be discontinued permanently. Among patients receiving adjuvant trastuzumab in trial B-31 (study 1), 30.5% required at least one dose delay because of asymptomatic decrease in LVEF or cardiac symptoms. In 16% of patients, trastuzumab therapy was discontinued because of substantial decline in LVEF or clinical evidence of myocardial dysfunction.

Patients receiving trastuzumab therapy for advanced or metastatic breast cancer, particularly those with preexisting cardiac dysfunction, should be monitored closely for signs of cardiotoxicity. Discontinuance of trastuzumab should be considered strongly in patients who develop a clinically important decrease in left ventricular function or congestive heart failure.

An independent committee reviewing cardiac data from clinical trials of trastuzumab used alone or in combination with chemotherapy for metastatic breast cancer found that, in most cases, cardiac dysfunction in patients receiving trastuzumab was similar to anthracycline-induced cardiomyopathy. Others report a lack of anthracycline-like ultrastructural changes and suggest a different mechanism for trastuzumab-induced cardiac toxicity. In clinical trials for metastatic breast cancer, cardiac dysfunction associated with trastuzumab typically responded to appropriate medical therapy, often including discontinuance of the drug. For the treatment of cardiac dysfunction, single-agent therapy with a diuretic or an angiotensin-converting enzyme (ACE) inhibitor often was used in patients receiving trastuzumab and paclitaxel whereas combination therapy with digoxin, a diuretic, and an ACE inhibitor typically was used in patients receiving trastuzumab with an anthracycline and cyclophosphamide.

Among patients for whom trastuzumab therapy is discontinued because of left ventricular dysfunction, close monitoring for evidence of clinical deterioration and further decline in left ventricular function is required. The safety of continuing or restarting treatment with the drug in patients who have developed trastuzumab-induced left ventricular cardiac dysfunction has not been fully evaluated. Some clinicians report reinitiation of therapy in patients with metastatic breast cancer following recovery from trastuzumab-induced cardiac dysfunction.

Cautions

Serious adverse effects, sometimes fatal, have occurred in patients receiving trastuzumab. Serious adverse effects associated with trastuzumab include cardiomyopathy; pulmonary toxicity such as respiratory failure, pneumonitis, and pulmonary infiltrates; infusion reactions such as anaphylaxis or angioedema; febrile neutropenia; and exacerbation of chemotherapy-induced neutropenia. Deaths associated with pulmonary reactions (including acute respiratory distress syndrome), infusion-related reactions, and hypersensitivity reactions (including fatal anaphylaxis) have been reported in patients receiving trastuzumab. Deaths caused by sepsis in patients with severe neutropenia have been reported when trastuzumab is used in combination with myelosuppressive chemotherapy. Another serious adverse effect associated with trastuzumab is cardiotoxicity, including ventricular dysfunction and congestive heart failure, which may be severe and occasionally disabling; the risk of cardiotoxicity increases substantially when the drug is combined with an anthracycline, and such combination therapy for use in metastatic breast cancer is *not* recommended by most experts.

Adverse effects are common with trastuzumab therapy, with the incidence of most effects generally increasing with combination versus monotherapy. The most common adverse effects associated with trastuzumab include fever, nausea, vomiting, infusion reactions, diarrhea, infections, increased cough, headache, fatigue, dyspnea, rash, neutropenia, anemia, and myalgia.

Data regarding serious adverse effects are based on experience in a total of 958 patients receiving trastuzumab alone or in combination with chemotherapy for metastatic breast cancer or other cancers in clinical trials. The incidence of adverse effects that occurred in at least 5% of patients receiving the drug or that occurred at increased incidence among patients receiving trastuzumab and chemotherapy versus chemotherapy alone is derived from data for a total of 586 patients with metastatic breast cancer (352 patients receiving trastuzumab as a single agent and 234 patients receiving trastuzumab in combination with chemotherapy).

Of 213 patients receiving trastuzumab as a single agent, about 3% discontinued the drug because of adverse effects. Of 91 patients receiving trastuzumab and paclitaxel, 6 patients (6.6%) discontinued trastuzumab because of an adverse effect, 3 of which were cardiac in origin. A higher percentage of patients (20/143 or 14%) receiving the drug in combination with an anthracycline and cyclophosphamide discontinued trastuzumab because of adverse effects, mostly cardiovascular in nature.

Limited data were collected for adverse effects in clinical trials of adjuvant trastuzumab for early breast cancer (studies 1 and 2). Unless otherwise noted, the incidence data for noncardiac adverse effects occurring in at least 2% of patients refer to grade 2–5 toxicities for study 1.

■ Respiratory Effects Trastuzumab can cause serious, sometimes fatal, pulmonary toxicity. Severe adverse respiratory effects, including acute respiratory distress syndrome, have been reported in patients receiving trastuzumab and, in some cases, have been fatal. Interstitial pneumonitis, sometimes fatal, was reported rarely in patients receiving adjuvant trastuzumab. Manifestations of severe adverse pulmonary reactions, which may occur as sequelae of infusion-related reactions (see Cautions: Infusion-related Effects), include dyspnea, wheezing, pneumonitis, pulmonary infiltrates, pleural effusions, noncardiogenic pulmonary edema, pulmonary insufficiency and hypoxia requiring supplemental oxygen or ventilatory support, acute respiratory distress syndrome, and pulmonary fibrosis. Patients with symptomatic intrinsic lung disease or extensive tumor involvement of the lungs, resulting in dyspnea at rest, experience more severe pulmonary toxicity associated with trastuzumab. (See Precautions and Contraindications.)

Among patients receiving trastuzumab and paclitaxel as adjuvant therapy for breast cancer, the most common pulmonary toxicity was dyspnea (study 1: 12%, study 2: 2.5%). Pneumonitis/pulmonary infiltrates and respiratory failure, sometimes fatal, also occurred in patients receiving trastuzumab and chemotherapy.

Among patients with metastatic breast cancer, increased cough occurred in 26 or 41% of patients receiving trastuzumab as a single agent or in combination with paclitaxel, respectively. Dyspnea and pharyngitis have been reported in 22 and 12%, respectively, of patients receiving trastuzumab monotherapy for metastatic breast cancer. Rhinitis and sinusitis have been reported in 14 and 9%, respectively, of patients receiving trastuzumab as a single agent and in 22 and 21%, respectively, of patients receiving trastuzumab and paclitaxel for metastatic breast cancer. Other adverse respiratory effects, including apnea, asthma, hypoxia, laryngitis, and pneumothorax, have been reported in patients receiving trastuzumab.

■ Infusion-related Effects Serious infusion-related reactions, sometimes fatal, have been reported infrequently in patients receiving trastuzumab. Severe infusion-related reactions include bronchospasm, hypoxia, and severe hypotension. In most patients experiencing such reactions, manifestations typically occurred with the first dose of trastuzumab, with onset generally occurring during or immediately following the infusion; however, the onset and clinical course were variable. In some patients, symptoms progressively worsened. In some patients, initial improvement was followed by marked clinical deterioration. Delayed adverse events with rapid clinical deterioration occurring following completion of trastuzumab infusion also has been reported. Fatal infusion-related reactions resulted in death within hours or days of the infusion. (See Infusion-related Toxicity under Dosage: Dosage Modification for Toxicity and Contraindications for Continued Therapy, in Dosage and Administration. Also see Infusion-related Effects under Cautions: Precautions and Contraindications.)

Other infusion-related symptoms, typically consisting of chills and/or fever, occurred in approximately 40% of patients with metastatic breast cancer in clinical trials during the first infusion of trastuzumab. Other manifestations of infusion reactions include nausea, vomiting, pain (including pain at tumor sites), rigors, headache, dizziness, dyspnea, hypotension, elevated blood pressure, rash, and asthenia. On second (or subsequent) infusions of trastuzumab administered as monotherapy or in combination with chemotherapy, infusion-related reactions occurred in 21 or 35% of patients, respectively, and were severe in 1.4% or 9% of patients, respectively.

■ Sensitivity Reactions Serious infusion-related reactions may manifest as hypersensitivity reactions, including anaphylaxis, angioedema, bronchospasm, and/or hypotension, in patients receiving trastuzumab. See Cautions: Infusion-related Effects.

Allergic reactions have occurred in 3% of patients receiving trastuzumab monotherapy and 8% of patients receiving trastuzumab and paclitaxel for metastatic breast cancer. Anaphylactoid reactions have been reported in patients receiving trastuzumab.

■ Hematologic Effects Hematologic toxicity occurs infrequently in patients receiving trastuzumab as a single agent. Grade 3 adverse hematologic effects, including leukopenia, anemia, and thrombocytopenia, each occurred in less than 1% of patients receiving trastuzumab monotherapy in clinical trials, and grade 4 hematologic toxicity was not reported.

Deaths caused by sepsis in patients with severe neutropenia have been reported when trastuzumab is used in combination with myelosuppressive chemotherapy for metastatic breast cancer. In controlled clinical trials, the incidence of septic death was not increased in patients receiving trastuzumab in combination with chemotherapy. Although the mechanism is not known, trastuzumab is thought to exacerbate chemotherapy-induced neutropenia. In randomized clinical trials in women with metastatic breast cancer, the incidences of moderate or severe neutropenia and of febrile neutropenia were higher in patients receiving trastuzumab in combination with myelosuppressive chemotherapy than in those receiving chemotherapy alone. In a randomized trial, moderate or severe neutropenia occurred more frequently in patients receiving trastuzumab in combination with myelosuppressive chemotherapy for metastatic breast cancer than in those receiving chemotherapy alone (32 versus 22%). The incidence of febrile neutropenia also was higher in patients receiving trastuzumab in combination with myelosuppressive chemotherapy for metastatic breast cancer than in those receiving chemotherapy alone (23 versus 17%). Among patients receiving adjuvant therapy for breast cancer, neutropenia occurred more frequently in patients receiving trastuzumab and chemotherapy than in those receiving chemotherapy alone (study 1: 7.1 versus 4.5%, grade 4–5 neutropenia in study 2: 2 versus 0.7%).

Leukopenia and anemia occurred in 24 and 14%, respectively, of patients receiving trastuzumab in combination with paclitaxel for metastatic breast cancer in a randomized trial. The incidence of leukopenia was increased in patients receiving trastuzumab combined with chemotherapy compared with those receiving chemotherapy alone (53 versus 37%) for metastatic breast cancer. The incidence of anemia was higher in patients receiving trastuzumab combined with chemotherapy compared with those receiving chemotherapy alone for metastatic breast cancer (30 versus 21%) or as adjuvant therapy for breast cancer (study 1: 13 versus 7%).

Other adverse hematologic effects reported in patients receiving trastuzumab in clinical trials include pancytopenia, acute leukemia (see Mutagenicity and Carcinogenicity), and coagulation disorder.

■ **Cardiovascular Effects** Deaths from cardiomyopathy have occurred in patients receiving trastuzumab. Trastuzumab can cause left ventricular myocardial dysfunction characterized by a decline in ejection fraction and manifestations of congestive heart failure. Cardiotoxicity manifested by dyspnea, increased cough, paroxysmal nocturnal dyspnea, peripheral edema, S_3 gallop, cardiomyopathy, congestive heart failure, and/or reduced ejection fraction (decrease of greater than 10%) has been observed in patients receiving trastuzumab. Cardiac dysfunction associated with trastuzumab may be severe and in some cases has resulted in disabling heart failure, mural thrombosis and stroke, and/or death. Trastuzumab also can cause asymptomatic decline in left ventricular ejection fraction. Volume overload and congestive heart failure have been reported as complications of nephrotic syndrome in patients receiving trastuzumab. (See Cautions: Renal and Genitourinary Effects.)

In patients receiving trastuzumab monotherapy for metastatic breast cancer in an open-label, phase 2 study, cardiac dysfunction including congestive heart failure occurred in 7% of patients, and class III or IV cardiac dysfunction (according to the New York Heart Association [NYHA] classification system with class IV being the most severe level of cardiac failure) was reported in 5% of patients. Among patients receiving a combination of trastuzumab and paclitaxel for metastatic breast cancer in a randomized, phase 3 trial, cardiac dysfunction including congestive heart failure was reported in 11% of patients, and 4% of patients experienced NYHA class III or IV cardiac dysfunction.

Among patients receiving adjuvant trastuzumab in 2 North American randomized trials, the cumulative incidence of class III or IV congestive heart failure or death from cardiac causes at 3 years was 4.1% in trial B-31 (study 1) and 2.9% in trial N9831 (study 2). The incidence of new-onset left ventricular dysfunction was approximately twofold higher in patients receiving trastuzumab and paclitaxel versus paclitaxel alone following adjuvant chemotherapy with doxorubicin and cyclophosphamide. About 50% of the adverse cardiac events among patients receiving trastuzumab were identified by the completion of paclitaxel therapy and about 90% were identified within 1 year of the completion of paclitaxel therapy. In an international randomized trial, the incidence of class III or IV congestive heart failure in patients receiving adjuvant trastuzumab was 0.5% at 1 year.

In a randomized trial, patients who received trastuzumab in combination with an anthracycline (rather than paclitaxel) for advanced or metastatic breast cancer had the highest incidence of cardiotoxicity; cardiac dysfunction including congestive heart failure occurred in 28% of patients, and 19% of patients developed NYHA class III or IV cardiac dysfunction. Because of the increased frequency and severity of cardiac toxicity, most experts believe that the clinical benefit obtained from the concomitant use of trastuzumab with an anthracycline and cyclophosphamide regimen does *not* outweigh the increased risk of toxicity, and combined therapy with an anthracycline is *not* recommended for the treatment of advanced or metastatic breast cancer.

For discussion of risks of cardiotoxicity, precautions and contraindications, and monitoring requirements in patients receiving trastuzumab therapy, see Cardiovascular Effects under Cautions: Precautions and Contraindications.

Among patients receiving trastuzumab and paclitaxel as adjuvant therapy for breast cancer, hot flushes (flashes) (study 1: 17%) have been reported. Among patients with metastatic breast cancer, tachycardia has been reported in 5% of patients receiving trastuzumab as a single agent and in 12% of patients receiving trastuzumab in combination with paclitaxel. Peripheral edema and edema occurred in 10 and 8%, respectively, of patients receiving trastuzumab alone for metastatic breast cancer. The incidence of thrombosis/embolism was higher in patients receiving trastuzumab and chemotherapy versus chemotherapy alone for metastatic breast cancer (study 3: 2 versus 0%) or as adjuvant therapy for breast cancer (study 1: 3 versus 1%). Other adverse cardiovascular effects reported in patients receiving trastuzumab in clinical trials include pericardial effusion, cardiac arrest, syncope, hemorrhage, shock, and arrhythmia.

■ **GI Effects** Diarrhea, typically mild to moderate in severity, occurred in 25 or 45% of patients receiving trastuzumab as a single agent or in combination with paclitaxel, respectively, for metastatic breast cancer. An increased incidence of diarrhea was observed in patients receiving trastuzumab in combination with chemotherapy compared with those receiving trastuzumab alone. Among patients with metastatic breast cancer, nausea and vomiting have been reported in 33 and 23%, respectively, of patients receiving trastuzumab as a single agent and in 51 and 37%, respectively, of patients receiving trastuzumab and paclitaxel; nausea in combination with vomiting occurred in 8% of patients receiving trastuzumab as a single agent in clinical trials. Some patients experiencing adverse GI effects of trastuzumab consequently had metabolic complications, such as dehydration and hypokalemia. Anorexia occurred in 14% of patients receiving trastuzumab alone and in 24% of patients receiving trastuzumab and paclitaxel for metastatic breast cancer.

Other adverse GI effects, including gastroenteritis, hematemesis, ileus, intestinal obstruction, colitis, esophageal ulcer, stomatitis, and pancreatitis, have been reported in patients receiving trastuzumab.

■ **Infectious Complications** Febrile neutropenia and infection with neutropenia resulting in death have been reported in patients receiving trastuzumab in combination with myelosuppressive chemotherapy. (See Cautions: Hematologic Effects.)

Among patients with metastatic breast cancer, infection has been reported in 20 or 47% of patients receiving trastuzumab as a single agent or in combination with paclitaxel, respectively. Among patients receiving trastuzumab and paclitaxel as adjuvant therapy for breast cancer, infection/febrile neutropenia (study 1: 22%, grade 3–5 infection/febrile neutropenia in study 2: 3%) has been reported. Compared with patients receiving chemotherapy alone, patients receiving trastuzumab combined with chemotherapy for metastatic breast cancer or as adjuvant therapy for early breast cancer experienced an increased incidence of infections (study 3: 46 versus 30%, study 1: 22 versus 14%). Upper respiratory tract infections, typically mild, and infections of indwelling catheters were the most commonly reported infectious complications in patients receiving trastuzumab for metastatic breast cancer. Infections of the upper respiratory tract, skin, and urinary tract were the most commonly reported infectious complications in patients receiving trastuzumab as adjuvant therapy for breast cancer. Urinary tract infection occurred in 5% of patients receiving trastuzumab monotherapy for metastatic breast cancer in clinical trials. Lymphangitis and cellulitis also have been reported in patients receiving the drug.

■ **Musculoskeletal Effects** Back pain has been reported in 22% of patients receiving trastuzumab monotherapy for metastatic breast cancer in clinical trials. Among patients with metastatic breast cancer, bone pain and arthralgia have occurred in 7 and 6%, respectively, of patients receiving trastuzumab as a single agent and in 24 and 37%, respectively, of patients receiving trastuzumab and paclitaxel. Among patients receiving trastuzumab and paclitaxel as adjuvant therapy for breast cancer, arthralgia (study 1: 31%, study 2: 11%) and myalgia (study 2: 10%) have been reported. Bone necrosis, pathologic fractures, and myopathy also have been reported in patients receiving trastuzumab.

■ **Dermatologic and Immunologic Reactions** Among patients receiving trastuzumab and paclitaxel as adjuvant therapy for breast cancer, rash/desquamation (study 1: 11%) and nail changes (study 2: 9%) have been reported. Among patients with metastatic breast cancer, rash has been reported in 18 or 38% of patients receiving trastuzumab as a single agent or in combination with paclitaxel, respectively. Acne and herpes simplex occurred in 11 and 12%, respectively, of patients receiving trastuzumab and paclitaxel, and each has been reported in 2% of patients receiving trastuzumab alone for metastatic breast cancer. Other adverse dermatologic effects, including herpes zoster and skin ulceration, have been reported in patients receiving trastuzumab.

Of 903 women receiving trastuzumab for metastatic breast cancer, human anti-human antibody (HAHA) to the drug has been detected in one patient, who had no allergic reactions.

■ **Flu-like Syndrome** Flu-like syndrome has occurred in about 10% of patients receiving trastuzumab alone or in combination with chemotherapy for metastatic breast cancer. Pain, asthenia, and abdominal pain have been reported in 47, 42, and 22%, respectively, of patients receiving trastuzumab monotherapy for metastatic breast cancer.

■ **Nervous System Effects** Among patients with metastatic breast cancer, paresthesia, which occurred in 48% of patients receiving trastuzumab and paclitaxel, occurred in 9% of patients receiving trastuzumab alone and 39% of those receiving paclitaxel alone. Peripheral neuritis and neuropathy have been reported in 2 and 1%, respectively, of patients receiving trastuzumab as a single agent and in 23 and 13%, respectively, of patients receiving trastuzumab and paclitaxel for metastatic breast cancer. A larger cumulative dose of paclitaxel given in conjunction with trastuzumab (approximately 20% greater than the cumulative dose in patients receiving paclitaxel alone) may have contributed to the increased incidence of paresthesia, peripheral neuritis, and neuropathy in these patients compared with those receiving paclitaxel alone.

Among patients with metastatic breast cancer, headache, insomnia, and dizziness have occurred in 26, 14, and 13%, respectively, of patients receiving trastuzumab monotherapy. Depression has been reported in 6% of patients receiving trastuzumab as a single agent and in 12% of patients receiving trastuzumab and paclitaxel for metastatic breast cancer. Among patients receiving trastuzumab and paclitaxel as adjuvant therapy for breast cancer, headache (study 1: 6%) and insomnia (study 1: 4%) have been reported. Other adverse neurologic effects, including ataxia, confusion, seizures, hydrocephalus, and manic reaction, have been reported in patients receiving trastuzumab.

■ Endocrine and Metabolic Effects Adverse endocrine and metabolic effects, including hypothyroidism, hypercalcemia, hypomagnesemia, hyponatremia, and hypoglycemia, have been reported in patients receiving trastuzumab. Growth retardation and weight loss also occurred in patients receiving the drug.

■ Hepatic Effects Ascites, hepatitis, and hepatic failure have been reported in patients receiving trastuzumab.

■ Ocular Effects Amblyopia has been reported in patients receiving trastuzumab.

■ Renal and Genitourinary Effects Nephrotic syndrome with pathologic evidence of glomerulopathy has been reported rarely in patients receiving trastuzumab. Onset has ranged from 4 to approximately 18 months following initiation of trastuzumab therapy. Pathologic findings have included membranous glomerulonephritis, focal glomerulosclerosis, and fibrillary glomerulonephritis, and complications have included volume overload and congestive heart failure. Renal failure has been reported in patients receiving trastuzumab.

Other adverse genitourinary effects reported in patients receiving trastuzumab include hematuria, hemorrhagic cystitis, hydronephrosis, and pyelonephritis.

■ Other Adverse Effects Among patients with metastatic breast cancer, accidental injury has been reported in 6% of patients receiving trastuzumab as a single agent and in 13% of patients receiving trastuzumab and paclitaxel. Among patients receiving trastuzumab and paclitaxel as adjuvant therapy for breast cancer, fatigue (study 1: 28%) has been reported. Other adverse effects occurring in patients receiving trastuzumab in clinical trials include radiation injury and deafness.

■ Precautions and Contraindications Serious adverse events, rarely fatal, including severe respiratory effects, such as acute respiratory distress syndrome (see Cautions: Respiratory Effects), severe infusion-related reactions (see Cautions: Infusion-related Effects), and severe hypersensitivity reactions, such as anaphylaxis (see Cautions: Sensitivity Reactions), have occurred in patients receiving trastuzumab. In most patients experiencing severe adverse reactions, manifestations typically occurred during or within 24 hours of the infusion of trastuzumab. In some cases, initial improvement in symptoms was followed by marked and delayed clinical deterioration, and a small number of patients died at home. Patients should be informed of the possibility of delayed severe reactions associated with trastuzumab therapy.

Trastuzumab should be administered with extreme caution in patients with preexisting pulmonary compromise, and the risks and benefits of therapy should be weighed carefully. Most patients experiencing fatal adverse reactions associated with trastuzumab had clinically important preexisting pulmonary compromise secondary to intrinsic lung disease and/or malignant pulmonary involvement.

Interruption or discontinuance of trastuzumab therapy is required in patients experiencing severe or life-threatening adverse reactions. (See Dosage Modification for Toxicity and Contraindications for Continued Therapy under Dosage and Administration: Dosage.)

Respiratory Effects Patients with either symptomatic intrinsic pulmonary disease (e.g., asthma, COPD) or extensive tumor involvement of the lungs (e.g., lymphangitic spread of tumor, pleural effusions, parenchymal masses) resulting in dyspnea at rest may be at increased risk of serious adverse pulmonary events associated with trastuzumab, and the manufacturer recommends *extreme caution* in such patients.

Infusion-related Effects Patients with preexisting pulmonary compromise may be at increased risk of serious infusion-related adverse effects associated with trastuzumab.

Sensitivity Reactions For administration in patients with known hypersensitivity to benzyl alcohol, the preservative in bacteriostatic water for injection (the diluent supplied by the manufacturer), trastuzumab should be reconstituted using sterile water for injection. (See Dosage and Administration: Reconstitution and Administration.)

Trastuzumab should be administered with caution in patients with known hypersensitivity to trastuzumab, Chinese Hamster Ovary (CHO) cell proteins, or any component of the formulation.

Cardiovascular Effects Because trastuzumab may cause serious adverse cardiovascular effects, including ventricular dysfunction and congestive heart failure, a thorough baseline cardiac evaluation including history, physical examination, and cardiac function tests (i.e., echocardiogram and/or MUGA scan) should be performed prior to initiating trastuzumab therapy.

Among patients with metastatic breast cancer, the risk of cardiac dysfunction including congestive heart failure associated with trastuzumab therapy may be increased with increased age, preexisting cardiac disease, or prior cardiotoxic therapy (e.g., anthracycline therapy or radiation therapy to the chest area). Potential benefit versus the increased risk of cardiac toxicity should be weighed carefully when deciding whether the use of trastuzumab is advisable in patients with preexisting cardiac disease.

Among patients receiving adjuvant therapy for breast cancer, the risk of symptomatic cardiomyopathy associated with trastuzumab may be increased in patients experiencing decline in left ventricular ejection fraction (LVEF) to below the lower limit of normal (following completion of treatment with doxorubicin and cyclophosphamide or during treatment with trastuzumab), patients with previous or concurrent use of antihypertensive medications, and geriatric patients. According to the exclusion criteria applied in the North American randomized trials, use of adjuvant trastuzumab therapy is *not* recommended in patients with angina pectoris requiring medication; arrhythmia requiring medication; a severe conduction abnormality; clinically important valvular disease; cardiomegaly on chest radiography; left ventricular hypertrophy on echocardiography; poorly controlled hypertension; clinically important pericardial effusion; or a history of myocardial infarction, congestive heart failure, or cardiomyopathy. Adjuvant trastuzumab therapy should be initiated only if the measurement of LVEF at baseline is within normal limits (at least 50%) and the decrease from the baseline value is less than 15 points following completion of adjuvant chemotherapy with doxorubicin and cyclophosphamide. Patients who develop clinical manifestations of cardiac toxicity during adjuvant chemotherapy with doxorubicin and cyclophosphamide should *not* receive trastuzumab. In clinical trials of adjuvant therapy for breast cancer, 6% of patients were unable to receive trastuzumab following completion of doxorubicin and cyclophosphamide therapy because of cardiac dysfunction.

Left ventricular function should be monitored frequently in patients receiving trastuzumab. For patients with preexisting cardiac dysfunction, more frequent monitoring is required. Monitoring will not identify all patients who will develop cardiac dysfunction.

In patients receiving adjuvant trastuzumab, cardiac function must be assessed at regular intervals using MUGA scan or echocardiogram performed at baseline (prior to adjuvant therapy with doxorubicin and cyclophosphamide), at the completion of adjuvant chemotherapy with doxorubicin and cyclophosphamide (immediately prior to initiation of trastuzumab therapy), at 3 months following the initiation of concomitant therapy with paclitaxel and trastuzumab, at 3 months following the initiation of trastuzumab monotherapy (upon completion of concomitant therapy with paclitaxel and trastuzumab), and at 3 months following the completion of trastuzumab monotherapy. Age and LVEF following adjuvant chemotherapy with doxorubicin and cyclophosphamide may be risk factors for symptomatic cardiac dysfunction in patients being considered for adjuvant therapy with trastuzumab.

A thorough cardiac assessment, including evaluation of left ventricular function, should be performed in candidates for trastuzumab therapy for advanced or metastatic breast cancer, and cardiac function should be monitored frequently in those receiving the drug. Following baseline echocardiogram or MUGA scan, clinicians recommend cardiac monitoring with either test as indicated by the presence of clinical manifestations of cardiac dysfunction or at regular intervals every 1–4 months according to the patient's age and risk of cardiac toxicity. *Extreme caution is advised during trastuzumab therapy for metastatic disease in patients with preexisting cardiac dysfunction.*

Because of the increased risk of cardiotoxicity, most experts generally do *not* recommend use of trastuzumab in combination with an anthracycline agent for the treatment of metastatic breast cancer.

Dispensing and Administration Precautions Trastuzumab (Herceptin®) should not be confused with ado-trastuzumab emtansine (Kadcyla®). Because of the similarity between the original generic name of Kadcyla® (trastuzumab emtansine) and the generic name for Herceptin® (trastuzumab), the US Food and Drug Administration (FDA) approved the addition of the prefix "ado" to the generic name for Kadcyla® (i.e., ado-trastuzumab emtansine). However, the potential exists for dispensing or prescribing errors involving these drugs. Such medication errors may be associated with severe toxicity or lack of appropriate therapy in patients who did not receive the intended drug. The manufacturer of ado-trastuzumab emtansine (Kadcyla®) states that this drug should *not* be substituted for or used with trastuzumab (Herceptin®). Therefore, extra care should be exercised to ensure the accuracy of prescriptions for trastuzumab (Herceptin®) and ado-trastuzumab emtansine (Kadcyla®). (See Special Alerts.)

■ Pediatric Precautions Safety and efficacy of trastuzumab in children younger than 18 years of age have not been established.

■ Geriatric Precautions Although safety and efficacy of trastuzumab in geriatric patients 65 years of age or older have not been established specifically, the manufacturer cautions that clinical data currently are insufficient to exclude the possibility of age-related differences during trastuzumab therapy. The risk of cardiotoxicity associated with trastuzumab is increased in geriatric patients compared with younger patients receiving either adjuvant therapy for early breast cancer or treatment for metastatic breast cancer.

■ Mutagenicity and Carcinogenicity Data from in vitro and in vivo tests of trastuzumab, including Ames tests, the micronucleus assay, and tests in human peripheral blood lymphocytes, have not shown any evidence of mutagenic activity.

The carcinogenicity of trastuzumab has not been evaluated. Acute leukemia and cervical cancer have been reported in patients receiving trastuzumab. Several cases of secondary leukemia have occurred in patients receiving trastuzumab.

■ Pregnancy, Fertility, and Lactation Oligohydramnios has been reported in women receiving trastuzumab during pregnancy. Placental transfer of trastuzumab has been observed in monkeys. Although reproduction studies in cynomolgus monkeys using trastuzumab dosages up to 25 times the weekly human maintenance dosage of 2 mg/kg have not revealed evidence of harm to the fetus, the important role of the *HER2* receptor in embryonic development of the cardiac and central nervous systems raises concerns about possible teratogenic effects of trastuzumab. The *HER2* receptor is expressed at high levels in many embryonic tissues, including cardiac and neural tissues, and death of embryos in early gestation has been observed in mice lacking the *HER2* protein. Further study is needed to determine whether trastuzumab has teratogenic effects in humans. The possibility that trastuzumab may persist in maternal tissues for up to 5–6 months after the last dose should be considered. There are no adequate and controlled studies to date using trastuzumab in pregnant women, and the drug should be used during pregnancy only when the potential benefits justify the possible risks to the fetus.

Reproduction studies in cynomolgus monkeys using trastuzumab dosages up to 25 times the weekly human maintenance dosage of 2 mg/kg have not revealed evidence of impaired fertility.

When trastuzumab was administered in lactating cynomolgus monkeys at dosages 25 times the usual human maintenance dosage of 2 mg/kg weekly, distribution of the drug in milk was demonstrated. No adverse effects on growth or development from birth to 3 months of age were observed in infant monkeys with measurable serum trastuzumab concentrations. It is not known whether trastuzumab is distributed into human milk. Because human IgG is distributed in milk, and because of the potential for absorption of trastuzumab and adverse reactions to the drug in nursing infants, women should be advised to discontinue nursing during trastuzumab therapy and for 6 months following the last dose of the drug.

Drug Interactions

Formal drug interaction studies of trastuzumab have not been conducted. However, the incidence of most common adverse effects of the drug has been increased in patients receiving combination chemotherapy. (See Cautions.)

■ **Anthracycline Antineoplastic Agents** The risk of trastuzumab-induced cardiotoxic effects is increased in patients receiving an anthracycline concomitantly. (See Cautions: Cardiovascular Effects.) Such combined therapy currently is *not* recommended by most experts for use in the treatment of metastatic breast cancer.

■ **Paclitaxel** In clinical studies, a 1.5-fold increase in mean trough serum concentrations of trastuzumab was reported when the drug was administered concomitantly with paclitaxel versus an anthracycline and cyclophosphamide. In primate studies, administration of trastuzumab in combination with paclitaxel resulted in a twofold decrease in trastuzumab clearance. The clinical importance of the interaction between trastuzumab and paclitaxel is not known.

Acute Toxicity

Limited information is available on the acute toxicity of trastuzumab. The acute lethal dose of trastuzumab in humans is not known. Overdosage has not been reported in clinical trials with patients receiving single doses of trastuzumab of up to 500 mg.

Pharmacology

Trastuzumab is an antineoplastic agent that inhibits proliferation of tumor cells that overexpress *HER2*. The *HER2* proto-oncogene (also known as c-*erb*B2 or *neu*) encodes a 185-kd transmembrane tyrosine kinase receptor known as $p185^{HER2}$ or human epidermal growth factor receptor 2 (*HER2*), which has partial homology with other members of the epidermal growth factor receptor family. Trastuzumab, a recombinant humanized murine monoclonal antibody, binds specifically to the extracellular domain of the *HER2* receptor or *HER2/neu* protein. The *HER2* receptor participates in receptor-receptor interactions that regulate cell differentiation, growth, and proliferation. Overexpression of the *HER2* receptor contributes to the process of neoplastic transformation. Results from in vitro assays and animal studies have shown that trastuzumab inhibits the proliferation of human tumor cells that overexpress *HER2/neu* protein. Trastuzumab-mediated antibody-dependent cellular cytotoxicity (ADCC) also has been demonstrated and, according to in vitro studies, occurs preferentially in cells that overexpress the *HER2* protein compared with cells that do not.

Amplification of the *HER2* oncogene and/or overexpression of the *HER2* protein occurs in 25–30% of node-positive or -negative primary breast cancers, and several studies have shown that *HER2* amplification and/or overexpression is an independent predictor of poor prognosis, including more rapid disease progression and shorter overall survival, in patients with node-positive breast cancer. Overexpression of this growth factor receptor also has been shown to be associated with other adverse prognostic factors in breast cancer, including advanced pathologic stage, DNA ploidy, increased S-phase fraction, high nuclear grade, absence of estrogen and progesterone receptors, and number of metastatic axillary lymph nodes.

Pharmacokinetics

Data from studies in patients with metastatic breast cancer receiving trastuzumab 10–500 mg once weekly by IV infusion over short periods indicate that the pharmacokinetics of the drug are dose dependent. Limited data suggest that the pharmacokinetics of trastuzumab are not affected by age or increased serum creatinine concentrations up to 2 mg/dL.

■ **Absorption** In patients with metastatic breast cancer receiving a loading dose of 4 mg/kg IV followed by a weekly maintenance dose of 2 mg/kg IV, peak and trough plasma concentrations of trastuzumab at steady state (between weeks 16 and 32) averaged approximately 123 and 79 mcg/mL, respectively. In patients with metastatic breast cancer receiving trastuzumab 500 mg once weekly by short-duration IV infusion, peak plasma concentrations of the drug averaged 377 mcg/mL.

Measurable serum concentrations of circulating extracellular domain of the *HER2* receptor (i.e., shed antigen) have been detected in some patients with tumors that overexpress *HER2/neu*. Shed antigen in concentrations of up to 1880 ng/mL (median: 11 ng/mL) was detected in baseline serum samples of 64% of patients (286/447) receiving a loading dose of trastuzumab 4 mg/kg IV followed by 2 mg/kg IV once weekly. Higher baseline concentrations of shed antigen were associated with lower trough serum concentrations of trastuzumab; however, with once-weekly dosing of trastuzumab, target serum concentrations of the drug were attained by week 6 in most patients with elevated serum concentrations of shed antigen.Concentration of shed antigen does not appear to affect tumor response to trastuzumab.

■ **Distribution** Following administration of trastuzumab by short-duration IV infusion, the mean apparent volume of distribution is about 44 mL/kg (approximately equal to serum volume). It is not known whether trastuzumab crosses the blood-brain barrier or distributes into the CSF. It also is not known whether trastuzumab crosses the placenta or distributes into milk in humans; however, placental transfer of trastuzumab and distribution of the drug into milk have been observed in monkeys.

■ **Elimination** The pharmacokinetics of trastuzumab are nonlinear; increased doses of the drug are associated with increased mean half-life and decreased clearance. In patients receiving a loading dose of trastuzumab 4 mg/kg IV followed by a weekly maintenance dose of 2 mg/kg IV, elimination half-life averaged 5.8 days (range: 1–32 days). Following IV infusion of 10 or 500 mg of trastuzumab, elimination half-life averaged 1.7 or 12 days, respectively. The metabolism of trastuzumab is not fully understood, but it appears that elimination of the drug would involve clearance of IgG through the reticuloendothelial system.

Chemistry and Stability

■ **Chemistry** Trastuzumab, a recombinant DNA-derived humanized anti-*HER2* monoclonal antibody, is an antineoplastic agent.

Trastuzumab is an IgG_1 kappa immunoglobulin containing human framework regions and the complementarity-determining regions of a murine antibody (4D5) that binds to *HER2/neu*, a transmembrane receptor protein that is overexpressed in selected cancer cells. The drug occurs as a sterile, lyophilized, white to pale yellow powder and is soluble in water; trastuzumab powder for injection also contains histidine monohydrochloride, histidine, *α,α*-trehalose dihydrate, and polysorbate (Tween®) 20. Following reconstitution as recommended with bacteriostatic water for injection containing benzyl alcohol (see Dosage and Administration: Reconstitution and Administration), solutions containing trastuzumab 21 mg/mL are clear to slightly opalescent and colorless to pale yellow and have a pH of about 6.

■ **Stability** Vials of trastuzumab should be stored at 2–8°C; when stored under recommended conditions, commercially available trastuzumab powder for injection should be stable up to the date of expiration marked on the vial.

Following reconstitution of the sterile powder with bacteriostatic water for injection containing benzyl alcohol (as supplied by the manufacturer), trastuzumab solutions are stable for 28 days when refrigerated at 2–8°C. If trastuzumab powder for injection is reconstituted with sterile water for injection (e.g., in patients with hypersensitivity to benzyl alcohol), the possibility of microbial contamination should be considered, and the manufacturer recommends that such solutions be used immediately and unused portions discarded. The manufacturer states that use of other diluents for the reconstitution of trastuzumab should be avoided. Trastuzumab solutions should not be frozen following reconstitution or dilution.

Reconstituted solutions of trastuzumab diluted in 0.9% sodium chloride injection are stable for no more than 24 hours when prepared and stored in polyvinyl chloride or polyethylene bags at 2–8°C. The manufacturer states that 5% dextrose injection should *not* be used as a diluent for trastuzumab solutions; diluents other than those recommended by the manufacturer may not maintain the stability or sterility of the antibody solution.

For further information on the handling of antineoplastic agents, see the ASHP Guidelines on Handling Hazardous Drugs at http://www.ahfsdruginformation.com.

Preparations

Trastuzumab (Herceptin®) should not be confused with ado-trastuzumab emtansine (Kadcyla®). (See Special Alerts.)

Excipients in commercially available drug preparations may have clinically important effects in some individuals; consult specific product labeling for details.

Trastuzumab

Parenteral

For injection, for IV infusion	440 mg	**Herceptin®** (supplied with 20 mL bacteriostatic water for injection containing 1.1% benzyl alcohol;), Genentech

†Use is not currently included in the labeling approved by the US Food and Drug Administration

Tretinoin

■ Tretinoin, a retinoid, is an antineoplastic agent.

Uses

■ **Acute Promyelocytic Leukemia** Tretinoin is used for remission induction in acute promyelocytic leukemia (APL), French-American-British classification M3 including the M3 variant, characterized by the presence of certain genetic markers (i.e., 15;17 chromosomal translocation and/or PML/RAR-α gene) in patients with relapsed or refractory disease following anthracycline-based chemotherapy or in patients for whom anthracycline therapy is contraindicated. Tretinoin also is added to induction with chemotherapy as initial† treatment for APL in patients with previously untreated disease.

Tretinoin is indicated for induction of remission, and patients with disease in remission following completion of induction therapy should receive consolidation and/or maintenance therapy for APL. For patients with APL that fails to respond or relapses following induction therapy with anthracycline-based therapy and tretinoin, induction therapy with arsenic trioxide is recommended. (See Arsenic Trioxide 10:00.)

APL is associated with a translocation between the long arms of chromosomes 15 and 17 [t(15;17)]. The 15;17 translocation results in fusion of the genes for promyelocytic leukemia (PML) and retinoic acid receptor-alpha (RAR-α), leading to 2 reciprocal fusion transcripts, PML/RAR-α and RAR-α/PML; the PML/RAR-α fusion protein is thought to play a role in leukemogenesis. Although therapy with tretinoin may be initiated based on the morphologic diagnosis of APL, cytogenetic evaluation to confirm presence of the 15;17 translocation should be performed. If this genetic marker is absent, molecular diagnostic testing for the PML/RAR-α fusion protein should be performed. The response rate to tretinoin has been determined only in patients with the 15;17 translocation and/or the PML/RAR-α gene, and alternative therapy should be considered in patients with APL lacking these genetic markers. Limited evidence indicates that response to tretinoin is poor in patients with a variant t(11;17) chromosomal abnormality.

Induction regimens are used to rapidly reduce the tumor burden to achieve complete remission, which generally is defined as less than 5% leukemic blast cells in the bone marrow and normalization of peripheral blood cell counts. Conventional induction therapy for APL consists of a combination of cytotoxic agents (i.e., an anthracycline and cytarabine), and results in a complete remission in about 60–80% of patients. The rate of early mortality is relatively high in patients with APL undergoing induction therapy, mainly secondary to intracranial or pulmonary hemorrhage in association with disseminated intravascular coagulation, fibrinolysis, and thrombocytopenia. Induction therapy with cytotoxic agents often initially worsens coagulopathy associated with APL, and aggressive replacement of platelets and clotting factors is necessary; although low-dose heparin therapy is used by some clinicians for anticoagulation, other clinicians do not recommend this approach. In contrast, induction therapy with tretinoin typically results in improvement of the coagulopathy associated with APL, and prophylactic heparin therapy generally is not required. However, tretinoin therapy is associated with complications including leukocytosis and a syndrome of respiratory distress described as the retinoic acid-APL syndrome.

The optimal postremission management of patients with APL receiving remission induction therapy with tretinoin has not been established. Patients with disease in complete remission should receive consolidation and/or maintenance therapy for APL following completion of induction therapy. Because of hypercatabolism of tretinoin with prolonged administration (see Pharmacokinetics), clinical resistance appears to result from continued therapy with the drug (see Pharmacology); however, the use of tretinoin in an intermittent maintenance regimen has been investigated.

Treatment for Relapsed or Refractory Disease The current indication for tretinoin is based principally on the results from an open-label, single-arm trial and on data from 2 cohorts of compassionate cases treated in multiple centers under the direction of the National Cancer Institute. All patients received tretinoin 45 mg/m² daily as a divided oral dose for up to 90 days or 30 days beyond attainment of a complete remission. In the clinical trial, tretinoin therapy was associated with a complete remission rate of 80% in the 20 patients with relapsed APL and 73% in the 15 patients with previously untreated APL; median survival was 10.8 months in the patients with relapsed disease. In the 2 cohorts of compassionate cases of APL, complete remission rates of 50–52% in patients with relapsed disease and 36–68% in patients with previously untreated disease were reported. The median time to achieve a complete remission was between 40–50 days (range: 2–120 days) in all patients studied. Most of the patients in these studies also received cytotoxic chemotherapy during the remission phase. The treatment outcomes observed with tretinoin in these patients compare favorably to the 30–50% complete remission rate and median survival of 6 months or less associated with cytotoxic chemotherapy alone in the treatment of relapsed APL.

Among 4 patients in whom cytogenetic analysis failed to detect the t(15;17) translocation, treatment with tretinoin resulted in a response in 3 patients. Although molecular genetic studies were not performed, these cases probably involved a masked translocation resulting in PML/RAR-α fusion. Responses to tretinoin have not been reported in cases of APL in which PML/RAR-α fusion has been shown to be absent. Although tretinoin has been used to induce second remissions in patients with APL that has relapsed following prior treatment with tretinoin, results have been inconsistent; continuous treatment with tretinoin results in resistance to the drug secondary to increased catabolism and decrease in plasma concentrations (see Pharmacokinetics), and response may be more likely for late relapse occurring after discontinuation of tretinoin therapy.

Limited data on the clinical use of tretinoin in children are available. (See Precautions and Contraindications: Pediatric Precautions.). A complete remission rate of 67% (8 of 10 males and 2 of 5 females) was reported in 15 pediatric patients (age range: 1–16 years) receiving tretinoin induction therapy for APL.

Initial Treatment for Newly Diagosed Disease Tretinoin is added to induction with chemotherapy as initial† treatment for acute promyelocytic leukemia in patients with previously untreated disease. Although tretinoin has not been shown to increase the complete remission rate or lower morbidity and mortality during induction therapy for APL compared with cytotoxic chemotherapy, the results of 2 large randomized trials have demonstrated that relapse-free (and, in one of the studies, overall) survival is prolonged in patients with previously untreated APL who receive tretinoin as a part of their treatment. In a randomized, multicenter trial in 346 patients with newly diagnosed APL, induction therapy with tretinoin was shown to be superior to induction therapy with standard chemotherapy (daunorubicin and cytarabine) with similar rates of complete remission and early mortality but prolonged disease-free and overall survival resulting from a reduced rate of relapse. Another randomized trial was terminated early when the addition of tretinoin to induction therapy with daunorubicin and cytarabine was shown to result in an increased rate of event-free survival. Long-term follow-up shows that the results of these randomized trials have been maintained.

Based on these findings, most clinicians recommend the addition of tretinoin to induction with chemotherapy as initial† treatment for acute promyelocytic leukemia. Although the optimal regimen for induction therapy has not been established, data from initial randomized trials suggests that tretinoin should be administered concurrently with anthracycline-based chemotherapy for newly diagnosed APL. In one of these randomized trials, the use of maintenance therapy (continuous low-dose chemotherapy with mercaptopurine and methotrexate) following induction and consolidation therapy for APL was shown to reduce the rate of relapse and increase the 2-year survival rate. Maintenance regimens including tretinoin have been shown to increase the rate of disease-free or event-free survival.

■ **Acne, Photoaging, and Other Dermatologic Conditions** **For topical uses, see Tretinoin 84:16.**

Dosage and Administration

■ **Administration** Tretinoin is administered orally. The effect of food on the absorption of tretinoin is not known; however, the absorption of other retinoids has been shown to be enhanced when administered with food.

■ **Dosage** ***Acute Promyelocytic Leukemia*** For the induction of remission in patients with APL, the recommended dosage of tretinoin is 45 mg/m² daily administered in 2 evenly divided doses. The manufacturer states that tretinoin therapy should be continued until 30 days after complete remission is achieved, or for a total of 90 days, whichever occurs first. Some clinicians report that tretinoin therapy should be continued until complete remission is achieved, or for a total of 90 days, whichever occurs first. Unless contraindicated, consolidation and/or maintenance chemotherapy for APL should be administered to all patients following induction therapy.

If tretinoin therapy has been initiated according to morphologic diagnosis of APL, but the presence of certain genetic markers (i.e., 15;17 chromosomal translocation and/or PML/RAR-α gene) is not confirmed in subsequent diagnostic studies and the disease is not responding, the drug should be discontinued and alternative treatment for acute myeloid leukemia should be considered.

Dosage Modification for Toxicity **Retinoic Acid-APL Syndrome.** Temporary discontinuance of tretinoin therapy should be considered in patients experiencing moderate or severe retinoic acid-APL syndrome. (See Retinoic Acid-APL Syndrome under Cautions: Adverse Effects.)

Hepatic Toxicity. Temporary discontinuance of tretinoin therapy should be considered in patients with serum transaminase concentrations exceeding 5 times the upper limit of normal.

Toxicity in Children. The manufacturer recommends increased caution in the use of tretinoin in pediatric patients. Dosage reduction may be considered for pediatric patients who experience serious or intolerable drug toxicity; however, the safety and efficacy of tretinoin dosages less than 45 mg/m² daily in pediatric patients have not been established.

Cautions

■ **Adverse Effects** Virtually all patients receiving tretinoin experience adverse effects, including headache, fever, weakness, and fatigue. The most common adverse effects of tretinoin therapy are similar to those reported in patients receiving high dosages of vitamin A. These adverse effects of tretinoin usually are reversible and do not require discontinuance of the drug. Severe adverse effects associated with tretinoin therapy include potentially fatal retinoic acid-APL syndrome (also known as APL differentiation syndrome) and rapidly evolving leukocytosis. Some adverse events, such as GI hemorrhage, cerebral hemorrhage, infections, disseminated intravascular coagulation, pneumonia, and septicemia, are common in patients with APL regardless of treatment.

The incidence of adverse effects associated with tretinoin is derived principally from data from 181 patients receiving the drug for up to 90 days (or 30 days beyond attainment of a complete response) in an uncontrolled clinical study or under a compassionate-use protocol.

Retinoic Acid-APL Syndrome Retinoic acid-APL (RA-APL) syndrome (also known as APL differentiation syndrome), characterized by fever, dyspnea, acute respiratory distress, weight gain, pulmonary infiltrates, pleural and pericardial effusions, edema, hepatic failure, renal failure, and multiorgan failure, occurs in approximately 25% of patients receiving tretinoin for the treatment of APL. RA-APL syndrome occasionally has been accompanied by impaired myocardial contractility and episodic hypotension and can occur with or without concomitant leukocytosis. In severe cases, progressive hypoxemia requiring endotracheal intubation and mechanical ventilation may occur, and deaths secondary to progressive hypoxemia and multiorgan failure have been reported. Onset of the syndrome generally is within the first month of treatment and can occur after the first dose of tretinoin. Manifestations suggestive of the RA-APL syndrome may occur in 60% or more of patients receiving tretinoin therapy for APL.

The cause of RA-APL syndrome is not known. Potential mechanisms of the syndrome include release of vasoactive cytokines, increased expression of adhesion molecules on myeloid cell surfaces (leading to enhanced cellular adherence to capillary endothelium and focal endothelial leakage), and development of migratory properties during leukemic cell differentiation.

Optimal treatment for RA-APL syndrome has not been established. However, high-dose corticosteroid treatment (e.g., dexamethasone 10 mg IV every 12 hours for at least 3 days or until resolution of symptoms) appears to reduce morbidity and mortality associated with the syndrome. High-dose corticosteroid treatment should be instituted immediately in patients with signs or symptoms suggestive of the syndrome (e.g., fever, dyspnea, weight gain, abnormal chest auscultatory findings, radiographic abnormalities) regardless of the leukocyte count. High-dose corticosteroid treatment of manifestations associated with RA-APL syndrome may be required in 60% or more of patients receiving tretinoin as induction therapy for APL. Patients successfully treated for RA-APL syndrome may experience a recurrence of the syndrome; if the syndrome recurs, another course of corticosteroid treatment should be initiated. Discontinuance of tretinoin therapy is not required in most patients during treatment for RA-APL syndrome; however, this condition may be fatal, so discontinuance of tretinoin therapy should be considered in patients experiencing moderate or severe RA-APL syndrome.

Hematologic Effects **Leukocytosis.** Rapidly evolving leukocytosis occurs in approximately 40% of patients receiving tretinoin. Rapidly evolving leukocytosis is associated with an increased risk of life-threatening complications in patients receiving tretinoin. Rarely, leukocytosis may exacerbate coagulopathy in patients with APL. Possible mechanisms leading to leukocytosis associated with tretinoin include a transient increase in survival of leukemic cells, "release" from the bone marrow, or mitosis in a cell population still capable of self-renewal (i.e., prior to its maturation to a stage at which it is no longer capable of further replication). Isolated cases of basophilia have been reported in patients receiving tretinoin.

The optimal management of leukocytosis associated with tretinoin has not been established. Treatment with high-dose steroids should be initiated immediately in patients with leukocytosis who develop signs or symptoms of RA-APL syndrome (see Cautions: Retinoic Acid-APL Syndrome). In patients with a baseline leukocyte count exceeding 5000/mm^3, or in patients who initially are leukopenic and subsequently develop a rapid increase in leukocyte count, some investigators routinely add chemotherapy agents to tretinoin treatment; the addition of such chemotherapy reportedly has been associated with a lower incidence of the RA-APL syndrome. According to the manufacturer, it may be appropriate to add full-dose chemotherapy (including an anthracycline unless contraindicated) to tretinoin therapy on day 1 or 2 in patients with a baseline leukocyte count exceeding 5000/mm^3; such chemotherapy may be initiated immediately in patients with a baseline leukocyte count less than 5000/mm^3 who subsequently develop a leukocyte count exceeding 6000/mm^3 by day 5, 10,000/mm^3 by day 10, or 15,000/mm^3 by day 28.

Hemorrhage. Hemorrhage has been reported in 60% of patients receiving tretinoin. In a randomized, multicenter trial comparing tretinoin with combination chemotherapy (daunorubicin and cytarabine) for remission induction in patients with APL, there was no significant difference in the incidence of severe hemorrhage associated with the 2 treatments.

Disseminated Intravascular Coagulation. Disseminated intravascular coagulation occurs in 26% of patients receiving tretinoin as induction therapy for APL. According to most clinicians, patients who develop disseminated intravascular coagulation should receive transfusions of platelets and fresh frozen plasma sufficient to maintain a platelet count of at least 50,000/mm^3 and a fibrinogen level of at least 100 mg/dL. Recommendations for additional treatment in this situation vary; some clinicians suggest use of heparin in patients with marked or persistent elevation of fibrin degradation products or thrombosis, and use of fibrinolytic inhibitors (e.g., aminocaproic acid) in patients with imminent or life-threatening retinal or intracranial hemorrhage.

Other Hematologic Effects. Bone marrow necrosis, sometimes fatal, has been reported in several patients receiving hydroxyurea during tretinoin therapy. (See: Drug Interactions: Hydroxyurea.) Thrombocytosis has been reported rarely in patients receiving tretinoin.

Infectious Complications Infection has been reported in 58% of patients receiving tretinoin for induction therapy of APL. Specific infections reported in patients receiving the drug include pneumonia in 14% of patients and cellulitis in 8% of patients. In a randomized, multicenter trial comparing tretinoin with combination chemotherapy (daunorubicin and cytarabine) for remission induction in patients with APL, the incidence of serious infections was greater in patients receiving chemotherapy (52%) than in those receiving tretinoin (25%).

Respiratory Effects Adverse respiratory effects have been observed frequently in patients receiving tretinoin and often occur as a manifestation of retinoic acid-APL syndrome. (See Cautions: Retinoic Acid-APL Syndrome.) In a randomized, multicenter trial comparing tretinoin with combination chemotherapy (daunorubicin and cytarabine) for remission induction in patients with APL, the incidence of severe pulmonary toxicity was greater in patients receiving tretinoin than in those receiving chemotherapy (21 versus 6%, respectively). According to the database for 181 patients receiving tretinoin, upper respiratory tract disorders, dyspnea, and respiratory insufficiency occurred in 63, 60, and 26%, respectively. Pleural effusion, rales, expiratory wheezing, lower respiratory tract disorders, and pulmonary infiltration have been reported in 20, 14, 14, 9, and 6% of patients, respectively. Other adverse respiratory effects, each reported in 3% of patients receiving tretinoin, include bronchial asthma, pulmonary edema, laryngeal edema, and unspecified pulmonary disease.

Metabolic Effects Reversible hypercholesterolemia and/or hypertriglyceridemia occur in up to 60% of patients receiving tretinoin. The clinical importance of transient elevations in cholesterol and triglycerides is not known; however, venous thrombosis and myocardial infarction have been reported in patients who otherwise are at low risk for these conditions. Weight gain has been reported in 23% of patients receiving tretinoin. Other adverse metabolic effects associated with tretinoin include acidosis and hypothermia, each occurring in 3% of patients. Hypercalcemia has been reported rarely in patients receiving the drug.

Hepatic Effects Adverse hepatic effects may occur as a manifestation of retinoic acid-APL syndrome in patients receiving tretinoin. (See Retinoic Acid-APL Syndrome under Cautions: Adverse Effects.) Elevations in liver function test results occur in 50–60% of patients receiving tretinoin. In most cases, discontinuance of tretinoin is not required, and liver function test abnormalities usually resolve during or after treatment. Temporary discontinuance of tretinoin should be considered in patients with serum transaminase concentrations exceeding 5 times the upper limit of normal. Other adverse hepatic effects reported in patients receiving tretinoin include hepatosplenomegaly in 9%, and hepatitis, ascites, and unspecified liver disorder, each in 3% of patients.

Nervous System Effects **Pseudotumor cerebri.** Pseudotumor cerebri (intracranial hypertension) has been reported in approximately 9% of patients receiving tretinoin. The risk of pseudotumor cerebri associated with the drug appears to be higher in pediatric patients. Patients receiving tretinoin who develop signs and symptoms of pseudotumor cerebri, such as papilledema, headache, nausea, vomiting, and visual disturbances, should be evaluated and treated appropriately; in some cases, narcotic analgesics, corticosteroids, and lumbar puncture may be required.

Headache. Headache occurs in 86% of patients receiving tretinoin. Headache associated with tretinoin typically occurs several hours after drug administration and usually responds to mild analgesics; tolerance to this adverse effect usually occurs with continued therapy.

Other Nervous System Effects. Cerebrovascular accident has been reported rarely in patients receiving tretinoin. Dizziness has been reported in 20%, and paresthesias in 17%, of patients receiving tretinoin. Anxiety, insomnia, depression, and confusion occurred in 17, 14, 14, and 11% of patients receiving the drug. Cerebral hemorrhage was reported in 9% of patients receiving tretinoin. Agitation and hallucinations have been reported in 9 and 6% of patients, respectively. Other adverse neurologic effects, each reported in 3% of patients receiving tretinoin, include abnormal gait, agnosia, aphasia, asterixis, cerebellar edema, cerebellar disorders, convulsions, coma, CNS depression, dysarthria, encephalopathy, facial paralysis, hemiplegia, hyporeflexia, hypotaxia, absent light reflex, neurologic reaction, spinal cord disorder, tremor, leg weakness, unconsciousness, dementia, forgetfulness, somnolence, and slow speech.

Dermatologic Effects **Dryness.** As with other retinoids, dryness of the skin and/or mucous membranes is common, occurring in 77% of patients receiving tretinoin. Dryness of the skin and mucous membranes can be treated with topical lubricants if necessary and usually does not require discontinuance or attenuation of tretinoin therapy.

Other Dermatologic Effects. Rash has been reported in 54% of patients receiving tretinoin. Pruritus and increased sweating each were observed in 20% of patients. Alopecia and skin changes each occurred in 14% of patients receiving the drug.

Sweet's syndrome (acute febrile neutrophilic dermatosis) and necrotizing vasculitis are uncommon adverse effects associated with tretinoin. Leukemia cutis (leukemic infiltration of the skin) has been reported in patients receiving tretinoin. Isolated cases of erythema nodosum also have been reported in patients receiving tretinoin. Genital ulceration and rare cases of vasculitis, mainly involving the skin, have been reported in patients receiving tretinoin.

GI Effects Nausea and vomiting occur in 57% of patients receiving tretinoin. GI hemorrhage and mucositis have been reported in 34 and 26%, respectively, of patients receiving the drug. Abdominal pain, diarrhea, and constipation have occurred in 31, 23, and 17% of patients, respectively. Anorexia and weight loss each have been reported in 17% of patients receiving tretinoin. Other adverse GI effects associated with tretinoin include unspecified GI disorder, dyspepsia, abdominal distension, and ulcer in 26, 14, 11, and 3% of patients, respectively.

Pancreatic Effects Pancreatitis has been reported rarely in patients receiving tretinoin.

Musculoskeletal Effects Bone pain was reported in 77% of patients with APL receiving tretinoin. Myalgia, flank pain, and bone inflammation have been observed in 14, 9, and 3%, respectively, of patients receiving the drug. Bone pain and arthralgia associated with tretinoin usually occur early in treatment and diminish with continued therapy. In some cases, treatment with parenteral opiate analgesics may be required for pain relief. Myositis associated with tretinoin has been reported rarely.

Cardiovascular Effects Cardiac failure occurred in 6% of patients receiving tretinoin, and cardiac arrest, myocardial infarction, stroke, and pulmonary hypertension each occurred in 3% of patients. There is a risk of arterial or venous thrombosis, involving any organ system, during the first month of tretinoin therapy. Cerebrovascular accident, myocardial infarction, and renal infarct have occurred in patients receiving tretinoin. Thromboembolic events, including fatal pulmonary embolism, have been reported in patients receiving tretinoin. In one patient receiving tretinoin, fatal thromboembolism occurred during concomitant therapy with an antifibrinolytic agent for the prophylaxis of hemorrhage associated with APL.

Peripheral edema occurs in 52% of patients receiving tretinoin. Chest discomfort, edema, arrhythmias, and flushing have been reported in 32, 29, 23, and 23% of patients, respectively. Hypotension and hypertension occurred in 14 and 11% of patients receiving tretinoin. Phlebitis has been reported in 11% of patients; other types of vasculitis have been reported rarely. Other adverse cardiovascular effects, each reported in 3% of patients receiving tretinoin, include cardiomegaly, heart murmur, ischemia, myocarditis, pericarditis, and secondary cardiomyopathy.

Renal Effects Adverse renal effects may occur as a manifestation of retinoic acid-APL syndrome in patients receiving tretinoin. (See Retinoic Acid-APL Syndrome under Cautions: Adverse Effects.) Renal insufficiency has been reported in 11% of patients receiving tretinoin, and acute renal failure and renal tubular necrosis each occurred in 3% of patients. Granulomatous tubulointerstitial nephritis has been reported in a patient receiving tretinoin as induction therapy for APL.

Genitourinary Effects Dysuria, urinary frequency, and enlarged prostate have been reported in 9, 3, and 3%, respectively, of patients receiving tretinoin. Scrotal and penile ulcerations also have been reported in patients receiving tretinoin.

Otic Effects Earache or a feeling of fullness in the ears occurred in 23% of patients receiving tretinoin. Hearing loss and other unspecified otic disorders have been reported in 6% of patients; irreversible hearing loss has occurred in less than 1% of patients.

Ocular Effects Visual disturbances and ocular disorders each have been reported in 17% of patients receiving tretinoin. Altered visual acuity and visual field defects were reported in 6 and 3% of patients, respectively.

Local Effects Injection site reactions have been observed in 17% of patients receiving tretinoin.

Other Adverse Effects Fever occurred in 83% of patients with APL receiving tretinoin. Malaise, shivering, and pain have been reported in 66, 63, and 37% of patients, respectively. Pallor was reported in 6% of patients receiving the drug. Lymphatic disorders (including cervical and tonsillar lymphadenopathy), facial edema, and fluid imbalance each have been reported in 6% of patients receiving tretinoin. Hyperhistaminemia and organomegaly rarely have been reported in patients receiving the drug.

■ Precautions and Contraindications

The manufacturer states that tretinoin should be administered only to patients with acute promyelocytic leukemia (APL). Because patients with APL are at high risk for medical complications in general and tretinoin can cause severe adverse reactions, this drug should be administered under the strict supervision of a qualified clinician experienced in the management of patients with acute leukemia and only when the potential benefits of tretinoin therapy are thought to outweigh the known adverse effects as well as other possible risks. In addition, appropriate diagnostic and treatment facilities must be readily available in case the patient develops severe toxicity, such as respiratory compromise. Patients receiving tretinoin should be observed closely for leukocytosis or respiratory compromise. Laboratory tests, including hematologic profile, coagulation parameters, liver function tests, and serum triglyceride and cholesterol concentrations should be monitored frequently in patients receiving tretinoin. Supportive care appropriate for patients with APL, such as prophylaxis for bleeding and prompt therapy for infection, should be maintained during tretinoin therapy.

Clinical manifestations associated with RA-APL syndrome (also known as APL differentiation syndrome), with or without leukocytosis, may occur in 60% or more of patients receiving tretinoin and require high-dose corticosteroid therapy. This syndrome, which can be fatal, occurs in about 25% of patients receiving tretinoin. Patients presenting with a high leukocyte count at diagnosis (i.e., exceeding 5000/mm^3) have an increased risk of a rapid further increase in leukocyte count. (See Retinoic Acid-APL Syndrome and Hematologic Effects, in Cautions.)

Tretinoin and other retinoids have been associated with pseudotumor cerebri, a form of intracranial hypertension, particularly in pediatric patients. (See: Cautions: Nervous System Effects.)

Liver function tests should be monitored carefully during tretinoin therapy. (See: Cautions: Hepatic Effects and Dosage: Dosage Modification for Toxicity: Hepatic Toxicity.) Frequent monitoring of serum cholesterol and triglyceride concentrations and clinical assessment of cardiac status is advised in patients receiving tretinoin regardless of history of cardiac conditions. (See Cardiovascular Effects and Metabolic Effects, in Cautions.)

Patients should be informed that their ability to drive or operate machinery may be impaired during tretinoin therapy, particularly if they are experiencing dizziness or severe headache.

Tretinoin is a known teratogen and special precautions and instruction are necessary in women of childbearing potential or pregnant women receiving the drug. Patients should be fully informed of the risks of fetal harm and contraceptive failure. (See: Cautions: Pregnancy, Fertility, and Lactation.)

Tretinoin is contraindicated in patients with known hypersensitivity to tretinoin, any of its components, or other retinoids or in patients who are sensitive to parabens, which are used as preservatives in commercially available tretinoin capsules.

Tretinoin therapy is *not* indicated in patients with subtypes of AML other than APL, and cytogenetic and molecular diagnostic studies should be performed to identify appropriate candidates.

■ Pediatric Precautions

The manufacturer states that safety and efficacy of tretinoin in infants younger than 1 year of age have not been established. Clinical data on the use of tretinoin in children are limited (see Uses: Acute Promyelocytic Leukemia). Tretinoin therapy is associated with severe headache and pseudotumor cerebri, requiring treatment with analgesics and lumbar puncture, in some pediatric patients. The manufacturer recommends increased caution in the use of tretinoin in pediatric patients. Dosage reduction may be appropriate for pediatric patients who experience severe adverse effects; however, the safety and efficacy of tretinoin dosages below 45 mg/m^2 daily have not been established in pediatric patients.

■ Geriatric Precautions

Approximately 20% of the patients enrolled in clinical studies of tretinoin were 60 years of age or older. Although no overall differences in efficacy or safety have been observed between geriatric and younger patients to date, the possibility that some older patients may exhibit increased sensitivity to the drug cannot be ruled out.

■ Mutagenicity and Carcinogenicity

Tretinoin was not mutagenic in the Ames test or the CHO/HGRPT gene mutation assay. In human diploid fibroblasts, a twofold increase in the sister chromatid exchange has been demonstrated. Clastogenic or aneuploidogenic effects were not demonstrated when tretinoin was tested in other chromosome aberration assays, including an in vitro assay in human peripheral lymphocytes and an in vivo mouse micronucleus assay.

Long-term studies to evaluate the carcinogenicity of tretinoin have not been performed to date. Therapy-related myelodysplasia, acute myeloid leukemia, or a combination of both has been reported in patients receiving tretinoin during induction and consolidation therapy for APL. When administered in mice at a dose of 30 mg/kg daily (about 2 times the recommended human dose on a mg/m^2 basis), tretinoin was associated with an increased rate of diethylnitrosamine-induced liver adenomas and carcinomas.

■ Pregnancy, Fertility, and Lactation

Pregnancy Tretinoin may cause fetal harm and the risk of birth of a severely deformed infant is high in pregnant women receiving the drug, but potential benefits may be acceptable in certain conditions despite possible risks to the fetus.

Experience with tretinoin administered to pregnant women is limited; however, increased spontaneous abortions and major fetal abnormalities have been documented in humans with the use of other retinoids. (See Cautions: Pregnancy, Fertility, and Lactation in Isotretinoin 84:92.) Reported defects, sometimes fatal, include abnormalities of the CNS, musculoskeletal system, external ear, eye, thymus, and great vessels, as well as facial dysmorphia, cleft palate, and parathyroid hormone deficiency. Low IQ scores (i.e., below 85), with or without obvious CNS abnormalities, also have been reported. According to the manufacturer, all fetuses exposed during pregnancy can be affected, and currently there is no antepartum method for determining whether a fetus is affected. In 2 women, tretinoin 45 mg/m^2 daily was administered during the second trimester of pregnancy, and both patients received consolidation chemotherapy after delivery. One woman delivered an infant at 30 weeks' gestation by cesarean section who required resuscitation for a cardiac arrhythmia followed by cardiac arrest. In the other case, no abnormalities were observed during pregnancy or at birth in twins born at 32 weeks' gestation; however, extensive vaginal and perineal ruptures led to severe perinatal and postnatal bleeding in the mother, and whether tretinoin therapy may have contributed to the fragility of the perineum and vagina and the severe bleeding during delivery is not known.

Tretinoin is teratogenic and embryotoxic in mice, rats, hamsters, rabbits, and pigtail monkeys. In all animals studied, the drug caused fetal resorptions and a decrease in live fetuses. Gross external, soft tissue, and skeletal deformities occurred at dosages exceeding 0.7 mg/kg daily, 2 mg/kg daily, or 7 mg/kg daily (approximately one-twentieth, one-fourth, and one-half the recommended human dosage on a mg/m² basis) in mice, rats, and hamsters, respectively, and at a dosage of 10 mg/kg daily (approximately 4 times the recommended human dosage on a mg/m² basis) in pigtail monkeys.

There are no adequate and well-controlled studies to date using tretinoin in pregnant women. There is a high risk of a severely deformed infant if tretinoin is administered to a pregnant woman. Tretinoin should be used during pregnancy only in life-threatening situations or severe disease for which safer drugs cannot be used or are ineffective. When the drug is administered during pregnancy or if the patient becomes pregnant while receiving the drug, the patient should be informed of the high risk of a severely deformed fetus, and the desirability of continuing or terminating the pregnancy should be discussed. Effective contraception must be used by all women during tretinoin therapy and for 1 month following discontinuance of the drug. Contraception must be used by all women receiving tretinoin (including those with a history of infertility or menopause) unless a hysterectomy has been performed. Unless abstinence is the chosen method, it is recommended that 2 reliable forms of contraception be used simultaneously. Progestin-only preparations (i.e., minipill) may be an inadequate method of contraception during tretinoin therapy. A reliable blood or urine pregnancy test with a sensitivity of at least 50 mIU/mL should be performed within 1 week prior to the initiation of tretinoin therapy. Whenever possible, initiation of therapy should be delayed until a negative pregnancy test result is obtained. When a delay is not possible, the patient should be placed on 2 reliable forms of contraception. Pregnancy testing and contraception counseling should be repeated monthly during tretinoin therapy.

Fertility When administered at dosages of up to 5 mg/kg daily (about two-thirds the recommended human dosage on a mg/m² basis), no adverse effects of tretinoin on fertility or reproductive performance were observed in rats. Minimal to marked testicular degeneration and increased numbers of immature spermatozoa were observed in dogs receiving tretinoin 10 mg/kg daily (about 4 times the equivalent human dosage in mg/m²) during a 6-week toxicology study.

Lactation It is not known whether tretinoin is distributed into milk. Because of the potential for serious adverse reactions to tretinoin in nursing infants, women should be advised to discontinue nursing during tretinoin therapy.

Drug Interactions

■ **Drugs Affecting Hepatic Microsomal Enzymes** Although specific studies have not been performed and the clinical importance has not been determined, concomitant use of drugs that affect cytochrome P-450 (CYP) hepatic microsomal enzymes, such as the CYP3A4, CYP2C8, and CYP2E isoenzymes, could alter the metabolism of tretinoin. Metabolism of tretinoin is mediated by CYP microsomal enzymes, and the possibility exists that drugs that induce these enzymes (e.g., rifampin, corticosteroids, phenobarbital, pentobarbital) may reduce plasma tretinoin concentrations. Conversely, concomitant use of tretinoin with drugs that inhibit the CYP enzymes (e.g., ketoconazole, cimetidine, erythromycin, verapamil, diltiazem, cyclosporine) may increase plasma tretinoin concentrations. Currently, it is not known whether concomitant use of drugs affecting the CYP enzyme system alters the efficacy or toxicity of tretinoin.

In a small number of patients receiving daily dosages of tretinoin for 4 consecutive weeks, oral administration of ketoconazole 400–1200 mg 1 hour prior to the tretinoin dose on day 29 was associated with a 72% increase in the mean area under the plasma concentration-time curve (AUC) for tretinoin.

■ **Hydroxyurea** Concurrent use of hydroxyurea, which is cytotoxic to cells in S phase, and tretinoin, which induces cells to enter the S phase, may cause a synergistic effect leading to massive cell lysis. Bone marrow necrosis, sometimes fatal, has been reported in patients receiving hydroxyurea during tretinoin therapy. Although some clinicians have administered hydroxyurea in conjunction with tretinoin therapy to reduce leukocytosis, the safety and efficacy of this practice have not been established, and caution is recommended in the use of hydroxyurea in patients receiving tretinoin.

■ **Agents Known to Cause Pseudotumor Cerebri/Intracranial Hypertension** Risk of pseudotumor cerebri (intracranial hypertension) is increased in patients receiving tretinoin. Concomitant use of other agents known to cause pseudotumor cerebri or intracranial hypertension, such as tetracyclines, may increase the risk of this condition in patients receiving tretinoin.

■ **Fibrinolytic Inhibitors** Fatal thrombotic complications have been reported rarely in patients receiving tretinoin and fibrinolytic inhibitors, such as tranexamic acid, aminocaproic acid, or aprotinin. Caution is advised when tretinoin is used concomitantly with antifibrinolytic agents.

■ **Vitamin A** The same as for other retinoids, tretinoin must *not* be used concomitantly with vitamin A because concomitant use could exacerbate symptoms of hypervitaminosis A.

Acute Toxicity

Limited information is available on the acute toxicity of tretinoin. The maximum tolerated dosage of the drug in patients with myelodysplastic syndrome or solid tumors is 195 mg/m² daily. The maximum tolerated dosage of tretinoin in pediatric patients is 60 mg/m² daily.

Symptoms of overdosage for other retinoids have been rapidly reversible without apparent residual effects and include transient headache, facial flushing, cheilosis, abdominal pain, dizziness, and ataxia. Treatment of tretinoin toxicity is primarily supportive, but patients experiencing an overdosage of the drug should receive care in a special hematologic unit.

Pharmacology

Although the precise mechanism(s) of action of tretinoin has not been fully elucidated, it is known that the drug is *not* a cytolytic agent. Tretinoin induces cellular differentiation and decreases the proliferation of acute promyelocytic leukemia (APL) cells. The PML/RAR-α fusion protein resulting from the 15; 17 chromosomal translocation appears to block myeloid differentiation at the promyelocyte stage, possibly by complexing and inactivating wild-type PML or by inhibiting the normal retinoic acid signaling pathway. In patients with APL who achieve a complete remission with tretinoin therapy, the drug causes an initial maturation of the primitive promyelocytes derived from the cellular leukemic clone followed by a repopulation of the bone marrow and peripheral blood by normal, polyclonal hematopoietic cells. Observations supporting cellular differentiation effects as a mechanism of tretinoin include the absence of bone marrow hypoplasia during induction, the appearance of immunophenotypically unique "intermediate cells" expressing both mature and immature cell surface antigens, and the presence of both Auer rods and the 15;17 translocation in morphologically mature granulocytes until a late stage of induction. The mechanism by which the population of malignant cells is eliminated is not fully understood but appears to involve apoptosis (programmed cell death). Following induction therapy, the PML/RAR-α fusion protein can be detected in the majority of patients, suggesting that tretinoin alone does not eradicate the leukemic clone.

Despite the high initial complete response rate, remissions induced and maintained by tretinoin alone in patients with APL are short (median: 3.5 months). Increased metabolism and clearance of tretinoin with prolonged administration leading to reduction in plasma concentrations of the drug may contribute to clinical resistance to tretinoin in patients with APL. However, decreased plasma concentrations may not necessarily indicate pharmacologic inactivity in other tissues; pseudotumor cerebri, an adverse effect associated with tretinoin, was observed in a patient in whom plasma concentrations of the drug were undetectable.

Pharmacokinetics

The pharmacokinetics of tretinoin have not been evaluated separately by gender or ethnic group.

■ **Absorption** Because an IV dosage form of tretinoin is not available, the pharmacokinetics of the drug (e.g., bioavailability, volume of distribution) have not been fully characterized. However, the results of some studies indicate that there is extensive intrapatient and interpatient variability.

Tretinoin is readily absorbed from the GI tract, and peak plasma concentrations are achieved in about 1–2 hours. The bioavailability of tretinoin has been estimated to be about 50%, and marked interpatient variation has been observed. In patients with APL who received a single oral dose of tretinoin 45 mg/m², peak plasma concentrations of tretinoin ranged from 95 to about 948 ng/mL. In a pharmacokinetic study involving children receiving single doses of tretinoin, peak plasma concentration and area under the plasma concentration-time curve (AUC) increased in a nonlinear manner relative to increases in dose.

Evidence suggests that tretinoin induces its own metabolism. (See Pharmacokinetics: Elimination.) During 1 week of continuous therapy, plasma concentrations of tretinoin decrease to an average of one-third of the plasma concentrations observed on the first day. In a small number of pediatric patients who received tretinoin daily for 28 days, the mean area under the plasma concentration-time curve on day 28 was approximately one-fifth that determined on day one.

The absorption of retinoids generally has been shown to be enhanced by coadministration with food; however, the effect of food on the absorption of tretinoin has not been evaluated. Because tretinoin is fat-soluble, some clinicians have suggested that a fat-restricted diet may cause reduced bioavailability of the drug.

■ **Distribution** Distribution of tretinoin into body tissues and fluids has not been fully characterized. The apparent volume of distribution of tretinoin has not been determined. Tretinoin does not appear to be distributed into the CSF and probably is not effective for treating leukemia in the CNS.

Plasma protein binding (principally to albumin) of tretinoin exceeds 95% and remains constant at plasma concentrations ranging from 10–500 ng/mL.

Oral tretinoin has been shown to cross the placenta in animal studies, and the drug is recognized as a potent teratogen. It is not known whether tretinoin distributes into milk.

■ **Elimination** In patients with APL receiving tretinoin orally, a terminal elimination half-life of 0.5–2 hours has been reported following initial dosing.

The precise metabolic pathway of tretinoin has not been fully elucidated. Although various metabolites have been identified, the activity of tretinoin results mainly from the parent drug. Stereoisomerization of tretinoin occurs in the liver, followed by oxidation. Cytochrome P-450 (CYP) isoenzymes (e.g., CYP3A4, CYP2C8, CYP2E) have been implicated in the oxidative metabolism of the drug. Metabolites are excreted as glucuronide conjugates in urine and bile. Metabolites of tretinoin that have been identified include 13-*cis* retinoic acid, 4-oxo *trans* retinoic acid, 4-oxo *cis* retinoic acid, and 4-oxo *trans* retinoic acid glucuronide.

Evidence suggests that tretinoin induces its own metabolism. In patients with APL receiving 45 mg/m^2 tretinoin daily, urinary excretion of 4-oxo *trans* retinoic acid glucuronide increased approximately tenfold over the course of 2–6 weeks of continuous therapy, suggesting that increased metabolism of tretinoin may be the primary mechanism leading to the decreased plasma drug concentrations observed during continued administration. Possible mechanisms for the increased clearance of tretinoin with continuous daily dosing of the drug include induction of CYP enzymes or oxidative cofactors and increased expression of cellular retinoic acid binding proteins. Increasing the dosage of tretinoin to compensate for the apparent autoinduction has not been shown to increase therapeutic response. Reduced plasma retinoid concentrations have been associated with relapse and clinical resistance, and some investigators suggest that the clinical failure of tretinoin may be related to a lack of sustained effective concentrations of the drug during prolonged treatment.

Following oral administration of radiolabeled tretinoin at doses of 2.75 and 50 mg, greater than 90% of the radioactivity was recovered in urine and feces. Based on pharmacokinetic data from 3 individuals, approximately 63% of radioactivity was excreted in urine within 72 hours, and 31% was recovered in feces within 6 days.

The effect of renal or hepatic impairment on the elimination of tretinoin has not been established.

Chemistry and Stability

■ **Chemistry** Tretinoin, a retinoid, is an antineoplastic agent. Tretinoin (all-*trans* retinoic acid) is chemically related to retinol (vitamin A). The drug occurs as a yellow to light orange crystalline powder. Inactive ingredients contained in commercially available tretinoin capsules include beeswax, butylated hydroxyanisole, edetate disodium, hydrogenated soybean oil flakes, hydrogenated vegetable oils, and soybean oil. The gelatin capsule shell contains glycerin, yellow iron oxide, red iron oxide, titanium dioxide, methylparaben, and propylparaben.

■ **Stability** Tretinoin capsules should be stored at 15–30°C and protected from light.

Preparations

Excipients in commercially available drug preparations may have clinically important effects in some individuals; consult specific product labeling for details.

Tretinoin

Oral		
Capsules	10 mg	**Vesanoid®**, Roche

†Use is not currently included in the labeling approved by the US Food and Drug Administration

Trifluridine and Tipiracil Hydrochloride

■ Trifluridine and tipiracil hydrochloride (trifluridine/tipiracil) is a fixed-combination antineoplastic agent containing the antimetabolite trifluridine (a thymidine-based nucleoside analog) and the thymidine phosphorylase inhibitor tipiracil; tipiracil enhances the oral bioavailability of trifluridine by inhibiting its metabolism by thymidine phosphorylase.

Uses

■ **Colorectal Cancer** The fixed combination of trifluridine and tipiracil hydrochloride (trifluridine/tipiracil) is used for the treatment of metastatic colorectal cancer in patients who previously received fluoropyrimidine-, oxaliplatin-, and irinotecan-containing regimens; a vascular endothelial growth factor inhibitor (anti-VEGF therapy); and, in those with tumors bearing the wild-type (nonmutated) *KRAS* gene, an epidermal growth factor receptor inhibitor (anti-EGFR therapy). In patients with previously treated metastatic colorectal cancer, trifluridine/tipiracil fixed-combination therapy has been shown to prolong overall and progression-free survival compared with placebo; however, overall response rates were low, suggesting that the drug's main effect was disease stabilization.

The current indication for trifluridine/tipiracil in the treatment of metastatic colorectal cancer is based principally on the results of a randomized, double-blind, placebo-controlled phase 3 study (RECOURSE) in patients with previously treated metastatic colorectal cancer. The primary measure of efficacy was overall survival. The median age of patients was 63 years; 49% of patients had wild-type *KRAS* and 51% had *KRAS* mutations.

Patients enrolled in the RECOURSE study had received at least 2 prior therapies for their disease; all patients had received previous treatment with fluoropyrimidine-, oxaliplatin-, and irinotecan-containing regimens. With one exception, all patients had previously received bevacizumab therapy. All except 2 patients with tumors bearing the wild-type *KRAS* gene had previously received panitumumab or cetuximab therapy. In addition, 17 or 20% of patients receiving trifluridine/tipiracil or placebo, respectively, had previously received regorafenib, an inhibitor of multiple receptor tyrosine kinases. Most patients (over 90%) enrolled in the study had disease refractory to fluoropyrimidine therapy during their last exposure to these drugs.

In the RECOURSE study, 800 patients were randomized (stratified by *KRAS* mutation status, time since diagnosis of initial metastasis, and geographic region) in a 2:1 ratio to receive either trifluridine/tipiracil (35 mg/m^2 [of trifluridine] orally twice daily after meals) or placebo on days 1–5 and 8–12 of each 28-day cycle; all patients received best supportive care. Treatment was continued until disease progression, death, or unacceptable toxicity occurred or treatment was discontinued for other reasons. The median duration of treatment was 6.7 weeks for patients receiving trifluridine/tipiracil and 5.7 weeks for those receiving placebo. At the time of the primary analysis, patients receiving trifluridine/tipiracil had a longer median overall survival (7.1 versus 5.3 months; hazard ratio for death: 0.68) and longer median progression-free survival (2 versus 1.7 months; hazard ratio for progression: 0.48) than those receiving placebo. Overall response rates were low (1.6 versus 0.4%, respectively) and were not substantially different between patients receiving trifluridine/tipiracil and those receiving placebo, suggesting that the drug's main effect in this patient population was disease stabilization; one patient (a placebo recipient) achieved a complete response. Results of a subgroup analysis (based on age, gender, geographic region, ECOG performance status, time since diagnosis of initial metastasis, number of metastatic sites, primary site of disease, disease refractory to fluoropyrimidine, number of prior therapies, prior use of regorafenib, and *KRAS* mutation status) suggested that the drug's effect on overall survival was consistent in most subgroups. Subgroup analysis suggested that the drug's effect on progression-free survival was consistent across all the subgroups.

For ophthalmic use of single-entity trifluridine as an antiviral agent, see Trifluridine 52:04.20.

Dosage and Administration

■ **General** Complete blood cell (CBC) counts should be obtained prior to initiation of each cycle and on day 15 of each cycle. Patients should have an absolute neutrophil count (ANC) of at least 1500/mm^3 and a platelet count of at least 75,000/mm^3 prior to each cycle.

■ **Administration** The fixed combination of trifluridine and tipiracil hydrochloride (trifluridine/tipiracil) is administered orally within 1 hour of completion of morning and evening meals. (See Description.)

Procedures for proper handling (e.g., use of gloves) and disposal of antineoplastic agents should be followed.

■ **Dosage** Dosage of the fixed combination of trifluridine and tipiracil hydrochloride is expressed in terms of the trifluridine content.

Each fixed-combination tablet of trifluridine and tipiracil hydrochloride contains 15 or 20 mg of trifluridine and 6.14 or 8.19 mg of tipiracil, respectively (equivalent to a molar ratio of 1:0.5).

Colorectal Cancer For the treatment of metastatic colorectal cancer in patients who previously received fluoropyrimidine-, oxaliplatin-, and irinotecan-containing regimens, anti-vascular endothelial growth factor (anti-VEGF) therapy, and, in those with tumors bearing the wild-type (nonmutated) *KRAS* gene, anti-epidermal growth factor receptor (anti-EGFR) therapy, the recommended dosage of trifluridine/tipiracil is 35 mg/m^2 (of trifluridine) twice daily on days 1–5 and days 8–12 of each 28-day cycle. Doses should be rounded to the nearest 5-mg increment and should *not* exceed 80 mg (of trifluridine). Therapy should be continued until disease progression or unacceptable toxicity occurs.

Dosage Modification for Toxicity When dosage modification is necessary, dosage of trifluridine/tipiracil should be reduced by 1 dose level in decrements of 5 mg/m^2 (of trifluridine) (from 35 to 30 mg/m^2, from 30 to 25 mg/m^2, from 25 to 20 mg/m^2); however, no more than 3 dosage adjustments are permitted. If a dose of 20 mg/m^2 is not tolerated, trifluridine/tipiracil should be discontinued.

Dosage of trifluridine/tipiracil should *not* be re-escalated following a dosage reduction.

Hematologic Toxicity. If uncomplicated grade 4 neutropenia (ANC less than 500/mm^3) or thrombocytopenia (platelet count less than 25,000/mm^3) delays initiation of a cycle by more than 1 week, trifluridine/tipiracil therapy should be withheld until ANC reaches or exceeds 1500/mm^3 and platelet counts reach or exceed 75,000/mm^3; the next cycle may then be initiated at 1 dose level lower than the previous dosage.

If grade 4 neutropenia occurs or platelet counts decrease to less than 50,000/mm^3 during a cycle, trifluridine/tipiracil therapy should be withheld; therapy may be resumed at 1 dose level lower than the previous dosage when ANC reaches or exceeds 1500/mm^3 and platelet counts reach or exceed 75,000/mm^3.

If febrile neutropenia occurs, trifluridine/tipiracil therapy should be withheld; therapy may be resumed at 1 dose level lower than the previous dosage when febrile neutropenia resolves.

Nonhematologic Toxicity. If grade 3 or 4 nonhematologic toxicity (excluding grade 3 nausea and/or vomiting controlled by antiemetic agents and grade 3 diarrhea responsive to antidiarrheal agents) occurs, trifluridine/tipiracil therapy should be withheld; therapy may be resumed at 1 dose level lower than the previous dosage when the toxicity improves to grade 1 or less.

■ **Special Populations** No dosage adjustment is necessary in patients with mild hepatic impairment. Safety and efficacy of trifluridine/tipiracil have not been established in patients with moderate or severe hepatic impairment. (See Hepatic Impairment under Warnings/Precautions: Specific Populations, in Cautions.)

No initial dosage adjustment is necessary in patients with mild or moderate renal impairment; however, patients with moderate renal impairment may be more likely to require dosage adjustment for toxicity since increased trifluridine/tipiracil-related toxicity has been observed in this patient population. Safety and efficacy of trifluridine/tipiracil have not been established in patients with severe renal impairment. (See Renal Impairment under Warnings/Precautions: Specific Populations, in Cautions.)

No initial dosage adjustment is necessary in geriatric patients. (See Geriatric Use under Warnings/Precautions: Specific Populations, in Cautions.)

Cautions

■ **Contraindications** The manufacturer states that there are no known contraindications to the use of the fixed combination of trifluridine and tipiracil hydrochloride (trifluridine/tipiracil).

■ **Warnings/Precautions** ***Hematologic Effects*** Severe and life-threatening myelosuppression (anemia, neutropenia, thrombocytopenia) has been reported in patients receiving trifluridine/tipiracil. In the RECOURSE study, grade 3 or 4 anemia, neutropenia, or thrombocytopenia occurred in 18, 38, or 5%, respectively, of patients receiving trifluridine/tipiracil and in 3, 0, or less than 1%, respectively, of those receiving placebo. Febrile neutropenia and fatal neutropenic infection occurred in 3.8 and 0.2%, respectively, of patients receiving trifluridine/tipiracil.

Complete blood cell (CBC) counts should be monitored prior to initiation of each cycle, on day 15 of each cycle, and as clinically indicated. Patients should have an absolute neutrophil count (ANC) of at least 1500/mm^3 and a platelet count of at least 75,000/mm^3 prior to each cycle. In patients who develop neutropenia or thrombocytopenia, temporary interruption of therapy, dosage reduction, or drug discontinuance may be required. (See Hematologic Toxicity under Dosage: Dosage Modification for Toxicity, in Dosage and Administration.)

Fetal/Neonatal Morbidity and Mortality There are no adequate and well-controlled studies of trifluridine/tipiracil in pregnant women; however, based on its mechanism of action and animal findings, trifluridine and tipiracil may cause fetal harm. Embryofetal toxicity (i.e., decreased fetal weight), teratogenicity (i.e., kinked tail, cleft palate, ectrodactyly, anasarca, great vessel and skeletal abnormalities), and lethality were observed in pregnant animals receiving trifluridine/tipiracil at exposure levels similar to or less than the human exposure at the recommended dosage.

Pregnancy should be avoided during trifluridine/tipiracil therapy. Women of childbearing potential should be advised to use an effective method of contraception while receiving trifluridine/tipiracil. Male patients should be advised to use an effective method of contraception while receiving trifluridine/tipiracil and for at least 3 months after discontinuance of therapy each time they have sexual contact with women of childbearing potential. If trifluridine/tipiracil is used during pregnancy or if the patient becomes pregnant while receiving the drug, the patient should be informed of the potential hazard to the fetus.

Specific Populations **Pregnancy.** Trifluridine/tipiracil may cause fetal harm if administered to pregnant women based on its mechanism of action and animal findings. (See Fetal/Neonatal Morbidity and Mortality under Cautions: Warnings/Precautions.)

Lactation. Trifluridine and tipiracil, or metabolites of these drugs, are distributed into milk in rats; it is not known whether trifluridine and tipiracil, or their metabolites, are distributed into milk in humans. Because of the potential for serious adverse reactions to trifluridine/tipiracil in nursing infants, women should be advised to discontinue nursing during therapy. Women may begin nursing 1 day after discontinuance of therapy. The effects of trifluridine and tipiracil, or metabolites of these drugs, on nursing infants or on the production of milk are unknown.

Pediatric Use. Safety and efficacy of trifluridine/tipiracil have not been established in pediatric patients.

Dental abnormalities (e.g., whitening, malocclusions, broken teeth) have been observed in animals receiving trifluridine/tipiracil at exposure levels approximately 0.33 times the human exposure at the recommended dosage.

Geriatric Use. In the RECOURSE study in patients with previously treated metastatic colorectal cancer, 44% of patients receiving trifluridine/tipiracil were 65 years of age or older and 7% were 75 years of age or older. No overall differences in efficacy were observed between geriatric and younger patients, but some grade 3 or 4 adverse effects (i.e., neutropenia, anemia, thrombocytopenia) occurred more frequently in geriatric patients.

Hepatic Impairment. The pharmacokinetic profile of trifluridine/tipiracil has not been fully established in patients with hepatic impairment.

In a population pharmacokinetic analysis, systemic exposure to trifluridine and tipiracil was similar in patients with mild hepatic impairment (total bilirubin concentration not exceeding the upper limit of normal [ULN] with AST concentration exceeding the ULN *or* total bilirubin concentration exceeding the ULN, but no more than 1.5 times the ULN, with any AST concentration) and those with normal hepatic function. No initial dosage adjustment of trifluridine or tipiracil is necessary in patients with mild hepatic impairment.

The pharmacokinetic profiles of trifluridine and tipiracil have not been established in patients with moderate or severe hepatic impairment (total bilirubin concentration exceeding 1.5 times the ULN with any AST concentration), and these patients were excluded from the RECOURSE study in patients with previously treated metastatic colorectal cancer.

Renal Impairment. The pharmacokinetic profile of trifluridine/tipiracil has not been fully established in patients with renal impairment.

In a population pharmacokinetic analysis, the estimated mean areas under the plasma concentration-time curve (AUCs) of trifluridine and tipiracil were increased by 31 and 34%, respectively, in patients with mild renal impairment (creatinine clearance of 60–89 mL/minute) and by 43 and 65%, respectively, in patients with moderate renal impairment (creatinine clearance of 30–59 mL/minute) compared with patients with normal renal function. No initial dosage adjustment of trifluridine or tipiracil is necessary in patients with mild to moderate renal impairment; however, dosage adjustment for toxicity may be necessary in patients with moderate renal impairment.

In the RECOURSE study in patients with previously treated metastatic colorectal cancer, grade 3 or greater adverse effects, serious adverse effects, and dose delays or reductions occurred more frequently in patients with moderate renal impairment compared with those with normal renal function or mild renal impairment.

The pharmacokinetic profiles of trifluridine and tipiracil have not been established in patients with severe renal impairment (creatinine clearance less than 30 mL/minute) or end-stage renal disease, and these patients were excluded from the RECOURSE study.

■ **Common Adverse Effects** Adverse effects reported in 5% or more of patients receiving trifluridine/tipiracil for the treatment of previously treated metastatic colorectal cancer and at an incidence more than 2% higher than that reported with placebo include asthenia/fatigue, nausea, loss of appetite, diarrhea, vomiting, infection (nasopharyngitis, urinary tract infection), abdominal pain, pyrexia, stomatitis, alopecia, and dysgeusia. Laboratory abnormalities reported in 10% or more of patients receiving trifluridine/tipiracil and more frequently with the fixed-combination drug than with placebo include anemia, neutropenia, and thrombocytopenia.

Drug Interactions

Trifluridine is a substrate of thymidine phosphorylase; the drug is not metabolized by cytochrome P-450 (CYP) isoenzymes. In vitro, trifluridine, tipiracil, and 5-(trifluoromethyl)uracil (the primary inactive metabolite of trifluridine) did not inhibit CYP isoenzymes or induce CYP isoenzymes 1A2, 2B6, or 3A4/5.

In vitro studies indicate that trifluridine is not a substrate or inhibitor of human hepatic uptake transport proteins or efflux transporters; however, in vitro data indicate that tipiracil is a substrate and inhibitor of organic cation transporter (OCT) 2 at concentrations of 3 or more times clinically relevant concentrations.

No formal drug interaction studies with the fixed combination of trifluridine and tipiracil hydrochloride (trifluridine/tipiracil) have been performed to date.

■ **Drugs Affected by Organic Cation Transporter** Limited data suggest that concomitant administration of trifluridine/tipiracil with OCT2 inhibitors (i.e., famotidine, metformin, ranitidine) does not result in clinically important changes in the pharmacokinetics of trifluridine or tipiracil.

Description

Trifluridine and tipiracil hydrochloride (trifluridine/tipiracil) is a fixed-combination antineoplastic agent containing the antimetabolite trifluridine (a thymidine-based nucleoside analog) and the thymidine phosphorylase inhibitor tipiracil; tipiracil enhances the oral bioavailability of trifluridine by inhibiting its metabolism by thymidine phosphorylase. Although initial development of trifluridine and fluorouracil occurred at approximately the same time, early clinical studies evaluating oncologic use of IV trifluridine were discontinued because of the drug's rapid metabolism by thymidine phosphorylase and severe adverse effects associated with the IV dosing schedule. When trifluridine was administered orally alone, plasma concentrations of the drug were very low, suggesting extensive first-pass metabolism in the liver and intestine. Subsequent development of an inhibitor of thymidine phosphorylase, tipiracil, resulted in enhanced oral bioavailability and maintenance of therapeutic plasma concentrations of trifluridine when the drugs were used concomitantly. In vivo, maximum antitumor activity and low trifluridine toxicity were achieved with a 1:0.5 molar ratio of trifluridine to tipiracil. Following oral administration of the drugs in this molar ratio as trifluridine/tipiracil (single dose containing 35-mg/m^2 of trifluridine), the area under the serum concentration-time curve (AUC) and peak plasma concentration of trifluridine exhibited less variability and were increased by 38- and 22-fold, respectively, compared with administration of trifluridine alone.

Trifluridine is converted intracellularly by thymidine kinase to trifluoromethyl deoxyuridine 5′-monophosphate (F_3dTMP), a reversible tight-binding inhibitor of thymidylate synthase (TS), and trifluoromethyl deoxyuridine 5′-triphosphate (F_3dTTP). These active metabolites interfere with DNA synthesis and inhibit the cell cycle via several mechanisms including inhibition of TS and incorporation of F_3dTTP into the DNA chain. In vitro, inhibition of TS declines rapidly following a trifluridine wash-out period; therefore, in contrast to fluorouracil, inhibition of TS is not the major mechanism by which trifluridine exerts antitumor activity. Preclinical studies suggest that the predominant mechanism by which trifluridine/tipiracil exerts antitumor activity is prolonged incorporation of trifluridine into tumor cell DNA. In vitro, F_3dTTP is incorporated into DNA to a substantially greater degree than fluorouracil (approximately 300-fold greater). Tipiracil may inhibit tumor angiogenesis via inhibition of thymidine phosphorylase (platelet derived endothelial cell growth factor-1 [PD-ECGF-1]), an enzyme with angiogenic properties; however, the clinical relevance of this finding has not been established. Trifluridine/tipiracil has demonstrated antitumor activity in mice bearing tumor xenografts that expressed mutated and wild-type (nonmutated) *KRAS*. Trifluridine/tipiracil also has demonstrated antitumor activity in mice bearing fluorouracil-sensitive and fluorouracil-resistant tumor xenografts.

Following oral administration of trifluridine/tipiracil as a single dose of 35 mg/m^2 (of trifluridine) in cancer patients, peak plasma concentrations of trifluridine occur in approximately 2 hours. With twice-daily dosing of trifluridine/tipiracil, the AUC of trifluridine increases more than proportionally with dose over the trifluridine dose range of 15–35 mg/m^2. Following repeated administration of trifluridine/tipiracil, accumulation of trifluridine (threefold and twofold increases in AUC and peak plasma concentrations, respectively), but no accumulation of tipiracil, was observed. Administration of trifluridine/tipiracil 35 mg/m^2 (of trifluridine) with a high-fat, high-calorie meal in cancer patients decreased peak plasma concentrations of trifluridine by 40% and systemic exposure and peak plasma concentrations of tipiracil by 45% compared with administration in the fasted state; however, systemic exposure of trifluridine was not affected. The manufacturer recommends administration of trifluridine/tipiracil within 1 hour of completion of morning and evening meals to reduce the risk of neutropenia associated with increased peak plasma concentrations of trifluridine. In vitro, trifluridine is highly bound (exceeding 96%) to plasma proteins, independent of drug concentrations and presence of tipiracil; however, tipiracil is less than 8% bound to plasma proteins. Following administration of trifluridine/tipiracil 35 mg/m^2 (of trifluridine) twice daily, the mean elimination half-lives of trifluridine and tipiracil at steady state are 2.1 and 2.4 hours, respectively. Trifluridine and tipiracil are not metabolized by cytochrome P-450 (CYP) pathways; trifluridine is metabolized mainly by thymidine phosphorylase to its primary inactive metabolite, 5-(trifluoromethyl)uracil. Following oral administration of trifluridine/tipiracil as a single dose of 60 mg (of trifluridine), 1.5% of the trifluridine/tipiracil dose was recovered in urine as unchanged trifluridine, 19.2% was recovered as 5-(trifluoromethyl)uracil, and 29.3% was recovered as unchanged tipiracil within 48 hours.

The pharmacokinetics of trifluridine and tipiracil do not appear to be affected substantially by age (33–82 years), gender, or ethnicity.

Advice to Patients

Importance of advising patients to take the fixed combination of trifluridine and tipiracil hydrochloride (trifluridine/tipiracil) exactly as prescribed. Importance of advising patients receiving 2 strengths of trifluridine/tipiracil to take the appropriate number of tablets of each strength.

Importance of advising patients to take trifluridine/tipiracil within 1 hour after completion of morning and evening meals. If a dose of trifluridine/tipiracil is missed or withheld, an additional dose should not be administered to replace the missed or withheld dose.

Importance of advising patients that individuals other than the patient should not handle trifluridine/tipiracil tablets without protection (e.g., gloves).

Importance of complete blood cell (CBC) count monitoring before and during trifluridine/tipiracil therapy. Importance of immediately reporting any manifestations of infection.

Importance of contacting a clinician if severe or persistent nausea, vomiting, diarrhea, or abdominal pain occurs.

Risk of fetal harm. Necessity of advising women of childbearing potential that they should use an effective method of contraception while receiving the drug. Necessity of advising men to use a condom during sexual encounters with women of childbearing potential; these contraceptive measures are required during and for at least 3 months after discontinuance of trifluridine/tipiracil therapy. If pregnancy occurs, advise pregnant women of potential risk to the fetus.

Importance of advising women to avoid breast-feeding while receiving trifluridine/tipiracil and for 1 day after discontinuance of therapy.

Importance of informing clinicians of existing or contemplated concomitant therapy, including prescription and OTC drugs and dietary or herbal supplements, as well as any concomitant illnesses.

Importance of informing patients of other important precautionary information. (See Cautions.)

Overview® (see Users Guide). For additional information on this drug until a more detailed monograph is developed and published, the manufacturer's labeling should be consulted. It is *essential* that the manufacturer's labeling be consulted for more detailed information on usual cautions, precautions, contraindications, potential drug interactions, laboratory test interferences, and acute toxicity. For further information on the handling of antineoplastic agents, see the ASHP Guidelines on Handling Hazardous Drugs at http://www.ahfsdruginformation.com.

Preparations

Excipients in commercially available drug preparations may have clinically important effects in some individuals; consult specific product labeling for details.

Trifluridine and Tipiracil Hydrochloride

Oral

Tablets, film-coated	Trifluridine 15 mg and Tipiracil Hydrochloride 6.14 mg (of tipiracil)	**Lonsurf®**, Taiho Oncology
	Trifluridine 20 mg and Tipiracil Hydrochloride 8.19 mg (of tipiracil)	**Lonsurf®**, Taiho Oncology

Vandetanib

■ Vandetanib, an inhibitor of multiple receptor tyrosine kinases, is an antineoplastic agent.

REMS

FDA approved a REMS for vandetanib to ensure that the benefits outweigh the risks. The REMS may apply to one or more preparations of vandetanib and consists of the following: elements to assure safe use and implementation system. See the FDA REMS page (https://www.accessdata.fda.gov/scripts/cder/rems/index.cfm). Also see Restricted Distribution Program under Dosage and Administration: General.

Uses

■ **Medullary Thyroid Cancer** Vandetanib is used for the treatment of symptomatic or progressive medullary thyroid cancer in patients with unresectable locally advanced or metastatic disease; vandetanib is designated an orphan drug by the US Food and Drug Administration (FDA) for the treatment of this cancer.

The current indication for vandetanib is based principally on the results of a randomized, double-blind, placebo-controlled, phase 3 study in patients with unresectable locally advanced or metastatic medullary thyroid cancer. In this study, 331 patients were randomized in a 2:1 ratio to receive either vandetanib (300 mg) or placebo once daily until disease progression occurred. Upon disease progression, patients were eligible to receive open-label vandetanib; 19 or 58% of patients initially randomized to receive vandetanib or placebo, respectively, opted to receive open-label vandetanib. The median duration of treatment during the randomized phase of the study was 90.1 weeks for vandetanib-treated patients and 39.9 weeks for placebo-treated patients. At the time of the primary analysis, patients receiving vandetanib experienced prolonged median progression-free survival (22.6 versus 16.4 months, although median progression-free survival has not been reached) and a higher overall objective response rate (partial responses) (44 versus 1%) compared with patients receiving placebo. Overall survival was not substantially different between treatment and placebo groups.

Use of vandetanib in patients with indolent, asymptomatic, or slowly progressing disease should be carefully considered because of the treatment-related risks of the drug. (See Cautions.)

Dosage and Administration

■ **General** Because diarrhea occurs frequently in patients receiving vandetanib, routine use of antidiarrheal agents is recommended.

Adverse effects may not resolve quickly because of the long half-life (19 days) of vandetanib. Patients should be monitored appropriately.

Restricted Distribution Program Because of the risk of QT prolongation, torsades de pointes, and sudden death, the US Food and Drug Administration (FDA) required and has approved a Risk Evaluation and Mitigation Strategy (REMS) for vandetanib. (See REMS.)

Under the terms of the REMS program, vandetanib is available only under a restricted distribution program (CAPRELSA® REMS Program). Prescribers and pharmacies must be certified with the CAPRELSA® REMS Program before they can prescribe or dispense vandetanib. To be certified, prescribers must review the educational materials, agree to comply with the REMS requirements, and enroll in the program. Pharmacies that dispense vandetanib must enroll in the program, train their pharmacy staff to verify that each prescription is written by a certified prescriber before dispensing the drug to the patient, and agree to comply with the REMS requirements. Clinicians may contact 800-236-9933 or visit http://www.caprelsarems.com for additional information and to enroll in the program.

■ **Administration** Vandetanib is administered orally without regard to meals. Vandetanib tablets should be swallowed whole and should *not* be crushed.

If vandetanib tablets cannot be swallowed whole, the manufacturer states that the tablet may be dispersed in a glass containing 60 mL (2 ounces) of noncarbonated water; no other liquids should be used. The water should be stirred (without crushing the tablet) for approximately 10 minutes until the tablet is dispersed (the tablet will not completely dissolve). The dispersion should be swallowed immediately; to ensure the full dose is administered, any residues in the glass should be mixed again with an additional 120 mL (4 ounces) of noncarbonated water and swallowed. The dispersion also may be administered through a nasogastric or gastrostomy tube.

Direct contact of crushed tablets with skin or mucous membranes should be avoided. If such contact occurs, the affected area should be washed thoroughly.

Procedures for proper handling and disposal of antineoplastic drugs should be followed when preparing or administering vandetanib.

■ Dosage

Medullary Thyroid Cancer The recommended adult dosage of vandetanib for the treatment of symptomatic or progressive medullary thyroid cancer in patients with unresectable locally advanced or metastatic disease is 300 mg once daily. Therapy should be continued for as long as the patient derives clinical benefit from the drug or until unacceptable toxicity occurs.

Dosage Modification for Toxicity If grade 3 or greater toxicity occurs, vandetanib therapy should be interrupted. When the toxicity resolves or improves to grade 1, vandetanib may be resumed at a reduced dosage. Dosage of vandetanib should be reduced in decrements of 100 mg daily (i.e., from 300 to 200 mg daily, from 200 to 100 mg daily).

Dosage Modification for Cardiovascular Toxicity. Vandetanib should be interrupted if the QT interval (corrected for heart rate using Fridericia's formula [QTcF]) exceeds 500 msec. When QTcF returns to less than 450 msec, vandetanib may be resumed at a reduced dosage.

If hypertension occurs, dosage reduction or temporary interruption of vandetanib therapy may be necessary to control blood pressure. If hypertension cannot be controlled, vandetanib should not be resumed.

Dosage Modification for Dermatologic Toxicity. If grade 3 or greater skin reactions occur, vandetanib therapy should be interrupted. When symptoms improve, consideration should be given to resuming vandetanib at a reduced dosage or permanently discontinuing therapy.

Dosage Modification for Diarrhea. If severe diarrhea occurs, vandetanib therapy should be interrupted. When diarrhea improves, vandetanib may be resumed at a reduced dosage.

■ Special Populations

No dosage adjustment is necessary in geriatric patients older than 65 years of age. The manufacturer makes no specific dosage recommendations in patients older than 75 years of age because data are limited in this population.

Vandetanib should *not* be used in patients with moderate (Child-Pugh class B) or severe (Child-Pugh class C) hepatic impairment because safety and efficacy have not been established in these patients. (See Hepatic Impairment under Warnings/Precautions: Specific Populations, in Cautions.)

The initial dosage of vandetanib αshould be reduced to 200 mg once daily in patients with moderate (creatinine clearance of 30–49 mL/minute) or severe (creatinine clearance less than 30 mL/minute) renal impairment. (See Renal Impairment under Warnings/Precautions: Specific Populations, in Cautions.)

Cautions

■ Contraindications

Congenital long QT syndrome.

■ Warnings/Precautions

Warnings Because of the risk of QT interval prolongation, torsades de pointes, and sudden death, the US Food and Drug Administration (FDA) required and has approved a Risk Evaluation and Mitigation Strategy (REMS) and a restricted distribution program for vandetanib. (See REMS and also see Restricted Distribution Program under Dosage and Administration: General.)

Prolongation of QT Interval and Torsades de Pointes. Vandetanib prolongs the QT interval in a concentration-dependent manner. Torsades de pointes, ventricular tachycardia, and sudden death have been reported in patients receiving vandetanib. In the phase 3 clinical study, patients randomized to receive vandetanib (300 once daily) had a mean increase in the QT interval (corrected for heart rate using Fridericia's formula [QTcF]) of 35 msec (range: 33–36 msec) from baseline; this increase in QTcF remained above 30 msec for the duration of the study (up to 2 years). In addition, an increase in QTcF of more than 60 msec from baseline occurred in 36% of patients receiving vandetanib, and QTcF exceeded 450 msec or 500 msec in 69 or 7% of patients, respectively.

Vandetanib should *not* be initiated in patients with QTcF exceeding 450 msec. The drug should *not* be used in patients who have a history of torsades de pointes, congenital long QT syndrome, bradyarrhythmias, or uncompensated heart failure, or in patients with electrolyte disturbances; hypocalcemia, hypokalemia, and/or hypomagnesemia must be corrected prior to administration of vandetanib. Vandetanib has not been evaluated in patients with ventricular arrhythmias or recent myocardial infarction (MI).

ECG, serum electrolytes (i.e., calcium, magnesium, potassium), and thyrotropin (thyroid-stimulating hormone, TSH) concentrations should be measured at baseline, at 2–4 weeks and 8–12 weeks after initiating vandetanib, and then every 3 months thereafter. Following dosage reduction for QT prolongation or therapy interruption lasting longer than 2 weeks, ECG should be monitored as described above. Serum potassium concentrations should be at least 4 mEq/L (within normal range), and serum magnesium and calcium concentrations should be maintained within normal ranges, to reduce the risk of QT interval prolongation. Concomitant use of vandetanib with drugs known to prolong the QT interval should be *avoided*. (See Drug Interactions: Drugs that Prolong the QT Interval.) If a drug known to prolong the QT interval must be administered, more frequent ECG monitoring is recommended.

Vandetanib therapy should be interrupted if QT_cF exceeds 500 msec. When QT_cF returns to less than 450 msec, vandetanib may be resumed at a reduced dosage. (See Dosage Modification for Toxicity under Dosage and Administration: Dosage.)

Sensitivity Reactions **Photosensitivity Reactions.** Photosensitivity reactions have been reported in 13% of patients receiving vandetanib in the phase 3 clinical study. In patients receiving vandetanib for malignancies other than medullary throid cancer (i.e., non-small cell lung cancer, hepatocellular carcinoma, brain tumor), photosensitivity reactions (including hyperpigmentation and erythematous edematous lesions) occurred within 3 weeks to 2 months after initiating vandetanib. Rashes improved after discontinuance of vandetanib and treatment with topical or systemic corticosteroids and oral antihistamines; however hyperpigmentation remained in all of the reported cases. (See Advice to Patients.)

Other Warnings and Precautions **Dermatologic Effects.** Mild to moderate skin reactions (i.e., rash, acne, dry skin, dermatitis, pruritus, other skin reactions [including palmar-plantar erythrodysesthesia syndrome]) have been reported in patients receiving vandetanib. Severe skin reactions (including Stevens-Johnson syndrome), some resulting in death, also have been reported with the drug. Treatment options for mild to moderate skin reactions included topical and systemic corticosteroids, oral antihistamines, and topical and systemic antibiotics. Treatment options for severe skin reactions included systemic corticosteroids and permanent discontinuance of vandetanib. If grade 3 or greater skin reactions occur, vandetanib therapy should be interrupted. When symptoms improve, consideration should be given to resuming vandetanib at a reduced dosage or permanently discontinuing therapy.

Pulmonary Effects. Interstitial lung disease or pneumonitis, sometimes fatal, has been reported in patients receiving vandetanib. The mechanism of action of this adverse effect is unknown; however, review of available data (including data in patients receiving vandetanib for non-small cell lung cancer†) suggested that Japanese ethnicity, history of smoking, coincidence of interstitial pneumonia, preexisting pulmonary fibrosis, male gender, and previous radiation or chemotherapy may be possible risk factors for developing interstitial lung disease.

Interstitial lung disease should be considered in patients presenting with nonspecific respiratory manifestations (e.g., hypoxia, pleural effusion, cough, dyspnea) and in whom infectious, neoplastic, and other causes have been excluded. If symptoms of interstitial lung disease are moderate, interruption of vandetanib therapy should be considered until symptoms improve; use of corticosteroids and antibiotics may be required. If symptoms of interstitial lung disease are severe, vandetanib should be discontinued, and use of corticosteroids and antibiotics may be required until symptoms resolve. Upon resolution of severe interstitial lung disease, permanent discontinuance of vandetanib should be considered.

Patients who develop radiologic changes suggestive of interstitial lung disease who have few or no symptoms may continue vandetanib therapy with close monitoring at the discretion of the clinician.

Cerebrovascular Events. Ischemic cerebrovascular events, sometimes fatal, have been reported with vandetanib. In the phase 3 clinical study, ischemic cerebrovascular events were observed more frequently with vandetanib compared with placebo (1.3 versus 0%); all ischemic cerebrovascular events reported in this study were grade 3. Vandetanib should be discontinued in patients who experience a severe ischemic cerebrovascular event. The safety of resumption of vandetanib therapy after resolution of an ischemic cerebrovascular event has not been studied.

Hemorrhage. Serious hemorrhagic events, sometimes fatal, have been reported with vandetanib. Vandetanib should *not* be used in patients with a recent history of hemoptysis (2.5 mL of red blood or more). Vandetanib should be discontinued in patients with severe hemorrhage.

Cardiovascular Effects. Heart failure, sometimes fatal, has been reported with vandetanib use. In the phase 3 clinical study, heart failure occurred in 0.9% of patients receiving vandetanib compared with 0% of those receiving placebo. Patients should be monitored for manifestations of heart failure. If heart failure occurs, discontinuance of vandetanib may be necessary; heart failure may not be reversible following discontinuance of vandetanib.

Hypertension and hypertensive crisis have been reported in 33% of patients receiving vandetanib. Blood pressure should be monitored in all patients and controlled as appropriate. Dosage reduction or temporary interruption of vandetanib therapy may be necessary. If hypertension cannot be controlled, vandetanib should *not* be resumed.

Diarrhea. Diarrhea has been reported in patients receiving vandetanib. In the phase 3 clinical study, diarrhea or colitis (all grades) was reported in 57% and grade 3–4 diarrhea or colitis was reported in 11% of patients receiving vandetanib. Routine use of antidiarrheal drugs is recommended during vandetanib therapy. Because diarrhea may cause electrolyte imbalances, and because QT interval prolongation has been reported in patients receiving vandetanib, the manufacturer recommends careful and more frequent monitoring of serum electrolytes and ECG in patients who develop diarrhea. (See Prolongation of QT Interval and Torsades de Pointes under Warnings/Precautions: Warnings, in Cautions.) If severe diarrhea occurs, vandetanib therapy should be interrupted. When symptoms improve, vandetanib should be resumed at a reduced dosage. (See Dosage Modification for Toxicity under Dosage and Administration: Dosage.)

Hypothyroidism. In the phase 3 clinical study in which 90% of enrolled patients had prior thyroidectomy, increases in the dosages of thyroid replacement therapy were required in 49% of patients receiving vandetanib compared with 17% of patients receiving placebo. TSH concentrations should be monitored at baseline, at 2–4 weeks and 8–12 weeks after initiating vandetanib, and then every 3 months thereafter. If manifestations of hypothyroidism occur, thyroid hormone concentrations should be examined, and thyroid replacement therapy should be adjusted accordingly.

Reversible Posterior Leukoencephalopathy Syndrome. Reversible posterior leukoencephalopathy syndrome (RPLS) has been reported in patients receiving vandetanib. RPLS should be considered in any patient presenting with seizures, headache, visual disturbances, confusion, or altered mental function. In clinical studies, 3 of the 4 patients who developed RPLS, including one pediatric patient, also had hypertension. Discontinuance of vandetanib should be considered if RPLS occurs.

Fetal/Neonatal Morbidity and Mortality. Vandetanib may cause fetal harm if administered to pregnant women; the drug has been shown to be embryotoxic, fetotoxic, and teratogenic in animals. Pregnancy should be avoided during therapy. If vandetanib is used during pregnancy or if the patient becomes pregnant while receiving the drug, the patient should be apprised of the potential fetal hazard. (See Advice to Patients.)

Ocular Effects. Blurred vision and corneal opacities (which can lead to halos and decreased visual acuity) have been reported in patients receiving vandetanib. It is not known whether corneal opacities will improve after discontinuance of vandetanib. Ophthalmologic examination, including slit lamp examinations, is recommended in patients who report visual changes. (See Advice to Patients.)

Specific Populations **Pregnancy.** Category D. (See Fetal/Neonatal Morbidity and Mortality under Warnings/Precautions: Other Warnings and Precautions, in Cautions.) (See Users Guide.)

Lactation. Vandetanib is distributed into milk in rats. It is not known whether vandetanib is distributed into human milk. Because of the potential for serious adverse reactions to vandetanib in nursing infants, a decision should be made whether to discontinue nursing or the drug, taking into account the importance of the drug to the woman.

Pediatric Use. Safety and efficacy of vandetanib have not been established in pediatric patients.

Geriatric Use. In the phase 3 clinical study in patients with medullary thyroid cancer, 18% of patients receiving vandetanib were 65 years of age or older while 3% were 75 years of age or older. No overall differences in safety or efficacy were observed between geriatric and younger patients. Data in patients older than 75 years of age are limited. (See Dosage and Administration: Special Populations.)

Hepatic Impairment. In a pharmacokinetic study in which a limited number of individuals received a single 800-mg dose of vandetanib, mean area under the plasma concentration-time curve (AUC) and clearance of the drug were comparable between individuals with mild (Child-Pugh class A), moderate (Child-Pugh class B), or severe (Child-Pugh class C) hepatic impairment and individuals with normal hepatic function. There are limited data in patients with serum bilirubin concentrations exceeding 1.5 times the upper limit of normal (ULN).

Because safety and efficacy of vandetanib have not been established, use of the drug is not recommended in patients with moderate or severe hepatic impairment.

Renal Impairment. In a pharmacokinetic study in which a limited number of individuals received a single 800-mg dose of vandetanib, mean AUC and clearance of the drug were comparable between individuals with mild renal impairment and individuals with normal renal function; however, in individuals with moderate or severe renal impairment, mean AUC of vandetanib was increased by 39 or 41%, respectively, compared with individuals with normal renal function.

Patients with moderate or severe renal impairment should receive a lower initial dosage of vandetanib (see Dosage and Administration: Special Populations); ECG should be monitored closely in these patients.

Vandetanib has not been evaluated systematically in patients with end-stage renal disease requiring dialysis.

■ **Common Adverse Effects** Adverse effects reported in more than 20% of patients receiving vandetanib include diarrhea, rash, acne, nausea, hypertension, headache, fatigue, decreased appetite, and abdominal pain. Other adverse effects reported in 10–15% of patients receiving vandetanib include dry skin, vomiting, asthenia, QT interval prolongation, photosensitivity reaction, insomnia, nasopharyngitis, dyspepsia, hypocalcemia, cough, pruritus, weight loss, proteinuria, and depression. Serious (grade 3 or 4) adverse effects reported in 5% or more of patients receiving vandetanib include diarrhea/colitis, hypertension/hypertensive crisis, QT interval prolongation, and fatigue.

Laboratory abnormalities reported in more than 20% of patients receiving vandetanib include decreased calcium concentrations, increased ALT concentrations, and decreased glucose concentrations.

Drug Interactions

■ **Drugs Affecting Hepatic Microsomal Enzymes** Concomitant use of vandetanib with a potent inhibitor of cytochrome P-450 (CYP) isoenzyme 3A4 (CYP3A4) (i.e., itraconazole) resulted in no clinically important interaction.

Inducers of CYP3A4 can alter plasma vandetanib concentrations. Concomitant use of vandetanib with potent CYP3A4 inducers (e.g., carbamazepine, dexamethasone, phenobarbital, phenytoin, rifabutin, rifampin, rifapentine) should be *avoided*. St. John's wort (*Hypericum perforatum*) may unpredictably decrease vandetanib exposure, and concomitant use of vandetanib with this agent also should be avoided.

■ **Drugs that Prolong the QT Interval** Concomitant use of vandetanib with drugs known to prolong the QT interval, including class Ia (e.g., disopyramide, procainamide, quinidine) and class III (e.g., amiodarone, sotalol, dofetilide) antiarrhythmic agents, some anti-infectives (e.g., clarithromycin, gatifloxacin, moxifloxacin), some antipsychotic agents (e.g., chlorpromazine, thioridazine, haloperidol, asenapine, olanzapine, paliperidone, pimozide, quetiapine, ziprasidone), some type 3 serotonin (5-HT_3) receptor antagonists used as antiemetic agents (e.g., dolasetron, granisetron, ondansetron), chloroquine, methadone, and tetrabenazine should be *avoided*. If a drug known to prolong the QT interval must be administered, more frequent ECG monitoring is recommended. (See Prolongation of QT Interval and Torsades de Pointes under Warnings/Precautions: Warnings, in Cautions.) If a 5-HT_3 receptor antagonist is clinically necessary, some clinicians prefer granisetron because its effects on ECG intervals are less pronounced than those observed with dolasetron or ondansetron.

Description

Vandetanib, an inhibitor of multiple receptor tyrosine kinases, is an antineoplastic agent. Receptor tyrosine kinases (RTKs) are involved in the initiation of various cascades of intracellular signaling events that lead to cell proliferation and/or influence processes critical to cell survival and tumor progression (e.g., angiogenesis, metastasis, inhibition of apoptosis), based on the respective kinase. Various tyrosine kinases and pathways are abnormally activated in medullary thyroid carcinoma cells (e.g., rearranged during transfection [RET] proto-oncogene signaling is associated with development of hereditary medullary thyroid cancer). *In vitro*studies have shown that vandetanib inhibits the activity of multiple receptor tyrosine kinases, including vascular endothelial growth factor receptors (i.e., VEGFR-1, VEGFR-2, VEGFR-3), members of the epidermal growth factor receptor (EGFR) family, RET, protein tyrosine kinase 6 (BRK), TIE2, members of the EPH receptor kinase family, and members of the Src family of tyrosine kinases. *In vivo*, vandetanib has been shown to reduce tumor cell-induced angiogenesis and tumor vessel permeability; the drug also has been shown to inhibit tumor growth and metastasis in mouse models of cancer. There is no evidence of a relationship between RET mutations and efficacy of vandetanib.

Vandetanib is partially metabolized by cytochrome P-450 (CYP) isoenzyme 3A4. Approximately 44 or 25% of an oral dose of the drug is excreted in feces or urine, respectively, as unchanged drug or metabolites. The terminal half-life of vandetanib is 19 days. Limited data indicate that systemic exposure to vandetanib is higher in Japanese and Chinese patients than in Caucasian patients receiving the same dose.

Advice to Patients

A copy of the manufacturer's patient information (medication guide) for vandetanib must be provided to all patients with each prescription of the drug. (See REMS and also see Restricted Distribution Program under Dosage and Administration: General.) Importance of patients reading the medication guide prior to initiation of therapy and each time the prescription is refilled.

Importance of not crushing vandetanib tablets. Importance of avoiding direct contact of crushed tablets with the skin or mucous membranes.

If a dose is missed, importance of not taking the missed dose if it is less than 12 hours before the next dose.

Risk of QT interval prolongation, torsades de pointes, ventricular tachycardia, and sudden death. Importance of regular monitoring of ECG and serum electrolytes. Importance of contacting clinician promptly if feelings of lightheadedness or faintness or an irregular heartbeat occurs.

Risk of photosensitivity/phototoxicity reactions. Importance of using sunscreen and protective clothing and limiting sun exposure during therapy and for at least 4 months after discontinuance of the drug.

Risk of severe adverse dermatologic effects. Importance of contacting clinician promptly if dermatologic manifestations (e.g., rash; acne; dry skin; itching; blisters on skin or in mouth; peeling; fever; muscle or joint aches; redness or swelling of face, hands, or soles of feet) occur.

Risk of interstitial lung disease. Importance of promptly reporting new or worsening respiratory manifestations (e.g., shortness of breath, persistent cough, fever).

Risk of diarrhea. Importance of using antidiarrheal drugs to manage symptoms; importance of contacting clinician if diarrhea becomes persistent or severe. Importance of contacting clinician for regular monitoring of serum electrolytes.

Risk of reversible posterior leukoencephalopathy syndrome (RPLS). Importance of contacting clinician promptly if seizures, headache, visual disturbances, confusion, or difficult thinking occurs.

Importance of women using an effective method of contraception while receiving vandetanib and for at least 4 months after discontinuance of therapy. Importance of discontinuing nursing while receiving vandetanib therapy.

Risk of blurred vision. Importance of avoiding driving a vehicle or operating machinery if blurred vision occurs.

Importance of informing clinician of existing or contemplated concomitant therapy, including prescription and OTC drugs and herbal supplements, as well as any concomitant illnesses (e.g., hepatic or renal impairment, cardiovascular disease).

Importance of informing patients of other important precautionary information. (See Cautions.)

Overview® (see Users Guide). For additional information on this drug until a more detailed monograph is developed and published, the manufacturer's labeling should be consulted. It is *essential* that the manufacturer's labeling be consulted for more detailed information on usual cautions, precautions, contraindications, potential drug interactions, laboratory test interferences, and acute toxicity. For further information on the handling of antineoplastics agents, see the ASHP Guidelines on Handling Hazardous Drugs at http://www.ahfsdruginformation.com.

Preparations

Distribution of vandetanib is restricted. (See REMS and also see Restricted Distribution Program under Dosage and Administration: General.)

Excipients in commercially available drug preparations may have clinically important effects in some individuals; consult specific product labeling for details.

Vandetanib

Oral		
Tablets, film-coated	100 mg	**Caprelsa**®, AstraZeneca
	300 mg	**Caprelsa**®, AstraZeneca

†Use is not currently included in the labeling approved by the US Food and Drug Administration

Selected Revisions September 2017, © Copyright, November 2011, American Society of Health-System Pharmacists, Inc.

Vemurafenib

PLX4032, RG7204, RO5185426

■ Vemurafenib, an inhibitor of b-Raf serine-threonine kinase with V600E mutation (BRAF V600E), is an antineoplastic agent.

Uses

■ **Melanoma** Vemurafenib is used for the treatment of unresectable or metastatic melanoma with BRAF V600E mutation. Vemurafenib is designated an orphan drug by the US Food and Drug Administration (FDA) for the treatment of this cancer. An FDA-approved diagnostic test (e.g., cobas® 4800 BRAF V600 Mutation Test) is required to confirm the presence of the BRAF V600E mutation prior to initiation of therapy.

The current indication for vemurafenib is based principally on the results of a randomized, open-label phase 3 study (BRIM-3) in patients with previously untreated, unresectable or metastatic melanoma. All patients in this study tested positive for the BRAF V600E mutation detected by the cobas® 4800 BRAF V600 Mutation Test. In this study, 675 patients were randomized in a 1:1 ratio to receive either vemurafenib (960 mg orally twice daily) or dacarbazine (1 g/m² IV every 3 weeks). Treatment was continued until disease progression or unacceptable toxicity occurred, or the patient withdrew from the study. The primary endpoints of this study were overall survival and progression-free survival. The median age of patients enrolled in the study was 54 years. Most of the patients had metastatic disease (95%).

A planned interim analysis for overall survival indicated a reduction in the risk of death by 63% and a higher rate of overall survival at 6 months of therapy in patients receiving vemurafenib than in those receiving dacarbazine (84 versus 64%). The median follow-up period at the time of the interim analysis was 3.8 months for those receiving vemurafenib and 2.3 months for those receiving dacarbazine. Because of the survival benefit observed at the interim analysis, study investigators permitted patients previously randomized to receive dacarbazine to cross over to open-label vemurafenib therapy. A final analysis for progression-free survival estimated a prolonged median progression-free survival (5.3 versus 1.6 months) and reduction in risk of either death or disease progression (74%) in patients receiving vemurafenib compared with those receiving dacarbazine. An updated overall survival analysis with a median follow-up of 13.4 months confirmed prolonged median overall survival (13.6 versus 10.3 months; hazard ratio for death: 0.47) in patients receiving vemurafenib compared with those receiving dacarbazine. Patients receiving vemurafenib also had a higher objective response rate (48.4 versus 5.5%) compared with those receiving dacarbazine; complete response was achieved in 0.9% of patients treated with vemurafenib compared with none treated with dacarbazine. A shorter median time to response (1.45 versus 2.7 months) also was observed in patients receiving vemurafenib compared with those receiving dacarbazine.

In a single-arm, multicenter, multinational phase 2 study, treatment with vemurafenib (960 mg orally twice daily) in patients with BRAF V600E mutation-positive, metastatic melanoma previously treated with systemic therapy (including interleukin-2 or standard chemotherapy) produced an overall response rate of 53% with a complete response reported in 6% and a partial response reported in 47% of these patients. At the time of the analysis, the median duration of response was 6.7 months and median overall survival was 15.9 months.

In a post-hoc analysis of the BRIM-3 study, median overall and progression-free survival were significantly longer in vemurafenib-treated patients compared with dacarbazine-treated patients in those whose melanoma harbored either the BRAF V600E or the less common BRAF V600K mutation. Vemurafenib currently is not indicated for the treatment of metastatic melanoma with BRAF V600K mutation.

Use of vemurafenib also was investigated in a single-arm, multicenter, open-label phase 2 study in patients with BRAF V600E mutation-positive melanoma with symptomatic or asymptomatic brain metastases. Patients in this study were enrolled in 2 cohorts: those with previously untreated brain metastases and those with previously treated brain metastases (i.e., resection, whole brain radiation therapy, stereotactic radiation therapy) and measurable disease progression. Patients enrolled in this study must have had at least one brain lesion 0.5 cm or greater in size, were receiving a stable or decreasing corticosteroid dosage, and had no history of BRAF or mitogen-activated extracellular signal-regulated kinase (MEK) inhibitor therapy. In this study, 146 patients received vemurafenib 960 mg orally twice daily until disease progression or unacceptable toxicity occurred. The primary measure of efficacy was overall intracranial response rate in the cohort of patients with previously untreated brain metastases (as evaluated by an independent review committee according to Response Evaluation Criteria in Solid Tumors [RECIST]). The median duration of follow-up was 9.6 months. In the cohort of patients with previously untreated brain metastases, the intracranial overall response rate was 18%; complete responses were achieved in 2% of patients. In the cohort of patients with previously treated brain metastases, the overall intracranial response rate was 18%; however, none of the patients in this cohort achieved a complete response. At the time of analysis, the median duration of response was 4.6 or 6.6 months in those with previously untreated or previously treated brain metastases, respectively.

The safety and efficacy of vemurafenib in patients with wild-type BRAF melanoma have not been established; use of vemurafenib is *not* indicated for use in these patients. (See Tumor Promotion in BRAF Wild-Type Melanoma under Warnings/Precautions: Other Warnings and Precautions, in Cautions.)

■ **Erdheim-Chester Disease** Vemurafenib is used for the treatment of Erdheim-Chester disease with BRAF V600 mutation. Vemurafenib is designated an orphan drug by the FDA for the treatment of this condition.

The current indication for vemurafenib in the treatment of Erdheim-Chester disease is based principally on the results of a single-arm, multicenter, open-label phase 2 study in a cohort of 22 patients with BRAF V600 mutation-positive Erdheim-Chester disease. In this study, patients received vemurafenib 960 mg orally twice daily. The primary measure of efficacy was overall response rate (as evaluated by the investigator according to RECIST). The median age of patients enrolled in the cohort of patients with Erdheim-Chester disease was 59 years; 55% were male and 68.2% had previously received systemic therapy.

The overall response rate for patients in the Erdheim-Chester disease cohort of this study was 54.5% with a median time to response of 11 months; complete response was achieved in one patient. The median duration of follow-up for the Erdheim-Chester disease cohort was 26.6 months. At the time of analysis, median duration of response had not been reached. At a median follow-up of 28.8 months, median progression-free survival and overall survival had not been reached. The rates of 2-year progression-free survival and overall survival were 83 and 95%, respectively.

Dosage and Administration

■ **General** Presence of the BRAF V600E mutation must be confirmed prior to initiation of therapy. (See Uses: Melanoma and also see Tumor Promotion in BRAF Wild-Type Melanoma under Warnings/Precautions: Other Warnings and Precautions, in Cautions.)

Restricted Distribution Program Vemurafenib can be obtained only through a restricted distribution program called Zelboraf Access Solutions®. Only designated pharmacies from a specialty pharmacy network will be authorized to dispense the drug. Specific information is available at https://www.genentech-access.com/hcp/brands/zelboraf.html.

■ **Administration** Vemurafenib is administered orally twice daily without regard to meals. Vemurafenib tablets should *not* be crushed or chewed.

If a dose of vemurafenib is missed, the dose may be taken up to 4 hours prior to the next dose to maintain the twice-daily dosing regimen. However, 2 doses should not be taken at the same time.

If vomiting occurs following administration of vemurafenib, a replacement dose should *not* be administered, and the next dose should be taken at the regularly scheduled time.

■ **Dosage** ***Melanoma*** The recommended adult dosage of vemurafenib for the treatment of unresectable or metastatic melanoma with BRAF V600E mutation is 960 mg twice daily. Therapy should be continued until disease progression or unacceptable toxicity occurs.

Erdheim-Chester Disease The recommended adult dosage of vemurafenib for the treatment of Erdheim-Chester disease with BRAF V600 mutation is 960 mg twice daily. Therapy should be continued until disease progression or unacceptable toxicity occurs.

In the principal efficacy study, the initial dosage of vemurafenib was 960 mg twice daily; however, 64 or 36% of patients required dosage reductions to 480 or 720 mg twice daily, respectively. The manufacturer states that efficacy of vemurafenib was maintained in patients requiring dosage reduction. The median duration of exposure to vemurafenib following dosage reduction to 480 or 720 mg twice daily was 236 or 77 days, respectively.

Dosage Modification **General Toxicity.** If intolerable grade 2 or any grade 3 toxicity occurs, vemurafenib therapy should be temporarily interrupted. When the toxicity resolves to grade 0 or 1, vemurafenib may be resumed at a reduced dosage of 720 mg twice daily. If the toxicity recurs at a dosage of 720 mg twice daily, therapy should be withheld again until the toxicity resolves to grade 0 or 1; therapy may then be resumed at a reduced dosage of 480 mg twice daily. If toxicity recurs at a dosage of 480 mg twice daily, treatment with vemurafenib should be permanently discontinued.

If grade 4 toxicity occurs, vemurafenib therapy should be permanently discontinued or interrupted until the toxicity resolves to grade 0 or 1; if clinically appropriate, therapy may then be resumed at a reduced dosage of 480 mg twice daily. If toxicity recurs at a dosage of 480 mg twice daily, treatment with vemurafenib should be permanently discontinued.

Dosages less than 480 mg twice daily are not recommended.

Prolongation of QT Interval. Vemurafenib therapy should be temporarily interrupted if the corrected QT interval (QT_c) exceeds 500 msec. When the QT_c interval decreases to 500 msec or less, the drug may be resumed at a reduced dosage. Vemurafenib should be permanently discontinued if the QT_c interval exceeds 500 msec and increases more than 60 msec from baseline despite correction of electrolyte abnormalities and other risk factors for QT prolongation (e.g., congestive heart failure, bradyarrhythmias).

ECGs and serum electrolyte concentrations (including concentrations of potassium, magnesium, and calcium) should be obtained prior to initiation or following dosage modification of vemurafenib or as clinically indicated. (See Prolongation of QT Interval under Warnings/Precautions: Other Warnings and Precautions, in Cautions.)

Development of New Primary Cutaneous Malignancies. No dosage adjustment is necessary in patients who develop new primary cutaneous malignancies.

Concomitant Use with Drugs and Foods Affecting Hepatic Microsomal Enzymes. Concomitant use of vemurafenib with drugs that are potent inducers of cytochrome P-450 (CYP) isoenzyme 3A4 should be avoided. If concomitant therapy with a potent CYP3A4 inducer cannot be avoided, the manufacturer recommends increasing the dosage of vemurafenib by 240 mg twice daily (e.g., from 960 mg twice daily to 1.2 g twice daily). When concomitant use of the potent CYP3A4 inducer is discontinued, the vemurafenib dosage should be returned (2 weeks after discontinuance of the CYP3A4 inducer) to the dosage used prior to initiation of the potent CYP3A4 inducer. (See Drug Interactions: Drugs and Foods Affecting Hepatic Microsomal Enzymes.)

■ **Special Populations** No initial dosage adjustment is necessary in patients with mild or moderate hepatic impairment. The manufacturer makes no specific dosage recommendations in patients with severe hepatic impairment because data are limited in this population. (See Hepatic Impairment under Warnings/Precautions: Specific Populations, in Cautions.)

No initial dosage adjustment is necessary in patients with mild or moderate renal impairment. The manufacturer makes no specific dosage recommendations in patients with severe renal impairment because data are limited in this population. (See Renal Impairment under Warnings/Precautions: Specific Populations, in Cautions.)

The manufacturer makes no specific dosage recommendations for geriatric patients. (See Geriatric Use under Warnings/Precautions: Specific Populations, in Cautions.)

Cautions

■ **Contraindications** The manufacturer states there are no known contraindications to the use of vemurafenib.

■ **Warnings/Precautions** ***Sensitivity Reactions*** **Hypersensitivity Reactions.** Serious hypersensitivity reactions (e.g., anaphylaxis, generalized rash and erythema, hypotension, drug reaction with eosinophilia and systemic symptoms [DRESS syndrome]) may occur during and upon reinitiation of vemurafenib therapy. Vemurafenib should be permanently discontinued in patients who experience a severe hypersensitivity reaction.

Photosensitivity Reactions. Photosensitivity reactions (mild to severe) have been reported in 33–49% of patients receiving vemurafenib in clinical trials. If intolerable grade 2 or greater reaction occurs, the dosage of vemurafenib should be reduced. (See Dosage Modification under Dosage and Administration: Dosage.)

Other Warnings and Precautions **Development of New Primary Malignancies.** In the phase 3 clinical trial evaluating vemurafenib in patients with unresectable or metastatic melanoma, cutaneous squamous cell carcinoma, keratoacanthoma, and melanoma were reported more frequently in patients receiving vemurafenib compared with those receiving dacarbazine. In this study, cutaneous squamous cell carcinoma and keratoacanthoma occurred in 24% of patients receiving vemurafenib compared with less than 1% of those receiving dacarbazine. In a phase 2 clinical trial in patients receiving the drug for metastatic melanoma, cutaneous squamous cell carcinoma and keratoacanthoma occurred in 24% of patients. In clinical trials, the median time to first appearance of cutaneous squamous cell carcinoma was 7–8 weeks. Approximately 33% of patients in a phase 3 clinical trial who had previously experienced cutaneous squamous cell carcinoma during vemurafenib treatment had more than one subsequent occurrence with median time between occurrences of 6 weeks. In clinical trials, skin lesions were excised and vemurafenib therapy was continued without dosage adjustment. In the phase 3 clinical trial, development of new primary malignant melanoma was reported in 2.1% of patients receiving vemurafenib compared with none of those receiving dacarbazine. In a clinical trial evaluating vemurafenib in patients with Erdheim-Chester disease, cutaneous squamous cell carcinoma and/or keratoacanthoma occurred in 40.9% of patients. In this trial, the median time to first appearance of cutaneous squamous cell carcinoma was 12.1 weeks.

In clinical trials, non-cutaneous squamous cell carcinoma of the head and neck (e.g., oropharyngeal squamous cell carcinoma) has been reported in less than 10% of patients receiving vemurafenib therapy. Progression of a preexisting chronic myelomonocytic leukemia with NRAS mutation also has been reported during postmarketing experience with the drug.

Although the mechanism for development of cutaneous squamous cell carcinoma has not been fully determined, it has been suggested that paradoxical activation of mitogen-activated protein kinase (MAPK) signaling may lead to accelerated growth of such skin lesions as well as development of other primary malignancies. MAPK-mediated events in wild-type BRAF cells have been observed in a study evaluating the pathology and immunohistochemistry of normal and proliferating skin lesions in patients receiving the weak b-Raf kinase inhibitor sorafenib. Another study performed a molecular analysis of DNA extracted from tumor specimens of patients receiving vemurafenib; results indicated that these patients have a secondary mutation (in addition to the BRAF V600E mutation) that appears to be activated by vemurafenib treatment. Some clinicians suggest that advanced age (i.e., 65 years of age or older), history of skin cancer, and chronic sun exposure may be risk factors for developing cutaneous squamous cell carcinoma. Some data suggest that mitogen-activated extracellular signal-regulated kinase (MEK) inhibitors (i.e., binimetinib, cobimetinib, trametinib) block the paradoxical activation of the MAPK pathway induced by BRAF inhibitors (i.e., vemurafenib, dabrafenib, encorafenib); therefore, combination therapy with a BRAF inhibitor and an MEK inhibitor may reduce the risk of developing cutaneous squamous cell carcinoma. Findings from a meta-analysis of randomized controlled studies that assessed the relative risk of development of cutaneous squamous cell carcinoma in cancer patients receiving a BRAF inhibitor indicate that the risk of cutaneous squamous cell carcinoma is higher in patients receiving a BRAF inhibitor than in patients receiving combination therapy with a BRAF inhibitor and an MEK inhibitor.

A dermatologic evaluation should be performed at baseline and every 2 months during therapy. Continued monitoring for 6 months following discontinuance of vemurafenib may be considered. Suspicious cutaneous lesions should be treated as appropriate and excised for pathologic evaluation. Close monitoring for signs and symptoms of development of new non-cutaneous squamous cell carcinoma or of other primary malignancies should be performed.

In clinical trials, myeloid neoplasms have been reported in patients with Erdheim-Chester disease receiving vemurafenib therapy. The manufacturer recommends monitoring complete blood cell (CBC) counts in patients with Erdheim-Chester disease and coexisting myeloid malignancies.

Tumor Promotion in BRAF Wild-Type Melanoma. In vitro, paradoxical activation of MAPK signaling and increased cell proliferation have been observed in wild-type BRAF cells exposed to BRAF inhibitors. Presence of the BRAF V600E mutation must be confirmed prior to initiation of therapy. (See Uses: Melanoma.)

Dermatologic Effects. Severe skin reactions (e.g., Stevens-Johnson syndrome, toxic epidermal necrolysis) have been reported with vemurafenib. If severe skin reactions occur, vemurafenib therapy should be permanently discontinued.

Prolongation of QT Interval. Vemurafenib prolongs the QT interval in a concentration-dependent manner. In a multicenter, open-label, phase 2 study, QT interval prolongation was evaluated in patients with BRAF V600E mutation-positive, metastatic melanoma who were receiving vemurafenib (960 mg twice daily). A maximum mean corrected QT (QT_c) interval change from baseline of 12.8 msec during the first month of treatment and 15.1 msec during the first 6 months of treatment was observed in these patients.

Vemurafenib should not be initiated in patients with electrolyte abnormalities unresponsive to corrective measures, QT_c intervals exceeding 500 msec, or congenital long QT syndrome. In addition, concomitant use of vemurafenib with drugs known to prolong the QT interval (e.g., class Ia and III antiarrhythmic agents) should be avoided. (See Drug Interactions: Drugs that Prolong the QT Interval.)

ECGs and serum electrolyte concentrations, including concentrations of potassium, magnesium, and calcium, should be obtained prior to initiation of therapy or following dosage modification for QT interval prolongation, and monitored 15 days following initiation of therapy, then monthly for the first 3 months of treatment, and then every 3 months thereafter or more often as clinically indicated.

Interruption or discontinuance of vemurafenib may be necessary if increases in the QT_c interval occur during therapy with the drug. (See Prolongation of QT Interval under Dosage: Dosage Modification, in Dosage and Administration.)

Hepatic Effects. Hepatic injury may occur during therapy with vemurafenib resulting in functional hepatic impairment, including coagulopathy or other organ dysfunction. In clinical trials, grade 3 and 4 elevations in aminotransferase (ALT or AST), bilirubin, and alkaline phosphatase concentrations have been reported in 0.9–2.9% of patients receiving vemurafenib. Serum aminotransferase, bilirubin, and alkaline phosphatase concentrations should be evaluated prior to initiation of therapy and monitored monthly during treatment or as clinically indicated. Laboratory abnormalities should be managed with dosage reduction, treatment interruption, or discontinuance. (See Dosage Modification under Dosage and Administration: Dosage.)

The safety and efficacy of vemurafenib used concomitantly with ipilimumab have not been established; however, grade 3 elevations in aminotransferase and bilirubin concentrations have occurred in the majority of patients receiving vemurafenib (720 or 960 mg twice daily) and ipilimumab (3 mg/kg) concurrently. (See Drug Interactions: Ipilimumab.)

Ocular Effects. Uveitis, blurry vision, and photophobia have been reported in patients receiving vemurafenib. In the phase 3 clinical trial evaluating vemurafenib in patients with previously untreated metastatic melanoma, uveitis, including iritis, occurred in 2.1% of patients receiving vemurafenib compared with none of those receiving dacarbazine. Monitoring for signs and symptoms of uveitis should be performed. In patients experiencing uveitis, therapy with ophthalmic corticosteroid and mydriatic preparations may be required. Retinal vein occlusion also has been reported in patients receiving the drug.

Fetal/Neonatal Morbidity and Mortality. There are no adequate and well-controlled studies of vemurafenib in pregnant women; however, based on its mechanism of action, vemurafenib may cause fetal harm. No evidence of developmental toxicity was observed in pregnant animals receiving vemurafenib at exposure levels equivalent to approximately 0.6–1.3 times the area under the concentration-time curve [AUC] at the recommended human dosage; however, these exposure levels to vemurafenib were not sufficient to fully evaluate its potential toxicity in pregnant women. In animals, fetal plasma concentrations of vemurafenib were 3–5% of maternal plasma concentrations, indicating that vemurafenib has the potential to cross the placenta.

Pregnancy should be avoided during vemurafenib therapy. Women of childbearing potential should be advised to use effective contraception during therapy and for 2 weeks after the last dose. If used during pregnancy or if the patient becomes pregnant while receiving the drug, the patient should be apprised of the potential fetal hazard.

Radiation Sensitization and Recall. Radiation sensitization and recall, sometimes severe or fatal, involving cutaneous and visceral organs have been reported during postmarketing experience in patients receiving vemurafenib prior to, during, or subsequent to radiation therapy. Fatal cases have been reported in patients with radiation sensitization or recall involving visceral organs. Patients receiving vemurafenib concomitantly or sequentially with radiation therapy should be closely monitored for signs and symptoms of radiation sensitization or recall.

Renal Effects. Renal failure, including acute interstitial nephritis and acute tubular necrosis, has been reported in patients receiving vemurafenib.

In the phase 3 clinical trial evaluating vemurafenib in patients with previously untreated metastatic melanoma, grade 1–2 elevations of serum creatinine (exceeding the upper limit of normal [ULN], but no more than 3 times the ULN) occurred in 26% of patients receiving vemurafenib compared with 5% of those receiving dacarbazine; grade 3–4 elevations of serum creatinine (exceeding 3 times the ULN) occurred in 1.2 or 1.1% of patients receiving vemurafenib or dacarbazine, respectively.

In a clinical trial evaluating vemurafenib in patients with Erdheim-Chester disease, grade 1–2 or 3 elevations of serum creatinine occurred in 86 or 9.1% of patients, respectively.

Serum creatinine concentrations should be evaluated at baseline and periodically during therapy.

Dupuytren Contracture and Plantar Fascial Fibromatosis. Dupuytren contracture and plantar fascial fibromatosis have been reported during postmarketing experience in patients receiving vemurafenib. The majority of cases have been mild to moderate in severity, but severe, disabling cases of Dupuytren contracture also have been reported.

Specific Populations **Pregnancy.** Vemurafenib may cause fetal harm if administered to pregnant women based on its mechanism of action. (See Fetal/Neonatal Morbidity and Mortality under Warnings/Precautions: Other Warnings and Precautions, in Cautions.)

Lactation. It is not known whether vemurafenib is distributed into milk in humans. Because of the potential for serious adverse reactions to vemurafenib in breast-fed infants, women should be advised not to breast-feed while receiving the drug and for 2 weeks after the last dose. The effects of the drug on breast-fed infants or on the production of milk are unknown.

Pediatric Use. Safety and efficacy of vemurafenib in pediatric patients have not been established.

Based on limited data in pediatric patients (range: 15–17 years of age) with unresectable or metastatic melanoma with BRAF V600 mutation, steady-state exposure of vemurafenib in pediatric patients was similar to that observed in adults. The maximum tolerated dosage of the drug has not been established in pediatric patients; however, no new adverse effects were observed in pediatric patients receiving vemurafenib dosages up to 960 mg twice daily.

Geriatric Use. Clinical studies of vemurafenib did not include sufficient numbers of patients 65 years of age or older to determine whether geriatric patients respond differently than younger adults. (See Dosage and Administration: Special Populations.)

Hepatic Impairment. In a population pharmacokinetic analysis, the clearance of vemurafenib was not affected in patients with mild or moderate hepatic impairment. Pharmacokinetic data in patients with severe hepatic impairment are limited; therefore, the drug should be used with caution in these patients. (See Dosage and Administration: Special Populations.)

Renal Impairment. In a population pharmacokinetic analysis, the clearance of vemurafenib was not affected in patients with mild or moderate renal impairment. Pharmacokinetic data in patients with severe renal impairment are limited; therefore, the drug should be used with caution in these patients. (See Dosage and Administration: Special Populations.)

■ **Common Adverse Effects** Adverse effects reported in 10% or more of patients receiving vemurafenib for the treatment of unresectable or metastatic melanoma include arthralgia, rash, alopecia, fatigue, photosensitivity reaction, nausea, pruritus, cutaneous squamous cell carcinoma, and skin papilloma.

Adverse effects reported in 20% or more of patients receiving vemurafenib for the treatment of Erdheim-Chester disease include arthralgia, maculopapular rash, alopecia, fatigue, QT interval prolongation, skin papilloma, diarrhea, hyperkeratosis, dry skin, palmar-plantar erythrodysesthesia syndrome, photosensitivity reaction, seborrheic keratosis, cough, cutaneous squamous cell carcinoma, hypertension, pruritus, peripheral sensory neuropathy, actinic keratosis, keratosis pilaris, nausea, melanocytic nevus, sunburn, papular rash, and vomiting.

Drug Interactions

In vivo studies indicate that vemurafenib is a moderate inhibitor of cytochrome P-450 (CYP) isoenzyme 1A2 and a weak inhibitor of CYP isoenzyme 2D6. In vitro studies suggest that vemurafenib is an inhibitor of CYP isoenzymes 1A2, 2A6, 2B6, 2C8, 2C9, 2C19, 2D6, and 3A4/5. Vemurafenib is an inhibitor and a substrate of CYP isoenzyme 3A4. In vitro studies indicate that vemurafenib is a substrate and an inhibitor of P-glycoprotein (P-gp) and breast cancer resistance protein (BCRP). Effects of potent CYP3A4 inhibitors or inducers on vemurafenib concentrations have not been evaluated in vivo.

■ **Drugs and Foods Affecting Hepatic Microsomal Enzymes** Concomitant use of vemurafenib with potent inhibitors of CYP3A4 may result in increased plasma concentrations of vemurafenib and an increased incidence of adverse effects. Concomitant use with potent CYP3A4 inhibitors (e.g., clarithromycin, indinavir, itraconazole, ketoconazole, nelfinavir, ritonavir, saquinavir, voriconazole) should be avoided, and selection of an alternative drug with no or minimal CYP3A4 inhibition potential is recommended.

Concomitant use of vemurafenib with potent inducers of CYP3A4 may result in decreased plasma concentrations of vemurafenib and reduced vemurafenib efficacy. When the potent CYP3A inducer rifampin (600 mg daily) was administered concomitantly with vemurafenib (single 960-mg dose), systemic exposure to vemurafenib was decreased by 40% and peak plasma concentrations were unchanged. Concomitant use with potent CYP3A4 inducers (e.g., carbamazepine, phenytoin, rifampin) should be avoided, and selection of an alternative drug with no or minimal CYP3A4 induction potential is recommended. If concomitant therapy with a potent CYP3A4 inducer cannot be avoided, the manufacturer recommends increasing the dosage of vemurafenib by 240 mg twice daily (e.g., from 960 mg twice daily to 1.2 g twice daily). When concomitant use of the potent CYP3A4 inducer is discontinued, the vemurafenib dosage should be returned (2 weeks after discontinuance of the CYP3A4 inducer) to the dosage used prior to initiation of the potent CYP3A4 inducer.

■ **Drugs Metabolized by Hepatic Microsomal Enzymes** Concomitant use of vemurafenib with CYP1A2 substrates may result in increased plasma concentrations of the CYP1A2 substrate and possible toxicity. When the CYP1A2 substrate caffeine was administered concomitantly with vemurafenib, the systemic exposure to caffeine increased by 2.6-fold. When the sensitive CYP1A2 substrate tizanidine (single 2-mg dose) was administered concomitantly with vemurafenib (960 mg twice daily), systemic exposure and peak plasma concentrations of tizanidine increased by 4.7- and 2.2-fold, respectively. Concomitant use of vemurafenib with CYP1A2 substrates that have a narrow therapeutic index should be avoided. If concomitant use cannot be avoided, dosage reduction of the CYP1A2 substrate should be considered, and patients should be closely monitored for adverse effects.

When the CYP2D6 substrate dextromethorphan was administered concomitantly with vemurafenib, the systemic exposure of dextromethorphan increased by 47%.

When the CYP3A4 substrate midazolam was administered concomitantly with vemurafenib, the systemic exposure of midazolam decreased by 39%.

When the CYP2C9 substrate warfarin was administered concomitantly with vemurafenib, the systemic exposure of *S*-warfarin increased by 18%.

When the CYP2C19 substrate omeprazole was administered concomitantly with vemurafenib, the systemic exposure of omeprazole was unchanged.

■ **Drugs Affected by Efflux Transport Systems** Concomitant use of vemurafenib with P-gp substrates may result in increased plasma concentrations of the P-gp substrate. When the sensitive P-gp substrate digoxin (single 0.25-mg dose) was administered concomitantly with vemurafenib (960 mg twice daily), systemic exposure and peak plasma concentrations of digoxin increased by 1.8- and 1.5-fold, respectively. Concomitant use of vemurafenib with P-gp substrates that have a narrow therapeutic index should be avoided. If concomitant use cannot be avoided, dosage reduction of the P-gp substrate should be considered.

■ **Drugs that Prolong the QT Interval** Concomitant use of vemurafenib with drugs known to prolong the QT interval, including class Ia (e.g., quinidine, procainamide) and class III (e.g., amiodarone, sotalol) antiarrhythmic agents, some antipsychotic agents (e.g., asenapine, chlorpromazine, haloperidol, olanzapine, paliperidone, pimozide, quetiapine, thioridazine, ziprasidone), some anti-infectives (e.g., gatifloxacin, moxifloxacin), and tetrabenazine, should be avoided. (See Prolongation of QT Interval under Warnings/Precautions: Other Warnings and Precautions, in Cautions.)

■ **Ipilimumab** Concomitant use of vemurafenib with ipilimumab resulted in increased aminotransferase and bilirubin concentrations in a majority of patients. (See Hepatic Effects under Warnings/Precautions: Other Warnings and Precautions, in Cautions.)

Description

Vemurafenib, a potent inhibitor of b-Raf serine-threonine kinase with V600E mutation (BRAF V600E), is an antineoplastic agent. Approximately 40–60% of cutaneous melanomas carry a BRAF mutation. The most common BRAF mutation is the substitution of glutamic acid for valine at codon 600 in exon 15 (BRAF V600E); a less frequently occurring BRAF mutation is the substitution of lysine for valine at codon 600 in exon 15 (BRAF V600K). The mutation of BRAF V600E activates the mitogen-activated protein kinase (MAPK) and extracellular-signal regulated kinase (ERK) signal transduction pathway, which enhances cell proliferation and tumor progression (e.g., metastasis). In vitro studies indicate that vemurafenib also inhibits other kinases such as c-Raf, a-Raf, wild-type b-Raf, SRMS, ACK1, MAP4K5, and FGR at similar concentrations at which inhibition of BRAF V600E occurs.

Clinical resistance to monotherapy with a BRAF inhibitor, generally occurring 6–7 months following initiation of therapy, has been attributed to several possible resistance mechanisms mostly relying on reactivation of the MAPK/ERK pathway. Complete inhibition of the MAPK/ERK pathway resulting in durable responses may be achieved with the use of combination therapy with a BRAF inhibitor (i.e., dabrafenib, encorafenib, vemurafenib) and an MEK inhibitor (i.e., binimetinib, cobimetinib, trametinib).

The bioavailability of vemurafenib is unknown. Following administration of vemurafenib within the dosage range of 240–960 mg, the drug exhibits linear pharmacokinetics and achieves steady-state concentrations within approximately 15–22 days. The median terminal half-life of vemurafenib in patients with unresectable melanoma is 57 hours. Following oral administration of a radiolabeled dose of vemurafenib, about 94% of the dose is recovered in feces and 1% is recovered in urine.

Systemic exposure to vemurafenib is increased when the drug is administered with a high-fat meal. Administration of a single dose of vemurafenib with a high-fat meal resulted in increases in systemic exposure or peak plasma concentrations of approximately fivefold or 2.5-fold, respectively. (See Dosage and Administration: Administration.)

Advice to Patients

Importance of advising patient to read the manufacturer's medication guide before beginning treatment and each time the prescription is refilled.

Patients should be instructed to take a missed dose as soon as it is remembered, but only if it can be taken at least 4 hours before the next scheduled dose.

If vomiting occurs following administration of vemurafenib, the next dose should be taken at the regularly scheduled time. A replacement dose should *not* be administered.

Necessity of advising women of childbearing potential to use effective contraception during therapy and for 2 weeks after the last dose. Importance of women informing clinicians immediately if they are or plan to become pregnant. Apprise patient of potential fetal hazard if used during pregnancy.

Importance of advising women to avoid breast-feeding while receiving vemurafenib and for 2 weeks after the last dose.

Importance of confirming that patients have melanomas testing positive for the BRAF V600E mutation using cobas® 4800 BRAF V600 Mutation Test or other FDA-approved diagnostic test prior to initiation of therapy with vemurafenib.

Risk of new primary cutaneous malignancies. Importance of contacting a clinician promptly if dermatologic changes (e.g., new wart, skin sore or reddish bump that bleeds or does not heal, or mole that changes in size or color) occur.

Risk of mild to severe photosensitivity reactions. Importance of using sunscreen and lip balm (minimum SPF of 30), wearing protective clothing, and avoiding sun exposure during therapy.

Risk of severe adverse dermatologic effects. Importance of contacting a clinician promptly if a skin rash occurs with symptoms such as blisters appearing on the skin or in the mouth; peeling of the skin; redness or swelling of the face, hands, or soles of the feet; or fever.

Risk of QT-interval prolongation, which may result in ventricular arrhythmias. Importance of informing clinicians immediately if an abnormal heartbeat or feelings of dizziness or faintness occur.

Risk of new primary malignant melanoma. Importance of contacting a clinician promptly if skin changes occur.

Risk of anaphylaxis or other serious hypersensitivity reactions during or upon reinitiation of vemurafenib therapy. Importance of advising patients to promptly notify their clinician if signs or symptoms of an allergic reaction occur during therapy, including rash, angioedema, difficulty breathing, tachycardia, throat tightness, or hoarseness.

Risk of hepatic injury resulting in functional hepatic impairment. Importance of advising patients to schedule periodic laboratory monitoring for hepatotoxicity and to report clinically relevant symptoms to their clinician.

Risk of adverse ocular effects. Importance of monitoring and contacting clinician promptly if ocular pain, swelling, redness, or blurred vision occurs.

Risk of radiation sensitization and recall in patients receiving vemurafenib prior to, during, or subsequent to radiation therapy. Importance of informing clinician of previous or planned radiation therapy.

Risk of renal failure. Importance of monitoring serum creatinine concentrations prior to and periodically during therapy.

Risk of Dupuytren contracture or plantar fascial fibromatosis. Importance of informing clinician if unusual thickening of palms or soles or inward tightening of the fingers occurs.

Importance of informing clinicians of existing or contemplated concomitant therapy, including prescription and OTC drugs and herbal supplements, as well as any concomitant illnesses (e.g., hepatic, renal, or cardiovascular disease, electrolyte abnormalities) or planned surgical, dental, or other medical procedures.

Importance of informing patients of other important precautionary information.

Overview® (see Users Guide). For additional information on this drug until a more detailed monograph is developed and published, the manufacturer's labeling should be consulted. It is *essential* that the manufacturer's labeling be consulted for more detailed information on usual cautions, precautions, contraindications, potential drug interactions, laboratory test interferences, and acute toxicity. For further information on the handling of antineoplastic agents, see the ASHP Guidelines on Handling Hazardous Drugs at http://www.ahfsdruginformation.com.

Preparations

Distribution of vemurafenib is restricted. (See Restricted Distribution Program under Dosage and Administration: General.)

Excipients in commercially available drug preparations may have clinically important effects in some individuals; consult specific product labeling for details.

Vemurafenib

Oral

Tablets, film-coated	240 mg	**Zelboraf®**, Genentech

Venetoclax

■ Venetoclax, a selective inhibitor of B-cell lymphoma 2 (BCL-2), is an antineoplastic agent.

Uses

■ **Chronic Lymphocytic Leukemia** Venetoclax is used for the treatment of chronic lymphocytic leukemia (CLL) with 17p deletion in patients who have received at least one prior therapy. The presence of the 17p deletion chromosomal abnormality should be confirmed by an FDA-approved diagnostic test prior to initiation of therapy. The accelerated approval of venetoclax for this indication is based on overall response rate. Continued approval may be contingent on verification and description of clinical benefit of venetoclax in confirmatory studies. Venetoclax has been designated an orphan drug by FDA for the treatment of CLL.

The current indication for venetoclax is based principally on the results of an open-label, noncomparative, phase 2 study in 106 adults with relapsed or refractory 17p deletion CLL (confirmed by the Vysis® fluorescent in situ hybridization [FISH] kit). Patients in this study had received a median of 2.5 prior therapies for their disease and had a median time since diagnosis of 79.4 months. The median age of patients was 67 years; 97% were Caucasian, 92% had a baseline ECOG performance status of 0 or 1, 50% had an absolute lymphocyte count of 25,000/mm^3 or greater, and 53% had one or more lymph nodes measuring 5 cm or greater. Venetoclax was administered at a dosage of 400 mg orally once daily (after an initial 5-week dose-escalation period) until disease progression or unacceptable toxicity occurred. Because of an increased risk of tumor lysis syndrome identified in an earlier study of venetoclax, the study protocol included a risk-based management plan for monitoring and prophylaxis of this condition. The primary end point of this study was overall response rate as assessed by an independent review committee using the 2008 updated International Workshop Criteria for CLL (IWCLL) National Cancer Institute-sponsored Working Group Guidelines. The overall response rate was 85%; complete remission or complete remission with incomplete bone marrow recovery was achieved in 8% of the patients. Among patients who achieved complete remission, 3 of 8 of these patients were minimal residual disease negative (defined as the presence of less than 0.01% CLL cells) in peripheral blood and bone marrow. At the time of analysis, the median duration of response had not been reached in this study; however, the median time to first response was 0.8 months.

Venetoclax also is being investigated in an ongoing open-label phase 2 study in patients with CLL whose disease has progressed following therapy with a B-cell antigen receptor (BCR) inhibitor, including ibrutinib and idelalisib.

Dosage and Administration

■ **General** Confirmation of the presence of the 17p deletion abnormality by an FDA-approved diagnostic test (e.g., Vysis® fluorescent in situ hybridization [FISH] kit) is necessary prior to initiating therapy with venetoclax. Because 17p deletion can be acquired, patients without this chromosomal abnormality at diagnosis should be retested at the time of relapse.

Prior to initiating venetoclax therapy, patients should be assessed for their risk of tumor lysis syndrome and given appropriate prophylaxis (e.g., adequate hydration and an antihyperuricemic agent) according to tumor burden at baseline. The manufacturer recommends the following guidelines for prophylaxis and monitoring of tumor lysis syndrome based on clinical trial data (see Table 1); patient comorbidities and other risk factors also should be considered when determining an appropriate prophylactic regimen. (See Tumor Lysis Syndrome under Cautions: Warnings/Precautions.) In patients with a high tumor burden at baseline, the first 20- and 50-mg dose of venetoclax should be administered in the hospital; subsequent doses may be given in the outpatient setting. Venetoclax dosage modifications may be necessary if laboratory evidence or clinical manifestations of tumor lysis syndrome occur during therapy. (See Dosage Modification for Tumor Lysis Syndrome under Dosage: Dosage Modification for Toxicity, in Dosage and Administration.)

Table 1. Recommended Prophylaxis and Monitoring for Tumor Lysis Syndrome

Tumor Burden	Prophylaxis	Monitoring
Low tumor burden: All lymph nodes with diameter of less than 5 cm *and* absolute lymphocyte count of less than 25,000/mm³	Oral hydration (1.5–2 L)[a,b] and allopurinol[c]	Assess blood chemistries (i.e., potassium, phosphorus, calcium, uric acid, creatinine) prior to, at 6–8 and 24 hours following the first 20- and 50-mg dose of venetoclax, and prior to each subsequent escalating dose (100, 200, and 400 mg)
Medium tumor burden: Any lymph node diameter of 5 cm to less than 10 cm or absolute lymphocyte count of 25,000/mm³ or greater	Oral hydration (1.5–2 L)[a,b] and allopurinol[c] Consider additional IV hydration	Assess blood chemistries (i.e., potassium, phosphorus, calcium, uric acid, creatinine) prior to, at 6–8 and 24 hours following the first 20- and 50-mg dose of venetoclax, and prior to each subsequent escalating dose (100, 200, and 400 mg) In patients with creatinine clearance less than 80 mL/minute prior to the first 20- and 50-mg dose, consider hospitalization for drug administration and more intensive hydration and monitoring (see the following recommendations for monitoring in the hospital)
High tumor burden: Any lymph node diameter of 10 cm or greater *or* any lymph node diameter of 5 cm or greater *and* absolute lymphocyte count of 25,000/mm³ or greater	Oral (1.5–2 L)[a,b] and IV (150–200 mL/hour as tolerated) hydration and allopurinol[c] Consider rasburicase if baseline uric acid concentrations are elevated	Hospitalize patient for the first 20- and 50-mg dose of venetoclax; assess blood chemistries (i.e., potassium, phosphorus, calcium, uric acid, creatinine) prior to and at 4, 8, 12, and 24 hours following each dose Administer subsequent escalating doses (100, 200, and 400 mg) in the outpatient setting; assess blood chemistries prior to and at 6–8 and 24 hours following each dose

[a] Administer IV hydration if oral hydration is not tolerated

[b] Begin oral hydration 2 days prior to initiating venetoclax, on the day of the first dose, and every time the dose is increased

[c] Initiate therapy with antihyperuricemic agent (e.g., allopurinol) 2–3 days prior to initiating venetoclax

■ **Administration** Venetoclax is administered orally once daily with a meal and a full glass of water at approximately the same time each day. (See Description.) Venetoclax tablets should be swallowed intact and should *not* be chewed, crushed, or broken.

■ **Dosage** ***Chronic Lymphocytic Leukemia*** For the treatment of chronic lymphocytic leukemia (CLL) with 17p deletion in patients who have received at least one prior therapy, the recommended adult dosage of venetoclax is 400 mg once daily; to minimize the risk of tumor lysis syndrome, venetoclax therapy should be initiated at a low dosage and increased gradually over 5 weeks to the recommended dosage according to the following schedule: 20 mg daily in the first week, 50 mg daily in the second week, 100 mg daily in the third week, 200 mg daily in the fourth week, and 400 mg daily thereafter.

Therapy should be continued until disease progression or unacceptable toxicity occurs.

Dosage Modification for Toxicity If adverse reactions occur during venetoclax therapy, temporary interruption of therapy, dosage reduction, and/or discontinuance of the drug may be necessary. If a dosage modification is needed, the manufacturer recommends that the current dose of venetoclax be reduced by one dose level (i.e., 400 mg to 300 mg; 300 mg to 200 mg; 200 mg to 100 mg; 100 mg to 50 mg; 50 mg to 20 mg; 20 mg to 10 mg); however, larger dose reductions may be required at the discretion of the clinician. If a dose reduction occurs during the initial dose-titration period, the reduced dose should be continued for 1 week before escalating back to the previous dose. If a dose reduction to less than 100 mg for more than 2 weeks is necessary, discontinuance of therapy should be considered.

If interruption of therapy is necessary for more than 1 week during the initial dose-titration period or for more than 2 weeks while receiving venetoclax 400 mg once daily, patients should be reassessed for their risk of tumor lysis syndrome to determine if a reduced dosage is necessary when resuming therapy.

Dosage Modification for Tumor Lysis Syndrome. If abnormalities in blood chemistry or symptoms consistent with tumor lysis syndrome occur, the next dose of venetoclax should be withheld. If resolution occurs within 24–48 hours of the last dose, therapy may be resumed at the same dosage; however, if laboratory abnormalities require more than 48 hours to resolve or if clinical tumor lysis syndrome (clinical sequelae may include acute renal failure, cardiac arrhythmias, sudden death, and/or seizures) occurs, venetoclax therapy should be resumed at a reduced dosage when resolution occurs. (See Tumor Lysis Syndrome under Cautions: Warnings/Precautions.)

Dosage Modification for Hematologic Toxicity. For the first occurrence of grade 3 or 4 neutropenia associated with fever or infection, or grade 4 hematologic toxicity (except for lymphopenia), venetoclax therapy should be interrupted and granulocyte colony-stimulating factor (G-CSF) considered if clinically indicated; when the toxicity resolves (i.e., improves to grade 1 or returns to baseline levels), therapy may be resumed at the same dosage. (See Neutropenia under Cautions: Warnings/Precautions.)

For subsequent occurrences of grade 3 or 4 neutropenia associated with fever or infection, or grade 4 hematologic toxicity (except for lymphopenia), venetoclax therapy should be interrupted and G-CSF administered if clinically indicated; when the toxicity resolves, therapy may be resumed at a reduced dosage.

Dosage Modification for Nonhematologic Toxicity. For the first occurrence of grade 3 or 4 nonhematologic toxicity, venetoclax therapy should be interrupted; when the toxicity resolves (i.e., improves to grade 1 or returns to baseline levels), therapy may be resumed at the same dosage.

For subsequent occurrences of grade 3 or 4 nonhematologic toxicity, venetoclax therapy should be interrupted; when the toxicity resolves, therapy may be resumed at a reduced dosage.

Dosage Modification for Concomitant Therapy If venetoclax is used concomitantly with a potent cytochrome P-450 (CYP) 3A inhibitor in patients who have completed the initial dose titration and are receiving a steady daily dose of venetoclax, dosage of venetoclax should be reduced by at least 75%. When the potent CYP3A inhibitor is discontinued, the dosage of venetoclax that was used prior to initiating the potent CYP3A inhibitor should be resumed after 2–3 days.

If venetoclax is used concomitantly with a moderate inhibitor of CYP3A or inhibitor of P-glycoprotein (P-gp), dosage of venetoclax should be reduced by at least 50%. When the moderate CYP3A inhibitor or P-gp inhibitor is discontinued, the dosage of venetoclax that was used prior to initiating the moderate CYP3A inhibitor or P-gp inhibitor should be resumed after 2–3 days. (See Drug Interactions.)

■ **Special Populations** No dosage adjustment is necessary in patients with mild (total bilirubin concentration not exceeding the upper limit of normal [ULN] with AST concentration exceeding the ULN *or* total bilirubin concentration exceeding the ULN, but no more than 1.5 times the ULN) or moderate (total bilirubin concentration exceeding 1.5 times the ULN, but no more than 3 times the ULN) hepatic impairment; however, patients with moderate hepatic impairment should be monitored for signs of toxicity during the initial 5-week titration period since increased venetoclax-related toxicity has been observed in these patients. Venetoclax has not been studied in patients with severe (total bilirubin concentration exceeding 3 times the ULN) hepatic impairment. (See Hepatic Impairment under Warnings/Precautions: Specific Populations, in Cautions.)

No dosage adjustment is necessary in patients with mild or moderate renal impairment (creatinine clearance of 30 mL/minute or greater). Venetoclax has not been studied in patients with severe renal impairment or in those requiring dialysis. (See Renal Impairment under Warnings/Precautions: Specific Populations, in Cautions.)

The manufacturer makes no specific dosage recommendations for geriatric patients. (See Geriatric Use under Warnings/Precautions: Specific Populations, in Cautions.)

Cautions

■ **Contraindications** Concomitant use of venetoclax and potent cytochrome P-450 (CYP) 3A inhibitors at initiation of therapy and during the initial dose-escalation period is contraindicated.

■ **Warnings/Precautions** ***Tumor Lysis Syndrome*** Tumor lysis syndrome, sometimes fatal or resulting in acute renal failure requiring dialysis, has been reported in patients with chronic lymphocytic leukemia (CLL) receiving venetoclax. The risk of tumor lysis syndrome generally is greatest when the drug is first administered and during the dose-escalation period; laboratory abnormalities consistent with tumor lysis syndrome that require prompt medical treatment may occur as early as 6–8 hours following the initial dose of venetoclax and after each dose increase. In the initial dose-finding studies of venetoclax, tumor lysis syndrome was reported in 12% of patients, including 2 deaths and 3 cases of acute renal failure. After adjusting the dosing regimen (to a longer dose-escalation period and reduced initial doses) and providing more intensive prophylactic and monitoring measures, the incidence was reduced to about 6% and was limited to laboratory evidence of tumor lysis syndrome only without any clinical sequelae. All patients experiencing tumor lysis syndrome had a lymph node diameter of 5 cm or greater or an absolute lymphocyte count of 25,000/mm^3 or greater.

Patients should be assessed for their risk of developing tumor lysis syndrome and receive appropriate interventions (e.g., prophylactic antihyperuricemic therapy, adequate hydration, monitoring) prior to and during venetoclax therapy. The risk is increased in patients with a high tumor burden. Renal impairment (creatinine clearance less than 80 mL/minute) or concomitant use of certain drugs (e.g., inhibitors of CYP3A or P-glycoprotein [P-gp]) may further increase this risk. (See Drug Interactions.) Tumor burden assessments, including radiographic evaluation (e.g., CT scan), and blood chemistries (i.e., potassium, phosphorus, calcium, uric acid, creatinine) should be performed and any abnormalities corrected prior to initiating venetoclax therapy and during the dose-escalation period. (See Dosage and Administration: General.) As the overall risk increases, more intensive measures (i.e., IV hydration, more frequent monitoring, hospitalization) should be employed.

If tumor lysis syndrome occurs, venetoclax therapy should be temporarily interrupted until resolution. Dosage reduction may be necessary when therapy is resumed. (See Dosage Modification for Tumor Lysis Syndrome under Dosage: Dosage Modification for Toxicity, in Dosage and Administration.)

Neutropenia Grade 3 or 4 neutropenia occurs commonly in patients receiving venetoclax. In clinical studies evaluating venetoclax in patients with previously treated CLL, grade 3 or 4 neutropenia occurred in 41% of patients receiving the drug.

Complete blood cell (CBC) counts should be monitored periodically during venetoclax therapy. In patients who develop hematologic toxicity, temporary interruption of therapy or dosage reduction may be required. (See Dosage Modification for Hematologic Toxicity under Dosage: Dosage Modification for Toxicity, in Dosage and Administration.) Use of hematopoietic growth factors (e.g., granulocyte colony-stimulating factor [G-CSF]) and/or anti-infective therapy should be considered.

Immunization Safety and efficacy of immunization with live, attenuated vaccines during or following venetoclax therapy have not been established. Immune response to vaccines may be reduced. The manufacturer recommends that live, attenuated vaccines be avoided prior to, during, and following venetoclax therapy until B-cell counts have recovered.

Fetal/Neonatal Morbidity and Mortality Based on its mechanism of action and animal findings, venetoclax may cause fetal harm. Embryofetal toxicity (i.e., postimplantation loss, decreased fetal weight) was observed in animals at venetoclax exposure levels equivalent to the human exposure at recommended dosages; no evidence of teratogenicity was observed.

Pregnancy should be avoided during venetoclax therapy. Women of childbearing potential should undergo pregnancy testing prior to initiating venetoclax therapy and use an effective method of contraception while receiving the drug and for at least 30 days after discontinuance of therapy. If venetoclax is used during pregnancy or if the patient becomes pregnant while receiving the drug, the patient should be apprised of the potential fetal hazard.

Impairment of Fertility Results of animal studies suggest that venetoclax may impair male fertility. In a fertility and early embryonic development study, degeneration of reproductive tissues (germ cell loss) was observed in male animals receiving venetoclax at exposure levels 0.5 times the human exposure at the recommended dosage. (See Advice to Patients.)

Treatment-related Mortality Increased mortality has been reported in clinical trials in patients with multiple myeloma receiving venetoclax in combination with bortezomib and dexamethasone; venetoclax is *not* currently FDA-labeled for use in patients with multiple myeloma. In a randomized, controlled phase 3 trial (BELLINI) that enrolled 291 patients with multiple myeloma, interim analyses indicated that the risk of death was increased by 103% in patients receiving venetoclax in combination with bortezomib and dexamethasone compared with those receiving bortezomib and dexamethasone. Because of these findings, the BELLINI trial was terminated at FDA's request. However, patients experiencing benefit from the drug may continue therapy with venetoclax in combination with bortezomib and dexamethasone, but only after the risks associated with use of the drug combination have been discussed completely with the patient and a new written informed consent has been obtained.

Specific Populations **Pregnancy.** There are no adequate and well-controlled studies of venetoclax in pregnant women; however, animal studies suggest that venetoclax may cause fetal harm. (See Fetal/Neonatal Morbidity and Mortality under Cautions: Warnings/Precautions.)

Lactation. It is not known whether venetoclax is distributed into milk. Because of the potential for serious adverse reactions to venetoclax in nursing infants, women should be advised to discontinue nursing during venetoclax therapy. The effects of the drug on nursing infants or milk production are unknown.

Pediatric Use. Safety and efficacy of venetoclax have not been established in pediatric patients.

Geriatric Use. In the principal clinical study evaluating efficacy of venetoclax in patients with previously treated 17p deletion CLL, 57% of patients were 65 years of age or older, and 17% were 75 years of age or older. In open-label studies evaluating safety of venetoclax in patients with previously treated CLL, 58% of patients were 65 years of age or older, and 17% were 75 years of age or older. No overall differences in efficacy or safety were observed between geriatric and younger patients.

Hepatic Impairment. Clinical studies have not been specifically conducted with venetoclax in patients with hepatic impairment; however, the drug is principally eliminated by the liver. In a population pharmacokinetic analysis, systemic exposure to venetoclax was similar in patients with mild (normal total bilirubin concentration with AST concentration exceeding the upper limit of normal [ULN] *or* total bilirubin concentration exceeding the ULN, but no more than 1.5 times the ULN) or moderate (total bilirubin concentration exceeding 1.5 times the ULN, but no more than 3 times the ULN) hepatic impairment and those with normal hepatic function. The pharmacokinetics of venetoclax have not been evaluated in patients with severe hepatic impairment (total bilirubin concentration exceeding 3 times the ULN).

Renal Impairment. Clinical studies have not been specifically conducted in patients with renal impairment. In a population pharmacokinetic analysis, systemic exposure to venetoclax was similar in patients with mild (creatinine clearance of 60–89 mL/minute) or moderate (creatinine clearance of 30–59 mL/minute) renal impairment compared with patients with normal renal function. The pharmacokinetics of venetoclax have not been evaluated in patients with severe renal impairment (creatinine clearance less than 30 mL/minute) or those requiring dialysis; however, substantial removal of the drug by dialysis is unlikely because of the drug's large volume of distribution and extensive protein binding.

Patients with reduced renal function (creatinine clearance less than 80 mL/minute) have an increased risk of tumor lysis syndrome; therefore, more intensive prophylaxis and monitoring may be necessary during initiation of venetoclax therapy. (See Dosage and Administration: General and also see Tumor Lysis Syndrome under Cautions: Warnings/Precautions.)

■ **Common Adverse Effects** Adverse effects reported in 10% or more of patients receiving venetoclax for the treatment of previously treated CLL include neutropenia, diarrhea, nausea, anemia, upper respiratory tract infection, thrombocytopenia, fatigue, pyrexia, headache, vomiting, constipation, nasopharyngitis, cough, peripheral edema, and back pain.

Laboratory abnormalities reported in more than 5% of patients receiving venetoclax include hyperkalemia, hyperphosphatemia, hypokalemia, hypocalcemia, hyperuricemia, and laboratory tumor lysis syndrome.

Drug Interactions

Venetoclax is metabolized principally by cytochrome P-450 (CYP) isoenzyme 3A4/5. In vitro studies indicate that venetoclax is a weak inhibitor of CYP isoenzymes 2C8 and 2C9 and uridine diphosphate-glucuronosyltransferase (UGT) 1A1; however, inhibition is not predicted to be clinically relevant because of high plasma protein binding. In vitro, venetoclax does not inhibit or induce CYP isoenzymes 1A2, 2B6, 2C19, 2D6, or 3A4 at clinically relevant concentrations. Venetoclax also does not inhibit UGT1A4, 1A6, 1A9, or 2B7 in vitro at clinically relevant concentrations.

In vitro, venetoclax is a substrate and inhibitor of P-glycoprotein (P-gp) and breast cancer resistance protein (BCRP) and a weak inhibitor of organic anion transport protein (OATP) 1B1. Venetoclax is not expected to inhibit OATP1B3, organic cation transporter (OCT) 1, OCT2, renal organic anion transporter (OAT) 1, OAT3, multidrug and toxic compound extrusion (MATE) 1, or MATE2K at clinically relevant concentrations.

■ **Drugs Affecting Hepatic Microsomal Enzymes** ***Inhibitors of CYP3A*** Concomitant use of venetoclax with potent or moderate inhibitors of CYP3A may result in increased peak plasma concentrations and systemic exposure (area under the concentration-time curve [AUC]) of venetoclax. Concomitant administration of the potent CYP3A, P-gp, and BCRP inhibitor ketoconazole (400 mg daily for 7 days) with venetoclax in patients with previously treated non-Hodgkin's lymphoma increased the peak plasma concentration and AUC of venetoclax by 2.3- and 6.4-fold, respectively.

Concomitant use of venetoclax with potent inhibitors of CYP3A (e.g., clarithromycin, conivaptan, indinavir, itraconazole, ketoconazole, lopinavir, posaconazole, ritonavir, voriconazole) during the initial dose-escalation period of venetoclax is contraindicated; however, the drugs may be used concomitantly, if necessary, once the dose titration has been completed and the patient is receiving a steady daily dose of venetoclax. Dosage of venetoclax should be reduced by at least 75% during concomitant therapy. If concomitant use of the potent CYP3A inhibitor is discontinued, the venetoclax dosage should be returned to the dosage used prior to initiation of the potent CYP3A inhibitor in 2–3 days.

Concomitant use of venetoclax with moderate inhibitors of CYP3A (e.g., ciprofloxacin, diltiazem, dronedarone, erythromycin, fluconazole, verapamil) should be avoided; selection of an alternative drug with no or minimal CYP3A inhibition potential should be considered. If concomitant use of a moderate CYP3A inhibitor cannot be avoided, the manufacturer recommends reducing the dosage of venetoclax by at least 50%; patients should be monitored closely for signs of venetoclax toxicity. If concomitant use of the moderate CYP3A inhibitor is discontinued, the venetoclax dosage should be returned to the dosage used prior to initiation of the moderate CYP3A inhibitor in 2–3 days.

The manufacturer states that grapefruit products, Seville oranges, and starfruit are known to inhibit CYP3A and should be avoided during venetoclax therapy.

Inducers of CYP3A Concomitant use of venetoclax with potent or moderate inducers of CYP3A may result in decreased peak plasma concentrations and AUC of venetoclax. Concomitant administration of the potent CYP3A inducer rifampin (600 mg daily for 13 days) with venetoclax (single 200-mg dose) in healthy individuals decreased the peak plasma concentration and AUC of venetoclax by 42 and 71%, respectively.

Concomitant use of venetoclax with potent (e.g., carbamazepine, phenytoin, rifampin, St. John's wort [*Hypericum perforatum*]) or moderate (e.g., bosentan, efavirenz, etravirine, modafinil, nafcillin) inducers of CYP3A should be avoided; selection of an alternative drug with no or minimal CYP3A induction potential should be considered.

■ **Drugs Affecting Efflux Transport Systems** Concomitant use of venetoclax with inhibitors of P-gp may result in increased peak plasma concentrations and AUC of venetoclax. Concomitant administration of the OATP1B1/1B3 and P-gp inhibitor rifampin (single 600-mg dose) with venetoclax (single 200-mg dose) in healthy individuals increased the peak plasma concentration and AUC of venetoclax by 106 and 78%, respectively.

Concomitant use of venetoclax with inhibitors of P-gp (e.g., amiodarone, azithromycin, captopril, carvedilol, cyclosporine, felodipine, quercetin, quinidine, ranolazine, ticagrelor) should be avoided; selection of an alternative drug with no or minimal P-gp inhibition potential should be considered. If concomitant use with a P-gp inhibitor cannot be avoided, the manufacturer recommends reducing the dosage of venetoclax by at least 50%; patients should be monitored closely for signs of venetoclax toxicity. If concomitant use of the P-gp inhibitor is discontinued, the venetoclax dosage should be returned to the dosage used prior to initiation of the P-gp inhibitor in 2–3 days.

■ **Substrates of Efflux Transport Systems** In vitro studies suggest that venetoclax may inhibit P-gp in the gut at clinically relevant concentrations; therefore, concomitant use of venetoclax with P-gp substrates with a narrow therapeutic index (e.g., digoxin, everolimus, sirolimus) should be avoided. If such concomitant therapy is necessary, the manufacturer recommends administering the substrate drug at least 6 hours prior to venetoclax.

■ **Drugs Affecting Gastric Acidity** In a population pharmacokinetic analysis, concomitant administration of gastric acid-reducing agents (e.g., antacids, histamine H_2-receptor antagonists, proton-pump inhibitors) with venetoclax did not result in clinically important changes in the bioavailability of venetoclax.

■ **Warfarin** Concomitant administration of venetoclax (single 400-mg dose) with warfarin sodium (5 mg) in 3 healthy individuals increased peak plasma concentrations and systemic exposure of warfarin by 18–28%. Because venetoclax was not dosed to steady state in this study, the manufacturer recommends close monitoring of the international normalized ratio (INR) in patients receiving warfarin.

■ **Vaccines** Live, attenuated vaccines should not be administered prior to, during, and following venetoclax therapy until B-cell recovery occurs. (See Immunization under Cautions: Warnings/Precautions.)

Description

Venetoclax is a potent and selective inhibitor of B-cell chronic lymphoma 2 (BCL-2); the drug is an antineoplastic agent. BCL-2, an anti-apoptotic protein, is overexpressed in CLL and mediates tumor cell survival and has been associated with resistance to chemotherapy. Following binding of venetoclax to BCL-2, displacement of pro-apoptotic proteins (e.g., BIM), mitochondrial outer membrane permeabilization, and caspase activation occur; these actions result in restoration of the intrinsic apoptotic pathway. In nonclinical studies, venetoclax demonstrated cytotoxic activity in tumor cells overexpressing BCL-2.

Venetoclax exhibits linear pharmacokinetics over a dose range of 150–800 mg. Peak plasma concentrations of the drug are achieved about 5–8 hours following oral administration under fed conditions. Administration of venetoclax with a low-fat or high-fat meal increased systemic exposure by approximately 3.4- or 5.2-fold, respectively, compared with the fasting state. Venetoclax is highly bound (over 99%) to plasma proteins. The mean terminal half-life of venetoclax is approximately 26 hours. Venetoclax is metabolized to its major metabolite (M27) mainly by cytochrome P-450 (CYP) isoenzyme 3A4/5. The major metabolite has demonstrated inhibitory activity against BCL-2 that is at least 58-fold lower than that of the parent drug. Following oral administration of a single radiolabeled dose of venetoclax, more than 99.9% of the radioactivity was recovered in feces (20.8% as unchanged drug) and less than 0.1% was recovered in urine within 9 days.

Population pharmacokinetic analyses indicate that age (25–88 years), gender, race, and body weight do not have clinically important effects on the clearance of venetoclax.

Advice to Patients

Importance of taking venetoclax exactly as prescribed with food and water. Avoid grapefruit products, Seville oranges, and starfruit while taking the drug.

Importance of storing venetoclax tablets in the original package during the initial 4 weeks of therapy.

Importance of advising patients to swallow venetoclax tablets whole and to not chew, crush, or break the tablets.

If a dose is missed, importance of advising patients to take it as soon as they remember and resume the next dose at the regularly scheduled time unless the dose was missed by more than 8 hours, in which case they should not take the missed dose. If a dose is vomited, importance of administering the next dose at the regularly scheduled time; an additional dose should not be administered to make up for a missed dose.

Risk of tumor lysis syndrome. Importance of maintaining scheduled appointments for blood work and other laboratory tests. Importance of immediately reporting any signs or symptoms of tumor lysis syndrome (e.g., fever, chills, nausea, vomiting, confusion, shortness of breath, seizure, arrhythmia, dark or cloudy urine, fatigue, muscle pain, joint discomfort). Importance of advising patients to maintain adequate hydration during venetoclax therapy. The recommended volume is 6–8 glasses (approximately 56 ounces) a day. Patients should start drinking water 2 days before initiating venetoclax, on the day of the first dose, and each time the dose is increased. (See Dosage and Administration: General.)

Risk of neutropenia. Importance of monitoring complete blood cell (CBC) counts periodically during venetoclax therapy. Importance of immediately reporting any signs or symptoms of infection (e.g., fever).

Importance of avoiding use of live vaccines prior to, during, and following venetoclax therapy until B-cell count recovery.

Risk of fetal harm. Necessity of advising women of childbearing potential that they should use an effective method of contraception while receiving the drug and for at least 30 days after discontinuance of therapy. Importance of women informing clinicians if they are or plan to become pregnant. If pregnancy occurs, advise pregnant women of potential risk to the fetus.

Risk of male infertility. Importance of advising men of reproductive potential to consider sperm banking.

Importance of advising women to avoid breast-feeding while receiving venetoclax.

Importance of informing clinicians of existing or contemplated concomitant therapy, including prescription and OTC drugs and dietary or herbal supplements (e.g., St. John's wort), as well as any concomitant illnesses.

Importance of informing patients of other important precautionary information. (See Cautions.)

Overview® (see Users Guide). For additional information on this drug until a more detailed monograph is developed and published, the manufacturer's labeling should be consulted. It is *essential* that the manufacturer's labeling be consulted for more detailed information on usual cautions, precautions, contraindications, potential drug interactions, laboratory test interferences, and acute toxicity. For further information on the handling of antineoplastic agents, see the ASHP Guidelines on Handling Hazardous Drugs at http://www.ahfsdruginformation.com.

Preparations

Excipients in commercially available drug preparations may have clinically important effects in some individuals; consult specific product labeling for details.

Venetoclax

Oral		
Tablets, film-coated	10 mg	**Venclexta®**, Genentech
	50 mg	**Venclexta®**, Genentech
	100 mg	**Venclexta®**, Genentech
Titration Pack	14 Tablets, Venetoclax 10 mg (Venclexta®)	**Venclexta® Starting Pack,** Genentech
	7 Tablets, Venetoclax 50 mg (Venclexta®)	
	7 Tablets, Venetoclax 100 mg (Venclexta®)	
	14 Tablets, Venetoclax 100 mg (Venclexta®)	

vinBLAStine Sulfate

Vincaleukoblastine Sulfate, VLB

■ Vinblastine sulfate, a naturally occurring vinca alkaloid, is an antineoplastic agent.

Uses

■ **Hodgkin's Disease** Vinblastine is used in combination chemotherapy for the treatment of Hodgkin's disease. Various regimens have been used in combination therapy and comparative efficacy is continually being evaluated. Vinblastine often is used with doxorubicin, bleomycin, and dacarbazine (known as the ABVD regimen) for the treatment of patients with Hodgkin's disease. The use of vinblastine in other combination regimens (e.g., Stanford V regimen: doxorubicin, bleomycin, vinblastine, vincristine, mechlorethamine, etoposide, and prednisone) for the treatment of advanced Hodgkin's disease is being investigated.

■ **Testicular Cancer** For the treatment of advanced nonseminomatous testicular carcinoma, combination chemotherapy regimens containing vinblastine, cisplatin, and bleomycin have been used; however, most clinicians recommend regimens containing cisplatin and bleomycin, in combination with etoposide rather than vinblastine, particularly because of the reduced risk of neuromuscular toxicity and evidence suggesting greater efficacy in poor-risk patients. A regimen of cisplatin, ifosfamide, and either vinblastine or etoposide currently is considered by most clinicians to be the standard initial salvage (i.e., second-line) regimen in patients with recurrent testicular cancer. The best combination or sequential therapy in the treatment of advanced nonseminomatous testicular tumors has not been established, and comparative efficacy is continually being evaluated.

■ **AIDS-related Kaposi's Sarcoma** Vinblastine sulfate has been used alone or in combination chemotherapy for the palliative treatment of AIDS-related Kaposi's sarcoma. Single-agent therapy with vinblastine is considered an alternative regimen for treatment of such sarcoma. Combination chemotherapy with a vinca alkaloid (vinblastine or vincristine) also has been a preferred regimen, but many clinicians currently consider a liposomal anthracycline (doxorubicin or daunorubicin) the first-line therapy of choice for advanced AIDS-related Kaposi's sarcoma (see Uses: AIDS-related Kaposi's Sarcoma in Doxorubicin 10:00 for overview and further discussion; also see Daunorubicin 10:00).

Combination chemotherapy with conventional antineoplastic agents (e.g., bleomycin, conventional doxorubicin, etoposide, vinblastine, vincristine) has been used for more advanced disease (e.g., extensive mucocutaneous disease, lymphedema, symptomatic visceral disease). However, the results of several randomized, multicenter trials indicate that patients receiving a liposomal anthracycline for the treatment of advanced AIDS-related Kaposi's sarcoma experience similar or higher response rates with a more favorable toxic effects profile than those receiving combination therapy with conventional chemotherapeutic agents.

■ **Bladder Cancer** Vinblastine is used in combination regimens with cisplatin and methotrexate, with or without doxorubicin, for the treatment of invasive and advanced bladder cancer†. (See Uses: Bladder Cancer, Cisplatin 10:00.)

■ **Non-small Cell Lung Cancer** Vinblastine used in combination with cisplatin and mitomycin (MVP) is an alternative regimen for the treatment of non-small cell lung cancer†. Currently preferred regimens for the treatment of advanced non-small cell lung cancer include the combination of cisplatin with another agent, such as paclitaxel, vinorelbine, or gemcitabine. (See Uses: Non-small Cell Lung Cancer in Cisplatin 10:00.)

■ **Melanoma** Vinblastine is used in combination regimens (e.g., cisplatin, vinblastine, and dacarbazine, with or without interferon alfa and aldesleukin) for the treatment of metastatic melanoma†. Evidence from large, randomized trials has not established the superiority of combination regimens compared with dacarbazine alone, and dacarbazine monotherapy currently is a systemic treatment of choice for metastatic melanoma. (See Uses: Metastatic Melanoma, in Dacarbazine 10:00.)

■ **Other Uses** Vinblastine sulfate is labeled for use in the palliative treatment of non-Hodgkin's lymphomas, including lymphocytic lymphoma (nodular and diffuse, poorly and well differentiated) and histiocytic lymphoma, and in advanced stages of mycosis fungoides; however, other agents currently are preferred for the treatment of these cancers. Vinblastine also is labeled for use in the treatment of Letterer-Siwe disease (histiocytosis X).

Single-agent vinblastine has been used for the treatment of classic Kaposi's sarcoma.

Vinblastine in combination with cisplatin and bleomycin has been used for the treatment of intracranial germ cell tumors†.

Although not as effective as for the previous indications, vinblastine also may be of some use in the palliative treatment of choriocarcinoma resistant to other chemotherapeutic agents and cancer of the breast which is unresponsive to appropriate endocrine surgery and hormonal therapy.

Vinblastine has been used in the treatment of immune thrombocytopenic purpura†. Slow IV infusions of vinblastine or the use of vinblastine-loaded platelets has reportedly been effective in some cases for the treatment of autoimmune hemolytic anemia†.

Dosage and Administration

■ **Reconstitution and Administration** Vinblastine sulfate is administered only by IV injection by individuals experienced in the administration of the drug. *Vinblastine sulfate is very irritating and must not be given IM, subcutaneously, or intrathecally. Intrathecal administration of vinblastine usually results in death.* When dispensed, the container or syringe holding the individual dose prepared for administration to the patient *must* be labeled with the statement **"Fatal if given intrathecally. For intravenous use only."** and enclosed in an overwrap (e.g., plastic bag or similar wrap with typed label) bearing the statements: **"Do not remove covering until moment of injection. Fatal if given intrathecally. For intravenous use only."**

In addition to the use of the warning labels and overwrap, other protective measures to prevent inadvertent intrathecal administration of vinblastine or other vinca alkaloids include: administering diluted vinca alkaloid solutions in minibags, preparing the medication at the time of administration, attaching a unique filter, dispensing the vinca alkaloid separately from all other medications, dispensing the vinca alkaloid directly to the individual who is administering the drug, conducting an independent check of the dose and route of administration for the drug both at the time of preparation and prior to administration of the drug, and administering the vinca alkaloid in a separate room from rooms where other medications are administered.

Management of patients mistakenly receiving intrathecal vinblastine is a medical emergency. Immediate neurosurgical intervention is required to prevent ascending paralysis leading to death. Unfortunately, the prognosis to date (principally with patients inadvertently administered vincristine intrathecally) generally has been poor despite immediate efforts at removing spinal fluid and flushing with lactated Ringer's injection, with such efforts failing to prevent ascending paralysis and death in almost all cases. In a very small number of patients, life-threatening paralysis and subsequent death have been averted; however, devastating neurologic sequelae, with limited recovery afterwards, have resulted. There are no published cases of survival following intrathecal administration of vinblastine to use as guidance for treatment. However, according to the published reports of survivors of inadvertent intrathecal administration of vincristine, treatment consists of immediate removal of as much CSF as safely possible via lumbar access, followed by insertion of an epidural catheter into the subarachnoid space via the intervertebral space above initial lumbar access and then CSF irrigation with lactated Ringer's solution. When available upon request, fresh frozen plasma (25 mL) should be added to every 1 liter of lactated Ringer's solution. An intraventricular drain or catheter should be inserted by a neurosurgeon, and CSF irrigation should be continued with fluid removal through the lumbar access connected to a closed drainage system. Lactated Ringer's solution should be given by continuous infusion at a rate of 150 mL/hour, or at a rate of 75 mL/hr when fresh frozen plasma has been added. The rate of infusion should be adjusted to maintain a CSF protein concentration of 150 mg/dL. Additional measures which also have been used but may not be essential include the administration of glutamic acid, leucovorin, and pyridoxine. Glutamic acid has been administered in a dose of 10 g given IV over 24 hours, followed by 500 mg orally 3 times daily for 1 month. Leucovorin has been administered as a 100-mg IV bolus followed by an infusion of 25 mg/hour for 24 hours, then 25 mg by IV bolus every 6 hours for 1 week. Pyridoxine hydrochloride 50 mg has been administered as an IV infusion over 30 minutes every 8 hours. The contribution of these additional therapies to the reduction of neurotoxicity is unclear.

Vinblastine sulfate powder is reconstituted by adding 10 mL of bacteriostatic sodium chloride injection containing benzyl alcohol as a preservative or 10 mL of sodium chloride injection (without preservatives) to a vial labeled as containing 10 mg of the drug to provide a solution containing 1 mg/mL. The manufacturers state that other diluents should not be used. The appropriate quantity of solution reconstituted from the powder or vinblastine sulfate injection may be injected into the tubing of a running IV infusion or directly into a vein over about a 1-minute period. To minimize the risk of extravasation and/or venous irritation, the manufacturers recommend that vinblastine sulfate not be diluted in large volumes of IV solution (i.e., 100–250 mL) or infused over long periods of time (i.e., from 30–60 minutes or longer); however, the drug has been diluted in larger volumes of IV solution and infused over periods of 3–8 hours in the treatment of refractory idiopathic thrombocytopenic purpura† or autoimmune hemolytic anemia†. Care should be taken to ensure that the needle or catheter is securely within the vein in order to avoid extravasation. The manufacturers recommend rinsing the syringe and needle with venous blood after administration of the drug and before withdrawal of the needle to further minimize the possibility of extravasation. If leakage occurs, the injection should be discontinued immediately and the remainder of the dose given through another vein; local treatment of the area of leakage may minimize discomfort and the possibility of cellulitis. (See Cautions: Local Effects.) Because of the enhanced possibility of thrombosis, vinblastine sulfate solutions should not be injected into an extremity with impaired or potentially impaired circulation caused by compression or invading neoplasm, phlebitis, or varicosity.

Vinblastine sulfate injection and solutions reconstituted from the powder should be inspected visually for particulate matter and discoloration whenever solution and container permit.

■ **Dosage** ***General Dosage*** Although various dosages have been used, the usual adult dosage of vinblastine sulfate recommended by the manufacturers for initiation of therapy is 3.7 mg/m^2 given as a single dose.

According to the manufacturer, a review of published literature from 1993–1995 indicates that the usual initial pediatric dosage varies depending on the schedule used and whether vinblastine is administered as a single agent or incorporated within a particular chemotherapeutic regimen. When used as monotherapy for the treatment of Letterer-Siwe disease (histiocytosis X), an initial vinblastine sulfate dosage of 6.5 mg/m^2 was reported. When used in combination with other chemotherapeutic agents for the treatment of Hodgkin's disease, an initial vinblastine sulfate dosage of 6 mg/m^2 was used. For the treatment of testicular germ cell carcinoma, an initial vinblastine sulfate dosage of 3 mg/m^2 has been used in a combination regimen.

Dosage Modification for Toxicity Subsequent dosage of vinblastine sulfate must be determined by the clinical and hematologic response and tolerance of the patient in order to obtain optimum therapeutic results with minimum adverse effects. Because of the possible leukopenic response that follows administration of vinblastine, the drug is given at intervals of *at least 7 days;* however, even if 7 days have elapsed, the next dose of vinblastine should not be given until the leukocyte count has returned to at least 4000/mm^3. Doses are usually increased at weekly intervals in increments of about 1.8 mg/m^2 in adults until the desired therapeutic response is obtained, the leukocyte count decreases to about 3000/mm^3, or a maximum weekly dose of 18.5 mg/m^2 is being administered to adults.

For most adult patients, the optimum weekly dose of vinblastine sulfate will be 5.5–7.4 mg/m^2; however, leukopenia (leukocyte count of 3000/mm^3) may occur in some patients with 3.7 mg/m^2 per week, whereas other patients may tolerate 18.5 mg/m^2 per week. Dosage is generally reduced in patients with recent exposure to radiation therapy or chemotherapy; single doses in these patients usually do not exceed 5.5 mg/m^2.

Dosage modifications in pediatric patients should be guided by hematologic tolerance.

Once the dose required to produce a leukocyte count of 3000/mm^3 has been determined, a maintenance dose of one increment (about 1.8 mg/m^2 in adults) *less than this amount* should be administered at weekly intervals. Thus, the patient receives the maximum dose of vinblastine sulfate that does not cause leukopenia (leukocyte count of 3000/mm^3 or less).

To ensure an adequate trial, vinblastine therapy must be continued for at least 4–6 weeks. Some experts advocate a trial of at least 12 weeks, particularly in patients with carcinomas.

Strict adherence to the recommended dosage interval is important. The use of small daily doses for prolonged periods (even if equivalent to the total weekly dosage) is not recommended because it has produced severe toxicity with little or no added therapeutic benefit. When doses several times the recommended weekly dosage were administered daily for long periods, seizures, permanent CNS damage, and death occurred. However, some clinicians believe that patients with rapidly progressing tumors with short generation times should receive large divided doses over several days, repeated as often as toxicity permits.

Maintenance Dosage The duration of maintenance therapy varies according to the disease being treated and the combination of chemotherapeutic agents being used. Some clinicians have reported successful maintenance with vinblastine sulfate doses administered at intervals as long as 3–8 weeks, but most reports indicate that patients frequently relapse if maintenance dosage intervals exceed 2 weeks. Clinicians should consult published protocols for the dosage of vinblastine and other chemotherapeutic agents and the method and sequence of administration. There are differences of opinion regarding the duration of maintenance therapy with the same protocol for a particular disease. Prolonged chemotherapy for maintaining remissions involves several risks, including life-threatening infectious diseases, sterility, and possibly the appearance of other neoplasms as a result of suppression of the immune system. In some disorders, survival following complete remission may not be as prolonged as that achieved with shorter periods of maintenance therapy. However, failure to provide maintenance therapy in some patients may lead to unnecessary relapse.

■ **Dosage in Renal and Hepatic Impairment** The effect of renal and/or hepatic impairment on the disposition of vinblastine has not been fully determined. Reduction of vinblastine dosage in patients with renal impairment does not appear to be necessary. Because the drug is extensively metabolized in the liver, doses of vinblastine should be reduced and the drug should be administered with caution in patients with hepatic impairment. A 50% reduction in vinblastine sulfate dose is recommended for patients with a direct serum bilirubin exceeding 3 mg/dL.

Cautions

In general, adverse reactions to vinblastine are dose related and reversible. Toxicity may be enhanced by the presence of hepatic insufficiency.

■ **Hematologic Effects** The major adverse effect of vinblastine is hematologic toxicity which occurs much more frequently than with vincristine therapy. Leukopenia (granulocytopenia) occurs most commonly and is usually the dose-limiting factor in vinblastine therapy; however, numerous patients have achieved a sustained remission without leukopenia. Leukopenia may not be a problem with small doses used for maintenance therapy; however, the possibility of a cumulative effect should be considered. The nadir in the leukocyte count usually occurs 4–10 days after administration of vinblastine. Recovery occurs rapidly, usually within another 7–14 days; however, following administration of high doses of vinblastine, recovery may take 21 days or more. The patient's hematologic status must be carefully monitored. (See Cautions: Precautions and Contraindications.)

Although thrombocytopenia is usually slight and transient, substantial platelet count depression may occur, particularly in patients who have received prior radiation therapy or chemotherapy. In patients whose bone marrow has been infiltrated with malignant cells, vinblastine may produce an abrupt fall in the leukocyte and thrombocyte counts. If this occurs, the manufacturers recommend that vinblastine therapy be discontinued; however, many clinicians consider it appropriate to continue vinblastine therapy in these patients if the drug is clearly destroying tumor cells in the bone marrow. Anemia also may occur in patients receiving vinblastine.

■ **Respiratory Effects** Acute shortness of breath and bronchospasm, which can be severe or life threatening, have occurred following administration of vinca alkaloids (e.g., vinblastine), and have been reported most frequently when mitomycin was administered concomitantly. Such reactions may occur a few minutes to several hours after administration of a vinca alkaloid or up to 2 weeks after a dose of mitomycin. Aggressive treatment may be required, particularly in patients with preexisting pulmonary dysfunction. Progressive dyspnea, which may require chronic therapy, can occur in patients receiving vinblastine; the drug should *not* be readministered to these patients.

■ **GI Effects** Nausea and vomiting are the most frequently occurring adverse GI effects of vinblastine. Nausea and vomiting usually last less than 24 hours, and are reported to be easily controlled by administration of antiemetics. Other adverse GI effects of vinblastine include anorexia, diarrhea, constipation, epigastric and abdominal pain, adynamic ileus, pharyngitis, stomatitis, vesiculation of the mouth, hemorrhagic enterocolitis, rectal bleeding, and bleeding from old peptic ulcers. GI symptoms, particularly constipation, abdominal pain, and adynamic ileus, may be related to the neurotoxicity of vinblastine. Stomatitis, although reversible, can be disabling.

■ **Nervous System Effects** Neurotoxicity occurs occasionally in patients receiving vinblastine, especially with high doses or prolonged therapy, but less frequently than with vincristine therapy. Neurotoxicity can be disabling. Adverse neurologic effects of vinblastine include numbness, paresthesia, peripheral neuropathy and neuritis, mental depression (usually 2–3 days after administration of the drug), loss of deep tendon reflexes, headache, malaise, weakness, dizziness, seizures, psychoses, severe face and jaw pain, severe immediate or delayed pain at the tumor site, bone pain, vocal cord paralysis, and dysfunction of the autonomic nervous system with such symptoms as urinary retention, sinus tachycardia, orthostatic hypotension, and tender parotid glands associated with dry mouth. In some studies, patients who showed marked neurotoxicity following vinblastine therapy later received vincristine without evidence of neuropathy. GI symptoms, headache, and paresthesia may appear 4–6 hours after administration of vinblastine and usually persist for 2–10 hours.

■ **Cardiovascular Effects** Hypertension is the most common adverse cardiovascular effect of vinblastine. Myocardial infarction, angina pectoris, and transient ECG abnormalities related to coronary ischemia have been reported rarely in patients receiving the drug. Caution is advised when using vinblastine in patients with ischemic cardiovascular disease, and care of this condition should be recommended. Cases of unexpected myocardial infarction and cerebrovascular accident have been reported in patients receiving vinblastine in combination with bleomycin and cisplatin. Raynaud's phenomenon has been reported in patients receiving vinblastine and bleomycin, with or without cisplatin; a few cases have been reported in patients receiving bleomycin alone.

■ **Local Effects** Vinblastine is a tissue irritant and may cause phlebitis and necrosis. Extravasation can result in pain and cellulitis. If extravasation of large amounts of the injection occurs, sloughing may result. Local reactions may be severe and can persist for several weeks to months. The manufacturers state that local injection of hyaluronidase and application of moderate heat may decrease local reactions resulting from extravasation; however, some clinicians prefer to treat extravasation with cold compresses, dilution with 0.9% sodium chloride injection, and/or local injection of hydrocortisone.

■ **Dermatologic Effects** Vinblastine-induced alopecia is common. Other adverse dermatologic effects occur infrequently following vinblastine therapy and include dermatitis and vesiculation of the skin, phototoxicity, and epilation. Epilation is partial and almost always reversible; in some cases, hair may regrow during maintenance therapy. Fever has also occurred in patients receiving vinblastine.

■ **Otic Effects** Eighth cranial nerve damage, which may be manifested by vestibular manifestations such as dizziness, nystagmus, and vertigo, and by auditory manifestations such as varying degrees of hearing impairment (including partial or total deafness) that may be temporary or permanent, has been reported in patients receiving vinca alkaloids. Vinca alkaloids should be used concomitantly with other potentially ototoxic drugs such as platinum-containing antineoplastic agents with extreme caution.

■ **Precautions and Contraindications** Vinblastine sulfate is a highly toxic drug with a low therapeutic index, and a therapeutic response is not likely to occur without some evidence of toxicity. The drug must be used only under constant supervision by clinicians experienced in therapy with cytotoxic agents. Patients and/or their parents or guardians should be advised of the possibility of adverse effects and associated manifestations.

Patients with cachexia or ulcerated areas of the skin may be more susceptible to the leukopenic effects of vinblastine; therefore, the drug should be administered with extreme caution to patients (especially geriatric patients) with these conditions.

Patients who receive myelosuppressive drugs experience an increased frequency of infections as well as possible hemorrhagic complications. Because these complications are potentially fatal, the patient should be instructed to notify the physician if fever, sore throat, or unusual bleeding or bruising occurs. Blood counts should be performed weekly or at least before administration of each dose of vinblastine. The manufacturers state that if the leukocyte count falls below 2000/mm^3, patients should be observed carefully for signs of infection. The effect of vinblastine on the erythrocyte count and hemoglobin is usually insignificant; however, it should be remembered that patients with malignant disease may exhibit anemia in the absence of any therapy.

Patients with preexisting pulmonary dysfunction may be particularly susceptible to severe or life-threatening pulmonary effects of vinblastine. (See Cautions: Respiratory Effects.)

Caution is advised when using vinblastine in patients with ischemic cardiovascular disease, and care of this condition should be recommended.

Care must be taken to avoid contact of vinblastine sulfate solutions with the eyes as severe irritation and possibly corneal ulceration can result; if contact occurs, the eye should be thoroughly washed with water immediately.

As a result of extensive purine catabolism accompanying rapid cellular destruction, hyperuricemia may occur in some patients receiving vinblastine, especially those with non-Hodgkin's lymphomas or leukemia. In some patients, uric acid nephropathy may result. These effects may be minimized by adequate hydration, alkalinization of the urine, and/or administration of allopurinol.

For additional information on precautions associated with the use of vinblastine, see Cautions: Hematologic Effects and Cautions: Local Effects.

Because of the hepatic metabolism and biliary excretion of vinblastine, some clinicians recommend reduced doses in patients with obstructive or hepatocellular jaundice. Metabolism of vinblastine via cytochrome P-450 (CYP) isoenzymes may be impaired in patients with hepatic dysfunction.

The manufacturers state that vinblastine is contraindicated in patients who are severely leukopenic. The manufacturers also state that the drug should not be administered in the presence of bacterial infections; infections should be controlled prior to initiation of vinblastine therapy.

■ **Pregnancy, Fertility, and Lactation** Although information on the use of vinblastine during pregnancy is limited, the drug may cause fetal toxicity when administered to pregnant women. The drug causes resorption of fetuses in animals and produces gross fetal abnormalities in surviving offspring. There are no adequate and controlled studies to date using vinblastine in pregnant women, and the drug should be used during pregnancy only in life-threatening situations or severe disease for which safer drugs cannot be used or are ineffective. Women of childbearing potential should be advised to avoid becoming pregnant while receiving the drug. When vinblastine is administered during pregnancy or the patient becomes pregnant while receiving the drug, the patient should be informed of the potential hazard to the fetus.

The effect of vinblastine on fertility in humans is not fully known. Aspermia has occurred in some individuals during vinblastine therapy. Reproduction studies in animals have revealed evidence of metaphase arrest and degenerative changes in germ cells.

It is not known whether vinblastine is distributed in milk. Because of the potential for serious adverse reactions to vinblastine in nursing infants, a decision should be made whether to discontinue nursing or the drug, taking into account the importance of the drug to the woman.

Drug Interactions

■ **Drugs Affecting Hepatic Microsomal Enzymes** Metabolism of vinca alkaloids (e.g., vincristine, vinblastine) is mediated by the cytochrome P-450 isoenzyme CYP3A, and caution should be exercised when vinca alkaloids are used concurrently with inhibitors of this isoenzyme.

Increased toxicity has been reported in patients receiving concomitant erythromycin and vinblastine.

Concomitant administration of vincristine and the antifungal agent itraconazole, a potent inhibitor of CYP3A, has been associated with earlier onset and/or increased severity of adverse neuromuscular effects, presumably because of inhibition of vincristine metabolism. In vitro studies demonstrate that antifungal agent voriconazole is a less potent inhibitor of CYP3A4 than ketoconazole or itraconazole. Because concomitant use of voriconazole or other azole antifungal agents may increase plasma concentrations of vinblastine and lead to neurotoxicity, dosage reduction of vinblastine should be considered. Patients receiving a vinca alkaloid and itraconazole or other azole antifungal agent concomitantly should be monitored for increases in and/or prolongation of the effects of the vinca alkaloid, including adverse effects such as peripheral neuropathy and ileus, and dosage of the vinca alkaloid should be reduced accordingly.

Because it is a potent CYP3A4 inhibitor, vinblastine may cause increased plasma concentrations of tolterodine during concomitant use; reduction to 50% of the recommended dose for tolterodine is recommended.

Caution and careful monitoring are advised during concomitant use of vinblastine and aprepitant, an antiemetic agent, which may inhibit or induce CYP3A.

■ **Ototoxic Drugs** Since varying degrees of permanent or temporary hearing impairment (including partial or total deafness) associated with eighth cranial nerve damage have been reported in patients receiving vinca alkaloids, vinblastine should be used concomitantly with other potentially ototoxic drugs such as platinum-containing antineoplastic agents with extreme caution.

■ **Phenytoin** In patients receiving phenytoin and combination regimens containing vinblastine, decreased serum concentrations of phenytoin and increased seizure activity have been reported, possibly as a result of decreased absorption and/or increased metabolism of phenytoin. The contribution of vinblastine to this interaction is uncertain; however, in patients receiving phenytoin and vinblastine concomitantly, serum concentrations of phenytoin should be monitored and dosage adjustments made as necessary.

Pharmacology

Although the mechanism of action has not been fully elucidated, vinblastine and other vinca alkaloids exert their cytotoxic effects by binding to tubulin, the protein subunit of the microtubules that form the mitotic spindle. The formation of vinblastine-tubulin complexes prevents the polymerization of the tubulin subunits into microtubules and induces depolymerization of microtubules resulting in inhibition of microtubule assembly and cellular metaphase arrest. In high concentrations, vinblastine also exerts complex effects on nucleic acid and protein synthesis. Vinblastine reportedly also interferes with amino acid metabolism by blocking cellular utilization of glutamic acid and thus inhibits purine synthesis, the citric acid cycle, and the formation of urea. Vinblastine exerts some immunosuppressive activity.

Pharmacokinetics

Vinblastine sulfate is unpredictably absorbed from the GI tract. Following IV administration, the drug is rapidly cleared from the blood and distributed into body tissues. Vinblastine crosses the blood-brain barrier poorly and does not appear in the CSF in therapeutic concentrations. Vinblastine is reported to be extensively metabolized, primarily in the liver, to desacetylvinblastine, which is more active than the parent compound on a weight basis. Metabolism of vinca alkaloids (e.g., vinblastine, vincristine) is mediated by the cytochrome P-450 isoenzymes in the CYP3A subfamily. The drug is excreted slowly in urine and in feces via the bile.

Chemistry and Stability

■ **Chemistry** Vinblastine sulfate, a naturally occurring vinca alkaloid, is an antimicrotubule antineoplastic agent. Vinblastine sulfate is the salt of a dimeric alkaloid isolated from *Cantharanthus roseus*. Vinblastine sulfate occurs as a white, off-white, or slightly yellow, hygroscopic, amorphous or crystalline powder and is freely soluble in water, soluble in methanol, and slightly soluble in ethanol. Vinblastine sulfate is insoluble in benzene, ether, and naphtha. Commercially available vinblastine sulfate powder occurs as a yellowish white solid having the characteristic appearance of a lyophilized preparation. Vinblastine sulfate injection is a clear, colorless solution with a pH of 3–5.5; the injection also contains sodium chloride and benzyl alcohol. Vinblastine reportedly has pK_as of 5.4 and 7.4.

■ **Stability** Vinblastine sulfate powder, vinblastine sulfate injection, and solutions of the drug are light-sensitive and must be protected from light. Vinblastine sulfate powder and injection should be refrigerated at 2–8°C. Following reconstitution of the powder with bacteriostatic sodium chloride injection which contains benzyl alcohol as a preservative, solutions of the drug have a pH of 3.5–5 and are stable for 28 days when refrigerated at 2–8°C. Sodium chloride injection (without preservatives) also may be used as a diluent. The manufacturer states that other diluents should *not* be used. When vinblastine sulfate powder is reconstituted with a diluent that does not contain a preservative, any unused portions of reconstituted solution of the drug should be discarded immediately.

For further information on the handling of antineoplastic agents, see the ASHP Guidelines on Handling Hazardous Drugs at http://www.ahfsdruginformation.com.

Preparations

Excipients in commercially available drug preparations may have clinically important effects in some individuals; consult specific product labeling for details.

vinBLAStine Sulfate

Parenteral

Injection, for IV use only	1 mg/mL*	**Vinblastine Sulfate Injection**
For injection, for IV use only	10 mg*	**Vinblastine Sulfate for Injection**

*available from one or more manufacturer, distributor, and/or repackager by generic (nonproprietary) name

†Use is not currently included in the labeling approved by the US Food and Drug Administration

vinCRIStine Sulfate Leurocristine Sulfate, Oncovin, LCR, VCR

■ Vincristine sulfate, a naturally occurring vinca alkaloid, is an antineoplastic agent.

Uses

Vincristine sulfate is commercially available in 2 types of formulations: conventional vincristine sulfate and liposomal vincristine sulfate. The efficacy and safety of vincristine for each indication is based on research and clinical experience using a specific formulation.

■ **Acute Lymphocytic Leukemia** ***Conventional Vincristine*** Conventional vincristine is used as a component of combination chemotherapeutic regimens for the induction of remissions of childhood or adult acute lymphocytic (lymphoblastic) leukemia (ALL). Various drugs have been used for combination chemotherapy of childhood and adult ALL, and comparative efficacy of these regimens is continually being evaluated. Additional therapy (e.g., intrathecal administration of methotrexate with or without intrathecal cytarabine and hydrocortisone, with or without systemic methotrexate and leucovorin rescue and/or cranial radiation in children; intrathecal methotrexate given alone or in conjunction with cranial radiation or high-dose systemic methotrexate and leucovorin rescue in adults) is needed for prophylaxis of CNS involvement (meningeal leukemia) in patients with ALL. Once remission has been attained, patients generally receive consolidation-intensification therapy and maintenance therapy. Other regimens are preferred in certain subsets of patients with ALL (e.g., B-cell ALL, T-cell ALL, Philadelphia chromosome-positive ALL). Certain patients with a poor prognosis or with a poor response to initial treatment may be candidates for hematopoietic stem cell transplantation. Specialized references and experts should be consulted for additional information.

Although conventional vincristine used with a corticosteroid such as prednisone results in high remission induction rates in children with ALL, addition of an asparaginase preparation and/or an anthracycline (e.g., daunorubicin) can improve both the rate and duration of remission and therefore such 3- or 4-drug regimens generally are preferred. (For additional information on the asparaginase component of ALL regimens, see Asparaginase [Erwinia chrysanthemi] 10:00.) The use of intensive induction regimens with 4 or more drugs, including conventional vincristine, an asparaginase preparation, a corticosteroid (e.g., prednisone), and an anthracycline (e.g., daunorubicin), with or without cyclophosphamide, may improve the rate of event-free survival but is associated with greater toxicity. An induction regimen containing 4 or more drugs does not appear to be necessary to achieve favorable outcomes in patients at low or standard risk of treatment failure provided adequate intensification therapy is provided following achievement of remission. Therefore, some clinicians reserve such regimens for patients with high-risk childhood ALL. However, other clinicians have elected to use a 4- or 5-drug induction regimen for all patients with childhood ALL regardless of presenting features. Maintenance therapy (e.g., methotrexate and mercaptopurine with or without pulses of conventional vincristine and prednisone) is administered for about 2–3 years.

Induction regimens for adult ALL typically include conventional vincristine, prednisone, and an anthracycline; some regimens also add other drugs, such as an asparaginase preparation or cyclophosphamide.

Liposomal Vincristine Liposomal vincristine is used for the treatment of Philadelphia chromosome-negative (Ph$^-$) relapsed or refractory ALL in patients in second or greater relapse or in those whose disease has progressed following at least 2 prior therapies. The drug has been designated an orphan drug by FDA for use in this condition. The accelerated approval of liposomal vincristine for this indication is based on overall response rate; continued approval for this indication may be contingent on verification and description of clinical benefit (e.g., overall survival) of liposomal vincristine in confirmatory studies.

The current indication for liposomal vincristine is based principally on the results of an open-label, noncomparative, phase 2 study in 65 adults with Ph$^-$ relapsed or refractory ALL. Patients were enrolled if they were in second or greater relapse or if their disease had relapsed or was refractory following at least 2 prior therapies. Patients enrolled in the study also were required to have achieved complete remission (defined as a leukemia-free interval lasting at least 90 days) after at least one prior therapy. In this study, patients received liposomal vincristine sulfate at a dosage of 2.25 mg/m^2 of vincristine sulfate by IV infusion over 60 minutes on days 1, 8, 15, and 22 of each 28-day cycle; concomitant therapy with systemic corticosteroids or hydroxyurea was not permitted beyond day 5 or 14, respectively, of the first cycle. The primary measure of efficacy was complete remission (CR) or complete remission with incomplete hematologic recovery (CRi) according to the International Working Group (IWG) response criteria. The median age of patients was 31 years; 85% of the patients had precursor B-cell ALL (pre-B-ALL), 15% had precursor T-cell ALL (pre-T-ALL), 48% had undergone hematopoietic stem cell transplantation prior to study entry, and 80% of the patients had residual neuropathy at baseline following prior therapy with conventional vincristine. Approximately one-half of patients had received 3 or more prior therapies for their disease; all of the enrolled patients received prior therapy with conventional vincristine and 45% were refractory to their most recent therapy prior to study entry. Overall, CR or CRi was reported in 15.4% of patients; 4.6% of patients achieved CR. At the time of analysis, the median duration of response from initial CR or CRi to date of documented relapse, death, or subsequent chemotherapy or stem-cell transplantation was 56 days.

■ **Acute Myeloid Leukemia** Conventional vincristine is used in various combination regimens for the treatment of acute myeloid (myelogenous, nonlymphocytic) leukemias (AML, ANLL), but the comparative efficacy of these combinations is continually being evaluated. (See Uses: Leukemias, in Cytarabine 10:00.)

■ **Hodgkin's Disease** Conventional vincristine is used as a component of various chemotherapeutic regimens for the treatment of Hodgkin's disease. Various drugs have been used for combination chemotherapy, and comparative efficacy of these regimens is continually being evaluated. Conventional vincristine is used in combination with bleomycin, etoposide, doxorubicin, cyclophosphamide, procarbazine and prednisone (in the increased-dose BEACOPP regimen) for the treatment of early or advanced Hodgkin's disease. Conventional vincristine also is used in combination with doxorubicin, bleomycin, vinblastine, mechlorethamine, etoposide, and prednisone (Stanford V regimen); mechlorethamine, procarbazine, doxorubicin, bleomycin, and prednisone (MOPP-ABV regimen); and cyclophosphamide, procarbazine, doxorubicin, bleomycin, vinblastine, dacarbazine, and prednisone (COPP-ABVD regimen) for the treatment of Hodgkin's disease.

■ **Non-Hodgkin's Lymphoma** Conventional vincristine is used as a component of combination chemotherapeutic regimens for the treatment of non-Hodgkin's lymphomas, and the comparative efficacy of various regimens is continually being evaluated. Conventional vincristine generally is used with cyclophosphamide and prednisone with or without doxorubicin (i.e., CHOP or CVP regimen); rituximab usually is administered with these regimens.

■ **Neuroblastoma** Conventional vincristine is used as a component of various chemotherapeutic regimens for the treatment of neuroblastoma.

■ **Rhabdomyosarcoma** Conventional vincristine is used as a component of combination chemotherapeutic regimens for the treatment of childhood rhabdomyosarcoma; conventional vincristine is commonly used with dactinomycin, with or without cyclophosphamide, as an adjunct to surgery and/or radiation therapy.

■ **Wilms' Tumor** Combination chemotherapy is superior to single-drug therapy as an adjunct to surgery and/or radiation therapy in prolonging relapse-free survival and overall survival in children with Wilms' tumor. Conventional vincristine is generally used with dactinomycin (with or without doxorubicin) or in combination with doxorubicin, cyclophosphamide, and etoposide for the treatment of Wilms' tumor.

■ **Brain Tumors** Conventional vincristine is used for the palliative treatment of various primary brain tumors†. Various regimens that typically include conventional vincristine and lomustine with another antineoplastic agent, such as procarbazine or cisplatin, or a corticosteroid (prednisone) have been used in the treatment of astrocytic tumors (e.g., glioblastoma multiforme and anaplastic astrocytoma), medulloblastoma, and oligodendroglioma. See Uses: Brain Tumors in Lomustine 10:00 for further discussion.

■ **AIDS-related Kaposi's Sarcoma** Conventional vincristine is used in combination chemotherapy for the palliative treatment of AIDS-related Kaposi's sarcoma†. Combination chemotherapy that includes a vinca alkaloid (vinblastine or conventional vincristine), conventional doxorubicin, and bleomycin has previously been a preferred regimen for the disease, but many clinicians currently consider a liposomal anthracycline (doxorubicin or daunorubicin) the first-line therapy of choice for advanced AIDS-related Kaposi's sarcoma (see Uses: AIDS-related Kaposi's Sarcoma in Doxorubicin 10:00 for overview and further discussion of therapy; also see Daunorubicin 10:00).

Combination chemotherapy with conventional antineoplastic agents (e.g., bleomycin, conventional doxorubicin, etoposide, vinblastine, conventional vincristine) usually has been used for more advanced disease (e.g., extensive mucocutaneous disease, lymphedema, symptomatic visceral disease). However, the results of several randomized, multicenter trials indicate that patients receiving a liposomal anthracycline for the treatment of advanced AIDS-related Kaposi's sarcoma experience similar or higher response rates with a more favorable toxic effects profile than those receiving combination therapy with conventional chemotherapeutic agents.

Conventional vincristine also has been used alone for the palliative treatment of AIDS-related Kaposi's sarcoma. In one study in patients with AIDS-related Kaposi's sarcoma who received a conventional vincristine dosage of 2 mg weekly for 2–5 weeks and then every 2 weeks thereafter as tolerated, partial or minor response was observed in about 61 or 39% of evaluable patients, respectively.

■ **Small Cell Lung Cancer** Conventional vincristine is used in combination with cyclophosphamide and doxorubicin (CAV) for the treatment of extensive-stage small cell lung cancer†. Survival outcomes are similar in patients with extensive-stage small cell lung cancer receiving CAV or cisplatin/etoposide. Conventional vincristine also has been used in combination with cyclophosphamide and etoposide for the treatment of extensive-stage small cell lung cancer†. Combination chemotherapy regimens have produced response rates of 70–85% and complete response rates of 20–30% in patients with extensive-stage disease; however, comparative efficacy is continually being evaluated. Because the current prognosis for small cell lung carcinoma is unsatisfactory regardless of stage and despite considerable diagnostic and therapeutic advances, all patients with this cancer are candidates for inclusion in clinical trials at the time of diagnosis.

■ **Other Uses** Conventional vincristine also is used as a component of combination chemotherapy for the treatment of osteosarcoma† (including Ewing's sarcoma†), multiple myeloma†, and choriocarcinoma†. Combination chemotherapy with conventional vincristine, cyclophosphamide, and prednisone, with or without doxorubicin, is used in the treatment of chronic lymphocytic leukemia (CLL)†. Combination chemotherapy with conventional vincristine, cisplatin, and fluorouracil is used in the treatment of hepatoblastoma†. Conventional vincristine combined with cyclophosphamide and dacarbazine is used for the treatment of pheochromocytoma†.

Conventional vincristine has been used in the treatment of immune thrombocytopenic purpura†. IV injections of the drug have also been used with some success for the treatment of thrombotic thrombocytopenic purpura†, and the use of vincristine-loaded platelets has reportedly been useful in some cases for the management of autoimmune hemolytic anemia†.

Dosage and Administration

■ **Reconstitution and Administration** Vincristine sulfate is commercially available in 2 types of formulations: conventional vincristine sulfate and liposomal vincristine sulfate (Marqibo®). The properties of vincristine may differ according to formulation, and the dosage and preparation for vincristine sulfate are specific to formulation. The manufacturer's instructions for the specific formulation should be consulted to ensure that the correct preparation procedure is followed.

Conventional and liposomal vincristine formulations are for IV use *only* and should be administered by individuals experienced in the administration of the drug. *Conventional and liposomal vincristine sulfate must not be given by other routes (e.g., IM, subcutaneously, intrathecally). Intrathecal administration of vincristine usually results in death.* When dispensed, the infusion bag or syringe holding the individual dose prepared for administration to the patient *must* be labeled with the statement **"For intravenous use only. Fatal if given by other routes."** The syringe *must* be enclosed in an overwrap bearing the statements: **"Do not remove covering until moment of injection. For intravenous use only. Fatal if given by other routes."**

In addition to use of the labels and overwrap, other protective measures to prevent inadvertent intrathecal administration of conventional or liposomal vincristine or other vinca alkaloids include: administration of the diluted drug in small-volume IV bags (i.e., minibags), preparing the medication at the time of administration, attaching a unique filter, dispensing the vinca alkaloid separately from all other medications, dispensing the vinca alkaloid directly to the individual who is administering the drug, conducting an independent check of the dose and route of administration for the drug both at the time of preparation and prior to administration of the drug, and administering the vinca alkaloid in a separate room from rooms where other medications are administered.

Management of patients mistakenly receiving intrathecal conventional or liposomal vincristine is a medical emergency. Unfortunately, the prognosis to date generally has been poor despite immediate efforts at removing spinal fluid and flushing with lactated Ringer's injection as well as other solutions, with such efforts failing to prevent ascending paralysis and death in almost all cases. In one case, progression of paralysis was stopped in an adult patient when the following treatment was initiated immediately after inadvertent intrathecal injection of conventional vincristine. Such treatment consisted of immediate removal of as much CSF as safely possible via lumbar access, followed by flushing of the subarachnoid space with lactated Ringer's solution infused continuously at a rate of 150 mL/hour through a catheter in a cerebral lateral ventricle and removal of fluid through a lumbar access. As soon as available, fresh frozen plasma (25 mL) diluted in 1 L of lactated Ringer's solution was infused through the cerebral ventricular catheter at a rate of 75 mL per hour with removal of fluid through the lumbar access. The rate of infusion was adjusted to maintain a CSF protein concentration of 150 mg/dL. Glutamic acid was administered in a dose of 10 g given IV over 24 hours, followed by 500 mg orally 3 times daily for 1 month or until stabilization of neurologic status. The role of glutamic acid in this treatment is uncertain.

Conventional Vincristine Sulfate Extra fluid should not be added to the vial containing conventional vincristine sulfate prior to removal of the dose. Conventional vincristine sulfate injection should be withdrawn from the vial into an accurate dry syringe, and the dose should be measured carefully. Extra fluid should not be added to the vial in an attempt to empty it completely.

Preparation of the conventional vincristine dose as a diluted solution in a minibag is recommended as a protective measure to prevent inadvertent intrathecal administration of the drug; however, if the drug is prepared as a diluted solution in a syringe, a 30-mL syringe is recommended. The larger volume of the diluted conventional vincristine solution and incompatible packaging make it less likely that the IV conventional vincristine dose will be confused with a drug that is intended for intrathecal use. For preparation in a minibag, the dose of conventional vincristine sulfate should be diluted with an appropriate volume of 0.9% sodium chloride injection to a final concentration of 0.0015–0.08 mg/mL. If the drug is prepared in a minibag or diluted in a 30-mL syringe, the dose should be administered by IV injection over 5–10 minutes in adults; in children, the dose should be administered at a slower rate. The Oncology Nursing Society (ONS) recommends that if a vesicant drug such as vincristine is administered by short infusion into a peripheral vein, an IV pump *not* be used in order to decrease pressure applied on the veins.

Conventional vincristine also has been diluted in a large volume of IV solution and administered as a slow IV infusion† (e.g., over 4–8 hours); continuous 4- or 5-day IV infusions† have also been used. Specialized references should be consulted for specific information on slow IV infusion of conventional vincristine.

For rapid IV ("bolus") injections, conventional vincristine sulfate injection must be administered through an intact, free-flowing IV needle or catheter. Care should be taken to ensure that the needle or catheter is securely within the vein to avoid extravasation. If leakage or swelling occurs, the injection should be discontinued immediately and the remainder of the dose given through another vein; local treatment of the area of leakage may minimize discomfort and the possibility of cellulitis. (See Cautions: Local Effects.) Conventional vincristine sulfate injection may be injected either directly into a vein or into the tubing of a running IV infusion; injection of the drug should be completed within 1 minute.

When conventional vincristine and asparaginase must be administered sequentially, the sequence of vincristine followed by asparaginase is recommended. (See Drug Interactions: Antineoplastic Agents.)

Liposomal Vincristine Sulfate Liposomal vincristine sulfate (Marqibo®) is commercially available as a 3-vial kit containing single-use vials of vincristine sulfate solution, sphingomyelin-cholesterol liposome suspension, and dibasic sodium phosphate solution. Preparation of liposomal vincristine sulfate suspension requires 60–90 minutes of dedicated and uninterrupted time because extensive monitoring of temperature and time is required during the process. Deviations from temperature control, timing, and preparation procedures may affect encapsulation of vincristine sulfate into the liposomes. If deviations in the preparation process occur, the components of the kit should be discarded and a new kit should be used to prepare liposomal vincristine sulfate.

Vincristine sulfate solution must be mixed with the sphingomyelin-cholesterol liposome suspension and dibasic sodium phosphate solution provided in the kit; the resultant liposomal vincristine sulfate injection concentrate must be diluted prior to IV infusion. For preparation of liposomal vincristine sulfate injection concentrate, equipment provided by the manufacturer (i.e., water bath or block heater, calibrated thermometer, electronic timer, tongs) must be used. Either the water bath or block heater (but not both) may be used to prepare liposomal vincristine sulfate injection concentrate. All steps required to mix and dilute the drug product should be performed *inside* the sterile area using strict aseptic technique since the injection does not contain any preservative or bacteriostatic agent. Each vial in the kit and the final diluted suspension for infusion should be inspected visually for particulate matter and discoloration prior to preparation and administration whenever solution and container permit; the vials and diluted suspension for infusion should *not* be used if foreign particles or precipitate is present.

Liposomal vincristine is administered by IV infusion over 1 hour. Liposomal vincristine should not be admixed with any other drug and should not be administered using an inline filter. Care should be taken to ensure that the venous access line is secure and free-flowing to avoid extravasation. If extravasation is suspected, the infusion should be discontinued immediately and local treatments considered. (See Cautions: Local Effects.)

Water Bath Preparation Instructions. The water bath should be prepared and maintained *outside* the sterile area. The water in the bath should be maintained at a minimum depth of 8 cm and at a temperature of 63–67°C (measured by the calibrated thermometer) throughout the preparation process. The calibrated thermometer should remain in the water bath throughout the preparation process. All steps required to mix and dilute the drug product should be performed *inside* the sterile area using strict aseptic technique.

For preparation of liposomal vincristine sulfate injection concentrate, a venting needle (or other suitable venting device) with a 0.2-μm filter should be inserted into the vial containing dibasic sodium phosphate solution with the point of the venting needle positioned well above the surface of the solution. A volume of 1 mL of sphingomyelin-cholesterol liposome suspension followed by 5 mL of vincristine sulfate solution should be injected into the vial. The venting needle should then be removed and the vial should be gently inverted 5 times to mix the 3 components; the vial should *not* be shaken. The neck of the vial containing the mixture of the 3 components should be fitted with the manufacturer-provided flotation ring, and then the vial should be placed in the water bath for 10 minutes; the temperature of the water bath and duration of flotation should be closely monitored using the calibrated thermometer and electronic timer. After 10 minutes, the vial should be removed from the water bath using tongs to prevent burns, and the flotation ring should be removed from the vial. The start time and temperature and the end time and temperature should be recorded on the liposomal vincristine sulfate injection concentrate overlabel immediately after the vial is placed into the water bath and upon removal, respectively. The vial exterior should be dried with a clean paper towel upon removal from the water bath, and then the overlabel should be affixed to the vial. The vial should be gently inverted another 5 times to mix the contents; the vial should *not* be shaken. The resultant liposomal vincristine sulfate injection concentrate contains vincristine sulfate 0.16 mg/mL and should be stored at room temperature (15–30°C) for no more than 12 hours. Liposomal vincristine sulfate injection concentrate should be allowed to come to room temperature (i.e., 15–30°C) over at least 30 minutes prior to dilution.

For preparation of the *final* diluted IV infusion of liposomal vincristine sulfate, a volume equivalent to the volume of the appropriate dose of liposomal vincristine sulfate should be withdrawn from an infusion bag containing 100 mL of 5% dextrose or 0.9% sodium chloride injection and discarded; the appropriate dose of liposomal vincristine sulfate injection concentrate is then withdrawn from the vial and added to the infusion bag to yield a final volume of 100 mL. The infusion bag label supplied by the drug's manufacturer should be completed and affixed to the bag. Infusion of the diluted drug should be completed within 12 hours of *initiation* of preparation of liposomal vincristine sulfate injection.

Block Heater Preparation Instructions. When a block heater is used for the preparation of liposomal vincristine sulfate injection concentrate, the block heater should be placed *outside* the sterile area. All steps required to mix and dilute the drug product should be performed *inside* the sterile area using strict aseptic technique.

For preparation of liposomal vincristine sulfate injection concentrate using a block heater, 3 heating blocks should be placed in the block heater with the block that will hold the vial containing the drug components placed between 2 blank blocks. The controller of the block heater should be set to 75°C and the temperature should be allowed to equilibrate to 73–77°C (measured by the calibrated thermometer) for 15 minutes. The temperature of the block heater should be maintained at 73–77°C throughout the preparation process. The calibrated thermometer should remain in the block heater throughout the preparation process.

For preparation of liposomal vincristine sulfate injection concentrate, a venting needle (or other suitable venting device) with a 0.2-μm filter should be inserted into the vial containing dibasic sodium phosphate solution with the point of the venting needle well above the surface of the solution. A volume of 1 mL of sphingomyelin-cholesterol liposome suspension followed by 5 mL of vincristine sulfate solution should be injected into the vial. The venting needle should then be removed and the vial should be gently inverted 5 times to mix the 3 components; the vial should *not* be shaken. The vial containing the mixture of the 3 components should be placed in the block heater for 18 minutes; the temperature of the block heater and duration in the block heater should be closely monitored using the calibrated thermometer and electronic timer. After 18 minutes, the vial should be removed from the block heater using tongs to prevent burns. The start time and temperature and the end time and temperature should be recorded on the liposomal vincristine sulfate injection concentrate overlabel immediately after the vial is placed into the block heater and upon removal, respectively. The vial should be gently inverted another 5 times to mix the contents; the vial should *not* be shaken. The resultant liposomal vincristine sulfate injection concentrate contains vincristine sulfate 0.16 mg/mL and should be stored at room temperature (15–30°C) for no more than 12 hours. Liposomal vincristine sulfate injection concentrate should be allowed to come to room temperature (i.e., 15–30°C) over at least 30 minutes prior to dilution.

For preparation of the *final* diluted IV infusion of liposomal vincristine sulfate, a volume equivalent to the volume of the appropriate dose of liposomal vincristine sulfate should be withdrawn from an infusion bag containing 100 mL of 5% dextrose or 0.9% sodium chloride injection and discarded; the appropriate dose of liposomal vincristine sulfate injection concentrate is then withdrawn from the vial and added to the infusion bag to yield a final volume of 100 mL. The infusion bag label supplied by the drug's manufacturer should be completed and affixed to the bag. Infusion of the diluted drug should be completed within 12 hours of *initiation* of preparation of liposomal vincristine sulfate injection.

■ **Dosage** ***Conventional Vincristine Sulfate*** Various conventional vincristine sulfate dosages have been used. Clinicians should consult published protocols for the dosage of conventional vincristine sulfate and other chemotherapeutic agents and the method and sequence of administration. The manufacturers of conventional vincristine sulfate recommend a usual adult dose of 1.4 mg/m^2 and a usual pediatric dose of 1.5–2 mg/m^2. For children weighing 10 kg or less, the manufacturers of conventional vincristine sulfate recommend that therapy be initiated at 0.05 mg/kg once weekly. Some clinicians recommend that adult doses not exceed 2 mg of conventional vincristine sulfate. Subsequent doses must be determined by the clinical and hematologic response and tolerance of the patient in order to obtain optimum therapeutic results with minimum adverse effects. Conventional vincristine is usually administered at weekly intervals. Small daily doses are not recommended because they produce severe toxicity with no added therapeutic benefit.

Liposomal Vincristine Sulfate For the treatment of Philadelphia chromosome-negative (Ph$^-$) relapsed or refractory ALL in patients in second or greater relapse or in those whose disease has progressed following at least 2 prior therapies, the recommended adult dosage of liposomal vincristine sulfate is 2.25 mg/m^2 of vincristine sulfate administered IV over 1 hour once weekly.

Dosage Modification for Toxicity **Neurologic Toxicity.** Careful monitoring for neurologic toxicity including clinical evaluation (e.g., history, physical examination) is advised, and dosage reduction may be necessary, particularly in patients with preexisting neuromuscular disease or in patients receiving other agents with neurotoxic potential. Adverse neurologic effects, such as neuritic pain or constipation, may lessen or disappear when the dosage of conventional vincristine is reduced.

If grade 3 peripheral neuropathy (severe symptoms resulting in interference with self-care activities of daily living) occurs in patients receiving liposomal vincristine, therapy with the drug should be withheld. If grade 3 peripheral neuropathy persists or worsens despite interruption of therapy, liposomal vincristine therapy should be discontinued. If peripheral neuropathy improves to grade 2 or less, liposomal vincristine therapy may be resumed at a reduced vincristine sulfate dosage (i.e., 2.25 mg/m^2 reduced to 2 mg/m^2).

If persistent grade 2 peripheral neuropathy (moderate symptoms resulting in interference with instrumental activities of daily living) occurs in patients receiving liposomal vincristine, therapy with the drug should be withheld. If grade 2 peripheral neuropathy worsens to grade 3 or 4 despite interruption of therapy, liposomal vincristine therapy should be discontinued. If the toxicity improves, liposomal vincristine therapy may be resumed at a reduced vincristine sulfate dosage (i.e., 2.25 mg/m^2 reduced to 2 mg/m^2).

If the patient has persistent grade 2 peripheral neuropathy at a reduced dosage of 2 mg/m^2, liposomal vincristine therapy should be withheld again for up to 7 days. If grade 2 peripheral neuropathy worsens despite interruption of therapy, liposomal vincristine therapy should be discontinued. If the toxicity improves to grade 1, liposomal vincristine therapy may be resumed at a further reduced vincristine sulfate dosage (i.e., 2 mg/m^2 reduced to 1.825 mg/m^2). If the patient has persistent grade 2 peripheral neuropathy at a dosage of 1.825 mg/m^2, liposomal vincristine therapy should be withheld again for up to 7 days. If grade 2 peripheral neuropathy worsens despite interruption of therapy, liposomal vincristine therapy should be discontinued. If the toxicity improves to grade 1, liposomal vincristine therapy may be resumed at a further reduced vincristine sulfate dosage (i.e., 1.825 mg/m^2 reduced to 1.5 mg/m^2).

Hematologic Toxicity. Complete blood cell (CBC) counts should be performed before the administration of each dose of conventional or liposomal vincristine.

Following administration of conventional vincristine, a decrease in leukocyte count or platelet count may occur, particularly in patients for whom previous therapy or disease has reduced bone marrow function. In patients with leukopenia or infectious complications, withholding of the next dose of conventional vincristine should be considered. Leukopenia may lessen or disappear when the dosage of conventional vincristine is reduced.

If grade 3 or 4 neutropenia, thrombocytopenia, or anemia occurs in patients receiving liposomal vincristine, dosage reduction or temporary interruption of liposomal vincristine therapy and supportive care measures should be considered.

Hepatic Toxicity. If hepatotoxicity occurs in patients receiving liposomal vincristine, dosage reduction or temporary interruption of liposomal vincristine therapy should be considered.

Pulmonary Toxicity. Conventional vincristine therapy should be discontinued in patients who develop progressive dyspnea.

Other Nonhematologic Toxicity. If fatigue occurs in patients receiving liposomal vincristine, dosage reduction, temporary interruption, or discontinuance of liposomal vincristine therapy should be considered.

■ **Dosage in Hepatic Impairment** A 50% reduction in conventional vincristine dose is recommended for patients with a direct serum bilirubin concentration exceeding 3 mg/dL or other evidence of clinically important hepatic impairment.

The manufacturer makes no specific recommendations regarding dosage of liposomal vincristine in patients with hepatic impairment. (See Pharmacokinetics.)

Cautions

In general, adverse reactions to vincristine are dose related and reversible.

The incidence of adverse effects associated with liposomal vincristine is based principally on clinical trial data for 83 patients with Philadelphia chromosome-negative (Ph$^-$) relapsed or refractory acute lymphocytic (lymphoblastic) leukemia (ALL) who received the drug at the recommended dosage. The most common adverse effects, each occurring in more than 30% of patients, included constipation, nausea, fever, fatigue, peripheral neuropathy, febrile neutropenia, diarrhea, anemia, decreased appetite, and insomnia. All patients receiving the drug experienced adverse effects; 96% of patients experienced grade 3 or greater adverse effects, and 76% experienced serious adverse effects, most commonly febrile neutropenia (21%), fever (13%), hypotension (7%), respiratory distress (6%), and cardiac arrest (6%). Dose reduction, delay, or omission occurred in 53% of patients, and 28% of patients discontinued therapy because of adverse events, including peripheral neuropathy (10%), leukemia-related effects (7%), and tumor lysis syndrome (2%).

■ **Nervous System Effects** The major and dose-limiting adverse effect of conventional and liposomal vincristine is neurotoxicity, the severity of which may vary greatly among patients. Adverse neuromuscular effects often occur in a sequence with early development of sensory impairment and paresthesia followed by neuritic pain and motor difficulties as therapy with conventional vincristine is continued. The most frequent neurotoxic manifestation is peripheral (mixed sensorimotor) neuropathy, which occurs in nearly every patient receiving conventional vincristine. In clinical trials in patients with ALL, peripheral neuropathy occurred in 39% of patients receiving liposomal vincristine and was grade 3 or greater in 17% of patients receiving the drug. The earliest and most consistent indication of peripheral neuropathy is asymptomatic depression of the Achilles reflex. Loss of other deep tendon reflexes occurs in most patients after 3 or more weekly doses of conventional vincristine, and peripheral paresthesias, especially numbness, pain, and tingling, are common. If prolonged or high-dose conventional vincristine therapy is given, wrist drop, foot drop, cranial nerve palsy, atrophy, cramps, ataxia, slapping gait, and difficulty in walking or inability to walk may occur. Cranial nerve palsies may account for headaches and jaw pain; jaw pain usually occurs within 24 hours after the first and/or second dose of conventional vincristine and rarely recurs. Pain in other areas, including pharyngeal, parotid gland, bone, back, or limb pain as well as myalgia, has been reported in patients receiving vincristine and may be severe. Cranial nerve palsies and muscular weakness involving the larynx may produce hoarseness and vocal cord paresis, including potentially life-threatening bilateral vocal cord paralysis, while those involving extrinsic eye muscles may cause ptosis, double vision, and optic and extraocular neuropathy. Optic atrophy with blindness or transient cortical blindness has been reported in patients receiving conventional vincristine. Peripheral neuritis (both mononeuritis and polyneuritis) and neuralgia also occur frequently in patients receiving conventional vincristine. Grade 3 or greater asthenia and muscle weakness have been reported during clinical trials in 5 and 1%, respectively, of patients with ALL receiving liposomal vincristine.

Vincristine also produces autonomic and CNS toxicity, although less frequently than peripheral neuropathy. Autonomic effects commonly include severe constipation or obstipation, abdominal cramps, bowel obstruction, and colonic pseudo-obstruction. Adynamic ileus, which mimics "surgical abdomen," is particularly likely to occur in young children. In clinical trials in patients with ALL, grade 3 or greater constipation occurred in 5% of patients receiving liposomal vincristine and grade 3 or greater ileus and colonic pseudo-obstruction occurred in 6% of patients receiving the drug. Constipation may take the form of upper-colon impaction, and a flat abdominal film may be used to facilitate diagnosis so the clinician is not misled by presentation of colicky abdominal pain coupled with an empty rectum. Constipation may be treated with high enemas and laxatives. A routine regimen (e.g., laxatives, enemas) to prevent constipation is recommended for patients receiving conventional or liposomal vincristine. When conventional vincristine is administered in single weekly doses, constipation usually persists less than 7 days; abdominal cramps and adynamic ileus in children usually also disappear in 1 week or less. Urinary tract disturbances including bladder atony, incontinence, urinary retention, nocturia, oliguria, dysuria, and polyuria also have been reported in patients receiving conventional vincristine. Whenever possible, other drugs known to cause urinary retention should be discontinued during the first few days following administration of conventional vincristine, particularly in geriatric patients. Other autonomic effects of vincristine include orthostatic hypotension, abnormal Valsalva response, defective sweating, and myoclonic jerks. CNS effects including episodes of altered consciousness and mental changes such as depression, agitation, insomnia, and hallucinations have been reported. Seizures (frequently accompanied by hypertension), progressive encephalopathy, respiratory difficulties, and coma also have occurred. Seizures followed by coma have been reported in several pediatric patients receiving conventional vincristine.

Neurotoxic effects of conventional or liposomal vincristine may be additive with those of other neurotoxic agents and spinal cord irradiation. Geriatric patients and those with underlying neurologic disease may be more susceptible than other patients to the neurotoxic effects of conventional or liposomal vincristine. No antidote to the neurotoxic effects of vincristine has been found to date. Most experts reduce the dose or discontinue the drug if depression of reflexes, paresthesia, and/or motor weakness develop. Sensory loss, paresthesia, difficulty in walking, slapping gait, loss of deep tendon reflexes, and/or muscle wasting may persist during conventional vincristine therapy. Generalized sensorimotor dysfunction may become increasingly severe with continued therapy with conventional vincristine. Recovery from neurotoxicity usually begins with the discontinuance of conventional vincristine. Paresthesia is the most readily reversible, followed by motor and sensory impairment. Although these symptoms resolve by about the sixth week following discontinuance of conventional vincristine therapy in most patients, some patients may experience neuromuscular problems for prolonged periods. Depressed deep tendon reflexes return slowly, if at all, and some patients experience minor neurologic symptoms up to several months after conventional vincristine has been discontinued.

■ **Respiratory Effects** Acute shortness of breath and bronchospasm, which can be severe or life threatening, have occurred following administration of vinca alkaloids (e.g., vincristine), being reported most frequently when mitomycin was used concomitantly with conventional vincristine. Such reactions may occur a few minutes to several hours after administration of a vinca alkaloid or up to 2 weeks after a dose of mitomycin. Progressive dyspnea, which may require chronic therapy, can occur in patients receiving conventional vincristine; the drug should not be readministered to these patients. In clinical trials in patients with ALL, respiratory distress or failure has been reported in 6 or 5%, respectively, of patients receiving liposomal vincristine.

■ **Dermatologic Effects** Alopecia is reported to occur in 20–70% of patients who receive conventional vincristine. Alopecia is reversible when conventional vincristine is discontinued. Regrowth of hair may occur even when conventional vincristine is continued in therapeutic doses. Rash has occurred occasionally in patients receiving conventional vincristine.

■ **Sensitivity Reactions** Allergic reactions, including anaphylaxis, rash, and edema, that were temporally related to conventional vincristine therapy have been reported in patients receiving the drug as part of combination chemotherapy regimens.

■ **Hematologic Effects** Hematologic toxicity produced by vincristine is less than that produced by most other antineoplastic agents; therefore, the drug is useful in patients with pancytopenia or in combination regimens. Anemia, leukopenia, and thrombocytopenia have been reported. Leukopenia usually persists less than 7 days when conventional vincristine is given in single weekly doses. In clinical trials in patients with ALL, grade 3 or greater anemia, neutropenia, and thrombocytopenia each have been reported in 17–18% of patients receiving liposomal vincristine, and grade 3 or greater febrile neutropenia has occurred in 31% of patients. An increase in the platelet count has been observed in some patients with thrombocytopenia after initiation of therapy with conventional vincristine before evidence of marrow remission is apparent.

■ **Local Effects** Vincristine is a tissue irritant and may cause phlebitis and necrosis. Extravasation results in pain and cellulitis. The manufacturers of conventional vincristine state that local injection of hyaluronidase and application of moderate heat may decrease local reactions resulting from extravasation; however, some clinicians prefer to treat extravasation with cold compresses, dilution with 0.9% sodium chloride injection or infiltration of sodium bicarbonate (5 mL of 8.4% injection), and/or local injection of hydrocortisone. The manufacturer of liposomal vincristine states that the infusion should be discontinued immediately if extravasation is suspected and local treatments should be considered.

■ **Cardiovascular Effects** Hypertension and hypotension have been reported in patients receiving vincristine. In clinical trials in patients with ALL, grade 3 or greater hypotension and cardiac arrest each have been reported in 6% of patients receiving liposomal vincristine. Coronary artery disease and myocardial infarction have occurred in patients receiving conventional vincristine in combination with other antineoplastic agents. Although a causal relationship has not been established, infarction was temporally related to administration of conventional vincristine in several patients, occurring within several hours after injection of the drug. Some conventional vincristine-treated patients who developed myocardial infarction had previously received radiation therapy to the mediastinal area, but infarction also has been reported in patients with no history of mediastinal radiation or risk factors associated with coronary artery disease.

■ **GI Effects** In addition to adverse GI effects of neurogenic origin associated with conventional or liposomal vincristine therapy (see Cautions: Nervous System Effects), local effects including nausea, vomiting, diarrhea, abdominal distention, stomatitis, and oral ulceration occur occasionally in patients receiving conventional vincristine. In clinical trials in patients with ALL, nausea, diarrhea and decreased appetite have been reported in 52, 37, and 33%, respectively, of patients receiving liposomal vincristine. Intestinal necrosis and/or perforation and anorexia also have been reported in patients receiving conventional vincristine.

■ **Otic Effects** Eighth cranial nerve damage, which may be manifested by vestibular manifestations such as dizziness, nystagmus, and vertigo, and by auditory manifestations such as varying degrees of hearing impairment (including partial or total deafness) that may be temporary or permanent, has been reported in patients receiving vinca alkaloids. The manufacturers of conventional vincristine state that the drug should be used concomitantly with other potentially ototoxic drugs such as platinum-containing antineoplastic agents with extreme caution.

■ **Endocrine Effects** A syndrome of inappropriate secretion of antidiuretic hormone (SIADH) has occurred rarely in patients receiving conventional vincristine therapy. The syndrome may be associated with the neurotoxicity of the drug, possibly resulting from a direct effect on the hypothalamus. In these patients, hyponatremia associated with increased urinary sodium excretion occurs without evidence of renal or adrenal disease, hypotension, dehydration, azotemia, or clinical edema. Fluid restriction produces improvement in sodium balance and facilitates the safe use of repeated courses of conventional vincristine in patients who experience this syndrome.

■ **Metabolic Effects** Tumor lysis syndrome may occur following rapid lysis of malignant cells. The risk of tumor lysis syndrome is increased in patients with non-Hodgkin's lymphomas or leukemia. Such patients should be monitored closely and appropriate precautions should be taken. In some patients, uric acid nephropathy may result. These effects may be minimized by adequate hydration, alkalinization of the urine, and/or administration of allopurinol.

■ **Hepatic Effects** Hepatic veno-occlusive disease, sometimes fatal, has been reported in patients receiving conventional vincristine, particularly in pediatric patients receiving conventional vincristine in combination with other chemotherapy agents. Hepatotoxicity, sometimes fatal, also has occurred in patients receiving liposomal vincristine. Grade 3 or greater elevations in AST concentrations have been reported during clinical trials in 6–11% of patients receiving liposomal vincristine.

■ **Other Adverse Effects** Other occasionally occurring adverse effects of conventional vincristine include fever and, at high doses, weight loss. In clinical trials in patients with ALL, fever and fatigue have occurred in 43 and 41%, respectively, of patients receiving liposomal vincristine and were grade 3 or greater in 15 and 12%, respectively, of patients receiving the drug. In these clinical trials, grade 3 or greater infections (e.g., pneumonia, septic shock, staphylococcal bacteremia) occurred in 40% of patients receiving liposomal vincristine and grade 3 or greater pain and abdominal pain each occurred in 8% of patients.

■ **Precautions and Contraindications** Vincristine is a highly toxic drug with a low therapeutic index, and a therapeutic response is not likely to occur without some evidence of toxicity. Vincristine must be used only under constant supervision by clinicians experienced in therapy with cytotoxic agents and should only be administered by individuals experienced in administration of the drug. (See Dosage and Administration: Reconstitution and Administration.) Patients and/or their parents or guardians should be advised of the possibility of adverse effects and associated manifestations.

Because of the hepatic metabolism and biliary excretion of vincristine, some clinicians recommend reduced doses in patients with obstructive jaundice or other hepatic impairment. Conventional and liposomal vincristine must be given with care, and dosage and toxicity monitored, particularly in patients receiving other neurotoxic drugs or those with preexisting neuromuscular disease. Complete blood cell (CBC) counts should be performed before the administration of each dose of conventional or liposomal vincristine. Serum concentrations of uric acid should be determined frequently during the first 3–4 weeks of therapy in patients receiving vincristine for the induction of remission in acute leukemia, and appropriate measures should be taken to prevent the occurrence of hyperuricemia related to the rapid lysis of leukemic cells. Because of the potential for hepatotoxicity, liver function tests should be monitored.

The manufacturer states that conventional vincristine is contraindicated in patients with the demyelinating form of Charcot-Marie-Tooth syndrome. Conventional vincristine also should not be administered to patients while they are receiving radiation therapy through ports that include the liver. Liposomal vincristine is contraindicated in patients with demyelinating conditions including Charcot-Marie-Tooth syndrome. Liposomal vincristine also is contraindicated in patients with known hypersensitivity to the conventional or liposomal drug or to any ingredient in the formulation.

Care must be taken to avoid contact of conventional vincristine sulfate solutions with the eye(s), as severe irritation or corneal ulceration (especially if the drug is administered under pressure) may result. If contact with the eye(s) occurs, the eye(s) should be washed immediately with copious amounts of water; patients should consult a clinician if ocular irritation persists.

■ **Pediatric Precautions** The manufacturer states that safety and efficacy of liposomal vincristine in pediatric patients have not been established.

■ **Geriatric Precautions** Vincristine should be used with caution in geriatric patients because of the greater frequency of decreased hepatic, renal, and/or cardiac function and of concomitant disease and drug therapy observed in this age group.

■ **Mutagenicity and Carcinogenicity** Genotoxicity has been demonstrated with conventional vincristine in some in vivo and in vitro studies; however, in vivo and in vitro tests have failed to demonstrate conclusively that vincristine is mutagenic. There was no evidence of carcinogenicity following intraperitoneal administration of conventional vincristine in rats and mice, but the study was limited. Patients receiving chemotherapy that included conventional vincristine and drugs known to be carcinogenic have developed secondary malignancies; however, the contribution of vincristine has not been determined. Formal carcinogenicity studies have not been conducted for conventional or liposomal vincristine.

■ **Pregnancy, Fertility, and Lactation** Vincristine can cause fetal toxicity when administered to pregnant women, but potential benefits from use of the drug may be acceptable in certain conditions despite the possible risks to the fetus. The drug can induce teratogenic and embryocidal effects in animals at doses that are not toxic to the pregnant animal. Dosages of conventional vincristine that caused resorption of 23–85% of fetuses in pregnant mice and hamsters produced fetal malformations that were present in surviving offspring. In 5 monkeys receiving single doses of conventional vincristine between days 27–34 of gestation, 3 fetuses were normal at term, while 2 had grossly evident malformations. Administration of liposomal vincristine to pregnant rats during organogenesis caused teratogenicity (skeletal and visceral malformations), decreased fetal weight, increased embryofetal deaths (resorptions, postimplantation losses), and decreased maternal body weight. Fetal malformations were observed in pregnant rats receiving liposomal vincristine at exposure levels that were approximately 20–40% of the human exposure at the recommended dosage. There are no adequate and controlled studies to date using conventional or liposomal vincristine in pregnant women, and the drugs should be used during pregnancy only in life-threatening situations or severe disease for which safer drugs cannot be used or are ineffective. Women of childbearing potential should be advised to avoid becoming pregnant while receiving conventional or liposomal vincristine. When conventional or liposomal vincristine is administered during pregnancy or the patient becomes pregnant while receiving the drug, the patient should be informed of the potential hazard to the fetus.

Reproduction studies in animals using conventional vincristine have not been performed to date; however, an animal toxicology study indicates that liposomal vincristine may impair male fertility, which is consistent with literature on conventional vincristine. Azoospermia and increased plasma concentrations of follicle-stimulating hormone have occurred in males who received combination chemotherapy that included conventional vincristine and prednisone with cyclophosphamide or mechlorethamine and procarbazine, and amenorrhea has occurred in females receiving chemotherapy that included conventional vincristine. The manufacturers state that irreversible azoospermia or amenorrhea is less likely when chemotherapy that includes conventional vincristine is administered in prepubertal patients. Epididymal aspermia and testicular degeneration and atrophy have occurred in rats receiving liposomal vincristine.

It is not known whether vincristine or its metabolites are distributed into milk. Because of the potential for serious adverse effects in nursing infants, a decision should be made whether to discontinue nursing or conventional or liposomal vincristine, taking into account the importance of the drug to the woman.

Drug Interactions

Formal studies of drug interactions have not been conducted for liposomal vincristine; however, liposomal vincristine is expected to interact with drugs known to interact with conventional vincristine.

■ **Phenytoin** Simultaneous administration of phenytoin (oral or IV) and combination chemotherapy containing conventional vincristine may reduce serum concentrations of phenytoin and increase seizure activity. The mechanism of this interaction may involve reduced absorption of phenytoin and an increase in the rate of its metabolism and elimination. (See Drug Interactions: Drugs Affecting Hepatic Microsomal Enzymes.)

■ **Antineoplastic Agents** When conventional vincristine and asparaginase must be administered sequentially, the sequence of conventional vincristine followed by asparaginase is recommended. Conventional vincristine should be administered 12–24 hours preceding administration of asparaginase to minimize toxicity; administration of asparaginase first may reduce hepatic clearance of vincristine and increase the severity of adverse effects of the drug.

Concomitant use of mitomycin and conventional vincristine may increase the risk of serious adverse respiratory effects, particularly in patients with preexisting pulmonary dysfunction. (See Cautions: Respiratory Effects.)

■ **Drugs Affecting Hepatic Microsomal Enzymes** Metabolism of vinca alkaloids is mediated by the cytochrome P-450 (CYP) isoenzyme 3A, and the possibility exists that potent inhibitors of this isoenzyme may impair metabolism of vinca alkaloids. Concomitant use of azole antifungal agents (e.g., itraconazole, ketoconazole, posaconazole, voriconazole) and vincristine may increase plasma concentrations of vincristine and has resulted in serious adverse effects, including neuropathy (peripheral, autonomic, and cranial neuropathy), seizures, hyponatremia or syndrome of inappropriate secretion of antidiuretic hormone (SIADH), and GI toxicity (including paralytic ileus); earlier onset and/or increased severity of adverse neuromuscular effects has occurred. Therefore, concomitant use of vincristine with potent CYP3A inhibitors (e.g., atazanavir, clarithromycin, indinavir, itraconazole, ketoconazole, nefazodone, nelfinavir, posaconazole, ritonavir, saquinavir, telithromycin, voriconazole) should be avoided. Azole antifungal agents should be used concomitantly with vincristine only in patients who have no alternative antifungal treatment options; if concomitant use cannot be avoided, patients should be monitored frequently for toxicity.

Concomitant use of vincristine with potent CYP3A inducers (e.g., carbamazepine, dexamethasone, phenobarbital, phenytoin, rifabutin, rifampin, rifapentine, St. John's wort [*Hypericum perforatum*]) should be avoided.

■ **Drugs Affecting or Affected by P-glycoprotein Transport** Vincristine is a P-glycoprotein (P-gp) substrate, and the possibility exists that potent inhibitors or inducers of P-gp may alter the pharmacokinetics or pharmacodynamics of vincristine. Concomitant use of vincristine with potent P-gp inhibitors or inducers should be avoided.

■ **Ototoxic Drugs** Since varying degrees of permanent or temporary hearing impairment associated with eighth cranial nerve damage have been reported in patients receiving vinca alkaloids, vincristine should be used concomitantly with other potentially ototoxic drugs such as platinum-containing antineoplastic agents with extreme caution.

Acute Toxicity

Overdosage with vincristine produces adverse effects that are mainly extensions of common adverse effects. Doses 10 times the usual recommended doses of conventional vincristine sulfate have been lethal in children younger than 13 years of age, and severe manifestations of toxicity have been apparent following administration of 3–4 mg/m^2 in this age group. Single doses of 3 mg/m^2 of conventional vincristine sulfate can be expected to produce severe toxic manifestations in adults. Increased severity of adverse effects may be experienced by patients with hepatic impairment characterized by decreased biliary excretion. Grade 3 motor neuropathy and grade 4 grand mal seizure, elevated concentrations of AST, and hyperbilirubinemia occurred following administration of 2.4 mg/m^2 of vincristine sulfate as the liposomal drug.

Following vincristine overdosage, supportive and symptomatic treatment should be initiated. Treatment should include the prevention of adverse effects resulting from the syndrome of inappropriate secretion of antidiuretic hormone (SIADH) (e.g., by restricting fluid intake and possibly by use of an appropriate diuretic); prophylactic administration of anticonvulsants; use of enemas to prevent ileus (in some cases, decompression of the GI tract may be necessary); monitoring of the cardiovascular system;

and daily blood counts to monitor the hematologic system and guide transfusion requirements. Studies in mice and a few case reports have suggested that administration of leucovorin calcium may be of some value in the management of vincristine overdosage. A suggested regimen is to administer leucovorin calcium 100 mg IV every 3 hours for 24 hours and then every 6 hours for at least 48 hours. Treatment with leucovorin calcium does not preclude the need for the usual treatment measures. Because only small amounts of vincristine are removed by hemodialysis, removal of the drug by this method is not likely to be helpful following overdosage.

In dogs pretreated with cholestyramine, fecal excretion of vincristine was increased; no published data are available regarding the use of cholestyramine as a possible antidote for vincristine overdosage in humans. No published data are available on the clinical outcome of oral ingestion of conventional vincristine. If oral ingestion of vincristine occurs, the stomach should be emptied immediately followed by oral administration of activated charcoal and a cathartic.

Pharmacology

Although the mechanism of action has not been fully elucidated, vincristine and other vinca alkaloids exert their cytotoxic effects by binding to tubulin, the protein subunit of the microtubules that form the mitotic spindle. The formation of vincristine-tubulin complexes prevents the polymerization of the tubulin subunits into microtubules and induces depolymerization of microtubules resulting in inhibition of microtubule assembly and cellular metaphase arrest. In high concentrations, the drug also exerts complex effects on nucleic acid and protein synthesis. Vincristine exerts some immunosuppressive activity.

Pharmacokinetics

■ **Absorption** Vincristine sulfate is unpredictably absorbed from the GI tract. Following rapid IV injection of a 2-mg dose of conventional vincristine sulfate in patients with normal renal and hepatic function, peak serum drug concentrations of approximately 0.19–0.89 μM occur immediately and the drug is rapidly cleared from serum. The area under the serum vincristine concentration-time curve has been shown to be increased following continuous IV infusion of conventional vincristine compared with rapid IV injection of the drug when comparable doses are administered. Following IV infusion over 1 hour of a 2.25-mg/m^2 dose of vincristine sulfate as the liposomal drug in patients with acute lymphocytic leukemia (ALL), peak concentrations of total vincristine sulfate average 1220 ng/mL and reflect liposome-encapsulated drug that may not be immediately bioavailable. Because clearance of the drug is slower following administration as liposomal vincristine, systemic exposure of the drug is increased relative to that of conventional vincristine.

■ **Distribution** Distribution of vincristine and its metabolites (and/or decomposition products) into human body tissues and fluids has not been fully characterized, but the drug is rapidly and apparently widely distributed following IV administration of conventional vincristine. Drug that is distributed into tissues is tightly but reversibly bound. Vincristine and its metabolites (and/or decomposition products) are rapidly and extensively distributed into bile, with peak biliary concentrations occurring within 2–4 hours after rapid IV injection of conventional vincristine. Vincristine and its metabolites (and/or decomposition products) cross the blood-brain barrier poorly following rapid IV injection of conventional vincristine and generally do not appear in the CSF in cytotoxic concentrations. It is not known whether vincristine and its metabolites are distributed into milk.

■ **Elimination** Following rapid IV injection of conventional vincristine, serum concentrations of the drug appear to decline in a triphasic manner. The terminal elimination half-life of conventional vincristine has ranged from 19–155 hours. Clearance of the drug is slower following administration as a liposome-encapsulated formulation compared with administration as a conventional formulation (345 versus 11,340 mL/hour).

The metabolic fate of vincristine has not been clearly determined; the drug appears to be extensively metabolized, probably in the liver by the cytochrome P-450 microsomal enzyme system, including CYP3A, but the extent of metabolism is not clear since the drug also apparently undergoes decomposition in vivo. In patients with hepatic impairment, metabolism of vincristine may be decreased. Vincristine and its metabolites (and/or decomposition products) are excreted principally in feces via biliary elimination. Following rapid IV injection of conventional vincristine in adults with normal renal and hepatic function, about 30% of a dose is excreted in feces within 24 hours and 70% within 72 hours; about 10% of a dose is excreted in urine within 24 hours, with very little urinary excretion occurring thereafter. Following IV administration of liposomal vincristine, the extent of urinary excretion (less than 8% of the administered dose within 96 hours) is similar to that of conventional vincristine. The effects of hepatic impairment on the elimination of vincristine and its metabolites (and/or decomposition products) have not been established, but individuals with decreased hepatic function may have impaired elimination. In a limited number of patients with melanoma and moderate hepatic impairment (Child-Pugh class B) secondary to liver metastases, dose-adjusted peak plasma concentrations and systemic exposure of liposomal vincristine were similar to those observed in patients with ALL and normal hepatic function.

Only small amounts of vincristine are removed by hemodialysis.

Chemistry and Stability

■ **Chemistry** Vincristine sulfate, a naturally occurring vinca alkaloid, is an antimicrotubule antineoplastic agent. Vincristine sulfate is the salt of a dimeric alkaloid isolated from *Catharanthus roseus*. Vincristine sulfate occurs as a white, off-white, or slightly yellow, hygroscopic, amorphous or crystalline powder and is freely soluble in water and slightly soluble in alcohol. Sulfuric acid, sodium hydroxide, acetic acid, and/or sodium acetate is added during the manufacture of conventional vincristine sulfate injection to adjust pH to 4–5 or 3.5–5.5 depending on the preparation; the injection also contains mannitol.

Liposomal vincristine sulfate (Marqibo®) is commercially available as a 3-vial kit containing single-use vials of vincristine sulfate solution, sphingomyelin-cholesterol liposome suspension, and dibasic sodium phosphate solution. When prepared as directed, vincristine sulfate liposome injection is a sterile, preservative-free, white to off-white suspension of vincristine sulfate encapsulated in sphingomyelin-cholesterol liposomes. Each mL of vincristine sulfate liposome injection contains 0.16 mg of vincristine sulfate; more than 95% of the drug is encapsulated in liposomes. The liposomes are composed of sphingomyelin and cholesterol in a molar ratio of approximately 60:40; the mean liposome diameter is approximately 100 nm. Vincristine sulfate liposome injection also contains dibasic sodium phosphate, sodium citrate, citric acid, mannitol, sodium chloride, and ethanol.

■ **Stability** Conventional vincristine sulfate solutions are light-sensitive and must be protected from light. Conventional vincristine sulfate injection should be refrigerated at 2–8°C; the vials should be stored in an upright position.

Commercially available liposomal vincristine sulfate (Marqibo®) kits containing single-use vials of vincristine sulfate solution, sphingomyelin-cholesterol liposome suspension, and dibasic sodium phosphate solution should be refrigerated at 2–8°C and should not be frozen. Once the 3 components have been admixed, the resultant liposomal vincristine sulfate injection concentrate may be stored at 15–30°C for up to 12 hours. Administration of the final diluted preparation of the drug should be completed within 12 hours of *initiation* of preparation of vincristine sulfate liposome injection.

When preparing a diluted solution, the manufacturer states that conventional vincristine sulfate injection should be mixed only with 0.9% sodium chloride injection or 5% dextrose injection; the drug should not be diluted in solutions that raise or lower the pH outside the range of 3.5–5.5.

Specialized references should be consulted for specific compatibility information. Doses of 0.5, 1, 2, or 3 mg of conventional vincristine sulfate diluted in 25 or 50 mL of 0.9% sodium chloride solution in small-volume IV bags (i.e., minibags) or in 20 mL of 0.9% sodium chloride solution in a 30-mL syringe remained stable when stored for 7 days at 4°C followed by 2 days at 23°C.

For further information on the handling of antineoplastic agents, see the ASHP Guidelines on Handling Hazardous Drugs at http://www.ahfsdruginformation.com.

Preparations

Excipients in commercially available drug preparations may have clinically important effects in some individuals; consult specific product labeling for details.

vinCRIStine Sulfate

Parenteral

Injection, for IV use only	1 mg/mL (1 and 2 mg)*	**Vincristine Sulfate Injection**

*available from one or more manufacturer, distributor, and/or repackager by generic (nonproprietary) name

vinCRIStine Sulfate Liposomal

Parenteral

Kit, for suspension, for injection, for IV infusion only	1 Vial, Injection, Vincristine Sulfate 5 mg/5 mL (for preparation of liposome-encapsulated vincristine sulfate suspension, 0.16 mg [of vincristine sulfate] per mL [5 mg]), 1 Vial, For injectable suspension, Sphingomyelin/Cholesterol Liposome 103 mg/mL (Sphingomyelin 73.5 mg/mL and Cholesterol 29.5 mg/mL) 1 Vial, Injection, Sodium Phosphate, Dibasic 355 mg/25mL	**Marqibo®** (available with flotation ring, vial overlabel, and infusion bag label), Spectrum

†Use is not currently included in the labeling approved by the US Food and Drug Administration

Vinorelbine Tartrate

Didehydrodeoxynorvincaleukoblastine

■ Vinorelbine, a semisynthetic vinca alkaloid, is an antineoplastic agent.

Uses

■ **Non-small Cell Lung Cancer** ***Adjuvant Therapy*** Cisplatin-containing chemotherapy, such as cisplatin in combination with vinorelbine, is used for the adjuvant treatment of completely resected non-small cell lung cancer†.

The use of cisplatin-containing adjuvant therapy prolongs survival in patients with completely resected non-small cell lung cancer. (Also see Uses: Non-small Cell Lung Cancer in Cisplatin 10:00.) In the International Adjuvant Lung Cancer Trial (IALT), 1867 patients with completely resected stage I, II, or III non-small cell lung cancer were assigned to receive either adjuvant chemotherapy (cisplatin with etoposide, or cisplatin with a vinca alkaloid) or observation. At 5 years, the rate of survival was higher among patients receiving cisplatin-based adjuvant therapy (44.5%) than among those assigned to observation (40.4%). Subset analysis of pooled abstracted data from 11 randomized trials including this one indicates that adjuvant therapy with cisplatin-based therapy prolongs survival in patients with completely resected non-small cell lung cancer.

Vinorelbine is used in combination with cisplatin as adjuvant therapy for completely resected non-small cell lung cancer. In a randomized trial (National Cancer Institute of Canada and Intergroup JBR10 study) involving 482 patients with completely resected stage IB or stage II non-small cell lung cancer, overall survival (94 versus 73 months) and relapse-free survival were prolonged in patients receiving adjuvant therapy with vinorelbine and cisplatin compared with those assigned to observation. Retrospective analysis of the data from this clinical trial showed that, despite receiving lower dose intensities of both drugs, patients older than 65 years experienced a survival benefit similar to that observed for all patients receiving adjuvant therapy with vinorelbine and cisplatin for non-small cell lung cancer. In the Adjuvant Navelbine International Trialist Association (ANITA) trial, which involved 840 patients with stage IB, II, or IIIA non-small cell lung cancer, median survival was prolonged (66 versus 44 months) in patients receiving adjuvant therapy with vinorelbine and cisplatin compared with those assigned to observation.

Analysis of pooled data for individual patients from 5 large randomized trials, including the IALT, JBR10, and ANITA studies, indicates that adjuvant treatment with cisplatin-based therapy prolongs survival in patients with completely resected non-small cell lung cancer. Subgroup analysis showed that survival benefit varies according to stage of disease; cisplatin-based adjuvant chemotherapy prolongs survival in patients with stage II or III disease, may benefit some patients with stage IB disease, and may not benefit patients with stage IA disease.

Therapy for Metastatic Disease Depending on the stage of disease and the performance status of the patient, vinorelbine is used either alone or in combination with cisplatin as first-line therapy in ambulatory patients for the palliative treatment of unresectable, advanced (stage III or IV) non-small cell lung cancer.

Although the drug is active alone in this cancer, use of vinorelbine in combination with cisplatin is preferred for the treatment of advanced non-small cell lung cancer in patients with good performance status because of improved response and survival. In the American Society of Clinical Oncology (ASCO) practice guidelines for the treatment of unresectable non-small cell lung cancer (NSCLC), an expert panel recommended 2-drug combination chemotherapy for patients with good performance status (ECOG/Zubrod performance status 0 or 1); for patients with ECOG/Zubrod performance status 2, or for geriatric patients, single-agent chemotherapy, such as vinorelbine alone, may be used. A European Experts Panel that convened in April 2003 also stated that single-agent therapy may be used in patients with advanced NSCLC and ECOG performance status 2. In patients with stage IV disease, quality-of-life considerations may prompt monotherapy with vinorelbine, and the manufacturer states that such monotherapy can be used for stage IV but not stage III non-small cell lung cancer.

Age alone should not deter the use of chemotherapy for the treatment of advanced non-small cell lung cancer in geriatric patients. Data from a randomized trial demonstrate a survival benefit among geriatric patients (70 years of age or older) receiving single-agent therapy with vinorelbine compared with those receiving supportive care alone. Subgroup analysis of a phase III randomized trial according to age and performance status indicates that among patients receiving cisplatin-based combination chemotherapy for advanced non-small cell lung cancer, fit older patients (i.e., 70 years of age or older with ECOG performance status of 0 or 1) had similar outcomes for response rate and survival as younger patients; older patients were more likely to have concomitant disease and had a higher incidence rate of certain drug-related toxicities. Results of a large randomized trial among geriatric patients (70 years of age or older) with advanced non-small cell lung cancer showed that combination therapy with vinorelbine and gemcitabine did not improve survival and caused greater toxicity than single-agent therapy with either vinorelbine or gemcitabine. Systemic therapy should be offered to geriatric patients with advanced non-small cell lung cancer; further study is needed to determine optimal therapy with single agents or combination regimens for such patients.

The combination of cisplatin with vinorelbine currently is a preferred regimen for the treatment of advanced non-small cell lung cancer.

In a randomized trial involving 612 patients with advanced non-small cell lung cancer, similar results were noted for response rate, median survival, and time to disease progression between 3 platinum-based regimens; adverse effects occurring more frequently in each group included neutropenia and nausea/vomiting in patients receiving vinorelbine and cisplatin, thrombocytopenia in those receiving gemcitabine and cisplatin, and peripheral neuropathy and alopecia in those receiving paclitaxel followed by carboplatin. In another randomized trial, response rates, median survival, and 1- and 2-year survival rates were similar in patients receiving either cisplatin and vinorelbine or carboplatin and paclitaxel for advanced non-small cell lung cancer; grade 3 or 4 leukopenia and neutropenia and grade 3 nausea and vomiting were more frequent in patients receiving vinorelbine and cisplatin whereas grade 3 peripheral neuropathy occurred more frequently in patients receiving paclitaxel and carboplatin.

In a randomized study, 432 patients with stage IIIb or IV non-small cell lung cancer receiving vinorelbine 25 mg/m^2 once weekly and cisplatin 100 mg/m^2 once every 4 weeks had a longer median survival (8 versus 6 months) and higher survival rate at 1 year (38 versus 22%) than those receiving cisplatin 100 mg/m^2 once every 4 weeks. Objective response rates of 19 and 8% were observed in patients receiving vinorelbine and cisplatin versus cisplatin alone. The incidence and severity of granulocytopenia was substantially higher in patients receiving combination therapy with vinorelbine and cisplatin than in those receiving cisplatin alone. Granulocyte-colony stimulating factor was administered in approximately one-third of patients receiving combination therapy to reduce the severity of myelosuppression associated with vinorelbine. All patients in the study had a WHO performance status of 0 or 1, and none had received prior chemotherapy.

In a randomized study of 612 patients with stage III or IV non-small cell lung cancer who had not received prior chemotherapy, higher response rates and longer survival times (albeit modestly improved) were observed in patients receiving vinorelbine and cisplatin compared with those receiving either vinorelbine alone or vindesine and cisplatin. All patients in this study had a WHO performance status of 0, 1, or 2. Patients were randomized to receive single-agent vinorelbine 30 mg/m^2 once weekly; vinorelbine 30 mg/m^2 once weekly and cisplatin 120 mg/m^{2}on days 1 and 29 and then once every 6 weeks; or vindesine 3 mg/m^2 once weekly for 7 weeks and then once every other week and cisplatin 120 mg/m^2 on days 1 and 29 then once every 6 weeks. Median survival times of 9.2, 7.4, or 7.2 months were observed in patients with advanced non-small cell lung cancer receiving vinorelbine and cisplatin, vindesine and cisplatin, or vinorelbine alone, respectively. Survival at 1 year was 35% in patients receiving vinorelbine and cisplatin, 27% in those receiving vindesine and cisplatin, and 30% in those receiving single-agent therapy with vinorelbine. The overall objective response rate (all partial responses) was 28% (based on intention-to-treat analysis) in patients receiving vinorelbine and cisplatin, 19% in those receiving vindesine and cisplatin, and 14% in those receiving vinorelbine alone.

Follow-up at 5 years indicates that survival is prolonged for patients receiving vinorelbine and cisplatin compared with either vindesine and cisplatin or vinorelbine alone. However, subgroup analysis suggests that this survival benefit is obtained only among patients with a WHO performance status of 0 or 1. Among patients with nonresectable non-small cell lung cancer who have a WHO performance status of 2, single-agent therapy with vinorelbine may be appropriate.

In a clinical trial in which 211 patients with stage IV non-small cell lung cancer were randomized on a 2:1 basis to receive vinorelbine 30 mg/m^2 once weekly or fluorouracil 425 mg/m^2 IV plus leucovorin 20 mg/m^2 IV daily for 5 days every 4 weeks, respectively, median survival time was 30 weeks for patients receiving vinorelbine compared with 22 weeks for those receiving fluorouracil with leucovorin. Combination therapy with fluorouracil and leucovorin was chosen as a control treatment because this regimen has a tolerable safety profile and its activity in non-small cell lung cancer is unknown. Because the median survival time in patients with non-small cell lung cancer who received the control treatment was comparable to that usually observed in patients with untreated disease, it appears that combination therapy with fluorouracil and leucovorin did not have a detrimental effect. All patients in the study had a Karnofsky performance status of 70 or higher and none had received prior chemotherapy. Survival at 1 year was 24% in patients receiving vinorelbine and 16% in patients receiving fluorouracil with leucovorin. Overall objective response rates (all partial responses) were 12 and 3% for vinorelbine and fluorouracil with leucovorin, respectively. Measurements of quality of life assessing role functioning, physical functioning, symptom distress, and global quality of life were similar in patients receiving either vinorelbine or combination therapy with fluorouracil and leucovorin.

■ **Breast Cancer** ***Vinorelbine and Trastuzumab for HER2-positive Metastatic Breast Cancer*** Combination therapy with vinorelbine and trastuzumab is being investigated as an active regimen for the treatment of HER2-overexpressing metastatic breast cancer†.

Monotherapy for Metastatic Breast Cancer Vinorelbine is used as monotherapy in the first-line or salvage (e.g., second-line or subsequent) treatment of metastatic breast cancer†.

First-line vinorelbine monotherapy produced a median objective response rate (complete and partial responses) of 44% (range: 35–52%) in women with advanced disease. The median duration of response and the median time to treatment failure were 8.5 (range: 4.3–9) and 5 (range: 4.4–6) months, respectively. Patients treated with vinorelbine had a median survival of 16 (range: 9.9–24) months.

Salvage (second-line or subsequent) chemotherapy with vinorelbine alone also has been employed in the treatment of metastatic breast cancer. When administered as salvage therapy, vinorelbine monotherapy produced a median objective response in 28% (range: 16–37%) of patients with advanced/ metastatic breast cancer that failed to respond to a previous cytotoxic chemotherapy regimen. The drug produced a median duration of response, time to treatment failure, and survival of 5 (range: 3.5–8.5), 3.8 (range: 3–4.5), and 11.7 (range: 7–24) months, respectively. Objective responses to vinorelbine have been observed in patients with metastatic breast cancer refractory to anthracyclines or taxanes.

In a randomized, active-control trial involving women with anthracycline-refractory metastatic breast cancer, vinorelbine's antitumor activity appeared superior to that of melphalan. Vinorelbine and melphalan produced objective responses in 16 and 9% of patients, respectively. Differences favoring vinorelbine were noted for median time to disease progression and treatment failure, median survival, and 1-year survival rates. The median time to disease progression and treatment failure was 3 or 2 months for patients receiving vinorelbine or melphalan, respectively, the median survival rate was 8.8 or 7.8 months, respectively, and the 1-year survival rate was 35.7 or 21.7%, respectively.

Vinorelbine has been administered in various regimens for the treatment of metastatic breast cancer, such as a short IV infusion once weekly, or a continuous IV infusion of up to 5 days in duration. The use of oral† vinorelbine (currently not commercially available in the US) also is being investigated in the treatment of metastatic breast cancer.

■ **Cervical Cancer** Vinorelbine is being investigated as an active agent in the treatment of metastatic or recurrent cervical cancer†. An objective response rate of 18% was reported in a small uncontrolled study of patients receiving vinorelbine as a single agent for advanced or recurrent squamous cell carcinoma of the cervix. The combination of vinorelbine with other antineoplastic agents (e.g., cisplatin) is being evaluated in patients with metastatic or recurrent cervical cancer. (See Uses: Cervical Cancer in Cisplatin 10:00 for an overview of therapy for cervical cancer.)

■ **Other Uses** Vinorelbine also is used in the treatment of adult soft tissue sarcomas† and esophageal cancer†.

Dosage and Administration

■ **Administration** Vinorelbine is administered only by IV injection into a free-flowing IV infusion or a large central vein, usually over a period of 6–10 minutes followed by flushing of the vein with a compatible IV solution, by individuals experienced in administration of the drug. The IV needle or catheter must be properly positioned before vinorelbine is injected. Improper administration of vinorelbine may result in extravasation of the drug causing local tissue necrosis and/or thrombophlebitis. Although vinorelbine also has been infused IV over 20–60 minutes via a peripheral vein or by rapid IV injection over 1–2 minutes, such methods of administration are *not* recommended because of the high rate of adverse local effects (e.g., phlebitis, erythema, venous discoloration, ulceration, pain) associated with this infusion rate and reports of severe back pain associated with rapid injection. Continuous IV infusions† of vinorelbine have been well tolerated, but additional study is needed to establish the role of such infusion in treating various cancers.

Vinorelbine tartrate is very irritating and must not be given IM, subcutaneously, or intrathecally. Intrathecal administration of other vinca alkaloids (i.e., vinblastine, vincristine) has resulted in death. When dispensed, the syringe containing the individual dose prepared for administration to the patient *must* be labeled with the statement: **"Warning: For IV use only. Fatal if given intrathecally."** The syringe must be enclosed in an overwrap (e.g., plastic bag or similar wrap with typed label) bearing the statements: **"Do not remove covering until moment of injection. Fatal if given intrathecally. For IV use only."**

In addition to the use of the warning labels and overwrap, other protective measures to prevent inadvertent intrathecal administration of vinorelbine or other vinca alkaloids include: administering diluted vinca alkaloid solutions in minibags, preparing the medication at the time of administration, attaching a unique filter, dispensing the vinca alkaloid separately from all other medications, dispensing the vinca alkaloid directly to the individual who is administering the drug, conducting an independent check of the dose and route of administration for the drug both at the time of preparation and prior to administration of the drug, and administering the vinca alkaloid in a separate room from rooms where other medications are administered.

Management of patients mistakenly receiving intrathecal vinorelbine is a medical emergency. Currently, there are no reports of patients mistakenly receiving intrathecal administration of vinorelbine. Unfortunately, the prognosis to date for patients inadvertently administered vincristine, another vinca alkaloid, intrathecally generally has been poor despite immediate efforts at removing spinal fluid and flushing with lactated Ringer's injection as well as other solutions, with such efforts failing to prevent ascending paralysis and death in almost all cases. In one case, progression of paralysis was stopped in an adult patient when the following treatment was initiated immediately after inadvertent intrathecal injection of vincristine. Such treatment consisted of immediate removal of as much CSF as safely possible via lumbar access, followed by flushing of the subarachnoid space with lactated Ringer's solution infused continuously at a rate of 150 mL/hour through a catheter in a cerebral lateral ventricle and removal of fluid through a lumbar access. As soon as available, fresh frozen plasma (25 mL) diluted in 1 L of lactated Ringer's solution was infused through the cerebral ventricular catheter at a rate of 75 mL/hour with removal of fluid through the lumbar access. The rate of infusion was adjusted to maintain a CSF protein concentration of 150 mg/dL. Glutamic acid was administered in a dose of 10 g given IV over 24 hours, followed by 500 mg orally 3 times daily for 1 month or until stabilization of neurologic status. The role of glutamic acid in this treatment is uncertain. There currently is no experience with this or any other treatment protocol in patients who mistakenly receive vinorelbine intrathecally.

Leakage of vinorelbine into surrounding tissue during IV administration of the drug can cause considerable irritation, local tissue necrosis, and/or thrombophlebitis. If extravasation occurs, the injection should be discontinued immediately, and any remaining portion of the dose should then be administered into another vein. The manufacturer states that there are no established guidelines for the treatment of extravasation injuries caused by vinorelbine and that institutional guidelines for extravasation injuries may be used. (See Cautions: Local Effects.)

Vinorelbine for injection concentrate must be diluted prior to injection into a free-flowing IV infusion or a large central vein. The manufacturer recommends diluting the concentrate in a syringe with 5% dextrose injection or 0.9% sodium chloride injection to a final vinorelbine concentration of 1.5–3 mg/mL *or* in an IV bag with 5% dextrose injection, 0.9% sodium chloride injection, 0.45% sodium chloride injection, 5% dextrose and 0.45% sodium chloride injection, Ringer's injection, or lactated Ringer's injection to a final vinorelbine concentration of 0.5–2 mg/mL. The diluted solution of vinorelbine should then be administered over a period of 6–10 minutes into the side port closest to the IV bag of a free-flowing IV infusion or into a large central vein followed by flushing with at least 75–125 mL of 0.9% sodium chloride injection or 5% dextrose injection over a period of 10 minutes.

Caution should be exercised in handling and preparing solutions of vinorelbine. Because skin reactions may occur with accidental exposure to vinorelbine, the manufacturer recommends the use of latex gloves when handling the drug. If vinorelbine tartrate injection or a solution of the drug comes in contact with the skin or mucosa, the affected area should be washed immediately and thoroughly with soap and water. Care must be taken to avoid contact of vinorelbine tartrate solutions with the eyes since severe irritation of the eye has been reported with accidental exposure to another vinca alkaloid; if contact occurs, the eye should be flushed thoroughly with water immediately.

Vinorelbine tartrate injection or solutions of the drug should be inspected visually for particulate matter and/or discoloration prior to administration.

■ **Dosage** Dosage of vinorelbine tartrate is expressed in terms of the base.

Adjustment of vinorelbine dosage in geriatric patients solely on the basis of age is not necessary.

Non-small Cell Lung Cancer **Combination Therapy.** For the treatment of non-small cell lung cancer in adults, IV vinorelbine 25 mg/m^2 once weekly may be administered in combination with IV cisplatin 100 mg/m^2 given once every 4 weeks. Dosage reductions for both vinorelbine and cisplatin typically were required (see Dosage Modification for Toxicity and Contraindications for Continued Therapy: Hematologic Toxicity). Another regimen for the treatment of non-small lung cancer in adults is IV vinorelbine 30 mg/m^2 administered once weekly in combination with cisplatin (120 mg/m^2 given on days 1 and 29 and then once every 6 weeks).

In a dose-ranging study, 32 patients with non-small cell lung cancer receiving vinorelbine 20, 25, or 30 mg/m^2 weekly plus cisplatin 120 mg/m^2 on days 1 and 29 then once every 6 weeks had a median survival of 10 months. No responses were observed in patients receiving the 20 mg/m^{2}dose; a response rate of 33% was observed in patients receiving a vinorelbine dose of either 25 or 30 mg/m^2.

According to ASCO practice guidelines, patients with unresectable stage III non-small cell lung cancer (NSCLC) who are candidates for combined chemotherapy and radiation should receive 2 to 4 cycles of initial platinum-based chemotherapy; no more than 4 cycles of chemotherapy are recommended. In patients with stage IV NSCLC, a maximum of 4 cycles of first-line chemotherapy should be administered if the disease is not responding to treatment, and a maximum of 6 cycles of chemotherapy should be administered if the disease responds to treatment.

Monotherapy. For the treatment of non-small cell lung cancer in adults, the manufacturer reports a usual initial dosage of single-agent vinorelbine of 30 mg/m^2 IV administered once weekly.

In clinical studies, dosages of vinorelbine have ranged from 15–30 mg/m^2 IV once weekly.

The optimum duration of vinorelbine therapy in patients with non-small cell lung cancer has not been determined, and in clinical trials, patients were treated with single-agent vinorelbine until the occurrence of either dose-limiting toxicity or progression of disease. According to ASCO practice guidelines, for patients with stage IV NSCLC, a maximum of 4 cycles of first-line chemotherapy should be administered if the disease is not responding to treatment, and a maximum of 6 cycles of chemotherapy should be administered if the disease responds to treatment.

Breast Cancer When used as first-line or salvage (second-line or subsequent) monotherapy in the treatment of advanced/ metastatic breast cancer†, vinorelbine has been infused IV over 20–60 minutes at initial doses of 20–30 mg/m^2 per week. The drug also has been administered at 30 mg/m^2 per week as a direct IV injection over 3–5 minutes or as a rapid IV dose. However, because of better local tolerance, the manufacturer currently recommends that vinorelbine usually be infused IV over 6–10 minutes. (See Dosage and Administration: Administration.) During the course of therapy, the dosing regimen generally was modified (e.g., dosing was delayed or doses were reduced) because of vinorelbine-induced toxicity.

Dosage Modification for Toxicity and Contraindications for Continued Therapy **Hematologic Toxicity.** Vinorelbine therapy should not be administered to patients with baseline granulocyte counts less than 1000 cells/ mm^3. In patients with a granulocyte count less than 1000 cells/ mm^3, the granulocyte count should be repeated in 1 week. If it is necessary to withhold vinorelbine doses for 3 consecutive weeks because of persistence of a granulocyte count less than 1000 cells/ mm^3, therapy with the drug should be discontinued. In patients with a granulocyte count of 1000–1499 cells/ mm^3, the vinorelbine dose should be reduced to 50% of the starting dose.

In patients who have experienced fever and/or sepsis because of granulocytopenia during vinorelbine therapy or in patients in whom the vinorelbine dose has been withheld for 2 consecutive weeks because of granulocytopenia, subsequent doses of vinorelbine should be reduced to 75% of the starting dose in patients with a granulocyte count of at least 1500 cells/ mm^{3}and to 37.5% of the starting dose in those with a granulocyte count of 1000–1499 cells/ mm^3. The vinorelbine dose should be withheld if the granulocyte count is less than 1000 cells/mm^3, and the granulocyte count should be repeated in 1 week. If it is necessary to withhold vinorelbine doses for 3 consecutive weeks because of persistence of a granulocyte count less than 1000 cells/mm^3, therapy with the drug should be discontinued.

Among patients receiving combination therapy with vinorelbine and cisplatin, blood counts should be checked weekly and dosage of vinorelbine and/ or cisplatin should be reduced according to hematologic toxicity. In a large randomized trial, most patients required a 50% dose reduction of vinorelbine at day 15 of each cycle and a 50% dose reduction of cisplatin by cycle 3.

In patients with concurrent hematologic toxicity and hepatic impairment, vinorelbine dosage should be adjusted to the lower dosage advised by these guidelines. (See Dosage and Administration: Dosage in Renal and Hepatic Impairment.)

Hepatic Toxicity. Dosage of vinorelbine should be reduced in patients who develop hyperbilirubinemia. (See Dosage and Administration: Dosage in Renal and Hepatic Impairment.) In patients with concurrent hepatic impairment and hematologic toxicity, vinorelbine dosage should be adjusted to the lower dosage advised by these guidelines.

Renal Toxicity. Reduction of vinorelbine dosage in patients with renal impairment does not appear to be necessary. When vinorelbine is used in combination with cisplatin, appropriate dosage reductions for cisplatin should be made in patients with renal impairment.

Neurologic Toxicity. If manifestations of moderate or severe (grade 2 or higher) neurotoxicity occur in patients receiving vinorelbine, therapy with the drug should be discontinued immediately.

■ **Dosage in Renal and Hepatic Impairment** The effect of renal and/or hepatic impairment on the disposition of vinorelbine has not been fully established. Reduction of vinorelbine dosage in patients with renal impairment does not appear to be necessary.

Because the drug is extensively metabolized in the liver, doses of vinorelbine should be reduced and the drug should be administered with caution in patients with hepatic impairment. In patients with total serum bilirubin concentration of 2 mg/dL or less, no dosage reduction is required. In patients with total serum bilirubin concentration of 2.1–3 mg/dL, vinorelbine dose should be reduced to 50% of the starting dose. In patients with total serum bilirubin concentration exceeding 3 mg/dL, vinorelbine dose should be reduced to 25% of the starting dose. In patients with concurrent hepatic impairment and hematologic toxicity, vinorelbine dosage should be adjusted to the lower dosage advised by these guidelines.

Cautions

A similar pattern of adverse effects is observed in patients receiving vinorelbine as a single agent or in combination therapy. Unless otherwise noted, incidence data for adverse effects are derived from data for 365 patients (222 patients with advanced breast cancer, 143 patients with non-small cell lung cancer) receiving vinorelbine as a single agent in 3 clinical studies. The dosing schedule in each study was vinorelbine 30 mg/m^2 once weekly.

■ **Hematologic Effects and Infectious Complications** The major and dose-limiting adverse effect of vinorelbine is myelosuppression, manifested principally by granulocytopenia and leukopenia. The incidence of myelosuppression does not appear to be influenced by age or prior exposure to chemotherapy. Granulocyte counts less than 2000 and 500/mm^3 occurred in 90 and 36% of patients, respectively. Leukopenia (less than 4000/mm^3) occurred in 92% of patients, and was severe (less than 1000 cells/mm^3) in 15% of patients. Leukopenia occurred at a similar rate in patients receiving vinorelbine and cisplatin in randomized trials (88 or 94%), but the rate of grade 3 or 4 leukopenia was higher (about 60%). Hospitalization for granulocytopenic complications (e.g., fever, sepsis, infection, pneumonia) occurred in 9% of patients. Hospitalization for documented sepsis was reported in about 4% of patients receiving vinorelbine either alone or with cisplatin. Septic death occurred in approximately 1% of patients.

The manufacturer states that, although the pharmacokinetics of vinorelbine are not influenced by the concurrent administration of cisplatin, the incidence of granulocytopenia is higher when vinorelbine is used in combination with cisplatin than when it is used as a single agent. In a clinical trial in which patients were randomized to receive single-agent vinorelbine or vinorelbine plus cisplatin, grade 3 or 4 granulocytopenia occurred more frequently with the combination (79%) than with single-agent vinorelbine (53%). In another randomized trial, grade 3 or 4 granulocytopenia occurred more frequently in those receiving vinorelbine and cisplatin (82%) than in those receiving cisplatin alone (5%); fever and/or sepsis related to granulocytopenia occurred in 11% of patients receiving combination therapy compared with 0% of patients receiving cisplatin alone, and 4 patients receiving vinorelbine and cisplatin died of granulocytopenia-related sepsis. In the same study, death from febrile neutropenia occurred in 3 patients receiving vinorelbine and cisplatin. Infection (unspecified type) was reported in 11% of patients receiving vinorelbine and cisplatin compared with less than 1% of those receiving cisplatin alone, and severe infection occurred in 6% of patients receiving combination therapy. Respiratory infection was reported in patients receiving vinorelbine and cisplatin (10%) or cisplatin alone (3%).

Vinorelbine-induced myelosuppression generally is reversible and does not appear to increase with cumulative exposure. Granulocyte nadirs generally occur between 7–10 days after dosing, and granulocyte count recovery usually occurs within the following 7–14 days. However, granulocytopenia may require dosage adjustment, treatment delay, or drug discontinuance. Among patients with non-small cell lung cancer receiving vinorelbine and cisplatin who experienced grade 3 or 4 granulocytopenia (1000/mm^3 or less) following the first course of therapy or who developed neutropenic fever between cycles of therapy, the use of granulocyte colony-stimulating factor (G-CSF) was permitted. At 24 hours following completion of chemotherapy, G-CSF 5 mcg/kg daily was initiated and continued until the total granulocyte count exceeded 1000/mm^3 on 2 successive determinations; G-CSF was not administered on the day of treatment. Some data suggest that the addition of filgrastim to vinorelbine therapy may reduce the duration and severity of granulocytopenia and/or allow dose intensification.

Anemia (hemoglobin less than 11 g/dL) was reported in 83% of patients, and was severe (hemoglobin less than 8 g/dL) in 9% of patients. Whole blood and/or packed red blood cells were administered to 18% of patients who received vinorelbine. Among patients with non-small cell lung cancer in a randomized trial, grade 3 or 4 anemia occurred more frequently in those receiving vinorelbine and cisplatin (24%) than in those receiving cisplatin alone (8%).

Thrombocytopenia (less than 100,000/mm^3) developed less frequently than granulocytopenia, neutropenia, or anemia, occurring in 5% of patients; severe thrombocytopenia (less than 50,000/mm^3) was reported in 1% of patients. In randomized trials, grade 3 or 4 thrombocytopenia was reported in 6% of those receiving vinorelbine and cisplatin compared with 2% of those receiving cisplatin alone, and in 4% of those receiving vinorelbine and cisplatin compared with 0% of those receiving vinorelbine alone.

■ **Nervous System Effects** Peripheral neuropathy, manifested by paresthesia and hypesthesia, occurred in 25% of patients, and was grade 3 or 4 in 1% and less than 1% of patients, respectively. Painful paresthesia with marked motor loss on the plantar surfaces has been reported rarely. Peripheral neuropathy may be related to cumulative dose and is generally reversible upon drug discontinuance.

In a randomized trial, the incidence of grade 3 or 4 peripheral numbness was higher in patients receiving vinorelbine and cisplatin than in those receiving cisplatin alone (2 versus 1%); paresthesias occurred in 17% of patients receiving combination therapy versus 10% of those receiving cisplatin alone. In another randomized study, the incidence of neurotoxicity (including peripheral neuropathy and constipation) was similar in patients receiving combination therapy with cisplatin and vinorelbine compared with those receiving single-agent vinorelbine (44%).

Loss of deep tendon reflexes occurred in less than 5% of patients. Myasthenia also has been reported. Adverse peripheral nervous system effects, including muscle weakness and gait disturbance, have been observed in patients with and without prior symptoms. Patients with preexisting neuropathy, regardless of etiology, or previous or concomitant exposure to neurotoxic agents (e.g., paclitaxel) may be at increased risk for adverse nervous system effects when receiving vinorelbine. (See Cautions: Precautions and Contraindications.)

Asthenia was reported in 36% of patients, and was grade 3 in 7% of patients. Fatigue occurred in 27% of patients receiving vinorelbine. Fatigue is usually mild to moderate in severity, although the frequency and severity tend to increase with dose or repeated drug administration. Malaise, fatigue, or lethargy was reported in 67% of patients receiving vinorelbine and cisplatin versus 49% of those receiving cisplatin alone. Dizziness, hyperalgesia, confusion, disorientation, hyporeflexia, insomnia, headache, generalized pain, pain in tumor-containing tissue, and back pain also have been reported. In a randomized trial, dizziness/vertigo was reported in patients receiving vinorelbine and cisplatin (9%) or cisplatin alone (3%).

Vestibular and auditory deficits have been reported in patients receiving vinorelbine, principally in those receiving cisplatin concomitantly. Taste alterations occurred at a similar rate among patients receiving vinorelbine and cisplatin versus cisplatin alone (17 versus 15%) in a randomized trial.

■ **Respiratory Effects** Cases of interstitial pulmonary changes and acute respiratory distress syndrome (ARDS), most of which were fatal, have been reported in patients receiving vinorelbine as monotherapy. The mean time to onset of symptoms was 1 week (range: 3–8 days) after vinorelbine administration. Patients who experience an increase in baseline pulmonary manifestations or the onset of new manifestations (e.g., dyspnea, cough, hypoxia) should undergo prompt evaluation.

Acute shortness of breath and severe bronchospasm have been reported infrequently following the administration of vinorelbine and other vinca alkaloids, usually when administered in combination with mitomycin. These adverse pulmonary events may require treatment with supplemental oxygen, bronchodilators, and/or corticosteroids, particularly in patients with preexisting pulmonary dysfunction.

Dyspnea was reported in 7% of patients, and was severe (grade 3 or 4) in 3% of patients. Shortness of breath was reported in 3% of patients, and was severe in 2% of patients. (See Cautions: Precautions and Contraindications.) Interstitial pulmonary changes, hypoxia, and pneumonia also have been reported. Adverse respiratory effects associated with hypersensitivity to vinorelbine also have been reported. Acute pulmonary reactions to vinorelbine usually resemble an allergic reaction and respond to bronchodilators. Subacute pulmonary reactions generally occur within 1 hour after vinorelbine administration and manifest as cough, dyspnea, hypoxemia, and interstitial infiltration. These reactions usually respond to corticosteroid administration.

■ GI Effects A fatal case of neutropenic enterocolitis (typhlitis) occurred in a patient following a single dose of vinorelbine.

Severe constipation (grade 3 or 4), paralytic ileus, and intestinal obstruction, necrosis, and perforation have been reported in patients receiving vinorelbine. In some cases, these events have been fatal.

Nausea was reported in 44% of patients receiving vinorelbine, and was grade 3 in 2% of patients. Antiemetic agents generally were not administered prophylactically in clinical trials, and serotonin type 3 (5-HT_3) receptor antagonists generally are not required for management of nausea and vomiting. Vomiting was reported in 20% of patients, and was grade 3 in 2% of patients. Nausea and vomiting usually occur within 24 hours of vinorelbine dosing. Nausea or vomiting each was reported at a similar rate (about 60%) in patients receiving vinorelbine and cisplatin or cisplatin alone in a randomized trial. In another randomized trial, grade 3 or 4 nausea and/or vomiting occurred more frequently in patients receiving vinorelbine and cisplatin (30%) than in those receiving vinorelbine alone (2%).

Constipation occurred in 35% of patients receiving vinorelbine, and was severe in 3% of patients. Constipation may cause treatment delay. Grade 3 or 4 constipation and/or paralytic ileus was reported in 3% of patients receiving vinorelbine and cisplatin and in 1% of patients receiving cisplatin. Diarrhea was reported in 17% of patients, and was grade 3 in 1% of patients. Similar or higher rates of diarrhea (17 or 25%) were reported in patients receiving vinorelbine and cisplatin in randomized trials. Anorexia occurred at a similar rate in patients receiving vinorelbine and cisplatin (46%) or cisplatin alone (37%); anorexia has been reported in patients receiving vinorelbine alone. Stomatitis also has been reported in patients receiving vinorelbine. Vomiting, diarrhea, anorexia, and stomatitis usually were mild or moderate in severity. In a randomized clinical trial, severe nausea and vomiting was reported in 30% of patients receiving vinorelbine concomitantly with cisplatin, compared with less than 2% of patients receiving single-agent vinorelbine. Duration of vinorelbine treatment, previous therapy with emetogenic agents, prior abdominal irradiation, and/or pathology of the abdominal cavity may increase the incidence and severity of GI adverse effects.

Dysphagia, mucositis, dyspepsia, epigastralgia, pancreatitis, esophagitis or radiation recall esophagitis, and abdominal pain also have been reported in patients receiving vinorelbine. Ischemic colitis occurred in a patient receiving vinorelbine and cisplatin.

■ Cardiovascular Effects Fatal cardiovascular effects have been reported rarely when vinorelbine was used with cisplatin.

In a randomized trial, 2 deaths related to myocardial ischemia and one death from massive stroke occurred in patients receiving vinorelbine and cisplatin.

Chest pain was reported in 5% of patients receiving vinorelbine in clinical trials. Most patients experiencing chest pain had a history of cardiovascular disease or tumor within the chest. Myocardial ischemia and infarction, and cardiogenic shock have been reported rarely. Flushing, hypertension, hypotension, vasodilation, tachycardia, and pulmonary edema also have been reported.

Thromboembolic adverse effects, including pulmonary embolus and deep venous thrombosis, have been reported in patients receiving vinorelbine, principally in those who were seriously ill and debilitated with known predisposing risk factors for these adverse effects. In a randomized trial, phlebitis/thrombosis/embolism occurred in 10% of those receiving vinorelbine and cisplatin versus less than 1% of those receiving cisplatin alone; these adverse effects were grade 3 or 4 in severity in 3% of those receiving combination therapy versus less than 1% of those receiving cisplatin alone. Central venous catheter thrombosis has been reported in patients receiving vinorelbine by continuous IV infusion.

■ Hepatic Effects Fatal hepatic failure has been reported in a patient receiving vinorelbine and gemcitabine.

Increased serum AST (SGOT) concentrations occurred in 67%, and increased serum total bilirubin concentrations occurred in 13% of patients. Increased serum ALT (SGPT) concentrations and increased serum alkaline phosphatase concentrations also have been reported. Transient elevations in hepatic enzymes generally were not associated with clinical symptoms. However, vinorelbine should be used with caution in patients with hepatic insufficiency, and dosage adjustment may be required. (See Dosage and Administration: Dosage in Renal and Hepatic Impairment.)

■ Dermatologic Effects Alopecia, manifested as a gradual thinning of hair, was reported in 12% of patients and was reversible. Total hair loss was uncommon. In a randomized trial, alopecia occurred more frequently in patients receiving vinorelbine and cisplatin (34%) than in those receiving cisplatin alone (14%); in another randomized trial, the incidence of alopecia was higher among patients receiving vinorelbine and cisplatin than in those receiving vinorelbine alone (51 versus 30%), including grade 3 or 4 alopecia (8 versus 2%). Radiation recall dermatitis has been reported.

Hand-foot syndrome, generally manifested as bilateral erythema of both the hands and feet, which responds to corticosteroids, has been reported in patients receiving vinorelbine by prolonged (96-hour) IV infusion; the mechanism of the reaction is unclear, but it appears to be dose related. In vitro, vinorelbine has been shown to stimulate histamine release from mast cells.

■ Local Effects Vinorelbine is a moderate vesicant. Injection site reactions and injection site pain occurred in 28 and 16% of patients, respectively. Injection site reactions, including reactions secondary to extravasation, usually were mild and were characterized by erythema, pain at the injection site, and vein discoloration; 5% were severe. Among patients receiving vinorelbine and cisplatin in randomized trials, injection site reactions occurred in 17% and were severe in up to 2% of patients. In clinical practice, injection site reactions also have been characterized by localized rash, urticaria, blister formation, and skin sloughing.

The incidence of injection site reactions may be dose related, and delayed onset of injection site reactions also has been reported. Chemical phlebitis along the vein proximal to the injection site was reported in 10% of patients receiving vinorelbine.

The incidence of adverse local reactions appears to be lower when vinorelbine is administered over 6–10 minutes rather than 20 minutes, and when the veins are flushed with 75–125 mL of IV fluid after the infusion is completed. The incidence of adverse local reactions also may be decreased by flushing the vein with 100 mL of fluid before administering vinorelbine and then flushing with an additional 400 mL of fluid following completion of the vinorelbine infusion. Dexamethasone has been added to the IV fluid used to flush the vein following completion of the vinorelbine infusion to help prevent adverse local reactions. Treatment of injection site reactions has included silver sulfadiazine, local hyaluronidase injection, warm compresses, and central venous catheter placement.

Supravenous hyperpigmentation at the infusion site and a localized necrotizing epidermal reaction each have been reported rarely.

■ Renal Effects Elevated serum creatinine concentration was reported in a randomized trial in 13% of patients receiving vinorelbine as a single agent versus 46% of patients receiving vinorelbine and cisplatin; in another randomized trial, elevated serum creatinine concentration occurred at a similar rate among patients receiving vinorelbine and cisplatin (37%) or cisplatin alone (28%).

■ Musculoskeletal Effects Jaw pain, myalgia, and arthralgia each have been reported in less than 5% of patients receiving vinorelbine. In a randomized trial, myalgia/arthralgia was reported in 12% of patients receiving vinorelbine and cisplatin versus 3% of patients receiving cisplatin alone. Myalgias generally are controlled with nonopioid analgesics but may require treatment delay until symptoms are relieved.

■ Sensitivity Reactions Rash has been reported in less than 5% of patients receiving vinorelbine. Systemic allergic reactions, including anaphylaxis, pruritus, urticaria, and angioedema also have been reported. Drug fever has been reported in patients receiving high doses of vinorelbine as a continuous infusion.

■ Other Effects Hemorrhagic cystitis and the syndrome of inappropriate ADH secretion each were reported in less than 1% of patients receiving vinorelbine. Electrolyte abnormalities, including hyponatremia with or without the syndrome of inappropriate ADH secretion, have been reported in seriously ill and debilitated patients receiving vinorelbine. Weight loss has been reported in 34% of patients receiving vinorelbine and cisplatin and in 21% of those receiving cisplatin alone in a randomized trial. Fever without infection occurred more frequently in patients receiving vinorelbine and cisplatin than in those receiving cisplatin alone (20 versus 4%). Hearing loss or impairment occurred at a similar rate (18%) among patients receiving either vinorelbine and cisplatin or cisplatin alone in a randomized trial; in another randomized trial, ototoxicity occurred in 10% of patients receiving vinorelbine and cisplatin versus 1% of patients receiving vinorelbine alone.

■ Precautions and Contraindications Vinorelbine is a toxic drug with a low therapeutic index, and a therapeutic response is not likely to occur without evidence of toxicity. The drug must be used only under constant supervision by clinicians experienced in therapy with cytotoxic agents and only when the potential benefits of vinorelbine therapy are thought to outweigh the possible risks. Most adverse effects of vinorelbine are reversible. When severe adverse effects occur during vinorelbine therapy, the drug should be discontinued or dosage reduced and appropriate measures initiated. Vinorelbine should be reinstituted with caution, if at all, with adequate consideration of further need for the drug, and with awareness of possible recurrence of toxicity. (See Dosage and Administration: Dosage: Dosage Modification for Toxicity and Contraindications for Continued Therapy.)

Administration of vinorelbine is contraindicated in patients with baseline granulocyte counts less than 1000 cells/mm^3, and the drug should be administered with extreme caution in patients whose bone marrow reserve may have been compromised by prior irradiation or chemotherapy, or in patients whose marrow function is recovering from the effects of previous chemotherapy. To monitor the occurrence of vinorelbine-induced myelosuppression, mainly granulocytopenia, which may be severe and result in infection, it is recommended that frequent peripheral blood cell counts with differentials be performed before administration of each vinorelbine dose and following discontinuance of therapy with the drug. Vinorelbine therapy should be withheld in patients with granulocyte counts less than 1000 cells/mm^3. Patients with severe vinorelbine-induced granulocytopenia should be monitored carefully for evidence of infection and/or fever. For further instructions regarding monitoring and dosage adjustment according to hematologic toxicity, see Dosage Modification for Toxicity: Hematologic Toxicity in Dosage and Administration: Dosage.

Prophylactic colony-stimulating factors have not been used routinely with vinorelbine. However, as clinically indicated, such hematopoietic agents may be used at recommended doses no sooner than 24 hours following completion of the administration of cytotoxic chemotherapy. Growth factors should not be administered in the 24-hour period preceding the administration of chemotherapy. Hematopoietic agents also may be indicated for the treatment of vinorelbine overdosage.

Patients should be informed that the major acute toxicities of vinorelbine are related to bone marrow toxicity, particularly granulocytopenia with increased susceptibility to infection, and should be advised to report fever or chills immediately. Patients also should be advised to contact their clinician if they experience increased shortness of breath, cough, or other new respiratory symptoms, or if they experience abdominal pain or constipation.

Administration of vinorelbine to patients who have received prior radiation therapy may result in radiation recall reactions, such as dermatitis and esophagitis.

Patients who have experienced neuropathy with previous drug therapy (e.g., paclitaxel-associated neuropathy) should be monitored for symptoms of neuropathy while receiving vinorelbine. Patients with a previous or preexisting neuropathy, regardless of etiology, as well as those receiving combination therapy with vinorelbine and paclitaxel, either concomitantly or sequentially, should be monitored for new or worsening signs and symptoms of neuropathy while receiving vinorelbine. For further instructions regarding dosage adjustment according to neurologic toxicity, see Dosage Modification for Toxicity: Neurologic Toxicity in Dosage and Administration: Dosage.

Acute shortness of breath and severe bronchospasm have been reported infrequently following the administration of vinorelbine and other vinca alkaloids, most commonly when these agents were used in combination with mitomycin. If a patient develops these adverse effects during administration of vinorelbine, appropriate therapy (e.g., supplemental oxygen, bronchodilators, corticosteroids) may be required, particularly in patients with preexisting pulmonary dysfunction.

Because severe irritation of the eye has been reported with accidental exposure to another vinca alkaloid, the manufacturer states that care must be taken to avoid contamination of the eyes with concentrations of vinorelbine used clinically. If ocular exposure occurs, the eye(s) should be thoroughly flushed with water immediately.

There is no evidence that the toxicity of vinorelbine is greater in patients with elevated serum hepatic enzyme concentrations, and no data are available regarding the use of the drug in patients with severe baseline cholestasis. Because vinorelbine is metabolized mainly in the liver and clinical experience with the drug in patients with severe liver disease is limited, vinorelbine should be administered with caution in patients with severe hepatic injury or impairment, and dosage reduction may be necessary. (See Dosage and Administration: Dosage in Renal and Hepatic Impairment.)

■ **Pediatric Precautions** Safety and efficacy of vinorelbine in children younger than 18 years of age have not been established. No meaningful clinical activity was demonstrated among 46 pediatric patients receiving vinorelbine (at dosages similar to those used in adults) for recurrent solid malignant tumors, including rhabdomyosarcoma/undifferentiated sarcoma, neuroblastoma, and CNS tumors; children experienced similar toxicities as adults.

■ **Geriatric Precautions** When the total number of patients studied in North American clinical trials of vinorelbine is considered, approximately one-third were 65 years of age or older. Although no overall differences in efficacy or safety were observed between geriatric and younger patients, and other clinical experience revealed no evidence of age-related differences, the possibility that some geriatric patients may exhibit increased sensitivity to the drug cannot be ruled out.

■ **Mutagenicity and Carcinogenicity** In in vivo studies, vinorelbine has been shown to cause chromosomal damage (polyploidy in bone marrow cells from Chinese hamsters and positive results of the micronucleus test in mice). The drug was not mutagenic in the Ames test, and results of the mouse lymphoma TK locus assay were inconclusive.

Studies to determine the carcinogenic potential of vinorelbine have not been performed to date.

■ **Pregnancy, Fertility, and Lactation** Vinorelbine can cause fetal toxicity when administered to pregnant women, but potential benefits from use of the drug may be acceptable in certain conditions despite the possible risks to the fetus. Vinorelbine has been shown to be embryotoxic and/or fetotoxic in mice and rabbits at single doses of 9 and 5.5 mg/m^2, respectively (one-third and one-sixth the usual human dose). At doses that were not toxic to the pregnant animal, fetal weight was reduced and ossification was delayed. Vinorelbine and fluorouracil were administered to 3 women with breast cancer during the second or third trimester of pregnancy. The infants were delivered at 34, 37, and 41 weeks' gestation and no chemotherapy-related adverse effects were observed except for anemia in one infant, which occurred 21 days after delivery. There are no adequate and controlled studies to date using vinorelbine in pregnant women. Vinorelbine should be used during pregnancy only in life-threatening situations or severe disease for which safer drugs cannot be used or are ineffective. When vinorelbine is administered during pregnancy or the patient becomes pregnant while receiving the drug, the patient should be informed of the potential hazard to the fetus. Women of childbearing potential should be advised to avoid becoming pregnant while receiving the drug.

Vinorelbine did not affect fertility when administered to rats on either a once-weekly (9 mg/m^2, approximately one-third the usual human dose) or alternate-day (4.2 mg/m^2, approximately one-seventh the usual human dose) schedule preceding and during mating. However, studies in rats using biweekly (i.e., once every 2 weeks) administration of vinorelbine for 13 or 26 weeks at doses of 2.1 and 7.2 mg/m^2 (approximately one-fifteenth and one-fourth the usual human dose, respectively) showed decreased spermatogenesis and prostate/seminal vesicle secretion.

It is not known whether vinorelbine is distributed in milk. Because many drugs are distributed in milk and because of the potential for serious adverse reactions to vinorelbine in nursing infants, nursing should be discontinued during vinorelbine therapy.

Drug Interactions

■ **Antineoplastic Agents** Acute pulmonary reactions have been reported in patients receiving vinorelbine or other vinca alkaloids (vinblastine, vincristine) in combination with mitomycin. (See Cautions: Respiratory Effects.) A higher incidence of grade 3 and 4 granulocytopenia has been reported in patients receiving combination therapy with vinorelbine and cisplatin than in those receiving vinorelbine alone. (See Cautions: Hematologic Effects and Infectious Complications.) Concomitant administration of vinorelbine and paclitaxel may be associated with an increased risk of neuropathy. (See Cautions: Nervous System Effects.)

■ **Drugs Affecting Hepatic Microsomal Enzymes** Metabolism of vinca alkaloids is mediated by the cytochrome P-450 (CYP) isoenzyme CYP3A, and inhibitors of this isoenzyme may impair the metabolism of vinca alkaloids. Caution is advised since concomitant administration of vinorelbine and inhibitors of isoenzyme CYP3A may cause earlier onset and/or increased severity of adverse effects.

Death occurred in a patient following chemotherapy with vinorelbine and cisplatin; an interaction between vinorelbine and itraconazole was cited as possible cause.

Concomitant use of itraconazole, a potent inhibitor of CYP3A, and another vinca alkaloid, vincristine, has been associated with earlier onset and/or increased severity of adverse neuromuscular effects, probably related to inhibition of vincristine metabolism. In vitro studies demonstrate that voriconazole is a less potent inhibitor of CYP3A4 than ketoconazole or itraconazole. Because concomitant use of voriconazole or other azole antifungal agents may increase plasma concentrations of vinca alkaloids, such as vinorelbine, and lead to neurotoxicity, dosage reduction of vinorelbine should be considered.

Caution and careful monitoring are advised during concomitant use of a vinca alkaloid and aprepitant, an antiemetic agent, which may inhibit or induce CYP3A4. In clinical studies, the dosage of vinorelbine was not adjusted during concomitant use of aprepitant.

■ **Ototoxic Drugs** Because vestibular deficits and varying degrees of permanent or temporary hearing impairment associated with damage of the eighth cranial nerve have been reported in patients receiving vinca alkaloids, vinorelbine should be used concomitantly with other potentially ototoxic drugs, such as platinum-containing antineoplastic agents, with extreme caution.

Acute Toxicity

■ **Manifestations** Overdosage with vinorelbine produces adverse effects that are mainly extensions of common adverse effects, including paralytic ileus, stomatitis, and esophagitis. Bone marrow aplasia, sepsis, and paresis also have been reported. Overdoses of up to 10 times the recommended dose of 30 mg/m^2 have been reported, and some fatalities have occurred. Death from multisystem failure caused by an overdose of vinorelbine has been reported in a patient receiving the drug in combination with cisplatin.

■ **Treatment** There is no known specific antidote for vinorelbine overdosage. Management of vinorelbine overdosage should consist of general supportive measures and symptomatic treatment, including blood transfusions, hematopoietic agents, and anti-infectives, when clinically indicated.

Pharmacology

Vinorelbine is an antimicrotubule antineoplastic agent. Microtubules are organelles that exist in a state of dynamic equilibrium with their components, tubulin dimers. They form an essential part of the mitotic spindle, participate in intracellular transport, and contribute to the cell's shape, rigidity, and motility.

Vinorelbine and other vinca alkaloids exert their cytotoxic effects by binding to tubulin, the protein subunit of the spindle microtubules. The formation of vinorelbine-tubulin complexes prevents the polymerization of the tubulin subunits into microtubules and induces depolymerization of microtubules resulting in inhibition of microtubule assembly and cellular metaphase arrest.

In addition to the antineoplastic effects of antimicrotubule activity, vinca alkaloids interfere with the microtubule-mediated movement of neurotransmitter substances along neuronal axons resulting in dose-limiting neurotoxicity. Although the depolymerizing action of vincristine, vinblastine, and vinorelbine on axonal microtubules is identical, this action occurs in vitro at higher concentrations of vinorelbine than these other vinca alkaloids, and in vitro studies suggest that vinorelbine has a higher affinity than these drugs for mitotic rather than axonal microtubules. In comparative clinical trials, vinorelbine was shown to be less neurotoxic than vindesine, another vinca alkaloid.

Like other vinca alkaloids, vinorelbine reportedly also interferes with amino acid, cyclic AMP, and glutathione metabolism; calmodulin-dependent Ca^{2+}-transport ATPase activity; cellular respiration; and nucleic acid and lipid biosynthesis.

Pharmacokinetics

■ **Absorption** Following IV administration, plasma concentrations of vinorelbine decline in a triphasic manner with an initial rapid decrease.

■ **Distribution** The initial rapid decline in plasma vinorelbine concentration following IV administration represents distribution of the drug to peripheral compartments. Following administration of vinorelbine 30 mg/m^2 IV over 15–20 minutes, a steady-state volume of distribution of 25.4–40.1 L/kg has been reported.

Vinorelbine demonstrates high binding to human platelets and lymphocytes. Binding of the drug to plasma constituents in patients with cancer ranges from 79.6–91.2%, and a free fraction of approximately 0.11 was observed in pooled human plasma over a concentration range of 234–1169 ng/mL. The presence of cisplatin, fluorouracil, or doxorubicin does not affect vinorelbine binding.

■ **Elimination** The 3 phases of plasma decline of vinorelbine concentrations represent an initial rapid decline in plasma concentrations caused by distribution of the drug to peripheral compartments followed by metabolism and excretion of the drug and a prolonged terminal phase because of relatively slow efflux of drug from peripheral compartments. A mean terminal elimination half-life of 27.7–43.6 hours and a mean plasma clearance of 0.97–1.26 L/hour per kg have been reported for vinorelbine.

Vinorelbine is extensively metabolized in the liver. The metabolism of vinca alkaloids (e.g., vinblastine, vincristine) is mediated by the cytochrome P-450 (CYP) isoenzymes in the CYP3A subfamily. Two metabolites of vinorelbine, vinorelbine *N*-oxide and deacetylvinorelbine, have been identified in human blood, plasma, and urine. Deacetylvinorelbine, the primary metabolite of vinorelbine in humans, has been shown to possess antitumor activity similar to the parent drug. However, therapeutic doses of vinorelbine result in very small, if any, quantifiable concentrations of either metabolite in blood or urine.

Following IV administration of radiolabeled vinorelbine, approximately 46% of the administered dose was recovered in the feces and 18% in the urine. In another study, approximately 11% of an administered IV dose of vinorelbine was excreted unchanged in the urine.

The effect of renal and/or hepatic impairment on the elimination of vinorelbine has not been evaluated. Limited data from pharmacokinetic studies indicate that the disposition of the drug in geriatric patients is similar to that observed in younger adults.

Chemistry and Stability

■ **Chemistry** Vinorelbine (didehydrodeoxynorvincaleukoblastine), a semisynthetic vinca alkaloid, is an antineoplastic agent. Like other vinca alkaloids, vinorelbine is a large dimeric asymmetric compound composed of a dihydroindole nucleus (vindoline), which is the major alkaloid present in the periwinkle (*Catharanthus roseus* [Apocynaceae]), and an indole nucleus (catharanthine), which is present in low concentrations in the plant. However, vinorelbine differs structurally from other currently available vinca alkaloids by the presence of substitutions on the catharanthine ring, rather than the vindoline ring, of the molecule.

Vinorelbine tartrate occurs as a white to yellow or light brown amorphous powder. The aqueous solubility of the drug exceeds 1000 mg/mL in distilled water. Commercially available vinorelbine tartrate injection occurs as a clear, colorless to pale yellow solution in water for injection and has a pH of approximately 3.5.

■ **Stability** Commercially available vinorelbine tartrate injection is stable until the date indicated on the package when stored unopened and refrigerated at 2–8°C and protected from light. Unopened vials of vinorelbine tartrate injection are stable at temperatures up to 25°C for up to 72 hours. Vinorelbine tartrate injection should not be frozen.

For further information on the handling of antineoplastic agents, see the ASHP Guidelines on Handling Hazardous Drugs at http://www.ahfsdruginformation.com.

Preparations

Excipients in commercially available drug preparations may have clinically important effects in some individuals; consult specific product labeling for details.

Vinorelbine Tartrate

Parenteral

For injection concentrate, for IV infusion only	10 mg (of vinorelbine)/mL (10 and 50 mg)	**Navelbine®**, Pierre Fabre **Vinorelbine Tartrate for Injection**

†Use is not currently included in the labeling approved by the US Food and Drug Administration

Vismodegib

■ Vismodegib, a hedgehog signaling pathway inhibitor, is an antineoplastic agent.

Uses

■ **Basal Cell Carcinoma** Vismodegib is used for the treatment of metastatic basal cell carcinoma. The drug also is used for the treatment of locally advanced basal cell carcinoma in patients whose disease has recurred following surgery, and in patients who are not candidates for surgery or radiation therapy.

In an open-label, multicenter, noncomparative study in 104 adults with basal cell carcinoma treated with vismodegib for a median duration of 10.2 months, objective response was observed in 30.3 or 42.9% of patients with metastatic or locally advanced disease, respectively. While a complete response was not observed in patients with metastatic disease, 20.6% of those with locally advanced disease achieved a complete response. Both cohorts had a median response duration of 7.6 months. Tumor response was evaluated in patients with metastatic disease using the Response Evaluation Criteria in Solid Tumors (RECIST) and in patients with locally advanced disease by measurement of externally assessable tumor (including scar), assessment of ulceration, radiographic assessment of target lesions (if appropriate), and tumor biopsy. Objective response in locally advanced disease was defined as lack of disease progression and at least one of the following: 30% or greater reduction in lesion size (i.e., sum of the longest diameter from baseline in target lesions as assessed by radiograph), 30% or greater reduction from baseline in the sum of the longest diameter in externally visible dimension of target lesions, or complete resolution of ulceration in all target lesions. Patients with such an objective response and no residual basal cell carcinoma (as determined by tumor biopsy) were considered to have a complete response. Disease progression was defined as a 20% or greater increase from nadir in the sum of the longest diameter in target lesions (as assessed by radiograph or external visualization), a new ulceration of target lesionspersisting for at least 2 weeks without evidence of healing, new lesions (identified by radiograph or physical examination), or progression of nontarget lesions using RECIST.

Dosage and Administration

■ **General** ***Restricted Distribution Program*** Vismodegib can be obtained only through a restricted distribution program called Erivedge Access Solutions®. Only designated pharmacies from a specialty pharmacy network will be authorized to dispense the drug. Specific information is available at http://www.erivedgeaccesssolutions.comor at 888-249-4918.

■ **Administration** Vismodegib is administered orally once daily without regard to meals. Capsules should be swallowed whole and not opened or crushed. In the event of a missed dose, therapy should be resumed with the next scheduled dose. Missed doses should not be replaced.

■ **Dosage** The recommended adult dosage for the treatment of metastatic or locally advanced basal cell carcinoma is 150 mg once daily until disease progression or unacceptable toxicity occurs.

■ **Special Populations** There are no special population dosage recommendations at this time.

Cautions

■ **Contraindications** Manufacturer states none known.

■ **Warnings/Precautions** ***Warnings*** **Fetal/Neonatal Morbidity and Mortality.** Vismodegib may cause fetal harm, including death or severe birth defects. Teratogenicity, embryotoxicity, and fetotoxicity have been demonstrated in animals at exposures lower than those achieved in humans at the recommended daily dosage. Fetal malformations in animals have included severe midline defects, craniofacial anomalies, open perineum, absent or fused digits, and other irreversible malformations. Fetal retardations and variations also have been observed.

Male and female patients should be advised of the risk of embryofetal death and severe birth defects. All patients should be counseled regarding pregnancy prevention and planning, including the need for effective contraception during and after therapy.

Pregnancy status should be verified in female patients with reproductive potential within 7 days prior to initiation of vismodegib therapy. In women with a negative pregnancy test, highly effective contraception (i.e., failure rate less than 1%) should be initiated prior to the first dose of vismodegib and continued during therapy and for 7 months following the last dose of the drug.

Male patients should be advised of the potential to expose female sexual partners to vismodegib through semen. Male patients, including those with a history of vasectomy, should use effective barrier methods of contraception (e.g., condoms with spermicide) during sexual intercourse with female partners while receiving vismodegib and for 2 months following the last dose of the drug.

If pregnancy occurs or is suspected in female patients during vismodegib therapy or within 7 months following completion of therapy or if female sexual partners of male patients are exposed to the drug during pregnancy, the patient should be apprised of the potential fetal hazard. Exposure during pregnancy should be reported to the manufacturer and pregnant women are encouraged to participate in the manufacturer's pregnancy pharmacovigilance program by calling 888-835-2555.

Other Warnings/Precautions **Blood Donation.** Patients should not donate blood or blood components while receiving vismodegib and for at least 7 months following the last dose of the drug.

Specific Populations **Pregnancy.** Category D. (See Fetal/Neonatal Morbidity and Mortality under Warnings/Precautions: Warnings, in Cautions.) (See Users Guide.)

Lactation. It is not known whether vismodegib is distributed into milk. Because of the potential for serious adverse reactions to vismodegib in nursing infants, a decision should be made whether to discontinue nursing or the drug, taking into account the importance of the drug to the woman.

Pediatric Use. Safety and efficacy have not been established in children.

Geriatric Use. There is insufficient experience in patients 65 years of age or older to determine whether geriatric patients respond differently than younger adults.

Hepatic Impairment. Safety and efficacy have not been established in patients with hepatic impairment.

Renal Impairment. Safety and efficacy have not been established in patients with renal impairment.

■ **Common Adverse Effects** Adverse effects reported in 10% or more of patients receiving vismodegib include muscle spasms, alopecia, dysgeusia, weight loss, fatigue, nausea, diarrhea, decreased appetite, constipation, arthralgia, vomiting, ageusia.

Amenorrhea of unknown reversibility also has been reported in premenopausal women receiving the drug.

Drug Interactions

Vismodegib is minimally metabolized by cytochrome P-450 (CYP) isoenzymes 2C9 and 3A4/5. Vismodegib is an inhibitor of CYP isoenzymes 2C8, 2C9, and 2C19 but does not induce CYP isoenzymes 1A2, 2B6, or 3A4/5.

In vitro data indicate that vismodegib is a substrate of P-glycoprotein (P-gp) and an inhibitor of breast cancer resistance protein (BCRP).

■ **Drugs Affecting Hepatic Microsomal Enzymes** Pharmacokinetic interactions are unlikely with drugs that induce or inhibit CYP isoenzymes. In clinical trials, steady-state plasma vismodegib concentrations were similar in patients receiving concomitant CYP3A4 inducers (i.e., carbamazepine, modafinil, phenobarbital) or CYP3A4 inhibitors (i.e., erythromycin, fluconazole).

■ **Drugs Metabolized by Hepatic Microsomal Enzymes** In a pharmacokinetic study in patients with cancer, concomitant use of rosiglitazone (a CYP2C8 substrate) and vismodegib did not alter systemic exposure to rosiglitazone.

■ **Inhibitors of P-glycoprotein Transport** Potential increased vismodegib exposure and toxicity when used concomitantly with inhibitors of P-gp (e.g., azithromycin, clarithromycin, erythromycin).

■ **Drugs Transported by Breast Cancer Resistance Protein** Potential pharmacokinetic interaction (e.g., increased plasma concentration of drugs transported by BCRP).

■ **Drugs Affecting Gastric Acidity** Potential for decreased vismodegib exposure when used concomitantly with agents that alter the pH of the upper GI tract (e.g., antacids, histamine H_2-receptor antagonists, proton-pump inhibitors). Clinical data are lacking, but increased dosages of vismodegib are unlikely to compensate for the interaction. The effect of concomitant use on efficacy of vismodegib is unknown.

■ **Hormonal Contraceptives** Pharmacokinetic interactions with oral contraceptives are unlikely. In a pharmacokinetic study in patients with cancer, concomitant use of vismodegib and an oral contraceptive containing ethinyl estradiol and norethindrone did not alter systemic exposure to the oral contraceptive components.

Description

Vismodegib is an antineoplastic agent that inhibits the hedgehog pathway by binding to and inhibiting smoothened, a transmembrane protein involved in hedgehog signal transduction. The hedgehog signaling pathway is a key regulator of cell growth during development that is generally inactive in adult tissues. Genetic mutations that allow for activation of the hedgehog pathway are often observed in patients with basal cell carcinoma. In patients with metastatic or locally advanced basal cell carcinoma, vismodegib therapy has been associated with tumor regression, stable disease, and down-regulation of glioma-associated protein 1 (GLI1) in normal skin and hair follicles.

Vismodegib is orally bioavailable (31.8%) with saturable absorption that is not affected by food. Increased steady-state exposure has not been observed with doses exceeding 150 mg. The drug is more than 99% bound to plasma proteins, particularly α_1-acid glycoprotein, but also albumin. Binding to α_1-acid glycoprotein is saturable and total plasma vismodegib concentrations correlate with plasma α_1-acid glycoprotein concentrations. While vismodegib is metabolized by cytochrome P-450 (CYP) isoenzymes 2C9 and 3A4/5, it is primarily excreted unchanged in the feces (82%) and to a lesser extent in the urine (4.4%).

Advice to Patients

Importance of patients reading the medication guide prior to initiation of therapy and each time the prescription is refilled.

Importance of women informing their clinician if they are or plan to become pregnant. Advise women to avoid pregnancy while receiving the drug. Advise patients to contact their clinician immediately if pregnancy is confirmed or suspected; advise pregnant women of risk to the fetus.

Importance of both women and men using effective methods of contraception during vismodegib therapy. Advise women to avoid pregnancy while receiving vismodegib and for at least 7 months after therapy with the drug is discontinued. Advise men to use condoms with spermicide while receiving the drug and for at least 2 months after therapy with the drug is discontinued.

Importance of women informing clinicians immediately if they are breastfeeding or plan to breast-feed. Advise women of the potential for serious adverse reactions from the drug in nursing infants.

Importance of patients not donating blood or blood components while receiving vismodegib and for at least 7 months after discontinuance of the drug.

Advise patients to swallow vismodegib capsules whole and not to crush or open capsules.

Advise patients not to replace any missed doses and to resume regular dosing schedule after a missed dose.

Importance of informing clinicians of existing or contemplated concomitant therapy, including prescription and OTC drugs and dietary or herbal supplements, as well as any concomitant illnesses.

Importance of informing patients of other important precautionary information. (See Cautions.)

Overview® (see Users Guide). For additional information on this drug until a more detailed monograph is developed and published, the manufacturer's labeling should be consulted. It is *essential* that the manufacturer's labeling be consulted for more detailed information on usual cautions, precautions, contraindications, potential drug interactions, laboratory test interferences, and acute toxicity.

Preparations

Distribution of vismodegib is restricted. (See Restricted Distribution Program under Dosage and Administration: General.)

Excipients in commercially available drug preparations may have clinically important effects in some individuals; consult specific product labeling for details.

Vismodegib

Oral		
Capsules	150 mg	**Erivedge®**, Genentech

Vorinostat

Suberoylanilide Hydroxamic Acid, SAHA

■ Vorinostat, a histone deacetylase (HDAC) inhibitor, is an antineoplastic agent.

Uses

■ **Cutaneous T-cell Lymphoma** Vorinostat is used for the treatment of skin manifestations of cutaneous T-cell lymphoma (CTCL) in patients who have progressive, persistent, or recurrent disease during or after 2 prior systemic therapies. Vorinostat is designated an orphan drug by the US Food and Drug Administration (FDA) for use in this condition.

Efficacy of vorinostat was evaluated in 2 open-label clinical trials in patients with refractory CTCL. In one multicenter study, 74 patients with CTCL who had received at least 2 prior systemic therapies, including bexarotene (unless the patient was not a candidate for or did not tolerate the drug), received vorinostat 400 mg orally once daily. Most (82%) of the patients had stage IIB or more advanced disease. Extent of disease was assessed using a modified Severity Weighted Assessment Tool (SWAT); complete clinical response was defined as no evidence of skin disease, and partial response was defined as a decrease of at least 50% from baseline in SWAT skin assessment score, with the respective response lasting at least 4 weeks. An overall objective response was reported in about 30% of patients receiving vorinostat. One patient with stage IIB CTCL achieved a complete clinical response. Median time to response was 55 days; however, in rare cases, up to 6 months of treatment was required to achieve an objective response. Median response duration was not reached but was estimated to exceed 6 months. Estimated median duration of response, with end of response defined as a 50% increase in SWAT score from the nadir, was 168 days, and median time to tumor progression was 202 days. Estimated median time to progression, with tumor progression defined as a 25% increase in SWAT score from the nadir, was 148 days for the overall population and 169 days for the 61 patients with stage IIB or more advanced CTCL. Response to prior systemic therapy did not appear to be predictive of response to vorinostat.

In a second open-label trial, 33 patients with CTCL refractory to at least one prior systemic therapy received one of the following oral vorinostat dosage regimens: 400 mg once daily (regimen 1); 300 mg twice daily 3 times weekly (regimen 2); or 300 mg twice daily for 14 days (induction therapy) followed by a 7-day rest and then, in those who had not achieved at least a partial response (defined as improvement in disease findings of at least 50% from baseline), maintenance therapy with vorinostat 200 mg twice daily (regimen 3). Extent of disease was assessed using the 7-point Physician's Global Assessment (PGA) scale. Overall objective response rates of about 24, 25, and 36%, respectively, were reported in the overall patient population, the 28 patients with stage IIB or more advanced disease, and the 11 patients with Sézary syndrome. No complete responses, defined as 100% clearing of all findings, were observed. Overall response rates for regimens 1, 2, and 3 were about 31, 9, and 33%, respectively. The median time to response in the 8 patients who responded to vorinostat was about 84 days (range: 25–153 days); median response duration and median time to progression were 106 (range: 66–136) and about 212 (range: 94–255) days, respectively. Compared with the 400-mg once-daily regimen, a dosage of 300 mg twice daily was associated with increased toxicity and no additional clinical benefit.

Dosage and Administration

■ **Administration** Vorinostat is administered orally once daily. The drug should be administered with food. The manufacturer states that vorinostat capsules should be swallowed whole and should not be opened or crushed. Exposure to crushed or broken capsules should be avoided. If the powder comes in direct contact with the skin or mucous membranes, the affected area should be washed thoroughly.

■ **Dosage** ***Adults*** **Cutaneous T-cell Lymphoma.** The recommended adult oral dosage of vorinostat for the treatment of skin manifestations of cutaneous T-cell lymphoma (CTCL) refractory to 2 prior systemic therapies is 400 mg once daily. In patients who do not tolerate a dosage of 400 mg once daily (e.g., because of anemia or thrombocytopenia), the manufacturer recommends reducing the dosage to 300 mg once daily. If needed, the dosage may be further reduced to 300 mg once daily for 5 consecutive days each week. The optimal duration of treatment has not been clearly established. In clinical trials, treatment generally was continued until evidence of disease progression or unacceptable toxicity was observed.

■ **Special Populations** No special dosage recommendations at this time. Information on the pharmacokinetics or use of vorinostat in patients with renal or hepatic impairment is not available, and the manufacturer currently makes no specific dosage recommendations for such patients.

Cautions

■ **Contraindications** The manufacturer states that there are no known contraindications to the use of vorinostat.

■ **Warnings/Precautions** ***Warnings*** **Fetal/Neonatal Morbidity and Mortality.** May cause fetal harm; teratogenicity demonstrated in animals. If used during pregnancy or if patient becomes pregnant, apprise of potential fetal hazard.

Major Toxicities **Thromboembolism.** Risk of pulmonary embolism and deep-vein thrombosis. Clinicians should be alert to signs and symptoms of such effects, especially in patients with a prior history of thromboembolic events.

Hematologic Effects. Risk of dose-related thrombocytopenia and anemia. Dosage should be adjusted or therapy discontinued if thrombocytopenia or anemia occurs. (See Dosage under Dosage and Administration.)

GI Effects. Risk of nausea, vomiting, and diarrhea; antiemetic and/or antidiarrheal agents may be required.

To prevent dehydration, fluid and electrolyte replacement should be administered. Preexisting nausea, vomiting, and diarrhea should be adequately controlled before initiating therapy.

Hyperglycemia. Risk of hyperglycemia. Serum glucose concentrations should be monitored, especially in patients with known or possible diabetes mellitus. Diet and/or antidiabetic therapy should be adjusted, if needed.

General Precautions **Adequate Patient Monitoring.** Complete blood cell counts and blood chemistries (including serum electrolyte [i.e., potassium, magnesium, calcium], glucose, and creatinine concentrations) should be monitored every 2 weeks for the first 2 months of therapy and monthly thereafter. Hypokalemia or hypomagnesemia should be corrected before initiation of therapy. Consideration should be given to monitoring serum potassium and magnesium in symptomatic patients (e.g., patients who develop nausea, vomiting, diarrhea, fluid imbalance, or cardiac symptoms).

Interactions with Other Histone Deacetylase Inhibitors. Concomitant use of vorinostat with other histone deacetylase (HDAC) inhibitors (e.g., valproic acid) may result in severe thrombocytopenia and GI bleeding. Platelet count should be monitored every 2 weeks during the first 2 months.

Specific Populations **Pregnancy.** Category D. (See Fetal/Neonatal Morbidity and Mortality under Cautions.)

Lactation. Not known whether vorinostat is distributed into human milk. Discontinue nursing or the drug.

Pediatric Use. Safety and efficacy have not been established in pediatric patients younger than 18 years of age.

Geriatric Use. No substantial differences observed in safety and efficacy relative to younger adults, but increased sensitivity cannot be ruled out.

Hepatic Impairment. Vorinostat has not been studied in patients with hepatic impairment. Since the drug is extensively metabolized, it should be used with caution in patients with hepatic impairment.

Renal Impairment. Vorinostat has not been studied in patients with renal impairment. Although vorinostat is not renally excreted, the manufacturer states that the drug should be used with caution in patients with preexisting renal impairment.

■ **Common Adverse Effects** Adverse effects occurring in 10% or more of patients receiving vorinostat include diarrhea, fatigue, nausea, dysgeusia, thrombocytopenia, anorexia, weight loss, muscle spasms, alopecia, dry mouth, increased serum creatinine concentrations, chills, vomiting, constipation, dizziness, anemia, decreased appetite, peripheral edema, headache, pruritus, cough, upper respiratory infection, and pyrexia.

Drug Interactions

Vorinostat is not metabolized by cytochrome P-450 (CYP) isoenzymes. Pharmacokinetic interactions are unlikely with drugs that are CYP enzyme inducers or inhibitors.

Vorinostat does not inhibit CYP isoenzymes in vitro at therapeutic serum concentrations. Pharmacokinetic interactions with drugs metabolized by these isoenzymes are unlikely.

■ **Anticoagulants** Potential prolongation of prothrombin time (PT) or international normalized ratio (INR) in patients receiving vorinostat concomitantly with coumarin-derivative antiacoagulants. PT and INR should be carefully monitored.

■ **Histone Deacetylase Inhibitors** Potential severe thrombocytopenia and GI bleeding in patients receiving vorinostat concomitantly with other histone deacetylase (HDAC) inhibitors (e.g., valproic acid). Platelet count should be monitored every 2 weeks for the first 2 months.

Description

Vorinostat, a histone deacetylase inhibitor, is an antineoplastic agent. The mechanism of the antineoplastic effect of vorinostat has not been fully characterized. Vorinostat inhibits the enzymatic activity of histone deacetylases HDAC1, HDAC2, and HDAC3 (Class I) and HDAC6 (Class II) at nanomolar concentrations. HDAC enzymes catalyze the removal of acetyl groups from the lysine residues of proteins, including histones and transcription factors. Overexpression of HDAC enzymes or aberrant recruitment of HDAC enzymes to oncogenic transcription factors causing hypoacetylation of core nucleosomal histones has been observed in some cancer cells. Hypoacetylation of histones is associated with a condensed chromatin structure and repression of gene transcription. Inhibition of HDAC activity allows for the accumulation of acetyl groups on the histone lysine residues, resulting in an open chromatin structure and transcriptional activation. In vitro, vorinostat causes the accumulation of acetylated histones and induces cell cycle arrest and/or apoptosis of some transformed cells.

Vorinostat is extensively metabolized to inactive metabolites, principally by glucuronidation and hydrolysis followed by β-oxidation. The drug is not metabolized by cytochrome P-450 (CYP) isoenzymes. In vitro studies indicate that vorinostat is not a substrate of human P-glycoprotein and does not inhibit the P-glycoprotein transport system. Vorinostat is excreted principally (about 35–52%) in urine as the 2 major, inactive metabolites. Only a small portion (less than 1%) of a dose is excreted in urine as unchanged drug.

Advice to Patients

Importance of informing clinicians of any history of pulmonary embolism, deep-vein thrombosis, or diabetes mellitus.

Risk of deep-vein thrombosis and pulmonary embolism. Importance of notifying a clinician immediately if sudden swelling in leg, leg pain or tenderness, increased warmth in area of swelling, skin redness, skin color change, sudden sharp chest pain, shortness of breath, cough with bloody secretions, sweating, rapid pulse, fainting, or anxiety occurs.

Importance of swallowing capsules whole and of not chewing or opening the capsules. If capsules are accidentally opened or crushed, importance of not touching capsules or powder contents. If powder contacts skin or eyes, importance of washing area well with plain water and informing a clinician.

Importance of taking vorinostat with food.

Importance of advising patient that if a dose of vorinostat is missed, it should be taken as soon as remembered. If it is close to the next dose, patients should be advised to take the drug at the regularly scheduled time.

Importance of contacting clinician, local emergency room, or poison control center immediately in case of overdosage.

Risk of nausea, vomiting, and diarrhea; dehydration may occur. Importance of drinking at least 2 L of liquids every day while taking the drug. Importance of informing clinician immediately if excessive vomiting or diarrhea occurs or if unable to eat or drink normally because of nausea, vomiting, or diarrhea.

Patients with high blood sugar (hyperglycemia) or diabetes mellitus should continue monitoring serum glucose concentrations; antidiabetic therapy may require adjustment by a clinician.

Importance of informing clinician if fatigue, pallor, shortness of breath, or unusual bruising develops.

Importance of informing patient that regular blood tests will be performed to check blood counts and chemistries during therapy.

Importance of women informing clinicians if they are or plan to become pregnant or plan to breast-feed. Advise pregnant women of risk to the fetus.

Importance of informing clinicians of existing or contemplated concomitant therapy, including prescription (e.g., valproic acid, anticoagulants) and OTC drugs and herbal supplements, as well as any concomitant illnesses.

Importance of informing patients of other important precautionary information. (See Cautions.)

Overview® (see Users Guide). For additional information on this drug until a more detailed monograph is developed and published, the manufacturer's labeling should be consulted. It is *essential* that the manufacturer's labeling be consulted for more detailed information on usual cautions, precautions, contraindications, potential drug interactions, laboratory test interferences, and acute toxicity.

Preparations

Excipients in commercially available drug preparations may have clinically important effects in some individuals; consult specific product labeling for details.

Vorinostat

Oral

Capsules	100 mg	**Zolinza®**, Merck

Ziv-aflibercept

■ Ziv-aflibercept, a recombinant humanized fusion protein, is a vascular endothelial growth factor A (VEGF-A), VEGF-B, and placental growth factor (PlGF) antagonist that is used as an antineoplastic agent.

The IV preparation of Zaltrap® (ziv-aflibercept) for use in the treatment of metastatic colorectal cancer contains the same drug as the intravitreal preparation of Eylea® (aflibercept), which is used in the treatment of macular degeneration. Because of the potential for medication errors, the US Food and Drug Administration (FDA) required the addition of a prefix to the nonproprietary (generic) name; FDA later approved the addition of the prefix "ziv" to the generic name of Zaltrap® (ziv-aflibercept) for the US market.

Uses

■ **Colorectal Cancer** Ziv-aflibercept is used in combination with fluorouracil, leucovorin, and irinotecan (FOLFIRI) for the treatment of metastatic colorectal cancer that is refractory to or has progressed following oxaliplatin-based chemotherapy.

The current indication for ziv-aflibercept in combination with FOLFIRI is based principally on the results of a randomized, double-blind, placebo-controlled, multinational phase 3 study (VELOUR) in adult patients with metastatic colorectal cancer whose disease was refractory to or had progressed during or within 6 months of oxaliplatin-based chemotherapy (with or without bevacizumab). In this study, 1226 patients were randomized in a 1:1 ratio to receive either ziv-aflibercept (4 mg/kg by IV infusion over 1 hour) in combination with FOLFIRI (irinotecan 180 mg/m^2 by IV infusion over 90 minutes with leucovorin 400 mg/m^2 by IV infusion over 2 hours, followed by fluorouracil 400 mg/m^2 by rapid IV injection ["bolus"], and then fluorouracil 2400 mg/m^2 by IV infusion over 46 hours) *or* placebo in combination with FOLFIRI. Treatment was repeated every 2 weeks and continued until disease progression or unacceptable toxicity occurred. The primary efficacy end point was overall survival. The median age of patients enrolled in the study was 61 years (range: 19–86 years). The majority (89–90%) of enrolled patients had received prior oxaliplatin-based chemotherapy for metastatic disease; 28% of patients had received bevacizumab in combination with prior oxaliplatin-based chemotherapy. The median duration of treatment was approximately 21 weeks for patients receiving ziv-aflibercept in combination with FOLFIRI (median of 7 cycles of ziv-aflibercept, 9 cycles overall) and approximately 18 weeks for patients receiving placebo in combination with FOLFIRI (8 cycles overall).

Analysis of data at a median follow-up of 22.3 months indicated that patients receiving ziv-aflibercept in combination with FOLFIRI had a longer median overall survival compared with those receiving placebo in combination with FOLFIRI (13.5 versus 12.1 months, respectively). The 2-year survival rate was 28% in patients receiving ziv-aflibercept in combination with FOLFIRI compared with 18.7% in those receiving placebo in combination with FOLFIRI. Treatment effects of ziv-aflibercept were consistent across various patient subgroups defined by age, gender, race, geographic region, number of organs with metastasis, liver metastasis, history of hypertension, and prior bevacizumab use. Although not statistically significant (and there were fewer patients in the bevacizumab subgroup), patients who previously received bevacizumab appeared to benefit less from ziv-aflibercept treatment; the hazard ratio for overall survival was 0.86 in patients who received prior bevacizumab and 0.79 in those without prior bevacizumab exposure. Patients randomized to receive ziv-aflibercept in combination with FOLFIRI had a longer median progression-free survival compared with those receiving placebo in combination with FOLFIRI (6.9 versus 4.7 months, respectively). In addition, patients receiving ziv-aflibercept in combination with FOLFIRI had a higher overall response rate compared with those receiving placebo in combination with FOLFIRI (19.8 versus 11.1%, respectively).

Dosage and Administration

■ **General** Ziv-aflibercept therapy should *not* be initiated in patients who have undergone surgery until after the surgical incision has fully healed. (See Surgery and Wound Healing Complications under Warnings/Precautions: Warnings, in Cautions.)

Clinicians should consult the respective manufacturers' labelings or published protocols for information on the dosage, method of administration, and administration sequence of other antineoplastic agents used in combination regimens.

■ **Administration** Ziv-aflibercept is administered by IV infusion over 1 hour. *The drug should not be administered by rapid IV injection, such as IV push or bolus.*

Ziv-aflibercept injection must be diluted prior to administration. Prior to dilution, ziv-aflibercept injection should be inspected visually for particulate matter and discoloration; if particulate matter or discoloration is evident, the solution should *not* be used. Ziv-aflibercept is diluted by adding the appropriate dose (4 mg/kg) of ziv-aflibercept injection concentrate (containing 25 mg/mL) to a diethylhexyl phthalate (DEHP) plasticized polyvinylchloride (PVC) or non-PVC polyolefin infusion bag containing the appropriate volume of 0.9% sodium chloride or 5% dextrose injection to yield a final concentration of 0.6–8 mg/mL. No other drug should be added to or administered in the same IV line with ziv-aflibercept infusion.

After dilution, ziv-aflibercept infusion solution should be administered by IV infusion through a 0.2-μm polyethersulfone filter; filters made of polyvinylidene fluoride (PVDF) or nylon should not be used. The diluted infusion solution should be administered through DEHP PVC, non-DEHP trioctyltrimellitate (TOTM) PVC, polypropylene, polyethylene-lined PVC, or polyurethane administration sets.

Any unused portion left in the vial or infusion bag should be discarded since ziv-aflibercept injection contains no preservative.

Diluted ziv-aflibercept infusion solution may be stored at 2–8°C for up to 4 hours. Unopened vials of ziv-aflibercept injection should be protected from light and stored in the original carton at 2–8°C.

■ **Dosage** ***Metastatic Colorectal Cancer*** For the treatment of metastatic colorectal cancer that is refractory to or has progressed following oxaliplatin-based chemotherapy, the recommended dosage of ziv-aflibercept is 4 mg/kg by IV infusion over 1 hour in combination with fluorouracil, leucovorin, and irinotecan (FOLFIRI; irinotecan 180 mg/m^2 by IV infusion over 90 minutes with leucovorin 400 mg/m^2 by IV infusion over 2 hours, followed by fluorouracil 400 mg/m^2 by rapid IV injection ["bolus], and then fluorouracil 2400 mg/m^2 by IV infusion over 46 hours). Ziv-aflibercept should be administered prior to the FOLFIRI regimen on the day of treatment. The ziv-aflibercept-FOLFIRI combination regimen should be repeated every 2 weeks and continued until disease progression or unacceptable toxicity occurs.

Dosage Modification for Toxicity If toxicities occur, temporary or permanent discontinuance of ziv-aflibercept may be required based on causality.

Ziv-aflibercept should be *discontinued* in patients who develop severe hemorrhage, GI perforation, compromised wound healing, fistula formation, hypertensive crisis or hypertensive encephalopathy, arterial thromboembolic events, nephrotic syndrome or thrombotic microangiopathy, or reversible posterior leukoencephalopathy syndrome (RPLS). (See Cautions: Warnings/Precautions.)

Ziv-aflibercept therapy should be *temporarily suspended* at least 4 weeks prior to elective surgery. Therapy also should be temporarily interrupted in patients who develop recurrent or severe hypertension or proteinuria. (See Hypertension and also Proteinuria under Dosage: Dosage Modification for Toxicity, in Dosage and Administration.) Ziv-aflibercept therapy should be delayed in patients with a neutrophil count of less than 1500/mm^3. (See Neutropenia and Neutropenic Complications under Warnings/Precautions: Other Warnings and Precautions, in Cautions.)

Hypertension. If recurrent or severe hypertension occurs, ziv-aflibercept therapy should be interrupted until hypertension is controlled; therapy may then be resumed at a *permanently* reduced dosage of 2 mg/kg. If hypertensive crisis or hypertensive encephalopathy occurs, treatment with ziv-aflibercept should be discontinued. (See Hypertension under Warnings/Precautions: Other Warnings and Precautions, in Cautions.)

Proteinuria. Ziv-aflibercept therapy should be interrupted for proteinuria of or exceeding 2 g per 24 hours and resumed when proteinuria declines below this level. If proteinuria recurs, therapy should be withheld again until proteinuria declines below 2 g per 24 hours; therapy may then be resumed at a *permanently* reduced dosage of 2 mg/kg. If nephrotic syndrome or thrombotic microangiopathy occurs, treatment with ziv-aflibercept should be discontinued. (See Proteinuria under Warnings/Precautions: Other Warnings and Precautions, in Cautions.)

■ **Special Populations** No dosage adjustment is required in geriatric patients. (See Geriatric Use under Warnings/Precautions: Specific Populations, in Cautions.)

The manufacturer makes no specific dosage recommendations for patients with hepatic or renal impairment. (See Hepatic Impairment and also Renal Impairment under Warnings/Precautions: Specific Populations, in Cautions.)

Cautions

■ **Contraindications** The manufacturer states there are no known contraindications to the use of ziv-aflibercept.

■ **Warnings/Precautions** ***Warnings*** **Hemorrhage.** Ziv-aflibercept is associated with an increased risk of hemorrhage, including severe and sometimes fatal hemorrhage. In the VELOUR study, bleeding or hemorrhage (all grades) was reported in 38% of patients receiving ziv-aflibercept in combination with fluorouracil, leucovorin, and irinotecan (FOLFIRI) compared with 19% of those receiving placebo in combination with FOLFIRI. Grade 3 or 4 hemorrhagic events (including GI hemorrhage, hematuria, and postprocedural hemorrhage) were reported in 3% of patients receiving ziv-aflibercept in combination with FOLFIRI compared with 1% of those receiving placebo in combination with FOLFIRI. Severe intracranial hemorrhage and pulmonary hemorrhage/hemoptysis, including fatal cases, have been reported in patients receiving ziv-aflibercept.

Patients should be monitored for signs and symptoms of bleeding. Ziv-aflibercept should *not* be initiated in patients with severe hemorrhage. Ziv-aflibercept should be discontinued if severe hemorrhage occurs during therapy with the drug.

GI Perforation. GI perforation, sometimes fatal, has been reported in patients receiving ziv-aflibercept. In phase 3 studies in patients with various cancers (i.e., colorectal, pancreatic, and lung cancer), GI perforation (all grades) was reported in 0.8% of patients receiving ziv-aflibercept compared with 0.3% of those receiving placebo; grade 3 or 4 GI perforation was reported in 0.8 or 0.2% of patients receiving ziv-aflibercept or placebo, respectively.

Patients should be monitored for signs and symptoms of GI perforation. Ziv-aflibercept should be discontinued if GI perforation occurs.

Surgery and Wound Healing Complications. Grade 3 compromised wound healing has been reported in 0.3% of patients receiving ziv-aflibercept in combination with FOLFIRI compared with none of those receiving placebo in combination with FOLFIRI.

Ziv-aflibercept therapy should be suspended at least 4 weeks prior to elective surgery. The drug should not be resumed until at least 4 weeks following major surgery and after the surgical incision has fully healed. In patients undergoing minor surgery (e.g., central venous access port placement, biopsy, tooth extraction), ziv-aflibercept may be initiated or resumed after the surgical incision has fully healed.

Ziv-aflibercept should be discontinued in patients with compromised wound healing.

Other Warnings and Precautions **Fistula Formation.** Fistula formation involving GI and non-GI sites has been reported in more patients receiving ziv-aflibercept compared with those receiving placebo. Fistula formation involving anal, enterovesical, enterocutaneous, colovaginal, and intestinal sites was reported in 1.5% of patients with metastatic colorectal cancer receiving ziv-aflibercept in combination with FOLFIRI compared with 0.5% of those receiving placebo in combination with FOLFIRI. Grade 3 GI fistula formation was reported in 0.3% of patients receiving ziv-aflibercept in combination with FOLFIRI compared with 0.2% of those receiving placebo in combination with FOLFIRI.

Ziv-aflibercept should be discontinued if fistula formation occurs.

Hypertension. Ziv-aflibercept is associated with an increased risk of grade 3 or 4 hypertension. In the VELOUR study, grade 3 hypertension (defined as requiring adjustment to existing antihypertensive therapy or treatment with more than one drug) was reported in 19% of patients receiving ziv-aflibercept in combination with FOLFIRI compared with 1.5% of those receiving placebo in combination with FOLFIRI. Grade 4 hypertension (hypertensive crisis) was reported in 0.2% of patients receiving ziv-aflibercept in combination with FOLFIRI compared with none of those receiving placebo in combination with FOLFIRI. Among patients experiencing grade 3 or 4 hypertension, 54% developed hypertension during the first 2 cycles of therapy. In a phase 1 study evaluating ziv-aflibercept over a dosage range of 0.3–7 mg/kg every 2 weeks, the median time to onset of hypertension was 3.5 days; hypertension was reversible or manageable following discontinuance of ziv-aflibercept or initiation of appropriate supportive measures.

Blood pressure should be monitored every 2 weeks or more frequently as clinically indicated during ziv-aflibercept therapy. If hypertension occurs, patients should be treated with appropriate antihypertensive therapy, and blood pressure should be monitored regularly. If hypertension recurs or becomes severe, temporary interruption of ziv-aflibercept therapy and subsequent dosage reduction is required. (See Hypertension under Dosage: Dosage Modification for Toxicity, in Dosage and Administration.) Ziv-aflibercept should be discontinued in patients who develop hypertensive crisis or hypertensive encephalopathy.

Ziv-aflibercept has not been evaluated in patients with New York Heart Association (NYHA) class III or IV heart failure.

Arterial Thromboembolic Events. Arterial thromboembolic events (including transient ischemic attacks, cerebrovascular accident, and angina pectoris) have been reported in more patients with metastatic colorectal cancer receiving ziv-aflibercept in combination with FOLFIRI compared with those receiving placebo in combination with FOLFIRI (2.6 versus 1.7%, respectively). Grade 3 or 4 arterial thromboembolic events were reported in 1.8% of patients receiving ziv-aflibercept in combination with FOLFIRI compared with 0.7% of those receiving placebo in combination with FOLFIRI.

Ziv-aflibercept should be discontinued in patients who experience an arterial thromboembolic event.

Proteinuria. Severe proteinuria, nephrotic syndrome, and thrombotic microangiopathy have been reported in more patients receiving ziv-aflibercept compared with those receiving placebo. In the VELOUR study, proteinuria occurred in 62% of patients receiving ziv-aflibercept in combination with FOLFIRI compared with 41% of those receiving placebo in combination with FOLFIRI. Grade 3 or 4 proteinuria was reported in 8% of patients receiving ziv-aflibercept in combination with FOLFIRI compared with 1% of those receiving placebo in combination with FOLFIRI. Nephrotic syndrome occurred in 0.5% of patients receiving ziv-aflibercept in combination with FOLFIRI compared with none of those receiving placebo in combination with FOLFIRI. Thrombotic microangiopathy has been reported in 3 of 2258 patients with cancer receiving ziv-aflibercept in various studies. In a phase 1 study evaluating ziv-aflibercept over a dosage range of 0.3–7 mg/kg every 2 weeks, the median time to onset of proteinuria was 15 days; proteinuria was reversible or manageable following discontinuance of ziv-aflibercept or initiation of appropriate supportive measures.

Urine dipstick and urinary protein to creatinine ratio should be monitored for the development or worsening of proteinuria during therapy. Patients with a urinary protein to creatinine ratio exceeding 1 should undergo further assessment with a 24-hour urine collection. Ziv-aflibercept therapy should be interrupted for proteinuria of or exceeding 2 g per 24 hours and resumed when proteinuria declines below this level. If proteinuria recurs, temporary interruption of ziv-aflibercept therapy and subsequent dosage reduction is required. (See Proteinuria under Dosage: Dosage Modification for Toxicity, in Dosage and Administration.)

Ziv-aflibercept should be discontinued in patients who develop nephrotic syndrome or thrombotic microangiopathy.

Neutropenia and Neutropenic Complications. Neutropenic complications (e.g., febrile neutropenia, neutropenic infection) have been reported in more patients receiving ziv-aflibercept compared with those receiving placebo. Grade 3 or 4 neutropenia occurred in 37% of patients with metastatic colorectal cancer receiving ziv-aflibercept in combination with FOLFIRI compared with 30% of those receiving placebo in combination with FOLFIRI. Grade 3 or 4 febrile neutropenia or neutropenic infection/sepsis was reported in 4 or 1.5%, respectively, of patients receiving ziv-aflibercept in combination with FOLFIRI compared with 2 or 1.2%, respectively, of those receiving placebo in combination with FOLFIRI.

Complete blood cell (CBC) counts, including differential, should be monitored at baseline and prior to initiation of each cycle of ziv-aflibercept. Therapy with ziv-aflibercept should be delayed until neutrophil counts are at least 1500/mm^3.

Diarrhea and Dehydration. Grade 3 or 4 diarrhea has been reported in more patients receiving ziv-aflibercept in combination with FOLFIRI compared with those receiving placebo in combination with FOLFIRI (19 versus 8%, respectively). Grade 3 or 4 dehydration has been reported in 4% of patients receiving ziv-aflibercept in combination with FOLFIRI compared with 1% of those receiving placebo in combination with FOLFIRI. Diarrhea is more likely to occur in patients 65 years of age or older.

Patients 65 years of age or older should be monitored more closely for diarrhea and dehydration. (See Geriatric Use under Warnings/Precautions: Specific Populations, in Cautions.)

Reversible Posterior Leukoencephalopathy Syndrome. Reversible posterior leukoencephalopathy syndrome (RPLS) has been reported in 0.5% of patients receiving ziv-aflibercept alone or in combination with chemotherapy.

If signs or symptoms of RPLS develop, diagnosis of RPLS should be confirmed by magnetic resonance imaging (MRI), and ziv-aflibercept therapy should be discontinued. Symptoms of RPLS usually resolve or improve within days, but some patients have experienced ongoing neurologic sequelae or death.

Immunogenicity. As with all therapeutic proteins, there is a potential for immunogenicity. In multiple studies in patients who received ziv-aflibercept for various malignancies, anti-product antibody formation occurred in 3.1% of patients receiving ziv-aflibercept compared with 1.7% of those receiving placebo. Among those patients who tested positive for anti-product antibodies, neutralizing antibodies were detected in 17 of 48 patients (35%) receiving ziv-aflibercept and in 2 of 40 patients (5%) receiving placebo. Mean free ziv-aflibercept trough concentrations were lower in patients with positive neutralizing antibodies than in the overall population; the clinical relevance of neutralizing antibodies is not known.

Because the observed incidence of antibody positivity may be influenced by several factors including sample handling, timing of sample collection, concomitant drug therapy, and underlying disease, comparison of the incidence of antibodies to ziv-aflibercept to that of other drugs may be misleading.

Specific Populations **Pregnancy.** Category C. (See Users Guide.) (See Advice to Patients.)

Lactation. It is not known whether ziv-aflibercept is distributed into milk in humans. Because of the potential for serious adverse reactions to ziv-aflibercept in nursing infants, a decision should be made whether to discontinue nursing or the drug, taking into account the importance of the drug to the woman.

Pediatric Use. Safety and efficacy of ziv-aflibercept have not been established in pediatric patients younger than 18 years of age.

Geriatric Use. In the VELOUR study, 34% of patients were 65 years of age or older and 5% were 75 years of age or older. Although no overall differences in efficacy (i.e., overall survival) were observed between geriatric and younger patients, the incidences of diarrhea, dizziness, asthenia, weight loss, and dehydration were higher among patients 65 years of age or older compared with younger patients. Geriatric patients should be monitored more closely for diarrhea and dehydration. (See Diarrhea and Dehydration under Warnings/Precautions: Other Warnings and Precautions, in Cautions.) Dosage adjustment is not required in patients 65 years of age or older.

Hepatic Impairment. The effects of hepatic impairment on the pharmacokinetics of ziv-aflibercept have not been formally studied. Analysis of population pharmacokinetic data from 1507 patients indicates that ziv-aflibercept exposure and clearance are similar between patients with mild (total bilirubin concentration exceeding 1–1.5 times the upper limit of normal [ULN] and any AST concentration) or moderate (total bilirubin concentration exceeding 1.5–3 times the ULN and any AST concentration) hepatic impairment and those with normal hepatic function. Data are not available for patients with severe hepatic impairment (total bilirubin concentration exceeding 3 times the ULN and any AST concentration).

Renal Impairment. The effects of renal impairment on the pharmacokinetics of ziv-aflibercept have not been formally studied. Analysis of population pharmacokinetic data indicates that ziv-aflibercept exposure and clearance are similar between patients with mild (creatinine clearance of 50–80 mL/minute), moderate (creatinine clearance of 30–50 mL/minute), or severe (creatinine clearance less than 30 mL/minute) renal impairment and those with normal renal function.

■ **Common Adverse Effects** The most common adverse effects reported in 20% or more of patients receiving ziv-aflibercept in combination with FOLFIRI and at an incidence that is at least 2% higher than that reported with placebo in combination with FOLFIRI include leukopenia, diarrhea, neutropenia, proteinuria, elevated aminotransferase (i.e., AST, ALT) concentrations, stomatitis, fatigue, thrombocytopenia, hypertension, weight loss, decreased appetite, epistaxis, abdominal pain, dysphonia, elevated serum creatinine concentration, and headache.

The most common grade 3 or 4 adverse effects reported in 5% or more of patients receiving ziv-aflibercept in combination with FOLFIRI and at an incidence that is at least 2% higher than that reported with placebo in combination with FOLFIRI include neutropenia, diarrhea, hypertension, leukopenia, stomatitis, fatigue, proteinuria, and asthenia.

Drug Interactions

No formal drug interaction studies have been performed to date.

■ **Antineoplastic Agents** Cross-study comparisons and population pharmacokinetic analyses indicate no clinically important pharmacokinetic interactions between ziv-aflibercept and irinotecan or between ziv-aflibercept and fluorouracil.

Description

Ziv-aflibercept, a recombinant humanized fusion protein, is a vascular endothelial growth factor A (VEGF-A), VEGF-B, and placental growth factor (PlGF) antagonist. The drug consists of VEGF-binding portions from the extracellular domains of human VEGF receptors 1 and 2 (VEGFR-1 and VEGFR-2), fused to the Fc portion of human immunoglobulin G_1 (IgG_1). The IV preparation of Zaltrap® (ziv-aflibercept) for use in the treatment of metatastic colorectal cancer contains the same drug as the intravitreal preparation of Eylea® (aflibercept), which is used in the treatment of macular degeneration. Because of the potential for medication errors, the US Food and Drug Administration (FDA) required the addition of a prefix to the nonproprietary (generic) name; FDA later approved the addition of the prefix "ziv" to the generic name of Zaltrap® (ziv-aflibercept) for the US market.

Ziv-aflibercept acts as a soluble decoy receptor that binds to VEGF-A, VEGF-B, and PlGF and inhibits their biologic activity. VEGF-A, VEGF-B, and PlGF are angiogenic factors that promote endothelial cell proliferation, survival, migration, and vascular permeability. Binding of ziv-aflibercept to VEGF-A, VEGF-B, and PlGF prevents these factors from binding to their endogenous receptors, reducing neovascularization and vascular permeability. The binding affinity of ziv-aflibercept for VEGF-A isoforms is higher than that of bevacizumab; ziv-aflibercept also is more potent than bevacizumab in inhibiting VEGF-1 and VEGFR-2 activation. Ziv-aflibercept has been shown to inhibit angiogenesis by inhibiting proliferation of endothelial cells in animals; the drug also has been shown to inhibit the growth of xenotransplanted colon tumors in mice.

Free ziv-aflibercept concentrations appear to exhibit linear pharmacokinetics over a dosage range of 2–9 mg/kg. Steady-state concentrations of free ziv-aflibercept are reached by the second dose. Following administration of ziv-aflibercept at a dosage of 4 mg/kg every 2 weeks, the accumulation ratio for free ziv-aflibercept is approximately 1.2; the elimination half-life of free ziv-aflibercept is approximately 6 days (range: 4–7 days).

Analysis of population pharmacokinetic data indicates that age, race, and gender have no clinically important effects on exposure to free ziv-aflibercept. However, a 29% increase in systemic exposure to the drug has been observed in patients weighing 100 kg or more compared with those weighing 50–100 kg.

Advice to Patients

Increased risk of severe bleeding. Importance of informing clinician of any episodes or symptoms of bleeding (e.g., lightheadedness).

Risk of wound healing complications. Importance of discussing with clinician prior to undergoing any surgery or procedures (including tooth extractions).

Risk of development or exacerbation of hypertension. Importance of receiving routine monitoring of blood pressure and informing clinician if blood pressure is elevated or if manifestations of hypertension (e.g., severe headache, lightheadedness, neurologic symptoms) occur.

Importance of informing clinician of severe diarrhea, vomiting, or severe abdominal pain.

Importance of informing clinician of fever or other signs and symptoms of infection.

Risk of arterial thromboembolic events.

Risk of fetal or neonatal toxicity. Necessity of advising women and men receiving ziv-aflibercept to use an effective method of contraception during and for at least 3 months after the last dose of ziv-aflibercept. Importance of immediately informing clinician if the patient or their partner becomes pregnant during therapy.

Importance of informing clinicians of existing or contemplated concomitant therapy, including prescription and OTC drugs, as well as any concomitant illnesses.

Importance of informing patients of other important precautionary information. (See Cautions.)

Overview® (see Users Guide). For additional information on this drug until a more detailed monograph is developed and published, the manufacturer's labeling should be consulted. It is *essential* that the manufacturer's labeling be consulted for more detailed information on usual cautions, precautions, contraindications, potential drug interactions, laboratory test interferences, and acute toxicity. For further information on the handling of antineoplastic agents, see the ASHP Guidelines on Handling Hazardous Drugs at http://www.ahfsdruginformation.com.

Preparations

Excipients in commercially available drug preparations may have clinically important effects in some individuals; consult specific product labeling for details.

Ziv-aflibercept (Recombinant)

Parenteral

Injection, for IV infusion only	25 mg/mL (100 and 200 mg)	**Zaltrap®**, Sanofi-Aventis

12:00 AUTONOMIC DRUGS*

§ Omitted from the print version of *AHFS Drug Information*® because of space limitations. This monograph is available on the *AHFS Drug Information*® website, http://ahfsdruginformation.com. Username: ahfs2020; Password: ASHP94498.

* Please see the full *AHFS Pharmacologic-Therapeutic Classification*© on p. viii. Not all classes are used in the printed edition.

Autonomic Drugs 12:00

Parasympathomimetic (Cholinergic) Agents 12:04

Donepezil Hydrochloride

■ Donepezil hydrochloride is a centrally active, reversible acetylcholinesterase inhibitor.

Uses

■ **Alzheimer's Disease** Donepezil hydrochloride is used for the palliative treatment of mild to moderate dementia of the Alzheimer's type (Alzheimer's disease, presenile or senile dementia). The rationale for use of donepezil in this condition is to potentially increase CNS acetylcholine concentrations, which can be deficient in patients with Alzheimer's disease (see Description). The current indication is based principally on 2 short-term (15 or 30 weeks), double-blind, placebo-controlled studies in patients with a diagnosis of Alzheimer's disease of mild to moderate severity. Both studies demonstrated clinically important but modest and variable improvement in cognitive function and clinician-rated global assessment of observed clinical change. However, as with tacrine (no longer available in the US), improvement associated with donepezil therapy was not maintained following discontinuance of the drug, suggesting that donepezil does not alter the underlying disease process of dementia.

The specific role of donepezil in the management of Alzheimer's disease, particularly long-term or in patients with severe disease, remains to be fully elucidated. In patients who received therapy with donepezil for at least 2 years in uncontrolled studies following their participation in placebo-controlled studies of the drug, improvement in cognitive function was maintained for an average of at least 40 weeks, with some benefit still evident after 2 years of follow-up. However, the cognitive abilities of patients receiving donepezil decline over time, although apparently to a lesser degree than in untreated patients.

The American Psychiatric Association (APA) and other experts (e.g., the American Geriatrics Society, the American Academy of Neurology) state that because anticholinesterase agents produce apparently modest improvement in some patients and because other established effective therapies are lacking, the use of an anticholinesterase agent (e.g., donepezil, galantamine, rivastigmine, tacrine [no longer available in the US]) to treat cognitive symptoms should be considered in the management of Alzheimer's disease in patients who are mildly or moderately impaired. Anticholinesterase therapy potentially may improve cognitive functioning or delay decline and also may enhance clinician and family assessments and activities of daily living in such patients, albeit modestly. Although comparative studies have not been performed to date, donepezil does not share the hepatotoxic potential of tacrine and may be preferable to tacrine as a first-line treatment because it can be administered once daily and does not require regular monitoring of liver function. The APA states that the limited potential benefits and the costs of therapy with anticholinesterase agents should be discussed with patients and their families. As the efficacy of such therapy is modest, therapeutic alternatives such as other drug therapy (e.g., vitamin E, selegiline), psychosocial interventions, participation in a study of investigational treatment, and/or no treatment, may be considered. Further study and clinical experience are needed to more fully elucidate the efficacy and safety of donepezil in the management of Alzheimer's disease.

In the 15- and 30-week, placebo-controlled studies upon which the current indication principally is based, donepezil therapy was associated with improvements in cognitive and overall functioning (e.g., as assessed by results of neuropsychological tests and clinicians' impression of change, respectively). Age, race, or gender did not predict response to donepezil therapy in these studies. Cognitive function was evaluated with the cognitive subscale of the Alzheimer's Disease Assessment Scale (ADAS cog), a multiple-item instrument that has been extensively validated in longitudinal cohorts of patients with Alzheimer's disease. ADAS cog measures elements of memory, orientation, attention, reasoning, language, and praxis. Scores on the ADAS cog range from 0–70, with increasing scores being indicative of increasing cognitive impairment. Although normal geriatric adults may have scores of 0 or 1, slightly higher scores are not unusual in adults without dementia. Patients recruited into the 2 controlled studies of donepezil had initial scores of approximately 26 (range: 4–61) on the ADAS cog. Longitudinal studies of ambulatory patients with mild to moderate Alzheimer's disease suggest that scores on the ADAS cog will increase (i.e., indicating a decline in cognitive function) by 6–12 points each year in such patients. A smaller annual change in scores is observed in patients with either very mild or very advanced Alzheimer's disease because the ADAS cog does not uniformly reflect cognitive change over the course of the disease. In clinical trials of donepezil, ADAS cog scores increased by approximately 2–4 points per year in patients who received placebo.

Overall clinical change in patients receiving donepezil or placebo was evaluated with a Clinician's Interview Based Impression of Change (CIBIC) that required use of information from caregivers (CIBIC plus). A variety of CIBIC formats have been used in clinical studies, and the various CIBIC formats may differ in terms of depth and structure. The CIBIC plus used in the studies of donepezil was a subjective, semistructured instrument intended to measure the patient's ability to function generally, cognitively, behaviorally, and in activities of daily living. Scores of 1, 4, or 7 on the CIBIC plus denote marked improvement, no change, or markedly worse, respectively.

In the 15- and 30-week controlled studies of donepezil, the treatments were administered for 12 or 24 weeks, respectively, followed by placebo washout periods of 3 or 6 weeks, respectively, to determine whether rebound effects would occur following discontinuance of the drug. Patients received 5 or 10 mg of donepezil hydrochloride or placebo once daily in these studies; patients who were assigned to receive the 10-mg dosage of donepezil hydrochloride initially received 5 mg daily for 7 days to minimize the likelihood of adverse cholinergic effects. In the 15-week study, the improvement from baseline in the ADAS cog score with donepezil compared with placebo averaged 2.7 or 3 points after 12 weeks of treatment with donepezil hydrochloride 5 or 10 mg daily, respectively; the difference in ADAS cog scores for the 2 dosages was not statistically significant. In this study, an improvement of 7 points in the ADAS cog score was attained at 12 weeks by a cumulative 14, 21, or 36% of patients who received placebo, 5 mg of donepezil hydrochloride, or 10 mg of donepezil hydrochloride once daily, respectively, while an improvement of 4 points was attained at 12 weeks by a cumulative 30, 49, or 57% of patients in these respective groups. Cognitive function was maintained (i.e., no change in ADAS cog score from baseline) at 12 weeks in a cumulative 72, 83, or 87% of patients who received placebo, 5 mg of donepezil hydrochloride, or 10 mg of donepezil hydrochloride once daily, respectively. In the 30-week study, improvement from baseline in ADAS cog score with donepezil compared with placebo averaged 2.8 or 3.1 points after 24 weeks of treatment with 5 or 10 mg daily, respectively, of donepezil hydrochloride; the difference in ADAS cog scores for the 2 dosages was not statistically significant. An improvement of 7 points from baseline in the ADAS cog score was attained at 24 weeks by a cumulative 8, 15, or 26% of patients who received placebo, 5 mg of donepezil hydrochloride, or 10 mg of donepezil hydrochloride once daily, respectively. Improvement of 4 points from baseline in the ADAS cog score was attained at 24 weeks by a cumulative 28, 40, or 58% of patients who received placebo, 5 mg of donepezil hydrochloride, or 10 mg of donepezil hydrochloride once daily, respectively. Cognitive function was maintained (i.e., no change in ADAS cog score from baseline) at 24 weeks in a cumulative 59, 83, or 82% of patients who received placebo, donepezil hydrochloride 5 mg, or donepezil hydrochloride 10 mg once daily, respectively.

Overall clinical improvement (as determined by the CIBIC plus assessment) also was observed in patients treated with donepezil in these 2 controlled studies. CIBIC plus scores attained in patients receiving 5 or 10 mg of donepezil hydrochloride once daily differed from placebo by 0.36 or 0.38 points, respectively, after 12 weeks of treatment in the 15-week study and by 0.35 or 0.39 points, respectively, after 24 weeks of treatment in the 30-week study. As with the ADAS cog scores, a dose-related effect of donepezil on overall clinical change in these studies was not established.

Following the 6-week placebo washout period in the 30-week study, scores on the ADAS cog for patients treated with donepezil or placebo were indistinguishable, indicating no evidence of an effect of donepezil on the underlying disease process in dementia. Results of neuropsychologic tests (i.e., ADAS cog, CIBIC plus, Mini-Mental State Examination [MMSE], and Clinical Dementia Rating [CDR]) performed 6 weeks after discontinuance of donepezil therapy did not show evidence of a rebound deterioration in cognitive symptoms.

Dosage and Administration

■ **Administration** Donepezil hydrochloride is administered orally as conventional or orally disintegrating tablets. The drug is administered once daily, usually in the evening at bedtime.Donepezil hydrochloride orally disintegrating tablets should be allowed to dissolve on the tongue and followed with water. Donepezil hydrochloride orally disintegrating and conventional film-coated tablets are bioequivalent. Because food does not affect the rate or extent of absorption of donepezil when administered as conventional film-coated tablets, the drug can be administered with or without food. The effect of food on absorption of donepezil after administration as orally disintegrating tablets has not been studied. However, the manufacturer states that any effects are expected to be minimal, and orally disintegrating tablets may be taken without regard to meals.

Donepezil should not be used in patients with known hypersensitivity to the drug or to piperidine derivatives.

As a cholinesterase inhibitor, donepezil hydrochloride may exaggerate the effects of succinylcholine-type muscle relaxants during anesthesia. Cholinesterase inhibitors such as donepezil may increase gastric acid secretion as a result of increased cholinergic activity. Therefore, although placebo-controlled studies have shown no increase in the incidence of peptic ulcer disease or GI bleeding with donepezil, the manufacturer states that patients receiving the drug, especially those at increased risk for developing ulcers (e.g., those with a history of peptic ulcer disease, those taking concurrent nonsteroidal anti-inflammatory agents), should be monitored carefully for symptoms of active or occult GI bleeding.

Cholinesterase inhibitors may produce vagotonic effects on the sinoatrial or atrioventricular nodes. These effects may be manifested as bradycardia or heart block in patients with or without known cardiac conduction abnormalities. In clinical trials, syncopal episodes were reported in 2 or 1% of patients receiving donepezil or placebo, respectively.

Cholinesterase inhibitors such as donepezil, because of their cholinomimetic actions, should be prescribed with caution in patients with a history of asthma or obstructive pulmonary disease.

Although not reported in clinical studies with donepezil, cholinomimetic agents may cause bladder outflow obstruction; urinary frequency was reported more often (in 2% more patients) with donepezil therapy than with placebo in clinical trials. In addition, these agents may have the potential to cause generalized seizures; however, seizure activity also may be a manifestation of Alzheimer's disease.

■ **Dosage** The manufacturer states that safety and efficacy of donepezil hydrochloride for any use in children have not been established. Dementia of the Alzheimer's type occurs principally in patients more than 55 years of age. The mean age of patients receiving donepezil in clinical studies was 73 years of age. For most adverse effects, there were no clinically important differences reported in patients 65 years of age or older compared with those younger than 65 years of age.

Alzheimer's Disease For the palliative treatment of mild to moderate dementia of the Alzheimer's type (Alzheimer's disease), the recommended initial dosage of donepezil hydrochloride is 5 mg daily. Donepezil hydrochloride dosages of 5 or 10 mg daily are both effective, but additional clinical benefit with the 10-mg dosage has not been demonstrated in controlled clinical studies. However, based on the ordering of treatment group mean ADAS cog scores and dose trend analyses from these studies, there is the possibility of additional benefit with the higher (10 mg) dosage in some patients.

The manufacturer states that use of the 10-mg daily dosage of donepezil hydrochloride depends on prescriber and patient preference. In controlled studies, the occurrence of adverse cholinergic effects was more likely in patients receiving 10 mg of donepezil hydrochloride daily following titration from 5 mg daily over a 1-week period, than in those who received 5 mg daily. However, adverse cholinergic effects with the 10-mg daily dosage of donepezil hydrochloride were no more frequent than with the 5-mg daily dosage when the dosage of donepezil hydrochloride increased from 5 to 10 mg over a 6-week period in uncontrolled studies. Therefore, because plasma concentrations of donepezil do not reach steady state for 15 days, and the occurrence of adverse effects may be influenced by the rate of increase in dosage, the daily administration of 10 mg of donepezil hydrochloride should not be considered until after the patient has received 5 mg daily for 4–6 weeks.

■ **Dosage in Renal and Hepatic Impairment** Limited data in a few patients with moderate to severe renal impairment (creatinine clearance less than 22 mL/minute per 1.73 m^2) indicate no difference in the clearance of donepezil compared with that in healthy individuals matched for age and gender, and the manufacturer makes no specific recommendation for dosage adjustment in patients with renal impairment.

Clearance of donepezil in a limited number of patients with stable alcoholic cirrhosis was reduced by 20% compared with that in healthy age- and gender-matched individuals; however, the manufacturer makes no specific recommendation for dosage adjustment in patients with hepatic disease.

Description

Donepezil hydrochloride, a piperidine derivative, is a centrally active, reversible inhibitor of acetylcholinesterase. The drug is structurally unrelated to other anticholinesterase agents (e.g., physostigmine).

The precise mechanism(s) of action of donepezil in patients with dementia of the Alzheimer's type (Alzheimer's disease) has not been fully elucidated. The drug is an anticholinesterase agent that binds reversibly with and inactivates cholinesterases (e.g., acetylcholinesterase), thus inhibiting hydrolysis of acetylcholine. As a result, the concentration of acetylcholine increases at cholinergic synapses. In vitro data and data in animals indicate that the anticholinesterase activity of donepezil is relatively specific for acetylcholinesterase in the brain compared with butyrylcholinesterase inhibition in peripheral tissues.

A deficiency of acetylcholine caused by selective loss of cholinergic neurons in the cerebral cortex, nucleus basalis, and hippocampus is recognized as one of the early pathophysiologic features of Alzheimer's disease associated with memory loss and cognitive deficits. Because the resultant cortical deficiency of this neurotransmitter is believed to account for some of the clinical manifestations of mild to moderate dementia, enhancement of cholinergic function with an anticholinesterase agent, such as donepezil, is one of the pharmacologic approaches to treatment. Because widespread degeneration of multiple central neuronal systems eventually occurs in patients with Alzheimer's disease, potentially beneficial effects of anticholinesterase agents theoretically would diminish as the disease process advances and fewer cholinergic neurons remain functioning.

SumMon® (see Users Guide). For additional information on this drug until a more detailed monograph is developed and published, the manufacturer's labeling should be consulted. It is *essential* that the labeling be consulted for detailed information on the usual cautions, precautions, and contraindications.

Preparations

Excipients in commercially available drug preparations may have clinically important effects in some individuals; consult specific product labeling for details.

Donepezil Hydrochloride

Oral		
Tablets, film-coated	5 mg	**Aricept®**, Eisai (also promoted by Pfizer)
	10 mg	**Aricept®**, Eisai (also promoted by Pfizer)
Tablets, orally disintegrating	5 mg	**Aricept®ODT**, Eisai (also promoted by Pfizer)
	10 mg	**Aricept®ODT**, Eisai (also promoted by Pfizer)

Galantamine Hydrobromide

■ Galantamine hydrobromide is a centrally active, reversible acetylcholinesterase inhibitor.

Uses

■ **Alzheimer's Disease** Galantamine hydrobromide is used for the palliative treatment of mild to moderate dementia of the Alzheimer's type (Alzheimer's disease). Efficacy has been demonstrated in 5 randomized, placebo-controlled studies of 3–6 months' duration in patients diagnosed with probable Alzheimer's disease utilizing a dual outcome assessment strategy; 4 of these studies utilized conventional tablets, and 1 study utilized extended-release capsules. Changes in cognitive performance were assessed by various instruments, including the cognitive subscale of the Alzheimer's Disease Assessment Scale (ADAS cog), and changes in overall clinical effects were assessed using the Clinician's Interview Based Impression of Change that required the use of caregiver information (CIBIC plus). (For additional information on ADAS cog and CIBIC plus, see Uses: Alzheimer's Disease in Donepezil Hydrochloride 12:04.) Overall, galantamine 8–16 mg twice daily (as conventional tablets) was found to be more effective than placebo for improvements in cognitive function and overall clinical status as assessed by the ADAS cog and CIBIC plus scales. In a 6-month study, galantamine 16–24 mg once daily (as extended-release capsules) was as effective as galantamine 8–12 mg twice daily (as conventional tablets) and more effective than placebo in improving cognitive function and overall daily function as assessed by the ADAS cog and Alzheimer's Disease Cooperative Study Activities of Daily Living (ADCS-ADL) scales, respectively; however, galantamine extended-release capsules were not more effective than placebo in improving overall clinical status (as assessed by the CIBIC plus scale). In a 6-month extension of a randomized, placebo-controlled study utilizing galantamine conventional tablets, clinical improvements were maintained over a 12-month study period in patients who continued to receive galantamine therapy. However, as with other anticholinesterase inhibitors (e.g., donepezil, tacrine), improvement associated with galantamine therapy was not maintained following discontinuance of the drug, suggesting that galantamine does not alter the underlying disease process of dementia.

For additional information on the management of Alzheimer's disease, see Uses in Tacrine 12:04.

■ **Mild Cognitive Impairment** Galantamine has been investigated in patients with mild cognitive impairment† who did not meet diagnostic criteria for Alzheimer's disease. However, the incidence of death in patients receiving galantamine was higher than the incidence in those receiving placebo in 2 randomized controlled studies in patients with mild cognitive impairment. (See Mortality under Warning/Precautions: Warnings, in Cautions.) Galantamine is *not* approved by the US Food and Drug Administration (FDA) for use in patients with mild cognitive impairment who do not have Alzheimer's disease; the manufacturer of galantamine does not intend to seek FDA approval for this indication.

Dosage and Administration

■ **Administration** Galantamine hydrobromide conventional tablets and oral solution are administered orally twice daily, preferably with morning and evening meals. Galantamine hydrobromide extended-release capsules are administered orally once daily in the morning, preferably with food. Administration of galantamine with food and use of a slow, 4-week interval escalation of dosages may reduce the incidence of adverse GI effects (e.g., nausea, vomiting).

The oral solution should be administered using the graduated pipette provided by the manufacturer, referring to the accompanying patient information for instructions. The appropriate dose should be diluted in 100 mL of a nonalcoholic beverage just prior to administration, stirring well and then consuming the entire mixture.

Dispensing and Administration Precautions Because similarity in spelling between Reminyl® (the former trade name for galantamine hydrobromide) and Amaryl® (the trade name for glimepiride, a sulfonylurea antidiabetic agent) previously has resulted in dispensing errors, the manufacturer of Reminyl® announced in April 2005 that the trade name for galantamine hydrobromide would be changed from Reminyl® to Razadyne® to avoid future dispensing errors. (See Dispensing and Administration Precautions under Warnings/Precautions: General Precautions, in Cautions.)

■ **Dosage** Dosage of galantamine hydrobromide is expressed in terms of galantamine. The recommended initial adult dosage of galantamine is 4 mg twice daily (as conventional tablets or oral solution) or 8 mg once daily (as extended-release capsules). The dosage may be increased after a minimum of 4 weeks to 8 mg twice daily (as conventional tablets or oral solution) or 16 mg once daily (as extended-release capsules). Subsequent increases to 12 mg twice daily (as conventional tablets or oral solution) or 24 mg once daily (as extended-release capsules) should be attempted after a minimum of 4 weeks of treatment at the previous dosage. Dosage increments should be based on clinical assessment of benefit and tolerance of the previous dosage. The recommended dosage of galantamine is 8–12 mg twice daily (as conventional tablets or oral solution); a dosage of 16–24 mg once daily (as extended-release capsules) was effective in clinical studies. Use of higher dosages (e.g., 16 mg twice daily) does not result in greater efficacy and is less well tolerated than lower dosages. If galantamine therapy has been interrupted for more than a few days for any reason and reinitiation of the drug is not contraindicated, therapy should be restarted using the lowest dosage and titrated upward to prior dosages.

■ **Special Populations** Use with caution in patients with mild to moderate hepatic or renal impairment. Dosage generally should not exceed 16 mg daily in patients with moderate hepatic (Child-Pugh score of 7–9) or moderate renal impairment. Use not recommended in patients with severe hepatic (Child-Pugh score of 10–15) or severe renal (creatinine clearance less than 9 mL/minute) impairment.

Cautions

■ **Contraindications** Known hypersensitivity to galantamine hydrobromide or any ingredient in the formulation.

■ **Warnings/Precautions** ***Warnings*** **Cardiovascular Effects.** Cholinesterase inhibitors such as galantamine may produce bradycardia, AV block, or other vagotonic effects on the heart. Although patients with supraventricular cardiac conduction abnormalities and those receiving concomitant therapy with drugs that substantially decrease heart rate appear to be at particular risk, these adverse cardiovascular effects may occur in any patient. In clinical studies, bradycardia or syncope was reported in 2–3 or 0.4–2.2%, respectively, of patients receiving up to 24 mg daily of galantamine compared with fewer than 1% of those receiving placebo.

Peptic Ulcers/GI Bleeding. Cholinesterase inhibitors such as galantamine may increase gastric acid secretion. Monitor closely for manifestations of active or occult GI bleeding, especially in patients at increased risk (e.g., history of ulcer disease, concomitant nonsteroidal anti-inflammatory agent [NSAIA] therapy).

Genitourinary Effects. Although not reported in clinical studies with galantamine, cholinomimetic agents may cause bladder outflow obstruction.

Nervous System Effects. Potential for increased risk of seizures secondary to cholinergic activity (seizures also may be a manifestation of Alzheimer's disease).

Respiratory Effects. Like other drugs that increase cholinergic activity, use with caution in patients with a history of severe asthma or obstructive pulmonary disease.

Mortality. In 2 controlled studies of 2 years' duration in patients with mild cognitive impairment who did *not* meet diagnostic criteria for Alzheimer's disease, the incidence of death in those randomized to receive galantamine was higher than in those randomized to receive placebo (10.2 per 1000 person-years compared with 0.7 per 1000 person-years, respectively). The deaths were attributed to various causes that would be expected in a geriatric population; approximately half of the deaths in patients receiving galantamine were attributed to vascular causes (i.e., myocardial infarction, stroke, sudden death). Although the difference in mortality was significant, it should be noted that the incidence of mortality in these 2 studies differs from the incidence observed in other placebo-controlled studies that evaluated galantamine. The incidence of death in placebo-treated patients with mild cognitive impairment was substantially lower than the incidence observed in clinical studies in placebo-treated patients with Alzheimer's disease (0.7 per 1000 person-years compared with 21–61 per 1000 person-years, respectively). In addition, the incidence of death in galantamine-treated patients with mild cognitive impairment was lower than the incidence observed in clinical studies in galantamine-treated patients with Alzheimer's disease (10.2 per 1000 person-years compared with 23–31 per 1000 person-years, respectively). In the studies in patients with mild cognitive impairment, no placebo-treated patient died after 6 months, an unexpected finding in this age group.

General Precautions **Dispensing and Administration Precautions.** Because of similarity in spelling between Reminyl® (the former trade name for galantamine) and Amaryl® (the trade name for glimepiride, a sulfonylurea antidiabetic agent), dispensing errors resulting in serious adverse events (e.g., severe hypoglycemia, death) have been reported. Therefore, in April 2005, the manufacturer of Reminyl® announced that the trade name for galantamine hydrobromide would be changed from Reminyl® to Razadyne® to avoid future dispensing errors.

Specific Populations **Pregnancy.** Category B. (See Users Guide.)

Lactation. Not known whether galantamine is distributed into milk; use in nursing women is not currently indicated.

Pediatric Use. Use not recommended.

Hepatic Impairment. Use not recommended in patients with severe hepatic impairment (Child-Pugh score of 10–15). Caution in patients with moderate hepatic impairment. (See Dosage and Administration: Special Populations.)

Renal Impairment. Use not recommended in patients with severe renal impairment (creatinine clearance less than 9 mL/minute). Caution in patients with moderate renal impairment. (See Dosage and Administration: Special Populations.)

■ **Common Adverse Effects** Adverse effects reported in 5% or more of patients receiving galantamine hydrobromide (as conventional tablets) and with an incidence of at least twice that of placebo include nausea, vomiting, diarrhea, anorexia, and weight decrease; adverse effects associated with galantamine hydrobromide extended-release capsules were similar to those reported with the conventional tablets. Most adverse effects associated with galantamine occurred during the upward titration of dosages. Administration of galantamine with food, use of antiemetic agents, and ensuring adequate fluid intake may reduce the impact of these adverse events.

Description

Galantamine hydrobromide, a phenanthrene alkaloid, is a reversible, competitive acetylcholinesterase inhibitor that is structurally unrelated to other acetylcholinesterase inhibitors (e.g, donepezil, rivastigmine, tacrine). The precise mechanism(s) of action of galantamine in patients with dementia of the Alzheimer's type (Alzheimer's disease) has not been fully elucidated. Galantamine is an anticholinesterase agent that binds reversibly with and inactivates acetylcholinesterase, thus inhibiting hydrolysis of acetylcholine and increasing the concentration of acetylcholine at cholinergic synapses. The drug also binds allosterically with nicotinic acetylcholine receptors and may potentiate the action of agonists (e.g., acetylcholine) at these receptors. Because a deficiency of acetylcholine caused by selective loss of cholinergic neurons in the cerebral cortex, nucleus basalis, and hippocampus is recognized as one of the early pathophysiologic features of Alzheimer's disease associated with memory loss and cognitive deficits, enhancement of cholinergic function with an anticholinesterase agent, such as galantamine, is one of the pharmacologic approaches to treatment. Galantamine's effect may diminish as the disease process advances and fewer cholinergic neurons remain functioning.

Galantamine is metabolized by hepatic cytochrome P-450 (principally CYP2D6 and 3A4) isoenzymes and by glucuronidation; the drug also is excreted unchanged in the urine.

Advice to Patients

Risk of adverse effects such as nausea, vomiting, anorexia, and weight loss. Importance of administering galantamine with food and ensuring adequate fluid intake.

Importance of beginning therapy at lowest dosage and gradually increasing back to prior dosage range if therapy is interrupted for any reason.

Importance of understanding the proper procedure for administering the oral solution, including review of the patient information provided by the manufacturer; advise that questions about administration should be directed to their pharmacist or clinician.

Importance of informing clinicians of existing or contemplated concomitant therapy, including prescription and OTC drugs.

Importance of women informing clinicians if they are or plan to become pregnant or plan to breast-feed.

Importance of informing patients of other important precautionary information. (See Cautions.)

Preparations

Excipients in commercially available drug preparations may have clinically important effects in some individuals; consult specific product labeling for details.

Galantamine Hydrobromide

Oral		
Capsules, extended-release	8 mg (of galantamine)	**Razadyne® ER**, Janssen
	16 mg (of galantamine)	**Razadyne® ER**, Janssen
	24 mg (of galantamine)	**Razadyne® ER**, Janssen
Solution	4 mg (of galantamine) per mL	**Razadyne®**, Janssen
Tablets, film-coated	4 mg (of galantamine)	**Razadyne®**, Janssen
	8 mg (of galantamine)	**Razadyne®**, Janssen
	12 mg (of galantamine)	**Razadyne®**, Janssen

†Use is not currently included in the labeling approved by the US Food and Drug Administration

Neostigmine Methylsulfate

■ Neostigmine methylsulfate is an anticholinesterase agent.

Uses

■ **Reversal of Neuromuscular Blockade** Neostigmine methylsulfate is used for reversal of the effects of nondepolarizing neuromuscular blocking agents (e.g., atracurium, cisatracurium, mivacurium, pancuronium, rocuronium, vecuronium) after surgery. An anticholinergic agent such as atropine sulfate or glycopyrrolate should be used in conjunction with neostigmine to minimize adverse muscarinic effects of the drug (e.g., bradycardia, bradyarrhythmias, increased secretions, bronchoconstriction).

Incomplete neuromuscular recovery after surgery can cause prolonged weakness of the upper airway muscles and associated complications (e.g., airway obstruction, aspiration, hypoxemia, pneumonia, atelectasis, respiratory failure). Anticholinesterase agents such as neostigmine are used to reverse the effects of nondepolarizing neuromuscular blocking agents and reduce the risk of postoperative residual neuromuscular blockade. Evidence supporting the efficacy of neostigmine methylsulfate for reversal of neuromuscular blockade is based principally on data from the published literature. In several randomized studies, neostigmine effectively reduced the time to recovery of neuromuscular blockade after surgery when compared with spontaneous recovery or placebo; all of the studies used a similar efficacy end point of a return of the train-of-four (TOF) twitch ratio to 0.9, which is the currently accepted standard for adequate recovery of neuromuscular function.

Anticholinesterase agents are not effective in reversing deep levels of neuromuscular blockade and generally should not be used until some degree of spontaneous recovery occurs (e.g., when there is a detectable twitch response to the first TOF stimulus). However, administration of these drugs to fully recovered patients should be avoided because of the possibility of paradoxical neuromuscular effects (e.g., weakness of upper airway muscles, increased airway collapsibility). (See Cautions: Precautions and Contraindications.) Anticholinesterase agents do not antagonize the phase I block of depolarizing neuromuscular blocking agents such as succinylcholine and should not be used to reverse the effects of these drugs. (See Drug Interactions: Neuromuscular Blocking Agents.)

■ **Myasthenia Gravis** Neostigmine (as neostigmine bromide) has been used in the symptomatic treatment of myasthenia gravis†, principally to improve muscle strength. However, an oral preparation (Prostigmin®) that was previously used for this indication no longer is commercially available in the US, and this is not an FDA-labeled use for the currently available parenteral injection. If an anticholinesterase agent is required for symptomatic treatment of myasthenia gravis, pyridostigmine generally is preferred because of its longer duration of action and reportedly lower incidence of adverse muscarinic effects. (See Pyridostigmine Bromide 12:04.)

Neostigmine also has been used for the diagnostic testing of myasthenia gravis, although edrophonium usually is preferred because of its rapid onset and short duration of effect. However, the longer duration of neostigmine compared with edrophonium may be particularly useful for diagnostic testing of myasthenia gravis in children and infants.

■ **GI Disorders** Neostigmine has been used for the treatment of acute colonic pseudo-obstruction or Ogilvie syndrome†, a GI motility disorder characterized by marked dilation of the colon in the absence of mechanical obstruction. Conservative therapy is considered the treatment of choice for this condition; however, there is some evidence suggesting that neostigmine may be an effective alternative for patients who fail to respond to conservative management. In several retrospective and prospective studies, IV administration of neostigmine produced rapid colonic decompression and improved symptoms of acute colonic pseudo-obstruction in such patients.

Neostigmine also has been used as a prokinetic agent in patients with postoperative ileus following surgery†; however, the adverse muscarinic effects of the drug (e.g., bradycardia, increased bronchial secretions) may limit its clinical usefulness in this setting.

Limited data suggest that neostigmine may be useful in the management of severe constipation in patients with thoracic spinal cord injury†.

Dosage and Administration

■ **Administration** Neostigmine methylsulfate is administered by slow IV injection (over a period of at least 1 minute). The drug also has been administered by IM or subcutaneous injection†, but the manufacturer of the currently available injectable preparation that is FDA-labeled for reversal of neuromuscular blocking agents states that the injection is for IV use only. Neostigmine has been administered orally† (as neostigmine bromide) for the management of myasthenia gravis; however, an oral dosage form no longer is commercially available in the US.

When used as a neuromuscular reversal agent, neostigmine should be administered only by trained clinicians experienced in the use of such agents. Patients must be well ventilated and have a patent airway prior to administration of neostigmine and until complete recovery of normal respiration. Continuous monitoring of neuromuscular function is recommended to ensure adequate reversal from the neuromuscular block. To exclude with certainty the possibility of residual paralysis, an objective (quantitative) method of monitoring such as peripheral nerve stimulation should be used in conjunction with other clinical assessments (e.g., observation of skeletal muscle tone, respiratory measurements). Adequate recovery of neuromuscular function generally is defined as a train-of-four (TOF) ratio of 0.9 in addition to the patient's ability to maintain satisfactory ventilation and a patent airway. Recovery times may vary based on the patient's medical condition and the duration of action of the specific neuromuscular blocking agent used.

■ **Dosage** ***Reversal of Neuromuscular Blockade*** Dosage of neostigmine methylsulfate should be based on individual patient requirements and response. A peripheral nerve stimulator capable of delivering a TOF stimulus should be used to determine when neostigmine should be administered and if additional doses are necessary. Neostigmine should be administered only after some degree of spontaneous recovery has occurred (i.e., at least 10% recovery of the first twitch response).

For reversal of the effects of nondepolarizing neuromuscular blocking agents after surgery, the manufacturer states that a neostigmine methylsulfate dose of 0.03–0.07 mg/kg given by slow IV injection usually is sufficient to achieve adequate recovery of neuromuscular function (i.e., TOF ratio of 0.9) within 10–20 minutes of administration. Selection of an appropriate dose should be based on the half-life of the neuromuscular blocking agent being reversed, degree of spontaneous recovery, and the need for rapid reversal. For reversal of neuromuscular blocking agents with a shorter half-life (e.g., rocuronium) or reversal of shallower blocks (i.e., when first twitch response is substantially greater than 10% of baseline or when a second twitch is present), the manufacturer recommends a neostigmine methylsulfate dose of 0.03 mg/kg. The higher dose of 0.07 mg/kg is recommended for reversal of longer-acting neuromuscular blocking agents (e.g., pancuronium, vecuronium), reversal of deeper blocks (i.e., when first twitch response is not substantially greater than 10% of baseline), or when more rapid recovery is needed. Although weight-based dosing of neostigmine methylsulfate is recommended by the manufacturer, the drug also has been administered in fixed IV doses of 0.5–2.5 mg for reversal of nondepolarizing neuromuscular blockade in adults. The recommended maximum total dose of neostigmine methylsulfate is 0.07 mg/kg or 5 mg, whichever is less; higher doses are unlikely to provide additional clinical benefit. The need for additional doses should be determined by TOF monitoring and the extent of recovery of neuromuscular function.

The manufacturer states that the same dosage recommendations in adults should be applied to pediatric patients since dosing requirements generally are similar between the two populations. Other experts have recommended IV neostigmine methylsulfate doses of 0.025–0.1 mg/kg in infants and 0.025–0.08 mg/kg in children for reversal of nondepolarizing neuromuscular blocking agents.

To counteract the adverse muscarinic effects of neostigmine methylsulfate, an IV anticholinergic agent (atropine sulfate or glycopyrrolate) should be administered prior to or concomitantly (in separate syringes) with neostigmine. In the presence of bradycardia, the anticholinergic agent should be given before neostigmine.

Myasthenia Gravis In adults with myasthenia gravis† who require parenteral therapy, some experts state that 0.5–2.5 mg of neostigmine methylsulfate may be administered by IV, IM, or subcutaneous injection every 1–3 hours as needed (up to a maximum dosage of 10 mg in 24 hours). In children, 0.01–0.04 mg/kg of neostigmine methylsulfate may be administered every 2–4 hours as needed by IM, IV, or subcutaneous injection. Because of the self-limiting nature of neonatal myasthenia gravis, the daily dosage in neonates should be gradually reduced until the drug can be withdrawn.

If neostigmine methylsulfate is used for diagnosis of myasthenia gravis in adults, a single IM dose of 0.02 mg/kg has been recommended; in children, a single IM dose of 0.025–0.04 mg/kg has been recommended for such use.

■ **Dosage in Renal and Hepatic Impairment** ***Reversal of Neuromuscular Blockade*** Dosage adjustments do not appear to be necessary in patients with hepatic impairment; however, such patients should be carefully monitored if neuromuscular blocking agents with hepatic elimination or active metabolites are administered because the effects of the neuromuscular blocking agent may be prolonged and persist beyond the effects of neostigmine.

Dosage adjustments do not appear to be necessary in patients with renal impairment; however, such patients should be closely monitored if renally eliminated neuromuscular blocking agents are administered because the effects of the neuromuscular blocking agent may persist beyond the effects of neostigmine.

■ **Dosage in Geriatric Patients** ***Reversal of Neuromuscular Blockade*** Although dosage adjustments are not required in geriatric patients, a longer period of monitoring is recommended in such patients. (See Cautions: Geriatric Precautions.)

Cautions

■ **Adverse Effects** Adverse effects of neostigmine methylsulfate generally are due to exaggerated pharmacologic effects of the drug, particularly at muscarinic-cholinergic receptors. Such adverse muscarinic effects include nausea, vomiting, diarrhea, miosis, excessive salivation and sweating, increased bronchial secretions, abdominal cramps, and bronchoconstriction. Cardiovascular effects such as bradycardia, hypotension, tachycardia, and cardiac arrhythmias also have been reported following parenteral administration of neostigmine methylsulfate. Stimulation of nicotinic-cholinergic receptors may produce weakness, muscle cramps, and fasciculation. Overdosage of neostigmine can cause cholinergic crisis and death. (See Acute Toxicity: Manifestations.)

Adverse muscarinic effects can be prevented or reduced by concomitant administration of an anticholinergic agent (e.g., atropine sulfate, glycopyrrolate); however, these symptoms may indicate neostigmine overdosage, and masking them with atropine may lead to inadvertent induction of cholinergic crisis.

■ Precautions and Contraindications Cholinergic crisis, a condition causing extreme muscle weakness, can occur in patients who receive an overdosage of neostigmine. Because manifestations can resemble myasthenic crisis in patients with myasthenia gravis, it is important to differentiate between the two conditions. (See Acute Toxicity: Manifestations.)

Because of the risk of blood pressure and heart rate complications, neostigmine should be used with caution in patients with certain cardiac conditions such as coronary artery disease, cardiac arrhythmias, or recent acute coronary syndrome. Patients with myasthenia gravis also may be at increased risk of cardiovascular complications. Concomitant use of an anticholinergic agent generally will minimize the risk of adverse cardiovascular effects associated with neostigmine; however, there have been some cases where the combination of neostigmine and atropine produced transient cardiac arrhythmias.

Neostigmine can cause paradoxical neuromuscular effects (e.g., weakness of upper airway muscles and increased airway collapsibility) if used in patients with complete or near complete neuromuscular recovery. Neuromuscular dysfunction and other postoperative respiratory complications have occurred when high doses of neostigmine were administered during minimal neuromuscular blockade. The dose of neostigmine methylsulfate should be reduced if neuromuscular recovery is almost complete.

Neostigmine is contraindicated in patients with known hypersensitivity to the drug; hypersensitivity reactions that have been reported include urticaria, angioedema, erythema multiforme, generalized rash, facial swelling, peripheral edema, pyrexia, flushing, hypotension, bronchospasm, bradycardia, and anaphylaxis. Because of the possibility of hypersensitivity, atropine and other drugs for the treatment of anaphylaxis should be readily available during administration. Neostigmine also is contraindicated in patients with peritonitis or mechanical obstruction of the intestinal or urinary tracts.

■ Pediatric Precautions Neostigmine may be used in pediatric patients of all ages to reverse the effects of nondepolarizing neuromuscular blocking agents after surgery. The available data indicate that efficacy and pharmacokinetics of neostigmine are similar across all pediatric age groups and also similar to those in adults when the same dosing guidelines are applied.

Based on limited data, neostigmine dosing requirements for reversal of neuromuscular blockade may be lower in infants and neonates than in older pediatric patients and adults; however, pediatric patients have a greater risk of incomplete reversal of neuromuscular blockade because of their decreased respiratory reserve. Therefore, the risks of administering higher doses of neostigmine (up to maximum recommended dosage) should not outweigh the risks associated with incomplete reversal in this age group.

Because pediatric patients, particularly neonates and infants, may be more sensitive to changes in heart rate, the effects of anticholinergic agents should be observed prior to administration of neostigmine to lessen the probability of bradycardia and hypotension.

■ Geriatric Precautions Because geriatric patients may have decreased renal function, neostigmine should be used with caution and increased monitoring in this age group. The duration of action of neostigmine is prolonged in geriatric patients; however, such patients also experience slower spontaneous recovery from neuromuscular blocking agents. Although dosage adjustments are not required in geriatric patients, these patients should be monitored for longer periods of time to ensure that additional doses of neostigmine are not necessary to adequately reverse neuromuscular blockade.

■ Mutagenicity and Carcinogenicity Neostigmine did not exhibit evidence of mutagenic or clastogenic potential when tested in vitro in bacterial and Chinese hamster ovary cell assays or in an in vivo mouse micronucleus assay.

■ Pregnancy, Fertility, and Lactation It is not known whether neostigmine can cause fetal harm when administered to pregnant women or affect reproductive capacity; the drug should be used during pregnancy only when clearly indicated. Animal reproduction studies have not been performed to date with the drug. Few data are available regarding the effects of cholinesterase inhibitors, including neostigmine, on the fetus because of the rarity of maternal conditions requiring the use of these drugs during pregnancy. Transient muscular weakness has occurred in 10–20% of neonates whose mothers received anticholinesterase drugs for the treatment of myasthenia gravis, although similar symptoms have also been reported in infants whose mothers were not treated with these drugs. Anticholinesterase drugs may induce premature labor when given IV to pregnant women near term.

It is not known whether neostigmine is distributed into human milk. Caution should be exercised when the drug is used in nursing women.

Drug Interactions

Drug interaction studies have not been conducted to date with neostigmine methylsulfate. Clinically important drug interactions are not likely to occur if neuromuscular monitoring is employed and both relaxants and reversal agents are titrated to effect.

■ Drugs Affecting Hepatic Microsomal Enzymes Neostigmine is metabolized by hepatic microsomal enzymes; caution is advised when used concomitantly with drugs that can alter the activity of these enzymes.

■ Neuromuscular Blocking Agents Neostigmine does not antagonize, and may in fact prolong, the phase I block of depolarizing muscle relaxants such as succinylcholine. Fully established phase II (desensitization) block can be reversed by neostigmine, but the individual variation in transition time between phases I and II and difficulty in accurately determining the stage of depolarizing neuromuscular block at any given time often make neostigmine administration ineffective or dangerous under these circumstances. Parenteral neostigmine effectively antagonizes the effect of nondepolarizing muscle relaxants (e.g., atracurium, cisatracurium, mivacurium, pancuronium, rocuronium, vecuronium), and this interaction is used to therapeutic advantage to reverse muscle relaxation after surgery. (See Uses: Reversal of Neuromuscular Blockade.)

■ Other Drugs Atropine antagonizes the muscarinic effects of neostigmine, and this interaction is utilized to counteract the muscarinic symptoms of neostigmine toxicity.

Acute Toxicity

■ Manifestations Neostigmine overdosage may induce cholinergic crisis, which is characterized by nausea, vomiting, diarrhea, excessive salivation and sweating, increased bronchial secretions, miosis, lacrimation, bradycardia or tachycardia, cardiospasm, bronchospasm, hypotension, incoordination, blurred vision, muscle cramps, weakness, fasciculation, and paralysis. Increasing muscle weakness can ultimately cause respiratory paralysis and death. Myasthenic crisis, a complication of myasthenia gravis, can also cause extreme muscle weakness and resemble cholinergic crisis. It is extremely important to differentiate between the two conditions since treatment methods differ considerably. Whereas more intensive anticholinesterase therapy is required in patients with myasthenic crisis, administration of higher doses of neostigmine can have serious consequences in patients with cholinergic crisis. The timing of the onset of weakness may indicate whether the crisis is the result of overdosage or underdosage of (or resistance to) anticholinesterase drugs. Weakness that begins approximately 1 hour after drug administration suggests overdosage, while weakness occurring 3 or more hours after drug administration is more likely to be due to underdosage or resistance. Edrophonium can be used to distinguish cholinergic crisis from myasthenic crisis. (See Edrophonium Chloride 36:56.)

■ Treatment In the treatment of neostigmine overdosage, maintaining adequate respiration is of primary importance. Ventilation should be assisted by artificial means and cardiac function monitored until spontaneous respiration is restored. Neostigmine should be discontinued immediately and atropine sulfate administered to control muscarinic symptoms. It should be kept in mind that, unlike muscarinic effects, the skeletal muscle effects and consequent respiratory paralysis which can occur following neostigmine overdosage are not alleviated by atropine.

Pharmacology

Neostigmine is an anticholinesterase agent; the drug inhibits the enzyme acetylcholinesterase, reducing the degradation of acetylcholine. By competing with acetylcholine for binding to acetylcholinesterase, neostigmine slows the rate of hydrolysis of acetylcholine. As a consequence, acetylcholine accumulates at cholinergic synapses, producing prolonged and exaggerated effects. Increased concentrations of acetylcholine at the neuromuscular junction compete with and reverse the effects of nondepolarizing neuromuscular blocking agents. In patients with myasthenia gravis, neostigmine enhances neuromuscular transmission, providing symptomatic improvement. Neostigmine stimulates both muscarinic and nicotinic receptors, producing generalized cholinergic effects including miosis, increased tonus of intestinal and skeletal musculature, constriction of bronchi and ureters, bradycardia, and stimulation of secretion by salivary and sweat glands. In addition, neostigmine has a direct cholinomimetic effect on skeletal muscle.

Because of its quaternary ammonium structure, moderate doses of neostigmine do not cross the blood-brain barrier to produce CNS effects. Extremely high doses, however, produce CNS stimulation followed by CNS depression, in addition to a depolarizing neuromuscular blockade, and may result in respiratory depression, paralysis, and death.

Pharmacokinetics

■ Absorption Neostigmine bromide is poorly absorbed from the GI tract after oral administration (an oral preparation no longer is commercially available in the US). Following a single 30-mg oral dose in fasting myasthenic patients, an estimated 1–2% of the dose was absorbed; peak plasma drug concentrations occurred within 1–2 hours after oral administration (with considerable individual variations) or within 30 minutes after IM injection. Effects of neostigmine on peristaltic activity begin 10–30 minutes after parenteral injection or 2–4 hours after oral administration. The maximal effects on skeletal muscle may occur within 20–30 minutes after parenteral administration; in most patients, the effects of neostigmine last for 2.5–4 hours after IM injection.

■ **Distribution** Because of its quaternary ammonium structure, neostigmine would not be expected to cross the placenta in therapeutic doses, nor has the drug been detected in human milk. However, placental transfer of pyridostigmine has been reported after large oral doses, and this possibility should be considered with neostigmine. Neostigmine is 15–25% bound to serum albumin.

■ **Elimination** Following administration of a single IV dose of neostigmine, the reported elimination half-life of the drug ranged from 24–113 minutes. Following IM administration, the elimination half-life reportedly ranged from 51–90 minutes. In a pharmacokinetic study in pediatric patients, half-life of neostigmine (administered as an IV infusion over 2 minutes) was approximately 39, 48, or 67 minutes in infants 2–10 months of age, children 1–6 years of age, or adults 29–48 years of age, respectively.

Neostigmine undergoes hydrolysis by cholinesterases to 3-hydroxyphenyltrimethylammonium (3-OH PTM), which in animals has activity similar to but much weaker than that of neostigmine. Neostigmine is also metabolized by microsomal enzymes in the liver. Radioisotope studies show the liver as the major site of uptake, although high concentrations of both 3-OH PTM and neostigmine occur in animal heart muscle. Neostigmine and 3-OH PTM are excreted by renal tubular secretion. Unchanged neostigmine and free and conjugated 3-OH PTM have been isolated from urine in animal studies; 3-OH PTM has been identified in human urine. About 80% of a single IM dose of neostigmine is excreted in urine in 24 hours, approximately 50% as unchanged drug and the remainder as metabolites.

Clearance of neostigmine is reduced in patients with renal impairment compared with individuals with normal renal function. In a study in patients with various states of renal function (normal, undergoing renal transplantation, or bilateral nephrectomy), elimination half-life of neostigmine was prolonged in anephric individuals.

Chemistry and Stability

■ **Chemistry** Neostigmine is a synthetic quaternary ammonium compound that is pharmacologically similar to pyridostigmine. Neostigmine methylsulfate occurs as a white crystalline powder, and is very soluble in water and soluble in alcohol. Commercially available neostigmine methylsulfate injections have a pH of 5.5.

■ **Stability** Neostigmine methylsulfate injection should be stored at controlled room temperature (20–25°C) but may be exposed to temperatures ranging from 15–30°C; the injection should be stored in the original carton until time of use and protected from light.

Preparations

Excipients in commercially available drug preparations may have clinically important effects in some individuals; consult specific product labeling for details.

Neostigmine Methylsulfate

Parenteral		
Injection	0.5 mg/mL*	**Bloxiverz®**, Eclat **Neostigmine Methylsulfate Injection**
	1 mg/mL*	**Bloxiverz®**, Eclat **Neostigmine Methylsulfate Injection**

*available from one or more manufacturer, distributor, and/or repackager by generic (nonproprietary) name

†Use is not currently included in the labeling approved by the US Food and Drug Administration

Selected Revisions September 2015, © Copyright, July 1977, American Society of Health-System Pharmacists, Inc.

Rivastigmine
Rivastigmine Tartrate

■ Rivastigmine is a centrally active, reversible cholinesterase inhibitor.

Uses

■ **Alzheimer's Disease** Rivastigmine is used orally and transdermally for the management of mild to moderate dementia of the Alzheimer's type (Alzheimer's disease). Efficacy of orally administered rivastigmine has been evaluated in 2 placebo-controlled clinical trials each of 26 weeks' duration utilizing a dual outcome assessment strategy; changes in cognitive performance were assessed by various instruments, including the cognitive subscale of the Alzheimer's Disease Assessment Scale (ADAS cog), and changes in overall clinical effects were assessed using the Clinician's Interview-Based Impression of Change (CIBIC) that required the use of caregiver information (CIBIC plus). (For additional information on ADAS cog and CIBIC plus, see Uses: Alzheimer's Disease in Donepezil Hydrochloride 12:04.) Two dosage ranges (1–4 and 6–12 mg daily administered orally) were used in each study. Rivastigmine 6–12 mg daily was found to be more effective than placebo or rivastigmine 1–4 mg daily in both studies for improvements in cognitive function and overall clinical status as assessed by the ADAS cog and CIBIC plus scales. A third placebo-controlled clinical trial utilizing forced titration to fixed dosages (3, 6, or 9 mg daily administered orally) was performed employing the same outcome assessment tools. Rivastigmine was more effective than placebo at the 2 higher dosages for mean change from baseline on the ADAS cog scores. However, no substantial differences were observed between any of the rivastigmine dosage groups and placebo when CIBIC plus scores were compared.

Rivastigmine transdermal system has been evaluated for the management of dementia of the Alzheimer's type in a single, placebo-controlled, international clinical trial of 24 weeks' duration utilizing a dual outcome assessment strategy; changes in cognitive performance were assessed by various instruments, including the cognitive subscale of ADAS cog, and changes in overall clinical effects were assessed using the Alzheimer's Disease Cooperative Study–Clinician's Global Impression of Change (ADCS-CGIC), which is a more standardized form of CIBIC plus. Study participants were randomized to receive a target dose of one transdermal system delivering rivastigmine 9.5 mg/24 hours, one system delivering 17.4 mg/24 hours, rivastigmine 6 mg orally twice daily, or placebo. The first 16 weeks of the study was a dosage escalation phase, with initial dosages of one transdermal system delivering 4.6 mg/24 hours applied once daily or 3 mg daily (administered as 1.5 mg orally twice daily) gradually increased over 16 weeks to the target dosage; the 16-week dose escalation phase was followed by an 8-week maintenance phase. Results of this study indicate that efficacy of a system delivering 9.5 mg/24 hours was similar to that of orally administered rivastigmine. At week 24, rivastigmine transdermal system delivering 9.5 mg/24 hours, the transdermal system delivering 17.4 mg/24 hours, and orally administered rivastigmine (6 mg twice daily) were more effective than placebo for mean change from baseline on the ADAS cog scores. In addition, rivastigmine transdermal system delivering 9.5 mg/24 hours and orally administered rivastigmine were more effective than placebo for mean change from baseline on the ADCS-CGIC scale; no substantial differences were observed between the transdermal system delivering 17.4 mg/ 24 hours and placebo on change on the ADCS-CGIC scale.

For additional information on the management of Alzheimer's disease, see Uses in Tacrine Hydrochloride 12:04.

■ **Dementia Associated with Parkinsonian Syndrome** Rivastigmine is used orally and transdermally for the management of mild to moderate dementia associated with Parkinson's disease. Dementia associated with Parkinson's disease generally is characterized by impairments in executive function, memory retrieval, and attention in patients with an established diagnosis of Parkinson's disease. However, the diagnosis of dementia associated with Parkinson's disease can be made without documenting these specific deficits in patients in whom a progressive dementia syndrome occurs at least 2 years after a diagnosis of Parkinson's disease has been made and in whom other causes of dementia have been ruled out.

Efficacy of orally administered rivastigmine has been evaluated for the management of dementia associated with idiopathic Parkinson's disease in a single, placebo-controlled, international clinical trial of 24 weeks' duration in patients with mild to moderate dementia with onset at least 2 years after the initial diagnosis of idiopathic Parkinson's disease. The first 16 weeks of the study was a dosage escalation phase, with initial dosages of 3 mg daily (administered orally as 1.5 mg twice daily) gradually increased by increments of 3 mg daily at intervals of at least 4 weeks up to a maximum dosage of 12 mg daily. The highest tolerated dosage was then maintained for the remainder of the study; dosages could be adjusted as needed because of adverse effects. The trial used a dual outcome assessment strategy; changes in cognitive performance were assessed by ADAS cog and changes in overall clinical effects were assessed using the Alzheimer's Disease Cooperative Study–Clinician's Global Impression of Change (ADCS-CGIC), which is a more standardized form of CIBIC plus. (For additional information on ADAS cog and CIBIC plus, see Uses: Alzheimer's Disease in Donepezil Hydrochloride 12:04.) Rivastigmine (mean final oral dosage 8.6 mg daily) was found to be more effective than placebo for improvements in cognitive performance and in overall clinical efficacy as assessed by the ADAS cog and ADCS-CGIC scales, respectively.

Dosage and Administration

■ **Administration** Rivastigmine tartrate is administered orally twice daily. Rivastigmine is administered percutaneously by topical application of a transdermal system.

When rivastigmine is administered orally, administration with food has been shown to reduce the rate and increase the extent of GI absorption, and administration of the drug in the morning and evening with food is recommended, since the incidence of adverse GI effects (e.g., nausea, vomiting) may be related to high peak plasma concentrations.

The oral solution and capsules may be interchanged at equal doses.

The oral solution should be administered using the oral dosing syringe according to the patient instructions provided by the manufacturer.

Patients receiving transdermal rivastigmine therapy or their caregivers should be carefully instructed in the use of the transdermal system. To expose the adhesive surface of the system, the protective liner should be peeled and discarded prior to administration. The transdermal system is applied topically to a dry, hairless area of intact skin, preferably the back, by firmly pressing the system with the adhesive side touching the skin; placement on the back is recommended to reduce the risk that the system could be removed by the patient. Alternatively, the transdermal system may be applied to the upper arm or chest. The rivastigmine transdermal system is worn continuously for 24 hours; subsequent systems are applied after removal of the previous system. To minimize and/or prevent potential skin irritation, each system should be applied to a different site, with an interval of at least 14 days between applications to a particular site. The application site should not be red, irritated, or cut. The transdermal system should not be applied to areas where the system might be rubbed off. If the system should inadvertently come off during the period of use, a new system may be applied; the application schedule employed should be continued.

■ Dosage Dosage of rivastigmine tartrate is expressed in terms of rivastigmine.

Alzheimer's Disease The recommended initial oral dosage of rivastigmine for the management of mild to moderate dementia of the Alzheimer's type in adults is 1.5 mg twice daily. If well tolerated, this dosage may be increased after a minimum of 2 weeks to 3 mg twice daily. Subsequent increases to 4.5 mg twice daily and then to 6 mg twice daily should be attempted after a minimum of 2 weeks of treatment at the previous dosage. In clinical studies, a dosage of 6–12 mg daily (administered as doses of 3–6 mg twice daily) was effective. There is evidence from placebo-controlled studies that dosages at the higher end of this range may be more beneficial. The maximum recommended dosage is 12 mg daily (administered as doses of 6 mg twice daily).

When transdermal rivastigmine is used for the management of mild to moderate dementia of the Alzheimer's type in adults, the recommended initial dosage is one system delivering 4.6 mg/24 hours applied once daily. If well tolerated, this dosage may be increased after a minimum of 4 weeks to one system delivering 9.5 mg/24 hours applied once daily. The maximum recommended daily dosage is 9.5 mg/24 hours.

If patients are unable to tolerate adverse effects associated with rivastigmine, the patient should be instructed to discontinue the drug for several doses and then resume therapy at the same or the immediately preceding (lower) dosage in the titration regimen. However, if therapy is interrupted for more than several days, the drug should be restarted using the recommended initial dosage (i.e., 1.5 mg twice daily or one system delivering 4.6 mg/24 hours applied once daily) and titration schedule until the previous maintenance dosage is reached to decrease the risk of severe vomiting and related sequelae (e.g., spontaneous esophageal rupture). Clinical experience with reinitiating rivastigmine therapy using dosages higher than the initial dosage recommended by the manufacturer is limited. (See Warnings: GI Effects.)

Transdermal Dosage in Patients Transferred from Oral Therapy. If the rivastigmine oral dosage has been less than 6 mg daily, the initial recommended dosage of the transdermal system is one system delivering 4.6 mg/24 hours applied once daily. If the rivastigmine oral dosage has been 6–12 mg daily, the initial recommended dosage of the transdermal system is one system delivering 9.5 mg/24 hours applied once daily. The first transdermal system should be applied the day after the last oral rivastigmine dose.

Dementia Associated with Parkinsonian Syndrome The recommended initial oral dosage of rivastigmine for the management of mild to moderate dementia associated with Parkinson's disease in adults is 1.5 mg twice daily. If well tolerated, this dosage may be increased after a minimum of 4 weeks to 3 mg twice daily. Subsequent increases to 4.5 mg twice daily and then to 6 mg twice daily should be attempted after a minimum of 4 weeks of treatment at the previous dosage. In the single controlled clinical study, a dosage of 3–12 mg daily (administered as doses of 1.5–6 mg twice daily) was effective.

When transdermal rivastigmine is used for the management of mild to moderate dementia associated with Parkinson's disease, the recommended initial dosage is one system delivering 4.6 mg/24 hours applied once daily. If well tolerated, this dosage may be increased after a minimum of 4 weeks to one system delivering 9.5 mg/24 hours applied once daily. The maximum recommended daily dosage is 9.5 mg/24 hours.

If patients are unable to tolerate adverse effects associated with rivastigmine, the patient should be instructed to discontinue the drug for several doses and then resume therapy at the same or the immediately preceding (lower) dosage in the titration regimen. However, if therapy is interrupted for more than several days, the drug should be restarted using the recommended initial dosage (i.e., 1.5 mg twice daily or one system delivering 4.6 mg/24 hours applied once daily) and titration schedule until the previous maintenance dosage is reached to decrease the risk of severe vomiting and related sequelae (e.g., spontaneous esophageal rupture). Clinical experience with reinitiating rivastigmine therapy using dosages higher than the initial dosage recommended by the manufacturer is limited. (See Warnings: GI Effects.)

Transdermal Dosage in Patients Transferred from Oral Therapy. If the rivastigmine oral dosage has been less than 6 mg daily, the initial recommended dosage of the transdermal system is one system delivering 4.6 mg/24 hours applied once daily. If the rivastigmine oral dosage has been 6–12 mg daily, the initial recommended dosage of the transdermal system is one system delivering 9.5 mg/24 hours applied once daily. The first transdermal system should be applied the day after the last oral rivastigmine dose.

■ Special Populations In clinical studies, oral clearance was reduced 60 or 65% after single or multiple doses, respectively, in patients with hepatic impairment. In patients with moderate or severe renal impairment, oral clearance was reduced 64% or *increased* 43%, respectively. The unexpected increase in clearance in patients with severe renal impairment has not been explained. However, the manufacturer states that dosage adjustment may not be necessary in patients with renal or hepatic impairment since the dosage of rivastigmine is individually titrated to adverse effect tolerability. The manufacturer currently makes no specific recommendations for dosage adjustment based on age, gender, or race.

Cautions

■ Contraindications Known hypersensitivity to rivastigmine or any ingredient in the formulation. Although there are no reports of cross-sensitivity to date, the manufacturer states that the drug also is contraindicated in patients with known hypersensitivity to other carbamates.

■ Warnings/Precautions ***Warnings*** **GI Effects.** Rivastigmine is associated with clinically important adverse GI effects, including nausea and vomiting, diarrhea, anorexia, and weight loss. In controlled trials, 47% of patients treated with oral rivastigmine in a dosage of 6–12 mg daily developed nausea, and 31% developed at least one episode of vomiting. In controlled trials that evaluated rivastigmine transdermal therapy, 7% of patients treated with the recommended dosage (one system delivering 9.5 mg/24 hours daily) developed nausea, and 6% developed vomiting. Discontinuance of rivastigmine because of nausea, vomiting, or anorexia was reported in 8, 5, or 3% of patients, respectively, receiving orally administered rivastigmine 6–12 mg daily in clinical studies.

Severe vomiting and spontaneous rupture of the esophagus (Boerhaave's syndrome) were reported in a patient who resumed therapy by erroneously taking a single higher than recommended initial dose (i.e., 4.5 mg administered orally) of rivastigmine after therapy had been interrupted for 8 weeks. Because these adverse effects may have been caused by the lack of titration of the drug, the manufacturer has recommended strict adherence to prescribed initial dosages and titration schedules, particularly when reinitiating therapy following temporary interruptions lasting longer than several days. (See Dosage and Administration: Dosage.)

Peptic Ulcers/GI Bleeding. Cholinesterase inhibitors such as rivastigmine may increase gastric acid secretion. Monitor closely for manifestations of active or occult GI bleeding, especially in patients at increased risk (e.g., history of ulcer disease, concomitant nonsteroidal anti-inflammatory agent [NSAIA] therapy).

Cardiovascular Effects. Since cholinesterase inhibitors may produce bradycardia or other vagotonic effects on the heart, rivastigmine should be used with caution in patients with sick sinus syndrome or other supraventricular cardiac conduction abnormalities.

Genitourinary Effects. Although not reported in clinical studies with rivastigmine, cholinomimetic agents may cause urinary obstruction.

Seizures. Potential for increased risk of seizures secondary to cholinergic activity (seizures also may be a manifestation of Alzheimer's disease).

Respiratory Effects. Like other drugs that increase cholinergic activity, use with caution in patients with a history of asthma or obstructive pulmonary disease.

General Precautions **Extrapyramidal Reactions.** Like other cholinomimetic agents, rivastigmine may exacerbate or induce extrapyramidal symptoms. Worsening in patients with Parkinson's disease, including an increased incidence or intensity of tremor, reported.

Effects on Ability to Drive and Use Heavy Machinery. Dementia may cause gradual impairment of ability to drive or operate heavy machinery; adverse effects (e.g., dizziness, asthenia, fatigue) of rivastigmine also may be detrimental to these functions. The ability to drive or use heavy machinery should be evaluated by the treating clinician on a routine basis.

Low-weight Individuals. When rivastigmine transdermal system is used, patients with body weight less than 50 kg may experience more adverse effects and may be more likely to discontinue therapy due to adverse effects. If the dosage exceeds the maximum recommended dosage, patient with low body weight should be closely supervised by the clinician.

Specific Populations **Pregnancy.** Category B. (See Users' Guide.)

Lactation. Not known whether rivastigmine is distributed into milk; use in nursing women is not recommended.

Pediatric Use. Currently not indicated.

■ Common Adverse Effects In clinical trials of oral rivastigmine in patients with dementia of the Alzheimer's type, adverse effects occurring in 5% or more of patients receiving rivastigmine and more than twice as frequently as among those receiving placebo included nausea, vomiting, anorexia, dyspepsia, and asthenia. Dizziness, diarrhea, headache, abdominal pain, accidental trauma, fatigue, insomnia, confusion, urinary tract infection, depression, malaise, somnolence, constipation, and anxiety occurred in at least 5% of patients receiving rivastigmine and more frequently than in patients receiving placebo in clinical studies in patients with dementia of the Alzheimer's type.

In clinical trials of oral rivastigmine in patients with dementia associated with Parkinson's disease, adverse effects occurring in 5% or more of patients receiving rivastigmine and more than twice as frequently as among those receiving placebo included nausea, vomiting, tremor, anorexia, and dizziness.

In a clinical trial that evaluated rivastigmine transdermal therapy in patients with dementia of the Alzheimer's type, nausea, vomiting, and diarrhea occurred in at least 5% of patients receiving rivastigmine (one system delivering 9.5 mg/

24 hours) and more frequently than in patients receiving placebo. Most patients experienced no, slight, or mild skin irritation.

Description

Rivastigmine tartrate, a carbamate derivative, is an intermediate-acting, reversible cholinesterase inhibitor that is structurally related to physostigmine but unrelated to donepezil or tacrine. The precise mechanism(s) of action of rivastigmine in patients with dementia of the Alzheimer's type (Alzheimer's disease) and dementia associated with Parkinson's disease has not been fully elucidated. The drug is an anticholinesterase agent that binds reversibly with and inactivates cholinesterases (e.g., acetylcholinesterase, butyrylcholinesterase), thus inhibiting hydrolysis of acetylcholine and increasing the concentration of acetylcholine at cholinergic synapses. The anticholinesterase activity of rivastigmine is relatively specific for brain acetylcholinesterase and butyrylcholinesterase compared with that in peripheral tissues. After a 6-mg oral dose administered twice daily, cholinesterase activity in CSF is inhibited for approximately 10 hours, with a maximum inhibition of about 60% at 5 hours after dosing.

Metabolism of rivastigmine is rapid and extensive and occurs principally via cholinesterase-mediated hydrolysis to the decarbamylated metabolite, which is tenfold less active than rivastigmine. The drug is only minimally metabolized by cytochrome P-450 (CYP) isoenzymes.

Advice to Patients

Importance of informing caregivers of potential for adverse effects such as nausea, vomiting, anorexia, and weight loss. Importance of caregivers monitoring for adverse effects and informing clinicians if they occur.

Importance of informing caregivers and patients that rivastigmine may exacerbate or induce extrapyramidal symptoms; worsening in patients with Parkinson's disease (including increased incidence or intensity of tremor) reported.

Importance of informing caregivers and patients that the ability to drive or use heavy machinery should be evaluated by the treating clinician on a routine basis.

Importance of taking oral formulations of rivastigmine with food.

Importance of following recommended procedure for administering rivastigmine oral solution and of reviewing the instruction sheet provided by the manufacturer.

Importance of following recommended procedure for administration, removal, and disposal of rivastigmine transdermal system and of reviewing the instruction sheet provided by the manufacturer.

Importance of informing caregivers and patients to avoid exposure of the transdermal system to external heat sources (e.g., excess sunlight, saunas, solariums) for extended periods of time.

Importance of *not* administering the next maintenance dosage of rivastigmine until a clinician is consulted if therapy has been interrupted for longer than several days.

Importance of informing clinicians of existing or contemplated concomitant therapy, including prescription and OTC drugs, as well as any concomitant illnesses.

Importance of women informing clinicians if they are or plan to become pregnant or plan to breast-feed.

Importance of informing patients of other precautionary information. (See Cautions.)

Overview (see Users Guide). For additional information until a more detailed monograph is developed and published, the manufacturer's labeling should be consulted. It is *essential* that the manufacturer's labeling be consulted for more detailed information on usual cautions, precautions, contraindications, potential drug interactions, laboratory test interferences, and acute toxicity.

Preparations

Excipients in commercially available drug preparations may have clinically important effects in some individuals; consult specific product labeling for details.

Rivastigmine

Topical		
Transdermal System	4.5 mg/24 hours (9 mg/5 cm²)	**Exelon®**, Novartis
	9.5 mg/24 hours (18 mg/10 cm²)	**Exelon®**, Novartis

Rivastigmine Tartrate

Oral		
Capsules	1.5 mg (of rivastigmine)	**Exelon®**, Novartis
	3 mg (of rivastigmine)	**Exelon®**, Novartis
	4.5 mg (of rivastigmine)	**Exelon®**, Novartis
	6 mg (of rivastigmine)	**Exelon®**, Novartis
Solution	2 mg (of rivastigmine) per mL	**Exelon®**, Novartis

ANTICHOLINERGIC AGENTS 12:08

ANTIMUSCARINICS/ANTISPASMODICS 12:08.08

Antimuscarinics/Antispasmodics General Statement

■ Antimuscarinics competitively inhibit the muscarinic effects of acetylcholine.

Uses

Antimuscarinics have been used as adjunctive therapy in the treatment of peptic ulcer disease and irritable bowel syndrome. The drugs also have been used in the treatment of a variety of other conditions (e.g., diarrhea, hyperhidrosis, overactive bladder) in which antimuscarinic effects might produce potential therapeutic benefit. There is a general lack of information from well-controlled studies to support their use in these conditions. In addition, adverse effects of antimuscarinics often limit or preclude their use and they generally have been replaced by other more effective and/or less toxic therapies. Glycopyrrolate is used via oral inhalation or nebulization for the long-term maintenance treatment of airflow obstruction. Ipratropium is used via oral inhalation or nebulization for the treatment and prevention of bronchospasm. Ipratropium also is used as a nasal spray for the symptomatic relief of rhinorrhea associated with allergic or nonallergic perennial rhinitis or the common cold. Tolterodine tartrate is used in the treatment of overactive bladder to manage symptoms such as urinary frequency, urgency, and urge incontinence.

Some antimuscarinics are or have been commercially available in combination with other antimuscarinics or with barbiturates, phenothiazines, or benzodiazepines or other anxiolytics. Some clinicians believe that sedatives and/or anxiolytic agents may have a beneficial supportive role in patients with irritable bowel syndrome who respond to sedatives or in some patients with peptic ulcer disease. However, there are no data from well-controlled studies that support the superiority of currently available fixed-ratio combination preparations over single-ingredient preparations. In addition, fixed-ratio combination preparations do not permit individual titration of dosages. Many such preparations no longer are commercially available.

■ **Peptic Ulcer Disease and GI Hypersecretory States** Some antimuscarinics (e.g., atropine, belladonna, clidinium, glycopyrrolate, methscopolamine, propantheline) have been used as adjunctive therapy for peptic ulcer disease. However, there are *no* conclusive data from well-controlled studies which indicate that, in usually recommended dosages, antimuscarinics aid in the healing, decrease the rate of recurrence, or prevent complications of peptic ulcers. The efficacy of antimuscarinics for the treatment of gastric ulcers has also been questioned by many clinicians. In addition, in patients with gastric ulcer, antimuscarinics may delay gastric emptying and result in antral stasis.

When used as adjunctive therapy in the treatment of peptic ulcer disease, none of the synthetic or semisynthetic antimuscarinics has been shown to be therapeutically superior to effective doses of any of the naturally occurring alkaloids (i.e., atropine, belladonna). Claims of specificity, increased efficacy, or improved tolerance reported for specific antimuscarinics usually arise from uncontrolled studies, use of ineffective dosages, or complete inactivity of the drug. Although minor differences in receptor-selectivity (organ-specificity) among the various drugs have been reported, resultant differences in adverse effects do not generally appear to be clinically important enough to warrant the preferential use of any one drug, and the cost of the drug to the patient may be an important consideration. If an antimuscarinic is indicated, some clinicians recommend that belladonna tincture be used, since it usually is the most economical and easily titrated of the currently available antimuscarinics.

Current epidemiologic and clinical evidence supports a strong association between gastric infection with *Helicobacter pylori* and the pathogenesis of duodenal and gastric ulcers; *H. pylori* infection usually is treated with a multiple-drug regimen that includes 2 or 3 anti-infectives (e.g., clarithromycin, amoxicillin, metronidazole, tetracycline or doxycycline, levofloxacin) and a proton-pump inhibitor (e.g., omeprazole) with or without a bismuth salt. Antimuscarinics are not included in American College of Gastroenterology (ACG) guidelines for the management of peptic ulcer disease and *H. pylori* infection.

Antimuscarinics have been administered before meals to prolong and potentiate the effects of postprandial antacid therapy. However, controlled studies have failed to demonstrate a substantial difference in gastric pH when combined antimuscarinic and antacid therapy was compared to antacid therapy alone. Some clinicians use an antimuscarinic in conjunction with a histamine H_2-receptor antagonist to potentiate the inhibitory effects on food-stimulated gastric acid secretion. A regimen that included antacids, an antimuscarinic, and a histamine H_2-receptor antagonist has also been used effectively to reduce gastric acidity.

Antimuscarinics (except those that act mainly as antispasmodics) have been used in the treatment of GI hypersecretory states (e.g., Zollinger-Ellison syndrome) in conjunction with a histamine H_2-receptor antagonist. However, other therapy (e.g., surgical resection of the gastrinoma, high-dosage proton-pump inhibitor therapy) currently is recommended. Antimuscarinics appear to prolong and/or augment the inhibitory effects of histamine H_2-receptor antagonists on gastrin- and pentagastrin-induced gastric acid secretion in patients with the

Zollinger-Ellison syndrome. In one study in patients with Zollinger-Ellison syndrome, 20 mg of oral isopropamide iodide (no longer commercially available in the US) given in conjunction with 600 mg of oral cimetidine hydrochloride reduced the rate of gastric acid secretion to less than 10% of the pretreatment basal secretion rate. In another study in patients with Zollinger-Ellison syndrome, propantheline 30 mg decreased gastric emptying and increased intragastric volume, but was ineffective in controlling gastric acid output or concentrations; when used in conjunction with cimetidine, oral combination therapy (propantheline 30 mg and cimetidine 300 mg) was effective in a patient who did not respond to cimetidine alone. In patients with the Zollinger-Ellison syndrome, a histamine H_2-receptor antagonist used in conjunction with an antimuscarinic may be more effective than an H_2-antagonist alone, especially in patients who fail to respond to usual dosages of an H_2-antagonist. Antimuscarinics should not be used alone to treat Zollinger-Ellison syndrome, since they may delay gastric emptying and produce gastric retention.

■ **Irritable Bowel Syndrome** Antimuscarinics, including those that act principally as antispasmodics, have been used in the treatment of irritable bowel syndrome; however, supportive evidence for the efficacy of these drugs is minimal. Many antimuscarinics in combination with phenobarbital were previously considered possibly or probably effective for the treatment of irritable bowel syndrome, but attempts to substantiate these claims of efficacy have generally failed and these combinations are generally considered as lacking substantial evidence of efficacy in the treatment of this condition.

The majority of patients with irritable bowel syndrome do not require drug therapy; placebo produces a satisfactory response in 35% or more of those treated. If used at all in patients with irritable bowel syndrome, antimuscarinics should usually be reserved for patients failing to respond to other therapies (e.g., diet, placebo, sedation, counseling, amelioration of environmental factors). However, antimuscarinics may provide symptomatic relief in patients with spastic colon in whom pain and/or constipation are major symptoms.

■ **Cardiac Disorders** Atropine sulfate is used in advanced cardiovascular life support (ACLS) for the management of symptomatic bradycardia and is considered the initial drug of choice in adults with unstable bradycardia (e.g., that which is accompanied by altered mental status, cardiac ischemia, acute heart failure, hypotension, or other signs of shock). In pediatric advanced life support (PALS), atropine is used for bradycardia secondary to increased vagal activity or primary atrioventricular (AV) block. Atropine was previously included in ACLS guidelines for the treatment of asystole or pulseless electrical activity (PEA) during cardiopulmonary resuscitation (CPR); however, routine use of the drug during cardiac arrest is no longer recommended because of the lack of evidence demonstrating clinical benefit. (See Uses: Advanced Cardiovascular Life Support and Bradyarrhythmias, in Atropine 12:08.08.)

Because atropine can increase conduction through the AV node, the drug also may be beneficial in the management of AV nodal block. However, atropine is not likely to be effective in patients with type II second-degree AV block or third-degree AV block, including third-degree AV block accompanied by a new wide QRS complex when the conduction block is at or below the His-Purkinje level.

Atropine's principal cardiac use in patients with myocardial infarction (MI) is for the management of sinus bradycardia. Sinus bradycardia caused by increased vagal tone commonly occurs after ST-segment-elevation MI (STEMI), especially in patients with an inferior infarction. However, some data and case reports indicate that atropine may increase ventricular irritability and that increased vagal tone is not necessarily harmful in patients with MI. In addition, uncontrolled atropine-induced tachycardia may increase the size of the infarct. Although some clinicians have questioned the usefulness of atropine in patients with MI, the drug is currently recommended in expert guidelines for the management of symptomatic or hemodynamically unstable sinus bradycardia during an acute MI. Atropine also has been used for the management of symptomatic type I second- or third-degree AV block in patients with acute MI; however, the incidence of abnormal conduction in STEMI patients has decreased considerably in the current reperfusion era. Other uses of atropine in the MI setting include treatment of sustained bradycardia and hypotension associated with nitroglycerin use, and treatment of nausea and vomiting associated with morphine use.

Antimuscarinics, principally atropine, also have been used in the diagnosis of sinus node dysfunction and in the evaluation of coronary artery disease during atrial pacing. Atropine also has been used to assist in the diagnosis of MI in patients with Wolff-Parkinson-White (WPW) syndrome by normalizing the QRS complex and facilitating ECG evaluation of the suspected infarction.

■ **Surgery** Antimuscarinics, particularly atropine, scopolamine, or glycopyrrolate, have been used effectively as preoperative medications. When used preoperatively, these drugs inhibit salivation and excessive secretions of the respiratory tract; however, the current practice of using thiopental (no longer commercially available in the US), halothane, or similar general anesthetics that do not stimulate the production of salivary and tracheobronchial secretions, rather than ether, has reduced the need to control excessive respiratory secretions during surgery. Scopolamine is also used preoperatively in conjunction with analgesics or sedatives to produce tranquilization and amnesia; however, benzodiazepines (e.g., diazepam, lorazepam) appear to produce a more rapid onset of and possibly more marked amnesia than does scopolamine, and benzodiazepines may be preferred by some clinicians as preoperative amnestic agents.

Although atropine and glycopyrrolate have been used prophylactically to prevent acid-aspiration pneumonitis during surgery, preoperative administration of atropine (0.4–0.6 mg IM) or glycopyrrolate (0.2–0.3 mg IM) has not been shown to be effective in increasing gastric pH or reducing gastric fluid volume. Neither the frequency nor the severity of acid-aspiration pneumonitis was reduced in several studies when the drugs were given prophylactically. In addition, by decreasing lower esophageal sphincter tone, antimuscarinics may increase the risk of regurgitation and subsequent aspiration during surgery.

Atropine and glycopyrrolate are used to prevent cholinergic effects during surgery, such as cardiac arrhythmias, hypotension, and bradycardia, which may result from traction on viscera (with resultant vagal stimulation), stimulation of the carotid sinus, or administration of drugs (e.g., succinylcholine).

Atropine, glycopyrrolate, and hyoscyamine are used concurrently with anticholinesterase agents (e.g., neostigmine, pyridostigmine) to block the muscarinic effects of these latter agents when they are used after surgery to reverse the effects of neuromuscular blocking agents. Atropine, glycopyrrolate, and hyoscyamine do not block the effects of anticholinesterase agents at the neuromuscular junction.

The transdermal scopolamine system is used for the prevention of nausea and vomiting associated with recovery from anesthesia and surgery. Although results of some clinical studies have indicated that the transdermal scopolamine system was more effective than placebo in preventing postoperative nausea and vomiting, results of other clinical studies have failed to demonstrate any benefit. Some clinicians believe that the transdermal scopolamine system has some efficacy in the prevention of postoperative nausea and vomiting, particularly when it is applied several hours prior to surgery.

■ **Genitourinary Tract Disorders** In patients with uninhibited or reflex neurogenic bladder, atropine, oxybutynin (see Oxybutynin Chloride 86:12), and propantheline have been effective in reducing the amplitude and frequency of uninhibited contractions of the bladder and in increasing bladder capacity. In addition, incontinence associated with uninhibited contractions is relieved and the volume of residual urine and the frequency of urination are returned to normal in these patients. The diagnosis of neurogenic bladder should be confirmed by cystometry and other appropriate diagnostic procedures before therapy with an antimuscarinic is initiated. In addition, the patient's response to therapy should be periodically evaluated by cystometry. Appropriate anti-infective therapy should be administered whenever urinary tract infection is present. Antimuscarinics are ineffective in the treatment of nonneurogenic nocturnal or functional enuresis. (See Pharmacology: Genitourinary Effects.)

Tolterodine tartrate is used in the treatment of overactive bladder to manage symptoms such as urinary frequency, urgency, and urge incontinence. (See Tolterodine Tartrate 86:12.) The drug is used for the management of symptoms associated with both neurogenic and nonneurogenic overactive bladder. Oxybutynin chloride is used in the treatment of overactive bladder for the relief of symptoms associated with voiding (e.g., urge urinary incontinence, urgency, frequency, urinary leakage, dysuria). Analysis of pooled data from comparative studies of 12 weeks' duration using tolterodine tartrate at a dosage of 2 mg twice daily and oxybutynin 5 mg 3 times daily indicated that tolterodine at this dosage was approximately equivalent to oxybutynin in decreasing the mean number of micturitions per 24 hours and the mean number of episodes of incontinence. Both drugs increased the mean volume voided per micturition, although the increase was greater with oxybutynin than with tolterodine. Some clinicians consider tolterodine to be less effective than older agents used for treatment of overactive bladder (e.g., oxybutynin), although it is better tolerated.

Oxybutynin also has been reportedly effective in relieving mild to moderate urinary tract discomfort resulting from prostatectomy, radiation therapy, or infection; however, controlled studies to determine the efficacy of this or other antimuscarinics in relieving urinary tract discomfort have not been conducted to date.

■ **Bronchospasm** Antimuscarinics (i.e., atropine, ipratropium) are potent bronchodilators. Atropine sulfate has been used effectively by oral inhalation or in a combined regimen of oral inhalation and IM injection to prevent antigen-, methacholine-, histamine-, or exercise-induced bronchospasm. Certain antimuscarinics (i.e., atropine or ipratropium) administered by oral inhalation have been shown to be effective bronchodilators in the treatment of chronic bronchitis and asthma, and atropine sulfate has been used by oral inhalation for the short-term treatment and prevention of bronchospasm associated with chronic bronchial asthma, bronchitis, and chronic obstructive pulmonary disease (COPD). The bronchodilator effect of orally inhaled atropine is similar to that of orally inhaled isoproterenol and, although its onset is delayed, its effect is more prolonged than that of orally inhaled isoetharine.

Glycopyrrolate is used alone or in fixed combination with other respiratory agents via oral inhalation or nebulization for the long-term maintenance treatment of airflow obstruction associated with COPD, including chronic bronchitis and emphysema. Ipratropium (a derivative of atropine) is used by oral inhalation for chronic treatment and prevention of bronchospasm associated with COPD, including bronchitis and emphysema. The efficacy of ipratropium in the management of COPD generally has been similar to or greater than that of β-adrenergic agonists (e.g., albuterol, metaproterenol) in comparative studies with oral inhalation or nebulization. Orally inhaled ipratropium does not appear to have substantial effects on sputum viscosity or volume or on mucociliary clearance.

Some clinicians state that repeated oral or parenteral administration of antimuscarinics to patients with chronic lung disease may be hazardous, since these drugs can reduce the volume and fluidity of bronchial secretions, obstruct airflow, and predispose these patients to infection; however, such hazards do not appear to be a substantial problem when the drugs are administered by oral inhalation.

■ **Other Uses** Antimuscarinics have been used in the treatment of GI hypermotility and diarrhea caused by reserpine, guanethidine, or cholinergic stimulation. Although antimuscarinics have been used in the treatment of diarrhea from other causes (e.g., ulcerative colitis, dysentery, shigellosis), they should be used with extreme caution, if at all, in patients with ulcerative colitis or GI infections. (See Cautions: Precautions and Contraindications.)

Antimuscarinics have been used in the management of parkinsonian syndrome and drug-induced extrapyramidal reactions. In general, the maximum therapeutic response attainable with antimuscarinics is in the range of 20–30% symptomatic improvement in 50–80% of parkinsonian patients. Although some antimuscarinics (e.g., trihexyphenidyl) continue to be used as initial therapy in mild cases of parkinsonian syndrome, in patients who do not tolerate other agents, or as adjunctive therapy to other agents, antimuscarinics generally have been replaced with dopaminergic drugs (e.g., levodopa, bromocriptine). Antimuscarinics may be especially useful in the treatment of excessive salivation associated with parkinsonian syndrome.

Parenterally administered antimuscarinics (e.g., atropine 1 mg IV, propantheline 30–60 mg IV or IM) have been used to facilitate hypotonic duodenography or contrast examination of the colon by reducing duodenal or colonic motility and spasm; however, glucagon appears to be more effective and generally is preferred in these examinations. Antimuscarinics also have been used to enhance visualization of esophageal varices during radiographic examinations and enhance visualization of the urinary tract in excretion urography.

Antimuscarinics have been used to decrease gastric and pancreatic secretions in the treatment of acute pancreatitis; however, there is little, if any, evidence that antimuscarinics improve the prognosis of the disease. It has been suggested that supportive measures and intensive care are probably more important determinants of prognosis than pharmacologic treatment.

Topically applied antimuscarinics have been used to inhibit muscarinic-mediated sweating; topical application of propantheline has been used effectively to treat plantar and palmar hyperhidrosis without adverse systemic effects.

Antimuscarinics also have been used effectively as prophylactic therapy in the prevention of motion sickness; of the currently available antimuscarinics, scopolamine appears to be the most effective. (See Scopolamine 12:08.08.)

In patients with myasthenia gravis, antimuscarinics have been used to minimize unwanted muscarinic effects (e.g., diarrhea, excessive salivation) of anticholinesterase agents (e.g., neostigmine). Although concomitant antimuscarinic and anticholinesterase therapy usually reduces muscarinic effects without interfering with the therapeutic effect of the anticholinesterase agent, antimuscarinics may mask the signs of anticholinesterase overdosage and prevent early detection of cholinergic crisis. Antimuscarinics, principally atropine, have also been used effectively to reverse the muscarinic effects associated with toxic exposure to organophosphate and carbamate anticholinesterase pesticides (e.g., parathion) and ingestion of cholinomimetic plants and fungi (e.g., *Amanita muscaria* mushroom) and drugs having cholinergic effects.

Glycopyrrolate oral solution is used for the symptomatic management of chronic severe drooling in certain pediatric patients with neurologic conditions (e.g., cerebral palsy) associated with problematic drooling.

Antimuscarinics have been used in combination with other drugs (e.g., antihistamines, bronchodilators, expectorants, vasoconstrictors) for the symptomatic treatment of cold and cough. However, there is no evidence from well-designed clinical studies to support their use in combination with other drugs for the management of cold and cough, and most cold and cough combination preparations that previously contained antimuscarinics have been reformulated without these drugs.

Ipratropium nasal spray is used for the symptomatic relief of rhinorrhea associated with allergic or nonallergic perennial rhinitis or the common cold. The drug generally does not relieve nasal congestion, sneezing, or postnasal drip associated with these conditions.

Hyoscyamine sulfate injection is used as an antidote in the treatment of cholinesterase inhibitor toxicity. Hyoscyamine sulfate oral and sublingual preparations also are used in the treatment of cholinesterase inhibitor toxicity.

Atropine combined with a cholinesterase reactivator (pralidoxime chloride) is used in the treatment of organophosphate pesticide poisoning and chemical warfare poisoning. (See Uses in Atropine 12:08.08.)

Antimuscarinics and antispasmodics have been used alone or in combination with phenobarbital in the treatment of infant colic. However, there is minimal evidence from well-designed clinical studies of the efficacy of these drugs in the management of this condition. Infant colic is considered a benign, self-limiting condition that tends to resolve spontaneously and not require medical treatment. Combination preparations are generally considered as lacking substantial evidence of efficacy in the treatment of infant colic.

Antimuscarinics also have been used in the treatment of other conditions (e.g., achalasia, biliary dyskinesia, dysmenorrhea, enuresis, urinary frequency) in which the various antimuscarinic effects of the drugs have been applied for potential therapeutic benefit. However, there is a general lack of information from well-designed clinical studies to support their use in the management of these conditions.

For ophthalmic uses of antimuscarinics, see the individual monographs in 52:24.

Dosage and Administration

■ **Administration** Antimuscarinics usually are administered orally. Atropine sulfate, dicyclomine hydrochloride, glycopyrrolate, hyoscyamine sulfate, propantheline bromide, and scopolamine hydrobromide also may be administered parenterally, although a parenteral preparation of propantheline bromide is no longer commercially available. Glycopyrrolate also may be administered by oral inhalation. Ipratropium bromide may be administered by oral inhalation or intranasally, and scopolamine may be administered topically. Atropine sulfate also has been administered by oral inhalation, but a solution of the drug for oral inhalation no longer is commercially available in the US.

When IV access is not readily available, atropine sulfate has been administered by intraosseous (IO) injection† in the setting of advanced cardiovascular life support (ACLS); onset of action and systemic concentrations are comparable to those achieved with venous administration. The drug also may be administered via an endotracheal tube when vascular access (IV or IO) is not possible; however, IV or IO administration is preferred because of more predictable drug delivery and pharmacologic effect.

■ **Dosage** Dosage of an antimuscarinic should be adjusted according to the patient's response and tolerance. Dosage usually is increased until adverse effects become intolerable; then, a slight reduction in dosage generally yields the maximum dosage tolerated by the patient. Dosages higher than those recommended by the manufacturers are often required to produce a therapeutic effect. Dosage may have to be increased if tolerance to the therapeutic and adverse effects of the drug develops.

Quaternary ammonium antimuscarinics are poorly absorbed orally and are much less effective orally than parenterally; higher oral than parenteral dosages are usually required to achieve the same effect.

Cautions

■ **Adverse Effects** Most adverse effects observed with antimuscarinics are manifestations of the pharmacologic effects of the drugs at muscarinic-cholinergic receptors and usually are reversible when therapy with the drug is discontinued. Antimuscarinics share the toxic potential of atropine, and the usual precautions associated with atropine therapy should be observed with these agents. The frequency and severity of adverse effects of antimuscarinics generally are dose related and adverse effects occasionally may be obviated by a reduction in dosage; however, dosage reduction also may eliminate any potential therapeutic effect of the drugs.

To some extent, adverse effects of antimuscarinics correlate with their structural class. Naturally occurring alkaloids possess the full range of antimuscarinic and antinicotinic activities of atropine and thus have the potential for producing adverse central and peripheral effects associated with atropine. Quaternary ammonium compounds are completely ionized at physiologic pH and are less lipid soluble than tertiary amine compounds. As a result, quaternary ammonium compounds are relatively less active orally than tertiary amine compounds and exhibit fewer effects in the CNS and the eye. Quaternary ammonium compounds generally have the greatest nicotinic (ganglionic) blocking activity of the antimuscarinics. Antimuscarinics that act principally as antispasmodics (e.g., dicyclomine, oxybutynin) have minimal antimuscarinic effects at usual dosages; however, as dosage is increased these drugs also may elicit various antimuscarinic effects. Differences in pharmacologic effects among the antimuscarinics may result in minor differences in adverse effects. (See Pharmacology.)

Adverse reactions frequently associated with the use of antimuscarinics include xerostomia (dry mouth), dry skin, blurred vision, cycloplegia, mydriasis, photophobia (especially with scopolamine), anhidrosis, urinary hesitancy and retention, tachycardia, palpitation, xerophthalmia, and constipation. These adverse effects may appear at therapeutic or subtherapeutic doses. In many patients, xerostomia is the dose-limiting adverse effect of antimuscarinics. Saliva substitutes (e.g., Xero-lube®) have been effective in alleviating xerostomia in patients taking drugs that produce this antimuscarinic effect.

Other reported adverse effects of antimuscarinics include increased ocular tension (especially in patients with angle-closure glaucoma), loss of taste, headache, nervousness, drowsiness, weakness, dizziness, flushing, insomnia, nausea, vomiting, and bloated feeling. Mental confusion and/or excitement also may occur, especially in geriatric patients. Abuse and/or dependence on dicyclomine for its anticholinergic effects has been reported rarely.

Some patients may exhibit excessive susceptibility to the effects of scopolamine and toxic symptoms may occur with therapeutic doses. Marked CNS disturbances, ranging from complete disorientation to an active delirium resembling that encountered in atropine overdosage may occur in these patients. Some patients may exhibit marked somnolence. Other manifestations may include dilated pupils, accelerated pulse rate, and dryness of mouth with a husky quality of the voice apparently caused by laryngeal paralysis. IM or IV administration of antimuscarinics may cause a temporary sensation of lightheadedness and local irritation.

Apparent hypersensitivity reactions have occurred in patients receiving antimuscarinic therapy. Parabens contained in multiple-dose vials of injectable antimuscarinics, lecithin in orally inhaled ipratropium, or other preservatives in antimuscarinic preparations may cause hypersensitivity reactions in patients allergic to these preservatives. Anaphylaxis, urticaria, rash that may progress to exfoliation, delayed hypersensitivity reactions, and various dermal manifestations also have been reported. As with other inhaled drugs for asthma, paradoxical bronchospasm has been reported in a few patients receiving ipratropium via nebulized solution or inhalation aerosol, although a causal relationship to the drug has not been definitely established.

Infants, patients with Down's syndrome (mongolism), and children with spastic paralysis or brain damage may be hypersensitive to antimuscarinic effects (e.g., mydriasis, positive chronotropic effect). Hypersensitivity to antimuscarinic effects of these drugs has also been reported in other patients.

■ **Precautions and Contraindications** Use of antimuscarinics in patients exposed to high environmental temperatures may result in heat prostration. In patients with fever, the risk of hyperthermia may be increased; therefore, antimuscarinics should be used with caution in patients who may be exposed to elevated environmental temperatures or in patients who are febrile. Patients should be advised of the risk of hyperthermia. Since antimuscarinics may produce drowsiness, dizziness, or blurred vision, patients should be warned not to engage in activities requiring mental alertness and/or visual acuity (e.g., operating a motor vehicle or other machinery, performing hazardous work) while taking these drugs.

Antimuscarinics should be used with caution in geriatric patients and children (see Cautions: Pediatric Precautions) since they may be more susceptible to adverse effects of these drugs. Antimuscarinics should also be used with caution in patients with hyperthyroidism, hepatic or renal disease, or hypertension. Antimuscarinics block vagal inhibition of the SA nodal pacemaker and thus should be used with caution in patients with tachyarrhythmias, congestive heart failure, or coronary artery disease. Systemically administered antimuscarinics should be used cautiously in debilitated patients with chronic pulmonary disease, since a reduction in bronchial secretions may lead to inspissation and formation of bronchial plugs; however, antimuscarinics have been used effectively as bronchodilators when administered via oral inhalation. (See Uses: Bronchospasm.) Antimuscarinics should be used with extreme caution in patients with autonomic neuropathy.

Antimuscarinics may produce a delay in gastric emptying with possible antral stasis in patients with gastric ulcer; therefore these drugs should be used cautiously in these patients. Antimuscarinics should be used with caution in patients with esophageal reflux or hiatal hernia associated with reflux esophagitis, since the drugs decrease gastric motility and relax the lower esophageal sphincter (decrease lower esophageal pressure); these effects promote gastric retention and aggravate reflux in these patients.

Antimuscarinics should be administered with extreme caution to patients with known or suspected GI infections (e.g., *Clostridium difficile*-associated diarrhea and colitis [also known as antibiotic-associated pseudomembranous colitis], shigellosis, dysentery), since these drugs may decrease GI motility and prolong symptomatology by causing retention of the causative organism or toxin(s). Because diarrhea may be an early symptom of incomplete intestinal obstruction, especially in patients with ileostomy or colostomy, antimuscarinics should also be used with extreme caution in patients with diarrhea. In addition, antimuscarinics may further aggravate the diarrhea. Antimuscarinics should be used with extreme caution in patients with mild to moderate ulcerative colitis, since antimuscarinics may suppress intestinal motility and produce paralytic ileus with resultant precipitation or aggravation of toxic megacolon; the drugs are contraindicated in patients with severe ulcerative colitis or toxic megacolon complicating ulcerative colitis. Antimuscarinics also are contraindicated in patients with obstructive disease of the GI tract (e.g., pyloroduodenal stenosis, achalasia), cardiospasm, paralytic ileus, or intestinal atony (especially in geriatric or debilitated patients).

Antimuscarinics are contraindicated in patients with known hypersensitivity to the drugs. The drugs also are contraindicated in patients with angle-closure glaucoma; however, antimuscarinics can be administered safely to patients with open-angle glaucoma who are being treated with miotics. Antimuscarinics should be used with extreme caution in patients with partial obstructive uropathy and are contraindicated in patients with obstructive uropathy (e.g., bladder neck obstruction caused by prostatic hypertrophy). Antimuscarinics are also contraindicated in patients with myasthenia gravis unless the antimuscarinic is used to reduce adverse muscarinic effects of an anticholinesterase agent (e.g., neostigmine). (See Uses: Other Uses.)

Antimuscarinics are contraindicated in patients with acute hemorrhage whose cardiovascular status is unstable.

■ **Pediatric Precautions** Antimuscarinics generally should be used with caution in infants, since there have been a few isolated reports of respiratory distress, seizures, asphyxia, muscular hypotonia, and coma in children 6 weeks of age or younger who received dicyclomine orally. These symptoms reportedly occurred within minutes of ingestion, lasted 20–30 minutes, and eventually resolved with no long-term sequelae. The manufacturer states that because of the timing and nature of these reactions, they probably resulted from local irritation and/or aspiration rather than a direct pharmacologic effect; however, caution should be exercised in this age group. The manufacturer of Bentyl® states that dicyclomine is contraindicated in infants younger than 6 months of age.

Safety and efficacy of clidinium (as a fixed-combination preparation with chlordiazepoxide hydrochloride), dicyclomine, homatropine, methscopolamine, propantheline, or tolterodine have not been established in children. Safety in children has been established for belladonna, glycopyrrolate, and hyoscyamine. Safety and efficacy of scopolamine soluble tablets and transdermal system in children have not been established. Safety in children 12 years of age or older has been established for ipratropium bromide. (See the individual monographs in 12:08.08.)

Because glycopyrrolate injection contains benzyl alcohol as a preservative, the manufacturer recommends that the drug not be used in neonates younger than 1 month of age. Although a causal relationship has not been established, administration of injections preserved with benzyl alcohol has been associated with toxicity in neonates. Toxicity appears to have resulted from administration of large amounts (i.e., 100–400 mg/kg daily) of benzyl alcohol in these neonates. Although use of drugs preserved with benzyl alcohol should be avoided in neonates whenever possible, the American Academy of Pediatrics (AAP) states that the presence of small amounts of the preservative in a commercially available injection should not proscribe its use when indicated in neonates.

■ **Pregnancy, Fertility, and Lactation** Reproduction studies with antimuscarinics have generally not been performed. Although some manufacturers state that uncontrolled clinical experience with the drugs (e.g., clidinium, glycopyrrolate, propantheline) has revealed no evidence of toxicity to the mother or fetus, there are no adequate and controlled studies to date using the drugs in pregnant women. Antimuscarinics should generally be used during pregnancy only when the potential benefits justify the possible risks to the fetus.

The effects of antimuscarinics on fertility in animals and humans have not been fully determined. Impotence has occurred during therapy with antimuscarinics. Antimuscarinics inhibit penile erection by blocking cholinergically mediated vasodilation, thereby preventing the increased blood flow to the sinuses (corpora cavernosa and corpus spongiosum) and the resultant penile rigidity that usually occurs during male sexual stimulation. Although studies in dogs indicate that high doses of glycopyrrolate diminish seminal secretion (emission), other evidence suggests that antimuscarinics block cholinergically induced depression of α-adrenergically mediated seminal secretion.

Although information indicating that antimuscarinics inhibit lactation and are distributed into milk is minimal and has been questioned, some manufacturers and clinicians state that these drugs should not be used in nursing women since infants may be particularly sensitive to antimuscarinic effects if the drugs were present in milk.

Drug Interactions

■ **Drugs with Anticholinergic Effects** Additive adverse effects resulting from cholinergic blockade (e.g., xerostomia, blurred vision, constipation) may occur when antimuscarinics are administered concomitantly with phenothiazines, amantadine, antiparkinsonian drugs, glutethimide, meperidine, tricyclic antidepressants, muscle relaxants, antiarrhythmic agents that possess anticholinergic activity (e.g., quinidine, disopyramide, procainamide), or some antihistamines (including meclizine). Patients receiving concomitant therapy with an antimuscarinic and any of these drugs may be at increased risk of developing adverse anticholinergic effects and should be informed of this possibility.

■ **Effects on GI Absorption of Drugs** By inhibiting the motility of the GI tract and prolonging GI transit time, antimuscarinics have the potential to alter GI absorption of various drugs.

In one study, propantheline bromide reduced the rate of absorption of acetaminophen while having little or no effect on the extent of absorption as determined by 24-hour urinary excretion. Propantheline (and probably other antimuscarinics) inhibits gastric emptying and thus apparently delays the delivery of acetaminophen to its site of absorption in the intestine. Although not specifically determined, antimuscarinics could potentially delay the onset of therapeutic effects (e.g., analgesia, antipyresis) of acetaminophen.

Concurrent administration of an antimuscarinic and levodopa may decrease the extent of absorption of levodopa in the small intestine by causing increased metabolism of levodopa in the stomach. If the antimuscarinic is discontinued without a concomitant reduction in levodopa dosage, toxicity may result from the increased absorption of levodopa.

Concurrent use of propantheline and slow-dissolving tablets of digoxin may result in increased serum digoxin concentrations. This interaction can be avoided by using digoxin oral solution or tablets that dissolve rapidly (e.g., Lanoxin®). Patients receiving an antimuscarinic and digoxin should be closely observed for signs of digitalis toxicity.

Because antimuscarinics may decrease gastric acid output and/or increase gastric pH, they may decrease the GI absorption of ketoconazole which depends on gastric acidity for dissolution and absorption. If concomitant therapy is necessary, the antimuscarinic should be given at least 2 hours after ketoconazole tablets.

Prior administration of propantheline bromide delayed the rate of absorption of riboflavin but increased the total amount absorbed, presumably by increasing the residence time of the drug at GI absorption sites.

■ **Antacids** Antacids may decrease the extent of absorption of some oral antimuscarinics when these drugs are administered simultaneously. Therefore, oral antimuscarinics should be administered at least 1 hour before antacids. Antimuscarinics may be administered before meals to prolong the effects of postprandial antacid therapy. However, controlled studies have failed to demonstrate a substantial difference in gastric pH when combined antimuscarinic and antacid therapy was compared with antacid therapy alone.

■ **Other Drugs** Concurrent administration of glycopyrrolate and a wax-matrix potassium chloride preparation (Slow-K®) increased the severity of potassium chloride-induced GI mucosal lesions (as determined endoscopically) compared with potassium chloride administration alone; antimuscarinics slow GI transit time and thus apparently potentiate the local GI mucosal effects of potassium chloride. Minimal endoscopic evidence of GI mucosal lesions was seen when glycopyrrolate was administered concurrently with a microencapsulated potassium chloride preparation (Micro-K®). Antimuscarinics should be used cautiously with potassium chloride preparations (especially wax-matrix preparations) and patients should be carefully monitored for evidence of GI mucosal lesions.

Concomitant administration of antimuscarinics and corticosteroids may result in increased intraocular pressure.

Caution should be exercised if scopolamine is administered concomitantly with other CNS depressants (e.g., sedatives, tranquilizers, alcohol).

Laboratory Test Interferences

Scopolamine (and probably other antimuscarinics) may interfere with the gastric secretion test.

Acute Toxicity

■ **Pathogenesis** Overdosage of antimuscarinics produces symptoms that are principally extensions of common adverse effects of the drugs. Single 10-mg oral doses of atropine may produce signs and symptoms of acute toxicity in adults; however, one adult male reportedly survived a single 1-g oral dose of the drug. Children may be more susceptible than adults to the toxic effects of atropine; deaths have been reported in children following ingestion of 10 mg of atropine.

The LD_{50} of hyoscyamine in rats is 375 mg/kg. The oral LD_{50} of methscopolamine bromide in rats is 1.4–2.6 g/kg. The oral LD_{50} of propantheline bromide in mice and rats is 780 mg/kg and 370 mg/kg, respectively.

■ **Manifestations** Acute overdosage with antimuscarinics produces both peripheral and CNS symptomatology. The quaternary ammonium compounds do not readily penetrate the CNS and thus exhibit minimal central effects even at toxic doses. Peripheral symptoms may include dilated and unreactive pupils; blurred vision; hot, dry, and flushed skin; dryness of mucous membranes; difficulty in swallowing; foul breath; diminished or absent bowel sounds; urinary retention; tachycardia; hyperthermia; hypertension; and increased respiratory rate. In addition to tachycardia, cardiac manifestations may include ECG abnormalities similar to those produced by quinidine toxicity (e.g., ventricular arrhythmias, extrasystoles); these abnormalities result from enhanced reentrant excitation secondary to reduced conduction velocity. Widening of the QRS complex, prolongation of the QT interval, and ST-segment depression may also be seen. Other peripheral signs and symptoms may include nausea, vomiting, and a scarlatiniform or maculopapular rash over the face, neck, and upper trunk. Acute overdosage with quaternary ammonium antimuscarinics may produce a curariform neuromuscular block and ganglionic blockade manifested as respiratory paralysis.

Acute overdosage with antimuscarinics generally produces CNS stimulation followed by depression. CNS manifestations may resemble acute psychosis characterized by various neuropsychiatric signs and symptoms including disorientation, incoherence, confusion, stupor, hallucinations (usually visual, but may also be auditory or tactile), delusions, paranoia, disturbed speech (e.g., dysarthria, pressure to keep talking), periods of hyperactivity (sometimes alternating with somnolence), anxiety, abnormal motor behavior (e.g., ataxia, incoordination), agitation, seizures, and restlessness. In severe overdosage, CNS depression, circulatory collapse, and hypotension may occur. Scopolamine may cause CNS excitement and delirium, especially in patients with painful conditions. Coma and skeletal muscle paralysis may also occur and may be followed by death from respiratory failure. Comatose patients may also exhibit clonic movements, upgoing plantar reflexes (positive Babinski sign), and hyperreflexia. Death has also reportedly resulted from hyperpyrexia (especially in children), cardiac depression, or from environmental exposure or drowning in patients who were delirious.

Blurred vision, numbness on the left side, cold fingertips, abdominal and flank pain, decreased appetite, dry mouth, and nervousness were reported in an adult who ingested 320 mg of dicyclomine hydrochloride daily for 4 days; these adverse effects resolved when the drug was discontinued.

It is necessary to distinguish the signs and symptoms of scopolamine overdosage from the withdrawal symptoms that are observed occasionally in patients who discontinue the transdermal scopolamine system. (See Adverse Effects: CNS Effects in the Cautions section of Scopolamine 12:08.08.) Although mental confusion and dizziness may be observed with both acute toxicity and withdrawal, patients with anticholinergic toxicity also may exhibit signs and symptoms including tachyarrhythmias, dry skin, and decreased bowel sounds, while bradycardia, headache, nausea, abdominal cramps, and sweating may suggest symptoms associated with scopolamine withdrawal.

■ **Treatment** Treatment of acute antimuscarinic overdosage consists of symptomatic and supportive therapy. Patients should be hospitalized and closely monitored, including continuous ECG monitoring. If the patient is conscious, has not lost the gag reflex, and is not having seizures, the stomach should be emptied immediately by inducing emesis. If emesis is unsuccessful or contraindicated, gastric lavage (preferably accompanied by instillation of activated charcoal) may be performed with a cuffed endotracheal tube, inflated and in place, to prevent aspiration of gastric contents. Saline cathartics may also be administered. In patients who exhibit manifestations of severe poisoning, use of exchange transfusions should be considered. Hemodialysis or peritoneal dialysis is apparently not useful.

Because physostigmine has the potential for producing severe adverse effects (e.g., seizures, asystole), routine use of physostigmine as an antidote for antimuscarinic overdosage is controversial. The American Psychiatric Association (APA) states that, unless contraindicated, use of physostigmine can be considered for severe cases of delirium induced by anticholinergics. (See Cautions: Precautions and Contraindications.) Many clinicians believe that the drug should be used only in the treatment of severe or life-threatening symptoms of anticholinergic toxicity (e.g., extensive delirium or agitation, hallucinations, hyperthermia, severe sinus or supraventricular tachycardia, seizures) in patients who fail to respond to alternative therapy. Relative contraindications to the use of physostigmine include asthma, gangrene, cardiovascular disease, and mechanical obstruction of the GI or genitourinary tract. Physostigmine should be used in these situations only if a life-threatening emergency occurs.

Delirium, hallucinations, coma, and cardiac arrhythmias often respond to physostigmine. Physostigmine will reverse supraventricular tachycardia produced by antimuscarinic overdosage. IV propranolol may be useful for treating supraventricular tachyarrhythmias unresponsive to physostigmine or when physostigmine is contraindicated. Physostigmine should not be used to treat cardiac conduction defects or ventricular tachyarrhythmias. Frequent administration of physostigmine may be necessary as it is short-acting and patients may suddenly relapse; however, excessive doses of physostigmine may produce cholinergic toxicity (e.g., bradycardia, increased salivation, diarrhea, seizures, respiratory arrest). If indicated, physostigmine salicylate usually is administered by slow IV injection. The usual initial adult dose is 2 mg. If there is no response, 1–2 mg may be given every 20 minutes until reversal of toxic antimuscarinic effects occurs or adverse cholinergic effects develop. If initial doses of the drug are effective, additional doses of 1–4 mg may be given every 30–60 minutes as necessary. The usual initial pediatric IV dose of physostigmine salicylate recommended by the manufacturer is 0.02 mg/kg. Additional doses may be repeated at 5- to 10-minute intervals until a response is obtained, adverse cholinergic effects develop, or a total dose of 2 mg has been administered; thereafter, the lowest effective dose may be repeated as necessary. Adverse effects of physostigmine (e.g., life-threatening bronchoconstriction, bradycardia, seizures) can be reversed with IV administration of 0.5–1 mg of atropine sulfate.

Fluid therapy and other standard treatments of shock should be administered as needed. Hyperthermia is usually treated with cold packs, mechanical cooling devices, or sponging with tepid water. Diazepam may be administered to control excitement, delirium, or other symptoms of acute psychosis. *Phenothiazines should not be used as they may contribute to anticholinergic effects.* Conjunctival application of pilocarpine may be used to counteract mydriasis. Maintenance of an adequate airway is important, and respiratory assistance may be necessary. If the patient is comatose, urinary catheterization should be performed to avoid urinary retention.

If overdosage of scopolamine occurs following application of multiple transdermal systems and/or ingestion of the transdermal system, measures to ensure that the patient has an adequate airway and to provide cardiac and respiratory support should be instituted, followed by rapid removal of all transdermal systems from the skin and/or mouth. If there is evidence of ingestion of the transdermal system, gastric lavage, endoscopic removal of the swallowed transdermal system, or administration of activated charcoal should be considered depending on the clinical situation. ECG and vital signs should be monitored continuously, IV access should be established, and oxygen should be administered if a serious overdosage has occurred or there are evolving signs of acute toxicity.

Manifestations of overdosage of illicit drugs (apparently mixed or "cut" with scopolamine) that were injected or "snorted" included lethargy, agitation, hallucinations, paranoia, tachycardia, mild hypertension, mydriasis, dry skin or mucous membranes, diminished or absent bowel sounds, and urinary retention. Following administration of parenteral naloxone by emergency room personnel, some patients with lethargy experienced agitation and combativeness. In some patients, manifestations of toxicity resolved with physostigmine and/or sedation (e.g., diazepam, lorazepam); however, physostigmine should be administered with extreme caution by health-care personnel experienced in the use of the drug, since severe adverse effects (e.g., seizures, bronchospasm, bradycardia) have been associated with its use. Assessment of the described cases of overdosage is difficult since manifestations of opiate overdosage (e.g., lethargy, respiratory depression, miosis) and those associated with overdosage of antimuscarinics, including scopolamine (e.g., mydriasis, flushing, dry skin and mucous membranes, absent bowel sounds, tachycardia, altered mental status), are different, and some manifestations may obscure the classic effects associated with overdosage of the individual drugs. Timely recognition of these toxicities is important; therefore, the US Centers for Disease Control and Prevention (CDC) states that all new cases of these overdosages should be reported promptly to the local poison control center and health department.

Pharmacology

■ **General Pharmacology** ***Antimuscarinics*** Antimuscarinics competitively inhibit the actions of acetylcholine or other cholinergic stimuli at autonomic effectors innervated by postganglionic cholinergic nerves, and to a lesser extent, on smooth muscles that lack cholinergic innervation. These drugs are referred to as antimuscarinics because at usual doses they principally antagonize cholinergic stimuli at muscarinic receptors and have little or no effect on cholinergic stimuli at nicotinic receptors. Antimuscarinics also have been referred to as anticholinergics (cholinergic blocking agents), but this term is appropriate only when it describes the antagonism of cholinergic stimuli at any cholinergic receptor, whether muscarinic or nicotinic. Since the functions antagonized by antimuscarinics principally are under the parasympathetic division of the nervous system, these drugs also have been referred to as parasympatholytics.

At autonomic ganglia, where cholinergic transmission involves nicotinic receptors, atropine or other tertiary amine antimuscarinics produce a partial cholinergic block only at relatively high doses. At the neuromuscular junction, where cholinergic receptors are principally or exclusively nicotinic, only extremely high doses of atropine or other tertiary amine antimuscarinics produce any degree of blockade. However, quaternary ammonium antimuscarinics generally possess varying degrees of nicotinic blocking activity and may interfere with ganglionic or neuromuscular transmission at doses that block muscarinic receptors. At high doses, quaternary ammonium antimuscarinics may produce substantial ganglionic blockade with resultant adverse effects (e.g., impotence, postural hypotension) and, in overdosage, they may cause a curariform neuromuscular block.

There are considerable differences among antimuscarinics in the degree to which various pharmacologic effects are produced; this may result in part from existence of 4 or more subtypes of muscarinic receptors. The convention commonly used to classify muscarinic receptors designates pharmacologically defined muscarinic receptor subtypes as M_1, M_2, M_3, and M_4. These correspond to the genetically cloned receptor subtypes m1–m4. Although a fifth muscarinic gene product (designated m5) has been cloned, no functional correlate for this receptor has been unambiguously demonstrated, and its pharmacology appears to differ from that of other muscarinic receptor subtypes. Determining the precise location and role of the muscarinic receptor subtypes has been difficult, since multiple subtypes may be expressed in a tissue or cell, and much research remains to be done.

Receptors at various sites are not equally sensitive to inhibitory effects of antimuscarinics; therefore, the degree of inhibition at each site is dose-dependent. In general, the relative sensitivity of physiologic functions, proceeding from the most sensitive, is as follows: secretions of the salivary, bronchial, and sweat glands; pupillary dilation, ocular accommodation, and heart rate; contraction of the detrusor muscle of the bladder and smooth muscle of the GI tract; and gastric secretion and motility. An antimuscarinic, in a dose sufficient to depress gastric secretion, will usually also inhibit other, more sensitive functions to some degree. Therefore, if antimuscarinics are used to decrease gastric secretions, they are very likely to cause dryness of the mouth (xerostomia) and interfere with visual accommodation, and possibly cause difficulty in urinating.

Antispasmodics Dicyclomine, oxybutynin, and tolterodine are structurally related to the antimuscarinics and are often referred to as antispasmodic or antimuscarinic-antispasmodic agents. Although the exact mechanism(s) of action of these drugs has not been established, they appear to act as nonselective smooth muscle relaxants. It has been suggested that they have a nonspecific direct action on smooth muscle. These drugs generally have little or no antimuscarinic activity, except at high doses, and little or no effect on gastric secretion. Oxybutynin exhibits one-fifth the anticholinergic activity but 4–10 times the antispasmodic activity of atropine on the rabbit detrusor muscle. Since dicyclomine and oxybutynin, like the antimuscarinics, have been used as adjunctive therapy for irritable bowel syndrome, they generally are included in discussions on antimuscarinics. (See Uses: Irritable Bowel Syndrome.)

In vitro, the relative binding affinity of tolterodine at the muscarinic receptors of the bladder is similar to that of oxybutynin, while at the muscarinic receptors in the parotid gland the potency of oxybutynin appears to be eightfold greater than that of tolterodine. Because tolterodine is used for the management of overactive bladder, it is described with other genitourinary smooth muscle relaxants. (See Tolterodine Tartrate 86:12.)

■ GI Effects Antimuscarinics have various antisecretory effects in the GI tract.

The drugs reduce the volume of saliva and produce xerostomia. Receptors mediating these salivary effects usually are more sensitive to antimuscarinic blockade than other muscarinic receptors (e.g., those mediating gastric secretion). Antimuscarinics also generally reduce the volume of gastric secretions; however, the concentration of gastric acid is not necessarily reduced. Secretion during the gastric and psychic phases of gastric acid secretion is decreased but not eliminated. The intestinal phase of gastric acid secretion also may be inhibited. Relatively large doses of antimuscarinics (i.e., more than 1 mg of atropine IV, 4 mg of glycopyrrolate orally, or 0.8 mg of hyoscyamine orally) usually are required to reduce gastric acid secretion. These doses generally decrease basal or nocturnal gastric acid secretion by about 50%, histamine- or pentagastrin-stimulated gastric acid secretion by about 40%, and food-stimulated gastric acid secretion by about 30%. These relatively large doses of antimuscarinics may eliminate fasting gastric acid secretion in healthy individuals; however, this action is less prominent in patients with peptic ulcers. In a study comparing oral doses of pirenzepine (not commercially available in the US) with hyoscyamine in healthy adults using a placebo-controlled baseline, pirenzepine (50 mg twice daily) and hyoscyamine (0.6 mg twice daily) reduced gastric acid secretion by 57 and 54%, respectively, and reduced pentagastrin-stimulated gastric secretion by 22 and 31%, respectively; neither drug showed a substantial effect on gastric emptying. Antimuscarinics generally do not appear to provide effective control of gastric acid secretion at doses that are devoid of substantial adverse effects. However, in one study in patients with duodenal ulcer, a single, oral, 15-mg dose of propantheline reduced food-stimulated gastric acid secretion to the same extent as a single, oral, 45-mg dose without the pronounced adverse effects of the higher dosage.

Gastric acid secretion stimulated by choline esters (e.g., methacholine, carbachol) or pilocarpine is completely blocked by atropine. Histamine-, alcohol-, or caffeine-stimulated gastric acid secretion is reduced but not abolished by atropine. Antimuscarinics may decrease the concentration of mucin and enzymes in GI secretions. Atropine and other antimuscarinics have little direct effect on pancreatic, biliary, or intestinal secretions, since these secretions are principally controlled by hormonal rather than vagal mechanisms. Although the exact mechanism of action has not been determined, it has been suggested that antimuscarinic-induced delayed emptying can delay the release of secretin by slowing the entry of the acid stimulus into the duodenum and that this may indirectly decrease the volume and activity of pancreatic secretions. Antimuscarinics (e.g., atropine, propantheline) have been shown to reduce the volume of amylase secretion in some patients whose pancreatic secretion was stimulated by secretin, secretin and insulin, or secretin and pancreozymin, and in some patients with acute pancreatitis; however, there has been little, if any, evidence that antimuscarinics improve the prognosis of acute pancreatitis.

Antisecretory effects of antimuscarinics apparently do not persist for any prolonged period (generally less than 48 hours) following discontinuance of the drugs.

Therapeutic doses of antimuscarinics produce prolonged inhibitory effects on the motility of the esophagus, stomach, duodenum, jejunum, ileum, and colon; these effects are characterized by a decrease in tone and in the amplitude and frequency of peristaltic contractions. Antimuscarinics prolong GI transit time and thus have the potential to alter absorption of other drugs. (See Drug Interactions: Effects on GI Absorption of Drugs.) Increases in GI tone and motility resulting from insulin-induced hypoglycemia, emotional stimulation, or the administration of morphine or parasympathomimetic drugs are usually readily inhibited by antimuscarinics; however, some increases in GI tone and motility are resistant to antimuscarinic inhibition (e.g., direct GI stimulation secondary to vasopressin or histamine). Antimuscarinics relax the lower esophageal sphincter with a resultant decrease in lower esophageal sphincter pressure. Antimuscarinics exert a weak antispasmodic action on the gallbladder and bile ducts which is usually insufficient for therapeutic effect. It has been suggested that drugs that act principally as antispasmodics decrease spasm of the smooth muscle of the GI tract through some direct action without producing antimuscarinic effects on salivary or gastric secretions; however, dosages required to decrease GI hypermotility are probably not devoid of antimuscarinic effects.

Although the mechanism of action has not been determined, atropine and propantheline have been shown to decrease gastric plasma protein loss in patients with giant hypertrophic gastritis (Menetrier's disease).

■ Genitourinary Effects Atropine and other antimuscarinics decrease the tone and amplitude of contractions of the ureters and bladder; however, cholinergic innervation is not completely blocked by these drugs. In addition, the bladder smooth muscle appears to be less sensitive to the antimuscarinic effects of these drugs than are other smooth muscles (e.g., GI). In healthy individuals, atropine (0.5 mg IM) has no effect on urinary bladder capacity, micturition pressure, or urethral pressure. In one study, 30 mg of propantheline IM had no effect on empty bladder tone or sphincter pressure; however, in most of these patients, this dose produced an increase in bladder capacity and completely abolished the micturition reflex resulting in urinary retention. In a cystometric study in patients with overactive bladder, tolterodine increased the volume at first bladder contraction, the residual volume, and the maximum cystometric capacity after 4 weeks of therapy. In patients with obstructive uropathy, antimuscarinics may cause urinary retention. (See Cautions: Precautions and Contraindications.)

Antimuscarinics exhibit more pronounced effects on neurogenic bladders. In patients with uninhibited or reflex neurogenic bladder, the amplitude and frequency of uninhibited contractions are reduced and bladder capacity is increased by atropine (1–4 mg orally or 1.2 mg IV) or propantheline (60–120 mg orally or 30–60 mg IV). In addition, incontinence associated with uninhibited contractions is relieved and volume of residual urine and frequency of urination are returned to normal in these patients. Cystometric studies in patients with uninhibited neurogenic or reflex neurogenic bladder indicate that oxybutynin increases urinary bladder capacity, diminishes the frequency of uninhibited contractions of the detrusor muscle, and delays the initial desire to void. These effects are more evident in individuals with uninhibited neurogenic bladder than in those with reflex neurogenic bladder. Antimuscarinics are ineffective in inhibiting nonneurogenic or functional enuresis. Tolterodine tartrate is used for the management of symptoms associated with both neurogenic and nonneurogenic overactive bladder.

Atropine (1.2 mg IV) produces dilation of the pelves, calyces, and ureters and has been used to enhance visualization of the urinary tract in excretion urography. Some antimuscarinics may inhibit penile erection and may produce impotence. (See Cautions: Pregnancy, Fertility, and Lactation.) Atropine does not appear to exert any substantial pharmacologic effect on the uterus. When given as a preanesthetic to women in labor, scopolamine does not appear to have any effect on the frequency or duration of uterine contractions during labor. Except in large doses, drugs that act principally as antispasmodics may decrease spasm of the smooth muscle of the ureters and uterus without producing usual antimuscarinic effects (e.g., mydriasis).

■ Cardiovascular Effects Cardiac effects of antimuscarinics are dose dependent. Average doses of antimuscarinics (e.g., 0.4–0.6 mg of atropine) may produce a slight decrease in heart rate attributable to central vagal stimulation which occurs prior to peripheral cholinergic blockade; the decrease in heart rate is more prominent with scopolamine (0.1–0.2 mg) than with atropine (0.4–0.6 mg). Larger doses of antimuscarinics (e.g., 1–2 mg of atropine) cause progressively increasing tachycardia by blocking normal vagal inhibition of the sinoatrial (SA) node. Cardiac effects of antimuscarinics are sometimes unpredictable and paradoxical, depending on the component of the specialized cardiac conduction system and of the myocardium showing the predominant effect and on the physiologic condition of the heart.

Atropine is the principal antimuscarinic studied for its cardiac effects and used for the diagnosis, evaluation, and treatment of cardiac disorders. Atropine has a positive chronotropic effect (increased sinoatrial [SA] node automaticity), accelerating sinus rate by direct parasympathetic blockade. Although atropine is effective in reversing sinus bradycardia secondary to extracardiac causes, it has little, if any, effect on sinus bradycardia caused by intrinsic disease of the SA node. Atropine has been shown to shorten SA-conduction time in healthy individuals and in patients with sinus bradycardia; however, its effect on refractoriness of atrial muscle has not been fully determined. Atropine stimulates the atrioventricular (AV) functional pacemaker in healthy individuals and in patients with sinus node disease and facilitates AV nodal conduction in individuals with a normal AV node. Atropine shortens AV nodal conduction time and decreases effective and functional refractory periods of the AV node. The effects of atropine on first-degree AV block are variable and unpredictable. Generally, type I second-degree AV block responds to atropine, while the drug is ineffective in type II second-degree AV block. Response to atropine of the subjunctional portion of the specialized cardiac conduction system (i.e., His-Purkinje system) is unpredictable.

Atrial arrhythmias, AV dissociation, ventricular tachycardia, and ventricular fibrillation may occur during antimuscarinic therapy. Young healthy adults appear to be more susceptible to these effects than other age groups because of an apparent increased importance of cardiac vagal tone in this age group. Antimuscarinics can reverse reflex vagal cardiac slowing or asystole such as that induced by inhalation of irritant vapors or by vagal stimulation (e.g., carotid sinus stimulation, pressure on the eyeball).

Antimuscarinics may cause cutaneous vasodilation, especially at toxic doses; this effect is sometimes referred to as atropine flush. It is not known if this vasodilation is a compensatory response to dissipate an increase in body temperature or a direct effect of the drugs on cutaneous blood vessels.

■ **Respiratory Tract Effects** Antimuscarinics reduce the volume of secretions from the nose, mouth, pharynx, and bronchi. Ipratropium, a derivative of atropine, inhibits secretions from the serous and seromucous glands lining the nasal mucosa when applied locally. Antimuscarinics cause relaxation of smooth muscles of the bronchi and bronchioles with a resultant decrease in airway resistance. Atropine and ipratropium are potent bronchodilators, particularly in large bronchial airways, and are especially effective in reversing bronchoconstriction induced by parasympathetic stimulation. The autonomic control of bronchoconstriction and the release of bronchoconstrictor substances from mast cells appear to be mediated by cyclic nucleotides. Antimuscarinics block acetylcholine-induced stimulation of guanyl cyclase and thus reduce tissue concentrations of cyclic guanosine monophosphate (cGMP), a mediator of bronchoconstriction. Although some clinicians caution against the use of antimuscarinics in asthmatic patients because of the drying effect of the drugs, orally inhaled atropine and ipratropium have been effective in preventing antigen-, methacholine-, and exercise-induced bronchospasm in these patients.

Atropine and scopolamine effectively reduce the incidence of laryngospasm that occurs during general anesthesia. They act indirectly by reducing secretions that may stimulate reflex laryngospasm; a direct blockade of laryngeal skeletal muscle does not appear to occur.

For additional information on the respiratory tract effects of antimuscarinics, see Pharmacology in Ipratropium Bromide 12:08.08.

■ **CNS Effects** With the exception of quaternary ammonium compounds and scopolamine, antimuscarinics stimulate the medulla and higher cerebral centers and exhibit CNS effects similar to those produced by antimuscarinics used in the treatment of parkinsonian syndrome (e.g., trihexyphenidyl). Cholinergic transmission in the CNS mainly involves nicotinic receptors in the spinal cord and both muscarinic and nicotinic receptors in the brain. CNS effects of usual doses of atropine and related drugs result from their central antimuscarinic actions and are usually confined to mild vagal stimulation with a resultant decrease in heart rate. At toxic doses, CNS effects (i.e., prominent central stimulation leading to restlessness, irritability, disorientation, hallucinations, and delirium) of atropine and related drugs probably result from antimuscarinic and other effects. Antimuscarinics appear to cause an increased release and turnover of acetylcholine in the CNS which may result in activation of nicotinic receptors in the brain. As the dose of antimuscarinic is progressively increased, stimulation eventually gives way to depression, coma, medullary paralysis, and death. Quaternary ammonium compounds do not readily penetrate the CNS and thus exhibit minimal central effects even at toxic doses.

Unlike atropine and most other antimuscarinics, scopolamine, at usual dosages, produces CNS depression manifested as drowsiness, euphoria, amnesia, fatigue, and dreamless sleep (with a reduction in rapid eye movement [REM] sleep). However, excitement, restlessness, hallucinations, or delirium may paradoxically occur, especially when scopolamine is used in the presence of severe pain. High doses of scopolamine produce CNS effects (e.g., restlessness, disorientation, irritability, hallucinations) similar to those produced by toxic doses of other antimuscarinics.

Although other antimuscarinics have been used in the prevention of motion sickness, it appears that scopolamine is most effective. Scopolamine apparently corrects some central imbalance of acetylcholine and norepinephrine that may occur in patients with motion sickness. It has been suggested that antimuscarinics may block the transmission of cholinergic impulses from the vestibular nuclei to higher centers in the CNS and from the reticular formation to the vomiting center; these effects result in prevention of motion-induced nausea and vomiting.

■ **Ophthalmic Effects** Antimuscarinics block the responses of the sphincter muscle of the iris and the ciliary muscle of the lens to cholinergic stimulation. Mydriasis and cycloplegia result from these ocular effects and result in a decrease in ocular accommodation. Antimuscarinics usually have little effect on intraocular pressure except in patients with angle-closure glaucoma in whom intraocular pressure may increase. Drugs that act principally as antispasmodics generally have little or no ocular effects at usual doses. For information on ophthalmic effects of topical antimuscarinics, see the individual monographs in 52:24.

■ **Other Effects** Antimuscarinics reduce the volume of perspiration by inhibiting sweat-gland secretions. In toxic doses, antimuscarinics may suppress sweating sufficiently to increase body temperature.

Pharmacokinetics

Little information is available on the pharmacokinetics of most antimuscarinics.

■ **Absorption** Generally, those antimuscarinics having a quaternary ammonium group are incompletely absorbed from the GI tract since they are completely ionized. Generally, the tertiary amine antimuscarinics are readily absorbed from the GI tract. Tolterodine is well absorbed following oral administration, and absorption of the drug is rapid, with maximum serum concentrations of tolterodine occurring usually within 1–2 hours after administration of a dose. The presence of food in the GI tract may affect absorption of antimuscarinics. Scopolamine is well absorbed percutaneously following topical application. (See Scopolamine 12:08.08.) Following IM administration, atropine and glycopyrrolate are rapidly absorbed, reportedly reaching peak concentrations 15–50 minutes and peak antimuscarinic effects 30–45 minutes after administration, respectively. Following oral inhalation of usual doses, limited amounts of atropine or ipratropium reach systemic circulation. Systemic absorption of ipratropium following administration as a nasal spray also is limited but exceeds that resulting from oral inhalation of the drug as a nebulized solution or aerosol.

■ **Distribution** Distribution of most antimuscarinics has not been determined. Atropine and glycopyrrolate are apparently rapidly distributed throughout the body since the drugs disappear rapidly from blood after IV administration. Glycopyrrolate is distributed into bile; however, it is not known if other antimuscarinics undergo similar distribution. Quaternary ammonium antimuscarinics exhibit poor lipid solubility; they do not readily cross the blood-brain barrier and thus exhibit minimal CNS effects. In addition, because of their poor lipid solubility, quaternary ammonium antimuscarinics do not readily penetrate the eye. Atropine and hyoscyamine readily cross the blood-brain barrier; other tertiary amine antimuscarinics apparently penetrate the CNS since central effects have been observed. Although atropine, glycopyrrolate, hyoscyamine, and scopolamine cross the placenta, it is not known whether other antimuscarinics cross the placenta. Although atropine has been stated to distribute into milk in small quantities, there are minimal data to support this statement. It is unlikely that quaternary ammonium antimuscarinics distribute into milk; however, studies to determine this have apparently not been conducted.

■ **Elimination** Elimination of most antimuscarinics has not been determined. Atropine is apparently metabolized in the liver to tropic acid, tropine (or a chromatographically similar compound), and possibly, esters of tropic acid and glucuronide conjugates. Oxybutynin and tolterodine are metabolized by the cytochrome P-450 microsomal enzyme system. Metabolites of other antimuscarinics also have been identified. (See the individual monographs in 12:08.08.) Propantheline bromide is extensively hydrolyzed in the upper small intestine; however, it is not known if other antimuscarinics undergo similar inactivation.

Antimuscarinics mainly are eliminated in the urine. The drugs generally are excreted in urine as unchanged drug and metabolites. Following IM administration of atropine, about 30–50% of a dose is excreted in urine unchanged; tropine, tropic acid, and other metabolites are also excreted in urine. Small amounts (up to 3% of a dose in one study) of atropine may also be eliminated as carbon dioxide in expired air. Following oral administration, substantial amounts of antimuscarinics (especially quaternary ammonium compounds) may be eliminated in feces as unabsorbed drug. It is not known whether tertiary amine or quaternary ammonium antimuscarinics are removed by peritoneal dialysis or hemodialysis; however, atropine apparently is not removed by hemodialysis.

Chemistry

Antimuscarinics competitively inhibit the muscarinic effects of acetylcholine. Atropine (*dl*-hyoscyamine) is the prototype of the antimuscarinics and many of the currently available antimuscarinics were developed as structural derivatives of atropine. However, other antimuscarinics have been synthesized that have little structural similarity to atropine, and other drugs with a variety of structural characteristics also exhibit antimuscarinic activity. Most antimuscarinics are aminoalcohols or their derivatives (usually esters or ethers), aminoamides, or other amines.

All commercially available antimuscarinics contain a cationic site at *X* which is important in determining antimuscarinic activity. This cationic site results from a nitrogen atom in the chemical substituent at *X* and exists in a tertiary or quaternary form. Although other drugs exhibit antimuscarinic activity without having a cationic site, they generally are less effective inhibitors of acetylcholine. The type of amine, tertiary or quaternary, is the most important structural characteristic of antimuscarinics in determining pharmacologic differences among the drugs; discussion of this structural characteristic as it affects the pharmacology, pharmacokinetics, and adverse effects of these drugs is included in the sections that follow.

Antimuscarinics usually are classified on the basis of their source (natural, semisynthetic, or synthetic) and/or on their cationic nature (tertiary amine or quaternary ammonium compounds). Antimuscarinics can be divided into 2 groups—*naturally occurring alkaloids and their semisynthetic derivatives* and *synthetic amine compounds.*

■ Naturally Occurring Alkaloids and Semisynthetic Derivatives

All commercially available naturally occurring alkaloids and their semisynthetic derivatives are aminoalcohol esters.

Table 1. Naturally Occurring Alkaloids and Semisynthetic Derivatives

Alkaloid	Type
atropine	*natural, tertiary amine*
belladonna	*natural, mixture of tertiary amine alkaloids*
homatropine	*semisynthetic, tertiary amine*
homatropine methylbromide	*semisynthetic, quaternary ammonium compound*
hyoscyamine	*natural, tertiary amine*
methscopolamine	*semisynthetic, quaternary ammonium compound*
scopolamine	*natural, tertiary amine*

Hyoscyamine and scopolamine are naturally occurring tertiary amines which are formed by combining tropic acid and tropine or scopine, respectively. Structurally, the integrity of the ester must be maintained for antimuscarinic activity; neither the free acid nor the free base exhibits substantial antimuscarinic activity. Presence of a free hydroxyl group in the acid portion of the ester also is important for antimuscarinic activity. Tropic acid contains an asymmetric carbon which results in optical isomers. Alkaloids containing these isomers differ in antimuscarinic activity and potency. Atropine is a racemic mixture of *d-* and *l*-hyoscyamine which is probably formed during the extraction process. *l*-Hyoscyamine possesses approximately twice the antimuscarinic potency of the racemic mixture (atropine). *d*-Hyoscyamine has essentially no peripheral antimuscarinic activity. *l*-Hyoscyamine is 8–50 times as potent in central antimuscarinic activity as *d*-hyoscyamine. *l*-Hyoscine (scopolamine) is more potent than *d*-hyoscine. Belladonna leaf is a mixture of hyoscyamine, scopolamine, and minor alkaloids. The principal alkaloid is hyoscyamine, which occurs as a racemic mixture (atropine). Pharmacologic activity of belladonna preparations results principally from the atropine content.

Homatropine occurs as a racemic mixture and is a semisynthetic tertiary amine derivative of mandelic acid and tropine. Methscopolamine bromide and homatropine methylbromide are the quaternary ammonium derivatives of scopolamine and homatropine, respectively; they differ structurally from their respective parent compounds by addition of a second methyl group at the nitrogen.

■ Synthetic Amine Compounds

Quaternary Ammonium Compounds

aclidinium	propantheline
clidinium	tiotropium
glycopyrrolate	umeclidinium
ipratropium	

Tertiary Amine Compounds

dicyclomine	tolterodine
oxybutynin	

Like the naturally occurring alkaloids and their semisynthetic derivatives, most synthetic tertiary amines and quaternary ammonium compounds are aminoalcohol esters; only tridihexethyl is not an ester. Because the structure-activity relationships of the synthetic amine compounds are complex, specialized references on medicinal chemistry should be consulted for more specific information.

For specific dosages, duration of therapy, and additional information on the chemistry and stability, pharmacokinetics, uses, cautions, acute toxicity, and drug interactions of antimuscarinics/antispasmodics, see the individual monographs in 12:08.08 and 86:12.

†Use is not currently included in the labeling approved by the US Food and Drug Administration

Aclidinium Bromide

■ Aclidinium bromide, a synthetic quaternary ammonium antimuscarinic agent, is a long-acting orally inhaled bronchodilator.

Uses

■ Bronchospasm *Chronic Obstructive Pulmonary Disease*

Aclidinium bromide is used as a bronchodilator for the long-term maintenance treatment of reversible bronchospasm associated with chronic obstructive pulmonary disease (COPD), including chronic bronchitis and/or emphysema. Orally inhaled aclidinium is *not* indicated for the initial treatment of acute exacerbations of COPD or for relief of acute symptoms (i.e., as rescue therapy for treatment of acute episodes of bronchospasm); a drug with a more rapid onset of action (e.g., a short-acting β_2-adrenergic agonist) may be preferred in such cases.

Efficacy of aclidinium has been evaluated in 3 randomized, double-blind, placebo-controlled studies of 12 or 24 weeks' duration in adults 40 years of age or older with moderate to severe COPD. In the Aclidinium in Chronic Obstructive Respiratory Disease I (ACCORD I) study, the primary efficacy outcome was the change from baseline in the morning predose trough forced expiratory volume in 1 second (FEV_1) (defined as the average of 2 predose FEV_1 measurements) at 12 weeks. In this study, aclidinium 400 mcg twice daily improved the change from baseline in trough FEV_1 by 124 mL compared with placebo at 12 weeks. In addition, the change from baseline in peak FEV_1 (i.e., the highest value observed within 3 hours of the postmorning dose) following twice-daily administration of aclidinium 400 mcg improved by 192 mL versus placebo after 12 weeks of treatment. In the Aclidinium to Treat Airway Obstruction in COPD Patients (ATTAIN) study, the primary efficacy outcome was the change from baseline in the morning predose trough FEV_1 at 24 weeks. In this study, aclidinium 400 mcg twice daily improved the change from baseline in trough FEV_1 by 128 mL compared with placebo at 24 weeks. In addition, the change from baseline in peak FEV_1 following administration of aclidinium 400 mcg twice daily improved by 209 mL versus placebo at 24 weeks. Such improvement in lung function was maintained with aclidinium throughout the 12-hour dosing interval and for treatment periods of up to 12 or 24 weeks with no evidence of tolerance.

In addition to improvements in lung function, clinical studies indicate that aclidinium improves health status and reduces COPD symptoms and possibly reduces the rate of exacerbations. In some studies, treatment with aclidinium also has been associated with a reduction in the need for supplemental short-acting β_2-agonists as rescue therapy for treatment of acute bronchospasm compared with placebo.

For additional information on the treatment of COPD, see Uses: Chronic Obstructive Pulmonary Disease, in Ipratropium Bromide 12:08.08.

Dosage and Administration

■ **General** Dosage of aclidinium bromide is expressed in terms of the salt. Although each actuation of the metered-dose inhaler contains 400 mcg of aclidinium bromide as an inhalation powder, the precise amount of drug delivered to the lungs with each activation of the Pressair® device depends on factors such as the patient's inspiratory flow rate and time. Using standardized in vitro testing at a flow rate of 63 L/minute, the Pressair® inhaler delivered 375 mcg of aclidinium bromide from the mouthpiece. The commercially available inhaler delivers 60 metered doses.

■ **Administration** Aclidinium bromide is administered by oral inhalation *only* using a specific breath-actuated, oral inhalation device (Pressair®) that delivers powdered drug.

Prior to use, the inhaler should be removed from the sealed pouch. The protective cap should be removed from the inhaler by lightly squeezing the arrows marked on each side of the cap and pulling outward. The patient should then hold the inhaler with the mouthpiece toward the face, but not inside the mouth, with the green button facing straight up; the inhaler should not be tilted. Before placing the inhaler in the mouth, the patient should completely depress and then release the green button on the inhaler and then check the colored control window to ensure that it has changed from red to green, indicating that the dose is ready for inhalation.

Before inhaling the dose, the patient should exhale as completely as possible, being careful not to exhale into the Pressair® device. The patient should then place the mouthpiece of the inhaler tightly between the lips and inhale quickly and deeply through the mouth. The patient should hear a click (indicating that the inhaler is being used correctly) during the inhalation and should continue inhaling. The green button should not be pressed or held down during the inhalation. After a complete inhalation, the patient should remove the inhaler from the mouth and hold their breath for as long as comfortable, then exhale slowly through the nose. While some patients may taste the drug delivered from the Pressair® device, they should be instructed not to use another dose even if they do not taste the drug. The patient should check the control window to ensure that it has changed from green to red, indicating that the full dose has been inhaled. If the control window is still green, the patient should attempt to inhale through the device again. If the patient is unable to inhale correctly after several attempts, the patient should contact their clinician. After the control window has turned red, the protective cap should be pressed back onto the mouthpiece of the inhaler.

The inhaler does not need to be cleaned. However, if desired, the outside of the mouthpiece can be wiped with a dry tissue or paper towel; water should *not* be used to clean the inhaler. The inhaler should be discarded when the dose indicator (showing the number of doses remaining in intervals of ten) reads zero, when the device locks out (i.e., the green button stays depressed), or 45 days after removal of the inhaler from the sealed pouch, whichever comes first. The inhaler also should be discarded if the device appears damaged or the protective cap is lost.

■ **Dosage** For the long-term management of reversible bronchospasm associated with chronic obstructive pulmonary disease (COPD), the usual dosage of aclidinium bromide in adults is 400 mcg (one inhalation) twice daily via the Pressair® device. Orally inhaled aclidinium should *not* be used for the treatment of acute episodes of bronchospasm.

■ **Special Populations** Dosage adjustment is not necessary in geriatric patients or patients with hepatic or renal impairment.

Cautions

■ **Contraindications** The manufacturer states that there are no known contraindications to the use of aclidinium.

■ **Warnings/Precautions** ***Sensitivity Reactions*** Immediate hypersensitivity reactions may occur after administration of aclidinium. If such a reaction occurs, the drug should be discontinued immediately and alternative therapy considered. Because of the structural similarity between atropine and aclidinium, patients with a history of hypersensitivity reactions to atropine should be monitored closely for hypersensitivity to aclidinium. Aclidinium also should be used with caution in patients with severe hypersensitivity to milk proteins, because the commercially available formulation of aclidinium inhalation powder contains lactose monohydrate (may include milk proteins).

Acute Bronchospasm Aclidinium bromide oral inhalation therapy is indicated for maintenance treatment of bronchospasm associated with chronic obstructive pulmonary disease (COPD); the drug is *not* indicated for treatment of acute bronchospasm (i.e., as rescue therapy).

Paradoxical Bronchospasm As with other inhaled agents, patients may develop paradoxical bronchospasm upon inhalation of aclidinium.

If paradoxical bronchospasm occurs, aclidinium should be discontinued immediately and alternative therapy considered.

Ocular Effects Aclidinium should be used with caution in patients with acute angle-closure glaucoma. The drug may worsen acute angle-closure glaucoma manifested by ocular pain or discomfort, blurred vision, visual halos, or colored images in association with red eyes from conjunctival congestion and corneal edema. Patients with such manifestations should consult a clinician immediately; miotic eye drops alone are not considered effective treatment for this condition.

Care should be taken to avoid contact of the drug with the eyes during oral inhalation. (See Advice to Patients.)

Genitourinary Effects Aclidinium should be used with caution in patients with urinary retention. Aclidinium may worsen symptoms and signs (e.g., urinary retention, dysuria) associated with prostatic hyperplasia or bladder neck obstruction. Patients who develop such manifestations should consult a clinician immediately.

Cardiovascular Effects In a study evaluating potential effects of aclidinium on the QT interval, effects on prolongation of the QT interval were not observed in healthy individuals. In addition, clinically important effects on cardiac rhythm (24-hour Holter monitoring) were not observed in patients with COPD receiving aclidinium in another clinical trial.

Analysis of pooled data from clinical studies suggests that aclidinium is not associated with an increased incidence of major adverse cardiovascular events in patients receiving the drug. The manufacturer of aclidinium is conducting a postmarketing study to further assess cardiovascular risk of the drug.

Specific Populations **Pregnancy.** Category C. (See Users Guide.)

Lactation. Aclidinium is distributed into milk in rats; it is not known whether the drug is distributed into milk in humans. The manufacturer recommends that orally inhaled aclidinium be used with caution in nursing women.

Pediatric Use. Safety and efficacy of oral inhalation of aclidinium have not been established in children. However, COPD does not generally occur in children.

Geriatric Use. No overall differences in safety and efficacy were observed in geriatric patients relative to younger adults, but increased sensitivity cannot be ruled out. Dosage adjustment is not necessary in geriatric patients.

Hepatic Impairment. Pharmacokinetics of aclidinium have not been evaluated in patients with hepatic impairment.

Renal Impairment. Clinically important differences in pharmacokinetics of aclidinium were not observed in patients with mild, moderate, or severe renal impairment compared with patients with normal renal function. The manufacturer states that dosage adjustment of aclidinium in patients with renal impairment is not necessary.

■ **Common Adverse Effects** Adverse events occurring in at least 3% of patients receiving aclidinium and at an incidence greater than with placebo include headache, nasopharyngitis, and cough.

Drug Interactions

No formal drug interaction studies have been performed with aclidinium to date. Results of in vitro studies suggest that aclidinium has limited potential to cause metabolic interactions with cytochrome P-450 (CYP) isoenzymes at plasma concentrations achieved clinically.

■ **Drugs Affecting or Metabolized by Hepatic Microsomal Enzymes** In vitro studies indicate that aclidinium and its major metabolites do not inhibit CYP isoenzymes 1A2, 2A6, 2B6, 2C8, 2C9, 2C19, 2D6, 2E1, 3A4/5, or 4A9/11 at concentrations up to 1000 times greater than the peak plasma concentrations achieved clinically. Therefore, clinically important pharmacokinetic interactions with drugs affecting or metabolized by the CYP isoenzyme system are unlikely.

■ **Anticholinergic Agents** Potential pharmacologic interaction (additive anticholinergic effects). The manufacturer states that concomitant use of aclidinium with other anticholinergic agents should be avoided.

■ **Other Drugs** Results of clinical studies indicate that concomitant administration of aclidinium with other drugs used in the treatment of COPD such as sympathomimetic bronchodilators (i.e., short-acting β_2-agonists), methylxanthines, and oral or inhaled corticosteroids was not associated with an increased incidence of adverse effects.

Description

Aclidinium bromide is a synthetic quaternary ammonium antimuscarinic agent for use as a long-acting, orally inhaled bronchodilator. The drug is a nonselective competitive antagonist at muscarinic (M_1–M_5) receptors. Aclidinium competitively and reversibly inhibits the actions of acetylcholine and other cholinergic stimuli at M_3 receptors in the smooth muscle of the respiratory tract leading to bronchodilation.

Most of a dose of orally inhaled aclidinium bromide is deposited in the oropharynx and swallowed. Aclidinium is expected to be minimally absorbed into systemic circulation whether the dose is deposited in the lungs or swallowed, since the drug undergoes rapid and extensive hydrolysis that occurs both chemically and enzymatically via esterases to inactive metabolites. Aclidinium and its metabolites are not expected to affect drugs metabolized by cytochrome P-450 isoenzymes at plasma concentrations achieved clinically. Approximately 0.1% of a dose is excreted in urine following oral inhalation. The effective half-life of aclidinium bromide is 5–8 hours following oral inhalation.

Advice to Patients

A copy of the manufacturer's patient information for aclidinium bromide should be provided to all patients each time the drug is dispensed. Importance of instructing patients to read the patient information prior to initiation of therapy and each time the prescription is refilled.

Importance of informing clinician of any history of hypersensitivity reactions to atropine or severe allergy to milk proteins.

Importance of adequate understanding of proper storage and inhalation techniques, including use of the inhalation delivery system (Pressair®).

Importance of advising patients that if a dose of aclidinium bromide is missed, the next dose should be taken at the regularly scheduled time; a double dose should not be administered to make up for a missed dose.

Importance of not using aclidinium therapy to relieve acute symptoms or exacerbations of chronic obstructive pulmonary disease (COPD).

Importance of avoiding inadvertent contact of the drug with the eyes since this may cause blurred vision and pupillary dilation.

Importance of informing clinician immediately if eye pain or discomfort, blurred vision, visual halos, or colored images in association with red eyes from conjunctival congestion or corneal edema occur.

Importance of discontinuing aclidinium and informing clinician if paradoxical bronchospasm occurs.

Importance of informing clinician immediately if urinary retention or dysuria occurs.

Importance of informing clinicians of existing or contemplated concomitant therapy, including prescription and OTC drugs (e.g., eye drops) and herbal supplements, as well as any concomitant illnesses (e.g., urinary retention, enlarged prostate, angle-closure glaucoma).

Importance of women informing clinicians if they are or plan to become pregnant or plan to breast-feed.

Importance of informing patients of other important precautionary information. (See Cautions.)

Overview® (see Users Guide). For additional information on this drug until a more detailed monograph is developed and published, the manufacturer's labeling should be consulted. It is *essential* that the manufacturer's labeling be consulted for more detailed information on usual cautions, precautions, contraindications, potential drug interactions, laboratory test interferences, and acute toxicity.

Preparations

Excipients in commercially available drug preparations may have clinically important effects in some individuals; consult specific product labeling for details.

Aclidinium Bromide

Oral Inhalation

Powder for Inhalation	400 mcg	**Tudorza® Pressair®**, Forest

Atropine
Atropine Sulfate

d,l-Hyoscyamine

■ Atropine (*dl*-hyoscyamine) is a naturally occurring tertiary amine antimuscarinic.

Uses

■ **Surgery** Atropine sulfate is used parenterally as a preoperative medication to inhibit salivation and excessive secretions of the respiratory tract (antisialagogue); however, the current surgical practice of using general anesthetics that do not stimulate the production of salivary and tracheobronchial secretions has reduced the need to control excessive respiratory secretions during surgery. Although atropine has been used prophylactically to prevent acid-aspiration pneumonitis during surgery, antimuscarinics, including atropine, have not been shown to be effective for this use.

Atropine also may be used to prevent other cholinergic effects during surgery, such as cardiac arrhythmias, hypotension, and bradycardia, which may result from excessive vagal stimulation, from stimulation of the carotid sinus, or as a pharmacologic effect of some drugs (e.g., succinylcholine). Atropine is administered concurrently with anticholinesterase agents (e.g., neostigmine, pyridostigmine) to block the adverse muscarinic effects of these latter agents when they are used after surgery to reverse the effects of neuromuscular blocking agents.

Atropine has been used prophylactically to prevent reflex bradycardia in pediatric patients undergoing emergency intubation; however, there is no evidence that atropine reduces the risk of cardiac arrest or improves survival in this setting. Because of the lack of supporting evidence, preintubation use of atropine is not routinely recommended, but may be considered in situations where there is an increased risk of bradycardia (e.g., when succinylcholine is used to facilitate intubation).

■ Advanced Cardiovascular Life Support and Bradyarrhythmias Atropine sulfate is used in advanced cardiovascular life support (ACLS) for the management of symptomatic bradycardia. The drug reverses cholinergically mediated decreases in heart rate, systemic vascular resistance, and blood pressure, and is considered the initial drug of choice in adults with unstable bradycardia (e.g., that which is accompanied by altered mental status, cardiac ischemia, acute heart failure, hypotension, or other signs of shock). In pediatric advanced life support (PALS), atropine is used for the treatment of bradycardia secondary to increased vagal activity or primary atrioventricular (AV) block when bradycardia persists despite initial management with adequate oxygenation, ventilation, and chest compressions (if indicated).

Atropine was previously included in ACLS guidelines for the treatment of asystole or pulseless electrical activity (PEA) during cardiopulmonary resuscitation (CPR); however, routine use of the drug during cardiac arrest is no longer recommended because of the lack of evidence demonstrating clinical benefit. High-quality CPR and defibrillation are integral components of ACLS and the only proven interventions to increase survival to hospital discharge. Other resuscitative efforts including drug therapy are considered secondary and should be performed without compromising the quality and timely delivery of chest compressions and defibrillation. The principal goal of pharmacologic therapy during cardiac arrest is to facilitate the return of spontaneous circulation (ROSC), and epinephrine is considered the drug of choice for this use. (See Uses: Advanced Cardiovascular Life Support and Cardiac Arrhythmias, in Epinephrine 12:12.12.)

Because atropine can increase conduction through the AV node, the drug also may be beneficial in the management of AV nodal block. However, atropine is not likely to be effective in patients with type II second-degree AV block or third-degree AV block, including third-degree AV block accompanied by a new wide QRS complex when the conduction block is at or below the His-Purkinje level; patients with these bradyarrhythmias are preferably treated with transcutaneous pacing or a rate-accelerating β-adrenergic drug (e.g., dopamine or epinephrine) until transvenous pacing can be performed. Atropine administration should not delay implementation of external pacing for patients with poor perfusion.

Atropine also is used in patients with acute myocardial infarction (MI) who develop symptomatic or hemodynamically unstable sinus bradycardia. Sinus bradycardia caused by increased vagal tone commonly occurs after ST-segment-elevation MI (STEMI), particularly in patients with an inferior infarction. Other uses of atropine in the MI setting include treatment of sustained bradycardia and hypotension associated with nitroglycerin use, and treatment of nausea and vomiting associated with morphine use. Although atropine was previously used for the management of symptomatic type I second- or third-degree AV block associated with MI, the incidence of abnormal conduction in STEMI patients has decreased considerably in the current reperfusion era.

Because heart rate is a major determinant of myocardial oxygen requirements, atropine should be used cautiously in the presence of acute myocardial ischemia or infarction. Excessive rate acceleration in patients with these conditions may worsen ischemia or increase the extent of infarction. In addition, ventricular fibrillation and tachycardia have occurred rarely following IV administration of atropine. Because transplanted hearts lack vagal innervation, atropine may *not* be effective in patients who have undergone cardiac transplantation. Paradoxical slowing of the heart rate and high-degree AV block have been reported in patients who have received atropine after cardiac transplantation.

■ Pesticide Poisoning Atropine is used to reverse the muscarinic effects associated with toxic exposure to organophosphate or carbamate anticholinesterase pesticides. For the treatment of toxic exposure to organophosphate pesticides, atropine may be used concomitantly with a cholinesterase reactivator (pralidoxime chloride). Concomitant therapy with pralidoxime chloride may not be necessary in patients with carbamate anticholinesterase pesticide poisoning. Antidotes such as atropine and pralidoxime should not be solely relied upon to provide complete protection against the toxic effects of insecticide poisoning and should be used in conjunction with other protective measures (e.g., decontamination, immediate evacuation, specialized masks and clothing) and treatments (e.g., an anticonvulsant for seizures). Some clinicians have suggested a challenge (test) dose of atropine to aid in the diagnosis of cholinergic poisoning†; failure of the test dose to elicit typical antimuscarinic effects (e.g., mydriasis, tachycardia, dry mucous membranes) strongly suggests the presence of organophosphate or carbamate poisoning.

■ Chemical Warfare Agent Poisoning Atropine is used concomitantly with a cholinesterase reactivator (pralidoxime chloride) for the treatment of nerve agent poisoning in the context of chemical warfare or terrorism. The most toxic of the known chemical warfare agents are the nerve agents. Most nerve agents are liquid at room temperature (although most are volatile at ambient temperatures, the term "nerve gas" is a misnomer); nerve agents are readily absorbed after inhalation of aerosols (e.g., following an explosion), ingestion, or dermal contact. Nerve agents (e.g., sarin, soman, tabun, VX [methylphosphonothioic acid]) are chemically similar to the organophosphate pesticides and exert their biologic effects by inhibiting acetylcholinesterase enzymes. Nerve agents alter cholinergic synaptic transmission at neuroeffector junctions (muscarinic effects), at skeletal myoneural junctions and autonomic ganglia (nicotinic effects), and in the CNS. Manifestations of nerve agent exposure include rhinorrhea, chest tightness, pinpoint pupils, dyspnea, excessive salivation and sweating, nausea, vomiting, abdominal cramps, involuntary defecation and/or urination, muscle twitching, confusion, seizures, flaccid paralysis, coma, respiratory failure, and death. While initial effects of nerve agent exposure depend on dose and route of exposure, signs and symptoms generally are similar regardless of the route of exposure. Manifestations may not be apparent until as long as 18 hours following dermal exposure, and CNS effects (e.g., fatigue, irritability, nervousness, memory impairment) may persist as long as 6 weeks following recovery from the acute effects of nerve agent exposure.

Initial management of nerve agent poisoning includes aggressive airway control and ventilation (administration of nebulized β-adrenergic agonist [e.g., albuterol] and antimuscarinics [e.g., ipratropium bromide] may be necessary), and administration of atropine and pralidoxime chloride. Diazepam may be needed for seizure control. Rapid decontamination using standard hazardous materials (HAZMAT) procedures is important to prevent further absorption by the victim and to prevent contamination of others (e.g., emergency personnel, health-care workers) by direct contact or off-gassing of nerve agents from contaminated clothing. Following initial therapy and decontamination, additional treatment with atropine and supportive measures in a hospital setting are likely to be necessary.

■ Mushroom Poisoning Atropine sulfate also is used for the treatment of muscarinic effects associated with toxic ingestion of mushrooms containing muscarine (e.g., certain members of the *Clitocybe* and *Inocybe* genera); however, substantial toxicity is uncommon and supportive symptomatic care (e.g., atropine) rarely is necessary.

■ GI Disorders Atropine sulfate has been used as an adjunct in the treatment of peptic ulcer disease; although synthetic or semisynthetic antimuscarinics, especially quaternary ammonium compounds, have generally replaced atropine in the treatment of peptic ulcer disease, none of these antimuscarinics has been shown to be therapeutically superior to atropine. (See Uses: Peptic Ulcer Disease and GI Hypersecretory States, in the Antimuscarinics/Antispasmodics General Statement 12:08.08) As with other antimuscarinics, there are no conclusive data from well-controlled studies which indicate that, in usually recommended dosage, atropine aids in the healing, decreases the rate of recurrence, or prevents complications of peptic ulcers. In addition, in patients with gastric ulcer, antimuscarinics may delay gastric emptying and result in antral stasis. With the advent of more effective therapies for the treatment of peptic ulcer disease, antimuscarinics have only limited usefulness in this condition. Current epidemiologic and clinical evidence supports a strong association between gastric infection with *Helicobacter pylori* and the pathogenesis of duodenal and gastric ulcers, and the American College of Gastroenterology (ACG), the National Institutes of Health (NIH), and most clinicians currently recommend that all patients with initial or recurrent duodenal or gastric ulcer and documented *H. pylori* infection receive anti-infective therapy for treatment of the infection. For a more complete discussion of *H. pylori* infection, including details about the efficacy of various regimens and rationale for drug selection, see Uses: *Helicobacter pylori* Infection, in Clarithromycin 8:12.12.92.

Atropine has been used in the treatment of functional disturbances of GI motility such as irritable bowel syndrome. As with other antimuscarinics, atropine has limited efficacy in the treatment of these disorders and should be used only if other measures (e.g., diet, sedation, counseling, amelioration of environmental factors) have been of little or no benefit.

Atropine has been used in the treatment of GI hypermotility and diarrhea caused by reserpine, guanethidine, or cholinergic stimulation. Although antimuscarinics have been used in the treatment of diarrhea from other causes (e.g., ulcerative colitis, dysentery, shigellosis, *Clostridium difficile*-associated diarrhea and colitis [also known as antibiotic-associated pseudomembranous colitis]), they should be used with extreme caution, if at all, in patients with these conditions. (See Cautions: Precautions and Contraindications, in the Antimuscarinics/Antispasmodics General Statement 12:08.08.)

■ Genitourinary Tract Disorders Atropine sulfate has been used as adjunctive therapy in the management of hypermotility disorders of the lower urinary tract. Although atropine may provide symptomatic relief, the underlying cause should be determined and specifically treated. Appropriate anti-infective therapy should be initiated whenever urinary tract infection is present. With the exception of uninhibited or reflex neurogenic bladder, there is generally little evidence to support the use of antimuscarinics in the treatment of various genitourinary disorders. (See Uses: Genitourinary Tract Disorders, in the Antimuscarinics/Antispasmodics General Statement 12:08.08.)

■ **Bronchospasm** Because atropine sulfate is a potent bronchodilator, the drug has been used by oral inhalation for the short-term treatment and prevention of bronchospasm associated with chronic bronchial asthma, bronchitis, and chronic obstructive pulmonary disease; however, a solution of the drug for oral inhalation no longer is commercially available in the US. (See Uses: Bronchospasm, in the Antimuscarinics/Antispasmodics General Statement 12:08.08.) Atropine has also been used as a drying agent in the relief of symptoms of acute rhinitis.

■ **Other Uses** Atropine sulfate has been used in combination with other drugs (e.g., antihistamines, vasoconstrictors) for the symptomatic relief of cold and cough.

Atropine sulfate has been used to facilitate hypotonic duodenography or contrast examination of the colon by reducing duodenal or colonic motility and spasm; however, glucagon appears to be more effective and is generally preferred in these examinations. Atropine also has been used to increase visualization of the urinary tract in excretion urography.

Atropine sulfate has been used in conjunction with morphine or other opiates for the symptomatic relief of biliary or renal colic; however, since antimuscarinics exert only a weak biliary antispasmodic action, these drugs should not be relied on in the treatment of biliary tract disease. Atropine has also been used to reduce pain and hypersecretion in pancreatitis; however, there is little, if any, evidence that antimuscarinics improve the prognosis of the disease. (See Uses: Other Uses, in the Antimuscarinics/Antispasmodics General Statement 12:08.08.)

For ophthalmic uses of atropine sulfate, see 52:24. For other uses of atropine sulfate, see Uses in the Antimuscarinics/Antispasmodics General Statement 12:08.08.

Dosage and Administration

■ **Administration** Atropine sulfate is administered by IM, subcutaneous, or direct IV administration. IV administration is preferred for the treatment of severe or life-threatening muscarinic effects.

Atropine also has been administered by intraosseous (IO) injection† in the setting of advanced cardiovascular life support (ACLS), generally when IV access is not readily available; onset of action and systemic concentrations are comparable to those achieved with venous administration.

Atropine may be administered via an endotracheal tube when vascular access (IV or IO) is not possible; however, IV or IO administration is preferred because of more predictable drug delivery and pharmacologic effect. (See Pharmacokinetics: Absorption.)

Atropine sulfate has been administered orally; however, an oral dosage form no longer is commercially available in the US.

Atropine sulfate has been administered by oral inhalation using a nebulizer solution; however, a solution for oral inhalation no longer is commercially available in the US.

Parenteral Administration **IM Administration.** Atropine is commercially available in a prefilled auto-injector (e.g., AtroPen®) for IM administration in the treatment of pesticide or nerve agent poisoning. The auto-injector should be used only by individuals who have received proper training in the recognition and treatment of pesticide poisoning. The AtroPen® auto-injector may be self-administered by the patient or caregiver in an out-of-hospital setting to facilitate the initial treatment of muscarinic poisoning (usually breathing difficulty secondary to increased secretions); however, definitive medical care should be sought immediately.

For *self-administration* or administration by a caregiver in an out-of-hospital setting in the event of pesticide or nerve agent poisoning, the appropriate dose of atropine injection (AtroPen®) should be injected IM into the anterolateral aspect of the thigh. For very thin patients and small children, the thigh should be bunched up (to provide a thicker injection area) prior to administration of the drug. For additional instructions on proper use of atropine auto-injectors, the manufacturer's instructions should be consulted.

IV Administration. Although at least one manufacturer recommends that atropine sulfate injection be administered slowly and with caution, the drug generally is given rapidly by direct IV injection since slow injection may cause a paradoxical slowing of the heart rate.

Atropine has occasionally been administered by IV infusion† for the management of muscarinic poisoning (e.g., organophosphate pesticides).

Endotracheal Administration For endotracheal administration, the appropriate dose of atropine sulfate should be diluted in 5–10 mL of sterile water or 0.9% sodium chloride injection in adults or followed by a flush with 5 mL of 0.9% sodium chloride injection in pediatric patients. Absorption of the drug may be greater when sterile water rather than 0.9% sodium chloride injection is used as the diluent (in adults).

■ **Dosage** Dosage of atropine sulfate should be individualized based on indication, patient characteristics, and response (e.g., heart rate, blood pressure); pediatric patients tend to be more susceptible than adults to the toxic effects of atropine overdosage.

Parenteral Dosage **Surgery.** For antisialagogue or antivagal effects during surgery, the usual initial adult dose of atropine sulfate is 0.5–1 mg by IV, IM, or subcutaneous injection 30–60 minutes prior to surgery; the dose may be repeated in 1–2 hours. Dosing in pediatric patients has not been well studied, but initial doses usually range from 0.01–0.03 mg/kg, administered 30–60 minutes prior to surgery; according to some clinicians, repeat doses may be given every 4–6 hours. Some clinicians recommend a minimum dose of 0.1 mg and maximum dose of 0.4 mg in children; however, doses up to 0.6 mg have been suggested in pediatric patients weighing more than 41 kg.

The American Heart Association (AHA) guidelines for pediatric advanced life support (PALS) recommend a preintubation atropine sulfate dose of 0.02 mg/kg administered IV in infants and children undergoing emergency intubation. Although a minimum dose of 0.1 mg was previously recommended because of concerns about paradoxical bradycardia, current evidence suggests that no minimum dose is necessary.

To block adverse muscarinic effects of anticholinesterase agents (e.g., neostigmine, pyridostigmine) when these agents are used to reverse the effects of neuromuscular blocking agents after surgery, the usual IV dose of atropine sulfate is 0.6–1.2 mg for each 0.5–2.5 mg of neostigmine methylsulfate or 10–20 mg of pyridostigmine bromide administered; atropine is administered concurrently with (but in a separate syringe) or a few minutes before the anticholinesterase agent. In the presence of bradycardia, atropine sulfate should be administered IV before the anticholinesterase agent to increase the pulse rate to about 80 beats/minute. Neonates and infants have been given a 0.02-mg/kg dose of atropine sulfate concomitantly with a 0.04-mg/kg dose of neostigmine methylsulfate. Children have been given a 0.01- to 0.04-mg/kg dose of atropine sulfate concomitantly with each 0.025- to 0.08-mg/kg dose of neostigmine methylsulfate.

Advanced Cardiovascular Life Support and Bradyarrhythmias. For the treatment of symptomatic bradycardia in adults, AHA recommends an initial atropine sulfate dose of 0.5 mg by direct IV injection; the dose may be repeated every 3–5 minutes up to a maximum of 3 mg. Doses less than 0.5 mg may cause paradoxical slowing of the heart rate. In previous ACLS guidelines, an atropine sulfate dosage of 1 mg every 3–5 minutes up to a total of 3 doses by IV or IO injection† was recommended for the treatment of asystole and slow pulseless electrical activity (PEA) in adults; however routine use of atropine during cardiac arrest is no longer recommended. (See Uses: Advanced Cardiovascular Life Support and Bradyarrhythmias.)

In PALS guidelines, an atropine sulfate dose of 0.02 mg/kg by IV or IO injection† (repeated once if needed) is recommended in infants and children with symptomatic bradycardia secondary to increased vagal activity or primary atrioventricular (AV) block; a minimum dose of 0.1 mg and a maximum single dose of 0.5 mg is recommended. Larger doses may be required in special resuscitation situations (e.g., organophosphate toxicity or exposure to nerve gas agents); smaller doses (i.e., less than 0.1 mg) may cause paradoxical bradycardia.

Hypotonic Radiography of the GI Tract. For hypotonic radiography of the GI tract (contrast examination of the duodenum or colon) in adults, the usual IM dose of atropine sulfate is 1 mg.

Pesticide Poisoning. Various atropine sulfate doses and dosing intervals have been recommended for the treatment of muscarinic toxicity resulting from exposure to organophosphate anticholinesterase pesticides; dosage requirements are based on the severity of poisoning and individual patient response.

The usual initial dose of atropine sulfate for the treatment of muscarinic toxicity resulting from exposure to organophosphate anticholinesterase pesticides in adults is 1–2 mg, preferably administered IV. Some clinicians recommend that additional 2-mg doses may be administered IM or IV every 5–60 minutes until muscarinic signs and symptoms subside. In severe cases, 2–6 mg may be given initially, preferably administered IV, and repeated doses given every 5–60 minutes until muscarinic signs and symptoms subside. Mildly symptomatic poisoning may respond to 1–2 mg for reversal of muscarinic toxicity whereas *moderate* poisoning commonly requires total doses up to 40 mg. Some experts state that for *severe* poisoning, 5-mg doses may be repeated every 2–3 minutes for stabilization. Cumulative doses up to 1 g in 24 hours or 11 g over a course of treatment have been used. Atropine sulfate also has been administered by IV infusion† at an initial rate of 0.5–1 mg/hour in adults for muscarinic poisoning; the infusion rate should be adjusted according to response. In severe cases, atropine therapy should be gradually withdrawn to avoid abrupt recurrence of symptoms (e.g., pulmonary edema). Similar doses of atropine sulfate may be used in the treatment of muscarinic toxicity resulting from exposure to carbamate anticholinesterase pesticides.

To facilitate out-of-hospital administration, atropine injection may be administered using the commercially available prefilled auto-injector (e.g., AtroPen®). For *self-administration* or administration by a caregiver, the dose of atropine (AtroPen®) is based on severity of symptoms. Atropine should be administered as soon as symptoms of organophosphate or carbamate poisoning (e.g., tearing, excessive oral secretions, wheezing, muscle fasciculations) appear. For the treatment of adults with 2 or more mild symptoms of pesticide exposure (e.g., miosis or blurred vision, tearing, runny nose, hypersalivation or drooling, wheezing, muscle fasciculations, nausea/vomiting) when such exposure is known or suspected, one 2-mg IM dose of atropine sulfate should be administered. If the patient develops any severe symptoms (behavioral changes, severe breathing difficulty, severe respiratory secretions, severe muscle twitching, involuntary defecation or urination, seizures, unconsciousness), two additional 2-mg IM doses should be administered in rapid succession 10 minutes after the first dose. It is preferable that an individual other than the patient administer the second and third doses. For the treatment of adults who are either unconscious or present with any severe symptoms, three 2-mg doses should be administered IM in rapid succession. Additional treatment (i.e., supportive measures, additional doses of atropine, pralidoxime for organophosphate exposure, an anticonvulsant [e.g., diazepam] for seizures) generally is needed, and such treatment should be carried out under the supervision of trained medical personnel.

In children, the usual IM or IV dose of atropine sulfate for the treatment of muscarinic toxicity resulting from exposure to organophosphate anticholinesterase pesticides is 0.05–0.1 mg/kg every 5–10 minutes until muscarinic signs and symptoms subside. The drug also has been given by IV infusion† at a rate of 0.025 mg/kg per hour; continuous infusions have been maintained for up to several weeks in severe cases. Similar doses of atropine sulfate may be used in the treatment of muscarinic toxicity resulting from exposure to carbamate anticholinesterase pesticides.

To facilitate out-of-hospital administration, atropine injection may be administered using the commercially available prefilled auto-injector (e.g., AtroPen®). The AtroPen® auto-injector containing atropine sulfate 0.25, 0.5, or 1 mg is intended for use in children weighing less than 7, 7–18, or 18–41 kg, respectively. When administered by a caregiver in an out-of-hospital setting, the dose of atropine (AtroPen®) is based on severity of symptoms and body weight. *Mild* symptoms of pesticide exposure include miosis or blurred vision, tearing, runny nose, hypersalivation or drooling, wheezing, muscle fasciculations, and nausea/vomiting. Treatment with atropine is indicated in infants and children with 2 or more mild symptoms of pesticide exposure when such exposure is known or suspected. *Severe* symptoms of pesticide exposure include behavioral changes, severe breathing difficulty, severe respiratory secretions, severe muscle twitching, involuntary defecation or urination, seizures, and unconsciousness. Treatment is indicated in infants and children who are unconscious or have any severe symptoms of pesticide exposure. Atropine should be administered as soon as symptoms of organophosphate or carbamate poisoning (e.g., tearing, excessive oral secretions, wheezing, muscle fasciculations) appear. See Table 1 for specific dosage recommendations. Additional treatment (i.e., supportive measures, additional doses of atropine, pralidoxime for organophosphate exposure, an anticonvulsant [e.g., diazepam] for seizures) generally is needed, and such treatment should be carried out under the supervision of trained medical personnel.

Table 1. Pediatric Dosage of Atropine Sulfate Administered by Auto-injector (AtroPen®) for Initial Treatment of Pesticide Poisoning

Child's Weight	Presenting Symptoms	IM Dosage
Less than 7 kg	Mild	0.25 mg initially; if any severe symptoms develop, inject two additional 0.25-mg doses in rapid succession 10 minutes after the first dose
	Severe	Three 0.25-mg doses in rapid succession
7–18 kg	Mild	0.5 mg initially; if any severe symptoms develop, inject two additional 0.5-mg doses in rapid succession 10 minutes after the first dose
	Severe	Three 0.5-mg doses in rapid succession
18–41 kg	Mild	1 mg initially; if any severe symptoms develop, inject two additional 1-mg doses in rapid succession 10 minutes after the first dose
	Severe	Three 1-mg doses in rapid succession
Greater than 41 kg	Mild	2 mg initially; if any severe symptoms develop, inject two additional 2-mg doses in rapid succession 10 minutes after the first dose
	Severe	Three 2-mg doses in rapid succession

A cholinesterase reactivator (e.g., pralidoxime) is administered concomitantly with antimuscarinic therapy for the treatment of toxic exposure to organophosphate pesticides. For the treatment of muscarinic toxicity resulting from carbamate exposure, pralidoxime generally is not used unless exposure also included an organophosphate or unless respiratory depression and muscle weakness are severe manifestations of intoxication.

Chemical Warfare Agent Poisoning. Various atropine sulfate doses and dosing intervals have been recommended for the treatment of muscarinic toxicity resulting from exposure to nerve agent poisoning; dosage requirements are based on the severity of poisoning and individual patient response.

The initial dose of atropine for the treatment of nerve agent (e.g., sarin, soman, tabun, VX [methylphosphonothioic acid]) poisoning in the context of chemical warfare or terrorism is based on the severity of symptoms (i.e., mild/moderate or severe) and the victim's age. Mild to moderate symptoms include localized sweating, muscle fasciculations, nausea, vomiting, weakness, dyspnea; severe symptoms include apnea, flaccid paralysis, seizures, and/or coma. When atropine is used for the immediate treatment of nerve agent poisoning in an out-of-hospital setting or in an emergency department, the drug is administered IM. The usual initial adult IM dose of atropine sulfate is 2–4 mg for those with mild to moderate symptoms and 5–6 mg for those with severe symptoms; frail geriatric patients with mild to moderate symptoms may receive atropine sulfate 1 mg and those with severe symptoms may receive atropine sulfate 2–4 mg.

Additional doses of atropine may be administered at 5- to 10-minute intervals until secretions have diminished and breathing is comfortable or airway resistance has returned to near normal. Some patients may require up to 15–20 mg of the drug within the first 3 hours, but most patients respond to less than 20 mg usually during the initial 24 hours. In a report of sarin poisoning, less than 20% of moderately symptomatic patients required more than 2 mg. Pralidoxime chloride is administered concomitantly with atropine. Diazepam may be administered for seizure control.

To facilitate out-of-hospital administration, atropine injection may be administered using the commercially available prefilled auto-injector (e.g., AtroPen®). For *self-administration* or administration by a caregiver in an out-of-hospital setting, the dose of atropine (AtroPen®) is based on severity of symptoms. Atropine should be administered as soon as symptoms of nerve agent poisoning (e.g., tearing, excessive oral secretions, wheezing, muscle fasciculations) appear. For the treatment of adults with 2 or more mild symptoms of exposure (e.g., miosis or blurred vision, tearing, runny nose, hypersalivation or drooling, wheezing, muscle fasciculations, nausea/vomiting) when such exposure is known or suspected, one 2-mg IM dose of atropine sulfate should be administered. If the patient develops any severe symptoms (behavioral changes, severe breathing difficulty, severe respiratory secretions, severe muscle twitching, involuntary defecation or urination, seizures, unconsciousness), two additional 2-mg IM doses should be administered in rapid succession 10 minutes after the first dose. It is preferable that an individual other than the patient administer the second and third doses. For the treatment of adults who are either unconscious or present with any severe symptoms, three 2-mg doses should be administered IM in rapid succession. Additional treatment (i.e., supportive measures, additional doses of atropine, pralidoxime, an anticonvulsant [e.g., diazepam] for seizures) generally is needed, and such treatment should be carried out under the supervision of trained medical personnel.

The usual initial IM dose of atropine sulfate for the treatment of nerve agent poisoning in children 0–2 years of age, 2–10 years of age, or older than 10 years of age with mild to moderate symptoms is 0.05 mg/kg, 1 mg, or 2 mg, respectively, and the usual initial dose for children 0–2 years of age, 2–10 years of age, or older than 10 years with severe symptoms is 0.1 mg/kg, 2 mg, or 4 mg, respectively. Children 0–2 years of age with mild to moderate or severe symptoms treated in an emergency department may receive atropine sulfate 0.02 mg/kg, administered IV.

To facilitate out-of-hospital administration for infants and children, atropine injection may be administered using the prefilled auto-injector (e.g., AtroPen®). The AtroPen® auto-injector containing atropine sulfate 0.25, 0.5, or 1 mg is intended for use in children weighing less than 7, 7–18, or 18–41 kg, respectively. When administered by a caregiver in an out-of-hospital setting, the dose of atropine (AtroPen®) is based on body weight and severity of symptoms. *Mild* symptoms of nerve agent exposure include miosis or blurred vision, tearing, runny nose, hypersalivation or drooling, wheezing, muscle fasciculations, and nausea/vomiting. Treatment with atropine is indicated in infants and children with 2 or more mild symptoms of nerve agent exposure when such exposure is known or suspected. *Severe* symptoms of nerve agent exposure include behavioral changes, severe breathing difficulty, severe respiratory secretions, severe muscle twitching, involuntary defecation or urination, seizures, and unconsciousness. Treatment is indicated in infants and children who are unconscious or have any severe symptoms of nerve agent exposure. Atropine should be administered as soon as symptoms of nerve agent poisoning (e.g., tearing, excessive oral secretions, wheezing, muscle fasciculations) appear. See Table 2 for specific dosage recommendations. Additional treatment (i.e., supportive measures, additional doses of atropine, pralidoxime, an anticonvulsant [e.g., diazepam] for seizures) generally is needed, and such treatment should be carried out under the supervision of trained medical personnel.

Table 2. Pediatric Dosage of Atropine Sulfate Administered by Auto-injector (AtroPen®) for Initial Treatment of Nerve Agent Poisoning

Child's Weight	Presenting Symptoms	IM Dosage
Less than 7 kg	Mild	0.25 mg initially; if any severe symptoms develop, inject two additional 0. 25-mg doses in rapid succession 10 minutes after the first dose
	Severe	Three 0. 25-mg doses in rapid succession
7–18 kg	Mild	0.5 mg initially; if any severe symptoms develop, inject two additional 0.5-mg doses in rapid succession 10 minutes after the first dose
	Severe	Three 0.5-mg doses in rapid succession
18–41 kg	Mild	1 mg initially; if any severe symptoms develop, inject two additional 1-mg doses in rapid succession 10 minutes after the first dose
	Severe	Three 1-mg doses in rapid succession
Greater than 41 kg	Mild	2 mg initially; if any severe symptoms develop, inject two additional 2-mg doses in rapid succession 10 minutes after the first dose
	Severe	Three 2-mg doses in rapid succession

Mushroom Poisoning. If atropine is needed for severe symptoms of mushroom poisoning (i.e., muscarine-containing *Clitocybes* and *Inocybes*) in adults, some experts recommend an IV dose of 1–2 mg (minimum of 0.1 mg), repeated and titrated as needed according to response. If needed for severe symptoms in pediatric patients, an IV dose of 0.02 mg/kg (minimum of 0.1 mg) is recommended, repeated and titrated as needed according to response.

Endotracheal Dosage **Advanced Cardiovascular Life Support and Bradyarrhythmias.** When atropine sulfate cannot be administered IV in emergent situations such as during ACLS, the drug may be administered via an endotracheal tube. Although the optimum endotracheal dose of atropine sulfate remains to be established, some experts state that typical doses of drugs administered via this route are 2–2.5 times those administered IV in adults and generally should be diluted in 5–10 mL of 0.9% sodium chloride or sterile water prior to direct injection into the endotracheal tube. One manufacturer recommends an endotracheal atropine sulfate dose of 1–2 mg (diluted in no more than 10 mL of sterile water or 0.9% sodium chloride injection) for the treatment of bradysystolic cardiac arrest in adults.

The optimum dose(s) of atropine sulfate administered via an endotracheal tube in pediatric patients remains to be established; PALS guidelines suggest an endotracheal atropine sulfate dose of 0.04–0.06 mg/kg (repeated once if necessary) for the treatment of pediatric bradycardia, with a minimum dose of 0.1 mg and a maximum single dose of 0.5 mg. Larger doses may be required in special resuscitation situations (e.g., organophosphate toxicity or exposure to nerve gas agents). If cardiopulmonary resuscitation (CPR) is in progress, chest compressions should be interrupted briefly to administer atropine. Following administration, the endotracheal tube should be flushed with 5 mL of 0.9% sodium chloride injection and followed by 5 consecutive positive-pressure ventilations.

Pesticide and Nerve Agent Poisoning. One manufacturer recommends an endotracheal atropine sulfate dose of 1–2 mg (diluted in no more than 10 mL of sterile water or 0.9% sodium chloride injection) in adults.

The recommended endotracheal dose of atropine sulfate for the treatment of insecticide or nerve agent poisoning in pediatric patients is 0.05–0.1 mg/kg given every 5–10 minutes until muscarinic signs and symptoms disappear. The dose should be diluted in 1–2 mL of 0.9% sodium chloride injection for endotracheal administration.

Cautions

For a complete discussion of cautions, precautions, and contraindications associated with atropine, see Cautions in the Antimuscarinics/Antispasmodics General Statement 12:08.08.

Pharmacology

As the prototype of the antimuscarinics, atropine exhibits the pharmacologic actions associated with this group of drugs. The pharmacologic activity of atropine results almost completely from *l*-hyoscyamine; *d*-hyoscyamine has essentially no antimuscarinic activity. As a racemic mixture, atropine possesses about 50% of the antimuscarinic potency of *l*-hyoscyamine. In terms of central antimuscarinic activity, *l*-hyoscyamine is 8–50 times as potent as *d*-hyoscyamine. In general, atropine is more potent than scopolamine in its antimuscarinic action on the heart and on bronchial and intestinal smooth muscle, and less potent than scopolamine in its antimuscarinic action on the iris, ciliary body, and certain secretory (salivary, bronchial, sweat) glands. In contrast to scopolamine, atropine stimulates the CNS in usual doses.

For a complete discussion of the pharmacologic effects of atropine, see Pharmacology in the Antimuscarinics/Antispasmodics General Statement 12:08.08.

Pharmacokinetics

■ **Absorption** Atropine is well absorbed from the GI tract. The drug appears to be absorbed principally from the upper small intestine. Atropine is also well absorbed following IM administration, oral inhalation, or endotracheal administration. Following oral administration of a single, radiolabeled, 2-mg dose of atropine in healthy, fasting adults, about 90% of the dose was absorbed. In this study, peak plasma concentrations were reached within 1 hour. Following IM administration, peak plasma concentrations are reached within 30 minutes. Following oral inhalation, atropine appears in serum within 15 minutes and peak concentrations are achieved within 1.5–4 hours. Endotracheal administration of the drug results in lower plasma concentrations than when the drug is given IV.

Atropine-induced inhibition of salivation occurs within 30 minutes or 30 minutes to 1 hour and peaks within 1–1.6 or 2 hours after IM or oral administration, respectively; inhibition of salivation persists for up to 4 hours. Atropine-induced increase in heart rate occurs within 5–40 minutes or 30 minutes to 2 hours and peaks within 20 minutes to 1 hour or 1–2 hours after IM or oral administration, respectively. Following IV administration of the drug, peak increase in heart rate occurs within 2–4 minutes. Low doses of the drug cause a paradoxical decrease in heart rate. The ocular effects of atropine are delayed following systemic administration; in one study, near point of accommodation was increased within 2 or 4 hours after IM administration of a single 3-mg dose or oral administration of a single 4-mg dose, respectively. Bronchodilation (as determined by forced expiratory volume in 1 second [FEV_1]) occurs within 15 minutes and is maximal within 15 minutes to 1.5 hours after oral inhalation of atropine. Based on peak inhibition of salivation in one study, 0.9–1.4 mg of orally administered drug was estimated to be approximately equivalent in effect to 0.6 mg administered IM.

■ **Distribution** Atropine is well distributed throughout the body. The drug crosses the blood-brain barrier. Following IV administration of a single 0.1 mg/kg dose of radiolabeled atropine in dogs, peak CSF concentrations of the drug were 10.3 ng/mL, about 90% of the peak serum concentration.

Atropine crosses the placental barrier. Following IV administration of a single 12.5 mcg/kg dose of atropine sulfate in pregnant women, mean fetal blood (from the placental side of the cord) concentrations of atropine were 1.2 times those of the mother between 5–15 minutes after administration of the drug. In another study, fetal venous blood (from the cord) concentrations of atropine were 12 and 93% of simultaneous maternal venous concentrations 1 and 5 minutes after administration of the drug, respectively; fetal arterial blood (from the cord) concentrations were approximately 50% of simultaneous fetal venous blood concentrations. Although atropine has been stated to distribute into milk in small quantities, there are minimal data to support this statement.

In one in vitro study, atropine was about 18% bound to serum albumin.

■ **Elimination** Atropine has a plasma half-life of about 2–3 hours. Following IM administration of atropine in one study, elimination of the drug (determined by urinary excretion of radiolabeled drug) appeared to be biphasic, with a half-life in the initial phase of about 2 hours and a half-life in the terminal phase of 12.5 hours or longer.

Atropine is metabolized in the liver to several metabolites including tropic acid, tropine (or a chromatographically similar compound), and, possibly, esters of tropic acid and glucuronide conjugates. Atropine is excreted mainly in urine. Approximately 77–94% of an IM dose of atropine is excreted in urine within 24 hours. About 30–50% of a dose is excreted in urine unchanged. In one study, about 50% of the dose was excreted in urine unchanged; about 33% as unknown metabolites, possibly esters of tropic acid; and less than 2% as tropic acid. In another study, tropine or a chromatographically similar compound was the major metabolite in urine. Small amounts of atropine may also be eliminated in expired air as carbon dioxide and in feces.

Chemistry and Stability

■ **Chemistry** Atropine (*dl*-hyoscyamine) is a naturally occurring tertiary amine antimuscarinic. Atropine is the prototype of the antimuscarinics. The drug may be prepared synthetically but is usually obtained by extraction from various members of the *Solanaceae* genus of plants including *Atropa belladonna* (deadly nightshade), *Datura stramonium* (Jimson weed), or *Duboisia myoporoides*.

Atropine is a racemic mixture of *d*- and *l*-hyoscyamine, a tertiary amine organic ester formed by combining tropine and tropic acid. It is not clear whether atropine occurs naturally as a racemic mixture in plant tissues or is formed during extraction, a process known to cause racemization. Atropine occurs as white crystals, usually needle-like, or a white, crystalline powder; it is optically inactive, but usually contains a slight excess of *l*-hyoscyamine. Atropine has solubilities of approximately 2.17 mg/mL in water and 0.5 g/mL in alcohol at 25°C. The drug has a pK_a of 9.8. Atropine injection is commercially available as a sterile solution of the drug in water for injection and contains a citrate buffer, glycerin, and phenol as a preservative.

Atropine sulfate occurs as colorless crystals or a white, crystalline powder. Atropine sulfate has solubilities of approximately 2 g/mL in water and 0.2 g/mL in alcohol at 25°C. Atropine sulfate injection is commercially available as a sterile solution of the drug in water for injection or 0.9% sodium chloride injection; sulfuric acid may be added to adjust the pH to 3–6.5. The injection may also contain a preservative.

■ **Stability** Atropine sulfate effloresces on exposure to dry air and is slowly affected by light. Atropine should be stored in tight, light-resistant containers. Atropine sulfate should be stored in tight containers. Atropine injection (AtroPen® Auto-Injector) should be stored at 25°C but may be exposed to temperatures ranging from 15–30°C. Atropine sulfate injections should be stored in single-dose or multiple-dose containers, preferably of USP Type I glass, at a temperature less than 40°C, preferably between 15–30°C; freezing of the injections should be avoided.

When admixed in the same syringe at room temperature, atropine sulfate injection is reported to be physically compatible for at least 15 minutes with the following injections: chlorpromazine hydrochloride, cimetidine hydrochloride, dimenhydrinate, diphenhydramine hydrochloride, droperidol, fentanyl citrate, glycopyrrolate, hydroxyzine hydrochloride, hydroxyzine hydrochloride with meperidine hydrochloride, meperidine hydrochloride, meperidine hydrochloride with promethazine hydrochloride (Mepergan®, no longer commercially available in the US), morphine sulfate, concentrated opium alkaloids hydrochlorides, pentazocine lactate, pentobarbital sodium, prochlorperazine edisylate, promazine hydrochloride, promethazine hydrochloride, propiomazine hydrochloride, or scopolamine hydrobromide. Atropine sulfate injection is also reported to be physically compatible with butorphanol tartrate injection. Since the compatibility of these and other admixtures with atropine sulfate injection depends on several factors (e.g., concentration of the drugs, resulting pH, temperature), specialized references should be consulted for specific compatibility information.

Atropine sulfate injection is reported to be physically incompatible with norepinephrine bitartrate, metaraminol bitartrate, and sodium bicarbonate injections. A haze or precipitate may form within 15 minutes when atropine sulfate injection is mixed with methohexital sodium solutions.

For further information on the chemistry, pharmacology, pharmacokinetics, uses, cautions, acute toxicity, drug interactions, and dosage and ad-

ministration of atropine sulfate, see the Antimuscarinics/Antispasmodics General Statement 12:08.08.

Preparations

Excipients in commercially available drug preparations may have clinically important effects in some individuals; consult specific product labeling for details.

Atropine

Powder

Parenteral

Injection	equivalent to Atropine Sulfate 0.25 mg/0.3 mL	**AtroPen® Auto-Injector** ("yellow label"), Meridian
	equivalent to Atropine Sulfate 0.5 mg/0.7 mL	**AtroPen® Auto-Injector** ("blue label"), Meridian
	equivalent to Atropine Sulfate 1 mg/0.7 mL	**AtroPen® Auto-Injector** ("dark red label"), Meridian
	equivalent to Atropine Sulfate 2 mg/0.7 mL	**AtroPen® Auto-Injector** ("green label"), Meridian

Atropine Sulfate

Powder*

Parenteral

Injection	0.05 mg/mL*	**Atropine Sulfate Injection**
	0.1 mg/mL*	**Atropine Sulfate Injection**
	0.4 mg/mL*	**Atropine Sulfate Injection**
	1 mg/mL*	**Atropine Sulfate Injection**

*available from one or more manufacturer, distributor, and/or repackager by generic (nonproprietary) name

†Use is not currently included in the labeling approved by the US Food and Drug Administration

Glycopyrrolate

Glycopyrronium Bromide

■ Glycopyrrolate is a synthetic quaternary ammonium antimuscarinic.

Uses

■ **Chronic Obstructive Pulmonary Disease** ***Glycopyrrolate*** Glycopyrrolate is used alone or in fixed combination with formoterol fumarate or indacaterol for the long-term maintenance treatment of airflow obstruction associated with chronic obstructive pulmonary disease (COPD), including chronic bronchitis and emphysema. Glycopyrrolate is *not* indicated for the treatment of acute bronchospasm.

Efficacy of glycopyrrolate oral inhalation powder has been evaluated in 2 randomized, double-blind, placebo-controlled, parallel-group trials in 867 adults 40 years of age or older with moderate to severe COPD. Patients were randomized to receive glycopyrrolate 15.6 mcg or placebo twice daily and were allowed to use their prescribed inhaled corticosteroid therapy. The primary outcome measure was the change from baseline in forced expiratory volume in 1 second (FEV_1) area under the curve (AUC) from 0–12 hours following the morning dose on day 85. In both trials, patients receiving glycopyrrolate experienced a greater change from baseline in FEV_1 AUC from 0–12 hours (treatment difference of 123–139 mL) compared with patients receiving placebo.

Efficacy of glycopyrrolate oral inhalation solution has been evaluated in 2 randomized, double-blind, placebo-controlled, parallel-group trials in adults 40 years of age or older with COPD. Patients also had preexisting or concurrent cardiovascular disease. Patients were randomized to receive glycopyrrolate (25 or 50 mcg) or placebo twice daily and were allowed to use their prescribed respiratory medications (i.e., long-acting β_2-adrenergic agonists, with or without inhaled corticosteroids, and short-acting antimuscarinics). The primary outcome measure was the change from baseline in trough FEV_1 on day 84. In both trials, patients receiving glycopyrrolate experienced a greater change from baseline in trough FEV_1 compared with patients receiving placebo; the change from baseline in trough FEV_1 in patients receiving glycopyrrolate 25 mcg twice daily was 89–92 mL greater than that in patients receiving placebo. The additional benefit observed with glycopyrrolate 50 mcg twice daily compared with 25 mcg twice daily was not sufficient to warrant use of the higher dosage.

Fixed Combination of Glycopyrrolate and Formoterol Fumarate Glycopyrrolate in fixed combination with formoterol fumarate (glycopyrrolate/formoterol) is used as an oral inhalation aerosol for the long-term maintenance treatment of airflow obstruction associated with COPD, including chronic bronchitis and emphysema. The fixed combination containing glycopyrrolate and formoterol fumarate is *not* indicated for the treatment of acute bronchospasm. The fixed combination also is *not* indicated for the treatment of asthma; safety and efficacy in asthma have not been established.

Efficacy of glycopyrrolate in fixed combination with formoterol fumarate has been evaluated in 2 randomized, double-blind, placebo-controlled, parallel-group studies of 24 weeks' duration in 3699 patients 40 years of age or older with moderate to very severe COPD. Patients were randomized to receive orally inhaled glycopyrrolate/formoterol (glycopyrrolate 18 mcg and formoterol fumarate 9.6 mcg), glycopyrrolate 18 mcg alone, formoterol fumarate 9.6 mcg alone, or placebo twice daily and were allowed to use their prescribed respiratory medications (i.e., inhaled corticosteroids and/or phosphodiesterase type 4 inhibitors). The primary outcome measure was change from baseline in trough FEV_1 at week 24. In both trials, the change from baseline in trough FEV_1 at 24 weeks was greater in patients receiving glycopyrrolate/formoterol compared with patients receiving either drug alone or placebo.

Fixed Combination of Glycopyrrolate and Indacaterol Glycopyrrolate in fixed combination with indacaterol (glycopyrrolate/indacaterol) is used as an oral inhalation powder for the long-term maintenance treatment of airflow obstruction associated with COPD, including chronic bronchitis and emphysema. The fixed combination containing glycopyrrolate and indacaterol is *not* indicated for the treatment of acute bronchospasm. The fixed combination is *not* indicated for the treatment of asthma; safety and efficacy in asthma have not been established.

Efficacy of glycopyrrolate in fixed combination with indacaterol has been evaluated in 2 randomized, double-blind, placebo- and active-controlled studies of 12 weeks' duration in 2038 patients 40 years of age or older with moderate to severe COPD. Patients were randomized to receive therapy with orally inhaled glycopyrrolate 15.6 mcg/indacaterol 27.5 mcg in fixed combination, glycopyrrolate 15.6 mcg alone, indacaterol 27.5 mcg alone, or placebo twice daily and were allowed to use their prescribed inhaled corticosteroid therapy. The primary outcome measure was the change from baseline in FEV_1 AUC from 0–12 hours following the morning dose on day 85. Following administration of orally inhaled glycopyrrolate 15.6 mcg in fixed combination with indacaterol 27.5 mcg twice daily, the change from baseline in FEV_1 AUC from 0–12 hours following the morning dose on day 85 was larger than that observed with either drug alone or placebo in both trials.

■ **Drooling** Glycopyrrolate oral solution is used for the symptomatic management of chronic severe drooling in pediatric patients 3–16 years of age with neurologic conditions (e.g., cerebral palsy) associated with problematic drooling.

In one randomized, placebo-controlled trial, 36 patients 3–16 years of age and 2 patients older than 16 years of age with cerebral palsy, mental retardation, or other neurologic conditions associated with problematic drooling (i.e., drooling in the absence of treatment so that clothing is damp approximately 5–7 days per week) achieved a clinical response (defined as at least a 3-point reduction in mean daily scores on the 9-point modified Teacher's Drooling Scale [mTDS]) following therapy with glycopyrrolate oral solution. Dosages of glycopyrrolate were titrated over a 4-week period to optimal patient response starting at 0.02 mg/kg 3 times daily with increasing dosage increments of approximately 0.02 mg/kg 3 times daily every 5–7 days, not to exceed the lesser of approximately 0.1 mg/kg 3 times daily or 3 mg per dose 3 times daily. Following 8 weeks of therapy, a positive response was observed in 75 or 11% of patients receiving glycopyrrolate oral solution or placebo, respectively.

■ **Peptic Ulcer Disease** Glycopyrrolate is used orally or parenterally as an adjunct in the treatment of peptic ulcer disease. Glycopyrrolate injection is used in patients with peptic ulcer disease when rapid antimuscarinic effect is desired or oral therapy is not tolerated. As with other antimuscarinics, there are no conclusive data from well-controlled studies which indicate that, in usually recommended dosage, glycopyrrolate aids in the healing, decreases the rate of recurrence, or prevents complications of peptic ulcers. In addition, in patients with gastric ulcer, antimuscarinics may delay gastric emptying and result in antral stasis. With the advent of more effective therapies for the treatment of peptic ulcer disease, antimuscarinics have only limited usefulness in this condition. (See Uses: Peptic Ulcer Disease and GI Hypersecretory States, in the Antimuscarinics/Antispasmodics General Statement 12:08.08)

■ **Surgery** Glycopyrrolate injection is used parenterally as a preoperative medication to inhibit salivation and excessive secretions of the respiratory tract; however, the current practice of using thiopental (no longer commercially available in the US), halothane, or similar general anesthetics that do not stimulate the production of salivary or tracheobronchial secretions has reduced the need to control excessive respiratory secretions during surgery. Although glycopyrrolate injection has been used prophylactically to prevent acid-aspiration pneumonitis during surgery, antimuscarinics, including glycopyrrolate, have not been shown to be effective for this use. Glycopyrrolate injection may be used to prevent cholinergic effects during surgery, such as cardiac arrhythmias, hypotension, and bradycardia, which may result from traction on viscera (with resultant vagal stimulation), stimulation of the carotid sinus, or administration of drugs (e.g., succinylcholine). Glycopyrrolate injection is administered concurrently with anticholinesterase agents (e.g., neostigmine, pyridostigmine) to block the adverse muscarinic effects of these latter agents when they are used after surgery to terminate curarization. Unlike atropine or hyoscyamine (tertiary amine antimuscarinics), glycopyrrolate (quaternary ammonium antimuscarinic) does not readily penetrate the CNS and therefore will not reverse the central effects of physostigmine. Because glycopyrrolate does not have appreciable CNS effects, it may be preferred in some patients. For further discussion on the use of glycopyrrolate injection in surgery, see Uses: Surgery, in the Antimuscarinics/Antispasmodics General Statement 12:08.08.

Dosage and Administration

■ **Administration** Glycopyrrolate is administered orally, IM, IV, or by oral inhalation.

Oral Administration Glycopyrrolate is administered orally as tablets or an oral solution.

When the oral solution is used, it should be administered at least 1 hour before or 2 hours after meals. An accurate measuring device must be used to administer the oral solution.

Parenteral Administration For preoperative IM administration, glycopyrrolate may be administered in the same syringe with other compatible preoperative medications.

For IV administration, glycopyrrolate may be given by direct IV injection. Alternatively, glycopyrrolate may be administered via the tubing of a running IV infusion of 0.9% sodium chloride. When used concomitantly with neostigmine, physostigmine, or pyridostigmine, glycopyrrolate may be administered IV simultaneously with the anticholinesterase agent via the same syringe. (See Chemistry and Stability: Stability.)

Because glycopyrrolate injection contains benzyl alcohol as a preservative, the manufacturer recommends that the drug not be used in neonates younger than 1 month of age. Although a causal relationship has not been established, administration of injections preserved with benzyl alcohol has been associated with toxicity in neonates. Toxicity appears to have resulted from administration of large amounts (i.e., 100–400 mg/kg daily) of benzyl alcohol in these neonates. Although use of drugs preserved with benzyl alcohol should be avoided in neonates whenever possible, the American Academy of Pediatrics (AAP) states that the presence of small amounts of the preservative in a commercially available injection should not proscribe its use when indicated in neonates.

Oral Inhalation via Dry-Powder Inhaler Glycopyrrolate oral inhalation powder (Seebri® Neohaler®) is administered by oral inhalation *only* using a special oral inhalation device (Neohaler®) that delivers powdered drug from capsules. Glycopyrrolate capsules for oral inhalation must not be taken orally (i.e., swallowed), as the intended effects on the lungs will not be obtained.

Glycopyrrolate in fixed combination with indacaterol (glycopyrrolate/indacaterol; Utibron® Neohaler®) is administered by oral inhalation *only* using a special oral inhalation device (Neohaler®) that delivers powdered drug from capsules. Glycopyrrolate/indacaterol capsules for oral inhalation must not be taken orally (i.e., swallowed), as the intended effects on the lungs will not be obtained.

The Neohaler® device should not be used to administer other drugs. The Neohaler® device provided with each new prescription of glycopyrrolate or glycopyrrolate/indacaterol should be used to administer the drug. The capsules containing oral inhalation powder should be stored in the foil-wrapped sealed blisters, and only one capsule should be removed immediately before use; any unused additional capsules that are exposed to air should be discarded.

To obtain optimal benefit, the patient should be given a copy of the patient information and instructions for use provided by the manufacturer. To use the Neohaler® device, the cap should be removed, then the inhaler should be opened by holding the base firmly and tilting the mouthpiece. One blister should be separated from the blister card by tearing along the perforation. The protective backing should be pulled away to expose one capsule immediately before use; the capsule should not be pushed through the foil to remove it from the blister. The capsule should be removed from the blister with dry hands and placed into the capsule chamber of the device; the capsule should not be placed into the mouthpiece of the device. The inhaler should be closed fully until a click is heard. The inhaler should be held upright with the mouthpiece pointing upward, and both piercing buttons should be pressed together firmly at the same time only once (a click will be heard), then the piercing buttons should be released fully. Piercing the capsule may produce very small pieces, which may pass into the mouth; the pieces should not cause any harm if swallowed or inhaled.

Before inhaling the dose, the patient should exhale completely, being careful not to exhale into the mouthpiece of the Neohaler® device. The inhaler device should be held horizontally (piercing buttons facing left and right) and the mouthpiece placed in the mouth, with the lips closed firmly around it. The patient should then inhale rapidly, but steadily and as deeply as possible, without pressing the piercing buttons. During inhalation, a whirring noise created by the capsule spinning around in the chamber should be heard; a sweet flavor also may be detected. The patient should continue holding their breath for at least 5–10 seconds or as long as comfortably possible while removing the inhaler from the mouth, and then should exhale. The inhaler should be opened to see if any powder is left in the capsule. If powder remains, the inhaler should be closed and the steps for inhaling the drug should be repeated. Most patients are able to empty the capsule with 1 or 2 inhalations. Coughing may occur soon after inhaling the dose; however, coughing does not interfere with delivery of the full dose as long as the capsule is empty. After inhaling the dose, the mouthpiece should be opened and the device tipped to dispose of the used capsule, then the inhaler should be closed and the cap replaced. Used capsules should not be left in the device.

If a whirring noise is not heard during inhalation of the drug, the capsule may be stuck in the capsule chamber. If this occurs, the inhaler should be opened and the capsule carefully loosened by tapping the base of the inhaler; the piercing buttons should not be pressed. The steps to inhale the drug should then be repeated.

Routine cleaning of the inhaler is not necessary; if desired, the mouthpiece may be cleaned inside and outside with a clean, dry, lint-free cloth, or a clean, dry, soft brush may be used to wipe the inhaler and remove any powder residue. The inhaler should be kept dry, and the device should not be taken apart.

Oral Inhalation via Solution Glycopyrrolate oral inhalation solution (Lonhala® Magnair®) is administered by oral inhalation via nebulization *only* using a special oral inhalation device (Magnair® nebulizer system). Glycopyrrolate solution for oral inhalation must not be injected or taken orally (i.e., swallowed), as the intended effects on the lungs will not be obtained.

The Magnair® nebulizer system should not be used to administer other drugs. The Magnair® nebulizer system provided in the starter kit and the replacement handset provided with each new prescription should be used to administer the drug. The single-dose vials of glycopyrrolate oral inhalation solution should be stored in the sealed foil pouch; any unused vials should be discarded 7 days after the pouch is first opened.

Prior to administration of glycopyrrolate oral inhalation solution for nebulization, the Magnair® nebulizer system should be assembled according to the manufacturer's directions and checked to ensure it is working properly. To obtain optimal benefit, the patient should be given a copy of the patient information and instructions for use provided by the manufacturer.

Immediately prior to use, the foil pouch should be opened and the two vials of oral inhalation solution removed and separated; one vial should be returned to the foil pouch and stored in the nebulizer system carrying bag. The vial to be used should be inserted into the bottom of the medication cap until it clicks. The medication cap with the vial should then be placed on top of the handset body (with the aerosol head already inserted without touching the part that pierces the vial) and turned in a clockwise direction until a click is heard. The notch in the medication cap should line up with the blue line on the handset body.

To administer the treatment, the mouthpiece should be inserted into the mouth and the on/off button on the controller pressed. During the treatment, which should take about 2–3 minutes, the patient should breathe normally through the mouthpiece. Care should be taken to avoid tilting the handset, loosening or removing the medication cap, or unclasping the handset body until the treatment is complete. At the end of the treatment, a beep will sound and the controller will shut off automatically. After each treatment, the manufacturer's instructions for cleaning the handset should be followed.

Oral Inhalation via Aerosol Glycopyrrolate in fixed combination with formoterol fumarate (glycopyrrolate/formoterol; Bevespi® Aerosphere®) is administered by oral inhalation using an oral aerosol inhaler with hydrofluoroalkane (HFA) propellant. The glycopyrrolate/formoterol oral inhalation aerosol should only be used with the actuator supplied with the product.

The aerosol inhaler should be primed by releasing 4 test sprays into the air (away from the face) before initial use, and shaken well before each test spray. If the inhaler has not been used for more than 7 days, the priming process should be repeated (using only 2 sprays rather than 4). To administer a dose, the cap should be removed from the mouthpiece. Before each inhalation, the inhaler must be shaken well. The inhaler should be held with the mouthpiece pointing towards the face while the patient exhales through the mouth as fully and comfortably as possible. The lips should be closed around the mouthpiece and the head tilted back, keeping the tongue below the mouthpiece. While inhaling slowly and deeply, the center of the dose indicator should be pressed down until the canister stops moving in the actuator and a spray has been released, then the dose indicator should be released. Following inhalation, the mouthpiece should be removed from the mouth and the breath held as long as comfortably possible (up to 10 seconds) then the patient should exhale gently. The process should be repeated for the second inhalation. The cap should be replaced on the mouthpiece immediately after use.

The Bevespi® Aerosphere® inhaler should be cleaned once weekly by removing the canister from the actuator; the canister should not be cleaned or allowed to get wet. The actuator should be held under warm running water for about 30 seconds. The actuator should then be turned upside down and water rinsed through the actuator again for about 30 seconds. The actuator should be allowed to dry overnight. When the actuator is dry, the canister should be pressed gently down into it; however, the canister should not be pressed down too hard since this may cause drug to be released. Priming of the inhaler should be repeated after each cleaning by shaking well and releasing 2 test sprays into the air away from the face. The inhaler should be discarded when the labeled number of inhalations has been used or within 3 months after removal from the foil pouch or when the dose indicator reads "0," whichever comes first. The canister should never be immersed in water to determine the amount of drug remaining in the canister ("float test").

■ **Dosage** Each capsule of glycopyrrolate oral inhalation powder (Seebri® Neohaler®) contains 15.6 mcg of glycopyrrolate. However, the actual amount of drug delivered to the lungs depends on factors such as the patient's inspiratory flow rate and inspiratory time. Under standardized in vitro testing at a fixed flow rate of 90 L/minute for 1.3 seconds, the Neohaler® device delivered 13.1 mcg from the 15.6-mcg capsule (equivalent to 12.5 mcg of glycopyrronium) from the mouthpiece.

Each capsule of glycopyrrolate/indacaterol oral inhalation powder (Utibron® Neohaler®) contains 15.6 mcg of glycopyrrolate and 27.5 mcg of indacaterol. However, the actual amount of drug delivered to the lungs depends on factors such as the patient's inspiratory flow rate and inspiratory time. Under standardized in vitro testing at a fixed flow rate of 90 L/minute for 1.3 seconds, the Neohaler® device delivered 12.8 mcg of glycopyrrolate (equivalent to 12.5 mcg of glycopyrronium) and 20.8 mcg of indacaterol from the mouthpiece.

Each single-dose vial of glycopyrrolate oral inhalation solution (Lonhala® Magnair®) contains 25 mcg of glycopyrrolate in 1 mL of solution. However, the actual amount of drug delivered to the lungs depends on patient factors. Under standardized in vitro testing, the Magnair® device delivered approximately 14.2 mcg of glycopyrrolate (equivalent to 11.4 mcg of glycopyrronium) from the mouthpiece.

After priming of the oral aerosol inhaler containing glycopyrrolate/formoterol, each actuation of the oral aerosol inhaler (Bevespi® Aerosphere®) delivers 10.4 mcg of glycopyrrolate (equivalent to 8.3 mcg of glycopyrronium) and 5.5 mcg of formoterol fumarate from the valve. Dosage is expressed in terms of drug delivered from the mouthpiece; each actuation of the inhaler delivers 9 mcg of glycopyrrolate (equivalent to 7.2 mcg of glycopyrronium) and 4.8 mcg of formoterol fumarate from the mouthpiece. The actual amount of drug delivered to the lungs depends on factors such as the patient's coordination between actuation of the device and inspiration through the delivery system. Commercially available glycopyrrolate/formoterol aerosol inhaler delivers 28 or 120 metered sprays per 5.9- or 10.7-g canister, respectively.

Chronic Obstructive Pulmonary Disease **Glycopyrrolate.** For the long-term management of airflow obstruction associated with chronic obstructive pulmonary disease (COPD), the usual dosage of glycopyrrolate oral inhalation powder in adults is 15.6 mcg (the contents of one capsule) twice daily via the Neohaler® device. More frequent administration or higher dosages are not recommended. Orally inhaled glycopyrrolate powder should *not* be used for the treatment of acute episodes of bronchospasm.

For the long-term management of airflow obstruction associated with COPD, the usual dosage of glycopyrrolate oral inhalation solution in adults is 25 mcg (the contents of one single-dose vial) twice daily via the Magnair® device. More frequent administration or higher dosages are not recommended. Orally inhaled glycopyrrolate solution should *not* be used for the treatment of acute episodes of bronchospasm.

Fixed Combination of Glycopyrrolate and Formoterol Fumarate. For the long-term management of airflow obstruction associated with COPD, the usual dosage of glycopyrrolate in fixed combination with formoterol fumarate in adults is 18 mcg of glycopyrrolate and 9.6 mcg of formoterol fumarate (two inhalations of preparation containing 9 mcg of glycopyrrolate and 4.8 mcg of formoterol fumarate) twice daily via the Aerosphere® device. More frequent administration or higher dosages are not recommended. Orally inhaled glycopyrrolate/formoterol should *not* be used for the treatment of acute episodes of bronchospasm.

Fixed Combination of Glycopyrrolate and Indacaterol. For the long-term management of airflow obstruction associated with COPD, the usual dosage of glycopyrrolate in fixed combination with indacaterol in adults is 15.6 mcg of glycopyrrolate and 27.5 mcg of indacaterol (the contents of one capsule) twice daily via the Neohaler® device. More frequent administration or higher dosages are not recommended. Orally inhaled glycopyrrolate/formoterol should *not* be used for the treatment of acute episodes of bronchospasm.

Drooling The initial recommended dosage of glycopyrrolate oral solution for the symptomatic management of chronic severe drooling in pediatric patients 3–16 years of age with neurologic conditions (e.g., cerebral palsy) associated with problematic drooling is 0.02 mg/kg 3 times daily; dosage may be titrated in increments of 0.02 mg/kg every 5–7 days based on therapeutic response and tolerance. During dosage titration, tolerability of the current dose should be reviewed with the patient's caregiver prior to each increase in dosage. The maximum recommended dosage is 0.1 mg/kg 3 times daily (not to exceed 1.5–3 mg per dose based on weight).

Peptic Ulcer Disease The usual initial oral dosage of glycopyrrolate tablets for the adjunctive treatment of peptic ulcer disease in adults is 1 mg 3 times daily, in the morning, early afternoon, and at bedtime. Some patients may require 2 mg at bedtime to ensure overnight control of symptoms. Alternatively, an oral dosage for adults of 2 mg 2 or 3 times daily, given at equally spaced intervals, may be used. A maintenance dosage of 1 mg twice daily is adequate in most adults. The maximum adult oral dosage is 8 mg daily.

The usual IM or IV dosage of glycopyrrolate for the adjunctive treatment of peptic ulcer disease in adults is 0.1 mg, administered every 4 hours, 3 or 4 times daily. When a more profound antimuscarinic effect is desired, 0.2 mg may be given IM or IV. Some patients may only require a single dose, and frequency of parenteral administration should be determined by the patient's response up to a maximum of 4 doses daily.

As with other antimuscarinics, higher than recommended dosage may be required for therapeutic effect in patients with peptic ulcer disease. Dosage should be carefully titrated until therapeutic effect is achieved or adverse effects become intolerable, using the lowest possible effective dosage.

Safety and efficacy of oral or parenteral glycopyrrolate for the treatment of peptic ulcer disease in pediatric patients have not been established; the tablets are not recommended in children younger than 12 years of age.

Surgery As a preoperative medication in adults or children 2 years of age and older, the usual dose of glycopyrrolate is 0.004 mg/kg, administered IM 30–60 minutes prior to the anticipated time of induction of anesthesia or at the time other preanesthetic medications (e.g., opiates, sedatives) are administered. Children 1–24 months of age may require a preoperative dose up to 0.009 mg/kg.

When intraoperative use of glycopyrrolate is necessary to prevent cholinergic effects during surgery in adults or children, the usual IV dose is 0.1 mg or 0.004 mg/kg (not to exceed 0.1 mg), respectively; if necessary, the dose may be repeated at 2- to 3-minute intervals. Because of the long duration of antimuscarinic effects of the preoperative dose, intraoperative doses of glycopyrrolate are rarely needed in children.

To block adverse muscarinic effects of anticholinesterase agents (i.e., neostigmine, pyridostigmine) when these agents are used to reverse the neuromuscular blockade produced by curariform agents in adults or children, the usual IV dose of glycopyrrolate is 0.2 mg for each 1 mg of neostigmine or 5 mg of pyridostigmine administered; glycopyrrolate is administered concurrently in the same syringe with the anticholinesterase agent. Some clinicians recommend that, in the presence of bradycardia, antimuscarinics be administered IV before the anticholinesterase agent to increase the pulse rate to about 80 beats/minute.

Pharmacokinetics

■ Absorption Glycopyrrolate, like other quaternary ammonium drugs, is incompletely absorbed from the GI tract since it is completely ionized; however, the rate and extent of absorption of glycopyrrolate following oral administration have not been fully characterized. Following administration of oral glycopyrrolate tablets in children, mean absolute bioavailability was low (about 3%) and variable (range 1–13%). The mean time to peak plasma glycopyrrolate concentrations following administration of the oral solution is about 3 hours. Administration with a high-fat meal has been shown to decrease the absorption of glycopyrrolate following administration of the oral solution; the oral solution should be administered at least 1 hour before or 2 hours after meals.

Following oral inhalation of glycopyrrolate powder via the Neohaler® device, the drug is rapidly absorbed with peak plasma concentrations occurring at 5 minutes. Following oral inhalation of the powder, the absolute bioavailability is about 40%, with 90% of systemic exposure resulting from lung absorption and 10% from GI absorption. Steady-state concentrations are achieved within 1 week with repeated once-daily oral inhalation; changes in glycopyrrolate pharmacokinetics over time have not been observed. Linear pharmacokinetics were observed following oral inhalation dosages of 31.2–249.6 mcg daily.

Following oral inhalation of glycopyrrolate solution via the Magnair® nebulizer system, the drug is rapidly absorbed with peak plasma concentrations occurring within 20 minutes. Steady-state plasma concentrations are achieved within 1 week of repeated twice-daily oral inhalation; 2- to 3-fold accumulation of systemic glycopyrrolate exposure has been observed at steady state following twice-daily dosing.

Following IV administration of glycopyrrolate, the drug has an onset of action of about 1 minute. Following IM injection, pharmacologic effects are evident within 15–30 minutes and peak within 30–45 minutes. The vagal blocking effects of the drug persist for 2–3 hours and inhibition of salivation persists for up to 7 hours after parenteral administration of the drug. Following oral administration, the anticholinergic effects of glycopyrrolate may persist for up to 8–12 hours.

■ Distribution Little information is available on the distribution of glycopyrrolate. Quaternary ammonium antimuscarinics are completely ionized and possess poor lipid solubility. Accordingly they do not readily penetrate the CNS or eye.

Following IV administration of glycopyrrolate in animals, the drug is rapidly distributed throughout the body with highest concentrations appearing in the stomach and intestine. Following IV administration of a single 0.1 mg/kg dose of radiolabeled glycopyrrolate in dogs, peak CSF concentrations of the drug were 0.9 ng/mL, about 10% of the peak serum concentration. Glycopyrrolate is distributed into bile. Following surgery for cholelithiasis in patients who had T-tube drains placed into the common bile duct, peak biliary concentrations of drug were reached within 30–60 minutes after IV administration and persisted for up to 48 hours in some patients.

In vitro, plasma protein binding of 38–41% has been reported at concentrations of 1–10 ng/mL following IV administration.

Glycopyrrolate crosses the placental barrier to a limited extent. Following IV administration of a single 0.1 mg/kg dose of radiolabeled drug in pregnant dogs, peak fetal concentrations were 0.63 ng/mL, about 4% of the peak maternal serum concentration. It is not known if glycopyrrolate distributes into milk.

■ Elimination Following IV administration of glycopyrrolate, serum concentrations of the drug decline rapidly, with less than 10% of the dose remaining in serum after 5 minutes and essentially no drug remaining during the period of 0.5–3 hours after administration. Following IV administration, the elimination half-life of glycopyrrolate is approximately 50 minutes, 19–99 minutes, and 22–130 minutes in adults, children, and infants, respectively. Following IM administration in adults, the elimination half-life is 33–75 minutes.

Following administration of the oral solution, a mean elimination half-life of 3 hours was reported.

Following oral inhalation of glycopyrrolate powder via the Neohaler® device, a mean elimination half-life of 33–53 hours was reported.

In vitro studies show glycopyrrolate hydroxylation resulting in a variety of mono- and bis-hydroxylated metabolites and direct hydrolysis resulting in the formation of a carboxylic acid derivative (M9). Multiple cytochrome P-450 (CYP) isoenzymes appear to contribute to the oxidative biotransformation of glycopyrrolate; hydrolysis to M9 is likely catalyzed by members of the cholinesterase family presystemically and/or via first-pass metabolism from the swallowed dose fraction of orally inhaled drug. Following repeated oral inhalation, glucuronide and/or sulfate conjugates, accounting for about 3% of the inhaled dose, were found in urine. Renal elimination of parent drug accounts for about 60–70% of systemically available glycopyrrolate following oral inhalation; active tubular secretion contributes to renal clearance. Nonrenal clearance is mainly thought to result from metabolism, with biliary clearance contributing a small role.

Small amounts of IV glycopyrrolate are metabolized to one or more metabolites. Glycopyrrolate is excreted mainly as unchanged drug in feces via biliary elimination and in urine. In adults, approximately 65–80% of an IV dose was eliminated in urine as unchanged drug. In animals, 70–90% of a dose was eliminated in feces. Following IV administration of the drug in patients who had undergone surgery for cholelithiasis, about 85% of the dose was excreted in urine within 48 hours and less than 5% of the dose was distributed into T-tube drainage of bile, principally as unchanged drug.

In patients undergoing renal transplantation receiving IV glycopyrrolate, the half-life was prolonged to 47 minutes compared with 19 minutes in healthy individuals. Elimination of glycopyrrolate appears to be severely impaired in patients with renal failure. In patients receiving glycopyrrolate by oral inhalation, total systemic glycopyrrolate exposure increased by up to 1.4- or 2.2-fold, respectively, in those with mild to moderate (estimated glomerular filtration rate [GFR] greater than or equal to 30 mL/minute) or severe to end-stage renal impairment (estimated GFR less than 30 mL/minute).

Pharmacokinetics of glycopyrrolate have not been evaluated in patients with hepatic impairment.

There is no evidence that age, body weight, race, gender, or smoking status has any effect on the pharmacokinetics of glycopyrrolate oral inhalation powder.

Chemistry and Stability

■ **Chemistry** Glycopyrrolate is a synthetic quaternary ammonium antimuscarinic. Glycopyrrolate is an aminoalcohol ester. The drug occurs as a white, crystalline powder and has solubilities of approximately 238 mg/mL in water and 33.3 mg/mL in alcohol at 25°C.

Commercially available glycopyrrolate for injection is a clear, colorless, sterile solution of the drug in water for injection. Sodium hydroxide and/or hydrochloric acid may be added during the manufacture of the injection to adjust the pH to 2–3. Commercially available glycopyrrolate injection also contains 0.9% benzyl alcohol as a preservative.

■ **Stability** Commercially available glycopyrrolate injection should be stored in single-dose or multiple-dose containers, preferably of USP Type I glass, at controlled room temperature between 20 and 25°C.

Glycopyrrolate is stable under ordinary conditions of temperature, heat, and light. The drug is most stable at an acid pH. Glycopyrrolate is unstable at a pH greater than 6. Ester hydrolysis is the major cause of decomposition of glycopyrrolate; the rate of hydrolysis increases with increasing pH.

Solutions containing glycopyrrolate concentrations of 0.8 mg/L are stable for 48 hours at room temperature in the following IV infusion solutions: 5% dextrose, 5% dextrose and 0.45% sodium chloride, 0.9% sodium chloride, or Ringer's injection.

The manufacturer of glycopyrrolate injection states that the drug is stable in dextrose 10% solution. In addition, the manufacturer states that glycopyrrolate may be administered via the tubing of a running IV infusion of 0.9% sodium chloride.

When combined in the same syringe, admixtures containing glycopyrrolate have been reported to be stable for 48 hours at room temperature with the following injections: atropine sulfate, chlorpromazine hydrochloride, codeine phosphate, diphenhydramine hydrochloride, droperidol, droperidol and fentanyl citrate (Innovar®, no longer commercially available in the US), hydromorphone hydrochloride, hydroxyzine hydrochloride, levorphanol tartrate, lidocaine hydrochloride, meperidine hydrochloride, meperidine hydrochloride and promethazine hydrochloride (Mepergan®, no longer commercially available in the US), morphine sulfate, neostigmine methylsulfate, oxymorphone hydrochloride, procaine hydrochloride (no longer commercially available in the US), prochlorperazine edisylate, promazine hydrochloride (no longer commercially available in the US), promethazine hydrochloride, propiomazine hydrochloride (no longer commercially available in the US), pyridostigmine bromide, scopolamine hydrobromide, triflupromazine hydrochloride (no longer commercially available in the US), or trimethobenzamide hydrochloride.

In addition, when combined in the same syringe, the manufacturer states that admixtures containing glycopyrrolate injection are reported to be stable with the following injections: butorphanol tartrate, fentanyl citrate, nalbuphine hydrochloride, and physostigmine salicylate.

Since the compatibility of these and other admixtures with glycopyrrolate depends on several factors (e.g., concentration of the drugs, resulting pH, temperature), specialized references should be consulted for the specific conditions of compatibility. Chloramphenicol, dexamethasone sodium phosphate, diazepam, dimenhydrinate, methohexital sodium, pentazocine lactate, pentobarbital sodium, secobarbital sodium, sodium bicarbonate, or thiopental sodium (no longer commercially available in the US) are incompatible with glycopyrrolate when combined in the same syringe. Glycopyrrolate is physically incompatible with drugs having an alkaline pH; a gas may evolve or precipitation may occur if the drugs are mixed. Admixture with other drugs or solutions that results in a pH greater than 6 (e.g., dexamethasone sodium phosphate, a buffered solution of lactated Ringer's injection) will usually cause rapid ester hydrolysis of glycopyrrolate; however, glycopyrrolate may be administered via the tubing of a running IV infusion of lactated Ringer's injection.

Commercially available glycopyrrolate tablets should be stored in tight containers at 20–25°C (may be exposed to 15–30°C).

Commercially available glycopyrrolate oral solution containing 1 mg of glycopyrrolate per 5 mL should be stored at 20–25°C (may be exposed to 15–30°C).

Commercially available dry-powder capsules for oral inhalation containing glycopyrrolate alone or in fixed combination with indacaterol (glycopyrrolate/indacaterol) should be stored at 25°C (may be exposed to 15–30°C). The capsules should be stored in the foil-sealed blisters until immediately before use. Only one capsule should be removed immediately before use or effectiveness of the drug may be reduced. Capsules should be discarded if opened and exposed to air (i.e., not used immediately).

Commercially available single-dose vials containing glycopyrrolate oral inhalation solution should be stored at 20–25°C. Single-dose vials should be stored in the protective foil pouch. After the pouch is opened, unused vials should be returned to the pouch for storage; any vials not used within 7 days of opening the pouch should be discarded. Any vial containing solution that is not colorless should be discarded.

Commercially available oral inhalation aerosol containing glycopyrrolate in fixed combination with formoterol fumarate (glycopyrrolate/formoterol) should be stored at 20–25°C (may be exposed to 15–30°C). The inhalation aerosol should be discarded 3 months after the foil pouch is opened or when the dose indicator reaches "0", whichever comes first.

For further information on chemistry, pharmacology, pharmacokinetics, uses, cautions, acute toxicity, drug interactions, and dosage and administration of glycopyrrolate, see the Antimuscarinics/Antispasmodics General Statement 12:08.08.

Preparations

Excipients in commercially available drug preparations may have clinically important effects in some individuals; consult specific product labeling for details.

Glycopyrrolate

Oral		
Solution	0.2 mg/mL	**Cuvposa**®, Merz
Tablets	1 mg*	**Glycopyrrolate Tablets**
		Robinul® (scored), Shionogi
	2 mg*	**Glycopyrrolate Tablets**
		Robinul® **Forte** (scored), Shionogi
Oral Inhalation		
Powder, for inhalation (contained in capsules)	15.6 mcg	**Seebri**® **Neohaler**®, Sunovion
Solution, for nebulization	25 mcg/mL	**Lonhala**® **Magnair**®, Sunovion
Parenteral		
Injection	0.2 mg/mL*	**Glycopyrrolate Injection**
		Robinul®, West-ward

*available from one or more manufacturer, distributor, and/or repackager by generic (nonproprietary) name

Glycopyrrolate Combinations

Oral Inhalation		
Aerosol	9 mcg with Formoterol Fumarate 4.8 mcg per metered spray	**Bevespi**® **Aerosphere**® (with hydrofluoroalkane propellant), AstraZeneca
Powder, for inhalation (contained in capsules)	15.6 mcg with Indacaterol 27.5 mcg	**Utibron**® **Neohaler**®, Sunovion

Ipratropium Bromide

■ Ipratropium bromide is a synthetic quaternary ammonium antimuscarinic.

Uses

■ **Bronchospasm** Ipratropium bromide is used for the symptomatic treatment of reversible bronchospasm that may occur in association with chronic obstructive pulmonary disease (COPD), including chronic bronchitis and emphysema. Ipratropium bromide in fixed combination with albuterol sulfate is used by oral inhalation for the symptomatic management of bronchospasm associated with COPD in patients who continue to have evidence of bronchospasm despite the regular use of an orally inhaled bronchodilator and who require a second bronchodilator. Ipratropium bromide also is used for the symptomatic treatment of bronchial asthma† and for the prevention of exercise-induced bronchospasm†, and also has been used as a bronchodilator in patients with cystic fibrosis†.

Chronic Obstructive Pulmonary Disease Ipratropium bromide is used as a bronchodilator for the long-term symptomatic treatment of reversible bronchospasm associated with COPD, including chronic bronchitis and emphysema. Orally inhaled ipratropium is not indicated as a single agent for the initial treatment of acute episodes of bronchospasm or acute exacerbations of COPD; a drug with a more rapid onset of action (e.g., a β_2-adrenergic agonist) may be preferred in such cases. (See Cautions: Precautions and Contraindications.) However, some clinicians consider combined therapy with a β_2-agonist bronchodilator and ipratropium to be useful in selected patients with acute exacerbations of COPD.

The efficacy of ipratropium has been similar to or greater than that of β_2-adrenergic agonists (e.g., albuterol, metaproterenol) in comparative studies in which these drugs were administered via metered-dose inhaler or nebulization. As orally inhaled ipratropium produces fewer adverse effects than these drugs, ipratropium is a first-line maintenance bronchodilator for relief of chronic (e.g., daily) symptoms of bronchospasm in patients with mild COPD. However, in a few long-term studies comparing ipratropium bromide and tiotropium bromide, another long-acting orally inhaled anticholinergic agent, ipratropium bromide (36 mcg 4 times daily) oral inhalation aerosol with chlorofluorocarbon (CFC) propellants (preparation with CFC propellants no longer commercially available in the US) was less effective than tiotropium (18 mcg once daily) in improving lung function (e.g., as determined by changes in forced expiratory volume in 1 second [FEV_1] and peak expiratory flow rate [PEFR]) in patients with COPD. (See Chronic Obstructive Pulmonary Disease under Uses: Bronchospasm, in Tiotropium Bromide 12:08.08.) Short-term (e.g., 3-month) controlled studies indicate that the fixed combination of albuterol and ipratropium results in greater bronchodilation following oral inhalation than either agent given alone in patients with COPD.

The efficacy and safety of ipratropium bromide with a hydrofluoroalkane propellant (Atrovent® HFA) have been shown to be comparable to that of ipratropium bromide with chlorofluorocarbon propellants (Atrovent®, no longer commercially available in the US) in patients with COPD. In 2 randomized, comparative clinical trials in patients with COPD, therapy with ipratropium bromide inhalation aerosol with a hydrofluoroalkane (HFA) propellant (Atrovent® HFA 34 or 68 mcg [dose delivered from the mouthpiece] 4 times daily) produced similar improvements in FEV_1 and forced vital capacity (FVC) over the 12-week study period and had similar adverse effects as therapy with ipratropium bromide with chlorofluorocarbon propellants (Atrovent® 36 mcg [dose delivered from the mouthpiece] 4 times daily). In one of these studies, the mean peak improvement in FEV_1 relative to baseline on day 85 of therapy (one of the primary end points) was 0.295 L after a single dose of Atrovent® HFA (34 mcg or 2 inhalations) compared with 0.14 L observed with placebo (HFA propellant vehicle only).

Administration of nebulized ipratropium generally is reserved for patients with severe disease who do not respond adequately to conventional therapy and for those who find it difficult or are unable to optimally inhale the drug orally via a metered-dose inhaler.

In the stepped-care approach to COPD drug therapy, mild intermittent symptoms and minimal lung impairment (e.g., FEV_1 at least 80% of predicted) can be treated with a short-acting selective inhaled β_2-agonist as needed during acute exacerbations, but use should not exceed 8–12 inhalations daily. Alternatively, some clinicians initiate therapy with ipratropium inhalation aerosol. Patients with COPD who receive orally inhaled ipratropium generally have an increase in FEV_1 (at its peak) of 0.15–0.36 L and a decrease in functional residual capacity of 0.3–0.6 L. Although ipratropium produces objective bronchodilation (i.e., increase in FEV_1 and FVC) in patients with COPD, a beneficial effect on subjective symptom or quality-of-life scores has not been demonstrated in short-term (e.g., 3-month) clinical studies, and current evidence indicates that ipratropium therapy does not alter the disease process (neither accelerates nor slows the age-related decline in FEV_1 associated with COPD).

Low- to high-dose ipratropium bromide (6–16 inhalations daily) can be added to therapy with a selective β_2-agonist in patients with mild to moderate symptoms of COPD, with the frequency of inhalation dosing with either agent not to exceed 4 times daily; the highest dosage of ipratropium bromide included in some guidelines for COPD exceeds the manufacturer's recommended maximum daily dosage (12 inhalations). Therapy with anticholinergic and/or β_2-adrenergic agonist bronchodilators increases airflow and exercise tolerance and reduces dyspnea in patients with symptoms of COPD, and these drugs are used in the long-term management of airflow limitation in such patients. The mean peak FEV_1 increase was 0.37 L following short-term (approximately 3 months) administration of the fixed combination of albuterol sulfate (180 mcg as albuterol base) and ipratropium bromide monohydrate (36 mcg) 4 times daily. The fixed combination of ipratropium and albuterol did not affect morning PEFR after short-term administration (i.e., less than 3 months) in these patients.

Current evidence indicates that concomitant or sequential administration of inhaled ipratropium and an inhaled β_2-adrenergic agonist in patients with COPD generally produces additional bronchodilation compared with that achieved with either agent alone. Although the improvement in bronchodilation produced by combined therapy with ipratropium and a β_2-adrenergic agonist often may not exceed that which could be achieved with larger dosages of either agent alone, the duration of bronchodilation appears to be increased with such concomitant therapy, and the potential for adverse effects also may be minimized. The sequence of administration of ipratropium and a short-acting β_2-agonist generally does not alter the effectiveness of the bronchodilating action.

Home management of COPD exacerbations involves increasing the dose and/or frequency of existing short-acting bronchodilator therapy, preferably with a B_2-adrenergic agonist. If response to a short-acting β_2-adrenergic agonist alone is inadequate, some clinicians recommend the addition of ipratropium. In a severe exacerbation treated at home, administration of these agents by nebulization or metered-dose inhalation with a spacer device may be used as needed for short-term therapy.

Following initiation of oxygen therapy in hospitalized patients with COPD, therapy with a short-acting β_2-adrenergic agonist and/or ipratropium (administered separately or in fixed combination) should be used for acute exacerbations of COPD, although the effectiveness of such combination therapy remains controversial.

Asthma Orally inhaled ipratropium bromide has been used effectively for the symptomatic treatment of acute or chronic bronchial asthma† and can potentiate the bronchodilatory effects of β_2-adrenergic agonists, but the precise role of the drug in the management of this condition remains to be more fully elucidated. Ipratropium is suggested by some experts as an alternative to short-acting inhaled β_2-agonists for relief of asthma symptoms, particularly in patients who experience adverse effects with β_2-adrenergic agonists. However, the efficacy of ipratropium in the long-term management of asthma has not been established. Because the onset of action of ipratropium is slower than that of β_2-adrenergic agonist bronchodilators and the peak bronchodilator effects generally are less pronounced, β_2-adrenergic agonist bronchodilators generally are preferred *initially* for the symptomatic relief of bronchospasm in patients with asthma. Current guidelines for the management of asthma and many clinicians recommend concomitant anti-inflammatory therapy with orally inhaled corticosteroids as first-line therapy for long-term management of asthma in adults and children whose symptoms are not controlled by intermittent use of a short-acting β_2-adrenergic agonist alone. For additional information on the stepped-care approach for drug therapy in asthma, see Asthma under Uses: Bronchospasm, in Albuterol 12:12.08.12.

Orally inhaled, selective short-acting β_2-adrenergic agonists currently are recommended by an expert panel of the National Asthma Education and Prevention Program (NAEPP) for prehospital management of asthma exacerbations (e.g., in emergency medicine facilities and/or ambulances). During prolonged emergency transport, NAEPP recommends that other asthma therapies such as ipratropium bromide and oral corticosteroids also be available for use. In patients with acute exacerbations of asthma†, ipratropium generally has been reserved for use as an adjunct to other therapy, usually in combination with a β_2-adrenergic agonist bronchodilator. Because of its delayed onset, ipratropium generally should not be used *alone* for the management of *acute* bronchospasm, particularly if a prompt response is required. Some clinicians suggest that *adjunctive* therapy with ipratropium be considered in the emergency department in patients with moderate or severe exacerbations (peak expiratory flow [PEF] 60–80% or less than 60%, respectively, of predicted or personal best) of asthma who fail to respond adequately to β_2-adrenergic agonists and corticosteroids. NAEPP recommends adjunctive therapy with ipratropium (via nebulization or a metered-dose inhaler) and oral corticosteroids in patients with severe asthma exacerbations (FEV_1 or PEF less than 40% of predicted or personal best) who fail to respond adequately to short-acting, inhaled β_2-agonists. In patients with impending respiratory failure in the emergency department, ipratropium in combination with a short-acting β_2-adrenergic agonist (via nebulization) and an IV corticosteroid is recommended. In certain children with acute exacerbations of asthma, some evidence suggests that orally inhaled ipratropium (via nebulization) in conjunction with an orally inhaled β_2-adrenergic agonist (via nebulization) may be more effective than therapy with the β_2-agonist alone; in one study in children with severe acute asthma, children with the most severe bronchospasm (defined as baseline FEV_1 not exceeding 30% of predicted) who received via nebulization repeated doses of ipratropium in conjunction with albuterol were less likely to require hospitalization or additional bronchodilator therapy than children receiving albuterol alone. However, ipratropium does not appear to confer additional benefit in children once they have been hospitalized and treated with an intensive regimen including a nebulized β_2-agonist and systemic corticosteroids. Based on such data in children, NAEPP recommends discontinuance of ipratropium upon hospitalization for severe asthma exacerbations for patients of all age groups.

The benefit of maintenance therapy with ipratropium in patients with chronic asthma† remains to be elucidated, but the drug may be useful as alternative therapy in adults experiencing adverse effects (e.g., tachycardia, arrhythmia, tremor) with a β_2-adrenergic agonist. Some experts currently consider orally inhaled anticholinergics to have a limited role or no role in the long-term management of asthma in children because of a lack of data on safety and efficacy.

Orally inhaled ipratropium may be particularly useful for preventing or reversing bronchospasm induced by β_2-adrenergic blocking agents† (e.g., propranolol) in asthmatic patients; β_2-adrenergic bronchodilators generally are ineffective for this indication in such patients.

Prevention of Exercise-Induced Bronchospasm Although orally inhaled ipratropium bromide has been effective in the prevention of exercise-induced asthma† in a limited number of patients, orally inhaled β_2-adrenergic agonists are considered first-line agents in the management of this condition.

Cystic Fibrosis Orally inhaled ipratropium bromide has produced bronchodilation (i.e., increase in FEV_1) in a limited number of patients with cystic fibrosis†, but additional studies are needed to determine the clinical usefulness of such therapy in these patients.

■ **Other Uses** Ipratropium also has been used in a limited number of patients to minimize increases in lung resistance following anesthetic induction and tracheal intubation†; to protect against bronchoconstriction in patients undergoing fiberoptic bronchoscopy†; and to improve pulmonary function in ventilator-dependent patients, including preterm infants†. In a few patients with COPD and myasthenia gravis, ipratropium has been used to counteract the bronchoconstriction and the increase in respiratory secretions associated with cholinesterase inhibitor (e.g., pyridostigmine) therapy† in these patients.

Ipratropium bromide is used as a 0.03% nasal spray for the symptomatic relief of rhinorrhea associated with allergic and nonallergic perennial rhinitis in adults and children 6 years of age or older. The drug also is used as a 0.06% nasal spray for the symptomatic relief of rhinorrhea associated with the common cold in adults and children 5 years of age or older.

Dosage and Administration

■ **Administration** Ipratropium bromide is administered by oral inhalation using an oral aerosol inhaler or via nebulization. Ipratropium bromide is administered in fixed combination with albuterol sulfate via a metered-dose aerosol inhaler or via nebulization. Patients should be advised that ipratropium must be used consistently throughout the course of therapy for maximum benefit. In addition, patients should be advised that the drug will *not* provide immediate symptomatic relief and should *not* be used for the relief of acute bronchospasm.

Oral Inhalation via Metered-Dose Aerosol **Ipratropium Bromide.** Patients should be instructed carefully in the use of the ipratropium bromide metered-dose inhaler. To obtain optimum results, patients also should be given a copy of the patient instructions provided by the manufacturer. The aerosol inhaler should be actuated twice prior to the initial use or if it has not been used for more than 3 days. To avoid inadvertent contact of the drug with the eyes and subsequent adverse effects, patients should be advised to close their eyes during inhalation of ipratropium aerosol; it also has been suggested that ipratropium aerosol not be administered using the open-mouth technique in patients at high risk for ocular toxicity. (See Cautions: Precautions and Contraindications and also see Cautions: Ocular Effects.)

After the patient exhales slowly and completely, the inhaler should be held upright and the mouthpiece of the inhaler placed well into the mouth with the lips closed firmly around it. The patient should then inhale slowly and deeply through the mouth while actuating the inhaler. After holding the breath for 10 seconds, the patient should remove the mouthpiece and exhale slowly. If additional inhalations are required, the patient should wait at least 15 seconds and repeat the procedure. The manufacturer recommends that the ipratropium oral inhaler be cleaned at least once a week by removing the canister and dust cap from the mouthpiece and rinsing the mouthpiece in warm water for at least 30 seconds; nothing other than water should be used to wash the mouthpiece. The mouthpiece should be dried by shaking off the excess water and allowing the mouthpiece to air dry. When the mouthpiece is dry, the mouthpiece and the canister should be reassembled; patients should make sure that the canister is fully inserted into the mouthpiece.

Ipratropium Bromide and Albuterol Sulfate. Patients should insert the metal canister into the clear end of the mouthpiece. The aerosol inhaler should be shaken well for at least 10 seconds immediately prior to use and should be actuated 3 times prior to the initial use or if it has not been used for more than 24 hours. The mouthpiece provided for the inhalation aerosol of ipratropium bromide and albuterol sulfate should not be used for other aerosol drugs. Prior to use, the orange dust cap should be removed and the mouthpiece should be checked for foreign objects. Patients should avoid spraying ipratropium bromide and albuterol sulfate inhalation aerosol into their eyes. To avoid inadvertent contact of the drug with the eyes and subsequent adverse effects (e.g., temporary blurred vision, precipitation or worsening of narrow-angle glaucoma, ocular pain), patients should be advised to close their eyes during inhalation of ipratropium bromide and albuterol sulfate aerosol. (See Cautions: Precautions and Contraindications and also see Cautions: Ocular Effects.)

The patient should exhale deeply within 30 seconds of shaking the aerosol inhaler and the mouthpiece of the inhaler should be placed into the mouth with the canister held upright. The patient should then inhale slowly and deeply through the mouth while actuating the inhaler. After holding the breath for 10 seconds, the patient should remove the mouthpiece and exhale slowly. If additional inhalations are required, the patient should wait approximately 2 minutes and repeat the procedure. The manufacturer recommends that the ipratropium bromide and albuterol sulfate oral inhaler mouthpiece be cleaned as needed by rinsing the mouthpiece in hot water. If soap is used, the mouthpiece should be rinsed thoroughly with plain water. When dry, the cap on the mouthpiece should be replaced when the inhaler is not in use.

Oral Inhalation via Nebulization **Ipratropium Bromide.** Prior to administration of ipratropium bromide inhalation solution for nebulization, the nebulizer manufacturer's information should be reviewed to ensure thorough familiarity with the use and maintenance of the nebulizer. For administration of ipratropium bromide alone via a nebulizer, the entire contents of the single-use vial of solution should be emptied into the nebulizer reservoir and the reservoir attached to the mouthpiece or face mask and to the compressor according to the manufacturer's instructions. When a face mask is used to deliver the drug during nebulization, care should be taken to avoid leakage around the mask because transient blurred vision and other adverse effects may result if the drug enters the eyes. (See Cautions: Ocular Effects.) To avoid inadvertent entry of drug into the eye, it may be preferable to administer nebulized ipratropium bromide using a mouthpiece rather than a face mask.

The patient should place the mouthpiece of the nebulizer between the teeth and on top of the tongue and close the lips firmly around it, taking care not to block the airflow from the mouthpiece with the tongue. The patient should then breathe through the mouthpiece as calmly, deeply, and evenly as possible until the nebulizer stops producing mist. The duration of treatment for oral inhalation of a full dose of ipratropium usually is about 5–15 minutes. The nebulizer should be cleaned after use according to the manufacturer's instructions.

Ipratropium bromide inhalation solution contains no preservatives; the manufacturer states that once the single-use vial is opened, the entire contents must be used or the remainder discarded. When ipratropium bromide is mixed extemporaneously in a nebulizer with albuterol sulfate, metaproterenol sulfate, or cromolyn sodium solution for oral inhalation, the resulting solutions are stable for 1 hour; the manufacturer states that the drug stability and safety of ipratropium bromide inhalation solution mixed with other drugs in a nebulizer have not been established.

Ipratropium Bromide and Albuterol Sulfate. Prior to administration of ipratropium bromide and albuterol sulfate inhalation solution for nebulization, the nebulizer manufacturer's information should be reviewed to assess any changes in administration. For administration of ipratropium bromide in fixed combination with albuterol sulfate (DuoNeb®) via a nebulizer, the entire contents of the single-use vial of solution should be emptied into the nebulizer reservoir and the reservoir attached to the mouthpiece or face mask and to the compressor according to the manufacturer's instructions.

The patient should place the mouthpiece of the nebulizer into the mouth. Alternatively, patients may put the face mask over the mouth and nose. The patient should then breathe through the mouth as calmly, deeply, and evenly as possible until the nebulizer stops producing mist. The duration of treatment for oral inhalation of a full dose of ipratropium and albuterol sulfate in fixed combination usually is about 5–15 minutes. The nebulizer should be cleaned after use according to the manufacturer's instructions.

■ **Dosage** ***Oral Inhalation via Metered-Dose Aerosol*** Dosage of ipratropium bromide oral inhalation aerosol (Atrovent® HFA) is expressed in terms of the monohydrate. Dosage of ipratropium bromide in fixed combination with albuterol sulfate is expressed in terms of the monohydrate and dosage of albuterol sulfate is expressed in terms of albuterol.

While some published studies and manufacturers have reported a dose of 20–21 mcg of ipratropium bromide per metered spray, this is the amount released from the valve stem during actuation of the inhaler; the dose of ipratropium bromide alone or in fixed combination with albuterol sulfate delivered to the patient through the mouthpiece (actuator) is approximately 17 or 18 mcg, respectively, per metered spray. The commercially available aerosols deliver 200 metered sprays per canister. The actual amount of drug delivered to the lung via a metered-dose aerosol inhaler may depend on patient factors, such as coordination between actuation of the device and inspiration through the delivery system. The inhaler should be discarded after 200 sprays have been used.

COPD. For the management of bronchospasm associated with COPD, the usual initial dosage of ipratropium bromide administered via a metered-dose aerosol (Atrovent® HFA) in adults is 34 mcg (2 inhalations) 4 times daily. If necessary, additional inhalations of ipratropium bromide may be used. The manufacturer of Atrovent® HFA states that the dosage of ipratropium bromide should not exceed 204 mcg (12 inhalations) in 24 hours, although some clinicians suggest that even higher dosages of ipratropium bromide (up to 6 inhalations 4 times daily) may be used without notable adverse effects. The manufacturer recommends that 15 seconds elapse between successive inhalations of ipratropium.

The usual initial dosage of ipratropium bromide administered in fixed combination with albuterol sulfate (90 mcg of albuterol base per inhalation) via a metered-dose aerosol (Combivent®) in adults is 36 mcg (2 inhalations) 4 times daily. If necessary, additional inhalations of ipratropium bromide combined with albuterol sulfate may be used. The manufacturer recommends that approximately 2 minutes elapse between successive inhalations of ipratropium in fixed combination with albuterol. Since fatalities have been reported in association with excessive use of inhaled β_2-adrenergic agents in patients with asthma, the manufacturer of the fixed combination of ipratropium bromide and albuterol sulfate recommends *not* exceeding 12 inhalations (216 mcg of ipratropium bromide) in 24 hours. (See Cautions: Precautions and Contraindications, in Albuterol Sulfate 12:12.08.12.)

When COPD symptoms are not controlled with ipratropium alone or in fixed combination with albuterol (e.g., if there is a need to increase the dose or frequency of administration of the drug), medical assistance should be sought immediately. The dose or frequency of administration of ipratropium alone or in fixed combination with albuterol should not be increased without consultation with a clinician.

Asthma. For initial management of severe asthma exacerbations† (forced expiratory volume in 1 second [FEV_1] or peak expiratory flow [PEF] of less than 40% of predicted or personal best) in the emergency department in adolescents 12 years of age or older† and adults receiving ipratropium bromide as the metered-dose aerosol (Atrovent® HFA), an expert panel of the National

Asthma Education and Prevention Program (NAEPP) recommends a dose of 136 mcg (8 inhalations, 17 mcg per inhalation) every 20 minutes as needed for up to 3 hours, given in conjunction with a short-acting inhaled β_2-adrenergic agonist (administered separately). In children younger than 12 years of age† with severe asthma exacerbations†, NAEPP recommends an ipratropium bromide dose of 68–136 mcg (4–8 inhalations, 17 mcg per inhalation) as the metered-dose aerosol every 20 minutes as needed for up to 3 hours, given in conjunction with a short-acting inhaled β_2-adrenergic agonist (administered separately).

For initial management of severe asthma exacerbations† (FEV_1 or PEF of less than 40% of predicted or personal best) in the emergency department in adolescents 12 years of age or older† and adults receiving the fixed combination of ipratropium bromide and albuterol sulfate (90 mcg of albuterol base per inhalation) as the metered-dose aerosol, NAEPP recommends an ipratropium bromide dose of 144 mcg (8 inhalations, 18 mcg per inhalation) every 20 minutes as needed for up to 3 hours. For initial management of severe asthma exacerbations† in children younger than 12 years of age†, NAEPP recommends an ipratropium bromide dose of 72–144 mcg (4–8 inhalations, 18 mcg per inhalation) every 20 minutes as needed for up to 3 hours.

Oral Inhalation via Nebulization Dosage of ipratropium bromide inhalation solution for nebulization is expressed in terms of anhydrous drug. Dosage of ipratropium bromide in fixed combination with albuterol sulfate (as albuterol base) for nebulization is expressed as the monohydrate. Using in vitro testing at an average flow rate of 3.6 L per minute for an average of 15 minutes or less, the Pari-LC Plus® nebulizer delivered at the mouthpiece approximately 46 or 42% of the original dosage of albuterol or ipratropium bromide, respectively.

COPD. For administration via a nebulizer, the usual dosage of ipratropium bromide in adults with COPD is 500 mcg 3 or 4 times daily (i.e., every 6–8 hours). To administer 500 mcg of the drug, the contents of a single-use vial (2.5 mL) of the commercially available 0.02% solution of ipratropium bromide may be used.

The usual dosage of ipratropium bromide in fixed combination with albuterol sulfate (as 2.5 mg of albuterol base) for nebulization (DuoNeb®) in adults with COPD is 500 mcg 4 times daily, with up to 2 additional inhalations allowed daily. The flow rate of the nebulizer should be adjusted so that the dose is delivered over a period of approximately 5–15 minutes. The manufacturer of DuoNeb® recommends *not* exceeding 6 inhalations daily since such dosages have not been studied for the treatment of COPD.

Asthma. For initial management of severe asthma exacerbations† in the emergency department, an expert panel of the NAEPP recommends an ipratropium bromide dosage of 500 mcg via nebulization every 20 minutes for 3 doses initially (i.e., for the first hour) in adults and adolescents 12 years of age or older† in conjunction with a short-acting inhaled β_2-adrenergic agonist. For initial management of severe asthma exacerbations† in children younger than 12 years of age†, 250–500 mcg of ipratropium bromide may be given via nebulization every 20 minutes for 3 doses initially (i.e., for the first hour), in conjunction with a short-acting inhaled β_2-adrenergic agonist. Alternatively, ipratropium bromide via nebulization may be used continuously for the first hour after admittance to the emergency department in patients with severe asthma exacerbations. If there is no improvement after the first hour of treatment, ipratropium bromide in conjunction with a short-acting inhaled β_2-adrenergic agonist may be continued for no more than 2 additional hours for a total duration of 3 hours in the emergency department, with the frequency of administration after the first hour based on improvement in airflow obstruction and other symptoms and occurrence of adverse effects. Similarly, if a severe exacerbation develops after the first hour of treatment with a short-acting β_2-adrenergic agonist and an oral corticosteroid, ipratropium bromide in conjunction with a short-acting inhaled β_2-adrenergic agonist may be initiated and continued for no more than 2 additional hours. If the patient is admitted to the hospital, ipratropium bromide should be discontinued since benefit of the drug in conjunction with short-acting inhaled β_2-adrenergic agonist therapy (e.g., albuterol) has not been established once patients with severe asthma exacerbations are hospitalized.

Cautions

Adverse effects reported with orally inhaled ipratropium bromide are similar to those reported with other antimuscarinic drugs; however, because of the drug's limited systemic absorption, oral inhalation of ipratropium bromide produces anticholinergic adverse effects (e.g., increased intraocular pressure, mydriasis, urinary retention) less frequently than systemically administered antimuscarinic drugs. For further information on adverse effects reported with antimuscarinics, see Cautions in the Antimuscarinics/Antispasmodics General Statement 12:08.08. In comparative clinical trials, adverse effects reported with ipratropium inhalation aerosol employing a hydrofluoroalkane (HFA) propellant (ipratropium HFA) were similar to those reported with the drug in a preparation containing chlorofluorocarbon (CFC) propellants (ipratropium CFC aerosol; no longer commercially available in the US).

Unless otherwise stated, adverse effects mentioned in the Cautions section are those reported in patients receiving orally inhaled (via metered-dose inhaler or nebulizer) ipratropium and may or may not be directly attributable to the drug.

Orally inhaled ipratropium therapy generally is well tolerated and has a low incidence of adverse effects. No additive effect on the incidence of adverse effects was observed after short-term oral inhalation therapy with the fixed combination of albuterol and ipratropium as an aerosol. In a large, uncontrolled study in seriously ill patients receiving ipratropium inhalation aerosol, about 7% of patients required discontinuance of the drug because of adverse effects. In controlled clinical studies with nebulized ipratropium, adverse effects resulting in discontinuance of the drug most frequently included respiratory effects such as bronchitis, dyspnea, and bronchospasm. In controlled clinical studies with orally inhaled ipratropium HFA via a metered-dose inhaler, the most frequent drug-related adverse effects included dry mouth and taste perversion.

■ **Respiratory Effects** Bronchitis or upper respiratory tract infection was reported in 14.6 or 13.2% of patients, respectively, receiving nebulized ipratropium in controlled studies, although these effects may not necessarily be attributable to the drug. Bronchitis or upper respiratory tract infection was reported in 12.3 or 10.9%, respectively, of patients receiving the fixed combination of albuterol and ipratropium inhalation aerosol. Bronchitis was reported in 10–23%, and upper respiratory tract infection in 9–34% of patients receiving ipratropium HFA inhalation aerosol in controlled clinical trials. Cough following inhalation of ipratropium CFC inhalation aerosol (no longer commercially available in the US) has been reported in about 4.6–5.9% of patients with chronic obstructive pulmonary disease (COPD) in controlled clinical studies, and in 4.2% of patients receiving the fixed combination of albuterol and ipratropium inhalation aerosol. Coughing or exacerbation of COPD symptoms has been reported in 3–5 or 8–23%, respectively, of patients receiving ipratropium HFA inhalation aerosol in controlled clinical trials. Exacerbation of respiratory symptoms occurred in about 2.4% of patients receiving ipratropium CFC aerosol (no longer commercially available in the US) in controlled studies and reportedly is more common in patients receiving nebulized dosages of 2 mg or more daily. Dyspnea, pharyngitis, or increase in sputum was reported in 9.6, 3.7, or 1.4% of patients, respectively, receiving nebulized ipratropium in controlled studies, while bronchospasm, sinusitis, or rhinitis each was reported in 2.3% of such patients. Dyspnea, pharyngitis, sinusitis, bronchospasm, or rhinitis was reported in 4.5, 2.2, 2.3, 0.3, or 1.1%, respectively, of patients receiving the fixed combination of ipratropium and albuterol inhalation aerosol in controlled studies. Dyspnea, rhinitis, or sinusitis has been reported in 7–8, 4–6, or 1–11%, respectively, of patients receiving ipratropium bromide HFA inhalation aerosol in clinical trials. Influenza was reported in 1.4% of patients receiving combined ipratropium and albuterol inhalation aerosol in controlled studies. Influenza-like symptoms occurred in 4–8% of patients receiving ipratropium HFA inhalation aerosol in clinical trials. Irritation from the aerosol occurred in about 2% of patients receiving ipratropium aerosol in controlled studies; drying of secretions or hoarseness was reported in 1% or less of patients receiving the aerosol. As with other inhaled drugs for asthma, paradoxical bronchospasm has been reported in a few patients receiving ipratropium nebulized solution, inhalation aerosol, or the fixed combination (with albuterol) inhalation aerosol, although a causal relationship to the drug has not been definitely established. (See Cautions: Dermatologic and Sensitivity Reactions.) Lower respiratory tract disorders or pneumonia was reported in 2.5 or 1.4% of patients, respectively, receiving orally inhaled albuterol and ipratropium in fixed combination. Nasal congestion or wheezing also has been reported in patients receiving the fixed combination of albuterol and ipratropium inhalation aerosol.

Unlike β_2-adrenergic agonists, inhalation of ipratropium does not aggravate hypoxemia in patients with airway obstruction.

■ **GI Effects** Dryness of the mouth, throat, or tongue occurred in up to 5% of patients receiving orally inhaled ipratropium CFC inhalation aerosol (no longer commercially available in the US) or ipratropium via nebulization; dry mouth reportedly occurs more frequently with nebulized dosages of 2 mg or more daily. Nausea, GI distress, or constipation has been reported in about 4.1, 2.4, or 0.9% of patients receiving the drug. Nausea has been reported in 2% of patients receiving the fixed combination of albuterol and ipratropium inhalation aerosol. Paralytic ileus, thirst, bad/bitter taste, mucosal ulcers, and reduced appetite have occurred rarely with ipratropium therapy. Diarrhea, dyspepsia, or vomiting has been reported in less than 2% of patients receiving combined albuterol and ipratropium inhalation aerosol. Dyspepsia, dry mouth, or nausea has been reported in 1–5, 2–4, or 4%, respectively, of patients receiving ipratropium HFA inhalation aerosol in clinical trials.

■ **Ocular Effects** Blurred vision/difficulty in accommodation has been reported in about 1% of patients receiving orally inhaled ipratropium. Burning eyes, mydriasis, temporary blurred vision, ocular pain (sometimes acute), conjunctival or corneal congestion associated with visual halos or colored images, or precipitation or worsening of angle-closure glaucoma also has been reported, probably because of inadvertent contact of the drug with the eyes during administration. Increased intraocular pressure (IOP) has been reported in patients with angle-closure glaucoma receiving nebulized solutions of ipratropium alone or combined with albuterol, apparently as a result of the drug solution escaping from the face mask and entering the eyes. (See Cautions: Precautions and Contraindications.) Increased IOP also has been reported with ipratropium inhalation aerosol and with concomitant administration of ipratropium aerosol (using the open-mouth technique) and nebulized albuterol. While blurred vision has been reported in children given nebulized ipratropium and albuterol via face mask, acute angle-closure glaucoma as a result of environmental exposure to these drugs apparently has not occurred in parents, nurses, or respiratory therapists caring for children undergoing such therapy.

■ Cardiovascular Effects Ipratropium inhalation aerosol and solution for nebulization appear to cause adverse cardiovascular effects less frequently than β_2-adrenergic agonists or theophylline. Palpitation has occurred in up to 3% of patients receiving orally inhaled ipratropium. Chest pain has been reported in 3.2%, and induction or aggravation of hypertension in about 1% of patients receiving nebulized ipratropium in controlled studies. Angina was reported in less than 2% of patients receiving the fixed-combination inhalation aerosol of albuterol and ipratropium in controlled studies. Extrasystole, tachycardia, vasodilation, and hypotension have been reported infrequently with orally inhaled ipratropium therapy. Hospitalizations for supraventricular tachycardia and atrial fibrillation occurred in 0.5% of patients receiving ipratropium inhalation aerosol.

Data from an observational study involving over 32,000 patients and another pooled analysis of 17 studies enrolling almost 15,000 patients have shown an increased risk of mortality and/or cardiovascular events (e.g., myocardial infarction, stroke, transient ischemic attacks) in patients receiving inhaled anticholinergic agents, including ipratropium. (See Cautions: Precautions and Contraindications.)

■ Nervous System Effects Because of the drug's low lipid solubility, orally inhaled ipratropium produces adverse nervous system effects less frequently than orally inhaled atropine or β_2-adrenergic agonists. Nervousness, dizziness, and headache have occurred in about 0.5–6.4% of patients receiving orally inhaled ipratropium CFC inhalation aerosol (no longer commercially available in the US). Headache or dizziness occurred in 6–7 or 3%, respectively, of patients receiving ipratropium HFA inhalation aerosol in clinical trials. Headache occurs more frequently in patients receiving nebulized ipratropium bromide in total dosages of 2 mg or more daily. Fatigue or insomnia has been reported in less than 1% of patients receiving the drug. Paresthesia, drowsiness, coordination difficulty, and tremor also have been reported; tremor occurs less frequently with ipratropium than with β_2-adrenergic agonists or theophylline. Weakness or CNS stimulation has been reported in patients receiving albuterol and/or ipratropium inhalation aerosol.

■ Dermatologic and Sensitivity Reactions Immediate hypersensitivity reactions, including rash, angioedema of the tongue, lips, and face, urticaria (including giant urticaria), laryngospasm, bronchospasm, oropharyngeal edema, and anaphylactic reaction, have been reported in patients receiving orally inhaled ipratropium, with positive results upon rechallenge in some cases. Many of these patients had a history of allergies to other drugs and/or foods, including peanuts and soybeans (soya lecithin is present as an excipient in the fixed-combination inhalation aerosol containing ipratropium and albuterol sulfate). Paradoxical bronchospasm has occurred occasionally with the use of ipratropium via nebulizer or oral aerosol. While it has been suggested that such bronchospasm may result from hypersensitivity to the active drug or other ingredients in the formulation, altered bronchial reactivity in atopic individuals with asthma, or the acidity of the nebulized solution, such reactions also have occurred following administration of isotonic, pH 7, preservative-free solutions of ipratropium.

Rash was reported in 1.2%, and urticaria in less than 3% of patients receiving orally inhaled ipratropium in controlled studies. Pruritus, flushing, or alopecia has been reported in less than 1% of patients receiving ipratropium aerosol. Contact dermatitis has occurred in at least one patient receiving nebulized ipratropium.

■ Genitourinary Effects Although no alteration in micturition function was observed in a controlled study in a small number of geriatric men receiving orally inhaled ipratropium, urinary retention/difficulty has been reported occasionally in patients receiving the drug. Urinary tract infection or dysuria also has been reported in patients receiving ipratropium.

■ Other Effects Pain, back pain, or flu-like symptoms have occurred in 4.1, 3.2, or 3.7% of patients, respectively, receiving nebulized ipratropium in controlled studies; arthritis has been reported in 0.9% of such patients. Back pain occurred in 2–7% of patients receiving ipratropium HFA inhalation aerosol in clinical trials. Pain or arthralgia also has been reported in 2.5 or less than 2% of patients, respectively, receiving albuterol and ipratropium in fixed combination in controlled studies. Tinnitus also has occurred with ipratropium therapy. Although a causal relationship has not been established, a slight elevation of serum ALT (SGPT) has been reported during therapy with the drug.

Long-term toxicology studies in monkeys using orally inhaled ipratropium bromide dosages of up to 1.6 mg daily for 6 months did not reveal gross or microscopic changes consistent with systemic anticholinergic activity. Food consumption was reduced and body weight decreased in purebred beagles given oral ipratropium bromide dosages of up to 75 mg/kg daily for 1 year.

■ Precautions and Contraindications Although the toxic potential of orally inhaled ipratropium generally is less than that of other antimuscarinics because of its poor systemic absorption, the usual precautions of antimuscarinic therapy should be considered during therapy with ipratropium (e.g., the drug should be used with caution in patients with angle-closure glaucoma, bladder neck obstruction or prostatic hyperplasia). (See Cautions in the Antimuscarinics/Antispasmodics General Statement 12:08.08.)

When the preparation containing ipratropium bromide in fixed combination with albuterol sulfate is used, the cautions, precautions, and contraindications applicable to albuterol sulfate should be considered. Adverse cardiovascular effects (e.g., alterations in heart rate, blood pressure, or other manifestations) have been noted with albuterol in fixed combination with ipratropium as an inhalation aerosol; the combination aerosol should be discontinued if such effects occur.

The manufacturer warns that orally inhaled ipratropium is *not* indicated for the *initial* treatment of acute episodes of bronchospasm when a rapid response is required. For additional information on the use of ipratropium in asthma, see Asthma under Uses: Bronchospasm. In addition, use of orally inhaled ipratropium as a *single* agent for the management of bronchospasm in patients experiencing an acute exacerbation of COPD has not been adequately studied, and an agent with a faster onset of action (e.g., a β_2-adrenergic agonist) may be preferred as *initial* therapy in such patients.

Patients should be reminded that orally inhaled ipratropium is not intended for occasional use; it should be used consistently throughout the course of therapy for maximum effectiveness. Patients should contact their clinician if symptoms of COPD are not relieved by ipratropium or if a previously effective dosage regimen fails to provide the usual relief (i.e., the frequency of administration of the drug needs to be increased). The dosage or frequency of administration of ipratropium inhalation aerosol should not be increased without consultation with a clinician.

Data from an observational study involving over 32,000 patients and another pooled analysis have shown an increased risk of mortality and/or cardiovascular events, including stroke or transient ischemic attacks, in patients receiving inhaled anticholinergic agents, including ipratropium. (See Cautions: Cardiovascular Effects.) While data are conflicting, a possible increased risk of stroke has also been identified from ongoing safety monitoring and pooled analysis of placebo-controlled trials in patients receiving another anticholinergic agent, tiotropium. However, preliminary analysis of a placebo-controlled trial in approximately 6000 patients with COPD did not reveal an increased risk of stroke with tiotropium bromide. FDA has not yet confirmed the results of these analyses and is currently reviewing postmarketing adverse event reports and preliminary results of a recently completed placebo-controlled trial to assess additional long-term safety data and further evaluate the risk of stroke with tiotropium.

As with other inhaled drugs, paradoxical bronchospasm has been reported in a few patients receiving ipratropium nebulized solution, inhalation aerosol, or the fixed-combination (with albuterol) inhalation aerosol, although a causal relationship to the drug has not been definitely established. Ipratropium should be discontinued immediately if bronchoconstriction occurs, and alternative therapy instituted.

Temporary blurred vision, mydriasis, ocular pain, conjunctival or corneal congestion associated with visual halos or colored images, or precipitation or worsening of angle-closure glaucoma may occur following inadvertent contact of ipratropium with the eyes; therefore, when the drug is administered via a nebulizer, procedures to minimize ocular exposure should be employed (e.g., using a mouthpiece rather than a face mask to deliver the drug). In addition, patients should be instructed to close their eyes during oral inhalation of ipratropium aerosol. Patients should contact their clinician immediately if ocular symptoms develop after use of ipratropium inhalation aerosol.

Orally inhaled ipratropium should be used with caution in patients with angle-closure glaucoma, although the drug has been used in patients with open-angle glaucoma without clinically important effects on pupil size, accommodation, visual acuity, or intraocular pressure (IOP). Since the risk of ocular toxicity of ipratropium is associated with local exposure of the eye to aerosolized/nebulized drug, care to avoid such exposure is particularly important in patients who are at increased risk from the ocular consequences of exposure. Therefore, some clinicians suggest that ipratropium aerosol should not be administered using the open-mouth technique in patients at high risk for ocular toxicity (e.g., those with angle-closure glaucoma). It also has been suggested that children with blindness (e.g., marked retinal detachment secondary to retinopathy of prematurity, infantile or childhood glaucoma, traumatic cataracts, or dislocation of the lens) should not receive ipratropium via nebulization.

The manufacturer states that ipratropium should be used with caution in patients with renal or hepatic impairment because the drug has not been evaluated systematically in these patient groups. Albuterol and ipratropium inhalation aerosol should be used with caution in patients with cardiovascular disorders (especially coronary insufficiency, cardiac arrhythmias, or hypertension), seizure disorders, hyperthyroidism, diabetes mellitus, and in those who are unusually responsive to β_2-adrenergic agents.

Ipratropium aerosol and inhalation solution for nebulization are contraindicated in patients with known hypersensitivity to the drug or any other component of the respective formulation, or to atropine or its derivatives. Ipratropium aerosol in fixed combination with albuterol sulfate also is contraindicated in patients with known hypersensitivity to soya lecithin or related food products, including soybeans and peanuts.

■ Pediatric Precautions The manufacturer states that safety and efficacy of orally inhaled ipratropium via a metered-dose inhaler in pediatric patients have not been established, although the drug has been used in such patients (generally in children with asthma) with no unusual risk. The safety and efficacy ipratropium bromide for oral inhalation via nebulization have not been established in patients younger than 12 years of age. The safety and efficacy of albuterol sulfate in fixed combination with ipratropium bromide for oral inhalation via nebulization have not been established in patients younger than 18 years of age.

■ Geriatric Precautions When the total number of patients studied in clinical trials of ipratropium HFA inhalation aerosol is considered, 57% were

65 years of age or older. No overall differences in efficacy or safety were observed between geriatric and younger patients in these studies.

Safety and efficacy of ipratropium bromide in fixed combination with albuterol sulfate inhalation solution in geriatric patients have not been specifically studied to date; however, in clinical studies of the combination for the treatment of bronchospasm, approximately 62% of the patients were 65 years of age or older and 19% were 75 years of age or older. Although no overall differences were observed between geriatric and younger patients in the safety and efficacy of the combination in clinical studies, the possibility that some older patients may exhibit increased sensitivity to the drug cannot be ruled out.

■ Mutagenicity and Carcinogenicity No evidence of mutagenicity was seen with ipratropium in an in vitro microbial mutagen test (Ames test), the mouse micronucleus test, or the mouse dominant lethal assay, nor did the drug induce chromosomal aberrations in the bone marrow of Chinese hamsters.

No evidence of carcinogenic potential was seen in rats or mice receiving oral ipratropium bromide at dosages up to 6 mg/kg daily for 2 years.

■ Pregnancy, Fertility, and Lactation Reproduction studies in mice, rats, and rabbits receiving oral ipratropium bromide dosages of 10, 1000, and 125 mg/kg daily (approximately 200, 40,000, and 10,000 times the maximum recommended human daily inhalation dosage on a mg/m^2 basis), respectively, and in rats or rabbits receiving orally inhaled ipratropium bromide dosages of 1.5 or 1.8 mg/kg (approximately 60 or 140 times the maximum recommended human daily inhalation dosage on a mg/m^2 basis), respectively, have not revealed evidence of harm to the fetus. There are no adequate and controlled studies to date using orally inhaled ipratropium in pregnant women, and the drug should be used during pregnancy only when clearly needed.

Reproduction studies in male and female rats using oral ipratropium bromide dosages up to 50 mg/kg daily have not revealed evidence of impaired fertility; however, the drug was associated with impaired fertility (i.e., increased resorption) when given at an oral dosage exceeding 90 mg/kg in rats (approximately 3600 times the maximum recommended human daily inhalation dosage on a mg/m^2 basis). As these results were not obtained at dosages and a route of administration that were clinically relevant, the manufacturer states that such embryotoxic effects in rats are not considered clinically important.

It is not known whether ipratropium is distributed into milk in humans, but highly lipophobic quaternary bases are distributed slowly and at low concentrations into milk. Because ipratropium is not well absorbed systemically following oral inhalation, the manufacturer states that ingestion of substantial amounts of the drug by an infant during breast-feeding is unlikely. The manufacturer recommends that orally inhaled ipratropium be used with caution in nursing women.

Drug Interactions

The manufacturer states that because of the limited systemic absorption and low plasma drug concentrations associated with oral inhalation of ipratropium, it is unlikely that the drug would interact with systemically administered drugs. The manufacturer states that patients taking ipratropium bromide in fixed combination with albuterol sulfate should not use other inhaled agents unless directed by a clinician.

Adverse drug interactions have not been reported with concomitant administration of orally inhaled ipratropium and a β-adrenergic agonist bronchodilator (e.g., albuterol, fenoterol [currently not commercially available in the US], isoproterenol, metaproterenol), theophylline derivatives, oral or inhaled corticosteroids, or cromolyn sodium in clinical studies in patients with chronic obstructive pulmonary disease (COPD) or asthma.

While concomitant inhalation of ipratropium and a β_2-adrenergic agonist may not always result in substantial additional bronchodilation compared with inhalation of either agent alone, such combined therapy usually increases the duration of bronchodilation. Concomitant administration of ipratropium and albuterol via nebulization has been reported to increase intraocular pressure (IOP) and precipitate acute angle-closure glaucoma in susceptible individuals (i.e., individuals with untreated or undiagnosed angle-closure glaucoma), probably as a result of inadvertent contact of the drugs with the eyes. (See Cautions: Ocular Effects.) Caution is advised if the fixed combination of albuterol and ipratropium inhalation aerosol is used concomitantly with other β_2-adrenergic agents since the risk for adverse cardiovascular effects increases.

Although ipratropium inhalation aerosol is minimally absorbed into the systemic circulation, there is some potential for additive interaction with concomitantly used antimuscarinic agents. Therefore, caution is advised when ipratropium aerosol is used concomitantly with other antimuscarinic agents.

For further information on drug interactions reported with antimuscarinics, see Drug Interactions in the Antimuscarinics/Antispasmodics General Statement 12:08.08.

Acute Toxicity

Toxicology studies in animals indicate that ipratropium exhibits a low order of toxicity compared with that of other anticholinergic and bronchospasmolytic agents.

■ Pathogenesis The acute lethal dose of ipratropium bromide in humans is not known. The manufacturer states that ipratropium overdosage as a result of oral inhalation or oral administration is unlikely because systemic absorption of the drug is minimal after inhalation or oral administration of up to 4- or 40-fold the recommended oral inhalation dose, respectively.

The IV LD_{50} of ipratropium bromide in dogs, male rats, female rats, female mice, or male mice is approximately 17.5–20, 16, 15.7, 15, or 12.3 mg/kg, respectively. The oral LD_{50} of ipratropium bromide in rats, mice, or dogs is 1700 mg/kg (approximately 68,000 times the maximum recommended human daily inhalation dosage on a mg/m^2 basis), in excess of 1 g/kg (approximately 20,000 times the maximum recommended human daily inhalation dosage on a mg/m^2 basis), or 400 mg/kg (approximately 53,000 times the maximum human daily inhalation dosage on a mg/m^2 basis), respectively. The subcutaneous LD_{50} of ipratropium bromide in male or female mice is approximately 300 or 340 mg/kg, respectively. The inhalation LD_{50} of ipratropium bromide is about 200 mg/kg in guinea pigs and about 1 mg/kg in monkeys. The oral lethal dose of ipratropium ranges from 1001–2010 mg/kg in mice (approximately 30,000 and 60,000 times the maximum recommended human daily inhalation dose on a mg/m^2 basis), from 1667–4000 mg/kg in rats (approximately 100,000 and 240,000 times the maximum recommended human daily inhalation dose on a mg/m^2 basis), and from 400–1300 mg/kg in dogs (approximately 80,000 and 260,000 times the maximum recommended human daily inhalation dose on a mg/m^2 basis). Death from ipratropium bromide overdosage in animals usually resulted from inhibition of ganglionic transmission, which produced curariform paralysis of skeletal muscle.

■ Manifestations In general, overdosage of ipratropium bromide may be expected to produce effects associated with antimuscarinic administration; however, the manufacturer states that because of the low systemic absorption of orally inhaled ipratropium bromide, acute overdosage of the drug is unlikely following oral administration or oral inhalation.

For further information on acute overdosage reported with antimuscarinics, see Acute Toxicity in the Antimuscarinics/Antispasmodics General Statement 12:08.08.

Pharmacology

Ipratropium generally exhibits pharmacologic actions similar to those of other antimuscarinics. Similar to atropine, ipratropium is a nonselective competitive antagonist at muscarinic receptors present in airways and other organs. The drug relaxes smooth muscles of bronchi and bronchioles by blocking acetylcholine-induced stimulation of guanyl cyclase and thus reducing formation of cyclic guanosine monophosphate (cGMP), a mediator of bronchoconstriction. Ipratropium generally exhibits greater antimuscarinic activity on bronchial smooth muscle than on secretory (e.g., salivary, gastric) glands.

Following IV administration in animals, the antimuscarinic activity of ipratropium (as measured by mydriasis, inhibition of salivary or gastric secretions, tachycardia, or spasmolysis) is similar to that of atropine; following oral administration, the antimuscarinic activity of ipratropium is only about 10–50% that of atropine. In animals, the relative bronchoselectivity of ipratropium is even more pronounced with oral inhalation of the drug than with IV administration.

■ Respiratory Effects Ipratropium is a potent bronchodilator, particularly in large bronchial airways; however, some evidence suggests that the drug also has bronchodilator activity in small airways. Bronchodilation results from relaxation of smooth muscles of the bronchial tree. The extent of bronchodilation produced by ipratropium appears to be determined by the level of cholinergic parasympathetic bronchomotor tone and by inhibition of bronchoconstriction resulting from neural reflex activation of cholinergic pathways. The importance of cholinergic tone and neural reflexes in producing bronchoconstriction in airway disease remains to be determined; however, limited evidence indicates that cholinergic tone may be increased in patients with chronic obstructive pulmonary disease (COPD). In animals, the bronchodilator activity of ipratropium is similar to or exceeds that of atropine or isoproterenol and exceeds that of albuterol or metaproterenol when these drugs are given via nebulization. In patients with COPD, ipratropium is at least as effective in producing bronchodilation as β-adrenergic agonists. Combined use of ipratropium and a β_2-adrenergic agonist (e.g., albuterol) results in greater bronchodilation than either drug alone.

Ipratropium decreases airway resistance as measured by forced expiratory volume in 1 second (FEV_1) and forced expiratory flow during the middle half of forced vital capacity (FEF_{25-75}). Following oral inhalation of ipratropium in patients with pulmonary disease, FVC and specific airway conductance may increase and residual volume (RV) may decrease. In dose-ranging studies with ipratropium bromide inhalation aerosol in patients with chronic bronchitis, maximal bronchodilator effects reportedly were evident with ipratropium bromide doses of 36 mcg. Limited data suggest that in patients with COPD, the optimum dose (as determined by maximal increases in FEV_1 and forced vital capacity [FVC]) of nebulized ipratropium bromide is about 400 mcg. A 36-mcg dose (2 inhalations) of ipratropium bromide administered via a metered-dose inhaler appears to produce bronchodilation (defined as area under the FEV_1 curve) similar to that produced by a 100-mcg dose of ipratropium bromide administered via a nebulizer.

While systemic administration of anticholinergic agents can reduce the volume and fluidity of bronchial secretions, orally inhaled ipratropium has little or no effect on respiratory secretions. Orally inhaled ipratropium does not appear to have any substantial effect on sputum viscosity or, unlike atropine, on mucociliary clearance. Ipratropium decreases ciliary activity in vitro but to a smaller extent than atropine. Volume of sputum usually remains unchanged during ipratropium therapy.

Various mechanisms appear to be involved in irritant-, histamine-, exercise-, or allergen-induced bronchoconstriction, and the protective effect of ipratropium against a bronchoconstrictor stimulus appears to depend in part on the extent to which bronchospasm is mediated by vagal reflexes. As expected, orally inhaled ipratropium reliably prevents bronchospasm induced by cholinergic agonists such as methacholine or acetylcholine in both healthy individuals and asthmatic patients. Ipratropium also prevents bronchospasm induced by irritants such as sulfur dioxide, ozone, or cigarette smoke in healthy individuals, but generally is less effective in asthmatic patients whose airways are more reactive to such stimuli. Although in some asthmatic patients ipratropium may be effective in preventing bronchospasm provoked by allergens, histamine, exercise, bradykinin, prostaglandin $F_{2\alpha}$, adenosine monophosphate, or substance P (a noncholinergic neurotransmitter), patients with asthma exhibit considerable interindividual variation in their response to ipratropium; asthmatic patients in whom bronchoconstriction is mediated principally by the vagal reflex may respond better to the drug than those in whom other mechanisms predominate. Usual doses of orally inhaled ipratropium bromide in asthmatic patients provide little or no protection against bronchospasm induced by serotonin or leukotrienes. However, the drug does appear to prevent bronchospasm induced by β_2-adrenergic blocking agents, pentamidine, or psychogenic stimuli. In patients with COPD, cholinergic bronchomotor tone is the principal determinant of reversible airway constriction. Therefore, while patients with asthma show a variable response to anticholinergic bronchodilators, patients with COPD generally respond to these agents.

Inhalation of ipratropium does not appear to produce clinically important alterations in arterial oxygen or carbon dioxide tension; however, slight increases or decreases in arterial oxygen tension and slight decreases in carbon dioxide tension have been observed in some patients receiving the drug. In a limited number of studies in healthy adults or patients with COPD, no adverse effects on arterial pH, pulmonary blood pressure, or pulmonary diffusing capacity were observed following oral inhalation of ipratropium.

Tolerance to the bronchodilating effect of orally inhaled ipratropium does not appear to develop with prolonged use; the bronchodilator effect has been maintained throughout at least 5 years of continuous use in some patients.

■ **Cardiovascular Effects** Oral inhalation of ipratropium has not produced appreciable changes in heart rate, blood pressure, or cardiac rhythm in healthy adults, healthy adults with experimentally induced pulmonary hypertension, or patients with COPD or hypertension. Slight decreases in heart rate, accompanied by increases in stroke volume and ejection fraction, have been observed in healthy adults receiving high doses (e.g., up to 2.4 mg) of ipratropium bromide via a metered-dose inhaler; however, cardiac output in these patients remained unchanged, and these cardiovascular effects do not appear to be clinically important.

■ **GI Effects** Although orally inhaled ipratropium appears to have minimal effect on salivary secretions, the drug has produced inhibition of salivary secretions in animals and in healthy adults when given IV. Following oral administration of 15 mg of ipratropium bromide in healthy adults, basal gastric acid secretion decreased by 50% and gastric pH increased from 2.5 to 5 within 1 hour.

■ **Ocular Effects** Following IV administration of ipratropium in animals, the mydriatic activity of the drug is similar to that of atropine. When given by oral inhalation, ipratropium does not appear to produce mydriasis, increased intraocular pressure (IOP), or changes in ocular function in children or in adults with normal IOP or open-angle or angle-closure glaucoma. However, increased IOP and other adverse ocular effects have been reported during treatment with the drug, as a result of inadvertent exposure of the eyes during oral inhalation of ipratropium alone or combined with albuterol. (See Cautions: Ocular Effects.) β_2-Adrenergic agonists such as albuterol increase production of aqueous humor which, in combination with restricted outflow caused by anticholinergic-associated pupillary dilatation, may increase IOP and lead to acute angle-closure glaucoma in susceptible individuals (i.e., individuals with untreated or undiagnosed angle-closure glaucoma).

■ **Nervous System Effects** Because of its low lipid solubility, ipratropium, unlike atropine, does not appear to cross the blood-brain barrier. Current evidence indicates that the drug produces little or no CNS stimulation.

Pharmacokinetics

■ **Absorption** Following oral inhalation, ipratropium bromide is only minimally absorbed into systemic circulation from the surface of the lungs or from the GI tract. Following oral inhalation of 2 mg of ipratropium bromide via nebulization in healthy adults, approximately 7% (range: 1.4–16.3%) of the dose was absorbed into systemic circulation. Concomitant oral inhalation of ipratropium and albuterol in a fixed-combination aerosol did not alter the systemic absorption of either component. Following oral inhalation of 555 mcg of radiolabeled ipratropium bromide in healthy adults, radioactivity was detected in blood within 2 minutes, indicating rapid buccal and/or pulmonary absorption; peak plasma concentrations of about 0.06 ng/mL (as total radioactivity) occurred in about 1–3 hours. Following oral inhalation of a single, higher-than-recommended dose (4 inhalations, total dose 68 mcg) of ipratropium bromide (with a hydrofluoroalkane [HFA] propellant), mean peak plasma concentrations of ipratropium in a limited number of adult or geriatric patients with chronic obstructive pulmonary disease (COPD) were 59 or 56 pg/mL, respectively. Following administration of a higher-than-recommended dosage (4 inhalations 4 times daily, 272 mcg total daily dosage) of ipratropium (with HFA propellant) for 1 week, mean peak plasma ipratropium bromide concentrations in adult or geriatric patients increased to 82 or 84 pg/mL, respectively. The trough concentration of ipratropium 6 hours after inhalation in adult and geriatric patients was 28 pg/mL at steady state. Following oral inhalation of the fixed combination of albuterol sulfate (180 mcg as albuterol base) and ipratropium bromide monohydrate (36 mcg), peak plasma concentration of ipratropium bromide remained below detectable limits (less than 100 pg/mL); peak plasma concentrations of albuterol of about 492 pg/mL occurred within 3 hours after administration. Although most of a dose of an orally inhaled drug is actually swallowed, the bronchodilating action of ipratropium appears to result from a local action of the portion of the dose that reaches the bronchial tree.

Following oral aerosol inhalation of 34 mcg of ipratropium bromide (with HFA propellant) in patients with COPD, bronchodilation (as determined by an increase of 15% or more in FEV_1) is evident within 14–17.5 minutes, is maximal within 1–2 hours, and generally persists for 2–4 hours. The onset to a 15% increase in FEV_1 after oral inhalation of albuterol sulfate (180 mcg as albuterol base) and ipratropium bromide monohydrate (36 mcg) in fixed combination in patients with COPD was 15 minutes; median time to peak FEV_1 was 1 hour. The median duration of bronchodilation was 4–5 hours with the fixed combination and 4 hours with ipratropium alone. In dose-ranging studies in patients with bronchospasm, ipratropium bromide doses of 36–72 mcg given via a metered-dose inhaler generally have provided optimal clinical benefit. Because penetration of orally inhaled particles into airways is impaired when airways are severely obstructed, some clinicians suggest that higher doses of ipratropium bromide may be needed for maximal effect in some patients (e.g., those with severe airway disease).

Following oral inhalation via nebulization of 400–600 mcg of ipratropium bromide, bronchodilation (defined as increases of 15% or more in FEV_1) usually is evident within 15–30 minutes with peak effect in approximately 1–2 hours. In a dose-response study in patients with COPD, the optimal dose of nebulized ipratropium bromide was about 400 mcg. Bronchodilation with nebulized ipratropium generally persists for 4–5 hours, but may last up to 7–8 hours in some patients. Following concomitant administration via nebulization of a β_2-adrenergic agonist (i.e., albuterol, metaproterenol) and ipratropium in patients with COPD, bronchodilation persists for 5–7 hours compared with 3–4 hours in patients given a β_2-adrenergic agonist alone.

Following oral administration of a single 30-mg dose of radiolabeled ipratropium bromide in healthy adults, peak plasma ipratropium bromide concentrations of about 25 ng/mL (as total radioactivity) occurred within 2–4 hours. However, peak plasma radioactivity following administration of radiolabeled ipratropium bromide appears to represent both the parent drug and its metabolites. Peak plasma drug concentrations of about 1 ng/mL (determined by a radioreceptor assay that does not measure metabolites of ipratropium bromide) occurred within 2 hours following administration of a single 10-mg oral dose of ipratropium bromide in healthy adults. In these individuals, approximately 3.3% (range: 0.9–6.1%) of the dose of ipratropium bromide was absorbed. Oral administration of 15 mg of ipratropium bromide appears to produce bronchodilation similar to that produced by 36 or 150 mcg of the drug given by oral aerosol inhalation or IV, respectively; plasma concentrations are approximately 1000 times higher following oral administration than following oral inhalation of equipotent doses. Plasma drug concentrations following oral inhalation of ipratropium bromide do not appear to correlate with pharmacologic effects.

■ **Distribution** Distribution of ipratropium bromide into human tissues and body fluids has not been elucidated. Quaternary ammonium antimuscarinics are completely ionized and possess poor lipid solubility; accordingly, they do not readily penetrate the CNS. Following IV administration of ipratropium bromide in rats, the drug is distributed throughout the body with highest concentrations appearing in the stomach, intestines, liver, and kidneys; the drug is minimally distributed into brain, lung, and muscle. High concentrations of ipratropium bromide in the gut in these animals may indicate biliary elimination or enterohepatic circulation.

Ipratropium bromide reportedly is 0–9% bound to plasma albumin and α_1-acid glycoproteins in vitro.

It is not known whether ipratropium bromide crosses the placenta or is distributed into milk.

■ **Elimination** Following IV administration of ipratropium bromide in healthy adults, plasma drug concentrations appear to decline in a biphasic manner. Using radiolabeled ipratropium bromide, an elimination half-life of about 2–4 hours (determined by measurement of total radioactivity) generally has been reported following administration of the drug orally, IV, or by oral inhalation in animals and healthy adults. However, this method measures both ipratropium bromide and its metabolites. Using a radioreceptor assay that measures only unchanged ipratropium bromide, the initial distribution-phase half-life ($t_{1/2\alpha}$) and the terminal elimination-phase half-life ($t_{1/2\beta}$) following a single 2-mg IV dose of the drug in healthy adults averaged about 0.07 and 1.6 hours, respectively.

The exact metabolic fate of ipratropium bromide has not been fully determined. Following oral or IV administration or oral inhalation, the drug is partially metabolized to at least 8 metabolites. Metabolism appears to involve only the tropic acid moiety and usually consists of hydrolysis and conjugation. The main metabolites appear to be *N*-isopropylnortropium methobromide, which is formed by enzymatic hydrolysis of the ester; α-phenylacrylic acid-*N*-isopropylnortropine-ester methobromide, which is formed by enzymatic loss of a water; and phenylacetic acid-*N*-isopropylnortropine-ester methobromide, which is formed by enzymatic loss of a CH_3OH-group. In vitro, these metabolites have minimal or no antimuscarinic activity.

After oral inhalation, oral administration, or IV injection of radiolabeled ipratropium bromide, unchanged drug recovered in urine within 4 hours (as total radioactivity) averaged 13, 24, or 50% of the dose, respectively. After administration of albuterol sulfate (180 mcg as albuterol base) and ipratropium bromide monohydrate (36 mcg) in fixed combination, 27.1% of the estimated mouthpiece dose is excreted unchanged in urine within 24 hours. Following oral administration or oral inhalation of ipratropium bromide in healthy adults, most of the dose is excreted in feces within 24 hours, principally as unchanged drug. In healthy individuals receiving 555 mcg of radiolabeled ipratropium bromide by oral inhalation, about 69 and 3.2% of the dose was excreted in feces and urine, respectively, within 6–7 days. Following administration of radiolabeled ipratropium bromide in healthy adults, about 9 or 72% of a single oral or IV dose, respectively, was excreted in urine, and about 89 or 6% of the oral or IV dose was excreted in feces within 5–7 days; most excretion occurred within 24 hours. Ipratropium bromide undergoes biliary elimination and/or enterohepatic circulation in animals and appears to undergo some biliary elimination in humans.

Chemistry and Stability

■ **Chemistry** Ipratropium bromide is a synthetic quaternary ammonium antimuscarinic agent. Ipratropium is the quaternary *N*-methyl isopropyl derivative of noratropine. The drug is commercially available as the monobromide monohydrate (i.e., ipratropium bromide) in an oral aerosol formulation and in a solution for nebulization. Ipratropium bromide is also available in fixed combination with albuterol sulfate in an oral aerosol formulation and in a solution for nebulization. However, potencies of the commercially available preparations differ, the aerosol being expressed in terms of the monohydrate and the solution for nebulization being expressed in terms of anhydrous drug.

Ipratropium bromide, which is hydrated, occurs as a white, bitter-tasting crystalline powder and has solubilities of 90 mg/mL in water and 28 mg/mL in alcohol. Like other quaternary ammonium compounds, ipratropium exists in an ionized state in aqueous solutions and is insoluble in lipophilic solvents such as ether, chloroform, and fluorocarbons. A 1% aqueous solution of ipratropium bromide has a pH of 5–7.5.

Ipratropium bromide inhalation aerosol is commercially available as a solution of the drug in a vehicle containing a hydrofluoroalkane (tetrafluoroethane) propellant, water, dehydrated alcohol, and anhydrous citric acid. For oral inhalation, ipratropium bromide in fixed combination with albuterol sulfate, is commercially available as an aerosol containing a microcrystalline suspension of the drug (as the monohydrate) in a vehicle of chlorofluorocarbon propellants (dichlorodifluoromethane, dichlorotetrafluoroethane, and trichloromonofluoromethane) and soya lecithin. Each actuation of the aerosol inhaler delivers 17 mcg of ipratropium bromide monohydrate from the mouthpiece. Each actuation of the combination aerosol inhaler delivers 18 mcg of ipratropium bromide monohydrate and 103 mcg of albuterol sulfate (equivalent to 90 mcg of albuterol base) from the mouthpiece.

For oral administration by nebulizer, ipratropium bromide is commercially available as a 0.02% solution (expressed in terms of anhydrous drug) in 0.9% sodium chloride; hydrochloric acid may be added to adjust the pH to 3.4 (3–4). Ipratropium bromide also is available in fixed combination with albuterol sulfate as a 0.017% solution (expressed in terms of the anhydrous drug) in sodium chloride; hydrochloric acid may be added to adjust the pH to 4. Each 3-mL unit-dose vial of ipratropium bromide in fixed combination with albuterol sulfate inhalation solution contains 0.5 mg of ipratropium bromide and 2.5 mg of albuterol (equivalent to 3 mg of albuterol sulfate). The commercially available solutions for nebulization are sterile, clear, colorless and do not contain preservatives.

■ **Stability** Commercially available ipratropium bromide alone or in fixed combination with albuterol sulfate oral inhalation aerosol should be stored at 25 °C but may be exposed to temperatures ranging from 15 to 30°C; exposure to excessive humidity should be avoided. For best results, the aerosol canister should be at room temperature before use; at colder temperatures, cooling of the propellants may decrease the internal pressure of the canister and result in delivery of particles too large to provide full therapeutic effect. Because the contents of ipratropium bromide inhalation aerosol are under pressure, the aerosol container should *not* be punctured, used or stored near heat or an open flame, or placed into a fire or incinerator for disposal; exposure to high temperatures (49°C) may cause the canister to burst. When stored as directed, commercially available ipratropium bromide inhalation aerosol is stable for 18 months from the date of manufacture.

Commercially available ipratropium bromide inhalation solutions for nebulization should be stored at 15–30°C and protected from light, preferably in the manufacturer-supplied foil pouch. The commercially available inhalation solution of ipratropium bromide in fixed combination with albuterol sulfate should be stored at 2–30°C and be protected from light, preferably in the manufacturer-supplied foil pouch. When stored as directed, ipratropium bromide inhalation solution has an expiration date of 18 months following the date of manufacture.

The manufacturer states that solutions containing ipratropium bromide and albuterol sulfate or metaproterenol sulfate for oral inhalation are stable for 1 hour when mixed extemporaneously in a nebulizer prior to administration. Ipratropium bromide oral inhalation solution also has been reported to be stable for 1 hour when mixed in a nebulizer with cromolyn sodium. The manufacturer states that the stability and safety of ipratropium bromide inhalation solution mixed with other drugs in a nebulizer have not been established.

For further information on the chemistry, pharmacology, pharmacokinetics, uses, cautions, acute toxicity, and drug interactions of ipratropium bromide, see the Antimuscarinics/Antispasmodics General Statement 12.08.08.

Preparations

Excipients in commercially available drug preparations may have clinically important effects in some individuals; consult specific product labeling for details.

Ipratropium Bromide

Oral Inhalation		
Aerosol	17 mcg per metered spray	**Atrovent® HFA** (with hydrofluoroalkane propellant), Boehringer Ingelheim
Solution, for nebulization	0.02%*	**Ipratropium Bromide Inhalation Solution**

*available from one or more manufacturer, distributor, and/or repackager by generic (nonproprietary) name

Ipratropium Bromide Combinations

Oral Inhalation Only		
Aerosol	18 mcg with Albuterol Sulfate 90 mcg (of albuterol) per metered spray	**Combivent®** (with chlorofluorohydrocarbon propellants), Boehringer Ingelheim
Solution, for nebulization	0.5 mg with Albuterol Sulfate 2.5 mg (of albuterol) per 3 mL*	**DuoNeb®**, Dey **Ipratropium Bromide and Albuterol Sulfate Inhalation Solution**

*available from one or more manufacturer, distributor, and/or repackager by generic (nonproprietary) name
†Use is not currently included in the labeling approved by the US Food and Drug Administration

Tiotropium Bromide

■ Tiotropium bromide, a synthetic quaternary ammonium antimuscarinic agent, is a long-acting orally inhaled bronchodilator.

Uses

■ **Bronchospasm** ***Chronic Obstructive Pulmonary Disease*** Tiotropium bromide is used as a bronchodilator alone or in fixed combination with olodaterol hydrochloride for the long-term maintenance treatment of reversible bronchospasm associated with chronic obstructive pulmonary disease (COPD), including chronic bronchitis and emphysema. Tiotropium bromide alone also is used to reduce exacerbations of COPD in patients with a history of such exacerbations. In patients with moderate to severe COPD (e.g., forced expiratory volume in 1 second [FEV_1] 30 to less than 80% of predicted or, alternatively, less than 60% of predicted) who have persistent symptoms not relieved by as-needed therapy with ipratropium and/or a selective, short-acting inhaled β_2-agonist, maintenance monotherapy with a long-acting bronchodilator (e.g., orally inhaled salmeterol, formoterol, or tiotropium) or an inhaled corticosteroid may be used, and a short-acting, selective inhaled β_2-agonist is used as needed for immediate symptom relief. Maintenance therapy with long-acting bronchodilators in patients with moderate to severe COPD is more effective and more convenient than regular therapy with short-acting bronchodilators. Data are insufficient to favor one maintenance monotherapy over another for use in such patients. Some clinicians recommend therapy with a combination of several long-acting bronchodilators such as tiotropium and a long-acting β-adrenergic agonist in selected patients with inadequate response. In patients with severe to very severe COPD (e.g., FEV_1 less than 30 to less than 50% of predicted), some clinicians recommend addition of an inhaled corticosteroid to maintenance therapy with one or more long-acting bronchodilators given separately or in fixed combination; however, the benefits of combination therapy over monotherapy have not been consistently demonstrated. If symptoms are not adequately controlled with inhaled corticosteroids and a long-acting bronchodilator or if limiting adverse effects occur, addition or substitution of extended-release oral theophylline may be considered. Orally inhaled tiotropium alone or in combination with olodaterol is *not* indicated for treatment of acute episodes of bronchospasm or acute deterioration of COPD; a drug with a more rapid onset of action (e.g., a short-acting β-adrenergic agonist) may be preferred in such cases.

Currently available data indicate that tiotropium improves lung function (e.g., as determined by FEV_1) in patients with COPD compared with ipratropium or placebo. Such improvement in lung function has been maintained throughout the 24-hour dosing interval and for treatment periods of up to 1 year with no evidence of tolerance. In some studies, treatment with tiotropium also has been associated with a reduction in the need for supplemental short-acting β_2 agonists compared with placebo.

In several long-term (e.g., 1-year) comparative studies in patients with COPD, orally inhaled tiotropium (18 mcg once daily) improved lung function (e.g., as determined by mean change in trough FEV_1, morning and evening peak expiratory flow rate [PEFR]) to a greater degree than ipratropium bromide (36 mcg 4 times daily) oral inhalation aerosol. In addition, treatment with tiotropium reduced dyspnea and the number of COPD exacerbations and increased the time to a first exacerbation compared with ipratropium bromide aerosol.

In two 6-month comparative trials in patients with COPD receiving either orally inhaled tiotropium (18 mcg once daily) or salmeterol (50 mcg twice daily), tiotropium was more effective in improving bronchodilation (e.g., FEV_1, evening PEFR) than salmeterol therapy or placebo. In addition, while tiotropium or salmeterol each reduced dyspnea and improved FEV_1 compared with placebo, tiotropium also was more effective than placebo in reducing COPD exacerbations and all-cause hospital admissions and improving quality-of-life scores in these trials.

The efficacy of tiotropium oral inhalation powder for reducing exacerbations in patients with COPD also has been studied in 2 randomized, placebo-controlled clinical trials: a 6-month trial including 1829 patients and a 4-year trial including 5992 patients. In the 4-year study, long-term effects on lung function and other outcomes also were evaluated. In both studies, patients were allowed to use their prescribed respiratory medications (e.g., short- and long-acting β-agonists, inhaled and systemic corticosteroids, theophyllines) except for inhaled anticholinergic agents. In the 6-month trial, COPD exacerbations were defined as a complex of respiratory symptoms (increase or new onset) including more than one of the following: cough, sputum, wheezing, dyspnea, or chest tightness with a duration of at least 3 days requiring treatment with antibiotics, systemic corticosteroids, or hospitalization. Patients were 40–90 years of age, 99% were male, and 91% were white, with a mean pre-bronchodilator FEV_1 of 36% of predicted (range: 8–93%). The primary end points were the proportion of patients with COPD exacerbations and the proportion of patients with hospitalization due to COPD exacerbations. The proportion of patients with COPD exacerbations was substantially lower in patients receiving tiotropium than in patients receiving placebo (27.9 versus 32.3%). The proportion of patients with hospitalization due to COPD exacerbations (7 or 9.5% in patients receiving tiotropium or placebo, respectively) was not substantially different in the 2 groups.

In the 4-year trial, patients were 40–88 years of age, 75% were male, and 90% were white with a mean pre-bronchodilator FEV_1 of 39% of predicted (range: 9–76%). The primary efficacy end points (i.e., yearly rate of decline in pre- and post-bronchodilator FEV_1) did not differ between the 2 study groups. However, improvements in trough (pre-dose) FEV_1 (adjusted means over time: 87–103 mL) were maintained over the 4 years of the study in patients receiving tiotropium. COPD exacerbations were a secondary end point in this trial and were defined as an increase or new onset of more than one of the following respiratory symptoms: cough, sputum, sputum purulence, wheezing, and dyspnea, with a duration of 3 or more days requiring treatment with antibiotics and/or systemic corticosteroids. The risk of exacerbation and of exacerbation-related hospitalization both were reduced by 14% in patients receiving tiotropium compared with those receiving placebo; in addition, median time to first exacerbation was longer in patients receiving tiotropium compared with placebo (16.7 versus 12.5 months). All-cause mortality was similar in patients receiving tiotropium or placebo.

In a long-term, randomized, double-blind, double-dummy, active-controlled trial (Tiotropium Safety and Performance in Respimat [TIOSPIR]) with an observation period of up to 3 years, all-cause mortality was found to be similar in patients receiving tiotropium oral inhalation powder compared with those receiving tiotropium oral inhalation solution.

Efficacy of tiotropium oral inhalation solution was based principally on 5 confirmatory, placebo- and active-controlled studies of 12–48 weeks' duration. In the randomized, double-blind, placebo- and/or active-controlled trials, efficacy of tiotropium oral inhalation solution was evaluated in 6614 patients with COPD; patients were 40 years of age or older, had a history of smoking greater than 10 pack-years, an FEV_1 of 60% of predicted or less, and a baseline FEV_1/forced vital capacity (FVC) of 0.7 or less. The primary outcome measure was the change from baseline in trough FEV_1. All study medications were administered once daily in the morning via the Respimat® inhaler. In these studies, trough FEV_1 was improved by 100–140 mL with tiotropium compared with placebo. In the 3 trials that evaluated COPD exacerbations, tiotropium oral inhalation solution at a dosage of 5 mcg once daily reduced the rate of exacerbations compared with placebo.

Efficacy of tiotropium in fixed combination with olodaterol hydrochloride was based principally on 2 dose-ranging studies of 4 weeks' duration and 2 confirmatory, active-controlled studies of 52 weeks' duration. In the 2 randomized, double-blind, active-controlled, parallel-group trials, efficacy of tiotropium in combination with olodaterol was evaluated in 5162 patients 40 years of age or older with moderate to very severe COPD. The primary outcome measures were the change from baseline in FEV_1 AUC from 0–3 hours and trough FEV_1 after 24 weeks of therapy. All study medications were administered once daily in the morning via the Respimat® inhaler. In these studies, FEV_1 AUC from 0–3 hours at 24 weeks was improved by 256–268 mL with orally inhaled tiotropium 5 mcg in combination with olodaterol 5 mcg compared with improvements of 139–165 or 133–136 mL with either tiotropium 5 mcg or olodaterol 5 mcg, respectively, alone. Trough FEV_1 at 24 weeks was improved by 136–145 mL with tiotropium in combination with olodaterol compared with improvements of 65–96 or 54–57 mL with either tiotropium or olodaterol, respectively, alone. The increased bronchodilator effects observed with tiotropium in combination with olodaterol were maintained throughout the 52-week studies. Patients receiving the fixed combination of tiotropium and olodaterol required less albuterol as rescue therapy compared with those receiving either tiotropium or olodaterol alone.

For additional information on the treatment of COPD, see Uses: Chronic Obstructive Pulmonary Disease, in Ipratropium Bromide 12:08.08.

Asthma Tiotropium bromide oral inhalation solution is used for the long-term maintenance treatment of reversible bronchospasm associated with asthma. Orally inhaled tiotropium solution is *not* indicated for the treatment of acute episodes of bronchospasm; a drug with a more rapid onset of action (e.g., a short-acting β-adrenergic agonist) should be used in such cases. Tiotropium bromide in fixed combination with olodaterol hydrochloride is *not* indicated for the treatment of asthma.

Efficacy of tiotropium oral inhalation solution for the treatment of persistent asthma in adults was based principally on 5 randomized, double-blind, placebo-controlled studies of 12–48 weeks' duration. In the randomized, double-blind, placebo- and/or active-controlled trials, efficacy of orally inhaled tiotropium solution was evaluated in 3476 patients 18–75 years of age with a diagnosis of asthma who were receiving baseline therapy with at least inhaled corticosteroids. The primary outcome measure in all of the studies was the change from baseline in peak FEV_1 at 0–3 hours at week 12 or 24. In 2 trials, an additional primary outcome measure was change from baseline in trough FEV_1 at week 24. Patients randomized to receive tiotropium oral inhalation solution received the drug once daily via the Respimat® inhaler. In these studies, peak FEV_1 at 0–3 hours was improved by 160–240 mL with tiotropium compared with placebo. In the 3 trials that evaluated orally inhaled tiotropium dosages of 2.5 or 5 mcg once daily, FEV_1 response was generally lower for the 5-mcg dose compared with the 2.5-mcg dose. Improvement in lung function with tiotropium compared with placebo was maintained for 24 hours. The bronchodilator effects of tiotropium 2.5 mcg once daily were apparent after the first dose; however, maximum bronchodilator effect was not achieved for up to 4–8 weeks.

Efficacy of tiotropium oral inhalation solution for the treatment of persistent asthma in pediatric patients was based on extrapolation of efficacy in adults and on several randomized, double-blind, placebo-controlled studies of 12–48 weeks' duration. The primary outcome measure in these studies was the change from baseline in peak FEV_1 at 0–3 hours at week 12 or 24. In adolescents, 2 clinical studies evaluated efficacy of orally inhaled tiotropium solution in 789 patients 12–17 years of age with a diagnosis of asthma who were receiving baseline therapy with at least inhaled corticosteroids. Patients randomized to receive tiotropium oral inhalation solution were administered 2.5 or 5 mcg of the drug once daily via the Respimat® inhaler. In these studies, peak FEV_1 at 0–3 hours was improved by 110–130 mL with tiotropium 2.5 mcg once daily compared with placebo.

In children, 2 clinical studies evaluated efficacy of tiotropium oral inhalation solution in 801 patients 6–11 years of age with a diagnosis of asthma who were receiving baseline therapy with at least inhaled corticosteroids. Patients randomized to receive tiotropium oral inhalation solution were administered 2.5 or 5 mcg of the drug once daily via the Respimat® inhaler. In the 48-week study, peak FEV_1 at 0–3 hours was improved by 170 mL with tiotropium 2.5 mcg once daily compared with placebo. The efficacy results from the 12-week study were not statistically significant.

Dosage and Administration

■ **General** Dosage of tiotropium bromide, which is commercially available as the monohydrate, is expressed in terms of anhydrous tiotropium.

Although each capsule under the foil lid of the blister strip contains 18 mcg of tiotropium as an inhalation powder, the precise amount of drug delivered to the lungs with each activation of the HandiHaler® device depends on factors such as the patient's inspiratory flow. Peak inspiratory flow through the HandiHaler® device also varies according to the exposure time of the capsule outside of the blister pack. Using standardized in vitro testing at a flow rate of 39 L/minute for 3.1 seconds, the HandiHaler® inhaler delivered a mean of 10.4 mcg of tiotropium per activation from the mouthpiece.

Each activation of the oral inhalation device containing tiotropium bromide oral inhalation solution (Spiriva® Respimat®) delivers 1.56 or 3.1 mcg of tiotropium bromide monohydrate (equivalent to 1.25 or 2.5 mcg, respectively, of tiotropium) from the mouthpiece. Each activation of the oral inhalation device containing tiotropium and olodaterol in fixed combination (Stiolto® Respimat®) delivers 3.1 mcg of tiotropium bromide monohydrate (equivalent to 2.5 mcg of tiotropium) and 2.7 mcg of olodaterol hydrochloride (equivalent to 2.5 mcg of olodaterol) from the mouthpiece. The precise amount of drug delivered to the lungs with each activation of the inhaler device depends on factors such as the patient's coordination between actuation of the inhaler and inspiration through the delivery system. Because the Respimat® inhaler mechanically releases the dose, the delivered dose is independent of the patient's inspiratory effort. The commercially available inhalers deliver 60 metered sprays (not including the initial priming actuations) equivalent to 30 doses (2 actuations per dose) of the drug.

■ **Administration** ***Oral Inhalation via Dry Powder Inhaler*** Tiotropium bromide dry-powder capsules are administered by oral inhalation *only* using a special oral inhalation device (HandiHaler®) that delivers powdered drug from capsules. Tiotropium bromide capsules for oral inhalation must not be taken orally, as the intended effects on the lungs will not be obtained.

To obtain optimal benefit, the patient should be given a copy of the patient instructions provided by the manufacturer. To use the inhaler, the dust cap of the inhaler should be opened by pressing the green piercing button. The dust cap on the side opposite the hinge on the gray base should be pulled upward to expose the mouthpiece. The mouthpiece of the inhaler should be opened by pulling the mouthpiece ridge upward on the side opposite the hinge on the gray base to expose the center chamber. The blister card should be carefully opened to expose only one capsule immediately before use. The capsule contains only a small amount of powder and should not be opened. The capsule should then be placed into the center chamber of the inhaler. After the capsule is loaded, the inhaler mouthpiece should be closed firmly until it snaps (clicks) into position; the dust cap is left open (up). Patients should push down on the mouthpiece ridge to make sure that the mouthpiece is seated in the gray base of the inhaler. While holding the inhaler with the seated mouthpiece upward, the green piercing button on the side of the inhaler should be completely depressed (green button is flush with the gray base of the inhaler) and then released. The button pierces the capsule and disperses the powdered drug upon inspiration; the piercing button should not be pressed more than one time and the HandiHaler® device should not be shaken. Piercing the capsule may produce small gelatin pieces, which may pass into the mouth or throat during inhalation of the drug; the gelatin pieces should not cause any harm.

Before inhaling the dose, the patient should exhale as completely as possible, being careful not to exhale into the HandiHaler® device. The inhaler device should be held along the sides of the gray base taking care not to block the air intake vents near the mouthpiece ridge. With the head kept level, the patient should place the mouthpiece of the inhaler between the lips (inhaler is in horizontal position) and inhale deeply and slowly through the inhaler at a rate sufficient to hear or feel the loaded capsule vibrate. Pressure from the inhalation will disperse drug from the center chamber into the air stream created by the patient's inhalation. After a complete inhalation, the patient should remove the inhaler from the mouth and hold their breath for a few seconds, then resume normal breathing. The patient should breathe out completely and inhale once again to ensure full delivery of the powder from the same loaded, pierced capsule. *The green piercing button should not be pressed again.* Upon completion of the second inhalation, the patient should open the mouthpiece and tip the inhaler device to dispose of the used capsule. The mouthpiece and dust cap of the inhaler device should then be closed.

If the patient does not feel or hear the capsule vibrate upon inhalation, the inhaler device should be tapped gently on a table while holding the device in an upright position. The patient then should check to see that the mouthpiece is properly seated in the gray base. The patient should attempt to inhale through the device again. If capsule vibration still cannot be heard or felt during inhalation, the capsule should be discarded and the base of the device should be opened by lifting the green piercing button; the center chamber should be checked for pieces of the capsule. The device should be turned upside down and gently but firmly tapped to remove any capsule pieces, then the clinician should be contacted for instructions. (See Advice to Patients.)

Dry-powder capsules for oral inhalation should be left in foil-sealed blisters until immediately before use. Used or unused dry-powder capsules should not be stored in the inhaler device. The foil of the blister pack should not be cut nor should sharp objects be used to remove the capsule selected for dosing. If additional capsules are inadvertently opened and exposed to air (i.e., not intended for immediate use), they should be discarded since the effectiveness of the drug in those capsules may be reduced.

If patients taking tiotropium do not experience an improvement in control of COPD, a clinician should make sure that the patient is inhaling the drug using the oral inhaler rather than swallowing the dry-powder capsules. (See Accidental Oral Ingestion under Warnings/Precautions, in Cautions.)

The HandiHaler® device should be cleaned as needed. The dust cap and mouthpiece should be opened, and then the base should be opened by lifting the green piercing button. Any capsule pieces or powder buildup in the center chamber should be tapped out. The inhaler should be rinsed with warm water (cleaning agents or detergents should not be used), pressing the green piercing button a few times so that the center chamber and piercing needle are under the running water to remove any remaining powder or capsule pieces. The inhaler should be dried thoroughly and the dust cap, mouthpiece, and gray base left open and fully spread out to air dry for 24 hours. A hair dryer should not be used to dry the device. The inhaler should not be used when wet. If needed, the outside of the mouthpiece may be cleaned with a clean, damp cloth.

Oral Inhalation via Metered-Dose Inhaler Tiotropium bromide solution is administered by oral inhalation using a specific inhaler (Spiriva® Respimat®) that delivers a metered-dose spray. Tiotropium bromide in fixed combination with olodaterol hydrochloride is administered by oral inhalation using a specific inhaler (Stiolto® Respimat®) that delivers a metered-dose spray. Both inhalers deliver the drugs in an aqueous solution and mechanically produce a fine aerosol mist from the orally inhaled solution. Tiotropium bromide alone or in fixed combination with olodaterol should be administered once daily at the same time every day.

Before first use of either Spiriva® Respimat® or Stiolto® Respimat®, the inhaler cartridge should be placed into the inhaler. The manufacturer's prescribing information should be consulted for detailed information on preparation of the inhalers. The discard date (3 months after the cartridge is inserted into the inhaler) should be written on the inhaler label.

After the cartridge has been inserted into either the Spiriva® Respimat® or the Stiolto® Respimat® inhaler, the unit must be primed prior to first use. Beginning with the inhaler held upright and the cap closed, the clear base should be turned in the direction of the black arrows on the label until a click is heard (one-half turn). The cap should then be flipped until it fully snaps open, the inhaler should be pointed away from the face, the dose release button pressed, and then the cap closed. These steps (turning the clear base until it clicks, opening the cap, actuating the inhaler, and replacing the cap) should be repeated until a spray is visible, and then for 3 additional times. The initial actuation step of the priming process (without the 3 additional repetitions) should be repeated after a period of nonuse (i.e., more than 3 days). If the inhaler is not used for more than 21 days, the entire initial priming process should be repeated.

To administer a dose of tiotropium alone or in fixed combination with olodaterol, the patient should hold the inhaler upright with the cap closed and turn the clear base in the direction of the black arrows on the label until a click is heard (one-half turn). The cap should be flipped until it snaps fully open. Before inhaling the dose, the patient should exhale slowly and completely. The patient should then close the lips around the end of the mouthpiece, without covering the air vents. With the inhaler pointing toward the back of the throat, the patient should press the dose release button while taking a slow, deep inhalation through the mouth; the patient should continue inhaling as long as possible. The patient should then hold the breath for 10 seconds (or as long as comfortable). This procedure should be repeated once more to administer the full dose (2 inhalations) of tiotropium alone or in combination with olodaterol. After the full dose is administered, the cap of the inhaler should be closed.

The mouthpiece of either the Spiriva® Respimat® or the Stiolto® Respimat® inhaler, including the metal part inside, should be cleaned using only a damp tissue or cloth at least once weekly. If the outside of the inhaler gets dirty, it can be wiped with a damp cloth. The function of the inhaler is not affected by minor discoloration in the mouthpiece.

■ **Dosage** ***Chronic Obstructive Pulmonary Disease*** For the long-term management of reversible bronchospasm associated with chronic obstructive pulmonary disease (COPD), the usual dosage of tiotropium oral inhalation powder in adults is 18 mcg (2 inhalations, the contents of one capsule) once daily via the HandiHaler® device. No more than one dose should be taken in a 24-hour period. Orally inhaled tiotropium powder should *not* be used for the treatment of acute episodes of bronchospasm.

For the long-term management of reversible bronchospasm associated with COPD, the usual dosage of tiotropium oral inhalation solution in adults is 5 mcg (2 inhalations of the 2.5 mcg per metered-dose spray) once daily via the Respimat® device. No more than one dose should be taken in a 24-hour period. Orally inhaled tiotropium solution should *not* be used for the treatment of acute episodes of bronchospasm.

Asthma For the long-term management of reversible bronchospasm associated with asthma, the usual dosage of tiotropium oral inhalation solution in patients 6 years of age or older is 2.5 mcg (2 inhalations of the 1.25 mcg per metered-dose spray) once daily via the Respimat® device. No more than one dose (2 inhalations) should be taken in a 24-hour period. Orally inhaled tiotropium solution should *not* be used for the treatment of acute episodes of bronchospasm.

■ **Special Populations** The manufacturer states that adjustment of tiotropium dosage is not necessary in geriatric patients or patients with hepatic or renal impairment. (See Renal Impairment under Warnings/Precautions: Specific Populations, in Cautions.)

Cautions

■ **Contraindications** Known hypersensitivity to tiotropium, ipratropium, or any ingredient in the formulation.

■ **Warnings/Precautions** ***Sensitivity Reactions*** Immediate hypersensitivity reactions, including angioedema (e.g., swelling of the lips, tongue, or throat), urticaria, rash, bronchospasm, anaphylaxis, or itching, may occur after administration of tiotropium. If such a reaction occurs, the drug should be discontinued immediately and alternative therapy considered.

Patients with a history of hypersensitivity reactions to atropine or its derivatives should be closely monitored for hypersensitivity reactions. In addition, tiotropium oral inhalation powder (Spiriva® HandiHaler®) should be used with caution in patients with severe hypersensitivity to milk proteins.

Use of Fixed Combinations When tiotropium is used in fixed combination with olodaterol, the usual cautions, precautions, contraindications, and interactions associated with olodaterol must be considered. Cautionary information applicable to specific populations (e.g., pregnant or nursing women, individuals with hepatic or renal impairment, geriatric patients) should be considered for each drug in the fixed combination.

Acute Bronchospasm Tiotropium bromide should *not* be used for the relief of acute symptoms (i.e., as rescue therapy for the treatment of acute episodes of bronchospasm).

Possible Increased Risk of Stroke, Mortality, and/or Cardiovascular Events While data are conflicting, a possible increased risk of stroke has been identified by the manufacturer from ongoing safety monitoring and pooled analysis of placebo-controlled trials in patients receiving tiotropium therapy. Other observational data have suggested an increased risk of mortality and/or cardiovascular events in patients receiving the drug.

Analysis of data on approximately 13,500 patients with COPD in 29 studies indicated a stroke case rate of 8 or 6 per 1000 patient-years of exposure in patients receiving tiotropium or placebo, respectively, representing an absolute excess risk of 2 additional strokes per 1000 patient-years. In addition, data from an observational study involving over 32,000 patients and another pooled analysis of 17 studies enrolling almost 15,000 patients have shown an increased risk of mortality and/or cardiovascular events in patients receiving inhaled anticholinergic agents, including tiotropium bromide. However, the results of a placebo-controlled trial (Understanding Potential Long-term Impacts on Function with Tiotropium [UPLIFT]) in approximately 6000 patients with COPD did not reveal an increased risk of stroke, myocardial infarction (MI), or cardiovascular death with tiotropium bromide. Based on a review of the UPLIFT trial, FDA has concluded that the available data do not support an association between the use of tiotropium oral inhalation powder and an increased risk of stroke, MI, or cardiovascular death.

An increased risk of mortality with tiotropium oral inhalation solution compared with placebo has been reported in some meta-analyses and data reviews; however, in a long-term, randomized, double-blind, double-dummy, active-controlled trial (Tiotropium Safety and Performance in Respimat [TIOSPIR]) with an observation period of up to 3 years, all-cause mortality was found to be similar in patients receiving tiotropium oral inhalation powder and those receiving tiotropium oral inhalation solution. In addition, no increased risk of death was observed in patients with a history of cardiac disease (including stable cardiac arrhythmias at baseline) receiving tiotropium oral inhalation solution compared with those receiving tiotropium oral inhalation powder.

Increases in corrected QT (QT_c) interval have been reported in patients receiving tiotropium oral inhalation powder. In a multicenter, randomized, double-blind trial in 198 patients with COPD, changes from baseline-corrected QT interval (using either the Bazett or Fridericia corrections) of 30–60 msec occurred in more patients receiving tiotropium compared with those receiving placebo. In other clinical trials, an effect of the drug on QT_c intervals was not observed. In a crossover, placebo-controlled study of tiotropium oral inhalation powder in healthy individuals, the maximum mean change from baseline in study-specific QT_c compared with placebo was 3.2 or 0.8 msec in patients receiving tiotropium 18 or 54 mcg, respectively.

Paradoxical Bronchospasm Acute paradoxical bronchospasm may occur. If such a reaction occurs, it should be treated immediately with a short-acting inhaled β_2-adrenergic agonist; tiotropium should be discontinued and alternative therapy considered.

Ocular Effects Tiotropium may worsen angle-closure glaucoma. The drug should be used with caution in patients with angle-closure glaucoma. If signs or symptoms of acute angle-closure glaucoma (e.g., ocular pain or discomfort, blurred vision, visual halos, or colored images in association with conjunctival congestion and corneal edema) occur, patients should consult a clinician immediately. (See Advice to Patients.) Miotic eye drops alone are not considered effective treatment for this condition.

Temporary blurring of vision or pupillary dilation may occur following inadvertent contact of tiotropium with the eyes. Care should be taken to avoid contact of the drug with the eyes during oral inhalation. (See Advice to Patients.)

Genitourinary Effects Urinary retention/difficulty or urinary tract infection has been reported with tiotropium therapy. Tiotropium may worsen symptoms and signs of urinary retention (e.g., dysuria); patients should be carefully monitored for such signs and symptoms, especially those with prostatic hyperplasia or bladder neck obstruction. A clinician should be consulted immediately if such effects occur. Tiotropium should be used with caution in patients with urinary retention.

Accidental Oral Ingestion Acute intoxication by inadvertent oral ingestion of the dry-powder capsules for oral inhalation is unlikely since tiotropium is not well absorbed systemically. Few patients have reported adverse effects following ingestion of the dry-powder capsules.

Specific Populations **Pregnancy.** Category C. (See Users Guide.) Limited human data regarding use of orally inhaled tiotropium solution during pregnancy are inadequate to inform a drug-associated risk. However, poorly or moderately controlled asthma during pregnancy may increase the maternal risk of preeclampsia and the infant's risk for prematurity, low birth weight, and small size for gestational age. The level of asthma control should be closely monitored in pregnant women and therapy adjusted as needed to maintain optimal control.

Animal studies have not revealed evidence of structural abnormalities at tiotropium dosages of approximately 790 or 8 times the maximum recommended human daily inhalation dosage administered to pregnant rats or rabbits, respectively, during the period of organogenesis. However, tiotropium administration resulted in fetal resorption, fetal loss, decreased number of live pups at birth, decreased mean pup weights, and delays in pup sexual maturation in rats receiving approximately 40 times the maximum recommended human daily inhalation dosage. In pregnant rabbits, tiotropium administration resulted in increased postimplantation fetal loss at dosages of approximately 430 times the maximum recommended human daily inhalation dosage. These adverse fetal effects were not observed at tiotropium dosages approximately 5 or 95 times the maximum recommended human daily inhalation dosage in pregnant rats and rabbits, respectively.

Lactation. Tiotropium is distributed into milk in rodents. The drug and/or its metabolites are present in milk of lactating rats at concentrations higher than those in plasma. It is not known whether tiotropium is distributed into milk in humans. Effects of the drug on breast-fed infants or milk production also are not known. The benefits of breast-feeding and the woman's clinical need for tiotropium should be considered along with any potential adverse effects on the breast-fed infant from the drug or from the underlying maternal condition. The manufacturer recommends that orally inhaled tiotropium be used with caution in nursing women.

Pediatric Use. Safety and efficacy of orally inhaled tiotropium powder have not been established in children younger than 18 years of age. Tiotropium oral inhalation powder is not indicated for use in pediatric patients.

Safety and efficacy of orally inhaled tiotropium solution for the treatment of asthma have been established in pediatric patients 6–17 years of age in several clinical trials up to 1 years' duration. In 3 of these trials, 327 adolescents 12–17 years of age with asthma received tiotropium oral inhalation solution at a dosage of 2.5 mcg once daily. In 3 additional studies, 345 patients 6–11 years of age with asthma received tiotropium oral inhalation solution at a dosage of 2.5 mcg once daily. Safety and efficacy of the drug in these pediatric patients were similar to the effects in patients 18 years of age or older with asthma receiving the drug.

Safety and efficacy of orally inhaled tiotropium solution have not been established in children younger than 6 years of age.

Geriatric Use. The frequency of dry mouth, constipation, and urinary tract infection increased with age in clinical trials of tiotropium. However, no overall differences in efficacy were observed in geriatric patients relative to younger adults. The manufacturer states that adjustment of tiotropium dosage in geriatric patients is not necessary.

Hepatic Impairment. The pharmacokinetics of tiotropium have not been studied in patients with hepatic impairment.

Renal Impairment. Since tiotropium is excreted predominantly by the kidneys, the manufacturer recommends that patients with moderate to severe renal impairment (creatinine clearance of less than 60 mL/minute) be monitored closely for anticholinergic effects while receiving tiotropium therapy.

■ **Common Adverse Effects** Adverse reactions occurring in at least 3% of patients with COPD receiving tiotropium oral inhalation powder in long-term clinical trials and at a frequency at least 1% greater than with placebo include upper respiratory tract infection, dry mouth, sinusitis, pharyngitis, urinary tract infection, chest pain (nonspecific), rhinitis, dyspepsia, headache, abdominal pain, edema (dependent), arthralgia, constipation, depression, insomnia, vomiting, infection, moniliasis, epistaxis, myalgia, and rash.

Adverse reactions occurring in more than 3% of patients with COPD receiving tiotropium oral inhalation solution in clinical trials and more frequently than with placebo include pharyngitis, cough, dry mouth, and sinusitis.

Adverse reactions occurring in more than 2% of patients with asthma receiving tiotropium oral inhalation solution in clinical trials and more frequently than with placebo include pharyngitis, headache, bronchitis, and sinusitis.

Adverse effects occurring in more than 3% of patients with COPD receiving tiotropium 5 mcg daily in fixed combination with olodaterol 5 mcg daily and more frequently than in patients receiving either drug alone include nasopharyngitis, cough, and back pain.

Drug Interactions

■ **Histamine H_2-Antagonists** Pharmacokinetic interaction (increased area under the concentration-time curve [AUC_{0-4h}], decreased renal clearance of IV tiotropium [not currently available in the US]) with concomitant cimetidine but not ranitidine. Pharmacokinetic interactions between tiotropium bromide and histamine H_2-antagonists not considered clinically important.

■ **Other Drugs** Tiotropium has been used concomitantly with sympathomimetic bronchodilators, methylxanthines, oral or inhaled corticosteroids, antihistamines, mucolytics, leukotriene modifiers, mast-cell stabilizers, and anti-IgE monoclonal antibody therapy without apparent increases in adverse effects. Use of tiotropium with other anticholinergic drugs (e.g., ipratropium) may cause increased anticholinergic effects, and is therefore not recommended by the manufacturer.

Description

Tiotropium bromide is a nonselective competitive antagonist at muscarinic (M_1–M_5) receptors. Tiotropium competitively and reversibly inhibits the actions of acetylcholine and other cholinergic stimuli at M_3 receptors in the smooth muscle of the respiratory tract, leading to bronchodilation.

Most of a dose of orally inhaled tiotropium powder is swallowed. The drug is minimally absorbed into systemic circulation from the GI tract (bioavailability administered as an oral solution is 2–3%); the fraction reaching the lungs (about 20%) appears to be readily absorbed. Following administration of the oral inhalation solution, approximately 33% of an inhaled dose reaches the systemic circulation. In a pharmacokinetic study in patients with chronic obstructive pulmonary disease (COPD), similar systemic exposure was observed following once-daily administration of the oral inhalation powder (18 mcg) or the oral inhalation solution (5 mcg). In patients with asthma, peak and total systemic exposure of the drug following oral inhalation of the solution is similar between adults and pediatric patients (6–17 years of age). Maximum bronchodilator effects may take up to 4–8 weeks of therapy in patients with asthma.

Following oral inhalation of tiotropium powder in young healthy individuals, approximately 14% of an administered dose is eliminated in urine, principally as unchanged drug. Urinary excretion of unchanged drug following oral inhalation of tiotropium powder in patients with COPD was 7% over 24 hours. Following oral inhalation of tiotropium solution 5 mcg once daily for 21 days in patients with COPD, approximately 19% of the dose was excreted in urine over 24 hours. Following administration of tiotropium solution 2.5 mcg in patients with asthma, approximately 13% of an inhaled dose was excreted unchanged in urine over 24 hours. Tiotropium is metabolized to a limited extent by the cytochrome P-450 (CYP) microsomal enzyme system, principally by isoenzymes 2D6 and 3A4.

Advice to Patients

Provide a copy of the manufacturer's patient information (medication guide) and instructions for use to all patients each time the drug is dispensed. Importance of instructing patients to read the medication guide prior to initiation of therapy and each time the prescription is refilled.

Importance of informing a clinician of allergies to any medications prior to initiation of tiotropium bromide therapy.

Importance of adequate understanding of proper storage, preparation, and inhalation techniques, including use of the inhalation delivery system (HandiHaler® or Respimat®).

Importance of instructing caregivers to assist children with use of the Respimat® inhalation device.

Importance of not using the HandiHaler® or Respimat® device to administer other drugs.

Importance of informing a clinician of faulty inhaler performance (i.e., failure to hear or feel capsule vibrate) when certain procedures (i.e., confirming that the mouthpiece is firmly seated in gray base, tapping inhaler gently on a table) do not improve inhaler (Handihaler®) performance.

Importance of storing tiotropium dry-powder capsules in sealed blisters and of removing only one capsule immediately before use; unused additional capsules that are exposed to air should be discarded.

Importance of avoiding contact of the drug with the eyes since this may cause blurred vision and pupillary dilation.

Importance of not using tiotropium therapy to relieve acute symptoms or exacerbations of asthma or chronic obstructive pulmonary disease (COPD).

Importance of advising patients with asthma that maximum benefits may only be apparent after 4–8 weeks of treatment with tiotropium inhalation solution (Spiriva® Respimat®).

Risk of immediate hypersensitivity reactions such as anaphylaxis, angioedema (e.g., swelling of the lips, tongue, or throat), urticaria, rash, bronchospasm, or itching. If such signs and/or symptoms occur, tiotropium should be discontinued immediately and a clinician consulted.

Risk of paradoxical bronchospasm. If paradoxical bronchospasm occurs, tiotropium should be discontinued.

Risk of worsening of angle-closure glaucoma. Importance of immediately informing a clinician if eye pain or discomfort, blurred vision, or visual halos or colored images in association with conjunctival congestion or corneal edema occur.

Importance of advising patients to use caution when engaging in activities (e.g., driving a vehicle, operating appliances or machinery) since the drug may cause dizziness or blurred vision.

Risk of worsening of urinary retention. Importance of immediately informing a clinician if symptoms of urinary retention (e.g., dysuria) occur.

Importance of keeping drug out of reach of children.

Importance of informing clinicians of existing or contemplated therapy, including prescription and OTC drugs (e.g., eye drops) and herbal supplements, as well as any concomitant illnesses (e.g., urinary difficulty, enlarged prostate, narrow angle glaucoma).

Importance of women informing clinicians if they are or plan to become pregnant or plan to breast-feed.

Importance of informing patients of other important precautionary information. (See Cautions.)

Overview® (see Users Guide). For additional information on this drug until a more detailed monograph is developed and published, the manufacturer's labeling should be consulted. It is *essential* that the manufacturer's labeling be consulted for more detailed information on usual cautions, precautions, contraindications, potential drug interactions, laboratory test interferences, and acute toxicity.

Preparations

Excipients in commercially available drug preparations may have clinically important effects in some individuals; consult specific product labeling for details.

Tiotropium Bromide

Oral Inhalation		
Powder for inhalation (contained in capsules)	18 mcg (of anhydrous tiotropium)	**Spiriva® HandiHaler®**, Boehringer Ingelheim, (comarketed by Pfizer)
Solution for inhalation	1.25 mcg (of tiotropium) per metered spray	**Spiriva® Respimat®**, Boehringer Ingelheim
	2.5 mcg (of tiotropium) per metered spray	**Spiriva® Respimat®**, Boehringer Ingelheim

Tiotropium Bromide Combinations

Oral Inhalation		
Solution for inhalation	2.5 mcg (of tiotropium) with Olodaterol Hydrochloride 2.5 mcg (of olodaterol) per metered spray	**Stiolto® Respimat®**, Boehringer Ingelheim

Selected Revisions October 2017,

Umeclidinium Bromide

■ Umeclidinium bromide, a synthetic quaternary ammonium antimuscarinic agent, is a long-acting orally inhaled bronchodilator.

Uses

■ **Bronchospasm** ***Chronic Obstructive Pulmonary Disease***

Umeclidinium Bromide Therapy. Umeclidinium bromide is used as a bronchodilator for the long-term maintenance treatment of reversible bronchospasm associated with chronic obstructive pulmonary disease (COPD), including bronchitis and/or emphysema. Orally inhaled umeclidinium is *not* indicated for the initial treatment of acute exacerbations of COPD or for relief of acute symptoms (i.e., as rescue therapy for treatment of acute episodes of bronchospasm).

Efficacy of umeclidinium has been evaluated in 2 randomized, double-blind, placebo-controlled studies of 12 or 24 weeks' duration in 1738 adults 40 years of age or older with moderate to severe COPD. In the 24-week trial, the primary efficacy outcome was the change from baseline in the predose trough forced expiratory volume in 1 second (FEV_1) (defined as the average of FEV_1 measurements obtained 23 and 24 hours after the previous dose) on day 169. In this study, umeclidinium 62.5 mcg once daily improved the change from baseline in trough FEV_1 by 115 mL compared with placebo on day 169. In addition, the mean change from baseline in peak FEV_1 (i.e., the highest value observed within 6 hours of a dose) following once-daily administration of umeclidinium 62.5 mcg improved by 126 and 130 mL versus placebo on day 1 or day 168, respectively. A greater proportion of patients receiving umeclidinium compared with placebo (42 versus 31%) also experienced a clinically meaningful improvement in a health-related quality of life analysis.

In the 12-week trial, the primary efficacy outcome was the change from baseline in the predose trough FEV_1 (defined as the average of FEV_1 measurements obtained 23 and 24 hours after the previous dose) on day 85. In this study, umeclidinium 62.5 mcg once daily improved the change from baseline in trough FEV_1 by 127 mL compared with placebo on day 85.

Safety and efficacy of umeclidinium bromide in comparison with other inhaled antimuscarinic agents in patients with COPD have not been determined.

For additional information on the treatment of COPD, see Uses: Chronic Obstructive Pulmonary Disease, in Ipratropium Bromide 12:08.08.

Umeclidinium Bromide and Vilanterol Trifenatate Fixed-combination Therapy. Umeclidinium bromide is used in fixed combination with vilanterol trifenatate (long-acting β_2-adrenergic agonist) as a bronchodilator for the long-term maintenance treatment of airflow obstruction associated with COPD, including chronic bronchitis and emphysema. Umeclidinium bromide in fixed combination with vilanterol trifenatate is *not* indicated for the treatment of acute bronchospasm or for the treatment of asthma†; the safety and efficacy of umeclidinium bromide in asthma† have not been established.

Efficacy of umeclidinium bromide in combination with vilanterol trifenatate has been evaluated in a randomized, double-blind, placebo-controlled study of 24 weeks' duration in adults 40 years of age or older with COPD. The primary efficacy outcome was the change from baseline in the trough FEV_1 on day 169. Following administration of orally inhaled umeclidinium 62.5 mcg in fixed combination with vilanterol 25 mcg once daily, the change from baseline in trough FEV_1 at 169 days improved by 52, 95, and 167 mL compared with umeclidinium alone, vilanterol alone, and placebo, respectively.

Dosage and Administration

■ **Administration** Umeclidinium bromide is administered by oral inhalation using a specific preloaded inhaler (Incruse® Ellipta®) that delivers powdered drug from foil-wrapped blisters. Umeclidinium bromide in combination with vilanterol trifenatate is administered by oral inhalation using a specific preloaded inhaler (Anoro® Ellipta®) that delivers a fixed combination of powdered umeclidinium bromide and vilanterol trifenatate from foil-wrapped blisters. Umeclidinium bromide alone or in fixed combination with vilanterol trifenatate should be administered once daily at the same time every day.

Before first use of either the Incruse® Ellipta® or Anoro® Ellipta® inhaler, the device should be removed from the foil tray and the enclosed desiccant should be discarded out of reach of children and pets. The date the tray is opened and the discard date (6 weeks after opening) should be written on the inhaler label. The number of doses remaining in the inhaler is displayed on the counter located on the front of the device. The cover of the inhaler should not be opened until immediately before use; to avoid wasting doses, the inhaler cover should not be closed again until the dose has been inhaled. When the cover of the inhaler is opened fully to expose the mouthpiece, a click should be heard. If the dose counter does not advance when the click is heard, the dose has not been properly prepared, and the patient should contact the clinician.

Before inhaling the dose, the patient should exhale completely, but should *not* exhale into the mouthpiece of the inhaler. The patient should then place the mouthpiece between the lips and inhale deeply through the inhaler with a steady, even breath; the patient should not inhale through the nose. The air vent on the inhaler should not be blocked while the dose is administered. The patient should remove the inhaler from the mouth, hold the breath for about 3–4 seconds (or as long as comfortable), and then exhale slowly and gently. While some patients may taste or feel a dose of drug delivered from the inhaler, patients should be instructed not to use another dose even if they do not perceive that the dose has been delivered. After the dose is administered, the inhaler should be closed by sliding the cover up and over the mouthpiece as far as possible.

The inhaler does not need to be cleaned after use. However, if desired, the mouthpiece can be cleaned with a dry tissue. The inhaler should be discarded when every blister has been used or 6 weeks after removal of the inhaler from the foil tray, whichever comes first.

■ **Dosage** Dosage of umeclidinium bromide is expressed in terms of umeclidinium.

Each foil-wrapped blister in the Incruse® Ellipta® inhaler device contains 74.2 mcg of umeclidinium bromide (equivalent to 62.5 mcg of umeclidinium). After the inhaler is activated, the powder within the blister is exposed and dispersed into the air stream created by the patient's inhalation. Using standardized in vitro testing at a flow rate of 60 L/minute for 4 seconds, the inhaler delivered 55 mcg of umeclidinium per blister. The precise amount of drug delivered to the lungs with each activation of the inhaler device depends on factors such as the patient's inspiratory flow. The commercially available inhaler delivers 30 doses (or 7 doses from the sample or institutional package).

Each foil-wrapped blister in the Anoro® Ellipta® inhaler device contains 74.2 mcg of umeclidinium bromide (equivalent to 62.5 mcg of umeclidinium) or 40 mcg of vilanterol trifenatate (equivalent to 25 mcg of vilanterol) (in separate blisters). After the inhaler is activated, the powder within a pair of blisters is exposed and dispersed into the air stream created by the patient's inhalation. Using standardized in vitro testing at a flow rate of 60 L/minute for 4 seconds, the inhaler delivered 55 mcg of umeclidinium and 22 mcg of vilanterol per pair of blisters. The precise amount of drug delivered to the lungs with each activation of the inhaler device depends on factors such as the patient's inspiratory flow. The commercially available inhaler delivers 30 doses (or 7 doses from the sample or institutional package).

Chronic Obstructive Pulmonary Disease **Umeclidinium Bromide Therapy.** For maintenance therapy of chronic obstructive pulmonary disease (COPD), the recommended dosage of umeclidinium in adults is 62.5 mcg of umeclidinium (1 inhalation) once daily via the Incruse® Ellipta® inhaler device. The drug should not be administered more frequently than once every 24 hours. If a dose of umeclidinium bromide is missed, the dose may be taken as soon as it is remembered. However, 2 doses should not be taken at the same time.

Umeclidinium Bromide and Vilanterol Trifenatate Fixed-combination Therapy. For maintenance therapy of COPD, the recommended dosage of umeclidinium in fixed combination with vilanterol in adults is 62.5 mcg of umeclidinium and 25 mcg of vilanterol (1 inhalation) once daily via the Anoro® Ellipta® inhaler device. The drug should not be administered more frequently than once every 24 hours. If a dose of umeclidinium in fixed combination with vilanterol trifenatate is missed, the dose may be taken as soon as it is remembered. However, 2 doses should not be taken at the same time.

■ **Special Populations** The manufacturer of umeclidinium bromide and umeclidinium in fixed combination with vilanterol trifenatate states that dosage adjustment is not required in geriatric patients or in patients with renal impairment or moderate hepatic impairment. (See Specific Populations under Cautions: Warnings/Precautions.)

Cautions

■ **Contraindications** Known hypersensitivity to umeclidinium bromide or any other ingredient in the commercially available formulation. Known severe hypersensitivity to milk proteins.

When umeclidinium bromide is used in fixed combination with vilanterol trifenatate, contraindications associated with vilanterol should be considered.

■ **Warnings/Precautions** ***Sensitivity Reactions*** Hypersensitivity reactions may occur after administration of umeclidinium bromide alone or in fixed combination with vilanterol trifenatate. Anaphylactic reactions have been reported following oral inhalation of other powder preparations containing lactose in patients with severe hypersensitivity to milk proteins; therefore, patients with severe milk protein allergy should not use umeclidinium bromide alone or in fixed combination with vilanterol trifenatate. (See Cautions: Contraindications.)

Use of Fixed Combinations When umeclidinium bromide is used in fixed combination with vilanterol trifenatate, the usual cautions, precautions, contraindications, and interactions associated with vilanterol trifenatate must be considered. Cautionary information applicable to specific populations (e.g., pregnant or nursing women, individuals with hepatic or renal impairment, or geriatric patients) should be considered for each drug in the fixed combination.

Deterioration of Disease and Acute Episodes Umeclidinium bromide alone or in fixed combination with vilanterol trifenatate should not be initiated in patients with acutely deteriorating chronic obstructive pulmonary disease (COPD), which may be life-threatening. Umeclidinium has not been studied in this patient population, and initiation of the drug in this setting is not appropriate.

Umeclidinium bromide alone or in fixed combination with vilanterol trifenatate should *not* be used for the relief of acute symptoms (i.e., as rescue therapy for the treatment of acute episodes of bronchospasm). Umeclidinium bromide alone or in fixed combination with vilanterol trifenatate has not been studied for the relief of acute symptoms and extra doses of the drug should not be used for this purpose. All patients receiving umeclidinium bromide alone or in fixed combination with vilanterol trifenatate should be provided with and instructed in the use of a short-acting, inhaled β_2-agonist.

COPD may deteriorate acutely over a period of hours or chronically over several days or longer. Failure to respond to a previously effective dosage of umeclidinium bromide alone or in fixed combination with vilanterol trifenatate or to a supplemental short-acting, inhaled β_2-agonist (e.g., increased need for additional short-acting, inhaled β_2-agonists) may indicate deterioration of COPD for which prompt medical attention is indicated. In this setting, immediate reevaluation of the patient and treatment regimen is required. Increasing the daily dosage of umeclidinium bromide alone or in fixed combination with vilanterol trifenatate to exceed the recommended dosage is not appropriate in this situation.

Paradoxical Bronchospasm As with other inhaled drugs, patients receiving umeclidinium bromide alone or in fixed combination with vilanterol trifenatate may develop paradoxical bronchospasm, which may be life-threatening.

If paradoxical bronchospasm occurs, it should be treated immediately with an inhaled, short-acting bronchodilator. Umeclidinium bromide alone or in fixed combination with vilanterol trifenatate should be discontinued immediately and alternative therapy instituted.

Ocular Effects Umeclidinium bromide alone or in fixed combination with vilanterol trifenatate should be used with caution in patients with acute angle-closure glaucoma. The drug may worsen acute angle-closure glaucoma manifested by ocular pain or discomfort, blurred vision, visual halos, or colored images in association with red eyes from conjunctival congestion and corneal edema. (See Advice to Patients.)

Genitourinary Effects Umeclidinium bromide alone or in fixed combination with vilanterol trifenatate should be used with caution in patients with urinary retention. Umeclidinium bromide alone or in fixed combination with vilanterol trifenatate may worsen symptoms and signs (e.g., urinary retention, dysuria) associated with prostatic hyperplasia or bladder neck obstruction. (See Advice to Patients.)

Cardiovascular Effects Atrial fibrillation was reported in less than 1% of patients receiving umeclidinium, but more frequently than with placebo, in clinical trials.

In a study evaluating potential effects of umeclidinium alone or in fixed combination with vilanterol on the QT interval, effects on prolongation of the QT interval were not observed in healthy individuals.

Specific Populations **Pregnancy.** Category C. (See Users Guide.)

There are no adequate and well-controlled trials with umeclidinium in pregnant women. Umeclidinium should be used during pregnancy only if the potential benefit outweighs the potential risk to the fetus.

There are no adequate and well-controlled trials with umeclidinium during labor and delivery. Umeclidinium should be used during labor only if the potential benefit outweighs the potential risk.

Lactation. Umeclidinium may be distributed into milk in rats; it is not known whether the drug is distributed into milk in humans. The manufacturer states that orally inhaled umeclidinium should be used with caution in nursing women. The manufacturer recommends that a decision be made whether to discontinue nursing or the drug, taking into account the importance of the drug to the woman.

Pediatric Use. Safety and efficacy of umeclidinium have not been established in children. The drug is not indicated for use in pediatric patients.

Geriatric Use. When the total number of patients studied in clinical trials of umeclidinium is considered, about 49% were 65 years of age or older, while 11% were 75 years of age or older. In clinical trials evaluating umeclidinium in fixed combination with vilanterol, approximately 29% of patients receiving the drug were 65 years of age or older, and about 7% were 75 years of age or older. Although no overall differences in efficacy or safety were observed between geriatric and younger patients in clinical trials, and other clinical experience revealed no evidence of age-related differences, the possibility that some older patients may exhibit increased sensitivity to the drug cannot be ruled out. Dosage adjustment is not necessary in geriatric patients.

Hepatic Impairment. No clinically important differences in umeclidinium pharmacokinetics were observed in patients with moderate hepatic impairment (Child-Pugh score of 7–9). Umeclidinium has not been studied in patients with severe hepatic impairment.

Renal Impairment. No clinically important differences in umeclidinium pharmacokinetics were observed in patients with severe renal impairment (creatinine clearance less than 30 mL/minute). Dosage adjustment is not necessary in patients with renal impairment.

■ **Common Adverse Effects** Adverse events occurring in 1% or more of patients with COPD receiving umeclidinium and at an incidence greater than placebo include nasopharyngitis, upper respiratory tract infection, cough, and arthralgia.

Adverse effects reported in 1% or more of patients with COPD receiving umeclidinium in fixed combination with vilanterol trifenatate include pharyngitis, sinusitis, lower respiratory tract infection, constipation, diarrhea, extremity pain, muscle spasms, neck pain, and chest pain.

Drug Interactions

Umeclidinium is a substrate of cytochrome P-450 (CYP) isoenzyme 2D6 and P-glycoprotein (P-gp).

■ **Drugs Affecting or Metabolized by Hepatic Microsomal Enzymes and/or the P-glycoprotein Transport System** No clinically important effect on umeclidinium exposure was observed in individuals who were poor-metabolizers of CYP2D6 substrates compared with ultrarapid, extensive, and intermediate metabolizers. (See Description.) Therefore, dosage adjustment is not required when umeclidinium is used concomitantly with CYP2D6 inhibitors.

Concomitant administration of verapamil 240 mg daily (a moderate P-gp inhibitor) resulted in a 1.4-fold increase in area under the plasma concentration-time curve (AUC) of umeclidinium; no effect on peak plasma concentration of umeclidinium was observed. Dosage adjustment of umeclidinium is not required with concomitant use.

■ **Anticholinergic Agents** Additive adverse anticholinergic effects may occur if umeclidinium is used concomitantly with other anticholinergic agents. The manufacturer states that concomitant use of umeclidinium with other anticholinergic agents should be avoided.

Description

Umeclidinium bromide is a synthetic quaternary ammonium antimuscarinic agent for use as a long-acting, orally inhaled bronchodilator. The drug is a nonselective competitive antagonist at muscarinic (M_1–M_5) receptors. Umeclidinium competitively and reversibly inhibits the actions of acetylcholine and other cholinergic stimuli at M_3 receptors in the smooth muscle of the respiratory tract leading to bronchodilation.

Umeclidinium exhibits linear pharmacokinetics over a dosage range of 62.5–500 mcg. Steady-state plasma umeclidinium concentrations are achieved within 14 days, with 1.8-fold accumulation, following repeated once-daily inhalation of umeclidinium. Peak plasma umeclidinium concentrations are reached within 5–15 minutes following oral inhalation; however, umeclidinium plasma concentrations may not predict therapeutic effect. Umeclidinium is mostly absorbed from the lungs after an orally inhaled dose, with minimal contribution from oral absorption. Umeclidinium is approximately 89% bound to human plasma proteins. Umeclidinium is metabolized, primarily by cytochrome P-450 (CYP) isoenzyme 2D6, and also is a substrate for the P-glycoprotein (P-gp) transporter.

Following repeated administration of umeclidinium 500 mcg (8 times the usual recommended dosage), no clinically important effect was observed on umeclidinium exposure in individuals who were poor-metabolizers of CYP2D6 substrates compared with healthy ultrarapid, extensive, and intermediate metabolizers.

The principal routes of metabolism are oxidation via hydroxylation and *O*-dealkylation followed by conjugation (e.g., glucuronidation); systemic exposure to metabolites with reduced or undetermined pharmacologic activity compared with the parent drug is low. Umeclidinium undergoes biliary elimination with excretion of 58 and 22% of a radiolabeled IV dose in feces and urine, respectively. Following oral administration, 92 and less than 1% of a radiolabeled dose of umeclidinium is excreted in feces and urine, respectively, suggesting negligible oral absorption. The effective half-life following once daily dosing of umeclidinium is 11 hours. Age, gender, weight, race, and use of inhaled corticosteroids have not been found to affect umeclidinium pharmacokinetics.

Advice to Patients

When umeclidinium bromide is used in fixed combination with vilanterol trifenatate, importance of informing patients of important cautionary information about vilanterol trifenatate.

A copy of the manufacturer's patient information for umeclidinium bromide or the medication guide for umeclidinium in fixed combination with vilanterol should be provided to all patients each time the drug is dispensed. Importance of instructing patients to read the patient information or medication guide prior to initiation of therapy and each time the prescription is refilled.

Importance of informing clinician of any history of hypersensitivity reactions to umeclidinium or severe allergy to milk proteins.

Importance of adequate understanding of proper storage and inhalation techniques, including use of the inhalation delivery systems.

Importance of advising patients that if a dose of umeclidinium alone or in fixed combination with vilanterol is missed, the dose should be taken as soon as it is remembered. Importance of not doubling the dose, and of not taking more than one dose in a 24-hour period.

Importance of all patients being provided with and instructed in the use of a short-acting, inhaled β_2-adrenergic agonist (e.g., albuterol) as supplemental therapy for acute symptoms.

Importance of contacting a clinician immediately if symptoms worsen or if the short-acting β_2-agonist becomes less effective or more inhalations than usual are required to relieve symptoms.

Importance of patients not discontinuing therapy without medical supervision, since symptoms may recur after discontinuance.

Importance of not using umeclidinium therapy to relieve acute symptoms or exacerbations of chronic obstructive pulmonary disease (COPD).

Importance of discontinuing umeclidinium and informing a clinician if paradoxical bronchospasm occurs.

Importance of informing a clinician immediately if eye pain or discomfort, blurred vision, visual halos, or colored images in association with red eyes from conjunctival congestion or corneal edema occur.

Importance of informing a clinician immediately if urinary retention or dysuria occurs.

Importance of informing clinicians of existing or contemplated concomitant therapy, including prescription and OTC drugs (e.g., eye drops) and herbal supplements, as well as any concomitant illnesses (e.g., urinary retention, enlarged prostate, angle-closure glaucoma).

Importance of women informing clinicians if they are or plan to become pregnant or plan to breast-feed.

Importance of informing patients of other important precautionary information. (See Cautions.)

Overview® (see Users Guide). For additional information on this drug until a more detailed monograph is developed and published, the manufacturer's labeling should be consulted. It is *essential* that the manufacturer's labeling be consulted for more detailed information on usual cautions, precautions, contraindications, potential drug interactions, laboratory test interferences, and acute toxicity.

Preparations

Excipients in commercially available drug preparations may have clinically important effects in some individuals; consult specific product labeling for details.

Umeclidinium Bromide

Oral Inhalation

Powder for inhalation	62.5 mcg (of umeclidinium) per inhalation	**Incruse® Ellipta®**, GlaxoSmithKline

Umeclidinium Bromide Combinations

Oral Inhalation

Powder for inhalation	62.5 mcg (of umeclidinium) with Vilanterol Trifenatate 25 mcg (of vilanterol) per inhalation	**Anoro® Ellipta®**, GlaxoSmithKline

†Use is not currently included in the labeling approved by the US Food and Drug Administration

SYMPATHOMIMETIC (ADRENERGIC) AGENTS 12:12

α-ADRENERGIC AGONISTS 12:12.04

Lofexidine Hydrochloride

■ Lofexidine hydrochloride is a selective central α_2-adrenergic agonist.

Uses

■ **Opiate Withdrawal** Lofexidine hydrochloride is used for mitigation of opiate withdrawal symptoms to facilitate abrupt opiate discontinuance.

In patients with opiate use disorder, opiate withdrawal management (also referred to as detoxification) generally involves short-term use of tapering dosages of buprenorphine (an opiate partial agonist) or methadone (a full opiate agonist) to reduce withdrawal symptoms. However, prescribing restrictions may limit use of these drugs, and α_2-adrenergic agonists (e.g., lofexidine, clonidine) also have been used for symptomatic relief of noradrenergic-mediated opiate withdrawal symptoms (e.g., lacrimation, sweating, shivering, rhinorrhea) in both inpatient and outpatient settings and may allow for withdrawal over a shorter period of time. The α_2-adrenergic agonists appear to be less effective than buprenorphine or methadone in the management of opiate withdrawal, and some experts suggest that α_2-adrenergic agonists may be most useful in withdrawal management as adjuncts to opiate agonists or partial agonists, to facilitate transition to opiate antagonist (naltrexone) treatment for relapse prevention, or in settings where therapy with opiate agonists or partial agonists is contraindicated, unacceptable, or unavailable. While α_2-adrenergic agonists relieve noradrenergic-mediated symptoms of opiate withdrawal, concomitant supportive therapy for other withdrawal symptoms (e.g., abdominal cramping, diarrhea, nausea and vomiting, muscle spasms, anxiety or restlessness, insomnia) may improve patient comfort, particularly in patients treated principally with an α_2-adrenergic agonist.

Although direct comparisons between lofexidine and clonidine are limited, results of several small comparative studies suggest that lofexidine and clonidine have similar efficacy in managing opiate withdrawal symptoms but lofexidine may be associated with less hypotension. However, the greater cost of lofexidine compared with off-label clonidine use also must be considered.

Because of the potential for hypotension and bradycardia, some experts state that α_2-adrenergic agonists are not drugs of choice for opiate withdrawal management in geriatric patients or patients with coronary insufficiency, ischemic heart disease, bradycardia, or cerebrovascular disease.

Lofexidine is not a treatment for opiate use disorder and should be used for mitigation of opiate withdrawal symptoms in patients with opiate use disorder only in conjunction with a comprehensive treatment program. Opiate withdrawal without subsequent maintenance treatment is associated with high rates of relapse. For most patients with opioid use disorder, maintenance treatment with buprenorphine or methadone or treatment with naltrexone for relapse prevention is superior to opiate withdrawal management.

In patients receiving long-term opiate analgesia, withdrawal symptoms generally are managed by slow tapering of the opiate analgesic dosage.

Clinical Experience The current indication for lofexidine is based principally on the results of 2 randomized, double-blind, placebo-controlled, phase 3 studies in a total of 866 adults who were physically dependent on short-acting opiates (e.g., heroin, hydrocodone, oxycodone) and receiving inpatient treatment for withdrawal management. In both studies, lofexidine was associated with a reduced severity of opiate withdrawal symptoms (as measured by the Short Opiate Withdrawal Scale of Gossop [SOWS-Gossop]) and higher treatment completion rates compared with placebo. The SOWS-Gossop is a patient-reported outcome instrument used to evaluate the severity of 10 specific opiate withdrawal symptoms; each symptom is evaluated on a scale of 0–3 (corresponding to a rating of none, mild, moderate, or severe), and the total score (range: 0–30) is equal to the sum of the individual item scores. Patients in these studies could receive other concomitant supportive therapy for opiate withdrawal symptoms (e.g., guaifenesin, antacids, docusate, psyllium hydrocolloid suspension, bismuth sulfate, acetaminophen, zolpidem). The studies excluded patients with uncontrolled arrhythmias, corrected QT (QT_c) interval prolongation (exceeding 450 msec in males or 470 msec in females), or other clinically important electrocardiographic (ECG) abnormalities; history of myocardial infarction; symptomatic hypotension, systolic blood pressure less than 95 mm Hg (study 1) or 90 mm Hg (study 2), or diastolic blood pressure less than 65 mm Hg (study 1); hypertension with blood pressure exceeding 155/95 mm Hg (study 1) or 160/100 mm Hg (study 2); symptomatic bradycardia or heart rate less than 55 beats/minute (study 1) or 45 beats/minute (study 2); or recent use of antihypertensive or antiarrhythmic agents.

In study 1, 602 patients were randomized to receive lofexidine 0.54 mg given 4 times daily, lofexidine 0.72 mg given 4 times daily, or placebo for 7 days in an inpatient setting. Patients who successfully completed days 1–7 of inpatient treatment were eligible to receive open-label treatment with lofexidine (up to 2.88 mg daily) for an additional 7 days (days 8–14). Mean SOWS-Gossop scores for days 1–7 were 6.5, 6.1, or 8.8 for patients receiving lofexidine 2.16 mg daily, lofexidine 2.88 mg daily, or placebo, respectively; 41, 40, or 28% of patients receiving these respective treatments completed 7 days of treatment.

In study 2, 264 patients were randomized to receive lofexidine 0.72 mg given 4 times daily or placebo for 5 days in an inpatient setting, followed by 2 additional days of placebo prior to discharge. Mean SOWS-Gossop scores for days 1–5 were 7 or 8.9 for patients receiving lofexidine or placebo, respectively; 49 or 33% of patients receiving these respective treatments completed 5 days of treatment.

Dosage and Administration

■ General Vital signs should be assessed prior to lofexidine dosing. Electrocardiographic (ECG) monitoring is recommended in certain patients at risk for QT interval prolongation. (See Hypotension, Bradycardia, and Syncope and also see QT Interval Prolongation under Cautions: Warnings/Precautions.)

■ Administration Lofexidine is administered orally 4 times daily (i.e., every 5–6 hours) without regard to meals.

■ Dosage Dosage of lofexidine hydrochloride is expressed in terms of lofexidine. Dosage of the drug also has been expressed in terms of the salt; 0.18 mg of lofexidine is equivalent to 0.2 mg of lofexidine hydrochloride.

The manufacturer states that the usual initial dosage of lofexidine for the mitigation of opiate withdrawal symptoms in adults is 2.16 mg daily administered in 4 divided doses of 0.54 mg every 5–6 hours during the period of peak withdrawal symptoms (generally the first 5–7 days following the last use of opiates), with dosage guided by symptoms and adverse effects. Lofexidine may be administered for up to 14 days, with dosage guided by symptoms. Single adult doses should not exceed 0.72 mg, and the total daily dosage should not exceed 2.88 mg.

Some experts recommend an initial lofexidine dosage of 0.36–0.54 mg twice daily and state that dosage may be increased as necessary and tolerated to a maximum of 2.16 mg daily administered in 2–4 divided doses for 7–10 days.

Dosage of lofexidine should be reduced or therapy with the drug should be interrupted or discontinued in individuals demonstrating greater sensitivity to its adverse effects. As opiate withdrawal symptoms wane, lower dosages of lofexidine may be appropriate.

When lofexidine therapy is discontinued, dosage of the drug should be reduced gradually (e.g., by 0.18 mg per dose every 1–2 days) over 2–4 days to minimize lofexidine withdrawal symptoms and rebound elevations in blood pressure. (See Symptoms Resulting from Abrupt Lofexidine Discontinuance under Cautions: Warnings/Precautions.)

■ Special Populations ***Hepatic Impairment*** In patients with mild hepatic impairment (Child-Pugh score 5–6), the recommended dosage of lofexidine is 0.54 mg 4 times daily. In patients with moderate hepatic impairment (Child-Pugh score 7–9), the recommended dosage of lofexidine is 0.36 mg 4 times daily. In patients with severe hepatic impairment (Child-Pugh score exceeding 9), the recommended dosage of lofexidine is 0.18 mg 4 times daily. (See Hepatic Impairment under Warnings/Precautions: Specific Populations, in Cautions.)

Renal Impairment The manufacturer provides no specific dosage recommendations for patients with mild renal impairment. In patients with moderate renal impairment (estimated glomerular filtration rate [eGFR] 30–89.9 mL/minute per 1.73 m^2), the recommended dosage of lofexidine is 0.36 mg 4 times daily. In patients with severe renal impairment or end-stage renal disease (eGFR less than 30 mL/minute per 1.73 m^2) or in patients receiving dialysis, the recommended dosage of lofexidine is 0.18 mg 4 times daily. Supplemental doses are not required following dialysis. Lofexidine may be administered without regard to the timing of dialysis. (See Renal Impairment under Warnings/Precautions: Specific Populations, in Cautions.)

Geriatric Patients Dosage adjustments similar to those recommended in patients with renal impairment should be considered in geriatric patients.

Cautions

■ Contraindications The manufacturer states there are no known contraindications to the use of lofexidine.

■ Warnings/Precautions ***Hypotension, Bradycardia, and Syncope*** Lofexidine can cause hypotension, bradycardia, and syncope. In a phase 3 study in patients receiving inpatient treatment for opiate withdrawal (study 1), hypotension, orthostatic hypotension, bradycardia, and syncope were reported in approximately 30, 35, 28, and 1%, respectively, of lofexidine-treated patients. The incidence of serious cardiovascular effects was higher in women than in men receiving lofexidine 2.88 mg daily (4 versus 1%); similarly, bradycardia and orthostatic hypotension necessitating drug discontinuance or withholding of doses also occurred more frequently in women than in men receiving lofexidine 2.88 mg daily.

Vital signs should be assessed prior to lofexidine dosing, and patients receiving the drug should be monitored for symptoms of bradycardia and orthostatic hypotension.

Patients receiving lofexidine should be informed of the risk of hypotension. Those receiving the drug in the outpatient setting should be capable of performing self-monitoring for hypotension, orthostasis, bradycardia, and associated symptoms, and should be instructed on measures for reducing the risk of serious consequences should these adverse effects occur. Patients receiving lofexidine in the outpatient setting should be instructed to withhold doses of lofexidine during symptomatic episodes of hypotension or bradycardia and to contact their health-care provider for guidance on dosage adjustment; following clinically important or symptomatic hypotension and/or bradycardia, the subsequent dose should be reduced in strength, delayed, or omitted. (See Advice to Patients.)

Use of lofexidine should be avoided in patients with severe coronary insufficiency, recent myocardial infarction, cerebrovascular disease, chronic renal failure, or marked bradycardia. To avoid the risk of excessive bradycardia and hypotension, concomitant use of lofexidine with drugs known to decrease heart rate or blood pressure also should be avoided.

QT Interval Prolongation Lofexidine prolongs the QT interval. In healthy individuals, single 1.44- or 1.8-mg doses of lofexidine produced a maximum mean change from baseline in QT interval (corrected for heart rate using Fridericia's formula [QT_cF]) of 14.4 or 13.6 msec, respectively. In a phase 3, placebo-controlled, dose-response study in opiate-dependent patients, lofexidine 2.16 or 2.88 mg daily was associated with a maximum mean change in QT_cF of 7.3 or 9.3 msec, respectively. Torsades de pointes with cardiac arrest (with successful resuscitation) has been reported during postmarketing experience.

Clinically important QT interval prolongation may occur in patients with hepatic or renal impairment. Administration of lofexidine in patients with hepatic or renal impairment was associated with prolongation of the corrected QT interval; such effects were more pronounced in those with severe impairment.

Electrocardiographic (ECG) monitoring is recommended in patients with heart failure, bradyarrhythmias, or hepatic or renal impairment, and in those receiving other drugs known to prolong the QT interval (e.g., methadone). (See Drug Interactions: Drugs that Prolong the QT Interval.) In patients with electrolyte abnormalities (e.g., hypokalemia, hypomagnesemia), the electrolyte abnormalities should be corrected prior to initiation of lofexidine therapy, and ECG monitoring should be performed upon initiation of lofexidine. Use of lofexidine should be avoided in patients with congenital long QT syndrome.

Concomitant Use of CNS Depressants Lofexidine potentiates the CNS depressive effects of benzodiazepines and also is expected to potentiate the CNS depressive effects of alcohol and other sedating drugs (e.g., barbiturates). (See Drug Interactions: CNS Depressants.)

Risk of Opiate Overdosage following Relapse to Opiate Use Patients who complete opiate discontinuance are likely to have a reduced tolerance to opiates and are therefore at an increased risk of fatal opiate overdosage should they resume opiate use. Patients and caregivers should be informed of this increased risk of overdosage. Lofexidine is not a treatment for opiate use disorder and should be used for mitigation of opiate withdrawal symptoms in patients with opiate use disorder only in conjunction with a comprehensive treatment program.

Symptoms Resulting from Abrupt Lofexidine Discontinuance Abrupt discontinuance of lofexidine can result in marked increases in blood pressure, with peak blood pressure values observed on the second day after abrupt discontinuance. A 50% reduction in lofexidine dosage one day prior to drug discontinuance resulted in a similar incidence and magnitude of blood pressure elevations as compared with abrupt discontinuance. Discontinuance of lofexidine also has been associated with diarrhea, insomnia, anxiety, chills, hyperhydrosis, and extremity pain.

When lofexidine therapy is discontinued, the dosage should be gradually reduced. (See Dosage and Administration: Dosage.) Symptoms related to drug discontinuance can be managed by resuming administration of the previous lofexidine dosage and subsequently tapering the dosage.

Specific Populations **Pregnancy.** Safety of lofexidine has not been established in pregnant women. Oral administration of lofexidine during the period of organogenesis in pregnant rats and rabbits resulted in reduced fetal weights, increased fetal resorption, and loss of litters at exposures less than those achieved in humans. When the drug was administered orally from the beginning of organogenesis through lactation, increased stillbirths, loss of litters, and decreased viability and lactation indices resulted, and offspring demonstrated delays in sexual maturation (both males and females), auditory startle, and surface righting.

Experts state that the recommended treatment of opiate dependence in pregnant women is maintenance treatment with buprenorphine or methadone; this approach is superior to medically supervised withdrawal because withdrawal is associated with high relapse rates and poorer outcomes.

Lactation. It is not known whether lofexidine or its metabolites are distributed into milk. The effects of lofexidine or its metabolites on breast-fed infants or on milk production also are unknown. Lofexidine is chemically and pharmacologically related to clonidine, which reaches high concentrations in milk and in breast-fed infants. Caution should be exercised if lofexidine is administered to a nursing woman, especially while breast-feeding a neonate or preterm infant; the developmental and health benefits of breast-feeding and the importance of the drug to the woman should be considered along with the potential adverse effects on the breast-fed child from the drug or from the underlying maternal condition.

Pediatric Use. Safety and efficacy of lofexidine have not been established in pediatric patients.

Geriatric Use. Safety and efficacy of lofexidine have not been established in geriatric patients. Caution should be exercised when lofexidine is used in patients older than 65 years of age. (See Geriatric Patients under Dosage and Administration: Special Populations.)

Hepatic Impairment. Hepatic impairment decreases elimination of lofexidine but has less effect on peak plasma concentrations than on systemic exposure (i.e., area under the plasma concentration-time curve [AUC]) of the drug following a single dose; dosage adjustment is recommended depending on the degree of hepatic impairment. (See Hepatic Impairment under Dosage and Administration: Special Populations.) Following administration of a single 0.36-mg dose of lofexidine, peak plasma concentration in patients with mild (Class-Pugh class A, score 5–6), moderate (Child-Pugh class B, score 7–9), or severe (Child-Pugh class C, score 10–15) hepatic impairment is 114, 117, or 166%, respectively, and systemic exposure is 117, 185, or 260%, respectively, compared with that in individuals with normal hepatic function. The half-life of the drug in these respective groups is 139, 281, or 401% of that in individuals with normal hepatic function.

Clinically important prolongation of the QT interval may occur in patients with hepatic impairment. QT interval prolongation was more pronounced in patients with severe hepatic impairment. ECG monitoring is recommended in patients with hepatic impairment.

Renal Impairment. Renal impairment decreases elimination of lofexidine but has less effect on peak plasma concentrations than on systemic exposure (AUC) of the drug following a single dose; dosage adjustment is recommended depending on the degree of renal impairment. (See Renal Impairment under Dosage and Administration: Special Populations.) Following administration of a single 0.36-mg dose of lofexidine, peak plasma concentration in patients with mild (estimated glomerular filtration rate [eGFR] 60–89 mL/minute per 1.73 m^2), moderate (eGFR 30–59 mL/minute per 1.73^2), or severe (eGFR 15–29 mL/minute per 1.73 m^2) renal impairment is 124, 117, or 154%, respectively, and systemic exposure is 144, 173, or 243%, respectively, compared with that in individuals with normal renal function (eGFR at least 90 mL/minute per 1.73 m^2). The half-life of the drug in these respective groups is 111, 145, or 157% of that in individuals with normal renal function.

In patients with end-stage renal disease receiving hemodialysis 3 times weekly, mean peak plasma concentration was similar to that in individuals with normal renal function matched for sex, age, and body mass index (BMI). Only a negligible fraction of a lofexidine dose is removed during a typical dialysis session. Decreases in lofexidine plasma concentrations occurring during a 4-hour dialysis session are transient, with a return to near predialysis concentrations within a few hours after completion of the dialysis session.

Clinically important prolongation of the QT interval may occur in patients with renal impairment. QT interval prolongation was more pronounced in patients with severe renal impairment. ECG monitoring is recommended in patients with renal impairment.

Pharmacogenomics and Poor CYP2D6 Metabolizers. Because increased systemic exposure to lofexidine is expected in patients who are poor metabolizers of cytochrome P-450 isoenzyme 2D6 (CYP2D6) substrates, these patients should be monitored for adverse effects (e.g., orthostatic hypotension, bradycardia). Lofexidine exposure in patients with the poor CYP2D6 metabolizer phenotype is expected to be similar to that observed in individuals receiving lofexidine concomitantly with a potent CYP2D6 inhibitor. (See Drug Interactions: Drugs Affecting Hepatic Microsomal Enzymes.)

■ **Common Adverse Effects** Adverse effects reported in clinical studies in 10% or more of opiate-dependent patients receiving lofexidine for mitigation of opiate withdrawal symptoms and occurring more frequently with lofexidine than with placebo include insomnia, orthostatic hypotension, bradycardia, hypotension, dizziness, somnolence, sedation, and dry mouth.

Drug Interactions

In vitro studies indicate that lofexidine is extensively metabolized, principally by cytochrome P-450 (CYP) isoenzyme 2D6 and to a lesser extent by CYP1A2 and CYP2C19. Lofexidine and/or its metabolites cause slight inhibition of CYP2D6, but are unlikely to induce or inhibit major CYP isoenzymes at clinically relevant concentrations. Results from an in vitro study suggest that lofexidine is not a substrate of P-glycoprotein (P-gp).

■ **Drugs Affecting Hepatic Microsomal Enzymes** Use of lofexidine in combination with CYP2D6 inhibitors may increase lofexidine exposure. When lofexidine is used concomitantly with CYP2D6 inhibitors, patients should be monitored for adverse effects (e.g., orthostatic hypotension, bradycardia).

Paroxetine Concomitant administration of lofexidine (single 0.36-mg dose) and the potent CYP2D6 inhibitor paroxetine (40 mg daily) in healthy individuals increased peak plasma concentration and systemic exposure of lofexidine by approximately 11 and 28%, respectively.

■ **Drugs Metabolized by Hepatic Microsomal Enzymes** Clinically important pharmacokinetic interactions of lofexidine with substrates of CYP2D6 are not expected.

■ **Cardiovascular Drugs** Concomitant use of lofexidine with drugs that are known to cause hypotension or bradycardia should be avoided.

■ **CNS Depressants** Lofexidine enhances the CNS depressive effects of benzodiazepines and also is expected to enhance the effects of other CNS depressants, such as alcohol, barbiturates, opiate agonists or partial agonists, and other sedating drugs.

■ **Drugs that Prolong the QT Interval** Lofexidine prolongs the QT interval. Electrocardiographic (ECG) monitoring is recommended when lofexidine is used concomitantly with other drugs that are known to prolong the QT interval.

■ **Tricyclic Antidepressants** Limited experience suggests that concomitant use of lofexidine with a tricyclic antidepressant may reduce the efficacy of lofexidine, resulting in exacerbation of opiate withdrawal symptoms.

Desipramine Addition of desipramine hydrochloride (75 mg daily) to lofexidine therapy in a patient with substance (opiate, alcohol, and stimulant) use disorder resulted in exacerbation of opiate withdrawal symptoms (e.g., marked insomnia, feeling cold, twitching, yawning, runny eyes), which was reflected in increasing Short Opiate Withdrawal Scale of Gossop (SOWS-Gossop) scores. Desipramine was discontinued after 2 doses, and opiate withdrawal symptoms abated over the next 24 hours.

■ **Buprenorphine** In patients receiving maintenance treatment with buprenorphine (16–24 mg daily), concomitant use of lofexidine (up to 2.88 mg daily) resulted in no pharmacokinetic or pharmacodynamic interaction.

In patients receiving maintenance treatment with buprenorphine (16–24 mg daily), concomitant use of lofexidine (2.88 mg daily) resulted in a maximum mean increase from baseline in QT interval (corrected for heart rate using Fridericia's formula [QT_cF]) of 15 msec.

■ **Methadone** Lofexidine and methadone both prolong the QT interval. (See Drug Interactions: Drugs that Prolong the QT Interval.) In patients receiving maintenance treatment with methadone hydrochloride (80–120 mg daily), concomitant use of lofexidine (2.88 mg daily) resulted in a maximum mean increase from baseline in QT_cF of 9.1 msec.

In patients receiving maintenance treatment with methadone hydrochloride (80–120 mg daily), concomitant use of lofexidine (up to 2.88 mg daily) did not alter the pharmacokinetics of methadone. Lofexidine concentrations may be slightly increased, but the increase in concentration is not expected to be clinically important at recommended dosages.

■ **Naltrexone** Concomitant administration of oral naltrexone hydrochloride (50 mg daily) with lofexidine (single 0.36-mg dose) in healthy individuals did not result in clinically important changes in lofexidine pharmacokinetics; however, at naltrexone steady state, peak plasma naltrexone and 6-β-naltrexol concentrations were delayed by 2–3 hours and overall exposure to the opiate antagonist was reduced slightly. Administration of oral naltrexone within 2 hours of lofexidine administration may result in reduced efficacy of naltrexone; however, this interaction is not expected if naltrexone is administered via nonoral routes.

Description

Lofexidine hydrochloride, a centrally acting α_2-adrenergic agonist that is structurally and pharmacologically related to clonidine, binds to receptors on adrenergic neurons, reducing the release of norepinephrine and decreasing sympathetic tone. Lofexidine decreases sympathetic neurotransmission from the locus ceruleus, which is responsible for many opiate withdrawal symptoms during acute withdrawal. It has been postulated that lofexidine's greater selectivity for the α_{2A}-adrenergic receptor may be responsible for its improved adverse effect profile (e.g., decreased incidence and severity of hypotension and sedation) compared with structurally similar clonidine. Lofexidine is not an effective antihypertensive agent and does not suppress psychological cravings.

Pharmacokinetics of lofexidine are dose proportional over the dosage range of 0.72–2.88 mg daily. Absolute oral bioavailability of the drug is approximately 72%; approximately 30% of an orally administered dose is converted to inactive metabolites on first pass through the liver. Peak plasma concentrations are achieved 3–5 hours after a single oral dose. Administration of lofexidine with a high-fat, high-calorie meal did not alter peak plasma concentration or area under the concentration-time curve (AUC), and only slightly delayed the median time to peak plasma concentration (from 5 hours to 6 hours). Lofexidine is approximately 55% bound to plasma proteins. The volume of distribution of the drug suggests extensive distribution into tissues. Lofexidine is extensively metabolized, principally by cytochrome P-450 (CYP) isoenzyme 2D6 and to a lesser extent by CYP1A2 and CYP2C19. Lofexidine and its metabolites are eliminated principally by the kidneys; 93.5% of an administered dose is excreted in urine (15–20% as unchanged drug) and 0.9% is excreted in feces. The elimination half-life is approximately 12 hours. The terminal half-life is approximately 11–13 hours following the initial dose and approximately 17–22 hours at steady state. Pharmacokinetics were similar in opiate-dependent patients and healthy individuals.

Advice to Patients

Importance of reading the patient information provided by the manufacturer.

Importance of informing patients that lofexidine may lessen, but not completely prevent, symptoms associated with opiate withdrawal syndrome (e.g., feeling sick, stomach cramps, muscle spasms or twitching, feeling cold, palpitations, muscular tension, aches and pains, yawning, runny eyes, sleep disturbances). Additional supportive measures may be recommended as needed.

Risk of hypotension and bradycardia. Importance of advising patients to be alert for any symptoms of hypotension, orthostasis, or bradycardia (e.g., dizziness, lightheadedness, feelings of faintness at rest or on abrupt standing); to avoid dehydration and overheating; and to rise carefully from a seated or supine position. Importance of instructing patients on how to reduce the risk of serious consequences if hypotension occurs (e.g., by sitting or lying down). Patients experiencing symptomatic episodes of hypotension, orthostasis, or bradycardia in the outpatient setting should be advised to withhold lofexidine and contact their clinician for instructions.

Patients receiving lofexidine in the outpatient setting should be advised to avoid driving, operating heavy machinery, or performing other hazardous activities until they know how the drug will affect them. Risk of increased CNS depression with concomitant use of benzodiazepines, alcohol, barbiturates, or other drugs with sedative effects.

Importance of advising patients to avoid abrupt discontinuance of therapy and to consult a clinician prior to discontinuing therapy.

Risk of opiate overdosage if opiate use is resumed following a period of nonuse (i.e., relapse). Importance of informing patients that they may be more sensitive to the effects of opiates and at greater risk of fatal overdosage if they resume opiate use after a period of nonuse.

Importance of women informing their clinicians if they are or plan to become pregnant or plan to breast-feed.

Importance of informing clinicians of existing or contemplated concomitant therapy, including prescription and OTC drugs and dietary or herbal supplements, as well as any concomitant illnesses (e.g., renal or hepatic impairment; cerebrovascular or cardiovascular disease).

Importance of informing patients of other important precautionary information. (See Cautions.)

Overview® (see Users Guide). For additional information on this drug until a more detailed monograph is developed and published, the manufacturer's labeling should be consulted. It is *essential* that the manufacturer's labeling be consulted for more detailed information on usual cautions, precautions, contraindications, potential drug interactions, laboratory test interferences, and acute toxicity.

Preparations

Excipients in commercially available drug preparations may have clinically important effects in some individuals; consult specific product labeling for details.

Lofexidine Hydrochloride

Oral

Tablets, film-coated	0.18 mg (of lofexidine)	**Lucemyra®**, US WorldMeds

Phenylephrine Hydrochloride

■ Phenylephrine hydrochloride is a sympathomimetic amine that predominantly acts by a direct effect on α_1-adrenergic receptors.

Uses

■ **Hypotension** Phenylephrine hydrochloride is used parenterally to increase blood pressure and provide hemodynamic support in the management of certain acute hypotensive states. Phenylephrine hydrochloride injection is labeled by the US Food and Drug Administration (FDA) for use in the setting of anesthesia or septic shock to treat clinically important hypotension resulting principally from vasodilation. Evidence supporting the use of IV phenylephrine is based on studies from the published literature, the majority of which were conducted in the perioperative setting. Only a few clinical studies have evaluated use of the drug in patients with septic shock. The available data clearly indicate that phenylephrine is effective in increasing and maintaining blood pressure in hypotensive patients. In patients who require vasopressor support, individual hemodynamic abnormalities must be identified and monitored so that therapy can be adjusted as necessary. If severe peripheral vasoconstriction exists, phenylephrine may be ineffective and have a deleterious effect by causing further reductions in plasma volume and blood flow to vital organs.

Hypotension During Anesthesia Phenylephrine hydrochloride is used for the *treatment* of hypotension during anesthesia. Studies performed in a variety of surgical settings have demonstrated that phenylephrine increases systolic and mean arterial blood pressures when administered IV (as a direct "bolus" injection or continuous infusion) following the development of hypotension in patients receiving neuraxial and/or general anesthesia. In many of these studies, the drug was used in low-risk pregnant women undergoing cesarean section with neuraxial anesthesia. Although ephedrine historically has been considered the vasopressor of choice for treatment of hypotension in obstetric anesthesia, phenylephrine is increasingly being used in this setting because of evidence suggesting that the drug may provide a more favorable fetal acid-base balance.

Phenylephrine also has been used for the *prevention* of hypotension in patients undergoing spinal anesthesia. However, routine prophylactic use of vasopressors has been questioned because hypotension does not always occur during spinal anesthesia and treatment can readily be instituted if necessary; some clinicians have suggested that vasopressors be administered prophylactically only in those cases in which a substantial decrease in blood pressure is expected.

Septic Shock Vasopressors are used in the management of vasodilatory shock, the most common form of which is septic shock, to restore blood pressure and tissue perfusion after initial fluid resuscitation is attempted. The Surviving Sepsis Campaign International Guidelines for Management of Sepsis and Septic Shock recommend norepinephrine as the first-line vasopressor of choice in adults with septic shock; if adequate blood pressure is not achieved, vasopressin or epinephrine may be added. Phenylephrine generally has been considered only in selected situations when norepinephrine cannot be used (e.g., because of tachyarrhythmias) or as salvage therapy when other treatment methods have failed. Although data are limited, studies have shown that phenylephrine increases mean arterial pressure in patients with septic shock; however, the regional hemodynamic effects of the drug (particularly in regards to renal blood flow and possible renal toxicity) have not been completely elucidated. (See Cautions: Adverse Effects.) Because of uncertainty regarding the clinical outcomes of phenylephrine therapy, experts currently state that use of the drug should be limited until more information is available.

Although vasopressors have been used in the management of other types of shock or shock-like states (e.g., hemorrhagic or cardiogenic shock), there is insufficient evidence to support the use of phenylephrine for blood pressure support in general shock settings, particularly those not associated with a vasodilatory component. If a vasopressor is required in these situations, norepinephrine usually is preferred.

■ **Prolongation of Spinal Anesthesia** Phenylephrine has been used as an additive to solutions of some local anesthetics to decrease the rate of vascular absorption of the anesthetic and prolong the duration of anesthesia†. The risk of systemic toxicity due to the local anesthetic is also decreased. (See Local Anesthetics, Parenteral, General Statement 72:00.) Phenylephrine is not as effective as epinephrine in prolonging local anesthesia but may be preferred when cardiostimulation is undesirable.

■ **Nasal Congestion** Phenylephrine hydrochloride is administered orally for *self-medication* as a nasal decongestant for temporary relief of nasal congestion associated with upper respiratory allergy (e.g., hay fever) or the common cold; the drug also is used to provide temporary relief of sinus congestion and pressure. Preparations containing phenylephrine in fixed combination with other agents (e.g., acetaminophen, chlorpheniramine, dextromethorphan, diphenhydramine, guaifenesin, pheniramine) are used for temporary relief of nasal/sinus congestion and/or other symptoms (e.g., rhinorrhea, sneezing, lacrimation, itching eyes, oronasopharyngeal itching, cough) associated with seasonal or perennial allergic rhinitis, other upper respiratory allergies, or the common cold. Because of state and federal actions restricting the sale and purchase of nonprescription preparations containing decongestants such as pseudoephedrine, ephedrine, or phenylpropanolamine (no longer commercially available in the US), some manufacturers reformulated various nonprescription pseudoephedrine-containing preparations by substituting phenylephrine for pseudoephedrine. (See Uses: Misuse and Abuse, in Pseudoephedrine 12:12.12.) However, few studies evaluating the efficacy of oral phenylephrine in the treatment of nasal congestion have been published, and efficacy of the drug at currently recommended oral dosages has been questioned by some clinicians.

Nasal decongestants, including phenylephrine, have been used for *self-medication* for the temporary relief of nasal congestion associated with sinusitis. However, prospective studies of nasal decongestants for this use are lacking, and data on their use as adjunctive therapy in the management of sinusitis are limited and controversial. Furthermore, evidence from an animal study indicated that topical nasal decongestants (i.e., oxymetazoline) may *increase* the degree of sinus inflammation, potentially delaying resolution of sinusitis. Because labeling for nonprescription (over-the-counter, OTC) nasal decongestant preparations previously included use for sinusitis, there were concerns that consumers would assume that nasal decongestants were effective in the treatment of sinusitis, thereby choosing *self-medication* over medical evaluation and definitive treatment by a clinician; such delay in medical evaluation could result in a lost opportunity for early diagnosis of another serious medical condition (e.g., bacterial sinusitis). The FDA no longer considers oral or topical nasal decongestants appropriate for *self-medication* of sinusitis. In October 2005, the agency issued a final rule, which was effective in 2007, that amended the final monograph for OTC nasal decongestant preparations to remove the indication for relief of nasal congestion associated with sinusitis from labeling and prohibited use of the term "sinusitis" elsewhere in labeling.

Phenylephrine also is applied topically to the nasal mucosa as a vasoconstrictor to relieve nasal congestion. (See Phenylephrine 52:32.)

■ **Hemorrhoids** Anorectal preparations (e.g., creams, gels, ointments, suppositories) containing phenylephrine hydrochloride are used *topically* or *rectally* to provide temporary symptomatic relief of external or internal hemorrhoids. When applied topically or rectally to the anorectal area, vasoconstrictors such as phenylephrine stimulate α-adrenergic receptors in the vascular beds with a resultant temporary constriction of arterioles and a modest and transient reduction in congestion (swelling) of hemorrhoidal tissues. Vasoconstrictors also may relieve anorectal pruritus, discomfort, and irritation, possibly in part secondary to some weak local anesthetic action; the mechanism of this local anesthetic effect is unknown. Phenylephrine also may relieve pruritus associated with histamine release. However, vasoconstrictors are expected to provide only partial relief of pruritus associated with hemorrhoids, and there are more effective agents for relief of anorectal itching. The presence of other ingredients in the formulation (e.g., protectants, local anesthetics, astringents, antipruritics, analgesics) may provide additional relief of these and other anorectal symptoms (e.g., discomfort, pain, burning) associated with hemorrhoids. Although locally applied vasoconstrictors have been shown to alter mucosal blood flow, safety and efficacy for *self-medication* control of minor hemorrhoidal bleeding have not been established. If minor bleeding is present, a clinician should be consulted promptly for advice because anorectal bleeding may be a sign of conditions ranging in seriousness from simple abrasions to cancer.

Effectiveness of topical or intrarectal therapy with phenylephrine for relief of symptoms secondary to swollen hemorrhoidal tissues is based on a predicted effect of the drug's vasoconstrictive activity in reducing capillary and arteriovenous congestion in the anorectal area rather than on specific efficacy studies. Effective dosage of anorectal therapy with the drug was based on predictions from established efficacy of local therapy for nasal congestion.

■ **Other Uses** **For the use of phenylephrine as a mydriatic, see Phenylephrine Hydrochloride 52:24. For the use of phenylephrine as a vasoconstrictor in the eye or mucosa, see Phenylephrine Hydrochloride 52:32.**

Dosage and Administration

■ **Administration** ***Parenteral Administration*** Phenylephrine hydrochloride injection concentrate is administered after dilution by direct IV ("bolus") injection or continuous IV infusion. The drug also has been administered by IM† or subcutaneous injection†. The route of administration should be determined by the specific clinical situation and needs of the individual patient. For treatment of hypotension during anesthesia, the manufacturers recommend administration of phenylephrine hydrochloride as an IV injection or continuous infusion; when used in the treatment of septic shock, the drug should be administered as a continuous IV infusion with no initial bolus dose.

Commercially available phenylephrine hydrochloride injection concentrate must be diluted with a compatible IV solution prior to administration as a direct IV ("bolus") injection or continuous infusion. To prepare solutions for direct IV injection, 1 mL of the commercially available phenylephrine hydrochloride injection containing 10 mg/mL should be withdrawn and diluted with 99 mL of 5% dextrose or 0.9% sodium chloride injection to provide a final concentration of 100 mcg/mL. To prepare solutions for continuous IV infusion, 1 mL of the commercially available phenylephrine hydrochloride injection containing 10 mg/mL should be withdrawn and added to 500 mL of 5% dextrose or 0.9% sodium chloride injection to provide a final concentration of 20 mcg/mL. Diluted solutions may be stored at room temperature for up to 4 hours or under refrigeration for up to 24 hours; any unused portions should be discarded.

Commercially available phenylephrine hydrochloride bulk vials are intended for use in a pharmacy admixture program for preparation of single doses to be dispensed to multiple patients. Each vial should be penetrated only one time with a suitable sterile transfer device or dispensing set. The pharmacy bulk vial should be discarded within 4 hours after initial entry.

Prior to administration, phenylephrine hydrochloride solutions should be inspected visually for particulate matter and discoloration; the drug should be discarded if the solution is colored, cloudy, or contains any particulate matter.

During IV administration of phenylephrine, intravascular volume depletion and acidosis should always be corrected if present. Blood pressure should be monitored and dosage of phenylephrine hydrochloride adjusted as necessary to achieve appropriate blood pressure goals. Care should be taken to avoid extravasation and the infusion site should be checked for free flow.

Oral Administration As a vasoconstrictor for the management of nasal congestion, phenylephrine is administered orally alone or as a fixed-combination decongestant preparation.

Topical and Rectal Administration As a vasoconstrictor for the management of hemorrhoidal symptoms, phenylephrine hydrochloride topical preparations are administered externally to the affected perianal area and rectal preparations are administered externally to the affected perianal area and/or intrarectally.

Topical preparations of phenylephrine hydrochloride that are labeled for external use only should be applied externally to the affected area and should *not* be administered inside the rectum by either using fingers or any mechanical device or applicator.

Rectal preparations of phenylephrine hydrochloride are labeled either for rectal use only (e.g., suppositories) or for external and/or intrarectal use only. When a special applicator such as a pile pipe or other mechanical device is used to administer the drug intrarectally, the applicator should be attached to the tube of drug and then the applicator should be lubricated well and gently inserted into the rectum; the applicator should be cleansed thoroughly after each use and stored according to the manufacturer's instructions. Such preparations should *not* be used if introduction of the applicator or device into the rectum causes additional pain; patients should be advised to consult a clinician promptly in such cases. The wrapper should be removed from suppositories prior to insertion into the rectum.

Patients receiving phenylephrine hydrochloride for the local management of hemorrhoids should be advised to cleanse the affected perianal area by patting with warm water and mild soap and rinsing thoroughly or with an appropriate cleansing wipe whenever practical. The area then should be dried by patting or blotting with toilet tissue or a soft cloth before application of the drug.

■ **Dosage** Phenylephrine hydrochloride should be administered in the lowest effective dosage for the shortest possible time. When used to increase blood pressure in patients with acute hypotensive states, dosage should be individualized based on the pressor response.

Hypotension During Anesthesia Various phenylephrine hydrochloride dosing regimens have been used for the treatment of hypotension during anesthesia; optimal dosage and method of administration remain to be established. Dosages currently recommended by the manufacturers are based on information from published studies.

For the treatment of hypotension during anesthesia in adults, the manufacturers recommend direct IV ("bolus") doses of phenylephrine hydrochloride ranging from 40–250 mcg; the usual initial dose is 50 or 100 mcg. One manufacturer states that additional IV bolus doses may be administered every 1–2 minutes as needed not to exceed a total dosage of 200 mcg; however, if blood pressure is below the target goal, a continuous IV infusion should be initiated. If phenylephrine hydrochloride is administered by continuous IV infusion, the manufacturers recommend infusion rates of 10–35 mcg/minute or 0.5–1.4 mcg/kg per minute. The infusion generally should be started at a low rate and titrated to effect. Other dosage regimens for phenylephrine hydrochloride have been recommended for the treatment of hypotension; in all situations, dosage should be titrated to effect and the patient should be closely monitored.

Some manufacturers state that total dosage of phenylephrine hydrochloride should not exceed 200 mcg (if given by direct IV injection) or 200 mcg/minute (if given by continuous IV infusion). Higher dosages do not necessarily produce incremental increases in blood pressure and may cause hypertension and reflex bradycardia.

Septic Shock When used in the treatment of septic shock, phenylephrine hydrochloride is administered by continuous IV infusion without an initial bolus dose. (See Dosage and Administration: Administration.) For the treatment of septic shock or other vasodilatory shock in adults, the manufacturer recommends that phenylephrine hydrochloride therapy be initiated at an infusion rate of 0.5–6 mcg/kg per minute; the rate of infusion should be adjusted to maintain the target blood pressure goal. Infusion rates higher than 6 mcg/kg per minute do not appear to provide substantial incremental increases in blood pressure.

Prolongation of Spinal Anesthesia To prolong spinal anesthesia†, 2–5 mg of phenylephrine hydrochloride has been added to the anesthetic solution, and has increased the duration of nerve block by as much as approximately 50%.

Vasoconstriction for Regional Anesthesia To produce vasoconstriction in regional anesthesia†, some clinicians state that the optimum concentration of phenylephrine hydrochloride is 0.05 mg/mL (1:20,000). Solutions have been prepared for regional anesthesia by adding 1 mg of phenylephrine hydrochloride to each 20 mL of local anesthetic solution. Some pressor response can be expected when at least 2 mg is injected.

Nasal Congestion Phenylephrine is administered orally as a nasal decongestant alone or in fixed combination with other drugs. The usual oral decongestant dosage of phenylephrine hydrochloride for *self-medication* in adults and children 12 years of age or older is 10 mg every 4 hours. The manufacturer states that no more than 6 doses should be administered in a 24-hour period. For *self-medication*, the manufacturer recommends that patients discontinue the drug and consult a clinician if symptoms persist more than 7 days or are accompanied by fever, or if nervousness, dizziness, or insomnia occurs.

Hemorrhoids When used topically or rectally as a vasoconstrictor for temporary relief of hemorrhoidal symptoms in adults and children 12 years of age and older, phenylephrine hydrochloride is used for *self-medication* as a cream, gel, ointment, or suppository containing 0.25% of the drug alone or in combination with other anorectal agents (e.g., protectants, local anesthetics, astringents, antipruritics, analgesics). Anorectal preparations of the drug usually are administered at bedtime, in the morning, and *after* bowel movements up to 4 times daily.

Patients should be advised not to exceed the recommended dosage of phenylephrine hydrochloride unless otherwise directed by a clinician. Although the systemic bioavailability of phenylephrine hydrochloride following local application to the anorectal area is not known, it is recommended that anorectal dosage for *self-medication* of hemorrhoids *not* exceed 2 mg daily (i.e., 0.5 mg 4 times daily) in order to minimize adverse systemic effects. It currently is not known whether higher dosages would provide additional benefit.

Patients should be advised to consult a clinician if the anorectal condition worsens or does not improve within 7 days or if bleeding occurs.

Cautions

■ Adverse Effects

Systemic Use Phenylephrine hydrochloride may cause restlessness, anxiety, nervousness, weakness, dizziness, precordial pain or discomfort, tremor, respiratory distress, pallor or blanching of the skin, or a pilomotor response. Injections of the drug may be followed by paresthesia in the extremities or a feeling of coolness in the skin. When 2 mg or more of phenylephrine hydrochloride is injected during regional local anesthesia, a pressor response may occur.

Overdosage of phenylephrine may cause a rapid rise in blood pressure and associated manifestations including headache, seizures, cerebral hemorrhage, palpitation, paresthesia, and vomiting. Hypertensive crisis also has been reported. Hypertension may be relieved by administration of an α-adrenergic blocking agent (e.g., phentolamine).

Phenylephrine can cause severe peripheral and visceral vasoconstriction, reduced blood flow to vital organs, decreased renal perfusion, and possibly reduced urine output and metabolic acidosis. In patients with septic shock, phenylephrine may increase the need for renal replacement therapy. Severe vasoconstrictive effects may be more likely to occur in patients with substantial peripheral vascular disease. In addition, prolonged use of phenylephrine may cause plasma volume depletion that may result in perpetuation or recurrence of hypotension when the drug is discontinued.

Phenylephrine can cause severe bradycardia and decreased cardiac output. Decreased cardiac output may be especially harmful to elderly patients and/or those with initially poor cerebral or coronary circulation. Bradycardia may be treated by administration of atropine. Because of its potent vasoconstricting effects, phenylephrine may precipitate angina in patients with a history of the condition or with severe atherosclerosis. The drug also increases cardiac work by increasing peripheral arterial resistance and may possibly induce or exacerbate heart failure. In addition, phenylephrine may increase pulmonary arterial pressure. In patients with autonomic dysfunction (e.g., those with spinal cord injuries), the blood pressure response to phenylephrine may be increased.

Phenylephrine may cause necrosis or sloughing of tissue if extravasation occurs during IV administration or following subcutaneous administration.

Anorectal Use When used in recommended dosages for local effect in anorectal disorders (e.g., hemorrhoids), adverse systemic effects of vasoconstrictors such as phenylephrine generally are minimal. Such effects, although unlikely, can include blood pressure elevation, cardiac arrhythmia or irregular heart rate, CNS disturbance or nervousness, tremor, sleeplessness, and aggravation of hyperthyroid symptoms.

Based on observations with local use for nasal congestion, prolonged local use of excessive anorectal dosages of vasoconstrictors will likely lead to rebound vasodilation and congestion. Less commonly, prolonged local use of excessive anorectal dosages of vasoconstrictors can lead to anxiety and paranoia.

Phenylephrine reportedly is less likely than other topical vasoconstrictors (e.g., ephedrine, epinephrine) to cause local irritation. Contact dermatitis has been reported following topical application of certain formulations of vasoconstrictors.

The possibility that topical anorectal application of vasoconstrictors if absorbed systemically in adequate amounts could interact with monoamine oxidase (MAO) inhibitors resulting in potentiated hypertensive effects should be considered. Such hypertensive potentiation could result in serious, potentially fatal effects such as cerebral hemorrhage or stroke. (See Anorectal Precautions and Contraindications under Cautions: Precautions and Contraindications.)

■ Precautions and Contraindications

Vasopressor therapy is *not* a substitute for replacement of blood, plasma, fluids, and/or electrolytes. Blood volume depletion should be corrected as fully as possible before or during administration with phenylephrine hydrochloride. In an emergency, the drug may be used as an adjunct to fluid volume replacement or as a temporary supportive measure to maintain coronary and cerebral artery perfusion until volume replacement therapy can be completed, but phenylephrine must *not* be used as sole therapy in hypovolemic patients. Hypoxia and acidosis, which also may reduce the effectiveness of phenylephrine, must be identified and corrected prior to or concurrently with administration of the drug.

Prolonged administration of vasopressors has caused edema, hemorrhage, focal myocarditis, subpericardial hemorrhage, necrosis of the intestine, or hepatic and renal necrosis; these effects have generally occurred in patients with severe shock and it is not clear if the drug or the shock state itself was the cause. Because phenylephrine can cause necrosis of the skin and subcutaneous tissue, care should be taken to avoid extravasation of the drug during IV administration and the infusion site should be checked for free flow.

As with other sympathomimetic drugs, phenylephrine hydrochloride should not be used for *self-medication* of nasal congestion in patients with thyroid disease, diabetes mellitus, hypertension, or heart disease without consulting a clinician. In addition, the drug should not be used for *self-medication* of nasal congestion in patients with difficulty urinating because of prostatic hypertrophy without consulting a clinician. Patients should be advised to discontinue the drug and consult a clinician if symptoms persist more than 7 days or are accompanied by fever, or if nervousness, dizziness, or insomnia develops during therapy. In addition, patients should be advised to avoid phenylephrine if they are currently receiving or have recently received (i.e., within 2 weeks) an MAO inhibitor.

When phenylephrine is used in combination with other drugs, the cautions applicable to all ingredients in the formulations should be kept in mind.

Commercially available formulations of phenylephrine hydrochloride injection may contain sodium metabisulfite, a sulfite that may cause allergic-type reactions, including anaphylaxis and life-threatening or less severe asthmatic episodes, in certain susceptible individuals. The overall prevalence of sulfite sensitivity in the general population is unknown but probably low; such sensitivity appears to occur more frequently in asthmatic than in nonasthmatic individuals. Some manufacturers state that phenylephrine is contraindicated in patients with hypersensitivity to the drug or any of its components.

Some clinicians consider severe coronary disease or cardiovascular disease (including myocardial infarction) to be contraindications to use of phenylephrine. Because of possible renal toxicity in patients with septic shock, renal function should be monitored during phenylephrine use in such patients.

Anorectal Precautions and Contraindications Unless otherwise directed by a clinician, patients should not receive external or rectal preparations of vasoconstrictors such as phenylephrine hydrochloride for *self-medication* of hemorrhoidal symptoms if they have cardiac disease, high blood pressure, thyroid disease, diabetes mellitus, or difficulty in urination secondary to prostatic hyperplasia. Patients also should be advised to consult a clinician before initiating *self-medication* with an anorectal preparation of the drug if they currently are receiving an antihypertensive agent or antidepressant (e.g., MAO inhibitor). For additional precautions associated with anorectal phenylephrine therapy, see Dosage and Administration.

■ Pediatric Precautions

The manufacturers state that safety and efficacy of parenteral preparations of phenylephrine hydrochloride have not been established in pediatric patients; however, the drug has been used in children for the treatment of hypotension during spinal anesthesia.

Overdosage and toxicity (including death) have been reported in children younger than 2 years of age receiving nonprescription (over-the-counter, OTC) preparations containing antihistamines, cough suppressants, expectorants, and nasal decongestants alone or in combination for relief of symptoms of upper respiratory tract infection. There is limited evidence of efficacy for these preparations in this age group, and appropriate dosages (i.e., approved by the US Food and Drug Administration [FDA]) have not been established. Therefore, FDA stated that nonprescription cough and cold preparations should not be used in children younger than 2 years of age; the agency continues to assess safety and efficacy of these preparations in older children. Meanwhile, because children 2–3 years of age also are at increased risk of overdosage and toxicity, some manufacturers of oral nonprescription cough and cold preparations agreed to voluntarily revise the product labeling to state that such preparations should not be used in children younger than 4 years of age. FDA recommends that parents and caregivers adhere to the dosage instructions and warnings on the product labeling that accompanies the preparation if administering to children and consult with their clinician about any concerns. Clinicians should ask caregivers about use of nonprescription cough and cold preparations to avoid overdosage. For additional information on precautions associated with the use of cough and cold preparations in pediatric patients, see Cautions: Pediatric Precautions in Pseudoephedrine 12:12.12.

■ Geriatric Precautions

Clinical studies of phenylephrine hydrochloride did not include sufficient numbers of patients 65 years of age and older to determine whether geriatric patients respond differently than younger patients. Clinical experience to date has not identified any differences in response between geriatric and younger patients. If phenylephrine is used in geriatric patients, dosage should be selected carefully, usually starting at the low end of the dosage range, since renal, hepatic, and cardiovascular dysfunction and concomitant disease or other drug therapy are more common in this age group.

■ **Pregnancy and Lactation** It is not known whether phenylephrine hydrochloride can cause fetal harm when administered to pregnant women; the drug should be used during pregnancy only if the potential benefit justifies the potential risk to the fetus. Animal studies suggest a potential for adverse cardiovascular effects to the fetus if the drug is administered IV during pregnancy. Administration of phenylephrine to patients in late pregnancy or labor may cause fetal anoxia and bradycardia by increasing contractility of the uterus and decreasing uterine blood flow.

In studies of IV phenylephrine in pregnant women undergoing cesarean delivery with neuraxial anesthesia, common adverse effects reported in the mother included nausea and vomiting, bradycardia, reactive hypertension, and transient arrhythmias. The drug did not appear to affect neonatal Apgar scores or umbilical artery blood-gas status.

If a vasopressor is used in conjunction with oxytocic drugs, the vasopressor effect is potentiated and may result in potentially serious adverse effects. (See Drug Interactions: Oxytocic Drugs.)

It is not known whether phenylephrine is distributed into human milk following parenteral administration. The drug should be used with caution in nursing women.

Drug Interactions

■ **α- and β-Adrenergic Blocking Agents** The effects of both phenylephrine and α-adrenergic blocking agents may be blocked when these drugs are administered concomitantly. The vasopressor response to phenylephrine is decreased by prior administration of an α-adrenergic blocking agent such as phentolamine mesylate. Phenothiazine drugs (e.g., chlorpromazine) and amiodarone also have some α-adrenergic blocking effects and can reduce the pressor effect of phenylephrine.

The pressor effects of phenylephrine may be increased with concomitant administration of β-adrenergic blocking drugs.

■ **Oxytocic Drugs** When a vasopressor (e.g., phenylephrine) is used in conjunction with oxytocic drugs, the pressor effect is potentiated, increasing the risk of hemorrhagic stroke. If phenylephrine is used during labor and delivery to correct hypotension or is added to a local anesthetic solution, the obstetrician should be cautioned that some oxytocic drugs may cause severe persistent hypertension and that rupture of a cerebral blood vessel may occur during the postpartum period.

■ **General Anesthetics** Rarely, administration of phenylephrine to patients who have received cyclopropane or halogenated hydrocarbon general anesthetics that increase cardiac irritability and seem to sensitize the myocardium to phenylephrine may result in arrhythmias. However, in usual therapeutic doses, phenylephrine is much less likely to produce arrhythmias than is norepinephrine or metaraminol.

■ **Monoamine Oxidase Inhibitors** The cardiac and pressor effects of phenylephrine are potentiated by prior administration of monoamine oxidase (MAO) inhibitors (e.g., selegiline) because the metabolism of phenylephrine is reduced. The potentiation is greater following oral administration of phenylephrine than after parenteral administration of the drug because reduction of the metabolism of phenylephrine in the intestine results in increased absorption of the drug. Oral administration of phenylephrine to patients receiving a MAO inhibitor should be avoided. Parenteral administration of phenylephrine to these patients, if unavoidable, should be undertaken with extreme caution and with low initial doses. Patients should consult a clinician before initiating anorectal phenylephrine therapy if they are receiving an MAO inhibitor. (See Anorectal Precautions and Contraindications under Cautions: Precautions and Contraindications.)

■ **Other Drugs** Other drugs that may potentiate the pressor effect of phenylephrine include α_2-adrenergic agonists (e.g., clonidine), tricyclic antidepressants, atropine sulfate, steroids, norepinephrine-reuptake inhibitors (e.g., atomoxetine), and ergot alkaloids (e.g., methylergonovine maleate). Other drugs that can antagonize the pressor effect of phenylephrine include phosphodiesterase (PDE) type 5 inhibitors, benzodiazepines, and antihypertensive agents.

Atropine sulfate blocks the reflex bradycardia caused by phenylephrine and enhances the pressor response to phenylephrine.

An excessive rise in blood pressure may occur if phenylephrine is administered to patients receiving a parenteral injection of an ergot alkaloid such as ergonovine maleate.

The possibility that digitalis can sensitize the myocardium to the effects of sympathomimetic drugs should be considered.

Administration of furosemide or other diuretics may decrease arterial responsiveness to vasopressors such as phenylephrine.

Pharmacology

Phenylephrine acts predominantly by a direct effect on α_1-adrenergic receptors. In therapeutic doses, the drug has no substantial stimulant effect on the β-adrenergic receptors of the heart (β_1-adrenergic receptors) but substantial activation of these receptors may occur when larger doses are given. Phenylephrine does not stimulate β-adrenergic receptors of the bronchi or peripheral blood vessels (β_2-adrenergic receptors). Phenylephrine also has an indirect effect by releasing norepinephrine from its storage sites. The main effect of phenylephrine at therapeutic doses is vasoconstriction.

■ **Cardiovascular Effects** Phenylephrine constricts both arterial and venous blood vessels, although its effects on arterial vessels are more pronounced. Systemic vascular resistance is increased, resulting in increased systolic blood pressure, diastolic blood pressure, and mean arterial pressure. Vasoconstriction occurs in most vascular beds, including renal, pulmonary, and splanchnic arteries, but minimal to no effect is observed on cerebral blood vessels. In some patients, phenylephrine can substantially reduce cardiac output, presumably due to increased afterload; however, the exact effects of the drug on global cardiac output depend on the dose and contributory effects of the arterial and venous vasculature. Although phenylephrine reduces venous compliance and can potentially increase venous return, accompanying increases in arterial and venous resistance can negate this potential benefit. Phenylephrine may reduce circulating plasma volume (especially with prolonged use) as a result of loss of fluid into the extracellular spaces caused by postcapillary vasoconstriction. In contrast to methoxamine, phenylephrine constricts coronary and pulmonary blood vessels. Pulmonary arterial pressure usually is increased; however, a decrease in pulmonary arterial pressure has occurred in some patients, probably because of decreased cardiac output secondary to reflex bradycardia. At clinically relevant doses, phenylephrine increases myocardial work and oxygen requirements.

Constriction of renal blood vessels by phenylephrine may decrease renal blood flow. In hypotensive patients, phenylephrine may initially decrease urine flow and excretion of sodium and potassium. If the patient is not hypovolemic, renal blood flow and glomerular filtration rate increase as the systemic blood pressure is raised toward normal levels; however, renal blood flow and glomerular filtration rate again decrease if blood pressure is further increased toward hypertensive levels.

Phenylephrine can cause reflex bradycardia because of increased vagal activity. In some patients, phenylephrine has caused a paradoxical increase in heart rate when administered to treat hypotension occurring after spinal anesthesia. Because of some β_1-adrenergic activity, phenylephrine can exert positive inotropic effects on the myocardium at doses greater than those usually used therapeutically. Rarely, the drug may increase myocardial excitability, causing arrhythmias such as atrioventricular nodal rhythm, premature ventricular beats, ventricular tachycardia, or ventricular extrasystoles.

Local vasoconstriction and hemostasis also occur following topical application or infiltration of phenylephrine into tissues. Like epinephrine, phenylephrine probably produces hemostasis in cases of small vessel bleeding but does not control bleeding from larger vessels. Following oral administration or topical application of phenylephrine to the mucosa, constriction of blood vessels in the nasal mucosa may relieve nasal congestion.

■ **Other Effects** In therapeutic doses, phenylephrine causes little if any CNS stimulation but may cause nervousness, restlessness, anxiety, dizziness, and tremor in some patients, especially after overdosage.

As a result of its effects on α-adrenergic receptors, phenylephrine may cause contraction of the pregnant uterus and constriction of uterine blood vessels; however, the vasoconstrictor effect may be overcome by an increase in maternal blood pressure.

Pharmacokinetics

■ **Absorption** Phenylephrine is completely absorbed following oral administration and undergoes extensive first-pass metabolism in the intestinal wall. The bioavailability of phenylephrine following oral administration is approximately 38% relative to IV administration. Because of extensive first-pass metabolism, there is considerable interindividual and possibly intraindividual variation in oral bioavailability of the drug. Following oral administration of phenylephrine (1 or 7.8 mg), peak serum concentrations occur at 0.75–2 hours.

To achieve cardiovascular effects, phenylephrine should be given parenterally. After IV administration, a pressor effect occurs almost immediately and persists for 15–20 minutes. After IM administration, a pressor effect occurs within 10–15 minutes and persists for 30 minutes to 1 or 2 hours. Occasionally, enough phenylephrine may be absorbed after oral inhalation to produce systemic effects. Following oral administration, nasal decongestion may occur within 15 or 20 minutes and may persist for 2–4 hours.

■ **Distribution** Phenylephrine undergoes rapid distribution into peripheral tissues; there is some evidence that the drug may be stored in certain organ compartments. The pharmacologic effects of phenylephrine are terminated at least partially by uptake of the drug into tissues. Penetration of phenylephrine into the brain appears to be minimal.

Phenylephrine does not appear to be distributed to any great extent into breast milk.

■ **Elimination** Phenylephrine undergoes extensive metabolism in the intestinal wall (first-pass) and in the liver. The principal routes of metabolism involve sulfate conjugation (primarily in the intestinal wall) and oxidative deamination (by monoamine oxidase [MAO]); glucuronidation also occurs to a lesser extent. The metabolites are not pharmacologically active.

Phenylephrine and its metabolites are excreted mainly in urine. Following oral or IV administration, approximately 80 or 86% of the dose, respectively, is excreted in urine within 48 hours, principally as metabolites; approximately 2.6% of an oral dose or 16% of an IV dose is excreted in urine as unchanged drug. The terminal elimination half-life of phenylephrine averages 2–3 hours following oral or IV administration. The observed effective half-life is approximately 5 minutes following IV infusion of the drug.

Clinical data regarding effects of renal or hepatic impairment on the pharmacokinetics of phenylephrine are limited. Because the majority of an oral dose is metabolized in the intestinal wall and a lower fraction in the liver, hepatic impairment is unlikely to result in major changes following oral administration; however, phenylephrine pharmacokinetics may be substantially altered following IV administration of the drug. Patients with hepatic cirrhosis may have a reduced response to phenylephrine, potentially requiring higher dosages of the drug. Patients with end-stage renal disease may have an increased response to phenylephrine, potentially requiring lower dosages of the drug.

Chemistry and Stability

■ **Chemistry** Phenylephrine is a sympathomimetic amine that is pharmacologically similar to methoxamine hydrochloride. Phenylephrine is commercially available as the hydrochloride. Phenylephrine hydrochloride is soluble in water and ethanol, and insoluble in chloroform and ethyl ether. Phenylephrine hydrochloride injection has a pH of 3–6.5. Commercially available phenylephrine hydrochloride injections may contain the antioxidant, sodium metabisulfite.

■ **Stability** Phenylephrine hydrochloride injection should be stored at 20–25°C, but may be exposed to temperatures ranging from 15–30°C; single-dose and pharmacy bulk vials should be kept in their original carton until time of use and protected from light.

Phenylephrine hydrochloride oral tablets should be stored at 15–25°C in a dry place. Phenylephrine hydrochloride injections should be stored at room temperature up to 30°C and protected from light.

Preparations

Excipients in commercially available drug preparations may have clinically important effects in some individuals; consult specific product labeling for details.

Phenylephrine Hydrochloride

Oral		
Tablets	10 mg	**Sudafed PE® Congestion,** McNeil
Parenteral		
Injection	10 mg/mL	**Vazculep®**, Eclat
		Phenylephrine Hydrochloride Injection
Topical		
Cream	0.25% with Glycerin 14.4%, Petrolatum 15%, and Pramokine 1%	**Preparation H®**, Pfizer
Gel	0.25% with Witch Hazel 50%	**Preparation H®**, Pfizer
Ointment	0.25% with Mineral Oil 14%, Petrolatum 71.9%	**Preparation H®**, Pfizer
Suppository	0.25% with Cocoa Butter 85.39%	**Preparation H®**, Pfizer

Phenylephrine Hydrochloride Combinations

Oral		
Capsules, (liquid-filled)	5 mg with Acetaminophen 325 mg and Dextromethorphan Hydrobromide 10 mg	**Vicks® DayQuil® Cold & Flu Relief LiquiCaps,** Procter & Gamble
For Solution	10 mg/packet with Acetaminophen 325 mg/packet and Pheniramine Maleate 20 mg/packet	**Theraflu® Cold & Sore Throat,** Novartis
	10 mg/packet with Acetaminophen 650 mg/packet and Dextromethorphan Hydrobromide 20 mg	**Theraflu® Daytime Severe Cold & Cough,** Novartis
	10 mg/packet with Acetaminophen 650 mg/packet and Pheniramine Maleate 20 mg/packet	**Theraflu® Flu & Sore Throat,** Novartis
	10mg/packet with Acetaminophen 650 mg/packet and Diphenhydramine Hydrochloride 25 mg	**Theraflu® Nighttime Severe Cold & Cough,** Novartis
	10 mg/packet with Dextromethorphan Hydrobromide 20 mg/packet and Pheniramine Maleate 20 mg/packet	**Theraflu® Cold & Cough,** Novartis
Solution	5 mg/15 mL with Acetaminophen 325 mg/15 mL and Dextromethorphan Hydrobromide 10 mg/15 mL	**Theraflu Warming Relief® Daytime Severe Cold & Cough,** Novartis
		Tylenol® Cold Multi-Symptom Daytime Citrus Burst® Liquid, McNeil
		Vicks® DayQuil® Cold & Flu Relief, Procter & Gamble
	5 mg/15 mL with Acetaminophen 325 mg/15 mL and Diphenhydramine Hydrochloride 12.5 mg/15 mL	**Theraflu® Warming Relief® Flu & Sore Throat,** Novartis
		Theraflu® Warming Relief® Nighttime Severe Cold & Cough, Novartis
	2.5 mg/5 mL with Acetaminophen 160 mg/5 mL and Chlorpheniramine Maleate 1 mg/5 mL	**Children's Tylenol® Plus Cold,** McNeil
	2.5 mg/5 mL with Acetaminophen 160 mg/5 mL and Chlorpheniramine Maleate 1 mg/5 mL, and Dextromethorphan Hydrobromide 5 mg/5mL	**Children's Tylenol® Plus Multi-Symptom Cold,** McNeil
	2.5 mg/5 mL with Acetaminophen 160 mg/5 mL and Diphenhydramine Hydrochloride 12.5 mg/5 mL	**Children's Tylenol® Plus Cold & Allergy,** McNeil
	2.5 mg/5 mL with Chlorpheniramine Maleate 1 mg/5 mL	**Triaminic® Cold & Allergy,** Novartis
	2.5 mg/5 mL with Dextromethorphan Hydrobromide 5 mg/5mL	**Children's Sudafed PE® Cold & Cough,** McNeil
		Triaminic® Day Time Cold & Cough, Novartis
	2.5 mg/5mL with Diphenhydramine Hydrochloride 6.25 mg/5 mL	**Triaminic® Night Time Cold & Cough,** Novartis
	2.5 mg/5 mL with Guaifenesin 50 mg/5mL	**Triaminic® Chest and Nasal Congestion,** Novartis
Tablets	5 mg with Acetaminophen 325 mg, Chlorpheniramine Maleate 2 mg, and Dextromethorphan Hydrobromide 10 mg	**Theraflu Warming Relief Caplets® Nighttime Multi-Symptom Cold,** Novartis
	5 mg with Acetaminophen 325 mg and Dextromethorphan Hydrobromide 10 mg	**Theraflu Warming Relief Caplets® Daytime Multi-Symptom Cold,** Novartis
	10 mg with Chlorpheniramine Maleate 4 mg	**Sudafed PE® Sinus + Allergy,** McNeil
Tablets, film-coated	5 mg with Acetaminophen 325 mg	**Excedrin® Sinus Headache,** Novartis
		Sudafed PE® Pressure + Pain Caplets, McNeil
	5 mg with Acetaminophen 325 mg, Chlorpheniramine Maleate 2 mg, and Dextromethorphan Hydrobromide 10 mg	**Tylenol® Cold Head Congestion Nighttime Cool Burst® Caplets,** McNeil
	5 mg with Acetaminophen 325 mg and Dextromethorphan Hydrobromide 10 mg	**Tylenol® Cold Head Congestion Daytime Cool Burst® Caplets,** McNeil
	5 mg with Acetaminophen 325 mg, Dextromethorphan Hydrobromide 10 mg, and Guaifenesin 100 mg	**Sudafed PE® Cold + Cough Caplets,** McNeil
	5 mg with Acetaminophen 325 mg, Dextromethorphan Hydrobromide 10 mg, and Guaifenesin 200 mg	**Tylenol® Cold Head Congestion Severe Cool Burst® Caplets,** McNeil
	5 mg with Acetaminophen 325 mg and Diphenhydramine Hydrochloride 12.5 mg	**Sudafed PE® Severe Cold Caplets,** McNeil
	5 mg with Guaifenesin 200 mg	**Sudafed PE® Non-Drying Sinus Caplets,** McNeil

†Use is not currently included in the labeling approved by the US Food and Drug Administration

β-ADRENERGIC AGONISTS 12:12.08

SELECTIVE β_1-ADRENERGIC AGONISTS 12:12.08.08

DOBUTamine Hydrochloride

■ Dobutamine hydrochloride is a synthetic sympathomimetic that is structurally related to dopamine and generally is considered a relatively selective β_1-adrenergic agonist.

Uses

■ **Cardiac Decompensation** Dobutamine hydrochloride is used for inotropic support in the short-term management of cardiac decompensation caused by depressed contractility from organic heart disease or cardiac surgical procedures. The drug may be ineffective in patients with marked mechanical obstruction such as severe valvular aortic stenosis.

Safety and efficacy of dobutamine or other cyclic AMP (cAMP)-dependent inotropic agents in the long-term (e.g., exceeding 48 hours) treatment of patients with congestive heart failure have not been established, irrespective of their route of administration. In controlled studies in patients with congestive heart failure using chronic oral therapy with cAMP-dependent inotropic agents, symptoms were not consistently alleviated, and an increased risk of hospitalization and death, particularly in patients with New York Heart Association (NYHA) class IV symptoms, was associated with such therapy.

Because positive inotropic agents have not demonstrated improved outcomes in patients with heart failure and can be potentially harmful (e.g., increased risk of arrhythmias), particularly when used long term, the American College of Cardiology Foundation (ACCF) and American Heart Association (AHA) recommend that these drugs be reserved for patients with severe systolic dysfunction who have low cardiac index and evidence of systemic hypoperfusion and/or congestion, or for palliative therapy in those with end-stage heart failure. To minimize the risk of adverse effects, the lowest possible dosage should be used and the patient should be evaluated regularly for the need for continued inotropic therapy.

When used for inotropic support in patients with myocardial dysfunction after cardiac surgery, dobutamine has been shown in clinical studies to effectively increase cardiac output; however, the effects of the drug on clinically important outcomes and survival are not known. Although some data indicate that dobutamine may be preferable to other catecholamines (e.g., dopamine) in the period immediately following cardiopulmonary bypass surgery, additional studies are needed.

Inotropic agents such as dobutamine also are used in the treatment of septic or cardiogenic shock to improve myocardial contractility and maintain systemic perfusion. The Surviving Sepsis Campaign International Guidelines for Management of Severe Sepsis and Septic Shock recommend a trial of dobutamine (alone or in addition to a vasopressor) in patients with septic shock if myocardial dysfunction is present, as evidenced by elevated cardiac filling pressures and low cardiac output, or if there is ongoing hypoperfusion despite adequate intravascular volume and mean arterial pressure. Although the manufacturers of dobutamine hydrochloride state that safety of the drug following myocardial infarction (MI) has not been established (see Cautions: Precautions and Contraindications), dobutamine often is used for temporary inotropic support in patients with cardiogenic shock, a condition caused principally by acute MI. Early revascularization is the standard of care in patients with cardiogenic shock; use of inotropes in this setting should be individualized and guided by hemodynamic monitoring.

■ **Advanced Cardiovascular Life Support** Inotropic agents such as dobutamine also have been used for postresuscitation stabilization† after cardiac arrest in patients who require additional support of cardiac output and blood pressure.

■ **Cardiac Diagnostic Testing** Dobutamine has been used as a pharmacologic stress test agent† during echocardiography in patients who are unable to undergo exercise testing. Dobutamine also has been used as an alternative to exercise stress testing in patients undergoing myocardial perfusion imaging†. However, coronary vasodilating agents (e.g., adenosine, dipyridamole, regadenoson) are the drugs of choice for this use; dobutamine generally is recommended only in patients who have contraindications (e.g., bronchospastic airway disease) to these vasodilators.

Dosage and Administration

■ **Administration** Dobutamine hydrochloride is administered by IV infusion using an infusion pump or other apparatus to control the flow rate. One manufacturer recommends that a precision volume-control IV set be used when administering the drug. Care should be taken to control the rate of infusion to prevent rapid IV ("bolus") administration.

Dobutamine also has been administered by intraosseous (IO) infusion† in the setting of advanced cardiovascular life support (ACLS), generally when IV access is not readily available; onset of action and systemic concentrations are comparable to those achieved with venous administration.

Commercially available dobutamine hydrochloride injection concentrate *must* be further diluted with a compatible IV solution (see Chemistry and Stability: Stability) before IV infusion; 20 mL of concentrate should be diluted in at least 50 mL of diluent and 40 mL of concentrate should be diluted in at least 100 mL of diluent. The concentration of dobutamine hydrochloride administered should be individualized according to dosage and fluid requirements of the patient; concentrations up to 5000 mcg/mL have been administered. Following dilution, solutions of dobutamine should be used within 24 hours.

Commercially available prediluted solutions of dobutamine hydrochloride in 5% dextrose injection should not be administered unless the solution is clear and the container is undamaged; unused portions should be discarded. The flexible containers should not be used in series connections, and additives should not be introduced into the injection containers.

Dobutamine injection should be inspected visually for particulate matter and discoloration prior to administration, whenever solution and container permit. Dobutamine hydrochloride solutions should not be admixed with alkalinizing substances (e.g., sodium bicarbonate) since the drug is inactivated in alkaline solution. One manufacturer states that dobutamine hydrochloride should not be used in conjunction with other drugs or solutions containing both sodium bisulfite and ethanol. The manufacturer's labeling should be consulted for proper methods of administration and other associated precautions.

■ **Dosage** Dosage of dobutamine hydrochloride is expressed in terms of dobutamine.

Cardiac Decompensation Individual response to dobutamine is variable, and infusion rate should be titrated to achieve the desired clinical response.

Dobutamine infusion should be initiated at a slow rate (e.g., 0.5–1 mcg/kg per minute) and carefully adjusted at intervals of a few minutes according to the patient's response as indicated by heart rate, blood pressure, urine flow, presence of ectopic heartbeats, and, whenever possible, by measurement of central venous or pulmonary capillary wedge pressure and cardiac output. Clinical studies have shown that the rate of infusion usually needed to increase cardiac output is 2–20 mcg/kg per minute. Rarely, infusion of doses as great as 40 mcg/kg per minute has been required.

When dobutamine is used in geriatric patients, the initial dosage usually should be at the low end of the dosage range and caution should be exercised since renal, hepatic, and cardiovascular dysfunction and concomitant disease or other drug therapy are more common in this age group than in younger patients.

Advanced Cardiovascular Life Support If dobutamine is used for postresuscitation stabilization† in adults following cardiac arrest, the usual initial dosage range is 5–10 mcg/kg per minute. In pediatric patients, the usual dosage range is 2–20 mcg/kg per minute by IV or IO infusion. Rate of infusion should be titrated based on cardiac output and blood pressure response.

Cautions

■ **Cardiovascular Effects** The principal adverse effects of dobutamine hydrochloride include ectopic heartbeats, increased heart rate, angina, chest pain, palpitation, and elevations in blood pressure. In most patients, heart rate increases 5–15 beats per minute and systolic blood pressure increases by 10–20 mm Hg. Occasionally, however, patients experience an increase in heart rate of 30 beats per minute or greater or an increase in systolic blood pressure of 50 mm Hg or greater. Patients with preexisting hypertension may be predisposed to developing an exaggerated pressor response. All of these adverse cardiovascular effects are usually dose related, and dosage should be reduced or temporarily discontinued if they occur. Rarely, dobutamine has caused ventricular tachycardia.

Precipitous decreases in blood pressure also have been described occasionally; blood pressure generally will return to baseline following dosage reduction or discontinuance of the infusion. However, intervention rarely may be required and the effects on pressure may not be readily reversible.

■ **Dermatologic and Sensitivity Reactions** Manifestations suggestive of hypersensitivity, including skin rash, fever, eosinophilia, and bronchospasm, have been reported occasionally in patients receiving dobutamine hydrochloride.

■ **Other Adverse Effects** Other less frequent adverse effects include nausea, vomiting, tingling sensation, paresthesia, dyspnea, headache, fever, and mild leg cramps; pruritus of the scalp during IV infusion of dobutamine has been reported in at least one patient. Isolated cases of thrombocytopenia have been reported. Like other drugs with β_2-agonist activity, dobutamine may produce slight decreases in serum potassium concentrations; hypokalemia may occur rarely. Inadvertent overdosage has also reportedly caused nervousness and fatigue. Phlebitis at the site of IV infusion of dobutamine has been reported occasionally. Inadvertent subcutaneous infiltration of dobutamine has caused local inflammatory changes and local pain without local ischemia; however, isolated cases of cutaneous necrosis have been reported.

■ **Precautions and Contraindications** Before administration of dobutamine, hypovolemia should be corrected with an appropriate plasma volume expander. The ECG, blood pressure and, when possible, cardiac output and pulmonary wedge pressure should be monitored. Because dobutamine increases atrioventricular conduction, patients with atrial fibrillation are at risk of developing a rapid ventricular response and, therefore, should be digitalized prior to administration of dobutamine. Experience with the use of dobutamine following acute myocardial infarction (MI) is limited. The possibility that dobutamine may intensify or extend myocardial ischemia has not been ruled out. Therefore, the drug should be used with extreme caution following MI.

Like other drugs with β_2-agonist activity, dobutamine may produce slight reductions in serum potassium concentrations and hypokalemia may occur rarely. Consideration should be given to monitoring serum potassium concentrations during dobutamine therapy.

Commercially available injections of dobutamine hydrochloride or dobutamine hydrochloride in 5% dextrose may contain sulfites that can cause allergic-type reactions, including anaphylaxis and life-threatening or less severe asthmatic episodes, in certain susceptible individuals. The overall prevalence of sulfite sensitivity in the general population is unknown but probably low; such sensitivity appears to occur more frequently in asthmatic than in nonasthmatic individuals.

Dobutamine is contraindicated in patients with idiopathic hypertrophic subaortic stenosis or with known hypersensitivity to the drug or any ingredient in the formulation.

■ **Pediatric Precautions** Some manufacturers state that safety and efficacy of dobutamine injection have not been evaluated in pediatric patients. Other manufacturers state that dobutamine increases cardiac output and systemic blood pressure in pediatric patients of all age groups. In premature neonates, however, dobutamine is less effective than dopamine in increasing systemic blood pressure without causing undue tachycardia and has not been shown to provide any additional benefit when administered to such infants who are already receiving optimal dopamine therapy.

■ **Geriatric Precautions** Clinical studies of dobutamine hydrochloride did not include sufficient numbers of patients 65 years of age and older to determine whether geriatric patients respond differently than younger patients. Clinical experience suggests that substantial hypotension associated with dobutamine therapy may occur more frequently in geriatric patients. One manufacturer of dobutamine hydrochloride in 5% dextrose recommends that if dobutamine is used in geriatric patients, the initial dosage usually should be at the low end of the dosage range, and caution should be exercised since renal, hepatic, and cardiovascular dysfunction and concomitant disease or other drug therapy are more common in this age group than in younger patients.

■ **Pregnancy, Fertility, and Lactation** Safe use of dobutamine during pregnancy has not been established. Reproduction studies in rats or rabbits (at up to or 2 times, respectively, the usual human dose on a mg/kg basis) have not revealed evidence of harm to the fetus. Dobutamine should be used in pregnant women only if clearly needed. The effect of dobutamine on labor and delivery is not known.

Studies to evaluate the potential of dobutamine to affect fertility have not been performed.

It is not known whether dobutamine is distributed into human milk. Because many drugs are distributed into human milk, caution should be exercised when dobutamine is administered to a nursing woman. If a nursing woman requires dobutamine therapy, breast-feeding should be discontinued for the duration of drug therapy.

Drug Interactions

In clinical studies, dobutamine hydrochloride was administered concomitantly with atropine, cardiac glycosides (digoxin), furosemide, heparin, lidocaine, morphine, nitroglycerin, isosorbide dinitrate, potassium chloride, folic acid, protamine, acetaminophen, or spironolactone with no evidence of any drug interactions.

■ **β-Adrenergic Blocking Agents** In animals, the cardiac effects of dobutamine are antagonized by β-adrenergic blocking agents such as propranolol and metoprolol, resulting in predominance of α-adrenergic effects and increased peripheral resistance.

■ **General Anesthetics** Ventricular arrhythmias have been reported in animals receiving usual doses of dobutamine during halothane or cyclopropane anesthesia; therefore, caution should be used when administering dobutamine to patients receiving these general anesthetics.

■ **Sodium Nitroprusside** Concomitant use of dobutamine and sodium nitroprusside may potentiate effects on cardiac output and pulmonary wedge pressure.

Pharmacology

Dobutamine hydrochloride directly stimulates β_1-adrenergic receptors and is generally considered a selective β_1-adrenergic agonist, but the mechanisms of action of the drug are complex. It is believed that the β-adrenergic effects result from stimulation of adenyl cyclase activity. In therapeutic doses, dobutamine also has mild β_2- and α_1-adrenergic receptor agonist effects, which are relatively balanced and result in minimal net direct effect on systemic vasculature. Unlike dopamine, dobutamine does not cause release of endogenous norepinephrine. The main effect of therapeutic doses of dobutamine is cardiac stimulation. While the positive inotropic effect of the drug on the myocardium appears to be mediated principally via β_1-adrenergic stimulation, experimental evidence suggests that α_1-adrenergic stimulation may also be involved and that the α_1-adrenergic activity results mainly from the (−)-stereoisomer of the drug.

The β_1-adrenergic effects of dobutamine exert a positive inotropic effect on the myocardium and result in an increase in cardiac output due to increased myocardial contractility and stroke volume in healthy individuals and in patients with congestive heart failure. Increased left ventricular filling pressure decreases in patients with congestive heart failure. In therapeutic doses, dobutamine causes a decrease in peripheral resistance; however, systolic blood pressure and pulse pressure may remain unchanged or be increased because of augmented cardiac output. With usual doses, heart rate is usually not substantially changed. Coronary blood flow and myocardial oxygen consumption are usually increased because of increased myocardial contractility.

Electrophysiologic studies have shown that dobutamine facilitates atrioventricular conduction and shortens or causes no important change in intraventricular conduction. The tendency of dobutamine to induce cardiac arrhythmias may be slightly less than that of dopamine and is considerably less than that of isoproterenol or other catecholamines. Pulmonary vascular resistance may decrease if it is elevated initially and mean pulmonary artery pressure may decrease or remain unchanged. Unlike dopamine, dobutamine does not seem to affect dopaminergic receptors and causes no renal or mesenteric vasodilation; however, urine flow may increase because of increased cardiac output.

Pharmacokinetics

■ **Absorption** Orally administered dobutamine hydrochloride is rapidly metabolized in the GI tract. Following IV administration, the onset of action of dobutamine occurs within 2 minutes. Peak plasma concentrations of the drug and peak effects occur within 10 minutes after initiation of an IV infusion. The effects of the drug cease shortly after discontinuing an infusion.

■ **Distribution** It is not known if dobutamine crosses the placenta or is distributed into milk.

■ **Elimination** The plasma half-life of dobutamine is about 2 minutes. Dobutamine is metabolized in the liver and other tissues by catechol-*O*-methyltransferase to an inactive compound, 3-*O*-methyldobutamine, and by conjugation with glucuronic acid. Conjugates of dobutamine and 3-*O*-methyldobutamine are excreted mainly in urine and to a minor extent in feces.

Chemistry and Stability

■ **Chemistry** Dobutamine is a synthetic sympathomimetic drug which is structurally related to dopamine. Dobutamine hydrochloride occurs as a white to off-white, crystalline powder and is sparingly soluble in water and in alcohol. Dobutamine has a pK_a of 9.4.

Dobutamine hydrochloride is commercially available as a sterile solution of the drug (a racemic mixture) in water for injection. Commercially available concentrates for injection contain sulfites. Hydrochloric acid and/or sodium hydroxide may be added during manufacture of the commercially available concentrate for injection to adjust the pH between 2.5–5.5.

Dobutamine hydrochloride also is commercially available as prediluted solutions of the drug in 5% dextrose. Hydrochloric acid and/or sodium hydroxide may be added during manufacture of dobutamine hydrochloride in 5% dextrose injection to adjust pH to approximately 3 (range: 2.5–5.5); sodium metabisulfite and edetate disodium dihydrate are added as stabilizers. The commercially available injections of the drug in 5% dextrose are sterile, nonpyrogenic solutions of dobutamine hydrochloride; the injections containing 1, 2, or 4 mg/mL of dobutamine have osmolarities of 263, 270, or 284 mOsm/L, respectively.

■ **Stability** Dobutamine hydrochloride for injection concentrate should be stored at 20–25°C.

Commercially available solutions of dobutamine hydrochloride in 5% dextrose should be protected from excessive heat or freezing and stored at room temperature (20–25°C); however, some manufacturers state that brief exposure of the solutions to temperatures up to 40°C does not adversely affect the products. Dobutamine hydrochloride for injection concentrate is compatible with the following IV solutions: 5 or 10% dextrose, 5% dextrose and 0.45 or 0.9% sodium chloride, 5% dextrose in lactated Ringer's, lactated Ringer's, 0.9% sodium chloride, Isolyte®-M with 5% dextrose, Normosol®-M in 5% dextrose, 20% Osmitrol®, or ⅙ *M* sodium lactate injection. Dobutamine hydrochloride solutions diluted for IV infusion should be used within 24 hours.

Because of potential physical incompatibilities, it is recommended that dobutamine hydochloride solutions not be admixed with other drugs. Solutions of the drug are incompatible with sodium bicarbonate injection or other strongly alkaline solutions and should not be used in conjunction with other drugs or diluents containing both sodium bisulfite and ethanol. Pink discoloration of solutions of dobutamine hydrochloride indicates slight oxidation of the drug; however, there is no important loss of potency if the drug is administered within the recommended time period. Unused portions of dobutamine hydrochloride solutions should be discarded.

Some commercially available preparations of dobutamine hydrochloride in 5% dextrose injection (e.g., Lifecare®) are provided in plastic containers fabricated from a specially formulated nonplasticized, thermoplastic co-polyester (CR3). Water can permeate from inside the container into the overwrap in amounts insufficient to affect the solution substantially. Solutions in contact with the plastic container also can leach out some of the chemical components in very small amounts; however, safety of the plastic has been confirmed with biological testing.

Preparations

Excipients in commercially available drug preparations may have clinically important effects in some individuals; consult specific product labeling for details.

DOBUTamine Hydrochloride

Parenteral

For injection concentrate, for IV infusion	12.5 mg (of dobutamine) per mL*	**DOBUTamine Hydrochloride Injection**

*available from one or more manufacturer, distributor, and/or repackager by generic (nonproprietary) name

DOBUTamine Hydrochloride in Dextrose

Parenteral

Injection, for IV infusion	1 mg (of dobutamine) per mL (250 or 500 mg) in 5% Dextrose*	**DOBUTamine in 5% Dextrose Injection** (Lifecare®; Viaflex®)
	2 mg (of dobutamine) per mL (500 mg) in 5% Dextrose*	**DOBUTamine in 5% Dextrose Injection** (Lifecare®; Viaflex®)
	4 mg (of dobutamine) per mL (1000 mg) in 5% Dextrose*	**DOBUTamine in 5% Dextrose Injection** (Lifecare®; Viaflex®)

*available from one or more manufacturer, distributor, and/or repackager by generic (nonproprietary) name

†Use is not currently included in the labeling approved by the US Food and Drug Administration

DOPamine Hydrochloride

■ Dopamine hydrochloride, an endogenous catecholamine that is the immediate precursor of norepinephrine, is a sympathomimetic agent with prominent dopaminergic and β_1-adrenergic effects at low to moderate doses and α-adrenergic effects at high doses.

Uses

■ **Shock** Dopamine hydrochloride is used as adjunctive therapy to correct hemodynamic imbalances (e.g., increase cardiac output and blood pressure) in the treatment of shock. In patients who require vasopressor support, individual hemodynamic abnormalities must be identified and monitored so that therapy can be adjusted as necessary.

Vasopressors such as dopamine are used in the management of shock to restore blood pressure and tissue perfusion after initial fluid resuscitation is attempted. The Surviving Sepsis Campaign International Guidelines for Management of Sepsis and Septic Shock recommend norepinephrine as the first-line vasopressor of choice in adults with septic shock; if adequate blood pressure is not achieved, vasopressin or epinephrine may be added. Although dopamine was used widely in the past as a first-line vasopressor agent in patients with septic shock, more recent evidence indicates that the drug is associated with a greater risk of adverse effects (e.g., arrhythmias) and possibly also an increased risk of death compared with norepinephrine. In a multicenter randomized study (Sepsis Occurrence in Acutely Ill Patients II [SOAP II]) comparing the effects of dopamine and norepinephrine in patients with septic, cardiogenic, or hypovolemic shock, no substantial difference in 28-day mortality was observed between the vasopressors; however, use of dopamine was associated with more arrhythmic events in the overall population and an increased rate of death in the subgroup of patients with cardiogenic shock. In current expert guidelines, dopamine is considered an alternative vasopressor to norepinephrine only in highly selected patients with septic shock (e.g., those with low risk of tachyarrhythmias and bradycardia).

Vasopressors also have been used to provide hemodynamic support in other types of shock (e.g., cardiogenic, hemorrhagic), generally as a temporary measure until the underlying cause can be treated. Some evidence suggests that early use of vasopressors in patients with hemorrhagic shock may be deleterious compared with aggressive fluid resuscitation; however, additional studies are needed to confirm this finding. Dopamine may be particularly useful in the management of cardiogenic shock (including that associated with acute myocardial infarction) because of the drug's net hemodynamic effects; however, some evidence (e.g., from the SOAP II study) suggests an increased risk of mortality compared with norepinephrine when used in patients with this type of shock. Early revascularization is the standard of care in patients with cardiogenic shock; use of vasopressors in this setting should be individualized and guided by hemodynamic monitoring. Some experts state that dopamine may be considered for the treatment of drug-induced hypovolemic shock when the patient is unresponsive to fluid volume expansion and inotropic and/or vasopressor support is required. The use of dopamine in low cardiac output syndrome following open heart surgery has been shown to increase long-term survival. However, because dobutamine lowers peripheral resistance over a wide dosage range, is not dependent on release of endogenous catecholamines for its effects, and is cardioselective, that drug may be preferable in the period immediately following cardiopulmonary bypass surgery.

Dopamine may increase cardiac output, blood pressure, and urine flow in patients with shock; however, the exact effects of the drug are dose related and based on the patient's clinical status at the time of administration. In low or intermediate doses, dopamine usually does not produce sufficient peripheral vasoconstriction to cause a rise in blood pressure; therefore, the dose should be rapidly increased until adequate blood pressure is obtained. If hypotension persists, a more potent vasoconstrictor such as norepinephrine may be required. Dopamine appears to be most effective when therapy is initiated shortly after the signs and symptoms of shock appear and before physiologic parameters such as blood pressure and myocardial function undergo severe deterioration and before urine flow has decreased to less than 0.3 mL/minute. However, the drug may increase urine flow, in some cases to normal levels, in patients with oliguria or anuria. Urine flow may also increase in patients with normal urine output and thereby reduce preexisting fluid accumulation.

An α-adrenergic blocking agent such as phentolamine may be used to counteract the peripheral vasoconstriction produced by high doses of dopamine. Concomitant use of dopamine and a diuretic such as hydrochlorothiazide or furosemide may produce diuresis in patients who do not respond to dopamine or a diuretic alone. However, because dopamine acts as a proximal-tubule diuretic, the increased solute delivery to the distal tubular cells may increase distal oxygen consumption and potentially increase the risk of renal medullary ischemia in patients at risk of renal failure.

■ **Advanced Cardiovascular Life Support** Dopamine is used in advanced cardiovascular life support (ACLS)† for the treatment of symptomatic bradycardia in adults, particularly if associated with hypotension; although not a first-line drug, dopamine may be considered in patients who are unresponsive to atropine therapy, or as a temporizing measure while awaiting availability of a pacemaker.

Dopamine also has been used during the resuscitation period for management of patients in cardiac arrest. High-quality cardiopulmonary resuscitation (CPR) and defibrillation are integral components of ACLS and the only proven interventions to increase survival to hospital discharge. Other resuscitative efforts, including drug therapy, are considered secondary and should be performed without compromising the quality and timely delivery of chest compressions and defibrillation. The principal goal of pharmacologic therapy during cardiac arrest is to facilitate the return of spontaneous circulation (ROSC), and epinephrine is considered the drug of choice for this use. Vasoactive drugs such as dopamine may be used for hemodynamic support following resuscitation from cardiac arrest. (See Uses: Advanced Cardiovascular Life Support and Cardiac Arrhythmias, in Epinephrine 12:12.12.)

■ **Acute Renal Failure** Previous data from animal studies and some clinical studies in a limited number of healthy or critically ill adults indicated that low-dose (e.g., less than 5 mcg/kg per minute) infusions of dopamine may increase renal and mesenteric perfusion and improve renal function as a result of selective stimulation of renal dopaminergic receptors and subsequent renal vasodilation. However, more recent studies have failed to demonstrate any benefit from such therapy, and routine use of low-dose ("renal dose") dopamine therapy for the prevention or amelioration of acute renal failure in critically ill patients is no longer recommended. In a randomized, double-blind, placebo-controlled study, adults in an intensive care unit (ICU) at risk for acute renal failure who received dopamine as a continuous, low-dose (2 mcg/kg per minute) infusion had similar peak serum creatinine concentrations during treatment, similar durations of ICU and hospital stay, and similar survival to ICU or hospital discharge compared with those receiving placebo. Other studies in patients at high risk for renal failure receiving low-dose dopamine infusions (generally less than 2–3 mcg/kg per minute) have demonstrated similar findings. In a study in a small number of hemodynamically stable, critically ill patients, infusion of dopamine 3 mcg/kg per minute increased creatinine clearance, diuresis, and fractional excretion of sodium; however, these beneficial effects (except for diuresis) generally diminished after 24 hours, indicating the possibility of tolerance to the effects of dopamine. In addition, alterations in clearance and metabolism in critically ill patients may result in high interindividual variability in plasma dopamine concentrations for a given infusion rate (dosage) of the drug, making it difficult or impossible to guarantee a selective effect of the drug in this patient population. Low-dose infusions of dopamine are not without risk and may be associated with adverse effects such as suppression of respiratory drive, increased cardiac output and myocardial oxygen consumption, arrhythmias, hypokalemia, hypophosphatemia, gut ischemia, and disruption of metabolic and immunologic homeostasis.

■ **Heart Failure** Dopamine is used for short-term inotropic support in patients with refractory heart failure† to maintain systemic perfusion and preserve end-organ function. Because positive inotropic agents have not demonstrated improved outcomes in patients with heart failure and can be potentially harmful (e.g., increased risk of arrhythmias), particularly when used long term, the American College of Cardiology Foundation (ACCF) and American Heart Association (AHA) recommend that these drugs be reserved for patients with severe systolic dysfunction who have low cardiac index and evidence of systemic hypoperfusion and/or congestion, or for palliative therapy in those with end-stage heart failure. To minimize the risk of adverse effects, the lowest possible dosage should be used and the patient should be evaluated regularly for the need for continued inotropic therapy.

Low-dose dopamine infusion has been used in combination with loop diuretics to augment diuresis and improve renal blood flow in patients with acute decompensated heart failure†; however, the currently available evidence does not support routine use of dopamine for this purpose. Although some studies have suggested that dopamine may prevent worsening of renal function related to diuretic use in patients with acute decompensated heart failure, more recent studies generally have not confirmed this benefit.

Dosage and Administration

■ **Administration** Dopamine hydrochloride is administered by IV infusion using an infusion pump or other apparatus to control the rate of flow. Precise control of the infusion rate is essential to avoid inadvertent administration of a bolus dose. To minimize the risk of necrosis, infusion of dopamine should be given into a large vein, preferably the antecubital vein. Less suitable veins (e.g., hand or ankle vein) should be used only when required, but the site should be switched to a preferred vein as soon as possible. *Care must be taken to avoid extravasation because local necrosis may result.* (See Cautions: Precautions and Contraindications.)

Dopamine also has been administered by intraosseous infusion† in the setting of advanced cardiovascular life support (ACLS), generally when IV access is not readily available; onset of action and systemic concentrations are comparable to those achieved with venous administration.

The commercially available dopamine hydrochloride injection concentrate *must* be diluted prior to administration; alternatively, commercially available solutions of dopamine hydrochloride in 5% dextrose may be used without dilution. The concentration of dopamine is dependent upon the dosage and fluid requirements of the individual patient. One suggested solution for infusion may be prepared by diluting 10 mL of the injection concentrate containing 40 mg of dopamine hydrochloride per mL (a total of 400 mg of dopamine hydrochloride) with either 250 or 500 mL of one of the following solutions: 0.9% sodium chloride, 5% dextrose, 5% dextrose with 0.9% sodium chloride, 5% dextrose with 0.45% sodium chloride, lactated Ringer's, 5% dextrose in lactated Ringer's, or ⅙ *M* sodium lactate; dilution with 250 mL of solution will yield a final concentration of 1600 mcg/mL and dilution with 500 mL of solution will yield a final concentration of 800 mcg/mL.

Dopamine hydrochloride injections should be inspected visually for discoloration and/or particulate matter prior to administration whenever solution and container permit. Solutions darker than slightly yellow or that are discolored in any other way should not be used. Dopamine in 5% dextrose should not be infused into an umbilical artery catheter. The drug should be administered via a controlled-infusion device (pump), preferably a volumetric pump; dopamine should not be administered using an ordinary, gravity-controlled IV administration set. Dopamine in 5% dextrose in flexible containers (e.g., LifeCare®) should not be used in series connections.

The manufacturer's prescribing information should be consulted for proper methods of administration and other associated precautions.

■ **Dosage** ***Shock*** The rate and duration of dopamine hydrochloride infusion should be individualized and carefully adjusted to achieve the desired hemodynamic and renal response as indicated by heart rate, blood pressure, urine flow, and, whenever possible, measurement of central venous or pulmonary wedge pressure and cardiac output.

Dopamine hydrochloride infusion is usually initiated at a rate of 2–5 mcg/kg per minute in patients who are likely to respond to modest increases in cardiac contractility and renal perfusion. The infusion rate may be increased by 1–4 mcg/kg per minute at 10- to 30-minute intervals until the optimal response is attained. In more severely ill patients, dopamine hydrochloride infusion should be initiated at a rate of 5 mcg/kg per minute, and increased gradually in increments of 5–10 mcg/kg per minute, up to 20–50 mcg/kg per minute as needed. Once optimal hemodynamic effects have been achieved, the lowest possible dosage that maintains these effects should be used. In general, most patients can be maintained at an infusion rate less than 20 mcg/kg per minute; however, infusion rates exceeding 50 mcg/kg per minute have been used safely in advanced states of circulatory decompensation.

In patients with occlusive vascular disease, some clinicians recommend that dopamine hydrochloride therapy be initiated with an infusion rate of 1 mcg/kg per minute or less because of the risk of local ischemia. Such patients should be monitored closely for any signs or symptoms of compromised circulation during the infusion; if this occurs, the rate should be decreased or the infusion discontinued.

Patients who have been receiving monoamine oxidase (MAO) inhibitors within the previous 2–3 weeks should receive initial doses of dopamine hydrochloride of no greater than 10% of the usual dose.

At high dosages in patients in whom unnecessary expansion of fluid volume is a concern, administration of a more concentrated solution of dopamine hydrochloride (concentrations as high as 3.2 mg/mL have been used) may be preferable to increasing the flow rate of a dilute solution. Urine output should be measured frequently when doses exceeding 50 mcg/kg per minute are employed. When adjusting dosage to obtain the desired systolic blood pressure, optimal dosage for renal response may be exceeded and urine output may decrease. If urine flow begins to decrease in the absence of hypotension, reduction of the rate of infusion should be considered.

If a disproportionate increase in diastolic pressure (i.e., a marked decrease in pulse pressure) is observed in patients receiving dopamine, the rate of dopamine infusion should be decreased, and the patient observed carefully for further evidence of predominant vasoconstrictor activity, unless such an effect is desired. (See Cautions: Precautions and Contraindications.) Dosage reduction also may be required if a decrease in established urine flow rate, increase in tachycardia, or new dysrhythmia occurs.

Studies have not been conducted to specifically inform dosage recommendations in pediatric patients; however, clinical experience indicates that dosing in pediatric patients is generally similar to that in adults.

The manufacturer states that if dopamine hydrochloride is used in geriatric patients, the initial dosage usually should be at the low end of the dosage range since renal, hepatic, and cardiovascular dysfunction and concomitant disease or other drug therapy are more common in this age group than in younger patients.

When discontinuing an infusion, it may be necessary to gradually decrease the dose of dopamine while expanding blood volume with IV fluids to prevent a recurrence of hypotension. In patients who have been receiving moderate to high doses of dopamine, some clinicians recommend that the final dosage should not be less than 5 mcg/kg per minute in order to avoid hypotension.

Advanced Cardiovascular Life Support When used in ACLS for the treatment of symptomatic bradycardia in adults†, the usual initial dosage range of dopamine hydrochloride is 2–10 mcg/kg per minute; dosage should be titrated according to patient response. Infusion rates exceeding 10 mcg/kg per minute are associated with vasoconstrictive effects. If used for postresuscitation stabilization in adults, a dopamine hydrochloride infusion rate of 5–10 mcg/kg per minute has been recommended.

If dopamine hydrochloride is used for postresuscitation stabilization in pediatric patients†, the usual IV or intraosseous† infusion rate is 2–20 mcg/kg per minute. Although dosages exceeding 5 mcg/kg per minute stimulate the cardiac β-adrenergic receptors, this effect may be reduced in infants. Infusion rates exceeding 20 mcg/kg per minute may result in excessive vasoconstriction.

Heart Failure In the short-term treatment of patients with severe, refractory heart failure†, some clinicians recommend that dopamine hydrochloride infusion be initiated at a rate of 0.5–2 mcg/kg per minute. The usual dosage range of dopamine hydrochloride in patients with heart failure is 5–10 mcg/kg per minute. Although dosages exceeding 5 mcg/kg per minute stimulate the cardiac β-adrenergic receptors, this effect may be reduced in patients with congestive heart failure.

To minimize the risk of adverse effects, the lowest possible dosage of dopamine should be used and the patient should be evaluated regularly for the need for continued inotropic therapy.

Cautions

■ **Adverse Effects** Dopamine hydrochloride may cause ectopic heartbeats, tachycardia, angina, palpitation, vasoconstriction, hypotension, dyspnea, nausea, vomiting, and headache. Other less frequent adverse effects include cardiac conduction abnormalities, widened QRS complex, bradycardia, hypertension, azotemia, anxiety, and piloerection. Ventricular arrhythmias may occur with very high doses. Dopamine may cause elevations in serum glucose although the concentrations usually do not rise above normal limits. A few cases of peripheral cyanosis also have been reported in patients receiving dopamine.

Gangrene of the extremities has occurred when high doses of dopamine were administered for prolonged periods and in patients with occlusive vascular disease receiving low doses of dopamine, and extravasation of dopamine may result in tissue necrosis and sloughing of surrounding tissues. (See Cautions: Precautions and Contraindications.)

■ **Precautions and Contraindications** Pressor therapy is *not* a substitute for replacement of blood, plasma, fluids, and/or electrolytes. Blood volume depletion should be corrected as fully as possible before dopamine therapy is instituted. In an emergency, the drug may be used as an adjunct to fluid replacement or as a temporary supportive measure to maintain coronary and cerebral artery perfusion until volume replacement can be completed, but dopamine must *not* be used as sole therapy in hypovolemic patients. Additional volume replacement may also be required during or after administration of the drug because of the effects of dopamine on urine flow. Monitoring of central venous pressure or left ventricular filling pressure may be helpful in detecting and treating hypovolemia; in addition, monitoring of central venous or pulmonary arterial diastolic pressure is necessary to avoid overloading the cardiovascular system, diluting serum electrolyte concentrations, and precipitating congestive heart failure or pulmonary edema. Hypoxia, hypercapnia, and acidosis (which may also reduce the effectiveness and/or increase the incidence of adverse effects of dopamine) must be identified and corrected prior to, or concurrently with, administration of the drug.

During administration of dopamine, blood pressure and urine flow and, when possible, cardiac output and pulmonary wedge pressure should be monitored. If excessive vasoconstriction (as indicated by a disproportionate increase in diastolic blood pressure and a decrease in pulse pressure), decreased urine output, increased heart rate, or an arrhythmia occurs, the rate of infusion of dopamine should be decreased or temporarily suspended and the patient should be observed closely. If blood pressure or urine output fails to respond to discontinuance of the drug, administration of a short-acting α-adrenergic blocking agent such as phentolamine should be considered. If hypotension occurs during dopamine infusion, the infusion rate should be increased rapidly in order to increase blood pressure. If hypotension persists, dopamine should be discontinued and a drug with greater vasoconstricting properties such as norepinephrine should be administered. When discontinuing an infusion, it may be necessary to decrease the dose of dopamine gradually while expanding blood volume with IV fluids to prevent a recurrence of hypotension. *Sudden* cessation of dopamine infusion may result in marked hypotension.

Patients with a history of occlusive vascular disease (e.g., atherosclerosis, arterial embolism, Raynaud's disease, cold injury, diabetic endarteritis, Buerger's disease) should be carefully monitored during dopamine therapy for decreased circulation to the extremities indicated by changes in color or temperature of the skin or pain in the extremities. If such manifestations occur, they may be corrected by decreasing the rate of infusion or discontinuing dopamine; however, these changes occasionally have persisted and progressed after discontinuing the drug. The potential benefits of continuing dopamine should be weighed against the possible risk of necrosis. Some clinicians recommend IV administration of 5–10 mg of phentolamine mesylate if discoloration of the extremities occurs. To reverse ischemia induced by dopamine†, 10 mg of chlorpromazine IV followed by a chlorpromazine infusion of 0.6 mg/minute has been used.

Caution should be used to avoid extravasation of the drug. Dopamine should be administered through a large vein whenever possible, preferably in the antecubital fossa rather than the hand or ankle. One manufacturer states that administration into an umbilical arterial catheter is not recommended. If larger veins are unavailable and the condition of the patient requires that the hand or ankle veins be used to administer dopamine, the injection site should be changed to a larger vein as soon as possible. The site of infusion should be continuously monitored for free flow. If extravasation occurs, 10–15 mL of 0.9% sodium chloride injection containing 5–10 mg of phentolamine mesylate should be infiltrated (using a syringe with a fine hypodermic needle) liberally throughout the affected area. Immediate and conspicuous local hyperemic changes occur if the area is infiltrated within 12 hours; therefore, phentolamine should be administered as soon as possible after extravasation is noted. In children, phentolamine mesylate doses of 0.1–0.2 mg/kg, up to a maximum of 10 mg per dose, may be administered.

Commercially available formulations of dopamine hydrochloride injection may contain sodium metabisulfate, a sulfite that may cause allergic-type reactions, including anaphylaxis and life-threatening or less severe asthmatic episodes, in certain susceptible individuals. The overall prevalence of sulfite sensitivity in the general population is unknown but probably low; such sensitivity appears to occur more frequently in asthmatic than in nonasthmatic individuals.

Dopamine should be used with caution in patients with ischemic heart disease. The drug is contraindicated in patients with pheochromocytoma and in patients with uncorrected tachyarrhythmias or ventricular fibrillation.

■ **Pediatric Precautions** The manufacturer states that safety and efficacy of IV dopamine infusions have not been established in children; however, the drug has been used in pediatric patients of all age groups from neonate onward. In pediatric patients, dopamine is recommended as an appropriate drug for the treatment of shock when the patient is unresponsive to fluids and systemic vascular resistance is low. Except for vasoconstrictive effects caused by inadvertent infusion of dopamine into the umbilical artery, adverse effects unique to the pediatric population have not been identified, nor have adverse effects identified in adults been found to be more common in pediatric patients. Although dopamine reportedly has been administered at rates as high as 125 mcg/kg per minute in some neonates, the usual dosage in children has been similar to that in adults on a mcg/kg per minute basis.

■ **Geriatric Precautions** Clinical studies of dopamine hydrochloride did not include sufficient numbers of patients 65 years of age and older to determine whether geriatric patients respond differently than younger patients. Clinical experience to date has not identified any differences in responses between geriatric and younger patients. If dopamine hydrochloride is used in geriatric patients, the initial dosage of the drug usually should be at the low end of the dosage range, and caution should be exercised since renal, hepatic, and cardiovascular dysfunction and concomitant disease or other drug therapy are more common in this age group than in younger patients.

■ **Mutagenicity and Carcinogenicity** In the Ames microbial (*Salmonella*) mutagen test (with or without metabolic activation), there was a reproducible dose-dependent increase in the number of revertant colonies with strains TA100 and TA98 at dopamine dosages approaching maximal solubility. However, such small increases were considered inconclusive evidence of mutagenicity. In a mammalian mutagenicity assay using L5178Y TK± mouse lymphoma cells, dopamine was associated with toxicity and increases in mutant frequencies at concentrations of 750 mcg/mL without metabolic activation and 3000 mcg/mL with activation. No increases in mutant frequencies occurred at lower concentrations. In the in vivo mouse and male rat bone marrow micronucleus tests, no clear evidence of clastogenic potential was found at IV dosages up to 224 and 30 mg/kg of dopamine hydrochloride, respectively.

Long-term studies in animals have not been performed to date to evaluate the carcinogenic potential of dopamine.

■ **Pregnancy and Lactation** Reproduction studies in rats and rabbits using IV dopamine hydrochloride dosages up to 6 mg/kg daily during organogenesis have not revealed evidence of teratogenicity or embryotoxicity; however, maternal toxicity (e.g., decreased body weight gain, death) was observed in rats. In a study in rats, subcutaneous dosages of 10 mg/kg for 30 days markedly prolonged metestrus and increased mean pituitary and ovary weights. After similar administration to pregnant rats, either throughout gestation or for 5 days beginning on day 10 or 15 of gestation, decreased body weight gain, increased mortality, and slight increases in cataract formation occurred in the offspring.

There are no adequate and well-controlled studies to date using dopamine hydrochloride in pregnant women, and the drug should be used during pregnancy only when the potential benefits justify the possible risks to the fetus. It is not known whether dopamine crosses the placenta. When dopamine is administered for advanced cardiovascular life support (ACLS) during cardiopulmonary resuscitation, the drug may decrease blood flow to the uterus; however, the woman must be resuscitated for survival of the fetus. If a vasopressor (e.g., dopamine) is used during labor in conjunction with oxytocic drugs, the vasopressor effect may be potentiated and result in severe hypertension. (See Drug Interactions: Oxytocic Drugs.)

It is not known whether dopamine is distributed into human milk. Because many drugs are distributed into milk, the drug should be used with caution in nursing women.

Drug Interactions

■ **Monoamine Oxidase Inhibitors** Because dopamine is metabolized by monoamine oxidase (MAO), the effects of the drug are prolonged and intensified by MAO inhibitors. Patients who have been receiving MAO inhibitors within the previous 2–3 weeks should receive initial doses of dopamine of no greater than 10% of the usual dose.

■ **α- and β-Adrenergic Blocking Agents** The cardiac effects of dopamine are antagonized by β-adrenergic blocking agents such as propranolol and metoprolol, and the peripheral vasoconstriction caused by high doses of dopamine is antagonized by α-adrenergic blocking agents. Dopamine-induced renal and mesenteric vasodilation is not antagonized by either α- or β-adrenergic blocking agents, but, in animals, is antagonized by haloperidol or other butyrophenones, phenothiazines, and opiates.

■ **General Anesthetics** Ventricular arrhythmias and hypertension may occur when usual doses of dopamine are administered during halothane (or other halogenated hydrocarbon) or cyclopropane anesthesia. Extreme caution should be used when administering dopamine to patients receiving these general anesthetics which increase cardiac irritability.

■ **Phenytoin** Administration of IV phenytoin to patients receiving dopamine has resulted in hypotension and bradycardia; some clinicians recommend that phenytoin be used with extreme caution, if at all, in patients receiving dopamine.

■ **Oxytocic Drugs** When a vasopressor agent (e.g., dopamine) is used in conjunction with oxytocic drugs, the pressor effect may be potentiated and result in severe hypertension.

■ **Other Drugs** The diuretic effects of low dosages of dopamine may be additive with or potentiated by diuretics (e.g., hydrochlorothiazide or furosemide). The pressor response of dopamine may be potentiated by tricyclic antidepressants. The concomitant use of dopamine with other vasopressors or vasoconstrictors (e.g., ergonovine) may result in severe hypertension.

Laboratory Test Interferences

Dopamine suppresses pituitary secretion of thyrotropin (thyroid-stimulating hormone, TSH), growth hormone, and prolactin.

Acute Toxicity

Acute overdosage of dopamine may result in excessive elevation of blood pressure. The rate of infusion of dopamine should be decreased or the drug should be discontinued temporarily until the patient is stabilized. Because of dopamine's short duration of action, these measures usually provide adequate management of toxicity. In cases of severe toxicity, administration of a short-acting α-adrenergic blocking agent (e.g., phentolamine) should be considered. (See Uses: Other Uses in Phentolamine 12:16.04.04.)

Pharmacology

Dopamine stimulates adrenergic receptors of the sympathetic nervous system. The drug principally has a direct stimulatory effect on β_1-adrenergic receptors, but also appears to have an indirect effect by releasing norepinephrine from its storage sites. Dopamine also appears to act on specific dopaminergic receptors in the renal, mesenteric, coronary, and intracerebral vascular beds to cause vasodilation. The drug has little or no effect on β_2-adrenergic receptors. In IV doses of 0.5–2 mcg/kg per minute, the drug acts predominantly on dopaminergic receptors; in IV doses of 2–10 mcg/kg per minute, the drug also stimulates β_1-adrenergic receptors. In higher therapeutic doses, α-adrenergic receptors are stimulated and the net effect of the drug is the result of α-adrenergic, β_1-adrenergic, and dopaminergic stimulation. The main effects of dopamine depend on the dose administered. In low doses, cardiac stimulation and renal vascular dilation occur and in larger doses vasoconstriction occurs. It is believed that α-adrenergic effects result from inhibition of the production of cyclic adenosine-3′,5′-monophosphate (cAMP) by inhibition of the enzyme adenyl cyclase, whereas β-adrenergic effects result from stimulation of adenyl cyclase activity.

The β_1-adrenergic effects of dopamine exert a positive inotropic effect on the myocardium and result in an increase in cardiac output because of increased myocardial contractility and stroke volume in healthy individuals and in patients with shock or congestive heart failure. Systolic blood pressure and pulse pressure may be increased as a result of increased cardiac output; however, peripheral vasodilation and the resulting decrease in peripheral resistance may counteract these effects. Blood pressure, therefore, may remain unchanged or be only slightly elevated. Heart rate is usually not substantially changed. Coronary blood flow and myocardial oxygen consumption are usually increased as a result of increased myocardial contractility. Like other catecholamines, dopamine may facilitate atrioventricular conduction and increase myocardial excitability; however, the tendency of dopamine to induce cardiac arrhythmias may be slightly greater than that of dobutamine but is considerably less than that of isoproterenol and other catecholamines. Dopamine has variable effects on pulmonary vascular resistance and pulmonary artery pressure.

In low to moderate doses, dopamine causes renal and mesenteric vasodilation which is not antagonized by either α- or β-adrenergic blocking agents, atropine, or antihistamines and is therefore presumed to be the result of an action on dopaminergic receptors. Renal vasodilation results in increased renal blood flow and glomerular filtration rate. Urine flow is variably affected, but usually increases. Sodium excretion may increase, even in the absence of increased renal blood flow. The renal effects of dopamine may be at least partly due to intrarenal vascular changes and/or an inhibition of renal tubular sodium reabsorption. The osmolality of the urine usually does not decrease with increased urinary output.

In high doses (within and above the therapeutic range), α-adrenergic effects become more prominent and may result in increased peripheral resistance and renal vasoconstriction. This vasoconstriction may decrease previously augmented renal blood flow and urine output. Blood flow to peripheral vascular beds may decrease while mesenteric blood flow is increased because of increased cardiac output; however, with increasing doses of dopamine, mesenteric blood flow also decreases. In the absence of severe volume depletion, both systolic and diastolic blood pressures are increased because of increased cardiac output and increased peripheral resistance. Left ventricular filling pressure may be increased or decreased in patients with congestive heart failure. Heart rate response is variable. Blood pressure may return to normal if hypotension initially existed and may increase to hypertensive levels with excessive doses.

Pharmacokinetics

■ **Absorption** Orally administered dopamine is rapidly metabolized in the GI tract. Following IV administration, the onset of action of dopamine occurs within 5 minutes, and the drug has a duration of action of less than 10 minutes.

■ **Distribution** Dopamine is widely distributed in the body but does not cross the blood-brain barrier to a substantial extent. The apparent volume of distribution of the drug in neonates ranges from 0.6–4 L/kg. It is not known if dopamine crosses the placenta.

■ **Elimination** Dopamine has a plasma half-life of about 2 minutes. In neonates, the elimination half-life of dopamine reportedly is 5–11 minutes.

Dopamine is metabolized in the liver, kidneys, and plasma by monoamine oxidase (MAO) and catechol-*O*-methyltransferase to the inactive compounds homovanillic acid (HVA) and 3,4-dihydroxyphenylacetic acid. In patients receiving MAO inhibitors, the duration of action of dopamine may be as long as 1 hour. About 25% of a dose of dopamine is metabolized to norepinephrine within the adrenergic nerve terminals.

Dopamine is excreted in urine principally as HVA and its sulfate and glucuronide conjugates and as 3,4-dihydroxyphenylacetic acid. A very small fraction of a dose is excreted unchanged. Following administration of radiolabeled dopamine, approximately 80% of the radioactivity reportedly is excreted in urine within 24 hours.

In critically ill infants and children, the clearance rate of dopamine reportedly ranges from 48–168 mL/kg per minute, with the higher values reported in the younger patients.

Chemistry and Stability

■ **Chemistry** Dopamine is an endogenous catecholamine that is the immediate precursor of norepinephrine. Dopamine hydrochloride occurs as a white to off-white, crystalline powder that may have a slight odor of hydrochloric acid. Dopamine hydrochloride is freely soluble in water and soluble in alcohol. Dopamine hydrochloride concentrate for injection may contain an antioxidant (e.g., sodium metabisulfite) and has a pH of 2.5–5.

Commercially available dopamine hydrochloride in dextrose injections are sterile, nonpyrogenic, isotonic solutions of the drug. Some commercially available dopamine hydrochloride injections containing 200, 400, or 800 mg in 250 mL of 5% dextrose injections have osmolarities of 261–270, 269–275, or 286–295 mOsm/L, respectively; hydrochloric acid and/or sodium hydroxide may have been added to adjust pH to 3.3–3.8 (range: 2.5–4.5).

■ **Stability** Commercially available dopamine hydrochloride injection is sensitive to and should be protected from light. Yellow, brown, or pink to purple discoloration of solutions containing dopamine hydrochloride indicates decomposition of the drug, and solutions that are darker than slightly yellow or discolored in any way should not be used. Commercially available dopamine hydrochloride injections should be stored at 20–25°C; the injections should not be frozen.

Some commercially available preparations of dopamine hydrochloride in 5% dextrose are provided in plastic containers. The amount of water that can permeate from the container into the overwrap is insufficient to significantly affect the injection. Solutions in contact with the plastic can leach out some of the chemical components in very small amounts; however, safety of the plastic has been confirmed during biological testing.

Dopamine hydrochloride is stable for at least 24 hours after dilution with the following solutions: 0.9% sodium chloride, 5% dextrose, 5% dextrose with 0.9% sodium chloride, 5% dextrose with 0.45% sodium chloride, lactated Ringer's, 5% dextrose in lactated Ringer's, or ⅙ *M* sodium lactate. Dopamine hydrochloride is incompatible with alteplase, amphotericin B, iron salts, oxidizing agents, and sodium bicarbonate and other alkaline solutions. In addition, commercially available dopamine hydrochloride injection should not be admixed with alkalinizing substances (e.g., sodium bicarbonate) since the drug is inactivated in alkaline solution. Specialized references should be consulted for specific compatibility information.

Preparations

Excipients in commercially available drug preparations may have clinically important effects in some individuals; consult specific product labeling for details.

DOPamine Hydrochloride

Parenteral		
Concentrate, for injection, for IV infusion	40 mg/mL*	DOPamine Hydrochloride Injection
	80 mg/mL*	DOPamine Hydrochloride Injection
	160 mg/mL*	DOPamine Hydrochloride Injection

*available from one or more manufacturer, distributor, and/or repackager by generic (nonproprietary) name

DOPamine Hydrochloride in Dextrose

Parenteral		
Injection, for IV infusion	0.8 mg/mL Dopamine Hydrochloride (200 or 400 mg) in Dextrose 5%*	**0.08% DOPamine Hydrochloride in 5% Dextrose Injection** (LifeCare®, Viaflex® Plus)
	1.6 mg/mL Dopamine Hydrochloride (400 or 800 mg) in Dextrose 5%*	**0.16% DOPamine Hydrochloride in 5% Dextrose Injection** (LifeCare®, Viaflex® Plus)
	3.2 mg/mL Dopamine Hydrochloride (800 mg) in Dextrose 5%*	**0.32% DOPamine Hydrochloride in 5% Dextrose Injection** (LifeCare®, Viaflex® Plus)

*available from one or more manufacturer, distributor, and/or repackager by generic (nonproprietary) name

†Use is not currently included in the labeling approved by the US Food and Drug Administration

Selected Revisions August 2017,

SELECTIVE β_2-ADRENERGIC AGONISTS 12:12.08.12

Albuterol Sulfate
Levalbuterol Hydrochloride
(*R*)-Salbutamol Hydrochloride
Levalbuterol Tartrate

■ Albuterol (a racemic mixture) and levalbuterol (the *R*-enantiomer) are synthetic sympathomimetic amines that stimulate β-adrenergic receptors. The drugs are relatively selective, short-acting β_2-adrenergic agonists.

Uses

■ **Bronchospasm** Albuterol sulfate is used orally or by oral inhalation for the symptomatic management of bronchospasm in patients with reversible, obstructive airway disease and by oral inhalation for the prevention of exercise-induced bronchospasm. Levalbuterol hydrochloride or levalbuterol tartrate is used by oral inhalation for the symptomatic management or prevention of bronchospasm in patients with reversible, obstructive airway disease. Albuterol sulfate in fixed combination with ipratropium bromide is used by oral inhalation for the symptomatic management of bronchospasm associated with chronic obstructive pulmonary disease (COPD) in patients who continue to have evidence of bronchospasm despite the regular use of an orally inhaled bronchodilator and who require a second bronchodilator.

Clinical studies in adults and children 4 years of age or older indicate that albuterol sulfate inhalation aerosol with a hydrofluoroalkane (HFA) propellant (e.g., Proventil® HFA, Ventolin® HFA) has bronchodilator efficacy similar to that of albuterol inhalation aerosol with chlorofluorocarbons (no longer commercially available in the US). In one short-term (3 weeks' duration), randomized, double-blind, placebo-controlled study in children 4 to 11 years of age with asthma, patients receiving albuterol sulfate HFA inhalation aerosol (i.e., ProAir® HFA) at dosages of 180 mcg 4 times daily showed greater improvement in FEV_1 compared with baseline than did patients receiving placebo. In this study, 42% of children receiving albuterol sulfate HFA inhalation aerosol achieved a 15% increase in FEV_1 within 30 minutes postdose on the first day of the trial.

Albuterol solution for nebulization is used for the symptomatic treatment and control of acute, potentially recurrent bronchospasm in patients with reversible obstructive airway disease, including those with bronchial asthma, chronic bronchitis, pulmonary emphysema, and cystic fibrosis. Administration of β-adrenergic agonist bronchodilators via nebulization generally is reserved for patients with severe disease who do not respond adequately to more conventional therapy and for patients (e.g., children) who find it difficult or are unable to optimally inhale the drug orally via an inhaler. In clinical studies of orally inhaled albuterol sulfate via nebulization in asthmatic children aged 3 years or older, improvement in indices of pulmonary function (FEV_1 or PEFR) occurred within 2–20 minutes following single doses of nebulized drug. Following oral inhalation of nebulized albuterol sulfate (0.1 mg/kg or higher), clinically important increases in FEV_1 (as measured by a 15% increase compared with baseline) have been observed for up to 6 hours in children 5–11 years of age. In a short-term (4-weeks' duration), randomized, double-blind, placebo-controlled study in children 6–12 years of age with mild to moderate asthma (mean baseline FEV_1 60–70% of predicted values) who received albuterol 0.63 or 1.25 mg 3 times daily via nebulization with or without corticosteroids, the mean percent change in the area under the FEV_1-time curve over 6 hours with albuterol exceeded that produced by placebo. The mean time to peak effect (as determined by increase in FEV_1) with both doses was approximately 30–60 minutes postdose; no diminution of effect was noted during the 4-week period of observation.

Levalbuterol hydrochloride solution for nebulization and levalbuterol tartrate inhalation aerosol are used as bronchodilators for the symptomatic management and prevention of bronchospasm in patients with reversible obstructive airway disease. Current evidence suggests that most, if not all, of the bronchodilatory activity of albuterol is attributable to levalbuterol (*R*-albuterol) and that the *S*-enantiomer may potentially detract from the efficacy of racemic albuterol. (See Pharmacology.)

Safety and efficacy of levalbuterol tartrate with an HFA propellant via a metered-dose inhaler for the treatment of asthma have been established in 3 randomized, double-blind, placebo- and active-controlled studies of 4–8 weeks' duration in adults and children 4 years of age or older. Levalbuterol (90 mcg) and racemic albuterol with an HFA propellant (180 mcg) were more effective than placebo in improving lung function (defined as mean peak percent change from baseline in FEV_1).

In a small, placebo-controlled, dose-ranging study in adults with mild to moderate asthma receiving single doses of orally inhaled levalbuterol (0.31, 0.63, or 1.25 mg) or racemic albuterol (2.5 mg) via nebulization, the bronchodilator response to the highest dosage of levalbuterol (1.25 mg) was clinically comparable to that with albuterol 2.5 mg over the 6-hour evaluation period, although the period during which the increase in FEV_1 exceeded 15% compared with baseline was slightly more prolonged with levalbuterol. Adverse systemic β-adrenergic effects were observed with both treatments and generally were dose-related for *R*-albuterol, although the 1.25-mg dosage of levalbuterol was associated with a slightly greater incidence of such adverse effects than the 2.5-mg dosage of albuterol.

In a short-term (4-weeks' duration), placebo-controlled study in adults and adolescents with moderate to severe asthma (mean baseline FEV_1 60% of predicted) who received levalbuterol 0.63 or 1.25 mg 3 times daily or albuterol 1.25 or 2.5 mg 3 times daily via nebulization, the mean peak change in FEV_1 with levalbuterol (*R*-albuterol) exceeded that produced by equivalent dosages of the drug given as racemic albuterol (50:50 mixture of *R*- and *S*-albuterol). This improvement in FEV_1 in all patients receiving levalbuterol exceeded that for the combined albuterol group after the first dose (day 1) but not at the end (day 29) of the study. Improvement in FEV_1 was greatest and of longest duration with the levalbuterol 1.25-mg dosage regimen on days 1 and 29, while efficacy of the levalbuterol 0.63-mg and albuterol 2.5-mg regimens was similar at all time points measured. All active treatments were associated with improvement in FEV_1 compared with placebo, and adverse effects of levalbuterol and albuterol were similar.

In a short-term (3-weeks' duration), randomized, double-blind, placebo-controlled study in children (6–11 years of age) with mild to moderate asthma (mean baseline FEV_1 73% of predicted) who received levalbuterol (0.31 or 0.63 mg 3 times daily) or racemic albuterol (1.25 or 2.5 mg 3 times daily) via nebulization in addition to existing therapy (e.g., inhaled corticosteroids), the mean peak change in FEV_1 with levalbuterol (*R*-albuterol) was similar to that produced by albuterol. All active treatments were associated with improvement in FEV_1 compared with placebo, and adverse effects of levalbuterol were less than that associated with albuterol.

Asthma **Considerations in Initiating Antiasthma Therapy.** In the current stepped-care approach to antiasthmatic drug therapy, asthma is classified according to severity upon initial presentation (intermittent asthma or mild, moderate, or severe persistent asthma) and also by response to treatment (i.e., asthma control). While classification of asthma severity is useful for determining initial treatment, disease severity may vary over time and with treatment; therefore, after therapy is initiated, periodic assessment of asthma control is emphasized for guiding treatment decisions. Current asthma management guidelines state that initial therapy for asthma should correspond to disease severity, with subsequent monitoring and adjustments in therapy to achieve and maintain control of asthma according to the goals of treatment. Asthma therapy is aimed at achieving and maintaining control of asthma by reducing ongoing impairment (e.g., prevention of chronic and troublesome symptoms, reducing use of reliever drugs, maintaining normal or near-normal lung function and activity levels) and risk of future events (e.g., exacerbations requiring systemic corticosteroids, treatment-related adverse effects). These 2 components of asthma control (i.e., current impairment and future risk) may respond differently to treatment.

The National Asthma Education and Prevention Program (NAEPP) classifies the levels of asthma control as well controlled, not well controlled, or very poorly controlled. In the stepped-care approach, the treatment step selected for asthma control in patients already receiving asthma therapy is based on the patient's current treatment and level of asthma control. Stepwise therapy is meant to assist, not replace, the clinical decision-making process in selecting therapy for individual patients. Once initiated, treatment is adjusted continuously according to changes in asthma control. Patients should be monitored every 2–6 weeks following initiation of therapy to ensure that asthma control is achieved. If asthma symptoms are not controlled with the current treatment regimen, treatment is stepped up until control is achieved. If an alternative treatment was used and produced an inadequate response, the preferred treatment should be used before stepping up to the next level of therapy. Regular monitoring at 1- to 6-month intervals, depending on the level of control, is recommended to ensure that control of asthma is maintained and that appropriate adjustments in therapy are made. When control has been maintained for at least 3 months, treatment intensity may be stepped down to find the lowest dosage and/or number of drugs required to maintain asthma control, with continued follow-up at 3-month intervals.

Drugs for asthma may be categorized as relievers (e.g., bronchodilators taken as needed for acute symptoms) or controllers (principally inhaled corticosteroids or other anti-inflammatory agents taken regularly to achieve long-term control of asthma).

Intermittent Asthma. A reliever drug such as a selective short-acting inhaled β_2-adrenergic agonist (e.g., albuterol, levalbuterol, pirbuterol), is recommended on an as-needed basis to control occasional acute symptoms (e.g., cough, wheezing, dyspnea) of short duration; such use of an inhaled short-acting β_2-agonist alone generally is sufficient as initial treatment for newly diagnosed patients whose asthma severity is initially classified as intermittent (e.g., patients with daytime symptoms of asthma not more than twice weekly and nocturnal symptoms not more than twice a month). Most experts consider short-acting inhaled β_2-adrenergic agonists to be drugs of choice for treating acute asthma symptoms and exacerbations and for preventing exercise-induced bronchospasm. Alternatives to short-acting inhaled β_2-agonists recommended by some clinicians for relief of acute asthma symptoms include an inhaled anticholinergic agent (e.g., ipratropium), a short-acting oral β_2-agonist, or a short-acting theophylline (provided extended-release theophylline is not already used), but these alternatives have a slower onset of action and/or a greater risk of adverse effects. Oral β_2-adrenergic agonist therapy is suggested for use principally in patients unable to use inhaled bronchodilators (e.g., young children). Other experts do not recommend oral β_2-agonists for relief of acute asthma symptoms. Use of short-acting inhaled β_2-agonists in asymptomatic asthma should be limited to pretreatment prior to exercise and, in intermittent asthma, should be limited to providing relief as symptoms develop; some clinicians state that patients requiring symptomatic relief more than twice weekly or repeatedly over 1 or 2 days should be evaluated for possible initiation of long-term controller therapy.

Mild Persistent Asthma. When control of symptoms deteriorates in patients with intermittent asthma and symptoms become persistent (e.g., daytime symptoms of asthma more than twice weekly but less than once daily, and nocturnal symptoms of asthma 3–4 times per month), current asthma management guidelines and most clinicians recommend initiation of a controller drug such as an anti-inflammatory agent, preferably a low-dose orally inhaled corticosteroid, (e.g., 88–264, 88–176, or 176 mcg of fluticasone propionate [or its equivalent] daily via a metered-dose inhaler in adolescents and adults, children 5–11 years of age, or children 4 years of age or younger, respectively) as first-line therapy for persistent asthma, supplemented by as-needed use of a short-acting, inhaled β_2-agonist. Alternatives to low-dose inhaled corticosteroids for mild persistent asthma include certain leukotriene modifiers (i.e., montelukast, zafirlukast), extended-release theophylline, or mast-cell stabilizers (i.e., cromolyn, nedocromil [preparations for oral inhalation no longer commercially available in the US]), but these therapies are less effective and generally not preferred as initial therapy. Some experts recommend that long-term control therapy be considered in infants and children 4 years of age or younger who have identifiable risk factors for asthma (e.g., parental history of asthma, clinician-diagnosed atopic dermatitis, sensitization to aeroallergens, or 2 of the following conditions: sensitization to foods, peripheral blood eosinophilia exceeding 4%, or wheezing unrelated to colds) and who in the previous year have had 4 or more episodes of wheezing that lasted more than 1 day and symptoms that affected sleep. Low-dose inhaled corticosteroids also are recommended as the preferred initial therapy in such children. Cromolyn sodium is suggested (based on extrapolation of data from studies in older children) or montelukast is recommended by some experts as an alternative, but not preferred, therapy in children 4 years of age or younger with mild persistent asthma. Other experts do not consider mast-cell stabilizers or extended-release theophylline to be acceptable alternatives to inhaled corticosteroids for routine use as initial long-term therapy in such patients.

Moderate Persistent Asthma. According to current asthma management guidelines, therapy with a long-acting inhaled β_2-agonist such as salmeterol or formoterol generally is recommended in adults and adolescents who have moderate persistent asthma and daily asthmatic symptoms that are inadequately controlled following addition of low-dose inhaled corticosteroids to as-needed inhaled β_2-agonist treatment. However, the NAEPP recommends that the beneficial effects of long-acting inhaled β_2-agonists should be weighed carefully against the increased risk (although uncommon) of severe asthma exacerbations and asthma-related deaths associated with daily use of such agents. (See Asthma-related Death and Life-threatening Events under Cautions: Respiratory Effects, in Salmeterol 12:12.08.12.) Current asthma management guidelines also state that an alternative, but equally preferred option for management of moderate persistent asthma that is not adequately controlled with a low dosage of inhaled corticosteroid is to increase the maintenance dosage to a medium dosage (e.g., exceeding 264 but not more than 440 mcg of fluticasone propionate [or its equivalent] daily via a metered-dose inhaler in adults and adolescents). Alternative less-effective therapies that may be added to a low dosage of an inhaled corticosteroid include oral extended-release theophylline or certain leukotriene modifiers (i.e., montelukast, zafirlukast).

Limited data are available in infants and children 11 years of age or younger with moderate persistent asthma, and recommendations of care are based on expert opinion and extrapolation from studies in adults. According to current asthma management guidelines, a long-acting inhaled β_2-agonist (e.g., salmeterol, formoterol), a leukotriene modifier (i.e., montelukast, zafirlukast), or extended-release theophylline (with appropriate monitoring) may be added to low-dose inhaled corticosteroid therapy in children 5–11 years of age. Because comparative data establishing relative efficacy of these agents in this age group are lacking, there is no clearly preferred agent for use as adjunctive therapy with a low-dose inhaled corticosteroid for treatment of asthma in these children. In children 5–11 years of age with moderate persistent asthma that is not controlled with a low dosage of an inhaled corticosteroid, another preferred option according to current asthma management guidelines is to increase the maintenance dosage of the inhaled corticosteroid to a medium dosage (e.g., exceeding 176 but not more than 352 mcg of fluticasone propionate [or its equivalent] daily via a metered-dose inhaler). In infants and children 4 years of age or younger with moderate persistent asthma that is not controlled by a low dosage of an inhaled corticosteroid, the only preferred option is to increase the maintenance dosage of the inhaled corticosteroid to a medium dosage (e.g., exceeding 176 but not more than 352 mcg of fluticasone propionate [or its equivalent] daily via a metered-dose inhaler).

Severe Persistent Asthma. Maintenance therapy with an inhaled corticosteroid at medium dosages or high dosages (e.g., exceeding 440 mcg of fluticasone propionate in adults and adolescents or 352 mcg of the drug in children 5–11 years of age [or its equivalent] daily via a metered-dose inhaler) and adjunctive therapy with a long-acting inhaled β_2-agonist is the preferred treatment according to current asthma management guidelines in adults and children 5 years of age or older with severe persistent asthma (i.e., continuous daytime asthma symptoms, nighttime symptoms 7 times per week). Such recommendations in children 5–11 years of age are based on expert opinion and extrapolation from studies in older children and adults. Alternatives to a long-acting inhaled β_2-agonist for severe persistent asthma in adults and children 5 years of age or older receiving medium-dose inhaled corticosteroids include extended-release theophylline or certain leukotriene modifiers (i.e., montelukast, zafirlukast), but these therapies are generally not preferred. Omalizumab may be considered in adults and adolescents with severe asthma with an allergic component who are inadequately controlled with high-dose inhaled corticosteroids and a long-acting β_2-agonist. In infants and children 4 years of age or younger with severe asthma, maintenance therapy with an inhaled corticosteroid at medium or high dosages (e.g., exceeding 352 mcg of fluticasone propionate [or its equivalent] daily via a metered-dose inhaler) and adjunctive therapy with either a long-acting inhaled β_2-agonist or montelukast is the only preferred treatment according to current asthma management guidelines. Recommendations for care of infants and children with severe asthma are based on expert opinion and extrapolation from studies in adolescents and adults.

Poorly Controlled Asthma. If asthma symptoms in adults and children 5 years of age or older with moderate to severe asthma are very poorly controlled (i.e., at least 2 exacerbations per year requiring oral corticosteroids) with low-to-high maintenance dosages of an inhaled corticosteroid and a long-acting inhaled β_2-agonist bronchodilator, a short course (3–10 days) of an oral corticosteroid may be added to gain prompt control of asthma. In infants and children 4 years of age or younger with moderate to severe asthma who are very poorly controlled (more than 3 exacerbations per year requiring oral corticosteroids) with medium to high maintenance dosages of an inhaled corticosteroid with or without adjunctive therapy (i.e., a long-acting inhaled β_2-agonist, montelukast), a short course (3–10 days) of an oral corticosteroid may be added to gain prompt control of asthma.

While clinical efficacy of oral corticosteroids as add-on therapy in adults and children 5 years of age or older with severe asthma who are inadequately controlled with a high-dose inhaled corticosteroid, intermittent oral corticosteroid therapy, and a long-acting inhaled β_2-agonist bronchodilator has not been established in randomized controlled studies, some experts suggest regular use of oral corticosteroids in such patients, based on consensus and clinical experience. Similarly, some experts, based on consensus and clinical experience, suggest regular use of oral corticosteroid therapy in infants and children 4 years of age or younger with severe asthma who are not controlled with a high-dose inhaled corticosteroid and either a long-acting inhaled β_2-agonist or montelukast and intermittent oral corticosteroid therapy. However, other experts do not consider regular use of oral corticosteroid therapy to be appropriate therapy in children with severely uncontrolled asthma. (See Asthma under Uses: Respiratory Diseases, in the Corticosteroids General Statement 68:04.)

When asthma symptoms at any stage are not controlled with maintenance therapy (e.g., inhaled corticosteroids) plus supplemental short-acting inhaled β_2-agonist bronchodilator therapy as needed (e.g., if there is a need to increase the dose or frequency of administration of the short-acting sympathomimetic agent), prompt reevaluation is required to adjust dosage of the maintenance regimen or institute an alternative maintenance regimen.

Home Management of Acute Asthma Exacerbations. For acute exacerbations of asthma, initial home treatment consists of use of an inhaled short-acting β_2-agonist (no more than 2 doses via a metered-dose inhaler with 2–6 inhalations per dose or via nebulization every 20 minutes). Patients who have exacerbations of less severity may require a reduced dosage of a short-acting β_2-agonist. If response is good (peak expiratory flow [PEF] returns to at least 80% of predicted value or personal best and response is maintained for 3–4 hours), therapy with a short-acting β_2-agonist should be continued every 3–4 hours for 24–48 hours, and a short course of an oral corticosteroid may be considered. If response is incomplete (PEF 50–79% of predicted value or personal best), therapy with an inhaled short-acting β_2-agonist should be continued, and an oral corticosteroid should be added. If patients have a poor response to bronchodilator therapy (PEF less than 50% of predicted value or personal best), administration of an inhaled short-acting β_2-agonist should be repeated immediately, and an oral corticosteroid should be added. (See Asthma under Uses: Respiratory Diseases, in the Corticosteroids General Statement 68:04.)

For management of exacerbations due to viral respiratory infections, a short-acting inhaled β_2-agonist every 4–6 hours for 24 hours (longer therapy requires consultation with a clinician) in patients with mild symptoms may be sufficient to control symptoms and improve lung function. If viral infection-associated exacerbations occur more frequently than every 6 weeks, use of long-term control therapy should be considered. If a viral respiratory infection provokes moderate to severe exacerbations, a short course of an oral corticosteroid should be considered. For those with a history of severe exacerbations associated with viral infections, initiation of oral corticosteroids should be considered at the first sign of infection.

Prehospital Management of Acute Asthma Exacerbations. Should the response to home-initiated drug therapy be incomplete (PEF 50–79% of predicted value or personal best) or poor (PEF less than 50% of predicted value or personal best) after short-acting β_2-agonist therapy, the patient should seek medical attention urgently (same day if response is incomplete) or proceed immediately to the emergency department of a hospital (if response is poor). Orally inhaled, selective short-acting β_2-adrenergic agonists (i.e., albuterol, levalbuterol, pirbuterol) currently are recommended by an expert panel of NAEPP for prehospital management of asthma exacerbations (e.g., in emergency medicine facilities and/or ambulances). A short-acting β_2-agonist should be administered via metered-dose inhaler or nebulization at a frequency not exceeding 3 doses every 20 minutes during the first hour, followed by 1 dose hourly thereafter; supplemental oxygen is also currently recommended. If a β_2-adrenergic agonist and appropriate administration devices are not available for prehospital management, subcutaneous epinephrine or terbutaline should be given for severe exacerbations. During prolonged emergency transport, NAEPP recommends that other asthma therapies such as ipratropium bromide and oral corticosteroids should also be available for use. In patients with acute exacerbations of asthma†, ipratropium generally has been reserved for use as an adjunct to other therapy, usually in combination with a β_2-adrenergic agonist bronchodilator. Because of its delayed onset, ipratropium generally should *not* be used *alone* for the management of acute bronchospasm, particularly if a prompt response is required.

Management of Acute Asthma Exacerbations in Acute Care Setting. In the emergency department, orally inhaled, selective β_2-adrenergic agonists via metered-dose inhaler or nebulization (not exceeding 3 doses every 20 minutes during the first hour) and supplemental oxygen currently also are recommended for asthma management in patients with mild to moderate acute exacerbations (FEV_1 or PEF at least 40% of predicted or personal best). If response to a β_2-adrenergic agonist in patients with mild to moderate asthma exacerbations is not immediate or if patients used oral corticosteroids as self-medication prior to hospitalization, systemic oral corticosteroids should be added to the regimen in the emergency department. Some clinicians suggest that *adjunctive* therapy with an inhaled anticholinergic bronchodilator (i.e., ipratropium) be considered in the emergency department in patients with moderate or severe exacerbations (PEF 60–80% or less than 60%, respectively, of predicted or personal best) of asthma who fail to respond adequately to β_2-adrenergic agonists and corticosteroids. NAEPP recommends adjunctive therapy with ipratropium (via nebulization or a metered-dose inhaler) and oral corticosteroids in patients with severe asthma exacerbations (FEV_1 or PEF less than 40% of predicted or personal best) in the emergency department who fail to respond adequately to short-acting, inhaled β_2-agonists. If the episode is severe, 1 dose of a short-acting β_2-agonist should be given and the patient should be assessed for potential hospitalization. Adjunctive therapy such as IV magnesium sulfate or a nebulization gas mixture of helium and oxygen (heliox) may be considered to decrease the likelihood of intubation, but intubation should not be delayed if the procedure is deemed necessary. In patients with impending respiratory failure, intubation and mechanical ventilation with 100% oxygen, a short-acting β_2-adrenergic agonist in combination with ipratropium via nebulization given hourly or continuously, and an IV corticosteroid should be administered in the emergency department. In certain children with acute exacerbations of asthma, some evidence suggests that an orally inhaled β_2-adrenergic agonist in conjunction with orally inhaled ipratropium (via nebulization) may be more effective than therapy with a β_2-agonist alone. In one study in children with severe acute asthma, children with the most severe bronchospasm (defined as baseline FEV_1 not exceeding 30% of predicted) who received repeated does of ipratropium in conjunction with albuterol were less likely to require hospitalization or additional bronchodilator therapy than children receiving albuterol alone. However, ipratropium does not appear to confer additional benefit in children once they have been hospitalized and treated with an intensive regimen including a nebulized β_2-agonist and systemic corticosteroids. Based on such data in children, NAEPP recommends discontinuance of ipratropium upon hospitalization for severe asthma exacerbations for patients of all age groups.

A repeat assessment of response should be made in all patients after the initial hour of intensive conventional treatment in the emergency department. In patients who have a moderate asthma exacerbation (FEV_1 or PEF of 40–69% of predicted or personal best) after the initial hour of intensive conventional treatment, an oral corticosteroid and an inhaled short-acting β_2-agonist (once every hour) should be continued for 1–3 hours provided there is improvement; assessment of response and decision to hospitalize the patient should be made in less than 4 hours after admittance to the emergency department. For severe asthma exacerbations not responding to 1 hour of intensive conventional therapy, oxygen and oral corticosteroids should be continued and an inhaled short-acting β_2-agonist and ipratropium should be administered via nebulization either continuously or hourly in the emergency department. Assessment of response in patients with severe asthma exacerbations should be repeated at 2 hours and discharge is appropriate in patients with a good response (FEV_1 or PEF at least 70% of predicted value or personal best that is sustained for 60 minutes after last treatment, normal physical examination). If response is incomplete (FEV_1 or PEF 40–69% of predicted or personal best and continuing mild to moderate symptoms), the decision to hospitalize the patient should be individualized.

Upon hospitalization, therapy with oxygen and an inhaled short-acting β_2-agonist should be continued, and therapy with oral corticosteroids should be continued or intensified (switched from oral to IV). Adjunctive therapies (e.g., magnesium sulfate, heliox) could be considered in patients with an incomplete response to several hours of intensive therapy. Patients admitted to the hospital should be reassessed at regular intervals. Patients with a poor response to such hospitalization and interventions (FEV_1 or PEF less than 40% of predicted or personal best) and those with an incomplete response after 6–12 hours of hospitalization should be admitted to an intensive care unit (ICU). Patients with a poor response to several hours of intensive therapy and patients with impending respiratory failure also should be admitted to an ICU. Upon ICU admission, therapy with ipratropium should be discontinued, but therapy with a short-acting β_2-agonist, an IV corticosteroid, and possible adjunctive therapy should be continued. Discharge is appropriate in hospitalized patients with a good response. Upon discharge, treatment with a short-acting β_2-agonist and an oral corticosteroid (3–10 days) should be continued and initiation of an inhaled corticosteroid should be considered.

Regular Use of Short-acting β_2-Agonists. Concerns about the safety of *regular* use of short-acting inhaled β_2-agonist bronchodilators for maintenance therapy of asthma have been raised by evidence from some studies suggesting increased morbidity and mortality in patients receiving long-term therapy with short-acting, inhaled β-agonists, particularly fenoterol (currently not commercially available in the US). Other studies in patients with mild or moderate asthma suggest that while regularly scheduled use of short-acting, inhaled β_2-agonists may not cause harm, such use does not appear to have demonstrable advantages compared with intermittent use and does not adequately control asthmatic symptoms, peak flow variability, or airway hyperresponsiveness. Suggested mechanisms for detrimental effects of regularly scheduled, inhaled β-agonist therapy include down-regulation of β-adrenergic receptors (tolerance) (see Cautions: Precautions and Contraindications), increased responsiveness of airways to allergens and exercise, genetic changes in β_2-agonist receptor gene, or increased airway accessibility to inhaled allergens, which may lead to increased airway inflammation and reactivity and worsening of asthma symptoms. The validity of the evidence from these studies has been criticized in terms of study design and/or interpretation of study findings and a causal relationship between inhaled β_2-agonist therapy and asthma mortality has not been proven. Current asthma management guidelines and many clinicians recommend anti-inflammatory therapy with an inhaled corticosteroid as first-line therapy for long-term control in patients with persistent asthma, supplemented by as-needed use of a short-acting, inhaled β_2-agonist. Regular, daily use of a short-acting, inhaled β_2-agonist generally is not recommended, and increased chronic use of such β_2-agonists more than twice weekly (excluding use for exercise-induced bronchospasm) or acute use (e.g., repeated use over more than 1–2 days) for asthma deterioration may indicate the need to initiate or increase long-term control therapy for asthma.

Exercise-Induced Bronchospasm Orally inhaled albuterol sulfate administered via a metered-dose aerosol is used as a bronchodilator in the prevention of exercise-induced bronchospasm. Most experts consider short-acting inhaled β_2-adrenergic agonists to be drugs of choice for prevention of exercise-induced bronchospasm. Treatment with a short-acting, inhaled β_2-agonist immediately before vigorous activity or exercise may be helpful for 2–3 hours. If symptoms occur during usual exercise or play activities, a step up in long-term control therapy is warranted.

In clinical studies of orally inhaled albuterol aerosol for the prevention of exercise-induced bronchospasm in adults and children, administration of the drug 15 minutes prior to exercise prevented bronchospasm as evidenced by maintenance of FEV_1 within 80% of baseline in most patients. In one placebo-controlled clinical study of orally inhaled albuterol sulfate aerosol (ProAir® HFA) for the prevention of exercise-induced bronchospasm in adults and adolescents 12 years of age or older, administration of the drug 30 minutes prior to exercise prevented bronchospasm as evidenced by maintenance of FEV_1 within 80% of baseline in most patients. In another study in adults, a similar prophylactic effect was observed despite repeated exercise challenge for up to 4 hours in the majority of patients and for 6 hours in approximately one third of such treated patients. In one study in asthmatic children, oral albuterol† was as effective as orally inhaled albuterol, both in ability to produce bronchodilation and to prevent exercise-induced bronchospasm; however, oral albuterol's bronchodilating effect was delayed and its effect on some measures of pulmonary function (i.e., forced expiratory flow during the middle half of forced vital capacity [$FEF_{25-75\%}$], maximum expiratory flow after 75% forced vital capacity [V_{25}]) following exercise was slightly less than that of orally inhaled albuterol.

■ Chronic Obstructive Pulmonary Disease

Regular use of selective, short-acting inhaled β_2-adrenergic agonists in the management of chronic obstructive pulmonary disease (COPD)†, in contrast to that in asthma, does not appear to be detrimental. However, as long-acting β_2-adrenergic agonists have become available for maintenance treatment of COPD, short-acting β_2-adrenergic agonists are used by some clinicians mainly to relieve acute symptoms of COPD. Albuterol is used in combination with other bronchodilators or alone† on an as-needed or regular (e.g., 4 times daily) basis for the management of mild to very severe COPD. Albuterol sulfate in fixed combination with ipratropium bromide is used as maintenance therapy of reversible bronchospasm associated with COPD in patients who continue to have evidence of bronchospasm despite regular use of an orally inhaled bronchodilator and who require a second bronchodilator. Therapy with anticholinergic and/or β-adrenergic agonist bronchodilators increases airflow and exercise tolerance and reduces dyspnea in patients with COPD.

In the stepped-care approach to drug therapy in patients with COPD, mild intermittent symptoms and minimal lung impairment (e.g., FEV_1 at least 80% of predicted) can be treated with a short-acting, selective inhaled β_2-agonist such as albuterol as needed for acute symptoms. Inhaled β_2-adrenergic agonists are preferred over oral β_2-agonist therapy for treatment of COPD. Oral β_2-adrenergic agonists have a slower onset of action and an increased incidence of adverse effects compared with inhaled therapy; the role of oral β_2-adrenergic agonists in treatment of COPD is limited.

In patients with moderate (e.g., FEV_1 50–80% of predicted) COPD who have persistent symptoms despite as-needed therapy with ipratropium or a selective inhaled β_2-agonist, maintenance treatment with a long-acting bronchodilator (e.g., formoterol, salmeterol, tiotropium) can be added and a short-acting, selective inhaled β_2-agonist be used as needed for immediate symptom relief. Maintenance treatment with long-acting bronchodilators is recommended in such patients as this therapy is more effective and convenient than regular use of short-acting bronchodilators. For patients not responding adequately to treatment following addition of a long-acting bronchodilator, a combination of several long-acting bronchodilators such as tiotropium and a long-acting β-adrenergic agonist may be used.

Maintenance therapy (e.g., 4 times daily) with a short-acting, selective inhaled β_2-agonist is not preferred but may be used in patients with persistent symptoms of COPD; such therapy should not exceed 6–12 inhalations daily. Current guidelines for the management of COPD state that low- to high-dose ipratropium (6–16 inhalations daily) can be added to therapy with a short-acting, selective inhaled β_2-agonist in patients with mild to moderate persistent symptoms of COPD, with the frequency of inhalation therapy with either agent not to exceed 4 times daily; the high dosage of ipratropium included in some guidelines for COPD exceeds the manufacturer's maximum recommended dosage (12 inhalations). Combining bronchodilators from different classes and with differing durations of action may increase the degree of bronchodilation with a similar or lower frequency of adverse effects. In several randomized, double-blind clinical trials, albuterol sulfate and ipratropium bromide in fixed combination for oral inhalation produced greater improvement in pulmonary function (i.e., mean FEV_1 compared with baseline) than either drug alone; the median duration of effect (as measured by FEV_1) was 4–5 hours for the fixed combination compared with 4 hours for ipratropium bromide and 3 hours for albuterol sulfate. For additional information on the use of albuterol and ipratropium in fixed combination for patients with COPD, see Uses: Chronic Obstructive Pulmonary Disease, in Ipratropium Bromide 12:08.08.

For treatment of severe to very severe COPD (e.g., FEV_1 30–50% of predicted or less, history of exacerbations), the addition of an inhaled corticosteroid to one or more long-acting bronchodilators given separately or in fixed combination may be needed. If symptoms are not adequately controlled with inhaled corticosteroids and a long-acting bronchodilator, or if limiting adverse effects occur, oral extended-release theophylline may be added or substituted.

Management of acute exacerbations of COPD at home is based initially on the same drugs used for management of the stable patient. A short-acting β_2-adrenergic agonist is the preferred bronchodilator for treatment of acute exacerbations of COPD. If response to a short-acting β_2-adrenergic agonist alone is inadequate, some clinicians recommend the addition of ipratropium. In a severe exacerbation (FEV_1 less than 50% of predicted) treated at home, administration of these agents by nebulization or metered-dose inhalation with a spacer device may be used as needed for short-term therapy. For more severe exacerbations of COPD (e.g., FEV_1 less than 50% of predicted), a short (e.g., 7–10 days) course of oral corticosteroids (e.g., equivalent to 30–40 mg of prednisone daily) can be added to bronchodilator therapy. If symptoms of COPD continue to deteriorate several hours after administration of oral corticosteroids (e.g., sudden development of resting dyspnea, cyanosis, peripheral edema, changes in mental status, inability to eat or sleep because of symptoms), the patient should be hospitalized. Following initiation of oxygen therapy in hospitalized patients, therapy with short-acting β_2-adrenergic agonist and/or ipratropium (administered separately or in fixed combination) should be used for acute exacerbations of COPD, although the effectiveness of such combination therapy remains controversial. Oral corticosteroids are especially helpful within the first 72 hours of an acute exacerbation and should be initiated early in the management of the hospitalized patient. If patients cannot tolerate oral corticosteroids, IV corticosteroids should be initiated. If necessary for severe exacerbations, appropriate anti-infective therapy can be initiated if indicated (purulent exacerbations).

■ **Other Uses** Orally inhaled albuterol has been used effectively to prevent or alleviate episodes of muscle paralysis in the treatment of some patients with hyperkalemic familial periodic paralysis†.

Dosage and Administration

■ **Administration** Albuterol sulfate is administered orally or by oral inhalation via a metered-dose inhaler or nebulization. Albuterol sulfate is administered in fixed combination with ipratropium bromide via a metered-dose aerosol inhaler or via nebulization. Levalbuterol hydrochloride is administered by oral inhalation via nebulization. Levalbuterol tartrate with hydrofluoroalkane (HFA) propellant is administered by oral inhalation via a metered-dose inhaler. To avoid microbial contamination, proper aseptic technique should be used when albuterol or levalbuterol is administered via nebulization. Albuterol sulfate extended-release tablets should not be chewed or crushed.

Oral Inhalation via Metered-Dose Aerosol **Albuterol Sulfate.** It is important that the patient receive careful instruction in the use of the metered-dose inhaler to obtain optimum results. Albuterol sulfate inhalation aerosol should only be used with the actuator supplied with the product. Before using, the inhaler must be shaken well. The aerosol inhaler should be test sprayed (3 times for ProAir® HFA, 4 times for Ventolin® HFA or Proventil® HFA) into the air (away from the face) before initial use or whenever it has not been used for a prolonged period of time (i.e., exceeding 2 weeks). The manufacturer of Ventolin® HFA states that the aerosol inhaler also should be test sprayed whenever it has been dropped.

After exhaling as completely as possible, the patient should place the mouthpiece of the inhaler well into the mouth and close the lips firmly around it. Then the patient should inhale deeply through the mouth while actuating the inhaler. After holding the breath for as long as possible, the patient should remove the mouthpiece from the mouth and exhale slowly. It is recommended that 1 minute elapse between inhalations of albuterol sulfate when a 2-inhalation dose is administered. Some clinicians recommend an interval of 10–20 minutes between the first and second inhalation of an orally inhaled sympathomimetic agent in order to increase bronchial penetration of the agent and bronchodilation.

The technique employed for administration of albuterol sulfate by oral inhalation via a metered-dose inhaler is similar in children to that in adults, since the smaller ventilatory capacity of children provides a proportionally smaller dose of the inhaled drug.

To clean the albuterol sulfate inhalation aerosol (Proventil® HFA, Ventolin® HFA, Proair® HFA) inhaler, the metal canister should be removed and the plastic mouthpiece of the actuator cleansed by running warm water through the top and bottom for 30 seconds at least once a week. The mouthpiece of albuterol sulfate inhalation aerosol should be shaken to remove excess water, then air dried thoroughly (e.g., overnight) before replacing the metal canister and mouthpiece cap. If the inhaler is to be used before it is completely dry, excess water should be shaken off, the canister replaced, the inhaler test sprayed once (Ventolin® HFA) or twice (Proventil® HFA, Proair® HFA) away from the face, and the prescribed dose taken. After such use, the mouthpiece should be rewashed and allowed to air dry. Proper cleaning of the albuterol sulfate inhaler (Proventil® HFA, Ventolin® HFA, Proair® HFA) mouthpiece will prevent medication build-up and blockage.

The 3.7- or 6.7-g canister of albuterol sulfate inhalation aerosol (Proventil® HFA) should be discarded after 100 or 200 sprays, respectively. The 18-g canister of albuterol sulfate inhalation aerosol (Ventolin® HFA) should be discarded after 200 sprays or 2 months after removal from the foil pouch, whichever occurs first. The 8.5-g canister of albuterol sulfate inhalation aerosol (Proair® HFA) should be discarded after 200 sprays. Patients should avoid spraying oral aerosols or oral inhalation solutions containing albuterol into the eyes. (See Cautions: Precautions and Contraindications.)

Levalbuterol Tartrate. Levalbuterol tartrate inhalation aerosol should be used only with the actuator provided by the manufacturer. Before using, the inhaler should be shaken well. The aerosol inhaler should be test sprayed (4 times, away from the face) before first use and whenever the inhaler has not been used for more than 3 days. Patients should avoid spraying levalbuterol inhalation aerosol into the eyes.

After exhaling slowly and completely, the mouthpiece of the inhaler should be placed well into the mouth with the lips closed around it. The patient should inhale slowly and deeply through the mouth and actuate the aerosol inhaler. The patient should withdraw the mouthpiece, hold the breath for 10 seconds, if possible, and exhale; 1 minute should elapse between inhalations from the aerosol inhaler.

To clean the metered-dose inhaler, the metal canister and blue mouthpiece (actuator) cap should be removed and cleansed by running warm water through the mouthpiece for 30 seconds at least once a week. The mouthpiece should be shaken to remove excess water and allowed to air dry thoroughly (e.g., overnight). After drying, the metal canister should be inserted into the mouthpiece and the mouthpiece cap replaced. Patients should not attempt to clean the metal canister or allow the canister to become wet. If the inhaler is to be used before it is completely dry, excess water should be shaken off, the canister replaced, and the inhaler tested by spraying twice (away from the face) before administering the dose. After such use, the mouthpiece should be rewashed and allowed to air dry. Proper cleaning of the mouthpiece will prevent medication build-up and blockage. If the actuator becomes blocked, medication should be removed by washing. The metal canister of levalbuterol should be discarded after 200 sprays have been delivered from the 15-g canister, as delivery of the correct dose of the drug cannot be ensured after the labeled number of actuations have been used.

Albuterol Sulfate and Ipratropium Bromide. Patients should insert the metal canister into the clear end of the mouthpiece. The aerosol inhaler should be shaken well for at least 10 seconds immediately prior to use and should be actuated 3 times prior to the initial use or if it has not been used for more than 24 hours. The mouthpiece provided for the inhalation aerosol of albuterol sulfate and ipratropium bromide should not be used for other aerosol drugs. Prior to use, the orange dust cap should be removed and the mouthpiece should be checked for foreign objects. Patients should avoid spraying albuterol sulfate and ipratropium bromide inhalation aerosol into their eyes. To avoid inadvertent contact of the drug with the eyes and subsequent adverse effects (e.g., temporary blurred vision, precipitation or worsening of angle-closure glaucoma, ocular pain), patients should be advised to close their eyes during inhalation of albuterol sulfate and ipratropium bromide aerosol. (See Cautions: Ocular Effects, in Ipratropium Bromide 12:08.08.)

The patient should exhale deeply within 30 seconds of shaking the aerosol inhaler and the mouthpiece of the inhaler should be placed into the mouth with the canister held upright. The patient should then inhale slowly and deeply through the mouth while actuating the inhaler. After holding the breath for 10 seconds, the patient should remove the mouthpiece and exhale slowly. If additional inhalations are required, the patient should wait approximately 2 minutes and repeat the procedure. The manufacturer recommends that the albuterol sulfate and ipratropium bromide oral inhaler mouthpiece be cleaned as needed by rinsing the mouthpiece in hot water. If soap is used, the mouthpiece should be rinsed thoroughly with plain water. When dry, the cap on the mouthpiece should be replaced when the inhaler is not in use.

Oral Inhalation via Nebulization **Albuterol Sulfate Concentrate.** For administration of albuterol sulfate via a nebulizer using the concentrate solution, an appropriate volume of concentrate solution should be drawn into the specially marked dropper supplied with each bottle and then emptied into the nebulizer reservoir, taking care not to touch the dropper to any surface, including the reservoir or associated ventilatory equipment. The appropriate amount of 0.9% sodium chloride solution is then added to the reservoir to provide a total diluted volume of 3 mL. If the albuterol sulfate concentrate solution changes color or becomes cloudy, it should not be used. For administration of single-use units of albuterol sulfate 0.5% concentrate solution for nebulization, the entire contents of the plastic vial should be emptied into the nebulizer reservoir and 2.5 mL of 0.9% sodium chloride solution should be added to provide a final volume of 3 mL.

Albuterol Sulfate or Levalbuterol Hydrochloride Single-Use Solutions. For administration of albuterol sulfate or levalbuterol hydrochloride solution for nebulization in single-use polyethylene units via a nebulizer, the entire contents of the single-use unit of solution should be emptied into the nebulizer reservoir and used immediately to avoid microbial contamination. If albuterol sulfate solution for nebulization (in single-use units) becomes discolored, it should not be used. Vials of levalbuterol hydrochloride solution for nebulization should be discarded if the solution is not colorless.

Following addition of the drug to the nebulizer reservoir, the reservoir is attached to the mouthpiece or face mask and to the compressor according to the manufacturer's instructions. The patient should place the mouthpiece of the nebulizer in his or her mouth or put on the nebulizer face mask. The patient should then breathe through the mouthpiece as calmly, deeply, and evenly as possible until the nebulizer stops producing mist. The duration of treatment for oral inhalation of a full dose of albuterol sulfate or levalbuterol hydrochloride usually is about 5–15 minutes. The nebulizer should be cleaned after use according to the manufacturer's instructions in order to avoid microbial contamination.

Albuterol Sulfate and Ipratropium Bromide. Prior to administration of albuterol sulfate and ipratropium bromide inhalation solution for nebulization, the nebulizer manufacturer's information should be reviewed to assess any changes in administration. For administration of albuterol sulfate in fixed combination with ipratropium bromide (DuoNeb®) via a nebulizer, the entire contents of the single-use vial of solution should be emptied into the nebulizer reservoir and the reservoir attached to the mouthpiece or face mask and to the compressor according to the manufacturer's instructions.

The patient should place the mouthpiece of the nebulizer into the mouth. Alternatively, patients may put the face mask over the mouth and nose. The patient should then breathe through the mouth as calmly, deeply, and evenly as possible until the nebulizer stops producing mist. The duration of treatment for oral inhalation of a full dose of albuterol sulfate and ipratropium in fixed combination usually is about 5–15 minutes. The nebulizer should be cleaned after use according to the manufacturer's instructions.

■ **Dosage** Dosage of albuterol sulfate is expressed in terms of albuterol. Dosage of levalbuterol hydrochloride or tartrate is expressed in terms of levalbuterol. Dosage of albuterol sulfate and levalbuterol must be carefully adjusted according to individual requirements and response. The albuterol oral aerosol inhalers deliver 90 mcg of albuterol from the mouthpiece per metered spray. The levalbuterol tartrate oral aerosol inhaler delivers 45 mcg of levalbuterol from the mouthpiece per metered spray. The oral aerosol inhaler containing albuterol sulfate and ipratropium bromide delivers 18 mcg of ipratropium bromide and 103 mcg of albuterol sulfate (equivalent to 90 mcg of albuterol) from the mouthpiece per metered spray. Using in vitro testing at an average flow rate of 3.6 L/minute for an average of 15 minutes, the Pari-LC Plus® nebulizer delivered at the mouthpiece approximately 46 or 42% of the original dosage of albuterol or ipratropium bromide, respectively. Using in vitro testing at an average flow rate of 3.6 L/minute for an average of 15 minutes or less, the Pari-LC Plus® nebulizer delivered at the mouthpiece approximately 43 or 39% of the original dosage of albuterol at the 1.25- or 0. 63-mg strength, respectively.

Commercially available albuterol sulfate aerosol with a hydrofluoroalkane (HFA) propellant delivers at least 200 metered sprays per 18-g (Ventolin® HFA), 6.7-g (Proventil® HFA), or 8.5-g (ProAir® HFA) canister, respectively. The commercially available aerosol inhaler containing albuterol sulfate in fixed combination with ipratropium bromide delivers 200 metered sprays per 14.7-g canister. The commercially available levalbuterol aerosol inhaler delivers 200 metered sprays per 15-g canister. The canister should be discarded after the labeled number of actuations have been used.

Oral Inhalation via Metered-Dose Aerosol **Albuterol Sulfate.** For the symptomatic relief of acute episodes of bronchospasm or prevention of asthmatic symptoms, the usual dosage of orally inhaled albuterol administered via a metered-dose aerosol for adults and children 4 years of age or older (Ventolin® HFA, Proventil® HFA, ProAir® HFA) is 180 mcg (2 inhalations) every 4–6 hours. Some experts suggest 180 mcg of albuterol every 4–6 hours for the treatment of acute episodes of bronchospasm in infants and children younger than 4 years of age†. In some patients, 90 mcg (1 inhalation) every 4 hours may be sufficient. Because of the greater frequency of decreased hepatic, renal, and/or cardiac function and of concomitant disease and drug therapy in geriatric patients, the manufacturers of Ventolin® HFA or ProAir® HFA inhalation aerosol suggest that patients in this age group receive initial dosages of the drug at the lower end of the usual range.

The manufacturers of albuterol sulfate inhalation aerosol state that more frequent administration or a larger number of inhalations of albuterol should not be used. However, for acute asthma exacerbations that are managed initially in the patient's home, some experts state that up to 2 doses (2–6 inhalations per dose) of a short-acting inhaled β_2-agonist may be administered via metered-dose inhaler 20 minutes apart. A lower dosage may be sufficient in patients who have less severe exacerbations. If response is good (peak expiratory flow [PEF] returns to at least 80% of predicted value or personal best and response is maintained for 3–4 hours), therapy with a short-acting β_2-agonist should be continued every 3–4 hours for 24–48 hours. If response is incomplete (PEF 50–79% of predicted or personal best), therapy with an inhaled short-acting β_2-agonist should be continued, and the patient should seek medical attention urgently (same day). If response is poor (PEF less than 50% of predicted value or personal best), treatment with the short-acting inhaled β_2-agonist should be repeated immediately (i.e., up to 2 additional doses [2–6 inhalations per dose] of the short-acting β_2-agonist should be administered via metered-dose inhaler 20 minutes apart). If respiratory distress is severe and not responsive to bronchodilator therapy, the patient should proceed immediately to the hospital emergency department for further management. For information on concurrent therapy in the treatment of acute exacerbations, see Asthma under Uses: Bronchospasm.

For treatment of acute mild to moderate asthma exacerbations (forced expiratory volume in 1 second [FEV_1] or PEF at least 40% of predicted value or personal best) in the emergency department in children 12 years of age or younger, some experts suggest 360–720 mcg (4–8 inhalations) of albuterol every 20 minutes for the first hour, followed by 360–720 mcg hourly for 1–4 hours. In adults and adolescents older than 12 years of age, some experts suggest 720 mcg of albuterol every 20 minutes for the first hour, followed by 720 mcg hourly for 1–4 hours. (For treatment of severe exacerbations, see Albuterol Sulfate under Dosage: Oral Inhalation via Nebulization, in Dosage and Administration and also see Albuterol Sulfate and Ipratropium Bromide under Dosage: Oral Inhalation via Nebulization, in Dosage and Administration.)

Current guidelines for the management of asthma do not recommend regular (e.g., 4 times daily) use of short-acting β_2-agonist oral inhalations as *maintenance* therapy for the control of asthma. Instead, use of short-acting inhaled β_2-agonists is recommended for acute relief of bronchospasm or to prevent exercise-induced bronchospasm. If control of mild asthma deteriorates and results in regular use of a short-acting β_2-agonist (i.e., 4 times daily), patients should be instructed to contact a clinician for reevaluation and possible institution of maintenance therapy. (See Asthma under Uses: Bronchospasm.) The safety of concomitant use of more than 8 inhalations per day of a short-acting β_2-adrenergic agonist with a long-acting orally inhaled β_2-agonist (i.e., salmeterol) has not been established. If the patient uses 4 or more inhalations per day of a short-acting β_2-agonist for 2 or more consecutive days or if more than 1 canister (200 inhalations per canister) of a short-acting β_2-agonist is required during an 8-week period, a clinician should be consulted for reevaluation of maintenance therapy.

For the prevention of exercise-induced bronchospasm, the usual dosage of albuterol inhalation aerosol with HFA propellant (Ventolin® HFA, Proventil® HFA, Proair® HFA) is 180 mcg (2 inhalations) given 15–30 minutes before exercise.

Levalbuterol Tartrate. For the treatment of acute episodes of bronchospasm or prevention of asthmatic symptoms, the usual initial dosage of orally inhaled levalbuterol tartrate via a metered-dose inhaler for adults and children 4 years of age or older is 90 mcg (2 inhalations) every 4–6 hours. A dosage of 45 mcg (1 inhalation) every 4 hours may be sufficient in some patients. More frequent administration or a larger number of inhalations of levalbuterol is not routinely recommended. Levalbuterol inhalation aerosol should be used with caution in patients with renal impairment receiving high dosages of the drug.

Albuterol Sulfate and Ipratropium Bromide. For the management of bronchospasm associated with chronic obstructive pulmonary disease (COPD), the usual initial dosage of albuterol sulfate (90 mcg of albuterol base per inhalation) in fixed combination with ipratropium bromide (18 mcg per inhalation) via a metered-dose inhaler (Combivent®) is 180 mcg (2 inhalations) 4 times daily. If necessary, additional inhalations may be used. Since fatalities have been reported in association with excessive use of inhaled β-adrenergic agonists in patients with asthma, the manufacturer recommends *not*exceeding 12 inhalations in 24 hours with the fixed combination of albuterol sulfate and ipratropium bromide. (See Cautions: Precautions and Contraindications.)

For initial management of severe asthma exacerbations† (FEV_1 or PEF of less than 40% of predicted or personal best) in the emergency department in adolescents 12 years of age or older† and adults receiving the fixed combination of albuterol sulfate (90 mcg of albuterol base per inhalation) and ipratropium bromide (18 mcg per inhalation) as the metered-dose aerosol, the National Asthma Education and Prevention Program (NAEPP) recommends an albuterol dosage of 720 mcg (8 inhalations) every 20 minutes as needed for up to 3 hours. For initial management of severe asthma exacerbations† in children younger than 12 years of age receiving the fixed combination of albuterol sulfate and ipratropium bromide†, NAEPP recommends an albuterol dosage of 360–720 mcg (4–8 inhalations) every 20 minutes as needed for up to 3 hours. If the patient is admitted to the hospital, treatment with ipratropium bromide should be discontinued, since the addition of ipratropium to albuterol has not been shown to provide additional benefit once the patient is hospitalized.

Oral Inhalation via Nebulization **Albuterol Sulfate.** For administration via a nebulizer, the initial dosage of albuterol for adults and for children 2–12 years of age who weigh at least 15 kg is 2.5 mg 3 or 4 times daily. Alternatively, children 2–12 years of age may receive a lower initial albuterol dosage of 0.63 or 1.25 mg 3 or 4 times daily. More frequent administration or a higher dosage is not recommended by the manufacturers. Some experts suggest that infants and children 4 years of age or younger or children 5–11 years of age may receive 0.63–2.5 mg 4–6 times daily or 1.25–5 mg 3–6 times daily, respectively, based on clinical trial data. In children 2–12 years of age weighing less than 15 kg who require less than 2.5 mg of albuterol per dose, albuterol 0.5% inhalation solution should be used to prepare the appropriate dose. Alternatively, in children 2–12 years of age in whom an albuterol dose of less than 2.5 mg per dose is desired, a single-use pediatric formulation containing 0.63 or 1.25 mg of albuterol per 3 mL may be used. Children 6–12 years of age with more severe asthma (baseline FEV_1 less than 60% predicted) or weight more than 40 kg, or children 11–12 years of age may achieve a better initial response with an albuterol dosage of 1.25 mg. The manufacturer states that the single-use pediatric formulation containing 0.63 or 1.25 mg of albuterol per 3 mL (Accuneb®) has not been studied in patients with acute exacerbations of asthma; use of a 2. 5-mg dose of albuterol administered using a more concentrated inhalation solution (0.083% solution containing 2.5 mg of albuterol per 3 mL) may be more appropriate for treating acute exacerbations, particularly in children 6 years of age or older.

The usual initial dosage of single-use albuterol inhalation solution via nebulization for the symptomatic relief of acute episodes of bronchospasm in adults and adolescents 12 years of age or older is 2.5 mg 3 or 4 times daily. In patients receiving nebulized albuterol, the flow rate of the nebulizer should be adjusted so that the albuterol is delivered over a period of approximately 5–15 minutes.

The manufacturers of albuterol inhalation solutions state that use of doses exceeding 2.5 mg or administering the drug more frequently than 4 times daily is not recommended and that medical assistance should be sought immediately if a previously effective dosage regimen fails to provide the usual relief. However, dosages (e.g., 5 mg 3–6 times daily†) of albuterol inhalation solution that exceed the manufacturer-recommended dosage have been used in adolescents and adults for treatment of acute asthma.

For acute asthma exacerbations in adults and adolescents 12 years of age or older that are managed initially in the patient's home, some experts state that up to 2 doses (2.5–5 mg per dose) may be administered via nebulization 20 minutes apart. A reduced dosage of a short-acting β_2-agonist may be sufficient in patients who have less severe exacerbations. If response is good (PEF returns to at least 80% of predicted value or personal best), therapy with a short-acting β_2-agonist should be continued every 3–4 hours for 24–48 hours. If response is incomplete (PEF 50–79% of predicted value or personal best), therapy with an inhaled short-acting β_2-agonist should be continued, and the patient should seek medical attention urgently (same day). If response is poor (PEF less than 50% of predicted value or personal best), treatment with the short-acting inhaled β_2-agonist should be repeated immediately (i.e., up to 2 additional treatments may be administered via nebulization 20 minutes apart). If respiratory distress is severe and not responsive to bronchodilator therapy, the patient should proceed immediately to the hospital emergency department for further management. For information on concurrent therapy in the treatment of acute exacerbations, see Asthma under Uses: Bronchospasm.

For treatment of acute mild to moderate asthma exacerbations in the emergency department in children younger than 12 years of age, some experts suggest 0.15 mg/kg of albuterol inhalation solution every 20 minutes for the first hour, followed by 0.15–0.3 mg/kg (not exceeding 10 mg) every 1–4 hours as needed. In adults and adolescents 12 years of age and older, some experts suggest 2.5–5 mg of albuterol every 20 minutes for the first hour, followed by 2.5–10 mg every 1–4 hours as needed.

For treatment of acute severe asthma exacerbations in the emergency department in children younger than 12 years of age, albuterol inhalation solution may be given continuously at a rate of 0.5 mg/kg per hour or intermittently at 0.15 mg/kg every 20 minutes for the first hour. If the exacerbation continues to be severe after the first hour, albuterol inhalation solution is given intermittently at 0.15–0.3 mg/kg (not exceeding 10 mg) every hour or continuously at a rate 0.5 mg/kg per hour. In adults or adolescents 12 years of age or older, albuterol inhalation solution may be given continuously at a rate of 10–15 mg per hour for the first hour or intermittently at 2.5–5 mg of albuterol every 20 minutes for the first hour. If the exacerbation continues to be severe after the first hour, albuterol inhalation solution is given intermittently at 2.5–10 mg every hour or continuously at 10–15 mg per hour.

Levalbuterol Hydrochloride. For administration via a nebulizer, the manufacturer states that the initial dosage of levalbuterol for the management of acute bronchospasm in children 6–11 years of age is 0.31 mg 3 times daily. For adults or adolescents 12 years of age or older, the initial dosage of levalbuterol is 0.63 mg 3 times daily (every 6–8 hours). Children 6–11 years of age with more severe asthma or those not responding adequately to the 0. 31-mg dose may benefit from a higher dosage; however, routine dosage should not exceed 0.63 mg 3 times daily. Some experts suggest use of levalbuterol 0.31–0.63 mg 3 times daily as needed in children as young as 5 years of age† with asthma. Patients 12 years of age or older with more severe asthma or those not responding adequately to the 0. 63-mg dose may benefit from a dosage of 1.25 mg 3 times daily as needed. Patients, including geriatric patients, receiving the higher dosage should be monitored closely for possible adverse systemic effects, and the risk versus benefit should be assessed carefully. The flow rate of the nebulizer should be adjusted so that the dose of levalbuterol is delivered over a period of approximately 5–15 minutes. Levalbuterol nebulization therapy should be continued as necessary to control recurrent bronchospasm. During acute exacerbations of asthma, most patients obtain optimum benefit when the solution for nebulization is used regularly rather than on-demand, at least initially.

Albuterol Sulfate and Ipratropium Bromide. For administration via a nebulizer, the dosage of albuterol sulfate (as albuterol base) in fixed combination with ipratropium bromide (0.5 mg) (DuoNeb®) in adults is 2.5 mg 4 times daily, with up to 2 additional inhalations allowed daily. The flow rate of the nebulizer should be adjusted so that the dose is delivered over a period of approximately 5–15 minutes. The manufacturer of DuoNeb® recommends *not* exceeding 6 inhalations daily since these dosages have not been studied for the treatment of COPD.

For initial management of severe asthma exacerbations† using the fixed combination of albuterol sulfate and ipratropium bromide in the emergency department, the NAEPP recommends 2.5 mg of albuterol sulfate (as albuterol base) in combination with 0.5 mg of ipratropium bromide every 20 minutes for 3 doses initially in adolescents 12 years of age or older† and adults. For initial management of severe asthma exacerbations† using the fixed combination of albuterol sulfate and ipratropium bromide in children younger than 12 years of age†, NAEPP recommends 1.25–2.5 mg of albuterol in fixed combination with ipratropium bromide (250–500 mcg) every 20 minutes for 3 doses initially. Alternatively, albuterol sulfate in fixed combination with ipratropium bromide may be used continuously via nebulization for the first 1 hour after admittance to the emergency department in patients with severe asthma exacerbations. If there is no improvement after the first hour of treatment, albuterol sulfate in fixed combination with ipratropium bromide may be continued for no more than 2 additional hours for a total duration of 3 hours of treatment. Similarly, if a severe exacerbation develops after the first hour of treatment with a short-acting β_2-agonist and an oral corticosteroid, albuterol sulfate in fixed combination with ipratropium bromide may be initiated and continued for no more than 2 additional hours. If the patient is admitted to the hospital, ipratropium bromide should be discontinued since benefit of the drug in addition to short-acting inhaled β_2-adrenergic agonist therapy (e.g., albuterol) has not been established once patients with severe asthma exacerbations are hospitalized.

Oral Dosage **Albuterol Sulfate.** The usual initial oral dosage of albuterol for adults and children 12 years of age or older is 2 or 4 mg 3 or 4 times daily as conventional tablets. Alternatively, adults and children 12 years of age or older may receive an initial oral dosage of 8 mg every 12 hours as extended-release tablets; in some patients (e.g., those with low body weight), 4 mg every 12 hours may be sufficient. Dosages exceeding 4 mg 4 times daily as conventional tablets or 8 mg twice daily as extended-release tablets should be used only when the patient fails to respond to the usual initial dosage. If necessary, dosage may be cautiously and gradually increased to a maximum of 8 mg 4 times daily as conventional tablets or 16 mg twice daily as extended-release tablets in adults and adolescents 12 years of age or older. When patients stabilized on conventional albuterol sulfate tablets are transferred to extended-release tablets, each 2 mg administered every 6 hours as conventional tablets is approximately equivalent to 4 mg every 12 hours as extended-release tablets.

The usual initial oral dosage of albuterol for children 6 to younger than 12 years of age is 2 mg 3 or 4 times daily as conventional tablets. Dosages exceeding 2 mg 4 times daily as conventional tablets should be used only when the patient fails to respond to the usual initial dosage. If necessary, dosage may be cautiously and gradually increased to a maximum of 24 mg daily (in divided doses) as conventional tablets. In children 6–12 years of age, the usual initial dosage of albuterol extended-release tablets (VoSpire ER®) is 4 mg every 12 hours. Dosage of albuterol given as extended-release tablets may be increased cautiously stepwise as tolerated to a maximum of 12 mg twice daily.

The usual initial oral dosage of albuterol as the oral solution (syrup) for children 6–14 years of age is 2 mg 3 or 4 times daily. In patients older than 14 years of age receiving the oral solution who fail to respond to the usual initial dosage, dosage may be cautiously and gradually increased to a maximum of 24 mg daily given in 4 divided doses. For children 2 to 6 years of age, the usual initial oral dosage is 0.1 mg/kg 3 times daily (not to exceed 2 mg 3 times daily) as the oral solution; in patients who fail to respond to the usual initial dosage, dosage may be gradually increased to 0.2 mg/kg 3 times daily (not to exceed 4 mg 3 times daily). The usual initial oral dosage of albuterol for adults or children older than 14 years of age is 2 or 4 mg 3 or 4 times daily as the oral solution. Subsequent dosage is adjusted according to the patient's tolerance and response. Dosages exceeding 4 mg 4 times daily as the oral solution should be used only when the patient fails to respond to the usual initial dosage. If necessary, dosage of albuterol oral solution may be cautiously and gradually increased to a maximum of 8 mg 4 times daily in adults and children older than 14 years of age.

In geriatric patients and those sensitive to sympathomimetic amines, the initial oral albuterol dosage is 2 mg 3 or 4 times daily as conventional tablets or oral solution; if necessary, dosage may be gradually increased to as much as 8 mg 3 or 4 times daily.

Cautions

Information on the adverse effects of orally inhaled albuterol and albuterol sulfate and conventional albuterol sulfate oral tablets has been obtained principally from clinical studies in adults and children 4 years of age or older with asthma who received the drug in short-term (e.g., 1–13-week) clinical trials. Information on the adverse effects of albuterol sulfate extended-release tablets has been obtained from clinical trials in adults and children 6 years of age or older. Adverse effects associated with oral dosage forms (i.e., conventional or extended-release tablets, oral solution) of albuterol generally are transient in nature and usually do not require discontinuance of therapy; in selected cases, oral dosage of albuterol may be reduced temporarily until the adverse effect has subsided, then increased in small increments until the optimum dosage is reached. Evidence principally from a short-term (4-week), comparative clinical trial in adults and adolescents with mild to moderate asthma suggest that levalbuterol hydrochloride, the *R*-enantiomer of albuterol, may be associated with somewhat fewer adverse β-adrenergic effects than racemic albuterol at dosages (0.63 mg of levalbuterol and 2.5 mg of albuterol) that provide equivalent bronchodilation.

The most common adverse effects of albuterol or levalbuterol are dose related and characteristic of sympathomimetic agents, although certain cardiovascular effects may occur less frequently with these drugs than with less receptor-selective agents. Tremor appears to be the most frequently reported adverse effect of albuterol, occurring in up to 20% of patients in clinical trials with various dosage forms of the drug. Other frequently reported adverse effects of albuterol include nervousness, nausea, tachycardia, palpitations, chest pain, shakiness, and dizziness. Limited data suggest that the incidence and nature of adverse effects in patients receiving albuterol sulfate oral inhalation aerosol containing the hydrofluoroalkane (HFA) propellant, a non-chlorofluorocarbon (CFC) propellant, (Proventil® HFA, Ventolin® HFA, ProAir® HFA), are similar to those in patients receiving albuterol oral inhalation aerosol containing CFC propellants (e.g., Ventolin®, no longer commercially available in the US).

Data from a short-term (4-week), comparative clinical trial in adults and adolescents with mild to moderate asthma suggest that nervousness and tremor are the most common, potentially drug-related adverse effects associated with levalbuterol hydrochloride oral inhalation for nebulization therapy. Discontinuance of therapy because of adverse effects in this trial was slightly more common in patients receiving levalbuterol 1.25 mg 3 times daily than with levalbuterol 0.63 mg 3 times daily, albuterol 2.5 mg 3 times daily, or placebo.

■ **Nervous System Effects** Tremor was reported in 20% of patients receiving albuterol sulfate conventional oral tablets or oral inhalation via nebulization in clinical trials, and in less than 15% of patients 12 years of age or older receiving either albuterol or isoproterenol oral inhalation aerosol in a comparative clinical trial. Tremor was reported in 10% of children 6–12 years of age receiving escalating dosages of albuterol (4–12 mg twice daily) as albuterol sulfate extended-release tablets in a dose-ranging trial and also in 10% of adults and older children receiving albuterol sulfate oral solution in other clinical trials. In controlled clinical trials, tremor was reported in 24.2% of adults receiving albuterol sulfate extended-release tablets. In these trials, the frequency of tremor appeared to increase with increasing patient age, with tremor occurring in 1.2, 2.6, 6.9, and 6.9% of patients 12–20, 21–30, 31–40, and 41–50 years of age, respectively. The overall incidence of tremor in patients receiving conventional or extended-release albuterol sulfate tablets in clinical trials reportedly has been similar. Tremor was reported in 8 or 7% of patients receiving albuterol inhalation aerosol or albuterol sulfate inhalation aerosol, respectively; in 1% of patients receiving albuterol sulfate oral inhalation powder (Rotacaps®; no longer commercially available in the US), and in less than 1% of children 4–11 years of age receiving albuterol inhalation aerosol in clinical trials. In a comparative clinical trial in adults and adolescents with mild to moderate asthma, tremor was reported in 6.8 or 0% of patients receiving orally inhaled levalbuterol 1.25 or 0.63 mg, respectively, 3 times daily via nebulization and in 2.7% of those receiving nebulized albuterol 2.5 mg 3 times daily. Hypertonia occurred in 2.7% of patients receiving the 2.5 mg dose of orally inhaled albuterol via nebulization and in 0% of those receiving either 1.25 or 0.63 mg of levalbuterol oral inhalation via nebulization. Tremor was reported in less than 2% of patients receiving levalbuterol inhalation solution via nebulization in overall clinical trials.

Nervousness was reported in 20% of patients receiving albuterol sulfate oral tablets in clinical trials. Nervousness was reported in 15% of children 2–6 years of age receiving the oral solution in clinical trials, while nervousness/shakiness was reported in 9% of adults and older children (6–14 years of age) receiving the oral solution. Nervousness was reported in 13% of children 6–12 years of age receiving escalating dosages of albuterol (4–12 mg twice daily) as albuterol sulfate extended-release tablets in a dose-ranging trial. Nervousness was reported in 8.5% of adults receiving albuterol sulfate extended-release tablets in controlled clinical trials. In a comparative trial, nervousness was reported in 2 or 6% of patients receiving extended-release or conventional albuterol sulfate tablets, respectively. Nervousness occurred in less than 10% of patients 12 years of age or older receiving albuterol and in less than 15% of those receiving isoproterenol oral inhalation aerosol in a comparative clinical trial. Nervousness was reported in 9 or 7% of patients receiving albuterol (no longer commercially available in the US) or albuterol sulfate aerosol, respectively, and in 4% of patients receiving nebulized albuterol sulfate in clinical trials. Nervousness was reported in 1% of adults and children 12 years of age or older receiving albuterol sulfate oral inhalation powder (Rotacaps®; no longer commercially available in the US) and 1% of children 4–11 years of age receiving albuterol oral inhalation aerosol in clinical trials. Nervousness was reported during postmarketing experience in patients receiving levalbuterol HFA oral inhalation aerosol.

Dizziness was reported in 7% of patients receiving albuterol sulfate inhalation solution via nebulization, 3% of patients (adults and children 6–14 years of age) receiving albuterol sulfate oral solution, 2% of patients receiving albuterol sulfate tablets, and in less than 1% of patients receiving albuterol sulfate inhalation powder (Rotacaps®; no longer commercially available in the US) in overall clinical trials. In another comparative trial in patients 12 years of age or older, dizziness occurred in less than 5% of patients receiving either albuterol (Ventolin®, no longer commercially available in the US) or isoproterenol oral inhalation aerosol. Dizziness also has been reported in patients receiving albuterol sulfate inhalation aerosol, occurring in 3% of patients receiving albuterol sulfate HFA inhalation aerosol (Proair® HFA) in a clinical trial. In one short-term (3-week) clinical trial in children 4–11 years of age receiving albuterol sulfate HFA inhalation aerosol (Proair® HFA), adverse nervous system effects occurred at a low incidence (less than 2% in patients receiving albuterol) and were comparable to those effects observed with adults and adolescents. In a short-term, comparative clinical trial in adults and adolescents with mild to moderate asthma, dizziness was reported in 1.4 or 2.7% of patients receiving 0.63 or 1.25 mg doses, respectively, of orally inhaled levalbuterol and in 0% of patients receiving albuterol sulfate inhalation solution via nebulization. In short-term comparative trials in adults and adolescents with asthma, dizziness was reported in 2.7% of patients receiving levalbuterol HFA inhalation aerosol and in 0.6% of patients receiving albuterol HFA inhalation aerosol.

Headache was reported in 7% of patients receiving albuterol sulfate tablets and in 4% of patients (adults and children 6–14 years of age) receiving albuterol sulfate oral solution in clinical trials. In a dose-ranging trial, headache was reported in 22% of children 6–12 years of age receiving escalating dosages of albuterol (4–12 mg twice daily) as albuterol sulfate extended-release tablets. Headache occurred in 18.8% of adults receiving albuterol extended-release tablets in controlled clinical trials. Headache occurred in 5% of children 4–12 years of age and in 2% of adults and older children receiving albuterol sulfate oral inhalation powder (Rotacaps®; no longer commercially available in the US) in clinical trials. Headache occurred in 7% of adults and adolescents 12 year of age or older receiving albuterol sulfate oral inhalation aerosol (Proair® HFA) in a clinical trial. Headache was reported in 3% of patients receiving nebulized albuterol sulfate inhalation solution and in 3% of children 4–11 years of age receiving albuterol oral inhalation aerosol in clinical trials.

Headache was reported in 7.6, 11.9, 9.4, or 3.3% of patients receiving orally inhaled levalbuterol 0.31 mg, levalbuterol 0.63 mg, albuterol 1.25 mg, or albuterol 2.5 mg 3 times daily via nebulization, respectively. In a short-term, comparative clinical trial in adults and adolescents with mild to moderate asthma, migraine was reported in 2.7 or 0% of patients receiving orally inhaled levalbuterol 1.25 or 0.63 mg 3 times daily, respectively, and in 0% of patients receiving orally inhaled albuterol 2.5 mg 3 times daily via nebulization. Headache has been reported with levalbuterol HFA inhalation aerosol during postmarketing experience. Migraine was reported in 1.7 or 0.9% of children receiving orally inhaled levalbuterol 0.63 or 1.25 mg 3 times daily, respectively, via nebulization.

Insomnia occurred in 11% of children 6–12 years of age receiving escalating dosages of albuterol (4–12 mg twice daily) as albuterol sulfate extended-release tablets in a dose-ranging trial. Insomnia was reported in 2.4% of adults receiving albuterol sulfate extended-release tablets in controlled clinical trials. Insomnia was reported in 2% of children 2–6 years of age receiving albuterol sulfate oral solution in clinical trials. Sleeplessness was reported in 1% of patients receiving nebulized albuterol and in less than 1% of patients receiving albuterol sulfate oral inhalation powder (Rotacaps®; no longer commercially available in the US) in clinical trials. Insomnia or sleeplessness was reported in 2% of patients receiving albuterol sulfate tablets; sleeplessness was reported in 1% and disturbed sleep was reported in less than 1% of adults and older children receiving albuterol sulfate oral solution in clinical trials. In a comparative trial, somnolence was reported in 2% of patients receiving either extended-release or conventional albuterol sulfate tablets.

Insomnia was reported in less than 2% of patients receiving orally inhaled levalbuterol via nebulization in clinical trials. Sleeplessness or CNS stimulation has been reported during postmarketing experience with levalbuterol HFA inhalation aerosol.

Inhalation site sensation was reported in 9 or 6%, and inhalation taste sensation in 3 or 4% of patients receiving albuterol (no longer commercially available in the US) or albuterol sulfate inhalation aerosol, respectively. Tinnitus, anxiety, ataxia, depression, somnolence, or hyperkinesia has been reported in less than 3% of patients receiving albuterol sulfate oral inhalation aerosol in clinical trials.

In overall clinical trials in patients receiving levalbuterol inhalation solution via nebulization, hypesthesia of the hand, anxiety, or paresthesia occurred in less than 2% of patients. In a short-term, comparative trial in adults and adolescents with mild to moderate asthma, anxiety was reported in 2.7 or 0% of patients receiving orally inhaled levalbuterol 1.25 or 0.63 mg 3 times daily, respectively, and in 0% of those receiving orally inhaled albuterol 2.5 mg 3 times daily via nebulization.

Hyperactivity was reported in 2% of adults and older children receiving albuterol sulfate oral solution, in 1% of children 4–11 years of age receiving albuterol oral inhalation aerosol, and in less than 1% of children 4–12 years of age receiving albuterol sulfate oral inhalation powder (Rotacaps®; no longer commercially available in the US) in clinical trials. In clinical trials with albuterol sulfate oral solution, excitement was noted more frequently in young children than in older children and adults, occurring in 20% of children 2–6 years of age and in 2% of adults and older children (6–14 years of age). Other adverse nervous system effects reported with albuterol sulfate oral solution in adults and older children (6–14 years of age) include irritable behavior and weakness in less than 1% of patients. Hyperkinesia was reported in 4%, and emotional lability or fatigue in 1% of children 2–6 years of age receiving the oral solution in clinical trials. Weakness was reported in 2%, and drowsiness, restlessness, or irritability were reported in less than 1% of patients receiving albuterol sulfate tablets in clinical trials. Agitation, nightmares, or aggressive behavior have been reported in 1% of children 4–11 years of age receiving albuterol oral inhalation aerosol in clinical trials. Lightheadedness was reported in less than 1% of patients receiving albuterol sulfate oral inhalation powder (Rotacaps®; no longer commercially available in the US) and in less than 1% of children 4–11 years of age receiving albuterol oral inhalation aerosol in clinical trials. Tinnitus has been reported in patients receiving albuterol sulfate oral tablets. Like other sympathomimetic agents, albuterol has been associated with vertigo or CNS stimulation.

■ **GI Effects** The most frequently reported adverse GI effect of albuterol is nausea. In a comparative, placebo-controlled trial, nausea was reported in 9 or 10% of patients receiving albuterol (no longer commercially available in the US) or albuterol sulfate oral inhalation aerosol, respectively; vomiting was reported in 2 or 7%, respectively, of these patients. Nausea was reported in 2% of patients receiving albuterol sulfate conventional oral tablets in clinical trials. Nausea or vomiting was reported in 4 or 2%, respectively, of adults receiving extended-release or albuterol sulfate conventional tablets in a clinical trial. Nausea or vomiting was reported in 4.2% of adults receiving albuterol sulfate extended-release tablets in placebo-controlled or comparative clinical trials. In a comparative trial, nausea was reported in less than 15% of patients 12 years of age or older receiving either albuterol or isoproterenol oral inhalation aerosol. Nausea and/or vomiting was reported in 6% of children 4–11 years of age receiving albuterol oral inhalation aerosol. Nausea and/or vomiting was reported in 4% of children 4–12 years of age receiving albuterol sulfate oral inhalation powder (Rotacaps®; no longer commercially available in the US) in clinical trials. Nausea was reported in 4% or less than 2% of patients receiving albuterol oral inhalation solution or levalbuterol inhalation solution via nebulization in clinical trials. Vomiting was reported in less than 2% of patients receiving levalbuterol inhalation solution via nebulization in clinical trials (and less frequently than with placebo). Vomiting was reported in 10.5 or 7.7% of children 4–11 years of age receiving levalbuterol HFA or albuterol HFA inhalation aerosol, respectively, in a controlled clinical trial.

Increased appetite has been reported in 3% of adults and older children (6–14 years of age) receiving albuterol sulfate oral solution in clinical trials. Anorexia occurred in 1% of children 2–6 years of age in clinical trials. Epigastric pain or stomachache was reported in less than 1% of patients receiving albuterol sulfate oral solution in clinical trials. GI symptoms, which appeared to occur more frequently in young children than in older children and adults, were reported in 2% of children 2–6 years of age receiving albuterol sulfate oral solution. Dyspepsia was reported in 1% of patients receiving orally inhaled albuterol via nebulization in clinical trials; dyspepsia also has been reported in 2% of patients receiving albuterol sulfate tablets. In a comparative trial, heartburn occurred in less than 5% of patients 12 years of age or older receiving either albuterol or isoproterenol oral inhalation aerosol. Stomachache occurred in 3%, and diarrhea or discoloration of teeth in 1% of children 4–11 years of age receiving albuterol oral inhalation aerosol. Diarrhea occurred in less than 3% of adults and adolescents 12 years of age or older receiving albuterol sulfate HFA (ProAir® HFA) inhalation aerosol in a clinical trial. Constipation or gastroenteritis occurred in less than 2% of adults and adolescents receiving albuterol sulfate HFA (ProAir® HFA) inhalation aerosol but more frequently than with placebo in a few controlled clinical trials. Diarrhea, dyspepsia, constipation, or nausea occurred in 1.8, 1.3, more than 1, or 1.4%, respectively, of patients receiving the fixed combination of albuterol sulfate and ipratropium bromide inhalation solution via nebulization in a controlled clinical trial. Overall, in clinical trials in patients receiving levalbuterol inhalation solution via nebulization, diarrhea, dry mouth, dry throat, dyspepsia, or gastroenteritis was reported in less than 2% of patients. Diarrhea occurred in 1.5, 6, 1.6, and 0% of children receiving orally inhaled levalbuterol 0.31 mg, levalbuterol 0.63 mg, albuterol 1.25 mg, or albuterol 2.5 mg 3 times daily via nebulization, respectively. Dry mouth, eructation, or flatulence has been reported in less than 3% of patients receiving albuterol sulfate oral inhalation aerosol in clinical trials. Stomachache or unusual taste each was reported in 2% and diarrhea was reported in less than 1% of children 4–12 years of age receiving albuterol sulfate oral inhalation powder (Rotacaps®; no longer commercially available in the US) in clinical trials; burning in the stomach, dry mouth, or bad taste each was reported in less than 1% of patients 12 years of age or older receiving albuterol sulfate inhalation powder. Glossitis was reported in less than 3% of adults and adolescents 12 years of age or older receiving albuterol sulfate HFA (ProAir® HFA) inhalation aerosol in a clinical trial. In one short-term (3-week) clinical trial in children 4–11 years of age receiving albuterol sulfate HFA inhalation aerosol (ProAir® HFA), adverse GI effects occurred at a low incidence (less than 2% of children receiving albuterol) and were comparable to those effects observed in adults and adolescents. Throat irritation, altered taste, tongue ulceration, and gagging have been reported during postmarketing experience with albuterol sulfate HFA (ProAir® HFA) inhalation aerosol.

■ Cardiovascular Effects Albuterol sulfate may be associated with clinically important cardiovascular effects, including tachycardia, increased or decreased blood pressure, and related symptoms.

Clinically important changes in systolic and diastolic blood pressure have occurred in individual patients and could be expected to occur in some patients after use of any β-adrenergic bronchodilator. Although such effects are uncommon after recommended dosages of albuterol or levalbuterol therapy, cardiovascular effects may require discontinuance of the drug. Data from a study in a limited number of patients with mild asthma and experimentally induced hypoxia suggest that administration of orally inhaled albuterol may be associated with potentially detrimental cardiovascular effects (e.g., peripheral vasodilation, possible pulmonary shunting) in hypoxic patients, reinforcing the importance of concomitantly administering oxygen in patients with acute severe asthma receiving β-agonist bronchodilators.

ECG changes, including flattening of the T wave, prolongation of the QT_c interval, and ST-segment depression, have been reported infrequently with β-agonist therapy; the clinical importance of these findings is unknown. Cardiac arrhythmias (including atrial fibrillation, supraventricular tachycardia, and extrasystoles) also have been reported with albuterol or levalbuterol therapy. ECG changes or abnormal ECG has been reported in less than 2% of patients receiving levalbuterol inhalation solution via nebulization in overall clinical trials.

Tachycardia or palpitations were reported in 5% of patients receiving albuterol sulfate oral tablets and 1% of patients receiving albuterol oral inhalation solution via nebulization in clinical trials. In children 6–12 years of age receiving escalating dosages of albuterol (4–12 mg twice daily) as albuterol sulfate extended-release tablets, tachycardia or palpitations each occurred in 8% of patients. Tachycardia occurred in 2.7% of adults receiving albuterol sulfate extended-release tablets in controlled clinical trials. Tachycardia or pallor was reported in 2 or 1%, respectively, of children 2–6 years of age in clinical trials; tachycardia occurred in 1% of children 6–14 years of age and adults receiving albuterol sulfate oral solution. In a short-term, comparative clinical trial in adults and adolescents with mild to moderate asthma, tachycardia was reported in 2.7, 2.8, or 2.7% of patients receiving orally inhaled levalbuterol 1.25 mg, levalbuterol 0.63 mg, or albuterol 2.5 mg 3 times daily, respectively, via nebulization. In one short-term (3-week) clinical trial in children 4–11 years of age receiving albuterol sulfate HFA inhalation aerosol (Proair® HFA), adverse cardiovascular effects occurred at a low incidence (less than 2% of children receiving albuterol) and were comparable to those effects observed in adults and adolescents. Palpitations have been reported with albuterol sulfate oral inhalation aerosol. In a comparative trial in patients 12 years of age or older, tachycardia was reported in 10% of patients receiving either albuterol or isoproterenol aerosol; palpitations were reported in less than 10% of patients receiving albuterol oral inhalation aerosol and in less than 15% of those receiving isoproterenol oral inhalation aerosol. Palpitations also were reported in less than 1% of patients receiving albuterol oral solution in clinical trials. Palpitations, tachycardia, arrhythmias, and hypertension have also been reported with the fixed combination of albuterol sulfate and ipratropium bromide inhalation aerosol or solution for nebulization. In one large, case-control study in patients with recently diagnosed COPD that evaluated the risk of cardiovascular, respiratory, and all-cause mortality and exposure to drugs used to treat COPD, use of ipratropium therapy alone within the previous 6 months was associated with an 11 and 34% increased risk of all-cause and cardiovascular mortality, respectively. Although use of ipratropium alone may have the potential for increasing the risk of mortality in patients with COPD, the possibility exists that some of this risk may be reduced by the concomitant use of other drugs for the treatment of COPD. (See Cautions: Cardiovascular Effects, in Ipratropium Bromide 12:08.08.)

As with other sympathomimetic agents, angina has been reported in patients receiving albuterol or levalbuterol therapy. Chest pain or edema was reported in less than 3% of patients receiving albuterol sulfate oral inhalation aerosol in clinical trials, and flushing or chest discomfort was reported in less than 1% of patients receiving albuterol sulfate conventional oral tablets. Chest pain also was reported in less than 1% of patients receiving albuterol oral solution in clinical trials. In a short-term, placebo-controlled trial in children with mild to moderate asthma, chest pain was reported in 1.7 or 0.9% of children receiving orally inhaled albuterol pediatric inhalation solution 0.63 or 1.25 mg 3 times daily via nebulization, respectively. Chest pain was reported in less than 2% of patients receiving orally inhaled levalbuterol via nebulization in clinical trials. Chest pain was reported in less than 3% of adults and adolescents 12 years of age or older receiving albuterol sulfate HFA (ProAir® HFA) inhalation aerosol in a clinical trial. Chest pain was reported in 2.6% of patients receiving the fixed combination of albuterol sulfate and ipratropium bromide inhalation solution via nebulization in a controlled clinical trial.

Hypertension has been reported in 1% or less than 2% of patients receiving albuterol sulfate or levalbuterol hydrochloride inhalation solution via nebulization, respectively, in clinical trials. Hypertension has been reported in less than 2% of adults and adolescents receiving levalbuterol HFA inhalation aerosol but more frequently than with placebo in a few controlled clinical trials. In a comparative trial, increased blood pressure was reported in less than 5% of patients 12 years of age or older receiving either albuterol or isoproterenol oral inhalation aerosol. In overall clinical trials with levalbuterol inhalation solution via nebulization, hypertension, hypotension, or syncope has been reported in less than 2% of patients.

■ Respiratory Effects Bronchospasm has been reported in 8%, and wheezing in 1%, of patients receiving albuterol sulfate inhalation solution via nebulization. Bronchospasm has been reported in 1% of patients 12 years of age or older receiving albuterol sulfate inhalation powder (Rotacaps®; no longer commercially available in the US) in clinical trials. Paradoxical bronchospasm, a potentially life-threatening event, has been reported with orally inhaled sympathomimetic amines, including orally inhaled albuterol or levalbuterol, albuterol sulfate oral solution, and extended-release albuterol tablets. When associated with inhaled formulations, paradoxical bronchospasm frequently occurs with the first use of a new canister or vial. (See Cautions: Precautions and Contraindications.) In overall clinical trials in patients receiving levalbuterol inhalation solution via nebulization, asthma exacerbation occurred in less than 2% of patients receiving the drug (and less frequently than with placebo). Asthma exacerbation occurred in 11.1 or 13% of children receiving orally inhaled albuterol 0.63 mg or 1.25 mg 3 times daily via nebulization, respectively. Asthma exacerbation occurred in 9.1, 9, 6.3, or 10% of patients receiving orally inhaled levalbuterol 0.31 mg, levalbuterol 0.63 mg, albuterol 1.25, or albuterol 2.5 mg 3 times daily via nebulization, respectively. Asthma exacerbation occurred in 9.4 or 7.3% of adults and adolescents receiving levalbuterol HFA or albuterol sulfate HFA inhalation aerosol, respectively, in controlled clinical trials. Asthma exacerbation, aggravated bronchospasm, or lack of efficacy has been reported during postmarketing experience in patients receiving albuterol sulfate HFA (ProAir® HFA) inhalation aerosol. Lung disorder has been reported in less than 2% of adults and adolescents receiving levalbuterol HFA inhalation aerosol but more frequently than with placebo in a few controlled clinical trials. Wheezing has been reported in less than 2% of patients receiving levalbuterol inhalation solution via nebulization (and less frequently than with placebo). Dyspnea was reported during postmarketing experience in patients receiving levalbuterol via nebulization. Dyspnea was reported in less than 3% of adults and adolescents 12 years of age or older receiving albuterol sulfate HFA (ProAir® HFA) inhalation aerosol in a clinical trial. In one short-term (3-week) clinical trial in children 4–11 years of age receiving albuterol sulfate HFA inhalation aerosol (Proair® HFA), adverse respiratory effects occurred at a low incidence (less than 2% of children receiving albuterol) and were comparable to those effects observed in adults and adolescents.

Cough occurred in 5% of patients 12 years of age or older receiving albuterol sulfate oral inhalation powder (Rotacaps®; no longer commercially available in the US) and in 4% of patients receiving albuterol oral inhalation solution via nebulization in clinical trials. Cough was reported in 2% of children 4–12 years of age receiving albuterol oral inhalation aerosol (no longer commercially available in the US) or albuterol sulfate oral inhalation powder (Rotacaps®; no longer commercially available in the US) and in less than 1% of patients receiving albuterol sulfate oral solution in clinical trials. In a short-term, comparative clinical trial in adults and adolescents with mild to moderate asthma, increased coughing occurred in 4.1 or 1.4% of patients receiving orally inhaled levalbuterol 1.25 or 0.63 mg 3 times daily, respectively, and in 2.7% of those receiving albuterol 2.5 mg 3 times daily via nebulization. However, in overall clinical trials with levalbuterol inhalation solution via nebulization, increased cough was reported in less than 2% of patients (and less frequently than with placebo). Increased cough was reported during postmarketing experience in patients receiving levalbuterol via nebulization.

Bronchitis was reported in 4 or 1.7% of patients receiving albuterol oral inhalation solution via nebulization or the fixed combination of albuterol sulfate and ipratropium bromide inhalation solution via nebulization, respectively, in clinical trials. In a short-term, placebo-controlled trial, bronchitis was reported in 1.7 or 0.9% of children receiving the pediatric albuterol inhalation solution 0.63 or 1.25 mg 3 times daily, respectively, via nebulization. In another short-term comparative trial in children 4–11 years of age, bronchitis was reported in 2.6% of children receiving levalbuterol HFA inhalation aerosol and in none of the children receiving albuterol HFA or placebo. Nasal congestion was reported in 2% of children 4–12 years of age receiving albuterol sulfate oral inhalation powder (Rotacaps®; no longer commercially available in the US) in clinical trials. Nasal congestion was reported in 1% of patients receiving nebulized albuterol inhalation solution, and pharyngitis was reported in less than 1% of such patients. Pharyngitis, lung disease, or pneumonia was reported in 4.4, 6.4, or 1.3% of patients receiving fixed combination of albuterol sulfate and ipratropium bromide inhalation solution via nebulization in a controlled clinical trial. Pharyngitis was reported in 3, 10.4, 0, or 6.7% of children receiving orally inhaled levalbuterol 0.31 mg, levalbuterol 0.63 mg, albuterol 1.25 mg, or albuterol 2.5 mg 3 times daily via nebulization, respectively. Pharyngitis was reported in 7.9 or 2.2% of adults and adolescents receiving levalbuterol HFA or albuterol HFA inhalation aerosol, respectively, in controlled clinical trials. In a short-term comparative trial in children 4–11 years of age, pharyngitis was reported in 6.6 or 12.8% of children receiving levalbuterol HFA or albuterol HFA inhalation aerosol, respectively. Pharyngitis was reported in 14% of adults and adolescents 12 years of age or older receiving albuterol sulfate HFA inhalation aerosol (Proair® HFA) in a clinical trial. Drying or irritation of the oropharynx has been reported during postmarketing experience in patients receiving levalbuterol inhalation aerosol.

Epistaxis occurred in 3% of children 4–11 years of age receiving albuterol oral inhalation aerosol, 2% of children 4–12 years of age receiving albuterol sulfate oral inhalation powder (Rotacaps®; no longer commercially available in the US), and 1% of patients receiving albuterol sulfate oral solution in clinical trials. Epistaxis occurred in less than 2% of adults and adolescents receiving levalbuterol HFA inhalation aerosol in a few controlled clinical trials. Turbinate edema was reported in 1.4 or 2.8% of patients receiving orally inhaled levalbuterol 1.25 or 0.63 mg 3 times daily via nebulization and in 0% of patients receiving albuterol sulfate inhalation solution via nebulization 3 times daily in a short-term, comparative trial. In a comparative trial, rhinitis was reported in 22 or 16% of patients receiving albuterol (no longer commercially available in the US) or albuterol sulfate inhalation aerosol (Proventil® HFA), respectively; upper respiratory tract infection was reported in 20 or 21%, and unspecified respiratory disorder in 4 or 6% of these respective patients. Rhinitis was reported in 5% of adults and adolescents 12 years of age or older receiving albuterol sulfate inhalation aerosol (Proair® HFA) in a clinical trial. Rhinitis was reported in 6.1, 10.4, 3.1, or 5% of children receiving orally inhaled levalbuterol 0.31 mg, levalbuterol 0.63 mg, albuterol 1.25 mg, or albuterol 2.5 mg 3 times daily via nebulization, respectively. Rhinitis was reported in 2.7, 11.1%, or 6.8% of patients receiving orally inhaled levalbuterol 1.25 mg, 0.63 mg, or albuterol 2.5 mg 3 times daily, respectively, via nebulization in a short-term, comparative trial. Rhinitis was reported in 7.4 or 2.2% of adults and adolescents receiving orally inhaled levalbuterol HFA or albuterol HFA inhalation aerosol, respectively, in a few short-term, comparative trials. Sinusitis occurred in 1.4, 4.2, or 2.7% of patients receiving levalbuterol 1.25 mg, 0.63 mg, or albuterol 2.5 mg 3 times daily, respectively, via nebulization, in this comparative trial.

Viral infection was reported in 6.9, 12.3, or 12.2% of patients receiving orally inhaled levalbuterol 1.25 or 0.63 mg or albuterol 2.5 mg 3 times daily, respectively, via nebulization, in this clinical trial. Viral infection was reported in less than 2% of adults and adolescents receiving levalbuterol HFA inhalation aerosol but more frequently than with placebo in a few controlled clinical trials.

Dysphonia or voice alterations have been reported in less than 3 or more than 1%, respectively, of patients receiving albuterol sulfate inhalation aerosol or the fixed combination of albuterol sulfate and ipratropium bromide inhalation solution via nebulization, respectively, in clinical trials. Throat irritation was reported in 6% of children 4–11 years of age receiving albuterol oral inhalation aerosol and in 2% of patients 12 years of age or older receiving albuterol sulfate oral inhalation powder (Rotacaps®; no longer commercially available in the US) in clinical trials. Increased hemoptysis in a patient with preexisting hemoptysis also has been reported with nebulized albuterol sulfate inhalation. Throat irritation or hoarseness each was reported in 2% of children 4–12 years of age receiving albuterol sulfate oral inhalation powder (Rotacaps®; no longer commercially available in the US) in clinical trials. Hoarseness also has been reported in patients receiving albuterol sulfate inhalation solution via nebulization or oral solution.

■ Dermatologic and Sensitivity Reactions Increased sweating has been reported in less than 3% of patients receiving albuterol sulfate oral inhalation aerosol, and sweating has been reported in less than 2% of patients receiving levalbuterol inhalation solution via nebulization and less than 1% of patients receiving albuterol sulfate oral solution in clinical trials. Erythema multiforme or Stevens-Johnson syndrome has been reported rarely with administration of oral albuterol sulfate in children. Acne or herpes simplex infection occurred in less than 2% of adults and adolescents receiving levalbuterol HFA inhalation aerosol and more frequently than with placebo in a few controlled clinical trials.

Allergic reactions were reported in 6 or 4% of patients receiving albuterol sulfate or albuterol inhalation aerosol, respectively, in a comparative, placebo-controlled trial. In a short-term, comparative trial in adults and adolescents with mild to moderate asthma, allergic reactions were reported in 2.7% of the patients receiving orally inhaled albuterol 2.5 mg 3 times daily and in 0 or 0% of patients receiving levalbuterol 1.25 or 0.63 mg 3 times daily, respectively, via nebulization. Allergic reactions were reported in 3.4 or 0.9% of children receiving orally inhaled pediatric formulation of albuterol 0.63 or 1.25 mg 3 times daily, respectively, via nebulization. Immediate hypersensitivity reactions, consisting of urticaria, angioedema, rash, bronchospasm, anaphylaxis, and/or oropharyngeal edema, have been reported rarely in patients receiving orally inhaled or oral albuterol therapy alone or in fixed combination with ipratropium bromide. Angioedema, anaphylaxis, rash, or urticaria has been reported during postmarketing experience with levalbuterol via nebulization. Urticaria has been reported in 0.9 or 1.7% of children receiving orally inhaled albuterol pediatric inhalation solution 0.63 or 1.25 mg 3 times daily, respectively, in a controlled clinical trial. Skin/appendage infections occurred in 1.7% of children receiving orally inhaled albuterol sulfate inhalation solution pediatric formulation 1.25 mg 3 times daily and in none of the children receiving 0.63 mg 3 times daily via nebulization. The potential for hypersensitivity should be considered in the clinical evaluation of patients who experience immediate hypersensitivity reactions (urticaria, angioedema, rash, bronchospasm, anaphylaxis, oropharyngeal edema).

■ Endocrine and Metabolic Effects Diabetes mellitus has been reported in less than 3% of patients receiving albuterol sulfate inhalation aerosol in clinical trials. Increased blood glucose has occurred following inhalation via nebulization of higher than recommended (i.e., 5–10 mg) doses of the drug. Large IV doses of albuterol (an IV dosage form of albuterol currently is not commercially available in the US) also have aggravated preexisting diabetes mellitus and ketoacidosis. In a short-term, comparative trial in adults and adolescents with mild to moderate asthma, levalbuterol hydrochloride or albuterol sulfate inhalation solution via nebulization produced comparable increases in plasma glucose concentration (mean change from baseline: 4.6–10.3 mg/dL) within 1 hour after administration of either agent; this effect diminished during continued therapy. In a short-term, placebo-controlled, comparative trial in children with mild to moderate asthma, a single dose of levalbuterol inhalation solution (0.31 mg) or placebo produced comparable increases in serum glucose concentration within 1 hour after administration, and these changes were less than those observed with racemic albuterol inhalation solution; this effect decreased during continued active therapy.

Albuterol and other β-adrenergic agonists may produce decreases in serum potassium concentration possibly through intracellular shunting, which has the potential to produce adverse cardiovascular effects. (See Cautions: Precautions and Contraindications.) Decreased serum potassium concentrations have occurred following inhalation of albuterol sulfate via nebulization in higher than recommended (i.e., 5–10 mg) doses or following repeated doses of 0.15 mg/kg in children aged 5–17 years; asymptomatic decline of 20–25% in serum potassium has been noted in these children. In a comparative clinical trial in adults and adolescents with mild to moderate asthma, small decreases in plasma potassium (0.2–0.3 mEq/L) were noted within 1 hour after administration of orally inhaled levalbuterol hydrochloride, albuterol sulfate, or placebo via nebulization; this effect diminished during continued therapy.

■ Musculoskeletal Effects Muscle cramp was reported in 3% of patients receiving albuterol sulfate oral tablets and in 1% of children 4–11 years of age receiving albuterol oral inhalation aerosol in clinical trials. Muscle cramps were reported during postmarketing experience with albuterol sulfate HFA (ProAir® HFA) inhalation aerosol. Muscle spasm was reported in less than 1% of patients receiving albuterol sulfate oral solution in clinical trials.

Flu-like syndrome was reported in 1.4, 4.2, or 2.7% of adults and adolescents receiving levalbuterol 1.25 mg or 0.63 mg or albuterol 2.5 mg 3 times daily, respectively, in a short-term, comparative trial. Rigors occurred in less than 3% of patients receiving albuterol sulfate oral inhalation aerosol in clinical trials. Leg cramps have been reported in less than 2% of patients receiving levalbuterol inhalation solution via nebulization in overall clinical trials and in 1.4, 2.7, or 0% of patients receiving orally inhaled albuterol sulfate 2.5 mg, levalbuterol 1.25 mg, or levalbuterol 0.63 mg, respectively, 3 times daily via nebulization in a short-term, comparative clinical trial. In a short-term comparative trial, back pain occurred in 2.7, 0, or 0% of patients receiving orally inhaled albuterol 2.5 mg 3 times daily or levalbuterol 1.25 or 0.63 mg 3 times daily, respectively, via nebulization. Back pain occurred in 2 or 4% of patients receiving albuterol (no longer commercially available in the US) or albuterol sulfate inhalation aerosol.

Pain was reported in 1.4–2.8 or 2.7% of patients receiving levalbuterol hydrochloride inhalation solution or albuterol sulfate inhalation solution via nebulization, respectively, in a comparative trial. Pain has been reported in 1.3% of patients receiving the fixed combination of albuterol sulfate and ipratropium bromide inhalation solution via nebulization. Pain was reported in 3, 1.5, 4.7, or 6.7% of children receiving orally inhaled levalbuterol 0.31 mg, levalbuterol 0.63 mg, albuterol 1.25 mg, or albuterol 2.5 mg 3 times daily via nebulization, respectively. Pain was reported in 4 or 3% of adults and adolescents (12 years of age or older) receiving levalbuterol tartrate HFA inhalation aerosol or albuterol sulfate HFA (ProAir® HFA) inhalation aerosol, respectively, in a few clinical trials. In one short-term (3-week) clinical trial in children 4–11 years of age receiving albuterol sulfate HFA inhalation aerosol (Proair® HFA), adverse musculoskeletal effects occurred at a low incidence (less than 2% of children receiving albuterol) and were comparable to those effects observed in adults and adolescents. Pooled data from clinical trials indicate that pain, leg cramps, or myalgia was reported in less than 2% of patients receiving levalbuterol inhalation solution via nebulization. Myalgia was reported in less than 2% of adults and adolescents receiving levalbuterol HFA inhalation aerosol and more frequently than with placebo in a few controlled clinical trials. Leg cramps also have been reported in 1.4% of patients receiving the fixed combination of albuterol sulfate and ipratropium bromide inhalation solution via nebulization.

■ **Ocular and Otic Effects** Conjunctivitis was reported in 1% of children 2–6 years of age receiving albuterol sulfate oral solution in clinical trials. Conjunctivitis was reported in less than 2% of adults and adolescents receiving levalbuterol HFA aerosol and more frequently than with placebo in a few controlled clinical trials. Dilated pupils were reported in less than 1% of patients receiving albuterol sulfate oral solution in clinical trials. Ocular pruritus occurred in less than 2% of patients receiving levalbuterol hydrochloride inhalation solution via nebulization in overall clinical trials. Temporary pupillary dilation, blurred vision, ocular pain, or precipitation or aggravation of angle-closure glaucoma may occur following inadvertent exposure of the eyes to nebulized albuterol sulfate in fixed combination with ipratropium bromide. (See Cautions: Ocular Effects, in Ipratropium Bromide 12:08.08.)

Ear pain was reported in less than 2% of adults and adolescents receiving levalbuterol HFA aerosol and more frequently than with placebo in a few controlled clinical trials. Ear disorder or ear pain was reported in less than 3% of adults and adolescents receiving albuterol sulfate HFA (ProAir® HFA) inhalation aerosol in a clinical trial. In one short-term (3-week) clinical trial in children 4–11 years of age receiving albuterol sulfate HFA inhalation aerosol (ProAir® HFA), adverse otic effects occurred at a low incidence (less than 2% of patients receiving albuterol) and were comparable to those effects observed in adults and adolescents. Otitis media occurred in 3.3% of children 6–11 years of age receiving orally inhaled albuterol inhalation solution 2.5 mg 3 times daily via nebulization and was not reported in children receiving orally inhaled levalbuterol inhalation solution in a controlled clinical trial.

■ **Genitourinary Effects** Urinary tract infection was reported in 4 or 3% of patients receiving albuterol (no longer commercially available in the US) or albuterol sulfate inhalation aerosol (Proventil® HFA), respectively, in a comparative trial; and fever in 2 or 6% of patients. Urinary tract infection was reported in less than 3% of adults and adolescents receiving another formulation of albuterol sulfate inhalation aerosol (ProAir® HFA) in a clinical trial. In one short-term (3-week) clinical trial in children 4–11 years of age receiving albuterol sulfate HFA inhalation aerosol (ProAir® HFA), adverse genitourinary effects occurred at a low incidence (less than 2% of children receiving albuterol) and were comparable to those effects observed in adults and adolescents. Urinary tract infection was reported in 1.6% of patients receiving the fixed combination of albuterol sulfate and ipratropium bromide inhalation solution via nebulization in a controlled clinical trial. Difficulty in micturition was reported in less than 1% of patients in clinical trials with albuterol sulfate tablets. Dysmenorrhea or vaginal moniliasis was reported in less than 2% of adults and adolescents receiving levalbuterol HFA inhalation aerosol and more frequently than with placebo in a few controlled clinical trials.

■ **Other Adverse Effects** Accidental injury was reported in 2.7, 0, or 0% of patients receiving orally inhaled levalbuterol 1.25 mg or 0.63 mg or albuterol 2.5 mg 3 times daily, respectively, via nebulization in a short-term, comparative clinical trial. Accidental injury was reported in 6.1, 4.5, 3.1, or 5% of children receiving orally inhaled levalbuterol 0.31 mg, levalbuterol 0.63 mg, albuterol 1.25 mg, or albuterol 2.5 mg 3 times daily via nebulization, respectively. Accidental injury was reported in 9.2 or 10.3% of children 4–11 years of age receiving orally inhaled levalbuterol HFA or albuterol HFA inhalation aerosol, respectively, in a controlled clinical trial. Accidental injury was reported in less than 3% of adults and adolescents 12 years of age or older receiving albuterol sulfate inhalation aerosol (ProAir® HFA) in a clinical trial. In one short-term (3-week) clinical trial in children 4–11 years of age receiving albuterol sulfate HFA inhalation aerosol (ProAir® HFA), adverse effects occurred at a low incidence (less than 2% of children receiving albuterol) and were comparable to those effects observed in adults and adolescents.

Fever was reported in 9.1, 3, 1.6, or 6.7% of children receiving orally inhaled levalbuterol 0.31 mg, levalbuterol 0.63 mg, albuterol 1.25 mg, or albuterol 2.5 mg 3 times daily via nebulization, respectively. Viral infection was reported in 7.6, 9, 4.7, or 8.3% of children receiving orally inhaled levalbuterol 0.31 mg, levalbuterol 0.63 mg, albuterol 1.25 mg, or albuterol 2.5 mg 3 times daily via nebulization, respectively. Infection was reported in less than 3% of adults and adolescents 12 years of age or older receiving albuterol sulfate inhalation aerosol in a clinical trial. Lymphadenopathy was reported in 3, 0, 1.6, or 0% of children receiving orally inhaled levalbuterol 0.31 mg, levalbuterol 0.63 mg, albuterol 1.25 mg, or albuterol 2.5 mg 3 times daily via nebulization, respectively. Otitis media occurred in 0.9 or 4.3% of children receiving orally inhaled albuterol inhalation solution pediatric formulation 0.63 or 1.25 mg 3 times daily via nebulization, respectively.

Flu syndrome occurred in 2.6% of children receiving orally inhaled albuterol sulfate inhalation solution pediatric formulation (0.63 or 1.25 mg 3 times daily) via nebulization. Flu syndrome occurred in less than 2% of adults and adolescents receiving orally inhaled levalbuterol HFA aerosol and more frequently than with placebo. Lymphadenopathy occurred in 0.9 or 2.6% of children receiving orally inhaled albuterol inhalation solution pediatric formulation 0.63 or 1.25 mg 3 times daily via nebulization, respectively. Cold symptoms occurred in 3.4% of children receiving orally inhaled albuterol sulfate inhalation solution pediatric formulation 0.63 mg 3 times daily and in none of the children receiving 1.25 mg 3 times daily via nebulization. Chills or lymphadenopathy has been reported in less than 2% of patients receiving levalbuterol inhalation solution via nebulization in overall clinical trials. Sweating has been reported in less than 2% of patients receiving orally inhaled levalbuterol via nebulization in clinical trials (and less frequently than with placebo).

Cyst or hematuria occurred in less than 2% of adults and adolescents receiving orally inhaled levalbuterol HFA inhalation aerosol in clinical trials but more frequently than with placebo in a few controlled clinical trials.

■ **Precautions and Contraindications** **Oral inhalation therapy with short-acting β_2-agonists is intended for the acute symptomatic relief of bronchospasm in reversible, obstructive airway disease, and should not be used regularly (e.g., 4 times daily) in asthmatic patients for *maintenance* therapy.** If control of mild asthma deteriorates and requires regular use of a short-acting β_2-agonist (i.e., 4 times daily), long-term maintenance therapy (e.g., inhaled corticosteroids) should be instituted; patients should be instructed to discontinue regular use of short-acting β_2-agonists and use them only for relief of acute asthma symptoms. (See Uses: Bronchospasm.) The safety of concomitant use of more than 8 inhalations per day of a short-acting β_2-adrenergic agonist with long-acting β_2-agonist (e.g., salmeterol) oral inhalation therapy has not been established. If the patient uses 4 or more inhalations per day of a short-acting β_2-agonist for 2 or more consecutive days or if more than 1 canister (200 inhalations per canister) of a short-acting β_2-agonist is required during an 8-week period, a clinician should be consulted for reevaluation of maintenance therapy.

When albuterol is used in fixed combination with ipratropium, the usual cautions, precautions, and contraindications associated with ipratropium must be considered in addition to those associated with albuterol. Adverse cardiovascular effects (e.g., alterations in heart rate, blood pressure, or other manifestations) have been reported with albuterol in fixed combination with ipratropium as an inhalation aerosol; the combination aerosol should be discontinued if such effects occur. (See Cautions in Ipratropium Bromide 12:08.08.) The safety of more than 12 inhalations daily of albuterol sulfate and ipratropium bromide in fixed combination as an oral inhalation aerosol (Combivent®) or more than 6 inhalations daily as an oral inhalation solution for nebulization (DuoNeb®) has not been studied, nor has the safety of extra doses of albuterol sulfate or ipratropium bromide given in addition to the recommended dosage.

Excessive or prolonged use of some sympathomimetic amine aerosols can lead to tolerance. Failure to respond to a previously effective dosage of albuterol alone or in combination with ipratropium may indicate seriously worsening asthma that requires reevaluation and possible institution of alternative regimens or therapy. Patients should be instructed to contact their clinician if decreased effectiveness of albuterol or levalbuterol occurs rather than to increase the dose or frequency of administration. Fatalities have occurred following excessive use of sympathomimetic amine oral inhalations. The exact cause of death is not known; however, it has been suggested that severe, acute asthmatic crisis and hypoxia may have occurred in some patients, followed by cardiac arrest. Some evidence indicates that administration of β-adrenergic agonists in hypoxemic patients with asthma may be associated with detrimental cardiovascular effects such as peripheral vasodilation and possible pulmonary shunting. (See Cautions: Cardiovascular Effects.)

Paradoxical bronchospasm that is potentially life-threatening may occur with the use of orally inhaled albuterol or levalbuterol. When associated with inhaled formulations, paradoxical bronchospasm frequently occurs with the first use of a new canister or vial. Paradoxical bronchospasm also may occur with orally administered conventional or extended-release albuterol sulfate tablets or albuterol sulfate oral solution. Although the mechanism(s) has not been fully elucidated, paradoxical bronchospasm has occurred occasionally with repeated or excessive use of orally inhaled sympathomimetic amines, especially isoproterenol. Rarely, a patient may develop acute bronchospasm immediately upon inhalation of a sympathomimetic drug preparation. Acute bronchospasm probably represents a hypersensitivity reaction to the active drug or an ingredient in the commercial product. Although it may not be possible to distinguish paradoxical bronchoconstriction or that associated with hypersensitivity to the drug or an ingredient in the formulation from worsening of the asthma, albuterol or levalbuterol should be discontinued immediately if bronchoconstriction occurs and alternative therapy instituted.

Therapy with albuterol may produce clinically important hypokalemia in some patients, possibly via intracellular shunting, which has the potential to produce adverse cardiovascular effects; the decrease usually is transient and usually does not require supplementation.

Albuterol or levalbuterol should be used with caution in patients with sensitivity to sympathomimetic amines, hyperthyroidism, diabetes mellitus, seizure disorders, or cardiovascular disorders including coronary insufficiency, cardiac arrhythmias, or hypertension. Albuterol preparations are contraindicated in patients with a known hypersensitivity to the drug, and specific dosage forms are contraindicated in patients with known hypersensitivity to any ingredient in the specific formulation. Albuterol sulfate in fixed combination with ipratropium bromide is contraindicated in patients with a history of hypersensitivity to soya lecithin or related food products such as soybeans or peanuts; atropine and its derivatives; or any other ingredient in the specific formulation. Levalbuterol is contraindicated in patients with a known hypersensitivity to the drug, racemic albuterol, or any other ingredient in the specific formulation.

■ **Pediatric Precautions** The safety and efficacy of orally inhaled albuterol sulfate aerosol with hydrofluoroalkane propellant have not been established in children younger than 4 years of age (Proair® HFA, Proventil HFA®, Ventolin® HFA). The safety and efficacy of orally inhaled albuterol sulfate via nebulization have not been established in children younger than 12 years of age, although albuterol has been used in these patients with no unusual risk. The manufacturers of some albuterol inhalation solutions for nebulization (AccuNeb®, albuterol inhalation solutions 0.083% from Dey and Roxane) state that the safety and efficacy have been established in pediatric patients aged 2–12 years and are based on studies in children 5–17 years of age and from published reports of trials of albuterol in pediatric patients 3 years of age or older. The safety and efficacy of these inhalation solutions for nebulization have not been established in children younger than 2 years of age; although such inhalation solutions have been used in these patients with no unusual risk. The safety and efficacy of orally inhaled levalbuterol hydrochloride via nebulization have not been established in children younger than 6 years of age, although the drug has been used in these patients with no unusual risk. The safety and efficacy of orally inhaled levalbuterol tartrate via a metered-dose inhaler have not been established in children younger than 4 years of age. The safety and efficacy of albuterol sulfate in fixed combination with ipratropium bromide for oral inhalation via nebulization have not been established in patients younger than 18 years of age, although the fixed combination has been used in these patients for management of asthma exacerbations with no unusual risk. The manufacturer states that safety and efficacy of albuterol sulfate in fixed combination with ipratropium bromide for oral inhalation via a metered-dose inhaler have not been established in children, although the fixed combination has been used in these patients with no unusual risk.

Safety and efficacy of albuterol conventional and extended-release tablets have not been established in children younger than 6 years of age. Use of extended-release albuterol sulfate tablets in children 6 years of age or older for the treatment of asthma is supported by safety and efficacy studies with extended-release tablets in adults, safety studies with extended-release tablets in this pediatric age group, and established use of conventional tablets in these children. The recommended dosage of extended-release tablets in pediatric patients is based on the recommended pediatric dosage for conventional tablets and on comparative pharmacokinetic studies in adults showing comparative bioavailability at steady state and reduced bioavailability after single-dose administration with extended-release albuterol tablets. (See Pharmacokinetics: Absorption.)

Careful titration of oral albuterol dosage is necessary in children younger than 6 years of age and may be achieved by use of the commercially available oral solution. Safety and efficacy of albuterol oral solution have not been established in children younger than 2 years of age. Some adverse reactions have occurred more frequently in children 2–6 years of age receiving albuterol sulfate oral solution than in adults and older children. (See Cautions.) However, in a clinical trial in children comparing albuterol oral inhalation aerosol with a tetrafluoroethane propellant (Proventil HFA®) and albuterol inhalation aerosol with a chlorofluorocarbon propellant (no longer commercially available in the US), the incidence of adverse effects was low and similar to that observed in adult trials.

■ **Geriatric Precautions** Data on the use of levalbuterol or albuterol inhalation aerosol in geriatric patients 65 years of age or older are limited and are insufficient to determine whether the efficacy and safety of levalbuterol are different in geriatric patients versus younger patients. Because of the greater frequency of decreased hepatic, renal, and/or cardiac function and of concomitant disease and drug therapy in geriatric patients, the manufacturers of albuterol sulfate and levalbuterol inhalation aerosol suggests that patients in this age group receive initial dosages of the drugs in the lower end of the usual range. (See Oral Inhalation via Metered-Dose Aerosol under Dosage and Administration: Dosage.)

Safety and efficacy of albuterol sulfate in fixed combination with ipratropium bromide inhalation solution in geriatric patients have not been specifically studied to date; however, in clinical studies of the combination for the treatment of bronchospasm, approximately 62% of the patients were 65 years of age or older and 19% were 75 years of age or older. Although no overall differences were observed between geriatric and younger patients in the safety and efficacy of the combination in clinical studies, the possibility that some elderly patients may exhibit increased sensitivity to the drug cannot be ruled out.

As albuterol and levalbuterol are substantially eliminated by the kidneys, the risk of toxic reactions may be greater in patients with renal impairment. Renal function should be assessed periodically in geriatric patients, as such patients are more likely to have decreased renal function.

■ **Mutagenicity and Carcinogenicity** There was no evidence of mutagenicity when albuterol sulfate was tested in the Ames test (with or without metabolic activation), in a mutation test with yeast, or in fluctuation assays (with metabolic activation) in strains of *Salmonella typhimurium* or *Escherichia coli*. Levalbuterol was not mutagenic when tested in the Ames test or the HRT forward gene mutation assay in Chinese hamster ovary cells. The clastogenic potential of levalbuterol has not been evaluated. Albuterol did not exhibit mutagenic potential in vitro in a forward mutation assay or in a gene conversion assay in *Saccharomyces cerevisiae* with or without metabolic activation. Albuterol was not clastogenic in a human peripheral blood lymphocyte assay or in the AH1 mouse micronucleus assay at intraperitoneal doses of up to 200 mg/kg.

The carcinogenic potential of levalbuterol alone has not been evaluated; however, the carcinogenic potential of racemic albuterol sulfate has been investigated. There is no evidence to date that albuterol is tumorigenic in humans; however, in one study in rats receiving 2, 10, and 50 mg/kg of albuterol (as albuterol sulfate) (e.g., approximately 0.5, 3, and 15 times, respectively, the maximum recommended daily oral dosage of albuterol in adults; 0.5, 2, and 10 times, respectively, the maximum daily oral dosage of albuterol in children; at least equivalent to the maximum recommended daily inhalation dosage of albuterol alone or in fixed combination with ipratropium bromide via nebulization on a mg/m^2 basis; at least twice the maximum recommended daily adult inhalation dosage of albuterol sulfate via nebulization on a mg/m^2 basis; 0.6, 3 and 15 times the maximum recommended daily pediatric inhalation dosage via nebulization on a mg/m^2 basis; 10, 50, and 250 times the maximum adult inhalation dosage of albuterol sulfate via nebulization for a 50 kg human; at least 14–15 times the maximum daily adult inhalation aerosol dosage; at least 6 times the maximum daily inhalation aerosol dosage in children on a mg/m^2 basis; or at least twice the maximum recommended daily adult inhalation dosage of levalbuterol on a mg/m^2 basis), the drug caused a dose-related increase in the incidence of benign leiomyomas of the mesovarium. In another study, this tumorigenic effect was blocked by concurrent administration of propranolol.

An 18-month study in mice revealed no evidence of tumorigenicity with albuterol at dietary dosages of up to 500 mg/kg daily (e.g., approximately 65 or 50 times the maximum recommended daily oral dosage for adults or children, respectively, on a mg/m^2 basis; 140 times the maximum recommended daily adult inhalation dosage of albuterol sulfate in fixed combination with ipratropium bromide via nebulization on a mg/m^2 basis; 140 or 200 times the maximum recommended daily adult inhalation dosage of albuterol sulfate via nebulization on a mg/m^2 basis; 75 times the maximum recommended daily pediatric inhalation dosage of albuterol sulfate via nebulization on a mg/m^2 basis; 1600–1700 times the maximum daily recommended adult inhalation aerosol dosage on a mg/m^2 basis; 800 times the maximum recommended daily pediatric inhalation aerosol dosage on a mg/m^2 basis; or approximately 260 times the maximum daily adult and pediatric inhalation dosage of levalbuterol on a mg/m^2 basis). In a 22-month study in hamsters, albuterol showed no evidence of tumorigenicity at dietary dosages of up to 50 mg/kg (e.g., approximately 8 or 7 times the maximum recommended daily oral dosage in adults or children, respectively, on a mg/m^2 basis, or approximately 35 times the maximum daily adult inhalation dosage of levalbuterol; 20 times the maximum recommended dosage of albuterol sulfate in fixed combination with ipratropium bromide via nebulization on a mg/m^2 basis; 20 or 25 times the maximum recommended daily adult inhalation dosage of albuterol sulfate via nebulization on a mg/m^2 basis; 10 times the maximum daily pediatric inhalation dosage of albuterol sulfate via nebulization on a mg/m^2 basis; 210–225 times the maximum recommended daily adult inhalation aerosol dosage on a mg/m^2 basis; 100–110 times the maximum recommended daily pediatric inhalation aerosol dosage on a mg/m^{2}basis). The relevance of these studies to humans is not known.

■ **Pregnancy, Fertility, and Lactation** Experts from the National Asthma Education and Prevention Program (NAEPP) state that maintaining adequate control of asthma during pregnancy is important for the health and well-being of the mother and the fetus. Because of the risks associated with asthma symptoms and exacerbations (e.g., increased perinatal mortality, preeclampsia, preterm birth, low birth weight during pregnancy, such experts consider use of antiasthmatic agents to be safer than the complications of inadequately controlled asthma. Albuterol is the preferred short-acting inhaled β_2-agonist because more data are available on use of albuterol in pregnant women than on use of other short-acting inhaled β_2-agonists, and such data indicate an excellent safety profile.

The manufacturers of albuterol or levalbuterol state that the drugs should be used during pregnancy only if the possible benefits outweigh the potential risks. During marketing experience with the drug, various congenital anomalies, including cleft palate and limb defects, have been reported in the children of patients being treated with albuterol; however, some women were receiving multiple medications during their pregnancies. Because no consistent pattern of congenital abnormality development can be discerned, a relationship between albuterol use and the development of congenital anomalies cannot be established. Large IV doses of albuterol have reportedly inhibited uterine contractions, and the drug has reportedly delayed preterm labor following oral administration. Serious adverse effects, including maternal pulmonary edema, have been reported during or following treatment of premature labor with β_2-agonists, including albuterol. There are currently no well-controlled studies to show that albuterol will stop preterm labor or prevent labor at term, and the risks versus benefits of tocolytic therapy with levalbuterol or albuterol have not been established. Albuterol or orally inhaled levalbuterol should be used with caution in pregnant women when needed for relief of bronchospasm during labor and only when the potential benefits are expected to clearly outweigh the possible risks, since the drugs may interfere with uterine contractility.

Albuterol has been shown to be teratogenic in mice and rabbits. Reproduction studies in mice given subcutaneous albuterol doses of 0.025, 0.25, or 2.5 mg/kg (approximately 0.003, 0.03, or 0.3 times, respectively, the maximum recommended daily oral dosage for adults; 0.125, 1.25, and 12.5 times the maximum recommended human albuterol single-use inhalation solution via nebulization; less than the maximum recommended adult daily inhalation solution dosage on a mg/m^2 basis; and up to 8 times the maximum recommended daily inhalation aerosol dosage on a mg/m^2 basis) showed cleft palate formation in 4.5% of fetuses at 0.25 mg/kg and in 9.3% of fetuses at 2.5 mg/kg (approximately equal to the maximum daily nebulized levalbuterol, albuterol sulfate, or albuterol sulfate/ipratropium bromide dosage in adults on a mg/m^2 basis); cleft palate did not occur in mice receiving 0.025 mg/kg of albuterol (representing less than the maximum daily adult inhalation dosage of albuterol sulfate alone via metered-dose inhalation or nebulization or in fixed combination with ipratropium bromide via nebulization on a mg/m^2 basis). Cleft palate also occurred in 30.5% of fetuses treated with 2.5 mg/kg of isoproterenol (positive control). A reproduction study with oral albuterol in rabbits revealed cranioschisis in 37% of fetuses at 50 mg/kg (approximately 25, 55, 60 or 80 times the maximum recommended daily adult oral albuterol sulfate dosage, albuterol sulfate/ipratropium bromide nebulized adult dosage, nebulized pediatric albuterol dosage or nebulized albuterol sulfate adult dosage, respectively, on a mg/m^2 basis; 630–680 times the maximum daily adult inhalation aerosol dosage; or 250 times the maximum albuterol inhalation solution dosage via nebulization for a 50-kg human). In a reproduction study in rats given albuterol sulfate aerosol containing a hydrofluoroalkane propellant by oral inhalation, the drug did not exhibit any teratogenic effects at 10.5 mg/kg daily (approximately 60–65 times the maximum recommended human daily inhalation dosage on a mg/m^2 basis). Safe use of the drug in pregnant women has not been established. A reproduction study in rabbits given oral levalbuterol dosages of up to 25 mg/kg (approximately 110 times the maximum recommended daily adult oral inhalation dosage on a mg/m^2 basis) revealed no evidence of teratogenicity.

Reproduction studies in rats given oral albuterol at dosages up to 50 mg/kg (representing 15 times the maximum recommended human daily oral dosage on a mg/m^2 basis; 25 times the maximum daily adult inhalation of albuterol sulfate in fixed combination with ipratropium bromide via nebulization on a mg/m^2 basis; 40 times the maximum daily adult inhalation dosage of albuterol sulfate via nebulization on mg/m^2 basis; 310–340 times the maximum recommended daily adult inhalation aerosol dosage of albuterol sulfate on a mg/m^2 basis; 30 times the maximum recommended daily pediatric inhalation dosage of albuterol via nebulization on a mg/m^2 basis; or 55 times the maximum recommended adult daily inhalation dosage of levalbuterol via nebulization) have revealed no evidence of albuterol- or levalbuterol-induced impaired fertility. It is not known whether albuterol or levalbuterol affects fertility in humans.

It is not known whether albuterol, albuterol sulfate, or levalbuterol is distributed into milk. Because of the potential for tumorigenicity shown for albuterol in animal studies, a decision should be made whether to discontinue nursing or albuterol or levalbuterol, taking into account the importance of the drug to the woman.

Drug Interactions

■ **Sympathomimetic Agents** The manufacturers state that albuterol sulfate or levalbuterol tartrate should not be administered by oral inhalation concurrently with other short-acting, orally inhaled sympathomimetic agents or epinephrine. Current guidelines for the management of asthma state that orally inhaled short-acting β_2-adrenergic agonists can be used in patients with moderate to severe asthma for short-term relief of acute bronchospasm that occurs despite maintenance therapy that includes adjunctive therapy with a long-acting, orally inhaled β_2-adrenergic agonist, (e.g., formoterol, salmeterol); successful clinical experience with concomitant use of orally inhaled short-acting (for intermittent acute relief) and long-acting (for additional control) β_2-adrenergic agonists is extensive. Salmeterol is a highly selective β_2-agonist, and certain cardiovascular effects (e.g., ventricular or nodal arrhythmias, severe tachycardia, anginal-type pain, myocardial ischemia) reported with less receptor-selective β-adrenergic agonists such as isoproterenol theoretically may occur less frequently, or not at all, with salmeterol. In addition, if other sympathomimetic agents are to be administered by any route in patients receiving orally inhaled albuterol or levalbuterol, the additional agents should be used with caution to avoid deleterious cardiovascular effects. The manufacturers also state that oral albuterol sulfate should not be administered concurrently with other oral sympathomimetic agents, since serious adverse cardiovascular effects may occur; however, this does not preclude the cautious use of an orally inhaled sympathomimetic agent in patients receiving oral albuterol sulfate. Such concomitant use must be individualized and should not be employed on a routine basis; if such concomitant use is regularly required, alternative therapy should be considered.

■ **Digoxin** Following single-dose IV or oral administration of albuterol to healthy individuals who had received digoxin for 10 days, a 16–22% decrease in serum digoxin concentration was observed. Although the clinical importance of these findings for patients receiving chronic albuterol or levalbuterol and digoxin therapy is unclear, patients receiving such concomitant therapy should have their serum digoxin concentration carefully evaluated.

■ **Other Drugs** Since albuterol may lower serum potassium concentration, care should be taken in patients also receiving other drugs that can lower serum potassium concentration, as the effects may be additive. The electrocardiographic changes and/or hypokalemia that may result from the administration of nonpotassium-sparing diuretics (such as loop or thiazide diuretics) may be aggravated by concomitant β-agonists, especially when the recommended dosage of the β-agonist is exceeded. Although the clinical importance of these effects is not known, caution is advised when administering β-agonists with nonpotassium-sparing diuretics.

The manufacturers state that the effects of albuterol or levalbuterol on the vascular system may be potentiated in patients receiving monoamine oxidase inhibitors or tricyclic antidepressants; therefore, albuterol or levalbuterol should be administered with extreme caution to patients receiving these drugs or within 2 weeks of discontinuation of such agents.

The action of albuterol or levalbuterol is antagonized by β-adrenergic blocking agents (e.g., propranolol). β-Adrenergic blocking agents not only block the pulmonary effects of β-agonists, but may produce severe bronchospasm in asthmatic patients; therefore, asthmatic patients should not normally be treated with β-adrenergic blocking agents. However, under certain circumstances (e.g., prophylaxis after myocardial infarction), there may be no acceptable alternatives to the use of β-adrenergic blocking agents in patients with asthma; cardioselective β-adrenergic blocking agents should be used with caution in these patients.

There is some evidence from animal studies that concomitant administration of a β-adrenergic agonist (e.g., isoproterenol) and a methylxanthine (aminophylline) may produce increased cardiotoxic effects (e.g., cardiac arrhythmias, sudden death, myocardial necrosis). Although such an interaction has not been established in humans, a few reports have suggested that such a combination may have the potential for producing cardiac arrhythmias. Further accumulation of clinical data is needed to determine whether this potential interaction exists in humans.

Acute Toxicity

■ **Pathogenesis** The oral LD_{50} of albuterol sulfate in mice exceeds 2 g/kg, which is approximately 200–6800 times the maximum recommended adult or pediatric daily dosage of albuterol sulfate (depending on dosage form) on a mg/m^2 basis. In mature rats, the subcutaneous median lethal dose of albuterol sulfate is approximately 450 mg/kg, which is approximately 90–3000 times the maximum recommended adult or pediatric daily dosage (depending on dosage form) on a mg/m^2 basis. In small young rats, the subcutaneous median lethal dose is approximately 2 g/kg, which is approximately 400–14,000 times the maximum recommended human daily dosage (depending on dosage form) on a mg/m^2 basis. In rats, the median IV lethal dose of levalbuterol hydrochloride is approximately 60 mg/kg (representing 900 times the maximum recommended daily adult inhalation dosage on a mg/m^2 basis, 430 times the maximum recommended pediatric inhalation dosage on a mg/m^2 basis). In mice, the median IV lethal dose of levalbuterol hydrochloride is approximately 66 mg/kg (representing approximately 70 times the maximum recommended daily adult inhalation solution dosage on a mg/m^2 basis, 500 times the maximum recommended daily adult inhalation dosage on a mg/m^2 basis, 230 times the maximum recommended daily pediatric inhalation dosage on a mg/m^2 basis). The median lethal dose of inhaled albuterol or levalbuterol has not been determined in animals. No fatalities occurred in dogs receiving orally inhaled levalbuterol via nebulization at dosages not exceeding 2.73 mg/kg (representing approximately 140 times the maximum recommended daily adult levalbuterol inhalation dosage on a mg/m^2 basis, 65 times the maximum recommended daily pediatric levalbuterol inhalation dosage on a mg/m^2 basis).

■ **Manifestations** The effects of overdosage of the fixed combination of albuterol sulfate and ipratropium bromide inhalation aerosol or solution are expected to be related principally to albuterol sulfate, as ipratropium bromide is not well absorbed following oral inhalation. Overdosage of oral albuterol or orally inhaled albuterol alone or in combination with ipratropium produces symptoms that are mainly extensions of common adverse effects of albuterol (e.g., seizures, hypotension or hypertension, arrhythmias, palpitation, nervousness, dizziness, fatigue, malaise, insomnia/sleeplessness, headache, tremor, dry mouth, nausea). In addition to exaggeration of common adverse effects, angina, tachycardia (with a heart rate of up to 200 bpm, including in children 2–12 years of age), and hypokalemia have occurred following overdosage. Cardiac arrest and even fatalities may occur following excessive use of sympathomimetic amine (including preparations containing albuterol) oral inhalations, oral solution, or extended-release tablets.

■ **Treatment** The manufacturers suggest that in case of overdosage with preparations containing albuterol or levalbuterol, the drug should be discontinued and appropriate symptomatic therapy initiated. The manufacturers also suggest that a relatively selective β_1-adrenergic blocking agent (e.g., metoprolol tartrate) may be used, if necessary, but only with extreme caution in asthmatic patients because an asthmatic attack may be induced. Evidence is insufficient to determine if dialysis is beneficial for the management of overdosage with levalbuterol, albuterol, or with the fixed combination of albuterol sulfate and ipratropium bromide inhalation solution.

Pharmacology

Albuterol stimulates β-adrenergic receptors and has little or no effect on α-adrenergic receptors. Like albuterol, levalbuterol is a relatively selective β_2-

adrenergic agonist. It is believed that β-adrenergic agonists stimulate the production of cyclic adenosine-3′,5′-monophosphate (AMP) by activation of the enzyme adenyl cyclase. Cyclic AMP appears to mediate numerous cellular responses. Increased intracellular cyclic AMP enhances the activity of cAMP-dependent protein kinase A, which inhibits the phosphorylation of myosin and lowers intracellular calcium concentrations, resulting in smooth muscle relaxation. Increased intracellular cyclic AMP concentrations also are associated with inhibition of the release of mediators from mast cells in the airways. Albuterol appears to have a greater stimulating effect on β-adrenergic receptors of the bronchial, uterine, and vascular smooth muscles (β_2 receptors) than on β-adrenergic receptors of the heart (β_1 receptors). However, β_2-adrenergic receptors also occur in the heart at concentrations of 10–50%. The main effect following oral inhalation or oral administration of albuterol is bronchodilation resulting from relaxation of smooth muscles from the trachea to the terminal bronchial tree; the drug also has some vasodilating effect on peripheral vasculature and may decrease diastolic blood pressure to a small extent. In a study in a limited number of asthmatic patients, administration of a single high dose of albuterol (800 mcg) via metered-dose aerosol during experimentally induced hypoxia (breathing a N_2/O_2 gas mixture) resulted in an appreciable decrease in peripheral vascular resistance and possible pulmonary shunting (as determined by a decrease in forearm vascular resistance) compared with patients on ambient air receiving a placebo aerosol. (See Cautions: Cardiovascular Effects.) In patients with reversible airway obstruction, albuterol decreases resistance of the airways as measured by pulmonary function tests such as the forced expiratory volume in 1 second (FEV_1) and the maximum mid-expiratory flow rate; the drug also increases vital capacity. In most comparative clinical trials, albuterol had more effect on bronchial smooth muscle relaxation and less cardiovascular effects than isoproterenol.

Oral or orally inhaled albuterol has a longer duration of action than isoproterenol and only occasionally causes cardiac stimulation. Bronchodilation produced by oral inhalation of usual doses of albuterol is equal to or greater than that produced by oral inhalation of usual doses of isoproterenol. Oral inhalation of usual doses of albuterol appears to be as effective as usual doses of metaproterenol in producing bronchodilation, with similar adverse effects. Although it has not been clearly established, the duration of action of albuterol may be slightly longer than that of metaproterenol. In one study, albuterol also appeared to have a longer duration of action than isoetharine following oral inhalation of doses of either drug that produced equivalent bronchodilation.

Levalbuterol exhibits about 2 or 100 times the in vitro binding affinity for β-adrenergic receptors of racemic (*R*, *S*-) or *S*-albuterol, respectively, and 2 times the muscle relaxant, including bronchorelaxant, effects of the racemic mixture. Some data indicate that the *S*-enantiomer does not contribute substantially to the bronchodilating effect of racemic albuterol but may have a detrimental effect on pulmonary function. Limited data suggest that the *S*-enantiomer of albuterol opposes the bronchodilatory effects of levalbuterol and may potentially exacerbate airway reactivity to various spasmogens by enhancing contractile responses. Although the clinical importance has not been established, tolerance to the bronchodilating effects of albuterol has been reported in healthy individuals and in patients with asthma. In contrast to isoproterenol, albuterol does not appear to decrease arterial oxygen tension. Albuterol may cause reflex tachycardia, especially with higher than usual doses. In a comparative study in healthy individuals and asthmatic patients receiving increasing doses of albuterol and isoproterenol inhalation aerosol, increases in heart rate observed after administration of albuterol were ½ to ¼ of that observed after administration of isoproterenol. In a comparative clinical trial, patients receiving a single dose of levalbuterol (1.25 mg) or albuterol (2.5 mg) via nebulization exhibited small, comparable increases in heart rate within 15 minutes of administration; this effect diminished during continued therapy. In a short-term (3 weeks) placebo-controlled, comparative clinical trial, children with mild to moderate asthma receiving a single-dose of levalbuterol inhalation solution (0.31 mg) or placebo exhibited small, comparable increases in heart rate within 30 minutes of administration, and these changes were less than those observed with albuterol inhalation solution (2.5 mg) given via nebulization; this effect diminished during continued therapy. A larger dose of levalbuterol inhalation solution (0.63 mg) or the smaller dose of albuterol inhalation solution (1.25 mg) exhibited equivalent increases in heart rate, greater increases in heart rate compared with placebo or the smaller dose of levalbuterol (0.31 mg), but less than those observed with albuterol inhalation solution at the 2.5-mg dose.

When administered concomitantly in patients with COPD, ipratropium and albuterol generally produce greater bronchodilation compared with that achieved with either agent alone. (See Uses: Chronic Obstructive Pulmonary Disease, in Ipratropium Bromide 12:08.08.)

β_2-Adrenergic stimulation promotes an intracellular shift of potassium from serum, possibly via stimulation of Na^+-K^+-ATPase, and thereby appears to decrease temporarily both elevated and normal potassium concentrations. Both IV (dosage form not currently commercially available in the US) and orally inhaled forms of albuterol have been shown to decrease serum potassium concentrations, which makes the drug potentially useful in the treatment of conditions associated with hyperkalemia (e.g., hyperkalemic familial periodic paralysis, adjunctively for acute episodes of hyperkalemia in patients with renal failure). In a comparative clinical trial, small, comparable decreases in plasma potassium concentrations were noted 1 hour after administration of a single dose of levalbuterol (1.25 mg) or albuterol (2.5 mg) via nebulization; this effect diminished during continued therapy. In a comparative, placebo-controlled clinical trial in children with mild to moderate asthma, small equivalent decreases in serum potassium concentrations were noted 1 hour after administration of a single dose of levalbuterol (0.31 or 0.63 mg) or albuterol at a dosage of 1.25 mg; these decreases were greater than those observed after administration of placebo but less than those observed after administration of albuterol (2.5 mg) via nebulization. By the end of the study, the decreases in serum potassium concentrations were similar in children receiving levalbuterol inhalation solution at either dose or albuterol inhalation solution at the 2.5-mg dose, but greater than placebo. In children receiving albuterol at the 1.25-mg dose, the decreases in serum potassium concentrations by the end of the study were less than those with levalbuterol at the 0.63-mg dose and similar to placebo.

Pharmacokinetics

The pharmacokinetic disposition of racemic albuterol is enantioselective, with the *R*-enantiomer (levalbuterol) generally having a more rapid clearance, a lower bioavailability, and a shorter half-life than *S*-albuterol.

■ **Absorption** Although albuterol appears to be absorbed from the respiratory tract over several hours following oral inhalation, this process has not been clearly characterized. Pharmacokinetic studies in asthmatic patients receiving albuterol sulfate inhalation solution indicate that less than 20% of a single dose of the drug is absorbed when administered by intermittent positive-pressure breathing (IPPB) or nebulization; the remainder of the dose was recovered from the nebulizer and apparatus and expired air. The amount delivered to the lungs depends on patient factors, the jet nebulizer used, and the compressor performance. It has been suggested that most of an orally inhaled dose of the drug is swallowed and absorbed from the GI tract; studies with isoproterenol indicate that less than 10% of an orally inhaled dose reaches the bronchial tree. In one study in a limited number of patients in whom a solution of radiolabeled albuterol was instilled directly into the bronchial tree via a bronchoscope, peak plasma radioactivity occurred within 10 minutes; however, following oral inhalation of albuterol in other studies, peak plasma albuterol concentrations occurred in 2–5 hours.

Bioavailability of levalbuterol is less than that of *S*-albuterol following administration of the enantiomers or racemic albuterol; in healthy individuals, the area under the blood concentration-time curve (AUC) for levalbuterol was about 5–7-fold less than that for the *S*-enantiomer. Population pharmacokinetic analysis of data from a clinical trial in children (6–11 years of age) receiving levalbuterol inhalation solution at a dosage of 0.63 mg or albuterol inhalation solution at a dosage of 1.25 mg indicates that peak plasma concentrations and AUC values of *R*-albuterol were similar. In a cross-study comparison of adults and adolescents 12 years of age or older and children (6–11 years of age) receiving a single dose of levalbuterol of 0.63 mg, peak plasma concentrations were similar. However, AUC values were 1.5-fold higher in children compared with values in adolescents and adults; these data support a lower dosage in children compared with adults. (See Levalbuterol under Dosage: Oral Inhalation Dosage, in Dosage and Administration.)

Population pharmacokinetic analysis of data from patients with asthma indicates that the mean exposure to levalbuterol (90 mcg) via aerosol inhalation of a formulation containing an HFA propellant was 13–16% less in adults and adolescents 12 years of age or older, or 30–32% less in children 4–11 years of age, than a comparable dose of albuterol (180 mcg) via aerosol inhalation of a formulation containing an HFA propellant. When compared with adults receiving a 90-mcg dose of levalbuterol via aerosol inhalation, the mean exposure (AUC) in pediatric patients was 17% lower.

Following administration of a 3-mg dose of albuterol via nebulization in adults, peak plasma albuterol concentrations of 2.1 ng/mL were reached within 0.5 hours. In a limited number of healthy adults receiving a single dose of albuterol (2.5 mg) or levalbuterol (1.25 mg) via nebulization, peak plasma concentrations of the *R*-enantiomer of albuterol were 1.1 or 0.8 ng/mL, respectively, at 0.2 hours. Peak plasma concentrations of *S*-albuterol following a single 2.5-mg dose of racemic albuterol via oral inhalation in healthy individuals reportedly are twice as high as those of the *R*-enantiomer (levalbuterol).

The propellant tetrafluoroethane is rapidly absorbed with time-to-peak plasma concentrations being extremely short. In a single-dose bioavailability study in healthy individuals receiving either metered-dose albuterol (no longer commercially available in the US) or albuterol sulfate inhalation aerosol, similar low blood concentrations of albuterol were observed with either formulation.

Following administration of a single 4-mg dose of albuterol as an oral solution in healthy individuals, peak plasma drug concentrations of 18 ng/mL are attained. In a limited number of healthy individuals, median peak plasma concentrations of *S*-albuterol and *R*-albuterol (levalbuterol) were 11.4 and 3.6 ng/mL, respectively, at 30–130 minutes following administration of racemic albuterol sulfate as an oral elixir. In healthy adults, steady-state plasma albuterol concentrations were reached within 2 days with either conventional albuterol tablets or extended-release tablets. In a dose-ranging study in adults, increases in plasma drug concentrations were dose-proportional with single 4- or 8-mg doses of albuterol extended-release tablets in the fasted state.

Albuterol sulfate is rapidly and well absorbed following oral administration. Oral bioavailability of extended-release albuterol sulfate tablets is about 80% that of conventional tablets when administered in single doses. Food reduces the rate of absorption of extended-release albuterol sulfate tablets. While studies with the extended-release tablets have not been conducted in pediatric patients, extrapolation of data from studies in adults also indicates similar bioavailability of conventional and extended-release tablets at steady state and reduced bioavailability with single-dose administration. Peak plasma albuterol concentrations occur within about 2.5 and 2 hours following administration of the conventional tablets and oral solution, respectively. Peak plasma albuterol concentrations occur within 6 hours following administration of albuterol extended-release tablets.

Bronchodilation begins within 5–15 minutes after oral inhalation of albuterol (no longer commercially available in the US) or albuterol sulfate via the metered-dose aerosol or via the special oral inhaler (Rotahaler®; no longer commercially available in the US) that delivers powdered drug from capsules, with peak effect in 0.5–3 hours, and generally persists 2–5 hours; in some patients, bronchodilation may persist up to 6 hours. Following oral inhalation of albuterol sulfate via the metered-dose inhaler (Proventil® HFA), the onset of appreciable bronchodilation (i.e., a 15% increase in forced expiratory volume in 1 second [FEV_1]) occurs within 6 minutes; mean time-to-peak bronchodilation occurs within 50–55 minutes. Bronchodilation persists for 3–6 hours. With administration of another albuterol sulfate metered-dose inhalation aerosol preparation (ProAir®HFA) in adults and adolescents (12–16 years of age), the median time to onset, time to peak effect, and duration of effect are 8.2 minutes, 47 minutes, and approximately 3 hours, respectively. Bronchodilation usually begins within 5 minutes following nebulization with albuterol; the peak effect occurs in approximately 1–2 hours and bronchodilation generally persists 3–4 hours, but occasionally up to 6 hours or longer. Bronchodilation persists for up to 8 hours in some patients receiving levalbuterol hydrochloride inhalation solution via nebulization. Because of the prompt onset of action and a lack of correlation between plasma albuterol concentrations and bronchodilation, it has been suggested that the bronchodilating effect of orally inhaled albuterol results from a local action.

Bronchodilation begins within 30 minutes after oral administration of conventional tablets, with peak effect in 2–3 hours, and may persist up to 4–6 hours. Following a single oral dose of albuterol as conventional tablets, bronchodilation has persisted for up to 8 hours in some patients. Extended-release tablets of albuterol sulfate have a duration of action of up to 12 hours. Albuterol sulfate oral solution has a duration of action of up to 6 hours.

Following administration of a single dose (90 mcg) of levalbuterol via aerosol inhalation in adolescents and adults (12–81 years of age) with asthma, the median time to achieve a 15% increase in FEV_1 compared with baseline with levalbuterol was about 5.5–10.2 minutes, and the median time to reach peak effects was about 76–78 minutes. The median duration of bronchodilation (as determined by an increase in FEV_1 of 15% or greater from baseline) after levalbuterol administration was approximately 3–4 hours; some patients exhibited bronchodilatory effects for up to 6 hours.

Following administration of a single dose (90 mcg) of levalbuterol via aerosol inhalation in children (4–11 years of age) with asthma, the median time to achieve a 15% increase in FEV_1 compared with baseline, time to peak effect, and duration of effect (maintenance of an increase in FEV_1 of at least 15% compared with baseline) were 4.5 minutes, 77 minutes, and 3 hours, respectively. Some pediatric patients may experience bronchodilatory effects up to 6 hours following levalbuterol inhalation aerosol administration.

The onset (time to a 15% increase in FEV_1 compared with baseline) and duration (maintenance of a more than 15% increase in FEV_1 compared with test day baseline) of bronchodilation obtained with levalbuterol also were similar to those obtained with racemic albuterol.

In a 4-week study in adults and adolescents 12 years of age or older with asthma, the mean time to achieve a 15% increase in FEV_1 from baseline with levalbuterol doses of 0.63 or 1.25 mg via nebulization was about 17 or 10 minutes, respectively, while the mean time to reach peak effects for both of these doses was about 1.5 hours after 4 weeks of treatment. The mean duration of bronchodilation (as determined by the period during which the increase in FEV_1 from baseline exceeded 15%) was approximately 5 or 6 hours after levalbuterol doses of 0.63 or 1.25 mg, respectively; some patients exhibited bronchodilator effects for up to 8 hours.

■ **Distribution** Results of animal studies indicate that albuterol crosses the blood-brain barrier, reaching the brain at concentrations that are approximately 5% of plasma concentrations. In glands outside the blood-brain barrier (pineal and pituitary glands), the drug achieves concentrations that are 100 times the concentrations achieved in whole brain. Albuterol apparently crosses the placenta, but it is not known whether albuterol is distributed into milk. Studies in pregnant rats given radiolabeled albuterol indicate that approximately 10% of the maternal dose is transferred to the fetus. Disposition in fetal lungs is comparable to that in maternal lungs, but fetal liver disposition is 1% that of the maternal liver concentrations.

■ **Elimination** Following oral inhalation of radiolabeled albuterol in patients with asthma in one study, total plasma radioactivity declined with a half-life of 1.7–7.1 hours. In another study in healthy individuals receiving albuterol sulfate inhalation aerosol (Proair® HFA) or another comparator albuterol sulfate HFA inhalation aerosol, the terminal plasma half-life of albuterol sulfate given as Proair® HFA inhalation aerosol was approximately 6 hours; no differences in pharmacokinetics were noted between the formulations. In healthy individuals, the plasma clearance of *R*-albuterol (levalbuterol) exceeded that of *S*-albuterol following IV or oral dosing of racemic albuterol. After oral inhalation of albuterol in healthy adults in another study, the elimination half-life of unchanged drug was determined indirectly to be 3.8 hours based on urinary excretion data. Following nebulization of albuterol sulfate in fixed combination with ipratropium bromide in healthy individuals at twice the recommended dosage (i.e., 5 mg of albuterol and 1 mg of ipratropium bromide), the half-life of albuterol averaged 6.7 hours. In a small pharmacokinetic study in healthy adults, the half-life of levalbuterol, the *R*-enantiomer of albuterol, was 3.3 hours after a single 1.25-mg nebulized dose and 4 hours following multiple dosing (1.25 mg given every 30 minutes for 4 doses) via nebulization. In another cumulative-dose study in patients with mild to moderate asthma receiving orally inhaled *R*-albuterol as either the single enantiomer (levalbuterol) or racemic albuterol, the half-life of *R*-albuterol or *S*-albuterol averaged about 3.5 or 5 hours, respectively. After oral administration of albuterol sulfate conventional or extended-release tablets, the plasma half-life of albuterol reportedly is 5–7.2 or 9.3 hours, respectively. Following oral administration of albuterol oral solution in healthy individuals, the half-life of albuterol is about 5 hours. The propellant tetrafluoroethane in albuterol sulfate aerosol (Proventil® HFA, Ventolin® HFA) is eliminated rapidly, as reflected by a short residence time; accumulation of the propellant does not occur.

Albuterol enantiomers are extensively metabolized in the intestinal wall and liver by sulfotransferase 1A3 (dopamine phenolsulfotransferase), mainly to albuterol 4′-*O*-sulfate which has little or no β-adrenergic stimulating effect and no β-adrenergic blocking effect. Following administration of racemic albuterol either IV or by oral inhalation following oral charcoal administration, the AUCs for the *S*-enantiomer were 3–4 fold higher than for the *R*-enantiomer. However, following administration of racemic albuterol orally or via inhalation without oral charcoal pretreatment, the AUCs for the *S*-enantiomer were 8–24 fold higher than the *R*-enantiomer. These data suggest that the *R*-enantiomer of albuterol is preferentially metabolized in the GI tract, presumably by sulfotransferase 1A3. in vitro studies in human liver cytosol preparations, the rate of sulfate conjugation of *R*-albuterol (levalbuterol) exceeded that of the *S*-enantiomer by a factor of 10–15. Unlike isoproterenol, albuterol is not metabolized by the enzyme catechol-*O*-methyltransferase and is not a substrate for catecholamine cellular uptake processes. Albuterol and its metabolites are rapidly excreted in urine and feces. After oral inhalation of albuterol in patients with asthma, approximately 70% of a dose is excreted in urine as unchanged drug and metabolites within 24 hours and 80–100% within 72 hours; about 30% of the dose is excreted in urine unchanged in 24 hours. Following nebulization of a 5-mg dose of albuterol in fixed combination with a 1-mg dose of ipratropium bromide, a mean of 8.4% of the administered dose of albuterol is excreted unchanged in urine. Following administration of albuterol sulfate (180 mcg as albuterol base) and ipratropium bromide (36 mcg) inhalation aerosol, 27.1% of the estimated mouthpiece dose of albuterol is excreted unchanged in urine within 24 hours. About 10% of an inhaled dose of albuterol may be excreted in feces. Following oral administration of albuterol sulfate to healthy individuals, about 76% of a single dose is excreted in urine within 72 hours, mainly as the major metabolite; about 4% of the dose is excreted in feces.

Pharmacokinetics of levalbuterol or albuterol sulfate (Proair® HFA) inhalation aerosol when administered as formulations containing an HFA propellant in patients with hepatic impairment have not been studied. In a small number of patients with renal impairment (creatinine clearance of 7–53 mL/minute), a 67% decline in albuterol clearance was reported, but half-life of the drug was not affected.

Chemistry and Stability

■ **Chemistry** Albuterol and levalbuterol are synthetic sympathomimetic amines. Albuterol occurs as a 50:50 racemic mixture of the *R*- and *S*-enantiomers and is commercially available as albuterol sulfate. Levalbuterol is the *R*-enantiomer of albuterol and is commercially available as levalbuterol hydrochloride or tartrate.

Albuterol sulfate occurs as a white to off-white crystalline powder and is soluble in water and slightly soluble in ethanol. Levalbuterol occurs as a clear and colorless solution for nebulization and is very soluble in water, having a solubility of 180 mg/mL in water. Albuterol has pK_a values of 9.3 and 10.3. Albuterol sulfate concentrate solution for nebulization and single-use albuterol sulfate inhalation solution for nebulization (e.g., Proventil®) are clear and colorless to light yellow. Albuterol sulfate in fixed combination with ipratropium bromide solution for nebulization in polyethylene unit-dose vials (DuoNeb®) is clear and colorless. Sulfuric acid is added during manufacture of albuterol sulfate inhalation solution and levalbuterol hydrochloride inhalation solution to adjust the pH to 3–5 and 3.3–4.5, respectively. Sodium hydroxide is added during the manufacture of albuterol sulfate oral solution to adjust the pH to 3.5–4.5. Hydrochloric acid is added during manufacture of fixed combination of albuterol sulfate and ipratropium bromide inhalation solution to adjust the pH to 4.

Albuterol sulfate metered-dose aerosols for oral inhalation are microcrystalline suspensions of the drugs in hydrofluoroalkane (HFA: tetrafluoroethane) propellants. The metered-dose aerosol containing albuterol sulfate in fixed combination with ipratropium bromide for oral inhalation is a microcrystalline suspension of the drugs in a vehicle of chlorofluorocarbon (CFCs: trichloromonofluoromethane, dichlorodifluoromethane, and dichlorotetrafluoroethane) propellants and soya lecithin. Albuterol sulfate oral solution (syrup) usually has a pH of 3.3–4. Each 1.2 mg of albuterol sulfate is approximately equivalent to 1 mg of albuterol.

Each mL of a single-use of albuterol sulfate inhalation solution 0.083% contains 0.83 mg of albuterol (equivalent to 1 mg of albuterol sulfate). Each mL of albuterol sulfate inhalation solution 0.5% contains 5 mg of albuterol (equivalent to 6 mg of albuterol sulfate). Each 3-mL unit-dose vial of albuterol sulfate in fixed combination with ipratropium bromide inhalation solution contains 2.5 mg of albuterol (equivalent to 3 mg of albuterol sulfate) and 0.5 mg of ipratropium bromide. Each 3-mL unit-dose ampul of levalbuterol inhalation solution contains either 0.31, 0.63, or 1.25 mg of levalbuterol equivalent to 0.36, 0.73 or 1.44 mg of levalbuterol hydrochloride, respectively.

■ **Stability** Preparations containing albuterol sulfate should be stored in well-closed, light-resistant containers. Albuterol sulfate inhalation aerosol with hydrofluoroalkane propellant (ProAir® HFA, Proventil® HFA, Ventolin® HFA) should be stored at 15–25°C. Failure to use these inhalers within these respective temperature ranges could result in delivery of improper doses. At temperatures below these ranges, cooling of the propellants can decrease internal pressure of the canister, which may result in delivery of particles too large to provide full therapeutic effect. A 5-minute cooling of inhalers to 0°C produced a mean decrease in peak propellant pressure of 28% (range: 20–38%); however, this effect was reversed when the canisters were warmed to room temperature. For best results, the canisters should be at room temperature before use. Because the contents of albuterol sulfate oral inhalers are under pressure, the aerosol containers should *not* be punctured, used or stored near heat or an open flame, or placed into a fire or incinerator for disposal. Exposure of the canisters to temperatures exceeding 49°C may cause them to burst.

The commercially available metered-dose inhaler containing albuterol sulfate and ipratropium bromide in fixed combination should be stored at 25°C, but may be exposed to temperatures ranging from 15–30°C; exposure to excessive humidity should be avoided. For best results, the canister should be at room temperature before use.

Albuterol sulfate inhalation solutions for nebulization should be stored at 2–25°C or 15–30°C depending on the manufacturer. The commercially available inhalation solution of albuterol sulfate and ipratropium bromide for nebulization in fixed combination should be stored at 2–30°C and protected from light, preferably in the manufacturer-supplied foil pouch. Albuterol sulfate oral inhalation concentrate solution (0.5%) should be discarded if the solution changes color or becomes cloudy. Albuterol sulfate solution for nebulization (in single-use units) should be discarded if it becomes discolored. The manufacturers states that the physical and chemical compatibility of albuterol sulfate or levalbuterol hydrochloride solution for nebulization when mixed with other drugs in a nebulizer have not been established. However, experts from the National Asthma Education and Prevention Program (NAEPP) state that albuterol sulfate solution for nebulization may be mixed with cromolyn sodium solution for nebulization, budesonide suspension for nebulization, or ipratropium bromide solution for nebulization.

Albuterol sulfate tablets should be stored at 15–30°C and protected from light. Albuterol sulfate extended-release tablets should be stored at 20–25 °C in a well-closed, light resistant container. Albuterol sulfate oral solution should be stored at 20–25°C or 2–30°C, depending on the manufacturer, in a tight, light-resistant container.

Unit-dose ampuls of levalbuterol hydrochloride inhalation solution in foil pouches should be stored between 20–25°C and protected from light. Once the foil pouch is opened, any ampuls remaining within the foil pouch should be used within 2 weeks. Ampuls removed from foil pouches should be protected from light and used within 1 week. Levalbuterol hydrochloride inhalation solution ampuls should be discarded if the solution is not colorless. Experts from the NAEPP state that levalbuterol hydrochloride solution for nebulization is compatible with budesonide suspension for nebulization.

Preparations

Excipients in commercially available drug preparations may have clinically important effects in some individuals; consult specific product labeling for details.

Albuterol Sulfate

Oral		
Solution	2 mg (of albuterol) per 5 mL*	**Albuterol Sulfate Syrup**
Tablets	2 mg (of albuterol)*	**Albuterol Sulfate Tablets**
	4 mg (of albuterol)*	**Albuterol Sulfate Tablets**
Tablets, extended-release	4 mg (of albuterol)*	**VoSpire®** **ER**, Dava
		Albuterol Sulfate Extended-Release Tablets
	8 mg (of albuterol)*	**VoSpire®** **ER**, Dava
		Albuterol Sulfate Extended-Release Tablets
Oral Inhalation		
Aerosol	90 mcg (of albuterol) per metered spray	**ProAir® HFA** (with hydrofluoroalkane propellant), Teva
		Proventil® HFA (with hydrofluoroalkane propellant), Schering
		Ventolin®† **HFA** (with hydrofluoroalkane propellant), GlaxoSmithKline
Solution, for nebulization	0.021% (of albuterol)*	**AccuNeb®** (available as TwistFlex® polyethylene vials), Dey
		Albuterol Sulfate Inhalation Solution
	0.042% (of albuterol)*	**AccuNeb®** (available as TwistFlex® polyethylene vials), Dey
		Albuterol Sulfate Inhalation Solution
	0.083% (of albuterol)*	**Albuterol Sulfate Inhalation Solution**
		Proventil®, Schering
Solution, concentrate, for nebulization	0.5% (of albuterol)*	**Albuterol Sulfate Inhalation Solution**

*available from one or more manufacturer, distributor, and/or repackager by generic (nonproprietary) name

Albuterol Sulfate Combinations

Oral Inhalation		
Aerosol	90 mcg (of albuterol) with Ipratropium Bromide 18 mcg per metered spray	**Combivent®** (with chlorofluorohydrocarbon propellants), Boehringer Ingelheim
Solution, for nebulization	2.5 mg (of albuterol) with Ipratropium Bromide 0.5 mg per 3 mL	**DuoNeb®**, Dey

Levalbuterol Hydrochloride

Oral		
Solution, for nebulization	0.103 mg (of levalbuterol) per mL (0.31 mg)	**Xopenex®** (available as polyethylene vials), Sepracor
	0.21 mg (of levalbuterol) per mL (0.63 mg)	**Xopenex®** (available as polyethylene vials), Sepracor
	0.417 mg (of levalbuterol) per mL (1.25 mg)	**Xopenex®** (available as polyethylene vials), Sepracor

Levalbuterol Tartrate

Oral Inhalation		
Aerosol	45 mcg (of levalbuterol) per metered spray	**Xopenex HFA®** (with hydrofluoroalkane propellant), Sepracor

†Use is not currently included in the labeling approved by the US Food and Drug Administration

Selected Revisions November 2014,

Arformoterol Tartrate

■ Arformoterol tartrate, a relatively selective long-acting β_2-agonist, is a bronchodilator.

Uses

■ **Bronchospasm** ***Chronic Obstructive Pulmonary Disease*** Arformoterol tartrate is used as a bronchodilator for the long-term symptomatic treatment of reversible bronchospasm associated with chronic obstructive pulmonary disease (COPD), including chronic bronchitis and emphysema. Orally inhaled arformoterol is not indicated for treatment of acute episodes of bronchospasm or acute exacerbations of COPD. Patients receiving arformoterol should not receive concomitant therapy with additional long-acting β_2-adrenergic agonists. When therapy with arformoterol is initiated, *regular* use of short-acting inhaled β_2-adrenergic agonists should be discontinued, and such agents should be used only for relief of acute symptoms of COPD that are not controlled by arformoterol.

Efficacy of orally inhaled arformoterol for the treatment of reversible bronchospasm associated with COPD has been established in 2 randomized, double-blind, multicenter, placebo- and active-controlled studies of 12 weeks' duration in patients with moderate to severe airflow obstruction (mean forced expiratory volume in 1 second [FEV_1] 42% of expected). While regular use of other bronchodilators was not permitted during these studies, patients receiving stable dosages of oral or inhaled corticosteroids, xanthines, or leukotriene-receptor antagonists continued to receive these drugs during the study along with as-needed rescue or supplemental therapy with orally inhaled albuterol and ipratropium. Arformoterol (15 or 25 mcg twice daily or 50 mcg once daily via nebulization) was as effective as salmeterol (42 mcg twice daily as the inhalation aerosol) in improving lung function (defined as percent change from baseline to 12 weeks in morning trough FEV_1) in patients with COPD. Arformoterol (all dosages studied) and salmeterol were more effective than placebo in improving lung function and reducing the need for supplemental or rescue medication. Dosages of arformoterol exceeding 15 mcg twice daily did not provide sufficient additional improvement in lung function to support use of such dosages.

Dosage and Administration

■ **General** When arformoterol therapy is initiated, *regular* use of short-acting, inhaled β_2-adrenergic agonists should be discontinued, and such agents should be used only for relief of acute symptoms of chronic obstructive pulmonary disease (COPD) that are not controlled by arformoterol.

Failure to respond to a previously effective dosage may indicate destabilization of COPD that requires reevaluation. Extra/increased doses of arformoterol should not be used in such situations. (See Acute Exacerbations of COPD under Cautions.)

■ **Administration** ***Oral Inhalation Solution*** Arformoterol should be administered by oral inhalation via nebulization twice daily (morning and evening) only. The inhalation solution should not be administered orally.

Arformoterol should be administered via a standard jet nebulizer connected to an air compressor. Safety and efficacy of arformoterol inhalation solution administered by a nebulizer other than the Pari-LC Plus® nebulizer or a compressor other than Pari Dura-Neb® 3000 compressor have not been established. Using in vitro testing at a mean flow rate of 3.3 L/minute for an average of 6 minutes or less, the Pari-LC Plus® nebulizer connected to a Pari Dura-Neb® 3000 compressor delivered approximately 27.6% of the original dose at the mouthpiece.

For administration of arformoterol inhalation solution for nebulization in single-use units, 1 vial should be opened and the entire contents of the vial squeezed into the nebulizer reservoir. The reservoir should be attached to the mouthpiece or face mask and to the compressor according to the manufacturer's instructions. The patient should place the nebulizer mouthpiece in the mouth or put on the nebulizer face mask and turn on the compressor. The patient then should breathe as calmly, deeply, and evenly as possible until the nebulizer stops producing mist, about 5–10 minutes. The nebulizer should be cleaned after use according to the manufacturer's instructions.

■ **Dosage** Dosage of arformoterol tartrate is expressed in terms of arformoterol.

Delivery of oral inhalation solution to the lungs depends on the type of jet nebulizers used, performance of the compressor, and other factors such as the patient's inspiratory flow. (See Administration under Dosage and Administration.)

For long-term symptomatic treatment of chronic obstructive pulmonary disease, the usual adult dosage of arformoterol is 15 mcg twice daily by oral inhalation via nebulization. Higher dosages provide no additional therapeutic benefit and may increase risk of adverse effects. Maximum recommended dosage is 30 mcg daily.

■ **Special Populations** Dosage adjustments are not required in geriatric patients, patients with renal or hepatic impairment, or those with deficient cytochrome P-450 (CYP) isoenzyme 2D6 or uridine disphosphoglucuronosyltransferase 1A1 activity. (See Elimination: Special Populations, under Pharmacokinetics.)

Cautions

■ **Contraindications** Known hypersensitivity to arformoterol, formoterol, or any ingredient in the formulation.

All long-acting β_2-adrenergic agonists, including arformoterol, are contraindicated in patients with asthma without concomitant use of long-term asthma controller therapy; safety and efficacy of arformoterol in patients with asthma† have not been established. (See Asthma-related Death under Warnings/Precautions: Warnings, in Cautions.)

■ **Warnings/Precautions** ***Warnings*** **Asthma-related Death.** Long-acting β_2-adrenergic agonists increase the risk of asthma-related death. All long-acting β_2-adrenergic agonists, including arformoterol, are contraindicated in patients with asthma without concomitant use of long-term asthma controller therapy. The safety and efficacy of arformoterol in patients with asthma† have not been established.

Data from a large placebo-controlled safety study (Salmeterol Multicenter Asthma Research Trial [SMART]) showed an increase in asthma-related deaths in patients receiving certain long-acting β_2-adrenergic agonists (e.g., salmeterol) in addition to usual asthma therapy. The increased risk of asthma-related death with salmeterol is considered a class effect of the long-acting β_2-adrenergic agonists, including arformoterol. However, no adequate studies have been conducted to determine whether the rate of asthma-related death is increased in patients receiving arformoterol. (See Advice to Patients.)

While data from currently available studies do not show an increased risk of asthma-related death with racemic formoterol, data from small clinical studies suggest that there is a higher incidence of serious asthma exacerbations with formoterol compared with placebo.

It is not known whether rate of death is increased in patients with chronic obstructive pulmonary disease (COPD) receiving arformoterol. Data from a large placebo-controlled study (TOwards a Revolution in COPD Health [TORCH]) evaluating survival in patients with COPD receiving salmeterol, fluticasone propionate, or both drugs over a 3-year period did not reveal an increased incidence of COPD-related or overall deaths in patients receiving salmeterol in addition to usual COPD therapy.

Acute Exacerbations of COPD. Therapy with arformoterol should not be initiated in patients with acutely deteriorating COPD, which may be life threatening; the drug is not indicated for treatment of acute episodes of bronchospasm (i.e., rescue therapy). Safety and efficacy of arformoterol for relief of acute symptoms of COPD have not been established.

Failure to respond to a previously effective dosage of arformoterol or to a supplemental short-acting β_2-agonist (e.g., increased need for additional short-acting β_2-agonist) may indicate substantially worsening COPD. COPD therapy should be reevaluated promptly. Extra doses of arformoterol alone or with other long-acting, inhaled β_2-adrenergic agonists (e.g., formoterol) should not be used for maintenance therapy of COPD or any other reason.

Cardiovascular Effects. Clinically important changes in systolic and/or diastolic blood pressure, heart rate, ECG (e.g., flattening of T wave, prolongation of QT_c interval, ST-segment depression) changes, and/or cardiovascular symptoms have been reported in patients receiving arformoterol. Such effects are uncommon with the recommended dosage; may require discontinuance of the drug.

Arformoterol should be used with caution in patients with cardiovascular disorders, especially coronary insufficiency, cardiac arrhythmias, or hypertension.

Excessive Dosages. Fatalities have been associated with excessive use of inhaled sympathomimetic drugs. Higher than recommended dosages of arformoterol should not be used.

Patients receiving arformoterol should not use additional arformoterol or other long-acting β_2-adrenergic agonists for maintenance treatment of COPD.

Sensitivity Reactions Immediate hypersensitivity reactions (e.g., anaphylactic reactions, urticaria, angioedema, rash, bronchospasm) have been reported in patients receiving arformoterol.

Major Toxicities **Paradoxical Bronchospasm.** Acute, life-threatening, paradoxical bronchospasm may occur in patients receiving arformoterol.

Therapy should be discontinued immediately if bronchospasm occurs and alternative therapy instituted.

General Precautions **Metabolic Effects.** Possible hypokalemia; may increase risk of adverse cardiovascular effects. Hypokalemia usually is transient, not requiring supplementation.

Clinically important changes in blood glucose concentrations are possible during long-term therapy at recommended dosage.

Arformoterol should be used with caution in patients with thyrotoxicosis.

Nervous System Effects. Arformoterol should be used with caution in patients with seizure disorders and those unusually responsive to sympathomimetic amines.

Specific Populations **Pregnancy.** Category C. (See Users Guide.)

Lactation. Distributed into milk in rats. It is not known whether arformoterol is distributed into human milk. Use caution.

Pediatric Use. Safety and efficacy not established in pediatric patients. COPD does not occur in children.

Geriatric Use. No substantial differences in safety and efficacy observed relative to younger adults, but increased sensitivity cannot be ruled out. Incidence of ventricular ectopy with arformoterol therapy in geriatric patients 65–75 years of age is comparable to that with placebo.

Hepatic Impairment. Because plasma concentrations of arformoterol may be increased in patients with hepatic impairment, use with caution and monitor patients closely. (See Absorption under Pharmacokinetics.)

■ **Common Adverse Effects** Pain (unspecified), chest pain, back pain, diarrhea, sinusitis, leg cramps, dyspnea, rash, flu syndrome, peripheral edema, lung disorder.

Drug Interactions

Arformoterol is minimally metabolized by cytochrome P-450 (CYP) 2D6 and 2C19 isoenzymes; does not inhibit CYP isoenzymes 1A2, 2A6, 2C9/10, 2C19, 2D6, 2E1, 3A4/5, or 4A9/11.

■ **Drugs Affecting Hepatic Microsomal Enzymes** CYP2D6 inhibitors: Pharmacokinetic interaction unlikely; arformoterol dosage adjustment not required.

■ **Drugs that Prolong QT Interval** Potential pharmacodynamic interaction (increased risk of ventricular arrhythmias). Use concomitantly with extreme caution.

■ **Specific Drugs** ***β-Adrenergic Blocking Agents*** Potential for antagonism of pulmonary effects, resulting in severe bronchospasm in patients with chronic obstructive pulmonary disease (COPD).

If concomitant therapy is necessary, consider cautious use of cardioselective β-adrenergic blockers without intrinsic sympathomimetic activity (e.g., metoprolol, atenolol, esmolol). Use low dosages of cardioselective β-adrenergic blockers initially and titrate upward with caution.

Corticosteroids Possible potentiation of hypokalemic effects.

Potassium-depleting Diuretics Potential for additive hypokalemia and/or ECG changes, especially when recommended β-agonist dosage is exceeded.

Use concomitantly with caution.

MAO Inhibitors or Tricyclic Antidepressants Possible potentiation of cardiovascular effects.

Use concomitantly with extreme caution.

Paroxetine Pharmacokinetic interaction unlikely with potent CYP2D6 inhibitors (e.g., paroxetine).

Arformoterol dosage adjustment not necessary.

Sympathomimetic Agents Potential additive pharmacologic effects. Use caution with concomitant sympathomimetic agents administered by any route.

Xanthine Derivatives Possible potentiation of hypokalemic effects.

Description

Arformoterol, a synthetic sympathomimetic amine, is a relatively selective long-acting β_2 agonist. Arformoterol is the *R, R*-enantiomer of formoterol, which occurs as a racemic mixture; only the *R, R*-enantiomer of formoterol is active. Arformoterol stimulates β_2-adrenergic receptors and apparently has little or no effect on β_1-adrenergic receptors. Arformoterol is twice as potent as racemic formoterol.

Arformoterol's β_2-adrenergic effects appear to result from stimulation of the production of cyclic adenosine-3,5-monophosphate (cAMP) by activation of adenyl cyclase. Increased concentrations of cAMP are associated with relaxation of bronchial smooth muscle and suppression of some aspects of inflammation, such as inhibition of release of proinflammatory mast-cell mediators (e.g., histamine, leukotrienes). Some studies in animals suggest that arformoterol inhibits allergen-induced infiltration of eosinophils into airways and reduces histamine-induced extravasation of plasma proteins (e.g., albumin).

Tolerance to the bronchoprotective effects of arformoterol (diminished effect on FEV_1) has been reported after 6 weeks of treatment, with loss of protection at the end of the 12-hour dosing period.

Arformoterol is extensively metabolized, mainly via glucuronidation by uridine disphosphoglucuronosyltransferase (UGT) isoenzymes and to a limited extent via *O*-demethylation by the cytochrome P-450 (CYP) isoenzymes 2D6 and 2C19.

Advice to Patients

A copy of the manufacturer's patient information (medication guide) for arformoterol must be provided to all patients each time the drug is dispensed. Importance of instructing patients to read the medication guide prior to initiation of therapy and each time the prescription is refilled.

Advise of increased risk of asthma†-related death with long-acting β_2-adrenergic agonists, such as arformoterol. None of the long-acting β_2-adrenergic agonists, including arformoterol, should be used in patients with asthma† without concomitant use of long-term asthma controller therapy.

Advise of potential for adverse effects, such as palpitations, rapid heart rate, tremor, nervousness, or chest pain.

Importance of adequate understanding of proper storage, preparation, and inhalation techniques, including use of nebulizer delivery system.

Importance of adherence to dosing schedules, including not exceeding recommended dosage or frequency of use unless otherwise instructed by clinician.

Importance of advising patient that if a dose of arformoterol is missed, the next dose should be taken at the regularly scheduled time; dose should not be doubled.

Importance of not discontinuing arformoterol therapy without medical supervision, as symptoms may worsen.

Importance of all patients being provided with and instructed in use of a short-acting, inhaled β_2-adrenergic bronchodilator as supplemental therapy for acute chronic obstructive pulmonary disease (COPD) symptoms.

Importance of discontinuing *regular* use of a short-acting, inhaled β-adrenergic bronchodilator when initiating maintenance therapy with arformoterol and instituting *intermittent* use of a short-acting bronchodilator (*not* arformoterol) to relieve acute symptoms of COPD.

Importance of not using arformoterol to relieve acute symptoms or exacerbations of COPD.

Importance of contacting clinician immediately if decreased effectiveness occurs and/or breathing problems worsen quickly; do not increase dose or frequency of administration or add therapy with other long-acting, inhaled β_2-adrenergic agonists.

Importance of contacting a clinician immediately if the short-acting β_2-adrenergic agonist becomes less effective (e.g., increased dosage or frequency of administration) for acute symptoms of COPD.

Importance of promptly contacting a clinician if symptoms of serious allergic reaction occur, including rash, hives, breathing problems, and swelling of face, mouth, or tongue.

Importance of women informing clinicians if they are or plan to become pregnant or plan to breast-feed.

Importance of informing clinicians of existing or contemplated concomitant therapy, including prescription and OTC drugs, vitamins, and herbal supplements, as well as any concomitant illnesses (e.g., heart problems, hypertension, seizures, thyroid disorders, diabetes mellitus, liver disorders).

Importance of informing patients of other important precautionary information. (See Cautions.)

Overview® (see Users Guide). For additional information on this drug until a more detailed monograph is developed and published, the manufacturer's labeling should be consulted. It is *essential* that the manufacturer's labeling be consulted for more detailed information on usual cautions, precautions, contraindications, potential drug interactions, laboratory test interferences, and acute toxicity.

Preparations

Excipients in commercially available drug preparations may have clinically important effects in some individuals; consult specific product labeling for details.

Arformoterol Tartrate

Oral Inhalation		
Solution, for Nebulization	7.5 mcg (of arformoterol) per mL	**Brovana®**, Sunovion

†Use is not currently included in the labeling approved by the US Food and Drug Administration

Selected Revisions August 2014,

Formoterol Fumarate

■ Formoterol fumarate, a synthetic sympathomimetic amine, is a relatively selective, long-acting β_2-agonist.

Uses

■ **Bronchospasm** Formoterol fumarate is used alone or in fixed combination with budesonide or glycopyrrolate for long-term maintenance treatment of bronchospasm or airflow obstruction associated with chronic obstructive pulmonary disease (COPD), including chronic bronchitis and emphysema. Formoterol fumarate also is used concomitantly with long-term asthma controller therapy, such as inhaled corticosteroids, as a long-acting bronchodilator for the prevention of bronchospasm in patients with reversible obstructive airway disease (e.g., asthma). Monotherapy with long-acting β_2-adrenergic agonists, such as formoterol, increases the risk of asthma-related death and may increase the risk of asthma-related hospitalization in pediatric and adolescent patients. (See Asthma-related Death and Serious Asthma-related Events under Warnings/Precautions: Warnings, in Cautions.) *Because of these risks, the use of formoterol alone for the treatment of asthma without concomitant use of long-term asthma controller therapy, such as inhaled corticosteroids, is contraindicated.* (See Cautions: Contraindications.) The fixed combination of formoterol fumarate and budesonide (formoterol/budesonide; Symbicort®) and fixed combination of formoterol fumarate and mometasone furoate (formoterol/mometasone; Dulera®) are used *only* in patients with asthma who have not responded adequately to long-term asthma controller therapy, such as inhaled corticosteroids, or whose disease severity warrants initiation of treatment with both an inhaled corticosteroid and a long-acting β_2-adrenergic agonist. Once asthma control is achieved and maintained, the patient should be assessed at regular intervals and therapy should be stepped down (e.g., discontinuance of formoterol or formoterol in fixed combination with budesonide), if possible without loss of asthma control, and the patient should be maintained on long-term asthma controller therapy, such as inhaled corticosteroids. Formoterol in fixed combination with budesonide should not be used in patients whose asthma is adequately controlled on a low or medium dosage of inhaled corticosteroids.

Formoterol fumarate alone or in fixed combination with budesonide, glycopyrrolate, or mometasone furoate is *not* indicated for the relief of acute bronchospasm and should *not* be initiated in patients with rapidly deteriorating or potentially life-threatening episodes of asthma or COPD. Use of long-acting β_2-adrenergic agonists with or without inhaled corticosteroids for acute exacerbations of COPD has not been evaluated. A short-acting inhaled β_2-adrenergic agonist should be used intermittently (as needed) for acute symptoms of asthma or COPD. (See Acute Exacerbations of Asthma or Chronic Obstructive Pulmonary Disease under Warnings/Precautions: Warnings, in Cautions.)

Asthma **Considerations in Initiating Antiasthma Therapy.** In the stepped-care approach to antiasthmatic drug therapy, asthma is classified according to severity upon initial presentation (intermittent asthma or mild, moderate, or severe persistent asthma) and also by response to treatment (i.e., asthma control). While classification of asthma severity is useful for determining initial treatment, disease severity may vary over time and with treatment; therefore, after therapy is initiated, periodic assessment of asthma control is emphasized for guiding treatment decisions. Asthma management guidelines state that initial therapy for asthma should correspond to disease severity, with subsequent monitoring and adjustments in therapy to achieve and maintain control of asthma according to the goals of treatment. Asthma therapy is aimed at achieving and maintaining control of asthma by reducing ongoing impairment (e.g., prevention of chronic and troublesome symptoms, reducing use of reliever drugs, maintaining normal or near-normal lung function and activity levels) and risk of future events (e.g., exacerbations requiring systemic corticosteroids, treatment-related adverse effects). These 2 components of asthma control (i.e., current impairment and future risk) may respond differently to treatment.

The National Asthma Education and Prevention Program (NAEPP) classifies the levels of asthma control as well controlled, not well controlled, or very poorly controlled. In the stepped-care approach, the treatment step selected for asthma control in patients already receiving asthma therapy is based on the patient's current treatment and level of asthma control. Stepwise therapy is meant to assist, not replace, the clinical decision-making process in selecting therapy for individual patients. Once initiated, treatment is adjusted continuously according to changes in asthma control. Patients should be monitored every 2–6 weeks following initiation of therapy to ensure that asthma control is achieved. If asthma symptoms are not controlled with the current treatment regimen, treatment is stepped up until control is achieved. If an alternative treatment was used and produced an inadequate response, the preferred treatment should be used before stepping up to the next level of therapy. Regular monitoring at 1- to 6-month intervals, depending on the level of control, is recommended to ensure that control of asthma is maintained and that appropriate adjustments in therapy are made. When control has been maintained for at least 3 months, treatment intensity may be stepped down to find the lowest dosage and/or number of drugs required to maintain asthma control, with continued follow-up at 3-month intervals.

Intermittent Asthma. Drugs for asthma may be categorized as relievers (e.g., bronchodilators taken as needed for acute symptoms) or controllers (principally inhaled corticosteroids or other anti-inflammatory agents taken regularly to achieve long-term control of asthma). A reliever drug such as a selective short-acting inhaled β_2-adrenergic agonist (e.g., albuterol, levalbuterol, pirbuterol) is recommended on an as-needed basis to control occasional acute symptoms (e.g., cough, wheezing, dyspnea) of short duration; such use of an inhaled short-acting β_2-agonist alone generally is sufficient as initial treatment for newly diagnosed patients whose asthma severity is initially classified as intermittent (e.g., patients with daytime symptoms of asthma not more than twice weekly and nocturnal symptoms not more than twice a month). Most experts consider short-acting inhaled β_2-adrenergic agonists to be drugs of choice for treating acute asthma symptoms and exacerbations and for preventing exercise-induced bronchospasm. Alternatives to short-acting inhaled β_2-agonists recommended by some clinicians for relief of acute asthma symptoms include an inhaled anticholinergic agent (e.g., ipratropium), a short-acting oral β_2-agonist, or a short-acting theophylline (provided extended-release theophylline is not already used), but these alternatives have a slower onset of action and/or a higher risk for adverse effects. Oral β_2-adrenergic agonist therapy is suggested for use principally in patients unable to use inhaled bronchodilators (e.g., young children). Other experts do not recommend oral β_2-agonists for relief of acute asthma symptoms. Use of short-acting inhaled β_2-agonists in asymptomatic asthma should be limited to pretreatment prior to exercise and, in intermittent asthma, should be limited to providing relief as symptoms develop; some clinicians state that patients requiring symptomatic relief more than twice weekly or repeatedly over 1 or 2 days should be evaluated for possible initiation of long-term controller therapy.

Mild Persistent Asthma. When control of symptoms deteriorates in mild intermittent asthma and symptoms become persistent (e.g., daytime symptoms of asthma more than twice weekly but less than once daily, and nocturnal symptoms of asthma 3–4 times per month), asthma management guidelines and most clinicians recommend initiation of a controller drug such as an anti-inflammatory agent, preferably a low-dose orally inhaled corticosteroid (e.g., 88–264, 88–176, or 176 mcg of fluticasone propionate [or its equivalent] daily via a metered dose inhaler in adults and adolescents, children 5–11 years of age, or children 4 years of age or younger, respectively) as first-line therapy for persistent asthma supplemented by as-needed use of a short-acting, inhaled β_2-agonist. Alternatives to low-dose inhaled corticosteroids for mild persistent asthma include certain leukotriene modifiers (i.e., montelukast, zafirlukast), extended-release theophylline, or mast-cell stabilizers (i.e., cromolyn, nedocromil [preparations for oral inhalation no longer commercially available in the US]), but these therapies are less effective and generally not preferred as initial therapy. Some experts recommend that long-term control therapy be considered in infants and young children who have identifiable risk factors for asthma and who in the previous year have had 4 or more episodes of wheezing that lasted more than 1 day and symptoms that affected sleep. Low-dose inhaled corticosteroids also are recommended as the preferred initial therapy in such children. Cromolyn sodium is suggested (based on extrapolation of data from studies in older children) or montelukast is recommended by some experts as alternative, but not preferred, therapy in children 4 years of age or younger with mild persistent asthma. Other experts do not consider mast cell stabilizers or extended-release theophylline to be acceptable alternatives to inhaled corticosteroids for routine use as initial long-term therapy in such patients.

Moderate Persistent Asthma. According to asthma management guidelines, therapy with a long-acting inhaled β_2-agonist, such as formoterol or salmeterol generally is recommended in adults and adolescents who have moderate persistent asthma and daily asthmatic symptoms that are inadequately controlled following addition of low-dose inhaled corticosteroids to as-needed short-acting inhaled β_2-agonist treatment. However, NAEPP recommends that the beneficial effects of long-acting inhaled β_2-agonists should be weighed carefully against the increased risk (although uncommon) of severe asthma exacerbations and asthma-related deaths associated with daily use of such agents. (See Uses: Bronchospasm and also see Asthma-related Death and Life-threatening Events under Cautions: Respiratory Effects, in Salmeterol 12:12.08.12.) Asthma management guidelines also state that an alternative, but equally preferred option for management of moderate persistent asthma that is not adequately controlled with a low dosage of inhaled corticosteroid is to increase the maintenance dosage to a medium dosage (e.g., exceeding 264 but not more than 440 mcg of fluticasone propionate [or its equivalent] daily via a metered-dose inhaler in adults and adolescents). Alternative less effective therapies that may be added to a low dosage of inhaled corticosteroid include an oral extended-release theophylline or certain leukotriene modifiers (i.e., montelukast, zafirlukast).

Limited data are available in infants and children 11 years of age or younger with moderate persistent asthma, and recommendations of care are based on expert opinion and extrapolation from studies in adults. According to asthma management guidelines, a long-acting inhaled β_2-agonist (e.g., formoterol, salmeterol), a leukotriene modifier (i.e., montelukast, zafirlukast), or extended-release theophylline (with appropriate monitoring) may be added to low-dose inhaled corticosteroid therapy in children 5–11 years of age. Because comparative data establishing relative efficacy of these agents in this age group are lacking, there is no clearly preferred agent for use as adjunctive therapy with a low-dose inhaled corticosteroid for treatment of asthma in these children. In children 5–11 years of age with moderate persistent asthma that is not controlled with a low dosage of an inhaled corticosteroid, another preferred option according to asthma management guidelines is to increase the maintenance dosage of the inhaled corticosteroid to a medium dosage (e.g., exceeding 176 but not more than 352 mcg of fluticasone propionate [or its equivalent] daily via a metered-dose inhaler). In infants and children 4 years of age or younger with moderate persistent asthma that is not controlled by a low dosage of an inhaled corticosteroid, the only preferred option is to increase the maintenance dosage of the inhaled corticosteroid to a medium dosage (e.g., exceeding 176 mcg but not more than 352 mcg of fluticasone propionate [or its equivalent] daily via a metered-dose inhaler).

Severe Persistent Asthma. Maintenance therapy with an inhaled corticosteroid at medium dosages or high dosages (e.g., exceeding 440 mcg of fluticasone propionate in adults and adolescents or 352 mcg in children 5–11 years of age [or its equivalent] daily via a metered-dose inhaler) and adjunctive therapy with a long-acting inhaled β_2-agonist is the preferred treatment according to asthma management guidelines in adults and children 5 years of age or older with severe persistent asthma (i.e., continuous daytime asthma symptoms, nighttime symptoms 7 times per week). Such recommendations in children 5–11 years of age are based on expert opinion and extrapolation from studies in adolescents and adults. Alternatives to a long-acting inhaled β_2-agonist for severe persistent asthma in adults and children 5 years of age or older receiving medium-dose inhaled corticosteroids include extended-release theophylline or certain leukotriene modifiers (i.e., montelukast, zafirlukast), but these therapies are generally not preferred. Omalizumab may be considered in adults and adolescents with severe asthma with an allergic component who are inadequately controlled with high-dose inhaled corticosteroids and a long-acting β_2-agonist. In infants and children 4 years of age or younger with severe asthma, maintenance therapy with an inhaled corticosteroid at medium or high dosages (e.g., exceeding 352 mcg of fluticasone propionate [or its equivalent] daily via a metered-dose inhaler) and adjunctive therapy with either a long-acting inhaled β_2-agonist or montelukast is the only preferred treatment according to asthma management guidelines. Recommendations for care of infants and children with severe asthma are based on expert opinion and extrapolation from studies in older children.

Poorly Controlled Asthma. If asthma symptoms in adults and children 5 years of age or older with moderate to severe asthma are very poorly controlled (i.e., at least 2 exacerbations per year requiring oral corticosteroids) with low to high maintenance dosages of an inhaled corticosteroid and a long-acting inhaled bronchodilator, a short course (3–10 days) of an oral corticosteroid may be added to gain prompt control of asthma. In infants and children 4 years of age or younger with moderate to severe asthma who are very poorly controlled (more than 3 exacerbations per year requiring oral corticosteroids) with medium to high maintenance dosages of an inhaled corticosteroid with or without adjunctive therapy (i.e., a long-acting inhaled β_2-agonist, montelukast), a short course (3–10 days) of an oral corticosteroid may be added to gain prompt control of asthma.

While clinical efficacy of oral corticosteroids as add-on therapy in adults and children 5 years of age or older with very severe asthma that is inadequately controlled with a high-dose inhaled corticosteroid, intermittent oral corticosteroid therapy, and a long-acting inhaled β_2-agonist bronchodilator has not been established in randomized controlled studies, some experts suggest regular use of oral corticosteroids in such patients, based on consensus and clinical experience. Similarly, some experts, based on consensus and clinical experience, suggest regular use of oral corticosteroid therapy in infants and children 4 years of age or younger with very severe asthma who are not controlled with high-dose inhaled corticosteroid and either a long-acting inhaled β_2-agonist or montelukast and intermittent oral corticosteroid therapy. However, other experts do not consider regular use of oral corticosteroid therapy to be appropriate therapy in children with severely uncontrolled asthma. (See Asthma under Uses: Respiratory Diseases, in the Corticosteroids General Statement 68:04.)

When asthma symptoms at any stage are not controlled with maintenance therapy (e.g., inhaled corticosteroids) plus supplemental short-acting inhaled β_2-agonist bronchodilator therapy as needed (e.g., if there is a need to increase the dose or frequency of administration of the short-acting sympathomimetic agent), prompt reevaluation is required to adjust dosage of the maintenance regimen or institute an alternative maintenance regimen. For additional details on the stepped-care approach to drug therapy in asthma, see Asthma under Uses: Bronchospasm, in Albuterol 12:12.08.12 and also see Asthma under Uses: Respiratory Diseases, in the Corticosteroids General Statement 68:04.

Clinical Experience with Formoterol Fumarate. While formoterol has a more rapid onset of action than salmeterol, the clinical importance of this difference in the treatment of asthma has not been established, and neither formoterol nor salmeterol should be used to relieve symptoms of acute asthma. (See Acute Exacerbations of Asthma or Chronic Obstructive Pulmonary Disease under

Warnings/Precautions: Warnings, in Cautions and also see Supplemental Therapy in Acute Asthma under Bronchospasm: Asthma, in Uses in Salmeterol 12:12.08.12.)

Results of several controlled, comparative studies in adolescents and adults with mild to moderate asthma (i.e., requiring daily use of short-acting inhaled β_2-adrenergic bronchodilators with or without orally inhaled corticosteroids or theophylline) indicate that therapy with orally inhaled formoterol fumarate (12 or 24 mcg twice daily) is more effective than therapy with orally inhaled albuterol (180 mcg 4 times daily) or placebo in controlling asthma symptoms (e.g., as determined by days free of asthma symptoms, presence of nocturnal asthma symptoms, nights without nocturnal awakenings), reducing the need for rescue medication (e.g., intermittent use of a short-acting, β_2-agonist bronchodilator to control asthma exacerbations), and improving lung function (e.g., as determined by mean peak expiratory flow rate [PEFR], forced expiratory volume in 1 second [FEV_1]). In a large clinical study in children (5–12 years of age) with persistent asthma who required concomitant therapy with an anti-inflammatory agent (i.e., cromolyn sodium, inhaled corticosteroid) and a daily inhaled bronchodilator (e.g., albuterol) at study entry, usual dosages of orally inhaled formoterol fumarate (12 mcg twice daily) were consistently more effective than placebo in improving pulmonary function (as measured by FEV_1 area under the curve [AUC]) on day 1 of treatment and at 12 weeks and 1 year. Anti-inflammatory agents were continued throughout the study. While regular use of bronchodilators was not permitted during the study, orally inhaled albuterol was used as supplemental therapy for acute symptoms of asthma. While comparative clinical data for formoterol and salmeterol are limited, the drugs appeared to have similar efficacy (in terms of PEFR values, use of rescue medication, and symptom control) and safety in a 6-month, randomized, open-label study in adults with reversible obstructive airways disease who received orally inhaled formoterol fumarate 12 mcg or salmeterol 50 mcg twice daily.

Clinical Experience with Fixed Combination of Formoterol Fumarate and Budesonide. In 2 randomized, double-blind, placebo-controlled clinical studies in patients 12 years of age or older with mild to severe asthma, orally inhaled formoterol/budesonide (9 mcg of formoterol fumarate and 160 or 320 mcg of budesonide twice daily) produced greater improvement in most indices of pulmonary function (e.g., mean percent change from baseline in FEV_1 or morning and evening PEFR) than either drug alone and similar efficacy as concurrent therapy with both drugs given as single-entity preparations.

In one randomized, double-blind, multicenter study, 184 pediatric patients 6 to younger than 12 years of age with asthma received orally inhaled formoterol/budesonide (9 mcg of formoterol fumarate and 160 mcg of budesonide twice daily) or orally inhaled single-entity budesonide 160 mcg twice daily. In patients receiving formoterol/budesonide, there was a substantial change in 1-hour post-dose FEV_1 at 12 weeks, which improved by 0.28 L from baseline in those receiving the fixed combination compared with 0.17 L in those receiving single-entity budesonide.

Clinical Experience with Fixed Combination of Formoterol Fumarate and Mometasone Furoate. In one randomized, double-blind, placebo-controlled, 26-week study in patients with asthma 12 years of age or older, orally inhaled formoterol/mometasone (2 inhalations of preparation containing 5 mcg of formoterol fumarate and 100 mcg of mometasone furoate twice daily) was compared with either mometasone furoate 100 mcg, formoterol fumarate 5 mcg, or placebo (2 inhalations administered twice daily). A co-primary efficacy end point in this study was the change from baseline in FEV_1 AUC from 0–12 hours. In this study, patients receiving formoterol/mometasone had substantially greater increases in FEV_1 AUC 0–12 hours at 12 weeks compared with those receiving single-entity mometasone furoate or placebo; such improvements were maintained over the 26-week study period. Another primary end point in this study was deterioration in asthma or reduction in lung function. Patients who received formoterol/mometasone had fewer reports of asthma deterioration compared with patients receiving single-entity formoterol fumarate.

In a randomized, double-blind, 12-week study in patients with asthma 12 years of age or older, orally inhaled formoterol/mometasone (2 inhalations of preparation containing 5 mcg of formoterol fumarate and 100 or 200 mcg of mometasone furoate administered twice daily) was compared with mometasone furoate 200 mcg (2 inhalations administered twice daily). Patients who received either dosage of the formoterol/mometasone fixed combination had substantially greater increases in mean FEV_1 from baseline and over 12 weeks compared with those receiving single-entity mometasone furoate.

Chronic Obstructive Pulmonary Disease Orally inhaled formoterol is used alone or in fixed combination with budesonide or glycopyrrolate as a bronchodilator for the long-term symptomatic treatment of airflow obstruction associated with COPD, including chronic bronchitis and emphysema.

In the stepped-care approach to drug therapy for COPD, mild, intermittent symptoms and minimal lung impairment (FEV_1 at least 80% of predicted) can be treated with a short-acting, selective inhaled β_2-adrenergic agonist (e.g., albuterol) as needed for acute symptoms. For the treatment of moderate to severe COPD (e.g., FEV_1 30 to less than 80% of predicted value) who have persistent symptoms despite as-needed therapy with ipratropium or a selective inhaled β_2-agonist, maintenance treatment with one or more long-acting bronchodilators (e.g., orally inhaled formoterol, salmeterol, tiotropium) can be added, and a short-acting, selective inhaled β_2-agonist used as needed for immediate symptom relief. Maintenance therapy with long-acting bronchodilators in patients with moderate to severe COPD is more effective and more convenient than regular use of short-acting bronchodilators.

Maintenance therapy (e.g., 4 times daily) with a short-acting, selective inhaled β_2-agonist is not preferred but may be used in patients with persistent symptoms of COPD; such therapy should not exceed 6–12 inhalations daily. Guidelines for the management of COPD state that low- to high-dose ipratropium (6–16 inhalations daily) can be added to therapy with a short-acting, selective β_2-agonist (as separate inhalations or in fixed combination) in patients with mild to moderate persistent symptoms of COPD, with the frequency of inhalation dosing with either agent not to exceed 4 times daily; the highest dosage of ipratropium included in some guidelines for COPD exceeds the manufacturer's maximum recommended daily dosage (12 inhalations). Combining bronchodilators from different classes and with differing durations of action may increase the degree of bronchodilation with a similar or lower frequency of adverse effects.

For patients not responding adequately to treatment with a long-acting bronchodilator, a combination of several long-acting bronchodilators, such as tiotropium and a long-acting β-adrenergic agonist, may be used. A short-acting bronchodilator may be used as needed for relief of acute symptoms that occur despite regular use of long-acting bronchodilators. For treatment of severe to very severe COPD (e.g., FEV_1 less than 30 to less than 50% of predicted, history of exacerbations), the addition of an inhaled corticosteroid to one or more long-acting bronchodilators given separately or in fixed combination may be needed. If symptoms are not adequately controlled with inhaled corticosteroids and a long-acting bronchodilator or if limiting adverse effects occur, oral extended-release theophylline may be added or substituted. For additional information on the stepped-care approach to drug therapy in COPD, see Chronic Obstructive Pulmonary Disease under Uses: Bronchospasm, in Ipratropium Bromide 12:08.08.

Clinical Experience with Formoterol Fumarate. In a long-term (12-month) controlled comparative study in patients with COPD, orally inhaled formoterol fumarate (12 mcg twice daily) produced greater bronchodilation (as measured by increases in area under the forced expiratory volume in 1 second [FEV_1]-time curve) than dose-adjusted oral extended-release theophylline (dosage adjusted to maintain plasma drug concentrations within the range of 8–20 mcg/mL) or placebo for a period of 12 hours following the morning dose. Approximately half of the patients in each group were receiving inhaled corticosteroids, which were continued during the study along with as-needed rescue therapy with inhaled albuterol. Therapy with formoterol also decreased mild exacerbations of COPD (defined as the number of days with at least 2 symptom scores of 2 or greater and/or a reduction in peak expiratory flow [PEF] exceeding 20%) and the use of supplemental (rescue) medication compared with oral extended-release theophylline or placebo.

In a similar short-term (12-week) controlled study in patients with COPD, orally inhaled formoterol fumarate (12 mcg twice daily), produced greater improvement in FEV_1 (for 12 hours following the dose), symptoms, and quality of life than inhaled ipratropium bromide (36 mcg 4 times daily) or placebo. Therapy with orally inhaled formoterol also decreased mild exacerbations of COPD (defined as the number of days with at least 2 symptom scores of 2 or greater and/or a reduction in peak expiratory flow [PEF] exceeding 20%) and the need for rescue therapy with a short-acting β_2-agonist (albuterol) compared with orally inhaled ipratropium or placebo. Compared with formoterol fumarate 12 mcg twice daily, a dosage of 24 mcg twice daily did not provide additional benefits on FEV_1 and other end points in these studies.

Clinical Experience with Fixed Combination of Formoterol Fumarate and Budesonide. In 2 randomized, double-blind, placebo-controlled studies of 6 or 12 months' duration in patients with COPD, orally inhaled formoterol/budesonide (9 mcg of formoterol fumarate and 320 mcg of budesonide twice daily) produced greater improvements in the mean percent change from baseline in predose FEV_1 compared with formoterol fumarate alone or placebo and in 1-hour postdose FEV_1 compared with budesonide alone or placebo. The formoterol/budesonide fixed combination given in a dosage of 9 mcg of formoterol fumarate and 160 mcg of budesonide twice daily did not produce greater improvements from baseline in predose FEV_1 than formoterol alone or placebo. Therefore, the higher dosage of formoterol/budesonide is the only recommended dosage for the treatment of airflow obstruction in COPD.

Clinical Experience with Fixed Combination of Formoterol Fumarate and Glycopyrrolate. In 2 randomized, double-blind, placebo-controlled, parallel group studies of 24 weeks' duration in 3699 adults 40 years of age or older with moderate to very severe COPD, orally inhaled formoterol/glycopyrrolate (9.6 mcg of formoterol fumarate and 18 mcg of glycopyrrolate twice daily) resulted in a larger increase in mean change from baseline in trough FEV_1 after 24 weeks compared with either drug alone or placebo. The mean peak FEV_1 improvement from baseline with the formoterol/glycopyrrolate fixed combination compared with placebo after 24 weeks was 291 and 267 mL, respectively. Overall, the need for rescue medication with orally inhaled albuterol also was reduced in patients treated with formoterol/glycopyrrolate compared with those receiving placebo.

Dosage and Administration

■ **Administration** ***Oral Inhalation*** **Formoterol Fumarate.** Formoterol fumarate oral inhalation solution (Perforomist®) is administered by oral inhalation using a standard jet nebulizer connected to an air compressor and equipped with a mouthpiece or face mask. Formoterol fumarate oral inhalation solution is available in single-dose vials that should be stored in the foil pouch provided by the manufacturer and removed immediately before use.

For administration of formoterol fumarate oral inhalation solution for nebulization, the entire contents of the 20-mcg vial should be squeezed into the nebulizer reservoir. The nebulizer reservoir should be connected to the mouthpiece or face mask, and then the nebulizer should be connected to the compressor. The patient should be seated in an upright, comfortable position and should inhale the medication as calmly, deeply, and evenly as possible through the mouth using the mouthpiece or face mask of the nebulizer until the nebulizer stops producing mist in the reservoir (average nebulization time is 9 minutes). The nebulizer should be cleaned after use according to the manufacturer's instructions. The safety and efficacy of formoterol fumarate oral inhalation solution delivered from a nebulizer other than the Pari-LC Plus® nebulizer or a compressor other than the PRONEB® Ultra compressor have not been established. Formoterol fumarate oral inhalation solution should *not* be mixed with other inhalation solutions or ingested.

Fixed Combination of Formoterol Fumarate and Budesonide. Formoterol fumarate dihydrate in fixed combination with budesonide (formoterol/budesonide; Symbicort®) is administered by oral inhalation using an oral aerosol inhaler with hydrofluoroalkane (HFA) propellant. Formoterol/budesonide inhalation aerosol should only be used with the actuator supplied with the product.

Before each inhalation of formoterol/budesonide, the inhaler must be shaken well for 5 seconds. The aerosol inhaler should be test sprayed twice into the air (away from the face) before initial use, and shaken well for 5 seconds before each spray. If the inhaler has not been used for more than 7 days or if the inhaler was dropped, the inhaler should be test sprayed twice into the air (away from the face) and shaken well for 5 seconds before each spray. Rinsing the mouth after inhalation of formoterol/budesonide inhalation aerosol and spitting out the water are advised. The mouthpiece of the inhaler should be wiped clean with a dry cloth every 7 days. The inhaler should be discarded when the labeled number of inhalations has been used or within 3 months after removal from the foil pouch. The canister should never be immersed in water to determine the amount of drug remaining in the canister ("float test").

Fixed Combination of Formoterol Fumarate and Glycopyrrolate. Formoterol fumarate in fixed combination with glycopyrrolate (formoterol/glycopyrrolate; Bevespi® Aerosphere®) is administered by oral inhalation using an oral aerosol inhaler with HFA propellant. Formoterol/glycopyrrolate inhalation aerosol should only be used with the actuator supplied with the product.

The aerosol inhaler should be primed by releasing 4 test sprays into the air (away from the face) before initial use, and shaken well before each spray. If the inhaler has not been used for more than 7 days, the priming process should be repeated (using only 2 sprays rather than 4).

To administer a dose of formoterol/glycopyrrolate, the cap should be removed from the mouthpiece. Before each inhalation, the inhaler must be shaken well. The inhaler should be held with the mouthpiece pointing towards the face while the patient exhales through the mouth as fully and comfortably as possible. The lips should be closed around the mouthpiece and the head tilted back, keeping the tongue below the mouthpiece. While inhaling slowly and deeply, the center of the dose indicator should be pressed down until the canister stops moving in the actuator and a spray has been released, then the dose indicator should be released. At the end of inhalation, the mouthpiece should be removed from the mouth and the breath held as long as comfortably possible (up to 10 seconds) then the patient should exhale gently. The process should be repeated for the second inhalation. The cap should be replaced on the mouthpiece immediately after use.

The Bevespi® Aerosphere® inhaler should be cleaned once weekly by removing the canister from the actuator; the canister should not be cleaned or allowed to get wet. The actuator should be held under warm running water for about 30 seconds. The actuator should then be turned upside down and water rinsed through the actuator again for about 30 seconds. The actuator should be allowed to dry overnight. When the actuator is dry, the canister should be pressed gently down into the actuator; the canister should not be pressed down too hard since this may cause drug to be released. Priming of the inhaler should be repeated after each cleaning by shaking well and releasing 2 test sprays into the air away from the face. The inhaler should be discarded 3 months after removal from the foil pouch or when the dose indicator reads "0," whichever comes first. The canister should never be immersed in water to determine the amount of drug remaining in the canister ("float test").

Fixed Combination of Formoterol Fumarate and Mometasone Furoate. Formoterol fumarate dihydrate in fixed combination with mometasone furoate (formoterol/mometasone; Dulera®) is administered by oral inhalation as an oral inhalation suspension using a metered-dose aerosol inhaler with HFA propellant. Formoterol/mometasone inhalation aerosol should only be used with the actuator supplied with the product.

The aerosol inhaler should be primed by releasing 4 test sprays into the air (away from the face) before initial use, and shaken well before each spray. If the inhaler has *not* been used for more than 5 days, it should be primed again by test spraying 4 times into the air (away from the face) and shaken well before each spray. Before each inhalation, the inhaler must be shaken well. Following each dose, the mouth should be rinsed thoroughly without swallowing. The mouthpiece of the inhaler should be wiped clean with a dry cloth every 7 days; water should not be used to clean the inhaler.

■ Dosage

Each 2-mL single-dose vial of formoterol fumarate oral inhalation solution contains 20 mcg of formoterol fumarate. The oral inhalation solution does not require dilution prior to administration by nebulization. The actual amount of drug delivered to the lungs will depend on patient factors and the type of nebulization system used and its performance.

Each actuation of the oral aerosol inhaler containing the fixed combination of formoterol fumarate dihydrate and budesonide delivers 5.1 mcg of formoterol fumarate dihydrate and 91 or 181 mcg of budesonide from the valve and delivers 4.5 mcg of formoterol fumarate dihydrate and 80 or 160 mcg of budesonide from the actuator per metered spray, depending on the preparation used. The strength of formoterol/budesonide preparations and dosage of the fixed combination are expressed in terms of drug delivered from the mouthpiece of the actuator. The actual amount of drug delivered to the lungs depends on factors such as the patient's coordination between the actuation of the inhaler and inspiration through the delivery system. The commercially available formoterol/budesonide aerosol inhaler delivers 60 metered sprays per 6- or 6.9-g canister and 120 metered sprays per 10.2-g canister.

After priming of the oral aerosol inhaler containing the fixed combination of formoterol fumarate and glycopyrrolate, each actuation of the oral aerosol inhaler (Bevespi® Aerosphere®) delivers 5.5 mcg of formoterol fumarate and 10.4 mcg of glycopyrrolate (equivalent to 8.3 mcg of glycopyrronium) from the valve. Dosage is expressed in terms of drug delivered from the mouthpiece; each actuation of the inhaler delivers 4.8 mcg of formoterol fumarate and 9 mcg of glycopyrrolate (equivalent to 7.2 mcg of glycopyrronium) from the actuator. The actual amount of drug delivered to the lungs depends on factors such as the patient's coordination between actuation of the device and inspiration through the delivery system. Commercially available formoterol/glycopyrrolate aerosol inhaler delivers 28 or 120 metered sprays per 5.9- or 10.7-g canister, respectively.

Each actuation of the oral aerosol inhaler containing the fixed combination of formoterol fumarate dihydrate and mometasone furoate delivers 5.5 mcg of formoterol fumarate dihydrate and 115 or 225 mcg of mometasone furoate from the valve and delivers 5 mcg of formoterol fumarate dihydrate and 100 or 200 mcg of mometasone furoate from the actuator per metered spray, depending on the preparation used. The strength of formoterol/mometasone preparations and dosage of the fixed combination are expressed in terms of drug delivered from the mouthpiece of the actuator. The actual amount of drug delivered to the lungs may depend on factors such as the patient's coordination between actuation of the device and inspiration through the delivery system. Commercially available formoterol/mometasone aerosol inhaler delivers 60 or 120 metered sprays per 8.8- or 13-g canister, respectively.

Asthma

Fixed Combination of Formoterol Fumarate and Budesonide. In asthmatic patients 12 years of age or older, the recommended initial dosage of the oral inhalation aerosol containing formoterol fumarate dihydrate in fixed combination with budesonide is based on the patient's asthma severity. The dosage of the formoterol/budesonide fixed combination in this age group is 9 mcg of formoterol fumarate dihydrate and 160 or 320 mcg of budesonide (2 inhalations of preparation containing 4.5 mcg of formoterol fumarate dihydrate and 80 or 160 mcg of budesonide) twice daily, given approximately 12 hours apart (morning and evening). In asthmatic patients 6 to younger than 12 years of age, the recommended initial dosage of formoterol/budesonide is 9 mcg of formoterol fumarate dihydrate and 160 mcg of budesonide (2 inhalations of preparation containing 4.5 mcg of formoterol fumarate dihydrate and 80 mcg of budesonide) twice daily, given approximately 12 hours apart (morning and evening). The maximum recommended dosage of formoterol/budesonide in asthmatic patients 12 years of age or older is 9 mcg of formoterol fumarate dihydrate and 320 mcg of budesonide (2 inhalations of preparation containing 4.5 mcg of formoterol fumarate dihydrate and 160 mcg of budesonide) twice daily. The maximum recommended dosage in asthmatic children 6 to younger than 12 years of age is 9 mcg of formoterol fumarate dihydrate and 160 mcg of budesonide (2 inhalations of preparation containing 4.5 mcg of formoterol fumarate dihydrate and 80 mcg of budesonide) twice daily. The manufacturer states that administration of formoterol/budesonide oral inhalation aerosol more frequently than twice daily or in excess of 2 inhalations twice daily is not recommended. Patients receiving formoterol/budesonide should not use additional long-acting β_2-agonists for any reason.

Improvement in asthma control following oral inhalation of formoterol/budesonide may occur within 15 minutes of initiating treatment, although maximum benefit may not be achieved for 2 weeks or longer after therapy initiation. Individual patients will experience a variable time to onset and degree of symptom relief. If control of asthma is inadequate after 1–2 weeks of therapy at the lower dosage, switching to a higher strength of the fixed combination (higher strengths contain higher dosages of budesonide only) may provide additional asthma control. If acute asthmatic symptoms arise despite therapy with formoterol in fixed combination with budesonide, a short-acting inhaled β_2-adrenergic agonist should be taken for immediate relief. Patients should be advised not to discontinue formoterol/budesonide without medical supervision, as symptoms may recur after treatment discontinuance. If a previously effective dosage of formoterol/budesonide fails to provide adequate asthma control, the therapeutic regimen should be reevaluated and additional therapeutic options should be considered (e.g., switching to a higher strength of the fixed combination [higher strengths contain higher dosages of budesonide only], adding additional inhaled corticosteroids, initiating systemic corticosteroids). (See Acute Exacerbations of Asthma or Chronic Obstructive Pulmonary Disease under Warnings/Precautions: Warnings, in Cautions.)

Fixed Combination of Formoterol Fumarate and Mometasone Furoate. In asthmatic patients 12 years of age or older, the recommended initial dosage of the oral inhalation aerosol containing formoterol fumarate dihydrate in fixed combination with mometasone furoate is based on the patient's asthma severity, previous asthma therapy (including previous inhaled corticosteroid dosage), current control of asthma symptoms, and risk of future asthma exacerbations.

In adults and adolescents 12 years of age or older, the dosage of the formoterol/mometasone fixed combination is 10 mcg of formoterol fumarate dihydrate and 200 or 400 mcg of mometasone furoate (2 inhalations of preparation containing 5 mcg of formoterol fumarate dihydrate and 100 or 200 mcg of mometasone furoate) twice daily. If control of asthma is inadequate after 2 weeks of formoterol/mometasone therapy at the lower dosage, switching to a higher strength of the fixed combination (higher strengths contain higher dosages of mometasone only) may provide additional asthma control. The maximum recommended dosage of formoterol/mometasone in asthmatic adults and adolescents 12 years of age or older is 10 mcg of formoterol fumarate dihydrate and 400 mcg of mometasone furoate twice daily.

Chronic Obstructive Pulmonary Disease **Formoterol Fumarate.** For maintenance therapy of airflow obstruction in patients with chronic obstructive pulmonary disease (COPD), the recommended dosage of formoterol fumarate oral inhalation solution is 20 mcg (entire contents of a single-dose vial) every 12 hours (morning and evening) by nebulization. The total daily dosage of formoterol fumarate oral inhalation solution should not exceed 40 mcg. If shortness of breath occurs despite therapy with formoterol oral inhalation solution, a short-acting inhaled β_2-adrenergic agonist should be taken for immediate relief.

Fixed Combination of Formoterol Fumarate and Budesonide. For maintenance therapy of airflow obstruction in patients with COPD, the recommended dosage of the oral inhalation aerosol containing formoterol fumarate dihydrate in fixed combination with budesonide in adults is 9 mcg of formoterol fumarate dihydrate and 320 mcg of budesonide (2 inhalations of preparation containing 4.5 mcg of formoterol fumarate dihydrate and 160 mcg of budesonide) twice daily (morning and evening). In clinical studies, lower dosages of formoterol/budesonide (i.e., 2 inhalations of preparation containing 4.5 mcg of formoterol fumarate dihydrate and 80 mcg of budesonide twice daily) did not produce greater improvements from baseline in predose FEV_1 than formoterol alone or placebo; therefore, such dosages are not recommended for the treatment of airflow obstruction in COPD.

If shortness of breath occurs despite therapy with the recommended dosage of formoterol/budesonide, a short-acting inhaled β_2-adrenergic agonist should be taken for immediate relief. Patients should be advised not to discontinue formoterol/budesonide without medical supervision, as symptoms may recur after treatment discontinuance. The manufacturer states that administration of formoterol/budesonide inhalation aerosol more frequently than twice daily or in excess of 2 inhalations twice daily is not recommended. Patients receiving formoterol/budesonide should not use additional long-acting β_2-agonists for any reason.

Fixed Combination of Formoterol Fumarate and Glycopyrrolate. For the long-term management of airflow obstruction associated with COPD, the usual dosage of formoterol fumarate in fixed combination with glycopyrrolate in adults is 9.6 mcg of formoterol fumarate and 18 mcg of glycopyrrolate (2 inhalations of preparation containing 4.8 mcg of formoterol fumarate and 9 mcg of glycopyrrolate) twice daily via the Aerosphere® device. More frequent administration or higher dosages are not recommended. Orally inhaled formoterol/glycopyrrolate should *not* be used for the treatment of acute episodes of bronchospasm.

■ **Special Populations** ***Hepatic Impairment*** The manufacturers of formoterol fumarate and formoterol fumarate in fixed combination with budesonide, glycopyrrolate, or mometasone furoate make no specific dosage recommendations for patients with hepatic impairment at this time. However, since formoterol fumarate, budesonide, and mometasone are cleared predominantly by the liver, impaired liver function theoretically may lead to accumulation of the drugs in plasma. Therefore, the manufacturers of formoterol fumarate in fixed combination with budesonide, glycopyrrolate, or mometasone furoate state that patients with hepatic disease should be closely monitored for signs of increased drug exposure.

Renal Impairment The manufacturers of formoterol fumarate and formoterol fumarate in fixed combination with budesonide, glycopyrrolate, or mometasone furoate make no specific dosage recommendations for patients with renal impairment at this time.

The manufacturer of formoterol fumarate in fixed combination with glycopyrrolate states that the preparation should be used in patients with severe renal impairment (i.e., creatinine clearance less than 30 mL/minute) or end-stage renal disease requiring dialysis only if expected benefits outweigh potential risks.

Geriatric Patients The manufacturers of formoterol fumarate and formoterol fumarate in fixed combination with budesonide, glycopyrrolate, or mometasone furoate state that dosage adjustment is not required in geriatric patients.

Cautions

■ **Contraindications** Formoterol fumarate and fixed combinations containing formoterol fumarate are contraindicated in patients hypersensitive to the drug or any ingredient in the formulation.

Because of the risk of asthma-related death and hospitalization, use of formoterol for the treatment of asthma without concomitant use of long-term asthma controller therapy, such as inhaled corticosteroids, is contraindicated. (See Asthma-related Death and Serious Asthma-related Events under Warnings/Precautions: Warnings, in Cautions and also see Uses: Bronchospasm.)

Formoterol fumarate in fixed combination with budesonide (formoterol/budesonide; Symbicort®) and formoterol fumarate in fixed combination with mometasone furoate (formoterol/mometasone; Dulera®) are contraindicated as primary treatment of status asthmaticus or other acute episodes of asthma or chronic obstructive pulmonary disease (COPD) when intensive measures are required.

Formoterol fumarate in fixed combination with glycopyrrolate (formoterol/glycopyrrolate; Bevespi® Aerosphere®) is not indicated for the treatment of asthma.

■ **Warnings/Precautions** ***Warnings*** **Use of Fixed Combinations.** When formoterol fumarate is used in fixed combination with budesonide, glycopyrrolate, or mometasone furoate, the usual cautions, precautions, contraindications, and interactions associated with budesonide, glycopyrrolate, or mometasone furoate must be considered.

Cautionary information applicable to specific populations (e.g., pregnant or nursing women, individuals with hepatic or renal impairment, geriatric patients) should be considered for each drug in the fixed combination.

Asthma-related Death and Serious Asthma-related Events. Monotherapy with long-acting β_2-adrenergic agonists, such as formoterol, increases the risk of asthma-related death. In addition, available data from controlled clinical trials suggest that use of long-acting β_2-adrenergic agonists as monotherapy increases the risk of asthma-related hospitalization in pediatric and adolescent patients. *Because of these risks, the use of long-acting β_2-adrenergic agonists, including formoterol, alone for the treatment of asthma without concomitant use of long-term asthma controller therapy, such as inhaled corticosteroids, is contraindicated.* (See Cautions: Contraindications.) However, FDA has concluded that there is no clinically important increased risk of serious asthma-related events, including hospitalization, intubation, or death, associated with concomitant use of long-acting β_2-adrenergic agonists (e.g., formoterol) and inhaled corticosteroids compared with inhaled corticosteroids alone based on the results of several large clinical studies. In addition, these studies showed that combination therapy with long-acting β_2-adrenergic agonists and inhaled corticosteroids was more effective in reducing the incidence of asthma exacerbations (i.e., events requiring use of systemic corticosteroids for at least 3 outpatient days or an asthma-related hospitalization or emergency department visit requiring use of systemic corticosteroids) compared with use of inhaled corticosteroids alone.

The formoterol/budesonide and formoterol/mometasone fixed combinations should be used *only* in patients with asthma who have not responded adequately to long-term asthma controller therapy, such as inhaled corticosteroids, or whose disease severity warrants initiation of treatment with both an inhaled corticosteroid and a long-acting β_2-adrenergic agonist. Once asthma control is achieved and maintained, the patient should be assessed at regular intervals and therapy should be stepped down (e.g., discontinuance of the long-acting β_2-adrenergic agonist), if possible without loss of asthma control, and the patient should be maintained on long-term asthma controller therapy, such as inhaled corticosteroids. Long-acting β_2-adrenergic agonists, including formoterol alone or in fixed combination with budesonide, should not be used in patients whose asthma is adequately controlled on a low or medium dosage of inhaled corticosteroids. In pediatric and adolescent patients with asthma who require the addition of a long-acting β_2-adrenergic agonist to inhaled corticosteroid therapy, a fixed-combination preparation containing both an inhaled corticosteroid and a long-acting β_2-adrenergic agonist generally should be used to ensure compliance with both drugs. (See Uses: Bronchospasm.)

Data from a large placebo-controlled study (Salmeterol Multi-center Asthma Research Trial ([SMART]) evaluating the safety of another long-acting β_2-adrenergic agonist, salmeterol, in patients with asthma showed an increase in asthma-related deaths in patients receiving salmeterol. (See Asthma-related Death and Life-threatening Events under Cautions: Respiratory Effects, in Salmeterol 12:12.08.12.) The increased risk of asthma-related death with salmeterol is considered a class effect of the long-acting β_2-adrenergic agonists, including formoterol. However, no adequate studies have been conducted to determine whether the rate of asthma-related death is increased with formoterol. Clinical studies with inhalation of formoterol as a dry powder suggest that the incidence of serious asthma exacerbations is increased in patients receiving formoterol compared with those receiving placebo, although the sample sizes in these studies were not adequate to quantify the precise differences between treatment groups.

In 4 randomized, double-blind, active-controlled clinical trials mandated by FDA, the risk of serious asthma-related events from use of inhaled corticosteroids alone compared with combined use of long-acting β_2-adrenergic agonists and inhaled corticosteroids was evaluated over 26 weeks in 41,297 patients with asthma (3 trials in adults and adolescents 12 years of age or older and one trial in children 4–11 years of age). The primary safety end point in all of these trials was serious asthma-related events, including hospitalization, intubation, and death; these events were reviewed by a blinded committee to determine if the events were asthma related. The 3 trials performed in adults and adolescents were designed to rule out a hazard ratio of 2, and the pediatric trial was designed to rule out a hazard ratio of 2.7; this objective was met in all 4 individual trials. The trials were not designed to rule out all risk for serious asthma-related events associated with long-acting β_2-adrenergic agonists in combination with inhaled corticosteroids compared with inhaled corticosteroids alone.

The safety studies in adults and adolescents included one trial comparing salmeterol and fluticasone propionate in fixed combination as the inhalation powder with fluticasone propionate oral inhalation powder alone, one trial comparing formoterol and mometasone furoate in fixed combination with mometasone furoate alone, and one trial comparing formoterol and budesonide in fixed combination with budesonide alone. In a meta-analysis combining data from these 3 trials, a hazard ratio of 1.1 for first serious asthma-related event in patients receiving fixed-combination therapy with long-acting β_2-adrenergic agonists and inhaled corticosteroids compared with patients receiving inhaled corticosteroids alone was reported. Subgroup analyses for gender, adolescents 12–17 years of age, Asian and African-American patients, and obese patients also showed no substantial increase in the risk of serious asthma-related events or asthma exacerbations in these populations.

The safety study in children 4–11 years of age included 6208 patients who were randomized to receive salmeterol and fluticasone propionate in fixed combination as the inhalation powder or fluticasone propionate inhalation powder alone. Serious asthma-related events were reported in 0.9% of patients receiving salmeterol and fluticasone in fixed combination and in 0.7% of patients receiving fluticasone alone, with an estimated hazard ratio for first event of 1.29 for the combination therapy compared with fluticasone alone. No asthma-related deaths or intubations were reported in either group of pediatric patients.

No adequate studies have been conducted to determine whether the rate of death is increased in patients with COPD receiving long-acting β_2-adrenergic agonists.

Acute Exacerbations of Asthma or Chronic Obstructive Pulmonary Disease. Substantially worsening or acutely deteriorating asthma may be a life-threatening condition. Formoterol oral inhalation therapy should not be initiated in patients with substantially worsening or acutely deteriorating asthma. Formoterol in fixed combination with budesonide, glycopyrrolate, or mometasone furoate should not be initiated in patients with rapidly deteriorating or potentially life-threatening episodes of asthma or COPD.

Failure to respond to a previously effective dosage of formoterol may indicate substantially worsening asthma or destabilization of COPD that requires prompt reevaluation. If inadequate control of symptoms persists with supplemental β_2-agonist bronchodilator therapy (i.e., if there is a need to increase the dose or frequency of administration of the short-acting, inhaled bronchodilator), prompt reevaluation of asthma or COPD therapy is required, with special consideration given to the possible need for anti-inflammatory treatment (e.g., corticosteroids); however, extra or increased doses of formoterol should *not* be used in such situations. If asthma deteriorates in patients receiving formoterol in fixed combination with budesonide or mometasone furoate, prompt reevaluation of asthma therapy is required, with special consideration given to the possible need for increasing the strength of the fixed combination (higher strengths contain higher dosages of budesonide or mometasone only), adding additional inhaled corticosteroids, or initiating systemic corticosteroids; patients should not increase the frequency of administration of formoterol/budesonide or formoterol/mometasone. If COPD deteriorates in patients receiving formoterol/glycopyrrolate, prompt reevaluation of COPD therapy is required.

Concomitant Anti-Inflammatory Therapy. The manufacturer states that there are no data demonstrating clinical anti-inflammatory effects of formoterol that could be expected to substitute for or allow reduction in the dosage of corticosteroids. Particular care is needed for patients who have been transferred from systemically active corticosteroids to orally inhaled corticosteroids since death resulting from adrenal insufficiency has occurred in some asthmatic patients during and after such transfer. (See Withdrawal of Systemic Corticosteroid Therapy under Warnings/Precautions: Warnings, in Cautions in Budesonide 68:04.)

Concomitant Short-Acting Bronchodilators. The manufacturer states that if patients are taking a short-acting, inhaled β_2-agonist bronchodilator on a regular basis (e.g., 4 times daily) at the time formoterol or formoterol in fixed combination with budesonide, glycopyrrolate, or mometasone is initiated, these patients should be instructed to discontinue the *regular* use of the short-acting agent and use it only for relief of acute asthma symptoms. *Regular* (e.g., daily) use of inhaled β_2-agonists does not adequately control asthma symptoms or airway hyperresponsiveness on a long-term basis and is not recommended by current asthma management experts.

Cardiovascular Effects. Formoterol, like other sympathomimetic amines, may increase heart rate or blood pressure. Although such effects are uncommon at recommended dosages, the drug may need to be discontinued if such cardiovascular effects occur.

Excessive Doses. Fatalities have been reported in association with excessive use of inhaled sympathomimetic drugs. (See Cautions, in Albuterol 12:12.08.12.)

Patients receiving formoterol alone or in fixed combination with budesonide, glycopyrrolate, or mometasone furoate should not use additional formoterol or other long-acting β_2-agonists for any reason.

Sensitivity Reactions **Immediate Hypersensitivity Reactions.** Anaphylactic reactions, urticaria, angioedema, rash, flushing, allergic dermatitis, and bronchospasm have been reported with oral inhalation therapy with formoterol alone or in fixed combination with budesonide, glycopyrrolate, or mometasone. Orally inhaled formoterol/glycopyrrolate should be discontinued immediately if such allergic reactions occur, particularly angioedema (e.g., difficulties with breathing or swallowing; swelling of the tongue, lips, or face), urticaria, or rash, and alternative therapy considered.

Major Toxicities **Paradoxical Bronchospasm.** As with other inhaled β_2-receptor agonists, a patient may develop acute bronchospasm, which may be life-threatening, immediately upon inhalation of formoterol. If paradoxical bronchospasm occurs, formoterol should be discontinued immediately and alternative therapy instituted.

General Precautions **Acute or Worsening Asthma or COPD.** Formoterol, alone or in fixed combination with budesonide or mometasone furoate, or other long-acting β_2-adrenergic agonists (e.g., salmeterol) should *not* be used to relieve symptoms of acute asthma. Formoterol alone or in fixed combination with glycopyrrolate should not be used to relieve symptoms of acutely deteriorating COPD.

Failure to respond to a previously effective dosage of formoterol may indicate substantially worsening asthma or destabilization of COPD that requires prompt reevaluation. If inadequate control of symptoms persists with supplemental β_2-agonist bronchodilator therapy (i.e., if there is a need to increase the dose or frequency of administration of the short-acting inhaled bronchodilator or if a substantial decrease in peak expiratory flow or other index of lung function occurs), immediate reevaluation of asthma therapy is required (e.g., adjusting the inhaled corticosteroid dosage or initiating systemic corticosteroids); however, extra or increased doses of formoterol should *not* be used in such situations. If asthma deteriorates in patients receiving formoterol in fixed combination with budesonide or mometasone furoate, prompt reevaluation of asthma therapy is required, with special consideration given to the possible need for increasing the strength of the fixed combination (higher strengths contain higher dosages of budesonide or mometasone only), adding additional inhaled corticosteroids, or initiating systemic corticosteroids; patients should not increase the frequency of administration of formoterol in fixed combination with budesonide or mometasone furoate.

Cardiovascular Effects. Although uncommon at recommended dosages, clinically important changes in systolic and/or diastolic blood pressure, heart rate, and ECG (e.g., flattening of the T wave, prolongation of the QT_c interval, ST-segment depression) have been associated with formoterol oral inhalation therapy and may necessitate discontinuance of the drug. Cardiovascular effects generally have resolved within a few hours.

Like other sympathomimetic amines, formoterol should be used with caution in patients with cardiovascular disorders, especially coronary insufficiency, cardiac arrhythmias, or hypertension; in patients with seizure disorders or thyrotoxicosis; and in those who are unusually responsive to sympathomimetic amines.

Metabolic and Electrolyte Effects. Clinically important changes in blood glucose and serum potassium have occurred infrequently during clinical studies with formoterol at recommended dosage.

Specific Populations **Pregnancy.** Category C. (See Users Guide.) Formoterol may interfere with uterine contractility; carefully weigh benefit versus risk in labor.

There is an increased risk of adverse perinatal outcomes (e.g., preeclampsia, premature birth, low birth weight, and neonates small for gestational age) in women with poorly or moderately controlled asthma. Pregnant women with asthma should be closely monitored and therapy adjusted as necessary to maintain optimal asthma control.

The effects of formoterol fumarate in fixed combination with budesonide, glycopyrrolate, or mometasone furoate during labor and delivery are not known. Because of the potential for β-agonist interference with uterine contractility, use of formoterol in fixed combination with budesonide, glycopyrrolate, or mometasone during labor should be restricted to those patients in whom the benefits clearly outweigh the risk.

Lactation. Formoterol is distributed into milk in rats; it is not known whether formoterol is distributed into human milk. Effects of formoterol fumarate on breast-fed infants or milk production also are not known.

The benefits of breast-feeding and the woman's clinical need for formoterol fumarate alone or in fixed combination with budesonide or mometasone should be considered along with any potential adverse effects on the breast-fed infant from the drug or from the underlying maternal condition.

Because many drugs are distributed into human milk, caution should be exercised when formoterol fumarate in fixed combination with glycopyrrolate is administered to nursing women. Since there are no data from controlled clinical studies, the manufacturer of formoterol/glycopyrrolate states that a decision should be made whether to discontinue nursing or the drug, taking into account the importance of the drug to the woman.

Pediatric Use. Formoterol fumarate oral inhalation solution (Perforomist®) and formoterol fumarate in fixed combination with glycopyrrolate (Bevespi® Aerosphere®) are not indicated for use in children. Safety and efficacy of these preparations in children have not been established.

Safety and efficacy of formoterol fumarate in fixed combination with budesonide (Symbicort®) in pediatric patients 12 years of age or older with asthma have been established in studies of up to 12 months' duration. Safety and efficacy of formoterol/budesonide in pediatric patients 6 to less than 12 years of age with asthma have been established in studies of up to 12 weeks' duration; however, the manufacturer states that safety and efficacy of the fixed-combination preparation in children younger than 6 years of age with asthma have not been established.

Safety and efficacy of formoterol fumarate in fixed combination with mometasone furoate (Dulera®) in pediatric patients 12 years of age or older with asthma have been established in studies of up to 12 months' duration.

Available data from controlled clinical trials suggest that monotherapy with long-acting β_2-adrenergic agonists increases the risk of asthma-related hospitalization in pediatric and adolescent patients. (See Asthma-related Death and Serious Asthma-related Events under Warnings/Precautions: Warnings, in Cautions.)

Geriatric Use. No substantial differences in safety and efficacy of formoterol alone or in fixed combination with budesonide, glycopyrrolate, or mometasone furoate have been observed in geriatric patients relative to younger adults. However, the manufacturers state that the possibility that some geriatric patients may exhibit increased sensitivity to formoterol or fixed combinations containing formoterol cannot be ruled out. (See Dosage and Administration: Special Populations.)

■ **Common Adverse Effects** Adverse effects occurring in 2% or more of adults in clinical trials receiving formoterol fumarate oral inhalation solution for the treatment of COPD include diarrhea, nausea, vomiting, nasopharyngitis, dry mouth, dizziness, and insomnia.

Adverse effects occurring in 3% or more of patients receiving formoterol fumarate in fixed combination with budesonide for the treatment of asthma include nasopharyngitis, headache, upper respiratory tract infection, pharyngolaryngeal pain, sinusitis, influenza, back pain, nasal congestion, stomach discomfort, vomiting, and oral candidiasis.

Adverse effects occurring in 3% or more of patients receiving formoterol fumarate in fixed combination with budesonide for the treatment of COPD include nasopharyngitis, oral candidiasis, bronchitis, sinusitis, and upper respiratory tract infection.

Adverse effects occurring in 2% or more of patients receiving formoterol fumarate in fixed combination with glycopyrrolate for the treatment of COPD and more frequently than in those receiving placebo include urinary tract infection and cough.

Adverse effects occurring in 3% or more of patients receiving formoterol fumarate in fixed combination with mometasone furoate for the treatment of asthma and more frequently than in those receiving placebo include nasopharyngitis, sinusitis, and headache.

Drug Interactions

The following information addresses potential interactions with formoterol fumarate. When formoterol fumarate is used in fixed combination with budesonide, glycopyrrolate, or mometasone furoate, interactions associated with budesonide, glycopyrrolate, and mometasone also should be considered. No formal drug interaction studies have been performed to date with the fixed-combination preparations containing formoterol fumarate and budesonide, glycopyrrolate, or mometasone.

■ **Drugs that Prolong QT Interval** Potential pharmacologic interaction (increased risk of ventricular arrhythmias and effects of formoterol on the cardiovascular system may be potentiated). Drugs that prolong the QT interval should be used concomitantly with formoterol with extreme caution.

■ **Sympathomimetic Agents** Potential additive pharmacologic and adverse effects. Additional sympathomimetic agents administered by any route should be used with caution.

■ **Xanthine Derivatives/Corticosteroids** Potential pharmacologic interaction (increased risk of hypokalemia).

■ **Non-potassium-sparing Diuretics** Potential additive ECG and/or hypokalemic effects, especially when the recommended dosage of the β-agonist is exceeded; the clinical importance is unknown. Concomitant administration of β-agonists and non-potassium-sparing diuretics should be used with caution.

■ **Monoamine Oxidase Inhibitors/Tricyclic Antidepressants** Potential pharmacologic interaction (effects of formoterol on the cardiovascular system may be potentiated). Formoterol should be used with extreme caution during concomitant therapy or within 2 weeks following discontinuance of a monoamine oxidase (MAO) inhibitor or tricyclic antidepressant.

■ **β-Adrenergic Blocking Agents** Potential pharmacologic interaction (antagonism). Cardioselective β-adrenergic blocking agents should be considered if concomitant therapy with formoterol is necessary.

Description

Formoterol fumarate is a synthetic sympathomimetic amine. Like salmeterol, formoterol is a long-acting, selective β_2-receptor agonist, and is structurally and pharmacologically similar to other selective β_2-adrenergic receptor agonists (e.g., albuterol, salmeterol). Formoterol occurs as a racemic mixture; only the *R,R* -enantiomer is active.

Formoterol stimulates β_2-adrenergic receptors and apparently has little or no effect on β_1- or α-adrenergic receptors. The drug's β-adrenergic effects appear to result from stimulation of the production of cyclic adenosine-3′,5′-monophosphate (cAMP) by activation of adenyl cyclase. Cyclic AMP mediates numerous cellular responses, and increased concentrations of cAMP are associated with relaxation of bronchial smooth muscle and suppression of some aspects of inflammation, such as inhibition of release of proinflammatory mast-cell mediators (e.g., histamine, leukotrienes). Some studies in patients with mild asthma and in animals suggest that formoterol inhibits allergen-induced infiltration of eosinophils into airways, and reduces extravasation of plasma proteins (e.g., albumin). However, current evidence indicates that formoterol, like salmeterol, does not possess clinically important anti-inflammatory effects.

Tolerance to the bronchoprotective effects of formoterol (diminished effect on FEV1) has been reported after prolonged (2 weeks) dosing at twice the recommended dose (24 mcg), with loss of protection at the end of the 12-hour dosing period.

Limited data suggest that formoterol has a more rapid onset of action than salmeterol but a similar duration of action and similar bronchodilatory effects.

Advice to Patients

When formoterol fumarate is used in fixed combination with budesonide, glycopyrrolate, or mometasone furoate, importance of informing patients of important cautionary information about budesonide, glycopyrrolate, or mometasone furoate.

A copy of the manufacturer's patient information (medication guide) for formoterol alone or in fixed combination with budesonide, glycopyrrolate, or mometasone furoate must be provided to all patients each time the drug is dispensed. Importance of instructing patients to read the medication guide prior to initiation of therapy and each time the prescription is refilled.

Importance of informing patients that monotherapy with long-acting β_2-adrenergic agonists, including formoterol, increases the risk of asthma-related death and may increase the risk of asthma-related hospitalization in pediatric and adolescent patients. Importance of informing patients that long-term asthma controller drugs must be continued when formoterol is added to the treatment regimen.

Importance of pediatric patients receiving therapy under adult supervision.

Importance of adequate understanding of proper storage, preparation, and inhalation techniques, including use of the oral inhalation delivery system.

Importance of correct procedure for administering formoterol alone or in fixed combination with budesonide, glycopyrrolate, or mometasone furoate and any concomitant therapy (e.g., a short-acting β_2-adrenergic agonist). Importance of not breathing into the inhaler.

Importance of adherence to dosing schedules of formoterol alone or in fixed combination with budesonide, glycopyrrolate, or mometasone furoate and any concomitant therapy, including not altering the dose or frequency of use of such drugs unless otherwise instructed by a clinician. Importance of advising patient that if a dose of formoterol alone or in fixed combination with budesonide, glycopyrrolate, or mometasone furoate is missed, the next dose should be taken at the regularly scheduled time; the dose should not be doubled.

Importance of informing patients of adverse effects associated with β_2-adrenergic agonists such as palpitations, chest pain, rapid heart rate, tremor, or nervousness.

Importance of understanding that formoterol-containing therapy does not relieve acute symptoms of asthma or COPD. Importance of all patients being provided with and instructed in the use of a short-acting, inhaled β_2-adrenergic bronchodilator as supplemental therapy for acute asthma or COPD symptoms.

Importance of discontinuing *regular* use of a short-acting, inhaled β-adrenergic bronchodilator when initiating therapy with formoterol and instituting *intermittent* use of a short-acting bronchodilator (*not* formoterol) to relieve acute symptoms of asthma. Importance of contacting a clinician if respiratory symptoms worsen or are not relieved by usual dosage of formoterol fumarate. Importance of contacting a clinician or obtaining medical care right away if 4 or more inhalations of a short-acting β_2-agonist are required daily for 2 or more consecutive days, an entire canister of the short-acting β_2-agonist is used in 8 weeks, peak flow meter results decrease, or asthma symptoms do not improve after 1 week of formoterol therapy.

Importance of instructing patients to seek emergency medical care if breathing problems worsen rapidly and usual doses of a short-acting bronchodilator do not relieve acute asthma or COPD symptoms.

Importance of advising patients who are receiving formoterol-containing preparations not to use additional formoterol or other long-acting inhaled β_2-adrenergic agonists for any reason.

Importance of patients not discontinuing formoterol-containing therapy and not discontinuing or reducing concomitant asthma therapy without medical supervision, since symptoms may worsen.

Importance of promptly contacting clinicians or seeking emergency medical care if symptoms of a serious allergic reaction (e.g., rash, hives, breathing problems, swelling of the face, tongue, or mouth) develop.

Importance of informing clinicians of existing or contemplated concomitant therapy, including prescription and OTC drugs and dietary or herbal supplements, as well as concomitant illnesses (e.g., heart disease, high blood pressure, seizures, thyroid problems, diabetes mellitus, drug or food allergies).

Importance of women informing clinicians if they are or plan to become pregnant or plan to breast-feed.

Importance of informing patients of other important precautionary information. (See Cautions.)

Overview (see Users Guide). For additional information until a more detailed monograph is developed and published, the manufacturer's labeling should be consulted. It is *essential* that the manufacturer's labeling be consulted for more detailed information on usual cautions, precautions, contraindications, potential drug interactions, laboratory test interferences, and acute toxicity.

Preparations

Excipients in commercially available drug preparations may have clinically important effects in some individuals; consult specific product labeling for details.

Formoterol Fumarate (Dihydrate)

Oral Inhalation		
Solution, for nebulization	10 mcg (of formoterol fumarate) per mL	**Perforomist®**, Mylan

Formoterol Fumarate Combinations

Oral Inhalation		
Aerosol	4.5 mcg (of formoterol fumarate dihydrate) with Budesonide 80 mcg per metered spray	**Symbicort®** (with hydrofluoroalkane propellant), AstraZeneca
	4.5 mcg (of formoterol fumarate dihydrate) with Budesonide 160 mcg per metered spray	**Symbicort®** (with hydrofluoroalkane propellant), AstraZeneca
	4.8 mcg (of formoterol fumarate) with Glycopyrrolate 9 mcg per metered spray	**Bevespi® Aerosphere®** (with hydrofluoroalkane propellant), AstraZeneca
	5 mcg (of formoterol fumarate dihydrate) with Mometasone Furoate 100 mcg per metered spray	**Dulera®** (with hydrofluoroalkane propellant), Merck
	5 mcg (of formoterol fumarate dihydrate) with Mometasone Furoate 200 mcg per metered spray	**Dulera®** (with hydrofluoroalkane propellant), Merck

Indacaterol Maleate

■ Indacaterol maleate, a synthetic sympathomimetic amine, is a relatively selective, long-acting β_2-agonist.

Uses

■ **Bronchospasm** ***Chronic Obstructive Pulmonary Disease*** Indacaterol maleate is used as a bronchodilator for the long-term maintenance treatment of airflow obstruction associated with chronic obstructive pulmonary disease (COPD), including chronic bronchitis and/or emphysema. Orally inhaled indacaterol is *not* indicated for treatment of acute deterioration of COPD or relief of acute symptoms (i.e., as rescue therapy for treatment of acute episodes of bronchospasm). (See Deterioration of Disease and Acute Episodes under Warnings/Precautions: Other Warnings/Precautions, in Cautions.)Orally inhaled indacaterol is *not* indicated for treatment of asthma†; the safety and efficacy of indacaterol in asthma† have not been established.

Efficacy of indacaterol has been evaluated in 6 randomized, double-blind, placebo- and active-controlled studies of 12, 26, or 52 weeks' duration in adults 40 years of age or older with COPD. In all studies, the primary efficacy outcome was the 24-hour postdose trough forced expiratory volume in 1 second (FEV_1) (defined as the average of two FEV_1 measurements taken 23 hours 10 minutes and 23 hours 45 minutes after the previous dose) following 12 weeks of treatment. In these studies, indacaterol (75, 150, 300, or 600 mcg once daily) was more effective than placebo in improving lung function (i.e., 24-hour postdose trough FEV_1) at 12 weeks. The 24-hour postdose trough FEV_1 after 12 weeks of treatment was 1.38–1.49 L in patients receiving indacaterol 75 mcg once daily compared with 1.26–1.35 L in those receiving placebo.

While indacaterol dosages of 75, 150, 300, and 600 mcg once daily were evaluated in clinical studies, the US Food and Drug Administration (FDA) approved only the 75-mcg once daily dosage of indacaterol for the long-term maintenance treatment of airflow obstruction associated with COPD, including chronic bronchitis and/or emphysema. Prior to FDA approval, the manufacturer submitted a new drug application (NDA) to FDA proposing indacaterol dosages of 150 and 300 mcg once daily.

Following clinical review, the FDA concluded that the proposed dosages of 150 and 300 mcg were higher than necessary and not supported by the submitted efficacy and safety data; the data did not show a meaningful efficacy difference between the proposed dosages and a lower dosage of 75 mcg. In addition, there were higher incidences of adverse cardiovascular and cerebrovascular effects in patients with COPD receiving indacaterol compared with those receiving placebo or formoterol, and also a higher rate of possible asthma-related deaths compared with salmeterol in patients with asthma† (see Asthma-related Death under Warnings/Precautions: Warnings, in Cautions).

As a result, the FDA did not approve the NDA, and required the manufacturer to evaluate the efficacy and safety of lower dosages. The manufacturer submitted a complete response and lowered the proposed dosages of indacaterol to 75 or 150 mcg once daily. The 150-mcg dosage was proposed to provide an additional benefit over the 75-mcg dosage in patients with more severe bronchial constriction mainly based on a pharmacodynamic modeling analysis. The FDA concluded that the modeling analysis did not provide substantial evidence to support that the 150-mcg dosage provided a clinically meaningful benefit over the 75-mcg dosage, and there were no data comparing the 2 dosages in the same clinical study to support such a proposed dosage recommendation. Therefore, the FDA concluded that the available data and overall risk-benefit assessment supported the use of indacaterol for the long-term maintenance treatment of airflow obstruction associated with COPD, including chronic bronchitis and/or emphysema, at a dosage of 75 mcg once daily. Based on these conclusions, only the 75-mcg dosage of indacaterol received FDA approval.

For additional information on the treatment of COPD, see Uses: Chronic Obstructive Pulmonary Disease, in Ipratropium Bromide 12:08.08.

Dosage and Administration

■ **Administration** Indacaterol maleate is administered by oral inhalation *only* using a specific oral inhalation device (Neohaler®) that delivers powdered drug from capsules. Indacaterol maleate should be administered once daily at the same time every day. Indacaterol maleate capsules for oral inhalation must *not* be swallowed, as the intended effects on the lungs will not be obtained.

To use the inhaler, the cap of the inhaler should be pulled off. The inhaler should be opened by holding the base of the inhaler and tilting the mouthpiece. The capsule should then be placed into the capsule chamber of the inhaler; the capsule should not be placed directly into the mouthpiece. After the capsule is loaded, the inhaler should be closed fully; a click should be heard as the inhaler closes. While holding the inhaler upright, both buttons should be pressed fully one time and then released; a click should be heard as the capsule is pierced. The piercing buttons should not be pressed more than one time.

Before inhaling the dose, the patient should exhale fully, being careful not to blow into the mouthpiece. The inhaler device should be held with the buttons to the left and right (not up and down); the patient should not press the piercing buttons again. The patient should place the mouthpiece of the inhaler between the lips and inhale rapidly and steadily, as deeply as possible through the inhaler to create a whirring noise. After a complete inhalation, the patient should continue to hold their breath for as long as comfortable while removing the inhaler from their mouth, and then breathe out. The patient should open the inhaler to see if any powder remains in the capsule; if so, the patient should close the inhaler, breathe out completely, and inhale once again. Most patients are able to empty powder from the capsule in 1 or 2 inhalations. Upon completion of the inhalation(s), the patient should open the mouthpiece again, remove the empty capsule by tipping the inhaler device, and then discard the empty capsule. The inhaler should then be closed and the cap replaced.

If the patient does not hear a whirring noise upon inhalation, the capsule may be stuck in the capsule cavity; if this occurs, the patient should open the inhaler and carefully loosen the capsule by tapping the base of the inhaler device. The patient should not press the piercing buttons to loosen the capsule.

Dry-powder capsules for oral inhalation should be stored in foil-sealed blisters until immediately before use. Used or unused dry-powder capsules should not be stored in the inhaler device. If additional capsules are inadvertently opened and exposed to air (i.e., not intended for immediate use), they should be discarded since the effectiveness of the drug in those capsules may be reduced.

The inhalation device should be kept dry and should *not* be washed. Cleaning the inhaler device is not necessary; however, if desired, a clean, dry, lint-free cloth or soft brush may be used to wipe the inhaler between uses.

■ **Dosage** Dosage of indacaterol maleate is expressed in terms of indacaterol. Although each capsule contains 75 mcg of indacaterol as a dry powder for oral inhalation, the precise amount of drug delivered to the lungs with each activation of the Neohaler® device depends on factors such as the patient's inspiratory flow rate and inspiratory time. Using standardized in vitro testing at a fixed flow rate of 60 L/minute for 2 seconds, the Neohaler® inhaler delivered 57 mcg of indacaterol per activation from the mouthpiece.

Chronic Obstructive Pulmonary Disease For the long-term maintenance treatment of airflow obstruction associated with chronic obstructive pulmonary disease (COPD), the usual dosage of indacaterol in adults is 75 mcg (contents of one capsule) once daily via the Neohaler® device. Indacaterol should not be used more frequently than one 75-mcg dose in a 24-hour period.

■ **Special Populations** Dosage adjustment is not required in geriatric patients, patients with mild or moderate hepatic impairment, or those with renal impairment. Data are not available in patients with severe hepatic impairment. (See Specific Populations under Cautions: Warnings/Precautions.) Dosage adjustment is not necessary based on the effect of age, gender, and weight on systemic exposure of orally inhaled indacaterol in patients with COPD.

Cautions

■ **Contraindications** All long-acting β_2-adrenergic agonists are contraindicated in patients with asthma without concomitant use of long-term asthma controller therapy; indacaterol is not indicated for the treatment of asthma†. (See Asthma-related Death under Warnings/Precautions: Warnings, in Cautions.)

■ **Warnings/Precautions** ***Warnings*** **Asthma-related Death.** Long-acting β_2-adrenergic agonists increase the risk of asthma-related death. All long-acting β_2-adrenergic agonists are contraindicated in patients with asthma without concomitant use of long-term asthma controller therapy. The safety and efficacy of indacaterol in patients with asthma† have not been established and the drug is not indicated for the treatment of asthma.

Data from a large placebo-controlled safety study (Salmeterol Multicenter Asthma Research Trial [SMART]) showed an increase in asthma-related deaths in patients receiving certain long-acting β_2-adrenergic agonists (e.g., salmeterol) in addition to usual asthma therapy. The increased risk of asthma-related death with salmeterol is considered a class effect of the long-acting β_2-adrenergic agonists, including indacaterol. However, no adequate studies have been conducted to determine whether the rate of asthma-related death is increased in patients receiving indacaterol. (See Advice to Patients.)

Serious asthma-related events, including death, have been reported in patients receiving indacaterol in clinical studies. However, these studies were inadequate to precisely quantify the differences in serious asthma exacerbation rates between treatment groups. In a 6-month, randomized, double-bind, active-controlled safety study in 805 adults with moderate to severe persistent asthma receiving indacaterol (300 or 600 mcg once daily) or salmeterol (50 mcg twice daily) concomitantly with inhaled corticosteroids, 2 respiratory-related deaths occurred in patients receiving indacaterol 300 mcg once daily; no deaths occurred in patients receiving indacaterol 600 mcg once daily or salmeterol. In addition, serious adverse effects related to asthma exacerbations occurred in 2 patients receiving indacaterol 300 mcg once daily, 3 patients receiving indacaterol 600 mcg once daily, and none of the patients receiving salmeterol.

It is not known whether the rate of death is increased in patients with chronic obstructive pulmonary disease (COPD) receiving long-acting β_2-adrenergic agonists, including indacaterol.

Other Warnings/Precautions **Deterioration of Disease and Acute Episodes.** Indacaterol therapy should not be initiated in patients with acutely deteriorating COPD, which may be life-threatening. Indacaterol has not been studied in this patient population. Use of indacaterol in this setting is not appropriate.

Indacaterol should *not* be used for the relief of acute symptoms (i.e., as rescue therapy for the treatment of acute episodes of bronchospasm). Indacaterol has not been studied for the relief of acute symptoms and extra doses of the drug should not be used for this purpose. Acute symptoms should be treated with a short-acting, inhaled β_2-agonist.

When indacaterol therapy is initiated in patients receiving short-acting, inhaled β_2-agonists on a regular basis (e.g., 4 times daily), *regular* use of the short-acting agent should be discontinued, and such agents should be used only for symptomatic relief of acute respiratory symptoms. All patients receiving indacaterol should be provided with and instructed in the use of a short-acting, inhaled β_2-agonist.

COPD may deteriorate acutely over a period of hours or chronically over several days or longer. Failure to respond to a previously effective dosage of indacaterol or to a supplemental short-acting, inhaled β_2-agonist (e.g., increased need for additional short-acting, inhaled β_2-agonists) may indicate deterioration of COPD for which prompt medical attention is indicated. In this setting, immediate reevaluation of the patient and treatment regimen is required. Increasing the daily dosage of indacaterol to exceed the recommended dosage is not appropriate in this situation.

Excessive Use and Use With Other Long-acting β_2-Adrenergic Agonists. As with other inhaled β_2-adrenergic agonists, indacaterol should not be used more frequently or at doses higher than recommended, nor should indacaterol be used concomitantly with other preparations containing long-acting β_2-adrenergic agonists, since overdosage may result.

Clinically important cardiovascular effects and fatalities have been reported in association with excessive use of inhaled sympathomimetic drugs.

Paradoxical Bronchospasm. As with other inhaled β_2-adrenergic agonists, patients receiving indacaterol may develop paradoxical bronchospasm, which may be life-threatening.

If paradoxical bronchospasm occurs, indacaterol should be discontinued immediately and alternative therapy instituted.

Cardiovascular Effects. Indacaterol, like other β_2-adrenergic agonists, may produce a clinically important cardiovascular effect in some patients as measured by increases in pulse rate, systolic or diastolic blood pressure, or cardiovascular symptoms. If such effects occur, discontinuance of indacaterol therapy may be required.

In addition, β_2-agonists have been reported to produce ECG changes, such as flattening of the T wave, prolongation of the corrected QT (QT_c) interval, and ST-segment depression; the clinical importance of these effects is unknown.

Indacaterol, like other sympathomimetic amines, should be used with caution in patients with cardiovascular disorders, especially coronary insufficiency, cardiac arrhythmias, or hypertension.

Metabolic and Electrolyte Effects. Indacaterol, like other sympathomimetic amines, should be used with caution in patients with thyrotoxicosis.

IV doses of the β_2-adrenergic agonist albuterol (IV preparation not commercially available in the US) have been reported to aggravate preexisting diabetes mellitus and ketoacidosis.

Inhalation of high dosages of β_2-adrenergic agonists may result in increased plasma glucose concentrations.

Clinically important decreases in serum potassium or changes in blood glucose concentrations have been reported infrequently during clinical studies with long-term indacaterol therapy and with similar incidence in patients receiving placebo. Indacaterol has not been studied in patients with inadequately controlled diabetes mellitus.

Clinically important hypokalemia may occur in some patients receiving β_2-adrenergic agonists, possibly through intracellular shunting, which may result in adverse cardiovascular effects. (See Cardiovascular Effects under Warnings/Precautions: Other Warnings/Precautions, in Cautions.) However, the decrease in serum potassium concentrations usually is transient and generally does not require supplementation.

Nervous System Effects. Indacaterol, like other sympathomimetic amines, should be used with caution in patients with seizure disorders and in those unusually responsive to sympathomimetic amines.

Specific Populations **Pregnancy.** Category C. (See Users Guide.)

The effects of indacaterol on preterm labor or labor at term are not known. Because of the potential for β-agonist interference with uterine contractility, use of indacaterol during labor should be restricted to those patients in whom the benefits clearly outweigh the risks.

Lactation. Indacaterol is distributed into milk in rats; it is not known whether indacaterol is distributed into human milk. Because many drugs are distributed into human milk, caution should be exercised when indacaterol is administered in nursing women.

Pediatric Use. Indacaterol is not indicated for use in pediatric patients. Safety and efficacy of indacaterol have not been established in pediatric patients.

Geriatric Use. In the pooled 3-month database of clinical studies evaluating indacaterol 75 mcg once daily, approximately 46.8% of patients receiving indacaterol were 65 years of age or older and about 12.7% were 75 years of age or older. No overall differences in efficacy were observed, and adverse effects were similar in patients 65 years of age or older compared with the overall patient population in the pooled 3-month database. Dosage adjustment of indacaterol is not required in geriatric patients.

Hepatic Impairment. No clinically important changes in peak plasma concentration or area under the serum concentration-time curve (AUC) were observed in patients with mild or moderate hepatic impairment. Protein binding also did not differ in patients with mild or moderate hepatic impairment compared with healthy individuals. Indacaterol has not been studied in patients with severe hepatic impairment. Dosage adjustment is not required in patients with mild or moderate hepatic impairment.

Renal Impairment. Indacaterol was not studied in patients with renal impairment because of the minimal contribution of urinary excretion to the total body elimination of the drug. Dosage adjustment is not required in patients with renal impairment.

■ **Common Adverse Effects** Adverse effects reported in more than 2% of patients receiving indacaterol 75 mcg once daily for up to 3 months in controlled clinical studies include cough, oropharyngeal pain, nasopharyngitis, headache, and nausea.

Drug Interactions

Based on in vitro studies, indacaterol is metabolized via hydroxylation (mainly by cytochrome P-450 [CYP] isoenzyme 3A4 and, to a lesser extent, by CYP isoenzymes 1A1 and 2D6), as well as via glucuronidation by uridine diphosphate-glucuronosyltransferase (UGT) 1A1. In addition, indacaterol is a low-affinity substrate of the efflux transporter P-glycoprotein (P-gp).

The manufacturer states that indacaterol is unlikely to substantially inhibit transporter proteins, such as multidrug resistance protein (MRP) 2, breast cancer resistance protein (BCRP), human organic cation transporters (hOCT) 1 and 2, or human multidrug and toxin extrusion (hMATE) transporters 1 and 2K, in vivo; indacaterol has negligible potential to induce MRP2.

■ **Drugs Affecting or Metabolized by Hepatic Microsomal Enzymes and/or the P-glycoprotein (P-gp) Transport System** Data from drug interaction studies of potent and specific inhibitors of CYP3A4 and P-gp (i.e., erythromycin, ketoconazole, ritonavir, verapamil) suggest that systemic clearance of indacaterol is influenced by changes in both CYP3A4 and P-gp activities; the 1.9-fold increase in the area under the serum concentration-time curve (AUC) of indacaterol caused by ketoconazole, a potent inhibitor of both CYP3A4 and P-gp, reflects the effect of maximum combined inhibition of CYP3A4 and P-gp (see Drug Interactions: Ketoconazole). However, dosage adjustment of indacaterol is not required in patients receiving such agents concomitantly with indacaterol 75 mcg once daily.

Results of in vitro studies indicate that indacaterol has negligible potential to cause metabolic interactions by inhibition or induction of CYP isoenzymes at concentrations achieved clinically.

Results of in vitro studies also indicate that indacaterol is unlikely to substantially inhibit transporter proteins, such as P-gp, in vivo; indacaterol has negligible potential to induce P-gp.

■ **Drugs Metabolized by Uridine Diphosphate-glucuronosyltransferase (UGT)** Results of in vitro studies indicate that indacaterol has negligible potential to cause metabolic interactions by induction of UGT1A1 at concentrations achieved clinically.

■ **Drugs that Prolong the QT Interval** Indacaterol, like other β_2-adrenergic agonists, should be used with extreme caution in patients receiving drugs known to prolong the corrected QT (QT_c) interval because of the increased risk of ventricular arrhythmias and because such drugs may potentiate the effects of adrenergic drugs on the cardiovascular system.

■ **β-Adrenergic Blocking Agents** Indacaterol and β-adrenergic blocking agents may interfere with the actions of each other when administered concomitantly. β-Adrenergic blocking agents not only block the therapeutic effects of β-adrenergic agonists, but also may produce severe bronchospasm in patients with chronic obstructive pulmonary disease (COPD). Patients with COPD usually should not be treated with β-adrenergic blocking agents. However, under certain circumstances (e.g., prophylaxis after myocardial infarction), there may be no acceptable alternatives to the use of β-adrenergic blocking agents in these patients; the use of cardioselective β-adrenergic blocking agents may be considered but these agents should be used concomitantly with caution.

■ **Corticosteroids** Concomitant use with corticosteroids may potentiate any hypokalemic effect of indacaterol. (See Metabolic and Electrolyte Effects under Warnings/Precautions: Other Warnings/Precautions, in Cautions.)

■ **Diuretics** Concomitant use with diuretics may potentiate any hypokalemic effect of indacaterol. (See Metabolic and Electrolyte Effects under Warnings/Precautions: Other Warnings/Precautions, in Cautions.)

The ECG and/or hypokalemic effects that may result from the administration of non-potassium-sparing diuretics (e.g., loop or thiazide diuretics) may be aggravated by concomitant β-agonists, especially when the recommended dosage of the β-agonist is exceeded; the clinical importance is unknown. β-agonists and non-potassium-sparing diuretics should be used concomitantly with caution.

■ **Erythromycin** Concomitant administration of indacaterol (single 300-mcg dose) and erythromycin (400 mg 4 times daily for 7 days) increased the AUC and peak plasma concentrations of indacaterol by 1.4- and 1.2-fold, respectively. Dosage adjustment of indacaterol is not required in patients receiving erythromycin concomitantly with indacaterol 75 mcg once daily.

■ **Ketoconazole** Concomitant administration of indacaterol (single 300-mcg dose) and ketoconazole (200 mg twice daily for 7 days) increased the AUC and peak plasma concentrations of indacaterol by 1.9- and 1.3-fold, respectively. Dosage adjustment of indacaterol is not required in patients receiving ketoconazole concomitantly with indacaterol 75 mcg once daily.

■ **Monoamine Oxidase Inhibitors** The manufacturer states that the effects of indacaterol on the cardiovascular system may be potentiated in patients receiving concomitant therapy with monoamine oxidase (MAO) inhibitors; therefore, indacaterol should be administered with extreme caution to patients receiving these drugs.

■ **Ritonavir** Concomitant administration of indacaterol (single 300-mcg dose) and ritonavir (300 mg twice daily for 7.5 days) increased the AUC of indacaterol by 1.7-fold; peak plasma concentrations of indacaterol were not affected. Dosage adjustment of indacaterol is not required in patients receiving ritonavir concomitantly with indacaterol 75 mcg once daily.

■ **Sympathomimetic Agents** If other sympathomimetic agents are to be administered by any route in patients receiving indacaterol, the additional agents should be used with caution because the sympathetic effects of indacaterol may be potentiated.

■ **Tricyclic Antidepressants** The manufacturer states that the effects of indacaterol on the cardiovascular system may be potentiated in patients receiving concomitant therapy with tricyclic antidepressants; therefore, indacaterol should be administered with extreme caution to patients receiving these drugs.

■ **Verapamil** Concomitant administration of indacaterol (single 300-mcg dose) and verapamil (80 mg 3 times daily for 4 days) increased the AUC and peak plasma concentrations of indacaterol by 2- and 1.5-fold, respectively. Dosage adjustment of indacaterol is not required in patients receiving verapamil concomitantly with indacaterol 75 mcg once daily.

■ **Xanthine Derivatives** Concomitant use with xanthine derivatives may potentiate any hypokalemic effect of indacaterol. (See Metabolic and Electrolyte Effects under Warnings/Precautions: Other Warnings/Precautions, in Cautions.)

Description

Indacaterol maleate, a synthetic sympathomimetic amine, is a relatively selective, long-acting β_2-agonist. Similar to the selectivity profile of formoterol, indacaterol has more than 24- or 20-fold greater agonist activity at β_2-adrenergic receptors compared with β_1- or β_3-adrenergic receptors, respectively; the clinical importance is unknown. The drug's β_2-adrenergic effects appear to result from stimulation of the production of cyclic adenosine-3′,5′-monophosphate (cAMP) by activation of adenyl cyclase. Increased concentrations of cAMP are associated with relaxation of bronchial smooth muscle. Indacaterol appears to inhibit immunoglobulin E (IgE)-dependent release of mediators (e.g., histamine) from human lung mast cells. Unlike salmeterol, indacaterol does not appear to antagonize the bronchorelaxant effect of short-acting, inhaled β_2-agonists.

Tolerance has not been observed with long-term indacaterol administration. In two 12-week clinical studies evaluating indacaterol, the improvement in lung function (as measured by forced expiratory volume in 1 second [FEV_1]) observed after 4 weeks of treatment was consistently maintained over the 12-week treatment period in both studies.

Indacaterol is metabolized via hydroxylation (mainly by cytochrome P-450 [CYP] isoenzyme 3A4 and, to a lesser extent, by CYP isoenzymes 1A1 and 2D6), as well as via glucuronidation by uridine diphosphate-glucuronosyltransferase (UGT) 1A1. In addition, indacaterol is a low-affinity substrate of the efflux transporter P-glycoprotein (P-gp). Indacaterol is eliminated mainly in feces and, to a lesser extent, in urine; at least 90% of a dose is recovered in feces and renal elimination accounts for about 2–6% of systemic clearance. About 54 and 23% of a dose of indacaterol is eliminated in feces as unchanged drug and hydroxylated indacaterol metabolites, respectively; generally, less than 2% of a dose is eliminated in urine as unchanged drug. The average terminal and effective half-lives of indacaterol are approximately 45.5–126 and 40–56 hours, respectively.

In a pharmacokinetic study of indacaterol in individuals with the UGT1A1 (TA)7/(TA)7 genotype (low UGT1A1 expression; also referred to as UGT1A1*28/*28) and the (TA)6/(TA)6 genotype, the steady-state area under the serum concentration-time curve (AUC) and peak plasma concentration of indacaterol were 1.2-fold higher in individuals with the (TA)7/(TA)7 genotype suggesting no relevant effect of the UGT1A1 genotype on indacaterol exposure.

Advice to Patients

A copy of the manufacturer's patient information (medication guide) for indacaterol should be provided to all patients each time the drug is dispensed. Importance of instructing patients to read the medication guide prior to initiation of therapy and each time the prescription is refilled.

Importance of informing patients that long-acting β_2-adrenergic agonists, such as indacaterol, increase the risk of asthma-related death and that indacaterol is not indicated for the treatment of asthma.

Importance of adequate understanding of proper storage, preparation, and inhalation techniques, including use of the inhalation delivery system (Neohaler®).

Importance of advising patients using indacaterol dry-powder capsules not to swallow the capsules or to use them with any capsule inhaler other than the Neohaler® device. Importance of advising patients not to use this inhaler with any other capsules. Importance of advising patients to use the new inhaler device provided with each new prescription.

Importance of adherence to dosing schedules, including not altering the dose or frequency of use unless otherwise instructed by a clinician.

Importance of advising patients that if a dose of indacaterol is missed, the dose should be taken as soon as it is remembered; importance of not taking more than one dose in a 24-hour period.

Importance of all patients being provided with and instructed in the use of a short-acting, inhaled β_2-adrenergic agonist (e.g., albuterol) as treatment for acute chronic obstructive pulmonary disease (COPD) symptoms.

Importance of discontinuing *regular* use of short-acting, inhaled β_2-agonists when initiating indacaterol and using short-acting, inhaled β_2-agonists to relieve acute symptoms.

Importance of not using indacaterol to relieve acute symptoms or exacerbations of COPD.

Importance of contacting a clinician immediately if symptoms worsen; the short-acting, inhaled β_2-agonist becomes less effective or more inhalations than usual are required; or a clinically important decline in lung function (as outlined by clinician) occurs.

Importance of advising patients receiving indacaterol not to use additional doses of the drug or other inhaled, long-acting β_2-adrenergic agonists because excessive use of sympathomimetic agents may result in substantial cardiovascular effects or death.

Importance of patients not discontinuing indacaterol therapy without medical supervision, since symptoms may recur after discontinuance.

Importance of informing patients of adverse effects associated with β_2-adrenergic agonists, such as palpitations, chest pain, rapid heart rate, tremor, or nervousness.

Importance of informing clinicians of existing or contemplated concomitant therapy, including prescription and OTC drugs, vitamins, and herbal supplements, as well as any concomitant illnesses (e.g., cardiac disorders, hypertension, seizures, thyroid disorders, diabetes mellitus, allergies to drugs or food).

Importance of women informing clinicians if they are or plan to become pregnant or plan to breast-feed.

Importance of informing patients of other important precautionary information. (See Cautions.)

Overview® (see Users Guide). For additional information on this drug until a more detailed monograph is developed and published, the manufacturer's labeling should be consulted. It is *essential* that the manufacturer's labeling be consulted for more detailed information on usual cautions, precautions, contraindications, potential drug interactions, laboratory test interferences, and acute toxicity.

Preparations

Excipients in commercially available drug preparations may have clinically important effects in some individuals; consult specific product labeling for details.

Indacaterol Maleate

Oral Inhalation

Powder for inhalation (contained in capsules)	75 mcg (of indacaterol)	**Arcapta® Neohaler®**, Novartis

†Use is not currently included in the labeling approved by the US Food and Drug Administration

Olodaterol Hydrochloride

■ Olodaterol hydrochloride, a synthetic sympathomimetic amine, is a relatively selective, long-acting β_2-adrenergic agonist.

Uses

■ **Bronchospasm** ***Chronic Obstructive Pulmonary Disease*** Olodaterol hydrochloride is used as a bronchodilator alone or in fixed combination with tiotropium bromide for the long-term maintenance treatment of airflow obstruction associated with chronic obstructive pulmonary disease (COPD), including chronic bronchitis and emphysema. Olodaterol hydrochloride alone or in combination with tiotropium bromide is *not* indicated for the treatment of acute bronchospasm or for the treatment of asthma†; the safety and efficacy of olodaterol in asthma† have not been established.

Efficacy of olodaterol has been evaluated in 4 randomized, double-blind, placebo- or placebo- and active-controlled studies of 48 weeks' duration in 3104 adults 40 years of age or older with moderate to severe COPD. The primary outcome measures were the change from baseline in forced expiratory volume in 1 second (FEV_1) area under the curve (AUC) from 0–3 hours and in trough FEV_1 after 12 weeks of therapy in 2 trials and after 24 weeks in the other 2 trials. Across these studies, orally inhaled olodaterol 5 mcg once daily improved FEV_1 AUC from 0–3 hours and trough FEV_1 at 12 weeks by 130–180 and 30–80 mL, respectively, compared with placebo; differences in FEV_1 AUC from 0–3 hours compared with placebo were demonstrated at 12 and 24 weeks in all 4 trials, and differences in trough FEV_1 compared with placebo were observed in 3 trials at 12 weeks and in all 4 trials at 24 weeks. Patients receiving olodaterol 5 mcg required less albuterol as rescue therapy compared with those receiving placebo. Olodaterol 5 mcg demonstrated a bronchodilatory treatment effect at 5 minutes after the first dose with a mean increase in FEV_1 of 110 mL compared with placebo.

While olodaterol doses of 2, 5, 10, and 20 mcg as well as various dosage regimens including once-daily or twice-daily dosing were evaluated in clinical studies, the US Food and Drug Administration (FDA)-approved labeling includes only the 5-mcg once-daily dosage of olodaterol for the long-term maintenance treatment of airflow obstruction associated with COPD. No additional benefit of olodaterol 20 mcg compared with the 10-mcg dose or olodaterol 10 mcg compared with the 5-mcg dose was observed. In addition, no additional benefit was observed with twice-daily compared with once-daily dosing of olodaterol.

The bronchodilatory profile of olodaterol 5 mcg over the 24-hour dosing interval was evaluated in 4 randomized, double-blind, placebo- and active-controlled crossover trials of 6 weeks' duration in 429 patients with moderate to severe COPD. The primary outcome measures were the change from baseline in FEV_1 AUC from 0–12 hours and change from baseline in trough FEV_1 AUC from 12–24 hours after 6 weeks of therapy. In these studies, orally inhaled olodaterol 5 mcg once daily improved FEV_1 AUC from 0–12 hours and FEV_1 AUC from 12–24 hours at 6 weeks by 150–200 and 110–150 mL, respectively, compared with placebo. Trough FEV_1 improved by 100–130 mL with olodaterol 5 mcg once daily compared with placebo at 6 weeks.

Efficacy of olodaterol in fixed combination with tiotropium bromide was based principally on 2 dose-ranging studies of 4 weeks' duration and 2 confirmatory, active-controlled studies of 52 weeks' duration. In the 2 randomized, double-blind, active-controlled, parallel-group trials, efficacy of olodaterol in combination with tiotropium was evaluated in 5162 patients 40 years of age or older with moderate to very severe COPD. The primary outcome measures were the change from baseline in FEV_1 AUC from 0–3 hours and trough FEV_1 after 24 weeks of therapy. All study medications were administered once daily in the morning via the Respimat® inhaler. In these studies, FEV_1 AUC from 0–3 hours at 24 weeks was improved by 256–268 mL with orally inhaled olodaterol 5 mcg in combination with tiotropium 5 mcg compared with improvements of 133–136 or 139–165 mL with either olodaterol 5 mcg or tiotropium 5 mcg, respectively, alone. Trough FEV_1 at 24 weeks was improved by 136–145 mL with olodaterol in combination with tiotropium compared with improvements of 54–57 or 65–96 mL with either olodaterol or tiotropium, respectively, alone. The increased bronchodilator effects observed with olodaterol in combination with tiotropium were maintained throughout the 52-week studies. Patients receiving the fixed combination of olodaterol and tiotropium required less albuterol as rescue therapy compared with those receiving either olodaterol or tiotropium alone.

For additional information on the treatment of COPD, see Uses: Chronic Obstructive Pulmonary Disease, in Ipratropium Bromide 12:08.08.

Dosage and Administration

■ **Administration** Olodaterol hydrochloride alone is administered by oral inhalation using a specific inhaler (Striverdi® Respimat®) that delivers a metered-dose spray. Olodaterol hydrochloride in fixed combination with tiotropium bromide is administered by oral inhalation using a specific inhaler (Stiolto® Respimat®) that delivers a metered-dose spray. Both inhalers deliver the drugs in an aqueous solution and mechanically produce a fine aerosol mist from the orally inhaled solution. Olodaterol hydrochloride alone or in fixed combination with tiotropium should be administered once daily at the same time every day.

Before first use of either Striverdi® Respimat® or Stiolto® Respimat®, the inhaler cartridge should be placed into the inhaler. The manufacturer's prescribing information should be consulted for detailed information on preparation of the inhalers. The discard date (3 months after the cartridge is inserted into the inhaler) should be written on the inhaler label.

After the cartridge has been inserted into either the Striverdi® Respimat® or the Stiolto® Respimat® inhaler, the unit must be primed prior to first use. Beginning with the inhaler held upright and the cap closed, the clear base should be turned in the direction of the black arrows on the label until a click is heard (one-half turn). The cap should then be flipped until it fully snaps open, the inhaler should be pointed away from the face, the dose release button pressed, and then the cap closed. These steps (turning the clear base until it clicks, opening the cap, actuating the inhaler, and replacing the cap) should be repeated until a spray is visible, and then for 3 additional times. The initial actuation step of the priming process (without the 3 additional repetitions) should be repeated after a period of nonuse (i.e., more than 3 days). If the inhaler is not used for more than 21 days, the entire initial priming process should be repeated.

To administer a dose of olodaterol alone or in fixed combination with tiotropium, the patient should hold the inhaler upright with the cap closed and turn the clear base in the direction of the black arrows on the label until a click is heard (one-half turn). The cap should be flipped until it snaps fully open. Before inhaling the dose, the patient should exhale slowly and completely. The patient should then close the lips around the end of the mouthpiece, without covering the air vents. With the inhaler pointing toward the back of the throat, the patient should press the dose release button while taking a slow, deep inhalation through the mouth; the patient should continue inhaling as long as possible. The duration of inhalation should be at least as long as the spray duration (1.5 seconds). The patient should then hold the breath for 10 seconds (or as long as comfortable). This procedure should be repeated once more to administer the full dose (2 inhalations) of olodaterol alone or in combination with tiotropium. After the full dose is administered, the cap of the inhaler should be closed.

The mouthpiece of either the Striverdi® Respimat® or the Stiolto® Respimat® inhaler, including the metal part inside, should be cleaned using only a damp tissue or cloth at least once weekly. If the outside of the inhaler gets dirty, it can be wiped with a damp cloth. The function of the inhaler is not affected by minor discoloration in the mouthpiece.

■ **Dosage** Dosage of olodaterol hydrochloride is expressed in terms of olodaterol. Each actuation of the Striverdi® Respimat® inhaler delivers 2.7 mcg of olodaterol hydrochloride (equivalent to 2.5 mcg of olodaterol). Dosage of the fixed combination is expressed in terms of drug delivered from the mouthpiece; each actuation of the Stiolto® Respimat® inhaler delivers 2.7 mcg of olodaterol hydrochloride (equivalent to 2.5 mcg of olodaterol) and 3.1 mcg of tiotropium bromide monohydrate (equivalent to 2.5 mcg of tiotropium) per metered spray. The precise amount of drug delivered to the lungs with each activation of the inhaler device depends on factors such as the patient's coordination between actuation of the inhaler and inspiration through the delivery system. Because the Respimat® inhaler mechanically releases the dose, the delivered dose is independent of the patient's inspiratory effort. The commercially available inhalers deliver 60 metered sprays (or 28 metered sprays from the institutional package) (not including the initial priming actuations) equivalent to 30 or 14 doses (2 actuations per dose) of the drug, respectively.

Chronic Obstructive Pulmonary Disease For maintenance therapy of chronic obstructive pulmonary disease (COPD), the recommended dosage of olodaterol in adults is 5 mcg (2 inhalations) once daily via the Striverdi® Respimat® inhaler device. The drug should be administered at the same time every day and no more than one dose (2 inhalations) should be administered in a 24-hour period.

For maintenance therapy of COPD, the recommended dosage of olodaterol in fixed combination with tiotropium bromide in adults is 5 mcg of olodaterol and 5 mcg of tiotropium (2 inhalations) once daily via the Stiolto® Respimat® inhaler device. The drug should be administered at the same time every day and no more than one dose (2 inhalations) should be administered in a 24-hour period.

■ **Special Populations** The manufacturer of olodaterol states that dosage adjustment is not required in geriatric patients or in patients with renal impairment or mild or moderate hepatic impairment. (See Specific Populations under Cautions: Warnings/Precautions.)

The manufacturer of olodaterol in fixed combination with tiotropium states that dosage adjustment is not required in geriatric patients or in patients with renal or hepatic impairment. However, patients with moderate to severe renal impairment should be monitored for anticholinergic effects. (See Specific Populations under Cautions: Warnings/Precautions.)

Cautions

■ **Contraindications** All long-acting β_2-adrenergic agonists are contraindicated in patients with asthma without concomitant use of long-term asthma controller therapy; olodaterol is not indicated for the treatment of asthma†. (See Asthma-related Death under Warnings/Precautions: Warnings, in Cautions.)

Olodaterol is contraindicated in patients with known hypersensitivity to the drug or any other ingredient in the commercially available formulation.

When olodaterol is used in fixed combination with tiotropium, contraindications associated with tiotropium should be considered.

Warnings/Precautions

Warnings

Use of Fixed Combinations. When olodaterol is used in fixed combination with tiotropium, the usual cautions, precautions, contraindications, and interactions associated with tiotropium must be considered. Cautionary information applicable to specific populations (e.g., pregnant or nursing women, individuals with hepatic or renal impairment, geriatric patients) should be considered for each drug in the fixed combination.

Asthma-related Death. Long-acting β_2-adrenergic agonists, such as olodaterol, increase the risk of asthma-related death. All long-acting β_2-adrenergic agonists are contraindicated in patients with asthma without concomitant use of long-term asthma controller therapy. In addition, available data from controlled clinical trials suggest that long-acting β_2-adrenergic agonists increase the risk of asthma-related hospitalization in pediatric and adolescent patients. The safety and efficacy of olodaterol in patients with asthma† have not been established and the drug is not indicated for the treatment of asthma.

Data from a large placebo-controlled safety study (Salmeterol Multicenter Asthma Research Trial [SMART]) showed an increase in asthma-related deaths in patients receiving certain long-acting β_2-adrenergic agonists (e.g., salmeterol) in addition to usual asthma therapy. (See Asthma-related Death and Life-threatening Events under Cautions: Respiratory Effects, in Salmeterol 12:12.08.12.) The increased risk of asthma-related death with salmeterol is considered a class effect of the long-acting β_2-adrenergic agonists, including olodaterol. However, no adequate studies have been conducted to determine whether the rate of asthma-related death is increased with olodaterol. The US Food and Drug Administration (FDA) is requiring manufacturers of long-acting β_2-adrenergic agonists to conduct additional clinical trials to further evaluate the safety of long-acting β_2-adrenergic agonists when used concomitantly with inhaled corticosteroids.

It is not known whether the rate of death is increased in patients with chronic obstructive pulmonary disease (COPD) receiving long-acting β_2-adrenergic agonists, including olodaterol.

Other Warnings/Precautions

Deterioration of Disease and Acute Episodes. Olodaterol should not be initiated in patients with acutely deteriorating COPD, which may be life-threatening. Olodaterol has not been studied in this patient population, and initiation of olodaterol in this setting is not appropriate.

Olodaterol should *not* be used for the relief of acute symptoms (i.e., as rescue therapy for the treatment of acute episodes of bronchospasm). Olodaterol has not been studied for the relief of acute symptoms and extra doses of the drug should not be used for this purpose. All patients receiving olodaterol should be provided with and instructed in the use of a short-acting, inhaled β_2-agonist.

When olodaterol is initiated in patients receiving short-acting inhaled β_2-agonists on a regular basis (e.g., 4 times daily), *regular* use of the short-acting agent should be discontinued, and such agents should be used only for symptomatic relief of acute respiratory symptoms.

COPD may deteriorate acutely over a period of hours or chronically over several days or longer. Failure to respond to a previously effective dosage of olodaterol or to a supplemental short-acting, inhaled β_2-agonist (e.g., increased need for additional short-acting, inhaled β_2-agonists) may indicate deterioration of COPD for which prompt medical attention is indicated. In this setting, immediate reevaluation of the patient and treatment regimen is required. Increasing the daily dosage of olodaterol to exceed the recommended dosage is not appropriate in this situation.

Excessive Use and Use With Other Long-acting β_2-Adrenergic Agonists. Clinically important cardiovascular effects and fatalities have been reported in association with excessive use of inhaled sympathomimetic drugs.

As with other inhaled β_2-adrenergic agonists, olodaterol should not be used more frequently or at dosages higher than recommended, or concomitantly with other preparations containing long-acting β_2-adrenergic agonists, since overdosage may result. Olodaterol should not be used with another preparation containing a long-acting β_2-agonist (e.g., arformoterol, formoterol, indacaterol, salmeterol, vilanterol) for any reason.

Paradoxical Bronchospasm. As with other inhaled drugs, patients receiving olodaterol may develop paradoxical bronchospasm, which may be life-threatening.

If paradoxical bronchospasm occurs, olodaterol should be discontinued immediately and alternative therapy instituted.

Cardiovascular Effects. Olodaterol, like other β_2-adrenergic agonists, may produce a clinically important cardiovascular effect in some patients as measured by increases in pulse rate, systolic or diastolic blood pressure, or symptoms of cardiovascular disease. If such effects occur, discontinuance of olodaterol therapy may be required.

In addition, β_2-adrenergic agonists have been reported to produce ECG changes, such as flattening of the T wave, prolongation of the corrected QT (QT_c) interval, and ST-segment depression; the clinical importance of these effects is unknown. Administration of larger than recommended dosages of orally inhaled olodaterol (10–50 mcg) in healthy individuals resulted in dose-related increases in the QT_c interval; maximum mean prolongation of the QT_c interval compared with placebo after baseline correction was 2.5–8.5 msec. Olodaterol, like other sympathomimetic amines, should be used with caution in patients with cardiovascular disorders, especially coronary insufficiency, cardiac arrhythmias, known prolongation of the QT interval, hypertrophic obstructive cardiomyopathy, or hypertension.

Clinically important effects on heart rate or premature beats were not reported in patients with COPD receiving olodaterol in clinical trials.

Metabolic and Electrolyte Effects. Olodaterol, like other sympathomimetic amines, should be used with caution in patients with thyrotoxicosis.

IV dosages of the β_2-adrenergic agonist albuterol (IV preparation not commercially available in the US) have been reported to aggravate preexisting diabetes mellitus and ketoacidosis. Inhalation of high doses of β_2-adrenergic agonists may cause hyperglycemia in some patients. Olodaterol has not been studied in patients with poorly controlled diabetes mellitus. Clinically important changes in serum glucose concentrations were infrequent in patients with COPD receiving long-term treatment with olodaterol in clinical trials, with an incidence similar to that observed in patients receiving placebo.

Clinically important hypokalemia, which may result in adverse cardiovascular effects, may occur in some patients receiving β_2-adrenergic agonists. (See Cardiovascular Effects under Warnings/Precautions: Other Warnings/Precautions, in Cautions.) However, the decrease in serum potassium concentrations usually is transient and generally does not require supplementation. In patients with severe COPD, hypokalemia may be potentiated by hypoxia or by concomitant treatment; increased susceptibility to arrhythmias may result.

Clinically important changes in serum potassium concentrations were infrequent in patients with COPD receiving long-term treatment with olodaterol in clinical trials, with an incidence similar to that observed in patients receiving placebo.

Nervous System Effects. Olodaterol, like other sympathomimetic amines, should be used with caution in patients with seizure disorders and in those unusually responsive to sympathomimetic amines.

Sensitivity Reactions. Immediate hypersensitivity reactions, including angioedema, may occur after administration of olodaterol. If a hypersensitivity reaction occurs, olodaterol should be discontinued immediately and alternative therapy considered.

Specific Populations

Pregnancy. Category C. (See Users Guide.)

The effects of olodaterol on labor and delivery are not known. Because of the potential for β-agonist interference with uterine contractility, use of olodaterol during labor should be restricted to those patients in whom the benefits clearly outweigh the risks.

Lactation. Olodaterol and/or its metabolites are distributed into milk in rats; it is not known whether olodaterol is distributed into human milk. Because many drugs are distributed into human milk, distribution of the drug and/or its metabolites into human milk is probable. The effects on nursing infants of maternal use of orally inhaled olodaterol have not been evaluated. Olodaterol should be used with caution in nursing women.

Pediatric Use. Olodaterol is not indicated for use in pediatric patients. Safety and efficacy of olodaterol have not been established in pediatric patients.

Geriatric Use. In clinical trials evaluating olodaterol in patients with COPD, approximately 45% of patients receiving the drug at the recommended dosage of 5 mcg daily were 65 years of age or older. In clinical trials evaluating olodaterol in fixed combination with tiotropium for COPD, approximately 40% of patients receiving the drug at the recommended daily dosage were 65 years of age or older, and about 9% were 75 years of age or older. No overall differences in safety and efficacy were observed between geriatric and younger adults. Dosage adjustment of olodaterol is not necessary in geriatric patients.

Hepatic Impairment. Pharmacokinetics of olodaterol were similar in patients with mild or moderate hepatic impairment compared with patients with normal hepatic function. Olodaterol has not been evaluated in patients with severe hepatic impairment. The manufacturer states that dosage adjustment is not required in patients with mild or moderate hepatic impairment.

Renal Impairment. Olodaterol concentrations are increased by approximately 40% in patients with severe renal impairment compared with patients with normal renal function; these increases are not considered clinically important. Olodaterol has not been evaluated in patients with mild or moderate renal impairment. The manufacturer states that dosage adjustment is not required in patients with renal impairment. However, patients with moderate to severe renal impairment who are receiving olodaterol in fixed combination with tiotropium should be monitored for anticholinergic effects.

Common Adverse Effects

Adverse effects reported in 2% or more of patients with COPD receiving olodaterol 5 mcg daily in controlled clinical studies and more frequently than in patients receiving placebo include nasopharyngitis, upper respiratory tract infection, bronchitis, cough, back pain, diarrhea, urinary tract infection, dizziness, rash, and arthralgia.

Adverse effects reported in more than 3% of patients with COPD receiving olodaterol 5 mcg daily in fixed combination with tiotropium 5 mcg daily and more frequently than in patients receiving either drug alone include nasopharyngitis, cough, and back pain.

Drug Interactions

Cytochrome P-450 (CYP) isoenzymes 2C9 and 2C8 are involved in the *O*-demethylation of olodaterol; isoenzyme 3A4 has a negligible role.

Uridine diphosphate glucuronosyltransferase (UGT) isoforms 2B7, 1A1, 1A7, and 1A9 are involved in the formation of olodaterol glucuronides.

Drugs Affecting or Metabolized by Hepatic Microsomal Enzymes

Concomitant use of ketoconazole (400 mg once daily for 14 days), a potent inhibitor of P-glycoprotein (P-gp) and an inhibitor of CYP isoenzymes 3A4, 2C8, and 2C9, resulted in a 1.7-fold increase in peak plasma concentrations and area under the plasma concentration-time curve (AUC) of olodaterol. Because olodaterol was evaluated in clinical trials of up to 1 year at twice the recommended dosage, the manufacturer states that no dosage adjustment is necessary when the drug is used concomitantly with ketoconazole. Concomitant use of fluconazole (400 mg once daily for 14 days), an inhibitor of CYP2C9, had no clinically important effect on systemic olodaterol exposure.

■ **Sympathomimetic Agents** Other orally inhaled preparations containing long-acting β_2-adrenergic agonists (e.g., arformoterol, formoterol, indacaterol, salmeterol, vilanterol) should not be used in patients receiving olodaterol.

Additional adrenergic agents administered by any route may potentiate the sympathomimetic effects of olodaterol. Such agents should be used with caution in patients receiving olodaterol.

■ **Drugs that Prolong the QT Interval** Olodaterol, like other β_2-adrenergic agonists, should be used with extreme caution in patients receiving drugs known to prolong the corrected QT (QT_c) interval (e.g., monoamine oxidase inhibitors, tricyclic antidepressants) because of the increased risk of ventricular arrhythmias and because such drugs may potentiate the effects of olodaterol on the cardiovascular system.

■ **β-Adrenergic Blocking Agents** β-Adrenergic blocking agents may interfere with the actions of olodaterol when the drugs are used concomitantly. Olodaterol also may interfere with the actions of β-adrenergic blocking agents when the drugs are used concomitantly. β-Adrenergic blocking agents not only block the therapeutic effects of β_2-adrenergic agonists, but also may produce severe bronchospasm in patients with chronic obstructive pulmonary disease (COPD). Patients with COPD usually should not be treated with β-adrenergic blocking agents. However, under certain circumstances (e.g., prophylaxis after myocardial infarction), there may be no acceptable alternatives to the use of β-adrenergic blocking agents in these patients; the use of cardioselective β-adrenergic blocking agents may be considered but olodaterol and β-adrenergic blocking agents should be used concomitantly with caution.

■ **Corticosteroids** Concomitant use with corticosteroids may potentiate any hypokalemic effect of olodaterol.

■ **Diuretics** Concomitant use of olodaterol with non-potassium-sparing diuretics (e.g., loop diuretics, thiazides) may increase the risk of ECG changes or hypokalemic effects. Although the clinical importance is not known, caution is recommended when these drugs are used concomitantly with olodaterol.

■ **Tiotropium** Concomitant use of tiotropium bromide, delivered as a fixed-dose combination with olodaterol for 21 days, had no clinically important effect on systemic exposure to olodaterol or tiotropium.

■ **Xanthine Derivatives** Concomitant use of xanthine derivatives may potentiate any hypokalemic effect of olodaterol.

Description

Olodaterol hydrochloride, a synthetic sympathomimetic amine, is a relatively selective, long-acting β_2-adrenergic agonist. In vitro studies have shown that olodaterol's agonist activity at β_2-adrenergic receptors is 241-fold and 2299-fold its activity at β_1-adrenergic and β_3-adrenergic receptors, respectively; the clinical importance of these findings is unknown. The drug's β_2-adrenergic effects appear to result from stimulation of the production of cyclic adenosine-3',5'-monophosphate (cAMP) by activation of adenyl cyclase. Increased concentrations of cAMP are associated with relaxation of bronchial smooth muscle and also may have an anti-inflammatory effect in immune cells (e.g., neutrophils, mast cells). Activation of β_2-adrenergic receptors may also reduce profibrotic activity in human lung fibroblasts.

Steady-state plasma olodaterol concentrations are achieved after 8 days of repeated once-daily inhalation of olodaterol; accumulation of olodaterol is up to 1.8-fold higher following repeated dosing compared with single-dose administration. Peak plasma olodaterol concentrations are reached within 10–20 minutes following oral inhalation. Absolute bioavailability of orally inhaled olodaterol is approximately 30%, principally due to absorption of the inhaled portion of the dose delivered to the lungs. Oral bioavailability of olodaterol is low (less than 1%). Bronchodilation generally persists for 24 hours. The binding, kinetic, and functional properties of olodaterol indicate that the drug forms a stable complex with β_2-adrenergic receptors, with a dissociation half-life of approximately 18 hours. Olodaterol is extensively distributed into tissue. Binding of olodaterol to plasma proteins is about 60% and is independent of drug concentration. Olodaterol is extensively metabolized by direct glucuronidation and *O*-demethylation followed by conjugation. Uridine diphosphate glucuronosyltransferase (UGT) isoforms 2B7, 1A1, 1A7, and 1A9 are involved in direct glucuronidation of the drug, and *O*-demethylation is mediated by cytochrome P-450 (CYP) isoenzymes 2C9 and 2C8, with a negligible contribution by CYP3A4. The unconjugated demethylated metabolite of olodaterol is the only identified metabolite that binds to β_2-receptors, and is not detectable in plasma after repeated inhalation of the recommended dosage of the drug. The effective half-life of orally inhaled olodaterol in patients with COPD receiving 5 mcg daily is 7.5 hours. Following oral administration, approximately 9 and 84% of a radiolabeled dose of olodaterol is excreted in urine and feces, respectively. Following oral inhalation, approximately 5–7% of an administered dose is excreted as unchanged drug in the urine.

Advice to Patients

A copy of the manufacturer's patient information (medication guide) and instructions for use for olodaterol should be provided to all patients each time the drug is dispensed. Importance of instructing patients to read the medication guide prior to initiation of therapy and each time the is refilled.

Importance of informing patients that long-acting β_2-adrenergic agonists, such as olodaterol, increase the risk of asthma-related death and that olodaterol is not indicated for the treatment of asthma.

Importance of adequate understanding of proper storage, preparation, and inhalation techniques, including use of the inhalation delivery system (Respimat®).

Importance of not using olodaterol to relieve acute symptoms of chronic obstructive pulmonary disease (COPD); extra doses should not be used for such symptoms.

Importance of advising patients that if a dose of olodaterol is missed, the dose should be taken as soon as it is remembered. Importance of not taking more than one dose (2 inhalations) in a 24-hour period.

Importance of all patients being provided with and instructed in the use of a short-acting, inhaled β_2-adrenergic agonist (e.g., albuterol) as supplemental therapy for acute symptoms.

Importance of discontinuing *regular* use of short-acting, inhaled β_2-agonists when initiating olodaterol and using short-acting, inhaled β_2-agonists to relieve acute symptoms.

Importance of contacting a clinician immediately if symptoms worsen, the short-acting β_2-agonist becomes less effective or more inhalations than usual are required to relieve symptoms, or a clinically important decline in lung function (as outlined by clinician) occurs.

Importance of advising patients receiving olodaterol not to use other long-acting, inhaled β_2-adrenergic agonists.

Importance of patients not discontinuing therapy without medical supervision, since symptoms may recur after discontinuance.

Importance of informing patients of adverse effects associated with β_2-adrenergic agonists such as palpitations, chest pain, tachycardia, tremor, or nervousness.

Importance of women informing clinicians if they are or plan to become pregnant or plan to breast-feed.

Importance of informing clinicians of existing or contemplated concomitant therapy, including and OTC drugs and dietary or herbal supplements, as well as any concomitant illnesses (e.g., cardiac disease, hypertension, seizures, thyroid disease, diabetes mellitus, allergies to drugs or food).

Importance of informing patients of other important precautionary information. (See Cautions.)

Overview® (see Users Guide). For additional information on this drug until a more detailed monograph is developed and published, the manufacturer's labeling should be consulted. It is *essential* that the manufacturer's labeling be consulted for more detailed information on usual cautions, precautions, contraindications, potential drug interactions, laboratory test interferences, and acute toxicity.

Preparations

Excipients in commercially available drug preparations may have clinically important effects in some individuals; consult specific product labeling for details.

Olodaterol Hydrochloride

Oral Inhalation

Solution for inhalation	2.5 mcg (of olodaterol) per metered spray	**Striverdi® Respimat®**, Boehringer Ingelheim

Olodaterol Hydrochloride Combinations

Oral Inhalation

Solution for inhalation	2.5 mcg (of olodaterol) with Tiotropium Bromide 2.5 mcg (of tiotropium) per metered spray	**Stiolto® Respimat®**, Boehringer Ingelheim

†Use is not currently included in the labeling approved by the US Food and Drug Administration

Salmeterol Xinafoate

■ Salmeterol xinafoate, a synthetic sympathomimetic amine, is a relatively selective, long-acting β_2-adrenergic agonist. The drug is structurally and pharmacologically similar to the short-acting β_2-adrenergic agonist albuterol.

Uses

■ **Bronchospasm** Salmeterol xinafoate is used only with concomitant long-term asthma controller therapy, such as inhaled corticosteroids, as a long-acting bronchodilator for the treatment of asthma and prevention of bronchospasm in patients with reversible obstructive airway disease, including symptoms of nocturnal asthma. Monotherapy with long-acting β_2-adrenergic agonists, such as salmeterol, increases the risk of asthma-related death and may increase the risk of asthma-related hospitalization in pediatric and adolescent patients. (See Asthma-related Death and Life-threatening Events under Cautions: Respiratory Effects.) *Because of these risks, the use of salmeterol for the treatment of asthma without concomitant use of long-term asthma controller therapy, such as inhaled corticosteroids, is contraindicated.* (See Cautions: Precautions and Contraindications.) Salmeterol is used only as additional therapy in patients with asthma who are currently receiving long-term asthma controller therapy, such as inhaled corticosteroids, but whose disease is inadequately controlled with such therapy. The fixed combination of salmeterol and fluticasone propionate is used only in patients with asthma who have not responded adequately to long-term asthma controller therapy, such as inhaled corticosteroids, or whose disease severity warrants initiation of treatment with both an inhaled corticosteroid and a long-acting β_2-adrenergic agonist. Once asthma control is achieved and maintained, the patient should be assessed at regular intervals and therapy should be stepped down (e.g., discontinuance of salmeterol), if possible without loss of asthma control, and the patient should be maintained on long-term asthma controller therapy, such as inhaled corticosteroids. *Salmeterol is not a substitute for corticosteroids; corticosteroid therapy should not be stopped or reduced in dosage when salmeterol is initiated.* (See Cautions: Precautions and Contraindications.) Salmeterol or salmeterol in fixed combination with fluticasone propionate should not be used in patients whose asthma is adequately controlled on a low or medium dosage of inhaled corticosteroids.

In pediatric and adolescent patients with asthma who require the addition of a long-acting β_2-adrenergic agonist to an inhaled corticosteroid, a fixed-combination preparation containing both an inhaled corticosteroid and a long-acting β_2-adrenergic agonist generally should be used to ensure compliance with both drugs. In cases where separate administration of long-term asthma controller therapy (e.g., inhaled corticosteroids) and a long-acting β_2-adrenergic agonist is clinically indicated, appropriate steps must be taken to ensure compliance with both treatment components. If compliance cannot be ensured, a fixed-combination preparation containing both an inhaled corticosteroid and a long-acting β_2-adrenergic agonist is recommended.

Salmeterol also is used for the prevention of exercise-induced bronchospasm. The use of salmeterol as a single agent for the prevention of exercise-induced bronchospasm may be clinically indicated in patients who do not have persistent asthma. In patients with persistent asthma, use of salmeterol for the prevention of exercise-induced bronchospasm may be clinically indicated; however, the treatment of asthma should include long-term asthma controller therapy, such as inhaled corticosteroids.

Salmeterol also is used as a bronchodilator for the long-term symptomatic management of reversible bronchospasm associated with moderate to severe (forced expiratory volume in 1 second [FEV_1] less than 80% predicted) chronic obstructive pulmonary disease (COPD), including chronic bronchitis and emphysema. Salmeterol in fixed combination with fluticasone propionate as the inhalation powder (Advair® Diskus®) is used for the maintenance treatment of airflow obstruction in patients with COPD, including chronic bronchitis and/or emphysema. Salmeterol in fixed combination with fluticasone propionate as the inhalation powder (Advair® Diskus®) also is used to reduce exacerbations of COPD in patients with a history of such exacerbations.

Salmeterol alone or in fixed combination with fluticasone propionate is *not* indicated for the relief of acute bronchospasm. A short-acting inhaled β_2-adrenergic agonist should be used intermittently (as needed) for acute symptoms of asthma or COPD.

Asthma **Considerations in Initiating Antiasthma Therapy.** In the current stepped-care approach to antiasthmatic drug therapy, asthma is classified according to severity upon initial presentation (intermittent asthma or mild, moderate, or severe persistent asthma) and also by response to treatment (i.e., asthma control). While classification of asthma severity is useful for determining initial treatment, disease severity may vary over time and with treatment; therefore, after therapy is initiated, periodic assessment of asthma control is emphasized for guiding treatment decisions. Current asthma management guidelines state that initial therapy for asthma should correspond to disease severity, with subsequent monitoring and adjustments in therapy to achieve and maintain control of asthma according to the goals of treatment. Asthma therapy is aimed at achieving and maintaining control of asthma by reducing ongoing impairment (e.g., prevention of chronic and troublesome symptoms, reducing use of reliever drugs, maintaining normal or near-normal lung function and activity levels) and risk of future events (e.g., exacerbations requiring systemic corticosteroids, treatment-related adverse effects). These 2 components of asthma control (i.e., current impairment and future risk) may respond differently to treatment.

The National Asthma Education and Prevention Program (NAEPP) classifies the levels of asthma control as well controlled, not well controlled, or very poorly controlled. In the stepped-care approach, the treatment step selected for asthma control in patients already receiving asthma therapy is based on the patient's current treatment and level of asthma control. Stepwise therapy is meant to assist, not replace, the clinical decision-making process in selecting therapy for individual patients. Once initiated, treatment is adjusted continuously according to changes in asthma control. Patients should be monitored every 2–6 weeks following initiation of therapy to ensure that asthma control is achieved. If asthma symptoms are not controlled with the current treatment regimen, treatment is stepped up until control is achieved. If an alternative treatment was used and produced an inadequate response, the preferred treatment should be used before stepping up to the next level of therapy. Regular monitoring at 1- to 6-month intervals, depending on the level of control, is recommended to ensure that control of asthma is maintained and that appropriate adjustments in therapy are made. When control has been maintained for at least 3 months, treatment intensity may be stepped down to find the lowest dosage and/or number of drugs required to maintain asthma control, with continued follow-up at 3-month intervals.

Intermittent Asthma. Drugs for asthma may be categorized as relievers (e.g., bronchodilators taken as needed for acute symptoms) or controllers (principally inhaled corticosteroids or other anti-inflammatory agents taken regularly to achieve long-term control of asthma). A reliever drug such as a selective short-acting inhaled β_2-adrenergic agonist (e.g., albuterol, levalbuterol, pirbuterol) is recommended on an as-needed basis to control occasional acute symptoms (e.g., cough, wheezing, dyspnea) of short duration; such use of an inhaled short-acting β_2-agonist alone generally is sufficient as initial treatment for newly diagnosed patients whose asthma severity is initially classified as intermittent (e.g., patients with daytime symptoms of asthma not more than twice weekly and nocturnal symptoms not more than twice a month). Most experts consider short-acting inhaled β_2-adrenergic agonists to be drugs of choice for treating acute asthma symptoms and exacerbations and for preventing exercise-induced bronchospasm. Alternatives to short-acting inhaled β_2-agonists recommended by some clinicians for relief of acute asthma symptoms include an inhaled anticholinergic agent (e.g., ipratropium), a short-acting oral β_2-agonist, or a short-acting theophylline (provided extended-release theophylline is not already used), but these alternatives have a slower onset of action and/or a higher risk for adverse effects. Oral β_2-adrenergic agonist therapy is suggested for use principally in patients unable to use inhaled bronchodilators (e.g., young children). Other experts do not recommend oral β_2-agonists for relief of acute asthma symptoms. Use of short-acting inhaled β_2-agonists in asymptomatic asthma should be limited to pretreatment prior to exercise and, in intermittent asthma, should be limited to providing relief as symptoms develop; some clinicians state that patients requiring symptomatic relief more than twice weekly or repeatedly over 1 or 2 days should be evaluated for possible initiation of long-term controller therapy.

Mild Persistent Asthma. When control of symptoms deteriorates in mild intermittent asthma and symptoms become persistent (e.g., daytime symptoms of asthma more than twice weekly but less than once daily, and nocturnal symptoms of asthma 3–4 times per month), current asthma management guidelines and most clinicians recommend initiation of a controller drug such as an anti-inflammatory agent, preferably a low-dose orally inhaled corticosteroid (e.g., 88–264, 88–176, or 176 mcg of fluticasone propionate or equivalent daily via a metered dose inhaler in adults and adolescents, children 5–11 years of age, or children 4 years of age or younger, respectively) as first-line therapy for persistent asthma, supplemented by as-needed use of a short-acting, inhaled β_2-agonist. Alternatives to low-dose inhaled corticosteroids for mild persistent asthma include certain leukotriene modifiers (i.e., montelukast, zafirlukast), extended-release theophylline, or mast-cell stabilizers (i.e., cromolyn, nedocromil [preparations for oral inhalation no longer commercially available in the US]), but these therapies are less effective and not preferred as initial therapy. Some experts recommend that long-term control therapy be considered in infants and young children who have identifiable risk factors for asthma and who in the previous year have had 4 or more episodes of wheezing that lasted more than 1 day and symptoms that affected sleep. Low-dose inhaled corticosteroids also are recommended as the preferred initial therapy in such children. Cromolyn sodium is suggested (based on extrapolation of data from studies in older children) or montelukast is recommended by some experts as alternative, but not preferred, therapy in children 4 years of age or younger with mild persistent asthma. Other experts do not consider mast cell stabilizers or extended-release theophylline to be acceptable alternatives to inhaled corticosteroids for routine use as initial long-term therapy in such patients.

Moderate Persistent Asthma. According to current asthma management guidelines, therapy with a long-acting inhaled β_2-agonist such as salmeterol or formoterol generally is recommended in adults and adolescents who have moderate persistent asthma and daily asthmatic symptoms that are inadequately controlled following addition of low-dose inhaled corticosteroids to as-needed inhaled β_2-agonist treatment. However, NAEPP recommends that the beneficial effects of long-acting inhaled β_2-agonists should be weighed carefully against the increased risk (although uncommon) of severe asthma exacerbations and asthma-related deaths associated with daily use of such agents. (See Asthma-related Death and Life-threatening Events under Cautions: Respiratory Effects and also see Uses: Bronchospasm.) Current asthma management guidelines also state that an alternative, but equally preferred option for management of moderate persistent asthma that is not adequately controlled with a low dosage of inhaled corticosteroid is to increase the maintenance dosage to a medium dosage (e.g., exceeding 264 but not more than 440 mcg of fluticasone propionate [or its equivalent] daily via a metered-dose inhaler in adults and adolescents). Alternative less effective therapies that may be added to a low dosage of inhaled corticosteroid include an oral extended-release theophylline or certain leukotriene modifiers (i.e., montelukast, zafirlukast).

Limited data are available in infants and children 11 years of age or younger with moderate persistent asthma, and recommendations of care are based on expert opinion and extrapolation from studies in adults. According to current asthma management guidelines, a long-acting inhaled β_2-agonist (i.e., salmeterol, formoterol), a leukotriene modifier (i.e., montelukast, zafirlukast), or extended-release theophylline (with appropriate monitoring) may be added to low-dose inhaled corticosteroid therapy in children 5–11 years of age. Because comparative data establishing relative efficacy of these agents in this age group are lacking, there is no clearly preferred agent for use as adjunctive therapy with a low-dose inhaled corticosteroid for treatment of asthma in these children. In children 5–11 years of age with moderate persistent asthma that is not controlled with a low dosage of an inhaled corticosteroid, another preferred option according to current asthma management guidelines is to increase the maintenance dosage of the inhaled corticosteroid to a medium dosage (e.g., exceeding 176 but not more than 352 mcg of fluticasone propionate [or its equivalent] daily via a metered dose inhaler). In infants and children 4 years of age or younger with moderate persistent asthma that is not controlled by a low dosage of an inhaled corticosteroid, the only preferred option is to increase the maintenance dosage of the inhaled corticosteroid to a medium dosage (e.g., exceeding 176 but not more than 352 mcg of fluticasone propionate [or its equivalent] daily via a metered-dose inhaler).

Severe Persistent Asthma. Maintenance therapy with an inhaled corticosteroid at medium dosages or high dosages (e.g., exceeding 440 mcg of fluticasone propionate in adults and adolescents or 352 mcg in children 5–11 years of age [or its equivalent] daily via a metered-dose inhaler) and adjunctive therapy with a long-acting inhaled β_2-agonist is the preferred treatment according to current asthma management guidelines in adults and children 5 years of age or older with severe persistent asthma (i.e., continuous daytime asthma symptoms, nighttime symptoms 7 times per week). Such recommendations in children 5–11 years of age are based on expert opinion and extrapolation from studies in adolescents and adults. Alternatives to a long-acting inhaled β_2-agonist for severe persistent asthma in adults and children 5 years of age or older receiving medium-dose inhaled corticosteroids include extended-release theophylline or certain leukotriene modifiers (i.e., montelukast, zafirlukast), but these therapies are generally not preferred. Omalizumab may be considered in adolescents and adults with severe asthma with an allergic component who are inadequately controlled with high-dose inhaled corticosteroids and a long-acting β_2-agonist. In infants and children 4 years of age or younger with severe asthma, maintenance therapy with an inhaled corticosteroid at medium or high dosages (e.g., exceeding 352 mcg of fluticasone propionate [or its equivalent] daily via a metered-dose inhaler) and adjunctive therapy with either a long-acting inhaled β_2-agonist or montelukast is the only preferred treatment according to current asthma management guidelines. Recommendations for care of infants and children with severe asthma are based on expert opinion and extrapolation from studies in older children.

Poorly Controlled Asthma. If asthma symptoms in adults and children 5 years of age or older with moderate to severe asthma are very poorly controlled (at least 2 exacerbations per year requiring oral corticosteroids) with low to high maintenance dosages of the inhaled corticosteroid and a long-acting inhaled β_2-agonist bronchodilator, a short course (3–10 days) of an oral corticosteroid may be added to gain prompt control of asthma. In infants and children 4 years of age or younger with moderate to severe asthma who are very poorly controlled (more than 3 exacerbations per year requiring corticosteroids) with medium to high maintenance dosages of an inhaled corticosteroid with or without adjunctive therapy (i.e., a long-acting inhaled β_2-agonist, montelukast), a short course (3–10 days) of an oral corticosteroid may be added to gain prompt control of asthma.

While clinical efficacy of oral corticosteroids as add-on therapy in adults and children 5 years of age or older with very severe asthma that is inadequately controlled with a high-dose inhaled corticosteroid, intermittent oral corticosteroid therapy, and a long-acting inhaled β_2-agonist bronchodilator has not been established in randomized controlled studies, some experts suggest regular use of oral corticosteroids in such patients, based on consensus and clinical experience. Similarly, some experts, based on consensus and clinical experience, suggest regular use of oral corticosteroid therapy in infants and children 4 years of age or younger with very severe asthma who are not controlled with high-dose inhaled corticosteroid and either a long-acting inhaled β_2-agonist or montelukast and intermittent oral corticosteroid therapy. However, other experts do not consider regular use of oral corticosteroid therapy to be appropriate therapy in children with severely uncontrolled asthma. (See Asthma under Uses: Respiratory Diseases, in the Corticosteroids General Statement 68:04.)

When asthma symptoms at any stage are not controlled with maintenance therapy (e.g., inhaled corticosteroids) plus supplemental short-acting inhaled β_2-agonist bronchodilator therapy as needed (e.g., if there is a need to increase the dose or frequency of administration of the short-acting sympathomimetic agent), prompt reevaluation is required to adjust dosage of the maintenance regimen or institute an alternative maintenance regimen. For additional details on the stepped-care approach to drug therapy in asthma, see Asthma under Uses: Bronchospasm, in Albuterol 12:12.08.12 and see also Asthma under Uses: Respiratory Diseases, in the Corticosteroids General Statement 68:04.

Clinical Experience with Salmeterol. The initial studies supporting the indication of salmeterol for the treatment of asthma did not require the regular use of inhaled corticosteroids. However, for the treatment of asthma, salmeterol currently is indicated only as concomitant therapy with long-term asthma controller therapy, such as inhaled corticosteroids. (See Uses: Bronchospasm and also see Asthma-related Death and Life-threatening Events under Cautions: Respiratory Effects.)

Results of a limited number of comparative studies suggest that salmeterol oral inhalation powder is more effective than orally inhaled albuterol or placebo in producing bronchodilation (e.g., as determined by mean peak expiratory flow rate) and reducing nighttime awakenings, and more effective than placebo in reducing the need for rescue medication (e.g., intermittent use of a short-acting, β_2-agonist bronchodilator to control asthma exacerbations). While published studies have reported a salmeterol dose of 25 mcg per inhalation of salmeterol aerosol alone (e.g., 50 mcg per 2 metered sprays) or in fixed combination with fluticasone propionate, this is the amount released during actuation from the valve stem; the dose delivered to the patient through the mouthpiece (actuator) is approximately 21 mcg per inhalation (e.g., 42 mcg per 2 metered sprays). In the Uses section, unless otherwise stated, the dose of salmeterol (as salmeterol xinafoate) administered as the aerosol is expressed in terms of the dose delivered from the mouthpiece.

In a clinical study in patients with mild to moderate asthma, some of whom were receiving concomitant therapy with orally inhaled corticosteroids, inhaled salmeterol powder 50 mcg twice daily was more effective than inhaled albuterol 180 mcg 4 times daily in improving pulmonary function (as measured by forced expiratory volume in 1 second [FEV_1] and PEFR), alleviating respiratory symptoms, and reducing the need for supplemental albuterol oral inhalations. In a 12-week comparative study in patients with mild to moderate persistent asthma who were symptomatic despite receiving low to intermediate dosages of inhaled corticosteroids, salmeterol inhalation powder (50 mcg twice daily) was more effective than montelukast (10 mg daily) in improving lung function (morning PEFR) and asthma symptoms. Data from comparative studies in patients receiving salmeterol inhalation aerosol (no longer commercially available in the US) versus orally inhaled terbutaline, cromolyn sodium, or nedocromil sodium (preparations for oral inhalation no longer commercially available in the US) or individualized oral extended-release theophylline therapy also suggest greater efficacy of salmeterol therapy.

Evidence from a limited number of comparative studies in patients with mild to moderate asthma, including those who did or did not receive concurrent inhaled corticosteroid therapy, suggests similar efficacy and safety of salmeterol oral inhalation powder administered via the Serevent® Diskus® device and orally inhaled salmeterol aerosol (no longer commercially available in the US). However, the manufacturer states that clinical equivalence of salmeterol oral inhalation powder and oral inhalation aerosol should not be assumed in all patient populations. In a short-term (12-week), randomized clinical trial in children 4–11 years of age with mild to moderate asthma who did or did not receive concurrent inhaled corticosteroid therapy, therapy with salmeterol oral inhalation powder (50 mcg twice daily) administered via the Serevent® Diskus® device (with or without concurrent inhaled corticosteroids) produced improvements in peak expiratory flow rate (36–39% postdose increase compared with baseline) and FEV_1 (32–33% postdose increase from baseline).

Prolonged use of some sympathomimetic amines (e.g., albuterol, isoproterenol, terbutaline) in the treatment of chronic asthma or COPD may lead to tolerance to the bronchodilating effects of these drugs, and it has been suggested that prolonged stimulation of β_2-adrenergic receptors by salmeterol may have a greater potential to induce tolerance to bronchodilation than short-acting β_2-agonists. However, in several studies of 1–12 months' duration in patients with mild to moderately severe asthma, salmeterol inhalation aerosol (no longer commercially available) remained effective over the study period as indicated by increases in FEV_1 and PEFR and decreases in diurnal variation in PEFR, asthma symptoms, frequency of asthma exacerbations, and the need for additional relief medication.

Because of its long duration of action, salmeterol may be particularly useful for the management of asthma in patients who have nocturnal symptoms despite maintenance therapy with inhaled or oral corticosteroids, extended-release theophylline, and/or other drug therapy. Comparative studies in patients with moderate asthma and nocturnal symptoms suggest that nocturnal symptoms or the need for nocturnal relief medications was decreased with orally inhaled salmeterol as compared with patients receiving placebo, orally inhaled albuterol, oral montelukast, oral extended-release theophylline, orally inhaled nedocromil sodium (preparations for oral inhalation no longer commercially available in the US), or orally inhaled cromolyn sodium. Combined data from 2 multicenter studies in patients with asthma indicate that the mean percentage of nights with no awakenings increased from 63 to 85% following 12 weeks of therapy with salmeterol oral inhalation powder and from 68 to 71% following 12 weeks of albuterol oral inhalation therapy.

In patients with moderate to severe asthma, combined therapy with inhaled salmeterol and inhaled corticosteroids has been instituted to promote greater control of asthma symptoms. In one clinical study in patients with mild to moderate asthma, the addition of salmeterol inhalation aerosol (no longer commercially available in the US) to therapy with an orally inhaled corticosteroid and an intermittent, short-acting β_2-agonist allowed a reduction in inhaled corticosteroid use while maintaining adequate asthma control.

In other clinical studies in patients with persistent asthma whose symptoms were not controlled by 336–1000 mcg/day of beclomethasone dipropionate, combined therapy with inhaled beclomethasone dipropionate (336–1000 mcg/day) and orally inhaled salmeterol aerosol with chlorofluorocarbon (CFC) propellant (42–84 mcg/day; CFC preparation no longer commercially available in the US) was more effective in improving lung function and in reducing the need for supplemental albuterol than therapy with higher dosages of beclomethasone dipropionate alone (672–2000 mcg/day).

Results from comparative clinical trials in patients with asthma not adequately controlled by 176 mcg/day of fluticasone propionate indicate that combined therapy with inhaled fluticasone propionate (176 mcg/day) and orally inhaled salmeterol aerosol with CFC propellant (84 mcg/day; CFC preparation no longer commercially available in the US) given separately was more effective in improving lung function and asthma symptoms and in reducing the need for supplemental albuterol than therapy with a higher dosage of fluticasone propionate (440 mcg/day). In addition, fewer patients receiving combined therapy experienced asthma exacerbations in these trials.

In several randomized, double-blind, placebo-controlled clinical trials in patients with mild to severe asthma, fluticasone propionate (100, 250, or 500 mcg) in fixed combination with salmeterol xinafoate (42 mcg as salmeterol) as the inhalation powder produced greater improvement in most indices of pulmonary function (e.g., mean percent change from baseline in FEV_1, morning FEV_1 or PEFR) than either drug alone and similar efficacy as concurrent therapy with both agents given separately. In several randomized, double-blind, comparative trials in patients with mild to moderate persistent asthma who were not optimally controlled on their current antiasthma therapy, the fixed combination of salmeterol (42 mcg twice daily) and fluticasone propionate (90, 230, or 460 mcg twice daily) with hydrofluoroalkane (HFA) propellant for oral inhalation via a metered-dose inhaler (Advair® HFA) produced greater improvement in indices of pulmonary function (e.g., mean percent change from baseline in FEV_1 or morning and evening PEFR) than either drug alone. In a comparative clinical trial in patients with asthma who were not controlled on high dosages of inhaled corticosteroids, salmeterol/fluticasone inhalation aerosol (salmeterol 42 mcg/fluticasone propionate 460 mcg twice daily) produced greater or similar improvement in morning PEFR than fluticasone inhalation aerosol (440 mcg twice daily) with CFC propellants (no longer commercially available in the US) or salmeterol/fluticasone inhalation powder (50 mcg of salmeterol and 500 mcg of fluticasone propionate twice daily), respectively.

Supplemental Therapy in Acute Asthma. Salmeterol has a delayed onset of action, and the drug (alone or in fixed combination with fluticasone propionate) should *not* be used for the relief of acute symptoms (i.e., as rescue therapy for the treatment of acute episodes of bronchospasm). In addition, salmeterol, alone or in fixed combination with fluticasone propionate, should not be *initiated* in patients during rapidly deteriorating or potentially life-threatening episodes of asthma since serious acute respiratory events, including fatalities, have been reported in such situations. (See Cautions: Precautions and Contraindications.)

All patients receiving salmeterol alone or in fixed combination with fluticasone propionate should be provided with and instructed in the use of a short-acting, inhaled β_2-adrenergic agonist (e.g., albuterol) as supplemental therapy for acute symptoms. The manufacturer states that when initiating salmeterol alone or in fixed combination with fluticasone propionate in patients who have been taking short-acting, oral or inhaled β_2-agonists on a regular basis (e.g., 4 times daily), these patients should be instructed to discontinue the *regular* use of the short-acting agent and to use short-acting, inhaled β_2-agonists, not salmeterol (alone or in fixed combination with fluticasone propionate), for relief of acute symptoms, such as shortness of breath. *Regular* (e.g., daily) use of short-acting inhaled β_2-agonists does not adequately control asthma symptoms or airway hyperresponsiveness on a long-term basis and is not recommended by current asthma management guidelines. If such symptoms are not controlled with salmeterol plus supplemental bronchodilator therapy (i.e., if there is a need to increase the dose or frequency of administration of the short-acting sympathomimetic agent), immediate reevaluation with reassessment of the treatment regimen is required, giving special consideration to the possible need for adding additional inhaled corticosteroids or initiating systemic corticosteroids; however, the dosage of salmeterol should *not* be increased in such situations. If asthma deteriorates in patients receiving salmeterol in fixed combination with fluticasone propionate, immediate reevaluation with reassessment of the treatment regimen is required, with special consideration given to the possible need for increasing the strength of the fixed combination (higher strengths contain higher dosages of fluticasone propionate only), adding additional inhaled corticosteroids, or initiating systemic corticosteroids. Patients should not increase the frequency of administration of the fixed combination. Patients receiving salmeterol alone or in fixed combination with fluticasone propionate should not use additional salmeterol or other long-acting inhaled β_2-agonists (e.g., arformoterol, formoterol) for any indication. (See Cautions: Precautions and Contraindications.)

Concerns about the safety of *regular* use of short-acting inhaled β_2-agonist bronchodilators for maintenance therapy of asthma have been raised by evidence from some studies suggesting increased morbidity and mortality in patients receiving long-term therapy with short-acting inhaled β-agonists, particularly fenoterol (currently not commercially available in the US). In a placebo-controlled, crossover study in which intermittent use of inhaled fenoterol was compared with regularly scheduled use of the drug, regular use over a 24-week period was associated with deterioration in asthma control as determined by peak expiratory flow rate (PEFR), symptoms, and use of additional inhaled bronchodilator. However, the design and interpretation of these study findings suggesting increased morbidity and mortality have been criticized, and reanalysis of these data demonstrated that the differences between treatment periods were small and unlikely to be clinically important. Data from case-control studies have been conflicting and have not demonstrated a causal relationship between inhaled β_2-agonist therapy and asthma mortality. An alternative hypothesis to explain the apparent association between inhaled β-agonist use and asthma mortality is that increased use of β-agonist therapy is a marker of severe asthma. While some studies in patients with mild or moderate asthma suggest that regularly scheduled use of short-acting, inhaled β_2-agonists may not cause harm, such use does not appear to have demonstrable advantages compared with intermittent use and does not adequately control asthmatic symptoms. Regular, daily use of a short-acting, inhaled β_2-agonist generally is not recommended, and increased chronic use of such β_2-agonists more than twice weekly (excluding use for exercise-induced bronchospasm) or acute use (e.g., repeated use over more than 1–2 days) for asthma deterioration may indicate the need to initiate or increase long-term control therapy for asthma.

Monotherapy with long-acting β_2-adrenergic agonists, such as salmeterol, increases the risk of asthma-related death and may increase the risk of asthma-related hospitalization in pediatric and adolescent patients. Data from a large study evaluating the safety of salmeterol in patients with asthma showed an increase in asthma-related deaths in patients receiving salmeterol, particularly in African-American patients. (See Asthma-related Death and Life-threatening Events under Cautions: Respiratory Effects and see Uses: Bronchospasm.)

Exercise-Induced Bronchospasm Salmeterol is used for the prevention of exercise-induced bronchospasm. However, most experts consider short-acting inhaled β_2-adrenergic agonists to be drugs of choice for prevention of exercise-induced bronchospasm. The manufacturer states that the use of salmeterol as a single agent for the prevention of exercise-induced bronchospasm may be clinically indicated in patients who do not have persistent asthma. The manufacturer also states that in patients with persistent asthma, the use of salmeterol for the prevention of exercise-induced bronchospasm may be clinically indicated; however, the treatment of asthma should include long-term asthma controller therapy, such as inhaled corticosteroids. Experts from the NAEPP state that frequent or chronic use of a long-acting inhaled β_2-agonist for exercise-induced bronchospasm should be discouraged. Such use may disguise poorly controlled persistent asthma, which should be managed with daily anti-inflammatory therapy.

Protection against exercise-induced bronchospasm has been noted in children (4–11 years of age) in controlled trials with salmeterol inhalation powder (50 mcg 0.5 hour prior to exercise); in 2 single-dose trials, protection against exercise-induced bronchoconstriction (as measured by a decrease in FEV_1 with exercise) lasted up to 11.5 hours following the dose. In 2 single-dose, comparative clinical trials in adults and adolescents, salmeterol inhalation aerosol with CFC propellant (42 mcg; CFC preparation no longer commercially available in the US) and inhalation powder (50 mcg) demonstrated similar efficacy and safety for the prevention of exercise-induced bronchospasm. However, continued dosing with salmeterol oral inhalation aerosol (42 mcg once or twice daily for 4 weeks) has been associated with loss or waning of protection against exercise-induced bronchospasm in some patients or a decreased duration of such protection.

Chronic Obstructive Pulmonary Disease Salmeterol is used as a bronchodilator for the long-term symptomatic treatment of reversible bronchospasm associated with COPD, including chronic bronchitis and emphysema. Salmeterol in fixed combination with fluticasone propionate as the inhalation powder (Advair® Diskus®) is used for the maintenance treatment of airflow obstruction in patients with COPD, including chronic bronchitis and/or emphysema. Salmeterol in fixed combination with fluticasone propionate as the inhalation powder (Advair® Diskus®) also is used to reduce exacerbations of COPD in patients with a history of such exacerbations. Because of its slow onset of action, orally inhaled salmeterol is *not* indicated as monotherapy for the initial treatment of acute episodes of bronchospasm or acute exacerbations of COPD; a drug with a shorter onset of action (e.g., a short-acting β_2-adrenergic agonist) may be preferred in such cases.

In the stepped-care approach to COPD drug therapy, mild, intermittent symptoms and minimal lung impairment (e.g., FEV_1 at least 80% of predicted) can be treated with a short-acting, selective inhaled β_2-adrenergic agonist (e.g., albuterol) as needed for acute symptoms. For the treatment of persistent symptoms not relieved by as-needed therapy with ipratropium or a short-acting, selective inhaled β_2-agonist in patients with moderate to severe COPD (e.g., FEV_1 30 to less than 80% of predicted value), a long-acting bronchodilator (e.g., orally inhaled salmeterol, formoterol, tiotropium) can be added and a short-acting, selective inhaled β_2-agonist used as needed for immediate symptom relief. Maintenance therapy with long-acting bronchodilators in patients with moderate to severe COPD is more effective and more convenient than regular use of short-acting bronchodilators.

Maintenance therapy (e.g., 4 times daily) with a short-acting, selective inhaled β_2-agonist is not preferred but may be used in patients with persistent symptoms of COPD; such therapy should not exceed 6–12 inhalations daily. Current guidelines for the management of COPD state that low- to high-dose ipratropium (6–16 inhalations daily) can be added to therapy with a short-acting, selective β_2-agonist (as separate inhalations or in fixed combination) in patients with mild to moderate persistent symptoms of COPD, with the frequency of inhalation dosing with either agent not to exceed 4 times daily; the high dosage of ipratropium included in some guidelines for COPD exceeds the manufacturer's maximum recommended dosage (12 inhalations). Combining bronchodilators from different classes and with differing durations of action may increase the degree of bronchodilation with a similar or lower frequency of adverse effects.

For patients not responding to treatment with a long-acting bronchodilator, a combination of several long-acting bronchodilators such as tiotropium and a long-acting β-adrenergic agonist may be used. A short-acting bronchodilator may be used as needed for relief of acute symptoms that occur despite regular use of long-acting bronchodilators. For treatment of severe to very severe COPD (e.g., FEV_1 less than 30 to less than 50% of predicted value, history of exacerbations), the addition of an inhaled corticosteroid to one or more long-acting bronchodilators given separately or in fixed combination may be needed.

If symptoms are not adequately controlled with inhaled corticosteroids and a long-acting bronchodilator or if limiting adverse effects occur, oral extended-release theophylline may be added or substituted. For additional details on the stepped-care approach for drug therapy in COPD, see Chronic Obstructive Pulmonary Disease under Uses: Bronchospasm, in Ipratropium Bromide 12:08.08.

Orally inhaled salmeterol therapy in patients with COPD generally has produced increases in peak FEV_1 averaging 7–20%. In a subset of patients from a short-term (i.e., 24-week) placebo-controlled study in patients with COPD, orally inhaled salmeterol inhalation powder produced improvement in FEV_1 that was apparent on the first day of treatment, sustained over the 12-hour dosing interval, and showed no loss of effectiveness over the study period.

In two 6-month comparative trials in patients with COPD, orally inhaled tiotropium (18 mcg once daily) was more effective in improving FEV_1 than salmeterol (42 mcg twice daily) inhalation aerosol (no longer commercially available in the US) after day 1 of therapy. In addition, while tiotropium or salmeterol each reduced dyspnea and improved FEV_1 compared with placebo, tiotropium also was more effective than placebo in reducing COPD exacerbations and all-cause hospital admissions and improving quality-of-life scores in these trials. In another 6-month, placebo-controlled study in patients with COPD, treatment with tiotropium (18 mcg once daily) was associated with greater improvement in bronchodilation (e.g., FEV_1, evening PEFR), dyspnea, and quality-of-life scores than salmeterol (42 mcg twice daily) oral inhalation aerosol.

In several randomized, double-blind, placebo-controlled studies of 6 or 12 months' duration in patients with COPD, orally inhaled salmeterol (50 mcg twice daily) in fixed combination with fluticasone propionate (250 or 500 mcg twice daily) as the inhalation powder (Advair® Diskus®) produced greater improvement in lung function (defined as predose or postdose FEV_1) than either drug alone or placebo. The improvement in lung function with salmeterol 50 mcg and fluticasone propionate 500 mcg in fixed combination was similar to that observed with salmeterol 50 mcg and fluticasone propionate 250 mcg in fixed combination. In two randomized, double-blind, placebo-controlled studies of 12 months' duration in patients with COPD, orally inhaled salmeterol (50 mcg twice daily) in fixed combination with fluticasone propionate (250 mcg twice daily) as the inhalation powder produced a greater reduction in the annual incidence of moderate/severe COPD exacerbations and exacerbations requiring treatment with oral corticosteroids compared with salmeterol alone. No studies have been conducted to directly compare the efficacy of salmeterol 50 mcg and fluticasone propionate 250 mcg in fixed combination with salmeterol 50 mcg and fluticasone propionate 500 mcg in fixed combination on exacerbations; however, in clinical studies, the reduction in exacerbations observed with salmeterol 50 mcg and fluticasone propionate 500 mcg in fixed combination was not greater than the reduction in exacerbations observed with salmeterol 50 mcg and fluticasone propionate 250 mcg in fixed combination. In a double-blind, placebo-controlled study of 3 years' duration in patients with COPD, orally inhaled salmeterol (50 mcg) in fixed combination with fluticasone propionate (500 mcg) as the inhalation powder did not improve all-cause mortality compared with either drug alone or placebo. Salmeterol 50 mcg and fluticasone propionate 250 mcg in fixed combination twice daily is the only recommended dosage for the treatment of COPD; an efficacy advantage of the higher dosage of the fixed combination containing 50 mcg of salmeterol and 500 mcg of fluticasone propionate over the lower dosage (50 mcg of salmeterol/250 mcg fluticasone propionate) has not been established.

Dosage and Administration

■ **Administration** Salmeterol xinafoate is administered by oral inhalation using a special preloaded oral inhaler (Serevent® or Advair® Diskus®, or AirDuo® RespiClick®) that delivers powdered drug alone or in fixed combination with fluticasone propionate. The manufacturer of the Diskus® devices states that spacer devices should not be used with Serevent® or Advair® Diskus®. The manufacturer of the RespiClick® device states that spacers or volume holding chambers should not be used with AirDuo® RespiClick®.

Salmeterol/fluticasone propionate inhalation aerosol (Advair® HFA) should only be used with the actuator supplied with the product. Before each inhalation, the inhaler must be shaken well for 5 seconds. The aerosol inhaler should be test sprayed 4 times into the air (away from the face) before initial use, and shaken well for 5 seconds before each spray. If the inhaler has not been used for more than 4 weeks or if the inhaler was dropped, the inhaler should be test sprayed twice into the air (away from the face) and shaken well for 5 seconds before each spray.

The cap covering the mouthpiece should be slipped off the mouthpiece; the strap on the cap will stay attached to the mouthpiece. The patient should look for foreign objects inside the inhaler prior to use, and should check to see that the canister is fully seated within the actuator. After exhaling as completely as possible, the patient should place the mouthpiece of the inhaler well into the mouth and close the lips firmly around it. Then the patient should inhale deeply through the mouth while actuating the inhaler. The patient should remove the mouthpiece from the mouth and hold the breath for as long as possible, up to 10 seconds, and exhale slowly. It is recommended that 30 seconds elapse between inhalations. Rinsing the mouth after inhalation of salmeterol/fluticasone propionate inhalation aerosol and spitting out the water are advised. The opening for the spray of the metal canister and the mouthpiece should be wiped with a dry cotton swab and dampened tissue, respectively, at least once a week after the evening dose. The actuator should be allowed to air-dry overnight. When the dose counter on the inhaler reads "020," the patient should contact the pharmacy for a refill or consult their clinician to determine whether a refill is needed. The inhaler should be discarded when the dose counter reads "000." The counter should never be altered or removed from the canister.

For administration of salmeterol xinafoate alone (Serevent®) or in combination with fluticasone propionate (Advair®) inhalation powder via the Diskus® device, the patient should hold the device in one hand, put the thumb of the other hand on the thumbgrip, and push the thumbgrip until the mouthpiece appears and snaps into position. The lever on the Diskus® should then be depressed in a direction away from the patient while the inhaler is held in a level, horizontal position; the lever pierces the foil blister and releases the powdered drug into an exit port. To avoid releasing and wasting additional doses of the drug, the patient should not tilt or close the Diskus® device, play with the lever, or advance the lever more than once at this point. A dose counter will advance each time the lever is depressed. Before inhaling the dose, the patient should exhale as completely as possible; the patient should *not* exhale into the Diskus® device because pressure from the exhalation will interfere with proper inhaler operation. The patient should then place the mouthpiece of the inhaler between the lips and inhale deeply and quickly through the inhaler with a steady, even breath; pressure from the inhalation will disperse drug from the exit port into the air stream created by the patient's inhalation. The patient should remove the inhaler from the mouth, hold his or her breath for 10 seconds (or as long as comfortable), and then exhale slowly. While most patients can taste or feel a dose of drug delivered from the Diskus® device, they should be instructed not to use another dose even if they do not perceive that the dose has been delivered. Rinsing the mouth after inhalation of salmeterol in fixed combination with fluticasone propionate is advised. The Diskus® device may be closed and reset for the next dose by sliding the thumbgrip towards the patient as far as it will go. The inhaler should not be washed but should be stored in a dry place away from direct heat or sunlight. The inhaler should be discarded when every blister has been used, or 4 or 6 weeks after removal of the Advair® Diskus® or Serevent® Diskus®, respectively, from its foil overwrap pouch. The inhaler should not be taken apart.

For instructions on use of the AirDuo® RespiClick® oral inhaler, the manufacturer's labeling should be consulted.

To obtain optimal benefit, the patient should be given a copy of the product-specific patient instructions and medication guide provided by the manufacturer. (See Asthma-related Death and Life-threatening Events under Cautions: Respiratory Effects.)

■ **Dosage** Dosage of salmeterol xinafoate is expressed in terms of salmeterol. Although each blister of the double-foil blister strip in the Serevent® Diskus® device contains 50 mcg of salmeterol as salmeterol xinafoate inhalation powder, the precise amount of drug delivered to the lungs with each activation of the Diskus® device depends on factors such as the patient's inspiratory flow. (See Chemistry and Stability: Chemistry.)

Each blister of the foil blister strip in the Advair® Diskus® device contains 50 mcg of salmeterol as salmeterol xinafoate and 100, 250, or 500 mcg of fluticasone propionate; however, the precise amount of each drug delivered to the lungs with each activation of the Diskus® device depends on factors such as the patient's inspiratory flow. (See Chemistry and Stability: Chemistry.)

Each actuation of the AirDuo® RespiClick® device contains 14 mcg of salmeterol as salmeterol xinafoate and 55, 113, or 232 mcg of fluticasone propionate; however, the precise amount of each drug delivered to the lungs with each actuation of the RespiClick® device depends on factors such as the patient's inspiratory flow.

Each actuation of the oral aerosol inhaler of the fixed combination of salmeterol and fluticasone propionate (Advair® HFA) delivers 50, 125, or 250 mcg of fluticasone propionate and 25 mcg of salmeterol from the valve. Dosages of salmeterol and fluticasone propionate in the fixed-combination inhalation aerosol are expressed in terms of drug delivered from the mouthpiece; each actuation of the inhaler delivers 45, 115, or 230 mcg of fluticasone propionate and 21 mcg of salmeterol from the mouthpiece. The commercially available inhalation aerosol of salmeterol in fixed combination with fluticasone propionate delivers 60 or 120 metered sprays per 8- or 12-g canister, respectively.

The manufacturer states that adjustment of salmeterol dosage alone or in fixed combination with fluticasone propionate is not necessary in geriatric patients.

Asthma **Salmeterol.** When salmeterol inhalation powder is administered via the Serevent® Diskus® device, the usual dosage in adults and children 4 years of age or older is 50 mcg (one inhalation) twice daily, given approximately 12 hours apart. If a dose of salmeterol is missed, the next dose should be taken at the regularly scheduled time; the dose should not be doubled. Higher dosages (e.g., 84 mcg of salmeterol twice daily as the inhalation aerosol; no longer commercially available in the US) have been used in some studies in patients with severe asthma, usually in conjunction with corticosteroids, cromolyn sodium, nedocromil sodium (preparations for oral inhalation no longer commercially available in the US), and/or theophylline; however, such dosages are more likely to be associated with adverse effects, and the manufacturer states that patients should not use more than 50 mcg (1 inhalation) twice daily of salmeterol. Patients receiving salmeterol should not use additional long-acting β_2-adrenergic agonists for any reason.

Patients should contact a clinician if asthma symptoms do not improve after 1 week of therapy. Failure to respond to a previously effective dosage of salmeterol may indicate destabilization of asthma that requires immediate medical attention and reevaluation of the therapeutic regimen. If symptoms arise in the period between doses, a short-acting, inhaled β_2-agonist should be used for immediate relief. However, increasing use of short-acting, inhaled β_2-agonists is a marker of deteriorating asthma; patients in this situation require immediate reevaluation with reassessment of the treatment regimen, giving special consideration to the possible need for adding additional inhaled corticosteroids or initiating systemic corticosteroids. Extra/increased doses of salmeterol should *not* be used in such situations. Patients should be advised to contact a clinician immediately if they experience decreasing effectiveness of short-acting, inhaled β_2-agonists, a need for more inhalations than usual of short-acting, inhaled β_2-agonists, or a substantial decrease in lung function as outlined by the clinician. Patients should adhere to dosing schedules, including not altering the dose or frequency of use of salmeterol unless otherwise instructed by a clinician. (See Cautions: Precautions and Contraindications.)

Salmeterol is not a substitute for inhaled or oral corticosteroids, and patients receiving corticosteroid therapy should be advised *not* to discontinue or alter the dosage of corticosteroids without consulting a clinician, even if the patient has subjective improvement after initiating therapy with salmeterol. When initiating therapy and throughout treatment with salmeterol in patients receiving oral or inhaled corticosteroids for treatment of asthma, patients must continue taking a suitable dosage of corticosteroids to maintain clinical stability even if they have subjective improvement as a result of initiation of salmeterol; any change in corticosteroid dosage should be made only after clinical evaluation. In addition, all patients with asthma should be advised that they *must* continue regular maintenance treatment with an inhaled corticosteroid if they are receiving salmeterol. Patients also should be advised not to discontinue salmeterol without medical supervision because symptoms may recur after treatment discontinuance. (See Cautions: Precautions and Contraindications.)

Salmeterol/Fluticasone Propionate Fixed-combination Therapy. In asthmatic patients 4–11 years of age who are inadequately controlled on an inhaled corticosteroid, the recommended dosage of the commercially available inhalation powder preparation containing salmeterol in fixed combination with fluticasone propionate (Advair® Diskus®) is 50 mcg of salmeterol and 100 mcg of fluticasone propionate (1 inhalation) twice daily, given approximately 12 hours apart.

In asthmatic patients 12 years of age or older, the recommended initial dosage of the commercially available inhalation powder preparation containing salmeterol in fixed combination with fluticasone propionate (Advair® Diskus®) is based on the patient's asthma severity and current asthma therapy, including the dosage of inhaled corticosteroids, as well as the patient's current control of asthma symptoms and risk of future exacerbations. The dosage of the inhalation powder fixed-combination preparation is 50 mcg of salmeterol and 100, 250, or 500 mcg of fluticasone propionate (1 inhalation) twice daily, given approximately 12 hours apart. The maximum recommended dosage of salmeterol in fixed combination is 50 mcg of salmeterol with 500 mcg of fluticasone propionate twice daily. The manufacturer states that administration of the inhalation powder of salmeterol in fixed combination with fluticasone more frequently than twice daily or exceeding 1 inhalation twice daily is not recommended.

When the fixed combination of salmeterol and fluticasone propionate is administered via the AirDuo® RespiClick® device in asthmatic patients 12 years of age or older, the recommended initial dosage is based on the patient's current asthma therapy and asthma severity. For patients with asthma not previously receiving inhaled corticosteroid therapy, the usual recommended initial dosage is 14 mcg of salmeterol and 55 mcg of fluticasone propionate (1 inhalation) twice daily, given approximately 12 hours apart at approximately the same time every day. For patients with asthma switching from another inhaled corticosteroid or fixed-combination therapy, the dosage strength should be selected based on the dosage strength of the previously inhaled corticosteroid alone or in combination as well as disease severity. For patients who do not respond to AirDuo® RespiClick® containing 14 mcg of salmeterol and 55 mcg of fluticasone propionate after 2 weeks of therapy, increasing the dosage may provide additional asthma control. If the dosage regimen does not provide adequate control of asthma, the regimen should be reevaluated and additional therapeutic options (e.g., replacing the current strength of the fixed combination with a higher strength [higher strengths contain higher dosages of fluticasone propionate only], using additional asthma controller therapy) should be considered. The maximum recommended dosage of salmeterol in fixed combination with fluticasone is 14 mcg of salmeterol and 232 mcg of fluticasone propionate twice daily. The manufacturer states that administration of the inhalation powder of salmeterol in fixed combination with fluticasone more frequently than twice daily or exceeding 1 inhalation twice daily is not recommended.

In asthmatic patients 12 years of age or older, the recommended initial dosage of the inhalation aerosol containing salmeterol in fixed combination with fluticasone propionate (Advair® HFA) is based on the patient's current asthma therapy, including the dosage of inhaled corticosteroids, as well as the patient's current control of asthma symptoms and risk of future exacerbations. The dosage of the inhalation aerosol fixed-combination preparation (Advair® HFA) is 42 mcg of salmeterol and 90, 230, or 460 mcg of fluticasone propionate (2 inhalations) twice daily, given approximately 12 hours apart. The maximum recommended dosage of salmeterol is 42 mcg in fixed combination with 460 mcg of fluticasone propionate (2 inhalations) twice daily. The manufacturer states that administration of salmeterol in fixed combination with fluticasone inhalation aerosol more frequently than twice daily or in excess of 2 inhalations twice daily is not recommended.

If control of asthma is inadequate after 2 weeks of therapy at the initial dosage, replacing the current strength of the fixed combination with a higher strength (higher strengths contain higher dosages of fluticasone propionate only) may provide additional asthma control. Patients receiving the fixed combination of salmeterol and fluticasone propionate twice daily should not use additional salmeterol or other long-acting β_2-adrenergic agonists (e.g., formoterol) for any reason, including the treatment of asthma or prevention of exercise-induced bronchospasm. If a dose of salmeterol in fixed combination with fluticasone is missed, the next dose should be taken at the regularly scheduled time; the dose should not be doubled. Patients also should be advised not to discontinue salmeterol in fixed combination with fluticasone propionate without medical supervision because symptoms may recur after treatment discontinuance. If a previously effective dosage of salmeterol in fixed combination with fluticasone fails to provide adequate improvement in asthma control, the therapeutic regimen should be reevaluated and additional therapeutic options should be considered (e.g., increasing the strength of the fixed combination [higher strengths contain higher dosages of fluticasone only], adding additional inhaled corticosteroids, initiating systemic corticosteroids). (See Cautions: Precautions and Contraindications.)

Exercise-Induced Bronchospasm For the prevention of exercise-induced bronchospasm, the usual dosage of salmeterol oral inhalation powder in adults and children 4 years of age or older is 50 mcg administered through the Serevent® Diskus® device at least 30 minutes before exercise. *Additional doses of salmeterol should not be used for 12 hours.* In addition, the manufacturer states that patients who are receiving salmeterol oral inhalation powder twice daily should *not* use additional salmeterol for the prevention of exercise-induced bronchospasm. Patients receiving salmeterol alone or in fixed combination with fluticasone propionate should not use additional salmeterol or other long-acting β_2-adrenergic agonists (e.g., formoterol) for any reason, including prevention of exercise-induced bronchospasm.

Chronic Obstructive Pulmonary Disease **Salmeterol.** For maintenance therapy of bronchospasm in patients with COPD (including chronic bronchitis and emphysema), the dosage of orally inhaled salmeterol given as the inhalation powder (Serevent® Diskus®) in adults is 50 mcg (1 inhalation) twice daily, given approximately every 12 hours. Higher dosages of salmeterol are more likely to be associated with adverse effects, and more frequent administration or administration of higher dosages (i.e., more than 1 inhalation twice daily) of the drug is not recommended by the manufacturer. Patients should not discontinue salmeterol without medical supervision because symptoms may recur after treatment discontinuance.

Salmeterol/Fluticasone Propionate Fixed-combination Therapy. For maintenance therapy of COPD, the recommended dosage of salmeterol in fixed combination with fluticasone propionate (Advair® Diskus®) in adults is 50 mcg of salmeterol and 250 mcg of fluticasone propionate (1 inhalation) twice daily, given approximately every 12 hours. If shortness of breath occurs between doses, an inhaled, short-acting β_2-adrenergic agonist may be administered for immediate relief. Higher dosages of salmeterol in fixed combination with fluticasone propionate (e.g., 50 mcg of salmeterol and 500 mcg of fluticasone propionate) do not result in additional benefit and are not recommended. Patients receiving salmeterol in fixed combination with fluticasone propionate should not use additional salmeterol or other long-acting β_2-adrenergic agonists (e.g., arformoterol, formoterol, indacaterol) for any reason, including the treatment of COPD. Patients should not discontinue salmeterol in fixed combination with fluticasone propionate without medical supervision because symptoms may recur.

■ **Dosage in Renal and/or Hepatic Impairment** The pharmacokinetics of salmeterol or salmeterol in fixed combination with fluticasone have not been studied in patients with hepatic impairment. Since salmeterol and fluticasone propionate are cleared predominantly by hepatic metabolism, impaired liver function theoretically may lead to accumulation of the drugs in plasma. Therefore, the manufacturers recommend that patients with hepatic disease be monitored closely while receiving salmeterol therapy.

The pharmacokinetics of salmeterol in fixed combination with fluticasone have not been studied in patients with renal impairment. Therefore, there are no specific dosage recommendations for such patients.

Cautions

Salmeterol xinafoate oral inhalation appears to be well tolerated when administered in recommended doses. However, monotherapy with long-acting β_2-adrenergic agonists, such as salmeterol, increases the risk of asthma-related death and may increase the risk of asthma-related hospitalization in pediatric and adolescent patients. (See Asthma-related Death and Life-threatening Events under Cautions: Respiratory Effects.) In general, adverse effects reported with salmeterol in controlled studies were similar in type and frequency to those reported with other selective β_2-adrenergic agonists (e.g., albuterol) or placebo. The most common adverse effects of salmeterol oral inhalation powder reported in controlled studies in patients with asthma include headache, influenza, nasal/sinus congestion, pharyngitis, rhinitis, and tracheitis/bronchitis. The most common adverse effects of salmeterol oral inhalation powder reported in controlled studies in patients with chronic obstructive pulmonary disease (COPD) include cough, headache, musculoskeletal pain, throat irritation, and viral respiratory infection. In children 4–11 years of age with mild to moderate asthma, currently available data on adverse effects of salmeterol inhalation powder are derived principally from 2 comparative, 12-week clinical trials with salmeterol (50 mcg twice daily) and albuterol inhalation powder (200 mcg 4 times daily). In adolescents and adults with mild to moderate asthma, currently available data on adverse effects of salmeterol inhalation powder are derived principally from 2 large, 12-week comparative trials with salmeterol (50 mcg twice daily) inhalation powder and albuterol (180 mcg 4 times daily) inhalation aerosol. For adverse effects reported with salmeterol therapy in the Cautions section, a causal relationship to the drug has not always been established.

■ **Cardiovascular Effects** Usual doses of salmeterol oral inhalation generally produce no apparent cardiovascular effects. However, salmeterol may produce a clinically important cardiovascular effect in some patients as measured by pulse rate, blood pressure, and/or cardiovascular symptoms. Although such effects are uncommon after administration of salmeterol at recommended dosages, if they occur, discontinuance of the drug may be needed. In addition, β_2-agonists have been reported to produce ECG changes, such as flattening of the T wave, prolongation of the QT_c interval, and ST segment depression; the clinical importance of these effects is unknown. Hypertension was reported in 4% of patients with COPD receiving salmeterol inhalation powder during clinical trials and also has been reported during postmarketing surveillance. Supraventricular tachycardia or atrial fibrillation has been reported with salmeterol inhalation powder during postmarketing surveillance. Pallor has been reported in 9% of adults and adolescents with asthma receiving salmeterol inhalation powder in clinical trials.

Nonsustained ventricular tachycardia among patients with COPD receiving salmeterol inhalation powder was reported in an incidence similar to that with placebo and fluticasone propionate. The incidence of clinically important ECG abnormalities indicating myocardial ischemia, ventricular hypertrophy, conduction abnormalities, or arrhythmias was lower in patients with COPD receiving salmeterol inhalation powder alone or in fixed combination with fluticasone propionate than in patients receiving placebo. ECG changes, including extrasystoles (supraventricular and ventricular premature complexes), also have been noted with salmeterol inhalation powder. Clinically important prolongation of the QT_c interval, which potentially can cause ventricular arrhythmias, has been associated with administration of large oral or inhaled doses (about 12–20 times the recommended dose) of salmeterol or other β_2-agonists. Fatalities also have been reported in association with excessive use of inhaled sympathomimetic drugs. (See Cautions: Precautions and Contraindications.) Cardiorespiratory arrest has been reported in a patient with COPD and preexisting alcoholic cardiomyopathy who had received usual dosages of orally inhaled salmeterol in conjunction with orally inhaled ipratropium and albuterol. Salmeterol is a highly selective β_2-agonist, and certain cardiovascular effects (e.g., ventricular or nodal arrhythmias, severe tachycardia, anginal-type pain, myocardial ischemia) reported with less receptor-selective β_2-adrenergic agonists such as isoproterenol theoretically may occur less frequently, or not at all, with salmeterol.

■ **Nervous System Effects** In clinical trials with salmeterol inhalation powder, headache was reported in 14% of patients with COPD, 13% of adults and adolescents with asthma, and 17% of children with asthma. Migraine has been reported in at least 1% of patients receiving salmeterol inhalation powder for the treatment of COPD. In clinical studies in adults and adolescents 12 years of age or older with asthma, sleep disturbances and paresthesia occurred more frequently in patients receiving salmeterol inhalation powder than those receiving placebo. Dizziness has been reported in 4% of patients receiving salmeterol inhalation powder for the treatment of COPD. Unrest, depression, anxiety, and vertigo also have been reported rarely with salmeterol oral inhalation therapy. Anxiety has been reported in at least 1% of patients receiving salmeterol inhalation powder for the treatment of COPD.

■ **Respiratory Effects** ***Asthma-related Death and Life-threatening Events*** Monotherapy with long-acting β_2-adrenergic agonists, such as salmeterol, increases the risk of asthma-related death. In addition, available data from controlled clinical trials suggest that monotherapy with long-acting β_2-adrenergic agonists increases the risk of asthma-related hospitalization in pediatric and adolescent patients. *Because of these risks, the use of long-acting β_2-adrenergic agonists, including salmeterol, alone for the treatment of asthma without concomitant use of long-term asthma controller therapy, such as inhaled corticosteroids, is contraindicated.* (See Cautions: Precautions and Contraindications.) However, FDA has concluded that there is no clinically important increased risk of serious asthma-related events, including hospitalization, intubation, or death, associated with concomitant use of long-acting β_2-adrenergic agonists (e.g., salmeterol) and inhaled corticosteroids compared with inhaled corticosteroids alone based on the results of several large clinical studies. In addition, these studies showed that combination therapy with long-acting β_2-adrenergic agonists and inhaled corticosteroids was more effective in reducing the incidence of asthma exacerbations (i.e., events requiring use of systemic corticosteroids for at least 3 outpatient days or an asthma-related hospitalization or emergency department visit requiring use of systemic corticosteroids) compared with use of inhaled corticosteroids alone.

Long-acting β_2-adrenergic agonists, including salmeterol, should only be used as additional therapy in patients with asthma who are currently receiving long-term asthma controller therapy, such as inhaled corticosteroids, but whose disease is inadequately controlled with such therapy. The fixed combination of salmeterol and fluticasone propionate should be used only in patients with asthma who have not responded adequately to long-term asthma controller therapy, such as inhaled corticosteroids, or whose disease severity warrants initiation of treatment with both an inhaled corticosteroid and a long-acting β_2-adrenergic agonist. Once asthma control is achieved and maintained, the patient should be assessed at regular intervals and therapy should be stepped down (e.g., discontinuance of the long-acting β_2-adrenergic agonist), if possible without loss of asthma control, and the patient should be maintained on long-term asthma controller therapy, such as inhaled corticosteroids. Long-acting β_2-adrenergic agonists, including salmeterol alone or in fixed combination with fluticasone propionate, should not be used in patients whose asthma is adequately controlled on a low or medium dosage of inhaled corticosteroids. In pediatric and adolescent patients with asthma who require the addition of a long-acting β_2-adrenergic agonist to inhaled corticosteroid therapy, a fixed-combination preparation containing both an inhaled corticosteroid and a long-acting β_2-adrenergic agonist generally should be used to ensure compliance with both drugs. (See Uses: Bronchospasm.)

Data from a large (approximately 26,000 patients) placebo-controlled study in patients receiving salmeterol xinafoate as part of an asthma treatment regimen showed an increase in asthma-related deaths in patients receiving salmeterol. In the Salmeterol Multi-center Asthma Research Trial (SMART), a 28-week safety study, patients received salmeterol 42 mcg or placebo via metered-dose aerosol with a chlorofluorocarbon (CFC) propellant (CFC preparation no longer commercially available in the US) twice daily in addition to their usual asthma therapy. The primary end point of the SMART study was the combined number of respiratory-related deaths and respiratory-related life-threatening experiences (intubation and mechanical ventilation). Secondary end points included asthma-related deaths and combined asthma-related deaths or life-threatening experiences. The risk of respiratory-related death or life-threatening experience (primary end point) was higher in patients receiving salmeterol versus placebo (relative risk: 1.4) in the SMART trial, although this difference was not statistically significant. However, analysis of secondary end points revealed a statistically significant greater risk for asthma-related death (relative risk: 4.37) or combined asthma-related death or life-threatening experience (relative risk: 1.71) with salmeterol therapy in the overall patient population compared with placebo. Results of a post hoc analysis also revealed a greater risk for asthma-related death (relative risk: 7.26) with salmeterol therapy in African-American patients (18% of study patients) and in patients not receiving concomitant inhaled corticosteroid therapy (53% of study patients) compared with placebo. A greater risk for asthma-related death (relative risk: 5.82) was observed in white patients (71% of the study population) receiving salmeterol therapy compared with placebo; no asthma-related deaths occurred in Hispanic or Asian subpopulations. Factors possibly contributing to the increased numbers of adverse events in African-American patients include the findings that these patients had more severe asthma at baseline than white patients and that fewer African-American than white patients were receiving concomitant inhaled corticosteroid therapy (38 versus 50%, respectively). Results of post hoc analyses in pediatric patients 12–18 years of age (12% of study patients) revealed that the rate of respiratory-related deaths and life-threatening experiences was similar in both the salmeterol and placebo groups (relative risk: 1); however, the rate of all-cause hospitalizations was higher in the salmeterol group compared with the placebo group (relative risk: 2.1). Because of the similar mechanism of action of long-acting β_2-adrenergic agonists, the findings of the SMART study are considered a class effect of these drugs.

A prior 16-week comparative study performed in the United Kingdom (Salmeterol Nationwide Surveillance [SNS] study) also reported a numerically, but not statistically significantly, higher incidence of asthma-related deaths in patients treated with salmeterol (42 mcg twice daily) compared with those receiving albuterol (180 mcg 4 times daily).

The SMART and SNS studies enrolled patients with asthma; no studies have been conducted that were adequate to determine whether the rate of death is increased in patients with COPD receiving long-acting β_2-adrenergic agonists.

In 4 randomized, double-blind, active-controlled clinical trials mandated by FDA, the risk of serious asthma-related events from use of inhaled corticosteroids alone compared with combined use of long-acting β_2-adrenergic agonists and inhaled corticosteroids was evaluated over 26 weeks in 41,297 patients with asthma (3 trials in adults and adolescents 12 years of age or older and one trial in children 4–11 years of age). The primary safety end point in all of these trials was serious asthma-related events, including hospitalization, intubation, and death; these events were reviewed by a blinded committee to determine if the events were asthma related. The 3 trials performed in adults and adolescents were designed to rule out a hazard ratio of 2, and the pediatric trial was designed to rule out a hazard ratio of 2.7; this objective was met in all 4 individual trials. The trials were not designed to rule out all risk for serious asthma-related events associated with long-acting β_2-adrenergic agonists in combination with inhaled corticosteroids compared with inhaled corticosteroids alone.

The safety studies in adults and adolescents included one trial comparing salmeterol and fluticasone propionate in fixed combination as the inhalation powder (Advair® Diskus®) with fluticasone propionate inhalation powder alone, one trial comparing formoterol and mometasone furoate in fixed combination with mometasone furoate alone, and one trial comparing formoterol and budesonide in fixed combination with budesonide alone. In a meta-analysis combining data from these 3 trials, a hazard ratio of 1.1 for serious asthma-related events in patients receiving fixed-combination therapy with long-acting β_2-adrenergic agonists and inhaled corticosteroids compared with patients receiving inhaled corticosteroids alone was reported. Subgroup analyses for gender, adolescents 12–17 years of age, Asian and African-American patients, and obese patients also showed no substantial increase in the risk of serious asthma-related events or asthma exacerbations in these populations.

The trial comparing salmeterol and fluticasone propionate in fixed combination as the inhalation powder (Advair® Diskus) with fluticasone propionate inhalation powder alone included 11,679 adults and adolescents 12 years of age or older with moderate to severe persistent asthma who had a history of asthma-related hospitalization or at least one asthma exacerbation in the previous year requiring treatment with systemic corticosteroids. Patients with a history of life-threatening or unstable asthma were excluded from the study. In this trial, serious asthma-related events were reported in 0.6% of patients in each treatment group, with a hazard ratio for first event for the combination therapy compared with fluticasone alone of approximately 1.

The safety study in children 4–11 years of age included 6208 patients who were randomized to receive salmeterol and fluticasone propionate in fixed combination as the inhalation powder (Advair® Diskus) or fluticasone propionate inhalation powder alone. Patients had a diagnosis of asthma and a history of at least one asthma exacerbation in the previous year requiring treatment with systemic corticosteroids; patients with life-threatening asthma were excluded from the study. Serious asthma-related events were reported in 0.9% of patients receiving salmeterol and fluticasone in fixed combination and in 0.7% of patients receiving fluticasone alone, with an estimated hazard ratio for first event of 1.29 for the combination therapy compared with fluticasone alone. No asthma-related deaths or intubations were reported in either group of pediatric patients.

Other Respiratory Effects Cough was reported in 5% of patients receiving salmeterol inhalation powder for the treatment of COPD. In clinical studies in adults and adolescents 12 years of age or older with asthma, sinus headache was reported more frequently in patients receiving salmeterol inhalation powder than those receiving placebo. Exacerbations of asthma have been reported in 4% of children and 3% of adults and adolescents receiving salmeterol inhalation powder for the treatment of asthma. Tracheitis/bronchitis or influenza occurred in 7 or 5%, respectively, of adults and adolescents receiving salmeterol inhalation powder. Nasal/sinus congestion or rhinitis occurred in 9 or 5%, respectively, of adults and adolescents with asthma receiving salmeterol inhalation powder. Nasal congestion or blockage, rhinitis, or sinusitis occurred in 4% of patients with COPD receiving salmeterol inhalation powder in clinical trials. Pharyngitis, sinusitis, upper respiratory tract infection, and cough occurred in at least 3% of adults and adolescents receiving salmeterol inhalation powder for the treatment of asthma in clinical trials but occurred less frequently than with placebo. However, throat irritation has been reported in 7% of patients with COPD receiving salmeterol inhalation powder in controlled clinical trials. Pharyngitis was reported in 6% of children with asthma receiving salmeterol inhalation powder in clinical trials. Lower respiratory tract signs and symptoms occurred in greater than 1% of children with asthma receiving salmeterol inhalation powder. Lower respiratory viral infection or lower respiratory tract signs and symptoms occurred in 5% or at least 1% of patients, respectively, receiving salmeterol inhalation powder for the treatment of COPD.

Upper airway symptoms of laryngeal spasm, irritation, or swelling, such as stridor or choking, and oropharyngeal irritation, have been reported during postmarketing experience with salmeterol oral inhalation therapy. As with other inhaled drugs, paradoxical bronchospasm, a potentially life-threatening event, also has occurred with salmeterol therapy. (See Cautions: Dermatologic and Sensitivity Reactions.)

Increased airway reactivity and variability or decreases in pulmonary function (e.g., as measured by PEFR or FEV_1), in some cases progressing to respiratory arrest or death, have been reported with regular use (e.g., 2 inhalations 4 times daily) of short-acting, inhaled β-agonists and also in some patients (generally with severe and/or deteriorating asthma) receiving salmeterol oral inhalation powder. Such detrimental effects may be related to down-regulation of β-adrenergic receptors (tolerance), increased responsiveness of airways to allergens and exercise, genetic changes in β_2-agonist receptor gene, or increased airway accessibility to inhaled allergens, which may lead to increased airway inflammation and reactivity and worsening of asthma symptoms. However, increased airway accessibility to inhaled allergens theoretically also would occur with long-acting bronchodilators such as extended-release theophylline.

■ **GI Effects** Hyposalivation, dyspepsia, oral (mouth/throat) candidiasis, or GI infections were reported in at least 1% of patients with COPD receiving salmeterol inhalation powder in clinical trials. In clinical studies in adults and adolescents 12 years of age or older with asthma, nausea has been reported more frequently in patients receiving salmeterol inhalation powder than those receiving placebo. Nausea and vomiting have been reported in 3% of patients receiving salmeterol inhalation powder for the treatment of COPD. In clinical studies in patients with asthma, GI signs and symptoms occurred in greater than 1% of children receiving salmeterol inhalation powder, while oral mucosal abnormality was reported more frequently in adults and adolescents 12 years of age or older receiving salmeterol inhalation powder than those receiving placebo.

■ **Metabolic and Electrolyte Effects** The manufacturer states that large IV doses of the β_2-adrenergic agonist albuterol (IV preparation not currently commercially available in the US) have aggravated preexisting diabetes mellitus and ketoacidosis.

The manufacturer states that clinically important and dose-related changes in blood glucose and/or serum potassium concentrations have been observed infrequently during clinical studies with salmeterol oral inhalation powder at recommended dosages. No clinically important changes in glucose or potassium concentrations were reported in clinical studies in patients with asthma receiving salmeterol oral inhalation powder. In addition, no clinically important changes in serum potassium concentrations were reported in clinical studies in patients with COPD receiving salmeterol oral inhalation powder at recommended dosages. Patients should inform their clinician of the presence of diabetes mellitus prior to initiation of therapy. Salmeterol and other β_2-adrenergic agonists may decrease serum potassium concentrations through increased intracellular uptake of potassium resulting from β_2-receptor mediated Na^+- K^+-ATPase activation in liver and skeletal muscle. Although such reductions potentially may cause adverse cardiovascular effects, the decreases usually are transient and supplemental potassium therapy generally is not required. Hyperglycemia occurred in at least 1% of patients receiving salmeterol inhalation powder for the treatment of COPD. The potential for hyperglycemia or hypokalemia with salmeterol therapy appears to be dose related. Tolerance to the hypokalemic effects of albuterol has been demonstrated but has not been reported to date with salmeterol therapy.

■ **Musculoskeletal Effects** Musculoskeletal pain occurred in 12% of patients receiving salmeterol inhalation powder for the treatment of COPD, and muscle cramps and spasms were reported in 3% of such patients with COPD. In clinical studies in patients with asthma, joint pain was reported more frequently in adults and adolescents 12 years of age or older receiving salmeterol inhalation powder than those receiving placebo, and arthralgia or arthritis occurred in greater than 1% of children receiving the inhaled powder in such trials. Arthralgia or arthritis; muscle, bone, or skeletal pain; musculoskeletal inflammation; or muscle stiffness, tightness, or rigidity has occurred in at least 1% of patients receiving salmeterol inhalation powder for the treatment of COPD in clinical trials.

■ **Dermatologic and Sensitivity Reactions** Immediate hypersensitivity reactions, including urticaria, angioedema, rash, and bronchospasm may occur following administration of salmeterol alone or salmeterol and fluticasone propionate in fixed combination. Anaphylactic reactions have been reported very rarely in patients with severe milk protein allergy after inhalation of powder products containing lactose; therefore, patients with severe milk protein allergy should not receive such products containing salmeterol or salmeterol and fluticasone in fixed combination. (See Cautions: Precautions and Contraindications.) Anaphylaxis also has been reported during postmarketing surveillance studies with the drug.

In clinical studies in adults and adolescents 12 years of age or older with asthma, contact dermatitis and eczema were reported more frequently in patients receiving salmeterol inhalation powder than those receiving placebo. Rash, photodermatitis, or urticaria was reported in 4, greater than 1, or 3%, respectively, of children receiving salmeterol inhalation powder in clinical trials. Rash was reported in at least 1% of patients receiving salmeterol inhalation powder for the treatment of COPD.

Although the mechanism(s) has not been fully elucidated, paradoxical bronchospasm (defined as a decrease of 20% or greater in PEFR) has occurred occasionally with repeated or excessive use of orally inhaled sympathomimetic amines (especially isoproterenol). Preliminary results of a controlled study in almost 12,000 patients demonstrated that paradoxical bronchospasm occurred less frequently with salmeterol oral inhalation than with placebo (either lecithin or oleic acid) given via metered-dose inhaler (no longer commercially available), suggesting that orally inhaled ingredients other than the active drug may be more likely to produce paradoxical bronchospasm.

■ **Other Adverse Effects** Dental discomfort and pain have been reported in at least 1% of patients receiving salmeterol inhalation powder for the treatment of COPD. In clinical studies in patients with asthma, ear symptoms have been reported in 4% of children, and localized aches and pains and fever of unknown origin have been reported more frequently in adults and adolescents 12 years of age or older receiving salmeterol inhalation powder than those receiving placebo. Otic manifestations have been reported in 3% of patients with COPD receiving salmeterol inhalation powder in clinical trials. Edema and swelling have been reported in at least 1% of patients receiving salmeterol inhalation powder for the treatment of COPD. Keratitis and conjunctivitis occurred in at least 1% of patients receiving salmeterol inhalation powder for the treatment of COPD. Pain also has been reported in at least 1% of such patients. Herniated disk has been reported in at least one patient receiving inhaled salmeterol, but a causal relationship to the drug has not been established. A reduction in platelet count has been reported during long-term (1 year) therapy with salmeterol oral inhalation, but platelet count remained within the normal range and the reduction was not associated with sequelae. Elevation of hepatic enzymes was reported in at least 1% of patients with asthma receiving salmeterol oral inhalation powder in clinical studies. However, these elevations were transient and did not lead to discontinuance from the studies.

■ **Precautions and Contraindications** When salmeterol is used in fixed combination with fluticasone propionate, the usual cautions, precautions, and contraindications associated with fluticasone propionate must be considered in addition to those associated with salmeterol.

Patients should be advised to read the product-specific medication guide, patient information, and/or instructions for use prior to initiating therapy with the drug and each time the prescription is refilled.

Patients should be informed that monotherapy with long-acting β_2-adrenergic agonists, such as salmeterol, increases the risk of asthma-related death and may increase the risk of asthma-related hospitalization in pediatric and adolescent patients. (See Asthma-related Death and Life-threatening Events under Cautions: Respiratory Effects.) Patients also should be informed that salmeterol should not be the only therapy used for the treatment of asthma and must only be used as additional therapy when long-term asthma controller therapy (e.g., inhaled corticosteroids) does not adequately control asthma symptoms. Patients should be advised that when salmeterol is added to their treatment regimen they must continue to use their long-term asthma controller drugs. (See Uses: Bronchospasm.)

Salmeterol, alone or in fixed combination with fluticasone propionate, should not be initiated in patients during rapidly deteriorating or potentially life-threatening episodes of asthma or COPD. Salmeterol alone or in fixed combination has not been studied in patients with acutely deteriorating asthma or COPD. Initiation of salmeterol in this setting is not appropriate. Serious acute respiratory events, including fatalities, have been reported when salmeterol has been initiated in patients with substantially worsening or acutely deteriorating asthma. In most cases, these adverse events have occurred in patients with severe asthma (e.g., those with a history of corticosteroid dependence, low pulmonary function, intubation, mechanical ventilation, frequent hospitalizations, previous life-threatening acute asthma exacerbations) and in some patients with acutely deteriorating asthma (e.g., patients with substantially increasing symptoms, increasing need for inhaled short-acting β_2-agonists, decreasing response to usual medications, increasing need for systemic corticosteroids, recent emergency room visits, deteriorating lung function). However, such events also have occurred in patients with less severe asthma. It was not possible from these reports to determine whether salmeterol contributed to these events.

Increasing use of short-acting, inhaled β_2-agonists is a marker of deteriorating asthma and failure to respond to a previously effective dosage regimen of salmeterol alone or in fixed combination with fluticasone propionate often is a sign of destabilization of asthma. In this situation in patients receiving salmeterol, the patient requires immediate reevaluation with reassessment of the treatment regimen, giving special consideration to the possible need to add additional inhaled corticosteroids or initiating systemic corticosteroids. If asthma deteriorates in patients receiving salmeterol in fixed combination with fluticasone, immediate reevaluation with reassessment of the treatment regimen is required, with special consideration given to the possible need for increasing the strength of the fixed combination (higher strengths contain higher dosages of fluticasone only), adding additional inhaled corticosteroids, or initiating systemic corticosteroids. However, extra/increased doses of salmeterol alone or in fixed combination with fluticasone propionate should *not* be used in such situations. Patients should be advised to contact a clinician immediately if they experience decreasing effectiveness of short-acting, inhaled β_2-agonists, a need for more inhalations than usual of short-acting, inhaled β_2-agonists, or a substantial decrease in lung function as outlined by the clinician. Patients should be advised not to discontinue therapy with salmeterol alone or in fixed combination with fluticasone without medical supervision since symptoms may recur following discontinuance.

Salmeterol has a delayed onset of action, and the drug alone or in fixed combination with fluticasone propionate should *not* be used for the relief of acute symptoms (i.e., as rescue therapy for the treatment of acute episodes of bronchospasm). A short-acting, inhaled β_2-agonist, not salmeterol (alone or in fixed combination with fluticasone propionate), should be used to relieve acute symptoms such as shortness of breath. All patients receiving salmeterol alone or in fixed combination with fluticasone propionate should be provided with and instructed in the use of a short-acting, inhaled β_2-agonist (e.g,. albuterol) for treatment of acute symptoms. When initiating salmeterol alone or in fixed combination with fluticasone in patients who have been taking short-acting, oral or inhaled β_2-agonists on a regular basis (e.g., 4 times daily), these patients should be instructed to discontinue the *regular* use of the short-acting agent.

Salmeterol is *not* a substitute for inhaled or oral corticosteroids, and patients receiving corticosteroid therapy should be advised *not* to discontinue or alter the dosage of corticosteroids without consulting a clinician, even if the patient has subjective improvement after initiating therapy with salmeterol, since worsening of asthma may occur. In addition, all patients with asthma should be advised that they *must* continue regular maintenance treatment with an inhaled corticosteroid if they are receiving salmeterol. The manufacturer states that there are no data demonstrating that salmeterol has a clinical anti-inflammatory effect such as that associated with corticosteroids. When initiating and throughout therapy with salmeterol in patients receiving oral or inhaled corticosteroids for treatment of asthma, patients must continue taking a suitable dosage of corticosteroids to maintain clinical stability even if they have subjective improvement as a result of initiation of salmeterol; any change in corticosteroid dosage should be made only after clinical evaluation. Salmeterol in fixed combination with fluticasone as the inhalation aerosol (Advair® HFA) should not be used to transfer patients from systemic corticosteroid therapy. Particular care is needed for patients who have been transferred from systemically active corticosteroids to inhaled corticosteroids since death resulting from adrenal insufficiency has occurred in patients with asthma during and after such transfer. (See Cautions: Precautions and Contraindications, in Beclomethasone Dipropionate 68:04.)

As with other inhaled β_2-adrenergic drugs, salmeterol, alone or in fixed combination with fluticasone propionate, should not be used more often or at higher than recommended dosages, or in conjunction with other preparations containing long-acting β_2-adrenergic agonists, since an overdose may result. Clinically important cardiovascular effects and fatalities have been reported in association with excessive use of inhaled sympathomimetic drugs. Patients receiving salmeterol alone or in fixed combination with fluticasone propionate should not use additional salmeterol or other long-acting β_2-adrenergic agonists (e.g., arformoterol, formoterol, indacaterol) for any reason, including prevention of exercise-induced bronchospasm or treatment of asthma or COPD.

Rarely, a patient may develop acute bronchospasm immediately upon inhalation of a sympathomimetic drug preparation. Acute bronchospasm probably represents a hypersensitivity reaction to the active drug or an ingredient in the formulation. Although it may not be possible to distinguish paradoxical bronchoconstriction or that associated with hypersensitivity to the drug or an ingredient in the formulation from worsening of the asthma, salmeterol alone or in fixed combination with fluticasone propionate should be discontinued immediately if paradoxical bronchospasm occurs. Paradoxical bronchospasm should immediately be treated with a short-acting inhaled bronchodilator, and alternative therapy should be instituted. Patients should inform their clinicians of allergic reactions to salmeterol-containing preparations, other agents, or foods (including milk proteins).

Salmeterol and other β_2-adrenergic agonists may produce substantial hypokalemia in some patients, which has the potential to produce adverse cardiovascular effects (e.g., arrhythmias); however, decreases in serum potassium usually are transient and generally do not require supplementation. (See Cautions: Metabolic and Electrolyte Effects.)

Excessive β_2-adrenergic stimulation has been associated with seizures, angina, hypertension or hypotension, tachycardia with rates up to 200 beats/minute, arrhythmias, nervousness, headache, tremor, palpitation, nausea, dizziness, fatigue, malaise, and insomnia (see Acute Toxicity: Manifestations). Therefore, salmeterol, like all preparations containing sympathomimetic amines, should be used with caution in patients with cardiovascular disorders, especially coronary insufficiency, cardiac arrhythmias, and hypertension; in patients with seizure disorders or thyrotoxicosis; and in those who are unusually responsive to sympathomimetic amines. Patients should be informed of adverse effects associated with β_2-agonists, such as palpitations, chest pain, rapid heart rate, tremor, or nervousness. Patients should inform their clinician of heart problems, hypertension, seizures, thyroid disorders, or diabetes mellitus prior to initiation of salmeterol-containing therapy. Patients receiving salmeterol oral inhalation should use other inhaled medications only as directed by their clinician.

The pharmacokinetics of salmeterol or salmeterol in fixed combination with fluticasone propionate have not been studied in patients with hepatic impairment. Because salmeterol and fluticasone propionate are metabolized predominantly in the liver and potentially may accumulate in the plasma of patients with hepatic impairment, such patients should be monitored closely while receiving such therapy. Patients should inform their clinician of liver dysfunction prior to initiation of therapy.

Clinicians should remain vigilant for the possible development of pneumonia in patients with COPD who are receiving the inhalation powder preparation containing salmeterol in fixed combination with fluticasone propionate (Advair® Diskus®), since the clinical features of pneumonia and COPD exacerbations frequently overlap. Lower respiratory tract infections, including pneumonia, have been reported in patients with COPD following the administration of inhaled corticosteroids, including fluticasone propionate and the inhalation powder preparation containing salmeterol in fixed combination with fluticasone propionate.

Because of the risk of asthma-related death and hospitalization, use of salmeterol for the treatment of asthma without concomitant use of long-term asthma controller therapy, such as inhaled corticosteroids, is contraindicated. (See Asthma-related Death and Life-threatening Events under Cautions: Respiratory Effects and also see Uses: Bronchospasm.) Salmeterol alone or in fixed combination with fluticasone propionate as the inhalation powder (Advair® Diskus®, AirDuo® RespiClick®) is contraindicated in patients with severe hypersensitivity to milk proteins. Salmeterol in fixed combination with fluticasone propionate as the inhalation aerosol (Advair® HFA) is contraindicated in patients with known hypersensitivity to the drugs or any ingredient in the formulation. Patients should inform their clinician of allergies to drugs or food prior to initiation of therapy. Salmeterol alone or in fixed combination with fluticasone propionate is contraindicated in the primary treatment of status asthmaticus or other acute episodes of asthma or COPD where intensive measures are required.

■ **Pediatric Precautions** Safety and efficacy of salmeterol oral inhalation powder in adolescents 12 years of age or older have been established based on adequate and well-controlled trials conducted in adults and adolescents. However, monotherapy with long-acting β_2-adrenergic agonists, such as salmeterol, increases the risk of asthma-related death. In addition, available data from controlled clinical trials suggest that monotherapy with long-acting β_2-adrenergic agonists increases the risk of asthma-related hospitalization in pediatric and adolescent patients. (See Asthma-related Death and Life-threatening Events under Cautions: Respiratory Effects.) In pediatric and adolescent patients with asthma who require the addition of a long-acting β_2-adrenergic agonist to an inhaled corticosteroid, a fixed-combination preparation containing both an inhaled corticosteroid and a long-acting β_2-adrenergic agonist generally should be used to ensure compliance with both drugs. (See Uses: Bronchospasm.)

Safety and efficacy of salmeterol oral inhalation powder in children 4–11 years of age with asthma have been evaluated for periods not exceeding 1 year, and current data suggest that such children may receive the same dosage as adults for the treatment of asthma or exercise-induced bronchospasm. Pediatric patients should receive salmeterol therapy under adult supervision. Use of salmeterol in fixed combination with fluticasone propionate inhalation powder (Advair® Diskus®) in children 4–11 years of age with asthma is supported by data from one clinical trial and from extrapolation of efficacy data from older patients. Data from a 12-week study in children (4–11 years of age) with persistent asthma who were symptomatic with low dosages of inhaled corticosteroids indicate that the safety profile of salmeterol inhalation powder (50 mcg) in fixed combination with fluticasone propionate (100 mcg) inhalation powder is similar to that of fluticasone propionate monotherapy.

Safety and efficacy of salmeterol in fixed combination with fluticasone propionate inhalation powder (Advair® Diskus®) in children younger than 4 years of age with asthma have not been established. Safety and efficacy of salmeterol in fixed combination with fluticasone propionate inhalation powder (AirDuo® RespiClick®) in children younger than 12 years of age have not been established. Safety and efficacy of salmeterol in fixed combination with fluticasone propionate inhalation aerosol (Advair® HFA) in children younger than 12 years of age have not been established. Data from a limited number of adolescents 12–17 years of age receiving salmeterol and fluticasone propionate inhalation aerosol in fixed combination suggest that safety and efficacy of the fixed combination are similar to those in adults.

■ **Geriatric Precautions** Data from trials in patients with COPD receiving salmeterol inhalation powder suggested a greater effect on FEV_1 in younger adults compared with geriatric patients. No apparent differences in the type or frequency of adverse effects were noted in geriatric patients with asthma receiving salmeterol alone or in fixed combination with fluticasone inhalation aerosol (Advair® HFA) or in those with COPD receiving salmeterol compared with those in the total population of patients in these studies. No overall differences in safety or efficacy were observed in geriatric patients receiving salmeterol in fixed combination with fluticasone propionate inhalation powder (AirDuo® RespiClick®) compared with younger adults. Clinical studies of salmeterol in fixed combination with fluticasone inhalation powder (Advair® Diskus®) or inhalation aerosol (Advair® HFA) for asthma did not include sufficient numbers of patients 65 years of age or older to determine whether geriatric patients respond differently than younger patients. In clinical studies of salmeterol in fixed combination with fluticasone inhalation powder for COPD, patients 65 years of age or older experienced a higher incidence of serious adverse effects compared with those younger than 65 years of age, although the distribution of adverse effects was similar in the two groups. The possibility of greater sensitivity of some older patients cannot be ruled out. As with other β_2-agonists, special caution should be observed when using salmeterol alone or in fixed combination with fluticasone in geriatric patients who have concomitant cardiovascular disease that could be adversely affected by this class of drugs. (See Cautions: Precautions and Contraindications.) Adjustment of salmeterol dosage alone or in combination with fluticasone propionate in geriatric patients solely on the basis of age is not necessary.

■ **Mutagenicity and Carcinogenicity** No evidence of mutagenicity was observed when salmeterol was tested in several in vitro systems, including microbial and mammalian gene mutation tests and in a cytogenic assay of human lymphocytes. In an in vivo rat micronucleus assay, salmeterol did not exhibit evidence of mutagenicity.

Dose-related increases in the incidence of smooth muscle hyperplasia, cystic glandular hyperplasia, uterine leiomyomas, and ovarian cysts occurred in mice given oral salmeterol dosages of at least 1.4 mg/kg (approximately 20 times the maximum recommended daily inhalation dosage for adults and children based on comparisons of the plasma area under the curve [AUC]) in an 18-month carcinogenicity study. In a 24-month study in rats given salmeterol orally and/or by inhalation, mesovarian leiomyomas and ovarian cysts occurred at dosages of at least 0.68 mg/kg (approximately 55 or 25 times the maximum recommended daily inhalation dosage for adults or children respectively, on a mg/m² basis). The findings of these studies in rodents are similar to those reported previously for other β-adrenergic agonist drugs; the relevance of these findings to human use is unknown. No carcinogenic effects were observed in mice given salmeterol in doses of 0.2 mg/kg (approximately 3 times the maximum recommended daily inhalation dosage for adults and children based on AUC comparisons) or in rats given 0.21 mg/kg (approximately 15 or 8 times the maximum recommended daily inhalation dosage for adults or children, respectively, on a mg/m² basis).

■ **Pregnancy, Fertility, and Lactation** There are no adequate and well-controlled studies of salmeterol in pregnant women. Because of the potential for β-agonist interference with uterine contractility, use of salmeterol during labor should be restricted to those patients in whom the benefits clearly outweigh the risks. The drug should be used during other stages of pregnancy only if the potential benefit justifies the potential risk to the fetus. Salmeterol in fixed combination with fluticasone propionate inhalation aerosol (Advair® HFA) should be used during pregnancy only if the potential benefit justifies the potential risk to the fetus. In pregnant women with poorly or moderately controlled asthma, there is an increased risk of adverse perinatal events such as preeclampsia in the mother, and prematurity, low birth weight, and small size for gestational age in the neonate. Pregnant women with asthma should be closely monitored and dosage of medications should be adjusted as needed to maintain optimal asthma control.

Reproduction studies in male and female rats using oral salmeterol dosages of up to 2 mg/kg daily (representing 160 times the recommended clinical dosage on a mg/m² basis) have not revealed evidence of harm to the fetus. Dutch rabbit fetuses exposed to oral salmeterol dosages of at least 1 mg/kg (representing 50 times the maximum recommended daily inhalation dosage based on comparison of AUC data) exhibited characteristic effects of β-receptor stimulation, including precocious eyelid openings, cleft palate, sternebral fusion, limb and paw flexures, and delayed ossification of the frontal cranial bones. No teratogenic effects were observed at oral salmeterol doses of 0.6 mg/kg (20 times the maximum recommended daily inhalation dosage based on comparison of AUC data). Delayed ossification of the frontal bones was seen in the fetuses of New Zealand White rabbits given oral salmeterol dosages of 10 mg/kg (representing 1600 times the maximum recommended daily inhalation dosage on a mg/m² basis). Extensive use of other β-agonists has provided no evidence that these class effects in animals are relevant to use in humans.

In reproduction studies in mice and rats, no evidence of an increased toxicity was associated with the use of salmeterol combined with fluticasone propionate when compared with toxicity observed from the components administered separately. Teratogenicity (i.e., cleft palate), fetal death, or increased implantation loss has been observed in mice receiving a subcutaneous dosage of 150 mcg/kg of fluticasone propionate (representing approximately less than the maximum recommended daily inhalation dosage in adults on a mcg/m² basis) combined with a 10 mg/kg oral dosage of salmeterol (representing approximately 410 times the maximum recommended daily inhalation dosage in adults on a mg/m² basis), but these effects did not occur when lower dosages of fluticasone propionate (up to 40 mcg/kg subcutaneously, representing less than the maximum recommended daily inhalation dosage in adults on a mcg/m² basis) were combined with lower dosages of salmeterol (up to 1.4 mg/kg orally, representing approximately 55 times the maximum recommended daily inhalation dosage in adults on a mg/m² basis). Reproduction studies in rats receiving subcutaneous dosages of fluticasone propionate of up to 30 mcg/kg (representing less than the maximum recommended daily inhalation dosage in adults on a mcg/m² basis) combined with dosages of up to 1 mg/kg of salmeterol (approximately 80 times the recommended daily inhalation dosage in adults on a mg/m² basis) did not reveal evidence of teratogenicity. Delayed ossification, changes in the occipital bone, umbilical hernia, decreased placental or fetal weight, and maternal toxicity have been observed in rats receiving subcutaneous dosages of fluticasone propionate 100 mcg/kg (representing less than the maximum recommended daily inhalation dosage in adults on a mcg/m² basis) combined with oral salmeterol dosages of 10 mg/kg (approximately 810 times the maximum recommended daily inhalation dosage in adults on a mg/m² basis).

Reproduction studies in rats given oral salmeterol dosages up to 2 mg/kg (approximately 160 times the maximum recommended daily inhalation dosage for adults on a mg/m² basis) have not revealed evidence of impaired fertility.

It is not known whether salmeterol xinafoate or fluticasone propionate is distributed into human milk. However, salmeterol is distributed into milk in rats. Corticosteroids, other than fluticasone propionate, are distributed into human milk. Effects of salmeterol xinafoate or fluticasone propionate on breast-fed infants or milk production also are not known. The benefits of breast-feeding and the woman's clinical need for salmeterol xinafoate or fluticasone propionate should be considered along with any potential adverse effects on the breast-fed infant from the drugs or from the underlying maternal condition. Since no data from controlled trials are available on the use of such preparations in nursing women, caution is advised if salmeterol alone or salmeterol in fixed combination with fluticasone propionate is administered in nursing women.

Drug Interactions

The following information addresses potential interactions with salmeterol. When salmeterol is used in fixed combination with fluticasone propionate, interactions associated with fluticasone propionate should be considered. No formal drug interaction studies have been performed to date with the fixed-combination preparations containing salmeterol and fluticasone propionate.

■ **Monoamine Oxidase Inhibitors and Tricyclic Antidepressants** The effects of salmeterol xinafoate on the vascular system may be potentiated in patients receiving concomitant therapy with monoamine oxidase (MAO) inhibitors or tricyclic antidepressants; therefore, salmeterol should be administered with extreme caution to patients being treated with these agents or to patients receiving salmeterol within 2 weeks of discontinuance of these agents.

■ **Drugs Affecting Hepatic Microsomal Enzymes** Salmeterol and fluticasone propionate are substrates for cytochrome P-450 (CYP) isoenzyme 3A4. The manufacturers state that the use of potent CYP3A4 inhibitors (e.g., atazanavir, clarithromycin, indinavir, itraconazole, ketoconazole, nefazodone, nelfinavir, ritonavir, saquinavir, telithromycin) with salmeterol is not recommended because of the increased potential for systemic adverse effects (e.g., cardiovascular effects such as QT_c prolongation, palpitations, or sinus tachycardia).

■ **Supplemental Short-Acting β_2-Adrenergic Agonists** In several 3-month clinical trials, adults and adolescents with asthma receiving therapy with salmeterol inhalation powder required an average of approximately 1.5 inhalations daily of a supplemental, short-acting β_2-adrenergic agonist. In patients receiving salmeterol inhalation powder, 26% required 8–24 inhalations daily of a supplemental, short-acting β_2-agonist on at least one occasion. Consistent use of greater than 4 inhalations daily of supplemental, short-acting β_2-agonist therapy was required in 9% of patients receiving orally inhaled salmeterol over the course of these trials. In trials that evaluated salmeterol inhalation powder and as-needed short-acting β_2-agonists, a few patients required an average of 8–11 inhalations of short-acting β_2-agonists daily; no increase in cardiovascular effects were noted. However, the safety of concomitant use of more than 8 inhalations of supplemental, short-acting β_2-agonist therapy daily with salmeterol inhalation therapy has not been established. In a moderate number of patients who experienced a worsening of asthma with salmeterol inhalation powder therapy, administration of albuterol by metered-dose inhaler or nebulizer (one dose in most patients) led to improvement in FEV_1 with no increase in the occurrence of cardiovascular adverse effects.

In two 6-month clinical trials, patients with chronic obstructive pulmonary disease (COPD) receiving therapy with salmeterol inhalation powder alone or in fixed combination with fluticasone propionate required an average of approximately 4 inhalations daily of a supplemental, rapid-acting β_2-adrenergic agonist. In COPD patients receiving salmeterol inhalation powder alone or in fixed combination with fluticasone propionate, 24 or 26%, respectively, required an average of 6 or more inhalations daily of a supplemental, rapid-acting β_2-agonist over the course of these trials; no increase in the frequency of adverse cardiovascular effects was noted.

■ **Cromolyn Sodium** In clinical studies, inhaled cromolyn sodium did not alter the safety profile of salmeterol oral inhalation when these drugs were administered concurrently.

■ **Theophyllines** There is some evidence from studies in animals that concomitant administration of sympathomimetic agents (e.g., isoproterenol) and aminophylline may produce increased cardiotoxic effects (e.g., arrhythmias and sudden death, with histologic evidence of myocardial necrosis). Although such an interaction has not been established in humans, a few reports have suggested that such a combination may have the potential for producing cardiac arrhythmias and death. However, in one study in patients receiving theophylline therapy, no evidence of increased cardiotoxic effects was noted when salmeterol aerosol (no longer commercially available) was added to theophylline therapy. In a number of clinical trials in patients with COPD, concurrent therapy with theophylline did not alter the adverse effect profile of salmeterol given alone or in fixed combination with fluticasone propionate.

■ **β-Adrenergic Blocking Agents** β-Adrenergic blocking agents not only block the pulmonary effects of β-adrenergic agonists (e.g., salmeterol), but also may produce severe bronchospasm in patients with asthma or COPD. Patients with asthma or COPD usually should not be treated with β-adrenergic blocking agents. However, under certain circumstances, there may be no acceptable alternatives to the use of β-adrenergic blocking agents in these patients; the use of cardioselective β-adrenergic blocking agents may be considered but should be used concomitantly with caution.

■ **Other Drugs** Since salmeterol may decrease serum potassium concentration, care should be taken in patients also receiving other drugs that can lower serum potassium concentration, such as non-potassium-sparing diuretics (loop or thiazide diuretics). ECG changes and/or hypokalemia that may result from the administration of non-potassium-sparing diuretics may be aggravated by concomitant β-agonist therapy, especially when the recommended dosage of the β-agonist is exceeded. Although the clinical importance of these effects is not known, caution is advised when administering salmeterol with non-potassium-sparing diuretics.

Acute Toxicity

■ **Pathogenesis** Rats and dogs survived inhalation doses of 2.9 and 0.7 mg/kg of salmeterol, respectively, representing approximately 240 or 190 times the maximum daily adult inhalation powder dosage, and 110 or 90 times the maximum daily pediatric inhalation powder dosage, respectively, on a mg/m² basis. No deaths occurred in mice and rats given oral salmeterol doses of 150 and 1000 mg/kg, respectively, representing 6100 or 81,000 times the maximum recommended human daily inhalation powder dosage in adults, and 2900 or 38,000 times the maximum recommended daily pediatric inhalation powder dosage, respectively, on a mg/m² basis.

In humans, single orally inhaled doses as high as 400 mcg have been studied and appeared to be relatively safe in short-term use. However, in a dose-response study in healthy men, single orally inhaled 400-mcg doses of salmeterol were associated with tremor, headache, increases in heart rate and blood glucose, and decreases in plasma potassium concentrations. Nonspecific T-wave changes and prolonged QT interval also were observed at this dose; patients receiving lower doses did not display ECG changes.

■ **Manifestations** The expected signs and symptoms associated with overdosage of orally inhaled salmeterol xinafoate are those of excessive β-adrenergic stimulation and/or occurrence or exaggeration of any of the following: tachycardia (with rates up to 200 beats/minute) and/or arrhythmia, nervousness, palpitation, nausea, dizziness, fatigue, malaise, seizures, angina, hypertension or hypotension, insomnia, dry mouth, tremor, headache, hypokalemia, hyperglycemia, and muscle cramps. Large IV doses of albuterol (dosage form currently not commercially available in the US) have been reported to exacerbate preexisting diabetes mellitus and ketoacidosis; the potential for salmeterol to cause such effects has not been determined. Large oral or inhaled doses of salmeterol (12–20 times the recommended dosage) have produced clinically important prolongation of the QT_c interval, which increases the risk for ventricular arrhythmias. Cardiac arrest and fatalities have occurred following excessive use of sympathomimetic pressurized aerosol medications, and may occur with overuse of salmeterol. However, cardiorespiratory arrest has been reported in at least one patient with chronic obstructive pulmonary disease (COPD) and pre-existing alcoholic cardiomyopathy receiving the recommended dosage of inhaled salmeterol in conjunction with usual dosages of ipratropium and albuterol. No cases of overdosage of salmeterol were reported during controlled studies with the orally inhaled drug. The safety of concomitant therapy with salmeterol and more than 8 inhalations per day of a short-acting β_2-agonist has not been established.

■ **Treatment** The manufacturer suggests that in case of salmeterol overdosage, therapy with salmeterol and all other β-adrenergic agonists be discontinued and appropriate symptomatic therapy initiated. The judicious use of a β-adrenergic blocking agent may be considered but only with extreme caution in asthmatic patients because such agents may induce an asthmatic attack. (See Drug Interactions: β-Adrenergic Blocking Agents.) Cardiac monitoring is recommended in cases of overdosage with salmeterol. The manufacturer states that there is insufficient evidence to determine if dialysis is effective for the treatment of salmeterol overdosage.

Pharmacology

Salmeterol xinafoate has pharmacologic actions similar to those of other selective β_2-adrenergic receptor agonists (e.g., albuterol). Salmeterol stimulates β_2-adrenergic receptors and apparently has little or no effect on α-, β_1-, or β_3-adrenergic receptors. In vitro and in vivo pharmacologic studies indicate that the selectivity of salmeterol for β_2- versus β_1-adrenergic receptors is greater than that of albuterol (e.g., approximately 50–60 times). It is believed that β-adrenergic effects result from stimulation of the production of cyclic adenosine-3′,5′-monophosphate (cAMP) by activation of the enzyme adenyl cyclase. Cyclic AMP appears to mediate numerous cellular responses, and increased concentrations of cAMP are associated with relaxation of bronchial smooth muscle, suppression of some aspects of inflammation, and stimulation of lung ciliary function.

The principal effect following oral inhalation of salmeterol and other β_2-adrenergic agonists is bronchodilation resulting from relaxation of smooth muscles of the bronchial tree. The delayed onset and prolonged duration of action of salmeterol may be the result of its slow cellular uptake and/or membrane translocation to the β_2 receptor, lipophilicity, and protracted binding at the β_2 receptor. Some evidence suggests that salmeterol binds reversibly to an active site on the β_2 receptor and irreversibly to an exosite, which may be a domain adjacent to the active site within the β_2 receptor in the lipid bilayer of the cell membrane. The persistence of salmeterol at the β_2 receptor is thought to be related to the binding of the oxyalkyl side chain of salmeterol to the exosite while the saligenin end of the molecule is free to dissociate from the active receptor site in the presence of β-adrenergic blocking agents. It has been suggested that the slow waning of the bronchodilatory effect of salmeterol is related to slow dissociation from the receptor or to turnover of the occupied β_2-adrenergic receptor protein.

■ **Respiratory Effects** Salmeterol relaxes bronchial smooth muscle by stimulating β_2-adrenergic receptors when administered by oral inhalation. In isolated bronchial smooth muscle tissue in which muscle tone was increased by a spasmogen (e.g., methacholine, prostaglandin $F_2\alpha$) or by electrical stimulation, salmeterol generally was more potent than albuterol and at least as potent as isoproterenol in relaxing smooth muscle. In patients with reversible airway obstruction, salmeterol decreases airway resistance (as measured by forced expiratory volume in 1 second [FEV_1], peak expiratory flow rate [PEFR], and vital capacity) and airway reactivity to histamine. Residual elevation of morning PEFR has been maintained for up to at least 1–6 days following completion of salmeterol therapy. In addition to bronchodilator activity, salmeterol and other inhaled β_2-agonists may affect clearance of pulmonary secretions by increasing the ciliary activity of airway epithelial cells.

Salmeterol inhibits the release of proinflammatory mediators associated with early-phase inflammatory response to allergen challenge (e.g., histamine, leukotrienes $C_4$and D_4, prostaglandin D_2) in human lung tissue and may thereby attenuate early- and late-phase-associated bronchoconstriction. Salmeterol also attenuates late-phase-associated vascular permeability, and inflammatory cell activation, migration, and recruitment. However, the extent of salmeterol's anti-inflammatory activity is not well characterized, and the lack of a consistent effect of the drug on inflammatory processes suggests that anti-inflammatory effects are of secondary or negligible importance in producing the clinical improvement noted in patients with asthma receiving the drug. Studies in animals and humans indicate that orally inhaled salmeterol inhibits extravasation of plasma proteins, neutrophils, and eosinophils associated with late-phase response to challenge with histamine, leukotriene B_4, antigen, endotoxin, granulocyte-macrophage colony-stimulating factor (GM-CSF), and platelet-activating factor. Some evidence indicates that salmeterol is as potent as isoproterenol and more potent than albuterol in inhibiting the release of these mediators and has a longer duration of anti-inflammatory action, including late-phase response to allergen challenge than either of these drugs. In addition, these anti-inflammatory effects have been reversed by pretreatment with β-adrenergic blocking agents (e.g., propranolol), suggesting that such effects may be mediated by β-adrenergic receptors. As inflammatory changes occur during periods of increased bronchial hyperresponsiveness, the degree of response to bronchoconstrictor stimuli has been used as an indirect measure of inflammation. In a few single-dose, placebo-controlled or comparative studies with albuterol, salmeterol decreased the degree of airway responsiveness to bronchoconstrictor stimuli (e.g., allergens, cold air). Whether these bronchoprotective effects of salmeterol are associated with sustained bronchodilation or anti-inflammatory effects has not been fully determined. The lack of activity of other β-adrenergic agonists on the late-phase response to allergen challenge may be related to their short duration of action.

Current evidence and experience indicate that prolonged therapy with salmeterol does not appear to be associated with development of tolerance to the bronchodilatory effects of the drug. However, conflicting data exist with regard to the development of tolerance to the drug's protective effects against bronchoconstrictor stimuli, and further study is needed to clarify the potential for development of tolerance to these effects of salmeterol.

■ **Cardiovascular Effects** Salmeterol, like other β_2-adrenergic agonists, can produce changes in heart rate and blood pressure. In several studies in asthmatic patients or healthy individuals receiving escalating doses of inhaled salmeterol (up to 84 mcg) or usual doses of inhaled albuterol (180 mcg), dose-related increases in heart rate of 3–16 beats/minute were noted with salmeterol but did not exceed those observed with albuterol therapy. The increase in heart rate observed in patients with asthma with salmeterol or albuterol therapy probably results either indirectly from peripheral vasodilation or directly from a chronotropic effect via β_2-receptors in the heart. In patients with chronic obstructive pulmonary disease (COPD) receiving orally inhaled salmeterol (50 mcg/dose) inhalation powder alone or in combination with fluticasone propionate, pulse rate or systolic or diastolic blood pressure was not affected.

In several studies in patients with asthma in which continuous electrocardiographic monitoring during 12- or 24-hour periods was performed during therapy with orally inhaled salmeterol (42 or 50 mcg twice daily) or albuterol (180 mcg 4 times daily), no clinically important dysrhythmias were noted. In several studies (24 weeks' duration) in patients with COPD in whom electrocardiographic monitoring was performed at weeks 12 and 24 of therapy with orally inhaled salmeterol inhalation powder (50 mcg twice daily) or placebo, the incidence of clinically important dysrhythmias was similar. In a clinical trial in patients with COPD who were receiving salmeterol inhalation powder, fluticasone inhalation powder, salmeterol in fixed combination with fluticasone propionate, or placebo, continuous ECG monitoring for 24 hours (prior to the first dose and after 4 weeks of therapy) did not reveal appreciable differences in ventricular or supraventricular arrhythmias or heart rate. The incidence of ventricular premature complexes with salmeterol, albuterol, or placebo in clinical studies generally has been similar. However at higher dosages, both salmeterol and albuterol administration have been associated with prolongation of the QT_c interval. Tolerance to the effects of salmeterol on the QT_c interval has been reported in healthy individuals receiving high dosages of the drug.

■ **Metabolic Effects** Administration of salmeterol and other β-adrenergic agonists may cause dose-related increases in blood glucose and/or decreases in serum potassium concentrations. (See Cautions: Metabolic and Electrolyte Effects.) Increases in blood glucose concentration may be caused by stimulation of glycogenolysis or gluconeogenesis through activation of β_2-receptors in skeletal muscle and liver; tolerance to this effect may occur with regular salmeterol treatment. Reductions in serum potassium concentration that occur during therapy with salmeterol and other β-adrenergic agonists may be related to β-adrenergic stimulation of cell membrane Na^+- K^+-ATPase, with increased intracellular shunting of potassium from blood into liver, skeletal muscle, and myocardium. Limited data in healthy individuals suggest that tolerance to the hypokalemic effects of high-dose salmeterol does not occur.

■ **Other Effects** Like other sympathomimetic amines, salmeterol may cause CNS stimulation and adverse nervous system effects. (See Cautions: Nervous System Effects.)

Pharmacokinetics

Limited data are available on the pharmacokinetics of salmeterol xinafoate after oral inhalation. Salmeterol xinafoate dissociates in solution to salmeterol and xinafoate moieties that are absorbed, distributed, metabolized, and excreted independently. The xinafoate moiety has no intrinsic pharmacologic activity. While commercially available salmeterol is administered as salmeterol xinafoate, dosages and drug concentrations are expressed in terms of salmeterol.

■ **Absorption** The absorption of salmeterol xinafoate from the respiratory tract following oral inhalation has not been fully characterized. Although it has been suggested that most of an orally inhaled drug actually is swallowed, the bronchodilating action of orally inhaled sympathomimetic agents is believed to result from a local action of the portion of the dose that reaches the bronchial tree. Systemic concentrations of salmeterol are low or undetectable after inhalation of the recommended dosage of the powder (50 mcg) twice daily and are not predictive of therapeutic effects. Delayed absorption was noted following oral administration of 1 mg of radiolabeled salmeterol (as salmeterol xinafoate) in a few healthy individuals; peak plasma salmeterol concentrations of about 600–650 pg/mL occurred at 45–75 minutes. Following repeated, twice-daily administration of 50 mcg of salmeterol as the oral inhalation powder in patients with asthma, salmeterol was detected in the plasma within 5–45 minutes; mean peak plasma concentrations of the drug were 167 pg/mL, and no accumulation was noted with repeated dosing.

Compared with short-acting β-agonists such as albuterol or isoproterenol, the onset and duration of bronchodilation with orally inhaled salmeterol are longer. Following administration of a single dose (50 mcg) of salmeterol oral inhalation powder in patients with asthma, most patients experienced clinically important improvement (as measured by a 15% improvement in FEV_1) within 1 hour. Maximum improvement in FEV_1 generally occurred within 3 hours, and clinically important improvement was maintained for 12 hours in most patients. Following administration of a single dose (50 mcg) of salmeterol oral inhalation powder in patients with chronic obstructive pulmonary disease (COPD), improvement in lung function (as measured by a 12% improvement in FEV_1 and at least 200 mL) occurred in 2 hours. Mean time to maximum improvement in FEV_1 occurred at 4.75 hours, and improvement was maintained for 12 hours. In the prevention of exercised-induced bronchospasm, salmeterol oral inhalation powder provided protection for up to about 9 hours in adolescents and adults and up to about 12 hours in children 4 to 11 years of age following a single 50- mcg dose 30 minutes prior to exercise.

■ **Distribution** Binding of salmeterol averages 96% in vitro to human plasma proteins over the concentration range of 8 ng/mL to 7.7 mcg/mL, which are concentrations greatly exceeding those achieved following usual doses of the drug. Salmeterol is bound to albumin and α_1-acid glycoprotein; the xinafoate moiety also is highly protein bound (exceeding 99%) to albumin.

The distribution of salmeterol into various human organs and tissues following oral inhalation has not been fully characterized. Results of studies in rats indicate that salmeterol crosses the blood-brain barrier in trace amounts.

It is not known if salmeterol and/or its metabolites cross the placenta in humans. Salmeterol crossed the placenta following oral administration in mice and rats. It also is not known if salmeterol is distributed into milk in humans; however the drug is distributed into milk in rats.

■ **Elimination** Salmeterol is extensively metabolized in the liver by hydroxylation and is eliminated predominantly in feces. In a few healthy individuals who received radiolabeled salmeterol 1 mg orally, approximately 25 and 60% of the dose were eliminated in urine and feces, respectively, 1–7 days after administration. Negligible amounts of unchanged salmeterol are detectable in urine or feces. A minor metabolite is formed by *o*-dealkylation of the phenylalkyl side chain. Following oral administration of salmeterol in healthy individuals, the terminal elimination half-lives of salmeterol and the xinafoate moiety are about 5.5 hours and 11–15 days, respectively.

Chemistry and Stability

■ **Chemistry** Salmeterol xinafoate is a long-acting, synthetic, sympathomimetic amine. The drug is structurally and pharmacologically similar to the short-acting β_2-adrenergic agonist albuterol. The pharmacologically active moiety of salmeterol contains a saligenin nucleus identical to that in albuterol. This polar nucleus reversibly attaches to the classic β_2-receptor binding site. Salmeterol differs structurally from albuterol in part by the presence of a long, *N*-substituted, phenylalkyl side chain. This substitution contributes to increased lipophilicity; greater bronchial tissue penetration; increased resistance to metabolism by catechol-*o*-methyltransferase (COMT); prolonged and selective binding to a second, nonpolar domain (exosite) on the β_2-receptor; and decreased clearance from the airways. The ether oxygen on the *N*-substituent facilitates binding of the substituent to the exosite portion of the β_2-adrenergic receptor protein.

Salmeterol is commercially available as the xinafoate salt, the racemic form of the 1-hydroxy-2-naphthoic acid salt of salmeterol. Both the *R*- and *S*- enantiomers of salmeterol are long acting. Available data suggest that the *S*-enantiomer of salmeterol does not antagonize the effects of the *R*-enantiomer and does not have pharmacologic effects that are different from those of the racemic mixture. Salmeterol xinafoate occurs as an off-white powder and has solubilities of approximately 40 mg/mL in methanol, 7 mg/mL in ethanol, 3 mg/mL in chloroform, 2–3 mg/mL in isopropanol, and 0.07–0.11 mg/mL in water.

Salmeterol xinafoate powder for oral inhalation is a powdered mixture of drug and lactose and is contained in a foil blister strip for use in a special oral inhaler device (Serevent® Diskus®). Salmeterol xinafoate also is commercially available in fixed combination with fluticasone propionate as a powder for oral inhalation (Advair® Diskus® or AirDuo® RespiClick®).With commercially available salmeterol inhalation powder delivered via the Serevent® Diskus®, Advair® Diskus®, or AirDuo® RespiClick® device, the amount of drug delivered to the lungs depends on factors such as the patient's inspiratory flow. Using standardized in vitro testing at a flow rate of 60 L per minute for 2 seconds, the Serevent® Diskus® device delivered 47 mcg of salmeterol per activation. Under similar conditions, the Advair®Diskus® device delivered 93, 233, and 465 mcg of fluticasone propionate and 45 mcg of salmeterol per activation from a Diskus® labeled as containing 100, 250, or 500 mcg of fluticasone propionate and 50 mcg of salmeterol. In adult patients with obstructive lung disease and severely compromised lung function (FEV_1 of 0.65 L or 20–30% of the predicted value), mean peak inspiratory flow through the Diskus® device was 82.4 L per minute for Serevent® and 82.4 L per minute for Advair®. In adults and adolescents with asthma, mean peak inspiratory flow through the

Diskus® device was 122.2 L per minute. In a group of children 4 years of age, mean peak inspiratory flow through the Diskus®device averaged 75.5 L per minute; in children 8 years of age, mean peak inspiratory flow averaged 107.3 L per minute. Based on in vitro modeling of these flow rates, a dose of approximately 46 mcg of salmeterol is emitted per activation of the Diskus® device. Results of standardized in vitro testing at a flow rate of 85 L per minute for 1.4 seconds indicated that the AirDuo® RespiClick® device delivered 49, 100, or 202 mcg of fluticasone propionate and 12.75 mcg of salmeterol per actuation from an oral inhaler labeled as containing 55, 113, or 232 mcg of fluticasone propionate and 14 mcg of salmeterol. In adult and adolescent patients with asthma, mean peak inspiratory flow through the RespiClick® device was 108.3 and 106.7 L per minute, respectively.

■ **Stability** The commercially available inhalation powder containing salmeterol xinafoate alone (Serevent®) or in fixed combination with fluticasone propionate (Advair® Diskus®) should be stored at room temperature (20–25°C) in a dry place away from direct heat and sunlight. The Serevent® Diskus® inhaler should be discarded 6 weeks after removal from the foil pouch or when every blister has been used (when the dose counter reads "0"), whichever comes first. The Advair® Diskus® inhaler should be discarded 1 month after removal from the foil pouch or when every blister has been used, whichever comes first.

The commercially available inhalation powder containing salmeterol in fixed combination with fluticasone propionate (AirDuo® RespiClick®) should be stored at 15–25°C in a dry place away from extreme heat, cold, and humidity. The inhaler should be discarded 30 days after opening the foil pouch or when the dose counter reads "0," whichever comes first.

The commercially available inhalation aerosol of salmeterol in fixed combination with fluticasone propionate (Advair® HFA) should be stored (with the mouthpiece down) at 20–25°C but may be exposed to temperatures ranging from 15–30°C. Because the contents of the aerosol oral inhaler are under pressure, the aerosol container should *not* be punctured, used or stored near heat or an open flame, or placed into a fire or an incinerator for disposal. Exposure of the canister to temperatures exceeding 49°C may cause the canister to burst. The inhaler should be discarded when the dose counter reads "0."

Salmeterol xinafoate oral inhalation powder (Serevent® Diskus®) is stable for 18 months from the date of manufacture.

Preparations

Excipients in commercially available drug preparations may have clinically important effects in some individuals; consult specific product labeling for details.

Salmeterol Xinafoate

Oral Inhalation

Powder	50 mcg (of salmeterol) per inhalation	**Serevent® Diskus®**, GlaxoSmithKline

Salmeterol Xinafoate Combinations

Oral Inhalation

Aerosol	21 mcg (of salmeterol) with Fluticasone Propionate 45 mcg per metered spray (from the actuator)	**Advair® HFA** (with hydrofluoroalkane propellant), GlaxoSmithKline
	21 mcg (of salmeterol) with Fluticasone Propionate 115 mcg per metered spray (from the actuator)	**Advair® HFA** (with hydrofluoroalkane propellant), GlaxoSmithKline
	21 mcg (of salmeterol) with Fluticasone Propionate 230 mcg per metered spray (from the actuator)	**Advair® HFA** (with hydrofluoroalkane propellant), GlaxoSmithKline
Powder	14 mcg (of salmeterol) with Fluticasone Propionate 55 mcg per inhalation	**AirDuo® RespiClick®**, Teva
	14 mcg (of salmeterol) with Fluticasone Propionate 113 mcg per inhalation	**AirDuo® RespiClick®**, Teva
	14 mcg (of salmeterol) with Fluticasone Propionate 232 mcg per inhalation	**AirDuo® RespiClick®**, Teva
	50 mcg (of salmeterol) with Fluticasone Propionate 100 mcg per inhalation	**Advair® Diskus®**, GlaxoSmithKline
	50 mcg (of salmeterol) with Fluticasone Propionate 250 mcg per inhalation	**Advair® Diskus®**, GlaxoSmithKline
	50 mcg (of salmeterol) with Fluticasone Propionate 500 mcg per inhalation	**Advair® Diskus®**, GlaxoSmithKline

Terbutaline Sulfate

■ Terbutaline sulfate is a synthetic sympathomimetic amine that stimulates β-adrenergic receptors less selectively than relatively selective β_2-agonists (e.g., albuterol).

Uses

■ **Bronchospasm** Terbutaline sulfate is used as a relatively short-acting bronchodilator in the symptomatic treatment of bronchial asthma and of reversible bronchospasm that may occur in association with chronic obstructive pulmonary disease (COPD), including chronic bronchitis and emphysema. Subcutaneous terbutaline is about as effective as an equal subcutaneous dose of epinephrine in improving pulmonary function. Orally administered terbutaline appears to have bronchodilator activity about equal to that of ephedrine; however, the onset of action is more rapid and duration of action is longer than that of ephedrine. Compared to oral metaproterenol, oral terbutaline has equal or slightly greater efficacy and a slower onset and longer duration of action.

Asthma **Intermittent Asthma.** In the stepped-care approach to antiasthmatic drug therapy, use of a selective short-acting inhaled β_2-adrenergic agonist (e.g., albuterol, levalbuterol, pirbuterol) on an as-needed basis to control occasional acute symptoms (e.g., cough, wheezing, dyspnea) of short duration is recommended for all patients with asthma; such use of an inhaled short-acting β_2-agonist alone generally is sufficient as initial treatment for newly diagnosed patients whose asthma severity is initially classified as intermittent (e.g., patients with daytime symptoms of asthma not more than twice weekly and nocturnal symptoms not more than twice a month). Most experts consider short-acting inhaled β_2-adrenergic agonists to be drugs of choice for treating acute asthma symptoms and exacerbations and for preventing exercise-induced bronchospasm. Less β_2-selective bronchodilators such as terbutaline generally are not recommended because of their potential to cause excessive cardiac stimulation, particularly at high doses. Alternatives to short-acting inhaled β_2-agonists recommended by some clinicians for relief of acute asthma symptoms include an inhaled anticholinergic agent (e.g., ipratropium), a short-acting oral β_2-agonist, or a short-acting theophylline (provided extended-release theophylline is not already used), but these alternatives have a slower onset of action and/or a greater risk of adverse effects. Oral β_2-adrenergic agonist therapy is suggested for use principally in patients unable to use inhaled bronchodilators (e.g., young children). Other experts do not recommend oral β_2-agonists for relief of acute asthma symptoms. Use of short-acting inhaled β_2-agonists in asymptomatic asthma should be limited to pretreatment prior to exercise and, in intermittent asthma, should be limited to providing relief as symptoms develop. Some clinicians state that patients requiring symptomatic relief more than twice weekly or repeatedly over 1 or 2 days should be evaluated for possible initiation of long-term controller therapy.

Mild Persistent Asthma. When control of symptoms deteriorates in patients with intermittent asthma and symptoms become persistent (e.g., daytime symptoms of asthma more than twice weekly but less than once daily, and nocturnal symptoms of asthma 3–4 times per month), current asthma management guidelines and most clinicians recommend initiation of a controller drug such as an anti-inflammatory agent, preferably a low-dose orally inhaled corticosteroid (e.g., 88–264, 88–176, or 176 mcg of fluticasone propionate [or its equivalent] daily via a metered-dose inhaler in adolescents and adults, children 5–11 years of age, or children 4 years of age or younger, respectively) as first-line therapy for persistent asthma, supplemented by as-needed use of a short-acting, inhaled β_2-agonist. Alternatives to low-dose inhaled corticosteroids for mild persistent asthma include certain leukotriene modifiers (i.e., montelukast, zafirlukast), extended-release theophylline, or mast-cell stabilizers (i.e., cromolyn, nedocromil [preparations for oral inhalation no longer commercially available in the US]), but these therapies are less effective and generally not preferred as initial therapy. Some experts recommend that long-term control therapy be considered in infants and children 4 years of age or younger who have identifiable risk factors for asthma and who in the previous year have had 4 or more episodes of wheezing that lasted more than 1 day and symptoms that affected sleep. Low-dose inhaled corticosteroids also are recommended as the preferred initial therapy in such children. Cromolyn is suggested (based on extrapolation of data from studies in older children) or montelukast is recommended by some experts as alternative, but not preferred, therapy in children 4 years of age or younger with mild persistent asthma. Other experts do not consider mast cell stabilizers or extended-release theophylline to be acceptable alternatives to inhaled corticosteroids for routine use as initial long-term therapy in such patients.

Moderate Persistent Asthma. According to current asthma management guidelines, therapy with a long-acting inhaled β_2-agonist such as salmeterol or formoterol generally is recommended in adults and adolescents who have moderate persistent asthma and daily asthmatic symptoms that are inadequately controlled following addition of low-dose inhaled corticosteroids to as-needed inhaled β_2-agonist treatment. However, the National Asthma Education and Prevention Program (NAEPP) recommends that the beneficial effects of long-acting inhaled β_2-agonists should be weighed carefully against the increased risk (although uncommon) of severe asthma exacerbations and asthma-related deaths associated with daily use of such agents. (See Asthma-related Death and Life-threatening Events under Cautions: Respiratory Effects, in Salmeterol 12:12.08.12.) Current asthma management guidelines also state that an alternative, but equally preferred option for management of moderate persistent asthma that is not adequately controlled with a low dosage of inhaled corticosteroid is to increase the maintenance dosage to a medium dosage (e.g., exceeding 264 but not more than 440 mcg of fluticasone propionate [or its equivalent] daily via a metered-dose inhaler in adults and adolescents). Alternative less effective therapies that may be added to a low dosage of inhaled corticosteroid include oral extended-release theophylline or certain leukotriene modifiers (i.e., montelukast, zafirlukast).

Limited data are available in infants and children 11 years of age or younger with moderate persistent asthma, and recommendations of care are based on expert opinion and extrapolation from studies in adults. According to current asthma management guidelines, a long-acting inhaled β_2-agonist (e.g., salmeterol, formoterol) a leukotriene modifier (i.e., montelukast, zafirlukast), or extended-release theophylline (with appropriate monitoring) may be added to low-dose inhaled corticosteroid therapy in children 5–11 years of age. Because comparative data establishing relative efficacy of these agents in this age group are lacking, there is no clearly preferred agent for use as adjunctive therapy with a low-dose inhaled corticosteroid for treatment of asthma in these children. In children 5–11 years of age with moderate persistent asthma that is not controlled with a low dosage of an inhaled corticosteroid, another preferred option according to current asthma management guidelines is to increase the maintenance dosage of the inhaled corticosteroid to a medium dosage (e.g., exceeding 176 but not more than 352 mcg of fluticasone propionate [or its equivalent] daily via a metered-dose inhaler). In infants and children 4 years of age or younger with moderate persistent asthma that is not controlled by a low dosage of an inhaled corticosteroid, the only preferred option is to increase the maintenance dosage of the inhaled corticosteroid to a medium dosage (e.g., exceeding 176 but not more than 352 mcg of fluticasone propionate [or its equivalent] daily via a metered-dose inhaler).

Severe Persistent Asthma. Maintenance therapy with an inhaled corticosteroid at medium dosages or high dosages (e.g., exceeding 440 mcg of fluticasone propionate in adults and adolescents or 352 mcg of the drug in children 5–11 years of age [or its equivalent] daily via a metered-dose inhaler) and adjunctive therapy with a long-acting inhaled β_2-agonist is the preferred treatment according to current asthma management guidelines in adults and children 5 years of age or older with severe persistent asthma (i.e., continuous daytime asthma symptoms, nighttime symptoms 7 times per week). Such recommendations in children 5–11 years of age are based on expert opinion and extrapolation from studies in older children and adults. Alternatives to a long-acting inhaled β_2-agonist for severe persistent asthma in adults and children 5 years of age or older receiving medium-dose inhaled corticosteroids include extended-release theophylline or certain leukotriene modifiers (i.e., montelukast, zafirlukast), but these therapies are generally not preferred. Omalizumab may be considered in adults and adolescents with severe asthma with an allergic component who are inadequately controlled with high-dose inhaled corticosteroids and a long-acting β_2-agonist. In infants and children 4 years of age or younger with severe asthma, maintenance therapy with an inhaled corticosteroid at medium dosages or high dosages (e.g., exceeding 352 mcg of fluticasone propionate [or its equivalent] daily via a metered-dose inhaler) and adjunctive therapy with either a long-acting inhaled β_2-agonist or montelukast is the only preferred treatment according to current asthma management guidelines. Recommendations for care of infants and children with severe asthma are based on expert opinion and extrapolation from studies in adolescents and adults.

Poorly Controlled Asthma. If asthma symptoms in adults and children 5 years of age or older with moderate to severe asthma are very poorly controlled (i.e., at least 2 exacerbations per year requiring oral corticosteroids) with low-to-high maintenance dosages of the inhaled corticosteroid and a long-acting inhaled β_2-agonist bronchodilator, a short course (3–10 days) of an oral corticosteroid may be added to gain prompt control of asthma. In infants and children 4 years of age or younger with moderate to severe asthma who are very poorly controlled (more than 3 exacerbations per year requiring oral corticosteroids) with medium-to-high maintenance dosages of an inhaled corticosteroid with or without adjunctive therapy (i.e., a long-acting inhaled β_2-agonist, montelukast), a short course (3–10 days) of an oral corticosteroid may be added to gain prompt control of asthma. For information concerning the regular use of oral corticosteroids in patients with very severe asthma, see Asthma under Uses: Bronchospasm, in Albuterol 12:12.08.12.

When asthma symptoms at any stage are not controlled with maintenance therapy (e.g., inhaled corticosteroids) plus supplemental short-acting inhaled β_2-agonist bronchodilator therapy as needed (e.g., if there is a need to increase the dose or frequency of administration of the short-acting sympathomimetic agent), prompt reevaluation is required to adjust dosage of the maintenance regimen or institute an alternative maintenance regimen. For additional information on the management of asthma, see Asthma under Uses: Bronchospasm, in Albuterol 12:12.08.12.

Acute Asthma Exacerbations. Orally inhaled selective β_2-adrenergic agonists currently are recommended for prehospital management of asthma exacerbations (e.g., in emergency medicine facilities and/or ambulances) and for asthma management in hospitalized patients. Subcutaneous terbutaline is reserved for prehospital management of severe asthma exacerbations when inhaled β_2-selective agents are not readily available. Subcutaneous terbutaline is not used routinely for the treatment of severe asthma exacerbations in hospitalized patients and has no proven advantage compared with oral inhalation of the drug (no longer commercially available in the US).

Regular Use of Short-acting β_2-Agonists. Concerns about the safety of *regular* use of short-acting inhaled β-agonist bronchodilators for maintenance therapy of asthma have been raised by evidence from some studies suggesting increased morbidity and mortality in patients receiving long-term therapy with short-acting, inhaled β-agonists, particularly fenoterol (currently not commercially available in the US). Other studies in patients with mild or moderate asthma suggest that while regularly scheduled use of short-acting, inhaled β_2-agonists may not cause harm, such use does not appear to have demonstrable advantages compared with intermittent use and does not adequately control asthmatic symptoms. Suggested mechanisms for detrimental effects of regularly scheduled, inhaled β-agonist therapy include down-regulation of β-adrenergic receptors (tolerance) (see Cautions: Precautions and Contraindications), increased responsiveness of airways to allergens and exercise, genetic changes in β_2-agonist receptor gene, or increased airway accessibility to inhaled allergens, which may lead to increased airway inflammation and reactivity and worsening of asthma symptoms. The validity of the evidence from studies suggesting increased morbidity and mortality has been criticized in terms of study design and/or interpretation of study findings and a causal relationship between inhaled β_2-agonist therapy and asthma mortality has not been proven. Current asthma management guidelines and many clinicians recommend concomitant anti-inflammatory therapy with an inhaled corticosteroid as first-line therapy for long-term control in patients with persistent asthma, supplemented by as-needed use of a short-acting, inhaled β_2-agonist. Regular, daily use of a short-acting, inhaled β_2-agonist generally is not recommended, and increased chronic use of such β_2-agonists more than twice weekly (excluding use for exercise-induced bronchospasm) or acute use (e.g., repeated use over more than 1–2 days) for asthma deterioration may indicate the need to initiate or increase long-term control therapy for asthma.

Chronic Obstructive Pulmonary Disease In contrast to asthma, regular use of selective inhaled β_2-adrenergic agonists in the management of chronic obstructive pulmonary disease (COPD) does not appear to be detrimental. However, as long-acting β_2-adrenergic agonists have become available for the treatment of COPD, short-acting β_2-adrenergic agonists are used by some clinicians mainly to relieve acute symptoms of COPD. In the stepped-care approach to drug therapy in patients with COPD, mild intermittent symptoms and minimal lung impairment (e.g., FEV_1 at least 80% of predicted) can be treated with a short-acting, selective inhaled β_2-agonist such as albuterol as needed during acute exacerbations. Inhaled β_2-adrenergic agonists are preferred over oral β_2-agonist therapy for treatment of COPD. Oral β_2-adrenergic agonists have a slower onset of action and an increased incidence of adverse effects compared with inhaled therapy; the role of oral β_2-adrenergic agonists in the treatment of COPD is limited.

In patients with moderate (e.g., FEV_1 50–80% of predicted) COPD who have persistent symptoms despite as-needed therapy with ipratropium or a selective inhaled β_2-agonist, maintenance treatment with one or more long-acting bronchodilators (e.g., salmeterol, formoterol, tiotropium) can be added and a short-acting, selective inhaled β_2-agonist can be used as needed for immediate symptom relief. Maintenance therapy with long-acting inhaled bronchodilators is recommended in such patients as this therapy is more effective and convenient than regular use of short-acting bronchodilators. For patients not responding adequately to treatment following addition of a long-acting bronchodilator, a combination of several long-acting bronchodilators such as tiotropium and a long-acting β-adrenergic agonist may be used.

Maintenance therapy (e.g., 4 times daily) with a short-acting, selective inhaled β_2-agonist is not preferred, but may be used in patients with persistent symptoms of COPD; such therapy should not exceed 6–12 inhalations daily. Current guidelines for the management of COPD state that low- to high-dose ipratropium (6–16 inhalations daily) can be added to therapy with a short-acting, selective inhaled β_2-agonist in patients with mild to moderate persistent symptoms of COPD, with the frequency of inhalation therapy with either agent not to exceed 4 times daily. Combining bronchodilators from different classes and with differing durations of action may increase the degree of bronchodilation with a similar or lower frequency of adverse effects.

For treatment of severe to very severe COPD (e.g., FEV_1 30–50% of predicted or less, history of exacerbations), the addition of an inhaled corticosteroid to one or more long-acting bronchodilators given separately or in fixed combination may be needed. If symptoms are not adequately controlled with inhaled corticosteroids and a long-acting bronchodilator or if limiting adverse effects occur, oral extended-release theophylline may be added or substituted.

For severe exacerbations of COPD, a short (e.g., 7–10 days) course of oral corticosteroids (e.g., equivalent to 30–40 mg of prednisone daily) can be added to bronchodilator therapy. For additional details on the treatment of COPD exacerbations, see Chronic Obstructive Pulmonary Disease under Uses: Bronchospasm, in Ipratropium 12:08.08.

■ **Preterm Labor** Terbutaline sulfate has been used IV† or subcutaneously in selected patients to inhibit uterine contractions in preterm labor† (tocolysis) and thus prolong gestation when such prolongation of intrauterine life would be expected to benefit pregnancy outcome. The American College of Obstetricians and Gynecologists (ACOG) considers terbutaline to be one of several possible tocolytic agents. Because of conflicting results, there is no clear first-line tocolytic agent. Although the US Food and Drug Administration (FDA) states that it may be clinically appropriate based on the clinician's judgment to administer terbutaline by injection in urgent and individual obstetrical situations in a hospital setting, the manufacturers and FDA warn that terbutaline sulfate injection is not FDA labeled for and should not be used for prolonged tocolysis (beyond 48–72 hours), and is contraindicated for such use, because of the potential for serious maternal cardiac effects and death. The manufacturers and FDA also warn that oral terbutaline sulfate is not FDA labeled for and should not be used for acute or maintenance tocolysis, and is contraindicated for such use, because it has not been shown to be effective and has similar safety concerns as terbutaline sulfate injection. Terbutaline sulfate (injection or oral tablets) should not be used for maintenance tocolysis, particularly in the outpatient or home setting. (See Cautions: Adverse Effects.)

While use of terbutaline sulfate may effectively delay delivery for about 48 hours, the principal goal of prolongation of gestation is to potentially reduce the incidence of neonatal death, preterm delivery, low-birthweight infants, respiratory distress syndrome, and long-term morbidity and mortality associated with prematurity, and there currently is insufficient evidence substantiating the efficacy of β-adrenergic tocolytic agents in this regard. Therefore, the main benefit currently derived from tocolytic therapy appears to be short term to forestall labor and provide time for patients to receive corticosteroids to increase fetal lung maturation and/or to be transferred to other (e.g., tertiary-care) facilities; any other potential benefits of prolonging pregnancy are unclear. (See Uses: Antenatal Uses in the Corticosteroids General Statement 68:04.)

Dosage and Administration

■ Administration Terbutaline sulfate is administered orally or subcutaneously (usually into the lateral deltoid area). Terbutaline sulfate also has been used IV† in selected patients to inhibit uterine contractions in preterm labor† (tocolysis). However, administration of parenteral terbutaline sulfate by routes or methods other than subcutaneous injection (e.g., IV) is not recommended by the manufacturers.

■ Dosage ***Bronchospasm*** **Oral Dosage.** The usual adult oral dosage of terbutaline sulfate is 5 mg 3 times daily administered at approximately 6-hour intervals while the patient is awake. The total dosage of terbutaline sulfate in adults should not exceed 15 mg within a 24-hour period. If disturbing adverse effects occur, dosage may be reduced to 2.5 mg 3 times daily.

The recommended dosage of terbutaline sulfate in children 12–15 years of age is 2.5 mg orally 3 times daily; the total dosage of terbutaline sulfate should not exceed 7.5 mg within a 24-hour period.

Subcutaneous Dosage. The usual subcutaneous dose of terbutaline sulfate in adults and adolescents 12 years of age and older is 0.25 mg injected into the lateral deltoid area. If substantial clinical improvement does not occur within 15–30 minutes, a second dose of 0.25 mg may be administered. If the patient fails to respond within another 15–30 minutes, other therapeutic measures should be considered. The manufacturer states that the total dosage of terbutaline sulfate should not exceed 0.5 mg subcutaneously within a 4-hour period.

In hospitalized children or adolescents older than 12 years of age with an asthma exacerbation, 0.25 mg of terbutaline sulfate every 20 minutes for a total of 3 doses has been suggested by some clinicians. In hospitalized children 12 years of age or younger† with an acute asthma exacerbation, 0.01 mg/kg has been given every 20 minutes for a total of 3 doses, then every 2–6 hours as needed.

Preterm Labor **IV Dosage.** For use as a tocolytic agent in the management of preterm labor†, the rate and duration of IV† infusions of terbutaline sulfate should be carefully adjusted according to the patient's response as indicated by uterine response, maternal blood pressure, and maternal and fetal heart rates. For acute tocolytic therapy, IV terbutaline sulfate has been initiated at a dosage of 2.5–20 mcg/minute. Dosage may be increased gradually as tolerated at 10- to 20-minute intervals until the desired effects are achieved. Effective maximum dosages have ranged from 17.5–30 mcg/minute, although higher maximum dosages (e.g., 70–80 mcg/minute) have been used cautiously in some patients. Terbutaline sulfate injection should *not* be used for prolonged tocolysis (beyond 48–72 hours). (See Uses: Preterm Labor and Cautions: Adverse Effects.)

Subcutaneous Dosage. For acute tocolytic therapy in the management of preterm labor†, subcutaneous terbutaline sulfate at a dosage of 0.25 mg every 0.3–3 hours has been recommended. If pulse rate exceeds 120 beats/minute, terbutaline sulfate therapy should be temporarily discontinued. (See Cautions: Adverse Effects.) Terbutaline sulfate injection should *not* be used for prolonged tocolysis (beyond 48–72 hours). (See Uses: Preterm Labor and Cautions: Adverse Effects.)

Cautions

■ Adverse Effects The most common adverse effects of terbutaline sulfate are dose related and characteristic of sympathomimetic agents. Adverse effects of terbutaline include tachycardia, nervousness, tremor, palpitation, dizziness, headache, nausea, vomiting, anxiety, restlessness, lethargy, drowsiness, weakness, flushes, sweating, chest discomfort, muscle cramps, and tinnitus. Seizures, hypersensitivity vasculitis, and elevations in liver enzymes have been reported rarely in patients receiving terbutaline sulfate. Seizures did not recur following discontinuance of the drug. Immediate hypersensitivity reactions and exacerbations of bronchospasm have been reported in patients receiving terbutaline. Pain at the injection site may occur in some patients receiving terbutaline subcutaneously. Adverse effects with usual oral or subcutaneous doses are generally transient and usually do not require treatment; however, the increase in heart rate may persist for a relatively long time.

ECG changes, including flattening of the T wave, prolongation of the corrected QT (QT_c) interval, and ST-segment depression, have been reported with β-agonist therapy; the clinical importance of these findings is unknown.

Serious adverse effects, including death, have been reported after administration of terbutaline sulfate in pregnant women. Such adverse effects in pregnant women include increased heart rate, transient hyperglycemia, hypokalemia, cardiac arrhythmias, pulmonary edema, and myocardial ischemia. In addition, increased fetal heart rate and neonatal hypoglycemia may occur as a result of maternal administration of terbutaline. In February 2011, the US Food and Drug Administration (FDA) reported the results of an analysis of postmarketing reports of maternal death and serious cardiovascular events submitted to the FDA Adverse Event Reporting System (AERS) associated with obstetric use of terbutaline. Between 1976 and 2009, 16 maternal deaths were reported to AERS. Of the 16 reports of maternal death, 3 involved outpatient use of terbutaline administered by a subcutaneous infusion pump, 9 involved use of oral terbutaline (2 cases of outpatient use and 7 cases of inpatient use) alone or in addition to subcutaneous or IV† terbutaline, and 4 involved subcutaneous, IV, or unknown routes of administration. Between January 1, 1998 and July 2009, 12 maternal cases of serious cardiovascular events, including cardiac arrhythmias, myocardial infarction, pulmonary edema, hypertension, and tachycardia, associated with use of terbutaline were reported to AERS. Among the 12 maternal cases of serious cardiovascular events were 3 cases involving use of terbutaline administered by a subcutaneous infusion pump and 5 cases involving use of oral terbutaline (3 cases of outpatient use and 2 cases of inpatient use) alone or in addition to subcutaneous terbutaline.

Based on these results and a review of the medical literature, the FDA has concluded that the risk of serious adverse events outweighs any potential benefit to pregnant women receiving prolonged tocolysis with terbutaline injection (beyond 48–72 hours) or acute or prolonged tocolysis with oral terbutaline. Because of the potential for serious maternal cardiac effects and death, the manufacturers and FDA warn that terbutaline sulfate injection is not FDA labeled for and should not be used for prolonged tocolysis (beyond 48–72 hours) and is contraindicated for such use. The manufacturers and FDA also warn that oral terbutaline sulfate is not FDA labeled for and should not be used for acute or maintenance tocolysis, and is contraindicated for such use. Terbutaline sulfate (injection or oral tablets) should not be used for maintenance tocolysis, particularly in the outpatient or home setting. Clinicians are encouraged to report adverse events involving terbutaline to the FDA MedWatch program. (See Uses: Preterm Labor.)

■ Precautions and Contraindications **Oral inhalation therapy with short-acting β_2-agonists is intended for the acute symptomatic relief of bronchospasm in reversible, obstructive airway disease, and should not be used regularly (e.g., 4 times daily) in asthmatic patients for *maintenance* therapy.** If control of mild asthma deteriorates and requires regular use of a short-acting β_2-agonist (i.e., 4 times daily), long-term maintenance therapy (e.g., inhaled corticosteroids) should be instituted. Patients with deteriorating asthma should be instructed to contact a clinician for reevaluation and possible institution of maintenance therapy. Patients should be instructed on the importance of adherence to dosing schedules, including not exceeding the recommended dose or frequency of use. Patients should use inhaled or other antiasthma agents only as directed by a clinician.

Failure to respond to a previously effective dosage of terbutaline may indicate seriously worsening asthma that requires reevaluation and possible institution of alternative regimens or therapy. Patients should be instructed to contact their clinician if decreased effectiveness of terbutaline occurs rather than increasing the dose or frequency of administration.

Terbutaline sulfate should be used with caution in patients with diabetes mellitus, hypertension, hyperthyroidism, a history of seizures, or cardiac disease, including those with ischemic heart disease, coronary insufficiency, or associated arrhythmias. Adverse cardiovascular effects may require discontinuance of the drug. Large IV† doses of terbutaline reportedly have aggravated preexisting diabetes and ketoacidosis; however, the clinical relevance of this finding to other dosage forms of the drug is unknown.

Therapy with β-adrenergic agonists may produce clinically important hypokalemia in some patients, possibly via intracellular shunting, which has the potential to produce adverse cardiovascular effects; the decrease usually is transient and usually does not require supplementation.

Use of terbutaline sulfate injection for prolonged tocolysis (beyond 48–72 hours) and use of oral terbutaline sulfate for acute or maintenance tocolysis are contraindicated. Terbutaline sulfate (injection or oral tablets) should not be used for maintenance tocolysis, particularly in the outpatient or home setting. (See Cautions: Adverse Effects and also Uses: Preterm Labor.)

Terbutaline sulfate also is contraindicated in patients who are known to be hypersensitive to sympathomimetic agents or any ingredient in the formulations.

■ Pediatric Precautions Some studies on the use of terbutaline sulfate in asthmatic children indicate that the drug may be a useful alternative to epinephrine in acute asthmatic attacks; however, pending accumulation of further data on the use of terbutaline in children, the drug is not recommended by the manufacturer for use in children younger than 12 years of age.

■ Geriatric Precautions Clinical studies of terbutaline did not include sufficient numbers of patients 65 years of age or older to determine whether geriatric patients respond differently than younger patients. While other clinical experience has not revealed age-related differences in response, drug dosage generally should be titrated carefully in geriatric patients, usually initiating therapy at the low end of the dosage range. The greater frequency of decreased hepatic, renal, and/or cardiac function and of concomitant disease and drug therapy observed in the elderly also should be considered.

■ **Pregnancy and Lactation** Although there are no adequate and controlled studies to date in humans, terbutaline sulfate has been associated with alterations in behavior and brain development, including decreased cellular proliferation and differentiation, in rat offspring when terbutaline was administered subcutaneously to dams during the late stage of the pregnancy and lactation period. Terbutaline exposures in rat dams were approximately 6.5 times the human exposure of an oral adult dosage of terbutaline sulfate 15 mg daily (on a mg/m^2 basis) and approximately 24–48 times the human exposure of a subcutaneous adult dosage of terbutaline sulfate 2–4 mg daily (on a mg/m^2 basis). In embryofetal developmental studies, teratogenic effects were not observed in offspring when pregnant rats and rabbits received terbutaline sulfate at oral dosages up to 50 mg/kg daily (approximately 32 and 65 times, respectively, the maximum recommended oral dosage for adults on a mg/m^2 basis; approximately 810 and 1600 times, respectively, the maximum recommended subcutaneous dosage for adults on a mg/m^2 basis).

Terbutaline sulfate injection is not FDA labeled for and should not be used for prolonged tocolysis (beyond 48–72 hours), and is contraindicated for such use. Oral terbutaline sulfate is not FDA labeled for and should not be used for acute or maintenance tocolysis, and is contraindicated for such use. Terbutaline sulfate (injection or oral tablets) should not be used for maintenance tocolysis, particularly in the outpatient or home setting. Serious adverse reactions, including death, have been reported after administration of terbutaline sulfate in pregnant women. Such adverse reactions in pregnant women include increased heart rate, transient hyperglycemia, hypokalemia, cardiac arrhythmias, pulmonary edema, and myocardial ischemia. In addition, increased fetal heart rate and neonatal hypoglycemia may occur as a result of maternal administration of terbutaline. The manufacturers state that terbutaline should be used with caution in pregnant women when needed for relief of bronchospasm during labor and only when the potential benefits are expected to clearly outweigh the possible risks. The manufacturers also state that terbutaline should be used during pregnancy only if the potential benefits justify the potential risks to the fetus. (See Cautions: Adverse Effects and Uses: Preterm Labor.)

Patients should be advised that serious adverse effects, including maternal cardiac effects and death, have been reported after prolonged use of terbutaline to manage preterm labor. Patients should be advised that there are serious situations where a clinician may decide that short-term use of terbutaline injection in the hospital setting may benefit a pregnant woman. Patients should be advised that oral terbutaline should not be used either to treat preterm labor or prevent recurrent preterm labor. (See Cautions: Adverse Effects and Uses: Preterm Labor.) Patients receiving terbutaline for another condition (e.g., asthma) should be advised to contact their clinician if they are or plan to become pregnant.

Terbutaline is distributed into milk, but in amounts generally considered insufficient to affect nursing infants; however, the drug should be used with caution in nursing women and only if the potential benefits justify the possible risks to the infant.

Drug Interactions

■ **Sympathomimetic Agents** Terbutaline sulfate should not be administered concurrently with other sympathomimetic agents because of the possibility of additive adverse cardiovascular effects; however, an aerosol bronchodilator of the adrenergic stimulant type may be used to relieve acute bronchospasm in patients receiving chronic oral terbutaline therapy.

■ **Theophylline Derivatives** There is some evidence from animal studies that concomitant administration of a sympathomimetic agent (e.g., terbutaline) and a theophylline derivative (e.g., aminophylline) may produce increased cardiotoxic effects. Although such an interaction has not been established in humans, a few reports have suggested that such a combination may have the potential for producing cardiac arrhythmias. Further accumulation of clinical data is needed to determine whether this potential interaction occurs in humans.

■ **Other Drugs** The effects of terbutaline on the vascular system may be potentiated in patients receiving monoamine oxidase inhibitors or tricyclic antidepressants; therefore, terbutaline should be administered with extreme caution to patients receiving these drugs or having recently received (i.e., within 2 weeks) such agents.

β-Adrenergic blocking agents such as propranolol not only block the pulmonary effects of β-agonists, but may produce severe bronchospasm in patients with asthma; therefore, these patients should not generally be treated with β-adrenergic blocking agents. However, under certain circumstances (e.g., prophylaxis after myocardial infarction), there may be no acceptable alternatives to the use of β-adrenergic blocking agents in patients with asthma; cardioselective β-adrenergic blocking agents without intrinsic sympathomimetic activity (e.g., metoprolol, atenolol, esmolol) should be used with caution in these patients. Low dosages of a cardioselective β-adrenergic blocker should be used initially.

Since terbutaline may lower serum potassium concentrations, care should be taken in patients also receiving other drugs that can lower serum potassium concentration, such as non-potassium-sparing diuretics (such as loop or thiazide diuretics). The electrocardiographic changes and/or hypokalemia that may result from the administration of non-potassium-sparing diuretics may be aggravated by concomitant β-agonists, especially when the recommended dosage of the β-agonist is exceeded. Although the clinical importance of these effects is not known, caution is advised when administering β-agonists with non-potassium-sparing diuretics.

Acute Toxicity

Limited information is available on the acute toxicity of orally administered terbutaline sulfate in humans. Overdosage of terbutaline would be expected to produce manifestations that are principally extensions of pharmacologic and adverse effects of the drug. Treatment of acute terbutaline overdosage consists of symptomatic and supportive therapy including cardiac and respiratory support. In the conscious patient, emesis should be induced followed by gastric lavage. If emesis cannot be induced (i.e., patient is unconscious), gastric lavage is indicated; an endotracheal tube with cuff inflated should be in place to prevent aspiration of gastric contents. Administration of activated charcoal may be considered. The patient should remain under medical supervision until symptoms have resolved.

Pharmacology

Terbutaline sulfate stimulates β-adrenergic receptors of the sympathetic nervous system and has little or no effect on α-adrenergic receptors. Data from in vitro and in vivo pharmacologic studies have demonstrated that terbutaline exerts a preferential effect on β_2-adrenergic receptors. Terbutaline stimulates β-adrenergic receptors less selectively than relatively selective β_2-agonists (e.g., albuterol). However, following subcutaneous administration of terbutaline in controlled clinical studies, no apparent preferential β_2-adrenergic effect was noted. It is believed that β-adrenergic agonists stimulate the production of cyclic adenosine-3′,5′-monophosphate (AMP) by activation of the enzyme adenyl cyclase, which appears to mediate numerous cellular responses, including bronchial smooth muscle relaxation and inhibition of the release of mediators from mast cells in the airways. The main effect of terbutaline is relaxation of smooth muscles of the bronchial tree and the peripheral vasculature. The drug significantly increases pulmonary flow rates as measured by pulmonary function tests such as the forced expiratory volume in 1 second (FEV_1). Terbutaline does not appear to cause changes in arterial oxygen tension.

Like metaproterenol and albuterol, terbutaline appears to have a greater stimulating effect on β-receptors of the bronchial, vascular, and uterine smooth muscles (β_2 receptors) than on the β-receptors of the heart (β_1 receptors). Terbutaline relaxes uterine smooth muscle and inhibits uterine contractions. (See Uses: Preterm Labor.) However, terbutaline may cause some cardiostimulatory effects and CNS stimulation. It is unclear whether the tachycardia that sometimes occurs with terbutaline is caused by β_1 stimulation or by a reflex response to blood pressure changes secondary to peripheral vasodilation.

Pharmacokinetics

■ **Absorption** About 30–50% of an oral dose of terbutaline sulfate is absorbed from the GI tract. The drug is well absorbed following subcutaneous administration. Following subcutaneous administration, clinically important increases in FEV_1 occur within 15 minutes, and maximum effects usually occur within 30–60 minutes. Clinically important bronchodilator activity may continue for 1.5–4 hours. Following oral administration, a change in flow rate usually occurs within 30 minutes; substantial clinical improvement in pulmonary function occurs within 1–2 hours and is maximal within 2–3 hours. Clinically important decreases in airway and pulmonary resistance may persist for 4 hours or longer following oral administration.

■ **Distribution** Terbutaline is apparently distributed into milk in concentrations at least as high as concurrent plasma concentrations; however, the amount distributed into milk is estimated to be less than 1% of a dose given to a nursing woman.

■ **Elimination** Terbutaline is partially metabolized in the liver, mainly to the inactive sulfate conjugate. Following parenteral administration, about 60% of a dose is excreted in urine unchanged, up to 3% of a dose is excreted in feces via the bile, and the remainder is excreted in urine as the conjugate. After oral administration, a larger proportion of a dose is excreted as the conjugate, indicating that metabolism of the drug may occur in the GI tract or during first pass through the liver. Excretion of the drug and its metabolites is essentially complete within 72–96 hours after a single parenteral or oral dose.

Following subcutaneous administration of terbutaline, mean terminal half-life is 5.7 hours. Following administration of a single oral dose in patients with asthma, the elimination half-life of terbutaline is approximately 3.4 hours.

Chemistry and Stability

■ **Chemistry** Terbutaline sulfate is a synthetic sympathomimetic amine that is similar to isoproterenol and metaproterenol in chemical structure and in pharmacologic action. The drug occurs as a white to gray-white crystalline powder that is odorless or has a faint odor of acetic acid and is soluble in water and 0.1 N hydrochloric acid, slightly soluble in methanol, and insoluble in chloroform. The commercially available terbutaline sulfate injection is a sterile, nonpyrogenic, aqueous solution; sodium chloride has been added to adjust tonicity. Hydrochloric acid also may be added to adjust pH of the injection to 4 (tonicity range: 3–5).

■ **Stability** Terbutaline sulfate is stable in solutions with a pH of 1–7 and is sensitive to excessive heat and light. Solutions of the drug should not be used if they are discolored. Terbutaline sulfate injection should be stored at 20–25°C and protected from light by storing in original carton until use. Terbutaline sulfate tablets should be stored at controlled room temperature (15–30°C); the tablets should be stored in tight, light-resistant containers.

Preparations

Excipients in commercially available drug preparations may have clinically important effects in some individuals; consult specific product labeling for details.

Terbutaline Sulfate

Oral		
Tablets	2.5 mg*	**Terbutaline Sulfate Tablets**
	5 mg*	**Terbutaline Sulfate Tablets**
Parenteral		
Injection, for subcutaneous use only	1 mg/mL*	**Terbutaline Sulfate Injection**

*available from one or more manufacturer, distributor, and/or repackager by generic (nonproprietary) name

†Use is not currently included in the labeling approved by the US Food and Drug Administration

Vilanterol Trifenatate

■ Vilanterol trifenatate, a synthetic sympathomimetic amine, is a relatively selective, long-acting β_2-adrenergic agonist.

Uses

■ **Bronchospasm** ***Chronic Obstructive Pulmonary Disease*** Vilanterol trifenatate is used in fixed combination with fluticasone furoate (a corticosteroid) or umeclidinium bromide (an antimuscarinic agent) as a bronchodilator for the long-term maintenance treatment of airflow obstruction associated with chronic obstructive pulmonary disease (COPD), including chronic bronchitis and emphysema. Vilanterol trifenatate in fixed combination with fluticasone furoate also is used to reduce exacerbations of COPD in patients with a history of such exacerbations. Vilanterol trifenatate in fixed combination with fluticasone furoate is *not* indicated for the treatment of acute bronchospasm. Vilanterol trifenatate in fixed combination with umeclidinium bromide is *not* indicated for the treatment of acute bronchospasm or for the treatment of asthma†.

Efficacy of vilanterol in combination with fluticasone furoate has been evaluated in 2 randomized, double-blind, placebo-controlled studies of 24 weeks' duration in adults 40 years of age or older with moderate to severe COPD. The primary efficacy outcomes were the weighted mean postdose (0–4 hours) forced expiratory volume in 1 second (FEV_1) on day 168 and the change from baseline in the trough FEV_1 on day 169. In these studies, orally inhaled vilanterol (25 mcg once daily) in fixed combination with fluticasone furoate (100 mcg once daily) improved postdose FEV_1 at 168 days by 173–214 mL compared with placebo and by 120–168 mL compared with fluticasone furoate alone. The change from baseline in trough FEV_1 improved by 115–144 mL compared with placebo at 169 days.

In 2 randomized, double-blind studies of 12 months' duration in patients with COPD and moderate to severe airflow obstruction, orally inhaled vilanterol (25 mcg once daily) in fixed combination with fluticasone furoate (100 mcg once daily) resulted in a decreased mean annual rate of COPD exacerbations compared with vilanterol alone (0.7–0.9 versus 1.05–1.14 exacerbations per year).

Efficacy of vilanterol in combination with umeclidinium bromide has been evaluated in a randomized, double-blind, placebo-controlled study of 24 weeks' duration in adults 40 years of age or older with COPD. The primary efficacy outcome was the change from baseline in the trough FEV_1 on day 169. Following administration of orally inhaled vilanterol 25 mcg in fixed combination with umeclidinium 62.5 mcg once daily, the change from baseline in trough FEV_1 at 169 days improved by 52, 95, and 167 mL compared with umeclidinium alone, vilanterol alone, and placebo, respectively.

For additional information on the treatment of COPD, see Uses: Chronic Obstructive Pulmonary Disease, in Ipratropium Bromide 12:08.08.

Dosage and Administration

■ **Administration** Vilanterol trifenatate in combination with fluticasone furoate is administered by oral inhalation using a specific preloaded inhaler (Breo® Ellipta®) that delivers a fixed combination of powdered vilanterol trifenatate and fluticasone furoate from foil-wrapped blisters. Vilanterol trifenatate in combination with umeclidinium bromide is administered by oral inhalation using a specific preloaded inhaler (Anoro® Ellipta®) that delivers a fixed combination of powdered vilanterol trifenatate and umeclidinium bromide from foil-wrapped blisters. Vilanterol trifenatate in fixed combination with fluticasone furoate or umeclidinium bromide should be administered once daily at the same time every day.

Before first use of either the Breo® Ellipta® or Anoro® Ellipta® inhaler, the device should be removed from the foil tray and the enclosed desiccant should be discarded out of reach of children and pets. The date the tray is opened and the discard date (6 weeks after opening) should be written on the inhaler label. The number of doses remaining in the inhaler is displayed on the counter located on the front of the device. The cover of the inhaler should not be opened until immediately before use; to avoid wasting doses, the inhaler cover should not be closed again until the dose has been inhaled. When the cover of the inhaler is opened fully to expose the mouthpiece, a click should be heard. If the dose counter does not advance when the click is heard, the dose has not been properly prepared, and the patient should contact the clinician.

Before inhaling the dose, the patient should exhale completely, but should *not* exhale into the mouthpiece of the inhaler. The patient should then place the mouthpiece between the lips and inhale deeply through the inhaler with a steady, even breath; the patient should not inhale through the nose. The air vent on the inhaler should not be blocked while the dose is administered. The patient should remove the inhaler from the mouth, hold the breath for about 3–4 seconds (or as long as comfortable), and then exhale slowly and gently. While some patients may taste or feel a dose of drug delivered from the inhaler, patients should be instructed not to use another dose even if they do not perceive that the dose has been delivered. After the dose is administered, the inhaler should be closed by sliding the cover up and over the mouthpiece as far as possible.

Rinsing the mouth with water (without swallowing) after inhalation of vilanterol in fixed combination with fluticasone furoate is advised.

The inhaler does not need to be cleaned after use. However, if desired, the mouthpiece can be cleaned with a dry tissue. The inhaler should be discarded when every blister has been used or 6 weeks after removal of the inhaler from the foil tray, whichever comes first.

■ **Dosage** Dosage of vilanterol trifenatate is expressed in terms of vilanterol.

Each foil-wrapped blister in the Breo® Ellipta® inhaler device contains 40 mcg of vilanterol trifenatate (equivalent to 25 mcg of vilanterol) or 100 mcg of fluticasone furoate (in separate blisters). After the inhaler is activated, the powder within a pair of blisters is exposed and dispersed into the air stream created by the patient's inhalation. Using standardized in vitro testing at a flow rate of 60 L/minute for 4 seconds, the inhaler delivered 22 mcg of vilanterol and 92 mcg of fluticasone furoate per pair of blisters. The precise amount of drug delivered to the lungs with each activation of the inhaler device depends on factors such as the patient's inspiratory flow. The commercially available inhaler delivers 30 doses (or 14 doses from the sample or institutional package).

Each foil-wrapped blister in the Anoro® Ellipta® inhaler device contains 40 mcg of vilanterol trifenatate (equivalent to 25 mcg of vilanterol) or 74.2 mcg of umeclidinium bromide (equivalent to 62.5 mcg of umeclidinium) (in separate blisters). After the inhaler is activated, the powder within a pair of blisters is exposed and dispersed into the air stream created by the patient's inhalation. Using standardized in vitro testing at a flow rate of 60 L/minute for 4 seconds, the inhaler delivered 22 mcg of vilanterol and 55 mcg of umeclidinium per pair of blisters. The precise amount of drug delivered to the lungs with each activation of the inhaler device depends on factors such as the patient's inspiratory flow. The commercially available inhaler delivers 30 doses (or 7 doses from the sample or institutional package).

Chronic Obstructive Pulmonary Disease **Vilanterol/Fluticasone Furoate Fixed-combination Therapy.** For maintenance therapy of chronic obstructive pulmonary disease (COPD), the recommended dosage of vilanterol in fixed combination with fluticasone furoate in adults is 25 mcg of vilanterol and 100 mcg of fluticasone furoate (1 inhalation) once daily via the Breo® Ellipta® inhaler device. The drug should not be administered more frequently than once every 24 hours. If a dose of vilanterol in fixed combination with fluticasone furoate is missed, the dose may be taken as soon as it is remembered. However, 2 doses should not be taken at the same time.

Vilanterol/Umeclidinium Bromide Fixed-combination Therapy. For maintenance therapy of COPD, the recommended dosage of vilanterol in fixed combination with umeclidinium in adults is 25 mcg of vilanterol and 62.5 mcg of umeclidinium (1 inhalation) once daily via the Anoro® Ellipta® inhaler device. The drug should not be administered more frequently than once every 24 hours. If a dose of vilanterol in fixed combination with umeclidinium bromide is missed, the dose may be taken as soon as it is remembered. However, 2 doses should not be taken at the same time.

■ **Special Populations** The manufacturer of vilanterol in fixed combination with fluticasone furoate states that dosage adjustment is not required in geriatric patients or in patients with hepatic or renal impairment. (See Specific Populations under Cautions: Warnings/Precautions.)

The manufacturer of vilanterol in fixed combination with umeclidinium bromide states that dosage adjustment is not required in geriatric patients or in patients with renal impairment or moderate hepatic impairment. (See Specific Populations under Cautions: Warnings/Precautions.)

Cautions

■ **Contraindications** Known hypersensitivity to vilanterol trifenatate or any other ingredient in the commercially available formulation. Known severe hypersensitivity to milk proteins.

When vilanterol trifenatate is used in fixed combination with fluticasone furoate or umeclidinium bromide, contraindications associated with fluticasone or umeclidinium should be considered.

■ **Warnings/Precautions** ***Use of Fixed Combinations***

Serious Asthma-related Events Monotherapy with long-acting β_2-adrenergic agonists, such as vilanterol, increases the risk of asthma-related death. In addition, available data from controlled clinical trials suggest that use of long-acting β_2-adrenergic agonists as monotherapy increases the risk of asthma-related hospitalization in pediatric and adolescent patients.

Data from a large placebo-controlled safety study (Salmeterol Multicenter Asthma Research Trial [SMART]) showed an increase in asthma-related deaths in patients receiving certain long-acting β_2-adrenergic agonists (e.g., salmeterol) in addition to usual asthma therapy. (See Asthma-related Death and Life-threatening Events under Cautions: Respiratory Effects, in Salmeterol 12:12.08.12.) The increased risk of asthma-related death with use of salmeterol as monotherapy is considered a class effect of the long-acting β_2-adrenergic agonists, including vilanterol. However, FDA has concluded that there is no clinically important increased risk of serious asthma-related events, including hospitalization, intubation, or death, associated with concomitant use of long-acting β_2-adrenergic agonists (e.g., vilanterol) and inhaled corticosteroids compared with inhaled corticosteroids alone based on the results of several large clinical studies. In addition, these studies showed that combination therapy with long-acting β_2-adrenergic agonists and inhaled corticosteroids was more effective in reducing the incidence of asthma exacerbations (i.e., events requiring use of systemic corticosteroids for at least 3 outpatient days or an asthma-related hospitalization or emergency department visit requiring use of systemic corticosteroids) compared with use of inhaled corticosteroids alone.

In 4 randomized, double-blind, active-controlled clinical trials mandated by FDA, the risk of serious asthma-related events from use of inhaled corticosteroids alone compared with combined use of long-acting β_2-adrenergic agonists and inhaled corticosteroids was evaluated over 26 weeks in 41,297 patients with asthma (3 trials in adults and adolescents 12 years of age or older and one trial in children 4–11 years of age). The primary safety end point in all of these trials was serious asthma-related events, including hospitalization, intubation, and death; these events were reviewed by a blinded committee to determine if the events were asthma related. The 3 trials performed in adults and adolescents were designed to rule out a hazard ratio of 2, and the pediatric trial was designed to rule out a hazard ratio of 2.7; this objective was met in all 4 individual trials. The trials were not designed to rule out all risk for serious asthma-related events associated with long-acting β_2-adrenergic agonists in combination with inhaled corticosteroids compared with inhaled corticosteroids alone.

The safety studies in adults and adolescents included one trial comparing salmeterol and fluticasone propionate in fixed combination as the inhalation powder with fluticasone inhalation powder alone, one trial comparing formoterol and mometasone furoate in fixed combination with mometasone furoate alone, and one trial comparing formoterol and budesonide in fixed combination with budesonide alone. In a meta-analysis combining data from these 3 trials, a hazard ratio of 1.1 for serious asthma-related events in patients receiving fixed-combination therapy with long-acting β_2-adrenergic agonists and inhaled corticosteroids compared with patients receiving inhaled corticosteroids alone was reported. Subgroup analyses for gender, adolescents 12–17 years of age, Asian and African-American patients, and obese patients also showed no substantial increase in the risk of serious asthma-related events or asthma exacerbations in these populations.

The safety study in children 4–11 years of age included 6208 patients who were randomized to receive salmeterol and fluticasone propionate in fixed combination as the inhalation powder or fluticasone propionate inhalation powder alone. Serious asthma-related events were reported in 0.9% of patients receiving salmeterol and fluticasone in fixed combination and in 0.7% of patients receiving fluticasone alone, with an estimated hazard ratio for first event of 1.29 for the combination therapy compared with fluticasone alone. No asthma-related deaths or intubations were reported in either group of pediatric patients.

Data are not available to determine whether the rate of death is increased in patients with chronic obstructive pulmonary disease (COPD) receiving long-acting β_2-adrenergic agonists, including vilanterol.

Deterioration of Disease and Acute Episodes Vilanterol in fixed combination with fluticasone furoate or umeclidinium bromide should not be initiated in patients with acutely deteriorating COPD, which may be life-threatening. Vilanterol has not been studied in this patient population, and initiation of vilanterol in this setting is not appropriate.

Vilanterol in fixed combination with fluticasone furoate or umeclidinium bromide should *not* be used for the relief of acute symptoms (i.e., as rescue therapy for the treatment of acute episodes of bronchospasm). Vilanterol in fixed combination with fluticasone furoate or umeclidinium bromide has not been studied for the relief of acute symptoms and extra doses of the drug should not be used for this purpose. All patients receiving vilanterol in fixed combination with fluticasone furoate or umeclidinium bromide should be provided with and instructed in the use of a short-acting, inhaled β_2-agonist.

When vilanterol in fixed combination with fluticasone furoate or umeclidinium bromide is initiated in patients receiving short-acting, oral or inhaled β_2-agonists on a regular basis (e.g., 4 times daily), *regular* use of the short-acting agent should be discontinued, and such agents should be used only for symptomatic relief of acute respiratory symptoms.

COPD may deteriorate acutely over a period of hours or chronically over several days or longer. Failure to respond to a previously effective dosage of vilanterol in fixed combination with fluticasone furoate or umeclidinium bromide or to a supplemental short-acting, inhaled β_2-agonist (e.g., increased need for additional short-acting, inhaled β_2-agonists) may indicate deterioration of COPD for which prompt medical attention is indicated. In this setting, immediate reevaluation of the patient and treatment regimen is required. Increasing the daily dosage of vilanterol in fixed combination with fluticasone furoate or umeclidinium bromide to exceed the recommended dosage is not appropriate in this situation.

Excessive Use and Use With Other Long-acting β_2-Adrenergic Agonists Clinically important cardiovascular effects and fatalities have been reported in association with excessive use of inhaled sympathomimetic drugs.

As with other inhaled β_2-adrenergic agonists, vilanterol should not be used more frequently or at dosages higher than recommended, or concomitantly with other preparations containing long-acting β_2-adrenergic agonists, since overdosage may result. Vilanterol in fixed combination with fluticasone furoate or umeclidinium bromide should not be used with another preparation containing a long-acting β_2-agonist (e.g., arformoterol, formoterol, indacaterol, olodaterol, salmeterol) for any reason.

Paradoxical Bronchospasm As with other inhaled drugs, patients receiving vilanterol in fixed combination with fluticasone furoate or umeclidinium bromide may develop paradoxical bronchospasm, which may be life-threatening.

If paradoxical bronchospasm occurs, it should be treated immediately with an inhaled, short-acting bronchodilator. Vilanterol in fixed combination with fluticasone furoate or umeclidinium bromide should be discontinued immediately and alternative therapy instituted.

Sensitivity Reactions Hypersensitivity reactions may occur after administration of vilanterol in fixed combination with fluticasone furoate or umeclidinium bromide. Anaphylactic reactions have been reported following oral inhalation of other powder preparations containing lactose in patients with severe hypersensitivity to milk proteins; therefore, patients with severe milk protein allergy should not use vilanterol in fixed combination with fluticasone furoate or umeclidinium bromide. (See Cautions: Contraindications.)

Hypersensitivity reactions including anaphylaxis, angioedema, rash, and urticaria have been reported during postmarketing surveillance of vilanterol in fixed combination with fluticasone furoate.

Cardiovascular Effects Vilanterol, like other β_2-adrenergic agonists, may produce a clinically important cardiovascular effect in some patients as measured by increases in pulse rate, systolic or diastolic blood pressure, or cardiac arrhythmias (e.g., supraventricular tachycardia, extrasystoles). If such effects occur, discontinuance of vilanterol therapy may be required.

In addition, β_2-adrenergic agonists have been reported to produce ECG changes, such as flattening of the T wave, prolongation of the corrected QT (QT_c) interval, and ST-segment depression; the clinical importance of these effects is unknown. Administration of large dosages of orally inhaled vilanterol in combination with fluticasone furoate (i.e., 4 times the recommended dosage of vilanterol, representing a systemic exposure 12-fold higher than that observed in patients with COPD) in healthy individuals resulted in clinically important prolongation of the QT_c interval, which may cause ventricular arrhythmias. Therefore, vilanterol, like other sympathomimetic amines, should be used with caution in patients with cardiovascular disorders, especially coronary insufficiency, cardiac arrhythmias, or hypertension.

No clinically important effects on heart rate, QT_c, or blood pressure were observed in patients with COPD receiving vilanterol alone or in combination with fluticasone furoate in clinical trials. No clinically important effects on cardiac rhythm were observed in patients with COPD receiving vilanterol in combination with umeclidinium bromide in clinical trials, and no clinically important effects on QT_c were observed in studies in healthy individuals.

Metabolic and Electrolyte Effects Vilanterol, like other sympathomimetic amines, should be used with caution in patients with thyrotoxicosis.

IV doses of the β_2-adrenergic agonist albuterol (IV preparation not commercially available in the US) have been reported to aggravate preexisting diabetes mellitus and ketoacidosis. β_2-Adrenergic agonists may cause transient hyperglycemia in some patients.

Clinically important hypokalemia, which may result in adverse cardiovascular effects, may occur in some patients receiving β_2-adrenergic agonists, possibly through intracellular shunting. (See Cardiovascular Effects under Warnings/Precautions: Other Warnings and Precautions, in Cautions.) However, the decrease in serum potassium concentrations usually is transient and generally does not require supplementation.

Changes in serum glucose or potassium concentrations were not observed in patients with COPD receiving vilanterol in fixed combination with fluticasone furoate or umeclidinium bromide in clinical trials of 6 or 12 months' duration.

Nervous System Effects Vilanterol, like other sympathomimetic amines, should be used with caution in patients with seizure disorders and in those unusually responsive to sympathomimetic amines.

Specific Populations **Pregnancy.** Category C. (See Users Guide.)

The effects of vilanterol on labor and delivery are not known. Because of the potential for β-agonist interference with uterine contractility, use of vilanterol during labor should be restricted to those patients in whom the benefits clearly outweigh the risks.

Lactation. It is not known whether vilanterol is distributed into human milk; however, other β_2-adrenergic agonists are distributed into human milk. The manufacturer recommends that vilanterol in fixed combination with fluticasone furoate or umeclidinium bromide should be used with caution in nursing women.

Pediatric Use. Vilanterol is not indicated for use in pediatric patients. Safety and efficacy have not been established in pediatric patients.

Geriatric Use. In clinical trials evaluating vilanterol in fixed combination with fluticasone furoate in patients with COPD, approximately 33% of patients receiving the drug were 65 years of age or older, and about 7% were 75 years of age or older. In clinical trials evaluating vilanterol in fixed combination with umeclidinium bromide in patients with COPD, approximately 29% of patients receiving the drug were 65 years of age or older, and about 7% were 75 years of age or older. Although no overall differences in safety and efficacy were observed between geriatric and younger adults, and other clinical experience revealed no evidence of age-related differences, the possibility that some geriatric patients may exhibit increased sensitivity to the drug cannot be ruled out. Dosage adjustment is not necessary in geriatric patients.

Hepatic Impairment. Following repeated daily dosing of vilanterol in fixed combination with fluticasone furoate for 7 days, no clinically important changes in peak plasma concentrations or area under the serum concentration-time curve (AUC) of vilanterol were observed in patients with mild, moderate, or severe hepatic impairment. However, increases of 34, 83, and 75% in AUC of fluticasone were observed in patients with mild, moderate, or severe hepatic impairment, respectively, compared with healthy individuals. Therefore, the manufacturer states that vilanterol in fixed combination with fluticasone furoate should be used with caution in patients with moderate or severe hepatic impairment. Dosage adjustment of vilanterol in fixed combination with fluticasone furoate is not required in patients with hepatic impairment.

Following administration of vilanterol in fixed combination with umeclidinium bromide, no clinically important changes in peak plasma concentrations or AUC of vilanterol or umeclidinium were observed in patients with moderate hepatic impairment. Therefore, the manufacturer states that dosage adjustment of vilanterol in fixed combination with umeclidinium is not required in patients with moderate hepatic impairment. Vilanterol in fixed combination with umeclidinium has not been studied in patients with severe hepatic impairment.

Renal Impairment. Following administration of vilanterol in fixed combination with fluticasone furoate or umeclidinium bromide, no clinically important increases in vilanterol, fluticasone, or umeclidinium exposure were observed in patients with severe renal impairment (creatinine clearance less than 30 mL/minute) compared with individuals with normal renal function. However, the AUC of vilanterol was 56% higher in individuals with severe renal impairment compared with those having normal renal function. The manufacturer states that dosage adjustment is not required in patients with renal impairment.

■ **Common Adverse Effects** Adverse effects reported in 3% or more of patients with COPD receiving vilanterol in fixed combination with fluticasone furoate in controlled clinical studies include nasopharyngitis, headache, upper respiratory tract infection, and oropharyngeal candidiasis.

Adverse effects reported in 1% or more of patients with COPD receiving vilanterol in fixed combination with umeclidinium bromide in controlled clinical studies include pharyngitis, sinusitis, lower respiratory tract infection, constipation, diarrhea, extremity pain, muscle spasms, neck pain, and chest pain.

Drug Interactions

Vilanterol is a substrate of cytochrome P-450 (CYP) isoenzyme 3A4 and P-glycoprotein (P-gp).

■ **Drugs Affecting or Metabolized by Hepatic Microsomal Enzymes and/or the P-glycoprotein Transport System** Concomitant use of vilanterol with potent inhibitors of CYP3A4 (e.g., clarithromycin, conivaptan, ketoconazole, indinavir, itraconazole, lopinavir, nefazodone, nelfinavir, ritonavir, saquinavir, telithromycin, troleandomycin, voriconazole) is expected to result in increased systemic exposure to vilanterol.

Concomitant administration of ketoconazole 400 mg daily resulted in a 65% increase in area under the serum concentration-time curve (AUC) of vilanterol; associated increases in β-agonist-related effects on heart rate or potassium concentrations were not observed. Caution should be exercised when vilanterol is used in patients receiving long-term therapy with ketoconazole or other potent CYP3A4 inhibitors.

Concomitant administration of multiple daily 240-mg doses of verapamil (a potent P-gp inhibitor and moderate CYP3A4 inhibitor) did not affect peak plasma concentrations or AUC of vilanterol in healthy individuals. Dosage adjustment of vilanterol is not required with concomitant use.

■ **Drugs that Prolong the QT Interval** Vilanterol, like other β_2-adrenergic agonists, should be used with extreme caution in patients who are receiving or have recently received (i.e., within 2 weeks) drugs known to prolong the corrected QT (QT_c) interval because of the increased risk of ventricular arrhythmias and because such drugs may potentiate the effects of adrenergic drugs on the cardiovascular system.

■ **β-Adrenergic Blocking Agents** β-Adrenergic blocking agents may interfere with the actions of vilanterol when the drugs are used concomitantly. β-Adrenergic blocking agents not only block the therapeutic effects of β_2-adrenergic agonists, but also may produce severe bronchospasm in patients with chronic obstructive pulmonary disease (COPD). Patients with COPD usually should not be treated with β-adrenergic blocking agents. However, under certain circumstances (e.g., prophylaxis after myocardial infarction), there may be no acceptable alternatives to the use of β-adrenergic blocking agents in these patients; the use of cardioselective β-adrenergic blocking agents may be considered but vilanterol and β-adrenergic blocking agents should be used concomitantly with caution.

■ **Diuretics** The ECG and/or hypokalemic effects that may result from the administration of non-potassium-sparing diuretics (e.g., loop or thiazide diuretics) may be aggravated by concomitant use of β-agonists, especially when the recommended dosage of the β-agonist is exceeded; the clinical importance is unknown. β-Agonists and non-potassium-sparing diuretics should be used concomitantly with caution.

■ **Monoamine Oxidase Inhibitors** The manufacturer states that the effects of vilanterol on the cardiovascular system may be potentiated in patients receiving concomitant therapy with monoamine oxidase (MAO) inhibitors; therefore, vilanterol should be used with extreme caution in patients who are receiving or have recently received (i.e., within 2 weeks) these drugs.

■ **Sympathomimetic Agents** Other preparations containing long-acting β_2-adrenergic agonists (e.g., arformoterol, formoterol, indacaterol, olodaterol, salmeterol) should not be used for any reason in patients receiving vilanterol in fixed combination with fluticasone furoate or umeclidinium bromide.

■ **Tricyclic Antidepressants** The manufacturer states that the effects of vilanterol on the cardiovascular system may be potentiated in patients receiving concomitant therapy with tricyclic antidepressants; therefore, vilanterol should be used with extreme caution in patients who are receiving or have recently received (i.e., within 2 weeks) these drugs.

Description

Vilanterol trifenatate, a synthetic sympathomimetic amine, is a relatively selective, long-acting β_2-adrenergic agonist. In vitro, the functional selectivity of vilanterol is similar to that of salmeterol; the clinical importance is unknown. The drug's β_2-adrenergic effects appear to result at least in part from stimulation of the production of cyclic adenosine-3′,5′-monophosphate (cAMP) by activation of adenyl cyclase. Increased concentrations of cAMP are associated with relaxation of bronchial smooth muscle. Vilanterol appears to inhibit release of mediators of immediate hypersensitivity from cells, especially mast cells.

Steady-state plasma vilanterol concentrations are achieved after 6 days of repeated once-daily inhalation of vilanterol in fixed combination with fluticasone furoate; accumulation of vilanterol is up to 2.4-fold higher following repeated dosing compared with single-dose administration. Steady-state plasma vilanterol concentrations are achieved within 14 days of repeated once-daily inhalation of vilanterol in fixed combination with umeclidinium bromide; accumulation of vilanterol is up to 1.7-fold higher following repeated dosing compared with single-dose administration. Peak plasma vilanterol concentrations are reached within 5–15 minutes following oral inhalation; however, vilanterol plasma concentrations may not predict therapeutic effect. Absolute bioavailability of orally inhaled vilanterol is approximately 27%, principally due to absorption of the inhaled portion of the dose delivered to the lungs. Oral bioavailability of the swallowed portion of an inhaled dose is low (less than 2%) because of extensive first-pass metabolism. Systemic exposure to vilanterol is 24% higher in patients with chronic obstructive pulmonary disease (COPD) compared with healthy individuals. Vilanterol is highly bound (approximately 94%) to human plasma proteins. Vilanterol is extensively metabolized, principally by cytochrome P-450 (CYP) isoenzyme 3A4, to metabolites with substantially reduced β_1- and β_2-agonist activity compared with the parent drug. The effective half-life for accumulation of vilanterol used in fixed combination with fluticasone in patients with COPD following multiple 25-mcg doses administered by oral inhalation is 21.3 hours. In one study in healthy individuals, the effective half-life for accumulation of vilanterol used in fixed combination with umeclidinium following oral inhalation of 25 or 100 mcg once daily for 10 days was 11–19 hours. Following oral administration, approximately 70 and 30% of a radiolabeled dose of vilanterol is excreted in urine and feces, respectively, mostly as metabolites.

Advice to Patients

When vilanterol trifenatate is used in fixed combination with fluticasone furoate or umeclidinium bromide, importance of informing patients of important cautionary information about fluticasone furoate or umeclidinium bromide.

A copy of the manufacturer's patient information (medication guide) and instructions for use for vilanterol in fixed combination with fluticasone furoate or umeclidinium bromide should be provided to all patients each time the drug is dispensed. Importance of instructing patients to read the medication guide prior to initiation of therapy and each time the prescription is refilled.

Importance of informing patients that monotherapy with long-acting β_2-adrenergic agonists, such as vilanterol, increases the risk of asthma-related death.

Importance of adequate understanding of proper storage, preparation, and inhalation techniques, including use of the inhalation delivery systems.

Importance of not using vilanterol in fixed combination with fluticasone furoate or umeclidinium bromide to relieve acute symptoms of chronic obstructive pulmonary disease (COPD); extra doses should not be used for such symptoms.

Importance of adherence to dosing schedules, including not altering the dose or frequency of use unless otherwise instructed by a clinician.

Importance of advising patients that if a dose of vilanterol in fixed combination with fluticasone furoate or umeclidinium bromide is missed, the dose should be taken as soon as it is remembered. Importance of not doubling the dose, and of not taking more than one dose in a 24-hour period.

Importance of all patients being provided with and instructed in the use of a short-acting, inhaled β_2-adrenergic agonist (e.g., albuterol) as supplemental therapy for acute symptoms.

Importance of discontinuing *regular* use of short-acting, inhaled β_2-agonists when initiating vilanterol in fixed combination with fluticasone furoate or umeclidinium bromide and using short-acting, inhaled β_2-agonists to relieve acute symptoms.

Importance of contacting a clinician immediately if symptoms worsen; the short-acting β_2-agonist becomes less effective or more inhalations than usual are required to relieve symptoms; or a clinically important decline in lung function (as outlined by clinician) occurs.

Importance of advising patients receiving vilanterol-containing preparations not to use additional vilanterol or other long-acting, inhaled β_2-adrenergic agonists for any reason.

Importance of patients not discontinuing therapy without medical supervision, since symptoms may recur after discontinuance.

Importance of informing patients of adverse effects associated with β_2-adrenergic agonists such as palpitations, chest pain, rapid heart rate, tremor, or nervousness.

Importance of advising patients that hypersensitivity reactions (e.g., anaphylaxis, angioedema, rash, urticaria) may occur following administration of vilanterol in fixed combination with fluticasone furoate; patients should be instructed to discontinue the drug if such reactions occur.

Patients with severe milk protein allergy should not use vilanterol in fixed combination with fluticasone furoate or umeclidinium bromide because of anaphylactic reactions reported in such patients following oral inhalation of other lactose-containing powder preparations.

Advise patients receiving orally inhaled vilanterol in fixed combination with fluticasone furoate to rinse their mouth with water (without swallowing) after each dose.

Importance of women informing clinicians if they are or plan to become pregnant or plan to breast-feed.

Importance of informing clinicians of existing or contemplated concomitant therapy, including and OTC drugs and dietary or herbal supplements, as well as any concomitant illnesses (e.g., cardiac disease, hypertension, seizures, thyroid disease, diabetes mellitus, allergies to drugs or food).

Importance of informing patients of other important precautionary information. (See Cautions.)

Overview® (see Users Guide). For additional information on this drug until a more detailed monograph is developed and published, the manufacturer's labeling should be consulted. It is *essential* that the manufacturer's labeling be consulted for more detailed information on usual cautions, precautions, contraindications, potential drug interactions, laboratory test interferences, and acute toxicity.

Preparations

Excipients in commercially available drug preparations may have clinically important effects in some individuals; consult specific product labeling for details.

Vilanterol Trifenatate Combinations

Oral Inhalation		
Powder for inhalation	25 mcg (of vilanterol) with Fluticasone Furoate 100 mcg per inhalation	**Breo® Ellipta®**, GlaxoSmithKline
Powder for inhalation	25 mcg (of vilanterol) with Umeclidinium Bromide 62.5 mcg (of umeclidinium) per inhalation	**Anoro® Ellipta®**, GlaxoSmithKline

†Use is not currently included in the labeling approved by the US Food and Drug Administration

α- and β-Adrenergic Agonists 12:12.12

ePHEDrine Hydrochloride
ePHEDrine Sulfate

■ Ephedrine is a sympathomimetic agent that occurs naturally in plants of the genus *Ephedra*; ephedrine stimulates both α- and β-adrenergic receptors.

Uses

■ **Hypotension During Anesthesia** Ephedrine is used parenterally as a vasopressor for the treatment of hypotension during anesthesia. Ephedrine sulfate injection is labeled by the US Food and Drug Administration (FDA) for the treatment of clinically important hypotension occurring in the setting of anesthesia. Because ephedrine sulfate injection was introduced into the US market before 1962 without an approved new drug application (NDA), some commercially available preparations may not be approved by the FDA.

Evidence supporting the efficacy of ephedrine for this indication is based principally on data from the published literature demonstrating that the drug increases systolic and mean arterial blood pressures when administered as a direct IV ("bolus") injection following the development of hypotension in patients undergoing neuraxial (spinal/epidural) and/or general anesthesia. In these studies, ephedrine was administered as either the sulfate or hydrochloride salt forms of the drug; however, only ephedrine sulfate is commercially available in the US as a parenteral preparation. Although IM use of ephedrine also has been evaluated in this setting, results of studies using IM ephedrine have been equivocal. The majority of patients who received ephedrine for the treatment of hypotension in these clinical studies were pregnant women undergoing cesarean section with neuraxial anesthesia. Although ephedrine historically has been considered the vasopressor of choice for the treatment of hypotension in obstetric anesthesia, there is some evidence suggesting that phenylephrine may provide a more favorable fetal acid-base balance. Experts currently recommend the use of either IV ephedrine or phenylephrine for the treatment of hypotension during neuraxial anesthesia; however, consideration should be given to selection of phenylephrine in the absence of maternal bradycardia because of improved fetal acid-base status in uncomplicated pregnancies.

Ephedrine also has been used with limited success for the prevention of hypotension† in patients undergoing spinal anesthesia; however, routine prophylactic use of vasopressors has been questioned because hypotension does not always occur during spinal anesthesia and treatment can readily be instituted if necessary. In addition, IV ephedrine has been associated with an increased incidence of hypertension when given prophylactically.

■ **Bronchospasm** ***Asthma*** Ephedrine is used orally as a bronchodilator for the symptomatic treatment of asthma. Preparations containing ephedrine hydrochloride or ephedrine sulfate in fixed-combination with guaifenesin are used as *self-medication* for the temporary relief of mild symptoms of intermittent asthma (e.g., wheezing, chest tightness, shortness of breath). Once a diagnosis of asthma has been confirmed by a clinician, use of a nonprescription (over-the-counter, OTC) bronchodilator may be appropriate in patients with mild symptoms of intermittent asthma; because asthma may be life-threatening, those with more severe asthma (i.e., persistent asthma) or worsening asthma (symptoms not relieved within 60 minutes or with maximum recommended dosages of ephedrine, increasing frequency of asthma attacks) should consult a clinician for other treatment options. A single-ingredient oral ephedrine sulfate preparation no longer is commercially available in the US. Ephedrine sulfate also has been used parenterally for the treatment of bronchial asthma; however, currently available parenteral preparations of the drug are not FDA-labeled for this use.

While oral ephedrine was once widely used for its bronchodilating effects in the management of reversible airway obstruction, the drug generally has been replaced by more selective and rapid-acting agents (e.g., inhaled β_2-adrenergic agonists); ephedrine is not recommended as a drug of choice for the rapid relief of asthma in current asthma management guidelines. In the stepped-care approach to antiasthmatic therapy, most experts currently recommend use of a selective, short-acting inhaled β_2-adrenergic agonist (e.g., albuterol, levalbuterol, pirbuterol) on an intermittent, as-needed basis in all patients with asthma to control acute symptoms (e.g., cough, wheezing, dyspnea). Alternatives to short-acting inhaled β_2-agonists recommended by some clinicians for relief of acute asthma symptoms include an inhaled anticholinergic agent (e.g., ipratropium), a short-acting oral β_2-agonist, or a short-acting theophylline (provided extended-release theophylline is not already used), but these alternatives have a slower onset of action and/or a greater risk of adverse effects.

Expectorants such as guaifenesin are used in combination with ephedrine to help loosen and thin bronchial secretions and facilitate the removal of mucous from bronchial passageways. However, use of expectorants in the management of asthma has been questioned by the FDA because of insufficient evidence supporting their use and inconsistency of such treatment with the pathogenesis of the disease. Increased sputum production is not a common feature of asthma; thus, patients with mild asthma (the population for whom self-medication with OTC drugs may be appropriate) generally do not require expectorant therapy. Furthermore, expectorants are not recommended in current asthma management guidelines. Based on these factors, FDA currently believes that there is no role for expectorants in the routine pharmacologic management of asthma and no longer considers the combination of an oral bronchodilator (i.e., ephedrine) and an expectorant (i.e., guaifenesin) rational therapy for patients with mild asthma.

Ephedrine also has been administered concomitantly with theophylline in the treatment of asthma; however, the combination of ephedrine and theophylline was shown in a study in asthmatic children to be no more effective than theophylline alone and was associated with an increased incidence of adverse effects.

■ **Nasal Congestion** Ephedrine has been administered orally as a nasal decongestant, but is of doubtful value when used for this condition. Extensive clinical experience indicates that ephedrine produces nasal decongestion when solutions of 0.5–3% (nasal solution no longer commercially available in the US) are applied topically to the nasal mucosa; however, controlled clinical studies supporting its effectiveness are lacking. Rebound congestion and tachyphylaxis may occur within a few days when ephedrine is used topically as a nasal decongestant.

As part of its ongoing review of OTC drug products, FDA has determined that any cough and cold preparation containing an oral bronchodilator active ingredient (e.g., ephedrine, ephedrine hydrochloride, ephedrine sulfate, racephedrine hydrochloride, or any other ephedrine salt) in combination with any analgesic, analgesic/antipyretic, anticholinergic, antihistamine, oral antitussive, or stimulant (e.g., caffeine) active ingredient generally is *not* recognized as safe and effective for *self-medication*. Such a combination is considered by the FDA to be a new drug and misbranded, and cannot be marketed for OTC cough and cold use unless it is the subject of an approved new drug application.

■ **Obesity** Because of its anorexigenic effects, ephedrine alone or combined with caffeine has been used for *self-medication* in the management of exogenous obesity†. (See Issues and Regulations Associated with Misuse and Abuse of Ephedrine-containing Preparations under Uses: Misuse and Abuse.)

Efficacy and safety of ephedrine and dietary supplements containing ephedra (a plant that contains several ephedrine alkaloids) have been assessed in numerous controlled studies involving several hundred individuals receiving the preparations for exogenous obesity†. Retrospective analysis of pooled data from these studies indicates that short-term (8 weeks up to 4 months) use of ephedrine (high doses), ephedrine combined with caffeine, or dietary supplements containing ephedra with or without herbs containing caffeine was associated with statistically significant, albeit modest, short-term weight loss when compared with placebo. The addition of caffeine to ephedrine moderately increases short-term weight loss. There is no evidence that the effect on short-term (up to 4–6 months) weight loss of dietary supplements containing ephedra combined with caffeine differs from that of ephedrine combined with caffeine; use of both drug combinations was associated with increased weight loss (about 0.9 kg more per month) compared with placebo. Safety and efficacy of *long-term* (i.e., more than 6 months) use of ephedrine for management of obesity have not been established. Because substantial weight loss (5–10% of baseline body weight) *and* long-term weight maintenance are necessary to improve health outcomes and reduce the risk of morbidities associated with obesity, the benefit of short-term weight loss associated with ephedrine or ephedra on health outcomes currently is not known. (See Issues and Regulations Associated with Misuse and Abuse of Ephedrine-containing Preparations under Uses: Misuse and Abuse.)

■ **Other Uses** Ephedrine has reportedly been used orally with good results for the management of peripheral edema secondary to diabetic neuropathy† in a few patients with type 1 diabetes mellitus.

Ephedrine has been used in patients with myasthenia gravis†. Limited data suggest that the drug may improve muscle weakness, fatigue, and quality of life in some patients with myasthenic conditions; however, randomized controlled studies are needed to further evaluate these potential benefits.

Ephedrine also has been used as a CNS stimulant in the treatment of narcolepsy† or depressive states†; however, the cardiovascular effects of the drug limit its usefulness in these conditions, and it has been largely replaced by other CNS stimulants.

Ephedrine sulfate also has been used in the treatment of Stokes-Adams disease†; when used for this condition, ephedrine provides a similar benefit to that of epinephrine.

■ **Misuse and Abuse** ***Enhancement of Athletic Performance*** Because of its stimulant effects, ephedrine has been misused and abused by athletes, bodybuilders, weight lifters, and others, including high school- and college-aged individuals engaged in sports. Evidence from several surveys indicates that about 4% of student athletes and 13–25% of individuals attending a gymnasium use ephedrine. (See Issues and Regulations Associated with Misuse and Abuse of Ephedrine-containing Preparations under Uses: Misuse and Abuse.)

Studies evaluating the safety and efficacy of dietary supplements containing ephedra for enhancement of athletic performance† are lacking. In addition, the few studies evaluating safety and efficacy of ephedrine for this use generally have included only a limited number of fit individuals (i.e., young male military recruits) and have assessed effects of ephedrine only for very short-term use (for immediate performance) rather than for long-term, repeated use as seen in the general population. These data support a modest effect of ephedrine used in combination with caffeine on very short-term athletic performance. Limited data also indicate that addition of caffeine to ephedrine is necessary for the modest enhancement of athletic performance. However, the effect of sustained use of ephedrine on improvement of athletic performance has not been assessed. Therefore, safety and efficacy of dietary supplements containing ephedrine or ephedra, as they have been used in the general population to promote enhancement of athletic performance, have not been established. (See Issues and Regulations Associated with Misuse and Abuse of Ephedrine-containing Preparations under Uses: Misuse and Abuse.)

CNS Stimulation Over-the-counter ephedrine has been abused by some users including adolescents and young adults for its CNS stimulating action. (See Issues and Regulations Associated with Misuse and Abuse of Ephedrine-containing Preparations under Uses: Misuse and Abuse.) Ephedrine (as the primary precursor) also has been used in the clandestine synthesis of methamphetamine (see Chronic Toxicity in the Amphetamines General Statement 28:20.04) and methcathinone (both potent CNS stimulants with great potential for habituation and physical and/or psychic dependence). Abuse of ephedrine has produced psychic dependence (characterized by compulsion, obsession, and preoccupation) and worsened mental disorders (e.g., depressive anxiety, thought disorders). Acute overdosage of the drug has been associated with tachycardia, difficulty in breathing, and death. (See Acute Toxicity.)

Issues and Regulations Associated with Misuse and Abuse of Ephedrine-containing Preparations Because use of dietary supplements that contain ephedrine or ephedra, alone or in combination with caffeine, may be associated with substantial adverse health effects and toxicity (see Dietary Supplements under Cautions: Adverse Effects), FDA issued a final regulation in February 2004 prohibiting the manufacturing, distribution, and sale of all dietary supplements containing ephedrine alkaloids after April 12, 2004. (See Regulations Governing Dietary Supplements under Adverse Effects: Dietary Supplements, in Cautions.) In April 2005, a federal judge in a Utah district court overturned part of the FDA ruling, declaring the agency could not ban the sale of dietary supplements containing ephedrine dosages of 10 mg or less without proving that such low dosages are unsafe; this ruling partially lifted FDA's ban, allowing products with 10 mg or less of active ingredient to return to the US market. However, in August 2006, a 3-judge panel of the US Court of Appeals for the 10th Circuit in Denver reversed the lower Utah district court decision and upheld FDA's final rule declaring all dietary supplements containing ephedrine alkaloids adulterated. FDA then reiterated its position that no dosage of dietary supplements containing ephedrine alkaloids is considered safe, and the sale of these products in the US is illegal and subject to FDA enforcement action.

Transactions (e.g., distribution, receipt, sale, use, importation, exportation) involving ephedrine-containing *drug* products also have been restricted under the Chemical Diversion and Trafficking Act of 1988, the Domestic Chemical Diversion Control Act of 1993, and the Comprehensive Methamphetamine Control Act of 1996 (MCA [US Public Law 104-237]). Under MCA, effective October 1997, 24 g of ephedrine (in terms of the base) was the limit for a single transaction for drug products containing ephedrine in combination with other drugs (regardless of the form in which these drugs are packaged) that could be sold by retail distributors (e.g., grocery stores, general merchandise stores, drug stores). As of October 1997, mail-order distribution of ephedrine-containing drug products must be reported monthly to the US Attorney General according to applicable regulations. In addition, under regulations finalized by the Drug Enforcement Administration (DEA), effective April 2002, nonprescription preparations containing ephedrine had to be stored behind the counter in retail settings that were open to the public to ensure that only employees have access to these products so that their availability to the general public could be more closely controlled.

Despite the enactment of MCA and other stringent laws, methamphetamine abuse remains a serious problem. In March 2006, the Combat Methamphetamine Epidemic Act (CMEA) of 2005 (Title VII of the USA Patriot Act Improvement and Reauthorization Act of 2005) was signed into law, which effectively amends the Federal Controlled Substances Act of 1970 to tighten control over the sale and distribution of nonprescription ephedrine and pseudoephedrine. This law creates a new class of products called "scheduled listed chemical products," which are defined in the law as products containing ephedrine, pseudoephedrine, or phenylpropanolamine (no longer commercially available in the US) or any salt, optical isomer, or salt of an optical isomer of these drugs that are lawful nonprescription products in the US, and sets additional requirements for their sale. Effective September 30, 2006, the law requires pharmacies and other retail distributors to store ephedrine- and pseudoephedrine-containing preparations behind the counter or in locked cabinets; requires purchasers to provide approved photographic identification and sign a written or electronic logbook for each purchase; requires pharmacies and other retail distributors to keep information about the purchasers (e.g., name, address, signature) and purchases (e.g., name of product, quantity sold, date and time of sale) for at least 2 years; and limits the amount of ephedrine that can be purchased to no more than 3.6 g per day or 9 g per month. The law exempts requirements of a written or electronic logbook for any purchase of single-dose packages that contain no more than 60 mg of pseudoephedrine; however, these single-dose packages also must be stored behind the counter. To comply with CMEA, pharmacies and other retail distributors selling preparations containing ephedrine are required to submit to the Attorney General a statement regarding self-certification and employee training on the requirements of this new law and to maintain records relating to such training at their place of operation. Additional information about legal and regulatory requirements under CMEA may be obtained at the website of the Office of Diversion Control of the US Drug Enforcement Administration (DEA) (http://www.deadiversion.usdoj.gov/), including specific requirements for various sellers (e.g., pharmacies, mail-order sellers) and employee training materials developed by DEA. (See Uses: Misuse and Abuse, in Pseudoephedrine 12:12.12.)

Use of ephedrine in some states may be subject to additional controls, since some states had restricted the prescription, dispensing, and distribution of ephedrine (e.g., as a controlled substance or a prescription drug) prior to passage of the federal law. For example, in the state of Oregon, legislation was enacted in August 2005 that required the Oregon State Board of Pharmacy to classify ephedrine, pseudoephedrine, and phenylpropanolamine as schedule III drugs by July 2006, which effectively moved these drugs from the nonprescription to the prescription-only category in that state. Where such state laws are more stringent than the provisions of CMEA, the state requirements also must be followed.

Dosage and Administration

■ **Administration** ***Oral Administration*** Ephedrine (as the hydrochloride or sulfate salt) is administered orally as fixed-combination preparations containing guaifenesin.

Parenteral Administration Ephedrine sulfate is administered by IV injection. The drug also has been administered by IM† or subcutaneous† injection.

Ephedrine sulfate injection (Akovaz®) is administered by direct IV ("bolus") injection. Prior to IV administration, the commercially available solution for injection must be diluted. The manufacturer recommends that a 5-mg/mL solution be prepared by diluting 1 mL of the 50-mg/mL injection concentrate with 9 mL of 0.9% sodium chloride injection or 5% dextrose injection. Vials of the drug are for single-use only; unused portions should be discarded.

Ephedrine sulfate injection should be inspected visually for particulate matter and discoloration prior to administration whenever solution and container permit.

■ **Dosage** Ephedrine is commercially available as ephedrine hydrochloride or ephedrine sulfate; dosage is expressed in terms of the salt.

Oral Dosage When ephedrine hydrochloride or ephedrine sulfate is administered orally for *self-medication* as a bronchodilator (in fixed combination with guaifenesin) in adults and children 12 years of age and older, the usual oral dosage is 12.5–25 mg every 4 hours as needed, not to exceed 150 mg in 24 hours. Ephedrine should be used in children younger than 12 years of age only under the direction of a clinician.

Parenteral Dosage When used as a pressor agent, ephedrine should be administered in the lowest effective dosage for the shortest possible time. The recommended initial adult dose of ephedrine sulfate for the treatment of clinically important hypotension during anesthesia is 5–10 mg by IV bolus injection; additional bolus doses should be administered as needed (up to a total dose of 50 mg) to achieve the desired blood pressure response. Other parenteral dosage regimens have been recommended in adults, including a dose of 5–25 mg by slow IV injection (repeated in 5–10 minutes if necessary) and an IM† or subcutaneous† dose of 25–50 mg.

In children†, parenteral ephedrine sulfate doses of 0.5 mg/kg or 16.7 mg/m^2 have been administered every 4–6 hours by subcutaneous† or IM† injection; however, safety and efficacy of ephedrine sulfate injection have not been established in pediatric patients.

When used parenterally to relieve severe, acute bronchospasm, ephedrine sulfate doses of 12.5–25 mg usually have been given in adults.

Cautions

■ **Adverse Effects** The CNS-stimulating effects of ephedrine may result in nervousness, anxiety, restlessness, or insomnia, especially with large doses. Vertigo also may occur. Prolonged abuse of ephedrine may cause symptoms of paranoid schizophrenia. Ephedrine also may cause headache, sweating, mild epigastric distress, anorexia, nausea, or vomiting.

Ephedrine increases the work of the heart and probably myocardial oxygen consumption. In patients with coronary insufficiency and/or ischemic heart disease, the drug can induce anginal pain. Ephedrine increases the irritability of the heart muscle and may alter the rhythmic function of the ventricles. Palpitation and tachycardia may result. Extrasystoles and potentially fatal arrhythmias including ventricular fibrillation may occur, especially in patients with organic heart disease or those receiving other drugs that sensitize the heart to arrhythmias including cardiac glycosides, cyclopropane, or halogenated hydrocarbon anesthetics. (See Drug Interactions.) Precordial pain also may occur following administration of ephedrine sulfate injection.

Acute urinary retention may occur in men with prostatism; increased vesicular sphincter tone may cause difficult and painful urination. Some patients may require catheterization.

Ephedrine may cause tachyphylaxis with repeated administration. Although tolerance to ephedrine may develop with prolonged or excessive usage, addiction to the drug does not occur. Temporary cessation of ephedrine and subsequent reinitiation of therapy restores the drug's effectiveness.

Dietary Supplements Ephedrine alkaloid-containing dietary supplements (frequently combined with caffeine) were previously promoted for various uses (e.g., weight loss, body building, energy enhancement, increased mental concentration, increased sexual sensations, euphoria, alternative to illicit drugs); although these products constituted less than 1% of all dietary supplement sales, they accounted for 64% of adverse events associated with dietary supplements. Use of ephedrine alkaloid-containing dietary supplements has been associated with a twofold to threefold increased risk of nausea, vomiting, adverse psychiatric effects (e.g., anxiety, mood changes), autonomic hyperactivity, and palpitations. Serious adverse effects (e.g., cardiovascular and nervous system effects) and deaths have been reported in individuals receiving ephedrine or ephedra-containing dietary supplements. Such adverse effects, including irregular heart rate, palpitations, increased blood pressure, chest pain, anxiety, nervousness, tremor, hyperactivity, headache, and insomnia, usually were associated with clinically serious conditions (e.g., myocardial infarction, stroke, psychoses, seizures, nephrolithiasis, death) and frequently were reported in young (i.e., 30 years of age or younger) to middle-aged adults (over 70% of whom were females) using the supplements, mainly for weight loss or energy enhancement. Many such adverse effects occurred within 2 weeks of first use, although they were reported on the first day of use in some cases. Most individuals who developed such adverse effects claim that they used the dietary supplements according to labeled instructions.

Source of Ephedrine in Dietary Supplements. The labeled source of ephedrine in dietary supplements varied from raw botanicals to powdered plant material, sometimes pharmaceutical ephedrine alkaloids, but mainly consisted of concentrated extracts of the amphetamine-like *Ephedra* species (usually listed on labels as ma huang, ephedra, Chinese ephedra, Ephedra sinica, ephedra herb powder, epitonin, ephedrine, or ephedrine alkaloids). Small amounts of ephedrine alkaloids also are found in *Sida cordifolia*. Plants of the genus *Ephedra* may contain ephedrine alkaloids as single ingredients; however, ephedrine alkaloids usually are combined with other compounds. Although some dietary supplements contained only *Ephedra* as a labeled ingredient, most dietary supplements contained other ingredients, many of which have known or suspected physiologic and pharmacologic activities that have the potential of interacting with ephedrine alkaloids and thus increasing their effects.

Regulations Governing Dietary Supplements. Although the quality and consistency of prescription and nonprescription drugs in the US generally are ensured by strict FDA regulations concerning drug uniformity, purity, and labeling accuracy, dietary supplements (e.g., herbal preparations, vitamins and minerals, amino acids, tissue extracts) are regulated as *foods* under the Dietary Supplement Health and Education Act (DSHEA) of 1994. Therefore, FDA bears the burden to prove that a marketed dietary supplement is unsafe when used according to the conditions of use on the label or as commonly consumed. These requirements are in contrast to FDA regulations concerning prescription and nonprescription drugs that stipulate that a drug has to be proven safe and effective (for a particular indication) before it is approved for marketing.

Serious adverse effects (e.g., cardiovascular and nervous system effects) and deaths have been reported with ephedrine or ephedra-containing dietary supplements. As a result, FDA has proposed strict regulations for these preparations since 1997 to protect the public health. In 1997, the agency proposed regulations to limit the amount of ephedrine alkaloids that dietary supplement preparations contain and to change labeling and marketing practices for these supplements. In 2001, FDA seized drug products containing synthetic ephedrine hydrochloride labeled as dietary supplements. In 2003, with the emergence of new scientific evidence (including approximately 18,000 adverse event reports received overall by FDA and a comprehensive evaluation of the scientific literature through 2002 conducted by the RAND corporation), FDA proposed additional changes to labeling to emphasize the risks of using ephedrine-containing dietary supplements. In addition, the agency also proposed rules to establish GMPs for all dietary supplements and issued warnings prohibiting manufacturers from making unsubstantiated efficacy claims (e.g., enhancement of athletic performance, street drug alternative) for these preparations.

In February 2004, FDA finally concluded that dietary supplements containing ephedrine alkaloids pose a risk of serious adverse events (e.g., heart attack, stroke, death), and that these risks are unreasonable in light of any benefits that may result from the use of these products. Therefore, the agency issued a final regulation declaring that dietary supplements containing ephedrine alkaloids are *adulterated* under the Federal Food, Drug, and Cosmetic Act. Under this rule, manufacturing, distribution, and sale of all dietary supplements containing ephedrine alkaloids (e.g., *Ephedra* spp. ["ma huang"], *Sida cordifolia*, *Pinellia* spp.) were prohibited after April 12, 2004. This regulation does not apply to traditional Chinese herbal remedies or products regulated as conventional foods (e.g., herbal teas). Ephedra is *not* generally recognized as safe for foods and not approved for use as a food additive.

In April 2005, about one year after issuance of FDA's final ruling, a federal judge in a Utah district court overturned part of the ruling, declaring that the agency cannot ban the sale of dietary supplements containing ephedrine dosages of 10 mg or less without proving that such low dosages are unsafe; this ruling partially lifted FDA's ban, allowing products with 10 mg or less of active ingredient to return to the US market. However, in August 2006, a 3-judge panel of the US Court of Appeals for the 10th Circuit in Denver reversed the lower Utah district court decision and upheld FDA's final rule declaring all dietary supplements containing ephedrine alkaloids adulterated. FDA then reiterated its position that no dosage of dietary supplements containing ephedrine alkaloids is considered safe, and the sale of these products in the US is illegal and subject to FDA enforcement action.

■ **Precautions and Contraindications** Ephedrine may cause hypertension. The drug should be used with caution in patients with hypertension, cardiovascular disease, angina, diabetes mellitus, hyperthyroidism, or prostatic hyperplasia, and in those receiving digoxin. An increased risk of hypertension has been observed in patients receiving ephedrine sulfate injection for the prevention of hypotension during anesthesia. Serious postpartum hypertension, in some cases resulting in stroke, has been reported in patients receiving a vasopressor (e.g., ephedrine) and an oxytocic agent (e.g., ergonovine, methylergonovine) concomitantly.

Patients considering *self-medication* with ephedrine as a bronchodilator should be advised that the drug be used only if they have been diagnosed by a clinician as having asthma, and that *self-medication* not be undertaken if they ever have been hospitalized for asthma or are currently receiving a prescription drug for the management of this condition unless otherwise directed by a clinician. These patients also should be advised not to use the drug if they have cardiovascular disease, hypertension, diabetes mellitus, thyroid disease, angle-closure (narrow-angle) glaucoma, seizures, a psychiatric or emotional condition, or difficulty urinating because of prostatic hyperplasia unless directed by a clinician. In addition, patients should be advised not to exceed recommended dosages or frequency of administration unless otherwise instructed by a clinician. Patients should contact their clinician if symptoms are not improved within 1 hour or become worse, more than the recommended dosage of ephedrine is required, or asthma attacks become more frequent (i.e., more than 2 asthma attacks in a week). Patients also should be cautioned that ephedrine can cause hypertension and tachycardia, which could increase the risk of cardiovascular disease, stroke, or death. Foods, beverages, and dietary supplements that contain stimulants (e.g., caffeine) should be avoided.

Prolonged use of parenteral ephedrine may produce a syndrome resembling an anxiety state. Tolerance to ephedrine also may develop with repeated administration of the drug; in some cases, effectiveness may return after the drug is temporarily withheld. If ephedrine sulfate injection is used for the treatment of hypotension during anesthesia, clinicians should be aware of the possibility of tachyphylaxis and be prepared to use an alternative vasopressor agent in the event that an unacceptable response to ephedrine occurs.

Because ephedrine is substantially excreted by the kidneys, patients with impaired renal function may eliminate the drug more slowly, consequently prolonging its pharmacologic effect and potentially increasing the risk of adverse effects. Patients with renal impairment should be carefully monitored after administration of the initial IV dose of ephedrine.

Misuse or abuse of ephedrine can result in potentially serious adverse effects. (See Uses: Misuse and Abuse.) Serious adverse effects also have been reported with dietary supplements containing ephedrine alkaloids. In February 2004, FDA issued a final regulation prohibiting the manufacturing, distribution, and sale of all dietary supplements containing ephedrine alkaloids (effective April 12, 2004). Effective August 2006, no dosage of dietary supplements containing ephedrine alkaloids is considered safe, and the sale of these products in the US is illegal and subject to FDA enforcement action. (See Dietary Supplements under Cautions: Adverse Effects.)

Some manufacturers state that ephedrine is contraindicated in patients with known hypersensitivity to the drug or other sympathomimetic agents, although allergic reactions to ephedrine are rare.

■ **Pediatric Precautions** Ephedrine sulfate injection is not FDA-labeled for use in pediatric patients. Although the drug has been used in children, safety and efficacy have not been established in this patient population.

Overdosage and toxicity (including death) have been reported in children younger than 2 years of age receiving nonprescription (over-the-counter, OTC) preparations containing antihistamines, cough suppressants, expectorants, and nasal decongestants alone or in combination for relief of symptoms of upper respiratory tract infection. There is limited evidence of efficacy for these preparations in this age group, and appropriate dosages (i.e., approved by the FDA) for the symptomatic treatment of cold and cough have not been established. Therefore, FDA stated that nonprescription cough and cold preparations should not be used in children younger than 2 years of age; the agency continues to assess safety and efficacy of these preparations in older children. Meanwhile, because children 2–3 years of age also are at increased risk of overdosage and toxicity, some manufacturers of oral nonprescription cough and cold preparations agreed to voluntarily revise the product labeling to state that such preparations should not be used in children younger than 4 years of age. FDA recommends that parents and caregivers adhere to the dosage instructions and warnings on the product labeling that accompanies the preparation if administering to children and consult with their clinician about any concerns. Clinicians should ask caregivers about use of nonprescription cough and cold preparations to avoid overdosage. For additional information on precautions associated with the use of cough and cold preparations in pediatric patients, see Cautions: Pediatric Precautions, in Pseudoephedrine 12:12.12.

■ **Geriatric Precautions** Clinical studies of ephedrine sulfate did not include sufficient numbers of patients 65 years of age and older to determine whether geriatric patients respond differently than younger patients. Clinical experience to date has not identified any differences in response between geriatric and younger patients. If ephedrine is used in geriatric patients, dosage should be selected carefully, usually starting at the low end of the dosage range, since renal, hepatic, and cardiovascular dysfunction and concomitant disease or other drug therapy are more common in this age group.

Ephedrine is known to be substantially excreted by the kidneys and the risk of ephedrine-induced adverse effects may be increased in patients with impaired renal function; because geriatric patients may have decreased renal function, it may be useful to monitor renal function in such patients.

■ **Pregnancy and Lactation** Animal reproduction studies have not been performed to date with ephedrine sulfate injection; it is not known whether the drug can cause fetal harm or miscarriage when administered during pregnancy. However, ephedrine has been used in pregnant women for the treatment of hypotension during spinal anesthesia, and the available data support the efficacy and safety of ephedrine sulfate injection for such use. There is some evidence indicating that fetal acidosis is more likely to occur with maternal administration of ephedrine compared with phenylephrine. Low umbilical artery pH (7.2 or less) has been reported at the time of delivery in neonates whose mothers were exposed to ephedrine. Newborn infants with such maternal exposure should be assessed for their acid-base status and monitored for signs and symptoms of metabolic acidosis.

Limited data indicate that ephedrine is distributed into human milk; however, there is no information regarding the effects of the drug on the breast-fed infant or on milk production. The known benefits of breast-feeding should be considered along with the mother's clinical need for ephedrine and any potential adverse effects of the drug or underlying maternal condition on the infant.

Drug Interactions

■ **α- and β-Adrenergic Blocking Agents** Administration of an α-adrenergic blocking drug reduces the vasopressor response to ephedrine. Phentolamine, by blocking the α-adrenergic effects of ephedrine, can cause vasodilation. However, because of the cardiac stimulating effects of ephedrine, a pressor response may be achieved if sufficient doses are administered.

As with other sympathomimetic drugs having cardiostimulating effects, administration of a β-adrenergic blocking drug such as propranolol may block the cardiac and bronchodilating effects of ephedrine.

Blood pressure should be monitored in patients receiving ephedrine concomitantly with an α- or β-adrenergic blocking agent.

■ **Cardiac Glycosides** Cardiac glycosides (e.g., digoxin) can sensitize the myocardium to the effects of sympathomimetic drugs and increase the risk of arrhythmias; patients receiving such concomitant therapy should be carefully monitored.

■ **Diuretics** Administration of furosemide or other diuretics may decrease arterial responsiveness to pressor drugs such as ephedrine.

■ **Epidural Anesthesia** Ephedrine may decrease efficacy of epidural blockade by facilitating the regression of sensory analgesia. Patients should be monitored for this effect and treated accordingly.

■ **General Anesthetics** Some manufacturers state that concurrent use of ephedrine with general anesthetics, especially cyclopropane or halogenated hydrocarbons, can sensitize the myocardium to the effects of ephedrine and possibly increase the risk of arrhythmias.

■ **Monoamine Oxidase Inhibitors** By increasing the quantity of norepinephrine in adrenergic nervous tissue, monoamine oxidase (MAO) inhibitors may potentiate the pressor effects of indirectly acting sympathomimetic drugs such as ephedrine. Potentiation is approximately the same following IV or oral administration of ephedrine. A hypertensive crisis and subarachnoid hemorrhage occurred in a patient receiving an MAO inhibitor after 50 mg of ephedrine was administered orally.

Blood pressure should be carefully monitored in patients receiving ephedrine and an MAO inhibitor concomitantly. Some manufacturers recommend that ephedrine not be used in patients currently receiving, or for 2 weeks after discontinuance of, an MAO inhibitor.

■ **Oxytocic Drugs** Concomitant use of a vasopressor (e.g., ephedrine) with an oxytocic drug (e.g., ergonovine, methylergonovine) may increase the pressor effect and cause severe postpartum hypertension, which may lead to stroke. Blood pressure should be carefully monitored in patients receiving such concomitant therapy.

■ **Rocuronium** Ephedrine may reduce the onset time of rocuronium-induced neuromuscular blockade for intubation when administered simultaneously with anesthetic induction.

■ **Theophylline** Concomitant use of ephedrine and theophylline may increase the frequency of nausea, nervousness, and insomnia. Patients receiving such concomitant therapy should be monitored for these symptoms and treated accordingly.

■ **Other Drugs** Other drugs that may potentiate the pressor effect of ephedrine include clonidine, propofol, and atropine. Other drugs that can antagonize the pressor effect of ephedrine include reserpine and quinidine. Blood pressure should be carefully monitored in patients receiving such concomitant therapy.

Acute Toxicity

■ **Manifestations** Overdosage of ephedrine can cause a rapid increase in blood pressure. Hypertension may develop initially, followed later by hypotension accompanied by anuria. Careful monitoring of blood pressure is recommended in the event of an overdosage. Another principal manifestation of ephedrine overdosage is the development of seizures. Acute overdosage of ephedrine also may result in nausea, vomiting, chills, cyanosis, irritability, nervousness, fever, suicidal behavior, tachycardia, dilated pupils, blurred vision, opisthotonos, spasms, pulmonary edema, gasping respirations, coma, and respiratory failure.

■ **Treatment** If respirations are shallow or cyanosis is present, one manufacturer recommends initiation of assisted respiration. In the presence of cardiovascular collapse, blood pressure should be maintained; however, vasopressors are contraindicated.

Parenteral antihypertensives may be administered at the discretion of the clinician for the management of severe hypertension. One manufacturer recommends administration of 5 mg of phentolamine mesylate diluted in 0.9% sodium chloride injection and administered slowly by IV injection; alternatively, 100 mg of the drug may be given orally (an oral dosage form of phentolamine is not commercially available in the US). Seizures may be controlled with diazepam; pyrexia may be managed with external cooling and IV dexamethasone (1 mg/kg administered slowly).

Pharmacology

Ephedrine stimulates both α- and β-adrenergic receptors through direct and indirect mechanisms. It is believed that β-adrenergic effects result from stimulation of the production of cyclic adenosine 3′,5′-monophosphate (cAMP) by activation of the enzyme adenyl cyclase, whereas α-adrenergic effects result from inhibition of adenyl cyclase activity. Ephedrine also exerts an indirect effect by releasing norepinephrine from its storage sites. With prolonged or excessive use, ephedrine may deplete norepinephrine stores in sympathetic nerve endings and tachyphylaxis may develop. Tachyphylaxis to the bronchial effects of the drug may also occur, but it is not the result of norepinephrine depletion. The main effects of therapeutic doses of ephedrine are relaxation of the smooth muscle of the bronchial tree, and when norepinephrine stores are not depleted, cardiac stimulation and increased systolic and usually increased diastolic blood pressure. Unlike epinephrine and norepinephrine, ephedrine produces bronchodilation and possibly increased blood pressure and has pronounced CNS activity following oral administration.

■ **Respiratory Effects** Ephedrine relaxes bronchial smooth muscle by stimulation of β_2-adrenergic receptors. Bronchodilation produced by oral ephedrine occurs more slowly, is less pronounced, and is more prolonged than that achieved with epinephrine administered subcutaneously or by oral inhalation.

■ **Cardiovascular Effects** The cardiovascular effects of ephedrine are mediated by its α- and β-adrenergic properties and the overall clinical response is based on the balance between α_1-mediated vasoconstriction, β_2-mediated vasoconstriction, and β_2-mediated vasodilation. Ephedrine increases heart rate, increases cardiac output, and variably increases peripheral vascular resistance, resulting in an increase in systemic blood pressure.

Ephedrine acts on β_1-adrenergic receptors in the heart, producing a positive inotropic effect on the myocardium when single low doses are administered. This effect contributes to, and may be principally responsible for, the pressor effects of the drug when venous return to the heart is adequate. Although the drug also produces a positive chronotropic effect through the sinoatrial node, this effect may be overcome by increased vagal activity occurring as a reflex to increased arterial blood pressure. Bradycardia, tachycardia, or unchanged heart rate has been reported. Cardiac output usually is increased, especially after IV administration. Because of its positive inotropic effects, ephedrine increases cardiac work and probably myocardial oxygen consumption, and usually increases pulmonary arterial pressure.

Ephedrine increases the irritability of the heart muscle and may alter the rhythmic function of the ventricles, especially when the heart has been sensitized to this action by other drugs including digitalis glycosides or certain anesthetics. Arrhythmias including ventricular tachycardia, extrasystoles, and fibrillation may result. As with epinephrine, arrhythmias may be more likely to occur if large doses are given or if the patient has acute myocardial infarction.

Ephedrine may dilate coronary blood vessels. As with epinephrine, coronary artery vasodilation may be indirect, caused by enhanced cardiac metabolism due to direct cardiac stimulation. Ephedrine may increase coronary artery blood flow; as with other sympathomimetic drugs, increased coronary blood flow may result from increased systemic blood pressure as well as indirect coronary artery vasodilation. However, decreased coronary artery blood flow has also been reported and the effects of the drug on coronary circulation may be dose dependent.

Like epinephrine, ephedrine can produce both vasodilation by its effect on β_2-adrenergic receptors and vasoconstriction by its effect on α-adrenergic receptors. The drug constricts arterioles in the skin, mucous membranes, and viscera, and dilates arterioles in the skeletal muscle. Either constriction or dilation of pulmonary and cerebral vessels may occur. Peripheral vascular resistance may be increased, decreased, or unchanged after administration of the drug. Conditions causing an increase or decrease in vascular resistance have not been identified. Pressor responses to parenteral ephedrine occur more slowly but are more prolonged than those achieved with epinephrine or norepinephrine. Increased blood pressure may be caused by vasoconstriction as well as by cardiac stimulation; however, when peripheral vascular resistance is decreased, elevation of blood pressure is due entirely to increased cardiac output. Ephedrine may constrict both arterial and venous blood vessels; peripheral venous pressure also is increased. Ephedrine may decrease circulating plasma volume. This may result from loss of fluid into extracellular spaces caused by postcapillary vasoconstriction.

Constriction of renal blood vessels by parenteral ephedrine decreases renal blood flow. In hypotensive patients, ephedrine may initially decrease urine flow and excretion of sodium and potassium. If the patient is not hypovolemic, renal blood flow and glomerular filtration rate increase as the systemic blood pressure is raised toward normal levels; however, renal blood flow and glomerular filtration rate again decrease if blood pressure is further increased toward hypertensive levels.

Ephedrine may constrict dilated blood vessels in the nasal mucosa and produce nasal decongestion following topical application; however, rebound congestion may occur. There is insufficient evidence that the drug is effective as a nasal decongestant when administered orally in usual doses.

■ **Other Effects** Ephedrine has CNS stimulating effects similar to those of amphetamines but less pronounced. (See Cautions: Adverse Effects.)

Ephedrine generally relaxes smooth muscles of the GI tract. Ephedrine contracts the urinary bladder trigone and sphincter; relaxation of the detrusor muscle is not prominent. (See Cautions: Adverse Effects.) The drug usually decreases the activity of the uterus; however, an excitatory effect has also been reported. Use of ephedrine during delivery to correct maternal hypotension resulting from spinal anesthesia may result in improved uterine blood flow. In experimental animals, the drug has corrected fetal hypoxia, hypercapnia, acidosis, and bradycardia resulting from maternal hypotension.

Blood glucose concentrations are not increased as much by ephedrine as by epinephrine, and usual doses of ephedrine are not likely to produce hyperglycemia. Ephedrine increases oxygen consumption and metabolic rate, probably as a result of central stimulation.

Administration of ephedrine to patients with myasthenia gravis may result in increased muscle strength. The mechanism by which ephedrine acts in these patients is not known.

Pharmacokinetics

■ **Absorption** Bronchodilation occurs within 15–60 minutes after oral administration of the drug and appears to persist for 2–4 hours. The duration of pressor and cardiac responses to ephedrine is 1 hour after IV administration of 10–25 mg or IM or subcutaneous administration of 25–50 mg and up to 4 hours after oral administration of 15–50 mg of the drug.

There appears to be a wide variation in ephedrine plasma concentrations associated with bronchodilation. In one study, therapeutic plasma concentrations were reported to range from 20 ng/mL to more than 80 ng/mL.

Following oral administration of ephedrine as conventional ephedrine hydrochloride capsules containing 25 mg of ephedrine base (no longer commercially available in the US) or as 3 dietary supplement preparations of *Ephedra* (a botanical source of ephedrine alkaloids referred to as ma huang, no longer commercially available in the US) assayed as containing the equivalent of 23.6, 25.6, or 27 mg of ephedrine base in a randomized, crossover pharmacokinetic study in healthy fasting adults, the absorption rate and area under the serum concentration-time curve (AUC) were similar among the 4 preparations, although the absorption of one of the dietary supplements and AUC of another differed substantially from the remaining preparations. Mean peak serum ephedrine concentrations of about 73.4, 86, and 100 ng/mL were achieved in about 3, 2.6, and 2.7 hours following oral administration of the 23.6-, 25.6-, or 27-mg dose of ephedrine, respectively, compared with a mean peak serum concentration of 86.5 ng/mL at about 2.81 hours with the 25-mg dose of ephedrine administered as the conventional capsules (no longer commercially available in the US). Most of these dietary supplements contained other ingredients besides ephedrine and these ingredients may have increased the rate but not the extent of absorption of ephedrine from the GI tract.

■ **Distribution** Ephedrine is presumed to cross the placenta and distribute into milk.

In one study in healthy fasting adults comparing oral administration of conventional ephedrine hydrochloride capsules (no longer commercially available in the US) with botanical preparations (ma huang, *Ephedra*, no longer commercially available in the US) containing the drug, the apparent steady-state volume of distribution ranged from about 220–240 L.

■ **Elimination** The metabolic pathway of ephedrine has not been completely elucidated. However, some data suggest that small quantities of ephedrine are slowly metabolized in the liver by oxidative deamination, demethylation, aromatic hydroxylation, and conjugation. The metabolites have been identified as *p*-hydroxyephedrine, *p*-hydroxynorephedrine, norephedrine, and conjugates of these compounds.

Ephedrine and its metabolites are excreted in urine. Most of the drug is excreted unchanged. The rate of urinary excretion of the drug and its metabolites is dependent upon urinary pH. In one study, 74–92% of an oral dose and 87–99% of an IV dose of 25 mg of ephedrine hydrochloride were excreted as ephedrine and 8–10% of the oral dose and 3–7% of the IV dose were excreted as norephedrine within 24 hours when the urine was acidified to pH 5 by administration of ammonium chloride. When the urine was alkalinized to pH 8 by administration of sodium bicarbonate, 22–35% of a 25-mg oral dose of ephedrine hydrochloride was excreted as ephedrine and 11–24% of this dose was excreted as norephedrine within 24 hours. Approximately 70–80% of a 25-mg oral dose of ephedrine sulfate was excreted in urine within 48 hours when the urine pH averaged 6.3. The ratio of ephedrine to norephedrine excreted in this study was not determined.

The elimination half-life of ephedrine has been reported to be about 3 hours when the urine is acidified to pH 5 and about 6 hours when urinary pH is about 6.3. In a study in healthy fasting adults comparing oral administration of conventional ephedrine hydrochloride capsules (no longer commercially available in the US) with botanical preparations (ma huang, *Ephedra*, no longer commercially available in the US) containing the drug, elimination half-life ranged from 4.85–6.47 hours, with apparent clearances of 25.5–34.1 L/hour; urinary pH was not reported.

Chemistry and Stability

■ **Chemistry** Ephedrine is a sympathomimetic drug that occurs naturally in plants of the genus *Ephedra*, most commonly *E. sinica*. *Ephedra* spp., known in traditional Chinese medicine as "ma huang," contains 6 ephedrine alkaloids (sometimes collectively referred to as "ephedra"), including ephedrine, pseudoephedrine, norephedrine, methylephedrine, norpseudoephedrine, and methylpseudoephedrine. The total ephedrine alkaloid content of *E. sinica* is approximately 1–2%, with ephedrine being the most abundant alkaloid. Although the content may vary between samples, ephedrine and pseudoephedrine together generally constitute more than 80% of the alkaloid content of the dried herb. In dietary supplements, the ephedrine alkaloid content was typically expressed as a standardized percentage of total herb content. However, results of one study evaluating the content of 20 dietary supplements labeled as containing botanical sources of ephedrine alkaloids indicate that considerable discrepancies exist between the labeled amount of ephedrine alkaloid content and the assayed amount, and that ephedrine alkaloid contents vary from lot to lot. (See Dietary Supplements under Cautions: Adverse Effects.) FDA issued a final regulation in February 2004 prohibiting the manufacturing, distribution, and sale of all dietary supplements containing ephedrine alkaloids after April 12, 2004. (See Regulations Governing Dietary Supplements under Adverse Effects: Dietary Supplements, in Cautions.)

Ephedrine is commercially available as the hydrochloride or sulfate salt. Ephedrine hydrochloride and ephedrine sulfate occur as fine, white, odorless crystals or powders. Ephedrine hydrochloride has solubilities of approximately 0.33 g/mL in water and 71 mg/mL in alcohol at 25°C. Ephedrine sulfate has solubilities of approximately 0.77 g/mL in water and 11 mg/mL in alcohol at 25°C. Ephedrine sulfate injection has a pH of 4.5–7.

■ **Stability** Ephedrine sulfate injection should be stored at 20–25°C but may be exposed to temperatures of 15–30°C. Ephedrine salts and preparations containing the drugs gradually decompose and darken on exposure to light and must be stored in light-resistant containers.

Ephedrine injections have been reported to be incompatible with various drugs, but the compatibility depends on several factors (e.g., concentration of the drugs, resulting pH, temperature). Specialized references should be consulted for specific compatibility information.

Preparations

Excipients in commercially available drug preparations may have clinically important effects in some individuals; consult specific product labeling for details.

ePHEDrine Hydrochloride

Powder*		

*available from one or more manufacturer, distributor, and/or repackager by generic (nonproprietary) name

ePHEDrine Sulfate

Parenteral		
Injection	50 mg/mL*	**Akovaz®**, Eclat
		ePHEDrine Sulfate Injection

*available from one or more manufacturer, distributor, and/or repackager by generic (nonproprietary) name

ePHEDrine Hydrochloride Combinations

Oral		
Tablets	12.5 mg with Guaifenesin 200 mg	**Ephed Plus®**, DMD
		Primatene®, Pfizer
	25 mg with Guaifenesin 200 mg	**Ephed Plus®**, DMD

ePHEDrine Sulfate Combinations

Oral		
Tablets	25 mg with Guaifenesin 400 mg	**Bronkaid® Caplets**, Bayer

†Use is not currently included in the labeling approved by the US Food and Drug Administration

EPINEPHrine racEPINEPHrine

Adrenaline
Racemic Epinephrine

■ Epinephrine is an endogenous catecholamine that is the active principle of the adrenal medulla; epinephrine acts directly on both α- and β-adrenergic receptors.

Uses

■ **Sensitivity Reactions** Epinephrine is the drug of choice in the emergency treatment of severe acute anaphylactic reactions, including anaphylactic shock. The drug is used to relieve clinical manifestations such as urticaria, pruritus, angioedema, hypotension, and respiratory distress, which may result from reactions to drugs, contrast media, latex, insect stings, foods (e.g., milk, eggs, fish, shellfish, peanuts, tree nuts), or other allergens, as well as from idiopathic or exercise-induced anaphylaxis. Epinephrine should be given to all patients with signs of systemic reactions, particularly hypotension, airway swelling, or breathing difficulty. Recommendations for the use of epinephrine in anaphylaxis are largely based on clinical pharmacology studies, observational studies, retrospective studies, and animal models; however, the available data provide compelling evidence to support the prompt use of epinephrine in patients with anaphylaxis. When administered at the recommended dosages and routes of administration, beneficial pharmacologic effects mediated by both the α- and β-adrenergic properties of the drug (e.g., increased blood pressure, increased force and rate of cardiac contraction, bronchodilation, decreased airway mucosal edema, and suppression of mediator release) are observed. Patients with anaphylactic shock may require rapid volume resuscitation and vasopressor therapy; epinephrine also is used for its vasopressor effects for the treatment of anaphylactic shock and cardiac arrest associated with anaphylaxis.

Epinephrine should be administered immediately by IM injection as soon as anaphylaxis is diagnosed or strongly suspected. Initial administration by IM injection is preferred, mainly because of safety considerations. Serious adverse effects have occurred after IV administration of epinephrine, in part because of confusion regarding correct dosages and routes of administration for the different indications (e.g., treatment of anaphylaxis versus treatment of cardiac arrest). (See Dosage and Administration: Administration.) However, IV administration of epinephrine may be necessary in extreme situations such as in anaphylactic shock, cardiac arrest, or in unresponsive or severely hypotensive patients who have failed to respond to multiple IM injections; close hemodynamic monitoring is critical during IV administration of the drug. Epinephrine also may be administered subcutaneously, but absorption and subsequent achievement of peak plasma concentrations after subcutaneous injection are slower and may be substantially delayed in patients with shock. Although oral inhalation has been recommended, the drug may be absorbed too slowly and/or inadequately to be effective in treating allergic manifestations other than laryngeal angioedema.

Cardiac arrest secondary to anaphylaxis should be managed with standard advanced cardiovascular life support (ACLS) measures; alternative vasoactive drugs (e.g., vasopressin, norepinephrine) may be considered in patients who do not respond to epinephrine, and other therapeutic agents such as antihistamines, inhaled β_2-adrenergic agents, and IV corticosteroids also may be useful. (See Uses: Advanced Cardiovascular Life Support and Cardiac Arrhythmias.)

Patients receiving β-adrenergic blocking agents have an increased incidence and severity of anaphylaxis, and may develop a paradoxical response to epinephrine; glucagon or ipratropium may be considered for the treatment of anaphylaxis in these patients.

■ **Advanced Cardiovascular Life Support and Cardiac Arrhythmias** Epinephrine is used for its α-adrenergic effects to increase blood flow and facilitate return of spontaneous circulation (ROSC) in patients with cardiac arrest. The drug may be administered by IV, intraosseous (IO)†, endotracheal, or intracardiac injection during cardiopulmonary resuscitation (CPR). The principal benefits of epinephrine in patients with cardiac arrest result from increases in aortic diastolic blood pressure and in coronary and cerebral perfusion pressure during resuscitation. The value and safety of the β-adrenergic effects of epinephrine are controversial because they may increase myocardial work and reduce subendocardial perfusion.

High-quality CPR and defibrillation are integral components of ACLS and the only proven interventions to increase survival to hospital discharge. Other resuscitative efforts, including drug therapy, are considered secondary and should be performed without compromising the quality and timely delivery of chest compressions and defibrillation. The principal goal of pharmacologic therapy during cardiac arrest is to facilitate ROSC, and epinephrine is considered the drug of choice for this use.

Despite epinephrine's widespread use in ACLS and evidence of beneficial physiologic effects in both animals and humans, there currently is no evidence demonstrating that the drug improves survival to hospital discharge. The current evidence does, however, support that the drug improves survival to hospital admission (when the arrest occurs outside of the hospital setting) and the potential for achieving ROSC. The American Heart Association (AHA) states that it is reasonable to administer epinephrine 1 mg IV/IO every 3–5 minutes during adult cardiac arrest. Although higher doses of epinephrine may increase the rate of ROSC, numerous studies comparing standard (1 mg) versus high-dose (e.g., 0.1–0.2 mg/kg) epinephrine have not demonstrated any advantage of the higher doses with regards to survival (i.e., survival to discharge with or without good neurologic recovery, survival to hospital admission). While high-dose epinephrine may improve coronary perfusion and increase vascular resistance to promote initial ROSC during cardiac resuscitation, these same effects may result in increased myocardial dysfunction and occasionally a severe hyperadrenergic state in the postresuscitation period. AHA does not recommend the routine use of high-dose epinephrine in cardiac arrest; however, high-dose epinephrine may be considered in certain circumstances (e.g., overdosage of β-adrenergic or calcium-channel blocking agents).

Management of cardiac arrest is based on the patient's arrest rhythm (i.e., ventricular fibrillation, pulseless ventricular tachycardia, pulseless electrical activity [PEA], or asystole). As the rhythm is likely to evolve over the course of resuscitation, the appropriate management strategy should be adapted accordingly. In adults with ventricular fibrillation or pulseless ventricular tachycardia resistant to initial CPR attempts and at least one defibrillation shock, epinephrine may be administered with the goal of increasing myocardial blood flow during CPR and achieving ROSC; however, the optimal timing of epinephrine administration, particularly in relation to defibrillation, is not known and may vary based on patient-specific factors and resuscitation conditions. In adults with asystole or PEA, epinephrine may be given as soon as feasible after the onset of cardiac arrest based on studies demonstrating improved survival to hospital discharge and increased ROSC when the drug was administered early during the course of treatment for a nonshockable rhythm. In previous ACLS guidelines, vasopressin was recommended as an alternative to epinephrine in the treatment of adult cardiac arrest; however, vasopressin has been removed from the current ACLS guideline because of equivalence of effect with epinephrine and efforts to simplify the management approach when therapies are found to be equivalent.

Once a patient achieves ROSC, appropriate postcardiac arrest care should be initiated immediately because of evidence indicating that systematic postresuscitation care can improve the likelihood of patient survival with good quality of life. Because hemodynamic instability is common after cardiac arrest, epinephrine infusion may be used in the postresuscitation period to optimize blood pressure, cardiac output, and systemic perfusion after ROSC. Epinephrine also may be used during the periarrest period in adults who require inotropic or vasopressor support, in particular for the treatment of symptomatic bradycardia; although not a first-line drug, epinephrine may be considered in patients who are unresponsive to atropine therapy, or as a temporizing measure while awaiting availability of a pacemaker.

In contrast to adults, cardiac arrest in infants and children is not usually precipitated by a primary cardiac cause, but is more often the result of progressive respiratory failure or shock. In addition to high-quality CPR, ventilation is extremely important in pediatric advanced life support (PALS) because of the high percentage of asphyxial arrests that occur in pediatric patients. Similar to adults, vasopressors are used during pediatric cardiac arrest to restore spontaneous circulation although no specific pediatric studies have demonstrated the effectiveness of any vasopressor in this setting. AHA states that it is reasonable to administer epinephrine during pediatric cardiac arrest. The drug also may be used for hemodynamic support during the postresuscitation period. Epinephrine also is used in the emergency treatment of infants and children with bradycardia and cardiopulmonary compromise (with a palpable pulse) and is included in current PALS guidelines for this use; epinephrine is recommended in this situation when bradycardia persists despite ventilation, oxygenation, and chest compressions. Drugs are rarely needed during the resuscitation of neonates; because hypoxemia and inadequate lung inflation are common causes of bradycardia in the newborn infant, establishing adequate ventilation is the most important corrective measure in these patients.

Epinephrine also has been used in the treatment of syncope resulting from atrioventricular (AV) nodal block. However, permanent pacemaker implantation is the treatment of choice for third-degree and advanced second-degree AV nodal block (complete heart block).

■ **Septic Shock** Epinephrine is used for the treatment of hypotension associated with septic shock, generally as a second-line agent.

Vasopressors such as epinephrine are used in the management of shock to restore blood pressure and tissue perfusion after initial fluid resuscitation is attempted. The Surviving Sepsis Campaign International Guidelines for Management of Sepsis and Septic Shock recommend norepinephrine as the vasopressor of choice in adults with septic shock; if adequate blood pressure is not achieved, epinephrine may be added. Epinephrine is a potent vasoconstrictor with predominantly β-adrenergic effects at low doses and α-adrenergic effects at higher doses. Epinephrine administration can be associated with an increased rate of arrhythmias, decreased splanchnic blood flow, and increased blood lactate concentrations. Despite these adverse effects, there is no clinical evidence indicating that the drug is associated with worse outcomes than norepinephrine, and therefore, some experts suggest that epinephrine should be considered when an additional agent is needed to maintain adequate blood pressure during septic shock. In a double-blind, randomized controlled study comparing the effects of epinephrine and norepinephrine in intensive care patients, including a subgroup with septic shock, no substantial difference in 28- or 90-day mortality or time to achieve mean arterial pressure (MAP) goals was observed between the treatment groups; however, 13% of patients who received epinephrine were withdrawn from the study as a result of lactic acidosis or tachycardia. In another study in patients with septic shock, there was no difference in all-cause mortality, hemodynamic stabilization, resolution of organ dysfunction, or adverse events between patients receiving epinephrine and those receiving norepinephrine plus dobutamine.

Epinephrine should not be used in cardiogenic shock because it increases myocardial oxygen demand, nor should it be used in hemorrhagic or traumatic shock.

■ **Local Vasoconstriction** Epinephrine may be added to solutions of some local anesthetics to decrease the rate of vascular absorption of the anesthetic, thereby localizing anesthesia and prolonging the duration of anesthesia; the risk of systemic toxicity from the local anesthetic is also decreased. (See Local Anesthetics, Parenteral 72:00.)

Epinephrine has been applied topically to control superficial bleeding from arterioles or capillaries in the skin, mucous membranes, or other tissues. Bleeding from larger vessels is not controllable by topical application of epinephrine.

■ **Premature Labor** Epinephrine has been used to relax uterine musculature and inhibit uterine contractions in premature labor; however, the cardiovascular effects and other adverse effects limit the usefulness of the drug for this purpose. (See Cautions: Pregnancy.) Other β-agonists (e.g., terbutaline) are preferred. Some manufacturers state that epinephrine injection should be avoided during the second stage of labor.

■ **Bronchospasm** ***Asthma*** Epinephrine and racepinephrine hydrochloride are used for the symptomatic treatment of asthma. Racepinephrine is commercially available as an oral bronchodilator for *self-medication* for the temporary relief of mild symptoms of intermittent asthma (e.g., wheezing, chest tightness, shortness of breath). Once a diagnosis of asthma has been confirmed by a clinician, use of a nonprescription (over-the-counter, OTC) bronchodilator may be appropriate in patients with mild intermittent asthma; because asthma may be life-threatening, those with more severe asthma (i.e., persistent asthma) or worsening asthma (symptoms not relieved within 20 minutes or with maximum recommended dosages, increasing frequency of asthma attacks) should consult a clinician for other treatment options. An epinephrine preparation for oral inhalation use no longer is commercially available in the US.

While orally inhaled epinephrine was once widely used for its bronchodilating effects in the management of reversible airway obstruction, the drug has been replaced by more selective and rapid-acting agents (e.g., inhaled β_2-adrenergic agonists), and epinephrine is not recommended as a drug of choice for the rapid relief of asthma in current asthma management guidelines. In the stepped-care approach to antiasthmatic therapy, most experts currently recommend use of a selective short-acting inhaled β_2-adrenergic agonist (e.g., albuterol, levalbuterol, pirbuterol) on an intermittent, as-needed basis to control acute symptoms (e.g., cough, wheezing, dyspnea). Less β_2-selective bronchodilators such as epinephrine generally are not recommended because of their potential to cause excessive cardiac stimulation (e.g., increased heart rate, myocardial irritability, increased oxygen demand), particularly at high doses. For information on the stepped-care approach for drug therapy in asthma, see Asthma under Uses: Bronchospasm, in Albuterol 12:12.08.12.

Epinephrine also has been used parenterally for the treatment of severe asthma. Subcutaneous or IM epinephrine is the drug of choice for acute asthma attacks potentially associated with anaphylaxis but otherwise is reserved for severe asthma exacerbations when inhaled or parenteral β_2-selective agents are not readily available or are ineffective. Subcutaneous administration of epinephrine also may be useful when tachypnea and low tidal volume may prevent effective therapy with an orally inhaled β_2-adrenergic agonist or when orally inhaled therapy is not effective. Epinephrine also has been used IV for the treatment of severe asthma exacerbations; however, there is no evidence that the drug improves outcomes when compared with the selective inhaled β_2-adrenergic agonists.

■ **Upper GI Hemorrhage** Epinephrine injection has been used as an endoscopic treatment modality for the management of acute nonvariceal upper GI bleeding†; when used for this purpose, a dilute solution of epinephrine (in 0.9% sodium chloride injection) is injected into and around the ulcer base during endoscopy to produce tamponade and achieve hemostasis. Such therapy should not be used alone and should be combined with an additional endoscopic hemostatic modality (e.g., clips, thermocoagulation).

For uses of epinephrine in the treatment of glaucoma or as a mydriatic, see 52:24. For use of epinephrine as a vasoconstrictor and hemostatic in the eye and mucosa, see 52:32.

Dosage and Administration

■ **Administration** *USP has changed its labeling standard for single-entity drug products to no longer allow the use of ratios to express drug concentrations. This labeling change was prompted by numerous reports of serious medication errors caused by confusion with different ratio expressions. Effective May 1, 2016, all single-entity preparations of epinephrine injection, USP should be labeled only in terms of strength per mL (i.e., mg/mL). While concentrations of some epinephrine preparations were historically expressed in ratios (e.g., 1:1000 or 1:10,000), such designation is no longer acceptable because of the risk of dosing errors.*

Epinephrine usually is administered by IM, subcutaneous, or IV injection, or by continuous IV infusion. Epinephrine also has been administered by intraosseous (IO) injection† in the setting of advanced cardiovascular life support (ACLS), generally when IV access is not readily available; onset of action and systemic concentrations are comparable to those achieved with venous administration. If vascular access (IV or IO) cannot be established during cardiac arrest, epinephrine may be administered endotracheally; however, this method of administration results in lower plasma concentrations compared with the same dose given intravascularly. Epinephrine also has been administered by intracardiac injection (into the left ventricular chamber) during cardiac arrest; however, this route of administration is not recommended in current ACLS guidelines.

The appropriate concentration and route of administration of epinephrine should be selected carefully; serious adverse effects (e.g., cerebral hemorrhage) have occurred after concentrated solutions of epinephrine intended for IM administration were administered IV. Because of the risks associated with IV use, epinephrine generally should be administered by the IV route only in extreme situations (such as in the treatment of septic or anaphylactic shock, cardiac arrest, or when the patient is unresponsive to multiple IM injections). Dilute solutions of epinephrine (e.g., 0.1 mg/mL) should always be used when administering the drug IV. Commercially available epinephrine solutions for IM or subcutaneous injection are tenfold more concentrated (1 mg/mL) and should not be administered IV without dilution.

Solutions of epinephrine should be inspected visually for particulate matter and discoloration prior to administration. Epinephrine injection must not be used if it is discolored or cloudy or contains any particulate matter.

Parenteral Administration **IM or Subcutaneous Administration.** Epinephrine injection solution containing epinephrine 1 mg/mL may be administered IM or subcutaneously, but IM injection into the buttock should be avoided. (See Cautions: Adverse Effects.) When used for the treatment of anaphylaxis, epinephrine should be administered by IM (preferred) or subcutaneous injection into the anterolateral aspect of the thigh; injection into or near smaller muscles (i.e., deltoid muscle) is not recommended because of possible differences in absorption. Following subcutaneous administration, absorption and subsequent achievement of peak plasma concentrations may be slower and substantially delayed if shock is present. Repeated injections of epinephrine should not be administered at the same site because of the risk of possible tissue necrosis due to vasoconstriction.

Epinephrine is commercially available in a prefilled auto-injector for the emergency treatment of allergic reactions. When IM or subcutaneous epinephrine is used for *self-medication*, patients and their caregivers should be instructed about proper administration techniques using the auto-injector provided by the manufacturer. Patients should seek immediate medical or hospital care in conjunction with self-administration of the drug. First aid providers should be familiar with auto-injectors in order to assist patients experiencing an anaphylactic reaction, and they should be able to administer epinephrine using an auto-injector if a patient is unable to self-administer the drug, provided that state law permits it and a valid prescription exists. When using the auto-injector, the appropriate weight-based dose should be injected IM or subcutaneously into the anterolateral aspect of the thigh. The injection may be administered through clothing if necessary. Some manufacturers recommend massaging the injection area for several seconds after the drug is administered. The auto-injectors are overfilled and most of the solution will remain in the device after injection of the appropriate dose; however, the auto-injector cannot be reused. The respective manufacturer's prescribing information should be consulted for additional instructions on use of prefilled epinephrine auto-injectors.

IV Administration. For IV administration, epinephrine is commercially available as a 0.1-mg/mL solution. This concentration also may be prepared by diluting the commercially available 1-mg/mL epinephrine injection with a suitable diluent. Various methods have been described for diluting epinephrine solutions for IV administration, and the manufacturers' information should be consulted for specific instructions. Commercially available epinephrine 1-mg/mL injection should not be administered IV unless the solution is further diluted.

In emergency situations, diluted solutions of epinephrine may be administered by slow IV injection or as a continuous IV infusion. Extreme caution is recommended when epinephrine is administered by direct IV injection since the risk of overdosage and adverse cardiovascular effects is substantially higher with such administration; the drug should be administered slowly with close hemodynamic monitoring.

During cardiac resuscitation, epinephrine may be administered IV into a central or peripheral line. IV access should be established and the drug administered without interrupting chest compressions. To ensure delivery of the drug into the central compartment, each dose of epinephrine given by *peripheral* injection should be followed by a 20-mL flush of IV fluid and the extremity should be elevated during and after drug administration. Although central venous access is advantageous because higher plasma drug concentrations can be achieved and physiologic monitoring for return of spontaneous circulation (ROSC) can be performed, placement of a central line can potentially interrupt cardiopulmonary resuscitation (CPR). Central line placement should be avoided in patients who are candidates for pharmacologic reperfusion (e.g., with thrombolytic therapy).

During resuscitation in infants and children, a peripheral IV line may be established if it can be done rapidly. Central venous access is not recommended as the initial route of vascular access during an emergency because of the expertise and time required for establishing a central line. If, however, both central and peripheral lines are available, the central venous route is preferred. Whereas venous access can be challenging in critically ill infants and children, IO access can be achieved rapidly with minimal complications.

To minimize the risk of necrosis, continuous IV infusions of epinephrine should be infused into a large vein. A catheter tie-in technique should be avoided because obstruction to blood flow around the tubing may cause stasis and increase local concentration of the drug. *Care must be taken to avoid extravasation because local necrosis may result.*

Endotracheal Administration If vascular access (IV or IO) is not possible during cardiac resuscitation, lipid-soluble drugs such as epinephrine may be administered via an endotracheal tube. However, studies have shown conflicting results regarding the effectiveness of endotracheal versus vascular administration of the drug. Epinephrine administered via an endotracheal tube should be diluted in 5–10 mL of 0.9% sodium chloride or sterile water in adults or flushed with a minimum of 5 mL of 0.9% sodium chloride injection in pediatric patients. Absorption of epinephrine, administered via endotracheal tube, may be increased by diluting the drug in sterile water instead of 0.9% sodium chloride.

Oral Inhalation Epinephrine and racepinephrine also have been administered via oral inhalation using a nebulizer, aerosol, or intermittent positive-pressure breathing (IPPB) apparatus for the treatment of asthma. However, an oral inhalation preparation of epinephrine is no longer commercially available in the US.

Topical Administration Solutions of epinephrine hydrochloride also are applied topically as a spray or on cotton or gauze to the skin, mucous membranes, or other tissues.

■ **Dosage** Dosage of epinephrine salts is expressed in terms of epinephrine. Dosage of racepinephrine hydrochloride is expressed in terms of racepinephrine; racepinephrine is about one-half as active as epinephrine.

Sensitivity Reactions **Adult Dosage.** For the emergency treatment of allergic reactions, including anaphylaxis, the usual adult dose of epinephrine is 0.2–0.5 mg (0.2–0.5 mL of a 1-mg/mL solution) administered IM or subcutaneously; the dose may be repeated every 5–15 minutes as necessary. A maximum single dose of 0.5 mg in adults is recommended. IM administration is preferred since absorption and subsequent achievement of peak plasma concentrations may be slower and substantially delayed following subcutaneous administration of the drug if shock is present.

For *self-administration* of epinephrine using a prefilled auto-injector (e.g., EpiPen®), an IM or subcutaneous dose of 0.3 mg is recommended. For severe persistent anaphylaxis, repeated doses may be needed; if more than 2 sequential doses are needed, subsequent doses should be administered under direct medical supervision.

In extreme circumstances (e.g., anaphylactic shock, cardiac arrest, or no response to initial IM injections), IV administration may be necessary since absorption of epinephrine may be impaired with subcutaneous or IM administration. The usual adult IV dose of epinephrine for the treatment of anaphylaxis ranges from 0.1 to 0.25 mg (1–2.5 mL of a 0.1-mg/mL solution); the dose may be repeated every 5–15 minutes as needed. Although there is no established dosage for continuous IV infusions of epinephrine, some studies have demonstrated efficacy at IV infusion rates of 2–15 mcg/minute, titrated based on severity of the reaction and clinical response.

Patients with anaphylaxis who respond to therapy require observation for possible recurrence even if there is an intervening asymptomatic period; length of observation time has not been established. Symptoms may recur within 1–36 hours after the initial reaction. The duration of direct observation and monitoring after an episode of anaphylaxis should be individualized based on the severity and duration of the anaphylactic event as well as other factors (e.g., response to treatment, pattern of previous anaphylactic reactions, comorbidities, patient reliability, access to medical care). Some experts suggest that patients with moderate to severe anaphylaxis should be observed for a minimum of 4–8 hours after treatment.

Pediatric Patients. For the treatment of anaphylaxis in pediatric patients, the recommended dose of epinephrine is 0.01 mg/kg (0.01 mL/kg of a 1-mg/mL solution) by IM or subcutaneous injection. Single IM or subcutaneous doses should not exceed 0.3–0.5 mg (depending on the patient's weight). The dose may be repeated every 5–15 minutes as necessary. Some clinicians state that doses may be repeated at 20-minute to 4-hour intervals depending on the severity of the condition and patient response.

For *self-administration* of epinephrine in children using a prefilled auto-injector, a dose of 0.15 or 0.3 mg, depending on body weight, should be injected IM or subcutaneously; 0.3 mg is recommended for patients weighing at least 30 kg and 0.15 mg is recommended for patients weighing 15–30 kg. If doses less than 0.15 mg are considered more appropriate, alternative injectable forms of the drug should be used. For severe persistent anaphylaxis, repeat doses may be needed; however, if more than 2 sequential doses of epinephrine are needed, subsequent doses should only be administered under direct medical supervision.

If IV administration is necessary for the treatment of anaphylaxis in pediatric patients, some clinicians recommend an initial IV epinephrine dose of 0.01 mg/kg (0.1 mL/kg of a 0.1-mg/mL solution). If repeated doses are required, a continuous IV infusion should be initiated at a rate of 0.1 mcg/kg per minute, and increased gradually to 1.5 mcg/kg per minute to maintain blood pressure. A slow, continuous, low-dose infusion is preferred to repeat IV injections because the drug may be titrated to effect.

Advanced Cardiovascular Life Support and Cardiac Arrhythmias

For ACLS during cardiac arrest, epinephrine preferably is administered IV but also may be instilled directly into the tracheobronchial tree via an endotracheal tube or administered by IO injection or intracardially. (See Dosage and Administration: Administration.) Although endotracheal administration of epinephrine is possible, IV or IO administration is preferred because of more predictable drug delivery and pharmacologic effect. IO administration of epinephrine may be particularly useful in children when IV access is not readily available.

Adult Dosage. When used for cardiac resuscitation in adults, epinephrine doses ranging from 0.1–1 mg have been used. In ACLS guidelines, a standard dosage of epinephrine (defined as 1 mg every 3–5 minutes by IV/IO injection) is recommended during adult cardiac arrest. Current evidence indicates that higher doses (e.g., 0.1–0.2 mg/kg) do not provide any benefits in terms of survival or neurologic outcomes compared with the standard dose and may be harmful.

The optimum dose of epinephrine during cardiac resuscitation has been a subject of controversy. Many clinicians had questioned the commonly used doses of 0.5–1 mg because of concern that these doses were not based on body weight, and thus may be lower than necessary for optimum cardiovascular effects. Interest in high doses of epinephrine was stimulated by animal studies indicating that such doses (e.g., 0.045–0.2 mg/kg) provided optimal improvement in hemodynamics, including ROSC, and timely achievement of successful cardiopulmonary resuscitation (CPR). Results of several clinical studies, including randomized controlled studies, found no substantial improvement in survival rates to hospital discharge nor trend for improved neurologic outcomes in patients with cardiac arrest receiving higher than usual doses of epinephrine, despite evidence of increased rates of ROSC and higher initial resuscitation rates with high-dose therapy. A retrospective study of functional neurologic outcomes (assessed by measurement of cerebral performance category) of patients with ventricular fibrillation who received high IV dosages of epinephrine during cardiac resuscitation found that such dosages were independently associated with unfavorable neurologic outcomes. Patients with unfavorable neurologic outcomes after resuscitation had received substantially higher median cumulative doses (i.e., 4 mg [range: 2–8 mg]) of epinephrine than those with favorable neurologic outcomes who received a median cumulative dose of 1 mg (range: less than 1–3 mg). These findings persisted after neurologic outcomes were stratified by duration of CPR and other potentially confounding conditions were considered. Based on the currently available evidence, the American Heart Association (AHA) states that it is reasonable to administer standard-dose epinephrine (1 mg every 3–5 minutes) during cardiac arrest in adults; high-dose epinephrine should not be used routinely, but may be considered in certain situations (e.g., overdosage of β-adrenergic or calcium-channel blocking agents).

The optimal timing of epinephrine administration, particularly in relation to defibrillation, is not known and may vary based on patient-specific factors and resuscitation conditions. In adults with asystole or pulseless electrical activity (PEA), epinephrine may be given as soon as feasible after the onset of cardiac arrest based on studies demonstrating improved survival to hospital discharge and increased ROSC when the drug was administered early during the course of treatment for a nonshockable rhythm.

If IV or IO access cannot be established during cardiac arrest, epinephrine may be administered via the endotracheal route. Although the optimal dose of epinephrine administered via an endotracheal tube remains to be established, some experts state that typical doses should be 2–2.5 times those administered IV.

If epinephrine is used for hemodynamic support following cardiac resuscitation, the usual IV dosage in adults is 0.1–0.5 mcg/kg per minute; the infusion rate should be titrated to patient response.

If epinephrine is used for the treatment of symptomatic bradycardia in adults, an initial infusion rate of 2–10 mcg/minute has been recommended and should be titrated to patient response. Intravascular volume and support should be assessed as needed.

Pediatric Dosage. When used for pediatric advanced life support (PALS), the usual IV or IO dose of epinephrine is 0.01 mg/kg (0.1 mL/kg of a 0.1-mg/mL solution), up to a maximum single dose of 1 mg, and the usual dose of epinephrine administered via an endotracheal tube is 0.1 mg/kg (0.1 mL/kg of a 1-mg/mL solution), up to a maximum single dose of 2.5 mg. The same IV, IO, or endotracheal dose should be repeated every 3–5 minutes if needed. Higher doses are not recommended because of the potential for harm, particularly in cases of asphyxia, and lack of survival benefit. AHA states, however, that high-dose epinephrine may be considered in exceptional circumstances (e.g., β-adrenergic blocking agent overdose).

In a prospective, randomized, double-blind study of 68 children who received either 0.01 mg/kg (standard dose) or 0.1 mg/kg (high dose) of epinephrine as rescue therapy for in-hospital cardiac arrest after failure of CPR and an initial dose of 0.01 mg/kg (standard dose) of epinephrine, high-dose rescue therapy was not associated with any benefits. High-dose epinephrine rescue therapy did not improve the survival rate at 24 hours compared with standard-dose therapy, and appeared to be harmful in children with asphyxia-precipitated cardiac arrest. In addition, a trend toward reduced rate of survival at 24 hours was observed among children who received high-dose therapy as compared with standard-dose therapy. Also, the rates of ROSC or survival to hospital discharge were not significantly different between the 2 groups.

For postresuscitation stabilization in pediatric patients, epinephrine may be administered by IV or IO infusion at a rate of 0.1–1 mcg/kg per minute; the rate of infusion should be adjusted based on patient response. Although low-dose IV infusions (less than 0.3 mcg/kg per minute) generally produce predominantly β-adrenergic effects, while higher-dose IV infusions (exceeding 0.3 mcg/kg per minute) generally result in α-adrenergic vasoconstriction, there is substantial interindividual variation in response, and infusion dosage should be titrated to the desired effect.

The usual neonatal IV dose of epinephrine is 0.01–0.03 mg/kg (0.1–0.3 mL/kg of a 0.1-mg/mL solution). AHA states that higher IV doses are not recommended; in pediatric and animal studies, administration of IV doses in the range of 0.1 mg/kg have been associated with exaggerated hypertension, decreased myocardial function, and worsening neurologic function. In addition, the sequence of hypotension followed by hypertension is likely to increase the risk of intracranial hemorrhage, especially in neonates. IV administration of epinephrine (0.01–0.03 mg/kg per dose) is the preferred route in neonates, since there are limited data available on endotracheal administration of epinephrine. If the endotracheal route is used, doses of 0.01 or 0.03 mg/kg will likely be ineffective. Although safety and efficacy have not been established, endotracheal administration of a higher dose (0.05–0.1 mg/kg) while IV access is being obtained may be considered.

In one retrospective study in children and neonates who received either mean doses of 0.01 mg/kg (standard dose) or 0.12 mg/kg (high dose) of epinephrine administered IV, via an endotracheal tube, or by IO infusion during CPR after cardiac arrest occurring during a hospital stay, high doses of the drug were not associated with improvements in rates of ROSC, short- or long-term survival rates, or overall outcome scores. In this study, the time to ROSC was substantially shorter in patients receiving standard doses of epinephrine than in those receiving higher doses. In addition, high-dose epinephrine may be associated with adverse effects such as increased myocardial oxygen consumption during cardiac resuscitation, a postarrest hyperadrenergic state with tachycardia, hypertension and ventricular ectopy, myocardial necrosis, and worse postarrest myocardial dysfunction. Additional clinical studies are needed to evaluate fully the optimum dosage regimen of epinephrine in pediatric patients.

For the emergency treatment of infants and children with bradycardia and cardiorespiratory compromise (with a palpable pulse), epinephrine may be given at a dose of 0.01 mg/kg (0.1 mL/kg of a 0.1-mg/mL solution) by IV/IO injection, and repeated every 3–5 minutes as needed; alternatively, an endotracheal dose of 0.1 mg/kg (0.1 mL/kg of a 1-mg/mL solution) may be given if IV/IO access is not available.

Septic Shock For the treatment of hypotension during septic shock in adults, the manufacturer suggests an IV infusion rate of 0.05–2 mcg/kg per minute. The infusion rate may be increased in increments of 0.05–0.2 mcg/kg per minute every 10–15 minutes to achieve the desired blood pressure goal. The duration of therapy or total dose required is not known; continuous epinephrine infusion may be necessary for several hours or days until the patient's hemodynamic status improves. If epinephrine is used in pediatric patients with septic shock, some clinicians have recommended an IV infusion rate of 0.05–0.3 mcg/kg per minute, titrated to effect.

When therapy is discontinued, the infusion rate should be decreased gradually (e.g., by reducing the infusion rate every 30 minutes over a 12- to 24-hour period).

Bronchospasm **Parenteral Dosage.** For the treatment of severe asthma exacerbations when orally inhaled, selective short-acting β_2-adrenergic agonists are not available, an expert panel of the National Asthma Education and Prevention Program (NAEPP) states that epinephrine 0.3–0.5 mg may be given subcutaneously every 20 minutes for 3 doses in adults and adolescents older than 12 years of age. Alternatively, some clinicians recommend a subcutaneous epinephrine dose of 0.01 mg/kg (using a 1-mg/mL solution), divided into 3 doses of approximately 0.3 mg each, administered at 20-minute intervals. For the treatment of severe asthma exacerbations in children 12 years of age or younger, 0.01 mg/kg of epinephrine (0.01 mL/kg using a 1-mg/mL solution), but no more than 0.3–0.5 mg per dose, may be administered by subcutaneous injection at 20-minute intervals for 3 doses.

For the treatment of bronchospasm in adults, some manufacturers recommend an epinephrine dose of 0.1–0.25 mg (1–2.5 mL of a 0.1-mg/mL solution) by slow IV injection. If IV administration of epinephrine is required for the management of asthma attacks in pediatric patients, some clinicians recommend a slow IV injection of 0.01 mg/kg in neonates and an initial IV dose of 0.05 mg (which may be repeated at 20- to 30-minute intervals) in infants.

Oral Inhalation Dosage. For the temporary relief of mild symptoms of intermittent asthma, the usual dose of 2.25% racepinephrine inhalation solution (equivalent to 1% epinephrine) in adults and children 4 years of age or older is 1–3 inhalations; doses should not be repeated more often than every 3 hours. Patients should be advised to seek medical assistance immediately if symptoms are not relieved within 20 minutes or become worse.

Local Vasoconstriction As a topical hemostatic, solutions containing epinephrine in concentrations of 0.002–0.1% have been sprayed or applied with cotton or gauze to the skin, mucous membranes, or other tissues. In conjunction with local anesthetics, epinephrine may be used in concentrations of 0.002–0.02 mg/mL. The most frequently used concentration is 0.005 mg/mL.

Cautions

■ Adverse Effects Epinephrine may cause fear, anxiety, tenseness, restlessness, headache, tremor, dizziness, lightheadedness, nervousness, sleeplessness, excitability, and weakness. In patients with parkinsonian syndrome, the drug increases rigidity and tremor. Patients with diabetes mellitus may experience transient increases in blood glucose concentrations. Epinephrine may aggravate or induce psychomotor agitation, disorientation, impaired memory, assaultive behavior, panic, hallucinations, suicidal or homicidal tendencies, and psychosis characterized by clear consciousness with schizophrenic-like thought disorder and paranoid delusions in some patients. Nausea, vomiting, sweating, pallor, respiratory difficulty, or respiratory weakness and apnea may also occur. It may be advisable to warn patients of possible adverse effects.

Epinephrine causes ECG changes including a decrease in T-wave amplitude in all leads in normal persons. Disturbances of cardiac rhythm and rate may result in palpitation and tachycardia. In patients with a perfusing rhythm, epinephrine may cause tachycardia, ventricular ectopy, tachyarrhythmias, hypertension, and vasoconstriction. In patients with coronary insufficiency and/or ischemic heart disease, epinephrine may aggravate or precipitate angina pectoris by increasing cardiac work and accentuating the insufficiency of the coronary circulation. Epinephrine can cause potentially fatal ventricular arrhythmias including fibrillation, especially in patients with organic heart disease or those receiving other drugs that sensitize the heart to arrhythmias. (See Drug Interactions.)

Epinephrine hydrochloride injection has been reported to cause syncope characterized by pallor, unconsciousness, and tachycardia in 4 children in doses varying from 0.05–0.2 mg subcutaneously. One of the children was later treated with 0.75 mg (0.15 mL of the longer-acting 5 mg/mL aqueous suspension, which is no longer commercially available in the US) subcutaneously with no such complication.

Overdosage or inadvertent IV injection of usual subcutaneous doses of epinephrine may cause hypertension. (See Acute Toxicity.) Subarachnoid hemorrhage and hemiplegia have resulted from hypertension, even following subcutaneous administration of usual doses. To avoid the possibility of dangerously high blood pressure from epinephrine therapy, blood pressure should be monitored closely during IV administration of the drug.

Epinephrine can cause tissue necrosis and sloughing at the site of injection as a result of local vasoconstriction. (See Cautions: Precautions and Contraindications.) Repeated injections of epinephrine can increase the risk of necrosis. Tissue necrosis may also occur in the extremities, kidneys, and liver. Fatal gas gangrene has occurred in patients receiving IM injection of epinephrine oil suspension (no longer available) in the buttocks. Gangrene of the lower extremities also may occur if epinephrine is infused into an ankle vein. It has been postulated that epinephrine-induced vasoconstriction reduces the oxygen tension of tissues, enabling anaerobic *Clostridium welchii* which may be present in the patient's feces and on the buttocks to multiply. IM injection of the drug into the buttocks should be avoided. If gas gangrene is suspected after epinephrine administration, treatment should be instituted immediately.

Prolonged use or overdosage of epinephrine can result in severe metabolic acidosis because of elevated blood concentrations of lactic acid. It has been proposed that epinephrine may cause hyperuricemia by its vasoconstrictor action in the kidneys; however, elevated BUN has been reported only rarely in cases of overdosage. IV use of epinephrine may initially constrict renal blood vessels and decrease urine formation.

Absorption of epinephrine from the respiratory tract following large doses by oral inhalation may result in adverse effects similar to those occurring after parenteral administration. Rarely, bronchial irritation and edema may occur. In some patients, severe prolonged asthma attacks may be precipitated. Rebound bronchospasm may occur when the effects of epinephrine end. Arterial oxygen tension, already reduced during asthmatic attacks, may be further reduced following oral inhalation of epinephrine. Dryness of pharyngeal membranes may follow oral inhalation and may be prevented by rinsing the mouth with water immediately after use of the drug. If epinephrine inhalation is inadvertently swallowed, epigastric pain may occur.

■ **Precautions and Contraindications** Vasopressor therapy is *not* a substitute for replacement of blood, plasma, fluids, and/or electrolytes. Blood volume depletion should be corrected as fully as possible before epinephrine therapy is instituted.

Because severe local adverse effects (e.g., tissue necrosis) may occur, extravasation of epinephrine infusions must be avoided. *The site of infusion should be checked frequently for free flow and the infused vein should be observed for blanching.* Infusion into leg veins, especially in geriatric patients or those with occlusive vascular diseases (e.g., atherosclerosis, arteriosclerosis, diabetic endarteritis, Buerger's disease) should be avoided. If blanching is observed in the infused vein, changing the infusion site periodically may be advisable. If extravasation occurs, 10–15 mL of sodium chloride solution containing 5–10 mg of phentolamine mesylate should be infiltrated (using a syringe with a fine hypodermic needle) liberally throughout the affected area, which is identified by a cold, hard, and pallid appearance. Immediate and conspicuous local hyperemic changes occur if the area is infiltrated within 12 hours; therefore, phentolamine should be administered as soon as possible after extravasation is noted.

Epinephrine should not be administered in the digits, hands, or feet. Accidental injection into the digits, hands, or feet may result in loss of blood flow to the affected area and has been associated with tissue necrosis.

Particular attention should be paid to the appropriate concentration and route of administration of epinephrine since serious adverse effects (e.g., cerebral hemorrhage) have occurred after concentrated solutions of epinephrine intended for IM administration were administered IV. Because of the risks associated with IV use, epinephrine generally should be administered by the IV route only in extreme situations (such as in the treatment of septic or anaphylactic shock, cardiac arrest, or when the patient is unresponsive to multiple IM injections). (See Dosage and Administration: Administration.)

Racepinephrine, a racemic mixture of epinephrine, shares the toxic potentials of epinephrine, and the usual precautions of epinephrine therapy should be observed. Adverse reactions to epinephrine may be most likely to occur in hypertensive or hyperthyroid patients, and the drug must be administered with extreme caution, if at all, to such patients. Epinephrine should be administered with caution to geriatric patients, patients with diabetes mellitus, hyperthyroidism, Parkinson's disease, pheochromocytoma, or cardiovascular diseases (including cardiac arrhythmias, coronary artery disease, and organic heart disease), and/or those with a history of sensitivity to sympathomimetic amines. Coronary insufficiency is usually considered to be a contraindication to parenteral use of the drug. The drug must be used cautiously in patients with bronchial asthma and emphysema who may also have degenerative heart disease. Epinephrine injection should be used with caution in patients with psychoneurotic disorders.

Some commercially available formulations of epinephrine hydrochloride or racepinephrine hydrochloride contain sulfites that can cause allergic-type reactions, including anaphylaxis and life-threatening or less severe asthmatic episodes, in certain susceptible individuals. The overall prevalence of sulfite sensitivity in the general population is unknown but probably low; such sensitivity appears to occur more frequently in asthmatic than in nonasthmatic individuals. The presence of sulfites in a parenteral epinephrine preparation and the possibility of allergic-type reactions should *not* deter use of the drug when indicated for the treatment of serious allergic reactions or for other emergency situations. Epinephrine is the preferred treatment for such conditions, and currently available alternatives to epinephrine may not be optimally effective. The possibility of adverse reactions to sulfite(s) contained in the preparation should be considered in asthmatic patients who show paradoxical worsening of respiratory function following use of the drug or whose symptoms worsen or in whom bronchodilatory response decreases with increasing use of the drug.

Patients considering *self-medication* with racepinephrine as a bronchodilator should be advised to use the drug only if they have been diagnosed by a clinician as having asthma; patients also should be advised that the drug should not be used for *self-medication* if they ever have been hospitalized for asthma or are currently receiving a prescription drug for the management of this condition unless otherwise directed by a clinician. These patients also should be advised not to use the drug if they have cardiovascular disease, hypertension, diabetes mellitus, thyroid disease, angle-closure (narrow-angle) glaucoma, seizures, a psychiatric or emotional condition, or difficulty urinating because of prostatic hypertrophy unless directed by a clinician. In addition, patients should be advised not to exceed recommended dosages or frequency of administration unless otherwise instructed by a clinician. Patients should contact their clinician if their symptoms are not relieved within 20 minutes or become worse, more than the recommended dosage is required, or asthma attacks become more frequent (i.e., more than 2 asthma attacks in a week). Patients should be cautioned that racepinephrine can cause hypertension and tachycardia, which could increase the risk of cardiovascular disease, stroke, or death. Foods, beverages, and dietary supplements that contain stimulants (e.g., caffeine) should be avoided.

There are no absolute contraindications to the use of epinephrine in life-threatening conditions. Relative contraindications to epinephrine include shock (other than anaphylactic and septic shock), known hypersensitivity to sympathomimetic amines, coronary insufficiency, and cardiac dilatation, as well as use in most patients with angle-closure glaucoma or organic brain damage. The drug is contraindicated for use during general anesthesia with agents such as cyclopropane and halogenated hydrocarbon anesthetics (e.g., halothane). (See Drug Interactions: General Anesthetics.) In conjunction with local anesthetics, epinephrine is contraindicated for use in certain areas (e.g., fingers, toes, ears).

■ **Pregnancy** Epinephrine usually inhibits spontaneous or oxytocin-induced contractions of the pregnant human uterus and may delay the second stage of labor. In dosages sufficient to reduce uterine contractions, the drug may cause a prolonged period of uterine atony with hemorrhage. If used during pregnancy, epinephrine may cause anoxia to the fetus and/or spontaneous abortion. When administered in advanced cardiovascular life support (ACLS) during cardiac resuscitation, epinephrine may decrease blood flow to the uterus; however, the woman must be resuscitated for survival of the fetus. Some manufacturers state that epinephrine should be avoided during the second stage of labor; parenteral administration of the drug to maintain blood pressure during spinal anesthesia for delivery can cause acceleration of fetal heart rate and should not be used in obstetric patients when maternal systolic/diastolic blood pressure exceeds 130/80 mm Hg. Epinephrine should be administered cautiously by oral inhalation to pregnant patients. Epinephrine should be used during pregnancy only if the potential benefits justify the possible risks to the fetus. There is some evidence to support that epidural administration of some local anesthetics (e.g., lidocaine) with epinephrine during labor is safe.

Drug Interactions

■ **Sympathomimetic Agents** Epinephrine must not be administered concomitantly with other sympathomimetic agents (e.g., isoproterenol) because of the possibility of additive effects and increased toxicity.

■ **α- and β-Adrenergic Blocking Agents** The cardiac and bronchodilating effects of epinephrine are antagonized by β-adrenergic blocking drugs such as propranolol, and the vasoconstriction and hypertension caused by high doses of epinephrine are antagonized by α-adrenergic blocking agents such as phentolamine. Because of their α-adrenergic blocking properties, ergot alkaloids can reverse the pressor response to epinephrine. Concomitant use of β-adrenergic blocking drugs (e.g., propranolol) may also potentiate the pressor effects of epinephrine.

■ **Cardiac Glycosides** Epinephrine should not be used in patients receiving excessive dosages of other drugs (e.g., cardiac glycosides) that can sensitize the heart to arrhythmias.

■ **Diuretics** Concomitant use of diuretics may antagonize the pressor effect and potentiate the arrhythmogenic effects of epinephrine. Some diuretics also may potentiate the hypokalemic effects of epinephrine.

■ **General Anesthetics** Administration of epinephrine in patients receiving cyclopropane or halogenated hydrocarbon general anesthetics that increase cardiac irritability and seem to sensitize the myocardium to epinephrine may result in arrhythmias including PVCs, tachycardia, or fibrillation. Epinephrine is contraindicated for use with chloroform, trichloroethylene, or cyclopropane and should be used cautiously, if at all, with other halogenated hydrocarbon anesthetics such as halothane. Epinephrine may not be absorbed rapidly enough to cause serious adverse effects when applied topically as a hemostatic in patients undergoing short surgical procedures such as tonsillectomy and adenoidectomy using halothane anesthesia. Prophylactic administration of lidocaine or prophylactic IV administration of propranolol 0.05 mg/kg may protect against ventricular irritability if epinephrine is used during anesthesia with a halogenated hydrocarbon anesthetic. In one study, arrhythmias occurring after parenteral use of epinephrine during general anesthesia responded promptly to IV propranolol 0.05 mg/kg.

■ **Hypotensive Agents** Epinephrine may antagonize the neuronal blockade produced by guanethidine (not commercially available in the US), resulting in loss of antihypertensive effectiveness. The vasopressor effect of epinephrine also may be antagonized by rapidly acting vasodilators (e.g., nitrates) and other antihypertensive agents.

■ **Monoamine Oxidase Inhibitors** Monoamine oxidase (MAO) is one of the enzymes responsible for epinephrine metabolism. The manufacturer states that epinephrine should be administered with caution in patients receiving an MAO inhibitor because severe, prolonged hypertension may result.

■ **Oxytocic Drugs** Concomitant use of epinephrine with oxytocics may result in severe, persistent hypertension.

■ **Other Drugs** Tricyclic antidepressants such as imipramine, some antihistamines (especially diphenhydramine, tripelennamine, and dexchlorpheniramine), and thyroid hormones may potentiate the effects of epinephrine, especially on heart rhythm and rate. Potentiation by tricyclic antidepressants or antihistamines may result from inhibition of tissue uptake of epinephrine or norepinephrine or by increased adrenoreceptor sensitivity to epinephrine. Concomitant use of catechol-*O*-methyltransferase (COMT) inhibitors (e.g., entacapone), clonidine, or doxapram also may potentiate the pressor effects of epinephrine and quinidine may potentiate the arrhythmogenic effects of epinephrine.

Concomitant use of corticosteroids or theophylline also may potentiate the hypokalemic effects of epinephrine.

Epinephrine should not be used to counteract circulatory collapse or hypotension caused by phenothiazines; a reversal of epinephrine's pressor effects resulting in further lowering of blood pressure may occur.

Because epinephrine may cause hyperglycemia, patients with diabetes mellitus receiving epinephrine may require increased dosage of insulin or oral hypoglycemic agents.

Acute Toxicity

■ **Pathogenesis** Autopsy findings in patients who died of epinephrine overdosage revealed evidence of circulatory collapse, and most organs and veins were congested with blood. In test animals, there is evidence that death is the result of respiratory arrest caused by hypertension. Death resulting from epinephrine overdosage may partially depend on factors other than the dose received; some patients have died following IV doses not exceeding 10 mg while others have survived doses as high as 30 mg IV or 110 mg subcutaneously.

■ **Manifestations and Treatment** After overdosage or inadvertent IV administration of usual subcutaneous doses of epinephrine, systolic and diastolic blood pressure rise sharply; venous pressure also rises. Cerebrovascular or other hemorrhage and hemiplegia may result, especially in geriatric patients. Because epinephrine is rapidly inactivated in the body, treatment of acute toxicity is mainly supportive. If necessary, the pressor effects of the drug may be counteracted by rapidly acting α-adrenergic blocking drugs such as phentolamine. Prolonged hypotension may follow, and another pressor agent such as norepinephrine may be required. Pulmonary edema may result from pulmonary arterial hypertension; administration of a rapidly acting α-adrenergic blocking drug and/or intermittent positive-pressure respiration may be required if pulmonary edema interferes with respiration. Respiratory difficulties including hyperventilation sometimes preceded by a brief period of apnea may also occur. Epinephrine overdosage causes transient bradycardia followed by tachycardia and may cause other potentially fatal cardiac arrhythmias. PVCs may appear within 1 minute after injection and may be followed by multifocal ventricular tachycardia (prefibrillation rhythm). Atrial tachycardia, occasionally accompanied by atrioventricular block, may occur after the drug's effects on the ventricles subside. Prolonged ECG changes and substantial changes in serum AST (SGOT) concentration were considered evidence of possibly permanent myocardial injury caused by overdosage of epinephrine in 2 patients. Arrhythmias, if they occur, may be counteracted by a β-adrenergic blocking drug such as propranolol. Kidney failure, metabolic acidosis, and cold, white skin may also occur.

Pharmacology

Epinephrine acts directly on both α- and β-adrenergic receptors of tissues innervated by sympathetic nerves except the sweat glands and arteries of the face. It is believed that β-adrenergic effects result from stimulation of the production of cyclic adenosine-3′,5′-monophosphate (AMP) by activation of the enzyme adenyl cyclase, whereas α-adrenergic effects result from inhibition of adenyl cyclase activity. The main effects of therapeutic parenteral doses of epinephrine are relaxation of smooth muscle of the bronchial tree, cardiac stimulation, and dilation of skeletal muscle vasculature.

■ **Respiratory Effects** Epinephrine relaxes bronchial smooth muscle by stimulation of β_2-adrenergic receptors and constricts bronchial arterioles by stimulation of α-adrenergic receptors when administered parenterally or by oral inhalation. In patients with bronchial constriction, the drug relieves bronchospasm, reduces congestion and edema, and increases tidal volume and vital capacity. However, decreased arterial oxygen tension may not be increased and may be further reduced. Respiration rate is increased briefly, but epinephrine has no clinical value as a respiratory stimulant. In some patients receiving the drug IV, respiratory stimulation may be preceded by a brief period of apnea, probably caused by a direct inhibition of the respiratory center.

Epinephrine inhibits histamine release and antagonizes the effect of the mediator on end organs. As a result, the drug may reverse bronchiolar constriction, vasodilation, and edema produced by this mediator.

■ **Cardiovascular Effects** Systemically absorbed epinephrine acts on β_1-adrenergic receptors in the heart producing a positive chronotropic effect through the sinoatrial node and a positive inotropic effect on the myocardium. Cardiac output, oxygen consumption, and the work of the heart are increased, and cardiac efficiency is decreased. Epinephrine increases the irritability of the heart muscle and often alters the rhythmic function of the ventricles, especially after large doses or when the heart has been sensitized to this action by other drugs including digitalis and certain anesthetics or by acute myocardial infarction. Arrhythmias including ventricular extrasystoles and fibrillation may result. In patients with cardiopulmonary arrest, epinephrine can convert asystole to sinus rhythm. Epinephrine has a direct constricting effect on coronary arteries, but this effect is overcome by indirect vasodilation caused by enhanced cardiac metabolism secondary to cardiac stimulation. As a result, coronary blood flow is increased. Cardiac stimulation produced by epinephrine increases left atrial pressure, and peripheral vasoconstriction causes redistribution of blood from the systemic to the pulmonary circulation. Pulmonary arterial hypertension and increased pulmonary capillary filtration pressure may occur; pulmonary edema may result.

Epinephrine constricts arterioles in the skin, mucous membranes, and viscera after parenteral administration by its effect on α-adrenergic receptors and reduces cutaneous blood flow, especially in the hands and feet. Topically applied epinephrine produces local vasoconstriction and hemostasis in bleeding from small vessels but does not control bleeding from larger vessels. Small doses of parenterally administered epinephrine dilate arterioles of the skeletal muscles as a result of stimulation of β-adrenergic receptors, whereas larger doses stimulate α-adrenergic receptors and cause constriction of these arterioles. With usual therapeutic doses of the drug, the dilator effects predominate; blood flow to the skeletal muscle is increased and total peripheral resistance is decreased. Systolic blood pressure is moderately increased, mainly because of increased cardiac output; however, diastolic blood pressure may be decreased as a result of vasodilation. Doses of epinephrine large enough to constrict blood vessels in the skeletal muscle, however, cause an increase in peripheral resistance and elevate both systolic and diastolic blood pressure. When the drug's effects on α-adrenergic receptors end, the effect on β-adrenergic receptors persists and hypotension may result.

Constriction of renal blood vessels by epinephrine, especially after IV administration, initially reduces renal blood flow and increases renal vascular resistance. Urine flow and excretion of sodium, potassium, and chloride are decreased. Renal blood flow and urine flow may then increase as a result of elevated blood pressure. Glomerular filtration rate is not greatly altered by the drug; alterations in electrolyte and water excretion may be caused by renal vascular changes, a direct tubular action, or an indirect effect through the posterior pituitary. Very large IV or intra-arterial doses of epinephrine may cause total renal shutdown which may be prolonged by trapping of the drug in the vessels as a result of vasoconstriction.

■ **Metabolic Effects** Epinephrine increases glycogenolysis in the liver, reduces glucose uptake by tissues, and inhibits insulin release in the pancreas, resulting in hyperglycemia. Muscle glycogenolysis also increases, and lactic acid blood concentrations are elevated. Transient hyperkalemia may also occur and may be followed by more prolonged hypokalemia. Epinephrine has calorigenic activity; oxygen consumption may increase by as much as 20–30% after parenteral administration of usual doses. Body temperature may be elevated, partly because of cutaneous vasoconstriction. Blood concentrations of free fatty acids are increased as a result of increased lipolysis in adipose tissue, and plasma concentrations of cholesterol, phospholipids, and low-density lipoproteins are also generally elevated. Fat may be deposited in muscles and liver.

■ **Other Effects** Epinephrine has no direct effect on cerebral arterioles or cerebral blood flow. However, elevations in cerebral blood flow and oxygen consumption may occur secondary to increased blood pressure. The drug is not a powerful CNS stimulant but may cause restlessness, apprehension, headache, and tremor, probably resulting from peripheral effects. In patients with parkinsonian syndrome, epinephrine increases rigidity and tremor by an unknown mechanism.

Epinephrine generally relaxes smooth muscles of the GI tract by stimulation of either α- or β-adrenergic receptors but contracts the pyloric and ileocecal sphincters by stimulation of α-adrenergic receptors. Because these effects are transient, inconsistent, and usually occur only with doses causing marked cardiovascular response, they have no therapeutic application.

The effects of epinephrine on the uterus are probably mediated through both α- and β-adrenergic receptors in the myometrium and vary with hormonal influences, the route of administration, and the dose given. The drug usually inhibits spontaneous or oxytocin-induced contractions of the pregnant human uterus and may delay the second stage of labor. Transient uterine hyperactivity frequently occurs after the drug is discontinued. In dosage sufficient to reduce uterine contractions, epinephrine may cause prolonged uterine atony with hemorrhage. Use of the drug during pregnancy may cause anoxia in the fetus.

Pharmacokinetics

■ **Absorption** Orally ingested epinephrine is rapidly metabolized in the GI tract and liver; pharmacologically active concentrations are not reached when the drug is given orally. Epinephrine is well absorbed after subcutaneous or IM injection; absorption can be hastened by massaging the injection site. Both rapid and prolonged absorption occur after subcutaneous injection of the longer-acting aqueous suspension (no longer commercially available in the US). Epinephrine also is absorbed following endotracheal administration, although serum concentrations achieved may be only 10% of those with an equivalent IV dose. After oral inhalation of epinephrine absorption is slight and the effects of the drug are restricted mainly to the respiratory tract. Absorption increases somewhat when larger doses are inhaled, and systemic effects may occur.

Epinephrine has a rapid onset and short duration of action when solutions of the drug are administered parenterally or by oral inhalation. Subcutaneous administration of epinephrine hydrochloride injection in patients with asthmatic attacks may produce bronchodilation within 5–10 minutes and maximal effects in about 20 minutes. Following subcutaneous injection of the longer-acting aqueous epinephrine suspension, the onset of action is as rapid as that occurring after subcutaneous administration of epinephrine hydrochloride aqueous injection; however, the effects are more prolonged and may persist for several hours. After oral inhalation of epinephrine, bronchodilation usually occurs within 1 minute.

■ **Distribution** Epinephrine crosses the placenta but not the blood-brain barrier. The drug is distributed into milk.

■ **Elimination** The pharmacologic actions of epinephrine are terminated mainly by uptake and metabolism in sympathetic nerve endings. Circulating drug is metabolized in the liver and other tissues by a combination of reactions involving the enzymes catechol-*O*-methyltransferase (COMT) and monoamine oxidase (MAO). The major metabolites are metanephrine and 3-methoxy-4-hydroxymandelic acid (vanillylmandelic acid, VMA) both of which are inactive. About 40% of a parenteral dose of epinephrine is excreted in urine as metanephrine, 40% as VMA, 7% as 3-methoxy-4-hydroxyphenoglycol, 2% as 3,4-dihydroxymandelic acid, and the remainder as acetylated derivatives. These metabolites are excreted mostly as the sulfate conjugates and, to a lesser extent, the glucuronide conjugates. Only small amounts of the drug are excreted unchanged.

Chemistry and Stability

■ **Chemistry** Epinephrine is an endogenous catecholamine which is the active principle of the adrenal medulla. Both the endogenous substance and the official preparation are the levorotatory isomer which is 15 times more active than is the dextrorotatory isomer. The drug is also commercially available as racepinephrine hydrochloride, which is a racemic mixture of the hydrochlorides of the enantiomorphs of epinephrine. Racepinephrine is about one-half as active as the levorotatory isomer.

Epinephrine may be obtained from the adrenal glands of animals or prepared synthetically; that obtained from animals may contain up to 4% norepinephrine. Epinephrine occurs as a white to nearly white, microcrystalline powder or granules. Epinephrine is only very slightly soluble in water and in alcohol but readily forms water soluble salts (such as the hydrochloride and bitartrate) with acids.

Racepinephrine hydrochloride occurs as a fine, white powder and is freely soluble in water and sparingly soluble in alcohol. Racepinephrine hydrochloride oral inhalation has a pH of 2–3.5.

■ **Stability** Epinephrine, epinephrine salts, racepinephrine hydrochloride, and preparations containing the drugs gradually darken on exposure to light and air and must be stored in tight, light-resistant containers. Epinephrine injection should be stored at room temperature (approximately 25°C). Freezing of racepinephrine hydrochloride oral inhalation should be avoided. In some commercially available injections, the air has been replaced with nitrogen to avoid oxidation. Withdrawal of doses from multiple-dose vials introduces air into the vials, subjecting the remaining epinephrine to oxidation. Oxidation of the drug imparts first a pink, then a brown color; epinephrine preparations must not be used if they have a pinkish or darker than slightly yellow color or contain a precipitate. Racepinephrine hydrochloride solutions must not be used if they are brown or contain a precipitate. Commercially available epinephrine preparations may contain a variety of preservatives including the antioxidants, sodium bisulfite or sodium metabisulfite, and bacteriostatic agents. Commercially available preparations vary in stability, depending on the form in which epinephrine is present and on the preservatives used. The manufacturer's directions should be followed with respect to storage requirements for each product.

Epinephrine is readily destroyed by oxidizing agents or alkalies including sodium bicarbonate, halogens, permanganates, chromates, nitrates, nitrites, and salts of easily reducible metals such as iron, copper, and zinc. Epinephrine injection has been reported to be physically incompatible with many drugs, but the compatibility depends on several factors (e.g., concentration of the drugs, specific diluents used, resulting pH, temperature). Specialized references should be consulted for specific compatibility information. Epinephrine may be mixed with 0.9% sodium chloride injection but is incompatible with 5% sodium chloride injection. Stability of epinephrine in 5% dextrose injection decreases when the pH exceeds 5.5.

Preparations

Effective May 1, 2016, a new USP labeling standard for Epinephrine Injection, USP has been implemented. Single-entity preparations of epinephrine injection will be expressed only in terms of strength per mL; use of ratios (e.g., 1:1000 or 1:10,000) to express concentrations is no longer acceptable. Epinephrine injection 1:1000 is equivalent to 1 mg/mL and epinephrine injection 1:10,000 is equivalent to 0.1 mg/mL.

Excipients in commercially available drug preparations may have clinically important effects in some individuals; consult specific product labeling for details.

EPINEPHrine

Parenteral		
Injection	0.1 mg/mL*	**EPINEPHrine Injection** (available in prefilled syringes)
	0.5 mg/mL	**EpiPen® Jr. Auto-Injector** (delivers a single 0.15-mg [0.3 mL] dose), Meridian
	1 mg/mL*	**Adrenaclick® Auto-Injector** (available in dose of 0.15 mg [0.15 mL] or 0.3 mg [0.3 mL]), Amedra
		Adrenalin®, Par
		Auvi-Q® Auto-Injector (available in dose of 0.15 mg [0.15 mL] or 0.3 mg [0.3 mL]), Sanofi-Aventis
		EPINEPHrine Injection
		EpiPen® Auto-Injector (delivers a single 0.3-mg [0.3 mL] dose), Meridian

*available from one or more manufacturer, distributor, and/or repackager by generic (nonproprietary) name

racEPINEPHrine Hydrochloride

Oral Inhalation		
Solution, for nebulization	2.25% (of racepinephrine)	**S2®**, Nephron Pharmaceuticals

†Use is not currently included in the labeling approved by the US Food and Drug Administration

Norepinephrine Bitartrate

l-Arterenol Bitartrate, Levarterenol Bitartrate, Noradrenaline Acid Tartrate

■ Norepinephrine bitartrate is identical to the endogenous catecholamine that is synthesized in the adrenal medulla and in sympathetic nervous tissue; norepinephrine predominantly acts by a direct effect on α-adrenergic receptors.

Uses

■ **Acute Hypotensive States** Norepinephrine bitartrate is used as adjunctive therapy to produce vasoconstriction and maintain blood pressure in the management of certain acute hypotensive states (e.g., pheochromocytomectomy, sympathectomy, poliomyelitis, spinal anesthesia, myocardial infarction, septicemia, blood transfusion, drug reactions). In patients who require vasopressor support, individual hemodynamic abnormalities must be identified and monitored so that therapy can be adjusted as necessary. If severe peripheral vasoconstriction exists, norepinephrine may be ineffective and may have a deleterious effect by causing further reductions in plasma volume and blood flow to vital organs.

Shock Vasopressors such as norepinephrine are used in the management of shock to restore blood pressure and tissue perfusion after initial fluid resuscitation is attempted. The Surviving Sepsis Campaign International Guidelines for Management of Sepsis and Septic Shock recommend norepinephrine as the first-line vasopressor of choice in adults with septic shock; if adequate blood pressure is not achieved, vasopressin or epinephrine may be added. Vasopressin also may be given in conjunction with norepinephrine to reduce dosage requirements of norepinephrine. Norepinephrine is a potent vasoconstrictor that increases mean arterial pressure (MAP) with minimal change in heart rate and cardiac output, and has been shown to preserve tissue perfusion when titrated to effect (i.e., MAP of at least 65 mm Hg). Although dopamine was used widely in the past as a first-line vasopressor agent in patients with septic shock, recent studies indicate that the drug is associated with a greater risk of adverse effects and possibly also an increased risk of death compared with norepinephrine. In a multicenter randomized study (Sepsis Occurrence in Acutely Ill Patients II [SOAP II]) comparing the effects of dopamine and norepinephrine in patients with shock (septic, cardiogenic, or hypovolemic), no substantial difference in 28-day mortality was observed between the vasopressors; however, use of dopamine was associated with more arrhythmias in the overall population and an increased rate of death in the subgroup of patients with cardiogenic shock.

Norepinephrine also has been used to provide vasopressor support in patients with other types of shock (e.g., cardiogenic, hemorrhagic), generally as a temporary measure until the underlying cause can be treated. Some evidence suggests that early use of vasopressors in patients with hemorrhagic shock may be deleterious; however, additional studies are needed to confirm this finding. The manufacturer states that norepinephrine should be used only as an emergency measure to maintain coronary and cerebral artery perfusion until blood volume replacement therapy can be completed in patients who are hypotensive from blood volume deficits. Early revascularization is the standard of care in patients with cardiogenic shock; use of vasopressors in this setting should be individualized and guided by hemodynamic monitoring.

Hypotension During Anesthesia Norepinephrine has been used to treat hypotension during spinal anesthesia, but other vasopressors with a longer duration of action such as phenylephrine are more commonly used.

■ **Advanced Cardiovascular Life Support** Norepinephrine has been used adjunctively in the management of cardiac arrest to restore and maintain adequate blood pressure after an effective heartbeat and ventilation have been established by other means. High-quality cardiopulmonary resuscitation (CPR) and defibrillation are integral components of advanced cardiovascular life support (ACLS) and the only proven interventions to increase survival to hospital discharge. Other resuscitative efforts, including drug therapy, are considered secondary and should be performed without compromising the quality and timely delivery of chest compressions and defibrillation. The principal goal of pharmacologic therapy during cardiac arrest is to facilitate the return of spontaneous circulation (ROSC), and epinephrine is considered the drug of choice for this use. Vasoactive drugs such as norepinephrine may be used for hemodynamic support following resuscitation from cardiac arrest. (See Uses: Advanced Cardiovascular Life Support and Cardiac Arrhythmias, in Epinephrine 12:12.12.)

■ **Prolongation of Anesthesia** Norepinephrine has been added to solutions of some local anesthetics to decrease the rate of vascular absorption of the anesthetic and prolong the duration of anesthesia†. Because norepinephrine is less potent than epinephrine and must be used in higher concentrations potentially causing greater risk of adverse effects, epinephrine is more commonly used for this purpose. (See Local Anesthetics, Parenteral, General Statement 72:00.)

Dosage and Administration

■ **Administration** Norepinephrine bitartrate is administered by IV infusion using an infusion pump or other apparatus to control the rate of flow. To minimize the risk of necrosis, infusion of the drug should be given into a large vein, particularly the antecubital vein of the arm, although some clinicians state that the femoral vein also may be used. The infusion should be administered through a plastic catheter inserted deep into the vein. A catheter tie-in technique should be avoided if possible because obstruction of blood flow around the tubing may cause stasis and increased local concentration of the drug. *Care must be taken to avoid extravasation because local necrosis may result.* (See Cautions: Precautions and Contraindications, for discussion on the prevention and treatment of the adverse effects of extravasation.)

Prior to administration, the commercially available concentrate for injection *must* be diluted with a dextrose-containing solution (5% dextrose injection, with or without 0.9% sodium chloride injection); dilution with 0.9% sodium chloride injection alone is not recommended because of possible loss of potency due to oxidation. The concentration of norepinephrine and the infusion rate depend on the drug and fluid requirements of the individual patient. The infusion solution is usually prepared by adding 4 mg of norepinephrine (4 mL of the commercially available injection) to 1 liter of a 5% dextrose-containing solution; the resultant solution contains 4 mcg/mL. A more dilute or concentrated solution may be prepared depending on the fluid requirements of the patient.

Solutions of norepinephrine should be inspected visually for particulate matter and discoloration prior to administration whenever solution and container permit. Norepinephrine bitartrate injection must not be used if it is discolored (e.g., pink, dark yellow) or contains any particulate matter. Contact of the drug with iron salts, alkalies, or oxidizing agents must be avoided. Norepinephrine should *not* be administered in the same IV line as alkaline solutions, which may inactivate the drug.

■ **Dosage** Dosage of norepinephrine bitartrate is expressed in terms of norepinephrine.

Acute Hypotensive States Norepinephrine should be administered in the lowest effective dosage for the shortest possible time.

For restoration of blood pressure in adults with acute hypotensive states, the usual initial dosage of norepinephrine is 8–12 mcg/minute. Alternatively, some clinicians have suggested an initial dosage of 0.5–1 mcg/minute, titrated to effect, patients with refractory shock may require 8–30 mcg/minute. If norepinephrine is used in pediatric patients, some clinicians have recommended an initial infusion rate of 0.05–0.1 mcg/kg per minute, titrated to effect (up to a maximum of 2 mcg/kg per minute).

The manufacturer recommends that if norepinephrine is used in geriatric patients, the initial dosage usually should be at the low end of the dosage range since renal, hepatic, and cardiovascular dysfunction and concomitant disease or other drug therapy are more common in this age group than in younger patients.

The effect of the initial dose on blood pressure should be carefully observed and the rate of flow adjusted to establish and maintain the desired blood pressure. The patient should not be left unattended and the infusion flow rate must be closely monitored. Blood pressure should be checked every 2 minutes from the time the norepinephrine infusion is started until the desired effect is achieved, then every 5 minutes while the drug is being infused. Blood pressure should be elevated to a low normal blood pressure sufficient to maintain circulation to vital organs. In previously normotensive patients, systolic blood pressure should be maintained at 80–100 mm Hg; in previously hypertensive patients, systolic blood pressure should be maintained at no more than 40 mm Hg below their preexisting systolic pressure. The average adult maintenance dosage of norepinephrine is 2–4 mcg/minute; however, there is wide variability in dosage range. A few hypotensive patients have required much larger dosages (as much as 68 mg of norepinephrine daily). In patients requiring very large dosages of norepinephrine, occult blood volume depletion should be suspected and corrected if necessary; central venous pressure monitoring is usually helpful in detecting and managing this situation.

Norepinephrine therapy should be continued until adequate blood pressure and tissue perfusion are maintained. In some cases of vascular collapse resulting from acute myocardial infarction, treatment has been required for up to 6 days. When therapy is discontinued, the infusion rate should be slowed gradually and abrupt withdrawal avoided. The patient should be observed carefully so that therapy may be resumed if the blood pressure falls too rapidly.

Advanced Cardiovascular Life Support If norepinephrine is used adjunctively to restore and maintain blood pressure during cardiac resuscitation in adults, the manufacturer states that the same dosage guidelines for the treatment of other acute hypotensive states should be followed. (See Acute Hypotensive States under Dosage and Administration: Dosage.)

For postresuscitation stabilization in pediatric patients†, norepinephrine has been administered at an infusion rate of 0.1–2 mcg/kg per minute, adjusted based on patient response.

Cautions

■ **Adverse Effects** Norepinephrine bitartrate may cause headache, anxiety, or respiratory difficulty. Overdosage or administration of usual doses to patients who are hypersensitive to the effects of norepinephrine (e.g., hyperthyroid patients) may result in photophobia, pallor, intense sweating, vomiting, retrosternal pain, and severe headache. Headache may be a symptom of hypertension.

Norepinephrine can cause severe peripheral and visceral vasoconstriction, reducing blood flow and tissue perfusion to vital organs and resulting in possible tissue hypoxia, lactic acidosis, and ischemic injury. These effects are most likely to occur in hypovolemic patients if plasma volumes are not adequately corrected. In addition, prolonged use of norepinephrine may cause plasma volume depletion, which may result in hypotension when the drug is discontinued in the absence of blood volume replacement.

Norepinephrine increases myocardial oxygen consumption and the work of the heart. Cardiac output may be decreased following prolonged use of the drug or administration of large doses because venous return to the heart may be diminished as a result of increased peripheral vascular resistance. Decreased cardiac output may be especially harmful to elderly patients or those with initially poor cerebral or coronary circulation. Norepinephrine may cause bradycardia, probably as a result of a reflex response to increased blood pressure, as well as potentially fatal cardiac arrhythmias, including ventricular tachycardia and ventricular fibrillation. Arrhythmias are especially likely to occur in patients with severe hypoxia, or hypercapnia, or those receiving other drugs which may increase cardiac irritability such as cyclopropane or halogenated hydrocarbon general anesthetics. (See Drug Interactions: General Anesthetics.)

Norepinephrine can cause tissue necrosis and sloughing at the site of injection as a result of local vasoconstriction. (See Cautions: Precautions and Contraindications.) Blanching of the infused vein due to constriction of the vasa vasorum also may occur, sometimes without obvious extravasation. Gangrene of the extremities has been reported rarely and has occurred in a lower extremity when norepinephrine was infused into an ankle vein.

Prolonged administration of norepinephrine has caused edema, hemorrhage, focal myocarditis, subpericardial hemorrhage, necrosis of the intestine, or hepatic and renal necrosis. These effects have generally occurred in patients with severe shock and it is not clear if the drug or the shock state itself was the cause.

■ **Precautions and Contraindications** Vasopressor therapy is *not* a substitute for replacement of blood, plasma, fluids, and/or electrolytes. Blood volume depletion should be corrected as fully as possible before norepinephrine therapy is instituted. In an emergency, the drug may be used as an adjunct to fluid volume replacement or as a temporary supportive measure to maintain coronary and cerebral artery perfusion until volume replacement therapy can be completed, but norepinephrine must *not* be used as sole therapy in hypovolemic patients. Additional volume replacement may also be required during or after administration of the drug, especially if hypotension recurs. Monitoring of central venous pressure may be helpful in detecting and treating hypovolemia; in addition, monitoring of central venous or pulmonary arterial diastolic pressure is necessary to avoid overloading the cardiovascular system and precipitating congestive heart failure. Hypoxia, hypercapnia, and acidosis, which may also reduce the effectiveness and/or increase the incidence of adverse effects of norepinephrine, must be identified and corrected prior to or concurrently with administration of the drug.

To avoid the possibility of dangerously high blood pressures from norepinephrine therapy, blood pressure should be monitored closely during administration of the drug. Headache may be a symptom of hypertension due to overdosage.

Because severe local adverse effects (e.g., tissue necrosis) may occur, extravasation of norepinephrine must be avoided. *The site of infusion should be checked frequently for free flow and the infused vein should be observed for blanching.* The risk of tissue damage is apparently very slight if the drug is infused through a plastic catheter deep into an antecubital vein. Infusion into leg veins, especially in geriatric patients or those with occlusive vascular diseases (e.g., atherosclerosis, arteriosclerosis, Buerger's disease) should be avoided. If blanching is observed in the infused vein or if therapy is to be prolonged, changing the infusion site periodically may be advisable. If extravasation occurs, 10–15 mL of sodium chloride solution containing 5–10 mg of phentolamine mesylate should be infiltrated (using a syringe with a fine hypodermic needle) liberally throughout the affected area, identified by a cold, hard, and pallid appearance. Immediate and conspicuous local hyperemic changes occur if the area is infiltrated within 12 hours; therefore, phentolamine should be administered as soon as possible after extravasation is noted.

Commercially available formulations of norepinephrine bitartrate injection contain sodium metabisulfite, a sulfite that may cause allergic-type reactions, including anaphylaxis and life-threatening or less severe asthmatic episodes, in certain susceptible individuals. The overall prevalence of sulfite sensitivity in the general population is unknown; such sensitivity appears to occur more frequently in asthmatic than in nonasthmatic individuals.

Unless necessary as a life-saving procedure, norepinephrine should not be given to patients with peripheral or mesenteric vascular thrombosis because ischemia may be increased and the area of infarction extended. Use of norepinephrine during anesthesia with cyclopropane or halogenated hydrocarbon general anesthetics is generally considered to be contraindicated because of the risk of inducing cardiac arrhythmias. (See Drug Interactions: General Anesthetics.) Use of the drug in patients with profound hypoxia or hypercapnia may be contraindicated for the same reason.

■ **Pediatric Precautions** The manufacturer states that safety and efficacy of norepinephrine in children have not been established. Norepinephrine has been used for postresuscitation stabilization in pediatric patients; however, there are no specific studies evaluating the benefit of any vasopressor after return of spontaneous circulation in pediatric patients. Norepinephrine also has been used in some children with septic shock depending on the specific hemodynamic state of the patient.

■ **Geriatric Precautions** Clinical studies of norepinephrine bitartrate did not include sufficient numbers of patients 65 years of age and older to determine whether geriatric patients respond differently than younger patients. Clinical experience to date has not identified any differences in responses between geriatric and younger patients. If norepinephrine is used in geriatric patients, dosage should be selected carefully, usually starting at the low end of the dosage range, since renal, hepatic, and cardiovascular dysfunction and concomitant disease or other drug therapy are more common in this age group. Norepinephrine infusions should not be administered into leg veins in geriatric patients. (See Cautions: Precautions and Contraindications.)

■ **Mutagenicity and Carcinogenicity** The mutagenic and carcinogenic potentials of norepinephrine have not been studied to date.

■ **Pregnancy, Fertility, and Lactation** Animal reproduction studies have not been performed with norepinephrine, and it also is not known whether the drug can cause fetal harm when administered to pregnant women or can affect reproduction capacity. The drug should be used during pregnancy only when clearly needed.

Studies to determine the potential effects of norepinephrine on fertility have not been performed to date.

It is not known whether norepinephrine is distributed into human milk. Because many drugs are distributed into milk, the manufacturer recommends that the drug be used with caution in nursing women.

Drug Interactions

■ **α- and β-Adrenergic Blocking Agents** In animals, most of the pressor response to norepinephrine bitartrate is eliminated by preadministration of an α-adrenergic blocking drug such as phentolamine. In humans, however, the addition of 5–10 mg of phentolamine to each liter of infusion fluid containing norepinephrine may prevent sloughing of tissue, if extravasation occurs, without altering the pressor effects of norepinephrine.

In animals, preadministration of a β-adrenergic blocking drug such as propranolol blocks the cardiac stimulating effects of norepinephrine. The possibility that administration of norepinephrine in patients receiving propranolol might result in higher elevations of blood pressure because of blockade of any β-mediated arteriolar dilation should be kept in mind.

■ **General Anesthetics** Administration of norepinephrine to patients who are receiving cyclopropane or halogenated hydrocarbon general anesthetics, which increase cardiac irritability, may result in arrhythmias. It has been recommended that if a pressor drug is required when these general anesthetics are used, one with minimal cardiac stimulating effects such as phenylephrine should be given.

■ **Other Drugs** Atropine sulfate blocks the reflex bradycardia caused by norepinephrine and enhances the pressor response to norepinephrine.

Tricyclic antidepressants (e.g., imipramine), some antihistamines (especially diphenhydramine), parenteral ergot alkaloids, or methyldopa may potentiate the pressor effects of norepinephrine, resulting in severe, prolonged hypertension. Norepinephrine should be given cautiously and in small doses to patients receiving these drugs. Potentiation may result from inhibition of tissue uptake of norepinephrine or by increased adrenoreceptor sensitivity to the drug. Monoamine oxidase (MAO) is one of the enzymes responsible for norepinephrine metabolism. Although some clinicians have reported that MAO inhibitors do not appear to potentiate the effects of norepinephrine to a clinically important extent, the manufacturer states that norepinephrine should be administered with extreme caution to patients receiving an MAO inhibitor because severe, prolonged hypertension may result.

Administration of furosemide or other diuretics may decrease arterial responsiveness to pressor drugs such as norepinephrine.

Pharmacology

Norepinephrine acts predominantly by a direct effect on α-adrenergic receptors. The drug also directly stimulates β_1-adrenergic receptors but not β_2-adrenergic receptors. It is believed that α-adrenergic effects result from inhibition of the production of cyclic adenosine-3′,5′-monophosphate (AMP) by inhibition of the enzyme adenyl cyclase, whereas β-adrenergic effects result from stimulation of adenyl cyclase activity. The main effect of therapeutic doses of norepinephrine is a clinically important increase in mean arterial pressure (MAP), with minimal change in heart rate or cardiac output.

■ **Cardiovascular Effects** Norepinephrine constricts both arterial and venous blood vessels through its effect on α-adrenergic receptors. Systemic vascular resistance is increased, resulting in increased systolic and diastolic blood pressure. Local vasoconstriction caused by the drug may result in hemostasis and/or necrosis. Norepinephrine may reduce circulating plasma volume (especially with prolonged use) as a result of loss of fluid into extracellular spaces caused by postcapillary vasoconstriction.

Norepinephrine induces vasoconstriction in most vascular beds, potentially reducing blood flow to the renal, splanchnic, and cutaneous vasculature. In hypotensive patients, norepinephrine may initially decrease urine flow and excretion of sodium and potassium. If the patient is not hypovolemic, renal blood flow and glomerular filtration rate increase as the systemic blood pressure is raised toward normal levels; however, renal blood flow and glomerular filtration rate again decrease if blood pressure is further increased toward hypertensive levels.

Norepinephrine acts on β_1-adrenergic receptors in the heart, producing a positive inotropic effect on the myocardium. Although the drug also produces a positive chronotropic effect through the sinoatrial node, this effect is overcome by increased vagal activity occurring as a reflex to increased arterial blood pressure; bradycardia usually results. The bradycardia is blocked by atropine. In hypotensive patients, cardiac output may be increased by the positive inotropic effect of norepinephrine and may contribute to the pressor effects of the drug. However, because of the reflex bradycardia, cardiac output may also be unchanged or decreased. A decrease in cardiac output may also occur following prolonged use of the drug or administration of large doses if venous return to the heart is diminished as a result of increased peripheral vascular resistance.

Norepinephrine has a direct local vasoconstricting effect on coronary arteries, but this effect is overcome by indirect coronary artery vasodilation caused by enhanced cardiac metabolism resulting from direct cardiac stimulation. In hypotensive patients, coronary artery blood flow is increased as a result of increased systemic blood pressure as well as secondary coronary artery vasodilation. In patients with acute myocardial infarction and hypotension, myocardial oxygenation may be increased in areas of the heart not damaged by infarction. However, because of its positive inotropic effects, norepinephrine increases myocardial oxygen consumption and the work of the heart and decreases cardiac efficiency. The myocardial oxygen deficit and extent of damage may be increased in some patients.

Norepinephrine may increase the irritability of the heart and may alter the rhythmic function of the ventricles, especially after large doses or when the heart has been sensitized to this action by drugs including digitalis or certain anesthetics or by acute myocardial infarction, hypoxia, or hypercapnia. Arrhythmias, including ventricular tachycardia and ventricular fibrillation, may result.

Norepinephrine has been reported to decrease cerebral blood flow and oxygen consumption. However, administration of the drug in patients with reduced cerebral blood flow due to hypotension or cerebrovascular insufficiency has resulted in increased cerebral blood flow secondary to increased blood pressure and cardiac output.

■ **Other Effects** Although norepinephrine has fewer CNS effects than does epinephrine, restlessness, headache, and tremor may occur in some patients.

Norepinephrine has less effect on metabolism than does epinephrine but can increase glycogenolysis and inhibit insulin release in the pancreas, resulting in hyperglycemia. Elevation of blood concentrations of lactic acid may result from increased glycogenolysis due to diminished tissue perfusion resulting from vasoconstriction as well as to the direct metabolic effects of the drug. Blood concentrations of free fatty acids may be increased as a result of increased lipolysis in adipose tissue; plasma concentrations of cholesterol may also be elevated. Other metabolic effects which may occur during norepinephrine therapy include increased oxygen consumption and elevation of body temperature.

Norepinephrine may slightly increase respiratory minute volume, but the drug has no clinical value as a respiratory stimulant. Some patients receiving the drug may experience brief apnea.

As a result of its effect on α-adrenergic receptors, norepinephrine may cause contraction of the pregnant uterus and constriction of uterine blood vessels; however, the vasoconstrictor effects may be overcome by an increase in maternal blood pressure.

Pharmacokinetics

■ **Absorption** Orally ingested norepinephrine is destroyed in the GI tract, and the drug is poorly absorbed after subcutaneous injection. After IV administration, a pressor response occurs rapidly. The drug has a short duration of action, and the pressor action stops within 1–2 minutes after the infusion is discontinued.

■ **Distribution** Norepinephrine localizes mainly in sympathetic nervous tissue. The drug crosses the placenta but not the blood-brain barrier.

■ **Elimination** The pharmacologic actions of norepinephrine are terminated primarily by uptake and metabolism in sympathetic nerve endings. The drug is metabolized in the liver and other tissues by a combination of reactions involving the enzymes catechol-*O*-methyltransferase (COMT) and monoamine oxidase (MAO). The major metabolites are normetanephrine and 3-methoxy-4-hydroxy mandelic acid (vanillylmandelic acid, VMA), both of which are inactive. Other inactive metabolites include 3-methoxy-4-hydroxyphenylglycol, 3,4-dihydroxymandelic acid, and 3,4-dihydroxyphenylglycol. Norepinephrine metabolites are excreted in urine primarily as the sulfate conjugates and, to a lesser extent, as the glucuronide conjugates. Only small quantities of norepinephrine are excreted unchanged.

Chemistry and Stability

■ **Chemistry** Norepinephrine is identical to the endogenous catecholamine that is synthesized in the adrenal medulla and in sympathetic nervous tissue. Both the endogenous substance and the drug are the levorotatory isomer which is several times more active than is the dextrorotatory isomer. Norepinephrine is commercially available as the bitartrate salt; however, potency is expressed in terms of norepinephrine. Norepinephrine bitartrate occurs as an odorless, white or faintly gray, crystalline powder and has solubilities of approximately 400 mg/mL in water and 3.33 mg/mL in alcohol at 25°C. The injection has a pH of 3–4.5. Norepinephrine bitartrate injection contains the antioxidant, sodium metabisulfite, and the air in the ampuls has been replaced with nitrogen to avoid oxidation.

■ **Stability** Norepinephrine bitartrate injection should be protected from light and stored at 20–25°C. Norepinephrine bitartrate is readily oxidized; both the drug and the injection gradually darken on exposure to light and air and must be stored in tight, light-resistant containers. Contact of the drug with iron salts, alkalies, or oxidizing agents must be avoided. Norepinephrine bitartrate injection must not be used if it is discolored (e.g., pink, dark yellow) or contains a precipitate.

The manufacturer states that for IV infusion norepinephrine should be diluted with 5% dextrose injection with or without sodium chloride to protect against loss of potency caused by oxidation during IV infusion; sodium chloride injection alone should not be used. Following dilution with 5% dextrose, IV infusions containing norepinephrine 2.5 or 4 mcg/mL have been reported to be stable for at least 24 hours at room temperature if the pH is approximately 5.6. Norepinephrine solutions containing 2.5 mcg/mL in 5% dextrose have been reported to lose 5% of their potency in 6 hours at pH 6.5 and in 4 hours at pH 7.5. It has been recommended that caution be used if norepinephrine is diluted with 5% dextrose injections with a pH of greater than 5.5–6. The manufacturer recommends that whole blood or plasma, if indicated during therapy with norepinephrine, be administered separately or via a Y-tube.

Preparations

Excipients in commercially available drug preparations may have clinically important effects in some individuals; consult specific product labeling for details.

Norepinephrine Bitartrate

Parenteral

For injection, concentrate, for IV infusion	1 mg (of norepinephrine) per mL*	**Levophed®**, Hospira **Norepinephrine Bitartrate Injection**

*available from one or more manufacturer, distributor, and/or repackager by generic (nonproprietary) name

†Use is not currently included in the labeling approved by the US Food and Drug Administration

Selected Revisions August 2017,

Pseudoephedrine Hydrochloride

Isoephedrine Hydrochloride

Pseudoephedrine Sulfate

■ Pseudoephedrine is a sympathomimetic agent that occurs naturally in plants of the genus *Ephedra*; the drug acts directly on both α- and, to a lesser degree, β-adrenergic receptors.

Uses

Pseudoephedrine is used as a nasal decongestant for *self-medication* for the temporary relief of nasal congestion associated with upper respiratory allergy and to provide temporary relief of sinus congestion and pressure. The drug also has been used for *self-medication* in the symptomatic prevention of otitic barotrauma† (aerotitis [barotitis] media). Pseudoephedrine also has been misused for clandestine synthesis of methamphetamine and methcathinone for illicit use.

■ **Nasal Congestion and Other Respiratory Conditions** Pseudoephedrine is used as a nasal decongestant for *self-medication* for the temporary relief of nasal congestion associated with upper respiratory allergy (e.g., hay fever) or the common cold; the drug also is used to provide temporary relief of sinus congestion and pressure. Preparations containing pseudoephedrine in fixed combination with other agents (e.g., acetaminophen, brompheniramine, chlorpheniramine, desloratadine, dextromethorphan, fexofenadine, guaifenesin, ibuprofen, loratadine, methscopolamine, triprolidine) are used for relief of nasal/sinus congestion and pressure and/or other symptoms (e.g., rhinorrhea, sneezing, lacrimation, itching eyes, oronasopharyngeal itching, cough, fever) associated with seasonal or perennial allergic rhinitis, nonallergic (vasomotor) rhinitis, other upper respiratory allergies, or the common cold.

In clinical studies, oral pseudoephedrine administered as single 60-mg doses was effective in relieving congestion. Unlike topically applied decongestants, pseudoephedrine produces little if any rebound congestion. In patients with otic inflammation or infection, the drug may be useful in opening obstructed eustachian ostia. Pseudoephedrine may be used as an adjunct to analgesics, antihistamines, antitussives, expectorants, or antibiotics when indicated.

Nasal decongestants, including pseudoephedrine, are labeled and have been used for *self-medication* for the temporary relief of nasal congestion associated with sinusitis. However, prospective studies of nasal decongestants for this use are lacking, and data on their use as adjunctive therapy in the management of sinusitis are limited and controversial. Furthermore, evidence from an animal study indicates that topical nasal decongestants (i.e., oxymetazoline) may *increase* the degree of sinus inflammation, potentially delaying resolution of sinusitis. Because current labeling for non (over-the-counter, OTC) nasal decongestant preparations includes use for sinusitis, there are concerns that consumers will assume that nasal decongestants are effective in the treatment of sinusitis, thereby choosing *self-medication* over medical evaluation and definitive treatment by a clinician; such delay in medical evaluation could result in a lost opportunity for early diagnosis of another serious medical condition (e.g., bacterial sinusitis). As a result, the US Food and Drug Administration (FDA) no longer considers oral or topical nasal decongestants appropriate for *self-medication* of sinusitis. In October 2005, the agency issued a final rule amending the final monograph for OTC nasal decongestant preparations to remove the indication for relief of congestion associated with sinusitis from labeling and prohibiting use of the term sinusitis elsewhere in labeling. The compliance date for preparations with annual sales less than $25,000 was October 11, 2007; the compliance date for all other preparations was April 11, 2007.

Although pseudoephedrine has been used in the symptomatic treatment of bronchial asthma and reversible bronchospasm, the drug appears to be ineffective as a bronchodilator.

As part of its ongoing review of over-the-counter drug products, the FDA has determined that pseudoephedrine in combination with caffeine is *not* generally recognized as safe and effective for over-the-counter use. Such a combination introduced or initially delivered for introduction into interstate commerce after October 29, 2001, is considered by the FDA to be a new drug and misbranded, and cannot be marketed for over-the-counter use unless it is the subject of an approved new drug application.

Although cough and cold preparations that contain nasal decongestants, antihistamines, cough suppressants, and/or expectorants commonly were used in pediatric patients younger than 2 years of age, systematic reviews of controlled trials have concluded that non (over-the-counter, OTC) cough and cold preparations are *no* more effective than placebo in reducing acute cough and other symptoms of upper respiratory tract infection in these patients. Furthermore, adverse events, including deaths, have been (and continue to be) reported in pediatric patients younger than 2 years of age receiving these preparations. (See Cautions: Pediatric Precautions.) Therefore, the US Centers for Disease Control and Prevention (CDC) state that, as an alternative to pseudoephedrine and other nasal decongestants, caregivers may consider using a rubber suction bulb to clear nasal congestion and using saline nasal drops or a cool-mist humidifier to soften secretions in infants.

■ **Otitic Barotrauma** Pseudoephedrine has been used orally for *self-medication* in the symptomatic prevention of otitic barotrauma† (aerotitis [barotitis] media). Otitic barotrauma, commonly known as middle ear squeeze, refers to tissue damage caused by failure of the middle ear to equilibrate its internal pressure to accommodate changes in atmospheric pressure (e.g., during descent of an aircraft, underwater diving, hyperbaric oxygenation). Clinical manifestations include a sensation of otic blockage or discomfort, otalgia, tinnitus, vertigo, and transient conductive hearing loss; these manifestations may be accompanied by tympanic membrane congestion or hemorrhage, hemotympanum, or membrane perforation or rupture. Although few controlled clinical studies have been conducted, oral (e.g., pseudoephedrine) or nasal (e.g., oxymetazoline) decongestants generally have been recommended for prevention or treatment of otitic barotrauma.

Prophylactic treatment with pseudoephedrine appears to be effective in preventing otitic barotrauma associated with *air travel* in adults†. In a randomized, double-blind, placebo-controlled study in a limited number of healthy adults with a history of otic discomfort during air travel, administration of extended-release pseudoephedrine hydrochloride (120 mg) at least 30 minutes before flight departure was associated with a lower incidence of otitic barotrauma; approximately 32% of individuals receiving pseudoephedrine reported manifestations of otitic barotrauma (e.g., blockage, hearing loss) compared with

62% of those receiving placebo. In a randomized, double-blind, comparative study, pseudoephedrine appeared to be more effective than oxymetazoline, which was no more effective than placebo, in reducing the incidence of otitic barotrauma. Manifestations of otitic barotrauma (e.g., otalgia, blockage) reportedly occurred in 34, 64, or 71% of healthy adults receiving extended-release pseudoephedrine hydrochloride (120 mg) tablets, oxymetazoline hydrochloride (0.05%) nasal spray, or placebo, respectively, at least 30 minutes before flight departure.

Efficacy of pseudoephedrine in preventing otitic barotrauma associated with *air travel* in children† has not been established. In a randomized, double-blind, placebo-controlled study in a limited number of children 6 months to 6 years of age, administration of pseudoephedrine hydrochloride oral solution (1 mg/kg) 30–60 minutes before flight departure did not decrease the incidence of otic pain during either ascent (4 vs 5% of children treated with pseudoephedrine or placebo, respectively) or descent (12 vs 13% of those receiving pseudoephedrine or placebo, respectively) of the aircraft. Furthermore, prophylactic treatment with pseudoephedrine was associated with a higher incidence of drowsiness during takeoff; drowsiness was reported in 60% of children receiving pseudoephedrine compared with 27% of those receiving placebo. Treatment with pseudoephedrine was not associated with drowsiness during descent or with excitability during ascent of the aircraft.

Limited data indicate that pseudoephedrine may be more effective than placebo in preventing otitic barotrauma associated with *underwater diving*†. In one randomized, double-blind, placebo-controlled study in a limited number of first-time underwater divers, approximately 8% of individuals receiving pseudoephedrine hydrochloride (60 mg) 30 minutes before diving reported otic discomfort and blockage compared with 32% of those receiving placebo.

Although additional study is needed, the limited data available suggest that pseudoephedrine may be useful in the symptomatic prevention of otitic barotrauma associated with aircraft descent or underwater diving in adults. However, evidence to support such use of intranasal oxymetazoline is lacking.

■ **Misuse and Abuse** Because pseudoephedrine has been used in the clandestine synthesis of methamphetamine and methcathinone, both CNS stimulants with great potential for habituation and physical and/or psychic dependence, the US enacted the Comprehensive Methamphetamine Control Act of 1996 (US Public Law 104-237) and later the Methamphetamine Anti-Proliferation Act (MAPA [US Public Law 106-310], title XXXVI of the Children's Health Act of 2000) to reduce the potential for misuse (diversion) of pseudoephedrine. MAPA, effective October 2001, limited retail sales (including mail-order distribution) of pseudoephedrine-containing drug products to 9 g (in terms of the base) for a single transaction and limited the package size to no more than 3 g of pseudoephedrine (in terms of the base). Neither law regulated "ordinary over-the-counter (OTC) pseudoephedrine drug products," which have been defined as products containing no more than 3 g of pseudoephedrine (in terms of the base), packaged in blister or unit-dose packs of 1 or 2 dosage units per pack or as packaged-size liquid preparations. As of October 1997, transactions of pseudoephedrine by mail-order pharmacies must be reported monthly to the US Attorney General according to applicable regulations.

Despite the enactment of MAPA, methamphetamine abuse remains a serious problem. In March 2006, the Combat Methamphetamine Epidemic Act (CMEA) of 2005 (Title VII of the USA Patriot Act Improvement and Reauthorization Act of 2005) was signed into law, which effectively amends the Federal Controlled Substances Act of 1970 to tighten control over the sale and distribution of non pseudoephedrine and ephedrine. This law created a new class of products called "scheduled listed chemical products," which are defined in the law as products containing pseudoephedrine, ephedrine, or phenylpropanolamine (no longer commercially available in the US) or any salt, optical isomer, or salt of an optical isomer of these drugs that are lawful non products in the US, and set additional requirements for their sale. Effective September 30, 2006, the law requires pharmacies and other retail distributors to store pseudoephedrine- and ephedrine-containing preparations behind the counter or in locked cabinets; requires purchasers to provide approved photographic identification and sign a written or electronic logbook for each purchase; requires pharmacies and other retail distributors to keep information about the purchasers (e.g., name, address, signature) and purchases (e.g., name of product, quantity sold, date and time of sale) for at least 2 years; and limits the amount that can be purchased to no more than 3.6 g per day or 9 g per month. The law exempts the requirements for a written or electronic log for any purchase of single-dose packages that contain no more than 60 mg of pseudoephedrine; however, these single-dose packages also must be stored behind the counter. To comply with CMEA, pharmacies and other retail distributors selling preparations containing pseudoephedrine are required to submit to the Attorney General a statement regarding self-certification and employee training on this new law and to maintain records relating to such training at their place of operation. Additional information about legal and regulatory requirements under CMEA may be obtained at the website of the Office of Diversion Control of the US Drug Enforcement Administration (DEA) (http://www.deadiversion.usdoj.gov/), including specific requirements for various sellers (e.g., pharmacies, mail-order sellers) and employee training materials developed by DEA.

Use of pseudoephedrine in some states may be subject to additional controls, since some states had restricted the , dispensing, and distribution of pseudoephedrine (e.g., as a controlled substance or a drug) prior to passage of the federal law. For example, in the state of Oregon, legislation was enacted in August 2005 that required the Oregon State Board of Pharmacy to classify pseudoephedrine, ephedrine, and phenylpropanolamine as schedule III drugs by July 2006, which effectively moved these drugs from the non to the -only category in that state. Where such state laws are more stringent than the provisions of CMEA, the state requirements also must be followed.

In response to such restrictions, some manufacturers have voluntarily reformulated various existing pseudoephedrine-containing preparations, replacing the pseudoephedrine component with other decongestants such as phenylephrine.

Dosage and Administration

■ **Administration** Pseudoephedrine hydrochloride and sulfate are administered orally.

Pseudoephedrine hydrochloride 240-mg extended-release tablets should be administered orally once daily and swallowed whole with water; the extended-release tablets should *not* be divided, crushed, chewed, or dissolved. Patients should be advised that the tablet does not completely dissolve and may be passed in the stool.

■ **Dosage** ***Nasal Congestion and Other Respiratory Conditions*** The usual dosage of pseudoephedrine hydrochloride for adults and children 12 years of age or older is 60 mg every 4–6 hours with a maximum of 240 mg daily.

Children 6–11 years of age may receive 30 mg of pseudoephedrine hydrochloride every 4–6 hours with a maximum dosage of 120 mg daily, and children 2–5 years of age may receive 15 mg every 4–6 hours with a maximum dosage of 60 mg daily. Alternatively, some pediatricians recommend 4 mg/kg or 125 mg/m^2 daily, given in 4 divided doses. For children younger than 2 years of age, a pediatrician should be consulted. Suggested dosages for children younger than 2 years of age† for some cough and cold preparations have been published in various references for prescribing and parenting. Using recommended dosages for adults and older children, some clinicians have extrapolated dosages for these preparations based on the weight or age of children younger than 2 years of age. However, these extrapolations were based on assumptions that pathology of the disease and pharmacology of the drugs are similar in adults and pediatric patients. There currently are *no* specific dosage recommendations (i.e., approved by US Food and Drug Administration [FDA]) for cough and cold preparations for this patient population. (See Cautions: Pediatric Precautions.)

When an extended-release preparation of pseudoephedrine hydrochloride is used, adults and children 12 years of age or older may receive 120 mg of the drug every 12 hours or 240 mg every 24 hours. The manufacturer recommends that this dosage not be exceeded.

For *self-medication*, the manufacturers recommend that patients discontinue the drug and consult a clinician if symptoms persist for longer than 7 days or are accompanied by fever. (See Cautions: Precautions and Contraindications.)

Otitic Barotrauma For *self-medication* to prevent otitic barotrauma†, pseudoephedrine hydrochloride has been given orally at a dosage of 120 mg (as the extended-release tablets) in adult air travelers or 60 mg in adult underwater divers; in clinical studies, the drug was administered 30 minutes before flight departure in air travelers or 30 minutes before diving in underwater divers.

Cautions

■ **Adverse Effects** Because pseudoephedrine is a sympathomimetic agent, the possibility of adverse effects associated with other sympathomimetic drugs, including fear, anxiety, tenseness, tremor, hallucinations, seizures, pallor, respiratory difficulty, dysuria, and cardiovascular collapse should be considered. Large doses of pseudoephedrine may cause lightheadedness, nausea, and/or vomiting.

■ **CNS Effects** Pseudoephedrine may cause mild CNS stimulation, especially in patients who are hypersensitive to the effects of sympathomimetic drugs. Nervousness, excitability, restlessness, dizziness, weakness, and insomnia may occur. Headache and drowsiness also have been reported.

■ **Cardiovascular Effects** Although oral administration of usual doses of pseudoephedrine to normotensive patients usually produces negligible pressor effects, the drug should be used with caution in hypertensive patients. Pseudoephedrine may increase the irritability of the heart muscle and may alter the rhythmic function of the ventricles, especially in large doses or when administered to patients who are hypersensitive to the myocardial effects of sympathomimetic drugs. Tachycardia or palpitation may occur. One patient who received 120 mg of pseudoephedrine hydrochloride every 4 hours developed multifocal premature ventricular contractions which disappeared within a few days after the drug was discontinued. In addition, pseudoephedrine may have precipitated an attack of atrial fibrillation in an infant. It was postulated that the patient may have had previously unsuspected idiopathic atrial fibrillation, and therefore may have been especially sensitive to the myocardial effects of the drug.

■ **Dermatologic and Sensitivity Reactions** Fixed dermatologic eruptions (erythematous nummular patches) developed in 2 patients after a combination containing 60 mg of pseudoephedrine hydrochloride and 2.5 mg of triprolidine hydrochloride was administered. Sensitivity testing indicated that pseudoephedrine was the cause of this reaction.

■ Ocular Effects In one patient with latent Horner's syndrome, administration of pseudoephedrine in combination with triprolidine caused anisocoria.

■ Precautions and Contraindications As with other sympathomimetic drugs, pseudoephedrine should not be used for *self-medication* in patients with hyperthyroidism, diabetes mellitus, hypertension, ischemic heart disease, or difficulty urinating secondary to prostatic hypertrophy without consulting a clinician. The drug should be used cautiously, and may be contraindicated, in patients who are hypersensitive to the effects of other sympathomimetic drugs. Pseudoephedrine is contraindicated in patients with severe hypertension, severe coronary artery disease, angle-closure glaucoma, or urinary retention. Pseudoephedrine also is contraindicated in patients currently receiving, or having recently received (i.e., within 2 weeks), a monoamine oxidase (MAO) inhibitor. (See Drug Interactions: Monoamine Oxidase Inhibitors.)

The possibility that pseudoephedrine hydrochloride 240-mg extended-release tablets rarely can cause GI obstruction, particularly in patients with severe narrowing of the esophagus, stomach, or intestine, should be considered. Patients with GI obstruction or narrowing should not use the 240-mg extended-release tablets without consulting a clinician.

Unless otherwise directed by a clinician, patients receiving pseudoephedrine for *self-medication* should be advised to discontinue the drug if nervousness, dizziness, or insomnia develops during therapy, *or* if symptoms persist for longer than 7 days or are accompanied by fever. Patients receiving pseudoephedrine hydrochloride 240-mg extended-release tablets should be advised to discontinue the drug and consult a clinician if persistent abdominal pain or vomiting occurs.

The potential for misuse or abuse of pseudoephedrine should be considered. (See Uses: Misuse and Abuse.)

When pseudoephedrine is used in fixed combination with other agents, the cautions, precautions, and contraindications associated with the concomitant agent(s) should be considered.

Individuals with phenylketonuria (i.e., homozygous genetic deficiency of phenylalanine hydroxylase) and other individuals who must restrict their intake of phenylalanine should be warned that each 15-mg chewable tablet of Sudafed® Children's Nasal Decongestant contains aspartame (NutraSweet®) which is metabolized in the GI tract to provide about 0.78 mg of phenylalanine following oral administration.

■ Pediatric Precautions The extended-release preparations containing 120 mg of pseudoephedrine hydrochloride or sulfate or 240 mg of pseudoephedrine hydrochloride should not be administered to patients younger than 12 years of age. An increased incidence of drowsiness was reported in children who received pseudoephedrine hydrochloride (1 mg/kg) compared with those who received placebo before air travel (60 vs 27%, respectively).

Death has been reported rarely in pediatric patients younger than 2 years of age receiving cough and cold preparations. In a report published by the US Centers for Disease Control and Prevention (CDC), cough and cold preparations were determined by medical examiners or coroners to be the underlying cause of death in 3 infants 6 months of age or younger during 2005. According to the report, all 3 of these infants had received and/or OTC preparations that contained pseudoephedrine, and 2 of the infants received preparations containing carbinoxamine. Postmortem examination revealed high blood concentrations of pseudoephedrine (i.e., 9–14 times higher than those achieved following administration of recommended dosages of pseudoephedrine in children 2–12 years of age) in all 3 of the infants, detectable blood concentrations of acetaminophen and dextromethorphan in 2 of the infants, and detectable blood concentrations of doxylamine in one of the infants. Because few data exist regarding the therapeutic or toxic concentrations of cough and cold medications in pediatric patients younger than 2 years of age and because there are no universally accepted criteria for attributing deaths to cough and cold preparations, the cause of death in these infants was based on the report of the medical examiner or coroner. However, the actual cause of death might have been overdosage of one drug, interaction of different drugs, an underlying medical condition, or a combination of drugs and underlying medical conditions. In addition to these 3 deaths, an estimated 1519 children younger than 2 years of age were treated in emergency departments in the US during 2004–2005 for adverse events, including overdoses, associated with cold and cough preparations.

The dosages at which cough and cold preparations can cause illness or death in pediatric patients younger than 2 years of age are not known, and there are no specific dosage recommendations (i.e., approved by the US Food and Drug Administration [FDA]) for the symptomatic treatment of cold and cough for patients in this age group. (See Dosage and Administration: Dosage.) Because of the absence of dosage recommendations, limited published evidence of effectiveness, and risks for toxicity (including fatal overdosage), FDA stated that non cough and cold preparations should not be used in children younger than 2 years of age; the agency continues to assess safety and efficacy of these preparations in older children. Meanwhile, because children 2–3 years of age also are at increased risk of overdosage and toxicity, some manufacturers of oral nonprescription cough and cold preparations agreed to voluntarily revise the product labeling to state that such preparations should not be used in children younger than 4 years of age. FDA recommends that parents and caregivers adhere to the dosage instructions and warnings on the product labeling that accompanies the preparation if administering to children and consult with their clinician about any concerns. Clinicians should ask caregivers about use of non cough and cold preparations to avoid overdosage.

■ Geriatric Precautions Geriatric patients may be especially sensitive to the effects of sympathomimetic amines. Overdosage of sympathomimetic amines in patients older than 60 years of age may cause hallucinations, CNS depression, seizures, and death. Extended-release preparations containing pseudoephedrine, therefore, should not be administered to these patients until safety has been established by administration of a short-acting preparation.

■ Pregnancy and Lactation Sympathomimetic amines have been shown to be teratogenic in some animal species. However, use of pseudoephedrine during pregnancy to date has not been definitely associated with any specific congenital malformations.

Pseudoephedrine distributes into and is concentrated in breast milk. About 0.5% of an oral dose is distributed into breast milk over 24 hours. In a limited study, milk-to-plasma concentration ratios were 3.3, 3.9, and 2.6 at 1, 3, and 12 hours, respectively, following administration of a single oral dose of the drug to nursing women. Although milk concentrations of pseudoephedrine are expected to be somewhat greater with multiple-dose administration of the drug, some experts state that the actual amounts of the drug distributed in breast milk are not high enough to warrant cessation of nursing. The American Academy of Pediatrics (AAP) states that no change in the nursing infant has been observed while the mother was ingesting pseudoephedrine and that the drug usually is compatible with breast-feeding.

Drug Interactions

■ Sympathomimetic Agents Pseudoephedrine should be administered with extreme caution, if at all, with other sympathomimetic agents because of the possibility of additive effects and increased toxicity.

■ Monoamine Oxidase Inhibitors Monoamine oxidase (MAO) inhibitors, by increasing the quantity of norepinephrine in adrenergic nervous tissue, potentiate the pressor effects of indirectly acting sympathomimetic drugs such as pseudoephedrine. Infrequently, a hypertensive crisis may result. Pseudoephedrine should therefore be *avoided* in patients receiving drugs with MAO inhibiting activity, or for 2 weeks after discontinuance of an MAO inhibitor.

■ Other Drugs One manufacturer states that β-adrenergic blocking drugs such as propranolol also may increase the pressor effects of pseudoephedrine and that pseudoephedrine may reduce the antihypertensive effects of reserpine, methyldopa, mecamylamine hydrochloride, and veratrum alkaloids.

Pharmacology

Pseudoephedrine acts directly on both α- and, to a lesser degree, β-adrenergic receptors. It is believed that α-adrenergic effects result from the inhibition of the production of cyclic adenosine-3′,5′-monophosphate (AMP) by inhibition of the enzyme adenyl cyclase, whereas β-adrenergic effects result from stimulation of adenyl cyclase activity. Like ephedrine, pseudoephedrine also has an indirect effect by releasing norepinephrine from its storage sites.

Pseudoephedrine acts directly on α-adrenergic receptors in the mucosa of the respiratory tract producing vasoconstriction that results in shrinkage of swollen nasal mucous membranes, reduction of tissue hyperemia, edema, and nasal congestion, and an increase in nasal airway patency; drainage of sinus secretions is increased. Sympathomimetic effects of pseudoephedrine presumably also may occur in other areas of the respiratory tract, including the eustachian tube; these effects may improve or maintain eustachian tube patency and allow equilibration of middle ear pressure during external atmospheric pressure changes (e.g., during descent of an aircraft, underwater diving, hyperbaric oxygenation).

Pseudoephedrine may relax bronchial smooth muscle by stimulation of β_2-adrenergic receptors; however, substantial bronchodilation has not been demonstrated consistently following oral administration of the drug.

Oral administration of usual doses of pseudoephedrine to normotensive patients usually produces negligible effect on blood pressure. Pseudoephedrine may increase the irritability of the heart muscle and may alter the rhythmic function of the ventricles, especially in large doses or after administration to patients such as those with cardiac disease who are hypersensitive to the myocardial effects of sympathomimetic drugs. Tachycardia, palpitation, and/or multifocal premature ventricular contractions may occur. (See Cautions: Cardiovascular Effects.)

Pseudoephedrine may cause mild CNS stimulation, especially in patients who are sensitive to the effects of sympathomimetic drugs. (See Cautions: CNS Effects.)

Pharmacokinetics

■ Absorption Pseudoephedrine is readily and almost completely absorbed from the GI tract and there is no evidence of first-pass metabolism. Following oral administration of a 60- or 120-mg dose of pseudoephedrine hydrochloride as an oral solution, peak plasma concentrations of about 180–300 or 397–422 ng/mL, respectively, were achieved in approximately 1.39–2 or 1.84–1.97 hours, respectively. Absorption from extended-release preparations is slower and peak plasma concentrations of the drug are achieved in about 3.8–6.1 hours. Following oral administration of single 30- or 60-mg doses of pseudoephedrine hydrochloride as a solution in pediatric patients (6–12 years of age), mean peak serum concentrations of 244 or 492 ng/mL, respectively, were achieved after 2.1 or 2.4 hours, respectively. Food delays absorption of the drug when administered as a solution, but appears not to have an effect on absorption when the drug is administered as extended-release preparations.

Plasma pseudoephedrine concentrations of 274 ng/mL have been associated with a mean nasal decongestant response of 57.2%. After oral administration of 60 mg of pseudoephedrine hydrochloride as tablets or oral solution, nasal decongestion occurs within 30 minutes and persists for 4–6 hours. Nasal decongestion may persist for 8 hours following oral administration of 60 mg and up to 12 hours following 120 mg of the drug in extended-release capsules.

■ **Distribution** Following oral administration of single 30- or 60-mg doses of pseudoephedrine hydrochloride as a solution in children (6–12 years of age), the mean apparent volume of distribution at steady-state was 2.6 or 2.4 L/kg, respectively.

Although specific information is lacking, pseudoephedrine is presumed to cross the placenta and to enter CSF. Pseudoephedrine distributes into breast milk; about 0.5% of an oral dose is distributed into breast milk over 24 hours.

■ **Elimination** Pseudoephedrine is incompletely metabolized (less than 1%) in the liver by *N*-demethylation to an inactive metabolite. The drug and its metabolite are excreted in urine; 55–96% of a dose is excreted unchanged.

Urinary pH can affect the elimination half-life of pseudoephedrine, prolonging it when alkaline (pH 8) and reducing it when acidic (pH 5). The elimination half-life of pseudoephedrine ranges from 3–6 or 9–16 hours when urinary pH is 5 or 8, respectively, while when urinary pH is 5.8, the elimination half-life of the drug ranges from 5–8 hours. In one study in children 6–12 years of age, the elimination half-life of pseudoephedrine averaged about 3 hours when urinary pH was 6.5. The rate of urinary excretion of pseudoephedrine is accelerated when urine is acidified to a pH of about 5 by prior administration of ammonium chloride. When the urine is alkalinized to a pH of about 8 by prior administration of sodium bicarbonate, some of the drug is reabsorbed in the kidney tubule and the rate of urinary excretion is slowed.

Renal clearance of pseudoephedrine is about 7.3–7.6 mL/minute per kg in adults. Following oral administration of a single 30- or 60-mg dose of pseudoephedrine hydrochloride given as an oral solution in children 6–12 years of age, total body clearance was faster than that reported in adults, averaging about 10.3 or 9.2 mL/minute per kg, respectively.

Chemistry and Stability

■ **Chemistry** Pseudoephedrine is a sympathomimetic drug that occurs naturally in plants of the genus *Ephedra*. The drug is a stereoisomer of ephedrine. Both naturally occurring pseudoephedrine and the official preparation are the dextrorotatory isomer. Pseudoephedrine is commercially available as the hydrochloride or sulfate salt. Pseudoephedrine hydrochloride is commercially available in single-ingredient preparations as well as in fixed-combination preparations; pseudoephedrine sulfate is commercially available in the US only in fixed-combination preparations. Pseudoephedrine hydrochloride and pseudoephedrine sulfate are available as fixed-combination preparations containing antihistamines, analgesics, antitussives, and/or expectorants. Pseudoephedrine hydrochloride occurs as fine, white to off-white crystals or powder having a faint, characteristic odor. The drug has solubilities of approximately 2 g/mL in water and 278 mg/mL in alcohol at 25°C. Pseudoephedrine sulfate occurs as a white, crystalline powder.

■ **Stability** Pseudoephedrine hydrochloride preparations generally should be stored at 15–30°C; the oral solution should be protected from light, and freezing should be avoided. Pseudoephedrine hydrochloride tablets should be stored in tight containers and oral solution in tight, light-resistant containers.

Preparations

Excipients in commercially available drug preparations may have clinically important effects in some individuals; consult specific product labeling for details.

Pseudoephedrine Hydrochloride

Powder*		
Oral		
Solution	15 mg/5 mL	**Children's Silfedrine®**, Silarx
		Children's Sudafed® Nasal Decongestant, McNeil
	30 mg/5 mL*	**Pseudoephedrine Hydrochloride Oral Solution**
Tablets	30 mg*	**Pseudoephedrine Hydrochloride Tablets**
		Sudafed® Congestion, McNeil
Tablets, extended release	120 mg*	**Pseudoephedrine Hydrochloride Extended Release Tablets**
Tablets, extended-release, film-coated	120 mg	**Pseudoephedrine Hydrochloride Extended Release Tablets**
		Sudafed® 12 Hour, McNeil
	240 mg	**Sudafed® 24 Hour**, McNeil

*available from one or more manufacturer, distributor, and/or repackager by generic (nonproprietary) name

Pseudoephedrine Hydrochloride Combinations

Oral		
Capsules, liquid-filled	30 mg with Ibuprofen 200 mg	**Advil® Cold & Sinus Liqui-Gels®**, Pfizer
Solution	15 mg/5 mL with Chlorpheniramine Maleate 1 mg/5 mL and Dextromethorphan Hydrobromide 5 mg/5mL	**Kidkare® Cough & Cold Liquid**, Rugby
Tablets	30 mg with Acetaminophen 325 mg	**Ornex® Caplets**, B.F. Ascher
	30 mg with Chlorpheniramine Maleate 2 mg and Ibuprofen 200 mg	**Advil® Allergy Sinus**, Pfizer
	30 mg with Ibuprofen 200 mg	**Advil® Cold & Sinus**, Pfizer
Tablets, extended-release	60 mg with Guaifenesin 600 mg	**Mucinex® D**, Reckitt Benekiser
	120 mg with Fexofenadine Hydrochloride 60 mg	**Allegra-D® 12 Hour**, Chattem
	240 mg with Fexofenadine Hydrochloride 180 mg	**Allegra-D® 24 Hour**, Chattem

Pseudoephedrine Sulfate Combinations

Oral		
Tablets, extended-release core (pseudoephedrine sulfate only)	120 mg with Desloratadine 2.5 mg	**Clarinex-D® 12 Hour**, Schering-Plough
	120 mg with Loratadine 5 mg	**Alavert® Allergy & Sinus D-12 Hour**, Pfizer
		Claritin-D® 12 Hour, Schering-Plough
	240 mg with Desloratadine 5 mg	**Clarinex-D® 24-Hour**, Schering-Plough
	240 mg with Loratadine 10 mg	**Claritin-D® 24 Hour**, Schering-Plough

†Use is not currently included in the labeling approved by the US Food and Drug Administration

SYMPATHOLYTIC (ADRENERGIC BLOCKING) AGENTS 12:16

α-ADRENERGIC BLOCKING AGENTS 12:16.04

NONSELECTIVE α-ADRENERGIC BLOCKING AGENTS 12:16.04.04

Phentolamine Mesylate

■ Phentolamine is an imidazoline α-adrenergic blocking agent.

Uses

Phentolamine is used mainly in the diagnosis of pheochromocytoma and to control or prevent paroxysmal hypertension immediately prior to or during pheochromocytomectomy.

■ **Diagnosis of Pheochromocytoma** Although no single chemical or pharmacological test is completely reliable, determinations of blood concentrations of catecholamines and/or urinary excretion of catecholamines or their metabolites are the safest and most reliable methods for the diagnosis of pheochromocytoma. The phentolamine test may be used when additional confirmatory evidence of pheochromocytoma is required and the potential benefits of the test outweigh the possible risks. (See Cautions: Adverse Effects.) The phentolamine test is more reliable in detecting pheochromocytomas in patients with sustained hypertension than in those with paroxysmal hypertension and is of no value in patients who are not hypertensive at the time of the test. Sudden and marked reduction in blood pressure following parenteral administration of phentolamine to a hypertensive patient suggests the presence of a pheochromocytoma. However, false-negative and false-positive responses to the phentolamine test occur frequently. (See Cautions: Precautions and Contraindications.)

■ **Hypertension in Pheochromocytoma** In patients with pheochromocytomas, phentolamine may be administered immediately prior to or during pheochromocytomectomy to prevent or control paroxysmal hypertension resulting from anesthesia, stress, or operative manipulation of the tumor.

For information regarding pheochromocytoma crisis, see Uses: Hypertensive Crises.

Although phentolamine has also been used for the medical management of patients with pheochromocytomas until surgery is performed and for prolonged treatment of hypertension caused by a pheochromocytoma not amenable to surgery, most clinicians consider phenoxybenzamine the drug of choice because it has a longer duration of action.

■ **Hypertensive Crises** Phentolamine mesylate also has been used to treat hypertensive crises or emergencies† (severe elevations in blood pressure exceeding 180/120 mm Hg accompanied by new or worsening target organ dysfunction) induced by catecholamine excess (e.g., pheochromocytoma, drug interactions with a monoamine oxidase [MAO] inhibitor, amphetamine overdosage, cocaine toxicity, clonidine withdrawal)†.

Phentolamine is not used in the treatment of essential hypertension because most patients become refractory to the antihypertensive effect of the drug and because of the high incidence of adverse GI effects. Although phentolamine has been used as adjunctive therapy in the treatment of peripheral vasospastic disorders†, the efficacy of the drug has not been established and the frequency of adverse effects limits its usefulness.

■ **Extravasation of Catecholamines** Phentolamine mesylate is used for the prevention and treatment of dermal necrosis and sloughing following IV administration or extravasation of norepinephrine. Phentolamine mesylate has also been used to prevent necrosis after extravasation of dopamine†.

■ **Myocardial Infarction** Phentolamine mesylate has been used IV to decrease the impedance to left ventricular ejection and the size of infarction in patients with myocardial infarction (MI) associated with left ventricular failure†. However, the manufacturers state that the drug is contraindicated in patients with MI and investigators do not recommend this therapy for routine use, since left ventricular function and the ECG must be monitored continuously.

■ **Erectile Dysfunction** Self-injection of small doses of phentolamine mesylate combined with papaverine hydrochloride into a corpus cavernosum of the penis has been effective for the treatment of erectile dysfunction† (impotence). Injection into a single cavernosum can increase tumescence (in both cavernosa because of cross circulation) and produce erection probably secondary to drug-induced increased arterial inflow and sinusoidal relaxation and decreased venous outflow (from increased venous resistance). The goal of such therapy is to provide an erection of adequate rigidity and duration to be sexually functional while avoiding prolonged erection or priapism. Intracavernosal papaverine (alone or combined with phentolamine and/or alprostadil) is one of the most effective and well-studied agents for the treatment of erectile dysfunction and has been in widespread clinical use. The combination has been effective in patients with neurogenic and/or limited vasculogenic impotence or with psychogenic impotence, but efficacy in those with a vasculogenic component of their impotence may be variable depending on the extent and type of vascular dysfunction. Erection, which can be potentiated by sexual arousal, usually occurs within 10 minutes after injection of the drugs and may persist for one to several hours; tolerance to the beneficial vascular effects of the drugs may occur during long-term use and may require an increase in dosage. Occasionally, priapism may occur. (See Cautions: Adverse Effects.)

Because of their convenience (e.g., ease of administration, patient and partner acceptance, and effectiveness in a broad range of patients), most experts (e.g., the American Urological Association [AUA]) currently recommend that selective phosphodiesterase (PDE) type 5 inhibitor therapy (sildenafil, tadalafil, vardenafil) be offered as first-line treatment of erectile dysfunction unless contraindicated. Intracavernosal therapy with papaverine and/or phentolamine generally is reserved for patients who do not respond to psychotherapy/behavioral therapy, vacuum constriction devices, and/or selective PDE type 5 inhibitors, and in whom attempts at identifying and modifying any drug-related (e.g., certain antihypertensive agents) or other potential reversible medical cause of erectile dysfunction have proved inadequate. Intracavernosal therapy or vacuum constriction devices generally are considered or attempted before resorting to more invasive (e.g., surgical) therapies. Ultimately, the choice of therapy for erectile dysfunction should be individualized, taking into account differences in response, tolerability and safety, administration considerations, cost and patient reimbursement factors, experience and judgment of the clinician, and individual patient and partner preference, expectations, and satisfaction.

Intracavernosal vasoactive therapy (e.g., papaverine, papaverine and phentolamine, alprostadil) is the most effective treatment for erectile dysfunction; however, it is invasive and associated with the highest risk of priapism. Clinician preference and experience often guide the initial treatment choice when intracavernosal therapy is indicated.

Additional study of the long-term safety and efficacy of intracavernous injection of vasoactive drugs for the treatment of erectile dysfunction is necessary and ongoing, particularly regarding the relative efficacy of single- versus multiple-drug therapy and the relative complications (e.g., penile scarring, penile fibrosis) and safety of each approach. Additional study also is needed to identify optimal patient education and follow-up support that might improve compliance and decrease dropout rates. Patients should be instructed to visit their clinician regularly (e.g., at 3-month intervals) for assessment of therapeutic benefit, including the need for possible dosage adjustment, and of potential adverse effects of their therapy.

Vasoactive therapy for erectile dysfunction should *not* be used in patients who might have conditions predisposing to priapism (e.g., sickle cell anemia or trait, multiple myeloma, leukemia), in those with anatomic deformation of the penis (e.g., angulation, cavernosal fibrosis, Peyronie's disease), or in men for whom sexual activity is inadvisable or contraindicated. In addition, vasoactive therapy should be discontinued in any patient who develops penile angulation, cavernosal fibrosis, or Peyronie's disease during therapy with the drug. One manufacturer also states that patients with penile implants should *not* be treated with vasoactive therapy for impotence.

Because of the risk of priapism and other potential complications (e.g., adverse morphologic penile effects such as fibrosis) associated with intercavernosal vasoactive therapy, such therapy is *not* recommended for simply enhancing erections in men who are not impotent†.

■ **Cocaine-induced Acute Coronary Syndrome** Phentolamine has been used as an adjunct in the management of cocaine overdose† to reverse coronary vasoconstriction.

■ **Other Uses** IV phentolamine has been used effectively to treat ventricular or supraventricular premature contractions†.

Dosage and Administration

■ **Reconstitution and Administration** Phentolamine mesylate may be administered by IM or IV injection. Phentolamine mesylate injection is reconstituted by adding 1 mL of sterile water for injection to the vial containing 5 mg of lyophilized drug. The resulting solution contains 5 mg of phentolamine mesylate per mL.

Phentolamine mesylate also has been administered by intracavernous injection† for the treatment of erectile dysfunction. (See Uses: Erectile Dysfunction.) Patients receiving the drug via intracavernosal injection should be advised of the potential for prolonged erections (priapism) and advised of steps to take in the event that this potentially serious adverse effect occurs. (See Adverse Effects: Adverse Intracavernosal Effects, in Cautions.)

■ **Dosage** ***Diagnosis of Pheochromocytoma*** For the diagnosis of pheochromocytoma, phentolamine mesylate may be administered IM or preferably IV. The usual adult IV or IM dose is 5 mg. Children may receive 1 mg IV or 3 mg IM. Alternatively, some clinicians have recommended an IV pediatric dose of 0.1 mg/kg or 3 mg/m². Before the drug is injected, the patient should rest in a supine position (preferably in a quiet, darkened room) until the blood pressure is stabilized and a basal level is established by blood pressure readings taken every 10 minutes for at least 30 minutes. When phentolamine mesylate is administered IV, injection of the drug should be delayed until the effect of the venipuncture on the blood pressure has passed; the drug should then be rapidly injected. In patients with a pheochromocytoma which is secreting epinephrine or norepinephrine, the response to IV injection of phentolamine mesylate is an immediate, marked decrease in both systolic and diastolic blood pressure. The maximum effect is usually obtained within 2 minutes after IV injection of the drug, and the blood pressure usually returns to pretest levels within 15–30 minutes. Therefore, blood pressure should be recorded immediately after the injection, at 30-second intervals for the first 3 minutes, and at 1-minute intervals for the next 7 minutes. Following IM injection, the maximum effect usually occurs within 20 minutes and persists for about 30–45 minutes. Blood pressure returns to pretest levels after 3–4 hours. After IM administration of phentolamine mesylate, blood pressure determinations should be made at 5-minute intervals for 30–45 minutes.

In the phentolamine test, a typical blood pressure response in patients with pheochromocytomas is a decrease in blood pressure of 60 mm Hg systolic and 25 mm Hg diastolic within 2 minutes after IV administration of the drug or within 20 minutes after IM administration. A blood pressure decrease of at least 35 mm Hg systolic and 25 mm Hg diastolic is considered a positive response and a positive test for pheochromocytoma. A negative response is indicated when the blood pressure is unchanged, elevated, or lowered less than 35 mm Hg systolic and 25 mm Hg diastolic.

Hypertension in Pheochromocytoma To reduce elevated blood pressure prior to surgical removal of a pheochromocytoma, 5 mg of phentolamine mesylate is given IM or IV 1–2 hours preoperatively to adults or 1 mg, 0.1 mg/kg, or 3 mg/m² is given IM or IV to children; the dose may be repeated if necessary. During surgery for pheochromocytoma, 5 mg of phentolamine mesylate may be given IV to adults as needed to prevent or control paroxysms of hypertension, tachycardia, respiratory depression, convulsions, or other effects of excessive epinephrine secretion due to manipulation of the tumor. For children, the IV dose of phentolamine mesylate during surgery is 1 mg, 0.1 mg/kg, or 3 mg/m². Postoperatively, norepinephrine may be administered to control hypotension which commonly follows removal of a pheochromocytoma; however, this hypotension is more often prevented by administration of blood, plasma, or 5% albumin in 0.9% sodium chloride injection to correct the reduced blood volume which may occur.

Hypertensive Crisis For hypertensive crisis resulting from catecholamine excess†, some experts recommend 5 mg administered as a rapid IV ("bolus") injection. Experts state that this dosage may be repeated every 10 minutes as necessary to achieve the desired blood pressure target.

If IV phentolamine is used in the management of a hypertensive crisis, patients who have hypertensive crisis *with* a compelling condition (e.g., aortic dissection, severe preeclampsia or eclampsia, pheochromocytoma crisis) should have their systolic blood pressure reduced to less than 140 mm Hg during the first hour and, in patients with acute aortic dissection, to less than 120 mm Hg within the first 20 minutes. The initial goal of such therapy in adults *without* a compelling condition is to reduce systolic blood pressure by no more than 25% within the first hour, followed by further blood pressure reduction *if stable* to 160/110 or 160/100 mm Hg within the next 2–6 hours, avoiding excessive declines in pressure that could precipitate renal, cerebral, or coronary ischemia. If this blood pressure is well tolerated and the patient is clinically stable, further gradual reductions toward normal can be implemented in the next 24–48 hours.

Extravasation of Catecholamines To treat dermal necrosis and sloughing following IV administration or extravasation of norepinephrine, 5–10 mg of phentolamine mesylate diluted in 10 mL of 0.9% sodium chloride injection is injected into the affected area within 12 hours. Immediate and conspicuous local hyperemic changes occur if the area is infiltrated within 12 hours, but such treatment is ineffective when given more than 12 hours after extravasation.

To prevent dermal necrosis and sloughing from IV administration or extravasation of norepinephrine, 10 mg of phentolamine mesylate may be added to each liter of IV fluids containing norepinephrine (the pressor effect of norepinephrine is unaffected).

To prevent tissue necrosis and sloughing following extravasation of dopamine injection, 10–15 mL of 0.9% sodium chloride injection containing 5–10 mg of phentolamine mesylate should be infiltrated (using a syringe with a fine hypodermic needle) liberally throughout the affected area, which is identified by coldness, hardness, and a pallid appearance. In children, phentolamine mesylate dosages of 0.1–0.2 mg/kg, up to a maximum of 10 mg per dose, may be administered. Immediate and conspicuous local hyperemic changes occur if the area is infiltrated within 12 hours.

Myocardial Infarction For the treatment of left ventricular failure secondary to acute myocardial infarction (MI)†, the adult IV dosage of phentolamine mesylate as an infusion has ranged from 0.17–0.4 mg/minute. Left ventricular function and the ECG must be monitored continuously.

Erectile Dysfunction When used for the treatment of erectile dysfunction† (impotence), self-injection into the corpus cavernosum of the penis of small doses of phentolamine mesylate (0.08–1.25 mg, but usually 0.5–1 mg) combined with papaverine hydrochloride (2.5–37.5 mg, but usually titrated up to 30 mg) have been effective. Erection, which can be potentiated by sexual arousal, usually occurs within 10 minutes after injection of the drugs and may persist for one to several hours; tolerance to the beneficial vascular effects of the drugs may occur during long-term use and may require an increase in dosage. Occasionally, priapism may occur. (See Cautions: Adverse Effects.)

Cautions

■ Adverse Effects

Phentolamine may cause acute and prolonged hypotension, tachycardia, cardiac arrhythmias, and angina, especially after parenteral administration. Myocardial infarction (MI) and cerebrovascular spasm or occlusion, usually in association with marked hypotension and a shock-like state, have been reported occasionally following parenteral administration of phentolamine. Deaths have occurred after IV administration of phentolamine for the diagnosis of pheochromocytoma.

Weakness, dizziness, flushing, orthostatic hypotension, and nasal congestion have been reported in patients receiving phentolamine. Adverse GI effects are common and include abdominal pain, nausea, vomiting, diarrhea, and exacerbation of peptic ulcer; these adverse effects generally prevent long-term administration of phentolamine.

Adverse Intracavernosal Effects Intracavernous injection† of combined phentolamine and papaverine for the treatment of impotence occasionally has caused priapism. Priapism is a medical emergency that could result in penile tissue damage and permanent loss of potency if not treated immediately, and therefore, patients should be advised to report promptly to their physician or, if unavailable, to seek alternative immediate medical attention if an erection that persists longer than 4 hours or that is extremely painful occurs. Management of priapism should be according to established medical practice, and has included aspiration of cavernosal blood and/or intracavernous injection of small doses of an α-adrenergic agonist (e.g., metaraminol, phenylephrine), or dopamine. Rarely, more radical therapy for priapism (e.g., cavernospongiosus or Winter's shunt) may be necessary, such as in patients with persistent priapism (e.g., for longer than 24 hours).

Other complications of intracavernous injection of combined phentolamine and papaverine have included transient pain, including referred pain to the glans, burning, and paresthesia. Penile ecchymosis has occurred in many patients, and superficial hematoma and bruising of the penis also have occurred. Fibrotic changes (e.g., induration, lumpy areas of the penis but not necessarily at the injection site), including bilateral fibrosis of the corpora cavernosa, also have been reported. Embolus in the glans has been reported rarely, and the development of priapism, deep vein thrombosis, and fatal pulmonary embolus occurred in one patient. Adverse systemic effects of the drugs (e.g., facial flushing, dizziness, decreased systemic blood pressure, metallic taste) also have occurred.

The risk of priapism, although reportedly uncommon, can be reduced by careful patient instruction and dosage titration.Alternatively, switching to another therapy (e.g., alprostadil) may provide better patient tolerance. Some clinicians also have used alprostadil in combination with papaverine and phentolamine in an attempt to potentiate their therapeutic activity, reduce the dose of each drug required, and decrease the risk of local pain, penile corporal fibrosis, fibrotic nodules, hypotension, and priapism associated with higher dosages. However, additional study is needed to elucidate the long-term safety and benefits of such combined therapy.

■ Precautions and Contraindications

If severe hypotension or other signs and symptoms of shock occur following administration of phentolamine, treatment must be vigorous and prompt. Therapy should include supportive measures and norepinephrine may be administered if necessary; epinephrine should not be given since it may cause a paradoxical fall in blood pressure. The manufacturer states that if cardiac arrhythmias occur during therapy with phentolamine, administration of digitalis glycosides should be deferred until the cardiac rhythm returns to normal.

False-negative responses to the phentolamine test may occur, especially in patients with paroxysmal hypertension or with a pheochromocytoma which is not secreting enough epinephrine or norepinephrine to elevate the blood pressure or to sustain an elevation. False-positive reactions occur more commonly than do false-negative responses and have occurred in patients with essential hypertension, in patients who have received sedatives, opiates, or antihypertensive drugs, and in patients with uremia. When practical, sedatives, analgesics, and all other medication should be withdrawn at least 24 hours (but preferably 48–72 hours) prior to the phentolamine test. Antihypertensive drugs should be withdrawn and the test should not be performed until blood pressure returns to pretreatment hypertensive levels; rauwolfia drugs should be withdrawn at least 4 weeks prior to testing.

The possibility that intracavernosal therapy for impotence could result in persistent priapism requiring medical and/or surgical intervention should be considered. (See Cautions: Adverse Effects.) Patients should be advised to contact their clinician if they develop a persistent (e.g., longer than 4 hours) erection during such therapy. The possibility that intracavernosal therapy may be problematic in patients receiving anticoagulants or who cannot tolerate transient hypotension and, because of the self-injection techniques involved, in those with poor manual dexterity, poor vision, or severe psychiatric disease also should be considered. For additional precautions and contraindications associated with vasoactive therapy in impotence, see Uses.

Phentolamine should be used with caution in patients with gastritis or peptic ulcer. Although the manufacturer states that phentolamine is contraindicated in patients with MI or a history of MI, coronary insufficiency, angina, or other evidence suggestive of coronary artery disease, results of some studies indicate that the drug may have a beneficial effect in patients with MI. (See Uses: Other Uses.) The drug is contraindicated in patients who are hypersensitive to phentolamine or to related drugs.

■ Mutagenicity and Carcinogenicity

Studies to determine the mutagenic and carcinogenic potentials of phentolamine mesylate have not been performed to date.

■ Pregnancy, Fertility, and Lactation

Reproduction studies in rats and mice using oral phentolamine mesylate dosages 24–30 times the usual daily human dosage (based on a 60-kg individual) have shown slightly decreased fetal growth and slight fetal skeletal immaturity (manifested by an increased incidence of incomplete or unossified calcanei and phalangeal nuclei of the hind limb and of incompletely ossified sternebrae). In rats receiving oral dosages 60 times the usual human daily dosage (based on a 60-kg individual), a slightly decreased rate of implantation occurred. In rabbits receiving oral dosages 20 times the usual human daily dosage (based on a 60-kg individual), embryonic and fetal development were not affected. No teratogenic or embryotoxic effects were observed in reproduction studies in rats, mice, and rabbits. At least one human death has been reported following the phentolamine test during pregnancy. There are no adequate and well-controlled studies using phentolamine in pregnant women, and the drug should be used during pregnancy only when the potential benefits outweigh the possible risks to the fetus.

Studies to determine the potential effects of phentolamine mesylate on fertility have not been performed to date.

It is not known whether phentolamine mesylate is distributed into milk. Because of the potential for serious adverse reactions to phentolamine mesylate in nursing infants, a decision should be made whether to discontinue nursing or the drug, taking into account the importance of the drug to the woman.

Pharmacology

Phentolamine inhibits responses to adrenergic stimuli by competitively blocking α-adrenergic receptors (primarily excitatory responses of smooth muscle and exocrine glands), but the action of the drug is relatively transient and α-adrenergic blockade is incomplete. Phentolamine has greater α-adrenergic blocking effects than does tolazoline. Phentolamine is more effective in antagonizing responses to circulating epinephrine and/or norepinephrine than in antagonizing responses to mediator released at the adrenergic nerve ending. The drug causes peripheral vasodilation and decreases peripheral resistance, primarily by direct relaxation of vascular smooth muscle, but α-adrenergic blockade also contributes to vasodilation. Phentolamine also stimulates β-adrenergic receptors and produces a positive inotropic and chronotropic effect on the heart and increases cardiac output.

Blood pressure response to phentolamine depends on the relative contributions of its vasodilating and cardiac stimulating effects. IV infusion of phentolamine mesylate 0.3 mg/minute may increase blood pressure because of a predominant inotropic effect, but with higher rates of administration vasodilation may predominate, decreasing blood pressure and masking the inotropic effect. Pulmonary vascular resistance and pulmonary arterial pressure are decreased. Cerebral blood flow is generally maintained. Usual doses of phentolamine lower blood pressure when it is maintained by circulating epinephrine or norepinephrine, but have little effect on the blood pressure of healthy individuals or patients with essential hypertension.

When phentolamine is administered IV to patients with acute myocardial infarction (MI) associated with hypertension and/or left ventricular failure, improvement in left ventricular performance results, with cardiac output, stroke index, heart rate, and cardiac index being increased and left ventricular filling pressure being decreased. In one study, IV phentolamine increased coronary blood flow in patients with recent MI. In animal studies, the drug prolonged the action potential duration and the effective refractory period and decreased conduction velocity.

Phentolamine dilates bronchial smooth muscle, presumably through stimulation of β-adrenergic receptors. The drug stimulates the smooth muscle of the GI tract, an effect which is blocked by atropine, and has a histamine-like effect which stimulates gastric secretion of both acid and pepsin. Large IV doses (40–50 mg) cause relaxation of the ureters.

Pharmacokinetics

The pharmacokinetics of phentolamine have not been determined. Phentolamine is only about 20% as active after oral administration as after parenteral administration. About 10% of a parenteral dose can be recovered in the urine as active drug; the fate of the remainder is not known. It is not known whether the drug crosses the placenta or appears in milk.

Chemistry and Stability

■ **Chemistry** Phentolamine is an imidazoline α-adrenergic blocking agent that is related structurally to tolazoline. Phentolamine mesylate occurs as a white or off-white, crystalline powder and has solubilities of approximately 1 g/mL in water and 250 mg/mL in alcohol at 25°C. The pK_a of phentolamine mesylate is 8.01. Following reconstitution of the commercially available lyophilized powder with sterile water for injection to a concentration of 5 mg/mL, phentolamine mesylate injection has a pH of 4.5–6.5.

■ **Stability** Phentolamine mesylate powder for injection should be stored at 15–30°C.

Following reconstitution of the commercially available lyophilized powder with sterile water for injection to a concentration of 5 mg/mL, phentolamine mesylate injection is stable for 48 hours at room temperature or 1 week at 2–8°C; however, the manufacturer recommends that the reconstituted injection be used immediately and not stored.

Following reconstitution of phentolamine mesylate lyophilized powder with 2 mL of commercially available papaverine hydrochloride injection (containing 30 mg/mL) and further dilution in 8 mL of the papaverine injection to provide an admixture containing 0.5 mg of phentolamine mesylate per mL and 30 mg of papaverine hydrochloride per mL, the resultant admixture had a pH of 3.6 and was stable for at least 30 days when stored in the papaverine vial at 5 or 25°C. It should be noted, however, that the manufacturer of papaverine hydrochloride injection recommends that the injection not be refrigerated since solubility of the drug is reduced at cold temperatures, possibly resulting in precipitation or crystallization. In addition, the possibility of microbial contamination of such admixtures during prolonged storage should be considered.

Preparations

Excipients in commercially available drug preparations may have clinically important effects in some individuals; consult specific product labeling for details.

Phentolamine Mesylate

Parenteral

For injection	5 mg*	**Phentolamine Mesylate for Injection**

*available from one or more manufacturer, distributor, and/or repackager by generic (nonproprietary) name

†Use is not currently included in the labeling approved by the US Food and Drug Administration

Selected Revisions April 2019,

SELECTIVE α_1-ADRENERGIC BLOCKING AGENTS 12:16.04.12

Alfuzosin Hydrochloride

■ Alfuzosin is an α_1-adrenergic blocking agent that exhibits selectivity for α_1-adrenergic receptors in the lower urinary tract (e.g., bladder base, bladder neck, prostate, prostatic capsule, prostatic urethra).

Uses

■ **Benign Prostatic Hyperplasia** Alfuzosin hydrochloride is used to reduce urinary obstruction and relieve associated manifestations in patients with symptomatic benign prostatic hyperplasia (BPH, benign prostatic hypertrophy). Alfuzosin relieves moderate to severe irritative (e.g., frequency, urgency, nocturia) and obstructive (e.g., hesitancy, interrupted or weak stream, sensation of incomplete bladder emptying or straining) manifestations and improves urinary flow rates in a substantial proportion of patients. Although drug therapy is not curative, α_1-adrenergic blocking agents (e.g., alfuzosin) may be a useful alternative to surgery, particularly in those who are awaiting or are unwilling to undergo surgical correction of the hyperplasia (e.g., via transurethral resection of the prostate [TURP]) or who are not candidates for such surgery.

Results of several controlled studies indicate that alfuzosin hydrochloride is more effective than placebo in the management of BPH. In addition, results of several comparative studies in patients with BPH suggest that the drug (as conventional formulations) is at least as effective as other α_1-adrenergic blocking agents (e.g., prazosin, tamsulosin). While symptomatic improvement has been maintained for up to 3 years of alfuzosin therapy in some patients, the long-term effects of α_1-adrenergic blocking agents on the need for surgery and on the frequency of developing BPH-associated complications such as acute urinary obstruction remain to be established.

Combination therapy with an α_1-adrenergic blocker and a 5α-reductase inhibitor (e.g., finasteride) has been more effective than therapy with either drug alone in preventing long-term BPH symptom progression; combined therapy also can reduce the risks of long-term acute urinary retention and the need for invasive therapy compared with α-blocker monotherapy.

For additional information on the use of α_1-blockers in the management of BPH, see Uses: Benign Prostatic Hyperplasia, in Doxazosin 24:20.

■ **Other Uses** The manufacturer states that alfuzosin hydrochloride should *not* be used in the management of hypertension.

Dosage and Administration

■ **General** Alfuzosin hydrochloride is administered orally. For the management of benign prostatic hyperplasia (BPH), the recommended adult dosage of alfuzosin hydrochloride is 10 mg once daily. Because the extent of absorption is decreased by 50% under fasting conditions, alfuzosin hydrochloride should be taken immediately after the same meal each day. The extended-release tablets should *not* be chewed or crushed.

■ **Special Populations** The manufacturer states that use of alfuzosin hydrochloride is contraindicated in patients with moderate to severe hepatic impairment. (See Hepatic Impairment under Cautions: Special Populations.) Pharmacokinetics of alfuzosin hydrochloride have not been studied in patients with mild hepatic impairment, and the manufacturer does not provide guidelines for dosage adjustment in such patients.

No dosage adjustment is necessary in patients with mild to moderate renal impairment (creatinine clearance of 30–80 mL/minute) nor in geriatric patients. Caution is advised if alfuzosin hydrochloride is used in patients with severe renal impairment (creatinine clearance less than 30 mL/minute). (See Renal Impairment under Cautions: Special Populations.)

Cautions

■ **Contraindications** Moderate or severe hepatic impairment (Child-Pugh class B or C).

Concomitant use with potent inhibitors of cytochrome P-450 (CYP) isoenzyme 3A4 (e.g., itraconazole, ketoconazole, ritonavir). (See Drug Interactions.)

Known hypersensitivity to alfuzosin hydrochloride or any ingredient in the formulation.

■ **Warnings/Precautions** ***Warnings*** **Postural Hypotension.** Like other α-adrenergic blocking agents, alfuzosin can cause postural hypotension with or without symptoms (e.g., dizziness), and the drug should be administered with caution to patients with symptomatic hypotension or patients who have had a hypotensive response to other drugs. During initiation of alfuzosin therapy, patients should be cautioned to avoid situations where injury could result if syncope occurs. If syncope occurs, the patient should be placed in a recumbent position and treated supportively as necessary.

General Precautions **Prostate Cancer.** Because manifestations of prostate cancer may mimic those of benign prostatic hyperplasia (BPH), the possibility of prostate cancer should be excluded prior to initiation of therapy.

Intraoperative Floppy Iris Syndrome. Intraoperative floppy iris syndrome (IFIS) has been observed during phacoemulsification cataract surgery in some patients currently receiving or previously treated with α_1-adrenergic blocking agents. IFIS is a variant of small pupil syndrome and is characterized by the combination of a flaccid iris that billows in response to intraoperative irrigation currents, progressive intraoperative miosis despite preoperative dilation with mydriatics, and potential prolapse of the iris toward the phacoemulsification incisions. Male patients being considered for cataract surgery should be advised to inform their ophthalmologist of current or prior therapy with α_1-adrenergic blockers, including alfuzosin. If a patient has received such agents, the ophthalmologist should be prepared to modify the surgical technique (e.g., through use of iris hooks, iris dilator rings, or viscoelastic substances) to minimize complications of IFIS. There does not appear to be a benefit from discontinuing α_1-blocker therapy prior to cataract surgery.

Prolongation of QT Interval. Prolongation of the QT interval has been observed with higher than recommended dosages of alfuzosin; however, development of atypical ventricular tachycardia (torsades de pointes) has not been reported to date in patients receiving the drug. The manufacturer states that the

QT-interval prolongation observed with higher than recommended dosages of the drug should be considered in clinical decisions regarding use of alfuzosin in patients with known prolongation of the QT interval and in those receiving drugs known to prolong the QT interval.

Angina Pectoris. If symptoms of angina pectoris develop or worsen in patients with coronary artery disease, alfuzosin should be discontinued.

Specific Populations **Pregnancy.** Category B. (See Users Guide) Alfuzosin is not intended for use in women.

Lactation. Alfuzosin is not intended for use in women.

Pediatric Use. Alfuzosin is not intended for use in children.

Geriatric Use. When the total number of patients studied in clinical trials of alfuzosin is considered, 48% were 65 years of age or older, while 11% were 75 years of age or older. Although no overall differences in efficacy or safety were observed between geriatric and younger patients, and other clinical experience revealed no evidence of age-related differences, the possibility that some older patients may exhibit increased sensitivity to the drug cannot be ruled out.

Hepatic Impairment. Apparent plasma clearance of alfuzosin is decreased in patients with moderate or severe hepatic impairment (Child-Pugh class B or C), resulting in 3- to 4-fold higher plasma concentrations of alfuzosin in these patients compared with healthy individuals. Alfuzosin is contraindicated in patients with moderate or severe hepatic impairment.

Renal Impairment. Systemic exposure to alfuzosin is increased by approximately 50% in patients with renal impairment (creatinine clearance less than 80 mL/minute) relative to those with normal renal function. In phase III studies, the safety profile of alfuzosin hydrochloride in patients with mild (creatinine clearance of 60–80 mL/minute) or moderate (creatinine clearance of 30–59 mL/minute) renal impairment was similar to that in patients with normal renal function (creatinine clearance exceeding 80 mL/minute). Safety data are available for only a limited number of patients with severe renal impairment (creatinine clearance less than 30 mL/minute). Therefore, the manufacturer recommends that alfuzosin be used with caution in patients with severe renal impairment.

■ **Common Adverse Effects** Adverse effects reported in 2% or more of patients receiving alfuzosin and at an incidence higher than that reported with placebo include dizziness, upper respiratory tract infection, headache, and fatigue.

Drug Interactions

■ **Drugs Affecting Hepatic Microsomal Enzymes** Pharmacokinetic interaction (increased plasma alfuzosin concentrations) with inhibitors of the cytochrome P-450 (CYP) 3A4 isoenzyme. Concomitant use of potent inhibitors of the CYP 3A4 isoenzyme (e.g., itraconazole, ketoconazole, ritonavir) with alfuzosin is contraindicated.

■ **Drugs that Prolong the QT Interval** Potential pharmacologic interaction (additive effect on QT interval prolongation). (See Prolongation of QT Interval under Cautions: Warnings.)

■ **α_1-Adrenergic Blocking Agents** Potential pharmacologic interaction (additive cardiovascular effects) with other α_1-adrenergic blocking agents. Concomitant use is not recommended by the manufacturer.

■ **Atenolol** Potential pharmacologic (additive cardiovascular effects) and pharmacokinetic (increased plasma concentrations of alfuzosin and atenolol) interactions.

■ **Diltiazem** Potential pharmacologic (additive cardiovascular effects) and pharmacokinetic (increased plasma concentrations of alfuzosin and diltiazem) interactions.

■ **Hydrochlorothiazide** No pharmacologic or pharmacokinetic interaction observed between hydrochlorothiazide and alfuzosin.

■ **Cimetidine** Potential pharmacokinetic interaction (increased plasma alfuzosin concentrations).

■ **Digoxin** Pharmacokinetic interaction unlikely.

■ **Warfarin** Pharmacologic interaction unlikely.

Description

Alfuzosin hydrochloride, a quinazoline-derivative α_1-adrenergic blocking agent, is structurally and pharmacologically related to doxazosin, prazosin, and terazosin and pharmacologically related to tamsulosin. Alfuzosin is a non-subtype-specific α_1-adrenergic blocking agent that exhibits selectivity for α_1-adrenergic receptors in the lower urinary tract (e.g., bladder base, bladder neck, prostate, prostatic capsule, prostatic urethra). Blockade of these adrenoreceptors can cause relaxation of smooth muscle in the bladder neck and prostate, resulting in improvement in urine flow and a reduction in symptoms of benign prostatic hyperplasia (BPH). Such effects generally are achieved with alfuzosin hydrochloride dosages that do not have clinically important effects on blood pressure or heart rate.

Alfuzosin is extensively metabolized in the liver via oxidation, *O*-demethylation, and/or *N*-dealkylation, principally by the cytochrome P-450 (CYP) 3A4 isoenzyme, to form pharmacologically inactive metabolites. Alfuzosin is not an inhibitor of CYP isoenzymes 1A2, 2A6, 2C9, 2C19, 2D6, or 3A4 nor an inducer of CYP isoenzymes 1A, 2A6, or 3A4.

Advice to Patients

Possible manifestations of postural hypotension (e.g., dizziness, syncope) at the beginning of alfuzosin therapy; importance of exercising caution while driving, operating machinery, or performing hazardous tasks following initiation of therapy.

Importance of taking the drug exactly as prescribed by the clinician (e.g., immediately after the same meal each day).

Importance of informing clinicians of existing or contemplated concomitant therapy, including prescription and OTC drugs, as well as any concomitant diseases.

Overview® (see Users Guide). For additional information on this drug until a more detailed monograph is developed and published, the manufacturer's labeling should be consulted. It is *essential* that the manufacturer's labeling be consulted for more detailed information on usual cautions, precautions, contraindications, potential drug interactions, laboratory test interferences, and acute toxicity.

Preparations

Excipients in commercially available drug preparations may have clinically important effects in some individuals; consult specific product labeling for details.

Alfuzosin Hydrochloride

Oral

Tablets, extended-release	10 mg	**Uroxatral®**, Sanofi-Aventis

Silodosin

■ Silodosin is a postsynaptic α_1-adrenergic blocking agent that exhibits selectivity for α_{1A}-adrenergic receptors located in the lower urinary tract (e.g., bladder base, bladder neck, prostate, prostatic capsule, prostatic urethra).

Uses

■ **Benign Prostatic Hyperplasia** Silodosin is used for the symptomatic management of benign prostatic hyperplasia (BPH, benign prostatic hypertrophy). Silodosin relieves moderate to severe irritative (e.g., frequency, urgency, nocturia) and obstructive (e.g., hesitancy, weak stream, sensation of incomplete bladder emptying) symptoms and improves urinary flow rates in patients with BPH. Because silodosin has produced a substantial improvement in some patients with severe manifestations of BPH, the drug may be a useful alternative to surgery, particularly in those who are awaiting surgical correction of the hyperplasia (e.g., via transurethral resection of the prostate [TURP]) or who are not candidates for such surgery.

Results of several controlled studies indicate that silodosin is more effective than placebo in the management of BPH. In addition, results of a comparative study in patients with BPH suggest that the drug is at least as effective as the α_1-adrenergic blocking agent tamsulosin. Symptomatic improvement has been maintained for up to 1 year of silodosin therapy in some patients.

Combination therapy with an α_1-adrenergic blocking agent (e.g., doxazosin) and a 5α-reductase inhibitor (e.g., finasteride) has been more effective than therapy with either drug alone in preventing long-term BPH symptom progression; combined therapy also can reduce the risks of long-term acute urinary retention and the need for invasive therapy compared with α-blocker monotherapy.

For additional information on the use of α_1-blockers in the management of BPH, see Uses: Benign Prostatic Hyperplasia, in Doxazosin 24:20.

■ **Other Uses** The manufacturer states that silodosin should *not* be used in the management of hypertension.

Dosage and Administration

■ **Administration** Silodosin is administered orally once daily with a meal. The manufacturer states that silodosin should be administered with a meal to reduce the risk of adverse effects.

■ **Dosage** The usual adult dosage of silodosin for the management of benign prostatic hyperplasia (BPH) is 8 mg once daily.

■ **Special Populations** The manufacturer states that use of silodosin is contraindicated in patients with severe hepatic impairment (Child-Pugh class C). (See Hepatic Impairment under Warnings/Precautions: Specific Populations, in Cautions.) No dosage adjustment is necessary in patients with mild or moderate hepatic impairment (Child-Pugh class A or B).

The manufacturer states that use of silodosin is contraindicated in patients with severe renal impairment (creatinine clearance less than 30 mL/minute). In patients with moderate renal impairment (creatinine clearance 30–50 mL/minute), the manufacturer recommends that the dosage be reduced to 4 mg once daily. (See Renal Impairment under Warnings/Precautions: Specific Populations, in Cautions.) No dosage adjustment is necessary in patients with mild renal impairment (creatinine clearance 50–80 mL/minute).

Cautions

■ **Contraindications** Severe hepatic impairment (Child-Pugh class C). Severe renal impairment (creatinine clearance less than 30 mL/minute).

Concomitant use with potent inhibitors of cytochrome P-450 (CYP) isoenzyme 3A4 (e.g., clarithromycin, itraconazole, ketoconazole, ritonavir). (See Drug Interactions.)

■ **Warnings/Precautions** ***Warnings*** **Orthostatic Hypotension.** Silodosin can cause orthostatic hypotension with or without symptoms (e.g., dizziness) during initiation of therapy. Like other α-adrenergic blocking agents, there is also potential for syncope to occur. During initiation of silodosin therapy, patients should exercise caution while driving, operating machinery, or performing hazardous tasks. (See Advice to Patients.)

General Precautions **Prostate Cancer.** Because manifestations of prostate cancer may mimic those of benign prostatic hyperplasia (BPH), the possibility of prostate cancer should be excluded prior to initiation of silodosin therapy.

Intraoperative Floppy Iris Syndrome. Intraoperative floppy iris syndrome (IFIS) has been observed during phacoemulsification cataract surgery in some patients currently receiving or previously treated with α_1-adrenergic blocking agents. IFIS is a variant of small pupil syndrome and is characterized by the combination of a flaccid iris that billows in response to intraoperative irrigation currents, progressive intraoperative miosis despite preoperative dilation with mydriatics, and potential prolapse of the iris toward the phacoemulsification incisions. Male patients being considered for cataract surgery should be advised to inform their ophthalmologist of current or prior therapy with α_1-adrenergic blockers, including silodosin. If a patient has received such agents, the ophthalmologist should consider use of corrective measures such as modification of the surgical technique through use of iris hooks or iris dilator rings or pharmacologic intervention with intracameral phenylephrine or preoperative administration of atropine. The benefit of discontinuing α_1-blocker therapy prior to cataract surgery has not been established.

Specific Populations **Pregnancy.** Category B. (See Users Guide.) Silodosin is not intended for use in women.

Lactation. Silodosin is not intended for use in women.

Pediatric Use. Silodosin is not intended for use in pediatric patients.

Geriatric Use. In clinical studies with silodosin, a higher incidence of orthostatic hypotension was reported in geriatric patients 65 years of age and older relative to younger adults. No other substantial differences in safety and efficacy were observed between geriatric and younger adults.

Hepatic Impairment. Dosage adjustment is not required in patients with mild or moderate hepatic impairment. Silodosin has not been studied in patients with severe hepatic impairment. Therefore, use of the drug is contraindicated in patients with severe hepatic impairment. (See Cautions: Contraindications.)

Renal Impairment. Silodosin should be used with caution in patients with moderate renal impairment. In one study, plasma concentrations and half-life of silodosin increased threefold and twofold, respectively, in individuals with moderate renal impairment compared with those having normal renal function. Therefore, dosage reduction is recommended for patients with moderate renal impairment (creatinine clearance 30–50 mL/minute). (See Dosage and Administration: Special Populations.) Use of the drug is contraindicated in patients with severe renal impairment. (See Cautions: Contraindications.)

■ **Common Adverse Effects** Adverse effects reported in 2% or more of patients receiving silodosin and at an incidence higher than that reported with placebo include retrograde ejaculation, dizziness, diarrhea, orthostatic hypotension, headache, nasopharyngitis, and nasal congestion.

Drug Interactions

■ **Drugs Affecting Hepatic Microsomal Enzymes** Pharmacokinetic interaction (increased plasma silodosin concentrations) with potent inhibitors of the cytochrome P-450 (CYP) 3A4 isoenzyme. Concomitant use of potent inhibitors of the CYP3A4 isoenzyme (e.g., clarithromycin, itraconazole, ketoconazole, ritonavir) with silodosin is contraindicated. The effect of moderate CYP3A4 inhibitors on silodosin pharmacokinetics has not been evaluated. Concomitant use of moderate CYP3A4 inhibitors (e.g., diltiazem, erythromycin, verapamil) may increase silodosin concentrations. Caution is advised and patients should be monitored for adverse effects when silodosin is used concomitantly with moderate CYP3A4 inhibitors, particularly those that also inhibit P-glycoprotein. (See Drug Interactions: Drugs Affecting or Affected by P-glycoprotein Transport.)

In vitro studies indicate that silodosin does not have the potential to inhibit or induce CYP isoenzymes.

■ **Drugs Affecting or Affected by P-glycoprotein Transport** Potential pharmacokinetic interaction (increased silodosin concentrations) with inhibitors of P-glycoprotein transport. Concomitant use of silodosin and ketoconazole (a CYP3A4 inhibitor and a P-glycoprotein inhibitor) resulted in substantially increased silodosin exposure. Studies evaluating concomitant use of silodosin and a potent P-glycoprotein inhibitor (e.g., cyclosporine) have not been conducted. Therefore, the manufacturer states that concomitant use of silodosin with a potent P-glycoprotein inhibitor is not recommended.

In vitro studies show that silodosin is a substrate for the P-glycoprotein transport system.

■ **Drugs Affecting Uridine Diphosphate-glucuronosyltransferase** Potential pharmacokinetic interaction (increased silodosin exposure) with drugs that are inhibitors of uridine diphosphate-glucuronosyltransferase (UGT) 2B7 (e.g., fluconazole, probenecid, valproic acid).

■ ***α*-Adrenergic Blocking Agents** Potential pharmacodynamic interaction (additive cardiovascular effects) with other α-adrenergic blocking agents. However, the interaction between silodosin and other α-adrenergic blocking agents has not been determined. Concomitant use is not recommended by the manufacturer.

■ **Antihypertensive Agents** Potential pharmacodynamic interaction between silodosin and antihypertensive agents. Although the interaction has not been evaluated in a clinical study, one-third of patients in studies with silodosin used antihypertensive agents concomitantly. The incidence of dizziness and orthostatic hypotension in the patients receiving concomitant therapy was higher than that reported in those receiving silodosin alone. Caution is advised and patients should be monitored for adverse effects when silodosin is used concomitantly with antihypertensive agents.

■ **Digoxin** Concomitant use of silodosin and digoxin in one study did not substantially alter the steady-state pharmacokinetics of digoxin. The manufacturer states that no dosage adjustment is required during concomitant use.

■ **Phosphodiesterase Inhibitors** Concomitant use of silodosin with a phosphodiesterase (PDE) type 5 inhibitor (i.e., sildenafil, tadalafil) in one study showed a greater number of orthostatic effects in the group receiving silodosin and a PDE type 5 inhibitor compared with those receiving silodosin alone. However, symptomatic orthostasis or dizziness was not reported in individuals receiving concomitant therapy.

Description

Silodosin, a trifluoroethoxy-phenoxyethyl amine derivative, is an α_1-adrenergic blocking agent that exhibits selectivity for postsynaptic α_{1A}-adrenergic receptors in the lower urinary tract (e.g., bladder base, bladder neck, prostate, prostatic capsule, prostatic urethra). Blockade of these adrenoreceptors can cause relaxation of smooth muscle in the bladder neck and prostate, resulting in improvement in urinary flow and a reduction in symptoms of benign prostatic hyperplasia (BPH). Such effects generally are achieved with silodosin dosages that do not have clinically important effects on blood pressure or heart rate. The higher affinity of silodosin for α_{1A}-adrenergic receptors in the lower urinary tract than for α_{1B}-adrenergic receptors in vascular smooth muscle may result in reduced incidence of cardiovascular effects (e.g., syncope, dizziness, hypotension).

Administration of silodosin with a moderate-fat, moderate-calorie meal in 3 studies decreased AUC by 4–49% and peak plasma concentrations by 18–43%. Administration of silodosin with a high-fat, high-calorie meal was not evaluated.

Silodosin undergoes extensive metabolism in the liver via glucuronidation, alcohol and aldehyde dehydrogenases, and cytochrome P-450 (CYP) 3A4 pathways. The primary active metabolite of silodosin, KMD-3213G, is formed via uridine diphosphate-glucuronosyltransferase (UGT) 2B7-mediated glucuronidation. Another major metabolite is KMD-3293, formed via alcohol and aldehyde dehydrogenases; this metabolite is not expected to contribute substantially to the pharmacologic activity of silodosin. Silodosin is not likely to inhibit CYP isoenzymes 1A2, 2A6, 2C9, 2C19, 2D6, 2E1, or 3A4 nor induce CYP isoenzymes 1A2, 2C8, 2C9, 2C19, or 3A4. Silodosin is also not an inducer of the P-glycoprotein transport system, but in vitro studies show that silodosin is a substrate for P-glycoprotein.

Advice to Patients

Possible manifestations of orthostatic hypotension (e.g., dizziness, syncope) following initiation of silodosin therapy, particularly in patients with hypotension or in those receiving antihypertensive agents; importance of exercising caution when driving, operating machinery, or performing hazardous tasks.

Importance of taking the drug exactly as prescribed by the clinician (i.e., once daily with a meal).

Risk of retrograde ejaculation; importance of advising patients that this common adverse effect does not pose a safety concern and is reversible upon discontinuance of therapy.

Risk of intraoperative floppy iris syndrome (IFIS); importance of male patients planning cataract surgery or other ophthalmic procedures to inform clinicians of current or prior therapy with α_1-adrenergic blocking agents.

Importance of informing clinicians of existing or contemplated concomitant therapy, including prescription and OTC drugs, as well as any concomitant diseases.

Importance of informing patients of other important precautionary information. (See Cautions.)

Overview® (see Users Guide). For additional information on this drug until a more detailed monograph is developed and published, the manufacturer's labeling should be consulted. It is *essential* that the manufacturer's labeling be consulted for more detailed information on usual cautions, precautions, contraindications, potential drug interactions, laboratory test interferences, and acute toxicity.

Preparations

Excipients in commercially available drug preparations may have clinically important effects in some individuals; consult specific product labeling for details.

Silodosin

Oral		
Capsules	4 mg	Rapaflo®, Watson
	8 mg	Rapaflo®, Watson

Tamsulosin Hydrochloride

■ Tamsulosin hydrochloride is an α_1-adrenergic blocking agent with selectivity for α_{1A}-adrenergic receptors, which are mainly located in nonvascular smooth muscle (e.g., prostate).

Uses

■ **Benign Prostatic Hyperplasia** Tamsulosin is used to reduce urinary obstruction and relieve associated manifestations in hypertensive or normotensive patients with symptomatic benign prostatic hyperplasia (BPH, benign prostatic hypertrophy). Tamsulosin relieves mild to moderate obstructive manifestations (e.g., hesitancy, terminal dribbling of urine, interrupted or weak stream, impaired size and force of stream, sensation of incomplete bladder emptying or straining) and improves urinary flow rates in a substantial proportion of patients and may be a useful alternative to surgery, particularly in those who are awaiting or are unwilling to undergo surgical correction of the hyperplasia (e.g., via transurethral resection of the prostate [TURP]) or who are not candidates for such surgery. Therapy with α_1-adrenergic blocking agents appears to be less effective in relieving irritative (e.g., nocturia, daytime frequency, urgency, dysuria) than obstructive symptomatology, although tamsulosin also has been shown to be effective in relieving irritative symptoms. In addition, therapy with α_1-adrenergic blocking agents generally can be expected to produce less subjective and objective improvement than prostatectomy, and periodic monitoring (e.g., performance of digital rectal examinations, serum creatinine determinations, serum prostate specific antigen [PSA] assays) is indicated in these patients to detect and manage other potential complications of or conditions associated with BPH (e.g., obstructive uropathy, prostatic carcinoma).

Results of several controlled studies indicate that tamsulosin is more effective than placebo and limited data suggest that the drug is at least as effective as other α_1-adrenergic blocking agents (e.g., doxazosin, prazosin, terazosin) in the management of BPH. While symptomatic improvement has been maintained for up to at least 60 weeks of tamsulosin therapy in some patients, the long-term effects of α-blockers on the need for surgery and on the frequency of developing BPH-associated complications such as acute urinary obstruction remain to be established. Although tamsulosin appears to be associated with a decreased incidence of adverse cardiovascular effects including hypotension, dizziness, and syncope, patients should be warned of the possibility of tamsulosin-induced postural dizziness and measures to take if it develops (e.g., sitting, lying down). During initiation of tamsulosin therapy, patients should be cautioned to avoid situations where injury could result if syncope occurs. If syncope occurs, the patient should be placed in a recumbent position and treated supportively as necessary.

Combination therapy with an α_1-blocker and 5α-reductase inhibitor (e.g., finasteride) has been more effective than therapy with either drug alone in preventing long-term BPH symptom progression; combined therapy also can reduce the risks of long-term acute urinary retention and the need for invasive therapy compared with α-blocker monotherapy.

For additional information on the use of α_1-blockers in the management of BPH, see Uses: Benign Prostatic Hyperplasia, in Doxazosin 24:20.

Allergic-type reactions, including skin rash, pruritus, urticaria, and angioedema of the tongue, lips, and face, have been reported in some patients with positive rechallenge of tamsulosin therapy.

The possibility of carcinoma of the prostate and other conditions associated with manifestations that mimic those of BPH should be excluded in any patient for whom tamsulosin therapy for presumed BPH is being considered.

The manufacturer states that tamsulosin should *not* be used in the management of hypertension.

Dosage and Administration

■ **Administration** Tamsulosin is administered orally. Because food may decrease peak plasma concentrations of tamsulosin and lengthen the time to achievement of peak plasma concentrations and decrease oral bioavailability of the drug, the manufacturer recommends that tamsulosin be taken 30 minutes after a meal; it is recommended that the drug be taken after the same meal each day. Patients should be advised that the capsules must be swallowed intact and *not* be opened, chewed, or crushed.

Risk of Intraoperative Floppy Iris Syndrome A condition termed intraoperative floppy iris syndrome (IFIS) has been observed during phacoemulsification cataract surgery in some patients receiving α_1-adrenergic blocking agents, including tamsulosin. IFIS is a variant of small pupil syndrome and is characterized by the combination of a flaccid iris that billows in response to intraoperative irrigation currents, progressive intraoperative miosis despite preoperative dilation with mydriatics, and potential prolapse of the iris toward the phacoemulsification incisions. Most reported cases of IFIS were in patients who continued α_1-blocker therapy at the time of cataract surgery. A few cases also were reported in patients who had discontinued such therapy prior to surgery, generally 2–14 days prior to surgery but occasionally 5 weeks to 9 months prior to surgery. The manufacturer of tamsulosin recommends that male patients being considered for cataract surgery be specifically questioned to ascertain whether they have received tamsulosin or other α_1-blockers. If a patient has received such agents, the ophthalmologist should be prepared to modify the surgical technique (e.g., through use of iris hooks, iris dilator rings, or viscoelastic substances) to minimize complications of IFIS. The benefit of discontinuing α_1-blockers, including tamsulosin, prior to cataract surgery has not been established.

■ **Dosage** The manufacturer states that safety and efficacy of tamsulosin in children younger than 18 years of age have not been established, and clinical experience in these patients is not available.

Benign Prostatic Hyperplasia For the management of benign prostatic hyperplasia (BPH), the usual initial adult dosage of tamsulosin is 0.4 mg once daily. About 2–4 weeks may be needed to adequately assess the response at this dosage. To achieve the desired improvement in symptoms and/or urinary flow rates, subsequent dosage may be increased to 0.8 mg daily as needed. If tamsulosin is discontinued for several days at either dosage (i.e., 0.4 or 0.8 mg daily), therapy with the drug should be reinstituted at the lower daily dosage. Although the elimination half-life may be slightly prolonged and intrinsic clearance of tamsulosin may be decreased in patients 55 years of age and older, the manufacturer makes no specific recommendations for dosage adjustment in such patients.

The manufacturer states that tamsulosin should not be used concomitantly with other α-adrenergic blocking agents.

■ **Dosage in Renal and Hepatic Impairment** Although protein binding of tamsulosin may be altered in patients with mild to moderate (i.e., creatinine clearance of 30–70 mL/minute per 1.73 m^2) or severe (i.e., creatinine clearance of 10 to less than 30 mL/minute per 1.73 m^2) renal impairment and in patients with moderate hepatic impairment resulting in changes of overall plasma concentrations of the drug, alterations in intrinsic clearance and concentrations of unbound tamsulosin do not appear to be substantial. Therefore, the manufacturer states that dosage adjustment in such patients is not necessary. However, tamsulosin has not been studied in patients with end-stage (i.e., creatinine clearance of less than 10 mL/minute per 1.73 m^2) renal disease.

Cautions

■ **Contraindications** Known hypersensitivity to tamsulosin or any ingredient in the formulation.

■ **Warnings/Precautions** ***Warnings*** **Postural Hypotension.** Potential for postural hypotension, dizziness, or vertigo; syncope may occur.

Priapism. Priapism reported rarely; treat promptly.

Sensitivity Reactions **Allergic Reactions.** Rash, pruritus, urticaria, and angioedema of the tongue, lips, and face reported; positive rechallenge in some patients.

Sulfa Sensitivity. Allergic reaction to tamsulosin reported rarely in patients with sulfa sensitivity. Use with caution in patients with serious or life-threatening sulfa sensitivity.

General Precautions **Prostate Cancer.** Exclude possibility of prostate cancer prior to initiation of therapy.

Intraoperative Floppy Iris Syndrome. Intraoperative floppy iris syndrome (IFIS) observed during phacoemulsification cataract surgery in some patients receiving α_1-adrenergic blocking agents, including tamsulosin. Most reported cases were in patients who continued such therapy at the time of cataract surgery.

Manufacturer recommends that male patients being considered for cataract surgery be specifically questioned to ascertain whether they have received tamsulosin or other α_1-blockers. If the patient has received α_1-blockers, the ophthalmologist should be prepared to modify the surgical technique (e.g., through use of iris hooks, iris dilator rings, or viscoelastic substances) to minimize complications of IFIS.

Benefit of discontinuing α_1-blockers prior to cataract surgery not established.

Specific Populations **Pregnancy.** Category B. Not indicated for use in women.

Lactation. Not indicated for use in women.

Pediatric Use. Not indicated for use in children.

Geriatric Use. No substantial differences in safety and efficacy relative to younger adults, but increased sensitivity cannot be ruled out.

■ **Common Adverse Effects** Headache, infection, asthenia, back pain, chest pain, dizziness, somnolence, insomnia, decreased libido, rhinitis, pharyngitis, increased cough, sinusitis, diarrhea, nausea, tooth disorder, abnormal ejaculation, blurred vision.

Description

Tamsulosin hydrochloride is a sulfamoylphenethylamine-derivative α_1-adrenergic blocking agent. Commercially available tamsulosin hydrochloride is a racemic mixture of 2 isomers. The drug is pharmacologically related to doxazosin, prazosin, and terazosin; however, unlike these drugs, tamsulosin has higher affinity and selectivity for α_{1A}-adrenergic receptors, which are mainly located in nonvascular smooth muscle (e.g., prostate), than for α_{1B}-adrenergic receptors located in vascular smooth muscle (e.g., internal iliac artery). Results of in vitro studies indicate that tamsulosin has 7–38 times greater affinity for α_{1A}-adrenoceptors than for α_{1B}-adrenoceptors; the drug has about 12 times greater affinity for α_1-adrenergic receptors in the prostate than for those in the aorta. Such selectivity of tamsulosin for α_{1A}-receptors may result in a reduced incidence of adverse cardiovascular effects (e.g., syncope, dizziness, hypotension). On a molar basis, the α_1-adrenergic receptor affinity of tamsulosin is about 6 times that of prazosin when tested in human prostatic tissue.

Because of the prevalence of α-receptors on the prostate capsule, prostate adenoma, and bladder trigone and the relative absence of these receptors on the bladder body, α-adrenergic blocking agents decrease urinary outflow resistance in men.

SumMon® (see Users Guide). For additional information on this drug until a more detailed monograph is developed and published, the manufacturer's labeling should be consulted. It is *essential* that the labeling be consulted for detailed information on the usual cautions, precautions, and contraindications.

Preparations

Excipients in commercially available drug preparations may have clinically important effects in some individuals; consult specific product labeling for details.

Tamsulosin

Oral		
Capsules	0.4 mg	**Flomax®**, Boehringer Ingelheim

SKELETAL MUSCLE RELAXANTS 12:20

CENTRALLY ACTING SKELETAL MUSCLE RELAXANTS 12:20.04

Cyclobenzaprine Hydrochloride

■ Cyclobenzaprine is a centrally acting skeletal muscle relaxant.

Uses

■ **Muscular Conditions** Cyclobenzaprine is used as an adjunct to rest and physical therapy for the relief of muscular spasm associated with acute, painful musculoskeletal conditions. Skeletal muscle relaxants generally appear to be more effective than placebo in providing symptomatic relief of acute low back pain, but are associated with a high incidence of adverse effects. Although comparative studies are limited, available data suggest that various skeletal muscle relaxants generally have similar efficacy for such use. Acute low back pain usually is a benign and self-limiting condition that improves spontaneously over time; if pharmacologic therapy is required, an analgesic agent such as acetaminophen or a nonsteroidal anti-inflammatory agent (NSAIA) generally is recommended as first-line therapy for most patients. Skeletal muscle relaxants (alone or in combination with analgesics) may be used as an option for short-term relief of acute low back pain; however, the possibility of adverse effects, particularly adverse CNS effects, should be considered. In general, skeletal muscle relaxants should be used with caution after weighing the potential risks against the benefits in individual patients.

Efficacy of cyclobenzaprine hydrochloride 10 mg initially was established in 8 controlled clinical studies comparing cyclobenzaprine, diazepam, and placebo for their effect on muscle spasm, local pain and tenderness, limitation of motion, and restriction in activities of daily living. Improvement in patients receiving cyclobenzaprine was substantially greater than in those receiving diazepam in 3 studies and was comparable to diazepam in the remaining 5 studies.

Efficacy of cyclobenzaprine hydrochloride 5 mg was evaluated in 2 controlled clinical studies; in one study patients received cyclobenzaprine hydrochloride 5 or 10 mg or placebo 3 times daily, and in the second study patients received 2.5 or 5 mg of the drug or placebo 3 times daily. In both studies, efficacy of cyclobenzaprine hydrochloride 5 mg was substantially greater than placebo for patient-assessed primary end points (i.e., global impression of change, medication helpfulness, and relief from starting backache) by the seventh day of treatment. In addition, cyclobenzaprine 5 mg was substantially more effective than placebo for a physician-assessed secondary end point (reduction in presence and extent of palpable muscle spasm). In the study comparing cyclobenzaprine 5 or 10 mg 3 times daily with placebo, both dosages of the drug were substantially more effective than placebo by the third or fourth day (48–72 hours after the first dose of medication) of treatment. The only efficacy-related difference between the 2 dosages was in onset of patient-rated relief from starting backache, which occurred after the third or fourth dose in patients receiving 5 mg but after the first 2 doses in patients receiving 10 mg. In the second study, the 2.5 mg dosage of cyclobenzaprine was no more effective than placebo.

Analysis of data from controlled studies indicates that an effective dosage of cyclobenzaprine may produce clinical improvement whether or not sedation occurs. A subanalysis of data from patients in both studies who received either cyclobenzaprine hydrochloride (5 mg 3 times daily) or placebo and did not report somnolence demonstrated a meaningful treatment effect for all primary efficacy variables for the 5-mg dose despite the absence of somnolence in these patients. The manufacturer states that no well-controlled clinical studies have been performed to determine whether cyclobenzaprine will enhance the clinical effects of aspirin or other analgesics or vice versa when such combinations are used to manage acute musculoskeletal conditions.

Some data suggest that cyclobenzaprine may be useful for the treatment of fibrositis†. Cyclobenzaprine is ineffective in the treatment of spasticity associated with cerebral or spinal disease or in children with cerebral palsy.

Dosage and Administration

■ **Administration** Cyclobenzaprine hydrochloride is administered orally.

■ **Dosage** ***Muscular Conditions*** The recommended oral dosage of cyclobenzaprine hydrochloride for most adults and adolescents 15 years of age and older is 5 mg 3 times daily. Depending on response, dosage may be increased to 10 mg 3 times daily. The manufacturer states that cyclobenzaprine should be used only for short periods (e.g., up to 2–3 weeks) because adequate evidence of effectiveness for more prolonged use is not available and because muscle spasm associated with acute, painful musculoskeletal conditions generally is of short duration and specific therapy for longer periods seldom is warranted.

Dosage in Hepatic Impairment The manufacturer states that cyclobenzaprine hydrochloride dosage should be initiated with caution and less frequent dosing should be considered in patients with mild hepatic impairment, beginning with a 5 mg dose and slowly titrating upward. Use of the drug is not recommended in patients with moderate or severe hepatic impairment.

Dosage in Geriatric Patients The manufacturer states that less frequent dosing should be considered in geriatric patients, initiating cyclobenzaprine hydrochloride with a 5 mg dose and titrating upward slowly.

Cautions

The most common adverse effects reported in patients receiving cyclobenzaprine in clinical studies were drowsiness, dry mouth, dizziness, fatigue, and headache. Cyclobenzaprine is closely related to the tricyclic antidepressants, and the possibility that cyclobenzaprine may cause adverse effects similar to those of the tricyclic antidepressants should be considered.

■ **Nervous System Effects** Drowsiness occurred in 29 or 38% of patients receiving cyclobenzaprine 5 or 10 mg, respectively, compared with 10% of those receiving placebo in controlled studies; drowsiness also was reported in 39 or 16% of patients receiving cyclobenzaprine 10 mg in controlled studies or during postmarketing surveillance, respectively. Dizziness occurred in 1–3% of patients receiving cyclobenzaprine 5 or 10 mg in controlled studies, and in 11 or 3% of patients receiving cyclobenzaprine 10 mg in clinical studies or during postmarketing surveillance, respectively. Fatigue occurred in 6% of patients receiving either 5 or 10 mg of cyclobenzaprine compared with 3% of those receiving placebo in controlled studies; fatigue or tiredness occurred in 1–3% of patients receiving 10 mg of the drug in controlled studies and in postmarketing surveillance.

Headache occurred in 5% of those receiving 5 or 10 mg of cyclobenzaprine and in 8% of those receiving placebo in controlled studies; headache occurred in 1–3% of patients receiving 10 mg of the drug in controlled studies and postmarketing surveillance. Irritability, decreased mental acuity, nervousness, asthenia, and confusion occurred in 1–3% of patients receiving 5 or 10 mg of cyclobenzaprine in controlled studies or during postmarketing surveillance in patients receiving 10 mg of the drug.

Malaise, seizures, ataxia, vertigo, dysarthria, hypertonia, tremors, disorientation, insomnia, depressed mood, abnormal sensations, anxiety, agitation, psychosis, abnormal thinking, abnormal dreaming, hallucinations, excitement, paresthesia, and diplopia were reported during postmarketing surveillance or in less than 1% of patients receiving 10 mg of the drug in controlled studies. Other adverse nervous system effects that have been reported in patients receiving other tricyclic drugs or rarely with cyclobenzaprine but for which a causal relationship with the drug could not be established include decreased or increased libido, abnormal gait, delusions, aggressive behavior, paranoia, peripheral neuropathy, Bell's palsy, alterations in EEG patterns, and extrapyramidal manifestations.

■ **GI Effects** Dry mouth occurred in 21 or 32% of patients receiving 5 or 10 mg, respectively, of cyclobenzaprine and in 7% of those receiving placebo in controlled studies. Dry mouth also occurred in 27 or 7% of patients receiving 10 mg of the drug in clinical studies or during postmarketing surveillance, respectively. Abdominal pain, acid regurgitation, dyspepsia, constipation, diarrhea, nausea, and unpleasant taste occurred in 1–3% of patients receiving 5 or 10 mg of cyclobenzaprine in controlled studies or during postmarketing surveillance in patients receiving 10 mg of the drug. Vomiting, anorexia, GI pain, gastritis, thirst, edema of the tongue, and flatulence were reported during postmarketing surveillance or in less than 1% of patients receiving 10 mg of the drug in controlled studies. Paralytic ileus, tongue discoloration, stomatitis, and parotid swelling were reported in patients receiving other tricyclic drugs or rarely with cyclobenzaprine, but a causal relationship with cyclobenzaprine could not be established.

■ Respiratory Effects Upper respiratory infection and pharyngitis occurred in 1–3% of patients receiving cyclobenzaprine 5 or 10 mg in controlled studies. Dyspnea was reported in patients receiving other tricyclic drugs or rarely with cyclobenzaprine, but a causal relationship with cyclobenzaprine could not be established.

■ Cardiovascular Effects Syncope, tachycardia, arrhythmia, vasodilation, palpitation, and hypotension were reported during postmarketing experience or in less than 1% of patients receiving cyclobenzaprine 10 mg in clinical studies; hypertension, myocardial infarction, heart block, and stroke have been reported in patients receiving other tricyclic drugs or rarely with cyclobenzaprine, but a causal relationship with cyclobenzaprine could not be established.

■ Dermatologic and Sensitivity Reactions Anaphylaxis, angioedema, pruritus, facial edema, urticaria, rash, and sweating occurred during postmarketing experience or in less than 1% of patients receiving cyclobenzaprine 10 mg in clinical studies; photosensitivity, and alopecia have been reported in patients receiving other tricyclic drugs or rarely with cyclobenzaprine, but a causal relationship with cyclobenzaprine could not be established.

■ Musculoskeletal Effects Local weakness and muscle twitching were reported during postmarketing experience or in less than 1% of patients receiving cyclobenzaprine 10 mg in clinical studies; myalgia was reported in patients receiving other tricyclic drugs or rarely with cyclobenzaprine, but a causal relationship with cyclobenzaprine could not be established.

■ Genitourinary Effects Urinary frequency and/or urinary retention were reported during postmarketing experience or in less than 1% of patients receiving cyclobenzaprine 10 mg in clinical studies; impaired urination, dilatation of the urinary tract, impotence, testicular swelling, gynecomastia, breast enlargement, and galactorrhea have been reported in patients receiving other tricyclic drugs or rarely with cyclobenzaprine, but a causal relationship with cyclobenzaprine could not be established.

■ Hematologic Effects Purpura, bone marrow depression, leukopenia, eosinophilia, and thrombocytopenia have been reported in patients receiving other tricyclic drugs or rarely with cyclobenzaprine, but a causal relationship with cyclobenzaprine could not be established.

■ Hepatic Effects Abnormal liver function and rarely, hepatitis, jaundice, and cholestasis were reported during postmarketing experience or in less than 1% of patients receiving cyclobenzaprine 10 mg in clinical studies.

■ Other Adverse Effects Blurred vision was reported in 1–3% of patients receiving cyclobenzaprine 10 mg in controlled studies or in postmarketing surveillance. Tinnitus and ageusia each have been reported during postmarketing surveillance or in less than 1% of patients receiving cyclobenzaprine 10 mg in controlled studies.

Elevation or reduction of blood glucose, weight gain or loss, syndrome of inappropriate antidiuretic hormone (SIADH), chest pain, and edema have been reported in patients receiving other tricyclic drugs or rarely with cyclobenzaprine, but a causal relationship with cyclobenzaprine could not be established.

■ Precautions and Contraindications Cyclobenzaprine shares the toxic and drug interaction potentials of the tricyclic antidepressants, and the usual precautions of tricyclic antidepressant therapy should be observed. (See Cautions and see Drug Interactions in the Tricyclic Antidepressants General Statement 28:16.04.28.) The possibility that cyclobenzaprine may cause other adverse effects similar to those of the tricyclic antidepressants should be kept in mind, especially when the dosage for musculoskeletal conditions is exceeded.

Cyclobenzaprine should be used with caution in patients with mild hepatic impairment, and its use is not recommended in patients with moderate or severe hepatic impairment. Plasma concentrations of cyclobenzaprine are increased in patients with hepatic impairment, and such patients generally are more susceptible to sedation caused by some drugs, including cyclobenzaprine. Therefore, when cyclobenzaprine is used in patients with mild hepatic impairment, dosage should be titrated carefully, usually initiating therapy at the low end of the dosage range. (See Dosage and Administration: Dosage in Hepatic Impairment.)

Because cyclobenzaprine has adverse anticholinergic effects, it should be used with caution in patients with a history of urinary retention, angle-closure glaucoma, or increased intraocular pressure or in patients receiving anticholinergic drugs. Patients should be warned that cyclobenzaprine may impair their ability to perform hazardous activities requiring mental alertness or physical coordination such as operating machinery or driving a motor vehicle, particularly when the drug is used with alcohol or other CNS depressants.

Cyclobenzaprine is contraindicated in patients with hyperthyroidism, congestive heart failure, arrhythmias, heart block or conduction disorders, known hypersensitivity to the drug or any ingredient in the formulation and in the acute recovery phase following myocardial infarction. Cyclobenzaprine also is contraindicated in patients receiving monoamine oxidase inhibitors and should not be used within 14 days following discontinuance of these agents.

■ Pediatric Precautions Safety and efficacy of cyclobenzaprine in children and adolescents younger than 15 years of age have not been established.

■ Geriatric Precautions Plasma concentrations of cyclobenzaprine and the frequency and severity of adverse effects, with or without other concomitantly used drugs, are increased in the elderly. Geriatric patients receiving cyclobenzaprine may be at increased risk for adverse CNS effects (e.g., hallucinations, confusion, sedation), adverse cardiovascular effects resulting in falls or other sequelae, and interactions with other drugs or diseases. Therefore, cyclobenzaprine should be used in the elderly only if clearly needed. Dosage should be titrated carefully in geriatric patients, initiating therapy at the low end of the dosage range. (See Dosage and Administration: Dosage in Geriatric Patients.)

■ Pregnancy, Fertility, and Lactation Reproduction studies in rats, mice, and rabbits using cyclobenzaprine doses up to 20 times the human dose have not revealed evidence of harm to the fetus. There are no adequate and controlled studies to date using cyclobenzaprine in pregnant women, and the drug should be used during pregnancy only when clearly needed.

Reproduction studies in rats, mice, and rabbits receiving cyclobenzaprine have not revealed evidence of impaired fertility.

It is not known whether cyclobenzaprine is distributed into milk; however, the drug is distributed into milk in rats. Because some related tricyclic antidepressants are distributed into milk, cyclobenzaprine should be used with caution in nursing women.

Drug Interactions

Cyclobenzaprine is structurally and pharmacologically related to tricyclic antidepressants and shares the drug interaction potentials of these drugs. For additional information on potential drug interactions of tricyclic antidepressants, see Drug Interactions in the Tricyclic Antidepressants General Statement 28:16.04.28.

■ Monoamine Oxidase Inhibitors Concomitant use of cyclobenzaprine or structurally similar tricyclic antidepressants with monoamine oxidase (MAO) inhibitors has resulted in hyperpyretic crisis, seizures, and death. Cyclobenzaprine is contraindicated in patients receiving MAO inhibitors and should not be used within 14 days following discontinuance of these drugs.

■ CNS Depressants Cyclobenzaprine may be additive with or may potentiate the action of other CNS depressants (e.g., alcohol, barbiturates). Cyclobenzaprine, especially when used concomitantly with alcohol or other CNS depressants, may impair the patient's ability to perform activities requiring mental alertness or physical coordination (e.g., operating machinery, driving a motor vehicle).

■ Tramadol Cyclobenzaprine and structurally similar tricyclic antidepressants may enhance the risk of seizures in patients receiving tramadol. For additional information about the risk of seizures in patients receiving these drugs, see Precautions and Contraindications: Seizures in Cautions in Tramadol 28:08.08.

■ Hypotensive Agents Cyclobenzaprine and structurally similar tricyclic antidepressants may block the hypotensive effects of guanethidine (no longer commercially available in the US) and other similarly acting drugs.

■ Nonsteroidal Anti-inflammatory Agents Concomitant use of cyclobenzaprine with diflunisal or naproxen reportedly was well tolerated and did not appear to result in any unexpected adverse effects. However, concomitant use of cyclobenzaprine with naproxen has been associated with an increased incidence of drowsiness. Plasma concentrations of aspirin or cyclobenzaprine were unaffected when the drugs were administered concomitantly. It has not been established whether combined therapy with cyclobenzaprine and aspirin (or other analgesics) will result in enhanced clinical efficacy.

Acute Toxicity

Because the management of overdose is complex and changing, clinicians should consult a poison control center for additional information on the management of cyclobenzaprine overdosage. Cyclobenzaprine is structurally related to and shares the toxic potentials of the tricyclic antidepressants. For additional information about pathogenesis, manifestations, and treatment of toxic doses of structurally similar tricyclic antidepressants, see Acute Toxicity in the Tricyclic Antidepressants General Statement 28:16.04.28.

■ Pathogenesis The manufacturer states that the acute oral LD_{50} of cyclobenzaprine is about 338 and 425 mg/kg in mice and rats, respectively.

■ Manifestations Manifestations of toxicity may develop rapidly after a cyclobenzaprine overdose, and rarely, death may occur. The most common toxic effects associated with cyclobenzaprine overdose are drowsiness and tachycardia; less frequent manifestations include tremor, agitation, coma, ataxia, hypertension, slurred speech, confusion, dizziness, nausea, vomiting, and hallucinations. Rarely, potentially serious effects may include cardiac arrest, chest pain, cardiac dysrhythmias, severe hypotension, seizures, and neuroleptic malignant syndrome.

■ **Treatment** Treatment of cyclobenzaprine overdosage, as in that of structurally similar tricyclic antidepressants, generally involves symptomatic and supportive care. Because of the potential for rapid clinical deterioration, cardiac function should be monitored, and IV access should be established; early endotracheal intubation and maintenance of an adequate airway are advised in patients with CNS depression and/or substantial ECG changes (e.g., wide-complex tachycardia).

The manufacturer states that all patients suspected of an overdose with cyclobenzaprine should receive GI decontamination, including gastric lavage; induction of emesis is contraindicated if consciousness is impaired. However, the management of overdose is complex and changing, and clinicians should consult a poison control center for additional information on the management of cyclobenzaprine overdosage, particularly in pediatric patients. Instillation of activated charcoal should occur in all adults and children suspected of cyclobenzaprine ingestion if an endotracheal tube with cuff inflated is in place to prevent aspiration of gastric contents. For additional information about specific treatment of cardiovascular and CNS disturbances associated with toxic doses of tricyclic compounds, including cyclobenzaprine, see Acute Toxicity: Treatment in the Tricyclic Antidepressants General Statement 28:16.04.28.

Pharmacology

Cyclobenzaprine is a CNS depressant that has sedative and skeletal muscle relaxant effects. The precise mechanism of action of the drug is not known. Cyclobenzaprine does not directly relax skeletal muscle and, unlike neuromuscular blocking agents, does not depress neuronal conduction, neuromuscular transmission, or muscle excitability.

Like the tricyclic antidepressants, cyclobenzaprine potentiates the effects of norepinephrine and has anticholinergic effects.

Pharmacokinetics

■ **Absorption** Orally administered cyclobenzaprine is well absorbed. Cyclobenzaprine undergoes enterohepatic circulation, and appears to be metabolized during its first pass through the GI tract and/or liver. Mean oral bioavailability of the drug is estimated to range from 33–55%. Following oral administration of a single 5- or 10-mg dose of cyclobenzaprine hydrochloride, peak plasma concentrations of 4.3 or 8.5 ng/mL, respectively, are attained in about 4 hours. When cyclobenzaprine is administered 3 times daily, steady-state plasma concentrations are attained within 3–4 days that are about fourfold greater than those after a single dose. In healthy individuals receiving the drug 3 times daily, a mean steady-state peak plasma cyclobenzaprine concentration of 14.9 or 25.9 ng/mL was achieved at 4 or 3.9 hours after administration of a 5 or 10 mg dose, respectively.

Values for steady-state mean area under the cyclobenzaprine concentration time curve (AUC) were about 1.7 times greater in male and female individuals 65 years of age and older than in younger adults. Mean AUCs in geriatric males were about 2.4 times greater than in younger males, and those in elderly females were about 1.2 times greater than in younger females. (See Cautions: Geriatric Precautions.)

Peak plasma cyclobenzaprine concentrations and AUCs in 15 patients with mild hepatic impairment (and one with moderate hepatic impairment) were twice those observed in healthy individuals. Insufficient data exist to establish the safety of cyclobenzaprine use in patients with moderate or severe hepatic impairment. (See Cautions: Precautions and Contraindications.)

■ **Distribution** Cyclobenzaprine is widely distributed into body tissues. It is not known if cyclobenzaprine is distributed into milk in humans; however, the drug is distributed into milk in rats. It is not known if cyclobenzaprine crosses the placenta. The drug is extensively (about 93%) bound to plasma protein.

■ **Elimination** Cyclobenzaprine is extensively metabolized by both oxidative and conjugative pathways. Hepatic cytochrome P-450 (CYP) 3A4, 1A2, and (to a lesser extent) 2D6 isoenzymes are responsible for oxidative *N*-demethylation of the drug. Orally administered cyclobenzaprine is excreted in urine principally as inactive glucuronide metabolites; less than 1% of the drug is excreted renally as unchanged drug. Elimination of the drug is slow; plasma clearance is 700 mL/minute per 1.73 m^2 and the effective elimination half-life is about 18 hours (range: 8–37 hours). Decreased clearance and increased plasma concentrations of the drug occur in the elderly and those with hepatic impairment. (See Cautions: Precautions and Contraindications and see Cautions: Geriatric Precautions.)

Chemistry and Stability

■ **Chemistry** Cyclobenzaprine is a centrally acting skeletal muscle relaxant that is structurally and pharmacologically related to the tricyclic antidepressants. Cyclobenzaprine hydrochloride occurs as a white to off-white, crystalline powder and is freely soluble in water and in alcohol. The drug has a pK_a of 8.47.

■ **Stability** Commercially available cyclobenzaprine hydrochloride tablets should be stored at a controlled room temperature of 25°C but may be exposed to temperatures ranging from 15–30°C.

For further information on cautions, acute toxicity, and drug interactions of cyclobenzaprine hydrochloride, see the Tricyclic Antidepressants General Statement 28:16.04.28.

Preparations

Excipients in commercially available drug preparations may have clinically important effects in some individuals; consult specific product labeling for details.

Cyclobenzaprine Hydrochloride

Oral

Tablets, film-coated	5 mg	**Flexeril®**, McNeil
	10 mg*	**Flexeril®**, McNeil

*available from one or more manufacturer, distributor, and/or repackager by generic (nonproprietary) name

†Use is not currently included in the labeling approved by the US Food and Drug Administration

tiZANidine Hydrochloride

■ Tizanidine hydrochloride, a centrally acting α_2-adrenergic agonist, is a skeletal muscle relaxant.

Uses

■ **Spasticity** Tizanidine is used alone or in conjunction with other standard therapies (e.g., baclofen) for the management of spasticity associated with cerebral or spinal injury. In these patients, tizanidine decreases the number and severity of spasms, alleviates clonus, and improves mobility to a greater extent than does placebo. Some evidence from comparative studies suggests that tizanidine may produce muscle weakness less frequently than other antispastic agents (e.g., baclofen, diazepam). The manufacturer states that because of its short duration of effect, tizanidine should be reserved for those daily activities and times when relief of spasticity is most important.

Efficacy for the management of spasticity has been demonstrated in 2 placebo-controlled, randomized studies in patients with multiple sclerosis or spinal cord injury. In these studies, patients 18–75 years of age received initial tizanidine hydrochloride dosages of 2 or 4 mg daily, which were titrated according to response and tolerance to a maximum of 36 mg (in up to 3 divided doses) daily over a 3-week period. Following initial dosage titration, tizanidine hydrochloride dosages averaged 30.7–31.1 mg daily. Based on changes in Ashworth scores (a 5-point rating scale for assessing muscle tone, with 0 representing normal muscle tone and 4 representing immobilization of the muscle by spasticity), reductions in muscle tone were greater with tizanidine than with placebo during dosage titration, plateau, and/or study end point assessments. Mean reductions from baseline in Ashworth scores at the end point assessment were 4.41 and 0.44 for the tizanidine and placebo groups, respectively, in one study and 4.4 and 1.2, respectively, in the other study. However, in the larger of these studies, reductions in muscle tone (primary outcome measure) with tizanidine were not associated with comparable improvements in secondary outcome measures such as muscle strength, the frequency of daytime muscle spasms, pain, or deep tendon reflex activity. Improvement in muscle tone with tizanidine therapy was not consistently associated with improvements in quality of life as determined by activities of daily living (ADL) assessment scores.

In comparative studies in patients with spasticity associated with multiple sclerosis or cerebrovascular disorders, principally stroke, tizanidine's ability to improve muscle tone has been shown to be similar to that of baclofen or diazepam. Combined analysis of data from studies of 4–8 weeks' duration indicated improvements in muscle tone, spasms, and clonus in about 50–67% of patients treated with any of these drugs, while improvement in muscle strength was noted in about 33% of such patients. In these studies, patients receiving tizanidine exhibited better retention of muscle strength than those receiving baclofen or diazepam, and the incidence of somnolence was somewhat lower with tizanidine than with diazepam.

Concomitant therapy with tizanidine and another antispastic agent (e.g., baclofen) reportedly may allow control of spasticity with lower dosages of each agent. However, it should be kept in mind that such concomitant therapy may cause additive sedative effects (see Drug Interactions: Alcohol and Other CNS Depressants); some clinicians suggest that tizanidine not be given concomitantly with benzodiazepines (e.g., diazepam).

Dosage and Administration

■ **General** Tizanidine hydrochloride is administered orally. Food has complex effects on the pharmacokinetics of tizanidine, and these effects differ between the commercially available capsule and tablet formulations. Clinically important differences (e.g., increased adverse effects, delayed or more rapid onset of activity) may be apparent when switching administration of capsules or tablets between fed and/or fasting states, switching between capsules and tablets in the fed state, or switching between administration of intact capsules and sprinkling capsule contents on applesauce. Clinicians should be thoroughly familiar with possible pharmacokinetic changes associated with these conditions. (See Description.)

Dosage of tizanidine hydrochloride is expressed in terms of tizanidine.

The dosage of tizanidine should be individualized according to the patient's requirements and response using the lowest dosage that produces optimum response without adverse effects. While single doses of tizanidine smaller than 8 mg have not been shown to be effective in controlled clinical studies, initiation of tizanidine therapy with single doses of 4 mg is recommended to minimize the incidence of common dose-related adverse effects (e.g., orthostatic hypotension). The dose can be repeated every 6–8 hours as needed for a maximum of 3 doses in 24 hours. Dosage of tizanidine may be increased gradually in increments of 2–4 mg daily until optimum therapeutic effects are obtained with tolerable adverse effects; optimum dosage generally can be attained over a period of 2–4 weeks.

Clinical experience is limited with single doses exceeding 8 mg or total daily dosages exceeding 24 mg, and the manufacturer states that there is essentially no experience with repeated single or total daily dosages exceeding 12 or 36 mg, respectively. The dosage of tizanidine in adults should not exceed 36 mg in any 24-hour period.

■ **Special Populations** Initiate with caution in patients with renal impairment (creatinine clearance less than 25 mL/minute). In these patients, the manufacturer recommends using smaller individual doses during dosage titration. If higher doses are needed, the manufacturer recommends increasing the amount of each individual dose rather than increasing the frequency of dosing.

Pharmacokinetics not studied in patients with hepatic impairment; however, tizanidine is known to undergo extensive first-pass hepatic metabolism. Therefore, the manufacturer recommends that the drug be avoided or used only with extreme caution in patients with hepatic impairment.

Although use of tizanidine ordinarily should be avoided in women taking oral contraceptives, if the drug is considered clinically necessary in such women, the initial dosage and rate of titration should be reduced. (See Drug Interactions: Oral Contraceptives.)

Cautions

■ **Contraindications** Concomitant therapy with ciprofloxacin or fluvoxamine. (See Drug Interactions.)

Known hypersensitivity to tizanidine hydrochloride or any ingredient in the formulation.

■ **Warnings/Precautions** ***Warnings*** **Limited Experience with Long-term Use of Higher Dosages.** Clinical experience with long-term use of tizanidine at single doses of 8–16 mg or total daily dosages of 24–36 mg is limited. Therefore, only adverse effects with a relatively high incidence are likely to have been identified in long-term clinical studies. (See Dosage and Administration.)

Hypotension. Hypotension was reported in two-thirds of patients treated with 8 mg of tizanidine in a single-dose study. Patients in the study had a 20% reduction in either diastolic or systolic blood pressures within 1 hour after dosing; hypotensive effects peaked 2–3 hours after dosing and were occasionally associated with bradycardia, orthostatic effects, dizziness, and, rarely, syncope. Tizanidine's hypotensive effect is dose related. The risk of marked hypotension may therefore be minimized by careful dosage titration; patients should be observed for manifestations of hypotension prior to dosage adjustment. (See Advice to Patients.)

Tizanidine should be used with caution in patients receiving concomitant antihyperdensive therapy. (See Drug Interactions: Hypotensive Agents.) Concomitant use of tizanidine and other α_2-adrenergic agonists (e.g., clonidine) is not recommended.

Because clinically important hypotension has been reported with concurrent use of either fluvoxamine or ciprofloxacin, these drugs are contraindicated in patients receiving tizanidine. (See Drug Interactions.)

Risk of Liver Injury. Liver injury (most often hepatocellular in type) has been reported occasionally. Elevations (i.e., exceeding 3 times the upper limit of normal, or 2 times the upper limit of normal if baseline levels were elevated) of ALT or AST have occurred in approximately 5% of patients receiving tizanidine in controlled clinical studies. Nausea, vomiting, anorexia, and jaundice occasionally have been reported in patients with elevated aminotransferase concentrations. Death associated with liver failure has been reported rarely.

Monitoring of serum aminotransferase concentrations should be performed prior to and during the first 6 months of treatment (e.g., at baseline and at 1, 3, and 6 months) and periodically thereafter based on clinical status. Tizanidine should be avoided or used only with extreme caution in patients with impaired hepatic function. (See Hepatic Impairment under Warnings/Precautions: Specific Populations, in Cautions.)

Sedation. Sedation was reported in 48% of patients receiving any dose of tizanidine in multiple-dose, controlled clinical studies. Sedation was rated as severe by 10% of these tizanidine-treated patients compared with less than 1% of patients receiving placebo. Risk of sedation appears to be dose related. Sedation may interfere with daily activity. During multiple-dose studies, the prevalence of sedation peaked following the first week of dosage titration, then remained stable for the duration of the maintenance treatment phase. In comparative studies with baclofen or diazepam, the incidence of somnolence/drowsiness in patients receiving tizanidine or baclofen (15–67%) was slightly lower than that in patients receiving diazepam (44–82%).

Hallucinations/Psychotic-like Symptoms. Hallucinations (formed, visual) or delusions were reported in 5 of 170 patients (3%) receiving tizanidine in 2 North American controlled studies. All of these cases occurred within the first 6 weeks of therapy. Psychoses associated with hallucinations have been reported in at least one patient.

Potential Interaction with Fluvoxamine or Ciprofloxacin. In pharmacokinetic studies, substantial increases in serum tizanidine concentrations were observed during concurrent administration of fluvoxamine or ciprofloxacin; potentiated hypotensive and sedative effects also were observed. Concurrent administration of tizanidine with either fluvoxamine or ciprofloxacin is contraindicated. (See Drug Interactions.)

Potential Interaction with Other CYP1A2 Inhibitors. Because of potential drug interactions, concurrent administration of tizanidine with other cytochrome P-450 (CYP) isoenzyme 1A2 (CYP1A2) inhibitors should ordinarily be avoided. However, if their concomitant use is considered clinically necessary, the drugs should be used with caution. (See Drug Interactions: Drugs Affecting or Metabolized by Hepatic Microsomal Enzymes.)

General Precautions **Cardiovascular Effects.** Prolongation of the QT interval and bradycardia were reported in chronic toxicity studies in animals at dosages equal to the maximum recommended human daily dosage on a mg/m² basis. ECG evaluation was not included in controlled clinical studies, but pulse rate reduction in association with decreases in blood pressure has been reported in patients receiving single doses of tizanidine.

Ocular Effects. Evidence of dose-related retinal degeneration and corneal opacities has been reported in animal studies at tizanidine dosages equivalent to approximately the maximum recommended human daily dosage on a mg/m² basis. Retinal degeneration and corneal opacities have not been reported to date in clinical studies.

Use in Women Taking Oral Contraceptives. Because drug interaction studies have demonstrated that concurrent use of tizanidine and oral contraceptives may substantially reduce the clearance of tizanidine, concomitant use should ordinarily be avoided. However, if the drug is considered clinically necessary, tizanidine dosage adjustment is recommended. (See Dosage and Administration: Special Populations and also see Drug Interactions: Oral Contraceptives.)

Discontinuance of Therapy. Tizanidine is pharmacologically related to clonidine, and rebound manifestations similar to those reported with abrupt withdrawal of clonidine therapy, including hypertension, tachycardia, hypertonia, tremor, and anxiety, have been reported upon sudden withdrawal of tizanidine therapy.

If tizanidine therapy is to be discontinued, dosage of the drug should be decreased gradually, particularly in patients who have been receiving high dosages for prolonged periods, to minimize the risk of withdrawal and rebound symptoms.

Specific Populations **Pregnancy.** Category C. (See Users Guide.)

Lactation. It is not known whether tizanidine is distributed into milk in humans. However, because it is lipid-soluble, tizanidine might be expected to pass into milk in humans. Tizanidine should be used with caution in nursing women.

Pediatric Use. Safety and efficacy not established in children.

Geriatric Use. The manufacturer states that clearance is decreased fourfold in this patient population. Tizanidine should be used with caution in geriatric patients.

Hepatic Impairment. Although the pharmacokinetics of tizanidine have not been evaluated in patients with hepatic impairment, the drug undergoes extensive first-pass metabolism in the liver. Therefore, hepatic impairment would be expected to have substantial effects on tizanidine pharmacokinetics. The manufacturer states that tizanidine ordinarily should be avoided or used only with extreme caution in patients with impaired hepatic function. (See Risk of Liver Injury under Warnings/Precautions: Warnings, in Cautions.)

Renal Impairment. Clearance of tizanidine reportedly is reduced by greater than 50% in patients with a creatinine clearance less than 25 mL/minute. Tizanidine should be used with caution in patients with renal impairment. Patients should be monitored closely for onset or increased severity of common adverse effects (e.g., dry mouth, somnolence, asthenia, dizziness) that may indicate potential overdosage. (See Special Populations under Dosage and Administration.)

■ **Common Adverse Effects** Adverse effects reported in greater than 2% of patients receiving tizanidine in multiple-dose, controlled clinical studies include dry mouth, somnolence, asthenia (weakness, fatigue, and/or tiredness), dizziness, urinary tract infection, infection, constipation, abnormal liver function test results (e.g., elevated ALT), vomiting, speech disorder, amblyopia (blurred vision), urinary frequency, flu symptoms, dyskinesia, nervousness, pharyngitis, and rhinitis. In addition, hypotension and bradycardia also have been reported in single-dose, placebo-controlled studies.

Drug Interactions

■ **Drugs Affecting or Metabolized by Hepatic Microsomal Enzymes** Potential pharmacokinetic interaction; decreased plasma clearance of tizanidine may occur when tizanidine is given concurrently with other inhibitors of cytochrome P-450 (CYP) isoenzyme 1A2, including acyclovir, antiarrhythmics (e.g., amiodarone, mexiletine, propafenone, verapamil), cimetidine, famotidine, fluvoxamine (see Drug Interactions: Fluvoxamine), fluoroquinolones (e.g., ciprofloxacin [see Drug Interactions: Ciprofloxacin]), oral contraceptives (see Drug Interactions: Oral Contraceptives), ticlopidine, and zileuton. Concomitant use ordinarily should be avoided; if considered clinically necessary, the drugs should be used with caution.

Tizanidine and its major metabolites are not likely to affect the metabolism of other drugs metabolized by CYP isoenzymes.

■ **Hypotensive Agents** Potential pharmacologic interaction (additive hypotensive effects) when used concomitantly with antihypertensive agents; should not be used with other α_2-adrenergic agonists (e.g., clonidine).

■ **Acetaminophen** Potential pharmacokinetic interaction (delayed time to peak plasma concentration of acetaminophen). Acetaminophen does not affect pharmacokinetics of tizanidine.

■ **Alcohol and Other CNS Depressants** Alcohol increased the areas under the plasma concentration-time curve (AUCs) and peak concentrations of tizanidine by approximately 20 and 15%, respectively; these changes were associated with an increase in adverse effects of tizanidine.

Potential pharmacologic interaction (additive CNS depression) with alcohol or other CNS depressants (e.g., baclofen, dantrolene, diazepam).

■ **Ciprofloxacin** Potential pharmacokinetic interaction; significantly increased plasma concentrations and AUCs of tizanidine have been observed with concomitant administration, resulting in increased risk of adverse cardiovascular (including substantial hypotension) and CNS (e.g., drowsiness, psychomotor impairment) effects associated with tizanidine use. Concomitant use of tizanidine and ciprofloxacin is contraindicated.

■ **Fluvoxamine** Potential pharmacokinetic interaction; significantly increased plasma concentrations, elimination half-life, and AUCs of tizanidine have been observed with concomitant administration, resulting in increased risk of adverse cardiovascular (including substantial hypotension) and CNS (e.g., drowsiness, psychomotor impairment) effects associated with tizanidine use. Concomitant use of tizanidine and fluvoxamine is contraindicated.

■ **Oral Contraceptives** Potential pharmacokinetic interaction; decreased plasma clearance (by up to 50%) of tizanidine reported with concomitant use. Although use of tizanidine ordinarily should be avoided in women taking oral contraceptives, if the drug is considered clinically necessary in such women, tizanidine dosage adjustment is recommended. (See Dosage and Administration: Special Populations.)

Description

Tizanidine hydrochloride, an imidazoline derivative, is a centrally acting α_2-adrenergic agonist with myotonolytic effects on skeletal muscle. Tizanidine is structurally and pharmacologically related to clonidine and other α_2-adrenergic agonists, but studies in animals indicate that tizanidine has one-tenth to one-fiftieth the potency of clonidine in lowering blood pressure. The exact mechanism of tizanidine in reducing muscle tone and spasm frequency is not clear. However, tizanidine reportedly decreases the frequency and amplitude of muscle spasms (tonic reflexes) that arise in response to muscle stretching in patients with various spinal cord lesions. The drug appears to reduce spasticity by increasing presynaptic inhibition of motor neurons, leading to reduced facilitation of spinal motor neurons and a resultant decrease in muscle tone. Tizanidine has its greatest effects on polysynaptic pathways, with no important effect on monosynaptic spinal reflexes. The drug does not have direct effects on skeletal muscle fibers or the neuromuscular junction. Tizanidine has been shown to have antinociceptive effects in animals, and some reports have suggested that it may improve pain associated with muscle spasm.

Tizanidine undergoes extensive first-pass hepatic metabolism. In fasting healthy individuals, peak plasma tizanidine concentrations are attained about 1 hour after administration of the commercially available capsules and tablets. The half-life of tizanidine averages about 2.5 hours. When tizanidine is administered as two 4-mg tablets with food, the mean peak plasma concentration is increased by about 30%, the median time to peak plasma concentration is increased from about 60 to about 85 minutes, and the extent of absorption is increased by about 30%.

When tizanidine is administered as the commercially available capsules, food decreases the mean peak plasma concentration by 20%, increases the median time to peak plasma concentration from about 1 hour to 3 hours, and increases the extent of absorption by about 10%. When given with food, the amount of tizanidine absorbed from the capsule is about 80% of the amount absorbed from the tablet. Administration of the capsule contents sprinkled on applesauce is not bioequivalent to administration of the intact capsule under fasting conditions and results in a 15–20% increase in peak plasma concentration and AUC and a 15-minute decrease in median lag time and time to achieve peak plasma concentration compared with administration of intact capsules while fasting.

Advice to Patients

Importance of advising patients of limited clinical experience with tizanidine with respect to both duration of therapy and the higher dosages necessary to reduce muscle tone.

Risk of marked orthostatic hypotension; importance of exercising caution when moving from a supine to a fixed upright position.

Risk of sedation, which may be additive when taken in conjunction with alcohol or other CNS depressants; importance of exercising caution when performing activities requiring alertness, including driving a motor vehicle or operating machinery.

Importance of not discontinuing tizanidine abruptly because of potential for rebound hypertension and tachycardia.

Importance of advising patients of potential changes in absorption profile and resulting changes in efficacy and adverse effect profile when taken with food.

Importance of informing clinicians of existing or contemplated concomitant therapy, including prescription and OTC drugs and herbal supplements, as well as any concomitant illnesses, and of informing clinicians or pharmacists whenever any drug is added or discontinued. Importance of not taking tizanidine concomitantly with either ciprofloxacin or fluvoxamine.

Importance of women informing clinicians if they are or plan to become pregnant or plan to breast-feed.

Importance of informing patients of other important precautionary information. (See Cautions.)

Overview® (see Users Guide). For additional information on this drug until a more detailed monograph is developed and published, the manufacturer's labeling should be consulted. It is *essential* that the manufacturer's labeling be consulted for more detailed information on usual cautions, precautions, contraindications, potential drug interactions, laboratory test interferences, and acute toxicity.

Preparations

Excipients in commercially available drug preparations may have clinically important effects in some individuals; consult specific product labeling for details.

tiZANidine Hydrochloride

Oral		
Capsules	2 mg (of tizanidine)	**Zanaflex®**, Acorda
	4 mg (of tizanidine)	**Zanaflex®**, Acorda
	6 mg (of tizanidine)	**Zanaflex®**, Acorda
Tablets	2 mg (of tizanidine)*	**Tizanidine Hydrochloride Tablets**
		Zanaflex® (scored), Acorda
	4 mg (of tizanidine)*	**Tizanidine Hydrochloride Tablets**
		Zanaflex® (scored), Acorda

*available from one or more manufacturer, distributor, and/or repackager by generic (nonproprietary) name

Selected Revisions August 2011, © Copyright, March 2003, American Society of Health-System Pharmacists, Inc.

DIRECT-ACTING SKELETAL MUSCLE RELAXANTS 12:20.08

Dantrolene Sodium

■ Dantrolene sodium is a direct-acting skeletal muscle relaxant.

Uses

■ **Spasticity** Dantrolene sodium is used orally in the management of spasticity resulting from upper motor neuron disorders such as multiple sclerosis, cerebral palsy, spinal cord injury, and stroke. Dantrolene is *not* indicated for the treatment of muscle spasms resulting from rheumatic disorders or musculoskeletal trauma and is ineffective in the management of amyotrophic lateral sclerosis.

Evidence supporting the use of dantrolene for spasticity is limited and the drug is associated with many adverse effects, some of which may be severe (e.g., hepatotoxicity). However, subtle but meaningful improvement (e.g., decrease in severity of spasticity, ability to resume daily function) may occasionally occur in some patients receiving the drug. In the management of spasticity, the manufacturer states that dantrolene is particularly useful in patients whose functional rehabilitation has been slowed by the sequelae of spasticity. For the drug to be beneficial, such patients must have presumably reversible spasticity where relief of spasticity will aid in restoring residual function. Although effective doses of dantrolene frequently cause muscle weakness, the patient may feel more confident in the use of his residual strength because of a parallel decrease in involuntary muscle activity. The desirability of long-term dantrolene therapy in ambulatory patients depends on the balance between the weakness and other adverse effects caused by the drug and the benefits obtained from its use. Adverse effects such as weakness may not be as important a consideration in paraplegic patients as in ambulatory patients.

There is presently no method of predicting which patients will benefit from dantrolene therapy; therefore, a therapeutic trial of the drug is necessary to determine the benefits to a specific individual. Many patients with chronic spasticity may not benefit from long-term (several months or longer) dantrolene therapy; however, the benefits may be considerable in some patients. Tolerance to the therapeutic effects of dantrolene apparently does not occur. Although the safety and efficacy of long-term therapy have not been established, long-term administration of dantrolene is considered justifiable if the drug produces a substantial reduction in painful and/or disabling spasticity or a reduction in the intensity of nursing care needed, or if annoying manifestations of spasticity are eliminated as judged by the patient. Subjective impressions of improvement noted by the physician, patient, or persons in close contact with the patient may sometimes be confirmed by withdrawal of the drug for 2–4 days. Observation of the patient for exacerbations of the condition during this time may demonstrate improvements which are otherwise difficult to document. Because of dantrolene's potential for causing liver damage, therapy with the drug should be continued only if it is clearly beneficial.

Compared with other drugs used for spasticity (e.g., baclofen, diazepam, tizanidine), dantrolene is a peripherally acting agent that exhibits direct effects on skeletal muscle; however, few controlled studies have been conducted comparing efficacy and tolerability of the various antispastic agents. In one study comparing dantrolene and diazepam in patients with multiple sclerosis, the drugs were about equally effective in relieving spasticity; diazepam was associated with more frequent CNS effects (e.g., drowsiness, incoordination, imbalance), while dantrolene was associated with more muscle weakness. Use of dantrolene in combination with other antispastic agents (e.g., diazepam) may produce better control of spasticity in some patients than either drug alone and enable a decrease in the dosage of either or both drugs. However, it should be considered that concomitant therapy may cause additive adverse effects. (See Cautions: Precautions and Contraindications.)

■ **Malignant Hyperthermia Crisis** IV dantrolene sodium is used with appropriate supportive measures in the management of fulminant hypermetabolism of skeletal muscle that is characteristic of malignant hyperthermia crisis, a rare inherited condition that can be triggered by certain inhaled anesthetic agents or succinylcholine. Dantrolene sodium for injectable suspension (Ryanodex®) has been designated an orphan drug by the FDA for this use. As soon as malignant hyperthermia crisis is recognized (i.e., tachycardia, tachypnea, central venous desaturation, hypercarbia, metabolic acidosis, skeletal muscle rigidity, increased utilization of anesthesia circuit carbon dioxide absorber, cyanosis and mottling of the skin, and, in many cases, fever), all anesthetic agents and other potential triggering agents (e.g., succinylcholine) should be discontinued immediately and IV dantrolene therapy initiated. IV dantrolene is used in conjunction with supportive measures, which include administering oxygen, treating metabolic acidosis, and instituting cooling procedures if necessary; urinary output and serum electrolytes should be monitored. The use of IV dantrolene in the management of malignant hyperthermia crisis is *not* a substitute for these supportive measures.

Since the combination of IV dantrolene and a calcium-channel blocking agent (e.g., diltiazem, verapamil) in anesthetized animals resulted in myocardial depression, ventricular fibrillation, and cardiovascular collapse in association with marked hyperkalemia, it is recommended that the combination of IV dantrolene and a calcium-channel blocking agent not be used during the management of malignant hyperthermia crisis. (See Drug Interactions: Calcium-Channel Blocking Agents.) If mannitol is used for the prevention or treatment of late renal complications of malignant hyperthermia, the amount of mannitol administered as part of the IV dantrolene formulation should be considered. When using the injectable suspension formulation of dantrolene sodium, a diuretic should be administered to prevent late kidney injury due to myoglobinuria because the amount of mannitol contained in the formulation is insufficient to maintain diuresis.

Following a malignant hyperthermia crisis, oral dantrolene is used for up to 3 days to prevent recurrence of manifestations of the condition; IV dantrolene may be used postoperatively for this purpose when oral therapy is not practical or feasible.

Dantrolene also has been used orally and/or IV prior to surgery to prevent or attenuate the development of malignant hyperthermia crisis in individuals thought to be at risk; however, prophylactic use of dantrolene no longer is recommended because of adverse effects and questionable benefit. Vital signs should be monitored in patients receiving dantrolene preoperatively, and the usual precautions associated with surgery in susceptible patients must still be employed since malignant hyperthermia may only be attenuated rather than prevented.

■ **Neuroleptic Malignant Syndrome** Although the manufacturer states that dantrolene currently is not indicated for the management of neuroleptic malignant syndrome (NMS)†, the drug has been used successfully in a limited number of patients with this syndrome. The manufacturer states that fatalities have occurred in patients with NMS despite therapy with the drug. Further study is needed to determine the efficacy and optimum dosage and route of administration of the drug in this condition.

■ **Other Uses** Dantrolene was also reportedly successful for the management of a fulminant hypermetabolic reaction induced by an acute overdosage of phenelzine†.

In one study, preoperative administration of dantrolene sodium substantially reduced the strength of succinylcholine-induced muscle fasciculations intraoperatively and decreased the incidence of postoperative muscle pain†.

Dosage and Administration

■ **Reconstitution and Administration** Dantrolene sodium is administered orally for the management of spasticity and its sequelae secondary to upper motor neuron disorders, and for prevention of the recurrence of malignant hyperthermia following initial IV therapy. For the acute management of malignant hyperthermia crisis, the drug is given by rapid IV injection. For preoperative prophylaxis of malignant hyperthermia in patients at risk, dantrolene may be administered orally or as an IV infusion.

For IV administration, dantrolene sodium is commercially available as a lyophilized drug for injection (e.g., Dantrium®, Revonto®, or generic equivalents) or a lyophilized drug for injectable suspension (Ryanodex®) that must be reconstituted. Reconstitution procedures differ based on the preparation; the manufacturer's prescribing information should be consulted for specific instructions on reconstitution, preparation, and administration of the drug. Because of the high pH of dantrolene sodium injection and the potential for tissue necrosis, care must be taken to avoid extravasation.

Dantrolene sodium for injection is reconstituted by adding 60 mL of sterile water for injection to the vial labeled as containing 20 mg of the drug and shaking the vial until the solution is clear. Bacteriostatic water for injection, 5% dextrose injection, or 0.9% sodium chloride injection should *not* be used. For IV infusion, the desired volume of reconstituted solution should be transferred to an appropriate-size empty sterile IV plastic bag for administration. Reconstituted solutions should not be transferred to large glass containers for prophylactic IV infusion therapy because precipitate formation has been observed with the use of some glass containers as reservoirs. Reconstituted and transferred solutions of dantrolene sodium should be inspected visually for particulate matter and discoloration prior to administration. Cloudy solutions or those containing a precipitate should not be used. Although reconstituted solutions are stable for 6 hours, it is recommended that IV infusions of the drug be prepared immediately before administration. Reconstituted solutions should be protected from light and stored at 15–30°C or 20–25°C depending on the preparation.

Dantrolene sodium for injectable suspension is reconstituted by adding 5 mL of sterile water for injection to the vial labeled as containing 250 mg of the drug and shaking the vial until an orange-colored uniform suspension is formed. No other solutions should be used for reconstitution. The reconstituted suspension should *not* be diluted or transferred to another container. After reconstitution, the drug is stable for 6 hours at 20–25°C and must be used within this time period. Reconstituted dantrolene sodium suspension may be administered into the IV catheter of a freely running IV infusion of 0.9% sodium chloride or 5% dextrose for injection, or into an indwelling catheter (after assuring its patency) without a freely running IV infusion. If an indwelling catheter is used, the line should be flushed to assure that there is no residual drug remaining in the catheter.

A suspension for oral administration of a single dose may be prepared by emptying the contents of an appropriate number of dantrolene sodium capsules into fruit juice or any liquid which would serve as a vehicle. For preparation of a suspension containing multiple doses, an appropriate number of capsules may be emptied into an acidic vehicle that has suspending properties. For example, 100 mL of a suspension containing 25 mg of dantrolene sodium per 5 mL can be prepared by suspending the contents of five 100-mg capsules in a small amount of simple syrup NF. A solution containing 150 mg of citric acid in 10 mL of water is added to this suspension followed by addition of a sufficient volume of simple syrup NF to make 100 mL. The suspension must be mixed thoroughly before use. This suspension is stable for 2 days when refrigerated. Alternatively, an oral suspension containing 5 mg/mL dantrolene sodium (using ten 50-mg capsules) in citric acid and Syrup BP with or without methyl hydroxybenzoate preservative may be prepared; the suspension is stable for 30 days if protected from light and stored under refrigeration (preferable) or at room temperature. Another extemporaneously prepared suspension of the drug in a methylcellulose-Syrup NF vehicle preserved with sodium benzoate has also been described; however, there are no published data on the stability of the suspension.

■ **Dosage** ***Spasticity*** **Adult Dosage.** Dosage of oral dantrolene sodium for the management of spasticity must be carefully adjusted according to the requirements and response of the patient, using the lowest dosage that produces optimal response without adverse effects. The manufacturer recommends a gradual dosage titration schedule in which each dosage level is maintained for 7 days to determine the patient's response. If no additional benefit is observed at the next higher dosage, dosage should be decreased to the previous lower dosage. Some patients will not respond until higher daily dosage is achieved, and therapy with doses administered 4 times daily may be necessary in some individuals. Because of the potential for liver toxicity with long-term use of oral dantrolene sodium, therapy should be discontinued if beneficial effects are not attained within 45 days.

For the management of spasticity in adults, the manufacturer recommends an initial oral dantrolene sodium dosage of 25 mg once daily for 7 days, followed by 25 mg 3 times daily for 7 days, then 50 mg 3 times daily for 7 days, and then 100 mg 3 times daily, if necessary. Some patients may require up to 100 mg 4 times daily, but dosages exceeding this should not be used.

Pediatric Dosage. For the management of spasticity in children 5 years of age or older, the manufacturer recommends an initial oral dantrolene sodium dosage of 0.5 mg/kg once daily for 7 days, followed by 0.5 mg/kg 3 times daily for 7 days, then 1 mg/kg 3 times daily for 7 days, and then 2 mg/kg 3 times daily, if necessary. Some patients may require up to 100 mg 4 times daily, but dosages exceeding this should not be used.

Malignant Hyperthermia Crisis For the management of malignant hyperthermia crisis, the minimum initial adult or pediatric dose of dantrolene sodium is 1 mg/kg administered by rapid IV injection. Continuous rapid IV injections should be administered as necessary until physiologic and metabolic abnormalities subside or a maximum total IV dosage of 10 mg/kg is reached. Reversal of malignant hyperthermia is usually achieved with an average total IV dosage of 2.5 mg/kg; however, the effective dosage will vary between patients based on their susceptibility to malignant hyperthermia, the amount and time of exposure to the triggering agent, and the rapidity of treatment. If physiologic and metabolic abnormalities reappear after initial control, the regimen may be repeated. To prevent recurrence of the manifestations of malignant hyperthermia following initial IV therapy for a crisis, the manufacturer states that oral dantrolene sodium dosages of 4–8 mg/kg daily should be administered in 4 divided doses for up to 3 days after the crisis. If oral therapy is not practical or feasible postoperatively, the drug may be given IV; the dose must be individualized, starting with 1 mg/kg or more as clinically indicated.

For the prevention of malignant hyperthermia in adults or children thought to be at risk of developing this condition, oral dantrolene sodium dosages of 4–8 mg/kg daily may be administered in 3 or 4 divided doses for 1–2 days prior to surgery, with the last dose being given approximately 3–4 hours prior to surgery with a small amount of water. Dosage may be adjusted within the recommended dosage range if adverse effects (e.g., skeletal muscle weakness, sedation, GI effects) occur. Alternatively, an IV dose of 2.5 mg/kg may be administered over a period of approximately 1 hour (if using Dantrium®, Revonto® or generic equivalents) or at least 1 minute (if using Ryanodex®), beginning about 1.25 hours before anticipated anesthesia or surgery; additional IV doses, which must be individualized, may be given intraoperatively if necessary (e.g., appearance of manifestations of malignant hyperthermia, prolonged surgery).

Other Uses To reduce succinylcholine-induced muscle fasciculations and postoperative muscle pain†, 100 mg of dantrolene sodium has been given orally 2 hours preoperatively in adults weighing less than 45 kg or 150 mg has been given in those weighing more than 45 kg.

Cautions

Adverse effects occur quite commonly in patients who receive dantrolene, and it should be considered that the long-term safety and efficacy of dantrolene have not been established. The serious adverse effects occurring occasionally with long-term oral dantrolene therapy (e.g., hepatitis, seizures, pleural effusion with pericarditis) have not been reasonably associated with short-term IV use of the drug to date.

The most common adverse effect of dantrolene is muscle weakness which rarely may result in slurring of speech, drooling, and enuresis. Other common adverse effects are drowsiness, dizziness, lightheadedness, diarrhea, nausea, malaise, and fatigue. These adverse effects are usually transient, lasting up to 4 days after the initiation of oral therapy or up to 2 days after IV administration of the drug, and are generally related to the rate of increase in dosage and total daily dosage. Severe weakness and/or diarrhea may necessitate decreasing the dosage or discontinuing the drug. If diarrhea recurs after reinstitution of dantrolene at a lower dosage, the drug should probably be discontinued permanently. Thrombophlebitis, tissue necrosis secondary to extravasation, urticaria and erythema, and injection site reactions (e.g., pain, erythema, swelling) also have occurred with IV administration of the drug. Adverse effects associated with the injectable suspension formulation of the drug (Ryanodex®) generally are similar to those experienced with other IV formulations; although results of a study in healthy individuals identified several adverse effects that were more frequent with Ryanodex® than with an older IV formulation of dantrolene sodium (Dantrium®), this finding was not considered to be clinically important.

■ **Hepatic Effects** Oral dantrolene therapy has caused abnormal liver function test results such as increased serum AST (SGOT), ALT (SGPT), alkaline phosphatase, LDH, BUN, and total serum bilirubin concentrations which, if detected early, return to normal when the drug is discontinued. In some patients, these abnormalities may be transient even when dantrolene is continued. Fatal or nonfatal hepatitis has occurred in patients receiving dantrolene and is apparently an idiosyncratic reaction. In about 60% of the cases, nausea, anorexia, vomiting, and abdominal discomfort precede the onset of hepatitis. Hepatomegaly and, rarely, splenomegaly also may occur.

Symptomatic hepatitis (fatal and nonfatal) has been reported at various dosages and following various durations of dantrolene therapy. Dantrolene-induced hepatitis occurs most frequently in patients receiving more than 300 mg daily for longer than 2 months, but even intermittent short courses of therapy with 800 mg or more daily markedly increase the risk of hepatotoxicity. Overt hepatitis has been observed most frequently between the third and twelfth month of therapy. The risk of dantrolene-induced hepatotoxicity is greatest in females, in patients older than 35 years of age, and in patients receiving other drugs (particularly estrogens) concomitantly. The risk of dantrolene-induced hepatotoxicity possibly may be increased in patients with baseline liver function test abnormalities and in geriatric patients. (See Cautions: Geriatric Precautions.)

■ **Musculoskeletal Effects** IV dantrolene therapy is associated with skeletal muscle weakness (e.g., loss of grip strength, leg weakness). Dysphagia also has been reported.

■ **GI Effects** In addition to diarrhea, other adverse GI effects that have been reported with oral dantrolene include anorexia, nausea, vomiting, gastric irritation, abdominal cramps, constipation (which rarely progresses to signs of intestinal obstruction), difficulty in swallowing, and GI bleeding. Severe constipation has occasionally resulted in abdominal distention and signs of bowel obstruction. These symptoms usually have responded to reduction of dosage and/or discontinuance of the drug. Although a causal relationship to dantrolene was not established, adynamic ileus and death occurred in one patient receiving the drug.

■ **Nervous System Effects** Adverse nervous system effects of oral dantrolene include speech disturbance, headache, visual disturbances including diplopia, alteration of taste, mental depression, confusion, auditory and visual hallucinations, increased nervousness, insomnia, drooling, and exacerbation or precipitation of seizures. In addition, drowsiness and dizziness have been associated with IV administration of dantrolene in healthy individuals. Concomitant use of dantrolene and other CNS depressants may cause additive CNS effects. (See Drug Interactions: CNS Depressants.)

■ **Urogenital Effects** Adverse urogenital effects of oral dantrolene include increased urinary frequency, urinary incontinence and/or nocturia, difficult urination and/or urinary retention, crystalluria, hematuria, and difficult erection.

■ **Dermatologic and Sensitivity Reactions** Adverse dermatologic effects of oral dantrolene include abnormal hair growth, acneiform rash, eczematoid eruption, pruritus, urticaria, and sweating. There have also been rare reports of urticaria and erythema possibly associated with IV dantrolene. Injection site reactions (pain, erythema, swelling), commonly due to extravasation, also have been reported with IV dantrolene. Pleural effusions with associated eosinophilia or with pericarditis have been reported with oral dantrolene, and anaphylaxis has been reported with both IV and oral dantrolene.

■ **Cardiovascular Effects** Adverse cardiovascular effects of oral dantrolene include tachycardia, erratic blood pressure, phlebitis, and heart failure.

■ **Respiratory Effects** Dantrolene therapy has been associated with respiratory depression, a feeling of suffocation, dyspnea, respiratory muscle weakness, and decreased inspiratory capacity. Rarely, pulmonary edema has developed during the treatment of malignant hyperthermia crisis in which the diluent volume and amount of mannitol associated with the IV dantrolene sodium dose may have contributed.

■ **Hematologic Effects** Adverse hematologic effects of oral dantrolene include aplastic anemia, anemia, leukopenia, lymphocytic lymphoma, and thrombocytopenia.

■ **Other Adverse Effects** Other reported adverse effects of oral dantrolene include backache, myalgia, excessive tearing, chills, and fever.

Chronic administration of high doses of dantrolene has caused reversible growth or weight depression and possible nephrotoxicity in some animal species.

■ **Precautions and Contraindications** Since dantrolene may cause severe hepatotoxicity, the manufacturer states that the drug should not be used in patients with conditions other than those for which such therapy is recommended. Serum AST (SGOT), ALT (SGPT), alkaline phosphatase, and total serum bilirubin concentrations should be determined prior to oral dantrolene therapy, and tests should be repeated periodically during therapy or whenever symptoms of hepatitis occur. If liver function test abnormalities occur alone, dantrolene should usually be discontinued; the drug should be continued or reinstituted only if major benefits occurred during dantrolene therapy. If symptoms of hepatitis are accompanied by liver function test abnormalities or jaundice, dantrolene should be discontinued. Dantrolene therapy has been resumed in a few patients who developed clinical and/or laboratory evidence of hepatotoxicity; if therapy is reinstituted, it should only be in patients who clearly need dantrolene and only after symptoms and laboratory abnormalities have cleared. The patient should be hospitalized and therapy should be initiated with very small doses and gradually increased with frequent monitoring of liver function; dantrolene should be discontinued immediately if signs of liver abnormality recur. Dantrolene should be used with particular caution in females, in patients older than 35 years of age, and in those receiving other drugs (especially estrogens) concomitantly, since the risk of hepatotoxicity may be increased in these groups of patients. The drug should be used with caution in patients with a history of previous liver disease or dysfunction.

Dantrolene should be used with caution in patients with severely impaired cardiac function due to myocardial disease or with impaired pulmonary function (particularly those with obstructive pulmonary disease). Patients should be monitored for adequate ventilation since respiratory muscle weakness and other respiratory effects may occur. Patients who engage in potentially hazardous activities requiring mental alertness or physical coordination such as operating machinery or driving a motor vehicle should be warned about possible weakness, drowsiness, or dizziness; since these effects may persist for up to 2 days following IV administration of dantrolene, patients should not drive a motor vehicle or engage in other potentially hazardous activities during such a time period. The drug should be administered with caution in patients receiving other drugs that can produce drowsiness (e.g., diazepam). Patients should be advised that decreased grip strength and leg muscle weakness, particularly upon walking down stairs, may be expected to occur postoperatively. Patients should not ambulate without assistance until normal strength and balance return. Caution should be employed at meals during the day(s) of dantrolene administration since choking and difficulty in swallowing have been reported. Dantrolene may cause photosensitivity reactions, so patients should be warned against excessive or unnecessary exposure to sunlight.

Dantrolene is contraindicated in patients who must utilize spasticity to maintain upright posture and balance in moving or when spasticity is utilized to obtain or maintain increased body function. The drug is also contraindicated in patients with upper motor neuron disorders and active hepatic disease such as hepatitis and cirrhosis. There are no contraindications to the use of IV dantrolene sodium in the prophylaxis or management of malignant hyperthermia crisis.

■ **Pediatric Precautions** The long-term safety of orally administered dantrolene sodium in children younger than 5 years of age has not been established. Before initiating long-term oral therapy in pediatric patients, the possibility that adverse effects may only become evident after many years should be weighed against the potential benefit to the patient.

■ **Geriatric Precautions** Clinical studies of dantrolene did not include sufficient numbers of patients 65 years of age and older to determine whether geriatric patients respond differently than younger patients. While other clinical experience has not revealed age-related differences in response or tolerance, dosage generally should be titrated carefully in geriatric patients, usually initiating therapy at the low end of the dosage range. The greater frequency of decreased hepatic, renal, and/or cardiac function and of concomitant disease and drug therapy observed in the elderly also should be considered. Spontaneous reports suggest that geriatric patients receiving oral dantrolene may have a higher risk of hepatic events with fatal outcomes; however, the majority of these reports were complicated by confounding factors (e.g., comorbid illnesses, concomitant use of hepatotoxic drugs).

■ **Mutagenicity and Carcinogenicity** Dantrolene sodium has produced positive results in microbial mutagen (Ames) tests using *Salmonella typhimurium* with and without liver metabolic activation.

One strain of female rats receiving oral dantrolene sodium dosages of 15, 30, and 60 mg/kg daily for 18 months showed an increased incidence of malignant and nonmalignant mammary tumors and, at the highest dosage level (approximately equal to the maximum recommended human daily dosage on a mg/m^2 basis) an increased incidence of hepatic lymphangiomas and angiosarcomas. The only drug-related effect seen in 30-month carcinogenicity studies in rats was a dose-related decrease in the time of onset of mammary and/or testicular tumors. Carcinogenic effects were not seen in mice receiving the drug. The relevance of these findings to human toxicity is not known.

■ **Pregnancy, Fertility, and Lactation** There are no adequate and well-controlled studies of dantrolene in pregnant women. The drug has been shown to be embryocidal in rabbits and to decrease pup survival in rats when given at doses 7 times the human oral dose. Dantrolene sodium readily crosses the placenta but, when given to pregnant women at term in a dosage of 100 mg daily, no adverse respiratory or neuromuscular effects were detected at low dose in neonates born to these women. Further studies are needed, particularly with higher dosages. Dantrolene should not be used in women who are or may become pregnant unless the possible benefits outweigh the potential risks to the fetus.

Dantrolene sodium administered to male and female rats at dose levels up to 45 mg/kg daily (approximately 1.4 times the maximum recommended human daily dosage on a mg/m^2 basis) showed no adverse effects on fertility or general reproductive performance.

Dantrolene is distributed into human milk. Because of the potential for serious adverse effects in nursing infants, a decision should be made whether to discontinue nursing or the drug, taking into account the importance of the drug to the woman.

Drug Interactions

■ **Drugs Affecting Hepatic Microsomal Enzymes** Dantrolene is metabolized by the liver, and it is theoretically possible that its metabolism may be enhanced by drugs known to induce hepatic microsomal enzymes. However, neither phenobarbital nor diazepam appears to affect dantrolene metabolism.

■ **Calcium-Channel Blocking Agents** While cardiovascular collapse following concomitant use of dantrolene and verapamil is rare, it has been reported in patients receiving such concomitant therapy. In anesthetized animals (e.g., swine, dogs), IV administration of dantrolene and a calcium-channel blocking agent (e.g., diltiazem, verapamil) has resulted in myocardial depression, ventricular fibrillation, and cardiovascular collapse in association with marked hyperkalemia. In addition, metabolic changes (i.e., hyperglycemia, hyperkalemia) accompanied by decreased cardiac output and metabolic acidosis have been reported following preoperative administration of IV dantrolene in at least one diabetic patient already receiving oral verapamil therapy. Consequently, concomitant use of dantrolene and a calcium-channel blocking agent during the management of malignant hyperthermia is not recommended by the manufacturers.

■ **CNS Depressants** Dantrolene may be additive with, or may potentiate the action of, other CNS depressants such as sedatives and tranquilizing agents. When dantrolene is used concomitantly with other CNS depressants, caution should be used to avoid excessive sedation.

■ **Estrogens** Hepatotoxicity has occurred more frequently in women over 35 years of age receiving concomitant dantrolene and estrogen therapy. Although the potential for an interaction between these agents has not been clearly established, caution should be observed if the 2 drugs are used concomitantly.

■ **Muscle Relaxants** Concomitant use of dantrolene and muscle relaxants may potentiate the neuromuscular block.

■ **Protein-Bound Drugs** Plasma protein binding of dantrolene is increased by tolbutamide and is decreased by warfarin and clofibrate, but does not appear to be substantially affected by diazepam or phenytoin.

■ **Vecuronium Bromide** Dantrolene reportedly potentiates vecuronium bromide-induced neuromuscular blockade.

Acute Toxicity

■ **Manifestations** Overdosage of dantrolene produces symptoms that include muscular weakness and alterations in the state of consciousness (e.g., lethargy, coma), vomiting, diarrhea, and crystalluria.

■ **Treatment** Overdosage of oral dantrolene sodium should be treated conservatively with supportive measures, gastric lavage, and close observation of the patient. An adequate airway should be maintained and artificial respiration facilities should be readily available. ECG monitoring and large quantities of IV fluids to avoid crystalluria should be instituted. The efficacy of dialysis in the treatment of dantrolene sodium overdosage is unknown.

Pharmacology

Dantrolene causes skeletal muscle relaxation through a direct effect on skeletal muscle. In vitro experiments on animal tissue indicate that the drug may act by reducing the release of calcium from the sarcoplasmic reticulum by the muscle action potential, resulting in a decreased response of the muscle to the action potential and a decreased muscle contraction. Therefore, in patients with upper motor neuron disorders, dantrolene decreases muscle contractions caused by direct stimulation as well as those mediated through monosynaptic and polysynaptic reflexes. In patients with anesthesia-induced malignant hyperthermia, the drug's interference with the release of calcium from the sarcoplasmic reticulum to the myoplasm may prevent the increase in myoplasmic calcium which activates the acute catabolism in the skeletal muscle cell. The drug has no effect on the electrical activity at the myoneural junction or within the muscle, nor does it affect the rate of acetylcholine synthesis or release. The extent of CNS involvement in muscle relaxation produced by dantrolene is not known. It has been postulated that adverse CNS effects such as drowsiness and dizziness may be caused indirectly as a result of decreased skeletal muscle activity. Dantrolene has little or no effect on the contraction of cardiac or intestinal smooth muscle, except possibly with higher concentrations than those required for effects on skeletal muscle contraction.

In patients with upper motor neuron disorders, the drug produces generalized, mild weakness of skeletal muscles, decreases the force of reflex muscle contractions, and decreases hyperreflexia, clonus, muscle stiffness, spasticity, and phasic involuntary movements. Improvement in motor performance of the upper extremities may occur as evidenced by decreased resistance to passive motion and increased active and passive range of motion.

Pharmacokinetics

■ **Absorption** Oral bioavailability of dantrolene sodium is 70%. The absorption half-life has been reported to average 1.1 hours in adults and 1.4 hours in children. In patients with upper motor neuron disorders, beneficial effects of dantrolene may not become apparent for a week or more after institution of therapy in the usual initial oral dosage. Therapeutically effective blood concentrations of dantrolene and its metabolites appear to vary with the individual, but have been reported to range from 100–600 ng/mL or more. The blood concentration which is attained after oral administration varies widely among patients, but peak concentrations are usually attained about 5 hours after oral administration. In a study in 6 patients who received a single 100-mg oral dose, peak blood concentrations ranged from 0.7–1.45 mcg/mL. When dantrolene is administered IV as recommended for prophylaxis, blood concentrations of the drug remain at approximately steady-state levels for 3 or more hours after the infusion is completed.

■ **Distribution** Substantial amounts of dantrolene are bound to plasma proteins, principally albumin. The drug readily crosses the placenta.

■ **Elimination** The plasma half-life of dantrolene in adults is 8.7 hours after a single 100-mg dose. In a study in children with chronic spasticity, the estimated plasma half-life was 7.3 hours after a single dose. The mean plasma half-life of IV dantrolene is variable (range: 4–11.4 hours) depending on the preparation.

Dantrolene is metabolized in the liver primarily to the 5-hydroxy derivative which is less active than the parent drug. Dantrolene is also metabolized by reductive pathways to the amino derivative which has considerably less skeletal muscle relaxant effect than does dantrolene; the amino derivative is acetylated to the acetamido derivative. Dantrolene also may undergo hydrolysis and subsequent oxidation to form nitrophenylfuroic acid. Dantrolene and its metabolites are excreted mainly in urine and bile.

Chemistry and Stability

■ **Chemistry** Dantrolene sodium is a hydantoin derivative which is chemically and pharmacologically unrelated to other skeletal muscle relaxants. Dantrolene sodium, which is commercially available as the hydrate, occurs as an orange powder and is slightly soluble in water. Dantrolene is a weak acid with a pK_a of about 7.5. The sodium salt of the drug hydrolyzes in aqueous solution to form a precipitate of dantrolene.

Sodium hydroxide is added during manufacture of the commercially available lyophilized powder for injection to adjust the pH. Each 20-mg vial of dantrolene sodium for injection also contains 3 g of mannitol. When reconstituted with 60 mL of sterile water for injection, the injection has a pH of about 9.5.

Sodium hydroxide or hydrochloric acid is added during manufacture of the commercially available lyophilized powder for injectable suspension to adjust the pH. Each 250-mg vial of dantrolene sodium for injectable suspension contains 125 mg of mannitol. When reconstituted with 5 mL of sterile water for injection, the suspension has a pH of about 10.3.

■ **Stability** Dantrolene sodium capsules should be stored at a controlled room temperature of 20–25°C. The powder for injection should be stored at controlled room temperature between 20–25°C, and the powder for injectable suspension should be stored at 20–25°C, but may be exposed to 15–30°C; prolonged exposure to light should be avoided.

Following reconstitution with 60 mL of sterile water for injection, dantrolene sodium injection (Dantrium®) is stable for 6 hours when stored at 15–30°C; Revonto® and generic equivalents are stable for 6 hours when stored at 20–25°C after reconstitution. Following reconstitution with 5 mL of sterile water for injection, dantrolene sodium injectable suspension (Ryanodex®) is stable for 6 hours when stored at 20–25°C. The reconstituted IV solution or suspension should be protected from direct light and used within 6 hours after reconstitution.

Dantrolene sodium injection is not compatible with 5% dextrose or 0.9% sodium chloride injection; however, the injectable suspension formulation of the drug is compatible with small amounts of 5% dextrose or 0.9% sodium chloride injection when administered into the IV catheter of a freely running IV infusion of these solutions.

Preparations

Excipients in commercially available drug preparations may have clinically important effects in some individuals; consult specific product labeling for details.

Dantrolene Sodium

Oral		
Capsules	25 mg*	**Dantrium®**, Par
		Dantrolene Sodium Capsules
	50 mg*	**Dantrium®**, Par
		Dantrolene Sodium Capsules
	100 mg*	**Dantrium®**, Par
		Dantrolene Sodium Capsules
Parenteral		
For injection	20 mg*	**Dantrium® Intravenous**, Par
		Dantrolene Sodium for Injection
		Revonto®, US WorldMeds
For injectable suspension	250 mg	**Ryanodex®**, Eagle

*available from one or more manufacturer, distributor, and/or repackager by generic (nonproprietary) name

†Use is not currently included in the labeling approved by the US Food and Drug Administration

GABA-DERIVATIVE SKELETAL MUSCLE RELAXANTS 12:20.12

Baclofen

■ Baclofen, a γ-aminobutyric acid (GABA) derivative, is a skeletal muscle relaxant and antispastic agent.

Uses

■ **Spasticity** Baclofen is used orally in the management of spasticity and its sequelae secondary to severe chronic disorders such as multiple sclerosis and other types of spinal cord lesions. For the drug to be beneficial, patients must have presumably reversible spasticity where relief of spasticity will aid in restoring residual function. In these patients, baclofen decreases the number and severity of spasms (particularly flexor spasms); alleviates associated pain, clonus, and muscle rigidity; and improves mobility to a greater extent than does placebo. In patients with multiple sclerosis, the drug produces little improvement in residual muscle function, but patient comfort is improved when the painful spasms are reversible. In one uncontrolled study, less than one-third of multiple sclerosis patients with urinary retention caused by bladder spasm showed decrease in urinary retention.

Although few controlled studies have been conducted comparing efficacy and tolerability of the various antispastic agents, available data suggest that oral baclofen appears to have similar efficacy to other commonly used oral agents (e.g., diazepam, tizanidine). In studies comparing doses of about 60 mg of baclofen daily to 30 mg of diazepam daily in patients with multiple sclerosis or spinal cord lesions, the drugs were equally effective in reducing the number and severity of muscle spasms; however, baclofen produced a lower incidence of sedation than did diazepam. In comparative studies in patients with spasticity associated with cerebral or spinal disorders, improvement in muscle tone occurred in a similar proportion of patients receiving baclofen, diazepam, or tizanidine. When spasticity cannot be adequately managed with oral antispastic agents, other interventions such as botulinum toxin injection, intrathecal baclofen, intrathecal injection of sclerosing agents (e.g., phenol), or surgery (e.g., rhizotomy, chordotomy) may be necessary.

Baclofen crosses the blood-brain barrier in only small amounts following oral administration. It has been suggested that administration of the drug at the spinal cord level (i.e., intrathecally) would increase drug efficacy while decreasing the dosage required and possibly the toxicity profile in patients with spasticity of spinal cord origin. While baclofen may be effective at relatively high *oral* dosages in some patients with spasticity of spinal cord origin, many other patients, particularly those with severe spasticity, do not respond adequately to and/or do not tolerate such therapy. Therefore, *intrathecal* baclofen may be a suitable alternative to ablative surgical or chemical procedures in patients who do not tolerate or respond adequately to oral therapy with the drug. (See Uses: Severe Spasticity.)

■ **Severe Spasticity** Baclofen usually is used *intrathecally* in the management of severe spasticity of *spinal cord origin* in patients who do not tolerate or respond adequately to oral therapy with the drug. Baclofen also is used intrathecally in the management of intractable spasticity secondary to severe chronic disorders such as multiple sclerosis and other types of spinal diseases such as spinal ischemia, spinal tumor, transverse myelitis, cervical spondylosis, and degenerative myelopathy. Baclofen is designated an orphan drug by the FDA for use in these conditions. The clinical goal of such therapy is to maintain muscle tone as close to normal as possible and to minimize the frequency and severity of spasms without inducing intolerable adverse effects. In controlled studies in patients with severe spasticity and spasms secondary to spinal cord injury or multiple sclerosis, single doses or 3-day continuous infusions of intrathecal baclofen were more effective than placebo in improving the Ashworth (rigidity) rating of spasticity and in reducing the frequency of spasms. During chronic intrathecal baclofen therapy, many patients experience improvement in activities associated with daily living, especially in self-care, transferring, bowel function, and urinary continence.

Baclofen also is used *intrathecally* in patients with spasticity of *cerebral origin*, including those with cerebral palsy and acquired brain injury. Baclofen injection is designated an orphan drug by the FDA for the management of spasticity in patients with cerebral palsy. The clinical goal of such therapy is to maintain muscle tone as close to normal as possible and to minimize the frequency and severity of spasms without inducing intolerable adverse effects or to titrate dosage of baclofen to the desired degree of muscle tone for optimal function. Results of one randomized, controlled, crossover study in patients with cerebral palsy indicate that intrathecal baclofen was more effective than placebo in reducing spasticity as measured by the Ashworth scale. In addition, results of a small (11 patients) controlled study in patients with brain injury indicate that intrathecal baclofen was more effective than placebo in reducing spasticity.

Patients with spasticity secondary to brain injury should wait at least one year after the injury before considering long-term intrathecal baclofen therapy.

■ **Other Uses** Baclofen has been used orally to reduce choreiform movements in patients with Huntington's chorea†, to reduce rigidity in patients with parkinsonian syndrome†, and to reduce spasticity in patients with cerebral lesions†, cerebral palsy†, or rheumatic disorders†; however, the drug has not been shown to produce a substantial degree of improvement in these patients. Oral baclofen also has been used to reduce spasticity in patients with cerebrovascular stroke†; however, therapy with the drug generally did not provide substantial improvement and was poorly tolerated. The manufacturer states oral baclofen is *not* indicated for use in patients with rheumatic disorders; use of oral baclofen also is not recommended in patients with stroke, cerebral palsy, or Parkinson's disease.

Although in one study oral baclofen reportedly improved behavior in patients with schizophrenic disorder† receiving other drugs concomitantly (e.g., phenothiazines), schizophrenic behavior worsened in other patients when baclofen was used alone. Preliminary data indicate that oral baclofen has beneficial effects in the treatment of trigeminal neuralgia† and may be synergistic with carbamazepine and phenytoin.

Dosage and Administration

■ **Administration** Baclofen is administered orally or intrathecally. Abrupt discontinuance of the drug, including inadvertent discontinuance of the intrathecal infusion, should be avoided because of the risk of precipitating withdrawal. (See Cautions: Precautions and Contraindications.) For intrathecal use, baclofen is administered as an additive-free injection by direct intrathecal injection (via lumbar puncture or catheter) over a period of at least 1 minute employing barbotage or by continuous intrathecal infusion into a lumbar intrathecal space via an implantable controlled-infusion device (pump). The manufacturer's labeling should be consulted for specialized administration techniques.

In the preparation of test doses of the drug for the purposes of drug-response screening prior to initiation of chronic intrathecal baclofen therapy, 1-mL ampuls containing 50 mcg of baclofen should be used without further dilution. For maintenance therapy in patients receiving concentrations of the drug other than the commercially available strengths (i.e., 0.5 or 2 mg/mL), baclofen for injection concentrate for intrathecal administration *must* be diluted. The concentrate *must* only be diluted with sterile, preservative-free 0.9% sodium chloride injection. The specific concentration that should be used depends on the total daily dosage required and the delivery rate of the pump. The manufacturer's manual should be consulted for specific recommendations.

As with other parenteral drug products, baclofen for injection concentrate and diluted solutions of the drug should be inspected visually for particulate matter and/or discoloration prior to administration, whenever solution and container permit.

Patients receiving intrathecal baclofen therapy must be monitored closely in a fully equipped and staffed environment during the initial test for responsiveness and dosage-titration period immediately following implantation of the pump. Resuscitative equipment should be immediately available for use in case of life-threatening or intolerable adverse effects.

■ Dosage

Spasticity **Oral Dosage.** Oral dosage of baclofen should be individualized according to the patient's requirements and response using the lowest dosage that produces optimum response. Initially, low oral dosages of the drug should be administered.

For the management of spasticity, the initial oral dosage of baclofen is 5 mg 3 times daily. Oral daily dosage may be increased by 15 mg at 3-day intervals (i.e., 5 mg 3 times daily for 3 days, then 10 mg 3 times daily for 3 days, then 15 mg 3 times daily for 3 days, then 20 mg 3 times daily for 3 days) until optimum effect is achieved (usually at dosages of 40–80 mg daily). In patients with psychiatric or brain disorders and in geriatric patients, oral dosage should be increased more gradually. In some patients, a smoother antispastic effect is obtained by administering the oral daily dosage in 4 divided doses. Some clinicians suggest that daily oral dosages of up to 150 mg are well tolerated and provide additional therapeutic benefit in some patients; however, the manufacturers state that total dosage should not exceed 80 mg daily (i.e., 20 mg 4 times daily). Some patients require 1–2 months of treatment for full benefit; however, the length of baclofen trial should be determined by the clinical state of the patient. If benefits are not evident after a reasonable trial, baclofen therapy should be discontinued by slowly reducing the daily dosage.

Severe Spasticity **Intrathecal Dosage.** Prior to implantation of the controlled-infusion device (e.g., Medtronic SynchroMed® pump) and initiation of chronic intrathecal baclofen therapy, the patient must exhibit a positive response (defined as a clinically important decrease in muscle tone and/or frequency and/or severity of spasms over a 4- to 8-hour observation period) to initial intrathecal baclofen test dose(s). Initially, a dose containing 50 mcg (1 mL of a 50-mcg/mL solution) of baclofen is administered into the intrathecal space by barbotage over a period of at least 1 minute. If response observed at 4–8 hours after the initial test dose is less than desired, a second injection containing 75 mcg (1.5 mL of a 50-mcg/mL solution) of baclofen may be administered 24 hours after the first dose. If response observed at 4–8 hours after the second test dose remains inadequate, a final injection containing 100 mcg (2 mL of a 50-mcg/mL solution) of baclofen may be administered 24 hours after the second dose. In pediatric patients, the initial test dose is the same as in adults (i.e., 50 mcg); however, in very small children, an initial dose of 25 mcg may be considered. Patients not responding to the 100-mcg intrathecal test dose of the drug are not considered candidates for chronic intrathecal baclofen therapy.

Following establishment of responsiveness to intrathecal baclofen and implantation of a compatible pump (e.g., SynchroMed® infusion system), the initial intrathecal dose of baclofen for the management of spasticity is twice the test dose that produced a positive response with a duration not exceeding 8 hours; this dose is infused intrathecally over 24 hours. For patients in whom a positive response to the test dose persisted for longer than 8 hours, the initial intrathecal dose is the same as the test dose that produced a positive response; this dose also is infused intrathecally over 24 hours. Dosage should not be increased within 24 hours after the initial intrathecal dose (i.e., until steady state is achieved). Following the initial infusion dose in adults with spasticity of *spinal cord origin,* the daily dose can be increased slowly by 10–30% increments at 24-hour intervals until the desired clinical response is achieved; in pediatric patients with spasticity of *spinal cord origin* and adult and pediatric patients with spasticity of *cerebral origin*, the daily dose can be increased slowly by 5–15% increments at 24-hour intervals until the desired clinical response is achieved. If no substantive increase in response is observed with upward titration of intrathecal baclofen dosage, the function of the pump and patency of the catheter should be checked.

Adjustment of maintenance dosage often is needed during the initial months of intrathecal baclofen therapy as the patient adjusts to changes in life-style secondary to relief of spasticity. During periodic refills of the pump, the 24-hour dose may be increased by up to 10–40% or up to 5–20% in patients with spasticity of spinal cord origin or those with spasticity of cerebral origin, respectively, as necessary to maintain adequate control of symptoms. In patients who develop intolerable adverse effects, the 24-hour maintenance dose can be decreased by 10–20%. During chronic therapy, gradual increases in dosage will be required in most patients to maintain optimal response. A sudden increase in dosage requirement should suggest the possibility of pump and/or catheter malfunction (i.e., catheter kink or dislodgement). In patients with spasticity of *spinal cord origin*, maintenance dosage during chronic intrathecal therapy has ranged from 12–2003 mcg daily, with most patients responding adequately to 300–800 mcg daily. There is only limited experience with intrathecal baclofen dosages of 1000 mcg daily or greater in these patients. In patients with spasticity of *cerebral origin*, maintenance dosage during chronic intrathecal therapy has ranged from 22–1400 mcg daily, with most patients responding adequately to 90–703 mcg daily. In clinical studies in patients with spasticity of cerebral origin, only about 2% of patients required daily dosages exceeding 1000 mcg daily.

Maintenance dosage recommendations for pediatric patients are similar to those for patients with spasticity of cerebral origin. Pediatric patients younger than 12 years of age may require lower daily dosages; in clinical trials, the maintenance daily dosage averaged 274 mcg daily (range: 24–1199 mcg daily). Dosage requirements for pediatric patients older than 12 years of age does not appear to be different from that for adult patients. Determination of optimum therapy requires individual titration. The lowest possible dosage that produces optimum response should be employed.

During prolonged intrathecal baclofen therapy for spasticity, approximately 5% of patients become refractory to increasing dosages of the drug. While experience currently is insufficient to make firm recommendations regarding amelioration of such tolerance, patients occasionally have been hospitalized and subjected to a "drug holiday" in which intrathecal dosage was decreased gradually over a 2- to 4-week period, during which baclofen therapy was alternated with other methods of spasticity management. After a few days, sensitivity to baclofen may return and continuous intrathecal baclofen therapy may be resumed at the previously effective initial dosage.

For patients achieving relatively satisfactory relief via continuous intrathecal infusion employing an implantable pump, further benefit may be possible with more complex dosing schedules. For example, patients who commonly experience an exacerbation of spasticity at night that disrupts sleep may require a 20% increase in the hourly infusion rate; such changes should be programmed to begin approximately 2 hours before the time of desired clinical benefit.

The manual provided by the manufacturer of the implantable infusion device (i.e., pump) must be consulted for additional information, including specific instructions and precautions for programming the pump and/or refilling the reservoir. Various pumps (with different reservoir volumes) and refill kits are available; clinicians must be familiar with these products in order to select the appropriate refill kit for the particular pump in use.

■ Dosage in Renal Impairment

Because baclofen is excreted principally in urine as unchanged drug, it may be necessary to reduce either oral or intrathecal dosage in patients with impaired renal function. (See Cautions: Precautions and Contraindications.)

Cautions

■ Adverse Effects

The most common adverse effect of *oral* baclofen therapy is transient drowsiness (10–63%); other common adverse effects of oral baclofen therapy include dizziness (5–15%), weakness (5–15%), and fatigue (2–4%).

The most common adverse effects of *intrathecal* baclofen therapy in patients with spasticity of *spinal cord origin* include somnolence, dizziness, nausea, hypotension, headache, seizures, and hypotonia. The most common adverse effects of *intrathecal* baclofen therapy in patients with spasticity of *cerebral origin* include agitation, constipation, somnolence, leukocytosis, chills, urinary retention, and hypotonia.

The incidence of adverse effects during oral administration of baclofen can be minimized by slowly increasing dosage to therapeutic levels. If adverse effects occur, they can be reduced by decreasing dosage. Psychiatric disturbances, including hallucinations, euphoria, mental excitation, depression, confusion or anxiety, occur most commonly in patients with psychiatric or brain disorders, including stroke, and in geriatric patients; any increase in oral dosage should be made slowly in these patients. Many adverse CNS and genitourinary effects also are symptoms of the underlying disease (i.e., multiple sclerosis, spinal cord lesions) and may not be related to baclofen therapy.

CNS Effects Neuropsychiatric disturbances reported during oral baclofen treatment include confusion, headache, insomnia, and, rarely, euphoria, excitement, depression, hallucinations, paresthesia, muscle pain, tinnitus, slurred speech, coordination disorder, tremor, rigidity, dystonia, ataxia, blurred vision, nystagmus, strabismus, miosis, mydriasis, diplopia, dysarthria, and seizures. Neuropsychiatric disturbances or adverse CNS effects reported during intrathecal baclofen treatment include hypotonia, somnolence, dizziness, paresthesia, hypertonia, headache, seizures, asthenia, confusion, speech disorder, coma, insomnia, anxiety, depression, abnormal thinking, tremor, agitation, dysautonomia, hallucinations, abnormal gait, amnesia, twitching, vasodilation, cerebrovascular accident, nystagmus, personality disorder, psychotic depression, cerebral ischemia, emotional lability, euphoria, ileus, drug dependence, incoordination, paranoid reaction, ptosis, akathisia, ataxia, opisthotonos, hysteria, insomnia, decreased reflexes, and vasodilation.

Genitourinary Effects Urinary frequency and, rarely, enuresis, urinary retention, dysuria, impotence, inability to ejaculate, nocturia, and hematuria have occurred during oral baclofen therapy. During intrathecal baclofen therapy, urinary retention or incontinence, impotence, urinary frequency, impaired urination, hematuria, kidney failure, abnormal ejaculation, kidney calculus, oliguria, and vaginitis have been reported.

In female rats, chronic administration of oral baclofen has caused a dose-related increase in the incidence of ovarian cysts and a less marked increase in enlarged or hemorrhagic adrenal glands. Ovarian cysts have been found by palpation in about 4% of multiple sclerosis patients receiving oral baclofen for up to 1 year, but these cysts spontaneously disappeared despite continued use of the drug in most patients. It should be noted, however, that ovarian cysts are estimated to occur spontaneously in approximately 1–5% of healthy females.

Cardiovascular Effects Adverse cardiovascular effects such as hypotension and, rarely, dyspnea, palpitation, chest pain, and syncope have occurred during oral baclofen therapy. Hypotension (including orthostatic hypotension), hypertension, dyspnea, bradycardia, palpitations, syncope, ventricular arrhythmia, deep thrombophlebitis, pallor, and tachycardia have been reported during intrathecal baclofen therapy.

GI Effects Adverse GI effects of oral baclofen therapy include nausea and constipation and, rarely, dry mouth, anorexia, taste disorders, abdominal pain, vomiting, diarrhea, and positive tests for occult blood in the stool. Nausea, vomiting, constipation, dry mouth, diarrhea, anorexia, increased salivation, flatulence, dysphagia, dyspepsia, gastroenteritis, fecal incontinence, GI hemorrhage, tongue disorder, and abdominal pain have been reported during intrathecal baclofen therapy.

Abrupt Withdrawal Abrupt discontinuance of oral baclofen therapy, regardless of the cause, has resulted in hallucinations and seizures. Abrupt discontinuance of intrathecal baclofen therapy has resulted in high fever, altered mental status, exaggerated rebound spasticity, and muscle rigidity that, in rare cases, have progressed to rhabdomyolysis, multisystem organ failure, and death. In most cases, manifestations of withdrawal appeared within hours to a few days following discontinuance of baclofen therapy. All patients receiving intrathecal baclofen therapy are potentially at risk for withdrawal. Early manifestations of intrathecal baclofen withdrawal may include return of baseline spasticity, pruritus, hypotension, and paresthesias. Clinical presentation of advanced intrathecal baclofen withdrawal syndrome may resemble autonomic dysreflexia, infection (sepsis), malignant hyperthermia, neuroleptic malignant syndrome (NMS), or other conditions associated with a hypermetabolic state or widespread rhabdomyolysis. (See Cautions: Precautions and Contraindications.) Baclofen therapy should be slowly discontinued to minimize the risk of withdrawal.

Death Although fatalities, including one case of unexpected death after administration of 3 test doses and 2 cases of sudden and unexpected death occurring within 2 weeks of pump implantation, have been reported rarely during the use of intrathecal baclofen therapy, the manufacturer states that a causal relationship to the drug could not be established.

Other Adverse Effects Rash, pruritus, ankle edema, excessive perspiration, weight gain, and nasal congestion have been reported during oral baclofen therapy. Increases in blood glucose concentration and serum AST (SGOT) and alkaline phosphatase concentrations also have been reported during oral therapy. During intrathecal baclofen therapy, accidental injury, death, pain, amblyopia, hypoventilation, peripheral edema, fever, pneumonia, urticaria, diplopia, back pain, pruritus, rash, sweating, alopecia, contact dermatitis, skin ulcer, chills, respiratory disorder, aspiration pneumonia, hyperventilation, apnea, pulmonary embolus, rhinitis, weight loss, albuminuria, dehydration, hyperglycemia, abnormal vision, abnormality of accommodation, photophobia, taste loss, tinnitus, suicide, hypothermia, neck rigidity, chest pain, chills, face edema, flu syndrome, anemia, carcinoma, malaise, leukocytosis, and petechial rash have been reported.

■ Precautions and Contraindications

Deteriorations in seizure control and EEG occasionally have been noted in epileptic patients receiving the drug; the epileptic patient's clinical state and EEG should be monitored at regular intervals during baclofen treatment.

Because baclofen may cause sedation and/or drowsiness, patients should be warned that therapy with the drug may impair their ability to perform hazardous activities requiring mental alertness or physical coordination such as operating machinery or driving a motor vehicle. In addition, additive CNS depression may occur when the drug is administered concomitantly with other CNS depressants, including alcohol. Oral or intrathecal baclofen should be used with caution, and it may be necessary to reduce dosage in patients with impaired renal function. The drug should be used with caution, with careful dosage titration, in patients who must use spasticity to maintain upright posture and balance in moving or when spasticity is used to obtain increased or optimal body function.

Patients with psychotic disorders, schizophrenia, or confusional states should be treated cautiously and kept under careful surveillance during intrathecal baclofen therapy, as exacerbations of these conditions have been reported following oral administration of the drug.

Intrathecal baclofen therapy should be instituted with caution in patients with a history of autonomic dysreflexia, since the presence of nociceptive stimuli or the abrupt withdrawal of therapy may precipitate an episode of dysreflexia.

The clinical goal of baclofen therapy is to maintain muscle tone as close to normal as possible and to minimize the frequency and severity of spasms without inducing intolerable adverse effects. It may be important to maintain some degree of muscle tone and allow occasional spasms to help support circulatory function, minimize the risk of development of deep-vein thrombosis, and optimize activities of daily living and ease of care.

If intrathecal baclofen therapy is to be employed, an attempt should be made to discontinue concomitant oral antispasmodic drugs, including oral baclofen, to avoid possible overdose and drug interactions, either prior to the screening phase or following implantation of the infusion device. Dosage reduction and discontinuance of concomitant oral antispasmodics should be employed slowly, and the patient should be monitored carefully; abrupt dosage reduction or discontinuance of concomitant antispasmodics should be avoided.

Patients undergoing pump implantation for the initiation of intrathecal baclofen therapy should be without concurrent infection, as the presence of infection may interfere with assessment of the patient's response to the baclofen test dose(s), increase surgical complications after pump implantation, and complicate attempts to adjust dosage.

Development of intrathecal mass at the tip of the implanted catheter, usually involving pharmacy compounded analgesic admixtures, has been reported in patients receiving long-term intrathecal baclofen therapy. The most common sequelae or manifestations associated with intrathecal mass include decreased therapeutic response (i.e., worsening spasticity, return of spasticity despite previous response, withdrawal symptoms, poor response to escalating doses, frequent or large dosage increases), pain, and neurologic deficit or dysfunction. Patients receiving intraspinal therapy should be carefully monitored for any new neurologic manifestations. If new neurologic manifestations suggestive of an intrathecal mass occur, a neurosurgical consultation should be considered, since many of the symptoms of inflammatory mass are similar to those observed in patients with severe spasticity. In some cases, performance of an imaging procedure may be appropriate to confirm or rule out the diagnosis of an intrathecal mass.

Because of the possibility of potentially life-threatening CNS depression, cardiovascular collapse, and/or respiratory failure, baclofen should be administered intrathecally only by qualified individuals familiar with the techniques of administration and patient management problems. When an implantable pump is used, familiarization with the device is essential, including specific instructions and precautions for programming the pump and refilling the reservoir. The patient, their caregivers, and health-care providers must receive adequate information regarding the risks of such therapy, including information on recognition and management of potential overdosage and proper care of the pump and catheter insertion site. Because of the risks involved, the initial test for responsiveness to intrathecal baclofen, implantation of the pump, and subsequent periods of dosage titration must be performed in a medically supervised setting that is adequately equipped for the management of potential complications; resuscitative equipment should be readily available. Filling of the drug reservoir of the device should be performed under aseptic conditions (to avoid bacterial contamination and serious infection) and only by fully trained and qualified personnel, following the directions provided by the device's manufacturer. The pump should be filled with extreme caution and should be refilled only through the reservoir refill septum of the device. If the reservoir refill septum is not properly accessed, inadvertent injection into the subcutaneous tissue can occur, possibly resulting in life-threatening overdosage or early depletion of the reservoir. Some pumps also are equipped with a catheter access port that allows direct access to the intrathecal catheter; direct injection into this catheter may cause life-threatening overdosage of the drug. During chronic therapy, care should be taken in employing the proper refill frequency so that depletion of the drug reservoir during use is avoided; symptoms of spasticity (e.g., rigidity) usually return within a few days if dosing is discontinued, and manifestations of withdrawal (e.g., hallucinations, seizures) could emerge. Careful patient monitoring is particularly important during the initial phase of pump use, dosage titration, and reservoir refilling so that an acceptable, reasonably stable response is ensured.

Abrupt discontinuance of oral baclofen therapy, regardless of the cause, has resulted in hallucinations and seizures. Abrupt discontinuance of intrathecal baclofen therapy has resulted in high fever, altered mental status, exaggerated rebound spasticity, and muscle rigidity that, in rare cases, have progressed to rhabdomyolysis, multisystem organ failure, and death. Common reasons for abrupt interruption of intrathecal baclofen therapy include malfunction of the catheter (particularly disconnection), low volume in the pump reservoir, end of pump battery life, and, possibly, human error. Cases of intrathecal mass at the tip of the implanted catheter (most of which involved pharmacy compounded analgesic admixtures) also have reportedly resulted in withdrawal symptoms. Therefore, the manufacturer states that careful attention to programming and monitoring of the infusion system, refill scheduling and procedures, and pump alarms is necessary to prevent abrupt discontinuance of intrathecal baclofen therapy. Patients and caregivers should be advised of the importance of keeping scheduled refill visits and should be informed of the early signs and symptoms of baclofen withdrawal. (See Abrupt Withdrawal under Cautions: Adverse Effects.) Special attention should be given to patients at apparent risk for withdrawal (e.g., spinal cord injury at the T6 level or above, communication difficulties, history of withdrawal symptoms from oral or intrathecal baclofen). Rapid, accurate diagnosis and treatment in an emergency room or intensive care setting are important in order to prevent the potentially life-threatening CNS and systemic effects of intrathecal baclofen withdrawal. Treatment of intrathecal baclofen withdrawal includes restoration of intrathecal baclofen at or near the dosage used prior to interruption of therapy. However, if reinstitution of intrathecal delivery is delayed, therapy with drugs that enhance GABA effects (e.g., oral or enteral baclofen; oral, enteral, or IV benzodiazepines) may prevent potentially fatal sequelae. However, the manufacturer states that oral or enteral baclofen alone should not be relied upon to halt the progression of intrathecal baclofen withdrawal.

Oral and intrathecal baclofen are contraindicated in patients with a history of hypersensitivity to the drug. Baclofen injection for intrathecal administration is not recommended or intended for IV, IM, subcutaneous, or epidural administration.

■ **Pediatric Precautions** The manufacturers state that safety of oral or intrathecal baclofen therapy in pediatric patients younger than 12 or 4 years of age, respectively, has not been established. Pediatric patients undergoing pump implantation for the initiation of intrathecal baclofen therapy should have sufficient body mass to accommodate the pump. Directions provided by the device's manufacturer should be consulted.

■ **Pregnancy and Lactation** Reproduction studies in rats receiving oral baclofen at a dosage approximately 13 or 3 times the maximum recommended human oral dosage on a mg/kg or mg/m² basis, respectively, demonstrated an increased incidence of omphaloceles (ventral hernias) in the fetuses; substantial reductions in food intake and weight gain occurred in pregnant rats receiving this dosage. An increased incidence of omphaloceles did not occur in mice or rabbit fetuses. An increased incidence of incomplete sternebral ossification occurred in the fetuses of rats receiving approximately 13 times the maximum recommended human dosage, and an increased incidence of unossified phalangeal nuclei of the forelimbs and hindlimbs occurred in the fetuses of rabbits receiving approximately 7 times the maximum recommended dosage. No teratogenic effects occurred in mice, although reduction in mean fetal weight with consequent delay in skeletal ossification occurred in offspring of mice receiving 17 or 34 times the human daily dosage of baclofen. There are no adequate and controlled studies using baclofen in pregnant women, and the drug should be used during pregnancy only when the potential benefits justify the possible risks to the fetus.

Baclofen is distributed into milk following oral administration; it not known whether the drug distributes into milk following intrathecal administration. At least one manufacturer states that nursing should not be undertaken by women receiving oral baclofen. Nursing should be undertaken by women receiving intrathecal baclofen only if the potential benefit justifies the potential risks to the infant.

Drug Interactions

Experience with concomitant use of intrathecal baclofen with other drugs is insufficient to predict specific drug-drug interactions.

■ **CNS Depressants** Concomitant use of baclofen with other CNS depressants (e.g., alcohol) may result in additive CNS depression.

■ **Morphine** Concomitant use of intrathecal baclofen with epidural morphine reportedly has resulted in hypotension and dyspnea.

Acute Toxicity

■ **Manifestations** Following ingestion of about 1 g of baclofen by a patient attempting suicide, reflexes were absent, and vomiting, muscle hypotonia, marked salivation, drowsiness, visual accommodation disorders, coma, respiratory depression, and seizures occurred. Serum lactic dehydrogenase and AST (SGOT) concentrations were also elevated. Supportive treatment consisted of endotracheal intubation and positive-pressure ventilation; after 3 days, some signs of muscle flaccidity still persisted. If oral baclofen overdosage occurs, the manufacturer recommends that the stomach be emptied promptly (i.e., by inducing emesis followed by gastric lavage) if the patient is alert. If the patient is obtunded, the airway should be secured with a cuffed endotracheal tube before beginning lavage, and adequate respiratory exchange should be maintained; induction of emesis and use of respiratory stimulants should be avoided.

Signs of intrathecal baclofen overdose may appear suddenly or over a period of time. Special attention must be given to recognizing the signs and symptoms of overdosage, particularly during the initial test for responsiveness, dosage titration, and reintroduction of therapy following temporary interruption. Acute, massive overdose may present as coma; in reports of coma resulting from overdose of intrathecal baclofen, the coma generally has been reversible following discontinuance of the infusion. Less sudden and/or less severe forms of overdose may present with drowsiness, lightheadedness, dizziness, somnolence, respiratory depression, hypothermia, seizures, rostral progression of hypotonia, and loss of consciousness progressing to coma persisting up to 72 hours. Should overdose appear likely, the patient should be taken immediately to a hospital for assessment and emptying of the pump reservoir. The manufacturer states that in cases reported to date, overdose generally has been related to pump malfunction, inadvertent subcutaneous injection, or dosing error; however, symptoms of overdose were reported in a baclofen-sensitive adult patient following intrathecal injection of a 25-mcg dose.

■ **Treatment** In the treatment of oral baclofen overdosage, immediate removal of the drug from the GI tract by emesis (if patient is conscious) or gastric lavage and maintenance of adequate respiratory exchange are recommended. If the patient is comatose, gastric lavage may be performed if an endotracheal tube with cuff inflated is in place to prevent aspiration of gastric contents. Respiratory stimulants should not be used.

There is no specific antidote for treating overdoses of baclofen intrathecal injection; however, any remaining baclofen solution in the pump should be removed as soon as possible and patients exhibiting respiratory depression should be intubated as necessary until the drug is eliminated.

If lumbar puncture is not contraindicated, consideration should be given to withdrawing 30–40 mL of CSF in order to reduce CSF baclofen concentration.

Pharmacology

Baclofen decreases the frequency and amplitude of muscle spasms (tonic reflexes) that arise in response to muscle stretching in patients with various spinal cord lesions. The drug simultaneously and equally suppresses cutaneous reflexes and muscle tone but only slightly depresses the amplitude of tendon jerks (phasic reflexes). The mechanism of action of baclofen is not completely understood, but the drug appears to act primarily at the spinal cord level. Apparently, baclofen predominantly inhibits spinal polysynaptic afferent pathways but may also inhibit monosynaptic afferent pathways to a lesser extent. The drug may inhibit monosynaptic and polysynaptic reflexes by acting as an inhibitory neuronal transmitter or by blocking excitatory synaptic transmission through hyperpolarization of afferent terminals. Because baclofen contains both GABA and phenylethylamine moieties, it has been postulated, but not proven, that the drug activates one of these putative inhibitory neurotransmitters. Baclofen has been shown to increase the metabolism of dopamine in animals but, in humans, CSF concentrations of 5-hydroxyindole acetic acid or dopamine metabolites are not altered by the drug. Because baclofen produces generalized CNS depression (e.g., sedation with tolerance, somnolence, ataxia, respiratory and cardiovascular depression), it has also been suggested that the drug may act at supraspinal sites.

Intrathecal administration of the drug in animals has been shown to increase antinociception and decrease muscle rigidity and spasticity.

Pharmacokinetics

■ **Absorption** Studies with radiolabeled baclofen have shown oral doses of 40 mg to be rapidly and almost completely absorbed from the GI tract, but there is relatively large intersubject variation in absorption and/or elimination. GI absorption of baclofen is reduced as dosage is increased. Serum concentrations required for therapeutic effects reportedly range from 80–395 ng/mL. Following oral administration of 40 mg of baclofen to healthy patients, peak blood concentrations of 500–600 ng/mL are reached in 2–3 hours and concentrations remain above 200 ng/mL for 8 hours. Beneficial effects of oral baclofen may not be immediately apparent; onset of therapeutic effect may vary from hours to weeks.

Following intrathecal administration of the drug, concurrent plasma baclofen concentrations are expected to be low (0–5 ng/mL); plasma concentrations of baclofen following intrathecal administration are 100 times lower than those achieved following oral administration. In pediatric patients 8–18 years of age who were receiving a continuous intrathecal infusion of baclofen at dosages of 77–400 mcg daily, plasma baclofen concentrations were near or below 10 mg/mL.

When baclofen is administered via intrathecal injection, the onset of action in adult patients generally is 0.5–1 hour following injection; peak spasmolytic effect is seen approximately 4 hours after dosing and effects may last 4–8 hours, although onset, peak, and duration of action are subject to interindividual variation, depending on the dose and severity of symptoms. Onset and duration of action and peak effects of baclofen in pediatric patients are similar to those reported in adult patients.

Following continuous intrathecal infusions of the drug, initial spasmolytic action is seen within 6–8 hours in adult patients; peak spasmolytic effect is observed within 24–48 hours. Pharmacokinetic data following continuous intrathecal infusion in pediatric patients currently are not available.

■ **Distribution** In animals, orally administered baclofen is widely distributed throughout the body, but only small amounts of the drug cross the blood-brain barrier.

Limited data suggest that a lumbar-cisternal gradient of approximately 4:1 is established along the neuroaxis during infusion of baclofen injection, based on simultaneous CSF sampling via lumbar and cisternal taps in a limited number of patients receiving continuous lumbar infusion of the drug at doses associated with therapeutic efficacy; however, there was wide interindividual variation. This gradient was not affected by patient position.

Baclofen crosses the placenta. Baclofen is distributed into milk following oral administration; it is not known whether the drug is distributed into milk following intrathecal administration.

At blood concentrations of 10 ng to 300 mcg/mL, 30% of baclofen is bound to serum proteins.

■ **Elimination** Baclofen has a serum half-life of 2.5–4 hours.

CSF clearance of baclofen following intrathecal administration via injection or continuous infusion approximates CSF turnover, suggesting that elimination of the drug occurs via bulk-flow removal of CSF. Following lumbar injection of the drug in doses of 50 or 100 mcg in a limited number of patients, the mean CSF elimination half-life was 1.51 hours for the first 4 hours following injection; mean CSF clearance of the drug was 30 mL/hour. Mean CSF clearance of the drug also was 30 mL/hour in a limited number of patients receiving the drug via continuous intrathecal infusion.

Only about 15% of a dose of the drug is metabolized in the liver, mostly by deamination. Baclofen is almost completely excreted within 72 hours following oral administration; 70–80% of the drug is excreted in urine unchanged or as metabolites and the remainder is excreted in the feces.

Chemistry and Stability

■ **Chemistry** Baclofen, the *p*-chlorophenyl derivative of γ-aminobutyric acid (GABA) containing a phenylethylamine moiety, is a skeletal muscle relaxant. Baclofen occurs as white to off-white crystals and is slightly soluble in water, very slightly soluble in methanol, and insoluble in chloroform. The drug has pK_a values of 5.4 and 9.5.

■ **Stability** Baclofen tablets should be stored in well-closed containers at 20–25°C.

Baclofen for injection concentrate for intrathecal administration is a sterile, nonpyrogenic, isotonic solution of the drug in water for injection. Each mL of the concentrate contains 0.39 mEq of sodium. Baclofen concentrate does not require refrigeration and is stable in solution at 37°C; however, the concentrate should not be stored at a temperature that exceeds 30°C and should not be frozen or autoclaved. The pH of the concentrate is 5–7. Because baclofen for injection concentrate contains no preservatives, each vial is intended for single use only; any unused solution should be discarded. Baclofen for injection concentrate is compatible with CSF, and must *only* be diluted with sterile, preservative-free 0.9% sodium chloride for injection.

Preparations

Excipients in commercially available drug preparations may have clinically important effects in some individuals; consult specific product labeling for details.

Baclofen

Oral		
Tablets	10 mg*	**Baclofen Tablets** (scored)
	20 mg*	**Baclofen Tablets** (scored)
Parenteral		
For injection concentrate, for intrathecal administration via compatible infusion device or for intrathecal injection	50 mcg/mL	**Gablofen®**, CNS Therapeutics **Lioresal® Intrathecal**, Medtronic
	0.5 mg/mL	**Gablofen®**, CNS Therapeutics **Lioresal® Intrathecal**, Medtronic
	2 mg/mL	**Gablofen®**, CNS Therapeutics **Lioresal® Intrathecal**, Medtronic

*available from one or more manufacturer, distributor, and/or repackager by generic (nonproprietary) name

†Use is not currently included in the labeling approved by the US Food and Drug Administration

NEUROMUSCULAR BLOCKING AGENTS 12:20.20

Neuromuscular Blocking Agents General Statement

■ Neuromuscular blocking agents are drugs that cause skeletal muscle relaxation and are classified as depolarizing or nondepolarizing (competitive) agents.

Uses

■ **Skeletal Muscle Relaxation** Neuromuscular blocking agents are used to produce skeletal muscle relaxation during surgery after general anesthesia has been induced. When neuromuscular blocking drugs are used to provide the necessary muscle relaxation during surgery, operating conditions may be improved and a lighter level of anesthesia may be used.

Neuromuscular blocking agents also are used to facilitate endotracheal intubation and prevent laryngospasm. A neuromuscular blocking agent with a rapid onset of action (e.g., succinylcholine, rocuronium) generally is preferred in emergency situations when rapid intubation (e.g., rapid sequence intubation) is required.

Neuromuscular blocking agents also have been used to facilitate mechanical ventilation in the intensive care unit (ICU). Long-term use of neuromuscular blocking agents in the ICU has been associated rarely with prolonged paralysis and/or skeletal muscle weakness. Whenever neuromuscular blocking agents are used in the ICU, the benefits versus risks of such therapy must be considered and patients should be assessed frequently to determine the need for continued paralysis. (See Cautions: Precautions and Contraindications.)

Neuromuscular blocking agents (generally succinylcholine) also have been used during electroconvulsive therapy† to reduce muscle contractions and reduce the risk of serious patient injury. In addition, neuromuscular blocking agents have been used for symptomatic control of muscular spasms in various seizure states† including tetanus, status epilepticus, drug intoxication, eclampsia, and those resulting from black widow spider bites. The drugs can modify the muscular component of these seizure states, but the underlying CNS process is unaffected. Management of these states should be directed to more specific modes of treatment of the underlying cause before a neuromuscular blocking agent is employed.

Neuromuscular blocking agents are classified as depolarizing or nondepolarizing based on their mechanism of action. (See Pharmacology.) Succinylcholine is the only currently available depolarizing neuromuscular blocking agent. Nondepolarizing neuromuscular blocking agents include atracurium, cisatracurium, pancuronium, rocuronium, and vecuronium; these drugs are further characterized based on their structure as a benzylisoquinolinium (atracurium, cisatracurium) or aminosteroid (rocuronium, vecuronium, pancuronium) compound.

The choice of a specific neuromuscular blocking agent should be individualized based on factors such as the clinical setting (surgical or ICU), duration of procedure, anesthetic technique, patient condition, and adverse effects and pharmacokinetic profile (onset and duration) of the drug. A neuromuscular blocking agent with a rapid onset of action (e.g., succinylcholine, rocuronium) is desirable for short procedures lasting less than 3 minutes. Because of its rapid onset (less than 1 minute after IV administration) and short duration of action (approximately 4–6 minutes), succinylcholine traditionally has been considered the drug of choice for rapid sequence intubation; however, the drug is associated with serious adverse effects (e.g., bradycardia, hyperkalemia, malignant hyperthermia). If succinylcholine cannot be used, rocuronium (which has the most similar pharmacokinetic profile) generally is recommended as an alternative. Clinical studies have shown that rocuronium can produce similar intubating conditions to succinylcholine when given in sufficient doses (e.g., at least 1 mg/kg); however, succinylcholine is more likely to achieve excellent intubating conditions and remains clinically superior to rocuronium with respect to its shorter duration of action. Vecuronium, atracurium, and cisatracurium have acceptable onsets of action and may be suitable for certain procedures depending on the urgency of the situation. Pancuronium is not appropriate for emergency intubation because of its slow onset and long duration of action, but may be used for other indications (e.g., mechanical ventilation) in which rapid onset and short duration of action are not as important. Although priming-dose regimens of nondepolarizing neuromuscular blocking agents have been used to accelerate the onset of these drugs, this technique is limited clinically because of the potential for respiratory compromise. The potential for neuromuscular blocking agents to cause adverse cardiovascular effects also should be considered in patients undergoing surgery; since rocuronium, cisatracurium, and vecuronium are associated with minimal cardiac effects, these drugs usually are preferred. Pancuronium has prominent vagolytic effects and generally should not be used in patients who cannot tolerate an increase in heart rate (e.g. those with cardiovascular disease). Cisatracurium or atracurium may be particularly useful in patients with renal or hepatic impairment since these drugs undergo Hofmann degradation and are not dependent on renal and hepatic pathways for elimination.

The criteria for selecting a neuromuscular blocking agent in the ICU differ from the criteria used during surgery. In the ICU, it is more important to consider a drug that does not accumulate with long-term use rather than a drug with a rapid onset and short duration of action. Cisatracurium and atracurium are less likely to accumulate with prolonged use because of their lack of dependence on renal and hepatic pathways for elimination, and therefore may be the preferred neuromuscular blocking agents in this setting.

Although the nondepolarizing agents and the depolarizing agents may be mutually antagonistic under some circumstances, various neuromuscular blocking agents are often used together. Succinylcholine, because of its short duration of action, may be used to facilitate intubation prior to a nondepolarizing agent; however, the effects of succinylcholine should be allowed to dissipate before the nondepolarizing agent is given. If tachyphylaxis develops to the effects of a depolarizing agent after prolonged or repeated administration, a nondepolarizing agent may be substituted to maintain neuromuscular blockade.

Since neuromuscular blocking agents have no known effect on consciousness, pain, or cerebration, these drugs should be used in conjunction with adequate levels of general anesthesia, and only after appropriate analgesics and sedatives are administered. To avoid distress to the patient, neuromuscular blocking agents generally should be administered only after unconsciousness has been induced.

Dosage and Administration

■ **Administration** Neuromuscular blocking agents are usually administered IV because of the need for careful control of their effects. For infants or other patients in whom a suitable vein is not accessible, succinylcholine may be administered IM. For specific procedures and techniques of administration, specialized references should be consulted.

■ **Dosage** Dosage of neuromuscular blocking agents must be carefully adjusted according to individual requirements and response and should be no larger than that necessary for adequate muscle relaxation. The use of a peripheral nerve stimulator (in conjunction with clinical assessments) is recommended to accurately monitor the degree of neuromuscular blockade and recovery, determine the need for additional doses, and minimize the possibility of overdosage.

Cautions

■ **Adverse Effects** Adverse effects of neuromuscular blocking agents consist principally of extensions of the pharmacologic actions of the drugs. The potential for adverse effects varies considerably among the different neuromuscular blocking agents depending on their affinity for extrajunctional cholinergic receptors.

Neuromuscular blocking agents can stimulate nicotinic and muscarinic receptors outside the neuromuscular junction, predominantly causing adverse cardiac effects. Among the nondepolarizing neuromuscular blocking agents, pancuronium is associated with the greatest potential for cardiac effects because of its affinity for muscarinic receptors in the parasympathetic and peripheral sympathetic nervous systems; tachycardia usually results from vagolytic and sympathomimetic effects. Rocuronium also exhibits some vagal blocking activity and has been associated with transient tachycardia. The remaining nondepolarizing neuromuscular blocking agents (cisatracurium, atracurium, vecuronium) have weaker affinities for these extrajunctional receptors and cause minimal or no clinically important cardiovascular effects at the recommended doses. While succinylcholine does not have a direct effect on the myocardium, the drug stimulates autonomic ganglia and muscarinic receptors, which can cause bradycardia. All of the neuromuscular blocking agents have histamine-releasing properties that can also result in hypotension and tachycardia; atracurium and succinylcholine have the greatest potential for histamine release, while pancuronium, cisatracurium, vecuronium, and rocuronium are associated with minimal or no histamine-releasing activity at the recommended doses.

Prolonged recovery of neuromuscular function after cessation of neuromuscular blocking drugs can occur due to accumulation of the neuromuscular blocking agent (or its metabolites) or concomitant use of certain drugs and appears to be more common with the longer-acting agents (e.g., pancuronium, vecuronium). Complications include various degrees of residual muscle weakness and/or paralysis, which can result in respiratory complications.

Hypersensitivity reactions, including anaphylaxis, have been reported rarely with all neuromuscular blocking agents; such reactions have been life-threatening or fatal in some cases.

Manifestations associated with histamine release (other than cardiac effects) may include cutaneous effects such as flushing, erythema, pruritus, urticaria, wheal formation, and pulmonary effects such as wheezing and bronchospasm. (See Pharmacology.)

Malignant hyperthermia is a rare but often fatal adverse reaction associated with the use of neuromuscular blocking agents and/or potent inhalation anesthetics. Succinylcholine and halothane are the agents most commonly associated with this condition. Heredity appears to be a factor in this reaction, because several families have been shown to have high incidence of hyperthermia. Malignant hyperthermia is manifested by a rapid, profound elevation in body temperature and sometimes extreme muscular rigidity unresponsive to the neuromuscular blocking agents. Because malignant hyperthermia can occur even in the absence of a recognized precipitating factor, clinicians should be vigilant for its possible development and prepared for its management in any patient undergoing general anesthesia. As soon as malignant hyperthermia is recognized, all anesthetic agents should be discontinued and IV dantrolene therapy initiated. IV dantrolene is used in conjunction with supportive measures which include administering oxygen, treating metabolic acidosis, and instituting cooling procedures if necessary; urinary output should be maintained and serum electrolytes should be monitored. Large IV doses of procainamide hydrochloride have also been reported to occasionally be effective in reversing the condition.

Prolonged or repeated use of depolarizing agents may produce tachyphylaxis and phase II blockade and, therefore, multiple fractional doses of these agents should generally not be used.

■ **Precautions and Contraindications** Because neuromuscular blocking agents can severely compromise respiratory function and cause respiratory paralysis if not used correctly, these drugs should be administered only by individuals who are experienced in their use and complications. For specific procedures and techniques of administration, specialized references should be consulted. Facilities and personnel necessary for intubation, administration of oxygen, and respiratory support should be immediately available whenever these agents are used. Dispensing and administration precautions (e.g., storage segregation, warning labels, access limitations) should be taken to ensure that neuromuscular blocking agents are not administered without adequate respiratory support. Affixing warning labels to storage containers and final administration containers is recommended to clearly communicate that respiratory paralysis can occur and ventilator support is required. The Institute for Safe Medication Practices (ISMP) recommends the following wording for these containers: "Warning: Paralyzing agent—causes respiratory arrest—patient must be ventilated". If respiratory paralysis occurs, primary attention should be given to reestablishment of adequate respiratory exchange by maintenance of an adequate airway, control of respiration, and oxygen administration. Ventilatory support should be continued until complete respiratory recovery is assured.

A reversal agent should be readily available during administration of the nondepolarizing neuromuscular blocking agents. Pharmacologic reversal may be needed during a failed intubation attempt or to accelerate postoperative recovery of neuromuscular function. Competitive blockade produced by the nondepolarizing agents may be antagonized by IV administration of cholinesterase inhibitors such as neostigmine methylsulfate, pyridostigmine bromide, or edrophonium chloride, which produce an excess of acetylcholine at the motor end-plate. An anticholinergic agent such as atropine or glycopyrrolate is often administered in conjunction with a cholinesterase inhibitor to counteract the adverse muscarinic effects (e.g., bradycardia, hypotension, salivation) of the cholinesterase inhibitor. Sugammadex, a selective relaxant binding agent, may be used to reverse the effects of rocuronium or vecuronium in adults after surgery. To minimize the risk of residual neuromuscular blockade, pharmacologic reversal should only be attempted after some degree of spontaneous recovery has occurred; patients should be monitored closely until adequate recovery of normal neuromuscular function is assured (i.e., ability to maintain satisfactory ventilation and a patent airway). No effective antagonist is available to reverse the characteristic phase I depolarization block produced by succinylcholine. However, depending on the dose and duration of succinylcholine administration, phase I block may transition to a phase II block. Fully established phase II block may occasionally be antagonized by the use of small, repeated doses of a cholinesterase inhibitor. Prolonged administration of the depolarizing agents may lead to desensitization of the motor end-plate resulting in a prolonged neuromuscular blockade unresponsive to the anticholinesterases.

In the intensive care setting, long-term use of neuromuscular blocking drugs to facilitate mechanical ventilation may be associated with prolonged paralysis and/or skeletal muscle weakness that may be noted first during attempts to wean such patients from the ventilator. Typically, such patients are receiving concurrent drug therapy (e.g., broad-spectrum anti-infectives, opiate agonists, corticosteroids) and may have electrolyte imbalances and/or diseases known to produce electrolyte imbalances, renal or hepatic impairment, hypoxic episodes of varying duration, acid-base imbalances, and/or extreme debilitation, any of which may enhance the effects of a neuromuscular blocking agent. Additionally, patients immobilized for extended periods of time frequently may develop symptoms consistent with disuse muscle atrophy. The recovery period may vary from regaining movement and strength in all muscles to initial recovery of the facial and small muscles of the extremities, followed by recovery of the remaining muscles. Rarely, recovery of muscle strength and movement may be over an extended period of time and may even require occasional rehabilitation. Therefore, when there is a need for long-term mechanical ventilation, the benefits of such therapy must be weighed against the risks. To reduce the possibility of prolonged neuromuscular blockade and other complications that might occur following long-term use of neuromuscular blocking drugs in intensive care settings, these drugs should be administered in carefully adjusted doses by or under the supervision of experienced clinicians familiar with appropriate peripheral nerve stimulator muscle monitoring techniques. Continuous monitoring of neuromuscular transmission should be considered during both therapy and recovery in patients receiving the drugs long term in the intensive care setting. Additional doses of neuromuscular blocking drugs should not be given before there is a definite response to nerve stimulation tests. If no response is elicited, administration of the drug should be discontinued until a response returns.

All neuromuscular blocking agents should be used with caution in patients with renal, hepatic, or pulmonary impairment, or respiratory depression, and in geriatric or debilitated patients. The drugs should be used with extreme caution, if at all, in patients with myasthenia gravis. Other conditions that are associated with increased response to the neuromuscular blocking agents are the myasthenic syndrome associated with lung cancer, dehydration, thyroid disorders, collagen diseases, porphyria, and familial periodic paralysis. Potent inhalation anesthetics and neuromuscular blocking agents should be avoided if possible in patients who have experienced malignant hyperthermia and in members of their families, and the possibility that this reaction could occur in any patient undergoing general anesthesia should be considered. (See Cautions: Adverse Effects.) During the first month of life, neonates are particularly sensitive to the action of most nondepolarizing agents and respond with prolonged neuromuscular blockade to usual doses of the drugs.

Because of the risk of anaphylaxis, appropriate precautionary measures (including the immediate availability of emergency treatment for anaphylaxis) should be taken whenever neuromuscular blocking agents are administered. Because of the potential for cross-sensitivity, particular caution should be taken in individuals who have previously experienced an anaphylactic reaction to any neuromuscular blocking agent (depolarizing or nondepolarizing).

Resistance to nondepolarizing neuromuscular blocking agents can develop in burn patients and may be substantial. The magnitude of resistance depends on the extent of thermal injury and elapsed time since the burn, with patients having burns that extend over 25–30% or more of body surface area being most likely to exhibit resistance (increasing with increased injury) and the resistance only becoming apparent 1 week or longer after the burn. Such resistance generally peaks 2 or more weeks after the burn, persists for several months or longer, and decreases gradually with healing. The mechanism of this resistance appears to be complex, and may involve pharmacokinetic, pharmacodynamic, and pathophysiologic factors. While reductions in the free (unbound)-fraction of circulating plasma concentrations of the drugs may contribute to this resistance, the magnitude of such resistance cannot be explained entirely by such alterations in protein binding of the drugs. It also has been suggested that changes in the number of acetylcholine receptors and/or in anticholinesterase activity may contribute to this resistance, but some evidence does not support this suggestion. Other mechanisms (e.g., circulating substances in plasma that bind to or inactivate the drugs) also have been suggested. The possible need for substantially increased doses of nondepolarizing agents in burn patients should be considered.

Succinylcholine should be used with caution in patients with electrolyte disturbances, especially hyperkalemia, and in digitalized patients because depolarizing agents may cause release of intracellular potassium into the plasma. The resulting hyperkalemia is particularly great in patients with severe burns or trauma, spinal cord injuries, or degenerative or dystrophic muscle diseases, and in paraplegic patients. Hypokalemia can lead to depressed membrane excitability of skeletal muscle and potentiate the effects of the nondepolarizing agents. When suspected of being abnormal, serum potassium concentrations should be determined before administering neuromuscular blocking agents. High magnesium concentrations partially block the release of ACh from the motor nerve ending and can potentiate the effects of both depolarizing and nondepolarizing agents. Hypocalcemia can increase the excitability of muscles and potentiate the effects of neuromuscular blocking agents, particularly the nondepolarizing agents.

Succinylcholine should be used with caution in patients with fractures or muscular spasms, as the initial muscle fasciculation caused by the drugs may result in additional trauma. Hypothermia tends to decrease the intensity and duration of a nondepolarizing block, but increases the intensity and duration of a depolarizing block; hyperthermia causes the opposite effects. Patients with severe hepatic impairment may have decreased plasma concentrations of pseudocholinesterase. In these patients, the duration of action of succinylcholine may be increased because of reduced metabolism.

■ **Pediatric Precautions** Some preparations of neuromuscular blocking agents may contain benzyl alcohol as a preservative. Although a causal relationship has not been established, administration of injections preserved with benzyl alcohol has been associated with toxicity in neonates. Toxicity appears to have resulted from administration of large amounts (i.e., 100–400 mg/kg daily) of benzyl alcohol in these neonates. Although use of drugs preserved with benzyl alcohol should be avoided in neonates whenever possible, the American Academy of Pediatrics states that the presence of small amounts of the preservative in a commercially available injection should not proscribe its use when indicated in neonates.

■ **Pregnancy** It is not known whether administration of neuromuscular blocking agents during vaginal delivery has immediate or delayed adverse effects on the fetus or whether it increases the likelihood that resuscitation of the neonate will be necessary. Neuromuscular blocking agents should be used with caution and dosage reduced as necessary in pregnant women receiving magnesium sulfate during delivery, since the neuromuscular blockade may be potentiated and its reversal impeded. Since neuromuscular blocking agents may cross the placenta, the possibility of respiratory depression in neonates should be considered following cesarean section in which a neuromuscular blocking agent is administered to the mother. Neuromuscular blocking agents should be used during pregnancy only when the potential benefits justify the possible risks to the fetus. Animal reproduction studies have not been performed with many neuromuscular blocking agents; however, some of the agents have been shown to be potentially teratogenic (e.g., atracurium).

Drug Interactions

Concurrent administration of several drugs has been reported to affect patient response to neuromuscular blocking agents.

■ **General Anesthetics** General anesthetics, particularly enflurane and isoflurane, and to a lesser extent, halothane, can potentiate the effects of nondepolarizing neuromuscular blocking agents. The response to depolarizing agents may also be affected, but to a lesser extent.

■ **Anti-infective Agents** Aminoglycoside antibiotics are believed to inhibit neuromuscular transmission. These drugs have been reported to increase or prolong skeletal muscle relaxation produced by the neuromuscular blocking agents when the antibiotics were administered parenterally or intraperitoneally during surgery and have reinstated neuromuscular blockade when administered parenterally postoperatively. Kanamycin, neomycin, and streptomycin appear to have the greatest potential for causing this effect. Potentiation of neuromuscular blockade has been reported following oral administration of some of the aminoglycoside antibiotics, but not as frequently as with parenteral use. The polymyxin antibiotics (polymyxin B sulfate, colistin, colistimethate sodium) and, to a lesser extent, another polypeptide antibiotic, capreomycin sulfate, and clindamycin and lincomycin have also been reported to potentiate effects of neuromuscular blocking agents. If any of these anti-infective agents is used before, during, or after surgical procedures in which a neuromuscular blocking agent is administered, the possibility of prolonged duration of neuromuscular blockade (or recurarization, particularly postoperatively) should be considered. Reversible cholinesterase inhibitors (edrophonium chloride, neostigmine methylsulfate) and IV calcium sometimes reverse neuromuscular blockade produced by neuromuscular blocking agents and potentiated by the aminoglycoside antibiotics. IV calcium (but not the cholinesterase inhibitors) has occasionally been successful in reversing neuromuscular blockade produced by neuromuscular blocking agents and potentiated by the polymyxins.

■ **Anticonvulsants** In patients receiving chronic therapy with carbamazepine or phenytoin, the duration of neuromuscular blockade with nondepolarizing agents may be shorter than anticipated and the degree of blockade for a given dose may be decreased. Therefore, such patients should be monitored closely for reduced effectiveness of nondepolarizing neuromuscular blocking agents and the dose (e.g., rate of IV infusion) adjusted accordingly. The mechanism of this resistance is not known, but receptor up-regulation may be a contributing factor.

■ **Diazepam** There have been conflicting reports concerning the effects of concurrent administration of diazepam and nondepolarizing neuromuscular blocking agents. Some reports indicate that IV diazepam may increase the intensity and duration of the neuromuscular blockade produced by gallamine (no longer commercially available in the US). Other studies have failed to confirm this interaction.

■ **Opiate Analgesics** The central respiratory depressant effects of the opiate analgesics can add to the respiratory depressant effects of the neuromuscular blocking agents. Extreme caution should be used when administering opiates during surgery or in the immediate postoperative period in patients who have received neuromuscular blocking agents.

■ **Potassium-depleting Agents** Potassium-depleting drugs such as the thiazide diuretics, furosemide, ethacrynic acid, chlorthalidone, the carbonic anhydrase inhibitors, amphotericin B, the corticosteroids, or corticotropin may cause prolonged neuromuscular blockade in patients receiving nondepolarizing agents.

■ **Other Drugs** Multiple doses of quinine or quinidine, β-adrenergic blocking agents (e.g., propranolol), and excessively high IV doses of lidocaine have been shown to potentiate the effects of both types of neuromuscular blocking agents. These drugs are believed to interfere with the ionic permeability of the post-junctional membrane. The drugs can cause apnea when given postoperatively to patients thought to have recovered from neuromuscular blockade and can increase neuromuscular blockade when given simultaneously with the neuromuscular blocking agents.

Parenteral administration of magnesium sulfate may raise serum magnesium concentrations sufficiently to potentiate the neuromuscular blocking agents. When magnesium sulfate is administered for the management of toxemia of pregnancy, the neuromuscular blockade induced by a blocking agent may be potentiated and its reversal impeded. If a neuromuscular blocking agent is used in a pregnant woman receiving magnesium sulfate, the drug should be used with caution and its dosage reduced as necessary.

Pharmacology

Neuromuscular blocking agents are drugs that cause skeletal muscle relaxation mainly by producing a decreased response to the neurotransmitter acetylcholine (ACh) at the neuromuscular junction of skeletal muscle. Based on the mechanism by which they decrease the effects of ACh, these drugs can be classified as depolarizing or nondepolarizing (competitive) neuromuscular blocking agents:

DEPOLARIZING AGENTS
Succinylcholine Chloride

NONDEPOLARIZING AGENTS
Atracurium Besylate
Cisatracurium Besylate
Pancuronium Bromide
Rocuronium Bromide
Vecuronium Bromide

Although depolarizing and nondepolarizing neuromuscular blocking agents have different mechanisms of action, the similarity of the end result of their pharmacologic actions and of their therapeutic uses permits their discussion as a class.

Neuromuscular blocking agents produce skeletal muscle paralysis mainly by causing a decreased response to ACh at the myoneural junction. At that site, the neurotransmitter normally produces electrical depolarization of the postjunctional membrane of the motor end-plate, leading to conduction of muscle action potential which in turn induces skeletal muscle contraction. The drugs also act prejunctionally on the motor neuron, although the importance of this action is unclear.

Nondepolarizing agents have a high affinity for ACh receptor sites and competitively block access of ACh to the motor end-plate of the myoneural junction. Nondepolarizing agents have little or no agonist activity. Thus, they may block the effects of both the small quantities of ACh that maintain muscle tone and the large quantities of ACh that produce voluntary skeletal muscle contraction, but they do not alter the resting electrical potential of the motor end-plate or cause muscular contractions. There is evidence that nondepolarizing agents also affect ACh release. It has been hypothesized that nondepolarizing agents bind to postjunctional ("curare") receptors and may thereby interfere with the sodium and potassium flux which is responsible for depolarization and repolarization of the membranes involved in muscle contraction. The degree to which each mechanism of action contributes to the clinical effect of the nondepolarizing agents is unclear and may vary with the specific drug.

Depolarizing agents have a high affinity for ACh receptor sites and like ACh produce depolarization of the motor end-plate at the myoneural junction. Immediately after a single IV dose of a depolarizing agent, transient twitching or fasciculation of the skeletal muscles occurs and is followed by muscle paralysis. Because of their high affinity for ACh receptors and their resistance to acetylcholinesterase, the depolarizing agents produce more prolonged depolarization at the motor end-plate than does ACh. The initial depolarization block is also known as a phase I block and is characterized by well-sustained muscular contractions following both fast (tetanic) and slow (twitch) electrical nerve stimulation; post-tetanic facilitation is absent. Cholinesterase inhibitors may potentiate phase I block and nondepolarizing agents reverse it. With prolonged or repeated administration of a depolarizing agent, the nature of the block changes to a phase II or desensitization block which resembles a nondepolarizing block. Phase II block is characterized by poorly sustained muscle contractions following both fast and slow electrical nerve stimulation and the presence of post-tetanic facilitation. The transition from a phase I to a phase II block is gradual and variable in time course among individuals in contrast to phase I block. Fully established phase II block can be reversed by cholinesterase inhibitors and potentiated by nondepolarizing agents. In neonates and patients with myasthenia gravis, depolarizing agents produce an immediate phase II block, bypassing phase I.

The first muscles to be affected following administration of a neuromuscular blocking agent are those producing fine, rapid movements such as those of the eyes, face, and neck. Muscles of the limbs, abdomen, and chest are affected next, and the diaphragm is affected last. Recovery of muscles generally occurs in the reverse order. Respiratory depression or apnea may result from involvement of the intercostal muscles and diaphragm. Relaxation of the muscles of the tongue, pharynx, and epiglottis may also completely close the airway.

By competing with ACh for cholinergic receptors at the autonomic ganglia, tubocurarine (no longer commercially available in the US) may further affect the autonomic nervous system and produce ganglionic blockade. It has been reported that succinylcholine stimulates the cardiac vagus and subsequently sympathetic ganglia. The histamine-releasing properties of the neuromuscular blocking agents vary according to the specific drug and dose employed. Tubocurarine appears to be a potent stimulator of histamine release; metocurine (no longer commercially available in the US) and succinylcholine also cause histamine release, but to a lesser extent. Atracurium is a less potent stimulator of histamine release than is tubocurarine. Pancuronium appears to release detectable amounts of histamine only at excessive dosages. Vecuronium, cisatracurium, and rocuronium appear to have little, if any, histamine-releasing activity at recommended doses. Neuromuscular blocking agents also exhibit cardiovascular effects to varying degrees. Neuromuscular blocking agents do not affect pain or other sensory perception.

Young and small children may generally require larger doses of neuromuscular blocking agents than adolescents and adults, when calculated on a weight basis, to achieve the same degree of neuromuscular blockade during comparable techniques of anesthesia. Factors that may influence dose-response relationships during childhood include age-related changes in the relative amount of muscle as a proportion of body weight, in renal function, and in the size of the extracellular fluid volume and the resultant apparent volume of distribution for neuromuscular blocking agents.

Pharmacokinetics

■ **Absorption** All neuromuscular blocking agents are poorly absorbed from the GI tract.

The onset of action varies among individual patients and with the various neuromuscular blocking agents and their route of administration, dosage, and the general anesthetic agent employed. In general, the first signs of neuromuscular blockade occur within approximately 2 minutes following IV administration of nondepolarizing agents and maximal effects occur in about 3–6 minutes; maximal effects of succinylcholine usually occur within 1 minute. The onset of action is slower and less predictable following IM administration than after IV injection and for this reason the IM route is seldom used. The duration of action of the individual agents varies widely. After a single dose, redistribution accounts for termination of action of most of the agents; however, after multiple doses, metabolism and excretion as well as further redistribution play a part in determining the duration of action.

■ **Distribution** After IV administration, the drugs are distributed in the extracellular fluid and rapidly reach their site of action at the motor end-plate of the myoneural junction. Most neuromuscular blocking agents cross the blood-brain barrier to a very small extent, if at all. Increased protein binding (possibly to α_1-acid glycoprotein) of nondepolarizing neuromuscular blocking agents with subsequent decreases in the free-fraction of circulating drug may occur in patients with burns.

Neuromuscular blocking agents may cross the placenta, especially during the first trimester of pregnancy.

■ **Elimination** Succinylcholine is metabolized rapidly by pseudocholinesterase and is excreted in urine as active and inactive metabolites and small amounts of unchanged drug. Pancuronium is eliminated mainly unchanged by the kidneys, although small amounts may be metabolized and some of the drug may be eliminated in the bile. Rocuronium is metabolized to a less active metabolite, 17-desacetyl-rocuronium, that is rarely detected in the plasma and urine, and is eliminated principally by the liver. Atracurium and cisatracurium undergo rapid metabolism via Hofmann elimination and via nonspecific enzymatic ester hydrolysis; the liver does not appear to play a major role in the metabolism of these drugs. Atracurium, cisatracurium, and their metabolites, including the metabolic products of Hofmann elimination and nonspecific enzymatic ester hydrolysis, are excreted principally in urine and also in feces via biliary elimination. The metabolic fate of vecuronium has not been fully characterized. In aqueous solution in vitro, vecuronium undergoes spontaneous deacetylation at the 3α- and/or 17β-positions to form the hydroxy derivatives. The extent of spontaneous deacetylation and/or metabolism of the drug in vivo in humans remains to be clearly determined. Vecuronium and its metabolite(s) appear to be excreted principally in feces via biliary elimination; the drug and its metabolite(s) are also excreted in urine.

Chemistry

Although neuromuscular blocking agents are structurally similar in that most contain quaternary ammonium groups, it is difficult to generalize about the structure-activity relationships of the neuromuscular blocking agents. The presence of multiple quaternary ammonium groups seems to increase each drug's affinity for its receptor sites.

For further information on chemistry and stability, pharmacology, pharmacokinetics, uses, cautions, acute toxicity, drug interactions, and dosage and administration of the neuromuscular blocking agents, see the individual monographs in 12:20.20.

†Use is not currently included in the labeling approved by the US Food and Drug Administration

Cisatracurium Besylate

■ Cisatracurium besylate, a benzylisoquinolone nondepolarizing neuromuscular blocking agent, is an isomer of atracurium.

Uses

■ **Skeletal Muscle Relaxation** Cisatracurium besylate is used to produce skeletal muscle relaxation during surgery after general anesthesia has been induced. The drug also is used to facilitate endotracheal intubation; however, a neuromuscular blocking agent with a rapid onset of action (e.g., succinylcholine, rocuronium) generally is preferred in emergency situations when rapid intubation is required. Cisatracurium is *not* recommended for rapid sequence intubation because of its intermediate onset of action.

Cisatracurium also is used to facilitate mechanical ventilation in the intensive care unit (ICU). The drug has been given as a continuous IV infusion for up to 6 days in this setting; longer durations of use have not been evaluated. Whenever neuromuscular blocking agents are used in the ICU, the benefits versus risks of such therapy must be considered and patients should be assessed frequently to determine the need for continued paralysis. (See Intensive Care Setting under Warnings/Precautions: General Precautions, in Cautions.)

Compared with other neuromuscular blocking agents, cisatracurium has an intermediate onset and duration of action. In clinical studies, cisatracurium was administered at a rate of infusion one-third that of atracurium and exhibited a similar time to spontaneous recovery. Studies comparing cisatracurium with vecuronium showed a longer duration of action and faster time to spontaneous recovery with cisatracurium. Cisatracurium has minimal, if any, cardiovascular effects and causes less histamine release than atracurium. Because cisatracurium (and atracurium) undergo Hofmann degradation and are not dependent on renal or hepatic pathways for elimination, these neuromuscular blocking agents may be particularly useful in patients with hepatic or renal impairment; some experts prefer the use of cisatracurium or atracurium if prolonged therapy is necessary in ICU patients with multiple organ dysfunction.

For additional information on uses and treatment principles of neuromuscular blocking agents, see Uses in the Neuromuscular Blocking Agents General Statement 12:20.20.

Dosage and Administration

■ **Administration** Cisatracurium is administered IV only.

Commercially available 20-mL single-dose vials of cisatracurium besylate containing 10 mg/mL are intended for intensive care unit (ICU) use *only.*

IV Administration The initial (intubating) dose of cisatracurium is administered by rapid IV injection; maintenance doses may be administered by intermittent IV injection or continuous IV infusion.

For continuous IV infusion, cisatracurium besylate injection should be diluted to the desired concentration (e.g., 0.1–0.4 mg/mL) in a compatible IV solution (5% dextrose, 0.9% sodium chloride, or 5% dextrose and 0.9% sodium chloride injection). Continuous IV infusions of cisatracurium have been administered for up to 3 hours without evidence of cumulative neuromuscular blocking effects; such administration has no effect on duration of blockade, provided partial recovery is allowed to occur between doses. The rate of spontaneous neuromuscular recovery following discontinuance of the infusion is likely to be comparable to the rate of recovery following administration of a single IV injection of the drug.

Cisatracurium besylate injection should be stored at 2–8°C and protected from light prior to use; the drug should not be frozen. Once removed from refrigeration, the injection should be used within 21 days, regardless of whether it was subsequently returned to refrigeration. Following dilution, the infusion solution should be used within 24 hours.

Rate of Administration. Initial (intubating) doses of cisatracurium are administered by direct IV injection, usually over 5–10 seconds.

Continuous IV infusion rates should be individualized based on patient requirements and response to peripheral nerve stimulation. (See Tables 1 and 2 for recommended rates of infusion.) Accurate dosage is best achieved using a precision infusion device.

Table 1. Infusion Rates Required to Deliver Selected Dosages of Cisatracurium from Solutions Containing 0.1 mg/mL of the Drug

	Drug Delivery Rate (mcg/kg per minute)				
	1	1.5	2	3	5
Weight (kg)	Infusion Delivery Rate (mL/hr)				
10	6	9	12	18	30
45	27	41	54	81	135
70	42	63	84	126	210
100	60	90	120	180	300

Table 2. Infusion Rates Required to Deliver Selected Dosages of Cisatracurium from Solutions Containing 0.4 mg/mL of the Drug

	Drug Delivery Rate (mcg/kg per minute)				
	1	1.5	2	3	5
Weight (kg)	Infusion Delivery Rate (mL/hr)				
10	1.5	2.3	3	4.5	7.5
45	6.8	10.1	13.5	20.3	33.8
70	10.5	15.8	21	31.5	52.5
100	15	22.5	30	45	75

Dispensing and Administration Precautions Neuromuscular blocking agents should be administered only by individuals who are adequately trained in their use and complications. For specific procedures and techniques of administration, specialized references should be consulted. Facilities and personnel necessary for intubation, administration of oxygen, and respiratory support should be immediately available whenever these drugs are used. In addition, a reversal agent should be readily available in the event of a failed intubation or to accelerate neuromuscular recovery after surgery. (See Dosage and Administration: Reversal of Neuromuscular Blockade.)

Because neuromuscular blocking agents can cause respiratory arrest, precautions (e.g., storage segregation, warning labels, access limitations) should be taken to ensure that these drugs are not administered without adequate respiratory support. Affixing warning labels to storage containers and final administration containers is recommended to clearly communicate that respiratory paralysis can occur and ventilator support is required. The Institute for Safe Medication Practices (ISMP) recommends the following wording for these containers: "Warning: Paralyzing agent—causes respiratory arrest—patient must be ventilated."

Neuromuscular blocking agents have no known effect on consciousness, pain, or cerebration, and should therefore be used in conjunction with adequate levels of anesthesia, and only after appropriate analgesics and sedatives are administered. To avoid distress to the patient, cisatracurium should be administered only after unconsciousness has been induced.

■ Dosage

Dosage of cisatracurium besylate is expressed in terms of cisatracurium.

Dosage of cisatracurium must be carefully adjusted according to individual requirements and response. The use of a peripheral nerve stimulator is recommended to accurately monitor the degree of neuromuscular blockade and recovery, determine the need for additional doses, and minimize the possibility of overdosage. (See Administration Precautions under Warnings/Precautions: Warnings, in Cautions.)

Skeletal Muscle Relaxation in Pediatric Patients **Initial (Intubating) Dose.** The recommended initial intubating dose of cisatracurium in infants 1–23 months of age when used concomitantly with halothane or opiate anesthesia is 0.15 mg/kg. This dose generally produces maximum neuromuscular blockade in about 2 minutes and clinically effective blockade for about 43 minutes.

The recommended initial intubating dose of cisatracurium in children 2–12 years of age when used concomitantly with halothane or opiate anesthesia is 0.1–0.15 mg/kg. A dose of 0.1 mg/kg administered under these conditions can be expected to produce maximum neuromuscular blockade in about 2.8 minutes and clinically effective blockade for about 28 minutes, and a dose of 0.15 mg/kg can be expected to produce maximum neuromuscular blockade in about 3 minutes and clinically effective blockade for about 36 minutes.

The manufacturer makes no specific dosage recommendations for adolescents 13 years of age or older.

Maintenance Dosage During Prolonged Surgical Procedures. After the initial intubating dose is administered, children 2 years of age or older may receive a continuous IV infusion of cisatracurium to maintain neuromuscular blockade during prolonged surgical procedures. The infusion should be initiated only after early spontaneous recovery from the initial dose is evident. The rate of infusion should be individualized based on patient response to peripheral nerve stimulation. An initial rate of 3 mcg/kg per minute may be necessary to rapidly counteract spontaneous neuromuscular recovery; thereafter, a rate of 1–2 mcg/kg per minute generally is sufficient to maintain neuromuscular blockade in the range of 89–99% in most pediatric patients receiving balanced anesthesia.

A reduction in the cisatracurium infusion rate by up to 30–40% may be necessary if steady-state anesthesia has been induced with enflurane or isoflurane; greater reductions may be required with prolonged durations of enflurane or isoflurane administration.

Skeletal Muscle Relaxation in Adults **Initial (Intubating) Dose.** The recommended initial (intubating) dose of cisatracurium in adults is 0.15 or 0.2 mg/kg depending on the desired time to intubation and duration of the procedure. When used concomitantly with balanced anesthesia, good to excellent intubating conditions generally occur within 2 minutes following a dose of 0.15 mg/kg or 1.5 minutes following a dose of 0.2 mg/kg. A dose of 0.15 mg/kg generally produces maximum neuromuscular blockade in approximately 3.5 minutes and clinically sufficient neuromuscular blockade for about 55 minutes, and a dose of 0.2 mg/kg generally produces maximum neuromuscular blockade in approximately 2.9 minutes and clinically sufficient neuromuscular blockade for about 65 minutes.

Maintenance Dosage During Prolonged Surgical Procedures. For maintenance of neuromuscular blockade during prolonged surgical procedures, additional cisatracurium doses of 0.03 mg/kg may be administered by intermittent IV injection in adults. The first maintenance dose generally is required within 40–50 or 50–60 minutes following an initial dose of 0.15 or 0.2 mg/kg, respectively. Each 0.03-mg/kg dose can provide approximately 20 minutes of additional neuromuscular blockade. Smaller or larger doses may be needed to provide shorter or longer durations of action.

Less frequent or lower doses of cisatracurium may be necessary when administered concomitantly with enflurane or isoflurane anesthesia during prolonged surgical procedures. No dosage adjustment appears to be necessary when the drug is administered shortly (e.g., within 15–30 minutes) after initiation of the inhalation anesthetic.

Alternatively, after the initial intubating dose is administered, patients may receive a continuous IV infusion of cisatracurium to maintain neuromuscular blockade during prolonged surgical procedures; the infusion should be initiated only after early spontaneous recovery from the initial dose is evident. Infusion rates should be individualized and adjusted based on patient response to peripheral nerve stimulation. An initial rate of 3 mcg/kg per minute may be necessary to rapidly counteract spontaneous recovery from neuromuscular blockade. Thereafter, a maintenance infusion rate of 1–2 mcg/kg per minute generally is sufficient to maintain neuromuscular blockade in the range of 89–99% in most patients receiving balanced anesthesia.

A reduction in the cisatracurium infusion rate by up to 30–40% may be necessary if steady-state anesthesia has been induced with enflurane or isoflurane; greater reductions may be required with prolonged durations of enflurane or isoflurane administration.

Maintenance Dosage in Intensive Care Setting. Cisatracurium may be administered by continuous IV infusion for maintenance of neuromuscular blockade during mechanical ventilation in the intensive care unit (ICU). The degree of neuromuscular blockade should be monitored with a peripheral nerve stimulator; additional doses should not be given before there is a definite response to nerve stimulation. (See Intensive Care Setting under Warnings/Precautions: General Precautions, in Cautions.)

In clinical studies, an average cisatracurium infusion rate of approximately 3 mcg/kg per minute was required for maintenance of neuromuscular blockade in mechanically ventilated adults in the ICU; however, dosage requirements may vary widely among patients and also may increase or decrease with time. In these studies, patients received up to 6 days of cisatracurium infusion; longer durations of use in the ICU have not been evaluated. Recovery of neuromuscular function (train-of-four [TOF] ratio of at least 0.7) generally occurred within approximately 50–55 minutes after the infusion was discontinued. Following neuromuscular recovery, administration of an IV ("bolus") dose of cisatracurium may be necessary to reestablish neuromuscular blockade prior to reinstitution of the infusion.

■ Reversal of Neuromuscular Blockade

Neuromuscular blockade induced by cisatracurium can be reversed by administering a cholinesterase inhibitor (e.g., neostigmine, pyridostigmine, edrophonium) in conjunction with an anticholinergic agent such as atropine or glycopyrrolate to block the adverse muscarinic effects of the cholinesterase inhibitor. *For specific information on the uses and dosage and administration of these other drugs, see the individual monographs.*

To minimize the risk of residual neuromuscular blockade, reversal should only be attempted after some degree of spontaneous recovery has occurred; patients should be closely monitored until adequate recovery of normal neuromuscular function is assured (i.e., ability to maintain satisfactory ventilation and a patent airway). Time to recovery of neuromuscular function is dependent upon the strength of neuromuscular blockade at the time of reversal.

■ Special Populations

Renal Impairment Since onset of complete neuromuscular blockade may be slower in patients with renal impairment, it may be necessary to extend the interval between administration of cisatracurium and the intubation attempt in such patients.

Geriatric Patients Since onset of complete neuromuscular blockade may be slower in geriatric patients, it may be necessary to extend the interval between administration of cisatracurium and the intubation attempt in such patients.

Burn Patients Substantially increased doses of cisatracurium may be required in burn patients due to the development of resistance. *However, there are no clinical studies to date in these patients, and no specific doses are recommended.* (See Burn Patients under Warnings/Precautions: General Precautions, in Cautions.)

Cardiopulmonary Bypass Patients with Induced Hypothermia The infusion rate of atracurium required to maintain adequate surgical relaxation during hypothermia (i.e., 25–28°C) is approximately 50% of the infusion rate necessary in normothermic patients; a similar reduction in the infusion rate of cisatracurium may be expected.

Other Populations A cisatracurium dose of 0.02 mg/kg or less is recommended along with monitoring of subsequent dosage adjustments in patients in whom potentiation of neuromuscular blockade or difficulties with reversal of blockade may occur (e.g., neuromuscular disease, carcinomatosis). (See Neuromuscular Diseases and also see Carcinomatosis under Warnings/Precautions: General Precautions, in Cautions.)

Cautions

■ Contraindications

Cisatracurium besylate is contraindicated in patients with known hypersensitivity to the drug or any of its components.

Multiple-dose vials of cisatracurium containing benzyl alcohol are contraindicated in premature infants. (See Pediatric Use under Warnings/Precautions: Specific Populations, in Cautions.)

■ Warnings/Precautions

Warnings Cisatracurium shares the toxic potentials of the nondepolarizing neuromuscular blocking agents, and the usual precautions of neuromuscular blocking agent administration should be observed. (See Cautions in the Neuromuscular Blocking Agents General Statement 12:20.20.)

Administration Precautions. When used inappropriately, neuromuscular blocking agents can severely compromise respiratory function and induce respiratory paralysis; special precautions should be taken during and after administration of these drugs. (See Dispensing and Administration Precautions under Dosage and Administration: Administration.) The degree of neuromuscular blockade produced by cisatracurium should be monitored with a peripheral nerve stimulator, particularly in patients with conditions that may potentiate (e.g., neuromuscular diseases) or cause resistance to (e.g., burns) the neuromuscular blocking effects of the drug.

Sensitivity Reactions **Hypersensitivity Reactions.** Serious hypersensitivity reactions, including anaphylaxis, have been reported rarely with all neuromuscular blocking agents; such reactions were life-threatening or fatal in some cases. Appropriate emergency treatment should be readily available whenever these drugs are administered. Because of the possibility of cross-sensitivity, cisatracurium should be used with caution in patients who have experienced previous anaphylactic reactions to other neuromuscular blocking agents (depolarizing or nondepolarizing). (See Cautions: Contraindications.)

General Precautions **Neuromuscular Diseases.** Patients with neuromuscular diseases (e.g., myasthenia gravis, Eaton-Lambert syndrome) may have an exaggerated response to cisatracurium. In such patients, the degree of neuromuscular blockade should be monitored with a peripheral nerve stimulator and dosage reduction is recommended. (See Other Populations under Dosage and Administration: Special Populations.)

Burn Patients. Resistance to nondepolarizing neuromuscular blocking agents, including atracurium, can develop in burn patients, particularly those with burns over 25–30% or more of body surface area. (See Cautions: Precautions and Contraindications, in the Neuromuscular Blocking Agents General Statement 12:20.20.)

Cisatracurium has not been studied in this population; however, based on its similarity to atracurium, the possible need for substantially increased doses should be considered in such patients.

Intensive Care Setting. Although the manufacturer states that continuous IV infusion of cisatracurium for up to 6 days in the intensive care unit (ICU) has been safely used in several studies, prolonged paralysis and/or muscle weakness have been reported with long-term administration of neuromuscular blocking agents.

Continuous monitoring of neuromuscular transmission with a peripheral nerve stimulator is recommended whenever cisatracurium is used in the ICU. Additional doses of cisatracurium or any other neuromuscular blocking agent should not be administered before there is a definite response to nerve stimulation tests. If no response is elicited, administration of the drug should be discontinued until a response returns.

Seizures have been reported rarely in patients receiving continuous IV infusions of atracurium for facilitation of mechanical ventilation in the ICU; these patients usually had predisposing factors (e.g., head trauma, cerebral edema, hypoxic encephalopathy, viral encephalitis, uremia). It is unclear whether laudanosine (a metabolite of atracurium and cisatracurium that produces CNS excitation at higher doses) contributes to CNS excitation.

Cardiovascular Effects. Cisatracurium has no clinically important effects on heart rate at recommended doses and exhibits minimal, if any, cardiovascular effects; therefore, the drug will not counteract the bradycardia induced by many anesthetic agents or by vagal stimulation.

Electrolyte Disturbances. Acid-base and/or serum electrolyte abnormalities may potentiate or antagonize the action of cisatracurium.

Hemiparesis and Paraparesis. Resistance to cisatracurium may develop in the affected limbs of patients with hemiparesis or paraparesis. To avoid inaccurate dosing, neuromuscular monitoring in the nonparetic limb is recommended.

Malignant Hyperthermia. Malignant hyperthermia is rarely associated with the use of neuromuscular blocking agents and/or potent inhalation anesthetics. In an animal study in susceptible swine, cisatracurium did not trigger malignant hyperthermia; however, the drug has not been studied in patients with increased susceptibility to this condition. Because malignant hyperthermia can occur even in the absence of a recognized precipitating factor, clinicians should be vigilant for its possible development and prepared to manage the condition in any patient undergoing general anesthesia.

Carcinomatosis. Because of possible exaggerated response to cisatracurium in patients with carcinomatosis, the degree of neuromuscular blockade should be monitored carefully with a peripheral nerve stimulator; dosage reduction is recommended. (See Other Populations under Dosage and Administration: Special Populations.)

Specific Populations **Pregnancy.** Category B. (See Users Guide.)

It is not known whether use of cisatracurium during labor, delivery, or cesarean section has any effects on the fetus.

Lactation. It is not known whether cisatracurium is distributed into milk. Because many drugs are distributed into human milk, caution is advised if the drug is used in nursing women.

Pediatric Use. Safety and efficacy of cisatracurium have not been established in neonates (younger than 1 month of age).

Each mL of cisatracurium besylate injection in multiple-dose vials contains 9 mg of benzyl alcohol. Although a causal relationship has not been established, administration of injections preserved with benzyl alcohol has been associated with toxicity in neonates. Toxicity appears to have resulted from administration of large amounts (i.e., 100–400 mg/kg daily) of benzyl alcohol in these neonates. Although use of drugs preserved with benzyl alcohol should be avoided in neonates whenever possible, the American Academy of Pediatrics (AAP) states that the presence of small amounts of the preservative in a commercially available injection should not proscribe its use when indicated in neonates. (See Caution: Contraindications.)

Pediatric patients may exhibit faster clearance of cisatracurium than adults. Onset of the drug is faster and duration is longer in pediatric patients compared with adults, and in infants compared with older children.

In clinical studies, tracheal intubation was facilitated more reliably in children 1–4 years of age when cisatracurium was used in conjunction with halothane than when used in conjunction with opiates and nitrous oxide.

Geriatric Use. No overall differences in safety and efficacy have been observed in geriatric patients relative to younger adults, but increased sensitivity of some older patients cannot be ruled out.

Minor alterations in cisatracurium pharmacokinetics (e.g., prolonged half-life, slower onset of action) have been observed in geriatric patients compared with younger individuals; however, these changes were not associated with substantial differences in recovery profile.

Cisatracurium half-life may be slightly prolonged in geriatric patients.

Hepatic Impairment. Minor alterations in cisatracurium pharmacokinetics have been observed in patients with end-stage liver disease compared with healthy adults; however, these changes were not associated with substantial differences in recovery profile.

Concentrations of cisatracurium metabolites may be increased after prolonged administration in patients with hepatic disease.

Renal Impairment. The pharmacokinetic/pharmacodynamic and recovery profile of cisatracurium in patients with renal impairment is similar to that in healthy adults. Concentrations of cisatracurium metabolites may be increased after prolonged administration in patients with renal failure.

■ Common Adverse Effects

Adverse effects were uncommon in clinical trials in patients who received cisatracurium in conjunction with anesthetic agents or other drugs (e.g., opiates, propofol) during surgery; no adverse effects were reported with an incidence exceeding 1% in these studies.

Similarly, adverse effects were uncommon in ICU patients receiving cisatracurium, but several cases of prolonged recovery were reported.

Drug Interactions

Concurrent administration of some drugs, including general anesthetics (e.g., enflurane, isoflurane), antibiotics (e.g., aminoglycosides, polymyxins), lithium, succinylcholine, magnesium salts, procainamide, and quinidine, may affect the neuromuscular blocking activity of cisatracurium besylate. *For additional information on potential drug interactions of cisatracurium, see Drug Interactions in the Neuromuscular Blocking Agents General Statement 12:20.20.*

■ Anticonvulsants

Resistance to the neuromuscular blocking effects of cisatracurium may occur in patients receiving long-term phenytoin or carbamazepine therapy. Because this may result in a shorter duration of neuromuscular block, higher infusion rates of cisatracurium may be required.

■ Anti-infective Agents

The possibility that some anti-infective agents (e.g., aminoglycosides, bacitracin, clindamycin, lincomycin, polymyxins, tetracyclines) may enhance the neuromuscular blocking effects of cisatracurium should be considered.

■ **General Anesthetics** Inhalation anesthetics (enflurane and isoflurane) are known to potentiate the effects of neuromuscular blocking agents. A reduction in cisatracurium dose and/or infusion rate may be necessary depending on the duration of administration of the inhalation anesthetic. (See Dosage and Administration: Dosage.)

■ **Lithium** The neuromuscular blocking effects of cisatracurium may be enhanced by lithium.

■ **Local Anesthetics** The neuromuscular blocking effects of cisatracurium may be enhanced by local anesthetics.

■ **Magnesium Salts** The neuromuscular blocking effects of cisatracurium may be enhanced by magnesium salts. Caution is advised and a reduction in cisatracurium dosage may be necessary.

■ **Nondepolarizing Neuromuscular Blocking Agents** Potency and duration of nondepolarizing neuromuscular blocking agents may be altered by concurrent or prior administration of other nondepolarizing agents. In clinical studies, vecuronium, pancuronium, or atracurium was administered following various degrees of recovery from cisatracurium-induced neuromuscular blockade without any evidence of interaction.

■ **Procainamide** The neuromuscular blocking effects of cisatracurium may be enhanced by procainamide.

■ **Propofol** Propofol has no apparent effect on the duration of neuromuscular blockade induced by cisatracurium. No dosage adjustment of cisatracurium is required.

■ **Quinidine** The neuromuscular blocking effects of cisatracurium may be enhanced by quinidine.

■ **Succinylcholine** Cisatracurium has been used safely following various degrees of recovery from succinylcholine-induced neuromuscular blockade. Prior administration of succinylcholine may decrease the time to maximum neuromuscular blockade with cisatracurium by about 2 minutes. Prior administration of succinylcholine does not appear to alter the duration of blockade induced by intermittent injections of cisatracurium; prior administration resulted in no change or only a slight increase in cisatracurium infusion requirements.

Description

Cisatracurium besylate is a nondepolarizing neuromuscular blocking agent that produces pharmacologic effects similar to those of other nondepolarizing neuromuscular blocking agents. (See Pharmacology in the Neuromuscular Blocking Agents General Statement 12:20.20.) Cisatracurium produces skeletal muscle relaxation by causing a decreased response to acetylcholine (ACh) at the myoneural (neuromuscular) junction of skeletal muscle. The drug exhibits a high affinity for ACh receptor sites and competitively blocks access of ACh to the motor end-plate of the myoneural junction, and may affect ACh release. Cisatracurium blocks the effects of both the small quantities of ACh that maintain muscle tone and the large quantities of ACh that produce voluntary skeletal muscle contraction. The drug does not alter the resting electrical potential of the motor end-plate or cause muscular contractions. The neuromuscular blocking potency of cisatracurium is approximately threefold that of atracurium. Cisatracurium exhibits minimal, if any, cardiovascular effects. The drug exhibits little histamine-releasing activity at usual therapeutic doses.

Cisatracurium has an intermediate onset and duration of action. Cisatracurium is rapidly metabolized via Hofmann elimination (independent of the liver) to form a monoquaternary acrylate metabolite (which undergoes nonspecific plasma esterase hydrolysis and subsequent Hofmann elimination) and laudanosine (which is demethylated and glucuronidated). Both metabolites lack neuromuscular blocking activity; laudanosine may have CNS excitatory activity when present in large amounts. Cisatracurium is eliminated principally by Hofmann elimination (77–80%) and to lesser extent by renal and hepatic elimination (20%). Metabolites of the drug are eliminated principally by renal and hepatic elimination. The elimination half-life of cisatracurium is approximately 22–30 minutes.

Advice to Patients

Importance of women informing clinicians if they are or plan to become pregnant or plan to breast-feed.

Importance of informing clinician of existing or contemplated concomitant therapy, including prescription and OTC drugs, as well as any concomitant illnesses (e.g., cardiovascular disease, neuromuscular disease).

Importance of informing patients of other important precautionary information. (See Cautions.)

Overview® (see Users Guide). For additional information on this drug until a more detailed monograph is developed and published, the manufacturer's labeling should be consulted. It is *essential* that the manufacturer's labeling be consulted for more detailed information on usual cautions, precautions, contraindications, potential drug interactions, laboratory test interferences, and acute toxicity.

Preparations

Excipients in commercially available drug preparations may have clinically important effects in some individuals; consult specific product labeling for details.

Cisatracurium Besylate

Parenteral		
Injection, for IV use only	2 mg (of cisatracurium) per mL	**Cisatracurium Besylate Injection**
		Nimbex®, Abbvie
	10 mg (of cisatracurium) per mL	**Cisatracurium Besylate Injection**
		Nimbex®, Abbvie

Rocuronium Bromide

■ Rocuronium bromide is an aminosteroid nondepolarizing neuromuscular blocking agent.

Uses

■ **Skeletal Muscle Relaxation** Rocuronium bromide is used to produce skeletal muscle relaxation during surgery after general anesthesia has been induced. Rocuronium also is used to facilitate endotracheal intubation (rapid sequence and routine tracheal intubation); while slightly slower than that of succinylcholine, the onset of action of rocuronium is more rapid than that of most other currently available nondepolarizing agents.

Rocuronium also is used to facilitate mechanical ventilation in the intensive care unit (ICU); however, the manufacturer states that prolonged use of the drug in this setting has not been evaluated. Whenever neuromuscular blocking agents are used in the ICU, the benefits versus risks of such therapy must be considered and patients should be assessed frequently to determine the need for continued paralysis. (See Intensive Care Setting under Warnings/Precautions: Other Warnings and Precautions, in Cautions.)

Compared with other neuromuscular blocking agents, rocuronium has a rapid onset and intermediate duration of action; the drug's rapid onset of effect is particularly desirable in emergency situations when rapid tracheal intubation is required. Succinylcholine traditionally has been considered the neuromuscular blocking agent of choice for rapid sequence intubation because of its rapid onset and short duration of action; however, the drug is associated with serious adverse effects (e.g., hyperkalemia, bradycardia, malignant hyperthermia). If succinylcholine cannot be used, rocuronium, which has the most similar pharmacokinetic profile, generally is recommended as an alternative. Clinical studies have shown that rocuronium can produce similar intubating conditions to succinylcholine when given in sufficient doses (e.g., at least 1 mg/kg); however, succinylcholine is more likely to achieve excellent intubating conditions and remains clinically superior to rocuronium with respect to its shorter duration of action.

For additional information on uses and treatment principles of neuromuscular blocking agents, see Uses in the Neuromuscular Blocking Agents General Statement 12:20.20.

Dosage and Administration

■ **Administration** Rocuronium bromide is administered IV only.

IV Administration The initial (intubating) dose of rocuronium is administered by rapid IV injection; maintenance doses may be administered by intermittent IV injection or continuous IV infusion.

For continuous IV infusion, rocuronium bromide injection should be diluted to the desired concentration (e.g., 0.5, 1, or 5 mg/mL) in a compatible IV solution (0.9% sodium chloride, 5% dextrose, 5% dextrose and 0.9% sodium chloride, lactated Ringer's, or sterile water for injection). The infusion solution should be used within 24 hours of preparation. Use of a controlled-infusion device is recommended to ensure precise control of the flow rate during continuous IV infusion of the drug. The rate of spontaneous neuromuscular recovery following discontinuance of the infusion is likely to be comparable to the rate of recovery following administration of a single IV injection of the drug.

Rocuronium bromide injection should be stored at 2–8°C prior to use; the drug should not be frozen. Once removed from refrigeration, the injection should be used within 60 days; opened vials of the drug should be used within 30 days. Following dilution, the infusion solution may be stored at room temperature for up to 24 hours.

Rocuronium should not be mixed in the same syringe nor administered simultaneously through the same needle as an alkaline solution.

If extravasation occurs, administration of the drug should be discontinued immediately and restarted in another vein.

Dispensing and Administration Precautions Neuromuscular blocking agents should be administered only by individuals who are adequately trained in their use and complications. For specific procedures and techniques of administration, specialized references should be consulted. Facilities and personnel necessary for intubation, administration of oxygen, and respiratory support should be immediately available whenever these drugs are used. In addition, a reversal agent should be readily available in the event of a failed intubation or to accelerate neuromuscular recovery after surgery. (See Dosage and Administration: Reversal of Neuromuscular Blockade.)

Because neuromuscular blocking agents can cause respiratory arrest, precautions (e.g., storage segregation, warning labels, access limitations) should be taken to ensure that these drugs are not administered without adequate respiratory support. Affixing warning labels to storage containers and final administration containers is recommended to clearly communicate that respiratory paralysis can occur and ventilator support is required. The Institute for Safe Medication Practices (ISMP) recommends the following wording for these containers: "Warning: Paralyzing agent—causes respiratory arrest—patient must be ventilated."

Neuromuscular blocking agents have no known effect on consciousness, pain, or cerebration, and should therefore be used in conjunction with adequate levels of anesthesia, and only after appropriate analgesics and sedatives are administered. To avoid distress to the patient, rocuronium should be administered only after unconsciousness has been induced.

■ **Dosage** Dosage of rocuronium bromide must be adjusted carefully according to individual requirements and response. The use of a peripheral nerve stimulator is recommended to accurately monitor the degree of neuromuscular blockade and recovery, determine the need for additional doses, and minimize the possibility of overdosage. (See Administration Precautions under Warnings/Precautions: Warnings, in Cautions.)

A reduction in the dosage of rocuronium bromide may be required in patients receiving general anesthetics (e.g., enflurane, isoflurane) that potentiate its neuromuscular blocking activity. Potentiation is minimal when rocuronium is administered prior to these anesthetics.

Adult Dosage The recommended initial (intubating) dose of rocuronium bromide in adults is 0.6 mg/kg. Following administration of this initial dose, neuromuscular blockade sufficient for intubation (80% or more blockade) is attained in about 1 minute (range: 0.4–6 minutes) and most patients have intubation completed within 2 minutes; maximum neuromuscular blockade generally occurs in less than 3 minutes. When used concomitantly with balanced anesthesia, this initial dose usually results in clinically sufficient neuromuscular blockade for about 31 minutes (range: 15–85 minutes). When used concomitantly with inhalation anesthetics, a longer duration of blockade is expected.

The manufacturer states that a lower initial rocuronium bromide dose of 0.45 mg/kg may be used, which can provide sufficient neuromuscular blockade for intubation in about 1.3 minutes, maximum blockade in approximately less than 4 minutes, and clinically sufficient blockade for about 22 minutes under balanced anesthesia. Spontaneous recovery may occur more rapidly with this lower initial dose. When administration of a larger initial dose is considered necessary, the manufacturer states that rocuronium bromide may be administered in initial doses of 0.9 or 1.2 mg/kg, providing clinically sufficient neuromuscular blockade for about 58 (range: 27–111) or 67 (range: 38–160) minutes, respectively.

For rapid sequence intubation, the manufacturer states that a rocuronium bromide dose of 0.6–1.2 mg/kg generally results in good to excellent intubating conditions in less than 2 minutes in most patients who are appropriately premedicated and adequately anesthetized. In clinical studies, the median dose of rocuronium bromide for rapid sequence intubation with etomidate as the induction agent was 1.19 mg/kg. Although a higher dose of rocuronium bromide (1.2 mg/kg) can produce a faster onset of action, higher doses do not necessarily produce better intubating conditions and may increase the duration of action.

For maintenance of neuromuscular blockade during prolonged surgical procedures, additional rocuronium bromide doses may be given by intermittent IV injection when recovery of neuromuscular function is evident. When used concomitantly with balanced anesthesia, additional rocuronium bromide doses of 0.1, 0.15, or 0.2 mg/kg administered at 25% recovery of control T1 (i.e., 3 twitches in a train-of-four [TOF]) can be expected to provide clinically sufficient neuromuscular blockade for about 12, 17, or 24 minutes, respectively. Alternatively, patients may receive a continuous IV infusion of rocuronium bromide at a rate of 10–12 mcg/kg per minute to maintain adequate neuromuscular blockade during surgery; the infusion should be initiated only after early spontaneous recovery from the initial dose is evident. The rate of infusion should be individualized based on patient response to peripheral nerve stimulation. In clinical studies, maintenance infusion rates of 4–16 mcg/kg per minute were required. A reduction in the rocuronium infusion rate by 30–50% may be necessary approximately 45–60 minutes following the initial intubating dose if steady-state anesthesia has been induced with enflurane or isoflurane. Additional direct IV ("bolus") doses of rocuronium may be necessary if the infusion is initiated after substantial return of neuromuscular function (more than 10% of control).

Pediatric Dosage The recommended initial (intubating) dose of rocuronium bromide in pediatric patients is 0.6 mg/kg. A lower initial dose of 0.45 mg/kg may be used depending on the anesthetic technique and patient age. Neonates tend to have lower dosage requirements than older children (2–11 years of age).

When used concomitantly with halothane anesthesia, a rocuronium bromide dose of 0.6 mg/kg generally produces good to excellent intubating conditions within approximately 60 seconds and clinically effective blockade for about 41 minutes (in children 3–12 months of age) or 26 minutes (in children 1–12 years of age). When used concomitantly with sevoflurane (induction) and isoflurane/nitrous oxide (maintenance) anesthesia in pediatric patients of any age, an initial rocuronium bromide dose of 0.45 or 0.6 mg/kg generally produces good to excellent intubating conditions within 75 seconds.

To maintain neuromuscular blockade when halothane is used as the anesthetic agent, additional rocuronium bromide doses of 0.075–0.125 mg/kg may be administered by intermittent IV injection upon return of T1 to 25% in pediatric patients 3 months of age through adolescence; doses in this range can be expected to provide clinical relaxation for 7–10 minutes. Alternatively, a continuous IV infusion may be initiated at a rate of 12 mcg/kg per minute upon return of T1 to 10% (i.e., one twitch present in a TOF).

To maintain neuromuscular blockade when sevoflurane is used for induction and isoflurane/nitrous oxide for maintenance of general anesthesia, additional rocuronium bromide doses of 0.15 mg/kg may be administered by intermittent IV injection at the reappearance of T3 in pediatric patients of all ages. Alternatively, a continuous IV infusion may be initiated at a rate of 7–10 mcg/kg per minute at the reappearance of T2.

More frequent administration of maintenance doses may be required in children 1–12 years of age compared with adults.

■ **Reversal of Neuromuscular Blockade** Neuromuscular blockade induced by rocuronium can be reversed by administering a cholinesterase inhibitor (e.g., neostigmine, pyridostigmine, edrophonium) in conjunction with an anticholinergic agent such as atropine or glycopyrrolate to block the adverse muscarinic effects of the cholinesterase inhibitor. Alternatively, sugammadex may be used for the reversal of rocuronium-induced neuromuscular blockade after surgery. *For specific information on the uses and dosage and administration of these other drugs, see the individual monographs.*

To minimize the risk of residual neuromuscular blockade, reversal should only be attempted after some degree of spontaneous recovery has occurred; patients should be closely monitored until adequate recovery of normal neuromuscular function is assured (i.e., ability to maintain satisfactory ventilation and a patent airway).

■ **Special Populations** An increased initial dose of rocuronium bromide may be required for rapid sequence induction in patients with ascites; however, doses higher than 0.6 mg/kg have not been evaluated. Once blockade is established, duration may be prolonged in such patients. (See Hepatic Impairment under Warnings/Precautions: Specific Populations, in Cautions.)

Dosage adjustment of rocuronium generally is not necessary in patients with renal impairment; however, dosage should be individualized in such patients because of wide interpatient variability.

Because metabolism of rocuronium does *not* depend on plasma cholinesterase (pseudocholinesterase), dosage adjustment is not necessary in patients with reduced activity of this enzyme.

Although the onset time of rocuronium may be delayed in patients with impaired circulation, larger than usual initial doses of the drug generally are not recommended; when feasible, more time should be allowed for the drug to achieve its effect in such patients.

Substantially increased doses may be required in burn patients due to the development of resistance.

In obese patients, the initial dose of rocuronium 0.6 mg/kg should be based on *actual* body weight. In clinical studies, patients were dosed according to actual body weight, and no substantial differences in rocuronium pharmacokinetics were observed in patients who were 30% or more above their ideal body weight.

Cautions

■ **Contraindications** Rocuronium is contraindicated in patients with known hypersensitivity to the drug or other neuromuscular blocking agents.

■ **Warnings/Precautions** ***Warnings*** Rocuronium shares the toxic potentials of the nondepolarizing neuromuscular blocking agents, and the usual precautions of neuromuscular blocking agent administration should be observed. (See Cautions in the Neuromuscular Blocking Agents General Statement 12:20.20.)

Administration Precautions. When used inappropriately, neuromuscular blocking agents can severely compromise respiratory function and induce respiratory paralysis; special precautions should be taken during and after administration of these drugs. (See Dispensing and Administration Precautions under Dosage and Administration: Administration.) The degree of neuromuscular blockade produced by rocuronium should be monitored with a peripheral nerve stimulator, particularly in patients with conditions that may potentiate (e.g., neuromuscular diseases) or cause resistance to (e.g., burns) the neuromuscular blocking effects of the drug.

Extravasation of rocuronium may cause local tissue irritation. (See Dosage and Administration: Administration.)

Sensitivity Reactions **Hypersensitivity Reactions.** Serious hypersensitivity reactions, including anaphylaxis, have been reported rarely with all neuromuscular blocking agents; such reactions were life-threatening or fatal in some cases. Appropriate emergency treatment should be readily available whenever these drugs are administered. Because of potential cross-sensitivity, rocuronium should be used with caution in patients who have experienced previous anaphylactic reactions to other neuromuscular blocking agents (depolarizing or nondepolarizing). (See Cautions: Contraindications.)

Other Warning and Precautions **Residual Paralysis.** Residual neuromuscular blockade after cessation of neuromuscular blocking drugs can occur as a result of accumulation of the neuromuscular blocking agent (or its metabolites) or concomitant use of certain drugs. Use of a reversal agent should be considered (see Dosage and Administration: Reversal of Neuromuscular Blockade) and patients should be extubated only when adequate recovery of neuromuscular function is assured.

Intensive Care Setting. Prolonged paralysis and/or muscle weakness or myopathy have been reported after long-term use of neuromuscular blocking agents to support mechanical ventilation in the intensive care unit (ICU).

Continuous monitoring of neuromuscular transmission with a peripheral nerve stimulator is recommended whenever rocuronium is used in the ICU. Additional doses of rocuronium or any other neuromuscular blocking agent should not be administered before there is a definite response to nerve stimulation tests.

Malignant Hyperthermia. Malignant hyperthermia is rarely associated with the use of neuromuscular blocking agents and/or potent inhalation anesthetics. In an animal study in susceptible swine, rocuronium did not trigger malignant hyperthermia; however, the drug has not been studied in patients with increased susceptibility to this condition. Because malignant hyperthermia can occur even in the absence of a recognized precipitating factor, clinicians should be vigilant for its possible development and prepared for its management in any patient undergoing general anesthesia.

Cardiovascular Effects. Patients with conditions that prolong circulation time (e.g., cardiovascular disease) may experience a delay in the onset time of rocuronium. (See Dosage and Administration: Special Populations.)

Rocuronium may increase pulmonary vascular resistance; caution is advised in patients with pulmonary hypertension or valvular heart disease. Transient tachycardia has been reported in some patients receiving the drug.

Conditions that May Potentiate or Cause Resistance to Neuromuscular Blocking Agents. The neuromuscular blocking effects of rocuronium may be potentiated in patients with debilitation, cachexia, or carcinomatosis or in those receiving certain concomitant drugs (e.g., enflurane, isoflurane, antibiotics, magnesium salts, lithium, local anesthetics, procainamide, quinidine). A reduction in rocuronium dosage may be required.

Conditions that may cause resistance to nondepolarizing neuromuscular blocking agents include burns, disuse atrophy, denervation, direct muscle trauma, and long-term use of carbamazepine, phenytoin, or neuromuscular blocking agents. (See Cautions: Precautions and Contraindications, in the Neuromuscular Blocking Agents General Statement 12:20.20.) An increase in rocuronium dosage may be required.

Neuromuscular Diseases. Patients with neuromuscular diseases (e.g., myasthenia gravis, Eaton-Lambert syndrome) may have an exaggerated response to rocuronium. The degree of neuromuscular blockade in such patients should be monitored with a peripheral nerve stimulator and a small test dose is recommended.

Electrolyte Disturbances. Increased or decreased neuromuscular blockade is possible in patients with electrolyte disturbances or acid/base abnormalities receiving rocuronium.

QT Interval Prolongation. Prolongation of the QT interval has been reported in pediatric patients receiving rocuronium and general anesthetics concomitantly.

Extravasation. Local irritation may occur during administration of rocuronium; if extravasation occurs, injection or infusion of the drug should be discontinued and restarted in another vein.

Specific Populations **Pregnancy.** Category C. (See Users Guide.)

Rocuronium has been used in a limited number of pregnant women undergoing cesarean section. The manufacturer states that the drug is not recommended for rapid sequence induction in patients undergoing cesarean section because of possible poor or inadequate intubating conditions.

Pediatric Use. Rocuronium has been evaluated in pediatric patients of all ages, including neonates, receiving sevoflurane and isoflurane/nitrous oxide anesthesia, and in pediatric patients 3 months to 14 years of age receiving halothane anesthesia. In pediatric patients receiving halothane anesthesia, transient increases in heart rate were observed following an intubating dose of rocuronium; this occurred mostly in patients who did not receive atropine.

Although not conclusively demonstrated, there is some evidence suggesting that concomitant use of general anesthetics with rocuronium can prolong the corrected QT (QT_c) interval in pediatric patients.

The manufacturer states that rocuronium is not recommended for rapid sequence intubation in pediatric patients.

Geriatric Use. Rocuronium has been evaluated in geriatric patients 65–80 years of age in clinical studies. Geriatric patients exhibited a slightly slower onset and increased duration of neuromuscular blockade with rocuronium compared with younger adults; however, recovery times were not prolonged. Other clinical experience has not revealed age-related differences in response among geriatric patients receiving the drug; however, the possibility of greater sensitivity of some older patients cannot be ruled out.

Hepatic Impairment. Rocuronium should be used with caution in patients with clinically important hepatic impairment since the drug is eliminated principally by the liver; duration of neuromuscular blockade and recovery times may be prolonged in such patients. Incomplete neuromuscular blockade has been reported in patients with cirrhosis, which is consistent with the increased volume of distribution observed in patients with substantial hepatic impairment. (See Dosage and Administration: Special Populations.)

Renal Impairment. Rocuronium is not substantially eliminated by the kidneys; the duration of neuromuscular blockade induced by the drug is not expected to be prolonged in patients with renal impairment. (See Dosage and Administration: Special Populations.)

No substantial differences in pharmacokinetics have been observed in patients with renal impairment relative to those with normal renal function.

■ **Common Adverse Effects** Adverse effects of rocuronium observed in 2% or more of patients in clinical studies were transient hypotension and hypertension.

Drug Interactions

Concurrent administration of some drugs, including general anesthetics (e.g., enflurane, isoflurane), antibiotics (e.g., aminoglycosides, polymyxins), lithium, succinylcholine, magnesium salts, procainamide, and quinidine, may affect the neuromuscular blocking activity of rocuronium. *For additional information on potential drug interactions of rocuronium, see Drug Interactions in the Neuromuscular Blocking Agents General Statement 12:20.20.*

■ **Anticonvulsants** Resistance to the neuromuscular blocking effects of rocuronium has been observed in patients receiving long-term phenytoin or carbamazepine therapy. Higher rocuronium infusion rates may be necessary in such patients.

■ **Anti-infective Agents** The possibility that some anti-infective agents (e.g., aminoglycosides, bacitracin, polymyxins, vancomycin, tetracyclines) may enhance the neuromuscular blocking effects of rocuronium should be considered. A reduction in the dose or infusion rate of rocuronium may be necessary in such patients.

■ **General Anesthetics** Enflurane and isoflurane may prolong the duration of initial and maintenance doses of rocuronium, with maintenance doses affected to a greater degree (prolonging the duration by 30–50%). Under enflurane or isoflurane anesthesia, infusion rate requirements of rocuronium are reduced by approximately 40%. Spontaneous recovery of neuromuscular function is prolonged by enflurane and isoflurane, but induced recovery (with a reversal agent) is minimally affected.

A reduction in the rocuronium dose and/or infusion rate may be necessary depending on when the drug is administered in relation to the inhalation anesthetic. Potentiation is minimal when rocuronium is administered prior to the inhalation anesthetic. (See Dosage and Administration: Dosage.)

■ **Lithium** The neuromuscular blocking effects of rocuronium may be enhanced by lithium. A reduction in the dose or infusion rate of rocuronium may be necessary.

■ **Local Anesthetics** The neuromuscular blocking effects of rocuronium may be enhanced by local anesthetics. A reduction in the dose or infusion rate of rocuronium may be necessary.

■ **Magnesium Salts** The neuromuscular blocking effects of rocuronium may be enhanced by magnesium salts. A reduction in rocuronium dosage may be necessary.

■ **Nondepolarizing Neuromuscular Blocking Agents** Interactions have not been observed between rocuronium and other nondepolarizing neuromuscular blocking agents.

■ **Procainamide** The neuromuscular blocking effects of rocuronium may be enhanced by procainamide. A reduction in the dose or infusion rate of rocuronium may be necessary.

■ **Propofol** Propofol has no apparent effect on the duration of neuromuscular blockade induced by rocuronium or on subsequent recovery of neuromuscular function.

■ **Quinidine** The neuromuscular blocking effects of rocuronium may be enhanced by quinidine. A reduction in the dose or infusion rate of rocuronium may be necessary.

Recurrent paralysis has occurred when quinidine was administered during recovery from muscle relaxants.

■ **Succinylcholine** Prior administration of succinylcholine has been reported to increase the duration of neuromuscular blockade produced by rocuronium; the effects of succinylcholine should be allowed to subside before administration of rocuronium.

Description

Rocuronium bromide is a nondepolarizing neuromuscular blocking agent that produces pharmacologic effects similar to those of other nondepolarizing neuromuscular blocking agents. (See Pharmacology in the Neuromuscular Blocking Agents General Statement 12:20.20.) Rocuronium produces skeletal muscle relaxation by causing a decreased response to acetylcholine (ACh) at the myoneural (neuromuscular) junction of skeletal muscle. The drug exhibits a high affinity for ACh receptor sites and competitively blocks access of ACh to the motor end-plate of the myoneural junction, and may affect ACh release.

Rocuronium has a rapid onset and intermediate duration of action. The onset of action is slower than that of succinylcholine but more rapid than that of most other currently available nondepolarizing agents. Rocuronium is metabolized to a less active metabolite, 17-desacetyl-rocuronium, that is rarely detected in the plasma and urine and is eliminated principally by the liver.

Rocuronium exhibits transient increases in heart rate and minimal histamine-releasing activity at usual therapeutic doses.

Advice to Patients

Importance of women informing clinicians if they are or plan to become pregnant or plan to breast-feed.

Importance of informing clinician of existing or contemplated concomitant therapy, including prescription and OTC drugs, as well as any concomitant illnesses (e.g., cardiovascular disease, neuromuscular disease).

Importance of informing patients of other important precautionary information. (See Cautions.)

Overview® (see Users Guide). For additional information on this drug until a more detailed monograph is developed and published, the manufacturer's labeling should be consulted. It is *essential* that the manufacturer's labeling be consulted for more detailed information on usual cautions, precautions, contraindications, potential drug interactions, laboratory test interferences, and acute toxicity.

Preparations

Excipients in commercially available drug preparations may have clinically important effects in some individuals; consult specific product labeling for details.

Rocuronium Bromide

Parenteral

Injection, for IV use only	10 mg/mL	**Rocuronium Bromide Injection**

Succinylcholine Chloride

Suxamethonium Chloride

■ Succinylcholine chloride is a depolarizing neuromuscular blocking agent.

Uses

■ **Skeletal Muscle Relaxation** Succinylcholine chloride is used to produce skeletal muscle relaxation during procedures of short duration such as endotracheal intubation after general anesthesia has been induced.

Because of its short duration of action, succinylcholine is generally considered the neuromuscular blocking agent of choice for procedures lasting less than 3 minutes. In addition, because of its rapid onset (less than 1 minute after IV administration) and short duration of action (approximately 4–6 minutes), succinylcholine traditionally has been considered the neuromuscular blocking agent of choice in emergency situations when rapid intubation (e.g., rapid sequence intubation) is required. However, the drug is associated with serious adverse effects (e.g., hyperkalemia, bradycardia, malignant hyperthermia), which can limit its use. Because of the risk of hyperkalemic rhabdomyolysis, cardiac arrest, and death, use of succinylcholine in pediatric patients should be restricted to those who require emergency intubation, those in whom an airway should be secured immediately (e.g., patients with laryngospasm, difficult airway, or full stomach), or those in whom a suitable vein is not accessible and IM administration is needed. (See Cautions: Pediatric Precautions.) If succinylcholine cannot be used, rocuronium (a nondepolarizing neuromuscular blocking agent with the most similar pharmacokinetic profile) generally is recommended as an acceptable alternative. Clinical studies have shown that rocuronium can produce similar intubating conditions to succinylcholine when given in sufficient doses (e.g., at least 1 mg/kg); however, succinylcholine is more likely to achieve excellent intubating conditions and remains clinically superior to rocuronium with respect to its shorter duration of action.

Succinylcholine also is used to provide skeletal muscle relaxation during mechanical ventilation; however, the drug is not used for prolonged neuromuscular blockade in the intensive care unit (ICU).

For additional information on uses and treatment principles of neuromuscular blocking agents, see Uses in the Neuromuscular Blocking Agents General Statement 12:20.20.

Dosage and Administration

■ **Reconstitution and Administration** Succinylcholine chloride usually is administered IV. For infants or older patients in whom a suitable vein is not accessible, the drug may be administered by IM injection. Because of a slower onset of effect (which can potentially compromise respiratory function), some clinicians recommend that IM administration be reserved for life-threatening situations.

For prolonged procedures, the manufacturer states that succinylcholine may be given by continuous IV infusion or intermittent IV injection. Continuous IV infusion of the drug is preferable to administration of repeated fractional doses because the latter method of dosing may lead to tachyphylaxis and prolonged apnea which may be difficult to reverse. However, some clinicians state that continuous IV infusion of succinylcholine also is limited clinically because of tachyphylaxis, potential conversion from phase I to phase II block, and the uncertain nature and prolongation of the blockade.

For continuous IV infusion, succinylcholine chloride usually is diluted to a concentration of 1–2 mg/mL (0.1–0.2%) with a compatible IV solution such as 5% dextrose injection or 0.9% sodium chloride injection. The 1-mg/mL concentration is usually used for optimum dosage control, but in patients in whom the amount of fluid should be limited, the 2-mg/mL concentration may be preferred. To provide a solution containing 1 or 2 mg/mL, 1 g of succinylcholine chloride injection may be added to 1 L or 500 mL of diluent, respectively. The infusion solution should be used within 24 hours of preparation. Use of a controlled-infusion device is recommended to ensure precise control of the flow rate during continuous IV infusion of the drug. Succinylcholine injections should not be admixed with alkaline (having a pH exceeding 8.5) solutions (e.g., barbiturates).

Dispensing and Administration Precautions Neuromuscular blocking agents should be administered only by individuals who are adequately trained in their use and complications. For specific procedures and techniques of administration, specialized references should be consulted. Facilities and personnel necessary for intubation, administration of oxygen, and respiratory support should be immediately available whenever these drugs are used.

Because neuromuscular blocking agents can cause respiratory arrest, precautions (e.g., storage segregation, warning labels, access limitations) should be taken to ensure that these drugs are not administered without adequate respiratory support. Affixing warning labels to storage containers and final administration containers is recommended to clearly communicate that respiratory paralysis can occur and ventilator support is required. The Institute for Safe Medication Practices (ISMP) recommends the following wording for these containers: "Warning: Paralyzing agent—causes respiratory arrest—patient must be ventilated".

Neuromuscular blocking agents have no known effect on consciousness, pain, or cerebration, and should therefore be used in conjunction with adequate levels of anesthesia and only after appropriate analgesics and sedatives are administered. To avoid distress to the patient, succinylcholine generally should be administered after unconsciousness has been induced; however, in emergency situations, the drug may be administered before a sedative has been given.

■ **Dosage** Dosage of succinylcholine must be carefully adjusted according to individual requirements and response. The use of a peripheral nerve stimulator is recommended during continuous IV infusion of the drug to accurately monitor the degree of neuromuscular blockade and recovery, detect the development of phase II block, and minimize the possibility of overdosage.

Test Dose To evaluate sensitivity to succinylcholine in patients with reduced plasma cholinesterase activity, a test dose of 5–10 mg of succinylcholine chloride is recommended; alternatively, a 1-mg/mL solution of the drug may be cautiously administered by slow IV infusion. In patients who metabolize succinylcholine normally, respiratory depression rarely occurs and, if it does, is transient and usually disappears in less than 5 minutes. Patients unable to metabolize the drug develop paralysis sufficient to permit endotracheal intubation; recovery generally occurs in 30–60 minutes. Apnea or prolonged muscle paralysis should be treated with controlled respiration.

Adult Dosage For short procedures, the manufacturer states that the usual adult IV dose of succinylcholine chloride is 0.6 mg/kg (range 0.3–1.1 mg/kg); following administration of this dose, neuromuscular blockade generally is attained in approximately 1 minute and persists for about 4–6 minutes. Because there is a wide variation in individual patient response, a test dose of succinylcholine chloride may be administered to determine the individual patient's sensitivity and recovery time. (See Test Dose under Dosage and Administration: Dosage.)

For rapid sequence intubation, the usual dose of succinylcholine chloride is 1.5 mg/kg; this dose generally produces an onset of effect within 45 seconds and a duration of paralysis of about 10 minutes.

For maintenance of neuromuscular blockade during prolonged procedures, succinylcholine chloride may be administered by continuous IV infusion, generally at a rate of 2.5–4.3 mg/minute in adults; the rate may range from 0.5–10 mg/minute depending on the response and requirements of the patient. Succinylcholine also may be administered by intermittent IV injection for maintenance of neuromuscular blockade during prolonged procedures; a dose of 0.3–1.1 mg/kg may be given initially in adults, followed by additional doses of 0.04–0.07 mg/kg as necessary to maintain adequate relaxation.

If IM administration is necessary, a succinylcholine chloride dose of up to 3–4 mg/kg may be given, but the total dose should not exceed 150 mg.

Pediatric Dosage The manufacturer states that the usual pediatric IV dose of succinylcholine chloride is 1–2 mg/kg (2 mg/kg for infants and small pediatric patients, and 1 mg/kg for older pediatric patients and adolescents). The possibility that succinylcholine may produce profound bradycardia or, rarely, asystole when administered by rapid IV injection in infants and children should be considered; as in adults, the risk of these effects increases with repeated doses, and pretreatment with atropine should be considered to reduce the risk of bradyarrhythmias.

Because of the risk of malignant hyperthermia, continuous IV infusions of succinylcholine are considered unsafe in neonates and children.

If IM administration is necessary, a succinylcholine chloride dose of up to 3–4 mg/kg may be given, but the total dose should not exceed 150 mg.

Cautions

■ **Adverse Effects** Succinylcholine may produce initial muscle fasciculation which may result in postoperative pain; jaw rigidity also has been reported.

Patients with decreased concentrations and/or activity of plasma pseudocholinesterase are especially sensitive to the action of succinylcholine and may experience prolonged respiratory depression and apnea after receiving the drug. (See Cautions: Precautions and Contraindications.) About 1 individual in 2800 has a genetic abnormality that causes the production of an atypical pseudocholinesterase which is incapable of rapidly hydrolyzing succinylcholine. These individuals are homozygous for this trait and invariably respond to administration of succinylcholine by prolonged muscle relaxation. Several other genetic variants also exist, some producing enzymes that hydrolyze succinylcholine at slower than normal rates than others that hydrolyze succinylcholine more rapidly than normal. Plasma pseudocholinesterase concentrations may also be decreased in patients with hepatocellular disease, malnutrition, severe anemia, severe dehydration, burns, cancer, collagen diseases, myxedema, or abnormal body temperature and in pregnant women. (See also Drug Interactions.)

While succinylcholine does not have a direct effect on the myocardium, the drug stimulates autonomic ganglia and muscarinic receptors. Bradycardia accompanied by hypotension and cardiac arrhythmias ranging from nodal rhythms and extrasystoles to bigeminy, atrioventricular block, and cardiac arrest may occur after succinylcholine administration. Cardiac effects also may result from vagal stimulation or from hyperkalemia, and are most common during halothane anesthesia, with repeated administration of succinylcholine, in children, or in patients with pheochromocytoma. Prior administration of atropine may inhibit vagal stimulation. Succinylcholine has also been reported to cause sinus tachycardia with hypertension and sympathetic ganglion stimulation.

Succinylcholine causes an increase in intraocular pressure which may be hazardous in patients with glaucoma or in those undergoing eye surgery and in patients with penetrating wounds of the eye. Although administration of a small dose of a nondepolarizing neuromuscular blocking agent prior to succinylcholine can prevent the rise in intraocular pressure, it may be preferable to use a nondepolarizing blocking agent alone in patients with these conditions of the eye. An increase in intragastric pressure secondary to fasciculation of the abdominal muscles has been reported. An increase in intragastric pressure may be prevented by the administration of a small dose of a nondepolarizing agent prior to succinylcholine. Enlargement of the salivary glands, excessive salivation, rash, hypersensitivity reactions (e.g., anaphylaxis) and, rarely, bronchospasm have also been reported in patients receiving succinylcholine. Premedication with a parasympatholytic agent such as atropine or scopolamine may be used to prevent excessive salivation.

Rarely, myoglobinuria and myoglobinemia have been reported after succinylcholine administration, particularly in children. These symptoms have sometimes been reported in conjunction with malignant hyperthermia and muscle rigidity. Administration of succinylcholine has been associated with acute onset of malignant hyperthermia; the risk of developing such hyperthermia increases with concomitant administration of inhalation anesthetics. (See Cautions: Adverse Effects in the Neuromuscular Blocking Agents General Statement 12:20.20.) Manifestations associated with histamine release also can occur. Hyperkalemia has been reported in several catabolic patients who had either massive tissue destruction or CNS injury with muscle wasting (e.g., those with extensive or severe burns, severe abdominal infections, tetanus, massive trauma, spinal cord injury, neuromuscular disease) who received succinylcholine. The precise time of onset and duration of the risk period are not known. It has been reported that skeletal muscle denervation hypersensitivity usually develops over several weeks; however, it can occur as early as 1–2 days after injury. Results of an animal study indicate that hyperkalemia developed 7 days after denervation when receiving succinylcholine. In humans, succinylcholine-associated hyperkalemia can persist for over 6 months after neural injury. The risk of hyperkalemia depends on the extent and location of injury, increases over time, and usually peaks 7–10 days after the injury.

Serious hypersensitivity reactions, including anaphylaxis, have been reported rarely with all neuromuscular blocking agents; such reactions have been life-threatening or fatal in some cases. Although uncommon, succinylcholine has the potential to release histamine and cause histamine-related manifestations (e.g., bronchospasm, flushing, hypotension).

■ **Precautions and Contraindications** Succinylcholine chloride shares the toxic potentials of the depolarizing neuromuscular blocking agents, and the usual precautions of neuromuscular blocking agent administration should be observed. (See Cautions in the Neuromuscular Blocking Agents General Statement 12:20.20.)

When used inappropriately, neuromuscular blocking agents can severely compromise respiratory function and induce respiratory paralysis. Special precautions should be taken during and after administration of these drugs. (See Dispensing and Administration Precautions under Dosage and Administration: Reconstitution and Administration.)

Immediately after administration of succinylcholine and during the fasciculation phase, slight increases in intracranial pressure may occur.

Some clinicians suggest that plasma pseudocholinesterase activity should be determined prior to administration of succinylcholine. The drug should be administered with extreme caution and in reduced doses, if at all, to patients with abnormally low pseudocholinesterase concentrations including those who are homozygous for the genetic trait that causes the production of an atypical pseudocholinesterase. If low pseudocholinesterase activity is suspected, a small test dose (5–10 mg) may be administered or relaxation may be produced by cautious IV infusion of a 0.1% solution of the drug. Apnea or prolonged muscle paralysis should be treated with controlled respiration. Administration of fresh whole blood or plasma has been reported to be of benefit in restoring pseudocholinesterase concentrations.

Succinylcholine should be used with extreme caution in patients with electrolyte imbalance, those receiving quinidine or cardiac glycosides, or those with suspected cardiac glycoside toxicity, since succinylcholine may induce serious cardiac arrhythmias or cardiac arrest in such patients. Succinylcholine should be used with extreme caution, if at all, during ocular surgery or in patients with glaucoma. The drug also should be used with extreme caution in patients with preexisting hyperkalemia or paraplegia and those with chronic abdominal infection, subarachnoid hemorrhage, degenerative or dystrophic neuromuscular disease, or conditions that may cause degeneration of central and peripheral nervous systems, since the potential of developing severe hyperkalemia is increased in such patients. Succinylcholine is contraindicated in patients with upper motor neuron injury, multiple trauma, extensive or severe burns, extensive denervation of skeletal muscle because of disease or injury to the CNS, since such patients tend to become severely hyperkalemic following succinylcholine administration which may result in cardiac arrest. (See Cautions: Adverse Effects.)

Since neuromuscular blocking agents have been reported to cause severe anaphylactic reactions, appropriate emergency treatment should be readily available whenever these drugs are administered. Because of potential cross-sensitivity, succinylcholine should be used with caution in patients who have experienced previous anaphylactic reactions to other neuromuscular blocking agents (depolarizing or nondepolarizing).

Succinylcholine is contraindicated in patients with known hypersensitivity to the drug, personal or familial history of malignant hyperthermia, or skeletal muscle myopathies.

■ **Pediatric Precautions** Acute rhabdomyolysis with hyperkalemia followed by ventricular dysrhythmias, cardiac arrest, and death has been reported rarely in apparently healthy children and adolescents receiving succinylcholine; subsequently it was observed that these children had undiagnosed skeletal muscle myopathy, most frequently Duchenne type muscular dystrophy. Peaked T-waves and sudden cardiac arrest within minutes of administration of succinylcholine may occur in apparently healthy children, usually males 8 years of age or younger, although this syndrome has been reported in some adolescents. Therefore, when an apparently healthy infant or child develops cardiac arrest shortly after administration of succinylcholine (supposedly not associated with inadequate ventilation, oxygenation, or overdosage of an anesthetic), treatment for hyperkalemia should be initiated immediately. Emergency measures for the treatment of hyperkalemia should include hyperventilation and IV administration of calcium, sodium bicarbonate, glucose, and insulin. Since this syndrome is characterized by an abrupt onset, standard resuscitative measures may be unsuccessful. Prolonged or unusual resuscitative measures have been successful in some patients. If signs of malignant hyperthermia are present, appropriate therapy should be instituted concurrently. Since it is difficult to identify which children and adolescents may be at risk of developing such a syndrome, it is recommended that a nondepolarizing neuromuscular blocking agent be used in these patients and succinylcholine be reserved for children and adolescents undergoing emergency intubation, for those in whom an airway should be secured immediately (e.g., those with laryngospasm, difficult airway, full stomach), or for those in whom a suitable vein is not accessible and IM administration is needed.

The possibility that succinylcholine may produce profound bradycardia or, rarely, asystole when administered by rapid IV injection in infants and children should be considered; as in adults, the risk of these effects increases with repeated doses, and pretreatment with atropine should be considered to reduce the risk of bradyarrhythmias.

■ **Geriatric Precautions** Clinical studies of succinylcholine did not include sufficient numbers of patients 65 years of age and older to determine whether geriatric patients respond differently than younger patients. While other clinical experience has not revealed age-related differences in response or tolerance, drug dosage generally should be titrated carefully in geriatric patients, usually initiating therapy at the low end of the dosage range. The greater frequency of decreased hepatic, renal, and/or cardiac function and of concomitant disease and drug therapy observed in the elderly also should be considered.

■ **Pregnancy and Lactation** Animal reproduction studies have not been performed to date with succinylcholine chloride. It is also not known whether the drug can cause fetal harm when administered to pregnant women. Pseudocholinesterase concentrations are decreased during pregnancy and for several days postpartum, and a higher proportion of patients may be expected to show sensitivity to succinylcholine when pregnant. Succinylcholine may be used to provide muscle relaxation during delivery by cesarean section. Although succinylcholine generally crosses the placenta in small amounts, residual neuromuscular blockade (apnea, flaccidity) may occur in the neonate after repeated administration of high doses to the mother or in the presence of atypical pseudocholinesterase in the mother. Succinylcholine should be used during pregnancy only when clearly needed.

It is not known whether succinylcholine is distributed into human milk, and the manufacturers recommend that the drug be used with caution in nursing women.

Drug Interactions

Cholinesterase inhibitors, particularly the irreversible organophosphate type, can substantially reduce the activity of plasma pseudocholinesterase. Prolonged apnea and death have occurred following administration of succinylcholine to patients who had received prolonged therapy with echothiophate iodide ophthalmic drops (no longer commercially available in the US). The possibility of reactions should be considered in patients receiving isofluorophate or demecarium bromide and in those who have recently been exposed to organophosphate insecticides. In high blood concentrations, procaine competes with succinylcholine for hydrolysis by pseudocholinesterase, and procaine should not be given IV concurrently with succinylcholine because prolonged apnea may result. In addition, promazine, oxytocin, certain anti-infective agents (excluding penicillins), chloroquine, quinine, terbutaline, β-adrenergic blocking agents, lidocaine, procainamide, quinidine, lithium carbonate, magnesium salts, metoclopramide, and inhalation anesthetics (e.g., isoflurane) may potentiate the neuromuscular blocking effect of succinylcholine. Several other drugs, including cyclophosphamide, oral contraceptives, corticosteroids, some monoamine oxidase inhibitors (e.g., phenelzine), pancuronium, neostigmine, phenothiazines, and thiotepa, have been reported to reduce plasma pseudocholinesterase concentrations and possibly enhance the neuromuscular blocking effects of succinylcholine. Although most of these reports are poorly documented and the clinical importance of their interaction with succinylcholine is unknown, caution should be used when administering these drugs simultaneously with succinylcholine.

Acute Toxicity

■ **Manifestations** The duration of neuromuscular blockade produced by an overdose of succinylcholine may be longer than that following usual doses, and skeletal muscle weakness, decreased respiratory reserve, low tidal volume, or apnea beyond the period of surgery and anesthesia may occur.

■ **Treatment** In succinylcholine overdosage, supportive and symptomatic treatment should be initiated. Maintenance of an adequate, patent airway and respiratory support are necessary until recovery of normal respiration is assured. Depending on the dose and duration of succinylcholine administration, the characteristic phase I depolarizing neuromuscular block may change to a superficially resembling, phase II nondepolarizing neuromuscular block.

Pharmacology

Succinylcholine produces pharmacologic effects similar to those of other depolarizing neuromuscular blocking agents. The drug possesses histamine-releasing properties. It has been reported that succinylcholine stimulates the cardiac vagus and subsequently sympathetic ganglia.

Succinylcholine causes a slight, transient increase in intraocular pressure immediately after injection and during the fasciculation phase, and the increase may persist after the onset of complete paralysis.

Pharmacokinetics

■ **Absorption** Succinylcholine has a rapid onset and a short duration of action. Following IV administration of 10–30 mg of succinylcholine chloride in healthy adults, complete muscle relaxation occurs within 0.5–1 minute, persists for about 2–3 minutes, and gradually dissipates within 10 minutes. The duration of action following a single IV dose appears to be determined by the rate of diffusion of the drug away from the motor end-plate rather than the elimination of the drug by enzymatic hydrolysis. After relatively stable blood concentrations are achieved, however, as with continuous infusion or multiple injections, the short duration of action of succinylcholine results from its rapid hydrolysis. Following IM administration the onset of action occurs in about 2–3 minutes and the duration of action ranges from 10–30 minutes. The duration of action is prolonged in patients with low plasma pseudocholinesterase concentrations.

■ **Distribution** Succinylcholine crosses the placenta, generally in small amounts.

■ **Elimination** Succinylcholine (succinyldicholine) is metabolized rapidly, mainly by plasma pseudocholinesterase, to succinylmonocholine and choline. Succinylmonocholine has only about one-twentieth the activity of succinylcholine and produces a nondepolarizing rather than a depolarizing block.

Succinylmonocholine is excreted partly in urine; the remainder of the metabolite is further broken down in the plasma, principally by alkaline hydrolysis to succinate and choline, which are inactive. Since hydrolysis of succinylmonocholine occurs relatively slowly, succinylmonocholine may occasionally accumulate and cause prolonged apnea, especially in patients with impaired renal function. Up to 10% of a dose of succinylcholine is excreted unchanged in urine.

Chemistry and Stability

■ **Chemistry** Succinylcholine chloride is a depolarizing neuromuscular blocking agent. The drug occurs as a white, odorless, crystalline powder and has solubilities of approximately 1 g/mL in water and 2.9 mg/mL in alcohol at 25°C. Succinylcholine chloride usually contains about 2 molecules of water of hydration, but its potency is labeled in terms of its anhydrous equivalent. Commercially available succinylcholine chloride injections are adjusted to pH 3–4.5 with hydrochloric acid or sodium hydroxide and may contain methylparaben and propylparaben as preservatives.

■ **Stability** Succinylcholine decomposes in solutions with pH greater than 4.5. Succinylcholine chloride injection is incompatible with alkaline solutions such as barbiturates; decomposition of succinylcholine chloride and precipitation of the barbiturate may occur if the drugs are mixed.

Succinylcholine chloride undergoes hydrolysis in aqueous solutions and the commercially available injections should be stored at 2–8°C to retard loss of potency. Multiple-dose vials of the injection are stable for up to 14 days at room temperature without substantial loss of potency.

For further information on chemistry, pharmacology, pharmacokinetics, uses, cautions, drug interactions, and dosage and administration of succinylcholine chloride, see the Neuromuscular Blocking Agents General Statement 12:20.20.

Preparations

Excipients in commercially available drug preparations may have clinically important effects in some individuals; consult specific product labeling for details.

Succinylcholine Chloride

Parenteral

Injection	20 mg/mL	**Anectine®**, Sandoz
		Quelicin®, Hospira

Vecuronium Bromide

■ Vecuronium bromide is an aminosteroid nondepolarizing neuromuscular blocking agent.

Uses

■ **Skeletal Muscle Relaxation** Vecuronium bromide is used to produce skeletal muscle relaxation during surgery after general anesthesia has been induced. The drug also is used to facilitate endotracheal intubation; however, a neuromuscular blocking agent with a more rapid onset of action (e.g., succinylcholine, rocuronium) generally is preferred in emergency situations when rapid intubation is required.

Vecuronium has produced adequate neuromuscular blockade in patients undergoing cesarean section, vagotomy, and other types of surgery, including otolaryngologic, cardiovascular (e.g., coronary artery bypass), facial, dental and oral, ophthalmic, orthopedic, abdominal (i.e., gynecologic, splenic, pancreatic, exploratory, and hernia procedures, as well as adrenalectomy, colostomy, sigmoidectomy, laparotomy, cholecystectomy, and gastrectomy), and routine minor procedures. The drug has also produced adequate blockade with minimal adverse effects in patients with renal or hepatic failure, critically ill or high-risk patients, and children 7 weeks of age and older.

Vecuronium also has been used to facilitate mechanical ventilation in the intensive care unit (ICU); however, the manufacturer states that insufficient data are available to support dosage recommendations for such use. Whenever neuromuscular blocking agents are used in the ICU, the benefits versus risks of such therapy must be considered and patients should be assessed frequently to determine the need for continued paralysis. (See Cautions: Precautions and Contraindications.)

Compared with other neuromuscular blocking agents, vecuronium has an intermediate onset and duration of action, and exhibits minimal cardiovascular effects. Because of its slow onset of paralysis, vecuronium is not suitable for rapid sequence intubation, but may be used for procedures requiring profound muscle relaxation for short durations (e.g., laryngoscopy, bronchoscopy) or for maintenance of neuromuscular blockade during the postintubation period. Although vecuronium is mostly metabolized, cumulative effects attributed to its active 3-desacetyl metabolite may occur in patients with renal or hepatic dysfunction. Because vecuronium has minimal effects on the heart, it may be a suitable neuromuscular blocking agent during surgery.

For additional information on uses and treatment principles of neuromuscular blocking agents, see Uses in the Neuromuscular Blocking Agents General Statement 12:20.20.

Dosage and Administration

■ **Reconstitution and Administration** Vecuronium bromide is administered IV only. The initial (intubating) dose is administered by rapid IV injection; maintenance doses may be administered by intermittent IV injection or by continuous IV infusion. *Vecuronium should not be administered by IM injection,* since there are no clinical data to support this route of administration.

While reactions associated with histamine release are unlikely with vecuronium, if the drug is used in patients in whom substantial histamine release would be particularly hazardous (e.g., patients with clinically important cardiovascular disease) or in patients with any history suggesting a greater risk of histamine release (e.g., a history of severe anaphylactoid reactions or asthma), it may be prudent to administer the drug slowly over a period of 1–2 minutes or longer and discontinue administration if any signs of histamine release occur.

For IV injection, commercially available vecuronium bromide for injection should be reconstituted with a compatible IV solution (e.g., 5% dextrose, 5% dextrose and 0.9% sodium chloride, 0.9% sodium chloride, lactated Ringer's, bacteriostatic water for injection). When reconstituted with bacteriostatic water for injection, the solution should be used within 5 days; when reconstituted with other compatible solutions, the solution should be used within 24 hours and any unused portions should be discarded. (See Chemistry and Stability: Stability.)

For continuous IV infusion, the reconstituted vecuronium solution should be further diluted to the desired concentration (usually 0.1 or 0.2 mg/mL) in a compatible IV infusion solution such as 5% dextrose, 5% dextrose and 0.9% sodium chloride, 0.9% sodium chloride, or lactated Ringer's. Use of a controlled-infusion device is recommended to ensure precise control of the flow rate during continuous IV infusion of the drug.

Reconstituted solutions of vecuronium and diluted solutions of the drug should be inspected visually for particulate matter and discoloration prior to administration whenever solution and container permit. Vecuronium should not be mixed in the same syringe nor administered simultaneously through the same needle as an alkaline solution (e.g., barbiturate solution). (See Chemistry and Stability: Stability.)

Dispensing and Administration Precautions Neuromuscular blocking agents should be administered only by individuals who are adequately trained in their use and complications. For specific procedures and techniques of administration, specialized references should be consulted. Facilities and personnel necessary for intubation, administration of oxygen, and respiratory support should be immediately available whenever these drugs are used. In addition, a reversal agent should be readily available in the event of a failed intubation or to accelerate neuromuscular recovery after surgery. (See Dosage and Administration: Reversal of Neuromuscular Blockade.)

Because neuromuscular blocking agents can cause respiratory arrest, precautions (e.g., storage segregation, warning labels, access limitations) should be taken to ensure that these drugs are not administered without adequate respiratory support. Affixing warning labels to storage containers and final administration containers is recommended to clearly communicate that respiratory paralysis can occur and ventilator support is required. The Institute for Safe Medication Practices (ISMP) recommends the following wording for these containers: "Warning: Paralyzing agent—causes respiratory arrest—patient must be ventilated."

Neuromuscular blocking agents have no known effect on consciousness, pain threshold, or cerebration, and should therefore be used in conjunction with adequate levels of anesthesia, and only after appropriate analgesics and sedatives are administered. To avoid distress to the patient, vecuronium should be administered only after unconsciousness has been induced.

■ Dosage

Dosage of vecuronium bromide must be carefully adjusted according to individual requirements and response. The use of a peripheral nerve stimulator is recommended to accurately monitor the degree of neuromuscular blockade and recovery, determine the need for additional doses, and minimize the possibility of overdosage.

The possible need for substantially increased doses of vecuronium bromide in burn patients should be considered. (See Cautions: Precautions and Contraindications.)

Initial Dose The usual initial (intubating) adult dose of vecuronium bromide is 0.08–0.1 mg/kg (1.4–1.75 times the dose necessary to induce 90% neuromuscular blockade). Following administration of this initial dose, endotracheal intubation for nonemergency surgical procedures can be performed within 2.5–3 minutes in most patients and maximum neuromuscular blockade generally occurs within 3–5 minutes. When used concomitantly with balanced anesthesia, this initial dose usually results in clinically sufficient neuromuscular blockade for about 25–30 minutes; spontaneous recovery to about 25% of baseline generally occurs within 25–40 minutes and is usually 95% complete 45–65 minutes after administration. When used concomitantly with inhalation anesthesia, this initial dose usually results in clinically sufficient neuromuscular blockade for 30–40 minutes. When administration of a larger initial dose is considered necessary, the manufacturer states that vecuronium bromide has been administered in initial doses ranging from 0.15–0.28 mg/kg in patients undergoing halothane anesthesia with minimal adverse cardiovascular effects as long as ventilation was adequately maintained. Although onset of action may be delayed with usual initial doses in patients with impaired circulation or in whom volume of distribution of the drug may be increased (e.g., patients with cardiovascular disease or edema), larger than usual initial doses are not recommended for these patients.

When vecuronium is used concomitantly with general anesthetics (e.g., enflurane, isoflurane, halothane) that potentiate its neuromuscular blocking activity, dosage of vecuronium bromide may need to be reduced. The manufacturer states that the initial adult dose of vecuronium bromide may be reduced by about 15% (i.e., to 0.06–0.085 mg/kg) when the drug is administered more than 5 minutes after administration of enflurane, isoflurane, or halothane has been initiated or after steady-state anesthesia has been achieved.

When used following succinylcholine, vecuronium bromide should be administered at a reduced initial dose and its administration should be delayed until the patient begins recovering from the neuromuscular blockade induced by succinylcholine. Following use of succinylcholine for endotracheal intubation in adults, a reduced initial vecuronium bromide dose of 0.05–0.06 mg/kg with balanced anesthesia or 0.04–0.06 mg/kg with inhalation anesthesia may be necessary.

Because even small doses of vecuronium may cause profound neuromuscular blockade in patients with neuromuscular diseases (e.g., myasthenia gravis, Eaton-Lambert syndrome), response should be monitored carefully with a peripheral nerve stimulator; use of a small test dose of vecuronium bromide (e.g., 0.005–0.02 mg/kg) may be of value in monitoring the response to administration of skeletal muscle relaxants in these patients.

Maintenance Dosage **Intermittent IV Injection.** For maintenance of neuromuscular blockade during prolonged surgical procedures in adults receiving balanced anesthesia, additional vecuronium bromide doses of 0.01–0.015 mg/kg may be administered by intermittent IV injection as necessary. In patients receiving inhalation anesthesia, the usual maintenance dose is 0.008–0.012 mg/kg, administered as necessary. The manufacturer states that a maintenance dose of 0.01 mg/kg during enflurane anesthesia is approximately equivalent to a dose of 0.015 mg/kg during balanced anesthesia. In patients undergoing balanced or inhalation anesthesia, the first maintenance dose of vecuronium bromide generally is necessary 25–40 minutes after administration of the initial dose. Because the drug lacks clinically important cumulative effects at usual doses, the manufacturer states that repeated maintenance doses of vecuronium bromide may be administered at relatively regular intervals, generally ranging from 12–15 minutes in patients undergoing balanced anesthesia and at slightly longer intervals in patients undergoing enflurane or isoflurane anesthesia. When longer intervals between doses are desirable, the size of each maintenance dose may be increased (i.e., to greater than 0.01–0.015 mg/kg).

Continuous IV Infusion. After the initial intubating dose is administered, patients may receive a continuous IV infusion of vecuronium to maintain neuromuscular blockade during prolonged surgical procedures; the infusion should be initiated approximately 20–40 minutes after administration of the initial dose when early spontaneous recovery from this dose is evident. The wide interindividual range in dosage requirements of vecuronium with continuous IV infusions requires that patients be very closely monitored to avoid excessive dosage when this method of administration is employed. Following rapid IV injection of an initial dose of vecuronium, required infusion rates of the drug initially decrease progressively and become relatively constant within 30–50 minutes. When administered by continuous IV infusion in adults, an initial vecuronium bromide infusion rate of 1 mcg/kg per minute is recommended by the manufacturer. Subsequently, the infusion rates should be adjusted to maintain 90% neuromuscular blockade; maintenance infusion rates of 0.8–1.2 mcg/kg per minute usually are adequate to maintain continuous neuromuscular blockade in most patients. Following rapid IV administration of an initial 0.1-mg/kg dose in a limited number of patients undergoing general surgery with nitrous oxide and halothane anesthesia, the rate of continuous IV infusion necessary to maintain 95% neuromuscular blockade at steady state ranged from approximately 0.55–1.67 mcg/kg per minute (mean: 1 mcg/kg per minute).

The rate of spontaneous recovery from vecuronium-induced neuromuscular blockade following discontinuance of the infusion is likely to be comparable to that following administration of a single IV injection of the drug.

When vecuronium is administered by IV infusion in patients receiving general anesthetics that potentiate its neuromuscular blocking activity, a reduction in the infusion rate of vecuronium bromide may be required. The manufacturer states that the infusion rate may need to be reduced by about 25–60% approximately 45–60 minutes following the initial IV dose when the drug is administered in the presence of steady-state anesthesia with enflurane or isoflurane. However, a reduction in the vecuronium bromide infusion rate may not be necessary in the presence of steady-state anesthesia with halothane.

The manufacturer states that prolonged use of continuous IV infusions of vecuronium during mechanical ventilation in the ICU has not been adequately studied to date to establish dosage recommendations for this use.

Pediatric Dosage Recommendations for initial and maintenance doses of vecuronium bromide administered by intermittent IV injection in pediatric patients 10–16 years of age and older are the same as those for adults. (See Initial Dose and Maintenance Dosage: Intermittent IV Injection under Dosage and Administration: Dosage.) Slightly higher initial doses of vecuronium bromide and more frequent administration of maintenance doses may be necessary in children 1–9 years of age than in older children and adults. Infants older than 7 weeks but less than 1 year of age appear to be more sensitive than adults to the neuromuscular blocking effects of vecuronium and may experience a longer period of time (about 1.5 times longer) to neuromuscular recovery; although these children may receive doses comparable to those used in adults, less frequent administration of maintenance doses may be necessary.

Safety and efficacy of vecuronium in children younger than 7 weeks of age have not been established. In addition, the manufacturer states that administration of the drug by continuous IV infusion has not been adequately studied to date to establish dosage recommendations for this route of administration in any pediatric age group.

■ Dosage in Renal and Hepatic Impairment

The manufacturer states that vecuronium is well tolerated and neuromuscular blockade induced by the drug is not substantially prolonged in patients with renal failure who are optimally prepared with dialysis prior to surgery; although experience with these patients is limited, most clinicians use the usual initial and maintenance doses of the drug, with the interval between doses based on careful monitoring of the patient. Since prolongation of blockade may occur in patients with severe renal failure (i.e., creatinine clearance less than 10 mL/minute) who are not optimally prepared with dialysis, the manufacturer cautions that a lower than usual initial dose of vecuronium bromide should be considered if emergency surgery is necessary in these patients; however, most clinicians believe that the usual initial dose can be administered, anticipating that the duration of blockade may be prolonged, with maintenance dosing adjusted carefully according to the patient's response.

Data currently are insufficient for specific dosage recommendations in patients with hepatic impairment. The duration of and rate of recovery from vecuronium-induced neuromuscular blockade appear to be prolonged in these patients. If vecuronium is used in patients with impaired hepatic function, some clinicians suggest that the usual initial dose of the drug may be given while others suggest giving a reduced initial dose; maintenance dosing (probably with reduced doses) would be adjusted carefully according to the patient's response.

■ **Reversal of Neuromuscular Blockade** Neuromuscular blockade induced by vecuronium can be reversed by administering a cholinesterase inhibitor (e.g., neostigmine, pyridostigmine, edrophonium) in conjunction with an anticholinergic agent such as atropine or glycopyrrolate to block the adverse muscarinic effects of the cholinesterase inhibitor. Alternatively, sugammadex may be used for the reversal of vecuronium-induced neuromuscular blockade after surgery. *For specific information on the uses and dosage and administration of these other drugs, see the individual monographs.*

To minimize the risk of residual neuromuscular blockade, reversal should only be attempted after some degree of spontaneous recovery has occurred; patients should be closely monitored until adequate recovery of normal neuromuscular function is assured (i.e., ability to maintain satisfactory ventilation and a patent airway).

Cautions

■ **Adverse Effects** Adverse effects of vecuronium bromide generally are manifestations of the usual pharmacologic actions of the nondepolarizing neuromuscular blocking agents, including skeletal muscle weakness or paralysis and respiratory insufficiency or apnea. However, the respiratory depression that occurs during or following anesthesia that includes vecuronium bromide may also result at least in part from concomitantly administered drugs, including opiate agonists, barbiturates, and other CNS depressants.

Prolonged to profound extensions of paralysis and/or muscle weakness as well as muscle atrophy have been reported after long-term use of the drug to support mechanical ventilation in intensive care settings. Prolonged paralysis has been associated with electrolyte disturbances (e.g., increased plasma magnesium concentrations), metabolic acidosis, and renal failure (which may result in high plasma concentrations of 3-desacetyl vecuronium); limited data indicate that prolonged paralysis may occur more frequently in female patients. (See Cautions: Precautions and Contraindications, in the Neuromuscular Blocking Agents General Statement 12:20.20.)

Following intradermal administration of vecuronium in several healthy individuals, minimal induration, redness, and itching, which are characteristic manifestations of cutaneous histamine release, have been observed, but these effects were less severe than those seen with other neuromuscular blocking agents. Rarely, hypersensitivity reactions associated with histamine release (e.g., bronchospasm, flushing, erythema, acute urticaria, hypotension, tachycardia) have been reported following IV administration of usual doses of the drug. Redness (flare) in skin proximal to the injection site, with subsequent urticaria, occurred in one patient following IV injection of vecuronium; subsequent intradermal testing with the drug produced a wheal and flare. In another patient, bronchospasm occurred following IV injection of the drug; subsequent intradermal testing with the drug was positive, although other immunologic studies, including basophil degranulation tests, revealed no evidence that the reaction was mediated by IgE or direct histamine release.

Cardiovascular effects, including changes in heart rate, cardiac index, cardiac output, filling pressure of the heart, mean systolic blood pressure, mean arterial pressure, and systemic vascular resistance, have been observed occasionally following administration of vecuronium; however, these effects appear to be minimal and transient. Some cardiovascular effects may be associated with endotracheal intubation rather than with the drug. Systolic blood pressure, diastolic blood pressure, and/or mean arterial pressure reportedly did not change substantially in healthy patients following administration of doses of vecuronium bromide up to 0.15 mg/kg (up to 3 times the doses necessary for clinical relaxation); heart rate remained unchanged or decreased by an average of up to 8% from baseline values. The drug did not produce changes in heart rate or rhythm, mean arterial pressure, central venous pressure, or pulmonary wedge pressure when administered in a dose of 0.28 mg/kg in patients undergoing preparation for coronary artery bypass surgery; systemic vascular resistance decreased 12% and cardiac output increased 9% in these patients. Vecuronium did not produce tachycardia or changes in blood pressure in several patients undergoing surgery for pheochromocytoma. In comatose patients not receiving anesthesia who were administered vecuronium bromide doses of 0.1 mg/kg, the drug did not increase heart rate or cardiac output; in doses of 0.3 mg/kg, the drug caused only a very slight, transient increase in heart rate and cardiac output.

Serious hypersensitivity reactions, including anaphylaxis, have been reported rarely with all neuromuscular blocking agents; such reactions were life-threatening or fatal in some cases.

■ **Precautions and Contraindications** Vecuronium bromide shares the toxic potentials of the nondepolarizing neuromuscular blocking agents, and the usual precautions of neuromuscular blocking agent administration should be observed. (See Cautions in the Neuromuscular Blocking Agents General Statement 12:20.20.)

When used inappropriately, neuromuscular blocking agents can severely compromise respiratory function and cause respiratory paralysis; special precautions should be taken during and after administration of these drugs. (See Dispensing and Administration Precautions under Dosage and Administration: Reconstitution and Administration.) The degree of neuromuscular blockade produced by vecuronium should be monitored with a peripheral nerve stimulator, particularly in patients with conditions that may potentiate (e.g., neuromuscular diseases) or cause resistance to (e.g., burns) the neuromuscular blocking effects of the drug.

Data from some clinical studies and intradermal skin testing indicate that histamine-like hypersensitivity reactions, including bronchospasm, flushing, redness, hypotension, and tachycardia, are *not* likely to occur following administration of vecuronium; however, this does not preclude the rare development of a hypersensitivity reaction and the possibility of histamine release should be considered. (See Pharmacology: Effects on Histamine.)

Since vecuronium exhibits minimal effects on heart rate, especially at recommended doses, the drug will not counteract the bradycardia induced by many anesthesia agents (e.g., high-dose fentanyl) or by vagal stimulation; as a result, bradycardia may be more common when vecuronium is used concomitantly during anesthesia with agents that may cause bradycardia than when certain other neuromuscular blocking agents are used concomitantly.

Many drugs administered during anesthesia are suspected of being capable of initiating the development of malignant hyperthermia. The manufacturer states that data from screening in susceptible animals are insufficient to determine whether vecuronium is capable of initiating the development of this condition. However, because malignant hyperthermia can occur even in the absence of a recognized precipitating factor, clinicians should be vigilant for its possible development and prepared for its management in any patient undergoing general anesthesia.

Resistance to nondepolarizing neuromuscular blocking agents, including vecuronium, can develop in burn patients and may be substantial. The magnitude of resistance depends on the extent of thermal injury and elapsed time since the burn. The possible need for substantially increased doses of vecuronium bromide in burn patients should be considered.

Vecuronium is well tolerated and neuromuscular blockade induced by the drug is not substantially prolonged in patients with renal dysfunction who have undergone adequate dialysis prior to surgery. Since blockade may be prolonged in patients with severe renal failure (i.e., creatinine clearance less than 10 mL/minute) who are undergoing emergency surgery and cannot be adequately prepared with dialysis preoperatively, the manufacturer cautions that a lower than usual initial dose of vecuronium bromide be considered in these patients. (See Dosage and Administration: Dosage in Renal and Hepatic Impairment.) The manufacturer also cautions that inadvertent overdosage in patients with renal dysfunction may be avoided by careful monitoring with a peripheral nerve stimulator.

Since the onset of neuromuscular blockade and maximum effect of vecuronium may be delayed secondary to impaired circulation or an increased volume of distribution of the drug, larger than usual doses of the drug are not recommended in patients with these conditions (e.g., patients with cardiovascular disease or edema) and caution should be used when administering a subsequent dose of the drug in such patients before the maximum effect of the initial dose is attained. Vecuronium should be administered with caution in patients with hepatic dysfunction (e.g., cirrhosis, cholestasis), since the drug appears to be eliminated principally via bile and recovery from neuromuscular blockade may be prolonged in these patients. The manufacturer cautions that inadvertent overdosage in patients with impaired circulation or hepatic dysfunction may be avoided by careful monitoring with a peripheral nerve stimulator.

Vecuronium should be administered with caution in severely obese patients; maintenance of an adequate airway and ventilation support prior to, during, and following administration of neuromuscular blocking agents may require particular care in these patients.

Patients with neuromuscular diseases (e.g., myasthenia gravis, Eaton-Lambert syndrome) may have an exaggerated response to vecuronium. In patients with neuromuscular diseases, the degree of neuromuscular blockade induced by vecuronium should be monitored with a peripheral nerve stimulator; use of a small test dose of the drug (e.g., 0.005–0.02 mg/kg) may be of value in monitoring the response to administration of skeletal muscle relaxants in these patients. The degree of neuromuscular blockade produced by vecuronium should also be monitored with a peripheral nerve stimulator in patients with severe electrolyte disturbances (i.e., hypermagnesemia, hypokalemia, hypocalcemia) or diseases that result in electrolyte disturbances (e.g., adrenal cortical insufficiency) and in patients with severe debilitation or carcinomatosis. *For other conditions associated with increased response to neuromuscular blocking agents, see Cautions: Precautions and Contraindications, in the Neuromuscular Blocking Agents General Statement 12:20.20.*

Long-term use of neuromuscular blocking agents to support mechanical ventilation in the intensive care unit (ICU) has been associated with prolonged paralysis and/or skeletal muscle weakness. Although confounding factors were present and a causal relationship has not been definitively established, the risks versus benefits of neuromuscular blockade should be considered whenever there is a need for long-term mechanical ventilation. Continuous monitoring of neuromuscular transmission with a peripheral nerve stimulator is recommended whenever vecuronium is used in the ICU. Additional doses of vecuronium or any other neuromuscular blocking agent should not be administered before there is a definite response to nerve stimulation tests. If no response is elicited, administration of the drug should be discontinued until a response returns.

Since neuromuscular blocking agents have been reported to cause severe anaphylactic reactions, appropriate emergency treatment should be readily available whenever these drugs are administered. Vecuronium is contraindicated in patients with known hypersensitivity to the drug. Because of the possibility of cross-sensitivity, vecuronium should be used with caution in patients who have experienced previous anaphylactic reactions to other neuromuscular blocking agents (depolarizing or nondepolarizing).

■ **Pediatric Precautions** Safety and efficacy of vecuronium in children younger than 7 weeks of age have not been established. The drug has been used safely and effectively in children older than 7 weeks of age who were undergoing surgery. Vecuronium bromide that has been reconstituted with bacteriostatic water for injection containing benzyl alcohol should *not* be used in neonates.

■ **Mutagenicity and Carcinogenicity** Long-term animal studies to determine the mutagenic and carcinogenic potentials of vecuronium bromide have not been performed to date.

■ **Pregnancy, Fertility, and Lactation** Animal reproduction studies have not been performed to date with vecuronium. It is not known whether administration of neuromuscular blocking agents during vaginal delivery has immediate or delayed adverse effects on the fetus or whether it increases the likelihood that resuscitation of the neonate will be necessary. Vecuronium should be used with caution and dosage reduced as necessary in pregnant women receiving magnesium sulfate during delivery, since the neuromuscular blockade may be potentiated and its reversal impeded. When vecuronium was administered to pregnant women during delivery by cesarean section, no adverse effects attributed to the drug were observed in neonates born to these women. In 2 limited studies, Apgar scores were 9 or greater at 5 minutes after birth in neonates born to women who received vecuronium bromide 0.04 or 0.06–0.08 mg/kg (after tracheal intubation with succinylcholine) during cesarean delivery. However, the drug crosses the placenta minimally, and the possibility of respiratory depression in neonates should be considered following cesarean section in which a neuromuscular blocking agent is administered to the mother. It is not known whether vecuronium can cause fetal harm when administered to pregnant women. The drug should be used during pregnancy only when clearly needed.

It is not known if vecuronium affects fertility.

Since it is not known if vecuronium is distributed into milk, the drug should be administered with caution to nursing women. However, since animal studies suggest that GI absorption of vecuronium is negligible, any drug that may be present in milk is not likely to be of any clinical importance to a nursing infant.

Drug Interactions

Concurrent administration of some drugs, including general anesthetics (i.e., enflurane, isoflurane, halothane), antibiotics (e.g., aminoglycosides, tetracyclines, bacitracin, polymyxins, clindamycin), skeletal muscle relaxants (e.g., succinylcholine, pancuronium), magnesium salts, and quinidine, may affect the neuromuscular blocking activity of vecuronium bromide. Concurrent administration of barbiturates, opiate agonists, nitrous oxide, or droperidol appears to have little effect on the intensity or duration of the neuromuscular blockade induced by vecuronium. **For additional information on potential drug interactions of vecuronium, see Drug Interactions in the Neuromuscular Blocking Agents General Statement 12:20.20.**

■ **General Anesthetics** Enflurane and isoflurane reportedly increase the potency and prolong the duration of the neuromuscular blockade induced by vecuronium by about 30–50%; halothane appears to have only a marginal effect on the potency and duration of neuromuscular blockade induced by vecuronium, prolonging the duration by about 20%. In a study comparing concomitant administration of vecuronium and either enflurane, isoflurane, or halothane with 60% nitrous oxide anesthesia, the ED_{50} (dose required to produce 50% suppression of the control twitch response) of vecuronium decreased by about 50, 33, or 18% when the MAC (minimal alveolar anesthetic concentration) of enflurane, isoflurane, or halothane anesthesia, respectively, was increased from 1.2 to 2.2. When the MAC of the inhalation anesthetic was increased to 2.2 in this study, the duration of neuromuscular blockade was increased twofold by enflurane but only minimally by isoflurane or halothane; the potentiating effect of an increasing MAC is markedly less for vecuronium than for pancuronium.

■ **Skeletal Muscle Relaxants** Administration of succinylcholine prior to vecuronium appears to increase the potency and prolong the duration of neuromuscular blockade induced by vecuronium. In one study, when a 0.04-mg/kg dose of vecuronium bromide was given 15 or 30 minutes after complete recovery from the blockade of a 1-mg/kg dose of succinylcholine, the duration of neuromuscular blockade to 90% recovery was about 26 minutes compared with 12 minutes when vecuronium was administered alone; the onset of blockade was more rapid in patients receiving vecuronium subsequent to succinylcholine. In another study, a 1-mg/kg dose of succinylcholine followed 9–14 minutes later by a 0.036-mg/kg dose of vecuronium bromide induced a 91% neuromuscular blockade compared with a 72–78% blockade when vecuronium was administered alone; the time for recovery from 25% to 75% of the control twitch tension was about 10 or 8 minutes in patients who received both succinylcholine and vecuronium or vecuronium alone, respectively. If succinylcholine is administered prior to vecuronium, the manufacturer states that administration of vecuronium should be delayed until the effects of succinylcholine begin to dissipate. The manufacturer states that the administration of vecuronium prior to succinylcholine in order to attenuate some of the adverse effects of succinylcholine has not been fully evaluated.

Concomitant use of vecuronium and other nondepolarizing neuromuscular blocking agents (e.g., pancuronium bromide) may result in additive or synergistic effects. The manufacturer states that data are insufficient to support concomitant administration of vecuronium and other nondepolarizing neuromuscular blocking agents. In healthy adults in one study, concomitant administration of vecuronium and pancuronium did not result in potentiation, whereas in another study concomitant administration of vecuronium and tubocurarine (no longer commercially available in the US) did result in potentiation.

■ **Anti-infective Agents** IV and/or intraperitoneal injection of high doses of certain anti-infective agents, including aminoglycosides, metronidazole, tetracyclines, bacitracin, clindamycin, lincomycin, and polymyxins (i.e., polymyxin B sulfate, colistin, sodium colistimethate), has been shown to induce neuromuscular blockade. If these anti-infective agents are used before, during, or after surgical procedures in which vecuronium is administered, the possibility of prolonged duration of neuromuscular blockade (or recurarization, particularly postoperatively) should be considered. For additional information, see Drug Interactions: Anti-Infective Agents, in the Neuromuscular Blocking Agents General Statement 12:20.20.

Intraoperative administration of acylaminopenicillins, including piperacillin, reportedly prolongs vecuronium-induced neuromuscular blockade, increasing the duration of skeletal muscle relaxation by an average of 40–55%. Acylaminopenicillins should be used perioperatively with caution in patients receiving vecuronium and the possibility of prolonged neuromuscular blockade should be considered.

■ **Other Drugs** When magnesium sulfate is administered for the management of toxemia of pregnancy, the neuromuscular blockade induced by vecuronium may be potentiated and its reversal impeded. If used in pregnant women receiving magnesium sulfate, vecuronium should be used with caution and its dosage reduced as necessary.

Experience with skeletal muscle relaxants other than vecuronium suggests that recurrence of paralysis may occur in patients following parenteral administration of quinidine during recovery from neuromuscular blockade. The manufacturer states that the possibility of recurrence of paralysis following parenteral administration of quinidine during recovery from vecuronium-induced neuromuscular blockade should be considered.

Although further documentation is needed, a difficult and prolonged recovery from vecuronium-induced neuromuscular blockade in a patient receiving IV verapamil suggests that calcium-channel blocking agents may be capable of prolonging the duration of neuromuscular blockade induced by vecuronium. Similarly, a prolonged duration of vecuronium-induced blockade was reported in a patient who received oral dantrolene preoperatively, but further evaluation of a potential interaction is needed.

Acute Toxicity

The manufacturer states that there has been no experience to date with overdosage following parenteral administration of vecuronium bromide. The possibility of overdosage can be minimized by assessing the vecuronium-induced effect on the response to peripheral nerve stimulation. (See Pharmacology: Neuromuscular Blockade.)

■ **Manifestations** Overdosage of vecuronium is likely to produce symptoms that are mainly extensions of the usual pharmacologic effects of the drug. The duration of neuromuscular blockade produced by an overdose of vecuronium may be longer than that following usual doses and skeletal muscle weakness, decreased respiratory reserve, low tidal volume, or apnea beyond the period of surgery and anesthesia may occur. A peripheral nerve stimulator should be used to monitor recovery from blockade and may be used to differentiate prolonged neuromuscular blockade from other causes of diminished respiratory reserve.

■ **Treatment** In vecuronium overdosage, supportive and symptomatic treatment should be initiated. An adequate, patent airway should be maintained, using assisted or controlled respiration as necessary. The possibility that other drugs (e.g., general anesthetics, opiate agonists, barbiturates) used during the surgical procedure may be wholly or partially responsible for respiratory depression should be considered. If cardiovascular support is necessary, treatment should include proper patient positioning, IV fluid administration, and, if necessary, use of vasopressors. Reversal of the neuromuscular blockade produced by vecuronium may be achieved by administration of a cholinesterase inhibitor such as neostigmine, pyridostigmine, or edrophonium. (See Dosage and Administration: Reversal of Neuromuscular Blockade.)

Pharmacology

■ **Neuromuscular Blockade** Vecuronium bromide is a nondepolarizing neuromuscular blocking agent that produces pharmacologic effects similar to those of other nondepolarizing neuromuscular blocking agents. (See Pharmacology in the Neuromuscular Blocking Agents General Statement 12:20.20.) On a weight basis, vecuronium bromide is about 1.2–1.7 or 4–5 times as potent as pancuronium bromide or atracurium besylate, respectively. The duration of neuromuscular blockade induced by initially equipotent doses of vecuronium bromide is about 33–50% or 25–33% that induced by pancuronium bromide or tubocurarine chloride (no longer commercially available in the US), respectively, and about 70–100% that induced by atracurium besylate. The neuromuscular blocking activity of vecuronium is enhanced in the presence of some inhalation general anesthetics (e.g., enflurane, isoflurane). (See Drug Interactions: General Anesthetics.)

The effects of patient age on vecuronium-induced neuromuscular blockade in adults remain to be clearly determined. The time of onset of neuromuscular blockade appears to be increased and the dose of vecuronium bromide necessary to maintain steady-state neuromuscular blockade and the rate of recovery appear to be decreased in older adults compared with younger adults. In one study in anesthetized patients younger than 40, 40–60, and older than 60 years of age, mean steady-state vecuronium bromide dosage requirements were approximately 3, 2.4, and 1.8 mg/m^2 per hour, respectively, and the mean times for the recovery of twitch height to 75% of the original twitch height were approximately 25, 31, and 60 minutes, respectively. However, other preliminary data suggest that vecuronium dosage requirements and the rate of recovery from neuromuscular blockade are similar in young and older adults. Further studies are needed to fully evaluate the effects of age on vecuronium-induced neuromuscular blockade in adults. Young (1–10 years of age) children may require slightly larger doses of vecuronium bromide than adolescents and adults, when calculated on a weight basis, to achieve the same degree of neuromuscular blockade during comparable techniques of anesthesia; however, children younger than 1 year of age may require smaller doses of the drug or doses similar to adults, administered at longer time intervals. (See Pediatric Dosage in Dosage and Administration: Dosage.)

The ED_{50} (dose required to produce 50% suppression of the control twitch response) of vecuronium bromide in patients undergoing balanced or nitrous oxide and halothane anesthesia reportedly ranges from 0.015–0.036 mg/kg. The manufacturer states that the ED_{90} (dose required to produce 90% suppression of the control twitch response) of the drug in patients undergoing balanced anesthesia averages 0.057 mg/kg; in several studies in patients undergoing balanced anesthesia, the ED_{90} has ranged from 0.043–0.062 mg/kg. The ED_{95} (dose required to produce 95% suppression of the control twitch response) of vecuronium bromide in patients undergoing balanced anesthesia has ranged from 0.037–0.065 mg/kg.

The ED_{50} in children 7–45 weeks, 1–9 years, and 10–17 years of age undergoing nitrous oxide and halothane anesthesia has reportedly averaged 0.0165, 0.019–0.033, and 0.023 mg/kg, respectively; the ED_{95} in children 2–9 and 10–17 years of age undergoing nitrous oxide and halothane anesthesia has reportedly averaged 0.06 and 0.045 mg/kg, respectively.

In animals, metabolic or respiratory acidosis substantially increases and metabolic alkalosis substantially decreases the intensity of vecuronium-induced neuromuscular blockade; respiratory alkalosis only slightly decreases the intensity of neuromuscular blockade. The effects of acid-base balance on vecuronium-induced neuromuscular blockade in humans have not been fully determined. In anesthetized patients receiving vecuronium by an infusion sufficient to produce a continual 50% depression of the control twitch tension, induced hypercapnia or hypocapnia decreased or increased twitch tension, respectively; however, changes in Pa_{CO_2} induced prior to administration of vecuronium had little effect on the maximal depression of twitch tension induced by the drug or the time necessary for spontaneous recovery from 25% to 75% of control twitch tension.

■ **Effects on Histamine** Vecuronium appears to have little histamine-releasing activity when administered at usual clinical doses. In studies comparing vecuronium bromide, atracurium besylate, metocurine iodide (no longer commercially available in the US), pancuronium bromide, and tubocurarine chloride (no longer commercially available in the US), vecuronium was the least potent stimulator of histamine release as determined by cutaneous reaction (i.e., induration, redness, itching) to intradermal injection of the drugs. While the risk of a histamine-induced sensitivity reaction to vecuronium appears to be low, anaphylaxis and anaphylactoid reactions have been reported rarely in patients receiving the drug. (See Cautions: Precautions and Contraindications.)

■ **Other Effects** Despite its steroidal structure, vecuronium apparently exhibits no hormonal activity.

The effect of vecuronium on intraocular pressure (IOP) in patients undergoing elective ophthalmic surgery has not been clearly determined. In one study, a 0.12-mg/kg dose of vecuronium bromide caused an additional reduction in IOP following an initial anesthesia-induced reduction, while in another study, a 0.1-mg/kg dose of the drug appeared to slightly reverse the initial anesthesia-induced reduction in IOP.

Vecuronium is about 10 times less potent than pancuronium bromide and about 1000 times more potent than succinylcholine chloride in its ability to inhibit plasma pseudocholinesterase; vecuronium's activity appears to be of no clinical importance. Although probably of no clinical relevance, vecuronium is also about 5 times more potent than pancuronium bromide or atracurium besylate in its ability to inhibit erythrocyte cholinesterase.

In animals, the effects of vecuronium on adrenergic receptors, cardiac muscarinic receptors, or norepinephrine reuptake mechanisms are minimal and occur only at dosages many times in excess of those required for neuromuscular blockade.

Unlike most other nondepolarizing neuromuscular blocking agents, vecuronium exhibits minimal cardiovascular effects. The drug does not appear to substantially affect heart rate or rhythm, systolic or diastolic blood pressure, mean arterial pressure, cardiac output, systemic vascular resistance, or pulmonary capillary wedge pressure. (See Cautions: Adverse Effects.) In animals, 50% vagal blockade occurs only at vecuronium bromide doses 50–80 times greater than those required for 50% neuromuscular blockade.

Pharmacokinetics

■ **Absorption** The onset and duration of and the rate of recovery from neuromuscular blockade induced by vecuronium bromide vary among individuals, are dose dependent, and may be altered by the anesthetic agent (e.g., enflurane, isoflurane, halothane) employed. (See Drug Interactions: General Anesthetics.) The onset and duration of and rate of recovery from neuromuscular blockade generally do not appear to be substantially altered by renal dysfunction; however, the duration of blockade may be prolonged in patients with severe renal impairment who have not undergone dialysis prior to surgery. The duration of and rate of recovery from neuromuscular blockade appear to be prolonged by hepatic dysfunction (i.e., cirrhosis, cholestasis). The duration of blockade may also be prolonged in patients undergoing cardiopulmonary bypass surgery under induced hypothermia.

As with other nondepolarizing neuromuscular blocking agents, the time from injection to maximum blockade decreases as the dose of vecuronium bromide increases. The manufacturer states that following IV administration of a vecuronium bromide dose of 0.08–0.1 mg/kg, neuromuscular blockade begins within 1 minute and is maximal at 3–5 minutes. Following concomitant administration of vecuronium bromide and halothane or nitrous oxide in adults, the time from injection to maximum blockade ranges from 3.3–6.7 minutes with doses of 0.01–0.05 mg/kg and 2.2–5.9 minutes with doses of 0.06–0.2 mg/kg. Following concomitant administration of a vecuronium bromide dose of 0.07 mg/kg and halothane and nitrous oxide anesthesia in children 7–45 weeks and 1–8 years of age, the time from injection to maximum blockade has reportedly averaged 1.5 and 2.4 minutes, respectively.

The duration of neuromuscular blockade increases as the dose of vecuronium bromide increases. In animals, the intensity of vecuronium-induced neuromuscular blockade has been shown to be increased by acidosis; however, the effects of acid-base balance on vecuronium-induced blockade in humans have not been fully determined. (See Pharmacology: Neuromuscular Blockade.) The duration of neuromuscular blockade induced by initially equipotent doses of vecuronium bromide is about 33–50% or 25–33% of that induced by pancuronium bromide or tubocurarine chloride (no longer commercially available in the US), respectively, and about 70–100% of that induced by atracurium besylate. The manufacturer states that the duration of clinically sufficient neuromuscular blockade (i.e., time from injection to 25% spontaneous recovery of control twitch response) induced by initial vecuronium bromide doses of 0.08–0.1 mg/kg under balanced (e.g., thiopental [no longer commercially available in the US], nitrous oxide, fentanyl) or halothane anesthesia is about 25–30 or 30–40 minutes, respectively. Following intubation with succinylcholine, the duration of clinically sufficient neuromuscular blockade of initial vecuronium bromide doses of 0.05–0.06 mg/kg under balanced anesthesia is 20–25 minutes and the duration of initial doses of 0.03–0.06 mg/kg under inhalation anesthesia is 25–30 minutes. In various studies, the duration of vecuronium-induced blockade (time from injection to 90% spontaneous recovery of control twitch response) under nitrous oxide, halothane, or enflurane anesthesia has reportedly averaged from 14–32 minutes with initial doses of approximately 0.01–0.05 mg/kg and 34–60 minutes with initial doses of approximately 0.06–0.12 mg/kg. In children 7–45 weeks and 1–8 years of age, the duration of blockade (time from injection to 90% spontaneous recovery of control twitch response) under halothane and nitrous oxide anesthesia has reportedly averaged 73 and 35 minutes, respectively, following administration of a vecuronium bromide dose of 0.07 mg/kg. The prolonged duration of action in children younger than 1 year of age appears to be related to the larger volume of distribution of, and possibly an increased sensitivity to, the drug in this age group. Repeated administration of maintenance doses of vecuronium bromide appears to have little, if any, cumulative effect on duration of the neuromuscular blockade. In addition, since the time necessary to recover from maintenance doses of the same size generally does not change with each additional dose, doses may be administered at relatively regular intervals with predictable neuromuscular blocking results; however, the interval between maintenance doses depends on the size of the dose and concomitant anesthesia.

Recovery from the neuromuscular blocking effects of vecuronium bromide occurs more rapidly than recovery from those of pancuronium bromide or tubocurarine chloride. Recovery from neuromuscular blockade may be enhanced slightly by alkalosis and prolonged by acidosis. The manufacturer states that the recovery time (the time necessary for spontaneous recovery of the twitch response from 25% to 75% of the control response) following administration of vecuronium bromide doses of 0.08–0.1 mg/kg under balanced or halothane anesthesia is about 15–25 minutes; the recovery time following initial doses of vecuronium bromide appears to be dose dependent. In children 7–45 weeks and 1–8 years of age, the recovery time following administration of a vecuronium bromide dose of 0.07 mg/kg under halothane and nitrous oxide anesthesia has reportedly averaged 20 and 9 minutes, respectively. Following administration of a single vecuronium bromide dose of 0.2 mg/kg in patients with cirrhosis, the recovery time reportedly averaged 44 minutes. Repeated administration of maintenance doses of vecuronium bromide appears to have little, if any, cumulative effect on the rate of recovery from neuromuscular blockade. The rate of recovery from vecuronium-induced blockade is more rapid than that from pancuronium-induced blockade and is similar to that from atracurium-induced blockade.

Good to excellent conditions for performing endotracheal intubation generally are present within 2.5–3.7 minutes after administration of a 0.08- to 0.1-mg/kg dose of vecuronium bromide in most patients; however, intubation has been performed successfully within 1.5–2.5 minutes in some patients after administration of 0.07- to 0.2-mg/kg doses of the drug.

In adults, mean plasma vecuronium concentrations of 0.09–0.14 and 0.2 mcg/mL at steady-state are reportedly associated with 50% and 90% neuromuscular blockade, respectively.

■ Distribution Distribution of vecuronium into human body tissues and fluids has not been fully characterized. Following IV administration, vecuronium appears to rapidly distribute into the extracellular space. Limited data indicate that the drug undergoes rapid and extensive hepatic extraction. Following administration of a single 0.025- to 0.28-mg/kg dose in adults with normal renal and hepatic function, the volume of distribution of vecuronium in the central compartment (V_c) and at steady-state (V_{ss}) reportedly ranges from 50–120 and 179–400 mL/kg, respectively. The V_c and V_{ss} averaged 50 and 200–210 mL/kg, respectively, following an initial 0.06-mg/kg dose and continuous infusion at 1 mcg/kg per minute in adults with normal renal and hepatic function undergoing inhalation or balanced anesthesia. The volume of distribution of vecuronium is increased in children younger than 1 year of age and may be decreased in geriatric patients; although not clearly established, the volume of distribution may be slightly increased in patients with renal failure.

Vecuronium is approximately 60–90% bound to plasma proteins; however, in one study, the drug was reportedly 30 and 24% bound to serum proteins in healthy patients and patients with cirrhosis, respectively. The wide range in reported values may have resulted from the different methods used to determine the extent of protein binding. Vecuronium crosses the placenta minimally; placental transfer of the drug appears to be about 50% that of pancuronium. Umbilical venous plasma concentrations of vecuronium were 11% of maternal concentrations at delivery in 2 limited studies in women undergoing cesarean section who received 0.04 or 0.06–0.08 mg/kg of vecuronium bromide after tracheal intubation with succinylcholine. It is not known if vecuronium distributes into milk.

■ Elimination Plasma concentrations of vecuronium generally appear to decline in a biphasic manner. In adults with normal renal function, the plasma half-life in the distribution phase ($t_{1/2\alpha}$) averages 3.3–9 minutes and in the terminal elimination phase ($t_{1/2\beta}$) averages 31–80 minutes. Some pharmacokinetic data indicate that plasma concentrations of vecuronium decline in a triphasic manner, with the drug undergoing a very rapid initial distribution. In adults with normal renal function, the plasma half-life in the initial distribution phase reportedly averages 1.1–3 minutes, the plasma half-life in the redistribution phase ($t_{1/2\alpha}$) reportedly averages 9–14 minutes, and the plasma half-life in the terminal elimination phase ($t_{1/2\beta}$) reportedly averages 58–103 minutes. In a few children 3–11 months or 1–5 years of age, the $t_{1/2\beta}$ of vecuronium reportedly averaged 65 or 41 minutes, respectively. The $t_{1/2\alpha}$ and $t_{1/2\beta}$ of vecuronium are not substantially altered in patients with renal failure, the $t_{1/2\alpha}$ averaging 4–11 minutes and the $t_{1/2\beta}$ averaging 68–97 minutes. In one study in patients with cirrhosis, the $t_{1/2\beta}$ averaged 84 minutes. The $t_{1/2\beta}$ is reportedly decreased to about 35–40 minutes during late pregnancy.

The metabolic fate of vecuronium in humans has not been fully characterized. In aqueous solution in vitro, vecuronium undergoes spontaneous deacetylation at the 3α- and/or 17β-positions to form the hydroxy derivatives. The neuromuscular blocking activity of the 3α-hydroxy derivative appears to be at least 50% that of the unchanged drug; in animals, equipotent doses of vecuronium bromide and the 3α-hydroxy derivative induce neuromuscular blockade of similar duration. In vitro, the 3α-hydroxy derivative undergoes rapid conversion to the 3α,17β-dihydroxy derivative. The 17β-hydroxy and 3α,17β-dihydroxy derivatives appear to have about 5 and 2% of the neuromuscular blocking activity of the unchanged drug, respectively. The extent of spontaneous deacetylation and/or metabolism of vecuronium in vivo in humans remains to be clearly determined.

Vecuronium and its metabolite(s) appear to be excreted principally in feces via biliary elimination; the drug and its metabolite(s) are also excreted in urine. Although only unchanged drug has been detected in plasma in patients receiving the drug as an adjunct to surgical anesthesia, up to 10% of a dose of vecuronium has been excreted in urine and 5–25% in bile as the 3α-hydroxy derivative in some patients. Another metabolite, 3-desacetyl vecuronium, has been detected rarely in plasma following prolonged clinical use of the drug in an intensive care setting. Studies in rabbits with orally administered drug indicate that enterohepatic circulation of vecuronium and its active metabolites probably does not occur. Approximately 20–30% (range: 3–36%) of an IV dose of vecuronium bromide is excreted in urine within 24 hours after administration in humans, principally as unchanged drug and to a lesser extent as the 3α-hydroxy derivative; most urinary excretion occurs within the first 4–6 hours. In patients with a T-tube in the common bile duct, 12–45% of an IV dose of vecuronium was reportedly excreted in bile within 18–42 hours after administration, almost completely as unchanged drug, with most biliary excretion occurring within the first 4–6 hours. Since excretion of the drug occurs mainly via biliary elimination, temporary or permanent exclusion of the liver in animals results in increased intensity and duration of the neuromuscular blockade induced by vecuronium bromide and prolongs recovery.

Total body clearance of vecuronium reportedly averages 2.9–6.4 mL/minute per kg in patients with normal renal function. Total body clearance reportedly averages 2.5–4.5 mL/minute per kg in patients with renal dysfunction and 0.97–2.7 mL/minute per kg in patients with hepatic dysfunction (i.e., cirrhosis, biliary obstruction).

The manufacturer states that the effect of hemodialysis or peritoneal dialysis on plasma concentrations of vecuronium and its metabolite(s) is unknown.

Chemistry and Stability

■ Chemistry Vecuronium bromide is a synthetic, nondepolarizing neuromuscular blocking agent. Vecuronium bromide differs structurally from pancuronium bromide only by the absence of an *N*-methyl group on the piperidine ring at position 2, resulting in a monoquaternary rather than bisquaternary compound. Vecuronium, like pancuronium bromide, contains the steroid or androstane nucleus.

Vecuronium bromide occurs as white to off-white or slightly pink crystals or crystalline powder and has solubilities of 9 and 23 mg/mL in water and in alcohol, respectively. The drug has a pK_a of 8.97 in distilled water at 25°C. The commercially available powders for injection occur as a lyophilized cake of very fine microscopic crystals. Anhydrous citric acid, anhydrous dibasic sodium phosphate, sodium hydroxide, and/or phosphoric acid are added during manufacture of the powders for injection to buffer and adjust the pH. Mannitol is also added during manufacture of the powders for injection to adjust tonicity. Following reconstitution with sterile water for injection, vecuronium bromide solutions containing 2 mg/mL are clear, colorless, and isotonic and have a pH of 4.

■ Stability Vecuronium bromide is unstable in the presence of bases and undergoes gradual hydrolysis in aqueous solutions, alcohol, and chlorinated hydrocarbons. Vecuronium bromide solutions should not be administered in the same syringe as an alkaline solution nor should vecuronium bromide and an alkaline solution be administered simultaneously through the same needle.

Commercially available vecuronium bromide powder for injection should be stored at 20–25°C and protected from light.

When reconstituted with 5% dextrose, 5% dextrose and 0.9% sodium chloride, 0.9% sodium chloride, or lactated Ringer's, resulting vecuronium bromide solutions are stable for 24 hours when refrigerated. Since vials of the drug do not contain a preservative and are designed for single use only, unused portions of the reconstituted solution should be discarded. Following reconstitution with bacteriostatic water for injection, vecuronium bromide solutions are stable for 5 days at room temperature or when refrigerated. Vecuronium bromide solutions are stable for 48 hours after reconstitution with sterile water for injection when stored in plastic or glass syringes at 2–8°C or 15–30°C, but the manufacturer recommends that they be used within 24 hours.

Vecuronium bromide is physically and chemically compatible with the following IV solutions: 5% dextrose, 0.9% sodium chloride, 5% dextrose and 0.9% sodium chloride, or lactated Ringer's.

For further information on chemistry, pharmacology, pharmacokinetics, uses, cautions, drug interactions, and dosage and administration of vecuronium bromide, see the Neuromuscular Blocking Agents General Statement 12:20.20.

Preparations

Excipients in commercially available drug preparations may have clinically important effects in some individuals; consult specific product labeling for details.

Vecuronium Bromide

Parenteral

For injection, for IV use only	10 mg*	**Vecuronium Bromide for Injection**
	20 mg*	**Vecuronium Bromide for Injection**

*available from one or more manufacturer, distributor, and/or repackager by generic (nonproprietary) name

16:00 BLOOD DERIVATIVES

Albumin Human *p. 1629*
Plasma Protein Fraction§

§ Omitted from the print version of *AHFS Drug Information*® because of space limitations. This monograph is available on the *AHFS Drug Information*® website, http://ahfsdruginformation.com. Username: ahfs2020; Password: ASHP94498.

BLOOD DERIVATIVES 16:00

Albumin Human

Normal Human Serum Albumin, Normal Serum Albumin (Human)

■ Albumin human, a protein colloid, is a sterile solution of serum albumin prepared by fractionating pooled plasma from healthy human donors.

Uses

■ **Hypovolemia** Albumin human solutions are used for plasma volume expansion and maintenance of cardiac output (fluid resuscitation) in the emergency treatment of hypovolemia (with or without shock) when urgent restoration of blood volume is indicated.

The goal of fluid resuscitation is to restore intravascular volume and preserve organ perfusion while minimizing fluid overload complications (e.g., pulmonary edema). Albumin human, a protein colloid, is one of several options that can be used to restore effective circulating volume. Other options include nonprotein colloids (e.g., hetastarch, dextran) and large volume crystalloids (e.g., lactated Ringer's, various sodium chloride-containing solutions). When used for fluid resuscitation, the beneficial effects of albumin human are thought to result principally from its contribution to colloid osmotic pressure (i.e., oncotic pressure).

Ongoing controversy exists regarding the optimum choice of fluid (i.e., crystalloids, albumin human, nonprotein colloids) for fluid resuscitation in emergency situations. Protocols used for fluid resuscitation, including the type of replacement fluid, vary widely among health-care facilities and may depend on the geographic area (e.g., country) where the patient is being treated. Some clinicians state that colloids such as albumin human are preferred because they offer therapeutic advantages over crystalloids, while others recommend use of crystalloids based on cost considerations and lack of established superiority of colloids. The potential advantages of colloids include greater retention in the intravascular space, more rapid and effective plasma volume expansion, and a reduced risk of pulmonary edema. However, such benefits are theoretical and have not been proven; in addition, the favorable oncotic gradients that colloids provide may be diminished in situations where there is endothelial damage and transcapillary leakage (e.g., in septic shock or burns). Clinical studies generally have not shown colloids to be more effective than crystalloids for fluid resuscitation, and costs associated with colloid administration are substantially higher than those associated with crystalloid administration.

Previous pooled analyses of randomized controlled clinical studies have questioned the role and safety of albumin human relative to other colloids and crystalloids in the management of critically ill patients, including those with hypovolemia. In a pooled analysis of 30 randomized, controlled clinical studies involving 1419 critically ill patients receiving albumin human or plasma protein fraction (with or without crystalloids) that was performed by the Cochrane Injuries Group Albumin Reviewers in 1998, there was no evidence that albumin human reduced mortality compared with control (crystalloid solution alone or no albumin human) in patients with hypovolemia, burns, or hypoproteinemia (hypoalbuminemia). Instead, this analysis revealed evidence suggesting that mortality risk actually may be increased by 6% overall with use of albumin human in these patients. An increased risk of mortality also was observed in each patient population, reaching statistical significance for patients with burns or hypoproteinemia. As a result of this analysis, the authors and others cautioned that recommendations for the use of albumin human in critically ill patients should be reevaluated, and such use should be undertaken only after careful consideration, weighing the potential benefits and risks. However, the findings of this study have been criticized for methodologic problems that limit clinical interpretation, and the clinical studies that were evaluated used many different end points, making it difficult to determine comparative efficacy and safety. In a larger, subsequent meta-analysis of 55 randomized, controlled trials comparing albumin human to crystalloid therapy, no albumin, or lower dosages of albumin in 3504 patients from a broad population (e.g., patients with trauma, burns, hypoalbuminemia, or ascites; high-risk neonates; surgery patients), there was no evidence of increased risk of death associated with use of albumin human.

To resolve conflicting evidence from meta-analyses, a large, multicenter randomized controlled study (the Saline versus Albumin Fluid Evaluation [SAFE] trial) was conducted comparing the effects of normal saline (0.9% sodium chloride) with albumin human in approximately 7000 adults in intensive care units (ICUs) who required fluid resuscitation. Pediatric patients, burn patients, and those who had undergone liver transplantation or cardiac surgery were excluded from the study. Eligible patients who had at least one objective sign of hypovolemia were randomized to receive either albumin human 4% solution (not commercially available in the US) or normal saline for 28 days in addition to maintenance fluids, specific replacement fluids, blood products, or other concurrent interventions as required. There was no difference in 28-day mortality (primary outcome), development of organ failure, length of hospital or ICU stay, duration of mechanical ventilation, or duration of renal replacement therapy between patients who received albumin human and those who received normal saline. Results generally were consistent across subgroups of patients with severe sepsis, trauma, and acute respiratory distress syndrome (ARDS; previously known as adult respiratory distress syndrome), although there was a slight trend towards increased mortality in patients with head trauma who received albumin human and a trend towards reduced mortality in those with severe sepsis who received albumin human. However, the study was not specifically designed to detect any clinically important differences between subgroups and results of such analysis should be interpreted with caution. Based on findings from the SAFE study, the US Food and Drug Administration (FDA) Blood Products Advisory Committee concluded in 2005, that the prior safety issues raised by the Cochrane Injuries Group had been resolved. In an updated meta-analysis performed by the Cochrane Albumin Reviewers, there was no difference in overall mortality between albumin human and normal saline in critically ill patients with hypovolemia, burns or hypoalbuminemia. There was a suggestion of a higher risk of death with albumin human in patients with burns and hypoalbuminemia (relative risk of 2.4 and 1.38, respectively), but not in patients with hypovolemia (relative risk of 1.01). The authors note that the estimate in hypovolemic patients was heavily influenced by results of the SAFE study.

Based on current evidence, albumin human appears to offer no advantage in terms of survival over crystalloids for fluid resuscitation, although the possibility of a modest benefit or harm cannot be excluded. Although results of a meta-analysis suggest that albumin human may provide a protective effect in reducing morbidity among acutely ill hospitalized patients, additional study is needed to substantiate these findings and more fully evaluate the effect of albumin human on other clinically important outcomes. Additional studies also are needed to evaluate the use of albumin human in specific groups who were excluded from the SAFE study (e.g., pediatric, burn, liver transplant, cardiac surgery patients).

Hemorrhagic Shock Albumin human is used for fluid resuscitation in patients with hemorrhagic shock.

Guidelines on use of albumin, nonprotein colloids, and crystalloids issued by the US University Health System (formerly Hospital) Consortium (UHC) in 2000 state that crystalloid solutions are preferred for initial fluid resuscitation in adults with hemorrhagic shock, but that nonprotein colloids may be considered if crystalloids (4 L) fail to produce an adequate response within 2 hours. These guidelines state that albumin human 5% solution may be used if nonprotein colloids are contraindicated.

Crystalloids and colloids should *not* be considered substitutes for blood or blood components when oxygen-carrying capacity is reduced and/or when replenishment of clotting factors or platelets is necessary. Transfusion with whole blood or packed red blood cells (RBCs) should be initiated as soon as possible when there is active hemorrhage and/or substantial anemia.

Nonhemorrhagic (Maldistributive) Shock Albumin human has been used for fluid resuscitation in patients with nonhemorrhagic (maldistributive) shock, including septic shock. Severe sepsis or septic shock with hypotension or signs of hypoperfusion requires early, vigorous fluid resuscitation to restore tissue perfusion and normalize oxidative metabolism.

The UHC guidelines state that crystalloids should be considered first-line treatment in adults with nonhemorrhagic (maldistributive) shock and that nonprotein colloids and albumin human should be used with caution in those with systemic sepsis. These guidelines also state that, in the presence of capillary leak with pulmonary and/or severe peripheral edema, use of up to 4 L of crystalloid solution is appropriate before using colloids. If albumin human is used for acute management of nonhemorrhagic shock, the possibility that it may have a potentially detrimental effect on edema in patients with increased capillary permeability or capillary leak should be considered.

Other experts state that either crystalloids or colloids can be used for fluid resuscitation in patients with septic shock. However, additional study is needed since there is no evidence-based support from prospective, randomized studies to clearly identify which type of fluid is superior for fluid resuscitation in patients with septic shock. Although there is some evidence that adult or pediatric patients with severe infection and shock who receive albumin human for fluid resuscitation have lower mortality compared with those who receive crystalloids, most studies to date comparing the relative efficacy of crystalloids, albumin human, and nonprotein colloids in patients with septic shock are hampered by difficulties in controlling the effects of concomitant therapy and were not designed or adequately powered to examine mortality as a primary outcome.

Thermal Injury Albumin human has been used for fluid resuscitation in burn patients.

Fluid resuscitation is an essential component of burn therapy; however, the optimum regimen of crystalloids, colloids, electrolytes, and fluid for the management of patients with thermal (burn) injuries has not been clearly established. There is ongoing controversy regarding the role of and most appropriate time to initiate colloids for fluid resuscitation in burn patients. Some clinicians believe that use of colloids during the initial hours after a burn is inappropriate because much of the volume is drawn into the interstitial space secondary to increased permeability of surrounding unburned tissue; others believe that colloids should be administered from the beginning of fluid resuscitation. In patients with thermal injury, crystalloids generally are recommended during the first 24 hours to reverse acute hypovolemia and maintain hemodynamic stability. Beyond 24 hours, use of colloids also may be employed to prevent hemoconcentration, combat electrolyte imbalances, and counteract the protein deficit that occurs in severe burns. To avoid complications of over-resuscitation ("fluid creep"), such as abdominal compartment syndrome and ARDS, the least amount of fluid necessary to maintain adequate organ perfusion should be used.

The UHC guidelines recommend that crystalloids be used for initial fluid resuscitation in adults with thermal injury, but state that nonprotein colloids may be added if burns extend over more than 30% of body surface area and more than 4 L of crystalloid solution has been administered 18–26 hours following initial injury. These guidelines state that albumin human may be considered if nonprotein colloids are contraindicated. Guidelines issued by the American Burn Association state that the addition of colloids to burn resuscitation protocols may be beneficial in terms of decreasing total fluid volume requirements, but randomized, controlled trials are needed to clearly establish other benefits.

Additional study is needed to determine the acute-phase and short-term differences between albumin human, crystalloids, and nonprotein colloids for fluid resuscitation in pediatric burn patients. Albumin human does not appear to decrease morbidity and mortality when used in pediatric burn patients and, depending on the preparation used, may result in aluminum accumulation in infants. (See Aluminum Content under Cautions: Precautions and Contraindications.)

■ **Kidney Disease** ***Nephrosis and Nephrotic Syndrome*** Albumin human is used as an adjunct to diuretic therapy to treat edema in patients with acute nephrosis refractory to cyclophosphamide and steroid therapy.

Cardinal features of nephrotic syndrome include albuminuria, hypoalbuminemia, and edema. Urinary albumin loss, with a resultant decrease in plasma oncotic pressure, was thought to be associated with the development of edema and secondary renal sodium retention. Additional evidence indicates that decreased hepatic production and increased renal catabolism are responsible for hypoalbuminemia, while renal sodium retention is responsible for edema. The principal goal of therapy for nephrotic syndrome is treatment of the underlying cause; when the cause does not respond to therapy, alleviation of pathophysiologic manifestations, including sodium retention and edema, is important.

Diuretic therapy is the treatment of choice for symptomatic management of nephrotic syndrome. The UHC guidelines recommend short-term adjunctive use of albumin human with diuretics in adults with nephrotic syndrome who have acute, severe peripheral and/or pulmonary edema that is unresponsive to diuretics alone; however, the possibility of a potentially detrimental effect on edema should be considered.

Albumin human has no role in the management of chronic nephrosis since parenteral albumin is rapidly excreted renally with no relief of the chronic edema or effect on the underlying renal lesion.

Hemodialysis Albumin human has been used as an adjunct to hemodialysis in long-term hemodialysis patients with oncotic or volume deficits or in those experiencing shock or hypotension who cannot tolerate substantial volumes of sodium chloride solutions.

Intradialytic hypotension, a complication of hemodialysis (especially in long-term hemodialysis patients), usually is managed by volume expansion through the use of crystalloids (e.g., 0.9% sodium chloride solutions, hypertonic sodium chloride solutions), nonprotein colloids, or albumin human. Some experts state that colloids may be preferred to crystalloids for dialysis-related hypotension and maintenance of hemodynamics in chronic dialysis patients. Others recommend 0.9% sodium chloride solution as first-line therapy if treatment of intradialytic hypotension is indicated in maintenance hemodialysis patients. This recommendation is based on results of a randomized, controlled study that indicated that albumin human 5% solution is not superior to 0.9% sodium chloride solution for treatment of symptomatic hypotension in maintenance hemodialysis patients with a previous history of intradialytic hypotension.

The UHC guidelines state that albumin human should not be used for intradialytic blood pressure support. If adults undergoing hemodialysis experience shock symptoms, the UHC guidelines state that crystalloid solutions are preferred for initial fluid resuscitation, but that nonprotein colloids may be considered if crystalloids (4 L) fail to produce an adequate response within 2 hours. These guidelines state that albumin human 5% solution may be used if nonprotein colloids are contraindicated.

Kidney Transplantation Albumin human has been used intraoperatively in conjunction with crystalloids for volume expansion in kidney transplant patients. However, there is no conclusive evidence from controlled, randomized studies that albumin human given during and/or after renal transplant surgery improves outcome.

■ **Liver Disease** ***Cirrhotic Ascites and Paracentesis*** Albumin human is used to prevent central volume depletion following paracentesis in adults with cirrhosis who require removal of large volumes of ascitic fluid.

Diet modification (e.g., sodium restricted to 2 g daily) combined with oral diuretic therapy is the first-line therapy for adults with cirrhosis and ascites. An initial large-volume paracentesis may be necessary in addition to sodium restriction and oral diuretic therapy if tense ascites is present in new-onset disease. In patients with refractory ascites (fluid overload unresponsive to sodium restriction and high-dose oral diuretic therapy or that recurs rapidly after paracentesis), serial therapeutic paracentesis may be indicated to control ascites. A single paracentesis involving removal of no more than 4–5 L of fluid usually can be performed safely without postparacentesis colloid support; however, when larger volumes (greater than 5 L) are removed, use of albumin human may be considered and usually is recommended to decrease the risk of postparacentesis circulatory dysfunction and maintain arterial blood volume. Nonprotein colloids also have been used for plasma expansion following paracentesis and have been recommended as alternatives to albumin human; however, some clinicians state that albumin human may be preferred since there is some evidence that the incidence of postparacentesis circulatory dysfunction following large-volume paracentesis may be less with albumin human than with some nonprotein colloids. The UHC guidelines and some clinicians state that when less than 3–5 L of ascites fluid has been removed and repletion of intravascular volume is of concern, adjunctive use of a crystalloid (e.g., sodium chloride solution) should be considered following paracentesis.

Although albumin human has been used alone (without large-volume paracentesis) in patients with cirrhosis in an attempt to control or prevent recurrence of ascites, guidelines issued by the American Association for the Study of Liver Diseases (AASLD) and UHC state that such use is not recommended. In addition, the UHC guidelines state that albumin human should not be used for the treatment of noncirrhotic postsinusoidal portal hypertension.

Despite the presence of hypoalbuminemia, albumin human has no role in the management of *chronic* cirrhosis†.

Hepatorenal Syndrome Albumin human has been used in conjunction with vasoconstrictors for the treatment of type I hepatorenal syndrome† in patients with cirrhosis. Type I hepatorenal syndrome is characterized by acute, rapidly progressing renal failure caused by intrarenal vasoconstriction and usually requires liver transplantation if not reversed. There is some evidence that use of regimens that include albumin human to expand intravascular volume and vasoconstrictors to increase vascular tone (e.g., terlipressin [not commercially available in the US], octreotide and midodrine, norepinephrine) in patients with rapidly progressing type I hepatorenal syndrome may improve renal function and delay the need for or improve outcomes after liver transplantation. Although additional study is needed, the AASLD and other experts state that a regimen of albumin human used in conjunction with vasoconstrictors (e.g., terlipressin, octreotide and midodrine) should be considered in the treatment of type I hepatorenal syndrome.

Data are limited regarding the use of albumin human alone or in conjunction with vasoconstrictors in the management of type II hepatorenal syndrome† (characterized by moderate and slowly progressive renal failure and typically associated with refractory ascites), and additional study is needed to determine if albumin human has a role in this form of the disease.

Spontaneous Bacterial Peritonitis Albumin human has been used as an adjunct to anti-infectives in the treatment of spontaneous bacterial peritonitis† in patients with cirrhosis and ascites.

Spontaneous bacterial peritonitis is a complication that can occur in patients with cirrhosis and ascites, develops without a contiguous source of infection (e.g., intestinal perforation, intra-abdominal abscess), requires prompt empiric anti-infective treatment, and may result in potentially fatal, progressive renal impairment or hepatorenal syndrome. There is some evidence that adjunctive use of albumin human for volume expansion in addition to appropriate anti-infective treatment in patients with spontaneous bacterial peritonitis may decrease the risk of renal impairment and death. Such use is controversial and additional study is needed. The AASLD recommends that albumin human be used in addition to appropriate anti-infective treatment (e.g., cefotaxime) in patients who have ascitic fluid polymorphonuclear (PMN) counts of 250 cells/mm^3 or higher and also have serum creatinine concentrations greater than 1 mg/dL, BUN greater than 30 mg/dL, or total bilirubin concentrations greater than 4 mg/dL.

Acute Liver Failure Albumin human has been used in patients with acute liver failure. In such patients, albumin human may provide a stabilizing effect and serve the dual purpose of supporting plasma colloid osmotic pressure as well as binding excess plasma bilirubin in the uncommon situation of rapid loss of liver function, with or without coma. Use of albumin human in patients with acute liver failure should be individualized based on the clinical situation. When fluid resuscitation is indicated in patients with acute liver failure, some experts recommend use of colloids (e.g., albumin human) instead of crystalloids.

Hepatic Resection Albumin human has been used for postoperative fluid support in patients undergoing hepatic resection†. Surgical resection of the liver results in substantial blood loss and, depending on the preoperative functional status of the liver, decreased albumin production capacity. The UHC guidelines state that crystalloids should be considered first-line therapy for maintenance of effective circulating volume following hepatic resection in adults and, if crystalloids have no effect and anemia and/or coagulopathy are present, then packed RBCs and fresh frozen plasma should be considered before use of albumin human. However, the UHC guidelines state that albumin human is appropriate to maintain effective circulation volume following major hepatic resection (more than 40%) in adults and also is indicated if clinically important edema develops secondary to use of crystalloids.

Liver Transplantation Albumin human has been used to control ascites and severe pulmonary and peripheral edema in liver transplant recipients†. Because of excessive blood loss, volume expanders such as crystalloids, blood products, nonprotein colloids, and albumin human may be required intraoperatively during liver transplantation. The UHC guidelines state that albumin human may be used in adult liver transplant recipients when serum albumin is less than 2.5 g/dL, pulmonary capillary wedge pressure is less than 12 mm Hg, and hematocrit exceeds 30%.

■ **Hypoproteinemia** Albumin human has been used in the management of severe hypoalbuminemia (with or without edema) in an attempt to restore serum albumin concentrations to within the normal range. However, in the absence of clinically important hypovolemia, albumin human should not be used to correct temporary protein deficits resulting from redistribution of albumin.

The principal goal of therapy in hypoproteinemia (hypoalbuminemia) is treatment of the underlying cause; albumin human may be used to provide symptomatic relief and prevent acute complications. Hypoproteinemia can occur in association with various clinical conditions (e.g., surgery, sepsis, chronic liver failure, chronic renal impairment) and is a result of inadequate production, increased catabolism, redistribution, and/or excessive loss of albumin. Use of albumin human in patients with severe hypoalbuminemia simply in an attempt to increase serum albumin concentrations to within the normal range (i.e., the patient does not exhibit manifestations of hypovolemia) cannot be recommended based on current evidence; instead, the cause of the underlying hypoalbuminemia should be identified and treated. To varying degrees, albumin human may relieve edema associated with hypoproteinemia by increasing colloid osmotic pressure and producing diuresis. However, if albumin human is administered to hypoproteinemic patients who do not have an accompanying volume deficit, there is a potential risk of fluid overload.

Albumin human should not be used for the treatment of hypoproteinemia associated with chronic cirrhosis, chronic nephrosis, malabsorption, protein-losing enteropathies, pancreatic insufficiency, or malnutrition, unless there is a concomitant indication that warrants use.

Although albumin human has been used to treat neonatal hypoalbuminemia†, data are insufficient to determine whether routine use of albumin human reduces mortality or morbidity in preterm neonates with hypoalbuminemia.

■ **Nutritional Support** Although there is some evidence suggesting that serum albumin concentration is an accurate measure of patient prognosis using indicators of morbidity and mortality, and that albumin concentrations can be safely and effectively restored using total parenteral nutrition (TPN) supplemented with albumin human, other evidence has led many clinicians to question the importance of albumin supplementation. Serum albumin concentration is a poor indicator of nutritional status and it may take several weeks to months to see an increase in the serum albumin concentration following adequate nutritional support. Albumin human is not recommended for use as a supplemental caloric protein source in patients requiring nutritional support. Iatrogenic elevation of serum albumin concentrations above 4 g/dL may increase the overall catabolic rate. In general, oral, enteral, and/or parenteral nutrition with amino acids and treatment of underlying disorders will restore plasma protein concentrations more effectively than albumin human. However, patients with diarrhea associated with enteral feeding intolerance may benefit from parenteral administration of albumin human if they have severe diarrhea (more than 2 L daily) and a serum albumin concentration less than 2 g/dL or if diarrhea occurs despite a trial of short-peptide and elemental formulas and other causes of diarrhea have been excluded.

■ **Neonatal Hyperbilirubinemia** In the treatment of neonatal hyperbilirubinemia, including hemolytic disease of the newborn (erythroblastosis fetalis), albumin human (20 or 25% solution) is used as an adjunct to exchange transfusions in an attempt to bind unconjugated bilirubin and decrease the risk of kernicterus. Albumin human has been administered prior to exchange transfusion (as a primer) or during the procedure (as a substitute for a portion of the blood) in infants with severe hemolytic disease of the newborn. Because there is some evidence that administration of albumin human prior to exchange transfusion is less efficient in bilirubin removal and may increase the risk of volume overload, the UHC guidelines recommend that albumin human be administered during the procedure if it is used as an adjunct to exchange transfusion. Albumin human should be used with caution in hypervolemic infants. (See Hypervolemia/Hemodilution under Cautions: Precautions and Contraindications.)

Albumin human should *not* be used if neonatal hyperbilirubinemia is treated using phototherapy without exchange transfusion.

Crystalloids and nonprotein colloids do not share the bilirubin-binding properties of albumin human and should *not* be considered alternatives for adjunctive treatment of hyperbilirubinemia in neonates.

■ **Ovarian Hyperstimulation Syndrome** Albumin human (20 or 25% solution) is used as a plasma expander for fluid management in the treatment of severe ovarian hyperstimulation syndrome (OHSS). Severe OHSS is a life-threatening complication of gonadotropin treatment characterized by growth of multiple large ovarian follicles with massive extravascular protein-rich fluid shift; this can lead to hypovolemia, hemoconcentration, ascites, oliguria, and electrolyte disturbances and may result in potentially fatal thromboembolic complications and acute respiratory distress syndrome. Albumin human 20 or 25% solution has been recommended in the treatment of severe OHSS if 0.9% sodium chloride solutions fail to achieve or maintain hemodynamic stability and adequate urine output.

Albumin human also has been investigated for prevention of severe OHSS in high-risk women undergoing ovulation induction†. However, additional study is needed to more fully evaluate the benefits and risks of albumin human for prevention of OHSS. One meta-analysis of 5 randomized, controlled clinical studies in high-risk women (i.e., younger than 35 years of age, multifollicular development, high serum estradiol concentrations, nonobesity, polycystic ovary disease) indicated that administration of a single IV infusion of albumin human 20 or 25% immediately before or after oocyte retrieval appeared to reduce the risk of severe OHSS in such patients. This meta-analysis indicated that use of albumin human in women at high risk may prevent 1 case of severe OHSS in every 18 women who receive such prophylaxis. However, other studies and meta-analyses evaluating use of albumin human for prevention of OHSS in high-risk women failed to demonstrate a statistically significant reduction in the occurrence of severe OHSS in those receiving albumin human.

■ **Acute Respiratory Distress Syndrome and Acute Lung Injury** Albumin human (20 or 25% solution) has been used in conjunction with a diuretic in the management of acute respiratory distress syndrome (ARDS, previously known as adult respiratory distress syndrome). However, use of albumin human in patients with ARDS is controversial because of the risk of aggravating interstitial fluid accumulation and other possible detrimental pulmonary effects. Although uncertainty exists regarding the precise indication for albumin human in patients with ARDS, some manufacturers state that albumin human may have a therapeutic effect if used in conjunction with a diuretic in patients with pulmonary overload accompanied by hypoalbuminemia.

Albumin human has been used in conjunction with furosemide in the management of hypoproteinemic patients with acute lung injury† (ALI) and has resulted in improved oxygenation and hemodynamic stability in some patients. Some experts state that conservative fluid management or restriction is appropriate for most patients with hemodynamically stable ALI/ARDS; however, although conclusive data are lacking, a regimen of colloids and diuretics may be considered in those with hypo-oncotic ALI/ARDS.

■ **Sequestration of Protein Rich Fluids** Albumin human has been used for volume and oncotic replacement in conditions associated with sequestration of protein rich fluid or third-spacing (e.g., acute peritonitis, pancreatitis, mediastinitis, extensive cellulitis).

Albumin human has been used as an adjunct to anti-infectives in the treatment of spontaneous bacterial peritonitis† in patients with cirrhosis and ascites. (See Spontaneous Bacterial Peritonitis under Uses: Liver Disease.)

Albumin human may be useful in the early treatment of shock associated with acute hemorrhagic pancreatitis or peritonitis.

The UHC guidelines state that albumin human is not recommended in the treatment of acute or chronic pancreatitis.

■ **Cardiac Surgery** Albumin human has been used as a pump prime for preoperative dilution of blood prior to cardiopulmonary bypass procedures, usually in conjunction with a crystalloid. However, studies generally have shown only marginal or no additional benefit when colloids were added to crystalloids in the preoperative regimen. The UHC guidelines state that crystalloids alone usually are the regimen of choice for priming cardiopulmonary bypass pumps, although use of nonprotein colloids in addition to crystalloids may be preferable in cases in which it is extremely important to avoid pulmonary shunting.

Albumin human also has been used in cardiac surgery patients to restore fluid balance during surgery and in the postoperative period. Although albumin human has been recommended prior to or during cardiopulmonary bypass and there is some evidence that use of albumin human in cardiopulmonary bypass patients is associated with less postoperative bleeding than use of hetastarch (a nonprotein colloid), there are no data establishing a clear benefit for use of albumin human over use of crystalloids alone. For postoperative volume expansion after cardiac surgery, the UHC guidelines state that crystalloids are preferred, followed in descending order of preference by nonprotein colloids and then albumin human.

■ **Neurosurgery and Cerebral Injury** Albumin human has been used for hemodilution to maintain or improve cerebral perfusion in the treatment of subarachnoid hemorrhage†, acute ischemic stroke†, traumatic brain injury†, and in other neurosurgical patients†. Various fluid protocols have been used in an attempt to prevent secondary ischemia after subarachnoid hemorrhage, severe ischemic stroke, or severe traumatic brain injury. Although improved clinical outcomes have been reported in some patients, results have been conflicting and there is no clear evidence to date from adequately controlled, randomized studies that hemodilution decreases mortality or improves functional outcome in survivors of acute ischemic stroke.

The UHC guidelines state that crystalloids are preferred for maintenance of cerebral perfusion pressure in the treatment of cerebral vasospasm associated with subarachnoid hemorrhage, cerebral ischemia, or head trauma in adults; however, if cerebral edema is a concern, albumin human 25% solution should be used. These guidelines state that patients with elevated hematocrits should receive crystalloids first to increase intravascular volume, creating a state of hypervolemia and hemodilution, and that those with hematocrits less than 30% should receive packed RBCs to increase the intravascular volume and maintain cerebral perfusion pressure. If volume therapy alone is inadequate to maintain cerebral perfusion pressure, vasopressor therapy may be necessary.

■ **Plasmapheresis** Albumin human is used in conjunction with large-volume plasma exchange as protein volume replacement in plasmapheresis† procedures involving exchange of more than 20 mL of plasma per kg in one session or more than 20 mL/kg weekly in multiple sessions. The UHC guidelines state that nonprotein colloids and crystalloids may substitute for some of the albumin human in therapeutic plasmapheresis procedures and should be considered cost-effective exchange media. Some evidence indicates that nonprotein colloids (e.g., hetastarch 3%) are comparably effective and tolerated relative to albumin for small- or large-volume plasma exchange.

■ **Erythrocyte Resuspension** Albumin human has been used to resuspend large volumes of previously frozen or washed RBCs prior to administration or during certain types of exchange transfusion to provide sufficient volume and/or avoid excessive hypoproteinemia during the transfusion.

Dosage and Administration

■ **Administration** Albumin human solutions are administered by IV infusion.

The concentration of albumin human administered (i.e., albumin human 5, 20, or 25% solution) depends on the fluid and protein requirements of the patient and is determined in part by whether there is a greater need for volume or oncotic replacement.

Albumin human 5% solutions usually are preferred in the treatment of acute blood volume deficits in the *absence* of adequate or excessive hydration.

Albumin human 20 or 25% solutions may be preferred when there is an oncotic deficit or when hypovolemia is long standing (e.g., due to treatment delay) and hypoalbuminemia exists in the *presence* of adequate or excessive hydration. Albumin human 20 or 25% solutions also are preferred when the drug is being used for its binding rather than oncotic effects (e.g., in the treatment of neonatal hyperbilirubinemia).

When used for the treatment of hypovolemia, albumin human solutions are most effective in well-hydrated patients. If the patient is dehydrated, albumin human 5% solution usually is preferred; if albumin human 20 or 25% solutions are used in dehydrated patients, additional crystalloids or other fluids should be administered.

IV Infusion Depending on the indication, protein and fluid requirements, sodium restrictions, and availability, commercially available albumin human solutions can be administered *undiluted* or can be further diluted in a compatible IV solution (e.g., 0.9% sodium chloride, 5% dextrose).

Whenever dilution of albumin human is considered necessary (e.g., to prepare a 5% solution from a 25% solution), **the oncotic and osmotic properties as well as the tonicity of the resultant dilution must be considered.**

Because of the risk of potentially life-threatening hemolysis, **albumin human must not be diluted using hypotonic solutions such as sterile water for injection.** (See Oncotic, Osmotic, and Tonicity Considerations under Cautions: Precautions and Contraindications.)

If necessary, albumin human 5% solutions may be prepared from albumin human 25% solutions by adding 1 volume of the 25% solution to 4 volumes of 0.9% sodium chloride injection or 5% dextrose injection. Since albumin human 25% solution diluted with 0.9% sodium chloride or 5% dextrose results in 5% dilutions that are approximately isotonic and iso-oncotic with citrated plasma, these diluents are preferred for such dilutions.

When sodium restriction is necessary, albumin human solutions should be administered either undiluted or diluted in a sodium-free carbohydrate solution such as 5% dextrose. However, because administration of large volumes of albumin human 5% prepared by diluting 25% solutions with 5% dextrose could result in hyponatremia and potentially serious adverse effects (e.g., cerebral swelling), 0.9% sodium chloride generally should be used as the preferred diluent when administration, particularly rapid administration, of large volumes is anticipated (e.g., during plasmapheresis or plasma exchange) and the fluid and electrolyte status of the patient permits.

Prior to administration, albumin human solution should be inspected visually for particulate matter and discoloration and should not be used if it appears turbid or contains sediment.

Albumin human should be used immediately after the vial or container is opened. Albumin human solutions should be discarded if more than 4 hours have elapsed since the container was first entered.

The manufacturers' prescribing information should be consulted for specific directions regarding use of IV administration sets and filters. Some manufacturers state that adequate filtration is required; other manufacturers state that filtration is not required.

Albumin human may be administered in conjunction with whole blood, plasma, or dextrose, sodium lactate, or sodium chloride injections. Albumin human should *not* be mixed with parenteral nutrient solutions, protein hydrolysates, amino acid solutions, or solutions containing alcohol. (See Chemistry and Stability: Stability.)

Rate of Administration. The rate of IV infusion of albumin human should be individualized based on the indication, concentration of albumin human solution used, and clinical status and response of the patient. The manufacturers' information should be consulted for specific information regarding recommended rates of administration.

When albumin human 5% solution is used for the treatment of hypovolemic shock in patients with greatly reduced blood volume, a rapid IV infusion rate may be necessary *initially* to provide clinical improvement and restore normal blood volume. However, in patients with a history of cardiac or vascular disease, some manufacturers suggest a slow infusion rate (e.g., 5–10 mL/minute) to avoid an increase in blood pressure that is too rapid. In patients with normal or slightly low blood volume, some manufacturers suggest that albumin human 5% solution should be administered at a rate of 1–2 mL/minute.

When albumin human 20 or 25% solution is used for the treatment of hypovolemic shock in patients with greatly reduced blood volume, a rapid IV infusion rate may be necessary *initially* to provide clinical improvement and restore normal blood volume. However, in patients with normal or slightly low blood volume, some manufacturers state that the IV infusion rate should not exceed 1 mL/minute since more rapid infusion rates may result in circulatory overload or pulmonary edema. A slower infusion rate also is recommended in patients with hypertension. When albumin human 20 or 25% solution is used in hypoproteinemic patients with approximately normal blood volume, a maximum infusion rate of 2 mL/minute (Plasbumin®-20, Plasbumin®-25) or 2–3 mL/minute (Albuminar®-25) has been recommended.

When albumin human solutions are used in pediatric patients, some manufacturers recommend that the IV infusion rate should be reduced to 25% of the usual adult rate.

■ **Dosage** Dosage of albumin human is variable and should be individualized based on the specific indication, concentration of albumin human solution used, and clinical status and response of the patient. The manufacturers' information should be consulted for specific dosage recommendations.

Predetermined formulas for dosage calculation generally are avoided since they assume that the same dose is appropriate for all patients. In the absence of active hemorrhage, total daily albumin dosage should not exceed the theoretical amount present in normal plasma volume (i.e., 2 g/kg body weight).

Response to therapy should be determined by factors such as hemodynamic response (e.g., blood pressure), degree of pulmonary congestion, and hematocrit. Serum protein concentrations usually do not need to be monitored during albumin human therapy, but may be useful in some cases of hypoproteinemia to estimate the total body albumin deficit and guide selection of dosage.

Osmotic Equivalence of Commercially Available Albumin Human Injections for IV Infusion

Albumin human injection for IV infusion	Osmotic equivalence
100 mL of 5% solution (5 g)	100 mL of normal human plasma
100 mL of 20% solution (20 g)	400 mL of normal human plasma
100 mL of 25% solution (25 g)	500 mL of normal human plasma

Hypovolemia **Adults.** When albumin human is used for the treatment of hypovolemic shock in adults, some manufacturers recommend the following initial dose. The dose may be repeated in 15–30 minutes if the response is inadequate.

Albumin human 5% solution: 12.5–25 g (250–500 mL of a 5% solution).

Albumin human 20% solution: 25 g (125 mL of a 20% solution).

Albumin human 25% solution: 25–50 g (100–200 mL of a 25% solution).

Pediatric Patients. Some manufacturers recommend that 25–50% of the usual initial adult dosage be used and adjusted according to the child's weight and clinical condition. The manufacturers' prescribing information should be consulted for specific dosing recommendations in children.

If albumin human is used for the treatment of hypovolemic shock in pediatric patients, some clinicians recommend a dose of 0.5–1 g/kg (maximum of 6 g/kg in 24 hours or 250 g in 48 hours).

Albumin human 5% solution: Some manufacturers recommend an initial dose of 0.5–1 g/kg or 2.5–12.5 g for the treatment of hypovolemia in pediatric patients. One manufacturer recommends a dose of 12–20 mL/kg for infants and young children and 250–500 mL for older children. The dose may be repeated after 15–30 minutes if the response is inadequate.

Albumin human 20% solution: One manufacturer recommends an initial dose of 0.5–1 g/kg or 2.5–12.5 g for the treatment of hypovolemia in pediatric patients. The dose may be repeated after 15–30 minutes if the response is inadequate.

Albumin human 25% solution: Some manufacturers recommend an initial dose of 0.5–1 g/kg or 2.5–12.5 g for the treatment of hypovolemia in pediatric patients. The dose may be repeated after 15–30 minutes if the response is inadequate.

Thermal Injury The optimum regimen of crystalloids, colloids, electrolytes, and fluid for the management of patients with thermal (burn) injuries has not been clearly established. In addition, the duration of replacement therapy in burn patients varies, depending on such factors as the extent of protein loss from renal excretion, denuded skin areas, and decreased albumin production.

A suggested goal of burn therapy is to maintain a plasma albumin concentration of 2–3 g/dL and plasma oncotic pressure of 20 mm Hg (equivalent to a total plasma protein concentration of 5.2 g/dL).

If albumin human is used in burn patients, one manufacturer recommends that large volumes of crystalloids be given initially to maintain plasma volume; after 24 hours, albumin human may be added using an initial dose of 25 g with dosage adjusted thereafter to maintain a plasma protein concentration of 2.5 g/dL or a serum protein concentration of 5.2 g/dL.

Kidney Disease **Acute Nephrosis.** If albumin human 20 or 25% solution is used as an adjunct to treat edema in the management of acute nephrosis, some manufacturers recommend a dosage of 20 or 25 g once daily for 7–10 days (in conjunction with an appropriate diuretic).

Hemodialysis. If albumin human 20 or 25% solution is used for the treatment of a volume or oncotic deficit in patients undergoing long-term hemodialysis or for the treatment of shock or hypotension in these patients, some manufacturers state that the usual dose is about 100 mL (the initial dose should not exceed 100 mL). Patients must be carefully monitored for signs of circulatory overload.

Liver Disease **Cirrhotic Ascites and Paracentesis.** If albumin human is used to prevent central volume depletion following large-volume paracentesis in adults with cirrhosis and ascites, the usual dose is 6–8 g per liter of ascitic fluid removed. A single paracentesis involving removal of no more than 4–5 L of fluid usually can be performed safely without colloid support; however, use of albumin human may be considered when larger volumes (greater than 5 L) are removed.

Hepatorenal Syndrome. Although albumin human used in conjunction with vasoconstrictors has been recommended for the treatment of type I hepatorenal syndrome† in patients with cirrhosis (see Hepatorenal Syndrome under Uses: Liver Disease), optimum regimens have not been identified.

If albumin human is used in conjunction with vasoconstrictors in adults with type I hepatorenal syndrome†, some experts recommend a dosage regimen that includes an initial dose of 1 g/kg (up to 100 g) of albumin human on day 1, followed by 20–40 g once daily. If a response is obtained, treatment should be continued until serum creatinine concentrations are less than 1.5 mg/dL. Albumin human may be discontinued if serum albumin concentrations exceed 4.5 g/dL and should be discontinued if pulmonary edema is present.

Spontaneous Bacterial Peritonitis. Although albumin human has been used as an adjunct to anti-infectives in the treatment of spontaneous bacterial peritonitis† in patients with cirrhosis and ascites, optimum regimens have not been identified.

The American Association for the Study of Liver Diseases (AASLD) recommends that adults with ascitic fluid polymorphonuclear (PMN) counts of 250 cells/mm^3 or higher and clinical suspicion of spontaneous bacterial peritonitis who also have serum creatinine concentrations greater than 1 mg/dL, BUN greater than 30 mg/dL, or total bilirubin concentrations greater than 4 mg/dL receive 1.5 g/kg of albumin human within 6 hours of detection and another dose of 1 g/kg on day 3.

Hypoproteinemia **Adults.** If albumin human 5% solution is used for the treatment of hypoproteinemia in adults, one manufacturer recommends a dose of 50–75 g.

If albumin human 20 or 25% solution is used for the treatment of hypoproteinemia in adults, some manufacturers recommend a daily dosage of 50–75 g (e.g., 250–375 mL of a 20% solution or 200–300 mL of a 25% solution). Larger amounts may be required in patients with severe hypoproteinemia who continue to lose albumin. Some manufacturers recommend a maximum dosage of 2 g/kg daily.

The total body albumin deficit (including hidden extravascular albumin deficiency) should be considered when determining the dosage of albumin human necessary to reverse hypoalbuminemia. When using serum albumin concentrations to estimate the protein deficit in hypoproteinemia, some manufacturers recommend that the body albumin compartment be calculated based on 80–100 mL/kg body weight to account for any hidden extravascular albumin deficits.

Pediatric Patients. If albumin human is used for the treatment of hypoproteinemia in pediatric patients, some clinicians recommend a dosage of 0.5–1 g/kg given by IV infusion over 0.5–2 hours and repeated once every 1–2 days as needed (maximum of 6 g/kg in 24 hours or 250 g in 48 hours).

For the treatment of hypoproteinemia in children, one manufacturer recommends that albumin human 20 or 25% be given in a dosage of 25 g daily. Larger amounts may be required in patients with severe hypoproteinemia who continue to lose albumin.

Neonatal Hyperbilirubinemia If albumin human 20 or 25% solution is used as an adjunct to exchange transfusions for the treatment of neonatal hyperbilirubinemia, including hemolytic disease of the newborn (erythroblastosis fetalis), the recommended dose is 1 g/kg. The dose of albumin human has been given prior to exchange transfusion (as a primer) or during the procedure (as a substitute for a portion of the blood). (See Uses: Neonatal Hyperbilirubinemia.)

Ovarian Hyperstimulation Syndrome If albumin human 20 or 25% solution is used for fluid management in the treatment of severe ovarian hyperstimulation syndrome (OHSS), one manufacturer recommends that 50–100 g be given by IV infusion over 4 hours every 4–12 hours as necessary.

Acute Respiratory Distress Syndrome If albumin human 20 or 25% solution is used in conjunction with a diuretic in the management of fluid overload in adults with acute respiratory distress syndrome (ARDS; previously known as adult respiratory distress syndrome), one manufacturer recommends that 25 g be given by IV infusion over 30 minutes and repeated at 8-hour intervals for 3 days, if necessary.

Cardiac Surgery The optimum fluid regimen to ensure adequate blood volume during cardiopulmonary bypass is unclear. (See Uses: Cardiac Surgery.) Some manufacturers recommend that albumin human and crystalloid pump prime solutions be adjusted to achieve a plasma albumin concentration of 2.5 g/dL and a hematocrit of 20%.

Erythrocyte Resuspension If albumin human 20 or 25% solution is used to resuspend red blood cells (RBCs) during certain types of exchange transfusion or to resuspend large volumes of previously frozen or washed RBCs, some manufacturers recommend that approximately 20–25 g of albumin be added per liter of isotonic suspended RBCs immediately prior to transfusion. Greater amounts may be required in patients with preexisting hepatic impairment or hypoproteinemia.

Cautions

■ **Adverse Effects** Although adverse effects occur infrequently in patients receiving albumin human, serious adverse effects (e.g., anaphylaxis, circulatory failure, cardiac failure, pulmonary edema), including some fatalities possibly related to albumin human, have been reported rarely.

The most common adverse effects reported in patients receiving albumin human include anaphylactoid reactions, fever, chills, rash, nausea, vomiting, tachycardia, and hypotension.

Anaphylaxis, urticaria, pruritus, angioneurotic edema, erythema or flushing, dysguesia, increased salivation, hyperhidrosis, headache, confusion, loss of consciousness, pulmonary edema, dyspnea, and bronchospasm have been reported during postmarketing surveillance.

Albumin human has variable effects on respiration, blood pressure, and heart rate. Hypotension, hypertension, circulatory failure, tachycardia, bradycardia, congestive heart failure, and cardiac failure have been reported. Rapid IV infusion of albumin human may cause vascular overload with resultant pulmonary edema. (See Hypervolemia/Hemodilution under Cautions: Precautions and Contraindications.)

Several cases of hemolysis (e.g., during or after plasmapheresis) and at least one death probably related to hemolysis have been reported following administration of as little as 270 mL of an albumin human 5% solution that had been prepared extemporaneously by diluting albumin human 25% with sterile water. Such dilutions are markedly hypotonic with respect to blood, with calculated resultant sodium concentrations of 26–32 mEq/L. (See Oncotic, Osmotic, and Tonicity Considerations under Cautions: Precautions and Contraindications.)

■ **Precautions and Contraindications** Albumin human is contraindicated in patients hypersensitive to albumin, any ingredient in the formulation, or any component of the container. (See Sensitivity Reactions under Cautions: Precautions and Contraindications.)

Albumin human is contraindicated in patients with severe anemia or with cardiac failure in the presence of normal or increased intravascular volume. Certain individuals are at particular risk of circulatory overload, including those with stabilized chronic anemia, congestive heart failure, or renal insufficiency. (See Hypervolemia/Hemodilution under Cautions: Precautions and Contraindications.)

Because of the risk of aluminum accumulation, the manufacturer states that Buminate® 25% should not be used in patients with chronic renal impairment. (See Aluminum Content under Cautions: Precautions and Contraindications.)

Use of sterile water for injection for dilution of commercially available albumin human solutions is contraindicated because of the risk of potentially life-threatening hemolysis and acute renal failure. (See Oncotic, Osmotic, and Tonicity Considerations under Cautions: Precautions and Contraindications.)

Risk of Transmissible Agents in Plasma-derived Preparations Because albumin human is prepared using pooled human plasma, it is a potential vehicle for transmission of human viruses (e.g., hepatitis A virus [HAV], hepatitis B virus [HBV], hepatitis C virus [HCV], human immunodeficiency virus [HIV]) and theoretically may carry a risk of transmitting the causative agent of Creutzfeldt-Jakob disease (CJD) or related agents such as variant CJD (vCJD). Although donor plasma is screened for certain viruses and all currently available albumin human preparations undergo viral elimination/inactivation processes (e.g., pasteurization) to further reduce the risk of transmission of infectious agents, a potential for transmission of infectious agents still remains.

Because no purification method has been shown to be totally effective in removing the risk of viral infectivity from plasma-derived preparations and because new blood-borne viruses or other disease agents may emerge that may not be removed or inactivated by the manufacturing processes currently used, clinicians should discuss the risks and benefits of albumin human with the patient. Any infection believed to have been transmitted by albumin human should be reported to the manufacturer.

Risk of Hepatitis and Human Immunodeficiency Virus Infection. Although albumin human is prepared from human plasma and is a potential vehicle for transmission of the causative agents of viral hepatitis and HIV infection, the risk of transmission of viral diseases with plasma-derived albumin human is considered extremely remote.

Studies using plasma-derived coagulation factor preparations indicate that improved donor screening practices and viral elimination/inactivation procedures (e.g., pasteurization) have resulted in plasma-derived preparations with greatly reduced risk for transmission of HBV, HCV, and HIV viruses. There have been no documented cases of transmission of enveloped viruses (including HBV, HCV, and HIV) or nonenveloped viruses (including HAV and parvovirus B19) associated with commercially available albumin human. However, transmission of nonenveloped viruses (HAV, parvovirus B19) has been documented following administration of plasma-derived coagulation factors. (See Risk of Transmissible Agents in Plasma-derived Preparations under Cautions: Precautions and Contraindications, in Antihemophilic Factor [Human] 20:28.16.)

Risk of Creutzfeldt-Jakob Disease or Variant Creutzfeldt-Jakob Disease. Because albumin human is prepared from human blood, it theoretically may carry a risk of transmitting the causative agent of Creutzfeldt-Jakob disease (CJD) or other related agents such as variant CJD (vCJD). CJD is a rare, but invariably fatal, degenerative disease of the CNS associated with a poorly understood transmissible agent. The nature of this agent is not completely known, but it is highly resistant to current methods of viral inactivation applied to plasma-derived products; the effect, if any, of fractionation procedures on the agent is not known. CJD may be acquired by exogenous (usually iatrogenic) exposure to infectious material or may be familial, caused by a genetic mutation of the prion protein gene. There is some evidence that infected individuals may harbor the causative agent for up to 30 years before becoming symptomatic. A variant of CJD (vCJD) was first identified in the United Kingdom in 1996. The clinical presentation and neuropathologic changes associated with vCJD are different than those of CJD and include an earlier age of onset, absence of diagnostic EEG changes, and detectable abnormal prion protein in lymphoid tissue.

There are no documented cases of CJD or vCJD transmitted through plasma-derived preparations (including plasma-derived albumin human) and the theoretical risk for transmission of CJD with commercially available albumin human is considered extremely remote. However, there have been 3 probable cases of vCJD acquired through transfusion of human red blood cells (RBCs) identified by an ongoing epidemiologic review being conducted in the United Kingdom. One of these patients developed symptoms of vCJD 6.5 or 7.8 years, respectively, after receiving non-leukodepleted RBCs from 2 different donors; the donors developed clinical symptoms approximately 40 and 21 months after donating. The third probable case of transfusion-associated vCJD had no clinical symptoms of the disease prior to death, but abnormal prion protein was found in postmortem lymphoid tissue (5 years after RBC transfusion); the donor involved in this case had made the RBC donation 18 months before the onset of their clinical symptoms. Although attempts to transmit CJD to nonhuman primates via blood transfusion have failed, bovine spongiform encephalopathy (BSE) has been transmitted to at least one sheep through blood transfusion.

CJD has been transmitted in humans by transplantation of cornea or dura mater from infected individuals, injection of growth hormone (somatropin) derived from human pituitary of infected individuals, or the reuse of surface EEG electrodes contaminated by use on an infected individual. The disease also has been transmitted experimentally in rodents and primates by intracerebral injection of the buffy coat cell portion of blood, homogenates of brain or cornea, whole blood, or untreated CSF from a known infected individual.

Certain lots of plasma products, including coagulation factors, albumin human, plasma protein fraction, and immune globulin IV (IGIV), produced from blood derived from donors with probable CJD were withdrawn from the market during 1995. Withdrawal of the implicated products was seen by the US Food and Drug Administration (FDA) as a prudent interim measure pending further analysis of the relative risks and benefits of such plasma products. A similar withdrawal of certain lots of Buminate® 25% was made by the manufacturer in 1997 when it was discovered that a healthy plasma donor who contributed to the plasma pools from which these lots of albumin human were derived had a history of having received a dura mater transplant; this was done as a precautionary measure only, since there was no evidence of CJD in the transplant donor and no cases of CJD associated with products derived from the transplant recipient's plasma.

Tests are being developed to detect CJD and vCJD infection in blood and plasma donors. Until such donor screening tests are available for these diseases, the FDA has recommended interim preventive measures that include specific guidelines for deferral of blood and plasma donors with possible exposure to CJD and vCJD that are based on geographic considerations and guidelines for product retrieval, quarantine, and disposition that are based on consideration of risk in the donor and product and the effect that withdrawals and deferrals might have on the supply of blood, blood components, and plasma derivatives.

For further information on CJD and vCJD precautions related to blood and blood products, the FDA's guidance for industry on this topic should be consulted (http://www.fda.gov/downloads/BiologicsBloodVaccines/GuidanceComplianceRegulatoryInformation/Guidances/UCM213415.pdf).

Risk of West Nile Virus. It is unlikely that West Nile Virus (WNV) could be transmitted through commercially available plasma-derived preparations since WNV is an enveloped virus, like HCV, which is known to be inactivated by the purification and viral elimination/inactivation procedures used in the manufacture of these preparations. However, there is evidence that WNV can be transmitted in transplanted organs (e.g., heart, liver, kidney) and blood products (e.g., whole blood, packed RBCs, fresh frozen plasma). WNV has been isolated from frozen plasma obtained from a blood donor subsequently found to have WNV, indicating that the virus can survive in frozen blood components.

Beginning in 2003, specific tests to screen donated blood for WNV became available in the US. The FDA also recommends additional measures to assess donor suitability to help screen out potential blood donors who have past or present manifestations that suggest WNV illness. These recommendations apply to whole blood and blood components intended for transfusion and blood components, including recovered plasma, source leukocytes, and source plasma intended for use in further manufacturing into injectable or noninjectable products.

Because of the possible transmission of WNV through organ transplants and blood transfusions, any case of WNV that occurs in a patient who received organs, blood, or blood products within the 8 weeks preceding onset of the illness should be reported to CDC through state and local health authorities and serum or tissue samples should be retained for later studies. In addition, cases of WNV infection occurring in blood or organ donors within 2 weeks after their donation should be reported to CDC.

For further information on WNV precautions related to blood and blood products, the FDA's guidance for industry on this topic should be consulted (http://www.fda.gov/downloads/BiologicsBloodVaccines/GuidanceComplianceRegulatoryInformation/Guidances/Blood/ucm080286.pdf).

Sensitivity Reactions If an allergic or hypersensitivity reaction (e.g., anaphylaxis) occurs or is suspected, albumin human should be discontinued immediately and appropriate therapy initiated as indicated. Epinephrine should be readily available in case acute hypersensitivity occurs.

Patients should be advised that albumin human should be discontinued immediately if allergic symptoms (e.g., rash, hives, itching, breathing difficulties, coughing, nausea, vomiting, decrease in blood pressure, increased heart rate) occur.

Latex Sensitivity. Some packaging components of certain albumin human preparations (e.g., Buminate® 5%, Buminate® 25%) contain natural latex proteins in the form of natural rubber latex. Health-care personnel should take appropriate precautions if these albumin human preparations are administered to individuals with a history of latex sensitivity.

Some individuals may be hypersensitive to natural latex proteins found in a wide range of medical devices, including packaging components, and the level of sensitivity may vary depending on the form of natural rubber present; rarely, hypersensitivity reactions to natural latex proteins have been fatal.

Hypervolemia/Hemodilution Hypervolemia may occur if the dosage and IV infusion rate of albumin human are not adjusted based on the patient's volume status. Rapid IV infusion of albumin human solutions may cause vascular overload.

Albumin human should be used with caution in conditions where hypervolemia and its consequences or hemodilution could represent a special risk for the patient (e.g., decompensated cardiac insufficiency, hypertension, esophageal varices, pulmonary edema, hemorrhagic diathesis, severe anemia, renal and postrenal anuria).

Albumin human should be administered with caution in patients with low cardiac reserve (e.g., cardiac disease) and in those who do not have albumin deficiency. Albumin human should be administered with great caution in patients with chronic anemia, hypertension, or renal insufficiency.

Patients should be closely observed for signs of increased venous pressure such as pulmonary edema.

At the first clinical sign of possible cardiovascular overload (e.g., headache, dyspnea, increased blood pressure, jugular venous distention, elevated central venous pressure, pulmonary edema), albumin human infusion should be immediately stopped and the patient reevaluated.

Hemodynamic Monitoring Hemodynamic performance should be monitored closely during albumin human therapy, and the patient evaluated for evidence of cardiac, respiratory, or renal failure or increasing intracranial pressure.

Arterial blood pressure and pulse rate, central venous pressure, pulmonary artery occlusion pressure, urine output, electrolytes, hemoglobin, and hematocrit should be monitored frequently.

In postoperative or injured patients, a rapid rise in blood pressure following administration of albumin human may reveal bleeding points that were not apparent at lower blood pressure. To prevent hemorrhage and shock, such patients should be observed carefully and treated appropriately.

Anemia and Coagulation Abnormalities If hemorrhage has occurred in a patient receiving albumin human, relative anemia may be present and should be controlled by supplemental administration of compatible whole blood or RBCs.

If comparatively large volumes of fluid are being replaced with albumin human, coagulation parameters and hematocrit must be monitored and adequate substitution of other blood constituents (coagulation factors, electrolytes, platelets, erythrocytes) ensured.

Electrolyte Imbalance Compared with albumin human 5% solution, albumin human 20 or 25% solutions are relatively low in electrolytes.

Electrolyte status should be monitored in patients receiving albumin human, and appropriate steps taken to restore or maintain electrolyte balance.

Commercially available albumin human preparations contain 130–160 mEq of sodium per liter.

Oncotic, Osmotic, and Tonicity Considerations When dilution of albumin human is necessary (e.g., to prepare a 5% solution from a 25% solution), **the oncotic and osmotic properties as well as the tonicity of the resultant dilution must be considered.** Because the membrane of erythrocytes is not perfectly semipermeable, it can permit the passage of water (solvent) molecules and solutes; as a result, solutions that are iso-osmotic with blood are not necessarily isotonic with blood. Substantially hypotonic solutions when admixed with erythrocytes result in the inward passage of water causing the cells to swell and finally burst (hemolyze), releasing hemoglobin. Such hemolysis occurs when erythrocytes are admixed in vitro with albumin human solutions containing less than 90 mEq of sodium per L; the risk of such hemolysis depends on the sodium concentration, not on the suspending medium (albumin) or cell concentration.

When albumin human 25% is diluted with 0.9% sodium chloride injection or 5% dextrose injection, resulting 5% dilutions are approximately isotonic and iso-oncotic with citrated plasma; therefore, these diluents are preferred if such dilutions are considered necessary (e.g., if commercially available albumin human 5% solution cannot be obtained). Although sterile water occasionally was used in the past to dilute albumin human solutions (e.g., to adjust the sodium content when restriction of intake of the electrolyte was considered necessary), sterile water must *not* be used to dilute albumin human. Depending on the relative proportions of albumin human and diluent, dilutions with sterile water may be dangerously hypotonic, carrying the risk of life-threatening hemolysis, particularly if large volumes of markedly hypotonic dilutions are inadvertently administered. Several cases of hemolysis (e.g., during or after plasmapheresis) and at least one death probably related to the hemolysis have been reported following administration of as little as 270 mL of an albumin human 5% solution that had been prepared by inappropriately diluting a 25% solution with sterile water. Such dilutions are markedly hypotonic with respect to blood, with calculated resultant sodium concentrations of 26–32 mEq/L. In the hypotonic environment, shearing forces produced by the plasmapheresis procedures may have contributed to hemolysis in these cases. Potentially life-threatening acute renal failure can result from the toxic effects of hemoglobin (released from hemolyzed erythrocytes) in the renal tubules.

Albumin human dilutions with substantially reduced tonicity should *not* be used as replacement fluids in plasmapheresis procedures or other situations where administration of large volumes and resultant replacement of a significant fraction of the patient's blood volume could result. When sodium restriction is necessary, 5% dextrose injection is the diluent of choice for albumin human solutions. However, because administration of large volumes of albumin human 5% solution prepared by diluting 25% solutions with 5% dextrose could result in hyponatremia and potentially serious adverse effects (e.g., cerebral swelling), 0.9% sodium chloride generally should be used as the preferred diluent when administration of large volumes is anticipated (e.g., during plasmapheresis or plasma exchange) and the fluid and electrolyte status of the patient permits, particularly if rapid infusion is expected. The use of more physiologic diluents (e.g., those closely resembling plasma) also has been suggested as an alternative for diluting albumin human for use in plasmapheresis or plasma exchange.

If sterile water is used for other situations to dilute albumin human (e.g., when only small volumes are to be infused) and unless other diluents are used concomitantly to raise the final tonicity to a clinically acceptable level, the resultant tonicity of the solution must be considered and any potential risks (e.g., hemolysis, acute renal failure) weighed carefully.

Aluminum Content Aluminum has been detected as a contaminant in albumin human solutions, and aluminum accumulation and associated toxicity (e.g., hypercalcemia, osteodystrophy with associated fracturing osteomalacia, severe progressive encephalopathy) have been reported in some patients with renal failure receiving albumin human (e.g., via plasmapheresis procedures).

The possibility that aluminum could accumulate in patients with impaired renal function should be considered.

Aluminum concentrations in albumin human solutions have varied widely from brand to brand and lot to lot, and reportedly may range up to 323–1830 mcg/L.

Because of the risk of aluminum accumulation, the manufacturer states that Buminate® 25% should not be used in patients with chronic renal impairment.

Certain commercially available albumin human preparations are labeled as containing no more than 200 mcg/L of aluminum (AlbuRx® 5 or 25%, Albutein® 5 or 25%, Plasbumin® 5, 20, or 25% [low aluminum formulations]). It has been suggested that preparations containing no more than 200 mcg/L of aluminum may be preferred in patients at high risk for aluminum toxicity (e.g., neonates, premature infants, geriatric adults, dialysis patients and others with impaired renal function, patients receiving total parenteral nutrition, burn patients).

■ **Pediatric Precautions** The manufacturers of Albuminar® and Plasbumin® state that safety and efficacy of albumin human have not been established in pediatric patients.

The manufacturers of Buminate® and Flexbumin® state that, although specific pediatric safety studies have not been performed, the safety of albumin human has been demonstrated in children receiving dosages appropriate for the child's body weight.

Some manufacturers state that data regarding use of albumin human in pediatric patients, including premature infants, are limited. Clinicians should weigh the benefits and risks and use albumin human in pediatric patients only when clearly needed.

Albumin human has been used as an adjunct to exchange transfusions in the treatment of neonatal hyperbilirubinemia, including hemolytic disease of the newborn (erythroblastosis fetalis), but should *not* be used if neonatal hyperbilirubinemia is treated using phototherapy without exchange transfusion. (See Uses: Neonatal Hyperbilirubinemia.) Albumin human should be used with caution in hypervolemic infants .

Some clinicians state that albumin human 25% solution is contraindicated in preterm infants because of the risk of intraventricular hemorrhage.

If albumin human is used in neonates or premature infants, a preparation with low aluminum may be preferred because of the risk of aluminum accumulation and associated toxicity. (See Aluminum Content under Cautions: Precautions and Contraindications.)

■ **Geriatric Precautions** Clinical studies of albumin human did not include sufficient numbers of geriatric patients 65 years of age or older to determine whether they respond differently than younger patients.

■ **Pregnancy, Fertility, and Lactation** ***Pregnancy*** Animal reproduction studies have not been performed with albumin human. It is not known whether albumin human can cause fetal harm when administered during pregnancy or during labor or delivery. Potential risks and benefits for the specific patient should be considered, and albumin human should be used in pregnant women or during labor and delivery only if clearly needed. One manufacturer states that there is no evidence for any contraindications specifically associated with reproduction, pregnancy, or the fetus.

Fertility It is not known whether albumin human can affect reproductive capacity.

Lactation It is not known whether albumin human is distributed into milk. Albumin human should be used with caution in breast-feeding women and only when clearly needed.

Drug Interactions

Specific drug interaction studies have not been performed using albumin human.

■ **Angiotensin-converting Enzyme Inhibitors** Patients receiving angiotensin-converting enzyme (ACE) inhibitors are at increased risk of atypical reactions (e.g., flushing, hypotension) to the drugs if they undergo therapeutic plasma exchange with albumin human replacement. It has been suggested that this interaction may result from prekallikrein activator (PKA, a metabolite of factor XII) present in albumin human, which activates prekallikrein to bradykinin; metabolism of bradykinin is inhibited by ACE inhibitors, thus resulting in accumulation of this naturally occurring vasoactive peptide. Because of the risk of atypical reactions, ACE inhibitors should be withheld for at least 24 hours prior to plasma exchange in which large volumes of albumin human are administered.

Pharmacology

Serum albumin is an important factor in the regulation of plasma volume and tissue fluid balance through its contribution to the colloid oncotic pressure of plasma. Albumin, a highly soluble globular protein with a relatively low molecular weight (66,500), exerts 70–80% of the colloidal oncotic pressure of normal plasma.

Albumin human 5% solution is iso-oncotic with normal human plasma and will expand circulating blood volume by an amount approximately equal to the volume infused. IV administration of concentrated albumin human solutions causes a shift of fluid from the interstitial spaces into the circulation. When used for the treatment of hypovolemia, albumin human solutions are most effective in well-hydrated patients. When administered IV to a well-hydrated patient, each volume of albumin human 20 or 25% solution draws about 2.5 or 3.5 volumes of additional fluid, respectively, into the circulation within 15 minutes, reducing hemoconcentration and blood viscosity. The extent and duration of volume expansion produced by albumin human is dependent on the initial blood volume. In patients with reduced circulating blood volumes (as from hemorrhage or loss of fluid through exudates or into extravascular spaces), hemodilution persists for many hours, but in patients with normal blood volume, excess fluid and protein are lost from the circulation within a few hours.

Although albumin is a protein, it provides only modest nutritive effect.

Albumin binds and functions as a carrier of intermediate metabolites (including bilirubin), trace metals, some drugs, dyes, fatty acids, hormones, and enzymes, thus affecting the transport, inactivation, and/or exchange of tissue products.

Chemistry and Stability

■ **Chemistry** Albumin human, a protein colloid, is a sterile solution of serum albumin prepared by fractionating pooled plasma from healthy human donors. Albumin human commercially available in the US meets standards established by the US Food and Drug Administration (FDA). No less than 96% of the total protein in the product is albumin.

Depending on the manufacturer, albumin human solutions occur as clear to slightly opalescent, pale straw to amber or brownish fluids which may have a slight greenish tint. The pH of albumin human solutions is adjusted to 6.4–7.4 with sodium carbonate, sodium bicarbonate, sodium hydroxide, and/or acetic acid. The commercially available preparations contain no preservatives or antimicrobial agents, but do contain stabilizers (e.g., caprylic acid, sodium caprylate, sodium acetyltryptophanate).

In the US, albumin human is commercially available as 5, 20, or 25% solutions; other concentrations (e.g., 4% solutions) are commercially available in other countries. Because of the risks associated with administration of hypotonic solutions, commercially available 5, 20, and 25% solutions of albumin human contain 130–160 mEq of sodium per liter. (See Oncotic, Osmotic, and Tonicity Considerations under Cautions: Precautions and Contraindications.) Albumin human 5% solutions are approximately isotonic and iso-oncotic with normal human plasma; albumin human 20 and 25% solutions are oncotically equivalent to approximately 4 and 5 times the volume of normal human plasma, respectively.

Plasma used for preparation of albumin human undergoes viral screening procedures, and albumin human is pasteurized at 60°C for 10–11 hours to reduce the viral infectious potential of the preparation. However, no method has been shown to be totally effective in removing the risk of viral infectivity from plasma-derived preparations. (See Risk of Transmissible Agents in Plasma-derived Preparations under Cautions: Precautions and Contraindications.)

■ **Stability** Albumin human solutions should be stored in tight containers at the temperature recommended by the manufacturer or indicated on the label and should be protected from light. Most commercially available 5, 20, or 25% solutions of albumin human should be stored at 30°C or less.

Albumin human solutions should not be frozen; solutions that have been frozen should not be used. Albumin human solutions should not be used if they appear turbid or contain sediment. The solutions do not contain preservatives and should not be used if more than 4 hours have elapsed since the vial or container was first entered.

Albumin human solutions may be used in conjunction with whole blood or plasma, or with dextrose, sodium lactate, or sodium chloride injections. However, albumin human solutions should not be mixed with parenteral nutrient solutions, protein hydrolysates, amino acid solutions, or solutions containing alcohol since protein precipitates may occur.

When albumin human 25% is diluted with 0.9% sodium chloride injection or 5% dextrose injection, resulting 5% dilutions are approximately isotonic and iso-oncotic with citrated plasma; therefore, these diluents are preferred for such dilutions. Sterile water for injection must *not* be used to dilute albumin human solutions. Depending on the relative proportions of albumin human and diluent, dilutions prepared with sterile water may be dangerously hypotonic, carrying the risk of life-threatening hemolysis, particularly if large volumes of markedly hypotonic dilutions are inadvertently administered. (See Oncotic, Osmotic, and Tonicity Considerations under Cautions: Precautions and Contraindications.) Sterile water is compatible with albumin human and can be a suitable diluent in *non*-clinical situations (e.g., for preparing dilutions to be used in *in vitro* laboratory procedures).

There are conflicting reports of the compatibility of albumin human with other IV infusion fluids; specialized references should be consulted for specific compatibility information.

Preparations

Excipients in commercially available drug preparations may have clinically important effects in some individuals; consult specific product labeling for details.

Albumin Human

Parenteral		
Injection, for IV infusion	50 mg/mL*	**Albuminar®-5**, CSL Behring
		AlbuRx®-5, CSL Behring
		Albumin Human 5%
		Albutein® 5%, Grifols
		Buminate® 5%, Baxter
		Plasbumin®-5, Talecris
	200 mg/mL*	**Albumin Human 20%**
		Plasbumin® -20, Talecris
	250 mg/mL*	**Albuminar®-25**, CSL Behring
		Albumin Human 25%
		Albutein® 25%, Grifols
		AlbuRx® 25, CSL Behring
		Buminate® 25%, Baxter
		Flexbumin® 25%, Baxter
		Plasbumin®-25, Talecris

*available from one or more manufacturer, distributor, and/or repackager by generic (nonproprietary) name

†Use is not currently included in the labeling approved by the US Food and Drug Administration

20:00 BLOOD FORMATION, COAGULATION, AND THROMBOSIS*

§ Omitted from the print version of *AHFS Drug Information* because of space limitations. This monograph is available on the *AHFS Drug Information* web site, http://www.ahfsdruginformation.com. See the Preface for details on accessing this site.
Username: ahfs2020; Password: ASHP94498

* Please see the full AHFS Pharmacologic-Therapeutic Classification© on *p. viii*. Not all classes are used in the printed edition.

ANTIANEMIA DRUGS 20:04

IRON PREPARATIONS 20:04.04

Iron Dextran

Iron-Dextran Complex

■ Iron dextran injection, a sterile, colloidal solution of ferric hydroxide or ferric oxyhydroxide in a complex with partially hydrolyzed low molecular weight dextran, corrects the erythropoietic abnormalities that are due to a deficiency of iron.

Uses

■ **Iron Deficiency Not Amenable to Oral Iron Therapy** Iron dextran is used in the treatment of iron deficiency when oral iron preparations are ineffective or cannot be used. There are relatively few indications for parenteral iron therapy. Occasionally, however, parenteral administration may be required in iron-deficient patients in whom oral administration of iron is infeasible or ineffective because of intolerance, poor absorption, GI disease, refusal or inability to take the oral medication, or when rapid replenishment of iron stores is necessary as in hypochromic anemia of infancy or the last trimester of pregnancy. In addition, most chronic kidney disease patients who receive therapy with erythropoiesis-stimulating agents (ESAs) (e.g., epoetin alfa, darbepoetin alfa) will require oral or parenteral iron therapy because of the dramatic decrease in iron stores associated with erythrocyte formation. In several randomized controlled studies comparing IV and oral administration of iron in patients with chronic kidney disease on hemodialysis, IV iron was superior to orally administered iron in increasing hemoglobin concentrations and/or minimizing the dosage of ESA required to maintain target hemoglobin levels; guidelines from the National Kidney Foundation Kidney Disease Outcomes Quality Initiative (NKF-KDOQI) state that the IV route is preferred for administration of iron in patients with chronic kidney disease undergoing hemodialysis. (See Uses: Anemia of Chronic Kidney Disease, in Epoetin Alfa 20:16.) The response to iron dextran is quantitatively similar to that produced by other iron preparations administered parenterally.

Since parenteral use of complexes of iron and carbohydrates has resulted in fatal anaphylactoid reactions, iron dextran should be used only in patients in whom a clearly established indication for parenteral iron therapy exists, confirmed by appropriate laboratory tests.

For additional information on the prevention and treatment of iron deficiency, including anemia, see Uses in Iron Preparations, Oral, 20:04.04.

Dosage and Administration

■ **Administration** Iron dextran injection is administered undiluted by *slow* (50 mg/minute or less if undiluted) IV injection; some preparations (i.e., INFeD®) also are FDA-labeled for IM injection. Iron dextran injection also has been diluted in 0.9% sodium chloride injection and administered by IV infusion† (e.g., over 1–6 hours).

Before administration of the first therapeutic dose of iron dextran, a test dose of iron should be given by the chosen route and appropriate method of administration. If iron dextran is to be administered IV, the manufacturer of INFeD® recommends that a test dose of 25 mg (0.5 mL) of iron dextran be given IV over at least 30 seconds; the manufacturer of Dexferrum® recommends a 25-mg (0.5 mL) test dose given IV over at least 5 minutes. If administered IM, a test dose of 25 mg (0.5 mL) of iron dextran (InFeD®) should be administered into the buttock using the IM injection technique recommended by the manufacturer. It has been recommended that the test dose and subsequent doses of iron dextran be administered by individuals trained to provide emergency treatment of serious allergic reactions should they occur and that immediate access to drugs and resuscitation equipment needed to treat such reactions be available. Although anaphylactic reactions usually are evident within a few minutes when they occur, it is recommended that a period of 1 hour or longer elapse before the remaining portion of the initial dose is given.

IV administration may be preferred to IM administration when there is insufficient muscle mass for IM administration, when there is impaired absorption from the muscle because of stasis or edema, when there is a possibility of uncontrolled IM bleeding (as in hemophilia), or when massive and prolonged parenteral therapy is indicated (as in chronic substantial blood loss), and to avoid the pain, irritation, and staining of the skin at the injection site secondary to IM administration. IM administration may be preferred when venous access is difficult or infeasible (e.g., in infants or in adults with poor veins).

For IM administration, the manufacturer of INFeD® recommends that iron dextran be injected deeply with a 2- or 3-inch, 19- or 20-gauge needle into the upper outer quadrant of the buttock only; the drug should never be administered into the arm or any other exposed area. When the drug is administered IM, if the patient is standing, the injection should be made in the buttock of the leg opposite the patient's weight-bearing leg; if supine, the patient should be in a lateral position with the injection site uppermost. To avoid injection or leakage into subcutaneous tissue, the Z-track technique of injection in which the subcutaneous tissue over the site of injection is firmly pushed aside before inserting the needle is recommended.

The manufacturers state that iron dextran should not be mixed with other drugs or added to parenteral nutrition solutions for IV infusion. Iron dextran solutions should be inspected visually for particulate matter and discoloration prior to administration whenever solution and container permit.

■ **Dosage** Dosage of iron dextran is expressed in terms of mg of elemental iron. Iron dextran injection contains the equivalent of 50 mg of elemental iron per mL.

Iron Deficiency Anemia Before initiating therapy for *iron deficiency anemia,* total iron requirements (allowing for storage iron) are calculated by using a dose formula or table. Calculations are based on the amount of iron needed to restore hemoglobin concentration to normal or near normal plus an additional amount to provide adequate replenishment of iron stores in most individuals with moderately or severely reduced levels of hemoglobin. In the formula recommended by the manufacturers, the total dose of iron dextran injection (in mL) containing the equivalent of 50 mg/mL of iron is calculated as follows:

$$[0.0442 \times (Hb_d - Hb_o) \times Wt] + (0.26 \times Wt) = \text{total dose of iron dextran injection (mL)}$$

Where Wt is the patient's lean body weight in kg, Hb_d is the *desired* hemoglobin concentration in g/dL (14.8 for patients weighing more than 15 kg and 12 for patients weighing 15 kg or less), Hb_o is the patient's *observed* hemoglobin concentration in g/dL, and (0.26 × lean body weight) is a factor that accounts for storage iron.

In patients with chronic kidney disease who are receiving supplemental therapy with an erythropoiesis-stimulating agent (ESA), sufficient iron should be administered to maintain certain indices of iron therapy (i.e., transferrin saturation and serum ferritin concentrations) at target levels; periodic monitoring of these iron indices is recommended, and the results should be used (in conjunction with hemoglobin concentrations and ESA dosage) to guide iron therapy.

Iron Replacement Secondary to Blood Loss For *iron replacement secondary to blood loss* (e.g., in patients with hemorrhagic diatheses or patients on long-term renal hemodialysis), total iron requirements are based on estimates of the amount of iron represented in the blood loss; the formula above for iron deficiency anemia is *not* applicable. Instead, the following formula, based on the approximation that 1 mL of normocytic, normochromic erythrocytes contains 1 mg of elemental iron, may be used to calculate the required total dosage in mL of iron dextran injection containing the equivalent of 50 mg of iron per mL:

0.02 × blood loss (in mL) × hematocrit (expressed as a decimal fraction) = total dosage of iron dextran injection in mL

IV Dosage Iron dextran may be injected IV, undiluted, at a slow, gradual rate not exceeding 50 mg of iron per minute (1 mL/minute). If adverse reactions to the test dose do not occur, subsequent IV doses may be increased to up to 100 mg of iron daily until the total calculated dose has been administered. The manufacturers recommend that the maximum daily IV dosage of *undiluted* iron dextran not exceed 25 mg (0.5 mL) of iron in infants weighing less than 5 kg; 50 mg (1 mL) of iron in children weighing less than 10 kg; and 100 mg (2 mL) of iron in other patients.

Although the manufacturers do not recommend dilution of iron dextran injection† or administration of the drug in single IV doses exceeding 100 mg†, numerous reports have been made in which the total dose of an iron dextran preparation was administered as a single dose either by direct IV injection or as an IV infusion. Large IV doses of iron dextran, such as those used in total-dose infusions†, reportedly have been associated with an increased frequency of adverse effects, especially delayed reactions (e.g., arthralgia, myalgia, fever). In the total-dose infusion technique, the total calculated dose of iron dextran is diluted in 250–1000 mL of 0.9% sodium chloride injection. The use of 5% dextrose injection instead of 0.9% sodium chloride injection has been reported to be associated with a higher incidence of local pain and phlebitis. With the total-dose infusion technique, if no reaction occurs after administration of a 25-mg IV test dose over 5 minutes, the remainder of the dose may be infused (e.g., over 1–6 hours). After the infusion is completed, the vein is often flushed with 0.9% sodium chloride injection.

IM Dosage Iron dextran labeled for IM use (i.e., INFeD®) may be injected IM daily or less frequently until the calculated amount has been given. If adverse reactions to the test dose do not occur, subsequent doses may be given. The manufacturer of INFeD® recommends that the maximum daily IM dosage of *undiluted* iron dextran not exceed 25 mg (0.5 mL) of iron in infants weighing less than 5 kg, 50 mg (1 mL) of iron in children weighing less than 10 kg, and 100 mg (2 mL) of iron in other patients.

Cautions

Sensitivity (e.g., anaphylactoid or anaphylactic) reactions appear to be the most common adverse effects of iron dextran, occurring with either IV or IM administration, and such reactions vary widely in severity and can be immediate or delayed. Incidences of such reactions are difficult to ascertain since some studies only reported severe or potentially serious reactions whereas others reported a wide range of severity. Sensitivity reactions may be severe enough to require discontinuance of iron dextran therapy and can be fatal. (See Cautions: Sensitivity Reactions.) Local reactions associated with IV or IM administration also appear to be relatively common. Adverse reactions associated with IV administration of the drug generally resemble those associated with IM administration. Large IV doses of iron dextran, such as those used in total-dose infusions, have been associated with an increased incidence of adverse effects, and such adverse effects frequently have been delayed (1–2 days).

■ **Sensitivity Reactions** Anaphylactic or anaphylactoid reactions to iron dextran, including fatal anaphylaxis, have been reported. These reactions occur most frequently within the first several minutes of administration and are generally characterized by sudden onset of respiratory difficulty (e.g., wheezing, bronchospasm, rigor, dyspnea, cyanosis), tachycardia, hypotension, respiratory arrest, and/or cardiovascular collapse. The manufacturers state that concomitant use of angiotensin-converting enzyme (ACE) inhibitors may increase the risk for reactions to iron dextran. The level of risk for anaphylactic-type reactions following exposure to specific iron dextran preparations is not known and may vary. Iron dextran preparations differ in chemical characteristics and may differ in clinical effects; the manufacturers state that such preparations are not clinically interchangeable.

Acute hypersensitivity reactions to iron dextran have been estimated to occur in 0.2–3% of patients. These reactions have been reported after administration of uneventful test doses of iron dextran as well as after therapeutic doses of the drug. Although it has been suggested that severe systemic reactions, including anaphylactoid reactions, are more common following IV rather than IM administration of iron dextran, the risk of severe systemic reactions following IV or IM administration has not been directly compared and there appears to be no well-substantiated evidence of a difference in the frequency of anaphylactoid reactions following either route of administration. The National Kidney Foundation Kidney Disease Outcomes Quality Initiative (NKF-KDOQI) guidelines state that direct observation of the patient after IV administration of an iron agent permits the most reliable assessment of the frequency of associated adverse drug reactions. Relatively large IV doses such as those employed with total-dose infusions have been associated with an increased risk of adverse effects, mainly delayed effects. The risk of anaphylactic or anaphylactoid reactions to iron dextran appears to be increased in patients with a positive history of drug allergy, particularly those with multiple drug allergies. Other hypersensitivity reactions may include sweating, dyspnea, urticaria, other rashes and pruritus, arthralgia, myalgia, and febrile episodes.

The mechanism of anaphylactic/anaphylactoid reactions to iron dextran has not been elucidated, but because of the rapid nature of their onset and similarity to anaphylactoid reactions observed with radiographic contrast media they probably result from a direct effect on mast cells and basophils leading to their degranulation and release of mediators (e.g., histamine). An immunoglobulin E-mediated reaction appears unlikely.

■ **Musculoskeletal and Delayed Adverse Effects** Large IV doses of iron dextran, such as those used in total-dose infusions†, may be associated with an increased frequency of adverse effects,especially delayed (1–2 days) reactions manifested by arthralgia, backache, myalgia, adenopathy, moderate to high fever, backache, chills, dizziness, headache, malaise, nausea, and/or vomiting. The onset of these adverse effects is usually 24–48 hours after administration of the drug, and the effects generally subside within 3–4 days. Delayed adverse effects have also occurred following IM administration and usually subsided within 3–7 days. The etiology of delayed adverse effects is not known, but the symptom complex resembles that of a serum sickness reaction. Patients with rheumatoid arthritis and possibly other inflammatory diseases (e.g., ankylosing spondylitis, lupus erythematosus) may be at particular risk for delayed reactions. IV administration of iron dextran has caused fever and exacerbation or reactivation of joint pain and swelling in patients with rheumatoid arthritis; in addition, exacerbation of ankylosing spondylitis in one patient and arthralgia, myalgia, erythema nodosum, and fever in a patient with lupus erythematosus have been reported. Such exacerbations of underlying inflammatory conditions may respond to nonsteroidal anti-inflammatory agent (NSAIA) therapy and may be prevented with corticosteroid pretreatment.

■ **Local Effects** Local reactions may occur at the injection site of iron dextran and are more common following IM administration. Local reactions at the injection site following IM injection include soreness or pain (in rare cases persisting longer than a year), inflammation, sterile abscesses, necrosis, atrophy, fibrosis, cellulitis, swelling, and harmless but persistent brown staining of the skin and/or underlying tissue. Phlebitis, pain along the course of the vein, and venospasm may occur following IV injection. Inadvertent intra-arterial injection of a 1-g undiluted dose over 20 minutes resulted in marked erythema, warmth, and tingling in the hand and arm distal to the brachial artery injection site during infusion.

■ **Cardiovascular Effects** Chest pain, chest tightness, shock, hypotension, hypertension, tachycardia, bradycardia, flushing, edema, cardiac arrest, thrombophlebitis, pulmonary embolus, and arrhythmias have occurred in patients receiving iron dextran. Flushing and hypotension may occur when the drug is administered IV too rapidly.

■ **GI Effects** Abdominal pain, dyspepsia, nausea, vomiting, diarrhea, metallic taste in the mouth, altered taste, and transient loss of taste perception have occurred in patients receiving iron dextran.

■ **Nervous System Effects** Headache, transient paresthesia, weakness, dizziness, faintness, syncope, unresponsiveness, disorientation, numbness, malaise, and seizures (which may accompany anaphylaxis) have been reported in patients receiving iron dextran.

■ **Hematologic Effects** Latent folic acid deficiency may occasionally become apparent in patients receiving iron dextran. Leukocytosis, frequently with fever, may occur. One case of leukocytosis was reported in a severely iron-deficient infant who received the drug. Purpura has also occurred.

■ **Other Adverse Effects** Other adverse effects of iron dextran include chills, shivering, regional lymphadenopathy (generally inguinal and associated with IM injection of the drug), and hematuria.

■ **Precautions and Contraindications** Because anaphylactic reactions to iron dextran, including fatal anaphylaxis, have been reported, an initial test dose should be administered prior to administration of the first therapeutic dose of the drug and the patient should be observed for manifestations of anaphylactic-type reactions. Because anaphylaxis and other hypersensitivity reactions have been reported after administration of uneventful test doses of iron dextran as well as after therapeutic doses of the drug, the manufacturers state that administration of subsequent test doses should be considered during iron dextran therapy. (See Dosage and Administration: Administration.) It is recommended that the test dose and subsequent doses of iron dextran be administered by personnel trained to provide emergency treatment and that appropriate resuscitation equipment and drugs for the treatment of a severe allergic or anaphylactic reaction (e.g., epinephrine) be readily available when iron dextran is administered. Patients receiving β-adrenergic blocking agents may not respond adequately to epinephrine, and use of isoproterenol or a similar β-adrenergic agonist may be required in these patients.

The fact that large IV doses of iron dextran, such as those used in total-dose infusions, have been associated with an increased incidence of adverse effects, especially delayed reactions, should be considered when evaluating the benefits and risks of such therapy. Patients should be advised of potential effects associated with the use of iron dextran.

Iron dextran should be used with caution in patients with a history of serious allergies and/or asthma. Iron dextran should be used with extreme caution in patients with serious impairment of hepatic function. Adverse effects following administration of iron dextran may exacerbate cardiovascular complications in patients with preexisting cardiovascular disease.

Extreme caution should also be used in administering the drug IV in patients with rheumatoid arthritis, since IV administration may cause fever and exacerbation or reactivation of joint pain and swelling in these patients; the possibility of an increased risk of delayed reactions (e.g., arthralgia, myalgia, fever) should also be considered in patients with other inflammatory diseases (e.g., ankylosing spondylitis, lupus erythematosus). (See Cautions: Musculoskeletal and Delayed Adverse Effects.)

Unwarranted administration of parenteral iron preparations may cause excess storage of iron and a syndrome similar to hemosiderosis in patients whose anemia is not attributable to iron deficiency (e.g., those with hemoglobinopathies and other refractory anemias that might be erroneously diagnosed as iron deficiency anemias).

Because iron can increase the pathogenicity of certain microorganisms and has been postulated as potentially adversely affecting prognosis in certain HIV-infected individuals, some clinicians recommend that HIV-infected individuals who do not have documented iron-deficiency anemia avoid iron supplementation for the management of HIV-associated anemia. *Iron dextran should not be administered concomitantly with oral iron preparations.* Determinations of hematologic response, such as serum ferritin, blood hemoglobin concentration, hematocrit, and reticulocyte count, should be performed periodically during the course of therapy with iron dextran. Serum ferritin has been shown to correlate with iron stores, at least in nonuremic patients; while a correlation between serum ferritin and iron stores has been reported in hemodialysis patients, other data suggest that elevated serum ferritin can result from hepatosplenic siderosis in some of these patients, and may not reliably indicate bone marrow iron stores.

Iron dextran should not be used during the acute phase of infectious renal disease. The drug is contraindicated in patients with any anemia other than iron deficiency anemia and in patients who are hypersensitive to iron dextran.

■ **Pediatric Precautions** The manufacturers state that the use of iron dextran in children younger than 4 months of age is not recommended. Use of IM iron dextran in neonates† in other countries (e.g., New Zealand) reportedly has been associated with an increased incidence of gram-negative sepsis, principally infections caused by *Escherichia coli*. However, the drug has been administered IV in a limited number of neonates in the US without evidence of unusual adverse effect or risk of sepsis.

■ **Carcinogenicity** IM administration of iron-carbohydrate complexes may be associated with a risk of carcinogenesis. Subcutaneous injection of very large doses of iron dextran or small doses injected repeatedly at the same site have been shown to produce sarcomas in mice, rats, rabbits, and possibly hamsters. Such tumors have not been produced in guinea pigs. Animal studies suggest that sarcomas may result from high tissue concentrations of iron remaining at the site of injection and that the latent period between administration of the drug and appearance of the tumor may be one-quarter to one-third of the life span of the particular species. Sarcoma at the site of injection has been reported rarely in patients approximately 4–14 years after receiving IM iron dextran or other complexes of iron and carbohydrates; however, a causal relationship has not been proven. Although the carcinogenic potential of iron dextran is generally considered remote by most authorities, it may require years before the carcinogenic potential in humans can be clearly defined.

■ **Pregnancy and Lactation** Reproduction studies in mice, rats, rabbits, dogs, and monkeys using iron dextran doses about 3 times the maximum human dose have shown the drug to be teratogenic and embryocidal. At doses equivalent to 50 mg/kg or less of iron, no consistent adverse fetal effects were observed in mice, rats, rabbits, dogs, or monkeys. At a total IV dose equivalent to 90 mg/kg of iron given over a 14-day period, fetal and maternal toxicity has been reported in monkeys; similar effects were observed in mice and rats with a single dose equivalent to 125 mg/kg of iron. In dogs and rats, fetal abnormalities were observed at doses equivalent to 250 mg/kg or higher of iron. The animals used in reproduction studies were not iron deficient. The effect of iron dextran on the human fetus is not known. Results of various studies in pregnant animals and humans have been inconclusive regarding placental transfer of intact iron dextran. Small amounts of iron apparently cross the placenta (the form in which it crosses the placenta has not been clearly established) and increase neonatal serum iron concentrations when iron dextran is administered within 2 weeks of delivery; however, no adverse effects on the neonate have been reported. There are no adequate and well-controlled studies using iron dextran in pregnant women, and the drug should be used during pregnancy only when the potential benefits justify the possible risks to the fetus.

Only traces of unmetabolized iron dextran are distributed into milk, but the drug should be used with caution in nursing women.

Laboratory Test Interferences

Large IV doses (250 mg or more of iron) of iron dextran may cause serum from blood samples obtained 4 hours after administration of the drug to have a brown color. The drug may cause falsely elevated values of serum bilirubin and falsely decreased values of serum calcium. Serum iron determinations (especially colorimetric assays) may not be meaningful for 3 weeks following the administration of iron dextran. Results of serum iron measurements obtained within 1–2 weeks of administration of large doses of the drug should be interpreted with caution. Serum ferritin concentrations peak approximately 7–9 days following an IV dose of iron dextran and slowly return to baseline over a period of about 3 weeks. Examination of the bone marrow for iron stores may not be meaningful for prolonged periods following iron dextran therapy because residual iron dextran may remain in the reticuloendothelial cells.

Prolongation of the partial thromboplastin time has been reported to occur after IV administration of iron dextran when the blood sample for the test is mixed with anticoagulant citrate dextrose solution. This interference apparently does not occur when anticoagulant sodium citrate solution is used. Blood typing and cross-matching are not affected by iron dextran.

Bone scans involving technetium Tc 99m diphosphonate have been reported to exhibit dense, crescentic areas of activity along the contour of the iliac crest, visualized 1–6 days after IM injections of iron dextran.Bone scans using imaging agents labeled with technetium Tc 99m, in the presence of high serum ferritin concentrations or following IV infusions of iron dextran, have been reported to show reduced bone uptake, marked renal activity, and excessive blood pool and soft tissue accumulation.

Acute Toxicity

The LD_{50} of iron dextran in mice is 500 mg/kg or greater. Overdosage of iron dextran is unlikely to be associated with any acute manifestations; however, dosage of the drug in excess of that required for restoration of hemoglobin and replenishment of iron stores may lead to hemosiderosis. Periodic monitoring of serum ferritin concentrations may be useful in recognizing a deleterious, progressive accumulation of iron resulting from impaired iron uptake from the reticuloendothelial system that may occur in some patients (e.g., those with chronic kidney disease, Hodgkin's disease, rheumatoid arthritis). Only negligible amounts of iron dextran are removed by hemodialysis.

Pharmacology

Iron is a constituent of hemoglobin, and administration of iron dextran corrects the erythropoietic abnormalities that are due to a deficiency of iron. Some iron also may be utilized for synthesis of myoglobin or nonhemoglobin heme units. In iron-deficient patients, reticulocytosis may begin by the fourth day following an IV infusion of the total calculated dose of iron dextran and reaches a maximum by about the tenth day. Iron does not stimulate erythropoiesis nor does it correct hemoglobin disturbances not caused by iron deficiency.

Administration of iron may reverse esophageal, gastric, and other tissue changes associated with iron deficiency. Iron therapy also relieves other symptoms associated with iron deficiency such as soreness of the tongue, cheilosis, dysphagia, and dystrophy of the nails and skin. Some of the toxic effects of iron dextran may be due to a pharmacologic or allergenic effect of dextran; however, conclusive studies have not been performed to establish the importance of this effect.

Pharmacokinetics

■ **Absorption** Following IM injection, iron dextran is absorbed from the site of injection principally through the lymphatic system. Absorption takes place in two stages. In the initial phase lasting about 3 days, a local inflammatory reaction facilitates passage of the drug from the site of IM injection into the lymphatic system. In the second, slower phase, iron dextran is ingested by macrophages, which then enter the lymphatic system and eventually the blood. Results of studies using radiolabeled iron dextran have shown that about 60% of an IM dose of iron dextran is absorbed after 3 days and up to 90% is absorbed after 1–3 weeks; the remainder is gradually absorbed over a period of several months or longer. Absorption of iron dextran from subcutaneous tissue is very slow, and the skin may be stained brown for up to 2 years if the drug is deposited in this tissue.

■ **Distribution** Following IM or IV injection, iron dextran is gradually cleared from the plasma by the reticuloendothelial cells of the liver, spleen, and bone marrow. Results of several studies indicate that a variable portion of an IV dose of iron dextran may be stored in an unusable form in bone marrow. Following IV doses containing more than 500 mg of elemental iron, the uptake of iron dextran by the reticuloendothelial system appears to be constant and amounts to 10–20 mg per hour. Reticuloendothelial cells separate iron from the iron dextran complex and the iron becomes a part of the body's total iron stores.

Ferric iron is gradually released into the plasma where it rapidly combines with transferrin and is carried to the bone marrow and incorporated into hemoglobin. Rate of incorporation of iron into hemoglobin is determined by the extent of iron deficiency, with greater rates of hemoglobin synthesis occurring in iron deficient patients than in normal or mildly anemic patients. Following an IV infusion of the total calculated dose of iron dextran in iron-deficient patients, the rate of increase in hemoglobin concentration appears to be most rapid during the first 1–2 weeks and ranges from 1.5–2.2 g/dL per week. Subsequently, hemoglobin concentration increases at a rate of 0.7–1.6 g/dL per week until normal hemoglobin concentrations are attained.

Small amounts of iron apparently reach the fetus following administration of iron dextran during pregnancy, but the form in which it crosses the placenta is not clearly established. Only traces of unmetabolized iron dextran are distributed into breast milk.

For additional information on the distribution of iron, see Pharmacokinetics: Distribution, in Iron Preparations, Oral, 20:04.04.

■ **Elimination** In doses of 500 mg or less, iron dextran plasma concentrations decrease exponentially with a half-life of about 6 hours. In studies in iron-deficient patients with coexistent end-stage renal disease and other clinical problems, the serum elimination half-life of iron averaged 58.9 hours (range: 9.4–87.4 hours) following IV administration of iron dextran; these studies measured the total serum iron directly as well as transferrin bound iron non-radioisotopically. It should be recognized that elimination of iron from serum, including elimination half-life, does *not* correspond to clearance of the mineral from the body.

Dextran, a polyglucose, is either metabolized or excreted. Only traces of unmetabolized iron dextran are excreted in urine, bile, or feces.

Iron dextran is negligibly removed by hemodialysis. Several dialyzer membranes have been studied (e.g., polysulphone, cuprophane, cellulose acetate, cellulose triacetate, polymethylmethacrilate, polyacrylonitrile), including those considered high efficiency and high flux.

Chemistry and Stability

■ **Chemistry** Iron dextran injection is a sterile, colloidal solution of ferric hydroxide or oxyhydroxide in a complex with partially hydrolyzed low molecular weight dextran. During the manufacture of iron dextran, polymerization occurs resulting in a complex with a molecular weight estimated to be approximately 165,000. Approximately 98–99% of the iron in iron dextran is present as a stable ferric-dextran complex; the remainder is present as a weak ferrous complex. Iron dextran injection occurs as a dark brown, slightly viscous liquid that is completely miscible with water and 0.9% sodium chloride injection. The commercially available injection of InFed® or Dexferrum® has a pH of 5.2–6.5 or 4.5–7, respectively; sodium hydroxide and/or hydrochloric acid may have been added to adjust pH.

■ **Stability** Iron dextran injection should be stored at a controlled room temperature of 20–25°C, with excursions permitted to 15–30°C.

Iron dextran injection has been reported to be physically incompatible with oxytetracycline and with sulfadiazine sodium in IV infusions.

Preparations

Excipients in commercially available drug preparations may have clinically important effects in some individuals; consult specific product labeling for details.

Iron Dextran

Parenteral		
Injection, for IV use	equivalent to 50 mg of elemental iron per mL	**Dexferrum®**, American Regent
Injection, for IV or IM use	equivalent to 50 mg of elemental iron per mL	**INFeD®**, Watson

†Use is not currently included in the labeling approved by the US Food and Drug Administration

Iron Preparations, Oral

■ Ferrous fumarate, ferrous gluconate, ferrous sulfate, carbonyl iron, and polysaccharide-iron complex are iron preparations that are commercially available in the US for oral administration in the prevention and treatment of iron deficiency.

Uses

■ **Iron Deficiency** Iron preparations are used for the prevention and treatment of iron deficiency. Iron will not correct hemoglobin disturbances caused by conditions other than iron deficiency but may cause iron toxicity or iron storage disease if used in these conditions. Iron also is not indicated for the treatment of anemia resulting from causes other than iron deficiency.

Ensuring adequate dietary iron intake is the principal means for primary prevention of iron deficiency in all age groups, reserving iron supplementation for individuals and groups at high risk of deficiency and/or in whom adequate dietary intake is unlikely to be achieved and iron therapy for those with presumed or established iron-deficiency anemia. Oral administration is the route of choice for iron therapy in most patients and for iron supplementation. Because they appear to be the most readily absorbed, ferrous salts are the iron preparations of choice. Since absorption of iron salts occurs maximally in the duodenum and proximal jejunum, extended-release or enteric-coated preparations should be used only if objective bioavailability data have shown the preparation to be effective and if the potential benefits outweigh the disadvantage of added cost.

Iron deficiency is the most common known nutritional deficiency. Deficiency of iron may result from inadequate ingestion, decreased absorption or utilization, abnormal blood losses (including menstruation), or increased requirements. When a diagnosis of iron deficiency is confirmed, a cause must be identified. Iron deficiency represents a spectrum ranging from iron depletion, which results in no physiologic impairment, to anemia, which affects the functioning of several organ systems. In depletion, the amount of stored iron is reduced but the amount of functional iron (e.g., in hemoglobin) may not be affected; if body requirements increase in depleted individuals, there are no stores from which to mobilize iron. Erythropoiesis in iron deficiency depletes iron stores and reduces transport iron further; GI absorption of iron is insufficient to replace the amount depleted or to provide the amount needed for growth and function. As a result, erythrocyte production is limited and erythrocyte protoporphyrin concentration increases secondarily. In iron-deficiency anemia, the most severe form of deficiency, the iron shortage results in inadequate production of iron-containing functional compounds, including hemoglobin; erythrocytes are microcytic and hypochromic. In the treatment of iron deficiency, administration of iron in combination with other minerals and/or vitamins has not been established as being superior to iron alone.

Risks and Prevalence of Iron Deficiency Despite recent improvements (e.g., secondary to increased use of iron-fortified formulas in nonbreast-fed infants), iron deficiency remains relatively prevalent in the US in adolescent girls and women of childbearing age and in infants. Considerable morbidity, particularly among young children and pregnant women, can result from iron deficiency, and efforts to prevent, detect, and treat iron deficiency should be heightened in the US, especially among such individuals and females of childbearing age. Because some developmental deficits in young children may not be fully reversible, the importance of primary prevention in this age group is particularly important.

Infants and Young Children. Iron-deficiency anemia can result in considerable morbidity in young children. In infants and preschool children up to 5 years of age, iron-deficiency anemia results in developmental delays and behavioral disturbances (e.g., decreased motor activity, social interaction, and attention to tasks). Such developmental delays may persist beyond 5 years of age into the school years if the iron deficiency is not reversed fully, and some developmental deficits may not be fully reversible even with iron therapy. The effects of *mild* iron-deficiency anemia on infant and early childhood development and behavior remain to be further elucidated. Iron-deficiency anemia also may enhance the risk of lead toxicity in children by increasing GI absorption of heavy metals, including lead. Iron-deficiency anemia in young children also may be associated with conditions (e.g., low birthweight, undernutrition, poverty, high blood lead concentrations) that independently affect development, and such potential confounding factors should be considered when interventions aimed at managing iron-deficiency anemia are developed and evaluated.

Rapid growth rate combined with frequently inadequate dietary iron intake places children younger than 2 years of age, particularly those 9–18 months of age, at the highest risk of any age group for iron deficiency.Iron stores of full-term infants generally meet iron requirements until 4–6 months of age, and iron-deficiency anemia generally does not become evident until about 9 months of age. However, iron stores can be depleted by 2–3 months of age in premature or low-birthweight infants secondary to lower iron stores at birth and more rapid growth during infancy, placing such infants at greater risk for iron deficiency than full-term infants with normal or high birthweight.

In the US, iron deficiency occurs in about 9% of children 12–36 months of age, in about one-third of whom the deficiency has progressed to anemia. The prevalence of iron deficiency is greater in children living at or below the poverty line than in those living above the poverty line and also is greater in blacks and Mexican-Americans than in white children.

The iron content and absorption efficiency of various milk sources and feeding practices are a strong predictor of iron nutritional status during the first year of life.

Breast milk has the highest percentage of bioavailable iron (about 50%), and breast milk and iron-fortified formula can provide adequate iron to meet an infant's iron requirements. However, the relatively high iron bioavailability of breast milk does not completely compensate for the relatively low iron content. Although iron-fortified formula has a relatively low iron bioavailability (about 4%), it has a substantially higher iron concentration than breast milk, which can compensate for differences in bioavailability.Nonfortified-formulas and whole cow's milk have an iron bioavailability of about 10% but relatively low iron concentrations (especially cow's milk).

Although most nonbreast-fed infants in the US appear to receive the recommended dietary allowance of iron through diet, 20–40% of infants fed nonfortified formula or whole cow's milk are at risk for iron deficiency by 9–12 months of age, while those fed mainly iron-fortified formula are unlikely to have deficiency (e.g., about an 8% risk). In addition, 15–25% of US breast-fed infants are at risk for iron deficiency by 9–12 months of age, and more than 50% of US children 1–2 years may not be receiving adequate dietary iron. Consumption of iron-fortified cereal can reduce the risk of iron deficiency in infants. Although the effect of prolonged exclusive breast-feeding on iron status remains unclear, limited evidence suggests that exclusive breast-feeding for longer than 7 months minimizes the risk of iron deficiency relative to breast-feeding that is supplemented by nonfortified foods beginning at 7 months of age or younger. Introduction of whole cow's milk before 1 year of age or consumption of more than 720 mL (24 oz) after the first year of life increases the risk of iron deficiency because such milk has little bioavailable iron, may displace the desire for foods with higher iron content, and may cause occult GI bleeding; goat's milk is likely to carry a similar risk because of similar iron composition to whole cow's milk, and soy milk (not iron-fortified soy-based formula) also should be avoided for the milk-based part of the diet before 12 months of age. Because iron-fortified formulas are readily available, do not cost much more than nonfortified formulas, and have few proven adverse effects other than dark stools, they are preferred for primary prevention of iron deficiency in nonbreast-fed or partially breast-fed infants younger than 1 year old as well as for weaning breast-fed infants in this age group; no common medical indication exists for the use of low-iron formulas.

The risk of iron deficiency declines after 24 months of age because growth velocity slows, the diet becomes more diversified, and iron stores start to accumulate. After 36 months of age, dietary iron and iron status usually are adequate. However, iron deficiency can develop in either age group as a result of limited access to food (e.g., because of low income or migrant or refugee status), a low-iron or other specialized diet, or a medical condition that affects iron status (e.g., inflammatory or bleeding disorders).

Females of Childbearing Age and Adolescents. In adolescents 12 up to 18 years of age, iron requirements and the risk of iron deficiency increase because of rapid growth. Among boys, the risk subsides after the peak pubertal growth period. However, among girls and women, menstruation increases the risk of iron deficiency throughout childbearing years. In addition, heavy menstrual blood loss (80 mL or more monthly) is an important risk factor for iron-deficiency anemia in women, affecting about 10% of such women in the US. Other risk factors for iron deficiency include use of an intrauterine device (secondary to increased menstrual blood loss), high parity, previous diagnosis of iron-deficiency anemia, and low iron intake. Oral contraceptive use is associated with a decreased risk of iron deficiency. Only about 25% of adolescent girls and women of childbearing age (12–49 years old) achieve the recommended dietary allowance of iron through diet, and 11% of nonpregnant women 16–49 years of age experience iron deficiency, in about 25–50% of whom the deficiency has progressed to anemia.

Pregnancy. During the first and second trimester of pregnancy, iron-deficiency anemia is associated with a twofold increased risk of premature delivery and a threefold increased risk of a low-birthweight delivery.Although iron supplementation during pregnancy has been shown to decrease the incidence of anemia, evidence on the effect of routine iron supplementation during pregnancy on adverse maternal and infant outcomes is inconclusive. Blood volume expands by about 35% during pregnancy, and growth of the fetus, placenta, and other maternal tissues increases the iron requirement threefold during the second and third trimesters of pregnancy to about 5 mg of iron daily. Although menstruation ceases and iron absorption increases during pregnancy, most pregnant women who do not use iron supplements to meet increased iron requirements cannot maintain adequate iron stores, particularly during the last 2 trimesters. Following delivery, iron in the fetus and placenta are lost to the woman, although some of the iron in the expanded blood volume may return to blood stores. Among low-income pregnant women enrolled in health programs in the US, the prevalence of iron-deficiency anemia is 9, 14, and 37% during the first, second, and third trimesters, respectively. While similar data currently are not available for all pregnant women in the US, the low dietary iron intake among US women of childbearing age, the high prevalence of iron deficiency and associated anemia among such women, and the increased iron requirements during pregnancy suggest that anemia during pregnancy may extend beyond low-income women. In addition, use of prenatal multivitamin and mineral supplements among African-Americans, native American and Alaskan Indians, women younger than 20 years of age, and those having less than a high school education is substantially lower than in the general US pregnant population.

The principal reasons for the current lack of widespread adoption of a recommended iron supplementation regimen during pregnancy in US women may include lack of health-care provider and patient perceptions that iron supplements improve maternal and infant outcomes, complicated dose schedules, and adverse effects (e.g., constipation, nausea, vomiting). However, adequate dietary iron intake and iron supplementation generally are recommended for primary prevention of iron deficiency during pregnancy. By employing low-dose (i.e., 30 mg of iron daily) regimens with simplified dose schedules (i.e., once-daily dosing), patient compliance may be improved; low-dose regimens have been shown to increase patient tolerance and are as effective as higher dosages (e.g., 60–120 mg iron daily) in preventing iron-deficiency anemia.

Other Adults. In adults 18 years of age and older, effects of iron-deficiency anemia on daily functioning may be less overt than in children. Such anemia in laborers (e.g., tea pickers, latex tappers, cotton mill workers) in developing countries can impair work capacity, which appears to be at least partially reversible with iron therapy. Whether iron-deficiency anemia in adults affects the capacity to perform less physically demanding labor that depends on sustained cognitive or coordinated motor function remains to be elucidated.Iron-deficiency anemia also can manifest as impaired exercise capacity, lethargy, and dyspnea. Skin, nail, and other epithelial changes of chronic iron deficiency include atrophic changes of the skin, nail changes such as koilonychia (spoon-shaped nails) that manifest as brittle flattened nails, angular stomatitis (i.e., painful fissuring at the angles of the lips), glossitis, and esophageal and pharyngeal webs with associated dysphagia.

Iron-deficiency anemia is uncommon in the US among males 18 years of age and older and among postmenopausal women. The incidence of this anemia in the US is 2% or less among males 20 years of age and older and 2% among postmenopausal women. Most adults in the US with iron-deficiency anemia have GI bleeding secondary to lesions (e.g., ulcers, tumors), and about two-thirds of anemia cases among men and postmenopausal women were attributable to chronic disease or inflammatory conditions; therefore, iron-deficiency anemia in adults, unlike that in children or women of childbearing age, appears to be caused principally by an underlying disease rather than by low iron intake.

■ Prevention and Treatment of Iron Deficiency

Primary prevention of iron deficiency involves ensuring adequate dietary intake of the mineral in all age groups, and selective use of iron supplementation (e.g., in individuals or groups at high risk or when adequate dietary intake is unlikely to be achieved). Primary prevention of iron deficiency is particularly important in children younger than 2 years of age and in women (including adolescents) of childbearing age, including those who are or who are not pregnant. Secondary prevention involves screening for, diagnosing, and treating iron deficiency.

Prevention of Deficiency

The normal US diet, which provides about 12 mg of iron per 2000 calories, is usually sufficient to maintain iron equilibrium in normal adult men and postmenopausal women. Fish, meat (especially liver), and fortified cereals and bread are the best dietary sources of iron. Dietary intake of iron is inadequate and prophylactic iron is required during the first year of life in infants whose diet consists largely of milk and in pregnant women; dietary iron may be marginal in menstruating women. Prophylactic iron therapy may also be required in chronic blood donors. Hemodialysis patients who are receiving therapy with an erythropoiesis-stimulating agent (ESA) (e.g., epoetin alfa, darbepoetin alfa) for anemia of chronic kidney disease may not respond adequately to oral iron therapy and may require parenteral (IV) iron replacement therapy. (See Treatment of Anemia, under Uses: Prevention and Treatment of Iron Deficiency.)

Infants and Young Children. Primary prevention of iron deficiency is most important in children younger than 2 years of age because this age group is at greatest risk for deficiency secondary to inadequate iron intake. To minimize the risk of iron deficiency in infants, exclusive breast feeding (without supplemental liquid, formula, or food) should be encouraged for 4–6 months after birth. In premature or low birthweight (less than 2.5 kg) breast-fed infants, prophylactic iron supplementation with 2–4 mg/kg (not exceeding 15 mg) daily should be initiated by at least 2 months, preferably at 1 month, of age.

When exclusive breast-feeding is stopped in full-term infants, an additional source of iron should be used (about 1 mg/kg daily of iron), preferably from supplementary foods (e.g., iron-fortified formula and/or cereals). In normal full-term infants, iron stores are usually adequate during the first few months of life, but prophylactic iron should be initiated when the infant is about 4–6 months of age. Infants who are not breast-fed or who are only partially breast-fed should receive prophylactic iron, preferably as iron-fortified formula, usually beginning at birth and continuing during the first year of life; iron-fortified formula should be the only type of infant formula used during this period, regardless of when formula-feeding is started. For breast-fed infants who receive insufficient iron from supplementary foods by 6 months of age (i.e., less than 1 mg/kg daily), iron supplementation (e.g., 1 mg/kg daily) is suggested. If breast-feeding is not possible, only iron-fortified formulas should be used during the first year of life, supplementing the formula with foods beginning at 4–6 months of age or once the extrusion reflex disappears.

To improve iron absorption, one feeding daily preferably should include foods rich in ascorbic acid (vitamin C) (e.g., fruits, vegetables, juices), by approximately 6 months of age, given with meals if possible. Plain pureed meats can be introduced to the diet after 6 months of age or when the infant is developmentally ready to consume such food. (See Cautions: Adverse Effects.) Although infants' iron requirements may be provided by use of iron-containing infant formulas or cereals, these preparations should not be relied upon to *treat* iron deficiency if it occurs. Consumption of regular cow's, goat's, or soy milk should be limited to 720 mL (24 oz) daily in children 1–5 years of age.

Older Children and Adolescents. Because of slight increases in iron requirements associated with increases in iron mass related to growth in body size, children and adolescents approximately 10 years of age and older may require prophylactic iron during the pubertal growth spurt and with the start of menstruation in females. However, most adolescents, including menstruating girls, do not require iron supplementation; instead, consumption of iron-rich foods and foods that enhance GI iron absorption should be encouraged.

Pregnant Women. Primary prevention of iron deficiency in pregnant women requires adequate dietary iron intake and iron supplementation. Although conclusive evidence of the benefits of *routine* iron supplementation for all women currently is lacking, routine prophylactic iron supplementation currently is recommended for all *pregnant* women because a large proportion of such women experience difficulty in maintaining iron stores during pregnancy, iron-deficiency anemia during pregnancy is associated with adverse outcomes, and such supplementation during pregnancy is not associated with important health risks.

Prophylactic iron supplementation during pregnancy should be initiated with oral, low-dose (30 mg daily) iron at the initial prenatal visit. Pregnant women also should be encouraged to consume iron-rich foods and foods that enhance GI iron absorption. Pregnant women with low-iron diets should be counseled about optimizing dietary iron intake. If no risk factors for iron deficiency are present at delivery, iron supplementation should be discontinued. Iron supplementation is particularly important for pregnant women who are vegetarians. Women at risk for anemia should be screened postpartum and treated as necessary.

Patients with Anemia of Chronic Kidney Disease. Almost all patients with chronic kidney disease who receive therapy with an ESA (e.g., epoetin alfa, darbepoetin alfa) will require iron therapy because of the dramatic decrease in iron stores associated with erythrocyte formation. Although chronic kidney disease patients with iron overload prior to starting ESA therapy may not require iron supplementation initially, profound iron deficiency may develop subsequently, so monitoring of serum and tissue iron stores is essential during therapy with the drug. Supplemental iron should be administered to prevent iron deficiency and to maintain adequate iron stores in patients with chronic kidney disease who are receiving ESA therapy. (See Uses: Anemia of Chronic Kidney Disease and also see Cautions: Precautions and Contraindications, in Epoetin Alfa 20:16.)

Most hemodialysis patients receiving ESAs require IV iron to maintain iron stores. (See Treatment of Anemia, under Uses: Prevention and Treatment of Iron Deficiency.) Even though a temporary improvement in hematocrit may occur with oral iron therapy, iron depletion resulting from blood loss exceeds the absorption of iron from oral supplements in most ESA-treated hemodialysis patients, and iron stores eventually decrease (as indicated by decreasing serum ferritin concentrations). As negative iron balance continues, iron stores decrease and become inadequate. Although GI absorption of iron does not appear to be impaired in patients with chronic kidney disease, only a small fraction of orally administered iron is absorbed even in individuals without the disease. Consequently, 200 mg of elemental iron (approximately two 325-mg tablets of ferrous fumarate or three 325-mg tablets of ferrous sulfate) ingested daily usually cannot meet the demands of epoetin alfa-induced erythropoiesis in hemodialysis-associated blood losses. Inadequate absorption of oral iron is exacerbated by the fact that patient compliance with oral iron regimens is often poor due to the inconvenience of dosing (i.e., 1 hour before or 2 hours after meals for optimal absorption), adverse effects such as GI irritation and constipation, and costs of therapy.

Some clinicians state that a small percentage of hemodialysis patients, and many predialysis or peritoneal dialysis patients, are able to maintain adequate iron stores using only oral iron supplements, perhaps as a result of augmented intestinal iron absorption, smaller blood losses, and/or lower epoetin alfa requirements.

Other Adults. Most nonpregnant women of childbearing age also do not require iron supplementation, but instead primary prevention of iron deficiency should be through dietary means, encouraging the consumption of iron-rich foods and foods that increase GI iron absorption. Although women with low-iron diets are at additional risk for iron deficiency, counseling such women about optimizing dietary iron intake can be sufficient. Men 18 years of age and older and postmenopausal women usually do not require iron supplementation.

Screening for Anemia

Routine screening currently is recommended by the US Centers for Disease Control (CDC) and American Academy of Pediatrics (AAP) for all infants and children from populations at high risk of iron-deficiency anemia (e.g., those from low-income families, children eligible for the Special Supplemental Nutrition program for Women, Infants, and Children [WIC], recently arrived refugees) beginning at 9–12 months of age and then 6 months later (i.e., at 15–18 months of age) and annually thereafter from 2–5 years of age. AAP also considers *routine* screening an option for all full-term infants, regardless of risk, beginning at 9–12 months of age and repeated 6 months later at 15–18 months of age; continued routine screening beyond this period is not recommended for the general pediatric population because few children older than 2 years of age develop iron deficiency.

Selective screening is recommended by CDC and AAP for selected individuals who reside in communities or under circumstances where the incidence of anemia is low (e.g., 5% or less) and there generally are good dietary practices relative to iron intake but who nonetheless are at risk for iron deficiency. Selective screening is targeted at subsets of children who have a less than satisfactory diet or have special health-care needs and should follow the same schedule as routine screening. Selective screening is recommended for premature or low-birthweight infants, infants fed a diet of nonfortified formula for longer than 2 months, infants introduced to cow's milk before 12 months of age, breast-fed infants whose supplementary diet does not provide adequate iron after 6 months of age, children who consume more than 720 mL (24 oz) of cow's milk daily, and those with special health-care needs such as conditions that interfere with iron absorption, chronic infection, inflammatory disorders, restricted (e.g., nonmeat) diets, or excessive blood loss from a wound, accident, or surgery. Although anemia screening before 6 months of age generally is of little value for detecting iron deficiency because iron stores are adequate for most infants, premature or low-birthweight infants who are not fed iron-fortified formula may benefit from beginning screening before 6 months of age. Children 2–5 years of age not previously identified as being at risk for iron deficiency should be assessed annually for risk factors (e.g., low-iron diet, limited access to food because of poverty or neglect, special health-care needs), screening those who have any such identifiable risk.

Because preadolescent school-age children 5 years of age and older in the US, other than those receiving a very restrictive diet, are at lower risk for iron deficiency than are younger children, *routine* screening for anemia in this age group is not recommended. Instead, anemia screening should be employed *selectively*. Children in this age group who consume a strict vegetarian diet should be screened for iron-deficiency anemia as should those with a history of iron-deficiency anemia, special health-care needs, or low iron intake. Likewise, adolescent males 12 up to 18 years of age generally should be screened selectively, although screening also can be considered during a routine physical examination that coincides with the peak growth period. Iron deficiency is particularly common in children consuming vegan diets, but is less common in lacto-ovo vegetarians.

All nonpregnant females should be screened for iron-deficiency anemia during all routine adolescent physical examinations and every 5–10 years throughout their childbearing years as part of routine health examinations. In addition, women with risk factors for anemia (e.g., extensive menstrual or other blood loss, low iron intake, history of iron-deficiency anemia) should be screened annually.

Pregnant women should be screened for iron-deficiency anemia during the initial prenatal visit. Postpartum women at risk for anemia also should be screened 4–6 weeks postpartum.

Routine screening for iron-deficiency anemia is not recommended for males 18 years of age and older or for postmenopausal women. Iron deficiency or anemia suspected or detected during routine medical examinations should be evaluated fully.

Treatment of Anemia Presumed or confirmed iron-deficiency anemia should be treated with iron, preferably with oral preparations in most patients. However, hemodialysis patients with anemia of chronic kidney disease who are receiving epoetin alfa may have an inadequate response to oral iron and may require parenteral (IV) iron supplementation. (See Patients with Anemia of Chronic Kidney Disease, under Prevention and Treatment of Iron Deficiency: Treatment of Anemia, in Uses.)

Infants and Young Children. Iron-deficiency anemia can be treated presumptively in infants and preschool-age children with 3 mg/kg daily of iron; the parent or guardian should be counseled about adequate diet to correct the underlying problem of low iron intake. If anemia is confirmed by a repeat screening 4 weeks later, dietary counseling should be reinforced and iron treatment should continue for 2 more months, at which time testing should be repeated. Hemoglobin and hematocrit should be reassessed 6 months after completion of successful iron treatment. If iron deficiency is not corrected after 4 weeks of iron treatment in the absence of acute illness (e.g., otitis, diarrhea, upper respiratory tract infection), further diagnostic measures (e.g., mean corpuscular volume [MCV], erythrocyte distribution width [RDW], serum ferritin concentration) should be performed to determine whether the anemia is secondary to iron deficiency.

Older Children and Adolescents. Preadolescent school-age children and adolescent boys up to 18 years of age can be treated presumptively for iron-deficiency anemia with a trial of iron; school-age children 5 up to 12 years of age can receive 60 mg of iron daily and adolescent boys can receive 120 mg daily. Follow-up and laboratory evaluation are the same as those for infants and preschool children. Menstruating adolescent girls 12 up to 18 years of age also can be treated presumptively for anemia with a trial of 60–120 mg of iron daily. Follow-up and laboratory evaluation are the same as those for infants and preschool children, except that iron treatment should continue for 2–3 months longer if anemia is confirmed. If iron deficiency is not corrected after 4 weeks of iron treatment in the absence of acute illness, further diagnostic measures (e.g., mean corpuscular volume [MCV], erythrocyte distribution width [RDW], serum ferritin concentration) should be performed to determine whether the anemia is secondary to iron deficiency.

Pregnant Women. Iron-deficiency anemia can be treated presumptively in pregnant women with 60–120 mg of iron daily. However, if the hemoglobin concentration is less than 9 g/dL or hematocrit is less than 27%, the woman should be referred for further evaluation to a clinician familiar with anemia during pregnancy. If after 4 weeks the anemia does not respond to iron treatment to a level appropriate for the stage of pregnancy despite compliance with an iron treatment regimen in the absence of an acute illness, further diagnostic measures (e.g., mean corpuscular volume [MCV], erythrocyte distribution width [RDW], serum ferritin concentration) should be performed to determine whether the anemia is secondary to iron deficiency. When hemoglobin concentration becomes normal for the stage of pregnancy, iron treatment should be decreased to 30 mg daily. If hemoglobin concentration exceeds 15 g/dL or hematocrit exceeds 45% during the second or third trimester, the woman should be evaluated for potential pregnancy complications related to poor blood volume expansion.

Iron-deficiency anemia in postpartum women should be treated the same as that in nonpregnant women of childbearing age.

Patients with Anemia of Chronic Kidney Disease. Iron supplementation is required in virtually all patients with chronic kidney disease who are undergoing hemodialysis, particularly those receiving ESAs, because of the blood losses associated with hemodialysis and the increased demands for iron resulting from ESA-induced erythropoiesis. While some clinicians state that a trial of oral iron therapy is acceptable in hemodialysis patients, orally administered iron has been reported to be ineffective in maintaining adequate iron stores in such patients. To maintain and achieve adequate hemoglobin concentrations in hemodialysis patients, most of these patients receiving ESAs will require IV iron on a regular basis. (See Uses: Anemia of Chronic Kidney Disease and also see Cautions: Precautions and Contraindications, in Epoetin Alfa 20:16.) Oral iron therapy is not indicated for chronic kidney disease patients who requires maintenance doses of IV iron.

In predialysis and peritoneal dialysis patients with minimal daily iron losses, provision of 200 mg of elemental oral iron per day may be sufficient to replace ongoing losses and support erythropoiesis.

If oral iron is used, some experts state that use of one of the ionic iron salts, such as iron sulfate, fumarate, or gluconate, is preferable since these salts are inexpensive and provide known amounts of elemental iron. Well-controlled studies have not documented that iron polysaccharide is better tolerated (i.e., the incidence of nausea, vomiting, or abdominal discomfort leading to discontinuance is not reduced) than other iron salts.

Other Adults. Nonpregnant women of childbearing age also can be treated presumptively for anemia with a trial of 60–120 mg of iron daily. Follow-up and laboratory evaluation are the same as those for infants and preschool children, except that iron treatment should continue for 2–3 months longer if anemia is confirmed. If iron deficiency is not corrected after 4 weeks of iron treatment in the absence of acute illness, further diagnostic measures (e.g., mean corpuscular volume [MCV], erythrocyte distribution width [RDW], serum ferritin concentration) should be performed to determine whether the anemia is secondary to iron deficiency. In women of African, Mediterranean, or Southeast Asian descent, mild anemia may be secondary to thalassemia minor or sickle-cell trait.

Dietary Requirements. The National Academy of Sciences (NAS) has issued a comprehensive set of Recommended Dietary Allowances (RDAs) as reference values for dietary nutrient intakes since 1941. In 1997, the NAS Food and Nutrition Board (part of the Institute of Medicine [IOM]) announced that they would begin issuing revised nutrient recommendations that would replace RDAs with Dietary Reference Intakes (DRIs). DRIs are reference values that can be used for planning and assessing diets for healthy populations and for many other purposes and that encompass the Estimated Average Requirement (EAR), the Recommended Dietary Allowance (RDA), the Adequate Intake (AI), and the Tolerable Upper Intake Level (UL).

The NAS has established an EAR and RDA for iron for adults, children and adolescents 1–18 years of age, and infants 7–12 months of age based on the need to maintain a normal functional iron concentration but only minimal stores. Physiologic requirements for absorbed iron were calculated by factorial modeling of the components of iron requirement. Components used as factors in the modeling include basal iron losses, menstrual losses, fetal requirements in pregnancy, increased requirement during growth for expansion of blood volume, and/or increased tissue and storage iron. An AI has been established for infants through 6 months of age based on the observed mean iron intake of infants fed principally human milk. (For a definition of Estimated Average Intake, Recommended Dietary Allowance, Adequate Intake, and other reference values for dietary nutrient intakes, see Uses: Dietary Requirements in Folic Acid 88:08.)

The principal goal of maintaining an adequate intake of iron in the US and Canada is to prevent the functional consequences of iron deficiency such as impaired physical work performance, developmental delay, cognitive impairment, or adverse pregnancy outcome. Adequate intake of iron usually can be accomplished through consumption of foodstuffs; however, women usually need iron supplementation during pregnancy. Iron is present in food as part of heme (meat, poultry, fish) or as nonheme iron (vegetables, fruits, milk, cereals). Most grain products in the US are fortified with iron, and about one-half of ingested iron is supplied by iron-fortified breads, cereals, and breakfast bars.

For specific information on currently recommended AI and RDAs of iron for various life-stage and gender groups, see Dosage: Dietary and Replacement Requirements, under Dosage and Administration.

Dosage and Administration

■ **Administration** Oral iron preparations generally should be taken between meals (e.g., 1 hour before or 2 hours after a meal) for maximum absorption but may be taken with or after meals, if necessary, to minimize adverse GI effects. Patients who have difficulty tolerating oral iron supplements also may benefit from smaller, more frequent doses, starting with a lower dose and increasing slowly to the target dose, trying a different form or preparation, or taking the supplement at bedtime.

■ **Dosage** Dosage of oral iron preparations should be expressed in terms of elemental iron. The elemental iron content of the various preparations is approximately:

Table 1.

Drug	Elemental Iron
ferric pyrophosphate	120 mg/g
ferrous gluconate	120 mg/g
ferrous sulfate	200 mg/g
ferrous sulfate, dried	300 mg/g
ferrous fumarate	330 mg/g
ferrous carbonate, anhydrous	480 mg/g
carbonyl iron	1000 mg/g[a]

[a] carbonyl iron is elemental iron, not an iron salt.

Treatment of Iron Deficiency In general, large oral doses of iron, based on calculated deficiency, must be given because of the incomplete and variable absorption of these preparations. The usual therapeutic dosage of elemental iron for adults is 50–100 mg 3 times daily. Smaller dosages (e.g., 60–120 mg daily) also have been recommended, and may be particularly useful for minimizing GI intolerance, but the possibility that iron stores will be replenished at a slower rate should be considered. Iron-deficient children should receive elemental iron in a dosage of 3–6 mg/kg daily given in 3 divided doses. In patients with chronic kidney disease undergoing hemodialysis and receiving epoetin alfa therapy, some experts currently recommend oral iron in a daily dosage of at least 200 mg of elemental iron for adults and 2–3 mg/kg for children and state that the daily dosage should be given in 2 or 3 divided doses. For additional information, see Prevention and Treatment of Iron Deficiency: Treatment of Anemia, in Uses.

With usual oral therapeutic dosages of iron salts, symptoms of iron deficiency usually improve within a few days, peak reticulocytosis occurs in 5–10 days, and the hemoglobin concentration rises after 2–4 weeks. Hemoglobin production usually increases at a rate of 100–200 mg/dL of blood daily; normal hemoglobin values are usually attained in 2 months unless blood loss continues. Because iron stores remain depleted, recurrence of anemia may result if iron therapy is discontinued at this time. In the treatment of severe deficiencies, iron therapy should be continued for approximately 6 months.

If a satisfactory response is not noted after 3 weeks of oral iron therapy, consideration should be given to the possibilities of patient noncompliance, simultaneous blood loss, additional complicating factors, or incorrect diagnosis.

Prevention of Iron Deficiency To prevent iron deficiency, pregnant women generally should receive daily iron supplementation sufficient to maintain the daily dietary iron intake at 30 mg. Normal full-term infants who are not breast-fed or are only partially breast-fed should receive supplemental iron, preferably as iron-fortified formula, in a dosage of 1 mg/kg daily starting at birth and continuing during the first year of life. Premature or low-birthweight infants require 2–4 mg/kg daily starting by at least 2 months, preferably at 1 month, of age. Infants of normal or low birthweight should not receive iron supplementation exceeding 15 mg daily. Children approximately 10 years of age and older who have begun their pubertal growth spurt may require daily iron supplementation of 2 and 5 mg daily in males and females, respectively. For additional information, see Prevention and Treatment of Iron Deficiency: Prevention of Deficiency, in Uses.

Dietary and Replacement Requirements The Adequate Intake (AI) (see Uses: Dietary Requirements) of iron currently recommended by the National Academy of Sciences (NAS) for healthy infants through 6 months of age is 0.27 mg daily. The Recommended Dietary Allowance (RDA) of iron currently recommended by NAS for healthy children 7–12 months of age, 1–3 years, 4–8 years, or 9–13 years of age is 11, 7, 10, or 8 mg daily, respectively. The RDA of iron for boys 14–18 years of age is 11 mg daily, and the RDA for girls 14–18 years of age is 15 mg daily. The RDA for healthy men of all ages (19–70 years of age and those older than 70 years of age) is 8 mg of iron daily. The RDA for healthy women 19–50 years of age is 18 mg of iron daily, and the RDA for healthy women 51–70 years of age and those older than 70 years of age is 8 mg daily.

The RDA of iron recommended by the NAS for pregnant women 14–50 years of age is 27 mg daily. The NAS recommends an RDA of 10 or 9 mg of iron daily for lactating women 14–18 or 19–50 years of age, respectively.

Cautions

■ GI Effects

Usual oral therapeutic dosages of iron preparations produce constipation, diarrhea, dark stools, nausea, and/or epigastric pain in approximately 5–20% of patients. GI intolerance of all iron preparations is mainly a function of the total amount of elemental iron per dose and of psychological factors. Adverse GI effects usually subside within a few days. If necessary, they can be reduced or eliminated by ingesting iron after meals instead of between meals, by reducing the daily dosage for a few days, or by decreasing the size of the individual dose and increasing the number of doses daily.

Claims for prolonged action and reduced incidence of adverse effects with extended-release and enteric-coated preparations are not well substantiated. The low incidence of adverse effects associated with these preparations may reflect the small amount of iron released or the low total dose of elemental iron.

Large amounts of iron exert a strong corrosive action on the GI mucosa. Administration of Fero-Gradumet® has resulted in a perforated jejunal diverticulum in at least one patient and a Meckel's diverticulum with localized gangrene in at least one other patient. Liquid iron preparations may temporarily stain dental enamel or the membrane covering the teeth of infants.

■ Hemosiderosis

Long-term administration of large amounts of iron may cause hemosiderosis clinically resembling hemochromatosis, which is a genetic condition characterized by excessive iron absorption, excess tissue iron stores, and potential tissue injury. Iron overload is particularly likely to occur in patients given excessive amounts of parenteral iron, in those taking both oral and parenteral preparations, and in patients with hemoglobinopathies or other refractory anemias that might be erroneously diagnosed as iron deficiency anemia. Iron overload is associated with an increased susceptibility to certain infections (e.g., those caused by *Vibrio vulnificus*, *Yersinia enterocolitica*, or *Y. pseudotuberculosis*). Iron overload also may adversely affect prognosis in patients infected with human immunodeficiency virus (HIV). Since there is no excretory mechanism for iron, therapeutic removal by repeated phlebotomy or long-term administration of deferoxamine is necessary to prevent or reverse tissue damage if hemosiderosis occurs.

■ Other Adverse Effects

Administration of iron preparations to premature infants who normally have low serum vitamin E concentrations may cause increased red cell hemolysis and hemolytic anemia. Therefore, vitamin E deficiency should also be corrected if possible. Because vitamin E may not be well absorbed from the GI tract in these infants and oral iron may reduce vitamin E absorption, IM administration of the vitamin may be advisable.

■ Precautions and Contraindications

Administration of iron for longer than 6 months should be avoided except in patients with continued bleeding, menorrhagia, or repeated pregnancies. Iron should not be used to treat hemolytic anemias unless an iron-deficient state also exists, since excess storage of iron with possible secondary hemochromatosis can result. Iron should not be administered to patients receiving repeated blood transfusions, since there is a considerable amount of iron in the hemoglobin of transfused erythrocytes. Some manufacturers state that iron preparations usually are contraindicated in patients with peptic ulcer, regional enteritis, or ulcerative colitis. Parenteral iron should not be administered concomitantly with oral iron therapy.

Although primary hemochromatosis has been considered a contraindication to iron preparations, there currently is no evidence that iron fortification of foods or the use of a recommended low-dose iron supplementation regimen during pregnancy is associated with increased risk for hemochromatosis-associated clinical disease. Even when dietary iron intake is approximately average, individuals with hemochromatosis-associated iron overload will require phlebotomy to reduce their iron stores.

Because accidental overdosage of iron-containing preparations is a leading cause of fatal poisoning in children younger than 6 years of age, patients should be advised to keep such preparations out of reach of children. If accidental overdosage occurs, a poison control center or clinician should be contacted immediately.

Because iron can increase the pathogenicity of certain microorganisms and has been postulated as potentially adversely affecting prognosis in certain HIV-infected individuals, some clinicians recommend that HIV-infected individuals who do not have documented iron-deficiency anemia avoid iron supplementation for the management of HIV-associated anemia.

Fergon® 225-mg tablets contain the dye tartrazine (FD&C yellow No. 5), which may cause allergic reactions including bronchial asthma in susceptible individuals. Although the incidence of tartrazine sensitivity is low, it frequently occurs in patients who are sensitive to aspirin.

Drug Interactions

■ Antacids and Other GI Drugs

Concurrent administration of antacids or aluminum-containing phosphate binders with oral iron preparations may decrease iron absorption. Antacids and oral iron preparations should be administered as far apart as possible.

Drugs such as H_2-receptor antagonists and proton-pump inhibitors increase gastric pH and possibly may decrease the GI absorption of oral iron preparations that depend on gastric acidity for dissolution and absorption. The clinical importance of this potential interaction has not been fully determined. Some clinicians recommend that oral iron preparations be given at least 1 hour prior to these drugs if concomitant therapy is necessary.

■ Methyldopa

Results of one crossover study in healthy adults indicate that concomitant administration of a single oral dose of ferrous sulfate (325 mg) or ferrous gluconate (600 mg) can decrease oral absorption of methyldopa (500 mg) by 61–73%. In addition, concomitant administration of either oral iron preparation appears to affect metabolism of methyldopa since there was a 79–88% decrease in urinary excretion of free methyldopa and an increase in urinary excretion of the sulfate conjugate of the drug. When oral ferrous sulfate therapy (325 mg every 8 hours) was initiated in hypertensive patients receiving chronic methyldopa therapy (250 mg 1–3 times daily or 500 mg 3 times daily), there was an increase in blood pressure during concomitant therapy and an decrease in blood pressure when the oral iron preparation was discontinued. Although further study is needed to evaluate the clinical importance of this drug interaction, the fact that oral iron preparations apparently can decrease the hypotensive effect of methyldopa probably should be considered in situations when the drugs might be used concomitantly (e.g., pregnant women being treated for hypertension, geriatric patients with hypertension).

■ Quinolones

Concomitant administration of oral preparations containing iron may interfere with oral absorption of some quinolone anti-infective agents (e.g., ciprofloxacin, norfloxacin, ofloxacin) resulting in decreased serum and urine concentrations of the quinolones. Therefore, oral preparations containing iron should not be ingested concomitantly with or within 2 hours of a dose of an oral quinolone. In one crossover study, concomitant administration of a single dose of oral ferrous sulfate complex with ofloxacin decreased the area under the concentration-time curve (AUC) of the anti-infective agent by 36%.

■ Tetracyclines

Oral administration of iron preparations inhibits absorption of tetracyclines from the GI tract and vice versa, leading to decreased serum concentrations of both the antibiotic and iron. If simultaneous administration of the drugs is necessary, patients should receive the tetracycline 3 hours after or 2 hours before oral iron administration.

■ **Thyroid Agents** Concomitant administration of ferrous sulfate (300 mg once daily) in patients with primary hypothyroidism receiving thyroxine replacement therapy (0.075–0.15 mg of l-thyroxine daily) resulted in an increase in serum concentrations of thyrotropin (thyroid-stimulating hormone, TSH) and increased signs and symptoms of hypothyroidism. Although the free thyroxine index (FTI) was decreased in some patients after 12 weeks of concomitant therapy, the extent of this reduction was not clinically important; free serum thyroxine concentration and resin triiodothyronine uptake (RT_3U) were not substantially affected by concomitant therapy. It has been suggested that thyroxine and ferrous sulfate (and possibly other oral iron preparations) may form an insoluble ferric-thyroxine complex in vivo resulting in decreased absorption of thyroxine. If concomitant administration of oral iron preparations and thyroxine replacement therapy is necessary (e.g., geriatric patients, premature infants, pregnant women), doses of the drugs probably should be administered at least 2 hours apart and thyroid function should be monitored.

■ **Vitamin C** Concurrent administration of more than 200 mg of ascorbic acid per 30 mg of elemental iron increases absorption of iron from the GI tract. However, most individuals are able to absorb orally ingested iron adequately without concurrent administration of ascorbic acid, and preparations containing iron and ascorbic acid may not contain sufficient quantities of ascorbic acid to substantially affect iron absorption. Inclusion of foods rich in vitamin C in the diet of infants has been suggested as a possible means of increasing GI iron absorption.

■ **Chloramphenicol** Response to iron therapy may be delayed in patients receiving chloramphenicol. Therefore, chloramphenicol therapy should be avoided, if possible, in patients with iron-deficiency anemia receiving iron therapy.

■ **Penicillamine** Orally administered iron decreases the cupruretic effect of penicillamine, probably by decreasing its absorption. Therefore, at least 2 hours should elapse between administration of penicillamine and iron.

Laboratory Test Interferences

Iron preparations color the feces black, and large amounts may interfere with tests used for detection of occult blood in the stools. The guaiac test occasionally yields false-positive tests for blood, whereas results with the benzidine test are not likely to be affected by iron medication.

Acute Toxicity

■ **Pathogenesis** Following acute overdosage, most iron preparations are probably equally toxic per unit of elemental iron. Some studies in animals suggest that carbonyl iron may be less toxic than iron salts because of the mechanism of absorption of carbonyl iron, but comparative studies between these formulations in humans generally are lacking. The acute lethal dose of elemental iron in humans is estimated to be 180–300 mg/kg. However, a dose of elemental iron as low as 30 mg/kg may be toxic in some individuals, and ingestion of doses as low as 60 mg/kg have resulted in death.

Iron is the most common cause of pediatric poisoning deaths reported to US poison control centers. In 1991, there were 5144 cases of accidental ingestion of oral iron preparations reported; 11 of these were fatal.Although many reported fatalities in children have been associated with accidental ingestion of 30 or more tablets of an oral iron preparation containing 60 mg of elemental iron per tablet (total dose 1.8 g or more of elemental iron), ingestion of as few as 5 or 6 tablets of a high-potency preparation could be fatal for a 10-kg child. Serious toxicity and/or death have occurred after accidental ingestion of oral iron preparations as well as multivitamin preparations (including prenatal vitamins) containing iron.

Toxicity occurring with acute iron overdosage results from a combination of the corrosive effects on the GI mucosa and the metabolic and hemodynamic effects caused by the presence of excessive elemental iron.

■ **Manifestations** The clinical course of acute iron poisoning has 4 distinct phases. Signs and symptoms may occur within 10–60 minutes or may be delayed several hours.

During the first phase, which may last 6–8 hours after ingestion, the patient experiences acute GI irritation including epigastric pain, nausea, vomiting, diarrhea of green and subsequently tarry stools, melena, and hematemesis which may be associated with drowsiness, pallor, cyanosis, lassitude, seizures, shock, and coma. Local erosion of the stomach and small intestine may result in increased iron absorption.

If death does not occur during the first phase, there may be a transient period of apparent recovery which may last up to 24 hours after ingestion (second phase). CNS abnormalities, metabolic acidosis, hepatic dysfunction or necrosis, renal failure, and bleeding diathesis occur during the third phase from 4–48 hours after ingestion and may progress to cardiovascular collapse, coma, and death.

Late complications of iron intoxication (fourth phase) occurring 2–6 weeks after overdosage include intestinal obstruction, pyloric stenosis, hepatic cirrhosis, or severe gastric scarring.

■ **Treatment** Careful assessment of the severity of acute iron poisoning (the patient's clinical status, based on the estimated amount of iron ingested, abdominal radiographs, and measurement of serum iron concentrations and iron binding capacity) is necessary to determine appropriate management of the patient and to avoid unnecessary treatment. Patients who develop vomiting, diarrhea, leukocytosis (leukocyte count exceeding 15,000/mm^3), hyperglycemia (blood glucose concentration exceeding 150 mg/dL), and/or an abdominal radiograph positive for iron within 6 hours of iron ingestion are likely to have a serum iron concentration exceeding 300 mcg/dL and to be at risk of serious toxicity, while those who do not develop any of these signs are unlikely to have a serum iron concentration exceeding 300 mcg/dL or to be at risk of toxicity requiring treatment. A negative deferoxamine challenge (see Deferoxamine Mesylate 64:00) or iron screening test obtained within 2 hours of ingestion also indicates that the patient has not ingested a clinically important amount of iron and probably does not require further assessment or treatment.

If ingestion exceeding 10 mg/kg of elemental iron has occurred within the previous 4 hours, the stomach should be emptied immediately by ipecac-induced emesis or, preferably, by lavage with a large bore tube. If the patient has had multiple episodes of vomiting, and especially if the vomitus contains blood, ipecac syrup should not be administered. Gastric lavage should be performed with tepid water or 1–5% sodium bicarbonate solution. Gastric lavage with disodium phosphate solution has also been used; however, administration of large volumes of this lavage solution has produced life-threatening hyperphosphatemia and hypocalcemia in some children. Although some clinicians suggest that use of sodium bicarbonate solution for gastric lavage generally appears to have no advantage compared with water for the treatment of iron overdose, the value of sodium bicarbonate solution in reducing iron absorption via formation of insoluble iron complexes remains to be established. Deferoxamine has also been used as an additive to gastric lavage solutions to chelate elemental iron in the GI tract; however, the efficacy of this procedure has not been clearly established. (See Deferoxamine Mesylate 64:00.) The possibility that gastric lavage may not remove enteric-coated and/or extended-release preparations should be considered. Whole gut lavage with 0.9% sodium chloride solution, administration of a saline cathartic, or surgical removal of iron tablets (which are visible in abdominal radiographs) may be required if other methods of removing the drug are unsuccessful. Hemodialysis is of little value in the treatment of iron intoxication.

When a potentially lethal dose of iron (180–300 mg/kg or more of elemental iron) has been ingested, serum iron concentrations exceed 400–500 mcg/dL or serum iron concentrations exceed total iron binding capacity, and/or the patient has severe symptoms of iron intoxication such as coma, shock, or seizures, chelation therapy with deferoxamine should be initiated. (See Deferoxamine Mesylate 64:00.) Supportive treatment including suction and maintenance of airway, correction of acidosis, and control of shock and dehydration with IV fluids or blood, oxygen, and vasopressors should be administered as required.

Pharmacology

Iron is present in all cells and has several vital functions. Ionic iron is a component of a number of enzymes necessary for energy transfer (e.g., cytochrome oxidase, xanthine oxidase, succinic dehydrogenase) and is also present in compounds necessary for transport and utilization of oxygen (e.g., hemoglobin, myoglobin). Cytochromes serve as a transport medium for electrons within cells. Hemoglobin is a carrier of oxygen from the lungs to tissues and myoglobin facilitates oxygen use and storage in muscle. Iron deficiency can interfere with these vital functions and lead to morbidity and mortality.

Administration of iron preparations corrects erythropoietic abnormalities caused by a deficiency of iron. Iron does not stimulate erythropoiesis nor does it correct hemoglobin disturbances not caused by iron deficiency. Administration of iron also relieves other manifestations of iron deficiency such as soreness of the tongue, dysphagia, dystrophy of the nails and skin, and fissuring of the angles of the lips.

Iron is vital for microorganisms such as bacteria, and the mineral plays a role both in bacterial pathogenicity and in host defense mechanisms. (See Cautions: Hemosiderosis.)

Pharmacokinetics

■ **Absorption** Regulation of iron balance occurs mainly in the GI tract through absorption. When GI absorption is normal, functional iron is maintained and there is a tendency to establish iron stores.

Absorption of iron is complex and is influenced by many factors including the form in which it is administered, the dose, iron stores, the degree of erythropoiesis, and diet. Oral bioavailability of iron can vary from less than 1% to greater than 50%, and the principal factor controlling GI iron absorption is the amount of iron stored in the body. GI absorption of iron increases when body iron stores are low and decreases when stores are sufficient or large. Increased erythrocyte production also can stimulate GI absorption of iron by severalfold.

Approximately 5–13% of dietary iron is absorbed in healthy individuals and about 10–30% in iron-deficient individuals. Among adults, dietary iron absorption averages approximately 6% for males and 13% for nonpregnant females of childbearing potential; the higher GI absorption efficiency in these women principally results from lower body stores secondary to menstruation and pregnancy. GI absorption of iron increases during pregnancy to compensate for tissue growth and blood loss at delivery and postpartum, but the extent of this increase is not well defined; as iron stores become replenished postpartum, GI iron absorption decreases. GI iron absorption also is increased in iron-deficient individuals. As much as 60% of a therapeutic dose of an iron salt may be absorbed in iron-deficient patients; however, absorption of inorganic iron is decreased when it is administered with many foods and with some drugs. (See Drug Interactions.)

Inorganic iron reportedly is absorbed up to twice as well as dietary iron. Although the precise form in which iron is absorbed has not been elucidated, ferrous iron appears to be most readily absorbed. Oral bioavailability of iron also depends on dietary composition. Heme iron, which is present in meat, poultry, and fish, is absorbed 2–3 times more readily than non-heme iron, which is present in plant-based and iron-fortified foods. GI absorption of iron can be enhanced by dietary heme iron and vitamin C and can be inhibited by polyphenols (e.g., from certain vegetables), tannins (e.g., from tea), phytates (e.g., from bran), and calcium (e.g., from dairy products). Vegetarian diets are low in heme iron, but iron bioavailability can be increased by including other sources of iron and enhancers of GI iron absorption. Prior to the introduction of solid foods into the diet, the amount of iron absorbed in infants depends on the amount of iron present in breast milk or formula.

Although absorption of iron can occur along the entire length of the GI tract, it is greatest in the duodenum and proximal jejunum and becomes progressively less distally. Enteric-coated and some extended-release preparations may transport iron past the duodenum and proximal jejunum, thus reducing iron absorption.

Following oral administration, carbonyl iron is dissolved in gastric secretions (i.e., hydrochloric acid) and converted to the hydrochloride salt prior to absorption from the stomach. The rate of absorption is affected by gastric acid production and the equilibrium between the formation of ionized iron and passage of the ionized iron to the intestine. Also affecting absorption is the particle size of carbonyl iron; a smaller particle size will be ionized more rapidly and thus absorbed more rapidly than formulations with a larger particle size.

The mechanisms involved in iron absorption have not been completely elucidated; however, two mechanisms, which are believed to operate simultaneously, appear to be involved. An active transport process with enzymatic or carrier characteristics occurs principally with normal dietary concentrations of iron; a first-order passive transport process occurs principally with doses of iron exceeding those in a normal diet.

■ **Distribution** Ferrous iron passes through GI mucosal cells directly into the blood and is immediately bound to transferrin. Transferrin, a glycoprotein β_1-globulin, transports iron to the bone marrow where it is incorporated into hemoglobin. When sufficient iron is present to meet the body's needs, most iron (greater than 70%) in the body is present as functional iron, with greater than 80% of functional iron existing in erythrocytes as hemoglobin and the rest existing in myoglobin and intracellular respiratory enzymes (e.g., cytochromes); less than 1% of total body iron is present in enzymes. The remainder of body iron is present as storage or transport iron. Total body iron is determined by intake, loss, and storage of the mineral.

Small excesses of iron within the villous epithelial cells are oxidized to the ferric state. Ferric iron combines with the protein apoferritin to yield ferritin and is stored in mucosal cells, which are exfoliated at the end of their life span and excreted in the feces. Ferritin, a soluble protein complex, is the principal storage form of iron (about 70% in men and 80% in women), with smaller amounts being stored in hemosiderin, an insoluble protein complex. Ferritin and hemosiderin are present principally in the liver, reticuloendothelial system, bone marrow, spleen, and skeletal muscle; small amounts of ferritin also circulate in plasma. When long-term negative iron balance occurs, iron stores are depleted before hemoglobin concentration is reduced or iron deficiency ensues. In women, the iron storage reserve tends to be substantially less than that in men (about 0.2–0.4 g versus 1–4 g of iron), and is even less in children. Total body iron in full-term infants with normal or high birthweight is relatively high (averaging 75 mg/kg), to which iron stores contribute about 25%. Premature or low-birthweight infants are born with the same ratio of total body iron to body weight, but the amount of stored iron is low because of low body weight.

The body of a healthy adult man contains approximately 3.8 g total or 50 mg/kg; that of an adult woman contains about 2.3 g total or 35–42 mg/kg. Iron exists in humans almost exclusively complexed to protein or in heme molecules. Approximately 70% is in hemoglobin, 25% in iron stores as ferritin and hemosiderin, 4% in myoglobin, 0.5% in heme enzymes, and 0.1% in transferrin. Erythrocyte formation and destruction is responsible for most iron turnover in the body. In adult males, about 95% of the iron required for erythropoiesis is recycled from the breakdown of erythrocytes and only 5% comes from oral intake. In infants, about 70% of iron required for erythropoiesis is recycled from the breakdown of erythrocytes and about 30% from oral intake.

About 0.15–0.3 mg of iron is distributed into milk daily.

Transfer of iron across the placenta is believed to be an active process since it occurs against a concentration gradient. The total iron requirement for pregnancy may be 440 mg to 1.05 g.

■ **Elimination** Iron metabolism occurs in a virtually closed system. Most of the iron liberated by destruction of hemoglobin is conserved and reused by the body. Daily excretion of iron in healthy men amounts to only 0.5–2 mg. This excretion occurs principally through feces and as desquamation of cells such as skin, GI mucosa, nails, and hair; only trace amounts of iron are excreted in bile and sweat.

Blood loss greatly increases iron loss. The average monthly loss of iron in normal menstruation is 12–30 mg, increasing the average iron requirement by 0.3–0.5 mg daily to compensate for this loss. The increased requirement secondary to pregnancy-associated tissue growth and blood loss at delivery and postpartum averages 3 mg daily over 280 days of gestation. In healthy individuals, trace amounts of blood are lost through physiologic GI loss secondary to normal turnover of intestinal mucosa. Pathologic GI blood loss occurs in infants and children sensitive to cow's milk and in adults secondary to peptic ulcer disease, inflammatory bowel syndrome, and GI cancer. Hookworm infections also are associated with blood loss.

Chemistry and Stability

■ **Chemistry** Ferrous fumarate, ferrous gluconate, ferrous sulfate, carbonyl iron, and polysaccharide-iron complex are commercially available in the US for oral administration in the prevention and treatment of iron deficiency. Ferric pyrophosphate and ferrous carbonate are available only as components of combination products.

Ferrous Fumarate Ferrous fumarate occurs as a reddish-orange to red-brown, odorless powder. It may contain soft lumps that produce a yellow streak when crushed. The drug is slightly soluble in water and very slightly soluble in alcohol.

Ferrous Gluconate Ferrous gluconate occurs as a yellowish-gray or pale greenish-yellow fine powder or granules with a slight odor of burned sugar. The drug is soluble in water with slight heating and practically insoluble in alcohol.

Ferrous Sulfate Ferrous sulfate occurs as pale bluish-green, odorless crystals or granules which have a saline, styptic taste. The drug is efflorescent in dry air. Ferrous sulfate is freely soluble in water and insoluble in alcohol. Dried ferrous sulfate, which contains 86–89% anhydrous ferrous sulfate, occurs as a grayish-white to buff-colored powder which dissolves slowly in water and is insoluble in alcohol. Ferrous sulfate contains 7 molecules of water of hydration; dried ferrous sulfate consists mainly of the monohydrate with varying amounts of the tetrahydrate.

Carbonyl Iron Carbonyl iron consists of microparticles of elemental iron; it is not an iron salt. Carbonyl iron is produced by a manufacturing process involving the controlled heating of vaporized iron pentacarbonyl, which is designed to result in the deposition of unchanged elemental iron as microscopic spheres of less than 5 μm in diameter. Carbonyl iron prepared for pharmaceutical or nutritional use in the US reportedly has an average particle size of 5–6 μm.

Polysaccharide-Iron Complex Polysaccharide-iron complex occurs as an amorphous brown powder and is very soluble in water and insoluble in alcohol.

■ **Stability** ***Ferrous Sulfate*** In moist air, ferrous sulfate rapidly oxidizes and becomes coated with brownish-yellow ferric sulfate which must not be used medicinally. The rate of oxidation is increased by the addition of alkali or by exposure to light.

Preparations

Excipients in commercially available drug preparations may have clinically important effects in some individuals; consult specific product labeling for details.

Carbonyl Iron

Oral		
Suspension	15 mg (of iron) per 1.25 mL	**Icar® Pediatric,** Hawthorn
Tablets	45 mg (of iron)	**Feosol® Caplets,** GlaxoSmithKline
Tablets, chewable	15 mg (of iron)	**Icar® Pediatric,** Hawthorn

Ferrous Fumarate

Oral		
Tablets	200 mg (66 mg iron)	**Ircon®**, Kenwood
	324 mg (106 mg iron)*	**Hemocyte®**, US Pharmaceutical
	325 mg (107 mg iron)*	**Ferrous Fumarate Tablets**
	350 mg (115 mg iron)	**Nephro-Fer®**, R&D Labs
Tablets, chewable	100 mg (33 mg iron)	**Feostat®**, Forest

*available from one or more manufacturer, distributor, and/or repackager by generic (nonproprietary) name

Ferrous Fumarate Combinations

Oral		
Capsules, extended-release	150 mg (50 mg iron) with Docusate Sodium 100 mg*	**Ferrous Fumarate with DSS® Timed Capsules,** Vita-Rx
Tablets, extended-release, film-coated	150 mg (50 mg iron) with Docusate Sodium 100 mg	**Ferro-DSS® Caplets®**, Time-Caps
		Ferro-Sequels®, Inverness

*available from one or more manufacturer, distributor, and/or repackager by generic (nonproprietary) name

Ferrous Gluconate

Powder		
Oral		
Tablets	225 mg (27 mg iron)	**Fergon®**, Bayer
		Ferrous Gluconate Tablets
	300 mg (35 mg iron)	**Ferrous Gluconate Tablets**
	320 mg (37 mg iron)*	
	325 mg (38 mg iron)*	

*available from one or more manufacturer, distributor, and/or repackager by generic (nonproprietary) name

Ferrous Sulfate

Powder		
Oral		
Solution	220 mg (44 mg iron) per 5 mL*	**Ferrous Sulfate Elixir**
	300 mg (60 mg iron) per 5 mL	**Ferrous Sulfate Solution**
	125 mg (25 mg iron) per mL*	**Fer-Gen-Sol® Drops,** Teva
		Fer-In-Sol® Drops, Mead Johnson
Tablets	195 mg (39 mg iron)*	**Mol-Iron®**, Schering-Plough
	300 mg (60 mg iron)*	**Feratab®**, Upsher-Smith
	325 mg (65 mg iron)*	
Tablets, enteric-coated	325 mg (65 mg iron)*	**Ferrous Sulfate Tablets EC**
Tablets, film-coated	325 mg (65 mg iron)	**Ferrous Sulfate Tablets**

*available from one or more manufacturer, distributor, and/or repackager by generic (nonproprietary) name

Ferrous Sulfate, Dried

Oral		
Capsules	190 mg (60 mg iron)	
Tablets	200 mg (65 mg iron)	**Feosol®**, GlaxoSmithKline
Tablets, extended-release	160 mg (50 mg iron)	**Slow FE®**, Novartis

Polysaccharide-iron Complex

Oral		
Capsules	150 mg (of iron)	**Ferrex®-150,** Breckenridge
		Fe-Tinic® 150, Ethex
		Hytinic®, Hyrex
		Niferex®-150, Ther-Rx
Solution	100 mg (of iron) per 5 mL	**Niferex® Elixir,** Ther-Rx
Tablets, film-coated	50 mg (of iron)	**Niferex®**, Ther-Rx

Oral iron preparations are also commercially available in combination with vitamins and minerals and oral contraceptives.

Selected Revisions October 2017,

Iron Sucrose

Iron Saccharate, Iron Sucron Complex

■ Iron sucrose, a polynuclear iron (III)-hydroxide sucrose complex, is used to replenish and maintain the total body content of iron and has pharmacologic actions similar to those of other parenteral iron preparations.

Uses

■ **Iron Deficiency Anemia in Patients with Chronic Kidney Disease** Iron sucrose injection is used for the treatment of iron deficiency anemia in patients with chronic kidney disease, including those who are undergoing dialysis (hemodialysis or peritoneal) and those who do not require dialysis. In several randomized controlled studies comparing IV and oral administration of iron in patients with chronic kidney disease undergoing hemodialysis, IV iron was superior to orally administered iron in increasing hemoglobin concentrations and/or minimizing the dosage of an erythropoiesis-stimulating agent (ESA) (e.g., epoetin alfa) required to maintain target hemoglobin levels; guidelines for the treatment of anemia of chronic kidney disease from the National Kidney Foundation Kidney Disease Outcomes Quality Initiative (NKF-KDOQI) state that the IV route is preferred for administration of iron in patients with chronic kidney disease undergoing hemodialysis. (See Uses: Iron Deficiency Anemia in Hemodialysis Patients Receiving Epoetin Alfa Therapy, in Sodium Ferric Gluconate 20:04.04.) Although published clinical studies do not permit a reliable comparison of iron sucrose with other parenteral iron preparations (e.g., iron dextran, sodium ferric gluconate), it has been suggested that these iron preparations may have comparable efficacy but different safety profiles. Available data suggest that iron sucrose and sodium ferric gluconate may be associated less frequently with serious adverse effects (e.g., hypersensitivity reactions) than iron dextran. (See Sensitivity Reactions under Warnings/Precautions: Warnings, in Cautions and also see Cautions: Sensitivity Reactions, in Sodium Ferric Gluconate 20:04.04.)

Efficacy and safety of iron sucrose injection for the treatment of iron deficiency anemia have been established in several open-label, multicenter clinical trials in patients with chronic kidney disease, both in dialysis-dependent (hemodialysis or peritoneal dialysis) adults and in adults who did not require dialysis (non-dialysis dependent). In dialysis-dependent patients, increases in mean hemoglobin, hematocrit, serum ferritin, and transferrin saturation (TSAT) from baseline were observed following iron sucrose therapy (e.g., consisting of 100-mg doses given at consecutive dialysis treatment sessions for a cumulative elemental iron dosage of 1 g); most patients in these studies were receiving an ESA prior to study enrollment and continued to receive such therapy at either the same dosage or an adjusted dosage based on study protocol or the investigator's discretion. In one of these studies, 66% of hemodialysis patients receiving iron sucrose therapy achieved a target hemoglobin concentration exceeding 11 g/dL within 5 weeks of completing iron sucrose therapy (the primary study end point); 78% of patients attained this target hemoglobin level at one or more intervals after the treatment period. Compared with a historical control group of patients with similar ferritin levels who were receiving epoetin alfa but who had not received IV iron for at least 2 weeks, patients receiving iron sucrose therapy in this study achieved greater increases in hemoglobin and hematocrit; the mean change in hemoglobin concentration at the 5-week follow-up evaluation was 1.2 or −0.1 g/dL for the iron sucrose or historical control group, respectively. In another study in patients with hemodialysis-dependent chronic kidney disease, substantial increases from baseline in mean hemoglobin (1.7 g/dL), hematocrit (5%), serum ferritin (434.6 ng/mL), and TSAT (14%) were observed by week 2 of the observation period and maintained at week 4 (the final evaluation). Results of a study comparing IV iron and an ESA with ESA therapy alone in patients undergoing peritoneal dialysis demonstrated superiority of the iron sucrose/ESA regimen compared with ESA alone in increasing mean hemoglobin concentrations from baseline. In a study conducted in non-dialysis-dependent chronic kidney disease patients, treatment with iron sucrose (with or without ESA therapy) was more effective than an oral iron preparation (i.e., ferrous sulfate) in increasing hemoglobin concentrations. Response to IV iron appears to be more vigorous in patients with TSATs less than 20% compared with those having higher TSATs.

Iron sucrose injection also is used as iron *maintenance* therapy in children with dialysis-dependent (hemodialysis or peritoneal dialysis) or non-dialysis-dependent chronic kidney disease. (See Pediatric Use under Warnings/Precautions: Specific Populations, in Cautions.)

Dosage and Administration

■ **General** Iron sucrose is administered by slow IV injection or IV infusion.

When given by IV injection, the drug is administered undiluted at a slow rate (e.g., over 2–5 minutes). (See Cardiovascular Effects under Warnings/Precautions: Warnings, in Cautions.)

When given by IV infusion, iron sucrose should be diluted in 0.9% sodium chloride injection; specific recommendations for dilution and administration of the drug by IV infusion vary depending on the intended patient population (e.g., hemodialysis-dependent adults, peritoneal dialysis-dependent adults, non-dialysis-dependent adults, pediatric patients). (See Dosage and Administration: Dosage.) Iron sucrose injection should not be mixed with other drugs or added to parenteral nutrition solutions for IV infusion. Iron sucrose injection and diluted solutions of the drug should be inspected visually for particulate matter and discoloration prior to administration whenever solution and container permit.

Although the manufacturer does not make any specific recommendations regarding a test dose of iron sucrose, test doses of 20–25 or 50 mg have been administered in some clinical trials. (See Sensitivity Reactions under Warnings/Precautions: Warnings, in Cautions.) The manufacturer states that personnel trained to provide emergency treatment and appropriate agents for the treatment of a severe allergic or anaphylactic reaction should be immediately available whenever iron sucrose is administered.

■ **Dosage** Dosage of iron sucrose is expressed in terms of mg of elemental iron. Iron sucrose injection contains the equivalent of 20 mg of elemental iron per mL.

For the treatment of iron deficiency anemia in hemodialysis-dependent adults with chronic kidney disease, the recommended dosage of iron sucrose is 100 mg administered by slow IV injection (over 2–5 minutes) or by IV infusion (diluted in a maximum of 100 mL of 0.9% sodium chloride injection) over at least 15 minutes during each consecutive hemodialysis session. Doses should be administered early during the dialysis procedure. A cumulative dose of 1 g of iron sucrose usually is required to achieve a favorable response in these patients.

In peritoneal dialysis-dependent adults with chronic kidney disease, a series of 3 doses of iron sucrose should be administered by IV infusion (diluted in a maximum of 250 mL of 0.9% sodium chloride injection) 14 days apart over a 28-day period. Patients should receive 300 mg of iron sucrose by IV infusion over 1.5 hours for the first 2 doses, followed by a dose of 400 mg administered over 2.5 hours.

For the treatment of iron deficiency anemia in adults with non-dialysis-dependent chronic kidney disease, the recommended dosage of iron sucrose is 200 mg administered by slow IV injection (over 2–5 minutes) or by IV infusion (diluted in a maximum of 100 mL of 0.9% sodium chloride injection and administered over 15 minutes) for a total of 5 doses; doses should be administered on 5 different occasions over a 14-day period. Iron sucrose also has been administered as a 2-dose regimen in a limited number of patients with non-dialysis-dependent chronic kidney disease; in this regimen, 500 mg of iron sucrose is administered by IV infusion (diluted in a maximum of 250 mL of 0.9% sodium chloride injection and administered over 3.5–4 hours) on days 1 and 14.

For iron *maintenance* therapy in children 2 years of age or older with hemodialysis-dependent chronic kidney disease, the recommended dosage of iron sucrose is 0.5 mg/kg (not to exceed 100 mg per dose) every 2 weeks for 12 weeks; doses may be administered undiluted by slow IV injection over 5 minutes or diluted in 25 mL of 0.9% sodium chloride injection and administered over 5–60 minutes.

For iron *maintenance* therapy in children 2 years of age or older with non-dialysis-dependent chronic kidney disease or peritoneal dialysis-dependent chronic kidney disease who are receiving supplemental erythropoiesis-stimulating agent (ESA) therapy, the recommended dosage of iron sucrose is 0.5 mg/kg (not to exceed 100 mg per dose) every 4 weeks for 12 weeks; doses may be administered undiluted by slow IV injection over 5 minutes or diluted in 25 mL of 0.9% sodium chloride injection and administered over 5–60 minutes.

If necessary, iron sucrose treatments may be repeated.

■ **Special Populations** Dosage should be selected carefully for geriatric patients 65 years of age and older because of limited experience with iron sucrose in these patients and the greater frequency of decreased hepatic, renal, and cardiac function and of concomitant disease and/or other drug therapies.

Cautions

■ **Contraindications** Known hypersensitivity to iron sucrose or any ingredient in the formulation.

■ **Warnings/Precautions** ***Warnings*** **Sensitivity Reactions.** Hypersensitivity reactions, including anaphylactic shock, loss of consciousness, collapse, hypotension, dyspnea, and seizures, have been reported in patients receiving iron sucrose therapy. In some cases, serious or fatal reactions have occurred. If hypersensitivity reactions or signs of intolerance develop during iron sucrose therapy, immediate drug discontinuance and medical intervention is required. Since hypersensitivity reactions associated with IV iron preparations tend to occur within 30 minutes after completion of an infusion, patients should be observed for at least this period of time until they are clinically stable. (See Dosage and Administration: General.)

Cardiovascular Effects. Iron sucrose may cause clinically important hypotension. Patients should be observed closely for signs and symptoms of hypotension during and following administration of the drug. Hypotension associated with IV administration of iron sucrose may be minimized by adhering to recommended total doses and rates of administration. (See Dosage and Administration.)

General Precautions **Iron Toxicity.** Because body iron excretion is limited and excessive iron in tissues can be hazardous, iron sucrose should not be administered to patients with evidence suggesting iron overload. Periodic monitoring of laboratory values indicative of iron storage in the body (e.g., transferrin saturation, serum ferritin concentrations, hemoglobin, hematocrit) may assist in the recognition of iron accumulation. Because transferrin saturation values increase rapidly after IV administration of iron sucrose, serum iron measurements should not be performed until at least 48 hours after the drug is administered.

Specific Populations **Pregnancy.** Category B. (See Users Guide.)

Lactation. It is not known whether iron sucrose is distributed into milk. Caution is advised if the drug is administered in nursing women.

Pediatric Use. Efficacy and safety of iron sucrose for iron maintenance therapy have been established in children 2 years of age or older with dialysis-dependent or non dialysis-dependent-chronic kidney disease. In a 12-week open-label, dose-ranging study in pediatric patients with chronic kidney disease (dialysis-dependent or non-dialysis dependent) who were receiving stable dosages of an erythropoiesis-stimulating agent (ESA), treatment with iron sucrose maintained hemoglobin concentrations between 10.5 and 14 g/dL in approximately 45–59% of the patients receiving 0.5, 1, or 2 mg/kg of the drug; a dose-response relationship was not demonstrated. Safety and efficacy of iron sucrose for iron *replacement* therapy in pediatric patients with chronic kidney disease have not been established.

Experience principally in another country revealed that 5 premature neonates (each weighing less than 1250 g) who received iron sucrose developed necrotizing enterocolitis; 2 of the 5 infants died during or following a period during which they received epoetin alfa, iron sucrose, and several other drugs concomitantly. A causal relationship to iron sucrose or any of the drugs could not be established.

Geriatric Use. Experience in those 65 years of age and older insufficient to determine whether they respond differently from younger adults; use caution in selecting and adjusting dosage. (See Dosage and Administration: Special Populations.)

Concomitant Disease States. Clinicians should consider that clinical studies in which the effects of iron sucrose were established generally excluded patients with serious underlying disease, inflammatory conditions, or active infections.

■ **Common Adverse Effects** Adverse effects occurring in 2% or more of patients receiving iron sucrose injection include diarrhea, nausea, vomiting, headache, dizziness, hypotension, pruritus, extremity pain, arthralgia, back pain, muscle cramp, injection site reactions, chest pain, and peripheral edema.

Drug Interactions

■ **Oral Iron Preparations** Potential pharmacokinetic interaction (reduced absorption of concomitantly administered oral iron).

Description

Iron sucrose (iron sucrose complex) is a polynuclear iron(III)-hydroxide sucrose complex with a molecular weight of approximately 34,000–60,000. Iron sucrose is used to replenish and maintain the total body content of iron and has pharmacologic actions similar to those of other parenteral iron preparations (e.g., iron dextran, sodium ferric gluconate). Unlike iron dextran, however, iron sucrose is free of ferrous ions and dextran polysaccharides, which are believed to be antigenic stimuli for anaphylactic reactions.

Following IV administration of iron sucrose, the drug is dissociated into iron and sucrose by the reticuloendothelial system. It has been suggested that the release of iron from iron sucrose is more rapid than that from iron dextran but less rapid than that from sodium ferric gluconate. In a limited number of hemodialysis patients receiving iron sucrose dosages equivalent to 100 mg of elemental iron 3 times weekly for 3 weeks, substantial increases in serum iron and serum ferritin and decreases in total iron binding capacity occurred within 4 weeks from initiation of iron therapy.

Advice to Patients

Risk of potentially fatal sensitivity (e.g., anaphylactoid) reactions. (See Sensitivity Reactions under Warnings/Precautions: Warnings, in Cautions.) Risk of hypotension. Importance of informing clinicians of existing or contemplated concomitant therapy, including prescription and OTC drugs.

Overview® (see Users Guide). For additional information on this drug until a more detailed monograph is developed and published, the manufacturer's labeling should be consulted. It is *essential* that the manufacturer's labeling be consulted for more detailed information on usual cautions, precautions, contraindications, potential drug interactions, laboratory test interferences, and acute toxicity.

Preparations

Excipients in commercially available drug preparations may have clinically important effects in some individuals; consult specific product labeling for details.

Iron Sucrose

Parenteral

For injection, for IV infusion	equivalent to 20 mg of elemental iron per mL	**Venofer®**, American Regent

Sodium Ferric Gluconate

■ Sodium ferric gluconate, a stable macromolecular complex composed of ferric oxide hydrate directly bonded to sucrose and chelated with gluconate, is used to replenish and maintain the total body content of iron and has pharmacologic actions similar to those of other parenteral iron preparations.

Uses

■ **Iron Deficiency Anemia in Hemodialysis Patients Receiving Epoetin Alfa Therapy** Sodium ferric gluconate is used for the treatment of iron deficiency anemia in adults and children 6 years of age or older with chronic kidney disease who are undergoing hemodialysis and receiving supplemental epoetin alfa therapy. Patients undergoing hemodialysis lose an estimated 1–3 g of iron annually as a result of blood loss from repeated laboratory tests, blood retention in the dialyzer equipment, and the bleeding diathesis associated with anticoagulants used during dialysis. In addition, epoetin alfa therapy results in an increased demand for iron by stimulating erythroid marrow; virtually all patients receiving epoetin alfa therapy will require supplemental iron therapy. (See Uses: Anemia of Chronic Kidney Disease, in Epoetin Alfa 20:16.) Orally administered iron has been reported to be ineffective in maintaining adequate iron stores in hemodialysis patients during epoetin alfa therapy. In several randomized controlled studies comparing IV and oral administration of iron in patients with chronic kidney disease undergoing hemodialysis, IV iron was found to be superior to orally administered iron in increasing hemoglobin concentrations and/or minimizing the dosage of an erythropoiesis-stimulating agent (ESA) (e.g., epoetin alfa) required to maintain target hemoglobin levels; guidelines for the treatment of anemia of chronic kidney disease from the National Kidney Foundation Kidney Disease Outcomes Quality Initiative (NKF-KDOQI) state that the IV route is preferred for administration of iron in patients with chronic kidney disease undergoing hemodialysis. The goal of iron therapy is achievement of the target hematocrit/hemoglobin with the lowest dosage of epoetin alfa necessary to stimulate erythropoiesis.

One of the most important factors in patient response to epoetin alfa therapy is iron status. Current evidence indicates that regular administration of parenteral iron improves the erythroid response to epoetin alfa and generally allows attainment of the target hematocrit at lower epoetin alfa dosages. In addition, appropriate use of iron therapy may minimize the fluctuation of hematocrit/hemoglobin concentrations compared with manipulation of epoetin alfa dosage as the principal means of managing anemia. (See Uses: Anemia of Chronic Kidney Disease, in Epoetin Alfa 20:16.)

The current FDA-labeled indication for sodium ferric gluconate in the treatment of iron deficiency anemia in hemodialysis patients receiving epoetin alfa is based principally on 2 clinical trials of approximately 50 days' duration in adults and one clinical trial in pediatric patients.

In a randomized, open-label study, patients undergoing chronic hemodialysis and receiving stable dosages of epoetin alfa were given an IV test dose of sodium ferric gluconate equivalent to 25 mg of elemental iron. Patients then received sodium ferric gluconate IV in either a low-dose (62.5 mg in 50 mL of 0.9% sodium chloride injection over 30 minutes) or high-dose (125 mg in 100 mL of 0.9% sodium chloride injection over 60 minutes) regimen for 8 doses during sequential dialysis sessions over a period of 16–17 days (cumulative dosage equivalent to 500 or 1000 mg, respectively, of elemental iron). Efficacy of iron replacement therapy in this study was evaluated based on a primary end point of change in hemoglobin from baseline to the last available observation through day 40. Patients receiving high-dose sodium ferric gluconate therapy had greater increases in hemoglobin, hematocrit, and iron saturation at all time points during the study than patients receiving low-dose sodium ferric gluconate or oral iron therapy. Fourteen days after completion of iron therapy, the mean change in hematocrit and hemoglobin in patients receiving high-dose sodium ferric gluconate therapy was 3.6% and 1.1 g/dL, respectively. Increases in hematocrit and hemoglobin in patients receiving low-dose sodium ferric gluconate therapy (1.4% and 0.3 g/dL, respectively) were similar to those in patients who received oral iron therapy (0.8% and 0.4 g/dL, respectively).

A smaller, nonrandomized study in iron-deficient hemodialysis patients receiving variable, cumulative doses of sodium ferric gluconate IV also demonstrated appreciable increases in hematocrit and hemoglobin compared with those produced by oral iron therapy. In this study, a total of 14 patients (37%) completed the study protocol (receiving at least 8 doses of either low- or high-dose IV sodium ferric gluconate); the remainder received less than 8 doses (32%) or had incomplete information on the sequence of dosing (32%). An unspecified number of patients also failed to receive the drug at consecutive dialysis sessions, and many received oral iron during the study.

In a randomized, open-label study in iron-deficient pediatric patients 6–15 years of age (mean age: 12 years) who were undergoing chronic hemodialysis and receiving stable dosages of epoetin alfa, sodium ferric gluconate in doses equivalent to 1.5 or 3 mg/kg of elemental iron (maximum dose of elemental iron not exceeding 125 mg) was administered IV in 25 mL of 0.9% sodium chloride injection over 1 hour during each of 8 sequential dialysis sessions. The primary end point in this study was change in hemoglobin from baseline to 2 weeks after the last dose of sodium ferric gluconate. Two weeks after completion of iron therapy, the mean change in hemoglobin in patients receiving 1.5 mg/kg or 3 mg/kg of elemental iron was 0.8 or 0.9 g/dL, respectively; increased hemoglobin concentrations were maintained at 4 weeks after the final dose of sodium ferric gluconate in both treatment groups. Patients receiving either dosage of sodium ferric gluconate had similar increases in hematocrit, iron saturation, serum ferritin levels, and reticulocyte hemoglobin content 2 weeks after completion of iron therapy.

Because of a lack of randomized, comparative studies, the relative efficacy of sodium ferric gluconate and other parenteral iron preparations (e.g., iron dextran) for the treatment of iron deficiency anemia in hemodialysis patients has not been clearly established. However, limited data suggest that sodium ferric gluconate may be associated with less frequent serious adverse effects (e.g., hypersensitivity reactions) than iron dextran. (See the introductory discussion under Cautions and see also Cautions: Sensitivity Reactions.)

■ **Iron Deficiency Anemia** Data regarding the safety and efficacy of sodium ferric gluconate injection for the prevention and/or treatment of iron deficiency anemia not associated with chronic kidney disease (e.g., anemia in HIV or cancer patients) generally are lacking. In a study in a limited number of pregnant women with iron deficiency anemia who did not benefit from or could not tolerate oral iron therapy, IV sodium ferric gluconate (mean cumulative dosage: 1 g) produced appreciable improvement in hematocrit, hemoglobin, and other indices of iron status; reported adverse effects (sinus tachycardia, palpitation, shortness of breath, hot flushes) generally were mild and transient.

For additional information on the prevention and treatment of iron deficiency anemia, see Uses in Iron Preparation, Oral, 20:04.04.

Dosage and Administration

■ **Administration** Sodium ferric gluconate is administered by IV infusion. The drug should be diluted in 0.9% sodium chloride injection and administered by slow IV infusion (e.g., over 1 hour). Sodium ferric gluconate also may be administered undiluted by slow IV injection at a rate of up to 12.5 mg/minute at the end of dialysis. Sodium ferric gluconate should be administered immediately after dilution; any unused portion of the diluted solution should be discarded.

A test dose equivalent to 25 mg of elemental iron, which has been diluted in 50 mL of 0.9% sodium chloride injection and given IV over 60 minutes, was recommended in the past by the manufacturer prior to administration of the first therapeutic dose of sodium ferric gluconate.

It has been suggested that administration of sodium ferric gluconate even at recommended dosage and infusion rates may result in adverse effects (e.g., hypotension, flushing) that have been attributed to oversaturation of transferrin and accompanying adverse effects. (See Acute Toxicity.) Although the cause of such adverse effects has not been fully elucidated, reducing the dose to 62.5 mg and infusing the drug over 4 hours has been shown to reduce the occurrence of adverse effects.

■ **Dosage** The dosage of sodium ferric gluconate is expressed in terms of mg of elemental iron. Sodium ferric gluconate injection contains the equivalent of 12.5 mg of elemental iron per mL.

For the treatment of iron deficiency in adults undergoing chronic hemodialysis who are receiving supplemental epoetin alfa therapy, the recommended dosage of sodium ferric gluconate is 125 mg administered by IV infusion over 1 hour. Most adults will require a minimum cumulative dose of 1 g of elemental iron, administered over 8 sessions at or during sequential dialysis treatments, to achieve a favorable hemoglobin or hematocrit response.

In patients with chronic kidney disease who are receiving supplemental therapy with an erythropoiesis-stimulating agent (ESA), sufficient iron should be administered to maintain selected indices of iron therapy (i.e., transferrin saturation [TSAT] and serum ferritin concentrations) at target levels; periodic monitoring of these iron indices is recommended, and the results should be used (in conjunction with hemoglobin concentrations and ESA dosage) to guide iron therapy. Once patients achieve TSAT levels of 20% or greater or serum ferritin concentrations of 100 ng/mL or greater, IV iron therapy with sodium ferric gluconate or other IV iron preparations should be continued at the lowest dose necessary to maintain target hematocrit/hemoglobin levels and iron stores within acceptable limits.

For the treatment of iron deficiency in children undergoing chronic hemodialysis who are receiving supplemental epoetin alfa therapy, the recommended dosage of sodium ferric gluconate is 1.5 mg/kg (up to 125 mg/dose) diluted in 25 mL 0.9% sodium chloride and administered by IV infusion over 1 hour during 8 sequential dialysis sessions.

Cautions

Current evidence suggests that sodium ferric gluconate is well tolerated. In a single-dose, post-marketing safety study, 11% of patients who received sodium ferric gluconate and 9.4% of patients who received placebo reported adverse reactions. The most frequent adverse reactions following sodium ferric gluconate were hypotension (2%); nausea, vomiting, and/or diarrhea (2%); pain (0.7%); hypertension (0.6%); allergic reaction (0.5%); chest pain (0.5%); pruritus (0.5%); and back pain (0.4%). Similar adverse reactions were seen following placebo administration. However, because of the high baseline incidence of adverse events in the hemodialysis patient population, insufficient number of exposed patients, and limitations inherent to the crossover, single-dose study design, no comparison of event rates between sodium ferric gluconate and placebo treatments can be made at this time.

Clinical experience with sodium ferric gluconate has been documented in over 1400 adults on hemodialysis, including 1097 treatment-naive individuals who received a single 125-mg dose of undiluted sodium ferric gluconate over 10 minutes during a postmarketing safety study. No test dose was used in this postmarketing study. From a total of 1498 adults in medical reports, North American trials, and postmarketing studies who received sodium ferric gluconate therapy, 12 patients (0.8%) experienced serious reactions that precluded further therapy with the drug.

In iron-deficient pediatric patients undergoing chronic hemodialysis and receiving stable dosages of epoetin alfa who received 1.5 or 3 mg/kg of sodium ferric gluconate IV during 8 sequential dialysis sessions, the most common adverse effects (whether or not drug related) occurring in at least 5% of patients were hypotension (35%), headache (24%), hypertension (23%), tachycardia (17%), vomiting (11%), fever (9%), nausea (9%), abdominal pain (9%), pharyngitis (9%), diarrhea (8%), infection (8%), rhinitis (6%), and thrombosis (6%). The incidences of the following adverse effects were higher with the 3-mg/kg versus the 1.5-mg/kg dosage of sodium ferric gluconate: hypotension (41 or 28%, respectively), tachycardia (21 or 13%, respectively), fever (15 or 3%, respectively), headache (29 or 19%, respectively), abdominal pain (15 or 3%, respectively), nausea (12 or 6%, respectively), vomiting (12 or 9%, respectively), pharyngitis (12 or 6%, respectively), and rhinitis (9 or 3%, respectively).

IV iron dextran preparations are associated with idiopathic sensitivity reactions. Although the mechanism of sensitivity reactions is unknown, it has been suggested that dextran polymers may be the antigenic stimulus for these reactions. (See Cautions: Sensitivity Reactions, in Iron Dextran 20:04.04.) Published clinical studies do not permit a reliable comparison of IV sodium ferric gluconate with IV iron dextran, but limited data suggest that sodium ferric gluconate, a compound devoid of dextran, may be associated with fewer sensitivity reactions than IV iron dextran. Sensitivity (e.g., anaphylactoid or anaphylactic) reactions appear to occur rarely with sodium ferric gluconate injection, and no fatalities associated with the use of sodium ferric gluconate have been reported. In addition, sodium ferric gluconate has been administered without incident to a limited number of hemodialysis patients who had experienced severe sensitivity reactions to iron dextran. However, sensitivity reactions to sodium ferric gluconate severe enough to require discontinuance of the drug have occurred. (See Cautions: Sensitivity Reactions.) In addition, rapid IV infusion of the drug has been associated with an increased incidence of acute iron toxicity manifested by flushing; pain in the chest, back, flank, or groin; and hypotension. (See Acute Toxicity.)

Unless otherwise stated in the Cautions section, adverse effects reported during therapy with sodium ferric gluconate may or may not be directly attributable to the drug.

■ Sensitivity Reactions The risk of acute anaphylactic reactions following administration of sodium ferric gluconate has been estimated to be 3.3 cases per million doses versus 8.7 cases per million doses for iron dextran based on retrospective analysis of adverse events data from use of sodium ferric gluconate in Germany and Italy or iron dextran in the United States. Although fatal hypersensitivity reactions did not occur during therapy with sodium ferric gluconate in clinical studies, the number of patients exposed to the drug during such studies may not have been sufficient to observe such reactions.

Of 88 patients in a randomized, controlled clinical trial of sodium ferric gluconate therapy, 3 patients (3.4%) experienced type III sensitivity reactions manifested by rash, pruritus, nausea, fatigue, and/or pain in the chest, abdomen, and flank that resulted in premature study discontinuance. These events were not dose-dependent and occurred in 2 cases following the first dose of sodium ferric gluconate and immediately after the IV test dose in the other incident. In addition, one case of a life-threatening hypersensitivity reaction, consisting of diaphoresis, nausea, vomiting, severe lower back pain, dyspnea, and wheezing, for 20 minutes, out of 1097 patients who received a single dose of sodium ferric gluconate has been observed in a postmarketing safety study, and 3 serious hypersensitivity reactions have been reported from the spontaneous reporting system in the US.

Serious adverse events that precluded further therapy with sodium ferric gluconate have been reported in 6 of 387 patients (1.6%) treated with the drug in clinical studies and in 9 of 1097 patients (0.8%) treated with the drug in a postmarketing safety study. During the postmarketing safety study, adverse reactions that, in the view of the investigator, precluded further administration of the drug because of drug intolerance included one life-threatening reaction, 6 allergic reactions (e.g., pruritus [2 cases], facial flushing, chills, dyspnea/chest pain, rash), and 2 other reactions (hypotension and nausea). Another 2 patients (0.2%) experienced allergic reactions not deemed to represent drug intolerance (nausea/malaise and nausea/dizziness) following administration of the drug. Anaphylactoid reaction, characterized by severe hypotension and paresthesias in the lips, fingers, and genitalia, also has been reported immediately following initiation of a slow infusion of sodium ferric gluconate in at least one patient; the reaction subsided completely within 1 hour. In clinical studies conducted in Europe, 2 of 226 hemodialysis patients (0.9%) experienced adverse events (malaise, heat, vomiting, loin pain, and/or intense epigastric pain lasting 3–4 hours) when treated with sodium ferric gluconate. These reactions recurred when patients were rechallenged with the drug and precluded further therapy. Since allergy histories of patients who experienced sensitivity reactions to sodium ferric gluconate were not reported in the literature, it is not known whether patients with a history of multiple drug allergies are at increased risk for adverse sensitivity reactions with sodium ferric gluconate as they are with iron dextran. The manufacturer states that the incidence of both drug intolerance and suspected allergic events following the first dose of sodium ferric gluconate administration in the postmarketing study was 2.8% in patients with prior iron dextran sensitivity and 0.8% in patients without prior iron dextran sensitivity. The one patient who experienced a life-threatening adverse event following administration of sodium ferric gluconate during the postmarketing study did have a previous severe anaphylactic reaction to both commercially available preparations of iron dextran (INFeD® and Dexferrum®).

Clinical studies of sodium ferric gluconate included 9 patients undergoing chronic hemodialysis who had a history of allergic reactions to iron dextran; 5 of these patients had a history of anaphylaxis to iron dextran. All patients were treated successfully with sodium ferric gluconate (1000 mg) given IV during each of 8 consecutive dialysis treatments, although one patient reported paresthesias within 1 hour of completing a full course of therapy with the drug.

For additional information on sensitivity reactions to sodium ferric gluconate, including that pertaining to this drug versus iron dextran, see the introductory discussion under Cautions.

■ Cardiovascular Effects The most common adverse cardiovascular effect associated with sodium ferric gluconate is hypotension, occurring in 29% of patients receiving the drug in clinical trials. Serious hypotensive events, accompanied by flushing in 2 cases, reportedly occurred in 3 of 226 hemodialysis patients (1.3%) treated with IV sodium ferric gluconate. Hypotensive episodes reported in clinical studies were not thought to be dose dependent since they occurred in 34 versus 36% of patients receiving 62.5 mg of sodium ferric gluconate IV over 30 minutes versus 125 mg IV over 60 minutes, respectively, and were comparable to those occurring in patients receiving oral iron therapy. However, rapid IV administration of sodium ferric gluconate has been associated with hypotensive episodes accompanied by flushing, lightheadedness, malaise, fatigue, weakness, or severe pain in the chest, back, flanks, or groin, which are unrelated to sensitivity reactions. These hypotensive episodes usually resolved within 1–2 hours following clinical interventions ranging from observation to volume expansion as warranted by the severity of the symptoms. Such hypotension and flushing have been attributed to oversaturation of transferrin and excessive free iron in the serum. Alternatively, it has been suggested that such transferrin oversaturation is unlikely because of the high binding coefficient of ferric iron in the sodium ferric gluconate complex; such adverse effects may instead result from direct chemical or mechanical stimulation of mast cells. Sodium ferric gluconate is intended to be administered during dialysis, during which many patients may experience transient hypotension. Administration of sodium ferric gluconate may augment hypotension caused by dialysis.

Hypertension, chest pain, syncope, tachycardia, and generalized edema have been reported in 13, 6, 5, and 5% of patients in clinical trials, respectively. In addition, bradycardia, angina pectoris, leg edema, myocardial infarction, vasodilation, or pulmonary edema occurred in more than 1% of patients receiving sodium ferric gluconate in clinical trials.

■ Nervous System Effects Dizziness, asthenia, headache, fatigue, and paresthesias are the most common adverse nervous system effects of sodium ferric gluconate, occurring in 13, 7, 7, 6, and 6% of patients, respectively. In addition, agitation, insomnia, or somnolence occurred in more than 1% of patients receiving sodium ferric gluconate in clinical trials. Lightheadedness, diplopia,malaise, and/or weakness have been reported rarely during therapy with sodium ferric gluconate in North American clinical trials and hypertonia and nervousness rarely were reported during postmarketing surveillance. Transient decreased level of consciousness without hypotension has been reported in at least one patient receiving the drug.

■ Respiratory Effects Dyspnea, coughing, and upper respiratory infection are the most common adverse respiratory effects of sodium ferric gluconate, occurring in 11, 6, and 6% of patients, respectively. Rhinitis or pneumonia occurred in more than 1% of patients receiving sodium ferric gluconate.

■ GI Effects Vomiting, nausea, and/or diarrhea are the most common adverse GI effects of sodium ferric gluconate, each occurring in 35% of patients. In addition, abdominal pain occurred in 6% of patients and nausea, rectal disorder, dyspepsia, eructation, GI disorder, flatulence, or melena occurred in more than 1% of patients receiving sodium ferric gluconate in clinical trials. Dry mouth was reported rarely during postmarketing surveillance.

■ Musculoskeletal Effects Generalized cramps and leg cramps are the most common adverse musculoskeletal effects of sodium ferric gluconate, occurring in 25 and 10% of patients, respectively. Myalgia, back pain, arm pain, or arthralgia occurred in more than 1% of patients receiving sodium ferric gluconate in clinical trials. Whether these events were dose dependent or delayed reactions similar to those observed with iron dextran has not been determined.

■ Renal and Electrolyte Effects Hyperkalemia occurred in 6% of patients receiving sodium ferric gluconate in clinical trials. In addition, hypokalemia or hypervolemia has been reported in more than 1% of patients receiving sodium ferric gluconate.

■ Hematologic Effects Abnormal erythrocytes occurred in 11% of patients receiving sodium ferric gluconate in clinical trials. In addition, anemia, leukocytosis, or lymphadenopathy occurred in more than 1% of patients receiving sodium ferric gluconate in clinical trials. Hemorrhage was reported rarely during postmarketing surveillance.

■ Other Adverse Effects Injection site reaction and fever have been reported in 33 and 5% of patients receiving sodium ferric gluconate in clinical trials, respectively. Other adverse effects reported in more than 1% of patients receiving sodium ferric gluconate in clinical trials include pain, otic disorder, increased sweating, conjunctivitis, abnormal vision, hypoglycemia, urinary tract infection, infection, rigors, chills, flu-like syndrome, sepsis, and carcinoma.

■ Precautions and Contraindications Unwarranted administration of parenteral iron preparations may cause excess storage of iron and possibly result in a syndrome similar to hemosiderosis, particularly in patients whose anemia is not attributable to iron deficiency (e.g., those with hemoglobinopathies or other refractory anemias that might be erroneously diagnosed as iron deficiency anemia). Periodic monitoring of laboratory values indicative of iron storage in the body (e.g., transferrin saturation, serum ferritin concentrations) may assist in the recognition of iron accumulation. Sodium ferric gluconate should not be administered to patients with iron overload.

Potentially fatal sensitivity (e.g. anaphylactic or anaphylactoid) reactions characterized by cardiovascular collapse, cardiac arrest, bronchospasm, oral or pharyngeal edema, dyspnea, angioedema, urticaria, or pruritus sometimes associated with pain and muscle spasm of the chest or back have been reported rarely in patients receiving sodium ferric gluconate; fatal immediate hypersensitivity reactions have been reported with other iron carbohydrate complexes. Serious anaphylactoid reactions require appropriate resuscitative measures. Although fatal reactions have not been observed with sodium ferric gluconate in clinical studies, insufficient numbers of patients may have been enrolled to observe such events. (See Caution: Sensitivity Reactions.) Although sodium ferric gluconate has been used successfully to treat iron deficiency anemia in a few hemodialysis patients with a history of allergic reactions to iron dextran, sodium ferric gluconate should be used with extreme caution in such patients (especially those who experienced life-threatening anaphylaxis or anaphylactoid reactions) since the drug itself is known to cause potentially life-threatening sensitivity reactions and the incidence of cross-reactivity between iron dextran and sodium ferric gluconate is unknown.

Hypotension not associated with sensitivity and accompanied by flushing, lightheadedness, malaise, fatigue, weakness, or severe pain in the chest, back, flanks, or groin has been associated with rapid IV administration of iron. Such reactions usually have resolved within 1–2 hours. Successful treatment of these reactions may include observation or, if symptoms are present, volume expansion.

Sodium ferric gluconate should not be used in patients with serum ferritin concentrations exceeding 1000 ng/mL. In addition, clinicians should consider that clinical studies in which the effects of sodium ferric gluconate were established excluded patients with serious underlying disease or inflammatory conditions. Sodium ferric gluconate is contraindicated in patients with any anemia not associated with iron deficiency, in patients who are hypersensitive to sodium ferric gluconate or any ingredients in the formulation, and in patients with evidence of iron overload.

■ **Pediatric Precautions** The safety and efficacy of sodium ferric gluconate in children younger than 6 years of age has not been established.

Sodium ferric gluconate contains benzyl alcohol, and the manufacturer states that the drug should not be used in neonates. Although a causal relationship has not been established, administration of injections preserved with benzyl alcohol has been associated with toxicity in neonates. Toxicity appears to have resulted from administration of large amounts (i.e., about 100–400 mg/kg daily) of benzyl alcohol in these neonates. Although use of drugs preserved with benzyl alcohol should be avoided in neonates whenever possible, the American Academy of Pediatrics (AAP) states that the presence of small amounts of the preservative in a commercially available injection should not proscribe its use when indicated in neonates.

■ **Geriatric Precautions** Clinical studies of sodium ferric gluconate did not include sufficient numbers of patients aged 65 years and older to determine whether they respond differently to the drug than do younger patients. Although other reported clinical experience has not revealed age-related differences in response or tolerance, drug dosage should be titrated carefully in geriatric patients, usually initiating therapy at the low end of the dosage range. The greater frequency of decreased hepatic, renal, and/or cardiac function and of concomitant disease and drug therapy observed in the elderly also should be considered.

■ **Mutagenicity and Carcinogenicity** No evidence of mutagenicity was seen when sodium ferric gluconate was evaluated in in vitro test systems (Ames test and rat micronucleus test). Long-term studies in animals to evaluate the carcinogenic potential of sodium ferric gluconate are ongoing.

■ **Pregnancy, Fertility, and Lactation** ***Pregnancy*** Reproductive studies in mice and rats using sodium ferric gluconate dosages up to 100 or 20 mg/kg daily, respectively, have not revealed evidence of harm to the fetus. These dosages were 1.3 or 3.24 times, respectively, the recommended human daily dosage of 125 mg or 92.5 mg/m^2 (based on a patient of average height weighing 50 kg and having a body surface area of 1.46 m^2). In a study involving 21 pregnant women who were treated with sodium ferric gluconate as an alternative to blood transfusions, dose-dependent adverse events occurred; these adverse events included sinus tachycardia, palpitations, shortness of breath, and hot flushes (flashes), which were transient and resolved spontaneously without treatment after a few minutes. There are no adequate and controlled studies to date using sodium ferric gluconate in pregnant women, and the drug should be used during pregnancy only when clearly needed.

Fertility Studies to assess the effects of sodium ferric gluconate on fertility in animals have not been conducted. However, the drug produced a clastogenic effect in an in vitro chromosomal aberration assay in Chinese hamster ovary cells.

Lactation Since it is not known whether sodium ferric gluconate is distributed into milk, the drug should be used with caution in nursing women.

Drug Interactions

■ **Angiotensin-converting Enzyme Inhibitors** Limited data suggest that concomitant administration of IV sodium ferric gluconate and oral enalapril may potentiate adverse effects associated with IV iron therapy. During a postmarketing safety study, one patient who was already receiving an ACE inhibitor had facial flushing immediately following exposure to sodium ferric gluconate. No hypotension occurred in this patient, and the event resolved rapidly and spontaneously without intervention other than drug withdrawal. However, hypotension (systolic blood pressure of 80 mm Hg), diffuse erythema, nausea, vomiting, and abdominal cramps have been reported in a few patients who received IV sodium ferric gluconate while receiving enalapril therapy. The onset of these adverse effects varied from immediately after administration of IV iron to a couple of hours or days following infusion of the drug. These reactions subsided within 20–30 minutes following prompt discontinuance of the IV iron infusion and IV administration of hydrocortisone. One patient, who agreed to discontinue enalapril therapy while on sodium ferric gluconate, was successfully treated again with sodium ferric gluconate; the other patients were not treated with IV iron therapy again but were able to continue enalapril therapy without further incident.

It has been suggested that Angiotensin-converting enzyme (ACE) inhibitors potentiate sensitivity reactions by decreasing the breakdown of kinins. In a postmarketing safety study in which 28% of the patients received concomitant ACE inhibitor therapy, the incidences of both drug intolerance or suspected allergic events following first dose administration of sodium ferric gluconate were 1.6% in patients with concomitant ACE inhibitor use compared with 0.7% in patients without concomitant ACE inhibitor use. The patient with a life-threatening event during the postmarketing study was not on ACE inhibitor therapy. Although this interaction appears to occur rarely, the potential seriousness of the interaction warrants caution when IV iron and ACE inhibitors are used together.

Acute Toxicity

Dosage of sodium ferric gluconate in excess of that required for restoration of hemoglobin and replenishment of iron stores may lead to hemosiderosis. Serum iron concentrations exceeding 300 mcg/dL (combined with transferrin oversaturation) may indicate iron toxicity, which is characterized by abdominal pain, diarrhea, or vomiting that progresses to pallor or cyanosis, lassitude, drowsiness, hyperventilation secondary to acidosis, and cardiovascular collapse. Symptoms following rapid IV infusion of sodium ferric gluconate have been reported rarely; such symptoms include flushing; chest, back, and loin pain; and hypotension. (See Cautions: Cardiovascular Effects.) Periodic monitoring of laboratory indices of iron storage (e.g., serum ferritin, transferrin saturation [TSAT]) may assist in recognition of iron accumulation. Sodium ferric gluconate should not be administered to patients with iron overload. Sodium ferric gluconate is not dialyzable.

Overdosage of sodium ferric gluconate in animals produced symptoms such as decreased activity, staggering, ataxia, increases in the respiratory rate, tremor, and convulsions. Deaths occurred with sodium ferric gluconate at elemental iron doses of 125, 78.8, 62.5, or 250 mg/kg in mice, rats, rabbits, or dogs, respectively.

Pharmacology

Sodium ferric gluconate is used to replenish and maintain the total body content of iron and has pharmacologic actions similar to those of iron dextran. Iron is essential for normal hemoglobin synthesis to maintain oxygen transport; iron also is necessary for the metabolism and synthesis of DNA and functions as a cofactor in various enzymatic processes.

The total body iron content of an adult ranges from 2–4 g with approximately two-thirds in hemoglobin and one-third in reticuloendothelial storage (liver, spleen, and bone marrow) and bound to tissue ferritin. The human body avidly conserves iron so that only about 1 mg (about 0.03% of total body stores) is excreted daily in healthy, nonmenstruating adults.

Iron deficiency anemia in patients with chronic kidney disease undergoing hemodialysis may result from various factors, including increased iron utilization (e.g., in patients receiving exogenous erythropoietin [epoetin alfa]), blood loss (e.g., from fistula, retention in dialyzer, hematologic testing, menses), decreased dietary intake or absorption, surgery, iron sequestration related to inflammatory processes, and malignancy. In addition, transferrin concentrations reportedly may be depressed in chronic kidney disease, resulting in subnormal iron uptake by cells. Administration of epoetin alfa increases red blood cell production and iron utilization, which may lead to absolute or functional iron deficiency.

Functional iron deficiency in patients with chronic kidney disease receiving epoetin alfa or in other patients with chronic blood loss refers to the condition where the body's demand for iron to maintain erythropoiesis exceeds the rate at which iron can be released from the reticuloendothelial system. Iron-replete hemodialysis patients reportedly have been shown to have decreased iron stores within 3 months of beginning epoetin alfa therapy. Because there is no widely available hematologic indicator of functional iron deficiency, the only way to determine its presence is to monitor the erythroid response to iron administration. Iron administration in hemodialysis patients with functional iron deficiency will result in an increase in hematocrit and/or hemoglobin levels despite a stable dose of epoetin alfa or can maintain a stable hematocrit and/or hemoglobin while allowing a reduction in epoetin alfa dosage. (See Uses: Iron Deficiency Anemia in Hemodialysis Patients Receiving Epoetin Alfa Therapy.)

Administration of iron may reverse esophageal, gastric, and other tissue changes associated with iron deficiency. Iron therapy also relieves other symptoms associated with iron deficiency, such as soreness of the tongue, cheilosis, dysphagia, and dystrophy of the nails and skin. Iron does not stimulate erythropoiesis nor does it correct hemoglobin disturbances not caused by iron deficiency.

Iron is vital for microorganisms such as bacteria, and the mineral plays a role both in bacterial pathogenicity and host defense mechanisms. (See Cautions: Hemosiderosis, in Iron Preparations, Oral.)

Pharmacokinetics

■ **Distribution** Following administration of IV iron, the metal is taken up by the reticuloendothelial system. Subsequently, ferric iron is gradually released into the plasma where it rapidly combines with transferrin and is carried to the bone marrow and incorporated into hemoglobin. Plasma transferrin is normally 30–40% saturated by iron; in iron deficiency, elevated transferrin concentrations maintain circulating iron concentrations despite a reduction in transferrin saturation (TSAT). In a limited number of healthy iron-deficient individuals who received multiple sequential single doses of either 125 mg/hour or 62.5 mg over 30 minutes of undiluted sodium ferric gluconate IV, approximately 80% of drug-bound iron was delivered to transferrin as a mononuclear ionic iron species within 24 hours of administration in each dosage regimen. Direct movement of iron from sodium ferric gluconate to transferrin, however, was not observed. In addition, mean peak transferrin saturation did not exceed 100% in these studies and returned to near baseline by 40 hours after administration of each dose regimen.

Preliminary pharmacokinetic data in a single hemodialysis patient and in a limited number of healthy iron-deficient individuals who received IV sodium ferric gluconate suggest an initial volume of distribution consistent with the vascular compartment, approximately 6 L.

■ **Elimination** Following IV injection of sodium ferric gluconate, the terminal elimination half-life of drug-bound iron varied by dose but not by rate of administration and was approximately 1 hour in healthy iron-deficient adults. The shortest terminal half-life (0.85 hours) occurred in adults administered 62.5 mg of the drug over 4 minutes and the longest terminal half-life (1.45 hours) occurred in adults administered 125 mg of the drug over 7 minutes. In addition, total clearance of sodium ferric gluconate was 3.02–5.35 L/hour and did not substantially vary by rate of administration. The terminal half-life following IV injection of 1.5 or 3 mg/kg sodium ferric gluconate in iron-deficient pediatric patients undergoing chronic hemodialysis was 2.0 or 2.5 hours, respectively. Pharmacokinetic studies in renally competent adults suggest that urinary excretion is not an important route of elimination of the drug in humans. In in vitro studies conducted with sodium ferric gluconate either undiluted or diluted in 0.9% sodium chloride injection or distilled water, less than 1% of the iron species in a dose of sodium ferric gluconate was removed during hemodialysis periods of up to 270 minutes using membranes with pore sizes corresponding to 12,000–14,000 daltons.

Iron metabolism occurs in a virtually closed system. Most of the iron liberated by destruction of hemoglobin is conserved and reused by the body. Daily excretion of iron in healthy men amounts to only 0.5–2 mg. This excretion occurs principally through feces and as desquamation of cells such as skin, GI mucosa, nails, and hair; only trace amounts of iron are excreted in bile and sweat. For additional information on the distribution of iron, see Pharmacokinetics: Elimination, in Iron Preparations, Oral 20:04.04.

Chemistry and Stability

■ **Chemistry** Sodium ferric gluconate is a stable macromolecular complex composed of ferric oxide hydrate directly bonded to sucrose and chelated with gluconate, which has a high affinity for ferric ions and enables the bridging of adjacent ferric oxide centers. Unlike iron dextran, sodium ferric gluconate is free of ferrous ion and dextran polysaccharides. The sodium ferric gluconate complex exists as a 2:1 molar ratio of iron to gluconate and has an apparent molecular weight of approximately 350,000.

Sodium ferric gluconate injection occurs as a deep-red, viscous solution that is completely miscible in water and 0.9% sodium chloride injection. The drug is negatively charged at alkaline pH and is present in solution with sodium cations. The commercially available injection is an alkaline aqueous solution with approximately 20% sucrose w/v in water for injection at a pH of 7.7–9.7. Each mL of sodium ferric gluconate injection contains 9 mg of benzyl alcohol as a preservative.

■ **Stability** Sodium ferric gluconate injection should be stored at 20–25°C, but may be exposed to temperatures ranging from 15–30°C. Sodium ferric gluconate injection should not be frozen. Sodium ferric gluconate injection should not be frozen.

The compatibility of sodium ferric gluconate injection with IV solutions other than 0.9% sodium chloride injection has not been evaluated. The manufacturer states that sodium ferric gluconate injection should not be mixed with other drugs or added to parenteral nutrition solutions for IV infusion.

Preparations

Excipients in commercially available drug preparations may have clinically important effects in some individuals; consult specific product labeling for details.

Sodium Ferric Gluconate

Parenteral

Injection, for IV use	equivalent to 12.5 mg of elemental iron per mL	**Ferrlecit®**, Sanofi-Aventis

ANTITHROMBOTIC AGENTS 20:12

ANTICOAGULANTS 20:12.04

COUMARIN DERIVATIVES 20:12.04.08

Warfarin Sodium

■ Warfarin sodium is a coumarin-derivative anticoagulant that alters the synthesis of blood coagulation factors II (prothrombin), VII (proconvertin), IX (Christmas factor or plasma thromboplastin component), and X (Stuart-Prower factor) in the liver by interfering with the action of vitamin K.

Uses

Warfarin is used for prophylaxis and/or treatment of venous thrombosis and its extension, prophylaxis and treatment of pulmonary embolism, prophylaxis and treatment of thromboembolic complications associated with atrial fibrillation and/or cardiac valve replacement, and as an adjunct in the treatment of coronary occlusion. The drug also is used to reduce the risk of death, reinfarction, and thromboembolic events such as stroke or systemic embolization following myocardial infarction (MI).

The most widely accepted indications for anticoagulant therapy include the treatment of venous thrombosis and pulmonary embolism and prevention of these conditions in high-risk patients, such as those with a history of thromboembolism, those undergoing certain types of major surgery, or those who require prolonged immobilization. Because the effects of warfarin are delayed and early full-dose anticoagulant therapy reduces the risk of extension or recurrence of venous thrombosis, a rapid-acting parenteral anticoagulant such as heparin (referring throughout this monograph to unfractionated heparin), a low molecular weight heparin, or fondaparinux is used for the initial treatment of venous thromboembolism. Warfarin generally is used for follow-up anticoagulant therapy after the effects of the initial parenteral anticoagulant have been established and when long-term anticoagulant therapy is indicated. Therapy with warfarin and the parenteral anticoagulant should be overlapped for a short period of time until the therapeutic effects of warfarin are achieved. (See Dosage and Administration: Dosage.)

■ **Deep-Vein Thrombosis and Pulmonary Embolism** ***Treatment and Secondary Prevention*** In the treatment of acute proximal deep-vein thrombosis (DVT) or pulmonary embolism (PE) (i.e., venous thromboembolism) in adults, the American College of Chest Physicians (ACCP) recommends that warfarin therapy be initiated concomitantly with a parenteral anticoagulant (heparin, a low molecular weight heparin, or fondaparinux). Warfarin should be initiated on the same day that the parenteral anticoagulant is started, and such therapy should be overlapped for at least 5 days and until a stable international normalized ratio (INR) of at least 2 has been maintained for 24 hours or longer. Anticoagulant therapy generally is not recommended for the treatment of isolated distal DVT unless symptoms are severe and there is a risk for thrombus extension. ACCP recommends a moderate intensity (target INR of 2.5, range 2–3) of warfarin anticoagulation in most patients for the treatment of DVT and PE. While use of either a lower intensity of anticoagulation (INR <2) or a higher intensity of anticoagulation (INR of 3–5) has been evaluated for these indications, both low-intensity and high-intensity anticoagulation appear to be less optimal than moderate-intensity warfarin; low-intensity warfarin is no safer than moderate-intensity warfarin, and high-intensity warfarin is associated with an increased incidence of bleeding complications.

In patients with venous thromboembolism, ACCP recommends that anticoagulant therapy be continued beyond the acute treatment period for at least 3 months, and possibly longer depending on the individual clinical situation (e.g., location of thrombi, presence or absence of precipitating factors, presence of cancer, patient's risk of bleeding). Warfarin generally is the preferred anticoagulant for long-term treatment of venous thromboembolism in patients without cancer; however, in patients with cancer, ACCP suggests the use of a low molecular weight heparin over warfarin because of certain factors in such patients that may affect warfarin therapy (e.g., possible reduced response to warfarin, drug interactions, need for invasive procedures that require reversal of anticoagulation). While several randomized, controlled studies of patients receiving warfarin indicate that recurrence of venous thromboembolism is less frequent with longer periods of anticoagulation (exceeding 6 months) compared with shorter periods (3–6 months), particularly in patients with idiopathic (i.e., unprovoked) venous thromboembolism, prolonged therapy with warfarin (in addition to increased intensity of anticoagulation) is associated with an increased risk of bleeding complications. Therefore, the shortest period of anticoagulant therapy deemed to be effective should be used, keeping in mind the high morbidity and mortality of undertreated venous thromboembolism. ACCP states that 3 months of anticoagulant treatment usually is sufficient in patients experiencing a proximal DVT or PE provoked by surgery or other transient risk factor. For those with an unprovoked thromboembolic event, anticoagulant therapy should be continued for at least 3 months; after this time, the risks versus benefits of extended therapy (defined by ACCP as treatment beyond 3 months without a scheduled stop date) should be evaluated in individual patients. In general, extended anticoagulant therapy is suggested in patients with unprovoked (idiopathic) DVT or PE who are at low risk of bleeding. Extended therapy is recommended by ACCP in cancer patients with acute venous thromboembolism because of the high risk of recurrence in these patients. Patients with acute upper-extremity DVT involving the axillary or more proximal veins also should receive anticoagulant therapy for at least 3 months. If the upper-extremity DVT is associated with a central venous catheter, anticoagulation should be continued as long as the catheter remains in place; if the catheter is removed, ACCP states that 3 months of anticoagulation is sufficient. For additional information on treatment of venous thromboembolism, consult the most recent ACCP Evidence-based Clinical Practice Guidelines on Antithrombotic Therapy and Prevention of Thrombosis available at http://www.chestnet.org.

Although warfarin therapy can be problematic in children for several reasons (e.g., dietary differences, compliance issues, monitoring difficulty, lack of a commercially available liquid preparation), the drug has been used in selected pediatric patients† with venous thromboembolism. Experience with warfarin in the pediatric population is mostly based on use of the drug in children older than 3 months of age; there is little efficacy or safety information in neonates. Heparin or a low molecular weight heparin generally is recommended for both the initial and ongoing treatment of venous thromboembolism in children. However, ACCP recommends that children with recurrent idiopathic venous thromboembolism receive indefinite treatment with warfarin. Unlike in adults, most episodes of venous thromboembolism in children are secondary to an identifiable risk factor such as the presence of a central venous access device (e.g., central venous catheter or umbilical venous catheter). In children with central venous catheter-related thromboembolism, ACCP recommends that the catheter be removed if no longer functioning or required; at least 3–5 days of therapeutic anticoagulation is suggested prior to its removal. If the central venous access device is required, ACCP suggests that anticoagulants be given until the catheter is removed. After the initial 3 months of therapy, use of prophylactic dosages of warfarin (target INR 1.5–1.9) or a low molecular weight heparin is suggested until the catheter is removed; however, if recurrent thromboembolism occurs, therapeutic-dose anticoagulation may be required.

Prophylaxis **Orthopedic Surgery.** ACCP recommends routine thromboprophylaxis (with a pharmacologic and/or mechanical method [e.g., intermittent pneumatic compression]) in all patients undergoing major orthopedic surgery, including total hip-replacement, total knee-replacement, and hip-fracture surgery, because of the high risk for postoperative venous thromboembolism; thromboprophylaxis should be continued for at least 10–14 days, and possibly for up to 35 days after surgery. Several antithrombotic agents (e.g., low molecular weight heparins, fondaparinux, low-dose heparin, warfarin, aspirin) are recommended by ACCP for pharmacologic thromboprophylaxis in patients undergoing major orthopedic surgery. Although ACCP suggests that a low molecular weight heparin generally is preferred because of its relative efficacy and safety and extensive clinical experience, alternative agents such as warfarin may be a reasonable choice in situations in which a low molecular weight heparin is not available or cannot be used (e.g., in patients with heparin-induced thrombocytopenia or in those who refuse or are uncooperative with subcutaneous injections). ACCP states that when selecting an appropriate thromboprophylaxis regimen, factors such as relative efficacy and bleeding risk as well as logistics and compliance issues should be considered. For additional information on the prevention of venous thromboembolism in patients undergoing major orthopedic surgery, consult the most recent ACCP Evidence-based Clinical Practice Guidelines on Antithrombotic Therapy and Prevention of Thrombosis available at http://www.chestnet.org.

Thromboprophylaxis in Pediatric Patients. Warfarin also has been used for primary thromboprophylaxis in children with ventricular assist devices† or with an arteriovenous fistula undergoing hemodialysis† and in children with certain medical conditions associated with a high risk of thrombosis (e.g., moderate or giant coronary aneurysms following Kawasaki disease†, primary pulmonary hypertension†).

■ Embolism Associated with Atrial Fibrillation

Warfarin is used for the prevention of stroke and systemic embolism in patients with atrial fibrillation. In several randomized, controlled studies in patients with chronic atrial fibrillation unrelated to rheumatic fever (i.e., nonvalvular atrial fibrillation), the incidence of thromboembolic events (e.g., transient ischemic attack [TIA], ischemic stroke) in patients anticoagulated with warfarin was substantially reduced compared with that in patients receiving placebo. ACCP, the American College of Cardiology (ACC), the American Heart Association (AHA), the American Stroke Association (ASA), and other experts currently recommend that antithrombotic therapy be administered to all patients with nonvalvular atrial fibrillation (i.e., atrial fibrillation in the absence of rheumatic mitral stenosis, a prosthetic heart valve, or mitral valve repair) who are considered to be at increased risk of stroke, unless such therapy is contraindicated.

Recommendations regarding choice of antithrombotic therapy in patients with atrial fibrillation are based on the patient's risk for stroke and bleeding. In general, oral anticoagulant therapy (traditionally warfarin) is recommended in patients with atrial fibrillation who have a moderate to high risk for stroke and acceptably low risk of bleeding, while aspirin or no antithrombotic therapy may be considered in patients at low risk of stroke. Although many risk stratification methods have been used, patients considered to be at increased risk of stroke generally include those with prior ischemic stroke or TIA, advanced age (e.g., 75 years or older), history of hypertension, diabetes mellitus, or congestive heart failure. In addition, population-based studies suggest that female sex is an important risk factor for stroke in patients with atrial fibrillation, particularly in patients 75 years of age or older, and AHA and the American Stroke Association (ASA) recommend the use of risk stratification tools that account for age- and sex-specific differences in stroke risk. One such tool is the CHA_2DS_2-VASc score, an extension of the $CHADS_2$ system (which considers the risk factors congestive heart failure, hypertension, age 75 years or older, diabetes mellitus, and prior stroke/TIA) that adds extra points for female sex (1 point); previous MI, peripheral arterial disease, or aortic plaque (1 point); and age 65–74 years (1 point) or 75 years or older (2 points). In a large drug registry study in Sweden, women had a greater reduction in stroke (60%) than men (40%) with warfarin therapy while the risk of major hemorrhage was similar between groups.

Although warfarin traditionally has been used for oral anticoagulation in patients with atrial fibrillation at increased risk of stroke, some experts suggest that non-vitamin K antagonist oral anticoagulants such as apixaban, dabigatran, or rivaroxaban may provide certain advantages over warfarin (e.g., rapid onset of action, predictable anticoagulant effect, no requirement for coagulation monitoring, less potential for drug-drug and drug-food interactions) and may be considered as alternative therapy in selected patients. (See Uses: Embolism Associated with Atrial Fibrillation, in Rivaroxaban 20:12.04.14.) Warfarin generally should remain the treatment of choice in patients with severe renal impairment pending clinical outcomes data with the non-vitamin K antagonist oral anticoagulants in such patients. AHA and ASA state that while clinical trials of non-vitamin K antagonist oral anticoagulants were not designed to determine differences in efficacy compared with warfarin in men versus women, apixaban, dabigatran, or rivaroxaban may be a useful alternative to warfarin for the prevention of stroke and systemic thromboembolism in women with paroxysmal or permanent atrial fibrillation and prespecified risk factors (according to CHA_2DS_2-VASc) who do not have a prosthetic heart valve or hemodynamically important valve disease, severe renal failure (creatinine clearance less than 15 mL/minute), lower body weight (less than 50 kg), or advanced liver disease (impaired baseline clotting function). When selecting an appropriate anticoagulant for patients with atrial fibrillation, experts recommend that the risks versus benefits of such therapy be considered for individual patients based on the absolute and relative risks of stroke and bleeding; patient compliance, preference, tolerance, and comorbidities; cost; availability of agents to reverse anticoagulant effects in case of bleeding complications; and other clinical factors such as renal function, availability of facilities to monitor INR, and degree of current INR control in patients already receiving warfarin.

Pooled analysis of data from a number of comparative studies evaluating therapy with warfarin and aspirin in patients with chronic atrial fibrillation demonstrate that warfarin therapy is more effective than aspirin (e.g., 75–325 mg daily) in reducing thromboembolic complications. In addition, warfarin therapy appears to have a therapeutic advantage over aspirin in preventing nonfatal stroke. However, the anticipated greater benefits of warfarin compared with aspirin must be weighed against the greater risk of bleeding and inconvenience of monitoring oral anticoagulation. Because the net clinical benefit with warfarin relative to aspirin appears to be greatest in patients with a high (and possibly also intermediate) risk of stroke, ACCP and other experts generally recommend the use of oral anticoagulation (e.g., warfarin targeted to an INR of 2–3) over aspirin in such patients. For patients at low risk of stroke, the expected benefits of warfarin may not outweigh the risks of bleeding, and thus, aspirin is preferred. AHA and ASA state that oral anticoagulation is not recommended in women 65 years of age or younger with atrial fibrillation and no other risk factors ($CHADS_2$ = 0 or CHA_2DS_2-VASc = 1); instead, antiplatelet therapy is a reasonable option in selected low-risk women.

Dual antiplatelet therapy with clopidogrel and aspirin was evaluated as a potential alternative to oral anticoagulation in a randomized controlled study in patients with atrial fibrillation at high risk of stroke. The study was terminated early because of clear evidence of superiority of warfarin over antiplatelet therapy for the primary outcome of stroke, systemic embolism, MI, or vascular death. Results of another study comparing dual antiplatelet therapy (clopidogrel and aspirin) with aspirin monotherapy in patients with atrial fibrillation who had an increased risk of stroke but were unable to take warfarin showed that the combination of clopidogrel and aspirin was more effective than aspirin in reducing the risk of nonfatal stroke; however, dual antiplatelet therapy was associated with an increased risk of bleeding. Based on these findings, ACCP and other experts recommend the use of clopidogrel and aspirin rather than aspirin alone as an alternative to oral anticoagulation in patients with atrial fibrillation at increased risk of stroke who cannot take or choose not to take oral anticoagulants for reasons other than concerns about major bleeding (e.g., those with difficulty maintaining stable INRs, compliance issues, dietary restrictions, or cost limitations). Because the risk of bleeding with combination aspirin and clopidogrel therapy is similar to the risk of bleeding with warfarin, such combination therapy is not recommended in patients with a hemorrhagic contraindication to warfarin.

Antiplatelet agents may be used in addition to warfarin in certain patients with atrial fibrillation who have coexisting conditions that warrant the use of antiplatelet therapy (e.g., patients with recent placement of an intracoronary stent or those experiencing an acute coronary syndrome).

While randomized clinical trials evaluating warfarin anticoagulation in patients with atrial fibrillation and prosthetic heart valves or rheumatic mitral valve disease have not been conducted, long-term warfarin therapy also is strongly recommended in such patients based on results of studies in patients who have atrial fibrillation *without* these coexisting conditions. The intensity of anticoagulation in patients with prosthetic heart valves should be based on the particular type of prosthesis but should not be less than that required to maintain an INR of 2.5; patients with prosthetic mechanical heart valves should have a target INR of at least 2.5. (See Uses: Thromboembolism Associated with Prosthetic Heart Valves.)

In patients with atrial fibrillation who have ischemic stroke or systemic embolism during warfarin anticoagulation at an INR of 2–3, ACC, AHA, and the European Society of Cardiology (ESC) suggest that it may be reasonable to increase the intensity of anticoagulation to a maximum target INR of 3–3.5; however, other experts state that data are lacking regarding the efficacy of increasing anticoagulation in providing future protection against thromboembolic events, and higher INRs are associated with an increased risk of bleeding.

The risk of thromboembolism in patients with atrial flutter is not as well established as it is in those with atrial fibrillation. In addition, many patients with atrial flutter have alternating periods of atrial fibrillation. Experts state that antithrombotic therapy in patients with atrial flutter generally should be managed in the same manner as in patients with atrial fibrillation.

■ **Cardioversion of Atrial Fibrillation** Use of warfarin is recommended to decrease the risk of embolization in patients undergoing pharmacologic or electrical cardioversion of atrial fibrillation.

Because the risk of thromboembolism appears to be greatest when atrial fibrillation has been present for more than 48 hours, recommendations for the use of anticoagulant therapy in such patients vary based on the duration of the arrhythmia. ACCP and other experts recommend that patients with atrial fibrillation of unknown or greater than 48 hours' duration who are to undergo elective cardioversion receive therapeutic anticoagulation (e.g., usually with warfarin) for at least 3 weeks prior to cardioversion; alternatively, a transesophageal echocardiography (TEE)-guided approach may be used. In patients who have atrial fibrillation of short duration (e.g., 48 hours or less), cardioversion usually is performed without prolonged warfarin anticoagulation or TEE prior to the procedure. After successful cardioversion to sinus rhythm, all patients should receive therapeutic anticoagulation for at least 4 weeks.

Experts suggest that patients with atrial flutter undergoing cardioversion be managed according to the same approach as that used in patients with atrial fibrillation.

■ **Embolism Associated with Valvular Heart Disease** Warfarin and/or aspirin is used to prevent thromboembolism associated with various types of valvular heart disease; the choice of antithrombotic therapy depends on balancing the risk of thromboembolism with the risk of hemorrhagic complications from antithrombotic therapy.

Analysis of data from trials evaluating thromboembolism in patients with nonvalvular atrial fibrillation indicate that oral anticoagulants are most effective in patients at highest risk for embolic events. Among the common types of valvular heart disease, rheumatic mitral valve disease is associated with the greatest risk of systemic thromboembolism, and the risk is further increased in patients with concurrent atrial fibrillation, left atrial thrombus, or a history of systemic embolism. Therefore, ACCP recommends warfarin anticoagulation (INR of 2–3) in such patients.

Patients with rheumatic mitral valve disease and in normal sinus rhythm who have a left atrial diameter exceeding 5.5 cm† also may be considered for oral anticoagulation with warfarin (target INR 2.5, range 2–3) because of their high likelihood of developing atrial fibrillation. Antithrombotic therapy usually is not required in patients with rheumatic mitral valve disease who are in normal sinus rhythm and have a left atrial diameter of less than 5.5 cm.

In selected patients with mitral valve prolapse who have atrial fibrillation (i.e., those 65 years of age or older or those with a mitral valve regurgitation murmur, hypertension, or a history of heart failure), prophylaxis with warfarin is recommended by ACC and AHA. Warfarin (INR of 2–3) also is recommended by ACC and AHA for prevention of thromboembolic events in patients with mitral valve prolapse and a history of stroke who have concomitant mitral valve regurgitation, atrial fibrillation, or left atrial thrombus.

Warfarin has been used in a limited number of patients undergoing percutaneous balloon mitral valvotomy† to prevent left atrial embolism. In patients who are being considered for percutaneous balloon mitral valvotomy who have TEE-confirmed left atrial thrombus, ACCP recommends postponing the procedure and administering warfarin (target INR 3, range 2.5–3.5) until confirmed thrombus resolution occurs. The procedure should not be performed if thrombus resolution does not occur with warfarin therapy.

Antithrombotic therapy generally should not be initiated in patients with infective endocarditis involving a native valve because of the risk of serious hemorrhage, including intracerebral hemorrhage, and lack of documented efficacy in such patients. In patients with a prosthetic valve who are already receiving warfarin therapy, ACCP suggests temporary discontinuance of the drug if infective endocarditis develops, and reinitiation of therapy once invasive procedures no longer are required and the patient is stabilized without signs of neurologic complications.

■ **Thromboembolism Associated with Prosthetic Heart Valves** Warfarin is used to reduce the incidence of thromboembolism (e.g., stroke) in patients with prosthetic mechanical or biological heart valves. The risk of systemic embolism is higher with mechanical than with bioprosthetic heart valves, higher with first-generation mechanical (e.g., caged ball, caged disk) valves than with newer mechanical (e.g., bileaflet, Medtronic Hall tilting disk) heart valves, higher with more than one prosthetic valve, and higher with prosthetic mitral than with aortic valves; risk also is higher in the first few days and months after valve insertion (before full endothelialization) and increases in the presence of atrial fibrillation.

All patients with mechanical heart valves require long-term warfarin therapy because of the high risk of thromboembolism with these valves, which appears to average 1–2% annually even with the use of warfarin. During the early postoperative period following insertion of a mechanical heart valve, ACCP suggests bridging anticoagulation with heparin or a low molecular weight heparin until the patient is stable on warfarin therapy. (See Initial Dosage under Dosage and Administration: Dosage.) Warfarin therapy also is suggested by ACCP in patients with bioprosthetic heart valves in the mitral position, at least for the first 3 months after valve insertion; after the first 3 months, patients may be switched to aspirin therapy provided they are in normal sinus rhythm. In patients with aortic bioprosthetic valves who are in sinus rhythm and have no other indications for warfarin therapy, aspirin generally is suggested for initial (e.g., first 3 months after valve insertion) and long-term antithrombotic therapy. However, long-term warfarin therapy (INR 2.5, range 2–3) may be indicated in some patients with bioprosthetic heart valves who have additional risk factors for thromboembolism (e.g., atrial fibrillation, prior thromboembolism, left ventricular dysfunction, hypercoagulable states).

In general, a target INR of 2.5 (range 2–3) is suggested with warfarin therapy in patients with a mechanical heart valve in the aortic position, while a higher intensity of anticoagulation (target INR of 3; range 2.5–3.5) is recommended in those with a mechanical heart valve in the mitral position. A higher intensity of warfarin anticoagulation also may be considered in patients with mechanical heart valves in both the aortic and mitral positions. (See Initial Dosage under Dosage and Administration: Dosage.)

Because warfarin therapy alone does not completely prevent thrombosis in patients with prosthetic heart valves, aspirin or dipyridamole has been used in conjunction with warfarin to reduce the incidence of thrombosis in these patients. The combination of warfarin and aspirin appears to be more effective than warfarin alone but may increase the risk of bleeding. In 2 studies comparing treatment with warfarin alone or in combination with 500-mg or 1-g daily doses of aspirin, patients receiving 1 g of aspirin daily had an increased risk of GI bleeding. In another study comparing treatment with warfarin alone or in combination with aspirin (500 mg daily) or dipyridamole (400 mg daily), the combination regimen with aspirin was associated with an increased risk of bleeding complications compared to the other regimens. In a randomized, placebo-controlled study in patients with prosthetic heart valves who were at high risk for systemic embolism, addition of delayed-release, enteric-coated aspirin (100 mg daily) to warfarin therapy (adjusted to maintain an INR of 3–4.5) resulted in a substantial reduction in major systemic embolism or death, particularly from vascular causes, compared with warfarin therapy alone. Although the risk of hemorrhagic complications with combined aspirin-warfarin therapy was considerably higher than that with warfarin alone (55% increase, principally in minor bleeding), combined therapy was associated with a 61% reduction in relative risk (compared with warfarin alone) for the combined end point of major systemic embolism, nonfatal intracranial hemorrhage, death from hemorrhage, and death from vascular causes. Based on the current evidence, ACCP recommends the addition of an antiplatelet agent such as low-dose aspirin (e.g., 50–100 mg daily) to warfarin therapy in all patients with mechanical heart valves who are at low risk of bleeding. In addition, combination therapy with aspirin and warfarin also is recommended by ACC/AHA in patients with bioprosthetic valves who have additional risk factors for thrombosis (e.g., atrial fibrillation, previous thromboembolism, left ventricular dysfunction, hypercoagulable condition).

■ **ST-Segment Elevation Myocardial Infarction** ***Secondary Prevention*** Warfarin is used for secondary prevention to reduce the risk of death, recurrent MI, and thromboembolic events such as stroke or systemic embolization after an acute ST-segment-elevation MI (STEMI). In general, antiplatelet therapy is preferred to the use of anticoagulants for secondary prevention and risk reduction in patients with atherosclerosis, including those with acute STEMI; however, warfarin in conjunction with low-dose aspirin is recommended in patients who have other compelling indications for anticoagulation therapy (e.g., atrial fibrillation, prosthetic heart valve, left ventricular thrombus or high risk for such thrombi, concomitant venous thromboembolic disease). Anticoagulant therapy with warfarin has been shown to reduce the risk of left ventricular thrombus formation and systemic embolization in patients with Q-wave (transmural) anterior STEMI.

Results of a few prospective studies and analysis of pooled data from other controlled trials suggest that long-term therapy (1–2 years or longer) with a coumarin derivative (e.g., warfarin) may be useful in selected patients for *secondary prevention* of death and/or nonfatal recurrent STEMI. In a randomized, placebo-controlled study in patients with acute STEMI, therapy with warfarin, initiated 2–4 weeks postinfarction and continued for an average of 37 months, was associated with reductions in the risk of death (24% reduction), nonfatal or fatal reinfarction (34% reduction), and total cerebrovascular events (55% reduction). In another placebo-controlled study in patients randomized to treatment with a coumarin anticoagulant (nicoumalone or phenprocoumon, not currently available in the US) within 6 weeks (usually within 2 weeks) after hospital discharge following acute STEMI, anticoagulant therapy was associated with statistically significant reductions in the risks of reinfarction (53% reduction) and cerebrovascular events (40% reduction); a reduction in the risk of death from any cause (10%) also occurred but was not statistically significant. In an open-label, randomized, comparative study in hospitalized patients with recent acute STEMI, long-term (approximately 4 years) therapy with warfarin alone or in combination with aspirin was more effective than aspirin therapy alone in reducing the incidence of the composite end point of death, nonfatal reinfarction, or thromboembolic stroke. The benefit of warfarin (dosage adjusted to achieve an INR of 2–2.5) in combination with aspirin (75 mg daily) or warfarin alone (dosage adjusted to achieve an INR of 2.8–4.2) compared with aspirin alone (160 mg daily) was restricted to reduction of nonfatal reinfarction and thromboembolic stroke; overall mortality was similar among the treatment groups.

The manufacturers and other experts currently recommend the use of warfarin (target INR 2–3) in conjunction with low-dose aspirin (not exceeding 100 mg daily) for at least 3 months following an acute STEMI in high-risk patients (e.g., those with a large anterior STEMI, substantial heart failure, intracardiac thrombus visible on transthoracic echocardiography, atrial fibrillation, history of previous thromboembolic event). For patients with an anterior STEMI and left ventricular thrombus (or at high risk for such thrombi) who undergo coronary artery stent placement, some experts suggest the use of warfarin in combination with low-dose aspirin and clopidogrel; the recommended duration of such triple antithrombotic therapy is dependent on whether the patient has a bare-metal or drug-eluting stent. Some experts state that triple antithrombotic therapy should be limited to clinical situations in which the risk of systemic or venous thromboembolism or stent thrombosis is considered to exceed the risk of bleeding. ACCP generally recommends a target INR of 2–3 in post-MI patients receiving triple antithrombotic therapy; other experts state that a lower target INR of 2–2.5 may be reasonable in such patients, although prospective data are lacking.

■ **Other Cardiovascular Disease** ACC and AHA recommend the use of anticoagulation in patients with heart failure who have persistent or paroxysmal atrial fibrillation or a prior thromboembolic event†. (See Uses: Embolism Associated with Atrial Fibrillation.) However, routine use of aspirin or warfarin for prevention of thromboembolic events is not recommended by ACC and AHA in patients who have heart failure without an ischemic etiology† (e.g., idiopathic, hypertensive) or in those who do not have atrial fibrillation or previous thromboembolism.

■ **Cerebral Embolism** Antiplatelet agents are considered preferable to oral anticoagulation for secondary prevention of noncardioembolic stroke in patients with a history of ischemic stroke or TIA. However, oral anticoagulation with warfarin or one of the non-vitamin K antagonist oral anticoagulants (e.g., apixaban, dabigatran, rivaroxaban) is recommended for secondary prevention in patients with TIAs or ischemic stroke and concurrent atrial fibrillation, provided no contraindications to therapy exist. (See Uses: Embolism Associated with Atrial Fibrillation.) Warfarin anticoagulation also is recommended for the prevention of recurrent stroke in patients at high risk for recurring cerebral embolism from other cardiac sources (e.g., prosthetic mechanical heart valves, anterior MI and left ventricular thrombus).

For arterial ischemic stroke associated with dissection or a cardioembolic cause in children†, ACCP suggests the use of warfarin as an option for long-term anticoagulation.

In patients with cryptogenic stroke and a patent foramen ovale or atrial septal aneurysm†, ACCP recommends aspirin therapy for secondary prophylaxis of such events; however, if recurrent events occur despite aspirin therapy or another condition requiring anticoagulation (e.g., DVT) exists in such patients, warfarin (target INR 2.5; range 2–3) is suggested over aspirin.

ACCP, AHA, and ASA state that oral anticoagulation with warfarin usually is recommended following initial therapy with heparin or a low molecular weight heparin in patients with acute cerebral venous sinus thrombosis†. Following low molecular weight heparin therapy during pregnancy in women with cerebral venous sinus thrombosis†, AHA and ASA recommend postpartum anticoagulation with warfarin (target INR of 2–3) as an alternative to low molecular weight heparin for at least 6 weeks (for a total minimum duration of 6 months of anticoagulant therapy). ACCP recommends initial therapy with heparin or a low molecular weight heparin followed by conversion to warfarin or continued therapy with a low molecular weight heparin for at least 3 months in children with cerebral venous sinus thrombosis† without substantial intracranial hemorrhage. If symptoms persist or there is continued occlusion of the cerebral venous sinuses, another 3 months of anticoagulant therapy is suggested. For additional information on the use of anticoagulants in pediatric patients with cerebral venous sinus thrombosis, consult the most recent ACCP Evidence-based Clinical Practice Guidelines on Antithrombotic Therapy and Prevention of Thrombosis available at http://www.chestnet.org.

■ **Arterial Occlusive Disease** Warfarin has been used in certain patients with peripheral arterial occlusive disease†. However, ACCP generally recommends the use of antiplatelet agents (aspirin or clopidogrel) rather than anticoagulants for the primary or secondary prevention of cardiovascular events in patients with peripheral arterial disease.

Extended anticoagulant therapy (e.g., with warfarin) is recommended by ACCP in all patients with chronic thromboembolic pulmonary hypertension.

■ **Heparin-Induced Thrombocytopenia** While warfarin should not be used for initial treatment of heparin-induced thrombocytopenia (HIT), the manufacturers and other clinicians state that therapy with the drug may be considered after platelet counts have normalized. Cases of venous limb ischemia, necrosis, and gangrene, sometimes resulting in amputation or death, have occurred in patients with HIT when heparin was discontinued and warfarin was initiated or continued. ACCP recommends against initiating warfarin in patients with strongly suspected or confirmed HIT until substantial platelet recovery occurs (e.g., platelet count of at least 150,000/mm^3); for patients already receiving warfarin at the time of diagnosis of HIT, use of vitamin K is suggested.

ACCP states that HIT should be treated initially with a nonheparin anticoagulant (e.g., lepirudin, argatroban). Conversion to warfarin therapy should be initiated with low dosages (maximum 5 mg daily) and only after substantial recovery from acute HIT has occurred. To avoid prothrombotic effects and ensure continuous anticoagulation, ACCP recommends that therapy with the nonheparin anticoagulant and warfarin be administered concurrently for at least 5 days and until the desired INR has been achieved. (See Initial Dosage under Dosage and Administration: Dosage)

Dosage and Administration

■ **Administration** ***Oral Administration*** Warfarin sodium is administered orally in a single, daily dose. Patients should adhere strictly to the prescribed dosage and schedule of warfarin. Patients should take warfarin tablets at the same time each day, with food or on an empty stomach. If a dose of warfarin is missed, or if an excess dose of warfarin is taken, patients should contact their clinician. The missed dose should be taken as soon as possible on the same day. However, a double dose of warfarin should not be taken the next day to make up for the missed dose.

IV Administration The drug also is administered by IV injection when warfarin therapy is indicated and oral administration is not feasible. The manufacturer of commercially available warfarin sodium for injection states that this preparation is not recommended for IM administration.

Warfarin sodium sterile, lyophilized powder for injection is reconstituted by adding 2.7 mL of sterile water for injection to a vial labeled as containing 5 mg of warfarin sodium. The resultant solution contains 2 mg of warfarin sodium per mL. The appropriate dose of warfarin sodium should be injected slowly (over 1–2 minutes) into a peripheral vein.

■ **Dosage** Warfarin is commercially available as oral tablets and as an injection. The drug is available as the sodium salt; dosage is expressed in terms of warfarin sodium.

Nonproprietary (generic) preparations of warfarin sodium are available, and the manufacturers warn that patients should be carefully instructed about what they are receiving so that overdosage from inadvertent simultaneous use of equivalent preparations is avoided.

Warfarin sodium dosage requirements vary greatly among individual patients, and dosage must be carefully individualized based on clinical and laboratory findings (i.e., determination of PT ratios/INRs) in order to obtain optimum therapeutic effects while minimizing the risk of hemorrhage. Pharmacogenomic factors (e.g., genetic variations in enzymes that metabolize warfarin or modulate its effect on clotting factor synthesis) also may be considered in determining the dosage of warfarin. (See Dosage: Factors Influencing Anticoagulant Response, under Dosage and Administration.) Dosage of warfarin sodium does not vary with the route of administration.

Laboratory Monitoring and Dosage Adjustment The prothrombin time (PT) is the most commonly used laboratory method for monitoring therapy with warfarin. Clotting times and bleeding times are not effective methods for monitoring therapy with the drugs. The PT is sensitive to plasma concentrations of functional blood coagulation factors II, V, VII, and X and, to a minor extent, fibrinogen; the test is not sensitive to decreased concentrations of functional factor IX. The PT does not measure antithrombogenic effects but may provide an indication of the risk of hemorrhage. Although results of the test are frequently reported as a percentage of the normal prothrombin activity, it is more satisfactory to report actual PT values in seconds of the sample being tested compared with that of a control sample (PT ratio). PT values depend on the procedures and reagents used for each test and are relevant only in the laboratory in which they are determined. Clinicians must understand the test procedures employed and methods of reporting results in order to monitor therapy.

Variability in PT values obtained from the same plasma sample occurs because of differences in the responsiveness (sensitivity) of commercial thromboplastins to the reduction in clotting factors induced by oral anticoagulants (e.g., warfarin). Therefore, a system of standardizing the reporting of PT values through determination of an international normalized ratio (INR) was introduced by the World Health Organization (WHO) and has been recommended by the American College of Chest Physicians (ACCP) and the National Heart, Lung, and Blood Institute (NHLBI). The INR is derived from calibrations of commercial thromboplastin reagents against an international reference preparation (IRP), a sensitive thromboplastin prepared from human brain tissue. For the 3 commercial rabbit brain thromboplastins currently used in North America, a PT value of 1.3–2 times the control PT value (i.e., PT ratio of 1.3–2) is equivalent to an INR of 2–4. For other thromboplastins, the INR can be calculated from the prothrombin time ratio determined using any local thromboplastin as follows:

$$\text{INR} = (\text{observed PT ratio})^{\text{ISI}}$$

where the ISI (international sensitivity index) is a calibration factor that is available from the manufacturers of the thromboplastin reagent. The ISI is a measure of the responsiveness of the individual thromboplastin to the reduction in vitamin K-dependent coagulation factors; the lower the ISI, the more responsive the reagent and the closer the derived INR will be to the observed prothrombin time ratio. Current data suggest that the ISIs of most thromboplastin reagents used in the US range from 1.8–2.8. The INR is the prothrombin time ratio that would be obtained if the WHO reference thromboplastin, which by definition has an ISI of 1, were used to assess prothrombin time.

The generally accepted therapeutic PT range has been 1.5–2.5 times the control value in seconds (PT ratio = 1.5–2.5) or 15–35% of the normal prothrombin activity; however, this range was determined from studies in which sensitive human brain thromboplastin was used. Recent studies with the less sensitive rabbit brain thromboplastin reagents currently used in the US indicate that a lower therapeutic range may be appropriate for most thromboembolic conditions and may minimize the risk of bleeding.

The INR should be determined regularly in all patients receiving warfarin. The manufacturers recommend that INR determinations be performed daily after initiation of warfarin therapy until the INR stabilizes in the therapeutic range. ACCP states that INR determinations usually are performed daily in hospitalized patients until the INR is in the therapeutic range for at least 2 consecutive days; in outpatients, initial INR determinations may be reduced from daily to every few days until a stable response has been achieved. The frequency of INR determinations should be based on clinical judgment and patient response, but generally is every 1–4 weeks. In patients with consistently stable INRs, ACCP has suggested an INR testing interval of up to 12 weeks.

For adequate anticoagulation control, additional INR determinations should be performed when different warfarin preparations (e.g., proprietary versus nonproprietary [generic]) are interchanged and when concomitant drug therapy is added, discontinued, or taken irregularly. Heparin prolongs the PT/INR, and caution should be observed in evaluating the INR and/or PT ratio in patients receiving concomitant therapy with warfarin and heparin. Valid PT/INR determinations can usually be made during concurrent heparin therapy if blood samples for the test are drawn at least 4–6 hours after an IV injection or 12–24 hours after a subcutaneous injection of heparin. The PT/INR may not be substantially prolonged by heparin when the drug is administered by continuous IV infusion and blood samples for the test may be obtained at any time during the infusion. Warfarin may prolong the activated partial thromboplastin time (aPTT), even in the absence of heparin. However, during initial therapy with warfarin, the interference with heparin anticoagulation is of minimal clinical importance.

Safety and efficacy of warfarin therapy can be improved by increasing the quality of laboratory control. Available data indicate that the proportion of time in the therapeutic INR range is increased in patients managed by anticoagulation clinics and patients in whom anticoagulation is managed with the assistance of computer programs compared with patients receiving usual monitoring by their primary care clinician. Self-management of warfarin therapy is suggested by ACCP as an alternative to outpatient INR monitoring in patients who are motivated and can demonstrate competency in self-management strategies, including the use of self-testing equipment.

Factors Influencing Anticoagulant Response A number of factors, including concomitant therapy with drugs or dietary or herbal supplements (see Drug Interactions) and changes in diet, environment (prolonged hot weather), physical state, and genetic variations in warfarin metabolism and/or sensitivity may alter an individual's response to warfarin therapy. Factors reported to *increase* response, prolong the PT/INR, and increase the risk of hemorrhage include vitamin K deficiency caused by decreased dietary intake, alterations in intestinal flora, or malabsorption states; scurvy; malnutrition or cachexia; small body size; hepatic dysfunction; moderate to severe renal impairment; hypermetabolic states such as fever or hyperthyroidism; infectious disease; carcinoma; collagen disease; congestive heart failure; diarrhea; biliary obstruction; old age; debility; menstruation and menstrual disorders; radiation therapy; initial hypoprothrombinemia; and decreased clearance of warfarin as a result of variations in genes responsible for warfarin metabolism.

Factors reported to *decrease* response to coumarin anticoagulants and shorten the PT/INR include increased intake or GI absorption of vitamin K; GI states that result in decreased anticoagulant absorption; diabetes mellitus; edema; hyperlipidemia; hypothyroidism; and visceral carcinoma. In addition, 2 types of resistance to warfarin have been reported. Rarely, familial resistance to warfarin, apparently resulting from variations in the anticoagulant-vitamin K receptor site, has been reported and appears to be inherited as an autosomal dominant trait. In individuals with familial resistance to warfarin, absorption and metabolism of the drugs are unaltered but 10–20 times the usual anticoagulant dosage may be required to achieve therapeutic effects. These patients also demonstrate increased sensitivity to antidotal effects of phytonadione. Another type of warfarin resistance appears to involve an increased rate of warfarin metabolism and excretion.

Pharmacogenomics. Variations in the genes responsible for warfarin metabolism or pharmacodynamic response may affect warfarin dosage requirements. Over 30% of European and Caucasian populations have one or more variant alleles encoding cytochrome P-450 (CYP) isoenzyme 2C9 (CYP2C9), the enzyme principally responsible for metabolism of *S*-warfarin, and such alleles are associated with reduced clearance of warfarin. (See Pharmacokinetics: Elimination.) Patients with one or more variant CYP2C9 alleles (e.g., CYP2C9*2, CYP2C9*3) are at increased risk of excessive anticoagulation (e.g., INR exceeding 3) and bleeding and require lower dosages of warfarin, particularly during initiation of therapy.

Warfarin inhibits vitamin K epoxide reductase, which is a vitamin K-cycle enzyme complex controlling the regeneration of reduced vitamin K from vitamin K epoxide. Reduced vitamin K is an essential cofactor involved in the formation of vitamin K-dependent clotting factors. (See Pharmacology.) Limited evidence suggests that variations in the gene that encodes vitamin K epoxide reductase, vitamin K epoxide reductase complex subunit 1 (VKORC1), may have an even larger impact on warfarin dosage than CYP2C9 genetic variations. Common polymorphisms in non-coding regions of the VKORC1 gene contribute substantially to warfarin dosage variability across the normal dosage range. Asians appear to be more sensitive than Caucasians to the anticoagulant effect of warfarin and may require lower initial and maintenance dosages. In an uncontrolled study in Chinese patients receiving warfarin for various indications and on a stable warfarin sodium dosage for at least 1 month, the average daily dosage required to maintain an INR of 2–2.5 was 3.3 mg. Age also was an important determinant of warfarin dosage (inverse correlation) in these patients, as were body weight and underlying disease (positive correlations). A single nucleotide polymorphism of VKORC1 that identifies a low-dose and a high-dose warfarin phenotype has been found to associate with optimal warfarin dosage in both European and Asian patients. The reduced average warfarin maintenance dosage requirement in Asian individuals is largely related to the relatively rare occurrence of the high-dose allele in this ethnic group.

Several dosing algorithms for warfarin have been developed that take into account genetic variations in CYP2C9 and VKORC1 genes and individual clinical factors (e.g., age, height, body weight, interacting drugs, indication for warfarin therapy). In one such model in Caucasian patients, approximately 30, 40, or 55% of the variability in warfarin dosage could be attributed to variations in the VKORC1 gene alone, variations in CYP2C9 and VKORC1 genes, or variations in both of these genes plus inclusion of individual clinical factors, respectively.

Laboratory tests (e.g., Nanosphere Verigene Warfarin Metabolism Nucleic Acid Test, Warfarin DoseAdvise® Genetic Test) currently are available to determine if patients have certain VKORC1 or CYP2C9 gene variants that may influence their response to warfarin. Clinicians may consider incorporating information obtained from genetic testing along with individual clinical factors to improve their estimate of initial warfarin dosage. The availability and reliability of genetic tests vary, and clinicians should check with their local or reference clinical laboratory to obtain more information about specific tests. Genetic information does not replace regular INR monitoring (see Dosage: Laboratory Monitoring and Dosage Adjustment, in Dosage and Administration), and results of genetic testing, which currently require several days to obtain, should not delay initiation of warfarin therapy.

Although limited data have suggested that genetic testing could improve safety and potentially lower costs associated with warfarin therapy by lowering the risk of bleeding or ischemic complications from inappropriate dosing, current evidence does not appear to support routine use of such testing. In addition, genetic testing has not been shown to be cost-effective. ACCP currently recommends against the routine use of genetic testing to guide initial dosage selection of warfarin.

Initial Dosage The appropriate initial dosage of warfarin varies widely among different patients; dosage must be individualized taking into account factors such as age, race, body weight, sex, genotype, concomitant drugs, and the specific indication being treated. In patients whose CYP2C9 and VKORC1 genotypes are not known, the manufacturers state that the usual initial dosage of warfarin sodium is 2–5 mg daily. For patients with known CYP2C9 and VKORC1 genotypes, the manufacturers suggest that *initial* dosage of warfarin may be determined based on expected *maintenance* dosages observed in clinical studies of patients with various combinations of these gene variants. (See Table 1.)

Table 1. Expected Daily *Maintenance* Dosages of Warfarin Sodium Based on CYP2C9 and VKORC1 Genotypes[a]

VKORC1	CYP2C9					
	*1/*1	*1/*2	*1/*3	*2/*2	*2/*3	*3/*3
GG	5–7 mg	5–7 mg	3–4 mg	3–4 mg	3–4 mg	0.5–2 mg
AG	5–7 mg	3–4 mg	3–4 mg	3–4 mg	0.5–2 mg	0.5–2 mg
AA	3–4 mg	3–4 mg	0.5–2 mg	0.5–2 mg	0.5–2 mg	0.5–2 mg

[a] Manufacturers suggest using these expected *maintenance* dosage ranges to estimate *initial* daily dosage of warfarin sodium in patients with known CYP2C9 and VKORC1 genotypes. Dosage ranges are derived from multiple published clinical studies. VKORC1-1639G > A (rs9923231) variant is used in this table; other co-inherited VKORC1 variants also may be important determinants of warfarin sodium dosage.

Routine use of warfarin loading doses is not recommended by the manufacturers because such practice may increase the risk of hemorrhage or other complications and does not offer more rapid protection against clot formation. However, there is some evidence suggesting that use of a 10-mg loading dose may be a safe and effective approach in reducing the time to therapeutic INR. ACCP therefore suggests that in patients sufficiently healthy to be treated as outpatients, an initial dosage of 10 mg daily for the first 2 days may be administered, with subsequent dosing based on INR determinations.

Smaller initial dosages (e.g., 2–5 mg of warfarin sodium daily) result in less fluctuation in the degree of anticoagulation and decrease the risk of hemorrhage. Low initial dosages should be considered for geriatric and/or debilitated patients. (See Cautions: Geriatric Precautions.) Lower initial dosages also should be considered in patients with certain genetic variations in CYP2C9 and/or VKORC1 gene(s), which are associated with reduced warfarin clearance or altered pharmacodynamic response. Asians also appear to require lower initial and maintenance dosages than Caucasians, resulting in part from such genetic variations. (See Pharmacogenomics under Dosage: Factors Influencing Anticoagulant Response, in Dosage and Administration.)

Transferring from Parenteral Anticoagulation to Warfarin. When warfarin is indicated for follow-up therapy after initial treatment with a parenteral anticoagulant (e.g., heparin, a low molecular weight heparin, fondaparinux), therapy with the parenteral anticoagulant is usually continued until an adequate response to warfarin is obtained as indicated by INR determinations. The manufacturers recommend that heparin and warfarin be used concurrently for at least 4–5 days until the desired INR has been attained, after which the parenteral anticoagulant may be discontinued. In adults with acute deep-vein thrombosis (DVT) or pulmonary embolism (PE), ACCP recommends that heparin, a low molecular weight heparin, or fondaparinux be used concurrently with warfarin for at least 5 days and until the INR is at least 2 for 24 hours or longer.

In children with venous thromboembolism in whom long-term warfarin therapy is being considered, warfarin should be initiated on the same day as heparin or a low molecular weight heparin, and such therapy should be overlapped for at least 5 days and until the INR is therapeutic.

When warfarin is indicated for follow-up therapy after a nonheparin anticoagulant (e.g., argatroban, lepirudin) in the treatment of heparin-induced thrombocytopenia (HIT), therapy with warfarin and the nonheparin anticoagulant should be overlapped for a minimum of 5 days until an adequate response to warfarin is obtained as indicated by INR determinations. Warfarin therapy should be initiated only after substantial recovery from acute HIT has occurred (i.e., platelet counts of at least 150,000/mm^3).

Conversion from anticoagulation with argatroban to warfarin is more complex than with other direct thrombin inhibitors (e.g., lepirudin) since combined therapy with argatroban and warfarin prolongs the INR beyond that produced by warfarin alone. The INR should be determined daily during concurrent argatroban and warfarin therapy. The manufacturer of argatroban recommends using the aPTT to monitor the effects of argatroban during conversion to warfarin.

For an argatroban infusion rate of 2 mcg/kg per minute, argatroban therapy should be discontinued when the INR on combined therapy exceeds 4. Overshooting the target INR should be avoided, as supratherapeutic INRs during concomitant therapy with direct thrombin inhibitors and warfarin have been associated with necrosis or gangrene of the skin or limbs. The INR should be determined 4–6 hours after discontinuance of argatroban infusion during warfarin monotherapy. If INR is below the desired therapeutic range, argatroban infusion should be resumed. Attempts to discontinue argatroban should be repeated daily and until the INR (4–6 hours after discontinuance of argatroban) on warfarin alone is in therapeutic range.

For argatroban infusion rates exceeding 2 mcg/kg per minute, the infusion rate should be reduced temporarily to 2 mcg/kg per minute, and the procedure just described should be reinstituted for conversion to therapy. INR should be repeated 4–6 hours after reduction of the argatroban infusion.

Maintenance Dosage Maintenance dosage of warfarin sodium varies greatly among patients and should be based on INR determinations. The manufacturers state that the usual maintenance dosage of warfarin sodium is 2–10 mg daily for patients in whom CYP2C9 and VKORC1 genotypes are not known. Although dosage requirements may remain constant in an individual patient, genetic variations in warfarin metabolism or sensitivity or changes in clinical state, concurrent drug therapy, or diet may necessitate adjustment of dosage. For patients with known CYP2C9 and VKORC1 genotypes, the manufacturers suggest expected maintenance dosages observed in clinical studies of patients with various combinations of these gene variants. (See Initial Dosage under Dosage and Administration: Dosage.) Lower initial and maintenance dosages should be considered for geriatric and/or debilitated patients. Because of inherited increased sensitivity and/or reduced metabolism of warfarin, Asians also appear to require lower initial and maintenance dosages of warfarin than Caucasians. Acquired or inherited warfarin resistance is rare but should be suspected if large daily dosages of warfarin sodium are required to maintain INR within a normal therapeutic range. (See Pharmacology.) Changes in anticoagulant dosage should be made in small increments, and patient response should be carefully monitored with clinical observation and INR determinations. If a previously stable patient presents with a single subtherapeutic or supratherapeutic INR (not exceeding 0.5 above or below the therapeutic range), ACCP suggests that the current dosage of warfarin be continued and the INR retested within 1–2 weeks.

The manufacturers state that warfarin dosage in pediatric patients varies based on age, with infants generally having the highest, and adolescents having the lowest dosage requirements to maintain therapeutic INRs. When warfarin is used in children†, a target INR range of 2–3 generally is suggested by ACCP for most indications except in the setting of prosthetic cardiac valves where adherence to the adult recommendations is suggested.

In general, for prophylaxis or treatment of DVT and PE or for prophylaxis in most patients with acute myocardial infarction (MI), atrial fibrillation, valvular heart disease, or *bioprosthetic* heart valves, many clinicians recommend adjustment of warfarin dosage to maintain a moderate intensity of anticoagulation (INR of 2–3). (See Treatment and Secondary Prevention under Uses: Deep-Vein Thrombosis and Pulmonary Embolism.) In contrast, a higher intensity of anticoagulation may be necessary in patients with first-generation or mitral prosthetic *mechanical* heart valves, and many clinicians suggest maintaining an INR of 2.5–3.5 in such patients. An INR exceeding 4 appears to provide no additional therapeutic benefit in most patients and is associated with a higher risk of bleeding complications.

When warfarin is used for the prevention of stroke and systemic embolism in patients with atrial fibrillation, the dosage should be adjusted to maintain a target INR of 2.5 (range 2–3). In patients with atrial fibrillation or atrial flutter who require prolonged anticoagulation prior to cardioversion, warfarin dosage usually is adjusted to achieve a target INR range of 2–3 for at least 3 weeks before and at least 4 weeks after pharmacologic or electrical cardioversion.

In patients with mitral valve disease associated with rheumatic fever who have concurrent atrial fibrillation, left atrial thrombus, or a history of systemic embolism (e.g., stroke), ACCP recommends warfarin anticoagulation adjusted to prolong the INR to a target of 2.5 (range 2–3). In patients with rheumatic mitral valve disease who have left atrial hypertrophy (left atrial diameter exceeding 5.5 cm) and normal sinus rhythm†, warfarin anticoagulation at a target INR of 2.5 (range 2–3) is suggested.

In patients being considered for percutaneous mitral valvotomy who have evidence of left atrial thrombus (confirmed by transesophageal echocardiography [TEE])†, ACCP recommends treatment with warfarin (target INR 3, range 2.5–3.5) and postponement of the procedure.

At least 3 months of warfarin (INR range of 2–3) and aspirin therapy (not exceeding 100 mg daily) is recommended following acute ST-segment elevation MI (STEMI) in patients who are at high risk of systemic or pulmonary embolism (e.g., large anterior STEMI, a history of previous thromboembolism, intracardiac thrombus, atrial fibrillation, or substantial heart failure).

For secondary prevention of cardioembolic cerebral ischemic events in patients with transient ischemic attacks or ischemic stroke and concurrent atrial fibrillation, warfarin anticoagulation to maintain a target INR of 2.5 (range 2–3) may be used long-term, provided no contraindications to therapy exist. In patients at high risk for recurrent stroke from other cardiac sources (e.g., anterior MI and left ventricular thrombus), ACCP recommends warfarin anticoagulation to maintain an INR of 2–3 with concomitant low-dose aspirin; the addition of clopidogrel is recommended in selected patients.

In patients with acute cerebral venous sinus thrombosis† provoked by a transient risk factor, AHA, the American Stroke Association (ASA), and other experts suggest continuation of anticoagulation with warfarin (after initial heparin or low molecular weight heparin therapy) for 3–6 months, with dosage adjusted to maintain a target INR of 2–3. In patients with unprovoked cerebral venous sinus thrombosis†, AHA and ASA suggest continuing warfarin therapy for 6–12 months (target INR of 2–3). Indefinite anticoagulation with warfarin may be considered following an initial episode of cerebral venous sinus thrombosis† in patients with severe thrombophilia and in patients with recurrent cerebral venous sinus thrombosis†, venous thrombosis occurring after acute cerebral venous sinus thrombosis†, or other permanent risk factors for recurrent thrombosis (target INR of 2–3).

Warfarin dosed to a target INR of 2.5 (range 2–3) also is recommended in patients with a patent foramen ovale and cryptogenic stroke† who have evidence of DVT.

Long-term warfarin anticoagulation is required in patients with mechanical heart valves. In general, a target INR of 2.5 (range 2–3) is suggested with warfarin therapy in patients with a mechanical heart valve in the aortic position, while a higher intensity of anticoagulation (target INR 3; range 2.5–3.5) is recommended in those with a mechanical heart valve in the mitral position. A higher intensity of warfarin anticoagulation also may be considered in patients with mechanical heart valves in both the aortic and mitral positions. ACCP recommends the addition of an antiplatelet agent such as low-dose aspirin (e.g., 50–100 mg daily) to warfarin therapy in all patients with mechanical heart valves who are at low risk of bleeding.

Warfarin therapy (target INR 2.5; range 2–3) is suggested by ACCP in patients with *bioprosthetic* heart valves in the mitral position, at least for the first 3 months after valve insertion; after the first 3 months, patients may be switched to aspirin therapy provided they are in normal sinus rhythm. However, long-term warfarin therapy (INR 2.5, range 2–3) may be indicated in some patients with *bioprosthetic* heart valves who have additional risk factors for thromboembolism (e.g., atrial fibrillation, prior thromboembolism, left ventricular dysfunction, hypercoagulable states); the addition of aspirin therapy also may be considered in such high-risk patients.

During the early postoperative period following insertion of a mechanical heart valve, ACCP suggests bridging anticoagulation with heparin or a low molecular weight heparin until the patient is stable on warfarin therapy. (See Initial Dosage under Dosage and Administration: Dosage.)

In patients with prosthetic heart valves who develop infective endocarditis, ACCP suggests temporary discontinuance of warfarin therapy at the time of presentation for treatment until it is clear that invasive procedures will not be required and the patient is stable without signs of neurologic complications.

For long-term control of HIT with or without thrombosis†, warfarin is administered for follow-up treatment after therapy with a nonheparin anticoagulant (e.g., argatroban, lepirudin). Conversion to warfarin therapy should be initiated only after substantial recovery from acute HIT has occurred (i.e., platelet counts at least 150,000/mm^3). Warfarin therapy should be overlapped with the nonheparin anticoagulant for a minimum of 5 days and until the INR is within the target therapeutic range.

The optimum duration of warfarin therapy must be determined by the condition being treated and its severity. For the treatment of DVT or PE, full-dose heparin, a low molecular weight heparin, or fondaparinux is used initially with warfarin until a stable INR is achieved, then warfarin generally is continued (with dosage adjusted to maintain an INR of 2–3) as follow-up anticoagulant therapy for at least 3 months. After 3 months, the risks versus benefits of extended therapy (defined by ACCP as treatment beyond 3 months without a scheduled stop date) should be evaluated in individual patients. (See Treatment and Secondary Prevention under Uses: Deep-Vein Thrombosis and Pulmonary Embolism.)

Although it has been suggested that there is an increased risk of thrombosis or rebound thromboembolism following abrupt discontinuance of warfarin therapy, some studies suggest that there is no increased incidence of arterial or venous thromboembolism when anticoagulant therapy is stopped abruptly rather than tapered over a few weeks.

Managing Anticoagulation in Patients Requiring Invasive Procedures Temporary interruption of long-term warfarin therapy may be required in patients undergoing surgery or other invasive procedures to minimize the risk of perioperative bleeding. The decision whether to interrupt therapy should be based on an assessment of the patient's risk for thromboembolism versus risk of perioperative bleeding, taking into account individual patient- and surgery-related factors. Temporary discontinuance of warfarin usually is required for major surgical or invasive procedures, but may not be necessary for minor procedures associated with a low risk of bleeding (e.g., minor dental procedures, minor dermatologic procedures, cataract surgery).

In patients who require temporary interruption of warfarin prior to surgery, ACCP recommends that the drug be discontinued approximately 5 days prior to surgery. Warfarin may be resumed approximately 12–24 hours postoperatively when adequate hemostasis is achieved. Bridging anticoagulation (administration of a short-acting anticoagulant consisting of a low molecular weight heparin or IV heparin during the period of interruption of warfarin therapy) may be considered in some patients who are at particularly high risk of thromboembolism without warfarin therapy. The decision to administer bridging anticoagulation should be individualized based on the patient's risk of thromboembolism versus risk of bleeding. ACCP states that bridging therapy generally is unnecessary for patients other than those at highest risk for stroke and/or venous thromboembolism (e.g., patients with mechanical heart valves, atrial fibrillation, or a venous thromboembolic event with additional risk factors for venous thromboembolism). For additional information on the perioperative management of patients receiving warfarin, including risk stratification methods, consult the most recent ACCP Evidence-based Clinical Practice Guidelines on Antithrombotic Therapy and Prevention of Thrombosis available at http://www.chestnet.org.

Cautions

■ **Hemorrhage** Hemorrhage, the most common adverse effect of coumarin-derivative anticoagulants (e.g., warfarin), is an extension of the pharmacologic action of the drugs and may range from minor local ecchymoses to major hemorrhagic complications, which occasionally result in death. Massive hemorrhage, if it occurs, most frequently involves the GI tract or genitourinary sites but may involve the spinal cord or cerebral, pericardial, pulmonary, adrenal, or hepatic sites. Although hemorrhage results principally from overdosage or excessive prolongation of the prothrombin time (PT), hemorrhagic complications may occur when the PT is in the usual therapeutic range and frequently result from the presence of occult lesions. Hemorrhage is more likely to occur during the initiation of warfarin therapy and with higher dosages (which result in higher international normalized ratios [INRs]). Risk factors for hemorrhage include a high intensity of anticoagulation (INR exceeding 4), patient age 65 years or older, highly variable INRs, history of GI bleeding, hypertension, cerebrovascular disease, serious heart disease, anemia, malignancy, trauma, renal insufficiency, concomitant drugs that may increase PT/INR response, and a long duration of warfarin therapy. (See Pharmacology and see Pharmacokinetics: Elimination.) Regular monitoring of INR should be performed in all patients receiving warfarin therapy. (See Dosage: Laboratory Monitoring and Dosage Adjustment, in Dosage and Administration.) Patients at high risk of bleeding may benefit from more frequent monitoring, use of lower dosages with careful dosage adjustment to the desired INR, and a shorter duration of therapy. A severe elevation (exceeding 50 seconds) in activated partial thromboplastin time (aPTT) with a PT ratio or INR in the desired range reportedly may suggest an increased risk of postoperative hemorrhage.

Hemorrhagic complications may be manifested by signs or symptoms that do not indicate obvious bleeding, such as paralysis; headache; pain in the chest, abdomen, joints, muscles, or other areas; dizziness; shortness of breath; difficulty breathing or swallowing; unexplained swelling; weakness; hypotension; or unexplained shock. Paralytic ileus and intestinal obstruction also have been reported from submucosal or intramural hemorrhage. The possibility of hemorrhage should be considered in any anticoagulated patient with complaints that do not indicate an obvious diagnosis. Adrenal hemorrhage with resultant acute adrenal insufficiency also has been reported during anticoagulant therapy. Anticoagulant therapy should be discontinued in patients who develop manifestations compatible with acute adrenal hemorrhage or insufficiency. Plasma cortisol concentrations should be measured immediately and vigorous therapy with IV corticosteroids instituted promptly; delay in initiation of such therapy while awaiting laboratory confirmation of the diagnosis may result in the patient's death.

The frequency and severity of hemorrhage may be minimized by careful clinical management of the patient, including frequent PT/INR determinations. (See Laboratory Monitoring and Dosage Adjustment under Dosage and Administration: Dosage.) Early manifestations of overdosage include microscopic or gross hematuria, melena, excessive uterine or menstrual bleeding, petechiae, ecchymoses, bleeding from gums or other mucous membranes, and oozing from nicks made while shaving. If any unexpected bleeding occurs during anticoagulant therapy, the patient's condition must be critically evaluated immediately.

In the treatment of overdosage or excessive prolongation of the INR, therapy should be determined by the severity of the effect, the urgency of the need to restore normal hemostasis, and whether or not therapy with the anticoagulant is to be maintained. The American College of Chest Physicians (ACCP) suggests the use of oral phytonadione in patients with an INR of greater than 10 and no evidence of bleeding; routine use of phytonadione generally is not recommended for INR values between 4.5 and 10 with no evidence of bleeding.

In patients with major bleeding associated with warfarin therapy, ACCP suggests the use of 4-factor prothrombin complex concentrate rather than fresh frozen plasma for rapid reversal of anticoagulation, with additional use of phytonadione (administered at a dosage of 5–10 mg by slow IV infusion). (See Phytonadione 88:24.) Several hours are usually required for the effects of phytonadione to occur whether the drug is administered orally or parenterally. Purified factor IX preparations (e.g., factor IX [human]) should not be used because they cannot increase the levels of prothrombin, factor VII, and factor X that are also depressed by warfarin treatment.

Phytonadione, if given in excessive dosage, may make the patient unresponsive for several days or weeks to subsequent warfarin therapy and probably should not be used in patients with minor hemorrhage in whom the drug must be continued.

■ **Necrosis** Potentially fatal tissue necrosis and/or gangrene of skin or other tissues with subcutaneous infarction, vasculitis, and local thrombosis have occurred rarely in patients receiving a coumarin derivative, including warfarin. This reaction, which can occur on the first exposure to these drugs or during a subsequent course of therapy, usually appears early (e.g., 1–10 days) after initiation of therapy; tissue damage occurs principally at sites of fat tissue such as the abdomen, breasts, buttocks, and thighs. Most cases of warfarin-induced necrosis have been reported in women. The necrotic lesions generally begin as painful, erythematous patches on the skin that progress rapidly to dark, hemorrhagic areas. Necrosis may involve skin, soft tissue, and muscle; gangrene and, frequently, infection follow. In severe cases, surgical debridement of the affected tissue, skin grafting, or amputation may be necessary.

Possible limb ischemia, necrosis, and gangrene may occur in patients with heparin-induced thrombocytopenia (HIT) when warfarin is substituted for heparin treatment or continued after heparin discontinuance. In some patients, amputation of the involved area and/or death have occurred. Warfarin should be used with caution. Clinicians should consider delaying warfarin therapy until thrombin generation is adequately controlled and thrombocytopenia has resolved (i.e., platelet counts at least 150,000/mm^3 and stable).

Patients with hereditary, familial, or clinical deficiencies of protein C or its cofactor, protein S, appear to have an increased risk of developing necrosis during warfarin therapy; however, necrosis can occur in the absence of protein C deficiency. It has been suggested that necrotic reactions occur because initiation of warfarin therapy causes plasma concentrations of protein C to decrease more rapidly than plasma concentrations of factors II, IX, and X. Protein C generally inhibits coagulation by inactivating factors V and VIII and facilitating fibrinolysis; therefore, a rapid decrease in plasma concentrations of protein C results in a hypercoagulable state. Warfarin-induced necrosis generally occurs when the hypercoagulable state is maximal. If necrosis occurs during therapy with warfarin, decisions regarding diagnostic testing and therapy must be made on an individualized basis. If necrosis is suspected to be induced by warfarin and is not associated with HIT, the drug should be discontinued, vitamin K (phytonadione) or fresh frozen plasma should be administered, and alternative anticoagulant therapy (e.g., heparin) should be considered both to treat the underlying thromboembolic disease and possibly to prevent additional microvascular thrombosis. (See Cautions: Precautions and Contraindications.) In addition, protein C concentrate or epoprostenol (prostacyclin) reportedly has been used with some success to treat warfarin-induced necrosis.

It has been suggested that if warfarin therapy is discontinued and heparin therapy initiated or continued before actual tissue necrosis occurs (e.g., at the first patient complaint of pain or discomfort in a particular skin area), it may be possible to limit the extent of tissue damage. In addition, initiation of anticoagulant therapy with heparin for 4–5 days before initiation of warfarin therapy or overlapping therapy with the 2 drugs for 5–6 days may minimize the risk of warfarin-induced necrosis.

■ **Purple Toes Syndrome and Cholesterol Microembolization** Some evidence suggests that anticoagulation with coumarin derivatives (e.g., warfarin) may enhance the release of atheromatous plaque fragments and increase the risk of complications; some cases have progressed to necrosis and death. The most common visceral organs involved are the kidneys, followed by the pancreas, spleen, and liver. A distinct syndrome resulting from microemboli to the feet is known as "purple toes syndrome." Purple toes syndrome usually occurs 3–10 weeks or later following initiation of therapy with warfarin or related compounds (e.g., dicumarol [no longer commercially available in the US]) This syndrome typically is characterized by a purplish or mottled discoloration of the plantar surfaces and sides of the toes, which blanches on moderate pressure and fades with elevation of the legs; other characteristics may include pain and tenderness of the toes and waxing and waning of the color over time. Although purple toes syndrome reportedly is reversible, discontinuance of warfarin therapy is recommended in patients who develop this complication; some cases of purple toes syndrome have progressed to gangrene or necrosis, requiring debridement of the affected area and/or amputation. Systemic atheroembolism may be characterized by a variety of other manifestations depending on the site of microembolization, including livedo reticularis, rash, gangrene, abrupt and intense pain in the leg, foot, or toes, foot ulcers, myalgia, penile gangrene, abdominal pain, flank or back pain, hematuria, renal insufficiency, hypertension, cerebral ischemia, spinal cord infarction, pancreatitis, symptoms simulating polyarteritis, or any other sequelae of vascular compromise caused by embolic occlusion.

■ **Other Adverse Effects** GI disturbances such as nausea, vomiting, anorexia, flatulence/bloating, abdominal cramps, and diarrhea have been reported occasionally in patients receiving a coumarin derivative. Dermatitis (including bullous eruptions), urticaria, rash, alopecia, fever, fatigue, lethargy, malaise, pain, headache, mouth ulcers, and leukopenia have been reported occasionally and agranulocytosis, nephropathy, and increased serum concentrations of AST (SGOT), ALT (SGPT), and alkaline phosphatase and bilirubin have been reported rarely. Dizziness, taste perversion, hypotension, anemia, pallor, angina syndrome, chest pain, loss of consciousness, syncope, coma, and cold intolerance also have been reported infrequently. Minor and severe allergic/hypersensitivity reactions, including anaphylactic reactions, also have been reported infrequently. Other adverse effects reported infrequently with coumarin derivatives include vasculitis, edema, hepatitis, cholestatic hepatic injury, jaundice, asthenia, pruritus, and paresthesia, including chills and feeling cold. Priapism has been reported rarely with coumarin derivatives, and tracheal or tracheobronchial calcification has been reported rarely during long-term warfarin therapy; however, a causal relationship between these effects and the drugs has not been established.

■ **Precautions and Contraindications** Warfarin should be used with increased caution in any condition where added risk of hemorrhage, necrosis, and/or gangrene is present. *All patients receiving warfarin should be under close medical supervision, and adequate laboratory facilities for monitoring therapy (e.g., using INR) and measures for treating hemorrhage must be available.* Patients must be carefully selected to ensure that they are cooperative and can communicate effectively with their clinician. Patients receiving warfarin should carry a notice stating that they are undergoing anticoagulant therapy so that medical and paramedical personnel are alerted in emergency situations. The manufacturers state that patients should be informed that all warfarin sodium preparations (proprietary and nonproprietary [generic]) represent the same drug and should not be taken concomitantly unless instructed otherwise by their clinician, since overdosage may result from inadvertent simultaneous use of equivalent preparations.

The manufacturers' patient medication guide should be available to all patients when their prescriptions for warfarin are issued.

Patients should avoid drastic changes in diet and should eat a balanced diet with a constant amount of vitamin K. Ingestion of large quantities of certain foods that contain a large amount of vitamin K (e.g., leafy green vegetables, certain vegetable oils) should be avoided. Patients should not attempt to diet during warfarin therapy without discussion with their clinician.

Patients should report any signs of bleeding (e.g., pain, swelling or discomfort; headaches, dizziness, or weakness; unusual bleeding or bruising, such as bruises that develop without known cause or grow in size), nosebleeds, bleeding gums, prolonged bleeding from cuts, increased menstrual flow or vaginal bleeding, pink or brown urine, red or black stools, bloody sputum, vomiting blood or material resembling coffee grounds) to clinicians immediately. Patients should inform their clinicians of coexisting conditions such as bleeding problems, propensity for falling, hepatic or renal dysfunction, high blood pressure, congestive heart failure, diabetes mellitus, and alcohol use or abuse. During warfarin therapy, patients should avoid activities or sports that could cause traumatic injury. Clinicians should be informed of falls or injuries, especially head injuries, during warfarin therapy.

Patients should report to their clinician symptoms of blood clots (e.g., pain, color, or temperature changes to any area of the body). Symptoms of purple toes syndrome (e.g., pain in toes, purple or dark toes) should be reported to a clinician immediately.

In patients with HIT and deep-vein thrombosis (DVT), ACCP and other clinicians recommend that warfarin therapy be delayed until thrombin generation is adequately controlled and thrombocytopenia has resolved (as indicated by evaluation of platelet count) because of the risk of venous limb ischemia, necrosis, and gangrene occurring when heparin treatment is discontinued and warfarin therapy started or continued in such patients. (See Cautions: Necrosis and see Uses: Heparin-Induced Thrombocytopenia.)

The decision to use warfarin in patients with the following conditions should be based on clinical judgment after weighing the risks and benefits of anticoagulant therapy: severe to moderate hepatic or renal impairment; infectious diseases (e.g., patients receiving antibiotic therapy) or disturbances of intestinal flora (e.g., sprue); surgery or trauma that may result in large, exposed raw surfaces or trauma that may result in internal bleeding; patients with indwelling catheters; severe to moderate hypertension; and vitamin C or vitamin K deficiency. Patients should inform their clinician of diarrhea, infections, or fevers that occur during warfarin therapy.

IM injections of concomitantly administered therapy should be administered in an upper extremity to permit easy access for manual compression, inspection for bleeding, and/or use of pressure bandages.

Patients with hereditary, familial, or clinical deficiencies of protein C or its cofactor, protein S, appear to have an increased risk of developing tissue necrosis during warfarin therapy, and the drug should be used with caution in patients with known or suspected deficiency in protein C-mediated anticoagulant response. (See Cautions: Necrosis.)

Numerous contraindications to therapy with coumarin-derivative anticoagulants (e.g., warfarin) have been recommended. In many instances, contraindications are relative rather than absolute. Contraindications should be evaluated for each patient giving consideration to the need for anticoagulant therapy, the risk of hemorrhage, the expected duration of therapy, patient reliability, and the availability of adequate laboratory facilities for patient monitoring. Since a high degree of patient cooperation is required for long-term or outpatient use of warfarin, senility, alcoholism, or psychosis may be relative contraindications to use of this drug.

Warfarin is contraindicated in patients who have hemorrhagic tendencies or blood dyscrasias. The drug also is contraindicated in patients with overt bleeding or active ulceration involving the GI, respiratory, or genitourinary tract; cerebrovascular hemorrhage; aneurysms (cerebral, dissecting aorta); pericarditis and pericardial effusions; bacterial endocarditis; eclampsia, preeclampsia, or threatened abortion; or malignant hypertension. Warfarin generally is contraindicated in patients with known hypersensitivity to the drug.

Warfarin generally is contraindicated in patients with recent or contemplated surgery of the eye or central nervous system and in those undergoing traumatic surgery resulting in large open surfaces. Many minor dental and surgical procedures, however, may be performed if necessary without undue risk of hemorrhage in patients receiving an anticoagulant if meticulous surgical hemostasis is maintained. Patients should inform their clinician of any planned surgeries or medical or dental procedures, as the dosage of warfarin may need to be adjusted or temporarily withheld. (See Managing Anticoagulation in Patients Requiring Invasive Procedures, under Dosage and Administration: Dosage.) The operative site should be sufficiently limited to permit effective use of local procedures for hemostasis (e.g., absorbable hemostatic agents, sutures, pressure dressings), if necessary. If anticoagulant therapy is administered prior to, during, or immediately following minor dental or surgical procedures, minimal anticoagulation should be maintained.

■ **Pediatric Precautions** The manufacturers of warfarin state that safety and efficacy of the drug in children younger than 18 years of age have not been established in randomized, controlled studies. However, the drug has been used in pediatric patients for prevention and treatment of thromboembolic events. Difficulty achieving and maintaining therapeutic INRs has been reported in pediatric patients, and more frequent determinations of INR are recommended in such patients because of possible changing warfarin requirements.

■ **Geriatric Precautions** Age reportedly does not substantially affect the pharmacokinetics of racemic warfarin, and the manufacturers state that the clearance of *S*-warfarin is similar in geriatric versus younger individuals. However, the clearance of *R*-warfarin appears to be slightly reduced in geriatric patients compared with that in younger individuals. In addition, geriatric patients appear to exhibit greater than expected anticoagulant responses (as determined by PT/INR values) to warfarin, and less warfarin is required to produce a therapeutic level of anticoagulation; the reason for this increased response has not been determined. Caution should be observed when warfarin is administered to geriatric or debilitated patients, particularly when the risk of hemorrhage is present.

Close monitoring of the INR also is recommended during warfarin therapy in geriatric patients 75 years or older with atrial fibrillation who are at high risk for thromboembolism because of the greater risk for hemorrhage in such patients. A large retrospective study suggests that the risks versus benefits of warfarin therapy for atrial fibrillation in geriatric patients 80 years of age or older may require more careful consideration. Reviews of medical records of patients with anticoagulant-associated intracerebral hemorrhage (AAICH) in a large US metropolitan area showed a substantial (approximately fivefold) increase in the annual incidence of this adverse event between 1988 and 1999 based on point estimates for the periods of January through December 1988, July 1993 through June 1994, and January through December 1999. The annual incidence of AAICH per 100,000 persons was 0.8 in 1988, 1.9 in 1993–1994, and 4.4 in 1999. Most notably, there was an even more marked increase in the rate of AAICH in patients 80 years of age or older, from 2.5 in 1988 to 45.9 in 1999. Most of this increase could be explained by an increase in warfarin use (as determined by records of warfarin shipments from wholesalers to pharmacies, clinics, and hospitals during the period studied); the annual incidences of cardioembolic ischemic stroke due to atrial fibrillation between 1993–1994 and 1999 did not change appreciably (22.0 and 20.6, respectively, per 100,000 persons). In geriatric patients, therapy with low initial and maintenance dosages of warfarin (e.g., dosage adjusted to maintain the INR at the lower end of the range of 2–3) is recommended by the manufacturers.

■ **Pregnancy and Lactation** ***Pregnancy*** Warfarin generally is considered contraindicated during pregnancy, although the drug has been used during the second trimester in certain pregnant women (e.g., those with older-generation prosthetic mechanical heart valves in the mitral position, patients with a history of thromboembolism) considered to be at very high risk for thromboembolism. If anticoagulant therapy is required in pregnant women, therapy with a low molecular weight heparin generally is recommended based on a more favorable adverse effect profile. (See Uses: Thromboembolism Associated with Prosthetic Heart Valves, in Enoxaparin 20:12.04.16.)

Potential risks of warfarin therapy to the fetus include bleeding and teratogenicity. Fetal or neonatal hemorrhage and intrauterine death have occurred, even when maternal PT values were within the generally accepted therapeutic range. Hypoplastic nasal structures and other abnormalities (e.g., stippled epiphyses) consistent with a diagnosis of chondrodysplasia punctata have occurred rarely in children whose mothers received warfarin during the first trimester of pregnancy. CNS abnormalities also have been reported, including dorsal midline dysplasia characterized by agenesis of the corpus callosum, Dandy-Walker malformation, and midline cerebellar atrophy. Ventral midline dysplasia, characterized by optic atrophy, and eye abnormalities have been observed. Mental retardation, blindness, and other CNS abnormalities have been reported in association with second- and third-trimester exposure to warfarin. Other teratogenic effects reported rarely following in utero exposure to the drug include urinary tract abnormalities (e.g., single kidney), asplenia, anencephaly, spina bifida, cranial nerve palsy, hydrocephalus, cardiac defects and congenital heart disease, polydactyly, deformities of toes, diaphragmatic hernia, corneal leukoma, cleft palate, cleft lip, schizencephaly, and microcephaly. Spontaneous abortion and stillbirth are known to occur, and the use of warfarin is associated with a higher risk of fetal mortality. Low birth weight and growth retardation also have been reported. Women should inform their clinicians if they are or plan to become pregnant. If a woman becomes pregnant while receiving warfarin, she should be apprised of the potential risks to the fetus.

ACCP, the American College of Cardiology (ACC), and the American Heart Association (AHA) state that there is some evidence suggesting that warfarin might not be fetopathic when administered during the first 6 weeks of pregnancy. If the decision is made to use warfarin during pregnancy, such as in women with mechanical heart valves, ACCP recommends that the drug be avoided during weeks 6–12 of gestation and close to term (to avoid anticoagulation of the fetus).

Women receiving long-term warfarin therapy should be counseled about the risks of pregnancy before pregnancy occurs. If pregnancy is still desired, ACCP suggests performing frequent pregnancy tests and substituting a low molecular weight heparin for warfarin when pregnancy is achieved.

Despite the risks of warfarin to the fetus, the drug has been used in pregnant women with prosthetic heart valves who are at an increased risk for valve thrombosis. The need for warfarin therapy must be critically evaluated in pregnant women and the risks of not administering the drug must be carefully weighed against the possible risks to both the mother and fetus. Heparin or low molecular weight heparin is considered safer for the fetus than warfarin but has been associated with an increased maternal risk for valve thrombosis, death, and major bleeding complications compared with anticoagulant therapy in women with prosthetic heart valves. Although a causal relationship has not been established and the number of patients involved appears to be small, cases of valve thrombosis resulting in death and/or requiring surgical intervention have been reported with at least one low molecular weight heparin (enoxaparin) during thromboprophylaxis in patients with prosthetic heart valves, including in pregnant women. (See Uses: Thromboembolism Occurring During Pregnancy, in Enoxaparin 20:12.04.16.) The possibility of inadequate dosing or use of an inappropriate target aPTT range may complicate the evaluation of this data; some experts state that low molecular weight heparin may provide adequate protection against valve thrombosis if closely monitored to maintain target anti-factor Xa concentrations. As no prospective, controlled clinical trials have been performed in pregnant women with prosthetic mechanical heart valves, optimal antithrombotic therapy remains to be established.

ACCP recommends several approaches to the management of pregnant women with prosthetic heart valves. One approach is to administer heparin therapy (i.e., adjusted-dose heparin or adjusted-dose low molecular weight heparin) during the first trimester followed by conversion to warfarin therapy at week 13, and reinitiation of heparin therapy close to term. (See Uses: Pregnant Women with Prosthetic Heart Valves, in Heparin 20:12.04.16.) The option to continue warfarin throughout pregnancy until close to delivery may be reasonable in patients judged to be at very high risk of thromboembolism (e.g., those with a history of thromboembolism, first-generation mechanical valve in the mitral position). Experts generally suggest a target INR of 3 (range 2.5–3.5) in most pregnant women with prosthetic mechanical heart valves receiving warfarin anticoagulation. Some clinicians suggest that pregnant women close to term (e.g., 2–3 weeks prior to planned delivery) who have prosthetic mechanical heart valves and who are receiving warfarin should have therapy switched to subcutaneous adjusted-dose heparin or adjusted-dose low molecular weight heparin in order to avoid bleeding complications in the neonate secondary to the trauma of delivery. In the absence of appreciable bleeding, combined therapy with heparin and warfarin may be resumed 4–6 hours after delivery in pregnant women with prosthetic heart valves. The decision whether to use heparin during the first trimester or continue oral anticoagulation throughout pregnancy should be made after full discussion with the patient and her partner of the risks associated with available anticoagulant therapies. Low-dose aspirin may be used in conjunction with anticoagulant therapy in pregnant women with prosthetic heart valves who are at high risk of thromboembolism, although such combination therapy increases the risk of hemorrhage.

For some pregnant women with inherited thrombophilias, postpartum anticoagulation with warfarin titrated to a target INR range of 2–3 is suggested. (See Uses: Thromboembolism During Pregnancy, in Heparin 20:12.04.16 and see Uses: Thromboembolism Occurring During Pregnancy, in Enoxaparin 20:12.04.16.)

Lactation Limited data suggest that warfarin is not distributed into breast milk, is not detectable in plasma of nursing infants, and has not produced substantial coagulation abnormalities in such infants. Based on limited available data, it is considered unlikely that maternal warfarin therapy would pose a substantial risk to healthy, full-term breast-feeding infants, and the American Academy of Pediatrics (AAP), ACCP and other clinicians consider maternal warfarin therapy to be compatible with breast-feeding. ACCP recommends that warfarin therapy be continued in nursing women who are already receiving such therapy. Women should inform their clinician if they are breast-feeding or plan to breast-feed. The manufacturers state that the decision to breast-feed while receiving warfarin anticoagulation should be made only after careful consideration of the available alternatives, and women who decide to breast-feed should be monitored very carefully so that recommended PT/INRs are not exceeded. Neonates are particularly sensitive to the effects of warfarin as a result of vitamin K deficiency. Infants should be monitored with coagulation tests and have their vitamin K status evaluated before being breast-fed by women taking warfarin. The effects of warfarin in premature infants have not been evaluated.

Drug Interactions

Concurrent administration of numerous drugs or dietary or herbal supplements has been reported to affect patient response to coumarin-derivative anticoagulants (e.g., warfarin). Drugs may *increase* patient sensitivity to warfarin by decreasing intestinal synthesis or absorption of vitamin K or affecting distribution of the vitamin; decreasing the rate of anticoagulant metabolism by competing for sites of metabolism or inhibiting the function or synthesis of metabolic enzymes; increasing affinity of the anticoagulant for receptor sites; decreasing synthesis and/or increasing catabolism of functional blood coagulation factors II, VII, IX, and X; interfering with other components of normal hemostasis such as platelet function or fibrinolysis; and by producing ulcerogenic effects. Drugs may competitively or noncompetitively interfere with protein binding of warfarin, producing increased concentrations of unbound anticoagulant and potentiation of anticoagulant effects. In some instances, this is only a temporary effect and a shortened plasma half-life of the anticoagulant results from an increased rate of metabolism and renal clearance of the anticoagulant, and the prothrombin time (PT) may return to therapeutic levels after several days of concomitant therapy. Certain drugs may *decrease* patient response to warfarin by decreasing absorption of the anticoagulant; increasing the rate of metabolism of the anticoagulant by enzyme induction; or by increasing synthesis of functional blood coagulation factors II, VII, IX, and X. Some dietary or herbal supplements contain naturally occurring coumarins or salicylates that may have anticoagulant, antiplatelet, or fibrinolytic effects; these supplements would be expected to increase the anticoagulant effects of concomitantly administered warfarin. Certain dietary or herbal supplements also may decrease response to warfarin, possibly as a result of induction of hepatic microsomal enzymes (e.g., St. John's wort) or because of procoagulant effects (e.g., coenzyme Q10).

Because of the complexity of individual patient sensitivity (e.g., genetic factors), multiple interacting mechanisms with some drugs, the dependency of the extent of the interaction on the dosage and duration of therapy, and the possible administration of several interacting drugs simultaneously, it is often difficult to predict the direction and degree of the ultimate effect of concurrent drug administration on anticoagulant response. Tables 2 and 3 show a list of drugs that reportedly may *increase* or *decrease* patient response to coumarin derivatives (e.g., warfarin).

Table 2. Drugs That May *Increase* Response to Coumarin Derivatives (e.g., Warfarin)

acetaminophen	ezetimibe	pantoprazole
*alcohol (acute intoxication)	fenofibrate	*pentoxifylline
allopurinol	fenoprofen calcium	phenylbutazone
aminosalicylic acid	fluoroquinolone anti-infectives	pravastatin
*amiodarone	fluoxetine	propafenone
anabolic steroids	flutamide	propoxyphene
argatroban	fluvastatin	propylthiouracil
aspirin	fluvoxamine	quinidine
atenolol	gefitinib	quinine
atorvastatin	gemfibrozil	*rabeprazole
azithromycin	glucagon	salicylates
bivalirudin	ibuprofen	sertraline
capecitabine	indomethacin	streptokinase
cefixime	influenza virus vaccine	sulfinpyrazone
celecoxib	isoniazid	sulfonamides
chloral hydrate	ketoprofen	sulindac
chloramphenicol	lansoprazole	tamoxifen
cimetidine	lepirudin	tetracycline
cisapride	lovastatin	thiazides
co-trimoxazole	meclofenamate	thyroid drugs
danazol	mefenamic acid	tramadol
diazoxide	methylthiouracil	tricyclic antidepressants
diflunisal	*metronidazole	*urokinase
*disulfiram	miconazole	valdecoxib
erythromycin	nalidixic acid	vitamin E
esomeprazole	neomycin (oral)	zafirlukast
ethacrynic acid	oxandrolone	zileuton

* concurrent use probably should be avoided, if possible

Table 3. Drugs that May *Decrease* Response to Coumarin Derivatives (e.g., Warfarin)

*alcohol (chronic alcoholism)	ethchlorvynol	raloxifene
aminoglutethimide	glutethimide	rifampin
atorvastatin	griseofulvin	spironolactone
*barbiturates	mercaptopurine	sucralfate
carbamazepine	methaqualone	trazodone
clozapine	nafcillin	vitamin K
corticosteroids	*oral contraceptives containing estrogen	
corticotropin	pravastatin	

* concurrent use probably should be avoided, if possible

Warfarin is metabolized by cytochrome P-450 (CYP) isoenzymes CYP2C9, 2C19, 2C8, 2C18, 1A2, and 3A4; the *S*-enantiomer is metabolized principally by CYP2C9, while the *R*-enantiomer is metabolized by CYP1A2 and 3A4. Because the *S*-enantiomer of warfarin is about 2–5 times more potent than *R*-warfarin, drugs that preferentially alter (i.e., increase or decrease) the metabolism of *S*-warfarin are more likely to be associated with alterations in PT or the international normalized ratio (INR). Drugs that *inhibit* CYP2C9, CYP1A2, or CYP3A4 can potentially *increase* exposure and response to warfarin; conversely, drugs that *induce* CYP2C9, CYP1A2, or CYP3A4 can potentially *decrease* exposure and response to warfarin. (See Table 4.) INR should be closely monitored in patients who initiate, discontinue, or change dosages of concomitant drugs that affect these CYP isoenzymes.

Table 4. CYP Interactions with Warfarin

Enzyme	Inhibitors*	Inducers*
CYP2C9	amiodarone, capecitabine, co-trimoxazole, etravirine, fluconazole, fluvastatin, fluvoxamine, metronidazole, miconazole, oxandrolone, sulfinpyrazone, tigecycline, voriconazole, zafirlukast	aprepitant, bosentan, carbamazepine, phenobarbital, rifampin
CYP1A2	acyclovir, allopurinol, caffeine, cimetidine, ciprofloxacin, disulfiram, enoxacin, famotidine, fluvoxamine, methoxsalen, mexiletine, norfloxacin, oral contraceptives, phenylpropanolamine, propafenone, propranolol, terbinafine, thiabendazole, ticlopidine, verapamil, zileuton	montelukast, moricizine, omeprazole, phenobarbital, phenytoin, cigarette smoking
CYP3A4	alprazolam, amiodarone, amlodipine, amprenavir, aprepitant, atorvastatin, atazanavir, bicalutamide, cilostazol, cimetidine, ciprofloxacin, clarithromycin, conivaptan, cyclosporine, darunavir/ritonavir, diltiazem, erythromycin, fluconazole, fluoxetine, fluvoxamine, fosamprenavir, imatinib, indinavir, isoniazid, itraconazole, ketoconazole, lopinavir/ritonavir, nefazodone, nelfinavir, nilotinib, oral contraceptives, posaconazole, ranitidine, ranolazine, ritonavir, saquinavir, telithromycin, tipranavir, voriconazole, zileuton	armodafinil, amprenavir, aprepitant, bosentan, carbamazepine, efavirenz, etravirine, modafinil, nafcillin, phenytoin, pioglitazone, prednisone, rifampin, rufinamide

* list of drugs is not all-inclusive

Risk of bleeding may be increased when warfarin is used concomitantly with other drugs that can also increase bleeding risk. (See Table 5.) Patients should be monitored closely whenever such drugs are used concomitantly with warfarin. While the manufacturers of warfarin state that NSAIAs, including selective cyclooxygenase-2 (COX-2) inhibitors, may be used with close monitoring in patients receiving warfarin, some experts (e.g., the American College of Chest Physicians [ACCP]) suggest that such concomitant therapy be avoided. NSAIAs can inhibit platelet aggregation and cause GI bleeding and peptic ulceration and/or perforation, in addition to specific drug interactions that might affect the PT. ACCP also suggests that concomitant administration of warfarin and antiplatelet agents should be avoided unless the benefit is known or is highly likely to be greater than the potential harm from bleeding; patients in whom benefit may potentially outweigh risk include those with mechanical heart valves, acute coronary syndrome, or patients who have undergone recent coronary artery stent placement or bypass surgery.

Table 5. Drugs that Can Increase Bleeding Risk

Drug Class	Specific Drugs
Anticoagulants	argatroban, dabigatran, bivalirudin, desirudin, heparin, lepirudin
Antiplatelet agents	aspirin, cilostazol, clopidogrel, dipyridamole, prasugrel, ticlopidine
Nonsteroidal anti-inflammatory agents	celecoxib, diclofenac, diflunisal, fenoprofen, ibuprofen, indomethacin, ketoprofen, ketorolac, mefenamic acid, naproxen, oxaprozin, piroxicam, sulindac
Serotonin-reuptake inhibitors	citalopram, desvenlafaxine, duloxetine, escitalopram, fluoxetine, fluvoxamine, milnacipran, paroxetine, sertraline, venlafaxine, vilazodone

Changes in INR have been reported in patients receiving certain antibiotics or antifungal agents concomitantly with warfarin; however, clinical pharmacokinetic studies have not shown consistent effects of these drugs on plasma concentrations of warfarin. The manufacturer states that INR should be monitored closely whenever any antibiotic or antifungal agent is initiated or discontinued in patients receiving warfarin.

Altered coagulation parameters and/or bleeding, sometimes fatal, have been reported in patients receiving capecitabine concomitantly with coumarin-derivative anticoagulants (e.g., warfarin). (See Drug Interactions: Anticoagulants, in Capecitabine 10:00.) In patients stabilized on coumarin-derivative anticoagulants, increased PT/INR and/or bleeding episodes have occurred within several days to months following initiation of capecitabine therapy; similar events have been reported in at least a few patients within 1 month following discontinuance of capecitabine. This increased anticoagulant response appears to occur because of inhibition of the CYP2C9 isoenzyme involved in warfarin metabolism by capecitabine. Age exceeding 60 years and a diagnosis of cancer may predispose patients to the development of coagulopathy. Capecitabine and warfarin should be used concomitantly with caution. If capecitabine is used concomitantly with warfarin, PT/INR should be monitored frequently in order to facilitate anticoagulant dosage adjustments if necessary.

Concurrent use of oxandrolone, an anabolic androgenic steroid, with warfarin may result in unexpectedly large increases in the PT/INR. In a study in healthy individuals, oxandrolone increased the mean half-life and area under the blood concentration-time curve (AUC) of warfarin (affecting both *S*- and *R*-enantiomers similarly); microscopic hematuria and/or gingival bleeding also occurred in some individuals. A reduction of 80–85% in the mean daily warfarin dosage was required in these individuals to maintain a target INR of 1.5. When oxandrolone therapy is initiated, changed, or discontinued in patients receiving warfarin, patients should be monitored closely for occult bleeding and with laboratory tests (i.e., PT/INR) in order to facilitate dosage adjustments as necessary and diminish the risk of serious bleeding.

In one study, administration of antacids containing magnesium hydroxide or aluminum hydroxide concomitantly with warfarin had no effect on absorption of the anticoagulant.

Concurrent administration of cholestyramine with warfarin results in decreased absorption of the anticoagulant. In addition, cholestyramine has been shown to decrease the plasma half-life of warfarin by interfering with enterohepatic circulation of the drug. However, because vitamin K absorption may also be decreased by cholestyramine, the net effect of concurrent anticoagulant and cholestyramine therapy is difficult to predict. Concurrent use of cholestyramine and warfarin probably should be avoided, if possible.

Concomitant use of lomitapide with warfarin resulted in increased exposure to warfarin and a 22% increase in INR. If lomitapide is used concomitantly with warfarin, the manufacturer of lomitapide states that INR should be monitored regularly, particularly following adjustments in lomitapide dosage, and dosage of warfarin should be adjusted as clinically indicated.

Chronic ingestion of large doses of acetaminophen has been reported to potentiate the effects of coumarin-derivative anticoagulants (e.g., warfarin). Conflicting data exist and the clinical importance of such an interaction has been questioned. Large dosages of acetaminophen (exceeding 1.5 g per day) may augment the anticoagulant effect of warfarin. In addition, results of an observational study in patients stabilized on warfarin therapy indicate an association between ingestion of even low to moderate dosages of acetaminophen (7 or more 325-mg tablets weekly) and excessively high INR values. Some clinicians suggest that additional monitoring of INR values may be prudent in patients receiving warfarin therapy following initiation of, and during sustained therapy with, large doses of acetaminophen. (See Drug Interactions: Anticoagulants, in Acetaminophen 28:08.92.)

Concomitant administration of vaginal miconazole creams or suppositories with acenocoumarol or warfarin for approximately 3 days has resulted in an increased PT/INR and/or bleeding. Additional monitoring of INR values and appropriate dosage adjustments may be required in patients receiving concomitant intravaginal miconazole therapy.

Some clinicians state that alcohol ingestion should be avoided in patients receiving warfarin. However, other clinicians suggest that patients receiving warfarin therapy may consume alcohol in small amounts (e.g., 1–2 drinks occasionally) but that chronic heavy consumption (e.g., defined as greater than 720 mL of beer, 300 mL of wine, or 60 mL of liquor daily) should be avoided. The effects of moderate alcohol consumption (e.g., 1–2 drinks daily) on adverse events or anticoagulation control in patients receiving long-term therapeutic anticoagulation with warfarin has not been well studied. In 2 studies in a small number of healthy young men, daily ingestion of 300-600 mL of wine in the fasting or unfasting state on a short-term basis (21 days) did not affect plasma warfarin concentrations or therapeutic hypoprothrombinemia (maintained at 25–35% of normal prothrombin activity as measured by one-stage prothrombin time). However, numerous patient-specific factors affect response to warfarin, including, age, vitamin K status, concomitant disease (e.g., hepatic dysfunction, fat malabsorption, hyperthyroidism, fever), and hereditary resistance; therefore, lack of evidence of a warfarin-alcohol interaction in healthy individuals may not preclude such interactions in individual patients. Acute ingestion of alcohol has been reported to enhance hypoprothrombinemia and prolong INR by inhibiting warfarin metabolism, reducing its clearance, and/or displacing it from plasma proteins, while long-term use of alcohol (e.g., chronic alcoholism) may reduce anticoagulant effects by inducing CYP isoenzymes (e.g., CYP2E1,

CYP3A4, CYP1A2) and warfarin metabolism. Alcohol also has antiplatelet effects that may increase bleeding risk with warfarin without affecting INR.

Dietary and herbal supplements also have been reported to increase or decrease the effects of warfarin, in some cases through CYP-mediated interactions (e.g., echinacea, grapefruit juice, gingko, goldenseal, St. John's wort). (See Tables 6 and 7.) In general, caution should be exercised when dietary or herbal supplements are used in patients receiving warfarin, and additional INR monitoring is recommended whenever these products are initiated or discontinued; limited information is available regarding the interaction potential of these products with warfarin.

Table 6. Dietary or Herbal Supplements that May *Increase* Response to Coumarin Derivatives (e.g., Warfarin)

agrimony	chamomile (German and Roman)	parsley
alfalfa	clove	passion flower
aloe gel	*cranberry	pau d'arco
Angelica sinensis (dong quai)	dandelion	policosanol
aniseed	fenugreek	poplar
arnica	feverfew	prickly ash (Northern)
asa foetida	garlic	quassia
aspen	German sarsaparilla	red clover
black cohosh	ginger	senega
black haw	*Ginkgo biloba*	sweet clover
bladder wrack (*Fucus*)	ginseng (*Panax*)	sweet woodruff
bogbean	horse chestnut	tamarind
boldo	horseradish	tonka beans
bromelains	inositol nicotinate	wild carrot
buchu	licorice	wild lettuce
capsicum	meadowsweet	willow
cassia	nettle	wintergreen
celery	onion	

Table 7. Dietary or Herbal Supplements that May *Decrease* Response to Coumarin Derivatives (e.g., Warfarin)

agrimony	goldenseal	St. John's wort
coenzyme Q_{10} (ubidecarenone)	mistletoe	yarrow
ginseng (*Panax*)		

Several case reports have suggested a possible interaction between warfarin and cranberry juice; in these reports, the effects of warfarin appeared to be potentiated by cranberry juice or a cranberry product, in some cases resulting in clinically important bleeding events. However, confounding factors were present in many of these cases and prospective controlled studies generally have not been able to confirm this interaction. Results of several studies, including a randomized, double-blind trial evaluating the effects of daily consumption of 240 mL of cranberry juice over a 2-week period in 30 patients stabilized on warfarin therapy, showed no evidence of any clinically important pharmacokinetic or pharmacodynamic interaction. The amounts of cranberry juice ingested varied among these studies, but generally were lower than those described in the case reports. It is possible that this interaction may be dose dependent, with response elicited by ingestion of large quantities of cranberry juice. Although available data do not appear to support a clinically important interaction between warfarin and cranberry juice, clinicians should be aware of the possibility of such an interaction and monitor closely for changes in INR and manifestations of bleeding in patients consuming cranberry juice concurrently with warfarin.

In addition to the drugs and other substances (e.g., dietary or herbal supplements, foods) mentioned above, many other drugs have been reported to alter the response to coumarin-derivative anticoagulants; however, either the clinical importance of these reports has not been established or the reports have not been substantiated. Caution must be observed when *any* drug is added to or deleted from the therapeutic regimen of a patient receiving warfarin; the PT should be determined more frequently than usual and appropriate dosage adjustments made. In addition, patients should be warned not to initiate or discontinue nonprescription drugs, herbal supplements, or drugs prescribed by other physicians without first informing their primary physician or pharmacist. Patients should inform their clinicians of existing or contemplated concomitant therapy, including prescription and OTC drugs and dietary and herbal supplements.

Laboratory Test Interferences

Warfarin may interfere with the Schack and Waxler ultraviolet method for serum theophylline determinations, resulting in falsely decreased concentrations.

Pharmacology

Warfarin is an indirect-acting anticoagulant. In addition to being used clinically, warfarin and other coumarin derivatives have been used as rodenticides and insecticides.

Coumarin derivatives such as warfarin alter the synthesis of blood coagulation factors II (prothrombin), VII (proconvertin), IX (Christmas factor or plasma thromboplastin component), and X (Stuart-Prower factor) in the liver by interfering with the action of reduced vitamin K, which is necessary for the γ-carboxylation of several glutamic acid residues in the precursor proteins of these coagulation factors. Warfarin decreases clotting factor synthesis by inhibiting the regeneration of reduced vitamin K from vitamin K epoxide via inhibition of warfarin's target enzyme, vitamin K epoxide reductase. Without reduced vitamin K as a cofactor for γ-glutamyl carboxylase, carboxylation of glutamic acid residues on coagulation factors II, VII, IX, and X cannot proceed and these proteins do not become fully functional coagulation factors. Certain variations in the gene (vitamin K epoxide reductase complex subunit 1 [VKORC1]) that encodes vitamin K epoxide reductase may be associated with lower hepatic expression of the gene and lower concentrations of reduced vitamin K. Patients with such variant genes are at increased risk of excessive anticoagulation (e.g., supratherapeutic INRs) and/or bleeding and require lower dosages of warfarin. Other genetic variations in the VKORC1 gene may contribute to warfarin resistance and increased warfarin dosage requirements. (See Pharmacogenomics under Dosage: Factors Influencing Anticoagulant Response, in Dosage and Administration.)

Plasma concentrations of vitamin K-dependent coagulation factors are physiologically decreased in neonates compared with adults, and the capacity of plasma from children receiving warfarin to generate thrombin is delayed and reduced compared with adults.

Warfarin also inhibits the anticoagulant proteins C and S. In adequate dosage, phytonadione (vitamin K_1) reverses the effect of coumarin derivatives on the hepatic synthesis of vitamin K-dependent coagulation factors. Unlike heparin, warfarin has no anticoagulant effect in vitro.

Because warfarin does not alter catabolism of blood coagulation factors, depletion of circulating functional vitamin K-dependent coagulation factors must occur before effects of the drug become apparent. Depletion of functional coagulation factor II, factor VII, Protein C, factor IX, Protein S, and factor X occurs in a sequential manner; the rate of depletion of these coagulation factors depends on their individual rates of degradation. Following initiation of warfarin therapy, blood concentrations of functional coagulation factor VII (plasma half-life of 4–7 hours) are depressed first, followed by those of factors IX (plasma half-life of 20–24 hours) and X (plasma half-life of about 48–72 hours), and finally factor II (plasma half-life of 60 hours or longer). When warfarin therapy is discontinued or phytonadione is administered, blood concentrations of functional vitamin K-dependent coagulation factors return to pretreatment concentrations.

The enantiomers of warfarin, which is commercially available as a racemic mixture, have different half-lives, potencies, routes of administration, and rates of elimination. The *S*-enantiomer of warfarin has 2–5 times the anticoagulant activity of the *R*-enantiomer. An anticoagulant effect generally occurs within 24 hours following administration of warfarin, but peak anticoagulant effects may be delayed for 72–96 hours. Antithrombogenic effects of warfarin generally occur only after concentrations of functional coagulation factors IX and X are diminished, which may not occur until 2–7 days following initiation of therapy.

Warfarin therapy inhibits thrombus formation when stasis is induced and may prevent extension of existing thrombi. The drugs have no direct effect on established thrombi and appear to have little if any effect on the pathogenesis of arterial thrombi that result from interaction of platelets with an abnormal vessel wall. Because warfarin affects synthesis of blood coagulation factors that are involved in both extrinsic and intrinsic coagulation, the drug prolongs both the prothrombin time (PT), which measures the integrity of the extrinsic system, and the activated partial thromboplastin time (aPTT), which measures the integrity of the intrinsic system.

Coumarin derivatives have been reported to increase plasma concentrations of antithrombin III (heparin cofactor), but the therapeutic importance of this effect is unclear. Various other pharmacologic effects have been attributed to coumarin derivatives; however, most of these reports have been based on animal studies and their clinical importance has not been established.

Pharmacokinetics

■ Absorption Warfarin sodium is rapidly and extensively absorbed from the GI tract, but considerable interindividual variation in absorption exists. Absorption of oral warfarin sodium is dissolution-rate controlled, and the rate and extent of absorption of the drug may vary from one commercially available tablet to another. Studies using warfarin sodium indicate that the rate, but not the extent, of absorption of the drug is decreased by the presence of food in the GI tract. Warfarin also is absorbed percutaneously, and severe toxicity has occurred from repeated skin contact with rodenticides containing the drug.

Peak plasma concentrations of warfarin usually are attained within 4 hours; studies in healthy individuals indicate that peak drug concentrations are achieved 90 minutes after administration. However, plasma warfarin concentrations are not necessarily related to antithrombogenic effects and are not useful determinants of anticoagulant dosage requirements. Peak plasma drug concentrations may be achieved earlier following IV administration of warfarin than with oral administration; however, IV administration does not result in an enhanced anticoagulant response or an earlier onset of anticoagulant effect.

Although, with adequate dosage, synthesis of vitamin K-dependent coagulation factors is affected soon after absorption of warfarin (e.g., within 24 hours), depletion of circulating functional coagulation factors must occur before therapeutic effects of the drug become apparent. Antithrombogenic effects may not occur until 2–7 days following initiation of warfarin therapy. Similarly, there is a period of latency following discontinuance of the drug until blood concentrations of functional vitamin K-dependent coagulation factors return to pretreatment levels. Onset of antithrombogenic effects is similar whether warfarin is administered orally, IM, or IV. Doses of warfarin exceeding those required to affect synthesis of coagulation factors IX and X will not hasten the onset of action but may prolong duration of action after the drug is discontinued.

■ **Distribution** Warfarin is 99% bound to plasma proteins, principally albumin. Uptake of the drug by erythrocytes is variable. Studies in animals indicate that in addition to the liver, the drug is distributed to lungs, spleen, and kidneys. Warfarin crosses the placenta, and fetal plasma drug concentrations may be equal to maternal plasma concentrations. Based on a one-compartment model and assuming complete bioavailability, the estimated volumes of distribution for *R*- and *S*-warfarin and racemic warfarin are similar.

Limited data suggest that warfarin is not distributed into milk in humans. In one study, warfarin was not detected in the milk of 13 nursing women or in the plasma of their breast-fed infants following 30- or 40-mg initial doses and daily maintenance dosage of 2–12 mg of the drug. (See Cautions: Pregnancy and Lactation.)

■ **Elimination** The effective elimination half-life of warfarin averages about 40 hours and shows considerable interindividual variation (range: 20–60 hours); plasma half-life of the drug generally is independent of dose. The clearance of the *R*-enantiomer of warfarin is about 50% that of the *S*-enantiomer; since the volumes of distribution of the enantiomers are similar, the half-life of *R*-warfarin (e.g., 37–89 hours) is longer than that of *S*-warfarin (e.g., 21–43 hours).

Racemic warfarin is stereoselectively metabolized by hepatic cytochrome P-450 (CYP) microsomal enzymes to inactive metabolites. The CYP isoenzymes involved in warfarin metabolism include CYP2C9, CYP2C19, CYP2C8, CYP2C18, CYP1A2, and CYP3A4. Individual patients vary greatly in the rate at which they metabolize warfarin. *R*-Warfarin is metabolized by CYP1A2 and CYP3A4 isoenzymes to diastereoisomeric alcohols, which are excreted principally in urine. The metabolites of *R*-warfarin have some anticoagulant activity but considerably less than the parent compound. *S*-Warfarin is metabolized principally by oxidation via the CYP2C9 isoenzyme to the inactive metabolite 7-hydroxywarfarin, which is excreted in bile. The CYP2C9 isoenzyme appears to be the principal hepatic cytochrome P-450 isoenzyme that modulates the in vivo anticoagulant activity of warfarin.

The degree of activity of the CYP2C9 isoenzyme is under genetic control and is subject to individual variation. Patients who are homozygous for the CYP2C9*1 (wild-type) allele (about 80% of Caucasians) have normal enzyme activity (i.e., extensive metabolizers), and standard warfarin dosing regimens are adequate in such patients. (See Dosage: Initial Dosage, in Dosage and Administration.) However, approximately 11 or 7% of Caucasians are intermediate (e.g., CYP2C9*2 allele) or poor (e.g., CYP2C9*3 allele) metabolizers of warfarin, respectively; clearance of *S*-warfarin, the predominant active form of the drug, is reduced in such patients. Therefore, patients with variant CYP2C9 alleles are at increased risk of bleeding and excessive anticoagulation (e.g., INR exceeding 3) and require lower dosages of warfarin, particularly during initiation of therapy. The CYP2C9*2 and CYP2C9*3 alleles reduce metabolism of warfarin by about 30–50 and 90%, respectively. Other CYP2C9 variant alleles associated with reduced enzymatic activity occur less frequently, including CYP2C9*5, CYP2C9*6, and CYP2C9*11 alleles in African populations and CYP2C9*5, CYP2C9*9, and CYP2C9*11 alleles in Caucasians.

Chemistry and Stability

■ **Chemistry** Warfarin is a synthetic 3-substituted derivative of 4-hydroxycoumarin.

Commercially available warfarin sodium is a racemic mixture of the 2 optical isomers of the drug. Warfarin sodium occurs as a white, odorless, crystalline powder that has a slightly bitter taste, is discolored by light, and is very soluble in water, freely soluble in alcohol, and very slightly soluble in chloroform or ether. Crystalline warfarin sodium is an isopropanol clathrate prepared from warfarin or amorphous warfarin sodium to eliminate trace impurities present in amorphous warfarin.

■ **Stability** Warfarin sodium is discolored by light. Warfarin sodium preparations should be protected from light and stored at controlled room temperature (15–30°C). Warfarin sodium tablets should be stored in tight, light-resistant containers; warfarin sodium for injection should be kept in its original carton until ready for use.

Following reconstitution of lyophilized warfarin sodium for injection with sterile water for injection, solutions containing 2 mg of warfarin sodium per mL have a pH of 8.1–8.3 and are stable for 4 hours at room temperature; the reconstituted solution should not be refrigerated. Any unused portion of the reconstituted solution should be discarded after 4 hours.

Preparations

Excipients in commercially available drug preparations may have clinically important effects in some individuals; consult specific product labeling for details.

Warfarin Sodium

Oral		
Tablets 1 mg*	**Coumadin**® (scored), Bristol-Myers Squibb	
	Jantoven® (scored), USL	
	Warfarin Sodium Tablets (scored)	
2 mg*	**Coumadin**® (scored), Bristol-Myers Squibb	
	Jantoven® (scored), USL	
	Warfarin Sodium Tablets (scored)	
2.5 mg*	**Coumadin**® (scored), Bristol-Myers Squibb	
	Jantoven® (scored), USL	
	Warfarin Sodium Tablets (scored)	
3 mg*	**Coumadin**® (scored), Bristol-Myers Squibb	
	Jantoven® (scored), USL	
	Warfarin Sodium Tablets (scored)	
4 mg*	**Coumadin**® (scored), Bristol-Myers Squibb	
	Jantoven® (scored), USL	
	Warfarin Sodium Tablets (scored)	
5 mg*	**Coumadin**® (scored), Bristol-Myers Squibb	
	Jantoven® (scored), USL	
	Warfarin Sodium Tablets (scored)	
6 mg*	**Coumadin**® (scored), Bristol-Myers Squibb	
	Jantoven® (scored), USL	
	Warfarin Sodium Tablets (scored)	
7.5 mg*	**Coumadin**® (scored), Bristol-Myers Squibb	
	Jantoven® (scored), USL	
	Warfarin Sodium Tablets (scored)	
10 mg*	**Coumadin**® (scored dye-free), Bristol-Myers Squibb	
	Jantoven® (scored), USL	
	Warfarin Sodium Tablets (scored)	
Parenteral		
For injection, for IV use only 5 mg	**Coumadin**®, Bristol-Myers Squibb	

*available from one or more manufacturer, distributor, and/or repackager by generic (nonproprietary) name

†Use is not currently included in the labeling approved by the US Food and Drug Administration

DIRECT THROMBIN INHIBITORS 20:12.04.12

Argatroban

■ Argatroban, a synthetic piperidinecarboxylic acid derivative of L-arginine, is an anticoagulant.

Uses

■ **Thrombosis Associated with Heparin-induced Thrombocytopenia** Argatroban is used for the prevention and treatment of thrombosis in patients with heparin-induced thrombocytopenia (HIT). The American College of Chest Physicians (ACCP) recommends the use of a nonheparin anticoagulant (e.g., lepirudin, argatroban) as an alternative to further use of unfractionated heparin or a low molecular weight heparin or the initiation/continuation of warfarin for the initial management of patients with HIT with or without thrombosis. Safety and efficacy of argatroban for this use are based principally on the results of 2 studies in which patients with HIT or heparin-induced thrombocytopenia and thrombosis syndrome (HITTS) receiving argatroban were compared with a historical control group that did not receive the drug. Patients receiving argatroban were given an initial infusion of 2 mcg/kg per minute, with titration up to 10 mcg/kg per minute to achieve an activated partial thromboplastin time (aPTT) of 1.5–3 times the baseline value (not to exceed 100 seconds). The historical control group consisted of patients who had been treated for HIT/HITTS according to the local standard of medical practice (i.e., discontinuance of heparin therapy and/or oral anticoagulation with warfarin) since no other therapy was available for HIT/HITTS at that time. Patients received argatroban therapy until clinical resolution of their underlying condition, appropriate anticoagulation with another drug, or for a maximum of 14 days. In the first study, patients received argatroban for an average of 6 days; follow-up after termination of argatroban therapy in this study averaged 30 days. Most patients in the 2 studies were transferred to oral anticoagulant therapy with warfarin, with argatroban continued concurrently with warfarin for 3–4 days.

In both studies, argatroban therapy was associated with a reduction in the incidence of the composite end point (all-cause death, all-cause amputation, or new thrombosis during the 37-day study period) as well as the individual end points (time to first end point event) in patients with HIT, HITTS, or combined

HIT/HITTS. A target aPTT of at least 1.5 times the baseline value was achieved with a mean argatroban infusion rate of 2 or 1.9 mcg/kg per minute in 76 or 81% of patients with HIT or HITTS, respectively, at the first assessment in one of the studies. Recovery of platelet count (defined as an increase in platelet count to greater than 100,000/ mm^{3}or at least 1.5 times greater than the baseline aPTT) occurred in greater than 69% of argatroban-treated patients overall (53% of patients with HIT and 58% of those with HITTS by study day 3) in this study.

For continued anticoagulation following argatroban therapy, conversion to oral anticoagulant therapy (e.g., warfarin) has been used. (See Conversion to Oral Anticoagulant Therapy under Dosage and Administration: Dosage.)

■ **Heparin-induced Thrombocytopenia in Patients Undergoing Percutaneous Coronary Intervention** Argatroban is used in patients undergoing percutaneous coronary intervention (PCI), including percutaneous transluminal coronary angioplasty (PTCA), coronary stent placement, and atherectomy, who have or are at risk for HIT. Several nonheparin anticoagulants (e.g., bivalirudin, argatroban, lepirudin) have been evaluated as a substitute for unfractionated heparin or low molecular weight heparin therapy in patients with HIT undergoing PCI. Among the different options, ACCP, the American College of Cardiology Foundation (ACCF), the American Heart Association (AHA), and the Society for Cardiovascular Angiography and Interventions (SCAI) recommend the use of bivalirudin or argatroban based on evidence from prospective studies; factors such as availability, cost, and ease of monitoring may influence choice of a particular agent. Although ACCP states that some patients with a history of HIT may be re-exposed to heparin in special circumstances, use of nonheparin anticoagulants generally is favored over re-exposure to heparin in patients with a history of HIT undergoing PCI.

Efficacy and safety of argatroban for this indication are based principally on the results of several prospective, historically controlled studies evaluating therapy with the drug in patients with current or prior HIT (with or without thrombosis) or heparin-dependent antibodies who were undergoing PCI. The historical control group (selected by retrospective review of patient records) consisted of patients without HIT undergoing PCI who had been treated with heparin. The rates of procedural success (defined as lack of death, emergency coronary artery bypass grafting, Q-wave myocardial infarction) were similar in patients receiving argatroban (98.2%) versus the control group (94.3%); no deaths were reported in either group. Patients received argatroban 350 mcg/kg as an IV loading dose followed by a maintenance infusion of 25 mcg/kg per minute to achieve a target activated clotting time (ACT) of 300–450 seconds; additional IV loading doses of 150 mcg/kg or adjustments in the maintenance infusion rate over the range of 15–40 mcg/kg per minute to achieve the target ACT were allowed. All patients also received oral aspirin 325 mg 2–24 hours before PCI. Patients requiring anticoagulation following PCI could receive additional argatroban via a maintenance infusion at 2.5–5 mcg/kg per minute, adjusted (but not exceeding 10 mcg/kg per minute) to achieve an aPTT of 1.5–3 times control (not exceeding 100 seconds).

■ **Other Uses** Argatroban has been used concomitantly with aspirin as an adjunct to thrombolysis in a limited number of patients with unstable angina and non-ST-segment elevation/non-Q-wave myocardial infarction† and during extracorporeal circulation in open-heart surgery†. However, ACCF/AHA state that monovalent direct thrombin inhibitors such as argatroban are ineffective antithrombotic agents compared with unfractionated heparin in patients with acute coronary syndromes, and therefore do not recommend their use in such patients. The manufacturer states that safety and efficacy of argatroban for cardiac indications other than PCI in patients with HIT have not been established. Argatroban reportedly has been used in patients with HIT undergoing hemodialysis† as an alternative to unfractionated heparin to prevent clotting in the hemodialysis circuit.

Dosage and Administration

■ **Reconstitution and Administration** Argatroban is administered by continuous IV infusion. The commercially available injection concentrate (100 mg/mL) *must* be diluted in 0.9% sodium chloride injection, 5% dextrose injection, or lactated Ringer's injection to a final concentration of 1 mg/mL prior to administration. The solution should be mixed by repeated inversion of the IV container for 1 minute. The argatroban IV solution may be slightly hazy just after preparation because of the formation of microprecipitates that rapidly dissolve upon further mixing.

Before administering argatroban, all parenteral anticoagulants must be discontinued and a baseline activated partial thromboplastin time (aPTT) obtained.

Properly prepared argatroban IV solutions are stable for 24 hours at room temperature or 48 hours under refrigeration. Argatroban solutions should not be exposed to direct sunlight.

■ **Dosage** ***Heparin-induced Thrombocytopenia*** For prevention or treatment of thrombosis in adults with heparin-induced thrombocytopenia (HIT), the recommended initial dosage of argatroban in patients without hepatic impairment is 2 mcg/kg per minute by continuous IV infusion. Standard initial infusion rates for adult patients without hepatic impairment are shown in the table.

Infusion Rate (mL/hour) for Argatroban Dosage of 2 mcg/kg per minute (1 mg/mL final concentration)

Body Weight (kg)	Dose (mcg/minute)	Infusion Rate (mL/hour)
50	100	6
60	120	7
70	140	8
80	160	10
90	180	11
100	200	12
110	220	13
120	240	14
130	260	16
140	280	17

In patients receiving argatroban for the prevention or treatment of thrombosis associated with HIT, therapy with the drug generally is monitored using the aPTT. A steady-state anticoagulant effect generally is achieved 1–3 hours after initiation of the argatroban infusion in patients with normal hepatic function. The aPTT should be determined 2 hours after initiation of the infusion and/or following each dosage adjustment to confirm that a target aPTT of 1.5–3 times the initial baseline aPTT (not to exceed 100 seconds) has been achieved. The infusion rate can be adjusted as clinically indicated to achieve the desired aPTT range but should not exceed 10 mcg/kg per minute. Patients with hepatic impairment may require a longer time and more dosage adjustments to achieve steady-state aPTT concentrations. To minimize the risk of thrombotic events (e.g., limb gangrene) during the transition to oral anticoagulant therapy (e.g., warfarin) in patients with HIT, the American College of Chest Physicians (ACCP) and other clinicians recommend that treatment with argatroban or other nonheparin anticoagulant be continued until platelet counts have recovered substantially to near-normal levels (i.e., to at least 150,000/mm^3) and are stable.

HIT in Patients Undergoing Percutaneous Coronary Intervention For prevention or treatment of thrombosis in patients with HIT undergoing percutaneous coronary intervention (PCI), the recommended initial loading dose of argatroban is 350 mcg/kg administered by slow IV injection (over 3–5 minutes) followed by continuous IV infusion at 25 mcg/kg per minute. Argatroban therapy prior to and during PCI generally is monitored using the activated clotting time (ACT). An ACT determination should be obtained 5–10 minutes after infusion of the loading dose, and the procedure may proceed once an ACT of greater than 300 seconds has been achieved. If the ACT value is below 300 seconds, an additional IV loading dose of 150 mcg/kg should be administered and the infusion rate increased to 30 mcg/kg per minute. If the ACT value is above 450 seconds, the infusion rate should be decreased to 15 mcg/kg per minute. If dissection, impending abrupt closure, or thrombus of the coronary artery occurs during the procedure, or if an ACT greater than 300 seconds cannot be maintained, additional direct IV injections of 150 mcg/kg may be administered and the infusion rate increased to 40 mcg/kg per minute. The ACT values should be determined 5–10 minutes after each additional direct injection or change in the infusion rate, and at the completion of the procedure. Once the target ACT (300–450 seconds) is achieved, the infusion should continue for the duration of the procedure; additional ACT values should be determined every 20–30 minutes during a prolonged procedure.

If a patient requires anticoagulation after PCI, argatroban may be continued, but at the infusion rate used in patients not undergoing PCI (2 mcg/kg per minute).

Conversion to Oral Anticoagulant Therapy For continued anticoagulation, warfarin may be initiated after beginning argatroban therapy. ACCP and other clinicians recommend that warfarin therapy be initiated only after substantial recovery from acute HIT has occurred (i.e., as indicated by platelet counts that have increased to at least 150,000/mm^3 and are stable) with argatroban therapy. When converting to oral anticoagulant therapy following argatroban infusion, such therapy should be initiated using modest dosages of warfarin (2.5–5 mg, maximum of 5 mg); a loading dose should not be used. To avoid prothrombotic effects and ensure continuous anticoagulation when initiating warfarin, argatroban and warfarin therapy should be overlapped. Daily international normalized ratio (INR) determinations are recommended during concomitant argatroban and warfarin therapy.

Combined therapy with argatroban and warfarin results in prolongation of the PT and INR beyond that produced by warfarin alone; the relationship between the INR on warfarin alone and that on combined warfarin-argatroban therapy depends on the dosage of argatroban and the international sensitivity index (ISI) of the thromboplastin reagent used for INR determinations. The expected INR on warfarin alone (INR_W) may be calculated from the INR on combined warfarin-argatroban therapy (INR_{WA}). The manufacturer's labeling should be consulted for detailed information regarding calculation of INR_W and conversion from combined warfarin-argatroban therapy to warfarin alone. However, with an argatroban infusion rate of 2 mcg/kg per minute, argatroban therapy generally can be discontinued when the INR on combined therapy (INR_{WA}) exceeds 4. However, overshooting the target INR should be avoided, as supratherapeutic INRs during concomitant therapy with direct thrombin inhibitors and warfarin have been associated with necrosis or gangrene of the skin or limbs. (See Cautions: Necrosis, in Warfarin 20:12.04.08.) The INR on warfarin alone should then be determined 4–6 hours after discontinuance of the argatroban infusion; if it is not within the desired therapeutic range for warfarin, the argatroban infusion should be resumed. This procedure (discontinuance of argatroban infusion, checking the INR on warfarin alone, and resumption of argatroban infusion) should be continued on a daily basis until the INR on warfarin alone (i.e., 4–6 hours after discontinuance of argatroban) is in the therapeutic range.

With argatroban infusions at rates exceeding 2 mcg/kg per minute, the relationship between INR on warfarin alone versus that on combined warfarin-argatroban therapy is less predictable. Therefore, the manufacturer states that the argatroban infusion rate should be temporarily reduced to 2 mcg/kg per minute and the INR on combined therapy calculated again 4–6 hours after such dosage reduction in order to predict the INR on warfarin therapy alone.

■ **Special Populations** Use of argatroban in patients with hepatic impairment requires dosage reduction and careful monitoring of the aPTT. For adults with HIT and moderate hepatic impairment, an initial dosage of 0.5 mcg/kg per minute is recommended based on the approximate fourfold decrease in argatroban clearance relative to that in individuals with normal hepatic function. Subsequent dosage may then be adjusted as clinically indicated. Use of high dosages of argatroban should be avoided in patients undergoing PCI who have clinically important hepatic disease or serum AST or ALT elevations 3 times the upper limit of normal or higher because such patients have not been studied in clinical trials with the drug.

No dosage adjustment is necessary because of impaired renal function or for geriatric patients.

The safety and efficacy of argatroban, including appropriate anticoagulation goals and duration of therapy, in pediatric patients have not been fully established. Dosing recommendations have been made based on limited pharmacokinetic data in 15 seriously ill pediatric patients (younger than 16 years of age) who received argatroban as an alternative to unfractionated heparin for conditions such as HIT, heparin-induced thrombocytopenia and thrombosis syndrome (HITTS), or suspected HIT. Reduced dosages are recommended in such patients due to the potential for decreased clearance of the drug. When used as an alternative to heparin in seriously ill pediatric patients with HIT or HITTS, the manufacturer recommends an initial argatroban dosage of 0.75 mcg/kg per minute in patients with normal hepatic function or 0.2 mcg/kg per minute in those with hepatic impairment. The aPTT should be determined 2 hours after initiation of the infusion and the dosage adjusted to achieve a target aPTT 1.5–3 times that of the initial baseline value (not exceeding 100 seconds). Subsequent dosage may be adjusted in increments of 0.1–0.25 mcg/kg per minute in pediatric patients without hepatic impairment, or in increments of 0.05 mcg/kg per minute or less in those with hepatic impairment; however, dosage adjustments should be individualized based on patient's clinical status, current dosage, and current and target aPTT.

Cautions

■ **Contraindications** Active major bleeding. Known hypersensitivity to argatroban or any ingredient(s) in the formulation.

■ **Warnings/Precautions** ***Warnings*** **Hematologic Effects.** Like other anticoagulants, argatroban should be used with extreme caution in disease states or circumstances where there is an increased risk of hemorrhage (e.g., severe hypertension; postlumbar puncture; spinal anesthesia; major surgery, particularly of the brain, spinal cord, or eye; GI ulceration; congenital or acquired bleeding disorders). All parenteral anticoagulants should be discontinued and a baseline activated partial thromboplastin time (aPTT) obtained before initiation of argatroban therapy in patients with heparin-induced thrombocytopenia (HIT) or heparin-induced thrombocytopenia and thrombosis syndrome (HITTS).

Hemorrhage in patients receiving argatroban can occur at any site in the body.Unexplained decreases in hematocrit, hemoglobin, or blood pressure may indicate hemorrhage. In the event of overdose or excessive anticoagulation, discontinue argatroban infusion, monitor aPTT and other coagulation tests (prothrombin time [PT], international normalized ratio [INR]), and provide symptomatic and supportive treatment. No specific antidote to argatroban is currently available. Argatroban is partially removed by hemodialysis; approximately 20% of the drug is cleared during a 4-hour period of hemodialysis (when given as a continuous infusion at 2 mcg/kg per minute prior to and during hemodialysis). Major hemorrhage (defined as overt and associated with a hemoglobin decrease of at least 2 g/dL [in nonsurgical patients] or at least 5 g/dL [in patients undergoing PCI], transfusion of at least 2 units, or bleeding that was intracranial, retroperitoneal, or into a major prosthetic joint) occurred in 5.3% of patients receiving argatroban in 2 clinical studies and in 6.7% of those (based on retrospective analysis) in a historical control group. Major hemorrhage (i.e., retroperitoneal or GI hemorrhage) occurred in 1.8% of patients with current or prior HIT/HITTS who received argatroban and underwent PCI. Intracranial hemorrhage did not occur in clinical studies of argatroban in nonsurgical patients with HIT/HITTS but has been reported with argatroban therapy for other conditions (e.g., patients with acute myocardial infarction [MI] receiving concomitant thrombolytic therapy, patients with stroke).

Sensitivity Reactions Documented or suspected sensitivity reactions (e.g., coughing, dyspnea, rash, bullous eruption, vasodilation) have been reported in approximately 14% of patients receiving argatroban for indications other than HIT/HITTS; these patients usually were receiving concomitant thrombolytic agents (e.g., streptokinase) or radiographic contrast media.

General Precautions **Hepatic Impairment.** Caution is advised in patients with hepatic dysfunction. (See Dosage and Administration: Special Populations.) Achievement of steady-state anticoagulation and reversal of the anticoagulant effect may require longer than 1–3 hours and 4 hours, respectively, because of the decreased clearance and increased elimination half-life of argatroban in such patients.

Laboratory Monitoring. aPTT is well correlated with the anticoagulant effects of argatroban at therapeutic dosages; following discontinuance of the drug, aPTT generally returns to normal values within 2–4 hours. PT, INR, activated clotting time (ACT), and thrombin time (TT) are also prolonged by argatroban, but therapeutic ranges for these tests have not been identified.

Concomitant Therapy. Concomitant therapy with argatroban and antiplatelet agents, thrombolytics, or other anticoagulants may increase the risk of hemorrhage. (See Drug Interactions.)

Conversion to Oral Anticoagulant Therapy. A combined effect on the INR occurs with coadministration of argatroban and warfarin, and the relationship between INR and bleeding risk is altered. Daily INR determinations are recommended during concomitant use of argatroban and warfarin. Continue to monitor the effects of argatroban using aPTT during conversion to warfarin. Argatroban therapy can be discontinued when the INR exceeds 4 with combined therapy. Repeat INR determinations 4–6 hours after discontinuance of the argatroban infusion should be within the desired therapeutic range for warfarin monotherapy. (See General Dosage: Conversion to Oral Anticoagulant Therapy, in Dosage and Administration.)

Specific Populations **Pregnancy.** Category B. (See Users Guide.)

Lactation. Distributed in milk in rats; not known whether argatroban distributed in milk in humans. Discontinue nursing or the drug because of potential risk in nursing infants.

Pediatric Use. Safety and efficacy of argatroban not fully established in pediatric patients; however, the drug has been evaluated in a limited number of seriously ill pediatric patients younger than 16 years of age with HIT or HITTS. In a small, multicenter open-label study, 18 seriously ill pediatric patients with a clinical condition requiring alternative nonheparin anticoagulation received argatroban at an initial dosage of 1 mcg/kg per minute titrated to maintain a target aPTT of 1.5–3 times the baseline value. During the 30-day study period, thrombotic events occurred in 5 patients and major bleeding (intracranial hemorrhage) was reported in 2 patients. All of the patients had serious comorbid conditions and were receiving multiple concomitant medications; most were diagnosed with documented or suspected HIT. Pharmacokinetic analysis of the data indicated that argatroban clearance was reduced by 50% in seriously ill pediatric patients compared with healthy adults and by approximately 80% in pediatric patients with elevated bilirubin concentrations compared to pediatric patients with normal bilirubin concentrations. Based on these results, reduced dosages of argatroban are recommended in pediatric patients. (See Dosage and Administration: Special Populations.)

Geriatric Use. No substantial differences in efficacy or safety relative to younger adults.

Hepatic Impairment. Dosage reduction recommended for patients with hepatic impairment. (See Dosage and Administration: Special Populations.)

■ **Common Adverse Effects** Adverse hemorrhagic effects reported in 2% or more of nonsurgical patients with HIT/HITSS receiving argatroban include major or minor GI bleeding, minor genitourinary bleeding or hematuria, minor decrease in hemoglobin/hematocrit, minor groin or brachial bleeding (e.g., catheter insertion site), and hemoptysis; nonhemorrhagic effects include dyspnea, hypotension, fever, diarrhea, sepsis, cardiac arrest, nausea, ventricular tachycardia, pain, urinary tract infection, vomiting, infection, pneumonia, atrial fibrillation, coughing, abnormal renal function, abdominal pain, and cerebrovascular disorder.

Other nonhemorrhagic adverse effects occurring in at least 2% of argatroban-treated patients with HIT/HITTS undergoing PCI include chest pain, back pain, headache, bradycardia, and myocardial infarction.

Drug Interactions

■ **Warfarin** Pharmacodynamic interaction (increased prothrombin time [PT] and international normalized ratio [INR] relative to warfarin alone).

■ **Heparin** Heparin is contraindicated in patients with heparin-induced thrombocytopenia (HIT). Prior to initiation of argatroban therapy, allow sufficient time for effect of heparin on activated partial thromboplastin time (aPTT) to decrease.

■ **Other Drugs Affecting Coagulation** Potential pharmacologic interaction (increased risk of hemorrhage) with concomitant use of thrombolytics, antiplatelet agents, or other anticoagulants. No pharmacokinetic or pharmacodynamic interaction demonstrated with low-dose oral aspirin (162.5 mg given 26 and 2 hours prior to argatroban infusion) or oral acetaminophen (1 g given every 6 hours for 5 doses beginning 12 hours prior to argatroban infusion). The manufacturer states that the safety and efficacy of concomitant therapy with argatroban and platelet glycoprotein (GP) IIb/IIIa-receptor antagonists has not been established.

■ **Other Drugs** No drug interactions have been observed between argatroban and digoxin or erythromycin, a potent inhibitor of CYP3A4/5.

Description

Argatroban, a synthetic piperidinecarboxylic acid derivative of L-arginine, is an anticoagulant. Commercially available argatroban is a racemic mixture of the *R*- and *S*-diastereoisomers in a ratio of approximately 65 to 35, with the *S*-isomer having about twice the thrombin-inhibitory potency of the *R*-isomer.

Argatroban is a highly selective and reversible, small-molecule direct thrombin inhibitor that binds rapidly to the catalytic site/apolar region of both circulating (free) and clot-bound thrombin. Inhibition of thrombin prevents various steps in the coagulation process (e.g., activation of factors V, VIII, and XIII and of protein C; conversion of fibrinogen to fibrin; platelet activation and aggregation). At infusion rates up to 40 mcg/kg per minute, argatroban produces dose-dependent increases in activated partial thromboplastin time (aPTT) and several other coagulation assays (activated clotting time [ACT], prothrombin time [PT], and thrombin time [TT]). (See General Precautions: Laboratory Monitoring, in Cautions.)

Argatroban is metabolized principally by the liver via hydroxylation and aromatization of the 3-methyltetrahydroquinoline ring. Argatroban does not appear to induce antibody formation to itself nor does it interact with heparin-induced antibodies. Age or gender does not appear to substantially influence the pharmacokinetics and pharmacodynamics of argatroban.

Advice to Patients

Importance of reporting any signs of bleeding (e.g., bruising, petechiae, hematuria) to clinician immediately.

Importance of women informing clinician if they are, or plan to become, pregnant or breast-feed.

Importance of informing clinician of existing or contemplated concomitant therapy, including prescription (e.g., anticoagulants) and OTC drugs.

Overview (see Users Guide). For additional information until a more detailed monograph is developed and published, the manufacturer's labeling should be consulted. It is *essential* that the manufacturer's labeling be consulted for more detailed information on usual cautions, precautions, contraindications, potential drug interactions, laboratory test interferences, and acute toxicity.

Preparations

Excipients in commercially available drug preparations may have clinically important effects in some individuals; consult specific product labeling for details.

Argatroban

Parenteral

For injection concentrate, for IV infusion only	100 mg/mL (250 mg)	**Argatroban Injection,** GlaxoSmithKline

†Use is not currently included in the labeling approved by the US Food and Drug Administration

Bivalirudin

Hirulog

■ Bivalirudin, a synthetic analog of hirudin, is an anticoagulant.

Uses

■ Acute Ischemic Complications of Percutaneous Coronary Intervention Bivalirudin is used as an anticoagulant with aspirin to reduce the risk of acute ischemic complications (e.g., death, myocardial infarction [MI], need for urgent revascularization procedures) in patients undergoing percutaneous coronary intervention (PCI), including those with unstable angina undergoing percutaneous transluminal coronary angioplasty (PTCA) and those undergoing PCI with "provisional" use of platelet glycoprotein (GP) IIb/IIIa-receptor inhibitors. In clinical trials, provisional use of GP IIb/IIIa-receptor inhibitors (as opposed to "planned" use) involved use of the drugs under the following circumstances: decreased coronary artery perfusion (TIMI grade 0–2 flow) or slow reflow, dissection with decreased perfusion, new or suspected thrombus, persistent residual stenosis, distal embolization, unplanned or suboptimal stent placement, side branch or abrupt vessel closure, clinical instability, or prolonged ischemia.

Use of a parenteral anticoagulant is recommended in all patients undergoing PCI to prevent thrombus formation at the site of arterial injury, the coronary guidewire, and in the catheters used for the procedure. Bivalirudin (with or without prior unfractionated heparin treatment) is recommended by the American College of Cardiology Foundation (ACCF), the American Heart Association (AHA), and the Society for Cardiovascular Angiography and Interventions (SCAI) as an appropriate choice of anticoagulant for this use; other options include unfractionated heparin, enoxaparin, fondaparinux, and argatroban. Current evidence suggests that bivalirudin may be associated with a lower risk of bleeding than a regimen of unfractionated heparin and a GP IIb/IIIa-receptor inhibitor; however, this benefit is reduced when a GP IIb/IIIa-receptor inhibitor is used concomitantly. Therefore, a strategy of provisional use of a GP IIb/IIIa-receptor inhibitor has become widely accepted in patients receiving bivalirudin during PCI.

Efficacy and safety of bivalirudin in patients with unstable angina undergoing PTCA are based on the results of 2 randomized, double-blind, multicenter studies indicating that bivalirudin is as effective as high-dose unfractionated heparin in such patients. In these comparative studies, patients received either bivalirudin (1 mg/kg) by direct IV injection followed by a 4-hour IV infusion of the drug (2.5 mg/kg per hour) and then a second IV infusion (0.2 mg/kg per hour) for up to 14–20 hours, or heparin sodium (175 units/kg) by direct IV injection followed by IV infusion of the drug (15 units/kg per hour) for up to 24 hours. All patients also received oral aspirin 300–325 mg before PTCA and daily thereafter. The rates of procedural failure (defined as death, MI, or clinical deterioration of cardiac origin requiring revascularization or placement of an aortic balloon pump or angiographic evidence of abrupt vessel closure) were similar in both treatment groups. In a subgroup of patients with postinfarction angina undergoing PTCA, bivalirudin was more effective than heparin in decreasing procedural failures.

Efficacy and safety of bivalirudin in selected patients (i.e., those without high-risk features) undergoing PCI are based principally on the results of a double-blind, multicenter study (REPLACE-2 trial) designed to demonstrate noninferiority of bivalirudin and provisional use of a GP IIb/IIIa-receptor inhibitor compared with heparin and routine use of a GP IIb/IIIa-receptor inhibitor. In this trial, low-risk patients with unstable or stable angina, positive ischemic stress test, or recent (within 7 days) MI who were undergoing PCI (i.e., stent placement, atherectomy, or angioplasty) received either bivalirudin (0.75 mg/kg by direct IV injection prior to PCI) followed by IV infusion of bivalirudin (1.75 mg/kg per hour for the duration of the procedure), or heparin sodium (single dose of 65 units/kg by direct IV injection). Patients receiving bivalirudin also received a GP IIb/IIIa-receptor inhibitor (abciximab 0.25 mg/kg by direct IV injection followed by IV infusion of 0.125 mcg/kg per minute [maximum 10 mcg/minute] for 12 hours, or eptifibatide 180 mcg/kg by direct IV injection for 2 doses given 10 minutes apart, then 2 mcg/kg per minute by IV infusion for 18 hours) if they developed one or more of the following complications during the study: prolonged ischemia, decreased perfusion (TIMI grade 0–2 flow) or slow reflow, dissection with decreased perfusion, new or suspected thrombus, persistent residual stenosis, distal embolism, unplanned or suboptimal stenting, side branch closure, abrupt closure, or other clinical instability. Such complications occurred in 12.7% of patients receiving bivalirudin, and GP IIb/IIIa-receptor inhibitor therapy was subsequently administered to 7.2% of patients (62.2% of eligible patients). Patients receiving heparin were given *routine* GP IIb/IIIa-receptor inhibitor therapy. All patients also received daily aspirin, and most patients (about 85%) received pretreatment with clopidogrel (300 mg up to 24 hour before the procedure followed by 75 mg daily for at least 30 days). The rates of the primary composite end point (defined as the 30-day incidence of death, MI, urgent repeat revascularization, or in-hospital bleeding) and secondary composite end point (defined as the 30-day incidence of death, MI, or urgent repeat revascularization) were similar in both treatment groups; long-term follow-up also revealed similar rates of death, MI, and repeat revascularization at 6 months or death at 12 months in both groups. Treatment with bivalirudin was associated with lower rates of in-hospital bleeding compared with heparin. These efficacy and safety outcomes have been confirmed in women, in whom major and minor bleeding is reduced with bivalirudin compared with heparin.

Bivalirudin is intended to be used with adjunctive aspirin in patients undergoing PTCA or PCI and has been studied only in such patients receiving concomitant aspirin. The manufacturer states that safety and efficacy of bivalirudin have not been established in patients with acute coronary syndromes who are *not* undergoing PTCA or PCI.

■ Heparin-induced Thrombocytopenia in Patients Undergoing Percutaneous Coronary Intervention Bivalirudin is used with aspirin in patients undergoing PCI who have, or are at risk for, heparin-induced thrombocytopenia (HIT) or heparin-induced thrombocytopenia with thrombosis syndrome (HITTS). Several nonheparin anticoagulants (e.g., bivalirudin, argatroban, lepirudin) have been evaluated as substitutes for unfractionated heparin or low molecular weight heparin therapy in patients with HIT undergoing PCI. Among the different options, the American College of Chest Physicians (ACCP) and ACCF/AHA/SCAI recommend the use of bivalirudin or argatroban in such patients based on evidence from prospective studies; factors such as availability, cost, and ease of monitoring may influence choice of a particular agent. Although ACCP states that some patients with a history of HIT may be re-exposed to heparin in special circumstances, use of nonheparin anticoagulants generally is favored over re-exposure to heparin in patients with a history of HIT undergoing PCI.

In an open-label study in patients with a history of HIT or HITTS or active HIT/HITTS who were undergoing PCI, 48 of 51 patients receiving bivalirudin therapy (0.75 or 1 mg/kg by direct IV injection followed by continuous IV infusion of 1.75 or 2.5 mg/kg per hour, respectively) had successful PCI outcomes (i.e., TIMI grade 3 flow and stenosis less than 50%). Most patients received concomitant aspirin or clopidogrel, and some patients received concomitant GP IIb/IIIa-receptor inhibitors.

■ Heparin-induced Thrombocytopenia in Patients Undergoing Cardiac Surgery Bivalirudin also is used as a substitute for heparin in patients with acute HIT who require cardiac surgery† (e.g., coronary artery bypass grafting [CABG]). ACCP suggests the use of bivalirudin in patients with HIT or subacute HIT (platelets have recovered, but HIT antibodies are still present) who require urgent cardiac surgery; bivalirudin is suggested over other nonheparin anticoagulant options mainly because of direct supporting evidence from prospective, multicenter studies.

Dosage and Administration

■ **Reconstitution and Administration** Bivalirudin is administered by direct IV injection followed by IV infusion. The drug should *not* be administered IM.

Bivalirudin lyophilized powder should be stored at 20–25°C but may be exposed to temperatures ranging from 15–30°C.

Commercially available bivalirudin powder for injection must be reconstituted and diluted before administration. The drug should be reconstituted by adding 5 mL of sterile water for injection to a vial labeled as containing 250 mg of bivalirudin to provide a solution containing 50 mg/mL. The vial should be gently swirled to aid reconstitution and inspected for any evidence of particulate matter. The reconstituted solution may be stored at 2–8°C for up to 24 hours. The contents of the vial must be diluted in 50 mL of 5% dextrose or 0.9% sodium chloride injection to yield a final concentration of 5 mg/mL. This diluted solution may be used to administer the appropriate bivalirudin dose as a direct IV injection or 4-hour IV infusion. If the low-rate infusion is administered, the reconstituted bivalirudin solution should be further diluted in 500 mL of 5% dextrose or 0.9% sodium chloride to yield a final concentration of 0.5 mg/mL. The manufacturer states that bivalirudin solutions with concentrations of 0.5–5 mg/mL are stable at room temperature for up to 24 hours. Any unused reconstituted solution remaining in the vial should be discarded.

■ **Dosage** ***Acute Ischemic Complications of Percutaneous Coronary Intervention*** For use as an anticoagulant in reducing the risk of acute ischemic complications (e.g., death, myocardial infarction [MI], need for urgent revascularization procedures) in patients undergoing percutaneous coronary intervention (PCI), including percutaneous transluminal coronary angioplasty (PTCA), the recommended dosage of bivalirudin is 0.75 mg/kg by direct IV injection followed by a continuous IV infusion of 1.75 mg/kg per hour for the duration of the procedure. An activated clotting time (ACT) (as measured by a Hemochron device) should be obtained 5 minutes after the initial loading dose and an additional direct IV dose of 0.3 mg/kg given if needed (e.g., if the ACT is less than 225 seconds). The infusion of bivalirudin may be continued for up to 4 hours after PCI/PTCA at the discretion of the clinician. After completion of the 4-hour infusion, an additional IV infusion of bivalirudin at 0.2 mg/kg per hour may be administered for up to 20 hours if needed.

Administration of a platelet glycoprotein (GP) IIb/IIIa-receptor inhibitor should be considered in patients with procedural complications ("provisional use"). (See Uses: Acute Ischemic Complications of Percutaneous Coronary Intervention.)

The manufacturer states that bivalirudin is intended for use with aspirin (300–325 mg daily). According to the American College of Cardiology Foundation (ACCF), the American Heart Association (AHA), and the Society for Cardiovascular Angiography and Interventions (SCAI), a lower dose of aspirin (e.g., 81–325 mg) may be administered prior to PCI in patients who are already receiving daily aspirin therapy. (See Percutaneous Coronary Intervention and Revascularization Procedures under Dosage: Thrombosis, in Dosage and Administration in Aspirin 28:08.04.24.) In addition to aspirin, concomitant therapy with a P2Y12 platelet adenosine diphosphate (ADP)-receptor antagonist (e.g., clopidogrel, prasugrel, ticagrelor) also is recommended in patients undergoing PCI with coronary artery stent placement. (See Non-ST-Segment-Elevation Acute Coronary Syndromes under Dosage and Administration: Dosage, in Clopidogrel Bisulfate 20:12.18.)

Heparin-induced Thrombocytopenia in Patients Undergoing Percutaneous Coronary Intervention For patients with heparin-induced thrombocytopenia (HIT) or heparin-induced thrombocytopenia with thrombosis syndrome (HITTS) undergoing PCI, the recommended dosage of bivalirudin is 0.75 mg/kg (using a *5-mg/mL* solution) by direct IV injection immediately before PCI, followed by 1.75 mg/kg per hour (using a *5-mg/mL* solution) by continuous IV infusion for the duration of the procedure. The infusion of bivalirudin may be continued for up to 4 hours after PCI at the discretion of the clinician. After completion of the 4-hour infusion, an additional IV infusion (using a *0.5-mg/mL* solution) of bivalirudin at 0.2 mg/kg per hour may be administered for up 20 hours if needed.

Heparin-induced Thrombocytopenia in Patients Undergoing Cardiac Surgery For patients with acute HIT who undergo cardiac surgery† without the use of cardiopulmonary bypass (i.e., "off-pump"), a bivalirudin dosage of 0.75 mg/kg by direct IV injection followed by 1.75 mg/kg per hour by continuous IV infusion to maintain an ACT exceeding 300 seconds has been used.

During cardiopulmonary bypass, an initial bivalirudin dosage of 1 mg/kg given by direct IV injection followed by continuous IV infusion at a rate of 2.5 mg/kg per hour has been used; additional direct IV doses of 0.1–0.5 mg/kg have been given if needed to maintain a 2.5-fold or greater prolongation of the baseline ACT. In addition, 50 mg of bivalirudin is added to the recirculating priming fluid of the cardiopulmonary bypass circuit. As bivalirudin is metabolized by proteolytic cleavage by thrombin in the blood, special maneuvers are needed to avoid stasis within the cardiopulmonary bypass circuit during and after surgery. (See Cardiovascular Effects under Warnings/Precautions: Warnings, in Cautions.)

■ **Special Populations** ***Renal Impairment*** Close monitoring of anticoagulation status (e.g., ACT results) is recommended in patients with renal impairment. Total body clearance is reduced by approximately 20% in patients with moderate or severe renal impairment and by 80% in dialysis-dependent patients; approximately 25% of the drug is removed by hemodialysis. Reduction of the initial loading dose of bivalirudin is not necessary in patients with renal impairment. However, patients with severe renal impairment (creatinine clearance less than 30 mL/minute) should have the continuous IV infusion rate reduced to 1 mg/kg per hour, and dialysis-dependent patients should have the infusion rate reduced to 0.25 mg/kg per hour (off dialysis).

Cautions

■ **Contraindications** Active major bleeding. Known hypersensitivity to bivalirudin or any ingredient in the formulation.

■ **Warnings/Precautions** ***Warnings*** **Hematologic Effects.** Like other anticoagulants, bivalirudin should be used with caution in patients with an increased risk of hemorrhage. Although most bleeding associated with bivalirudin occurs at the site of arterial puncture in patients undergoing percutaneous transluminal coronary angioplasty (PTCA), hemorrhage can occur at any site during therapy. Unexplained decreases in hematocrit, hemoglobin, or blood pressure may indicate hemorrhage. If severe hemorrhage occurs, bivalirudin should be discontinued. Major hemorrhage (e.g., intracranial or retroperitoneal bleeding, clinically overt bleeding with a hemoglobin concentration decrease of at least 3 g/dL or requiring transfusion of at least 2 units of blood) occurred in 3.7% of patients with unstable angina undergoing PTCA receiving bivalirudin compared with 9.3% of those who received heparin in clinical studies. Major hemorrhage occurred in 2.3% of patients undergoing percutaneous coronary intervention (PCI) who were receiving bivalirudin with or without a platelet glycoprotein (GP) IIb/IIIa-receptor inhibitor and in 4% of such patients receiving heparin and a GP IIb/IIIa-receptor inhibitor.

Cardiovascular Effects. As an increased risk of potentially fatal thrombosis has been associated with use of bivalirudin during vascular brachytherapy procedures, the drug should be used with caution during such procedures. Catheter function should be assessed frequently by attempting to aspirate blood, and patency should be ensured by repeated flushing. Conditions promoting stasis within the catheter or circulatory system should be minimized.

When bivalirudin is used for intraoperative anticoagulation in patients with heparin-induced thrombocytopenia (HIT) undergoing cardiac surgery†, care must be taken to avoid formation of clots due to degradation of bivalirudin in areas of blood stasis. Special maneuvers are needed to avoid stasis within the cardiopulmonary bypass circuit during and after cardiac surgery.

Sensitivity Reactions **Hypersensitivity.** Although 2 patients in clinical studies had positive bivalirudin antibody tests, neither patient developed clinically apparent allergic or anaphylactic reactions. Nine additional patients who had positive test results were negative on repeat testing.

General Precautions **Factors Increasing Risk of Hemorrhage.** The risk of major bleeding events was increased with bivalirudin and concomitant heparin, warfarin, thrombolytic, or GP IIb/IIIa-receptor inhibitor therapy in clinical trials. (See Cautions: Common Adverse Effects.)

Caution should be used in patients with disease states associated with an increased risk of hemorrhage.

Brachytherapy Procedures. The manufacturer states that caution should be used when bivalirudin is used during vascular brachytherapy procedures because of an increased risk of thrombosis. (See Cardiovascular Effects under Warnings/Precautions: Warnings, in Cautions.)

Specific Populations **Pregnancy.** Category B. (See Users Guide.)

Lactation. Not known whether bivalirudin is distributed into milk; caution if used in nursing women.

Pediatric Use. Safety and efficacy not established in children.

Geriatric Use. In clinical trials, geriatric patients experienced more bleeding complications than younger adults.

Renal Impairment. Dosage adjustment (infusion dosage) recommended for patients with severe renal impairment. (See Renal Impairment under Dosage and Administration: Special Populations.)

■ **Common Adverse Effects** In a randomized, multicenter study, major hemorrhagic events occurred less frequently in patients undergoing PCI who were receiving bivalirudin with or without provisional GP IIb/IIIa-receptor inhibitor therapy compared with unfractionated heparin and routine GP IIb/IIIa-receptor inhibitor therapy. (See Hematologic Effects under Warnings/Precautions: Warnings, in Cautions.)

Nonhemorrhagic adverse effects reported in at least 5% of patients with unstable angina undergoing PTCA who were receiving bivalirudin in clinical trials include back pain, pain (unspecified), nausea, headache, hypotension, injection site pain, insomnia, hypertension, vomiting, pelvic pain, anxiety, bradycardia, dyspepsia, abdominal pain, fever, nervousness, and urinary retention. The incidence of these adverse effects was similar to that observed in patients receiving unfractionated heparin and routine GP IIb/IIIa-receptor inhibitor therapy.

Nonhemorrhagic adverse effects reported in at least 2% of patients undergoing PCI who were receiving bivalirudin and provisional GP IIb/IIIa-receptor inhibitor therapy in a large clinical trial include back pain, angina pectoris, pain, hypotension, nausea, injection site pain, headache, and chest pain; these adverse events occurred with similar frequency in patients receiving unfractionated heparin and routine GP IIb/IIIa-receptor inhibitor therapy.

Drug Interactions

■ **Drugs Inhibiting Coagulation** Potential pharmacologic interaction (increased risk of hemorrhage) when bivalirudin is used concomitantly with drugs inhibiting coagulation (e.g., aspirin, heparin, warfarin, GP IIb/IIIa-receptor inhibitors, thrombolytics). No data are available on the use of bivalirudin with plasma expanders such as dextran.

Description

Bivalirudin, a synthetic 20-amino acid peptide analog of naturally occurring hirudin, is an anticoagulant. Hirudin is the polypeptide that is responsible for the anticoagulant properties of the saliva of the medicinal leech (*Hirudo medicinalis*).

Bivalirudin is a specific and reversible direct thrombin inhibitor that binds to the catalytic site and the anion-binding exosite of circulating and clot-bound thrombin. Inhibition of thrombin prevents various steps in the coagulation process (e.g., activation of factors V, VIII, and XIII; conversion of fibrinogen to fibrin; platelet activation and aggregation). These effects of bivalirudin are reversed as thrombin slowly cleaves the bivalirudin-Arg_3-Pro_4 bond, resulting in recovery of thrombin active site function.

The onset of anticoagulant effect is immediate following direct IV injection of bivalirudin. Bivalirudin therapy prolongs several coagulation assays, including the activated clotting time (ACT), activated partial thromboplastin time (aPTT), thrombin time (TT), and prothrombin time (PT). Coagulation times return to the normal range approximately 1–2 hours after discontinuance of the drug.

Advice to Patients

Importance of reporting any signs of bleeding (e.g., bruising, petechiae, hematuria) to clinicians immediately. Importance of informing clinicians of any history of bleeding disorders or impaired renal function.

Importance of women informing clinician if they are or plan to become pregnant or plan to breast-feed.

Importance of informing clinician of existing or contemplated concomitant therapy, including prescription and OTC drugs.

Overview® (see Users Guide). For additional information until a more detailed monograph is developed and published, the manufacturer's labeling should be consulted. It is *essential* that the manufacturer's labeling be consulted for more detailed information on usual cautions, precautions, contraindications, potential drug interactions, laboratory test interferences, and acute toxicity.

Preparations

Excipients in commercially available drug preparations may have clinically important effects in some individuals; consult specific product labeling for details.

Bivalirudin

Parenteral

For injection, for IV infusion	250 mg	**Angiomax®**, Medicines Company

†Use is not currently included in the labeling approved by the US Food and Drug Administration

Selected Revisions September 2017,

Dabigatran Etexilate Mesylate

■ Dabigatran etexilate mesylate, a synthetic reversible direct thrombin inhibitor, is an anticoagulant.

Uses

■ **Embolism Associated with Atrial Fibrillation** Dabigatran etexilate mesylate is used to reduce the risk of stroke and systemic embolism in patients with nonvalvular atrial fibrillation. Some evidence suggests that dabigatran at a dosage of 150 mg twice daily may produce similar or superior outcomes in such patients compared with warfarin. Dabigatran should *not* be used in patients with prosthetic mechanical heart valves because of an increased risk of serious thromboembolic and bleeding events with such therapy; use of the drug also is not recommended in patients with other forms of valvular disease, including those with bioprosthetic heart valves. (See Patients with Prosthetic Heart Valves under Warnings/Precautions: Other Warnings and Precautions, in Cautions.)

The American College of Chest Physicians (ACCP), the American College of Cardiology (ACC), the American Heart Association (AHA), the American Stroke Association (ASA), and other experts currently recommend that antithrombotic therapy be administered to all patients with nonvalvular atrial fibrillation (i.e., atrial fibrillation in the absence of rheumatic mitral stenosis, a prosthetic heart valve, or mitral valve repair) who are considered to be at increased risk of stroke, unless such therapy is contraindicated. Recommendations regarding choice of antithrombotic therapy in patients with atrial fibrillation are based on the patient's risk for stroke and bleeding. In general, oral anticoagulant therapy (traditionally warfarin) is recommended in patients at moderate to high risk of stroke and acceptably low risk of bleeding, while aspirin or no antithrombotic therapy may be considered in patients at low risk of stroke. Although many risk stratification methods have been used, patients considered to be at increased risk of stroke generally include those with prior ischemic stroke or transient ischemic attack (TIA), advanced age (e.g., 75 years or older), history of hypertension, diabetes mellitus, or congestive heart failure. In addition, population-based studies suggest that female sex is an important risk factor for stroke in patients with atrial fibrillation, particularly in patients 75 years of age or older, and AHA and ASA recommend the use of risk stratification tools that account for age- and sex-specific differences in stroke risk. One such tool is the CHA_2DS_2-VASc score, an extension of the $CHADS_2$ system (which considers the risk factors congestive heart failure, hypertension, age 75 years or older, diabetes mellitus, and prior stroke/TIA) that adds extra points for female sex (1 point); previous myocardial infarction, peripheral arterial disease, or aortic plaque (1 point); and age 65–74 years (1 point) or 75 years or older (2 points).

The risk of thromboembolism in patients with atrial flutter is not as well established as it is in those with atrial fibrillation. In addition, many patients with atrial flutter have alternating periods of atrial fibrillation. Experts state that antithrombotic therapy in patients with atrial flutter generally should be managed in the same manner as in patients with atrial fibrillation.

Although warfarin traditionally has been used for oral anticoagulation in patients with atrial fibrillation at increased risk of stroke, some experts suggest that non-vitamin K antagonist oral anticoagulants such as dabigatran may provide certain advantages over warfarin (e.g., rapid onset of action, predictable anticoagulant effect, no requirement for coagulation monitoring, less potential for drug-drug and drug-food interactions) and may be considered as alternative therapy in selected patients. Some clinicians suggest that patients with the potential to benefit from dabigatran therapy compared with warfarin include warfarin-naive patients, those with difficulty maintaining therapeutic anticoagulation with warfarin, and those taking multiple drugs that may interact with warfarin. Warfarin may continue to be preferred in patients with severe renal insufficiency or liver disease, those with a history of dyspepsia or GI ulcer, those with hemodynamically important valvular heart disease or a prosthetic heart valve, those already achieving excellent control of anticoagulation with warfarin (e.g., international normalized ratio [INR] in therapeutic range more than 70% of the time), and those unwilling to commit to a twice-daily dosing regimen. Based on limited data, dabigatran also has been suggested as a reasonable alternative to warfarin in patients suitable for outpatient therapy who require more rapid therapeutic anticoagulation than that provided by warfarin (e.g., patients undergoing cardioversion for atrial fibrillation). However, because of the lack of direct, comparative studies, the relative efficacy and safety of dabigatran and other non-vitamin K antagonist oral anticoagulants (e.g., apixaban, edoxaban, rivaroxaban) used for the prevention of stroke in patients with nonvalvular atrial fibrillation remains to be fully elucidated. Some evidence from indirect comparisons suggests that there may be important differences (e.g., bleeding risk) between these agents; however, results of such analyses should be interpreted with caution because of possible confounding factors (e.g., differences in study design and methods, patient populations, and anticoagulation control). AHA and ASA state that while clinical trials of non-vitamin K antagonist oral anticoagulants were not designed to determine differences in efficacy compared with warfarin in men versus women, apixaban, dabigatran, or rivaroxaban may be a useful alternative to warfarin for the prevention of stroke and systemic thromboembolism in women with paroxysmal or permanent atrial fibrillation and prespecified risk factors (according to CHA_2DS_2-VASc) who do not have a prosthetic heart valve or hemodynamically important valve disease, severe renal failure (creatinine clearance less than 15 mL/minute), lower body weight (less than 50 kg), or advanced liver disease (impaired baseline clotting function). When selecting an appropriate anticoagulant for patients with atrial fibrillation, experts recommend that the risks versus benefits of such therapy be considered for individual patients based on absolute and relative risks of stroke and bleeding; patient compliance, preference, tolerance, and comorbidities; cost; availability of agents to reverse anticoagulant effects in case of bleeding complications; and other clinical factors such as renal function, availability of facilities to monitor INR, and degree of current INR control in patients already receiving warfarin. For additional information on antithrombotic therapy in patients with atrial fibrillation, see Uses: Embolism Associated with Atrial Fibrillation in Warfarin 20:12.04.08.

In a multinational, randomized, noninferiority study (Randomized Evaluation of Long-term Anticoagulation Therapy [RE-LY]) in adults with nonvalvular atrial fibrillation, therapy with dabigatran etexilate 150 or 110 mg twice daily was noninferior to adjusted-dose warfarin (target INR 2–3) with respect to the primary efficacy outcome of stroke or systemic embolism. In addition, the 150-mg dosage of dabigatran etexilate was superior to warfarin with regard to occurrence of stroke or systemic embolism, and the 110-mg dosage was superior to warfarin with regard to incidence of major bleeding. The net clinical benefit outcome, a measure of overall benefit to risk, was similar for both dosages of dabigatran etexilate.

In the RE-LY study, 18,113 adults with paroxysmal, persistent, or permanent atrial fibrillation and at least one additional risk factor for stroke (i.e., a history of stroke, transient ischemic attack, or systemic embolism; left ventricular ejection fraction less than 40%; symptomatic heart failure as defined by New York Heart Association [NYHA] class 2 or higher; age 75 years or older; age 65 years or older with diabetes mellitus, coronary artery disease, or hypertension) received dabigatran etexilate (110 or 150 mg twice daily) in a blinded fashion or adjusted-dose warfarin (target INR 2–3) in an unblinded fashion. The study population was principally white (70%) and male (64%), with a mean age of 71 years and a Congestive Heart Failure, Hypertension, Age, Diabetes, Stroke (doubled) ($CHADS_2$) score of 2.1. Approximately 20% of patients in each group continued aspirin throughout a median of 2 years of follow-up. Study exclusions included, but were not limited to, patients with valvular heart disease, recent stroke, increased risk of hemorrhage, renal impairment (creatinine clearance less than 30 mL/minute), or active liver disease.

The primary efficacy outcome of stroke (hemorrhagic or ischemic) or systemic embolism occurred substantially less frequently in patients receiving dabigatran etexilate 150 mg twice daily compared with adjusted-dose warfarin therapy (annualized rate of 1.11 or 1.69% of patients, respectively; relative risk reduction of 35%). In addition, compared with warfarin, therapy with dabigatran etexilate 150 mg twice daily was associated with reductions in ischemic and hemorrhagic stroke (relative risk reductions of 24 and 74%, respectively). Major hemorrhage occurred at a similar rate with dabigatran etexilate 150 mg twice daily versus warfarin.

In patients receiving dabigatran etexilate 110 mg twice daily, stroke or systemic embolism occurred with a frequency similar to that with warfarin (annualized rate of 1.53 or 1.69% of patients receiving dabigatran or warfarin, respectively). However, hemorrhagic stroke and major hemorrhage each occurred less frequently in those receiving dabigatran etexilate 110 mg compared with warfarin (relative risk reductions of 69 and 20%, respectively). Stroke or systemic embolism occurred less frequently with dabigatran etexilate 150 mg twice daily than with 110 mg twice daily (annualized rate of 1.1 or 1.53% of patients, respectively; relative risk reduction of 28%). Rates of hemorrhagic stroke and major hemorrhage were similar in the 2 dabigatran groups. In patients receiving warfarin, anticoagulation was maintained within the therapeutic range a mean 64% of the time during the study.

The rate of myocardial infarction was higher with dabigatran etexilate 150 or 110 mg than with warfarin (0.81, 0.82, or 0.64% per year, respectively; relative risk of 1.27 or 1.29 for the 150- or 110-mg dosages, respectively, versus warfarin), but these differences were not statistically significant.

While both a 150- and a 110-mg dosage of dabigatran etexilate were evaluated in the RE-LY study, the US Food and Drug Administration (FDA) approved only the 150-mg dosage of dabigatran etexilate for stroke risk reduction in patients with nonvalvular atrial fibrillation. Prior to FDA approval, some clinicians expressed interest in using the 110-mg dosage in specific patient populations, such as those that may be at greater risk of bleeding or, at lower risk of embolic events, or those who experienced bleeding when receiving the 150-mg dosage. FDA concluded that in patients who experienced major bleeding during the RE-LY study and who continued or resumed study medication, the risk of a repeat major bleeding event was similar among all 3 treatment groups. According to FDA, the appropriate population for the 110-mg dosage has not been identified. Because of superior efficacy with the 150-mg dosage and concern that a 110-mg dosage could potentially be overused and subsequently result in underdosing of many patients, FDA approved only the 150-mg dosage for stroke risk reduction in patients with nonvalvular atrial fibrillation. Approval of the 75-mg dosage for patients with severe renal impairment (creatinine clearance 15–30 mL/minute) was based on pharmacokinetic modeling using pharmacokinetic data from RE-LY and a smaller study in individuals with renal impairment.

Based on the results of a payer-perspective analysis that used data principally from the RE-LY study, therapy with dabigatran etexilate 150 mg twice daily, may be a cost-effective alternative to adjusted-dose warfarin in patients 65 years of age or older who are at high risk for stroke ($CHADS_2$ score of 1 or greater). In this analysis, therapy with dabigatran etexilate 150 mg twice daily resulted in an additional 0.56 quality-adjusted life-years (QALY) at an estimated cost of $45,372 (in 2008 dollars) per QALY gained compared with warfarin. Varying the cost of dabigatran had the greatest effect on cost effectiveness in this analysis. In another cost-effectiveness analysis based on RE-LY that considered patients with an average risk of major hemorrhage of about 3% per year, dabigatran etexilate 150 mg twice daily was found to be cost effective compared with warfarin (i.e., less than $50,000 per QALY gained versus warfarin) in patients with atrial fibrillation at high risk of stroke (i.e. $CHADS_2$ score of 3 or greater) unless INR control with warfarin was excellent (time in the therapeutic range exceeding 72.6%), while warfarin was cost effective compared with dabigatran in moderate-risk patients with atrial fibrillation unless risk of major bleeding was high or INR control was poor (time in the therapeutic range less than 57.1%).

Dabigatran also has been used for the prevention of stroke and systemic embolism in patients undergoing cardioversion for atrial fibrillation†. ACCP, ACC, AHA, and other experts recommend that patients with atrial fibrillation/atrial flutter who are to undergo elective cardioversion (pharmacologic or electrical) receive therapeutic anticoagulation for at least 3 weeks prior to the procedure. Although warfarin traditionally has been used for precardioversion anticoagulation, some data suggest that dabigatran may be as effective and safe as warfarin in preventing the risk of stroke and systemic embolism. Dabigatran is recommended by ACCP as an acceptable choice for precardioversion anticoagulation in patients with atrial fibrillation lasting more than 48 hours or of unknown duration; prolonged precardioversion anticoagulation generally is not required in patients with atrial fibrillation of short duration (e.g., 48 hours or less).

Based on the results of a randomized, open-label trial (RE-ALIGN), dabigatran should *not* be used for the prevention of stroke or other major thromboembolic events in patients with mechanical prosthetic heart valves. (See Patients with Prosthetic Heart Valves under Warnings/Precautions: Other Warnings and Precautions, in Cautions.) In this trial, patients received dabigatran (150, 220, or 300 mg twice daily) or adjusted-dose warfarin therapy (target INR of 2–3 or 2.5–3.5 depending on risk factors and position [aortic or mitral] of the mechanical heart valve). The trial was terminated early because of a substantially increased rate of stroke, myocardial infarction, and valve thrombosis in patients receiving dabigatran compared with those receiving warfarin; dabigatran-treated patients also had a higher risk of major bleeding, predominantly after valve surgery.

■ **Deep-Vein Thrombosis and Pulmonary Embolism** ***Treatment and Secondary Prevention*** Dabigatran is used for the treatment of acute deep-vein thrombosis (DVT) and/or pulmonary embolism (PE) following initial treatment with a parenteral anticoagulant for 5–10 days. The drug also is used as extended therapy (secondary prevention) to reduce the risk of recurrent DVT and PE in patients who have been treated previously for the acute venous thromboembolic event.

Dabigatran is recommended by ACCP as an acceptable option for long-term anticoagulant therapy in patients with acute proximal DVT of the leg and/or PE. In such patients, ACCP recommends that anticoagulant therapy be continued beyond the acute treatment period for at least 3 months, and possibly longer depending on the individual clinical situation (e.g., location of thrombi, presence or absence of precipitating factors, presence of cancer, patient's risk of bleeding). Although dabigatran may offer some advantages over existing anticoagulant drugs for the treatment of venous thromboembolism (e.g., oral administration, no requirement for routine coagulation monitoring, minimal drug and food interactions), ACCP generally suggests the use of warfarin or a low molecular weight heparin rather than dabigatran for long-term anticoagulant therapy pending additional data and experience with dabigatran. The relative efficacy and safety of dabigatran versus other non-vitamin K antagonist oral anticoagulants (e.g., apixaban, rivaroxaban) for the treatment of venous thromboembolism remains to be established in controlled, comparative trials. For additional information on treatment of venous thromboembolism, consult the most recent ACCP Evidence-based Clinical Practice Guidelines on Antithrombotic Therapy and Prevention of Thrombosis available at http://www.chestnet.org.

Efficacy and safety of dabigatran for the acute treatment and secondary prevention of DVT and/or PE has been established principally in 4 randomized, double-blind studies. In 2 identically designed studies (RE-COVER and RE-COVER II) in more than 5000 patients with symptomatic acute proximal DVT or PE who were treated initially with a parenteral anticoagulant (e.g., unfractionated heparin, low molecular weight heparin) for 5–10 days, dabigatran was shown to be noninferior to warfarin in preventing recurrent thromboembolic events over a mean treatment period of approximately 6 months (based on similar rates of the primary composite outcome of fatal or symptomatic nonfatal PE or symptomatic recurrent DVT) and was associated with a lower risk of clinically relevant bleeding. In both studies, patients received either dabigatran etexilate 150 mg twice daily or adjusted-dose warfarin (target INR 2–3). Patients who received warfarin in the RE-COVER and RE-COVER II studies had INRs within the therapeutic range (2–3) an average of 60 and 57% of time, respectively, which improved over the course of treatment from 53 or 51%, respectively, in the first month to 66 or 62%, respectively, in the last month.

Efficacy and safety of extended use of dabigatran for reducing the risk of recurrent DVT and/or PE (secondary prevention) has been established principally in an active-control (RE-MEDY) and a placebo-control (RE-SONATE) study. Dabigatran was shown to be noninferior to warfarin and superior to placebo in reducing the risk of recurrent DVT and PE in these studies. Patients in the studies had completed at least 3 months of initial anticoagulant therapy for an acute venous thromboembolic event prior to enrollment; the studies included some patients who previously had received dabigatran in the RE-COVER and RE-COVER II studies. In the RE-MEDY study, patients received either dabigatran etexilate (150 mg twice daily) or warfarin (with dose adjusted to achieve a target INR of 2–3) for a median duration of approximately 17.8 months; in the RE-SONATE study, patients received either dabigatran etexilate (150 mg twice daily) or placebo for a median duration of approximately 6 months. In patients receiving warfarin in the RE-MEDY study, the average time in the therapeutic INR range was 62%. Although the criteria for noninferiority of dabigatran compared with warfarin was met in this study, there were some limitations associated with the statistical analysis (e.g., large noninferiority margin, upper limit of confidence interval close to noninferiority margin). With respect to safety, dabigatran was associated with a lower risk of major or clinically relevant bleeding compared with warfarin, but a higher risk of bleeding compared with placebo.

Prophylaxis **Major Orthopedic Surgery.** Dabigatran is used for the prevention of DVT and PE in patients undergoing hip-replacement surgery. Dabigatran has also been used for the prevention of venous thromboembolism in patients undergoing total knee-replacement surgery†. ACCP recommends routine thromboprophylaxis (with a pharmacologic and/or mechanical [e.g., intermittent pneumatic compression] method) in all patients undergoing major orthopedic surgery because of the high risk for postoperative venous thromboembolism; thromboprophylaxis should be continued for at least 10–14 days, and possibly for up to 35 days after surgery. ACCP considers dabigatran an acceptable option for pharmacologic thromboprophylaxis in patients undergoing total hip- or knee-replacement surgery, although ACCP states that a low molecular weight heparin generally is preferred because of its relative efficacy and safety and extensive clinical experience. Dabigatran may be a reasonable choice in situations in which a low molecular weight heparin is not available or cannot be used (e.g., in patients with heparin-induced thrombocytopenia, in those who refuse or are uncooperative with subcutaneous injections). ACCP states that when selecting an appropriate thromboprophylaxis regimen, factors such as relative efficacy and bleeding risk as well as logistics and compliance issues should be considered. For additional details on prevention of venous thromboembolism in patients undergoing major orthopedic surgery, consult the most recent ACCP Evidence-based Clinical Practice Guidelines on Antithrombotic Therapy and Prevention of Thrombosis available at http://www.chestnet.org.

Efficacy and safety of dabigatran for the prevention of postoperative DVT and PE in patients undergoing hip-replacement surgery are based principally on the results of 2 randomized, double-blind, active-controlled studies (RE-NOVATE and RE-NOVATE II). In these studies, dabigatran was noninferior to enoxaparin in preventing venous thromboembolism in patients undergoing elective total hip-replacement surgery (based on similar rates of the primary composite end point of confirmed venous thromboembolism [proximal or distal DVT on venogram, confirmed symptomatic DVT, or confirmed PE] and all cause death) and was associated with similar rates of bleeding. Patients in these studies received a single dose of dabigatran 75 mg (administered 1–4 hours after surgery) followed by dabigatran 150 mg daily; a single dose of dabigatran 110 mg (administered 1–4 hours after surgery) followed by dabigatran 220 mg daily; or subcutaneous enoxaparin 40 mg daily starting the evening before surgery for a median duration of 33 days. For efficacy evaluation, all patients underwent bilateral venography of the lower extremities within 24 hours after the last dose of the study drug unless an end point event occurred earlier in the trial. The primary composite end point occurred in 6–7.7% of patients receiving dabigatran 220 mg daily and 6.7–8.8% of patients receiving enoxaparin therapy. Dabigatran was generally well tolerated across all studies, and rates of major bleeding or any bleeding event were generally similar between treatment groups.

■ **Cerebral Embolism** Antiplatelet agents are considered preferable to oral anticoagulant therapy for secondary prevention of noncardioembolic stroke in patients with a history of ischemic stroke or TIA. However, ACCP recommends oral anticoagulation (e.g., warfarin, dabigatran) for secondary prevention of cardioembolic stroke in patients with TIAs† or ischemic stroke† and concurrent atrial fibrillation; among the anticoagulant options, ACCP suggests the use of dabigatran (150 mg twice daily) over warfarin.

Dosage and Administration

■ **General** Routine laboratory monitoring of coagulation status is not required in patients receiving dabigatran etexilate mesylate. However, in certain situations, such as in the case of overdosage or in patients with hemorrhagic or thromboembolic complications or those requiring emergency surgery, it may be useful to assess the degree of anticoagulation. When necessary, the manufacturer states that the ecarin clotting time (ECT) or the activated partial thromboplastin time (aPTT) may be used to assess the anticoagulant effects of dabigatran; however, results of such tests should be interpreted with caution. It has been suggested that the thrombin time (TT) may be a useful test to detect the presence of any dabigatran in plasma because of its high sensitivity at low concentrations of the drug; however, changes in the TT also should be interpreted with caution if this test is used for monitoring anticoagulation with dabigatran. Use of the prothrombin time (PT)/international normalized ratio (INR) should be avoided since this test is relatively insensitive to the effects of dabigatran and results may be unreliable.

Renal function should be assessed prior to treatment initiation, during treatment in clinical situations that may be associated with a decline in renal function, and at least annually during treatment in patients older than 75 years of age or in those with a creatinine clearance less than 50 mL/minute.

■ **Administration** Dabigatran is administered orally without regard to meals.

To minimize potential product breakdown and loss of potency due to moisture, dabigatran capsules should be dispensed only in the manufacturer's original bottle with desiccant cap; the capsules should not be repackaged. If more than one bottle is dispensed, the patient should be advised to open only one bottle at a time. The manufacturer recommends that capsules in the bottle be used within 4 months after first opening the bottle. Patients should be advised about special storage and handling requirements for dabigatran etexilate. (See Advice to Patients.)

Capsules should be swallowed whole with a full glass of water; chewing, breaking, or opening the capsules may result in increased systemic exposure to the drug. A missed dose should be taken as soon as it is remembered on the same day. However, a missed dose should be skipped if it cannot be taken at least 6 hours before the next scheduled dose; doses should *not* be doubled.

■ **Dosage** Dosage of dabigatran, which is commercially available as dabigatran etexilate mesylate, is expressed in terms of the prodrug, dabigatran etexilate.

Embolism Associated with Atrial Fibrillation For reducing the risk of stroke and systemic embolism in patients with nonvalvular atrial fibrillation, the recommended dosage of dabigatran etexilate in adults with a creatinine clearance exceeding 30 mL/minute is 150 mg orally twice daily.

Deep-Vein Thrombosis and Pulmonary Embolism **Treatment and Secondary Prevention.** For the treatment and reduction in the risk of recurrence (secondary prevention) of acute deep-vein thrombosis (DVT) and/or pulmonary embolism (PE), the recommended dosage of dabigatran etexilate in adults with a creatinine clearance exceeding 30 mL/minute is 150 mg orally twice daily, after 5–10 days of parenteral anticoagulation.

The optimum duration of anticoagulant therapy should be determined by the individual clinical situation (e.g., location of thrombi, presence or absence of precipitating factors for thrombosis, presence of cancer, risk of bleeding). In general, the American College of Chest Physicians (ACCP) states that anticoagulant therapy should be continued beyond the acute treatment period for at least 3 months and possibly longer in patients with a high risk of recurrence and low risk of bleeding.

Thromboprophylaxis in Hip-Replacement Surgery. For the prevention of DVT and PE in patients who have undergone hip-replacement surgery, the recommended dosage of dabigatran etexilate in adults with a creatinine clearance exceeding 30 mL/minute is 110 mg administered as a single dose 1–4 hours after surgery (provided hemostasis has been achieved), followed by 220 mg once daily. If dabigatran therapy is not initiated on the day of surgery, dabigatran treatment should be initiated at a dosage of 220 mg once daily after hemostasis has been achieved. The manufacturer recommends a treatment duration of 28–35 days for patients who have undergone hip-replacement surgery. ACCP recommends at least 10–14 days of antithrombotic therapy, possibly up to 35 days, for patients undergoing major orthopedic surgery.

Transferring from Therapy with Other Anticoagulants When switching to dabigatran therapy from warfarin, dabigatran should be initiated after warfarin has been discontinued and the INR is less than 2.

When switching to dabigatran therapy in patients receiving *intermittently dosed* parenteral anticoagulants (e.g., enoxaparin), the first dose of dabigatran should be administered within 2 hours prior to what would have been the time of the next scheduled intermittent parenteral dose.

When switching to dabigatran therapy in patients receiving parenteral anticoagulants by *continuous* infusion, dabigatran should be initiated at the time the infusion is discontinued.

Transferring to Therapy with Other Anticoagulants When switching from dabigatran to warfarin therapy, warfarin should be initiated prior to dabigatran discontinuance. For patients with a creatinine clearance of 50 mL/minute or greater, warfarin should be started 3 days prior to dabigatran discontinuance. For patients with a creatinine clearance of 30–50 mL/minute, warfarin should be started 2 days prior and for patients with a creatinine clearance of 15–30 mL/minute, warfarin should be started 1 day prior to discontinuance of dabigatran. The manufacturer states that dosing recommendations are not available for patients with a creatinine clearance of less than 15 mL/minute. Because assessment of INR is unreliable in patients receiving dabigatran, the therapeutic effects of warfarin are more accurately reflected by INR measurements taken 2 or more days after dabigatran discontinuance.

When switching from dabigatran to therapy with a parenteral anticoagulant, dabigatran should be discontinued prior to initiating parenteral therapy. For patients with a creatinine clearance of 30 mL/minute or greater, the parenteral anticoagulant should be started 12 hours after the last dose of dabigatran. If the creatinine clearance is less than 30 mL/minute, the parenteral anticoagulant should be started 24 hours after the last dose of dabigatran. Dosing recommendations are not available for patients with a creatinine clearance of less than 15 mL/minute.

Managing Anticoagulation in Patients Requiring Invasive Procedures When possible, dabigatran therapy should be withheld prior to invasive or surgical procedures because of the increased risk of bleeding. For patients with a creatinine clearance of 50 mL/minute or greater, the manufacturer recommends withholding therapy beginning 1–2 days prior to the procedure. For patients with a creatinine clearance of less than 50 mL/minute, dabigatran should be withheld beginning 3–5 days prior to the procedure. However, withholding therapy for longer periods should be considered in patients who may require complete hemostasis (e.g., prior to major surgery, spinal puncture, placement of spinal or epidural catheter or port). (See Risk of Thrombosis Following Premature Discontinuance of Anticoagulation under Warnings/Precautions: Warnings, in Cautions.) When surgery cannot be delayed, the increased risk of bleeding with dabigatran therapy should be weighed against the urgency of the intervention. Idarucizumab, a specific reversal agent for dabigatran, can be used in case of emergency surgery or procedures when reversal of dabigatran's anticoagulant effect is needed. Dabigatran therapy can be reinitiated 24 hours after administration of idarucizumab; resumption of anticoagulant therapy should be considered as soon as medically appropriate. (See Bleeding under Warnings/Precautions: Other Warnings and Precautions, in Cautions.) For further information on idarucizumab, see Idarucizumab 20:28:92.

■ **Special Populations** ***Renal Impairment*** **Embolism Associated with Atrial Fibrillation.** In patients with severe renal impairment (creatinine clearance of 15–30 mL/minute), the manufacturer recommends that dosage of dabigatran etexilate be reduced to 75 mg orally twice daily. Patients with severe renal impairment were not included in the RE-LY study; therefore, dosage recommendations in this population are based on pharmacokinetic modeling. For patients with a creatinine clearance less than 15 mL/minute or who are receiving hemodialysis, the manufacturer states that dosage recommendations cannot be provided.

Concomitant use of the P-glycoprotein inhibitors dronedarone and ketoconazole (systemic) in patients with moderate renal impairment (creatinine clearance of 30–50 mL/minute) is expected to increase dabigatran exposure to a similar extent as that observed in patients with severe renal impairment; therefore, the manufacturer recommends that the dosage of dabigatran be reduced to 75 mg twice daily in patients with moderate renal impairment receiving such concomitant therapy. (See Drugs Affecting P-glycoprotein Transport under Warnings/Precautions: Other Warnings and Precautions, in Cautions.) Dosage adjustments are not necessary when dabigatran is administered concomitantly with the P-glycoprotein inhibitors verapamil, amiodarone, quinidine, clarithromycin, and ticagrelor in patients with moderate renal impairment. Concomitant use of dabigatran with P-glycoprotein inhibitors should be avoided in patients with severe renal impairment (creatinine clearance of 15–30 mL/minute).

Treatment and Secondary Prevention of Deep-Vein Thrombosis and Pulmonary Embolism. The manufacturer of dabigatran states that dosage recommendations cannot be provided for patients with a creatinine clearance of 30 mL/minute or less or for those receiving dialysis.

Concomitant use of P-glycoprotein inhibitors should be avoided in patients with a creatinine clearance less than 50 mL/minute. (See Drugs Affecting P-glycoprotein Transport under Warnings/Precautions: Other Warnings and Precautions, in Cautions.)

Thromboprophylaxis in Hip-Replacement Surgery. The manufacturer of dabigatran states that dosage recommendations cannot be provided for patients with a creatinine clearance of 30 mL/minute or less or for those receiving dialysis.

Concomitant use of P-glycoprotein inhibitors should be avoided in patients with a creatinine clearance less than 50 mL/minute. (See Drugs Affecting P-glycoprotein Transport under Warnings/Precautions: Other Warnings and Precautions, in Cautions.)

Cautions

■ **Contraindications** Active pathologic bleeding. History of serious hypersensitivity reaction to dabigatran etexilate mesylate (e.g., anaphylaxis, anaphylactic shock). Patients with mechanical prosthetic heart valves.

■ **Warnings/Precautions** ***Warnings*** **Risk of Thrombosis Following Premature Discontinuance of Anticoagulation.** Premature discontinuance of any oral anticoagulant, including dabigatran, in the absence of adequate alternative anticoagulation increases the risk of thrombotic events. If discontinuance of dabigatran is required for reasons other than pathologic bleeding or completion of a course of therapy, administration of an alternative anticoagulant should be considered. When transitioning patients from one anticoagulant therapy to another, it is important to ensure continuous anticoagulation while minimizing the risk of bleeding.

Spinal/Epidural Hematoma. Patients receiving anticoagulants are at risk of developing an epidural or spinal hematoma when concomitant neuraxial (epidural/spinal) anesthesia or spinal puncture is employed; such complications can result in long-term or permanent paralysis. The risk of these complications is increased by postoperative use of indwelling epidural catheters for administration of analgesia or by concomitant use of drugs affecting hemostasis, such as nonsteroidal anti-inflammatory agents (NSAIAs), platelet-aggregation inhibitors, or other anticoagulants. Risk also may be increased in patients with a history of traumatic or repeated epidural or spinal punctures, spinal deformity, or spinal surgery.

To reduce the risk of bleeding with concurrent use of dabigatran and neuraxial anesthesia or spinal puncture procedures, clinicians should carefully consider the pharmacokinetic profile of dabigatran in relation to timing of such procedures. Insertion or removal of an epidural catheter or lumbar puncture is best performed when the anticoagulant effect of dabigatran is minimal; however, the optimal timing to achieve a sufficiently low anticoagulant effect in individual patients is not known.

Patients receiving dabigatran in the setting of epidural or spinal anesthesia should be monitored frequently for signs and symptoms of neurologic impairment (e.g., midline back pain; numbness, tingling, or weakness in lower limbs; bowel or bladder dysfunction). If spinal hematoma is suspected, urgent diagnosis and treatment is necessary; spinal cord decompression should be considered even though it may not prevent or reverse neurologic sequelae. Clinicians should consider the potential benefits versus risks of spinal/epidural anesthesia or spinal puncture in patients receiving or being considered for anticoagulant therapy.

Other Warnings and Precautions **Bleeding.** Dabigatran increases the risk of hemorrhage and may cause serious, sometimes fatal bleeding. In the Randomized Evaluation of Long-term Anticoagulation Therapy (RE-LY) study, life-threatening bleeding (i.e., fatal bleeding, symptomatic intracranial bleeding, hemoglobin decrease of 5 g/dL or greater, hypotension requiring IV inotropic agents, transfusion of 4 or more units of blood, surgical intervention required) occurred at a rate of 1.5% per year in patients receiving dabigatran etexilate 150 mg twice daily versus 1.8% per year with adjusted-dose (target international normalized ratio [INR] 2–3) warfarin therapy. Major bleeding (i.e., hemoglobin decrease of at least 2 g/dL, transfusion of 2 or more units of packed red blood cells, bleeding into a critical organ/area, and/or fatal outcome) was similar in patients receiving dabigatran 150 mg twice daily compared with those receiving adjusted-dose warfarin therapy (approximately 3.5 or 3.6% per year, respectively); however, there was a trend towards a higher incidence of major bleeding with dabigatran therapy for patients 75 years of age and older. Dabigatran therapy was associated with substantially lower rates of life-threatening bleeding, intracranial bleeding, and combined major or minor bleeding compared with warfarin in the RE-LY study. However, the rate of GI bleeding, including major GI bleeding, was substantially higher with dabigatran etexilate 150 mg twice daily compared with warfarin. Rates of major bleeding or clinically relevant bleeding with dabigatran were lower or similar to those with warfarin in the randomized, controlled studies in patients with acute deep-vein thrombosis (DVT) and/or pulmonary embolism (PE) (RE-COVER and RE-COVER II). In these studies, GI bleeding occurred in 3.1% of patients receiving dabigatran etexilate 150 mg twice daily versus 2.4% of those receiving warfarin. In the RE-NOVATE and RE-NOVATE II studies in patients undergoing hip-replacement surgery, major bleeding occurred in 1.4–2% of patients receiving dabigatran 220 mg daily and 0.9–1.6% of patients receiving enoxaparin therapy. The rate of major GI bleeding in patients receiving dabigatran and enoxaparin was the same (0.1%) and the rate of any GI bleeding was 1.4 and 0.9% for dabigatran- and enoxaparin-treated patients, respectively. In longer-term studies in which patients received extended treatment with dabigatran for acute venous thromboembolism (RE-MEDY, RE-SONATE), major or clinically relevant bleeding occurred less frequently with dabigatran than with warfarin, but more frequently with dabigatran than with placebo. The rate of any GI bleeding with dabigatran therapy in these studies was 0.7–3.1%.

In December 2011, the US Food and Drug Administration (FDA) initiated a safety review of dabigatran following reports of a large number of serious, sometimes fatal bleeding events with the drug during postmarketing experience. As part of this review, FDA conducted an observational cohort study in more than 134,000 Medicare patients 65 years of age or older with atrial fibrillation, comparing rates of intracranial bleeding, major GI bleeding, and other adverse outcomes (i.e., ischemic stroke, myocardial infarction, death) in new users of dabigatran versus new users of warfarin. Dabigatran was associated with a higher risk of major GI bleeding, but a lower risk of intracranial hemorrhage, ischemic stroke, and death; rates of myocardial infarction were similar between the 2 groups. These findings generally were consistent with those of the RE-LY study. However, with regard to major GI bleeding, discrepant results have been reported in other studies, including a previous FDA study that found a lower rate of GI bleeding with dabigatran versus warfarin using data from the Mini-Sentinel Program. While this variability may be due, in part, to age differences in the patient populations studied (e.g., older versus younger population) or other potential confounding factors, FDA is continuing to investigate the reasons for this disparity. FDA currently believes that the benefits of dabigatran continue to outweigh its potential risks when used appropriately according to the manufacturer's prescribing information. Patients should continue to take dabigatran as prescribed unless otherwise instructed by a clinician; careful attention to dosing recommendations is advised, particularly in patients with renal impairment, to reduce the risk of bleeding.

Risk factors for hemorrhage include concomitant use of other drugs that generally increase bleeding risk (e.g., antiplatelet agents, heparin, thrombolytic therapy, chronic use of NSAIAs) and renal impairment. Overdosage also may lead to hemorrhagic complications.

Patients developing manifestations of blood loss (e.g., decrease in hemoglobin, decrease in hematocrit, hypotension) should have such manifestations promptly evaluated; evaluation of renal function also should be considered. Dabigatran should be discontinued in patients with active pathologic bleeding and appropriate therapy instituted. However, minor or "nuisance" bleeding is a common occurrence in patients receiving any anticoagulant and should not readily lead to treatment discontinuance. (See Risk of Thrombosis Following Premature Discontinuance of Anticoagulation under Warnings/Precautions: Warnings, in Cautions.)

Ecarin clotting time (ECT) or activated partial thromboplastin time (aPTT) may be used when necessary to assess the degree of anticoagulation from dabigatran therapy. Management of bleeding complications should be individualized according to the severity and location of hemorrhage. Idarucizumab, a recombinant humanized monoclonal antibody fragment, is a specific reversal agent that is used to neutralize the anticoagulant effect of dabigatran in patients with life-threatening or uncontrolled bleeding or a need to undergo an emergency surgery/urgent procedure. Idarucizumab has been shown to reverse the anticoagulant effects of dabigatran within minutes after administration. Idarucizumab can be used in conjunction with supportive measures (e.g., maintenance of adequate diuresis, mechanical compression, surgical hemostasis, volume replacement, blood products), which should be considered as medically appropriate. For further information on idarucizumab, see Idarucizumab 20:28:92. While clinical experience supporting the use of hemodialysis is limited, dabigatran is dialyzable and approximately 49–57% of the drug is removed over 4 hours using a high-flux dialyzer at a blood flow rate of 200 or 300 mL/minute; however, redistribution of the drug may occur after completion of dialysis, and the individual response to dialysis is likely to vary based on patient-specific characteristics. Limited experimental (in vitro and animal) data and case studies support the administration of anti-inhibitor coagulant complex (e.g., Feiba® VH or Feiba® NF; also known as activated prothrombin complex concentrate), factor VIIa (recombinant), or concentrates of coagulation factors II, IX, or X, but efficacy and safety of these agents have not been evaluated in clinical studies of patients receiving dabigatran. In a study in a limited number of healthy individuals, use of a nonactivated 4-factor prothrombin complex concentrate (PCC) failed to reverse the anticoagulant effect of dabigatran as measured by aPTT, ECT, or thrombin time (TT). Protamine sulfate and vitamin

K are not expected to affect the anticoagulant activity of dabigatran. Administration of platelet concentrates may also be considered in cases of thrombocytopenia or when long-acting antiplatelet drugs have been used. In the event of an overdosage, activated charcoal may be used if administered early (e.g., within 1–2 hours) after ingestion.

Patients with Prosthetic Heart Valves. Findings from a randomized, controlled study (RE-ALIGN) indicate an increased risk of thromboembolic events (valve thrombosis, stroke, transient ischemic attack, myocardial infarction) and major bleeding (principally postoperative pericardial effusions) with dabigatran compared with warfarin therapy in patients with mechanical prosthetic heart valves. (See Uses: Embolism Associated with Atrial Fibrillation.) Such thromboembolic and bleeding events were observed in patients with recently implanted as well as older (implanted more than 3 months prior to study entry) prosthetic valves. Based on these findings, the FDA and manufacturer state that dabigatran is contraindicated in patients with prosthetic mechanical heart valves. Patients with a mechanical heart valve who are currently receiving dabigatran therapy should be promptly transitioned to another anticoagulant. (See Advice to Patients.) Dabigatran should not be discontinued without guidance from a healthcare professional as sudden discontinuance may increase the risk of stroke and thromboembolism. (See Risk of Thrombosis Following Premature Discontinuance of Anticoagulation under Warnings/Precautions: Warnings, in Cautions.)

Data are lacking in patients with other forms of valvular heart disease, such as those with bioprosthetic heart valves, and dabigatran is not recommended in such patients.

Drugs Affecting P-glycoprotein Transport. Concomitant use of agents that *induce* P-glycoprotein transport (e.g., rifampin) reduces systemic exposure to dabigatran and generally should be avoided during dabigatran therapy. (See Rifampin under Drugs Affecting P-glycoprotein Transport, in Drug Interactions.)

Concomitant use of agents such as dronedarone and ketoconazole (systemic) that *inhibit* P-glycoprotein transport in patients with renal impairment may increase systemic exposure to dabigatran; therefore, dosage reduction or avoidance of such concomitant therapy is recommended in these situations. (See Dronedarone and also see Ketoconazole under Drugs Affecting P-glycoprotein Transport: Inhibitors of P-glycoprotein Transport, in Drug Interactions and also see Dosage and Administration: Special Populations.)

Sensitivity Reactions **Hypersensitivity Reactions.** Anaphylactic reactions, anaphylactic shock, allergic edema, urticaria, rash, and pruritus were reported in less than 0.1% of patients receiving dabigatran during the RE-LY study. In addition, angioedema has been reported during postmarketing experience with the drug.

Specific Populations **Pregnancy.** Category C. The American College of Chest Physicians (ACCP) recommends that dabigatran be avoided in pregnant women because of a lack of data and experience.

Safety and efficacy of dabigatran during labor and delivery have not been established; risks of bleeding and of stroke with dabigatran use in this setting should be considered.

Lactation. It is not known whether dabigatran is distributed into milk. Because of the potential for serious adverse reactions to dabigatran in nursing infants, a decision should be made whether to discontinue nursing or the drug, taking into account the importance of the drug to the woman. ACCP recommends that anticoagulants other than dabigatran be used in nursing women.

Pediatric Use. Safety and efficacy of dabigatran have not been established in pediatric patients.

Geriatric Use. In the RE-LY study, 82% of patients were 65 years of age or older, and 40% were 75 years of age or older. Risk of bleeding increases with age.

Hepatic Impairment. In patients with moderate hepatic impairment (Child-Pugh class B), large interpatient variability was apparent, but no consistent change in exposure or pharmacodynamic response was observed. Patients with active liver disease were excluded from the RE-LY study.

Renal Impairment. Dabigatran exposure and anticoagulant effects are increased in patients with renal impairment. Renal function should be assessed prior to initiation of dabigatran therapy and periodically thereafter as clinically appropriate. Dosage adjustments may be necessary depending on the patient's degree of renal impairment. (See Dosage and Administration: Special Populations.) Concomitant use of dabigatran and P-glycoprotein inhibitors is expected to further increase exposure to dabigatran in patients with renal impairment. (See Drug Interactions: Drugs Affecting P-glycoprotein Transport.) In patients who develop acute renal failure during dabigatran therapy, the drug should be discontinued and alternative anticoagulants considered.

■ **Common Adverse Effects** Adverse effects reported in more than 15% of patients receiving dabigatran during the RE-LY study include hemorrhage and gastritis-like symptoms (i.e., gastroesophageal reflux disease [GERD], esophagitis, erosive gastritis, gastric hemorrhage, hemorrhagic gastritis, hemorrhagic erosive gastritis, GI ulcer).

Drug Interactions

■ **Drugs Affecting or Metabolized by Hepatic Microsomal Enzymes** Pharmacokinetic interaction is unlikely. Dabigatran etexilate mesylate is not a substrate, inducer, or inhibitor of cytochrome P-450 (CYP) isoenzymes.

The concomitant use of a CYP3A4 isoenzyme substrate (atorvastatin) and dabigatran did not have clinically relevant effects on the pharmacokinetics of either drug. Also, the concomitant use of a CYP2C9 substrate (diclofenac) and dabigatran did not have clinically relevant effects on the pharmacokinetics of either drug.

■ **Drugs Affecting P-glycoprotein Transport** Dabigatran etexilate is a substrate for the P-glycoprotein transport system; pharmacokinetic interactions may occur with drugs that affect P-glycoprotein transport.

Inducers of P-glycoprotein Transport Concomitant use of dabigatran with P-glycoprotein inducers (e.g., rifampin) may reduce systemic exposure to dabigatran. Concomitant use generally should be avoided.

Rifampin. Administration of rifampin 600 mg daily for 7 days followed by a single dose of dabigatran resulted in decreases of 66 and 67% in dabigatran area under the plasma concentration-time curve (AUC) and peak plasma concentration, respectively. Within 7 days of rifampin discontinuance, dabigatran exposure approached levels expected without concurrent use of rifampin. Concomitant use should be avoided.

Inhibitors of P-glycoprotein Transport Concomitant use of P-glycoprotein transport inhibitors and dabigatran in patients with renal impairment is expected to increase systemic exposure to dabigatran compared with that resulting from either factor alone. Recommendations regarding such concomitant therapy are based on the degree of renal impairment and clinical situation (e.g., stroke prophylaxis in patients with nonvalvular atrial fibrillation versus treatment of venous thromboembolism). (See Dosage and Administration: Special Populations.)

Amiodarone. Administration of a single 600-mg oral dose of amiodarone with dabigatran resulted in 58 and 50% increases in dabigatran AUC and peak plasma concentration, respectively. This increase in systemic exposure was accompanied by a 65% increase in renal clearance of dabigatran. Because of the long half-life of amiodarone, increased renal clearance of dabigatran may persist after amiodarone discontinuance. Pharmacokinetics of amiodarone were not altered. Analysis of patient data from the Randomized Evaluation of Long-term Anticoagulation Therapy (RE-LY) study did not identify important changes in dabigatran trough concentrations in patients receiving dabigatran and amiodarone concurrently. Dosage adjustments are not necessary with concomitant use. However, such concomitant therapy should be avoided in patients with severe renal impairment (creatinine clearance 15–30 mL/minute) who are receiving dabigatran for stroke prophylaxis and in patients with a creatinine clearance less than 50 mL/minute who are receiving dabigatran for treatment or secondary prevention of venous thromboembolism or for thromboprophylaxis following hip-replacement surgery. (See Dosage and Administration: Special Populations.)

Clarithromycin. Concomitant use of clarithromycin and dabigatran had no effect on systemic exposure to either drug. Dosage adjustments are not necessary with concomitant use. However, such concomitant therapy should be avoided in patients with severe renal impairment (creatinine clearance 15–30 mL/minute) who are receiving dabigatran for stroke prophylaxis and in patients with a creatinine clearance less than 50 mL/minute who are receiving dabigatran for treatment or secondary prevention of venous thromboembolism or for thromboprophylaxis following hip-replacement surgery. (See Dosage and Administration: Special Populations.)

Dronedarone. Concomitant use of dronedarone and dabigatran resulted in a 70–140% increase in systemic exposure to dabigatran. Administration of dronedarone 2 hours after dabigatran was associated with a smaller increase (30–60%) in systemic exposure to dabigatran. In patients with a creatinine clearance of at least 50 mL/minute receiving dabigatran for thromboprophylaxis following hip-replacement surgery, it may be helpful to separate the timing of administration of dabigatran and dronedarone by several hours. Dosage reduction is recommended in patients with nonvalvular atrial fibrillation and moderate renal impairment (creatinine clearance 30–50 mL/minute) receiving such concomitant therapy. (See Dosage and Administration: Special Populations.) Concomitant use of dronedarone should be avoided in patients with severe renal impairment (creatinine clearance 15–30 mL/minute) receiving dabigatran for stroke prophylaxis and in patients with a creatinine clearance less than 50 mL/minute who are receiving dabigatran for treatment or secondary prevention of venous thromboembolism or for thromboprophylaxis following hip-replacement surgery.

Ketoconazole. Administration of a single oral 400-mg dose of ketoconazole or multiple oral doses of ketoconazole (400 mg daily) with dabigatran resulted in increases of 138 and 135% in dabigatran AUC and peak plasma concentration, respectively. Following multiple doses of ketoconazole (400 mg daily), the AUC and peak plasma concentrations of dabigatran were increased by 153 and 149%, respectively. In patients with a creatinine clearance of at least 50 mL/minute receiving dabigatran for thromboprophylaxis following hip-replacement surgery, it may be helpful to separate the timing of administration of dabigatran and ketoconazole by several hours. Dosage reduction is recommended in patients with nonvalvular atrial fibrillation and moderate renal impairment (creatinine clearance 30–50 mL/minute) receiving such concomitant therapy. (See Dosage and Administration: Special Populations.) Concomitant use of dronedarone should be avoided in patients with severe renal impairment (creatinine clearance 15–30 mL/minute) receiving dabigatran for stroke prophylaxis and in patients with a creatinine clearance less than 50 mL/minute who are receiving dabigatran for treatment or secondary prevention of venous thromboembolism or for thromboprophylaxis following hip-replacement surgery.

Quinidine. Concomitant use of quinidine (200 mg every 2 hours for 5 doses) on the third day of dabigatran administration resulted in increases of 53 and 56% in dabigatran AUC and peak plasma concentration, respectively. Dosage adjustments are not necessary with concomitant use. However, such concomitant therapy should be avoided in patients with severe renal impairment (creatinine clearance 15–30 mL/minute) who are receiving dabigatran for stroke prophylaxis and in patients with a creatinine clearance less than 50 mL/minute who are receiving dabigatran for treatment or secondary prevention of venous thromboembolism or for thromboprophylaxis following hip-replacement surgery. (See Dosage and Administration: Special Populations.)

Ticagrelor. Concomitant administration of ticagrelor and dabigatran modestly increases plasma concentrations of dabigatran; the magnitude of increase is dependent on the dosage and timing of dabigatran administration. When dabigatran etexilate (110 mg twice daily) was administered concurrently with ticagrelor (90 mg twice daily), the steady-state AUC and peak plasma concentration of dabigatran increased by 26% and 29%, respectively. Concurrent administration of dabigatran with a 180 mg-loading dose of ticagrelor resulted in an increase of 49 and 65% in steady-state dabigatran AUC and peak plasma concentration, respectively. However, when ticagrelor 180 mg was given 2 hours after dabigatran, the AUC and peak plasma concentration of dabigatran at steady state increased by only 27 and 24%, respectively. Dosage adjustments are not necessary with concomitant use. However, such concomitant therapy should be avoided in patients with severe renal impairment (creatinine clearance 15–30 mL/minute) who are receiving dabigatran for stroke prophylaxis and in patients with a creatinine clearance less than 50 mL/minute who are receiving dabigatran for treatment or secondary prevention of venous thromboembolism or for thromboprophylaxis following hip-replacement surgery. (See Dosage and Administration: Special Populations.)

Verapamil. Concomitant administration of verapamil and dabigatran may result in increased dabigatran AUC and peak plasma concentration. The extent of interaction depends on the verapamil formulation and timing of administration. The greatest increase in these parameters was observed when a single dose of immediate-release verapamil was given 1 hour prior to dabigatran, resulting in a 2.4-fold increase in dabigatran AUC. Administration of verapamil 2 hours after dabigatran administration resulted in negligible changes in dabigatran AUC. Analysis of data from the RE-LY study did not identify important changes in dabigatran trough concentrations in patients receiving dabigatran and verapamil concurrently. Dosage adjustments are not necessary with concomitant use. However, such concomitant therapy should be avoided in patients with severe renal impairment (creatinine clearance 15–30 mL/minute) who are receiving dabigatran for stroke prophylaxis and in patients with a creatinine clearance less than 50 mL/minute who are receiving dabigatran for treatment or secondary prevention of venous thromboembolism or for thromboprophylaxis following hip-replacement surgery. (See Dosage and Administration: Special Populations.)

■ **Drugs Affecting Gastric pH** Dabigatran is available in a capsule formulation containing drug pellets with a tartaric acid core that provides a microacidic environment for enhanced drug absorption. Because the absorption of dabigatran etexilate is dependent on an acidic gastric pH, concurrent use with drugs that increase gastric pH may decrease systemic exposure to dabigatran. Clinical studies indicate that ranitidine does not alter the pharmacokinetic parameters of dabigatran but that pantoprazole has the potential to decrease systemic exposure to dabigatran by up to 30%. However, the pharmacokinetics of pantoprazole or ranitidine were not altered by concomitant use with dabigatran. Analysis of pharmacokinetic data from the RE-LY study indicates that concurrent use with histamine H_2-receptor antagonists or proton-pump inhibitors does not appreciably alter trough dabigatran plasma concentrations.

■ **Drugs Affecting Hemostasis** The risk of bleeding may be increased when other agents that increase bleeding risk (e.g., antiplatelets, thrombolytics, heparin, chronic nonsteroidal anti-inflammatory agents) are used in patients receiving dabigatran. Patients should be monitored for manifestations of bleeding (e.g., decrease in hemoglobin/hematocrit, hypotension), and such manifestations should be promptly evaluated. (See Bleeding under Warnings/Precautions: Other Warnings and Precautions, in Cautions.)

When a single dose of dabigatran was administered 24 hours after completion of 3 days of therapy with enoxaparin sodium (40 mg subcutaneously once daily), dabigatran exposure and pharmacodynamic assessments (effects on activated thromboplastin time [aPTT], ecarin clotting time [ECT], or diluted thrombin time [dTT]) were not altered.

Concurrent administration of clopidogrel (as a 300- or 600-mg loading dose) and dabigatran resulted in increases of 30 and 40% in dabigatran AUC and peak plasma concentration, respectively. Pharmacokinetics of clopidogrel were not affected. The pharmacodynamic effects of clopidogrel (i.e., prolongation of capillary bleeding times, inhibition of platelet aggregation) or dabigatran (i.e., effects on aPTT, ECT, thrombin time) were not altered with concurrent administration when compared with monotherapy.

In the RE-LY trial, the risk of bleeding was increased approximately twofold when dabigatran was used concomitantly with either aspirin or clopidogrel compared with dabigatran monotherapy. The observed increase in risk was similar to that observed in patients randomized to warfarin and concomitantly receiving aspirin or clopidogrel when compared with warfarin alone.

Dabigatran has the potential to increase international normalized ratio (INR). When switching from dabigatran therapy to warfarin, the INR is more reflective of warfarin's effects when dabigatran has been discontinued for at least 2 days. (See Transferring to Therapy with Other Anticoagulants under Dosage and Administration: Dosage.)

■ **Digoxin** Pharmacokinetic interaction is unlikely. No meaningful alterations in pharmacokinetics of digoxin or dabigatran were observed with concurrent use.

Description

Dabigatran etexilate mesylate is a selective, competitive, reversible direct thrombin inhibitor. Dabigatran prevents thrombus formation by binding the catalytic site of free and clot-bound thrombin, thereby inhibiting conversion of fibrinogen to fibrin. Dabigatran also inhibits thrombin-mediated platelet aggregation.

Dabigatran is commercially available as dabigatran etexilate mesylate, an inactive ester prodrug that is rapidly and incompletely absorbed and subsequently hydrolyzed by esterases to dabigatran, the principal active moiety. Dabigatran exhibits linear, dose-dependent pharmacokinetics. Following oral administration of dabigatran etexilate, the absolute bioavailability of dabigatran is approximately 3–7%. Peak plasma concentrations are attained within 2 hours of oral administration and correlate with peak pharmacodynamic effects. Dabigatran undergoes conjugation to several acyl glucuronides that exhibit similar activity to dabigatran and account for approximately 20% of total plasma dabigatran concentrations. Dabigatran is approximately 35% protein bound in plasma. Systemically available dabigatran is primarily (80%) eliminated unchanged in the urine and the terminal half-life of dabigatran averages 12–17 hours. Steady state is achieved within 3 days when the drug is given 3 times daily. Dabigatran area under the concentration-time curve (AUC) and peak plasma concentrations are increased and half-life is prolonged in patients with renal impairment.

Dabigatran prolongs thrombin time (TT) and ecarin clotting time (ECT) linearly over the range of therapeutic plasma concentrations and prolongs activated partial thromboplastin time (aPTT) in a curvilinear manner. However, while dabigatran may contribute to an elevated international normalized ratio (INR), this is a relatively insensitive measure of dabigatran activity. Thrombin time may be too sensitive to be clinically useful; however, a diluted TT assay currently in clinical development may potentially allow for measurement of plasma dabigatran concentrations. While routine laboratory monitoring of anticoagulation status is not required during dabigatran therapy, the preferred and more sensitive method for assessing anticoagulation status is ETC. Alternatively, aPTT may be used as a qualitative measure of anticoagulation when ECT is unavailable. In healthy individuals, plasma dabigatran concentrations did not correlate linearly with aPTT, but were extremely low when aPTT was less than 1, while an aPTT exceeding 1 indicated the presence of dabigatran in plasma. With a dabigatran etexilate dosage of 150 mg twice daily, median peak aPTT is approximately 2 times control, and the median trough value (12 hours postdose) is approximately 1.5 times control. In the RE-LY study, the median trough aPTT and ECT in patients receiving dabigatran etexilate 150 mg twice daily was 52 and 63 seconds, respectively.

Advice to Patients

Risk of bleeding. Patients should seek emergency medical care if they experience manifestations of *serious* bleeding (e.g., unusual bruising, including bruises with unknown cause or that enlarge; pink or brown urine; red or black, tarry stool; coughing up blood; vomiting blood; vomitus with the appearance of coffee grounds).

Patients should consult healthcare provider if they experience other manifestations of bleeding (e.g., pain, swelling, or discomfort in a joint; headaches; dizziness; weakness; recurrent nose bleeds; unusual bleeding from the gums; prolonged bleeding from a cut; heavier than normal menstrual or vaginal bleeding).

Importance of advising patients who have had neuraxial anesthesia or spinal puncture to monitor for manifestations of spinal or epidural hematoma (e.g., back pain, tingling or numbness in lower limbs, muscle weakness, stool or urine incontinence), particularly if they are receiving concomitant nonsteroidal anti-inflammatory agents (NSAIAs), platelet-aggregation inhibitors, or other anticoagulants; importance of immediately contacting a clinician if any of these symptoms occur.

Risk of adverse GI reactions. Patients should consult healthcare provider if they experience dyspepsia, burning, nausea, abdominal pain/discomfort, epigastric discomfort, or indigestion.

Patients should inform healthcare provider that they are taking dabigatran before scheduling any invasive or dental procedure.

Importance of informing healthcare provider if patient has had or plans to have a heart valve replacement.

Importance of swallowing capsules whole with a full glass of water, without opening, chewing, or otherwise emptying the contents of the capsule. Do *not* sprinkle contents of capsules on food or into a beverage; also some clinicians state that capsule contents should not be placed in a nasogastric or gastric feeding tube.

Importance of taking dabigatran exactly as prescribed. Do not stop taking dabigatran without discussing with prescriber.

Instruct patients to take a missed dose as soon it is as remembered on the same day, but only if it can be taken at least 6 hours prior to the next scheduled dose.

Importance of informing patient of special storage and handling requirements for dabigatran. The drug should be stored only in the original container (bottle or blister package) and protected from moisture; capsules should not be stored in pill boxes or organizers. Remove only one capsule from the bottle at a time, right before use; close the bottle tightly immediately after use. When more than one bottle is dispensed, the patient should be advised to open only one bottle at a time. For blister packages, do not open or puncture the blister until time of use. The manufacturer currently states that dabigatran capsules should be used within 4 months after the bottle is first opened. (See Dosage and Administration: Administration.)

Importance of providing patient a copy of manufacturer's patient information.

Importance of women informing their clinician if they are or plan to become pregnant or plan to breast-feed.

Importance of informing clinicians of existing or contemplated concomitant therapy, including prescription (e.g., dronedarone, systemic ketoconazole) and OTC drugs and dietary or herbal supplements, as well as any concomitant illnesses (e.g., cardiovascular disease, kidney disease).

Importance of informing patients of other important precautionary information. (See Cautions.)

Overview® (see Users Guide). For additional information on this drug until a more detailed monograph is developed and published, the manufacturer's labeling should be consulted. It is *essential* that the manufacturer's labeling be consulted for more detailed information on usual cautions, precautions, contraindications, potential drug interactions, laboratory test interferences, and acute toxicity.

Preparations

Excipients in commercially available drug preparations may have clinically important effects in some individuals; consult specific product labeling for details.

Dabigatran Etexilate Mesylate

Oral		
Capsules	75 mg (of dabigatran etexilate)	Pradaxa®, Boehringer Ingelheim
	110 mg (of dabigatran etexilate)	Pradaxa®, Boehringer Ingelheim
	150 mg (of dabigatran etexilate)	Pradaxa®, Boehringer Ingelheim

†Use is not currently included in the labeling approved by the US Food and Drug Administration

DIRECT FACTOR XA INHIBITORS 20:12.04.14

Apixaban

■ Apixaban, an oral, reversible, direct activated factor X (factor Xa) inhibitor, is an anticoagulant.

Uses

■ Embolism Associated with Atrial Fibrillation Apixaban is used to reduce the risk of stroke and systemic embolism in patients with nonvalvular atrial fibrillation. Current evidence suggests that apixaban is more effective than aspirin or warfarin in reducing the risk of these thromboembolic events in patients with atrial fibrillation and at least one additional risk factor for stroke, with a similar risk of bleeding complications as aspirin and a lower risk than with warfarin.

Data are lacking on the use of apixaban in patients with prosthetic heart valves, and the manufacturer recommends that the drug not be used in such patients. (See Patients with Prosthetic Heart Valves under Warning/Precautions: Other Warnings/Precautions, in Cautions.)

The American College of Chest Physicians (ACCP), the American College of Cardiology (ACC), the American Heart Association (AHA), the American Stroke Association (ASA), and other experts currently recommend that antithrombotic therapy be administered to all patients with nonvalvular atrial fibrillation (i.e., atrial fibrillation in the absence of rheumatic mitral stenosis, a prosthetic heart valve, or mitral valve repair) who are considered to be at increased risk of stroke, unless such therapy is contraindicated. Recommendations regarding choice of antithrombotic therapy are based on the patient's risk for stroke and bleeding. In general, oral anticoagulant therapy (traditionally warfarin) is recommended in patients with atrial fibrillation who have a moderate to high risk for stroke and acceptably low risk of bleeding, while aspirin or no antithrombotic therapy may be considered in patients at low risk of stroke. Although many risk stratification methods have been used, patients considered to be at increased risk of stroke generally include those with prior ischemic stroke or transient ischemic attack (TIA), advanced age (e.g., 75 years or older), history of hypertension, diabetes mellitus, or congestive heart failure. In addition, population-based studies suggest that female sex is an important risk factor for stroke in patients with atrial fibrillation, particularly in patients 75 years of age or older, and AHA and ASA recommend the use of risk stratification tools that account for age- and sex-specific differences in stroke risk. One such tool is the CHA_2DS_2-VASc score, an extension of the $CHADS_2$ system (which considers the risk factors congestive heart failure, hypertension, age 75 years or older, diabetes mellitus, and prior stroke/TIA) that adds extra points for female sex (1 point); previous myocardial infarction, peripheral arterial disease, or aortic plaque (1 point); and age 65–74 years (1 point) or 75 years or older (2 points).

The risk of thromboembolism in patients with atrial flutter is not as well established as it is in those with atrial fibrillation. In addition, many patients with atrial flutter have alternating periods of atrial fibrillation. Experts state that antithrombotic therapy in patients with atrial flutter generally should be managed in the same manner as in patients with atrial fibrillation.

Warfarin traditionally has been used for oral anticoagulation in patients with atrial fibrillation at increased risk of stroke; however, experts currently state that non-vitamin K antagonist oral anticoagulants such as apixaban may provide advantages over warfarin (e.g., potentially less major bleeding risk, rapid onset of action, predictable anticoagulant effect, no requirement for coagulation monitoring, less potential for drug-drug and drug-food interactions). The non-vitamin K antagonist oral anticoagulants may be particularly useful in patients at moderate to high risk of stroke who are unable to comply with warfarin monitoring requirements or in whom a consistent therapeutic response to warfarin has not been achieved (e.g., because of drug or food interactions), while warfarin may continue to be preferred in patients who have well-controlled international normalized ratios (INRs) (e.g., INR in therapeutic range more than 70% of the time) and are compliant with regular laboratory monitoring. Warfarin generally should remain the treatment of choice in patients with severe renal impairment pending clinical outcomes data with the non-vitamin K antagonist oral anticoagulants in these patients. Because of the lack of direct comparative studies, the relative efficacy and safety of apixaban and other non-vitamin K antagonist oral anticoagulants (e.g., dabigatran, edoxaban, rivaroxaban) used for the prevention of stroke in patients with nonvalvular atrial fibrillation has not been fully elucidated.

Some evidence from indirect comparisons suggests that there may be important differences (e.g., bleeding risk) among the non-vitamin K antagonist oral anticoagulants; however, results of such analyses should be interpreted with caution because of possible confounding factors (e.g., differences in study design and methods, patient populations, and anticoagulation control). AHA and ASA state that while clinical trials of non-vitamin K antagonist oral anticoagulants were not designed to determine differences in efficacy compared with warfarin in men versus women, apixaban, dabigatran, or rivaroxaban may be a useful alternative to warfarin for the prevention of stroke and systemic thromboembolism in women with paroxysmal or permanent atrial fibrillation and prespecified risk factors (according to CHA_2DS_2-VASc) who do not have a prosthetic heart valve or hemodynamically important valve disease, severe renal failure (creatinine clearance less than 15 mL/minute), lower body weight (less than 50 kg), or advanced liver disease (impaired baseline clotting function). When selecting an appropriate anticoagulant for patients with atrial fibrillation, experts recommend that the risks versus benefits of such therapy be considered for individual patients based on the absolute and relative risks of stroke and bleeding; patient compliance, preference, tolerance, and comorbidities; cost; availability of agents to reverse anticoagulant effects in case of bleeding complications; and other clinical factors such as renal function, availability of facilities to monitor INR, and degree of current INR control in patients already receiving warfarin. For additional information on antithrombotic therapy in patients with atrial fibrillation, see Uses: Embolism Associated with Atrial Fibrillation in Warfarin 20:12.04.08.

Efficacy and safety of apixaban for the prevention of stroke and systemic embolism in patients with nonvalvular atrial fibrillation were evaluated in a multinational, randomized, double-blind study (Apixaban for Reduction in Stroke and Other Thromboembolic Events in Atrial Fibrillation [ARISTOTLE]) that was designed to demonstrate noninferiority of apixaban compared with warfarin. The study included a total of 18,201 adults with nonvalvular atrial fibrillation and at least one additional risk factor for stroke (i.e., prior stroke, TIA, or systemic embolism; age 75 years or older; arterial hypertension requiring treatment; diabetes mellitus; symptomatic heart failure as defined by New York Heart Association [NYHA] class 2 or higher; left ventricular ejection fraction of 40% or less). At baseline, patients had a mean Congestive Heart Failure, Hypertension, Age, Diabetes, Stroke (doubled) (i.e., $CHADS_2$) score of 2.1; 19% had a history of a previous embolic event (stroke, TIA, or non-CNS systemic embolism), and 57% had been previously treated with warfarin or another vitamin K antagonist prior to study entry. Patients received apixaban at a dosage of 5 mg orally twice daily (or a reduced dosage of 2.5 mg twice daily in patients with at least 2 of the following characteristics: age of 80 years or older, body weight of 60 kg or less, serum creatinine concentration of 1.5 mg/dL or higher) or warfarin in a dosage adjusted to achieve an INR of 2–3. Approximately 5% of patients in the apixaban group received the reduced dosage of the drug. The primary efficacy outcome of the study was a composite of stroke (ischemic or hemorrhagic) or systemic embolism, and the primary safety end point was major bleeding as defined by the International Society of Thrombosis and Hemostasis (ISTH) criteria; all-cause mortality was evaluated as a secondary outcome. Although the study was designed principally to test for noninferiority of apixaban compared with warfarin in reducing the rate of stroke or systemic embolism, a sequential testing strategy was employed where superiority testing was performed on the key outcome measures if noninferiority was achieved; all efficacy analyses were conducted in the intent-to-treat (per randomization) population.

Results of the study indicated that apixaban was not only noninferior, but also was superior to warfarin in reducing the risk of stroke and systemic embolism. After a median follow-up of 1.8 years, the rate of the primary outcome of stroke or systemic embolism was substantially lower in patients receiving apixaban than in those receiving warfarin (annual rate of 1.27 and 1.6%, respectively; relative risk reduction of 21%). Superiority of apixaban over warfarin was largely attributed to a reduction in the risk of hemorrhagic stroke and ischemic stroke with hemorrhagic conversion; there was no difference in the incidence of purely ischemic strokes between the treatment groups. With respect to the primary safety outcome, apixaban also demonstrated superiority over warfarin; major bleeding, including intracranial hemorrhage, occurred at a substantially lower rate in patients receiving apixaban than in those receiving warfarin (annual rate of 2.13 and 3.09%, respectively; relative risk reduction of 31%). In addition, a significant reduction in all-cause mortality was observed with apixaban versus warfarin therapy (annual rate of 3.52 and 3.94%, respectively), which was primarily due to a reduction in cardiovascular-related deaths. The beneficial effects of apixaban over warfarin on stroke risk reduction, major bleeding, and all-cause mortality were consistent across a variety of patient subgroups defined by geographic region, prior warfarin use, age, baseline body weight, $CHADS_2$ scores, renal function, apixaban dosage, type of atrial fibrillation, history of stroke or TIA, and aspirin use at randomization.

Patients who received warfarin in the ARISTOTLE study had an INR within therapeutic range 62% of the time, which is comparable to or better than that reported in other trials of non-vitamin K antagonist oral anticoagulants (e.g., dabigatran, rivaroxaban). Some clinicians have criticized this level of INR control as not being reflective of current practice and suggest that the benefits of apixaban may be less pronounced when compared with patients who achieve better warfarin control (e.g., INR in therapeutic range at least 70% of the time). However, in a subanalysis of the ARISTOTLE study, the benefits of apixaban relative to warfarin appeared to be consistent regardless of the quality of INR control (based on center-level comparison).

Apixaban was evaluated in another randomized double-blind study (Apixaban Versus Acetylsalicylic Acid to Prevent Stroke [AVERROES]) for the prevention of stroke in patients with atrial fibrillation and at least one additional risk factor for stroke (i.e., prior stroke or TIA; age 75 years or older; arterial hypertension requiring treatment; diabetes mellitus requiring treatment; symptomatic heart failure as defined by NYHA class 2 or higher; left ventricular ejection fraction of 35% or less; documented peripheral arterial disease); the study compared apixaban (5 mg twice daily or 2.5 mg twice daily in selected patients) with aspirin (81–324 mg daily) in such patients who had failed or were considered unsuitable for vitamin K antagonist therapy by their clinician. Approximately 5600 patients were included; a major reason for warfarin unsuitability in these patients was difficulty or anticipated difficulty maintaining therapeutic INRs. The AVERROES study was terminated early after a planned interim analysis demonstrated a clear benefit of apixaban over aspirin in reducing the risk of stroke without substantially increasing the risk of bleeding. After a mean follow-up of 1.1 years, the rate of the primary outcome of stroke (ischemic or hemorrhagic) or systemic embolism was substantially lower in patients receiving apixaban than in those receiving aspirin (annual rate of 1.6 and 3.7%, respectively; relative risk reduction of 55%). Although a modest increase in the risk of major bleeding was observed with apixaban versus aspirin, the difference was not statistically significant. The observed benefits of apixaban over aspirin in this study were consistent across major subgroups of patients.

■ Deep-Vein Thrombosis and Pulmonary Embolism

Prophylaxis **Major Orthopedic Surgery.** Apixaban is used for the prevention of postoperative deep-vein thrombosis (DVT), which may lead to pulmonary embolism (PE), in patients who have undergone total hip- or knee-replacement surgery. Evidence from randomized, controlled studies suggests that apixaban (2.5 mg twice daily) is more effective than once-daily subcutaneous enoxaparin sodium (40 mg once daily) in reducing the risk of venous thromboembolism in patients undergoing total hip- or knee-replacement surgery, without increasing bleeding risk. Noninferiority of apixaban (2.5 mg twice daily) and the currently recommended US dosing regimen for subcutaneous enoxaparin sodium in knee-replacement surgery (30 mg twice daily) was not established in a controlled study comparing these 2 anticoagulant regimens, although clinically relevant bleeding rates in this study were lower with apixaban. Data currently are lacking on the efficacy and safety of apixaban in patients undergoing hip-fracture surgery.

ACCP recommends routine thromboprophylaxis in all patients undergoing major orthopedic surgery, including total hip- or knee-replacement surgery, because of the high risk of postoperative venous thromboembolism. According to ACCP, thromboprophylaxis with an appropriate antithrombotic agent or an intermittent pneumatic compression device should be continued for at least 10–14 days, and potentially for up to 35 days after surgery in all patients undergoing major orthopedic surgery. Apixaban is considered by ACCP and other clinicians to be an acceptable option for pharmacologic thromboprophylaxis in patients undergoing total hip- or knee-replacement surgery. Although ACCP states a low molecular weight heparin generally is preferred for this use because of relative efficacy and safety and extensive clinical experience, apixaban may be a reasonable choice in situations in which a low molecular weight heparin is not available or cannot be used (e.g., in patients with a history of heparin-induced thrombocytopenia or in those who refuse or are uncooperative with subcutaneous injections). When selecting an appropriate thromboprophylaxis regimen for patients undergoing major orthopedic surgery, factors such as relative efficacy and bleeding risk as well as logistics and compliance issues should be considered. For additional details on prevention of venous thromboembolism in patients undergoing major orthopedic surgery, consult the most recent ACCP Evidence-based Clinical Practice Guidelines on Antithrombotic Therapy and Prevention of Thrombosis available at http://www.chestnet.org.

Apixaban was evaluated for the prevention of venous thromboembolism following total hip- or knee-replacement surgery in 3 multicenter randomized double-blind studies known as the ADVANCE (Apixaban Dose Orally versus Anticoagulation with Enoxaparin) studies. In these studies, apixaban was compared with subcutaneous enoxaparin therapy in patients undergoing elective total knee-replacement (ADVANCE 1 and 2) or total hip-replacement surgery (ADVANCE 3). The primary efficacy end point in all 3 studies consisted of a composite of asymptomatic and symptomatic DVT, nonfatal PE, and all-cause mortality; the primary safety outcome was bleeding. These studies were designed principally to test for noninferiority of apixaban compared with enoxaparin in reducing the rate of the primary efficacy end point; superiority testing was performed if noninferiority was achieved. In all 3 studies, apixaban was administered orally at the same dosage (2.5 mg twice daily, initiated 12–24 hours after surgery), but dosage and timing of enoxaparin sodium administration varied between the studies. In ADVANCE 1, enoxaparin sodium was administered at a dosage of 30 mg twice daily (initiated 12–24 hours after surgery), while in ADVANCE 2 and 3, enoxaparin sodium was administered at a dosage of 40 mg once daily (initiated 12 hours before surgery and continued after surgery according to the investigator's standard of care). Anticoagulant prophylaxis (with apixaban or enoxaparin) was continued postoperatively for 10–14 days in the knee-replacement studies and for 32–38 days in the hip-replacement study. These studies demonstrated that apixaban was more effective than enoxaparin sodium 40 mg once daily in reducing the risk of venous thromboembolism without increasing the risk of bleeding; the improved efficacy of apixaban over enoxaparin was due principally to a reduction in asymptomatic proximal DVT. When compared with enoxaparin sodium 30 mg twice daily (the approved US regimen for enoxaparin thromboprophylaxis after knee-replacement surgery) in the ADVANCE 1 study, apixaban did not meet the noninferiority criteria for the primary efficacy outcome, although apixaban was associated with lower rates of clinically relevant bleeding.

Treatment and Secondary Prevention Apixaban is used for the treatment of acute DVT and/or PE and for reduction in the risk of recurrent DVT and PE (secondary prevention) following initial anticoagulant therapy.

Efficacy and safety of apixaban for the treatment of acute DVT and/or PE has been established in a randomized, controlled study (Apixaban for the Initial Management of Pulmonary Embolism and Deep-Vein Thrombosis as First-Line Therapy [AMPLIFY]) in more than 5000 adults with symptomatic proximal DVT and/or PE. In this study, therapy with apixaban (10 mg orally twice daily for 7 days, followed by 5 mg twice daily for 6 months) was noninferior to conventional anticoagulant therapy (subcutaneous enoxaparin sodium 1 mg/kg every 12 hours for at least 5 days with overlapping warfarin therapy until INR was therapeutic (2 or greater), followed by daily warfarin therapy adjusted to maintain an INR of 2–3 and continued for 6 months) in reducing the incidence of the primary efficacy outcome (composite of symptomatic recurrent venous thromboembolism [defined as fatal or nonfatal PE and DVT] or death related to venous thromboembolism) and superior to the conventional regimen in reducing the incidence of major bleeding. The primary efficacy outcome occurred in 2.3% of patients receiving apixaban and 2.7% of those receiving the conventional regimen, and major bleeding occurred in 0.6 and 1.8% of patients in these respective groups (relative risk reduction of 69%).

Efficacy and safety of apixaban for reducing the risk of recurrent deep-vein thrombosis and pulmonary embolism (i.e., secondary prevention) has been established in another randomized, placebo-controlled study (AMPLIFY-EXT) in approximately 2500 patients who had received 6–12 months of anticoagulant therapy for venous thromboembolism. Some patients in the AMPLIFY-EXT study (approximately one-third) were participants in the AMPLIFY study who had received apixaban or enoxaparin and warfarin therapy and in whom clinicians were uncertain about the need for continuing anticoagulation. In the AMPLIFY-EXT study, extended treatment with apixaban 2.5 or 5 mg twice daily for 1 year reduced the incidence of the primary efficacy outcome (composite of symptomatic recurrent venous thromboembolism [defined as fatal and nonfatal PE and DVT] or death from any cause) without increasing the rate of major bleeding. The 2.5-mg (thromboprophylactic) and 5-mg (treatment) dosages of apixaban used in the extension study showed similar efficacy, and rates of adverse events in the 2 treatment groups were similar to those with placebo. The incidence of thromboembolism in the placebo group in the extension study was 8.8%, indicating an appreciable continuing risk of recurrent venous thromboembolism in the study population following an initial 6–12 months of anticoagulant therapy. Patients with provoked venous thromboembolism related to a transient risk factor (e.g., surgery) were not enrolled in the AMPLIFY and AMPLIFY-EXT studies unless they had another irreversible risk factor requiring 6 months of anticoagulant treatment (e.g., prior venous thromboembolism, immobilization, history of or active cancer, known prothrombotic genotype). In addition, these studies included relatively few patients with cancer, low body weight (less than 60 kg), or renal insufficiency (creatinine clearance less than 50 mL/minute); additional data on efficacy and safety of apixaban therapy in such patients with venous thromboembolism are needed. The relative efficacy and safety of apixaban versus other non-vitamin K antagonist oral anticoagulants (e.g., dabigatran, rivaroxaban) for the treatment of venous thromboembolism remains to be established in controlled, comparative trials.

The manufacturer states that apixaban is not recommended *as initial therapy* (as an alternative to heparin) in patients with PE who have hemodynamic instability or who may receive thrombolytic therapy or undergo pulmonary embolectomy.

Acute Medical Illness Current evidence suggests that extended treatment with apixaban is *not* superior to short-term treatment with subcutaneous enoxaparin for thromboprophylaxis in patients with acute medical illness† and is associated with a small but statistically significant increase in the risk of major bleeding. In a randomized, double-dummy placebo-controlled study (Apixaban Dosing to Optimize Protection from Thrombosis [ADOPT]), patients with an acute medical illness (e.g., congestive heart failure, respiratory failure) and moderately to severely restricted mobility received apixaban 2.5 mg twice daily for 30 days or subcutaneous enoxaparin sodium 40 mg once daily for 6–14 days or until hospital discharge; treatment was initiated within 72 hours of hospital admission. The primary efficacy outcome was the 30-day composite of death related to venous thromboembolism, PE, symptomatic DVT, or asymptomatic proximal-leg DVT (determined by systematic bilateral compression ultrasonography on day 30); the primary safety outcome was major bleeding. In approximately 4500 evaluable patients, the primary efficacy outcome occurred in 2.71% of those receiving apixaban and 3.06% who received enoxaparin (13% relative risk reduction with apixaban), a difference that was not statistically significant. However, the rapid increase in the rate of thromboembolic events following discontinuance of enoxaparin treatment suggests the benefits of some type of extended thromboembolism prophylaxis in this patient population; additional study and experience are needed. Apixaban therapy was associated with an increased risk of major bleeding; by day 30, major bleeding had occurred in 0.47% of the patients in the apixaban group and in 0.19% of the enoxaparin-treated patients (2.58-fold risk increase with apixaban).

■ **Acute Coronary Syndrome** Current evidence suggests that addition of apixaban to standard antiplatelet therapy (e.g., aspirin, clopidogrel) does *not* substantially reduce the rate of recurrent ischemic events in patients with acute coronary syndrome† (ACS) and may increase the risk of major, sometimes fatal, bleeding. In a randomized, phase 2, dose-ranging study (Apixaban for Prevention of Acute Ischemic and Safety Events [APPRAISE]), approximately 1700 patients with recent ST-segment elevation or non-ST-segment elevation ACS received apixaban (2.5 mg twice daily, 10 mg once daily, 10 mg twice daily, or 20 mg once daily) or placebo. Nearly all patients also received aspirin (up to 165 mg daily), and 76% of patients also received clopidogrel according to clinician discretion. The primary outcome of the study was major bleeding or clinically relevant nonmajor bleeding. The 2 higher-dose arms of apixaban therapy were discontinued early because of excess total bleeding events. Compared with placebo, apixaban (2.5 mg twice daily or 10 mg once daily for approximately 6 months) increased bleeding in a dose-dependent fashion. There was a trend toward fewer ischemic events (cardiovascular death, myocardial infarction, severe recurrent ischemia, ischemic stroke) in patients given apixaban; overall ischemic event rates and bleeding events in the apixaban group were greater in patients receiving dual antiplatelet therapy (adjunctive aspirin plus clopidogrel) compared with those receiving only adjunctive aspirin. In a follow-up randomized, phase 3 trial (APPRAISE-2), high-risk patients with ACS received apixaban (5 mg twice daily or a reduced dosage of 2.5 mg twice daily in those with a creatinine clearance less than 40 mL/minute) or placebo as adjuncts to antiplatelet therapy with aspirin with or without a P2Y12-receptor antagonist (e.g., clopidogrel, prasugrel, ticagrelor) for prevention of recurrent ischemic events. The trial was stopped early because of excess bleeding, including intracranial and fatal bleeding events, when apixaban was given in conjunction with dual antiplatelet therapy, without evidence of efficacy.

Dosage and Administration

■ **General** Routine coagulation monitoring (e.g., prothrombin time [PT], activated partial thromboplastin time [aPTT], international normalized ratio [INR]) is not necessary with apixaban therapy because of the drug's predictable pharmacokinetic and pharmacodynamic effects. However, in certain situations, such as in the case of overdosage or in patients with hemorrhagic or thromboembolic complications or those requiring emergency surgery, it may be useful to assess the degree of anticoagulation. Although apixaban produces concentration-dependent increases in aPTT, PT, INR, and the Heptest (used to measure inhibition of exogenous activated factor X [factor Xa]), these tests generally are not useful for monitoring the anticoagulant effects of apixaban because of a high degree of inconsistency and variability in results. A chromogenic anti-factor Xa assay (Rotachrom® Heparin chromogenic assay) was used during the apixaban development program to measure the effect of apixaban on factor Xa activity. Although the chromogenic assay appears to correlate well with apixaban activity and may produce less variable results than other coagulation tests, a standardized assay specifically calibrated for apixaban currently is not available in most healthcare facilities. The manufacturer does not recommend use of this chromogenic assay for assessing the anticoagulant effects of apixaban.

Apixaban is administered orally twice daily without regard to food. In patients who are unable to swallow whole tablets, apixaban 2.5- or 5-mg tablets may be crushed and suspended in water, 5% dextrose in water, or apple juice, or mixed with applesauce and promptly administered orally. Alternatively, apixaban tablets may be crushed and suspended in 60 mL of water or 5% dextrose in water and promptly delivered through a nasogastric feeding tube. Crushed apixaban tablets are stable in water, dextrose 5% in water, apple juice, or applesauce for up to 4 hours.

If a dose is missed, the missed dose should be taken as soon as possible on the same day, followed by resumption of the regular twice-daily dosing schedule; the dose should not be doubled to make up for the missed dose. (See Advice to Patients.)

■ **Dosage** ***Embolism Associated with Atrial Fibrillation*** The recommended dosage of apixaban to reduce the risk of stroke and systemic embolism in adults with nonvalvular atrial fibrillation is 5 mg twice daily.

Dosage should be reduced to 2.5 mg twice daily in patients with at least 2 of the following characteristics that can increase drug exposure and thus, increase the risk of bleeding: age 80 years or older, body weight of 60 kg or less, or serum creatinine concentration of 1.5 mg/dL or greater. (See Dosage and Administration: Special Populations.)

Deep-Vein Thrombosis and Pulmonary Embolism **Thromboprophylaxis in Hip- or Knee-Replacement Surgery.** For the prevention of deep-vein thrombosis (DVT) and associated pulmonary embolism (PE) in patients who have undergone hip- or knee-replacement surgery, the recommended dosage of apixaban is 2.5 mg twice daily. The initial dose should be administered at least 12–24 hours after surgery, provided hemostasis has been established. The recommended duration of apixaban therapy is 35 days for patients undergoing hip-replacement surgery and 12 days for patients undergoing knee-replacement surgery. In clinical studies, the initial dose of apixaban was administered 12–24 hours after wound closure, and treatment was continued postoperatively for 10–14 days after knee-replacement surgery and for 32–38 days after hip-replacement surgery.

Treatment and Secondary Prevention. For the treatment of acute DVT and/or PE, the recommended dosage of apixaban is 10 mg twice daily for 7 days, followed by 5 mg twice daily; in the principal efficacy trial, apixaban therapy was administered for 6 months. For reduction in the risk of recurrent DVT and PE (secondary prevention) in patients who have received at least 6 months of initial anticoagulant therapy, the recommended dosage of apixaban is 2.5 mg twice daily.

Transitioning to or from Other Anticoagulant Therapy When transitioning from warfarin to apixaban therapy, the manufacturer states that warfarin should be discontinued and apixaban initiated as soon as the INR is less than 2.

When transitioning from apixaban to warfarin therapy, INR measurements may not be useful for determining an appropriate dose of warfarin because apixaban also can prolong the INR. The manufacturer suggests that apixaban be discontinued and a parenteral anticoagulant and warfarin initiated simultaneously at the time of the next scheduled dose of apixaban; the parenteral anticoagulant can then be discontinued once an acceptable INR is achieved with warfarin. Some clinicians have suggested other strategies for transitioning from non-vitamin K antagonist oral anticoagulants (e.g., apixaban, rivaroxaban) to warfarin based on the patient's creatinine clearance and the warfarin start date.

When transitioning to or from therapy with anticoagulants other than warfarin, the manufacturer recommends discontinuing the current anticoagulant and initiating the other anticoagulant at the time of the next scheduled dose of the current anticoagulant.

Managing Anticoagulation in Patients Requiring Invasive Procedures Apixaban therapy should be temporarily interrupted prior to elective surgery or other invasive procedure to decrease the risk of bleeding; the recommended time interval for discontinuance is based on the anticipated risk of bleeding associated with the procedure and the elimination half-life of the drug. For procedures associated with a moderate to high risk of unacceptable or clinically important bleeding, the manufacturer recommends that apixaban be discontinued at least 48 hours prior to the procedure; some experts suggest a longer time interval for discontinuance (e.g., 5 days prior to a scheduled procedure) to ensure that apixaban has been completely eliminated. For procedures associated with a low risk of bleeding or bleeding in a noncritical location that can be easily controlled, the manufacturer recommends that apixaban be discontinued at least 24 hours prior to the procedure. Bridging anticoagulation generally is not required prior to the procedure or during the 24–48 hours after stopping apixaban. Apixaban therapy should be resumed postoperatively as soon as adequate hemostasis has been established; although experience is limited, some experts suggest that timing of reinitiation be based on procedural bleeding risk and hemostasis.

Coadministration with Dual Inhibitors of Cytochrome P-450 Isoenzyme 3A4 and P-glycoprotein In patients receiving apixaban dosages exceeding 2.5 mg twice daily (e.g., 5 mg twice daily) who are on concomitant therapy with drugs that are potent inhibitors of both cytochrome P-450 (CYP) isoenzyme 3A4 and P-glycoprotein (P-gp) (e.g., ketoconazole, itraconazole, ritonavir), the dosage of apixaban should be reduced by 50% (e.g., from 5 mg twice daily to 2.5 mg twice daily). Patients who are already receiving an apixaban dosage of 2.5 mg twice daily should avoid concomitant use with such potent dual inhibitors of CYP3A4 and P-gp. (See Drug Interactions: Drugs Affecting P-glycoprotein Transport and CYP3A4.)

■ **Special Populations** ***Hepatic Impairment*** No dosage adjustment is necessary in patients with mild hepatic impairment (Child-Pugh class A). Because of limited experience, the manufacturer states that dosage recommendations cannot be provided in patients with moderate hepatic impairment (Child-Pugh class B). Data are lacking on the use of apixaban in patients with severe hepatic impairment (Child-Pugh class C), and the manufacturer states that use of apixaban is not recommended in this population. (See Hepatic Impairment under Warnings/Precautions: Specific Populations, in Cautions.)

Renal Impairment The manufacturer states that dosage adjustment of apixaban based solely on renal impairment (including patients with end-stage renal disease [ESRD] who are maintained on intermittent hemodialysis) is not necessary; however, in patients with nonvalvular atrial fibrillation, a reduced dosage of 2.5 mg twice daily is recommended in those with an elevated serum creatinine concentration of 1.5 mg/dL or greater if they also are 80 years of age or older and/or weigh 60 kg or less. (See Renal Impairment under Warnings/Precautions: Specific Populations, in Cautions.) The manufacturer states that these dosage recommendations are based on pharmacokinetic and pharmacodynamic (anti-factor Xa activity) data in ESRD patients maintained on hemodialysis; such patients were not studied in clinical efficacy and safety trials of apixaban.

In patients with renal impairment (including ESRD patients maintained on hemodialysis) who are receiving apixaban for the prevention of DVT and associated PE following hip- or knee-replacement surgery or for the treatment or secondary prevention of DVT or PE, the manufacturer states that no dosage adjustments are necessary. The manufacturer states this recommendation is based on pharmacokinetic and pharmacodynamic (anti-factor Xa activity) data in ESRD patients maintained on hemodialysis; such patients were not studied in clinical efficacy and safety trials of apixaban.

Geriatric Patients The manufacturer states that dosage adjustment based solely on age is not necessary in geriatric patients 65 years of age or older; however, a reduced dosage of 2.5 mg twice daily is recommended in patients 80 years of age or older with nonvalvular atrial fibrillation if they also weigh 60 kg or less and/or have a serum creatinine concentration of 1.5 mg/dL or greater.

Body Weight The manufacturer states that dosage adjustment based solely on body weight is not necessary; however, a reduced dosage of 2.5 mg twice daily is recommended in patients with nonvalvular atrial fibrillation who weigh 60 kg or less if they also are 80 years of age or older and/or have a serum creatinine concentration of 1.5 mg/dL or greater.

Although extremes of body weight (less than 50 kg or more than 120 kg) may alter peak plasma concentrations of and systemic exposure to apixaban, the manufacturer states that no dosage adjustment is necessary based on extremes of body weight. In the principal efficacy study, patients with high body weight (exceeding 120 kg) had decreased drug exposure (approximately 25% lower), but this did not result in loss of efficacy.

Race/Ethnicity The manufacturer states that no dosage adjustment is necessary based on race or ethnicity.

Cautions

■ **Contraindications** Active pathologic bleeding.

Severe hypersensitivity reaction (e.g., anaphylactic reactions) to apixaban.

■ **Warnings/Precautions** ***Warnings*** **Risk of Thrombosis Following Premature Discontinuance of Anticoagulation.** Premature discontinuance of any oral anticoagulant, including apixaban, in the absence of adequate alternative anticoagulation increases the risk of thrombotic events (e.g., stroke). An increased incidence of stroke was observed during the transition from apixaban to warfarin in clinical trials in patients with atrial fibrillation. If discontinuance of apixaban is required for reasons other than pathologic bleeding or completion of a course of therapy, anticoagulant coverage with an alternative anticoagulant should be considered. When transitioning patients from one anticoagulant therapy to another, it is important to ensure continuous anticoagulation while minimizing the risk of bleeding. Particular caution is advised when switching patients from a factor Xa inhibitor to warfarin therapy because of the slow onset of action of warfarin. (See Transitioning to or from Other Anticoagulant Therapy under Dosage and Administration: Dosage.) Patients should be advised about the importance of adhering to the therapeutic regimen and instructed on steps to take if doses are missed. (See Advice to Patients.)

Spinal/Epidural Hematoma. Patients receiving anticoagulants are at risk of developing an epidural or spinal hematoma when concomitant neuraxial (epidural/spinal) anesthesia or spinal puncture is employed; such complications can result in long-term or permanent paralysis. The risk of these complications is increased by postoperative use of indwelling epidural catheters for administration of analgesia or by concomitant use of drugs affecting hemostasis, such as nonsteroidal anti-inflammatory agents (NSAIAs), platelet-aggregation inhibitors, or other anticoagulants. Risk also may be increased in patients with a history of traumatic or repeated epidural or spinal punctures, spinal deformity, or spinal surgery.

Removal of an indwelling epidural or intrathecal catheter should be delayed for at least 24 hours after a dose of apixaban, and at least 5 hours should elapse following removal of the catheter prior to administration of the next apixaban dose. If traumatic puncture occurs, the administration of apixaban should be delayed for 48 hours.

Patients receiving apixaban in the setting of epidural or spinal anesthesia should be monitored frequently for manifestations of neurologic impairment (e.g., numbness or weakness of the legs, bowel or bladder dysfunction). If neurologic compromise is noted, urgent diagnosis and treatment are necessary. Clinicians should consider the potential benefits versus risks of neuraxial intervention in patients who are currently receiving or will receive anticoagulant prophylaxis.

Sensitivity Reactions **Hypersensitivity.** Hypersensitivity reactions, including skin rash, allergic edema, and anaphylactic reactions, have been reported in less than 1% of patients receiving apixaban. (See Cautions: Contraindications.)

Other Warnings and Precautions **Bleeding.** Apixaban increases the risk of hemorrhage and can cause serious, potentially fatal, bleeding. The drug should be discontinued if active pathological hemorrhage occurs. (See Cautions: Contraindications and also see Advice to Patients.) However, minor or "nuisance" bleeding is a common occurrence in patients receiving any anticoagulant and should not readily lead to treatment discontinuance. (See Risk of Thrombosis Following Premature Discontinuance of Anticoagulation under Warnings/Precautions: Warnings, in Cautions.)

In the principal efficacy study of apixaban in patients with nonvalvular atrial fibrillation (ARISTOTLE), major bleeding occurred at an annual rate of 2.13% (327 out of 9088 patients) in patients who received the drug, although the rate was substantially lower with apixaban than with warfarin therapy (rate of 2.13% per year versus 3.09% per year). In this study, bleeding was assessed according to the International Society on Thrombosis and Hemostasis (ISTH) criteria, which defines major bleeding as clinically overt bleeding that is accompanied by one or more of the following events: decrease in hemoglobin of at least 2 g/dL, transfusion of at least 2 units of packed red blood cells, bleeding at a critical site (i.e., intracranial, intraspinal, intraocular, pericardial, intraarticular, intramuscular with compartment syndrome, or retroperitoneal) or resulting in death. Concomitant use of aspirin increased the risk of bleeding in patients receiving apixaban from 1.8 to 3.4% per year, and concomitant use of aspirin and warfarin increased the bleeding risk from 2.7 to 4.6% per year.

Risk of bleeding may be increased in patients with renal impairment and in those receiving concomitant therapy with drugs that affect hemostasis (e.g., aspirin or other antiplatelet drugs, fibrinolytics, heparin or other anticoagulants, selective serotonin reuptake inhibitors, serotonin norepinephrine reuptake inhibitors, chronic use of NSAIAs) or drugs that are inhibitors of both P-glycoprotein (P-gp) and cytochrome P-450 (CYP) isoenzyme 3A4. (See Drug Interactions.)

Apixaban therapy should be temporarily interrupted prior to any elective surgery or other invasive procedure to reduce the risk of bleeding. (See Managing Anticoagulation in Patients Requiring Invasive Procedures under Dosage and Administration: Dosage.)

Factor Xa (recombinant), inactivated-zhzo (also known as andexanet alfa), a recombinant modified human factor Xa protein, is a specific reversal agent for the anticoagulant effects of apixaban. Data from clinical trials indicate that factor Xa (recombinant), inactivated-zhzo is effective in rapidly reversing the anticoagulant effects of apixaban (as measured by anti-factor Xa activity, unbound anticoagulant concentration, and thrombin generation). The safety of factor Xa (recombinant), inactivated-zhzo has not been established in patients who have experienced a thromboembolic event or disseminated intravascular coagulation (DIC) within 2 weeks prior to the life-threatening bleeding event requiring treatment with the drug or in those who have received prothrombin complex concentrate (PCC), recombinant factor VIIa, or whole blood products within 7 days prior to the bleeding event. For further information on factor Xa (recombinant), inactivated-zhzo, see the monograph on Factor Xa (Recombinant), Inactivated-zhzo 20:28:92. If a serious bleeding event occurs during therapy, apixaban should be discontinued and appropriate supportive measures provided.

Limited data suggest that procoagulant reversal agents such as PCCs, activated PCC (also known as anti-inhibitor coagulant complex), or factor VIIa (recombinant) may be considered for immediate reversal of anticoagulation; however, efficacy and safety of these agents have not been established in clinical studies of patients receiving apixaban. In a clinical study in healthy individuals receiving apixaban dosed to steady state, endogenous thrombin potential (ETP) returned to pre-apixaban concentrations 4 hours after the initiation of a 30-minute PCC IV infusion, compared to 45 hours with placebo. When PCCs are used, monitoring for the anticoagulation effect of apixaban using a clotting test (prothrombin time [PT], international normalized ratio [INR], activated partial thromboplastin time [aPTT]) or anti-factor Xa activity is not useful and is not recommended. Because this study was conducted in healthy individuals, caution should be used in extrapolating these findings to clinical practice. Protamine sulfate and vitamin K are not expected to affect the anticoagulant activity of apixaban. There is no experience with antifibrinolytic agents (tranexamic acid, aminocaproic acid) or systemic hemostatics (desmopressin, aprotinin [no longer commercially available in the US]) in patients receiving apixaban, and such drugs are not expected to be effective as reversal agents. Because of high plasma protein binding, apixaban is not expected to be dialyzable. In the event of an overdosage, activated charcoal may be used to decrease plasma concentrations of apixaban more rapidly.

Patients with Prosthetic Heart Valves. Safety and efficacy of apixaban have not been established in patients with prosthetic heart valves, and use of apixaban is not recommended in such patients.

Specific Populations **Pregnancy.** Data are lacking on the use of apixaban in pregnant women. Animal studies have not demonstrated any evidence of fetotoxic effects; however, increased maternal bleeding was observed when apixaban was administered to pregnant animals at doses ranging from 1–19 times the human exposure at the maximum recommended dose. Apixaban use during labor or delivery in women who are receiving neuraxial anaesthesia may result in epidural or spinal hematomas. (See Spinal/Epidural Hematoma under Warnings/Precautions: Warnings, in Cautions.) Use of a shorter-acting anticoagulant should be considered as delivery approaches.

Lactation. Apixaban is distributed into milk in rats; it is not known whether the drug is distributed into human milk. The effects of apixaban on the breast-fed infant or on milk production are unknown. The manufacturer states that breast-feeding is not recommended during treatment with apixaban.

Pediatric Use. Safety and efficacy have not been established in pediatric patients younger than 18 years of age

Geriatric Use. No substantial differences in efficacy and safety were observed in geriatric patients 65 years of age or older relative to younger adults in clinical trials. In clinical trials of apixaban in patients with nonvalvular atrial fibrillation or deep-vein thrombosis/pulmonary embolism, no clinically important differences in efficacy or safety were observed among different age groups. Pharmacokinetic effects (systemic exposure and peak plasma concentrations) of apixaban were similar in patients 65 years of age or older and younger adults (18–40 years of age) receiving the drug.

Hepatic Impairment. Pharmacokinetic (systemic exposure and peak plasma concentrations) and pharmacodynamic (inhibition of factor Xa activity) effects of apixaban do not appear to be substantially altered in patients with mild or moderate hepatic impairment. (See Dosage and Administration: Special Populations.) Patients with moderate hepatic impairment may have intrinsic coagulation abnormalities that can affect response to apixaban therapy; however, the impact of this effect is not clear.

Data are lacking in patients with severe hepatic impairment, and the manufacturer recommends that apixaban not be used in such patients.

Renal Impairment. Pharmacokinetic (systemic exposure and peak plasma concentrations) and pharmacodynamic (inhibition of factor Xa activity) effects of apixaban do not appear to be substantially altered in patients with renal impairment (mild, moderate, or severe) compared with those with normal renal function. Although results of a pharmacokinetic study showed an approximate 44% increase in systemic exposure to apixaban in patients with severe renal impairment (i.e., creatinine clearance of 15 mL/minute) compared with those with normal renal function, this degree of change was considered to be modest. In the principal clinical study of the drug, patients with moderate to severe renal impairment had higher rates of bleeding regardless of treatment (apixaban or warfarin). Dosage adjustment based on renal function alone does not appear to be necessary, but is recommended in patients with nonvalvular atrial fibrillation and renal impairment who meet additional criteria for dosage modification. (See Dosage and Administration: Special Populations.)

Race/Ethnicity. Pharmacokinetics of apixaban do not appear to be substantially altered by race or ethnicity. In several studies in which healthy individuals of different ethnic or racial origins (Caucasian, Asian, and African-American) received apixaban, pharmacokinetic parameters (e.g., peak plasma concentrations, half-life, time to steady state) of the drug were similar regardless of race or ethnicity.

■ **Common Adverse Effects** Bleeding was the most common adverse effect reported in clinical trials of apixaban.

Drug Interactions

■ **Drugs Affecting or Metabolized by Hepatic Microsomal Enzymes** Apixaban is metabolized principally by cytochrome P-450 (CYP) isoenzyme 3A4/5, and to a lesser extent by CYP isoenzymes 1A2, 2C8, 2C9, 2C19, and 2J2. Although pharmacokinetic interactions are possible with drugs that inhibit or induce CYP3A4/5, in vitro studies indicate that the potential may be low because of apixaban's multiple routes of elimination. (See Drug Interactions: Drugs Affecting P-glycoprotein Transport and CYP3A4.)

In vitro studies indicate that apixaban does not inhibit CYP isoenzymes 1A2, 2A6, 2B6, 2C8, 2C9, 2D6, 3A4/5, or 2C19 nor induce CYP isoenzymes 1A2, 2B6, or 3A4/5; therefore, pharmacokinetic interactions are not expected with drugs that are metabolized by these isoenzymes.

■ **Drugs Affecting P-glycoprotein Transport** Apixaban is a substrate of the efflux transporter P-glycoprotein (P-gp); inhibitors or inducers of this transport protein may potentially alter apixaban exposure. (See Drug Interactions: Drugs Affecting P-glycoprotein Transport and CYP3A4.) Apixaban does not substantially inhibit P-gp.

■ **Drugs Affecting P-glycoprotein Transport and CYP3A4** Since apixaban is a substrate of both P-gp and CYP3A4, concomitant use of drugs that inhibit P-gp and CYP3A4 can increase exposure (peak plasma concentrations and area under the plasma concentration-time curve [AUC]) to apixaban and increase the risk of bleeding. In patients receiving apixaban dosages exceeding 2.5 mg twice daily (e.g., 5 mg twice daily), the dosage of apixaban should be reduced by 50% (e.g., from 5 mg twice daily to 2.5 mg twice daily) if concomitant therapy with potent dual inhibitors of P-gp and CYP3A4 (e.g., itraconazole, ketoconazole, ritonavir) is administered. In patients already receiving apixaban 2.5 mg twice daily, concomitant administration of potent dual inhibitors of P-gp and CYP3A4 should be avoided. While clarithromycin is an inhibitor of P-gp and a strong CYP3A4 inhibitor, pharmacokinetic data suggest that no dosage adjustment is necessary with concomitant use of apixaban and clarithromycin. Concomitant administration of other, less potent inhibitors of CYP3A4 and P-gp (e.g., diltiazem, naproxen) also may increase exposure to apixaban..

Conversely, drugs that induce P-gp and CYP3A4 can reduce plasma concentrations of apixaban and increase the risk of stroke. Concomitant use of apixaban and potent dual inducers of P-gp and CYP3A4 (e.g., carbamazepine, phenytoin, rifampin, St. John's wort [*Hypericum perforatum*]) should be avoided.

Diltiazem Concomitant administration of apixaban and diltiazem (a moderate CYP3A4 and weak P-gp inhibitor) increased AUC and peak plasma concentrations of apixaban by 1.4- and 1.3-fold, respectively.

Ketoconazole Concomitant administration of apixaban and ketoconazole (a strong inhibitor of both P-gp and CYP3A4) substantially increased the AUC and peak plasma concentration of apixaban by 2- and 1.6-fold, respectively. Dosage of apixaban should be reduced to 2.5 mg twice daily with such concomitant therapy. (See Dosage and Administration: Dosage.) Concomitant use of apixaban and ketoconazole should be avoided in patients who have 2 or more of the following characteristics: age 80 years or older, body weight 60 kg or less, serum creatinine concentration of 1.5 mg/dL or greater.

Naproxen Concomitant administration of apixaban and naproxen (a P-gp inhibitor) increased AUC and peak plasma concentrations of apixaban by 1.5- and 1.6-fold, respectively.

Apixaban did not substantially alter the pharmacokinetics of naproxen; however, a 50–60% increase in anti-factor Xa activity was observed with such concomitant therapy.

Rifampin Concomitant administration of apixaban and rifampin (a strong inducer of both P-gp and CYP3A4) decreased AUC and peak plasma concentrations of apixaban by 54 and 42%, respectively; concomitant use of these drugs should be avoided.

■ **Drugs Affecting Hemostasis** Concomitant use of apixaban and drugs that affect hemostasis (e.g., aspirin or other antiplatelet drugs, heparin or other anticoagulants, fibrinolytics, selective serotonin-reuptake inhibitors [SSRIs], selective serotonin- and norepinephrine-reuptake inhibitors [SNRIs], nonsteroidal anti-inflammatory agents [NSAIAs]) increases the risk of bleeding.

■ **Amiodarone** Efficacy and safety end points for apixaban compared with warfarin did not appear to be altered by concomitant administration of amiodarone in the principal efficacy study of apixaban in patients with nonvalvular atrial fibrillation.

■ **Aspirin** In the principal efficacy study of apixaban, bleeding risk was increased in patients who received concomitant apixaban and aspirin therapy. Additionally, a placebo-controlled study of patients with acute coronary syndromes was terminated early after an increased risk of bleeding was observed in patients receiving apixaban in combination with aspirin and clopidogrel.

In drug interaction studies in healthy individuals, apixaban did not substantially alter the pharmacokinetics of aspirin, and a pharmacodynamic interaction was not observed with such concomitant therapy.

■ **Atenolol** Concomitant administration of apixaban and atenolol in healthy individuals did not appreciably alter the pharmacokinetics of either drug.

■ **Clopidogrel** No pharmacodynamic interactions (e.g., anti-factor Xa activity) were observed with concomitant apixaban and clopidogrel therapy. However, a placebo-controlled study (APPRAISE-2) of patients with acute coronary syndromes was terminated early after an increased risk of bleeding was observed in patients receiving apixaban in combination with aspirin and clopidogrel.

■ **Digoxin** In drug interaction studies conducted in healthy individuals, apixaban did not substantially alter the pharmacokinetics of digoxin.

■ **Enoxaparin** In a study in healthy individuals, concomitant administration of apixaban and enoxaparin had no effect on the pharmacokinetics of apixaban, but had an additive effect on anti-factor Xa activity. The increased pharmacodynamic effect was considered to be modest. When administration of apixaban and enoxaparin was separated by 6 hours in this study, the additive effect on anti-factor Xa activity was attenuated.

■ **Famotidine** Famotidine did not substantially alter the pharmacokinetics of apixaban in healthy individuals.

■ **Prasugrel** Concomitant administration of apixaban and prasugrel in healthy individuals did not appreciably alter the pharmacokinetics of either drug.

Description

Apixaban is an oral, reversible, direct activated factor X (factor Xa) inhibitor. Factor Xa plays a central role in the blood coagulation cascade by serving as the convergence point for the intrinsic and extrinsic pathways; inhibition of coagulation factor Xa prevents conversion of prothrombin to thrombin, resulting in decreased thrombin generation and thrombus development. Unlike fondaparinux, heparin, and the low molecular weight heparins, apixaban binds directly to the active site of factor Xa with high affinity and selectivity, and does not require a cofactor (antithrombin III) for its antithrombotic activity. Apixaban inhibits free and clot-bound factor Xa and prothrombinase activity.

Apixaban exhibits linear, dose-proportional pharmacokinetics for oral doses up to 10 mg. The absolute bioavailability of the drug is approximately 50%, and peak plasma concentrations are reached approximately 3–4 hours after oral administration. Following oral administration of 10 mg of apixaban as 2 crushed 5-mg tablets suspended in 30 mL of water, bioavailability was similar to that after 2 intact 5-mg tablets taken orally. Following oral administration of 10 mg of apixaban as 2 crushed 5-mg tablets mixed with 30 g of applesauce, the peak plasma concentration and bioavailability of apixaban were decreased by 20 and 16%, respectively. Following administration via a nasogastric feeding tube of a single crushed 5-mg tablet suspended in 60 mL of 5% dextrose in water, bioavailability of the drug is similar to that of a whole tablet taken orally.

Apixaban has a total clearance of approximately 3.3 L/hour. Despite a short clearance half-life of about 6 hours, the apparent half-life of apixaban is longer (about 12 hours) following repeated administration because of prolonged absorption. Absorption of apixaban occurs throughout the GI tract, with about 55% of the drug absorbed in the distal small intestine and ascending colon. Food does not appear to affect the pharmacokinetics (systemic exposure and peak plasma concentrations) or pharmacodynamics of apixaban.

Apixaban is eliminated via multiple pathways, including hepatic metabolism by the cytochrome P-450 (CYP) enzyme system and through intestinal, biliary, and renal excretion; approximately 25% of an administered dose is eliminated renally. No active circulating metabolites have been identified. Approximately 87% of the drug is bound to plasma proteins. QT-interval prolongation has not been observed with apixaban doses up to 50 mg. Apixaban inhibits factor Xa activity, and prolongs prothrombin time (PT), activated partial thromboplastin time (aPTT), and the international normalized ratio (INR) in a concentration-dependent manner.

Advice to Patients

Importance of patients taking the drug exactly as prescribed and not discontinuing therapy without first consulting a clinician. Importance of advising patients how to take the drug if they cannot swallow whole tablets or if they require a nasogastric tube.

Importance of advising patients that if a dose is missed, to take it as soon as possible on the same day and then resume the regular twice-daily dosing schedule; the missed dose should not be doubled.

Importance of informing patients that they may bruise and/or bleed more easily and that a longer than normal time may be required to stop bleeding when taking apixaban; clinicians should advise patients on how to recognize signs and symptoms of bleeding. Importance of patients informing clinicians immediately about any unusual bleeding or bruising during therapy.

Importance of advising patients who have had neuraxial anesthesia or spinal puncture to monitor for manifestations of spinal or epidural hematoma (e.g., numbness or weakness of legs, bowel or bladder dysfunction), particularly if they are receiving concomitant nonsteroidal anti-inflammatory agents (NSAIAs), platelet-aggregation inhibitors, or other anticoagulants; importance of patient immediately seeking emergency medical attention if any of these symptoms occur.

Importance of patients informing clinicians (e.g., physicians, dentists) that they are receiving apixaban therapy before scheduling any surgery or invasive procedures, including dental procedures.

Importance of women informing clinicians if they are or plan to become pregnant or plan to breast-feed.

Importance of informing clinicians (e.g., physicians, dentists) of existing or contemplated concomitant therapy, including prescription and OTC drugs and herbal supplements.

Importance of informing patients of other important precautionary information. (See Cautions.)

Overview® (see Users Guide). For additional information on this drug until a more detailed monograph is developed and published, the manufacturer's labeling should be consulted. It is *essential* that the manufacturer's labeling be consulted for more detailed information on usual cautions, precautions, contraindications, potential drug interactions, laboratory test interferences, and acute toxicity.

Preparations

Excipients in commercially available drug preparations may have clinically important effects in some individuals; consult specific product labeling for details.

Apixaban

Oral		
Tablets	2.5 mg	**Eliquis®**, Bristol-Myers Squibb
	5 mg	**Eliquis®**, Bristol-Myers Squibb

†Use is not currently included in the labeling approved by the US Food and Drug Administration

Betrixaban Maleate

■ Betrixaban maleate, an oral, direct activated factor X (Xa) inhibitor, is an anticoagulant.

Uses

■ **Deep-Vein Thrombosis and Pulmonary Embolism *Prophylaxis*** **Acute Medical Illness.** Betrixaban is used for the prevention of venous thromboembolism in patients hospitalized for an acute medical illness who are at risk for thromboembolic complications due to moderately or severely restricted mobility and other risk factors for venous thromboembolism.

Treatment decisions regarding the use of prophylactic anticoagulants in acutely ill hospitalized patients should include an assessment of the patient's individual risk of venous thromboembolism and risk of bleeding. In general, pharmacologic thromboprophylaxis is recommended only in patients who are considered to be at high risk of venous thromboembolism because the risk-to-benefit trade-off between the reduction in venous thromboembolic events and bleeding is considered to be more favorable in such patients. Factors that should be considered when choosing an appropriate anticoagulant include patient preference, compliance, ease of administration, and costs associated with the individual agents. The American College of Chest Physicians (ACCP) recommends the use of anticoagulant thromboprophylaxis in acutely ill, hospitalized medical patients at increased risk of thrombosis who are not actively bleeding and do not have an increased risk of bleeding. Continued thromboprophylaxis is suggested for 6–21 days until full mobility is restored or hospital discharge, whichever comes first; extended prophylaxis beyond these periods generally is not recommended because of data suggesting an unfavorable benefit-to-risk ratio with regard to bleeding complications with extended prophylaxis. However, currently available evidence suggests that extended-duration (35–42 days) betrixaban may be more effective than standard-duration (6–14 days) enoxaparin in reducing the risk of venous thromboembolism in hospitalized patients with acute medical illness and reduced mobility, at the cost of an increase in nonmajor but not major bleeding. For additional information on thromboprophylaxis in patients with acute medical illness, see Medical Conditions Associated with Thromboembolism under Deep-Vein Thrombosis and/or Pulmonary Embolism: Prophylaxis, in Uses in Enoxaparin 20:12.04.16.

Efficacy and safety of extended-duration oral betrixaban compared with standard-duration subcutaneous enoxaparin for thromboprophylaxis in acutely ill medical patients were evaluated in a randomized, double-blind, active-controlled, double-dummy trial (Acute Medically Ill Venous Thromboembolism Prevention with Extended-Duration Betrixaban [APEX]) in more than 7500 hospitalized adults (mean and median ages: 76.4 and 77 years, respectively). Patients eligible for the trial were hospitalized (expected duration at least 3 days) for an acute medical illness (e.g., heart failure [45%], infection without septic shock [29%], acute respiratory failure [12%], acute ischemic stroke [11%], acute rheumatic disorders [3%]) and had moderately or severely reduced mobility (for at least 24 hours) and at least one of the following additional risk factors for venous thromboembolism: (1) age 75 years or older; (2) age 60 through 74 years and an elevated serum D-dimer concentration (at least twice the upper limit of normal); or (3) age 40 through 59 years, an elevated serum D-dimer concentration (at least twice the upper limit of normal), and a history of venous thromboembolism or cancer. Patients were randomly assigned to receive betrixaban (160-mg loading dose on day 1, then 80 mg daily for 35–42 days) plus subcutaneous enoxaparin placebo for 6–14 days, or subcutaneous enoxaparin (40 mg once daily for 6–14 days) plus oral betrixaban placebo for 35–42 days. However, patients with severe renal impairment (creatinine clearance 15–29 mL/minute) received a reduced dosage of betrixaban (loading dose of 80 mg followed by a maintenance dosage of 40 mg once daily) or enoxaparin (20 mg subcutaneously once daily), and patients who were taking a potent P-glycoprotein (P-gp) inhibitor (i.e., amiodarone, verapamil, quinidine) received a reduced dosage of betrixaban (loading dose of 80 mg followed by a maintenance dosage of 40 mg once daily).

After approximately 35% enrollment of patients, the trial protocol was altered using a US Food and Drug Administration (FDA)-approved "enrichment strategy" in an attempt to better demonstrate the drug's efficacy in patients at high risk for venous thromboembolism by modifying entry criteria to require the presence of an elevated D-dimer level or an age of at least 75 years. The statistical analysis plan also was modified by establishing 2 cohorts of patients within the overall trial population. Cohort 1 consisted of patients with an elevated baseline D-dimer concentration (at least 2 times the upper limit of normal [ULN]). Cohort 2 included the patients in cohort 1 plus those who were 75 years of age and older. The primary efficacy outcome was the composite of the occurrence of asymptomatic proximal deep-vein thrombosis (DVT) between day 32 and day 47, symptomatic proximal or distal DVT, symptomatic nonfatal pulmonary embolism (PE), or venous thromboembolism-related death between day 1 and day 42. Efficacy outcomes were analyzed in a fixed hierarchical sequence such that a statistically significant difference with respect to the primary efficacy outcome had to be demonstrated in cohort 1 before applying statistical testing of the same outcome in cohort 2 and, subsequently, in the overall population; i.e., if betrixaban was not found superior to enoxaparin with respect to the primary efficacy outcome in cohort 1, all subsequent analyses (i.e., in cohort 2 and the overall population) were considered exploratory.

The median duration of active treatment was 36 days in the betrixaban group and 9 days in the enoxaparin group. In cohort 1 (patients with baseline elevated D-dimer), there was no statistically significant difference between extended-duration betrixaban and standard-duration enoxaparin with respect to the primary composite efficacy outcome (event rates of 6.9 and 8.5%, respectively; relative risk of 0.81 for betrixaban). Therefore, interpretation of subsequent analyses was regarded as exploratory according to the prespecified trial protocol. Results of exploratory analyses of the primary efficacy outcome in cohort 2 and the overall trial population were consistent with a lower risk of venous thromboembolism with betrixaban extended-duration therapy compared with standard-duration enoxaparin therapy (relative risk of 0.8 for betrixaban in cohort 2; relative risk of 0.76 for betrixaban in the overall trial population). A post hoc analysis by study drug dosage suggested that the benefit of betrixaban was confined to patients who received the full-dose betrixaban regimen (160-mg loading dose, 80-mg daily maintenance dosage); rates of venous thromboembolism in patients who required a reduced dosage of betrixaban (80-mg loading dose, then 40 mg daily) due to severe renal impairment or concomitant use of a P-gp inhibitor were similar to those in the enoxaparin arm of the trial.

The risk of major bleeding among those who received betrixaban or enoxaparin therapy was similar. Clinically important nonmajor bleeding episodes occurred more often in patients receiving betrixaban therapy than in those receiving enoxaparin; however, most of the nonmajor bleeds that occurred in the betrixaban group were mild to moderate in severity, and the majority did not require medical intervention. (See Bleeding under Warnings/Precautions: Other Warnings and Precautions, in Cautions.)

Safety and efficacy of betrixaban have not been established in patients with prosthetic heart valves.

Dosage and Administration

■ **General** Routine coagulation monitoring is not necessary during betrixaban therapy because of the drug's predictable pharmacokinetic and pharmacodynamic effects. However, in certain situations, such as in the case of overdosage or in patients with hemorrhagic or thromboembolic complications, it may be useful to assess the degree of anticoagulation. Anti-factor Xa assays may be used to measure the effect of betrixaban on factor Xa activity. Use of prothrombin time (PT), activated partial thromboplastin time (aPTT), dilute thrombin time (dTT) or thrombin time (TT) assays, or heparin-specific assays (e.g., activated clotting time [ACT]) are not recommended.

■ **Administration** Betrixaban is administered orally with food. If a dose of betrixaban is missed, the missed dose should be taken as soon as possible on the same day, followed by resumption of the regular schedule; the dose should not be doubled to make up for the missed dose.

■ **Dosage** Dosage of betrixaban maleate is expressed in terms of betrixaban.

Deep-Vein Thrombosis and Pulmonary Embolism **Thromboprophylaxis for Acute Medical Illness.** For the prevention of venous thromboembolism in patients hospitalized for an acute medical illness who are at risk for thromboembolic complications, the recommended dosage of betrixaban is 160 mg *as a single loading dose*, followed by 80 mg once daily. The recommended duration of betrixaban therapy is 35–42 days.

■ **Special Populations** ***Hepatic Impairment*** Use of betrixaban should be avoided in patients with hepatic impairment. (See Hepatic Impairment under Warnings/Precautions: Specific Populations, in Cautions.)

Renal Impairment Dosage adjustments of betrixaban are not needed in patients with a creatinine clearance of 30 mL/minute or greater. A reduced dosage of 80 mg *as a single loading dose*, followed by 40 mg once daily, is recommended in patients with a creatinine clearance of 15–29 mL/minute. (See Renal Impairment under Warnings/Precautions: Specific Populations, in Cautions.)

Patients Receiving P-glycoprotein Inhibitors A reduced betrixaban dosage of 80 mg *as a single loading dose*, followed by 40 mg once daily, is recommended in patients currently receiving or initiating therapy with a P-glycoprotein (P-gp) inhibitor. (See Drug Interactions: Drugs Affecting P-glycoprotein Transport.)

Cautions

■ **Contraindications** Active pathologic bleeding.

Severe hypersensitivity reaction to betrixaban.

■ **Warnings/Precautions** ***Warnings*** **Spinal/Epidural Hematoma.** Patients receiving anticoagulants are at risk of developing an epidural or spinal hematoma when concomitant neuraxial (epidural/spinal) anesthesia or spinal puncture is employed; such complications can result in long-term or permanent paralysis. The risk of these adverse events is increased by use of indwelling epidural catheters or by concomitant use of drugs affecting hemostasis, such as nonsteroidal anti-inflammatory agents (NSAIAs), platelet-aggregation inhibitors, or other anticoagulants. Risk also may be increased in patients with a history of traumatic or repeated epidural or spinal punctures, spinal problems, or spinal surgery.

Removal of an epidural catheter should be delayed for at least 72 hours following a dose of betrixaban, and at least 5 hours should elapse following removal of the catheter before administration of the next betrixaban dose. If traumatic puncture occurs, administration of betrixaban should be delayed for 72 hours.

Patients receiving betrixaban in the setting of epidural or spinal anesthesia or lumbar puncture should be monitored frequently for manifestations of neurologic impairment (e.g., numbness or weakness of the legs, bowel or bladder dysfunction). If neurologic compromise is noted, urgent diagnosis and treatment are necessary. Clinicians should consider the potential benefits versus risks of neuraxial intervention in patients who are currently receiving or will receive anticoagulant prophylaxis.

Sensitivity Reactions **Hypersensitivity.** At least one serious adverse reaction associated with moderate hypersensitivity to betrixaban has been reported. (See Cautions: Contraindications.)

Other Warnings and Precautions **Bleeding.** Betrixaban increases the risk of hemorrhage and can cause serious or fatal bleeding. Bleeding complications were the most common adverse effects of betrixaban reported in the APEX trial. In that trial, bleeding that required drug discontinuance occurred in 2.4% of patients receiving betrixaban and 1.2% of those receiving enoxaparin. In the overall population evaluated for safety (which included events that occurred up to 7 days after the last dose of study drug), the principal safety outcome (occurrence of major bleeding, defined as clinically overt bleeding that resulted in death, involved a critical site [i.e., intraocular, intracranial, intraspinal, IM with compartment syndrome, retroperitoneal, intra-articular, pericardial], was associated with a fall in hemoglobin of at least 2 g/dL within 48 hours of an overt bleeding event, or required transfusion of at least 2 units of whole blood or packed red blood cells) in patients who received betrixaban or enoxaparin therapy was similar (event rate 0.67 versus 0.57%, respectively). There was one case of fatal bleeding in each treatment group. The incidence of clinically important nonmajor bleeding episodes (defined as overt bleeding not meeting the criteria for major bleeding but associated with medical intervention, unscheduled contact with a physician, discontinuance of the study drug [permanent or temporary], or associated with patient discomfort) was 2.45 versus 1.02% in patients receiving betrixaban versus enoxaparin therapy, respectively. The secondary safety outcome, major bleeding or clinically relevant nonmajor bleeding, occurred almost twice as often in the betrixaban group compared with the enoxaparin group in the overall safety population (relative risk 1.97 for betrixaban). However, most of the nonmajor bleeds that occurred in the betrixaban group were mild to moderate in severity and generally did not require medical intervention.

Risk of bleeding may be increased in patients with severe renal impairment (creatinine clearance 15–29 mL/minute computed by the Cockcroft-Gault method using actual body weight) and in those receiving concomitant therapy with drugs that affect hemostasis or drugs that are inhibitors of P-glycoprotein (P-gp). (See Drug Interactions.) Clinicians should evaluate any signs and symptoms of blood loss in patients receiving betrixaban therapy and consider the need for blood replacement. Betrixaban should be discontinued if active pathologic hemorrhage occurs. (See Cautions: Contraindications.)

There is no specific antidote or reversal agent for betrixaban; it is not known whether betrixaban is removed by hemodialysis. Protamine sulfate, vitamin K, and tranexamic acid are not expected to reverse the anticoagulant activity of betrixaban. The anticoagulant effect of betrixaban may persist for at least 72 hours after the last dose.

Specific Populations **Pregnancy.** There are no adequate or well-controlled studies of betrixaban in pregnant women. In animal reproduction studies, betrixaban administered to pregnant rats and rabbits during organogenesis at a dosage of up to 44 times the recommended human dosage (80 mg once daily) was not associated with adverse fetal developmental effects; however, maternal toxicity (i.e., hemorrhage) was observed. Treatment with betrixaban is likely to increase the risk of hemorrhage during pregnancy and delivery. Betrixaban should be used during pregnancy only if the potential benefits justify the potential risks to the mother and fetus. The risk of bleeding and stroke in pregnant women also should be considered.

Lactation. Data are lacking on the presence of betrixaban in human milk, the effects on the breast-fed infant, or the effects of the drug on milk production. The developmental and health benefits of breast-feeding should be considered along with the mother's clinical need for betrixaban and any potential adverse effects on the breast-fed infant from betrixaban or from the underlying maternal condition.

Pediatric Use. Safety and efficacy have not been established in pediatric patients.

Geriatric Use. In the APEX trial, 90% of patients were 65 years of age or older, and 68.6% were 75 years of age or older. No clinically important differences in efficacy or safety were observed in older relative to younger adults in this trial.

Hepatic Impairment. Safety and efficacy of betrixaban have not been established in patients with hepatic impairment. Due to the potential for intrinsic coagulation abnormalities, the use of betrixaban in patients with hepatic impairment is not recommended.

Renal Impairment. Betrixaban exposure is increased in patients with renal impairment. In a study in individuals with various degrees of renal function (computed by the Cockcroft-Gault method using actual body weight), betrixaban area under the concentration-time curve (AUC) was increased by 1.89-, 2.27-, and 2.63-fold in those with mild (estimated glomerular filtration rate [eGFR] of 60–89 mL/minute per 1.73 m^2), moderate (eGFR of 30–59 mL/minute per 1.73 m^2), or severe (eGFR of 15–29 mL/minute per 1.73 m^2) renal impairment, respectively, compared with values in healthy individuals. Patients with severe renal impairment who are receiving betrixaban may have an increased risk of bleeding events; such patients should be monitored closely and evaluated for any manifestations of blood loss.

Dosage of betrixaban should be reduced in patients with severe renal impairment. (See Renal Impairment under Dosage and Administration: Special Populations.) Use of betrixaban should be avoided in patients with severe renal impairment (creatinine clearance 15–29 mL/minute) who are receiving P-gp inhibitors.

■ **Common Adverse Effects** Bleeding is the most common adverse effect reported with betrixaban, occurring in more than 5% of patients receiving the drug in clinical trials.

Drug Interactions

Betrixaban is minimally metabolized (less than 1%) by cytochrome P-450 (CYP) isoenzymes 1A1, 1A2, 2B6, 2C9, 2C19, 2D6, and 3A4. Betrixaban is neither an inducer nor inhibitor of CYP isoenzymes.

■ **Drugs Affecting P-glycoprotein Transport** Betrixaban is a substrate of the efflux transporter P-glycoprotein (P-gp); inhibitors of this transport protein (e.g., amiodarone, azithromycin, clarithromycin, ketoconazole, verapamil) may increase betrixaban exposure. For patients receiving concomitant therapy with a P-gp inhibitor, the dosage of betrixaban should be reduced to *an initial loading dose of 80 mg* followed by 40 mg once daily. Use of betrixaban should be avoided in patients with severe renal impairment (creatinine clearance 15–29 mL/minute) who are receiving P-gp inhibitors.

Ketoconazole Following concomitant use of betrixaban (single 40-mg dose) with ketoconazole (200 mg twice daily for 5 days), betrixaban peak plasma concentration and area under the concentration-time curve (AUC) were increased by approximately 2.3-fold.

Verapamil Following concomitant use of betrixaban (single 40-mg dose) with extended-release verapamil (once-daily regimen), betrixaban peak plasma concentration and AUC were increased by approximately 4.7- and 3-fold, respectively.

■ **Drugs Affecting Gastric Acidity** Concomitant use of betrixaban (40 mg) with esomeprazole or an antacid containing aluminum hydroxide and magnesium hydroxide did not affect bioavailability of or exposure to betrixaban.

■ **Drugs Affecting Hemostasis** Concomitant use of betrixaban and drugs that affect hemostasis (e.g., aspirin or other nonsteroidal anti-inflammatory agents [NSAIAs] or antiplatelet drugs, heparin, other anticoagulants, thrombolytic agents, selective serotonin-reuptake inhibitors [SSRIs], selective serotonin- and norepinephrine-reuptake inhibitors [SNRIs]) increases risk of bleeding. Patients receiving such concomitant therapy who experience any manifestations of bleeding should be promptly evaluated. (See Bleeding under Warnings/Precautions: Other Warnings and Precautions, in Cautions.)

■ **Digoxin** Concomitant use of betrixaban (80 mg daily) with digoxin, a substrate of P-gp, did not affect the bioavailability of or exposure to either drug.

Description

Betrixaban maleate is an oral, direct activated factor X (Xa) inhibitor. Factor Xa plays a central role in the blood coagulation cascade by serving as the convergence point for the intrinsic and extrinsic pathways; inhibition of coagulation factor Xa by betrixaban prevents conversion of prothrombin to thrombin and subsequent thrombus formation. Betrixaban selectively blocks the active site of factor Xa, inhibiting both free and platelet-bound factor Xa within the prothrombinase complex. Unlike heparin and the low molecular weight heparins, betrixaban binds directly to the active site of factor Xa without the need for a cofactor (e.g., antithrombin III). Betrixaban inhibits factor Xa with 86,000-fold greater selectivity than other biologically important serine proteases (e.g., thrombin). Some data indicate that an 80-mg daily dose of betrixaban reduces thrombin generation to a level similar to warfarin therapy adjusted to an international normalized ratio (INR) of 2–3.

Betrixaban is rapidly absorbed following oral administration, with an estimated bioavailability of about 34%. Peak plasma concentrations of betrixaban are obtained 3–4 hours following oral administration, which coincides with betrixaban's peak effect (i.e., maximal inhibition of thrombin generation). The presence of food decreases peak plasma concentration and systemic exposure to betrixaban by approximately 60% compared with the fasting state. The effect of food on the pharmacokinetics of betrixaban can be observed for up to 6 hours following a meal. Steady state is achieved in 6 days when the drug is given without an initial loading dose.

Unchanged betrixaban is the predominant form of betrixaban found in human plasma. Betrixaban is mainly metabolized by cytochrome P-450 (CYP)-independent plasma hydrolysis, forming 2 major inactive metabolites. Less than 1% of the minor metabolites are formed via metabolism by CYP isoenzymes 1A1, 1A2, 2B6, 2C9, 2C19, 2D6, and 3A4. Betrixaban is 60% bound to plasma proteins in vitro. The effective and terminal half-lives of the drug are about 19–27 and 37 hours, respectively. The drug is mainly excreted in bile and has low renal excretion. Following oral administration, approximately 85% of an administered dose of betrixaban is excreted in feces and 11% is excreted in urine.

In a study evaluating the effect of betrixaban on the QT interval, a concentration-dependent increase in the QT interval corrected for rate (QT_c) was observed. A QT_c prolongation of 4 msec is predicted for an 80-mg dose of betrixaban and a prolongation of 13 msec is predicted for a supratherapeutic dose (associated with a 4.7-fold increase in exposure) of betrixaban.

Advice to Patients

Importance of informing patients to take betrixaban with food.

Importance of advising patients that if a dose is missed, it should be taken as soon as possible on the same day and the regular dosing schedule should be resumed the following day; the dose should not be doubled to replace a missed dose.

Importance of informing patients that they may bruise and/or bleed more easily and that a longer than normal time may be required for bleeding to stop when taking betrixaban. Importance of informing clinicians about any unusual bleeding or bruising during therapy. Importance of patients informing clinicians immediately and of seeking emergency care if they experience signs and symptoms of blood loss.

Importance of patients informing clinicians (e.g., physicians, dentists) that they are receiving betrixaban therapy before any surgery or invasive procedures, including dental procedures, are scheduled.

Importance of advising patients that the risk of bleeding is greater in people who have severe renal impairment.

Importance of advising patients who have had neuraxial anesthesia or spinal puncture to monitor for manifestations of spinal or epidural hematoma (e.g., numbness or weakness of the legs, bowel or bladder dysfunction); importance of immediately contacting a clinician if any of these symptoms occur.

Importance of women immediately informing clinicians if they are or plan to become pregnant or plan to breast-feed.

Importance of informing clinicians (e.g., physicians, dentists) of existing or contemplated concomitant therapy, including prescription and OTC drugs and herbal supplements.

Importance of informing patients of other important precautionary information. (See Cautions.)

Overview® (see Users Guide). For additional information on this drug until a more detailed monograph is developed and published, the manufacturer's labeling should be consulted. It is *essential* that the manufacturer's labeling be consulted for more detailed information on usual cautions, precautions, contraindications, potential drug interactions, laboratory test interferences, and acute toxicity.

Preparations

Excipients in commercially available drug preparations may have clinically important effects in some individuals; consult specific product labeling for details.

Betrixaban Maleate

Oral		
Capsules	40 mg (of betrixaban)	**Bevyxxa®**, Portola Pharmaceuticals
	80 mg (of betrixaban)	**Bevyxxa®**, Portola Pharmaceuticals

Edoxaban Tosylate

■ Edoxaban tosylate, an oral, direct, activated factor X (Xa) inhibitor, is an anticoagulant.

Uses

■ **Embolism Associated with Atrial Fibrillation** Edoxaban tosylate is used to reduce the risk of stroke and systemic embolism in patients with nonvalvular atrial fibrillation. Current evidence suggests that edoxaban is at least as effective as well-controlled warfarin therapy in the prevention of stroke and systemic embolism and is associated with a lower risk of bleeding and cardiovascular death than warfarin. However, the benefit of edoxaban in reducing ischemic stroke appears to be strongly dose- and plasma-concentration dependent, and the drug should not be used in patients with a creatinine clearance exceeding 95 mL/minute because of an increased risk of ischemic stroke in such patients. (See Reduced Efficacy in Nonvalvular Atrial Fibrillation Patients with Creatinine Clearance Exceeding 95 mL/minute under Warnings/Precautions: Warnings, in Cautions.)

The American College of Chest Physicians (ACCP), the American College of Cardiology (ACC), the American Heart Association (AHA), the American Stroke Association (ASA), and other experts currently recommend that antithrombotic therapy be administered to all patients with nonvalvular atrial fibrillation (i.e., atrial fibrillation in the absence of rheumatic mitral stenosis, a prosthetic heart valve, or mitral valve repair) who are considered to be at increased risk of stroke, unless such therapy is contraindicated. Recommendations regarding choice of antithrombotic therapy are based on a patient's relative risk for stroke and bleeding. In general, oral anticoagulant therapy (traditionally warfarin) is recommended in patients who have a moderate to high risk for stroke and acceptably low risk of bleeding, while aspirin or no antithrombotic therapy may be considered in patients at low risk of stroke. Although many risk stratification methods have been used, patients considered to be at increased risk of stroke generally include those with prior ischemic stroke or transient ischemic attack (TIA), advanced age (e.g., 75 years or older), history of hypertension, diabetes mellitus, or congestive heart failure. In addition, population-based studies suggest that female sex is an important risk factor for stroke in patients with atrial fibrillation, particularly in patients 75 years of age or older, and AHA and ASA recommend the use of risk stratification tools that account for age- and sex-specific differences in stroke risk. One such tool is the CHA_2DS_2-VASc score, an extension of the $CHADS_2$ system (which considers the risk factors congestive heart failure, hypertension, age 75 years or older, diabetes mellitus, and prior stroke/TIA) that adds extra points for female sex (1 point); previous myocardial infarction, peripheral arterial disease, or aortic plaque (1 point); and age 65–74 years (1 point) or 75 years or older (2 points).

The risk of thromboembolism in patients with atrial flutter is not as well established as it is in those with atrial fibrillation. In addition, many patients with atrial flutter have alternating periods of atrial fibrillation. Experts state that antithrombotic therapy in patients with atrial flutter generally should be managed in the same manner as in patients with atrial fibrillation.

Although warfarin traditionally has been used for oral anticoagulation in patients with atrial fibrillation at increased risk of stroke, non-vitamin K antagonist oral anticoagulants such as edoxaban may provide certain advantages over warfarin (e.g., rapid onset of action, predictable anticoagulant effect, no requirement for coagulation monitoring, less potential for drug-drug and drug-food interactions), and are considered by some experts to be useful alternatives to warfarin in selected patients. The non-vitamin K antagonist oral anticoagulants may be particularly useful in patients at moderate to high risk of stroke who are unable to comply with warfarin monitoring requirements or in whom a consistent therapeutic response to warfarin has not been achieved (e.g., because of drug or food interactions), while warfarin may continue to be preferred in patients who are optimally managed with well-controlled international normalized ratios (INRs) (e.g., INR in therapeutic range more than 70% of the time). Warfarin generally should remain the treatment of choice in patients with severe renal impairment pending clinical outcomes data with the non-vitamin K antagonist oral anticoagulants in these patients. Because of the lack of direct, comparative studies, the relative efficacy and safety of the non-vitamin K antagonist anticoagulants (e.g., apixaban, dabigatran, edoxaban, rivaroxaban) for the prevention of stroke in patients with nonvalvular atrial fibrillation remain to be fully elucidated. Some evidence from indirect comparisons suggests that there may be important differences (e.g., bleeding risk) between these agents; however, results of such analyses should be interpreted with caution because of possible confounding factors (e.g., differences in study design and methods, patient populations, and anticoagulation control). Selection of an appropriate anticoagulant for patients with nonvalvular atrial fibrillation should be individualized based on the absolute and relative risks of stroke and bleeding; costs; patient compliance, preference, tolerance, and comorbidities; and other clinical factors such as renal function and degree of INR control if the patient has been taking warfarin. For additional information on antithrombotic therapy in patients with atrial fibrillation, see Uses: Embolism Associated with Atrial Fibrillation in Warfarin 20:12.04.08.

Efficacy and safety of edoxaban for the prevention of stroke and systemic embolism in patients with nonvalvular atrial fibrillation have been established in a randomized, double-blind, double-dummy trial (Effective Anticoagulation with Factor Xa Next Generation in Atrial Fibrillation-Thrombolysis in Myocardial Infarction 48 [ENGAGE AF-TIMI 48]). In this trial, edoxaban was compared with warfarin in 21,105 patients with nonvalvular atrial fibrillation who were at moderate-to-high risk of stroke (Congestive Heart Failure, Hypertension, Age, Diabetes, Stroke [doubled] [i.e., $CHADS_2$] score of at least 2). Patients received one of 2 fixed dosages of edoxaban (30 or 60 mg daily) or warfarin (dosage-adjusted to achieve therapeutic INR of 2–3) for a median of 2.5 years; for those in the edoxaban treatment groups, dosage was reduced by 50% (from 60 to 30 mg or 30 to 15 mg) if any of the following conditions anticipated to increase drug exposure, and thus bleeding, were present: estimated creatinine clearance of 30–50 mL/minute, body weight of 60 kg or less, or concomitant use of the potent P-glycoprotein inhibitors verapamil, quinidine, or dronedarone.

Edoxaban was noninferior to warfarin in preventing stroke and systemic embolism and was associated with lower rates of bleeding. At a median follow-up of 2.8 years, both dosage regimens of edoxaban demonstrated noninferiority to warfarin for the primary composite outcome of time to first occurrence of stroke (ischemic or hemorrhagic) or a systemic embolic event; annualized rates of the primary end point were 1.5% with warfarin, 1.61% with edoxaban 30 mg, and 1.18% with edoxaban 60 mg. The effect of edoxaban on the primary outcome was attributable principally to a marked reduction in hemorrhagic stroke; the rate of ischemic stroke was similar between edoxaban 60 mg and warfarin, and substantially higher with edoxaban 30 mg than with warfarin. The primary efficacy analysis was performed on the modified intent-to-treat population, which included all patients who underwent randomization and received at least one dose of study drug during the treatment period. In a prespecified superiority analysis that was subsequently conducted on the intent-to-treat population, both dosage regimens of edoxaban failed to demonstrate superiority over warfarin in reducing the rate of stroke or systemic embolism. With regard to the primary safety end point in this trial, major bleeding was substantially reduced with edoxaban (at both dosage levels) compared with warfarin. Other bleeding end points (i.e., intracranial bleeding, life-threatening bleeding, clinically relevant nonmajor bleeding) also favored edoxaban, with the exception of GI bleeding, which occurred at a higher rate in patients receiving the 60-mg dose of edoxaban compared with warfarin. The reduction in major bleeding with edoxaban compared with warfarin was even greater in patients who required a reduction in edoxaban dosage, and no apparent loss of efficacy was observed.

The comparison between edoxaban and warfarin in the ENGAGE AF-TIMI 48 trial was based on well-controlled warfarin therapy; patients who received warfarin achieved a mean time in the therapeutic INR range (2–3) of 65%, which is higher than that reported with warfarin anticoagulation in other trials of non-vitamin K antagonist anticoagulants (e.g., dabigatran, apixaban, rivaroxaban) in patients with nonvalvular atrial fibrillation (e.g., 55–64%).

At the end of the ENGAGE AF-TIMI 48 trial, patients were switched to open-label anticoagulant therapy with the use of a transition plan that was specifically incorporated into the protocol to minimize the risk of stroke due to inadequate anticoagulation. (See Risk of Thrombosis Following Premature Discontinuance of Therapy under Warnings/Precautions: Warnings, in Cautions.) The transition plan included a period of overlap between edoxaban (at half the initial dosage used in the controlled trial) and warfarin until a therapeutic INR of 2 was achieved or for 14 days (whichever occurred first) in patients who switched from edoxaban to warfarin therapy. Similar rates of stroke and bleeding were observed across all treatment groups during the 30-day period following the end of the trial.

A strong relationship between plasma concentrations of edoxaban and the drug's effectiveness was observed in the ENGAGE AF-TIMI 48 trial. Patients who received the low dosage of edoxaban (30 mg daily) had a 64% higher rate of ischemic stroke compared with those who received the high dosage of the drug (60 mg daily). Because plasma edoxaban concentrations are affected by renal function, patients with good renal function are likely to have a lesser response to edoxaban due to lower plasma concentrations at a given dosage than those with mildly impaired renal function. When results of the ENGAGE AF-TIMI 48 trial were evaluated based on creatinine clearance, the relative benefits of edoxaban versus warfarin in reducing the rate of ischemic stroke decreased as renal function improved to the point where warfarin was more effective than edoxaban at creatinine clearances exceeding 95 mL/minute. Based on these findings, edoxaban should not be used in patients with a creatinine clearance exceeding 95 mL/minute. (See Reduced Efficacy in Nonvalvular Atrial Fibrillation Patients with Creatinine Clearance Exceeding 95 mL/minute under Warnings/Precautions: Warnings, in Cautions.)

Safety and efficacy of edoxaban have not been established in patients with mechanical heart valves or moderate to severe mitral stenosis; the drug is not recommended in such patients. (See Patients with Prosthetic Heart Valves or Mitral Stenosis under Warnings/ Precautions: Other Warnings and Precautions, in Cautions.)

■ Deep-Vein Thrombosis and Pulmonary Embolism *Treatment*

Edoxaban is used for the treatment of deep-vein thrombosis (DVT) and/or pulmonary embolism (PE) following initial treatment with a parenteral anticoagulant for 5–10 days.

Efficacy and safety of edoxaban for this use have been established in a randomized, double-blind noninferiority trial (Hokusai VTE) in more than 8000 adults with acute venous thromboembolism. In this trial, edoxaban demonstrated noninferiority to warfarin in reducing the risk of recurrent venous thromboembolism and was associated with substantially reduced rates of clinically important bleeding. The relative efficacy and safety of edoxaban versus other non-vitamin K antagonist oral anticoagulants (e.g., apixaban, dabigatran, rivaroxaban) for the treatment of venous thromboembolism remain to be established.

The Hokusai VTE trial was conducted in a broad population of patients with acute venous thromboembolism, including those with provoked (i.e., associated with a temporary risk factor) or unprovoked venous thromboembolism, and those with severe PE. All patients received initial therapy with heparin (enoxaparin or unfractionated heparin) on an open-label basis for at least 5 days; blinded treatment consisted of either edoxaban (60 mg daily, initiated after the heparin regimen was discontinued) or warfarin (initiated concurrently with heparin and dose-adjusted to achieve a therapeutic INR of 2–3), which was continued for a total of 3–12 months depending on the clinical situation. For those in the edoxaban treatment group, dosage was reduced to 30 mg daily if any of the following conditions anticipated to increase drug exposure, and thus bleeding, were present: estimated creatinine clearance of 30–50 mL/minute, body weight of 60 kg or less, or concomitant use of the potent P-glycoprotein inhibitors verapamil, quinidine, azithromycin, clarithromycin, erythromycin, oral itraconazole, or oral ketoconazole. The primary composite end point of DVT or nonfatal or fatal PE occurred in 3.2% of patients receiving edoxaban and 3.5% of those receiving warfarin during the 12-month trial period. The primary efficacy analysis was performed on a modified intent-to-treat population, which included all patients who underwent randomization and received at least one dose of study drug during the treatment period. With respect to the primary safety outcome, clinically relevant major or nonmajor bleeding occurred less frequently in patients receiving edoxaban than those receiving warfarin (8.5 versus 10.3%). Among patients who required a dosage reduction of edoxaban, bleeding rates were decreased without an apparent loss of efficacy. Patients who received warfarin in the trial achieved a median time in therapeutic INR range (2–3) of 65.6%.

Dosage and Administration

■ **General** Prior to initiating therapy with edoxaban tosylate, renal function should be assessed. Creatinine clearance should be calculated using the Cockcroft-Gault method as dosage recommendations for edoxaban are based on estimated creatinine clearance. Patients with nonvalvular atrial fibrillation who have a creatinine clearance exceeding 95 mL/minute should not receive the drug because of evidence indicating that efficacy may be reduced in such patients. (See Reduced Efficacy in Nonvalvular Atrial Fibrillation Patients with Creatinine Clearance Exceeding 95 mL/minute under Warnings/Precautions: Warnings, in Cautions.)

Routine coagulation monitoring (e.g., prothrombin time [PT], activated partial thromboplastin time [aPTT], international normalized ratio [INR]) is not necessary during edoxaban therapy because of the drug's predictable pharmacokinetic and pharmacodynamic effects. However, in certain situations, such as in the case of overdosage or in patients with hemorrhagic or thromboembolic complications or those requiring emergency surgery, it may be useful to assess the degree of anticoagulation. Although edoxaban has been shown to produce concentration-dependent increases in aPTT, PT, and INR, these tests are not useful for monitoring the anticoagulant effects of edoxaban because of a high degree of inconsistency, insensitivity, and variability in results.

■ **Administration** Edoxaban is administered orally without regard to food. (See Description.)

If a dose of edoxaban is missed, the missed dose should be taken as soon as possible on the same day, followed by resumption of the regular schedule; the dose should not be doubled to make up for the missed dose.

■ **Dosage** Dosage of edoxaban tosylate monohydrate is expressed in terms of edoxaban.

Embolism Associated with Atrial Fibrillation For the prevention of stroke and systemic embolism in adults with nonvalvular atrial fibrillation who have a creatinine clearance of 51–95 mL/minute, the recommended initial dosage of edoxaban is 60 mg once daily. Dosage should be reduced to 30 mg daily in patients with creatinine clearance of 15–50 mL/minute. (See Dosage and Administration: Special Populations.) The drug should *not* be used in patients with creatinine clearance exceeding 95 mL/minute.

Deep-Vein Thrombosis and Pulmonary Embolism **Treatment.** The recommended dosage of edoxaban for the treatment of deep-vein thrombosis (DVT) and/or pulmonary embolism (PE) is 60 mg once daily following 5–10 days of initial therapy with a parenteral anticoagulant.

Dosage should be reduced to 30 mg once daily in patients with creatinine clearance of 15–50 mL/minute, body weight of 60 kg or less, and/or in those receiving concomitant therapy with certain drugs that are potent P-glycoprotein inhibitors. In the Hokusai VTE trial, dosage of edoxaban was reduced in patients receiving concomitant therapy with verapamil, quinidine, or short-term treatment with azithromycin, clarithromycin, erythromycin, oral ketoconazole, or oral itraconazole. (See P-glycoprotein Inhibitors under Drug Interactions: Drugs Affecting Efflux Transport Systems.)

The optimum duration of anticoagulant therapy should be determined by the individual clinical situation (e.g., location of thrombi, presence or absence of precipitating factors for thrombosis, presence of cancer, risk of bleeding). In general, the American College of Chest Physicians (ACCP) states that anticoagulant therapy for venous thromboembolism should be continued beyond the acute treatment period for at least 3 months and possibly longer in patients with a high risk of recurrence and low risk of bleeding.

Transitioning from Other Anticoagulant Therapy When transitioning from a vitamin K antagonist (e.g., warfarin) to edoxaban therapy, the manufacturer states that the vitamin K antagonist should be discontinued and edoxaban initiated as soon as the INR is 2.5 or less. When transitioning from other oral anticoagulants, the current anticoagulant should be discontinued and edoxaban initiated at the time of the next scheduled dose of the other anticoagulant.

When transitioning from a low molecular weight heparin to edoxaban, the low molecular weight heparin should be discontinued and edoxaban initiated at the time of the next scheduled dose of the low molecular weight heparin. In patients currently receiving heparin by continuous IV infusion, the heparin infusion should be discontinued and edoxaban initiated 4 hours later.

Transitioning to Other Anticoagulant Therapy When transitioning from edoxaban to warfarin therapy, a parenteral or oral conversion strategy can be used. In the parenteral method, edoxaban is discontinued and a parenteral anticoagulant and warfarin are initiated simultaneously at the time of the next scheduled dose of edoxaban; the parenteral anticoagulant is then discontinued once a stable INR of at least 2 is reached. The oral conversion strategy is similar to the end-of-trial transition plan that was used in the ENGAGE AF-TIMI trial and involves the use of a half-dose edoxaban bridging regimen with overlapping warfarin therapy. In this method, the current dose of edoxaban is decreased by 50% (60 to 30 mg or 30 to 15 mg) and warfarin is initiated simultaneously. The 2 drugs are administered concomitantly until a stable INR of at least 2 is achieved; once this occurs, edoxaban should be discontinued and warfarin continued. INR values should be monitored at least once a week, with testing performed just prior to the daily dose of edoxaban to minimize the effect of the drug on the INR.

When transitioning from edoxaban to other anticoagulants, including parenteral anticoagulants or non-vitamin K-antagonist oral anticoagulants, edoxaban should be discontinued and the other anticoagulant initiated at the time of the next scheduled dose of edoxaban.

Managing Anticoagulation in Patients Requiring Invasive Procedures To minimize the risk of bleeding, edoxaban should be temporarily discontinued at least 24 hours prior to surgery or other invasive procedure. If surgery cannot be delayed, the potential increased risk of bleeding should be weighed against the urgency of the intervention. Edoxaban may be resumed postoperatively as soon as adequate hemostasis has been established; decisions regarding when to restart therapy should take into account the onset of the drug's pharmacodynamic effects (1–2 hours). If oral administration is not possible, a parenteral anticoagulant should be administered in the interim until edoxaban therapy can be resumed. (See Risk of Thrombosis Following Premature Discontinuance of Therapy under Warnings/Precautions: Warnings, in Cautions.)

■ **Special Populations** ***Hepatic Impairment*** No dosage adjustment is necessary in patients with mild (Child-Pugh class A) hepatic impairment. Use of edoxaban is not recommended in patients with moderate (Child-Pugh class B) or severe (Child-Pugh class C) hepatic impairment. (See Hepatic Impairment under Warnings/Precautions: Specific Populations, in Cautions.)

Renal Impairment Dosage of edoxaban should be reduced to 30 mg once daily in patients with a creatinine clearance of 15–50 mL/minute, regardless of indication. The drug is not recommended in patients with a creatinine clearance of less than 15 mL/minute. (See Renal Impairment under Warnings/Precautions: Specific Populations, in Cautions.)

Body Weight Edoxaban exposure is increased in patients with low body weight (less than 60 kg), which may increase the risk of bleeding. The manufacturer makes no dosage adjustment recommendations based on weight in patients with nonvalvular atrial fibrillation. When used for the treatment of venous thromboembolism, dosage of edoxaban should be reduced to 30 mg once daily in patients who weigh 60 kg or less.

Cautions

■ **Contraindications** Active pathologic bleeding.

■ **Warnings/Precautions** ***Warnings*** **Reduced Efficacy in Nonvalvular Atrial Fibrillation Patients with Creatinine Clearance Exceeding 95 mL/minute.** Edoxaban tosylate should not be used in patients with nonvalvular atrial fibrillation who have a creatinine clearance exceeding 95 mL/minute; the manufacturer states that alternative anticoagulants should be used in such patients. Reduced antithrombotic efficacy was observed in the principal efficacy trial of the drug (ENGAGE AF-TIMI 48) in patients with nonvalvular atrial fibrillation who had a creatinine clearance exceeding 95 mL/minute. In particular, the rate of ischemic stroke was substantially increased in such patients who were receiving edoxaban 60 mg daily compared with warfarin-treated patients who had a similar level of renal function. (See Uses: Embolism Associated with Atrial Fibrillation.)

Risk of Thrombosis Following Premature Discontinuance of Therapy. Premature discontinuance of any anticoagulant therapy, including edoxaban, in the absence of adequate alternative anticoagulation increases the risk of thromboembolic events. When transitioning patients from one anticoagulant therapy to another, it is important to ensure continuous anticoagulation while minimizing the risk of bleeding. Particular caution is advised when switching patients from a factor Xa inhibitor to warfarin therapy because of the slow onset of action of warfarin.

If discontinuance of edoxaban is required for reasons other than pathologic bleeding or completion of a course of therapy, coverage with an alternative anticoagulant should be considered. (See Dosage and Administration: Dosage.) Patients should be advised about the importance of adhering to the therapeutic regimen and instructed on steps to take if doses are missed. (See Advice to Patients.)

Spinal/Epidural Hematoma. Patients receiving anticoagulants are at risk of developing an epidural or spinal hematoma when concomitant neuraxial (epidural/spinal) anesthesia or spinal puncture is employed; such complications can result in long-term or permanent paralysis. The risk of these adverse events is increased by use of indwelling epidural catheters or by concomitant use of drugs affecting hemostasis, such as nonsteroidal anti-inflammatory agents (NSAIAs), platelet inhibitors, or other anticoagulants. Risk also may be increased in patients with a history of traumatic or repeated epidural or spinal punctures or a history of spinal deformity or spinal surgery.

Although optimal timing between the administration of edoxaban and neuraxial procedures is not known, the manufacturer states that removal of an indwelling epidural or intrathecal catheter should be delayed for at least 12 hours after the last administered dose of edoxaban, and at least 2 hours should elapse following removal of the catheter prior to administration of the next edoxaban dose.

Patients receiving edoxaban in the setting of epidural or spinal anesthesia should be monitored frequently for manifestations of neurologic impairment (e.g., numbness or weakness of the legs, bowel or bladder dysfunction). If neurologic compromise is noted, urgent diagnosis and treatment are necessary. Clinicians should consider the potential benefits versus risks of neuraxial intervention in patients who are currently receiving or will receive anticoagulants.

Other Warnings and Precautions **Bleeding.** Edoxaban increases the risk of hemorrhage and can cause serious, potentially fatal, bleeding. Patients should be promptly evaluated if any manifestations of blood loss occur during therapy. The drug should be discontinued if active pathological bleeding occurs. (See Cautions: Contraindications.) However, minor or "nuisance" bleeding is a common occurrence in patients receiving any anticoagulant and should not readily lead to treatment discontinuance. (See Risk of Thrombosis Following Premature Discontinuance of Therapy under Warnings/Precautions: Warnings, in Cautions.)

Bleeding complications were the most common adverse effects of edoxaban in clinical trials. In the principal efficacy trial of edoxaban in patients with nonvalvular atrial fibrillation (ENGAGE AF-TIMI 48), major bleeding (i.e., clinically overt bleeding at a critical organ/site or accompanied by a hemoglobin decrease of at least 2 g/dL when adjusted for transfusions or fatal bleeding) occurred at a rate of 2.75% per year with edoxaban 60 mg and 1.61% per year with edoxaban 30 mg; these rates were substantially lower than the rate of major bleeding in patients who received warfarin (3.43% per year). The rate of major GI bleeding was substantially higher with edoxaban 60 mg compared with warfarin (1.51 versus 1.23%), but the lower dosage of edoxaban (30 mg) was associated with the lowest rate of major GI bleeding (0.82%). In a dose-ranging study in patients with atrial fibrillation receiving edoxaban daily in 1 or 2 divided doses (twice-daily dosing currently not FDA-labeled), trough edoxaban concentrations and the frequency of bleeding complications were higher with 30 mg twice daily than with 60 mg once daily. In the Hokusai VTE trial in patients with acute venous thromboembolism, clinically relevant bleeding (major or nonmajor) occurred in 8.5% of patients receiving edoxaban 60 mg, which was substantially lower than the rate in patients receiving warfarin (10.3%).

Risk of bleeding may be increased in patients with renal impairment, low body weight (e.g., less than 60 kg), or in those receiving concomitant drugs that affect hemostasis (e.g., aspirin or other antiplatelet drugs, other anticoagulants, chronic use of NSAIAs). (See Drug Interactions.) Edoxaban therapy should be temporarily interrupted prior to surgery or other invasive procedure to minimize the risk of bleeding. (See Managing Anticoagulation in Patients Requiring Invasive Procedures under Dosage and Administration: Dosage.)

There is no specific reversal agent for edoxaban; anticoagulant effects can be expected to persist for approximately 24 hours after the drug is discontinued. Preliminary findings from a study in healthy individuals suggest that prothrombin complex concentrate (PCC) may be an effective reversal agent for edoxaban. In this study, administration of a 4-factor PCC reversed the effects of edoxaban 60 mg in a dose-dependent manner. At the highest dose studied (50 unit/kg), the PCC completely reversed bleeding duration and endogenous thrombin potential and partially reversed prothrombin time. Protamine sulfate, vitamin K, and tranexamic acid are not expected to be effective in reversing the anticoagulant effects of edoxaban. Edoxaban is not appreciably removed by dialysis.

Patients with Prosthetic Heart Valves or Mitral Stenosis. Safety and efficacy of edoxaban have not been evaluated in patients with mechanical heart valves or moderate to severe mitral stenosis; use of the drug is not recommended in such patients.

Specific Populations **Pregnancy.** Category C. (See Users Guide.)

There are no adequate or well-controlled studies of edoxaban in pregnant women. In animal studies, edoxaban was not teratogenic at exposure levels 49 times the maximum recommended human dose; however, fetotoxic effects, including gallbladder abnormalities, postimplantation pregnancy loss, spontaneous abortion, decreased live fetuses, and decreased fetal weight, occurred at maternally toxic doses. Edoxaban should be used during pregnancy only if the potential benefits justify the potential risks to the fetus.

Lactation. Edoxaban is distributed into milk in rats; it is not known whether the drug is distributed into human milk. Because of the potential for serious adverse reactions to edoxaban in nursing infants, the manufacturer states that a decision should be made whether to discontinue nursing or the drug, taking into account the importance of the drug to the woman.

Pediatric Use. Safety and efficacy of edoxaban have not been established in pediatric patients.

Geriatric Use. No substantial differences in efficacy and safety have been observed in geriatric patients 65 years of age or older relative to younger adults in clinical trials of edoxaban. In the ENGAGE AF-TIMI 48 trial, 74% of patients were 65 years of age or older, and 41% were 75 years of age or older. In the Hokusai VTE trial, 32% of patients were 65 years of age or older, and 14% were 75 years of age or older.

Hepatic Impairment. Mild (Child-Pugh class A) or moderate (Child-Pugh class B) hepatic impairment does not appear to affect pharmacokinetics or pharmacodynamics of edoxaban. Data on the drug are lacking in patients with severe hepatic impairment (Child-Pugh class C). (See Dosage and Administration: Special Populations.)

Edoxaban should not be used in patients with moderate or severe hepatic impairment because of the possibility of intrinsic coagulation abnormalities in such patients.

Renal Impairment. Edoxaban is eliminated renally. (See Description.) Clearance of edoxaban is decreased, and consequently, plasma concentrations are increased in patients with renal impairment. In a dedicated pharmacokinetic study in individuals with various degrees of renal dysfunction, systemic exposure of edoxaban was increased by 32, 74, and 72% in those with creatinine clearances of 51–79 mL/minute, 30–50 mL/minute, and less than 30 mL/minute, respectively, compared with that in individuals with normal renal function (creatinine clearance of at least 80 mL/minute). Systemic exposure of edoxaban was increased by 93% in patients undergoing peritoneal dialysis. Patients with creatinine clearance less than 15 mL/minute were not evaluated.

Renal function should be evaluated prior to initiating edoxaban therapy and periodically thereafter when clinically indicated. Assessment of renal function should include calculation of estimated creatinine clearance using the Cockcroft-Gault method. Recommendations regarding use and dosage of edoxaban are based on creatinine clearance. (See Dosage and Administration.) As renal function improves, plasma concentrations of edoxaban may decrease and potentially decrease efficacy of the drug. (See Reduced Efficacy in Nonvalvular Atrial Fibrillation Patients with Creatinine Clearance Exceeding 95 mL/minute under Warnings/Precautions: Warnings, in Cautions.)

Hemodialysis does not substantially contribute to clearance of edoxaban. Following a 4-hour hemodialysis session, total drug exposure was reduced by less than 7%.

■ **Common Adverse Effects** In studies in patients with nonvalvular atrial fibrillation, the most common adverse effects of edoxaban were bleeding and anemia. In studies in patients with acute venous thromboembolism, the most common adverse effects of the drug were bleeding, rash, abnormal liver function tests, and anemia.

Drug Interactions

■ **Drugs Affecting or Metabolized by Hepatic Microsomal Enzymes** Edoxaban tosylate is minimally metabolized by cytochrome P-450 (CYP) 3A4; drug interactions are unlikely with inhibitors or inducers of this isoenzyme.

In vitro studies indicate that edoxaban does not inhibit the major CYP isoenzymes (CYP1A2, 2A6, 2B6, 2C8/9, 2C19, 2D6, 2E1, or 3A4) nor induce CYP1A2 or CYP3A4; drug interactions involving these pathways are unlikely.

■ **Drugs Affecting Efflux Transport Systems** Edoxaban is a substrate of the efflux transporter P-glycoprotein, but does not appear to be a substrate of other major uptake transporters such as organic anion transporters OAT1 and OAT3, organic cation transporter OCT2, or organic anion transporting polypeptide OATP1B1. In vitro studies indicate that edoxaban does not induce the P-glycoprotein transporter. In addition, the drug does not substantially inhibit P-glycoprotein, OAT1, OAT3, OCT1, OCT2, OATP1B1, or OATP1B3.

P-glycoprotein Inhibitors Concomitant use of edoxaban with P-glycoprotein inhibitors may potentially increase edoxaban exposure; the potential for clinically important effects depends on the degree of P-glycoprotein inhibition. Drug interaction studies have demonstrated substantially increased peak plasma concentrations and systemic exposure of edoxaban when coadministered with the following potent P-glycoprotein inhibitors: ketoconazole, quinidine, verapamil, erythromycin, cyclosporine, and dronedarone. Concomitant administration of edoxaban with amiodarone, also a potent P-glycoprotein inhibitor, increased systemic exposure of edoxaban to a more modest extent. When coadministered with drugs with weaker affinity for the P-glycoprotein transporter (e.g., atorvastatin, digoxin), pharmacokinetics of edoxaban were only slightly altered.

The manufacturer states that based on criteria used in clinical studies, dosage of edoxaban should be reduced in patients with acute venous thromboembolism who are receiving certain P-glycoprotein inhibitors; in the Hokusai VTE trial, dosage of edoxaban was reduced for concomitant therapy with verapamil, quinidine, azithromycin, clarithromycin, erythromycin, oral itraconazole, and oral ketoconazole. (See Dosage and Administration: Dosage.) In patients with nonvalvular atrial fibrillation, no edoxaban dosage adjustment is necessary for concomitant P-glycoprotein inhibitors since patients in whom such dosages were adjusted in the ENGAGE AF-TIMI 48 trial had lower plasma edoxaban concentrations than those who received the full dosage of the drug.

P-glycoprotein Inducers Concomitant use of edoxaban with P-glycoprotein inducers may potentially decrease edoxaban exposure. Systemic exposure of edoxaban was substantially reduced when the drug was coadministered with rifampin, a known P-glycoprotein inducer; the manufacturer states that concomitant use of edoxaban and rifampin should be avoided.

■ **Drugs Affecting Hemostasis** Concomitant use of drugs that affect hemostasis (e.g., aspirin or other antiplatelet agents, other anticoagulants, fibrinolytics, nonsteroidal anti-inflammatory agents [NSAIAs]) can increase the risk of bleeding associated with edoxaban. (See Bleeding under Warnings/Precautions: Other Warnings and Precautions, in Cautions.)

Anticoagulant Agents When edoxaban was administered concomitantly with enoxaparin, no substantial changes in the pharmacokinetics of either drug were observed.

Because of the risk of bleeding, long-term concomitant use of edoxaban and other anticoagulants is not recommended; however, short-term concomitant therapy may be necessary in patients transitioning from one anticoagulant to another.

Antiplatelet Agents In a study in healthy individuals, bleeding time was increased by approximately twofold from baseline when edoxaban and aspirin (100 or 325 mg) were administered concomitantly relative to administration of either drug alone. The higher dose of aspirin (325 mg) increased peak plasma concentrations and systemic exposure of edoxaban, but the lower aspirin dose did not affect pharmacokinetics of edoxaban. The anticoagulant effects of edoxaban (i.e., activated partial thromboplastin time [aPTT], prothrombin time [PT], international normalized ratio [INR], anti-factor Xa activity, intrinsic factor Xa activity) were not altered by aspirin.

In clinical studies, patients who received edoxaban and aspirin concurrently had increased rates of clinically relevant bleeding; patients requiring chronic treatment with aspirin during edoxaban therapy should be carefully monitored for bleeding.

NSAIAs In a study in healthy individuals, concomitant administration of edoxaban and naproxen (500 mg) increased bleeding time by approximately twofold from baseline relative to administration of either drug alone. Naproxen did not alter the pharmacokinetics or anticoagulant effects (i.e., as indicated by aPTT, PT, INR, anti-factor Xa activity, intrinsic factor Xa activity) of edoxaban.

In clinical studies, patients who received edoxaban and NSAIAs concurrently had increased rates of clinically relevant bleeding; patients requiring long-term treatment with an NSAIA during edoxaban therapy should be carefully monitored for bleeding.

■ **Amiodarone** Peak plasma concentrations and systemic exposure of edoxaban increased by approximately 66 and 40%, respectively, when the drug was administered concomitantly with amiodarone. (See Drug Interactions: Drugs Affecting Efflux Transport Systems.)

■ **Atorvastatin** Peak plasma concentrations of edoxaban were decreased by 14.2% and systemic exposure increased by 1.7% when the drug was administered concomitantly with atorvastatin. (See Drug Interactions: Drugs Affecting Efflux Transport Systems.)

■ **Azole Antifungals** Peak plasma concentrations and systemic exposure of edoxaban were substantially increased with concomitant administration of ketoconazole. Dosage of edoxaban should be reduced when administered concomitantly with oral itraconazole or oral ketoconazole in patients with venous thromboembolism. (See Drug Interactions: Drugs Affecting Efflux Transport Systems.)

■ **Cyclosporine** Peak plasma concentrations and systemic exposure of edoxaban were substantially increased with concomitant administration of cyclosporine. (See Drug Interactions: Drugs Affecting Efflux Transport Systems.)

■ **Digoxin** In healthy individuals, concomitant administration of edoxaban and digoxin did not substantially affect peak plasma concentrations or systemic exposure of edoxaban. Although peak plasma concentrations of digoxin were increased by 28%, such concentrations remained within the established therapeutic range. Clinically important changes in the pharmacodynamics of either drug were not observed.

■ **Dronedarone** Dronedarone increased peak plasma concentrations and systemic exposure of edoxaban by approximately 46 and 85%, respectively. (See Drug Interactions: Drugs Affecting Efflux Transport Systems.)

■ **Esomeprazole** Peak plasma concentrations of edoxaban were decreased with concomitant administration of esomeprazole; however, systemic exposure of edoxaban was not substantially affected.

■ **Macrolide Antibiotics** Peak plasma concentrations and systemic exposure of edoxaban were substantially increased with concomitant administration of erythromycin. Dosage of edoxaban should be reduced when the drug is administered concomitantly with erythromycin, azithromycin, or clarithromycin in patients with venous thromboembolism. (See Drug Interactions: Drugs Affecting Efflux Transport Systems.)

■ **Quinidine** Quinidine increased peak plasma concentrations and systemic exposure of edoxaban by approximately 85 and 77%, respectively, but edoxaban did not affect pharmacokinetics of quinidine. Dosage of edoxaban should be reduced when the drug is administered concomitantly with quinidine in patients with venous thromboembolism. (See Drug Interactions: Drugs Affecting Efflux Transport Systems.)

■ **Verapamil** Verapamil increased peak plasma concentrations and systemic exposure of edoxaban by approximately 53%; pharmacokinetic parameters of verapamil were altered to only a slight extent. Dosage of edoxaban should be reduced when the drug is administered concomitantly with verapamil in patients with venous thromboembolism. (See Drug Interactions: Drugs Affecting Efflux Transport Systems.)

Description

Edoxaban tosylate monohydrate, an oral, direct activated factor X (Xa) inhibitor, is an anticoagulant. Factor Xa plays a central role in the blood coagulation cascade by serving as the convergence point for the intrinsic and extrinsic pathways; inhibition of coagulation factor Xa by edoxaban prevents conversion of prothrombin to thrombin and subsequent thrombus formation. The drug binds directly and selectively to factor Xa without the need for a cofactor (e.g., antithrombin III), and inhibits both free and prothrombinase-bound factor Xa as well as thrombin-induced platelet aggregation.

Edoxaban inhibits factor Xa activity, and prolongs prothrombin time (PT), activated partial thromboplastin time (aPTT), and the international normalized ratio (INR) in a dose-dependent manner. A rapid and predictable anticoagulant effect is demonstrated by linear correlations between plasma edoxaban concentrations and coagulation parameters.

Edoxaban exhibits dose-proportional pharmacokinetics over the dosage range of 10–150 mg daily. The drug is rapidly absorbed following oral administration, with peak plasma concentrations occurring within 1–3 hours. The absolute bioavailability of the drug is approximately 62%. It is not known whether the bioavailability is altered when edoxaban tablets are crushed and/or mixed with food, liquids, or administered through feeding tubes. Food delays absorption, but does not substantially alter systemic exposure of edoxaban. Approximately 50% of edoxaban is excreted unchanged in urine; the remainder is metabolized (minimally by hydrolysis, conjugation, and cytochrome P-450 [CYP] 3A4) and eliminated through biliary and intestinal routes. The terminal half-life of edoxaban is approximately 10–14 hours. Edoxaban is approximately 55% bound to plasma proteins. Systemic exposure of the drug is increased in patients with renal impairment and low body weight, but does not appear to be affected by age, gender, or race/ethnicity.

Advice to Patients

Importance of patients taking edoxaban tosylate exactly as prescribed and not discontinuing therapy without first consulting a clinician.

Importance of informing patients that they may bruise and/or bleed more easily and that a longer than normal time may be required to stop bleeding when taking edoxaban. Importance of informing clinicians about any unusual bleeding or bruising during therapy.

Importance of advising patients that if a dose is missed, it should be taken as soon as possible on the same day and the regular dosing schedule should be resumed the following day. A dose should not be doubled to make up for a missed dose.

Importance of advising patients undergoing neuraxial anesthesia or spinal puncture procedures to monitor for manifestations of spinal or epidural hematoma (e.g., tingling or numbness in lower limbs, muscle weakness, back pain, stool or urine incontinence); importance of immediately contacting a clinician if any of these symptoms occur.

Importance of patients informing clinicians that they are receiving edoxaban therapy before scheduling any medical, surgical, or invasive procedure, including dental procedures.

Importance of women immediately informing clinicians if they are or plan to become pregnant or plan to breast-feed.

Importance of informing clinicians of existing or contemplated concomitant therapy, including prescription and OTC drugs and herbal supplements.

Importance of informing patients of other important precautionary information. (See Cautions.)

Overview® (see Users Guide). For additional information on this drug until a more detailed monograph is developed and published, the manufacturer's labeling should be consulted. It is *essential* that the manufacturer's labeling be consulted for more detailed information on usual cautions, precautions, contraindications, potential drug interactions, laboratory test interferences, and acute toxicity.

Preparations

Excipients in commercially available drug preparations may have clinically important effects in some individuals; consult specific product labeling for details.

Edoxaban Tosylate

Oral

Tablets	15 mg (of edoxaban)	**Savaysa®**, Daiichi Sankyo
	30 mg (of edoxaban)	**Savaysa®**, Daiichi Sankyo
	60 mg (of edoxaban)	**Savaysa®**, Daiichi Sankyo

Rivaroxaban

■ Rivaroxaban, an oral, direct activated factor X (Xa) inhibitor, is an anticoagulant.

Uses

■ **Embolism Associated with Atrial Fibrillation** Rivaroxaban is used to reduce the risk of stroke and systemic embolism in patients with nonvalvular atrial fibrillation. Current evidence suggests that rivaroxaban is no less effective than warfarin for prevention of stroke and systemic embolism in patients with nonvalvular atrial fibrillation and does not increase the risk of major bleeding relative to warfarin. However, there are limited data on the relative efficacy of rivaroxaban and warfarin for the reduction of stroke and systemic embolism when warfarin anticoagulation is well controlled. Efficacy of rivaroxaban for the prevention of postcardioversion stroke and systemic embolism in patients with atrial fibrillation has not been established. Efficacy and safety of the drug in patients with prosthetic heart valves also have not been established. (See Patients with Prosthetic Heart Valves under Warnings/Precautions: Other Warnings and Precautions, in Cautions.)

The American College of Chest Physicians (ACCP), the American College of Cardiology (ACC), the American Heart Association (AHA), the American Stroke Association (ASA), and other experts currently recommend that antithrombotic therapy be administered to all patients with nonvalvular atrial fibrillation (i.e., atrial fibrillation in the absence of rheumatic mitral stenosis, a prosthetic heart valve, or mitral valve repair) who are considered to be at increased risk of stroke, unless such therapy is contraindicated. Recommendations regarding choice of antithrombotic therapy are based on the patient's risk for stroke and bleeding. In general, oral anticoagulant therapy is recommended in patients with atrial fibrillation who have a moderate to high risk for stroke and acceptably low risk of bleeding, while aspirin or no antithrombotic therapy may be considered in patients at low risk of stroke. Although many risk stratification methods have been used, patients considered to be at increased risk of stroke generally include those with prior ischemic stroke or transient ischemic attack (TIA), advanced age (e.g., 75 years or older), history of hypertension, diabetes mellitus, or congestive heart failure. In addition, population-based studies suggest that female sex is an important risk factor for stroke in patients with atrial fibrillation, particularly in patients 75 years of age or older, and AHA and ASA recommend the use of risk stratification tools that account for age- and sex-specific differences in stroke risk. One such tool is the CHA_2DS_2-VASc score, an extension of the $CHADS_2$ system (which considers the risk factors congestive heart failure, hypertension, age 75 years or older, diabetes mellitus, and prior stroke/TIA) that adds extra points for female sex (1 point); previous myocardial infarction, peripheral arterial disease, or aortic plaque (1 point); and age 65–74 years (1 point) or 75 years or older (2 points).

The risk of thromboembolism in patients with atrial flutter is not as well established as it is in those with atrial fibrillation. In addition, many patients with atrial flutter have alternating periods of atrial fibrillation. Experts state that antithrombotic therapy in patients with atrial flutter generally should be managed in the same manner as in patients with atrial fibrillation.

Warfarin traditionally has been used for oral anticoagulation in patients with atrial fibrillation at increased risk of stroke; however, experts currently state that non-vitamin K antagonist oral anticoagulants such as rivaroxaban provide advantages over warfarin (e.g., potentially less major bleeding risk, rapid onset of action, predictable anticoagulant effect, no requirement for coagulation monitoring, less potential for drug-drug and drug-food interactions). Rivaroxaban may be particularly useful in patients at moderate to high risk of stroke who are unable to comply with warfarin monitoring requirements or in whom a consistent therapeutic response to warfarin cannot be achieved (e.g., because of drug or food interactions), while warfarin may continue to be preferred in patients who have well-controlled international normalized ratios (INRs) (e.g., INR in the therapeutic range more than 70% of the time) and are compliant with regular laboratory monitoring. However, because of the lack of direct, comparative studies, the relative efficacy and safety of rivaroxaban and other non-vitamin K antagonist oral anticoagulants (e.g., apixaban, dabigatran, edoxaban) used for the prevention of stroke in patients with nonvalvular atrial fibrillation has not been fully elucidated. Some evidence from indirect comparisons suggests that there may be important differences (e.g., bleeding risk) between these agents; however, results of such analyses should be interpreted with caution because of possible confounding factors (e.g., differences in study design and methods, patient populations, and anticoagulation control). AHA and ASA state that while clinical trials of non-vitamin K antagonist oral anticoagulants were not designed to determine differences in efficacy compared with warfarin in men versus women, apixaban, dabigatran, or rivaroxaban may be a useful alternative to warfarin for the prevention of stroke and systemic thromboembolism in women with paroxysmal or permanent atrial fibrillation and prespecified risk factors (according to CHA_2DS_2-VASc) who do not have a prosthetic heart valve or hemodynamically important valve disease, severe renal failure (creatinine clearance less than 15 mL/minute), lower body weight (less than 50 kg), or advanced liver disease (impaired baseline clotting function).

When selecting an appropriate anticoagulant in patients with atrial fibrillation, the relative risks versus benefits should be considered for individual patients based on factors such as the absolute and relative risks of stroke and bleeding; patient compliance, preference, tolerance, and comorbidities; cost; availability of agents to reverse anticoagulant effects in case of bleeding complications; and other clinical factors such as renal function, availability of facilities to monitor INR; and degree of current INR control in patients already receiving warfarin. For additional information on antithrombotic therapy in patients with atrial fibrillation, see Uses: Embolism Associated with Atrial Fibrillation in Warfarin 20:12.04.08.

Efficacy and safety of rivaroxaban for the prevention of stroke and systemic embolism in patients with nonvalvular atrial fibrillation were evaluated in a randomized, double-blind, noninferiority study (ROCKET AF) in approximately 14,000 adults with nonvalvular atrial fibrillation who were considered to be at moderate to high risk of stroke (defined as having a history of stroke, TIA, non-CNS systemic embolism, or at least 2 of the following additional risk factors: age 75 years or older, hypertension, heart failure or left ventricular ejection fraction of 35% or less, or diabetes mellitus). The study population consisted principally of Caucasian men with a mean age of 71 years and a mean Congestive Heart Failure, Hypertension, Age, Diabetes, Stroke (doubled) (i.e., $CHADS_2$) score of 3.5; approximately 55% of patients had a history of stroke, TIA, or non-CNS systemic embolism. Patients received either rivaroxaban (20 mg once daily for those with a creatinine clearance of at least 50 mL/minute or 15 mg once daily for those with a creatinine clearance of 30–49 mL/minute) or adjusted-dose warfarin (titrated to an international normalized ratio [INR] of 2–3) for a median duration of 590 days; median follow-up was 707 days.

The primary composite end point of the study was the incidence of stroke (hemorrhagic or ischemic) and non-CNS systemic embolism. The primary efficacy analysis was performed in the per-protocol (as-treated) population, which included all patients who received at least one dose of a study drug, did not have a major protocol violation, and were followed for events while receiving a study drug or within 2 days after discontinuance of the drug. Outcome analyses also were performed in the intent-to-treat (per-randomization) population, which included all patients who underwent randomization and were followed for events during treatment or following premature discontinuance, and the safety population, which included all patients who received at least one dose of a study drug and were followed for events while they were receiving study drug or within 2 days after discontinuation, regardless of protocol adherence. Testing for superiority was performed if noninferiority was achieved.

Rivaroxaban was noninferior to warfarin for the primary composite outcome of time to first occurrence of stroke or non-CNS systemic embolism; noninferiority was demonstrated in both the per-protocol and intent-to-treat populations. Efficacy of rivaroxaban was consistent across a variety of patient subgroups, including in those with renal insufficiency, different $CHADS_2$ scores, prior warfarin use, and history of stroke. Superiority of rivaroxaban over warfarin was not demonstrated in the intent-to-treat population in this study; the rate of stroke or non-CNS systemic embolism with rivaroxaban therapy was no different than that observed with warfarin therapy (annualized event rate of 2.1 and 2.4% of patients, respectively). However, superiority of rivaroxaban over warfarin was shown in the as-treated safety population. This difference in the results of superiority testing may be explained by the inclusion of embolic events in patients who discontinued drug treatment prematurely as well as those occurring during study drug treatment in the intent-to-treat population, while analysis of the per-protocol population only included events that occurred during drug treatment and for 2 days after drug discontinuance. In addition, a requirement for anticoagulation following study drug discontinuance was not specified in the ROCKET AF protocol; however, patients in the warfarin group generally continued to receive warfarin after the treatment portion of the study, while those who had received rivaroxaban during the treatment portion were switched to warfarin without a period of overlap and therefore were not adequately anticoagulated until a therapeutic INR with warfarin was obtained. During the 28 days following the end of the study, a higher incidence of stroke was observed in patients who had received rivaroxaban compared with those who had received warfarin. (See Risk of Thrombosis Following Premature Discontinuance of Anticoagulation under Warnings/Precautions: Warnings, in Cautions.) There was no statistically significant difference in the risk of major and nonmajor clinically important bleeding between the treatment groups, although intracranial and fatal bleeding occurred less frequently in patients receiving rivaroxaban.

Patients who received warfarin in the ROCKET AF study had INRs within the therapeutic range of 2–3 only 55% of the time on average, which is lower than that reported with warfarin anticoagulation in other trials of non-vitamin K antagonist oral anticoagulants (e.g., dabigatran, apixaban) in patients with atrial fibrillation (e.g., 62–64%). It has been suggested that this difference may be explained in part by the inclusion of a higher-risk patient population in the ROCKET AF trial or to geographic variations among the study sites with respect to warfarin anticoagulation management skills. Therefore, data currently are insufficient to establish the relative efficacy of rivaroxaban and warfarin for the reduction of stroke and systemic embolism when warfarin therapy is well controlled.

■ Deep-Vein Thrombosis and Pulmonary Embolism

Prophylaxis **Major Orthopedic Surgery.** Rivaroxaban is used for the prevention of postoperative deep-vein thrombosis (DVT), which may lead to pulmonary embolism (PE), in patients undergoing total hip- or knee-replacement surgery.

ACCP recommends routine thromboprophylaxis in all patients undergoing major orthopedic surgery, including total hip- or knee-replacement surgery, because of the high risk of postoperative venous thromboembolism. According to ACCP, thromboprophylaxis with an appropriate antithrombotic agent or an intermittent pneumatic compression device should be continued for at least 10–14 days and possibly for up to 35 days after surgery. ACCP and other clinicians consider rivaroxaban to be an acceptable option for pharmacologic thromboprophylaxis in patients undergoing total hip- or knee-replacement surgery, although ACCP suggests that a low molecular weight heparin generally is preferred because of its relative efficacy and safety and extensive clinical experience. Rivaroxaban may be a reasonable choice in situations in which a low molecular weight heparin is not available or cannot be used (e.g., in patients with heparin-induced thrombocytopenia or in those who refuse or are uncooperative with subcutaneous injections). ACCP states that when selecting an appropriate thromboprophylaxis regimen, factors such as relative efficacy and bleeding risk as well as logistics and compliance issues should be considered. For additional details on prevention of venous thromboembolism in patients undergoing major orthopedic surgery, consult the most recent ACCP Evidence-based Clinical Practice Guidelines on Antithrombotic Therapy and Prevention of Thrombosis available at http://www.chestnet.org.

Efficacy and safety of rivaroxaban for the prevention of postoperative venous thromboembolism after major orthopedic surgery are based principally on the results of 4 randomized, double-blind, double-dummy trials known as the RECORD (Regulation of Coagulation in Orthopedic Surgery to Prevent Deep-vein Thrombosis and Pulmonary Embolism) trials. In these trials, rivaroxaban was more effective than subcutaneous enoxaparin in preventing venous thromboembolism in patients undergoing elective total hip-replacement

(RECORD 1 and 2) or total knee-replacement (RECORD 3 and 4) surgery and was associated with similar rates of bleeding. The primary efficacy and safety end points in all 4 trials were identical; however, there were differences with respect to dosage and duration of enoxaparin therapy. Patients received oral rivaroxaban (10 mg once daily initiated at least 6–8 hours after surgery) or subcutaneous enoxaparin sodium (40 mg once daily initiated 12 hours before surgery and resumed 6–8 hours after wound closure in RECORD 1, 2, and 3, or 30 mg twice daily initiated 12 hours before surgery and resumed 12–24 hours after wound closure in RECORD 4). Treatment generally was continued for 31–39 days in the hip-replacement trials and for 10–14 days in the knee-replacement trials. However, in RECORD 2, the duration of active drug treatments was different; rivaroxaban was administered for 31–39 (mean 33.5) days (with placebo injection for 10–14 days) while enoxaparin was administered for 10–14 (mean 12.4) days (with placebo tablets for 31–39 days).

In all 4 RECORD trials, the incidence of the composite primary outcome of DVT (symptomatic or venographic), nonfatal PE, and all-cause mortality was substantially lower in patients receiving rivaroxaban than in those receiving enoxaparin. Treatment with rivaroxaban resulted in relative risk reductions for venous thromboembolism of 70 and 79%, respectively, in patients undergoing hip replacement in RECORD 1 and 2, and relative risk reductions of 49 and 31%, respectively, in patients undergoing knee replacement in RECORD 3 and 4. Rivaroxaban was generally well tolerated across all trials and rates of major bleeding or any bleeding event were generally similar between treatment groups.

Some clinicians have suggested that the observed differences in outcome between the rivaroxaban and enoxaparin groups in the RECORD trials were influenced by differences in dosage and/or duration of enoxaparin therapy. In RECORD 1–3, an enoxaparin sodium dosage of 40 mg once daily was used, while the preferred dosage for thromboprophylaxis after hip-replacement surgery and the only recommended dosage for knee-replacement surgery in the US is 30 mg every 12 hours (i.e., twice daily), which was used only in the RECORD 4 trial. In addition, enoxaparin was given for an average of approximately 2 weeks versus approximately 5 weeks for rivaroxaban in the RECORD 2 trial. It has been suggested that use of a potentially suboptimal enoxaparin sodium dosage of 40 mg daily in RECORD 1–3 and an unequal (shorter) duration of enoxaparin therapy in RECORD 2 may have contributed to the increased risk of the primary efficacy end point with enoxaparin in these trials. In addition, in RECORD 3, which employed the 40-mg once-daily dosage of enoxaparin sodium in patients undergoing total knee replacement, there was an absolute risk difference of 9.2% favoring rivaroxaban for the primary end point (any DVT, nonfatal PE, and all-cause mortality in the modified intent-to-treat population), while in RECORD 4, which employed the US FDA-labeled enoxaparin sodium dosage of 30 mg every 12 hours for the same indication, the absolute risk difference favoring rivaroxaban for the same primary end point was only 3.2%. In an attempt to account for differences in study design among the RECORD trials, an analysis of pooled data that used only the period of active treatment common to all 4 trials (the 12 ± 2 days in which enoxaparin was administered) as the primary efficacy end point was performed; results of this analysis supported those of the individual trials with regard to the greater efficacy of rivaroxaban versus enoxaparin for reduction of total venous thromboembolism.

In the RECORD trials, use of a definition of major bleeding that did not include surgical site bleeding unless it necessitated reoperation or resulted in death may have resulted in a more conservative estimate of bleeding risk in these trials than in other comparative studies of other non-vitamin K antagonist oral anticoagulants and enoxaparin. Differences in the timing of initiation of rivaroxaban and enoxaparin therapy (preoperatively in RECORD 1–3; 6–8 hours postoperatively for rivaroxaban versus 12–24 hours postoperatively for enoxaparin in RECORD 4) potentially could have affected relative bleeding risk. The overall incidence of major bleeding in the RECORD trials was low (less than 1%), and these trials were not designed with enough statistical power to demonstrate differences in the end point of major bleeding. However, there was a trend toward increased bleeding events (numerically more frequent) with rivaroxaban in the RECORD trials. In a pooled analysis of data from all 4 trials, a small but statistically significant increase in the end point of major plus clinically relevant nonmajor bleeding was demonstrated for rivaroxaban versus enoxaparin in the total treatment duration pool; however, analysis of the active treatment pool at day 12±2 (i.e., the enoxaparin-controlled period common to all 4 RECORD studies) did not reveal a statistically significant difference in bleeding between the 2 groups.

The manufacturer states that rivaroxaban is not recommended acutely (as an alternative to heparin) in patients with PE who have hemodynamic instability or who may receive thrombolytic therapy or undergo pulmonary embolectomy. (See Patients with Pulmonary Embolism under Warnings/Precautions: Other Warnings and Precautions, in Cautions.)

Treatment and Secondary Prevention Rivaroxaban is used for the initial treatment of acute DVT and/or PE. The drug also is used beyond the initial 6 months of treatment to reduce the risk of recurrent venous thromboembolic events (secondary prevention) in patients with DVT and/or PE.

Rivaroxaban is recommended by ACCP and other experts as an acceptable option for initial and long-term anticoagulant therapy in patients with acute proximal DVT of the leg and/or PE. In such patients, ACCP recommends that anticoagulant therapy be continued beyond the acute treatment period for at least 3 months, and possibly longer depending on the individual clinical situation (e.g., location of thrombi, presence or absence of precipitating factors, presence of cancer, patient's risk of bleeding). Rivaroxaban may offer some advantages over other anticoagulant drugs for the treatment of venous thromboembolism (e.g., oral administration, no requirement for routine coagulation monitoring, minimal drug and food interactions). The relative efficacy and safety of rivaroxaban versus other non-vitamin K antagonist oral anticoagulants (e.g., apixaban, dabigatran) for the treatment of venous thromboembolism remains to be fully elucidated. For additional information on treatment of venous thromboembolism, consult the most recent ACCP Evidence-based Clinical Practice Guidelines on Antithrombotic Therapy and Prevention of Thrombosis available at http://www.chestnet.org.

In 2 randomized, open-label, noninferiority studies (EINSTEIN DVT and EINSTEIN PE) designed to evaluate efficacy and safety of rivaroxaban for the initial treatment and secondary prevention of venous thromboembolism, treatment with rivaroxaban was noninferior to therapy with enoxaparin and a vitamin K antagonist in preventing recurrent thromboembolic events. Patients in the studies were given either rivaroxaban (15 mg twice daily for 3 weeks, followed by 20 mg once daily) or a standard anticoagulant regimen consisting of enoxaparin sodium (1 mg/kg subcutaneously twice daily for at least 5 days), followed by a vitamin K antagonist (warfarin or acenocoumarol adjusted to maintain an INR of 2–3). The average duration of therapy in both treatment groups was approximately 200 days. The primary efficacy outcome in these studies was a composite of symptomatic recurrent DVT or nonfatal or fatal PE. The primary efficacy outcome (based on the intent-to-treat population) occurred in 2.1 or 3% of patients receiving rivaroxaban or standard therapy, respectively, in the EINSTEIN DVT study, and in 2.1 or 1.8% of patients receiving rivaroxaban or standard therapy, respectively, in the EINSTEIN PE study. The incidence of major and clinically relevant nonmajor bleeding was similar between the treatment groups.

In a double-blind, placebo-controlled extension study (EINSTEIN EXT) in patients who had already completed a course of anticoagulant therapy with rivaroxaban or a vitamin K antagonist, continued treatment with rivaroxaban was substantially more effective than placebo in reducing the rate of recurrent DVT, nonfatal PE, or fatal PE. Patients in the extension study received rivaroxaban 20 mg daily or placebo for an additional 6 or 12 months (average duration of 190 days). Recurrent thromboembolism occurred in 1.3% of patients receiving rivaroxaban compared with 7.1% of those receiving placebo. Major bleeding occurred in 0.7% of patients in the rivaroxaban group and in none of the patients in the placebo group.

In the Reduced-dosed Rivaroxaban in the Long-term Prevention of Recurrent Symptomatic Venous Thromboembolism (EINSTEIN CHOICE) study in patients requiring extended anticoagulation following an acute venous thromboembolic event, continued treatment with a prophylactic dose of rivaroxaban (10 mg once daily) was substantially more effective than low-dose aspirin (100 mg once daily) in reducing the risk of a recurrent thromboembolic event (DVT or PE), without a substantial increase in bleeding, in patients who had already completed a course of anticoagulant therapy. Patients in this study had been treated previously with a vitamin K antagonist or a direct oral anticoagulant agent (e.g., dabigatran, rivaroxaban, apixaban, edoxaban) for a provoked or unprovoked venous thromboembolism (51% DVT only, 33% PE only, 16% combined DVT and PE). Patients entered into the study received 10 or 20 mg of rivaroxaban or 100 mg of aspirin (enteric-coated) once daily for up to 1 year following the initial 6–12 months of anticoagulant therapy. Patients who required extended anticoagulation therapy at therapeutic doses or antiplatelet therapy were excluded from this study. The primary efficacy outcome was a composite of symptomatic, recurrent fatal or nonfatal venous thromboembolism and unexplained death, and the main safety outcome was major bleeding.

Compared with low-dose aspirin, rivaroxaban 10 or 20 mg once daily reduced the relative risk of recurrent venous thromboembolism or unexplained death by approximately 70%. A primary efficacy outcome event occurred in 13 of 1127 patients (1.2%) who were receiving the 10-mg daily dosage of rivaroxaban compared with 50 of 1131 patients (4.4%) who were receiving aspirin. An increased incidence of bleeding, including major and clinically important nonmajor bleeding, was observed in patients who received continued treatment with rivaroxaban at a treatment dosage (20 mg once daily) compared with those who received a prophylactic dosage of rivaroxaban (10 mg once daily) or aspirin (100 mg once daily). Major bleeding occurred in 5 or 6 patients (0.4 or 0.5%) in the 10- or 20-mg rivaroxaban group compared with 3 patients (0.3%) in the aspirin group.

Additional studies and experience are needed to evaluate the efficacy and safety of rivaroxaban for the treatment of cancer-related venous thromboembolism; relatively few patients with cancer were included in the principal efficacy studies evaluating rivaroxaban for the treatment and secondary prevention of venous thromboembolism.

■ Chronic Coronary Artery Disease or Peripheral Artery Disease

Rivaroxaban is used in conjunction with aspirin to reduce the risk of major cardiovascular events (e.g., cardiovascular death, myocardial infarction [MI], stroke) in patients with chronic coronary artery disease (CAD) or peripheral artery disease (PAD).

Efficacy and safety of rivaroxaban for this indication are based principally on the results of a randomized, double-blind, study known as the COMPASS (Cardiovascular Outcomes for People using Anticoagulation Strategies) study. In this study, adults (mean age: 68 years) with established CAD and/or PAD (91% had CAD, 27% had PAD, 18% had both) who received rivaroxaban (2.5 mg orally twice daily) in conjunction with aspirin (100 mg once daily) had better cardiovascular outcomes at the cost of an increase in major bleeding events compared with those receiving aspirin alone. Treatment with 5 mg of rivaroxaban twice daily alone was not superior to aspirin alone in terms of cardiovascular outcomes and was associated with an increase in major bleeding.

Patients in this study received rivaroxaban 2.5 mg orally twice daily plus aspirin 100 mg once daily, rivaroxaban 5 mg orally twice daily, or aspirin 100 mg once daily. The primary efficacy end point was the composite of cardiovascular death, stroke, or MI, and the primary safety outcome included fatal bleeding, symptomatic bleeding into a critical organ, bleeding into a surgical site requiring reoperation, and bleeding that led to hospitalization. Secondary efficacy end points included the composite of ischemic stroke, MI, acute limb ischemia, or death from coronary heart disease; the composite of ischemic stroke, MI, acute limb ischemia, or cardiovascular death; and death from any cause.

The incidence of the composite primary outcome of cardiovascular death, stroke, or MI was 24% lower in patients receiving rivaroxaban 2.5 mg twice daily in conjunction with aspirin than in those receiving aspirin alone (event rate 4.1 versus 5.4%). The beneficial effects of rivaroxaban plus aspirin therapy were observed early and the study was terminated early; the mean duration of follow-up was 23 months. Major bleeding occurred in substantially more patients receiving rivaroxaban 2.5 mg twice daily in conjunction with aspirin compared with aspirin alone (event rate 1.6 versus 0.9%). The secondary composite outcome of ischemic stroke, MI, acute limb ischemia, or death from coronary heart disease occurred in fewer patients who received rivaroxaban 2.5 mg twice daily in conjunction with aspirin than in those who received aspirin alone (event rate 3.6 versus 4.9%). The secondary outcome of ischemic stroke, MI, acute limb ischemia, or cardiovascular death also occurred in fewer patients receiving rivaroxaban 2.5 mg twice daily in conjunction with aspirin compared with those who received aspirin alone (event rate 4.3 versus 5.7%). All-cause mortality was higher among those who received aspirin alone compared with those who received rivaroxaban 2.5 mg twice daily in conjunction with aspirin (event rate 4.1 versus 3.4%).

Dosage and Administration

■ **General** Routine coagulation monitoring (e.g., prothrombin time [PT], activated partial thromboplastin time [aPTT], international normalized ratio [INR]) is not necessary during rivaroxaban therapy because of the drug's predictable pharmacokinetic and pharmacodynamic effects. However, in certain situations, such as in the case of overdosage or in patients with hemorrhagic or thromboembolic complications, it may be useful to assess the degree of anticoagulation. It has been suggested that the PT test may be used to assess rivaroxaban plasma concentrations since the drug prolongs PT in a concentration-dependent manner; however, PT test results may vary depending on the type of reagent and may not be a reliable indicator of the degree of anticoagulation with rivaroxaban. The INR is calibrated specifically for vitamin K antagonists (e.g., warfarin) and should not be used to monitor the effects of rivaroxaban.

■ **Administration** Rivaroxaban is administered orally. The manufacturer states that the 15- or 20-mg tablets should be taken with food; the 2.5- or 10-mg tablet may be administered with or without food. If a 2.5-mg dose of rivaroxaban is missed, the patient should take a single 2.5-mg dose as recommended at the next scheduled time. If a dose is missed in patients receiving a dosage of 10, 15, or 20 mg once daily, the missed dose should be taken immediately. The dose should not be doubled within the same day to make up for a missed dose. If a dose is missed in patients receiving a dosage of 15 mg twice daily, a dose of rivaroxaban should be taken immediately upon remembering; if necessary, two 15-mg tablets may be taken at the same time to ensure full intake of the 30-mg daily dose. The regular twice-daily dosing schedule should then be resumed the following day. (See Advice to Patients.)

In patients who are unable to swallow whole tablets, rivaroxaban tablets may be crushed and mixed with applesauce immediately before administration. When given orally as a crushed 15- or 20-mg tablet, the dose of rivaroxaban should be followed immediately by food. In patients requiring a nasogastric or gastric feeding tube, after confirming placement of the tube, rivaroxaban tablets should be administered by crushing and suspending the drug in 50 mL of water; enteral feeding via the tube should immediately follow administration of the 15- or 20-mg tablet. Crushed rivaroxaban tablets are stable in water or in applesauce for up to 4 hours.

Because of the possibility of reduced absorption and thereby reduced drug exposure, rivaroxaban should *not* be administered by a method that could deposit the drug distal to the stomach. (See Description.)

■ **Dosage** ***Embolism Associated with Atrial Fibrillation*** For reduction of the risk of stroke and systemic embolism in adults with nonvalvular atrial fibrillation, the recommended dosage of rivaroxaban in patients without renal impairment (creatinine clearance exceeding 50 mL/minute) is 20 mg once daily with the evening meal.

Deep-Vein Thrombosis and Pulmonary Embolism **Thromboprophylaxis in Hip- or Knee-Replacement Surgery.** For prophylaxis of deep-vein thrombosis (DVT) and associated pulmonary embolism (PE) in adults who have undergone hip- or knee-replacement surgery, the recommended dosage of rivaroxaban is 10 mg once daily. The initial dose should be administered at least 6–10 hours after surgery, provided hemostasis has been established. The recommended duration of rivaroxaban therapy is 35 days for patients undergoing hip-replacement surgery and 12 days for patients undergoing knee-replacement surgery.

Treatment and Secondary Prevention. The recommended dosage of rivaroxaban for the *treatment* of acute DVT and/or PE is 15 mg orally twice daily for the first 21 days, followed by 20 mg once daily taken at approximately the same time every day with food. The initial twice-daily dosing regimen provides higher trough drug concentrations and may be associated with improved thrombus regression compared with a once-daily regimen.

To reduce the risk of recurrent venous thromboembolism (*secondary prevention*) after an initial 6 months or more of standard anticoagulant (e.g,. vitamin K antagonist, direct-acting oral anticoagulant) treatment in patients at continued risk for DVT and/or PE, the recommended dosage of rivaroxaban is 10 mg once daily taken at approximately the same time every day with or without food.

The optimum duration of anticoagulant therapy should be determined by the individual clinical situation (e.g., location of thrombi, presence or absence of precipitating factors for thrombosis, presence of cancer, risk of bleeding). In general, the American College of Chest Physicians (ACCP) states that anticoagulant therapy should be continued beyond the acute treatment period for at least 3 months and possibly longer in patients with a high risk of recurrence and low risk of bleeding.

Chronic Coronary Artery Disease or Peripheral Artery Disease To reduce the risk of major cardiovascular events (e.g., cardiovascular death, myocardial infarction [MI], stroke) in patients with chronic coronary artery disease (CAD) or peripheral artery disease (PAD), the recommended dosage of rivaroxaban is 2.5 mg *twice* daily in conjunction with aspirin 75–100 mg *once* daily with or without food.

Transitioning to and from Rivaroxaban Therapy When switching from warfarin to rivaroxaban therapy, the manufacturer states that warfarin should be discontinued and rivaroxaban initiated as soon as the INR is less than 3 to avoid periods of inadequate anticoagulation. When transitioning to rivaroxaban from therapy with other anticoagulants (e.g., low molecular weight heparin, oral anticoagulant other than warfarin), the initial dose of rivaroxaban should be administered within 2 hours of the next scheduled evening dose of the other anticoagulant, and the other anticoagulant should be discontinued. When transitioning to rivaroxaban from heparin given by continuous IV infusion, the heparin infusion should be discontinued and rivaroxaban initiated at the same time.

The manufacturer states that data from clinical trials currently are not available to guide conversion from rivaroxaban to warfarin therapy. A suggested approach is to discontinue rivaroxaban and simultaneously initiate a parenteral anticoagulant and warfarin at the time the next scheduled dose of rivaroxaban would have been administered. Because rivaroxaban may affect INR, INR measurements may not be useful in determining an appropriate dose of warfarin during conversion. When converting from rivaroxaban to an oral or parenteral anticoagulant with a rapid onset of action, rivaroxaban should be discontinued and the first dose of the other anticoagulant should be administered at the time of the next scheduled dose of rivaroxaban.

Managing Anticoagulation in Patients Requiring Invasive Procedures If temporary discontinuance of anticoagulation is necessary prior to surgery or other invasive procedures to reduce the risk of bleeding, the manufacturer recommends that rivaroxaban be discontinued at least 24 hours prior to the procedure. In deciding whether a procedure should be delayed until 24 hours after the last dose of rivaroxaban, the increased risk of bleeding should be weighed against the urgency of the intervention. If rivaroxaban is discontinued prior to surgery or other invasive procedure, the drug should be resumed postoperatively as soon as adequate hemostasis has been established; if oral anticoagulation is not possible, use of a parenteral anticoagulant should be considered. (See Risk of Thrombosis Following Premature Discontinuance of Anticoagulation under Warnings/Precautions: Warnings, in Cautions.)

■ **Special Populations** ***Hepatic Impairment*** Use of rivaroxaban should be avoided in patients with moderate (Child-Pugh class B) or severe (Child-Pugh class C) hepatic impairment or with any hepatic disease associated with coagulopathy; systemic exposure and risk of bleeding may be increased in such patients. (See Hepatic Impairment under Warnings/Precautions: Specific Populations, in Cautions.)

Renal Impairment **Embolism Associated with Atrial Fibrillation.** For patients with a creatinine clearance of 50 mL/minute or less, the recommended dosage of rivaroxaban is 15 mg once daily with the evening meal. Renal function should be periodically assessed as clinically indicated (i.e., more frequently in situations where renal function may decline) and therapy adjusted accordingly. Dosage adjustment or discontinuance of rivaroxaban should be considered if acute renal failure develops.

In the ROCKET AF trial, serum concentrations of rivaroxaban and clinical outcomes were similar in patients with moderate renal impairment (creatinine clearance of 30–50 mL/minute) receiving rivaroxaban 15 mg once daily compared with those with normal renal function receiving rivaroxaban 20 mg once daily. Although patients with creatinine clearance of 30 mL/minute or less were not studied, the manufacturer states that a rivaroxaban dosage of 15 mg once daily in such patients is expected to result in serum concentrations similar to those observed in patients with moderate renal impairment. (See Renal Impairment under Warnings/Precautions: Specific Populations, in Cautions.)

Thromboprophylaxis in Hip- or Knee-Replacement Surgery. Use of rivaroxaban should be avoided in patients with severe renal impairment (creatinine clearance less than 30 mL/minute) undergoing hip- or knee-replacement surgery because of an expected increase in rivaroxaban exposure and pharmacodynamic effects in this patient population. Rivaroxaban should be discontinued if acute renal failure develops.

Treatment and Secondary Prevention of Venous Thromboembolism. Rivaroxaban should not be used for the treatment or secondary prevention of venous thromboembolism or for long-term thromboembolic risk reduction in patients with creatinine clearance less than 30 mL/minute because of an expected increase in rivaroxaban exposure and pharmacodynamic effects in such patients.

Chronic Coronary Artery Disease or Peripheral Artery Disease. The manufacturer states that dosage adjustments based on creatinine clearance are not needed when rivaroxaban is used to reduce the risk of major cardiovascular events in patients with CAD or PAD. (See Renal Impairment under Warnings/Precautions: Specific Populations, in Cautions.)

Body Weight Dosage adjustments based on weight are not likely to be necessary. Extremes in body weight in patients weighing less than 50 kg or more than 120 kg did not influence rivaroxaban exposure.

Pregnant Women An appropriate dosage of rivaroxaban in pregnant women has not been established.

Cautions

■ **Contraindications** Active pathologic bleeding.

Severe hypersensitivity reaction to rivaroxaban.

■ **Warnings/Precautions** ***Warnings*** **Risk of Thrombosis Following Premature Discontinuance of Anticoagulation.** Premature discontinuance of any oral anticoagulant, including rivaroxaban, in the absence of adequate alternative anticoagulation increases the risk of thrombotic events (e.g., stroke). An increased incidence of stroke was observed during the transition from rivaroxaban to warfarin in clinical trials (e.g., ROCKET AF) in patients with atrial fibrillation. In the ROCKET AF trial, rivaroxaban-treated patients generally were switched to warfarin without a period of concurrent administration of warfarin and rivaroxaban, so that they were not adequately anticoagulated until attaining a therapeutic international normalized ratio (INR). If discontinuance of rivaroxaban is required for reasons other than pathologic bleeding or completion of a course of therapy, anticoagulant coverage with an alternative anticoagulant should be considered. When transitioning patients from one anticoagulant therapy to another, it is important to ensure continuous anticoagulation while minimizing the risk of bleeding. Particular caution is advised when switching patients from a factor Xa inhibitor to warfarin therapy because of the slow onset of action of warfarin. (See Transitioning to and from Rivaroxaban Therapy under Dosage and Administration: Dosage.)

Spinal/Epidural Hematoma. Patients receiving anticoagulants are at risk of developing an epidural or spinal hematoma when concomitant neuraxial (epidural/spinal) anesthesia or spinal puncture is employed; such complications can result in long-term or permanent paralysis. Epidural and subdural hematomas have been reported during postmarketing experience in patients receiving rivaroxaban. The risk of these adverse events is increased by use of indwelling epidural catheters or by concomitant use of drugs affecting hemostasis, such as nonsteroidal anti-inflammatory agents (NSAIAs), platelet-aggregation inhibitors, or other anticoagulants. Risk also may be increased in patients with a history of traumatic or repeated epidural or spinal punctures, spinal deformity, or spinal surgery.

To reduce the risk of bleeding with concurrent use of rivaroxaban and neuraxial anesthesia or spinal puncture procedures, clinicians should carefully consider the pharmacokinetic profile of the anticoagulant. Insertion or removal of an epidural catheter or lumbar puncture is best performed when the anticoagulant effect of rivaroxaban is minimal. Although the optimal timing between the administration of rivaroxaban and neuraxial procedures is not known, the following recommendations should be considered. At least 2 half-lives of the drug (i.e., 18 hours in patients 20–45 years of age and 26 hours in patients 60–76 years of age) should elapse following administration of a rivaroxaban dose prior to removal of an indwelling epidural or intrathecal catheter, and at least 6 hours should elapse following removal of the catheter before the next dose is administered. If traumatic puncture occurs, administration of rivaroxaban should be delayed for 24 hours.

Patients receiving rivaroxaban in the setting of epidural or spinal anesthesia or lumbar puncture should be monitored frequently for manifestations of neurologic impairment (e.g., midline back pain; numbness, tingling, or weakness in lower limbs; bowel or bladder dysfunction). If spinal hematoma is suspected, urgent diagnosis and treatment are necessary; spinal cord decompression should be considered even though it may not prevent or reverse neurologic sequelae. Clinicians should consider the potential benefits versus risks of neuraxial intervention in patients who are currently receiving or will receive anticoagulant prophylaxis.

Sensitivity Reactions **Hypersensitivity.** Hypersensitivity reactions, including anaphylaxis, have been reported during postmarketing experience in patients receiving rivaroxaban to reduce the risk of deep-vein thrombosis (DVT). (See Cautions: Contraindications.)

Other Warnings and Precautions **Bleeding.** Rivaroxaban increases the risk of hemorrhage and can cause serious or fatal bleeding. Bleeding complications were the most common adverse effects of rivaroxaban reported in clinical trials. In the ROCKET AF trial in patients with nonvalvular atrial fibrillation, bleeding that required permanent drug discontinuance occurred in 4.3% of patients receiving rivaroxaban and 3.1% of those receiving warfarin. The rate of major bleeding (defined as clinically overt bleeding that resulted in death, involved a critical site [i.e., intracranial, intraspinal, intraocular, pericardial, intraarticular, intramuscular with compartment syndrome, or retroperitoneal], was associated with a fall in hemoglobin of at least 2 g/dL or required transfusion of at least 2 units of whole blood or packed red blood cells, or resulted in permanent disability) was similar between the rivaroxaban and warfarin treatment groups in the ROCKET AF trial (5.6 and 5.4%, respectively); however, decreases in hemoglobin concentration of at least 2 g/dL, bleeding requiring transfusion, and major bleeding from a GI site were more common in patients receiving rivaroxaban.

In the RECORD trials in patients undergoing orthopedic surgery, major bleeding (defined as fatal bleeding, bleeding into a critical organ, bleeding requiring reoperation, or extra-surgical site bleeding that was clinically overt and was associated with a fall in hemoglobin of at least 2 g/dL or that required transfusion of at least 2 units of whole blood or packed red blood cells) was reported in 0.3% of patients who received rivaroxaban 10 mg once daily and 0.2% of those who received enoxaparin. Although bleeding rates were comparable between rivaroxaban and enoxaparin in these trials, comparison of bleeding rates in the RECORD trials with those of other trials involving non-vitamin K antagonist oral anticoagulants and enoxaparin may be confounded by the use of different definitions for major bleeding. In the EINSTEIN DVT and EINSTEIN PE studies evaluating rivaroxaban for the treatment of venous thromboembolism, rates of major bleeding and clinically relevant nonmajor bleeding were similar between patients receiving rivaroxaban and those receiving enoxaparin plus a vitamin K antagonist; in the EINSTEIN EXT study in which rivaroxaban was compared with placebo, there was a slight increase in major and clinically relevant nonmajor bleeding with rivaroxaban therapy.

When deciding whether to use rivaroxaban in patients with an increased risk of bleeding (e.g., congenital or acquired bleeding disorders; active ulceration, hemorrhagic stroke, uncontrolled arterial hypertension, diabetic retinopathy; recent brain, spinal, or ophthalmic surgery), clinicians should weigh the risk of bleeding against the risk of thrombotic events. Patients with any manifestations of blood loss during rivaroxaban therapy should be promptly evaluated. Rivaroxaban should be discontinued if active pathologic hemorrhage occurs. (See Cautions: Contraindications.) However, minor or "nuisance" bleeding is a common occurrence in patients receiving any anticoagulant and should not readily lead to treatment discontinuance. (See Risk of Thrombosis Following Premature Discontinuance of Anticoagulation under Warnings/Precautions: Warnings, in Cautions.)

Risk of bleeding may be increased in patients with renal impairment and in those receiving concomitant therapy with drugs that affect hemostasis (e.g., aspirin or other NSAIAs, fibrinolytics, selective serotonin- and norepinephrine-reuptake inhibitors [SNRIs], selective serotonin-reuptake inhibitors [SSRIs], thienopyridines, other antithrombotic agents) or drugs that are inhibitors of both P-glycoprotein (P-gp) and cytochrome P-450 (CYP) isoenzyme 3A4 (e.g., ketoconazole, ritonavir). Patients with renal impairment taking P-gp inhibitors and weak to moderate CYP3A4 inhibitors may have substantial increases in exposure to rivaroxaban, which may increase bleeding risk. (See Drug Interactions and also see Renal Impairment under Warnings/Precautions: Specific Populations, in Cautions.)

Because of the risk of pregnancy-related hemorrhage and/or emergent delivery, rivaroxaban should be used with caution in pregnant women. (See Pregnancy under Warnings/Precautions: Specific Populations, in Cautions.) Pregnant women who receive rivaroxaban should be promptly evaluated if any manifestations of blood loss occur, such as a decline in hemoglobin and/or hematocrit, hypotension, or fetal distress.

Factor Xa (recombinant), inactivated-zhzo (also known as andexanet alfa), a recombinant modified human factor Xa protein, is a specific reversal agent for the anticoagulant effects of rivaroxaban. Data from clinical trials indicate that factor Xa (recombinant), inactivated-zhzo is effective in rapidly reversing the anticoagulant effects of rivaroxaban (as measured by anti-factor Xa activity, unbound anticoagulant concentration, and thrombin generation). The safety of factor Xa (recombinant), inactivated-zhzo has not been established in patients who have experienced a thromboembolic event or disseminated intravascular coagulation (DIC) within 2 weeks prior to the life-threatening bleeding event requiring treatment with the drug, or in those who have received prothrombin complex concentrate (PCC), recombinant factor VIIa, or whole blood products within 7 days prior to the bleeding event. For further information on factor Xa (recombinant), inactivated-zhzo, see the monograph on Factor Xa (Recombinant), Inactivated-zhzo 20:28:92. The manufacturer states that rivaroxaban should be discontinued and appropriate treatment initiated if bleeding associated with overdosage occurs. Because of high plasma protein binding, rivaroxaban is not expected to be dialyzable.

Procoagulant reversal agents such as PCC, anti-inhibitor coagulant complex (also known as activated PCC), or factor VIIa (recombinant) may be considered for immediate reversal of the anticoagulant effect of rivaroxaban; however, data from clinical studies are limited. In a randomized, double-blind, placebo-controlled study in 12 healthy men receiving rivaroxaban 20 mg twice daily, administration of a single dose of a 4-factor PCC (50 units/kg by IV infusion) immediately and completely reversed the anticoagulant effects of rivaroxaban as assessed by the prothrombin time and endogenous thrombin potential (ETP). Because the study was conducted in healthy individuals, caution should be used in extrapolating these findings to clinical practice. Protamine sulfate and vitamin K are not expected to affect the anticoagulant activity of rivaroxaban, and there is no experience with antifibrinolytic agents (tranexamic acid, aminocaproic acid) or systemic hemostatics (desmopressin, aprotinin [no longer commercially available in the US]) in patients receiving rivaroxaban.

Patients with Prosthetic Heart Valves. Safety and efficacy of rivaroxaban have not been established in patients with prosthetic heart valves, and the manufacturer states that the drug is not recommended in such patients.

Patients with Pulmonary Embolism. The manufacturer states that rivaroxaban is not recommended *as initial therapy* (as an alternative to heparin) in patients with pulmonary embolism who have hemodynamic instability or who may receive thrombolytic therapy or undergo pulmonary embolectomy.

Specific Populations **Pregnancy.** There are no adequate or well-controlled studies of rivaroxaban in pregnant women. In animal reproduction studies, pronounced maternal bleeding, postimplantation pregnancy loss, and fetotoxic effects have been observed. Because of the risks associated with rivaroxaban during pregnancy (e.g., hemorrhage, emergent delivery), the manufacturer states that the drug should be used with caution in pregnant women and only if the potential benefits justify the potential risks to the mother and fetus. Based on the pharmacologic activity of factor Xa inhibitors and the potential to cross the placenta, bleeding may occur at any site in the fetus and/or neonate. The American College of Chest Physicians (ACCP) recommends that rivaroxaban be avoided in pregnant women. Women of childbearing potential should discuss pregnancy planning with their clinician prior to initiating rivaroxaban therapy. Rivaroxaban dosing in pregnancy has not been studied.

Lactation. Rivaroxaban is distributed into human milk. The effects of rivaroxaban on the breast-fed infant or on milk production are unknown. The benefits of breast-feeding and the clinical need for rivaroxaban in the woman should be considered along with any potential adverse effects on the breast-fed infant from the drug or from the underlying maternal condition. ACCP recommends that anticoagulants other than rivaroxaban be used in nursing women.

Pediatric Use. Safety and efficacy have not been established in pediatric patients younger than 18 years of age.

Geriatric Use. No substantial differences in efficacy were observed in geriatric patients 65 years of age or older relative to younger adults in clinical trials. Although thrombotic and bleeding events occurred at a higher rate in older patients, the risk-to-benefit profile was favorable in all age groups.

Hepatic Impairment. Results of a pharmacokinetic study indicate that rivaroxaban exposure (area under the plasma concentration-time curve [AUC] and peak plasma concentrations) and pharmacodynamic effects (inhibition of factor Xa activity and prolongation of prothrombin time [PT]) are increased in patients with moderate hepatic impairment (Child-Pugh class B). Clinically important changes in pharmacokinetics or pharmacodynamics of rivaroxaban were not observed in patients with mild hepatic impairment (Child-Pugh class A). The safety and pharmacokinetics of rivaroxaban in patients with severe hepatic impairment (Child-Pugh class C) have not been established. Patients with substantial liver disease (hepatitis or cirrhosis) were excluded from the major efficacy trials of rivaroxaban.

Rivaroxaban should not be used in patients with moderate or severe hepatic impairment or with any hepatic disease associated with coagulopathy.

Renal Impairment. Clearance of rivaroxaban is decreased in patients with renal impairment, resulting in increased systemic exposure and pharmacodynamic effects. Rivaroxaban should be discontinued in patients who develop acute renal failure.

In a study in individuals with various degrees of renal function, rivaroxaban AUC was increased by 44, 52, or 64% in those with mild (creatinine clearance of 50–79 mL/minute), moderate (creatinine clearance of 30–49 mL/minute), or severe (creatinine clearance of 15–29 mL/minute) renal impairment, respectively, compared with individuals with normal renal function (creatinine clearance of at least 80 mL/minute). Increased pharmacodynamic effects (PT prolongation, factor Xa inhibition) also were observed with decreasing renal function.

In patients with nonvalvular atrial fibrillation, renal function should be assessed periodically and dosage of rivaroxaban adjusted accordingly. More frequent monitoring may be necessary in situations in which renal function may be expected to decline. Patients with moderate renal impairment (creatinine clearance of 30–50 mL/minute) who received a reduced dosage of rivaroxaban (15 mg once daily) had clinical outcomes similar to those in patients with normal renal function who received a dosage of 20 mg once daily. The manufacturer states that in patients with end-stage renal disease (ESRD) maintained on intermittent dialysis, a rivaroxaban dosage of 15 mg once daily will result in rivaroxaban concentrations and pharmacodynamic activity similar to those observed in the ROCKET AF trial. It is unknown whether these concentrations will lead to similar stroke reduction and bleeding risk as was seen in the ROCKET AF trial. (See Embolism Associated with Atrial Fibrillation under Special Populations: Renal Impairment, in Dosage and Administration.)

In an analysis of pooled data from RECORD trials 1–3, bleeding risk was not increased in patients with creatinine clearance of 30–50 mL/minute, but a possible increase in total venous thromboembolism was observed in this population. Patients with creatinine clearance of 30–50 mL/minute receiving rivaroxaban therapy for prophylaxis of DVT following hip- or knee-replacement surgery should be observed closely and promptly evaluated if any manifestations of bleeding occur. Rivaroxaban should not be used in such patients with creatinine clearance of less than 30 mL/minute because of a risk of increased exposure to the drug, which may increase risk of bleeding.

Patients with creatinine clearance less than 30 mL/minute were excluded from the EINSTEIN studies evaluating the use of rivaroxaban for treatment of venous thromboembolism; the manufacturer states that rivaroxaban should not be used in such patients because of an expected increase in drug exposure and pharmacodynamic effects.

In patients with a creatinine clearance of 30 mL/minute or less but not on dialysis, a rivaroxaban dosage of 2.5 mg twice daily is expected to result in rivaroxaban exposure similar to that observed in patients with moderate renal impairment whose efficacy and safety outcomes were similar to those with preserved renal function. The manufacturer states that in patients with ESRD maintained on intermittent hemodialysis, administration of rivaroxaban 2.5 mg twice daily in conjunction with aspirin will result in rivaroxaban concentrations and pharmacodynamic activity similar to those observed in patients with moderate renal impairment in the COMPASS study. It is not known whether these concentrations will lead to similar cardiovascular risk reduction and bleeding risk as was seen during the COMPASS study.

Patients with renal impairment receiving concomitant therapy with drugs that are combined P-gp and moderate CYP3A4 inhibitors may experience a substantial increase in rivaroxaban exposure, which may increase risk of bleeding. (See Drug Interactions: Drugs Affecting P-glycoprotein Transport and CYP3A4.)

■ **Common Adverse Effects** Bleeding was the most common adverse effect reported in clinical trials of rivaroxaban, occurring in more than 5% of patients receiving the drug.

Drug Interactions

■ **Drugs Affecting or Metabolized by Hepatic Microsomal Enzymes** Rivaroxaban is metabolized by cytochrome P-450 (CYP) isoenzymes 3A4/5 and 2J2; inhibitors or inducers of these enzymes may potentially alter rivaroxaban exposure. (See Drug Interactions: Drugs Affecting P-glycoprotein Transport and CYP3A4.)

In vitro studies indicate that rivaroxaban does not inhibit CYP1A2, 2C8, 2C9, 2C19, 2D6, 2J2, and 3A4 nor induce CYP1A2, 2B6, 2C19, and 3A4; therefore, drug interactions involving these pathways are unlikely.

■ **Drugs Affecting Efflux Transport Systems** Rivaroxaban is a substrate of the efflux transporter P-glycoprotein (P-gp); inhibitors or inducers of this transport protein may potentially alter rivaroxaban exposure. (See Drug Interactions: Drugs Affecting P-glycoprotein Transport and CYP3A4.) In vitro data indicate a low inhibitory potential of rivaroxaban for this transport protein.

Rivaroxaban is a substrate of the efflux transporter ABCG2 (breast cancer resistance protein [BCRP]); inhibitors or inducers of this transport protein may potentially alter rivaroxaban exposure. In vitro data indicate a low inhibitory potential of rivaroxaban for this transporter.

■ **Drugs Affecting P-glycoprotein Transport and CYP3A4** Concomitant use of rivaroxaban with drugs that inhibit both P-gp and CYP3A4 (e.g., erythromycin, ketoconazole, ritonavir) increases exposure to rivaroxaban and may increase the risk of bleeding. A substantial increase in rivaroxaban exposure may increase risk of bleeding; however, the extent of this interaction appears to be related to the degree of P-gp or CYP3A4 inhibition, and in some cases the increased exposure may not have a substantial effect on bleeding. Concomitant use of rivaroxaban and combined P-gp and potent CYP3A4 inhibitors such as ketoconazole, itraconazole, lopinavir/ritonavir, ritonavir, and conivaptan should be avoided. When clinical data suggest that increased rivaroxaban exposure is unlikely to affect bleeding, such as in the case of concomitant clarithromycin, no special precautions are necessary for concomitant use with drugs that are combined P-gp and CYP3A4 inhibitors.

Combined P-gp and potent CYP3A4 inducers (e.g., carbamazepine, phenytoin, rifampin, St. John's wort [*Hypericum perforatum*]) may decrease exposure to rivaroxaban, resulting in possible reduced efficacy; such concomitant use should be avoided.

In a post hoc analysis of the ROCKET AF trial, concomitant use of verapamil or diltiazem (combined P-gp and moderate CYP3A inhibitors) was not associated with an increased risk of stroke or non-CNS embolism or the composite outcome of nonmajor clinically relevant or major bleeding; however, there was an increased risk of major bleeding and intracranial hemorrhage. In a case-cohort analysis, coadministration of rivaroxaban with diltiazem did not result in an increased rate of bleeding. In a pharmacokinetic trial, administration of a single dose of rivaroxaban in conjunction with multiple doses of erythromycin (a combined P-gp and moderate CYP3A4 inhibitor) to patients with mild (creatinine clearance of 50–79 mL/minute) or moderate (creatinine clearance of 30–49 mL/minute) renal impairment resulted in a 76 or 99% increase in drug exposure and a 56 or 64% increase in peak plasma concentrations, respectively. Similar trends in pharmacodynamic effects also were observed. The manufacturer states that rivaroxaban should not be used in patients with creatinine clearances of 15–79 mL/minute who are receiving concomitant therapy with a combined P-gp and moderate CYP3A4 inhibitor unless the potential benefits justify the potential risks.

■ **Drugs Affecting Gastric Acidity** Concomitant administration of a single 30-mg dose of rivaroxaban with ranitidine (150 mg twice daily) or an antacid containing aluminum hydroxide and magnesium hydroxide (10 mL) did not affect bioavailability of or exposure to rivaroxaban. Concomitant administration of a single 20-mg dose of rivaroxaban and omeprazole (40 mg once daily for 5 days) also did not affect the pharmacokinetics of rivaroxaban.

■ **Drugs Affecting Hemostasis** Concomitant use of rivaroxaban and drugs that affect hemostasis (e.g., platelet-aggregation inhibitors, other antithrombotic agents, fibrinolytics, aspirin or other nonsteroidal anti-inflammatory agents [NSAIAs], selective serotonin- and norepinephrine-reuptake inhibitors [SNRIs], selective serotonin-reuptake inhibitors [SSRIs]) increases risk of bleeding. Patients receiving such concomitant therapy should be promptly evaluated if manifestations of bleeding occur.

Anticoagulants Because of an increased risk of bleeding, use of other anticoagulants should be avoided in patients receiving rivaroxaban unless the benefits outweigh the risks. (See Bleeding under Warnings/Precautions: Other Warnings and Precautions, in Cautions.)

Concomitant administration of a single 40-mg dose of enoxaparin sodium with rivaroxaban 10 mg resulted in an additive effect on antifactor Xa activity; enoxaparin did not affect the pharmacokinetics of rivaroxaban. Administration of a single 15-mg dose of warfarin sodium with rivaroxaban 5 mg resulted in additive effects on factor Xa inhibition and prothrombin time; warfarin did not affect the pharmacokinetics of rivaroxaban.

Nonsteroidal Anti-inflammatory Agents Patients receiving concomitant therapy with rivaroxaban and NSAIAs, including aspirin, should be promptly evaluated if any manifestations of blood loss occur.

In a single-dose drug interaction study in healthy men, concomitant administration of rivaroxaban 15 mg and naproxen (500 mg daily for 2 days) did not result in any substantial pharmacokinetic or pharmacodynamic interaction; although bleeding time was slightly increased, this was not considered clinically important.

In a single-dose study in healthy men, concurrent administration of aspirin and rivaroxaban 15 mg resulted in a slightly increased bleeding time compared with administration of aspirin alone, but did not affect the inhibitory effects of aspirin on platelet aggregation. No substantial change in pharmacokinetics or pharmacodynamics of rivaroxaban was observed. In the ROCKET AF trial, concomitant use of aspirin was identified as an independent risk factor for major bleeding.

Platelet-aggregation Inhibitors Patients receiving concomitant therapy with rivaroxaban and clopidogrel or other platelet-aggregation inhibitors (see Nonsteroidal Anti-inflammatory Agents under Drug Interactions: Drugs Affecting Hemostasis) should be promptly evaluated if any manifestations of blood loss occur. In 2 drug interaction studies in which healthy individuals received clopidogrel (300-mg loading dose followed by 75 mg daily) and a single 15-mg dose of rivaroxaban concomitantly, bleeding time was increased to 45 minutes (approximately twice the maximum increase observed with either drug alone) in approximately 30–45% of these individuals; no change in pharmacokinetics of either drug was observed.

■ **Antiarrhythmic Agents** Concomitant administration of rivaroxaban and amiodarone (a combined P-gp and weak CYP3A4 inhibitor) did not increase the risk of bleeding in patients with mild renal impairment. Concomitant administration of rivaroxaban and dronedarone (a combined P-gp and moderate CYP3A4 inhibitor) may increase rivaroxaban exposure in patients with renal impairment.

■ **Atorvastatin** A substantial pharmacokinetic interaction was not observed with concomitant administration of rivaroxaban (20 mg) and atorvastatin (20 mg once daily) in a study in healthy individuals. However, in the RECORD trials, the incidence of major or nonmajor clinically relevant bleeding was increased in patients receiving the combination of rivaroxaban and a statin compared with those receiving enoxaparin and a statin (23 or 18%, respectively).

■ **Azole Antifungals** Concomitant administration of rivaroxaban and ketoconazole (400 mg once daily) (a combined P-gp and potent CYP3A4 inhibitor) increased steady-state exposure (area under the plasma concentration-time curve [AUC]) and peak plasma concentrations of rivaroxaban by 160 and 70%, respectively. Concomitant use of ketoconazole should be avoided in patients receiving rivaroxaban. Because of the potential for substantially increased rivaroxaban exposure which may increase risk of bleeding, concomitant use of rivaroxaban and itraconazole (a combined P-gp and potent CYP3A4 inhibitor) also should be avoided.

Concomitant administration of a single dose of rivaroxaban and fluconazole (a moderate CYP3A4 inhibitor) increased AUC and peak plasma concentrations of rivaroxaban by 40 and 30%, respectively.

■ **Digoxin** A substantial pharmacokinetic interaction was not observed with concomitant administration of rivaroxaban (20 mg) and digoxin (0.375 mg once daily) in healthy individuals.

■ **HIV Protease Inhibitors** AUC and peak plasma concentrations of rivaroxaban were increased substantially (by 150 and 60%, respectively) when administered concurrently with ritonavir; similar increases in pharmacodynamic effects also were observed.

Because of the potential for substantially increased rivaroxaban exposure which may increase risk of bleeding, concomitant use of rivaroxaban with ritonavir, lopinavir/ritonavir, or indinavir should be avoided.

■ **Macrolide Antibiotics** Concomitant administration of a single dose of rivaroxaban with clarithromycin increased AUC and peak plasma concentrations of rivaroxaban by 50 and 40%, respectively. Both single-dose AUC and peak plasma concentrations of rivaroxaban were increased by 30% when administered concomitantly with erythromycin. The manufacturer states the increase in rivaroxaban exposure with concomitant clarithromycin use is not expected to increase risk of bleeding; therefore, no special precautions are necessary with concomitant administration of clarithromycin and rivaroxaban. The manufacturer states that erythromycin should not be used concomitantly with rivaroxaban in patients with moderate renal impairment. (See Drug Interactions: Drugs Affecting P-glycoprotein and CYP3A4.)

■ **Midazolam** A substantial pharmacokinetic interaction was not observed with concomitant administration of rivaroxaban (20 mg) and midazolam (single dose of 7.5 mg) in healthy individuals.

■ **Protein-bound Drugs** Interactions between rivaroxaban and other highly protein-bound drugs such as phenytoin or aspirin are likely.

■ **Rifampin** Concomitant administration of rifampin (a combined P-glycoprotein and potent CYP3A4 inducer) titrated up to a dosage of 600 mg once daily and a single 20-mg dose of rivaroxaban (with food) decreased AUC and peak plasma concentrations of rivaroxaban by 50 and 22%, respectively; similar decreases in pharmacodynamic effects also were observed. Because of the potential for reduced efficacy of rivaroxaban, concomitant use of rifampin should be avoided.

Description

Rivaroxaban, an oral, direct activated factor X (Xa) inhibitor, is an anticoagulant. Factor Xa plays a central role in the blood coagulation cascade by serving as the convergence point for the intrinsic and extrinsic pathways; inhibition of coagulation factor Xa by rivaroxaban prevents conversion of prothrombin to thrombin and subsequent thrombus formation. Rivaroxaban inhibits both free and prothrombinase-bound factor Xa. Unlike fondaparinux, heparin, and the low molecular weight heparins, rivaroxaban binds directly to the active site of factor Xa without the need for a cofactor (e.g., antithrombin III). Rivaroxaban inhibits factor Xa with more than 100,000-fold greater selectivity than other biologically important serine proteases (e.g., thrombin, trypsin, plasmin, factor VIIa, factor IXa, urokinase [no longer commercially available in the US], activated protein C).

Rivaroxaban exerts predictable pharmacokinetic and pharmacodynamic effects over a dose range of 5–80 mg. The drug inhibits factor Xa activity and prolongs prothrombin time (PT), activated partial thromboplastin time (aPTT), and HepTest (an indirect measure of factor Xa activity) in a dose-dependent manner.

Rivaroxaban is rapidly and well absorbed following oral administration, with an estimated bioavailability of about 80–100% for the 2.5- and 10-mg doses and 66% for the 20-mg dose. Peak plasma concentrations of rivaroxaban are obtained 2–4 hours following oral administration. The presence of food delays time to peak concentration and increases systemic exposure to rivaroxaban 20 mg but does not appear to have a substantial effect on systemic exposure to the 2.5- or 10-mg dose. Absorption of rivaroxaban is dependent on the site of release in the GI tract; exposure to the drug is reduced when the drug is released into the proximal small intestine (e.g., via feeding tube) and further reduced in the distal small intestine or ascending colon.

When administered as crushed tablets orally or via a nasogastric or gastric feeding tube, rivaroxaban is stable in applesauce or water for up to 4 hours. In vitro data indicate that the drug is not adsorbed to PVC or silicone nasogastric tubing when administered as a suspension in water. (See Dosage and Administration: Administration.) Following oral administration of a crushed 20-mg tablet in applesauce to healthy individuals, mean area under the plasma concentration-time curve (AUC) and mean peak plasma concentrations of rivaroxaban were comparable to those following administration of whole tablets; however, after administration of the crushed tablet in water via nasogastric tube followed by a liquid meal, mean AUC was comparable to that with a whole oral tablet but mean peak plasma concentrations were 18% lower.

Rivaroxaban undergoes oxidative degradation by cytochrome P-450 (CYP) isoenzymes 3A4/5 and 2J2 and hydrolysis; metabolites are subsequently eliminated through renal and fecal/biliary routes. No major circulating metabolites have been identified in plasma. Rivaroxaban is extensively bound (approximately 92–95%) to plasma proteins, mainly to albumin. Terminal elimination half-life of the drug is about 5–9 hours in healthy individuals 20–45 years of age. Following oral administration, approximately one-third of an absorbed dose of rivaroxaban is excreted unchanged in urine, with the remaining two-thirds excreted as inactive metabolites in both urine and feces. In a phase 1 study, approximately 66% of a radiolabeled dose of rivaroxaban was eliminated renally (36% as unchanged drug) and 28% was eliminated in feces (7% as unchanged drug). No substantial accumulation of the drug occurs with repeated dosing. QT-interval prolongation has not been observed with rivaroxaban.

Advice to Patients

Importance of patients taking the drug exactly as prescribed and not discontinuing therapy without first consulting a clinician. Patients with atrial fibrillation should take rivaroxaban once daily with the evening meal. Patients should be advised to take the 15- or 20-mg tablets with food at approximately the same time every day.

Patients who cannot swallow tablets whole should be advised to crush a 15- or 20-mg tablet of rivaroxaban and combine the drug with a small amount of applesauce immediately before administration, followed by food. For patients requiring a nasogastric (NG) or gastric feeding tube, the patient or caregiver should be instructed to crush the tablet and mix it with a small amount of water before administration via the tube, followed immediately by enteral feeding.

Importance of advising patients that if a dose is missed, it should be taken as soon as possible on the same day and then the regular dosing schedule resumed the following day. If a patient is taking a dosage of 15 mg twice daily and misses a dose, two 15-mg tablets may be taken at the same time to ensure full intake of the 30-mg daily dosage. (See Dosage and Administration: Administration.)

In patients who are at a continued risk of recurrent deep-vein thrombosis (DVT) and/or pulmonary embolism (PE) after at least 6 months of initial anticoagulant treatment, importance of advising such patients to take rivaroxaban 10 mg once daily with or without food.

Importance of advising patients who have had neuraxial anesthesia or spinal puncture to monitor for manifestations of spinal or epidural hematoma (e.g., back pain; tingling, numbness, or weakness in lower limbs; bowel or bladder incontinence), particularly if they are receiving concomitant nonsteroidal anti-inflammatory agents (NSAIAs) or platelet-aggregation inhibitors; importance of immediately contacting a clinician if any of these symptoms occur.

Importance of informing patients that they may bruise and/or bleed more easily and that a longer than normal time may be required to stop bleeding when taking rivaroxaban. Importance of informing clinicians about any unusual bleeding or bruising during therapy.

Importance of patients informing clinicians (e.g., physicians, dentists) that they are receiving rivaroxaban therapy before scheduling any surgery or invasive procedures, including dental procedures.

Importance of not administering rivaroxaban to patients with prosthetic heart valves.

Importance of women immediately informing clinicians if they are or plan to become pregnant or plan to breast-feed. Women of childbearing potential should discuss pregnancy planning with their clinician prior to receiving rivaroxaban. Importance of pregnant women immediately reporting any bleeding or symptoms of blood loss to a clinician.

Importance of informing clinicians of existing or contemplated concomitant therapy, including prescription and OTC drugs and herbal supplements.

Importance of informing patients of other important precautionary information. (See Cautions.)

Overview® (see Users Guide). For additional information on this drug until a more detailed monograph is developed and published, the manufacturer's labeling should be consulted. It is *essential* that the manufacturer's labeling be consulted for more detailed information on usual cautions, precautions, contraindications, potential drug interactions, laboratory test interferences, and acute toxicity.

Preparations

Excipients in commercially available drug preparations may have clinically important effects in some individuals; consult specific product labeling for details.

Rivaroxaban

Oral		
Tablets	2.5 mg	Xarelto®, Janssen
	10 mg	Xarelto®, Janssen
	15 mg	Xarelto®, Janssen
	20 mg	Xarelto®, Janssen

Selected Revisions October 2019.

HEPARINS 20:12.04.16

Dalteparin Sodium

Heparin Fragment KABI 2165

■ Dalteparin sodium, a low molecular weight heparin prepared by nitrous acid degradation of heparin (referring throughout this monograph to unfractionated heparin) of porcine intestinal mucosa origin, is an anticoagulant.

Uses

Dalteparin is used concurrently with aspirin and/or other therapy (e.g., nitrates, β-adrenergic blockers, clopidogrel, platelet glycoprotein [GP] IIb/IIIa-receptor inhibitors) to reduce the risk of acute cardiac ischemic events (death and/or myocardial infarction [MI]) in patients with unstable angina or non-ST-segment-elevation myocardial infarction (NSTEMI) (i.e., non-ST-segment-elevation acute coronary syndromes [NSTE ACS]). Dalteparin also is used for the prevention of deep-vein thrombosis (DVT), which may lead to pulmonary embolism (PE) in patients undergoing hip-replacement surgery, patients undergoing general (e.g., abdominal, gynecologic, urologic) surgery, and in patients with acute medical conditions (e.g., cancer, bedrest, heart failure, severe lung disease) and severely restricted mobility who are at risk for thromboembolic complications.

The use of a low molecular weight heparin such as dalteparin also is suggested by the American College of Chest Physicians (ACCP) as first-line or alternative therapy for prevention of venous thromboembolism in selected patients undergoing intracranial neurologic surgery† or spinal surgery†; in patients with major trauma†, including brain injury, acute spinal injury, and traumatic spine injury; selected cancer patients; and in patients with acute ischemic stroke†. Therapy with a low molecular weight heparin also has been recommended in selected patients for prevention of embolism associated with atrial fibrillation or atrial flutter† or thromboembolism associated with prosthetic heart valves† and for prevention or treatment of thromboembolism during pregnancy†. Although a causal relationship has not been established and the number of patients involved appears to be small, cases of valve thrombosis resulting in death (including maternal and fetal deaths) and/or requiring surgical intervention have been reported with at least one low molecular weight heparin (enoxaparin) during thromboprophylaxis in some patients (including pregnant women) with prosthetic heart valves; insufficient data, underlying conditions, and the possibility of inadequate anticoagulation also complicate evaluation of these events. However, ACCP suggests that in the absence of definitive data regarding optimal therapy in pregnant patients with prosthetic heart valves and the associated risks of withholding antithrombotic therapy, use of a low molecular weight heparin at a dosage adjusted to maintain the manufacturer-recommended peak anti-factor Xa concentrations 4 hours postinjection appears reasonable in such patients. (See Uses: Thromboembolism Associated with Prosthetic Heart Valves, in Enoxaparin 20:12.04.16.) The manufacturer of dalteparin states that the drug has not been studied systematically in patients with prosthetic heart valves. For further details on the use of low molecular weight heparins in various thromboembolic conditions, see Uses in Enoxaparin 20:12.04.16.

The usual precautions and contraindications associated with heparin anticoagulation should be followed in patients for whom dalteparin therapy is considered. (See Cautions.)

■ **Unstable Angina and Non-ST-Segment-Elevation Myocardial Infarction** Dalteparin is used concurrently with aspirin and/or other standard therapy (e.g., nitrates, β-adrenergic blockers, clopidogrel, GP IIb/IIIa-receptor inhibitors) to reduce the risk of acute cardiac ischemic events (death and/or MI) in patients with unstable angina or NSTEMI (i.e., non-ST-segment-elevation acute coronary syndromes [NSTE ACS]).

If a low molecular weight heparin is selected for initial parenteral anticoagulation in patients with NSTE ACS, the American Heart Association (AHA) and American College of Cardiology Foundation (ACCF) guidelines recommend the use of enoxaparin; other parenteral anticoagulants with established efficacy include heparin, bivalirudin (only in patients who are being managed with an early invasive strategy), and fondaparinux. For additional information on the use of low molecular weight heparins in the management of NSTE ACS, see Uses: Non-ST-Segment-Elevation Acute Coronary Syndromes, in Enoxaparin 20:12.04.16.

In several large placebo-controlled trials (Fragmin during Instability in Coronary Artery Disease [FRISC], Fragmin and Fast Revascularization during Instability in Coronary Artery Disease [FRISC II]) in patients who recently experienced unstable angina or NSTEMI (within 48–72 hours of treatment), therapy with dalteparin sodium (120 units/kg every 12 hours subcutaneously for 5–6 days followed by 5000–7500 units once or twice daily for 1.5–3 months) reduced the combined incidence of death or nonfatal MI (Q-wave MI) at 6 and 30 days. However, when a secondary end point was included, the need for revascularization after 40 days, the reduction in the frequency of the combined outcome of death, nonfatal MI, and need for revascularization persisted with dalteparin compared with placebo but was apparent only in nonsmokers (80% of the sample). Patients in the FRISC trial included those with acute coronary syndromes at low to high risk of ischemic complications; patients in the FRISC II trial included those at intermediate to high risk for ischemic complications, including those undergoing PCI.

All patients in clinical trials of dalteparin for NSTE ACS received concomitant therapy with aspirin; the benefit of aspirin for secondary prevention of ischemic events in patients with unstable angina has been demonstrated in several studies and pooled analyses of data.

■ **Deep-Vein Thrombosis and/or Pulmonary Embolism** ***Prophylaxis*** **Hip-Replacement, Knee-Replacement, or Hip-Fracture Surgery.** Dalteparin is used for the prevention of DVT, which may lead to PE, in patients undergoing hip-replacement surgery. Low molecular weight heparins also have been used for thromboprophylaxis in patients undergoing other types of major orthopedic procedures such as total knee-replacement† and hip-fracture surgery†. ACCP recommends routine thromboprophylaxis (with a pharmacologic and/or mechanical [e.g., intermittent pneumatic compression] method) in all patients undergoing major orthopedic surgery, including total hip-replacement, total knee-replacement, and hip-fracture surgery, because of the high risk for postoperative venous thromboembolism; thromboprophylaxis should be continued for at least 10–14 days, and possibly for up to 35 days after surgery. Several antithrombotic agents (e.g., low molecular weight heparins, fondaparinux, low-dose heparin, warfarin, aspirin) are recommended by ACCP for pharmacologic thromboprophylaxis in patients undergoing major orthopedic surgery. Among the different options, ACCP suggests that a low molecular weight heparin generally is preferred because of its relative efficacy and safety and extensive clinical experience; alternative agents may be considered in situations in which a low molecular weight heparin is not available or cannot be used (e.g., in patients with heparin-induced thrombocytopenia [HIT] or in those who refuse or are uncooperative with subcutaneous injections). ACCP states that when selecting an appropriate thromboprophylaxis regimen, factors such as relative efficacy and bleeding risk as well as logistics and compliance issues should be considered. For additional information on the prevention of venous thromboembolism in patients undergoing major orthopedic surgery, consult the most recent ACCP Evidence-based Clinical Practice Guidelines on Antithrombotic Therapy and Prevention of Thrombosis available at http://www.chestnet.org.

Data from several comparative clinical trials indicate that dalteparin is more effective than warfarin in preventing thromboembolic events in patients undergoing hip-replacement surgery. In a comparative short-term study (beginning preoperatively and continued for up to 9 days postoperatively) in patients undergoing hip-replacement surgery and receiving thromboprophylaxis with dalteparin sodium (2500 units subcutaneously 2 hours preoperatively followed by 2500 units on the evening of surgery, then 5000 units once daily on the first and subsequent postoperative days) or warfarin (5–7.5 mg on the evening before and after surgery followed by a daily dosage adjusted to achieve a target international normalized ratio [INR] of 2.5), postoperative DVT or proximal DVT (determined by venography) occurred in 15 or 5% of patients treated with dalteparin versus 26 or 8% of patients treated with warfarin, respectively. The incidence of PE was similar in each treatment group. In another short-term study (duration of therapy 4–8 days postoperatively) in patients undergoing hip-replacement surgery who received either preoperative dalteparin (within 2 hours before surgery), postoperative dalteparin (at least 4 hours after surgery), or postoperative warfarin, initiation of dalteparin at either time was more effective than warfarin (dosage adjusted to maintain an INR of 2–3) in preventing DVT or proximal DVT (as determined by venography). In addition, symptomatic DVT occurred less frequently in patients treated with preoperative dalteparin than with warfarin.

In another short-term comparative study (therapy beginning preoperatively and continuing for up to 9 days postoperatively) with dalteparin sodium (5000 units initiated the evening before surgery and once daily thereafter) and subcutaneous, fixed low-dose heparin sodium (5000 units 3 times daily, initiated 2 hours preoperatively), the incidence of DVT was similar in both treatment groups. The incidence of proximal (thigh) DVT and PE was lower in patients receiving dalteparin than in those receiving low-dose heparin.

Some evidence suggests that extended prophylaxis† with a low molecular weight heparin (i.e., for up to 35 days post-surgery) may provide additional protection against thromboembolism in patients undergoing total hip- or total knee-replacement surgery†. While the manufacturer states that the usual duration of dalteparin therapy following hip-replacement surgery is 5–10 days, with administration for up to 14 days in clinical trials, ACCP suggests extended prophylaxis for up to 35 days in patients undergoing major orthopedic surgery.

General/Abdominal Surgery. Dalteparin is used for the prevention of postoperative DVT, which may lead to PE, in patients undergoing general (e.g., abdominal) surgery who are at risk for thromboembolic complications. According to the manufacturer, abdominal surgery patients who are considered to be at risk for thromboembolic complications include individuals who are 40 years of age or older, obese, or undergoing major surgical procedures (defined as surgery requiring general anesthesia that exceeds 30 minutes in duration) and those with additional risk factors such as malignancy or a history of DVT or PE; however, other risk factors also may apply depending on the risk stratification method used. In general, clinicians should consider a combination of patient- and procedure-specific factors when determining a patient's level of risk of thromboembolism.

ACCP recommends pharmacologic (e.g., a low molecular weight heparin) and/or nonpharmacologic/mechanical (e.g., intermittent pneumatic compression) methods of thromboprophylaxis in patients undergoing general surgery, including abdominal, GI, gynecologic, and urologic surgery, according to the patient's level of risk for thromboembolism and bleeding. In general, pharmacologic prophylaxis is recommended in patients with high (and possibly moderate) risk of venous thromboembolism who do not have a high risk of bleeding, while mechanical methods are suggested in patients who require thromboprophylaxis but have a high risk of bleeding. If pharmacologic thromboprophylaxis is used in patients undergoing general surgery, ACCP states that a low molecular weight heparin or low-dose heparin is preferred; however, when these agents are contraindicated or not available, aspirin or fondaparinux may be considered. Because the risk of venous thromboembolism is particularly high in patients undergoing abdominal or pelvic surgery for cancer, extended (4 weeks) prophylaxis with a low molecular weight heparin is recommended in such patients. ACCP states that the same recommendations for the use of antithrombotic agents in general surgery patients can be applied to patients undergoing bariatric surgery, vascular surgery, and plastic and reconstructive surgery. For additional information on the prevention of venous thromboembolism in patients undergoing general surgery, consult the most recent ACCP Evidence-based Clinical Practice Guidelines on Antithrombotic Therapy and Prevention of Thrombosis available at http://www.chestnet.org.

Based on indirect evidence from patients undergoing general surgery, use of thromboprophylaxis following cesarean section may be beneficial in patients with additional risk factors (e.g., immobility, previous thromboembolic event, thrombophilia) for venous thromboembolism. If pharmacologic prophylaxis is used in patients undergoing cesarean section, ACCP states that a low molecular heparin generally is preferred over heparin because of its favorable safety profile.

In a placebo-controlled, double-blind study in patients at risk for thromboembolic complications undergoing major abdominal surgery in whom prophylaxis was initiated 1–2 hours prior to surgery and continued for 5–10 days, thromboembolic events (i.e., proximal or distal DVT detected by radioisotope leg scan and/or PE detected by perfusion lung scan) occurred in 4.4% of patients treated with dalteparin sodium 2500 units daily versus 17.6% of placebo-treated patients. Dalteparin was particularly effective in reducing the incidence of venous thrombosis in patients undergoing surgery for malignant disease. Comparative studies indicate that subcutaneous dalteparin sodium (2500 units daily) is at least as effective as subcutaneous heparin sodium (5000 units twice daily) in preventing thromboembolic events in at-risk patients undergoing abdominal surgery. In one study, thromboembolic events occurred in 3.9 or 4% of patients receiving these dosages of dalteparin or heparin, respectively.

There is some evidence that efficacy of dalteparin is dose dependent. In one study, dalteparin sodium 5000 units daily was more effective in preventing thrombotic complications than dalteparin sodium 2500 units daily in patients undergoing abdominal surgery for malignant disease. In this study, thromboembolic events occurred in 15.1% of such patients receiving dalteparin sodium 2500 units daily versus 9.3% of patients receiving dalteparin sodium 5000 units daily when prophylaxis was initiated the night before surgery and continued for 7 days. Despite the doubling of dosage, however, the incidence of bleeding events in patients receiving dalteparin sodium 5000 units daily was only slightly higher (but not significantly so) than that in those receiving the lower dosage.

Medical Conditions Associated with Thromboembolism. Dalteparin is used for the prevention of DVT, which may lead to PE, in patients whose mobility is severely restricted during acute illness.

In a placebo-controlled, short-term (14 days), double-blind study in acutely ill medical patients with severely impaired mobility, therapy with subcutaneous dalteparin sodium (5000 units once daily) decreased the incidence of the primary efficacy end point at day 21 from approximately 5% in patients receiving placebo to about 2.8% in patients receiving dalteparin (relative risk reduction of 45%). The primary efficacy end point included confirmed symptomatic DVT or PE, asymptomatic proximal DVT detected by compression ultrasound, or sudden death. Patients were eligible for study entry if they had acute congestive heart failure, acute respiratory failure, infection without septic shock, acute rheumatologic disorders, or inflammatory bowel disease and required a hospital stay of at least 4 days. Patients without congestive heart failure or acute respiratory failure were required to have at least one additional risk factor for thromboembolism, including age 75 years and older, cancer, history of venous thromboembolism, obesity, varicose veins or chronic venous insufficiency, hormone replacement therapy, or myeloproliferative syndrome. There was no difference in overall mortality between the 2 groups. Major bleeding episodes occurred in 9 (0.49%) or 3 patients (0.16%) receiving dalteparin or placebo, respectively.

Treatment decisions regarding the use of prophylactic anticoagulants in acutely ill hospitalized patients should include an assessment of the patient's individual risk of venous thromboembolism and risk of bleeding. In general, pharmacologic thromboprophylaxis is recommended only in patients who are considered to be at high risk of venous thromboembolism because the risk-to-benefit trade-off between the reduction in venous thromboembolic events and bleeding is considered to be more favorable in such patients. Factors that should be considered when choosing an appropriate anticoagulant include patient preference, compliance, ease of administration, and local cost considerations. ACCP recommends the use of anticoagulant thromboprophylaxis (e.g., a low molecular weight heparin) in acutely ill, hospitalized medical patients at increased risk of thrombosis who are not actively bleeding and do not have an increased risk of bleeding. Continued thromboprophylaxis is suggested for 6–21 days until full mobility is restored or hospital discharge, whichever comes first; extended prophylaxis beyond these periods generally is not recommended. Risk of venous thromboembolism in critically ill patients in an intensive care unit (ICU) varies depending on their acute or chronic conditions (e.g., sepsis, congestive heart failure) and ICU-specific exposures and events (e.g., surgery, immobilization, mechanical ventilation, central venous catheters). A low molecular weight heparin is suggested by ACCP as an option for pharmacologic thromboprophylaxis in critically ill patients who are not actively bleeding and do not have risk factors for bleeding.

Risk of venous thromboembolism is particularly high in patients with cancer. Routine pharmacologic thromboprophylaxis generally is not recommended in cancer patients in the outpatient setting who have no additional risk factors for venous thromboembolism; however, ACCP suggests the use of prophylactic-dose low molecular weight heparin or low-dose heparin in cancer outpatients with solid tumors who have additional thromboembolic risk factors and are at low risk of bleeding.

Cardiac Surgery. Because the risk of venous thromboembolism in most patients undergoing cardiac surgery† is considered to be moderate, mechanical methods of prophylaxis (preferably with an intermittent pneumatic compression device) generally are recommended over pharmacologic prophylaxis. However, ACCP states that use of a pharmacologic agent (e.g., a low molecular weight heparin) may be considered in cardiac surgery patients with a complicated postoperative course.

Thoracic Surgery. Pharmacologic thromboprophylaxis with a low molecular weight heparin or low-dose heparin is recommended by ACCP in patients undergoing thoracic surgery† who are at high risk of venous thromboembolism, provided risk of bleeding is low.

Neurosurgery. Patients undergoing craniotomy, especially for malignant disease, are considered to be at high risk of venous thromboembolism. Although low molecular weight heparins have been used for the prevention of venous thromboembolism in such patients, the benefits of pharmacologic prophylaxis may be outweighed by the possible increased risk of intracranial hemorrhage. ACCP suggests the use of a mechanical method of prophylaxis (preferably intermittent pneumatic compression) in craniotomy patients; for patients considered to be at *very* high risk for thromboembolism, such as those undergoing craniotomy for malignant disease†, a pharmacologic method (e.g., a low molecular weight heparin) may be added once adequate hemostasis has been established and the risk of bleeding decreases.

In patients undergoing spinal surgery†, a mechanical method of thromboprophylaxis (preferably intermittent pneumatic compression) also is suggested, with possible addition of pharmacologic prophylaxis (e.g., a low molecular weight heparin) in high-risk patients (e.g., those with malignancy or those undergoing surgery with a combined anterior-posterior approach) once adequate hemostasis is established and risk of bleeding decreases.

Trauma. In general, some form of thromboprophylaxis (with either a low molecular weight heparin, low-dose heparin, or a mechanical method) is suggested by ACCP in all patients with major trauma†. For major trauma patients at high risk of venous thromboembolism, including those with acute spinal cord injury, traumatic brain injury, or spinal surgery for trauma†, ACCP suggests the use of both a pharmacologic and mechanical method of prophylaxis, unless contraindications exist.

Treatment and Secondary Prevention

Venous Thromboembolism in Patients with Cancer. Dalteparin is used for the *extended* (6 months' duration) treatment of symptomatic venous thromboembolism (DVT and/or PE) in patients with cancer to reduce the recurrence (secondary prevention) of venous thromboembolism. Warfarin generally is the preferred anticoagulant for long-term treatment of venous thromboembolism in patients without cancer; however, in patients with cancer, ACCP suggests the use of a low molecular weight heparin over warfarin because of a possible reduced response to warfarin therapy in such patients. (See Treatment and Secondary Prevention under Uses: Deep-vein Thrombosis and Pulmonary Embolism, in Warfarin Sodium 20:12.04.08.) ACCP suggests extended anticoagulant therapy (beyond 3 months) in cancer patients with acute venous thromboembolism because of the high risk of recurrence in these patients.

Acute Venous Thromboembolism. The manufacturer states that dalteparin is not indicated for the *acute* treatment of venous thromboembolism†. However, low molecular weight heparins, including dalteparin†, are recommended by ACCP as an appropriate choice of anticoagulant for the initial treatment of acute proximal DVT or PE†. In adults with venous thromboembolism, ACCP recommends that anticoagulant therapy be continued beyond the acute treatment period for at least 3 months, and possibly longer depending on factors such as the location of thrombi (e.g., distal versus proximal vein), presence of a risk factor (e.g., surgery, cancer), and the patient's risk of bleeding. When warfarin therapy is being considered for long-term treatment of acute venous thromboembolism, the drug should be initiated concurrently with a parenteral anticoagulant (e.g., dalteparin), and such concurrent therapy should be continued for at least 5 days and until the INR is at least 2 for 24 hours or longer. Anticoagulant therapy generally is not recommended in patients with isolated distal DVT† unless symptoms are severe and there is a risk for thrombus extension.

Analysis of pooled data from numerous comparative randomized clinical studies suggests that a low molecular weight heparin is at least as effective as heparin in the treatment of acute DVT or PE and further outpatient prevention of recurrent venous thromboembolism. However, a low molecular weight heparin may offer certain advantages over heparin, such as more convenient administration and less risk of HIT. ACCP generally suggests the use of a low molecular weight heparin or fondaparinux rather than heparin for the initial treatment of acute venous thromboembolism in adults. Low molecular weight heparins and fondaparinux are considered to be comparable in efficacy and safety; therefore, the choice between these agents should be dictated by local considerations such as cost, availability, and familiarity of use. Heparin may be preferred in patients with renal impairment. In addition, ACCP states that IV heparin is preferred over subcutaneous therapies in patients with PE in whom thrombolytic therapy is being considered or if there is a concern about the adequacy of subcutaneous absorption.

For additional information on treatment of venous thromboembolism, consult the most recent ACCP Evidence-based Clinical Practice Guidelines on Antithrombotic Therapy and Prevention of Thrombosis available at http://www.chestnet.org.

Venous Thromboembolism in Pediatric Patients. Low molecular weight heparins also have been used for the treatment and secondary prevention of venous thromboembolism in pediatric patients†. Unlike in adults, most episodes of venous thromboembolism in children are secondary to an identifiable risk factor such as the presence of a central venous access device (e.g., central venous catheter or umbilical venous catheter). Recommendations regarding the use of antithrombotic therapy in children generally are based on extrapolation from adult guidelines. A low molecular weight heparin or heparin is recommended by ACCP for both the initial and ongoing treatment of venous thromboembolism in children. Potential advantages of low molecular weight heparins include reduced need for monitoring, lack of drug or dietary interactions, reduced risk of HIT, and possible reduced risk of osteoporosis. In children with central venous catheter-related thromboembolism, ACCP recommends that the catheter be removed if no longer functioning or required; at least 3–5 days of therapeutic anticoagulation is suggested prior to its removal. If the central venous access device is required, ACCP suggests that anticoagulants be given until the catheter is removed. For additional information on treatment of venous thromboembolism in neonates and children, consult the most recent ACCP Evidence-based Clinical Practice Guidelines on Antithrombotic Therapy and Prevention of Thrombosis available at http://www.chestnet.org.

■ Superficial Vein Thrombosis

Low molecular weight heparins also have been used for the treatment of superficial vein thrombosis (superficial thrombophlebitis)†. ACCP suggests the use of prophylactic dosages of a low molecular weight heparin or fondaparinux for 45 days in patients with superficial vein thrombosis of at least 5 cm in length.

■ Renal Vein Thrombosis

A low molecular weight heparin is suggested by ACCP as a possible treatment option in selected neonates with renal vein thrombosis†; however, use of anticoagulant therapy is controversial for the treatment of renal vein thrombosis.

■ Acute Ischemic Stroke

Although therapeutic-dose anticoagulation has been used in patients with acute ischemic stroke†, there is strong evidence that such treatment is associated with worse outcomes than aspirin therapy in terms of increased mortality and rates of nonfatal major extracranial bleeding. Therefore, ACCP recommends early treatment (within 48 hours) with aspirin over therapeutic anticoagulation to prevent recurrent cerebral thromboembolism in patients with acute ischemic stroke or TIA. (See Uses: Thrombosis, in Aspirin 28:08.04.24.) However, heparin anticoagulants (i.e., low molecular weight heparins or heparin) may be used in prophylactic dosages for thromboprophylaxis in some patients with acute ischemic stroke; those with additional risk factors for venous thromboembolism are more likely to benefit from such prophylaxis. ACCP suggests that thromboprophylaxis with either a low molecular weight heparin (in prophylactic dosages), subcutaneous heparin, or intermittent pneumatic compression devices be used in patients with acute ischemic stroke† and restricted mobility. Among the anticoagulant options, ACCP suggests the use of a low molecular weight heparin over heparin. Prophylactic-dose heparin (heparin or a low molecular weight heparin) usually is initiated within 48 hours of the onset of stroke and is continued throughout the hospital stay until the patient regains mobility; such heparin therapy should not be given within the first 24 hours after administration of thrombolytic therapy.

A low molecular weight heparin is recommended as an option for the initial management of acute arterial ischemic stroke in children† until dissection and embolic causes have been excluded. When dissection or cardioembolic causes have been excluded, daily aspirin therapy (in prophylactic dosages) is suggested for a minimum of 2 years; if arterial ischemic stroke is associated with dissection or a cardioembolic origin, ACCP suggests continued anticoagulant therapy (e.g., with a low molecular weight heparin). In children with acute arterial ischemic stroke secondary to non-Moyamoya vasculopathy, ACCP recommends ongoing antithrombotic therapy (e.g., with a low molecular weight heparin) for 3 months. Antithrombotic therapy generally is not recommended in neonates experiencing a first occurrence of arterial ischemic stroke in the absence of a cardioembolic origin; however, ACCP states that anticoagulant therapy (e.g., with a low molecular weight heparin) may be considered in neonates with a first episode of arterial ischemic stroke associated with a documented cardioembolic source.

■ Thromboembolism during Pregnancy

Low molecular weight heparins are used during pregnancy for prevention and treatment of venous thromboembolism† or for prevention and treatment of systemic embolism associated with prosthetic mechanical heart valves†. For information on the use of low molecular weight heparins in pregnant women with prosthetic heart valves, see Uses: Thromboembolism Associated with Prosthetic Heart Valves.

ACCP states that a low molecular weight heparin (rather than heparin or warfarin) is the anticoagulant of choice for prevention and treatment of thromboembolism during pregnancy. In pregnant women with an acute venous thromboembolic event, subcutaneous low molecular weight heparin is recommended for initial *treatment* and for *secondary prevention* throughout the remainder of the pregnancy. ACCP suggests that anticoagulant therapy be continued for at least 6 weeks postpartum (for a minimum total duration of 3 months) to prevent recurrence of venous thromboembolism.

Recommendations regarding the use of anticoagulant prophylaxis during the antepartum period in pregnant women who have a history of thromboembolism† are based on the patient's risk for recurrent events. In general, prophylaxis (e.g., with a low molecular weight heparin) is suggested only in those at moderate to high risk of recurrent thromboembolism (e.g., those with a single episode of unprovoked venous thromboembolism, pregnancy- or estrogen-related venous thromboembolism, history of multiple unprovoked events). Postpartum thromboprophylaxis† for 6 weeks is suggested in all pregnant women with a prior venous thromboembolic event; a low molecular weight heparin (in prophylactic or intermediate dosages) or warfarin (INR 2–3) may be used for such prophylaxis.

The presence of hereditary thrombophilias substantially increases the risk of pregnancy-related venous thromboembolism, and a family history of venous thromboembolism further increases this risk by twofold to fourfold. Homozygous genetic mutations for factor V Leiden or prothrombin G20210A are associated with the highest risks of thromboembolism in pregnant women. ACCP therefore suggests antepartum prophylaxis with a low molecular weight heparin (in prophylactic or intermediate dosages) in pregnant women with homozygous genetic mutations for factor V Leiden or prothrombin G20210A who have no personal history of venous thromboembolism, but have a family history of venous thromboembolism†; continued prophylaxis with a low molecular weight heparin or warfarin is suggested for 6 weeks postpartum. For pregnant women with homozygous genetic mutations for factor V Leiden or prothrombin G20210A with no individual or family history of venous thromboembolism†, clinical vigilance is suggested during the antepartum period, followed by postpartum prophylaxis with a low molecular weight heparin or warfarin. Antepartum prophylaxis is not recommended in pregnant women with other types of thrombophilias who have no history of venous thromboembolism; however, postpartum prophylaxis is suggested in such women who have a family history of venous thromboembolism.

Anticoagulation with subcutaneous heparin or a low molecular weight heparin is used in combination with low-dose aspirin for prevention of pregnancy loss in women with antiphospholipid antibody (APLA) syndrome in whom recurrent pregnancy loss (3 or more) has occurred†.

To avoid an unwanted anticoagulant effect on the fetus during delivery, therapy with a low molecular weight heparin should be discontinued at least 24 hours prior to induction of labor or cesarean section (or expected time of neuraxial anesthesia). If an at-term woman is at very high risk for recurrent venous thromboembolism (e.g., occurrence of proximal DVT or PE within the past 2 weeks), IV heparin may be initiated at this time and then discontinued 4–6 hours prior to the expected time of delivery. (See Dosage and Administration: Dosage, and see Cautions: Pregnancy and Lactation, in Warfarin 20:12.04.08.) For additional information on the use of antithrombotic therapy during pregnancy, consult the most recent ACCP Evidence-based Clinical Practice Guidelines on Antithrombotic Therapy and Prevention of Thrombosis available at http://www.chestnet.org.

■ Cardioversion of Atrial Fibrillation/Flutter Low molecular weight heparins also have been used for the prevention of stroke and systemic embolism in patients with atrial fibrillation undergoing electrical or pharmacologic cardioversion†. Because the risk of thromboembolism appears to be greatest when atrial fibrillation has been present for more than 48 hours, recommendations for the use of anticoagulant therapy in such patients vary based on the duration of the arrhythmia. ACCP and other experts recommend that patients with atrial fibrillation of unknown or greater than 48 hours' duration who are to undergo elective cardioversion receive therapeutic anticoagulation (e.g., usually with warfarin) for at least 3 weeks prior to cardioversion; an alternative strategy is to use a transesophageal echocardiography (TEE)-guided approach in which patients receive therapeutic anticoagulation with a low molecular weight heparin or heparin at the time of TEE and undergo cardioversion within 24 hours if no thrombus is detected. Patients with atrial fibrillation of short duration (e.g., 48 hours or less) usually do not require prolonged anticoagulation or TEE prior to cardioversion; instead, ACCP suggests that such patients receive therapeutic anticoagulation (e.g., with a low molecular weight heparin or heparin) at presentation, followed by immediate cardioversion. In patients requiring urgent cardioversion because of hemodynamic instability, initiation of a parenteral anticoagulant (e.g., IV heparin or a low molecular weight heparin) in therapeutic doses is suggested prior to cardioversion, if possible; however, initiation of the anticoagulant must not delay any emergency intervention. After successful cardioversion to sinus rhythm, experts recommend that all patients receive therapeutic anticoagulation for at least 4 weeks.

In patients undergoing cardioversion for atrial flutter†, experts state that the same approach to thromboprophylaxis should be used as for those with atrial fibrillation.

■ Thromboembolism Associated with Prosthetic Heart Valves A low molecular weight heparin or heparin is used during conversion to maintenance therapy with oral anticoagulants (e.g., warfarin) to reduce the incidence of thromboembolism (e.g., stroke) in patients with prosthetic mechanical heart valves†. In the absence of a bleeding risk, ACCP suggests bridging anticoagulation (administration of a low molecular weight heparin in either prophylactic or therapeutic dosages or heparin in prophylactic dosages) during the early postoperative period after insertion of a mechanical heart valve until an adequate response to warfarin is obtained. (See Dosage and Administration: Dosage.) In patients with a mechanical heart valve in whom therapy with warfarin must be temporarily discontinued (e.g., those undergoing major surgery), bridging anticoagulation with a low molecular weight heparin or heparin also is suggested in selected patients (e.g., those at high risk of thromboembolism). (See Uses: Thromboembolism Associated with Prosthetic Heart Valves, in Warfarin 20:12.04.08.)

Women with mechanical prosthetic heart valves may be at even higher risk for thromboembolism during pregnancy; thrombosis of prosthetic heart valves, sometimes resulting in death of the mother and/or fetus, has occurred in some pregnant women receiving prophylaxis with a low molecular weight heparin (enoxaparin). Although a causal relationship has not been established and the number of patients involved appears to be small, these deaths may have been related to therapeutic failure or inadequate anticoagulation. Experts state that definitive recommendations about optimal antithrombotic therapy in pregnant women with prosthetic mechanical heart valves† currently are not possible because of a lack of properly designed studies but that fixed-dose low molecular weight heparin or low-dose, poorly controlled heparin therapy is *not* effective in preventing systemic embolism in such patients. Although the manufacturer of dalteparin states that the drug has not been studied systematically in patients with prosthetic heart valves, ACCP and other clinicians state that the use of aggressive, adjusted-dose therapy with a low molecular weight heparin (i.e., given twice daily and adjusted to maintain the manufacturer-recommended peak anti-factor Xa concentrations 4 hours postinjection) may be a reasonable approach in pregnant women with prosthetic mechanical heart valves. (See Uses: Thromboembolism Associated with Prosthetic Heart Valves, in Enoxaparin 20:12.04.16.)

■ Cerebral Venous Sinus Thrombosis ACCP as well as ACC, AHA, and the American Stroke Association (ASA) suggest use of a low molecular weight heparin or heparin for the treatment of acute cerebral venous sinus (sinovenous) thrombosis† in adults; such therapy should be continued until the patient is stable. The patient's therapy may then be converted from heparin to coumarin anticoagulant therapy. AHA and ASA state that it is reasonable to use a low molecular weight heparin in full doses rather than heparin for treatment of acute cerebral venous sinus thrombosis during pregnancy. In addition, AHA and ASA suggest that prophylaxis with a low molecular weight heparin during pregnancy and the postpartum period is reasonable in women with a history of cerebral venous sinus thrombosis.

In children with cerebral venous sinus thrombosis† without substantial intracranial hemorrhage, initial anticoagulation with a low molecular weight heparin or heparin is recommended, followed by a low molecular weight heparin or warfarin for at least 3 months. Another 3 months of anticoagulation is suggested if symptoms persist or there is continued occlusion of the cerebral venous sinuses. Although the evidence is not as compelling as for children without substantial hemorrhage, ACCP also suggests that anticoagulation may be used for the treatment of cerebral venous sinus thrombosis in children with substantial hemorrhage. Low molecular weight heparins also are suggested by ACCP as a treatment option for neonates with cerebral sinovenous thrombosis†. For additional information on the use of anticoagulants in children with cerebral venous sinus thrombosis, consult the most recent ACCP Evidence-based Clinical Practice Guidelines on Antithrombotic Therapy and Prevention of Thrombosis available at http://www.chestnet.org.

■ Perioperative Antithrombotic Prophylaxis Low molecular weight heparins are used in the perioperative management of patients who require temporary interruption of long-term warfarin therapy for surgery or other invasive procedures†. Perioperative use of a low molecular weight heparin or IV heparin during the period of interruption of warfarin therapy (bridging anticoagulation†) is recommended by ACCP in some patients with venous thromboembolism, atrial fibrillation, or prosthetic mechanical heart valves depending on their risk of developing thromboembolism without warfarin therapy. In general, bridging anticoagulation is suggested in such patients who are considered to be at particularly high risk of developing thromboembolism. The decision to administer bridging anticoagulation should be individualized based on the patient's risk of thromboembolism versus bleeding. For additional information on the perioperative management of antithrombotic therapy, consult the most recent ACCP Evidence-based Clinical Practice Guidelines on Antithrombotic Therapy and Prevention of Thrombosis available at http://www.chestnet.org.

Dosage and Administration

■ Administration Dalteparin sodium is administered by deep subcutaneous injection; *it must not be given IM*. Patients should be sitting or supine during administration of the drug. Injections may be made into the U-shaped area around the navel, the upper outer aspect of the thigh, or the upper outer quadrangle of the buttock; injection sites should be alternated daily. When injecting dalteparin into the area around the navel or the thigh, the needle should be inserted into a skin fold created by the thumb and forefinger; the skin should be held until the needle is withdrawn. When injecting dalteparin, the entire length of the needle should be inserted at a 45–90° angle. The injection is commercially available in prefilled syringes equipped with a 27-gauge ½-inch needle.

In general, dalteparin should not be mixed with other injections or infusions unless specific compatibility data are available that support such mixing.

■ Dosage *Dosages for dalteparin sodium or other low molecular weight heparins and for heparin cannot be used interchangeably on a unit-for-unit (or mg-for-mg) basis.*

Dosage of dalteparin sodium is expressed in anti-factor Xa international units (IU, units). Each mg of dalteparin sodium is equivalent to 156.25 units.

Dosage adjustment and routine monitoring of coagulation parameters generally are not necessary if recommended regimens are followed. Monitoring of anti-factor Xa levels may be helpful in certain high-risk patient groups, such as pregnant women with mechanical prosthetic heart valves and pediatric patients receiving therapeutic dosages of low molecular weight heparins.

If a low molecular weight heparin is used for anticoagulation in pregnant women with mechanical prosthetic heart valves, frequent monitoring of peak and trough anti-factor Xa concentrations should be used to assess anticoagulation and dosage adjusted as necessary. (See Patients with Mechanical Prosthetic Heart Valves under Warnings/Precautions: Warnings, in Cautions in Enoxaparin 20:12.04.16.) The American College of Chest Physicians (ACCP) and other clinicians recommend twice-daily dosing of low molecular weight heparins in pregnant women, at least initially, because of the altered pharmacokinetics of these drugs in such women.

If a low molecular weight heparin is used for anticoagulation in children,

ACCP suggests that dosage of the drug be adjusted to a target anti-factor Xa level of 0.5–1 units/mL based on a sample taken 4–6 hours following subcutaneous administration, or 0.5–0.8 units/mL based on a sample taken 2–6 hours following subcutaneous administration.

In general, when warfarin is used for follow-up therapy after dalteparin, therapy with the 2 drugs is overlapped until an adequate response to warfarin is obtained, as indicated by international normalized ratio (INR) determinations. (See Dosage and Administration: Dosage, in Warfarin 20:12.04.08.) ACCP recommends that dalteparin and warfarin be used concurrently for a minimum of 5 days and until the INR is at least 2 for 24 hours or longer.

Unstable Angina and Non-ST-Segment-Elevation Myocardial Infarction For reducing the risk of ischemic complications in patients with unstable angina or non-ST-segment-elevation myocardial infarction (i.e., non-ST-segment-elevation acute coronary syndromes), the usual dosage of dalteparin sodium is 120 units/kg (up to a maximum of 10,000 units) every 12 hours by subcutaneous injection. Concurrent aspirin therapy is recommended in all patients except when contraindicated. Anticoagulant therapy should be administered as soon as possible after hospital admission. Treatment should continue until the patient is clinically stabilized, generally for 5–8 days.

Prevention of Deep-Vein Thrombosis and/or Pulmonary Embolism **Hip-Replacement Surgery.** For the prevention of postoperative deep-vein thrombosis (DVT), which may lead to pulmonary embolism (PE), in patients undergoing hip-replacement surgery, several dosing options are recommended by the manufacturer for dalteparin therapy. The drug may be initiated either before or after surgery. With preoperative administration, the manufacturer states that a dose of 5000 units of dalteparin sodium may be given 10–14 hours before surgery (the evening prior to the procedure), followed by a second dose of 5000 units 4–8 after surgery (or later if hemostasis has not been achieved). An alternative, manufacturer-recommended preoperative regimen is 2500 units given within 2 hours before surgery, followed by a second dose of 2500 units 4–8 hours after surgery (or later if hemostasis has not been achieved). With postoperative administration, a dose of 2500 units of dalteparin sodium may be given 4–8 hours *after* surgery (or later if hemostasis has not been achieved). ACCP states that risk of bleeding is closely associated with the timing of initiation of thromboprophylaxis around surgery. Although administration times closer to surgery have been recommended by the manufacturer for the first dose of dalteparin sodium, ACCP recommends that low molecular weight heparins be initiated at least 12 hours preoperatively or at least 12 hours postoperatively in patients undergoing major orthopedic surgery. Dalteparin sodium therapy should be continued throughout the postoperative period at a dosage of 5000 units once daily, generally for 5–10 days; ACCP recommends a minimum of 10–14 days of thromboprophylaxis, with extended prophylaxis suggested for up to 35 days on an outpatient basis.

General/Abdominal Surgery. For the prevention of postoperative DVT in patients undergoing general (e.g., abdominal) surgery who are at risk for thromboembolic complications, the usual dosage of dalteparin sodium is 2500 units daily by subcutaneous injection. The initial dose should be given 1–2 hours before surgery, followed by daily administration of the same dosage throughout the postoperative period, generally for 5–10 days, until the risk of DVT has diminished.

A higher dalteparin dosage is recommended in patients undergoing abdominal surgery associated with a high risk of thromboembolism (e.g., surgery for malignant disease). In such patients, a dosage of 5000 units of dalteparin sodium once daily is recommended; the initial dose should be administered the evening prior to surgery, followed by daily administration of 5000 units throughout the postoperative period. Alternatively, in patients with malignancy, 2500 units of dalteparin sodium may be administered subcutaneously 1–2 hours prior to surgery, followed 12 hours later by a second dose of 2500 units, then 5000 units once daily throughout the postoperative period. With either dosing regimen, the manufacturer states that the usual duration of thromboprophylaxis is 5–10 days. Because the risk of venous thromboembolism is particularly high in patients undergoing abdominal or pelvic surgery for cancer, ACCP recommends that therapy with a low molecular weight heparin be continued for up to 4 weeks in such patients.

Medical Conditions Associated with Thromboembolism. For prevention of venous thromboembolism in acutely ill medical patients with severely restricted mobility, the usual dosage of dalteparin sodium is 5000 units once daily. The duration of prophylaxis in clinical trials was 12–14 days.

Extended Treatment of Venous Thromboembolism in Cancer Patients For the extended treatment of symptomatic venous thromboembolism (DVT and/or PE) in patients with cancer to reduce recurrence (secondary prevention), the manufacturer recommends an initial dalteparin sodium dosage of 200 units/kg once daily (based on total body weight) for the first 30 days of treatment, followed by a dosage of approximately 150 units/kg once daily for up to 6 months; the total daily dosage should not exceed 18,000 units. Safety and efficacy of treatment beyond 6 months have not been evaluated in cancer patients with acute symptomatic venous thromboembolism.

The daily dosage of dalteparin sodium should be reduced by 2500 units in patients with thrombocytopenia (platelet counts of 50,000–100,000/mm^3) until platelet counts recover to at least 100,000/mm^3. If platelet counts decrease to less than 50,000/mm^3, therapy should be discontinued until recovery of platelet count to at least 50,000/mm^3.

Treatment and Prevention of Thromboembolism During Pregnancy For the initial treatment of acute venous thromboembolic events in pregnant women†, dalteparin sodium at a dosage of 200 units/kg daily in 1 or 2 divided doses is recommended by ACCP and should be continued throughout the remainder of the pregnancy. Anticoagulation should be continued postpartum for at least 6 weeks (minimum total duration of 3 months).

If dalteparin sodium is used for postpartum prophylaxis in pregnant women with a prior venous thromboembolic event†, a prophylactic (e.g., 5000 units once daily) or intermediate (e.g., 5000 units every 12 hours) dosage is suggested.

In pregnant women receiving long-term coumarin anticoagulation (e.g., warfarin)†, ACCP suggests the use of a low molecular weight heparin throughout pregnancy given in a weight-adjusted dosage (e.g., dalteparin sodium 100 units/kg twice daily or dalteparin sodium 200 units/kg once daily) or 75% of a weight-adjusted dosage, followed by postpartum resumption of long-term coumarin anticoagulation.

If dalteparin sodium is used for primary prevention of venous thromboembolism in pregnant women with certain high-risk thrombophilias†, a prophylactic (e.g., 5000 units once daily) or intermediate (e.g., 5000 units every 12 hours) dosage is suggested.

In women with antiphospholipid antibody (APLA) syndrome†, antepartum administration of a low molecular weight heparin in prophylactic dosages combined with low-dose aspirin (75–100 mg daily) is recommended by ACCP.

To avoid an unwanted anticoagulant effect on the fetus during delivery, therapy with a low molecular weight heparin should be discontinued at least 24 hours prior to induction of labor or cesarean section. If an at-term woman is at very high risk for recurrent venous thromboembolism (e.g., occurrence of proximal DVT within the past 2 weeks), IV heparin may be initiated at this time and then discontinued 4–6 hours prior to the expected time of delivery.

Cardioversion of Atrial Fibrillation/Flutter If dalteparin sodium is used for the prevention of stroke and systemic embolism in patients undergoing cardioversion for atrial fibrillation or atrial flutter†, administration of full-treatment dosages used for venous thromboembolism is recommended.

Perioperative Antithrombotic Prophylaxis If dalteparin is used for bridging anticoagulation in patients who require temporary interruption of warfarin therapy during surgery or other invasive procedure†, ACCP recommends the use of therapeutic dosages (e.g., dalteparin sodium 100 units/kg twice daily or 200 units/kg once daily) because of more extensive data and experience; however, other dosage regimens have been used.

ACCP suggests that the last preoperative dose of dalteparin sodium be given approximately 24 hours prior to surgery to allow sufficient time for anticoagulant effects to dissipate. Postoperative anticoagulation should be administered with caution and only when hemostasis has been achieved because of the potential for bleeding at the surgical site. In patients undergoing procedures associated with a high risk of bleeding, ACCP suggests delaying the resumption of therapeutic-dose dalteparin until 48–72 hours after surgery when adequate hemostasis has been achieved.

■ **Dosage in Renal and Hepatic Impairment** Dosage adjustment guidelines for dalteparin sodium in patients with renal or hepatic impairment have not been established. However, the manufacturer recommends caution in using the drug in patients with severe renal or hepatic insufficiency. Anti-factor Xa levels may be monitored to determine appropriate dosage in high-risk patients, such as pregnant women, patients with severe renal impairment, patients at extremes of weight, or if abnormal coagulation parameters or bleeding occurs during therapy. Limited evidence indicates that elimination of the drug may be delayed in patients with chronic renal insufficiency requiring hemodialysis. ACCP suggests that dosages of low molecular weight heparins be reduced in patients with severe renal impairment (creatinine clearance less than 30 mL/minute).

Cautions

Dalteparin generally is well tolerated. Although adverse reactions to dalteparin generally are mild, discontinuance has been required in approximately 1–5% of patients receiving the drug in clinical trials, principally because of hemorrhagic complications. The incidence of minor hemorrhagic complications with dalteparin is similar to or lower than that with heparin. The most frequent adverse effect of dalteparin is hematoma at the injection site.

■ **Spinal/Epidural Hematomas** Spinal or epidural hemorrhage and subsequent hematomas can occur with concurrent use of low molecular weight heparins or heparinoids and neuraxial (spinal/epidural) anesthesia or spinal puncture procedures. (See Cautions: Precautions and Contraindications.)

■ **Other Hematologic Effects** The incidence of hemorrhagic complications during dalteparin therapy is low. The incidence of hemorrhage may increase with higher doses of the drug; however, in patients with malignancy undergoing abdominal surgery, a significant increase in hemorrhage was not observed in patients receiving dalteparin sodium 5000 units compared with those receiving dalteparin sodium 2500 units or low-dose heparin. In a clinical trial in patients undergoing surgery for malignancy, the incidence of hemorrhagic events was 4.6% in those receiving dalteparin sodium 5000 units once daily and 3.6% in those receiving 2500 units once daily (the difference was not significant). In a subgroup of patients undergoing surgery for malignancy in a similar trial, the incidence of hemorrhagic events was 3.2 or 2.7% in patients receiving dalteparin sodium 5000 units once daily or heparin sodium 5000 units twice daily, respectively.

Major hemorrhagic events (e.g., intracranial hemorrhage, a hemoglobin decrease of at least 2 g/dL with an observed bleeding site, hemorrhage associated with death, or hemorrhage requiring a blood transfusion or drug discontinuance) in patients with acute coronary syndromes occurred in 1, 1, or 0.5% of patients receiving dalteparin subcutaneously, heparin IV and subcutaneously, or placebo injection subcutaneously, respectively, in controlled clinical trials. In several comparative clinical trials in patients undergoing hip-replacement surgery, major hemorrhagic events occurred in 2.5–3.6, 0.4–3.1, or 4.3% of patients receiving subcutaneous dalteparin, oral warfarin, or subcutaneous heparin, respectively. In a clinical trial in acutely ill medical patients with severely restricted mobility, major hemorrhagic events occurred in 0.49 or 0.16% of patients receiving dalteparin or placebo, respectively. Major hemorrhagic events in patients receiving dalteparin and undergoing hip-replacement surgery included wound hematoma (reoperation was required in at least one patient), bleeding from the operative site, intraoperative bleeding as a result of vessel damage, and GI bleeding.

The most frequent adverse hematologic effect of dalteparin is hematoma at the injection site, which occurred in 0.2–7.1% of patients receiving the drug in clinical trials. In comparison, hematoma at the injection site was reported in 1.1–9.5% of patients receiving heparin and 1.1% of patients receiving placebo in these clinical trials. In patients undergoing hip-replacement surgery, hematoma at the injection site was reported in 1.1–2.9 or 10.1% of patients receiving subcutaneous dalteparin or heparin, respectively. Wound hematomas occurred in 0.1–3.4, 1.2–3.9, or 2.6% of patients receiving dalteparin, heparin, or placebo, respectively, in these clinical trials. Wound hematomas occurred in 2.2% of patients undergoing hip-replacement surgery receiving dalteparin, and in none of the patients receiving heparin or warfarin in these clinical trials.

In clinical trials in patients undergoing abdominal surgery, postoperative transfusions were required in 5.7–8.7 or 12.1–15.9% of patients receiving dalteparin sodium 2500 or 5000 units once daily, respectively. In these trials in patients undergoing abdominal surgery, postoperative transfusions were required in 7.1 or 7.9–12.7% of patients receiving placebo or heparin sodium 5000 units twice daily, respectively. Reoperation because of hemorrhage was required in 0.5–1.3% of patients undergoing abdominal surgery receiving dalteparin in these clinical trials, and in 0.4–0.8 or 1.3% of patients receiving heparin or placebo, respectively. Postoperative hemorrhage, injection site bruising, perioperative hemorrhage, gastric hemorrhage, vaginal hemorrhage, and hematuria also have been reported with dalteparin in patients undergoing abdominal surgery. In clinical trials in patients undergoing hip-replacement surgery, hematuria was reported in 2.9 or 1.8% of patients receiving subcutaneous dalteparin or oral warfarin, respectively.

Thrombocytopenia with platelet counts less than 50,000/mm^3 was reported in less than 1% of patients receiving dalteparin for noncancer indications in clinical trials. In the clinical trial in patients with cancer receiving extended dalteparin therapy (i.e., up to 6 months) for acute symptomatic venous thromboembolism, thrombocytopenia with platelet counts less than 50,000 or less than 100,000/mm^3 occurred in 6.5 or 13.6%, respectively, of patients who received the drug; dosage reduction or treatment interruption was necessary in such patients. Thrombocytopenia with thrombosis, amputation, and death, also has been reported. (See Cautions: Precautions and Contraindications.)

■ **Dermatologic and Sensitivity Reactions** Allergic reactions (including pruritus, rash, fever, injection site reactions, and bullous eruptions) and skin necrosis have occurred rarely in patients receiving dalteparin. Anaphylactoid reactions also have been reported in patients receiving the drug.

■ **Local Effects** Injection site pain occurred in 12% of patients undergoing hip-replacement surgery receiving dalteparin and in up to 13% of patients receiving heparin in clinical trials. Injection site pain occurred in up to 4.5% of patients undergoing abdominal surgery receiving dalteparin and in up to 11.8% of patients receiving heparin in clinical trials. Hematoma at the injection site also has been reported. (See Cautions: Hematologic Effects.) Hyperkalemia also has been reported with dalteparin.

■ **Hepatic Effects** Asymptomatic increases in serum AST (SGOT) and ALT (SGPT) concentrations exceeding 3 times the upper limit of normal have been reported in 1.7 and 4.3%, respectively, of patients receiving dalteparin. Similar increases in serum aminotransferase concentrations also have occurred in patients receiving other low molecular weight heparins or heparin. These elevations are completely reversible and rarely associated with increases in serum bilirubin concentration.

■ **Precautions and Contraindications** The possibility of an underlying bleeding disorder should be ruled out before initiating dalteparin therapy. The usual precautions and contraindications associated with heparin anticoagulant therapy should be followed in patients for whom dalteparin therapy is considered. Dalteparin should be used with extreme caution in patients with an increased risk of hemorrhage. Factors that may increase the risk of hemorrhage during dalteparin therapy include severe uncontrolled hypertension, bacterial endocarditis, congenital or acquired bleeding disorders, active ulceration and angiodysplastic GI disease, hemorrhagic stroke, or recent brain, spinal, or ophthalmologic surgery.

As with other anticoagulants, bleeding may occur at any site during dalteparin therapy. If severe hemorrhage or dalteparin overdosage occurs, protamine sulfate should be administered immediately. To largely neutralize the effects of dalteparin following overdosage, the dose of protamine sulfate is determined by the administered dose of the low molecular weight heparin, the time elapsed since the drug was given, and blood coagulation studies. The dose of protamine sulfate to be given should be equal to that of the administered dalteparin dose if dalteparin was administered in the previous 8 hours (i.e., 1 mg of protamine sulfate should be given to neutralize 100 anti-factor Xa units of dalteparin sodium). If more than 8 hours has elapsed since dalteparin was administered, an infusion of 0.5 mg of protamine sulfate may be given for each 100 anti-factor Xa units of dalteparin sodium administered. If the activated partial thromboplastin time (aPTT) measured 2–4 hours after the first protamine infusion remains prolonged, a second dose of 0.5 mg of protamine sulfate may be given for each 100 anti-factor Xa units of dalteparin sodium administered. Protamine administration may not be required if more than 12 hours has elapsed since administration of dalteparin. However, even after higher dosages of protamine sulfate, the aPTT may remain more prolonged than would be the case following treatment of overdosage of conventional heparin since anti-factor Xa activity is never completely neutralized. A maximum of about 60–75% of anti-factor Xa activity is neutralized with protamine sulfate administration for overdosage of dalteparin.

Concurrent use of a low molecular weight heparin or heparinoid (e.g., danaparoid [no longer commercially available in the US]) with neuraxial (spinal/epidural) anesthesia or spinal puncture procedures has been associated with epidural or spinal hematomas. More than 15 cases of spinal/epidural hematoma associated with the concurrent use of dalteparin and neuraxial anesthesia have been reported since market introduction of the drug in 1985. Hematomas occurring in some of these patients have resulted in neurologic injury, including long-term or permanent paralysis. The risk of these adverse events is increased by the use of indwelling epidural catheters for administration of analgesia or the concomitant use of drugs that affect hemostasis, such as nonsteroidal anti-inflammatory agents (NSAIAs), platelet-aggregation inhibitors, or other anticoagulants. The risk also appears to be increased by a history of traumatic or repeated epidural or spinal puncture, spinal surgery, or spinal deformity.

The risk of spinal bleeding applies to all anticoagulants when used in conjunction with neuraxial anesthesia or spinal puncture. Prior to performing a spinal or epidural procedure, healthcare professionals should determine as part of a preprocedure checklist whether a patient is receiving anticoagulants. In addition, clinicians should carefully consider the timing of spinal catheter placement and removal in relation to anticoagulant use, considering both the dosage and pharmacokinetic properties (e.g., elimination half-life) of the anticoagulant. Patients receiving dalteparin thromboprophylaxis prior to surgery can be assumed to have altered coagulation; to minimize the risk of bleeding, the manufacturer recommends that the first postoperative dose (2500 units) be administered 6–8 hours after surgery and that the second dose (2500 or 5000 units) be administered no sooner than 24 hours after the first dose.

Insertion or removal of an epidural catheter or lumbar puncture is best performed when the anticoagulant effect of dalteparin is minimal. Although the optimal timing between the administration of dalteparin and neuraxial procedures is not known, the following guidelines are recommended. In patients receiving low (prophylactic) dosages of dalteparin sodium (2500 or 5000 units once daily), insertion or removal of a spinal catheter should be delayed for at least 12 hours after a dose of dalteparin is administered. In patients receiving higher (treatment) dosages of dalteparin sodium (200 units/kg once daily or 120 units/kg twice daily), a delay of at least 24 hours is recommended between the dalteparin dose and catheter placement/removal. In patients with renal impairment (creatinine clearance less than 30 mL/minute), a doubling of the recommended time delays (i.e., at least 24 hours after the prophylactic dosage and at least 48 hours after the treatment dosage) is recommended to account for possible prolonged elimination of dalteparin in such patients. The manufacturer suggests that while a specific recommendation cannot be made, administration of dalteparin should be delayed for at least 4 hours after catheter removal, taking into account a patient's risk of bleeding versus thrombosis in the context of the procedure and other patient risk factors.

Patients receiving low molecular weight heparins or heparinoids in the setting of epidural or spinal anesthesia or lumbar puncture should be monitored frequently for signs and symptoms of neurologic impairment (e.g., midline back pain, numbness or weakness in lower limbs, bowel or bladder dysfunction). If spinal hematoma is suspected, urgent diagnosis and treatment is necessary; spinal cord decompression should be considered even though such treatment may not prevent or reverse neurologic sequelae. The manufacturer and some experts recommend against the concomitant use of a low molecular weight heparin and other drugs affecting hemostasis (e.g., aspirin, NSAIAs, platelet-aggregation inhibitors, other anticoagulants) in patients receiving spinal anesthesia. The decision to implement thromboprophylaxis with a low molecular weight heparin in the presence of an indwelling epidural catheter should be made with extreme care. Clinicians should fully consider the potential benefits versus risks of spinal or epidural anesthesia or spinal puncture in patients receiving or being considered for thromboprophylaxis with anticoagulants.

Thrombocytopenia of any degree occurring in patients receiving dalteparin should be monitored closely. Heparin-induced thrombocytopenia (HIT) also can occur with the administration of dalteparin. For patients with HIT with or without thrombosis, nonheparin anticoagulants such as lepirudin or argatroban are recommended; continued use of a low molecular weight heparin is contraindicated in such patients.

Because of an increased risk of bleeding, dalteparin should be used with care in patients receiving oral anticoagulants and/or platelet-aggregation inhibitors.

Because serum aminotransferase determinations are important in the differential diagnosis of myocardial infarction (MI), liver disease, and pulmonary emboli, elevation of these enzymes during dalteparin therapy should be interpreted with caution.

Dalteparin is contraindicated in patients with known hypersensitivity to the drug or to heparin or pork products. Dalteparin also is contraindicated in patients with active major bleeding or a history of HIT or HIT with thrombosis. In patients undergoing epidural/neuraxial anesthesia, use of dalteparin for the treatment of unstable angina or non-ST-segment elevation MI or for prolonged prophylaxis of venous thromboembolism is contraindicated.

■ **Pediatric Precautions** Safety and efficacy of dalteparin in children have not been established.

Each mL of Fragmin® (dalteparin sodium injection) in multiple-dose vials contains 14 mg of benzyl alcohol as a preservative. Although a causal relationship has not been established, administration of injections preserved with benzyl alcohol has been associated with toxicity in neonates. Toxicity appears to have resulted from administration of large amounts (i.e., 100–400 mg/kg daily) of benzyl alcohol in these neonates, principally associated with the use of bacteriostatic 0.9% sodium chloride intravascular flush or endotracheal tube lavage solutions. The American Academy of Pediatrics (AAP) states that use of preservative-containing flush solutions (i.e., with benzyl alcohol) clearly should be avoided in neonates; however, the presence of small amounts of benzyl alcohol in a commercially available injection should not proscribe its use in neonates. Because benzyl alcohol may cross the placenta, the manufacturer states that dalteparin in multiple-dose vials should not be used in pregnant women.

■ **Geriatric Precautions** While safety and efficacy of dalteparin in geriatric patients have not been established specifically, a large proportion of patients treated with the drug for prevention of postoperative deep-vein thrombosis (DVT) have been 65 years of age or older and dosage adjustments based on age were not made. In addition, limited evidence indicates that the pharmacokinetics of dalteparin are similar in geriatric and younger adults. However, geriatric patients may have decreased renal function and because patients with severe renal impairment may be at increased risk of dalteparin-induced toxicity. Careful attention to dosing intervals and concomitant agents (particularly antiplatelet agents) is advised, particularly in geriatric patients with low body weight (less than 45 kg) and in patients predisposed to decreased renal function.

■ **Mutagenicity and Carcinogenicity** Dalteparin did not exhibit any evidence of mutagenicity in vitro in the Ames test, mouse lymphoma cell forward mutation test, or human lymphocyte chromosomal aberration test, or in vivo in the mouse micronucleus test.

Studies have not been performed to date to evaluate the carcinogenic potential of dalteparin.

■ **Pregnancy, Fertility, and Lactation** Reproduction studies using dalteparin sodium at IV doses up to 2400 units/kg (14,160 units/m^2) in pregnant rats and 4800 units/kg (40,800 units/m^2) in pregnant rabbits did not reveal any evidence of impaired fertility or fetal harm. Dalteparin has been used in a limited number of women during the second and/or third trimester of pregnancy for the prevention and treatment of DVT without detectable placental transfer or evidence of adverse fetal effects or unusual adverse maternal effects. However, there are no adequate and controlled studies to date using dalteparin in pregnant women, and the drug should be used during pregnancy only when clearly needed. Although a causal relationship has not been established, valve thrombosis and maternal and fetal deaths have occurred in some pregnant women with prosthetic heart valves who were receiving thromboprophylaxis with a low molecular weight heparin (e.g., enoxaparin), and the manufacturer of dalteparin states that the drug has not been studied systematically in patients with prosthetic heart valves. (See Uses: Thromboembolism During Pregnancy, in Enoxaparin 20:12.04.16.)

Reproduction studies in male and female rats using subcutaneous dalteparin sodium doses up to 1200 units/kg (7080 units/m^2) did not reveal any evidence of impaired fertility or reproductive performance.

Small amounts of dalteparin appear to be distributed into breast milk. Although one study estimated that such distribution is not clinically important, the manufacturer states that the drug should be used with caution in nursing women. The American College of Chest Physicians (ACCP) recommends that low molecular weight heparins be continued in nursing women who are already receiving such therapy.

Description

Dalteparin, a depolymerized heparin prepared by nitrous acid degradation of heparin of porcine intestinal mucosa origin, is an anticoagulant. Dalteparin is commercially available as the sodium salt. The average molecular weight of dalteparin is approximately one-third to one-half that of heparin (5000 [90% of which ranges between 2000–000] versus 12,000 daltons); therefore, dalteparin is referred to as a low molecular weight heparin.

At a given level of anti-factor Xa activity, dalteparin has less effect on thrombin than does heparin. The manufacturer states that, at recommended dosages, dalteparin does not substantially affect platelet aggregation, fibrinolysis, global clotting function tests (i.e., prothrombin time, thrombin time, activated partial thromboplastin time), or lipoprotein lipase. Compared with heparin, dalteparin has greater bioavailability (based on anti-factor Xa activity) after subcutaneous administration and a longer half-life, allowing less frequent administration.

The molecular weight, pharmacokinetics, and in vitro and in vivo activity of dalteparin differ from those of other low molecular weight heparins or heparin; therefore, the drugs are not interchangeable on a unit-for-unit (or mg-for-mg) basis.

SumMon® (see Users Guide). For additional information on this drug until a more detailed monograph is developed and published, the manufacturer's labeling should be consulted. It is *essential* that the labeling be consulted for detailed information on the usual cautions, precautions, and contraindications concerning potential drug interactions and/or laboratory test interferences and for information on acute toxicity.

Preparations

Excipients in commercially available drug preparations may have clinically important effects in some individuals; consult specific product labeling for details.

Dalteparin Sodium (Porcine)

Parenteral		
Injection, for subcutaneous use only	2500 units/0.2 mL	**Fragmin®** (available as single-dose prefilled syringes), Pfizer
	5000 units/0.2 mL	**Fragmin®** (available as single-dose prefilled syringes), Pfizer
	7500 units/0.3 mL	**Fragmin®** (available as single-dose prefilled syringes), Pfizer
	10,000 units/0.4 mL	**Fragmin®** (available as single-dose prefilled syringes), Pfizer
	12,500 units/0.5 mL	**Fragmin®** (available as single-dose prefilled syringes), Pfizer
	15,000 units/0.6 mL	**Fragmin®** (available as single-dose prefilled syringes), Pfizer
	18,000 units/0.72 mL	**Fragmin®** (available as single-dose prefilled syringes), Pfizer
	10,000 units/ mL	**Fragmin®** (available as single-dose graduated syringes), Pfizer
	95,000 units/9.5 mL (10,000 units/mL)	**Fragmin®** (available as multiple-dose vial), Pfizer
	25,000 units/mL	**Fragmin®** (available as multiple-dose vial), Pfizer
	95,000 units/3.8 mL (25,000 units/mL)	**Fragmin®** (available as multiple-dose vial), Pfizer

†Use is not currently included in the labeling approved by the US Food and Drug Administration

Selected Revisions October 2017, © Copyright, June 1996, American Society of Health-System Pharmacists, Inc.

Enoxaparin Sodium LMWH

■ Enoxaparin, a low molecular weight heparin prepared by alkaline degradation of unfractionated benzylated heparin ("unfractionated heparin" is subsequently referred to throughout this monograph as "heparin") of porcine intestinal mucosa origin, is an anticoagulant.

Uses

Enoxaparin is used for the prevention of postoperative deep-vein thrombosis (DVT), which may lead to pulmonary embolism (PE), in patients undergoing hip- or knee-replacement surgery, patients undergoing general (e.g., abdominal, gynecologic, urologic) surgery, and in patients with acute medical conditions and severely restricted mobility who are at risk for thromboembolic complications. Enoxaparin is used concurrently with warfarin in hospitalized patients for the treatment of DVT with or without PE and in outpatients for the treatment of acute DVT *without* accompanying PE. Enoxaparin also is used concurrently with aspirin and/or other therapy (e.g., nitrates, β-adrenergic blockers, clopidogrel, platelet glycoprotein [GP] IIb/IIIa-receptor inhibitors) for the prevention of ischemic events (e.g., myocardial infarction [MI]) associated with unstable angina or non-ST-segment-elevation MI (NSTEMI) (i.e., non-ST-segment-elevation acute coronary syndromes [NSTE ACS]). Enoxaparin also is used for the treatment of patients with acute ST-segment-elevation MI (STEMI) receiving thrombolysis and being managed medically or with percutaneous coronary intervention (PCI).

The use of a low molecular weight heparin such as enoxaparin also is suggested by the American College of Chest Physicians (ACCP) for prevention of venous thromboembolism in patients with major trauma†, including brain injury, acute spinal injury, and traumatic spine injury; in selected patients undergoing intracranial neurologic surgery† (e.g., craniotomy for malignant disease); selected cancer patients; and in patients with acute ischemic stroke†. Therapy with a low molecular weight heparin also has been recommended for the prevention and treatment of thromboembolism during pregnancy and for prevention of embolism in selected patients with atrial fibrillation or atrial flutter† who require prolonged (exceeding 1 week) interruption of oral anticoagulant therapy for diagnostic or surgical procedures or during shorter periods of interrupted therapy in high-risk patients (e.g., those with mechanical prosthetic heart valves†). Although a causal relationship has not been established and the number of patients involved appears to be small, cases of valve thrombosis resulting in death (including maternal and fetal deaths) and/or requiring surgical intervention have been reported with enoxaparin prophylaxis in patients (including pregnant women) with prosthetic heart valves; insufficient data, underlying conditions, and the possibility of inadequate anticoagulation also complicate evaluation of these events. (See Patients with Mechanical Prosthetic Heart Valves under Warnings/Precautions: Warnings, in Cautions.)

The usual precautions and contraindications associated with heparin anticoagulation should be followed in patients for whom enoxaparin therapy is considered. (See Cautions.)

■ Deep-Vein Thrombosis and/or Pulmonary Embolism

Prophylaxis **General/Abdominal Surgery.** Enoxaparin is used for the prevention of postoperative DVT, which may lead to PE, in patients undergoing general (e.g., abdominal) surgery who are at risk for thromboembolic complications. ACCP recommends pharmacologic (e.g., low molecular weight heparin) and/or nonpharmacologic/mechanical (e.g., intermittent pneumatic compression) methods of thromboprophylaxis in patients undergoing general surgery, including abdominal, GI, gynecologic, and urologic surgery, according to the patient's level of risk for thromboembolism for thromboembolism for thromboembolism and bleeding. In general, pharmacologic prophylaxis is recommended in patients with high (and possibly moderate) risk of venous thromboembolism who do not have a high risk of bleeding, while mechanical methods are suggested in patients who require thromboprophylaxis but have a high risk of bleeding. If pharmacologic prophylaxis is used in patients undergoing general surgery, ACCP states that a low molecular weight heparin or low-dose heparin is preferred, but when these agents are contraindicated or not available, aspirin or fondaparinux may be considered. Because the risk of venous thromboembolism is particularly high in patients undergoing abdominal or pelvic surgery for cancer, extended (4 weeks) prophylaxis with a low molecular weight heparin is recommended in such patients. ACCP states that the same recommendations for the use of antithrombotic agents in general surgery patients can be applied to patients undergoing bariatric surgery, vascular surgery, and plastic and reconstructive surgery. For additional information on the prevention of venous thromboembolism in patients undergoing general surgery, consult the most recent ACCP Evidence-based Clinical Practice Guidelines on Antithrombotic Therapy and Prevention of Thrombosis available at http://www.chestnet.org.

In a large trial comparing enoxaparin sodium (40 mg subcutaneously once daily) with heparin sodium (5000 units subcutaneously every 8 hours) administered 2 hours prior to initiation of GI, urologic, or gynecologic surgery in cancer patients and continuing for a maximum of 12 days after surgery, enoxaparin and heparin demonstrated similar efficacy in preventing thromboembolic events (DVT, PE, or death associated with thromboembolism), with these events occurring in 10.1 or 11.3% of patients receiving enoxaparin or heparin, respectively (based on intent-to-treat analysis). Data from another large trial of similar design and treatment duration in patients undergoing colorectal surgery (one-third of whom had cancer) also indicate similar efficacy for enoxaparin sodium (40 mg daily given subcutaneously) or heparin sodium (5000 units subcutaneously every 8 hours); thromboembolic events occurred in 7.1 or 6.7% of patients receiving enoxaparin or heparin, respectively (based on intent-to-treat analysis).

Hip-Replacement, Knee-Replacement, or Hip-Fracture Surgery. Enoxaparin is used during and following hospitalization for the prevention of postoperative DVT, which may lead to PE, in patients undergoing hip-replacement surgery. The drug also is used for the prevention of postoperative DVT and/or PE in patients undergoing knee-replacement surgery. Low molecular weight heparins, including enoxaparin, also have been used for thromboprophylaxis in patients undergoing hip-fracture surgery†. ACCP recommends routine thromboprophylaxis (with a pharmacologic and/or mechanical method [e.g., intermittent pneumatic compression]) in all patients undergoing major orthopedic surgery, including total hip-replacement, total knee-replacement, and hip-fracture surgery, because of the high risk for postoperative venous thromboembolism; thromboprophylaxis should be continued for at least 10–14 days, and possibly for up to 35 days after surgery. Several antithrombotic agents (e.g., low molecular weight heparins, fondaparinux, low-dose heparin, warfarin, aspirin) are recommended by ACCP for pharmacologic thromboprophylaxis in patients undergoing major orthopedic surgery. Among the different options, ACCP suggests that a low molecular weight heparin generally is preferred because of its relative efficacy and safety and extensive clinical experience; alternative agents may be considered in situations in which a low molecular weight heparin is not available or cannot be used (e.g., in patients with heparin-induced thrombocytopenia [HIT] or in those who refuse or are uncooperative with subcutaneous injections). ACCP states that when selecting an appropriate thromboprophylaxis regimen, factors such as relative efficacy and bleeding risk as well as other logistics and compliance issues should be considered. For additional information on the prevention of venous thromboembolism in patients undergoing orthopedic surgery, consult the most recent ACCP Evidence-based Clinical Practice Guidelines on Antithrombotic Therapy and Prevention of Thrombosis available at http://www.chestnet.org.

In a study in patients undergoing hip-replacement surgery in whom prophylaxis was initiated 12–24 hours postoperatively and continued for 10–14 days, DVT occurred in 10% of patients treated with enoxaparin sodium 30 mg twice daily versus 46% of placebo-treated patients. Limited data from comparative studies suggest that enoxaparin has efficacy similar to or exceeding that of heparin in preventing DVT in patients undergoing hip-replacement surgery. In a large dose-ranging study in patients undergoing hip-replacement surgery and receiving prophylactic enoxaparin sodium 10 mg once daily, 30 mg twice daily (every 12 hours), or 40 mg once daily 24–48 hours following surgery and continuing for 7–11 days, the incidence of DVT was 25, 11, or 14%, respectively. Thus, therapy with 40 mg of enoxaparin sodium daily is an alternative to 30 mg of enoxaparin sodium twice daily in patients undergoing hip-replacement surgery.

In a double-blind study in patients undergoing knee-replacement surgery in whom prophylaxis was initiated 12–24 hours postoperatively and continued for up to 15 days, DVT occurred in 11% of patients treated with enoxaparin sodium 30 mg twice daily versus 62% of placebo-treated patients. Limited data from an unblinded comparative study suggest that enoxaparin sodium (30 mg subcutaneously every 12 hours) has efficacy similar to or exceeding that of heparin sodium (5000 units subcutaneously every 8 hours) in preventing DVT in patients undergoing knee-replacement surgery.

Some evidence suggests that extended prophylaxis† with a low molecular weight heparin (i.e., for up to 35 days post-surgery) may provide additional protection against thromboembolism in patients undergoing total hip- or total-knee replacement surgery. The risk of DVT is greater for the first several months following hip- or knee-replacement surgery compared with general surgery. While the manufacturer states that the usual duration of enoxaparin therapy following hip- or knee-replacement surgery is 7–10 days, with up to 14 days administered in clinical trials, ACCP suggests extended prophylaxis for up to 35 days in patients undergoing major orthopedic surgery. Results from several placebo-controlled trials that included an extended treatment phase in outpatients with a hip prosthesis who had received short-term prophylaxis with enoxaparin sodium while hospitalized (40 mg once daily initiated 12 hours prior to surgery and continued for 10–15 days) indicate that extended prophylaxis with enoxaparin sodium (40 mg once daily for 3 additional weeks) decreased the incidence of DVT, including asymptomatic thrombosis (as determined by venography), compared with placebo. In one controlled trial in outpatients who had a normal phlebogram at study entry, DVT occurred in 7% of patients receiving extended therapy with enoxaparin compared with 20% of patients receiving placebo; PE was not detected. In another placebo-controlled trial in patients who had no clinical evidence of venous thromboembolism at study entry, DVT (as determined by venography) occurred in 16% of patients receiving extended enoxaparin therapy versus 34% of those receiving placebo; most thromboembolic events were asymptomatic. Broader inclusion criteria of one trial may have contributed to the relatively greater incidence of later thromboembolic events in these patients with a hip prosthesis receiving extended enoxaparin therapy.

Medical Conditions Associated with Thromboembolism. Enoxaparin is used for the prevention of DVT, which may lead to PE in patients whose mobility is severely restricted during acute illness.

In a large, placebo-controlled trial in hospitalized patients with acute illness (e.g., congestive heart failure, acute or chronic respiratory failure/insufficiency, acute infection, acute rheumatic disorder, acute arthritic episodes involving the lower extremities) reported to be at moderate risk for thromboembolism (e.g., patients who were immobilized for more than 3 days were excluded), venous thromboembolic events (DVT, PE, and death associated with thromboembolism) between days 1 and 14 (the primary outcome) occurred in 4.4% of patients treated with enoxaparin sodium (40 mg twice daily given subcutaneously for 6–14 days) versus 11.9% of patients receiving placebo (based on intent-to-treat analysis). Therapy with enoxaparin sodium at a dosage of 20 mg twice daily was no more effective than placebo in these patients.

Treatment decisions regarding the use of prophylactic anticoagulants in acutely ill hospitalized patients should include an assessment of the patient's individual risk of venous thromboembolism and risk of bleeding. In general, pharmacologic thromboprophylaxis is recommended only in patients who are considered to be at high risk of venous thromboembolism because the risk-to-benefit trade-off between the reduction in venous thromboembolic events and bleeding is considered to be more favorable in such patients. Factors that should be considered when choosing an appropriate anticoagulant include patient preference, compliance, ease of administration, and costs associated with the individual agents. ACCP recommends the use of anticoagulant thromboprophylaxis (e.g., a low molecular weight heparin) in acutely ill, hospitalized medical patients at increased risk of thrombosis who are not actively bleeding and do not have an increased risk of bleeding. Continued thromboprophylaxis is suggested for 6–21 days until full mobility is restored or hospital discharge, whichever comes first; extended prophylaxis beyond these periods generally is not recommended. Risk of venous thromboembolism in critically ill patients in an intensive care unit (ICU) varies depending on their acute or chronic conditions (e.g., sepsis, congestive heart failure), specific exposures, and circumstances (e.g., surgery, immobilization, mechanical ventilation, central venous catheters). A low molecular weight heparin is suggested by ACCP as an option for pharmacologic thromboprophylaxis in critically ill patients who are not actively bleeding and do not have risk factors for bleeding.

Risk of venous thromboembolism is particularly high in patients with cancer. Routine pharmacologic thromboprophylaxis generally is not recommended in cancer patients in the outpatient setting who have no additional risk factors for venous thromboembolism; however, ACCP suggests the use of prophylactic-dose low molecular weight heparin or low-dose heparin in cancer outpatients with solid tumors who have additional thromboembolic risk factors and are at low risk of bleeding.

Treatment and Secondary Prevention **Deep-vein Thrombosis and/or Pulmonary Embolism.** Enoxaparin is used concurrently with warfarin for the treatment of DVT with or without PE in hospitalized patients and also in outpatients for the treatment of acute DVT *without* PE.

Low molecular weight heparins are recommended by ACCP as an appropriate choice of anticoagulant for the initial treatment of acute proximal DVT and/or PE. When warfarin therapy is being considered for the long-term treatment of venous thromboembolism, the drug should be initiated concurrently with enoxaparin, and such therapy should be continued for at least 5 days and until the international normalized ratio (INR) is at least 2 for 24 hours or longer. (See Treatment of Venous Thromboembolism under Dosage and Administration: Dosage.) Anticoagulant therapy generally is not recommended for the treatment of isolated distal DVT unless symptoms are severe and there is a risk for thrombus extension.

Analysis of pooled data from numerous comparative randomized clinical studies suggests that a low molecular weight heparin is at least as effective as heparin in the treatment and further outpatient prevention (secondary prevention) of recurrent venous thromboembolism. However, a low molecular weight heparin may offer certain advantages over heparin such as more convenient administration and less risk of HIT. ACCP generally suggests the use of a low molecular weight heparin or fondaparinux rather than heparin for the initial treatment of acute venous thromboembolism. Low molecular weight heparins and fondaparinux are considered to be comparable; therefore, the choice between these agents should be dictated by local considerations such as cost, availability, and familiarity of use. Heparin may be preferred in patients with renal impairment. In addition, ACCP states that IV heparin should be considered over subcutaneous therapies (e.g., subcutaneous low molecular weight heparin) in patients with PE in whom thrombolytic therapy is being considered or if there is a concern about the adequacy of subcutaneous absorption.

In patients with venous thromboembolism, ACCP recommends that anticoagulant therapy be continued beyond the acute treatment period for at least 3 months, and possibly longer depending on the location of thrombi (e.g., distal versus proximal vein), presence of a reversible, provoking risk factor (e.g., surgery), presence of cancer, and the patient's risk of bleeding. Warfarin generally is the preferred anticoagulant for long-term treatment of venous thromboembolism in patients without cancer; however, in patients with cancer, ACCP suggests the use of a low molecular weight heparin over warfarin because of a possible reduced response to warfarin therapy in such patients. (See Treatment and Secondary Prevention under Uses: Deep-Vein Thrombosis and Pulmonary Embolism, in Warfarin Sodium 20:12.04.08.) For additional information on treatment of venous thromboembolism, consult the most recent ACCP Evidence-based Clinical Practice Guidelines on Antithrombotic Therapy and Prevention of Thrombosis available at http://www.chestnet.org.

Data from several comparative trials evaluating therapy with enoxaparin sodium (1 mg/kg twice daily or 1.5 mg/kg daily for a minimum of 5 days) or adjusted-dose heparin sodium (dosage adjusted to prolong the aPTT between 55 and 85 seconds) in patients with acute lower extremity DVT with or without PE indicate that enoxaparin is as effective as adjusted-dose heparin in the prevention of recurrent thromboembolic events (i.e., DVT, PE). Warfarin was initiated within 72 hours of initiation of enoxaparin or adjusted-dose heparin and was continued for 90 days. In one of the comparative trials, patients with uncomplicated acute DVT received adjusted-dose heparin as inpatients or enoxaparin with the option of home therapy. Patients were included in the study only if their condition warranted home treatment or early hospital discharge (within 4 days of admittance); most patients screened did not meet patient selection criteria and were excluded from study entry.

■ **Non-ST-Segment-Elevation Acute Coronary Syndromes**

Enoxaparin is used concurrently with aspirin and/or other therapy (e.g., nitrates, β-adrenergic blocking agents [β-blockers], clopidogrel, GP IIb/IIIa-receptor inhibitors) to reduce the risk of acute cardiac ischemic events (death and/or MI) in patients with non-ST-segment-elevation acute coronary syndromes (NSTE ACS). Patients with NSTE ACS have either unstable angina or NSTEMI; because these conditions are part of a continuum of acute myocardial ischemia and have indistinguishable clinical features upon presentation, the same initial treatment strategies are recommended. The American Heart Association/American College of Cardiology (AHA/ACC) guideline for the management of patients with NSTE ACS recommends an early invasive strategy (angiographic evaluation with the intent to perform revascularization procedures such as PCI with coronary artery stent implantation or coronary artery bypass grafting [CABG]) or an ischemia-guided strategy (initial medical management followed by cardiac catheterization and revascularization if indicated) in patients with definite or likely NSTE ACS; standard medical therapies for all patients should include a β-blocker, antiplatelet agents, anticoagulant agents, nitrates, and analgesic agents regardless of the initial management approach.

All patients with NSTE ACS should receive immediate antiplatelet therapy (e.g., aspirin, clopidogrel). An anticoagulant agent should be added to antiplatelet therapy as soon as possible after presentation. Initial parenteral anticoagulants with established efficacy in patients with NSTE ACS include enoxaparin, heparin, bivalirudin (only in patients who are being managed with an early invasive strategy), and fondaparinux.

Data from several trials comparing a low molecular weight heparin (e.g., enoxaparin, dalteparin) with heparin in patients with NSTE ACS indicate that low molecular weight heparins are at least as effective as heparin in preventing MI and death during the acute phase (e.g., first week) of therapy. While some patients with unstable angina in these trials had a low risk of further ischemic complications (e.g., effort angina only, no ECG changes indicative of myocardial ischemia), most patients studied were at intermediate to high risk of further ischemic complications.

In the acute phase (first 14 days after hospitalization) of a large comparative trial (Efficacy and Safety of Subcutaneous Enoxaparin in Non-Q-wave Coronary Events [ESSENCE]) evaluating short-term therapy with aspirin and enoxaparin sodium (1 mg/kg twice daily) or heparin sodium (loading dose of 5000 units, then a continuous infusion adjusted to maintain the aPTT between 55 and 85 seconds) for a median duration of 2.6 days (range: 2–8 days) in patients with acute coronary syndromes (unstable angina, NSTEMI), the frequency of the combined outcome of death, nonfatal MI, or recurrent angina was reduced in patients receiving enoxaparin compared with heparin. Combined end points in this study occurred in about 16.5 or 19.8% of patients receiving enoxaparin or heparin, respectively, at 14 days. The incidence of these end points increased to about 19.8 or 23.4% in those receiving enoxaparin or heparin, respectively, at 30 days and to about 32 or 35.7% of those receiving enoxaparin or heparin, respectively, at 1 year: differences in these combined end points were statistically significant at all these evaluation time points. Urgent revascularization procedures were performed less frequently in patients receiving enoxaparin (6.3%) than heparin (8.2%) at 30 days after initiation of treatment. Of the combined end points, reduction of recurrent angina was most striking with enoxaparin therapy. When the incidence of death or MI was considered separately, the effect of enoxaparin on these remaining end points was similar to heparin.

In another comparative trial (Thrombolysis in Myocardial Infarction [TIMI] 11B) evaluating enoxaparin sodium (30 mg loading dose followed by 1 mg/kg twice daily [every 12 hours] for approximately 5 days) and heparin sodium (70 units/kg loading dose followed by an infusion with dosage adjusted to maintain the aPTT between 1.5–2.5 times the control value for 3 days), the combined incidence of death, nonfatal MI, or need for urgent revascularization was 12.4% in those receiving enoxaparin and 14.5% in those receiving heparin at 8 days; the relative risk reduction in these end points was 14.6%. The effect of trial therapies of unequal duration on the observed outcome is uncertain.

In a randomized, open-label comparative (SYNERGY) study in approximately 10,000 high-risk patients with non-ST-segment elevation acute coronary syndromes, therapy with enoxaparin was noninferior to therapy with heparin in terms of the incidence of the combined outcome of all-cause death or nonfatal MI at 30 days (primary efficacy end point). The primary efficacy end point occurred in 14% of patients receiving enoxaparin sodium (1 mg/kg subcutaneously every 12 hours) versus 14.5% of patients receiving heparin sodium (60 units/kg by direct IV ["bolus"] injection followed by initial infusion of 12 units/kg per hour with subsequent dosage adjustment to achieve an aPTT of 1.5–2 times the upper limit of normal or 50–70 seconds). Patients were intended to be treated with an early invasive strategy, and most received concomitant therapy with aspirin (162–325 mg daily) and GP IIb/IIIa-receptor inhibitors. Approximately 47% of total patients underwent PCI and 19% had surgical revascularization procedures. Major bleeding (defined as intracranial bleeding or a decrease of at least 5 g/dL in hemoglobin or at least 15% in hematocrit, according to TIMI criteria) occurred more frequently in enoxaparin-treated patients and was related principally to CABG.

Enoxaparin also has been administered by direct IV injection† in patients with NSTE ACS undergoing PCI to prevent thrombus formation at the site of arterial injury, the coronary guidewire, and in the catheters used for the procedure. If therapy with subcutaneous enoxaparin is initiated prior to PCI ("upstream"), an additional IV dose may be required at the time of PCI based on the timing of the last administered subcutaneous dose. (See Non-ST-Segment-Elevation Acute Coronary Syndromes under Dosage and Administration: Dosage.)

■ **ST-Segment-Elevation Myocardial Infarction** Enoxaparin is used as adjunctive therapy in the management of acute ST-segment-elevation MI (STEMI) in patients receiving thrombolysis and being managed medically or with PCI. When used in conjunction with aspirin, enoxaparin has been shown to reduce the rate of a composite end point of recurrent MI or death in such patients.

The current standard of care in patients with STEMI is timely reperfusion (with primary PCI or thrombolytic therapy). Adjunctive therapy with anticoagulant (e.g., heparin) and antiplatelet (e.g., aspirin and clopidogrel) agents should be used during and after successful coronary artery reperfusion for the prevention of early reocclusion and death, unless contraindicated. (See Uses: Acute Ischemic Complications of ST-Segment-Elevation Myocardial Infarction, in Heparin 20:12.04.16.) Adjunctive use of a low molecular weight heparin (e.g., enoxaparin, dalteparin) in patients with STEMI has been associated with improvement in short-term clinical outcomes (e.g., death, reinfarction, recurrent ischemia) with generally similar rates of bleeding complications compared with adjunctive heparin or placebo in a few studies.

ACCF and AHA state that patients with STEMI undergoing thrombolytic therapy should receive an anticoagulant (e.g., heparin, enoxaparin, fondaparinux) for a minimum of 48 hours, and preferably for the duration of the index hospitalization, up to 8 days or until revascularization is performed. Enoxaparin is preferred over heparin if extended anticoagulation is necessary beyond 48 hours.

Efficacy of enoxaparin as adjunctive therapy in the management of acute STEMI has been established in more than 20,000 patients with acute STEMI who were scheduled to undergo thrombolytic therapy with tenecteplase, alteplase, reteplase, or streptokinase. In a multicenter, randomized, double-blind, double-dummy, parallel-group study (Enoxaparin and Thrombolysis Reperfusion for Acute Myocardial Infarction treatment-Thrombolysis in myocardial infarction 25 [EXTRACT-TIMI 25]), treatment with adjunctive enoxaparin was more effective than adjunctive heparin (17% relative risk reduction) in reducing the rate of the composite efficacy end point of death from any cause or nonfatal recurrent MI at 30 days; the treatment benefit of enoxaparin emerged after 48 hours and was observed both in patients who were managed medically as well as those managed with PCI. The benefit of enoxaparin on the primary efficacy end point during the first 30 days of treatment was maintained over a 12-month follow-up period; however, there was no additional reduction in recurrent MI after 30 days and no mortality reduction at 1 year. In addition, an increased risk of major bleeding (including intracranial hemorrhage) was observed in patients receiving enoxaparin compared with those in patients receiving heparin. Careful patient selection is needed to ensure that the benefits of enoxaparin outweigh the increased risk of bleeding associated with the drug.

In the EXTRACT-TIMI 25 study, enoxaparin was given in an initial dose of 30 mg by direct IV injection in conjunction with a 1-mg/kg subcutaneous dose, followed by 1 mg/kg every 12 hours by subcutaneous injection for patients younger than 75 years of age, or in a dosage of 0.75 mg/kg every 12 hours by subcutaneous injection without an initial direct IV dose for patients 75 years of age or older; heparin was administered in an initial dose of 60 units/kg (maximum 4000 units) by direct IV injection followed by continuous IV infusion of 12 units/kg per hour. All patients received aspirin (150–325 mg initially, then 75–325 mg daily) for at least 30 days. Enoxaparin was administered throughout the index hospitalization period (mean treatment duration of 6.6 days), while heparin was administered for at least 48 hours (mean duration of 54 hours). The relatively longer duration of enoxaparin treatment compared with that of heparin and a possible rebound increase in thrombotic events following discontinuance of heparin therapy may have contributed to the treatment differences in this study.

In patients with STEMI who are subsequently undergoing PCI, enoxaparin is administered initially by direct IV injection to prevent thrombus formation at the site of arterial injury, the coronary guidewire, and in the catheters used for the procedure. (See ST-Segment-Elevation Myocardial Infarction under Dosage and Administration: Dosage.) There is less experience with the use of enoxaparin in the setting of primary PCI† in patients with STEMI. (See Uses: Acute Ischemic Complications of Percutaneous Coronary Intervention, in Heparin 20:12.04.16.)

■ Superficial Vein Thrombosis Low molecular weight heparins also have been used for the treatment of superficial vein thrombosis (superficial thrombophlebitis)†. ACCP suggests the use of prophylactic dosages of a low molecular weight heparin or fondaparinux for 45 days in patients with superficial vein thrombosis of at least 5 cm in length.

■ Cardiac Surgery Because the risk of venous thromboembolism in most patients undergoing cardiac surgery† is considered to be moderate, mechanical methods of prophylaxis (preferably with an intermittent pneumatic compression device) generally are recommended over pharmacologic prophylaxis. However, ACCP states that use of a pharmacologic method (e.g., a low molecular weight heparin) may be considered in cardiac surgery patients with a complicated postoperative course.

■ Thoracic Surgery Pharmacologic thromboprophylaxis with a low molecular weight heparin or low-dose heparin is recommended by ACCP in patients undergoing thoracic surgery† who are at high risk of venous thromboembolism, provided risk of bleeding is low.

■ Neurosurgery Patients undergoing craniotomy, especially for malignant disease, are considered to be at increased risk of venous thromboembolism. Although low molecular weight heparins have been used for the prevention of venous thromboembolism in such patients, the benefits of pharmacologic prophylaxis may be outweighed by the possible increased risk of intracranial hemorrhage. ACCP suggests the use of a mechanical method of prophylaxis (preferably intermittent pneumatic compression) in craniotomy patients; for patients considered to be at *very* high risk for thromboembolism, such as those undergoing craniotomy for malignant disease†, a pharmacologic method (e.g., low molecular weight heparin) may be added once adequate hemostasis has been established and the risk of bleeding decreases.

In patients undergoing spinal surgery†, a mechanical method of thromboprophylaxis (preferably intermittent pneumatic compression) also is suggested, with possible addition of pharmacologic prophylaxis (e.g., low molecular weight heparin) in high-risk patients (e.g., those with malignancy or those undergoing surgery with a combined anterior-posterior approach) once adequate hemostasis is established and risk of bleeding decreases.

■ Trauma In general, some form of thromboprophylaxis (with a low molecular weight heparin, low-dose heparin, or a mechanical method) is suggested by ACCP in all patients with major trauma†. For major trauma patients at high risk of venous thromboembolism, including those with acute spinal cord injury, traumatic brain injury, or spinal surgery for trauma, ACCP suggests the use of both a pharmacologic and mechanical method of prophylaxis, unless contraindications exist.

■ Renal Vein Thrombosis Renal vein thrombosis† is the most common cause of spontaneous venous thromboembolism in neonates. Although use of anticoagulant therapy for treatment of renal vein thrombosis remains controversial, low molecular weight heparins are suggested by ACCP as a possible treatment option in selected neonates.

■ Acute Ischemic Stroke Although therapeutic-dose anticoagulation has been used in patients with acute ischemic stroke†, there is strong evidence that such treatment is associated with worse outcomes than aspirin therapy in terms of increased mortality and rates of nonfatal major extracranial bleeding. Therefore, ACCP recommends early treatment (within 48 hours) with aspirin over therapeutic anticoagulation to prevent recurrent cerebral thromboembolism in patients with acute ischemic stroke or TIA. (See Uses: Thrombosis, in Aspirin 28:08.04.24.)

Heparin anticoagulants (i.e., low molecular weight heparins or heparin) have been used for thromboprophylaxis in patients with acute ischemic stroke; those with additional risk factors for venous thromboembolism are more likely to benefit from such prophylaxis. ACCP suggests that thromboprophylaxis with a low molecular weight heparin (in prophylactic dosages), subcutaneous heparin, or intermittent pneumatic compression devices be administered to patients with acute ischemic stroke† and restricted mobility. Among the anticoagulant options, ACCP suggests the use of a low molecular weight heparin over heparin. Prophylactic-dose heparin (heparin or a low molecular weight heparin) usually is initiated within 48 hours of the onset of stroke and is continued throughout the hospital stay until the patient regains mobility; such heparin therapy should not be given within the first 24 hours after administration of thrombolytic therapy.

A low molecular weight heparin also is recommended by ACCP as an option for the initial management of acute arterial ischemic stroke in children† until dissection and embolic causes have been excluded. When dissection or cardioembolic causes have been excluded, daily aspirin therapy (in prophylactic dosages) is suggested for a minimum of 2 years; if arterial ischemic stroke is associated with dissection or a cardioembolic origin, ACCP suggests continued anticoagulant therapy (e.g., with a low molecular weight heparin). In children with acute arterial ischemic stroke secondary to non-Moyamoya vasculopathy†, ACCP recommends ongoing antithrombotic therapy (e.g., with a low molecular weight heparin) for 3 months. Antithrombotic therapy generally is not recommended in neonates experiencing a first occurrence of arterial ischemic stroke in the absence of a cardioembolic origin; however, ACCP states that anticoagulant therapy (e.g., with a low molecular weight heparin) may be considered in neonates with a first episode of arterial ischemic stroke associated with a documented cardioembolic source†.

■ Thromboembolism During Pregnancy Low molecular weight heparins are used during pregnancy for prevention and treatment of venous thromboembolism† or for prevention and treatment of systemic embolism associated with prosthetic mechanical heart valves†. Low molecular weight heparins also may be used in combination with aspirin for the prevention of recurrent pregnancy loss in women with antiphospholipid antibodies†. Pregnancy is associated with a hypercoagulable state and an increased risk of thromboembolism, and pregnant women with thromboembolic disease or hereditary or acquired thrombophilias are at greater risk for fetal loss as a result of stillbirth, spontaneous abortion, or premature delivery. For information on the use of low molecular weight heparins in pregnant women with prosthetic mechanical heart valves†, see Uses: Thromboembolism Associated with Prosthetic Heart Valves.

ACCP states that a low molecular weight heparin (rather than heparin or warfarin) is the anticoagulant of choice for prevention and treatment of thromboembolism during pregnancy. In pregnant women with an acute venous thromboembolic event†, subcutaneous low molecular weight heparin is recommended for initial *treatment* and *secondary prevention* throughout the remainder of the pregnancy. ACCP suggests that anticoagulant therapy be continued (for at least 6 weeks postpartum and a minimum total duration of 3 months) to prevent recurrence of venous thromboembolism.

Recommendations regarding the use of anticoagulant prophylaxis during the antepartum period in pregnant women who have a history of thromboembolism† are based on the patient's risk for recurrent events. In general, thromboprophylaxis (e.g., with a low molecular weight heparin) is suggested only in those at moderate to high risk of recurrent thromboembolism (e.g., those with a single episode of unprovoked venous thromboembolism, pregnancy- or estrogen-related venous thromboembolism, history of multiple unprovoked events). Postpartum thromboprophylaxis† for 6 weeks is suggested in all pregnant women with a prior venous thromboembolic event; a low molecular weight heparin (in prophylactic or intermediate dosages) or warfarin (INR 2–3) may be used for such prophylaxis.

The presence of hereditary thrombophilias substantially increases the risk of pregnancy-related venous thromboembolism, and a family history of venous thromboembolism further increases this risk by twofold to fourfold. Homozygous genetic mutations for factor V Leiden or prothrombin G20210A are associated with the highest risks of thromboembolism in pregnant women. ACCP therefore suggests antepartum prophylaxis with a low molecular weight heparin (in prophylactic or intermediate dosages) in pregnant women with homozygous genetic mutations for factor V Leiden or prothrombin G20210A who have no personal history of venous thromboembolism, but have a family history of venous thromboembolism†; continued prophylaxis with a low molecular weight heparin or warfarin is suggested for 6 weeks postpartum. For pregnant women with homozygous genetic mutations for factor V Leiden or prothrombin

G20210A with no individual or family history of venous thromboembolism†, clinical vigilance is suggested during the antepartum period, followed by postpartum prophylaxis with a low molecular weight heparin or warfarin. Antepartum prophylaxis is not recommended in pregnant women with other types of thrombophilias who have no history of venous thromboembolism; however, postpartum prophylaxis is suggested in such women who have a family history of venous thromboembolism†.

Anticoagulation with subcutaneous heparin or a low molecular weight heparin is used in combination with low-dose aspirin for prevention of pregnancy loss in women with antiphospholipid antibodies (APLA) syndrome in whom recurrent (3 or more) pregnancy loss has occurred†.

To avoid an unwanted anticoagulant effect on the fetus during delivery, therapy with a low molecular weight heparin should be discontinued at least 24 hours prior to induction of labor or cesarean section (or expected time of neuraxial anesthesia). If an at-term woman is at very high risk for recurrent venous thromboembolism (e.g., occurrence of proximal DVT or PE within the past 2 weeks), IV heparin may be initiated at this time and then discontinued 4–6 hours prior to the expected time of delivery. (See Dosage and Administration: Dosage and see Cautions: Pregnancy and Lactation, in Warfarin 20:12.04.08.)

For additional information on the use of antithrombotic therapy during pregnancy, consult the most recent ACCP Evidence-based Clinical Practice Guidelines on Antithrombotic Therapy and Prevention of Thrombosis available at http://www.chestnet.org.

■ **Cardioversion of Atrial Fibrillation/Flutter** Low molecular weight heparins also have been used for the prevention of stroke and systemic embolism in patients with atrial fibrillation undergoing electrical or pharmacologic cardioversion†. Because the risk of thromboembolism appears to be greatest when atrial fibrillation has been present for more than 48 hours, recommendations for the use of anticoagulant therapy in such patients vary based on the duration of the arrhythmia. ACCP and other experts recommend that patients with atrial fibrillation of unknown or greater than 48 hours' duration who are to undergo elective cardioversion receive therapeutic anticoagulation (e.g., usually with warfarin) for at least 3 weeks prior to cardioversion; an alternative strategy is to use a transesophageal echocardiography (TEE)-guided approach in which patients receive therapeutic anticoagulation with a low molecular weight heparin or heparin at the time of TEE and undergo cardioversion within 24 hours if no thrombus is detected. Patients with atrial fibrillation of short duration (e.g., 48 hours or less) usually do not require prolonged anticoagulation or TEE prior to cardioversion; instead, ACCP suggests that such patients receive therapeutic anticoagulation (e.g., with a low molecular weight heparin or heparin) at presentation, followed by immediate cardioversion. In patients requiring urgent cardioversion because of hemodynamic instability, initiation of a parenteral anticoagulant (e.g., IV heparin or a low molecular weight heparin) in therapeutic doses is suggested prior to cardioversion, if possible; however, initiation of the anticoagulant must not delay any emergency intervention. After successful cardioversion to sinus rhythm, experts recommend that all patients receive therapeutic anticoagulation for at least 4 weeks.

In patients undergoing cardioversion for atrial flutter†, experts state that the same approach to thromboprophylaxis should be used as for those with atrial fibrillation.

■ **Thromboembolism Associated with Prosthetic Heart Valves** A low molecular weight heparin or heparin is used during conversion to maintenance therapy with oral anticoagulants (e.g., warfarin) to reduce the incidence of thromboembolism (e.g., stroke) in patients with prosthetic mechanical heart valves†. In the absence of a bleeding risk, ACCP suggests bridging therapy (administration of a low molecular weight heparin in either prophylactic or therapeutic dosages or heparin in prophylactic dosages) during the early postoperative period after insertion of a mechanical heart valve until an adequate response to warfarin is obtained. (See Dosage and Administration: Dosage.) In patients with a mechanical heart valve in whom therapy with warfarin must be temporarily discontinued (e.g., those undergoing major surgery), bridging anticoagulation with a low molecular weight heparin or heparin also is suggested in selected patients (e.g., those at high risk of thromboembolism). (See Uses: Thromboembolism Associated with Prosthetic Heart Valves, in Warfarin 20:12.04.08.)

Pregnant women with prosthetic mechanical heart valves† may be at even higher risk for thromboembolism; thrombosis of prosthetic heart valves has occurred in some pregnant women receiving enoxaparin prophylaxis and in some cases has resulted in maternal and/or fetal death. Although a causal relationship has not been established and the number of patients involved appears to be small, these deaths may have been related to therapeutic failure or inadequate anticoagulation. Experts state that definitive recommendations about optimal antithrombotic therapy in pregnant women with prosthetic mechanical heart valves currently are not possible because of a lack of properly designed studies but that fixed-dose low molecular weight heparin or adjusted-dose, poorly controlled heparin therapy is *not* effective in preventing systemic embolism in such patients. ACCP and other clinicians state that in the absence of definitive data regarding optimal therapy and because of the associated risks of withholding antithrombotic therapy in pregnant women with prosthetic mechanical heart valves†, the use of aggressive, adjusted-dose therapy with a low molecular weight heparin (i.e., given twice daily and adjusted to maintain the manufacturer-recommended peak anti-factor Xa concentration at 4 hours post-injection) or high-dose subcutaneous heparin therapy (i.e., given every 12 hours and adjusted to maintain the mid-interval aPTT at least twice the control value or corresponding to an anti-factor Xa concentration of 0.35–0.7 units/mL) appears reasonable in such patients. Another option recommended in pregnant women with prosthetic mechanical heart valves is use of subcutaneous low molecular weight heparin or heparin until week 13 of pregnancy (i.e., because of teratogenicity concerns with warfarin), changing to warfarin until close to term to avoid anticoagulation of the fetus, and then resuming low molecular weight heparin or heparin; oral anticoagulation may be resumed postpartum in women requiring continuing anticoagulant therapy. The option to continue warfarin throughout pregnancy (until close to term) may be reasonable in patients judged to be at very high risk of thromboembolism (e.g., those with a history of thromboembolism, those with an older-generation mechanical valve in the mitral position). (See Cautions: Pregnancy and Lactation, in Warfarin 20:12.04.08.) In high-risk women with mechanical heart valves, ACCP suggests addition of aspirin (75–100 mg daily) to any of these anticoagulant regimens to reduce the risk of thrombosis.

Use of enoxaparin for thromboprophylaxis in pregnant women and other patients with mechanical prosthetic heart valves has not been adequately studied and a clinical consensus regarding optimal therapy remains to be established. (See Patients with Mechanical Prosthetic Heart Valves under Warnings/Precautions: Warnings, in Cautions.) The pharmacokinetics of low molecular weight heparins differ in pregnant versus nonpregnant women because of changes in volume of distribution resulting in increased plasma volume, decreased half-life, and changes in renal clearance. If enoxaparin is used for anticoagulation in pregnant women with mechanical prosthetic heart valves, frequent monitoring of peak and trough anti-factor Xa levels and dosage adjustments may be required to ensure consistent anticoagulation.

■ **Venous Thromboembolism in Pediatric Patients** Low molecular weight heparins also have been used for the treatment and secondary prevention of venous thromboembolism in pediatric patients†. Unlike in adults, most episodes of venous thromboembolism in children are secondary to an identifiable risk factor such as the presence of a central venous access device. Recommendations regarding the use of antithrombotic therapy in children generally are based on extrapolation from adult guidelines. A low molecular weight heparin or heparin is recommended by ACCP for both the initial and ongoing treatment of venous thromboembolism in children. Potential advantages of low molecular weight heparins include reduced need for monitoring, lack of drug or dietary interactions, reduced risk of HIT, and possible reduced risk of osteoporosis. In children with central venous catheter-related thromboembolism, ACCP recommends that the catheter be removed if no longer functioning or required; at least 3–5 days of therapeutic anticoagulation is suggested prior to its removal. If the central venous access device is required, ACCP suggests that anticoagulants be given until the catheter is removed. For additional information on treatment of venous thromboembolism in neonates and children, consult the most recent ACCP Evidence-based Clinical Practice Guidelines on Antithrombotic Therapy and Prevention of Thrombosis available at http://www.chestnet.org.

■ **Cerebral Venous Sinus Thrombosis** ACCP as well as ACC, AHA, and the American Stroke Association (ASA) suggest the use of heparin or a low molecular weight heparin for the treatment of acute cerebral venous sinus (sinovenous) thrombosis† in adults; such therapy should be continued until the patient is stable. The patient's therapy may then be converted from heparin to coumarin anticoagulant therapy. AHA and ASA state that it is reasonable to use a low molecular weight heparin in full doses rather than heparin for treatment of acute cerebral venous sinus thrombosis during pregnancy. In addition, AHA and ASA suggest that prophylaxis with a low molecular weight heparin during pregnancy and the postpartum period is reasonable in women with a history of cerebral venous sinus thrombosis.

In children with cerebral venous sinus thrombosis† without substantial intracranial hemorrhage, initial anticoagulation with a low molecular weight heparin or heparin is recommended, followed by a low molecular weight heparin or warfarin for at least 3 months. Another 3 months of anticoagulation is suggested if symptoms persist or there is continued occlusion of the cerebral venous sinuses. Although the evidence is not as compelling as for children without substantial hemorrhage, ACCP also suggests that anticoagulation may be used for the treatment of cerebral venous sinus thrombosis in children with substantial hemorrhage. Low molecular weight heparins also are suggested by ACCP as a treatment option for neonates with cerebral sinovenous thrombosis. For additional information on the use of anticoagulants in pediatric patients with cerebral venous sinus thrombosis, consult the most recent ACCP Evidence-based Clinical Practice Guidelines on Antithrombotic Therapy and Prevention of Thrombosis available at http://www.chestnet.org.

■ **Perioperative Antithrombotic Prophylaxis** Low molecular weight heparins are used during temporary interruption of long-term warfarin therapy for surgery or other invasive procedures†. Perioperative use of a low molecular weight heparin or IV heparin during the period of interruption of warfarin therapy (bridging anticoagulation†) is recommended by ACCP in some patients with venous thromboembolism, atrial fibrillation, or mechanical prosthetic heart valves depending on their risk of developing thromboembolism. In general, bridging anticoagulation is suggested in such patients who are considered to be at particularly high risk of venous thromboembolism. The decision to administer bridging anticoagulation should be individualized based on the patient's risk of thromboembolism versus risk of bleeding. For additional information on the perioperative management of antithrombotic therapy, consult the most recent ACCP Evidence-based Clinical Practice Guidelines on Antithrombotic Therapy and Prevention of Thrombosis available at http://www.chestnet.org.

Dosage and Administration

■ **Reconstitution and Administration** Enoxaparin sodium is administered by deep subcutaneous injection; *it must not be given IM.* In selected patients with acute ST-segment-elevation myocardial infarction (STEMI), enoxaparin is given as an initial direct IV ("bolus") injection followed by subcutaneous administration. Enoxaparin also has been administered by direct IV injection† in selected patients with unstable angina or non-ST-segment-elevation myocardial infarction (NSTEMI) undergoing percutaneous coronary intervention (PCI). Patients should be supine during administration of the drug.

To avoid loss of drug when using the 30- or 40-mg prefilled syringes, the manufacturer states that air should not be expelled from the syringe prior to injection.

When injecting enoxaparin subcutaneously, the entire length of the needle should be inserted into a skin fold created by the thumb and the forefinger; the skin fold should be held until the needle is withdrawn. Injections should be made into the left and right anterolateral and posterolateral abdominal wall; injection sites should be alternated frequently. To minimize bruising, injection sites should not be massaged after injection.

■ **Dosage** *Dosages for enoxaparin sodium or other low molecular weight heparins or heparin sodium cannot be used interchangeably on a unit-for-unit (or mg-for-mg) basis.* Enoxaparin sodium has an approximate anti-factor Xa activity of 100 units/mg according to the World Health Organization (WHO) First International Low Molecular Weight Heparin Reference Standard.

The possibility of an underlying bleeding disorder should be ruled out before initiating enoxaparin therapy. Since coagulation parameters are insensitive for monitoring enoxaparin activity, routine monitoring of coagulation parameters generally is not required. In pregnant patients, patients at extremes of weight, or if abnormal coagulation parameters, appreciable renal impairment, or bleeding should occur, anti-factor Xa levels may be used to monitor the anticoagulant effects of enoxaparin. (See Dosage and Administration: Special Populations.)

If enoxaparin is used for anticoagulation in pregnant women with mechanical prosthetic heart valves, frequent monitoring of peak and trough anti-factor Xa concentrations should be used to assess anticoagulation and dosage adjusted as necessary. (See Patients with Mechanical Prosthetic Heart Valves under Warnings/Precautions: Warnings, in Cautions.) The American College of Chest Physicians (ACCP) and other clinicians recommend twice-daily dosing of low molecular weight heparins in pregnant women, at least initially, because of the altered pharmacokinetics of these drugs in such women.

If a low molecular weight heparin is used for anticoagulation in children, ACCP suggests that dosage of the drug be adjusted to a target anti-factor Xa level of 0.5–1 units/mL based on a sample taken 4–6 hours, or 0.5–0.8 units/mL based on a sample taken 2–6 hours, following subcutaneous administration.

In general, when warfarin is used for follow-up therapy after enoxaparin, therapy with the 2 drugs is overlapped until an adequate response to warfarin is obtained, as indicated by international normalized ratio (INR) determinations. (See Dosage and Administration: Dosage, in Warfarin 20:12.04.08.) ACCP recommends that enoxaparin and warfarin be used concurrently for a minimum of 5 days and until the INR is at least 2 for 24 hours or longer.

Prevention of Venous Thrombosis and Pulmonary Embolism

General/Abdominal Surgery. For prevention of postoperative deep-vein thrombosis (DVT), which may lead to pulmonary embolism (PE), in patients undergoing general surgery, including abdominal, gynecologic, or urologic surgery, who are at risk for thromboembolic complications (e.g., those with malignancy, history of DVT or PE, or obesity, or patients older than 40 years of age or undergoing major surgery under general anesthesia lasting longer than 30 minutes), the manufacturer recommends an enoxaparin sodium dosage of 40 mg once daily by subcutaneous injection. The initial dosage should be given 2 hours prior to surgery. Enoxaparin should be administered throughout the postoperative period, generally for 7–10 days; however, the manufacturer states that treatment with enoxaparin has been well tolerated for up to 12 days in patients undergoing abdominal surgery in clinical trials. Because the risk of venous thromboembolism is particularly high in patients undergoing abdominal or pelvic surgery for cancer, ACCP recommends that therapy with a low molecular weight heparin be continued for up to 4 weeks in such patients.

Hip- or Knee-Replacement Surgery. For the prevention of postoperative DVT, which may lead to PE, in patients undergoing hip-replacement or knee-replacement surgery, the manufacturer recommends an enoxaparin sodium dosage of 30 mg twice daily (every 12 hours) by subcutaneous injection beginning 12–24 hours postoperatively, provided hemostasis has been established. Alternatively, in patients undergoing hip-replacement surgery, the manufacturer states that an enoxaparin sodium dosage of 40 mg once daily (every 24 hours) by subcutaneous injection beginning 12 (±3) hours preoperatively may be considered, based on dose-comparison data indicating that a dosage of 40 mg once daily may be as effective as 30 mg twice daily (every 12 hours) in preventing DVT in such patients. ACCP states that risk of bleeding is closely associated with the timing of initiation of thromboprophylaxis around surgery and recommends that a low molecular weight heparin be initiated at least 12 hours preoperatively or at least 12 hours postoperatively in patients undergoing major orthopedic surgery.

Enoxaparin should be administered throughout the postoperative period, generally for 7–10 days, until the risk of DVT has diminished; ACCP recommends a minimum of 10–14 days of thromboprophylaxis, with extended prophylaxis suggested for up to 35 days on an outpatient basis. The manufacturer states that treatment with enoxaparin for up to 14 days has been well tolerated in clinical trials. Following the initial phase of thromboprophylaxis during the acute postoperative period in patients undergoing hip-replacement surgery, the manufacturer recommends continued prophylaxis with enoxaparin sodium 40 mg once daily given subcutaneously for 3 weeks.

Medical Conditions Associated with Thromboembolism. For prevention of DVT, which may lead to PE, in patients whose mobility is severely restricted during acute illness (e.g., cancer, heart failure, severe lung disease, those confined to bedrest), the manufacturer recommends an enoxaparin sodium dosage of 40 mg daily, usually given for 6–11 days; however, the manufacturer states that treatment with the drug for up to 14 days has been well tolerated in clinical trials. ACCP suggests against the use of extended thromboprophylaxis beyond the period of patient immobilization or acute hospitalization in acutely ill medical patients because of an increased risk of bleeding and the burden and costs of daily injections.

Treatment of Venous Thromboembolism For the treatment of uncomplicated DVT without PE, outpatient therapy with enoxaparin may be considered in selected patients. In patients who can be treated at home, the usual dosage of enoxaparin sodium for the treatment of DVT is 1 mg/kg twice daily given subcutaneously.

In patients with acute DVT with or without PE who are not candidates for outpatient antithrombotic therapy, the usual dosage of enoxaparin sodium is 1 mg/kg twice daily or 1.5 mg/kg once daily administered subcutaneously at the same time every day. Warfarin therapy generally is given for follow-up treatment, initiated together with enoxaparin on the first treatment day; therapy with the 2 drugs should be overlapped for a minimum of 5 days and until an adequate response to warfarin is obtained as indicated by an INR of at least 2 for 24 hours or longer. Enoxaparin may be discontinued after overlap with warfarin, generally after a total of 7 days of enoxaparin treatment. The manufacturer states that treatment with enoxaparin for up to 17 days has been well tolerated in clinical trials.

Non-ST-Segment-Elevation Acute Coronary Syndromes For reducing the risk of ischemic complications (e.g., cardiac death or nonfatal myocardial infarction [MI]) in patients with non-ST-segment-elevation acute coronary syndromes (NSTE ACS; unstable angina or NSTEMI) who are receiving concurrent therapy with aspirin (e.g., 75–325 mg once daily), the usual dosage of enoxaparin sodium is 1 mg/kg every 12 hours by subcutaneous injection. Anticoagulant therapy should be administered as soon as possible after hospital admission. Treatment with enoxaparin should continue for a minimum of 2 days until the patient is clinically stabilized, generally for 2–8 days; however, the manufacturer states that treatment with enoxaparin for up to 12.5 days has been well tolerated in clinical trials.

The American College of Cardiology Foundation (ACCF), American Heart Association (AHA), and the Society for Cardiovascular Angiography and Interventions (SCAI) state that it is reasonable to administer enoxaparin sodium (e.g., 0.5–0.75 mg/kg *by direct IV injection*†) for prevention of thrombus formation during PCI in patients with NSTE ACS who have not received prior anticoagulant therapy. In patients with NSTE ACS in whom subcutaneous enoxaparin has been initiated prior to PCI ("upstream"), ACCF/AHA/SCAI state that an additional 0.3-mg/kg dose of enoxaparin sodium should be given *by direct IV injection* at the time of PCI if fewer than 2 prior therapeutic (e.g., 1 mg/kg) subcutaneous doses of enoxaparin sodium have been given or if the last subcutaneous dose of the drug was administered 8–12 hours before PCI†. To minimize the possibility of bleeding associated with vascular (e.g., vascular access sheath) instrumentation (e.g., PCI) during treatment of unstable angina or NSTEMI, strict adherence to dosage intervals of subcutaneous enoxaparin and precautions in the removal of the vascular access sheath should be observed. The next dose of enoxaparin sodium should be given no sooner than 6–8 hours after removal of the vascular access sheath; ACCF/AHA/SCAI suggest removal of femoral sheaths when the activated clotting time (ACT) falls to less than 150–180 seconds or when the activated partial thromboplastin time (aPTT) falls to less than 50 seconds. Careful monitoring of vascular access sites for signs of bleeding or hematoma formation should be undertaken after removal of the vascular sheath and during treatment with enoxaparin.

ST-Segment-Elevation Myocardial Infarction In patients with acute STEMI who are younger than 75 years of age, an initial direct IV injection of enoxaparin sodium 30 mg plus a 1-mg/kg subcutaneous dose is recommended by the manufacturer, followed by enoxaparin sodium 1 mg/kg every 12 hours by subcutaneous injection; a maximum of 100 mg is recommended for each of the first 2 subcutaneous doses. A reduced dosage, without an initial IV dose, is recommended in patients 75 years of age or older. (For dosage recommendations in patients 75 years of age and older, see Geriatric Patients under Dosage and Administration: Special Populations.) Aspirin (75–325 mg once daily) should be administered in conjunction with enoxaparin therapy unless contraindicated. When used with thrombolytic therapy, enoxaparin therapy should be initiated between 15 minutes before and 30 minutes after the start of thrombolytic therapy. The manufacturer states that the optimal duration of enoxaparin treatment is not known, but is likely to be more than 8 days since therapy was continued for 8 days or until hospital discharge in clinical trials.

In patients with acute STEMI undergoing PCI, the manufacturer recommends administration of an additional 0.3-mg/kg dose of enoxaparin sodium by direct IV injection during PCI if the last subcutaneous dose of enoxaparin sodium was administered more than 8 hours before balloon inflation; otherwise, no additional dose is recommended.

Treatment and Prevention of Thromboembolism During Pregnancy In pregnant women with an acute venous thromboembolic event†, enoxaparin sodium 1 mg/kg twice daily is recommended for initial treatment and should be continued throughout the remainder of the pregnancy. Anticoagulation should be continued postpartum for at least 6 weeks (for a minimum total duration of 3 months).

If enoxaparin sodium is used for postpartum prophylaxis in pregnant women with a prior venous thromboembolic event†, a prophylactic (e.g., 40 mg once daily) or intermediate dosage (e.g., 40 mg every 12 hours) is suggested.

In pregnant women already receiving long-term coumarin anticoagulation (e.g., warfarin)†, ACCP suggests the use of a low molecular weight heparin throughout pregnancy given in a weight-adjusted dosage (e.g., enoxaparin sodium 1 mg/kg every 12 hours) or 75% of a weight-adjusted dosage, followed by postpartum resumption of long-term coumarin anticoagulation.

If enoxaparin sodium is used for primary prevention of venous thromboembolism in pregnant women with certain high-risk thrombophilias†, a prophylactic (e.g., 40 mg once daily) or intermediate (e.g., 40 mg every 12 hours) dosage is suggested.

In women with antiphospholipid antibodies (APLA) syndrome†, antepartum administration of a low molecular weight heparin in prophylactic dosages combined with low-dose aspirin (75–100 mg daily) is recommended by ACCP.

In pregnant women with mechanical prosthetic heart valves†, ACCP recommends therapy with a low molecular weight heparin throughout pregnancy or, alternatively, a low molecular weight heparin until the 13th week of pregnancy, substitution of warfarin until close to delivery, then resumption of low molecular weight heparin therapy. If a low molecular weight heparin is used, the drug should be administered in a twice-daily subcutaneous dosage adjusted to maintain anti-factor Xa levels of 0.7–1.2 units/mL 4 hours after dosing.Twice-daily administration is recommended, at least initially, because of altered pharmacokinetics of these drugs in pregnant women. Long-term anticoagulation should be resumed in the postpartum period. (See Patients with Mechanical Prosthetic Heart Valves under Warnings/Precautions: Warnings, in Cautions.)

To avoid an unwanted anticoagulant effect on the fetus during delivery, therapy with a low molecular weight heparin should be discontinued at least 24 hours prior to induction of labor or cesarean section. If an at-term woman is at very high risk for recurrent venous thromboembolism (e.g., occurrence of proximal DVT within the past 2 weeks), IV heparin may be initiated at this time and then discontinued 4–6 hours prior to the expected time of delivery.

Cardioversion of Atrial Fibrillation/Flutter If enoxaparin sodium is used for the prevention of stroke and systemic embolism in patients undergoing cardioversion for atrial fibrillation or atrial flutter†, administration of full-treatment dosages used for venous thromboembolism is recommended.

Perioperative Antithrombotic Prophylaxis If enoxaparin is used for bridging anticoagulation in patients who require temporary interruption of warfarin therapy during surgery or other invasive procedure†, ACCP recommends the use of therapeutic dosages (e.g., enoxaparin sodium 1 mg/kg twice daily or 1.5 mg/kg once daily) because of more extensive data and experience; however, other dosage regimens have been used.

ACCP suggests that the last preoperative dose of enoxaparin sodium be given approximately 24 hours prior to surgery to allow sufficient time for anticoagulant effects to dissipate. Postoperative anticoagulation should be administered with caution and only when hemostasis has been achieved because of the potential for bleeding at the surgical site. In patients undergoing procedures associated with a high risk of bleeding, ACCP suggests delaying the resumption of therapeutic-dose enoxaparin until 48–72 hours after surgery when adequate hemostasis has been achieved.

■ **Special Populations** ***Renal Impairment*** The manufacturer recommends caution in using enoxaparin in patients with renal impairment since elimination of the drug may be delayed. Patients with renal impairment should be carefully monitored for signs and symptoms of bleeding. In addition, anti-factor Xa levels may be used to monitor the anticoagulant effect of enoxaparin in patients with substantial renal impairment. No dosage adjustment is recommended in patients with mild (creatinine clearance 50–80 mL/minute) or moderate (creatinine clearance 30–50 mL/minute) renal impairment. However, dosage should be adjusted in patients with severe renal impairment (creatinine clearance less than 30 mL/minute).

For prevention of postoperative DVT in patients with severe renal impairment (creatinine clearance less than 30 mL/minute) undergoing abdominal or hip or knee-replacement surgery, the recommended dosage of enoxaparin sodium is 30 mg once daily given subcutaneously.

For prevention of DVT in patients with severe renal impairment and restricted mobility during an acute illness, the recommended dosage of enoxaparin sodium is 30 mg once daily given subcutaneously.

For reducing the risk of ischemic complications in patients with unstable angina or non-ST-segment-elevation MI (NSTEMI) and severe renal impairment who are receiving concurrent aspirin, the recommended dosage of enoxaparin sodium is 1 mg/kg once daily subcutaneously.

For the treatment of acute ST-segment-elevation MI (STEMI) in patients with severe renal impairment (creatinine clearance less than 30 mL/minute) who are younger than 75 years of age, the recommended initial dose of enoxaparin sodium is 30 mg as a single *direct IV* dose plus a 1-mg/kg *subcutaneous* dose; treatment should continue with a dosage of 1 mg/kg once daily (maximum of 100 mg per dose for each of the first 2 subcutaneous doses) given by subcutaneous injection with concurrent aspirin therapy (75–325 mg daily).

For the treatment of acute STEMI in patients with severe renal impairment (creatinine clearance less than 30 mL/minute) who are 75 years of age or older, the recommended initial dose of enoxaparin sodium is 1 mg/kg once daily (maximum of 75 mg per dose for each of the first 2 doses) given by subcutaneous injection with concurrent aspirin therapy (75–325 mg daily); no initial IV dose should be given.

For treatment of DVT with or without PE in patients with severe renal impairment, the recommended dosage of enoxaparin sodium is 1 mg/kg once daily given subcutaneously, when used in conjunction with warfarin therapy.

Geriatric Patients For the treatment of acute STEMI in patients 75 years of age or older, the recommended dosage of enoxaparin sodium is 0.75 mg/kg every 12 hours (not to exceed 75 mg per dose for the first 2 doses) by subcutaneous injection; an initial IV dose should not be given.

Pregnant Patients The manufacturer and some clinicians state that if enoxaparin is used in pregnant women with mechanical prosthetic heart valves, anti-factor Xa levels should be used to monitor the anticoagulant effect of enoxaparin, and enoxaparin sodium dosage should be adjusted as needed. ACC and AHA suggest that if a low molecular weight heparin is used in pregnant women with a mechanical prosthetic heart valve, the dosage should be adjusted to maintain anti-factor Xa levels of 0.7–1.2 units/mL 4 hours after administration.

Low Body Weight Increased exposure to enoxaparin has been observed in patients with low body weight (less than 45 kg in women or less than 57 kg in men); all such patients should be carefully monitored for signs and symptoms of bleeding.

Obese Patients Safety and efficacy of thromboprophylactic dosages of enoxaparin in patients with a body mass index (BMI) greater than 30 kg/m^2 have not been established and there is no consensus on how dosage should be adjusted in such patients; these patients should be closely observed for signs and symptoms of thromboembolism during therapy.

Cautions

■ **Contraindications** Known hypersensitivity to enoxaparin, heparin, pork products, or any other ingredient (e.g., benzyl alcohol preservative in multiple-dose vials) in the formulation; active major bleeding; or thrombocytopenia associated with a positive in vitro test for antiplatelet antibodies in the presence of the drug.

■ **Warnings/Precautions** ***Warnings*** **Spinal/Epidural Hematomas.** Concurrent use of a low molecular weight heparin or heparinoid (e.g., danaparoid [no longer commercially available in the US]) with neuraxial (spinal/epidural) anesthesia or spinal puncture procedures has been associated with epidural or spinal hematomas. Hematomas occurring in such patients have resulted in neurologic injury, including long-term or permanent paralysis. The risk of these adverse events is increased by the use of indwelling epidural catheters for administration of analgesia or by the concomitant use of drugs that affect hemostasis, such as nonsteroidal anti-inflammatory agents (NSAIAs), platelet-aggregation inhibitors, or other anticoagulants. The risk also appears to be increased by a history of traumatic or repeated epidural or spinal puncture, spinal surgery, or spinal deformity. It is important to note that the risk of spinal hematoma applies to all anticoagulants when used in conjunction with neuraxial anesthesia or spinal puncture.

The US Food and Drug Administration (FDA) states that cases of epidural or spinal hematomas continue to be reported in patients receiving enoxaparin in the setting of neuraxial procedures. Between July 20, 1992 and January 31, 2013, at least 100 confirmed or probable cases of spinal/epidural hematoma associated with the concurrent use of enoxaparin thromboprophylaxis and neuraxial anesthesia were reported to FDA by the manufacturer. Risk factors that were present in many of these cases included female gender, older age (65 years of age or older), concomitant use of drugs affecting hemostasis, indwelling epidural catheter, epidural technique, twice-daily versus once-daily administration of enoxaparin, and underlying medical conditions with increased risk of hemorrhage. To address this safety concern, the FDA has recommended additional safety measures.

Prior to performing a spinal or epidural procedure, healthcare professionals should determine as part of a preprocedure checklist whether a patient is receiving anticoagulants. In addition, clinicians should carefully consider the timing of spinal catheter placement and removal in relation to anticoagulant use, considering both the dosage and pharmacokinetic properties (e.g., elimination half-life) of the anticoagulant. Insertion or removal of a epidural catheter or lumbar puncture is best performed when the anticoagulant effect of enoxaparin is minimal. Although the optimal timing between the administration of enoxaparin and neuraxial procedures is not known, the following guidelines are recommended. In patients receiving low (prophylactic) dosages of enoxaparin sodium (30 mg once or twice daily or 40 mg once daily), insertion or removal of a spinal catheter should be delayed for at least 12 hours after a dose of enoxaparin. In patients receiving higher (treatment) dosages of enoxaparin sodium (0.75 mg/kg twice daily, 1 mg/kg twice daily, or 1.5 mg/kg once daily), a delay of at least 24 hours is recommended between the enoxaparin dose and catheter placement/removal; if the patient is receiving a twice-daily treatment regimen, the second dose should be omitted to allow for a longer delay. In patients with renal impairment (creatinine clearance less than 30 mL/minute), a doubling of the recommended time delays is recommended to account for possible prolonged elimination of enoxaparin in such patients. The manufacturer suggests that clinicians consider delaying administration of enoxaparin for at least 4 hours after catheter removal, taking into account the patient's risk of bleeding versus thrombosis.

Patients receiving a low molecular weight heparin or heparinoid in the setting of epidural or spinal anesthesia or lumbar puncture should be monitored frequently for manifestations of neurologic impairment (e.g., midline back pain, numbness or weakness in lower limbs, bowel or bladder dysfunction). If spinal hematoma is suspected, urgent diagnosis and treatment is necessary; spinal cord decompression should be considered even though it may not prevent or reverse neurologic sequelae. Some experts recommend against the concomitant use of a low molecular weight heparin with other drugs affecting hemostasis (e.g., aspirin, NSAIAs, platelet-aggregation inhibitors, other anticoagulants) in patients receiving spinal anesthesia. Clinicians should fully consider the potential benefits versus risks of spinal or epidural anesthesia or spinal puncture in patients receiving or being considered for thromboprophylaxis with anticoagulants.

Other Warnings Related to Hemorrhage. Like other anticoagulants, enoxaparin should be used with extreme caution in patients with an increased risk of hemorrhage (e.g., bacterial endocarditis; congenital or acquired bleeding disorders; active ulceration and angiodysplastic GI disease; hemorrhagic stroke; recent brain, spinal, or ophthalmic surgery; concomitant platelet inhibitor therapy). The manufacturer states that the drug also should be used with care in patients with a bleeding diathesis, uncontrolled arterial hypertension, history of recent GI ulceration, diabetic retinopathy, or hemorrhage. Patients with low body weight or renal impairment should be monitored carefully for signs and symptoms of bleeding; dosage adjustment may be necessary in such patients. (See Renal Impairment and also Low Body Weight under Dosage and Administration: Special Populations.) Major hemorrhage (e.g., intracranial or retroperitoneal bleeding) has occurred in patients receiving enoxaparin, and fatalities have occurred. Bleeding can occur at any site during therapy. Hemorrhage should be seriously considered in anticoagulated patients with unexplained decreases in hematocrit or blood pressure.

To minimize risk of bleeding following percutaneous revascularization procedures (i.e., PCI), clinicians should adhere precisely to the recommended dosing intervals for enoxaparin. (See Dosage and Administration: Dosage.) Recommendations for the timing of sheath removal is based on the method of post-PCI arterial closure. If a closure device is used, the sheath may be removed immediately; however, if manual compression is used, the sheath should be removed 6 hours after the last dose of enoxaparin. In patients in whom enoxaparin therapy will be continued, the next scheduled dose should be given no sooner than 6–8 hours after sheath removal. The site of the procedure should be closely monitored for signs of bleeding or hematoma formation; it is important that hemostasis be achieved at the puncture site after PCI.

Thrombocytopenia. Moderate thrombocytopenia (platelet counts between 50,000 and 100,000/mm^3) was reported in 1.3% of patients in clinical studies, and severe thrombocytopenia (platelet counts less than 50,000/mm^3) was reported in 0.1% of patients. Heparin-induced thrombocytopenia (HIT) can occur with the administration of enoxaparin; some cases of thrombocytopenia have been complicated by organ infarction with secondary organ dysfunction or limb ischemia, and deaths have resulted. Enoxaparin should be used with extreme caution in patients with a history of HIT. Thrombocytopenia of any degree should be monitored closely, and enoxaparin should be discontinued if platelet counts fall below 100,000/mm^3. For patients with HIT with or without thrombosis, nonheparin anticoagulants such as lepirudin or argatroban are recommended; continued use of a low molecular weight heparin is contraindicated. (See Cautions: Contraindications.)

Patients with Mechanical Prosthetic Heart Valves. The use of enoxaparin for prophylaxis of thromboembolism in patients with mechanical prosthetic heart valves has not been adequately studied, and a clinical consensus regarding optimal therapy remains to be established. Valve thrombosis that was fatal (including maternal and fetal death) or potentially fatal and/or required surgical intervention has been reported during prophylaxis with enoxaparin in some patients (including pregnant women) with mechanical prosthetic heart valves. (See Uses: Thromboembolism During Pregnancy.) Insufficient data, the presence of underlying conditions, and the possibility of inadequate anticoagulation complicate the evaluation of these events in such patients. However, women with mechanical prosthetic heart valves may be at higher risk for thromboembolism during pregnancy.

The manufacturer and some clinicians currently state that if enoxaparin is used in pregnant women with mechanical prosthetic heart valves, frequent monitoring of peak and trough anti-factor Xa concentrations and adjustment of enoxaparin sodium dosage may be necessary. The American College of Chest Physicians (ACCP) currently recommends use of aggressive, adjusted-dose subcutaneous low molecular weight heparin (i.e., given twice daily and adjusted to maintain the manufacturer-recommended peak anti-factor Xa concentrations 4 hours postinjection) in pregnant women with mechanical prosthetic heart valves. Although empiric, the therapeutic monitoring recommendation for anti-factor Xa concentrations is based on differences in the pharmacokinetics of low molecular weight heparins that occur during pregnancy and is aimed at attempting to ensure that dosage is adjusted appropriately to ensure consistent anticoagulation. The American College of Cardiology (ACC) and American Heart Association (AHA) suggest that the dosage of a low molecular weight heparin should be adjusted to maintain anti-factor Xa levels of 0.7–1.2 units/mL 4 hours after administration in pregnant women with mechanical prosthetic heart valves and that a low molecular weight heparin should not be used in such women unless anti-factor Xa levels are monitored 4–6 hours after administration of the drug.

Sensitivity Reactions Hypersensitivity reactions, including anaphylactoid reactions, pruritus, urticaria, vesiculobullous rash, and rare cases of hypersensitivity cutaneous vesiculitis, have occurred.

General Precautions The usual precautions and contraindications associated with heparin anticoagulant therapy should be followed in patients for whom enoxaparin therapy is considered. Periodic complete blood cell counts, including platelet counts, and stool occult blood tests are recommended during use of enoxaparin.

As with other anticoagulants, bleeding may occur at any site during enoxaparin therapy. Women treated with a low molecular weight heparin with or without a GP IIb/IIIa-receptor inhibitor prior to PCI appear to experience more bleeding complications than do men. An unexpected decrease in hematocrit or blood pressure may indicate hemorrhage and should prompt evaluation to determine a bleeding site. To largely neutralize the effects of enoxaparin following overdosage, the dose of protamine sulfate is determined by the administered dose of the low molecular weight heparin, the time elapsed since the drug was given, and blood coagulation studies. The dose of protamine sulfate to be given should be equal to that of the administered enoxaparin sodium dose if enoxaparin was administered in the previous 8 hours (i.e., 1 mg of protamine sulfate should be given to neutralize 1 mg of enoxaparin sodium). If more than 8 hours has elapsed since enoxaparin was administered, an infusion of 0.5 mg of protamine sulfate may be given for each 1 mg of enoxaparin sodium administered. If the activated partial thromboplastin time (aPTT) measured 2–4 hours after the first protamine infusion remains prolonged, a second dose of 0.5 mg of protamine sulfate may be given for each 1 mg of enoxaparin sodium administered. Protamine administration may not be required if more than 12 hours has elapsed since administration of enoxaparin. However, even after higher dosages of protamine sulfate, the aPTT may remain more prolonged than would be the case following treatment of overdosage of conventional heparin since anti-factor Xa activity is never completely neutralized. A maximum of about 60% of anti-factor Xa activity is neutralized with protamine sulfate administration for overdosage of enoxaparin.

Specific Populations **Pregnancy.** Category B. (See Users Guide.) There are no adequate and well-controlled studies of enoxaparin in pregnant women. However, available data in humans and animals indicate that enoxaparin does not cross the placenta and has not shown evidence of teratogenicity or fetotoxicity. In a review of approximately 600 retrospectively followed pregnancies in women exposed to enoxaparin, the incidences of congenital anomalies did not exceed what would be expected in the general population. Maternal and neonatal hemorrhage did occur in some of the followed pregnancies.

Pregnancy alone is associated with an increased risk of thromboembolism, which is even higher in women with a history of thromboembolism and certain high-risk pregnancy conditions, including hereditary or acquired thrombophilias and the presence of a mechanical prosthetic heart valve. Some clinicians recommend frequent monitoring of anti-factor Xa concentrations and adjustment of enoxaparin sodium dosage in pregnant women with mechanical prosthetic heart valves to ensure a consistent anticoagulant effect.

All patients receiving anticoagulants such as enoxaparin, including pregnant women, are at risk for bleeding. Hemorrhage can occur at any site and may lead to death of mother and/or fetus. Pregnant women receiving enoxaparin should be apprised of the potential hazards to the mother and fetus associated with enoxaparin use during pregnancy, and such women should be carefully monitored for evidence of bleeding or excessive anticoagulation. As delivery approaches, use of a shorter-acting anticoagulant should be considered.

Lactation. It is not known whether enoxaparin is distributed into milk; because many drugs are distributed into human milk and because of the potential for serious adverse reactions to enoxaparin in nursing infants, a decision should be made whether to discontinue nursing or the drug, taking into account the importance of the drug to the woman.

ACCP recommends that low molecular weight heparins be continued in nursing women who are already receiving such therapy; small amounts of low molecular weight heparins have been detected in the milk of nursing women but are not likely to be clinically important.

Pediatric Use. Safety and efficacy not established in children younger than 18 years of age. Each mL of enoxaparin sodium injection in multiple-dose vials contains 15 mg of benzyl alcohol as a preservative. Although a causal relationship has not been established, administration of injections preserved with benzyl alcohol has been associated with toxicity in neonates. Toxicity appears to have resulted from administration of large amounts (i.e., about 100–400 mg/kg daily) of benzyl alcohol in these neonates. Because benzyl alcohol may cross the placenta, the manufacturer states that enoxaparin in multiple-dose vials should be used with caution and only if clearly needed in pregnant women.

Geriatric Use. No substantial differences in efficacy relative to younger adults. In geriatric patients, a higher incidence of bleeding complications has been observed following administration of enoxaparin sodium at a dosage of 1.5 mg/kg once daily or 1 mg/kg every 12 hours, and the risk of bleeding complications increases with age. Enoxaparin should be used with care in geriatric patients, and careful attention to dosing intervals and concomitant medications (particularly antiplatelet drugs) is advised. Monitoring (e.g., using anti-Factor Xa assay) of geriatric patients with low body weight (less than 45 kg) and those predisposed to decreased renal function should be considered.

■ **Common Adverse Effects** Adverse effects occurring in at least 2% of patients receiving enoxaparin for hip/knee replacement, abdominal, or colorectal surgery or treatment of deep-vein thrombosis (DVT) include hemorrhage (including at the injection site), anemia, ecchymosis, thrombocytopenia, hematuria, fever, nausea, diarrhea, peripheral or unspecified edema, dyspnea, injection site pain, or confusion.

Drug Interactions

■ **Drugs Affecting Hemostasis** Potential pharmacodynamic interaction (increased risk of bleeding) when enoxaparin is used with drugs inhibiting coagulation (e.g., anticoagulants, platelet aggregation inhibitors [e.g., salicylates or other nonsteroidal anti-inflammatory agents, dipyridamole, sulfinpyrazone]). The manufacturer recommends that such drugs be discontinued prior to initiating enoxaparin therapy since concomitant use of enoxaparin with these agents may increase the risk of hemorrhage. If concomitant use of enoxaparin and drugs that affect hemostasis is considered essential, careful clinical and laboratory monitoring is advised.

Description

Enoxaparin, a depolymerized heparin prepared by alkaline degradation of benzylated heparin of porcine intestinal mucosa origin, is an anticoagulant. Enoxaparin is commercially available as the sodium salt. The average molecular weight of enoxaparin is approximately one-third that of heparin (4500 vs 12,000 daltons); therefore, enoxaparin is referred to as a low molecular weight heparin.

Enoxaparin has an approximate anti-factor Xa activity of 100 units/mg according to the World Health Organization (WHO) First International Low Molecular Weight Heparin Reference Standard. At a given level of anti-factor Xa activity, enoxaparin has less effect on thrombin than does heparin. However, enoxaparin administration has been associated with a prolongation of some global clotting function tests (i.e., thrombin time, activated partial thromboplastin time [aPTT]) by up to 1.8 times the control value. In patients receiving enoxaparin sodium (1 mg/kg of the 100 mg/mL concentration subcutaneously every 12 hours) in a large clinical trial, the aPTT was 45 seconds or less in most treated patients. The manufacturer states that enoxaparin sodium in a concentration of 150 mg/mL is projected to produce anticoagulant activities similar to those of 100 or 200 mg/mL concentrations of the drug, although the 150 mg/mL concentration has not been studied clinically. Compared with heparin, enoxaparin has greater bioavailability (based on anti-factor Xa activity) after subcutaneous administration and a longer half-life, allowing less frequent administration.

The molecular weight, pharmacokinetics, and in vitro and in vivo activity of enoxaparin differ from those of heparin or other low molecular weight heparins; therefore, the drugs are not interchangeable on a unit-for-unit (or mg-for-mg) basis.

Advice to Patients

Importance of advising patients who have had neuraxial anesthesia or spinal puncture to monitor for manifestations of spinal or epidural hematoma (e.g., midline back pain, numbness or weakness in lower limbs, bowel and/or bladder dysfunction), particularly if they are receiving concomitant nonsteroidal anti-inflammatory agents (NSAIAs), platelet-aggregation inhibitors, or other anticoagulants; importance of immediately contacting a clinician if any of these symptoms occur.

Importance of informing patients that concomitant use of aspirin and other NSAIAs can increase risk of bleeding, and to discontinue use of these drugs whenever possible.

If enoxaparin therapy is to be continued after hospital discharge, importance of instructing patient on proper administration of the drug, including injection technique.

Importance of informing patients that they may bruise and/or bleed more easily and that a longer than normal time may be required to stop bleeding when taking enoxaparin. Importance of patients reporting any unusual bleeding, bruising, or signs of thrombocytopenia (e.g., dark red spots under skin) to their clinician.

Importance of patients informing clinicians (including dentists) that they are receiving enoxaparin therapy before scheduling any invasive procedures.

Importance of informing clinicians of existing or contemplated concomitant therapy, including prescription and OTC drugs.

Importance of women informing clinicians if they are or plan to become pregnant or plan to breast-feed.

Advise of potential hazards to fetus and mother if enoxaparin is administered during pregnancy.

Importance of informing patients of other precautionary information. (See Cautions.)

Overview® (see Users Guide). For additional information until a more detailed monograph is developed and published, the manufacturer's labeling should be consulted. It is *essential* that the labeling be consulted for detailed information on the usual cautions, precautions, contraindications, potential drug interactions, and acute toxicity.

Preparations

Excipients in commercially available drug preparations may have clinically important effects in some individuals; consult specific product labeling for details.

Enoxaparin Sodium (Porcine)

Parenteral		
Injection, for subcutaneous use	10 mg/0.1 mL (30, 40, 60, 80, and 100 mg)*	**Enoxaparin Sodium Injection**
		Lovenox® (available as prefilled disposable syringes), Sanofi-Aventis
	15 mg/0.1 mL (120 and 150 mg)*	**Enoxaparin Sodium Injection**
		Lovenox® (available as disposable prefilled syringes), Sanofi-Aventis
	300 mg/3 mL*	**Enoxaparin Sodium Injection**
		Lovenox®, Sanofi-Aventis

*available from one or more manufacturer, distributor, and/or repackager by generic (nonproprietary) name

†Use is not currently included in the labeling approved by the US Food and Drug Administration

Heparin Sodium

■ Heparin, an anionic, sulfated glycosaminoglycan anticoagulant present in mast cells, acts as a catalyst to markedly accelerate the rate at which antithrombin III (heparin cofactor) neutralizes thrombin and activated coagulation factor X (factor Xa). Unless otherwise specified in this monograph, the term "heparin" refers to unfractionated heparin, not low molecular weight heparin or both types of heparin.

Uses

Heparin is used for prophylaxis and treatment of venous thrombosis and its extension; prophylaxis of postoperative deep-vein thrombosis and pulmonary embolism in patients undergoing major abdominal or thoracic surgery who are at risk for thromboembolism; prophylaxis and treatment of pulmonary embolism; treatment of embolization associated with atrial fibrillation or atrial flutter and/or prosthetic heart valve replacement; treatment of acute and chronic consumptive coagulopathies (disseminated intravascular coagulation [DIC]); and prophylaxis and treatment of peripheral arterial embolism. Heparin is also used to prevent activation of the coagulation mechanism as blood passes through an extracorporeal circuit in dialysis procedures and during arterial and cardiac surgery. In addition, the drug is used as an in vitro anticoagulant in blood transfusions. Heparin also has been used as adjunctive antithrombotic therapy in patients with unstable angina, non-ST-segment-elevation myocardial infarction (NSTEMI), or ST-segment-elevation myocardial infarction (STEMI).

Heparin or a low molecular weight heparin is used when a rapid anticoagulant effect is required. A coumarin anticoagulant (e.g., warfarin) is generally used for follow-up anticoagulant therapy after the effects of therapy with full-dose heparin or a low molecular weight heparin have been established and when long-term anticoagulant therapy is appropriate. When warfarin is administered for follow-up treatment after full-dose heparin, therapy with warfarin and heparin should be overlapped for a short period of time. (See Dosage and Administration: Dosage.)

■ **Deep-Vein Thrombosis and Pulmonary Embolism** *Treatment* Heparin is used for the treatment of deep-vein thrombosis or pulmonary embolism. For the initial treatment of proximal deep-vein thrombosis or pulmonary embolism in adults, full-dose heparin generally is administered by continuous IV infusion; alternatively, subcutaneous heparin (given initially in a weight-based dosage) may be used, with or without monitoring. If warfarin is being considered for long-term anticoagulant therapy, the drug should be initiated on the same day as heparin, and such therapy should be overlapped for a minimum of 5 days and until the international normalized ratio (INR) is at least 2 for 24 hours or longer.

The American College of Chest Physicians (ACCP) recommends the use of heparin as an appropriate choice of anticoagulant for the initial treatment of acute proximal deep-vein thrombosis or pulmonary embolism; other options include a low molecular weight heparin or fondaparinux. Among the different anticoagulant options, fondaparinux or a low molecular weight heparin generally is preferred to heparin because of more convenient administration and less risk of heparin-induced thrombocytopenia (HIT). Heparin may be preferred in patients with renal impairment. In addition, ACCP states that IV heparin should be considered over subcutaneous therapies in patients with pulmonary embolism in whom thrombolytic therapy is being considered or if there is a concern about the adequacy of subcutaneous absorption. For additional information on treatment of venous thromboembolism in adults, consult the most recent ACCP Evidence-based Clinical Practice Guidelines on Antithrombotic Therapy and Prevention of Thrombosis available at http://www.chestnet.org.

After full-dose heparin therapy, warfarin or a low molecular weight heparin generally is administered as follow-up anticoagulant therapy for at least 3 months in patients with venous thromboembolism. (See Treatment and Secondary Prevention under Uses: Deep-Vein Thrombosis and Pulmonary Embolism, in Warfarin 20:12.04.08.)

Heparin also may be used for the treatment of venous thromboembolism in pediatric patients. Unlike in adults, most episodes of venous thromboembolism in children are secondary to an identifiable risk factor such as the presence of a central venous access device. Recommendations regarding the use of antithrombotic therapy in children generally are based on extrapolation from adult guidelines. Heparin or a low molecular weight heparin is recommended by ACCP for both the initial and ongoing treatment of venous thromboembolism in children. In children with central venous catheter-related thromboembolism, ACCP recommends that the catheter be removed if no longer functioning or required; at least 3–5 days of therapeutic anticoagulation is suggested prior to its removal. If the central venous access device is required, ACCP suggests that anticoagulants be given until the catheter is removed. For additional information on treatment of venous thromboembolism in neonates and children, consult the most recent ACCP Evidence-based Clinical Practice Guidelines on Antithrombotic Therapy and Prevention of Thrombosis available at http://www.chestnet.org.

Prophylaxis **General Surgery.** Fixed low-dose subcutaneous heparin therapy is used for prevention of postoperative deep-vein thrombosis and pulmonary embolism in patients undergoing general (e.g., abdominal) surgery who are at risk of thromboembolism.

ACCP recommends pharmacologic (e.g., low-dose heparin) and/or nonpharmacologic/mechanical (e.g., intermittent pneumatic compression) methods of thromboprophylaxis in patients undergoing general surgery, including abdominal, GI, gynecologic, and urologic surgery, according to the patient's level of risk for thromboembolism and bleeding. In general, pharmacologic prophylaxis is recommended in patients with high (and possibly moderate) risk of venous thromboembolism who do not have a high risk of bleeding, while mechanical methods are suggested in patients who require thromboprophylaxis but have a high risk of bleeding. If pharmacologic thromboprophylaxis is used in patients undergoing general surgery, ACCP states that low-dose heparin or a low molecular weight heparin is preferred, but when these agents are contraindicated or not available, aspirin or fondaparinux may be considered. ACCP states that the same recommendations for the use of antithrombotic agents in general surgery patients can be applied to patients undergoing bariatric surgery, vascular surgery, and plastic and reconstructive surgery. For additional information on the prevention of venous thromboembolism in patients undergoing general surgery, consult the most recent ACCP Evidence-based Clinical Practice Guidelines on Antithrombotic Therapy and Prevention of Thrombosis available at http://www.chestnet.org.

Cardiac Surgery. Because the risk of venous thromboembolism in most patients undergoing cardiac surgery is considered to be moderate, mechanical methods of prophylaxis generally are recommended over pharmacologic prophylaxis in such patients. However, ACCP states that use of a pharmacologic method (e.g., low-dose heparin) may be considered in cardiac surgery patients with a complicated postoperative course.

Thoracic Surgery. Heparin is used for the prevention of postoperative venous thromboembolism in patients undergoing major thoracic surgery. Pharmacologic thromboprophylaxis with low-dose heparin or a low molecular weight heparin is recommended by ACCP in patients undergoing thoracic surgery who are at high risk of venous thromboembolism, provided risk of bleeding is low.

Neurosurgery. Patients undergoing craniotomy, especially for malignant disease, are considered to be at high risk of venous thromboembolism. Although low-dose heparin has been used for the prevention of venous thromboembolism in such patients, the benefits of pharmacologic prophylaxis may be outweighed by the possible increased risk of intracranial hemorrhage. ACCP suggests the use of a mechanical method of prophylaxis (preferably intermittent pneumatic compression) in craniotomy patients; for patients considered to be at *very* high risk for thromboembolism, such as those undergoing craniotomy for malignant disease†, a pharmacologic method (e.g., low-dose heparin) may be added once adequate hemostasis has been established and the risk of bleeding decreases.

In patients undergoing spinal surgery, a mechanical method of thromboprophylaxis (preferably intermittent pneumatic compression) also is suggested, with possible addition of pharmacologic prophylaxis (e.g., heparin) in high-risk patients (e.g., those with malignancy or those undergoing surgery with a combined anterior-posterior approach) once adequate hemostasis is established and risk of bleeding decreases.

Trauma. In general, some form of thromboprophylaxis (with low-dose heparin, a low molecular weight heparin, or a mechanical method) is suggested by ACCP in all patients with major trauma†. For major trauma patients at high risk of venous thromboembolism, including those with acute spinal cord injury, traumatic brain injury, or spinal surgery for trauma, ACCP suggests the use of both a pharmacologic and mechanical method of prophylaxis, unless contraindications exist.

Orthopedic Surgery. Low-dose heparin has been used for the prevention of venous thromboembolism in patients undergoing major orthopedic surgery (total hip-replacement†, total knee-replacement†, or hip-fracture surgery†). ACCP recommends routine thromboprophylaxis (with a pharmacologic and/or mechanical method) in all patients undergoing major orthopedic surgery because of the high risk for postoperative venous thromboembolism; thromboprophylaxis should be continued for at least 10–14 days, and possibly for up to 35 days after surgery. Several antithrombotic agents (e.g., low molecular weight heparins, fondaparinux, low-dose heparin, warfarin, aspirin) are recommended by ACCP for pharmacologic thromboprophylaxis in patients undergoing major orthopedic surgery. Although ACCP suggests that a low molecular weight heparin generally is preferred because of its relative efficacy and safety and extensive clinical experience, alternative agents may be considered in situations in which a low molecular weight heparin is not available or cannot be used. ACCP states that when selecting an appropriate thromboprophylaxis regimen, factors such as relative efficacy and bleeding risk as well as logistics and compliance issues should be considered. For additional information on the prevention of venous thromboembolism in patients undergoing major orthopedic surgery, consult the most recent ACCP Evidence-based Clinical Practice Guidelines on Antithrombotic Therapy and Prevention of Thrombosis available at http://www.chestnet.org.

Perioperative Management of Antithrombotic Therapy. Heparin is used in the perioperative management of patients who require temporary interruption of long-term warfarin therapy for surgery or other invasive procedures. Perioperative use of IV heparin or a low molecular weight heparin (bridging anticoagulation) is recommended by ACCP in some patients with venous thromboembolism, atrial fibrillation, or mechanical prosthetic heart valves depending on their risk of developing thromboembolism during temporary interruption of oral anticoagulant therapy. Long-term therapy with warfarin should be resumed postoperatively when adequate hemostasis is achieved. For additional information on the perioperative management of antithrombotic therapy, consult the most recent ACCP Evidence-based Clinical Practice Guidelines on Antithrombotic Therapy and Prevention of Thrombosis available at http://www.chestnet.org).

Medical Conditions Associated with Thromboembolism. Heparin has been used for the prevention of deep-vein thrombosis and pulmonary embolism in acutely ill hospitalized medical patients and in those with medical conditions associated with a high risk of thromboembolism (e.g., cancer). Treatment decisions regarding the use of prophylactic anticoagulants in such patients should include an assessment of the patient's individual risk of venous thromboembolism and risk of bleeding. In general, pharmacologic thromboprophylaxis is recommended only in patients who are considered to be at high risk of venous thromboembolism because the risk-to-benefit trade-off between the reduction in venous thromboembolic events and bleeding is considered to be more favorable in such patients. Factors that should be considered when choosing an appropriate anticoagulant include patient preference, compliance, ease of administration, and local cost considerations. ACCP recommends the use of anticoagulant thromboprophylaxis (e.g., low-dose heparin) in acutely ill, hospitalized medical patients at increased risk of thrombosis who are not actively bleeding and do not have an increased risk of bleeding. Continued thromboprophylaxis is suggested for 6–21 days until full mobility is restored or hospital discharge, whichever comes first; extended prophylaxis beyond these periods generally is not recommended. Risk of venous thromboembolism in critically ill patients in an intensive care unit (ICU) varies depending on their acute or chronic conditions (e.g., sepsis, congestive heart failure) and ICU-specific exposures and events (e.g., surgery, immobilization, mechanical ventilation, central venous catheters). Low-dose heparin is suggested by ACCP as an option for pharmacologic thromboprophylaxis in critically ill patients who are not actively bleeding and do not have risk factors for bleeding.

Risk of venous thromboembolism is particularly high in patients with cancer. Routine pharmacologic thromboprophylaxis generally is not recommended in cancer patients in the outpatient setting who have no additional risk factors for venous thromboembolism; however, ACCP suggests the use of low-dose heparin or a low molecular weight heparin for prophylaxis in cancer outpatients with solid tumors who have additional thromboembolic risk factors and are at low risk of bleeding.

Thromboembolism During Pregnancy. Heparin has been used for the prevention and treatment of venous thromboembolism during pregnancy. Because of a more favorable safety profile, ACCP generally recommends the use of a low molecular weight heparin (rather than heparin or warfarin) for the prevention and treatment of thromboembolism during pregnancy. (See Uses: Thromboembolism Occurring During Pregnancy, in Enoxaparin 20:12.04.16.) If adjusted-dose subcutaneous heparin is used during pregnancy, ACCP states that the drug should be discontinued at least 24 hours prior to induction of labor or cesarean section to avoid an unwanted anticoagulant effect on the fetus during delivery. Women at very high risk for recurrent venous thromboembolism (e.g., occurrence of proximal deep-vein thrombosis or pulmonary embolism within 2 weeks of delivery) may have therapy switched to therapeutic dosages of IV heparin, which should then be discontinued 4–6 hours prior to the expected time of delivery.

For information on the prevention of other pregnancy complications with heparin, see Uses: Complications of Pregnancy.

Prophylaxis for Other Conditions. Heparin (in therapeutic dosages), followed by warfarin, is recommended by ACCP as an option for thromboprophylaxis in children following Fontan surgery†.

■ **Cardioversion of Atrial Fibrillation/Flutter** Heparin has been used to reduce the risk of stroke and systemic embolism in patients with atrial fibrillation undergoing electrical or pharmacologic cardioversion. Therapeutic anticoagulation with heparin or a low molecular weight heparin may be used in patients in whom prolonged anticoagulation (e.g., with warfarin for at least 3 weeks) prior to cardioversion is not necessary or not possible; in these situations, heparin or a low molecular weight heparin generally is administered at the time of transesophageal echocardiography (TEE) or at presentation (for those with atrial fibrillation of 48 hours or less), followed by cardioversion. In patients requiring urgent cardioversion because of hemodynamic instability, initiation of IV heparin or a low molecular weight heparin also is suggested, if possible; however, such therapy should not delay any emergency intervention.

In patients undergoing cardioversion for atrial flutter, experts state that the same approach to thromboprophylaxis should be used as for those with atrial fibrillation.

■ **Thromboembolism Associated with Prosthetic Heart Valves**

Overview Heparin is used during conversion to maintenance therapy with warfarin to reduce the incidence of thromboembolism (e.g., stroke) in patients with prosthetic mechanical heart valves, including in pregnant women. In the absence of a bleeding risk, ACCP suggests bridging anticoagulation (administration of a low molecular weight heparin in either prophylactic or therapeutic dosages or IV heparin in prophylactic dosages) during the early postoperative period after insertion of a mechanical heart valve until the patient is stable on warfarin therapy. (See Dosage and Administration: Dosage.) In patients with a mechanical heart valve in whom therapy with warfarin must be temporarily discontinued (e.g., those undergoing major surgery), substitution with a low molecular weight heparin or heparin is recommended in selected patients (e.g., those at high risk of thromboembolism). (See Uses: Thromboembolism Associated with Prosthetic Heart Valves, in Warfarin 20:12.04.08.)

Patients with Prosthetic Heart Valves Undergoing Surgical Procedures In patients with a prosthetic heart valve receiving long-term oral antithrombotic therapy (e.g., warfarin) who require surgical procedures, the risk of perioperative bleeding should be weighed against the increased risk of thromboembolism that may occur as a result of discontinuance of oral antithrombotic therapy. The American College of Cardiology (ACC) and American Heart Association (AHA) state that perioperative use of heparin should be considered for noncardiac surgery, invasive procedures, or dental procedures in patients with prosthetic heart valves who are at high risk for thrombosis without oral antithrombotic therapy; such patients include those with any mechanical mitral valve or a mechanical aortic valve with additional risk factors. In such high-risk patients, heparin should be initiated after discontinuance of warfarin therapy when the INR is below 2 (approximately 48 hours before surgery). Heparin should be discontinued 4–6 hours before the procedure and then reinitiated as early as possible after surgery once hemostasis has been established. Therapy with heparin should then be continued until the patient has achieved therapeutic anticoagulation on warfarin therapy (as assessed by the INR).

Pregnant Women with Prosthetic Heart Valves Since no controlled, prospective clinical trials have been performed in pregnant women with prosthetic mechanical heart valves, the optimal antithrombotic therapy in such women remains to be established. Women with prosthetic mechanical heart valves may be at even higher risk for thromboembolism during pregnancy. The risk of valve thrombosis in pregnant women with prosthetic mechanical heart valves is lowest with the use of warfarin. However, warfarin crosses the placenta and is associated with adverse embryopathic and fetopathic effects, prematurity, stillbirths, and spontaneous abortions, with the risk of embryopathy being highest during weeks 6–12 of gestation. (See Cautions: Pregnancy and Lactation, in Warfarin 20:12.04.08.) Heparin does not cross the placenta and is considered safer to the fetus than warfarin; however, use of heparin has been associated with an increased maternal risk for valve thrombosis, death, and major bleeding complications. In addition, thrombosis of prosthetic heart valves, resulting in maternal and/or fetal death in some cases, has occurred in some pregnant women receiving prophylaxis with a low molecular weight heparin (enoxaparin). (See Uses: Thromboembolism Associated with Prosthetic Heart Valves, in Enoxaparin 20:12.04.16.) The decision whether to use heparin during the first trimester or continue warfarin throughout pregnancy should be made after full discussion of the risks of anticoagulant therapies with the patient. ACCP states that in the absence of definitive data regarding optimal therapy and because of the associated risks of withholding antithrombotic therapy in pregnant women with prosthetic mechanical heart valves, the use of aggressive, adjusted-dose therapy with subcutaneous low molecular weight heparin (i.e., adjusted to maintain the manufacturer's peak anti-factor Xa concentrations at 4 hours postinjection) or adjusted-dose subcutaneous heparin sodium therapy (i.e., 17,500–20,000 units every 12 hours initially and adjusted to maintain the mid-interval aPTT at least twice the control value or corresponding to an anti-factor Xa concentrations of 0.35–0.7 units/mL) appears reasonable in such patients. Aspirin (75–100 mg daily) during the second and third trimesters of pregnancy may be used in conjunction with anticoagulant therapy to further reduce the incidence of valvular thrombosis in these high-risk women. Another option recommended in pregnant women with prosthetic mechanical heart valves is use of subcutaneous heparin or low molecular weight heparin as described above until week 13 of pregnancy (i.e., because of teratogenicity concerns with warfarin), changing to warfarin until close to term (middle of the third trimester) to avoid anticoagulation of the fetus, and then resuming low molecular weight heparin or heparin until 24 hours prior to induction of labor or cesarean section in order to avoid bleeding complications in the neonate secondary to the trauma of delivery. In pregnant women at very high risk of thromboembolism, including those with a history of thromboembolism or a first-generation mechanical mitral valve, ACCP states that use of warfarin throughout pregnancy, with substitution of heparin or low molecular weight heparin close to delivery, may be justified after a thorough discussion of the potential risks and benefits of such therapy with the patient. Oral anticoagulation with warfarin may be resumed postpartum once adequate hemostasis has been established in women requiring continuing anticoagulant therapy. (See Cautions: Pregnancy and Lactation, in Warfarin 20:12.04.08.)

■ **Arterial Thromboembolism** Full-dose heparin therapy has been used to reduce the extent of ischemic injury in patients with acute arterial emboli or thrombosis; however, ACCP states that formal studies demonstrating improved outcomes have not been conducted. In patients with limb ischemia secondary to arterial emboli or thrombosis, immediate systemic anticoagulation with heparin to prevent thrombotic propagation is suggested by ACCP.

For neonates and children requiring cardiac catheterization via an artery, thromboprophylaxis with IV heparin is recommended. If femoral artery thrombosis occurs following cardiac catheterization, initial treatment with therapeutic-dose IV heparin is recommended, followed by subsequent conversion to a low molecular weight heparin or continued treatment with heparin to complete 5–7 days of therapeutic anticoagulation.

■ **Disseminated Intravascular Coagulation** Heparin is used for the diagnosis and treatment of acute and chronic consumptive coagulopathies, including DIC. The use of heparin in patients with DIC is controversial. Generally, the underlying cause of the DIC episode should be determined and corrected. However, if the underlying cause is not evident or cannot readily be corrected, some clinicians recommend the use of heparin. Heparin appears to be most effective in the treatment of DIC when gross thrombosis or purpura fulminans is present; however, the drug appears to have little effect on the overall mortality associated with acute DIC.

■ **Thrombosis Associated with Indwelling Venous or Arterial Devices** Heparin lock flush solution is used to maintain patency of indwelling peripheral or central venipuncture devices designed for intermittent injections and/or blood sampling; the flush solution should not be used for anticoagulant therapy. Although such flush solutions generally contain low concentrations of heparin sodium (e.g., 10 or 100 units/mL) in 0.9% sodium chloride injection or other IV fluid, the optimum concentration of heparin sodium, and whether the drug is even needed in all circumstances, for maintaining patency of indwelling venipuncture devices have not been established. Since the optimum concentration of heparin sodium for maintaining patency in indwelling venipuncture devices has not been established, use of the lowest concentration shown to be effective (e.g., 10 units/mL) has been suggested when such heparin-containing flush solutions are deemed necessary. Heparin has no fibrinolytic activity and will not lyse existing clots; therefore, thrombolytic agents (e.g., urokinase [no longer commercially available in the US]) rather than heparin would be appropriate for catheters with preexisting obstruction with blood or fibrin.

Evidence principally in adults and to a limited extent in children, including pooled analysis of data from various studies, indicates that heparin-containing solutions are *no more effective* than 0.9% sodium chloride injection *alone* for maintaining patency of venipuncture devices in *peripheral veins when blood is not aspirated into the device*, and some clinicians state that *routine* use of heparin-containing flush solutions may not be advisable because of heparin-associated drug-drug incompatibilities, laboratory test interferences, and rare but potentially serious adverse effects. (See Chemistry and Stability: Stability and see Cautions: Hematologic Effects.) It also has been suggested that the type of solution used to maintain venipuncture device patency may not be as important as the positive pressure maintained in the IV line by the capped (sealed) injection device, which appears to prevent blood reflux and clot formation in the device. In several randomized, double-blind studies in which peripherally placed venipuncture devices composed of fluoroethylene propylene (FEP-Teflon®) principally were used, use of 0.9% sodium chloride injection for flushing indwelling venipuncture devices was associated with patency rates similar to those achieved with flush solutions containing 10 or 100 units/mL of heparin sodium, and the frequency of phlebitis with the use of these solutions also was similar. Therefore, some clinicians state that the use of 0.9% sodium chloride injection alone is sufficient to maintain patency of venipuncture devices, at least those made of FEP-Teflon® when such devices are placed in peripheral veins and used for intermittent IV access. Limited data in children also suggest no difference between 0.9% sodium chloride injection alone or with heparin sodium 10 units/mL in maintaining peripheral IV catheter patency, although additional controlled studies in larger numbers of patients are needed to evaluate more fully the potential risks and benefits of using heparinized versus non-heparinized flush solutions routinely for peripheral venipuncture devices in children and infants.

There is some evidence suggesting that heparin-containing flush solutions *are more effective* than 0.9% sodium chloride injection alone in maintaining patency of *indwelling venipuncture devices used to obtain blood specimens* and of *catheters used for arterial access* (arterial lines). Therefore, pending further study, it has been suggested that flush solutions containing heparin be used for maintaining catheter patency in these situations.

For primary thromboprophylaxis of central venous access devices in children, ACCP states that intermittent or continuous infusions of heparin or 0.9% sodium chloride injection generally are used.

Neonates and children with peripheral arterial catheters should receive thromboprophylaxis with continuous infusions of low concentrations of heparin. If arterial thrombosis of the catheter occurs, ACCP suggests immediate removal of the catheter; anticoagulant therapy with heparin may be considered as an option for the treatment of symptomatic catheter-related thromboembolism. ACCP also suggests that neonates with umbilical arterial catheters receive thromboprophylaxis with low-dose heparin infusion through the catheter to maintain patency.

■ **Acute Ischemic Complications of ST-Segment Elevation Myocardial Infarction** Heparin is used as adjunctive therapy in the management of acute ST-segment-elevation MI (STEMI). The current standard of care in patients with STEMI is timely reperfusion (with primary percutaneous coronary intervention [PCI] or thrombolytic therapy). Adjunctive therapy with anticoagulant (e.g., heparin) and antiplatelet (e.g., aspirin and clopidogrel) agents should be used during and after successful coronary artery reperfusion for the prevention of early reocclusion and death. The American College of Cardiology Foundation (ACCF) and AHA state that patients with STEMI undergoing thrombolytic therapy should receive an anticoagulant (e.g., heparin, enoxaparin, fondaparinux) for a minimum of 48 hours, and preferably for the duration of the index hospitalization, up to 8 days or until revascularization is performed. Enoxaparin is preferred over heparin if extended anticoagulation is necessary beyond 48 hours. Heparin also is used for anticoagulation therapy during PCI. (See Uses: Acute Ischemic Complications of Percutaneous Coronary Intervention.)

Combined analysis of results from 3 large, randomized comparative studies in patients with suspected acute MI who received thrombolytic therapy (i.e., anistreplase [no longer commercially available in the US], recombinant tissue-type plasminogen activator [rt-PA], or streptokinase [no longer commercially available in the US]) plus low-dose aspirin with or without subcutaneous heparin sodium (12,500 units initiated approximately 4 or 12 hours after thrombolytic therapy and usually continued for 1 week or until hospital discharge) indicated that adjunctive therapy with heparin reduced early (i.e., during heparin treatment) reinfarction and death; however, mortality at long-term follow-up (e.g., at 7 weeks or 6 months) was not different in these studies, and the addition of heparin was associated with an increased risk of bleeding, including cerebral hemorrhage. It should be noted that therapy with heparin in most patients in these studies was not given IV nor was it initiated as early in the course of treatment as was the case in most other studies in which mortality with rt-PA (e.g., alteplase) therapy was examined.

Current evidence from studies in which IV heparin has been administered *simultaneously* with thrombolytic therapy, including results of a multicenter study in more than 41,000 patients with acute MI (GUSTO-1), suggests that conjunctive therapy with IV heparin, in addition to aspirin, is effective in reducing reocclusion following thrombolytic therapy for acute MI. In addition, results of a pooled analysis of data from 300 studies of thrombolytic treatment for acute MI indicated a reduction in mortality for thrombolytic regimens including rt-PA but not for those including streptokinase (no longer commercially available in the US) or anistreplase (no longer commercially available in the US) when regimens in which early conjunctive heparin (initiated before or with thrombolytic agents) was used were compared with those in which late therapy with heparin (initiated after termination of thrombolytic therapy) was used; these data are consistent with results of the GUSTO-1 study demonstrating a mortality benefit for IV alteplase plus simultaneous IV heparin compared with streptokinase-heparin regimens. However, some evidence suggests a narrow margin of safety for upward adjustment of heparin dosage, and the need for serial monitoring of aPTT, in patients receiving heparin concurrently with thrombolytic therapy for acute MI. In 2 multicenter, randomized studies designed to compare IV heparin with IV hirudin (an antithrombin inhibitor) as early (within 1 hour following thrombolysis) adjunctive therapy to thrombolytic agents (rt-PA or streptokinase) and aspirin in patients with acute MI, administration of IV heparin in weight-adjusted dosages approximately 20% higher than the dosages used in the GUSTO-1 study was associated with a marked increase in the risk of hemorrhagic stroke, and recruitment of patients into the studies was halted prematurely. In addition, major hemorrhage appeared to be associated with prolonged aPTT values (i.e., those above the target aPTT range of 60–90 seconds [generally 2–3 times the control value]), especially during the first 12 hours following thrombolysis.

■ **Acute Ischemic Complications of Percutaneous Coronary Intervention** Heparin also is used to reduce the risk of ischemic complications in patients undergoing PCI. Adjunctive therapy with heparin is recommended in addition to aspirin, a GP IIb/IIIa-receptor inhibitor (i.e., abciximab, eptifibatide) and/or a P2Y12 receptor-antagonist (e.g., clopidogrel) for patients undergoing such procedures. Use of a parenteral anticoagulant is recommended in patients undergoing PCI to prevent thrombus formation at the site of arterial injury, the coronary guidewire, and in the catheters used for the procedure. IV heparin is recommended by the ACCF, AHA, and the Society for Cardiovascular Angiography and Interventions (SCAI) as an appropriate choice of anticoagulant for use during PCI. The activated clotting time (ACT) generally has been used to assess the degree of heparin anticoagulation in patients undergoing PCI; however, the utility of ACT monitoring recently has been questioned because a clear relationship between ACT values and clinical outcomes has not been demonstrated.

Heparin used in conjunction with GP IIb/IIIa-receptor inhibitors has further reduced the incidence of ischemic complications of PCI compared with heparin alone. Since GP IIb/IIIa-receptor inhibitors may have additive effects on ACT in patients receiving one of these drugs with heparin, the dosage of heparin required to maintain an appropriate ACT during such concurrent therapy may be lower than with heparin monotherapy. Full-dose anticoagulation is no longer used after successful PCI procedures. In most cases, the femoral sheath is removed when the ACT falls to less than 150–180 seconds or when the aPTT decreases to less than 50 seconds.

Results of clinical trials indicate that direct thrombin inhibitors (e.g., argatroban) are at least as effective as heparin in reducing the risk of acute ischemic complications (e.g., death, MI, need for urgent revascularization procedures) in patients undergoing PCI. For patients with HIT or a history of HIT undergoing urgent PCI, ACCF, AHA, and ACCP state that bivalirudin or argatroban may be used in place of heparin. (See Uses: Acute Ischemic Complications of Percutaneous Coronary Intervention, in Bivalirudin 20:12.04.12.)

■ **Cardiac and Arterial Vascular Surgery** Heparin is used for the prevention of blood clotting in arterial and cardiac surgery.

During cardiac surgery, heparin is commonly used to prevent coagulation in the cardiopulmonary bypass circuit and in the operative field. ACCP states that a nonheparin anticoagulant (e.g., bivalirudin) may be used in place of heparin in patients with acute HIT or subacute HIT (platelets have recovered, but HIT antibodies are still present) who require urgent cardiac surgery. Because HIT antibodies are transient, patients with a history of HIT may be re-exposed to heparin in special circumstances. ACCP states that short-term use of heparin may be appropriate in patients with a remote (more than 3 months) history of HIT and no detectable antibodies who require cardiac surgery.

■ **Acute Ischemic Complications of Non-ST-Segment-Elevation Acute Coronary Syndromes** Heparin is used in the management of non-ST-segment-elevation acute coronary syndromes (NSTE ACS)†. Patients with NSTE ACS have either unstable angina or non-ST-segment-elevation MI (NSTEMI); because these conditions are part of a continuum of acute myocardial ischemia and have indistinguishable clinical features upon presentation, the same initial treatment strategies are recommended. The AHA/ACC guideline for the management of patients with NSTE ACS recommends an early invasive strategy (angiographic evaluation with the intent to perform revascularization procedures such as PCI with coronary artery stent implantation or coronary artery bypass grafting [CABG]) or an ischemia-guided strategy (initial medical management followed by cardiac catheterization and revascularization if indicated) in patients with definite or likely NSTE ACS; standard medical therapies for all patients should include a β-adrenergic blocking agent (β-blocker), antiplatelet agents, anticoagulant agents, nitrates, and analgesic agents regardless of the initial management approach.

All patients with NSTE ACS should receive immediate antiplatelet therapy (e.g., aspirin, clopidogrel) unless contraindicated or not tolerated. (See Non-ST-Segment-Elevation Acute Coronary Syndromes under Uses: Acute Coronary Syndromes, in Clopidogrel 20:12.18.) An anticoagulant agent should be added to antiplatelet therapy as soon as possible after presentation. Initial parenteral anticoagulants with established efficacy in patients with NSTE ACS include enoxaparin, heparin, bivalirudin (only in patients who are being managed with an early invasive strategy), and fondaparinux. Fondaparinux is preferred over heparin therapy in patients with an increased risk of bleeding. Heparin anticoagulation should be continued for 48 hours or until PCI is performed. In patients who will undergo CABG and who are already receiving heparin, the drug should be continued during surgery. Patients receiving other anticoagulants (enoxaparin, fondaparinux, or bivalirudin) in whom CABG is to be performed should discontinue the anticoagulant and initiate heparin during the surgery. For recommendations regarding the use of heparin in patients with NSTE ACS undergoing PCI, see Uses: Acute Ischemic Complications of Percutaneous Coronary Intervention.

In patients in whom conservative medical therapy is selected as a postangiographic management strategy, recommendations for continued antiplatelet and anticoagulant therapy generally are based on the presence of coronary artery disease. ACC, AHA, and ACCF state that the optimum duration of heparin therapy has not been established; in clinical trials, the drug generally was administered for 2–5 days.

Current evidence indicates that heparin given by continuous IV infusion can reduce the incidence of acute MI, death, and recurrent refractory angina pectoris in patients with NSTE ACS†.

Early initiation of therapy with IV heparin appears to be necessary for beneficial effects in patients with unstable angina since initiation of the drug more than 24 hours following onset of symptoms has failed to reduce the incidence of adverse coronary events (e.g., angina, MI). In clinical studies in patients with acute unstable angina, data suggest that continuous IV infusion of heparin is more effective than intermittent IV administration, possibly because of inadequate anticoagulation achieved with the latter method.

■ **Cerebral Thromboembolism** Although therapeutic-dose anticoagulation has been used in patients with acute ischemic stroke, there is strong evidence that such treatment is associated with worse outcomes than aspirin therapy in terms of increased mortality and rates of nonfatal major extracranial bleeding. Therefore, ACCP recommends early treatment (within 48 hours) with aspirin over therapeutic anticoagulation to prevent recurrent cerebral thromboembolism in patients with acute ischemic stroke or transient ischemic attacks (TIA). (See Uses: Thrombosis, in Aspirin 28:08.04.24.) However, heparin anticoagulants (i.e., low molecular weight heparins or heparin) may be used in prophylactic dosages for thromboprophylaxis in some patients with acute ischemic stroke; those with additional risk factors for venous thromboembolism are more likely to benefit from such therapy. ACCP suggests that thromboprophylaxis with a low molecular weight heparin (in prophylactic dosages), subcutaneous heparin, or an intermittent pneumatic compression device be used in patients with acute ischemic stroke and restricted mobility. Among the anticoagulant options, ACCP suggests the use of a low molecular weight heparin over heparin. Prophylactic-dose heparin or a low molecular weight heparin usually is initiated within 48 hours of the onset of stroke and is continued throughout the hospital stay until the patient regains mobility; such heparin therapy should not be given within the first 24 hours after administration of thrombolytic therapy.

Heparin is recommended by ACCP as an option for the initial treatment of acute arterial ischemic stroke in children† until dissection and embolic causes have been excluded. When dissection or cardioembolic causes have been excluded, daily aspirin therapy (in prophylactic dosages) is suggested for a minimum of 2 years. In children with acute arterial ischemic stroke secondary to non-Moyamoya vasculopathy†, ACCP recommends ongoing antithrombotic therapy (e.g., with heparin) for 3 months. In neonates, antithrombotic therapy generally is not recommended for a first occurrence of arterial ischemic stroke in the absence of a cardioembolic origin; however, ACCP states that heparin may be considered in neonates with a first episode of arterial ischemic stroke associated with a documented cardioembolic source.

Heparin or a low molecular weight heparin is suggested for the treatment of acute cerebral venous sinus thrombosis† in adults. Heparin or a low molecular weight heparin also is recommended for the initial treatment of cerebral venous sinus thrombosis without substantial intracranial hemorrhage in children†, followed by continued treatment with a low molecular weight heparin or warfarin for at least 3 months; another 3 months of anticoagulation is suggested if symptoms persist or there is continued occlusion of the cerebral venous sinuses. Although the evidence is not as compelling as for children without substantial hemorrhage, ACCP also suggests that anticoagulation may be used for the treatment of cerebral venous sinus thrombosis in children with substantial hemorrhage. For additional information on the use of anticoagulants in children with cerebral venous sinus thrombosis, consult the most recent ACCP Evidence-based Clinical Practice Guidelines on Antithrombotic Therapy and Prevention of Thrombosis available at http://www.chestnet.org.

■ **Renal Vein Thrombosis** Renal vein thrombosis† is the most common cause of spontaneous venous thromboembolism in neonates. Although use of anticoagulant therapy for this condition remains controversial, heparin is suggested by ACCP as a possible treatment option for neonates with renal vein thrombosis.

■ **Complications of Pregnancy** Heparin should be used during pregnancy† only when clearly needed, weighing carefully the potential benefits versus the possible risks to the mother (e.g., bleeding, osteopenia/osteoporosis) and fetus (e.g., bleeding at the uteroplacental junction [heparin does not cross the placenta], complications secondary to maternal bleeding). (See Cautions: Pregnancy, Fertility, and Lactation.) Heparin has been used in combination with aspirin for the prevention of complications of pregnancy† (e.g., pregnancy loss in women with a history of antiphospholipid syndrome and recurrent fetal loss). The presence of maternal antiphospholipid antibodies is associated with an increased risk of thrombosis and pregnancy loss. Data from several small comparative studies indicate that combined prophylaxis with heparin and low-dose aspirin is more effective than aspirin alone or aspirin combined with a corticosteroid in preventing recurrent pregnancy loss (fetal death, miscarriage), preeclampsia, or premature delivery in women with antiphospholipid syndrome (Hughes syndrome). A systematic review in more than 800 pregnant women with antiphospholipid antibodies and a history of fetal loss supports the finding that combined prophylaxis with heparin and aspirin is superior to aspirin alone in reducing incidence of pregnancy loss. The beneficial effect of such prophylactic therapy may result from aspirin-induced suppression of thromboxane A_2-mediated vasospasm, ischemia, and thrombosis in the placental vasculature and by heparin-induced anticoagulation combined with binding to phospholipid antibodies that protects the trophoblast from antibody attack and thus promotes successful implantation in early pregnancy.

ACCP recommends that women with antiphospholipid antibody (APLA) syndrome in whom recurrent (3 or more) pregnancy loss has occurred should receive antepartum prophylactic or intermediate dosages of subcutaneous heparin in conjunction with low-dose aspirin. Alternatively, therapy with a low molecular weight heparin instead of heparin may be considered.

Because of experience in women with antiphospholipid syndrome, heparin and aspirin (often combined with immune globulin) also have been used to prevent venous thromboembolism and early pregnancy loss in women who have undergone in vitro fertilization†. However, current evidence suggests that the overall absolute risk of symptomatic thrombosis appears to be low in women undergoing in vitro fertilization. Therefore, ACCP recommends against routine thromboprophylaxis in most women undergoing assisted reproduction.

■ **Anticoagulation in Blood Transfusions, Blood Samples, and Other Procedures** Heparin is used as an in vitro anticoagulant in blood transfusions, extracorporeal circulation, and dialysis procedures.

Dosage and Administration

■ **Administration** *USP has changed its labeling standard for Heparin Sodium Injection, USP and Heparin Lock Flush Solution, USP to require that carton and container labels for these products clearly state the strength of the entire container (amount of heparin per total volume of container), followed in close proximity by the strength per mL in parentheses. The labeling change eliminates the need to calculate the total amount of heparin in a product containing more than 1 mL and thus reduces the chance of a dosing error. The new labeling standard for heparin was effective as of May 1, 2013. Clinicians should check the label on all heparin products to confirm the correct formulation and strength prior to dispensing and administering the drug.*

For full-dose therapy, heparin is administered by IV infusion, intermittent IV injection, or deep subcutaneous (intrafat) injection. For fixed low-dose therapy, heparin usually is administered by deep subcutaneous injection. *Heparin should not be administered IM because of the frequency of irritation, pain, and hematoma at the injection site.*

IV Administration Heparin lock flush solution is *not* intended for systemic anticoagulation. Conversely, heparin injection should not be used as a catheter lock flush solution.

For full-dose therapy, many clinicians advocate continuous IV infusion of heparin rather than intermittent IV injection because of a more constant degree of anticoagulation and a lower incidence of bleeding complications. To avoid fluctuations in the rate of administration and minimize the risk of overdosage, IV infusions of full doses of heparin should be administered with a constant-rate infusion pump if possible.

Heparin solutions for IV infusion may be prepared by diluting the drug in a compatible IV solution; when heparin is added to an IV solution, it is recommended that the container be inverted at least 6 times to ensure adequate mixing and prevent pooling of the drug in the solution. Alternatively, commercially available solutions of heparin in 0.45 or 0.9% sodium chloride injection or in 5% dextrose injection may be used. When one of the commercially available IV infusion solutions of heparin is used, accompanying labeling should be consulted for proper methods of administration and associated precautions.

Intermittent IV injections of heparin may be given undiluted or diluted with 50–100 mL of 0.9% sodium chloride injection.

Heparin injections and solutions for infusion and heparin lock flush solutions should be inspected visually for particulate matter and discoloration prior to administration whenever solution and container permit; the injection or solution should not be used if it is discolored, unclear, or contains a precipitate. However, slight discoloration does not alter potency.

Subcutaneous Administration Deep subcutaneous injections of heparin should be made with a 25- or 26-gauge ½- or ⅝-inch needle above the iliac crest or into the abdominal fat layer to minimize tissue trauma; abdominal injections should not be made within 2 inches of the umbilicus. The tissue around the injection site should be grasped creating a tissue roll and the needle inserted quickly into the elevated tissue perpendicular to the skin surface. Finger pressure on the tissue roll should be reduced slightly and the solution fully injected. The needle should be rapidly withdrawn while simultaneously releasing the tissue roll and gentle pressure should be applied to the area for 5–10 seconds. Injection sites should not be massaged before or after injection, and sites should be changed for each dose to prevent the development of a massive hematoma. It has been recommended that the plunger of the syringe not be pulled back to see if a vessel has been entered; however, most clinicians state that although it is not necessary, there is no reason why aspiration cannot be performed to determine if a blood vessel has been entered prior to injection of the solution.

Laboratory Monitoring of Therapy The activated partial thromboplastin time (aPTT) is the most commonly used laboratory method for monitoring full-dose heparin therapy. The activated coagulation time (ACT) may also be used and is especially convenient for monitoring the degree of anticoagulation in patients undergoing extracorporeal circulation because the test can be performed at bedside. Although the whole blood clotting time (Lee-White clotting time) was used in the past to monitor full-dose heparin therapy, the test is rarely used now because it is less convenient and less reproducible than are other available coagulation tests. The generally accepted therapeutic range for the aPTT during full-dose IV or subcutaneous heparin therapy is 1.5–2 times the control value in seconds, and the generally accepted therapeutic range for the ACT is 2.5–3 times the control value in seconds. However, in some patients at high risk for thromboembolic events (e.g., pregnant women with mechanical heart valves) an aPTT of at least 2 times the control value has been used. When full-dose heparin therapy is administered by continuous IV infusion, coagulation tests should be performed prior to initiation of therapy, approximately every 4 hours during the early stages of therapy, and daily thereafter. When full-dose heparin therapy is administered by intermittent IV injection or deep subcutaneous injection, coagulation tests should be performed prior to each dose (or 4–6 hours following the dose for deep subcutaneous injection) during the early stages of therapy, and at appropriate intervals thereafter. Laboratory monitoring of coagulation tests is not usually performed when fixed low-dose subcutaneous heparin therapy is used because currently available coagulation tests are generally unaffected or only minimally prolonged. Regardless of the route of administration, it is recommended that platelet counts and hematocrit be monitored and tests for occult blood in the stool be performed periodically during the entire course of heparin therapy.

■ **Dosage** Dosage of heparin sodium is expressed in USP units. USP units and international units (IU, units) for heparin sodium are equivalent.

Dosage requirements for full-dose heparin sodium therapy vary greatly among individual patients, and dosage should be carefully individualized based on clinical and laboratory findings in order to obtain optimum therapeutic effects without incurring hemorrhage. (See Laboratory Monitoring of Therapy under Dosage and Administration: Administration.) Because of a lack of adequate and well-controlled studies of heparin in pediatric patients, dosage recommendations in this population generally are based on clinical experience. Geriatric patients (older than 60 years of age) may require a lower dosage of heparin sodium. (See Cautions: Geriatric Precautions.)

The optimum duration of heparin therapy for thrombotic disorders has not been definitely established and must be determined by the condition being treated and its severity. Full-dose heparin is generally continued for at least 5 days in patients with acute venous thrombosis or pulmonary embolism, and for 2 days in patients with myocardial infarction (MI)†. A coumarin anticoagulant (e.g., warfarin) generally is administered for follow-up treatment after full-dose heparin, and therapy with the 2 drugs is usually overlapped for 4–5 days until an adequate response to the coumarin derivative is obtained (e.g., as indicated by INR values exceeding 2 on two consecutive days). (See Laboratory Test Interferences: Prothrombin Time.) Several manufacturers recommend abrupt discontinuance of heparin without tapering in patients who have an adequate therapeutic response to a coumarin derivative. However, concern exists that abrupt discontinuance of heparin may result in a high-risk period for rebound thrombosis, although recommendations to reduce this risk remain to be established. In the absence of such recommendations, some clinicians recommend that heparin infusions be reduced in a gradual fashion such as by reducing the rate by 50% over 6 hours and then discontinuing over the next 12 hours.

Treatment of Venous Thromboembolism **Adults.** For *full-dose continuous IV infusion therapy* for the treatment of venous thrombosis and pulmonary embolism in a 68-kg adult, some manufacturers recommend an initial heparin sodium loading dose of 5000 units given by IV injection, followed by a continuous infusion of 20,000–40,000 units in 1 L of 0.9% sodium chloride injection or other compatible IV solution over 24 hours. The American College of Chest Physicians (ACCP) suggests that therapy with IV heparin sodium may be initiated in a weight-adjusted dosage (loading dose of 80 units/kg followed by a continuous infusion of 18 units/kg per hour) or a fixed dosage (loading dose of 5000 units, followed by a continuous IV infusion of 1000 units/hour). Although the aPTT can be used to monitor either dosage regimen, ACCP states that there is no evidence suggesting that monitoring improves clinical outcomes.

For *full-dose intermittent IV therapy* in a 68-kg adult for the treatment of venous thromboembolism and pulmonary embolism, some manufacturers recommend an initial loading dose of 10,000 units of heparin sodium (either undiluted or diluted in 50 or 100 mL of 0.9% sodium chloride injection), followed by 5000–10,000 units every 4–6 hours.

For *full-dose subcutaneous therapy* in a 68-kg adult, some manufacturers recommend an initial heparin sodium dose of 5000 units by IV injection, then 10,000–20,000 units in a concentrated solution injected subcutaneously for 1 dose, followed by subcutaneous injection of 8000–10,000 units as a concentrated solution every 8 hours or 15,000–20,000 units as a concentrated solution every 12 hours. In patients receiving subcutaneous heparin sodium for the treatment of venous thromboembolism in the outpatient setting, ACCP and some manufacturers suggest the use of weight-based dosing (initial dose of 333 units/kg, followed by a dosage of 250 units/kg twice daily) without monitoring rather than a fixed dosage or a weight-adjusted dosage with monitoring.

In patients in whom long-term warfarin therapy will subsequently be prescribed, ACCP recommends initiating warfarin and heparin together on the first treatment day and overlapping therapy with the 2 drugs for a minimum of 5 days and until the international normalized ratio (INR) is at least 2 for 24 hours or longer.

When converting to oral dabigatran therapy in patients currently receiving heparin therapy by continuous IV infusion, the first dose of dabigatran should be administered, followed immediately by discontinuance of the heparin infusion; for patients currently receiving intermittently dosed IV heparin therapy, oral dabigatran should be initiated within 2 hours prior to what would have been the time of the next scheduled heparin dose.

Pediatric Patients. Dosage recommendations in the pediatric population generally are based on clinical experience because of a lack of adequate and well-controlled studies of heparin in these patients. In children receiving full-dose (therapeutic) heparin therapy, ACCP suggests that dosage be titrated to achieve an anti-factor Xa concentration of 0.35–0.7 units/mL or to prolong the aPTT to a corresponding anti-factor Xa range or to a protamine titration range of 0.2–0.4 units/mL. Because clinical outcome studies have not been conducted in children, the therapeutic range for heparin in neonates and children is mostly derived from experience in adults. Following initial heparin therapy in children with an acute venous thromboembolic event, a low molecular weight heparin or a coumarin anticoagulant (e.g., warfarin) may be initiated, or the patient may continue to receive heparin for ongoing therapy. In children with venous thromboembolism in whom warfarin therapy will subsequently be prescribed, ACCP recommends initiating warfarin on the first treatment day and overlapping therapy with warfarin and heparin for a minimum of 5 days and until the INR is at least 2 for 24 hours or longer.

An initial heparin sodium loading dose of 75–100 units/kg (by direct IV injection over 10 minutes) has been suggested in children based on some data indicating that such doses may be more likely to result in therapeutic aPTT values. Following the initial loading dose, a maintenance IV infusion of 25–30 units/kg per hour in infants or 18–20 units/kg per hour in children older than 1 year of age is suggested. The appropriate maintenance dosage of heparin sodium appears to be age dependent, with infants under the age of 2 months having the highest requirements (e.g., average of 28 units/kg per hour) and older children having lower requirements (e.g., average of 20 units/kg per hour in children older than 1 year of age); some experts suggest using a dosage of 18 units/kg per hour in older children. Although not preferred, a maintenance heparin sodium dosage of 75–100 units/kg every 4 hours by intermittent IV administration has been used. ACCP states that the initial dosing strategy in children should be individualized based on consideration of risk factors for bleeding and thrombosis; in general, loading doses should be withheld or reduced if there are substantial bleeding risks, and long-term use of heparin should be avoided in children.

Thromboprophylaxis in General Surgery For *fixed low-dose prophylaxis* of postoperative deep-vein thrombosis in general surgery patients, the most widely used dosage of heparin sodium has been 5000 units administered subcutaneously 2 hours prior to surgery and every 8–12 hours after surgery for 7 days or until the patient is fully ambulatory, whichever is longer. If clinical evidence of thromboembolism develops despite fixed low-dose prophylaxis, full-dose IV or subcutaneous heparin should be initiated.

Acute Ischemic Complications of ST-Segment-Elevation Myocardial Infarction As adjunctive therapy with fibrin-selective thrombolytic agents (e.g., alteplase, tenecteplase, reteplase) in patients with ST-segment-elevation MI (STEMI)†, the American College of Cardiology Foundation (ACCF) and the American Heart Association (AHA) recommend IV heparin sodium given in an initial loading dose of 60 units/kg (maximum 4000 units) followed by a continuous infusion of 12 units/kg per hour (maximum 1000 units/hour), adjusted to maintain a therapeutic aPTT of 1.5–2 times the control value or 50–70 seconds for 48 hours or until revascularization.

In patients with acute MI and concurrent atrial fibrillation, ACCF, AHA, and the Heart Rhythm Society (HRS) recommend continuous IV infusion or intermittent subcutaneous injection of heparin sodium in a dosage sufficient to prolong the aPTT to 1.5–2 times the control value.

Acute Ischemic Complications of Percutaneous Coronary Intervention In patients undergoing percutaneous coronary intervention (PCI) who are *not* receiving concurrent antiplatelet therapy with a GP IIb/IIIa-receptor inhibitor and who have not received prior anticoagulant therapy, ACCF, AHA, and the Society for Cardiovascular Angiography and Interventions (SCAI) suggest administration of a loading dose of 70–100 units/kg of heparin sodium by direct IV injection to achieve an ACT of 250–300 seconds with the HemoTec device or 300–350 seconds with the Hemochron device. If prior anticoagulant therapy has been administered in such patients, additional heparin sodium doses (e.g., 2000–5000 units) should be given as needed to achieve an ACT of 250–300 seconds with the HemoTec device or 300–350 seconds with the Hemochron device. In patients undergoing PCI who are receiving concurrent therapy with a GP IIb/IIIa-receptor inhibitor and who have not received prior anticoagulant therapy, use of a lower dose of concurrent heparin sodium (50–70 units/kg IV loading dose) targeted to an ACT of 200–250 seconds is suggested. If prior anticoagulant therapy has been administered in such patients, additional heparin sodium doses (e.g., 2000–5000 units) should be given as needed to achieve an ACT of 200–250 seconds. Lower dosages of heparin may be used in women and geriatric patients undergoing PCI, particularly when heparin is combined with GP IIb/IIIa-receptor inhibitors. Heparin sodium should be discontinued after successful PCI procedures; in most cases, the femoral sheath is removed when the ACT falls to less than 150–180 seconds or when the aPTT decreases to less than 50 seconds.

Acute Ischemic Complications of Non-ST-Segment-Elevation Acute Coronary Syndromes Adjusted-dose heparin sodium (e.g., 60 units/kg [maximum 4000 units] loading dose followed by continuous IV infusion of 12 units/kg per hour [maximum 1000 units/hr]) is recommended by ACCF, AHA, and ACC to maintain the aPTT between 1.5–2 times the control value in patients with non-ST-segment-elevation acute coronary syndromes (NSTE ACS; unstable angina or non-ST-segment-elevation MI [NSTEMI]) in addition to aspirin and/or clopidogrel. Therapy should be initiated as soon as possible upon presentation. Optimum duration of therapy has not been established; in clinical trials, heparin was continued for 2–5 days.

Disseminated Intravascular Coagulation When heparin is used for the treatment of disseminated intravascular coagulation (DIC), some clinicians recommend heparin sodium doses of 50–100 units/kg for adults and 25–50 units/kg for children given by IV infusion or IV injection every 4 hours. If there is no improvement after 4–8 hours, the drug should be discontinued.

Cardiac Surgery The initial dose of heparin sodium recommended by the manufacturers for adults undergoing total body perfusion for open-heart surgery is not less than 150 units/kg. A heparin sodium dose of 300 units/kg is frequently used for procedures estimated to last less than 1 hour and 400 units/kg for those procedures estimated to last longer than 1 hour. Some clinicians recommend that heparin sodium dosage during cardiopulmonary bypass procedures be adjusted to prolong the ACT to 480–600 seconds. In extracorporeal dialysis procedures, the equipment manufacturer's operating instructions should be followed carefully; if manufacturer's instructions are not available, an initial heparin sodium dose of 25–30 units/kg, followed by an infusion of 1500–2000 units/hour is suggested based on pharmacodynamic data.

Cardioversion of Atrial Fibrillation If heparin is used for the prevention of stroke and systemic embolism in patients undergoing cardioversion for atrial fibrillation or atrial flutter†, the use of full venous thromboembolism treatment dosages is recommended.

Thromboembolism During Pregnancy When heparin is used for thromboprophylaxis during pregnancy†, the drug is usually administered 2–3 times daily in a prophylactic dosage (fixed-dose) or intermediate dosage (dosage adjusted to target a specific anti-factor Xa level). When used in therapeutic dosages, heparin usually is administered by continuous IV infusion with doses adjusted to achieve a target therapeutic aPTT or by twice-daily subcutaneous injection in doses sufficient to achieve a therapeutic aPTT 6 hours after injection.

In women with antiphospholipid antibody (APLA) syndrome and a history of multiple pregnancy losses, antepartum administration of subcutaneous heparin sodium in a prophylactic or intermediate dosage has been recommended; low-dose aspirin (75–100 mg daily) should be administered in conjunction with heparin.

ACCF/AHA/HRS state that administration of heparin may be considered during the first trimester and last month of pregnancy in patients with atrial fibrillation and additional risk factors for thromboembolism. Heparin sodium may be administered by continuous IV infusion in a dosage sufficient to maintain the aPTT at least 1.5–2 times the control value. Alternatively, 10,000–20,000 units of heparin sodium may be given subcutaneously every 12 hours with dosage adjusted to maintain the mid-interval aPTT (6 hours after the dose) at 1.5–2 times the control value. Coumarin anticoagulant therapy (e.g., warfarin) may be considered during the second trimester in pregnant women with atrial fibrillation who have a high risk for thromboembolism.

If subcutaneous heparin sodium is used for the prevention of thromboembolism in pregnant women with prosthetic mechanical heart valves, the drug should be initiated in high dosages (17,500–20,000 units every 12 hours) and adjusted to maintain the mid-interval aPTT at least twice the control value or an anti-factor Xa concentration of 0.35–0.7 units/mL throughout pregnancy. Alternatively, 17,500–20,000 units of heparin sodium may be administered every 12 hours and adjusted to maintain the mid-interval aPTT at least twice the control value or an anti-factor Xa concentration of 0.35–0.7 units/mL until week 13 of pregnancy; subsequently, therapy is switched to warfarin until close to delivery when heparin may be resumed.

Perioperative Management of Antithrombotic Therapy If heparin is used for bridging anticoagulation in patients who require temporary interruption of warfarin therapy during surgery or other invasive procedure, ACCP recommends the use of therapeutic dosages (e.g., continuous infusion of heparin adjusted to maintain an aPTT of approximately 1.5–2 times the control value) because of more extensive data and experience; however, other dosage regimens have been used. ACCP suggests that heparin be discontinued approximately 4–6 hours prior to surgery to allow sufficient time for anticoagulant effects to dissipate. Postoperative anticoagulation should be administered with caution and only when hemostasis has been achieved because of the potential for bleeding at the surgical site.

Anticoagulation in Blood Transfusions and Blood Samples When heparin sodium is used as an in vitro anticoagulant in blood transfusions, 7500 units of the drug is usually added to 100 mL of 0.9% sodium chloride injection and 6–8 mL of this solution is added to each 100 mL of whole blood. When heparin sodium is used as an in vitro anticoagulant for blood samples, 70–150 units is added to each 10–20 mL of whole blood.

Thrombosis Associated with Indwelling Venous or Arterial Devices When a heparin-containing flush solution is used to maintain patency of indwelling venipuncture devices, a quantity of heparin lock flush solution (e.g., containing 10 or 100 units of heparin sodium per mL) sufficient to fill the device is injected into the lumen of the device after each use, after designated intervals (if the device is not used in the interim), or as necessary. While it has been reported that each dose of the solution will maintain anticoagulation within the lumen of the device for up to 4 hours, longer intervals between instillations of the flush solution (generally every 8–12 hours) are commonly employed when the device is not being used more frequently, and flushing with 0.9% sodium chloride injection alone at such intervals also appears to be effective in maintaining patency in venipuncture devices into which blood is not aspirated, at least those placed peripherally.

When a drug that is incompatible with heparin is to be administered via a venipuncture device in which a heparin-containing flush solution is used, the entire device should be flushed with 0.9% sodium chloride injection prior to and immediately after the incompatible drug is administered. Another dose of heparin lock flush solution may be injected into the device after the second saline flush. When the indwelling venipuncture device is used for repeated withdrawal of blood samples for laboratory analysis and the presence of heparin or 0.9% sodium chloride is likely to interfere with or alter results of the analysis, heparin lock flush solution should be cleared from the device by aspirating and discarding it from the device before withdrawing the blood sample. After the blood sample is drawn, another dose of heparin lock flush solution should be injected into the device.

Following injection of heparin lock solution from a single-dose vial into an indwelling venipuncture device, unused portions of the solutions should be discarded. The device manufacturer's instructions should be consulted for specific directions. Multiple-dose vials are available for repeated use. Since repeated injections of small doses of heparin sodium can alter aPTT results, it is recommended that a baseline aPTT value be obtained prior to insertion of an indwelling venipuncture device.

In neonates and children requiring cardiac catheterization via an artery†, ACCP recommends a heparin sodium dose of 100 units/kg as a direct IV injection. Additional doses may be required in prolonged procedures.

For thromboprophylaxis in neonates with a central venous access device†, ACCP recommends the use of heparin sodium 0.5 units/kg per hour as a continuous infusion.

For thromboprophylaxis of umbilical arterial catheters in neonates†, ACCP suggests the use of low-dose heparin sodium infusion (0.25–1 unit/mL) for a total dosage of 25–200 units/kg per day.

For thromboprophylaxis in neonates and children with peripheral arterial catheters, administration of heparin sodium by continuous IV infusion in low dosages (5 units/mL at 1 mL/hour) is recommended by ACCP.

Cautions

■ **Hematologic Effects** Hemorrhage, the major adverse effect of heparin, is an extension of the pharmacologic action of the drug and may range from minor local ecchymoses to major hemorrhagic complications. Rarely, hemorrhagic complications may result in death. Bleeding complications occur in approximately 1.5–20% of patients receiving heparin. Major bleeding episodes occur more frequently with full-dose than with low-dose heparin and have been reported more frequently with intermittent IV injection than with continuous IV infusion of the drug. The incidence of major bleeding appears to be similar among patients receiving heparin by continuous IV infusion or subcutaneously. Pooled data from a number of clinical trials evaluating IV heparin for the treatment of venous thromboembolism indicate that the rates of major bleeding range from 0–7% and fatal bleeding from 0–2%. In patients with ischemic coronary syndromes, the incidence of major bleeding ranges from 0–6.3% during the initial 8 days of treatment and from 0.3–3.2% during subsequent long-term therapy (approximately 0.25–3 months). Hemorrhage also has been reported occasionally with repeated administration of heparin lock flush solutions containing low concentrations of heparin sodium (e.g., 10–100 units/mL).

Patients with renal failure or with a history of recent surgery or trauma may be at increased risk of bleeding complications during therapy with heparin. There is some evidence that the risk of heparin-induced hemorrhage may be higher in patients older than 60 years of age, especially in women. Bleeding may occur at any site, and some hemorrhagic complications may be difficult to detect. GI or urinary tract bleeding during therapy with heparin may indicate the presence of occult lesions. Adrenal hemorrhage with acute adrenal insufficiency has occurred during therapy with heparin. Retroperitoneal hemorrhage has been reported in patients receiving anticoagulant therapy, and potentially fatal ovarian (corpus luteum) hemorrhage has also occurred in some women of reproductive age who received short- or long-term anticoagulant therapy. The frequency and severity of heparin-associated hemorrhage may be minimized by careful clinical management of the patient. (See Cautions: Precautions and Contraindications.)

Pooled analyses of data from comparative clinical trials evaluating heparin and low molecular weight heparins for the treatment of venous thromboembolism or ischemic coronary syndromes indicate that use of low molecular weight heparin does not result in an increased risk of major bleeding compared with heparin.

Two forms of acute thrombocytopenia have been reported with heparin. In some patients, thrombocytopenia appears to be caused by a direct, nonimmunologic effect on circulating platelets. In others, the reaction is immune mediated (heparin-induced thrombocytopenia [HIT]) and caused by the development of IgG antibodies to an immune complex that forms between heparin and platelet factor 4; these antibody-bound immune complexes bind to IgG receptors on the surface of platelets, resulting in platelet activation and increased thrombin generation. Thrombocytopenia has been reported with both low-dose and full-dose heparin therapy and does not appear to be dose related. Thrombocytopenia, including accompanying intracranial bleeding and GI hemorrhage, has been reported in patients receiving less than 500 units of heparin sodium daily via heparin lock flush solution. Although the reported incidences are variable (e.g., 0–30%), thrombocytopenia has occurred in about 15% of patients treated with heparin sodium prepared from bovine lung tissue and in about 5% of those treated with heparin sodium prepared from porcine intestinal mucosa. Thrombocytopenia, if it occurs, usually develops 1–20 days after initiation of therapy. Immune-mediated HIT usually is evident 5–10 days after exposure to heparin, but can occur more rapidly (e.g., within 24 hours) in patients with recent exposure (e.g., within the previous 3 months) to the drug or appear as late as several weeks after discontinuance of therapy. Mild thrombocytopenia (platelet count greater than 100,000/mm^3) may remain stable or even reverse with continued heparin therapy. However, thrombocytopenia of any degree should be monitored closely since HIT can sometimes lead to the development of serious, sometimes fatal, thrombotic events. Heparin therapy should generally be discontinued if substantial thrombocytopenia (platelet count less than 100,000/mm^3) or HIT (with or without thrombosis) occurs.

HIT is a serious complication of heparin therapy that can lead to life- or limb-threatening venous and arterial thrombosis (e.g., cerebral vein thrombosis, limb ischemia, acute myocardial infarction [MI], stroke, gangrene of the extremities [possibly requiring amputation], mesenteric thrombosis). Localized or disseminated thromboses associated with HIT have occurred in patients receiving heparin, even in the low concentrations used in heparin lock flush solution. HIT-associated thrombosis develops as a result of in vivo platelet aggregation induced by heparin and can occur at almost any vascular location. (See Cautions: Precautions and Contraindications.)

■ Sensitivity Reactions Allergic reactions to heparin occur rarely. Hypersensitivity, which can be generalized, may be manifested by chills, fever, pruritus, urticaria, asthma, rhinitis, lacrimation, headache, nausea, vomiting, and anaphylactoid reactions including shock. Allergic vasospastic reactions have been reported with heparin. These reactions, if they occur, generally develop 6–10 days after initiation of heparin and last 4–6 hours. The reactions frequently occur in a limb where an artery has been recently catheterized. The affected limb is painful, ischemic, and cyanosed. If heparin is continued, generalized vasospasm with cyanosis, tachypnea, feelings of oppression, and headache may occur. Protamine sulfate has no effect on these reactions.

Itching and burning, especially of the plantar side of the feet, has occurred during heparin therapy and may be caused by a similar allergic vasospastic reaction. Chest pain, hypertension, arthralgia, and/or headache have also been reported in the absence of definite peripheral vasospasm.

■ Local Effects Deep subcutaneous injection of heparin may rarely cause local irritation, erythema, mild pain, hematoma, ulceration, or cutaneous and subcutaneous necrosis (sometimes requiring skin grafts). Local irritation and erythema also have been reported with heparin lock flush solution. Histamine-like reactions have also been reported at the site of injection. A slightly lower incidence of local reactions has been reported following deep subcutaneous injection of heparin calcium (no longer commercially available in the US) than that reported following deep subcutaneous injection of equal doses of heparin sodium; this may be due to the smaller volume of heparin calcium required.

■ Hepatic Effects Increased serum concentrations of AST (SGOT) and ALT (SGPT), without increased serum concentrations of bilirubin or alkaline phosphatase, have been reported in a high percentage of patients following subcutaneous or IV administration of heparin; transient increases in serum LDH concentrations have also occurred in some patients receiving the drug. Increased concentrations of AST and ALT have also been reported following administration of heparin to healthy individuals. A reversible cholestatic reaction without jaundice, manifested by increased serum aminotransferase (ALT, AST) and alkaline phosphatase concentrations, also has been reported in a few patients receiving heparin therapy. It is not known whether elevated serum aminotransferases in patients receiving heparin represent hepatic toxicity, drug-induced laboratory test interference, or nonspecific stimulation of hepatic enzymes. (See Laboratory Test Interferences.) Since aminotransferase determinations are important in the differential diagnosis of MI, liver disease, and pulmonary emboli, elevation of these enzymes during heparin therapy should be interpreted with caution.

■ Other Adverse Effects Osteoporosis and spontaneous fractures of the vertebral column have been reported rarely in patients receiving large daily dosages (10,000 units or more) of heparin sodium for 3 months or longer. Suppression of aldosterone synthesis; priapism; delayed, transient alopecia; and rebound hyperlipemia following discontinuance of heparin therapy have also been reported rarely in patients receiving the drug.

■ Precautions and Contraindications All patients should be screened prior to initiation of heparin therapy to rule out bleeding disorders. In preoperative patients, the prothrombin time (PT), activated partial thromboplastin time (aPTT), hematocrit, and platelet count should be determined prior to surgery; coagulation tests should be normal or only slightly elevated before low-dose heparin therapy is instituted. Although monitoring of blood coagulation tests is useful for assuring adequate dosage during full-dose heparin therapy, coagulation test results do not always correlate with the frequency of bleeding complications. Heparin should be used with extreme caution whenever there is an increased risk of hemorrhage. Factors reported to increase the risk of hemorrhage during heparin therapy include concurrent administration of some drugs (see Drug Interactions); subacute bacterial endocarditis; arterial sclerosis; dissecting aneurysm; increased capillary permeability; presence of inaccessible ulcerative GI lesions; diverticulitis; ulcerative colitis; hemorrhagic blood dyscrasias (e.g., hemophilia, some vascular purpuras, thrombocytopenia); menstruation; ovulation; threatened abortion; severe renal, hepatic, or biliary disease; hypertension; indwelling catheters; eye, brain, or spinal cord surgery; continuous tube drainage of the stomach or small intestine; and spinal tap or spinal anesthesia.

If hemorrhage occurs, heparin should be discontinued immediately. Nosebleed, hematuria, or tarry stools may be noted as the first sign of bleeding or overdosage; easy bruising or petechiae may precede frank bleeding. Discontinuance of heparin will usually correct minor bleeding or overdosage within a few hours. If severe hemorrhage or overdosage occurs, protamine sulfate should be administered immediately. (See Protamine Sulfate 20:28.08.) Blood transfusions may also be required in patients with massive blood loss. If signs and symptoms of acute adrenal hemorrhage and insufficiency occur, plasma cortisol concentrations should be measured and vigorous therapy with IV corticosteroids should be initiated after discontinuing heparin. Initiation of corrective therapy should not depend on laboratory confirmation of the diagnosis, since any delay in an acute situation may be fatal.

Heparin is contraindicated in patients with severe thrombocytopenia or a history of HIT or HIT with thrombosis. If HIT with or without thrombosis is diagnosed or strongly suspected during heparin therapy, all sources of heparin (including heparin flushes) should be discontinued and an alternative (nonheparin) anticoagulant (e.g., argatroban, bivalirudin) substituted. Conversion to warfarin therapy (for longer-term anticoagulation) should be initiated only after substantial recovery from acute HIT has occurred (i.e., platelet counts at least 150,000/mm^3) with a nonheparin anticoagulant. The manufacturer recommends against future use of heparin in patients who experience HIT, particularly within 3–6 months following the event and if HIT antibodies are still present. HIT with or without thrombosis also can occur up to several weeks following discontinuance of heparin therapy. Patients who are found to have thrombocytopenia or thrombosis after discontinuance of heparin should be evaluated for HIT and HIT with thrombosis. Although there is some uncertainty regarding the risk-to-benefit ratio of platelet count monitoring in patients receiving heparin, the American College of Chest Physicians (ACCP) suggests that platelet counts may be monitored in those who are considered to be at high risk (higher than 1%) of developing HIT; for those considered to be at low risk (less than 1%), platelet count monitoring generally is not recommended.

Patients with familial antithrombin III deficiency may appear to be resistant to the effects of heparin, since adequate levels of antithrombin III are necessary for the drug's anticoagulant effect. Increased resistance to the antithrombotic effects of heparin has been reported in febrile patients, in postoperative patients, and in some patients with MI, pulmonary embolism, thrombophlebitis, infections with thrombosing tendencies, or extensive thrombotic disorders, especially in conjunction with malignant neoplasms. This phenomenon appears to be caused by alterations in the physiology of the patient and pharmacokinetics of the drug, and larger doses of heparin may be required during initial therapy to achieve an anticoagulant response in these patients.

Fatal medication errors have occurred as a result of confusion between different formulations of heparin, in particular with heparin sodium injection and catheter lock flush vials. At least 3 infant deaths have been reported following inadvertent administration of heparin sodium injection 10,000 units/mL instead of HEP-LOCK U/P (heparin lock flush solution) 10 units/mL. Heparin sodium injection should not be used as a catheter lock flush product. To minimize the risk of medication errors, clinicians should take appropriate measures to carefully distinguish between heparin formulations and review all labels for correct drug name, strength, and volume prior to dispensing and administering the drug. Dispensing errors involving heparin sodium injection and HEP-LOCK U/P should be reported to the manufacturer (800-ANA-Drug or 800-262-3784) or the FDA MedWatch program by phone (800-FDA-1088 or online at https://www.accessdata.fda.gov/scripts/medwatch/medwatch-online.htm.

Heparin is generally contraindicated in patients who are hypersensitive to the drug or to pork products. Patients with documented hypersensitivity to heparin should be given the drug only in clearly life-threatening situations.

Heparin is contraindicated in patients with uncontrollable bleeding, unless such bleeding is secondary to disseminated intravascular coagulation. The drug is also contraindicated whenever suitable blood coagulation tests cannot be performed at required intervals; however, this is not generally a contraindication for fixed low-dose heparin therapy, since monitoring of coagulation tests is not usually required when fixed low-dose therapy is used in patients with normal coagulation parameters.

Some commercially available formulations of heparin sodium injection contain sodium metabisulfite, a sulfite that can cause allergic-type reactions, including anaphylaxis and life-threatening or less severe asthmatic episodes, in certain susceptible individuals. The overall prevalence of sulfite sensitivity in the general population is unknown but probably low; such sensitivity appears to occur more frequently in asthmatic than in nonasthmatic individuals.

When heparin is used in combination with dihydroergotamine, the usual cautions, precautions, and contraindications associated with dihydroergotamine must be considered in addition to those associated with heparin. The potential risk of arterial vasospasm should be considered in patients receiving combined therapy with these drugs. For a more complete discussion, see Cautions in Dihydroergotamine Mesylate 12:16.

■ Pediatric Precautions There are no adequate and well-controlled studies evaluating the use of heparin in pediatric patients.

Some commercially available heparin sodium injections and heparin lock flush solutions contain benzyl alcohol as a preservative. Although a causal relationship has not been established, administration of injections preserved with benzyl alcohol has been associated with serious toxicity (e.g., "gasping syndrome") in pediatric patients. Toxicity appears to result from administration of large amounts (i.e., about 100–400 mg/kg daily) of benzyl alcohol in these patients, and may be more likely to occur in neonates and low-birthweight infants. When heparin sodium injection is required in neonates and infants, the manufacturer states that a preservative-free formulation should be used. When heparin lock flush is required in neonates, a preservative-free formulation should be used. The American Academy of Pediatrics (AAP) states that use of preservative-containing flush solutions (i.e., with benzyl alcohol) clearly should be avoided in neonates; however, the AAP further states that the presence of small amounts of the preservative in a commercially available injection should not proscribe its use in neonates. Although the recommended dosage range for heparin includes amounts of benzyl alcohol well below that associated with the "gasping syndrome," the minimum amount of benzyl alcohol at which toxicity may occur is unknown. If other benzyl alcohol-containing preparations are to be used in a patient, clinicians should take into account the total daily metabolic load of benzyl alcohol from all sources.

Fatalities have occurred in pediatric patients, including neonates, as a result of medication dispensing errors. Clinicians should take appropriate precautions when dispensing and administering the drug. (See Cautions: Precautions and Contraindications.)

The use of heparin to maintain patency of umbilical-artery catheters reportedly has been associated with an increased risk of germinal matrix-intraventricular hemorrhage in low-birthweight neonates; however, a causal relationship has not been definitely established, and well-controlled studies are needed to further evaluate this finding. Because of the potential risk of systemic anticoagulation, heparin lock flush solutions containing heparin sodium 100 units/mL should be avoided in neonates and in infants who weigh less than 10 kg. Caution also is advised when using heparin lock flush solutions containing 10 units/mL in premature infants who weigh less than 1 kg and are receiving frequent flushes.

■ **Geriatric Precautions** A higher incidence of bleeding has been reported in patients older than 60 years of age, especially women. Clinical studies indicate that lower dosages of heparin may be appropriate in these patients. (See Dosage and Administration: Dosage.)

■ **Pregnancy, Fertility, and Lactation** Increased fetal resorptions have been observed in animals when heparin was administered during the period of organogenesis in dosages higher than the maximum human dosage; there are no adequate and well-controlled studies to date using heparin in pregnant women. Published reports have not shown any evidence of a teratogenic potential or other adverse fetal effects when the drug is used during pregnancy; because heparin does not cross the human placenta, any fetal complications that may occur are likely to be related to other indirect factors (e.g., severe maternal disease).

Long-term (e.g., longer than 1 month) heparin therapy during pregnancy can result in maternal osteopenia and osteoporosis, and prophylactic calcium and vitamin D supplementation has been suggested to reduce this risk. At least one case of fatal cerebral hemorrhage has occurred in a woman receiving heparin and aspirin to prevent pregnancy loss following in vitro fertilization. (See Uses: Complications of Pregnancy.)

Heparin should be used during pregnancy only if the potential benefits justify the potential risks to the fetus; if needed, use of a preservative (benzyl alcohol)-free formulation is recommended. When anticoagulant therapy is required in pregnant women, ACCP generally recommends the use of a low molecular weight heparin because of a more favorable adverse effect profile. For information on the prophylactic use of heparin to improve pregnancy outcomes in certain women at risk (e.g., those with antiphospholipid syndrome), see Uses: Complications of Pregnancy.

Because of its high molecular weight, heparin is not likely to be distributed into human milk; any heparin that is ingested during breastfeeding would not be absorbed by a nursing infant. However, if benzyl alcohol is present in maternal serum, it is likely to distribute into human milk and be absorbed by a nursing infant. The manufacturer recommends caution if heparin is used in nursing women. ACCP recommends that heparin be continued in nursing women who are already receiving such therapy.

If heparin therapy is required in nursing women, use of a preservative (benzyl alcohol)-free formulation is recommended.

Drug Interactions

■ **Drugs Affecting Platelet Function** Drugs that affect platelet function (e.g., aspirin and other nonsteroidal anti-inflammatory agents, dextran, dipyridamole, phenylbutazone [no longer commercially available in the US], hydroxychloroquine, GP IIb/IIIa-receptor inhibitors such as abciximab, eptifibatide, and tirofiban) may increase the risk of hemorrhage and should be used with caution in patients receiving heparin.

■ **Thrombolytic Agents** Concomitant therapy with heparin and/or platelet-aggregation inhibitors has been used with thrombolytic agents to prevent reocclusion following lysis of coronary artery thrombi. However, since such therapy has not been shown to be of unequivocal benefit and may increase the risk of bleeding complications, use of anticoagulants concomitantly with thrombolytic therapy should be individualized and careful monitoring is advised. Some evidence suggests a narrow margin of safety for upward adjustment of heparin dosage, and the need for serial monitoring of activated partial thromboplastin time (aPTT), in patients receiving heparin concurrently with thrombolytic therapy for acute myocardial infarction (MI). (See Uses: Acute Ischemic Complications of ST-Segment-Elevation Myocardial Infarction.)

■ **Dihydroergotamine Mesylate** When used in combination with heparin, dihydroergotamine appears to potentiate the antithrombogenic effects of heparin by helping to reduce factors that contribute to venous thrombus formation. As a result of its vasoconstrictor effect, dihydroergotamine accelerates venous return, reduces venous stasis and pooling, and may also indirectly help to prevent damage to venous endothelium caused by excessive dilation. Therefore, concomitant use of dihydroergotamine and heparin may help to prevent deep-vein thrombosis.

Concomitant subcutaneous administration of dihydroergotamine mesylate with heparin sodium does not appear to affect the pharmacokinetics of heparin. Concomitant subcutaneous administration of the drugs reportedly decreases peak plasma concentrations of dihydroergotamine and decreases the rate of absorption of dihydroergotamine compared with administration of dihydroergotamine alone; however, the area under the concentration-time curve of dihydroergotamine is generally unaffected.

■ **Other Drugs** Although some reports suggest that IV nitroglycerin may antagonize the anticoagulant effect of heparin when these drugs are administered concomitantly, such antagonism has not been confirmed in other studies. Limited data suggest that nitroglycerin-induced heparin resistance, if it occurs, may be manifested only at high nitroglycerin dosages or infusion rates (e.g., greater than 350 mcg/minute) and may possibly be related to a nitroglycerin-induced abnormality in antithrombin III (heparin cofactor). Further study is required to confirm possible IV nitroglycerin-induced heparin resistance in patients receiving these drugs concomitantly and, if confirmed, to elucidate the potential clinical importance of such an interaction. Meanwhile, it has been suggested that patients receiving heparin and IV nitroglycerin concomitantly be monitored closely to avoid inadequate anticoagulation.

Cardiac glycosides, nicotine, quinine, tetracyclines, and antihistamines reportedly may interfere with the anticoagulant effect of heparin. Although there is some experimental evidence that heparin may antagonize the action of corticosteroids, corticotropin, and insulin, these effects have not been definitely established.

The anticoagulant effect of heparin is enhanced by concurrent treatment with antithrombin III (human) in patients with familial antithrombin III deficiency. To avoid bleeding, at least one manufacturer recommends a reduced dosage of heparin during concurrent treatment with antithrombin III.

Laboratory Test Interferences

■ **Prothrombin Time** Heparin prolongs the prothrombin time (PT), and caution should be observed in evaluating the test in patients receiving a coumarin or indandione derivative and heparin. Valid PT determinations can usually be made during concurrent therapy if blood samples for the test are drawn at least 4–6 hours after an IV dose or 12–24 hours after a subcutaneous dose of heparin. The PT may not be significantly prolonged by heparin when the drug is administered by continuous IV infusion and blood samples for the test can usually be obtained at any time during the infusion.

■ **Other Laboratory Tests** Heparin reportedly interferes with the sulfobromophthalein test by increasing the color intensity of the dye in serum and causing a shift in the absorption peak from 580 to 595 nm.

Heparin interferes with competitive protein binding methods for serum thyroxine determinations resulting in falsely elevated concentrations. Radioimmunoassay and protein bound iodine methods do not appear to be affected by heparin.

When heparin is used as an in vitro anticoagulant, leukocyte counts should be done within 2 hours after addition of heparin. Heparinized blood should not be used for erythrocyte sedimentation rates, platelet counts, or erythrocyte fragility tests and is unsuitable for tests involving complement or isoagglutinins.

Heparin may cause false elevations in plasma AST (SGOT) concentrations using an Ektachem dry-chemistry system analyzer. Since aminotransferase determinations are important in the differential diagnosis of myocardial infarction (MI), liver disease, and pulmonary emboli, elevation of these enzymes during heparin therapy should be interpreted with caution.

Pharmacology

■ **Anticoagulant Effect** Heparin acts as a catalyst to markedly accelerate the rate at which antithrombin III (heparin cofactor) neutralizes thrombin and activated coagulation factor X (Xa). Antithrombin III generally neutralizes these coagulation factors by slowly and irreversibly complexing stoichiometrically with them; however, in the presence of heparin, it neutralizes these factors almost instantaneously. Although the exact mechanism of action has not been fully elucidated, heparin apparently binds to antithrombin III and induces a conformational change in the molecule which promotes its interaction with thrombin and factor Xa. In the presence of heparin, antithrombin III also neutralizes activated coagulation factors IX, XI, XII, and plasmin.

With low-dose heparin therapy (see Dosage and Administration: Dosage), anticoagulation appears to result from neutralization of factor Xa which prevents the conversion of prothrombin to thrombin. Low doses of heparin have very little effect on thrombin and exert a measurable antithrombogenic effect only if thrombin formation has not already occurred. With full-dose heparin therapy (see Dosage and Administration: Dosage), anticoagulation appears to result primarily from neutralization of thrombin which prevents the conversion of fibrinogen to fibrin. Full-dose heparin therapy also prevents the formation of a stable fibrin clot by inhibiting activation of fibrin stabilizing factor. In contrast to coumarin and indandione derivatives, heparin has an anticoagulant effect both in vitro and in vivo. Low-dose or full-dose heparin therapy inhibits thrombus formation when stasis is induced, and full-dose therapy may prevent extension of existing thrombi. Heparin has no fibrinolytic activity and cannot lyse established thrombi.

In adequate dosage, protamine sulfate neutralizes the anticoagulant effect of heparin. Although there is no significant difference in the anticoagulant effectiveness between heparin derived from porcine intestinal mucosa or bovine lung tissue, slightly different amounts of protamine sulfate are required to neutralize one unit of heparin calcium (no longer commercially available in the US) derived from porcine intestinal mucosa or one unit of heparin sodium derived from bovine lung tissue or porcine intestinal mucosa. (See Protamine Sulfate 20:28.08.)

Because heparin acts on blood coagulation factors that are involved in both extrinsic and intrinsic coagulation, full-dose heparin therapy produces prolongation of several coagulation assays including the activated coagulation time (ACT), activated partial thromboplastin time (aPTT), plasma recalcification time, prothrombin time (PT), thrombin time, and whole blood clotting time. Coagulation test results are generally unaffected or only minimally prolonged by low-dose heparin therapy. Heparin sodium lock flush solution does not induce systemic anticoagulant effects when administered in single doses of 10 or 100 units/mL to maintain the patency of IV injection devices.

■ **Other Effects** In vivo, heparin clears lipemic plasma by stimulating the release and/or activation of lipoprotein lipase which hydrolyzes triglycerides to free fatty acids and glycerol. This effect may occur following doses of heparin that are smaller than those required to produce anticoagulant effects. Rebound hyperlipemia has been reported following a period of heparin-induced plasma clearing. Protamine sulfate inhibits the plasma-clearing effect of heparin.

Heparin has been reported to increase, decrease, or have no effect on platelet adhesiveness, aggregation, and release reaction. Many reports are based on in vitro studies that were performed under various conditions, and results do not necessarily correspond to in vivo effects of heparin on platelets. (See Cautions: Hematologic Effects.) Various other pharmacologic actions including anti-inflammatory, diuretic, antimetastatic, antiviral, and antienzymatic effects have been attributed to heparin; however, most of these reports are based on animal studies and their clinical importance has not been established.

Pharmacokinetics

■ **Absorption** Heparin is not absorbed from the GI tract and must be administered parenterally. The onset of anticoagulant activity is immediate following direct IV injection or the start of continuous IV infusion of full doses of heparin. There may be considerable interpatient variation in the extent of absorption following deep subcutaneous injection of heparin; however, onset of activity usually occurs within 20–60 minutes. Results of preliminary studies indicate that the rate and extent of absorption are lower following deep subcutaneous injection of heparin calcium (no longer commercially available in the US) than following deep subcutaneous injection of equal doses of heparin sodium.

Plasma heparin concentrations may be increased and activated partial thromboplastin times (aPTTs) may be more prolonged in geriatric adults (older than 60 years of age) compared with younger adults.

■ **Distribution** Heparin appears to be extensively bound to low-density lipoprotein, globulins, and fibrinogen. The drug does not cross the placenta and is not distributed into milk.

■ **Elimination** The plasma half-life of heparin averages 1–2 hours in healthy adults. However, the half-life of the drug increases with increasing doses. Following IV administration of heparin sodium 100, 200, or 400 units/kg, the plasma half-life of the drug averages 56, 96, and 152 minutes, respectively. Several studies using heparin sodium have shown that the drug has a shorter plasma half-life in patients with pulmonary embolism than in healthy individuals or patients with other thrombotic disorders. The plasma half-life of the drug is also decreased in patients with liver impairment but may be prolonged in cirrhotic patients. In anephric patients or patients with severe renal impairment, the half-life of heparin may be slightly prolonged.

The metabolic fate of heparin has not been fully elucidated, but the drug appears to be removed from the circulation mainly by the reticuloendothelial system and may localize on arterial and venous endothelium. Although there is no reproducible evidence, it has been suggested that heparin may be partially metabolized in the liver to uroheparin, which is partially desulfated heparin. A small fraction of each dose of heparin appears to be excreted in urine as unchanged drug. Heparin is not removed by hemodialysis.

Chemistry and Stability

■ **Chemistry** Heparin is an anionic, sulfated glycosaminoglycan present in mast cells. Heparin is a heterogeneous molecule with an average molecular weight of about 12,000. Heparin is commercially available as the sodium salt. Heparin sodium is prepared from either porcine intestinal mucosa or bovine lung tissue.

In most countries, potency of heparin is determined using a World Health Organization (WHO) reference standard and is expressed in international units. In the US, the potency of heparin previously was standardized according to a USP reference standard that was expressed in USP Heparin Units and required a potency of not less than 140 units/mg of heparin. On October 1, 2009, USP implemented a new reference standard for heparin to ensure the purity, consistency, and safety of heparin-containing products in the US supply chain. This new compendial standard was developed largely in response to a heparin contamination problem that occurred in 2007–2008. Included in the updated standard is a new potency test method (chromogenic anti-Factor IIa test) that can detect impurities in heparin preparations and a new potency reference standard that will harmonize the USP Heparin Unit with the WHO international unit. As a result of these changes, heparin produced under the new USP standard is approximately 10% less potent, unit for unit, than heparin prepared under the previous USP standard. (See Dosage and Administration: Dosage.) A revised potency limit of not less than 180 Heparin Units per mg also has been established by USP.

Heparin sodium (the calcium salt of heparin is no longer commercially available in the US) occurs as a white or pale-colored, amorphous, hygroscopic powder that may have a faint odor and is soluble in water and practically insoluble in alcohol. Heparin sodium injection is a clear, colorless to slightly yellow solution with a pH of 5–8; sodium hydroxide and/or hydrochloric acid may have been added to adjust the pH. Heparin lock flush solution is a sterile isotonic or hyperosmotic solution of heparin sodium injection adjusted to a pH of 5–7.5 with sodium hydroxide and/or hydrochloric acid. Some commercially available heparin sodium injections or flush solutions have been made isotonic by the addition of sodium chloride and may contain benzyl alcohol or methylparaben and propylparaben as preservatives.

Commercially available solutions of heparin sodium in 0.45% sodium chloride, 0.9% sodium chloride, or 5% dextrose injection have osmolalities of 155, 378, or 287 mOsm/L, respectively.

■ **Stability** Most commercially available heparin sodium injections and lock flush solutions should be stored at a temperature of 20–25°C. Commercially available injections of heparin sodium in 5% dextrose or in 0.45 or 0.9% sodium chloride should be stored at 20–25°C and protected from freezing.

Commercially available premixed IV solutions with heparin sodium injection are provided in containers fabricated from specially formulated PVC. Water can permeate from inside the containers into the overwrap, but not in amounts sufficient to substantially affect the solution. Solutions in contact with the plastics can leach out some of their chemical components in very small amounts within the expiration period of the injection; however, safety of the plastics has been confirmed in animals according to USP biological tests for plastic containers.

Heparin is strongly acidic and reacts with certain basic compounds resulting in a loss of pharmacologic activity. Although results of some compatibility studies are conflicting, heparin has been reported to be stable for 24 hours at room temperature in lactated Ringer's injection. Heparin should not be mixed with ciprofloxacin, doxorubicin, droperidol, or mitoxantrone since a precipitate may be formed. Heparin is potentially physically and/or chemically incompatible with other drugs, but the compatibility depends on several factors (e.g., concentration of the drugs, specific diluents used, resulting pH, temperature). Specialized references should be consulted for specific information on the stability and compatibility of heparin.

Preparations

Effective May 1, 2013, a new USP labeling standard for Heparin Sodium Injection, USP and Heparin Lock Flush Solutions, USP was implemented. The labels for these products now state the strength of the entire container (amount of heparin per total volume of container), followed in close proximity by the strength per mL in parentheses.

Excipients in commercially available drug preparations may have clinically important effects in some individuals; consult specific product labeling for details.

Heparin Sodium

Parenteral		
Injection (porcine intestinal mucosa)	1000 units/mL*	**Heparin Sodium Injection**
	5000 units/mL*	**Heparin Sodium Injection**
	10,000 units/mL*	**Heparin Sodium Injection**
	20,000 units/mL*	**Heparin Sodium Injection**
Solution, lock flush (porcine intestinal mucosa)	10 units/mL (10, 20, 30, 50, 100, 300 units)*	**Heparin Lock Flush Solution**
	100 units/mL (100, 200, 300, 500, 1000, 3000 units)*	**Heparin Lock Flush Solution**

*available from one or more manufacturer, distributor, and/or repackager by generic (nonproprietary) name

Heparin Sodium (Preservative-free)

Parenteral		
Injection (porcine intestinal mucosa)	1000 units/mL*	**Heparin Sodium Injection,** Pfizer
	10,000 units/mL*	**Heparin Sodium Injection**
Solution, lock flush (porcine intestinal mucosa)	10 units/mL (10, 30, 50, or 100 units)*	**HepFlush®-10,** APP Pharmaceuticals
		Heparin Lock Flush Solution
	100 units/mL (100, 300 or 500 units)*	**Heparin Lock Flush Solution**

*available from one or more manufacturer, distributor, and/or repackager by generic (nonproprietary) name

Heparin Sodium in Dextrose

Parenteral		
Injection, for IV infusion (porcine intestinal mucosa)	40 units/mL (20,000 units) Heparin Sodium in 5% Dextrose*	**Heparin Sodium 20,000 units in 5% Dextrose Injection**
	50 units/mL (12,500 units) Heparin Sodium in 5% Dextrose*	**Heparin Sodium 12,500 units in 5% Dextrose Injection**
	50 units/mL (25,000 units) Heparin Sodium in 5% Dextrose*	**Heparin Sodium 25,000 units in 5% Dextrose Injection**
	100 units/mL (10,000 units) Heparin Sodium in 5% Dextrose*	**Heparin Sodium 10,000 units in 5% Dextrose Injection**
	100 units/mL (25,000 units) Heparin Sodium in 5% Dextrose*	**Heparin Sodium 25,000 units in 5% Dextrose Injection**

*available from one or more manufacturer, distributor, and/or repackager by generic (nonproprietary) name

Heparin Sodium in Sodium Chloride

Parenteral		
Injection, for IV infusion (porcine intestinal mucosa)	2 units/mL (1000 units) Heparin Sodium in 0.9% Sodium Chloride*	**Heparin Sodium 1000 units in 0.9% Sodium Chloride Injection**
	2 units/mL (2000 units) Heparin Sodium in 0.9% Sodium Chloride*	**Heparin Sodium 2000 units in 0.9% Sodium Chloride Injection**
	50 units/mL (12,500 units) Heparin Sodium in 0.45% Sodium Chloride*	**Heparin Sodium 12,500 units in 0.45% Sodium Chloride Injection**
	50 units/mL (25,000 units) Heparin Sodium in 0.45% Sodium Chloride*	**Heparin Sodium 25,000 units in 0.45% Sodium Chloride Injection**
	100 units/mL (25,000 units) Heparin Sodium in 0.45% Sodium Chloride*	**Heparin Sodium 25,000 units in 0.45% Sodium Chloride Injection**

*available from one or more manufacturer, distributor, and/or repackager by generic (nonproprietary) name

†Use is not currently included in the labeling approved by the US Food and Drug Administration

ANTICOAGULANTS, MISCELLANEOUS 20:12.04.92

Fondaparinux Sodium

Fondaparin Sodium

■ Fondaparinux sodium, a synthetic activated factor X (Xa) inhibitor, is an anticoagulant.

Uses

■ **Venous Thrombosis and Pulmonary Embolism** ***Prophylaxis***

Hip- Fracture, Hip-Replacement, or Knee-Replacement Surgery. Fondaparinux sodium is used for the prevention of postoperative deep-vein thrombosis (DVT), which may lead to pulmonary embolism (PE), in patients undergoing hip-fracture, hip-replacement, or knee-replacement surgery. The American College of Chest Physicians (ACCP) recommends routine thromboprophylaxis (with a pharmacologic and/or mechanical [e.g., intermittent pneumatic compression] method) in all patients undergoing major orthopedic surgery, including total hip-replacement, total knee-replacement, and hip-fracture surgery, because of the high risk for postoperative venous thromboembolism; thromboprophylaxis should be continued for at least 10–14 days, and possibly for up to 35 days after surgery. Several antithrombotic agents (e.g., low molecular weight heparins, fondaparinux, low-dose heparin ["heparin" referring throughout this monograph to unfractionated heparin], warfarin, aspirin) are recommended by ACCP for pharmacologic thromboprophylaxis in patients undergoing major orthopedic surgery. Among the different options, ACCP suggests that a low molecular weight heparin generally is preferred because of its relative efficacy and safety and extensive clinical experience; alternative agents (e.g., fondaparinux) may be considered in situations in which a low molecular weight heparin is not available or cannot be used (e.g., in patients with heparin-induced thrombocytopenia). ACCP states that when selecting an appropriate thromboprophylaxis regimen, factors such as relative efficacy and bleeding risk as well as logistics and compliance issues should be considered. For additional details on the prevention of venous thromboembolism in patients undergoing major orthopedic surgery, consult the most recent ACCP Evidence-based Clinical Practice Guidelines on Antithrombotic Therapy and Prevention of Thrombosis available at http://www.chestnet.org.

Results of several randomized, double-blind, multicenter studies in patients undergoing hip-fracture, hip-replacement, or knee-replacement surgery indicate that subcutaneous fondaparinux sodium (2.5 mg once daily, usually initiated about 6 hours after surgery and continued for about 7 days) is more effective than subcutaneous enoxaparin (40 mg once daily given 12 hours prior to surgery and continued for about 7 days, or 30 mg every 12 hours given 12 hours prior to surgery or 12–24 hours after surgery and continued for about 7 days) in preventing venous thromboembolism in the short term (up to postoperative day 11). Pooled analysis of data from these studies indicate that the cumulative incidence of venous thromboembolism (i.e., venographically determined asymptomatic or symptomatic DVT and/or documented symptomatic PE) up to day 11 of therapy (the primary end point) was lower with fondaparinux than with enoxaparin therapy (overall relative risk reduction exceeding 50%). Asymptomatic DVT comprised most of the reduction in venous thromboembolic events observed with fondaparinux. Patients with such events usually received anticoagulant therapy at therapeutic dosages, thus reducing the development of subsequent symptoms. In these studies, approximately 19–20% of patients undergoing knee-replacement surgery, 25–28 and 52% of those undergoing hip-replacement surgery, and 56–59% of those undergoing hip-fracture surgery received prolonged anticoagulant prophylaxis (principally with a heparin preparation or oral anticoagulant according to the clinician's discretion) during the follow-up period (after treatment with one of the study drugs), and the incidence of symptomatic venous thromboembolism (a secondary end point) was similar in both treatment groups by day 49 of follow-up. Differences in efficacy and safety between fondaparinux and enoxaparin in clinical studies may have been influenced by differences in the drugs' selectivity of factor Xa inhibition, onset and duration of anticoagulant effect, dosage, and time of initiation of prophylaxis after surgery. In patients undergoing knee-replacement surgery, the incidence of major bleeding complications (see Hematologic Effects under Warnings/Precautions: Warnings, in Cautions) was substantially greater with fondaparinux (2.1%) than with enoxaparin therapy (0.2%).

In a dose-ranging study in patients undergoing hip-replacement surgery, the efficacy of fondaparinux was dose-dependent as indicated by rates of venous thromboembolism of 11.8, 6.7, 1.7, 4.4, or 0% (intent-to-treat analysis) with subcutaneous fondaparinux sodium dosages of 0.75, 1.5, 3, 6, or 8 mg daily, respectively. In this study, fondaparinux sodium dosages of 1.5 or 3 mg resulted in lower rates of venous thromboembolism (6.7 or 1.7%, respectively) than enoxaparin at a dosage of 30 mg every 12 hours (9.4%), while the incidence of major bleeding in patients receiving 1.5 or 3 mg of fondaparinux sodium was lower than or similar to that, respectively, in patients receiving enoxaparin.

Fondaparinux also is used for extended prophylaxis (for up to 35 days postoperatively) in patients undergoing hip-fracture surgery. In a randomized, double-blind study in patients who had undergone hip-fracture surgery and had received short-term prophylaxis with fondaparinux sodium (2.5 mg once daily for 6–8 days perioperatively), extended prophylaxis with the drug (2.5 mg once daily for an additional 19–23 days) decreased the incidence of venous thromboembolism (defined as DVT, PE, or both) by about 96% compared with placebo. DVT occurred in 1.4% of patients receiving extended therapy with fondaparinux compared with 33.9% of patients receiving placebo; PE occurred in 3 patients receiving placebo but in none of those receiving fondaparinux. Major bleeding occurred in 2.4% of fondaparinux-treated patients compared with 0.6% of those receiving placebo. In general, extended thromboprophylaxis is suggested by ACCP for all patients undergoing major orthopedic surgery.

General Surgery. Fondaparinux also is used for the prevention of postoperative venous thromboembolism in patients undergoing general (e.g., abdominal) surgery who are at risk for thromboembolic complications. ACCP recommends pharmacologic and/or nonpharmacologic/mechanical (e.g., intermittent pneumatic compression) methods of thromboprophylaxis in patients undergoing general surgery, including abdominal, GI, gynecologic, and urologic surgery, according to the patient's level of risk for thromboembolism and bleeding. In general, pharmacologic prophylaxis is recommended in patients with high (and possibly moderate) risk of venous thromboembolism who do not have a high risk of bleeding, while mechanical methods are suggested in patients who require thromboprophylaxis but have a high risk of bleeding. If pharmacologic prophylaxis is used in patients undergoing general surgery, ACCP states that a low molecular weight heparin or low-dose heparin is preferred, but when these agents are contraindicated or not available, aspirin or fondaparinux may be considered. ACCP states that the same recommendations for the use of antithrombotic agents in general surgery patients can be applied to patients undergoing bariatric surgery, vascular surgery, and plastic and reconstructive surgery. For additional information on the prevention of venous thromboembolism in patients undergoing general surgery, consult the most recent ACCP Evidence-based Clinical Practice Guidelines on Antithrombotic Therapy and Prevention of Thrombosis available at http://www.chestnet.org.

In a double-blind, comparative study evaluating fondaparinux (2.5 mg subcutaneously once daily starting postoperatively) and dalteparin (5000 units subcutaneously once daily postoperatively, with an initial 2500-unit dose preoperatively and postoperatively) for 7 days in patients at risk for thromboembolic complications undergoing abdominal surgery, the incidence of thromboembolic events (i.e., venogram-positive DVT, symptomatic DVT, and/or PE) was similar in patients treated with dalteparin (6.1%) or fondaparinux (4.6%).

Medical Conditions Associated with Thromboembolism. ACCP recommends the use of fondaparinux as an option for pharmacologic thromboprophylaxis in acutely ill, hospitalized medical patients at increased risk of thrombosis. Treatment decisions regarding the use of prophylactic anticoagulants in acutely ill hospitalized patients should include an assessment of the patient's individual risk of venous thromboembolism and risk of bleeding. In general, pharmacologic thromboprophylaxis is recommended only in patients who are considered to be at high risk of venous thromboembolism because the risk-to-benefit tradeoff between the reduction in venous thromboembolic events and bleeding is considered to be more favorable in such patients. Factors that should be considered when choosing an appropriate anticoagulant include patient preference, compliance, ease of administration, and costs associated with the individual agents.

Treatment **Deep-Vein Thrombosis and Pulmonary Embolism.** Fondaparinux is used in conjunction with warfarin for the treatment of DVT and for the treatment of acute PE when initial therapy is administered in the hospital. Warfarin should be initiated as soon as possible (e.g., on the first day that fondaparinux is administered) and such therapy should be overlapped for at least 5 days and until the international normalized ratio (INR) is at least 2 for 24 hours or longer. Fondaparinux is recommended by ACCP as an appropriate choice of anticoagulant for the initial treatment of acute proximal DVT or PE; other options include IV or subcutaneous heparin or a low molecular weight heparin. Among the different anticoagulant options, fondaparinux or a low molecular weight heparin generally is preferred to heparin because of more convenient administration and less risk of heparin-induced thrombocytopenia. Fondaparinux is considered to be comparable to low molecular weight heparins; therefore, the choice between these agents should be dictated by local considerations such as cost, availability, and familiarity of use. Heparin may be preferred in patients with renal impairment. In addition, ACCP states that use of IV heparin is preferred in patients with pulmonary embolism in whom thrombolytic therapy is being considered or if there is a concern about the adequacy of subcutaneous absorption. For additional information on treatment of venous thromboembolism, consult the most recent ACCP Evidence-based Clinical Practice Guidelines on Antithrombotic Therapy and Prevention of Thrombosis available at http://www.chestnet.org.

In a randomized, double-blind study in patients with acute lower extremity DVT without PE, treatment with fondaparinux sodium (5, 7.5, or 10 mg once daily subcutaneously based on patient weight) or enoxaparin sodium (1 mg/kg every 12 hours subcutaneously) for an average of approximately 7 days (until the INR exceeded 2 with vitamin K antagonist therapy, or a minimum of 5 days) demonstrated similar efficacy in the prevention of recurrent thromboembolic events (i.e., recurrent DVT, nonfatal or fatal PE) during the 3-month study period. Recurrent thromboembolism occurred in 3.9% of patients receiving fondaparinux compared with 4.1% of those receiving enoxaparin; major bleeding occurred in 1.1 or 1.2%, respectively, of these patients. Approximately one-third of patients received some or all of their treatment out of the hospital (i.e., at home).

In a randomized, open-label study in patients with acute symptomatic PE, treatment with fondaparinux sodium (5, 7.5, or 10 mg once daily subcutaneously based on patient weight) or heparin sodium (5000 units by direct IV injection followed by a continuous IV infusion to maintain an aPTT of 1.5–2.5 times the control value) for an average of approximately 6.5–7 days (until the INR exceeded 2 with vitamin K antagonist therapy, or a minimum of 5 days) demonstrated similar efficacy in the prevention of recurrent thromboembolic events (i.e., new or recurrent DVT, nonfatal or fatal PE) during the 3-month study period. Recurrent thromboembolism occurred in 3.8% of patients receiving fondaparinux compared with 5% of those receiving heparin; major bleeding occurred in 1.3 or 1.1%, respectively, of these patients. About 14.5% of fondaparinux-treated patients were discharged early from the hospital and continued to receive treatment as outpatients; the rate of recurrent thromboembolism was low (3.2%) in these patients and no major bleeding episodes occurred.

Superficial Thrombophlebitis. Fondaparinux also has been used for the treatment of superficial vein thrombosis (or thrombophlebitis)†. ACCP suggests the use of prophylactic dosages of fondaparinux sodium (2.5 mg daily for 45 days) or a low molecular weight heparin for 45 days in patients with superficial vein thrombosis of at least 5 cm in length, with fondaparinux being the preferred agent.

■ **ST-Segment-Elevation Myocardial Infarction** Fondaparinux has been used as an adjunct to thrombolysis in patients with acute ST-segment-elevation myocardial infarction (STEMI)†. The current standard of care in patients with STEMI is timely reperfusion (with primary percutaneous coronary intervention [PCI] or thrombolytic therapy). Adjunctive therapy with anticoagulant (e.g., heparin) and antiplatelet (e.g., aspirin and clopidogrel) agents should be used during and after successful coronary artery reperfusion for the prevention of early reocclusion and death, unless contraindicated. The American College of Cardiology Foundation (ACCF) and American Heart Association (AHA) state that patients with STEMI undergoing thrombolytic therapy should receive an anticoagulant (e.g., heparin, enoxaparin, fondaparinux) for a minimum of 48 hours, and preferably for the duration of the index hospitalization, up to 8 days or until revascularization is performed.

Fondaparinux should not be used as the sole anticoagulant to support PCI because of the risk of catheter thrombosis; an additional anticoagulant with anti-factor IIa (antithrombin) activity should be administered during the procedure.

■ **Non-ST-Segment-Elevation Acute Coronary Syndromes** Fondaparinux has been used as an alternative to heparin or a low molecular weight heparin in the management of non-ST-segment-elevation acute coronary syndromes (NSTE ACS)† in patients being managed conservatively or with invasive procedures (e.g., PCI, coronary artery bypass grafting [CABG], coronary artery stent implantation).

Patients with NSTE ACS have either unstable angina or NSTEMI; because these conditions are part of a continuum of acute myocardial ischemia and have indistinguishable clinical features upon presentation, the same initial treatment strategies are recommended. The American Heart Association/American College of Cardiology (AHA/ACC) guideline for the management of patients with NSTE ACS recommends an early invasive strategy (angiographic evaluation with the intent to perform revascularization procedures such as PCI with coronary artery stent implantation or CABG) or an ischemia-guided strategy (initial medical management followed by cardiac catheterization and revascularization if indicated) in patients with definite or likely NSTE ACS; standard medical therapies for all patients should include a β-adrenergic blocking agent (β-blocker), antiplatelet agents, anticoagulant agents, nitrates, and analgesic agents regardless of the initial management approach.

All patients with NSTE ACS should receive immediate antiplatelet therapy (e.g., aspirin, clopidogrel). An anticoagulant agent should be added to antiplatelet therapy as soon as possible after hospital admission. Initial parenteral anticoagulants with established efficacy in patients with NSTE ACS include enoxaparin, heparin, bivalirudin (only in patients who are being managed with an early invasive strategy), and fondaparinux. Fondaparinux is preferred over heparin therapy in patients with an increased risk of bleeding. If PCI is performed while a patient is receiving fondaparinux, an additional anticoagulant with anti-factor IIa (antithrombin) activity should be administered because of the risk of catheter thrombosis.

■ **Percutaneous Coronary Intervention** Use of a parenteral anticoagulant is recommended in patients undergoing PCI† to prevent thrombus formation at the site of arterial injury, the coronary guidewire, and in the catheters used for the procedure. Although fondaparinux has been used for anticoagulation during PCI, the drug should not be used as the sole anticoagulant during the procedure. An increased risk of catheter-related thrombosis has been observed in patients receiving fondaparinux alone during primary PCI; therefore, additional use of an anticoagulant possessing anti-factor IIa (antithrombin) activity is recommended. To date, the only anticoagulant that has been administered during PCI in patients receiving fondaparinux initially for the treatment of NSTE ACS has been heparin; however, experts state that the safety of this practice has not been fully established. There is some evidence suggesting that clinical outcomes may be improved when fondaparinux is replaced during PCI with standard dosages of heparin.

■ **Thrombosis Associated with Heparin-induced Thrombocytopenia** Fondaparinux has been used for the treatment of heparin-induced thrombocytopenia† (HIT) and heparin-induced thrombocytopenia and thrombosis syndrome† (HITTS). ACCP recommends the use of a nonheparin anticoagulant as an alternative to heparin in patients with HIT with or without thrombosis. Although limited data suggest that fondaparinux may be effective in the management of HIT or HITTS, ACCP recommends the use of other direct thrombin inhibitors such as lepirudin and argatroban because of more extensive data and a higher quality of evidence.

In patients with a previous history of HIT† who require treatment for acute thrombosis that is not related to HIT, ACCP suggests the use of fondaparinux at full treatment dosages until transition to warfarin can be achieved. Compared with heparin or low molecular weight heparins, fondaparinux may be less likely to exacerbate HIT in patients with preexisting platelet-activating antibodies.

Dosage and Administration

■ **Administration** Fondaparinux sodium is administered by subcutaneous injection; *it must not be given IM*. Fondaparinux also has been administered by direct IV injection† initially in the treatment of acute ST-segment-elevation myocardial infarction (STEMI)†. For ease of administration, patients should be sitting or supine during administration of the drug. Administration should be made into fatty tissue, alternating injection sites (e.g., between left and right anterolateral or posterolateral abdominal wall) daily. Insert the entire length of the needle into a skin fold created by the thumb and forefinger, hold the skin fold, and push the plunger of the syringe the full length of the syringe barrel. Once the plunger is released, the needle automatically withdraws from the skin and retracts into the security sleeve. Fondaparinux injection should not be mixed with other injections or infusions.

■ **Dosage** *Dosages for fondaparinux sodium, heparin, heparinoids, and low molecular weight heparins cannot be used interchangeably on a unit-for-unit (or mg-for-mg) basis, as they differ in manufacturing process, anti-factor Xa and antithrombin activity, and dosage.*

Dosage of fondaparinux sodium is expressed in terms of the salt.

The possibility of an underlying bleeding disorder should be ruled out before initiating fondaparinux therapy. Since global clotting function tests such as prothrombin time (PT) or activated partial thromboplastin time (aPTT) are relatively insensitive measures of fondaparinux sodium activity, routine monitoring of such parameters is not required.

Venous Thrombosis and Pulmonary Embolism **Prevention.** For prevention of postoperative deep-vein thrombosis (DVT) and pulmonary embolism (PE) in *adults weighing 50 kg or more* (see Cautions: Contraindications) who have undergone hip-fracture, hip-replacement, or knee-replacement, or abdominal surgery, the usual recommended dosage of fondaparinux sodium is 2.5 mg once daily by subcutaneous injection. The manufacturer recommends that the initial dose be given no earlier than 6–8 hours after surgery, provided hemostasis has been established; the American College of Chest Physicians (ACCP) states that the initial dose may be given either 6–8 hours after surgery or the next day following major orthopedic procedures. Administration of fondaparinux earlier than 6 hours after surgery has been associated with an increased risk of major bleeding. Fondaparinux should be administered throughout the postoperative period, generally for 5–9 days, until the risk of DVT has diminished. Extended thromboprophylaxis for up to 35 days is recommended in patients undergoing hip-fracture surgery, and suggested for patients undergoing other major orthopedic procedures.

Treatment. For the treatment of acute symptomatic DVT or PE, the usual dosage of fondaparinux sodium given by subcutaneous injection is 5 mg once daily in patients with low body weight (less than 50 kg), 7.5 mg once daily in patients with a body weight of 50–100 kg, or 10 mg once daily in patients with a body weight of greater than 100 kg. Warfarin therapy generally is given in conjunction with fondaparinux therapy, and therapy with the 2 drugs is overlapped until an adequate response to warfarin is obtained as indicated by prothrombin time (PT) determinations to achieve an international normalized ratio (INR) of 2–3 for at least 24 hours. The manufacturer states that concurrent administration of warfarin should be initiated as soon as possible (usually with 72 hours of initiation of fondaparinux therapy); ACCP recommends that warfarin be initiated on the first day of treatment with fondaparinux in patients with acute DVT or PE. The usual duration of therapy with fondaparinux is 5–9 days; up to 26 days of fondaparinux has been administered.

ST-Segment-Elevation Myocardial Infarction When used in the management of acute STEMI†, the initial dose of fondaparinux (2.5 mg) is given by direct IV injection, followed by 2.5 mg subcutaneously given once daily for the duration of hospitalization or up to 8 days or until revascularization.

Non-ST-Segment-Elevation Acute Coronary Syndromes Fondaparinux sodium has been administered in a dosage of 2.5 mg subcutaneously once daily in patients with non-ST-segment-elevation acute coronary syndromes (NSTE ACS)†. Although the optimum duration of therapy has not been established, fondaparinux generally is continued for the duration of hospitalization (up to 8 days) in patients managed medically. If the patient is to undergo coronary artery bypass grafting (CABG), fondaparinux should be discontinued 24 hours prior to such surgery. (See Percutaneous Coronary Intervention under Dosage and Administration: Dosage.)

Percutaneous Coronary Intervention In patients receiving fondaparinux prior to percutaneous coronary intervention (PCI), additional treatment with an IV anticoagulant possessing anti-factor IIa (antithrombin) activity should be administered during PCI; when managing these patients, clinicians should consider whether platelet glycoprotein (GP) IIb/IIIa-receptor inhibitor therapy has been administered.

■ **Special Populations** ***Hepatic Impairment*** The manufacturer states that no dosage adjustment is required in patients with mild to moderate hepatic impairment; the pharmacokinetics of fondaparinux have not been studied in patients with severe hepatic impairment. Because patients with hepatic impairment may be at increased risk of hemorrhage, such patients should be monitored closely for signs and symptoms of bleeding during fondaparinux therapy.

Renal Impairment Fondaparinux is contraindicated in patients with severe renal impairment (creatinine clearance less than 30 mL/minute) since the drug is eliminated principally by the kidney and such patients are at increased risk for major bleeding episodes. The manufacturer currently makes no specific recommendations for dosage modifications in patients with other degrees of renal impairment, although caution should be exercised.

Low Body Weight Fondaparinux sodium should be used with caution and at a low dosage (5 mg once daily) for the treatment of DVT or PE in patients with low body weight (less than 50 kg). Use of fondaparinux is contraindicated in patients with low body weight (less than 50 kg) undergoing hip-fracture, hip-replacement, knee-replacement, or abdominal surgery since therapy in such patients was associated with an increased incidence of major bleeding.

Cautions

■ **Contraindications** Fondaparinux is contraindicated in patients with severe renal impairment (creatinine clearance less than 30 mL/minute). The drug also is contraindicated in patients undergoing hip-fracture, hip-replacement, knee-replacement, or abdominal surgery who weigh less than 50 kg because of the increased risk of major bleeding in such patients. Known hypersensitivity to fondaparinux sodium; history of serious hypersensitivity reactions such as angioedema and anaphylactoid/anaphylactic reactions; active major bleeding, bacterial endocarditis, or thrombocytopenia associated with a positive in vitro test for antiplatelet antibody (heparin-induced thrombocytopenia [HIT]) in the presence of the drug) also are contraindications to use of the drug.

The manufacturer states that the usual precautions and contraindications associated with anticoagulant therapy should be followed in patients for whom fondaparinux therapy is considered.

■ **Warnings/Precautions** ***Warnings*** **Spinal/Epidural Hematoma.** Concurrent use of a low molecular weight heparin, heparinoid (e.g., danaparoid [no longer commercially available in the US]), or fondaparinux with neuraxial (epidural/spinal) anesthesia or spinal puncture procedures has been associated with epidural or spinal hematomas. Hematomas occurring in such patients have been associated with neurologic injury, including long-term or permanent paralysis. The risk of these adverse events is increased by use of indwelling epidural catheters for administration of analgesia or by concomitant use of drugs affecting hemostasis, such as nonsteroidal anti-inflammatory agents (NSAIAs), platelet-aggregation inhibitors, or other anticoagulants. The risk also appears to be increased by a history of traumatic or repeated epidural or spinal puncture, spinal surgery, or spinal deformity. The optimal timing between the administration of fondaparinux and neuraxial procedures is not known.

Patients should be monitored frequently for manifestations of neurologic impairment (e.g, midline back pain; numbness, tingling, or weakness in the lower limbs; bowel or bladder dysfunction). If neurologic compromise is noted, urgent treatment is necessary. Clinicians should fully consider potential benefits versus risks of spinal or epidural anesthesia or spinal puncture in patients who are currently receiving or will receive fondaparinux; some experts suggest that anticoagulant prophylaxis with fondaparinux be avoided in patients receiving epidural analgesia.

Hematologic Effects. Like other anticoagulants, fondaparinux should be used with extreme caution in patients with an increased risk of hemorrhage (e.g., congenital or acquired bleeding disorders; active ulceration and angiodysplastic GI disease; hemorrhagic stroke; uncontrolled arterial hypertension; diabetic retinopathy; recent brain, spinal, or ophthalmic surgery). Recommended regimens for administration of fondaparinux should be adhered to, particularly with respect to timing of the first dose after surgery; in clinical studies of hip-fracture, hip-replacement, knee-replacement, or abdominal surgery, administration of fondaparinux earlier than 6 hours following surgery was associated with an increased risk of major bleeding episodes. Analysis of all randomized, controlled perioperative prophylaxis studies in patients undergoing hip-fracture, hip-replacement, or knee-replacement surgery indicates that most (75% or more) major bleeding episodes occurred during the first 4 days following surgery.

In randomized clinical studies evaluating use of fondaparinux for the prevention of postoperative venous thromboembolism, major bleeding occurred at a higher rate among patients with a body weight of less than 50 kg compared with those weighing 50 kg or more. Fondaparinux should not be used for prophylaxis of venous thromboembolism in patients undergoing hip-fracture, hip-replacement, knee-replacement, or abdominal surgery who weigh less than 50 kg. The drug should be used with caution in the treatment of deep-vein thrombosis (DVT) or pulmonary embolism (PE) in patients who weigh less than 50 kg.

Periodic routine blood counts, including platelet counts, and tests for occult blood in stool are recommended during fondaparinux therapy. If overdosage associated with bleeding complications occurs, discontinue fondaparinux and initiate appropriate therapy. There is no specific antidote for fondaparinux overdosage; however, some data suggest that clearance of fondaparinux may increase by 20% in patients undergoing chronic intermittent hemodialysis.

Because of the increased risk of hemorrhage, fondaparinux should not be used for prophylaxis or treatment of venous thromboembolism in patients with severe renal insufficiency (creatinine clearance less than 30 mL/minute) and should be used with caution in patients with moderate renal insufficiency (creatinine clearance 30–50 mL/minute).

Concurrent use of drugs that increase risk of bleeding should be avoided in patients receiving fondaparinux unless they are essential for management of the underlying condition (e.g., concomitant use of vitamin K antagonists for treatment of venous thromboembolism). (See Drug Interactions: Drugs Affecting Hemostasis.)

Moderate thrombocytopenia (platelet counts of 50,000–100,000/mm^3) was reported in 3% of patients receiving the recommended dosage of fondaparinux sodium in clinical studies of hip-fracture, hip-replacement, knee-replacement, or abdominal surgery, and severe thrombocytopenia (platelet counts less than 50,000/mm^3) was reported in 0.2% of such patients. Moderate thrombocytopenia was reported in 0.5% of patients receiving fondaparinux for the treatment of DVT or PE in clinical studies, and severe thrombocytopenia was reported in 0.04% of such patients. The manufacturer recommends that thrombocytopenia of any degree be monitored closely and that fondaparinux be discontinued if platelet counts fall below 100,000/mm^3. Fondaparinux does not interact with platelet factor 4 or platelets, and some clinicians state that the drug is unlikely to cause HIT; however, isolated cases of thrombocytopenia with thrombosis resembling HIT have been reported during postmarketing experience. Although a direct causal relationship to fondaparinux has not been established, the manufacturer states that fondaparinux should be used with caution in patients with a history of HIT.

Patients with Prosthetic Heart Valves. Cases of valve thrombosis resulting in death and/or requiring surgical intervention have been reported with at least one low molecular weight heparin (enoxaparin) during thromboprophylaxis in some patients with prosthetic heart valves; some of these cases included pregnant women, and maternal and/or fetal deaths have been reported. (See Uses: Thromboembolism Associated with Prosthetic Heart Valves, in Enoxaparin 20:12.04.16.) The manufacturer of fondaparinux states that the drug has not been studied in patients with prosthetic heart valves and that no information is available on the safety of fondaparinux in such patients.

Sensitivity Reactions Serious hypersensitivity reactions, including angioedema and anaphylactoid/anaphylactic reactions, have been reported during postmarketing experience in patients receiving fondaparinux. (See Contraindications.)

Latex Sensitivity. Some packaging components (e.g., needle covers) of fondaparinux contain natural latex proteins in the form of dry natural rubber (latex). Some individuals may be hypersensitive to natural latex proteins found in a wide range of medical devices, including such packaging components, and the level of sensitivity may vary depending on the form of natural rubber present; rarely, hypersensitivity reactions to natural latex proteins have been fatal. The needle cover of the diluent syringe provided with fondaparinux contains dry natural rubber (latex), and should not be handled by individuals sensitive to latex.

Specific Populations **Pregnancy.** Category B. (See Users Guide.)

Lactation. Fondaparinux is distributed into milk in rats. The manufacturer states that caution is advised if the drug is used in nursing women. The American College of Chest Physicians (ACCP) suggests the use of anticoagulants other than fondaparinux in nursing women.

Pediatric Use. Safety and efficacy not established in children younger than 17 years of age.

Geriatric Use. Use with caution in geriatric patients older than 75 years of age. No substantial differences in efficacy relative to younger adults; however, major bleeding or other serious adverse effects occurred more frequently in patients 75 years of age or older than in younger adults. Fondaparinux is substantially eliminated by the kidneys. Because geriatric patients may have decreased renal function, monitoring renal function in such patients may be useful. Careful attention to fondaparinux sodium dosage and cautious use of concomitant therapy (particularly platelet-aggregation inhibitors) is advised.

Hepatic Impairment. Following a single 7.5-mg dose in patients with moderate hepatic impairment, changes in baseline activated partial thromboplastin time (aPTT), prothrombin time (PT), international normalized ratio (INR), and antithrombin III were similar to those in patients with normal hepatic function; however, risk of hemorrhage (e.g., mild hematomas at blood sampling or injection site) was increased in patients with moderate hepatic impairment. The effects of severe hepatic impairment on the pharmacokinetics of fondaparinux have not been evaluated.

Renal Impairment. Anticoagulant effects of fondaparinux may persist (e.g., for longer than 2–4 days) after drug discontinuance in patients with renal impairment, and risk of hemorrhage is increased with fondaparinux therapy in such patients. Use with caution in those with moderate renal impairment (creatinine clearance 30–50 mL/minute); contraindicated in patients with severe renal impairment (creatinine clearance less than 30 mL/minute). Renal function should be assessed periodically (e.g., serum creatinine determinations) in patients receiving fondaparinux therapy and the drug discontinued immediately in patients who develop severe renal impairment during therapy.

■ **Common Adverse Effects** Hip-fracture, hip-replacement, or knee-replacement surgery: Adverse effects occurring in at least 2% of patients in clinical trials included anemia, fever, nausea, edema, constipation, rash, vomiting, insomnia, increased wound drainage, hypokalemia, urinary tract infection, dizziness, purpura, hypotension, confusion, bullous eruption, urinary retention, hematoma, major bleeding, diarrhea, dyspepsia, postoperative hemorrhage, and headache.

Treatment of DVT or PE: Adverse effects occurring in at least 2% of patients in clinical trials included constipation, headache, insomnia, fever, nausea, urinary tract infection, and coughing.

Abdominal surgery: Adverse effects occurring in at least 2% of patients in clinical trials included post-operative wound infection, postoperative hemorrhage, fever, surgical site reaction, anemia, hypertension, pneumonia, and vomiting.

Drug Interactions

■ **Drugs Affecting Hemostasis** Potential pharmacodynamic interaction (increased risk of bleeding) when fondaparinux is used with drugs affecting hemostasis, such as oral anticoagulants (e.g., warfarin) or platelet-aggregation inhibitors (e.g., salicylates, nonsteroidal anti-inflammatory agents [NSAIAs]). In clinical studies, concomitant administration of warfarin, aspirin, and piroxicam did not substantially affect the pharmacokinetics and pharmacodynamics of fondaparinux. In addition, no clinically important effect of fondaparinux on the pharmacodynamics of warfarin, aspirin, or piroxicam was detected. The manufacturer recommends that drugs affecting hemostasis (i.e., oral anticoagulants such as warfarin and/or drugs that affect platelet function, including aspirin, salicylate salts, and other NSAIAs) be discontinued prior to initiating fondaparinux therapy since concomitant use of fondaparinux and these agents may increase the risk of hemorrhage. If concomitant use of fondaparinux and drugs that affect hemostasis is considered essential, careful clinical and laboratory monitoring (e.g., for signs and symptoms of bleeding) is advised.

■ **Digoxin** Pharmacokinetic/pharmacodynamic interaction unlikely.

■ **Drugs Metabolized by Hepatic Microsomal Enzymes** Pharmacokinetic interaction unlikely. Weak inhibitor of cytochrome P-450 isoenzymes 2A6, 1A2, 2C9, 2C19, 2D6, 3A4, and 3E1 in vitro.

■ **Protein-bound Drugs** Pharmacokinetic interaction unlikely.

Description

Fondaparinux sodium, a synthetic activated factor X (Xa) inhibitor, is an anticoagulant. Fondaparinux, a pentasaccharide, is a synthetic analog of the minimal binding sequence on antithrombin III (heparin cofactor) that is required for anticoagulant activity. Fondaparinux is commercially available as the decasodium salt.

Antithrombin III generally neutralizes coagulation factor Xa, thrombin, and other coagulation factors, but these reactions are slow in the absence of heparin or fondaparinux. Fondaparinux accelerates the rate at which antithrombin neutralizes factor Xa by inducing a conformational change in antithrombin. This conformational change increases the affinity of antithrombin III for factor Xa, a key enzyme in the coagulation cascade. With fondaparinux therapy, anticoagulation appears to result from rapid inhibition of factor Xa by antithrombin III (about 300-fold greater than innate activity), which inhibits the conversion of prothrombin to thrombin and subsequent thrombus formation.

Unlike heparin, which interacts with many plasma components, fondaparinux binds selectively to antithrombin III. Because of its small molecular size, fondaparinux cannot bind simultaneously to antithrombin III and thrombin and therefore is unable to inactivate thrombin itself. At the recommended dosage, fondaparinux does not affect fibrinolytic activity and cannot lyse established thrombi. Fondaparinux generally does not affect platelet function or global clotting function tests (e.g., prothrombin time [PT], bleeding time, activated partial thromboplastin time [aPTT]) when administered at the recommended dosage. Compared with heparin, fondaparinux has greater bioavailability (based on anti-factor Xa activity) after subcutaneous administration (absolute bioavailability 100%) and a longer half-life (about 17–21 hours), allowing once-daily administration. Fondaparinux is eliminated principally as unchanged drug in urine and must be used with caution in patients with moderate renal impairment and not at all in patients with severe renal impairment. (See Renal Impairment under General Precautions: Specific Populations, in Cautions.) In addition, total clearance of fondaparinux is reduced by approximately 30% in patients weighing less than 50 kg. (See Cautions: Contraindications.)

The activity of fondaparinux sodium is measured based on plasma drug concentrations quantified by anti-Factor Xa activity using fondaparinux as the calibrator. The international standards for heparin and low molecular weight heparins are not appropriate calibrators for fondaparinux sodium activity, which is expressed in mg and cannot be compared with the activities of heparin or low molecular weight heparins.

Advice to Patients

Importance of advising patients who have had neuraxial anesthesia or spinal puncture to monitor for manifestations of spinal or epidural hematoma (e.g., back pain; numbness, tingling, or weakness in lower limbs; loss of bowel or bladder control), particularly if they are receiving concomitant nonsteroidal anti-inflammatory agents (NSAIAs), platelet-aggregation inhibitors, or other anticoagulants; importance of immediately contacting a clinician if any of these symptoms occur.

Importance of informing patients that concomitant use of aspirin or other NSAIAs can increase risk of bleeding, and to discontinue use of these drugs whenever possible.

If fondaparinux therapy is to be continued after hospital discharge, importance of instructing patient on proper administration of the drug, including injection technique.

Importance of informing patients that they may bruise and/or bleed more easily and that a longer than normal time may be required to stop bleeding when taking fondaparinux. Importance of patients reporting any unusual bleeding, bruising, or signs of thrombocytopenia (e.g., dark red spots under skin) to their clinician.

Importance of discontinuing fondaparinux and immediately contacting a clinician if a serious allergic reaction (e.g., swelling of the face or mouth, difficulty swallowing or breathing) occurs while taking the drug.

Importance of patients informing clinicians (including dentists) that they are receiving fondaparinux therapy before scheduling any invasive procedures.

Importance of women informing clinicians if they are, or plan to become, pregnant or plan to breast-feed.

Importance of informing clinicians of existing or contemplated concomitant therapy, including prescription and OTC drugs.

Importance of informing patients of other important precautionary information. (See Cautions.)

Overview® (see Users Guide). For additional information on this drug until a more detailed monograph is developed and published, the manufacturer's labeling should be consulted. It is *essential* that the manufacturer's labeling be consulted for more detailed information on usual cautions, precautions, contraindications, potential drug interactions, laboratory test interferences, and acute toxicity.

Preparations

Excipients in commercially available drug preparations may have clinically important effects in some individuals; consult specific product labeling for details.

Fondaparinux Sodium

Parenteral		
Injection, for subcutaneous use	2.5 mg/0.5 mL	**Arixtra**® (available as a 0.5-mL, disposable prefilled syringe), **GlaxoSmithKline**
	5 mg/0.4 mL	**Arixtra**® (available as a 0.4-mL, disposable prefilled syringe), **GlaxoSmithKline**
	7.5 mg/0.6 mL	**Arixtra**® (available as a 0.6-mL, disposable prefilled syringe), **GlaxoSmithKline**
	10 mg/0.8 mL	**Arixtra**® (available as a 0.8-mL, disposable prefilled syringe), **GlaxoSmithKline**

†Use is not currently included in the labeling approved by the US Food and Drug Administration

PLATELET-AGGREGATION INHIBITORS 20:12.18

Abciximab

■ Abciximab, a platelet aggregation inhibitor, has been referred to as a platelet glycoprotein (GP) IIb/IIIa-receptor inhibitor.

Uses

■ **Acute Ischemic Complications of Percutaneous Coronary Intervention** Abciximab is used with anticoagulant therapy (e.g., heparin [referring throughout this monograph to unfractionated heparin], low molecular weight heparin), aspirin, and a P2Y12 platelet adenosine diphosphate (ADP)-receptor antagonist (e.g., clopidogrel, prasugrel, ticagrelor) as an adjunct to percutaneous coronary intervention (PCI) for the prevention of acute cardiac ischemic complications in patients undergoing PCI and in patients with unstable angina or non-ST-segment-elevation myocardial infarction (NSTEMI) (i.e., non-ST-segment-elevation acute coronary syndromes [NSTE ACS]) who have not responded to conventional medical therapy and who are scheduled to undergo PCI within 24 hours. Despite advances in percutaneous revascularization techniques, abrupt closure of a coronary vessel that occurs during PCI still is associated with substantial morbidity (e.g., myocardial infarction [MI]). Platelet glycoprotein (GP) IIb/IIIa-receptor inhibitors such as abciximab are used to minimize PCI-related ischemic complications and improve the risk-benefit ratio of these procedures. Studies involving abciximab or another GP IIb/IIIa-receptor inhibitor (i.e., eptifibatide) have demonstrated consistent reductions in the risk of composite ischemic events (death, MI, need for revascularization procedures) at 30 days in patients undergoing PCI.

Several meta-analyses of studies indicate that adjunctive therapy with a GP IIb/IIIa-receptor inhibitor can reduce the incidence of cardiac ischemic events, including subsequent MI and death, both in patients with NSTE ACS undergoing PCI and in patients without these conditions undergoing PCI. While benefits of GP IIb/IIIa-receptor inhibitors on mortality principally occur early during therapy (i.e., the first 48–96 hours), much of the drugs' absolute benefit on ischemia, including reductions in nonfatal MI, is maintained at 30 days and in some cases up to 6 months.

Abciximab (in conjunction with heparin regimens and aspirin) has been evaluated in a number of phase III trials in patients undergoing PCI (i.e., balloon angioplasty, atherectomy, or coronary artery stent placement). In the Evaluation of c7E3 to Prevent Ischemic Complications (EPIC) trial, patients undergoing percutaneous transluminal coronary angioplasty (PTCA) or atherectomy who were considered at high risk for abrupt closure of the treated coronary vessel were randomized to receive an abciximab IV loading dose (0.25 mg/kg), an abciximab loading dose (0.25 mg/kg) followed by IV infusion of abciximab (10 mcg/minute) for 12 hours, or placebo. Patients considered at high risk for abrupt closure of angioplasty-treated coronary blood vessels include those with NSTE ACS, those with acute ST-segment-elevation MI (STEMI) within 12 hours of the onset of symptoms, and those in whom angioplasty of an infarct-related lesion is scheduled to occur within 7 days following MI. Other patients considered at high risk for abrupt closure of angioplasty-treated coronary blood vessels are those with 2 type B (as classified by the American College of Cardiology/American Heart Association [ACC/AHA] Subcommittee on PTCA) lesion-specific characteristics in the artery to be dilated; one type B lesion characteristic in a woman 65 years of age or older or in a patient with diabetes mellitus; or one ACC/AHA-classified type C lesion characteristic in the artery to be dilated. Results from the EPIC study demonstrated a 4.5% lower incidence (8.3 versus 12.8%) of primary end-point events (i.e., death, MI, or the need for urgent intervention for recurrent ischemia) at 30 days in patients receiving abciximab loading dose plus infusion compared with patients in the placebo group. Reduction in primary end-point events with abciximab loading dose plus infusion therapy was maintained during long-term follow-up as indicated by absolute reductions of 8.1 and 6.1% in the incidence of primary end-point events at 6 months and 3 years, respectively, compared with placebo.

In the Evaluation in PTCA to Improve Long-Term Outcome with Abciximab GP IIb/IIIa Blockade (EPILOG) trial, a broad population of patients undergoing PCI was randomized to receive placebo plus standard-dose, weight-adjusted heparin; abciximab plus standard-dose, weight-adjusted heparin; or abciximab plus low-dose, weight-adjusted heparin. Patients with MI and NSTE ACS meeting the high-risk criteria used in the EPIC trial were excluded. The dosage regimen of abciximab used in the EPILOG trial consisted of a 0.25 mg/kg loading dose and a 0.125 mcg/kg per minute (up to a maximum of 10 mcg/minute) infusion, weight-adjusted in patients weighing up to 80 kg. The incidence of death or MI within 30 days was lower in both abciximab groups (4.2 and 3.8% in the standard- and low-dose heparin groups, respectively) compared with the placebo group (9.1%). Reductions in primary composite end-point events (i.e., death, MI, or any revascularization as well as death, MI, or urgent revascularization) with abciximab therapy were maintained at 6 months and 1 year. The risk of death occurring within 1 year of follow-up was increased in patients with elevations in the cardiac (MB) fraction of creatine kinase (CK, creatine phosphokinase, CPK) during either the periprocedural period (initial 24 hours) or first 30 days of follow-up.

In another study, the C7E3 Anti-Platelet Therapy in Unstable Refractory Angina (CAPTURE) trial, abciximab therapy was evaluated in patients with NSTE ACS not responding to conventional medical therapy (defined as at least one episode of myocardial ischemia despite bed rest and at least 2 hours of therapy with IV heparin and oral or IV nitrates) who were scheduled to undergo PCI within 24 hours. Patients were randomized to receive either placebo or abciximab (0.25 mg/kg loading dose plus infusion of 10 mcg/minute for 18–24 hours prior to PCI and continuing until 1 hour after completion of the intervention). Patients also were treated with standard-dose, weight-adjusted heparin and oral or IV nitrates. Data from the CAPTURE trial indicated that the incidence of primary end-point events (i.e., death, MI, or urgent intervention) at 30 days was lower (11.3 versus 15.9%) in patients treated with abciximab compared with patients in the placebo group.

In the Evaluation of Platelet IIb/IIIa Inhibitor for Stenting (EPISTENT) study in a large number of patients undergoing urgent or elective PCI with either coronary artery stenting or balloon angioplasty, therapy with abciximab (0. 25-mg/kg IV loading dose up to 60 minutes before either procedure, followed by an infusion of 0.125 mcg/kg per minute for 12 hours) reduced the incidence of composite clinical ischemic events (i.e., death, MI or reinfarction, repeat revascularization) at 30 days compared with that observed with placebo therapy with stenting. All patients received adjunctive therapy with aspirin (325 mg given 2 hours prior to the procedure and daily thereafter); ticlopidine (250 mg twice daily), if given, was administered to patients receiving stent implantation prior to therapy with abciximab or placebo. Low-dose, weight-adjusted heparin sodium injection (70 units/kg) was given initially to patients receiving abciximab with additional injections given to achieve and maintain an activated clotting time (ACT) of at least 200 seconds, and standard-dose, weight-adjusted heparin sodium injection (100 units/kg) was given initially to patients receiving stenting without abciximab, with additional injections given to achieve and maintain an ACT of at least 300 seconds.

At 6-months follow-up of the EPISTENT trial, the incidence of the composite clinical events (death, MI, urgent revascularization) was appreciably lower in those receiving stent implantation and abciximab (6.4%) compared with those receiving balloon angioplasty and abciximab (9.2%) or those receiving stent implantation and placebo therapy (12.1%). At 1 year of follow-up, the composite of clinical events followed were expanded to include all infarct-related artery revascularizations, urgent and nonurgent, as well as mortality and MI. The incidence of composite of clinical events at 1 year was appreciably lower in the group receiving stent implantation and abciximab (20.1%) than in the group receiving stent implantation and placebo (24%) or in the group undergoing balloon angioplasty and abciximab (25.3%). However, some of the efficacy in reduction in clinical end-point events observed with patients undergoing stent implantation may have been the result of ticlopidine pretreatment in these patients.

Pooled analysis of the EPIC, EPILOG, and EPISTENT studies indicate that abciximab is as effective in reducing ischemic complications of PCI in women as in men. Although other GP IIb/IIIa-receptor inhibitors have been shown to be safe and effective in women during PCI, data from a large (approximately 5000 patients, 27% women) randomized, double-blind trial evaluating abciximab and tirofiban in patients with non-ST-segment-elevation acute coronary syndromes showed that abciximab was more effective than tirofiban in preventing ischemic complications (i.e., composite end point of death, nonfatal MI, and urgent target-vessel revascularization) of PCI at 30 days. Such effects were observed regardless of gender. However, the benefit of abciximab in reducing ischemic complications at 6 months was not maintained.

Randomized controlled studies, including a meta-analysis of 16 randomized trials involving approximately 10,000 patients with STEMI undergoing primary PCI, generally have failed to demonstrate benefits of GP IIb/IIIa-receptor blockade similar to those observed in patients with NSTE ACS. The American College of Cardiology Foundation (ACCF), AHA, the Society for Cardiovascular Angiography and Interventions (SCAI), and other experts currently do not recommend the *routine* use of GP IIb/IIIa-receptor inhibitors in patients with STEMI undergoing PCI; however, selective use of these drugs as an adjunct to heparin may be reasonable in certain high-risk patients (e.g., those with large anterior MI and/or large thrombus). Studies evaluating the use of GP IIb/IIIa-receptor inhibitors in patients with NSTE ACS undergoing PCI have demonstrated reductions in ischemic outcomes, particularly in patients with high-risk features (e.g., elevated troponin); therefore, ACCF/AHA/SCAI states that it may be useful to administer a GP IIb/IIIa-receptor inhibitor at the time of PCI as an adjunct to heparin therapy in such high-risk patients who are not receiving bivalirudin and who are not adequately pretreated with clopidogrel. Regarding the choice of a GP IIb/IIIa-receptor inhibitor in patients undergoing PCI, abciximab, "double-bolus" eptifibatide (i.e., two 180-mcg/kg direct IV injections given 10 minutes apart), and high-dose tirofiban (25 mcg/kg given by direct IV injection) all have been shown to produce a high degree of platelet inhibition and reduce ischemic complications.

■ **Non-ST-Segment-Elevation Acute Coronary Syndromes** Although abciximab has been used in patients with unstable angina or NSTEMI (i.e., non-ST-segment-elevation acute coronary syndromes [NSTE ACS]) who were managed with conservative medical therapy only†, the manufacturer and some clinicians state that the safety and efficacy of abciximab have not been established in such patients who are *not* undergoing PCI. The American College of Chest Physicians (ACCP) states that a clear risk-benefit ratio has not been established for the use of GP IIb/IIIa-receptor inhibitors in patients with ACS who are not routinely scheduled for early revascularization.

Based on the results of the Global Use of Strategies to Open Occluded Coronary Arteries IV-Acute Coronary Syndromes (GUSTO IV-ACS) study, abciximab is not recommended as initial treatment in patients with NSTE ACS, except when the coronary anatomy is known and PCI is planned within 24 hours. In this large, multicenter study, use of abciximab in patients with NSTE ACS who did not undergo early cardiac catheterization was not associated with a reduction in mortality or nonfatal MI at 30 days, the primary end point of the study.

Although GP IIb/IIIa-receptor inhibitor therapy has been used in conjunction with aspirin prior to diagnostic angiography ("upstream") in patients with unstable angina or NSTEMI in whom an invasive management strategy is planned, IV eptifibatide or tirofiban is the preferred GP IIb/IIIa-receptor inhibitor for this use; abciximab is recommended only if there is no appreciable delay before angiography and PCI is likely to be performed.

Dosage and Administration

Treatment with abciximab should be undertaken only by clinicians qualified to appropriately manage therapy and possible complications of therapy (e.g., bleeding events, thrombocytopenia, possible hypersensitivity reactions), and only when adequate diagnosis and treatment facilities are readily available. Because efficacy of abciximab has not been demonstrated in patients in whom percutaneous coronary intervention (PCI) has failed, infusion of the drug should be discontinued in such cases. Administration of abciximab and heparin should be discontinued immediately if serious bleeding, which cannot be controlled by compression, occurs. Because hypersensitivity reactions have occurred with the administration of protein solutions such as abciximab and may occur at any time during the administration of the drug, drugs for the treatment of hypersensitivity reactions (e.g., epinephrine, dopamine, theophylline, antihistamines, corticosteroids) should be immediately available. If symptoms of an allergic reaction or anaphylaxis occur, abciximab should be discontinued immediately and appropriate resuscitative measures initiated.

■ **Administration** Abciximab is administered by direct IV injection and by IV infusion using a controlled-infusion device (infusion pump). The manufacturer recommends that abciximab injection be filtered prior to administration of the direct IV dose, prior to dilution of the infusion dose, and during infusion using a sterile, non-pyrogenic, low protein-binding filter (0.2 or 5 μm). The solution for continuous IV infusion is prepared by diluting the necessary amount of abciximab injection in an appropriate container of 0.9% sodium chloride or 5% dextrose injection. No other drug should be added to or administered in the same IV line with abciximab injection or infusion. The manufacturer states that no incompatibilities have been observed between abciximab solutions and glass bottles or polyvinyl chloride bags and administration sets. Abciximab is supplied in single-use vials that should be stored at 2–8°C, should not be frozen or shaken, and should not be used beyond the expiration date.

■ **Dosage** In clinical trials of abciximab therapy, most patients received adjunctive antithrombotic therapy with aspirin (325 mg 2 hours prior to the procedure and then once daily) and IV heparin. The safety and efficacy of abciximab therapy without concomitant aspirin and heparin remain to be established.

When used as an adjunct to PCI for the prevention of acute cardiac ischemic complications, the manufacturer and some clinicians recommend an initial dose of abciximab of 0.25 mg/kg administered by direct IV injection over at least 1 minute given 10–60 minutes prior to PCI. Following administration of the initial loading dose, abciximab is infused IV at a rate of 0.125 mcg/kg per minute (to a maximum of 10 mcg/minute) for 12 hours, after which the remaining infusion solution should be discarded.

For information on the risk of bleeding during coronary artery bypass grafting (CABG) following abciximab administration, see Cautions: Hematologic Effects. When used in patients with non-ST-segment-elevation acute coronary syndromes not responding to conventional medical therapy in whom PCI is planned within 24 hours, the recommended dose of abciximab is 0.25 mg/kg administered by direct IV injection over at least 1 minute followed by an IV infusion of 10 mcg/minute for 18–24 hours, concluding 1 hour after the procedure.

Adjunctive Antithrombotic Therapy Adjunctive antithrombotic therapy with aspirin and heparin was used in most patients receiving abciximab in clinical trials. In pivotal studies (i.e., the EPIC trial, the EPILOG trial, the CAPTURE trial, and the EPISTENT trial), aspirin was given in a dosage of 325 mg 2 hours prior to PCI and continued once daily thereafter. The American College of Cardiology Foundation (ACCF)/American Heart Association (AHA)/Society for Cardiovascular Angiography and Interventions (SCAI) recommends that aspirin 325 mg be given prior to PCI in patients not already receiving maintenance therapy with aspirin. Patients already receiving maintenance therapy with aspirin should receive a dose of 81–325 mg of aspirin before the procedure. For additional details regarding aspirin dosage regimens in patients undergoing PCI, see Percutaneous Coronary Intervention and Revascularization Procedures under Dosage: Thrombosis, in Dosage and Administration, in Aspirin 28:08.04.24.

In addition to aspirin, ACCF/AHA/SCAI recommends administration of a loading dose of a P2Y12 platelet adenosine diphosphate (ADP)-receptor antagonist (clopidogrel, prasugrel, or ticagrelor) in patients with acute coronary syndromes undergoing PCI with stent placement.

Since abciximab and other GP IIb/IIIa-receptor inhibitors may have additive effects on activated clotting time (ACT) in patients receiving one of these drugs concomitantly with heparin, the dosage of heparin sodium required to maintain an appropriate ACT during such concomitant therapy may be lower than with heparin monotherapy. Clinical experience from the EPILOG and EPISTENT studies, studies with other GP IIb/IIIa-receptor inhibitors (e.g., eptifibatide), and current ACCF/AHA/SCAI guidelines suggest that use of lower dosages of concomitant IV heparin sodium (e.g., 50–70 units/kg) given 6 hours prior to PCI and targeted to an ACT of at least 200 seconds may provide similar reductions in ischemic coronary events as dosages for higher target ACTs with less risk of major bleeding. In clinical studies, patients received 70 units/kg of heparin sodium if baseline ACT was less than 150 seconds, 50 units/kg if baseline ACT was 150–199 seconds, or no heparin sodium if baseline ACT exceeded 200 seconds. Additional heparin sodium injections (20 units/kg) were given in such studies to maintain an ACT of at least 200 seconds during the procedure. In patients who have received prior therapy with heparin before PCI, ACCF/AHA/SCAI states that additional heparin sodium injections should be administered during the procedure as needed. After uncomplicated PCI, discontinuance of the heparin infusion generally is recommended. In clinical studies, the femoral sheath was removed within 6 hours if the ACT was less than 175 seconds or the activated partial thromboplastin time (aPTT) was 50 seconds or less. If prolonged heparin therapy or delayed sheath removal was considered necessary, heparin was adjusted to a target aPTT of 55–75 seconds.

Cautions

■ **Hematologic Effects** The most frequent and potentially severe adverse effect of abciximab therapy is bleeding. Bleeding is an extension of the pharmacologic action of the drug and may range from minor local petechiae to major hemorrhagic complications; rarely, hemorrhagic complications may result in death. Almost all patients receiving abciximab in pivotal studies (i.e., the EPIC trial, the EPILOG trial, the CAPTURE trial, and the EPISTENT trial) received concomitant therapy with heparin and/or aspirin; therefore, the incidence of bleeding complications attributable solely to abciximab is difficult to determine.

In the EPIC trial, in which a non-weight-adjusted, standard-dose heparin regimen was used, a higher incidence of major bleeding, minor bleeding, and transfusion of blood products was reported in patients treated with abciximab compared with the placebo group. Results from the EPILOG and EPISTENT trials demonstrated that bleeding can be reduced through the use of low-dose, weight-adjusted heparin regimens, adherence to stricter anticoagulation guidelines, early femoral arterial sheath removal, careful patient and access site management, and weight-adjustment of the abciximab infusion dose.

In the EPIC study, bleeding was classified as major or minor according to the criteria of the Thrombolysis in Myocardial Infarction (TIMI) study group. Major bleeding was defined as intracranial bleeding or a decrease in hemoglobin concentration exceeding 5 g/dL, while minor bleeding was identified as spontaneous gross hematuria, spontaneous hematemesis, observed blood loss with a decrease in hemoglobin concentration exceeding 3 g/dL, or a decrease in hemoglobin concentration of at least 4 g/dL without an identified bleeding site.

Bleeding episodes occurred more frequently in patients receiving abciximab injection and infusion than in those receiving either abciximab injection and placebo infusion or placebo injection and infusion. Major bleeding events occurred in about 10.6 or 3.3% of patients receiving abciximab injection and infusion or placebo injection and infusion, respectively. Patients receiving abciximab had a higher incidence of major bleeding events at GI, genitourinary, retroperitoneal, and other sites than those receiving placebo. About 70% of patients who experienced major bleeding episodes while receiving abciximab had bleeding at the arterial access site in the groin.

In the CAPTURE trial, which incorporated weight-adjustment of the standard heparin dose, the incidence of major bleeding in patients treated with abciximab was reduced to 3.8%. The EPILOG and EPISTENT trials included the use of weight-adjusted low- or standard-dose heparin regimens, weight-adjusted abciximab infusion regimens, adherence to strict anticoagulation guidelines, and specific patient management measures designed to reduce the risk of bleeding. In these trials, the incidence of major bleeding was comparable in abciximab-treated patients and in patients receiving placebo and standard-dose heparin. The initial heparin sodium injection administered to patients in the low-dose arm of the EPILOG and EPISTENT trials was 70 units/kg with additional injections as necessary to maintain an ACT of at least 200 seconds. The initial heparin sodium injection administered to patients in the standard-dose arm of the EPILOG and EPISTENT trials was 100 units/kg with additional injections as necessary to maintain an ACT of at least 300 seconds.

Although data are limited, abciximab treatment was not associated with excess major bleeding in patients who underwent coronary artery bypass grafting (CABG). In the EPIC, CAPTURE, EPILOG, and EPISTENT studies in patients experiencing restenosis after PTCA or directional atherectomy and undergoing CABG, the incidence (3–5% in the EPIC trial, 1– 2% in the CAPTURE, EPILOG, and EPISTENT trials) of CABG-associated major bleeding events was similar in all treatment groups, and limited data indicate that abciximab treatment administered during the initial revascularization procedure was not associated with an increased number of major bleeding episodes in patients subsequently undergoing CABG. Some patients with prolonged bleeding times received platelet transfusions to correct prolonged bleeding times before undergoing CABG.

Subgroup analysis in the EPIC and CAPTURE trials indicated that major bleeding *not* associated with CABG occurred more frequently in patients weighing 75 kg or less who received abciximab. Major bleeding episodes *not* associated with CABG occurred in about 11 or 3% of patients receiving abciximab injection and continuous infusion or placebo injection and continuous infusion, respectively, in the EPIC trial. Major bleeding *not* associated with CABG was reduced in the CAPTURE trial to 3.8 or 1.9% of those receiving abciximab or placebo and standard-dose heparin, respectively. In the EPILOG and EPISTENT trials, the combined incidence of major bleeding *not* associated with CABG was further reduced to 1.9, 0.8, or 1% in those receiving abciximab and standard-dose heparin, abciximab and low-dose heparin, or placebo and standard-dose heparin.

The total incidence of intracranial hemorrhage or nonhemorrhagic stroke in the 4 trials (EPIC, CAPTURE, EPILOG, EPISTENT) was similar. Among the patients receiving abciximab, the rate of hemorrhagic stroke in patient receiving standard-dose heparin in the EPIC, CAPTURE, and EPILOG trials was higher than in those receiving low-dose heparin in the EPILOG and EPISTENT trials. In a pooled analysis of data from the EPIC, EPILOG, and EPISTENT studies, abciximab was not associated with an increase in major bleeding complications in women undergoing primary PCI for ST-segment elevation myocardial infarction (STEMI). However, use of GP IIb/IIIa-receptor inhibitors during PCI after failed thrombolytic therapy has been associated with an increased incidence of bleeding, especially in women and geriatric patients.

Minor bleeding episodes *not* associated with CABG occurred in about 16.8 or 9.2% of patients receiving abciximab injection and infusion or placebo injection and infusion, respectively, in the EPIC trial. In the CAPTURE trial, the incidence of minor bleeding *not* associated with CABG was 4.8% in patients receiving abciximab and standard-dose heparin and 2% in patients receiving placebo and standard-dose heparin. The incidence of minor bleeding *not* associated with CABG in the EPILOG and EPISTENT trials was increased in patients receiving standard-dose, weight-adjusted heparin and abciximab compared with placebo and standard-dose heparin (7.6 versus 2.6%) but was not substantially increased in patients treated with abciximab and low-dose, weight-adjusted heparin (3.2%).

Adverse hematologic effects with abciximab therapy have been severe enough to require blood or platelet transfusions. In the EPIC study, transfusion of red blood cells was required substantially more often in patients receiving one of the abciximab regimens than in those receiving placebo, and the 12-hour infusion was discontinued prematurely in about 16, 12, or 7% of patients receiving abciximab injection and infusion, abciximab injection and placebo infusion, or placebo injection and infusion, respectively. The manufacturer states that transfusions, including packed red blood cells or whole blood were required in 7.8% of patients in the EPIC study receiving abciximab injection and infusion and 2% of patients receiving placebo injection and infusion for bleeding *not* associated with CABG. The need for red blood cell transfusion was reduced further in the CAPTURE trial to 2.4 or 1.4% in patients receiving abciximab and standard-dose heparin or placebo and standard-dose heparin, respectively. Pooled data from the EPILOG and EPISTENT trials indicate that the incidence of red blood cell transfusion in patients *not* undergoing CABG was 0.8% in patients receiving abciximab and standard-dose heparin, 0.5% in patients receiving abciximab and low-dose heparin, and 0.9% in patients receiving placebo and standard-dose heparin.

Decreases in platelet count or thrombocytopenia occurs occasionally (2.3% overall) after therapy with platelet glycoprotein (GP) IIb/IIIa-receptor inhibitors. Thrombocytopenia associated with administration of a GP IIb/IIIa-receptor inhibitor generally occurs within hours or days after administration of the drug. In the EPIC study, patients receiving IV injection and infusion of abciximab experienced thrombocytopenia and required platelet transfusions more frequently than those receiving IV injection and infusion of placebo. Platelet counts decreased to less than 100,000/mm^3 in 2.6–5.2% or 2.5–3% of patients receiving abciximab injection and infusion in the EPIC and CAPTURE trials or the EPILOG and EPISTENT trials, respectively. Severe thrombocytopenia (reduction in platelet count to less than 50,000/mm^3) occurred in 0.9–1.7 or 0.4–1% of patients receiving abciximab injection and infusion in EPIC and CAPTURE trials or in the EPILOG and EPISTENT trials, respectively. Transfusion of platelets was required in 2.1–5.5 or 0.9–1.1% of patients receiving abciximab injection and infusion in the EPIC and CAPTURE trials or in the EPILOG and EPISTENT trials, respectively. In a registry study of patients receiving a second or subsequent course of abciximab therapy, the incidence of thrombocytopenia or profound thrombocytopenia (less than 20,000/mm^3) was 5 or 2%, respectively. Factors associated with an increased risk of thrombocytopenia include a history of thrombocytopenia with prior use of abciximab, readministration within 30 days, or detection of human anti-chimeric antibodies prior to readministration. A preliminary report based on pooled data from clinical trials indicates that the incidence of thrombocytopenia is not appreciably different among GP IIb/IIIa-receptor inhibitors (i.e., abciximab, eptifibatide, tirofiban), although the absolute risk of thrombocytopenia appears to increase (but not synergistically) with concomitant use of heparin. However, severe thrombocytopenia (i.e., platelet count less than 20,000/mm^3) has been reported more frequently with abciximab than with tirofiban.

Anemia occurred in 1.2% of patients receiving abciximab injection and infusion and in 0.4% of those receiving placebo injection and infusion in the EPIC study. Leukocytosis occurred in 1% of patients receiving abciximab injection and infusion versus 0.1% of those receiving placebo injection and infusion. Hemolytic anemia or petechiae each occurred in 0.3% of patients receiving abciximab injection and infusion; these effects occurred with similar frequency in patients receiving placebo injection and infusion.

■ **Nervous System Effects** Hypoesthesia, involving principally the extremities, occurred in 1 or 0.3% of patients in the EPIC study receiving rapid IV injection and continuous IV infusion of abciximab or rapid IV injection and continuous IV infusion of placebo, respectively. Confusion was reported in 0.6% of patients receiving abciximab injection and infusion but in no patients receiving placebo injection and infusion. Pain, involving principally the extremities, occurred in 3.4% of patients receiving abciximab injection and infusion and in 2.6% of those receiving placebo injection and infusion. Abnormal thinking occurred in 2.1%, dizziness in 1.8%, coma in 0.4%, and insomnia in 0.3% of patients receiving abciximab injection and infusion in the EPIC study, frequencies that were similar to those at which these effects occurred with placebo injection and infusion.

■ **GI Effects** Nausea occurred in 18.4% of patients receiving abciximab by rapid IV injection and continuous IV infusion and in 16% of those receiving placebo by rapid IV injection and continuous IV infusion in the EPIC study. Vomiting occurred in 11.4% of patients receiving abciximab injection and infusion and in 9% of those receiving placebo injection and infusion. Diarrhea, constipation, or ileus occurred in 0.9, 0.3, or 0.3%, respectively, of patients receiving abciximab injection and infusion, and at similar frequencies in patients receiving placebo injection and infusion.

■ **Cardiovascular Effects** Hypotension occurred in 21% of patients receiving abciximab by rapid IV injection and continuous IV infusion and in 12% of those receiving placebo by rapid IV injection and continuous IV infusion in the EPIC study; hypotension often was related to bleeding complications associated with abciximab therapy. Peripheral edema occurred in 1.6% of patients receiving abciximab injection and infusion and in 0.4% of those receiving placebo injection and infusion. Bradycardia occurred in 5.2% of patients receiving abciximab injection and infusion and in 2.9% of those receiving placebo injection and infusion.

Atrial fibrillation or flutter occurred in 3.5%, vascular disorder in 1.8%, pulmonary edema in 1.5%, complete AV block in 1.3%, supraventricular tachycardia in 1%, weak pulse in 1%, palpitation in 0.7%, intermittent claudication in 0.4%, pericardial effusion in 0.4%, limb embolism in 0.3%, pulmonary embolism in 0.3%, brain ischemia in 0.3%, and ventricular arrhythmia in 0.3% of patients receiving abciximab injection and infusion in the EPIC study; the frequencies of these adverse effects were similar to those among patients receiving placebo injection and infusion.

■ **Respiratory Effects** Pleural effusion or pleurisy occurred in 1.3% of patients receiving abciximab by rapid IV injection and continuous IV infusion and in 0.2% of those receiving rapid IV injection and continuous IV infusion of placebo in the EPIC study. Pneumonia occurred in 1% of patients receiving abciximab injection and infusion and in 0.4% of those receiving placebo injection and infusion.

Pulmonary alveolar hemorrhage in association with hypoxemia, alveolar infiltrates on chest radiograph, hemoptysis, or an unexplained decrease in hemoglobin has been reported rarely with use of abciximab.

■ **Musculoskeletal Effects** Myopathy occurred in 0.4%, and myalgia in 0.3% of patients receiving abciximab by rapid IV injection and continuous IV infusion in the EPIC study, frequencies that were similar to those at which these effects occurred with rapid IV injection and continuous IV infusion of placebo.

■ **Genitourinary Effects** Urinary tract infection occurred in 1.9%, urinary retention in 0.4%, and abnormal renal function in 0.3% of patients receiving abciximab by rapid IV injection and continuous IV infusion in the EPIC study; these effects occurred at similar frequencies in patients receiving rapid IV injection and continuous IV infusion of placebo.

■ **Dermatologic and Sensitivity Reactions** Pruritus occurred in 0.3% of patients receiving rapid IV injection and continuous IV infusion of abciximab in the EPIC study, but at a frequency that was similar to that reported with placebo injection and infusion.

Anaphylactic reactions have been reported rarely during postmarketing experience in patients receiving abciximab.

Readministration of abciximab may result in the formation of positive human antichimeric antibodies (HACA) that could potentially cause allergic or hypersensitivity reactions, including anaphylaxis. In the EPIC, EPILOG, and CAPTURE trials, positive HACA responses occurred in 5.8% of patients receiving a first abciximab injection; however, no increase in the incidence of allergic or hypersensitivity reactions in patients receiving abciximab was observed. In a registry study of patients receiving repeat courses of abciximab therapy, positive HACA after the first exposure to abciximab was associated with an increased incidence and severity of thrombocytopenia. Positive HACA responses following initial, second, and fourth or greater exposures occurred in 6, 27, and 44%, respectively. Positive HACA status in this study was not associated with serious allergic or anaphylactic reactions.

Data on the incidence of positive HACA are based on the results from an enzyme-linked immunosorbent assay (ELISA); these results are highly dependent on the sensitivity and specificity of the ELISA assay. Other factors that may influence the observed incidence of positive results for antibody include the manner in which samples are handled, timing of sample collection, concomitant therapy with other drugs, and underlying disease. Therefore, comparing the incidence of antibodies to abciximab versus that with other drugs may be misleading. Development of antibodies to other currently available GP IIb/IIIa-receptor inhibitors (i.e., tirofiban, eptifibatide) has not been reported to date, but very few patients have received the drugs on more than one occasion. No evidence of delayed-type hypersensitivity or antigenicity with eptifibatide was noted in studies in mice and guinea pigs.

■ **Other Adverse Effects** Abnormal vision occurred in 0.7% of patients receiving abciximab by rapid IV injection and continuous IV infusion and in 0.1% of those receiving placebo by rapid IV injection and continuous IV infusion in the EPIC study. Dysphonia and cellulitis each occurred in 0.3% of patients receiving abciximab injection and infusion and with similar frequency in patients receiving placebo injection and infusion.

■ **Precautions and Contraindications** The administration of abciximab is associated with an increased frequency of major bleeding complications (e.g., retroperitoneal bleeding, spontaneous GI and genitourinary bleeding, arterial access site bleeding). Therefore, treatment with abciximab should be undertaken only by clinicians qualified to appropriately manage therapy and possible complications of therapy, and only when adequate diagnostic and treatment facilities are readily available. Bleeding with GP IIb/IIIa-receptor inhibitors can be reduced by adherence to strict anticoagulation guidelines, the use of a short course of low-dose, weight-adjusted heparin, early arterial sheath removal, and careful patient and access site management. Prior to administration of abciximab, preexisting hemostatic abnormalities should be identified by obtaining a platelet count, prothrombin time, activated clotting time (ACT), and activated partial thromboplastin time (aPTT). During and following treatment with abciximab, platelet counts, and the extent of heparin anticoagulation (as assessed by ACT or aPTT) should be monitored closely. Based on the results of clinical trials, the manufacturer has established laboratory parameter guidelines to minimize the risk of bleeding. When abciximab treatment is initiated 18–24 hours prior to percutaneous coronary intervention, the aPTT should be maintained between 60–85 seconds during infusion of abciximab and heparin. The manufacturer and some clinicians state that during percutaneous coronary intervention, an ACT exceeding 200 seconds should be maintained. (See Adjunctive Antithrombotic Therapy under Dosage and Administration: Dosage.) The manufacturer recommends discontinuance of heparin immediately after the percutaneous coronary intervention and removal of the arterial sheath within 6 hours following the procedure. If anticoagulation is continued following percutaneous coronary intervention, the aPTT should be maintained between 55–75 seconds. In addition, arterial sheath removal should not be attempted unless aPTT is 50 seconds or less or ACT is 150–180 seconds approximately 6 hours after PCI. Also, careful monitoring of all potential bleeding sites, including catheter insertion sites, needle puncture (e.g., IV, IM, lumbar, subcutaneous, intradermal) sites, cutdown sites, and GI, genitourinary, and retroperitoneal sites, should be undertaken during and following treatment with abciximab.

Bleeding associated with abciximab may occur at any site but usually involves the arterial access site for cardiac catheterization and internal sites (e.g., GI, genitourinary, or retroperitoneal bleeding). In the EPIC study, patient weight was inversely related to the number of major bleeding episodes in patients receiving abciximab. The risk of abciximab-induced hemorrhage appears to be greatest in patients weighing less than 75 kg, those older than 65 years, those with a history of prior GI disease, and those receiving concomitant treatment with thrombolytic agents; the increased risk of major bleeding episodes in such patients should be weighed against the anticipated benefits of abciximab therapy. Patients undergoing PTCA or atherectomy in whom an increased risk of bleeding, which may be additive to that of abciximab therapy, also may exist include those undergoing one of these procedures within 12 hours of the onset of symptoms of myocardial infarction (MI), those undergoing a prolonged (exceeding 70 minutes) procedure, and those in whom the procedure fails. Heparin anticoagulation also may contribute to the risk of bleeding in patients undergoing PTCA or atherectomy who are receiving abciximab. The manufacturer states that any occurrence of serious bleeding that cannot be controlled by pressure on the bleeding site should result in discontinuance of abciximab and concomitantly administered heparin therapy.

To minimize the increased possibility of bleeding associated with the use of abciximab, particularly at the site of femoral vascular catheter placement for arterial access, the manufacturer states that precautions in placement, maintenance, and removal of the vascular access catheter should be observed. Placement of a femoral *venous* catheter should be avoided if possible. Only the anterior wall of the femoral artery should be punctured; a Seldinger (through and through) technique for puncture of the artery should be avoided. Complete bed rest is required while the vascular access catheter is in place, with the head of the bed elevated no more than 30°, and the limb in which the vascular access catheter was inserted should be restrained in a straight position. Frequent assessment of the vascular access catheter insertion site and monitoring of the distal pulse in the leg(s) in which the catheter was inserted should be undertaken throughout the period that the catheter is in place and for 6 hours after its removal; any hematoma should be measured and monitored for enlargement. Pressure (e.g., using manual compression or a mechanical hemostatic device) should be applied to the femoral artery for at least 30 minutes after catheter removal; after hemostasis, a pressure dressing should be applied. The patient should be restricted to bed rest for 6–8 hours after removal of the vascular access catheter or discontinuance of abciximab, or 4 hours following discontinuance of heparin, whichever occurs later.

In general, arterial or venous punctures, IM injections, urinary catheterization, nasotracheal intubation, placement of nasogastric tubes, and use of automatic blood pressure cuffs should be minimized. Establishment of IV access at noncompressible sites (e.g., in subclavian or jugular veins) should be avoided, an indwelling venipuncture device (e.g., heparin lock) should be considered for drawing blood, documentation and monitoring of vascular puncture sites should occur, and dressings should gently and carefully be removed. The manufacturer states that abciximab and any concomitant heparin should be discontinued if serious bleeding that is not controllable with pressure occurs. The manufacturer also states that an Ivy bleeding time should be determined in the event of uncontrolled bleeding or the need for surgery (especially major procedures required within 48–72 hours of treatment with abciximab).

Because thrombocytopenia has been reported with the use of abciximab, platelet counts should be determined prior to treatment with abciximab, at 2–4 hours following the initial rapid IV dose, and at 24 hours following initiation of abciximab therapy or prior to discharge of the patient, whichever occurs first. Patients experiencing an acute decrease in platelet count (e.g., a decrease to less than 100,000/mm^3, or a decrease of at least 25% from pretreatment values) should have additional platelet counts performed. Platelet count monitoring should continue until platelet counts return to normal. These platelet counts should be drawn in separate tubes containing edetate disodium (EDTA), citrate, or heparin to exclude pseudothrombocytopenia caused by an in vitro anticoagulant interaction. A low platelet count in the presence of EDTA but not in the presence of heparin and/or citrate supports a diagnosis of pseudothrombocytopenia. The possibility of heparin-induced thrombocytopenia also should be considered in the differential diagnosis of thrombocytopenia in patients receiving GP IIb/IIIa-receptor inhibitors concomitantly with heparin. The manufacturer states that if true thrombocytopenia is verified, abciximab should be discontinued immediately and the condition appropriately monitored and treated. The manufacturer states that based on preliminary evidence, platelet transfusions may at least partly restore platelet function. In the EPIC study, heparin and aspirin administration were discontinued in patients whose platelet counts decreased to 60,000/mm^3, and platelets were transfused if platelet counts decreased to less than 50,000/mm^3. Daily platelet counts were obtained for thrombocytopenic patients in this study until the platelet count returned to normal. However, further study is required to clarify the role of platelet transfusions in patients experiencing thrombocytopenia associated with abciximab administration.

Although interactions of abciximab with other drugs have not been studied systematically, drugs that affect hemostasis, including heparin, oral anticoagulants, thrombolytic agents, and drugs with antiplatelet activity (e.g., nonsteroidal anti-inflammatory agents, dipyridamole, ticlopidine), may be associated with an increased risk of bleeding and should be used with caution when administered concomitantly with abciximab. Although there is limited information on the concomitant use of abciximab with thrombolytic agents, caution should be exercised when such drugs are used with abciximab because of concern about synergistic effects on bleeding.

Major bleeding episodes occurred in 5 of 11 patients in the EPIC study who received low-molecular-weight dextran (usually for deployment of a coronary stent, for which oral anticoagulants were also given) concomitantly with abciximab, while none of 5 patients receiving low molecular weight dextran concomitantly with placebo experienced major bleeding. The manufacturer states that administration of abciximab is contraindicated when IV dextran is administered prior to PTCA or atherectomy or when such use is contemplated.

Administration of abciximab may result in human antichimeric antibody (HACA) formation. Limited evidence suggests that chimeric 7E3 Fab (abciximab) is far less immunogenic than murine 7E3 Fab, and the response to abciximab therapy of some patients with high pretreatment HACA assay reactivity was no different than those with low pretreatment HACA assay reactivity. Patients with HACA titers may have allergic or hypersensitivity reactions (including anaphylaxis) if abciximab is readministered. Readministration of abciximab also may result in thrombocytopenia or diminished effect of abciximab in patients with HACA titers. Anaphylaxis may occur at any time during the administration of abciximab; if anaphylaxis occurs, the drug should be discontinued immediately and appropriate resuscitative measures initiated.

Because abciximab increases the risk of bleeding, the drug is contraindicated in patients with active internal bleeding; recent (within 6 weeks) clinically important GI or genitourinary bleeding; bleeding diathesis; thrombocytopenia (platelet count less than 100,000/mm³); recent (within 6 weeks) major surgery or trauma; intracranial neoplasm, arteriovenous malformation, or aneurysm; or severe uncontrolled hypertension. The drug also is contraindicated in patients receiving IV dextran prior to PTCA or atherectomy or in whom use of IV dextran during PTCA or atherectomy is planned, and in patients who have received oral anticoagulants within the previous 7 days unless their prothrombin time is 1.2 times the control value or less. Abciximab is contraindicated in patients with a history of cerebrovascular accident (CVA) in the preceding 2 years or those with serious CVA-associated residual neurologic deficit, in those with a presumed or documented history of vasculitis, and in those with a known hypersensitivity to any component of the commercially available preparation or to murine proteins.

■ **Pediatric Precautions** Safety and efficacy of abciximab in patients younger than 18 years of age have not been established.

■ **Geriatric Precautions** No overall differences in safety or efficacy were observed among geriatric patients 65 to younger than 75 years of age in a number of premarketing clinical trials. Clinical experience in geriatric patients 75 years of age or older is inadequate to determine whether such patients respond differently than younger patients.

■ **Mutagenicity and Carcinogenicity** No evidence of mutagenicity was demonstrated by abciximab in in vitro or in vivo mutagenicity studies.

No long-term studies in animals have been performed to determine the carcinogenic potential of abciximab.

■ **Pregnancy, Fertility, and Lactation** Animal reproduction studies have not been performed with abciximab, and it is also not known whether the drug can cause fetal harm when administered to pregnant women. Abciximab should be used during pregnancy only when clearly needed.

Studies have not been conducted to date to determine whether abciximab affects fertility in males or females.

It is not known whether abciximab is distributed into human milk, or if the drug is absorbed systemically after ingestion. Because many drugs are distributed into human milk, caution should be exercised when abciximab is administered to a nursing woman.

Description

Abciximab is the Fab fragment of the chimeric human-murine monoclonal immunoglobulin antibody 7E3. Abciximab binds selectively to platelet glycoprotein (GP) IIb/IIIa receptors and inhibits platelet aggregation. Abciximab also binds to the vitronectin receptor located on platelets and vascular endothelial and smooth muscle cells.

SumMon® (see Users Guide). For additional information on this drug until a more detailed monograph is developed and published, the manufacturer's labeling should be consulted. It is *essential* that the labeling be consulted for information on the usual cautions, precautions, and contraindications concerning potential drug interactions and/or laboratory test interferences and for information on acute toxicity.

Preparations

Excipients in commercially available drug preparations may have clinically important effects in some individuals; consult specific product labeling for details.

Abciximab

Parenteral

Injection, for IV use	2 mg/mL (10 mg)	**ReoPro®, Lilly**

†Use is not currently included in the labeling approved by the US Food and Drug Administration

Selected Revisions September 2017, © Copyright, June 1995, American Society of Health-System Pharmacists, Inc.

Cangrelor Tetrasodium

■ Cangrelor tetrasodium, a nonthienopyridine, reversible P2Y12 platelet adenosine diphosphate (ADP)-receptor antagonist, is a platelet-activation and -aggregation inhibitor.

Uses

■ **Acute Ischemic Complications of Percutaneous Coronary Intervention** Cangrelor tetrasodium is used as an adjunct to percutaneous coronary intervention (PCI) to reduce the risk of periprocedural myocardial infarction (MI), repeat coronary revascularization, and stent thrombosis in patients who have not been treated with another P2Y12-receptor antagonist and are not being given a platelet glycoprotein IIb/IIIa-receptor (GP IIb/IIIa) inhibitor.

Dual-drug antiplatelet therapy with a P2Y12-receptor antagonist and aspirin is part of the current standard of care in patients with acute coronary syndromes (ACS). Current guidelines from the American College of Cardiology Foundation (ACCF), American Heart Association (AHA), and the Society for Cardiovascular Angiography and Interventions (SCAI) generally recommend that patients with ACS undergoing PCI with stent placement (bare-metal or drug-eluting) be given an oral loading dose of ticagrelor, clopidogrel, or prasugrel followed by maintenance therapy with one of these agents for at least 12 months (unless the risk of bleeding outweighs the anticipated net benefit of therapy); low-dose aspirin also should be given concomitantly and continued indefinitely in such patients. Potential advantages of cangrelor compared with current oral thienopyridine antiplatelet agents include more rapid onset and offset of effect and less interindividual variability in antiplatelet effect (i.e., compared with clopidogrel) due to its availability for IV use, absence of need for hepatic conversion to an active form, short biologic half-life, and reversibility of binding to the P2Y12 platelet receptor. It has been suggested that cangrelor may be of particular benefit in patients in whom oral administration is problematic (e.g., those who are intubated, patients with shock, cardiac arrest, nausea/vomiting) and in those who have bleeding complications with PCI and/or are candidates for emergent invasive procedures such as coronary artery bypass grafting (CABG). Currently available evidence suggests that cangrelor is more effective than clopidogrel in reducing the rate of acute ischemic cardiovascular events in patients with ACS undergoing PCI, at the cost of an increase in mild but not major bleeding. However, the precise role of cangrelor in the management of ACS remains to be established. Efficacy of cangrelor in improving cardiovascular outcomes in ACS has been variable, possibly due to methodologic and reporting issues in some clinical trials (e.g., difficulties in diagnosing reinfarction due to the definition used for periprocedural MI). The benefits of cangrelor over clopidogrel in the pivotal clinical trial appear to be based principally on a reduction in the rate of acute (within 48 hours following PCI) periprocedural MI; cangrelor did not decrease the rate of death. In addition, data are lacking on the relative efficacy and safety of cangrelor compared with prasugrel or ticagrelor, other P2Y12-receptor antagonists that have been more effective than clopidogrel in patients with ACS undergoing PCI.

The current indication for cangrelor as an adjunct to prevent acute ischemic complications of PCI is based principally on the results of a randomized, double-blind placebo-controlled trial (Clinical Trial Comparing Cangrelor to Clopidogrel Standard of Care Therapy in Subjects Who Require PCI [CHAMPION PHOENIX]) in patients with ACS undergoing PCI, which evaluated whether more rapid inhibition of platelet aggregation with IV cangrelor at the time of PCI would reduce the rate of periprocedural thrombotic events compared with a drug having a less rapid antiplatelet effect (oral clopidogrel). The trial consisted of 11,145 patients with coronary atherosclerosis who required PCI for stable angina, non-ST-segment elevation MI (NSTEMI), or ST-segment elevation MI (STEMI) and who did not receive previous treatment with an antiplatelet agent. Patients receiving cangrelor were given 30 mcg/kg by rapid IV injection followed by an IV infusion of 4 mcg/kg per minute for 2 hours or until the conclusion of PCI, whichever was longer. These patients then received oral clopidogrel 600 mg at the end of the cangrelor infusion. Patients receiving clopidogrel were given a loading dose of 300 or 600 mg as per institutional protocol shortly before or shortly after PCI. All patients were required to receive concomitant treatment with aspirin (75–325 mg daily, continued indefinitely) and clopidogrel (75 mg daily) during the first 48 hours after randomization. The choice of periprocedural anticoagulant (bivalirudin, unfractionated heparin, or fondaparinux) was at the discretion of the treating physician. GP IIb/IIIa inhibitors were allowed only as rescue therapy during PCI to treat new or persistent thrombus formation, slow or no re-flow side branch compromise, dissection, or distal embolization. The primary efficacy end point in the modified intention-to-treat population was the composite rate of death from any cause, MI, ischemia-driven revascularization, or stent thrombosis in the 48 hours after randomization. The primary safety end point was severe bleeding at 48 hours postrandomization not related to CABG, according to the Global Use of Strategies to Open Occluded Coronary Arteries (GUSTO) criteria.

Cangrelor substantially reduced the occurrence of the primary composite end point assessed at 48 hours after randomization compared with clopidogrel (event rate 4.7 versus 5.9%, 22% reduction) in the CHAMPION PHOENIX trial. The benefit of cangrelor was attributable principally to a reduction in the rate of MI (3.7 or 4.6% with cangrelor or clopidogrel, respectively). However, stent thrombosis at 48 hours postrandomization (the key secondary end point) was also reduced with cangrelor, particularly intraprocedural stent thrombosis. The benefits of cangrelor on these primary and secondary end points was maintained at 30 days. Cangrelor did not reduce the risk of death. Efficacy of cangrelor did not appear to be substantially affected by age, gender, race, or certain prior comorbid conditions (e.g., prior transient ischemic attack [TIA]/stroke, diabetes mellitus) according to subgroup analyses. While approximately 25% of patients in the clopidogrel group received a less-than-optimal 300-mg oral clopidogrel loading dose (a 600-mg loading dose is recommended in current ACS guidelines for patients undergoing PCI), subgroup analyses revealed similar results after stratification by loading dose. The use of rescue therapy with a GP IIb/IIIa inhibitor was substantially less frequent in the cangrelor group compared with the clopidogrel group (2.3 versus 3.5% of patients). The rate of severe bleeding was not substantially increased with cangrelor using the GUSTO bleeding criteria, although the rate of major bleeding events was substantially higher with cangrelor therapy when assessed using the more sensitive

Acute Catheterization and Urgent Intervention Triage Strategy (ACUITY) criteria (4.3 versus 2.5%). Rates of adverse effects related to treatment were low in both groups, although transient dyspnea was more frequent in patients receiving cangrelor.

Two trials evaluating the use of cangrelor in patients undergoing PCI (Cangrelor Versus Standard Therapy to Achieve Optimal Management of Platelet Inhibition in Patients Undergoing PCI [CHAMPION PCI] and Cangrelor Versus Standard Therapy to Achieve Optimal Management of Platelet Inhibition [CHAMPION PLATFORM]) were conducted prior to CHAMPION PHOENIX but were terminated early for futility. In these trials, cangrelor did not substantially reduce the incidence of the primary end point (death from any cause, MI, or ischemia-driven revascularization) compared with clopidogrel. It has been suggested that the lack of a substantial difference in the primary end point in the CHAMPION PLATFORM and CHAMPION PCI trials may have been related to trial design and reporting issues. In particular, these trials relied heavily on elevation of biomarker levels (e.g., myocardial creatine kinase [CK-MB], troponin) to define periprocedural MI, which made it difficult to discriminate between events occurring before or after randomization, especially in patients with initially elevated biomarkers. In addition, in the CHAMPION PLATFORM trial, administration of the clopidogrel loading dose was delayed until after PCI, although immediate administration of a loading dose of a P2Y12-receptor antagonist is currently recommended in guidelines for management of ACS in patients undergoing PCI. The CHAMPION PHOENIX trial was designed using a new primary end point (which included stent thrombosis) and a more accurate definition of MI (which included ECG changes, presence of ischemic symptoms and angiographic complications, as well as changes in biomarkers).

A pooled analysis of all three CHAMPION trials demonstrated a reduction of 19% in the primary end point (as defined in CHAMPION PHOENIX) with cangrelor compared with clopidogrel at 48 hours and 30 days. Mild bleeding events according to ACUITY and GUSTO criteria were more frequent in patients receiving cangrelor compared with those receiving clopidogrel.

Dosage and Administration

■ **Reconstitution and Administration** Cangrelor tetrasodium is administered by rapid IV ("bolus") injection (over less than 1 minute) from the prepared IV infusion bag via manual IV push or infusion pump, followed by IV infusion using a dedicated IV line. Rapid IV injection of the drug should be completed before the start of percutaneous coronary intervention (PCI). The continuous infusion should be initiated immediately after rapid IV injection of the drug and should be continued for at least 2 hours or for the duration of PCI, whichever is longer.

Cangrelor lyophilized powder for injection should be stored at 20–25°C but may be exposed to temperatures ranging from 15–30°C. Lyophilized cangrelor for injection must be reconstituted and diluted before administration. The drug is reconstituted by adding 5 mL of sterile water for injection to a vial labeled as containing 50 mg of cangrelor. The vial should be gently swirled to aid reconstitution and inspected for any evidence of particulate matter. The reconstituted drug should be further diluted immediately by withdrawing the contents of the vial and adding to 250 mL of 5% dextrose or 0.9% sodium chloride injection to yield a final cangrelor concentration of 200 mcg/mL. This diluted solution is stable for up to 12 hours in 5% dextrose and 24 hours in 0.9% sodium chloride at 20–25°C.

■ **Dosage** Dosage of cangrelor tetrasodium is expressed in terms of cangrelor. Cangrelor is intended to be given to patients prior to percutaneous coronary intervention (PCI) in conjunction with other standard-of-care therapy (e.g., aspirin, anticoagulants). Upon discontinuance of the cangrelor infusion, patients should be transitioned to an oral P2Y12 platelet adenosine diphosphate (ADP)-receptor antagonist to maintain platelet inhibition.

Acute Ischemic Complications of Percutaneous Coronary Intervention For reducing the risk of periprocedural myocardial infarction (MI), repeat coronary revascularization, and stent thrombosis in patients undergoing PCI, the recommended initial adult dosage of cangrelor is 30 mcg/kg administered by rapid IV ("bolus") injection (over less than 1 minute) prior to PCI, followed immediately by an IV infusion of 4 mcg/kg per minute for at least 2 hours or for the duration of PCI, whichever is longer.

Transitioning to Oral Therapy. To maintain platelet inhibition after discontinuance of the cangrelor infusion, an oral P2Y12-receptor antagonist (clopidogrel, prasugrel, or ticagrelor) should be administered. If ticagrelor is used, a 180-mg dose of the drug may be administered at any time during cangrelor infusion or immediately after the infusion is discontinued. If clopidogrel or prasugrel is used, clopidogrel 600 mg or prasugrel 60 mg may be administered immediately after discontinuance of cangrelor. Clopidogrel or prasugrel should not be administered during the cangrelor infusion. (See Drug Interactions: Thienopyridine Antiplatelet Agents.)

■ **Special Populations** ***Renal Impairment*** No dosage adjustment is required for patients with renal impairment.

Hepatic Impairment Safety and efficacy of cangrelor have not been established in patients with hepatic impairment. However, the metabolism of cangrelor is not dependent on hepatic function, so dosage adjustment is not required for patients with hepatic impairment. (See Hepatic Impairment under Warnings/Precautions: Specific Populations, in Cautions.)

Cautions

■ **Contraindications** Cangrelor is contraindicated in patients with substantial active bleeding and in those with known hypersensitivity to the drug or any ingredient in the formulation.

■ **Warnings/Precautions** ***Bleeding*** Like other antiplatelet agents, cangrelor increases the risk of bleeding, which may be serious. In the CHAMPION PHOENIX trial, bleeding events of all severities were somewhat more common with cangrelor than with clopidogrel. In clinical trials, bleeding events in patients receiving cangrelor were mild, generally consisting of hematoma, ecchymosis, and oozing at the puncture site. In the CHAMPION PHOENIX trial, the rate of severe bleeding (per the Global Use of Strategies to Open Occluded Coronary Arteries [GUSTO] criteria) was not substantially increased by cangrelor, although the rate of major bleeding according to more sensitive criteria (Acute Catheterization and Urgent Intervention Triage Strategy [ACUITY]) was substantially higher with cangrelor than with clopidogrel (4.3 versus 2.5%). The increase in major bleeding with the ACUITY criteria was attributable to a greater incidence of hematoma at the site of vascular access in patients receiving cangrelor.

Cangrelor should not be used in patients with substantial active bleeding. (See Cautions: Contraindications.) The antiplatelet effects of cangrelor are negligible 1 hour after discontinuance of the infusion.

Sensitivity Reactions **Hypersensitivity.** Hypersensitivity reactions (e.g., anaphylaxis, bronchospasm, angioedema, stridor) have been reported with cangrelor therapy. (See Cautions: Contraindications.)

Specific Populations **Pregnancy.** Category C. (See Users Guide.) There are no adequate and well-controlled studies of cangrelor in pregnant women. Cangrelor did not produce malformations in rat or rabbit reproduction studies and is not considered to be a teratogen. In embryofetal development studies in animals, cangrelor produced dose-related fetal growth retardation in rats at plasma concentrations approximately 5 times lower than those achieved during percutaneous coronary intervention (PCI) at the maximum recommended human dose; in addition, the drug increased incidences of abortion and intrauterine losses in rabbits at plasma concentrations approximately 12 times higher than those achieved during PCI at the maximum recommended human dose.

Lactation. It is not known whether cangrelor is distributed into human milk. Because of the potential for serious adverse reactions to cangrelor in nursing infants, a decision should be made whether to discontinue nursing or the drug, taking into account the importance of the drug to the woman.

Pediatric Use. Safety and efficacy of cangrelor have not been established in pediatric patients.

Geriatric Use. In the CHAMPION PHOENIX trial, 18% of the patients were 75 years of age or older. No overall differences in safety or efficacy were observed between these patients and those younger than 75 years of age.

Renal Impairment. Although dosage adjustment is not required because of renal impairment (see Renal Impairment under Dosage and Administration: Special Populations), worsening renal function has been reported in some patients with existing severe renal impairment (creatinine clearance less than 30 mL/minute) who received cangrelor in clinical trials.

Hepatic Impairment. Safety and efficacy of cangrelor have not been established in patients with hepatic impairment. However, hepatic impairment is not expected to affect the pharmacokinetics of the drug because the metabolism of cangrelor is not dependent on hepatic function.

■ **Common Adverse Effects** The most common adverse effect of cangrelor reported in clinical trials was bleeding. Cases of transient dyspnea were also reported during clinical trials.

Drug Interactions

■ **Drugs Metabolized by Hepatic Microsomal Enzymes** In vitro studies suggest that neither cangrelor tetrasodium nor its major metabolites inhibit activity of the hepatic cytochrome P-450 (CYP) isoenzymes at therapeutic concentrations. Therefore, cangrelor is not expected to interact with drugs metabolized by these microsomal enzymes.

■ **Aspirin** Concomitant administration of cangrelor and aspirin in healthy individuals did not substantially affect the pharmacokinetics or pharmacodynamics of cangrelor.

■ **Nitroglycerin** Concomitant administration of cangrelor and nitroglycerin in healthy individuals did not substantially affect the pharmacokinetics or pharmacodynamics of cangrelor.

■ **Ticagrelor** The antiplatelet effect of a ticagrelor loading dose was not altered substantially when ticagrelor was administered during cangrelor infusion. No interaction was observed between ticagrelor and cangrelor because of the longer half-life of ticagrelor.

■ **Thienopyridine Antiplatelet Agents** Concomitant administration of cangrelor with the thienopyridine antiplatelet drugs clopidogrel or prasugrel decreases the antiplatelet effect of clopidogrel and prasugrel by blocking P2Y12-receptor binding of the active metabolites of these drugs. Oral maintenance antiplatelet therapy with clopidogrel or prasugrel should not be administered until the cangrelor infusion has been discontinued.

■ **Other Antiplatelet or Antithrombotic Agents** Concomitant administration of cangrelor and unfractionated heparin did not substantially affect the pharmacokinetics or pharmacodynamics of cangrelor. In clinical trials, cangrelor has been administered concomitantly with bivalirudin and low molecular weight heparin without clinically detectable interactions.

Description

Cangrelor tetrasodium is a nonthienopyridine, direct-acting, P2Y12 platelet adenosine diphosphate (ADP)-receptor antagonist. Unlike the thienopyridine prodrugs clopidogrel and prasugrel but like ticagrelor, cangrelor does not require hepatic transformation to exert its pharmacologic effects. Cangrelor, like ticagrelor, binds reversibly to the P2Y12 platelet ADP receptor, preventing signal transduction of the cyclic adenosine monophosphate (cAMP) pathway. This action results in reduced exposure of fibrinogen binding sites to the platelet glycoprotein IIb/IIIa complex and subsequent inhibition of platelet activation and aggregation.

After administration of a 30-mcg/kg IV loading dose followed by a 4-mcg/kg per minute IV infusion, peak plasma concentrations of cangrelor are reached within 2 minutes. Unlike clopidogrel, cangrelor does not require metabolic activation and as a result is not associated with interindividual variability in plasma concentrations. Cangrelor is deactivated rapidly in circulation by dephosphorylation to its primary metabolite, a nucleoside, which has negligible antiplatelet activity. Cangrelor is eliminated principally in urine (58% of the dose) and to a lesser extent in feces (35%). Because of its short half-life (3–6 minutes) and reversible binding to the P2Y12 receptor, cangrelor has a rapid offset of effect that allows recovery of platelet function within 1 hour after cessation of IV infusion.

Advice to Patients

Importance of women informing clinician if they are or plan to become pregnant or plan to breast-feed. Importance of informing clinician of existing or contemplated concomitant therapy, including prescription and OTC drugs, as well as any concomitant diseases. Importance of informing patients of other important precautionary information. (See Cautions.)

Overview® (see Users Guide). For additional information until a more detailed monograph is developed and published, the manufacturer's labeling should be consulted. It is *essential* that the manufacturer's labeling be consulted for more detailed information on usual cautions, precautions, contraindications, potential drug interactions, laboratory test interferences, and acute toxicity.

Preparations

Excipients in commercially available drug preparations may have clinically important effects in some individuals; consult specific product labeling for details.

Cangrelor Tetrasodium

Parenteral

For injection, for IV use	50 mg (of cangrelor)	**Kengreal®**, Medicines Company

Clopidogrel Bisulfate

■ Clopidogrel bisulfate, a thienopyridine P2Y12 platelet adenosine diphosphate (ADP)-receptor antagonist, is a platelet-aggregation inhibitor.

REMS

FDA approved a REMS for clopidogrel to ensure that the benefits outweigh the risks. However, FDA later rescinded REMS requirements. See the FDA REMS page (https://www.accessdata.fda.gov/scripts/cder/rems/index.cfm).

Uses

■ Reduction of Cardiovascular and Cerebrovascular Events

Clopidogrel bisulfate is used to reduce the risk of cardiovascular or cerebrovascular events (myocardial infarction [MI], stroke, and vascular death) in patients with atherosclerosis documented by recent ischemic stroke, recent MI, or established peripheral arterial disease (secondary prevention). Results of a large, randomized study (Clopidogrel versus Aspirin in Patients at Risk of Ischemic Events [CAPRIE] study) suggest that clopidogrel is more effective than aspirin in reducing the risk of such cardiovascular or cerebrovascular events and has a similar overall safety profile. However, because of cost considerations, many clinicians state that aspirin should remain the drug of choice for most patients requiring long-term antiplatelet therapy for coronary artery disease, and recommend clopidogrel as an alternative in those who are unable to take aspirin because of intolerance or contraindications (e.g., allergy).

The American College of Chest Physicians (ACCP) recommends long-term antiplatelet therapy with either aspirin (75–100 mg daily) or clopidogrel (75 mg daily) in patients with established coronary artery disease (i.e., patients more than 1 year after an acute coronary syndrome (ACS), with prior revascularization, coronary stenosis greater than 50% by coronary angiogram, and/or evidence of cardiac ischemia on diagnostic testing). Long-term antiplatelet therapy also is recommended for the secondary prevention of stroke in patients with a history of noncardioembolic stroke or transient ischemic attacks (TIAs). In such patients, ACCP states that clopidogrel, aspirin, aspirin in combination with extended-release dipyridamole, or cilostazol are all acceptable options for long-term antithrombotic therapy. Based on a somewhat greater risk reduction for stroke, ACCP states that clopidogrel or the combination of aspirin with dipyridamole may be preferred over the other options for secondary prevention of noncardioembolic stroke; however, ACCP judges the evidence supporting this recommendation to be moderate in quality. Oral anticoagulation (e.g., warfarin, dabigatran) rather than antiplatelet therapy is recommended for the secondary prevention of cardioembolic stroke in patients with a history of ischemic stroke or TIA and concurrent atrial fibrillation; however, in patients who cannot or choose not to take oral anticoagulants (e.g., those with difficulty maintaining stable international normalized ratios [INRs], compliance issues, dietary restrictions, cost limitations), dual antiplatelet therapy with clopidogrel and aspirin is recommended.

ACCP and other experts also recommend antiplatelet therapy for the prevention of cardiovascular events and mortality in patients with peripheral arterial disease. Aspirin generally is suggested as the antiplatelet drug of choice for primary prophylaxis in patients with asymptomatic peripheral arterial disease. For the secondary prevention of cardiovascular events in patients with symptomatic peripheral arterial disease, including those with intermittent claudication, critical limb ischemia, or prior lower extremity procedures (e.g., peripheral artery percutaneous transluminal angioplasty, peripheral artery bypass graft surgery, amputation), long-term treatment with clopidogrel 75 mg daily or aspirin 75–100 mg daily is recommended; the addition of cilostazol may be considered in patients with refractory intermittent claudication. Dual antiplatelet therapy with clopidogrel and aspirin generally is not suggested in any of these patients with the exception of those receiving below-the-knee prosthetic bypass grafts. Clopidogrel also is recommended as an option for long-term antiplatelet therapy in patients with symptomatic carotid stenosis†, including in patients who are intolerant of aspirin and those who have undergone recent carotid endarterectomy.

Efficacy of clopidogrel for reduction of the risk of atherosclerotic events has been established in a multicenter, randomized, controlled study (the CAPRIE trial) in patients with atherosclerotic disease (recent [within 6 months] ischemic stroke, recent [within 35 days] MI, or symptomatic peripheral arterial disease) who received clopidogrel 75 mg once daily or aspirin 325 mg daily for an average of 1.6 years (maximum 3 years). The primary analysis of efficacy was based on the first occurrence of a new cardiovascular event (i.e., fatal or nonfatal ischemic stroke or MI, other vascular death) in all patients receiving clopidogrel or aspirin. The annual cardiovascular event rate in patients receiving clopidogrel was 5.32% compared with 5.83% in those receiving aspirin, representing an 8.7% decrease in the annual risk of a new cardiovascular event for clopidogrel-treated patients. The difference in overall risk of cardiovascular events was apparent early in the study and was maintained throughout the 3-year follow-up period. While the study was not designed to evaluate relative benefit of clopidogrel versus aspirin among patients in specific disease subgroups, most of the risk reduction associated with clopidogrel therapy occurred in patients with peripheral arterial disease, who experienced a statistically significant 23.8% decrease in risk compared with those in the same subgroup who received aspirin. Patients in the stroke subgroup who received clopidogrel experienced a relative risk reduction of 7.3%, while those in the MI subgroup experienced a relative risk reduction of −3.7% (*increased* relative risk compared with aspirin); neither of these relative-risk reductions was statistically significant.

Therapy with clopidogrel plus aspirin for prevention of ischemic events in a broad population of patients with established cardiovascular disease or multiple risk factors for atherosclerosis was evaluated in the CHARISMA (Clopidogrel for High Atherothrombotic Risk and Ischemic Stabilization, Management, and Avoidance) trial. In this large, randomized, double-blind, parallel-group study, therapy with clopidogrel (75 mg daily) and low-dose aspirin (75–162 mg daily) for approximately 2 years was not significantly more effective than low-dose aspirin alone in reducing the rate of the composite primary end point of MI, stroke, or death from cardiovascular causes. In addition, the combination of clopidogrel and aspirin was associated with an increased rate of moderate to severe bleeding.

■ Acute Coronary Syndromes Clopidogrel is used in combination with aspirin for the reduction of cardiovascular and cerebrovascular events in patients with non-ST-segment-elevation ACS (NSTE ACS), including unstable angina and non-ST-segment-elevation MI (NSTEMI). The drug is used in such patients who are to be managed medically or with coronary revascularization (percutaneous coronary intervention [PCI] with or without coronary artery stenting or coronary artery bypass grafting [CABG]). In patients in whom elective CABG is planned, it is recommended that clopidogrel be withheld for at least 5 days (the duration of effect of clopidogrel) since the drug, when added to aspirin treatment, increases the risk of bleeding during major surgery.

Clopidogrel also is used in combination with aspirin to reduce the rate of ischemic cardiovascular events (e.g., death, reinfarction, stroke) in patients with ST-segment-elevation MI (STEMI).

Dual-drug antiplatelet therapy with a P2Y12 platelet adenosine diphosphate (ADP)-receptor antagonist (e.g., clopidogrel, prasugrel, ticagrelor) and aspirin is part of the current standard of care in patients with ACS. The American Heart Association (AHA), the American College of Cardiology Foundation (ACCF), the Society for Cardiovascular Angiography and Interventions (SCAI), and ACCP recommend antiplatelet therapy with a P2Y12-receptor antagonist (clopidogrel, prasugrel, or ticagrelor) in conjunction with aspirin for treatment and secondary prevention in patients with ACS. These experts generally recommend ticagrelor or clopidogrel as the P2Y12-receptor antagonist in patients with ACS who are treated medically without stent placement; because prasugrel has been studied principally in patients undergoing planned percutaneous coronary intervention (PCI), recommendations for the use of this drug are restricted to that population. In patients being managed medically, therapy with a P2Y12-receptor antagonist should be continued for up to 12 months, while aspirin should be continued indefinitely. In patients undergoing PCI with stent placement (bare-metal or drug-eluting), a loading dose of ticagrelor, clopidogrel, or prasugrel is recommended, followed by maintenance therapy with one of these agents for at least 12 months (unless the risk of bleeding outweighs the anticipated net benefit of therapy); aspirin should be continued indefinitely in such patients. While current ACCF/AHA guidelines make no recommendations regarding the P2Y12-receptor antagonist of choice in patients with ACS, ACCP suggests the use of ticagrelor over clopidogrel, regardless of whether PCI is performed. When selecting an appropriate antiplatelet regimen for patients with ACS, clinicians should consider individual risks of ischemia and bleeding as well as the specific characteristics (e.g., adverse effects, drug interaction potential) of the drugs.

The efficacy of pretreatment with clopidogrel prior to diagnostic cardiac catheterization is controversial; while some studies have suggested a benefit in terms of decreased platelet aggregation and lower rates of periprocedural MI with clopidogrel pretreatment, other studies have found no such benefit. The potential benefit of pretreatment with clopidogrel should be balanced against the increased risk of bleeding should emergency CABG be needed. If clopidogrel is given at hospital admission or diagnosis of ACS and the patient is subsequently scheduled for CABG, the drug should be temporarily discontinued for at least 5 days prior to the procedure.

In patients with ACS who have indications for anticoagulation (e.g., atrial fibrillation, left ventricular dysfunction, cerebral emboli, extensive wall-motion abnormality, mechanical heart valves), the addition of warfarin (INR 2–3) to antiplatelet therapy is recommended; in some cases, triple antithrombotic therapy (warfarin, low-dose aspirin, and clopidogrel) is suggested. However, such triple-drug antithrombotic regimens† are associated with an increased risk of bleeding, and patients should be monitored closely. Triple antithrombotic therapy with clopidogrel, aspirin, and warfarin is suggested by ACCP in patients with anterior MI and left ventricular thrombus (or at high risk for such thrombi) undergoing stent implantation; the recommended duration of such triple therapy is dependent on whether the patient has a bare-metal or drug-eluting stent.

Non-ST-Segment-Elevation Acute Coronary Syndromes Patients with NSTE ACS have either unstable angina or NSTEMI; because these conditions are part of a continuum of acute myocardial ischemia and have indistinguishable clinical features upon presentation, the same initial treatment strategies are recommended. The American Heart Association/American College of Cardiology (AHA/ACC) guideline for the management of patients with NSTE ACS recommends an early invasive strategy (angiographic evaluation with the intent to perform revascularization procedures such as PCI with coronary artery stent implantation or CABG) or an ischemia-guided strategy (initial medical management followed by cardiac catheterization and revascularization if indicated) in patients with definite or likely NSTE ACS; standard medical therapies for all patients should include a β-adrenergic blocking agent (β-blocker), antiplatelet agents, anticoagulant agents, nitrates, and analgesic agents regardless of the initial management approach. Aspirin is the mainstay of antiplatelet therapy and should be administered as soon as possible after presentation in all patients with NSTE ACS unless contraindicated and continued indefinitely; in addition, a P2Y12-receptor antagonist (e.g., clopidogrel, ticagrelor) should be administered for up to 12 months.

Efficacy of clopidogrel for the long-term reduction of cardiovascular events in patients with NSTE ACS has been established in a randomized, controlled study (the Clopidogrel in Unstable Angina to Prevent Recurrent Ischemic Events [CURE] trial) in patients who received clopidogrel (75 mg once daily) or placebo in addition to aspirin (75–325 mg daily) and other standard therapy (e.g., heparin) for 3–12 months. Some evidence suggests that aspirin and clopidogrel may have synergistic antithrombotic effects related to their different mechanisms of action. In the CURE study, the combined incidence of cardiovascular death, nonfatal MI, or stroke, and the combined incidence of these 3 types of events plus refractory ischemia in the clopidogrel group were reduced compared with these outcomes in the placebo group. Clopidogrel therapy also was associated with reductions in the incidences of refractory or severe ischemia, heart failure, and (during the initial period of hospitalization) revascularization procedures. In this study, aspirin and clopidogrel or placebo were administered to patients within 24 hours of symptom onset and for 3–12 months (mean: 9 months) thereafter. Although no substantial increase in life-threatening bleeding episodes occurred with clopidogrel and aspirin therapy, major bleeding (principally GI hemorrhage and bleeding at recent arterial puncture sites) was more common in patients receiving clopidogrel and aspirin (3.7%) than in patients receiving aspirin and placebo (2.7%). While clopidogrel has been administered concomitantly with aspirin for up to 1 year in clinical studies, the manufacturer states that nonsteroidal anti-inflammatory agents (NSAIAs) should be used with caution in patients receiving clopidogrel. (See Drug Interactions: Nonsteroidal Anti-inflammatory Agents.)

ST-Segment-Elevation Myocardial Infarction The current standard of care in patients with STEMI is timely reperfusion (with primary PCI or thrombolytic therapy). Adjunctive therapy with anticoagulant (e.g., heparin) and antiplatelet (e.g., aspirin and clopidogrel) agents should be used during and after successful coronary artery reperfusion for the prevention of early reocclusion and death, unless contraindicated. Results of randomized, controlled studies indicate that clopidogrel produces reductions in mortality and vascular events beyond those of low-dose aspirin and other standard therapy (e.g., thrombolytic agents, heparin) in patients with acute STEMI, including those undergoing subsequent PCI. In patients taking clopidogrel in whom CABG is planned, ACCP suggests that the drug be withheld for at least 5 days prior to surgery. (See Managing Antiplatelet Therapy in Patients Requiring Invasive Procedures under Dosage and Administration: Dosage.)

In a randomized, controlled study in approximately 3500 patients with STEMI who were scheduled to receive therapy with a thrombolytic agent, unfractionated heparin or a low molecular weight heparin when appropriate, and aspirin (Clopidogrel as Adjunctive Reperfusion Therapy [CLARITY] study), addition of clopidogrel (300-mg loading dose followed by 75 mg once daily) was associated with a 36% reduction in the risk of the primary composite end point (occluded infarct-related artery at angiography 2–8 days later or death or recurrent MI prior to angiography); at 30 days, clopidogrel therapy had reduced the composite end point of cardiovascular death, recurrent MI, or recurrent ischemia requiring urgent revascularization by 20%. Rates of major bleeding, including intracranial hemorrhage, were similar with or without adjunctive clopidogrel therapy. In a prospective analysis of a subset of patients from the CLARITY study who underwent PCI after angiography (PCI-Clopidogrel as Adjunctive Reperfusion Therapy [CLARITY] study), pretreatment before PCI with clopidogrel (300-mg loading dose followed by 75 mg once daily) in addition to initial standard therapy (e.g., thrombolytic agents, aspirin) during hospitalization for acute STEMI was associated with a reduction of 38% in recurrent MI and stroke compared with standard therapy; considering cardiovascular events before and after PCI through 30 days after randomization in patients undergoing coronary artery stenting, adjunctive clopidogrel therapy reduced cardiovascular death, MI, and stroke by 41%.

In the Clopidogrel and Metoprolol in Myocardial Infarction Trial (COMMIT) in approximately 45,000 patients with acute STEMI, treatment with clopidogrel (75 mg once daily without a loading dose) in addition to aspirin (162 mg daily) beginning at hospital admission and continuing during hospitalization for up to 4 weeks (mean treatment duration: 14.9 days) was associated with a 9% reduction in death, reinfarction, or stroke (the primary composite end point) compared with aspirin therapy. In addition, death from any cause was reduced by 7%, and fatal or nonfatal reinfarction by 14%, in patients receiving adjunctive clopidogrel. Clopidogrel treatment was associated with a small increase in minor bleeding but no excess in major (i.e., transfused, cerebral, or fatal) bleeding complications.

In patients with STEMI who have undergone diagnostic cardiac catheterization and in whom PCI is planned†, experts recommend a loading dose of a P2Y12-receptor antagonist (e.g., clopidogrel, prasugrel, ticagrelor) before or at the time of PCI in conjunction with aspirin therapy. Therapy with a P2Y12-receptor antagonist should be continued for at least 12 months after stent (bare-metal or drug-eluting) placement, unless the risk of bleeding outweighs the anticipated net benefit of therapy; aspirin should be continued indefinitely in such patients. Clopidogrel also has been used in patients with STEMI who are receiving delayed PCI after receiving a thrombolytic agent.

The American Diabetes Association (ADA) suggests that clopidogrel may be used for prevention of a first MI (*primary prevention*†) as an alternative to aspirin in aspirin-allergic patients with type 1 or type 2 diabetes mellitus who are at high risk for cardiovascular events (i.e., family history of CHD, smoking, hypertension, obesity, albuminuria, elevated blood cholesterol or triglyceride concentrations).

■ **Prevention of Stent Thrombosis** Clopidogrel has been used in combination with aspirin (dual-drug therapy) to prevent stent thrombosis following implantation of coronary artery stents†.

Compared with bare-metal stents, implantation of drug-eluting stents has been associated with a reduction in the frequency of restenosis and repeat revascularization without evidence of excess MI or death in randomized controlled trials evaluated for US Food and Drug Administration (FDA) approval of these stents (in clinically stable patients without other serious medical conditions who had newly diagnosed coronary lesions less than 28–30 mm in length). Previous recommendations based on clinical trials in such patients advised dual-drug therapy with aspirin and a thienopyridine derivative (i.e., clopidogrel, ticlopidine) for at least 3 or 6 months following implantation of a sirolimus- or paclitaxel-eluting stent, respectively. However, with expanded use of drug-eluting stents to include patients with high-risk coronary lesions and coexisting medical conditions (e.g., diabetes, renal dysfunction), an increase in the incidence of late (e.g., 1–12 months or more post-implantation) stent thrombosis has been noted in patients with drug-eluting stents compared with bare-metal stents, often coincident with discontinuance of clopidogrel after initially recommended durations of dual-drug antiplatelet therapy.

Conflicting data have been reported regarding the risks of cardiovascular events in patients receiving drug-eluting stents, which may be related to variable definitions of stent thrombosis and differences in patient characteristics and coronary lesions in the populations studied. Some observational studies have indicated an increased risk of late cardiovascular events (e.g., death or death and MI) in patients with drug-eluting stents following discontinuance of dual-drug antiplatelet therapy with aspirin and clopidogrel, or just the clopidogrel component of such therapy. In a study in patients who had stopped taking clopidogrel (75 mg once daily) after 6 months but continued low-dose aspirin therapy (100 mg daily) and were without major adverse events 6 months after stent placement, the incidence of late cardiac events (defined as cardiac death or documented nonfatal MI in months 7–18 of follow-up) was higher in patients with drug-eluting stents versus bare-metal stents (4.9 versus 1.3% of patients, respectively). Thrombosis-related events, including late stent thrombosis and death related to stent thrombosis or target-vessel MI, were twice as frequent in patients with drug-eluting stents versus bare-metal stents (2.6 versus 1.3%, respectively). Overall rates of cardiac death and nonfatal MI during the entire 18-month follow-up period (6 months of clopidogrel therapy and 1 year of subsequent aspirin therapy) were not different in patients with either type of stent. Target vessel revascularizations related to restenosis were less frequent in patients with drug-eluting stents. In another observational study, patients with drug-eluting stents who were event-free (no death, MI, or revascularization) and who reported continued clopidogrel use at 6 or 12 months after stent implantation had lower rates of death, nonfatal MI, or the combined end point of death or MI at 24 months' follow-up than patients with drug-eluting stents who did not report continued use of clopidogrel. In contrast, rates of these cardiac events at 24 months in patients with bare-metal stents were similar regardless of reported clopidogrel use. A subgroup analysis by reported aspirin use did not alter the effect of clopidogrel on cumulative rates of death or combined death or MI in patients with drug-eluting stents except that event rates were lower.

A pooled analysis of data from a large patient records database in Sweden covering 3 years of follow-up revealed an increased rate of death beginning 6 months after stent implantation in patients with drug-eluting stents compared with bare-metal stents. An increase of 18% in the relative long-term risk of death was found in patients with drug-eluting stents at 3 years, corresponding to an absolute increase in the risk of death of 0.5% per year after the initial 6 months. However, results of 2 pooled analyses of data from randomized controlled trials that served as the basis for approval of drug-eluting stents in the US indicate a similar incidence of death or MI over long-term follow-up (4 years) in patients with sirolimus- or paclitaxel-eluting stents compared with bare-metal stents. Another pooled analysis of data from 14 randomized trials that included patients with high-risk features (e.g., diabetes, prior MI, long or complex coronary lesions) who received sirolimus-eluting or bare-metal stents also found similar outcomes with respect to the risk of death or the combined risk of death or MI. While the overall incidence of stent thrombosis was not increased with sirolimus-eluting versus bare-metal stents over the entire period of follow-up (approximately 1–5 years) in this analysis, the risk of stent thrombosis was greater with the drug-eluting stents after the first year following stent implantation (0.6 or 0.05% with the sirolimus-eluting or bare-metal stent, respectively), which coincided with the protocol-specified discontinuance of dual-drug antiplatelet therapy in these trials.

Because of evidence suggesting an increased incidence of late stent thrombosis and cardiovascular events (e.g., cardiac death, nonfatal MI) in patients with drug-eluting stents following discontinuance of dual-drug antiplatelet therapy with aspirin and clopidogrel, or just the clopidogrel component of such therapy, a broad range of experts recommend that patients who have undergone placement of a drug-eluting stent and who are not at high risk for bleeding receive clopidogrel for at least 12 months in conjunction with low-dose aspirin therapy. Current expert guidelines recommend a treatment duration of at least 12 months for patients with any type of coronary artery stent (bare-metal or drug-eluting). While a minimum duration of therapy of 1 month may be acceptable in patients receiving a bare-metal stent for a non-ACS indication, clopidogrel should ideally be given up to 12 months for these patients as well unless the patient is at increased risk of bleeding; in such a case, clopidogrel should be administered for a minimum of 2 weeks. There is some evidence suggesting that an even longer duration of dual antiplatelet therapy (for more than 12 months) may be beneficial in some patients with drug-eluting stents to reduce the risk of late stent thrombosis and other cardiovascular events, but such prolonged therapy may be associated with an increased risk of bleeding.

In a randomized, placebo-controlled, double-blind study (Dual Antiplatelet Therapy [DAPT] study), patients who received 30 months of dual antiplatelet therapy (aspirin plus clopidogrel or prasugrel) following placement of a drug-eluting stent had substantially reduced rates of stent thrombosis and major adverse cardiovascular and cerebrovascular events compared with those who received 12 months of dual antiplatelet therapy. Preliminary data from the study indicated that a longer duration of therapy was associated with a higher incidence of moderate to severe bleeding and also an unexpected finding of an increased rate of noncardiovascular mortality (principally related to trauma or cancer); however, these adverse mortality findings were not observed during FDA's final review of the DAPT study and other randomized, controlled clinical studies. FDA review of the DAPT study and additional long-term studies of clopidogrel, including meta-analyses conducted by FDA, concluded that there is no evidence of either a harmful or beneficial effect of clopidogrel on all-cause mortality or cancer-related deaths in a population with, or at risk for, coronary artery disease. The results of the FDA-conducted meta-analyses indicated that long-term (12 months or longer) dual antiplatelet therapy with clopidogrel and aspirin does not appear to change the overall risk of death when compared to short-term (6 months or less) clopidogrel and aspirin therapy, or aspirin alone. Additionally, there was no apparent increase in the risks of cancer-related deaths or cancer-related adverse effects with such long-term treatment.

Because of the potentially life-threatening consequences of premature discontinuance of dual-drug antiplatelet therapy in patients with drug-eluting stents, AHA/ACC/SCAI, the American College of Surgeons, and the American Dental Association currently state that implantation of a drug-eluting stent should be performed only in patients who can tolerate and are highly likely to comply with such prolonged combination therapy. For management of patients with coronary stents who require additional invasive procedures, see Managing Antiplatelet Therapy in Patients Requiring Invasive Procedures, under Dosage and Administration: Dosage.

■ **Chronic Stable Angina** Clopidogrel may be used as an alternative to aspirin in patients with symptomatic chronic stable angina† who cannot tolerate aspirin. In certain high-risk patients, combination therapy with aspirin and clopidogrel may be beneficial.

■ **Embolism Associated with Atrial Fibrillation and/or Valvular Heart Disease** Clopidogrel has been used in combination with aspirin as an alternative to warfarin anticoagulation for the prevention of stroke and systemic embolism in patients with atrial fibrillation†. Dual antiplatelet therapy with clopidogrel and aspirin was evaluated as a potential alternative to warfarin in a randomized controlled study in patients with atrial fibrillation at high risk of stroke. The study was terminated early because of clear evidence of superiority of warfarin over antiplatelet therapy for the primary outcome of stroke, systemic embolism, MI, or vascular death. Results of another study comparing dual antiplatelet therapy (clopidogrel and aspirin) with aspirin monotherapy in patients with atrial fibrillation who had an increased risk of stroke but were unable to take warfarin showed that the combination of clopidogrel and aspirin was more effective than aspirin in reducing the risk of stroke; however, dual antiplatelet therapy was also associated with an increased risk of bleeding. Based on these findings, ACCP and other experts recommend the use of clopidogrel and aspirin rather than aspirin alone as an alternative to oral anticoagulation in patients with atrial fibrillation at increased risk of stroke who cannot or choose not to take oral anticoagulants for reasons other than concerns about major bleeding (e.g., those with difficulty maintaining stable INRs, compliance issues, dietary restrictions, cost limitations). Because the risk of bleeding with combination aspirin and clopidogrel therapy is similar to the risk of bleeding with warfarin, such combination therapy is not recommended in patients with a hemorrhagic contraindication to warfarin.

In patients with atrial fibrillation and mitral stenosis† who cannot or choose not to take warfarin therapy (for reasons other than concerns about major bleeding), ACCP recommends combination therapy with aspirin and clopidogrel rather than aspirin alone.

While the risk of thromboembolism in patients with atrial flutter is not as well established as it is in those with atrial fibrillation, the risk has been estimated to be less than that for atrial fibrillation but greater than that for sinus rhythm. In addition, many patients with atrial flutter have alternating periods of atrial fibrillation. Experts state that antithrombotic therapy in patients with atrial flutter generally should be managed in the same manner as in patients with atrial fibrillation.

Dosage and Administration

■ **Administration** Clopidogrel bisulfate is administered orally. Food does not affect systemic exposure to the active metabolite of clopidogrel, and the drug may be administered without regard to meals. Dosage of clopidogrel bisulfate is expressed in terms of clopidogrel.

■ **Dosage** Pharmacogenomic factors can influence response to clopidogrel; the manufacturer states that an appropriate dosage of clopidogrel has not been determined in patients who are poor metabolizers based on their cytochrome P-450 (CYP) 2C19 genotype and who may have a diminished response to the drug because of reduced formation of the active metabolite. (See Reduced Efficacy Associated with Impaired CYP2C19 Function under Warnings/Precautions: Warnings, in Cautions.)

Reduction of Cardiovascular and Cerebrovascular Events In patients with established peripheral arterial disease or a history of recent myocardial infarction (MI) or stroke, the recommended dosage of clopidogrel for reducing the risk of fatal or nonfatal MI, stroke, or vascular death in adults is 75 mg once daily.

Acute Coronary Syndromes **Non-ST-Segment-Elevation Acute Coronary Syndromes.** In patients with non-ST-segment-elevation acute coronary syndromes (NSTE ACS), an initial loading dose of 300 mg of clopidogrel is recommended by the manufacturer, followed by 75 mg once daily given concomitantly with aspirin.

Although the optimal loading dose of clopidogrel in patients with NSTE ACS undergoing percutaneous coronary intervention (PCI) is uncertain, some experts suggest a loading dose of 600 mg, administered as early as possible prior to or at the time of the procedure in conjunction with aspirin; clopidogrel should then be continued at a maintenance dosage of 75 mg once daily for at least 12 months. There appears to be no benefit in increasing the clopidogrel loading dose to 900 mg in patients undergoing PCI. The manufacturer states that the optimal duration of clopidogrel therapy in patients with ACS is unknown; experts recommend that clopidogrel be administered for up to 12 months in patients with NSTE ACS being managed medically, and for at least 12 months in those undergoing PCI with coronary artery stent placement; aspirin should be continued indefinitely.

In patients who have indications for anticoagulation (e.g., atrial fibrillation, anterior MI and left ventricular thrombus or at high risk for left ventricular thrombosis), the addition of warfarin (international normalized ratio [INR] 2–

3) to antiplatelet therapy is recommended by some experts during the period of greatest risk.

For information on the dosage of aspirin used as adjunctive antithrombotic therapy in the management of NSTE ACS, see Non-ST-Segment-Elevation Acute Coronary Syndromes under Dosage: Thrombosis, in Dosage and Administration in Aspirin 28:08.04.24.

ST-Segment-Elevation Myocardial Infarction. In patients with acute ST-segment-elevation MI (STEMI), the manufacturer recommends a clopidogrel dosage of 75 mg once daily in conjunction with aspirin. The manufacturer states that clopidogrel may be initiated with or without a loading dose in patients with STEMI.

In patients with STEMI who are receiving thrombolytic therapy (e.g., alteplase), experts recommend a clopidogrel loading dose of 300 mg in patients 75 years of age or younger; a loading dose is not recommended in patients older than 75 years of age. Clopidogrel therapy should be initiated prior to or with the thrombolytic agent and continued for at least 14 days and up to 1 year at a maintenance dosage of 75 mg daily.

In patients with STEMI who will undergo primary PCI†, a clopidogrel loading dose of 600 mg, administered as soon as possible before or at the time of PCI, is recommended; therapy should be continued with a maintenance dosage of 75 mg daily. A higher loading dose of 900 mg does not appear to provide additional benefit in patients undergoing PCI. Patients undergoing delayed PCI after initial thrombolytic therapy should continue to receive a clopidogrel maintenance dosage of 75 mg daily if a loading dose was previously administered with thrombolytic therapy; if a loading dose was not previously administered, a loading dose of 300 or 600 mg (depending on the timing of PCI in relation to thrombolytic therapy) is recommended.

The manufacturer states that the optimal duration of clopidogrel therapy in patients with ACS is unknown. In general, dual antiplatelet therapy (e.g., clopidogrel and aspirin) should be continued for up to 12 months following ACS, and possibly longer in patients undergoing PCI with stent placement.

In patients who have indications for anticoagulation (e.g., atrial fibrillation, anterior MI and left ventricular thrombus or at high risk for left ventricular thrombosis), the addition of warfarin (INR 2–3) is recommended by some experts during the period of greatest risk.

For information on the dosage of aspirin used as adjunctive antithrombotic therapy in the management of STEMI, see Coronary Artery Disease and Myocardial Infarction under Dosage: Thrombosis, in Dosage and Administration in Aspirin 28:08.04.24.

Managing Antiplatelet Therapy in Patients Requiring Invasive Procedures The American College of Chest Physicians (ACCP) states that the decision to interrupt antiplatelet therapy prior to surgery or other invasive procedures should be individualized based on assessment of the patient's risks of thromboembolism and perioperative bleeding. The possible increased risk of stent thrombosis also should be considered when making decisions regarding the perioperative management of patients with coronary artery stents. (See Risks of Discontinuance of Therapy under Warnings/Precautions: Other Warnings and Precautions, in Cautions.)

Antiplatelet agents generally should be discontinued prior to surgery or other invasive procedures to minimize the risk of perioperative bleeding. The manufacturer states that in patients requiring an invasive procedure in whom an antiplatelet effect is not desired, clopidogrel should be temporarily discontinued 5 days prior to the procedure and resumed as soon as possible.

In patients receiving dual antiplatelet therapy (e.g., aspirin and clopidogrel) who require coronary artery bypass grafting (CABG), interruption of clopidogrel therapy is recommended at least 5 days prior to surgery. However, aspirin generally should be continued around the time of surgery in such patients.

In patients receiving dual antiplatelet therapy (e.g., aspirin and clopidogrel) who require surgery within 6 weeks of bare-metal stent implantation or within 6 months of drug-eluting stent implantation, ACCP suggests continuation of dual antiplatelet therapy in the periprocedural period. If therapy with clopidogrel is interrupted prior to nonelective major surgery to reduce the risk of excessive bleeding, the American College of Cardiology (ACC)/American Heart Association (AHA)/Society for Cardiovascular Angiography and Interventions (SCAI) recommends that aspirin be continued if at all possible and clopidogrel be restarted as soon as possible after the procedure because of concerns about late stent thrombosis.

■ **Special Populations** No dosage adjustments are necessary in geriatric patients or in those with hepatic impairment.

Cautions

■ **Contraindications** Known hypersensitivity to clopidogrel or any ingredient in the formulation. Presence of active pathological bleeding (e.g., peptic ulcer, intracranial hemorrhage).

■ **Warnings/Precautions** ***Warnings*** **Reduced Efficacy Associated with Impaired CYP2C19 Function.** Clopidogrel is a prodrug that requires activation by the cytochrome P-450 (CYP) enzyme system to produce its pharmacologically active metabolite. (See Description.) Production of the active metabolite and response to clopidogrel may be reduced by genetic polymorphism of CYP2C19, one of the key enzymes involved in the metabolic activation of clopidogrel, or concurrent use of drugs (e.g., omeprazole, esomeprazole) that inhibit CYP2C19. Use of alternative clopidogrel dosing strategies or other antiplatelet therapy options (e.g., prasugrel, ticagrelor) should be considered in patients who are identified as potential poor metabolizers of CYP2C19.

Specific variant alleles of CYP2C19 (e.g., CYP2C19*2, CYP2C19*3) have been associated with reduced metabolism of and diminished antiplatelet response to clopidogrel; while data on clinical outcomes are conflicting, higher rates of major adverse cardiovascular events (e.g., death, myocardial infarction, stroke, stent thrombosis) have been reported in patients receiving recommended dosages of clopidogrel who possess such variant alleles compared with those who have normal CYP2C19 activity. (See Description.) The impact of CYP2C19 metabolizer status on the pharmacokinetic and antiplatelet response to clopidogrel was evaluated in a randomized, crossover study in healthy individuals. Individuals were classified into one of 4 groups according to their CYP2C19 metabolizer phenotype (ultrarapid, extensive, intermediate, or poor metabolizer). Individuals in each group received either a 300-mg loading dose of clopidogrel followed by 75 mg daily or a 600-mg loading dose followed by 150 mg daily, with crossover to the alternate clopidogrel regimen after 5 days. Exposure to the active metabolite of clopidogrel was decreased and inhibition of platelet response was diminished in poor metabolizers compared with the other CYP2C19 metabolizer groups. When poor metabolizers received the higher-dose regimen of clopidogrel (600 mg loading dose followed by 150 mg daily), active metabolite exposure and antiplatelet response increased relative to that with the lower-dose regimen. Retrospective analyses of clopidogrel-treated patients from 2 large randomized, controlled studies (The Clopidogrel for High Atherothrombotic Risk and Ischemic Stabilization, Management, and Avoidance [CHARISMA] trial and Trial to Assess Improvement with Prasugrel-Thrombolysis in Myocardial Infarction [TRITON-TIMI 38]) and several published cohort studies have shown higher rates of adverse cardiovascular events (death, myocardial infarction, stroke) or stent thrombosis in patients with impaired CYP2C19 metabolizer status (intermediate or poor) compared with that in extensive metabolizers.

Genetic tests are available to identify a patient's CYP2C19 genotype and can be used to help individualize and optimize clopidogrel therapy. While such tests are considered appropriate for patients currently receiving or considering treatment with clopidogrel, ACCF/AHA states that the predictive value of pharmacogenomic testing is very limited at this time and the need for pharmacogenetic testing should be determined on an individual basis. Management options in patients who are identified as poor metabolizers of CYP2C19 include the use of higher dosages of clopidogrel or the use of alternative P2Y12 receptor antagonists (e.g., prasugrel, ticagrelor) that have not been shown to be affected by CYP2C19 genetic polymorphism; however, ACCF/AHA states that the relative efficacy and safety of these alternative treatment strategies remains to be determined. Although preliminary data indicate that higher initial and maintenance clopidogrel dosages (e.g., 600-mg loading dose followed by 150 mg daily) or administration of additional loading doses may improve the antiplatelet response in poor metabolizers, the manufacturer states that the appropriate dosage of clopidogrel in such patients has not been established in clinical outcome trials. When considering the use of alternative antiplatelet agents, clinicians should balance the anticipated greater benefits of these agents against the possible increased risk of bleeding, and also consider the patient populations in whom the drugs have been used.

Concurrent use of clopidogrel and omeprazole, a potent inhibitor of CYP2C19, also has been shown to reduce the antiplatelet effects of clopidogrel. Although the clinical importance of this interaction has not been fully elucidated, some evidence suggests that concurrent use of clopidogrel and omeprazole may result in reduced efficacy of clopidogrel in preventing cardiovascular events. A similar reduction in antiplatelet activity has been observed when esomeprazole was used concurrently with clopidogrel. Concomitant use of other drugs that inhibit CYP2C19 also may decrease the response to clopidogrel. (See Drug Interactions: Drugs Affecting or Metabolized by Hepatic Microsomal Enzymes.)

Other genetic variants of CYP isoenzymes (e.g., CYP2C19*17, CYP2B6) also may affect response to clopidogrel.

Other Warnings and Precautions **Bleeding.** Clopidogrel increases the risk of bleeding. The drug should be discontinued at least 5 days prior to surgery or coronary artery bypass grafting (CABG), if antiplatelet effect is undesirable. (See Managing Antiplatelet Therapy in Patients Requiring Invasive Procedures under Dosage and Administration: Dosage.) If bleeding occurs, hemostasis may be restored with exogenous administration of platelets; however, platelet transfusions within 4 hours of a loading dose of clopidogrel or within 2 hours of a maintenance dose may have reduced effectiveness. Withholding a dose is unlikely to resolve a bleeding episode or prevent bleeding associated with an invasive procedure because of clopidogrel's prolonged effects on platelet inhibition.

In patients with transient ischemic attacks (TIAs) or stroke who are at high risk for recurrent ischemic events, the combination of clopidogrel and aspirin has *not* been shown to be more effective than clopidogrel alone but has been associated with an increase in major bleeding.

Thienopyridines do not appear to cause GI ulcers or erosions, but their antiplatelet effects may promote bleeding at the site of preexisting lesions associated with use of aspirin or nonsteroidal anti-inflammatory agents or *H. pylori* infection. Current ACCF/ACG/AHA guidelines recommend prophylactic use of a proton-pump inhibitor to reduce the risk of ulcer complications and GI bleeding in patients receiving clopidogrel and aspirin therapy who have additional GI risk factors. However, the possibility of reduced antiplatelet effects should be considered when clopidogrel is used concomitantly with a proton-pump inhibitor (e.g., omeprazole, esomeprazole). (See Drug Interactions: Proton-Pump Inhibitors.)

Risks of Premature Discontinuance of Therapy. In general, treatment with a thienopyridine derivative should not be discontinued prematurely because of the increased risk of cardiovascular events. If clopidogrel must be temporarily discontinued (e.g., prior to surgery), therapy should be reinitated as soon as possible. Patients should be advised to *never* stop clopidogrel therapy without first consulting the prescribing clinician. Prior to scheduling an invasive procedure, patients should inform their clinicians (including dentists) that they are currently taking clopidogrel, and clinicians performing the invasive procedure should consult with the prescribing clinician before advising patients to discontinue therapy.

Premature discontinuance of dual-drug antiplatelet therapy with a thienopyridine derivative (e.g., clopidogrel, prasugrel) and aspirin in patients with coronary artery stents, particularly discontinuance of clopidogrel therapy in patients with drug-eluting stents, has been associated with stent thrombosis, often leading to myocardial infarction (MI) and/or death. (See Uses: Prevention of Stent Thrombosis.) Before implantation of a drug-eluting stent, patients should be carefully assessed regarding the likelihood of compliance with prolonged (e.g., at least 12 months) dual-drug antiplatelet therapy (i.e., aspirin and a thienopyridine derivative); strong consideration should be given to avoiding use of a drug-eluting stent in patients who are not expected to comply. In addition, patients should be educated before discharge about the reasons they have been prescribed the drugs and the substantial risks associated with premature discontinuance of dual-drug antiplatelet therapy. Superficial or "nuisance" bleeding is common in patients receiving dual-drug antiplatelet therapy after drug-eluting stent implantation and may be a reason for premature discontinuation of clopidogrel. In a single-center observational study in 2360 patients who underwent drug-eluting stent implantation, 11.1% of patients who were receiving dual-drug antiplatelet therapy discontinued clopidogrel prematurely as a result of superficial bleeding. The American College of Cardiology Foundation/American College of Gastroenterology/American Heart Association (ACCF/ACG/AHA) states that concomitant use of proton-pump inhibitors may reduce GI symptoms (e.g., dyspepsia) associated with antiplatelet agents and thereby prevent patients from discontinuing their antiplatelet treatment. (See Drug Interactions: Proton-Pump Inhibitors.) Patients should be advised to *never* stop taking dual-drug antiplatelet therapy without first consulting with their cardiologist, even if instructed to do so by another health-care professional (e.g., dentist). In patients who are likely to require invasive or surgical procedures within 12 months of drug-eluting stent implantation, implantation of a bare-metal stent or balloon angioplasty with provisional stent placement should be considered instead.

Health-care professionals who perform invasive or surgical procedures and are concerned about periprocedural or postprocedural bleeding must understand the potentially catastrophic consequences of premature discontinuance of thienopyridine derivative (i.e., clopidogrel, ticlopidine) therapy in patients with drug-eluting stents. If issues about a patient's antiplatelet therapy are unclear, such professionals should contact the patient's cardiologist to discuss optimal patient management. Elective procedures with substantial bleeding risk should be deferred until 12 months of dual-drug antiplatelet therapy has been completed. For non-elective procedures that mandate discontinuance of thienopyridine-derivative therapy, aspirin should be continued if at all possible and the thienopyridine derivative (i.e., clopidogrel, ticlopidine) restarted as soon as possible after the procedure because of concerns about late stent thrombosis.

Thrombotic Thrombocytopenic Purpura. Thrombotic thrombocytopenic purpura (TTP) has been reported rarely with clopidogrel, sometimes after short exposure (less than 2 weeks) to the drug. TTP is characterized by thrombocytopenia, microangiopathic hemolytic anemia (schistocytes on peripheral blood smear), neurologic findings, renal dysfunction, and fever. TTP is a potentially fatal condition that requires urgent referral to a hematologist for prompt treatment (e.g., plasmapheresis).

Specific Populations

Pregnancy. Category B. (See Users Guide.)

Lactation. Clopidogrel is distributed into milk in rats; not known whether the drug is distributed into milk in humans. Discontinue nursing or the drug because of potential for severe adverse effects in infants.

Pediatric Use. Safety and efficacy of clopidogrel have not been established in patients younger than 21 years of age. However, the drug has been used for thromboprophylaxis in children†; regular monitoring of liver and renal function is recommended. In neonates and infants† up to 24 months of age with systemic to pulmonary artery shunts or other cardiac conditions predisposing to thrombosis, clopidogrel 0.2 mg/kg daily for 1–4 weeks achieved similar inhibition of platelet aggregation as a 75-mg daily dosage in adults; no serious hemorrhagic events were reported.

Geriatric Use. No difference in platelet aggregation has been observed in patients 75 years of age or older compared with younger healthy individuals. In the CURE trial, geriatric patients (65 years of age or older) were at greater risk for thrombotic events and major bleeding compared with younger patients. However, in the COMMIT study evaluating patients with ST-segment-elevation MI (STEMI), the efficacy and safety of clopidogrel in preventing ischemic events was independent of age. Dosage adjustment based solely on age does not appear to be necessary in geriatric patients.

Hepatic Impairment. Inhibition of ADP-induced platelet aggregation in patients with severe hepatic impairment appears to be similar to that observed in healthy individuals.

Renal Impairment. Experience is limited in patients with moderate (creatinine clearance of 30–60 mL/minute) or severe (creatinine clearance of 5–15 mL/minute) renal impairment. Inhibition of ADP-induced platelet aggregation may be decreased by 25% in such patients.

■ Common Adverse Effects

Adverse effects occurring in at least 2.5% of patients with recent MI, stroke, or established peripheral arterial occlusive disease receiving clopidogrel in the CAPRIE study included chest pain, accidental injury, influenza-like symptoms, pain, fatigue, edema, hypertension, headache, dizziness, abdominal pain, dyspepsia, diarrhea, nausea, hypercholesterolemia, arthralgia, back pain, purpura (bruising), epistaxis, depression, upper respiratory tract infection, dyspnea, rhinitis, bronchitis, coughing, rash, pruritus, and urinary tract infection. In this study, rash and diarrhea were reported more frequently with clopidogrel therapy while patients receiving aspirin experienced indigestion/nausea/vomiting, GI hemorrhage, or abnormal liver function more frequently. Rash classified as severe was more common with clopidogrel therapy, while GI hemorrhage classified as severe was more common in patients receiving aspirin.

Adverse effects occurring in at least 2% of patients with non-ST-segment-elevation acute coronary syndrome (NSTE ACS) receiving clopidogrel and aspirin in the CURE study included chest pain, headache, dizziness, abdominal pain, dyspepsia, or diarrhea. In this study, the incidence of major bleeding (principally GI hemorrhage and bleeding at puncture sites), including life-threatening bleeding, was substantially greater in patients receiving clopidogrel and aspirin than in those receiving placebo and aspirin (3.7 and 2.7%, respectively); the incidence of life-threatening bleeding (2.2 and 1.8%, respectively) was similar.

In the COMMIT study in patients with STEMI, the incidence of major bleeding (intracranial hemorrhage or bleeding associated with a decrease in hemoglobin concentrations exceeding 5 mg/dL) was similar in patients receiving clopidogrel and aspirin and in those receiving placebo and aspirin (1.3 and 1.1%, respectively); the incidence of fatal bleeding (0.8 and 0.6%, respectively) also was similar. Only limited safety data were collected in the COMMIT study.

The incidence of severe neutropenia (neutrophil count less than 450/mm^3) was similar in patients receiving clopidogrel or aspirin (0.05 or 0.04%, respectively) in the CAPRIE study and much lower than that reported with ticlopidine therapy (0.8%). In the CURE study, the incidence of neutropenia was similar in patients receiving clopidogrel and aspirin or placebo and aspirin (0.08 or 0.1%, respectively).

Drug Interactions

■ Drugs Affecting or Metabolized by Hepatic Microsomal Enzymes

Potential pharmacokinetic interaction (clopidogrel-induced inhibition of the cytochrome P-450 [CYP] 2C9 isoenzyme [CYP2C9] at high drug concentrations in vitro).

Drugs that inhibit CYP2C19 decrease plasma concentrations of the active metabolite of clopidogrel and reduce its antiplatelet effects. (See Drug Interactions: Proton-Pump Inhibitors.) Concomitant use of drugs that are known to be potent inhibitors of CYP2C19 activity (e.g., omeprazole, esomeprazole) should be avoided in patients receiving clopidogrel.

■ Cilostazol

Potential additive inhibition of platelet aggregation. Caution is advised; bleeding times should be monitored during concurrent administration.

Pharmacokinetic interaction unlikely.

■ Nonsteroidal Anti-inflammatory Agents

Potential pharmacodynamic interaction (increased risk of bleeding).

■ Warfarin

Potential pharmacodynamic interaction (increased risk of bleeding). Caution is advised.

■ Proton-Pump Inhibitors

Potential pharmacokinetic interaction (decreased plasma concentrations of the active metabolite of clopidogrel) and pharmacodynamic interaction (reduced antiplatelet effects) with certain proton-pump inhibitors. Because the antiplatelet activity of clopidogrel (a prodrug) is dependent on biotransformation, principally by CYP2C19, of the prodrug to an active metabolite, concurrent use of drugs such as omeprazole or esomeprazole that inhibit CYP2C19 reduces plasma concentrations of the active metabolite and potentially could reduce clinical efficacy. (See Drug Interactions: Drugs Affecting or Metabolized by Hepatic Microsomal Enzymes and also see Reduced Efficacy Associated with Impaired CYP2C19 Function under Warnings/Precautions: Warnings, in Cautions.) Some experts state that additional data from large, prospective trials are needed to fully elucidate the clinical consequences, if any, of the observed interaction between clopidogrel and certain proton-pump inhibitors. The American College of Cardiology Foundation (ACCF) and the American Heart Association (AHA) state that although proton-pump inhibitors (e.g., omeprazole) can affect clopidogrel metabolism and result in diminished antiplatelet activity in vitro, these pharmacokinetic effects do not appear to be associated with worse clinical outcomes. If concomitant proton-pump inhibitor therapy is considered necessary, use of an agent with little or no CYP2C19-inhibitory activity should be considered.

Proton-pump inhibitors vary in their potency for inhibiting CYP2C19. The change in inhibition of adenosine diphosphate (ADP)-induced platelet aggregation associated with concomitant use of proton-pump inhibitors is related to the change in exposure to the active metabolite of clopidogrel. In pharmacokinetic and pharmacodynamic studies in healthy individuals, dexlansoprazole,

lansoprazole, or pantoprazole had less effect on the antiplatelet activity of clopidogrel than did omeprazole or esomeprazole. Pharmacokinetic and pharmacodynamic data from these interaction studies suggested that of these proton-pump inhibitors, dexlansoprazole had the least potential to interact with clopidogrel. In these studies, the observed effects of dexlansoprazole, lansoprazole, or pantoprazole on exposure to the active metabolite of clopidogrel and on clopidogrel-induced platelet inhibition were not considered clinically important, and the manufacturers of dexlansoprazole, lansoprazole, and pantoprazole state that no adjustment of clopidogrel dosage is required if clopidogrel is used concomitantly with FDA-labeled dosages of these proton-pump inhibitors. Omeprazole and esomeprazole substantially reduce the antiplatelet activity of clopidogrel; therefore, concomitant use of omeprazole or esomeprazole with clopidogrel should be avoided. (For additional information, see Drug Interactions: Clopidogrel in the individual monographs for proton-pump inhibitors in 56:28.36.)

The decision to use any proton-pump inhibitor concomitantly with clopidogrel should be based on the assessed risks and benefits in individual patients. The American College of Cardiology Foundation/American College of Gastroenterology/American Heart Association (ACCF/ACG/AHA) states that use of a proton-pump inhibitor concomitantly with dual antiplatelet therapy may provide the optimal balance of risk and benefit in patients with acute coronary syndrome (ACS) who have a history of upper GI bleeding since such a history is the strongest and most consistent risk factor for GI bleeding in patients receiving antiplatelet therapy. Among stable patients with a history of GI bleeding who undergo coronary revascularization and receive a coronary stent, ACCF/ACG/AHA states that the risk/benefit tradeoff may favor concomitant use of dual antiplatelet therapy and a proton-pump inhibitor. ACCF/ACG/AHA also states that the risk reduction with proton-pump inhibitors is substantial in patients with risk factors for GI bleeding (e.g., advanced age; concomitant use of warfarin, corticosteroids, or nonsteroidal anti-inflammatory agents [NSAIAs]; *H. pylori* infection) and may outweigh any potential reduction in the cardiovascular efficacy of antiplatelet treatment associated with a drug–drug interaction. In contrast, patients without these risk factors for GI bleeding receive little if any absolute risk reduction from proton-pump inhibitor therapy, and the risk/benefit balance may favor use of antiplatelet therapy without a concomitant proton-pump inhibitor.

In a crossover clinical trial in healthy individuals who received clopidogrel (a 300-mg loading dose, followed by 75 mg daily) alone or with a high dosage of omeprazole (80 mg administered at the same time as the clopidogrel dose) for 5 days, exposure to the active metabolite of clopidogrel was decreased by 46 and 42% on days 1 and 5, respectively, when the drugs were administered simultaneously. In addition, mean inhibition of platelet aggregation was reduced by 47 and 30% at 24 hours and on day 5, respectively. When administration of the 2 drugs (at the same dosages) was separated by 12 hours in another study, results were similar in terms of reduced exposure to the active clopidogrel metabolite and reduced platelet inhibition. The effects of a lower dosage of omeprazole on inhibition of platelet aggregation have not been established. When a higher dosage of clopidogrel was administered concomitantly with omeprazole, an increase in antiplatelet response was observed; however, an appropriate dosage regimen has not been established. Concomitant use of clopidogrel and omeprazole also has been associated with substantially decreased antiplatelet effects as determined by vasodilator-stimulated phosphoprotein (VASP) phosphorylation. The potential for such interactions must be considered for any drug that inhibits CYP2C19.

Results of several large observational studies suggest that concomitant therapy with clopidogrel and omeprazole (or potentially other proton-pump inhibitors) can reduce the effectiveness of clopidogrel in preventing cardiovascular events. However, conflicting data have been reported, including results of a prematurely discontinued randomized controlled trial suggesting no effect of concomitant clopidogrel–proton-pump inhibitor therapy on cardiovascular outcomes; given the limitations of observational studies (possibility of confounding factors such as comorbid conditions, unreported use of aspirin or OTC proton-pump inhibitors), the clinical importance of this interaction has been questioned. Pharmacokinetic/pharmacodynamic studies conducted by the manufacturer indicate that administration of the drugs at separate times (e.g., 12 hours apart) will *not* prevent the interaction.

Some clinicians suggest that an antacid or a histamine H_2-receptor antagonist (ranitidine, famotidine, nizatidine) may be considered as an alternative to therapy with a proton-pump inhibitor, although such agents may not be as effective as a proton-pump inhibitor in providing gastric protection. However, cimetidine should *not* be used as alternative therapy since it is a potent CYP2C19 inhibitor. There currently is no evidence that histamine H_2-receptor antagonists (other than cimetidine) or other drugs that reduce gastric acid (e.g., antacids) interfere with the antiplatelet effects of clopidogrel.

Several observational studies involving large numbers of patients suggest that proton-pump inhibitors reduce the effectiveness of clopidogrel in preventing cardiovascular events. In a case-control study in patients 66 years of age or older, concomitant use of clopidogrel and a proton-pump inhibitor that inhibits CYP2C19 (omeprazole, lansoprazole, rabeprazole) was associated with a 40% greater risk of recurrent myocardial infarction within 90 days of hospital discharge; this effect was not seen with pantoprazole, which does not inhibit CYP2C19. In 2 retrospective cohort studies involving more than 30,000 patients, the incidence of major adverse cardiovascular events (e.g., hospitalization for stroke, angina, myocardial infarction, coronary artery bypass grafting, urgent target vessel revascularization, death) in patients receiving clopidogrel for 12 months following stent placement was higher in those who were also prescribed a proton-pump inhibitor than in those who did not receive a proton-pump inhibitor. A subgroup analysis in one of these studies revealed that each proton-pump inhibitor (omeprazole, esomeprazole, pantoprazole, lansoprazole) was individually associated with an increased risk of cardiovascular events. In other retrospective cohort studies in patients with acute coronary syndrome (ACS), concomitant use of clopidogrel and a proton-pump inhibitor was associated with a significantly higher rate of adverse cardiovascular events (e.g., death or rehospitalization for ACS, coronary stent placement) versus administration of clopidogrel alone.

Data discounting the clinical importance of a clopidogrel–proton-pump inhibitor interaction also have been reported. In a study evaluating health insurance records of more than 18,500 patients 65 years of age or older who had received clopidogrel with or without proton-pump inhibitor therapy, a slightly increased risk of myocardial infarction or death was observed in patients receiving clopidogrel concurrently with a proton-pump inhibitor, but the finding was not statistically significant. In a post hoc analysis of a large randomized study evaluating a clopidogrel loading dose in patients prior to PCI (Clopidogrel for the Reduction of Events During Observation [CREDO]), use of a proton-pump inhibitor was independently associated with an increased risk of a cardiovascular event (e.g., death, myocardial infarction, stroke) regardless of whether patients received clopidogrel therapy. Post-hoc analysis of another large randomized controlled study (Trial to Assess Improvement with Prasugrel-Thrombolysis in Myocardial Infarction [TRITON-TIMI 38]) also found no clinically meaningful interaction between clopidogrel and a proton-pump inhibitor. In the only randomized, placebo-controlled trial (Clopidogrel Optimization of Gastrointestinal EveNTs [COGENT] trial) to date evaluating potential clinical outcomes of the clopidogrel–proton-pump inhibitor interaction, no effect of such concomitant therapy on the rate of cardiovascular events was found in patients receiving an investigational fixed-dose combination of clopidogrel and omeprazole or clopidogrel without a proton-pump inhibitor; however, interpretation of the data is limited due to premature termination of the study, insufficient statistical power, and incomplete follow-up.

Description

Clopidogrel bisulfate, a thienopyridine derivative structurally and pharmacologically related to ticlopidine, is a platelet-aggregation inhibitor. Clopidogrel is a prodrug with its platelet-aggregation inhibitory activity dependent on hepatic transformation to an active thiol metabolite.

Biotransformation occurs through a 2-step process where clopidogrel is initially oxidized to a 2-oxo-clopidogrel intermediate metabolite, then subsequently metabolized to the active thiol metabolite. This metabolic pathway has been shown to be mediated by several cytochrome P-450 isoenzymes (e.g., CYP2C19, CYP3A, CYP2B6, CYP1A2). In particular, the CYP2C19 isoenzyme is involved in the formation of both the active metabolite and the 2-oxo-clopidogrel intermediate. Genetic polymorphism of CYP2C19 can affect the pharmacokinetic and pharmacodynamic response to clopidogrel. Patients with at least one loss-of-function variant CYP2C19 allele (e.g., CYP2C19*2, CYP2C19*3) are described as poor or intermediate metabolizers of clopidogrel and have been shown to have lower plasma concentrations of active metabolite and diminished antiplatelet response, which in turn can lead to a higher incidence of major adverse cardiovascular events. (See Reduced Efficacy Associated with Impaired CYP2C19 Function under Warnings/Precautions: Warnings, in Cautions.) The prevalence of reduced-function CYP2C19 genotypes in the general population differs according to race and ethnicity; an estimated 2% of whites, 4% of blacks, and 14% of Chinese are poor CYP2C19 metabolizers.

Clopidogrel is an ADP-receptor antagonist; the active metabolite of clopidogrel binds selectively and noncompetitively to a low-affinity, P2Y12 ADP-receptor binding site on the surface of platelets, thereby inhibiting ADP binding to the receptor and subsequent activation of the platelet glycoprotein (GP IIb/IIIa) complex necessary for fibrinogen-platelet binding. Clopidogrel also inhibits ADP-mediated release of platelet dense granule (e.g., ADP, calcium, and serotonin) and alpha granule (e.g., fibrinogen and thrombospondin) contents that augment platelet aggregation. The low-affinity ADP receptor is irreversibly modified by the drug, so platelets exposed to clopidogrel remain affected for the remainder of their lifespan (about 7–10 days). Unlike aspirin, thienopyridine platelet-aggregation inhibitors such as clopidogrel and ticlopidine do not inactivate platelet cyclooxygenase to prevent synthesis of prostaglandin endoperoxides and thromboxane A.

Clopidogrel is rapidly absorbed after oral administration; at least 50% of an oral dose is absorbed. Peak plasma concentrations of the active metabolite occur approximately 30–60 minutes following an oral dose. When clopidogrel 75 mg is administered daily, inhibition of platelet aggregation is apparent on the first day of therapy, with 40–60% inhibition being achieved at steady state between days 3–7. Following discontinuance of the drug, platelet aggregation and bleeding time generally return to baseline values within about 5 days.

Advice to Patients

Importance of counseling patients about the potential risks versus benefits of clopidogrel. Importance of patients taking the drug exactly as prescribed and not discontinuing therapy without first consulting the prescribing clinician. Importance of informing patients that they may bruise and/or bleed more easily and a longer than normal time may be required to stop bleeding when taking clopidogrel. Importance of informing clinicians about any unanticipated, prolonged, or excessive bleeding, or blood in urine or stool.

Risk of thrombotic thrombocytopenic purpura (TTP); importance of advising patients to immediately seek medical attention if they experience manifestations such as fever, weakness, extreme skin paleness, purple skin patches, yellowing of the skin or eyes, or neurologic changes that cannot otherwise be explained.

Before implantation of a drug-eluting stent, determine likelihood of patient compliance with at least 12 months of aspirin–clopidogrel combination therapy; importance of informing patients prior to hospital discharge about risks associated with premature discontinuance of such combination therapy. Importance of informing clinicians (e.g., physicians, dentists) about clopidogrel therapy before any surgery is scheduled; clinician performing invasive procedure should consult with prescribing clinician before discontinuing clopidogrel.

Importance of informing clinicians of existing or contemplated concomitant therapy, including prescription and OTC drugs, particularly omeprazole (including Prilosec OTC®) or esomeprazole and drugs that affect bleeding (e.g., warfarin, nonsteroidal anti-inflammatory agents). (See Drug Interactions: Proton-Pump Inhibitors and Drug Interactions: Nonsteroidal Anti-inflammatory Agents.) Importance of women informing clinicians if they are or plan to become pregnant or plan to breast-feed. Importance of informing patients of other important precautionary information. (See Cautions.)

Overview® (see Users Guide). For additional information on this drug until a more detailed monograph is developed and published, the manufacturer's labeling should be consulted. It is *essential* that the manufacturer's labeling be consulted for more detailed information on usual cautions, precautions, contraindications, potential drug interactions, laboratory test interferences, and acute toxicity.

Preparations

Excipients in commercially available drug preparations may have clinically important effects in some individuals; consult specific product labeling for details.

Clopidogrel Bisulfate

Oral		
Tablets	75 mg (of clopidogrel)	**Plavix®**, Sanofi-Aventis (also promoted by Bristol-Myers Squibb)
	300 mg (of clopidogrel)	**Plavix®**, Sanofi-Aventis (also promoted by Bristol-Myers Squibb)

†Use is not currently included in the labeling approved by the US Food and Drug Administration

Eptifibatide

■ Eptifibatide, a selective platelet-aggregation inhibitor, has been referred to as a platelet glycoprotein (GP) IIb/IIIa-receptor inhibitor.

Uses

■ **Non-ST-Segment-Elevation Acute Coronary Syndromes** Eptifibatide is used with anticoagulant therapy (e.g., heparin [referring throughout this monograph to unfractionated heparin], low molecular weight heparin), aspirin, and a P2Y12 platelet adenosine diphosphate (ADP)-receptor antagonist (e.g., clopidogrel, prasugrel, ticagrelor) to reduce the risk of acute cardiac ischemic events (death and/or myocardial infarction [MI]) in patients with unstable angina or non-ST-segment-elevation MI (NSTEMI) (i.e., non-ST-segment-elevation acute coronary syndromes [NSTE ACS]), both in patients who are to receive medical management and those undergoing percutaneous coronary intervention (PCI). In clinical trials of eptifibatide, NSTE ACS was defined by prolonged symptoms of cardiac ischemia (at least 10 minutes' duration within the previous 24 hours) that were associated with *transient* ST-segment changes (ST elevation of 0.6–1 mm or ST depression exceeding 0.5 mm), T-wave inversion (exceeding 1 mm), or increased cardiac (MB) fraction of creatine kinase (CK, creatine phosphokinase, CPK); patients who had MI associated with Q waves or *persistent* (30 minutes' duration or longer) ST-segment elevation exceeding 1 mm were not included in these studies. NSTEMI and unstable angina clinically may be indistinguishable at initial presentation and are managed similarly. Almost all patients in clinical trials of eptifibatide received concomitant therapy with aspirin and IV heparin, and the efficacy and safety of eptifibatide without adjunctive aspirin and/or heparin therapy have not been established.

Platelet glycoprotein (GP) IIb/IIIa-receptor inhibitors are used as an adjunct to standard therapeutic measures for managing NSTE ACS. These measures include therapy with aspirin and a P2Y12-receptor antagonist (e.g., clopidogrel, prasugrel, ticagrelor), nitrates (e.g., nitroglycerin), anticoagulant therapy (e.g., low molecular weight heparins, heparin), and β-blockers followed by either conservative medical management or early aggressive management, such as angiographic evaluation and revascularization procedures (e.g., PCI, coronary artery bypass grafting [CABG], coronary artery stent implantation) as required. Several meta-analyses of studies indicate that adjunctive therapy with a GP IIb/IIIa-receptor inhibitor can reduce the incidence of cardiac ischemic events, including subsequent MI and death in patients with NSTE ACS. Benefits of GP IIb/IIIa-receptor inhibitors on mortality principally occur early during therapy (i.e., the first 48–96 hours).

The benefit of aspirin for secondary prevention of ischemic events in patients with unstable angina has been demonstrated in several studies and pooled analyses. Many clinicians recommend that all patients with NSTE ACS receive aspirin as soon as possible after hospital admission and then continued indefinitely unless they have documented hypersensitivity or other definite contraindication (e.g., active or recent major bleeding, peptic ulcer disease). (See Non-ST-Segment-Elevation Acute Coronary Syndromes under Thrombosis: Coronary Artery Disease and Myocardial Infarction, in Uses, in Aspirin 28:08.04.24.) The American College of Cardiology Foundation (ACCF) and the American Heart Association (AHA) state that in patients with NSTE ACS in whom an initial invasive management strategy is planned, an additional antiplatelet agent (either clopidogrel or a GP IIb/IIIa-receptor inhibitor given IV) should be administered prior to diagnostic angiography ("upstream") as an adjunct to aspirin therapy. Eptifibatide or tirofiban is the preferred GP IIb/IIIa-receptor inhibitor for this use; abciximab is indicated only if there is no appreciable delay before angiography and PCI is likely to be performed. The American College of Chest Physicians (ACCP) states that a clear risk-benefit ratio has not been established for the use of GP IIb/IIIa-receptor inhibitors in patients with ACS who are not routinely scheduled for early revascularization.

In patients with NSTE ACS with elevated troponin concentrations who were managed with conservative medical therapy, GP IIb/IIIa-receptor inhibitors were equally effective in men and women. However, in women with NSTE ACS who are not at high risk for acute cardiac ischemic events (e.g., no elevated troponin concentrations) and are managed with a conservative strategy, eptifibatide and tirofiban appear to show little benefit and may possibly have detrimental effects; these agents are not recommended by AHA in women at lower risk for adverse cardiac events.

The current labeled indication for eptifibatide in patients with NSTE ACS is based principally on the results of a large, international, placebo-controlled study, the Platelet Glycoprotein IIb/IIIa in Unstable Angina: Receptor Suppression Using Integrilin Therapy (PURSUIT) study. In the PURSUIT study, therapy with eptifibatide (180-mcg/kg IV loading dose followed by continuous IV infusion of 2 mcg/kg per minute until hospital discharge or initiation of CABG, up to 72 hours or a maximum of 96 hours in patients undergoing PCI) reduced the combined incidence of death or nonfatal MI at 30 days (the primary composite clinical end point).

Beneficial effects of eptifibatide in the PURSUIT study were evident within 72 hours of initiating the infusion and persisted for up to 6 months (based on ischemic events evaluated by a blinded clinical events committee for the first 30 days and on investigator-reported events thereafter up to 6 months). The combined incidence of death or nonfatal MI in the overall study was reduced from 7.6% to 5.9% at 3 days, from 11.6% to 10.1% at 7 days, from 15.7% to 14.2% at 30 days, and from 13.6% to 12.1% at 6 months. This absolute reduction of approximately 1.5% in clinical events was maintained at all time points measured, while relative reductions in risk declined from 22% at 3 days to 12.9 and 9.6% at 7 and 30 days, respectively. The decline in relative benefit over time is related to the continued random occurrence of ischemic events in both placebo and treatment groups after achievement of a constant absolute risk reduction with eptifibatide therapy. The incidences of the individual end points of death or new MI for eptifibatide or placebo were not different at 30 days, although MI was less frequent with eptifibatide therapy at 96 hours.

Most patients in the PURSUIT study received adjunctive therapy with oral aspirin (75–325 mg once daily) and IV or subcutaneous heparin. In patients receiving medical management alone (i.e., those not undergoing PCI), heparin sodium (generally an IV loading dose of 5000 units followed by IV infusion of 1000 units per hour) was given to maintain a target activated partial thromboplastin time (aPTT) of 50–70 seconds. Patients undergoing PCI were given IV heparin (loading dose followed by IV infusion) to maintain an activated clotting time (ACT) of 300–350 seconds. (See Dosage and Administration: Dosage.)

The efficacy of eptifibatide in the PURSUIT study varied according to use of concomitant therapy or procedures and by gender, age, and geographic region. In this study, about 13% of patients underwent PCI during infusion of eptifibatide, while the remainder received medical management alone. For patients who underwent early PCI (within 72 hours after randomization) during eptifibatide infusion, the reduction in adverse ischemic events (nonfatal MI only) was evident prior to the procedure (i.e., during medical management). Patients undergoing early PCI experienced a 5.1% absolute reduction (31% relative reduction) in the combined clinical end point of death or nonfatal MI at 30 days; reduction in this clinical end point also was maintained over 6 months. Of those who received medical management alone, the incidence of clinical events was not appreciably reduced (1.1% absolute reduction, 7% relative reduction).

Subgroup analyses in the PURSUIT study suggested that patients who used aspirin prior to (within 2 weeks of) study entry were less likely to have had a MI (versus unstable angina) at study enrollment but more likely to have worse long-term outcomes (death or MI) than patients who reported no prior aspirin use; however, there was no evidence that prior aspirin use influenced the efficacy of eptifibatide.

The effects of eptifibatide therapy in the PURSUIT study did not appear to be influenced by patient age, but in patients outside North America the drug appeared less beneficial in women than in men. Results were heterogenous among patients in the various geographic regions (US and Canada, Western

Europe, Eastern Europe, Latin America) of the study, possibly because of the practice-based nature of the study and the diverse pharmacologic and regional interventional strategies used to manage NSTE ACS. Patients treated in the US, who were the most homogeneous large subgroup in the study with regard to baseline characteristics (except ethnic background) and approach to patient management, achieved greater benefit than the overall study population. Eptifibatide therapy was associated with less benefit than placebo in women in Latin America and Eastern and Western Europe, while in the US and Canada men and women achieved similar benefit. These findings may reflect genuine biologic interactions between eptifibatide and gender, interactions between eptifibatide and international differences in concomitant therapy (e.g., timing and rate of interventions employed) given to men and women, or chance occurrences; the relative contributions of these possible factors are unknown.

■ **Acute Ischemic Complications of Percutaneous Coronary Intervention** Eptifibatide also is used with anticoagulant therapy (e.g., heparin, low molecular weight heparin), aspirin, and a P2Y12-receptor antagonist (e.g., clopidogrel, prasugrel, ticagrelor) to reduce the risk of acute ischemic complications (death, MI, and/or the need for urgent revascularization procedures) in patients undergoing PCI, including coronary artery stenting. Despite advances in percutaneous revascularization techniques, abrupt closure of a coronary vessel that occurs during PCI still is associated with substantial morbidity (e.g., MI). GP IIb/IIIa-receptor inhibitors such as eptifibatide are used to minimize PCI-related ischemic complications and improve the risk-benefit ratio of these procedures. Studies involving eptifibatide or another GP IIb/IIIa-receptor inhibitor (i.e., abciximab) have demonstrated consistent reductions in the risk of composite ischemic events (death, MI, need for revascularization procedures) at 30 days in patients with or without NSTE ACS undergoing PCI.

The current labeled indication for eptifibatide in patients undergoing PCI is based principally on the results of large, multicenter, placebo-controlled studies in patients undergoing PCI alone in the Integrilin to Minimize Platelet Aggregation and Coronary Thrombosis-II (IMPACT-II) study or with coronary artery stenting in the Enhanced Suppression of the Platelet IIb/IIIa receptor with Integrilin Therapy (ESPRIT) study. In the IMPACT-II study, therapy with eptifibatide (135-mcg/kg IV loading dose immediately before PCI, followed by 0.5–0.75 mcg/kg per minute by continuous IV infusion for 20–24 hours after PCI) reduced the combined incidence of death, nonfatal MI, or the need for urgent intervention at 30 days (the primary composite clinical end point) in patients undergoing elective, urgent, or emergency PCI (e.g., balloon angioplasty, directional atherectomy, transluminal extraction catheter atherectomy, rotational ablation angioplasty, excimer-laser angioplasty). All patients received adjunctive therapy with aspirin (75–325 mg given 1–24 hours prior to the procedure), and IV heparin sodium (an IV loading dose of 100 units/kg prior to initiation of the study drug followed by up to 2000 units of heparin sodium every 15 minutes by IV injection) was given to achieve and maintain an ACT of 300–350 seconds. The primary clinical end point of death, nonfatal MI (defined as an increase in the cardiac MB fraction of creatine kinase to 3 times the upper limit of normal or development of Q waves of at least 0.04 seconds' duration in 2 or more contiguous ECG leads), or urgent intervention (e.g., abrupt closure of a coronary artery followed by CABG, coronary artery stent implantation, repeat PCI) occurred in approximately 6.6% of patients receiving the lower-dose regimen of eptifibatide (135-mcg/kg IV loading dose and 0.5 mcg/kg per minute by IV infusion) versus 9.6% of placebo recipients (31% relative reduction in clinical events) at 24 hours, and in 9.1 or 11.6% of patients receiving the lower-dose regimen of eptifibatide or placebo, respectively, at 30 days (22% relative reduction in clinical events). However, for patients receiving any amount of study drug (excluding those who did not receive study drug or coronary intervention), the decrease in ischemic complications at 30 days was statistically significant only in the low-dose group (those receiving the 135-mcg/kg IV loading dose and 0.5 mcg/kg per minute infusion). There was no clustering of ischemic events in the 24–48 hours after discontinuance of the eptifibatide infusion, indicating no rebound effect associated with termination of eptifibatide therapy. Most clinical end-point events (63%) reported in the IMPACT-II study occurred within the first 6 hours after coronary intervention.

Unexpected findings in the IMPACT-II study include the inability to prospectively determine outcome according to risk (i.e., the beneficial effect of eptifibatide was more pronounced in low-risk than in high-risk patients) and the lack of a dose-response effect with eptifibatide therapy (i.e., no improvement in clinical efficacy with the higher-dose compared with the lower-dose regimen, and no reduction in bleeding risk with the lower-dose regimen). Because the assay used to determine inhibition of platelet aggregation and adjust eptifibatide dosage in the IMPACT-II study involved anticoagulation with citrate (which binds calcium), binding of eptifibatide to the GP IIb/IIIa-receptor was exaggerated relative to that occurring at physiologic concentrations of calcium. Use in subsequent studies (e.g., PURSUIT) of the anticoagulant D-phenylalanyl-L-propyl-L-arginine chloromethyl ketone (PPACK), which does not affect extracellular calcium concentrations in ex vivo platelet-aggregation assays, indicates that inhibition of platelet aggregation may not have been optimal at the eptifibatide dosages employed in the IMPACT-II study. (See Pharmacology.) An alternative explanation for the lack of improved outcome with the higher infusion rate of eptifibatide in the IMPACT-II trial may be the likelihood that the IV loading dose, rather than the infusion rate, was the principal determinant of plasma eptifibatide concentration at the time of greatest risk of ischemic events (within 6 hours after initiation of therapy).

In a subsequent multicenter placebo-controlled study (ESPRIT) in which the dosage of eptifibatide (2 IV loading doses of 180 mcg/kg given 10 minutes apart with a continuous infusion of 2 mcg/kg per minute initiated after the first loading dose) was 3–4 times higher than that in the IMPACT-II study in patients undergoing non-urgent coronary artery stenting, therapy with the drug reduced the primary end point (the combined incidences of death, nonfatal MI, and urgent target-vessel revascularization or rescue therapy with open-label drug for thrombotic complications of PCI) at 30 days and 1 year. All patients received adjunctive therapy with aspirin, clopidogrel, or ticlopidine, and IV heparin sodium (60 units/kg) was given as an IV loading dose followed by additional doses (10–40 units/kg) to achieve and maintain an ACT of 200–300 seconds. The combined clinical end point occurred in 7.5% of patients receiving eptifibatide versus 11.7% of placebo recipients, respectively, at 30 days. However, use of rescue therapy for threatened thrombotic complications (e.g., abrupt vessel closure, no reperfusion, coronary thrombosis) is likely to have reduced composite clinical end-point events in the placebo group. Benefits of eptifibatide appeared to be maintained during long-term follow-up as indicated by attainment of the primary end point in 14.3 or 18.5% of eptifibatide or placebo recipients, respectively, at 6 months and in 17.5 or 22.1% of eptifibatide or placebo recipients, respectively, at 1 year.

Randomized controlled studies, including a meta-analysis of 16 randomized trials involving approximately 10,000 patients with ST-segment-elevation MI (STEMI) undergoing primary PCI, generally have failed to demonstrate benefits of GP IIb/IIIa-receptor blockade similar to those observed in patients with NSTE ACS. ACCF, AHA, the Society for Cardiovascular Angiography and Interventions (SCAI), and other experts currently do not recommend the *routine* use of GP IIb/IIIa-receptor inhibitors in patients with STEMI undergoing PCI; however, selective use of these drugs as an adjunct to heparin may be reasonable in certain high-risk patients (e.g., those with large anterior MI and/or large thrombus). Studies evaluating the use of GP IIb/IIIa-receptor inhibitors in patients with NSTE ACS undergoing PCI have demonstrated reductions in ischemic outcomes, particularly in patients with high-risk features (e.g., elevated troponin); therefore, ACCF/AHA/SCAI states that it may be useful to administer a GP IIb/IIIa-receptor inhibitor at the time of PCI as an adjunct to heparin therapy in such high-risk patients who are not receiving bivalirudin and who are not adequately pretreated with a P2Y12-receptor antagonist. Regarding the choice of GP IIb/IIIa-receptor inhibitor in patients undergoing PCI, abciximab, "double-bolus" eptifibatide (i.e., two 180-mcg/kg direct IV injections given 10 minutes apart), and high-dose tirofiban (25 mcg/kg given by direct IV injection) all have been shown to produce a high degree of platelet inhibition and reduce ischemic complications.

■ **Adjunctive Therapy During Thrombolysis to Prevent Reocclusion** Eptifibatide has been administered concomitantly with a thrombolytic agent (e.g., alteplase, tenecteplase) in a limited number of patients to prevent coronary artery reocclusion† after an acute MI. However, the appropriate dosage of adjunctive eptifibatide therapy in terms of efficacy and bleeding complications (see Drug Interactions: Thrombolytic Therapy) in such patients has not been established, and studies to date have not been of sufficient size to detect differences in clinical outcomes such as survival.

Dosage and Administration

■ **Administration** Eptifibatide is administered by IV injection followed by IV infusion using a controlled-infusion device (e.g., pump). For IV injection, the appropriate dose of eptifibatide is withdrawn from the 10-mL vial containing the drug solution and administered undiluted IV over 1–2 minutes. The solution for continuous IV infusion should be administered directly from the 100-mL vial after spiking the vial with a vented infusion set. Care should be taken to center the spike within the circle on the stopper top. Any drug solution remaining after IV injection or infusion of the appropriate dose of eptifibatide should be discarded.

Parenteral eptifibatide solutions should be inspected visually for particulate matter and discoloration prior to administration whenever solution and container permit.

■ **Dosage** In clinical trials of eptifibatide therapy, most patients received adjunctive antithrombotic therapy with aspirin (75–325 mg daily) and IV heparin sodium. The safety and efficacy of eptifibatide therapy without concomitant aspirin and heparin remains to be established.

Non-ST-Segment-Elevation Acute Coronary Syndromes For reducing the risk of death and/or myocardial infarction (MI) in patients with unstable angina or non-ST-segment-elevation myocardial infarction (NSTEMI) (i.e., non-ST-segment-elevation acute coronary syndromes [NSTE ACS]) who have normal renal function, the recommended initial adult dosage of eptifibatide is 180 mcg/kg given as an IV loading dose over 1–2 minutes as soon as possible following diagnosis, followed by continuous IV infusion of 2 mcg/kg per minute until hospital discharge or initiation of coronary artery bypass grafting (CABG), or for up to 72 hours. In the PURSUIT study, bleeding occurred more frequently in both the placebo and treatment groups in patients undergoing CABG, and the incidence of major bleeding was not different between the groups. However, the manufacturer states that eptifibatide therapy should be discontinued prior to CABG.

The manufacturer states that if a patient with NSTE ACS is to undergo percutaneous coronary intervention (PCI) while receiving eptifibatide, the infusion should be continued at the same rate either up to hospital discharge or for up to 18–24 hours after the procedure, whichever comes first, for a maximum of 96 hours of therapy.

Adjunctive Antithrombotic Therapy. Adjunctive antithrombotic therapy with aspirin and heparin was used in most patients with NSTE ACS receiving eptifibatide therapy in clinical trials. The manufacturer of eptifibatide recommends an initial aspirin dosage of 160–325 mg daily in patients with NSTE ACS. For additional details regarding aspirin dosage regimens in patients with ACS, see Non-ST-Segment-Elevation Acute Coronary Syndromes under Dosage: Thrombosis, in Dosage and Administration in Aspirin 28:08.04.24.

In patients *not* undergoing PCI, the initial dosage of heparin sodium is based on patient weight and subsequently adjusted to a target activated partial thromboplastin time (aPTT) of 50–70 seconds. The manufacturer states that if patient weight is 70 kg or greater, an IV loading dose of 5000 units of heparin sodium should be administered followed by continuous IV infusion of 1000 units per hour. In patients weighing less than 70 kg, an IV loading dose of heparin sodium 60 units/kg should be given followed by infusion of 12 units/kg per hour.

In patients with NSTE ACS who undergo PCI, multiple IV injections of heparin sodium are administered based on activated clotting time (ACT) determinations during PCI to achieve and maintain an ACT of at least 200 seconds. Since eptifibatide and other GP IIb/IIIa-receptor inhibitors may have additive effects on ACT in patients receiving one of these drugs concomitantly with heparin, the dosage of heparin required to maintain an appropriate ACT during such concomitant therapy may be lower than with heparin monotherapy.

Clinical experience from other studies with GP IIb/IIIa-receptor inhibitors (e.g., abciximab) and current American College of Cardiology Foundation (ACCF)/American Heart Association (AHA)/Society for Cardiovascular Angiography and Interventions (SCAI) guidelines suggest that use of lower dosages of concomitant IV heparin sodium (e.g., 50–70 units/kg) given 6 hours prior to PCI and targeted to an ACT of at least 200 seconds may provide similar reductions in ischemic coronary events as dosages for higher target ACTs with less risk of major bleeding.

Percutaneous Coronary Intervention For reducing the risk of acute ischemic complications (death, MI, and/or the need for urgent revascularization procedures) in patients undergoing PCI, the manufacturer and some clinicians state that the initial adult dosage of eptifibatide in patients with normal renal function consists of an IV loading dose of 180 mcg/kg given immediately before PCI, followed in 10 minutes by a second 180-mcg/kg IV dose; in addition, a continuous IV infusion of 2 mcg/kg per minute should be initiated immediately after the first loading dose. The IV infusion should be continued until hospital discharge or for up to 18–24 hours, whichever comes first. A minimum infusion period of 12 hours is recommended in patients undergoing PCI. The manufacturer states that eptifibatide therapy should be discontinued prior to CABG.

Adjunctive Antithrombotic Therapy. Adjunctive antithrombotic therapy with aspirin and heparin was used in most patients receiving eptifibatide in clinical trials. In the IMPACT-II study, aspirin was given in a dosage of 75–325 mg 1–24 hours prior to PCI. In patients undergoing PCI, ACCF/AHA/SCAI recommends that aspirin 325 mg be given prior to PCI in patients not already receiving maintenance therapy with aspirin. Patients already receiving maintenance therapy with aspirin should receive a dose of 81–325 mg of aspirin before the procedure. For additional details regarding aspirin dosage regimens in patients undergoing PCI, see Percutaneous Coronary Intervention and Revascularization Procedures under Dosage: Thrombosis, in Dosage and Administration, in Aspirin 28:08.04.24.

In patients undergoing PCI with stent placement, a loading dose of a P2Y12 platelet adenosine diphosphate (ADP)-receptor antagonist (clopidogrel, prasugrel, or ticagrelor) also is recommended.

Since eptifibatide and other GP IIb/IIIa-receptor inhibitors may have additive effects on ACT in patients receiving one of these drugs concomitantly with heparin, the dosage of heparin sodium required to maintain an appropriate ACT during such concomitant therapy may be lower than with heparin monotherapy. The manufacturer recommends a heparin sodium dose of 60 units/kg given by direct ("bolus") IV injection within 6 hours prior to PCI. Additional injections of heparin sodium should be given during PCI to maintain an ACT of 200–300 seconds. In patients who have received prior therapy with heparin before PCI, ACCF/AHA/SCAI states that additional heparin sodium injections should be administered during the procedure as needed.

Postprocedural use of heparin generally is not recommended while GP IIb/IIIa-receptor inhibitor therapy is given.

■ **Dosage in Renal and Hepatic Impairment** Results of a small pilot study in patients with mild to moderate renal impairment (as determined by a reduction in creatinine clearance of 30 mL/minute from normal) revealed no apparent differences in mean pharmacokinetic parameters between renally impaired patients and healthy individuals. However, other data in patients with moderate to severe renal impairment (creatinine clearance less than 50 mL/minute) indicate a reduction of approximately 50% in eptifibatide clearance and a doubling of plasma drug concentrations. In vitro studies indicate that eptifibatide may be removed from plasma by dialysis.

Dosage adjustment is not necessary in patients with mild to moderate renal impairment (i.e., those with creatinine clearance of at least 50 mL/minute). However, patients with NSTE ACS who have a creatinine clearance of less than 50 mL/minute (using Cockcroft-Gault equation) should receive a 180-mcg/kg IV loading dose of eptifibatide as soon as possible following diagnosis followed by IV infusion of 1 mcg/kg per minute.

In patients undergoing PCI who have a creatinine clearance of less than 50 mL/minute, an IV loading dose of 180 mcg/kg of eptifibatide should be given immediately prior to PCI followed by IV infusion of the drug at 1 mcg/kg per minute; a second IV loading dose of 180 mcg/kg should be given 10 minutes after the first loading dose.

Information on the pharmacokinetics or use of eptifibatide in patients with hepatic impairment is not available, and the manufacturer currently makes no specific dosage recommendations for such patients. Patients with hepatic disease severe enough to produce alterations in the synthesis of coagulation factors were excluded from clinical trials of eptifibatide, and use of the drug is contraindicated in such patients.

Cautions

The incidence of adverse effects with eptifibatide therapy is based principally on data from 2 large, placebo-controlled studies, the PURSUIT study in patients with unstable angina or non-ST-segment-elevation myocardial infarction (NSTEMI) (i.e., non-ST-segment-elevation acute coronary syndromes [NSTE ACS]) and the IMPACT-II study in patients undergoing percutaneous coronary intervention (PCI). Patients in the PURSUIT study received 180 mcg/kg of eptifibatide as an IV loading dose followed by either 1.3 or 2 mcg/kg per minute by continuous IV infusion for up to 72–96 hours; patients in the IMPACT-II study received 135 mcg/kg of the drug as an IV loading dose immediately before PCI, followed by either 0.5 or 0.75 mcg/kg per minute by continuous IV infusion for 20–24 hours. (See Uses.) Almost all patients receiving eptifibatide in clinical studies received concomitant therapy with heparin and/or aspirin; therefore, the incidence of bleeding complications attributable solely to eptifibatide is difficult to determine. Because of the different eptifibatide dosage regimens used in the PURSUIT and IMPACT-II studies, data from these studies were not pooled.

The most frequent and severe adverse effect of eptifibatide therapy is bleeding. Bleeding complications, which usually are minor and develop at vascular access (e.g., femoral puncture) sites (e.g., in patients undergoing PCI), have been reported in 35–75% of patients receiving various dosages of eptifibatide in clinical studies. Bleeding is an extension of the pharmacologic action of eptifibatide and was classified in clinical trials principally according to criteria of the Thrombolysis in Myocardial Infarction (TIMI) study groups. Minor bleeding generally was defined as spontaneous gross hematuria or spontaneous hematemesis; observed blood loss with a decrease in hemoglobin concentration of 3–5 g/dL or a reduction in hematocrit of at least 10%; or a decrease of 4–5 g/dL or 12–15% in hemoglobin or hematocrit, respectively, with no identifiable bleeding site. Major bleeding was defined as intracranial hemorrhage or overt bleeding associated with a hemoglobin or hematocrit decrease of at least 5 g/dL or at least 15%, respectively.

In clinical trials, administration of eptifibatide was associated with an increase in major and minor bleeding complications compared with placebo. The overall incidence of major and minor bleeding according to TIMI criteria in the PURSUIT study was 23.5% compared with an incidence of 40–70% in smaller studies. Bleeding of any severity was reported in about 15–60% of patients receiving placebo (i.e., heparin and aspirin therapy alone). Bleeding episodes resulted in discontinuance of eptifibatide in 8, 4.6, or 3.5% of patients receiving the drug in the PURSUIT, ESPRIT, or IMPACT-II study, respectively.

■ **Hematologic Effects** Major bleeding events occurred in 4.4 or 4.7% of evaluable patients receiving eptifibatide 0.5 or 0.75 mcg/kg per minute, respectively, by IV infusion following an IV loading dose of 135 mcg/kg in the IMPACT-II study; major bleeding occurred in 10.5 or 10.8% of those receiving 1.3 or 2 mcg/kg per minute, respectively, of eptifibatide following an IV loading dose of 180 mcg/kg in the PURSUIT study. Major bleeding occurred in 1.3 or 0.4% of those receiving eptifibatide (2 IV loading doses of 180 mcg/kg each given 10 minutes apart followed by continuous infusion of 2 mcg/kg per minute initiated after the first loading dose) or placebo in the ESPRIT study, respectively. The incidence of bleeding increased as the activated clotting time (ACT) increased (mean ACT of 284 seconds) in those receiving eptifibatide. At the lower ACTs achieved in the ESPRIT trial, the incidence of bleeding was lower than that observed in the IMPACT-II and PURSUIT studies. The incidence of major bleeding with eptifibatide was similar to that with placebo in the IMPACT-II study and modestly increased compared with placebo in the PURSUIT study. The overall incidence of major bleeding was higher in the PURSUIT study than in the IMPACT-II study because coronary artery bypass grafting (CABG) was more commonly employed in the PURSUIT study (15.5% incidence within 30 days) than in the IMPACT-II study (4.3%); major bleeding was minimal (0.6%) in patients receiving medical management alone in the PURSUIT trial. However, bleeding episodes in patients who underwent CABG were not more frequent in patients receiving eptifibatide than in placebo recipients in either study.

In the PURSUIT and ESPRIT studies, the greatest increase in major bleeding with eptifibatide therapy compared with placebo was bleeding at the femoral vascular access site (2.8 and 1.3%, respectively, in the PURSUIT study and 0.8 and 0.1%, respectively, in the ESPRIT study) associated with PCI; oropharyngeal (principally gingival), genitourinary, GI, and retroperitoneal bleeding also were more common with eptifibatide therapy than with placebo. GI, pulmonary, and retroperitoneal hemorrhage, including fatalities, have been reported during postmarketing experience with eptifibatide given concomitantly with heparin and aspirin. Among patients experiencing major bleeding in the IMPACT-II study, an increase in bleeding with eptifibatide versus placebo was demonstrated only for bleeding at the femoral vascular access site (3.2 versus 2.8%, respectively). In the PURSUIT and ESPRIT studies, patient weight was inversely related to the number of major bleeding episodes in patients receiving eptifibatide; this relationship was not found in the IMPACT-II study.

Adverse hematologic effects with eptifibatide therapy have been severe enough to require blood or platelet transfusions. In the IMPACT-II study, the incidences of major bleeding events and transfusions (including whole blood, packed red blood cells, fresh frozen plasma, cryoprecipitate, platelets, and autotransfusion) were similar in patients receiving eptifibatide or placebo, while minor bleeding events were more common with eptifibatide therapy. Bleeding or thrombocytopenia requiring transfusions in the IMPACT-II study occurred in about 5.5 or 5.8% of patients receiving eptifibatide 0.5 or 0.75 mcg/kg per minute, respectively, following an IV loading dose of 135 mcg/kg, compared with about 5.1% of patients receiving placebo injection and infusion (based on treated-as-randomized analysis). In the PURSUIT study, transfusions were required in 12.8% of patients receiving eptifibatide and in 10.4% of patients receiving placebo. In the ESPRIT study, transfusions were required in 1.5% of patients receiving eptifibatide and in 1.1% of those receiving placebo.

Minor bleeding episodes occurred in about 11.7 or 14.2% of patients receiving 0.5 or 0.75 mcg/kg per minute, respectively, of eptifibatide following an IV loading dose of 135 mcg/kg in the IMPACT-II study, and in 10.5 or 13.1% of those receiving 1.3 or 2 mcg/kg per minute, respectively, following an IV loading dose of 180 mcg/kg in the PURSUIT study. Minor bleeding episodes occurred in 3 or 2% of patients receiving eptifibatide or placebo, respectively, in the ESPRIT study.

Decreases in platelet count or thrombocytopenia occur occasionally (2.3% overall) after therapy with GP IIb/IIIa-receptor inhibitors. Thrombocytopenia associated with administration of a GP IIb/IIIa-receptor inhibitor generally occurs within hours or days after administration of the drug. The incidence of thrombocytopenia (defined as a platelet count less than 100,000/mm^3 or a decrease of at least 50% in platelet count from baseline) and the need for platelet transfusions were similar in patients receiving eptifibatide in several clinical trials (IMPACT-II, PURSUIT, pilot studies) and in patients receiving placebo. In the ESPRIT study, the incidence of thrombocytopenia was 1.2 or 0.6% among patients receiving eptifibatide or placebo, respectively. A preliminary report based on pooled data from clinical trials indicates that the incidence of thrombocytopenia is not appreciably different among GP IIb/IIIa-receptor inhibitors (i.e., abciximab, eptifibatide, tirofiban), although the absolute risk of thrombocytopenia appears to increase (but not synergistically) with concomitant use of heparin. However, severe thrombocytopenia (i.e., platelet count less than 20,000 per mm^3) has been reported more frequently with abciximab than with eptifibatide. In the large PURSUIT study, the incidence of profound thrombocytopenia (defined as a platelet count less than 20,000/mm^3) was small (0.2%) in patients receiving eptifibatide, but greater than the incidence in those receiving placebo (less than 0.1%).

■ **Sensitivity Reactions** Anaphylaxis was reported in 7 patients (0.16%) receiving an eptifibatide infusion rate of 2 mcg/kg per minute, respectively, following an IV loading dose of 180 mcg/kg in the PURSUIT study and in 7 patients (0.15%) receiving placebo in this study; none of the patients receiving eptifibatide and one patient receiving placebo in the IMPACT-II study developed anaphylaxis. Allergic reactions were reported in 2 patients (0.19%) receiving eptifibatide and in one patient (0.1%) receiving placebo in the ESPRIT study. Of those who received eptifibatide in the PURSUIT study, the drug was discontinued in 3 patients (0.05%). In patients undergoing PCI and receiving the drug in the IMPACT-II study, eptifibatide therapy was discontinued in 2 patients (0.04%) because of allergic reactions.

While therapy with some platelet-aggregation inhibitors (e.g., abciximab) has been associated with development of antibodies to the drug, development of antibodies against eptifibatide has not been reported to date. No evidence of delayed-type hypersensitivity or antigenicity with eptifibatide was noted in studies in mice and guinea pigs. The low molecular weight of eptifibatide may account for its lack of antigenicity. Some clinicians suggest that the lack of antigenicity of eptifibatide and the rapidly reversible binding of the drug to platelets compared with abciximab may account for the relative lack of thrombocytopenia observed with eptifibatide.

■ **Cardiovascular Effects** Most adverse effects of eptifibatide other than bleeding in clinical trials were cardiovascular in nature and were typical of patients with unstable angina; the incidence of most of these effects, with the exception of hypotension, was similar in patients receiving eptifibatide or placebo.

Hypotension occurred in 7% of patients receiving eptifibatide and 6% of those receiving placebo in the PURSUIT study.

Stroke, including primary hemorrhagic stroke, cerebral infarction, or infarction with hemorrhagic conversion, occurred in 0.5% of patients receiving an eptifibatide infusion rate of 1.3 mcg/kg per minute following an IV loading dose of 180 mcg/kg in the PURSUIT study and in 0.5% of patients receiving an infusion rate of 0.5 mcg/kg per minute following an IV loading dose of 135 mcg/kg in the IMPACT-II study. The overall incidence of stroke was 0.7% in patients receiving an eptifibatide infusion rate of 2 mcg/kg per minute following an IV loading dose of 180 mcg/kg in the PURSUIT study and in 0.7% of patients receiving an infusion rate of 0.75 mcg/kg per minute following an IV loading dose of 135 mcg/kg in the IMPACT-II study. Hemorrhagic stroke occurred in 2 patients (0.19%) receiving eptifibatide and in one patient (0.1%) receiving placebo in the ESPRIT study.

Therapy with GP IIb/IIIa receptor inhibitors, including eptifibatide, has not been associated with an increased risk of intracranial hemorrhage. The incidence of stroke was similar among patients receiving eptifibatide or placebo in either the PURSUIT or IMPACT-II study. Most strokes occurring in these studies were nonhemorrhagic (thromboembolic) in nature (i.e., cerebral infarctions). Cerebral infarction occurred in one patient (0.1%) receiving eptifibatide in the ESPRIT study. The incidence of intracranial hemorrhage in the IMPACT-II study was low (0.1–0.2%) and also was similar in patients receiving eptifibatide or placebo. Cerebral hemorrhage, sometimes resulting in death, has been reported with eptifibatide, principally in combination with heparin and aspirin, during postmarketing experience. Adverse cardiovascular effects leading to discontinuance of eptifibatide therapy occurred in 0.3 or 1.4% of patients receiving the drug in the PURSUIT or IMPACT-II study, respectively.

■ **Other Adverse Effects** Serious adverse effects of eptifibatide other than bleeding occurred in 19% of patients receiving either eptifibatide or placebo, respectively, in the PURSUIT study and in 7 or 6% of patients receiving the drug or placebo, respectively, in the ESPRIT study. Other adverse effects in the PURSUIT study occurring in at least 0.1% of patients and leading to discontinuance of eptifibatide involved the digestive system (0.1%), hemic/lymphatic system (0.1%), nervous system (0.3%), urogenital system (0.1%), and whole body (0.2%); these adverse effects resulted in discontinuance of therapy in a similar percentage of placebo recipients. In patients undergoing PCI who received eptifibatide in the IMPACT-II study, adverse effects other than bleeding that resulted in discontinuance of drug therapy occurred in the following body systems: whole body (0.3% of patients), digestive system (0.2%), hemic/lymphatic system (0.2%), nervous system (0.3%), and respiratory system (0.1%).

■ **Precautions and Contraindications** The administration of eptifibatide in patients with NSTE ACS is associated with a small increase in the frequency of major bleeding compared with heparin and aspirin therapy alone. Bleeding with platelet glycoprotein (GP IIb/IIIa)-receptor inhibitors can be reduced by adherence to strict anticoagulation guidelines, the use of a short course of low-dose, weight-adjusted heparin, early arterial sheath removal, and careful patient and access site management. Prior to administration of eptifibatide, preexisting hemostatic and renal abnormalities should be identified by obtaining a prothrombin time (PT), serum creatinine, hematocrit or hemoglobin, and activated partial thromboplastin time (aPTT). In patients receiving heparin concomitantly with eptifibatide, the extent of heparin anticoagulation (as assessed by activated clotting time [ACT] or aPTT) should be monitored closely to minimize bleeding. The aPTT should be maintained at 50–70 seconds unless PCI is to be performed. In addition, the ACT should be measured in patients undergoing PCI. Current guidelines of the ACCP, ACC, and AHA and risk-benefit analyses in trials with GP IIb/IIIa-receptor inhibitors suggest that heparin sodium dosing should be adjusted to maintain the ACT at 200 seconds or greater during PCI in patients receiving GP IIb/IIIa-receptor inhibitors. (See Dosage and Administration: Dosage.) Routine use of postprocedural heparin is not recommended while GP IIb/IIIa-receptor inhibitor therapy is given. After PCI, the aPTT should be checked prior to arterial sheath removal, and the sheath should not be removed unless the aPTT is less than 45 seconds or the ACT is less than 150–180 seconds. The manufacturer recommends that concomitant thrombolytic therapy be used with caution.

Platelet counts should be determined prior to treatment with eptifibatide and periodically (e.g., daily) during concomitant eptifibatide and heparin therapy. The manufacturer states that there is no clinical experience with the use of eptifibatide in patients who have platelet counts less than 100,000/mm^3 and that the drug should be used with caution in such patients. Abciximab, another GP IIb/IIIa-receptor inhibitor, has been associated with pseudothrombocytopenia caused by an in vitro anticoagulant (edetate disodium [EDTA]) interaction. Some clinicians suggest that a peripheral-blood smear be examined for the presence of platelet clumping or that blood for platelet counts be drawn into separate tubes containing EDTA, citrate, or heparin to exclude pseudothrombocytopenia in patients receiving eptifibatide. The possibility of heparin-induced thrombocytopenia also should be considered in the differential diagnosis of thrombocytopenia in patients receiving GP IIb/IIIa-receptor inhibitors concomitantly with heparin. If true thrombocytopenia (platelet count less than 100,000/mm^3) is verified, eptifibatide should be discontinued and the condition appropriately monitored and treated. Thrombocytopenia is usually reversible following discontinuance of GP IIb/IIIa-receptor inhibitors and anticoagulant (heparin) therapy; however, platelet transfusions should be considered for the management of severe thrombocytopenia.

To minimize the possibility of bleeding associated with the use of eptifibatide, particularly at the site of femoral artery sheath placement, precautions in the placement, maintenance, and removal of the vascular access sheath should be observed. Placement of a femoral venous sheath should be avoided if possible. When inserting the femoral artery sheath, care should be taken so that only the anterior wall of the femoral artery is punctured; a Seldinger (through and through) technique for puncture of the artery should be avoided. Appropriate precautions should be observed while the vascular access sheath is in place (e.g., complete bed rest, elevation of the head of the bed not exceeding 30°, restraint of the limb in which the vascular access sheath is inserted, frequent monitoring of the vascular access site and the distal pulse in the involved limb). The femoral artery sheath may be removed during treatment with eptifibatide, provided that at least 3–4 hours have elapsed since heparin therapy was discontinued and its effects largely reversed (as indicated by an aPTT of less than 45 seconds or an ACT of less than 150–180 seconds). Early removal of femoral sheaths (4–6 hours after PCI) was encouraged in patients receiving PCI in both the PURSUIT and IMPACT-II studies while the study drug was being infused.

Both heparin and eptifibatide therapy should be discontinued and sheath hemostasis achieved with standard compressive techniques at least 4 hours before hospital discharge. Pressure (e.g., using manual compression or a mechanical hemostatic device) should be applied to the femoral artery for at least 20–30 minutes after sheath removal; after hemostasis, a pressure dressing should be applied. Any hematoma that forms should be measured and monitored for enlargement.

Careful monitoring of all potential bleeding sites should be undertaken during and following treatment with platelet aggregation inhibitors. Needle punctures (e.g., arterial, IM, IV, lumbar, subcutaneous, intradermal), cutdown sites, and use of nasotracheal intubation, nasogastric tubes, urinary catheterization, and automatic blood pressure cuffs should be minimized during and following treatment with eptifibatide. Establishment of IV access at noncompressible sites (e.g., in subclavian or jugular veins) should be avoided; an indwelling venipuncture device (e.g., heparin lock) should be considered for drawing blood; documentation and monitoring of vascular puncture sites should occur; and dressings should be removed gently and carefully. The manufacturer states that any occurrence of serious bleeding that cannot be controlled by pressure on the bleeding site should result in discontinuance of eptifibatide and concomitantly administered heparin therapy.

Because eptifibatide increases the risk of bleeding, the drug is contraindicated in patients with a history of bleeding diathesis or active abnormal bleeding (e.g., elevated hemostatic indices, recent noncompressible vascular punctures GI or genitourinary bleeding) within the previous 30 days. A low hematocrit value (less than 30%) at baseline could represent recent undetected bleeding, and patients with such values may not be able to tolerate additional bleeding episodes; eptifibatide should not be used in these patients. Eptifibatide also is contraindicated in patients with severe uncontrolled hypertension (systolic blood pressure exceeding 200 mm Hg or diastolic blood pressure exceeding 110 mm Hg with antihypertensive therapy); recent (within 6 weeks) major surgery; history of stroke within 30 days or any history of hemorrhagic stroke; current or planned therapy with another GP IIb/IIIa-receptor inhibitor; and patients receiving renal dialysis. No data are available on the use of eptifibatide in patients with serum creatinine concentrations of 4 mg/dL or greater; the dosage should be reduced in patients with serum creatinine concentrations between 2–4 mg/dL. (See Dosage in Renal and Hepatic Impairment under Dosage and Administration: Dosage.)

Eptifibatide also is contraindicated in patients with known hypersensitivity to any component of the commercially available preparation.

■ **Pediatric Precautions** Safety and efficacy of eptifibatide in pediatric patients have not been determined.

■ **Geriatric Precautions** Safety and efficacy of eptifibatide in geriatric patients have not been specifically studied to date; however, in clinical studies of eptifibatide involving over 14,000 patients up to 94 years of age, approximately 45% of the patients were 65 years of age or older, and 12% were 75 years of age or older. Clinical experience generally has not revealed age-related differences in efficacy with eptifibatide therapy. However, the incidence of bleeding complications in clinical trials was higher in geriatric than in younger patients receiving either placebo or eptifibatide in clinical trials. No dosage adjustment was made for geriatric patients in the principal clinical trials (PURSUIT, IMPACT II), but patients older than 75 years of age had to weigh at least 50 kg to be enrolled in the PURSUIT study because of a concern for an increased risk of bleeding in those weighing less than that. (See Cautions: Hematologic Effects.)

■ **Mutagenicity and Carcinogenicity** No evidence of mutagenicity was seen at the chromosomal or gene level when eptifibatide was evaluated in several in vitro and in vivo test systems. The drug was not genotoxic in the Ames microbial mutagen test, mouse micronucleus test, or mouse lymphoma cell forward mutation assay. Eptifibatide did not demonstrate any potential to induce chromosomal aberrations in human lymphocytes.

Since eptifibatide is designed to be used in acute-care settings, long-term studies in animals to evaluate the carcinogenic potential of eptifibatide have not been performed and are not planned.

■ **Pregnancy, Fertility, and Lactation** Reproduction studies using continuous IV infusion of eptifibatide dosages at a total daily dosage of up to 72 mg/kg in pregnant rats and up to 36 mg/kg in pregnant rabbits (either dosage representing about 4 times the recommended maximum daily human dosage based on body surface area) have not revealed evidence of harm to the fetus. However, since animal reproduction studies are not always predictive of human response and there are no adequate or controlled studies to date using eptifibatide in pregnant women, eptifibatide should be used during pregnancy only when clearly needed.

Reproduction studies in male and female rats using eptifibatide dosages up to 72 mg/kg daily (about 4 times the maximum recommended human daily dosage) by continuous IV infusion have not revealed evidence of impaired fertility.

Since it is not known if eptifibatide is distributed into milk, the drug should be used with caution in nursing women.

Drug Interactions

■ **Drugs Affecting Platelet Function** Limited data from preclinical and clinical studies in patients receiving eptifibatide (0.5 mcg/kg per minute by IV infusion) alone or concomitantly with aspirin, heparin, or both drugs suggest no substantial pharmacokinetic or pharmacodynamic interactions (e.g., additive effects on platelet-aggregation inhibition) between eptifibatide and aspirin. While coadministration of eptifibatide and aspirin resulted in up to a fivefold increase in bleeding time compared with baseline values, similar increases in bleeding time were observed with aspirin and placebo. Nevertheless, since eptifibatide inhibits platelet aggregation, caution should be observed when the drug is used with other drugs that affect hemostasis, including thrombolytic agents, oral anticoagulants, nonsteroidal anti-inflammatory agents (NSAIAs), or dipyridamole. (See Drug Interactions: Thrombolytic Therapy and also see Drug Interactions: Anticoagulants.) However, clopidogrel or ticlopidine was used routinely with eptifibatide in a large clinical, multicenter study (Enhanced Suppression of the Platelet IIb/IIIa Receptor with Integrilin Therapy [ESPRIT]) in patients undergoing coronary artery stent placement.

To minimize potentially additive pharmacologic effects, the manufacturer of eptifibatide states that concomitant therapy with other platelet glycoprotein (GP IIb/IIIa)-receptor inhibitors (e.g., abciximab, tirofiban) should be avoided.

■ **Thrombolytic Therapy** Eptifibatide has been administered concomitantly with thrombolytic agents (e.g., alteplase, streptokinase, tenecteplase) in a limited number of patients with acute myocardial infarction (MI) to reduce the risk of reocclusion of the infarct-related artery. (See Uses: Adjunctive Therapy During Thrombolysis to Prevent Reocclusion.) Some clinicians suggest that use of short-acting platelet-aggregation inhibitors such as eptifibatide concomitantly with thrombolytic therapy may provide optimal benefit while minimizing the risk of bleeding. However, use after thrombolysis of drugs that affect platelet function may increase the risk of bleeding complications, including those requiring blood transfusions, associated with thrombolytic therapy and has not been shown to be unequivocally effective to date; therefore, use of eptifibatide with thrombolytic therapy should be considered investigational and should be undertaken with caution.

In a small, placebo-controlled trial and dose-ranging study in patients with acute MI, combined therapy with eptifibatide (up to 180 mcg/kg as an IV loading dose followed by continuous infusion of 0.75 mcg/kg per minute for 24 hours) and alteplase (accelerated, weight-adjusted IV infusion up to 100 mg) was not associated with an increased incidence of major bleeding or transfusions compared with alteplase monotherapy. However, in another study in patients with acute MI receiving streptokinase (1.5 million units IV over 60 minutes) and eptifibatide (up to 180 mcg/kg as an IV loading dose followed by continuous infusion of 2 mcg/kg per minute for 72 hours), the higher infusion rates of eptifibatide (1.3 and 2 mcg/kg per minute) were associated with an increase in bleeding and the need for blood transfusion compared with streptokinase monotherapy. In the IMPACT-II study, 2 of 15 patients who received a thrombolytic agent concomitantly with eptifibatide (135 mcg/kg as an IV loading dose followed by 0.5 mcg/kg per minute by IV infusion) had a major bleeding episode, while 10 of 40 patients who received thrombolytic therapy and eptifibatide (180 mcg/kg as an IV loading dose followed by 2 mcg/kg per minute by IV infusion) in the PURSUIT study experienced major bleeding.

■ **Anticoagulants** Concomitant use of platelet-aggregation inhibitors and an anticoagulant (particularly in high dosages) may increase the risk of hemorrhage, and careful monitoring for bleeding is necessary, especially at arterial puncture sites. Eptifibatide and concomitant heparin therapy should be discontinued immediately and appropriate therapy (e.g., protamine sulfate in patients receiving heparin) instituted as necessary if serious bleeding occurs (e.g., bleeding not controlled by pressure). In healthy individuals, enoxaparin sodium (1 mg/kg subcutaneously every 12 hours for 4 doses) did not alter the pharmacokinetics or pharmacodynamics (platelet aggregation) of eptifibatide. The manufacturer states that caution should be employed when using eptifibatide with oral anticoagulants.

In almost all patients receiving eptifibatide for non-ST-segment-elevation acute coronary syndromes or in patients undergoing percutaneous coronary intervention (PCI), heparin (generally combined with aspirin) has been administered before and during eptifibatide therapy to reduce the risk of coronary artery occlusion or new thrombi formation. When eptifibatide was given alone or in combination with heparin in a limited number of healthy individuals at eptifibatide infusion rates exceeding 0.5 mcg/kg per minute or for durations exceeding 6 hours, bleeding time was prolonged approximately twofold or greater; smaller dosages infused over 90 minutes had minimal effects on bleeding time.

Laboratory Test Interferences

In blood samples, binding of eptifibatide to the GP IIb/IIIa-receptor and the drug's subsequent inhibitory activity on platelet aggregation are dependent on the free calcium concentration, and therefore the type of anticoagulant used in the sample. In the IMPACT-II study, the assay used to determine inhibition of platelet aggregation involved anticoagulation with sodium citrate, which removes calcium bound to the GP IIb/IIIa receptor and results in enhanced binding of eptifibatide to the receptor. Therefore, the inhibitory activity of eptifibatide is overestimated in blood samples collected in citrate relative to that in samples anticoagulated with PPACK. (See Uses: Acute Ischemic Complications of Percutaneous Coronary Intervention.)

Acute Toxicity

Limited information is available on the acute toxicity of eptifibatide. In general, overdosage of eptifibatide in humans may be expected to produce effects that are extensions of the pharmacologic and adverse effects of the drug, predominantly bleeding. (See Cautions: Hematologic Effects.) A small number of patients in each of the major clinical studies (IMPACT-II, PURSUIT) received doses of eptifibatide by IV injection and/or infusion that were more than twice those recommended or that were identified by study investigators as an overdose; none of these individuals had intracranial hemorrhage or other major bleeding.

In acute toxicity studies in animals (rats, rabbits, or monkeys) given 45 mg/kg of eptifibatide (about 2–5 times the maximum recommended daily human dose based on body surface area) over 90 minutes by continuous IV infusion, loss of righting reflex, dyspnea, ptosis, and decreased muscle tone were observed in rabbits, and petechial hemorrhages in the femoral and abdominal areas were observed in monkeys; no manifestations of toxicity were observed in rats given this dose of eptifibatide. In short-term toxicology studies (14–28 days) in monkeys, continuous IV infusion of eptifibatide in dosages exceeding 5 mcg/kg per minute produced contusions, hemorrhage, and petechial hemorrhages, resulting in anemia in some animals. At a dosage of 50 mcg/kg per minute, bleeding, decreased concentrations of plasma proteins, anemia, and death occurred. These effects were not observed in monkeys given eptifibatide 5 mcg/kg per minute (representing 1.1 times the mean steady-state plasma concentrations in patients undergoing PCI and receiving the recommended dosing regimen) in the IMPACT-II study.

Pharmacology

■ Platelet Aggregation and Thrombosis Eptifibatide is a selective, competitive, reversible inhibitor of platelet aggregation that is used to prevent acute ischemic complications associated with non-ST-segment-elevation acute coronary syndromes (NSTE ACS) and/or percutaneous coronary intervention (PCI). Because of its mechanism of action, eptifibatide, like abciximab and tirofiban, has been referred to as a platelet glycoprotein (GP) IIb/IIIa-receptor inhibitor. Platelet adhesion, activation, and aggregation are key processes leading to the formation of platelet-rich ("white") coronary artery thrombi and the development of ACS and ischemic complications associated with PCI. White thrombus formation is triggered by vascular injury (e.g., from PCI procedures), plaque rupture, or denudation of endothelium that exposes the subendothelial matrix of the vessel to circulating platelets. Upon exposure of the vessel subendothelium, potent thrombogenic stimuli (e.g., thrombin, collagen) present in both subendothelium and plaque, and/or high-shear stress, stimulate platelet adhesion and activation.

Activated platelets release intracellular granules consisting of vasoactive substances that are part of an autostimulatory loop for platelet aggregation; these vasoactive substances include thromboxane A_2, serotonin, and adenosine diphosphate (ADP); adhesive glycoproteins such as fibrinogen, fibronectin, and von Willebrand's factor; and plasminogen activator inhibitor-1 (PAI-1). Regardless of the initial stimulus for platelet activation, the final common pathway to platelet aggregation and thrombosis involves activation of the receptor function of the platelet glycoprotein (GP) IIb/IIIa complex (also known as $\alpha_{IIb}\beta_3$). GP IIb/IIIa receptors on the surface of activated platelets undergo a conformational change to accept soluble fibrinogen, von Willebrand's factor, and other ligands (e.g., fibronectin, vitronectin, thrombospondin). Some of these adhesive ligands form cross-links to GP IIb/IIIa receptors on the surface of adjacent activated platelets, causing aggregation and white thrombus formation. In addition, fibrinogen bound to the vessel wall or to other platelet aggregates can activate GP IIb/IIIa receptors on unstimulated platelets and recruit these platelets to growing white thrombi.

Progression of unstable angina or non-ST-segment-elevation myocardial infarction (NSTEMI) to ST-segment-elevation myocardial infarction (STEMI) or sudden death occurs when obstructive platelet-rich thrombi grow to become occlusive thrombi in the absence of perfusion beyond the obstruction through collateral blood vessels. Fibrin and erythrocytes comprise the outer layer of occlusive red thrombi that are formed on the surface of the platelet-rich inner core of the thrombus. While thrombolytic therapy effectively dissolves the occluding fibrin-rich portion of the thrombus, this process releases clot-bound thrombin and re-exposes the underlying disrupted plaque, which releases potent thrombogenic stimuli. This newly released thrombin then activates platelets, leading to platelet aggregation. In addition, activated platelets secrete a variety of factors associated with rethrombosis and thrombin production (e.g., PAI-1, fibrinogen, factor V) and bind factors Xa, VIIIa, and IXa, which are involved in further thrombin production. Platelet reactivity also may increase after thrombolysis. Use of platelet-aggregation inhibitors such as eptifibatide concomitantly with thrombolytic therapy may counter the thrombogenic activity of these agents and minimize the risk of reocclusion.

■ Inhibition of Platelet Aggregation Eptifibatide reversibly inhibits platelet aggregation by preventing the binding of fibrinogen, von Willebrand factor, and other adhesive ligands to resting and active GP IIb/IIIa receptors. Inhibition of platelet aggregation by eptifibatide occurs in a dose- and concentration-dependent manner via an increase in GP IIb/IIIa-receptor occupancy (as determined by ex vivo platelet aggregation assay with the direct thrombin inhibitor D-phenylalanyl-L-propyl-L-arginyl chloromethyl ketone [PPACK]). Some platelet-aggregation inhibitors such as aspirin, ticlopidine, and clopidogrel prevent platelet activation in response to one or more agonists (thromboxane A_2, adenosine diphosphate); agonists not affected by these drugs may continue to induce platelet aggregation. However, GP IIb/IIIa-receptor inhibitors such as abciximab, eptifibatide, and tirofiban prevent platelet aggregation regardless of the initial stimulus. In vitro studies indicate that eptifibatide is not effective in displacing fibrinogen cross-links from GP IIb/IIIa-receptors in platelet-rich thrombi when the bond between fibrinogen and GP IIb/IIIa becomes irreversible.

Following a single 180-mcg/kg IV dose of eptifibatide in healthy individuals or patients with NSTE ACS and/or those undergoing PCI, platelet aggregation was inhibited by greater than 90% within 15 minutes at physiologic calcium concentrations based on ex vivo platelet-aggregation assays using PPACK as the anticoagulant. Inhibition of platelet aggregation by eptifibatide also may depend on the degree of initial platelet activation, which may be influenced by concurrent disease states. In an ex vivo study, the concentration of eptifibatide needed to inhibit 50% of ADP-induced platelet aggregation was lowest in healthy men, higher in patients undergoing PCI, and highest in patients with NSTE ACS, perhaps reflecting differences in existing platelet activation. The pharmacodynamics of eptifibatide do not appear to be affected by age; differences in pharmacodynamic effects among ethnic groups have not been assessed.

■ Hemostatic Effects Since the effect of eptifibatide on platelet aggregation is rapidly reversible following cessation of the infusion, the drug has a modest effect on hemostatic indices (e.g., bleeding times) and platelet function. Normal hemostasis is restored more rapidly than with abciximab, a monoclonal antibody that dissociates very slowly from the GP IIb/IIIa-receptor.

When eptifibatide was administered alone or in combination with heparin in clinical trials, bleeding time was prolonged approximately twofold. At steady-state plasma eptifibatide concentrations in patients with NSTE ACS (who received a 180-mcg/kg IV loading dose followed by IV infusion of 2 mcg/kg per minute) or who were undergoing PCI (who received a 135-mcg/kg IV loading dose followed by IV infusion of 0.5 mcg/kg per minute) and also were receiving concomitant aspirin and heparin, bleeding time was prolonged up to 5 times the control value. Ex vivo ADP-induced platelet aggregation using PPACK in patients with NSTE ACS was restored toward baseline values (i.e., to less than 50% inhibition) within 4 hours after cessation of an eptifibatide infusion (180-mcg/kg IV loading dose followed by IV infusion of 2 mcg/kg per minute for 72–96 hours); 6 hours after discontinuance of the eptifibatide infusion, bleeding time averaged 1.4 times the control value. Data from an ex vivo platelet aggregation assay in these patients indicated a GP IIb/IIIa-receptor occupancy of less than 60% 8 hours after discontinuance of the eptifibatide infusion.

When administered alone, eptifibatide usually does not affect prothrombin time (PT) or activated partial thromboplastin time (aPTT).

■ Effect of Calcium Concentration on Platelet-Aggregation Assays The reported inhibitory effect of eptifibatide on platelet aggregation depends on the free calcium concentration (and therefore the type of anticoagulant used) in the samples to be assayed, which is negatively correlated with the inhibitory activity and can affect interpretation of results of platelet function tests. (See Laboratory Test Interferences.)

Pharmacokinetics

The pharmacokinetics of eptifibatide in healthy individuals are linear, and plasma concentrations are proportional to dose following IV loading doses of 90–250 mcg/kg and IV infusion rates of 0.5–3 mcg/kg per minute. Concomitant administration of aspirin or heparin does not appear to affect the pharmacokinetics of eptifibatide, nor does gender.

■ Absorption With recommended IV loading and maintenance infusions of eptifibatide, peak plasma drug concentrations occur within 5 minutes of IV injection and steady-state drug concentrations are attained within 4–6 hours. Following IV administration of an eptifibatide loading dose of 135 mcg/kg and an IV infusion of 0.5 mcg/kg per minute for 20–24 hours, plasma drug concentrations at steady state averaged 291 ng/mL in patients undergoing percutaneous coronary intervention (PCI). In geriatric patients with coronary artery disease, plasma concentrations are increased compared with those in younger adults. Following IV administration of an eptifibatide loading dose of 180 mcg/kg and IV infusion of 2 mcg/kg per minute for 24 or 72 hours, steady-state plasma drug concentrations (as determined using population pharmacokinetic methods) in patients with non-ST-segment-elevation acute coronary syndromes (NSTE ACS) or those undergoing PCI reportedly averaged 2.2 or 1.5 mcg/mL, respectively. In healthy individuals receiving eptifibatide infusion rates of 0.5–2 mcg/kg per minute for 24 hours, steady-state plasma drug concentrations reportedly average approximately 0.3–1.1 mcg/mL. In patients with moderate to severe renal impairment (estimated Cl_{cr} less than 50 mL/minute), steady-state plasma concentrations double.

Eptifibatide has a rapid onset and short duration of action; maximal inhibition of platelet aggregation occurs within 15 minutes after initiation of therapy and is rapidly reversible. Within 4 hours after cessation of drug infusion, platelet aggregation returned to greater than 50% of baseline in patients with NSTE ACS receiving recommended dosages of eptifibatide (180-mcg/kg IV loading dose followed by infusion of 2 mcg/kg per minute) and to less than 30% of peak values in patients undergoing PCI and receiving recommended dosages of the drug (135-mcg/kg IV loading dose followed by infusion of 0.5 mcg/kg per minute). Platelet aggregation usually returns toward normal within 4–8 hours after discontinuing eptifibatide in patients with NSTE ACS or ST-segment-elevation myocardial infarction (STEMI).

■ **Distribution** Eptifibatide is approximately 25% bound to plasma proteins, principally (9–16%) to albumin. The volume of distribution of eptifibatide in patients with coronary artery disease is about 185–260 mL/kg and is somewhat higher (220–270 mL/kg) in healthy individuals. It is not known whether eptifibatide is distributed into milk in humans.

■ **Elimination** Eptifibatide is eliminated by renal and nonrenal mechanisms. The drug appears to undergo rapid and nonmetabolic degradation in the urinary bladder after its elimination from plasma. Eptifibatide is metabolized principally through deamidation to a metabolite that has approximately 41% of the platelet-aggregation inhibitory activity of the parent compound, and through formation of other more polar metabolites. Approximately 27% of a dose of eptifibatide is broken down in plasma into naturally occurring amino acids; no major non-amino acid metabolites have been detected in plasma in humans. Following IV administration of a single, ^{14}C-radiolabeled dose of eptifibatide (135 mcg/kg) in healthy men, 34, 19, and 13% of the radioactivity was recovered in urine within the first 24 hours as parent compound, deamidated metabolite, and polar metabolites (as detected by radiochromatography), respectively. In healthy men receiving a single, radiolabeled IV dose of the drug (135 mcg/kg), 98, 1.5, and 0.8% of the dose was recovered in urine, feces, and breath carbon dioxide, respectively. In vitro studies indicate that eptifibatide is not extensively bound to plasma proteins; therefore, the drug may be removed from plasma by hemodialysis.

Plasma concentrations of eptifibatide decline in a biexponential manner following IV injection or infusion of the drug. The half-life of eptifibatide in patients with coronary artery disease averages 2.5–2.8 hours. In healthy individuals, half-life of the drug reportedly averages 0.83–2.4 hours. Clearance of eptifibatide in patients with coronary disease is 55–80 mL/kg per hour; clearance of the drug is twofold higher in healthy individuals. Plasma clearance of eptifibatide is proportional to body weight and estimated creatinine clearance and inversely proportional to age. Following a single IV dose of ^{14}C-radiolabeled eptifibatide (135 mcg/kg) in healthy men, renal clearance averaged approximately 40–50% of total body clearance. Clearance is reduced by 50% in patients with moderate to severe renal impairment (estimated Cl_{cr} less than 50 mL/minute). Total body clearance in geriatric patients with coronary artery disease is lower than that in younger adults.

Chemistry and Stability

■ **Chemistry** Eptifibatide, a synthetic cyclic heptapeptide, is a selective platelet-aggregation inhibitor. Eptifibatide, like abciximab and tirofiban, has been referred to as a platelet glycoprotein (GP) IIb/IIIa-receptor inhibitor. The drug is similar in structure to barbourin, a peptide constituent of the venom of the southeastern pigmy rattlesnake, *Sistrurus m. barbouri*.

Eptifibatide is composed of 6 amino acids and a mercaptopropionyl (desamino cysteinyl) residue with an interchain disulfide bridge between the cysteine amide and the mercaptopropionyl moieties. The active domain of eptifibatide contains a modified lysine-glycine-aspartate (KGD) amino acid sequence similar to the physiologic arginine-glycine-aspartate (RGD) sequence in von Willebrand's factor, vitronectin, fibrinogen, and fibronectin, adhesive ligands that bind to platelet glycoprotein (GP) IIb/IIIa receptors on activated platelets and cause platelet aggregation. The substitution of lysine for arginine on the binding site in eptifibatide increases the selectivity of binding to the GP IIb/IIIa receptor.

Commercially available eptifibatide injection is a clear, colorless, sterile solution of the drug in sterile water for injection; sodium hydroxide and citric acid have been added to adjust the pH to 5.25. Eptifibatide is insoluble in nonpolar solvents such as hexane (0.02 mg/mL), but is freely soluble in polar aqueous solvents and in highly polar solvents such as dimethyl sulfoxide (exceeding 400 mg/mL). Eptifibatide has pK_as of 4 and exceeding 12.5.

■ **Stability** Eptifibatide should be refrigerated at between 2–8°C and protected from light until administration. Commercially available eptifibatide injection has an expiration date of 24 months following the date of manufacture when stored as directed. The injection may be transferred to room temperature storage (15–30°C) for a period not to exceed 2 months. When stored at room temperature, the injection container should be marked to indicate that any unused vials should be discarded after 2 months or by the manufacturer's labeled expiration date (whichever comes first). The manufacturer states that vials of the injection that have been left unrefrigerated only for a brief period (i.e., the vial is still cool to the touch) may be returned to refrigeration without the need to alter the expiration date.

The manufacturer states that eptifibatide is chemically and physically compatible (i.e., no evidence of precipitation, color or pH change, or loss of potency) with, and may be administered in the same IV line as alteplase, atropine, dobutamine, heparin, lidocaine, meperidine, metoprolol, midazolam, morphine, nitroglycerin, or verapamil. Eptifibatide is chemically/physically incompatible with furosemide (i.e., precipitate formation within 1 hour of mixing, exceeding 40% loss of furosemide potency at 24 hours, and decrease in pH from about 8.9 to 5.4), and these drugs should *not* be administered through the same IV line. Eptifibatide may be administered in the same IV line with 0.9% sodium chloride injection or 0.9% sodium chloride and 5% dextrose injection. With either vehicle, the infusion may contain up to 60 mEq/L of potassium chloride. No incompatibilities have been observed between eptifibatide and IV administration sets, and no data are available concerning the compatibility of eptifibatide with polyvinyl chloride (PVC) bags.

Preparations

Excipients in commercially available drug preparations may have clinically important effects in some individuals; consult specific product labeling for details.

Eptifibatide

Parenteral		
Injection, for IV Use	2 mg/mL (20 mg)	Integrilin®, Schering
	0.75 mg/mL (75 mg)	Integrilin®, Schering

†Use is not currently included in the labeling approved by the US Food and Drug Administration

Selected Revisions September 2017,

Prasugrel Hydrochloride

■ Prasugrel hydrochloride, a thienopyridine P2Y12 platelet adenosine diphosphate (ADP)-receptor antagonist, is a platelet-activation and -aggregation inhibitor.

Uses

■ **Acute Coronary Syndromes** ***Patients Undergoing Percutaneous Coronary Intervention*** Prasugrel hydrochloride is used in combination with aspirin for the reduction of thrombotic cardiovascular events (e.g., stent thrombosis, myocardial infarction [MI]) in patients with acute coronary syndrome (ACS) undergoing percutaneous coronary intervention (PCI). Prasugrel is used in patients with unstable angina or non-ST-segment-elevation MI (NSTEMI) undergoing PCI and in patients with ST-segment-elevation MI (STEMI) managed with primary or nonprimary/delayed (i.e., after medical treatment for STEMI) PCI.

Dual-drug antiplatelet therapy with a P2Y12 platelet adenosine diphosphate (ADP)-receptor antagonist (e.g., clopidogrel, prasugrel, ticagrelor) and aspirin is part of the current standard of care in patients with ACS. The American Heart Association (AHA), the American College of Cardiology Foundation (ACCF), the Society for Cardiovascular Angiography and Interventions (SCAI), and the American College of Chest Physicians (ACCP) recommend antiplatelet therapy with a P2Y12-receptor antagonist (clopidogrel, prasugrel, or ticagrelor) in conjunction with aspirin for treatment and secondary prevention in patients with ACS. These experts generally recommend ticagrelor or clopidogrel as the P2Y12-receptor antagonist in patients with ACS who are treated medically without stent placement; because prasugrel has been studied principally in patients undergoing planned PCI, recommendations for the use of this drug are restricted to that population. In patients undergoing PCI with stent placement (bare-metal or drug-eluting), a loading dose of ticagrelor, clopidogrel, or prasugrel is recommended, followed by maintenance therapy with one of these agents for at least 12 months (unless the risk of bleeding outweighs the anticipated net benefit of therapy); aspirin should be continued indefinitely in such patients. There is some evidence suggesting that a longer duration of dual antiplatelet therapy (for more than 12 months) may be beneficial in some patients with drug-eluting stents to reduce the risk of late stent thrombosis and other cardiovascular events, but such prolonged therapy may be associated with an increased risk of bleeding and other adverse effects. (See Discontinuance of Therapy under Warnings/Precautions: Warnings, in Cautions.)

Current ACCF/AHA guidelines make no recommendations regarding the P2Y12-receptor antagonist of choice in patients with ACS. Unlike clopidogrel, genetic polymorphism of the cytochrome P-450 (CYP) 2C19 isoenzyme does not appear to affect the pharmacodynamic or clinical response to prasugrel; therefore, some experts recommend the use of prasugrel as an alternative to clopidogrel in patients who are identified as potential poor metabolizers of clopidogrel. In preclinical and early clinical studies, prasugrel inhibited platelet aggregation more potently and rapidly than standard or higher dosages of clopidogrel and was associated with less interpatient variability in antiplatelet effects. Such improved inhibition of platelet aggregation was associated with reduced ischemic events (e.g., reductions in stent thrombosis and MI) in a large prospective randomized study of patients with ACS undergoing PCI; however, these benefits were accompanied by an increased risk of bleeding. When considering the use of prasugrel over other P2Y12-receptor antagonists, clinicians should balance the anticipated greater benefits with prasugrel against the increased risk of bleeding, and also consider the patient populations in whom the drugs have been used. Some evidence suggests that certain patient populations (e.g., those with diabetes or previous MI) are more likely to benefit from prasugrel's greater inhibition of platelet aggregation, while others (e.g., geriatric patients, those with low body weight or history of stroke/transient ischemic attack [TIA]) may experience harm.

Because of the substantial risk of serious bleeding, prasugrel should not be initiated in patients who are likely to undergo urgent coronary artery bypass grafting (CABG); when possible, therapy with the drug should be discontinued at least 7 days prior to any surgery. (See Bleeding, under Warnings/Precautions: Warnings, in Cautions.) In addition, prasugrel should not be used in patients with a history of TIA or stroke. (See Cautions: Contraindications.)

The current indication for prasugrel is based principally on results of a multicenter, randomized, double-blind parallel group study (Trial to Assess Improvement in Therapeutic Outcomes by Optimizing Platelet Inhibition with Prasugrel-Thrombolysis in Myocardial Infarction [TRITON-TIMI 38]) comparing efficacy and safety of prasugrel and clopidogrel in 13,608 patients with moderate- to high-risk ACS undergoing planned PCI. Patients with unstable angina or NSTEMI were eligible if they had ischemic manifestations lasting 10 minutes or more within 72 hours prior to randomization, a TIMI risk score of at least 3, and either ST-segment deviation of at least 1 mm or elevated levels of a cardiac biomarker of necrosis; patients with STEMI were enrolled within 12 hours of symptom onset if primary PCI was planned or within 14 days after receiving medical treatment for STEMI (nonprimary/delayed PCI). Patients received either clopidogrel (300-mg loading dose followed by 75 mg daily) or prasugrel (60-mg loading dose followed by 10 mg daily) for 6–15 months. The loading dose of the study drug was administered anytime between randomization and 1 hour after the patient was transferred from the cardiac catheterization laboratory; most patients (approximately 75%) received the study drug after the first coronary guidewire was placed or within 1 hour of PCI. Patients were required to receive concomitant treatment with aspirin 75–325 mg daily; other standard therapies (e.g., heparin, platelet glycoprotein [GP] IIb/IIIa-receptor inhibitors) were given at the discretion of the treating clinician. Most patients (94%) received at least one intracoronary stent.

Treatment with prasugrel resulted in a 19% relative reduction in the composite primary end point of cardiovascular death, nonfatal MI, or nonfatal stroke compared with clopidogrel; such benefits were apparent within 3 days and persisted throughout the duration of the study (median 14.5 months). The reduction in the primary end point was largely driven by a substantial reduction in MI (new or recurrent) with little or no difference in the incidence of stroke or cardiovascular death (other than from MI) between groups. Reductions in the rate of stent thrombosis and urgent target-vessel revascularization also favored prasugrel. Stent thrombosis was substantially reduced with prasugrel in patients who received at least one intracoronary stent irrespective of the stent type (bare-metal or drug-eluting).

The benefit of prasugrel in reducing ischemic events in the TRITON-TIMI 38 study was accompanied by an increased risk of bleeding. Major and minor bleeding complications, including life-threatening and fatal bleeding, occurred more frequently in patients receiving prasugrel compared with clopidogrel. (See Bleeding under Warnings/Precautions: Warnings, in Cautions.) When efficacy and bleeding end points were combined, the net clinical benefit (defined as death from any cause, nonfatal MI, nonfatal stroke, or non-CABG-related nonfatal TIMI major hemorrhage) favored prasugrel over clopidogrel in the overall study population, but not in all subgroups. In post hoc analyses, patients 75 years of age or older, those weighing less than 60 kg, and those with previous stroke or TIA were identified as subgroups experiencing no net clinical benefit and possibly harm with such therapy. In patients with diabetes mellitus, however, a trend towards greater efficacy of prasugrel compared with nondiabetics was noted without a relative increase in major bleeding. Results of such subgroup analyses should be considered exploratory and should be interpreted with caution.

The prasugrel dosage regimen used in the TRITON-TIMI 38 study (60-mg loading dose, 10 mg daily maintenance dosage) has been shown to produce substantially greater and more consistent inhibition of platelet aggregation than that produced by a clopidogrel loading dose of 600 mg and maintenance dosage of 150 mg daily, dosages higher than current FDA-labeled loading and maintenance dosages. In addition, while it is generally recommended that antiplatelet agents be administered promptly upon presentation or diagnosis in patients with ACS, administration of prasugrel and clopidogrel in the TRITON-TIMI 38 study was delayed until after coronary anatomy was determined to be appropriate for PCI. Therefore, this study does not provide information on the comparative efficacy and safety of clopidogrel and prasugrel in dosages that provide equivalent inhibition of platelet aggregation, nor does it directly address the potential effects on efficacy of routine pretreatment with clopidogrel or prasugrel before diagnostic cardiac catheterization.

Increased risk of bleeding is a concern in patients receiving antiplatelet agents who require urgent CABG. Because most patients with ACS are managed without CABG, pretreatment with prasugrel may be considered prior to performing diagnostic coronary angiography in patients who are not likely to undergo CABG. The potential benefits of pretreatment should be balanced against the risk of surgical bleeding in patients who may subsequently require CABG.

Dosage and Administration

■ **Administration** Prasugrel hydrochloride is administered orally without regard to meals. Dosage of prasugrel hydrochloride is expressed in terms of prasugrel.

■ **Dosage** ***Acute Coronary Syndromes*** **Patients Undergoing PCI.** For the reduction of thrombotic cardiovascular events in patients with an acute coronary syndrome (ACS) undergoing percutaneous coronary intervention (PCI), the manufacturer recommends a loading dose of 60 mg of prasugrel, followed by 10 mg once daily. Aspirin (75–325 mg daily) should be given concomitantly. The majority of patients in the TRITON-TIMI 38 study received the loading dose of prasugrel after the first coronary guidewire was placed or within 1 hour of PCI. The American College of Cardiology Foundation (ACCF) and the American Heart Association (AHA) recommend that the loading dose of prasugrel be initiated as soon as possible or at the time of PCI in patients with ST-segment-elevation myocardial infarction (STEMI) undergoing *primary* PCI. Experts state that a prasugrel loading dose of 60 mg is reasonable in patients undergoing delayed PCI after initial thrombolytic therapy who did not previously receive a loading dose of clopidogrel; prasugrel should not be administered sooner than 24 hours after a fibrin-specific thrombolytic agent.

A prasugrel maintenance dosage of 5 mg daily may be considered in patients weighing less than 60 kg, although safety and efficacy of this lower dosage has not been established. (See Bleeding under Warnings/Precautions: Warnings, in Cautions.)

The optimum duration of prasugrel therapy has not been determined. However, in patients undergoing PCI with stent implantation, premature discontinuance of any antiplatelet therapy (i.e., aspirin, a P2Y12-receptor antagonist) increases the risk of stent thrombosis, myocardial infarction, and death; therefore, long-term (e.g., at least 12 months) dual antiplatelet therapy is recommended in such patients unless the risk of bleeding outweighs the anticipated net benefit. (See Discontinuance of Therapy under Warnings/Precautions: Warnings, in Cautions.)

Adjunctive Antithrombotic Therapy. Adjunctive antithrombotic therapy with daily aspirin (e.g., 75–325 mg) is recommended in all patients with ACS, including those undergoing PCI. For additional information on the dosage of aspirin used as adjunctive antithrombotic therapy in the management of ACS, see Dosage and Administration in Aspirin 28:08.04.24.

Discontinuance in Patients Undergoing Invasive Procedures Thienopyridines, including prasugrel, should be discontinued prior to elective surgery. In patients who require elective coronary artery bypass grafting (CABG), discontinuance of prasugrel therapy is recommended at least 7 days prior to surgery. Prasugrel should not be initiated in those who are likely to undergo emergent CABG. To minimize the risk of adverse cardiac events, thienopyridines, including prasugrel, and other antiplatelet therapy should be resumed as soon as possible after temporary discontinuance of therapy for adverse effects or invasive procedures. (See Discontinuance of Therapy under Warnings/Precautions: Warnings, in Cautions.)

■ **Special Populations** No dosage adjustment necessary in patients with renal impairment.

No dosage adjustment necessary in patients with mild to moderate hepatic impairment (Child-Pugh Class A and B). Not studied in patients with severe hepatic disease.

Not known whether dosage adjustments based on age, weight or other patient characteristics will maintain effectiveness of prasugrel while decreasing risk of bleeding.

Cautions

■ **Contraindications** Presence of active pathological bleeding (e.g., peptic ulcer, intracranial hemorrhage).

History of transient ischemic attack (TIA) or stroke.

■ **Warnings/Precautions** ***Warnings*** **Bleeding.** Use of prasugrel is associated with a risk of serious, sometimes fatal bleeding. Major bleeding (defined as intracranial hemorrhage or clinically overt bleeding associated with a decline in hemoglobin concentration of at least 5 g/dL) and minor bleeding (defined as overt bleeding with a decrease in hemoglobin concentration of at least 3 g/dL but less than 5 g/dL) were more frequent in patients receiving prasugrel versus clopidogrel in the TRITON-TIMI 38 study. Major hemorrhage not related to coronary artery bypass grafting (CABG) occurred in 2.4% of patients receiving prasugrel compared with 1.8% of those receiving clopidogrel; this included higher rates of life-threatening and fatal bleeding. Life-threatening bleeding occurred mostly at GI, intracranial, retroperitoneal, or puncture sites. CABG-related major bleeding occurred in 13.4% of patients receiving prasugrel versus 3.2% of those receiving clopidogrel. (See Bleeding Related to Coronary Artery Bypass Grafting under Warnings/Precautions: Warnings, in Cautions.) Subgroup analysis indicated that patients 75 years of age or older, those weighing less than 60 kg, and those with prior stroke or TIA had higher rates of bleeding than patients without these characteristics. Additional risk factors for bleeding include recent trauma, recent surgery (e.g., CABG), recent or recurrent GI bleeding, active peptic ulcer disease, severe hepatic impairment, and concurrent use of drugs that increase risk of bleeding (e.g., oral anticoagulants, sustained use of nonsteroidal anti-inflammatory agents, thrombolytic agents).

Prasugrel should not be used in patients who are actively bleeding and/or who have a history of stroke or TIA. The drug also should not be initiated in those who are likely to undergo emergent CABG. Bleeding should be suspected in any patient who is hypotensive and has recently undergone coronary angiography, percutaneous coronary intervention (PCI), CABG, or any other surgical procedure, even if there are no overt manifestations of bleeding. Risk of bleeding appears to be highest in the first several days of therapy. If possible, bleeding should be managed without discontinuing prasugrel; premature discontinuance is associated with an increased risk of subsequent cardiovascular events. (See Discontinuance of Therapy under Warnings/Precautions: Warnings, in Cautions.) If bleeding occurs, platelet transfusions may be given to restore homeostasis; however, such transfusions may be less effective within 6 hours of a loading dose or 4 hours of a maintenance dose. Withholding a dose of prasugrel is unlikely to resolve a bleeding episode or prevent bleeding associated with an invasive procedure because of the drug's prolonged inhibitory effects on platelet aggregation.

Cerebrovascular Events. In the TRITON-TIMI 38 study, patients with a history of TIA or ischemic stroke had no evidence of a clinical benefit from prasugrel and a strong trend towards a higher rate of major bleeding compared with clopidogrel. In this subgroup, a higher incidence of stroke was observed during treatment with prasugrel compared with clopidogrel (6.5 or 1.2%, respectively). In patients without such a history, the incidence of stroke was similar (0.9 or 1%, respectively) between treatment groups. Strokes occurring in patients receiving prasugrel were both thrombotic and hemorrhagic, while those reported with clopidogrel were all thrombotic. Based on these findings, prasugrel should not be initiated in patients with a history of stroke or TIA and generally should be discontinued in those who experience an adverse cerebrovascular event during therapy.

Bleeding Related to Coronary Artery Bypass Grafting. Risk of bleeding is increased in patients receiving prasugrel who undergo CABG. (See Bleeding under Warnings/Precautions: Warnings, in Cautions.) CABG-related major and minor bleeding events occurred more frequently in patients receiving prasugrel than with clopidogrel in the TRITON-TIMI 38 study (14.1 versus 4.5%, respectively). Bleeding was reported in 26.7 or 5% of those who received prasugrel or clopidogrel, respectively, within 3 days prior to CABG. Although the bleeding risk decreased in both groups when the last dose of study drug was given 4–7 days prior to surgery, the incidence of bleeding remained comparatively higher in the prasugrel-treated group (11.3 versus 3.4%, respectively). Prasugrel should not be initiated in patients who are likely to undergo urgent CABG. In patients scheduled for CABG, prasugrel should be discontinued at least 7 days prior to surgery. CABG-related bleeding may be treated with blood product transfusions (e.g., packed red blood cells, platelets); however, platelet transfusions within 6 hours of a loading dose or 4 hours of a maintenance dose of prasugrel may be less effective in restoring homeostasis.

Discontinuance of Therapy. Prasugrel should be discontinued in patients who develop active bleeding, stroke, or TIA during therapy. (See Cautions: Contraindications.) The drug also should be discontinued prior to elective surgery to minimize risk of bleeding, but should be reinitiated postoperatively as soon as possible (e.g., once adequate hemostasis has been established).

In general, treatment with a thienopyridine derivative should not be discontinued prematurely, particularly in the first few weeks after an acute coronary syndrome (ACS), because of the subsequent increased risk of cardiovascular events. Premature discontinuance of any antiplatelet therapy (e.g., thienopyridine derivative, aspirin) in patients undergoing PCI and coronary artery stent placement has been associated with an increased risk of stent thrombosis, myocardial infarction (MI), and/or death. Because of the risk of late stent thrombosis and other cardiovascular events in patients with drug-eluting stents, experts recommend at least 12 months of dual antiplatelet therapy in such patients. (See Uses: Prevention of Stent Thrombosis, in Clopidogrel Bisulfate 20:12.18.) Some evidence suggests that an even longer duration of dual antiplatelet therapy (for more than 12 months) may be beneficial in some patients with drug-eluting stents. Preliminary results of the DAPT (Dual Antiplatelet Therapy) study, a randomized, placebo-controlled, double-blind study, found that patients who received 30 months of dual antiplatelet therapy (aspirin plus clopidogrel or prasugrel) following placement of a drug-eluting stent had substantially reduced rates of stent thrombosis and major adverse cardiovascular and cerebrovascular events compared with those who received 12 months of dual antiplatelet therapy. However, the longer duration of therapy was associated with a higher incidence of moderate to severe bleeding and also an unexpected finding of an increased rate of noncardiovascular mortality (principally related to trauma or cancer). In November 2014, FDA issued a drug safety communication to alert health care professionals about these findings. At this time, the FDA has not reached any conclusions about the results of the DAPT study and is continuing to evaluate the information as well as other available data. FDA currently believes that the benefits of prasugrel continue to outweigh its potential risks when used appropriately according to the manufacturer's prescribing information; patients should continue to take prasugrel as directed and clinicians should not change their current prescribing practices at this time.

Patients should be advised to *never* stop prasugrel without first consulting their prescribing clinician, even if instructed by another health-care professional (e.g., dentist) to stop such therapy. Prior to scheduling an invasive procedure, patients should inform their clinicians (including dentists) that they currently are taking prasugrel, and clinicians performing the invasive procedure should consult with the prescribing clinician before discontinuing prasugrel therapy. If prasugrel must be temporarily discontinued because of an adverse event, therapy should be reinstituted as soon as possible.

Thrombotic Thrombocytopenic Purpura. Thrombotic thrombocytopenic purpura (TTP) has been reported rarely with use of thienopyridine derivatives, sometimes after brief exposure (less than 2 weeks). TTP is a potentially fatal condition that is characterized by thrombocytopenia, microangiopathic hemolytic anemia (schistocytes on peripheral blood smear), neurologic findings, renal dysfunction, and fever. Urgent treatment (e.g., plasmapheresis) is required in patients who develop TTP.

Specific Populations **Pregnancy.** Category B. (See Users Guide.)

Lactation. Prasugrel metabolites are distributed into milk in rats; not known whether the drug is distributed into milk in humans. The drug should be used in nursing women only if the anticipated benefits to the mother outweigh potential risks to the infant.

Pediatric Use. Safety and efficacy have not been established in pediatric patients.

Geriatric Use. Geriatric patients, particularly those 75 years of age and older, appear to be at greater risk of bleeding (including fatal bleeding) with prasugrel therapy compared with younger patients. In the TRITON-TIMI 38 trial, about 39% of patients were 65 years of age or older and 13% were 75 years of age or older. Risk of bleeding increased with advancing age in both prasugrel and clopidogrel treatment groups. Among patients 75 years of age or older, fatal bleeding was more common with prasugrel than with clopidogrel (1 or 0.1%, respectively); symptomatic intracranial hemorrhage also was reported more frequently with prasugrel (0.8 or 0.3%, respectively). Mean exposure to the active metabolite of prasugrel is approximately 19% higher in patients 75 years or older compared with younger patients. Prasugrel generally should be avoided in patients 75 years of age or older because of a higher risk of bleeding and uncertain efficacy, but use may be considered in certain patients with high-risk conditions (e.g., diabetes, previous MI) in whom a greater net clinical benefit has been demonstrated.

Hepatic Impairment. Pharmacokinetics of prasugrel's active metabolite and its inhibition of platelet aggregation are similar in patients with mild to moderate hepatic impairment (Child-Pugh Class A and B) and healthy individuals. The pharmacokinetics and pharmacodynamics of the drug have not been specifically studied in patients with severe hepatic impairment; however, such patients generally are at higher risk of bleeding.

Renal Impairment. Pharmacokinetics of prasugrel's active metabolite and its inhibition of platelet aggregation in patients with moderate renal impairment (creatinine clearance of 30–50 mL/minute) are similar to that observed in healthy individuals. In patients with end-stage renal impairment, exposure to the active metabolite was decreased to about half that of healthy individuals and those with moderate renal impairment.

Low Body Weight. In the TRITON-TIMI 38 study, patients with low body weight (less than 60 kg) had an increased exposure to the active metabolite of prasugrel and an increased risk of bleeding. Clearance of prasugrel's active metabolite appears to increase exponentially with increasing body weight. (See Bleeding under Warnings/Precautions: Warnings, in Cautions.)

■ **Common Adverse Effects** Bleeding, including life-threatening and fatal bleeding events, was the most commonly reported adverse effect in the TRITON-TIMI 38 study. Other nonhemorrhagic treatment-related adverse effects reported in at least 2.5% of patients in the TRITON-TIMI 38 study included hypertension, hypercholesterolemia/hyperlipidemia, headache, back pain, dyspnea, nausea, dizziness, cough, hypotension, fatigue, noncardiac chest pain, atrial fibrillation, bradycardia, leukopenia (white blood cells less than 4000/mm³), rash, pyrexia, peripheral edema, extremity pain, and diarrhea.

Drug Interactions

■ **Drugs Affecting Gastric Acidity** May be used concomitantly with proton pump inhibitors and histamine H_2-receptor antagonists. Maximum plasma concentrations of the active metabolite of prasugrel are decreased by 14 or 29% with ranitidine or lansoprazole, respectively, but systemic exposure of this metabolite is unaffected. In a pharmacokinetic study in healthy adults, concomitant daily administration of a single loading dose of prasugrel 60 mg with lansoprazole 30 mg decreased systemic exposure and peak plasma concentrations of prasugrel's active metabolite but did not affect inhibition of platelet aggregation.

■ **Drugs Affecting or Metabolized by Hepatic Microsomal Enzymes** Prasugrel is metabolized by the cytochrome P-450 (CYP) microsomal enzyme system, principally by isoenzymes 3A4 and 2B6, and to a lesser extent by isoenzymes 2C9 and 2C19. In vitro studies indicate that prasugrel is not likely to inhibit CYP isoenzymes 1A2, 2C9, 2C19, 2D6, and 3A or induce CYP isoenzymes 1A2 or 3A. Prasugrel is a weak inhibitor of CYP2B6.

Clinically important drug interactions mediated by CYP isoenzymes are considered unlikely with prasugrel. Studies have shown that if one of the CYP isoenzymes involved in the metabolism of prasugrel is inhibited, others remain capable of forming the active metabolite. CYP3A4 inhibitors such as verapamil, diltiazem, indinavir, ciprofloxacin, clarithromycin, and grapefruit juice are not expected to have a substantial effect on the pharmacokinetics of prasugrel's active metabolite. In healthy individuals receiving prasugrel, concomitant administration of ketoconazole (a potent inhibitor of CYP3A4) decreased maximum concentrations of prasugrel's active metabolite by 34–46%, but did not alter systemic exposure or degree of inhibition of platelet aggregation. Similarly, CYP3A4 inducers (e.g., rifampin, carbamazepine) are not expected to substantially alter the pharmacokinetic or pharmacodynamic response to prasugrel; concomitant administration of rifampin, a potent inducer of CYP3A4 and CYP2B6, did not affect formation of the active prasugrel metabolite nor its ability to inhibit platelet aggregation. Concomitant administration of prasugrel and drugs principally metabolized by CYP2B6 (e.g., halothane, cyclophosphamide, propofol, nevirapine) may increase plasma concentrations and exposure of the concomitant drug; however, clinically important interactions are not expected because of weak inhibition of CYP2B6.

■ **Digoxin** May be administered concomitantly. Prasugrel is not an inhibitor of the P-glycoprotein transport system and is not expected to affect clearance of digoxin.

■ **HMG-CoA Reductase Inhibitors (Statins)** May be used concomitantly without dosage adjustments. Coadministration of prasugrel and atorvastatin 80 mg daily had little effect on exposure to the active prasugrel metabolite and no effect on inhibition of platelet aggregation.

■ **Nonsteroidal Anti-inflammatory Agents** Increased risk of bleeding with concomitant long-term use of aspirin or other nonsteroidal anti-inflammatory agents (NSAIAs).

■ **Thrombolytic Agents** Increased risk of bleeding with concomitant use.

■ **Warfarin** Increased risk of bleeding in patients receiving concomitant therapy with warfarin. Bleeding time substantially prolonged with concomitant administration of a single 15-mg dose of warfarin.

■ **Other Antiplatelet or Antithrombotic Agents** The manufacturer states that prasugrel may be administered concomitantly with aspirin, heparin, and GP IIb/IIIa-receptor inhibitors. Concomitant use of prasugrel and aspirin 150 mg daily increased bleeding time compared with use of either drug alone, but inhibition of platelet aggregation was not altered. In a study in healthy individuals, concomitant use of prasugrel and aspirin 325 mg daily resulted in greater inhibition of platelet aggregation, but the combination was well tolerated; no clinically important bleeding events occurred. When a single IV dose of unfractionated heparin sodium 100 units/kg was given concomitantly with prasugrel, bleeding time was increased without any associated changes in coagulation or inhibition of platelet aggregation.

Although evidence from drug interaction studies generally is lacking, increased risk of bleeding is likely with concomitant use of prasugrel and other antiplatelet or antithrombotic agents; caution is advised.

Description

Prasugrel hydrochloride, a thienopyridine derivative structurally and pharmacologically related to clopidogrel, is a platelet-activation and aggregation inhibitor. Like clopidogrel, prasugrel is a prodrug that requires hepatic transformation to an active metabolite (R-138727) in order to exert its pharmacologic effect on the P2Y12 platelet adenosine diphosphate (ADP) receptor. Compared with clopidogrel, prasugrel inhibits ADP-mediated platelet aggregation more rapidly, more consistently, and to a greater extent; inhibition of platelet aggregation is at least 30% greater with prasugrel than with standard dosages of clopidogrel. The increased potency of prasugrel appears to be a result of more efficient conversion of the prodrug to its active metabolite. Genetic polymorphisms of cytochrome P-450 (CYP) isoenzymes (e.g., CYP2B6, CYP2C9, CYP2C19, CYP3A5) do not appear to affect the pharmacologic or clinical response to prasugrel.

Prasugrel is a P2Y12 platelet ADP-receptor antagonist; the active metabolite binds irreversibly to the P2Y12 class of ADP receptors on the surface of platelets, thereby inhibiting ADP-dependent platelet activation and aggregation for the life of the platelet (approximately 7–10 days). Following a 60-mg loading dose of prasugrel, at least 50% inhibition of platelet aggregation is achieved at 1 hour in approximately 90% of patients. Approximately 70% inhibition of platelet aggregation is achieved at steady state within 3–5 days with prasugrel 10 mg daily. The maximum inhibition of platelet aggregation attained with a 60-mg loading dose of prasugrel is about 80%. Platelet aggregation gradually returns to baseline values within 5–9 days following discontinuance of the drug. The relationship between inhibition of platelet aggregation and clinical activity of prasugrel has not been established.

Prasugrel is rapidly and completely (at least 79% of a dose) absorbed from the GI tract following oral administration. Once absorbed, the drug is rapidly hydrolyzed by esterases to an inactive thiolactone that is subsequently metabolized to the active metabolite (R-138727) by CYP enzymes (principally by 3A4 and 2B6, and to a lesser extent by 2C9 and 2C19). Compared with clopidogrel, which undergoes a 2-step oxidative process, prasugrel requires only a single step for metabolic activation; this may explain its faster onset of action. Peak plasma concentrations of the active metabolite of prasugrel are reached approximately 30 minutes after an oral dose, and there is no evidence of accumulation with repeated administration. The active metabolite of prasugrel is approximately 98% bound to human albumin. Administration of a high-fat or high-caloric meal to healthy individuals did not affect exposure to the active metabolite but decreased peak plasma concentrations by 49% and delayed time to peak concentration from 0.5 to 1.5 hours.

The manufacturer states that the elimination half-life of prasugrel's active metabolite (R-138727) averages about 7 hours (range: 2–15 hours), although a half-life of 3.7 hours has been reported in some studies. However, inhibition of platelet aggregation following prasugrel administration persists for about 96 hours. Prasugrel is eliminated principally in urine (68%) and to a lesser extent in feces (27%) as inactive metabolites. Dialysis is not expected to remove the active metabolite.

Advice to Patients

Importance of counseling patients about potential risks versus benefits of prasugrel.

Importance of informing patients that they will bruise and/or bleed more easily and that a longer than usual time will be required to stop bleeding when taking prasugrel. Importance of patients informing clinicians about any unexpected, prolonged, or excessive bleeding, or blood in urine or stool.

Importance of patients taking prasugrel exactly as prescribed and not discontinuing therapy without first consulting the prescribing clinician.

Importance of informing clinicians (e.g., physicians, dentists) about prasugrel therapy before any invasive procedure or surgery is scheduled. Clinician performing invasive procedure should consult with prescribing clinician before discontinuing prasugrel.

Risk of thrombotic thrombocytopenic purpura (TTP); importance of advising patients to immediately seek medical attention if they experience manifestations such as fever, weakness, extreme skin paleness, purple skin patches, yellowing of the skin or eyes, or otherwise unexplained neurologic changes.

Importance of informing clinicians of existing or contemplated concomitant therapy, including prescription and OTC drugs, particularly drugs that affect bleeding risk (e.g., warfarin, nonsteroidal anti-inflammatory agents).

Importance of women informing clinicians if they are or plan to become pregnant or plan to breast-feed.

Importance of informing patients of other important precautionary information. (See Cautions.)

Overview® (see Users Guide). For additional information on this drug until a more detailed monograph is developed and published, the manufacturer's labeling should be consulted. It is *essential* that the manufacturer's labeling be consulted for more detailed information on usual cautions, precautions, contraindications, potential drug interactions, laboratory test interferences, and acute toxicity.

Preparations

Excipients in commercially available drug preparations may have clinically important effects in some individuals; consult specific product labeling for details.

Prasugrel Hydrochloride

Oral

Tablets	5 mg (of prasugrel)	**Effient®**, Eli Lilly and Company (also promoted by Daiichi Sankyo Inc.)
	10 mg (of prasugrel)	**Effient®**, Eli Lilly and Company (also promoted by Daiichi Sankyo Inc.)

Selected Revisions October 2017, © Copyright, December 2010, American Society of Health-System Pharmacists, Inc.

Ticagrelor

■ Ticagrelor, a nonthienopyridine, reversible, P2Y12 platelet adenosine diphosphate (ADP)-receptor antagonist, is a platelet-activation and -aggregation inhibitor.

Uses

■ **Acute Coronary Syndrome** Ticagrelor is used in combination with aspirin to reduce the risk of thrombotic cardiovascular events (e.g., cardiovascular death, myocardial infarction [MI]) in patients with an acute coronary syndrome (unstable angina, non-ST-segment-elevation MI [NSTEMI], or ST-segment-elevation MI [STEMI]) who are to be managed medically or with an invasive strategy (percutaneous coronary intervention [PCI] with or without coronary artery stent placement, coronary artery bypass grafting [CABG]). In a large, randomized study (The Study of Platelet Inhibition and Patient Outcomes [PLATO]) in patients with an acute coronary syndrome (ACS), ticagrelor was more effective than clopidogrel in reducing the rate of the composite end point of cardiovascular death, MI, or stroke without increasing the risk of major bleeding over that observed with clopidogrel. The benefits of ticagrelor over clopidogrel consisted principally of reductions in cardiovascular death and MI; there was no difference in the rate of stroke. Ticagrelor also was associated with a reduction in the rate of stent thrombosis in those undergoing PCI and a reduction in death from any cause. In this and other clinical studies, ticagrelor was given in conjunction with aspirin therapy.

Dual-drug antiplatelet therapy with a P2Y12-receptor antagonist (e.g., clopidogrel, prasugrel, ticagrelor) and aspirin is part of the current standard of care in patients with ACS. The American College of Cardiology Foundation (ACCF), the American Heart Association (AHA), the Society for Cardiovascular Angiography and Interventions (SCAI), the American College of Chest Physicians (ACCP), and other experts recommend antiplatelet therapy with a P2Y12-receptor antagonist and aspirin for treatment and secondary prevention of ACS. These experts generally recommend ticagrelor or clopidogrel as the P2Y12-receptor antagonist in patients with ACS who are treated medically without stenting; because prasugrel has been studied principally in patients undergoing planned PCI, recommendations for the use of this drug are restricted to that population. In patients with ACS who are being managed medically, therapy with a P2Y12 receptor antagonist should be continued for up to 12 months, while aspirin should be continued indefinitely. In patients undergoing PCI with stent placement (bare-metal or drug-eluting), a loading dose of ticagrelor, clopidogrel, or prasugrel is recommended, followed by maintenance therapy with one of these agents for at least 12 months (unless the risk of bleeding outweighs the anticipated net benefit of therapy); aspirin also should be continued indefinitely in such patients.

The relative role of ticagrelor versus other P2Y12-receptor antagonists in the management of ACS remains to be fully established. While current ACCF/AHA guidelines make no recommendations regarding the P2Y12-receptor antagonist of choice, ACCP suggests the use of ticagrelor over clopidogrel in patients with ACS (who are or are not undergoing PCI). The European Society of Cardiology (ESC) generally recommends ticagrelor or prasugrel over clopidogrel in patients with non-ST-segment elevation ACS; according to ESC, clopidogrel should be considered an alternative in such patients unable to receive ticagrelor or prasugrel therapy. Other clinicians state that because of its reversibility and faster offset of action, ticagrelor may be preferred over the irreversible P2Y12-receptor antagonists (clopidogrel, prasugrel) in patients with ACS who are being managed with an early invasive strategy (e.g., those in whom coronary anatomy has not been determined and who are likely to undergo CABG); switching from clopidogrel or prasugrel to ticagrelor therapy 5–7 days prior to CABG is considered reasonable in such patients. Ticagrelor also may be a reasonable alternative in patients who are nonresponsive to clopidogrel based on studies demonstrating that ticagrelor not only inhibits platelet aggregation in clopidogrel nonresponders, but also produces greater inhibition of platelet aggregation than clopidogrel in patients who remain responsive to clopidogrel. When selecting an appropriate antiplatelet regimen for the management of patients with ACS, clinicians should consider individual risks of ischemia and bleeding as well as the specific characteristics (e.g., adverse effects, drug interaction potential) of the drugs.

The current indication for ticagrelor is based principally on an international, randomized, double-blind study (PLATO) in more than 18,000 patients hospitalized for ACS. The study compared efficacy and safety of ticagrelor versus clopidogrel in reducing the rate of death from vascular causes, nonfatal MI (excluding silent MI), or nonfatal stroke in these patients. Because the study was designed to evaluate patients at hospital presentation or diagnosis ("upstream"), patients with various types of ACS were enrolled, including those with NSTEMI in whom conservative or invasive management was planned and those with STEMI undergoing primary PCI. Approximately 50% of patients were pretreated with clopidogrel prior to randomization; PCI was performed in about 64% of the patients and approximately 10% underwent CABG. Within 24 hours of symptom onset and before PCI, patients received either ticagrelor (180-mg loading dose followed by 90 mg twice daily) or clopidogrel (300-mg loading dose followed by 75 mg daily) in addition to aspirin and other standard therapy; treatment was continued for at least 6 months up to a maximum of 12 months. Those undergoing PCI received an additional loading dose of study drug at the time of PCI (90 mg of ticagrelor if more than 24 hours had passed since the initial loading dose or 300 mg of clopidogrel at the investigator's discretion). Aspirin was administered to all patients in the study at a recommended loading dose of 160–500 mg and daily maintenance dosage of 75–100 mg; higher maintenance dosages (e.g., 325 mg daily for 6 months following stent placement) were permitted based on clinician judgment.

In the PLATO study, ticagrelor substantially reduced the rate of the primary composite end point of cardiovascular death, nonfatal MI, or nonfatal stroke compared with clopidogrel. The primary outcome occurred in 9.8% of patients receiving ticagrelor compared with 11.7% of those receiving clopidogrel, a relative risk reduction of 16%. The difference in treatment effect was apparent by 30 days and maintained throughout the 12-month study period. The benefit associated with ticagrelor was based on a reduction in the incidence of cardiovascular death and MI, but not stroke. Although the overall rate of stroke was similar between the treatment groups, hemorrhagic strokes were more frequent in patients receiving ticagrelor. Among patients who received a coronary artery stent during the study, the rate of stent thrombosis was substantially lower with ticagrelor than with clopidogrel regardless of the type of stent (bare-metal or drug-eluting) implanted. In addition, death from any cause was reduced with ticagrelor (1.4% absolute reduction, 22% relative reduction). Some experts state, however, that additional study is needed to confirm this mortality benefit since all-cause mortality was not evaluated as a primary outcome in the PLATO study. The overall rate of major bleeding was similar for patients who received ticagrelor or clopidogrel; however, ticagrelor was associated with a higher incidence of non-CABG related major bleeding, including fatal intracranial bleeding.

In the PLATO study, clinical outcomes with ticagrelor generally were consistent across subgroups of patients with ACS regardless of whether a conservative or invasive management strategy was employed and regardless of the type of antiplatelet therapy received prior to the index ACS event. However, the benefits of ticagrelor appeared to be reduced in patients enrolled in North America compared with those enrolled in other regions. Results of additional statistical analyses of a variety of baseline and procedural differences between the US and non-US regions identified aspirin maintenance dosage as a possible factor accounting for this regional discrepancy. These analyses showed that ticagrelor was associated with a more favorable response than clopidogrel in patients receiving low (100 mg or less daily) maintenance dosages of aspirin. This was seen in both US and non-US patients; however, substantially more (about 54%) US patients were treated with aspirin dosages exceeding 300 mg daily, whereas patients in other countries rarely (only about 2% of patients) received such high aspirin dosages. Because of inherent limitations of subgroup analyses and the possibility that the effect of aspirin dosage on ticagrelor outcome could be due to chance, these findings should be interpreted with caution. Nevertheless, the manufacturer states that aspirin dosage should be limited to 75–100 mg daily in patients receiving ticagrelor; higher dosages do not have an established benefit in the management of ACS and may be associated with reduced efficacy of ticagrelor.

Dosage and Administration

■ **Administration** Ticagrelor is administered orally without regard to meals. If a dose is missed, the next dose should be taken at the regularly scheduled time; the dose should not be doubled unless directed by the prescribing clinician.

Prescribing and Dispensing Precautions Prescribing and dispensing errors have been reported because of similarities in the spelling and pronunciation of Brilinta® (the trade name for ticagrelor) and Brintellix® (the former trade name for vortioxetine hydrobromide, an antidepressant agent). To avoid such errors, the manufacturer of Brintellix® changed the trade name for vortioxetine hydrobromide from Brintellix® to Trintellix®, which became commercially available in June 2016. (See Prescribing and Dispensing Precautions under Warnings/Precautions: Other Warnings and Precautions, in Cautions.)

■ **Dosage** ***Acute Coronary Syndrome*** For the reduction of thrombotic cardiovascular events in patients with an acute coronary syndrome (ACS), an initial ticagrelor loading dose of 180 mg is recommended, followed by a maintenance dosage of 90 mg twice daily. Aspirin should be administered concomitantly, with an initial loading dose (usually 325 mg) followed by a maintenance dosage of 75–100 mg daily. (See Adjunctive Aspirin Therapy under Dosage: Acute Coronary Syndrome, in Dosage and Administration.)

The manufacturer makes no specific recommendations regarding duration of ticagrelor therapy; however, the drug was administered for up to 12 months in the PLATO study. In general, long-term antiplatelet therapy is recommended in patients with coronary artery stents to prevent ischemic events. The American Heart Association (AHA), American College of Cardiology Foundation (ACCF), and other experts recommend continuation of dual-drug antiplatelet therapy (aspirin plus clopidogrel, prasugrel, or ticagrelor) for at least 12 months following placement of a bare-metal or drug-eluting stent.

Switching Therapy from Clopidogrel to Ticagrelor. Patients may be transitioned directly from clopidogrel to ticagrelor therapy without interruption in antiplatelet effects. In clinical trials, patients who were switched from clopidogrel to ticagrelor received an initial loading dose of ticagrelor regardless of whether a previous loading dose of clopidogrel was given. Therefore, the manufacturer states that patients who have already received a loading dose of clopidogrel may subsequently receive ticagrelor at the recommended dosage (initial loading dose of 180 mg, followed by 90 mg twice daily).

Adjunctive Aspirin Therapy. Adjunctive antithrombotic therapy with aspirin is recommended in all patients with ACS, including those undergoing percutaneous coronary intervention (PCI). Aspirin should be administered as soon as possible after hospital presentation and continued indefinitely in those who are able to tolerate it. For additional information on use of aspirin as adjunctive antithrombotic therapy in the management of ACS, see Unstable Angina and Non-ST-Segment Elevation Myocardial Infarction and also see Coronary Artery Disease and Myocardial Infarction under Dosage: Thrombosis, in Dosage and Administration in Aspirin 28:08.04.24.

The optimal maintenance dosage of aspirin in patients with ACS has not been established; recommendations vary from 75–162 mg daily in current clinical practice guidelines. However, since aspirin dosages exceeding 100 mg daily have been associated with reduced effectiveness of ticagrelor, the manufacturer recommends that ticagrelor be administered with aspirin maintenance dosages of 75–100 mg daily. (See Uses: Acute Coronary Syndrome and also see Reduced Efficacy with Higher Aspirin Dosages under Warnings/Precautions: Warnings, in Cautions.)

Discontinuance in Patients Undergoing Invasive Procedures Antiplatelet agents generally should be discontinued prior to surgery or other invasive procedures to minimize the risk of perioperative bleeding. Whenever feasible, ticagrelor should be discontinued at least 5 days prior to any surgery (e.g., coronary artery bypass grafting [CABG]) and resumed as soon as possible. If urgent CABG is required, ACCF and AHA state that ticagrelor should be discontinued at least 24 hours before the procedure. In the PLATO study, ticagrelor was discontinued 24–72 hours prior to CABG surgery and was associated with bleeding rates comparable to those observed with clopidogrel being withheld for 5 days.

The American College of Chest Physicians (ACCP) states that the decision to interrupt antiplatelet therapy prior to surgery or other invasive procedures should be individualized based on assessment of the patient's risks of thromboembolism and perioperative bleeding. The possible increased risk of stent thrombosis also should be considered when making decisions regarding the perioperative management of patients with coronary artery stents. (See Discontinuance of Therapy under Warnings/Precautions: Other Warnings and Precautions, in Cautions.)

■ **Special Populations** No dosage adjustments are necessary in patients with renal impairment or mild hepatic impairment (Child-Pugh class A). (See Hepatic Impairment under Warnings/Precautions: Specific Populations, in Cautions.)

Dosage adjustments based on body weight, ethnicity, gender, age, or smoking status are not required.

Cautions

■ **Contraindications** History of intracranial hemorrhage. Active pathologic bleeding (e.g., peptic ulcer, intracranial hemorrhage). Severe hepatic impairment.

■ **Warnings/Precautions** ***Warnings*** **Bleeding.** Like other antiplatelet agents, ticagrelor increases the risk of bleeding, which may be serious and sometimes fatal. When all major and minor bleeding events are considered, the overall risk of bleeding is somewhat greater with ticagrelor than with clopidogrel. The increased risk principally involves major bleeding events not related to coronary artery bypass grafting (CABG). In the PLATO study, total (major and minor) non-CABG-related bleeding occurred in 8.7% of patients who received ticagrelor compared with 7% of those who received clopidogrel. In addition, there was a small but statistically significant increase in the rate of fatal intracranial bleeding with ticagrelor versus clopidogrel; fatal bleeding of other types was not increased. Many of the bleeding events occurred early, at the time of coronary angiography, percutaneous coronary intervention (PCI), CABG, or other procedures, but the risk persisted throughout therapy.

Although major CABG-related bleeding occurred at a very high rate in the PLATO study, such bleeding rates were similar with ticagrelor or clopidogrel therapy. In addition, there was no difference in major bleeding between the treatment groups when antiplatelet therapy was discontinued 5 days or less prior to CABG surgery, suggesting that the pharmacokinetic advantages of ticagrelor (i.e., faster offset of action, reversibility) do not translate into a lower risk of bleeding in patients undergoing CABG.

Ticagrelor should not be used in patients who are actively bleeding or who have a history of intracranial hemorrhage. (See Cautions: Contraindications.) The drug also should not be initiated in patients who are likely to undergo urgent CABG. Risk factors for bleeding generally include advanced age, history of bleeding disorders, performance of percutaneous invasive procedures, and concurrent use of drugs that increase risk of bleeding (e.g., anticoagulants, thrombolytic agents, high dosages of aspirin, long-term use of nonsteroidal anti-inflammatory agents [NSAIAs]). Whenever possible, ticagrelor should be discontinued at least 5 days prior to surgery or other invasive procedures. Bleeding should be suspected in any patient receiving ticagrelor who is hypotensive and has recently undergone coronary angiography, PCI, CABG, or any other invasive procedure, even if no overt manifestations of bleeding are present. If possible, bleeding should be managed without discontinuing ticagrelor since premature discontinuance of such therapy may be associated with an increased risk of subsequent cardiovascular events. (See Discontinuance of Therapy under Warnings/Precautions: Other Warnings and Precautions, in Cautions.)

Reduced Efficacy with Higher Aspirin Dosages. A reduced response to ticagrelor was observed in patients receiving aspirin maintenance dosages exceeding 100 mg daily in the PLATO study. (See Uses: Acute Coronary Syndrome.) After the initial loading dose, ticagrelor should be used in conjunction with an aspirin maintenance dosage of 75–100 mg daily; the manufacturer states that higher maintenance dosages should be avoided. (See Adjunctive Aspirin Therapy under Dosage: Acute Coronary Syndrome, in Dosage and Administration.)

Other Warnings and Precautions **Dyspnea.** In clinical studies, dyspnea was reported more frequently with ticagrelor than with clopidogrel (13.8 versus 7.8% of patients, respectively, in the PLATO study). In most cases, dyspnea was mild to moderate in severity and resolved without further intervention. Although the mechanism of this adverse effect is unknown, it is thought to be an adenosine-mediated response. Ticagrelor does not appear to have adverse effects on cardiac or pulmonary function. Pulmonary function testing in a subset of patients from the PLATO study revealed no substantial difference in forced expiratory volume in 1 second (FEV_1) in those who received ticagrelor versus those who received clopidogrel.

Patients who develop any new, prolonged, or worsening dyspnea during ticagrelor therapy should be evaluated to rule out any associated underlying conditions. If dyspnea appears to be related to ticagrelor, the manufacturer states that no specific treatment is required and the drug may be continued without interruption.

Discontinuance of Therapy. In general, treatment with ticagrelor should not be discontinued prematurely because this increases the risk of cardiovascular events. Premature discontinuance of antiplatelet therapy (e.g., P2Y12 adenosine diphosphate [ADP]-receptor antagonists, aspirin) in patients with coronary artery stents has been associated with an increased risk of ischemic cardiovascular events (e.g., stent thrombosis, myocardial infarction [MI], death). If temporary discontinuance of ticagrelor is necessary such as prior to elective surgery or for management of bleeding, the drug should be restarted as soon as possible.

Patients should be advised to never stop taking ticagrelor without first consulting the prescribing clinician, even if instructed by another clinician (e.g., dentist) to stop such therapy. Prior to scheduling an invasive procedure, patients should inform clinicians (including dentists) that they are currently taking ticagrelor and clinicians performing the invasive procedure should consult with the prescribing clinician before discontinuing such therapy.

Cardiovascular Effects. Bradyarrhythmias, including ventricular pauses, have occurred in patients receiving ticagrelor. In the PLATO study, Holter monitor-detected ventricular pauses of at least 3 seconds were reported more frequently during the first week of therapy in patients receiving ticagrelor than in those receiving clopidogrel (5.8 versus 3.6%, respectively). There was no difference in the overall risk of clinically important bradycardic effects (e.g., syncope, need for pacemaker insertion) between the treatment groups. Ventricular pauses were mostly asymptomatic and attributed to sinoatrial nodal suppression.

Patients with a baseline increased risk of bradycardia (e.g., those with sick sinus syndrome, second- or third-degree AV block, syncope due to bradycardia without a pacemaker) were excluded from the PLATO study; therefore, some clinicians recommend that ticagrelor be used with caution in such patients.

Prescribing and Dispensing Precautions. Because of similarities in the spelling and pronunciation of Brilinta® (the trade name for ticagrelor) and Brintellix® (the former trade name for vortioxetine hydrobromide, an antidepressant agent), prescribing and dispensing errors have been reported to FDA for these drugs. As of June 2015, FDA had received 50 medication error reports describing trade name confusion with Brilinta® and Brintellix®. In most cases, Brintellix® was mistaken for Brilinta®. The wrong drug was actually dispensed in 12 of the reported cases of name confusion; however, none of the reports indicated that a patient ingested the wrong drug. To avoid future prescribing and dispensing errors, FDA approved a change in the trade name for vortioxetine in May 2016; the manufacturer of Brintellix® (vortioxetine hydrobromide) changed the trade name to Trintellix®, which became commercially available under this trade name in June 2016. To reduce the risk of medication errors (e.g., during the transition period to the new name), FDA recommends that clinicians include both the trade (brand) and generic (nonproprietary) names of the drug and the indication for use as well as the correct dosage and directions for use in each prescription. In addition, patients should be advised to check their prescriptions to ensure that the correct drug was dispensed and to carefully read the medication guide provided with their prescriptions.

Specific Populations **Pregnancy.** Category C. (See Users Guide.)

Lactation. Ticagrelor is distributed into milk in rats; it is not known whether the drug or its metabolites are distributed into human milk. Because of the potential for serious adverse effects in nursing infants, a decision should be made whether to discontinue nursing or the drug, taking into account the importance of the drug to the woman.

Pediatric Use. Safety and efficacy have not been established in patients younger than 18 years of age.

Geriatric Use. Of the total number of patients enrolled in the PLATO trial, 43% were 65 years of age or older and 15% were 75 years of age or older. No overall differences in efficacy or safety, including the risk of bleeding, were observed between geriatric and younger patients; however, increased sensitivity in some older individuals cannot be ruled out.

Age does not appear to substantially affect the pharmacokinetics of ticagrelor.

Hepatic Impairment. Ticagrelor has not been systematically evaluated in patients with moderate or severe hepatic impairment. Because the drug is metabolized by the liver, there is a potential for increased exposure and risk of bleeding in patients with impaired hepatic function. Ticagrelor is contraindicated in patients with severe hepatic impairment; use of the drug in those with moderate hepatic impairment should be considered carefully after weighing the risks and benefits of treatment.

Ticagrelor may be used in patients with mild hepatic impairment without the need for dosage adjustments. In a pharmacokinetic/pharmacodynamic study, systemic exposure to ticagrelor was slightly higher in individuals with mild (Child-Pugh class A) hepatic impairment compared with those with normal hepatic function; however, no clinically important effects of such impairment were observed.

Renal Impairment. No substantial differences in pharmacokinetics or clinical efficacy of ticagrelor have been observed in patients with renal impairment versus those with normal renal function.

Approximately 25% of patients enrolled in the PLATO study had chronic kidney disease (creatinine clearance less than 60 mL/minute); dosage reductions based on renal function were not required to prevent major bleeding. Data are lacking on the use of ticagrelor in patients undergoing dialysis.

■ **Common Adverse Effects** Adverse effects reported in 3% or more of patients receiving ticagrelor in clinical studies include bleeding, dyspnea, headache, cough, dizziness, nausea, atrial fibrillation, hypertension, noncardiac chest pain, diarrhea, back pain, hypotension, fatigue, and chest pain.

Drug Interactions

■ **Drugs Affecting Hemostasis** Risk of bleeding may be increased when ticagrelor is used concomitantly with drugs that affect hemostasis (e.g., anticoagulants, thrombolytics, high doses of aspirin, chronic nonsteroidal anti-inflammatory agents [NSAIAs]). (See Bleeding under Warnings/Precautions: Warnings, in Cautions.)

Efficacy of ticagrelor may be affected by aspirin maintenance dosage. (See Drug Interactions: Aspirin.)

■ **Drugs Affecting or Metabolized by Hepatic Microsomal Enzymes** Ticagrelor is metabolized principally by the cytochrome P-450 (CYP) 3A4 isoenzyme, and to a lesser extent by CYP3A5. In vitro studies indicate that ticagrelor and its major active metabolite are weak inhibitors of CYP3A4/5 and potential activators of CYP3A5. Ticagrelor does not appear to inhibit CYP 1A2, 2C19, or 2E1.

Concomitant use of ticagrelor with potent CYP3A inhibitors (e.g., atazanavir, clarithromycin, indinavir, itraconazole, ketoconazole, nefazodone, nelfinavir, ritonavir, saquinavir, telithromycin, voriconazole) may result in substantially increased exposure to ticagrelor and possible increased risk of bleeding; such concomitant use should be avoided. Moderate CYP3A inhibitors (e.g., diltiazem) also may increase ticagrelor exposure, but to a lesser extent; therefore, these drugs may be used with ticagrelor without any dosage adjustments. Concomitant use of ticagrelor with potent inducers of CYP3A (e.g., carbamazepine, dexamethasone, phenobarbital, phenytoin, rifampin) may result in substantially reduced plasma concentrations and possible reduced efficacy of ticagrelor; such concomitant use should be avoided.

Ticagrelor may increase serum concentrations of drugs metabolized by CYP3A4 (e.g., lovastatin, simvastatin). In some cases, reduced dosages of the CYP3A4 substrate may be required. (See Drug Interactions: HMG-CoA Reductase Inhibitors [Statins].)

■ **Drugs Affecting or Affected by P-glycoprotein Transport** Ticagrelor is a substrate and weak inhibitor of the P-glycoprotein transport system. Increased serum concentrations of P-glycoprotein substrates (e.g., digoxin) are possible when these drugs are used concomitantly with ticagrelor; appropriate laboratory and/or clinical monitoring is recommended.

■ **Aspirin** When ticagrelor is used in conjunction with aspirin maintenance dosages exceeding 100 mg daily, efficacy of ticagrelor may be reduced. (See Reduced Efficacy with Higher Aspirin Dosages under Warnings/Precautions: Warnings, in Cautions)

Aspirin does not appear to substantially affect the pharmacokinetics of ticagrelor.

■ **Desmopressin** Desmopressin does not appear to affect peak concentrations of or systemic exposure to ticagrelor; no dosage adjustment is necessary when these drugs are used concomitantly.

■ **Digoxin** Concomitant administration of ticagrelor and digoxin did not substantially affect pharmacokinetics of digoxin; therefore, these drugs may be used concomitantly without dosage adjustments. However, because of the possibility of increased digoxin concentrations as a result of P-glycoprotein inhibition, serum digoxin concentrations should be monitored during initiation of and following any change in ticagrelor therapy.

■ **HMG-CoA Reductase Inhibitors (Statins)** Concomitant administration of ticagrelor and simvastatin (a CYP3A4 substrate) resulted in substantially increased exposure to simvastatin and its active metabolite. If ticagrelor is used concomitantly with simvastatin or lovastatin, the manufacturer states that dosage of the statin should not exceed 40 mg daily.

Concomitant administration of ticagrelor and atorvastatin did not substantially affect the pharmacokinetics of atorvastatin; therefore, these drugs may be used concomitantly without dosage adjustments.

■ **Ketoconazole** Concomitant use of ketoconazole 200 mg twice daily and ticagrelor substantially increased peak plasma concentrations of and systemic exposure to ticagrelor. Concomitant use of ticagrelor and ketoconazole should be avoided.

■ **Oral Contraceptives** In healthy women receiving stable dosages of an oral contraceptive containing ethinyl estradiol and levonorgestrel, administration of ticagrelor (90 mg twice daily) increased peak plasma concentrations of and systemic exposure to the estrogen component, but did not alter the pharmacokinetics of levonorgestrel. Ticagrelor is not expected to affect contraceptive efficacy; therefore, no dosage adjustment is necessary when the drug is administered with levonorgestrel or ethinyl estradiol.

■ **Proton-pump Inhibitors** Ticagrelor may be used concomitantly with proton-pump inhibitors. In a clinical study in patients with acute coronary syndrome (ACS), concomitant administration of ticagrelor with a proton-pump inhibitor did not affect the platelet response to ticagrelor.

■ **Rifampin** Concomitant administration of ticagrelor and rifampin 600 mg once daily substantially decreased peak plasma concentrations of and systemic exposure to ticagrelor. Concomitant use of ticagrelor and rifampin should therefore be avoided.

■ **Tolbutamide** Concomitant administration of ticagrelor and tolbutamide did not substantially affect pharmacokinetics of tolbutamide; therefore, the drugs may be used concomitantly without dosage adjustments.

■ **Other Concomitant Therapy** Ticagrelor may be administered in conjunction with heparin, platelet glycoprotein (GP) IIb/IIIa-receptor inhibitors, β-adrenergic blocking agents, angiotensin-converting enzyme (ACE) inhibitors, and angiotensin II receptor antagonists.

Concomitant administration of ticagrelor with heparin or enoxaparin did not affect peak plasma concentrations of or systemic exposure to ticagrelor; therefore, no dosage adjustments are required when these drugs are used concomitantly.

Description

Ticagrelor, a cyclopentyltriazolopyrimidine derivative, is a nonthienopyridine, P2Y12 platelet adenosine diphosphate (ADP)-receptor antagonist. In contrast to the thienopyridines (e.g., clopidogrel, prasugrel), ticagrelor binds reversibly to the P2Y12 ADP receptor and does not require hepatic transformation to exert its pharmacologic effect. Ticagrelor exhibits noncompetitive and reversible binding to the P2Y12 platelet ADP receptor, preventing signal transduction of the cyclic adenosine monophosphate (cAMP) pathway. This results in reduced exposure of fibrinogen binding sites to the platelet glycoprotein (GP) IIb/IIIa complex and subsequent inhibition of platelet activation and aggregation. In addition to platelet ADP-receptor blockade, ticagrelor inhibits reuptake of adenosine into erythrocytes, a mechanism that may account for some of the beneficial cardiovascular effects of the drug, while potentially contributing to some of its adverse effects (e.g., dyspnea, ventricular pauses).

Compared with clopidogrel, ticagrelor produces more rapid and effective inhibition of platelet aggregation and has a faster offset of action. In a 6-week randomized study comparing the antiplatelet effects of ticagrelor with clopidogrel in patients with stable coronary artery disease, higher and more consistent levels of platelet-aggregation inhibition as assessed by light transmission aggregometry were achieved with ticagrelor (180-mg loading dose followed by 90 mg twice daily) compared with clopidogrel (600-mg loading dose followed by 75 mg once daily). Following discontinuance of therapy, the offset of antiplatelet effect occurred at a faster rate with ticagrelor than with clopidogrel. The mean maximal inhibition of platelet aggregation following the last dose of study drug was higher with ticagrelor than clopidogrel initially, but approached equivalent levels after 24 hours. In patients receiving ticagrelor, inhibition of platelet aggregation returned to baseline levels 5 days after the last dose was administered. Maximum inhibition of platelet aggregation with ticagrelor is observed approximately 2 hours after a dose and is maintained for at least 8 hours. Patients who transition from clopidogrel to ticagrelor therapy appear to achieve additional inhibition of platelet aggregation (absolute increase of 26.4%). The relationship between inhibition of platelet aggregation and bleeding or thrombotic risk of either drug is not known.

Ticagrelor is rapidly absorbed following oral administration. The drug is metabolized principally by cytochrome P-450 (CYP) isoenzyme 3A4 to an active metabolite that has similar antiplatelet activity as the parent drug. Plasma concentrations of ticagrelor and its active metabolite increase in a dose-dependent manner with peak concentrations achieved within approximately 1.5 and 2.5 hours, respectively. Ticagrelor is primarily eliminated in the feces and to a lesser extent in urine; less than 1% of a dose is recovered in urine as the parent drug and active metabolite. The mean terminal half-lives of ticagrelor and its active metabolite reportedly are about 7 and 9 hours, respectively. Both ticagrelor and its active metabolite are extensively (more than 99%) bound to human plasma proteins. Administration with a high-fat meal increases systemic exposure of ticagrelor by 21% and decreases peak plasma concentrations of the active metabolite by 22%, but has no effect on peak plasma concentrations of ticagrelor or on systemic exposure to the active metabolite.

Genetic polymorphism of the CYP2C19 isoenzyme does not appear to affect the pharmacodynamic or clinical response to ticagrelor. In 2 genotype studies, ticagrelor demonstrated greater inhibition of platelet aggregation than clopidogrel regardless of CYP2C19 genotype or metabolizer status; in contrast, patients with a loss-of-function CYP2C19 variant had reduced antiplatelet effects during clopidogrel therapy. In addition, results of a genetic substudy of the PLATO trial showed that clinical outcomes with ticagrelor (reduction in the risk of cardiovascular death, myocardial infarction [MI], or stroke) were superior to those with clopidogrel irrespective of CYP2C19 polymorphism.

Advice to Patients

Importance of patients taking ticagrelor exactly as prescribed and not discontinuing therapy without first consulting the prescribing clinician. Importance of reviewing with clinician how to resume therapy in the event of a missed dose. (See Dosage and Administration: General.) Importance of patients reading the medication guide prior to initiation of therapy and each time the prescription is refilled.

Importance of advising patients to check their prescription carefully to ensure that they have received the correct drug; prescribing and dispensing errors have been reported due to similarities in the spelling and pronunciation of Brilinta® (the trade name for ticagrelor) and Brintellix® (the former trade name for vortioxetine hydrobromide, an antidepressant agent; trade name was changed to Trintellix® in May 2016). (See Prescribing and Dispensing Precautions under Warnings/Precautions: Other Warnings and Precautions, in Cautions.)

Importance of patients informing clinicians (e.g., physicians, dentists) about ticagrelor therapy before any surgery or dental procedure is performed. Clinicians performing any invasive procedure should consult with the prescribing clinician before discontinuing ticagrelor.

Importance of informing patients not to take aspirin dosages exceeding 100 mg daily; patient also should be advised to not take any other aspirin-containing drugs.

Importance of informing patients that they will bruise and/or bleed more easily and that a longer than usual time will be required to stop bleeding when taking ticagrelor. Importance of patients informing clinicians about any unexpected, prolonged, or excessive bleeding, or blood in urine or stool.

Importance of informing patients that ticagrelor can cause dyspnea; patient should be advised to contact their clinician if they experience any unexpected dyspnea.

Importance of informing clinicians of existing or contemplated concomitant therapy, including prescription and OTC drugs, particularly drugs that affect bleeding risk (e.g., heparin, warfarin).

Importance of women informing clinicians if they are or plan to become pregnant or plan to breast-feed.

Importance of informing patients of other important precautionary information. (See Cautions.)

Overview® (see Users Guide). For additional information on this drug until a more detailed monograph is developed and published, the manufacturer's labeling should be consulted. It is *essential* that the manufacturer's labeling be consulted for more detailed information on usual cautions, precautions, contraindications, potential drug interactions, laboratory test interferences, and acute toxicity.

Preparations

Excipients in commercially available drug preparations may have clinically important effects in some individuals; consult specific product labeling for details.

Ticagrelor

Oral		
Tablets	90 mg	**Brilinta®**, AstraZeneca

Ticlopidine Hydrochloride

■ Ticlopidine, a thienopyridine derivative P2Y12 platelet adenosine diphosphate (ADP)-receptor antagonist, is a platelet-aggregation inhibitor.

Uses

■ **Prevention of Thrombotic Stroke** Ticlopidine is used to reduce the risk of fatal or nonfatal thrombotic stroke in patients who have had either a previous completed thrombotic stroke or stroke precursors (e.g., transient ischemic attack [TIA], transient monocular or partial blindness [amaurosis fugax], reversible ischemic neurologic deficit, minor stroke). Because of the risk of life-threatening adverse hematologic effects, including neutropenia and/or agranulocytosis, thrombotic thrombocytopenic purpura (TTP), and aplastic anemia, the manufacturer states that the drug should be reserved for patients who are unable to tolerate or are sensitive to aspirin or who have failed to respond to aspirin therapy where indicated to prevent stroke; the manufacturer further states that ticlopidine is contraindicated in patients with preexisting hematopoietic disorders such as neutropenia or thrombocytopenia or a history of either thrombotic thrombocytopenic purpura or aplastic anemia. The manufacturer also states that the drug should *not* be used in patients with a hemostatic disorder, active pathologic bleeding (e.g., bleeding peptic ulcer, intracranial bleeding), or severe hepatic impairment. The American College of Chest Physicians (ACCP) states that use of ticlopidine for the secondary prevention of stroke has become severely limited because of the risk of serious adverse effects and the availability of safer antiplatelet agents (e.g., clopidogrel).

Ticlopidine has been shown in 2 randomized, double-blind studies to reduce the risk of stroke and other vascular outcomes compared with aspirin or placebo in patients with stroke precursors or in those who had experienced an atherothrombotic stroke. Subgroup analyses of one of these studies suggested that the beneficial effects of ticlopidine relative to aspirin were more pronounced in nonwhite, predominantly African American patients. However, serious adverse effects, such as neutropenia and TTP, were reported with ticlopidine in these studies.

■ **Prevention of Coronary Artery Stent Thrombosis** Ticlopidine also is used as an adjunct to aspirin therapy to reduce the incidence of subacute stent thrombosis after percutaneous coronary intervention (PCI) with successful coronary artery stent placement. Because of the risk of serious adverse effects (e.g., thrombocytopenia, neutropenia, thrombotic thrombocytopenic purpura) associated with ticlopidine, use of the drug for the prevention of coronary artery stent thrombosis largely has been replaced by other antiplatelet agents. ACCP and other experts currently recommend dual-drug antiplatelet therapy with other P2Y12 platelet adenosine diphosphate (ADP)-receptor antagonists (e.g., clopidogrel, prasugrel, ticagrelor) and aspirin in patients undergoing PCI with stent placement.

In comparative clinical trials in patients undergoing stent implantation, therapy with ticlopidine hydrochloride (250 mg twice daily) plus aspirin (100 mg twice daily to 325 mg daily) was associated with a lower incidence of recurrent cardiovascular events (e.g., stent thrombosis resulting in death, myocardial infarction [MI], the need for repeat coronary angioplasty, or coronary artery bypass grafting [CABG]) than therapy with aspirin alone or combined with anticoagulants (e.g., warfarin).

Dosage and Administration

■ **Administration** Ticlopidine hydrochloride is administered orally. The drug should be taken with food to maximize GI absorption and tolerance.

■ **Dosage** ***Prevention of Thrombotic Stroke*** For reducing the risk of fatal or nonfatal stroke in adults, the usual dosage of ticlopidine hydrochloride is 250 mg twice daily. The safety and efficacy of this dosage in geriatric patients appear to be similar to those in younger adults, and clinical trials establishing the efficacy of the usual dosage principally involved the elderly; however, the possibility that some geriatric patients may exhibit increased sensitivity to ticlopidine hydrochloride cannot be excluded. The manufacturer states that the efficacy of dosages other than the usual adult dosage has not been studied in controlled clinical trials.

Therapy with ticlopidine hydrochloride has been continued for at least up to 5.8 years in some patients.

Prevention of Coronary Artery Stent Thrombosis When ticlopidine hydrochloride is used as an adjunct to aspirin to prevent subacute stent thrombosis in adults undergoing coronary stent placement, the usual initial dosage recommended by the manufacturer is 250 mg twice daily in conjunction with antiplatelet dosages of aspirin; therapy is initiated after successful stent implantation and continued for 30 days.

If ticlopidine is used in combination with aspirin as the thienopyridine-derivative component of dual-drug antiplatelet therapy following drug-eluting stent (DES) implantation, it is critical that combined therapy with ticlopidine and aspirin be continued for at least 12 months to minimize the risk of potentially catastrophic stent thrombosis. (See Myocardial Infarction under Dosage: Acute Coronary Syndrome, in Dosage and Administration in Clopidogrel Bisulfate 20:12.18.)

■ **Dosage in Renal and Hepatic Impairment** In patients with renal impairment, reduction of ticlopidine hydrochloride dosage or discontinuance of the drug may be necessary if hemorrhagic or hematopoietic complications occur. In controlled clinical trials, no unexpected adverse effects were observed in patients with mild renal impairment receiving usual dosages of the drug, but the manufacturer states that there has been no experience in patients with more severe degrees of impairment.

The manufacturer currently states that use of ticlopidine hydrochloride in patients with severe hepatic impairment is contraindicated, since experience to date in such patients is limited and they may be at risk for bleeding diathesis.

Cautions

Adverse effects of ticlopidine are relatively frequent, with more than 50% of patients in controlled clinical trials reporting at least one adverse effect while receiving the drug over study periods ranging up to 5.8 years. Most adverse effects are mild in severity and occur early in the course of treatment (i.e., within the first 3 months); however, some adverse effects may become evident for the first time only after several months of therapy. In comparative studies, ticlopidine generally appeared to be more poorly tolerated overall than aspirin, with diarrhea and rash occurring with ticlopidine at about twice the rates reported with aspirin; only adverse GI effects typically associated with nonsteroidal anti-inflammatory agent (NSAIA) therapy (e.g., GI pain or bleeding, peptic ulcer) occurred more frequently with aspirin than with ticlopidine.

The most serious adverse effects of ticlopidine involve the hematologic system, principally neutropenia, which may be life-threatening. The most frequently reported adverse effects of ticlopidine involve the GI tract. The most frequent adverse effects in controlled clinical trials were diarrhea, nausea, dyspepsia, and rash; these effects occurred more often in whites and women. In controlled clinical trials, 21% of patients discontinued ticlopidine therapy because of adverse effects. The most common adverse effects resulting in drug discontinuance were nausea, vomiting, diarrhea, GI pain, rash, and neutropenia.

■ **Hematologic Effects** The most serious adverse hematologic effects of ticlopidine are neutropenia (absolute neutrophil count [ANC] less than 1200 neutrophils/mm^3), agranulocytosis, thrombotic thrombocytopenic purpura (TTP), and aplastic anemia. The incidence of ticlopidine-induced neutropenia, TTP, or aplastic anemia peaks about 4–6, 3–4, or 4–8 weeks, respectively, following initiation of therapy; the incidence of these hematologic effects declines thereafter. Only in a few instances have these hematologic adverse effects occurred more than 3 months after initiation of ticlopidine therapy. Risk factors for development of these adverse hematologic effects have not been identified; however, data from a large clinical trial suggest that the risk of adverse effects, including severe neutropenia, with ticlopidine therapy may be reduced (and beneficial effects on stroke reduction more pronounced) in nonwhite (e.g., African American) patients. (See Uses: Prevention of Thrombotic Stroke.) Fever may be a clinical manifestation indicative of neutropenia, TTP, or aplastic anemia. Neutropenia occurred in 2.4% of stroke patients receiving the drug in controlled clinical trials. Hematologic status must be carefully monitored in patients receiving ticlopidine. (See Cautions: Precautions and Contraindications.)

The onset of neutropenia may be sudden. Mild to moderate neutropenia (ANC of 451–1200 neutrophils/mm^3) occurred in 1.6% of patients and severe neutropenia (ANC less than 450 neutrophils/mm^3) in 0.8% of patients receiving ticlopidine in controlled clinical trials. In patients with mild to moderate neutropenia, neutrophil counts usually recover within a few days of discontinuing ticlopidine, but neutropenia may be transient and may not necessarily require discontinuance of the drug. Severe neutropenia usually occurs within 3 weeks to 3 months after initiating ticlopidine therapy (but may occur later), may be idiosyncratic and not dose related, and can be detected with regular hematologic monitoring. The bone marrow usually shows a reduction in myeloid precursors, principally those associated with arrest of maturation of the granulocytic cell line. Neutropenia usually is not severe, often being relieved by a temporary reduction in dosage, but discontinuance of ticlopidine therapy was required in 1.3% of patients in controlled clinical trials. Neutrophil counts usually return to normal within 1–3 weeks when ticlopidine therapy is immediately discontinued following detection of neutropenia. However, neutropenia has been reported rarely following ticlopidine discontinuance and rarely has been fatal.

Thrombocytopenia (platelet count less than 80,000 cells/mm^3) may occur rarely in isolation or in conjunction with neutropenia, TTP, or aplastic anemia in patients receiving ticlopidine. If thrombocytopenia occurs, ticlopidine therapy should be discontinued. (See Cautions: Precautions and Contraindications.) Rarely, immune thrombocytopenia and thrombotic thrombocytopenic purpura have occurred and in some cases were fatal. TTP is characterized by thrombocytopenia, microangiopathic hemolytic anemia (fragmented red blood cells [schistocytes] on peripheral blood smear), neurologic changes, renal dysfunction, and fever. Clinical symptoms may precede laboratory evidence of TTP, but manifestations of the adverse effect can occur in any order. Based on an annual estimated patient exposure of 2–4 million and assuming an event reporting rate of 10%, the incidence of ticlopidine-associated TTP may be as high as one case in every 2000–4000 patients exposed. However, in a retrospective postmarketing surveillance study in patients undergoing percutaneous transluminal coronary angioplasty (PTCA) and coronary artery stenting, TTP was diagnosed in 0.02% of patients an average of 25 days after initiation of ticlopidine therapy in patients receiving the drug for an average of 22 days.

Purpura is a common adverse hematologic effect of ticlopidine, occurring in 2.2% of patients receiving the drug in controlled clinical trials. Rarely, purpura has resulted in discontinuance of ticlopidine.

Adverse hematologic effects occurring occasionally with ticlopidine therapy include increased bleeding, spontaneous posttraumatic bleeding, perioperative bleeding (including perioperative GI bleeding), ecchymosis, epistaxis, hematuria, conjunctival hemorrhage, unspecified bleeding disorders, easy bruisability, petechiae, GI hemorrhage, gingival bleeding, menorrhagia, and intracerebral bleeding or hemorrhage. Intracerebral hemorrhage rarely has been fatal. Hemolytic anemia with reticulocytosis, aplastic anemia (sometimes fatal), agranulocytosis (sometimes fatal), eosinophilia, pancytopenia (sometimes fatal), thrombocytosis, leukemia, and bone marrow depression each have been reported rarely. Aplastic anemia is characterized by anemia, thrombocytopenia, and neutropenia together with evidence of depression of myeloid precursors on bone marrow examination. Patients may exhibit manifestations suggestive of infection in association with low leukocyte and platelet counts. The incidence of aplastic anemia usually peaks after about 4—8 weeks of therapy. Based on an annual estimated patient exposure of 2–4 million and assuming an event reporting rate of 10%, the incidence of ticlopidine-associated aplastic anemia may be as high as one case in every 4000–8000 patients exposed.

■ **GI Effects** Adverse GI effects accounted for 30–40% of reported adverse effects, and usually occurred within the first 3 months of ticlopidine therapy, were usually mild in severity, tended to occur more frequently in geriatric patients, and often disappeared within 1–2 weeks despite continued therapy. The most common adverse GI effect of ticlopidine is diarrhea, which occurred in 12.5% of patients receiving the drug in controlled clinical trials. Diarrhea may be accompanied by abdominal cramps and is the most frequent adverse effect requiring discontinuance of therapy, resulting in ticlopidine discontinuance in 6.3% of patients receiving the drug in controlled clinical trials. Diarrhea may be alleviated by a temporary reduction in dosage. If diarrhea is severe or persistent, ticlopidine therapy should be discontinued. In some cases of severe or bloody diarrhea in clinical trials, colitis subsequently was diagnosed.

Other adverse GI effects of ticlopidine include nausea and dyspepsia, each of which occurred in 7% of patients receiving the drug in controlled clinical trials. GI pain occurred in 3.7% of patients receiving ticlopidine in controlled clinical trials. Nausea, dyspepsia, and GI pain resulted in drug discontinuance in 2.6%, 1.1%, and 1.9%, respectively, of patients receiving the drug in controlled clinical trials. Vomiting, which occurred in 1.9% of patients, flatulence, which occurred in 1.5% of patients, and anorexia, which occurred in 1% of patients, also have been reported with ticlopidine therapy in controlled clinical trials. Vomiting resulted in drug discontinuance in 1.4% of patients. Flatulence and anorexia occasionally have resulted in drug discontinuance. GI fullness, gastritis, and peptic ulcer have been reported rarely.

■ **Dermatologic and Sensitivity Reactions** Rash is the most common adverse dermatologic effect of ticlopidine, occurring in approximately 5% of patients receiving the drug in controlled clinical trials. The rash may be maculopapular or urticarial and often is associated with pruritus. Pruritus occurred in 1.3% of patients receiving ticlopidine in controlled clinical trials. Rash resulted in discontinuance of ticlopidine therapy in 3.4% of patients and pruritus in 0.8% of patients receiving the drug in controlled clinical trials. Rash usually occurs within 3 months of initiating ticlopidine therapy (average onset of 11 days), and resolves within several days with drug discontinuance. Ticlopidine therapy can often be reinstituted following resolution without rash recurrence. Urticaria has been reported occasionally. Vasculitis, erythema, angioedema, allergic pneumonitis, systemic lupus erythematosus with positive antinuclear antibody (ANA) titer, serum sickness, anaphylaxis, and severe rashes, including Stevens-Johnson syndrome, erythema multiforme, and exfoliative dermatitis, each have been reported rarely.

■ **Hepatic Effects** Elevations in serum alkaline phosphatase concentration (to greater than 2 times the upper limit of normal) occurred in 7.6% of patients and AST (SGOT) concentrations (to greater than 2 times the upper limit of normal) occurred in 3.1% of patients receiving ticlopidine in controlled clinical trials. These elevations generally occurred within 1–4 months of therapy. No progressive increases were observed, but most patients with these abnormalities discontinued therapy. Elevations in serum transaminase and bilirubin concentrations (up to and exceeding 10 times the upper limit of normal) have been reported rarely during postmarketing experience. Abnormal liver function test results occurred in 1% of patients and resulted in discontinuance of ticlopidine therapy in 0.7% of patients in controlled clinical trials. Increased or decreased serum bilirubin concentration, increased serum γ-glutamyltransferase (γ-glutamyltranspeptidase, GT, GGTP) concentration, hepatitis, hepatocellular jaundice, cholestatic jaundice, severe cholestasis, cholestatic hepatitis, hepatic failure, and hepatic necrosis each have been reported rarely. Granulomatous hepatitis also has been reported; a causal relationship to the drug has not been established.

■ **Nervous System Effects** Dizziness occurred in approximately 1% of patients receiving ticlopidine in controlled clinical trials and resulted in drug discontinuance in 0.4% of patients. Headache and asthenia each occasionally occurred in patients receiving the drug in controlled clinical trials. Peripheral neuropathy, pain, and tinnitus each have been reported rarely.

■ **Metabolic Effects** Increases in total serum cholesterol concentrations usually occur with ticlopidine therapy. Serum total cholesterol concentrations increase by 8–10% within 1 month of initiating therapy and persist for the duration of treatment. Such increases were not associated with liver dysfunction or an increase in vascular ischemic events. Increases in serum triglyceride concentrations also may occur with ticlopidine therapy. Ratios of lipoprotein subfractions are unchanged.

■ **Other Effects** Renal failure, nephrotic syndrome, acute interstitial nephritis, hyponatremia, sepsis, arthropathy, and myositis each have been reported rarely in patients receiving ticlopidine.

■ **Precautions and Contraindications** Because ticlopidine may cause life-threatening adverse effects, the potential benefit of therapy with the drug must be carefully weighed against the possible risks involved, and the patient should be apprised of the risks. Ticlopidine should be reserved for patients who are unable to tolerate or do not respond adequately to aspirin therapy where indicated to prevent stroke.

Because ticlopidine may cause severe neutropenia and/or agranulocytosis, as well as other hematologic abnormalities (see Cautions: Hematologic Effects), which may be life-threatening, it is essential that complete blood counts (including platelet count) and leukocyte differentials be performed prior to initiation of therapy and every 2 weeks to the end of the third month of therapy in patients receiving the drug. The manufacturer states that more frequent monitoring, and monitoring after the first 3 months of therapy, is necessary only in patients with clinical manifestations (e.g., suggestive of or consistent with infection) or laboratory evidence (e.g., neutrophil count less than 70% of the baseline count, decrease in hematocrit or platelet count) that suggest incipient adverse hematologic effects. The possibility of thrombotic thrombocytopenic purpura (TTP) should be considered in any patient receiving ticlopidine who develops fever, weakness, pallor, petechiae or purpura, dark urine, jaundice, neurologic changes, and/or acute, unexplained decreases in hemoglobin or platelet count, particularly during the 3 months following initiation of therapy. In such patients, a peripheral blood smear revealing fragmented red blood cells (schistocytes) should be considered presumptive evidence of TTP. The possibility of aplastic anemia should be investigated in any patient receiving ticlopidine who has evidence of a simultaneous decrease in platelet and leukocyte counts. If laboratory testing confirms neutropenia (less than 1200 cells/mm^3), TTP, aplastic anemia, or thrombocytopenia (less than 80,000 platelets/mm^3), ticlopidine therapy should be discontinued immediately. Because some cases of immune thrombocytopenia and TTP in patients receiving ticlopidine have been fatal, careful attention to diagnosis must be made to guide treatment. With prompt treatment (often including plasmapheresis), 70–80% of patients with TTP will survive with minimal or no sequelae. Prompt treatment of aplastic anemia, which may include use of hematopoietic agents, can minimize the mortality associated with aplastic anemia. When ticlopidine therapy is immediately discontinued following detection of neutropenia, neutrophil counts usually return to normal within 1–3 weeks, but fatalities have been reported rarely. Because of the long plasma half-life of ticlopidine, the manufacturer recommends that complete blood counts (including platelet count) and leukocyte differential should be performed for at least 2 weeks following discontinuance of ticlopidine in any patient who discontinues the drug for any reason within the first 3 months of therapy. Ticlopidine is contraindicated in patients with preexisting hematopoietic disorders such as neutropenia and thrombocytopenia or a history of either TTP or aplastic anemia.

In patients with coronary artery stents, particularly those with drug-eluting stents, premature discontinuance of therapy with a thienopyridine derivative (e.g., clopidogrel, ticlopidine) and aspirin has been associated with stent thrombosis with potentially fatal sequelae. Before implantation of a drug-eluting stent, patients should be assessed for likelihood of compliance with prolonged dual-drug antiplatelet therapy; strong consideration should be given to avoiding use of a drug-eluting stent in patients who are not expected to comply. In patients who are likely to require invasive or surgical procedures within 12 months after drug-eluting stent implantation, implantation of a bare-metal stent or use of balloon angioplasty with provisional stent implantation should be considered instead. Clinicians performing invasive procedures must understand the consequences of premature discontinuance of thienopyridine derivative therapy in patients with drug-eluting stents. If issues about a patient's antiplatelet therapy are unclear (e.g., concern about periprocedural bleeding), such professionals should contact the patient's cardiologist. Elective procedures with substantial bleeding risk should be deferred until dual-drug antiplatelet therapy has been completed. For nonelective procedures that mandate discontinuance of thienopyridine-derivative therapy, aspirin therapy should be continued if at all possible, and the thienopyridine derivative restarted as soon as possible after the procedure.

Because ticlopidine increases serum total cholesterol and triglyceride concentrations (see Cautions: Metabolic Effects), these effects should be considered when the drug is used in patients in whom such effects may be clinically important.

The tolerability and safety of concomitant therapy with ticlopidine and heparin, oral anticoagulants, or fibrinolytic agents have not been established. If a patient receiving any of these agents is to be transferred to therapy with ticlopidine, these agents should be discontinued before ticlopidine is administered.

Ticlopidine should be used with caution in patients who may be at risk for increased bleeding from trauma, surgery, or other pathologic conditions. If elective surgery is planned for patients receiving ticlopidine and it is desired that the platelet-aggregation inhibiting effects of the drug be avoided, ticlopidine should be discontinued 10–14 days prior to surgery to minimize excessive surgical bleeding. In patients with prolonged bleeding time, IV methylprednisolone (20 mg) can normalize such prolongation within 2 hours of administration. Platelet transfusions also can be considered for reversing the effects of ticlopidine on bleeding; administration of platelets should be avoided in patients who developed thrombotic thrombocytopenic purpura secondary to ticlopidine therapy, as such transfusions may accelerate thrombosis in these patients.

Because ticlopidine prolongs template bleeding time, the drug should be used with caution in patients who have lesions with a propensity to bleed (e.g., peptic ulcers). In addition, drugs that may cause such lesions should be used with caution in patients receiving ticlopidine. Aspirin reportedly does not appear to affect ticlopidine-mediated inhibition of adenosine diphosphate (ADP)-induced platelet aggregation, although ticlopidine can potentiate aspirin-mediated inhibition of collagen-induced platelet aggregation. While one manufacturer states that long-term concomitant use of aspirin and ticlopidine is not recommended, a thienopyridine derivative (i.e., clopidogrel) has been used as an adjunct to aspirin therapy for at least 12 months following PCI and intracoronary stenting. (See Uses: Prevention of Coronary Artery Stent Thrombosis.) Ticlopidine is contraindicated in patients with a hemostatic disorder or active pathologic bleeding (e.g., bleeding peptic ulcer, intracranial bleeding).

Because ticlopidine therapy may result in elevations of liver function test results, including serum alkaline phosphatase, transaminase, and, rarely, bilirubin concentrations, monitoring of hepatic function, including ALT (SGPT), AST (SGOT), and γ-glutamyltransferase concentrations, should be considered when hepatic dysfunction is suspected, especially during the first 4 months of therapy.

Because clinical experience with ticlopidine in patients with concurrent systemic disease is limited, the drug should be used with caution in patients with any systemic disease or condition that may alter metabolism of the drug. Dosage of drugs metabolized by hepatic microsomal enzymes with low therapeutic ratios or being administered to patients with hepatic impairment may require adjustment when initiating or discontinuing concomitant therapy with ticlopidine. Ticlopidine should be used with caution in patients with moderate to severe renal impairment, since decreased plasma clearance, increased AUC values, and prolonged bleeding times can occur in such patients. Reduction of ticlopidine dosage or discontinuance of the drug in patients with renal impairment may be necessary if hemorrhagic or hematopoietic complications occur. (See Dosage and Administration: Dosage in Renal and Hepatic Impairment.) Because ticlopidine is metabolized in the liver, dosage of ticlopidine or concomitantly administered drugs that are metabolized in the liver may require adjustment when starting or stopping therapy. Ticlopidine is contraindicated in patients with severe hepatic impairment, since experience in these patients is limited and they may be at risk for bleeding diathesis.

Patients receiving ticlopidine should be informed of the necessity of routine laboratory testing (e.g., complete blood counts, leukocyte differential, platelet counts) for the assessment of hematologic status. Patients receiving ticlopidine should be informed that neutropenia, thrombotic thrombocytopenic purpura (TTP), aplastic anemia, or thrombocytopenia can occur with the drug, especially during the first 3 months of therapy, and that severe neutropenia can result in an increased risk of infection. They also should be advised that it is critically important to undergo the scheduled hematologic tests in order to detect neutropenia, TTP, aplastic anemia, or thrombocytopenia. Patients should be advised regarding manifestations of infection and to contact their clinician if any indication of infection such as fever, chills, and sore throat develops or worsens during therapy with the drug. Patients should be advised to discontinue ticlopidine therapy immediately and contact their clinician if any manifestations suggestive of aplastic anemia (e.g., fever, weakness, pallor, bruising, bleeding from gums or nose, excessive fatigue) or TTP (e.g., fever, weakness, difficulty speaking, seizures, jaundice, dark or bloody urine, pallor, petechiae) occur. Patients also should be informed of the increased risk of bleeding and prolonged time to stop bleeding with ticlopidine and that they should report any unusual bleeding to their clinician. Patients should inform their clinicians and dentists that they are receiving ticlopidine prior to scheduling of any surgery or prescription of any new drug. Patients should be advised of possible adverse effects of ticlopidine including severe or persistent diarrhea, rash, subcutaneous bleeding, or any signs of cholestasis, including yellow skin or sclera, dark urine, or light colored stools, and should be advised to report the appearance of any of these signs or symptoms immediately to their clinician. Patients should be instructed to take ticlopidine with food to minimize GI discomfort.

Ticlopidine is contraindicated in patients with known hypersensitivity to the drug.

■ **Pediatric Precautions** Safety and efficacy of ticlopidine hydrochloride in children younger than 18 years of age have not been established.

■ **Geriatric Precautions** The manufacturer states that total plasma clearance of ticlopidine is somewhat lower and trough plasma concentrations are increased in geriatric patients. A large proportion of patients studied in controlled clinical trials of ticlopidine for stroke prevention were geriatric; 45% were older than 65 years of age and 12% were older than 75 years of age. Although no overall differences in efficacy or safety were observed between geriatric and younger patients, and other clinical experience revealed no evidence of age-related differences, the possibility that some older patients may exhibit increased sensitivity to the drug cannot be ruled out. Except for dyspepsia, adverse GI effects of ticlopidine tend to occur more frequently in geriatric patients.

■ **Mutagenicity and Carcinogenicity** Ticlopidine was not mutagenic in vitro in the Ames test, rat hepatocyte DNA-repair assay, and Chinese hamster fibroblast chromosomal aberration test. The drug also was not mutagenic in vivo in the mouse spermatozoid morphology test, Chinese hamster micronucleus test, and Chinese hamster bone marrow cell sister chromatid exchange test.

Ticlopidine hydrochloride was not tumorigenic when administered to rats for 2 years at dosages up to 100 mg/kg daily (610 mg/m^2; 14 times the recommended clinical human dosage on a mg/kg basis for a 70-kg individual and 2 times the clinical human dosage on a mg/m^2 basis for an individual with a body surface area of 1.73 m^2). Ticlopidine hydrochloride also was not tumorigenic when administered to mice for 78 weeks at dosages up to 275 mg/kg daily (1180 mg/m^2; 40 times the recommended clinical human dosage on a mg/kg basis and 4 times the clinical human dosage on a mg/m^2 basis).

■ **Pregnancy, Fertility, and Lactation** In reproduction studies, ticlopidine hydrochloride dosages of 400 mg/kg daily in rats, 200 mg/kg daily in mice, and 100 mg/kg daily in rabbits produced maternal toxicity as well as fetal toxicity, but there was no evidence of teratogenicity. There are no adequate and controlled studies to date using ticlopidine in pregnant women, and the drug should be used during pregnancy only when clearly needed.

Reproduction studies in male and female rats using oral ticlopidine hydrochloride dosages up to 400 mg/kg daily have not revealed evidence of impaired fertility.

Ticlopidine is distributed into milk in rats. It is not known whether ticlopidine is distributed into human milk. Because of the potential for serious adverse reactions to ticlopidine in nursing infants, a decision should be made whether to discontinue nursing or the drug, taking into account the importance of the drug to the woman.

Description

Ticlopidine, a thienopyridine-derivative P2Y12 platelet adenosine diphosphate (ADP)-receptor antagonist structurally and pharmacologically related to clopidogrel, is a platelet-aggregation inhibitor. While some in vitro data suggest that ticlopidine may be a prodrug, no specific metabolite(s) responsible for pharmacologic and therapeutic activity has been identified to date.

SumMon® (see Users Guide). For additional information on this drug until a more detailed monograph is developed and published, the manufacturer's labeling should be consulted. It is *essential* that the labeling be consulted for detailed information on the usual cautions, precautions, and contraindications concerning potential drug interactions and/or laboratory test interferences and for information on acute toxicity.

Preparations

Excipients in commercially available drug preparations may have clinically important effects in some individuals; consult specific product labeling for details.

Ticlopidine Hydrochloride

Oral

Tablets, film-coated	250 mg*	**Ticlopidine Hydrochloride**

*available from one or more manufacturer, distributor, and/or repackager by generic (nonproprietary) name

Tirofiban

■ Tirofiban hydrochloride, a selective, competitive platelet-aggregation inhibitor, has been referred to as a platelet glycoprotein (GP) IIb/IIIa-receptor inhibitor.

Uses

■ **Non-ST-Segment-Elevation Acute Coronary Syndromes** Tirofiban is used with anticoagulant therapy (e.g., heparin [referring throughout this monograph to unfractionated heparin], low molecular weight heparin), aspirin, and a P2Y12 platelet adenosine diphosphate (ADP)-receptor antagonist (e.g., clopidogrel, prasugrel, ticagrelor) to reduce the risk of acute cardiac ischemic events (death and/or myocardial infarction [MI]) in patients with unstable angina or non-ST-segment-elevation MI (NSTEMI) (i.e., non-ST-segment-elevation acute coronary syndromes [NSTE ACS]), both in patients who are to receive medical management and those undergoing percutaneous coronary intervention (PCI) (e.g., percutaneous transluminal coronary angioplasty [PTCA], stent placement, atherectomy). The goal of therapy in these patients is to maintain myocardial perfusion by inhibiting further platelet aggregation and thus preventing the progression of a nonocclusive thrombus to an occlusive thrombus. In clinical trials of tirofiban, NSTE ACS was defined by prolonged symptoms of cardiac ischemia (at least 10 minutes' duration within the previous 12–24 hours) occurring at rest or with minimal exertion that were associated with *transient* ST-segment changes (i.e., elevation or depression), T-wave inversion, or increased cardiac [MB] fraction of creatine kinase [CK, creatine phosphokinase, CPK]); patients who had MI associated with Q waves or *persistent* ST-segment elevation (exceeding 20 minutes) were not included in these studies. NSTEMI and unstable angina clinically may be indistinguishable at initial presentation and are managed similarly. Most of the patients in clinical trials of tirofiban received concomitant therapy with aspirin and IV heparin, and the efficacy and safety of tirofiban without adjunctive heparin and/or aspirin therapy have not been established.

Platelet glycoprotein (GP) IIb/IIIa-receptor inhibitors are used as an adjunct to standard therapeutic measures for managing NSTE ACS. These measures include therapy with aspirin and a P2Y12-receptor antagonist (e.g., clopidogrel, prasugrel, ticagrelor), nitrates (e.g., nitroglycerin), anticoagulant therapy (e.g., low molecular weight heparin, heparin), and β-blockers followed by either conservative medical management or early aggressive management, such as angiographic evaluation and revascularization procedures (e.g., PCI, coronary artery bypass grafting [CABG], coronary artery stent implantation) as required. Several meta-analyses of studies indicate that adjunctive therapy with a GP IIb/IIIa-receptor inhibitor can reduce the incidence of cardiac ischemic events, including subsequent MI and death, in patients with NSTE ACS. The benefits of GP IIb/IIIa-receptor inhibitors on mortality principally occur early during therapy (i.e., the first 48–96 hours).

The benefit of aspirin for secondary prevention of ischemic events in patients with NSTE ACS has been demonstrated in several studies and pooled analyses. Many clinicians recommend that all patients with NSTE ACS receive aspirin as soon as possible after hospital admission and then continued indefinitely unless they have documented hypersensitivity or other definite contraindications (e.g., active or recent major bleeding, peptic ulcer disease). (See Non-ST-Segment-Elevation Acute Coronary Syndromes under Thrombosis: Coronary Artery Disease and Myocardial Infarction, in Uses in Aspirin 28:08.04.24.) The American College of Cardiology Foundation (ACCF) and the American Heart Association (AHA) state that in patients with NSTE ACS in whom an initial invasive management strategy is planned, an additional antiplatelet agent (either clopidogrel or a GP IIb/IIIa-receptor inhibitor given IV) should be administered prior to diagnostic angiography ("upstream") as an adjunct to aspirin therapy. Eptifibatide or tirofiban is the preferred GP IIb/IIIa-receptor inhibitor for this use; abciximab is indicated only if there is no appreciable delay before angiography and PCI is likely to be performed.

Randomized controlled studies, including a meta-analysis of 16 randomized trials involving approximately 10,000 patients with ST-segment-elevation MI (STEMI) undergoing primary PCI, generally have failed to demonstrate benefits of GP IIb/IIIa-receptor blockade similar to those observed in patients with NSTE ACS. ACCF, AHA, the Society for Cardiovascular Angiography and Interventions (SCAI), and other experts currently do not recommend the *routine* use of GP IIb/IIIa-receptor inhibitors in patients with STEMI undergoing PCI; however, selective use of these drugs as an adjunct to heparin may be reasonable in certain high-risk patients (e.g., those with large anterior MI and/or large thrombus). Studies evaluating the use of GP IIb/IIIa-receptor inhibitors in patients with NSTE ACS undergoing PCI have demonstrated reductions in ischemic outcomes, particularly in patients with high-risk features (e.g., elevated troponin); therefore, ACCF/AHA/SCAI states that it may be useful to administer a GP IIb/IIIa-receptor inhibitor at the time of PCI as an adjunct to heparin therapy in such high-risk patients who are not receiving bivalirudin and who are not adequately pretreated with clopidogrel. Regarding the choice of GP IIb/IIIa-receptor inhibitor in patients undergoing PCI, abciximab, "double-bolus" eptifibatide (i.e., two 180-mcg/kg direct IV injections given 10 minutes apart), and high-dose tirofiban (25 mcg/kg by direct IV injection) all have been shown to produce a high degree of platelet inhibition and reduce ischemic complications.

In patients with NSTE ACS with elevated troponin concentrations who were managed with conservative medical therapy, GP IIb/IIIa-receptor inhibitors were equally effective in men and women. However, in women with NSTE ACS who are not at high risk for acute cardiac ischemic events (e.g., no elevated troponin concentrations) and are managed with a conservative strategy, eptifibatide and tirofiban appear to show little benefit and may possibly have detrimental effects; these agents are not recommended by AHA in women at lower risk for adverse cardiac events.

The current labeled indication for tirofiban is based principally on the results of 3 large, randomized controlled studies evaluating the efficacy of tirofiban alone or in combination with heparin in patients with NSTE ACS, including those who subsequently underwent PCI. All patients in these studies also received aspirin (300–325 mg daily) for at least 48 hours after randomization (indefinitely in some patients) or within 12 hours prior to PCI unless the drug was contraindicated. In the Platelet Receptor Inhibition in Ischemic Syndrome Management in Patients Limited by Unstable Signs and Symptoms [PRISM-PLUS]) study, therapy with tirofiban (IV loading dose of 0.4 or 0.6 mcg/kg per minute given over 30 minutes followed by continuous IV infusion of 0.1 mcg/kg per minute for 48–108 hours) plus adjusted-dose heparin reduced the incidence of ischemic events compared with adjusted-dose heparin alone in patients with NSTE ACS. All patients received aspirin 325 mg daily unless the drug was contraindicated. Patients who received medical management alone (i.e., those not undergoing PCI) were given an IV loading dose of heparin sodium (5000 units) followed by an IV infusion (1000 units/hour) that was titrated to a target activated partial thromboplastin time (aPTT) of twice the control value. In patients undergoing PCI after at least 48 hours of medical management, the infusion of heparin sodium or heparin placebo was discontinued and an IV loading dose of heparin sodium (5000–7500 units) was administered, followed by an IV infusion (1000 units/hour) that was titrated with additional IV injections of heparin sodium as needed. Overall, patients in each group received the study drug(s) for an average of about 71 hours. Patients undergoing PCI received the study drug(s) for an average of 76 hours, of which an average of 15.4 hours was after PCI.

Beneficial effects of therapy with tirofiban and heparin were evident within 48 hours of initiating the tirofiban infusion and persisted for up to 6 months. The combined incidence of nonfatal MI or death at 48 hours in patients receiving tirofiban plus heparin was reduced by 66% (from 2.6 to 0.9%). The combined incidence of death, nonfatal MI, or refractory ischemia at 7 days (the primary composite end point) in patients receiving tirofiban plus heparin was reduced by 32% (from 17.9% to 12.9%); relative reductions of 47 and 30% occurred in the individual incidences of MI and refractory ischemia, respectively. The incidences of the composite end point at 30 days and 6 months, which also included hospital readmissions for unstable angina in patients receiving tirofiban and heparin, were reduced by 22% (from 22.3% to 18.5%) and 19% (from 32.1% to 27.7%), respectively, compared with heparin therapy alone. Data from a substudy of patients in PRISM-PLUS indicate that troponin I concentrations, a sensitive marker of myocardial injury or ischemia, were reduced to a greater extent in patients receiving tirofiban and heparin than in those receiving heparin alone. In another substudy of PRISM-PLUS, a reduction in angiographically evident thrombus formation was accompanied by an increase in blood flow to the affected coronary artery in patients receiving tirofiban and heparin. The incidence of major hemorrhage was similar in patients receiving tirofiban plus heparin (4%) or heparin alone (3%). Death occurred in 1.9% of each study group; no intracranial hemorrhages or hemorrhage-related deaths occurred in either group.

An initial third arm of the PRISM-PLUS study that included patients receiving tirofiban alone (without heparin) was discontinued prematurely because of unexpected excess mortality at 7 days (4.6%) compared with that in patients receiving heparin alone (1.1%); however, similar increases in the incidences of refractory ischemia, MI, or the composite end point did not occur. Also, another randomized study (Platelet Receptor Inhibition in Ischemic Syndrome Management [PRISM]) in which tirofiban therapy was compared with heparin therapy in patients with NSTE ACS demonstrated reductions in the composite end point of death, MI, or refractory ischemia at 48 hours and in mortality at 30 days. The PRISM-PLUS study included more high-risk patients than did the PRISM study (based on a higher percentage of patients with baseline ST-segment changes on ECG), and it has also been suggested that the large proportion (70%) of patients receiving IV heparin prior to randomization in the PRISM-PLUS study may have increased the likelihood of heparin rebound (i.e., ischemic events, including death, associated with recent or current heparin therapy in patients receiving concomitant aspirin). It has been suggested that the small number of events involved (16 of 345 patients receiving tirofiban alone versus 4 of 350 receiving heparin alone) also makes it possible that the higher incidence of death in PRISM-PLUS in patients receiving tirofiban alone compared with that in the PRISM study was attributable to chance. However, other variables potentially influencing the efficacy of tirofiban monotherapy (without heparin) include differences in the severity of NSTE ACS; the extent of use of PCI, angiography, or CABG; and the duration of the tirofiban infusion. Alternatively, concomitant thrombin inhibition (e.g., heparin, a low molecular weight heparin) may be needed for optimal efficacy of tirofiban, especially in high-risk patients with more severe NSTE ACS. Pooled analysis of data from the PRISM and PRISM-PLUS studies reportedly indicates that the effect of tirofiban therapy alone on mortality at 7 and 30 days was comparable to that of heparin therapy alone.

The efficacy of tirofiban in reducing composite clinical events associated with NSTE ACS in the PRISM-PLUS study was not affected by age or gender; the effect of race on efficacy could not be determined from the small number of non-white patients studied. Subgroup analyses indicated that beneficial effects of tirofiban and aspirin and heparin were particularly evident in patients receiving β-adrenergic blocking agents prior to study entry; benefit appeared to be consistent for all other factors studied (e.g., age, gender prior treatment with aspirin or heparin). While evaluation of patients who did or did not undergo PCI was not based on a randomized cohort, the incidence of the composite end point at 30 days in patients undergoing PCI was reduced from 15.3% in patients receiving heparin alone to 8.8% in patients receiving tirofiban and heparin (45% reduction).

In the Platelet Receptor Inhibition in Ischemic Syndrome Management

[PRISM] study, therapy with tirofiban (IV loading dose of 0.6 mcg/kg per minute for 30 minutes followed by continuous IV infusion of 0.15 mcg/kg per minute for 48 hours) reduced the incidence of ischemic events compared with heparin sodium therapy (5000 units IV loading dose followed by 1000 units per hour for 48 hours, adjusted to achieve an aPTT of twice the control value). All patients received aspirin 300–325 mg before randomization and daily thereafter for at least 48 hours unless contraindicated. Approximately 25% of the patients in the PRISM study had evidence of NSTEMI, while 30% had no electrocardiographic evidence of cardiac ischemia (ST-segment depression).

Beneficial effects of tirofiban were apparent during infusion of the drug but diminished thereafter. The combined incidence of death, nonfatal MI, or refractory ischemia at 48 hours (the primary composite end point) was reduced by 33% in patients receiving tirofiban compared with those receiving heparin; reductions in the incidence of these end-point events at 7 and 30 days (10 and 8%, respectively) were no longer statistically significant. However, the effect of tirofiban on survival became more pronounced with time; death was less common at 30 days (risk reduction of 38%) in tirofiban-treated patients than in those who received heparin (2.3 versus 3.6% of patients, respectively). In patients treated with medical therapy alone (i.e., not undergoing PCI), the rate of death or MI at 30 days was reduced by 42% (from 6.2%, with heparin to 3.6% with tirofiban). The incidence of major bleeding was similar in both treatment groups.

In the Randomized Efficacy Study of Tirofiban for Outcome and Restenosis (RESTORE) study, therapy with tirofiban (IV loading dose of 10 mcg/kg followed by continuous IV infusion of 0.15 mcg/kg per minute for 36 hours, beginning immediately prior to coronary intervention) reduced the incidence of early ischemic events in patients at high risk for abrupt closure of the affected coronary artery who underwent urgent or emergency PCI, although this reduction was not sustained. Patients considered at high risk for abrupt closure of coronary blood vessels included those with NSTE ACS or acute STEMI. All patients were receiving adjunctive therapy with low-dose aspirin (325 mg within 12 hours before the procedure) and heparin sodium (IV loading dose of 10,000 units in patients weighing at least 70 kg or 150 units/kg in those weighing less than 70 kg) prior to PCI. Additional heparin sodium was administered during the procedure as required to maintain an activated clotting time (ACT) of 300–400 seconds; heparin generally was discontinued after completion of PCI.

Beneficial effects of tirofiban were most apparent during infusion of the drug and for several days after drug administration but declined thereafter. The relative risk reduction in the primary composite clinical end point of death, nonfatal MI, or additional surgical interventions (e.g., recurrent ischemia, complications, or procedural failure of initial PCI necessitating CABG, coronary artery stent implantation, or repeat PCI) at 48 hours was 38% (from 8.7% in placebo recipients to 5.4% in those receiving tirofiban); however, the reduction in these clinical events was no longer statistically significant at 30 days (16% relative risk reduction) or 6 months (11% relative risk reduction), principally because of nonemergency CABG and repeat PCI procedures. In an angiographic substudy of the RESTORE study, tirofiban had no effect on the angiographic measurements of restenosis at 6 months. The incidence of major bleeding complications or thrombocytopenia were similar in patients receiving tirofiban or placebo.

Dosage and Administration

■ Administration Tirofiban hydrochloride is administered by IV infusion using either the diluted injection concentrate or the premixed injection in plastic (IntraVia™) containers. *Tirofiban hydrochloride injection concentrate for IV infusion must be diluted to the same concentration as the premixed injection (50 mcg/mL of tirofiban) before administration.* The injection concentrate is prepared for infusion by withdrawing and discarding 50 or 100 mL of solution from a 250- or 500-mL bag, respectively, of 0.9% sodium chloride or 5% dextrose injection and replacing this volume with 50 mL (12.5 mg of tirofiban) or 100 mL (25 mg of tirofiban) of tirofiban hydrochloride injection to achieve a final tirofiban concentration of 50 mcg/mL. The solution should be mixed well prior to infusion. Any unused drug solution should be discarded.

The plastic container of the premixed injection may be somewhat opaque because of moisture absorption during sterilization; this opacity will diminish gradually. The container of the premixed injection should be checked for minute leaks by firmly squeezing the bag. The premixed injection should be discarded if the seal is not intact, leaks are found, or the solution is cloudy or contains a precipitate. Additives should not be introduced into the injection container. The plastic IV containers should not be used in series connections with other plastic containers, since such use could result in air embolism from residual air being drawn from the primary container if the first container is empty.

In clinical trials, almost all patients receiving tirofiban also received concomitant aspirin and/or heparin. Tirofiban and heparin may be administered through the same IV line.

Parenteral tirofiban hydrochloride solutions should be inspected visually for particulate matter and discoloration prior to administration whenever solution and container permit.

■ Dosage Dosage of tirofiban hydrochloride is expressed in terms of tirofiban.

Non-ST-Segment-Elevation Acute Coronary Syndromes For reducing the risk of death, nonfatal myocardial infarction (MI), and/or refractory ischemia/repeat revascularization procedures in patients with non-ST-segment-elevation acute coronary syndromes (NSTE ACS) who are receiving medical therapy alone, an IV loading dose consisting of 0.4 mcg/kg of tirofiban per minute for 30 minutes is given as soon as possible after diagnosis, followed by continuous IV infusion of tirofiban 0.1 mcg/kg per minute for at least 24–48 hours. Patients receiving tirofiban who undergo percutaneous coronary intervention (PCI) should receive the same IV loading dose of tirofiban (0.4 mcg/kg per minute for 30 minutes) followed by continuous IV infusion of 0.1 mcg/kg per minute given during angiography and for 12–24 hours after angioplasty or atherectomy. In the PRISM-PLUS study, the tirofiban infusion was continued in combination with heparin for 48–108 hours. In patients who require coronary artery bypass grafting (CABG), tirofiban should be discontinued at least 4–6 hours before the procedure. While females and geriatric patients had a higher incidence of adverse effects (both hemorrhagic and nonhemorrhagic) in clinical trials of tirofiban (see Cautions), the manufacturer does not recommend dosage adjustments for tirofiban in female or geriatric patients.

Adjunctive Antithrombotic Therapy. Adjunctive antithrombotic therapy with aspirin and heparin was used in most patients with NSTE ACS receiving tirofiban therapy in clinical trials. In the 3 large, randomized controlled studies evaluating the efficacy of tirofiban, patients received aspirin (300–325 mg daily) for at least 48 hours after randomization or within 12 hours prior to PCI, unless the drug was contraindicated; some patients received aspirin indefinitely. For additional details regarding aspirin dosage regimens in patients with ACS, see Non-ST-Segment-Elevation Acute Coronary Syndromes under Dosage: Thrombosis, in Dosage and Administration in Aspirin 28:08.04.24.

The American College of Cardiology Foundation (ACCF), American Heart Association (AHA), and Society of Cardiovascular Angiography and Interventions (SCAI) recommend that aspirin 325 mg be given prior to PCI in patients not already receiving maintenance therapy with aspirin. Patients already receiving maintenance therapy with aspirin should receive a dose of 81–325 mg of aspirin before the procedure. For additional details regarding aspirin dosage regimens in patients undergoing PCI, see Percutaneous Coronary Intervention and Revascularization Procedures under Dosage: Thrombosis, in Dosage and Administration in Aspirin 28:08.04.24.

In addition to aspirin, ACC/AHA/SCAI recommends administration of a loading dose of a P2Y12 platelet adenosine diphosphate (ADP)-receptor antagonist (clopidogrel, prasugrel, or ticagrelor) in patients undergoing PCI with stent placement.

In clinical trials with tirofiban in patients *not* undergoing PCI, an initial 5000-unit IV loading dose of heparin sodium was given, followed by IV infusion of 1000 units/hour and dosage titration to achieve a target activated partial thromboplastin time (aPTT) of twice the control value. In patients undergoing PCI after at least 48 hours of medical management with tirofiban and heparin in the PRISM-PLUS study, an IV loading dose of heparin sodium (5000–7500 units) was administered, followed by an IV infusion (1000 units/hour) that was titrated to an aPTT approximately 2 times the control value with additional IV injections of heparin sodium as needed. In the RESTORE trial, patients at high risk for abrupt closure of the affected coronary artery who underwent urgent or emergency PCI received heparin sodium as an IV loading dose (10,000 units in patients weighing at least 70 kg or 150 units/kg in those weighing less than 70 kg) prior to PCI. Additional heparin sodium was administered during the procedure as required to maintain an activated clotting time (ACT) of 300–400 seconds; heparin generally was discontinued after completion of PCI. Since tirofiban and other GP IIb/IIIa-receptor inhibitors may have additive effects on ACT in patients receiving one of these drugs concomitantly with heparin, the dosage of heparin required to maintain an appropriate ACT during such concomitant GP IIb/IIIa-receptor inhibitor therapy may be lower than with heparin monotherapy. Clinical experience from other studies with GP IIb/IIIa-receptor inhibitors (e.g., abciximab) and expert guidelines suggest that use of lower dosages of concomitant IV heparin sodium (e.g., 50–70 units/kg) given 6 hours prior to PCI and targeted to an ACT of at least 200 seconds may provide similar reductions in ischemic coronary events as dosages for higher target ACTs with less risk of major bleeding. In women and geriatric patients undergoing PCI and receiving adjunctive therapy with a GP IIb/IIIa-receptor inhibitor and heparin, a lower dosage of heparin should be considered to decrease the risk of minor bleeding that has been observed compared with that in men.

Postprocedural use of heparin generally is not recommended while GP IIb/IIIa-receptor inhibitor therapy is given.

■ Dosage in Renal and Hepatic Impairment Plasma clearance of tirofiban may be decreased substantially (more than 50%) in patients with severe renal impairment (i.e., creatinine clearance of 30 mL/minute or less), including patients requiring hemodialysis. These patients should receive half the usual rate of infusion of tirofiban.

In patients with mild to moderate hepatic impairment, plasma clearance of tirofiban is similar to that in healthy individuals; information on plasma clearance in patients with severe hepatic impairment is not available since these patients were excluded from participation in clinical trials of tirofiban. Metabolism of tirofiban appears to be limited, and the manufacturer does not make specific recommendations for dosage adjustment in patients with hepatic impairment.

Cautions

The most frequent and severe adverse effect of tirofiban therapy is bleeding. Bleeding is an extension of the pharmacologic action of tirofiban and was classified in clinical trials principally according to criteria of the Thrombolysis in Myocardial Infarction (TIMI) study groups. Minor bleeding generally was defined as spontaneous gross hematuria, hematemesis, hemoptysis, or observed blood loss with a decrease in hemoglobin concentration exceeding 3 but less than 5 g/dL; major bleeding was defined as intracranial bleeding, cardiac tamponade, or a hemoglobin decrease exceeding 5 g/dL with or without an observed bleeding site. Almost all patients receiving tirofiban in clinical trials received concomitant therapy with heparin and/or aspirin; therefore, the contribution of tirofiban to the incidence of bleeding complications in these trials is difficult to determine.

Approximately 30% of patients in clinical trials of tirofiban were female, and 43% were older than 65 years of age. Patients in these trials received tirofiban for up to 116 hours. Females (compared with males) and geriatric (compared with younger) patients receiving tirofiban plus heparin or heparin alone had a higher incidence of adverse effects (both hemorrhagic and nonhemorrhagic). However, the incremental risk of hemorrhage and the incidence of nonhemorrhagic adverse effects in patients treated with tirofiban and heparin versus heparin alone were comparable regardless of age or gender. The incidence of adverse effects was not affected by race or the presence of underlying hypertension, diabetes mellitus, or hypercholesterolemia.

■ Hematologic Effects ***Effects on Hemostasis*** Administration of tirofiban is associated with a small increase in major and minor bleeding complications compared with heparin and/or aspirin therapy. Major bleeding events (as defined by TIMI criteria) occurred in about 1.4 or 0.8% of patients receiving tirofiban plus heparin or heparin monotherapy, respectively, in the PRISM-PLUS study, in about 2.4 or 2.1% of patients receiving tirofiban plus heparin or heparin monotherapy, respectively, in the RESTORE study, and in 0.4% of each respective treatment group in the PRISM study. Major bleeding episodes, including fatalities, have been reported during postmarketing experience. Bleeding complications resulted in discontinuance of tirofiban in 3.5 or 1.3% of patients receiving tirofiban plus heparin or heparin alone, respectively, in PRISM-PLUS. Spontaneous (i.e., unrelated to catheter or other puncture sites) bleeding occurred at retroperitoneal, genitourinary, or GI sites in 0, 0.1, or 0.1%, respectively, of patients during therapy with tirofiban plus heparin in the PRISM-PLUS study, and in 0.6%, 0%, or 0.2%, respectively, of patients receiving this drug combination in the RESTORE study. During postmarketing experience, pulmonary (alveolar) hemorrhage, spinal-epidural hematoma, and hemopericardium have been reported in patients receiving tirofiban. Blood transfusions were required in 4 versus 2.8% of patients receiving tirofiban and heparin or heparin alone, respectively, in the PRISM-PLUS study and in 4.3 versus 2.5% of patients receiving these respective therapies in the RESTORE study.

Most major bleeding in clinical trials of tirofiban occurred at the arterial access site for femoral sheath placement in patients undergoing revascularization procedures. In patients undergoing PCI (e.g., percutaneous transluminal coronary angioplasty [PTCA]) in the PRISM-PLUS study, the incidences of major bleeding prior to PCI, following angiography (performed in 89.8% of the patients), and following PCI were 0.3, 1.3, and 2.5%, respectively, in patients receiving tirofiban plus heparin and 0.1, 0.7, and 2.2%, respectively, in patients receiving heparin monotherapy. The incidence of major bleeding (in some instances possibly reflecting hemoglobin decreases related to hemodilution rather than actual bleeding) in patients receiving tirofiban plus heparin or heparin monotherapy and undergoing coronary artery bypass grafting (CABG) within 1 day of discontinuance of study drug was 17.2 or 35.4%, respectively, in the PRISM-PLUS study and 25 or 37.5%, respectively, in the RESTORE study.

Therapy with GP IIb/IIIa-receptor inhibitors, including tirofiban, has not been associated with an increased risk of intracranial hemorrhage. Intracranial hemorrhage occurred in 0.1 or 0.3% of patients receiving tirofiban and heparin or heparin alone, respectively, in the RESTORE study, and was not reported in patients receiving these therapies in the PRISM-PLUS study. The incidence of intracranial hemorrhage in patients receiving tirofiban or heparin in the PRISM study was 0.1% in each group. Retroperitoneal bleeding or hemopericardium has been reported during postmarketing experience in patients receiving tirofiban.

Minor bleeding episodes occurred in about 10.5 or 8% of patients receiving tirofiban plus heparin or heparin monotherapy, respectively, in the PRISM-PLUS study and in 12 or 6.3% of patients receiving tirofiban plus heparin or heparin alone, respectively, in the RESTORE study.

Other Hematologic Effects Decreases in platelet count or thrombocytopenia occurs occasionally (2.3% overall) after therapy with GP IIb/IIIa-receptor inhibitors. Thrombocytopenia associated with administration of a GP IIb/IIIa-receptor inhibitor generally occurs within hours or days after administration of the drug. Decreases in platelet counts have been observed in patients with no prior history of thrombocytopenia following readministration of GP IIb/IIIa-receptor inhibitors. Severe thrombocytopenia (i.e., platelet count less than 20,000/mm³) has been reported more frequently with abciximab than with tirofiban. However, a preliminary report based on pooled data from clinical trials indicates that the incidence of thrombocytopenia is not appreciably different among GP IIb/IIIa-receptor inhibitors (i.e., abciximab, eptifibatide, tirofiban), although the absolute risk of thrombocytopenia appears to increase (but not synergistically) with concomitant use of heparin. In controlled clinical trials of tirofiban, the incidence of thrombocytopenia (defined as platelet counts less than 90,000/mm³) was increased in patients receiving tirofiban plus heparin (1.5%) compared with heparin monotherapy (0.6%), respectively; reductions in platelet count to less than 50,000/mm³) were observed in 0.3 or 0.1% of patients receiving tirofiban plus heparin or heparin alone, respectively, in clinical trials. In the PRISM study, the incidence of thrombocytopenia also was increased in patients receiving tirofiban versus those receiving heparin; platelet counts returned to normal several days after cessation of therapy without any other clinical sequelae. Decreased platelet counts associated with chills and a low-grade fever have been reported with tirofiban during postmarketing experience.

Reductions in hemoglobin or hematocrit were reported in 2.1 or 2.2%, respectively, of patients receiving tirofiban plus heparin and in 3.1 or 2.6%, respectively, of patients receiving heparin in controlled clinical trials. Microscopic hematuria or occult blood in the stool was noted in 10.7 or 18.3%, respectively, of patients receiving tirofiban plus heparin and in 7.8 or 12.2%, respectively, of those receiving heparin monotherapy in clinical trials.

■ Cardiovascular Effects Adverse cardiovascular effects that occurred in greater than 1% of patients receiving tirofiban plus heparin in clinical trials were bradycardia (4%) or dissection of the coronary artery (5%). Edema/swelling or vasovagal reactions were reported in 2% of patients receiving tirofiban and heparin in these trials.

■ Dermatologic and Sensitivity Reactions Sweating was reported in 2% of patients receiving tirofiban and heparin in controlled clinical trials. Anaphylaxis and/or urticaria requiring discontinuance of therapy was not reported in clinical trials of tirofiban, but anaphylaxis and other severe allergic reactions have been reported during postmarketing experience. Such reactions have occurred on the first day of tirofiban infusion, during initial treatment, and during readministration of the drug. Some severe allergic reactions have been associated with severe thrombocytopenia (platelet counts less than 10,000/mm³).

Therapy with some platelet-aggregation inhibitors (e.g., abciximab) has been associated with development of antibodies to the drug; limited information indicates that no antibodies to tirofiban have developed, but very few patients have received the drug on more than one occasion. However, as a nonpeptide GP IIb/IIIa-receptor inhibitor, tirofiban is expected to be less immunogenic than the monoclonal antibody abciximab.

■ Other Adverse Effects Pelvic pain occurred in 6%, leg pain in 3%, and dizziness in 3% of patients receiving tirofiban plus heparin in clinical trials. Other adverse effects reported in greater than 1% of patients receiving tirofiban plus heparin in clinical trials include headache, nausea, and fever.

■ Precautions and Contraindications The administration of tirofiban in patients with non-ST-segment-elevation acute coronary syndromes (NSTE ACS) has been associated with a small increase in the frequency of major bleeding compared with heparin and aspirin therapy alone. Bleeding with platelet glycoprotein (GP) IIb/IIIa-receptor inhibitors can be reduced by adherence to strict anticoagulation guidelines, the use of a short course of low-dose, weight-adjusted heparin, and in patients undergoing PCI, early arterial sheath removal and careful patient and access site management. Prior to administration of tirofiban, preexisting hemostatic abnormalities should be identified by obtaining determinations of hematocrit and hemoglobin; these parameters should then be monitored within 6 hours following the loading infusion and at least daily thereafter during therapy. In patients receiving heparin concomitantly with tirofiban, the extent of heparin anticoagulation (as assessed by activated clotting time [ACT] or aPTT) should be monitored closely to minimize bleeding, which may be potentially life-threatening. The aPTT should be monitored 6 hours after the start of the heparin infusion and be maintained at 50–70 seconds or approximately 2 times the control value unless PCI is to be performed. In addition, the ACT should be measured in patients undergoing PCI.Current guidelines of the American College of Chest Physicians (ACCP) and other experts and risk-benefit analyses in trials with GP IIb/IIIa-receptor inhibitors suggest that heparin dosing should be adjusted to maintain the ACT at 200 seconds or greater during PCI in patients receiving GP IIb/IIIa-receptor inhibitors. (See Adjunctive Antithrombotic Therapy under Dosage: Non-ST-Segment-Elevation Acute Coronary Syndromes, in Dosage and Administration.) Routine use of postprocedural heparin generally is not recommended during GP IIb/IIIa-receptor inhibitor therapy. After PCI, the aPTT should be checked prior to arterial sheath removal, and the sheath should not be removed unless the aPTT is less than 45 seconds or the ACT is less than 180 seconds. Tirofiban should be used with caution in patients with hemorrhagic retinopathy, anemia (hemoglobin concentration less than 10–12 g/dL) and in those requiring chronic hemodialysis.

Platelet counts should be determined prior to treatment with tirofiban and periodically (e.g., within the first 6 hours of the loading infusion and daily thereafter) during concomitant tirofiban and heparin therapy. should be used with caution in patients with a platelet count less than 150,000/mm³. If a patient experiences a reduction in platelet count to less than 90,000/mm³, additional platelet counts should be performed to exclude the possibility of pseudothrombocytopenia. The possibility of heparin-induced thrombocytopenia also should be considered in the differential diagnosis of thrombocytopenia in patients receiving GP IIb/IIIa-receptor inhibitors concomitantly with heparin. If thrombocytopenia is confirmed, tirofiban should be discontinued and the condition appropriately monitored and treated. Thrombocytopenia is usually reversible following discontinuance of GP IIb/IIIa-receptor inhibitors and anticoagulant (heparin) therapy; however, platelet transfusions should be considered for the management of severe thrombocytopenia.

To minimize the possibility of bleeding associated with the use of tirofiban, particularly at the site of femoral artery sheath placement in patients undergoing PCI, precautions in the placement, maintenance, and removal of the vascular access sheath should be observed. Placement of a femoral *venous* sheath should be avoided if possible. When inserting the femoral artery sheath, care should be taken so that only the anterior wall of the femoral artery is punctured; a Seldinger (through and through) technique for puncture of the artery should be avoided. Appropriate precautions should be observed while the vascular access sheath is in place (e.g., complete bed rest, elevation of the head of the bed no more than 30°, restraint of the limb in which the vascular access sheath is inserted, frequent monitoring of the vascular access site and the distal pulse in the involved limb). The femoral artery sheath may be removed during treatment with tirofiban, provided at least 3–4 hours have elapsed since heparin therapy was discontinued and its effects largely have reversed (as indicated by an aPTT of less than 45 seconds or an ACT of less than 180 seconds).

Both heparin and tirofiban therapy should be discontinued and sheath hemostasis achieved with standard compressive techniques at least 4 hours before hospital discharge. Pressure (e.g., using manual compression or a mechanical hemostatic device) should be applied to the femoral artery for at least 20–30 minutes after sheath removal; after hemostasis, a pressure dressing should be applied. Any hematoma that forms should be measured and monitored for enlargement.

Careful monitoring of all potential bleeding sites should be undertaken during and following treatment with platelet aggregation inhibitors. Needle punctures (e.g., arterial, IM, IV, lumbar, subcutaneous, intradermal), cutdown sites, and use of nasotracheal intubation, nasogastric tubes, urinary catheterization, and automatic blood pressure cuffs should be minimized during and following treatment with tirofiban. Establishment of IV access at noncompressible sites (e.g., in subclavian or jugular veins) should be avoided; an indwelling venipuncture device (e.g., heparin lock) should be considered for drawing blood; documentation and monitoring of vascular puncture sites should occur; and dressings should gently and carefully be removed. The manufacturer states that any occurrence of serious bleeding that cannot be controlled by pressure on the bleeding site should result in discontinuance of tirofiban and concomitantly administered heparin therapy.

Because tirofiban increases the risk of bleeding, the drug is contraindicated in patients with active internal bleeding (including microscopic hematuria or a positive test for occult fecal blood) or a history of bleeding diathesis (e.g., GI or genitourinary bleeding, elevated hemostatic indices, recent noncompressible vascular punctures) within the previous 30 days; a history of intracranial hemorrhage, intracranial neoplasm, arteriovenous malformation, or aneurysm; a history of thrombocytopenia following prior exposure to tirofiban; history of stroke within 30 days or any history of hemorrhagic stroke; recent (within 1 month) major surgery or severe physical trauma; history, symptoms, or findings suggestive of aortic dissection; severe uncontrolled hypertension (systolic or diastolic blood pressure exceeding 180 or 110 mm Hg, respectively); concomitant therapy with another parenteral GP IIb/IIIa-receptor inhibitor; or acute pericarditis. Tirofiban also is contraindicated in patients with a known hypersensitivity to any component of the commercially available preparation.

■ Pediatric Precautions Safety and efficacy of tirofiban in pediatric patients younger than 18 years of age have not been determined.

■ Geriatric Precautions Safety and efficacy of tirofiban in geriatric patients have not been specifically studied to date; however, in large clinical trials, approximately 43% of patients were 65 years of age or older, while 11.7% were 75 years of age or older. Clinical experience generally has not revealed age-related differences in response to tirofiban therapy. Plasma clearance of tirofiban is about 19–26% lower in geriatric patients (exceeding 65 years of age) with coronary artery disease than in younger patients. While the incidence of bleeding complications was higher in geriatric patients receiving either heparin plus tirofiban or heparin monotherapy, the incremental risk of bleeding among patients receiving these 2 regimens was similar regardless of age. The overall incidence of nonhemorrhagic adverse effects was higher in older patients compared with younger patients receiving either treatment regimen (heparin or tirofiban plus heparin). In the RESTORE study, the loading dose of IV heparin was weight-adjusted in patients weighing less than 70 kg because of concern for an increased risk for bleeding in these patients. However, the manufacturer recommends no dosage adjustment for tirofiban in geriatric patients.

■ Mutagenicity and Carcinogenicity No evidence of mutagenicity was seen at the chromosomal or gene level when tirofiban was evaluated in several in vitro and in vivo test systems. The drug was not directly genotoxic in the in vitro alkaline elution or chromosomal aberration assay. Tirofiban did not induce chromosomal aberrations in bone marrow cells of male mice given the drug IV at dosages of up to 5 mg/kg daily (about 3 times the maximum recommended daily human dosage based on body surface area).

Studies have not been performed to date to evaluate the carcinogenic potential of tirofiban.

■ Pregnancy, Fertility, and Lactation Reproduction studies using IV tirofiban dosages of up to 5 mg/kg daily in rats and rabbits (representing about 5 and 13 times, respectively, the recommended maximum daily human dosage based on body surface area) have not revealed evidence of harm to the fetus. However, animal reproduction studies are not always predictive of human response. There are no adequate or controlled studies to date using tirofiban in pregnant women, and the drug should be used during pregnancy only when clearly needed.

Reproduction studies of tirofiban in male and female rats given up to 5 mg/kg daily IV (representing about 5 times the recommended maximum daily human dosage based on body surface area) have not revealed evidence of impaired fertility or reproductive performance.

It is not known if tirofiban is distributed into milk in humans; however, the drug is distributed into milk in rats. Because of the potential for serious adverse effects in nursing infants, a decision should be made whether to discontinue nursing or tirofiban, taking into account the importance of the drug to the woman.

Drug Interactions

■ Drugs Affecting Hemostasis Almost all patients receiving tirofiban in clinical trials have received concomitant therapy with heparin and/or aspirin, and such concomitant therapy has been associated with a small increase in bleeding complications compared with that in patients receiving aspirin and heparin alone. (See Effects on Hemostasis under Cautions: Hematologic Effects.) Caution should be observed when tirofiban is used with other drugs that affect hemostasis, including thrombolytic agents, oral anticoagulants (e.g., warfarin), nonsteroidal anti-inflammatory agents (NSAIAs), dipyridamole, ticlopidine, and clopidogrel; some clinicians also recommend against concomitant use of tirofiban and IV dextran.

In several studies evaluating pharmacokinetic and pharmacodynamic interactions with tirofiban in healthy individuals, the pharmacokinetics of tirofiban were not affected by pretreatment with aspirin (325 mg administered 1 and 24 hours prior to tirofiban) or ticlopidine (200 mg once daily for 4 days). However, aspirin or ticlopidine may enhance the inhibition of platelet aggregation produced by tirofiban. In healthy individuals and in patients with non-ST-segment-elevation acute coronary syndromes (NSTE ACS), bleeding time was prolonged by the combination of tirofiban and aspirin compared with tirofiban or aspirin therapy alone; aPTT was not affected (compared with baseline values). (See Pharmacology.)

No information is available concerning the use of tirofiban concomitantly with thrombolytic agents.

■ Other Drugs Data from a large clinical study (the PRISM study) indicate that concomitant administration of tirofiban and levothyroxine or omeprazole was associated with a higher clearance of tirofiban; the clinical importance of this effect is not known. Concomitant administration of the following drugs in the same study was not associated with clinically important effects on the plasma clearance of tirofiban: acebutolol, acetaminophen, alprazolam, amlodipine, aspirin preparations, atenolol, bromazepam, captopril, diazepam, digoxin, diltiazem, docusate sodium, enalapril, furosemide, glyburide, heparin, insulin, isosorbide, lorazepam, lovastatin, metoclopramide, metoprolol, morphine, nifedipine, nitrate preparations, oxazepam, potassium chloride, propranolol, ranitidine, simvastatin, sucralfate, or temazepam.

Acute Toxicity

Limited information is available on the acute toxicity of tirofiban. In general, overdosage of tirofiban in humans may be expected to produce effects that are extensions of the pharmacologic and adverse effects of the drug, predominantly bleeding. (See Cautions: Hematologic Effects.) The most frequently reported manifestation of overdosage was bleeding, principally minor bleeding at mucocutaneous and cardiac catheterization sites. Inadvertent overdosage with tirofiban has occurred in doses of up to twice those recommended for an IV loading infusion and up to 9.8 times higher than the recommended maintenance infusion dosage of 0.15 mcg/kg per minute. In the event of overdosage, tirofiban therapy should be discontinued or the dosage adjusted and the patient's clinical status monitored as appropriate. Tirofiban is removed by hemodialysis.

Pharmacology

■ Platelet Aggregation and Thrombosis Tirofiban is a selective, competitive, reversible inhibitor of platelet aggregation that is used in combination with heparin to reduce the risk of acute ischemic events (death and/or myocardial infarction [MI]) associated with non-ST-segment-elevation acute coronary syndromes (NSTE ACS), including those undergoing percutaneous coronary intervention (PCI) (e.g., percutaneous transluminal coronary angioplasty [PTCA], atherectomy). Because of its mechanism of action, tirofiban, like abciximab and eptifibatide, has been referred to as a platelet glycoprotein (GP) IIb/IIIa-receptor inhibitor. Platelet adhesion, activation, and aggregation are key processes leading to the formation of platelet-rich ("white") coronary artery thrombi and the development of acute coronary artery syndromes and ischemic complications associated with PCI. White thrombus formation is triggered by vascular injury (e.g., from PCI procedures), plaque rupture, or denudation of endothelium that exposes the subendothelial matrix of the vessel to circulating platelets. Upon exposure of the vessel subendothelium, potent thrombogenic stimuli (e.g., thrombin, collagen) present in both subendothelium and plaque, and/or high-shear stress, stimulate platelet adhesion and activation.

Activated platelets release intracellular granules consisting of vasoactive substances that are part of an autostimulatory feedback loop for platelet aggregation; these substances include thromboxane A_2, serotonin, and adenosine diphosphate (ADP); adhesive glycoproteins such as fibrinogen, fibronectin, and von Willebrand's factor; and plasminogen activator inhibitor-1 (PAI-1). Regardless of the initial stimulus for platelet activation, the final common pathway to platelet aggregation and thrombosis involves activation of the receptor function of the GP IIb/IIIa complex (also known as $\alpha_{IIb}\beta_3$). Inactive GP IIb/IIIa receptors undergo a conformational change on the surface of activated platelets to accept soluble fibrinogen, von Willebrand's factor, and other ligands (e.g., fibronectin, vitronectin, thrombospondin). Some of these adhesive ligands form cross-links to other GP IIb/IIIa on surfaces of adjacent activated platelets, causing aggregation and white thrombus formation. In addition, fibrinogen bound to the vessel wall or to other platelet aggregates can activate GP IIb/IIIa receptors on unstimulated platelets and recruit these platelets to growing white thrombi.

Progression of NSTE ACS to ST-segment-elevation MI (STEMI) or sudden death occurs when obstructive platelet-rich thrombi grow to become occlusive thrombi in the absence of adequate perfusion beyond the obstruction through collateral blood vessels. Fibrin and erythrocytes comprise the outer layer of occlusive red thrombi that are formed on the surface of the platelet-rich inner core of the thrombus. While thrombolytic therapy effectively dissolves the occluding fibrin-rich portion of the thrombus, this process releases clot-bound thrombin and re-exposes the underlying disrupted plaque, which rereleases potent thrombogenic stimuli. These newly released thrombogenic stimuli then activate platelets, leading to platelet aggregation. In addition, activated platelets secrete a variety of factors (e.g., PAI-1, fibrinogen, factor V) associated with rethrombosis or thrombin production and bind factors Xa, VIIIa, and IXa, which are involved in further thrombin production. Platelet reactivity also may increase after thrombolysis. It has been suggested that use of platelet-aggregation inhibitors concomitantly with thrombolytic therapy may counter the thrombogenic activity of these agents and minimize the risk of reocclusion.

■ **Inhibition of Platelet Aggregation** Tirofiban reversibly inhibits platelet aggregation by preventing the binding of fibrinogen, von Willebrand's factor, and other adhesive ligands to resting and active GP IIb/IIIa receptors. Inhibition of platelet aggregation by tirofiban and other GP IIb/IIIa-receptor inhibitors occurs in a dose- and concentration-dependent manner via an increase in GP IIb/IIIa receptor occupancy (as determined by the ex vivo platelet aggregation assay for tirofiban using sodium citrate as the anticoagulant in blood samples); platelet aggregation is nearly completely abolished at receptor occupancy exceeding 80%. Sodium citrate reportedly does not affect binding of tirofiban to the GP IIb/IIIa receptor. Some platelet-aggregation inhibitors such as aspirin, ticlopidine, and clopidogrel prevent platelet aggregation by preventing platelet activation in response to one or more agonists (e.g., thromboxane A_2, adenosine diphosphate); agonists not affected by these drugs may continue to induce platelet aggregation. However, GP IIb/IIIa-receptor inhibitors such as abciximab, eptifibatide, and tirofiban prevent platelet aggregation regardless of the initial stimulus. Some in vitro data suggest that inhibition of platelet aggregation by tirofiban can be overcome by an increase in the concentration of fibrinogen, indicating reversible, competitive binding to the GP IIb/IIIa receptor. However, tirofiban or other GP IIb/IIIa-receptor inhibitors do not appear to be effective in displacing fibrinogen cross-links from GP IIb/IIIA receptors in established thrombi when the bond between fibrinogen and GP IIb/IIIa receptors becomes irreversible.

In vitro binding studies in platelets and human endothelial cells demonstrate that tirofiban is selective in binding to the platelet GP IIb/IIIa receptor; concentrations of the drug needed to inhibit the attachment of human endothelial cells to vitronectin or fibronectin receptors are approximately 1000-fold or greater than those required for inhibiting the attachment of platelets to fibrinogen.

Following the recommended IV loading infusion of tirofiban (0.4 mcg/kg per minute for 30 minutes) in patients with NSTE ACS receiving concomitant heparin and aspirin, inhibition of platelet aggregation exceeded 90% at the end of the infusion. Addition of heparin to tirofiban therapy (0.1 mcg/kg per minute by IV infusion) does not alter the percentage of individuals with platelet aggregation inhibition exceeding 70%.

■ **Hemostatic Effects** Since the effect of tirofiban on platelet aggregation is rapidly reversible following cessation of the infusion, the drug has a modest effect on hemostatic indices (e.g., bleeding times). Normal hemostasis is restored more rapidly than with abciximab, a monoclonal antibody that dissociates very slowly from the GP IIb/IIIa receptor.

In healthy individuals and patients with coronary artery disease, tirofiban prolongs bleeding time in a dose-dependent manner. Following administration of tirofiban as a loading infusion (0.4 mcg/kg per minute for 30 minutes) concomitantly with heparin and aspirin in patients with NSTE ACS, bleeding time was prolonged to 2.9 times that of baseline values. During continuous infusion of tirofiban (0.1 mcg/kg per minute) with concomitant heparin and aspirin in patients with NSTE ACS, bleeding time exceeded 20–30 minutes. However, in patients with NSTE ACS receiving heparin titrated to an aPTT twice the control value, addition of tirofiban did not alter the aPTT. When administered without heparin in patients with NSTE ACS in several large clinical trials (the Platelet Receptor Inhibitor in Ischemic Syndrome Management in Patients Limited by Unstable Signs and Symptoms [PRISM-PLUS] study and the Platelet Receptor Inhibition in Ischemic Syndrome Management [PRISM] study), tirofiban and aspirin prolonged bleeding time to less than 20 minutes and aPTT was not affected (compared with baseline values). In patients with coronary artery disease receiving tirofiban, ex vivo adenosine diphosphate (ADP)-induced platelet aggregation using sodium citrate as an anticoagulant in blood samples was restored toward baseline values in approximately 90% of patients within 4–8 hours after discontinuance of the infusion.

Pharmacokinetics

The pharmacokinetics of tirofiban are linear, and plasma concentrations are proportional to dose following IV infusions of 0.05–0.4 mcg/kg per minute for 1 hour or 0.1–0.2 mcg/kg per minute for 4 hours in healthy individuals. Concomitant administration of aspirin or ticlopidine does not appear to affect the pharmacokinetics of tirofiban. (See Drug Interactions: Drugs Affecting Hemostasis.)

■ **Absorption** Information concerning plasma concentrations resulting from recommended loading and maintenance infusion dosages of tirofiban is not available. In a study in healthy individuals, plasma tirofiban concentrations of 10.9 and 20.7 ng/mL were reported after infusion of 0.1 mcg/kg per minute of tirofiban for 1 and 4 hours, respectively.

Tirofiban has a rapid onset and short duration of action. In patients with non-ST-segment-elevation acute coronary syndromes (NSTE ACS) receiving the recommended tirofiban regimen consisting of an IV loading infusion of 0.4 mcg/kg per minute for 30 minutes followed by 0.1 mcg/kg per minute for up to 48 hours, approximately 90% inhibition of ex vivo adenosine diphosphate (ADP)-induced platelet aggregation was achieved by the end of the loading infusion, with inhibition persisting for the duration of the maintenance infusion. Platelet function returned to near baseline levels in approximately 90% of these patients within 4–8 hours following discontinuance of the tirofiban infusion.

In a randomized study in a limited number of patients with NSTE ACS undergoing PCI, administration of the recommended regimen of tirofiban (0.4 mcg/kg per minute IV for 30 minutes followed by 0.1 mcg/kg per minute by IV infusion) for 20–24 hours was associated with a delayed onset and reduced intensity of platelet-aggregation inhibition (as measured by rapid platelet function assay [RPFA] or light transmission aggregometry using 20 μmol ADP) compared with that produced by recommended regimens of abciximab (0.25-mg/kg IV loading dose followed by 0.125 mcg/kg per minute, up to a maximum infusion rate of 10 mcg/minute, for 12 hours) or eptifibatide (180-mcg/kg IV loading dose followed by 2 mcg/kg per minute by IV infusion for 20–24 hours). The delayed onset of action of tirofiban was attributed to its comparatively long loading infusion duration (30 minutes) since in another study, maximal inhibition of platelet aggregation (96%) occurred within 5 minutes after infusion of a 10-mcg/kg IV loading dose over 3 minutes. The diminished intensity of platelet-aggregation inhibition was related in part to the strength of the agonist (20 μM) used in the platelet-aggregation assay, which is identical to that used in clinical trials of abciximab and eptifibatide but exceeds the concentration used in clinical trials of tirofiban (5 μM).

■ **Distribution** Tirofiban is approximately 65% bound to plasma proteins, and protein binding is independent of plasma drug concentration over the range of 0.01–25 mcg/mL. The steady-state volume of distribution of tirofiban ranges from 22–42 L. It is not known whether tirofiban is distributed into milk or crosses the placenta in humans; however, the drug is distributed into milk in rats and crosses the placenta in pregnant rats and rabbits.

■ **Elimination** Following administration in healthy individuals, plasma concentrations of tirofiban decline in a biphasic manner. The half-life of tirofiban averages approximately 1.2–2 hours. Tirofiban is cleared from the plasma mainly by renal excretion; metabolism of the drug appears to be limited.

About 65 and 25% of a single dose of tirofiban is excreted in urine and feces, respectively, principally as unchanged parent drug. Plasma clearance of tirofiban in healthy individuals ranges from 213–314 mL/minute, with renal clearance accounting for 39–69% of plasma clearance. In patients with coronary artery disease, the plasma clearance of tirofiban ranges from 152–267 mL/minute and does not appear to be influenced by gender or race; renal clearance in these patients accounts for 39% of plasma clearance. Plasma clearance is about 19–26% lower in geriatric patients (those exceeding 65 years of age) with coronary artery disease than in younger patients. Plasma clearance appears to be independent of dose in healthy individuals and is not appreciably affected by mild to moderate hepatic insufficiency. In patients with renal impairment (creatinine clearance less than 30 mL per minute), including those requiring hemodialysis, plasma clearance of tirofiban is decreased by greater than 50% compared with that in individuals with normal renal function. Tirofiban is removed by hemodialysis.

Chemistry and Stability

■ **Chemistry** Tirofiban hydrochloride, a synthetic nonpeptide tyrosine derivative, is a selective, competitive platelet-aggregation inhibitor. Tirofiban, like abciximab and eptifibatide, has been referred to as a platelet glycoprotein (GP) IIb/IIIa-receptor inhibitor.

Tirofiban is produced by the addition of an *n*-butylsulfonyl group to the C-terminus and a 4-(piperidin-4-yl)butyloxy group to the *N*-terminus of tyrosine; these modifications increase the potency of the drug's inhibitory effect on platelet aggregation.

The final step in platelet aggregation involves the binding of fibrinogen to the activated, membrane-bound platelet glycoprotein complex, GP IIb/IIIa, principally through a recognition site on the C-terminal peptide of the γ chain of fibrinogen that is structurally similar to the amino acid sequence arginine-glycine-aspartate (RGD). Other adhesive glycoproteins (e.g., von Willebrand's factor, fibronectin, vitronectin) appear to bind to activated GP IIb/IIIa through the RGD sequence. Unlike other GP IIb/IIIa-receptor inhibitors such as abciximab, which is an antibody to the GP IIb/IIIa receptor, and eptifibatide, which is a peptide mimetic of the GP IIb/IIIa receptor binding site, tirofiban is a nonpeptide amino acid derivative that mimics the geometric, stereotactic, and charge characteristics of the RGD binding site on the GP IIb/IIIa receptor. Molecular modeling studies suggest that the piperidine nitrogen of tirofiban replaces the basic guanidino moiety of arginine, the aromatic ring of tyrosine replaces the glycine residue, and the tyrosine carboxyl group substitutes for the carboxyl group of aspartic acid on the GP IIb/IIIa receptor binding site. In addition, the butylsulfonyl group of tirofiban appears to enhance potency of the drug by interacting with another site (exosite) on the GP IIb/IIIa receptor to which peptide mimetics (e.g., eptifibatide) do not bind.

Tirofiban is commercially available as the hydrochloride salt, which is monohydrated; potency of tirofiban hydrochloride is expressed in terms of tirofiban, calculated on the anhydrous basis.

Tirofiban hydrochloride monohydrate occurs as a white to off-white powder and is very slightly soluble in water and freely soluble (exceeding 100 mg/mL) in alcohol. The drug has pK_a values of 3.6 and 11.1. Tirofiban hydrochloride is commercially available as a clear, colorless, sterile injection concentrate and as a clear, sterile premixed IV solution in water for injection that has been made iso-osmotic with sodium chloride. Tirofiban hydrochloride injections contain sodium citrate dihydrate and citric acid anhydrous as buffers; the injections contain no preservatives. Sodium hydroxide and/or hydrochloric acid may be added during manufacture to adjust the pH of the injections to 5.5–6.5. When tirofiban hydrochloride injection concentrate is diluted extemporaneously with 0.9% sodium chloride or 5% dextrose injection, the pH of the resulting IV solution is approximately 6. The osmolality of tirofiban hydrochloride injection concentrate after dilution or of the premixed IV solution is approximately 280 or 300 mOsm/kg, respectively.

Each mL of tirofiban hydrochloride injection concentrate contains 0.281 mg of tirofiban hydrochloride monohydrate equivalent to 0.25 mg of tirofiban base (250 mcg/mL of tirofiban). Each 500 mL of tirofiban hydrochloride injection premixed contains 28.09 mg of tirofiban hydrochloride monohydrate equivalent to 25 mg of tirofiban base (50 mcg/mL of tirofiban).

■ **Stability** Commercially available premixed tirofiban hydrochloride in 0.9% sodium chloride injection is provided in a flexible plastic (Intravia®) container fabricated from specially formulated, multilayered plastic (PL 2408). Premixed tirofiban hydrochloride injection or injection concentrate is stable for 18 or 24 months, respectively, following the date of manufacture when stored unopened as directed. Solutions in contact with the plastic container can leach out some of the container's chemical components in very small amounts within the expiration period of the injection; however, safety of the plastic container materials has been supported by USP biological tests.

Dopamine, lidocaine, potassium chloride, and famotidine injection may be administered in the same IV line with tirofiban hydrochloride injection; tirofiban should not be administered in the same IV line as diazepam.

Unused portions of tirofiban hydrochloride IV solutions should be discarded since these solutions contain no preservatives. Tirofiban hydrochloride injections should be stored at a temperature between 15 and 30°C and should be protected from light during storage; freezing should be avoided.

Preparations

Excipients in commercially available drug preparations may have clinically important effects in some individuals; consult specific product labeling for details.

Tirofiban Hydrochloride

Parenteral

For injection, concentrate, for IV infusion	250 mcg (of tirofiban) per mL (5 and 12.5 mg)	**Aggrastat®**, Medicure

Tirofiban Hydrochloride in Sodium Chloride

Parenteral

Injection, for IV infusion	50 mcg (of tirofiban) per mL (12.5 mg) in 0.9% Sodium Chloride	**Aggrastat® Premixed in Iso-osmotic Sodium Chloride Injection** (in IntraVia® flexible container), Medicure

Selected Revisions September 2017, © Copyright, January 2000, American Society of Health-System Pharmacists, Inc.

Vorapaxar Sulfate

■ Vorapaxar sulfate, a protease-activated receptor-1 (PAR-1) antagonist, is a platelet-aggregation inhibitor.

Uses

■ **Cardiovascular Risk Reduction in Established Atherosclerotic Disease** Vorapaxar sulfate is used for secondary prevention to reduce the risk of thrombotic cardiovascular events (e.g., cardiovascular death, myocardial infarction [MI], stroke, urgent coronary revascularization) in patients with a history of MI or in those with peripheral arterial disease (PAD). The drug should be used in conjunction with aspirin and/or clopidogrel; data are lacking on the use of vorapaxar in combination with other antiplatelet agents (e.g., prasugrel, ticagrelor) or as monotherapy. Efficacy and safety of vorapaxar have been established in patients with stable atherosclerotic disease (with a prior MI or with PAD); there currently is no evidence that the drug's benefits outweigh its risks in patients with acute coronary syndrome (ACS). (See Uses: Acute Coronary Syndrome.) Vorapaxar should not be used in patients with a history of stroke, transient ischemic attack (TIA), or intracranial hemorrhage because of an increased risk of intracranial hemorrhage observed in this population in clinical trials. (See Bleeding, under Warnings/Precautions: Warnings, in Cautions.)

The American Heart Association (AHA), American College of Cardiology Foundation (ACCF), American College of Chest Physicians (ACCP), and other experts recommend long-term antiplatelet therapy (e.g., aspirin and/or clopidogrel) for secondary prevention of recurrent thrombotic events in patients with established coronary artery disease. Long-term antiplatelet therapy (e.g., clopidogrel, aspirin) also is recommended for secondary prevention of cardiovascular events in patients with symptomatic PAD, including those with intermittent claudication, critical limb ischemia, or prior lower extremity procedures (e.g., revascularization, amputation). For additional information on the use of aspirin and clopidogrel for secondary prevention of cardiovascular events, see Uses: Reduction of Cardiovascular and Cerebrovascular Events, in Clopidogrel Bisulfate 20:12.18 and also see Secondary Prevention of Cardiovascular and Cerebrovascular Events under Thrombosis: Coronary Artery Disease and Myocardial Infarction, in Uses, in Aspirin 28:08.04.24.

Vorapaxar is used as an adjunct to aspirin and/or clopidogrel to provide further risk reduction in the long-term management of patients with established atherosclerotic disease. Addition of vorapaxar in such patients has been shown to reduce the rate of cardiovascular events (e.g., cardiovascular death, MI, stroke, urgent coronary revascularization), but these benefits were achieved at a cost of increased bleeding; in particular, the rate of intracranial hemorrhage was increased in patients with a history of stroke. Because of this tradeoff in potential risk versus benefit, appropriate patient selection is required to balance the incremental benefits of the drug against the increased risk of bleeding; certain patients (e.g., those with a history of MI who are at high risk of recurrence but low risk of bleeding and who have not had a previous stroke or TIA) may have the most potential for experiencing net clinical benefits from vorapaxar therapy. (See Bleeding under Warnings/Precautions: Warnings, in Cautions.) Whether vorapaxar plus aspirin and/or clopidogrel has any benefits over antiplatelet regimens that include prasugrel or ticagrelor instead of clopidogrel in patients with coronary artery disease has not been established, and the overall risk-benefit of vorapaxar in routine clinical practice remains to be fully elucidated.

Efficacy and safety of vorapaxar have been established in a multicenter, randomized, double-blind, placebo-controlled study (Thrombin Receptor Antagonist in Secondary Prevention of Atherothrombotic Ischemic Events-Thrombolysis in Myocardial Infarction 50 [TRA 2°P-TIMI 50]) in 26,449 patients with established atherosclerosis who were receiving standard antiplatelet therapy (almost exclusively aspirin with or without clopidogrel). The study included 3 cohorts of patients with atherosclerosis (those with a history of MI or a history of ischemic stroke within the past 2 weeks to 12 months and those with a current diagnosis of symptomatic PAD); aspirin was administered in the majority (94%) of these patients, and a thienopyridine (almost exclusively clopidogrel) was administered in 78, 37, and 24% of patients with MI, PAD, and stroke, respectively. While the study was not designed to evaluate the relative benefits and risks of vorapaxar in individual patient subgroups, a substantially increased risk of intracranial hemorrhage was identified at a median follow-up of 2 years in patients receiving vorapaxar (2.08 mg once daily) who had a history of stroke (2.4% with vorapaxar versus 0.9% with placebo). Due to this safety concern, the data and safety monitoring board recommended discontinuance of vorapaxar in all patients with previous stroke, and the protocol was subsequently amended. The protocol-defined primary end point in the TRA 2°P-TIMI 50 study was the composite of cardiovascular death, MI, stroke, and urgent coronary revascularization, and the protocol-defined major secondary end point was the composite of cardiovascular death, MI, and stroke. However, in the published study, the investigators reversed the hierarchy of these end points for data analysis based on the results of another study involving vorapaxar (Thrombin Receptor Antagonist for Clinical Event Reduction in Acute Coronary Syndrome [TRACER]). Therefore, in the published TRA 2°P-TIMI 50 study, the primary end point for data analysis is reported as the composite of cardiovascular death, MI, and stroke, and the major secondary end point is reported as the composite of cardiovascular death, MI, stroke, and urgent coronary revascularization.

At 3 years, vorapaxar reduced the occurrence of the protocol-defined primary composite end point of cardiovascular death, MI, stroke, and urgent coronary revascularization compared with placebo; Kaplan-Meier event rates for the primary composite end point were 11.2 and 12.4% for vorapaxar and placebo, respectively, (12% relative reduction) in the overall population (all randomized patients), and 10.1 and 11.8%, respectively, (17% relative reduction) in the cohort of patients without a history of stroke or TIA. The effects of vorapaxar on the primary composite end point were driven largely by a reduction in the rate of MI, with no difference in mortality observed between the treatment groups. For the protocol-defined major secondary end point (composite of cardiovascular death, MI, and stroke), Kaplan-Meier event rates were 9.3 and 10.5% for vorapaxar and placebo, respectively, (13% relative reduction) in all randomized patients and 7.9 and 9.5%, respectively, (20% relative reduction) in the cohort of patients without a history of stroke or TIA. The effects of vorapaxar on the primary and secondary end points were maintained for the duration of the study (median follow-up 2.5 years, up to 4 years).

Results of subgroup analyses in the TRA 2°P-TIMI 50 study suggest that the cardiovascular benefits of vorapaxar may be more pronounced in post-MI patients than in those with PAD. In a prespecified subgroup analysis of post-MI patients (including those with prior MI or TIA), the primary composite end point of cardiovascular death, MI, stroke, and urgent coronary revascularization was substantially reduced with vorapaxar versus placebo, which was consistent with the overall study results. Patients with PAD did not derive a statistically significant benefit from vorapaxar in terms of this primary cardiovascular end point but did experience improvements in manifestations of peripheral vascular disease (e.g., limb ischemia, need for peripheral revascularization). In another subgroup analysis of the overall study population, patients weighing less than 60 kg who received vorapaxar therapy had an increased risk of moderate or severe bleeding without apparent reductions in the primary composite efficacy end point, suggesting an unfavorable risk-to-benefit ratio for vorapaxar therapy in such patients. Pending confirmation in additional studies, findings from these subgroup analyses should be interpreted with caution because of the possibility of differences due to chance resulting from the large number of analyses and other limitations (e.g., small number of patients in the PAD cohort).

The benefits of vorapaxar in the TRA 2°P-TIMI 50 study were accompanied by an increased risk of bleeding. Moderate to severe bleeding, including fatal and nonfatal intracranial hemorrhage, were reported more frequently in patients receiving vorapaxar than those receiving placebo; after patients with a history of stroke or TIA were excluded, the bleeding risk was attenuated. (See Bleeding, under Warnings/Precautions: Warnings, in Cautions.)

■ **Acute Coronary Syndrome** Vorapaxar also has been used in patients with acute coronary syndrome (ACS)†; however, current evidence (e.g., results of the TRACER study) suggests that addition of the drug to standard antiplatelet therapy in such patients does not reduce the rate of ischemic events but substantially increases the risk of clinically important bleeding. Therefore, many clinicians currently advise against the use of vorapaxar in patients with ACS.

Efficacy of vorapaxar in the ACS setting was evaluated in a multinational, randomized, double-blind study (TRACER) in 12,944 high-risk patients with non-ST-segment elevation ACS. Patients received vorapaxar (loading dose followed by 2.08 mg daily [2.5 mg of vorapaxar sulfate]) or placebo in addition to standard antiplatelet therapy (aspirin and/or clopidogrel). At a median follow-up of 502 days, the primary composite end point of cardiovascular death, MI, stroke, recurrent ischemia requiring hospitalization, or urgent coronary revascularization occurred at a similar rate in patients receiving vorapaxar or placebo (18.5 or 19.9%, respectively). However, vorapaxar was associated with substantially higher rates of moderate or severe bleeding (using criteria from Global Utilization of Streptokinase and Tissue Plasminogen Activator for Occluded Arteries [GUSTO]), including at least a twofold increased rate of intracranial hemorrhage compared with placebo, and the bleeding risk increased incrementally over time. The TRACER study was terminated early before completion of the planned follow-up period, largely based on this increased bleeding risk.

Dosage and Administration

■ **Administration** Vorapaxar sulfate is administered orally without regard to food.

■ **Dosage** Dosage of vorapaxar sulfate is expressed in terms of vorapaxar.

Cardiovascular Risk Reduction in Established Atherosclerotic Disease The recommended dosage of vorapaxar is 2.08 mg once daily for secondary prevention of thrombotic cardiovascular events in adults with a history of myocardial infarction (MI) or with peripheral arterial disease (PAD). Aspirin and/or clopidogrel should be administered concomitantly according to their given indications or current standards of care. For additional information on the dosages of aspirin and clopidogrel used for secondary prevention in patients with atherosclerotic disease, see Coronary Artery Disease and Myocardial Infarction under Dosage: Thrombosis, in Dosage and Administration in Aspirin 28:08.04.24 and Reduction of Cardiovascular and Cerebrovascular Events under Dosage and Administration: Dosage, in Clopidogrel 20:12.18.

Managing Antiplatelet Therapy in Patients Requiring Invasive Procedures The American College of Chest Physicians (ACCP) states that the decision to interrupt antiplatelet therapy prior to surgery or other invasive procedure should be individualized based on an assessment of the patient's risks of thromboembolism and perioperative bleeding. In the TRA 2°P-TIMI 50 study, investigators were encouraged not to discontinue treatment with the study drug prior to surgery (e.g., coronary artery bypass grafting [CABG]). The manufacturer states that any decision regarding surgery or other invasive procedure requires clinical judgment and consideration of patient-specific information, which may include factors such as the type of procedure, risk and potential consequences of bleeding, and the pharmacologic properties of vorapaxar.

For additional information on the perioperative management of antithrombotic therapy, consult the most recent ACCP Evidence-based Clinical Practice Guidelines on Antithrombotic Therapy and Prevention of Thrombosis available at http://www.chestnet.org.

■ **Special Populations** No dosage adjustment is necessary in patients with mild or moderate hepatic impairment; use is not recommended in patients with severe hepatic impairment. (See Hepatic Impairment, under Warnings/Precautions: Special Populations, in Cautions.)

No dosage adjustment is necessary in patients with renal impairment, including those with end-stage renal disease. (See Renal Impairment, under Warnings/Precautions: Special Populations, in Cautions.)

No dosage adjustments are necessary based on age, race, gender, or weight.

Cautions

■ **Contraindications** History of stroke, transient ischemic attack (TIA), or intracranial hemorrhage.

Active pathological bleeding (e.g., intracranial hemorrhage, peptic ulcer).

■ **Warnings/Precautions** ***Warnings*** **Bleeding.** As with other antiplatelet agents, vorapaxar increases the risk of bleeding, including intracranial hemorrhage and fatal bleeding. Bleeding complications were the most common adverse effects of vorapaxar in clinical trials. In these trials, patients received vorapaxar in addition to aspirin with or without clopidogrel. In the full population of the TRA2°P-TIMI 50 secondary prevention study, moderate or severe bleeding occurred more frequently with vorapaxar than with placebo (4.2 versus 2.5% of patients, respectively, a 66% increase); this included a twofold higher rate of intracranial hemorrhage with vorapaxar versus placebo (1 versus 0.5% of patients, respectively). The rate of fatal bleeding was similar between the vorapaxar and placebo groups (0.3 and 0.2% of patients, respectively). Bleeding was assessed according to the GUSTO (Global Utilization of Streptokinase and Tissue Plasminogen Activator for Occluded Arteries) criteria, which defines moderate bleeding as bleeding without hemodynamic compromise but requiring transfusion of whole blood or packed red blood cells; and severe bleeding as fatal bleeding, intracranial bleeding, or bleeding with hemodynamic compromise requiring intervention. Patients with a history of stroke had substantially higher rates of intracranial hemorrhage with vorapaxar, which led to premature discontinuance of the drug in such patients. After these patients and those with prior TIA were excluded from the study, bleeding rates were attenuated but remained comparatively higher with vorapaxar than placebo; in the FDA-labeled population (i.e., post-MI patients or those with peripheral arterial disease [PAD] who did not have a history of stroke or TIA), there was a 55% increase in moderate or severe bleeding (not related to coronary artery bypass grafting [CABG]) with vorapaxar compared with placebo (3.7 versus 2.4% for moderate or severe bleeding, and 0.6 versus 0.4% for intracranial hemorrhage).

Vorapaxar should not be used in patients who are actively bleeding or have a history of stroke, TIA, or intracranial hemorrhage; the drug should be discontinued if any of these events occur during therapy. (See Cautions: Contraindications.) Because risk of bleeding with vorapaxar increases in proportion to a patient's underlying bleeding risk, patients should be evaluated for their baseline bleeding risk prior to initiating therapy. Risk factors for bleeding generally include advanced age, low body weight (e.g., less than 60 kg), renal or hepatic impairment, history of bleeding disorders, and concomitant use of drugs that can increase bleeding risk (e.g., anticoagulants, fibrinolytics, nonsteroidal anti-inflammatory agents [NSAIAs], selective serotonin- and norepinephrine-reuptake inhibitors [SNRIs], selective serotonin-reuptake inhibitors [SSRIs]). (See Drug Interactions: Drugs Affecting Hemostasis.) Bleeding should be suspected in any patient who is hypotensive and has recently undergone coronary angiography, percutaneous coronary intervention (PCI), CABG, or other surgical procedures. If bleeding occurs during vorapaxar therapy, standard treatment measures should be employed. Withholding a dose for a brief period is unlikely to resolve an acute bleeding episode because of the drug's prolonged half-life and effects on platelet inhibition; substantial inhibition of platelet aggregation exists 4 weeks after discontinuance of vorapaxar. There is no known agent for reversing the antiplatelet effects of vorapaxar and the drug is not expected to be dialyzable because of high plasma protein binding.

Other Warnings and Precautions **Concomitant Use of Potent Cytochrome P-450 (CYP) 3A Inhibitors or Inducers.** Vorapaxar should not be used concomitantly with drugs that are potent inhibitors or inducers of CYP3A. (See Drug Interactions: Drugs Affecting or Metabolized by Hepatic Microsomal Enzymes.)

Specific Populations **Pregnancy.** Category B. (See Users Guide.)

Data from developmental toxicity studies in animals indicate that vorapaxar is predicted to have a low probability for causing adverse fetal effects (e.g., malformations, embryo-fetal toxicities) or maternal toxicity when administered during pregnancy. There are no adequate and well-controlled studies of the drug in pregnant women. Vorapaxar should be used during pregnancy only if the potential benefits justify the potential risks to the fetus.

Lactation. Vorapaxar is distributed into milk in rats; it is not known whether the drug or its metabolites are distributed into human milk. Because of the potential for serious adverse effects from vorapaxar in nursing infants, a decision should be made whether to discontinue nursing or the drug.

Pediatric Use. Safety and efficacy of vorapaxar have not been established in pediatric patients.

Geriatric Use. In the principal efficacy study of vorapaxar in patients with established atherosclerosis, no overall differences in safety or efficacy were observed between geriatric patients 65 years of age or older and younger adults. The relative risk of bleeding with vorapaxar compared with placebo in this study was similar across all age groups. However, since risk of bleeding is generally increased in geriatric patients regardless of treatment, age should be considered prior to initiating vorapaxar therapy.

Hepatic Impairment. Hepatic impairment does not appear to substantially affect the pharmacokinetics of vorapaxar or its main active metabolite (M20). In a single-dose open-label study, peak plasma concentrations and systemic exposure of vorapaxar generally were similar between healthy individuals and patients with various degrees of hepatic impairment (mild, moderate, or severe). However, interpretation of the results in patients with severe hepatic impairment is limited because of the small sample size.

The manufacturer states that use of vorapaxar in patients with severe hepatic impairment is not recommended because of the inherent increased risk of bleeding in such patients.

Renal Impairment. Vorapaxar is minimally excreted in the urine; renal impairment does not appear to have a clinically important effect on the pharmacokinetics or pharmacodynamics of the drug. (See Description.) In a single-dose open-label study, plasma concentration-time profiles and platelet inhibitory effects of vorapaxar were similar in healthy individuals and patients with end-stage renal disease undergoing hemodialysis. Patients with a wide range of renal function were included in the primary efficacy study of vorapaxar.

Race/Ethnicity. Pharmacokinetics and pharmacodynamics of vorapaxar do not appear to be substantially affected by race or ethnicity.

■ **Common Adverse Effects** Bleeding was the most common adverse effect reported in clinical trials of vorapaxar.

Adverse effects other than bleeding reported in at least 2% of patients receiving vorapaxar in clinical trials and at a rate at least 10% higher than with placebo include anemia; depression; and rashes, eruptions, and exanthemas.

Drug Interactions

■ **Drugs Affecting or Metabolized by Hepatic Microsomal Enzymes** Vorapaxar is metabolized by cytochrome P-450 (CYP) 3A4 and 2J2; drugs that inhibit or induce these enzymes can increase or decrease vorapaxar concentrations, respectively. In vitro studies indicate that vorapaxar and its active metabolite do not inhibit or induce major CYP isoenzymes.

CYP3A Inhibitors Potent inhibitors of CYP3A (e.g., ketoconazole, itraconazole, posaconazole, clarithromycin, nefazodone, ritonavir, saquinavir, nelfinavir, indinavir, boceprevir, telaprevir, telithromycin, conivaptan) may substantially increase vorapaxar concentrations and possibly increase the risk of bleeding; concomitant use of these drugs should be avoided. In a study in which vorapaxar was coadministered with a potent CYP3A inhibitor (ketoconazole), peak plasma concentrations and systemic exposure of vorapaxar were increased by approximately twofold. Although the increased drug exposure did not have a substantial effect on bleeding, the study was conducted in healthy individuals who were not receiving other concomitant antiplatelet agents typical of the target patient population.

Data from phase 3 clinical studies suggest that clinically important pharmacokinetic interactions are unlikely with weak to moderate inhibitors of CYP3A.

CYP3A Inducers Potent inducers of CYP3A (e.g., rifampin, carbamazepine, St. John's Wort, phenytoin) may decrease plasma concentrations of vorapaxar and possibly reduce efficacy of the drug; concomitant use of these drugs should be avoided. In a study in healthy individuals, coadministration of vorapaxar and a potent CYP3A inducer (rifampin) reduced peak plasma concentrations and systemic exposure of vorapaxar by approximately 50%.

CYP2C8/9 Substrates Vorapaxar does not appear to substantially affect the pharmacokinetics of drugs metabolized by CYP2C8 (e.g., rosiglitazone) or CYP2C9 (warfarin).

■ **Drugs Affected by Efflux Transport Systems** Vorapaxar is a weak inhibitor of the P-glycoprotein (P-gp) transport system and may potentially increase plasma concentrations of drugs that are P-gp substrates. When vorapaxar was used concomitantly with a known P-gp substrate (digoxin), peak plasma concentrations of digoxin were substantially increased, but systemic exposure to the drug was unaffected. No dosage adjustments are necessary when vorapaxar and digoxin are administered concomitantly.

In vitro studies indicate that vorapaxar is not likely to cause clinically important inhibition of organic anion-transporting polypeptides (OATP) 1B1 and 1B3, organic anion transporters (OAT) 1 and 3, organic cation transporter (OCT) 2, and the breast cancer resistance protein (BCRP).

■ **Drugs Affecting Hemostasis** Concomitant use of vorapaxar with drugs that affect hemostasis (e.g., anticoagulants, fibrinolytics, selective serotonin-reuptake inhibitors [SSRIs], selective serotonin- and norepinephrine-reuptake inhibitors [SNRIs], nonsteroidal anti-inflammatory agents [NSAIAs]) can increase the risk of bleeding associated with vorapaxar.

Anticoagulants Clinically important pharmacokinetic and pharmacodynamic interactions between warfarin (a CYP2C9 substrate) and vorapaxar do not appear to be likely. In healthy individuals, concomitant administration of the drugs did not substantially alter pharmacokinetic parameters (plasma concentration-time profiles, peak plasma concentrations, systemic exposure) of warfarin. Changes observed in the anticoagulant effects of warfarin were not considered to be clinically meaningful.

Because of the potential for increased bleeding, use of warfarin or other anticoagulants should be avoided in patients receiving vorapaxar.

Antiplatelet Agents Vorapaxar is intended for use as an adjunct to therapy with aspirin and/or clopidogrel, and these drugs were used concomitantly as part of double or triple antiplatelet therapy in studies evaluating efficacy and safety of vorapaxar. However, the possibility that the risk of bleeding may be increased with concomitant antiplatelet therapy should be considered.

Although pharmacokinetic interactions between prasugrel and vorapaxar have not been observed, clinical experience with the use of vorapaxar in conjunction with antiplatelet agents other than aspirin and clopidogrel is very limited. (See Uses: Cardiovascular Risk Reduction in Established Atherosclerotic Disease.)

Specific studies evaluating potential pharmacokinetic interactions between clopidogrel and vorapaxar have not been conducted.

■ **Antacids** Concomitant administration of vorapaxar with an antacid containing aluminum hydroxide and magnesium carbonate (Gaviscon® Extra Strength liquid) resulted in slightly decreased peak plasma concentrations and systemic exposure of vorapaxar. No dosage adjustment is necessary.

■ **Proton-pump Inhibitors** Peak plasma concentrations and systemic exposure of vorapaxar were not substantially affected by concomitant administration of the proton-pump inhibitor pantoprazole. No dosage adjustment is necessary.

■ **Rosiglitazone** Concomitant administration of vorapaxar and rosiglitazone (a CYP2C8 substrate) did not substantially alter peak plasma concentrations or systemic exposure of rosiglitazone. No dosage adjustment is necessary.

Description

Vorapaxar sulfate, a protease-activated receptor-1 (PAR-1) antagonist, is a platelet-aggregation inhibitor. The drug inhibits platelet aggregation by a different mechanism than that of aspirin or thienopyridine P2Y12 platelet adenosine diphosphate (ADP)-receptor antagonists (e.g., clopidogrel, prasugrel); vorapaxar binds selectively to PAR-1, the primary thrombin receptor expressed on human platelets, resulting in potent inhibition of thrombin-mediated platelet aggregation. While binding of vorapaxar to the PAR-1 receptor is reversible, the drug's long half-life makes its inhibitory effects on platelet aggregation essentially irreversible.

Vorapaxar produces rapid and prolonged dose-dependent inhibition of thrombin-induced and thrombin receptor agonist peptide (TRAP)-induced platelet activation in vitro. Following administration of the recommended daily dosage of 2.08 mg, consistent and complete (defined as at least 80%) inhibition of TRAP-induced platelet aggregation has been demonstrated within 7 days of initiating therapy. After the drug is discontinued, platelet-inhibitory effects can be expected to persist at a level of 50% inhibition for about 4 weeks. Vorapaxar does not inhibit platelet activation induced by ADP, collagen, or arachidonic acid; the drug also does not affect standard coagulation tests (thrombin time [TT], prothrombin time [PT], activated partial thromboplastin time [aPTT], activated clotting time [ACT], and ecarin clotting time [ECT]). Vorapaxar has no effect on the QT interval corrected for rate (QT_c) in single doses of up to 48 times the recommended dose.

The pharmacokinetic disposition of vorapaxar is characterized by rapid and essentially complete absorption and rapid distribution, followed by slow elimination. Following oral administration, peak plasma concentrations occur within approximately 60 minutes (range 1–2 hours). Vorapaxar exposure is approximately dose proportional following single doses of up to 16 times the recommended dose. Administration with a high-fat meal moderately decreased peak plasma concentrations and delayed time to peak concentrations of vorapaxar, but did not substantially alter systemic exposure to the drug. (See Dosage and Administration: Administration.) Vorapaxar is metabolized by cytochrome P-450 (CYP) 3A4 and CYP2J2. The major circulating monohydroxy metabolite, M20, is pharmacologically active and accounts for approximately 20% of total drug exposure. Elimination occurs principally by hepatobiliary excretion as metabolites; no unchanged vorapaxar is detected in urine. Following oral administration of radiolabeled vorapaxar, approximately 58 and 25% of the dose is detected in feces and urine, respectively. The effective half-life of vorapaxar is 3–4 days and apparent terminal half-life of the drug and its active circulating metabolite is approximately 8 days (range 5–13 days). Vorapaxar is extensively distributed, and both vorapaxar and its active metabolite are extensively (99% or greater) bound to human plasma proteins (e.g., albumin).

Advice to Patients

Importance of advising patients to read the manufacturer's patient information (medication guide).

Importance of counseling patients about the potential risks versus benefits of vorapaxar.

Importance of taking vorapaxar exactly as prescribed and not discontinuing therapy without first consulting the prescribing clinician.

Importance of informing patients that they may bruise and/or bleed more easily (e.g., nosebleeds) when taking vorapaxar and that bleeding may take longer than usual to cease; these effects may be present for 4 weeks after vorapaxar is discontinued. Patients should be advised to report to their clinicians any unexpected, prolonged, or excessive bleeding.

Importance of informing clinicians (e.g., physicians, dentists) about vorapaxar therapy before any invasive procedure or surgery is scheduled. Clinicians performing invasive procedures should consult with prescribing clinician before discontinuing vorapaxar.

Importance of informing clinicians of existing or contemplated concomitant therapy, including prescription drugs, dietary supplements, and OTC drugs, particularly drugs that affect bleeding risk (e.g., warfarin, nonsteroidal anti-inflammatory agents [NSAIAs]).

Importance of women informing clinicians if they are or plan to become pregnant or plan to breast-feed.

Importance of informing patients of other important precautionary information. (See Cautions.)

Overview® (see Users Guide). For additional information on this drug until a more detailed monograph is developed and published, the manufacturer's labeling should be consulted. It is *essential* that the manufacturer's labeling be consulted for more detailed information on usual cautions, precautions, contraindications, potential drug interactions, laboratory test interferences, and acute toxicity.

Preparations

Excipients in commercially available drug preparations may have clinically important effects in some individuals; consult specific product labeling for details.

Vorapaxar Sulfate

Oral		
Tablets	2.08 mg (of vorapaxar)	**Zontivity®**, Merck

†Use is not currently included in the labeling approved by the US Food and Drug Administration

THROMBOLYTIC AGENTS 20:12.20

Alteplase

rt-PA, t-PA (Recombinant), t-PA

■ Alteplase, a biosynthetic (recombinant DNA origin) form of the enzyme human tissue-type plasminogen activator (t-PA), is a thrombolytic agent.

Uses

■ **Acute Myocardial Infarction** Alteplase, a recombinant tissue-type plasminogen activator, is used as a thrombolytic agent for reperfusion therapy in patients with acute myocardial infarction (MI). The term MI is used when there is evidence of myocardial necrosis in the setting of acute myocardial ischemia. MI is further distinguished based on the presence or absence of ST-segment elevation on ECG. Because patients with ST-segment-elevation MI (STEMI) typically have complete arterial occlusion, immediate reperfusion therapy is required. Reperfusion may be achieved with a pharmacologic (e.g., thrombolytic therapy) or mechanical (percutaneous coronary intervention [PCI]) strategy.

Almost all clinical studies to date of tissue-type plasminogen activator (t-PA) in patients with acute MI have been conducted using either the predominantly two-chain (prepared by Genentech roller-bottle method but not currently available) form of recombinant t-PA (rt-PA) that was used in early clinical studies or the currently marketed, predominantly one-chain form of rt-PA (alteplase) (prepared by Genentech suspension-culture methods); the manufacturer states that all Genentech-sponsored studies of rt-PA initiated since August 1985 have used the predominantly one-chain form. Therefore, unless otherwise specified, the term rt-PA in the Uses section refers to studies in which either alteplase or predominantly two-chain rt-PA was evaluated.

Choice of Coronary Reperfusion Strategy The principal goal of therapy in patients with STEMI is to reestablish coronary blood flow; therefore, the current standard of care in such patients is timely reperfusion (with primary PCI or thrombolytic therapy). Because of a demonstrated mortality benefit and lower rates of reinfarction with PCI compared with thrombolytic therapy, primary PCI is the preferred reperfusion strategy when it can be performed in a timely manner by experienced clinicians. Due to the limited number of PCI-capable facilities in the US, thrombolytic therapy is considered an acceptable alternative. Experts state that the appropriate and timely use of any form of reperfusion is likely more important than the choice of therapy.

The benefits of thrombolytic therapy in patients with STEMI are well established. When rt-PA is used by IV infusion in selected patients with acute MI, thrombolysis occurs usually within 1 hour after initiation of the IV infusion. The resulting reperfusion can limit infarct size, improve ventricular function (e.g., decrease ventricular arrhythmias), and reduce the incidence of congestive heart failure, cardiogenic shock, and death.

The American College of Cardiology Foundation (ACCF)/American Heart Association (AHA) guideline for the management of STEMI states that reperfusion therapy should be administered to all eligible patients with STEMI and onset of ischemic symptoms within the previous 12 hours. The appropriate reperfusion method (thrombolytic therapy or PCI) should be selected based on a risk-benefit analysis that incorporates the time from onset of MI symptoms, the clinical and hemodynamic status of the patient, presence of comorbidities (e.g., severe heart failure), bleeding risk, contraindications, and the availability (and timeliness) of PCI. Primary PCI is the preferred method of reperfusion when it can be performed in a timely manner. Thrombolytic therapy is recommended when it is anticipated that PCI cannot be performed within 120 minutes of first medical contact. Initial thrombolytic therapy is most appropriate for those patients with low bleeding risk who present early after symptom onset (less than 2–3 hours) to a non-PCI-capable hospital and who have longer delays to PCI. If therapy with rt-PA is selected, it should be instituted as soon as possible after acute MI since the potential clinical benefit diminishes as the time period from symptom onset to initiation of therapy increases. The greatest benefits of thrombolytic therapy in terms of reductions in mortality and morbidity have been observed when such therapy was initiated within the first 12 hours after symptom onset. Appreciable improvement of ventricular function (as assessed by left ventricular ejection fraction or regional wall motion), reduction in infarct size, and reduction in the incidence of congestive heart failure have been apparent when rt-PA was initiated within 6 hours of the onset of symptoms of MI, although the greatest clinical benefit has been observed when therapy was initiated earlier. ACCF and AHA recommend that thrombolytic therapy be administered within 30 minutes of hospital arrival.

Standard therapeutic measures for management of MI should be instituted concomitantly with rt-PA therapy. (See Uses: Acute Ischemic Complications of ST-Segment-Elevation Myocardial Infarction in Heparin 20:12.04.16 and see Secondary Prevention of Cardiovascular Events under Thrombosis: Coronary Artery Disease and Myocardial Infarction, in Uses in Aspirin 28:08.04.24.) In all patients receiving rt-PA, the potential risk of serious hemorrhage must be weighed against the possible benefit of therapy with the drug. (See Cautions: Effects on Hemostasis and also see Cautions: Precautions and Contraindications.)

Adjunctive Anticoagulant and Antiplatelet Therapy Adjunctive therapy with anticoagulant (e.g., heparin) and antiplatelet (e.g., aspirin and clopidogrel) agents should be used during and after successful coronary artery reperfusion for the prevention of early reocclusion and death, unless contraindicated. Coronary artery reocclusion (which often is not clinically evident) occurs in an appreciable number of patients after IV thrombolytic therapy. (See Uses: Prevention of Reocclusion After Thrombolysis.) Concomitant therapy with heparin and/or platelet-aggregation inhibitors has been used in most clinical studies with rt-PA to prevent reocclusion following lysis of coronary artery thrombi. While such concomitant therapy may increase the risk of bleeding complications, (see Cautions: Effects on Hemostasis and also see Drug Interactions: Anticoagulants and also Drugs Affecting Platelet Function) evidence suggests that early infarct-artery patency can be enhanced with the use of IV heparin as an adjunct to thrombolytic therapy. The use of platelet glycoprotein (GP IIb/IIIa)-receptor inhibitors does not appear to provide additional benefit over thrombolytic therapy alone and may increase the risk of bleeding. ACCF and AHA recommend that patients with STEMI undergoing thrombolytic therapy should receive an anticoagulant (e.g., heparin, enoxaparin, fondaparinux) for a minimum of 48 hours, and preferably for the duration of the index hospitalization, up to 8 days or until revascularization is performed. Aspirin should be initiated and continued indefinitely and clopidogrel therapy should be administered for at least 14 days (and up to 1 year) in all patients with STEMI who receive thrombolytic therapy.

Coronary Artery Patency The overall rate of coronary artery reperfusion or patency after rt-PA administration exceeds that of placebo or IV streptokinase (no longer commercially available in the US). Reperfusion after thrombolytic therapy may be evidenced by appearance of arrhythmias, relief of chest pain, and/or early peaking of serum concentrations of AST (SGOT) and the cardiac fraction (MB fraction) of creatine kinase (CK, creatine phosphokinase, CPK); however, these are not definitive measures of recanalization. Creatine kinase concentrations usually return to baseline levels rapidly after reperfusion. Beneficial effects of rt-PA therapy on ventricular function or mortality generally have been limited to patients with infarct-related coronary arteries that became patent with therapy. Analyses of data from an angiographic substudy of patients in the GUSTO-I trial indicate that "normal" perfusion (TIMI grade 3 flow) in an infarct-related artery at 90 minutes post-thrombolysis was associated with a lower 30-day mortality rate regardless of the thrombolytic agent used; these data support the "open-artery" hypothesis regarding early restoration of coronary artery patency and subsequent mortality reduction beyond that expected from preservation of left ventricular function (myocardial salvage) alone. Some evidence suggests that while the early benefit of infarct-artery patency occurs as a result of myocardial salvage, the late mortality benefit occurs independent of improvements in ventricular function. This late benefit appears to result from a reduction of scar formation and from attenuation of ventricular dilation and infarct remodeling, particularly in areas of the myocardium that depend on collateral circulation.

The extent of coronary recanalization after rt-PA therapy generally has been shown to be dose dependent. In studies employing pretreatment angiography to confirm coronary artery occlusion, rt-PA in dosages of 40–100 mg administered IV over 1–3 hours was associated with reperfusion after approximately 45–90 minutes in about 60–75% of infarct-related coronary arteries; at these dosages, coronary artery patency rates in studies not employing pretreatment angiography have been similar or somewhat higher. However, patency rates may overestimate efficacy because of failure to exclude patients with patent infarct-related coronary arteries or early spontaneous recanalization. In dose-ranging studies conducted before the second phase of the Thrombolysis in Myocardial Infarction (TIMI) trial (TIMI-2), intravenous infusion of alteplase at a dose of 150 mg over 5–8 hours was associated with patency rates of 75% at 90 minutes. However, because an increased incidence of life-threatening intracranial bleeding was noted at this dose, the maximum recommended total dose was reduced to 100 mg. (See Cautions: Effects on Hemostasis and also see Cautions: Precautions and Contraindications.) In phase 1 of the TIMI trial, a comparative trial of intravenous rt-PA and streptokinase in which *both* pretreatment and post-treatment angiography were used, the rate of reperfusion during the first 90 minutes after initiating therapy in patients with total or subtotal coronary artery occlusion was twice as high for rt-PA as for streptokinase (62% versus 31%, respectively). Although the average time from symptom onset until initiation of thrombolytic therapy was 4.75 hours in this study, the proportion of coronary arteries reperfused was greater for rt-PA than for streptokinase regardless of the time from symptom onset. An analysis of the combined results of the TIMI-1 trial and another randomized comparative trial also showed that the rate of coronary artery patency or reperfusion was greater with rt-PA than with streptokinase in patients treated both within 3 hours of symptom onset and 3–6 hours after onset of symptoms. These findings appear to confirm in vitro evidence indicating that the fibrinolytic efficacy of rt-PA is relatively unaffected by the age of a thrombus; however, delayed initiation of thrombolytic therapy is associated with a decreased likelihood of beneficial cardiac effects, regardless of the thrombolytic agent used.

Effects on Mortality Reduction Several controlled studies have demonstrated a survival benefit in patients with acute MI receiving alteplase. In a large, placebo-controlled, multicenter study (Anglo-Scandinavian Study of Early Thrombolysis; ASSET), patients with acute MI who received alteplase 100 mg IV over a 3-hour period (an initial 10-mg loading dose followed by infusions of 50, 20, and 20 mg/hour during hours 1, 2, and 3, respectively) within 5 hours of onset of symptoms had a 26% reduction in mortality (death occurred in 9.8% of placebo-treated patients versus 7.2% of patients who received alteplase) at 1 month after discharge. The mortality reductions in patients treated within 3 hours or between 3–5 hours of symptom onset (e.g., chest pain) were similar, and the overall mortality reduction in the ASSET study is similar to that in patients receiving streptokinase within 6 hours of symptom onset in several large studies. In another study, the mortality rates in patients receiving alteplase 100 mg IV over 3 hours versus placebo were 2.8 versus 5.7% (51% mortality reduction) at 14 days and 5.1 versus 7.9% (36% mortality reduction) at 3 months; patients treated within 3 hours of onset of symptoms had 14-day and 3-month mortality reductions of 82% and 59%, respectively. All patients in this study received concomitant therapy for 10–22 days after admission with heparin by continuous IV infusion and low-dose aspirin every other day; low-dose aspirin can independently reduce mortality after acute MI and may have contributed to the mortality reductions in this study.

In 2 randomized, multicenter studies, more than 20,000 patients with acute evolving MI received either alteplase 100 mg IV over 3 hours or streptokinase 1.5 million units over 30–60 minutes, with or without subcutaneous heparin therapy (starting 12 hours after initiation of thrombolytic therapy). In-hospital mortality rates for the combined studies were low and similar in all 4 treatment groups: 9.2, 8.7, 7.9, or 9.2% in patients receiving either alteplase plus heparin, alteplase alone, streptokinase plus heparin, or streptokinase alone, respectively. Aspirin therapy (300–325 mg daily) and atenolol 5–10 mg IV was also administered to all study patients who had no specific contraindications to such therapy; aspirin and atenolol were given to approximately 96 and 23% of patients, respectively, in each treatment group. Although the overall incidence of complications and adverse effects was low, stroke was reported more often with alteplase than with streptokinase therapy (1.3 and 1% of patients, respectively), while major bleeding occurred more frequently in streptokinase-treated patients; streptokinase and heparin were both independently associated with an increased risk of bleeding. Adjunctive therapy with subcutaneous heparin (12,500 units twice daily during hospitalization) did not appear to provide additional benefit in patients receiving thrombolytic therapy since the incidences of stroke and reinfarction were similar whether or not concomitant heparin therapy was given.

Improved survival with a thrombolytic regimen containing alteplase compared with streptokinase-containing regimens has been demonstrated in a multicenter study in more than 41,000 patients with acute MI (Global Utilization of Streptokinase and Tissue Plasminogen Activator for Occluded Coronary Arteries [GUSTO-1]). In the GUSTO-1 study, patients were randomized to receive 1 of 4 thrombolytic regimens: alteplase (maximum dose: 100 mg) in an "accelerated-dose" schedule (i.e., total dose administered IV over 1.5 rather than the usual 3 hours, with two-thirds of the dose given in the first 30 minutes) in conjunction with *simultaneously initiated* IV heparin therapy; streptokinase (1.5 million units over 1 hour) with IV heparin; streptokinase (1.5 million units over 1 hour) with subcutaneously administered heparin; or combined alteplase and streptokinase with IV heparin. Therapy with IV heparin (5000 units by rapid injection, then 1000–1200 units/hour) was initiated at the same time as thrombolytic therapy, while subcutaneously administered heparin (12,500 units twice daily) was begun 4 hours after initiation of thrombolytic therapy. In the combined alteplase-streptokinase regimen, streptokinase was given in a dosage of 1 million units over 1 hour; alteplase was administered in a dosage of 1 mg/kg (up to 90 mg) over 1 hour, with 10% of the dose given initially by rapid IV injection. The mortality rates at 30 days for the groups receiving streptokinase and subcutaneous heparin, streptokinase and IV heparin, accelerated-dose alteplase and IV heparin, and the combined alteplase-streptokinase regimen with IV heparin were 7.2, 7.4, 6.3, and 7%, respectively. The difference in these rates represent a 14% reduction in mortality with the accelerated-dose alteplase regimen compared with both streptokinase-only regimens and a 10% reduction compared with the combined alteplase-streptokinase regimen; there was no difference in 30 day-mortality between the 2 streptokinase-only regimens. Although hemorrhagic stroke occurred more frequently in patients receiving the accelerated-dose alteplase or combined alteplase-streptokinase regimens, the risk of the combined end point of death or disabling stroke was reduced with the accelerated-dose alteplase regimen compared with the streptokinase-only regimens, resulting in a net benefit of alteplase versus the other regimens.

Results of the GUSTO-1 study support previous data from smaller studies that demonstrated an association between early and complete coronary artery patency, improved left ventricular function, and increased survival after acute MI. In a subset of patients enrolled in the GUSTO-1 study who were randomly assigned to undergo coronary artery angiography at 90 minutes, 180 minutes, 24 hours, or 5–7 days after initiation of thrombolytic therapy, the rate of patency of the infarct-related artery and the percentage of patients with normal blood flow through that artery at 90 minutes was higher in the group given accelerated-dose alteplase with IV heparin than in those receiving other thrombolytic regimens; patency rates were similar for all groups at 180 minutes. Measures of left ventricular function paralleled the rate of patency at 90 minutes; ventricular function was best in the group given accelerated-dose alteplase with heparin and in patients with normal flow through the infarct-related artery regardless of treatment group. Likewise, mortality at 30 days was lowest (4.4%) among patients with normal blood flow in the infarct-related artery at 90-minute angiography and highest (8.9%) among those with no coronary blood flow in that artery. Failure of the combined alteplase-streptokinase regimen to produce an early patency rate similar to that of the accelerated-dose alteplase regimen has been attributed to the use of only a small initial rapid-injection dose of alteplase in the combined regimen.

Results from 2 large, comparative clinical trials (International Joint Efficacy Comparison of Thrombolytics [INJECT] trial, Global Utilization of Strategies to Open Occluded Coronary Arteries-III [GUSTO-III] trial) in patients with acute MI suggest similar effects of accelerated-dose alteplase (given as a 15-mg IV loading dose followed by 0.75 mg/kg [up to 50 mg] over 30 minutes, then 0.5 mg/kg [up to 35 mg] over 60 minutes), reteplase (2 doses of 10 units each given 30 minutes apart by direct IV injection), or streptokinase (1.5 million units IV over 60 minutes) on reduction of short-term (30 or 35 days) or long-term (6 months or 1 year) mortality. While previous studies had demonstrated improved coronary artery patency with reteplase compared with alteplase, analysis of more than 15,000 patients receiving the drugs in the GUSTO-III trial revealed very similar 30-day mortality rates (7.47 or 7.24% with reteplase or alteplase therapy, respectively); the incidences of other cardiovascular events, including stroke, bleeding, and intracranial hemorrhage, also were similar. The INJECT trial was not designed to demonstrate superiority of reteplase or streptokinase on reduction of mortality in patients with MI, only therapeutic equivalence; a trial in a larger number of patients would be required to demonstrate superiority of either agent. The occurrence of certain secondary clinical end points (i.e., stroke, reinfarction) was similar among patients with acute MI receiving any of the evaluated thrombolytic agents in these trials. The incidence of congestive heart failure also was lower in patients receiving reteplase than in those receiving streptokinase in the INJECT trial, and was similar among patients receiving reteplase or alteplase in the GUSTO-III trial. All patients in these trials received adjunctive antithrombotic therapy with aspirin (160–350 mg initially followed by 75–350 mg daily) and unfractionated heparin (5000 units by direct IV injection prior to reteplase administration, followed by 1000 units hourly by continuous IV infusion for at least 24 hours). Overall clinical outcomes also were improved with alteplase compared with anistreplase (no longer commercially available in the US), although the difference in mortality rate at 6 weeks was not statistically significant.

Choice of Thrombolytic Agent The relative role of alteplase versus other thrombolytic agents in acute evolving MI remains to be fully elucidated. Many clinicians suggest that the particular thrombolytic agent used is less important for patient survival than reducing the delay in initiating treatment in patients with MI. ACCF and AHA recommend the use of a fibrin-specific thrombolytic agent (e.g., alteplase, reteplase, tenecteplase).

Prevention of Reocclusion after Thrombolysis Reocclusion of the infarct-related coronary artery following therapy with rt-PA generally has occurred in approximately 10–20% of patients, although higher reocclusion rates (up to 45%) have been reported. The reocclusion rate reported after rt-PA therapy for acute MI varies considerably but appears to be similar to or greater than that reported for streptokinase or urokinase (both no longer commercially available in the US). The rate of reocclusion is greater with a standard infusion of alteplase than with an accelerated infusion. Reocclusion usually occurs in the first 24 hours after thrombolysis, but may occur within 30 minutes after completion of the infusion and be clinically silent; late reocclusion (e.g., 4–10 days or longer after thrombolytic therapy) also can occur. The rate of reocclusion appears to depend principally on the degree of residual stenosis of the affected coronary artery, but also may be influenced by other factors, such as fluctuations in coronary blood flow during infusion of the thrombolytic agent, induction of a transient procoagulant state or possible platelet activation during thrombolytic therapy, the dosage and duration of the infusion of the thrombolytic agent, subsequent therapeutic measures (e.g., anticoagulant and/or platelet-aggregation inhibitor therapy), and the timing of angiography after thrombolytic therapy. (See Pharmacology: Other Effects on Hemostasis.) In one study, all patients who developed reocclusion did so within 1 hour after discontinuance of the t-PA infusion when the plasma t-PA concentration had declined to less than 0.7 mcg/mL. However, in other studies, plasma rt-PA concentrations as low as 0.45 mcg/mL have been associated with prevention of reocclusion after thrombolytic therapy in patients with MI.

Several therapeutic measures (e.g., anticoagulation and/or antiplatelet therapy, prolonged infusion of the thrombolytic agent, or mechanical or surgical revascularization procedures) have been used to reduce the incidence of reocclusion after coronary artery thrombolysis with rt-PA. Anticoagulant therapy (e.g., heparin and/or oral anticoagulants) has been used concomitantly with and/or subsequent to rt-PA therapy in most patients treated for acute MI in clinical studies. Platelet-aggregation inhibitors (e.g., aspirin) and P2Y12-receptor antagonists (e.g., clopidogrel) also have been administered before, during, or after rt-PA therapy in many patients for secondary prevention of recurrent ischemic events. In addition, a vitamin K antagonist (i.e., warfarin) is recommended in patients who have other indications for anticoagulation, such as atrial fibrillation, mechanical heart valves, venous thromboembolism, or hypercoagulable disorders. (See Secondary Prevention under Uses: ST-Segment-Elevation Myocardial Infarction, in Warfarin 20:12.04.08.)

Since a substantial degree of coronary artery stenosis often remains even after successful thrombolysis and the presence of residual thrombus strongly predisposes to reocclusion, PCI also has been used after thrombolysis in an effort to maintain coronary artery patency and reduce the risk of reinfarction and recurrent ischemia.

■ **Pulmonary Embolism** Alteplase is used in adults for lysis of acute pulmonary emboli involving obstruction of blood flow to a lobe or multiple segments of the lungs, and for lysis of pulmonary emboli accompanied by unstable hemodynamics (i.e., when blood pressure cannot be maintained without supportive measures). rt-PA, including alteplase, has been administered IV or via the pulmonary artery† in patients with acute pulmonary embolism. In a comparative study in adults with symptoms of pulmonary embolism of less than 2 weeks (usually less than 5 days) duration, 100 mg of alteplase infused over 2 hours produced moderate or marked lysis of pulmonary emboli (as documented by pulmonary angiography at 2 hours) in 59% of patients compared with 13% receiving urokinase. Improvement in lung perfusion scans 24 hours after alteplase therapy was similar to that produced by a 24-hour IV infusion of urokinase, although the biological activity of the alteplase dosage substantially exceeded that of the urokinase dosage.

Use of systemic thrombolytic therapy in the treatment of pulmonary embolism remains controversial, in part because it has not been definitely established in randomized controlled trials that thrombolytic therapy ultimately decreases mortality or prevents recurrent pulmonary embolism and because of the high risk of bleeding associated with such therapy. The American College of Chest Physicians (ACCP) generally recommends against the use of systemic thrombolytic therapy in most patients with acute pulmonary embolism; however, in such patients with associated hypotension (e.g., systolic blood pressure less than 90 mmHg), thrombolytic therapy may provide some benefit in terms of a reduction in mortality, and is suggested by ACCP as a possible treatment option in patients without a high risk of bleeding. For additional information on treatment of pulmonary embolism, consult the most recent American College of Chest Physicians Evidence-based Clinical Practice Guidelines on Antithrombotic Therapy and Prevention of Thrombosis available at http://www.chestnet.org.

The optimal therapeutic regimen for rt-PA in patients with pulmonary embolism has not been established. In IV dosages of 40–100 mg over 2–7 hours or via the pulmonary artery in dosages of 30 or 50 mg over 1.5 or 2 hours, respectively, with or without concomitant heparin therapy, rt-PA produces clot lysis within 2–6 hours in more than 80% of patients with angiographically documented pulmonary emboli. However, substantial hemodynamic and angiographic improvement with such dosages of rt-PA has not been universally observed. Lysis of pulmonary emboli with rt-PA generally has been associated with early hemodynamic improvement and reversal of right ventricular dysfunction, and IV infusion appears to be as effective as administration via the pulmonary artery. Rapid IV injection† (e.g., over 2 minutes) of rt-PA also has been used effectively in a limited number of patients for the treatment of acute pulmonary embolism. Further comparative studies are needed to establish the efficacy, safety, and optimum dosage of rt-PA compared with heparin or comparable therapeutic dosages of streptokinase or urokinase , and to determine the effects of the therapies on morbidity and mortality, in the treatment of acute pulmonary embolism.

■ **Acute Ischemic Stroke** Alteplase is used in the management of acute ischemic stroke for improving neurologic recovery and reducing the incidence of disability. Current data from randomized, placebo-controlled studies and pooled analyses of such studies indicate that prompt initiation of alteplase treatment (within at least 3 hours but up to 4.5 hours following onset of stroke symptoms†) can result in long-term (e.g., 3-month) improvements in residual neurologic deficit, disability, and functional outcome following acute ischemic stroke with no net change in mortality. However, *because benefit from thrombolytic therapy decreases substantially with time, such therapy should be administered as soon as possible following onset of stroke symptoms to obtain optimal benefit*; experts recommend a "door-to-needle" time (i.e., from arrival at the treating facility until injection of alteplase) of no more than 1 hour. Treatment with alteplase in these studies has been associated with an increased incidence of intracranial hemorrhage, and careful diagnosis and patient selection are necessary to minimize the risk of hemorrhage and maximize benefit in patients with acute ischemic stroke. Therapy with alteplase in acute ischemic stroke should be initiated only in patients carefully selected according to history and physical examination and in whom intracranial hemorrhage has been excluded by cranial computed tomography (CT) scan or other diagnostic imaging method sensitive for the presence of hemorrhage. Reassurance regarding the safety and efficacy of alteplase in clinical practice is provided by the results of large phase 4 studies that included a variety of treatment centers, including academic and community hospitals with frequent and infrequent use of thrombolytic agents; a multicenter study (Safe Implementation of Thrombolysis in Stroke-Monitoring Study) in almost 6500 patients found incidences of symptomatic intracranial hemorrhage and 3-month mortality similar to or lower than those in placebo-controlled trials of alteplase given within 3 hours of symptom onset in acute stroke based on analyses of pooled data from those trials. Postmarketing surveillance and pooled analyses of data including a randomized trial in which alteplase was administered within 3–4.5 hours of symptom onset also indicate no increase in outcomes (risk of symptomatic intracranial hemorrhage, mortality, functional independence) compared with that in randomized trials in which the drug was given within 3 hours of symptom onset.

Current evidence from randomized studies and pooled analyses of data indicate that initiation of alteplase up to 4.5 hours following the onset of symptoms of stroke provides a net benefit in terms of reducing disability, and the American Heart Association/American Stroke Association (AHA/ASA) and other experts currently recommend administration of alteplase within up to 3–4.5 hours of the onset of symptoms in eligible patients. The importance of administering thrombolytic therapy as soon as possible after symptom onset is indicated by the results of a pooled analysis of data from 6 randomized, placebo-controlled trials of alteplase therapy in acute ischemic stroke, which found that such therapy was almost twice as effective when administered within 0–1.5 hours following onset of stroke symptoms (odds of a favorable outcome at 3 months: 2.81) as when administered 1.5–3 hours following onset of symptoms (odds of a favorable outcome at 3 months: 1.6). Based on a subsequent pooled analysis of data that also included a randomized study in which alteplase was administered up to 4.5 hours after symptom onset, it was estimated that substantial benefit was attained in 1 of 3 patients receiving the drug within 0–3 hours and in 1 of 6 patients receiving the drug within 3–4.5 hours after symptom onset. The safety of alteplase treatment administered more than 4.5 hours after symptom onset, in dosages higher than 0.9 mg/kg and without careful blood-pressure management, has not been established; a pooled analysis of data from several randomized trials of alteplase in acute ischemic stroke suggests that administration of the drug more than 4.5 hours following onset of stroke symptoms may even be associated with an increased risk of mortality.

ACCP, AHA, and ASA state that intra-arterial infusion† of alteplase may be used within 6 hours of symptom onset† in patients not otherwise eligible for IV thrombolysis who have middle cerebral artery occlusion†. Although studies demonstrating the benefits of intra-arterial thrombolysis exclusively enrolled patients with middle cerebral artery occlusions, ACCP states that the results can be generalized to acute occlusions of any proximal cerebral blood vessel because of similar pathophysiology and accessibility. AHA and ASA suggest that intra-arterial infusion of alteplase is reasonable in patients who have contraindications to IV thrombolysis (e.g., recent surgery); however, these experts state that the availability of intra-arterial thrombolysis generally should not preclude the use of IV alteplase in otherwise eligible patients. AHA and ASA do not recommend the use of thrombolytic therapy in patients with major early ischemic changes on baseline CT scan (defined as clearly identifiable hypodensity involving more than one-third of the middle cerebral artery territory). The manufacturer states that safety and efficacy of treatment with alteplase in patients with minor neurologic deficit or with rapidly improving symptoms prior to initiation of alteplase treatment have not been evaluated and such treatment is not recommended.

Several randomized, controlled trials in patients with acute ischemic stroke individually have failed to show statistically significant benefits of alteplase therapy in reducing disability from stroke; possible reasons for such findings include a lack of statistical power (e.g., small sample size), inclusion of patients who received the drug up to 6 hours after symptom onset or had less severe strokes, and/or choice of end points. Analyses of pooled data from these trials indicated that benefit from treatment decreased as time from stroke onset to start of treatment increased. In a subsequent 2-part, randomized, placebo-controlled study conducted by the National Institute of Neurological Disorders and Stroke (NINDS) rt-PA Stroke Study Group, treatment with alteplase (0.9 mg/kg IV to a maximum dose of 90 mg) was associated with improved functional outcome in adults with acute ischemic stroke who received the drug within 3 hours of symptom onset. All patients had CT scans at 24 hours and at 7–10 days after the onset of stroke and when clinical findings suggested intracranial hemorrhage. Blood pressure was carefully monitored and controlled (systolic and diastolic blood pressure maintained at 185 and 110 mm Hg, respectively, or less) in the study, and concomitant administration of aspirin or heparin was not allowed. In part 1 of the NINDS study, which evaluated neurologic improvement at 24 hours after stroke onset, the proportion of patients with an improvement of at least 4 points in the NIH Stroke Scale (NIHSS) or complete recovery (NIHSS score = 0) was not significantly different with alteplase or placebo treatment, although NIHSS scores suggested improvement in the condition of alteplase-treated patients at 3 months. This long-term (3-month) clinical benefit of alteplase treatment was confirmed in part 2 of the NINDS study; patients receiving alteplase were at least 30% more likely to have minimal or no disability at 3 months (as determined by median scores on the Barthel Index, Modified Rankin Scale, Glasgow Outcome Scale, and NIHSS) than those receiving placebo. In part 2, the favorable outcome of minimal or no disability occurred in at least 11% more patients treated with alteplase than in those receiving placebo. Alteplase treatment resulted in a more favorable outcome than placebo regardless of the type of stroke diagnosed at study entry or of prior aspirin use.

Combined analysis of the incidences of all-cause, 90-day mortality, intracranial hemorrhage, and new ischemic stroke for patients in both parts of the NINDS study indicated a significant increase in intracranial hemorrhage, particularly symptomatic intracranial hemorrhage within 36 hours, with alteplase therapy compared with placebo. The total incidence of intracranial hemorrhage during the study follow-up period was 15.4 or 6.4% with alteplase or placebo, respectively. Symptomatic intracranial hemorrhage (defined as the occurrence of sudden clinical worsening followed by subsequent verification of intracranial hemorrhage on CT scan) occurred in 8 versus 1.3% of alteplase- or placebo-treated patients, respectively, while symptomatic intracranial hemorrhage within 36 hours after the onset of stroke was found in 6.4 versus 0.6% of these respective groups. The incidence of asymptomatic intracranial hemorrhage (defined as intracranial hemorrhage detected on a routine repeat CT scan without preceding clinical worsening) was similar among patients receiving alteplase (7.4%) or placebo (5.1%), as was the incidence of new ischemic stroke at 3 months (5.8 versus 4.5% with alteplase or placebo, respectively). Alteplase therapy was not associated with increases in the incidences of 90-day mortality or severe disability compared with placebo.

There was a trend toward increased risk of symptomatic intracranial hemorrhage within the first 36 hours in patients with severe neurologic deficit (e.g., NIHSS score exceeding 22) or those of advanced age (e.g., patients greater than 77 years of age). Similar trends were observed for total intracranial hemorrhage and all-cause, 90-day mortality in these patients. When risk was assessed by the combination of death and severe disability in these patients, there was no difference between placebo and alteplase groups. Analyses of efficacy suggested a reduced but still favorable clinical outcome for alteplase-treated patients with severe neurologic deficit or advanced age on pretreatment evaluation.

In another randomized, placebo-controlled, phase 3 trial (ECASS-3), patients with acute ischemic stroke who received alteplase (0.9 mg/kg IV to a maximum dose of 90 mg) within up to 4.5 hours† following onset of stroke symptoms (median time: 3 hours 59 minutes following onset of symptoms) had more favorable clinical outcomes than those receiving placebo, and overall results with regard to efficacy and safety were consistent with those of an earlier trial (NINDS study) indicating efficacy of alteplase given within 3 hours of onset of stroke symptoms. The primary efficacy end point in the ECASS-3 trial, disability at day 90 (defined as a modified Rankin scale score of 0 or 1, indicating a favorable outcome of minimal or no disability) was achieved in 52.4 or 45.2% of those receiving alteplase or placebo, respectively. Alteplase recipients also had a 28% greater likelihood of attaining a favorable outcome in terms of a global composite secondary efficacy end point that assessed the patient's ability to return to an independent lifestyle. As in other trials of alteplase therapy for acute ischemic stroke, the incidence of symptomatic intracranial hemorrhage was higher with alteplase therapy (2.4%) than with placebo (0.2%); however, mortality was similar between the groups (7.7 or 8.4% with alteplase therapy or placebo, respectively). The incidence of intracranial hemorrhage was not substantially increased despite allowing the use of subcutaneous heparin to prevent deep-vein thrombosis in the first 24 hours after alteplase treatment, an exclusion criterion in earlier trials. Patient selection criteria for the ECASS-3 trial were similar to those of earlier trials of alteplase in acute ischemic stroke (e.g., NINDS) except that patients older than 80 years of age, those with severe stroke (a baseline National Institutes of Health Stroke Scale score exceeding 25), and those with a history of both stroke and diabetes were excluded. Therefore, some clinicians recommend close adherence to the ECASS-3 inclusion and exclusion criteria when treating patients with onset of stroke symptoms between 3 and 4.5 hours.

■ **Arterial Thrombosis and Embolism** rt-PA has been administered by selective intra-arterial injection in a limited number of adults for lysis of arterial occlusions† in peripheral vessels and bypass grafts. Angiographic and clinical improvement generally have occurred in more than 80% of patients treated with dosages of 0.05–0.1 mg/kg per hour, or even lower dosages (e.g., 0.02 mg/kg per hour) in a few patients, for 1–8 hours; however, most patients with acute arterial occlusion require further therapeutic intervention after thrombolysis. ACCP suggests the use of intra-arterial thrombolytic therapy in patients with acute limb ischemia due to arterial emboli or thrombosis; however, surgical reperfusion is preferred over thrombolytic therapy. If thrombolytic therapy is used in such patients, ACCP suggests that a recombinant tissue plasminogen activator (e.g., alteplase) or urokinase is preferred. In neonates and children with limb- or organ-threatening (via proximal extension) femoral artery thrombosis who fail to respond to initial treatment with unfractionated heparin, thrombolytic therapy is recommended unless such therapy is contraindicated. Like other thrombolytic agents, rt-PA probably should be avoided in patients with arterial emboli originating from the left side of the heart (e.g., in patients with mitral stenosis accompanied by atrial fibrillation or those with left ventricular thrombi) because of the potential risk of new embolic episodes, including those involving cerebral vessels. (See Cautions: Other Adverse Effects.)

■ **Occluded Catheters** Alteplase is used to restore patency to central venous catheters obstructed by a thrombus (assessed by the ability to withdraw blood). Causes of catheter dysfunction other than thrombus formation, such as catheter malposition, mechanical failure, constriction by a suture, lipid deposits, or drug precipitates, should be considered before instillation of alteplase. Pooled results of a placebo-controlled study and a large open-label study indicate that about 68% of central venous catheters occluded for less than 14 days were cleared (as determined by the successful withdrawal of 3 mL of blood and infusion of 5 mL of saline through the catheter) with a single dose of alteplase (2 mg) and about 88% of occluded catheters were cleared after a second dose of alteplase, administered 120 minutes after the first dose. The incidence of recurrent catheter dysfunction within 30 days after treatment was 26%. Restoration of catheter function was similar among all catheter types studied (single, double, or triple lumen; implanted ports). Results of an open-label study evaluating the efficacy of the drug in restoring catheter function in pediatric patients (2 weeks to 17 years of age) indicate that 83% of the occluded catheters (defined by the inability to withdraw at least 3 mL of blood from the catheter in children weighing at least 10 kg or at least 1 mL in children weighing less than 10 kg) were cleared with up to 2 doses of alteplase (2 mg/2 mL in children weighing at least 30 kg or 110% of the estimated lumen volume not to exceed 2 mg/2 mL in children weighing less than 30 kg) in up to 120 minutes postdose.

Alteplase has been used for clearing totally or partially occluded hemodialysis access catheters†. Studies of alteplase in patients with occluded hemodialysis catheters have evaluated similar dosing regimens as those currently used for clearing central venous catheters.

■ **Other Uses** rt-PA has been used for lysis of subocclusive intracoronary thrombi in a small number of patients with unstable angina pectoris†. Additional studies are needed to elucidate the role, including the relative benefits and risks, of rt-PA in the management of this condition.

Although thrombolytic agents have been used for the treatment of acute proximal deep-vein thrombosis†, anticoagulant therapy generally is recommended as the treatment of choice for venous thromboembolism. rt-PA also has been administered intraocularly for dissolution of fibrin after intraocular surgery†. Additional studies are necessary to determine the role of therapy with rt-PA in patients with these and other thromboembolic conditions.

rt-PA has been used for the treatment of cardiac arrest associated with acute pulmonary embolism†. Some evidence from nonrandomized observational studies suggests that systemic thrombolysis may improve return of spontaneous circulation (ROSC) and short-term mortality in patients with cardiac arrest associated with pulmonary embolism; earlier administration (rather than after initial failure of standard advanced cardiovascular life support [ACLS] measures) appears to be associated with improved outcomes.

Dosage and Administration

■ **Reconstitution and Administration** Alteplase is administered by IV infusion and by intracatheter instillation into occluded central venous catheters (Cathflo® Activase®, and the manufacturer states that the drug is intended for this method of administration only. The drug preferably should be administered via a controlled-infusion device using separate IV tubing. Alteplase also has been administered by intracoronary† injection, selective intra-arterial† infusion, and intraocularly† via intracameral injection in a limited number of patients.

Alteplase is reconstituted by adding 50 mL of sterile water for injection without preservatives to a vial labeled as containing 50 mg of drug using a large-bore (e.g., 18-gauge) needle and directing the stream of diluent into the lyophilized plug of powder; diluents other than sterile water for injection without preservatives should *not* be used for reconstitution. (See Chemistry and Stability: Stability.) The resultant solution contains approximately 1 mg of alteplase per mL. If foaming (usually slight) occurs during reconstitution, the vial should be left undisturbed for several minutes after addition of the diluent to allow dissipation of any large bubbles. The reconstituted solution may be used as reconstituted (1 mg/mL) or may be further diluted just prior to administration to a concentration of approximately 0.5 mg/mL using 0.9% sodium chloride injection or 5% dextrose injection; more dilute solutions should *not* be used since precipitation of the drug may occur at concentrations less than 0.5 mg/mL. Other infusion solutions, including sterile water for injection without preservatives or preservative-containing solutions, should not be used for dilution of the reconstituted solution. During dilution of the reconstituted solution, the solution should be mixed with gentle swirling and/or slow inversion of the infusion container; excessive agitation should be avoided. The manufacturer's labeling should be consulted for information on the reconstitution and dilution of vials labeled as containing 100 mg of the drug and for detailed instructions on preparing doses of alteplase for IV infusion.

Alteplase powder for restoring patency of central venous catheters (Cathflo® Activase®) is reconstituted by adding 2.2 mL of sterile water for injection to a vial labeled as containing 2 mg of alteplase to provide a concentration of 1 mg/mL. Bacteriostatic water for injection should *not* be used as a diluent. If foaming (usually slight) occurs during reconstitution, the vial should be left undisturbed for several minutes after addition of the diluent to allow dissipation of any large bubbles.

Reconstituted solutions of alteplase should be inspected visually for particulate matter and discoloration before further dilution or administration whenever solution and container permit. Because alteplase powder for injection or intracatheter instillation and reconstituted and diluted solutions of the drug contain no preservatives, the solutions preferably should be prepared immediately before use, but may be used for up to 8 hours after reconstitution or dilution; any unused solution should be discarded.

Administration into Occluded Central Venous Catheters When Cathflo® Activase® is used to restore patency of central venous catheters, 2 mL (i.e., 2 mg of alteplase) of the reconstituted solution is used for each catheter clearing process in patients weighing at least 30 kg. In patients weighing less than 30 kg, 110% of the internal lumen volume is instilled into the occluded catheter up to a maximum of 2 mL.

■ **Dosage** Dosage of alteplase usually is expressed in mg of drug but also may be expressed in international units (IU, units); each mg is equivalent to 580,000 units.

Acute Myocardial Infarction Alteplase therapy should be initiated *as soon as possible* after the onset of symptoms of myocardial infarction (MI) since potential clinical benefit diminishes as the time period to initiation of therapy increases. (See Uses: Acute Myocardial Infarction.) Some experts recommend that thrombolytic therapy be administered within 30 minutes of hospital arrival.

Various dosage regimens have been employed in patients treated with rt-PA for lysis of coronary artery thrombi. Alteplase may be administered by IV infusion over 3 hours or as an "accelerated" infusion over 1.5 hours. Controlled studies comparing clinical outcomes with these regimens have not been performed. However, pooled analyses of data from thrombolytic trials indicate that an accelerated infusion of alteplase is associated with greater rates of patency of the infarct-related artery than with a standard 3-hour infusion, and some experts consider the accelerated infusion regimen of alteplase to be the preferred method of administration. Although a dose of 150 mg of alteplase was used in early studies with the drug, this dose should *not* be used for the treatment of acute MI because of its association with an increased incidence of intracranial bleeding.

3-Hour Infusion. For lysis of coronary artery thrombi associated with acute MI, the usual adult dose of alteplase currently recommended is 100 mg (58 million units) IV over a 3-hour period, given as an initial 60-mg (34.8 million units) lytic dose during the first hour (of which 6–10 mg is infused rapidly over 1–2 minutes) and a subsequent maintenance infusion at a rate of 20 mg (11.6 million units) per hour for the next 2 hours. For adults weighing less than 65 kg (lean or actual body weight, whichever is less), a dose of 1.25 mg/kg may be infused IV over 3 hours as an initial lytic dose of 0.75 mg/kg during the first hour (of which 0.045–0.075 mg/kg is infused rapidly over 1–2 minutes) and a subsequent maintenance infusion at a rate of 0.25 mg/kg per hour for the next 2 hours.

Accelerated Infusion. When administered as an accelerated infusion for lysis of coronary artery thrombi associated with MI, the dose of alteplase is based on patient weight but should not exceed 100 mg. In adults weighing more than 67 kg, the usual dose of alteplase is 100 mg given by IV infusion; an initial 15-mg dose is given by rapid IV injection (e.g., over 1–2 minutes) followed by 50 mg IV over the next 30 minutes then 35 mg IV over the next hour. In patients weighing 67 kg or less, an initial 15-mg dose of alteplase is given by rapid IV injection (e.g., over 1–2 minutes), followed by 0.75 mg/kg (not to exceed 50 mg) over the next 30 minutes then 0.5 mg/kg (not to exceed 35 mg) over the next hour. The manufacturer states that the safety and efficacy of alteplase given by accelerated infusion has only been evaluated with concomitant heparin and aspirin administration. Although a dose of 150 mg of alteplase was used in early studies with the drug, this dose is no longer recommended because of its association with an increased incidence of intracranial bleeding.

Acute Pulmonary Embolism Various dosage regimens of rt-PA, including alteplase, have been used in adults for the management of acute pulmonary embolism, and the optimal dosage regimen for rt-PA in patients with this condition has not been established. For lysis of acute pulmonary emboli involving obstruction of blood flow to a lobe or multiple segments of the lungs, the usual adult dose of alteplase currently recommended is 100 mg (58 million units) IV over a 2-hour period. The manufacturer states that heparin should be instituted or reinstituted near the end of or immediately following the alteplase infusion when the activated partial thromboplastin time (aPTT) or thrombin time returns to twice the normal value or less. Alteplase also has been infused via the pulmonary artery† in adults in dosages of 30 or 50 mg over 1.5 or 2 hours, respectively, with concomitant heparin therapy. Lysis of pulmonary emboli usually has occurred within 2–6 hours after initiation of the IV or intra-arterial infusion, and IV infusion of the drug appears to be as effective as administration via the pulmonary artery.

Acute Ischemic Stroke For the treatment of acute ischemic stroke, the recommended dosage of alteplase is 0.9 mg/kg (up to a maximum dose of 90 mg) given by IV infusion over 1 hour, with 10% of the dose administered initially by rapid IV infusion over 1 minute. *The dosage of alteplase for the treatment of acute ischemic stroke should not exceed 0.9 mg/kg (maximum 90 mg).* For optimum benefit, alteplase should be administered as soon as possible, within at least 3–4.5 hours following onset of stroke symptoms. Heparin anticoagulation that produces an elevated aPTT should not be used within 48 hours of the use of alteplase. Administration of aspirin within 24 hours of the use of a thrombolytic agent is not recommended by AHA and the American Stroke Association (ASA). In patients with acute ischemic stroke who have not received recent anticoagulation therapy (e.g., oral anticoagulants, heparin), therapy with alteplase may be initiated prior to coagulation study results. However, infusion of alteplase should be discontinued if pretreatment coagulation study results are abnormal (as indicated by an INR exceeding 1.7, a prothrombin time exceeding 15 seconds, or an elevated aPTT).

Arterial Thrombosis and Embolism For lysis of arterial occlusion† in a peripheral vessel or bypass graft, alteplase usually has been infused intra-arterially in a dosage of 0.05–0.1 mg/kg per hour for 1–8 hours, although there is limited evidence that even lower dosages (e.g., 0.02 mg/kg per hour over 1–7 hours) may be effective. Regardless of the regimen used, however, some patients with acute arterial occlusion require further therapeutic intervention after thrombolysis.

Occluded Catheters To clear an occluded central venous IV catheter, 2 mg of alteplase in 2 mL of sterile water for injection is administered into the occluded catheter in patients weighing at least 30 kg. In patients weighing less than 30 kg, a volume of the alteplase solution equal to 110% of the internal lumen volume of the catheter should be instilled, up to a maximum of 2 mg of alteplase in 2 mL of solution. After at least 30 minutes of dwell time, catheter function is assessed by attempting to aspirate blood. When patency is restored, 4–5 mL of blood in patients weighing at least 10 kg or 3 mL of blood in patients weighing less than 10 kg should be aspirated to remove all drug and residual clot. An aspiration attempt may be repeated at 120 minutes of dwell time, and a second injection of alteplase (2 mg for a total of 4 mg) may be necessary in resistant cases. The American College of Chest Physicians (ACCP) suggests that a second dose of alteplase may be administered after 30 minutes of dwell time if the catheter remains occluded. The catheter should then be gently irrigated with 0.9% sodium chloride injection. If catheter patency is not successfully established after 2 doses of alteplase, ACCP suggests radiologic imaging to rule out a catheter-related thrombus.

When alteplase has been used to clear occluded hemodialysis access catheters†, several regimens have been employed. In a limited number of studies, 1–2 mg of alteplase were injected directly into the occluded catheter and allowed to remain for at least 30 minutes of dwell time. Catheter function was assessed by measurement of blood flow rate at the next hemodialysis session; blood flow rates of 200–300 mL/minute indicated successful restoration of patency of the hemodialysis access catheter. Some patients required additional intracatheter instillations of alteplase for reocclusion of hemodialysis access catheters after successful establishment of patency. Some clinicians have used 2 mg of alteplase in a total volume of 2 mL by direct injection into the catheter after a hemodialysis session and then aspirated the lumen contents before the next hemodialysis session in patients with indwelling catheters. Other clinicians have infused 2.5–5 mg of alteplase over 2–3 hours in each access port in patients with occluded hemodialysis catheters.

Cautions

The incidence of adverse effects associated with the intracatheter instillation of alteplase is not affected by age or gender. For adverse effects reported with alteplase therapy in the Cautions section, a causal relationship to the drug has not always been established. The most frequent and severe adverse effect of rt-PA therapy, including alteplase, is hemorrhage.

■ **Effects on Hemostasis** Almost all patients receiving rt-PA, including alteplase, in clinical studies have received concomitant therapy with heparin and/or platelet-aggregation inhibitors; therefore, the incidence of bleeding complications attributable solely to rt-PA is difficult to determine. Bleeding during rt-PA therapy occurs most frequently at sites of vascular access (e.g., insertion sites of arterial or venous catheters, venipuncture sites) and generally is not severe enough to require blood transfusion; avoidance of invasive procedures lessens the risk of hemorrhage associated with rt-PA therapy. Extravasation of alteplase during IV infusion of the drug can cause ecchymosis and/or inflammation. Management consists of terminating the infusion at that IV site and application of local therapy.

The hemostatic status of the patient may be more profoundly altered with rt-PA therapy than with heparin or coumarin-derivative anticoagulant therapy. Evidence from clinical trials indicates that the incidence of hemorrhagic complications associated with rt-PA therapy is similar to that observed with streptokinase (no longer commercially available in the US) or urokinase (no longer commercially available in the US) therapy, even though the extent of systemic fibrinogenolysis appears to be less with rt-PA. (See Pharmacology: Fibrinolytic Effects.) Although rt-PA is a relatively fibrin-selective thrombolytic agent, no currently available thrombolytic agent can discriminate between fibrin in pathologic thrombi and fibrin in hemostatic plugs. Therefore, bleeding from sites of percutaneous trauma occurs frequently, and bleeding related to lysis of fibrin clots at hidden sites of vascular injury also would be expected during rt-PA therapy. In addition, rt-PA administration has been associated with the production of fragment X, an intermediary fibrin/fibrinogen degradation product that forms clots more susceptible to plasmin lysis than those formed by fibrin; thus, it has been suggested that dissolution of hemostatic plugs into which fragment X has been incorporated may account in part for bleeding complications observed with rt-PA therapy.

Severe spontaneous (i.e., unrelated to catheter or other puncture sites) bleeding, including cerebral, retroperitoneal, genitourinary, respiratory tract, and GI bleeding, has occurred during rt-PA therapy and can be fatal (e.g., secondary to cerebral hemorrhage or other serious internal hemorrhage). Upper airway hemorrhage (sometimes fatal) at the site of traumatic intubation in patients with orolingual angioedema has been reported rarely with alteplase therapy. Less severe spontaneous bleeding, such as superficial hematoma or ecchymoses, hematuria, hemoptysis, epistaxis, and gingival bleeding, also can occur in patients receiving rt-PA. Painful purpuric lesions at the site of prior cutaneous trauma have been reported in at least one patient receiving the drug.

Limited evidence suggests that patients with prolongation of template bleeding time after rt-PA therapy may be at increased risk of serious spontaneous bleeding. Concomitant therapy with anticoagulants (e.g., heparin) or platelet-aggregation inhibitors may contribute to bleeding observed with rt-PA therapy.

The risk of alteplase-induced intracranial (e.g., cerebral) bleeding appears to be dose-related and is increased in patients receiving an IV dose of 150 mg compared with lower doses (e.g., 100 mg); therefore, use of a 150-mg dose currently is *not* recommended. In the Thrombolysis and Angioplasty in Myocardial Infarction (TAMI) study, there was a 0.5% incidence of life-threatening intracranial hemorrhage in patients receiving alteplase 150 mg IV over 5–8 hours. However, in a pilot study prior to the second phase of the Thrombolysis in Myocardial Infarction (TIMI-2) trial in which the same dose of alteplase (150 mg) was infused IV over 6 hours, intracranial bleeding occurred in approximately 1.5–1.6% of patients. Because the incidence of intracranial hemorrhage in previous studies using predominantly two-chain rt-PA (prepared by Genentech roller-bottle method but not currently available) or alteplase (which is the predominantly one-chain form of rt-PA) was approximately 0.3–0.5%, the maximum dose of alteplase was reduced to 100 mg in subsequent studies, and more stringent exclusion criteria were established (i.e., patients with a history of cerebrovascular disease or severe hypertension were excluded). Follow-up data in patients receiving the 100-mg dose of rt-PA in the TIMI trial indicate a substantial reduction in the incidence of intracranial hemorrhage (0.6% incidence) compared with that in patients receiving 150 mg. Differences in the reported incidence of intracranial hemorrhage in various clinical trials of thrombolytic therapy may reflect inconsistent use of techniques (e.g., computed tomography) capable of distinguishing between hemorrhagic and occlusive stroke. The incidence of stroke (all etiologies) in several large controlled studies of patients with acute myocardial infarction (MI) receiving thrombolytic agents has ranged from approximately 0.5–1%, which is similar to or less than that in patients receiving placebo in most of these studies. In evaluating the potential for intracranial hemorrhage in patients treated with alteplase, consideration should be given to evidence from large studies indicating that the incidence of stroke in patients with acute MI not treated with thrombolytic agents is approximately 1–2%. Intracranial hemorrhage and other major bleeding complications may be more common in geriatric patients and in patients with a history of cerebrovascular accident or severe or poorly controlled hypertension, and thrombolytic therapy should be initiated only after careful screening for contraindications such as previous neurologic events, severe hypertension, and potential bleeding sites. (See Cautions: Precautions and Contraindications.)

Although a few studies have reported a correlation between reduction in fibrinogen concentrations or elevation in fibrin/fibrinogen degradation products and bleeding, laboratory monitoring of the effect of thrombolytic agents on the hemostatic system generally has not been useful for predicting bleeding complications associated with such therapy. Clotting rate assays that measure only intact, rapidly coagulable fibrin (e.g., Clauss method) may underestimate the clotting ability of the blood because the limited fibrinogen breakdown produced by alteplase often produces only slowly coagulable degradation products (e.g., fragments X and Y) that are not measured by these assays, rather than incoagulable final fibrin/fibrinogen degradation products (FDPs). Therefore, if hemostatic indices are monitored during alteplase therapy, an assay that measures both intact fibrinogen and slowly coagulable fibrin degradation products (e.g., Ratnoff and Menzie method) may provide a better indication of total blood clotting activity. Since fibrinogen degradation resulting from in vitro activation of plasminogen by rt-PA may occur in blood samples obtained from patients receiving pharmacologic doses of the drug, blood samples for analysis of coagulation indices should be collected with a serine protease inhibitor such as aprotinin (150–200 units/mL) or D-phenylalanyl-L-prolyl-L-arginine chloromethyl ketone hydrochloride (PPACK). Activation of plasminogen to plasmin by high concentrations of t-PA also may occur during freezing and thawing of blood samples. Therefore, plasma for determination of plasminogen concentrations should be separated promptly from erythrocytes and frozen rapidly to prevent falsely low assay results. PPACK rather than aprotinin is preferred for use in blood samples that also will be used for determination of plasma plasminogen concentrations, since aprotinin interferes with the results of this assay.

Histopathologic studies in patients treated with thrombolytic therapy versus coronary angioplasty alone for acute MI indicate that thrombolytic therapy and/or the reperfusion produced by such therapy may predispose to hemorrhagic MI, which may in part explain the lack of clinical improvement in ventricular function in some patients receiving thrombolytic agents.

■ **Hypersensitivity Reactions** Since t-PA is a naturally occurring substance, it generally is not considered immunogenic, and sustained antibody formation has not been documented to date in patients receiving alteplase. However, detectable levels of antibody against alteplase have been found in a few patients receiving the drug, although subsequent (12 days to 10 months later) antibody determinations were negative. Studies evaluating antibody formation in patients receiving intracatheter instillation of alteplase have not been performed. Allergic-type reactions (e.g., anaphylactoid reaction, laryngeal edema, orolingual angioedema, rash, urticaria) have been reported with IV alteplase therapy, but not with intracatheter instillation of the drug. The onset of orolingual angioedema occurs during and up to 2 hours after infusion of alteplase. In many instances, such patients were receiving concomitant angiotensin-converting enzyme (ACE) inhibitors. When such reactions occur, they usually respond to conventional therapy. (See Cautions: Precautions and Contraindications.) There is only limited experience with repeated courses of alteplase therapy. It is not known whether the risk of an immunologic reaction is increased with repeated administration of alteplase, and use of alteplase in patients who previously received the drug should be undertaken with caution. If an anaphylactoid reaction occurs during administration of alteplase, the infusion should be discontinued immediately. Appropriate therapy for the management of the reaction should be instituted with IV or intracatheter instillation of alteplase.

■ **Arrhythmias** Rapid lysis of coronary artery thrombi by thrombolytic agents may be associated with reperfusion-related atrial and/or ventricular arrhythmias. Arrhythmias most commonly associated with reperfusion include accelerated idioventricular rhythm and ventricular premature complexes and, less frequently, ventricular fibrillation; atrial premature complexes, atrial fibrillation, junctional rhythm, ventricular tachycardia, and sinus bradycardia also have been observed. Reperfusion-related arrhythmias usually are transient, but immediate treatment occasionally may be required. The appearance of these arrhythmias, along with reduction in chest pain and in ST-segment elevation, has been used as a noninvasive indicator of successful reperfusion following thrombolytic therapy. However, information to date suggests that the accuracy of noninvasive measurements in predicting coronary artery patency is insufficient for routine use in clinical decision making. Patients receiving rt-PA, including alteplase, for acute MI should be monitored carefully for possible arrhythmias during and immediately after administration of the drug, and appropriate antiarrhythmic therapy for bradycardia and/or ventricular irritability should be available during administration of the drug.

AV block or cardiac arrest has been reported in patients with acute MI receiving alteplase in clinical trials and during postmarketing surveillance.

■ **Other Adverse Effects** Nausea and/or vomiting, hypotension, and fever have been reported in patients receiving rt-PA, including alteplase. These effects frequently are observed in patients with MI and may or may not be attributable to the drugs.

Cerebral infarction, possibly resulting from partial lysis and embolization of an intraventricular thrombus, has occurred in at least one patient after repeated therapy with rt-PA following a short period (i.e., 3 days) without heparin therapy. The thrombus in this patient may have formed in a documented dyskinetic portion of the left ventricle. New ischemic stroke, which may be potentially fatal, has been reported in patients with an acute ischemic stroke receiving alteplase in clinical trials or during postmarketing surveillance. Therefore, it is important that the benefits versus risks of rt-PA therapy be carefully considered, particularly when the potential for acute intraventricular thrombus exists. (See Cautions: Precautions and Contraindications.) Cholesterol crystal embolization and associated serious complications in the absence of antecedent invasive vascular procedures have been reported rarely in patients receiving thrombolytic therapy, including alteplase. This serious condition, which can be fatal, also is associated with invasive vascular procedures (e.g., cardiac catheterization, angiography, vascular surgery) and/or anticoagulant therapy. Clinical features of cholesterol embolization may include livedo reticularis, "purple toe" syndrome, acute renal failure, gangrenous digits, hypertension, pancreatitis, MI, cerebral infarction, spinal cord infarction, retinal artery occlusion, bowel infarction, and rhabdomyolysis. Potentially fatal adverse effects, such as thromboembolism or recurrent thromboembolic events (myocardial reinfarction, recurrent ischemia, or pulmonary re-embolization) have occurred in patients with acute MI or pulmonary embolism receiving alteplase in clinical trials or during postmarketing surveillance. Subclavian and upper extremity deep-vein thrombosis has been reported in patients receiving alteplase to restore patency of occluded IV catheters. These thromboses may have been related to the underlying disease process, the presence of a long-term indwelling catheter, or to the drug. A pediatric patient who had an indwelling ventral venous catheter for 2 years experienced rupture of the lumen of the catheter upon instillation of alteplase.

Catheter-related sepsis occurred in a small number of patients receiving alteplase to restore patency of occluded IV catheters. Sepsis occurred within 15 minutes to 3 days after treatment with alteplase in adult patients, and these patients had positive catheter or peripheral blood cultures within 24 hours after symptom onset. Sepsis occurred in 3 pediatric patients 2–44 hours after treatment with alteplase. All of these patients had evidence of infection prior to intracatheter instillation of alteplase. An additional pediatric patient developed fever and lethargy requiring anti-infectives within 1 day of intracatheter instillation of the drug. Instillation of alteplase into infected catheters may spread a localized infection into the systemic circulation.

Thrombocytopenia has been reported in a few patients treated with rt-PA for acute MI; however, the role, if any, of rt-PA in the development of thrombocytopenia is uncertain because most of these patients were receiving multiple drugs, including heparin, and other predisposing factors were present in some patients.

Other potentially fatal adverse cardiovascular, respiratory, or cerebrovascular effects have occurred in patients with acute MI, pulmonary embolism, or acute ischemic stroke receiving alteplase in clinical trials or during postmarketing experience. Cardiovascular effects such as cardiogenic shock, heart failure, myocardial rupture, electromechanical dissociation, pericardial effusion, pericarditis, mitral regurgitation, or cardiac tamponade have occurred in patients with acute MI receiving alteplase. Pleural effusion has been reported in patients with pulmonary embolism receiving alteplase. Hypotension, pulmonary edema, or fever has been reported in patients with either acute MI or pulmonary embolism receiving alteplase. Cerebral edema or herniation or seizures have been reported in patients with acute ischemic stroke receiving alteplase.

Precautions and Contraindications

The overall clinical status and history of the patient must be assessed carefully before initiation of alteplase therapy, and the anticipated benefits weighed against the possible risks of therapy with the drug. In addition to the precautions that follow, the section in Cautions on Effects on Hemostasis should be reviewed for further precautionary information associated with the use of alteplase.

Most clinicians do not recommend routine monitoring of hemostatic indices such as fibrinogen concentrations or thrombin times during therapy with rt-PA, including alteplase, for acute MI, although monitoring hemostatic function has been suggested for patients who exhibit bleeding. Some clinicians state that determination of plasma fibrinogen also may be useful after discontinuance of thrombolytic therapy for correcting potential hemostatic abnormalities before anticipated surgery or other invasive procedures; monitoring of other coagulation indices (e.g., activated partial thromboplastin time) may be indicated for adjusting subsequent anticoagulant therapy.

The possibility of bruising or hematoma formation, especially after IM injections, is high during rt-PA therapy. Careful selection of patients for rt-PA therapy and monitoring of all potential bleeding sites (e.g., sites of all venous cutdowns, arterial and venous punctures, needle punctures) in patients receiving the drug are required to minimize the risk of bleeding. IM injections and nonessential handling of the patient should be avoided, and invasive venous procedures, including venipunctures, should be performed carefully and as infrequently as possible. If bleeding from the site of an invasive procedure or other trauma is not serious, rt-PA may be continued while closely observing the patient; local measures such as application of pressure should be initiated immediately. Arterial and venous invasive procedures in areas that are inaccessible to manual compression (e.g., internal jugular or subclavian punctures) should be avoided before and during alteplase therapy; if an arterial puncture is absolutely essential, it should be performed by a clinician experienced in the procedure, preferably using an artery in an upper extremity (e.g., radial or brachial). Pressure should be applied to the puncture site for at least 30 minutes, followed by application of a pressure dressing and frequent inspection of the puncture site for evidence of bleeding.

If serious spontaneous bleeding occurs, therapy with rt-PA and any concomitant anticoagulants should be discontinued immediately and appropriate hemostatic therapy initiated as needed; simply reducing the rate of infusion of rt-PA usually will not stop bleeding. If serious bleeding at a critical location (e.g., intracranial, GI, retroperitoneal, pericardial) occurs with intracatheter instillation of alteplase, therapy with the drug should be discontinued immediately and the drug should be withdrawn from the catheter. Plasma volume expanders other than dextrans may be used to replace blood volume deficits; if blood loss has been extensive, administration of packed red blood cells is preferred to whole blood. Administration of fresh frozen plasma or cryoprecipitate also may be indicated. Some clinicians recommend therapy with an antifibrinolytic agent such as aminocaproic acid or tranexamic acid in cases of life-threatening bleeding (e.g., intracranial hemorrhage); however, the efficacy of such therapy has not been established to date.

Patients should be monitored during and several hours following alteplase infusion for signs of orolingual angioedema. If such a reaction occurs in a patient receiving alteplase, the patient should be given appropriate therapy (e.g., antihistamines, epinephrine, IV corticosteroids) and consideration should be given to discontinuing the drug.

In patients with suspected acute pulmonary embolism, the diagnosis should be confirmed objectively using pulmonary angiography or a noninvasive procedure such as lung scanning. It should be kept in mind that treatment of pulmonary embolism with rt-PA, including alteplase, may not constitute adequate therapy of underlying deep-vein thrombosis, and the potential risk of reembolization resulting from lysis of deep venous thrombi should be considered.

Blood pressure should be monitored frequently and controlled during and following the administration of alteplase for the management of acute ischemic stroke. In the NINDS study, blood pressure was monitored for 24 hours and was actively controlled (systolic and diastolic blood pressure maintained at 185 and 100 mm Hg, respectively, or less) during this period with appropriate medication. The concomitant use of aspirin or heparin during the first 24 hours after symptom onset was not allowed in the NINDS study. Administration of aspirin within 24 hours of the use of thrombolytic agents is not recommended by the American Heart Association (AHA) and American Stroke Association (ASA). In the management of acute ischemic stroke, alteplase therapy can be initiated prior to the availability of coagulation study results in patients without recent use of oral anticoagulants or heparin. However, infusion of the drug should be discontinued in patients in whom a pretreatment prothrombin time exceeding 15 seconds, an INR exceeding 1.7, or an elevated aPTT is identified.

Treatment of patients with acute ischemic stroke with alteplase should be limited to facilities that can provide appropriate evaluation and management of intracranial hemorrhage. In the differential diagnosis of acute ischemic stroke, care must be taken in making an accurate diagnosis in patients with blood glucose abnormalities (i.e., blood glucose less than 50 mg/dL or exceeding 400 mg/dL).

In acute ischemic stroke, neither the incidence of intracranial hemorrhage nor the benefits of therapy are known in patients treated with alteplase more than 3 hours after the onset of symptoms. *Therefore, treatment of patients with acute ischemic stroke more than 3 hours after symptom onset generally is not recommended.* In addition, the American College of Chest Physicians (ACCP) does not recommend alteplase therapy in patients with symptoms of ischemic stroke of unknown duration. However, in carefully selected patients with evidence of middle cerebral artery occlusion (as demonstrated by angiograms) and no signs of major early infarction (as demonstrated on a CT scan), intra-arterial thrombolytic therapy may be administered to patients within 6 hours of symptom onset.

Alteplase therapy for acute MI or pulmonary embolism is contraindicated in patients with active internal bleeding, history of cerebrovascular accident or intracranial hemorrhage, intracranial neoplasm, aneurysm, or recent intracranial or intraspinal surgery or trauma (closed head trauma, facial trauma). The drug also is contraindicated in patients with known bleeding diathesis, arteriovenous malformation, severe uncontrolled hypertension, or suspected aortic dissection.

Alteplase therapy for acute ischemic stroke is contraindicated in patients with evidence of intracranial hemorrhage on pretreatment evaluation, suspicion of subarachnoid hemorrhage, recent (within 3 months) intracranial or intraspinal surgery, or serious head trauma or recent previous stroke, history of intracranial hemorrhage, uncontrolled hypertension at time of treatment (e.g., systolic or diastolic blood pressure exceeding 185 or 110 mm Hg, respectively), hypertension requiring aggressive treatment, seizure at onset of stroke, active internal bleeding, recent (within 3 weeks) GI or urinary tract hemorrhage, or intracranial neoplasm, arteriovenous malformation, or aneurysm. In addition, some clinicians do not consider use of alteplase in patients with abnormal blood glucose concentrations (i.e., less than 50 mg/dL or greater than 400 mg/dL), pregnant women, recent lumbar puncture, or post-MI pericarditis. Alteplase also is contraindicated in patients with acute ischemic stroke who have a known bleeding diathesis, including but not limited to patients currently receiving oral anticoagulants (e.g., warfarin sodium) who have a prothrombin time exceeding 15 seconds or an INR exceeding 1.7, those in whom heparin has been administered within 48 hours preceding the onset of stroke and who have an elevated activated partial thromboplastin time (aPTT) on pretreatment evaluation, and those who have platelet counts less than 100,000/mm^3.

The risks of therapy with alteplase for any approved indication in patients with any of the following conditions are increased and should be weighed against the potential benefits: recent major surgery (e.g., coronary artery bypass, obstetric delivery, organ biopsy, previous puncture of noncompressible vessels), cerebrovascular disease, hypertension (systolic blood pressure of 175 mm Hg or more and/or diastolic blood pressure of 110 mm Hg or more); high likelihood of left heart thrombus (e.g., mitral stenosis with atrial fibrillation, profound left ventricular dyskinesia), acute pericarditis, subacute bacterial endocarditis, hemostatic defects (e.g., those secondary to severe hepatic or renal disease), substantial liver dysfunction, recent (within 6 months) internal (e.g., GI or genitourinary) bleeding, or recent (within the last 2–4 weeks) trauma. Other relative contraindications to thrombolytic therapy include active peptic ulcer and traumatic or prolonged chest compression (cardiopulmonary resuscitation [CPR] lasting more than 10 minutes). The risks of alteplase therapy for any approved indication also should be weighed against the anticipated benefits in patients with diabetic hemorrhagic retinopathy or other hemorrhagic ophthalmic conditions, septic thrombophlebitis, or an occluded arteriovenous cannula at a seriously infected site; geriatric patients older than 75 years of age; patients receiving concurrent therapy with oral anticoagulants (e.g., warfarin); pregnant women (See Cautions: Pregnancy, Fertility, and Lactation); and those with any other condition in which bleeding constitutes a substantial hazard or would be particularly difficult to manage because of its location. Menstruation generally should not be considered a contraindication to thrombolytic therapy.

The manufacturer and other clinicians state that the risks of alteplase therapy for the treatment of acute ischemic stroke may be increased and should be weighed against anticipated benefits in patients with severe neurologic deficit (e.g., NIH Stroke Scale [NIHSS] score greater than 22) on pretreatment evaluation (because of an increased risk of intracranial hemorrhage in such patients) and in patients with major early infarct signs on CT scan (e.g., substantial edema, mass effect, midline shift). However, AHA and ASA state that thrombolytic therapy almost always should *not* be administered to patients with major early infarct signs (greater than one-third of the middle cerebral artery territory and clearly identifiable hypodensity on CT scan).

Pediatric Precautions

Safety and efficacy of IV infusion of alteplase in children have not been established. However, the drug has been used with some success in a few infants and children with thrombosis of the vena cava, aorta, or peripheral arteries; successful lysis of pulmonary emboli without bleeding complications also has been reported in at least one child with angiographically documented pulmonary emboli of undetermined duration who received 0.1 mg/kg of alteplase per hour for 11 hours via the pulmonary artery†. Thrombolytic therapy generally is not recommended for the treatment of venous thromboembolism in neonates and children unless vessel occlusion is life-threatening and/or causes organ dysfunction. If thrombolysis is required, ACCP states that alteplase is the drug of choice.

Use of thrombolytic therapy in children with arterial ischemic stroke is not recommended by ACCP outside of a research setting.

Safety and efficacy of intracatheter instillation of alteplase for the restoration of central venous catheters in pediatric patients (2 weeks to 17 years) is similar to that observed in adults.

Mutagenicity and Carcinogenicity

Alteplase did not exhibit mutagenic potential in in vitro chromosomal aberration studies in human lymphocytes or in microbial (Ames) test systems with or without metabolic activation at concentrations of 6.25–50 mcg/mL. Cytotoxicity (evidenced by a decrease in mitotic index) was apparent only after prolonged (i.e., for 48–72 hours) exposure at 50 mcg/mL, the highest concentration tested. Long-term studies in animals to determine the carcinogenic potential of alteplase have not been performed to date. There was no evidence of tumorigenic effects or effects on tumor metastases in short-term studies in animals.

■ **Pregnancy, Fertility, and Lactation** Although no adequate studies have been performed in pregnant women, animal reproduction studies indicate that IV alteplase has been embryocidal in rabbits given the drug at a dosage of 3 mg/kg, representing approximately 2 times the human dosage used for the treatment of acute MI. Alteplase should be used during pregnancy only when clearly needed. Some clinicians consider the use of alteplase for ischemic stroke to be contraindicated in pregnant women. However, therapy with rt-PA followed by IV heparin treatment has been used successfully for lysis of pulmonary emboli in a pregnant woman with congenital antithrombin III deficiency. Approximately 20 hours following discontinuance of rt-PA therapy, at week 35 of pregnancy, the patient delivered a male infant by cesarean section. No placental bleeding occurred and the infant showed no signs of bleeding, but he died later from complications related to respiratory distress syndrome. Another pregnant woman with massive pulmonary embolism and circulatory shock at week 31 of pregnancy who was treated successfully with rt-PA (10 mg/hour for 4 hours followed by 2 mg/hour for 1.5 hours) delivered an otherwise healthy premature infant 48 hours following thrombolytic therapy.

It is not known whether the drug can affect fertility.

It is not known whether alteplase is distributed into milk, and the drug should be used with caution in nursing women.

Drug Interactions

The interaction of alteplase with other cardioactive or cerebroactive drugs has not been studied. In addition to bleeding associated with heparin and vitamin K antagonists (e.g., warfarin), drugs that alter platelet function (e.g., aspirin, dipyridamole, abciximab) may increase the risk of bleeding if administered prior to, during, or after alteplase therapy.

■ **Thrombolytic Agents** In vitro clot lysis studies have failed to show substantial synergistic effects with t-PA and an investigational plasminogen activator, single-chain urokinase plasminogen activator (scu-PA, prourokinase). However, in animals, simultaneous administration of t-PA and scu-PA in a molar ratio of 1:3 demonstrated synergistic thrombolytic effects without associated systemic fibrinogen breakdown. Synergistic thrombolysis also has been observed in preliminary studies in patients with acute myocardial infarction (MI) who received predominantly two-chain rt-PA (no longer currently available in the US) and recombinant scu-PA in doses of each approximately one-fourth the usual doses. Concomitant administration of t-PA and urokinase (no longer commercially available in the US) has been associated with synergistic thrombolytic effects in animals. However, in a study in patients with acute MI, combined use of alteplase and urokinase was not associated with synergistic thrombolysis, although a substantial reduction in the rate of reocclusion after coronary thrombolysis did occur and was not accompanied by an increase in bleeding complications. Further studies are needed to determine the efficacy and safety of alteplase therapy combined with other thrombolytic agents in patients with acute MI.

■ **Anticoagulants** In almost all patients receiving alteplase for the treatment of acute MI in clinical studies, heparin, followed by oral anticoagulants in some cases, has been administered before, during, and/or after alteplase therapy to reduce the risk of coronary artery reocclusion. However, concomitant use of alteplase and an anticoagulant may increase the risk of hemorrhage, and careful monitoring for bleeding is necessary, especially at arterial puncture sites. Anticoagulant therapy should be discontinued immediately and appropriate therapy (e.g., protamine sulfate in patients receiving heparin) instituted as necessary if serious bleeding occurs.

■ **Drugs Affecting Platelet Function** Platelet-aggregation inhibitors (e.g., aspirin, clopidogrel) also have been administered after alteplase therapy for the treatment of acute MI to reduce the risk of reocclusion of the infarct-related artery. Drugs that affect platelet function (e.g., aspirin, dipyridamole, abciximab) may increase the risk of bleeding if administered prior to, during, or after alteplase therapy.

In patients with acute stroke, the American Heart Association (AHA) and the American Stroke Association (ASA) do not recommend administration of aspirin within 24 hours of the use of a thrombolytic agent, as such adjunctive use of aspirin may increase the risk of bleeding from thrombolytic agents.

Acute Toxicity

Limited information is available on the acute toxicity of alteplase. In acute toxicity studies in animals, no unusual toxicities were observed beyond expected effects of alteplase on coagulation (e.g., dose-dependent depletion of coagulation proteins and production of fibrin degradation products [FDPs]). In subacute toxicity studies, decreased hemoglobin and hematocrit with a compensatory reticulocytosis were noted.

In general, overdosage of alteplase in humans may be expected to produce effects that are extensions of the pharmacologic and adverse effects of the drug, predominantly effects on hemostasis. (See Cautions: Effects on Hemostasis.)

Pharmacology

Alteplase, a recombinant DNA-derived form of human tissue-type plasminogen activator (t-PA), is a thrombolytic agent. Most studies of the pharmacology of t-PA have been performed using t-PA derived from human melanoma cell cultures or predominantly two-chain (prepared by Genentech roller-bottle method but not commercially available) recombinant t-PA (rt-PA). The amino acid sequence and biological properties of human melanoma cell t-PA are similar or identical to those of endogenous human t-PA from uterine tissue, and the amino acid sequence of alteplase is identical to that of human melanoma cell t-PA; therefore, differences between alteplase and human uterine tissue or melanoma cell t-PA apparently relate to variability in the carbohydrate moieties of the molecules. In the Pharmacology section, unless otherwise specified, the physiologic and pharmacologic effects of exogenously administered alteplase or other forms of rt-PA and endogenous human t-PA will be discussed in terms of endogenous human t-PA.

■ **Effects on Fibrinolytic System** In contrast to anticoagulants, which prevent propagation of thrombi, t-PA and other plasminogen activators such as streptokinase and urokinase (urinary-type plasminogen activator, u-PA) promote thrombolysis by hydrolyzing the arginine^{560}-valine^{561} peptide bond in plasminogen to form the active proteolytic enzyme plasmin. Plasmin is a relatively nonspecific serine protease that is capable of degrading fibrin, fibrinogen, and other procoagulant proteins, such as factors V, VIII, and XII.

During physiologic fibrinolysis, the activity of circulating plasmin is inhibited rapidly (half-life approximately 100 msec) by α_2-antiplasmin (α_2-plasmin inhibitor). Inhibitors such as α_2-macroglobulin, antithrombin III, and α_1-antitrypsin also react with plasmin, but more slowly, and are important particularly when systemic activation of large amounts of plasmin results in depletion of α_2-antiplasmin. The fibrinolytic activity of plasmin is maintained within the thrombus but minimized systemically because plasminogen is incorporated selectively into the thrombus when it is formed and because the active site and lysine-binding sites of plasminogen (and thus plasmin) at which fibrin binds are the same sites at which α_2-antiplasmin binds. Fibrin-bound plasmin within the thrombus, therefore, is relatively protected from inactivation by α_2-antiplasmin, although cross-linking of α_2-antiplasmin to fibrin renders the fibrin clot less susceptible to fibrinolysis by plasmin. Thrombolytic agents such as streptokinase and urokinase (no longer commercially available in the US) activate both fibrin-bound and circulating plasminogen indiscriminately; systemic activation of plasminogen results in the release of large amounts of plasmin into the circulation. Excess plasmin eventually depletes α_2-antiplasmin, leading to a "systemic lytic state" that is characterized by marked systemic fibrinogenolysis and degradation of other plasma procoagulant proteins.

Unlike streptokinase and urokinase, t-PA is a relatively fibrin-selective plasminogen activator. During in vitro and physiologic fibrinolysis, endogenous one-chain t-PA binds to fibrin and is converted rapidly to the two-chain form, which suggests that fibrinolysis from one-chain t-PA results principally from the action of the two-chain form. In the presence of fibrin, both one- and two-chain forms of t-PA have similar fibrinolytic and plasminogen-activating properties, although in the absence of fibrin, one-chain t-PA has substantially less activity. After binding to fibrin, t-PA acquires a high affinity for plasminogen. The binding of t-PA and plasminogen to the fibrin clot is associated with a conformational change in either t-PA or plasminogen. This binding increases the availability of plasminogen locally, which results in more efficient (several-hundred- to 1000-fold) activation of plasminogen at the fibrin surface than that occurring in circulation. In vitro studies suggest that the enhanced activation of plasminogen by one- or two-chain t-PA in the presence of fibrin is related to the increased affinity of fibrin-bound t-PA for plasminogen and to an increased catalytic efficiency which, for one-chain t-PA, appears to be associated with its conformational change upon binding to fibrin and confers enzymatic activity similar to that of the two-chain form. Inactivation by α_2-antiplasmin of plasmin generated at the fibrin surface within the thrombus occurs 100-fold more slowly (half-life approximately 10 seconds) than inactivation of circulating plasmin because the binding sites of α_2-antiplasmin on plasmin are occupied by fibrin. Thus, the sequentially formed ternary complex between t-PA, fibrin, and plasminogen facilitates localization of fibrinolytic activity to the site of the thrombus. However, the clot-selectivity of exogenously administered t-PA, including alteplase, is relative rather than absolute.

Dosages of exogenously administered t-PA required for rapid coronary artery reperfusion in patients with acute myocardial infarction (MI) may produce plasma t-PA concentrations 1000 times greater than physiologic levels; such concentrations overwhelm circulating inhibitors of t-PA and elicit variable degrees of fibrinogenolysis. Large doses and/or prolonged infusions of t-PA can produce a systemic lytic state, but usual therapeutic dosages of the drug result in less extensive fibrinogen breakdown and less accumulation of final fibrin/fibrinogen degradation products (i.e., fragments D and E) in plasma than usual therapeutic dosages of streptokinase or urokinase. Although a systemic lytic state generally is considered undesirable because of the associated impairment in hemostasis, some evidence suggests that some degree of fibrinogenolysis, with inhibition of fibrin production and/or interference with platelet function by circulating fibrin/fibrinogen degradation products, may enhance the efficacy of thrombolytic therapy by preventing rapid reformation of thrombi at sites of ongoing thrombolysis.

In clinical studies in patients with acute MI, the extent of systemic fibrinogenolysis produced by alteplase was less than that produced by the predominantly two-chain rt-PA (prepared by the Genentech roller-bottle method but not currently available) at dosages producing comparable rates of thrombolysis. This dissociation between thrombolytic and fibrinogenolytic effects appears to be attributable to the shorter plasma half-life of alteplase since both dosage of alteplase and duration of plasma concentrations of the drug may influence its fibrinogenolytic effects. Decreases of about 16–36% in plasma fibrinogen occur 3–6 hours after IV infusion in patients receiving 1.25 mg/kg or a total dose of 80–100 mg of alteplase. At these doses, plasminogen concentrations decreased by 25–49% 3–6 hours after IV infusion of 80 mg or 1–1.25 mg/kg of alteplase.

Failure of thrombolysis after administration of rt-PA, including alteplase, may be related to inadequate plasma concentrations of t-PA, inadequate duration of therapy, poor access to the site of the thrombus, deficiency of plasminogen, organization of the thrombus, absence of a thrombus, rupture of the coronary intimal plaque, or an intrinsic fibrinolytic defect; it also has been suggested that elevated concentrations of specific plasminogen activator inhibitors (e.g., PAI-1) identified in some men with MI occurring at an early age may attenuate the response to rt-PA and possibly contribute to the risk of coronary reocclusion.

For unexplained reasons, some patients with high plasma t-PA concentrations experience negligible fibrinogen breakdown, while others have extensive fibrinogenolysis in the presence of relatively low t-PA concentrations. Substantial interindividual variation in the response of the fibrinolytic system to alteplase has been observed, and it has been suggested that variability in the type of fibrinogen assay used may have confounded interpretation of the extent of fibrinogenolysis attributable to alteplase therapy. Use of assays that measure total clottable proteinrather than fibrinogen indicates that t-PA administration is associated with the formation of intermediary fibrinogen degradation products, principally fragment X, which are slowly clottable and form clots of less tensile strength than those formed by fibrin. Fragment X is not measured by fibrinogen assays based on coagulation rate, but some evidence suggests that its incorporation into hemostatic plugs may in part contribute to bleeding associated with rt-PA therapy. (See Cautions: Effects on Hemostasis.)

Although t-PA is cleared from the circulation rapidly, recovery from associated hemostatic defects depends on slower, thrombolytic agent-independent processes such as clearance of plasmin and fibrin/fibrinogen degradation products and synthesis of new clotting proteins.

Fibrinolytic activity after alteplase administration appears to be more intense and prolonged than that after streptokinase, probably because of sustained activity of alteplase bound to fibrin in the thrombus. Lysis of fibrin thrombi (as indicated by elevations in cross-linked fibrin degradation products and B-β-15-42 fibrinopeptide) has been detected up to 7 hours after discontinuance of alteplase infusion.

The activity of t-PA can be inhibited by one or more fast-acting plasminogen-activator inhibitors (e.g., PAI-1). In vitro evidence suggests that thrombin may regulate fibrinolytic activity by stimulating the release of PAI-1 and subsequently modulating its activity; the activity of the inhibitor appears to be inversely related to the concentration of thrombin. Low concentrations of these fast-acting inhibitors are present in healthy individuals but may be increased substantially in patients with certain diseases, such as venous thromboembolism or ischemic heart disease. Low t-PA activity, resulting mainly from elevated concentrations of PAI-1 and partially from impaired t-PA release, has been observed in patients with acute MI and in young men with recurrent infarction, especially in association with hypertriglyceridemia. This finding suggests that reduced fibrinolytic activity associated with elevated PAI-1 concentrations may be important in the pathogenesis of MI.

The thrombolytic efficacy and fibrin selectivity of both natural and recombinant human t-PA have been demonstrated in animal studies involving pulmonary embolism, venous thrombosis, or coronary artery thrombosis. In these studies, t-PA induced thrombolysis without substantial activation of circulating plasminogen, degradation of fibrinogen, or clinically evident bleeding. Timely reperfusion produced by t-PA after experimentally induced coronary artery thrombosis in animals has been associated with restoration of myocardial intermediary metabolism and substantial myocardial tissue salvage. In rabbits with experimentally induced jugular vein thrombosis, the extent of t-PA-induced thrombolysis depended mainly on the dose of t-PA and the delivery of the drug to the site of the thrombus; the age of the thrombus was a much less important determinant. In this study, t-PA was 5- to 10-fold more potent than urokinase, successfully lysing urokinase-resistant clots as old as 7 days. There also is limited evidence in humans to suggest that age of the thrombus is a much less important determinant of successful lysis with t-PA than these other factors.

■ **Other Effects on Hemostasis** Thrombolytic therapy paradoxically may transiently activate the coagulation system, which may decrease the patency of successfully reperfused infarct-related arteries in patients with acute MI. Some of the hemostatic markers (e.g., fibrinopeptide A, prothrombin fragments, thrombin-antithrombin complex) associated with thrombin activity or generation were increased for up to 1 day after initiation of thrombolytic therapy in patients with acute MI; plasma kallikrein (involved in the contact phase system of coagulation) concentrations also increased within 3 hours of initiation of thrombolytic therapy.

Studies in vitro and in animals indicate that t-PA and generated plasmin are associated with variable effects on platelets. Platelet activation has occurred in animals treated with t-PA or streptokinase and also has been reported in humans treated with streptokinase; this effect of plasminogen activators is transient and has been suggested to be a factor predisposing to reocclusion after thrombolytic therapy. However, prolonged exposure of platelets to plasmin or exposure to low concentrations of plasmin in vitro is associated with attenuated platelet aggregation. In addition, in vitro studies indicate that t-PA at pharmacologically achievable concentrations also may cause disaggregation of platelets, an effect that is potentiated by aspirin; platelets also may potentiate the activation of plasminogen by t-PA. In vitro studies indicate that t-PA also activates platelet- and thrombospondin-bound plasminogen, which may affect platelet-mediated hemostasis. Some clinicians suggest that these interactions of t-PA and platelets may contribute to lysis of platelet thrombi and subsequent bleeding in patients receiving therapeutic dosages of the drug. Platelets have been found to contain both activators of plasminogen and inhibitors of t-PA, and it has been suggested that the concentration of, and duration of exposure to, plasmin may be factors determining whether inhibition or stimulation of platelet aggregability occurs.

In vitro evidence indicates that t-PA binds to human endothelial cells and selectively activates plasminogen also bound to these cells; these effects may influence hemostasis and/or thrombosis at the vascular endothelial surface. t-PA forms circulating complexes with the first component of complement (C1) and also may activate the complement system in patients with MI. However, the importance of t-PA's effects on the complement system has not been established.

■ **Other Effects** There is limited evidence from animal studies that t-PA may have a cardioprotective effect independent of thrombolysis, but conflicting data have been reported, and additional study is necessary.

Pharmacokinetics

Pharmacokinetic data on exogenously administered tissue-type plasminogen activator (t-PA) consist of studies in which either alteplase or predominantly two-chain (prepared by Genentech roller-bottle method but not currently available) recombinant DNA-derived t-PA (rt-PA) was used; information on the pharmacokinetics of alteplase, which is predominantly one-chained, is derived from data in a relatively limited number of individuals.

Although an enzyme-linked immunosorbent assay (ELISA) specific for free (active) t-PA has been developed, most studies of the pharmacokinetics of rt-PA have used immunoradiometric or ELISA assays that measure concentrations of total (free and that complexed with inhibitors) t-PA. In addition, these assays apparently measure both endogenous t-PA and exogenously administered t-PA; however, pharmacologic dosages of rt-PA infused IV over 90 minutes produce plasma t-PA concentrations approximately 1000 times greater than endogenous t-PA levels, so the contribution of endogenous t-PA to plasma concentrations should be minimal. In the Pharmacokinetics section, unless otherwise specified, alteplase or rt-PA concentrations are expressed in terms of total t-PA.

■ **Absorption** Alteplase is not absorbed after oral administration and must be administered parenterally. A study in animals indicates that absorption of rt-PA is negligible when the drug is administered alone by IM injection, although absorption was facilitated to a limited extent by concomitant IM injection of rt-PA and hydroxylamine hydrochloride along with electrical stimulation of the muscle.

Endogenous t-PA in plasma exists in free form and in circulating complexes with plasma protease inhibitors, including PAI-1, α_2-antiplasmin, C_1-esterase inhibitor, and α_1-antitrypsin. Basal plasma concentrations of endogenous t-PA in healthy individuals are very low, averaging approximately 4–6 ng/mL; only about one-third of this represents free t-PA. Various physical and hormonal stimuli, including exercise, venous occlusion, and vasoactive substances such as epinephrine, vasopressin, desmopressin, niacin, or alcohol, increase endogenous t-PA concentrations.

Both the thrombolytic and fibrinolytic effects of alteplase appear to be dose dependent. In patients receiving maintenance IV infusions of alteplase, a plateau plasma t-PA concentration of 0.45 mcg/mL appeared to prevent coronary artery reocclusion after successful thrombolysis, while a plateau concentration of 0.34 mcg/mL did not. Although the extent of fibrinogenolysis in patients receiving alteplase appears to be dose dependent, laboratory indices of hemostatic function generally have not been useful for predicting the incidence of bleeding complications in patients receiving alteplase. (See Cautions: Effects on Hemostasis.)

Plasma t-PA concentrations in patients receiving alteplase generally are proportional to the rate of IV infusion. Plasma t-PA concentrations reported after alteplase administration in patients with acute myocardial infarction (MI) show considerably more interindividual variability than those in healthy individuals, possibly because of differences in hepatic blood flow and metabolism. In healthy individuals and in patients with acute MI, mean peak plasma concentrations following IV infusion of alteplase 7–11 mcg/kg per minute for 30–90 minutes (0.25- to 1-mg/kg doses) ranged from 0.7–1.8 mcg/mL; plateau plasma t-PA concentrations during a maintenance IV infusion of alteplase of approximately 2–3.3 mcg/kg per minute for 4–6 hours ranged from 0.34–0.45 mcg/mL.

■ **Distribution** It is not known whether alteplase crosses the placenta or distributes into milk or the CNS. The total volume of distribution of alteplase in patients with acute MI averages 27–53 L. The volume of distribution of alteplase in the central compartment (V_c) averages 3.2–6.6 L in patients with acute MI, and reportedly ranges from 1.7–6.1 L in patients with vascular thrombo-occlusive disease. In healthy men, V_c and the volume of distribution at steady state (V_{ss}) reportedly average approximately 3.9–4.3 and 7.2–12 L, respectively.

■ **Elimination** The mechanisms involved in the elimination of t-PA from blood are poorly understood. t-PA appears to be cleared principally by the liver, which subsequently releases degradation products into the blood. Animal studies indicate that at usual pharmacologic dosages initial rapid plasma clearance of t-PA occurs via a nonsaturable process in the liver (probably in the hepatocyte) that is not influenced by glomerular filtration rate (GFR); however, some evidence indicates that both active-site inhibition and the nature and extent of glycosylation influence t-PA's clearance from plasma. t-PA appears to be cleared principally as the free form (not complexed with an inhibitor). Because of the short half-life of t-PA, continuous infusion of the drug is probably necessary to achieve in vivo thrombolysis. Plasma clearance of t-PA after alteplase administration has ranged from 520–1000 mL/minute in patients with acute MI, and a mean plasma clearance of approximately 550 mL/minute has been reported in patients with thrombo-occlusive disease receiving the drug. In healthy men, mean plasma alteplase clearances of 690–730 mL/minute have been reported. More than 50% of t-PA is cleared from plasma within 5 minutes after discontinuance of an IV infusion of alteplase, and approximately 80% is cleared within 10 minutes.

The half-life of t-PA, like that of many other plasma proteins, is inversely proportional to body weight in animals. The decline in plasma t-PA concentrations following IV infusion of alteplase is biphasic, indicating that the pharmacokinetics of exogenously administered t-PA is adequately described by a two-compartment pharmacokinetic model. In a study in patients with MI, the half-lives of alteplase in the initial distribution phase ($t_{1/2\alpha}$) and in the terminal elimination phase ($t_{1/2\beta}$) averaged 3.6–4.6 and 39–53 minutes, respectively; mean $t_{1/2\alpha}$ and $t_{1/2\beta}$ averaged 4.4 and 26.5 minutes, respectively, in patients with thrombo-occlusive disease. In healthy men receiving alteplase, $t_{1/2\alpha}$ and $t_{1/2\beta}$ averaged 3.3–4.2 and 26–36 minutes, respectively. Limited evidence in animals suggests that the elimination half-life of t-PA may be prolonged in patients with severely impaired hepatic function and/or hepatic blood flow.

The excretion characteristics of alteplase and its degradation products have not been fully elucidated. There is limited evidence from healthy adults receiving radiolabeled human melanoma cell t-PA that exogenously administered t-PA is excreted mainly in urine, with about 80% of total radioactivity being excreted within 18 hours.

Chemistry and Stability

■ **Chemistry** Alteplase, a biosynthetic (recombinant DNA origin) form of the enzyme human tissue-type plasminogen activator (t-PA), is a thrombolytic agent. The drug is prepared from cultures of genetically modified mammalian (Chinese hamster ovary) cells using recombinant DNA technology. These cells have been modified by the addition of plasmids that incorporate genes for human t-PA synthesis. The plasmid for alteplase is synthesized using the complementary DNA (cDNA) for human t-PA obtained from the Bowes human melanoma cell line. Alteplase has an amino acid sequence identical to that of human melanoma t-PA, with possible differences only in the nature of the carbohydrate moieties.

Endogenous human t-PA is a glycosylated, trypsin-like serine protease (enzymatic glycoprotein) secreted principally by vascular endothelial cells. Endogenous human t-PA is secreted as a one-chain polypeptide, which may be cleaved at the arginine^{275}-isoleucine^{276} peptide bond by several endogenous proteases, including plasmin, tissue kallikrein, activated factor X (factor Xa), and trypsin, to form a two-chain derivative.

The two-chain t-PA molecule consists of a heavy chain beginning at the amino-terminal part of the molecule and a lighter chain arising from the carboxyl-terminal end; the chains are connected by a disulfide bond. The heavy or A chain contains 2 kringle regions (triple disulfide loops each consisting of approximately 82 amino acids) that are homologous with kringles found in prothrombin, single-chain urinary-type plasminogen activator (scu-PA, prourokinase), plasminogen, and urokinase (urinary-type plasminogen activator, u-PA). The light or B chain of t-PA contains the catalytic (active) site, which converts plasminogen to plasmin; this chain consists of histidine, aspartic acid, and serine residues and is structurally similar to the B chains of other serine proteases such as trypsin, elastase, urokinase (no longer commercially available in the US), plasmin, and thrombin. The primary structures of t-PA and high-molecular-weight urokinase are similar with the exception of a 43-amino acid "finger" region on the A chain of t-PA, which is homologous with the region in fibronectin responsible for its affinity for fibrin. Both the second kringle region and the "finger" region on the A chain of t-PA appear to be necessary for binding of t-PA to fibrin (i.e., fibrin selectivity); other portions of the molecule also may influence fibrin binding affinity.

The complete structure of human t-PA, as determined from the cDNA for t-PA expressed in *E. coli*, consists of a polypeptide of 562 amino acids, which includes a leader sequence of 35 amino acids and a mature protein of 527 amino acids. The mature t-PA protein contains 35 cysteine residues and 4 potential *N*-glycosylation sites at asparagine residues 117, 184, 218, and 448. Human t-PA has a molecular weight of approximately 70,000 to 72,000. Two variant forms (types I and II) of human t-PA that differ in carbohydrate composition and molecular weight have been identified by structural analyses of human melanoma cell t-PA and rt-PA. Type I melanoma cell t-PA is glycosylated at positions 117, 184, and 448, contains approximately 12.8% carbohydrate by weight, and has a molecular weight of approximately 63,000 to 70,000; type II melanoma cell t-PA has carbohydrate moieties at positions 117 and 448 only, contains approximately 7.1% carbohydrate by weight, and has a molecular weight approximately 2000–3000 less than that of type I t-PA. The variant glycosylation site is on the second kringle of the t-PA molecule. The asparagine residue at position 218 apparently is not glycosylated in either of the variant forms, presumably because the presence of a proline residue at this site prevents carbohydrate attachment. Removal of the carbohydrate moieties on human melanoma cell t-PA does not appear to affect the fibrin-binding or plasminogen-activating properties of the enzyme, although type II melanoma cell t-PA reportedly is more fibrin selective in its activation of plasminogen in vitro than is the type I form.

Commercially available alteplase is a glycosylated, predominantly (60–80%) one-chain form of t-PA consisting of 527 amino acids and 3 carbohydrate side chains. The carbohydrate moiety at asparagine residue 117 is a high-mannose oligosaccharide, while the oligosaccharides at asparagine residues 184 and 448 are of the fucosylated complex type; alteplase consists of both type I and type II forms of t-PA and contains approximately 7–10% carbohydrate by weight. The polypeptide portion of the alteplase molecule has an amino acid composition identical to that of human melanoma cell t-PA and a molecular weight of 59,000; the average molecular weight contributed by the carbohydrate moieties is 8000. The total molecular weight of alteplase ranges from 65,000 to 70,000, which reflects variations in the weights of the carbohydrate moieties.

Alteplase is commercially available as a white to off-white or white to pale yellow (Cathflo® Activase®), lyophilized powder. Phosphoric acid is added during manufacture to adjust pH. When reconstituted as directed with sterile water for injection, solutions containing 1 mg/mL of alteplase are colorless to pale yellow and transparent and have a pH of approximately 7.3. The drug itself is practically insoluble in water, having a solubility of less than 0.4 mcg/mL at pH 6 and 20°C. However, the presence of arginine in the commercially available powder for injection increases the aqueous solubility of alteplase substantially. Phosphoric acid and/or sodium hydroxide may be added before lyophilization to adjust pH. When reconstituted as directed with sterile water for injection, solutions containing 1 mg/mL of alteplase are colorless to pale yellow and transparent, and have a pH of approximately 7.3 and an osmolality of approximately 215 mOsm/kg. The powder for injection also contains arginine and polysorbate (Tween®) 80.

Potency of alteplase is determined using an in vitro clot lysis assay and is expressed in international units (IU; units) as tested against the WHO t-PA standard (purified from cultured human melanoma cells), which has an assigned potency of 850 units/ampul (425,000 units/mg). Each mg of commercially available alteplase has a potency of 580,000 units (range: 550,000 to 667,000 units).

■ **Stability** Alteplase powder for injection or for intracatheter instillation should be protected from excessive exposure to light and the IV injection should be stored at a room temperature of 15–30°C or refrigerated at 2–8°C. Alteplase lyophilized powder for intracatheter instillation should be refrigerated at 2–8°C. When stored as recommended, alteplase powder for injection has an expiration date of 2 years after the date of manufacture.

Alteplase is stable in solution over a pH range of 5–7.5. Alteplase powder for injection or intracatheter instillation contains no preservatives; when reconstituted with sterile water for injection, the solutions contain no preservatives and should be stored at 2–30°C and used within 8 hours. The drug is incompatible with bacteriostatic water for injection since the preservatives contained in this diluent can interact with the alteplase molecule. Following reconstitution with sterile water for injection and further dilution in 0.9% sodium chloride injection or 5% dextrose injection, solutions containing alteplase 0.5 mg/mL are stable for up to 8 hours at room temperatures not exceeding 30°C or when refrigerated; unused portions should be discarded after this time period. Exposure to light does not affect the stability of reconstituted or diluted solutions of the drug. Other solutions, including sterile water for injection or preservative-containing solutions, should *not* be used for further dilution of reconstituted alteplase, nor should any drug be admixed with alteplase. However, lidocaine hydrochloride, metoprolol tartrate, or propranolol hydrochloride reportedly is physically and/or chemically compatible when administered via a Y-site into the tubing of a freely flowing solution of alteplase in 5% dextrose or 0.9% sodium chloride injection.

Preparations

Excipients in commercially available drug preparations may have clinically important effects in some individuals; consult specific product labeling for details.

Alteplase (Recombinant DNA Origin)

Parenteral

For injection, for IV infusion	50 mg	**Activase®** (with sterile water for injection diluent), Genentech
	100 mg	**Activase®** (with sterile water for injection diluent), Genentech
For solution, for IV catheter clearance	2 mg	**Cathflo® Activase®**, Genentech

†Use is not currently included in the labeling approved by the US Food and Drug Administration

HEMATOPOIETIC AGENTS 20:16

Darbepoetin Alfa

■ Darbepoetin alfa, a biosynthetic (recombinant DNA origin) form of the glycoprotein hormone erythropoietin, is a hematopoietic agent that principally affects erythropoiesis.

Uses

■ **Anemia of Chronic Kidney Disease** Darbepoetin alfa is used for the treatment of anemia associated with chronic kidney disease (CKD) in patients who currently are undergoing dialysis and in those who do not yet require maintenance dialysis (predialysis patients). Clinical studies indicate that the drug increases and/or maintains hemoglobin concentrations in both dialysis-dependent and predialysis patients with CKD. Some evidence suggests that in patients with CKD who are undergoing hemodialysis or peritoneal dialysis, once-weekly IV or subcutaneous administration of darbepoetin alfa maintains hemoglobin concentrations as safely and effectively as equivalent doses of epoetin alfa administered 2 or 3 times weekly by the same route. In addition, administration of darbepoetin alfa once every other week appears to have similar efficacy as equivalent doses of subcutaneous epoetin alfa administered once weekly.

In a multicenter, double-blind, noninferiority study in adults with CKD undergoing hemodialysis who were stable on epoetin alfa, substitution of IV darbepoetin alfa given once weekly (median weekly dosage of 0.53 mcg/kg) was as effective as continuing IV epoetin alfa therapy (3 times weekly) in maintaining hemoglobin within a range of 9–13 g/dL. In an open-label, randomized study in predialysis or dialysis-dependent pediatric patients 1–18 years of age with CKD who were stable on epoetin alfa therapy, a median subcutaneous or IV weekly dosage of darbepoetin alfa of 0.41 mcg/kg was required to maintain hemoglobin concentrations within the target range of 10–12.5 g/dL when substituted for epoetin alfa. Studies have not evaluated the use of darbepoetin alfa as *initial* treatment of anemia associated with CKD in pediatric patients.

Results of controlled studies in patients with CKD indicate that erythropoiesis-stimulating agents (ESAs), including darbepoetin alfa, may increase the risk for death, stroke, and serious cardiovascular events when targeted to achieve hemoglobin concentrations exceeding 11 g/dL. (See Increased Mortality and Cardiovascular and Thromboembolic Effects under Warnings/Precautions: Warnings, in Cautions.) The US Food and Drug Administration (FDA) has issued a series of public health advisories regarding these risks associated with ESAs and has recommended more conservative dosing of these drugs in patients with CKD. (See Anemia of Chronic Kidney Disease under Dosage and Administration: Dosage and also see Cardiovascular Precautions and Contraindications under Cautions: Precautions and Contraindications, in Epoetin Alfa 20:16.) Clinicians should weigh the potential benefits of ESA therapy in reducing the need for red blood cell transfusions against the risk of serious cardiovascular events in patients with CKD. Treatment should be individualized and the lowest possible ESA dosage that will reduce the need for red blood cell transfusions should be used.

Darbepoetin alfa is *not* intended for patients with CKD who require *acute* correction of severe anemia; the drug should *not* be used as a substitute for emergency transfusion.

■ **Anemia in Patients with Nonmyeloid Malignancies** ***Chemotherapy-induced Anemia*** Darbepoetin alfa is used for the treatment of chemotherapy-induced anemia in patients with nonmyeloid malignancies in whom chemotherapy is planned for at least 2 additional months. Therapy with darbepoetin alfa or other ESAs should be initiated only when the hemoglobin concentration is less than 10 g/dL and should be discontinued after completion of a course of myelosuppressive chemotherapy. The manufacturer states that darbepoetin alfa is not indicated for use in patients receiving hormonal agents, biologic products, or radiation therapy unless they also are receiving concomitant myelosuppressive chemotherapy.

Use of ESAs has been associated with shortened overall survival and/or an increased risk of tumor progression or recurrence in clinical studies in patients with breast, non-small cell lung, head and neck, lymphoid, or cervical cancer. *ESAs are not indicated for patients with chemotherapy-induced anemia in whom the anticipated outcome of chemotherapy is cure of the underlying malignancy.* ESAs have not been shown to improve outcomes of cancer chemotherapy (e.g., in terms of greater tumor shrinkage, delayed tumor progression, increased survival). (See Increased Mortality and Tumor Progression under Warning/Precautions: Warnings, in Cautions.) In addition, ESAs do not improve quality of life, fatigue, or well-being, in patients with chemotherapy-induced anemia. *Darbepoetin alfa is not indicated in patients with cancer and anemia who are not receiving cancer chemotherapy.* (See Chronic Anemia Associated with Malignancy under Uses: Anemia in Cancer Patients.)

Safety and efficacy of darbepoetin alfa given once weekly for chemotherapy-induced anemia were established in a randomized, placebo-controlled, double-blind, multinational study of 12 weeks' duration in anemic (hemoglobin concentration not exceeding 11 g/dL) patients with small cell or non-small cell lung cancer who were receiving a platinum-based chemotherapy regimen. In this study, 26% of patients receiving darbepoetin alfa (2.25 mcg/kg once weekly) required blood transfusions between week 5 (day 29) and the end of treatment compared with 50% of those receiving placebo.

Safety and efficacy of darbepoetin alfa given once every 3 weeks for the treatment of chemotherapy-induced anemia (hemoglobin concentration less than 11 g/dL) were established in a randomized, double-blind, double-dummy multinational, noninferiority study of 15 weeks' duration in patients with nonmyeloid malignancies who were receiving chemotherapy. Fixed-dose subcutaneous darbepoetin alfa in a dosage of 500 mcg once every 3 weeks was as least as effective as 2.25 mcg/kg given once weekly in reducing red blood cell transfusion requirements in such patients. In this study, 23% of patients receiving darbepoetin alfa once every 3 weeks required at least one red blood cell transfusion between week 5 (day 29) and the end of treatment compared with 28% of patients receiving the drug once weekly. Dosage of darbepoetin alfa was reduced by 40% of the previous dosage if hemoglobin concentrations increased by more than 1 g/dL in a 14-day period. Dosage reductions were required in 71 or 77% of patients receiving darbepoetin alfa once every 3 weeks or weekly, respectively.

The effects of darbepoetin alfa on overall survival were evaluated in a randomized placebo-controlled study in anemic (hemoglobin concentrations 9–13 g/dL) patients with previously untreated advanced-stage small cell lung cancer receiving platinum and etoposide chemotherapy. Treatment with darbepoetin alfa 300 mcg once weekly for the first 4 weeks followed by 300 mcg once every 3 weeks in such patients did not prolong overall survival compared with placebo.

Darbepoetin alfa is *not* intended for patients with chemotherapy-induced anemia who require *acute* correction of severe anemia; the drug should *not* be used as a substitute for emergency transfusion.

Chronic Anemia Associated with Malignancy Randomized controlled studies in patients with certain types of cancer and associated anemia who were *not* receiving cancer chemotherapy or radiation therapy† indicate that *ESAs may decrease overall survival in such patients.* In addition, ESA therapy did not reduce red blood cell transfusion requirements in these patients. The manufacturers of darbepoetin alfa and epoetin alfa state that ESAs are *not* indicated for use in anemic patients with active malignant disease who are *not* receiving cancer chemotherapy. (See Hematologic Precautions and Contraindications under Cautions: Precautions and Contraindications, in Epoetin Alfa 20:16.)

Dosage and Administration

■ **Administration** Darbepoetin alfa is administered by IV or subcutaneous injection; subcutaneous injections are preferred by some clinicians for predialysis and peritoneal dialysis patients because of the lack of existing accessible IV sites in such patients. The manufacturer recommends IV administration in patients with chronic kidney disease (CKD) undergoing hemodialysis. Patients who self-administer darbepoetin alfa should be instructed on proper administration of the drug and advised to follow the manufacturer's "Patient Instructions for Use".

Because of its longer plasma half-life, darbepoetin alfa should be administered less frequently than epoetin alfa. Patients being switched from epoetin alfa to darbepoetin alfa should receive darbepoetin alfa by the same route of administration (IV or subcutaneous) that they were receiving epoetin alfa. Patients receiving epoetin alfa 2 or 3 times weekly should be switched to darbepoetin alfa once weekly, and those receiving epoetin alfa once weekly should be switched to darbepoetin alfa once every 2 weeks. The first dose of darbepoetin alfa should be administered in place of epoetin alfa at the time of the next scheduled dose.

Darbepoetin alfa should *not* be diluted or administered in conjunction with other drug solutions. Commercially available prefilled syringes and single-use vials of darbepoetin alfa should *not* be exposed to light, frozen, or shaken prior to use; if shaken or frozen, the product should not be used. Unused portions of the single-use vials or prefilled syringes of darbepoetin alfa should be discarded and vials should not be reentered. Contents of vials and prefilled syringes of darbepoetin alfa should be inspected visually for discoloration and/or particulate matter prior to administration; if either is present, the solution should be discarded.

Iron status (i.e., transferrin saturation, serum ferritin concentration) should be evaluated prior to and during therapy in patients receiving darbepoetin alfa. Supplemental iron therapy should be initiated if serum ferritin concentration is less than 100 mcg/L or transferrin saturation is less than 20%. The manufacturer states that the majority of patients with CKD will require supplemental iron during the course of ESA therapy. Prior to initiating darbepoetin alfa therapy, other causes of anemia (e.g., vitamin deficiency, metabolic or chronic inflammatory conditions, bleeding) should be corrected or excluded.

■ **Dosage** ***Anemia of Chronic Kidney Disease*** Hemoglobin concentrations should be monitored at least weekly following initiation of darbepoetin alfa therapy and after each dosage adjustment until stable, then at least monthly thereafter. In controlled trials of patients with CKD, administration of ESAs to achieve hemoglobin concentrations exceeding 11 g/dL did not provide additional benefit beyond that achieved with lower hemoglobin targets and was associated with a greater risk of death, stroke, and serious adverse cardiovascular events; no trial to date has identified a target hemoglobin concentration, ESA dosage, or dosing strategy that does not increase these risks. (See Increased Mortality and Cardiovascular and Thromboembolic Effects under

Warnings/Precautions: Warnings, in Cautions.) The potential benefits of darbepoetin alfa in decreasing transfusion requirements should be weighed against the increased risk of death and other serious adverse cardiovascular events in this patient population.

Dosage of darbepoetin alfa should be individualized, and the lowest possible dosage sufficient to reduce the need for red blood cell transfusions should be used. FDA and the manufacturer state that patients with CKD *on dialysis* should have darbepoetin alfa therapy initiated when their hemoglobin concentration is less than 10 g/dL. If hemoglobin concentration approaches or exceeds 11 g/dL in such patients, dosage should be reduced or therapy interrupted. FDA and the manufacturer also state that consideration should be given to initiating darbepoetin alfa therapy in patients with CKD *not on dialysis* only when their hemoglobin concentration is less than 10 g/dL and the following 2 conditions also apply: the rate of hemoglobin decline indicates the likelihood of requiring a transfusion, and a goal of therapy is to reduce the risk of alloimmunization and/or other risks associated with red blood cell transfusions. If hemoglobin concentration exceeds 10 g/dL in such patients, dosage should be reduced or therapy interrupted.

For the treatment of anemia associated with CKD in dialysis-dependent patients, the recommended initial adult dosage of darbepoetin alfa is 0.45 mcg/kg administered IV or subcutaneously once weekly or 0.75 mcg/kg administered IV or subcutaneously once every 2 weeks as appropriate. In CKD patients *not* on dialysis, the recommended initial adult dosage of darbepoetin alfa is 0.45 mcg/kg administered IV or subcutaneously once every 4 weeks as appropriate.

For conversion of epoetin alfa therapy to darbepoetin alfa in adults and pediatric patients older than 1 year of age with CKD *on dialysis*, the manufacturer recommends the following initial dosage of darbepoetin alfa based on the weekly epoetin alfa dosage at the time of substitution. These dosage guidelines cannot be used to accurately estimate the once-monthly dosage of the drug in patients *not* on dialysis.

Table 1.

Previous Weekly Epoetin Alfa Dosage (units/week)	Initial Adult Weekly Darbepoetin Alfa Dosage (mcg/week)	Initial Pediatric Weekly Darbepoetin Alfa Dosage (mcg/week)
<1,500	6.25	—[a]
1,500–2,499	6.25	6.25
2,500–4,999	12.5	10
5,000–10,999	25	20
11,000–17,999	40	40
18,000–33,999	60	60
34,000–89,999	100	100
≥90,000	200	200

[a] For pediatric patients receiving a weekly epoetin alfa dosage of <1500 units/week, data are insufficient to determine initial darbepoetin alfa dosage.

Subsequent dosage of darbepoetin alfa should be adjusted based on hemoglobin concentrations. Factors including the rate of increase or decrease in hemoglobin concentrations, responsiveness to the ESA, and hemoglobin concentration variability also should be considered when determining whether a dosage adjustment is needed; a single hemoglobin excursion may not require a dosage change. Frequent dosage adjustments should be avoided.

If the hemoglobin concentration increases rapidly (e.g., by more than 1 g/dL in any 2-week period), dosage of darbepoetin alfa should be reduced by 25% or more as necessary to reduce the risk of a rapid response. However, if the hemoglobin concentration has not increased by more than 1 g/dL after 4 weeks of therapy, dosage of darbepoetin alfa should be increased by 25%. Dosage increases should not be made more frequently than once every 4 weeks. If an adequate response to darbepoetin alfa is not obtained over a 12-week period of escalating dosages, the patient should be evaluated for other causes of anemia; further dosage increases are not likely to improve patient response and may increase the risks of therapy. (See Lack or Loss of Response to Therapy under Warnings/Precautions: General Precautions, in Cautions and also see Increased Mortality and Cardiovascular and Thromboembolic Effects under Warnings/Precautions: Warnings, in Cautions.) The lowest dosage of darbepoetin alfa that will maintain a hemoglobin concentration sufficient to reduce the need for red blood cell transfusions should be used in such patients, and if responsiveness does not improve, the drug should be discontinued.

Chemotherapy-induced Anemia in Patients with Nonmyeloid Malignancies Therapy with darbepoetin alfa should only be initiated in cancer patients with hemoglobin concentrations of less than 10 g/dL and in whom a minimum of 2 additional months of chemotherapy is planned. Hemoglobin concentrations should be monitored weekly following initiation of therapy and after each dosage change until stable and sufficient to minimize the need for red blood cell transfusions. *Therapy with darbepoetin alfa or other ESAs should be discontinued in patients with cancer following completion of a chemotherapy course.*

For the treatment of chemotherapy-induced anemia in patients with nonmyeloid malignancies, the recommended initial adult dosage of darbepoetin alfa is 2.25 mcg/kg administered subcutaneously once weekly or 500 mcg administered subcutaneously once every 3 weeks until completion of a course of myelosuppressive chemotherapy. Dosage should be adjusted to achieve and maintain the lowest hemoglobin concentration sufficient to avoid the need for red blood cell transfusion.

The manufacturer states that the once-weekly dosage of darbepoetin alfa may be increased up to 4.5 mcg/kg weekly if the patient's hemoglobin concentration has increased by less than 1 g/dL and remains below 10 g/dL after 6 weeks of therapy; no dosage adjustment is recommended in patients receiving the every-3-week dosage regimen if such a response is not obtained. If patients receiving the once-weekly or every-3-weeks dosage regimen experience hemoglobin concentration increases of more than 1 g/dL in any 2-week period or achieve a hemoglobin concentration sufficient to avoid the need for red blood cell transfusions, dosage of darbepoetin alfa should be decreased by 40%. If the hemoglobin exceeds a concentration needed to avoid red blood cell transfusion in patients receiving either dosing schedule, administration of darbepoetin alfa should be withheld until the hemoglobin concentration decreases to a concentration at which transfusions may be required. At this point, therapy should be reinitiated at a dosage 40% below the previous dosage. If response to darbepoetin alfa is not satisfactory after 8 weeks of therapy (i.e., continuing need for red blood cell transfusions, low hemoglobin concentrations), the drug should be discontinued. *Therapy with darbepoetin alfa or other ESAs should be discontinued in patients with cancer following completion of a chemotherapy course.*

Darbepoetin alfa and other ESAs are *not* indicated for use in anemic patients with active malignant disease who are not receiving cancer chemotherapy. (See Hematologic Precautions and Contraindications under Cautions: Precautions and Contraindications, in Epoetin Alfa 20:16.)

■ **Special Populations** No special population dosage recommendations at this time.

Cautions

■ **Contraindications** Uncontrolled hypertension.

Pure red cell aplasia (PRCA) that begins after treatment with darbepoetin alfa or other erythropoietin proteins.

Serious allergic reactions to darbepoetin alfa.

■ **Warnings/Precautions** ***Warnings*** **Increased Mortality and Cardiovascular and Thromboembolic Effects.** Therapy with darbepoetin alfa and other erythropoiesis-stimulating agents (ESAs) has been shown to increase the risk of death and serious cardiovascular events (e.g., myocardial infarction, stroke, congestive heart failure, hemodialysis graft occlusion) when targeted to achieve hemoglobin concentrations exceeding 11 g/dL in patients with chronic kidney disease (CKD). (See Increased Mortality and Thromboembolic Effects under Cautions: Cardiovascular Effects, in Epoetin Alfa 20:16.) An increase in hemoglobin concentration exceeding 1 g/dL in a 2-week period also may contribute to these risks. Patients with CKD and an insufficient response to ESA therapy may be at even greater risk for cardiovascular events and death than other patients.

Data from several controlled clinical studies in patients with CKD comparing higher ESA hemoglobin target concentrations (13–14 g/dL) to lower targets (9–11.3 g/dL) indicate that an increased risk of death, myocardial infarction, stroke, congestive heart failure, hemodialysis vascular access thrombosis, and other thromboembolic events occurred in the higher target hemoglobin groups. In one of these studies, a randomized, double-blind, placebo-controlled study (Trial to Reduce Cardiovascular Events with Aranesp Therapy [TREAT]) in patients with type 2 diabetes mellitus, anemia, and nondialysis-dependent CKD, treatment with darbepoetin alfa targeted to yield a hemoglobin concentration of 13 g/dL failed to reduce the overall rates of the primary cardiovascular and renal composite end points, but was associated with an increased risk of stroke compared with placebo (annualized stroke rate of 2.1 versus 1.1%, respectively). This increased risk was documented despite use of a conservative dosing strategy and measures designed to ensure gradual increases and avoidance of overshoots and oscillations in hemoglobin concentrations. In this study, the relative risk of stroke was particularly high in patients with a prior history of stroke (annualized stroke rate of 5.2 in the darbepoetin alfa-treated group versus 1.9% in the placebo-treated group). Results of 2 randomized prospective studies in patients with CKD receiving another ESA (epoetin alfa) also demonstrated an increased risk of adverse cardiovascular outcomes; both trials were terminated early due to adverse safety findings of a higher incidence of mortality or a major cardiovascular event (death, myocardial infarction, stroke, hospitalization for congestive heart failure) in those randomized to higher (13.5–14 g/dL) versus lower (10–11.3 g/dL) hemoglobin targets.

An increased incidence of thromboembolic events (e.g., pulmonary embolism, thromboembolism, thrombophlebitis [deep and/or superficial], thrombosis), some serious and life-threatening, also has been observed in cancer patients receiving darbepoetin alfa or other ESAs (epoetin alfa). The incidences of fatal thromboembolic/vascular events and overall mortality reportedly were higher in women with metastatic breast cancer who received an epoetin alfa preparation with a goal of achieving and maintaining hemoglobin concentrations of 12–14 g/dL (hematocrit: 36–42%).

An increased incidence of deep-vein thrombosis has been observed in patients undergoing orthopedic surgical procedures and receiving an ESA (epoetin alfa) to reduce allogeneic red blood cell transfusion requirements. Increased mortality associated with thrombotic events also has been reported with epoetin alfa in patients undergoing coronary artery bypass graft surgery (CABG)†. *Darbepoetin alfa is not labeled by the US Food and Drug Administration*

(FDA) for reduction of the need for red blood cell transfusions in patients undergoing surgery. (See Increased Mortality and Thromboembolic Effects under Cautions: Cardiovascular Effects, in Epoetin Alfa 20:16.)

Increased Mortality and Tumor Progression. ESA therapy has been associated with increased mortality and risk of tumor progression or recurrence in patients with cancer. Epoetin alfa, another ESA, shortened overall survival and increased deaths attributed to disease progression in women with metastatic breast cancer receiving cancer chemotherapy and shortened time to tumor progression in patients with advanced head and neck cancer receiving radiation therapy. Shortened overall survival was also noted in patients with lymphoid malignancy receiving darbepoetin alfa and cancer chemotherapy. Overall and progression-free survival rates were numerically lower in women with early breast cancer receiving neo-adjuvant cancer treatment and in patients with cervical cancer receiving cancer chemotherapy and radiation therapy with darbepoetin alfa or epoetin alfa therapy, respectively, targeted to hemoglobin concentrations of 12–14 g/dL. A higher locoregional failure rate or shortened locoregional progression-free survival was observed in patients with squamous cell carcinoma of the head and neck receiving radiation therapy and darbepoetin alfa or epoetin beta (not currently available in the US). In addition, patients with cancer-related anemia and non-small-cell lung cancer or nonmyeloid malignancy who were *not* receiving cancer chemotherapy or radiation therapy had an increased risk of death and no reduction in transfusion requirements while receiving epoetin alfa or darbepoetin alfa, respectively; *ESAs are not currently FDA-labeled for use in patients with cancer-related anemia who are not receiving myelosuppressive chemotherapy.* FDA and the manufacturers of ESAs currently recommend that ESAs *not* be used in patients in whom the anticipated outcome of cancer chemotherapy is cure of the underlying malignancy. (See Hematologic Precautions and Contraindications under Cautions: Precautions and Contraindications, in Epoetin Alfa 20:16.)

Hypertension and Seizures. Blood pressure may increase during treatment with darbepoetin alfa. In clinical studies, approximately 40% of patients with CKD required initiation or intensification of antihypertensive therapy during the early phase of darbepoetin alfa treatment. Use of darbepoetin alfa is contraindicated in patients with uncontrolled hypertension; blood pressure should be adequately controlled prior to initiation of therapy. If blood pressure becomes difficult to control, dosage of darbepoetin alfa should be reduced or therapy withheld.

Darbepoetin increases the risk of seizures in patients with CKD. Hypertensive encephalopathy and seizures also have been observed in patients with CKD treated with darbepoetin alfa. Blood pressure and the presence of premonitory neurologic symptoms should be closely monitored in patients receiving the drug, particularly during the first several months of therapy. (See Risk Evaluation and Mitigation Strategy under Advice to Patients.)

Pure Red Cell Aplasia. Pure red cell aplasia (PRCA) and severe anemia with or without other cytopenias in association with neutralizing antibodies to endogenous erythropoietin have been reported during postmarketing experience in patients receiving ESAs, including darbepoetin alfa. PRCA occurred predominantly in patients with CKD receiving ESAs subcutaneously. However, antibody-mediated PRCA resulting in transfusion-dependent anemia also has been reported in patients receiving ESAs for the treatment of anemia related to hepatitis C therapy (currently not an FDA-labeled indication for darbepoetin alfa). Darbepoetin alfa therapy should be withheld in any patient who develops severe anemia and low reticulocyte counts; patient should be evaluated for the presence of neutralizing antibodies to erythropoietin. The manufacturer should be contacted (1-800-77AMGEN) to perform assays for binding and neutralizing antibodies. Darbepoetin alfa should be permanently discontinued in any patient who develops PRCA following treatment with darbepoetin alfa or other erythropoietin proteins and such patients should not be switched to another ESA.

Sensitivity Reactions **Hypersensitivity Reactions.** Serious allergic reactions, including anaphylaxis, angioedema, bronchospasm, skin rash, and urticaria, may occur with darbepoetin alfa. If a serious allergic or anaphylactic reaction occurs, the drug should be discontinued immediately and appropriate treatment provided.

Latex Sensitivity. The needle cover of the prefilled syringe contains natural latex proteins in the form of dry natural rubber (latex). Individuals sensitive to latex should not handle the needle cover. Rarely, hypersensitivity reactions to natural latex proteins have been fatal.

General Precautions **Lack or Loss of Response to Therapy.** A lack or loss of response to darbepoetin alfa should prompt evaluation for potential causative factors (e.g., iron deficiency, infection, inflammation, bleeding). If typical causes are excluded, the patient should be evaluated for evidence of pure red cell aplasia (PRCA). In the absence of PRCA, dosage recommendations for the management of patients with an insufficient response to darbepoetin alfa therapy should be followed. Patients with CKD and an insufficient response to ESA therapy may be at even greater risk for cardiovascular events and death than other patients. (See Increased Mortality and Cardiovascular and Thromboembolic Effects under Warnings/Precautions: Warnings, in Cautions.)

Patient Monitoring. Iron stores should be evaluated in all patients prior to and periodically during darbepoetin alfa therapy. Supplemental iron therapy is recommended for patients whose serum ferritin concentration is below 100 mcg/L or whose serum transferrin saturation is below 20%. The majority of patients with CKD will require supplemental iron during the course of ESA therapy. For further information on the use of supplemental iron therapy in patients receiving recombinant erythropoietin therapy, see Uses: Iron Deficiency Anemia in Hemodialysis Patients Receiving Epoetin Alfa Therapy, in Sodium Ferric Gluconate 20:04.04.

Hemoglobin concentrations should be monitored weekly following initiation of darbepoetin alfa therapy and after each dosage change until stable and sufficient to minimize RBC transfusions. Subsequent monitoring of hemoglobin concentrations may be performed less frequently provided hemoglobin concentrations remain stable; the manufacturer recommends at least monthly monitoring in patients with CKD.

Dialysis Management. Patients undergoing dialysis may require adjustments in their dialysis prescriptions following initiation of darbepoetin alfa. Darbepoetin alfa may increase heparin anticoagulation requirements to prevent clotting of the extracorporeal circuit in patients receiving hemodialysis. (See Increased Mortality and Cardiovascular and Thromboembolic Effects under Warnings/Precautions: Warnings, in Cautions.)

Specific Populations **Pregnancy.** Category C. (See Users Guide.)

Women who become pregnant during darbepoetin alfa therapy are encouraged to enroll in the manufacturer's pregnancy surveillance program by calling 800-772-6436.

Lactation. Not known whether darbepoetin alfa is distributed into milk. Caution is advised if the drug is administered in nursing women.

Pediatric Use. Safety and efficacy of darbepoetin alfa in the initial treatment of anemic pediatric patients with CKD have not been established. Safety and efficacy of transitioning to darbepoetin alfa therapy from epoetin alfa in pediatric CKD patients older than 1 year of age are similar to that in adults. Safety and efficacy of transitioning from another erythropoietin have not been established in pediatric patients younger than 1 year of age. Safety and efficacy of darbepoetin alfa in pediatric cancer patients have not been established.

Geriatric Use. No substantial differences in safety and efficacy of darbepoetin alfa relative to younger adults, but increased sensitivity cannot be ruled out.

Hepatic Impairment. Darbepoetin should be used with caution in patients with hepatic impairment.

■ **Common Adverse Effects** Adverse effects occurring in at least 5% of adult CKD patients receiving darbepoetin alfa in clinical studies include hypertension, dyspnea, peripheral edema, cough, procedural hypotension, angina pectoris, vascular access complications, fluid overload, rash/erythema, and arteriovenous graft thrombosis. No important differences in incidence of adverse effects have been observed between patients receiving darbepoetin alfa and those receiving other recombinant erythropoietins in clinical studies.

The most commonly reported adverse effects in a study in pediatric patients with CKD receiving darbepoetin alfa included hypertension, injection site pain, rash, and convulsions.

Adverse effects occurring in at least 1% of adults with cancer receiving darbepoetin alfa in clinical studies include abdominal pain, edema, and thrombovascular events (myocardial infarction, pulmonary embolism, cerebrovascular accidents, CNS hemorrhage).

Drug Interactions

No formal drug interaction studies have been performed.

Description

Darbepoetin alfa, a biosynthetic (recombinant DNA origin) form of the glycoprotein hormone erythropoietin, is a hematopoietic agent that principally affects erythropoiesis. Darbepoetin alfa differs structurally from the endogenous hormone and epoetin alfa by the addition of 2 carbohydrate chains. This structural modification results in an increased molecular weight, increased sialic acid content, a more negative charge, and an approximately threefold longer terminal half-life compared with epoetin alfa, which allows for less frequent administration of the drug.

Like epoetin alfa, darbepoetin alfa has pharmacologic actions identical to those of the endogenous hormone. (See Pharmacology, in Epoetin Alfa 20:16.)

Advice to Patients

Importance of reading the manufacturer's medication guide prior to initiating darbepoetin alfa therapy and at regular intervals while receiving the drug. Importance of informing patients about the increased risks of death, serious cardiovascular effects (e.g., myocardial infarction, stroke, heart failure), thromboembolic events, or shortened overall survival and/or tumor progression or recurrence in certain patient populations. Importance of informing patients that an anticoagulant may be used as prophylaxis for thromboembolism if patients undergo surgery. (See Increased Mortality and Cardiovascular and Thromboembolic Effects and see Increased Mortality and Tumor Progression, under Warnings/Precautions: Warnings, in Cautions.) Importance of informing patients that darbepoetin alfa does not improve symptoms of anemia or health-related quality of life, including effects on fatigue, energy, strength, or well-being in patients with chemotherapy-induced anemia.

Importance of providing information on proper preparation and administration techniques for patients or caregivers who will be administering the drug and advising such individuals to follow the manufacturer's "Patient Instructions for Use." Importance of taking darbepoetin alfa exactly as prescribed. Importance of contacting a clinician immediately if more than the prescribed dose is taken or if a dose is missed.

Importance of discontinuing darbepoetin alfa when cancer chemotherapy is completed. Importance of recognizing and reporting serious allergic reactions (e.g., whole body rash, shortness of breath, wheezing, decreases in blood pressure, swelling around mouth or eyes, rapid pulse, sweating). Importance of immediately reporting signs or symptoms of blood clots such as chest pain, worsening of shortness of breath, pain of the legs with or without swelling, a cool or pale arm or leg, sudden difficulty walking, dizziness, loss of consciousness, loss of balance or coordination, sudden confusion, difficulty speaking or understanding others' speech, difficulty seeing, or blood clots in hemodialysis vascular access ports. Importance of contacting a clinician immediately if seizures occur. Importance of contacting a clinician if symptoms of severe anemia such as unusual tiredness, lack of energy, dizziness, or fainting occur.

Importance of adherence to antihypertensive treatment and dietary restrictions. Importance of regular monitoring of blood pressure and hemoglobin concentration and of keeping appointments for determination of hemoglobin concentrations.

Importance of patients contacting a clinician if any new-onset seizures, premonitory symptoms, or change in seizure frequency occurs.

Importance of patients informing clinician of latex allergy. Importance of informing patients that the needle cover of the prefilled darbepoetin alfa syringe contains natural dry rubber.

Importance of women informing clinicians if they are or plan to become pregnant or plan to breast-feed. Importance of informing clinicians of existing or contemplated concomitant therapy, including prescription and OTC drugs, as well as any concomitant illnesses (e.g., heart disease, high blood pressure, history of seizures or stroke, allergies to latex).

Importance of informing patients of other important precautionary information. (See Cautions.)

Overview® (see Users Guide.). For additional information on this drug until a more detailed monograph is developed and published, the manufacturer's labeling should be consulted. It is *essential* that the manufacturer's labeling be consulted for more detailed information on usual cautions, precautions, contraindications, potential drug interactions, laboratory test interferences, and acute toxicity.

Preparations

Excipients in commercially available drug preparations may have clinically important effects in some individuals; consult specific product labeling for details.

Darbepoetin Alfa

Parenteral

For injection	25 mcg/0.42 mL	Aranesp® (available as single-dose prefilled syringes), Amgen
	25 mcg/mL	Aranesp® (available as single-dose vials), Amgen
	40 mcg/0.4 mL	Aranesp® (available as single-dose prefilled syringes), Amgen
	40 mcg/mL	Aranesp® (available as single-dose vials), Amgen
	60 mcg/0.3 mL	Aranesp® (available as single-dose prefilled syringes), Amgen
	60 mcg/mL	Aranesp® (available as single-dose vials), Amgen
	100 mcg/0.5 mL	Aranesp® (available as single-dose prefilled syringes), Amgen
	100 mcg/mL	Aranesp® (available as single-dose vials), Amgen
	150 mcg/0.3 mL	Aranesp® (available as single-dose prefilled syringes), Amgen
	150 mcg/0.75 mL	Aranesp® (available as single-dose vials), Amgen
	200 mcg/0.4 mL	Aranesp® (available as single-dose prefilled syringes), Amgen
	200 mcg/mL	Aranesp® (available as single-dose vials), Amgen
	300 mcg/0.6 mL	Aranesp® (available as single-dose prefilled syringes), Amgen
	300 mcg/mL	Aranesp® (available as single-dose vials), Amgen
	500 mcg/mL	Aranesp® (available as single-dose prefilled syringes), Amgen

†Use is not currently included in the labeling approved by the US Food and Drug Administration

Eltrombopag Olamine

■ Eltrombopag olamine is a small-molecule thrombopoietin-receptor agonist.

Uses

■ **Idiopathic Thrombocytopenic Purpura** Eltrombopag olamine is used for the treatment of chronic idiopathic thrombocytopenic purpura (ITP; also known as immune thrombocytopenic purpura) in patients who have had an inadequate response to corticosteroids, immunoglobulins, or splenectomy and in whom the degree of thrombocytopenia and clinical status increase bleeding risk. Eltrombopag should not be used to normalize platelet counts since excessive increases in platelet count may increase the risk of thromboembolic complications. The drug is not indicated for the treatment of thrombocytopenia associated with myelodysplastic syndrome or thrombocytopenia associated with any condition other than chronic ITP. In addition, eltrombopag is not indicated for the treatment of thrombocytopenia in patients with chronic liver disease.

Safety and efficacy of eltrombopag for the treatment of chronic ITP have been established in 2 randomized, double-blind, placebo-controlled studies and an open-label extension study. Patients in the 2 randomized studies had an inadequate therapeutic response to corticosteroids, immunoglobulins, rituximab, cytotoxic agents, danazol, azathioprine, or splenectomy and had platelet counts of 30,000/mm³ or less prior to study entry. In study 1, patients received eltrombopag 50 mg or placebo daily for 6 weeks. In study 2, patients received 30, 50, or 75 mg of eltrombopag or placebo daily for a total of 6 weeks. Patients in study 2 who had received a stable maintenance regimen of immunosuppressive therapy (principally corticosteroids) for at least 1 month prior to study entry were allowed to continue such therapy at stable (unchanged) dosages throughout the study period. The primary objective in both studies was the achievement of a platelet count of 50,000/mm³ or greater; treatment was discontinued if the platelet count exceeded 200,000/mm³. The median baseline platelet count was 18,000/mm³ in both studies; the median durations of treatment in study 1 and 2 were 42 and 43 days, respectively. Based on a daily dosage of 50 mg, 59–70% of patients receiving eltrombopag versus 11–16% of those receiving placebo achieved a platelet count of 50,000/mm³ or greater in the 2 randomized studies. Increases in platelet count generally were detected within a week after initiation of eltrombopag therapy and a maximum response occurred within 2 weeks. A subset analysis performed in study 1 revealed no difference in response to eltrombopag based on splenectomy status or the use of concomitant drugs for ITP.

Bleeding was assessed in both studies using the World Health Organization (WHO) bleeding scale (grade 0 = no bleeding, grade 1 = petechiae, grade 2 = mild blood loss, grade 3 = gross blood loss, grade 4 = debilitating blood loss). In study 1, fewer bleeding episodes (all WHO grades) were reported during the treatment period (day 1 through 43) for patients treated with eltrombopag compared with placebo (61 versus 79%). After discontinuance of therapy, platelet counts returned to baseline values and the percentage of patients experiencing a grade 1–4 bleeding event increased between days 50 and 85 (post-treatment phase). In study 2, in which patients received 30, 50, or 75 mg of eltrombopag or placebo daily, the incidence of bleeding (all WHO grades) during treatment was 14% in the placebo group and 17, 7, or 4% in the groups receiving 30, 50, or 75 mg, respectively, of eltrombopag.

Patients were eligible to receive eltrombopag during an open-label extension study (EXTEND) following their original participation in a randomized trial in an attempt to reduce the eltrombopag dosage or eliminate the need for concomitant ITP treatment. The median daily dosage of eltrombopag after 6 months was 50 mg. During the extension study, platelet counts were 74,000/mm³, 67,000/mm³, and 95,000/mm³ at 3, 6, and 9 months, respectively, on a median daily dosage of 50 mg. Based on preliminary data from an updated interim analysis of 207 enrolled patients in the EXTEND study, 79% of patients achieved a platelet count of 50,000/mm³ or greater, and 24% of patients who received eltrombopag for at least 25 weeks maintained a platelet count above 50,000/mm³ continuously for at least 25 weeks. Platelet counts remained at a median of 50,000/mm³ or greater during the 44-week observation period of the study except for 3 instances, when platelet count declined but remained above a median of 40,000/mm³. Approximately 31% of evaluable patients (65/207 patients) treated with eltrombopag were receiving concomitant ITP therapy at the time of enrollment in the EXTEND study; a sustained reduction in dosage or discontinuance of other ITP therapy(s) was successful in 35% (23 out of 65) of these patients.

Dosage and Administration

■ **General** Dosage of eltrombopag olamine is expressed in terms of eltrombopag. Eltrombopag should not be given more often than once daily. The maximum daily dosage should not exceed 75 mg.

The drug should be administered 1 hour before or 2 hours after a meal because food may decrease the rate and extent of absorption. In addition, the drug should *not* be administered within 4 hours of other drugs, food, or supplements that contain polyvalent cations (e.g., iron, calcium, aluminum, magnesium, selenium, zinc). Since calcium-containing food (e.g., dairy products) is more frequently consumed at breakfast, it has been suggested that eltrombopag be taken in the evening, if possible, unless patients are also taking an antacid preparation containing polyvalent cations at that time.

■ **Administration** Eltrombopag is administered orally.

■ **Dosage** The usual initial adult dosage of eltrombopag is 50 mg daily. For patients of East Asian ancestry or those with moderate or severe hepatic insufficiency, the usual initial dosage is 25 mg daily.

Dosage of eltrombopag should be adjusted to achieve and maintain a platelet count of 50,000/mm^3 or greater. If the platelet count is less than 50,000/mm^3 after at least 2 weeks of eltrombopag treatment, daily dosage should be increased by 25 mg, up to a maximum daily dosage of 75 mg. If the platelet count has not reached a level sufficient to avoid a clinically important bleeding episode after 4 weeks at the maximum daily dosage, eltrombopag should be discontinued.

The daily dosage should be reduced by 25 mg if the platelet count is between 200,000/mm^3 and 400,000/mm^3 at any time during eltrombopag therapy; a follow-up assessment should be performed 2 weeks later to assess the effect of the lower dosage before additional dosage adjustments are made. Eltrombopag therapy should not be administered if the platelet count exceeds 400,000/mm^3. If therapy is interrupted, the platelet count should be assessed twice weekly and eltrombopag should be resumed at a dosage reduced by 25 mg daily once the platelet count is less than 150,000/mm^3. If the platelet count is persistently elevated (e.g., exceeding 400,000/mm^3 after 2 weeks at the lowest dosage), the manufacturer recommends that eltrombopag be discontinued permanently.

Dosage Modification for Hepatotoxicity Because of a risk of hepatotoxicity with eltrombopag therapy, liver function tests (i.e., serum ALT [SGPT], AST [SGOT], and bilirubin) should be performed prior to initiating therapy, every 2 weeks during the dosage adjustment phase, and then monthly once a stable dosage has been achieved. If serum bilirubin is elevated, a fractionated bilirubin concentration also must be obtained. Patients who develop liver function test abnormalities should have these tests repeated within 3–5 days to confirm the results; if an abnormality is confirmed, liver function tests should be monitored weekly until the abnormality resolves, stabilizes, or returns to baseline. Eltrombopag therapy should be discontinued if serum ALT concentrations increase to 3 times the upper limit of normal (ULN) or higher and are progressive, persist for 4 weeks or longer, or are accompanied by an increased direct bilirubin concentration or clinical symptoms of hepatotoxicity or hepatic decompensation.

■ **Special Populations** The manufacturer recommends that the initial dosage of eltrombopag be reduced to 25 mg daily in patients with moderate or severe hepatic impairment. (See Hepatic Impairment under Warnings/Precautions: Specific Populations, in Cautions.)

The manufacturer recommends that the initial dosage of eltrombopag be reduced to 25 mg daily in patients of East Asian ancestry (e.g., Chinese, Japanese, Taiwanese, or Korean). (See East Asian Ancestry under Warnings/Precautions: Specific Populations, in Cautions.)

The safety and efficacy of eltrombopag in patients with varying degrees of impaired renal function have not been established. The manufacturer recommends close monitoring of patients with impaired renal function.

Cautions

■ **Contraindications** The manufacturer states there are no known contraindications to the use of eltrombopag olamine.

■ **Warnings/Precautions** ***Warnings*** **Hepatotoxicity.** Eltrombopag may cause hepatic and biliary impairment. Grade 2 (or less) abnormalities in serum ALT, AST, and bilirubin concentrations have been reported in 10% of patients receiving the drug. Grade 4 (National Cancer Institute Common Terminology Criteria for Adverse Events [NCI CTCAE] toxicity scale) elevations in serum liver enzymes, as well as worsening of underlying cardiopulmonary disease and subsequent death, were reported in one patient receiving eltrombopag. Liver function tests (e.g., serum ALT, AST, and bilirubin concentrations) should be evaluated prior to starting therapy and monitored every 2 weeks during the initial dosage adjustment phase, then monthly thereafter once a stable dosage has been achieved. If serum bilirubin concentration is elevated, a fractionated measurement must be obtained. If liver function tests are abnormal, the tests should be repeated again within 3–5 days; if the abnormalities persist, liver function tests should be monitored on a weekly basis until the abnormality resolves, stabilizes, or returns to a baseline value. Eltrombopag should be discontinued if serum ALT (SGPT) levels increase to 3 times the upper limit of normal (ULN) or greater and are progressive, persistent (for at least 4 weeks), or are accompanied by an increased direct bilirubin concentration or clinical symptoms of hepatotoxicity or hepatic decompensation.

Retreatment with eltrombopag after discontinuance for hepatotoxicity is not recommended. However, the manufacturer suggests that retreatment *may* be considered if the anticipated clinical benefit of eltrombopag outweighs the potential risk of hepatotoxicity. If treatment is reinitiated, the manufacturer recommends that serum ALT, AST, and bilirubin concentrations be evaluated weekly during the dosage adjustment phase. If abnormal liver function tests persist, worsen, or recur, eltrombopag should be permanently discontinued.

Other Warnings/Precautions **Bone Marrow Reticulin Deposition and Bone Marrow Fibrosis.** Thrombopoietin (TPO)-receptor agonists increase the risk of development or progression of reticulin fiber deposition within the bone marrow, thereby increasing the risk for bone marrow fibrosis or myelofibrosis. In the extension study, 7 patients had evidence of reticulin fiber deposition confirmed by bone marrow biopsy, including 2 patients with collagen fiber deposition. The presence of fiber deposition in the bone marrow was not associated with cytopenia and did not result in the discontinuance of eltrombopag. Clinical studies have not excluded a risk for bone marrow fibrosis with cytopenias in patients receiving eltrombopag.

A peripheral blood smear should be evaluated prior to starting eltrombopag therapy and monthly thereafter once a stable dosage has been achieved. Examination of the peripheral blood smear should include establishment of a baseline level of cellular morphologic abnormalities; monthly evaluations should include examinations for new or worsening morphologic abnormalities (e.g., teardrop or nucleated erythrocytes or immature leukocytes). A complete blood count (CBC) also should be performed monthly to evaluate new or worsening cytopenias. If a new or worsening morphologic abnormality or cytopenia develops, eltrombopag should be discontinued and a bone marrow biopsy, with additional staining for fibrosis, should be considered.

Thrombocytopenia and Hemorrhage Following Eltrombopag Discontinuance. Thrombocytopenia may occur after the discontinuance of eltrombopag and may be more severe than prior to therapy. Worsening of thrombocytopenia may increase the risk of bleeding, especially if eltrombopag is discontinued while the patient is receiving concomitant antiplatelet or anticoagulation therapy. In clinical studies, a transient decrease in platelet count to levels lower than baseline was reported in 10% of patients following discontinuance of eltrombopag. Serious hemorrhagic events occurring within 1 month of discontinuance of eltrombopag and requiring the use of additional ITP therapy were reported in 3 patients with severe thrombocytopenia in clinical studies.

Following discontinuance of eltrombopag, a CBC with platelet count should be performed weekly for at least 4 weeks. Additional ITP therapy should be considered for worsening thrombocytopenia.

Thrombosis/Thromboembolism. An excessive increase in platelet count resulting from excessive dosages of eltrombopag or medication errors resulting in excessive dosages may be associated with the development of thrombosis or a thromboembolic complication. In the controlled clinical studies and extension study, a total of 8 patients receiving eltrombopag experienced a thrombotic or thromboembolic complication. Thrombosis also may occur even with normal or low platelet counts. Eltrombopag should be used with caution in patients with known risk factors for thromboembolism (e.g., factor V Leiden, antithrombin III [ATIII] deficiency, antiphospholipid syndrome). To minimize the risk for a thrombotic or thromboembolic complication, eltrombopag should *not* be used to normalize platelet counts, and should only be used to maintain a platelet count of 50,000/mm^3 or greater according to the dosage adjustment guidelines. (See Dosage and Administration: Dosage.)

Thrombosis of the portal venous system has been reported in patients with thrombocytopenia associated with chronic liver disease receiving eltrombopag. The ELEVATE study, a randomized, double-blind, placebo-controlled, multinational study, was conducted to assess the safety and efficacy of eltrombopag to reduce the need for platelet transfusion in thrombocytopenic patients with chronic liver disease prior to undergoing an elective invasive procedure. The study was terminated early because an imbalance of thrombosis of the portal venous system was noted in patients receiving eltrombopag compared with those receiving placebo. In the study, thrombocytopenic patients with chronic liver disease of diverse etiology were randomized to receive eltrombopag 75 mg or placebo for 14 days prior to an elective invasive procedure. Portal venous thrombosis occurred in 4% of patients receiving eltrombopag and in 1% of patients receiving placebo. Platelet counts exceeded 200,000/mm^3 in 5 of the 6 patients who received eltrombopag and experienced portal venous thrombosis. Eltrombopag is *not* indicated for the treatment of thrombocytopenia in patients with chronic liver disease.

Malignancy. Eltrombopag stimulates the TPO receptor present on the surface of hematopoietic cells and may possibly increase the risk for progression to a hematologic malignancy, especially in patients with myelodysplastic syndrome (MDS). In randomized, controlled clinical studies, no hematologic cancers were reported in patients receiving eltrombopag for a maximum of 6 weeks; however, one case of non-Hodgkin's lymphoma was reported in the prolonged extension study. Eltrombopag should not be used to treat or correct thrombocytopenia related to an underlying hematologic cause (e.g., myelodysplasia) or resulting from chemotherapy; eltrombopag should only be used for thrombocytopenia associated with chronic ITP.

Cataracts. Cataracts developed or worsened in 5% of patients receiving eltrombopag in controlled clinical studies. In the extension study, cataracts worsened or developed in 4% of patients who underwent ocular exams prior to eltrombopag therapy. A baseline ocular examination should be performed prior to eltrombopag therapy; while on therapy, patients should be monitored periodically for signs and symptoms of cataracts.

Laboratory Monitoring. A CBC, including platelet count and peripheral blood smear, should be obtained prior to starting therapy, weekly during the dosage adjustment phase, then monthly once a stable dosage has been achieved. Baseline peripheral blood smears should establish the presence and extent of red and white cell abnormalities. Once eltrombopag is discontinued, a CBC with platelet count should be evaluated weekly for at least 4 weeks to monitor for worsening thrombocytopenia.

Serum ALT, AST, and bilirubin concentrations should be evaluated prior to starting therapy and every 2 weeks during the dosage adjustment phase, then monthly once a stable dosage has been achieved. If serum bilirubin is elevated, a fractionated bilirubin concentration also must be obtained. Patients who develop liver function test abnormalities should have these tests repeated within

3–5 days to confirm the results; if an abnormality is confirmed, liver function tests should be monitored weekly until the abnormality resolves, stabilizes, or returns to baseline. Eltrombopag therapy should be discontinued if indications of important hepatic abnormalities occur. (See Hepatotoxicity under Warnings/Precautions: Warnings, in Cautions.)

Specific Populations **Pregnancy.** Category C. (See Users Guide.)

May cause fetal harm; embryolethality and reduced fetal weights reported in rats at maternally toxic dosages (7 times the human clinical exposure based on area under the plasma concentration-time curve [AUC]). No adequate and well-controlled studies in humans. Eltrombopag should be used in pregnant women only if the anticipated clinical benefit outweighs the potential risk to the fetus.

To monitor maternal-fetal outcomes of pregnant women exposed to eltrombopag, a pregnancy registry has been established. Clinicians are encouraged to enroll pregnant women receiving eltrombopag in the registry; women also may enroll themselves in the registry by calling 888-825-5249.

Lactation. It is not known whether eltrombopag is distributed into human milk. Discontinue nursing or the drug, taking into account the importance of the drug to the woman.

Pediatric Use. Safety and efficacy not established in pediatric patients younger than 18 years of age.

Geriatric Use. No substantial differences in safety and efficacy in geriatric patients 65 years of age or older relative to younger adults, but increased sensitivity cannot be ruled out.

Hepatic Impairment. The AUC for eltrombopag was 41% higher in patients with mild hepatic impairment; in patients with moderate to severe hepatic impairment, AUC was increased by 80–93% compared with that in individuals with normal hepatic function. A corresponding reduction (50%) in clearance of eltrombopag was reported in patients with moderate and severe hepatic impairment.

The manufacturer recommends that the initial dosage of eltrombopag be reduced to 25 mg daily for patients with moderate or severe hepatic impairment. Eltrombopag should be used with caution in patients with hepatic disease, and patients should be monitored carefully.

Thrombosis of the portal venous system has been reported in patients with thrombocytopenia and chronic liver disease receiving eltrombopag. (See Thrombosis/Thromboembolism under Warnings/Precautions: Other Warnings/Precautions, in Cautions.) Eltrombopag is *not* indicated for the treatment of thrombocytopenia in patients with chronic liver disease. To minimize the risk for a thrombotic or thromboembolic complication, eltrombopag should *not* be used to normalize platelet counts, but should only be used to maintain a platelet count of 50,000/mm^3 or greater according to the dosage adjustment guidelines. (See Dosage and Administration: Dosage.)

Renal Impairment. Safety and efficacy of eltrombopag in patients with varying degrees of renal function have not been established.

Patients with impaired renal function should be closely monitored while receiving eltrombopag.

East Asian Ancestry. The AUC for eltrombopag was approximately 70% higher in patients with East Asian ancestry (i.e., Japanese, Chinese, Taiwanese, or Korean) compared with non-Asian (predominantly Caucasian) patients. Pharmacodynamic responses to eltrombopag also were enhanced in East Asian patients. The manufacturer recommends an initial daily dosage of 25 mg in patients of East Asian ancestry.

■ **Common Adverse Effects** Adverse events reported in patients receiving eltrombopag at a frequency higher than with placebo in controlled clinical studies include nausea, vomiting, menorrhagia, myalgia, paresthesia, cataract, dyspepsia, ecchymosis, thrombocytopenia, increased serum transaminases (ALT, AST), and conjunctival hemorrhage. The most common adverse events reported with eltrombopag in the extension study were headache, upper respiratory tract infection, diarrhea, and nasopharyngitis.

Drug Interactions

Eltrombopag olamine is metabolized by the cytochrome P-450 (CYP) 1A2 and 2C8 isoenzymes and also undergoes glucuronidation by uridine diphosphate-glucuronosyltransferase (UGT) 1A1 and 1A3 isoenzymes. Eltrombopag is an inhibitor of the CYP2C8 and CYP2C9 isoenzymes and the organic anion-transporting polypeptide (OATP) 1B1.

Eltrombopag also inhibits uridine diphosphate-glucuronosyltransferase (UGT) isoenzymes 1A1, 1A3, 1A4, 1A6, 1A9, 2B7, and 2B15.

■ **Drugs Affecting or Metabolized by Hepatic Microsomal Enzymes** Substrates of CYP2C8 or CYP2C9: Potential pharmacokinetic interaction resulting in altered metabolism of CYP2C8 or CYP2C9 substrates. In a clinical study, administration of eltrombopag (75 mg once daily) for 7 days to healthy male individuals did not demonstrate inhibition or induction of the metabolism of a combination of probe substrates for CYP1A2 (caffeine), CYP2C19 (omeprazole), CYP2C9 (flurbiprofen), or CYP3A4 (midazolam). Probe substrates for CYP2C8 were not evaluated in this study.

Moderate to strong inhibitors of CYP1A2 (e.g., ciprofloxacin, fluvoxamine) or CYP2C8 (e.g., gemfibrozil, trimethoprim): Potential pharmacokinetic interaction resulting in increased systemic exposure to eltrombopag. Use with caution.

Moderate to strong inducers of CYP1A2 (e.g., tobacco, omeprazole) or CYP2C8 (e.g., rifampin): Potential pharmacokinetic interaction resulting in decreased systemic exposure to eltrombopag.

■ **Drugs Transported by Organic Anion-transporting Polypeptide 1B1** Substrates of organic anion-transporting polypeptide (OATP) 1B1: Potential pharmacokinetic interaction (increased concentrations of concomitantly administered OATP1BI substrates [e.g., benzylpenicillin, atorvastatin, fluvastatin, pravastatin, rosuvastatin, methotrexate, nateglinide, repaglinide, rifampin]). Consider reduction of OATP1B1 substrate dosage if manifestations of excessive systemic exposure to these drugs occur.

The area under the plasma concentration-time curve (AUC) and peak plasma concentration of rosuvastatin increased by 55 and 103%, respectively, with administration of a single 10-mg dose of rosuvastatin in healthy adults receiving 75 mg of eltrombopag daily for 5 days. In clinical trials, a 50% reduction in rosuvastatin dosage was recommended for patients receiving concomitant eltrombopag.

■ **Drugs Affecting or Metabolized by Uridine Diphosphate-glucuronosyltransferase (UGT)** Substrates of UDP-glucuronosyltransferases (UGTs): Potential pharmacokinetic interaction resulting in increased systemic exposure to multiple UGT substrates, including acetaminophen, opioid narcotics, and nonsteroidal anti-inflammatory agents. Use with caution.

Moderate to strong inhibitors of UGT1A1 or UGT1A3: Potential pharmacokinetic interaction resulting in increased systemic exposure to eltrombopag. Use with caution.

■ **Polyvalent Cations** Eltrombopag chelates polyvalent cations (e.g., iron, calcium, aluminum, magnesium, selenium, zinc) found in food, mineral supplements, and antacids. Plasma concentration of eltrombopag was reduced by 70% in patients receiving concomitant antacid therapy containing aluminum hydroxide, magnesium carbonate, and sodium alginate; a 59% reduction in AUC for eltrombopag was reported in association with a high-calcium, high-fat breakfast. Patients should avoid medications and foods containing polyvalent cations, including antacids, dairy products, and mineral supplements, for 4 hours before and after each dose of eltrombopag.

Description

Eltrombopag olamine is a small-molecule, nonpeptide, thrombopoietin (TPO)-receptor agonist. Eltrombopag interacts with the transmembrane domain of the TPO receptor, initiating a cascade of intracellular signaling events leading to proliferation and differentiation of bone marrow progenitor cells within the megakaryocytic lineage and subsequently increasing the production of platelets.

Eltrombopag (up to 150 mg daily for 5 days) did not demonstrate QT or QT corrected for rate (QT_c)-interval prolonging effects in a randomized, crossover study with placebo and positive (moxifloxacin) controls in healthy adults.

Advice to Patients

Importance of carefully reading patient information (medication guide) provided by the manufacturer before initiating therapy, and each time prescription is refilled.

Importance of informing patients that risks associated with long-term administration of eltrombopag are not known.

Importance of understanding the goal of therapy is to achieve and maintain a platelet count of 50,000/mm^3 or greater to reduce the risk of bleeding, not to normalize platelet count.

Risk of hepatic failure; importance of immediately reporting symptoms suggestive of jaundice (e.g., yellowing of skin or eyes), unusual darkening of urine, unusual fatigue, or right-upper quadrant (i.e., stomach area) pain to clinician.

Risk of worsening thrombocytopenia with possible bleeding shortly following discontinuance of eltrombopag, compared with such risks prior to starting therapy; increased risk if receiving concomitant anticoagulant or antiplatelet drugs.

Risk of reticulin fiber formation in bone marrow with possible progression to bone marrow fibrosis.

Increased risk of thrombosis or thromboembolism with high platelet counts resulting from excessive eltrombopag dosage. Risk of thrombosis even with normal or low platelet counts. Importance of immediately reporting symptoms suggestive of thrombosis (e.g., swelling, pain, or tenderness in leg) to clinician.

Increased risk of developing a hematologic malignancy, especially in patients with myelodysplastic syndrome (MDS).

Importance of avoiding situations or medications that may increase risk of bleeding.

Risk of new or worsened cataracts.

Importance of taking eltrombopag on an empty stomach (i.e., 1 hour before or 2 hours after a meal). Importance of avoiding foods, supplements, and drugs that contain polyvalent cations (e.g., iron, calcium, aluminum, magnesium, selenium, zinc) for 4 hours before and after taking eltrombopag.

Importance of informing clinicians of existing or contemplated concomitant therapy, including prescription and OTC drugs, as well as concomitant illnesses.

Importance of women informing clinicians if they are or plan to become pregnant or plan to breast-feed. (See Pregnancy under Warnings/Precautions: Specific Populations, in Cautions.)

Importance of informing patients of other important precautionary information. (See Cautions.)

Overview® (see Users Guide). For additional information on this drug until a more detailed monograph is developed and published, the manufacturer's labeling should be consulted. It is *essential* that the manufacturer's labeling be consulted for more detailed information on usual cautions, precautions, contraindications, potential drug interactions, laboratory test interferences, and acute toxicity.

Preparations

Excipients in commercially available drug preparations may have clinically important effects in some individuals; consult specific product labeling for details.

Eltrombopag Olamine

Oral		
Tablet	25 mg (of eltrombopag)	**Promacta®**, GlaxoSmithKline
	50 mg (of eltrombopag)	**Promacta®**, GlaxoSmithKline
	75 mg (of eltrombopag)	**Promacta®**, GlaxoSmithKline

Epoetin Alfa

Erythropoietin Human Glycoform α (Recombinant), EPO, rHuEPO-α

■ Epoetin alfa, a biosynthetic form of the glycoprotein hormone erythropoietin, is a hematopoietic agent that principally affects erythropoiesis.

Uses

■ **Anemia of Chronic Kidney Disease** Epoetin alfa is used for the treatment of anemia associated with chronickidney disease, including that in patients undergoing dialysis and in those who do not yet require maintenance dialysis (predialysis patients), to reduce the need for red blood cell transfusions; epoetin alfa has been designated an orphan drug by the US Food and Drug Administration (FDA) for this use. Clinical studies indicate that epoetin alfa increases and/or maintains hemoglobin concentrations and hematocrit and decreases the need for transfusions in dialysis-dependent patients with chronic kidney disease as well as in those who do not yet require maintenance dialysis (predialysis patients). While some evidence indicates that therapy with epoetin alfa also is associated with subjective improvements in these patients, including a perceived general increase in feeling of well-being and quality of life, the manufacturer states that the drug has not been shown to improve quality of life, fatigue, or patient well-being. Most patients with anemia of chronic kidney disease, whether anephric or transfusion dependent, appear to respond to therapy with the drug, and other palliative therapies for this disorder (e.g., red blood cell transfusions, androgens) have limited efficacy and/or are associated with more serious adverse effects. Therefore, many clinicians currently consider epoetin alfa first-line therapy for appropriately selected patients with anemia of chronic kidney disease. The manufacturer and some authorities recommend that the drug be used in patients with end-stage renal disease who currently are undergoing hemodialysis or peritoneal dialysis therapy and also in predialysis patients with chronic kidney disease who have a hematocrit less than 30% or hemoglobin concentration less than 10 g/dL.

Some evidence suggests that in patients with chronic kidney disease who are undergoing hemodialysis or peritoneal dialysis, once weekly IV or subcutaneous administration of darbepoetin alfa maintains hemoglobin concentrations as safely and effectively as equivalent doses of epoetin alfa administered 2 or 3 times weekly by the same route. In addition, administration of darbepoetin alfa once every other week appears to have similar efficacy as equivalent doses of subcutaneous epoetin alfa administered once weekly. (See Uses: Anemia of Chronic Kidney Disease, in Darbepoetin Alfa 20:16.)

Results of controlled studies in patients with chronic kidney disease indicate that erythropoiesis-stimulating agents (ESAs), including epoetin alfa, may increase the risk for death, stroke, and serious cardiovascular events when targeted to achieve hemoglobin concentrations exceeding 11 g/dL. (See Cautions: Cardiovascular Effects.) FDA has issued a series of public health advisories regarding these risks associated with ESAs and has recommended more conservative dosing of these drugs in patients with chronic kidney disease. (See Anemia of Chronic Kidney Disease under Dosage and Administration: Dosage and also see Cardiovascular Precautions and Contraindications under Cautions: Precautions and Contraindications.) Clinicians should weigh the potential benefits of ESA therapy in reducing the need for red blood cell transfusions against the risk of serious cardiovascular events in patients with chronic kidney disease. Treatment should be individualized and the lowest possible ESA dosage that will reduce the need for red blood cell transfusions should be used.

Therapy with epoetin alfa is *not* intended for patients with chronic kidney disease who require *acute* correction of severe anemia; the drug should *not* be used as a substitute for emergency transfusion.

Potentially serious adverse effects (e.g., hypertension, thromboembolic events, seizures) and death, possibly related to excessively rapid correction or overcorrection of anemia, have been reported occasionally with epoetin alfa. Frequent and close monitoring of hemoglobin concentrations and blood pressure is indicated in all patients receiving epoetin alfa, and care should be exercised to avoid overly rapid increases in, or overcorrection of, hemoglobin concentrations. (See Cardiovascular Precautions and Contraindications under Cautions: Precautions and Contraindications.)

One of the most important factors in patient response to epoetin alfa therapy is iron status. With the reversal of anemia, iron and ferritin concentrations will decrease dramatically as reticulocytes are formed and released. Patients with low serum iron and ferritin concentrations will have a decreased response to epoetin alfa, with minimal or absent bone marrow response and a minimal to absent rise in hematocrit/erythrocyte count. In patients with normal ferritin concentrations and transferrin saturation (determined by dividing the serum iron concentration in mcg/dL by total iron-binding capacity in mcg/dL and multiplying by 100) less than 20%, a functional iron deficiency may develop as a result of the inability to mobilize iron stores rapidly enough to support increased erythropoiesis. This results from the demand for hemoglobin synthesis by epoetin alfa exceeding the ability of the reticuloendothelial system to release iron to transferrin.

Prior to and during epoetin alfa therapy, the patient's iron status, including transferrin saturation and serum ferritin concentrations, should be evaluated. Supplemental iron therapy should be administered when transferrin saturation is less than 20% or when serum ferritin concentration is less than 100 ng/mL. It has been suggested that patients with low baseline iron profiles (e.g., serum ferritin concentrations less than 100 ng/mL) at the beginning of therapy be supplemented with oral or parenteral iron to achieve adequate blood concentrations for erythropoiesis. Patients with adequate iron stores should be maintained on oral iron supplementation if possible; virtually all patients with chronic kidney disease receiving epoetin alfa therapy will require supplemental iron therapy. Oral maintenance dosages of 200–975 mg daily of ferrous sulfate (40–195 mg of elemental iron) have been suggested in patients receiving therapy with epoetin alfa.

Orally administered iron has been reported to be ineffective in maintaining adequate iron stores in hemodialysis patients during epoetin alfa therapy, and guidelines for the treatment of anemia of chronic kidney disease from the National Kidney Foundation Dialysis Outcomes Quality Initiative (NKF-DOQI) currently recommend regular use of IV iron (i.e., small doses given weekly to replace predicted blood loss) to prevent functional (and absolute) iron deficiency and improve erythropoiesis in most hemodialysis patients receiving epoetin alfa therapy. (See Uses: Iron Deficiency Anemia in Hemodialysis Patients Receiving Epoetin Alfa Therapy, in Sodium Ferric Gluconate 20:04.04.)

The anemia of chronic kidney disease is characterized by decreased hematocrit, hemoglobin concentration, and an inappropriately low serum erythropoietin concentration. Erythrokinetic studies demonstrate that total erythrocyte mass, erythron transferrin uptake, and erythrocyte survival are reduced in these patients. Treatment with epoetin alfa appears to improve anemic status and increase transferrin uptake; however, erythrocyte survival does not appear to be affected.

Hemodialysis Patients Epoetin alfa is administered by IV or subcutaneous injection to stimulate erythropoiesis in patients with inadequate production of, or decreased response to, endogenous erythropoietin. In clinical studies of patients with chronic kidney disease on dialysis, epoetin alfa dosages of 50–150 units/kg 3 times weekly produced dose-dependent increases in hemoglobin concentrations and decreased the need for red blood cell transfusions. After 3 months of epoetin alfa therapy, more than 95% of transfusion-dependent patients with chronic kidney disease were able to maintain a stablehemoglobin concentration without further need of transfusion. The rate and extent of rise in hemoglobin concentration generally are dose dependent over a dosage range of 75–4500 units/kg of epoetin alfa per week. Epoetin alfa generally induces erythropoiesis within 1–6 weeks in patients with chronic kidney disease who have severe anemia (hematocrit less than 25%); increases in reticulocyte count may be observed within 10 days. Less than 6% of patients treated with the drug fail to respond with an increase in hematocrit. Increases in hematocrit may persist up to 6 weeks after cessation of long-term epoetin alfa therapy; however, such increases are related principally to the increase in mature circulating erythrocytes. Reticulocyte count decreases dramatically following discontinuance of epoetin alfa therapy, indicating a decrease in the formation and release of new erythrocytes.

Other palliative therapies for anemia of chronic or end-stage kidney disease include androgens (e.g., nandrolone, testosterone) and red blood cell-containing products. Adverse events associated with red blood cell transfusions include transfusion reactions, potential infectious complications (e.g., hepatitis B; non-A, non-B hepatitis [including hepatitis C]; cytomegalovirus; human immunodeficiency virus [HIV] infection), iron overload, depression of residual endogenous erythropoietin secretion, and sensitization of the recipient to serum histocompatibility antigens (leading to development of cytotoxic antibodies and possible increased risk of renal allograft rejection). Disadvantages of androgen therapy include pain upon administration (usually via IM injection), hirsutism and virilization in female patients, acne, premature epiphyseal closure in children, priapism in males, elevation of serum triglycerides, hepatic dysfunction, and suboptimal and delayed (i.e., up to several months) patient response.

Although there is some evidence suggesting that increases in erythrocyte count, hematocrit, and hemoglobin concentration associated with epoetin alfa therapy may decrease fatigue and increase work capacity and exercise tolerance (as evidenced by increased oxygen consumption in treadmill and bicycle ergometry tests), the manufacturer states that the drug has not been shown to improve quality of life, fatigue, or patient well-being. In addition, improvement in CNS function and cognitive ability (as evidenced by decreases in the latency of the P_3 wave on the EEG [indicative of increased attention span, memory, and efficiency of cognitive function], and increases in visual, conceptual, visual-conceptual tracking, and evoked potential measurements) have been noted.

Subjective benefits reported by patients receiving epoetin alfa therapy include improvement in sleep habits, sexual function, and tolerance to cold; decreased dyspnea and pruritus; improved appetite and taste perception; and a perceived general increase in feeling of well-being and quality of life (as determined by patient interviews and standardized questionnaires). Patients with anemia-induced Raynaud's syndrome (particularly of the hands and upper extremities) have a decrease in or cessation of symptoms after correction of hematocrit with epoetin alfa therapy; in addition, digital perfusion is improved in these patients. Decreases in anginal symptoms and tachycardia, diminished cardiomegaly, and improved amino acid and/or protein metabolism, with improved wound healing, improved skin color and hair thickness, and increased fingernail growth and hardness, also have been reported with epoetin alfa therapy.

Hematopoietic response to epoetin alfa therapy in anephric and/or transfusion-dependent patients is similar to or greater than that in other anemic patients undergoing hemodialysis. In several multicenter studies, therapy with epoetin alfa 80–300 units/kg 2 or 3 times weekly increased hematocrit from pretreatment levels averaging 17–23% to posttreatment levels of 29–36% in both transfusion-dependent and -independent patients; mean hemoglobin concentration also increased from 6 g/dL to 9–12 g/dL at these dosages.

The erythropoietic response to epoetin alfa appears to be dose dependent; however, the rate and extent of hemoglobin concentration increase are subject to interpatient variability. In a combined phase I and II clinical trial of epoetin alfa in patients with chronic kidney disease undergoing hemodialysis, dosages of 15–500 units/kg IV 3 times weekly resulted in dose-dependent increases in hematocrit; at the 500-unit/kg dose, increase in hematocrit averaged 10% over a 3-week period. No consistent erythropoietic responses have been observed in hemodialysis patients treated with epoetin alfa in doses less than 15 units/kg per dose. In hemodialysis patients receiving maintenance therapy with epoetin alfa, IV dosages of at least 50 units/kg 3 times weekly generally have been required to achieve consistent increases in hematocrit. Up to 65% of treated patients in the largest US multicenter study maintained a hemoglobin concentration of 11.7 g/dL with epoetin alfa dosages not exceeding 100 units/kg 3 times weekly; approximately 10% of patients required 25 units/kg or less 3 times weekly and another 10% required more than 200 units/kg 3 times weekly to maintain their hemoglobin at this level. Higher IV dosages reportedly have been required in some chronic kidney disease patients with concurrent diseases.

In a multicenter study in hemodialysis patients, response to epoetin alfa therapy was independent of baseline hemoglobin, age, weight, and/or duration of dialysis; however, the time required to achieve target hemoglobin concentration appeared to correlate with the baseline hemoglobin concentration. Initial dosages of 24 units/kg 3 times weekly were doubled every 2 weeks until a 10% increase in baseline hemoglobin concentration occurred.

Administration of epoetin alfa, with or without phlebotomy, has reduced iron and ferritin stores in hemodialysis patients with iron overload and associated hemosiderosis secondary to multiple red blood cell transfusions. In one study, concomitant use of epoetin alfa and therapeutic phlebotomy reduced iron stores by an average of 1.6 g over 18 weeks in patients with iron overload, while iron store reductions averaged only 150 mg in patients with normal iron status who received epoetin alfa therapy without phlebotomy; similar relative decreases in serum ferritin also were noted. Reductions in serum ferritin and iron concentrations and in liver density as evidenced by computed tomography (CT) scan also have been observed after 1 year of epoetin alfa therapy in other studies. Porphyria cutanea tarda has improved with epoetin alfa therapy in a few patients undergoing long-term hemodialysis or peritoneal dialysis, allowing use of therapeutic phlebotomy in some patients. Further study is needed to determine the role of epoetin alfa in the amelioration of iron overload in patients with these conditions.

Predialysis Patients Epoetin alfa dosages of 50–150 units/kg 3 times weekly also have produced dose-dependent increases (e.g., up to 2% weekly) in hemoglobin concentrations in patients with chronic kidney disease who have become anemic secondary to their disease state but who do not yet require maintenance dialysis therapy (predialysis patients), including in renal transplant patients experiencing chronic kidney rejection. A similar dose-dependent increase in hemoglobin concentration has been observed in these patients whether the hormone was administered IV or by subcutaneous injection. Administration of the hormone with subsequent correction of the anemia does not appear to adversely affect the progression of chronic kidney disease or renal hemodynamics in predialysis patients. Although a substantial number of predialysis patients in placebo-controlled studies have required initiation of dialysis therapy within 6 months of initiating treatment with epoetin alfa, eventual progression to end-stage renal disease is expected in such patients and the rate of decline in renal function (as measured by serial determinations of the reciprocal of the serum creatinine concentration or of glomerular filtration rate using an iothalamate technique) did not change appreciably with improvement in the hematocrit in these patients. Epoetin alfa maintenance dosage requirements in these patients also were similar both before and after initiation of hemodialysis.

Placebo-controlled trials of epoetin alfa therapy in predialysis patients demonstrated a dose-related increase in hematocrit from pretreatment means of 27–32% to posttreatment means of 35–40% in 8–12 weeks; this response was observed with dosages of 50–150 units/kg subcutaneously or IV 3 times weekly. Patients given placebo exhibited little or no response. In one randomized, placebo-controlled trial, erythrocyte mass increased by approximately 40% in treated patients, with a concurrent decrease in plasma volume; total blood volume remained unchanged. Initial erythropoietic response to epoetin alfa treatment was observed after 2–4 weeks of therapy, with continued increases in hematocrit and erythrocyte mass thereafter. Also, an increase in exercise tolerance (as evidenced by improved maximal oxygen consumption) was seen in epoetin alfa-treated patients compared with those receiving placebo. Improvement in quality of life in predialysis patients is similar to that in hemodialysis patients treated with the drug.

Patients Undergoing Renal Transplantation Data from a limited number of patients who have undergone renal transplantation following treatment with epoetin alfa suggest that therapy with the drug does not adversely affect renal engraftment, although renal artery thrombosis occurring soon after transplantation and resulting in loss of the graft has been reported in at least one such patient. It has been suggested that the drug be discontinued at the time of organ transplant, or at least within 2 weeks of renal engraftment, to prevent the risk of excessive erythrocytosis and possible resultant adverse effects. A slight delay in onset of graft function following transplantation has been reported in a limited number of patients treated preoperatively with epoetin alfa compared with the onset of graft function in untreated allograft recipients; however, no difference in graft function was evident between treated and untreated patients 3 weeks after transplantation, and the role of the drug and/or increased preoperative hematocrit in this delay is uncertain. In addition, it has been suggested that the potential for finding a compatible graft may be increased in patients treated with epoetin alfa compared with untreated patients because of reduced need for blood transfusions and, therefore, decreased exposure of the patient to foreign histocompatibility antigens and resultant sensitization.

Peritoneal Dialysis Patients In patients on continuous ambulatory peritoneal dialysis (CAPD), response to epoetin alfa therapy appears to be even more rapid than in those patients on hemodialysis. This rapid response may be related to the relatively less severe anemia in CAPD patients, their higher baseline erythropoietin concentrations, and/or their lack of blood loss related to the dialysis procedure. Subcutaneous injection of 50–150 units/kg of epoetin alfa 2 or 3 times weekly have produced increases in hemoglobin concentration of up to 0.5 g/dL weekly and have alleviated the need for blood transfusions in some CAPD patients. Response of CAPD patients who self-administer the drug subcutaneously reportedly is similar to that in patients receiving the drug IV. Some clinicians suggest that initial subcutaneous epoetin alfa dosages of 50 units/kg 3 times weekly be used in CAPD patients to prevent excessively rapid correction of hemoglobin concentrations and/or hematocrit. Hemoglobin concentrations in CAPD patients have been maintained at 11–11.5 g/dL with epoetin alfa dosages averaging 25 units/kg (range: 12.5–75 units/kg) subcutaneously 2 or 3 times weekly; a comparable population of hemodialysis patients required a median of 48 units/kg (range: 24–192 units/kg) IV 3 times weekly to maintain hemoglobin at the same concentration.

Some evidence suggests that administration of epoetin alfa via peritoneal dialysis solutions† can produce meaningful increases in hemoglobin, although the bioavailability of the hormone when given by this route is low (range: 2.5–14%). However, other studies have shown little to no effect on hematocrit when the drug was given by this method of administration.

■ **Anemia in HIV-infected Patients** ***Zidovudine-induced Anemia*** Epoetin alfa is used for the treatment of anemia associated with zidovudine therapy in patients with HIV infection.* The drug is indicated in such patients with endogenous serum erythropoietin concentrations of 500 milliunits/mL or less who are receiving zidovudine therapy in dosages not exceeding 4.2 g per week. Epoetin alfa has been designated an orphan drug by the FDA for use in this condition. Current evidence indicates that addition of epoetin alfa to the zidovudine regimen generally increases and/or maintains hemoglobin concentration and hematocrit and decreases the need for red blood cell transfusions in selected patients with the disease without an increase in adverse effects. Preliminary data suggest that anemia in HIV-infected patients not receiving zidovudine also may respond to therapy with recombinant human erythropoietin, and epoetin alfa also has been designated an orphan drug by the FDA for such use. (See Anemia in HIV-infected Patients Not Receiving Zidovudine under Uses: Anemia in HIV-infected Patients.) Therapy with epoetin alfa is *not* intended for patients who require *acute* correction of severe anemia; the drug should *not* be used as a substitute for emergency transfusion.

Anemia in HIV-infected patients may be related to drug therapy (e.g., zidovudine) used to treat the disease as well as to the disease itself and/or its complications. Zidovudine, a nucleoside antiviral agent, may adversely affect both erythrocyte and leukocyte counts. (See Cautions: Hematologic Effects, in Zidovudine 8:18.08.20.) Zidovudine-induced anemia appears to result from impaired erythrocyte maturation. The anemia generally is macrocytic and megaloblastic; however, a normocytic anemia associated with erythroid hypoplasia or aplasia also has been reported. In addition, the serum of HIV-infected individuals has been shown to suppress hematopoiesis in vitro, indicating possible direct bone marrow suppression by the infection. Zidovudine-treated HIV-infected patients may be anemic despite increased endogenous serum erythropoietin concentrations, sometimes requiring transfusions on a regular basis to maintain adequate hematocrit levels. Opportunistic infections (e.g., cytomegalovirus, cryptococcosis, histoplasmosis) associated with acquired immunodeficiency syndrome (AIDS) also may suppress bone marrow function, and poor nutrition and/or poor GI absorption may lead to decreased vitamin

B_{12} concentrations, adding a nutritional component to the anemia. In addition, other drugs used in the treatment of opportunistic infections (e.g., co-trimoxazole) and blood loss from disease-related thrombocytopenia, accelerated erythrocyte destruction, and frequent phlebotomy may contribute to the anemia.

In controlled studies, addition of epoetin alfa in initial dosages of 100 units/kg IV 3 times weekly to the zidovudine regimen significantly increased the hemoglobin concentration compared with placebo in anemic HIV-infected patients with endogenous serum erythropoietin concentrations not exceeding 500 milliunits/mL; patients with higher baseline endogenous erythropoietin concentrations generally did not respond to the drug. Correction of the anemia, occasionally in conjunction with a minimal decrease in zidovudine dosage, resulted in a decrease of approximately 40% in the number of red blood cell transfusions required by patients with endogenous pretreatment serum erythropoietin concentrations not exceeding 500 milliunits/mL, whereas transfusion requirements generally increased in placebo-treated patients. When treated with epoetin alfa, 43% of patients who previously were transfusion dependent became transfusion independent after 2–3 months of therapy, compared with 18% of transfusion-dependent patients receiving placebo.

While some evidence suggests that quality of life may improve as a result of improvement in the anemia, particularly in those whose hematocrit increases to at least 38% independent of transfusion or zidovudine dosage reduction, the manufacturers state that epoetin alfa has not been shown to improve quality of life, fatigue, or patient well-being.

Epoetin alfa has been used effectively with concomitant filgrastim (a recombinant human granulocyte colony-stimulating factor; G-CSF) therapy in a limited number of patients to ameliorate the hematologic toxicity (severe anemia and/or granulocytopenia) associated with zidovudine therapy in HIV-infected patients since epoetin alfa alone cannot ameliorate the granulocytopenia and filgrastim alone does not appear to have a clinically important effect on erythropoiesis. In a study in adults with HIV infection and substantial bone marrow suppression, filgrastim therapy was administered initially to increase the neutrophil count and epoetin alfa therapy was then added to increase hemoglobin concentration after the neutrophil count had normalized; zidovudine therapy subsequently was reinstituted and, in some patients, was given concomitantly with both hematopoietic growth factors. While the neutrophil count decreased substantially (compared with the initial filgrastim-induced increase) following initiation of epoetin alfa therapy and again when zidovudine was reinitiated, counts still remained substantially above baseline values during continued filgrastim therapy, and such combined therapy permitted resumption of full-dose zidovudine therapy in many patients who had developed intolerance. However, while epoetin alfa dosages averaging 240 units/kg IV 3 times weekly effectively increased serum hemoglobin concentration to more than 15 g/dL while zidovudine therapy was withheld, the drug only partially ameliorated the anemia once zidovudine (1–1.2 g daily) therapy was reinstituted, and most patients required red blood cell transfusions. Like epoetin alfa, current evidence suggests that filgrastim does not adversely affect HIV replication nor interfere with the antiviral activity of zidovudine.

Anemia in HIV-infected Patients Not Receiving Zidovudine Epoetin alfa also has been used to treat anemia associated with HIV infection in patients *not* receiving zidovudine†; decreases in transfusion requirements and increases in hematocrit associated with epoetin alfa therapy in these patients appear to be similar to those in HIV-infected patients receiving zidovudine. A normocytic, normochromic, sometimes transfusion-dependent anemia develops in up to 80% of patients with HIV infection who are not receiving zidovudine. Despite a normal endogenous serum erythropoietin concentration, such patients have an inappropriately low reticulocyte count; however, the serum erythropoietin concentration also may be inappropriately low for the degree of anemia present. Severity of the anemia seems to correlate with the degree of disease progression. Further studies are needed to determine more fully the usefulness of epoetin alfa in HIV-infected patients not receiving zidovudine therapy and to fully elucidate the risks and benefits of such therapy. (See Cautions: Precautions and Contraindications.)

■ **Anemia in Patients with Nonmyeloid Malignancies** ***Chemotherapy-induced Anemia*** Epoetin alfa is used for the treatment of chemotherapy-induced anemia in patients with nonmyeloid malignanciesin whom chemotherapy is planned for at least 2 additional months. Therapy with epoetin alfa or other ESAs should be initiated only when the hemoglobin concentration is less than 10 g/dL and should be discontinued after completion of a course of myelosuppressive chemotherapy. The manufacturers state that epoetin alfa is not indicated for use in patients receiving hormonal agents, biologic products, or radiation therapy unless they also are receiving concomitant myelosuppressive chemotherapy. Epoetin alfa also is *not* intended for patients who require *acute* correction of severe anemia; the drug should *not* be used as a substitute for emergency transfusion.

Use of ESAs has been associated with shortened overall survival and/or an increased risk of tumor progression or recurrence in clinical studies in patients with breast, non-small cell lung, head and neck, lymphoid, or cervical cancer. *ESAs are not indicated for patients with chemotherapy-induced anemia in whom the anticipated outcome of chemotherapy is cure of the underlying malignancy.* (See Cautions: Increased Mortality and Tumor Progression and also see Hematologic Precautions and Contraindications under Cautions: Precautions and Contraindications.) ESAs have not been shown to improve outcomes of cancer chemotherapy (e.g., in terms of greater tumor shrinkage, delayed tumor progression or recurrence, increased survival). In addition, ESAs do not improve quality of life, fatigue, or well-being in patients with chemotherapy-induced anemia. *Epoetin alfa also is not indicated in patients with cancer and anemia who are not receiving cancer chemotherapy.* (See Chronic Anemia Associated with Malignancy under Uses: Anemia in Cancer Patients.)

In a series of placebo-controlled, double-blind studies in 131 anemic cancer patients who were receiving antineoplastic agent therapy (59 were receiving concomitant chemotherapy regimens containing cisplatin and 72 were receiving concomitant chemotherapy regimens not containing cisplatin), epoetin alfa therapy (150 units/kg subcutaneously 3 times weekly for 12 weeks) resulted in a decrease in red blood cell transfusion requirements from week 5 through the end of the study. The combined proportion of patients transfused during this period (i.e., includes only those who remained on study beyond week 6) was 22 or 43% in those receiving epoetin alfa or placebo, respectively. Baseline endogenous serum erythropoietin concentrations varied among patients in these studies; approximately 75% of patients had pretreatment serum erythropoietin concentrations less than 132 milliunits/mL and approximately 4% had pretreatment concentrations exceeding 500 milliunits/mL. In general, patients with lower pretreatment erythropoietin concentrations responded better to epoetin alfa than those with higher pretreatment concentrations. In a separate placebo-controlled, double-blind study in a total of 344 adult cancer patients with anemia due to concomitant myelosuppressive chemotherapy, 14% of patients receiving epoetin alfa (40,000 units by subcutaneous injection once weekly) required a red blood cell transfusion between weeks 5 and 16 or the last day on study compared with 28% of those receiving placebo. Blood transfusion requirements were reduced with epoetin alfa relative to placebo in those who received a cisplatin-containing chemotherapy regimen (15 versus 39% of patients transfused) as well as in those who received a regimen without cisplatin (14 versus 26% of patients transfused).

In a randomized placebo-controlled, double-blind study in children and young adults (5–18 years of age) with anemia who were receiving chemotherapy regimens for the treatment of various childhood malignancies (e.g., Hodgkin's lymphoma, non-Hodgkin's lymphoma, acute lymphocytic leukemia, solid tumors), 51% of patients receiving epoetin alfa required red blood cell transfusions from week 5 through the end of the study compared with 69% of those receiving placebo. Epoetin alfa therapy did not result in improvements in health-related quality of life.

Chronic Anemia Associated with Malignancy Although epoetin alfa has been used for the treatment and prevention of the normocytic, normochromic anemia associated with malignancy†, results of randomized controlled studies in patients with certain types of cancer and associated anemia who were not receiving cancer chemotherapy or radiation therapy† indicate that *ESAs may decrease overall survival in such patients*. In addition, ESA therapy did not reduce red blood cell transfusion requirements in these patients. (See Hematologic Precautions and Contraindications under Cautions: Precautions and Contraindications.) The manufacturers of epoetin alfa and darbepoetin alfa state that ESAs are *not* indicated for use in anemic patients with active malignant disease who are *not* receiving cancer chemotherapy.

■ **Preoperative Use in Patients Undergoing Surgery** ***Reduction of Allogeneic Red Blood Cell Transfusion Requirements in Anemic Surgery Patients*** Epoetin alfa is used perioperatively to reduce the need for allogeneic red blood cell transfusions in anemic patients (hemoglobin concentrations exceeding 10 but not exceeding 13 g/dL) who are scheduled to undergo elective, noncardiac, nonvascular surgery. Epoetin alfa is indicated for such surgical patients at high risk for perioperative blood loss, but is not indicated in those who are willing to donate autologous blood prior to surgery. *An increased incidence of thromboembolic events (e.g., deep-vein thrombosis) has been observed in patients who received epoetin alfa preoperatively to reduce the need for allogeneic blood transfusions and who were not receiving prophylactic anticoagulation; administration of antithrombotic prophylaxis is strongly recommended in patients receiving ESAs for this indication.* (See Increased Mortality and Thromboembolic Effects under Cautions: Cardiovascular Effects.) Epoetin alfa is *not* intended for patients who require *acute* correction of severe anemia; the drug should *not* be used as a substitute for emergency transfusion.

Safety and efficacy of epoetin alfa for the reduction of allogeneic blood transfusion requirements have been evaluated in a placebo-controlled, double-blind study involving 316 patients scheduled for major, elective orthopedic hip or knee surgery who were expected to require 2 or more units of blood and who were unable or unwilling to participate in an autologous blood donation program. Patients were randomized to receive epoetin alfa (300 units/kg), epoetin alfa (100 units/kg), or placebo given by subcutaneous injection once daily for 10 days prior to surgery, on the day of surgery, and for 4 days after surgery; all patients received oral iron and a low-dose postoperative warfarin regimen. While patients with pretreatment hemoglobin concentrations ranging from exceeding 10 but not exceeding 13 g/dL who received the 300-unit/kg dosage regimen of epoetin alfa had a reduced risk of allogeneic red blood cell transfusions, there was no evidence of benefit in those with higher pretreatment hemoglobin concentrations (exceeding 13 but not exceeding 15 g/dL). Because there were too few patients enrolled with pretreatment hemoglobin concentrations of 10 g/dL or less, the effects of preoperative epoetin alfa treatment on transfusion requirements in these patients could not be determined. In the group of patients with pretreatment hemoglobin concentrations exceeding 10 but not exceeding 13 g/dL, the mean number of units transfused was 0.45 in those who received the 300-unit/kg epoetin alfa regimen, 0.42 units in those who received the 100-unit/kg epoetin alfa regimen, and 1.14 units in those who received placebo. In addition, mean hemoglobin, hematocrit, and reticulocyte counts increased substantially during the presurgical period in those who received epoetin alfa.

Use of epoetin alfa for preoperative treatment of anemic patients also has been evaluated in an open-label, parallel-group trial enrolling 145 patients with pretreatment hemoglobin concentrations of 10–13 g/dL who were scheduled for major orthopedic hip or knee surgery and who were not participating in an autologous blood donation program; all patients received oral iron and appropriate pharmacologic anticoagulation therapy. In this study, patients were randomized to receive epoetin alfa in a regimen of 600 units/kg once-weekly for 3 weeks prior to surgery and on the day of surgery or a regimen of 300 units/kg once daily for 10 days prior to surgery, on the day of surgery, and for 4 days after surgery. The mean increase in hemoglobin from pretreatment to presurgery was greater and the mean increase in absolute reticulocyte count was less in patients receiving the once-weekly regimen than in those receiving the daily regimen; however, the mean number of units of blood transfused per patient was approximately 0.3 units in both treatment groups, and mean hemoglobin concentrations throughout the postsurgical period were similar in both groups.

Autologous Blood Donation Epoetin alfa has been used prior to elective surgery to increase the volume of blood available for autologous donation†, particularly for procedures in which the potential for substantial blood loss exists (e.g., hip or knee replacement). However, the relative merits of using epoetin alfa for aggressive autologous blood harvesting (i.e., exceeding 4 units of blood per patient) prior to surgery have been questioned by some clinicians. The manufacturer states that epoetin alfa is *not* indicated in anemic patients who are willing to donate autologous blood prior to surgery.

■ **Anemia associated with Rheumatoid Arthritis and Rheumatic Disease** Limited data suggest that epoetin alfa may be useful and relatively safe in selected patients for treating the anemia associated with rheumatoid arthritis and/or rheumatic disease†; however, further study and long-term experience are needed to elucidate fully the efficacy of the drug in patients with these conditions. Although patients with anemia secondary to rheumatic disease may have normal to increased endogenous serum concentrations of erythropoietin, bone marrow responsiveness to the hormone is decreased.

■ **Anemia of Prematurity** Therapy with epoetin alfa may be beneficial in the treatment of anemia of prematurity†, a condition in premature neonates of unclear etiology and characterized by low hematocrit, decreased reticulocyte index, and an inappropriately low serum erythropoietin concentration relative to the severity of anemia. While asymptomatic premature neonates may require no treatment for this condition, those with pulmonary disease, tachypnea, tachycardia, apnea, and/or impaired growth may require transfusion of whole blood and/or red blood cells, which may further suppress endogenous erythropoietin production. Epoetin alfa or beta therapy combined with iron supplementation has reduced transfusion requirements and increased hematocrit during the first several weeks of life. In a limited number of premature neonates with a baseline hematocrit averaging 26.3% (range: 22–31%), hematocrit increased to a mean value of 29.6% (range: 24–35%) following 3 weeks of therapy with epoetin alfa 25–100 units/kg subcutaneously 3 times weekly. Although it appears that epoetin therapy is beneficial in this condition, particularly in low-birthweight neonates without concurrent severe illness, optimal patient selection criteria remain to be more fully elucidated. Epoetin also has been used effectively in a few infants to treat delayed hyporegenerative anemia of Rh hemolytic disease†, an anemia characterized by low endogenous erythropoietin production but highly erythropoietin-responsive erythroid progenitors.

■ **Sickle Cell Anemia** Limited animal data suggest that high, intermittent doses of epoetin alfa can increase fetal hemoglobin concentrations; since such increases have been shown to inhibit erythrocyte sickling, it has been suggested that therapy with the drug potentially could be beneficial in patients with sickle cell anemia†. However, limited study of high-dose (e.g., up to 3000 units/kg once weekly) epoetin alfa either alone or in combination with hydroxyurea (which also stimulates fetal hemoglobin synthesis) in patients with sickle cell anemia has indicated no discernible beneficial effect of epoetin alfa on fetal hemoglobin, and the uncertain benefits of epoetin alfa therapy in this condition must be weighed against the potential for intravascular sickling that may accompany an increased erythrocyte count.

■ **Myelodysplastic Syndrome** Epoetin alfa has been used in a limited number of patients with myelodysplastic syndromes, and has been designated an orphan drug by the FDA for use in this condition; however, IV dosages of up to 1600 units/kg twice weekly have been associated with relatively limited response rates, and effects of the hormone on nonerythroid cell lines and potential risks of leukemic transformation require further elucidation. *ESAs, including epoetin alfa, have been shown to increase the risk of death and tumor progression or recurrence in anemic patients with certain types of cancer receiving ESA therapy.* (See Hematologic Precautions and Contraindications under Cautions: Precautions and Contraindications.)

■ **Other Uses** Epoetin alfa also has been used in a limited number of patients with Gaucher's disease†, Castleman's disease†, the anemia of prolonged *acute* renal failure†, and in high dosages for the correction of ineffective hematopoiesis associated with paroxysmal nocturnal hemoglobinuria†; however, further study and experience are needed to determine the usefulness, if any, of the drug in these conditions.

■ **Misuse and Abuse** Because of the ergogenic effects of epoetin alfa therapy (i.e., increases in erythrocyte count, hematocrit, hemoglobin concentration, and oxygen-carrying capacity of blood), the potential exists for abuse of the drug by athletes, especially those participating in high-aerobic demand, endurance-type events. Effects of epoetin alfa would be expected to be similar to those of homologous or autologous red blood cell transfusions ("blood doping"), which have been used by athletes to increase cardiac output, maximal oxygen uptake capacity of blood, and aerobic exercise endurance by increasing arterial blood oxygen content; effects may be particularly evident in individuals with greater initial aerobic fitness. Such use would be difficult to detect since there is no reliable way to distinguish epoetin alfa from the endogenous hormone using readily available drug-screening methods (e.g., immunoradiometric assay).

Since epoetin alfa produces dose-related increases in hematocrit, administration of the drug in athletes with normal hematocrits could result in dangerously high hematocrits and/or hemoglobin concentrations; such increases could continue even after discontinuance of the drug. Systematic studies to determine the risks of potential misuse and abuse of epoetin alfa have not been performed to date, but evidence from legitimate medical use of the drug indicates that adverse effects involving the cardiovascular system (e.g., thromboembolic events) potentially could be observed. *Results of several controlled studies indicate that ESAs, including epoetin alfa, may increase the risk of death and serious cardiovascular events in certain patients when therapy is targeted to hemoglobin concentrations exceeding 11 g/dL.* (See Cautions: Cardiovascular Effects and also see Cautions: Hematologic Effects.) The harmful effects of the drug on hematocrit may be compounded by dehydration, especially in athletes participating in highly competitive, aerobic events. While abuse of epoetin alfa has been implicated in the deaths of several athletes, no direct causal relationship to administration of the drug has been established. The manufacturers of epoetin alfa and medical and sports experts, including the US and International Olympic Committees and the National Collegiate Athletic Association, consider the use of epoetin alfa to enhance athletic ergogenic potential inappropriate and unacceptable because its use by athletes is contrary to the rules and ethical principles of athletic competition.

Dosage and Administration

■ **Administration** Epoetin alfa is administered by IV or subcutaneous injection.

In patients undergoing hemodialysis, the manufacturers recommend that epoetin alfa be given IV rather than subcutaneously because of reports of pure red cell aplasia associated with the latter route of administration. (See Cautions: Immunogenicity.) Alternatively, epoetin alfa has been injected into the venous return line of the dialysis tubing following dialysis to eliminate the need for additional venous access. However, to prevent the drug from adhering to the tubing, some clinicians suggest that the dose be injected while blood is still in the line and that the line then be flushed with 0.9% sodium chloride injection. Epoetin alfa also has been administered through the arteriovenous (AV) fistula† following completion of dialysis and disconnection of the dialyzer unit, although special care is recommended to preserve graft function.

Epoetin alfa may be given IV or subcutaneously in predialysis patients with chronic kidney disease, in patients undergoing continuous ambulatory peritoneal dialysis (CAPD), or in HIV-infected patients receiving zidovudine. IV administration of the drug has been used successfully in patients receiving at-home hemodialysis. However, subcutaneous administration may be preferred when feasible because of comparative ease and practicality of administration, the ability of the patient to self-administer the drug, and the reduced cost for special equipment and trained personnel. Aggregate data from studies evaluating the efficacy of subcutaneous versus IV administration of epoetin alfa suggest that target hematocrit/hemoglobin levels are maintained with lower weekly dosages of epoetin alfa (15–50% lower) when the drug is given subcutaneously. In addition, some clinicians suggest that subcutaneous injection is preferred in predialysis patients because repeated IV administration of the drug may interfere with the integrity of the peripheral vascular system, posing a threat to future hemodialysis access.

Iron status (i.e., transferrin saturation, serum ferritin concentration) should be evaluated prior to and during therapy in patients receiving epoetin alfa. Supplemental iron should be initiated if serum ferritin concentration is less than 100 ng/mL or transferrin saturation is less than 20%. The manufacturer states that the majority of patients with chronic kidney disease will require supplemental iron during the course of ESA therapy. Prior to initiating epoetin alfa therapy, other causes of anemia (e.g., vitamin deficiency, metabolic or chronic inflammatory conditions, bleeding) should be corrected or excluded.

Patients who self-administer epoetin alfa should be instructed regarding proper dosage and administration of the drug and advised to follow the manufacturer's "Patient Instructions for Use". Patients should take epoetin alfa only as prescribed and should contact a clinician immediately if the prescribed dosage is exceeded or a dose is missed. Patients with chemotherapy-induced anemia should be informed that epoetin alfa therapy should be discontinued when chemotherapy is stopped. Patients should be instructed carefully regarding aseptic technique and regarding the importance of proper disposal and should be cautioned against the reuse of needles, syringes, and unused portions of the single-dose formulation. Patients also should be advised regarding the manifestations of sensitivity reactions (e.g., whole body rash, shortness of breath, wheezing, decreases in blood pressure, swelling around mouth or eyes, rapid pulse, sweating) and appropriate actions to take should such manifestations develop.

Vials of epoetin alfa should not be shaken or frozen, and should be discarded if subjected to these conditions. For IV or subcutaneous use, the appropriate dose of the drug should be withdrawn from the vial into the syringe for administration. Once the dose has been withdrawn from the vial, it should be administered promptly. (See Chemistry and Stability: Stability.)

Epoetin alfa injection generally should not be mixed with other drug solutions. However, the manufacturer states that the preservative-free formulation from single-use vials may be admixed in equal parts (in a 1:1 ratio) in a syringe with bacteriostatic 0.9% sodium chloride injection (preserved with benzyl alcohol) at the time of administration; presence of the benzyl alcohol may ameliorate local discomfort associated with subcutaneous injection of the drug. Because of the risks associated with benzyl alcohol, epoetin alfa injection that has been admixed with injection solutions containing benzyl alcohol should not be used in neonates, infants, pregnant women, and nursing women. Contents of vials of epoetin alfa should be inspected visually for discoloration and/or particulate matter prior to administration whenever solution and container permit; if either is present, the solution should be discarded.

■ **Dosage** ***Anemia of Chronic Kidney Disease*** Hemoglobin concentrations should be monitored at least weekly following initiation of epoetin alfa therapy and after each dosage adjustment until stable, then at least monthly thereafter. In controlled trials of patients with chronic kidney disease, administration of ESAs to achieve hemoglobin concentrations exceeding 11 g/dL did not provide additional benefit beyond that achieved with lower hemoglobin targets and was associated with a greater risk of death and serious adverse cardiovascular events; no trial to date has identified a target hemoglobin concentration, ESA dosage, or dosing strategy that does not increase these risks. (See Cautions: Cardiovascular Effects.) The potential benefits of epoetin alfa in decreasing transfusion requirements should be weighed against the increased risk of death and other serious adverse cardiovascular events in this patient population.

Dosage of epoetin alfa should be individualized, and the lowest possible dosage sufficient to reduce the need for red blood cell transfusions should be used. FDA and the manufacturer state that patients with chronic kidney disease *on dialysis* should have epoetin alfa therapy initiated when their hemoglobin concentration is less than 10 g/dL. If hemoglobin concentration approaches or exceeds 11 g/dL in such patients, epoetin alfa dosage should be reduced or therapy interrupted. FDA and the manufacturer also state that consideration should be given to initiating epoetin alfa therapy in patients with chronic kidney disease *not on dialysis* only when their hemoglobin concentration is less than 10 g/dL and the following 2 conditions also apply: the rate of hemoglobin decline indicates the likelihood of requiring a transfusion, and a goal of therapy is to reduce the risk of alloimmunization and/or other risks associated with red blood cell transfusions. If hemoglobin concentration exceeds 10 g/dL in such patients, dosage should be reduced or therapy interrupted.

Initial Dosage. For the treatment of anemia associated with chronic kidney disease in adults, the manufacturer recommends an initial epoetin alfa dosage of 50–100 units/kg IV or subcutaneously 3 times weekly. In pediatric patients 1 month of age or older receiving dialysis, the recommended initial dosage of epoetin alfa is 50 units/kg 3 times weekly. In geriatric patients, individualized dosing is recommended to maintain target hemoglobin concentrations.

Dosage Adjustment. Dosage of epoetin alfa should be adjusted based on hemoglobin concentrations. Factors including the rate of increase or decrease in hemoglobin concentration, responsiveness to the ESA, and hemoglobin concentration variability should be considered when determining whether a dosage adjustment is needed; a single hemoglobin excursion may not require a dosage change. Frequent dosage adjustments should be avoided.

If the hemoglobin concentration increases rapidly (e.g., by more than 1 g/dL in any 2-week period), dosage of epoetin alfa should be reduced by 25% or more as necessary to reduce the risk of a rapid response. However, if the hemoglobin concentration has not increased by more than 1 g/dL after 4 weeks of therapy, dosage of epoetin alfa should be increased by 25%. Dosage increases should not be made more frequently than once every 4 weeks. If an adequate response to epoetin alfa is not obtained over a 12-week period of escalating dosages, the patient should be evaluated for other causes of anemia; further dosage increases are not likely to improve patient response and may increase the risks of therapy. (See Other Precautions and Contraindications under Cautions: Precautions and Contraindications.) The lowest dosage of epoetin alfa that will maintain a hemoglobin concentration sufficient to reduce the need for red blood cell transfusions should be used in such patients, and if responsiveness does not improve, the drug should be discontinued.

In clinical studies, patients with chronic kidney disease on dialysis responded to epoetin alfa with clinically important increases in hemoglobin concentration, and over 95% of patients were red blood cell transfusion-independent after 3 months of therapy.

Zidovudine-associated Anemia in HIV-infected Patients **Initial Therapy.** For the treatment of anemia associated with zidovudine therapy in adults with human immunodeficiency virus (HIV) infection who have endogenous serum erythropoietin concentrations not exceeding 500 milliunits/mL and who are receiving zidovudine dosages not exceeding 4.2 g/week, the recommended initial dosage of epoetin alfa is 100 units/kg IV or subcutaneously 3 times weekly. HIV-infected patients with endogenous pretreatment (pretransfusion) serum erythropoietin concentrations not exceeding 500 milliunits/mL who are receiving weekly cumulative zidovudine dosages not exceeding 4.2 g are more likely to respond to epoetin alfa therapy than patients with higher endogenous pretreatment erythropoietin concentrations (i.e., exceeding 500 milliunits/mL).

Dosage Adjustment. Hemoglobin concentrations should be monitored at least weekly following initiation of therapy and after each dosage adjustment until concentrations are stable and sufficient to minimize the need for red blood cell transfusions. If hemoglobin has not increased after 8 weeks of therapy, the dose of epoetin alfa given 3 times weekly may be increased by approximately 50–100 units/kg at 4- to 8-week intervals until an adequate hemoglobin concentration is obtained or a dose of 300 units/kg is reached. If hemoglobin concentration does not increase after 8 weeks of treatment with epoetin alfa 300 units/kg 3 times weekly, the drug should be discontinued. If hemoglobin concentrations exceed 12 g/dL at any time during therapy, treatment should be withheld until the hemoglobin decreases to less than 11 g/dL; therapy may then be resumed at a dosage 25% less than the previous dosage.

HIV-infected pediatric patients with zidovudine-induced anemia, 8 months to 17 years of age, reportedly have received epoetin alfa dosages of 50–400 units/kg subcutaneously or IV 2 or 3 times weekly.

Chemotherapy-Induced Anemia in Patients with Nonmyeloid Malignancies Therapy with epoetin alfa should only be initiated in cancer patients who have hemoglobin concentrations of less than 10 g/dL and in whom a minimum of 2 additional months of chemotherapy is planned upon initiation of epoetin alfa. The lowest possible epoetin alfa dosage sufficient to avoid red blood cell transfusions should be used. Hemoglobin concentrations should be monitored weekly following initiation of therapy and after each dosage change until stable and sufficient to minimize the need for red blood cell transfusions. *Therapy with epoetin alfa or other ESAs should be discontinued in patients with cancer following completion of a chemotherapy course.*

3-Times-Weekly Dosing. For the treatment of chemotherapy-induced anemia in adults with cancer, the usual dosage of epoetin alfa is 150 units/kg subcutaneously 3 times weekly. If the hemoglobin concentration has increased by less than 1 g/dL after the initial 4 weeks of therapy and remains below 10 g/dL, dosage of the drug should be increased to 300 units/kg 3 times weekly. If response to epoetin alfa is not satisfactory (i.e., continuing need for red blood cell transfusion, low hemoglobin concentrations) after 8 weeks of therapy, the drug should be discontinued.

If the hemoglobin concentration reaches a level sufficient to avoid the need for red blood cell transfusion or increases by more than 1 g/dL in any 2-week period, dosage of the drug should be decreased by 25%. If hemoglobin *exceeds* a concentration needed to avoid red blood cell transfusions, doses of epoetin alfa should be withheld until the hemoglobin decreases to a concentration at which transfusions may be required. When epoetin alfa therapy is reinitiated, dosage of the drug should be 25% below the previous dosage.

Once-Weekly Dosing. When once-weekly dosing of epoetin alfa is indicated for chemotherapy-induced anemia in adults with cancer, the recommended initial dosage of epoetin alfa is 40,000 units subcutaneously once weekly. If the hemoglobin concentration has increased by less than 1 g/dL after the initial 4 weeks of therapy and remains below 10 g/dL, the epoetin alfa dosage should be increased to 60,000 units weekly. If response to epoetin alfa is not satisfactory after 8 weeks of therapy, the drug should be discontinued.

If epoetin alfa therapy produces a very rapid hemoglobin response (e.g., an increase exceeding 1 g/dL in any 2-week period) or if hemoglobin reaches a concentration sufficient to avoid the need for red blood cell transfusions, the dosage of epoetin alfa should be reduced by 25%. If the hemoglobin *exceeds* a concentration needed to avoid red blood cell transfusions, administration of the drug should be withheld temporarily until hemoglobin falls to a concentration at which transfusions may be required, at which point therapy should be reinstituted at a dosage 25% below the previous dosage.

For the treatment of chemotherapy-induced anemia in pediatric cancer patients 5–18 years of age, the recommended initial dosage of epoetin alfa is 600 units/kg IV once weekly. If the hemoglobin has increased by less than 1 g/dL after 4 weeks and remains below 10 g/dL, the weekly dosage should be increased to 900 units/kg IV (maximum 60,000 units weekly). If epoetin alfa therapy produces a very rapid hemoglobin response (e.g., an increase exceeding 1 g/dL in any 2-week period) or if hemoglobin reaches a concentration sufficient to avoid the need for red blood cell transfusions, epoetin alfa dosage should be reduced by 25%. If hemoglobin *exceeds* a concentration needed to avoid red blood cell transfusions, administration of the drug should be withheld temporarily until the hemoglobin falls to a concentration at which transfusions may be required, at which point therapy should be resumed at a dosage 25% below the previous dosage. If the response to epoetin alfa is not satisfactory after 8 weeks of therapy, the drug should be discontinued.

Dosage requirements in geriatric patients with chemotherapy-induced anemia appear to be similar to those in younger adults.

Reduction of Allogeneic Blood Transfusion Requirements in Anemic Surgery Patients When epoetin alfa is used perioperatively to reduce the need for allogeneic red blood cell transfusions in adults with hemoglobin concentration exceeding 10 but not exceeding 13 g/dL who are scheduled to undergo elective, noncardiac, nonvascular surgery, the recommended dosage is 300 units/kg given by subcutaneous injection once daily for 10 days prior to surgery, on the day of surgery, and for 4 days after surgery. Alternatively, epoetin alfa can be given subcutaneously in a regimen of 600 units/kg once weekly for 3 weeks prior to surgery (i.e., days 21, 14, and 7 before surgery), with an additional dose given on the day of surgery. In clinical studies, dosing requirements in geriatric patients receiving the 3-times-weekly or once-weekly regimen were similar to those in younger adults. Prophylaxis for deep-vein thrombosis is strongly recommended during therapy.

Cautions

The most frequent and serious adverse effects of epoetin alfa therapy in patients with chronic kidney disease are related to the rate and extent of increase of the erythrocyte count and hemoglobin; therefore, excessively rapid correction or overcorrection of the anemia should be avoided. *Evidence from controlled clinical trials indicates that therapy with epoetin alfa and other erythropoiesis-stimulating agents (ESAs) may increase the risk of death and serious cardiovascular events when targeted to hemoglobin concentrations exceeding 11 g/dL in patients with chronic kidney disease.* (See Cardiovascular Precautions and Contraindications under Cautions: Precautions and Contraindications.)

Epoetin alfa has been used principally in patients with chronic kidney disease undergoing hemodialysis, and many of the adverse effects reported with epoetin alfa therapy appear to be attributable to correction of the anemia or to the patient's disease rather than to the drug itself.

■ **Cardiovascular Effects** ***Increased Mortality and Thromboembolic Effects*** Therapy with epoetin alfa and other ESAs has been shown to increase the risk of death and serious and life-threatening cardiovascular events (e.g., myocardial infarction, stroke, congestive heart failure, hemodialysis vascular access thrombosis) when targeted to achieve hemoglobin concentrations exceeding 11 g/dL in patients with chronic kidney disease. An increase in hemoglobin concentration exceeding 1 g/dL in a 2-week period also may contribute to these risks. Patients with chronic kidney disease and an insufficient hemoglobin response to ESA therapy may be at greater risk for cardiovascular events and mortality than other patients. An increased risk of death and/or serious adverse cardiovascular events also have been observed in controlled clinical trials of epoetin alfa in patients with cancer and in those undergoing coronary artery bypass graft surgery (CABG), as well as an increased risk of deep-vein thrombosis in patients undergoing orthopedic surgery.

Data from several controlled clinical studies in patients with chronic kidney disease comparing higher ESA hemoglobin target concentrations (13–14 g/dL) to lower targets (9–11.3 g/dL) indicate that an increased risk of death, myocardial infarction, stroke, congestive heart failure, hemodialysis vascular access thrombosis, and other thromboembolic events occurred in the higher target hemoglobin groups. In one of the studies, a randomized, open-label study (Correction of Hemoglobin and Outcomes in Renal Insufficiency [CHOIR]) in patients with chronic kidney disease who were not receiving dialysis, therapy with epoetin alfa targeted to a hemoglobin concentration of 13.5 g/dL (high-hemoglobin group) was associated with an increased incidence of the primary composite end point of death, myocardial infarction, hospitalization for congestive heart failure (without renal replacement therapy), or stroke compared with that in patients treated to a target hemoglobin of 11.3 g/dL (low-hemoglobin group); the trial was terminated early as a result of these safety findings. More patients in the high-hemoglobin group (54.8%) than in the low-hemoglobin group (48.5%) had at least one serious adverse event. Improvements in quality of life were similar in both groups. At the end of the study, hemoglobin concentrations averaged 12.6 and 11.3 g/dL in the high- and low-hemoglobin groups, respectively. The mean weekly dosage of epoetin alfa required to maintain hemoglobin at target concentrations in the high-hemoglobin group (11,215 units) was almost twice that in the low-hemoglobin group (6276 units).

In another study (Normal Hematocrit Study [NHS]), hemodialysis patients with clinically evident cardiac disease (ischemic heart disease, congestive heart failure) who received epoetin alfa with a goal of achieving and maintaining a target hemoglobin concentration of 14 g/dL had increased mortality compared with that in similar patients treated to a target hemoglobin concentration of 10 g/dL; the trial was terminated early as a result of these safety findings. The incidence of nonfatal myocardial infarction, vascular access thrombosis, and other thromboembolic events was also higher in those treated to a target hemoglobin concentration of 14 g/dL.

In a randomized, double-blind, placebo-controlled study (Trial to Reduce Cardiovascular Events with Aranesp Therapy [TREAT]) in patients with type 2 diabetes mellitus, anemia, and non-dialysis-dependent chronic kidney disease, treatment with another ESA, darbepoetin alfa, targeted to a hemoglobin concentration of 13 g/dL failed to reduce the overall rates of the primary cardiovascular and renal composite end points, but was associated with an increased risk of stroke compared with placebo (annualized stroke rate of 2.1 versus 1.1%, respectively). This increased risk was documented despite use of a conservative dosing strategy and measures designed to ensure gradual increases and avoidance of overshoots and oscillations in hemoglobin concentrations. The relative risk of stroke was particularly high in patients with a prior history of stroke compared with those who received placebo (annualized stroke rate of 5.2 versus 1.9%, respectively).

The increased risk of adverse cardiovascular/thromboembolic outcomes with hemoglobin targets exceeding 12 g/dL also is supported by the results of a pooled analysis of data from randomized controlled trials in over 5000 patients with chronic kidney disease. In this analysis, the risk of all-cause mortality was higher (by about 20%) in patients receiving ESAs (epoetin alfa, epoetin beta [not commercially available in the US], darbepoetin alfa) targeted to a hemoglobin of 12–16 g/dL than in those receiving ESA therapy targeted to a lower hemoglobin range. The risk of other outcomes such as arteriovenous access thrombosis and poorly controlled blood pressure also were increased in the high-hemoglobin group.

In another randomized, open-label study in patients with stage 3 or 4 chronic kidney disease and mild-to-moderate anemia (hemoglobin 11–12.5 g/dL) who did not require dialysis, therapy with epoetin beta (currently not commercially available in the US) designed to normalize hemoglobin concentrations (treatment initiated immediately and targeted to a hemoglobin concentration of 13–15 g/dL) did not reduce the incidence of the primary composite end point (time to occurrence of a first cardiovascular event, including sudden death, myocardial infarction, acute heart failure, stroke, transient ischemic attack, angina pectoris resulting in hospitalization for at least 24 hours or prolongation of hospitalization, complication of peripheral vascular disease [amputation or necrosis], or cardiac arrhythmia resulting in hospitalization for at least 24 hours) compared with less-intensive epoetin beta therapy (targeted to a hemoglobin concentration of 10.5–11.5 g/dL and initiated only after hemoglobin had decreased to less than 10.5 g/dL) after 3 years of observation. Quality of life was improved in patients receiving therapy to normalize hemoglobin concentrations compared with those receiving less-intense epoetin beta therapy, but dialysis was required in more patients receiving hemoglobin normalization therapy.

An increased incidence of thromboembolic events, some serious and life-threatening, also has been observed in patients with cancer receiving ESAs. In a randomized, controlled study in patients with metastatic breast cancer who were receiving cancer chemotherapy, mortality was higher in patients receiving weekly epoetin alfa therapy (targeted to a hemoglobin of 12–14 g/dL or a hematocrit of 36–42%) versus placebo. The study was terminated early when interim results showed a higher mortality (8.7 or 3.4% with epoetin alfa or placebo, respectively) and a higher rate of fatal thrombotic events (1.1 or 0.2% with epoetin alfa or placebo, respectively) after 4 months. Based on Kaplan-Meier estimates, the proportion of these patients who survived 1 year after randomization was lower in the epoetin alfa group than in the placebo group (70% vs 76%).

An increased incidence of deep-vein thrombosis also has been observed in patients undergoing orthopedic surgical procedures and receiving epoetin alfa to reduce allogeneic red blood cell transfusion requirements, and the manufacturers state that antithrombotic prophylaxis is strongly recommended when ESAs are used in such patients. In a randomized, open-label, controlled study in adults undergoing spinal surgery and not receiving prophylactic anticoagulation, deep-vein thrombosis (as determined by color flow duplex imaging or clinical symptoms) occurred more frequently in patients who received epoetin alfa 600 units/kg (7, 14, and 21 days prior to surgery and on the day of surgery for a total of 4 doses) in addition to standard of care treatment (4.7%) than in patients who received standard of care treatment alone (2.1%). In addition, 12 patients in the epoetin alfa group had other thrombotic vascular events compared with 7 patients receiving only standard of care treatment. Patients in the study had baseline hemoglobin concentrations between 10 and 13 g/dL and received manufacturer-recommended dosages of epoetin alfa.

In a placebo-controlled study in patients undergoing coronary artery bypass graft surgery† (CABG), 7 deaths occurred in patients treated with perioperative epoetin alfa versus no deaths among those receiving placebo. Deaths that occurred during the time of epoetin alfa therapy (4 of 7 deaths) were associated with thromboembolic events. The manufacturer states that epoetin alfa is *not* indicated in patients undergoing cardiac or vascular surgery.

Hypertension The most frequent adverse effect observed in patients receiving epoetin alfa for anemia of chronic kidney disease is development or exacerbation of hypertension. The risk of hypertensive episodes is greatest in patients with chronic kidney disease who have preexisting hypertension or a history of hypertensive disease. Patients with extremely low baseline hematocrits (e.g., less than 22%) also may be at risk for the development of hypertension. The risk of hypertensive episodes appears to be low to nonexistent in patients with normal renal function compared with that in patients receiving the drug for anemia of chronic kidney disease; similar hypertensive episodes have been reported in patients with chronic kidney disease following red blood cell transfusions. Although a direct causal relationship to the drug has not been established, hypertensive encephalopathy with or without subsequent seizures of the tonic-clonic type has been reported with increases in blood pressure in chronic kidney disease patients receiving epoetin alfa, and correction of anemia should be performed slowly to minimize the risk of such complications. HIV-infected patients receiving epoetin alfa for zidovudine-induced anemia appear to be at minimal risk for epoetin alfa-induced hypertension.

The etiology of the hypertension reported in patients receiving epoetin alfa therapy is unclear; however, it usually is noted within the first 3 months of therapy and may be related to the rate or extent of increase in hematocrit. A decrease in compensatory vasodilation of the vascular system associated with increases in hematocrit and correction of anemia, either by transfusion or epoetin alfa therapy, may result in an increase in total peripheral resistance. An increase in the viscosity of whole blood, but not plasma, with increases in hematocrit and/or erythrocyte count and possibly platelet count, also has been implicated in the increase in total peripheral resistance. Limited in vitro evidence suggests that increased circulating hemoglobin binds to or chemically inactivates a vascular endothelium-derived relaxant factor (possibly nitric oxide), which blocks the vasodilatory effects of this factor in vivo and produces a rebound vasoconstriction; however, the clinical importance, if any, of this effect has not been established. Most evidence suggests that epoetin alfa does not possess direct vasopressor effects.

Limited evidence suggests that cautious adjustment of dialysis or "dry" weight (e.g., weight after correction of clinical volume overload and optimization of sitting blood pressure without inducing orthostatic hypotension) may result in decreased plasma volume and prevention or control of adverse hypertensive effects of epoetin alfa in patients with chronic kidney disease. However, such adjustments should be performed carefully to prevent hypovolemia and, preferably, prior to initiating epoetin alfa therapy.

Approximately 25–30% of chronic kidney disease patients will either develop or experience an exacerbation of hypertension during therapy with epoetin alfa, particularly during the early phase of therapy when hematocrit is rising. In a multicenter trial in patients with chronic kidney disease on hemodialysis, 32% of those receiving epoetin alfa developed an increase in diastolic blood pressure of at least 10 mm Hg or required an increase in the dosage of their antihypertensive medication. In several studies, pathologic increases in blood pressure occurred at hematocrit levels exceeding 30%. In patients with documented hypertension, lower initial dosages of epoetin alfa should be employed to allow for a gradual increase in hematocrit (i.e., achieving suggested target hematocrit over a period of 3–4 months). Limited evidence suggests that by slowly correcting the anemia, the sequelae of accelerated hypertension (e.g., seizures, hypertensive encephalopathy, pulmonary edema) may be reduced. It also has been suggested that the anemia in patients with preexisting hypertension be corrected to a lower target hematocrit (e.g., 30%) or hemoglobin concentration to prevent these sequelae. Management of persistently high blood pressure in patients receiving epoetin alfa may require initiation or increased dosage of antihypertensive therapy, control of weight with fluid and sodium restriction or modification of the dialysis regimen, phlebotomy (in cases of hypertension associated with excessively high hematocrit), and/or a decrease in the dosage or temporary or permanent withdrawal of epoetin alfa therapy.

Thrombosis at Vascular Access Sites An increased incidence of partial or complete clotting at the site of vascular access (arteriovenous [AV] fistula) has been observed in renal dialysis patients receiving epoetin alfa. A direct correlation between an epoetin alfa-induced increase in hematocrit and the rate of thrombotic events has not been shown, and little to no change in activated partial thromboplastin time (aPTT) and prothrombin time (PT) or fibrinogen concentration has been reported in patients or healthy individuals receiving the drug. However, thrombotic complications have been attributed to epoetin alfa-induced increases in erythrocyte count and whole blood viscosity in up to 13% of patients undergoing hemodialysis. In one patient whose AV fistula had been functional for 10 years, AV thrombosis occurred following an increase in hematocrit from 18% to 40% with epoetin alfa therapy. Vascular access clotting has been reported to occur in about 8% of patients receiving epoetin alfa therapy, and heparin anticoagulation requirements during dialysis may be increased in patients receiving epoetin alfa. While most patients require only modest increases in heparin dosage to prevent clotting complications, dosage increases of up to twofold reportedly have been required in some patients.

■ **Increased Mortality and Tumor Progression** Therapy with erythropoiesis-stimulating agents (ESAs) has been associated with increased mortality and risk of tumor progression or recurrence in patients with cancer. Epoetin alfa therapy resulted in shortened overall survival and increased deaths attributed to disease progression in women with metastatic breast cancer receiving cancer chemotherapy and a shortened time to tumor progression in patients with advanced head and neck cancer receiving radiation therapy. Shortened overall survival also was noted in patients with lymphoid malignancy receiving cancer chemotherapy and another ESA, darbepoetin alfa. Overall and progression-free survival rates were numerically lower in women with early breast cancer receiving neo-adjuvant cancer treatment and in women with cervical cancer receiving cancer chemotherapy and radiation therapy with darbepoetin alfa or epoetin alfa therapy, respectively, targeted to hemoglobin concentrations of 12–14 g/dL. A higher locoregional failure rate or shortened locoregional progression-free survival was observed in patients with squamous cell carcinoma of the head and neck receiving radiation therapy and darbepoetin alfa or epoetin beta (not currently available in the US). In addition, patients with cancer-related anemia and non-small-cell lung cancer or nonmyeloid malignancy who were *not* receiving cancer chemotherapy or radiation therapy had an increased risk of death and no reduction in transfusion requirements while receiving epoetin alfa or darbepoetin alfa targeted to hemoglobin concentrations of 12–14 or 12–13 g/dL, respectively; *ESAs are not currently FDA-labeled for use in patients with cancer-related anemia who are not receiving myelosuppressive chemotherapy.* FDA and the manufacturers of ESAs currently recommend that ESAs *not* be used in patients in whom the anticipated outcome of chemotherapy is cure of the underlying malignancy. (See Hematologic Precautions and Contraindications under Cautions: Precautions and Contraindications.)

■ **Hematologic Effects** Marked thrombocytosis has occurred rarely in patients receiving epoetin alfa. In several hemodialysis patients treated with usual dosages of epoetin alfa, temporary withdrawal of the drug and initiation of low-dose (100 mg/day) aspirin therapy were required. However, cases of thrombocytosis not requiring treatment also have been reported.

Porphyria has been reported during postmarketing experience with epoetin alfa.

Pure red cell aplasia (PRCA) and severe anemia have been reported in patients receiving epoetin alfa therapy. (See Cautions: Immunogenicity.)

■ **Nervous System Effects** Seizures (tonic-clonic [grand mal]) have been reported occasionally in patients receiving epoetin alfa. Risk of seizures is increased in patients with chronic kidney disease; in clinical trials, up to 5% of dialysis patients treated with epoetin alfa experienced seizures, more frequently within the first 3 months of therapy. In most cases, seizures have been attributed to a precipitous rise in blood pressure associated with overly rapid correction of hematocrit; an associated hypertensive encephalopathy also has been described. (See Hypertension under Cautions: Cardiovascular Effects.) Similar seizure activity has been observed in patients with chronic kidney disease receiving transfusions for correction of hematocrit. In some cases, seizure activity may be preceded by severe headache and increased blood pressure, and may occur as single episodes of the tonic-clonic type not requiring specific treatment. If seizures develop during epoetin alfa therapy, the etiology of the seizure should be determined and the drug discontinued if hematocrit is elevated and hypertension is present. Therapy with epoetin alfa generally has been resumed in such patients without recurrence of seizure activity; however, discontinuance of the drug has been required in some cases.

Headache, which may be temporally related to infusion of epoetin alfa and may reflect an acute or chronic increase in blood pressure, has been reported in patients with chronic kidney disease and in patients receiving the drug for zidovudine-induced anemia. Headache also has been reported in cancer patients on chemotherapy and in those undergoing surgery.

Although visual hallucinations have been reported in a limited number of patients receiving epoetin alfa for the anemia of renal failure, a direct causal relationship to the drug has not been established.

■ **Renal and Electrolyte Effects** Predialysis increases in serum concentrations of potassium, BUN, creatinine, uric acid, and phosphate have been reported with epoetin alfa therapy, especially in patients with chronic electrolyte abnormalities. It is unclear whether such increases are related to increased hemoglobin concentration, decreased efficiency of hemodialysis resulting from increased hematocrit (see Cautions: Effects on Dialyzer Function), or lifestyle changes (e.g., increased appetite) brought about by the feeling of well-being associated with correction of anemia. A decrease in potassium and phosphate clearance in patients on hemodialysis has been associated with increasing hematocrit to greater than 35% with epoetin alfa therapy, while a decrease in dialyzer creatinine clearance has been associated with increasing hemoglobin concentration (e.g., from 7.5 g/dL to 10 g/dL). Most of these changes respond to dietary modification, administration of phosphate-binding antacids, adjustments in dialysis time or other dialysis parameters, use of a larger surface-area dialyzer, or adjusting the electrolyte concentrations of the dialysis fluid.

Severe, recurrent hyperkalemia has been reported infrequently with epoetin alfa and has been implicated as the cause of death in at least one patient. Hyperkalemia may be caused by increased dietary intake of potassium associated with epoetin alfa-induced improvement in appetite, decreased dialyzer efficiency, or release of potassium into plasma from the increased erythrocyte load during dialysis. Modifications in dialysis frequency and dialysis fluid and use of nutritional counseling may be required for the treatment and/or prevention of hyperkalemia in epoetin alfa-treated patients; administration of cationic exchange resins (e.g., sodium polystyrene sulfonate) also has been effective in acute and long-term treatment of hyperkalemia in such patients.

In patients experiencing hyperphosphatemia, an increase in calcium-phosphate product associated with joint pain, inflammation, swelling, and periarticular calcification has been observed.

■ **Effects on Dialyzer Function** Although limited evidence suggests that decreases in hemodialyzer efficiency associated with increased hematocrit may be compensated for by adjusting dialyzer parameters (e.g., increasing high-efficiency hemodialysis prescription by 10–15% as the hematocrit approaches 40%), the circuit pressures and dialyzer function of high-flux or high-efficiency dialysis theoretically could be incompatible with the increased blood viscosity and hematocrit resulting from epoetin alfa therapy. Dialyzer fiber clotting and erythrocyte damage may occur as a result of interactions between increased blood viscosity and shear forces from the high flow rates used in these types of dialyzers; however, patients treated with epoetin alfa have undergone high-flux dialysis without serious complications when the hematocrit was maintained below 35%. Increased dialyzer fiber clotting also has been observed in patients not treated with epoetin alfa whose hematocrits exceeded 30%; slight increases in the heparin dosage administered during dialysis may be required to counteract this effect.

Although some studies have demonstrated little or no decrease in dialyzer clearance of urea and creatinine in hemodialysis patients treated with epoetin alfa, other studies indicate a decrease in hemodialyzer efficiency with increasing hematocrit, especially with regard to clearance of potassium and phosphate. (See Cautions: Renal and Electrolyte Effects.) In patients undergoing continuous ambulatory peritoneal dialysis (CAPD) who are treated with epoetin alfa, dialysis efficiency has been reported to increase (possibly because of increased vascular perfusion of the peritoneal cavity), decrease, or remain unchanged.

■ **Flu-like Syndrome** A flu-like syndrome has been reported in patients receiving epoetin alfa, principally with IV infusion of the drug, but also with subcutaneous administration. This flu-like syndrome is characterized by the development of transient diaphoresis, chills, shivering, malaise, feeling of cold or warmth, myalgia, bone pain and arthralgia of the limbs and pelvis, generalized aches and pains (including chest, back, and/or flank pain), fever,paresthesias, and/or abdominal pain/cramps. The reaction reportedly appears within 90–120 minutes of initiating the infusion and lasts for 2–12 hours. Although therapy with epoetin alfa has been discontinued in a few patients because of this adverse effect, the reaction generally is self-limiting and does not require dosage modification or preclude continued administration of the drug. To minimize the occurrence of this flu-like syndrome, some clinicians suggest administration of aspirin or acetaminophen prior to injection of the drug and a reduction in the infusion rate during administration.

■ **Immunogenicity** As with all therapeutic proteins, there is the potential for immunogenicity with epoetin alfa therapy. The observed incidence of antibody positivity in an assay may be influenced by several factors including assay methodology, sample handling, timing of sample collection, concomitant medications, and underlying disease. For these reasons, comparison of the incidence of antibodies to epoetin alfa with the incidence of antibodies to other products may be misleading.

Cases of pure red cell aplasia and severe anemia, with or without other cytopenias, have been associated with neutralizing antibodies in patients receiving erythropoiesis-stimulating agents (ESAs), including epoetin alfa. These cases have been observed predominantly in patients treated with subcutaneous ESAs for chronic kidney disease but also have been reported in patients receiving ESAs for anemia related to treatment of hepatitis C virus (HCV) infection (currently not an FDA-labeled indication for epoetin alfa). (See Immunologic Precautions and Contraindications under Cautions: Precautions and Contraindications.)

■ **Sensitivity Reactions** Serious allergic reactions, including anaphylaxis, angioedema, bronchospasm, skin rash, and urticaria, may occur with epoetin alfa. Urticarial reactions occurring within 48 hours of first exposure to the epoetin alfa vehicle have been described in 2 HIV-infected individuals, one receiving the drug and one receiving placebo (vehicle alone); reactions reportedly have occurred in at least one patient who did not have HIV infection. Skin tests revealed wheal and flare reactivity to the study formulation and a negative saline control. Such sensitivity may be related to albumin human present in the formulation, HIV-induced immunosuppression, or previous exposure to blood products.

■ **Other Adverse Effects** Nausea, vomiting, diarrhea, edema, arthralgias, and fatigue have been reported in more than 5% of chronic kidney disease patients receiving epoetin alfa. Difficulty in maintaining ideal or "dry" post-dialysis weight, cramps, night sweats, visual disturbances, exacerbation of acne, skin rash and urticaria (including petechial urticaria), petechial purpura, pruritus, transient local pain and/or stinging at the subcutaneous injection site, volume overload, shortness of breath, and conjunctival inflammation, redness, and/or injection have been reported infrequently.

An increase in unconjugated bilirubin (possibly associated with increased erythrocyte load and hemolysis) has been reported in some studies but not in others. In one hemodialysis patient with Coats-type retinitis pigmentosa who was treated with the recombinant hormone, subretinal neovascularization of the right eye was noted; however, a direct causal relationship to the drug was not established, and treatment was continued without further ocular complications. Aggravation of splenomegaly has been reported occasionally in patients receiving the drug for anemia of myeloproliferative disorders.

Adverse effects reported in 1% or more of HIV-infected individuals receiving epoetin alfa include pyrexia, cough, rash, urticaria, respiratory congestion, pulmonary embolism, and local reaction (e.g., burning, pain) at the site of injection.

Adverse effects reported in 5% or more of cancer patients receiving epoetin alfa include nausea, vomiting, myalgia, arthralgia, stomatitis, cough, weight decrease, leukopenia, bone pain, rash, hyperglycemia, insomnia, headache, depression, dysphagia, hypokalemia, and thrombosis.

The US Centers for Disease Control (CDC) has determined that an outbreak of 21 episodes of bacteremia or pyrogenic reactions reported at a US dialysis center was the result of extrinsic contamination of epoetin alfa. Contrary to manufacturer recommendations, personnel at this dialysis center collected and pooled unused portions of epoetin alfa remaining in single-dose vials and transferred these portions into common vials for use in other patients. This practice was linked to extrinsic bacterial contamination of the drug. Commercially available single-dose vials of epoetin do not contain a preservative, and sterility can no longer be guaranteed once such vials are entered. Preservative-free, single-dose vials of epoetin alfa should be entered only once and unused portions remaining in the vials should be discarded.

■ **Precautions and Contraindications** ***Administration Precautions and Contraindications*** Patients must be given a copy of and instructed to read the medication guide prior to initiating epoetin alfa therapy and each time the drug is dispensed. Patients who self-administer epoetin alfa should be instructed carefully regarding proper, safe use of the drug, including information on aseptic technique, on storage and disposal of the drug and administration equipment, and on recognition and management of sensitivity reactions. Patients should take epoetin alfa exactly as prescribed and should contact a clinician immediately if more than the prescribed dose is taken or if a dose is missed. Patients should discontinue therapy with epoetin alfa when cancer chemotherapy is completed. Clinicians should advise patients of appropriate actions to take if adverse effects occur.

Hematologic Precautions and Contraindications An increased risk of death and/or tumor progression or recurrence has been reported in patients with breast, head and neck, non-small cell lung, lymphoid, and cervical cancer who were receiving therapy with ESAs. (See Cautions: Increased Mortality and Tumor Progression.) FDA and the manufacturers of ESAs currently recommend that ESAs *not* be used in patients in whom the anticipated outcome of cancer chemotherapy is cure of the underlying malignancy. In addition, patients with cancer-related anemia who were *not* receiving cancer chemotherapy (*not* an FDA-labeled indication for epoetin alfa or darbepoetin alfa in such patients) had an increased risk of death and no reduction in transfusion requirements while receiving an ESA. (See Cautions: Hematologic Effects.) The manufacturers and other clinicians recommend individualized titration of epoetin alfa dosages to achieve and maintain hemoglobin concentrations sufficient to avoid the need for red blood cell transfusions. Patients with cancer receiving epoetin alfa or other ESAs (e.g., darbepoetin alfa) should be advised of the increased risk of tumor progression or recurrence and/or death with such therapy and that ESA therapy should be discontinued when chemotherapy is stopped.

Hemoglobin concentrations should be determined at least once a week following initiation of epoetin alfa therapy and after each dosage change until stabilized; subsequent monitoring of hemoglobin concentrations should be performed at regular intervals (manufacturer recommends at least monthly in patients with chronic kidney disease). A complete blood cell count, including reticulocyte count, blood cell differential, platelet count, and determination of erythrocyte indices (Wintrobe indices), should be performed regularly. To avoid overly rapid increases in or overcorrection of hemoglobin, the manufacturers and other clinicians recommend adherence to the suggested dosing schedule and recommendations for dosage adjustment. If the increase in hemoglobin concentration exceeds 1 g/dL in any 2-week period or approaches or exceeds 11 g/dL in patients with chronic kidney disease *on dialysis*, exceeds 10 g/dL in patients with chronic kidney disease *not on dialysis*, exceeds 12 g/dL in patients with zidovudine-induced anemia, or exceeds a concentration sufficient to avoid red blood cell transfusions in patients with chemotherapy-induced anemia, the dosage of epoetin alfa should be reduced to minimize the possibility of adverse effects, including an increased risk of death, exacerbation of hypertension or other serious cardiovascular events, and tumor progression or recurrence. (See Cautions: Cardiovascular Effects and also see Cautions: Increased Mortality and Tumor Progression.)

Evaluation of iron stores, including transferrin saturation (serum iron divided by total iron binding capacity) and serum ferritin, should be performed both prior to and periodically (i.e., once a month for 3 months, then every other month) during epoetin alfa therapy. To support erythropoiesis, some clinicians suggest that serum ferritin concentration should be at least 100 mcg/L and transferrin saturation should be at least 20%; at lower transferrin saturations and ferritin concentrations, it is recommended that patients receive parenteral iron supplementation. (See Uses: Anemia of Chronic Kidney Disease.) Virtually all chronic kidney disease patients will require supplementation with oral or parenteral iron to increase or maintain iron stores while receiving epoetin alfa. Patients with iron overload prior to starting therapy with the drug may not require such supplementation initially as the shift of excess iron from tissues and/or the reticuloendothelial system occurs; however, profound iron deficiency may develop subsequently, so monitoring of serum and tissue iron stores is essential during epoetin alfa therapy.

To prevent potential exacerbation of thrombocytosis, some clinicians suggest that epoetin alfa therapy be used with caution in patients with a high baseline platelet count (e.g., exceeding 500,000/mm^3).

Cardiovascular Precautions and Contraindications Because current evidence indicates that correction of hemoglobin to concentrations exceeding 11 g/dL may increase the risk of death and serious cardiovascular events in patients with chronic kidney disease, dosing of ESAs, including epoetin alfa, should be individualized, and the lowest dosage sufficient to reduce the need for red blood cell transfusions should be used. (See Increased Mortality and Thromboembolic Effects under Cautions: Cardiovascular Effects.) Patients should inform clinicians of any heart disease or history of stroke prior to initiation of therapy. Patients with chronic kidney disease receiving epoetin alfa or other ESAs (e.g., darbepoetin alfa) should be advised of the increased risks of death and serious cardiovascular events (e.g., myocardial infarction, stroke, heart failure, thrombosis) associated with such therapy titrated to achieve hemoglobin concentrations exceeding 11 g/dL. Patients with chemotherapy-induced anemia should be advised that the lowest dosage of epoetin alfa required to avoid the need for red blood cell transfusions should be used and that epoetin alfa therapy should be discontinued when a course of chemotherapy is stopped. Patients should be advised of the importance of regular laboratory tests for hemoglobin during therapy and instructed to keep all appointments for monitoring hemoglobin concentrations.

Patients should be advised that ESA therapy increases the risk of venous thrombosis and that an anticoagulant may be used as prophylaxis for thromboembolism if patients undergo surgery. Patients should contact their clinician immediately if any signs or symptoms of blood clots occur, including chest pain, worsening of shortness of breath, pain in the legs with or without swelling, a cool or pale arm or leg, sudden difficulty walking, dizziness or loss of consciousness, loss of balance or coordination, sudden confusion, difficulty speaking or understanding others' speech, difficulty seeing, or blood clots in hemodialysis vascular access ports.

Frequent, periodic monitoring of blood pressure (up to 3 times weekly) is indicated in all patients receiving epoetin alfa, including dialysis and nondialysis patients and cancer patients, since development of hypertension may be associated with the rate or extent of increase in hemoglobin. Blood pressure monitoring is particularly important in patients with an underlying history of hypertension or cardiovascular disease. Patients should monitor their blood pressure daily, if appropriate, and contact their clinician if results are outside the range established for the patient. While development or exacerbation of hypertension generally does not occur during epoetin alfa therapy in previously normotensive, HIV-infected individuals with zidovudine-induced anemia, and hypertension has been reported only rarely during epoetin alfa therapy in cancer patients, uncontrolled hypertension in *any* patient should be treated adequately prior to initiation of therapy with epoetin alfa. Some clinicians state that therapy with epoetin alfa should not be initiated in patients with a baseline systolic pressure exceeding 180 mm Hg or a diastolic pressure exceeding 90–100 mm Hg. Patients should inform clinicians of a history of high blood pressure prior to initiation of epoetin alfa therapy or if increases in blood pressure occur during therapy.

Up to 25% of patients receiving dialysis will require initiation of antihypertensive therapy or an increase in the dosage of such therapy following initiation of epoetin alfa therapy. Patients should be advised of the importance of compliance with antihypertensive therapy and dietary restrictions. If blood pressure becomes difficult to control despite otherwise adequate therapy (e.g., antihypertensive drugs, dietary restrictions) or if the patient develops hypertensive encephalopathy, the dosage of epoetin alfa should be reduced or therapy with the drug withheld until blood pressure is controlled.

Increased mortality was observed in a study in patients without chronic kidney disease undergoing coronary artery bypass† who received epoetin alfa. Because 4 out of the 7 deaths that occurred in 126 patients were associated with thromboembolic events reported during drug administration, the manufacturers recommend that clinicians weigh the anticipated benefits of epoetin alfa therapy against the potential for increased risks associated with therapy in patients at risk for thrombosis. The manufacturers state that ESAs (e.g., epoetin alfa, darbepoetin alfa) are not indicated in patients undergoing cardiac or vascular surgery.

Some clinicians suggest that therapy with epoetin alfa be initiated cautiously (e.g., at half the usual dosage with slower upward dosage escalation and more frequent monitoring of hematocrit than usual) in patients with documented unstable angina or history of recent myocardial infarction. The possibility exists that the increased hematocrit and potential associated increase in blood viscosity resulting from epoetin alfa may lead to a decrease in myocardial oxygen delivery, with subsequent deterioration of cardiovascular status. Patients with preexisting vascular disease also should be monitored closely for the development of adverse effects with epoetin alfa therapy.

Neurologic Precautions and Contraindications Since seizures have developed during therapy with epoetin alfa, especially during the first 3 months in dialysis patients who had rapid increases in hematocrit, patients should be monitored closely for premonitory neurologic symptoms during the first several months of epoetin alfa therapy. Patients should be instructed to inform clinicians of a history of seizures prior to initiation of therapy. During epoetin alfa therapy, patients should promptly contact a clinician if any new-onset seizures, premonitory symptoms, or change in seizure frequency occurs.

Renal and Electrolyte Precautions and Contraindications Renal function (as evaluated by measurement of BUN and serum creatinine concentration) and fluid and electrolyte balance (as determined by results of blood chemistry tests, especially serum potassium, phosphate, and uric acid) should be monitored in all chronic kidney disease patients receiving epoetin alfa, not just in those undergoing dialysis. This precaution may be particularly important in patients predisposed to hyperkalemia (e.g., chronic kidney disease patients).

Compliance with concurrent drug therapy (especially antihypertensive therapy) and dietary restrictions should be encouraged in chronic kidney disease patients receiving epoetin alfa therapy. Such patients whose diet is unrestricted are at increased risk for hyperkalemia, and at least one associated fatality has been reported.

Hemodialysis patients receiving epoetin alfa therapy who have a history of problems maintaining patency of vascular access sites should have the function of their access site regularly assessed. The benefit of therapy with epoetin alfa should be weighed against the potential risk of losing the site of vascular access. (See Increased Mortality and Thromboembolic Effects under Cautions: Cardiovascular Effects.)

Reevaluation of the dialysis regimen may be necessary in some patients receiving epoetin alfa because of the effects of such therapy on dialyzer function and the efficiency of regular and/or high-flux dialysis. (See Cautions: Effects on Dialyzer Function.) Patients who undergo dialysis only occasionally may require an increase in the number or duration of dialysis sessions, and heparin dosage during dialysis also may require upward adjustment.

Immunologic Precautions and Contraindications Pure red cell aplasia (PRCA) and severe anemia with or without other cytopenias, in association with neutralizing antibodies to native erythropoietin, have been reported in patients treated with ESAs, including epoetin alfa. PRCA occurred predominantly in patients with chronic kidney disease receiving ESAs subcutaneously. However, antibody-mediated PRCA resulting in transfusion-dependent anemia also has been reported in patients receiving ESAs for the treatment of anemia related to hepatitis C therapy (not an FDA-labeled indication for epoetin alfa). The manufacturers recommend that epoetin alfa therapy be withheld in any patient who develops severe anemia and low reticulocyte counts; patient should be evaluated for the presence of neutralizing antibodies to erythropoietin. Patients should contact a clinician if symptoms of severe anemia such as unusual tiredness, lack of energy, dizziness, or fainting occur. The manufacturers of epoetin alfa should be contacted (Janssen Biotech [formerly Centocor Ortho Biotech] at 800-457-6399, Amgen at 800-772-6436) to perform assays for binding and neutralizing antibodies. Epoetin alfa should be discontinued permanently in patients who develop PRCA during therapy . The drug is contraindicated in patients who develop PRCA following treatment with epoetin alfa or other erythropoietin proteins.

Other Precautions and Contraindications Because epoetin alfa contains albumin, a derivative of human blood, it carries an extremely remote risk for transmission of human viruses. A theoretical risk for transmission of the causative agent of Creutzfeldt-Jakob disease (CJD) also is considered extremely remote. No cases of transmission of viral diseases or CJD have ever been identified for albumin.

Severe allergic reactions, including anaphylactic reactions, angioedema, respiratory symptoms, skin rash, and urticaria, may occur in patients receiving epoetin alfa therapy. Epoetin alfa therapy should be discontinued immediately and appropriate therapy initiated if a serious allergic or anaphylactic reaction occurs; the drug should not be reinitiated. Patients experiencing symptoms of serious allergic reactions, including whole-body rash; shortness of breath; wheezing, dizziness, or fainting because of a drop in blood pressure; swelling around mouth or eyes; rapid pulse; or sweating, should contact a clinician or emergency medical personnel immediately.

Patients who fail to respond or experience a loss of hemoglobin response to epoetin alfa should be evaluated for causative factors. Conditions that may diminish or block the effects of epoetin alfa include states of acute or chronic inflammation, infection, neoplastic disease or malignancy, underlying myelodysplastic disorders, marrow suppression from uremia, aluminum overload (possibly by interfering with iron bioavailability), hyperparathyroidism/osteitis fibrosa cystica, hypersplenism, acute or chronic blood loss, erythrocyte enzyme abnormalities (e.g., pyruvate kinase deficiency), iron deficiency, and/or folic acid or vitamin B_{12} deficiency. It is especially important to consider the possibility of diminished response in patients with an acute or chronic infection or in those undergoing surgery, both states of acute inflammation.

If none of these conditions exists and the patient is still refractory to epoetin alfa therapy, the patient should be evaluated for evidence of PRCA. In the absence of PRCA, dosage recommendations for the management of patients with an insufficient response to epoetin alfa therapy should be followed. Patients with chronic kidney disease and an insufficient response to ESA therapy may be at even greater risk for cardiovascular events and death than other patients.

Epoetin alfa has not been shown in controlled clinical trials to improve symptoms of anemia, quality of life, fatigue, or patient well-being.

Epoetin alfa is contraindicated in patients with uncontrolled hypertension and in those who develop pure red cell aplasia (PRCA) following treatment with epoetin alfa or other erythropoietin protein drugs. The use of epoetin alfa also is contraindicated in patients with serious allergic reactions to the drug. The commercially available multidose vial of epoetin alfa containing benzyl alcohol is contraindicated in neonates, infants, pregnant women, and nursing women; when treating such patients, single-dose vials of the drug should be used and should not be admixed with bacteriostatic saline containing benzyl alcohol. (See Cautions: Pediatric Precautions.)

■ **Pediatric Precautions** Safety and efficacy of epoetin alfa for the treatment of anemia associated with chronic kidney disease requiring dialysis in pediatric patients younger than 1 month of age have not been established. In pediatric patients with chronic kidney disease on dialysis, the pattern of most adverse events was similar to that found in adults. Safety and efficacy of epoetin alfa have not been established in pediatric patients with chronic kidney disease not on dialysis.

Safety and efficacy of epoetin alfa have not been established in pediatric patients with HIV infection.

Epoetin alfa has been used in pediatric patients for the treatment of anemia associated with other conditions, including zidovudine-induced anemia (infants and children 8 months to 17 years of age were studied), chemotherapy-related anemia, and anemia of prematurity†. Safety and efficacy of epoetin alfa have been established for the treatment of chemotherapy-induced anemia in patients 5 years of age or older. (See Chemotherapy-induced Anemia under Uses: Anemia in Cancer Patients.) Studies indicate that adverse effects of epoetin alfa in pediatric cancer patients are similar to those experienced in adults. Results of studies in patients 2.5–18 years of age and in premature neonates suggest that the safety and efficacy of the hormone are similar to those in adults.

Limited data from a study in preterm, very low birth-weight neonates receiving IV erythropoetin indicate that volume of distribution and clearance of the drug were approximately 1.5–2 and 3 times higher, respectively, than in healthy adults.

Commercially available multidose vials of epoetin alfa contain benzyl alcohol as a preservative. Although a causal relationship has not been established, administration of injections preserved with benzyl alcohol has been associated with neurologic and other toxicity in neonates. Such toxicities include a potentially fatal "gasping syndrome" characterized by central nervous system depression, metabolic acidosis, gasping respirations, and high concentrations of benzyl alcohol and its metabolites in blood and urine. Other manifestations may include gradual neurologic deterioration, seizures, intracranial hemorrhage, hematologic abnormalities, skin breakdown, hypotension, bradycardia, cardiovascular collapse, and hepatic or renal failure. Toxicity appears to have resulted from administration of large amounts (i.e., 100–400 mg/kg daily) of benzyl alcohol in these neonates. Premature or low-birthweight infants also appear to be at increased risk. Use of drugs preserved with benzyl alcohol should be avoided in neonates and infants whenever possible. Epoetin alfa from multidose vials or epoetin alfa from single-dose vials admixed with bacteriostatic saline preserved with benzyl alcohol should not be used in neonates or infants.

■ **Geriatric Precautions** While safety and efficacy of epoetin alfa have not been established specifically in geriatric patients, a large proportion of patients treated with the drug for anemia associated with chronic kidney disease have been 65 years of age or older. In geriatric patients with anemia associated with chronic kidney disease, no overall differences in safety and efficacy have been observed relative to younger adults. In geriatric patients with anemia due to concomitant chemotherapy or in those undergoing elective surgery, no overall differences in safety and efficacy have been observed relative to younger adults; dosing requirements generally were similar between the 2 populations. Data are insufficient in HIV-infected patients 65 years of age or older receiving epoetin alfa for zidovudine-induced anemia to determine whether geriatric patients respond differently than younger adults. Because of a general increased risk of renal and/or cardiovascular complications in geriatric patients, careful monitoring of blood chemistry and blood pressure may be necessary.

■ **Mutagenicity and Carcinogenicity** Epoetin alfa does not induce bacterial gene mutation (Ames test), chromosomal aberrations in mammalian cells, micronuclei in mice, or gene mutation at the hypoxanthine-guanine phosphoribosyltransferase (HGPRT) locus. In a study of predialysis patients treated with epoetin alfa, bone marrow aspirate examination showed no evidence of karyotypic abnormalities in the cells nor any indicated increase in the rate of sister chromatid exchange after 8 weeks of therapy.

The carcinogenic potential of epoetin alfa has not been evaluated to date. However, epoetin alfa and other erythropoiesis-stimulating agents (ESAs) have been shown to shorten the time to tumor progression or recurrence and shorten survival in patients with cancer. (See Cautions: Increased Mortality and Tumor Progression.)

■ **Pregnancy, Fertility, and Lactation** Although there are no adequate and controlled studies to date of epoetin alfa use during pregnancy, the drug has been used in a limited number of pregnant women with anemia. Adverse pregnancy outcomes, including prenatal complications (i.e., polyhydramnios, intrauterine growth restriction) and at least 1 case of congenital deformity following first trimester exposure, have been reported. The manufacturer states that due to the limited number of exposed pregnancies and the presence of multiple confounding factors (e.g., concomitant medications or other maternal conditions), such data cannot be used to reliably estimate the frequency or absence of adverse pregnancy outcomes. Single-dose formulations of epoetin alfa should be used during pregnancy only when the potential benefits justify the possible risks to the fetus. Women who become pregnant during epoetin alfa therapy are encouraged to enroll in the manufacturers' Pregnancy Surveillance Program by calling 1-800-772-6436.

In teratogenicity studies of female rats given 500 units/kg of epoetin alfa IV after the period of organogenesis, there was a decrease in body weight gain, delayed appearance of abdominal hair, delayed eyelid opening, delayed ossification, and a decrease in the number of caudal vertebrae in the pups; the dose given in these studies was approximately fivefold higher than the clinical recommended starting dose, depending on treatment indication. No evidence of teratogenicity was observed in pregnant rats and rabbits exposed to epoetin alfa IV (up to 500 units/kg daily) during the period of organogenesis. Postnatal observations of the *live* first-generation and second-generation offspring of these female rats revealed no epoetin alfa-related adverse effects.

In fertility studies in rats, epoetin alfa doses of 100 and 500 units/kg caused slight increases in pre-implantation loss, post-implantation loss, and a decreased incidence of live fetuses; it is not clear whether these effects reflect a drug effect on the uterine environment or on the conceptus.

Since it is not known whether epoetin alfa is distributed into human milk, the drug should be used with caution in nursing women. When therapy with epoetin alfa is needed in nursing women, a benzyl alcohol-free formulation should be used.

Results of studies in animals are equivocal as to whether the drug crosses the placenta.

Because of a potential risk of neurologic and other toxicity in neonates exposed to benzyl alcohol, epoetin alfa from multidose vials (with benzyl alcohol preservative) or from single-dose vials admixed with bacteriostatic saline containing benzyl alcohol should not be used in pregnant or nursing women. When epoetin alfa therapy is needed during pregnancy or nursing, use of a benzyl alcohol-free formulation is recommended.

Drug Interactions

Systematic drug interaction studies have not been performed with epoetin alfa. Patients receiving multiple drugs concurrently with epoetin alfa should be observed carefully for potential adverse effects.

■ **Androgens** Since androgens have been shown to increase the sensitivity of erythroid progenitors to endogenous erythropoietin and possibly stimulate residual endogenous erythropoietin secretion, these drugs have been used as an adjunct to epoetin alfa therapy in a few patients to decrease the total amount of epoetin alfa required for the amelioration of anemia. Weekly IM administration of 100 mg of nandrolone decanoate in a limited number of men with chronic kidney disease increased the response to low dosages of epoetin alfa (i.e., a total of 2000 units IV 3 times weekly), improving the hematocrit response from 27.5% in patients on low-dose therapy alone to 33% in concomitantly treated patients. However, androgen therapy alone is associated with substantial adverse effects, and comparative, controlled studies are needed to establish the potential benefits and risks of combined therapy with androgens and epoetin alfa.

■ **Desmopressin** Concurrent therapy with epoetin alfa and desmopressin has resulted in an additive effect on reduction of bleeding time in a patient with end-stage renal disease who was receiving epoetin alfa for correction of uremia-induced increased bleeding time and epistaxis. Bleeding time had decreased from a baseline value exceeding 45 minutes to 22, 19, or 14 minutes when the patient was treated with epoetin alfa, conjugated estrogens, or desmopressin, respectively. When epoetin alfa and desmopressin were used simultaneously, the bleeding time decreased to 10 minutes.

■ **Other Drugs** Probenecid has been shown to inhibit renal tubular secretion of endogenous erythropoietin in animals. The relevance of this finding in humans is not known, but the possibility of such an interaction should be considered when epoetin alfa and probenecid are given concomitantly.

Acute Toxicity

Limited data are available on the acute toxicity of epoetin alfa. In acute toxicity studies in animals, no unusual toxicities beyond expected effects of epoetin alfa on erythropoiesis (e.g., dose-dependent increases in hematocrit and hemoglobin concentration) were observed.

Severe hypertension has been observed following overdosage of epoetin alfa. Potential overcorrection of hematocrit may be reversed expeditiously by phlebotomy. Dosage of epoetin alfa should be reduced, therapy discontinued, and/or phlebotomy performed if hemoglobin concentrations increase above desired levels. (See Dosage and Administration: Dosage.)

Pharmacology

Epoetin alfa is a hematopoietic agent that principally influences erythropoiesis. Most studies of the pharmacology of epoetin alfa have been performed using the recombinant glycoprotein hormone. The amino acid sequence and biologic properties of epoetin alfa are identical to those of endogenous human erythropoietin extracted from the urine of patients with aplastic anemia. In the Pharmacology section, unless otherwise specified, the physiologic and pharmacologic effects of endogenous human erythropoietin and exogenously administered epoetin alfa or other erythropoietin human preparations will be discussed in terms of endogenous human erythropoietin.

Endogenous human erythropoietin, a growth factor, is a glycosylated protein hormone that appears to be secreted principally by renal peritubular interstitial cells outside the tubular basement membrane in the cortex and outer medulla of the kidney; however, approximately 10% is produced in the liver and possibly in other extrarenal sites in adults. Fetal erythropoietin production occurs mainly in the liver. Secretion of the hormone occurs principally in response to reductions in arterial and/or venous oxygen tension and tissue oxygenation in the kidney; some evidence suggests that an oxygen-sensitive heme protein may be involved in the regulatory mechanism(s), the location of which remains to be determined.

Patients with chronic or end-stage renal disease develop normocytic, normochromic anemia and have inappropriately low reticulocyte counts principally because of a relative lack of erythropoietin, the glycoprotein hormone that regulates erythropoiesis.This erythropoietin deficiency appears to be secondary to decreased functional kidney mass available to produce the hormone. A defect in the bone marrow response to erythropoietin and accelerated erythrocyte destruction secondary to uremia also may contribute to the anemia associated with chronic kidney disease. Although small amounts of erythropoietin are produced by diseased renal tissue and by the liver and other extrarenal sites, these quantities usually are not adequate to support optimal erythropoiesis, especially during stress or acute blood loss. Anephric patients, relying solely on extrarenal production of erythropoietin, will demonstrate more severe anemia than other patients with renal failure. Following renal transplantation in patients with end-stage renal disease, increases in endogenous erythropoietin concentrations adequate to support erythropoiesis are observed. Patients with renal failure secondary to polycystic kidney disease may not be severely anemic; in fact, these patients may have a relative polycythemia because the considerably increased mass of their kidneys may produce physiologic or supraphysiologic amounts of erythropoietin. Patients with renal artery stenosis also exhibit enhanced secretion of the hormone.

Various uremic toxins (e.g., parathyroid hormone [parathyrin], polyamines) have been implicated in the etiology of the anemia of chronic kidney disease, including decreased production of erythropoietin by the kidney, the blunted response to the hormone of erythroid progenitors (especially the erythroid burst-forming units [BFU-E]) in bone marrow, and the increased fragility and shortened survival of erythrocytes already in circulation. Other possible factors contributing to the anemia related to dialysis or end-stage renal disease include erythrocyte damage or hemolysis from the dialysis procedure or from loss of blood in the dialyzer or dialysis tubing; increased occult blood loss and uremic bleeding; nutritional deficits from dialysis clearance of water-soluble vitamins (e.g., folic acid, vitamin B_{12}); iron deficiency from blood loss, decreased dietary intake, or decreased GI absorption; aluminum toxicity; hypervitaminosis A; hypersplenism; excessive parathyroid hormone concentrations with consequent replacement of bone marrow with fibrous tissue (osteitis fibrosa cystica); and repeated phlebotomy for laboratory tests. When patients with end-stage renal failure begin peritoneal dialysis or hemodialysis, their anemia improves; although not proven, this improvement may be secondary to increased clearance of erythropoiesis-inhibiting toxins. Patients undergoing continuous ambulatory peritoneal dialysis (CAPD) generally have less severe anemia than do patients undergoing hemodialysis, possibly because of decreased iatrogenic blood loss, improved clearance of uremic toxins, and/or increased erythropoietin production compared with hemodialysis patients.

In patients with human immunodeficiency virus (HIV) infection who develop anemia associated with zidovudine therapy, response to therapy with erythropoietin appears to depend on the endogenous serum erythropoietin concentration prior to treatment. Patients with an endogenous serum erythropoietin concentration not exceeding 500 milliunits/mL who are receiving zidovudine dosages not exceeding 4.2 g per week appear to be more responsive to the hormone than those with higher pretreatment serum erythropoietin concentrations; pooled analysis of data from several studies suggested no hematologic benefit from erythropoietin therapy in patients with baseline values exceeding 500 milliunits/mL. In such patients with a baseline endogenous erythropoietin concentration not exceeding 500 milliunits/mL, response to epoetin generally does not appear to be dose dependent, although some patients may show improved response with increasing dosages.

In patients with nonmyeloid malignancies who have chemotherapy-induced anemia, epoetin alfa has been shown to decrease transfusion requirements after the first month of therapy (i.e., during the second and third month of therapy).

■ **Hematologic Effects** ***Effects on Erythropoiesis*** Erythropoietin induces the production of erythrocytes (i.e., stimulates erythropoiesis) principally by stimulating the proliferation and differentiation of committed erythroid precursors (i.e., burst-forming units-erythroid [BFU-E], colony-forming units-erythroid [CFU-E]); CFU-E appear to be more sensitive and dependent on the effects of erythropoietin than BFU-E, responding in vitro to erythropoietin concentrations much lower than those required to stimulate BFU-E. Other marrow precursors, including colony-forming units (CFU)-megakaryocytic (CFU-MK), CFU-granulocytic-monocytic (CFU-GM), and pluripotent stem cells also may be increased with in vivo administration of erythropoietin. Stimulation of CFU-E and BFU-E appears to be direct, while stimulation of CFU-MK and CFU-GM may occur as indirect feedback responses. Both erythroblasts and reticulocytes, the direct precursors (immature forms) of erythrocytes, are increased by erythropoietin as a result of its action on CFU-E and BFU-E. The hormone also stimulates the release of reticulocytes from bone marrow, and the synthesis of cellular hemoglobin is increased as a result of enhanced differentiation of CFU-E into erythroblasts.

In general, no changes in erythrocyte indices (e.g., mean corpuscular volume, erythrocyte width) are seen in patients receiving erythropoietin therapy, although increases in mean corpuscular hemoglobin (MCH), mean corpuscular hemoglobin concentration (MCHC), and mean corpuscular volume (MCV) have occurred in some patients. In particular, patients with iron overload prior to initiation of erythropoietin therapy may experience an increase in MCV, the cause of which has not been fully elucidated to date. The effects of erythropoietin therapy in reversing shortened erythrocyte survival in uremic patients have been variable; limited evidence suggests that osmotic fragility of erythrocytes from hemodialysis patients decreases and erythrocyte half-life increases after erythropoietin therapy in predialysis patients, while other studies have demonstrated no such effects.

The usual serum concentration of endogenous erythropoietin in healthy individuals with normal hematocrit is 4–30 milliunits/mL; the erythropoietic response in patients with hypoxia, severe anemia from blood loss, or aplastic anemia may be associated with erythropoietin concentrations up to 1000 times greater than these concentrations. Most patients with anemia associated with chronic kidney disease cannot mount this same erythropoietic response and have an inappropriately low serum erythropoietin concentration for the degree of anemia present.

Erythropoietin appears to bind to 2 types of polypeptide receptors in erythroid progenitor cells—one high affinity and one low affinity— or possibly to different low- and high-affinity portions or chains of a receptor complex. Some data suggest that binding of the erythropoietin molecule to the receptor may stimulate nucleic acid synthesis and subsequent cell division in erythroid progenitor cells, although it also has been suggested that the hormone may prevent apoptosis (programmed cell death) in such erythroid cells, allowing them to proceed with mitosis and terminal differentiation. Following receptor binding, erythropoietin apparently is internalized and metabolized by the target cell. Erythropoietin receptors are of the hormone-receptor variety but are not cross-reactive with any other hormone (e.g., insulin) or growth factor (e.g., colony-stimulating factors, various interleukins, transferrin). Binding sites for erythropoietin have been identified in in vitro studies of isolated CFU-Es. Erythropoietin apparently does not bind to mature erythrocytes, granulocytes, monocytes, or plasma cells. In vitro studies have demonstrated receptors for erythropoietin in both human and animal placental tissue that may be similar to the erythroid cell receptor.

Plasma iron and ferritin concentrations decrease with new erythrocyte formation as a result of iron incorporation into these cells and subsequent mobilization of tissue iron stores. Intracellular free calcium concentrations have increased with addition of erythropoietin to bone marrow and cord blood erythroblast cultures; such increases in calcium may possibly initiate intracellular mechanisms for erythrocyte proliferation and differentiation.

Increases in erythron transferrin uptake parallel the increases in reticulocyte count and erythrocyte mass in both dialysis-dependent and predialysis patients who respond to erythropoietin therapy.

Other Hematologic Effects The biologic effects of erythropoietin are noted principally on erythrocyte precursors and their progeny. No meaningful increase in leukocyte or macrophage count occurs with endogenous secretion or exogenous administration of the hormone, although minimal increases in megakaryocytic and myeloid precursors have been reported. The leukocyte differential also does not appear to be affected by the hormone. Variable effects of erythropoietin on platelet production have been reported. Increased platelet count appears more likely when higher initial doses of the hormone are used, although it also has been suggested that such increases may reflect a reactive thrombocytosis associated with iron deficiency.

Packed erythrocyte volume, or total mass of erythrocytes in whole blood, increases during erythropoietin therapy. A corresponding decrease in plasma volume also may be seen, so total blood volume remains essentially unchanged.

The viscosity of whole blood, but not plasma, can increase with erythropoietin therapy and is accompanied by an increase in hematocrit. Treatment with the hormone also has been shown to induce an increase in erythrocyte aggregation at low and high shear (flow stress) rates, particularly in patients with increased baseline fibrinogen concentration.

■ **Cardiovascular Effects** Limited data indicate that hemodynamic changes associated with erythropoietin-induced increases in hemoglobin concentration may result in improved cardiovascular function in patients with chronic kidney disease; however, other studies have shown no clinically important changes in hemodynamic function with such therapy. Decreases in cardiomegaly and left ventricular mass have been reported in patients with chronic kidney disease receiving erythropoietin therapy. Results of some studies indicate that increased hemoglobin concentrations associated with erythropoietin therapy may produce variable effects on cardiac output, cardiac index, and stroke volume; other studies have demonstrated minimal or no effect of the hormone on ejection fraction, myocardial contractility, and mean end-diastolic volume.

Increases in peripheral vascular resistance have been reported in anemic patients whose condition was successfully treated with erythropoietin; this may be related to the compensatory vasodilation resulting from the anemia. Little or no effect on the renin-angiotensin-aldosterone system has been reported in patients receiving erythropoietin therapy. Decreases in atrial natriuretic factor (ANF) and 6-keto-prostaglandin $F_{1\alpha}$ (a prostaglandin metabolite) have been reported in patients receiving erythropoietin therapy; however, the importance of these findings currently is unknown.

■ **Other Effects** A reduction in bleeding time toward normal may occur in patients with chronic kidney disease treated with exogenous erythropoietin and may be similar to that occurring with blood transfusion. This reduction in bleeding time is evidenced by increases in platelet adhesion. Concomitant desmopressin therapy may have an additive effect on improvement of the hemostatic defect in patients with end-stage renal disease. (See Drug Interactions: Desmopressin.)

Successful reversal of anemia with exogenous erythropoietin in patients undergoing long-term hemodialysis has been shown to normalize elevated prolactin concentrations; such elevations have been implicated in decreased libido and sexual function in these patients. Improvement in sexual activity in chronic kidney disease patients treated with erythropoietin has been attributed to both the decrease in serum prolactin concentration and the overall increase in the patient's quality of life secondary to the reversal of anemia. Improvement of male sexual function in such patients also may be related to an increase in serum testosterone concentration, which may occur as a result of decreased serum prolactin concentrations and/or increases in hematocrit.

While limited animal data suggest that administration of exogenous erythropoietin does not suppress the production of endogenous hormone, limited evidence in humans receiving exogenous erythropoietin suggests that such suppression indeed may occur.

In a limited number of chronic kidney disease patients with uremic pruritus, low-dose erythropoietin therapy resulted in a decrease in plasma histamine concentration with subsequent decreases in pruritus; the mechanism of this effect of exogenous erythropoietin on plasma histamine is unclear.

Although uremic patients may have substantial dyslipidemia, limited data indicate that exogenous erythropoietin does not affect such abnormalities in the blood lipid profile. Plasma norepinephrine concentrations have increased in a limited number of patients treated with erythropoietin, which theoretically could be implicated as a cause of increased total peripheral resistance and/or blood pressure in such patients.

Pharmacokinetics

Early pharmacokinetic studies of erythropoietin in animals and humans employed impure, endogenously derived preparations and imprecise assay methods. In more recent studies, highly purified preparations, including recombinant epoetin preparations, and more sensitive and/or specific assays (e.g., radioimmunoassay [RIA], enzyme-linked immunosorbent assay [ELISA]) have been used. Unless otherwise specified, studies described in the Pharmacokinetics section employed epoetin alfa or another recombinant preparation (e.g., epoetin beta, not commercially available in the US), and serum concentrations of the hormone were determined via RIA and are expressed in terms of erythropoietin.

RIA and ELISA measure both endogenous erythropoietin and exogenously administered epoetin alfa; however, pharmacologic dosages of epoetin alfa administered IV or subcutaneously result in serum concentrations that exceed endogenous erythropoietin concentrations by approximately 10- to 100-fold, so the contribution of endogenous erythropoietin to total serum hormone concentrations probably should be minimal unless relatively low doses (e.g., 50 units/kg) of epoetin alfa are administered. If such low doses are used and particularly with subcutaneous administration of epoetin alfa, the relative contribution of the endogenous hormone to the total serum hormone concentration must be taken into account when evaluating the pharmacokinetics of epoetin alfa. Usual endogenous serum concentrations of erythropoietin measured via RIA in healthy adults have been reported to range from 4–30 milliunits/mL.

There is limited evidence that an immunologic cross-reactant may be present in the serum of certain individuals, resulting in falsely elevated concentrations of erythropoietin determined by RIA. It also has been suggested, but not confirmed, that RIA may measure biologically inactive asialylated epoetin. Bioassays that measure only biologically active hormone are more difficult to perform and may be less sensitive than RIA. ELISA also has been used, but additional experience is necessary to establish the relative usefulness of various assay methods for erythropoietin.

The pharmacokinetics of epoetin alfa in children and adolescents appear to be similar to that of adults. Limited data are available in neonates. The pharmacokinetics of the drug in patients infected with the human immunodeficiency virus (HIV) have not been determined to date.

The relationship, if any, between the pharmacokinetics and pharmacodynamics of epoetin alfa remains to be established.

■ **Absorption** Because of its protein nature, epoetin alfa is destroyed in the GI tract and must be administered parenterally (e.g., via IV infusion, subcutaneous injection, intraperitoneal instillation). Systemic absorption of epoetin alfa is delayed and incomplete following subcutaneous injection or intraperitoneal instillation. However, while serum concentrations peak sooner and are substantially higher with IV than subcutaneous injection of epoetin alfa, they are less sustained, and the IV route of administration generally offers no clinical advantage over the subcutaneous route except in patients with existing accessible IV sites (e.g., hemodialysis patients). In fact, limited evidence suggests that subcutaneous injection of epoetin alfa 3 times weekly can produce a hemoglobin response similar to that with IV administration but at lower dosages; other evidence indicates that dosages of epoetin alfa required for maintenance therapy generally are lower with subcutaneous than IV injection. The decreased and variable systemic absorption of subcutaneously administered epoetin alfa relative to IV administration may result from the lipophilicity and/or relatively large size of the molecule; degradation by peptidases in the skin also may be responsible. With usual epoetin alfa dosages of 50–300 units/kg 3 times weekly given either subcutaneously or IV, detectable serum concentrations of erythropoietin are maintained for at least 24 hours.

Serum erythropoietin concentrations exhibit considerable interindividual variation with a given epoetin alfa dose and route of administration. Peak serum erythropoietin concentrations following IV administration of 80, 120, or 150 units/kg of epoetin alfa reportedly range from 1200–1800, 3200–4700, or 3000–5000 milliunits/mL, respectively, in patients with chronic kidney disease; in healthy adults, peak serum concentrations following IV administration of 150 or 300 units/kg of the drug average 3500 or 7300 milliunits/mL, respectively. Peak serum erythropoietin concentrations after subcutaneous injection of 50, 150, or 300 units/kg of epoetin alfa in healthy individuals averaged 36 (corrected for endogenous serum erythropoietin concentration), 144–226, or 285–288 milliunits/mL. Peak serum erythropoietin concentrations are achieved within 4–24 hours following subcutaneous injection of usual therapeutic doses of epoetin alfa, and serum erythropoietin concentrations generally remain above baseline for 2–4 days. Following IV doses of 50–300 units/kg of exogenous erythropoietin, serum erythropoietin concentrations generally decline to baseline concentrations within 1–3 days.

Serum erythropoietin concentrations peak sooner but are substantially lower following intraperitoneal instillation compared with subcutaneous injection, at least when the drug is administered via a dialysis solution. In addition, systemic absorption following intraperitoneal administration via a dialysis solution is substantially lower than that following IV administration. The bioavailability of epoetin alfa following subcutaneous or intraperitoneal (via a dialysis solution) administration reportedly ranges from 10–49 or 2.5–14%, respectively. Although such data suggest that intraperitoneal administration of epoetin alfa would be impractical, limited evidence in animals and humans suggests that systemic bioavailability following intraperitoneal instillation can be increased substantially (e.g., to 40%) by administering the drug into an empty peritoneal cavity; additional study is needed to determine the clinical feasibility of administering the drug by this method. In a study in patients undergoing continuous ambulatory peritoneal dialysis (CAPD), peak serum drug concentrations following a single IV or subcutaneous dose of 300 units/kg of epoetin alfa averaged 7688 or 484 milliunits/mL, respectively, and 108 or 170 milliunits/mL with intraperitoneal instillation (via a dialysis solution) for 4 or 12 hours (dwell time), respectively. Peak serum erythropoietin concentrations in these CAPD patients were achieved within 24–36 or 8–12 hours after subcutaneous or intraperitoneal administration, respectively. Systemic absorption (as determined by area under the serum concentration-time curve [AUC]) during the first 24 hours after intraperitoneal dosing was approximately 25–33% of that after subcutaneous injection.

Peak serum drug concentrations following subcutaneous injection of epoetin alfa appear to be reduced (by up to 40–70% compared with the first-dose peak) with multiple-dose administration of the drug. Limited evidence suggests that bioavailability of the drug following subcutaneous administration into the thigh is increased compared with subcutaneous administration into the arm or abdomen.

■ **Distribution** The distribution of epoetin alfa and the endogenous hormone in humans remains to be fully elucidated. Epoetin alfa appears to distribute into a single compartment with an apparent volume of distribution that approximates or slightly exceeds plasma volume (about 4–5% of body weight). Thus, extravascular distribution of the drug and endogenous hormone appears to be relatively minor. In both healthy individuals and dialysis patients, the volume of distribution has been estimated to be 21–80 mL/kg following a single IV dose, and 57–107 or 42–70 mL/kg at the start of multiple-dose therapy or after normalization of hematocrit (98–378 days), respectively; distribution characteristics of epoetin alfa are similar in predialysis patients. In preterm neonates, the volume of distribution is approximately 1.5–2 times higher than in healthy adults. Little, if any, accumulation of the drug appears to occur at dosages of 50–150 units/kg given IV or subcutaneously 3 times weekly or at dosages of 40,000 units weekly given subcutaneously. However, drug accumulation may occur following multiple subcutaneous doses because of prolonged absorption.

In contrast to apparent distribution characteristics in humans, extravascular distribution of epoetin alfa and the endogenous hormone appears to be substantially greater in animals. Epoetin alfa has been shown to distribute into the liver, kidney, spleen, lung, and bone marrow in animals. Desialylated epoetin alfa appears to undergo extensive extravascular distribution. In animals, 85, 9, 4, and 2% of extravascular desialylated drug reportedly distributes into the liver, kidney, lung, and spleen, respectively.

Results of studies in animals are equivocal regarding the potential for epoetin alfa to cross the placenta, although in vitro evidence suggests erythropoietin receptors are present in placental tissue of some animals. It is not known whether the drug distributes into milk in humans.

■ **Elimination** The elimination characteristics of epoetin alfa and endogenous erythropoietin in humans remain to be fully established. Most currently available information on the elimination of the hormone comes from animal studies, and the relevance of these findings in humans is unclear. Serum concentrations appear to decline principally in a monoexponential (first-order) fashion,although biexponential elimination from serum has been described in animals and occasionally in humans, particularly at relatively low dosages. The elimination half-life of epoetin alfa following IV administration in healthy individuals and in adults and children with chronic kidney disease ranges from 4–16 hours. There is some evidence that the elimination half-life of epoetin alfa may increase with increasing dosage, but a reduction in half-life during continuous dosing also has been reported. The half-life of epoetin alfa is similar in adults older or younger than 65 years of age. In patients with impaired renal function, a prolongation in elimination half-life relative to that in patients with normal renal function may occur; however, the elimination half-life does not appear to be affected by hemodialysis. The elimination characteristics of epoetin alfa appear to be similar in patients undergoing hemodialysis or peritoneal dialysis.

With continuous dosing at IV doses of 15–500 units/kg administered up to 3 times weekly, the elimination half-life of epoetin alfa may decrease over time. In patients undergoing hemodialysis, mean elimination half-life was reduced by 20–40% after several weeks to months of such dosing; no further reductions generally were observed beyond 3–4 months of continued therapy. Similar reductions in half-life with multiple dosing have been observed in predialysis patients; the mean half-life of the drug decreased by 40% after 8 weeks of therapy in one study. Although it has been suggested that this decrease in half-life may be related to increased clearance of the drug as more erythroid precursors are formed and increased numbers of erythropoietin receptors are made available, other studies have not found reductions in elimination half-life after continuous dosing.

Serum clearance of epoetin alfa in patients undergoing CAPD averages 0.05 mL/minute per kg (range: 0.03–0.09 mL/minute per kg). Total body clearance of the drug after IV administration in healthy men has been estimated to be about 14 mL/minute. In preterm neonates, the clearance of epoetin alfa is approximately 3 times higher than in healthy adults.

The metabolic fate of endogenous erythropoietin and the recombinant hormone (i.e., epoetin alfa) is poorly understood. Although some in vitro and animal data suggest that the kidney may be involved in erythropoietin metabolism, limited evidence in humans suggests otherwise. It also has been suggested that the physicochemical characteristics of the glycoprotein would impede access to potential sites of renal metabolism, thus limiting any contribution of the kidney in the degradation of the endogenous and recombinant hormones. Current evidence from studies in animals suggests that hepatic metabolism contributes only minimally to elimination of the *intact* hormone, but desialylated epoetin alfa (i.e., terminal sialic acid groups removed) appears to undergo substantial hepatic clearance via metabolic pathways and/or binding. Desialylation and/or removal of the oligosaccharide side chains of erythropoietin appear to occur principally in the liver; bone marrow also may have a role in catabolism of the hormone. Elimination of desialylated drug by the kidneys, bone marrow, and spleen also may occur; results of animal studies suggest that proximal renal tubular secretion may be involved in renal elimination.

Approximately 10% or less of an administered dose of recombinant epoetin alfa is excreted unchanged in urine, which is similar to the elimination characteristics of the endogenous hormone. The effect of hepatic impairment on elimination of the hormone has not been elucidated.

Elimination of epoetin alfa is similar in patients with varying degrees of renal failure, suggesting predominantly nonrenal mechanisms of elimination. Total body clearance of epoetin alfa in patients with varying degrees of renal failure averages 0.09 mL/minute per kg (range: 0.06–0.12 mL/minute per kg). In patients undergoing CAPD receiving IV epoetin alfa, peritoneal clearance (based on quantity of drug found in the dialysate within 24 hours) was 1.7–3% of the administered dose.

Epoetin alfa apparently is not removed by hemodialysis; in fact, postdialysis serum concentrations of the hormone may exceed predialysis concentrations because of removal of excess extracellular fluid. Removal of the hormone from systemic circulation into peritoneal dialysate is small and contributes minimally to overall elimination of the drug.

Chemistry and Stability

■ **Chemistry** Epoetin alfa, a biosynthetic form of the glycoprotein hormone erythropoietin, is a hematopoietic agent that principally affects erythropoiesis. The drug is prepared from cultures of genetically modified mammalian (Chinese hamster ovary) cells using recombinant DNA technology. These cells have been modified by the addition of plasmids that incorporate the human erythropoietin gene, which was isolated from human fetal liver cells.

Epoetin alfa and some other epoetin preparations (e.g., epoetin beta, epoetin gamma, neither of which is commercially available in the US) have amino acid sequences and pharmacologic actions identical to those of the endogenous hormone; however, differences in the nature and composition of the carbohydrate moieties may exist and are the main factors that distinguish recombinant from endogenous preparations and that characterize various recombinant epoetin preparations. No assays currently are readily available to distinguish the endogenous from recombinant forms of erythropoietin. Currently available epoetin alfa preparations (Epogen®, Amgen; Procrit®, Ortho Biotech) are derived from the same source and are identical in composition.

The principal gene product of endogenous human erythropoietin is a 193-amino acid monomeric polypeptide, which includes a hydrophobic *N*-terminus leader sequence of 27 amino acids. This leader sequence is cleaved during secretion of the hormone to form a highly glycosylated, 166-amino acid hormonal peptide. However, both endogenous human erythropoietin extracted from urine of patients with aplastic anemia and recombinant preparations of the hormone lack a carboxy-terminal arginine residue, which apparently is cleaved from the hormonal peptide post-translationally by a carboxypeptidase in mammalian cells to form the 165-amino acid active hormone. Urinary human erythropoietin occurs as a mixture of 2 forms, α and β. Each form has the same functional polypeptide portion and produces the same in vivo response. The distinguishing characteristic of the α and β forms is the overall carbohydrate composition; the α form of urinary erythropoietin appears to have a greater percentage of *N*-acetylneuraminic acid in its carbohydrate portion.

Endogenous erythropoietin and recombinant preparations of the hormone generally have molecular weights of approximately 30,000 (e.g., epoetin alfa has a molecular weight of 30,400 $\pm$ 400 daltons), although molecular weights of up to 39,000 have been reported for glycosylated erythropoietin preparations, in part because of variations in assay techniques and/or variations in the composition and weight of the carbohydrate moieties. The molecular weight of the functional, 165-amino acid erythropoietin protein (excluding carbohydrate moieties) is approximately 18,400 daltons. Epoetin alfa contains 2 internal disulfide bonds linking positions 7 and 161 and positions 29 and 33; these bonds are necessary for the hormone's biologic activity.

Both endogenous human erythropoietin and epoetin derived from mammalian cell cultures are glycosylated by one *O*-linked oligosaccharide and 3 *N*-linked, complex, polyantennary saccharides containing $\alpha 2\rightarrow 3$-linked terminal sialic acid residues (derivatives and esters of *N*-acetylneuraminic acid), with and without repeating *N*-acetyllactosaminyl units. Glycosylation appears to be important for prolonging the half-life of the hormone but not for biologic activity. The carbohydrate side chains in epoetin alfa represent approximately 40% of the molecular mass. Although the individual carbohydrate chains may differ in structure and degree of sialylation, the carbohydrate residues of the recombinant hormone are essentially identical to those of the human urinary-derived endogenous hormone.

Production of erythropoietin in the mammalian cell line allows for glycosylation of the preparation. While enzymatic removal of any or all of the carbohydrate side chains or production of the nonglycosylated recombinant hormone in *Escherichia coli* or yeast results in a preparation with little or no in vivo activity, endogenous or recombinant erythropoietin with partial or complete desialylation of the carbohydrate side chains retains 50–60% of its in vitro activity. In addition, certain asialylated forms of erythropoietin possess increased in vitro activity relative to intact erythropoietin, possibly because of reduced negative charge and/or steric hindrance with resultant increased receptor-binding capability. Complete removal of the core (i.e., asparagine-linked) portions of the saccharide chains of erythropoietin leads to an almost total loss of in vitro activity, possibly because of loss of the molecule's active conformation. The carbohydrate portions may protect the molecule from intracellular and/or hepatic degradation and increase its half-life in vivo; partially desialylated erythropoietin undergoes hepatic degradation in animals because desialylation exposes galactose residues that bind to galactose receptors on hepatic cells. It also has been suggested that glycosylation of the molecule may contribute to its nonimmunogenicity, since other nonglycosylated recombinant proteins (e.g., insulin human, interferon) exhibit epitopes that may be a principal cause of antibody formation; epitopes present on epoetin alfa reportedly are identical to those found on human erythropoietin.

Epoetin alfa is commercially available as a sterile, preservative-free solution and as a sterile solution preserved with benzyl alcohol 1%. Both injections occur as colorless solutions and contain sodium chloride to adjust tonicity and sodium citrate or sodium phosphate and citric acid as a buffer; they also contain albumin human. The preservative-free injection has a pH of 6.6–7.2, and the preserved injection has a pH of 5.8–6.4. The pK_a of epoetin alfa ranges from 4.5–5.5, and its isoelectric point reportedly ranges from 3.5–4.

Biologic activity of epoetin alfa is determined by measuring incorporation of radiolabeled iron into heme of cultured rat bone marrow cells in vitro and by the in vivo exhypoxic polycythemic mouse bioassay; potency of the recombinant preparation has been expressed in units of activity per mg of protein as tested against the WHO second International Reference Preparation of human urinary erythropoietin. The specific activity of epoetin alfa has been reported to be approximately 210,000 units/mg of protein or 129,000 units/mg of total weight based on comparison with the second International Reference Standard.

■ **Stability** Commercially available epoetin alfa injection should be refrigerated at 2–8°C, protected from light, and should not be frozen. Exposure to light for periods less than 24 hours reportedly does not affect the color, clarity, or potency of the injection. Epoetin alfa injection also should not be shaken, since denaturation of the protein with resultant loss of biologic activity may occur; however, a small amount of flocculation in solution reportedly does not affect potency. When stored as directed, commercially available preservative-free or preserved epoetin alfa injection has an expiration date of 2 or 3 years, respectively, following the date of manufacture.

Preservative-free vials of epoetin alfa injection are intended for withdrawal of only a single dose; once such vials have been entered, unused portions should be discarded. (See Cautions: Other Adverse Effects.) In addition, once the preservative-free solution has been withdrawn from the vial into a syringe for administration, it should be used promptly. The manufacturers state that preservative-free solutions of epoetin alfa in concentrations of 2000 or 10,000 units/mL are stable for 2 weeks when refrigerated or stored at controlled room temperature in plastic tuberculin syringes; however, because of the absence of preservatives, the possibility of microbial contamination must be considered. The preservative-free and preserved injections should be inspected visually for particulate matter and/or discoloration whenever solution and container permit and should be discarded if either is present.

Commercially available multidose vials of epoetin alfa injection should be stored at 2–8°C after initial entry and between doses. The multidose vials should be discarded 21 days after initial entry.

Epoetin alfa injections should not be administered through the same IV tubing as other drugs. The manufacturers and some clinicians state that commercially available epoetin alfa injection generally should not be diluted further prior to administration nor transferred to other containers and/or admixed with other drugs or IV solutions because albumin human, which is present in the injection as a carrier protein, reportedly can adsorb to polyvinyl chloride (PVC) containers and tubing and thus allow disruption of the integrity of the solution.However, epoetin alfa that has been diluted aseptically in the original single-use, 10,000-unit vial with an appropriate volume of bacteriostatic sodium chloride injection to produce an epoetin alfa concentration of 4000 units/mL has been reported to be microbiologically and chemically stable for up to at least 12 weeks. In addition, preservative-free epoetin alfa injection from single-use vials may be diluted with equal parts of bacteriostatic 0.9% sodium chloride injection (preserved with benzyl alcohol) at the time of subcutaneous administration; however, risks are associated with use of benzyl alcohol in neonates, infants, pregnant women, and nursing women.

Preparations

Excipients in commercially available drug preparations may have clinically important effects in some individuals; consult specific product labeling for details.

Epoetin Alfa (Recombinant DNA Origin)

Parenteral

Injection, for IV or subcutaneous use	2000 units/mL	**Epogen®**, Amgen
		Procrit®, Janssen Biotech (formerly Centocor Ortho Biotech)
	3000 units/mL	**Epogen®**, Amgen
		Procrit®, Janssen Biotech (formerly Centocor Ortho Biotech)
	4000 units/mL	**Epogen®**, Amgen
		Procrit®, Janssen Biotech (formerly Centocor Ortho Biotech)
	10,000 units/mL	**Epogen®**, Amgen
		Procrit®, Janssen Biotech (formerly Centocor Ortho Biotech)

20,000 units/mL	**Epogen**®, Amgen
	Procrit®, Janssen Biotech (formerly Centocor Ortho Biotech)
40,000 units/mL	**Epogen**®, Amgen
	Procrit®, Janssen Biotech (formerly Centocor Ortho Biotech)

†Use is not currently included in the labeling approved by the US Food and Drug Administration

Filgrastim, Filgrastim-sndz, Tbo-filgrastim

Granulocyte Colony-Stimulating Factor, G-CSF, Recombinant Methionyl Human G-CSF, Filgrastim-sndz, Tbo-filgrastim

■ Filgrastim, filgrastim-sndz, and tbo-filgrastim are biosynthetic (recombinant DNA origin) hematopoietic agents (human granulocyte colony-stimulating factors [G-CSF]) that principally affect the proliferation and differentiation of neutrophils within the bone marrow and possibly other sites (e.g., spleen).

Filgrastim-sndz is biosimilar to filgrastim (Neupogen®). The US Food and Drug Administration (FDA) defines a biosimilar as a biological that is highly similar to an FDA-licensed reference biological with the exception of minor differences in clinically inactive components and for which there are no clinically meaningful differences in safety, purity, or potency. The claim of biosimilarity is based on a totality-of-evidence approach, which includes consideration of data from analytical, animal, and clinical studies. Therefore, biosimilarity of 2 drugs may be established even when there are formulation or minor structural differences or minor differences in rates of adverse effects between the drugs as long as these differences are not clinically meaningful. Clinical studies for demonstration of biosimilarity include assessment of immunogenicity and pharmacokinetics/pharmacodynamics and address at least one indication licensed for the reference biological. Biosimilars are approved through an abbreviated licensure pathway that establishes biosimilarity between the proposed biological and the reference biological but does not independently establish safety and effectiveness of the proposed biological.

While filgrastim-sndz is biosimilar to the reference biological, filgrastim (Neupogen®), these drugs are *not* interchangeable; instead, they are considered therapeutic alternatives. The possibility that variations in manufacturing may result in differences in efficacy and safety in longer-term studies of biosimilars cannot be excluded; postmarketing safety studies and surveillance of filgrastim-sndz are ongoing. Biosimilarity of filgrastim-sndz and filgrastim (Neupogen®) was established by evaluating structural and functional similarity through advanced analytical studies and pharmacokinetic/pharmacodynamics studies. A clinical safety and efficacy study in breast cancer patients confirmed biosimilarity.

Filgrastim and tbo-filgrastim are structurally and pharmacologically similar drugs that contain a related drug substance. Tbo-filgrastim was licensed by FDA through a biologics license application (BLA), *not* as a biosimilar to filgrastim; at the time of tbo-filgrastim's submission for approval, FDA had not finalized a process for approving biosimilars. The American Society of Clinical Oncology (ASCO) currently states that choice of a G-CSF (e.g., filgrastim, filgrastim-sndz, tbo-filgrastim) for the treatment of febrile neutropenia should be determined based upon convenience, cost, and the clinical situation.

Filgrastim also is commercially available covalently bound to monomethoxy polyethylene glycol (PEG) (i.e., pegfilgrastim). For information on pegfilgrastim, see Pegfilgrastim 20:16.

In this monograph, unless otherwise stated, the term "filgrastim products" refers to filgrastim (the reference drug), filgrastim-sndz (the biosimilar), or both drugs.

Uses

Filgrastim or filgrastim-sndz is used to decrease the incidence of infection (as manifested by febrile neutropenia) in patients with nonmyeloid malignancies receiving myelosuppressive cancer chemotherapy; to reduce the time to neutrophil recovery and the duration of fever following induction or consolidation chemotherapy in patients with acute myeloid leukemia (AML); and to reduce the incidence and duration of sequelae of neutropenia (e.g., fever, infections, oropharyngeal ulcers) in symptomatic patients with congenital, cyclic, or idiopathic neutropenia. Filgrastim or filgrastim-sndz also is used to reduce the duration of neutropenia and neutropenia-related clinical sequelae (e.g., febrile neutropenia) in patients undergoing autologous or allogeneic bone marrow transplantation (BMT), to mobilize hematopoietic progenitor cells into peripheral blood for collection by leukapheresis, and to accelerate myeloid engraftment following autologous peripheral blood progenitor cell (PBMC) transplantation. Filgrastim is used to increase survival in patients with hematopoietic syndrome of acute radiation syndrome following acute exposure to myelosuppressive doses of radiation. Filgrastim also has been used to increase neutrophil counts in patients with myelodysplastic syndrome (MDS)† or aplastic anemia† and to correct or minimize neutropenia and/or drug-induced neutropenia in a variety of patients, including those with hairy cell leukemia† or human immunodeficiency virus (HIV) infection†. Filgrastim is designated an orphan drug by FDA for the treatment of neutropenia associated with BMT, for mobilization of PBPs for collection in patients who will receive myeloablative or myelosuppressive cancer chemotherapy, for the treatment of patients with severe chronic neutropenia (absolute neutrophil count [ANC] less than 500/mm^3), for the treatment of MDS, for the treatment of patients at risk of developing myelosuppression after a radiologic or nuclear incident, for the treatment of amyotrophic lateral sclerosis (ALS), and for the treatment of HIV-infected patients who, in addition, are afflicted with cytomegalovirus retinitis and are being treated with ganciclovir. Additionally, filgrastim is designated an orphan drug by FDA for the reduction in duration of neutropenia, fever, antibiotic use, and hospitalization following induction and consolidation treatment for AML.

Biosimilarity of filgrastim-sndz to filgrastim has been established; therefore, FDA considers that no clinically meaningful differences exist between filgrastim-sndz and filgrastim with respect to efficacy.

Tbo-filgrastim is used to reduce the duration of severe neutropenia in patients with nonmyeloid malignancies receiving myelosuppressive cancer chemotherapy associated with a clinically important risk of febrile neutropenia.

■ **Cancer Chemotherapy-induced Neutropenia** Filgrastim, filgrastim-sndz, or tbo-filgrastim is used for the management of chemotherapy-induced neutropenia in patients receiving myelosuppressive cancer chemotherapy that is associated with a clinically important risk of febrile neutropenia; in clinical studies, filgrastim decreased the risk of infectious complications (as manifested by febrile neutropenia) and tbo-filgrastim reduced the duration of severe neutropenia in such patients. Myelosuppression is a major factor contributing to infection, morbidity (including that requiring hospitalization), and mortality in patients with malignancies undergoing chemotherapy and is a major dose-limiting factor in many such chemotherapy regimens. While filgrastim therapy generally produces a beneficial effect on neutrophil recovery in patients with chemotherapy-induced neutropenia, substantial, cost-effective clinical benefit, including possible effects on survival and quality of life, may be more difficult to establish. Such benefit appears particularly difficult to establish if filgrastim therapy is reserved for active *treatment* of neutropenia and fever (i.e., after the onset of febrile neutropenia) rather than for prophylactic therapy (i.e., in the absence of fever or other manifestations of infection). Some evidence suggests that filgrastim can be cost-effective, at least in certain patient groups, but additional study is needed to define further patient selection criteria. Some clinicians caution that further study is needed before *routine* use of filgrastim can be recommended as a primary part of myelosuppressive chemotherapy regimens. Current guidelines for the use of colony-stimulating factors (CSFs) in adults with solid tumors or nonmyeloid malignancies (e.g., lymphoma) recommend that CSFs be administered prophylactically based upon a patient's risk of developing febrile neutropenia following chemotherapy, taking into account the type of cancer, chemotherapy regimen, patient risk factors, and treatment intent. Based on the chemotherapy regimen and patient-related risk factors, prophylaxis generally is recommended for patients designated to be in an overall high-risk group (exceeding 20% risk of febrile neutropenia) and can be considered for those in an intermediate-risk group (10–20% risk) if risk is due to patient risk factors and not the chemotherapy regimen; prophylaxis generally is not recommended for those in the low-risk group (less than 10% risk). There is currently no consensus nomogram for assessment of the risk of developing febrile neutropenia; clinical judgment should be exercised.

In patients with nonmyeloid malignancy undergoing myelosuppressive chemotherapy, prophylactic use of filgrastim generally has ameliorated or occasionally prevented associated neutropenia and has decreased the incidence and/or duration of fever and infectious episodes, the frequency and/or duration of hospitalization, and requirements for anti-infective therapy.While further study is needed to evaluate whether use of filgrastim therapy in patients with nonmyeloid malignancy can enhance the efficacy of myelosuppressive chemotherapy or shorten the duration of chemotherapy needed, the drug's ameliorative effects on neutropenia have decreased the need to withhold courses and/or reduce dosages of chemotherapy in some patients and also have permitted dose intensification in some. However, the magnitude of response may show considerable interindividual variation, in part because of underlying patient differences (e.g., extent of prior radiation therapy and chemotherapy, underlying conditions and patient status, chemotherapy regimen employed). Some evidence suggests that prophylactic use of filgrastim can be cost-effective, at least in certain patient groups, but additional study is needed to further define patient selection criteria.

Studies have found that certain chemotherapy agents and regimens, as well as the delivered dose intensity, are important predictors of febrile neutropenia and febrile neutropenia-related hospitalizations. Antineoplastic agents such as anthracyclines (e.g., doxorubicin), taxanes (e.g., docetaxel), alkylating agents (e.g., cyclophosphamide), and topoisomerase inhibitors (e.g., etoposide) as well as gemcitabine and vinorelbine have been associated with myelosuppression. In adults receiving chemotherapy for a solid tumor or nonmyeloid malignancy, guidelines recommend that CSFs be administered prophylactically when the risk of febrile neutropenia is high (exceeding 20%) and if equally effective treatments that do not require CSF support are unavailable. Prophylaxis should be initiated in the first cycle and continued through subsequent cycles of chemotherapy. Prophylactic administration of CSFs is recommended for any patient considered at high risk, regardless of whether the treatment is intended to be curative, to prolong survival, or to manage symptoms. For patients receiving chemotherapy regimens who have an intermediate risk of febrile neutropenia (10–20%), prophylactic use of CSFs can be considered, especially if the increased risk is due to patient factors (e.g., older than 65 years of age, coexisting illness) instead of the chemotherapy regimen. Guidelines also recommend considering previous cytotoxic or radiation therapy, preexisting tumor-related neutropenia or bone marrow involvement, reduced performance status, reduced nutritional status, advanced cancer, impaired renal or hepatic function, and the presence of open sores when estimating a patient's overall risk of febrile neutropenia. Prophylaxis is generally not recommended for patients with a low risk (less than 10%) of febrile neutropenia. Secondary prophylaxis with CSFs is recommended in patients who have experienced a neutropenic complication from a previous chemotherapy cycle (for which primary prophylaxis was not received), in whom a reduced chemotherapy dose or treatment delay would compromise disease-free or overall survival or treatment outcomes. While it has been suggested that filgrastim may prove useful as an adjunct to empiric anti-infective therapy ("rescue treatment") in patients who develop febrile neutropenia secondary to chemotherapy-induced myelosuppression†, and then prophylactically to prevent subsequent episodes, the efficacy of such therapy has not been fully evaluated.

Efficacy of filgrastim has not been established in patients receiving antineoplastic therapy that is associated with delayed myelosuppression (e.g., nitrosourea derivatives) or in those receiving mitomycin or myelosuppressive doses of antimetabolites (e.g., cytarabine, fluorouracil); however, studies are ongoing.

Prophylactic filgrastim therapy has been used effectively to accelerate the recovery of neutrophil counts following a variety of myelosuppressive chemotherapy regimens in adults with small cell lung carcinoma. In a randomized, placebo-controlled study in patients with small cell lung carcinoma receiving 1–6 courses of chemotherapy with etoposide (120 mg/m^2 on days 1–3 of each course), cyclophosphamide (1 g/m^2 on day 1 of each course), and doxorubicin (50 mg/m^2 on day 1 of each course), the incidence, severity, and duration of severe neutropenia (ANC less than 500/mm^3) were lower in patients receiving filgrastim (4–8 mcg/kg [230 mcg/m^2] daily given subcutaneously for 4–17 consecutive days starting on day 4 after chemotherapy) compared with those receiving placebo. Patients receiving filgrastim had a 57% rate of severe neutropenia whereas patients receiving placebo had a 77% rate; the median duration of severe neutropenia in cycle 1 was reduced in patients receiving filgrastim compared with those receiving placebo (2 or 6 days, respectively). The mean and median severities of neutropenia (as measured by the ANC nadir) during the first cycle of therapy were 496/mm^3 (range: 0–1878/mm^3) and 72/mm^3 (range: 0–7912/mm^3), respectively, in patients receiving filgrastim and 204/mm^3 (range: 0–1157/mm^3) and 38/mm^3 (range: 0–9525/mm^3), respectively, in those receiving placebo; the ANC nadir occurred at a mean of 10 or 12 days in patients receiving filgrastim or placebo, respectively. In addition, patients receiving filgrastim had a lower incidence of infection (event rate 40 or 76%) and lower overall duration of infection (as manifested by febrile neutropenia), and required fewer episodes of hospitalization and fewer days of IV antibiotic therapy compared with patients receiving placebo; no differences in survival or disease progression were evident.

Prophylactic filgrastim therapy also has been used effectively to accelerate the recovery of neutrophil counts following a variety of chemotherapy regimens (some of which included use of methotrexate, doxorubicin, vinblastine, cisplatin, or melphalan) in adults with other types of malignancies, including advanced pulmonary carcinoma, bladder carcinoma, transitional cell carcinoma of the urothelium, testicular carcinoma, prostatic carcinoma, breast carcinoma, ovarian carcinoma, neuroblastoma, and non-Hodgkin's lymphoma. The drug effectively decreased the severity and duration of severe neutropenia in these patients and decreased the duration of hospitalization and requirements for anti-infective therapy; the drug also may decrease the frequency and severity of mucositis. Filgrastim therapy has been used with some success to accelerate neutrophil recovery in children with advanced-stage neuroblastoma receiving chemotherapy. When used in these children, the drug has reduced the duration of severe neutropenia and decreased the incidence of hospitalization for fever with neutropenia. The drug also has been used effectively to reduce the duration of neutropenia and incidence of febrile neutropenia in a limited number of children 7 months to 15 years of age receiving chemotherapy for various other malignancies (e.g., acute lymphocytic leukemia, Wilms' tumor, lymphoma, rhabdomyosarcoma, Hodgkin's disease, CNS tumor).

Filgrastim has been used in conjunction with empiric anti-infective therapy for the treatment of cancer chemotherapy-induced febrile neutropenia†. In one randomized, double-blind, placebo-controlled study in patients with nonmyeloid malignancies who developed febrile neutropenia following chemotherapy, filgrastim therapy (initiated within 12 hours of empiric anti-infective therapy) reduced the median duration of severe neutropenia and the time to resolution of febrile neutropenia by 1–2 days compared with use of empiric anti-infective therapy alone. However, filgrastim therapy did not have a clinically important impact on the duration of fever or median duration of hospitalization required. In a meta-analysis evaluating the use of CSFs in combination with antibiotics compared with antibiotic use alone for the treatment of chemotherapy-induced neutropenia, duration of hospitalization and time to neutrophil recovery were reduced in patients who received CSFs. No improvement in overall survival was seen with the therapeutic use of CSFs. It has been recommended that patients who have received prophylactic treatment with CSFs and develop febrile neutropenia should continue receiving the same CSF. CSFs should not be routinely used as adjunctive treatment with antibiotic therapy for patients with fever and neutropenia. For patients who have not received prophylaxis and develop febrile neutropenia, therapy with CSFs may be considered if certain risk factors that indicate an increased risk of infection-related complications or poor outcomes are present (e.g., patients older than 65 years of age, sepsis syndrome, ANC less than 100/mm^3, anticipated or prolonged neutropenia [exceeding 10 days], pneumonia, invasive fungal infections or other clinically documented infections, hospitalization, prior episodes of febrile neutropenia).

Efficacy of tbo-filgrastim was established in a multicenter, randomized study in 348 chemotherapy-naive adults with advanced (high-risk stage II, stage III, or stage IV) breast cancer receiving initial chemotherapy with doxorubicin 60 mg/m^2 and docetaxel 75 mg/m^2. Patients were randomly assigned to receive tbo-filgrastim, placebo, or a filgrastim preparation not available in the US; however, demonstration of efficacy is based only on the comparison between tbo-filgrastim and placebo. The study drug was initiated one day after chemotherapy at a dosage of 5 mcg/kg once daily by subcutaneous injection, and continued for at least 5 days up to a maximum of 14 days or until a post-nadir ANC of at least 10,000/mm^3 was achieved. The mean duration of severe neutropenia in the first chemotherapy cycle (primary efficacy end point) was substantially reduced in patients receiving tbo-filgrastim compared with that in placebo recipients (1.1 or 3.8 days, respectively).

■ **Leukemias** Filgrastim or filgrastim-sndz is used to reduce the time to neutrophil recovery and the duration of fever following induction or consolidation chemotherapy in adults with acute myeloid leukemia (AML).

A double-blind, multicenter trial of over 500 patients (mean age: 54 years; range: 16–89 years) who had completed a course of standard induction chemotherapy (daunorubicin, cytarabine, and etoposide) for newly diagnosed AML randomized patients to receive either filgrastim (5 mcg/kg daily) or placebo initiated 24 hours after the last dose of chemotherapy. Therapy was continued until neutrophil recovery (ANC 1000/mm^3 for 3 consecutive days or 10,000/mm^3 for 1 day) or for a maximum of 35 days. Filgrastim therapy decreased the median time to ANC recovery and the median duration of fever, anti-infective use, and hospitalization as compared with placebo following induction chemotherapy. In patients treated with filgrastim, the median time from initiation of chemotherapy to ANC recovery (ANC of at least 500/mm^3) was 20 days, as compared to 25 days in patients receiving placebo. The median duration of fever was reduced by 1.5 days, and there were reductions in the duration of IV anti-infective use, including systemic antifungal (amphotericin B) therapy, and hospitalization in treated patients. During consolidation chemotherapy, patients treated with filgrastim also experienced reductions in the incidence of severe neutropenia, time to neutrophil recovery, incidence and duration of fever, and the durations of IV anti-infective use and hospitalization. There were no differences between filgrastim- or placebo-treated groups in terms of complete remission rate (69 or 68%, respectively), median time to disease progression in all patients randomized (165 or 186 days, respectively), or median overall survival (380 or 425 days, respectively). Filgrastim did not appear to affect prognosis of patients with AML. Other reports of filgrastim therapy in patients receiving induction or consolidation chemotherapy for AML also showed decreased time to ANC recovery, sustained increase in ANC, decreased incidence and duration of fever, and decreased use of IV anti-infectives; the effects of the drug on hospitalization were less clear. Filgrastim appeared to have no adverse effects on duration of complete remission or survival.

Use of filgrastim in patients with acute leukemia has been considered controversial since results of in vitro studies indicate that certain leukemic cell lines have receptors for granulocyte CSF (G-CSF) and that the survival, proliferation, and differentiation of the cells are supported by CSFs. (See Pharmacology.) In studies in patients with relapsed or refractory AML or acute lymphocytic (lymphoblastic) leukemia (ALL) or patients with leukemia associated with myelodysplastic syndrome, the period of neutrophil recovery was shorter and the incidence of infectious complications was lower in patients who received filgrastim after induction therapy than in those who did not receive the drug. Although there was no evidence that filgrastim accelerated regrowth of leukemic cells, regrowth of leukemic blasts in the bone marrow did occur during filgrastim therapy in a few patients with acute leukemia associated with myelodysplastic syndromes; it is unclear whether this regrowth would have occurred even without filgrastim therapy. While it has been suggested that filgrastim may be a useful antileukemic agent secondary to its stimulation of leukemic differentiation or of proliferation of malignant leukemic cells, thereby increasing their sensitivity to cancer chemotherapy, it also has been suggested that such stimulation also might accelerate the malignancy. Therefore, some experts have stated that use of filgrastim in patients with myeloid leukemias should be considered investigational and should be undertaken with great caution. Some guidelines state the use of CSFs may be considered in patients with AML during induction therapy for patients who are septic and have a life-threatening infection in an attempt to shorten the duration of neutropenia. Data are lacking on whether CSFs have a positive or negative impact on long-term outcome if used during consolidation therapy. CSFs are not routinely recommended in post-remission therapy, except in life-threatening infections or when manifestations of sepsis are present and leukemia is believed to be in remission.

Filgrastim has been used effectively to increase neutrophil counts in a limited number of patients with hairy cell leukemia (leukemic reticuloendotheliosis) complicated by severe neutropenia†. The ANC normalized in these patients within 1–2 weeks following initiation of filgrastim therapy (approximately 1–7 mcg/kg given once daily by subcutaneous injection for 2–12 weeks). Although it has been suggested that filgrastim may become a useful adjunct to current therapy (e.g., cladribine, interferon alfa, pentostatin) for hairy cell leukemia, further study is needed to more fully evaluate efficacy and safety of filgrastim in these patients.

■ **Autologous and Allogeneic Bone Marrow Transplantation** Filgrastim or filgrastim-sndz is used to reduce the duration of neutropenia and neutropenia-related clinical sequelae (e.g., febrile neutropenia) in patients with nonmyeloid malignancies undergoing myeloablative cancer chemotherapy followed by bone marrow transplantation (BMT). When used following autologous BMT in adults with various nonmyeloid malignancies, non-Hodgkin's lymphoma, Hodgkin's disease, or ALL, filgrastim therapy effectively shortened the duration of severe neutropenia, decreased the median duration of infectious episodes and anti-infective therapy required, and shortened the median duration of hospitalization required. Filgrastim therapy also has effectively shortened the duration of severe neutropenia when used in a limited number of adults with myeloid† and nonmyeloid malignancies undergoing allogeneic BMT. However, because filgrastim generally does not completely prevent severe neutropenia nor shorten its duration sufficiently to reduce the incidence of infection associated with myeloablative therapy, benefit of the drug may be reflected principally in reducing the duration of fever, anti-infective therapy, and hospitalization. Filgrastim therapy has been associated with a reduced frequency and severity of mucositis in patients undergoing autologous BMT.

In one randomized, controlled study in patients with non-Hodgkin's lymphoma or Hodgkin's disease undergoing autologous BMT, the median time to neutrophil recovery (defined as the first of 3 consecutive days when neutrophil counts were 500/mm^3 or greater) was 10 days in patients who received filgrastim therapy (10 or 20 mcg/kg daily by continuous subcutaneous infusion) compared with 18 days in patients who received placebo. The median duration of febrile neutropenia was 5 days in those who received filgrastim compared with 13.5 days in those who received placebo. When filgrastim therapy was used in a nonrandomized study in patients with non-Hodgkin's lymphoma, Hodgkin's disease, ALL, or germ cell tumor undergoing autologous BMT, the average time to neutrophil recovery was 11 days. In another randomized, controlled trial, patients with non-Hodgkin's lymphoma or Hodgkin's disease undergoing autologous BMT received filgrastim 10 or 30 mcg/kg daily as a 24-hour continuous IV infusion (starting 24 hours after bone marrow infusion for a maximum of 28 days) or no filgrastim. A substantial reduction in the median duration of severe neutropenia (ANC less than 500/mm^3) was demonstrated in patients who received filgrastim therapy compared with that in patients who received no filgrastim (11 or 23 days, respectively). In one randomized, placebo-controlled trial in adults with myeloid† and nonmyeloid malignancies undergoing allogeneic BMT, the median duration of severe neutropenia and time to neutrophil recovery (absolute neutrophil count of 500/mm^3 or greater) were 15 and 16 days, respectively, in patients who received filgrastim (300 mcg/m^2 daily) compared with 19 and 21 days, respectively, in patients who received placebo.

When filgrastim or filgrastim-sndz is used in patients who have undergone BMT, a complete blood cell count (CBC) and platelet count should be performed frequently during therapy to monitor myeloid recovery. (See Cautions: Precautions and Contraindications.)

■ Peripheral Blood Progenitor Cell Transplantation Filgrastim or filgrastim-sndz is used for mobilization of hematopoietic progenitor cells into peripheral blood for collection by leukapheresis. Filgrastim mobilization allows for the collection of increased numbers of progenitor cells capable of engraftment compared with collection without mobilization.

Use of filgrastim for mobilization of PBPs has been evaluated in several clinical trials in patients with non-Hodgkin's lymphoma, Hodgkin's disease, ALL, breast cancer, and germ-cell tumor. Filgrastim generally was administered for 6–7 days and leukapheresis was performed on days 5, 6, and 7 (except for a limited number of patients who received apheresis on days 4, 6, and 8). Filgrastim also was administered to these patients following autologous PBPC transplantation of the filgrastim-mobilized leukapheresis product until a sustainable ANC (500/mm^3 or greater) was attained. Engraftment was evaluated in 64 patients who underwent transplantation using filgrastim-mobilized autologous hematopoietic progenitor cells and approximately 3% of these patients did not achieve the criteria for engraftment as defined by a platelet count of at least 20,000/mm^3 by 28 days. The rate of engraftment following filgrastim-mobilized PBPC transplantation without filgrastim therapy following the procedure has not been studied.

In a randomized study in patients with Hodgkin's disease or non-Hodgkin's lymphoma undergoing myeloablative cancer chemotherapy, autologous transplantation of filgrastim-mobilized PBPCs followed by filgrastim therapy (n=27) was compared with autologous BMT followed by filgrastim therapy (n=31). The median time to sustained ANC of 500/mm^3 or greater was 11 or 14 days in those who received autologous PBPC or autologous BMT, respectively. Patients who received autologous PBPC required fewer days of platelet transfusions; the median duration of platelet transfusions after grafting was 6 days in those who received PBPC versus 10 days in those who received autologous BMT. In addition, patients who received autologous PBPCs had fewer days of erythrocyte transfusions and a shorter duration of hospitalization. While filgrastim therapy may be effective for mobilization of PBPC, the optimum schedule for such therapy, the duration of engraftment with PBPC transplantation, and the potential of circulating malignant cells to propagate the malignancy remain to be established.

■ Congenital, Cyclic, and Idiopathic Neutropenias Filgrastim or filgrastim-sndz is used to reduce the incidence and duration of sequelae of neutropenia (e.g., fever, infections, oropharyngeal ulcers) in symptomatic patients with congenital neutropenia, cyclic neutropenia, and acquired idiopathic neutropenia. These severe chronic neutropenias are characterized by a selective decrease in the number of circulating neutrophils and an enhanced susceptibility to bacterial infections. Therapy in patients with severe chronic neutropenia previously relied principally on supportive care alone. While filgrastim can produce sustained amelioration of the underlying neutropenia in certain patients with these conditions, neutrophil counts decrease to pretreatment levels shortly after discontinuance of therapy with the drug.

Further study is needed to determine whether long-term maintenance therapy with filgrastim will maintain neutrophil counts in patients with primary neutropenias without substantial adverse effects. Limited evidence suggests that the beneficial effects associated with filgrastim-induced amelioration of neutropenia in these patients results in a decrease in infectious morbidity and also may be associated with improved quality of life. Results of a few comparative studies indicate that filgrastim may be more effective than sargramostim (a recombinant GM-CSF) for the treatment of primary neutropenia, including congenital neutropenia, since filgrastim increases the neutrophil count without causing eosinophilia.

When used in adults and children 4 months to 19 years of age with severe congenital neutropenia (Kostmann syndrome), cyclic neutropenia, or idiopathic neutropenia, filgrastim therapy has increased neutrophil counts, reduced the incidence and duration of infectious episodes and fever, and reduced the incidence of oropharyngeal ulcers and requirements for anti-infective therapy in these patients. In many patients with cyclic neutropenia, the average neutrophil count is 10–12 times higher during filgrastim therapy and the neutropenic cycle length is shortened from 21 to 14 days; this is associated with a reduction in the frequency of infectious episodes and a reduction in the severity of symptoms of infection and inflammation. In addition to ameliorating neutropenia, the drug increases the amplitude and frequency of cycling in circulating progenitor cell numbers in these patients, suggesting a stem cell effect.

Prior to initiation of filgrastim therapy, it is essential that the diagnosis of severe chronic neutropenia be confirmed with serial CBCs and platelet counts and an evaluation of bone marrow morphology and karyotype. Use of filgrastim prior to confirmation of severe chronic neutropenia could impair diagnostic efforts and interfere with or delay evaluation and treatment of an underlying condition other than severe chronic neutropenia. When filgrastim is used for chronic therapy in symptomatic patients with congenital, cyclic, or idiopathic neutropenia, CBCs with differential and platelet counts should be monitored during the initial 4 weeks of therapy and during the first 2 weeks following any dosage adjustment. After the patient is clinically stable, a CBC with differential and platelet count should be performed monthly during the first year of treatment. Thereafter, if the patient is clinically stable, less frequent routine monitoring has been recommended. (See Cautions: Precautions and Contraindications.)

Filgrastim therapy also has been used effectively to increase the neutrophil count in a few children 19 months to 21 years of age with glycogen storage disease type Ib†. Filgrastim has been used in at least one 3-month old child for the treatment of neutropenia associated with sepsis†.

■ Hematopoietic Syndrome of Acute Radiation Syndrome Filgrastim is used to increase survival in patients who have been acutely exposed to myelosuppressive doses of radiation. Acute radiation syndrome occurs following intense, whole or substantial partial body radiation of doses exceeding 1 Gy and is characterized by adverse effects on the hematopoietic, GI, central nervous, and cutaneous systems. The hematopoietic syndrome of acute radiation syndrome results from rapid bone marrow ablation, causing pancytopenia, and without treatment, leads to death from infection and/or hemorrhage. Medical management of patients with acute radiation syndrome includes early use of hematopoietic cytokines, antibiotics, and transfusion support. Prevention and management of infection is the mainstay of therapy. When administered at 24 hours following total body irradiation, filgrastim substantially enhanced survival in nonhuman primates; studies have not been conducted in humans for ethical reasons.

Safety and efficacy of filgrastim for the treatment of hematopoietic syndrome of acute radiation syndrome has been established by efficacy studies conducted in animals and data supporting the use of filgrastim for other FDA-labeled indications. In a randomized, blinded, placebo-controlled trial, rhesus monkeys were exposed to total body irradiation at a dose that would be lethal in 50% of animals (7.4 Gy delivered at 0.8 Gy/minute) by 60 days of follow-up. Starting 1 day after irradiation, animals received daily subcutaneous injections of placebo or filgrastim (10 mcg/kg). Treatment was discontinued if the ANC was 1000/mm^3 or greater for 3 consecutive days, the ANC was 10,000/mm^3 or greater for more than 2 consecutive days within days 1–5 of the trial, or if the ANC was 10,000/mm^3 or greater at any time after day 5 of the trial. Medical management consisting of IV fluids, antibiotics, blood transfusions, and other support was also provided as needed based upon prespecified criteria. Filgrastim therapy substantially reduced 60-day mortality in the irradiated rhesus monkeys compared with placebo (event rate 21 or 59%). The duration of ANC less than 100/mm^3 and less than 500/mm^3 was reduced from 12.3 and 18.6 days, respectively, in the animals receiving placebo therapy to 10.4 and 14.3 days, respectively, with filgrastim treatment. While filgrastim substantially decreased the duration of neutropenia, the ANC nadir was not affected. Febrile neutropenia was experienced by 79.2% of animals receiving filgrastim therapy compared with 90.9% of animals receiving placebo.

■ Myelodysplastic Syndromes and Aplastic Anemia Filgrastim has been used to increase neutrophil counts in adults with MDS†. While filgrastim has shown some promise for this use, safety and efficacy of the drug in the treatment of neutropenia associated with myelodysplastic disorders have not been established and use of the drug generally should be limited to experts in such therapy. Filgrastim has effectively increased neutrophil counts in patients with MDS classified as refractory anemia (RA), refractory anemia with ringed sideroblasts (RARS), refractory anemia with excess blasts (RAEB), or refractory anemia with excess blasts in transformation (RAEB-T). However, there appears to be considerable interindividual variation in filgrastim dosage required for the neutrophil response, and prolonged maintenance therapy with the drug is necessary since neutrophil counts return to pretreatment levels within 1–4 weeks after filgrastim is discontinued. In some patients with MDS, there was a reduced need for red blood cell transfusions during filgrastim therapy; no clinically important effects on lymphocyte, monocyte, platelet, or eosinophil counts were apparent.

Whether use of filgrastim in patients with MDS will alter (either increase or decrease) the rate of progression to acute myeloid (myelogenous, nonlymphocytic) leukemia (AML, ANLL) or affect the usually fatal outcome of the disease is unclear and requires further study. The rate of progression to AML in untreated patients with MDS is approximately 10–20%, 40–50%, and 60–75% in those with RA, RAEB, and RAEB-T, respectively. There is concern, but no clear evidence indicated to date, that use of filgrastim may stimulate progression to AML in patients with MDS since in vitro evidence indicates that the drug can stimulate the growth of myeloid leukemic blast cells and because an increase in the percentage of leukemic blasts in the bone marrow has occurred in some patients with MDS receiving the drug. Although sargramostim (a recombinant GM-CSF) also has been used in the treatment of MDS, the relative efficacy of these two hematologic growth factors in patients with MDS has not been evaluated to date in controlled studies.

Filgrastim has been used with some success to increase the neutrophil count in a limited number of children 1–17 years of age† with moderate to severe aplastic anemia†. However, patients with aplastic anemia generally have variable responses to hematopoietic growth factors, and patients with severe neutropenia (neutrophil counts less than 300/mm^3) may not respond to the drugs because of the absence of circulating hematopoietic progenitor cells. Further study is needed to evaluate the use of filgrastim in aplastic anemia and to determine the long-term safety and efficacy of the drug in these patients; pending accumulation of such data, this use generally should be limited to experts in such therapy. In addition, the role of filgrastim versus sargramostim (a recombinant GM-CSF) in patients with aplastic anemia remains to be elucidated. There is some concern that, while filgrastim therapy may decrease mortality associated with infectious complications in patients with aplastic anemia, these patients may be at increased risk for the development of myelodysplasia and progression to leukemia. Although further study is needed, there is some evidence that patients with aplastic anemia who do not respond to filgrastim alone may respond to the drug if another growth factor (e.g., interleukin-1, interleukin-2, or interleukin-3 [multi-GSF]) is administered initially to increase the level of circulating hematopoietic progenitor cells to a level sufficient for filgrastim to be effective. In a patient with severe aplastic anemia that did not respond to filgrastim alone, administration of interleukin-3 (5 mcg/kg daily for 20 days) prior to filgrastim appeared to effectively increase the level of circulating hematopoietic progenitor cells so that filgrastim could restore granulopoiesis; use of interleukin-3 prior to use of filgrastim had no effect on cells other than neutrophils, and the patient continued to need regular red blood cell and platelet transfusions.

■ Neutropenia Associated with HIV Infection and Antiretroviral Therapy Filgrastim has been used in some patients with HIV infections in an effort to correct or minimize HIV-associated neutropenia and/or drug-induced neutropenia†. When used in patients with HIV infection, filgrastim has effectively increased neutrophils and monocytes, but has had no clinically important effect on the number of erythrocytes, platelets, lymphocytes, eosinophils, or basophils. Some clinicians state that use of filgrastim to increase neutrophil counts in HIV-infected patients in an attempt to reduce the risk of bacterial infections in these patients can be considered. However, more data are needed to fully determine the benefit of filgrastim therapy in neutropenic patients with HIV infection.

Filgrastim has been effective when used alone or in conjunction with epoetin alfa (a recombinant erythropoietin) in adults with acquired immunodeficiency syndrome (AIDS) or AIDS-related complex (ARC) to ameliorate the hematologic toxicity (severe anemia and/or granulocytopenia) associated with zidovudine therapy†. Epoetin alfa alone has been shown to be effective in ameliorating the anemia but not the granulocytopenia associated with zidovudine therapy. In a study in adults with HIV infection and substantial bone marrow suppression, filgrastim therapy was administered initially to increase the neutrophil count and epoetin alfa therapy was then added to increase the hemoglobin concentration after the neutrophil count had normalized; zidovudine therapy was then reinstituted and, in some patients, was given concomitantly with both hematopoietic growth factors. While the neutrophil count decreased substantially (compared with the initial filgrastim-induced increase) following initiation of epoetin alfa therapy and again when zidovudine was reinitiated, counts still remained substantially above baseline values during continued filgrastim therapy, and such combined therapy permitted resumption of full-dose zidovudine therapy in many patients who had developed intolerance. Although further study is needed, there has been no evidence to date that use of filgrastim adversely affects HIV replication or interferes with the antiretroviral effects of zidovudine. Studies are ongoing to evaluate the use of filgrastim in children to minimize the hematologic toxicity of zidovudine. In addition, studies are ongoing to determine whether filgrastim and/or other hematologic growth factors can minimize hematologic toxicity associated with other anti-infective agents used in patients with HIV infection (e.g., ganciclovir, co-trimoxazole, sulfadoxine and pyrimethamine).

■ Amyotrophic Lateral Sclerosis Filgrastim has been used in a limited number of patients in an attempt to delay or slow progression of ALS†. Mouse models and preliminary human exposure data have suggested that treatment with G-CSF may have neuroprotective effects, possibly via modulation of the inflammatory pathway, an antiapoptotic effect on glial and/or neural cells, or functional stimulation and differentiation of neural stem cells. Results of a few small studies in patients with ALS suggest that G-CSF therapy may delay functional decline; however, other studies have reported no beneficial effects. In a randomized, double-blind, placebo-controlled pilot trial in 10 patients with ALS, a reduction in structural disintegration of white matter tracts was observed in ALS patients treated with filgrastim 10 mcg/kg daily subcutaneously on days 1–10 and 20–25. No substantial differences were found between treatment groups in clinical tests and brain volumetry from baseline to day 100; however, a reduction in structural disintegration of white matter tracts in patients treated with filgrastim was observed. Additional study and experience are needed to evaluate the potential benefits of filgrastim in patients with ALS.

■ Other Uses Filgrastim has been used effectively in a limited number of patients with nonmalignant conditions† who developed neutropenia while receiving various myelosuppressive drugs. The drug has been used effectively in at least one patient who developed bone marrow toxicity while receiving methotrexate treatment for rheumatoid arthritis. The drug also has been used effectively in a few patients for the management of agranulocytosis associated with clozapine, methimazole,captopril, procainamide, gold, phenothiazine, azathioprine, ticlopidine hydrochloride, phenobarbital, phenytoin, ciprofloxacin, cefuroxime, chloramphenicol, or sulfasalazine therapy and for mesalazine-associated neutropenia. In addition, filgrastim therapy appeared to accelerate bone marrow recovery in one patient who developed pancytopenia following colchicine overdosage.

Dosage and Administration

■ Administration ***Filgrastim or Filgrastim-sndz*** Depending on the indication for use, filgrastim or filgrastim-sndz may be administered by IV infusion or by subcutaneous injection. Filgrastim has also been administered by continuous subcutaneous infusion†. Subcutaneous injection is the most convenient for self-administration of filgrastim and is especially useful when prolonged maintenance therapy with the drug is necessary. Recommended sites for subcutaneous injection of filgrastim or filgrastim-sndz include the outer area of the upper arms, abdomen (except for the 2-inch area around the navel), front of middle thighs, and the upper outer areas of the buttocks. Injection sites should be rotated daily; any area that is tender, red, bruised, scaly, hard, or has stretch marks or scars should be avoided. Filgrastim-sndz prefilled syringes may not accurately measure volumes less than 0.3 mL; due to the potential for dosing errors, direct administration of a volume of filgrastim-sndz less than 0.3 mL is not recommended. When administered by IV infusion in patients with cancer chemotherapy-induced neutropenia, the manufacturers recommend that infusions of filgrastim or filgrastim-sndz be given over 15–30 minutes or by continuous infusion. In patients who have undergone bone marrow transplantation (BMT), the manufacturers recommend that filgrastim or filgrastim-sndz be given by IV infusion over a period not exceeding 24 hours. When administered by continuous subcutaneous infusion† for either use, filgrastim has been infused over 24 hours. For extended IV or subcutaneous infusions†, a controlled-infusion device generally is employed.

If required, filgrastim or filgrastim-sndz may be diluted in 5% dextrose injection. For IV infusion, filgrastim has been diluted in 50–100 mL of 5% dextrose injection. However, the manufacturers state that dilutions of filgrastim or filgrastim-sndz injection to a final concentration of less than 5 mcg/mL are not recommended. For continuous subcutaneous infusion†, filgrastim has been diluted in 10–50 mL of 5% dextrose injection and infused subcutaneously at a rate not exceeding 10 mL/24 hours. When filgrastim or filgrastim-sndz is diluted to produce a final concentration of less than 15 mcg/mL, it is recommended that albumin human be added to the infusion solution to a final concentration of 2 mg/mL (0.2%) to minimize adsorption of the drug to infusion containers or equipment. Diluted solutions of filgrastim or filgrastim-sndz can be stored at room temperature for up to 24 hours (including time during room temperature storage of the infusion solution and duration of the infusion). (See Chemistry and Stability: Stability.)

Filgrastim and filgrastim-sndz injections should *not* be diluted with 0.9% sodium chloride injection because precipitation may occur.

Filgrastim and filgrastim-sndz injections should *not* be shaken. (See Chemistry and Stability: Stability.) Prefilled syringes of filgrastim or filgrastim-sndz are for single-use only; any unused portions should be discarded. In addition, vials of filgrastim are intended for withdrawal of only a single dose; therefore, the manufacturer recommends that the vial not be reentered after initial withdrawal of a dose, and unused portions should be discarded and not saved for future use.

Prior to administration, solutions of filgrastim or filgrastim-sndz should be inspected visually for particulate matter or discoloration whenever solution and container permit. If particulates or discoloration is evident, the solution should not be used.

Filgrastim and filgrastim-sndz may be self-administered. If it is determined that the patient or their caregiver can safely and effectively administer filgrastim or filgrastim-sndz in the home, they should be given the patient information provided by the manufacturer and should receive careful instruction on the proper dosage and administration of the drug, including aseptic techniques. They also should be carefully instructed on the proper, safe disposal of needles, syringes, and unused drug.

Because many antineoplastic agents target rapidly proliferating cells, filgrastim or filgrastim-sndz should *not* be administered within 24 hours before or after therapy with myelosuppressive chemotherapy.

Tbo-filgrastim Tbo-filgrastim is administered by subcutaneous injection. Recommended sites for injection include the upper back portion of the upper arms, abdomen (except for the 2-inch area around the navel), front of middle thighs, or the upper outer areas of the buttocks. Injection sites should be rotated daily; any area that is tender, red, bruised, hard, or has stretch marks or scars should be avoided.

Tbo-filgrastim injection should *not* be shaken. (See Chemistry and Stability: Stability.) Prefilled syringes of tbo-filgrastim are for single-use only; any unused portions should be discarded.

Prior to administration, solutions of tbo-filgrastim should be inspected visually for particulate matter or discoloration whenever solution and container permit. If particulates or discoloration is evident, the solution should not be used.

Tbo-filgrastim may be self-administered. If it is determined that the patient or their caregiver can safely and effectively administer tbo-filgrastim at home, they should be given the patient information provided by the manufacturer and should receive careful instruction on the proper dosage and administration of the drug, including aseptic techniques. They also should be carefully instructed on the proper, safe disposal of needles, syringes, and unused drug.

Because many antineoplastic agents target rapidly proliferating cells, tbo-filgrastim should *not* be administered within 24 hours before therapy with such drugs. In addition, the first dose of tbo-filgrastim should be administered no earlier than 24 hours following myelosuppressive chemotherapy. In patients receiving tbo-filgrastim, a complete blood cell count (CBC) should be monitored prior to therapy and twice weekly thereafter until neutrophil counts have recovered. (See Cautions: Precautions and Contraindications.)

■ **Dosage** ***Cancer Chemotherapy-induced Neutropenia*** **Filgrastim or Filgrastim-sndz.** When filgrastim or filgrastim-sndz is used to decrease the incidence of infectious complications in patients receiving myelosuppressive cancer chemotherapy, dosage of the drug should be individualized since dosage requirements, including the duration of filgrastim or filgrastim-sndz therapy, may vary depending on the type and dosage of myelosuppressive chemotherapy regimen employed.

The recommended initial filgrastim or filgrastim-sndz dosage in patients receiving myelosuppressive chemotherapy is 5 mcg/kg once daily administered by subcutaneous injection, short (15–30 minutes) IV infusion, or continuous IV infusion. Filgrastim and filgrastim-sndz should be administered at least 24 hours after cytotoxic chemotherapy; it should *not* be administered within the 24-hour period before such chemotherapy. (See Filgrastim or Filgrastim-sndz under Dosage and Administration: Administration.) If the time to response or magnitude of neutrophil response is inadequate after 5–7 days of filgrastim therapy, dosage may be increased in increments of 5 mcg/kg with each chemotherapy cycle; dosage increases should be based on the duration and severity of the absolute neutrophil count (ANC) nadir associated with chemotherapy. A transient increase in neutrophil count is typically seen 1–2 days after initiation of filgrastim or filgrastim-sndz therapy. Therefore, to ensure a sustained therapeutic response, therapy with filgrastim or filgrastim-sndz should be continued for up to 2 weeks until the ANC reaches 10,000/mm^3 following the expected chemotherapy-induced ANC nadir. There is no evidence to date that filgrastim or filgrastim-sndz dosages that increase the ANC beyond 10,000/mm^3 result in any additional clinical benefit. Because the duration of neutropenia often increases with each cycle of chemotherapy, longer periods of filgrastim therapy may be required for later chemotherapy cycles than for early cycles.

Tbo-filgrastim. The recommended dosage of tbo-filgrastim for the management of cancer chemotherapy-induced neutropenia is 5 mcg/kg once daily administered by subcutaneous injection. Therapy should be continued until after the expected chemotherapy-induced neutrophil nadir and until the ANC has recovered to within the normal range.

Bone Marrow Transplantation **Filgrastim or Filgrastim-sndz.** When used to reduce the duration of neutropenia and neutropenia-related clinical sequelae (e.g., febrile neutropenia) in patients with nonmyeloid malignancies undergoing myeloablative cancer chemotherapy followed by BMT, the recommended initial dosage of filgrastim or filgrastim-sndz is 10 mcg/kg once daily given by IV infusion over a period not exceeding 24 hours. The first dose of filgrastim or filgrastim-sndz should be administered at least 24 hours after cytotoxic chemotherapy and at least 24 hours after BMT. This initial dosage is continued until the ANC has remained at greater than 1000/mm^3 for 3 consecutive days, at which time dosage should be reduced to 5 mcg/kg daily. If the ANC remains greater than 1000/mm^3 for an additional 3 consecutive days when the lower dosage is used, filgrastim or filgrastim-sndz may be discontinued. If discontinuance of filgrastim or filgrastim-sndz results in a decrease in the ANC to less than 1000/mm^3, the drug should be reinitiated at a dosage of 5 mcg/kg once daily. If the ANC decreases to less than 1000/mm^3 at any time when the 5-mcg/kg daily dosage is being used, dosage should be increased to 10 mcg/kg once daily and the preceding steps repeated.

Peripheral Blood Progenitor Cell Transplantation **Filgrastim or Filgrastim-sndz.** When filgrastim or filgrastim-sndz is used to mobilize hematopoietic progenitor cells into peripheral blood for collection by leukapheresis, the recommended dosage is 10 mcg/kg once daily given by subcutaneous injection. The manufacturers recommend that filgrastim or filgrastim-sndz be administered for at least 4 days prior to the first leukapheresis to collect peripheral blood progenitor cells (PBPCs) and continued until the last leukapheresis is performed. The optimal duration of filgrastim or filgrastim-sndz administration and the optimal schedule for PBPC collection have not been established; however, in clinical studies, administration of filgrastim for 6–7 days with leukaphereses performed on days 5, 6, and 7 was found to be safe and effective. Neutrophil counts should be monitored after 4 days of filgrastim or filgrastim-sndz therapy and filgrastim or filgrastim-sndz should be discontinued if the leukocyte count increases to more than 100,000/mm^3.

In clinical studies in patients who received filgrastim for PBPC mobilization, the drug also was administered following reinfusion of the PBPC collection in a dosage of 5–24 mcg/kg daily until a sustainable ANC (500/mm^3 or greater) was attained.

Congenital, Cyclic, and Idiopathic Neutropenias **Filgrastim or Filgrastim-sndz.** Filgrastim or filgrastim-sndz therapy should be initiated in patients with severe chronic neutropenia only after a diagnosis of congenital, cyclic, or idiopathic neutropenia has been confirmed and other diseases associated with neutropenia have been excluded. For the treatment of congenital neutropenia, the manufacturers recommend an initial filgrastim or filgrastim-sndz dosage of 6 mcg/kg administered twice daily by subcutaneous injection. For the treatment of cyclic or idiopathic neutropenia, the manufacturers recommend an initial dosage of 5 mcg/kg administered once daily by subcutaneous injection. Dosage requirements generally are higher in patients with congenital neutropenia than in patients with cyclic neutropenia or idiopathic neutropenia.

Long-term daily administration of filgrastim or filgrastim-sndz is required to maintain clinical benefit. The manufacturers recommend that the patient's clinical course and ANC be used to evaluate efficacy of filgrastim or filgrastim-sndz therapy and adjust dosage of the drug. In a postmarketing surveillance study, the median daily dosage of filgrastim in patients with congenital neutropenia was 6 mcg/kg. In clinical studies in adults and children with congenital neutropenia, filgrastim dosages of 2–60 mcg/kg daily, individualized according to neutrophil count, have been administered by subcutaneous injection or by IV infusion over 30 minutes. Rarely, patients with congenital neutropenia have required filgrastim dosages of 100 mcg/kg daily or greater. In a postmarketing surveillance study, the median daily dosage of filgrastim in patients with cyclic or idiopathic neutropenia was 2.1 or 1.2 mcg/kg, respectively. In adults and children with cyclic neutropenia or idiopathic neutropenia, filgrastim dosages of 0.5–11.5 mcg/kg daily, individualized according to neutrophil response, have been given by subcutaneous injection or by IV infusion over 30 minutes. Filgrastim dosage in patients with severe chronic neutropenia should be reduced if the ANC is persistently greater than 10,000/mm^3.

Hematopoietic Syndrome of Acute Radiation Syndrome **Filgrastim.** When filgrastim is used to increase survival in patients acutely exposed to myelosuppressive doses of radiation, the recommended dosage is 10 mcg/kg once daily given by subcutaneous injection. Filgrastim therapy should be initiated as soon as possible after suspected or confirmed exposure to radiation doses exceeding 2 Gy. A patient's absorbed radiation dose (i.e., level of radiation exposure) should be estimated based upon information from public health authorities, biodosimetry, or clinical findings (e.g., time to onset of vomiting, lymphocyte depletion kinetics). Filgrastim therapy should be continued until the ANC remains greater than 1000/mm^3 for 3 consecutive CBCs or exceeds 10,000/mm^3 after a radiation-induced nadir. Administration of filgrastim should not be delayed if results of a CBC are not readily available.

Myelodysplastic Syndromes **Filgrastim.** When used to increase neutrophil counts in patients with myelodysplastic syndrome (MDS)†, filgrastim dosages of 0.3–10 mcg/kg have been given once daily by subcutaneous injection or dosages of 50–400 mcg/m^2 have been given once daily by IV infusion over 30 minutes; dosage was individualized according to response. However, safety and efficacy of filgrastim in the treatment of neutropenia associated with myelodysplastic disorders have not been established, and additional study is needed to evaluate more fully the role of filgrastim in patients with MDS and to determine optimum dosage ranges for the drug in these patients.

Neutropenia Associated with HIV Infection **Filgrastim.** If filgrastim is used in neutropenic individuals with human immunodeficiency virus (HIV) infection in an attempt to reduce the risk of bacterial infections†, some clinicians recommend that adults or adolescents receive a dosage of 5–10 mcg/kg given by subcutaneous injection once daily for 2–4 weeks.

Cautions

Filgrastim, filgrastim-sndz, and tbo-filgrastim generally are well tolerated, and only rarely have adverse effects been severe enough to require discontinuance of therapy. The most common and consistent adverse effect attributed to filgrastim, filgrastim-sndz, or tbo-filgrastim therapy in patients with cancer chemotherapy-induced neutropenia is bone pain.

In patients with chemotherapy-induced neutropenia receiving filgrastim therapy, the adverse effects reported with at least a 5% higher incidence compared with placebo include thrombocytopenia, nausea, pyrexia, chest pain, pain, fatigue, back pain, arthralgia, bone pain, dizziness, cough, dyspnea, rash, and increases in serum LDH and alkaline phosphatase. Patients who received filgrastim therapy following induction chemotherapy for acute myeloid leukemia (AML) reported at least a 2% higher incidence of epistaxis, back pain, pain in extremity, erythema, and maculopapular rash compared with placebo-treated patients. In patients who receive filgrastim following bone marrow transplantation (BMT), the most frequently reported adverse effects with at least a 5% higher incidence compared with patients receiving no filgrastim are rash and hypersensitivity. Adverse effects in patients receiving intensive chemotherapy followed by autologous BMT with at least a 5% higher incidence in filgrastim-treated patients compared with patients receiving no filgrastim include thrombocytopenia, anemia, hypertension, sepsis, bronchitis, and insomnia. Adverse effects reported most frequently in patients who receive filgrastim for mobilization of hematopoietic progenitor cells into peripheral blood include bone pain, pyrexia, headache, and an increase in serum alkaline phosphatase. In patients who have received filgrastim therapy for severe chronic neutropenia (congenital, cyclic, or idiopathic), adverse effects occurring with at least a 5% higher incidence compared with that in patients receiving no filgrastim include arthralgia, bone pain, back pain, muscle spasms, musculoskeletal pain, pain in extremity, splenomegaly, anemia, upper respiratory tract infection, urinary tract infection, epistaxis, chest pain, diarrhea, hypoesthesia, and alopecia.

Information on safety and efficacy of filgrastim generally has been obtained from clinical studies in patients with malignancy who received the drug following multiple-drug cytotoxic chemotherapy regimens; most adverse effects reported in these patients were those usually associated with the underlying malignancy or with the chemotherapy regimen the patient had been receiving. Adverse effects reported in at least a 2% higher incidence with filgrastim than with placebo that may be associated with the sequelae of the underlying malignancy or cytotoxic chemotherapy include anemia, constipation, diarrhea, oral pain, vomiting, asthenia, malaise, peripheral edema, decreased hemoglobin, decreased appetite, oropharyngeal pain, alopecia, and transfusion reactions. Because filgrastim is used in patients with serious underlying disease and because many adverse effects that have been reported in patients receiving the drug also occur in patients not receiving the drug, a causal relationship between filgrastim therapy and these adverse effects is not clear.

Based on demonstration of biosimilarity, FDA considers that no clinically meaningful differences in safety exist between filgrastim-sndz and filgrastim. Similar frequencies of adverse effects have been observed for filgrastim-sndz and filgrastim.

Safety of tbo-filgrastim is based principally on data from 3 randomized clinical trials in patients receiving myeloablative chemotherapy for breast cancer, lung cancer, or non-Hodgkin's lymphoma; the most frequent treatment-related adverse effect observed in these patients was bone pain, which occurred at an overall incidence of about 3.4% in the first treatment cycle.

■ **Effects on the Spleen** ***Splenic Rupture*** Splenic rupture, including some fatalities, has been reported following administration of filgrastim products.

No cases of splenic rupture were reported in clinical trials of tbo-filgrastim. (See Precautions and Contraindications.)

Splenomegaly Splenomegaly has been reported occasionally in patients receiving filgrastim, principally in those with congenital or cyclic neutropenia who had received long-term therapy with the drug. Results of magnetic resonance imaging (MRI) in some of these patients indicated that spleen sizes during filgrastim therapy were 17–95% larger than pretreatment sizes. Increases in spleen size were not associated with clinical manifestations in most patients and partially resolved in some patients during continued therapy with the drug.

■ **Respiratory Effects** Acute respiratory distress syndrome (ARDS) has been reported in patients receiving filgrastim products. Although no cases of ARDS have been reported to date with tbo-filgrastim, the possibility that such a risk could occur should be considered.

Alveolar hemorrhage, manifesting as pulmonary infiltrates and hemoptysis, has been reported following administration of filgrastim products for peripheral blood progenitor cell (PBPC) mobilization in healthy donors (currently not an FDA-labeled indication for filgrastim or filgrastim-sndz). Hemoptysis resolved in these individuals upon discontinuance of therapy.

■ **Sickle Cell Disease** Sickle cell crisis, sometimes fatal, has been reported in patients with sickle cell trait or sickle cell disease receiving filgrastim products. Although no cases of sickle cell crisis have been identified with tbo-filgrastim to date, patients included in the principal clinical studies of the drug were not screened for sickle cell disease; therefore, the effect of tbo-filgrastim in patients with sickle cell disease could not be assessed.

■ **Glomerulonephritis** Glomerulonephritis has been reported in patients receiving filgrastim products. The diagnosis of glomerulonephritis in these cases has been based upon azotemia, hematuria, proteinuria, and renal biopsy. Glomerulonephritis generally resolved after dose reduction or discontinuance of filgrastim. In patients receiving filgrastim or filgrastim-sndz in whom glomerulonephritis is suspected, dosage reduction or interruption of therapy should be considered.

■ **Capillary Leak Syndrome** Capillary leak syndrome has been reported after administration of granulocyte colony-stimulating factor (G-CSF), including with filgrastim products, and is characterized by hypotension, hypoalbuminemia, edema, and hemoconcentration. Episodes vary in frequency and severity, and may be life-threatening if treatment is delayed. Patients who develop symptoms of capillary leak syndrome should be closely monitored and receive standard symptomatic treatment, which may also include a need for intensive care.

■ **Musculoskeletal Effects** In some phase 2 and 3 trials in patients with cancer chemotherapy-induced neutropenia, medullary bone pain was reported in 24% of patients overall receiving filgrastim. This adverse effect appears to be dependent on the dose and/or route of administration, occurring in about 40% of those receiving IV filgrastim dosages of 20–100 mcg/kg daily and less frequently (e.g., in 22% of patients) in those receiving lower dosages subcutaneously (3–10 mcg/kg daily). The bone pain variously has been characterized as pulsating deep pain; pressure in the lower back, ribs, pelvis, or sternum; or mild, nonspecific aches. In most reported cases, bone pain appeared to occur at sites containing bone marrow (e.g., sternum, spine, pelvis, long bone) in the 2- to 3-day period preceding the increase in peripheral neutrophil count and to be particularly severe in patients with marked leukocytosis. In clinical trials evaluating patients with malignancy undergoing mobilization of autologous PBPCs with filgrastim for collection by leukapheresis, musculoskeletal and connective tissue disorders occurred in approximately 30% of patients. Arthralgia, bone pain, back pain, musculoskeletal pain, pain in extremity, and muscle spasms were also reported in patients receiving daily filgrastim for severe chronic neutropenia.

Filgrastim-induced bone pain usually is mild to moderate in severity and usually can be effectively prevented or treated with nonopiate oral analgesics (e.g., acetaminophen). However, bone pain occasionally may be severe enough to require use of opiate analgesics and rarely may require discontinuance of filgrastim. Bone pain generally resolves spontaneously with continued filgrastim therapy or disappears shortly after filgrastim therapy is completed.

■ **GI Effects** Adverse GI effects, including nausea, vomiting, and abdominal pain, have been reported in patients receiving filgrastim; however, it is unclear whether these effects were caused by the drug. In 3 randomized, double-blind, placebo-controlled studies in adults with small cell lung carcinoma or non-Hodgkin's lymphoma and cancer chemotherapy-induced neutropenia, nausea occurred in 43% of patients receiving filgrastim and 32% of patients receiving placebo. The incidence of constipation, diarrhea, oral pain, vomiting, decreased appetite, and oropharyngeal pain was higher in patients treated with filgrastim compared with placebo; however, these effects may be attributable to the sequelae of underlying malignancy or cytotoxic chemotherapy. A causal relationship with the drug has not been established.

■ **Dermatologic and Sensitivity Reactions** Transient, generalized rash has been reported occasionally in patients receiving filgrastim. In controlled clinical studies in adults with small cell lung carcinoma or non-Hodgkin's lymphoma and cancer chemotherapy-induced neutropenia, rash was reported in 14% of patients receiving the drug and 5% of patients receiving placebo. In BMT patients, the incidence of rash and hypersensitivity was higher in patients receiving filgrastim compared with placebo. In a controlled clinical study in adults with AML and chemotherapy-induced neutropenia, erythema and maculopapular rash were reported more frequently in patients who received filgrastim compared with placebo. Although a causal relationship is unclear, generalized pruritus and exacerbation (e.g., bullous pyoderma gangrenosum) of preexisting eczema or preexisting psoriasis have been reported rarely in patients with chemotherapy-induced neutropenia receiving filgrastim and may require discontinuance of the drug.

Cutaneous vasculitis, which may be indicated by purpura or erythema, has been reported in patients receiving filgrastim products, and leukocytoclastic vasculitis of the lower extremities has been reported in at least 2 patients receiving the drug. Cutaneous vasculitis has been reported most frequently in patients with severe chronic neutropenia receiving long-term filgrastim therapy and generally has been described as moderate or severe in intensity. Filgrastim or filgrastim-sndz should be withheld in patients who develop cutaneous vasculitis and may be restarted at a reduced dosage when symptoms resolve and the absolute neutrophil count (ANC) has decreased. Acute neutrophilic dermatosis (Sweet's syndrome) occurred during filgrastim therapy in a patient with hairy cell leukemia who had preexisting cutaneous vasculitis and also occurred during therapy with the drug in another patient who had been receiving chemotherapy for breast cancer. In several of these cases, adverse cutaneous effects appeared to be related to high neutrophil counts and resultant infiltration at sites of vascular inflammation that occurred as a result of filgrastim therapy. It has been suggested that patients receiving filgrastim be monitored for adverse cutaneous effects and that the drug be used with caution in patients with preexisting autoimmune or inflammatory dermatologic conditions.

Serious allergic reactions, including anaphylaxis, have been reported in patients receiving filgrastim products. Most reported events have occurred following initial exposure. Symptomatic treatment should be provided to patients who have an allergic reaction; these reactions can recur within days after discontinuance of initial antiallergy therapy. These reactions may include rash, facial edema, wheezing, dyspnea, hypotension, and tachycardia. The administration of antihistamines, corticosteroids, bronchodilators, and/or epinephrine may reduce the severity of these reactions. Filgrastim, filgrastim-sndz, or tbo-filgrastim therapy should be permanently discontinued in patients who develop serious allergic reactions. In at least 2 patients, anaphylactoid reactions appeared to be temporally related to filgrastim administration, but the patients were receiving numerous other drugs concomitantly and it is unclear whether filgrastim was the causative agent of the reaction.

Allergic reactions also have been reported in patients receiving tbo-filgrastim; in clinical trials, at least 1 patient experienced a bronchospastic allergic reaction during the first cycle of chemotherapy, which was observed after the tenth dose of tbo-filgrastim.

The needle covers of prefilled syringes of filgrastim and filgrastim-sndz contain natural latex proteins in the form of dry natural rubber (latex). Some individuals may be hypersensitive to natural latex proteins found in a wide range of medical devices, including such packaging components, and the level of sensitivity may vary depending on the form of natural rubber present; rarely, hypersensitivity reactions to natural latex proteins have been fatal.

■ **Local Reactions** Subcutaneous injection or infusion of filgrastim may result in minor bruising, inflammation, or bleeding, and continuous IV infusion may result in inflammation at the site of administration. If adverse local effects occur, they generally persist for less than 2 days. To minimize adverse local reactions, the site of administration of filgrastim should be changed frequently.

■ **Hematologic and Cytogenetic Effects** Marked leukocytosis (leukocyte counts of 100,000/mm³ or greater) has been reported occasionally in cancer patients receiving filgrastim or tbo-filgrastim. Leukocytosis was observed in approximately 2% of patients with cancer chemotherapy-induced neutropenia receiving filgrastim dosages exceeding 5 mcg/kg daily and appeared to be dose and/or route dependent. In clinical studies, leukocytosis was reported in less than 1% of patients with nonmyeloid malignancies receiving tbo-filgrastim. Although the degree of leukocytosis observed in these patients has not been associated with clinically important adverse effects other than bone pain, the manufacturers of filgrastim and filgrastim-sndz recommend that leukocyte counts be monitored to avoid any potential complications of excessive leukocytosis. Dosages of filgrastim or filgrastim-sndz that increase the ANC beyond 10,000/mm³ may not result in any additional clinical benefit.

A decrease in hemoglobin was observed in patients with malignancy who received myelosuppressive chemotherapy followed by filgrastim treatment; however, this effect may be associated with the sequelae of the underlying malignancy or cytotoxic chemotherapy treatment. The incidence of epistaxis was higher in patients with AML and severe chronic neutropenia receiving filgrastim therapy compared with patients who received no filgrastim. Thrombocytopenia has been reported in patients receiving filgrastim, principally in those receiving high dosages (e.g., greater than 10 mcg/kg) of the drug. In some patients, thrombocytopenia was severe enough to require administration of platelets. In patients with malignancy receiving myelosuppressive chemotherapy, thrombocytopenia occurred in 38% of patients who received filgrastim therapy compared with 29% of those who received placebo. Patients receiving intensive chemotherapy followed by autologous BMT who received filgrastim therapy had at least a 5% higher incidence of thrombocytopenia compared with patients who received no filgrastim. Platelet counts should be closely monitored in patients receiving filgrastim or filgrastim-sndz, and such patients should be advised to report unusual bleeding or bruising to their clinician.

Although anemia has been reported in some patients with chemotherapy-induced neutropenia receiving filgrastim, a causal relationship to the drug has not been established, and the anemia may have been an adverse effect of the chemotherapy regimens the patients were receiving. Anemia has been reported in at least a 5% higher incidence in filgrastim-treated patients with malignancy receiving myelosuppressive chemotherapy, those with severe chronic neutropenia, or those undergoing BMT compared with patients receiving placebo.

Cytogenetic abnormalities, myelodysplastic syndrome (MDS), and AML have been reported in patients, including children, receiving filgrastim products for severe chronic neutropenia. The risk of developing MDS or AML appears to be limited to patients with congenital neutropenia. The effect of filgrastim products on the development of cytogenetic abnormalities and the effect of continued therapy with the drug in patients with such abnormalities is unknown. Because AML and cytogenetic abnormalities have been reported in patients with severe chronic neutropenia who have not received filgrastim therapy, it is unclear whether these effects are related to chronic daily filgrastim therapy or the natural history of severe chronic neutropenia. Myelodysplasia and progression to acute myelomonocytic leukemia also have occurred in several children with aplastic anemia within 6–15 months of initiation of filgrastim therapy and acute myeloblastic leukemia developed in a patient with Hodgkin's disease within 6 weeks after initiation of filgrastim therapy.

■ **Effects on Uric Acid and Serum Enzyme Concentrations** Mild to moderate increases in serum concentrations of uric acid, LDH, alkaline phosphatase, and leukocyte alkaline phosphatase (LAP) have been reported in patients receiving filgrastim following cytotoxic cancer chemotherapy. These increases were transient and appeared to correspond to the therapeutic response to filgrastim and the resultant increase in neutrophil count and increase in cell turnover. An increase in serum concentrations of alkaline phosphatase also has occurred in patients with malignancy undergoing autologous PBPC collection who are receiving filgrastim.

Concentrations of LAP increase as peripheral neutrophil counts increase, and LAP concentrations in patients receiving filgrastim may be 10 or more times higher than baseline values. In one study, LAP concentrations averaged 6 units prior to initiation of filgrastim therapy and 190 units during the period of therapeutic response to the drug. Because only mature polymorphonuclear cells and bands have moderate levels of LAP, increases in serum LAP probably result from production of functionally mature cells; however, it is unclear whether filgrastim might also directly induce production of this enzyme.

■ **Immunogenicity** As with all therapeutic proteins, there is a potential for immunogenicity with filgrastim, filgrastim-sndz, or tbo-filgrastim therapy; however, the incidence of antibody development in patients receiving these drugs has not been adequately determined. Available data suggest that a small proportion of patients receiving filgrastim develop binding antibodies to filgrastim. The nature and specificity of these antibodies have not been adequately studied. In clinical studies, anti-filgrastim antibodies were detected in approximately 3% of patients receiving filgrastim; none of these antibodies were neutralizing. Cytopenias resulting from an antibody response to exogenous growth factors have rarely been reported in patients treated with other recombinant growth factors.

No clinically meaningful differences have been found between filgrastim-sndz and filgrastim with respect to antidrug antibody response resulting from administration of these drugs.

Although binding or neutralizing antibodies to tbo-filgrastim did not appear to develop during treatment in the principal efficacy study of the drug, the antibody assays used were not considered to be reliable; therefore, further study is needed to determine the immunogenicity potential of tbo-filgrastim.

■ **Other Adverse Effects** In BMT patients receiving filgrastim, hypertension and insomnia have also been reported. Although a flu-like syndrome has been reported occasionally in patients receiving another CSF (sargramostim, a recombinant granulocyte-macrophage CSF [GM-CSF]), this syndrome has not been reported to date in patients receiving filgrastim.

A single case of angina pectoris occurring in a patient receiving a high-dose combination of filgrastim and cancer chemotherapy as a preparatory regimen for autologous peripheral blood stem-cell transplant has been reported.

In controlled clinical studies in patients with malignancy and chemotherapy-induced neutropenia, the incidence of alopecia was at least 5% higher in patients receiving filgrastim therapy compared with those receiving placebo. In these studies fever, fatigue, dyspnea, cough, chest pain, and unspecified pain occurred in 12–48% of patients receiving filgrastim and 6–29% of patients receiving placebo. In some patients, fatigue, diaphoresis, and other subjective complaints of discomfort were associated with marked leukocytosis.

■ **Precautions and Contraindications** Complete blood cell counts (CBCs), including platelet counts, should be performed prior to initiation of filgrastim, filgrastim-sndz, or tbo-filgrastim therapy and routinely during therapy to monitor myeloid recovery and avoid the potential complications of excessive leukocytosis and/or thrombocytopenia. (See Cautions: Hematologic and Cytogenic Effects.) The manufacturers recommend that these hematologic tests be performed prior to cancer chemotherapy and twice weekly in patients receiving filgrastim, filgrastim-sndz, or tbo-filgrastim for management of chemotherapy-induced neutropenia. CBC and platelet count should be monitored frequently in patients receiving filgrastim or filgrastim-sndz following bone marrow transplantation. In patients with severe chronic neutropenia receiving filgrastim, CBCs with differential and platelet counts should be monitored during the initial 4 weeks of therapy as well as during the first 2 weeks following any dosage adjustment; once the patient is clinically stable, hematologic monitoring may be performed on a monthly basis during the first year of treatment, then less frequent routine monitoring is recommended. In patients acutely exposed to myelosuppressive doses of radiation (hematopoietic syndrome of acute radiation syndrome) receiving filgrastim, a CBC should be obtained at baseline and then every third day until the ANC remains greater than 1000/mm³ for 3 consecutive days. Filgrastim therapy results in a shift to the left (toward progenitor cells) in leukocyte differentials; promyelocytes and myeloblasts may be present on the differentials. When filgrastim is used in patients with chemotherapy-induced neutropenia, the ANC nadir occurs sooner, the duration of severe neutropenia is decreased, and there is accelerated recovery of neutrophil counts compared with patients not receiving the drug. Regular monitoring of leukocyte counts is recommended during filgrastim therapy to avoid excessive leukocytosis. It is recommended that filgrastim be discontinued if the ANC exceeds 10,000/mm³ after the ANC nadir has occurred; dosages that increase the ANC to such levels may not result in any additional clinical benefit but might be associated with an increased risk of toxicity (e.g., bone pain).

Because splenic rupture has been reported in individuals receiving filgrastim products, patients receiving filgrastim, filgrastim-sndz, or tbo-filgrastim who experience left upper abdominal and/or shoulder tip pain should be evaluated for the presence of splenomegaly or splenic rupture. In addition, the manufacturer of tbo-filgrastim states that the drug should be discontinued if these symptoms occur.

ARDS has been reported in patients receiving filgrastim products. Patients receiving filgrastim, filgrastim-sndz, or tbo-filgrastim who develop fever, lung infiltrates, or respiratory distress should be evaluated for the presence of ARDS. If ARDS occurs during filgrastim, filgrastim-sndz, or tbo-filgrastim therapy, the manufacturers state that the drug should be discontinued.

Sickle cell crisis has been reported in patients with sickle cell trait or sickle cell disease receiving filgrastim products. Prior to administering filgrastim, filgrastim-sndz, or tbo-filgrastim in patients with sickle cell disease, the potential risks and benefits of therapy should be considered. The manufacturer of tbo-filgrastim states that the drug should be discontinued in patients who experience a sickle cell crisis.

Although filgrastim, filgrastim-sndz, and tbo-filgrastim are growth factors that principally affect the proliferation and differentiation of neutrophils, the possibility that the drugs could act as growth factors for any tumor type cannot be excluded. Because some malignant myeloid cells have receptors for G-CSF (see Pharmacology) and because the clinical importance of these receptors has not been determined, extreme caution regarding the use of filgrastim in patients with any malignancy having myeloid characteristics (e.g., AML) had been recommended by the manufacturer and some experts in the past; however, the drug currently is used in patients with AML receiving induction or consolidation chemotherapy without evidence of a negative effect on the disease (e.g., proliferation of the leukemic clone). In a randomized study evaluating the effects of filgrastim versus placebo in patients undergoing remission induction for AML, there was no difference in remission rate and overall survival (See Uses: Leukemias). The manufacturers state that the safety of filgrastim products in chronic myeloid leukemia (CML) or MDS has not been established. Tbo-filgrastim is not FDA-labeled for use in patients with myeloid malignancies or myelodysplasia.

Patients with severe chronic neutropenia have developed cytogenetic abnormalities, transformation to MDS, and AML during therapy with filgrastim products. Abnormal cytogenetics and MDS have been associated with the development of myeloid leukemia. Because the effect of filgrastim products on the development of abnormal cytogenetics and the effect of continued therapy in patients with abnormal cytogenetics or MDS are unknown, the risks and benefits of continuing filgrastim therapy should be carefully considered if a patient with severe chronic neutropenia develops abnormal cytogenetics or myelodysplasia during filgrastim therapy. Routine CBC monitoring is recommended in all patients with severe chronic neutropenia receiving filgrastim therapy. Therapy with filgrastim or filgrastim-sndz should be initiated in patients with severe chronic neutropenia only after a diagnosis of congenital, cyclic, or idiopathic neutropenia has been confirmed and other diseases associated with neutropenia have been excluded. Safety and efficacy of filgrastim, filgrastim-sndz, and tbo-filgrastim in the treatment of neutropenia caused by other hematopoietic disorders (e.g., MDS) have not been established.

Although solid tumor progression has not been reported to date in patients receiving filgrastim, the drug's effect on tumor growth has not been directly assessed in clinical trials and requires further study. The fact that therapy-stimulated tumor progression is difficult to distinguish from the natural history of tumors should be kept in mind during filgrastim therapy.

When filgrastim or filgrastim-sndz is used for mobilization of hematopoietic progenitor cells, tumor cells may be released from the marrow and subsequently collected in the leukapheresis product. The effect of reinfusion of tumor cells has not been well studied and the limited data available to date are inconclusive.

Safety and efficacy of filgrastim or filgrastim-sndz doses administered concomitantly with radiation therapy or concomitantly with doses of cytotoxic chemotherapy have not been established. Because rapidly dividing myeloid cells may be particularly sensitive to cytotoxic chemotherapy, filgrastim, filgrastim-sndz, or tbo-filgrastim should not be administered during the 24 hours before or after administration of cytotoxic chemotherapy. (See Drug Interactions: Antineoplastic Agents.) Filgrastim and filgrastim-sndz should not be administered concomitantly with radiation therapy.

Serious allergic reactions, including anaphylaxis, can occur with filgrastim, filgrastim-sndz, or tbo-filgrastim therapy. If any manifestations of serious hypersensitivity (e.g., whole body rash, swelling, dizziness, dyspnea, tachycardia) occur with filgrastim, filgrastim-sndz, or tbo-filgrastim therapy, the drug should be permanently discontinued. Administration of antihistamines, corticosteroids, bronchodilators, and/or epinephrine may reduce the severity of reactions. Filgrastim and filgrastim-sndz are contraindicated in patients with a history of serious allergic reactions to human G-CSF such as filgrastim or pegfilgrastim products. Tbo-filgrastim should not be used in any patient with a history of serious allergic reactions to filgrastim or pegfilgrastim.

■ **Pediatric Precautions** Filgrastim has been used in children and adolescents without unusual adverse effects. The pharmacokinetics of filgrastim in pediatric patients after cancer chemotherapy are similar to those in adults receiving the same weight-normalized doses, suggesting no age-related differences in pharmacokinetics of filgrastim products. The use of filgrastim to increase survival in pediatric patients acutely exposed to myelosuppressive doses of radiation is based on studies conducted in animals and clinical data supporting the use filgrastim in other FDA-labeled indications.

Cytogenetic abnormalities and transformation to MDS and AML have occurred during filgrastim therapy in pediatric patients with congenital types of neutropenia (Kostmann's syndrome, congenital agranulocytosis, Schwachman-Diamond syndrome). The relationship between these events and filgrastim therapy is unknown.

Filgrastim dosages of 5–15 mcg/kg daily have been used in children with advanced-stage neuroblastoma without unusual adverse effects and a dosage of 5 mcg/kg daily also has been well tolerated in children 7 months to 15 years of age with various other malignancies (e.g., acute lymphocytic leukemia, Wilms' tumor, lymphoma, rhabdomyosarcoma, CNS tumor). Follow-up from a postmarketing surveillance study indicates that long-term therapy with filgrastim (i.e., up to 5 years) does not result in alterations in height and weight. Based on limited data from children with severe chronic neutropenia who were followed for 1.5 years, there is no evidence that filgrastim therapy results in alterations in sexual maturation or endocrine function. When filgrastim was given to children 1–17 years of age with aplastic anemia in dosages of 400 mcg/m^2 daily by IV infusion, the only adverse effect reported was a mild increase in serum alkaline phosphatase concentration. There has been at least one report of palpable splenomegaly and hepatosplenomegaly in pediatric patients receiving filgrastim. Decreased bone density and osteoporosis have been reported in pediatric patients receiving chronic treatment with filgrastim products.

The use of filgrastim-sndz in pediatric patients has been extrapolated from pediatric data and information from the reference biological, filgrastim (Neupogen®). Filgrastim-sndz prefilled syringes may not accurately measure volumes less than 0.3 mL; due to the potential for dosing errors, direct administration of a volume of filgrastim-sndz less than 0.3 mL is not recommended.

The manufacturer states that safety and efficacy of tbo-filgrastim have not been established in pediatric patients younger than 18 years of age.

■ **Geriatric Precautions** Safety and efficacy profiles in geriatric individuals are similar to those in younger adults receiving filgrastim or tbo-filgrastim following myelosuppressive cancer chemotherapy. Clinical studies of filgrastim for other indications (e.g., bone marrow transplantation, PBPC mobilization, severe chronic neutropenia) did not include a sufficient number of individuals 65 years of age or older to determine whether geriatric patients respond differently to the drug than younger adults.

■ **Mutagenicity and Carcinogenicity** Filgrastim was not mutagenic in studies performed with or without metabolic activation. The drug can stimulate proliferation of leukemic progenitor cells and induce differentiation of some leukemic cells in vitro. Filgrastim also can stimulate the growth of clonogenic cells of certain malignant cell lines in vitro (e.g., human myeloid leukemia, colon adenocarcinoma, small cell lung cancer). Therefore, while the carcinogenic potential of filgrastim has not been elucidated to date, the possibility that filgrastim could stimulate the growth of any tumor type cannot be excluded. (See Cautions: Precautions and Contraindications.)

Studies to determine the carcinogenic or mutagenic potential of tbo-filgrastim have not been conducted to date; however, similar to filgrastim, there is a possibility that tbo-filgrastim may act as a growth factor for any tumor type.

■ **Pregnancy, Fertility, and Lactation** Although there are no adequate and controlled studies to date in humans, both filgrastim and tbo-filgrastim have been shown to cause adverse embryofetal effects in animals. These drugs should be used during pregnancy only when the potential benefits justify the possible risks to the fetus. Women who become pregnant during filgrastim therapy should be encouraged to enroll in the manufacturers' Pregnancy Surveillance Program by calling 1-800-77-AMGEN (1-800-772-6436).

Adverse effects were observed in pregnant rabbits receiving filgrastim dosages 2–10 times the usual human dosage. In pregnant rabbits showing signs of maternal toxicity, reduced embryofetal survival (at 20 and 80 mcg/kg daily) and increased abortions (at 80 mcg/kg daily) were observed. While there was no evidence of maternal or fetal effects in pregnant rats receiving filgrastim dosages of 575 mcg/kg daily in some reproduction studies, a delay in external differentiation (detachment of auricles and descent of testes) and slight growth retardation were observed in offspring of pregnant rats receiving at least 20 mcg/kg daily in other studies; a slightly decreased rate of survival was observed in offspring of pregnant rats receiving 100 mcg/kg daily.

Adverse embryofetal findings observed in pregnant rabbits exposed to tbo-filgrastim included increased spontaneous abortions, post-implantation loss, decreased litter size and fetal weight, and fetal malformations (e.g., malformed hindlimbs and cleft palate); such effects were observed at dosages (100 mcg/kg daily) corresponding to systemic exposures of approximately 50–90 times the exposure in patients treated with the usual clinical dosage (5 mcg/kg daily).

Reproduction studies in male or female rats have not revealed evidence of impaired fertility in males or females at filgrastim doses up to 500 mcg/kg.

It is not known whether filgrastim, filgrastim-sndz, or tbo-filgrastim is distributed into milk. Because many drugs are distributed into milk, filgrastim, filgrastim-sndz, and tbo-filgrastim should be used with caution in nursing women. Women who breastfeed while receiving filgrastim are encouraged to enroll in Amgen's Lactation Surveillance Program by calling 1-800-77-AMGEN (1-800-772-6436).

Drug Interactions

■ **Antineoplastic Agents** The safety and efficacy of concomitant administration of doses of filgrastim with doses of myelosuppressive antineoplastic agents have not been established. Because filgrastim stimulates proliferation of neutrophil precursors and because many antineoplastic agents target rapidly proliferating cells, filgrastim, filgrastim-sndz, or tbo-filgrastim should not be administered within 24 hours before or after a dose of one of these agents. When filgrastim is administered following myelosuppressive cancer chemotherapy, most reported adverse effects are similar to those usually reported following the chemotherapy regimen alone. However, because filgrastim therapy may allow use of higher doses of some antineoplastic agents or decreased intervals between chemotherapy cycles, patients receiving filgrastim therapy may receive higher cumulative dosages of the antineoplastic agents than patients not receiving the drug and may be at increased risk for thrombocytopenia, anemia, or nonhematologic adverse effects associated with the chemotherapy regimen.

The manufacturer of filgrastim states that efficacy of the drug has not been evaluated to date in patients receiving antineoplastic therapy associated with delayed myelosuppression (e.g., nitrosourea derivatives) or in those receiving mitomycin or myelosuppressive doses of antimetabolites (e.g., cytarabine, fluorouracil); however, studies are ongoing.

■ **Other Drugs** The manufacturer of tbo-filgrastim states that drugs that may potentiate the myeloproliferative effects (e.g., potentiation of neutrophil release) (e.g., lithium) should be used with caution in patients receiving tbo-filgrastim.

Specific drug interaction studies have not been performed to date with filgrastim, filgrastim-sndz, or tbo-filgrastim. The manufacturer states that filgrastim has been administered concurrently with various other drugs (e.g., anti-infective agents, benzodiazepines, zidovudine, epoetin alfa, analgesics) without evidence of clinically important drug interactions.

Laboratory Test Interferences

Increased hematopoietic activity of the bone marrow has been associated with transient positive bone-imaging changes. The possibility of such interference should be considered when interpreting results of bone-imaging tests in patients receiving filgrastim, filgrastim-sndz, or tbo-filgrastim.

Acute Toxicity

Limited information is available on the acute toxicity of filgrastim in humans. Overdosage of the drug would be expected to produce manifestations that are principally extensions of the pharmacologic and common adverse effects of the drug. The maximum tolerated dosage of filgrastim products in humans has not been determined. Some patients have received filgrastim dosages of up to 115–138 mcg/kg daily without clinically important toxic effects; however, the usually recommended dosage of the drug is considerably lower. (See Dosage and Administration: Dosage.)

Pharmacology

Filgrastim, filgrastim-sndz, and tbo-filgrastim are hematopoietic agents that principally influence leukopoiesis. The drugs appear to elicit the same pharmacologic effects produced by endogenous human granulocyte colony-stimulating factor (G-CSF). Endogenous G-CSF, a growth factor, is a lineage-restricted CSF that principally affects the proliferation, differentiation, and activation of committed progenitor cells of the neutrophil-granulocyte lineage. In addition, endogenous G-CSF enhances certain functions of mature neutrophils, including phagocytosis, chemotaxis, and antibody-dependent cellular cytotoxicity (ADCC). Despite extensive data concerning the effects of CSFs on myeloid progenitor and mature cells in vitro and concerning in vivo effects in animals and in healthy individuals and patients, the physiologic roles of CSFs are complex and have not been fully elucidated.

In healthy adults, circulating levels of endogenous G-CSF generally are less than 100 pg/mL and, in most individuals, are below the limits of detection of currently used immunoassays. Endogenous G-CSF may be increased to detectable levels in patients with bacterial infections or certain disease states and in patients under stress conditions (e.g., following cytotoxic cancer chemotherapy), but the stimulus for such increases is not necessarily dependent on baseline leukocyte counts. In a study that used an enzyme-linked immunosorbent assay (ELISA) capable of detecting human G-CSF levels as low as 50 pg/mL, all 10 healthy adults 24–44 years of age had undetectable serum concentrations of endogenous G-CSF and patients with acute myeloid leukemia, acute lymphocytic leukemia, or undifferentiated leukemia had serum concentrations that ranged from 50–3000 pg/mL. In patients with cytotoxic chemotherapy-induced neutropenia, endogenous levels of G-CSF reportedly are highest during the neutrophil nadir and decrease as the neutrophil count increases. In patients with infection, endogenous levels of G-CSF reportedly are highest during the acute phase of the infection.

Endogenous human G-CSF is produced by monocytes, fibroblasts, and endothelial cells and, although further study is needed to support the hypothesis, it has been suggested that both intrinsic and extrinsic pathways control secretion of human G-CSF from these cells. The intrinsic control may involve a feedback system that regulates G-CSF levels based on the level of circulating neutrophils; the extrinsic control may function in response to infection and inflammation with certain mediators (e.g., endotoxin, tumor necrosis factor) directly stimulating producer cells to secrete G-CSF.

Like endogenous G-CSF, filgrastim, filgrastim-sndz, and tbo-filgrastim appear to act directly on neutrophil progenitor target cells (granulocyte colony-forming units [CFU-G]) by binding to G-CSF receptors on their cell surfaces. How this binding to receptors results in the various intracellular events necessary to affect proliferation, differentiation, and cell function has not been fully elucidated to date. Results of studies using murine hematopoietic cells indicate that G-CSF receptors are present on all cells of the neutrophil-granulocyte lineage, including myeloblasts and mature neutrophils, but such receptors are absent from eosinophils and lymphocytes. The number of receptors per cell increases with the degree of maturation of the cell; mature neutrophils have 2–3 times more receptors than band forms or metamyelocytes. Certain monocytic cells appear to possess small numbers of G-CSF receptors; such receptors are absent from cells in the erythroid and megakaryocytic lineages. Although the clinical importance is unclear, G-CSF receptors also have been found on certain leukemic cell lines (including some human myeloid leukemia cells), cell lines derived from human small cell carcinoma, human placenta and trophoblastic cells, and human vascular endothelial cells.

■ **Effects on Neutrophil Maturation and Neutrophil Levels** Following subcutaneous or IV administration of filgrastim in patients with cancer chemotherapy-induced neutropenia, there is an initial (within 5–60 minutes) decrease in the absolute neutrophil count (ANC) to below baseline levels. Within 1–4 hours after administration, however, the neutrophil count begins to increase rapidly and generally exceeds baseline levels within 24 hours. The initial decrease in neutrophil count may occur because of margination of neutrophils to blood vessel walls, and the subsequent increase may occur as the result of demargination and mobilization of mature neutrophils from the bone marrow and/or other tissues. The increase in neutrophil count in response to filgrastim generally is dose dependent. Following discontinuance of the drug in patients with chemotherapy-induced neutropenia, a 50% decrease in the ANC generally occurs within 24 hours and the ANC returns to pretreatment levels within 1–7 days.

While proliferation appears to be stimulated by filgrastim in all stages of granulopoiesis, a substantial portion of the increased production appears to result from increased input of precursor cells into the myeloblast compartment. Other factors contributing to the neutrophilia induced by filgrastim include a substantial (e.g., ninefold) increase in neutrophil production rate, with several extra amplification divisions during neutrophil development, and a shortening (e.g., from the usual 4 or 5 days to 1 day) of the time required for neutrophil precursors to mature and appear in circulation. The life cycle of circulating neutrophils does not appear to be affected, nor does the frequency of progenitor cells per nucleated marrow cell appear to be increased, although biopsy evidence of increased cellularity suggests that the absolute number of progenitor cells in marrow may be increased.

In healthy individuals, the increase in ANC is sustained throughout the period of filgrastim administration, although transient decreases generally continue to be observed with each dose. In patients with chemotherapy-induced neutropenia, filgrastim reduces the duration and severity of neutropenia but generally does not eliminate the ANC nadir. In a study in patients with small cell lung cancer receiving myelosuppressive chemotherapy, the ANC nadir persisted for 10–15 days in patients not receiving filgrastim but for only 2–3 days in those receiving the drug. The increase in ANC results principally from an increase in mature segmented polymorphonuclear granulocytes, although there may be some increase in band forms, particularly at relatively high doses. Leukocyte differentials performed during filgrastim therapy usually demonstrate a shift to the left (toward progenitor cells), and promyelocytes and myeloblasts may be present, especially during neutrophil recovery following the chemotherapy-induced ANC nadir.

Filgrastim cannot increase neutrophil counts in the absence of progenitor target cells capable of responding to the drug, and the magnitude of the neutrophil response depends on the absolute numbers of target cells available. Patients who previously have received prolonged chemotherapy or excessive radiation generally are less responsive to filgrastim than those who have not received such treatment. Studies in patients with chemotherapy-induced neutropenia and patients with cyclic neutropenia or myelodysplastic syndromes receiving filgrastim indicate that the time to neutrophil response and the percentage of patients responding to the drug are not age dependent since geriatric patients (those 65 years of age or older) appear to respond the same as younger adults.

■ **Effects on Neutrophil Function** Results of in vitro studies evaluating the neutrophils produced in response to filgrastim therapy indicate that these cells have a normal survival time and function normally, at least in terms of phagocytic activity and chemotaxis. Neutrophils harvested from patients with various cancers (e.g., small cell lung carcinoma, transitional cell carcinoma of the urothelium) receiving filgrastim are at least as functionally active as those harvested from healthy individuals not receiving the drug. Although the clinical importance is unclear, morphologic changes in neutrophils have been reported during filgrastim therapy, including the appearance of Dohle bodies, toxic granulations, vacuolation, hypersegmentation, and decreased nuclear lobulation.

Results of in vitro studies indicate that filgrastim, like endogenous G-CSF, enhances certain end-cell functions of normal, mature neutrophils, including phagocytosis, chemotaxis, production of superoxide anions, priming of the cellular metabolism associated with respiratory burst, and antibody-dependent cellular cytotoxicity (ADCC). During bacterial infection, filgrastim-induced increases in neutrophil response at the site of infection are thought to improve host defenses by decreasing the bacterial burden, limiting bacterial proliferation, and reducing their dissemination from the original focus. The drug, unlike granulocyte-macrophage CSF (GM-CSF), appears to stimulate rather than inhibit neutrophil migration. Filgrastim also enhances chemotaxis of monocytes in vitro but not that of large lymphocytes or endothelial cells.

In vitro exposure of normal neutrophils to filgrastim results in a dose-dependent increase in ADCC against various target cells. In some studies, filgrastim appeared to enhance neutrophil ADCC toward cells inoculated with human immunodeficiency virus (HIV). In a study using MOLT-3A cells inoculated with HIV-1 (strain HTLV-IIIB), neutrophils obtained from both healthy individuals and patients with acquired immunodeficiency syndrome (AIDS) that were exposed to filgrastim had higher levels of neutrophil cytotoxicity toward the virus-infected cells than neutrophils not exposed to filgrastim.

■ **Effects on Other Cells** Although filgrastim principally affects neutrophils, results of some in vitro and in vivo studies indicate that the drug may have some effects on other leukocytes as well as other cells. In some patients, parenteral administration of filgrastim results in an initial, transient decrease in monocyte counts to below baseline levels similar to that seen with neutrophils.

In patients receiving low doses of filgrastim (e.g., 3 mcg/kg or less), monocyte counts return only to pretreatment levels. However, in some patients receiving higher doses of the drug (e.g., 10 mcg/kg or greater), lymphocyte and monocyte counts may increase beyond baseline values. Absolute monocyte counts may be up to 10 times higher than baseline levels in some patients receiving relatively high filgrastim doses (e.g., 60 mcg/kg); however, the percentage of monocytes in the leukocyte differential usually is within the normal range. Filgrastim does not appear to have any in vitro or in vivo effects on eosinophils or basophils; absolute eosinophil and basophil counts generally are unchanged during filgrastim therapy.

Although the clinical importance has not been determined, a transient dose-dependent decrease in platelet count has been reported in some patients receiving filgrastim. In these patients, platelets reached a nadir approximately 10 days after initiation of filgrastim therapy but returned to pretreatment levels despite continued therapy with the drug.

Results of in vitro studies indicate that erythroid precursors do not have G-CSF receptors and that filgrastim has no direct effect on these cells. However, a dose-dependent increase in erythroid precursors and/or erythrocytes occasionally has been observed in patients receiving filgrastim, and a decreased need for red blood cell transfusions has been reported in some patients with myelodysplastic syndrome receiving the drug. In addition, there is some evidence that filgrastim induces a shift in erythropoiesis from the marrow to the spleen. It has been suggested that filgrastim therapy may induce the production of another hematopoietic growth factor that causes these effects. Filgrastim does not appear to have any consistent effect on hemoglobin levels or hematocrit.

Although the clinical importance is unclear, results of in vitro studies using mouse leukemia and human promyelocytic leukemia cell lines indicate that filgrastim can stimulate proliferation of leukemic progenitor cells and induce differentiation of some leukemic cells.

Filgrastim reportedly may have an effect on the migration and proliferation of human endothelial cells; further study is needed to evaluate the validity and clinical importance, if any, of this reported effect. In one study, however, the drug did not affect migration of these cells.

Results of an in vitro study suggest that filgrastim does not stimulate the replication of HIV in vitro; however, there is some evidence that other hematologic growth factors (e.g., GM-CSF, macrophage-CSF, interleukin-3 [multicolony-stimulating factor; multi-CSF]) may stimulate replication of some strains of HIV in vitro. It has been suggested that the effects of these growth factors on HIV replication may vary depending on the cell culture system used for testing, and further study is needed to evaluate more fully the effects of filgrastim on HIV replication.

Other Effects At the maximum recommended IV dose of 5 mcg/kg, tbo-filgrastim was not shown to prolong the QT interval to any clinically relevant extent.

Pharmacokinetics

Filgrastim exhibits nonlinear pharmacokinetics. However, the contributions of endogenous granulocyte colony-stimulating factor (G-CSF) and remaining questions about the elimination characteristics of the drug complicate interpretation of pharmacokinetic data. Through the establishment of biosimilarity, filgrastim and filgrastim-sndz have been shown to exhibit equivalent dose-dependent pharmacokinetics.

■ **Absorption** Filgrastim is rapidly absorbed following subcutaneous injection, and peak serum concentrations of the drug generally are attained within 4–5 hours following rapid subcutaneous injection. Rapid subcutaneous injection of a single 3.45- or 11.5-mcg/kg dose of filgrastim results in peak serum concentrations averaging 4 or 49 ng/mL, respectively, within 2–8 hours; serum concentrations of the drug exceed 10 ng/mL for 8–16 hours after a single subcutaneous dose of 10 mcg/kg or more. G-CSF absorption has been described as a composite of zero-order and first-order processes. Most of the drug is absorbed through zero-order processes presumably through the lymphatic system. The absolute bioavailability of filgrastim after subcutaneous administration is 60–70%.

IV infusion of filgrastim over 30 minutes in single doses of 50, 100, 200, or 400 mcg/m^2 in adults with advanced pulmonary carcinoma or non-Hodgkin's lymphoma results in peak serum concentrations of 11.8, 25.8–55, 71.1–82, or 133.2–204 mcg/mL, respectively. Continuous IV infusion of 20 mcg/kg of filgrastim over 24 hours results in mean and median serum concentrations of approximately 48 and 56 ng/mL, respectively. The manufacturer states that there is no evidence of accumulation of filgrastim when daily dosages of 20 mcg/kg are given by continuous IV infusion for 11–20 days.

Following subcutaneous administration of tbo-filgrastim 5 mcg/kg in patients with cancer, the median time to peak plasma concentrations of the drug was approximately 4–6 hours; no evidence of accumulation was observed with repeated dosing. The absolute bioavailability of tbo-filgrastim following subcutaneous injection of a dose of 5 mcg/kg in healthy individuals is approximately 33%. The AUC and peak plasma concentrations of tbo-filgrastim were greater and more variable in patients with cancer compared with those in healthy individuals.

■ **Distribution** Filgrastim is rapidly distributed in animals, appearing in highest concentrations in bone marrow, adrenal glands, kidney, and liver. The volume of distribution of filgrastim following a single IV or subcutaneous dose reportedly averages 150 mL/kg (range: 46–384 mL/kg) in both healthy individuals and patients with cancer. It is not known whether filgrastim is distributed into cerebrospinal fluid. It also is not known whether filgrastim or filgrastim-sndz is distributed into milk in humans. There have been reports of transplacental passage of filgrastim products in pregnant women when administered within 30 hours of preterm delivery.

It is not known whether tbo-filgrastim distributes into milk in humans.

■ **Elimination** Filgrastim is eliminated by both renal elimination and specific degradation by G-CSF receptors and neutrophil elastase. Clearance is dependent on filgrastim concentration and neutrophil count; G-CSF receptor-mediated clearance is saturated by high concentrations of filgrastim and is diminished by neutropenia.

Studies using filgrastim or lenograstim (mammalian-derived recombinant G-CSF) indicate that the half-life of G-CSF shows considerable interindividual variation. It is unclear whether this occurs because of variations in clearance mechanisms or differences in the disease states of study patients. Some data indicate that serum filgrastim concentrations decline in a biphasic manner following single IV doses. In a limited number of adults with various malignancies, the distribution half-life of filgrastim has ranged from 0.13–1.1 hours and the terminal elimination half-life has ranged from 1.8–7.2 hours. It has been proposed that clearance is initially mediated by the binding of filgrastim to G-CSF receptors. When filgrastim binding sites become saturated, clearance of filgrastim decreases and elimination then occurs mostly via renal elimination. The manufacturer states that the elimination half-life of filgrastim following subcutaneous or IV administration averages 3.5 hours (range: 0.77–8.5 hours) in healthy individuals or patients with cancer and that the half-life of the drug following a single parenteral dose is comparable to that reported following IV doses of the drug given once daily for 2 weeks.

The median elimination half-life of tbo-filgrastim in patients with cancer receiving chemotherapy is 3.2–3.8 hours; in healthy individuals, median half-life of the drug was approximately 8.9 hours.

Chemistry and Stability

■ **Chemistry** Filgrastim, filgrastim-sndz, and tbo-filgrastim, human granulocyte colony-stimulating factors (G-CSF), are biosynthetic hematopoietic agents that principally affect the proliferation and differentiation of neutrophils within the bone marrow and possibly other sites (e.g., spleen). Filgrastim, filgrastim-sndz, and tbo-filgrastim are structurally and pharmacologically similar drugs that contain a related drug substance. The drugs are prepared using recombinant DNA technology and cultures of *Escherichia coli* that have been genetically modified to incorporate the human G-CSF gene. Endogenous human G-CSF is a glycoprotein hormone produced by monocytes, fibroblasts, and endothelial cells. (See Pharmacology.)

Filgrastim, filgrastim-sndz, and tbo-filgrastim are polypeptides containing 175 amino acids with molecular weights of 18,800 daltons. The molecular structure of filgrastim, filgrastim-sndz, and tbo-filgrastim consists of an amino acid sequence identical to that of endogenous human G-CSF, but differs from the endogenous glycoprotein by the addition of an *N*-terminal methionine and the absence of glycosylation. Because of these differences, these agents also have been referred to as recombinant methionyl human G-CSF (r-metHuG-CSF). The terminal methionine is necessary for expression of the G-CSF gene in *E. coli*. The physiologic and/or clinical relevance of glycosylation in biosynthetic CSFs is unclear and remains to be more fully elucidated. Glycosylation does not appear to be necessary for in vitro or in vivo activity since the absence of glycosylation does not affect binding of CSFs to receptors on target cells. Studies with other biosynthetic CSFs (e.g., granulocyte-macrophage CSF [GM-CSF]) suggest that the degree of glycosylation may affect pharmacokinetics, antigenicity, and adverse effects; however, the relevance of these findings to biosynthetic G-CSFs remains to be established. Filgrastim is prepared from a master seed lot of *E. coli* containing the gene for r-metHuG-CSF. The drug is purified from these cultures using conventional means and then allowed to oxidize to its native state; affinity chromatography is used in the final purification process.

Filgrastim is commercially available in single-use prefilled syringes and single-use vials. Commercially available filgrastim injection occurs as a clear, colorless, preservative-free solution. The injection is formulated in a sodium acetate buffer and contains mannitol and polysorbate (Tween®) 80. Filgrastim has an aqueous solubility of at least 10 mg/mL.

Filgrastim-sndz is commercially available in single-dose prefilled syringes; filgrastim-sndz is a clear, colorless to slightly yellowish, preservative-free solution.

Tbo-filgrastim is commercially available in single-use prefilled syringes; tbo-filgrastim injection is a clear, colorless, preservative-free solution.

Potency of filgrastim is determined using a cell mitogenesis assay and is expressed in terms of units per mg of protein. The commercially available injection has a specific activity of 1 ($\pm$ 0.6) $\times$ 10^8 units/mg of protein. When the cell mitogenesis assay is used, activity is defined in terms of the amount of filgrastim required for 50% of maximal incorporation of radiolabeled thymidine in mouse bone marrow cells. Alternatively, each 50 units of activity can be defined as the amount of filgrastim required for 50% of maximal stimulation of colony formation by normal bone marrow cells.

■ **Stability** Commercially available filgrastim or filgrastim-sndz injection should be refrigerated at 2–8°C and should not be frozen. Prior to administration, filgrastim or filgrastim-sndz should be removed from refrigeration and allowed to reach room temperature for approximately 30 minutes. Filgrastim may aggregate if frozen or if stored at temperatures exceeding 30°C. If filgrastim or filgrastim-sndz injection is inadvertently frozen, the drug should be thawed in the refrigerator prior to administration and drug that is frozen more than once should be discarded. In addition, shaking of filgrastim or filgrastim-sndz should be avoided. The transport of filgrastim via a pneumatic tube has not been studied. Filgrastim and filgrastim-sndz injections contain no preservatives. Filgrastim and filgrastim-sndz injections are stable for up to 24 hours at room temperature (provided the solution is clear, not cloudy, and contains no precipitate); however, the manufacturers state that any prefilled syringe or vial left at room temperature for longer than 24 hours should be discarded. Filgrastim may be stable for more prolonged periods at such temperatures, but the manufacturer should be consulted for specific stability information. When stored at 2–8°C, commercially available filgrastim injection has an expiration date of 2 years following the date of manufacture. Filgrastim injection should be stored in the original carton and protected from direct sunlight but does not need to be protected from normal room light. Filgrastim-sndz should also be stored in the original carton and protected from light.

Tbo-filgrastim injection should be stored in the refrigerator at 2–8°C and protected from light. Shaking of the injection should be avoided. The injection may be removed from the refrigerator and kept at room temperature (23–27°C) for a single period of up to 5 days; if not used within 5 days, the injection may be returned to the refrigerator until the expiration date. Stability studies have shown that exposure to temperatures of −1 to −5°C for up to 72 hours or −15 to −25°C for up to 24 hours does not adversely affect the stability of tbo-filgrastim. Tbo-filgrastim injection contains no preservatives; any unused portions of the prefilled syringes should be discarded after use.

Information on the physical and/or chemical compatibility of filgrastim with IV infusion equipment or solutions is limited. Commercially available filgrastim injection is stable over the pH range of 3.8–4.2; the drug is stable at neutral pH for only a very limited time period. The manufacturers state that, if required, filgrastim or filgrastim-sndz injection may be diluted with 5% dextrose (with or without 0.2% albumin human added); however, the injection should not be diluted with 0.9% sodium chloride injection since precipitation may occur. Filgrastim and filgrastim-sndz injections contain no preservatives and solutions that have been diluted in 5% dextrose injection should be stored at 2–8°C and used within 24 hours to minimize the possibility of bacterial contamination. To minimize adsorption of filgrastim or filgrastim-sndz to infusion containers or equipment, albumin human should be added to the infusion solution to a final concentration of 2 mg/mL (0.2%) whenever filgrastim or filgrastim-sndz is diluted to a concentration of 5–15 mcg/mL in 5% dextrose injection. The manufacturers state that dilution of filgrastim or filgrastim-sndz injection to a final concentration of less than 5 mcg/mL is not recommended.

When diluted in 5% dextrose injection with or without human albumin, filgrastim or filgrastim-sndz is compatible with glass or with plastics commonly used in the manufacture of syringes, IV bags, infusion sets, and IV pump cassettes, including polyvinyl chloride, polyolefin, and polypropylene. Undiluted filgrastim injection is stable in Becton-Dickinson tuberculin syringes for up to 24 hours at 15–30°C or for up to 7 days when refrigerated at 2–8°C; however, to reduce the possibility of bacterial contamination, filgrastim in syringes should be stored at 2–8°C and used within 24 hours.

Filgrastim or filgrastim-sndz is incompatible with and should *not* be diluted in solutions containing 0.9% sodium chloride injection.

Preparations

Excipients in commercially available drug preparations may have clinically important effects in some individuals; consult specific product labeling for details.

Filgrastim (Recombinant DNA Origin)

Parenteral

Injection, for IV or subcutaneous use	300 mcg/mL (300 and 480 mcg)	**Neupogen®** (available in single-dose vials), Amgen
	600 mcg/mL (300 and 480 mcg)	**Neupogen®** (available in prefilled syringes with UltraSafe® needle guard), Amgen

Filgrastim-sndz (Recombinant DNA Origin)

Parenteral

Injection, for IV or subcutaneous use	600 mcg/mL (300 and 480 mcg)	**Zarxio®** (available in prefilled syringes with UltraSafe Passive® needle guard), Sandoz

Tbo-filgrastim (Recombinant DNA Origin)

Parenteral

Injection, for subcutaneous use	600 mcg/mL (300 and 480 mcg)	**Granix®** (available in prefilled syringes with or without UltraSafe Passive® needle guard), Teva

†Use is not currently included in the labeling approved by the US Food and Drug Administration

Oprelvekin

Recombinant Interleukin-11, rhIL-11

■ Oprelvekin, a biosynthetic (recombinant DNA-derived) form of human interleukin-11 (IL-11), is a thrombopoietic growth factor that principally affects megakaryocytopoiesis.

Uses

■ **Chemotherapy-induced Thrombocytopenia** Oprelvekin is used for prevention of severe thrombocytopenia in adults with nonmyeloid malignancies receiving myelosuppressive antineoplastic therapy; oprelvekin has been designated an orphan drug by the US Food and Drug Administration (FDA) for this use.

Oprelvekin reduces the need for platelet transfusions following myelosuppressive chemotherapy. The drug is indicated for patients at high risk (as judged by the clinician) of developing severe chemotherapy-induced thrombocytopenia.

Oprelvekin is *not* indicated for use in patients undergoing *myeloablative* chemotherapy†. (See Fluid Retention under Cautions.)

The efficacy of oprelvekin has not been established in patients receiving chemotherapy regimens of more than 5 days' duration or regimens associated with delayed myelosuppression (e.g., nitrosoureas, mitomycin-C)†.

Dosage and Administration

■ **Administration** ***Subcutaneous Administration*** Administer by subcutaneous injection daily. Administer at approximately the same time each day.

Administer as a single injection into the abdomen, thigh, hip, or upper arm. Rotate injection sites. Do not rub injection sites.

Initiate oprelvekin 6–24 hours following completion of chemotherapy. Safety and efficacy of administering immediately prior to or concurrently with chemotherapy, or at the time of the expected platelet nadir, has not been established.

If a dose is missed, resume the next scheduled dose at the appropriate time; do *not* double a dose.

Oprelvekin is intended for use under the guidance and supervision of a clinician, but may be *self-administered* if the clinician determines that the patient and/or caregiver is competent to prepare and safely administer the drug.

Consult the manufacturer's labeling for specific instructions on reconstitution, dilution, and administration.

Reconstitution. Reconstitute a vial labeled as containing 5 mg of oprelvekin powder for injection with 1 mL of sterile water for injection to provide a solution containing oprelvekin 5 mg/mL.

During reconstitution, direct diluent toward the side of the vial. Gently swirl to dissolve the powder; do *not* shake.

Vials are for single use only; discard any unused solution after withdrawal of dose and do not re-enter or reuse vial.

Administer as soon as possible or within 3 hours after reconstitution.

■ **Dosage** ***Adults*** The recommended dosage of oprelvekin in patients with chemotherapy-induced thrombocytopenia is 50 mcg/kg daily given subcutaneously. Administer the first dose 6–24 hours following completion of chemotherapy and continue therapy until platelet counts are at least 50,000/mm^3. Do not exceed 21 days of treatment per chemotherapy cycle.

Discontinue oprelvekin at least 2 days prior to the next cycle of chemotherapy.

■ **Prescribing Limits** ***Adults*** There is limited experience with doses exceeding 50 mcg/kg; such doses may be associated with an increased risk of cardiovascular events. (See Cardiovascular Effects under Cautions.)

The recommended maximum duration of therapy for each course of treatment is 21 days.

The safety and efficacy of more than 6 cycles of oprelvekin treatment following a chemotherapy cycle has not been established.

■ **Special Populations** ***Renal Impairment*** Reduce the dosage of oprelvekin to 25 mcg/kg daily in patients with severe renal impairment (creatinine clearance less than 30 mL/minute, as estimated from serum creatinine).

Cautions

■ **Contraindications** Known hypersensitivity to oprelvekin or any ingredient in the formulation.

■ **Warnings/Precautions** ***Warnings*** **Fluid Retention.** Fluid retention, usually a result of increased sodium and water retention, has been reported. Clinical manifestations range from mild to moderate peripheral edema to more severe conditions (e.g., pulmonary edema, capillary leak syndrome, atrial arrhythmias, development or exacerbation of pleural or pericardial effusion). Fluid retention usually develops within the first few weeks of therapy and may continue for the duration of therapy. In most cases, edema is self-limiting and resolves within several days after drug discontinuance.

Serious, sometimes fatal, cases of fluid retention have been reported in patients who received oprelvekin following bone marrow transplantation. Do *not* use oprelvekin in patients undergoing myeloablative chemotherapy.

Increased plasma volume may result in decreased concentrations of serum proteins (e.g., albumin, transferrin, gamma globulin) and serum calcium.

Use with caution in patients who have heart failure or who may be susceptible to developing heart failure (e.g., history of heart failure even if well compensated and receiving appropriate medical management). Also, use caution in those with other conditions or treatments that may precipitate or exacerbate fluid retention (e.g., pleural effusions, aggressive hydration, concomitant drugs known to cause edema). Closely monitor fluid status and initiate appropriate treatment if fluid imbalance occurs. Monitor preexisting fluid collections (e.g., pericardial effusions, ascites) and consider drainage if indicated.

Monitor fluid and electrolyte status carefully in patients receiving maintenance therapy with diuretics. Sudden death has occurred in at least 2 patients who developed severe hypokalemia (less than 3 mEq/L) while receiving diuretic therapy concomitantly with ifosfamide and oprelvekin.

Hematologic Effects. Moderate decreases in hemoglobin, hematocrit, and red blood cells have been reported, principally because of fluid retention and hemodilution. (See Fluid Retention under Cautions.) Such effects usually manifest within 3–5 days following initiation of therapy and reverse over approximately 1 week upon drug discontinuance. Monitor complete blood cell counts prior to chemotherapy and periodically during therapy.

Reversible increases in plasma fibrinogen (e.g., twofold increase), haptoglobin, and other acute-phase reactants (e.g., C-reactive protein) have been observed. Increased concentrations of Von Willebrand factor (with normal multimer pattern) also have been reported in healthy individuals who received oprelvekin.

Cardiovascular Effects. An increased risk of cardiovascular events (e.g., arrhythmias, myocardial infarction, stroke, cardiomegaly, pulmonary edema) has been reported with oprelvekin therapy.

Atrial arrhythmias (fibrillation or flutter) have been reported in about 10–15% of patients receiving oprelvekin, in some cases resulting in stroke. Such arrhythmias usually are transient and convert to normal sinus rhythm spontaneously or with rate-control therapy. Cardiac arrest also has been reported, but a causal relationship to the drug is uncertain.

Ventricular arrhythmias, generally occurring within 2–7 days of initiation, have been reported during postmarketing experience.

Use with caution in patients with a history of cardiac arrhythmias, including atrial and ventricular arrhythmias. Carefully consider potential risks versus benefits of therapy. Doses exceeding 50 mcg/kg may increase the risk of adverse cardiovascular effects.

Cerebrovascular Effects. Stroke has been reported in association with atrial arrhythmias. (See Cardiovascular Effects under Cautions.) Risk may be increased in those with a history of stroke or transient ischemic attack.

Ocular Effects. Oprelvekin therapy has been associated with possible development or worsening of papilledema, which generally resolves upon drug discontinuance. This risk may increase with high dosages (e.g., exceeding 50 mcg/kg daily). A higher incidence of papilledema has been observed in children (16%) compared with adults (1%) in clinical trials. (See Pediatric Use under Cautions.) Use with caution in patients with preexisting papilledema or CNS tumors.

Other visual disturbances, including blurred vision, optic neuropathy, and blindness, have been reported.

Renal Effects. Renal failure has been reported during postmarketing experience in patients who received oprelvekin following bone marrow transplantation. Do *not* use oprelvekin in patients undergoing *myeloablative* chemotherapy.

Sensitivity Reactions **Hypersensitivity Reactions.** Serious hypersensitivity reactions, including anaphylaxis and shock, have been reported during postmarketing experience. Reported reactions include edema of the face, tongue, or larynx; dyspnea; wheezing; chest pain; hypotension (including shock); dysarthria; loss of consciousness; mental status changes; rash; urticaria; flushing; and fever. Such reactions can occur after initial administration or at any time during therapy. Take appropriate precautionary measures in case of hypersensitivity reactions (e.g., ensure immediate availability of antihistamines, epinephrine, oxygen, corticosteroids).

Advise patient regarding potential manifestations of hypersensitivity for which they should seek immediate medical attention. (See Advice to Patients.) Permanently discontinue therapy if allergic or hypersensitivity-type reactions occur.

Antibody Formation. Development of antibodies to oprelvekin has been reported infrequently; the clinical importance is unknown.

General Precautions **Laboratory Monitoring.** Perform CBC prior to chemotherapy and at regular intervals during therapy. (See Hematologic Effects under Cautions.)

Monitor platelet counts at time of the expected nadir and continue monitoring until platelet counts recover to at least 50,000/mm^3.

Monitor fluid status. (See Fluid Retention under Cautions.)

Monitor electrolytes in those receiving concomitant diuretic therapy. (See Fluid Retention under Cautions.)

Specific Populations **Pregnancy.** Category C. (See Users Guide.)

Lactation. It is not known whether oprelvekin is distributed into milk. Because of the potential for serious adverse reactions to oprelvekin in nursing infants, a decision should be made whether to discontinue nursing or the drug, taking into account the importance of the drug to the woman.

Pediatric Use. Safety and efficacy have not been established in children younger than 12 years of age. Restrict use to clinical trial settings in pediatric patients, especially in those younger than 12 years of age.

Oprelvekin therapy has been evaluated in a limited number of patients 8 months to 18 years of age. Pharmacokinetic studies suggest higher than recommended dosages may be necessary to achieve therapeutic effect in children and adolescents; however, dosages exceeding 50 mcg/kg daily have been associated with an increased risk of adverse effects (i.e., papilledema, periosteal bone changes.)

Tachycardia, conjunctival injection, cardiomegaly, periosteal changes, and papilledema have been reported more frequently in children than in adults. (See Ocular Effects under Cautions.)

Long-term effects of oprelvekin on bone growth and development in children have not been established. Limited data in animals suggest possible adverse effects on bone, joints, and tendons (e.g., thickening of femoral and tibial growth plates, joint and tendon fibrosis, periosteal hyperostosis).

Geriatric Use. Select dosage with caution because of greater frequency of decreased renal function in geriatric patients. (See Renal Impairment under Cautions.)

Renal Impairment. Renal impairment may result in possible increased serum concentrations and systemic exposure to oprelvekin. Reduce dosage in patients with severe renal impairment (creatinine clearance less than 30 mL/minute). (See Renal Impairment under Dosage and Administration.)

A substantial decrease in hemoglobin has been observed on day 2 of oprelvekin therapy in patients with any degree of renal impairment. (See Hematologic Effects under Cautions.)

The effects of oprelvekin on fluid retention in patients with renal impairment have not been established; carefully monitor fluid balance in such patients. (See Fluid Retention under Cautions.)

■ **Common Adverse Effects** Adverse effects reported in at least 10% of patients receiving oprelvekin in clinical trials and more often than with placebo include edema, tachycardia, palpitations, atrial fibrillation/flutter, oral moniliasis, dyspnea, pleural effusions, and conjunctival injection.

Drug Interactions

Drug interactions with oprelvekin have not been fully elucidated; in vitro and nonclinical in vivo studies suggest that the drug is not metabolized by cytochrome P-450 (CYP) enzymes.

■ **Diuretics** Severe hypokalemia resulting in death has occurred rarely in cancer patients receiving oprelvekin with chronic diuretic therapy and high doses of ifosfamide. Closely monitor fluid and electrolytes in patients receiving oprelvekin and chronic diuretic therapy.

■ **Filgrastim (G-CSF)** No adverse interactions observed with concomitant use.

■ **Sargramostim (GM-CSF)** Clinical studies are not available to assess potential interactions between oprelvekin and sargramostim. Limited data in animals suggest no evidence of adverse interactions with concomitant use.

Pharmacokinetics

■ **Absorption** ***Bioavailability*** Absolute bioavailability >80% with sub-Q administration in healthy adults.

Relative bioavailability of a 50-mcg/kg sub-Q dose was 65% compared with same dose given IV.

Peak plasma concentrations attained within 2–3 hours following single sub-Q dose.

Onset Platelet counts begin to increase in dose-dependent manner 5–9 days following daily sub-Q administration.

Duration Platelet counts continue to increase for up to 7 days following drug discontinuance and return to normal within 14 days.

Special Populations In patients with severe renal impairment (Cl_{cr} <30 mL/minute), mean AUC and peak plasma concentrations are approximately 2.6- and 2.2-fold higher, respectively, than in individuals with normal renal function. Clearance in severe renal impairment approximately 40% of that observed in individuals with normal renal function. No substantial change in pharmacokinetic parameters observed in patients with mild or moderate renal impairment compared with those with normal renal function.

In infants, children, and adolescents 8 months to 18 years of age receiving a 50 mcg/kg dose, mean AUC approximately half that observed in adults. Limited data suggest children <12 years of age may not achieve adequate plasma concentrations with recommended dosages (50 mcg/kg daily). (See Pediatric Use under Cautions.)

■ **Distribution** ***Extent*** Not known whether oprelvekin crosses the placenta or is distributed into milk.

May distribute through lymphatic system before entering systemic circulation. Rapidly distributes into highly perfused organs.

■ **Elimination** ***Metabolism*** Metabolic fate of oprelvekin not fully elucidated, but presumed to be extensively metabolized or degraded.

Elimination Route Excreted principally in urine; only small amounts of parent drug recovered.

Half-life Terminal half-life: Approximately 7 hours.

No evidence of drug accumulation following multiple sub-Q doses.

Special Populations Clearance higher in infants and children 8 months to 11 years of age than in adolescents and adults ≥12 years of age. (See Pediatric Use under Cautions.)

Description

■ **Actions** Oprelvekin is a thrombopoietic growth factor structurally and functionally similar to endogenous human interleukin-11 (IL-11). Oprelvekin lacks only the amino-terminal proline residue of endogenous IL-11. Oprelvekin exhibits no measurable difference in biologic activity in vivo or in vitro compared with endogenous IL-11.

Oprelvekin stimulates multiple stages of the hematopoietic pathway. The drug binds directly to IL-11 receptors on myeloid progenitor cell surfaces and stimulates production of erythrocytes, platelets, neutrophils, and macrophages within the bone marrow.

Oprelvekin principally affects megakaryocytopoiesis. The drug produces a dose-dependent increase in platelet counts by stimulating the proliferation and differentiation of megakaryocyte progenitor cells in synergy with other growth factors (e.g., interleukin-3 [IL-3], thrombopoietin [TPO], stem cell factor [SCF]).

Nonhematologic effects of oprelvekin include regulation of intestinal epithelium growth, inhibition of adipogenesis, stimulation of synthesis of acute phase reactants, modulation (e.g., inhibition) of pro-inflammatory cytokines, and stimulation of osteoclastogenesis and neurogenesis.

Advice to Patients

Risk of cardiovascular effects; importance of immediately informing clinician if symptoms of atrial arrhythmia (e.g., rapid heart rate, palpitations) or stroke occur.

Risk of fluid retention; importance of immediately informing clinician if swelling in hands or feet, rapid weight gain, shortness of breath, or difficulty breathing occurs; importance of informing clinician of preexisting heart failure or concurrent therapy with medications that can cause fluid retention.

Importance of recognizing symptoms of allergic or hypersensitivity reactions (e.g., swelling of the face, tongue, or throat; tightness in throat; difficulty breathing, swallowing, or talking; shortness of breath; wheezing; chest pain; lightheadedness; loss of consciousness; confusion; drowsiness; rash; itching; hives; flushing; fever), and immediately informing clinician if any of these symptoms occur.

Risk of papilledema; importance of patient and/or caregiver immediately informing clinician if headache or visual impairment (e.g., blurry vision, blindness) occurs.

Importance of informing clinician if any swelling or bruising persists at injection site.

Importance of providing copy of manufacturer's patient information to patient if drug is being self-administered. Instruct patient and/or caregiver regarding proper dosage and administration of oprelvekin, including use of aseptic technique and safe disposal of needles and syringes (e.g., using puncture-resistant container).

Importance of not taking a double dose to make up for a missed dose but instead taking the next scheduled dose at appropriate time.

Importance of women informing clinicians if they are or plan to become pregnant or plan to breast-feed.

Importance of informing clinicians of existing or contemplated concomitant therapy (e.g., diuretics), including prescription and OTC drugs as well as any concomitant illnesses (e.g., heart failure, renal impairment, papilledema).

Importance of informing patients of other important precautionary information (e.g., likelihood of developing anemia). (See Cautions.)

Overview® (see Users Guide). For additional information on this drug until a more detailed monograph is developed and published, the manufacturer's labeling should be consulted. It is *essential* that the manufacturer's labeling be consulted for more detailed information on usual cautions, precautions, contraindications, potential drug interactions, laboratory test interferences, and acute toxicity.

Preparations

Excipients in commercially available drug preparations may have clinically important effects in some individuals; consult specific product labeling for details.

Oprelvekin (Recombinant DNA Origin)

Parenteral		
For injection, for subcutaneous use only	5 mg	Neumega® (available with 1 mL sterile water for injection diluent), Wyeth

†Use is not currently included in the labeling approved by the US Food and Drug Administration

Pegfilgrastim

■ Pegfilgrastim, a covalent conjugate of filgrastim and monomethoxypolyethylene glycol, is a biosynthetic hematopoietic agent that principally affects the proliferation and differentiation of neutrophils within the bone marrow.

Uses

■ **Chemotherapy-Induced Neutropenia** Pegfilgrastim is used to decrease the risk of infectious complications (as manifested by febrile neutropenia) in patients with nonmyeloid malignancies receiving myelosuppressive antineoplastic therapy that is associated with a clinically important risk of severe neutropenia with fever. Efficacy of pegfilgrastim has been evaluated in 2 randomized, double-blind, active-control studies in patients with metastatic breast cancer receiving doxorubicin 60 mg/m² and docetaxel 75 mg/m² every 21 days for up to 4 cycles. Based on evidence from studies of filgrastim indicating that a correlation exists between duration of severe neutropenia and incidence of febrile neutropenia, efficacy of pegfilgrastim was demonstrated by establishing comparability between pegfilgrastim and filgrastim therapy with respect to the mean number of days of severe neutropenia. In the 2 studies of pegfilgrastim, the incidence, severity, and duration of severe neutropenia (absolute neutrophil count [ANC] less than 500/mm³) were similar in patients receiving a single fixed (6 mg) or weight-adjusted (100 mcg/kg) subcutaneous dose of pegfilgrastim on day 2 of each chemotherapy cycle or daily subcutaneous injections of filgrastim (5 mcg/kg) starting on day 2 of each chemotherapy cycle and continuing for up to 14 days. In these studies, the mean duration of severe neutropenia during the first chemotherapy cycle was 1.7–1.8 or 1.6 days in patients receiving pegfilgrastim or filgrastim, respectively, and febrile neutropenia occurred in 10–20% of patients receiving either pegfilgrastim or filgrastim. In the absence of growth factor support, febrile neutropenia or severe neutropenia has been reported in 30–40 or 100%, respectively, of patients receiving similar chemotherapy regimens, with severe neutropenia having a mean duration of 5–7 days.

The manufacturer states that efficacy of pegfilgrastim has not been established in patients receiving antimetabolites such as fluorouracil (see Drug Interactions), in those receiving antineoplastic agents that are associated with delayed myelosuppression (e.g., nitrosourea derivatives, mitomycin), or in those receiving radiation therapy.

Dosage and Administration

■ **General** Pegfilgrastim is administered by subcutaneous injection. Commercially available prefilled syringes of pegfilgrastim should be stored at 2–8°C in the carton to protect the solution from light. Pegfilgrastim injection should not be frozen; however, pegfilgrastim that inadvertently has been frozen can be thawed in a refrigerator before administration. Pegfilgrastim should be discarded if frozen a second time. Prior to administration, pegfilgrastim syringes may be allowed to reach room temperature for a maximum of 48 hours but should be protected from light during that period of time. The injection should not be shaken. Commercially available prefilled syringes of pegfilgrastim should be inspected visually for particulate matter and discoloration prior to administration. Pegfilgrastim should not be administered if discoloration or particulates are observed.

For the treatment of chemotherapy-induced neutropenia, the recommended adult dosage of pegfilgrastim is a single 6-mg injection administered subcutaneously once per chemotherapy cycle. Dosage of pegfilgrastim does not need to be modified based on body weight. Pegfilgrastim should *not* be administered during the 14 days before or 24 hours after administration of cytotoxic chemotherapy.

■ **Special Populations** No special population dosage recommendations at this time.

Cautions

■ **Contraindications** Known hypersensitivity to pegfilgrastim, filgrastim, any ingredient in the formulation, or proteins derived from *Escherichia coli*.

■ **Warnings/Precautions** *Warnings* **Splenic Rupture.** Although not reported to date in patients receiving pegfilgrastim, rare cases of splenic rupture (including some fatalities) have been reported following administration of filgrastim for peripheral blood progenitor cell (PBPC) mobilization in both healthy donors and patients with cancer. Pegfilgrastim has not been evaluated for mobilization of PBPCs and should not be used for this purpose. Patients receiving pegfilgrastim who experience left upper abdominal or shoulder tip pain should be evaluated for the presence of splenomegaly or splenic rupture.

Respiratory Effects. Although not reported to date in patients receiving pegfilgrastim, adult respiratory distress syndrome (ARDS) has been reported in neutropenic patients with sepsis receiving filgrastim. It has been postulated that an influx of neutrophils into sites of inflammation in the lungs may have caused such disease. Neutropenic patients receiving pegfilgrastim who develop fever, lung infiltrates, or respiratory distress should be evaluated for the presence of ARDS. If ARDS occurs, pegfilgrastim should be discontinued and/or withheld until ARDS has resolved, and patients should receive appropriate treatment for this condition.

Sickle Cell Disease. Although not reported to date in patients receiving pegfilgrastim, severe sickle cell crisis (which has been fatal in at least one case) has been reported in patients with sickle cell disease (specifically, homozygous sickle cell anemia, sickle cell-hemoglobin C disease, and sickle cell-β+-thalassemia disease) who received filgrastim for PBPC mobilization or following chemotherapy. Pegfilgrastim should be used with caution in patients with sickle cell disease, and only after careful consideration of the potential risks and benefits. Patients with sickle cell disease who receive pegfilgrastim should be well hydrated and monitored for the occurrence of sickle cell crisis. If severe sickle cell crisis occurs, supportive care should be initiated, and interventions to ameliorate the underlying event (e.g., therapeutic red blood cell exchange transfusion) should be considered.

Sensitivity Reactions Although not observed in clinical trials of pegfilgrastim, sensitivity reactions, including anaphylaxis, rash, and urticaria, have been reported in patients receiving initial or subsequent doses of filgrastim. In some cases, symptoms have recurred with rechallenge, suggesting a causal relationship. If serious sensitivity reactions occur, immediate medical intervention and drug discontinuance are required. Pegfilgrastim is contraindicated in patients with known hypersensitivity to pegfilgrastim or filgrastim.

General Precautions **Administration.** Because rapidly dividing myeloid cells may be particularly sensitive to cytotoxic chemotherapy, pegfilgrastim should not be administered during the 14 days before or 24 hours after administration of cytotoxic chemotherapy. (See Dosage and Administration: General.)

Potential Effect on Malignant Cells. Because some tumor cells (including some lines of myeloid, T-lymphoid, lung, head and neck, and bladder tumor cells) have receptors for granulocyte colony-stimulating factor (G-CSF), the possibility that pegfilgrastim could act as a growth factor for any tumor type cannot be excluded. Use of the drug in patients with myeloid malignancies or myelodysplastic syndrome (MDS) has not been studied.

Laboratory Monitoring. Complete blood cell and platelet counts should be performed prior to administration of chemotherapy to assess the patient's hematologic status and ability to tolerate myelosuppressive chemotherapy. Regular monitoring of hematocrit and platelet count also is recommended by the manufacturer.

Immunogenicity. Available data indicate that a small proportion of patients receiving pegfilgrastim or filgrastim have developed binding antibodies to the drug; however, the nature and specificity of those antibodies have not been adequately studied. Development of neutralizing antibodies in patients receiving pegfilgrastim has not been reported to date.

Specific Populations **Pregnancy.** Category C. (See Users Guide.)

Lactation. Not known whether pegfilgrastim is distributed into milk. Caution is advised if the drug is administered in nursing women.

Pediatric Use. Safety and efficacy of pegfilgrastim have not been established in pediatric patients. The manufacturer states that the commercially available 6-mg fixed-dose prefilled syringe should not be used in infants, children, or adolescents weighing less than 45 kg.

Geriatric Use. No substantial differences in safety and efficacy relative to younger adults, but clinically relevant differences cannot be ruled out.

■ **Common Adverse Effects** Adverse effects reported in approximately 15–72% of patients receiving pegfilgrastim or filgrastim include nausea, fatigue, alopecia, diarrhea, vomiting, constipation, fever, anorexia, skeletal pain, headache, taste perversion, dyspepsia, myalgia, insomnia, abdominal pain, arthralgia, generalized weakness, peripheral edema, dizziness, granulocytopenia, stomatitis, mucositis, and neutropenic fever. These adverse effects generally were attributed to the underlying malignancy or to concomitant cytotoxic chemotherapy. The most common adverse effect attributed to pegfilgrastim in clinical trials was mild-to-moderate medullary bone pain, which occurred in 26% of patients receiving pegfilgrastim and in a comparable percentage of patients receiving filgrastim and resulted in use of opiate or nonopiate analgesics in less than 6 or approximately 12% of those who experienced this adverse effect, respectively.

Drug Interactions

No formal drug interaction studies have been performed.

■ **Antineoplastic Agents** Concomitant use of pegfilgrastim and fluorouracil or other antimetabolites has not been evaluated in patients. In animal studies, increased mortality has been reported in mice administered pegfilgrastim at 0, 1, and 3 days prior to fluorouracil administration; administration of pegfilgrastim 24 hours following fluorouracil administration did not adversely affect survival.

■ **Lithium** Potential pharmacologic interaction (potentiation of neutrophil release); more frequent monitoring of neutrophil counts is recommended.

Description

Pegfilgrastim, a covalent conjugate of filgrastim (a human granulocyte colony-stimulating factor [G-CSF]) and monomethoxypolyethylene glycol (PEG), is a biosynthetic hematopoietic agent that principally affects the proliferation and differentiation of neutrophils within the bone marrow. Filgrastim used in the manufacture of pegfilgrastim is produced using recombinant DNA technology and cultures of*Escherichia coli* that have been genetically modified to incorporate the human G-CSF gene and is identical to that contained in commercially available filgrastim (recombinant DNA origin) (Neupogen®). Studies on cellular proliferation, receptor binding, and neutrophil function demonstrate that filgrastim and pegfilgrastim have the same mechanism of action.

As a result of conjugation with PEG, renal clearance of the drug is delayed and the plasma half-life is increased from about 3.5 hours (reported for filgrastim) to about 15–80 hours, and the PEG-conjugated drug can be administered once per chemotherapy cycle. Pegfilgrastim exhibits nonlinear, dose-dependent pharmacokinetics in cancer patients. The level of circulating neutrophils in the body affects serum clearance of pegfilgrastim, resulting in a rapid decline in serum concentrations of the drug with resolution of neutropenia; the mechanism of this effect involves receptor binding.

Advice to Patients

Importance of recognizing and reporting adverse effects of pegfilgrastim (e.g., sensitivity reactions). Importance of adherence to the treatment regimen, including regular monitoring of blood counts. Importance of clinicians providing appropriate instruction on the proper use of pegfilgrastim, including a copy of the patient instructions provided by the manufacturer, to patients and/or their caregivers who are allowed to administer the drug in a home setting.

Importance of women informing clinicians if they are or plan to become pregnant or to breast-feed. Importance of informing clinicians of existing or contemplated concomitant therapy, including prescription and OTC drugs, as well as concomitant illnesses.

Overview® (see Users Guide). For additional information on this drug until a more detailed monograph is developed and published, the manufacturer's labeling should be consulted. It is *essential* that the manufacturer's labeling be consulted for more detailed information on usual cautions, precautions, contraindications, potential drug interactions, laboratory test interferences, and acute toxicity.

Preparations

Excipients in commercially available drug preparations may have clinically important effects in some individuals; consult specific product labeling for details.

Pegfilgrastim

Parenteral		
Injection, for subcutaneous use	6 mg/0.6 mL	**Neulasta®** (available in prefilled disposable syringes), Amgen

Plerixafor

■ Plerixafor, a CXCR4 chemokine-receptor antagonist, is a hematopoietic stem cell mobilizer.

Uses

■ **Peripheral Blood Progenitor Cell Transplantation.** Plerixafor is used in combination with filgrastim (G-CSF) to mobilize hematopoietic stem cells into peripheral blood for collection (e.g., via leukapheresis as CD34+ peripheral blood progenitor cells [PBPCs]) and subsequent autologous transplantation in patients with non-Hodgkin's lymphoma or multiple myeloma. Safety and efficacy of plerixafor were established in two phase 3, randomized, placebo-controlled studies in patients with non-Hodgkin's lymphoma (OPTIMIZE I study) or multiple myeloma (OPTIMIZE II study) who were undergoing autologous hematopoietic stem cell transplantation. Patients were excluded in both studies if they had either undergone a prior hematopoietic stem cell transplantation (autologous or allogeneic) or if they had previously failed to achieve an adequate PBPC collection. In both studies, patients received plerixafor in combination with filgrastim or filgrastim alone (with placebo). Filgrastim 10 mcg/kg daily was given subcutaneously in the morning for 4 days prior to the initial apheresis session. Treatment with subcutaneous plerixafor 0.24 mg/kg or placebo was initiated in the evening on the fourth day of filgrastim therapy, approximately 11 hours prior to apheresis. These plerixafor and filgrastim regimens were then administered daily with planned apheresis sessions for up to 4 days or until the target collection of PBPCs was achieved. In the study in patients with non-Hodgkin's lymphoma (n=298), 59% of patients receiving plerixafor and filgrastim achieved a target collection goal of at least 5 million PBPCs/kg in 4 or fewer apheresis sessions compared with only 20% of those receiving filgrastim plus placebo. Patients receiving the combination therapy achieved the target goal for PBPC collection after a median of 3 days; the median time to reach the target PBPC collection goal was not evaluable for the filgrastim-placebo group. In the study in patients with multiple myeloma (n=302), a target collection goal of at least 6 million PBPCs/kg in 2 or fewer apheresis sessions was achieved by 72% of patients receiving plerixafor and filgrastim compared with 34% of those receiving filgrastim plus placebo; approximately 87 or 56% of patients had achieved a target collection goal of at least 6 million PBPCs/kg after 4 or fewer apheresis sessions in the combination and filgrastim-placebo groups, respectively. The median time for achieving the target collection goal in this study was 1 day versus 4 days for the plerixafor-filgrastim and filgrastim-placebo groups, respectively. In both studies, the times to engraftment for both neutrophils and platelets following autologous transplantation and myeloablative chemotherapy were similar in both treatment groups.

Dosage and Administration

■ **Administration** Plerixafor is administered by subcutaneous injection. The drug is available in single-use vials; any unused portion should be discarded.

■ **Dosage** The recommended adult dosage of plerixafor is 0.24 mg/kg (based on actual body weight) daily for up to 4 consecutive days. Plerixafor is given concomitantly with filgrastim as part of the hematopoietic stem cell mobilization regimen. Treatment with plerixafor should only begin *after* the patient has received the initial 4 doses of filgrastim. Plerixafor should be administered in the evening, approximately 11 hours prior to a scheduled apheresis session; the filgrastim dose should be administered in the morning prior to apheresis.

Dosage may be increased according to changes in weight, but the maximum dosage should not exceed 40 mg once daily.

■ **Special Populations** The manufacturer recommends a reduced dosage of 0.16 mg/kg (a 33% reduction in usual dosage) in patients with moderate to severe renal impairment (i.e., creatinine clearance of 50 mL/minute or less). If the creatinine clearance is 50 mL/minute or less, the maximum daily dosage should not exceed 27 mg once daily. The manufacturer states that information on the use of plerixafor in patients requiring hemodialysis is insufficient to allow dosage recommendations in such patients.

No dosage adjustments are required in geriatric patients based solely on age.

Cautions

■ **Contraindications** The manufacturer states there are no contraindications to the use of plerixafor.

■ **Warnings/Precautions** ***Tumor Cell Mobilization*** Plerixafor may cause mobilization of leukemic cells with subsequent contamination of the final apheresis product. Therefore, plerixafor is not recommended as part of a hematopoietic stem cell mobilization regimen in patients with leukemia.

Plerixafor also may cause mobilization of tumor cells from the marrow into the peripheral circulation with unintentional collection into the apheresis product. The effect of potential reinfusion of tumor cells has not been well studied.

Hematologic Effects Concomitant administration of plerixafor and filgrastim results in an increase in peripheral leukocytes, including an increase in hematopoietic stem or CD34$^+$ cells. Total white blood cell (WBC) count, including neutrophil count, should be monitored during plerixafor/filgrastim treatment. If the peripheral neutrophil count exceeds 50,000 cells/mm^3, clinical judgment should be used when considering the administration of plerixafor.

Thrombocytopenia has been reported with plerixafor. Platelet counts should be monitored in patients receiving plerixafor who then undergo subsequent apheresis.

Splenomegaly and Splenic Rupture Splenomegaly (i.e., increased spleen weights), associated with extramedullary hematopoiesis, has been observed in animals receiving prolonged (2–4 weeks) therapy with higher doses of plerixafor (fourfold higher than recommended human dose based on body surface area). The effect of plerixafor on spleen size has not been established in humans. Splenomegaly and splenic rupture have been reported in patients with myelodysplastic syndrome, amyloidosis, and in patients with both hematologic and solid tumors who received filgrastim (or pegfilgrastim) alone for the treatment of neutropenia or in conjunction with autologous stem cell transplantation. At least one case of splenic rupture has been reported in a patient with multiple myeloma who received the combination of filgrastim and sargramostim. Patients receiving plerixafor/filgrastim therapy who experience left upper abdominal pain and/or scapular or shoulder pain should be evaluated for splenic integrity (and possible rupture).

Fetal /Neonatal Morbidity and Mortality May cause fetal harm; teratogenicity and embryolethality demonstrated in rats receiving plerixafor, mainly at doses approximately 10 times the recommended human dose (0.24 mg/kg) on a mg/m^2 basis. No adequate and well-controlled studies in humans. Pregnancy should be avoided during plerixafor therapy. If used during pregnancy or if patient becomes pregnant while receiving the drug, the patient should be apprised of the potential hazard to the fetus.

Specific Populations **Pregnancy.** Category D. (See Users Guide). (See Fetal/Neonatal Morbidity and Mortality, under Cautions: Warnings/Precautions.)

Lactation. It is not known if plerixafor is distributed into human milk. Because many drugs are distributed into human milk and because of the potential for serious adverse effects of plerixafor in nursing infants, a decision should be made whether to discontinue nursing or the drug, taking into the account the importance of the drug to the woman.

Pediatric Use. Safety and efficacy not established in pediatric patients younger than 18 years of age.

Geriatric Use. No substantial differences in safety or efficacy relative to younger adults, but increased sensitivity cannot be ruled out.

Hepatic Impairment. No dosage modification recommended.

Renal Impairment. The manufacturer recommends a reduced dosage of 0.16 mg/kg (33% reduction in dosage) in patients with moderate to severe renal impairment (i.e., creatinine clearance of 50 mL/minute or less). If the creatinine clearance is 50 mL/minute or less, the maximum daily dosage should not exceed 27 mg once daily. The manufacturer makes no specific dosage recommendations in patients undergoing hemodialysis due to insufficient information in this population. No specific recommendations for dosage modification in geriatric patients with normal renal function (i.e., creatinine clearance exceeding 50 mL/minute using Cockcroft-Gault formula).

■ **Common Adverse Effects** The most common adverse events (occurring in at least 5% of patients in controlled clinical trials) reported with the combination of plerixafor and filgrastim included diarrhea, nausea, injection site reactions, fatigue, headache, arthralgia, dizziness, vomiting, flatulence, and insomnia.

Drug Interactions

In vitro studies indicate that plerixafor is not a substrate, inhibitor, or inducer of cytochrome P-450 (CYP) isoenzymes. Therefore, interactions with plerixafor and other drugs involving CYP isoenzymes are unlikely.

At in vitro concentrations similar to those achieved clinically, plerixafor did not act as a substrate or inhibitor of P-glycoprotein.

Because plerixafor is excreted principally by the kidneys, concurrent administration of drugs that reduce renal function or compete for active tubular secretion may potentially increase concentrations of plerixafor or the coadministered drug. The effects of coadministration of plerixafor with drugs that are excreted by the kidneys or known to affect renal function have not been established.

Description

Plerixafor, a CXCR4 chemokine-receptor antagonist, prevents the binding of stromal cell-derived factor-1α (SDF-1α) to the CXCR4 chemokine receptor. CXCR4 and SDF-1α together play a role in the trafficking of hematopoietic stem cells, specifically to promote their homing to and retention within the bone marrow. By disrupting the interaction between SDF-1α and its receptor, plerixafor interferes with the retention of hematopoietic stem cells in the bone marrow matrix. Subsequently, increased numbers of CD34+ hematopoietic progenitor cells are mobilized or released from the bone marrow, resulting in peripheral leukocytosis. Mobilized CD34+ cells are then collected by apheresis and used as a stem-cell infusion to promote engraftment following high-dose chemotherapy associated with autologous stem-cell transplantation.

In a study in healthy individuals, plerixafor did not prolong QT-interval or corrected QT-interval, Bazett's formula (QT$_c$), at single doses up to 0.4 mg/kg (producing peak concentrations approximately 1.8-fold higher than those produced by the usual dose of 0.24 mg/kg).

Advice to Patients

Importance of reporting symptoms of systemic reactions (e.g., urticaria, periorbital swelling, dyspnea, hypoxia) that develop within 30 minutes following plerixafor administration.

Importance of reporting any symptoms of a vasovagal reaction, such as orthostatic hypotension or syncope, that develop during or shortly after (e.g., within 1 hour) plerixafor administration.

Importance of reporting itching, rash, or reaction at the site of the injection. Such reactions may be treated with an OTC drug after consultation with a healthcare provider.

Risk of adverse GI effects (e.g., diarrhea, nausea, vomiting, flatulence, abdominal pain). Importance of advising patients how to manage GI effects and of reporting severe GI toxicity with plerixafor therapy.

Importance of informing clinicians of existing or contemplated concomitant therapy, including prescription and OTC drugs, as well as concomitant illnesses.

Importance of women informing clinicians if they are or plan to become pregnant or plan to breast-feed; necessity for clinicians to advise women of childbearing potential to avoid pregnancy during therapy. If patient becomes pregnant during therapy with plerixafor, advise about risk to fetus. (See Fetal/Neonatal Morbidity and Mortality, under Cautions: Warnings/Precautions.)

Importance of informing patients of other important precautionary information. (See Cautions.)

Overview® (see Users Guide). For additional information on this drug until a more detailed monograph is developed and published, the manufacturer's labeling should be consulted. It is *essential* that the manufacturer's labeling be consulted for more detailed information on usual cautions, precautions, contraindications, potential drug interactions, laboratory test interferences, and acute toxicity.

Preparations

Excipients in commercially available drug preparations may have clinically important effects in some individuals; consult specific product labeling for details.

Plerixafor

Parenteral

Injection, for subcutaneous use	20 mg/mL	**Mozobil®**, Genzyme

romiPLOStim

■ Romiplostim, a biosynthetic (recombinant DNA-derived) Fc-peptide fusion protein, is a thrombopoietin-receptor agonist.

REMS

FDA approved a REMS for romiplostim to ensure that the benefits outweigh the risks. The REMS may apply to one or more preparations of romiplostim and consists of the following: communication plan. See the FDA REMS page (https://www.accessdata.fda.gov/scripts/cder/rems/index.cfm).

Uses

■ **Idiopathic Thrombocytopenic Purpura** Romiplostim is used for the treatment of chronic idiopathic thrombocytopenic purpura (ITP; also known as immune thrombocytopenic purpura) in patients who have had an inadequate response to corticosteroids, immunoglobulins, or splenectomy and in whom the degree of thrombocytopenia and clinical status increase bleeding risk. Romiplostim should not be used to normalize platelet counts, since excessive increases in platelet count may increase the risk of thromboembolic complications. The drug is not indicated for the treatment of thrombocytopenia associated with myelodysplastic syndrome or thrombocytopenia associated with any condition other than chronic ITP.

Safety and efficacy of romiplostim for the treatment of chronic ITP were established in 2 double-blind, placebo-controlled studies and an open-label extension study. In studies 1 (nonsplenectomized patients) and 2 (splenectomized patients), patients with chronic ITP who had received prior therapy with corticosteroids, immunoglobulins, rituximab, cytotoxic agents, danazol, or azathioprine and had a platelet count of 30,000/mm^3 or less prior to study entry were randomized (2:1) to receive 24 weeks of therapy with romiplostim or placebo, with dosage adjusted to maintain a platelet count of 50,000–200,000/mm^3. Patients receiving corticosteroids, azathioprine, or danazol at study entry were allowed to continue these therapies at stable dosages throughout the studies. The primary objective was achievement of a durable platelet response, defined as a platelet count of 50,000/mm^3 or greater during at least 6 of the last 8 weeks of treatment without the need for rescue therapy (i.e., corticosteroids, immune globulin IV, platelet transfusions, Rh_o(D) immune globulin) at any time.

Among nonsplenectomized patients, a durable platelet response was achieved in 61% of those receiving romiplostim versus 5% of those receiving placebo. Among splenectomized patients, a durable platelet response was achieved in 38% of those receiving romiplostim versus none of those receiving placebo.

Severe, life-threatening, or fatal bleeding events occurred in 7% of patients receiving romiplostim compared with 12% of those receiving placebo in the 2 double-blind studies; 1 patient receiving romiplostim died from an intracranial hemorrhage after starting aspirin therapy to treat thrombosis and subsequently discontinuing romiplostim.

Patients were eligible to receive romiplostim during the open-label extension study if their platelet count decreased to 50,000/mm^3 or less following discontinuance of the assigned treatment at the end of the double-blind studies. Most patients in the extension study achieved a median platelet count of 50,000/mm^3 after receiving 1–3 doses of romiplostim. Based on interim follow-up results in 142 patients in the extension study who received romiplostim for up to 156 weeks (approximately 3 years), 87% achieved a platelet response during a mean treatment period of 69 weeks; responding patients sustained a platelet response for approximately 67% of the time while on treatment. A platelet response was defined as a platelet count equal to or exceeding 50,000/mm^3 that was at least twofold higher than the baseline platelet count and did not require the use of rescue therapy within the previous 8 weeks. Median platelet counts rose rapidly during the first 4 weeks of romiplostim treatment and more gradually through week 16; thereafter, the median platelet count remained between 61,000 and 149,000/mm^3 through week 144. Additional rescue ITP treatment was required by 36% of patients at some time during the study. Approximately 23% of the patients treated with romiplostim were receiving concomitant ITP treatment at baseline; discontinuance of other ITP therapy was feasible in 50% of patients and an additional 34% of patients had a 25% dosage reduction of their other ITP therapy. Severe bleeding events were reported in 8.5% of patients, most of which occurred within the first 24 weeks of treatment. The platelet count obtained around the time of the bleeding events was less than 30,000/mm^3 for all but one event.

Dosage and Administration

■ **General** Romiplostim should be administered by a clinician; the drug should *not* be self-administered by the patient.

Because injection volumes of the drug may be very small, romiplostim should be administered using a syringe calibrated in increments of 0.01 mL. Extra care should be exercised to ensure the accuracy of the administered dose because of the potential for serious adverse effects following administration of excessive doses.

Romiplostim may be used with other drugs to treat ITP such as corticosteroids, danazol, azathioprine, immune globulin IV (IGIV), and Rh_o(D) immune globulin. If the platelet count increases to 50,000/mm^3 or greater, the manufacturer states that medical therapies for ITP may be reduced or discontinued.

■ **Reconstitution and Administration** Romiplostim is administered by subcutaneous injection.

Romiplostim lyophilized powder is supplied in single-use vials containing 375 mcg (to deliver 250 mcg) or 625 mcg (to deliver 500 mcg) of the drug. Lyophilized romiplostim should be reconstituted using only sterile water for injection *without* preservatives; bacteriostatic water for injection should *not* be used. The powder is reconstituted by adding 0.72 or 1.2 mL of preservative-free sterile water for injection to a vial labeled as containing 250 or 500 mcg, respectively, of romiplostim. The vial should be gently swirled and inverted to facilitate dissolution, which generally takes less than 2 minutes; the vial should not be shaken or vigorously agitated. Reconstitution of the lyophilized drug as directed provides a clear and colorless solution containing 250 or 500 mcg per 0.5 or 1 mL, respectively, for subcutaneous administration.

Reconstituted solutions should be protected from light and stored at 25°C or refrigerated at 2–8°C for up to 24 hours prior to administration. No more than one dose should be administered from each single-use vial; any unused portions of the solution should be discarded.

■ **Dosage** The recommended initial dosage of romiplostim is 1 mcg/kg weekly based on actual body weight. Romiplostim dosage is adjusted at weekly intervals in increments of 1 mcg/kg (up to a maximum dosage of 10 mcg/kg weekly) until a platelet count of at least 50,000/mm^3 is achieved. Dosage should be reduced by 1 mcg/kg weekly if the platelet count exceeds 200,000/mm^3 for 2 consecutive weeks. Romiplostim should not be administered if the platelet count exceeds 400,000/mm^3; the platelet count should be assessed weekly and romiplostim should be resumed at a dosage reduced by 1 mcg/kg weekly once the platelet count is less than 200,000/mm^3. Romiplostim should be discontinued if, after 4 weeks of therapy at the maximum recommended dosage of 10 mcg/kg weekly, the platelet count has not increased to a level sufficient to avoid clinically important bleeding.

Complete blood cell count (CBC), including platelet count and peripheral blood smear, should be monitored weekly until a stable platelet count (50,000/mm^3 or greater for at least 4 weeks without dosage adjustment) has been achieved; CBC, including platelet count and peripheral blood smear, should be monitored at least monthly thereafter. Because of the potential for worsening thrombocytopenia following discontinuance of romiplostim, CBC, including platelet count, should be monitored weekly for at least 2 weeks after drug discontinuance.

Cautions

■ **Contraindications** The manufacturer states that there are no known contraindications to the use of romiplostim.

■ **Warnings/Precautions** ***Bone Marrow Reticulin Deposition and Bone Marrow Fibrosis*** Thrombopoietin (TPO)-receptor agonists increase the risk of development or progression of reticulin fiber deposition within the bone marrow, thereby increasing the risk for bone marrow fibrosis or myelofibrosis. Reticulin fiber deposition was reported in 10 of 271 patients receiving romiplostim in controlled clinical studies, leading to discontinuance of romiplostim in 4 patients; dosages of at least 5 mcg/kg were used in all 10 patients and 6 of these patients received dosages of at least 10 mcg/kg. In a subset of patients who had prospectively planned bone biopsies performed at baseline and during follow-up in an extension study, no evidence of reticulin staining was detected in 5 of 6 patients; however, one patient had evidence of mild reticulin staining after 3 months of romiplostim therapy. In addition, 8 cases of positive or increased bone marrow reticulin were spontaneously reported and characterized predominantly as mild to moderate or as a low-grade change; however, no evidence of collagen formation or clonal abnormalities was reported in the subset of patients who underwent additional testing (e.g., trichrome staining, immunophenotyping, and cytogenetic studies). In 4 patients identified retrospectively who had an increase in bone marrow reticulin compared with baseline, evidence of grade 1–2 reticulin changes were detected in 3 of 4 patients receiving maximum dosages of 9–18 mcg/kg following discontinuance of romiplostim; one case of a grade 4 finding (e.g., areas of collagen deposition) was reported in a single patient receiving a maximum dosage of 9 mcg/kg. Another patient with ITP and hemolytic anemia developed marrow fibrosis with collagen during the romiplostim extension study. Clinical studies of romiplostim have not excluded the risk of development of bone marrow fibrosis with cytopenias.

A peripheral blood smear should be evaluated prior to starting romiplostim therapy and monthly thereafter once a stable dosage has been achieved. Examination of the peripheral blood smear should include establishment of a baseline level of cellular morphologic abnormalities and monthly evaluations to detect new or worsening morphologic abnormalities (e.g., teardrop or nucleated erythrocytes or immature leukocytes). A complete blood cell count (CBC) also should be performed monthly to evaluate new or worsening cytopenias. If a new or worsening morphologic abnormality or cytopenia develops, romiplostim should be discontinued and a bone marrow biopsy, with additional staining for fibrosis, should be considered.

Thrombocytopenia Following Romiplostim Discontinuance Thrombocytopenia may occur after discontinuance of romiplostim and may be more severe than prior to therapy. Worsening of thrombocytopenia may increase the risk of bleeding, especially if romiplostim is discontinued while patients are receiving concomitant antiplatelet or anticoagulation therapy. In clinical studies, a transient decrease in platelet count from baseline was reported in 7% of patients (4 of 57) following discontinuance of romiplostim; the worsened thrombocytopenia subsequently resolved within 14 days.

Following discontinuance of romiplostim, a CBC including platelet count should be performed weekly for at least 2 weeks. Additional ITP therapy should be considered for worsening thrombocytopenia.

Thrombosis or Thromboembolism An excessive increase in platelet count resulting from excessive dosages of romiplostim may be associated with the development of thrombosis or a thromboembolic complication. In randomized, controlled studies, the incidence of thrombotic/thromboembolic events was similar between romiplostim and placebo. In the single-arm extension study, thrombotic complications were reported in 4.9% of patients, with most cases (8 of 12) occurring when the platelet count was less than 400,000/mm^3 within 2 weeks before or after the occurrence of a thrombotic event. Preexisting risk factor(s) for thrombosis were identified for most (6 of 7) patients in the extension study who experienced a serious thrombotic complication. To minimize the risk of developing a thrombotic or thromboembolic complication, romiplostim should *not* be used to normalize platelet counts, but should only be used to maintain a platelet count of 50,000/mm^3 or greater according to the dosage adjustment guidelines.

Malignancy Romiplostim stimulates the TPO receptor present on the surface of hematopoietic cells and may possibly increase the risk for a hematologic malignancy, especially in patients with myelodysplastic syndrome (MDS). In randomized, placebo-controlled studies, the incidence of hematologic malignancy with romiplostim treatment was low and similar to that with placebo. In a single-arm study of 44 patients with myelodysplastic syndrome receiving romiplostim, 11 cases (25%) of possible disease progression were reported; 4 patients in this study were confirmed to have progression to acute myelogenous leukemia (AML) during follow-up. Romiplostim should not be used to treat or correct thrombocytopenia related to an underlying hematologic cause (e.g., myelodysplasia) or resulting from chemotherapy; romiplostim should only be used for thrombocytopenia associated with chronic ITP.

Laboratory Monitoring A CBC, including platelet count and peripheral blood smear, should be obtained prior to starting therapy and repeated weekly during the dosage adjustment phase, then monthly once a stable dosage has been achieved. Baseline peripheral blood smears should establish the presence and extent of red blood cell and leukocyte abnormalities. Once romiplostim is discontinued, a CBC with platelet count should be evaluated weekly for at least 2 weeks to monitor for worsening thrombocytopenia.

Lack or Loss of Response In cases of lack of response (i.e., hyporesponsiveness) or failure to maintain a platelet response, an evaluation of possible causative factors, including the presence of neutralizing antibodies to romiplostim or evidence of bone marrow fibrosis, should be considered. Blood samples for detection of antibody formation can be sent to Amgen to determine if antibodies to either romiplostim or TPO are present.

If the platelet count does not increase to a sufficient level after 4 weeks of treatment at the highest recommended dosage of 10 mcg/kg weekly, the manufacturer recommends that romiplostim be discontinued.

Immunogenicity Detection of antibodies to both romiplostim and TPO were evaluated in 236 ITP patients before and after treatment with romiplostim. At baseline, 7% of patients tested positive for antibodies to romiplostim; 5% had evidence of antibodies against TPO. After romiplostim treatment, 10% of patients had developed binding antibodies to romiplostim and 5% had developed binding antibodies to TPO. There was no evidence of cross-reactivity between the anti-romiplostim and the anti-TPO antibodies. Across all studies, the incidence of anti-romiplostim *neutralizing* antibodies was 0.4% (1 of 236 patients); no anti-TPO *neutralizing* antibodies were detected. No clinical impact on safety or efficacy was observed in patients who tested positive for antibodies.

Specific Populations **Pregnancy.** Category C. (See Users Guide.) No adequate and well-controlled studies in humans. However, thrombocytosis, postimplantation loss, and increased pup mortality have been reported in animals. Romiplostim should only be used in pregnant women if the anticipated clinical benefit outweighs the potential risk to the fetus.

To monitor maternal-fetal outcomes of pregnant women exposed to romiplostim, a pregnancy registry has been established. Clinicians are encouraged to register pregnant women receiving romiplostim in the registry; women also may enroll themselves in the registry by calling 1-887-Nplate1 (1-887-675-2831).

Lactation. It is not known if romiplostim is distributed into human milk; however, human immunoglobulin G antibody (IgG) is distributed into milk. Published data suggest that antibodies contained in breast milk do not enter neonatal and infant circulation in substantial amounts. Because many drugs are distributed into human milk and because of the potential for serious adverse reactions to romiplostim in nursing infants, a decision should be made whether to discontinue nursing or the drug, taking into account the importance of the drug to the woman.

Pediatric Use. Safety and efficacy have not been established in children younger than 18 years of age.

Geriatric Use. No substantial differences in safety and efficacy in geriatric patients 65 years of age or older relative to younger adults, but increased sensitivity cannot be ruled out.

Hepatic Impairment. Safety and efficacy in patients with hepatic impairment not studied specifically to date. Use with caution.

Renal Impairment. Safety and efficacy in patients with renal impairment not specifically studied to date. Use with caution.

■ **Common Adverse Effects** Adverse events reported in at least 10% of patients receiving romiplostim include arthralgia, dizziness, insomnia, myalgia, extremity pain, and abdominal pain. The most common adverse events reported with romiplostim during the extension study were headache, nasopharyngitis, confusion, and fatigue.

Drug Interactions

No formal drug interaction studies have been performed with romplostim.

Description

Romiplostim, a biosynthetic (recombinant DNA-derived) Fc-peptide fusion protein, is a thrombopoietin receptor agonist. Romiplostim binds to the thrombopoietin receptor (also known as cMp1) and activates intracellular transcriptional pathways leading to increased platelet production. Romiplostim is produced by recombinant DNA technology in *Escherichia coli* and contains 2 identical single-chain subunits, each consisting of human immunoglobulin IgG_1 Fc domain covalently linked at the C-terminus to a peptide containing 2 thrombopoietin receptor-binding domains. Romiplostim has no amino acid sequence homology to endogenous thrombopoietin.

Advice to Patients

Importance of providing patient with a copy of the manufacturer's patient information (medication guide) prior to each dose of romiplostim. Importance of carefully reading the medication guide before initiating therapy and prior to receiving each dose.

Importance of understanding that the goal of therapy is to achieve and maintain a platelet count of at least 50,000/mm^3 to reduce the risk of bleeding, not to normalize platelet counts.

Risk of worsening thrombocytopenia with possible bleeding following discontinuance of romiplostim compared with the risk prior to starting therapy; increased risk if patient is receiving concomitant anticoagulant or antiplatelet drugs.

Risk of reticulin fiber formation in bone marrow with possible progression to bone marrow fibrosis.

Risk of thrombosis or thromboembolism.

Risk of progression of underlying myelodysplastic syndrome (MDS) or hematologic malignancy.

Risk of adverse events associated with long-term administration not fully known.

Importance of avoiding situations or drug therapies that may increase risk of bleeding.

Importance of informing clinicians of existing or contemplated concomitant therapy, including prescription and OTC drugs and herbal supplements, as well as any concomitant illnesses.

Importance of women informing clinicians if they are or plan to become pregnant or plan to breast-feed. (See Pregnancy under Warnings/Precautions: Special Populations, in Cautions.)

Importance of informing patients of other important precautionary information. (See Cautions.)

Overview® (see Users Guide). For additional information on this drug until a more detailed monograph is developed and published, the manufacturer's labeling should be consulted. It is *essential* that the manufacturer's labeling be consulted for more detailed information on usual cautions, precautions, contraindications, potential drug interactions, laboratory test interferences, and acute toxicity.

Preparations

Excipients in commercially available drug preparations may have clinically important effects in some individuals; consult specific product labeling for details.

romiPLOStim

Parenteral

For injection, for subcutaneous use	375 mcg (to deliver 250 mcg)	**Nplate®**, Amgen
	625 mcg (to deliver 500 mcg)	**Nplate®**, Amgen

Selected Revisions August 2014,

Sargramostim

Granulocyte-Macrophage Colony-Stimulating Factor, GM-CSF, Recombinant Human GM-CSF, rHuGM-CSF

■ Sargramostim, a human granulocyte-macrophage colony-stimulating factor (GM-CSF), is a biosynthetic hematopoietic agent that affects the proliferation and differentiation of a variety of hematopoietic progenitor cells.

Uses

Sargramostim is used to accelerate myeloid recovery in adults undergoing autologous or allogeneic bone marrow transplantation (BMT), to mobilize hematopoietic progenitor cells into peripheral blood for collection by leukapheresis, and to accelerate myeloid engraftment following autologous peripheral blood progenitor cell (PBPC) transplantation. The drug also is used in an attempt to prolong survival in adults who have undergone allogeneic or autologous BMT and in whom engraftment is delayed or has failed and is used to accelerate neutrophil recovery and reduce the incidence of severe and life-threatening infections following induction chemotherapy in adults 55 years of age or older with acute myeloid (myelogenous, nonlymphocytic) leukemia (AML, ANLL). Sargramostim is designated an orphan drug by the US Food and Drug Administration (FDA) for use in BMT patients for the management of neutropenia associated with BMT, the promotion of early engraftment, and the treatment of delayed or failed engraftment and for use in patients with AML to reduce neutropenia and leukopenia and increase survival. Sargramostim also has been used in an effort to increase leukocyte counts in adults with myelodysplastic syndrome† (MDS) or aplastic anemia† and to correct or minimize neutropenia and/or drug-induced neutropenia in a variety of patients, including those with human immunodeficiency virus (HIV) infection† or congenital, cyclic, or acquired neutropenias†.

■ **Autologous Bone Marrow Transplantation** Sargramostim is used to accelerate myeloid recovery in adults with non-Hodgkin's lymphoma (NHL), acute lymphocytic (lymphoblastic) leukemia (ALL), or Hodgkin's disease undergoing cytotoxic chemotherapy and autologous bone marrow transplantation (BMT). Results of placebo-controlled studies in patients with lymphoid malignancy (non-Hodgkin's lymphoma, ALL) indicate that sargramostim therapy following autologous BMT effectively shortens the time to myeloid engraftment resulting in certain clinical benefits such as decreased duration of post-BMT infectious episodes, decreased requirements for anti-infective therapy, and decreased duration of hospitalization. In these studies, the median time to myeloid engraftment (defined as an absolute neutrophil count [ANC]of 500/mm^3 or more) following BMT was 18 days in those receiving sargramostim and 24 days in those receiving placebo. The median duration of infectious episodes (defined as fever and neutropenia; 2 positive blood cultures of the same organism; fever exceeding 38°C and one positive blood culture; or clinical evidence of infection) and hospitalization was 1 and 25 days, respectively, in patients receiving sargramostim and 4 and 31 days, respectively, in those receiving placebo. When sargramostim therapy was used following autologous BMT in patients with Hodgkin's disease, there also was a trend toward earlier myeloid engraftment compared with patients receiving placebo; however, the median time to engraftment in these patients generally is 6 days longer than the median time to engraftment in patients with non-Hodgkin's lymphoma or ALL.

Neutropenia still occurs in most patients during the first week following autologous BMT despite use of sargramostim therapy, and patients may be at substantial risk for infection during this time. Because sargramostim therapy generally does not completely prevent severe neutropenia following autologous BMT and may not shorten its duration sufficiently to reduce the incidence of infection associated with myeloablative therapy in all patients, benefit of the drug may be reflected principally in reducing the duration of fever, anti-infective therapy, and hospitalization. Results of uncontrolled studies indicate that sargramostim therapy following BMT is more effective in accelerating myeloid recovery in patients who receive bone marrow that is either unpurged or purged by anti-B lymphocyte monoclonal antibodies than in patients who receive bone marrow that is chemically purged. Patients who receive chemically purged bone marrow may not respond to sargramostim therapy if the chemical agents cause a clinically important decrease in the number of responsive hematopoietic progenitors. However, if the bone marrow purging process preserves a sufficient number of progenitors (i.e., more than 1.2×10^4 per kg), sargramostim therapy may provide a beneficial effect on myeloid engraftment. Patients who previously have received extensive radiation therapy or have been exposed to multiple myelotoxic agents may have a limited response to sargramostim therapy following autologous BMT. (See Drug Interactions: Myelosuppressive Therapy and Antineoplastic Agents.)

Results of a follow-up analysis of patients with non-Hodgkin's lymphoma, ALL, or Hodgkin's disease who received sargramostim to accelerate myeloid recovery following cytotoxic chemotherapy and BMT indicate that up to 30–40 months after the procedure patients who received the drug had no increased risk of graft failure, leukemogenesis, relapse, or death compared with those who received placebo. Sargramostim therapy appeared to cause no long-term deleterious effects on bone marrow function and had no appreciable effect on disease-free survival or overall survival. The only factors in these patients that appeared to be associated with a high risk of relapse over time or death were a diagnosis of lymphoid leukemia and/or undergoing BMT while in resistant relapse.

■ **Allogeneic Bone Marrow Transplantation** Sargramostim is used to accelerate myeloid recovery in patients undergoing allogeneic BMT from HLA-matched related donors. Sargramostim has been shown to safely and effectively accelerate myeloid engraftment, reduce the incidence of bacteremia and other infections, and shorten the median duration of hospitalization in these patients.

Preliminary studies evaluating use of sargramostim in patients undergoing allogeneic BMT were performed in a limited number of adults with chronic myelogenous leukemia (CML), AML, ALL, or severe aplastic anemia undergoing allogeneic BMT from HLA-matched siblings or unrelated donors†. In a phase I/II study in patients undergoing allogeneic BMT from HLA-matched siblings, patients who received methotrexate and cyclosporine for graft-versus-host disease prophylaxis were less responsive to sargramostim therapy than those who received prednisone and cyclosporine; patients in the latter group had fewer febrile days and were discharged sooner than patients who received methotrexate.

Efficacy of sargramostim has been evaluated in a prospective, randomized, placebo-controlled phase III study in 109 patients with myeloid malignancies (AML, CML), lymphoid malignancies (ALL, NHL), Hodgkin's disease, multiple myeloma, myelodysplastic disease, or aplastic anemia who received allogeneic BMT from HLA-matched related donors. Compared with the group that received placebo, patients who received sargramostim had a shorter time to neutrophil engraftment (ANC of 500/mm^3 or greater) and a shorter duration of hospitalization. The time to myeloid engraftment was 13 days in those who received sargramostim versus 17 days in those who received placebo. The number of patients who developed bacteremia and documented infections was lower in the sargramostim group compared with the placebo group. In addition, the incidence of grade 3/4 mucositis was lower and the median duration of post-transplant IV anti-infective therapy and median time to last platelet and red blood cell transfusion were shorter in patients who received sargramostim. There was no difference in the incidence or severity of graft-versus-host disease, relapse rate, or survival between patients who received sargramostim and those who received placebo.

Further study is needed to evaluate efficacy of sargramostim for use in patients receiving allogeneic BMT from unrelated donors†. In one phase II study in patients who received allogeneic BMT from unrelated donors†, sargramostim therapy (250 mcg/m^2 daily given by IV infusion over 2 hours beginning within 2 hours after allogeneic BMT and continued for 20–27 days), fewer infections occurred following BMT in patients who received the drug; however, sargramostim therapy did not have a clinically important effect on neutrophil recovery and it is unclear whether the decrease in infections was related directly to the drug.

Although there is a theoretical concern that biosynthetic GM-CSF therapy may increase graft failure or exacerbate graft-versus-host disease in patients undergoing allogeneic BMT, there is no evidence to date that use of sargramostim or regramostim in these patients increases the incidence of graft rejection or the incidence and/or severity of acute graft-versus-host disease.

■ **Peripheral Blood Progenitor Cell Transplantation** Sargramostim is used for mobilization of hematopoietic progenitor cells into peripheral blood for collection by leukapheresis and also is used to accelerate myeloid engraftment following autologous peripheral blood progenitor cell (PBPC) transplantation. Sargramostim mobilization allows for the collection of increased numbers of progenitor cells capable of engraftment compared with collection without mobilization. When these increased numbers of cells are transplanted following myeloablative chemotherapy, more rapid engraftment can occur reducing the need for supportive care. Use of sargramostim following autologous PBPC transplantation further accelerates myeloid reconstitution.

A retrospective review of data from patients with cancer (i.e., lymphoma, breast cancer, other malignancies) undergoing PBPC collection and autologous transplantation at a single US transplant center was conducted and data obtained from 4 groups of patients who received sargramostim for PBPC mobilization (n=196) were compared with data from an historical control group of patients who received nonmobilized PBPCs (n=100). Patients who received sargramostim were enrolled in several sequential trials and cohorts differed in sargramostim dosage (125 or 250 mcg/m^2 daily), route of administration of the drug (continuous IV infusion or subcutaneous injection), and use of sargramostim following PBPC transplantation. Leukaphereses were initiated for all mobilization groups after the leukocyte count reached 10,000/mm^3 and continued until both a minimum number of mononucleated cells (MNCs) were collected (6.5 or 8×10^8/kg) and a minimum number of phereses (5–8) were performed. Patients who received the higher dosage of sargramostim (250 mcg/m^2 daily) by either IV infusion or subcutaneous injection exhibited the most marked effects in terms of mobilization and posttransplant engraftment. PBPCs collected from patients who received sargramostim mobilization at this dosage had higher numbers of granulocyte-macrophage colony-forming units (CFU-GM) than those collected without mobilization. After collections were thawed, the mean CFU-GM content was 11.41×10^4/kg in those who received mobilization compared with 0.96×10^4/kg for nonmobilized patients. A similar difference was observed in the mean number of erythrocyte burst-forming units (BFU-E) collected in mobilized patients (23.96×10^4/kg) compared with nonmobilized patients (1.63×10^4/kg). Following autologous PBPC transplantation, the time to myeloid engraftment (ANC exceeding 500/mm^3) was shorter in those who received sargramostim mobilization and the time between transplantation and last platelet transfusion also was shorter in these patients. Administration of sargramostim following PBPC transplantation further accelerated neutrophil recovery. The median time to myeloid engraftment was 29 days in patients who did not receive sargramostim mobilization, 21 days in those who received sargramostim for PBPC mobilization but did not receive the drug following the PBPC transplantation, and 12 days in those who received sargramostim for mobilization and following transplantation. Mobilized patients had fewer days to the last red blood cell transfusion and a shorter duration of hospitalization than nonmobilized patients.

A retrospective review of data from patients undergoing PBPC transplantation at another transplant center was evaluated to determine the effect of different dosages of sargramostim on mobilization of PBPC. Sargramostim was administered by subcutaneous injection in a dosage of 250 mcg/m^2 once daily (n=10) or twice daily (n=21) until completion of aphereses. Apheresis was started on day 5 of sargramostim administration and continued until the targeted MNC count (9×10^8) or CD34$^+$ cell count (1×10^6/kg) was collected. There was no difference in CD34$^+$ cell count in patients receiving sargramostim once or twice daily and the median time to myeloid engraftment (ANC greater than 500/mm^3) was 12 days and the median time to platelet recovery (platelet count greater than 25,000/mm^3) was 23 days. Studies comparing mobilized patients to nonmobilized patients and to an historical group of BMT patients indicate that there is no difference in median survival time.

■ Bone Marrow Transplantation Failure or Engraftment Delay Sargramostim is used in an attempt to prolong survival in adults who have undergone allogeneic or autologous BMT and in whom engraftment is delayed or has failed. The drug also has been used in a limited number of patients with delayed engraftment following PBPC transplantation†. Patients with delayed engraftment following BMT may have a prolonged period of severe myelosuppression and an increased risk of infectious complications, including severe or fatal infections.

Use of sargramostim therapy in patients with engraftment delay or failure appears to safely and effectively prolong survival (in the presence or absence of infection). Efficacy of sargramostim has been evaluated in studies in patients with lymphoid or myeloid leukemia, non-Hodgkin's lymphoma, Hodgkin's disease, aplastic anemia, myelodysplasia, or nonhematologic malignancy who had a delay in engraftment (ANC less than 100/mm^3 by day 28 after transplantation), a delay in engraftment (ANC less than 100/mm^3 by day 21) with evidence of active infection, or loss of marrow graft after a transient engraftment (manifested as an average ANC of more than 500/mm^3 for at least 1 week followed by loss of engraftment with an ANC less than 500/mm^3 for at least 1 week beyond day 21 after transplantation). In patients with graft failure following autologous or allogeneic BMT, those receiving sargramostim had an increased rate of survival at 100 days compared with historical controls who did not receive the drug, and the median survival was twice that of historical controls. The median survival in patients with autologous or allogeneic failure was 474 or 97 days, respectively, in those who received sargramostim and 161 or 35 days, respectively, in historical controls who did not receive the drug. This increased survival generally occurred as a result of accelerated neutrophil recovery, which was associated with a decreased incidence of infectious complications.

Sargramostim therapy appears to be most effective in prolonging survival in patients with one or more of the following characteristics: autologous BMT failure or engraftment delay, no previous total body irradiation, a malignancy other than leukemia, and/or a multiple organ failure score of 2 or less (i.e., 0, 1, or 2 dysfunctional organ systems). In one study, patients with graft failure following BMT with autologous bone marrow that was either unpurged or purged using monoclonal antibodies generally responded to sargramostim therapy; however, patients with graft failure following BMT with autologous bone marrow that had been chemically purged (i.e., with perfosfamide (4- hydroperoxycyclophosphamide) or etoposide) did not respond to sargramostim therapy. There was no evidence that sargramostim therapy exacerbated graft-versus-host disease.

■ Acute Myelogenous Leukemia Sargramostim is used to accelerate neutrophil recovery and reduce the incidence of severe and life-threatening infections following induction chemotherapy in adults 55 years of age or older with acute myelogenous leukemia (AML). Safety and efficacy of sargramostim in patients with AML who are younger than 55 years of age have not been determined. Use of biosynthetic GM-CSFs in patients with acute leukemia has been controversial since results of in vitro studies indicate that certain leukemic cell lines have receptors for GM-CSF and that these drugs may have a stimulatory effect on leukemic blast cells in vitro. (See Pharmacology.) In a phase III randomized, placebo-controlled study in adults 55–70 years of age with newly diagnosed AML, use of sargramostim shortened the period of neutrophil recovery and improved the outcome of infectious complications following induction therapy with daunorubicin and cytarabine. The incidence of severe infections and deaths associated with the infections was reduced in patients who received sargramostim. In addition, disease outcome did not appear to be adversely affected by sargramostim therapy; however, further study is needed to assess the effect of the drug on response or survival. The median duration of absolute neutrophil count (ANC) less than 500/mm^3 or 1000/mm^3 was 13 or 14 days, respectively, in patients receiving sargramostim and 16 or 21 days, respectively, in those receiving placebo; there was no difference in duration of platelet counts less than 20,000/mm^3 or requirements for red blood cell transfusions. Although sargramostim therapy accelerated neutrophil recovery following 1 or 2 cycles of induction chemotherapy in adults with AML, the drug did not shorten the duration of neutropenia following cytarabine consolidation therapy in these patients.

Other biosynthetic GM-CSFs, molgramostim and regramostim, also have been used in adults with relapsed or refractory ALL or newly diagnosed or relapsed AML. When molgramostim was used in conjunction with remission induction therapy in patients with newly diagnosed AML, there was no clear evidence of accelerated neutrophil recovery or a decreased incidence of infection in these patients compared with use of induction therapy alone. In addition, in some patients, use of molgramostim appeared to decrease the in vivo sensitivity of AML blast cells to the chemotherapy regimen used (daunorubicin, cytarabine); it is unclear whether this effect was related to the effect of GM-CSF on the blast cells or was related to an effect on the pharmacokinetics of the chemotherapy agents. When molgramostim was used in patients with ALL, the drug appeared to effectively increase neutrophil counts without increasing the number of ALL blast cells.

While it has been suggested that biosynthetic GM-CSFs may be useful antileukemic agents secondary to their stimulation of leukemic differentiation or of proliferation of malignant leukemic cells, thereby increasing sensitivity of the cells to chemotherapy, such stimulation also might accelerate the malignancy. Therefore, some experts currently state that use of sargramostim in the treatment of myeloid leukemias should be considered investigational and undertaken with caution.

■ Myelodysplastic Syndromes and Aplastic Anemia Sargramostim has been used in an effort to increase leukocyte counts in some adults with myelodysplastic syndrome† (MDS) classified as refractory anemia (RA), refractory anemia with excess blasts (RAEB), or refractory anemia with excess blasts in transformation (RAEB-T). While the drug has shown some promise for this use, further study is needed to evaluate the benefits and risks of biosynthetic GM-CSF therapy in patients with MDS; pending accumulation of such data, this use generally should be limited to protocol conditions. MDS is a heterogeneous group of disorders and several factors (e.g., biologic characteristics of the leukemic clone, presence of an abnormal karyotype, or high initial leukemia burden) may result in considerable variation in response to sargramostim therapy. Use of sargramostim therapy in patients with MDS generally results in an increase in the absolute number of granulocytes and monocytes in most patients and an increase in the absolute number of eosinophils and lymphocytes in many patients. Although an increase in platelets and/or reticulocytes is evident in a few patients with MDS receiving sargramostim, platelet and reticulocyte counts are unaffected in most patients and the need for red blood cell transfusions generally is unchanged during therapy with the drug. Prolonged maintenance therapy with sargramostim appears necessary in patients with MDS since leukocyte counts return to pretreatment levels within 2–10 days after sargramostim is discontinued.

Whether use of sargramostim in patients with MDS will alter (either increase or decrease) the rate of progression to AML or affect the usually fatal outcome of the disease is unclear and requires further study. The rate of progression to AML in untreated patients with MDS is approximately 10–20%, 40–50%, or 60–75% in those with RA, RAEB, or RAEB-T, respectively. There is concern, but no clear evidence indicated to date, that use of biosynthetic GM-CSFs may stimulate progression to AML in patients with MDS since in vitro evidence indicates that the drugs can stimulate the growth of myeloid leukemic blast cells and because an increase in the percentage of leukemic blasts in both bone marrow and peripheral blood has occurred in some patients with MDS receiving sargramostim. Although filgrastim (a biosynthetic G-CSF) also has been used in the treatment of MDS, the relative efficacy of these two hematologic growth factors has not been evaluated to date in controlled studies.

Sargramostim has been used with some success in an effort to increase leukocyte counts in a limited number of adults and adolescents 15 years of age or older with moderate to severe aplastic anemia†. Other biosynthetic GM-CSFs, molgramostim and regramostim, also have been used with some success in the treatment of aplastic anemia in adults and children 1 year of age and older†. Use of biosynthetic GM-CSFs in these patients resulted in an increase in ANCs that was sustained throughout the period of treatment and a transient increase in absolute eosinophil counts; most patients also had an increase in monocyte and lymphocyte counts. Erythrocyte and platelet counts and transfusion requirements generally were unaffected, although a few patients had increases in hemoglobin concentrations and/or platelet counts. In a limited number of patients, low doses of molgramostim (approximately 20–25% lower than those used in other studies) appeared to be effective in increasing neutrophil counts in a some patients with aplastic anemia when used alone or in conjunction with epoetin alfa (a recombinant erythropoietin); addition of epoetin alfa to the regimen resulted in an increase in the hemoglobin level in addition to an increase in the neutrophil count. Further study is needed to evaluate more fully use of sargramostim in aplastic anemia and to determine the optimum dosage and long-term safety and efficacy of the drug in these patients; pending accumulation of such data, this use generally should be limited to protocol conditions. Studies are ongoing to determine whether the increase in neutrophil counts resulting from GM-CSF therapy is associated with a decrease in infection and/or increased survival in patients with aplastic anemia.

■ Neutropenia associated with HIV Infection and Antiretroviral Therapy Sargramostim and other biosynthetic GM-CSFs (molgramostim, regramostim) have been used in patients with human immunodeficiency virus (HIV) infection in an effort to correct or minimize HIV-associated neutropenia† and/or for the treatment of drug-induced neutropenia (e.g., neutropenia associated with use of zidovudine, interferon alfa, and/or cytotoxic chemotherapy) in HIV-infected patients†. When used in patients with HIV infection, biosynthetic GM-CSFs effectively increase the number of neutrophils, monocytes, and eosinophils in most patients; however, the drugs appear to have no consistent effect on the absolute number of lymphocytes nor on the ratio of helper/inducer ($CD4^+$, $T4^+$) to suppressor/cytotoxic ($CD8^+$, $T8^+$) T cells.

There has been some concern about use of sargramostim or other biosynthetic GM-CSFs in patients with HIV infection since results of some in vitro studies indicate that, unlike filgrastim (a biosynthetic G-CSF), GM-CSFs can stimulate replication of some strains of HIV in vitro. (See Pharmacology: Effects on Other Cells.) However, there is no evidence to date that HIV-infected patients are at risk of increased viral load or clinical deterioration if sargramostim is used concomitantly with zidovudine. Further study is needed to determine the effect of concomitant use of sargramostim with nucleoside reverse transcriptase inhibitors and other antiretroviral agents (e.g., HIV protease inhibitors, nonnucleoside reverse transcriptase inhibitors). There is some evidence from in vitro studies that biosynthetic GM-CSFs may enhance the antiretroviral effect of zidovudine. (See Drug Interactions: Antiretroviral Agents.)

Studies are ongoing to evaluate the use of sargramostim in adults or children to minimize the hematologic toxicity of zidovudine. Studies also are ongoing to determine whether sargramostim and/or other hematologic growth factors can minimize hematologic toxicity associated with other anti-infective agents used in patients with HIV infection (e.g., ganciclovir, co-trimoxazole, sulfadoxine, pyrimethamine).

■ **Congenital, Cyclic, and Acquired Neutropenias** Sargramostim has been used with variable success in an effort to increase neutrophil counts in patients with various primary neutropenias, including congenital neutropenia†, acquired idiopathic neutropenia†, and glycogen storage disease type Ib†. In addition, another biosynthetic GM-CSF, molgramostim, has been used with some success in patients with congenital neutropenia, cyclic neutropenia, acquired idiopathic neutropenia, or autoimmune neutropenia. While biosynthetic GM-CSFs may ameliorate the underlying neutropenia in certain patients with these conditions, this effect is unpredictable and not all patients with primary neutropenias respond to the drugs. Filgrastim (a biosynthetic G-CSF) has effectively increased neutrophil counts in some patients with severe congenital neutropenia, chronic idiopathic neutropenia, or cyclic neutropenia who did not respond to sargramostim therapy. In addition, it has been suggested that filgrastim may be more effective than sargramostim or other biosynthetic GM-CSFs in the treatment of primary neutropenia since filgrastim therapy results in more consistent increases in the neutrophil count and does not cause eosinophilia.

In a study in children 1–19 years of age with severe congenital neutropenia (Kostmann syndrome), sargramostim therapy resulted in an increase in the absolute granulocyte count in all patients. However, an increase in the ANC occurred in only one patient; in most patients, the increase in granulocytes during sargramostim therapy resulted from an increase in eosinophils or monocytes rather than neutrophils. When sargramostim was used in a few patients with glycogen storage disease type Ib, neutrophil counts increased during therapy with the drug and there was a decrease in inflammatory bowel symptoms. Use of sargramostim in a patient with idiopathic neutropenia also resulted in an increase in the neutrophil count. Molgramostim has effectively increased the neutrophil count in some patients with cyclic neutropenia, congenital neutropenia, and autoimmune neutropenia. However, when used in a patient with acquired neutropenia, molgramostim was ineffective in increasing the neutrophil count; the patient subsequently received filgrastim, which effectively increased the neutrophil count.

■ **Chemotherapy-induced Neutropenia** Biosynthetic GM-CSFs have been used in patients with malignancies receiving myelosuppressive antineoplastic therapy in an attempt to increase neutrophil counts and decrease the risk of infectious complications†. Myelosuppression is a major factor contributing to infection, morbidity (including that requiring hospitalization), and mortality in patients with malignancies undergoing chemotherapy and is a major dose-limiting factor in many chemotherapy regimens. Sargramostim has been used prophylactically (i.e., in the absence of fever or other manifestations of infection) in a limited number of children with refractory solid tumors who were receiving myelosuppressive therapy†. Use of sargramostim in these children ameliorated the chemotherapy-induced neutropenia and decreased the frequency and/or duration of hospitalization and requirements for anti-infective therapy. Although there are no controlled studies to date evaluating efficacy of sargramostim in decreasing the risk of infectious complications in patients with malignancy undergoing cytotoxic chemotherapy, several studies have been performed using molgramostim or regramostim in patients with various malignancies, including non-Hodgkin's lymphoma, small cell lung cancer, sarcoma, urothelial tumors, germ cell tumors, breast cancer, ovarian carcinoma, and colon cancer. Results of studies using molgramostim or regramostim indicate that biosynthetic GM-CSF therapy produces a beneficial effect on neutrophil recovery in patients with chemotherapy-induced neutropenia and may decrease the duration of hospitalization and requirements for anti-infective therapy in some patients. However, substantial, cost-effective clinical benefit, including possible effects on survival and quality of life, may be more difficult to establish. Such benefit appears particularly difficult to establish if CSF therapy is reserved for active treatment of neutropenia and fever rather than for prophylactic therapy. Some evidence suggests that CSFs (e.g., filgrastim) can be cost-effective, at least in certain patient groups, but additional study is needed to define further patient selection criteria.

Although use of biosynthetic GM-CSFs in patients with chemotherapy-induced neutropenia appears promising and may decrease the need to withhold courses and/or reduce dosages of chemotherapy and also may permit dose intensification in some patients, further study is needed to evaluate use of sargramostim in these patients. The fact that GM-CSF therapy is associated with intermittent low-grade fevers in a large percentage of patients(see Cautions: Flu-like Syndrome) should be considered if sargramostim is used in patients with chemotherapy-induced neutropenia since this adverse effect of the drug could complicate decision-making concerning use of empiric anti-infective agent therapy in these patients. Filgrastim (a biosynthetic G-CSF) has been used more extensively to date than biosynthetic GM-CSFs in patients with chemotherapy-induced neutropenia. In addition, intermittent low-grade fevers have not been reported to date with filgrastim therapy.

■ **Other Uses** Biosynthetic GM-CSFs have been used to increase neutrophil counts in patients with cytomegalovirus (CMV) infection who develop neutropenia while receiving ganciclovir†. Although further study is needed, preliminary review of an ongoing phase II study evaluating use of combined ganciclovir and biosynthetic GM-CSF compared with the use of ganciclovir alone in patients with HIV infection and CMV retinitis suggests that patients who receive GM-CSF have fewer and less severe neutropenic episodes and shorter intervals when ganciclovir therapy must be interrupted because of severe neutropenia compared with patients who receive the antiviral agent alone.Sargramostim effectively increased the neutrophil count in at least one patient with CMV interstitial pneumonitis who developed ganciclovir-associated neutropenia. Molgramostim has been used effectively in at least one renal transplant patient with CMV infection and ganciclovir-associated neutropenia and one patient with dyskeratosis congenita who developed neutropenia while receiving ganciclovir for the treatment of CMV. While the precise role of GM-CSF therapy in such patients remains to be established and additional experience is needed, some clinicians state that this use is promising.

Biosynthetic GM-CSFs also have been used with some success in an attempt to increase neutrophil counts in a few patients with other nonmalignant conditions† who developed neutropenia while receiving myelosuppressive drugs. However, pending further accumulation of data, many clinicians state that use of the drugs in any of the following conditions generally should be considered investigational and confined to research protocols.

Sargramostim and molgramostim have been used effectively in several patients to hasten recovery from sulfasalazine-associated agranulocytosis†; biosynthetic GM-CSFs also have been used effectively to treat methimazole-associated agranulocytosis in at least one patient with hyperthyroidism†. In at least one patient with adult-onset juvenile rheumatoid arthritis, a biosynthetic GM-CSF appeared to effectively treat aplastic anemia associated with the use of gold therapy.

Biosynthetic GM-CSFs have been used in a limited number of patients with rheumatoid arthritis for the treatment of neutropenia associated with Felty's syndrome or large granular lymphocytic leukemia†. In at least one patient with Felty's syndrome, molgramostim therapy resulted in an increase in neutrophil count and appeared to contribute to resolution of an infectious complication; use of GM-CSF in another patient with Felty's syndrome reportedly was associated with a flare-up of arthritis.

In at least one patient with aplastic anemia who had unremitting psoriasis of more than 40 years' duration, GM-CSF therapy initiated for the treatment of the anemia apparently contributed to remission of the dermatologic condition†.

Dosage and Administration

■ **Reconstitution and Administration** Sargramostim is administered by IV infusion or subcutaneous injection. Subcutaneous injection is the most convenient for self-administration and is especially useful when prolonged maintenance is necessary.

Sargramostim should be administered under the guidance and supervision of a clinician, but may be *self-administered*outside of a hospital or medical office setting (e.g., at home) if the clinician determines that the patient and/or caregiver is competent to prepare and safely administer the drug. If home use is prescribed, patients and/or caregivers should be instructed on proper dosage, reconstitution procedures, and administration of the drug. They should also be cautioned against reuse of syringes and needles and diluent and instructed on proper disposal of such equipment using puncture-resistant containers.

Commercially available sargramostim lyophilized powder should be reconstituted prior to administration by adding 1 mL of sterile or bacteriostatic water for injection to a vial labeled as containing 250 mcg of the drug to provide a solution containing 250 mcg/mL. During reconstitution, the diluent should be directed at the side of the vial and the contents gently swirled to avoid foaming during dissolution; the vial should not be shaken and excessive or vigorous agitation should be avoided. To ensure the correct final concentration, care should be used to eliminate any air bubbles from the needle hub of the syringe containing the diluent.

For subcutaneous injection, sargramostim injection or reconstituted solutions of sargramostim should be administered without further dilution. For IV infusion, sargramostim injection or reconstituted solutions of sargramostim may be further diluted in 0.9% sodium chloride injection. If the final concentration of the sargramostim solution will be less than 10 mcg/mL, albumin human should be added to the 0.9% sodium chloride injection to a final concentration of 1 mg/mL (0.1%) to minimize adsorption of the drug to the components of the drug delivery system. This can be accomplished by adding 1 mg of albumin human per 1 mL of the infusion solution (e.g., dilute 1 mL of 5% albumin human in 50 mL of 0.9% sodium chloride injection).

IV infusions of sargramostim generally are infused over 2–4 hours. The drug also has been administered by IV infusion over 30–60 minutes or over 5–12 hours or by continuous IV infusion over 24 hours. Sargramostin should *not* be infused using an in-line membrane filter since adsorption of the drug could occur.

Sargramostim lyophilized powder contains no preservatives. The manufacturer recommends that sargramostim solutions be refrigerated and any unused solutions reconstituted with sterile water for injection be discarded after 6 hours; solutions reconstituted with bacteriostatic water for injection should be discarded if not used within 20 days. (See Chemistry and Stability: Stability.) Commercially available vials of sargramostim lyophilized powder are intended for single use only and should not be reentered or reused.

Prior to administration, solutions of sargramostim should be inspected visually for particulate matter and/or discoloration and discarded if either is present.

■ **Dosage** The fact that the various biosynthetic GM-CSFs have different specific activities and potencies when considered on a weight-to-weight basis should be considered if published clinical studies are consulted for dosage information on sargramostim. Because of differences in glycosylation, dosages of molgramostim (bacteria-derived, nonglycosylated GM-CSF) or regramostim (mammalian-derived, glycosylated GM-CSF) used in clinical studies should *not* be considered appropriate dosages for sargramostim (yeast-derived, glycosylated GM-CSF). Sargramostim currently is the only biosynthetic GM-CSF commercially available in the US.

If a severe adverse reaction occurs during sargramostim therapy, the dosage can be reduced or the drug temporarily discontinued until the reaction abates; if blast cells appear or disease progression occurs, sargramostim therapy should be discontinued. (See Cautions: Precautions and Contraindications.) If the absolute neutrophil count exceeds 20,000/mm^3, sargramostim therapy should be interrupted or the daily dose reduced by half.

Patients Undergoing Bone Marrow Transplantation When sargramostim is used to accelerate myeloid recovery in patients with non-Hodgkin's lymphoma, acute lymphocytic (lymphoblastic) leukemia, or Hodgkin's disease undergoing autologous bone marrow transplantation (BMT) or patients undergoing allogeneic BMT from HLA-matched related donors, the recommended dosage is 250 mcg/m^2 given once daily by IV infusion over 2 hours. Sargramostim therapy should be started 2–4 hours after BMT infusion (but no sooner than 24 hours after the last course of radiation therapy or the last dose of chemotherapy). Sargramostim therapy should not be initiated until the post-transplantation absolute neutrophil count (ANC) is less than 500/mm^3 and should be continued until the ANC is greater than 1500/mm^3 for 3 consecutive days. If a severe adverse reaction occurs, dosage can be reduced 50% or the drug temporarily discontinued until the reaction abates. Sargramostim should be discontinued immediately if blast cells appear or disease progression occurs.

Peripheral Blood Progenitor Cell Transplantation When sargramostim is used to mobilize hematopoietic progenitor cells into peripheral blood for collection by leukapheresis, the recommended dosage is 250 mcg/m^2 given by continuous IV infusion over 24 hours or by subcutaneous injection once daily. This dosage should be continued throughout the period of peripheral blood progenitor cell (PBPC) collection. The optimal schedule for PBPC collection has not been established; however, in clinical studies, PBPC collection usually was started by day 5 and performed daily until protocol-specified targets were achieved (see Uses: Peripheral Blood Progenitor Cell Transplantation). Sargramostim dosage should be reduced 50% if the leukocyte count increases to more than 50,000/mm^3. If adequate numbers of progenitor cells are not collected, other mobilization therapy should be considered.

When sargramostim is used to accelerate myeloid engraftment following autologous PBPC transplantation, the recommended dosage is 250 mcg/m^2 daily given by continuous IV infusion over 24 hours or by subcutaneous injection once daily beginning immediately following infusion of PBPC and continuing until the ANC is greater than 1500/mm^3 for 3 consecutive days.

Bone Marrow Transplantation Failure or Engraftment Delay When sargramostim is used in patients who have undergone allogeneic or autologous BMT and in whom engraftment is delayed or has failed, the recommended initial dosage is 250 mcg/m^2 given once daily by IV infusion over 2 hours. Sargramostim therapy is continued for 14 consecutive days in these patients and then discontinued for 7 consecutive days. If after this 7-day period engraftment has not occurred, a second 14-day course of sargramostim therapy can be given. If engraftment still has not occurred after the second course of therapy, a third 14-day course of the drug may be given after a 7-day interval using a dosage of 500 mcg/m^2 given once daily by IV infusion over 2 hours. If no improvement is observed after the third course of sargramostim therapy, it is unlikely that further dose escalation will be beneficial. If a severe adverse reaction occurs, dosage can be reduced 50% or the drug temporarily discontinued until the reaction abates. Sargramostim should be discontinued immediately if blast cells appear or disease progression occurs.

Acute Myelogenous Leukemia When sargramostim is used to accelerate neutrophil recovery following induction chemotherapy in adults 55 years of age or older with acute myelogenous leukemia, the recommended initial dosage is 250 mcg/m^2 given once daily by IV infusion over 4 hours. Sargramostim therapy should be started on approximately day 11 or 4 days following completion of induction therapy and should be used only if the bone marrow is hypoplastic with less than 5% blasts on day 10. If a second cycle of induction chemotherapy is necessary, sargramostim therapy should be started approximately 4 days after completion of chemotherapy and used only if the bone marrow is hypoplastic with less than 5% blasts. Sargramostim therapy should be continued until the absolute neutrophil count (ANC) is greater than 1500/mm^3 for 3 consecutive days or continued for a maximum of 42 days. The drug should be discontinued immediately if leukemia regrowth occurs. If a severe adverse reaction to sargramostim occurs, dosage should be reduced by 50% or the drug discontinued temporarily until the reaction abates. To avoid potential complications of excessive leukocytosis, CBCs should be performed twice weekly during sargramostim therapy and the drug temporarily discontinued or dosage redcued by 50% if the ANC exceeds 20,000/mm^3.

Myelodysplastic Syndromes and Aplastic Anemia When used to increase neutrophil counts in adults with myelodysplastic syndrome (MDS)†, sargramostim dosages of 15–500 mcg/m^2 have been given once daily by IV infusion over 1–12 hours or dosages of 30–500 mcg/m^2 have been given by continuous IV infusion over 24 hours. When used in adults with moderate to severe aplastic anemia†, sargramostim has been given in a dosage of 15–480 mcg/m^2 by IV infusion over 1–12 hours or in a dosage of 120–500 mcg/m^2 by continuous IV infusion over 24 hours. Additional study is needed to evaluate more fully the role of sargramostim in patients with MDS or aplastic anemia and to determine optimum dosage of the drug for these patients.

Neutropenia associated with HIV Infection If sargramostim is used in neutropenic individuals with human immunodeficiency virus (HIV) infection in an attempt to reduce the risk of bacterial infections†, some clinicians recommend that adults or adolescents receive a dosage of 250 mcg/m^2 given by IV infusion or subcutaneous injection once daily for 2–4 weeks.

Cautions

Sargramostim generally is well tolerated at usually recommended dosages. Adverse effects reported most frequently in patients receiving sargramostim include mild to moderate fever, asthenia, chills, headache, nausea, diarrhea, myalgia, and bone pain. Many of these adverse effects appear to be dose related and are reversible when sargramostim is discontinued. Patients should be informed of the most common and potentially serious adverse effects associated with sargramostim. Information on safety and efficacy of biosynthetic GM-CSFs generally has been obtained from clinical studies in patients with malignancy or other serious underlying disease who received a wide range of dosages of various biosynthetic GM-CSF formulations. Because many adverse effects that have been reported in patients receiving biosynthetic GM-CSFs also occur in patients not receiving the drugs, the causal relationship between the drugs and many of these adverse effects is not clear. In placebo- controlled studies in autologous bone marrow or peripheral stem cell transplant recipients, only diarrhea, asthenia, rash, and malaise occurred in sargramostim-treated patients at a frequency that exceeded that of placebo recipients by at least 5%. In a placebo-controlled study in adults 55–70 years of age with acute myelogenous leukemia, adverse effects associated with the skin were the only reactions reported more frequently in those receiving sargramostim.

The fact that some adverse effects reported in clinical studies may be related to the specific GM-CSF formulation used should be considered. The various biosynthetic GM-CSF formulations studied include sargramostim (yeast-derived, glycosylated GM-CSF), molgramostim (bacteria-derived, nonglycosylated GM-CSF), and regramostim (mammalian-derived, glycosylated GM-CSF); in some studies, it is unclear which biosynthetic GM-CSF was used. Although it has been suggested that sargramostim may be associated with a lower incidence of adverse effects than either molgramostim or regramostim, there have been no controlled studies directly comparing the safety and efficacy of the various biosynthetic GM-CSFs. Sargramostim currently is the only biosynthetic GM-CSF commercially available in the US.

An increased incidence of syncope with or without hypotension has been reported in temporal association with administration of sargramostim as a previously available injection containing the preservative edetate disodium (EDTA). A similar increase in such effects has not been observed with the commercially available lyophilized powder for injection that does not contain EDTA. Because of the potential for increased adverse effects, the manufacturer has withdrawn EDTA-containing sargramostim injection from the US market and reformulated the injection without EDTA. (See Preparations.)

■ **Flu-like Syndrome** A flu-like syndrome has been reported in many patients receiving sargramostim or other biosynthetic GM-CSF. Manifestations include mild to moderate fever, fatigue, malaise, asthenia, chills, headache, myalgia, and GI complaints. These manifestations generally are controllable with antipyretics and analgesics and disappear following completion or discontinuance of biosynthetic GM-CSF therapy. In controlled studies in adults undergoing autologous bone marrow transplantation or peripheral blood progenitor cell (PBPC) transplantation, asthenia and malaise occurred in 66 and 57%, respectively, of patients receiving sargramostim and in 51% of patients receiving placebo.

Intermittent low-grade fever (38–40°C), which may be associated with chills and/or rigors, has been reported in a large percentage of patients receiving sargramostim or other biosynthetic GM-CSF; in many cases, it was unclear whether fever during GM-CSF therapy was related to the drug or to infection in the neutropenic patients receiving the drug. This may complicate decision-making concerning use of empiric anti-infective agent therapy in these patients.

In controlled studies in adults undergoing autologous bone marrow transplantation or PBPC transplantation, fever occurred in 95% of patients receiving sargramostim and 96% of patients receiving placebo. Some clinicians suggest that fever that occurs with the first dose of biosynthetic GM-CSF, appears during the rapid increase in leukocyte count in the absence of systemic symptoms of infection, and resolves during continued treatment with the drug or within 24 hours after completion of GM-CSF therapy is probably related to the drug. Fever usually responds to treatment with acetaminophen or a nonsteroidal anti-inflammatory agent, although pretreatment with one of these agents may or may not prevent its development. Occasionally, opiate agonists have been used to manage severe shaking chills and rigors.

■ **Respiratory Effects** Various adverse respiratory effects have been reported in patients receiving biosynthetic GM-CSFs. Pulmonary infiltrates, pleural effusion, dyspnea, interstitial pneumonitis, lung disorder, and sequestration of granulocytes in the pulmonary circulation have been reported in patients receiving sargramostim. Acute bronchospasm, pulmonary infiltrates, pleuritis, pleural effusions, and diffuse alveolar hemorrhage have been reported in some patients receiving molgramostim; hypoxemia, dyspnea, bilateral pleural effusion, pulmonary infiltration, and pulmonary emboli have been reported rarely in patients receiving regramostim.

A severe first-dose reaction, characterized by respiratory distress, transient hypoxia, and symptomatic hypotension with flushing, fever, musculoskeletal aches or pains, tachycardia, bradycardia, dyspnea, involuntary leg spasms, nausea, and vomiting, has occurred in some patients receiving molgramostim or regramostim. This reaction generally occurs within 15 minutes to 3 hours after the first dose and may resolve within 2–4 hours. Severity of the reaction does not appear to be dose related; however, the reaction may appear more quickly with higher dosage than with lower dosage. In addition, first-dose reactions generally are more severe and have been reported more frequently with IV than with subcutaneous administration of molgramostim or regramostim. The first-dose reaction may recur with the first dose of each cycle of therapy, and patients who have had the reaction are at increased risk for subsequent reactions with future use of the drugs.

Although individual manifestations of the first-dose reaction (e.g., pulmonary infiltrates, hypotension with flushing and syncope, tachycardia, bone pain) have been reported following initiation of sargramostim therapy, severe first-dose reactions like those reported with molgramostim and regramostim have not been reported to date with sargramostim. In reported cases of hypotension with flushing and syncope following administration of the first dose of sargramostim, symptoms resolved with symptomatic treatment and did not recur with subsequent doses in the same cycle of treatment. If a first-dose reaction occurs, it should be treated empirically with oxygen, IV fluids, and acetaminophen or a nonsteroidal anti-inflammatory agent. Limited evidence has failed to show a benefit of pretreatment with acetaminophen, nonsteroidal anti-inflammatory agents, corticosteroids, and/or histamine H_1 and H_2 antagonists prior to initiation of molgramostim or regramostim therapy in an attempt to prevent the first-dose reaction. In some cases, the onset was delayed and the number and severity of manifestations were decreased when the drug was administered by subcutaneous injection rather than IV infusion.

■ **Fluid Retention** Edema, capillary leak syndrome, and pleural and/or pericardial effusion have been reported in patients receiving sargramostim, and use of the drug in patients with preexisting pleural and/or pericardial effusions may aggravate fluid retention. In controlled studies in adults undergoing autologous bone marrow transplantation or PBPC transplantation, peripheral edema occurred in 11% of patients receiving sargramostim (250 mcg/m^2 daily by IV infusion over 2 hours) and 7% of those receiving placebo; pleural or pericardial effusions occurred in 1–4% of those receiving the drug and 0–1% of those receiving placebo. Capillary leak syndrome appears to occur in less than 1% of patients receiving sargramostim. Fluid retention associated with or aggravated by sargramostim therapy generally is reversible when dosage is reduced or therapy with the drug is interrupted; improvement generally occurs regardless of whether diuretic therapy is initiated. Manifestations of fluid retention also have been reported in patients receiving molgramostim or regramostim.

The mechanism of fluid retention and capillary leak syndrome during biosynthetic GM-CSF therapy is unclear; however, these adverse effects appear to be dose related and may also be related to the route of administration of the drugs. It has been suggested that fluid retention during GM-CSF therapy may be mediated indirectly by tumor necrosis factor since GM-CSF has been shown to enhance neutrophil production of tumor necrosis factor in vitro and increase levels of tumor necrosis factor in patients receiving the drug.

■ **Dermatologic and Sensitivity Reactions** Rash has been reported in patients receiving sargramostim. In controlled studies in adults undergoing autologous bone marrow transplantation or PBPC transplantation, rash occurred in 44% of patients receiving sargramostim and 38% of those receiving placebo. Rash, pruritus, and generalized edema and erythema also have been reported in patients receiving molgramostim or regramostim and occasionally have been severe enough to require discontinuance of the drugs. In some patients, rash that developed during molgramostim therapy was described as raised, erythematous eczematous eruptions associated with pruritus and was followed by marked desquamation after discontinuance of the drug; in other patients, rash was described as diffuse erythematous areas resembling viral exanthema. Occasionally, such eruptions may persist for several weeks after discontinuance of GM-CSF therapy. Severe, generalized pruritus that did not respond to systemic antihistamine or topical corticosteroid therapy has occurred in several patients receiving molgramostim. Some evidence suggests that generalized rash may be more common following IV than subcutaneous administration. Atopic dermatitis, leucocytoclastic vasculitis, and necrotizing vasculitis also have been reported rarely in patients receiving biosynthetic GM-CSFs; in a patient who received molgramostim, hypersensitivity vasculitis with dyspnea, fever, and arthralgia appeared to be temporally associated with administration of the drug. In at least one case, leucocytoclastic vasculitis during regramostim therapy appeared to be related to high neutrophil counts and enhanced adherence of the cells to vascular endothelium. Some clinicians suggest that biosynthetic GM-CSFs be used with caution in patients with preexisting autoimmune or inflammatory dermatologic conditions.

Development of anti-GM-CSF antibodies has been reported occasionally in patients receiving sargramostim or molgramostim. In a study in patients with a variety of underlying diseases who received multiple courses of sargramostim by continuous IV infusion or subcutaneous injection over a 28- to 84-day period, neutralizing antibodies developed in 2.3% of patients. Patients who developed antibodies to GM-CSF in this study had impaired hematopoiesis prior to administration of sargramostim and the effect of antibody development on normal hematopoiesis could not be assessed. In another study, anti-GM-CSF antibodies developed in 4 out of 16 patients receiving sargramostim and were detectable within 7 days after initiation of therapy with the drug; in vitro evaluation of these antibodies indicated that they were cross-reactive with molgramostim but not regramostim. Anti-GM-CSF antibodies developed in 1 out of 75 patients with Crohn's disease receiving sargramostim by subcutaneous injection; such patients had normal hematopoiesis and were not taking any other immunosuppressive drugs. The clinical importance of these anti-GM-CSF antibodies has not been determined to date and it is unclear whether their presence could adversely affect efficacy of sargramostim. Therefore, the possibility that formation of anti-GM-CSF antibodies during sargramostim therapy theoretically could result in drug-induced neutropenia, neutralization of endogenous GM-CSF activity, or decreased effectiveness of sargramostim should be considered.

The manufacturer states that serious allergic or anaphylactic reactions have been reported in patients receiving sargramostim; the rate of occurrence of anti-GM-CSF antibodies in these patients has not been assessed. If any serious allergic or anaphylactic reaction occurs during sargramostim therapy, the drug should be discontinued immediately and appropriate therapy initiated.

■ **Local Reactions** Mild phlebitis has been reported rarely in patients receiving sargramostim by IV infusion and has also been reported in patients receiving IV regramostim. Although not reported to date with sargramostim, thrombosis at the IV catheter tip or site of administration has been reported rarely in patients receiving IV molgramostim or IV regramostim. It has been suggested that such thrombosis may occur because high concentrations of biosynthetic GM-CSF at the site cause local accumulation of activated neutrophils that bind and damage vascular endothelium and promote thrombus formation. IV administration of molgramostim or regramostim also has resulted in local erythema, rash, and pruritus at the site of injection in a high percentage of patients. In some patients, IV administration of molgramostim resulted in erythematous macules and papules (with or without pruritus) that lasted 3–4 weeks after discontinuance of the drug.

Subcutaneous injection of biosynthetic GM-CSFs has been associated with transient, erythematous eruptions and induration at the site of administration; however, it is unclear whether any specific derivative is associated with this adverse effect more frequently than the others. In a study in patients receiving regramostim by subcutaneous injection, local reactions occurred at the injection site in almost all patients. In another study in patients receiving molgramostim by subcutaneous injection, local erythema and tenderness occurred in 42% of patients. In some patients, erythematous lesions occur after each subcutaneous dose of biosynthetic GM-CSF, and even may recur at previous sites of injection not proximal to the current site; in other patients, the lesions occur only after initial injections. These lesions generally last 3–5 days, and results of skin biopsies indicate the presence of nonspecific perivascular lymphocytic infiltrates with large numbers of eosinophils. In at least one patient receiving molgramostim, severe necrotizing vasculitis occurred at the site of subcutaneous injection.

■ **GI Effects** Adverse GI effects, including nausea, vomiting, and abdominal cramps, have been reported in patients receiving sargramostim; however, it is unclear whether these effects were related to therapy with the drug. In controlled studies in adults undergoing autologous bone marrow transplantation or PBPC transplantation, nausea, diarrhea, vomiting, anorexia, GI disorder, GI hemorrhage, and stomatitis occurred in 24–90% of patients receiving sargramostim and 29–96% of those receiving placebo. Diarrhea was the only adverse GI effect that was reported more frequently in patients receiving sargramostim than in patients receiving placebo.

■ **Hematologic Effects** Sargramostim therapy may result in a rapid rise in leukocyte count. Marked leukocytosis (leukocyte counts of 100,000/mm^3 or greater) has been reported occasionally in patients receiving usual dosage of the drug (i.e., 250 mcg/m^2 daily). Excessive blood counts generally return to normal or baseline levels within 3–7 days following interruption of sargramostim therapy. The manufacturer recommends that leukocyte counts be monitored in patients receiving sargramostim to avoid any potential complications of excessive leukocytosis and that adjustment in dosage be made accordingly. (See Cautions: Precautions and Contraindications.) Sargramostim therapy causes a dose-related eosinophilia and monocytosis in many patients. Eosinophil and monocyte counts may be 2–6 times higher than pretreatment levels; in some patients, eosinophilia may be substantial, reaching levels associated with hypereosinophilic syndrome. Despite such increases, however, eosinophilia and monocytosis have not been associated with clinically important adverse effects, and eosinophil and monocyte counts rapidly return to pretreatment levels after sargramostim therapy is discontinued.

Various effects on platelet counts have been reported in patients receiving biosynthetic GM-CSFs. In most patients receiving biosynthetic GM-CSFs, platelet counts are not affected substantially. In some patients, there is an initial decrease in platelets during the first 5 days of therapy and then a return to pretreatment levels during the next 5–10 days; in addition, thrombocytopenia has been reported during concurrent radiation therapy. However, in some patients receiving molgramostim or regramostim, platelet counts increased during therapy with the drug. In addition, some patients who require platelet transfusions prior to initiation of GM-CSF therapy may exhibit a decreased need for such transfusions during therapy with the drug. Although a causal relationship was not established, one patient with a history of idiopathic thrombocytopenic purpura developed thrombocytopenia during molgramostim therapy; platelet counts returned to pretreatment levels after molgramostim was discontinued and several platelet transfusions had been given.

Although not reported to date with sargramostim, hemolysis and positive direct antiglobulin (Coombs') test results developed in at least one patient receiving molgramostim. Accelerated hemolysis also has been reported during GM-CSF therapy in at least one patient with a history of hemolytic anemia; it was suggested that accelerated hemolysis in this patient occurred as the result of macrophage stimulation by GM-CSF and resultant increased phagocytosis of erythrocytes.

■ **Cardiovascular Effects** Adverse cardiac effects have been reported in some patients receiving sargramostim, especially in those with a prior history of cardiac disease. Transient, reversible, supraventricular arrhythmia has been reported occasionally in patients receiving sargramostim; chest pain and reversible complete left bundle-branch block have been reported rarely. Although a causal relationship was not established, acute, aseptic, transudative pericardial effusion and hydrocephalus have been reported in at least one patient who received sargramostim. Chest (e.g., pericardial) pain, supraventricular tachyarrhythmia, pericarditis, and transient atrial fibrillation also have been reported in patients receiving molgramostim. Although a causal effect was not definitely established, molgramostim therapy appeared to contribute to the development of Loeffler's endocarditis in at least one patient receiving the drug.

■ **Musculoskeletal Effects** Mild to moderate bone pain has been reported in patients receiving sargramostim or molgramostim. Pain generally occurred in the lower back, pelvis, ribs, sternum, spine, shoulder, or hips, started within 20 minutes following administration of the drug, and lasted about 30 minutes. Bone pain was severe enough to require use of analgesics in some patients. Bone pain appeared to be related to the leukocyte count and resolved when the count decreased. If an analgesic is required for the treatment of musculoskeletal effects or bone pain during sargramostim therapy, acetaminophen or ibuprofen generally is effective; however, opiate analgesics have been used in some patients.

In at least 2 patients receiving regramostim, exacerbation of rheumatoid arthritis occurred within 1 day after initiation of therapy with the drug. Manifestations in these patients included increased stiffness and joint pain and appeared to be associated with an acute-phase response mediated by the release of cytokines (e.g., tumor necrosis factor, interleukin-6, C-reactive protein) stimulated by GM-CSF therapy.

■ **Other Adverse Effects** Fainting and dizziness have been reported with sargramostim. Mild, transient increases in serum concentrations of LDH and alkaline phosphatase have been reported in a few patients receiving sargramostim or molgramostim.

In uncontrolled clinical trials, increased concentrations of serum creatinine, bilirubin, and hepatic enzymes have been reported during sargramostim therapy in some patients with preexisting renal or hepatic impairment; concentrations returned to pretreatment levels following dosage reduction or discontinuance of the drug. (See Cautions: Precautions and Contraindications.) In controlled clinical trials, however, the incidence of renal and hepatic dysfunction in patients receiving sargramostim was similar to that in patients receiving placebo. Transient, dose-related increases in serum concentrations of AST (SGOT), ALT (SGPT), and γ-glutamyltransferase (γ-glutamyltranspeptidase, GGT, GGTP) have been reported in patients receiving molgramostim.

Although a causal relationship to the drug was not clearly established, molgramostim therapy was associated with reversible thyroid dysfunction, including goiter, hypothyroidism, or hyperthyroidism, in at least 2 patients with preexisting antibodies to thyroid peroxidase. It has been suggested that the drug may have caused an autoimmune thyroiditis similar to that reported with interferon alfa.

Levels of certain cytokines (e.g., tumor necrosis factor, C-reactive protein) may be increased during therapy with biosynthetic GM-CSFs. In a study in patients receiving regramostim by subcutaneous injection, there was a dose-related increase in levels of tumor necrosis factor and C-reactive protein in patients receiving the drug; levels of these cytokines returned to pretreatment levels after discontinuance of the drug.

■ **Precautions and Contraindications** Complete blood cell counts (CBCs) and platelet counts should be performed prior to initiation of sargramostim therapy and routinely (e.g., twice weekly) during therapy to avoid the potential complications of excessive leukocytosis and/or thrombocytosis. (See Cautions: Hematologic Effects.) Sargramostim therapy results in a rapid increase in leukocyte counts and a shift to the left (toward progenitor cells) in leukocyte differentials. The manufacturer recommends that if the absolute neutrophil count (ANC) exceeds 20,000/mm^3 or if the platelet count exceeds 500,000/mm^3, sargramostim therapy be temporarily discontinued or the dosage reduced by 50%. The decision to interrupt therapy or reduce sargramostim dosage should be based on the clinical condition of the patient; excessive blood cell counts usually return to normal or baseline levels within 2–10 days following interruption of sargramostim therapy. If blast cells appear on the leukocyte differential, sargramostim therapy should be discontinued.

Sargramostim should be used with caution in patients with preexisting fluid retention, pulmonary infiltrates, or congestive heart failure. Because edema, capillary leak syndrome, and pleural and/or pericardial effusion have been reported in patients receiving sargramostim, the possibility that the drug may aggravate fluid retention in patients with preexisting pleural and pericardial effusions or may precipitate such retention in patients without such preexisting conditions should be considered. In addition, some clinicians suggest that body weight and hydration status be monitored during therapy with the drug.

Sargramostim should be used with caution in patients with preexisting lung disease and/or hypoxia. Because sequestration of granulocytes in the pulmonary circulation and dyspnea have been reported in patients receiving sargramostim, special attention should be given to respiratory symptoms that develop during or immediately following administration of the drug. If patients develop dyspnea during administration of sargramostim, the rate of IV infusion should be decreased by 50%; oxygen should be used to provide symptomatic relief if necessary. If respiratory symptoms worsen despite a reduction in the IV infusion rate, sargramostim should be discontinued.

Because adverse cardiac effects, including transient, reversible, supraventricular arrhythmia, have been reported in some patients receiving sargramostim, the drug should be used with caution in patients with preexisting cardiac disease.

Although sargramostim is a growth factor that principally stimulates normal myeloid precursors, the possibility that the drug could act as a growth factor for any tumor type, particularly myeloid malignancies, cannot be excluded. Because of the possibility that the drug could potentiate tumor growth, sargramostim should be used with caution in patients with any malignancy with myeloid characteristics. Although sargramostim has been used in patients with myelodysplastic syndromes (MDS)† or acute myelogenous leukemia (AML) without evidence of increased relapse rates, regrowth of leukemic cells and an increase in leukemic blasts have occurred in a few patients with AML who were receiving the drug. The manufacturer states that sargramostim may be administered to those patients with MDS or AML who experience graft failure or delay in engraftment after bone marrow ablation and transplantation. Progression of the underlying neoplastic disease has not been observed to date in patients with non-Hodgkin's lymphoma, acute lymphocytic leukemia (ALL), or Hodgkin's disease receiving sargramostim, and the 24-month relapse rate in patients receiving sargramostim is similar to that in patients receiving placebo. If disease progression should be detected during sargramostim therapy in patients with non-Hodgkin's lymphoma, ALL, or Hodgkin's disease, the drug should be discontinued.

Limited data from in vitro studies suggest that tumor cells may be released into the leukapheresis product when sargramostim is used for mobilization of hematopoietic progenitor cells and that these cells may be reinfused into the patient during autologous PBPC transplantation. The effect of reinfusion of tumor cells has not been well studied and data are inconclusive to date.

Although a direct causal relationship between sargramostim and adverse renal or hepatic effects has not been established, the manufacturer recommends that renal and/or hepatic function be monitored every other week whenever sargramostim is used in patients with preexisting renal and/or hepatic impairment.

Sargramostim is contraindicated in patients with excessive (i.e., 10% or more) leukemic myeloid blasts in the bone marrow or peripheral blood.

Sargramostim is contraindicated in patients with known hypersensitivity to the drug or any ingredient in the formulation. The drug also is contraindicated in patients with known hypersensitivity to yeast-derived products.

■ **Pediatric Precautions** Although safety and efficacy of sargramostim in children have not been fully evaluated, the drug has been used in children 4 months to 18 years of age without unusual adverse effects. Sargramostim has been given IV in dosages of 60–1500 mcg/m^2 daily or subcutaneously in dosages of 4–1500 mcg/m^2 daily in such children. In controlled studies in children receiving sargramostim in a dosage of 250 mcg/m^2 daily given by IV infusion over 2 hours, the types and frequency of adverse effects were similar to those reported in adults receiving the drug. Although further study is needed, there is some evidence that children can tolerate higher dosages of biosynthetic GM-CSF than adults when the drugs are used to treat chemotherapy-induced neutropenia.†

The manufacturer states that commercially available sargramostim injection containing 1.1% benzyl alcohol and sargramostim lyophilized powder that is reconstituted with bacteriostatic water for injection containing 0.9% benzyl alcohol should *not* be administered to neonates. Although a causal relationship has not been established, administration of injections preserved with benzyl alcohol has been associated with toxicity in neonates. Toxicity appears to have resulted from administration of large amounts (i.e., 100–400 mg/kg daily) of benzyl alcohol in these neonates. Although use of drugs preserved with benzyl alcohol should be avoided in neonates whenever possible, the American Academy of Pediatrics (AAP) states that the presence of small amounts of the preservative in a commercially available injection should not proscribe its use when indicated in neonates.

■ **Geriatric Precautions** Safety and efficacy of sargramostim in geriatric patients have not been specifically studied to date. Clinical trial experience in patients 65 years of age or older is limited to those with AML. In a randomized controlled study of sargramostim therapy in patients with AML, approximately 42% of the 52 patients enrolled were 65–70 years of age. Although no apparent differences in safety and efficacy were observed relative to younger adults 55–64 years of age, the possibility that some older patients may exhibit greater sensitivity to the drug cannot be ruled out.

■ **Mutagenicity and Carcinogenicity** In vitro studies indicate that sargramostim can stimulate proliferation of leukemic progenitor cells and induce differentiation of some leukemic cells. Therefore, while the carcinogenic potential of sargramostim has not been elucidated to date, concerns that the drug could stimulate the growth of any tumor type, particularly myeloid malignancies, currently exist. (See Cautions: Precautions and Contraindications.)

■ **Pregnancy, Fertility, and Lactation** Animal reproduction studies have not been performed with sargramostim. It is not known whether the drug can cause fetal harm when administered to pregnant women. There are no adequate and controlled studies to date using sargramostim in pregnant women, and the drug should be used during pregnancy only when clearly needed. Women of childbearing potential should be advised of the potential risks to the fetus.

It is not known whether the drug can affect fertility or reproduction capacity.

It is not known whether sargramostim is distributed into milk. Because many drugs are distributed into milk, sargramostim should be used in nursing women only if clearly needed.

Drug Interactions

■ **Myelosuppressive Therapy and Antineoplastic Agents** The safety and efficacy of concomitant administration of doses of sargramostim with radiation therapy or with doses of myelosuppressive antineoplastic agents have not been established. Because sargramostim stimulates proliferation of hematopoietic progenitor cells and because radiation therapy and many antineoplastic agents target rapidly proliferating cells, doses of sargramostim should not be administered within 12 hours before or after radiation therapy or within 24 hours before or after a dose of a myelosuppressive antineoplastic agent.

Patients undergoing autologous bone marrow transplantation who previously have received extensive radiation therapy to hematopoietic sites for the treatment of primary disease of the abdomen or chest or have been exposed to multiple myelotoxic agents (e.g., alkylating agents, anthracycline antibiotics, antimetabolites) may have a limited response to sargramostim therapy.

In at least one in vitro study, pretreatment of leukemic blasts with GM-CSF appeared to enhance the cytotoxicity of cytarabine against these cells. This appparently occurred in part because exposure to GM-CSF resulted in an increase in the proportion of leukemic cells in the S phase and increased uptake of the antineoplastic agent drug by the cells. The clinical importance of this in vitro effect is unclear.

■ **Drugs with Myeloproliferative Effects** Because specific studies have not been performed to date to evaluate the additive effects of myeloproliferative drugs, drugs that theoretically could potentiate the myeloproliferative effects of sargramostim (e.g., lithium, corticosteroids) should be used with caution in patients receiving the drug.

■ **Antiretroviral Agents** Although the clinical importance is unclear, results of in vitro studies indicate that biosynthetic GM-CSFs may potentiate the antiretroviral activity of zidovudine against human immunodeficiency virus (HIV). In in vitro studies using monocyte/macrophage cell cultures, the presence of GM-CSF markedly enhanced the antiretroviral effect of zidovudine against HIV-1 (strain HTLV-IIIB) and a monocytotropic strain of HIV type 1. A synergistic effect between GM-CSF and zidovudine also was evident in vitro in monocytic U-937 cells inoculated with HIV-1 (strain HTLV-IIIB). The mechanism of this synergistic effect has not been determined but may result from enhanced entry of the antiretroviral agent into infected cells and/or enhanced conversion of zidovudine monophosphate into the metabolically active triphosphate derivative. The fact that conflicting results have been obtained from studies evaluating the in vitro effects of biosynthetic GM-CSFs on replication of HIV when used alone and the fact that GM-CSFs appear to stimulate replication of some strains of HIV in vitro in certain cell cultures should be considered if sargramostim is used in patients with HIV infection. (See Pharmacology: Effects on Other Cells.) Studies are ongoing to evaluate safety and efficacy of concomitant therapy with biosynthetic GM-CSFs and zidovudine in patients with HIV infection. (See Uses: HIV-infected Individuals.)

In in vitro studies using monocyte/macrophage cell cultures, the synergism demonstrated between zidovudine and GM-CSF against HIV was not evident when other nucleoside reverse transcriptase inhibitors (didanosine) were tested.

Acute Toxicity

Limited information is available on the acute toxicity of sargramostim in humans. Overdosage of sargramostim would be expected to produce manifestations that are principally extensions of the pharmacologic and common adverse effects of the drug. The maximum tolerated dosage of sargramostim in humans has not been determined. When some patients received sargramostim dosages up to 100 mcg/kg daily (4000 mcg/m^2 daily or 16 times the usual recommended dosage) by continuous IV infusion for 7–18 days, leukocyte counts were increased up to 200,000/mm^3 and various adverse effects, including dyspnea, malaise, nausea, fever, rash, sinus tachycardia, headache, and chills, occurred; these adverse effects disappeared after the drug was discontinued.

If overdosage of sargramostim occurs, the drug should be discontinued immediately and the patient monitored carefully for respiratory symptoms and leukocytosis.

Pharmacology

Sargramostim is a hematopoietic agent that principally influences leukopoiesis. The drug appears to elicit the pharmacologic effects usually produced by endogenous human granulocyte-macrophage colony-stimulating factor (GM-CSF). Endogenous GM-CSF, a growth factor, is a multilineage colony-stimulating factor that principally affects the proliferation, differentiation, and activation of granulocytes and macrophages by inducing partially committed progenitor cells (i.e., neutrophils, monocytes/macrophages, dendritic cells derived from myeloid cell lines) to divide and differentiate in the granulocyte-macrophage pathways. In addition, in conjunction with other growth factors, endogenous GM-CSF stimulates the proliferation of several other cell types including eosinophils, megakaryocytes, erythroid progenitors, and mast-cell precursors. Endogenous GM-CSF also enhances certain functions of mature neutrophils and monocytes, including chemotaxis, phagocytosis, and antibody-dependent cellular cytotoxicity (ADCC). Despite extensive data concerning the effects of colony-stimulating factors (CSFs) on myeloid progenitor and mature cells in vitro and concerning in vivo effects in animals and in healthy individuals and patients, the physiologic roles of endogenous CSFs have not been fully elucidated.

In healthy adults, adults with leukemia or aplastic anemia, and children with malignancy, circulating levels of endogenous GM-CSF generally are below the limits of detection of currently used immunoassays. In a study that used an enzyme-linked immunosorbent assay (ELISA) capable of detecting human GM-CSF levels as low as 0.1 ng/mL, 80% of the healthy adults 22–63 years of age tested had undetectable serum concentrations of endogenous GM-CSF; the remaining healthy adults had GM-CSF concentrations of 0.2–0.66 ng/mL.

Endogenous human GM-CSF is produced by both hematologic and tissue cells including fibroblasts, T cells, macrophages, and endothelial cells. The mechanisms that control production and secretion of GM-CSF from these cells have not been fully elucidated. Presence of several factors, including interleukin-1 (lymphocyte-activating factor), tumor necrosis factor, and endotoxin, appears to stimulate production and release of endogenous GM-CSF from various cells. Nonimmune activation of fibroblasts and endothelial cells and immune activation of T cells appear to lead to synthesis and release of GM-CSF. Although it has been suggested that a feedback mechanism based on the level of circulating neutrophils regulates production of another growth factor, endogenous granulocyte CSF (G-CSF), there is no evidence that endogenous levels of GM-CSF increase in response to severe neutropenia.

Endogenous GM-CSF acts on various progenitor target cells including colony-forming units-granulocytic (CFU-G), colony-forming units macrophagic (CFU-M), colony-forming units-granulocytic-monocytic (CFU-GM), colony-forming units-granulocytic-erythrocytic-monocytic-megakaryocytic (CFU-GEMM), colony-forming units-eosinophilic (CFU-Eo), colony-forming units-megakaryocytic (CFU-M), colony-forming units-blastic (CFU-Blast), and burst-forming units-erythroid (BFU-E). Endogenous GM-CSF and the various biosynthetic GM-CSFs, including sargramostim (yeast-derived, glycosylated GM-CSF), molgramostim (bacteria-derived, nonglycosylated GM-CSF), and regramostim (mammalian-derived, glycosylated GM-CSF), have similar mechanisms of action. Like endogenous GM-CSF, sargramostim and other biosynthetic GM-CSFs appear to act directly on target cells by binding to GM-CSF-specific receptors on their cell surfaces. How this binding to receptors results in the various intracellular events necessary to affect proliferation, differentiation, and cell function has not been fully elucidated to date. Although glycosylation is not necessary for binding of CSFs to receptors on target cells, the degree of glycosylation may affect the biologic activity of GM-CSFs by reducing receptor binding affinity. Endogenous GM-CSF is variably glycosylated, partly depending on its cell of origin, and each of the biosynthetic GM-CSFs differs in the degree of glycosylation. Although the clinical importance is unclear, heavily glycosylated GM-CSFs appear to have lower receptor affinity than less heavily glycosylated or nonglycosylated GM-CSFs because of lower kinetic association binding rates.

The GM-CSF receptor binding site on target cells appears to be complex and is composed of at least 2 subunits. The α subunit is a low-affinity receptor site. The β subunit cannot bind GM-CSF when expressed alone but acts as a high-affinity receptor site when expressed in conjunction with the α subunit; the β subunit is cross-reactive and also binds interleukin-3 (multicolony-stimulating factor, multi-CSF). GM-CSF receptors are present on all cells of the neutrophil, monocyte, and eosinophil lineages; mature cells generally have fewer receptors than more premature and progenitor cells. Neutrophils contain only the α/β complex and therefore have only high-affinity receptors. Although the clinical importance is unclear, GM-CSF receptors also have been found on certain leukemic cell lines (including some derived from human myeloid leukemia cells), cell lines derived from human small cell lung carcinoma, osteogenic sarcoma, breast carcinoma, and malignant melanoma cells as well as human placenta and human vascular endothelial cells.

■ **Effects on Leukocyte Maturation and Leukocyte Levels** Following IV or subcutaneous administration of sargramostim or another biosynthetic GM-CSF in patients with malignancy and/or neutropenia, there is an initial (within 5–45 minutes) transient decrease in the absolute leukocyte count to below baseline levels and a decrease in levels of circulating neutrophils, monocytes, and eosinophils. Within 2–6 hours, neutrophil counts and monocyte counts return to baseline levels or above. The initial decrease in leukocytes may occur because of margination of neutrophils and monocytes and sequestration within the lungs, and the subsequent increase may occur because of demargination. The increase in leukocyte count in response to biosynthetic GM-CSF therapy generally is dose dependent and biphasic. In most patients, there is an initial plateau in leukocyte counts that is achieved after 3–7 days of biosynthetic GM-CSF therapy. This initial plateau is followed by a slight decrease (despite continued GM-CSF therapy) and a second increase and plateau occurring 4–5 days after the first plateau. It has been suggested that the initial increase in leukocyte count represents redistribution of cells from the bone marrow after maturation, shortened maturation time, enhanced demargination of intravascular neutrophils, and inhibited extravascular migration of neutrophils; the second increase probably occurs because of an increase in the proliferative fraction of hematopoietic cells within the bone marrow. Alternatively, it has been suggested that the second peak in neutrophil response occurs because GM-CSFs induce production of other factors (e.g., interleukin-3, interleukin-5) that function in conjunction with GM-CSF to augment the leukocyte response. Following discontinuance of biosynthetic GM-CSF therapy, leukocyte counts return to pretreatment levels within 2–10 days.

Biosynthetic GM-CSFs alter the kinetics of myeloid progenitor cells within the bone marrow causing rapid entry of cells into the cell cycle and decreasing the cell cycle time. There is a marked increase in the proportion of immature cells within the bone marrow and in the pool of committed progenitors and morphologically identifiable granulopoietic precursors actively synthesizing DNA (S phase of the cell cycle). Biosynthetic GM-CSFs principally affect cells in the granulocyte-macrophage lineage. In patients receiving low doses of biosynthetic GM-CSFs, the leukocyte response is composed principally of neutrophils; at higher concentrations, the leukocyte response also involves proliferation of monocytes and eosinophils. Leukocyte differentials performed during biosynthetic GM-CSF therapy usually demonstrate a shift to the left (toward progenitor cells), and myelocytes, promyelocytes, and myeloblasts may be present. Regardless of the dosage, absolute lymphocyte and basophil counts generally are unaffected by biosynthetic GM-CSF therapy. Although the drugs do not directly affect lymphocyte precursors, it has been suggested that biosynthetic GM-CSFs may stimulate release of other factors that do affect lymphocyte proliferation.

Patients who previously received extensive radiation therapy to hematopoietic sites or have been exposed to multiple myelotoxic agents (e.g., alkylating agents, anthracycline antibiotics, antimetabolites) generally are less responsive to biosynthetic GM-CSF therapy than those who have not received such treatment. Studies in patients with chemotherapy-induced neutropenia and patients with cyclic neutropenia, myelodysplastic syndromes (MDS), or aplastic anemia receiving sargramostim indicate that the time to granulocyte response and the percentage of patients responding to the drug are not age dependent since geriatric patients (those 65 years of age or older) appear to respond the same as younger adults.

■ **Effects on Leukocyte Function** Results of in vitro studies evaluating the leukocytes produced in response to sargramostim or other biosynthetic GM-CSFs indicate that these cells function normally. However, although the clinical importance is unclear, neutrophils from patients receiving biosynthetic GM-CSFs may exhibit reduced migration. GM-CSFs, unlike filgrastim (a biosynthetic G-CSF), may inhibit rather than stimulate neutrophil migration in vitro and in vivo, especially at high dosage. Results of some in vitro studies indicate that neutrophils exposed to GM-CSFs for short periods of time (less than 30 minutes) exhibit enhanced directed chemotaxis whereas prolonged exposure of the cells to GM-CSFs results in decreased random migration but may not affect directed chemotaxis. Morphologic changes in neutrophils have been reported during biosynthetic GM-CSF therapy, including toxic granulations, cytoplasmic vacuolization, and hypersegmentation of polymorphonuclear neutrophils (PMNs).

Results of in vitro studies indicate that sargramostim and other biosynthetic GM-CSFs, like endogenous GM-CSF, enhance certain functions of normal, mature neutrophils, eosinophils, basophils, and macrophages. Biosynthetic GM-CSFs enhance oxidative metabolism of neutrophils, phagocytosis, eosinophil cytotoxicity, antibody-dependent cellular cytotoxicity (ADCC), chemotaxis, and hydrogen peroxide production. The drugs appear to enhance neutrophilic lysozymal secretion and complement-mediated neutrophilic and eosinophilic phagocytosis of microorganisms and to promote the killing of antibody-coated tumor cells and intracellular organisms including *Leishmania*, *Trypanosoma cruzi*, and *Mycobacterium avium* complex. GM-CSFs appear to affect monocytes by increasing the number of surface membrane receptors on the cells, enhancing respiratory burst activity, and enhancing antimicrobial and cytotoxic activity. The in vitro fungicidal activity of monocytes against *Candida albicans*, *Histoplasma capsulatum*, and *Cryptococcus neoformans* also is enhanced by GM-CSFs. In addition, studies using sargramostim in patients with neoplastic diseases indicate that the drug activates the antitumor potential of peripheral blood monocytes by increasing monocyte ADCC and the secretion of tumor necrosis factor and interferon. There is some evidence from one in vitro study that GM-CSFs may prolong survival of PMNs by inhibiting programmed cell death.

■ **Effects on Other Cells** Endogenous GM-CSF and biosynthetic GM-CSFs initiate proliferation in erythroid and megakaryocytic lineages; however, other factors are necessary for production of mature cells in these lineages. The percentage of BFU-E in the S phase generally is increased during biosynthetic GM-CSF therapy; however, the absolute number of reticulocytes in the peripheral circulation generally is unchanged. Variable effects on platelet counts have been reported in patients receiving biosynthetic GM-CSFs. In some patients, platelets decrease slightly during the first 5 days of therapy and then return to pretreatment levels during the next 5–10 days; in other patients, there is an increase in platelets.

Although the clinical importance is unclear, results of in vitro studies using human myelocytic leukemia cell lines adapted to grow in culture indicate that sargramostim can stimulate proliferation of leukemic progenitor cells and induce differentiation of some leukemic cells. In vitro, biosynthetic GM-CSFs promote monocyte antitumor effects; these effects may be mediated at least in part by a mechanism involving tumor necrosis factor. However, in one in vitro study using tumor cells taken from patients with various tumor types, sargramostim did not appear to stimulate or inhibit solid tumor growth.

There is some in vitro evidence that biosynthetic GM-CSFs may stimulate replication of some strains of human immunodeficiency virus (HIV). However, a few studies attempting to confirm this have given conflicting results and the clinical importance of this in vitro effect is unclear. In in vitro studies using monocyte/macrophage cell cultures, biosynthetic GM-CSF enhanced replication of HIV-1 (strain HTLV-IIIB) and a monocytotropic strain of HIV-1 (HTLV-III$_{\text{Ba-L}}$). It has been suggested that the in vitro effects of GM-CSF on HIV replication may depend on the specific cell culture system used for testing and/or the state of cellular differention or number of cellular receptors for GM-CSF present. There have been some reports of increased serum HIV p24 core antigen levels in HIV-infected patients receiving sargramostim; however, these reports generally involved patients who were not receiving concurrent antiretroviral therapy. There is no evidence to date that HIV-infected patients are at risk of increased viral load or clinical deterioration if sargramostim is used concomitantly with zidovudine; however, clinical trials are needed to fully determine the safety and efficacy of concurrent therapy with sargramostim and antiretroviral agents, including zidovudine.

Pharmacokinetics

Information on the pharmacokinetics of sargramostim is limited. The pharmacokinetics of sargramostim after parenteral administration reportedly are best described by a 2-compartment, first-order model. However, the contributions of endogenous GM-CSF and remaining questions about the elimination characteristics of sargramostim complicate interpretation of pharmacokinetic data.

Although there are several published studies on the pharmacokinetics of other biosynthetic GM-CSFs, including molgramostim (bacteria-derived, nonglycosylated GM-CSF) and regramostim (mammalian-derived, glycosylated GM-CSF), results of these studies cannot necessarily be extrapolated to sargramostim (yeast-derived, glycosylated GM-CSF) since each of these biosynthetic GM-CSFs differs in the degree of glycosylation, which may affect pharmacokinetics. Studies in rats indicate that the rate and extent of distribution of biosynthetic GM-CSFs into fluids and tissues, but not the rate of renal clearance of the drugs, varies depending on the degree of glycosylation. In studies comparing the pharmacokinetics of molgramostim and regramostim following subcutaneous injection in healthy adults or adults with malignant lymphomas, the nonglycosylated derivative was absorbed more rapidly and to a greater extent than the glycosylated derivative and also was cleared more rapidly. It is not known whether these pharmacokinetic differences result solely from differences in glycosylation or whether these differences have any effect on the in vivo activity of the various derivatives.

The manufacturer states that, based on statistical evaluation of the area under the concentration-time curve (AUC) in healthy adult males, 250-mcg/m^2 doses of sargramostim given as the commercially available injection are bioequivalent to 250-mcg/m^2 doses given as a solution prepared using the commercially available lyophilized powder of the drug.

■ **Absorption** Following IV infusion over 2 hours of 250-mcg/m^2 doses of sargramostim in healthy adults, peak serum concentrations of GM-CSF were attained during or immediately after completion of the infusion and averaged 5 ng/mL in those who received the commercially available sargramostim injection and 5.4 ng/mL in those who received solutions prepared using the commercially available lyophilized powder of the drug.

Sargramostim is rapidly absorbed following subcutaneous injection and peak serum concentrations of the drug generally are attained within 1–4 hours following rapid subcutaneous injection. In a limited number of healthy adults, subcutaneous injection of 250 mcg/m^2 of sargramostim resulted in peak GM-CSF serum concentrations 1–3 hours after the dose that averaged 1.5 ng/mL;

serum concentrations remained detectable for up to 6 hours after the dose. Following rapid subcutaneous injection of 125-mcg/m^2 doses of sargramostim every 12 hours in several adults with myelodysplastic syndromes, serum concentrations of the drug 5 minutes after injection ranged from 0.055–0.45 ng/mL, peak serum concentrations ranged from 0.35–3.9 ng/mL, and serum concentrations 6 hours after injection ranged from 0.15–2.7 ng/mL.

Studies using molgramostim indicate that there is considerable interindividual variation in peak serum concentrations and AUCs of the drug attained with a given dose and that the pharmacokinetics may vary depending on the route of administration; it is unclear whether this also occurs with sargramostim. In studies in adults with malignancies who received low doses of molgramostim, peak serum concentrations and AUCs of the drug were higher following IV administration than following rapid subcutaneous injection of equivalent doses. It was suggested that bioavailability following subcutaneous injection may be lower than that following IV administration because of irreversible binding of the drug to subcutaneous tissues. However, differences in bioavailability were not as apparent when larger doses of molgramostim were administered, and it is possible that a saturable clearance mechanism may be present that rapidly clears the drug from serum when low doses are administered subcutaneously.

■ **Distribution** Studies in mice using murine GM-CSF indicate that the hematopoietic agent is distributed into various tissues including liver, spleen, and kidney. It is not known whether sargramostim is distributed into cerebrospinal fluid. In a patient receiving regramostim, GM-CSF was undetectable in a cerebrospinal fluid sample obtained 18 hours after initiation of therapy with the drug.

It is not known whether sargramostim crosses the placenta or is distributed into milk.

■ **Elimination** Serum concentrations of sargramostim appear to decline in a biphasic manner. However, the elimination characteristics of the drug, including possible metabolic pathways and/or excretion mechanisms, remain to be more fully elucidated.

In healthy adults who received sargramostim by IV infusion over 2 hours, the elimination half-life of the drug was approximately 1 hour. In a study in several patients receiving a sargramostim dosage of 500–750 mcg/m^2 by IV infusion over 2 hours, the distribution half-life of the drug was approximately 12–17 minutes and the elimination half-life was approximately 2 hours. In patients 2–21 years of age with cancer, the elimination half-life of sargramostim was 1.6–2.8 hours following IV infusion over 2 hours.

Studies using molgramostim indicate that this nonglycosylated derivative has a distribution half-life of 5–15 minutes and an elimination half-life of 0.2–2.5 hours following rapid IV injection. Following IV infusion of molgramostim over 20–120 minutes, the drug has an elimination half-life ranging from 0.6–9.1 hours. In some studies using molgramostim, there was evidence of a saturable clearance mechanism for the drug.

The metabolic fate of sargramostim has not been fully elucidated to date, and it is not known whether the drug is metabolized or how it is eliminated from the body. Sargramostim has been detected in urine following IV infusion or rapid subcutaneous injection. In healthy adults who received sargramostim doses of 250 mcg/m^2 by IV infusion over 2 hours or by subcutaneous injection, clearance of the drug averaged 420–431 mL/minute per m^2 or 529–549 mL/minute per m^2, respectively. In a study in patients 21 years of age or younger with cancer who received a sargramostim dosage of 500–1250 mcg/m^2 daily by IV infusion over 2 hours, the clearance rate of the drug ranged from 41–252 mL/minute per m^2.

Chemistry and Stability

■ **Chemistry** Sargramostim, a human granulocyte-macrophage colony-stimulating factor (GM-CSF), is a biosynthetic hematopoietic agent that affects the proliferation and differentiation of a variety of hematopoietic progenitor cells. The drug is prepared using recombinant DNA technology and a yeast expression system that utilizes *Saccharomyces cerevisiae*. Endogenous human GM-CSF is a glycoprotein hormone produced by T cells, macrophages, fibroblasts, and endothelial cells. (See Pharmacology.)

Sargramostim is a single-chain, glycosylated polypeptide containing 127 amino acids and is characterized by equal proportions of 3 primary molecular species having molecular weights of 19,500, 16,800, and 15,500 daltons. Sargramostim has an amino acid sequence identical to that of endogenous human GM-CSF except that the drug contains a leucine instead of a proline at position 23 and may have a different carbohydrate moiety. Since sargramostim is produced using *S. cerevisiae*, it is termed yeast-derived recombinant human GM-CSF (rHuGM-CSF).

In addition to sargramostim, several other biosynthetic GM-CSFs have been produced and studied, including molgramostim (Leucomax®, Schering-Plough/Sandoz; not currently commercially available in the US) and regramostim (Sandoz; not currently commercially available in the US). Molgramostim is bacteria-derived recombinant GM-CSF prepared using *Escherichia coli* and regramostim is mammalian-derived recombinant GM-CSF prepared using Chinese hamster ovary (CHO) cells. Each of these biosynthetic GM-CSFs differs in the degree of glycosylation; molgramostim is not glycosylated, sargramostim is glycosylated at *N*- and *O*-linked glycosyl sites, and regramostim is glycosylated at *O*- and *N*-linked glycosyl sites with nonhuman mammalian carbohydrate chains. The physiologic and/or clinical relevance of these differences in glycosylation in biosynthetic CSFs is unclear and remains to be more fully elucidated. Glycosylation does not appear to be necessary for in vitro or in vivo activity of biosynthetic GM-CSFs; however, the degree of glycosylation may affect the rate of binding of GM-CSFs to receptors on target cells and may also affect pharmacokinetics, antigenicity, and adverse effects. In addition, because of differences in glycosylation, the various biosynthetic GM-CSFs have different specific activities and potencies when considered on a weight-to-weight basis.

Sargramostim is commercially available as a clear, colorless solution for IV infusion or subcutaneous injection containing 500 mcg of sargramostim per mL with 1.1% benzyl alcohol. The commercially available injection has a pH of 6.7–7.7. Sargramostim also is commercially available as a sterile, white, lyophilized powder containing no preservatives. Following reconstitution of the lyophilized powder with sterile or bacteriostatic water for injection as directed, solutions containing 250 mcg of sargramostim per mL are clear and colorless and have a pH of 7.1–7.7. Each mL of commercially available sargramostim injection and each mL of sargramostim reconstituted as directed from the lyophilized powder also contains 40 mg of mannitol, 10 mg of sucrose, and 1.2 mg of tromethamine. Sargramostim has an aqueous solubility exceeding 12 mg/mL at 2–8°C.

Potency of sargramostim is determined using a normal human bone marrow colony-forming assay and is expressed in terms of units per mg of protein as tested against the WHO first International Reference Standard. Commercially available sargramostim has a specific activity of approximately 5.6×10^6 units/mg of protein.

■ **Stability** Commercially available sargramostim injection and the lyophilized powder should be refrigerated at 2–8°C. The injection should not be frozen or shaken; the manufacturer states that there are no known deleterious effects of freezing on the powder. When stored at 2–8°C, the lyophilized powder is stable for 24 months following the date of manufacture.

Following reconstitution with sterile or bacteriostatic water for injection or further dilution in 0.9% sodium chloride injection or 5% dextrose injection, sargramostim solutions should be refrigerated at 2–8°C and should not be frozen. Following reconstitution with sterile water for injection or bacteriostatic water for injection, sargramostim solutions containing 250 mcg/mL retain potency for 30 days at 2–8°C or 25°C. The manufacturer, however, currently recommends that solutions reconstituted with sterile water for injection be used as soon as possible following reconstitution and discarded if not used within 6 hours and that solutions reconstituted with bacteriostatic water for injection be discarded if not used within 20 days. Solutions of the drug that have been reconstituted with bacteriostatic water for injection have been reported to meet USP criteria for preservative effectiveness and, when transferred aseptically to 1-mL plastic syringes, are stable for 14 days at 2–8°C.

Following reconstitution, sargramostim solutions may be diluted in 0.9% sodium chloride. To prevent adsorption of the drug to plastic or glass infusion containers or equipment, albumin human should be added to the infusion solution to a final concentration of 1 mg/mL (0.1%) whenever sargramostim is diluted to a concentration less than 10 mcg/mL. Reconstituted solutions of sargramostim that are diluted further in 50 mL of 0.9% sodium chloride injection in PVC bags to concentrations of 2.5 (with albumin human 0.1%), 8 (with albumin human 0.1%), or 12 mcg/mL are stable for 48 hours when refrigerated or stored at ambient temperatures. To reduce the possibility of bacterial contamination, the manufacturer recommends that any reconstituted and/or diluted solutions of sargramostim, including previously reconstituted solutions mixed with freshly reconstituted solutions be discarded if not used within 6 hours.

Information on the physical and/or chemical compatibility of sargramostim with other drugs is limited, and the manufacturer states that sargramostim should not be admixed with other drugs. Several in vitro studies have been done to assess the visual compatibility of sargramostim mixed in a 1:1 ratio with various drugs, including anti-infective agents, antineoplastic agents, heparin sodium, analgesics, and total parenteral nutrition solutions. Although there was no obvious evidence of physical incompatibility between sargramostim and some of these drugs, particulate formation was evident with certain combinations and further study is needed to evaluate more fully the physical and/or chemical compatibility of sargramostim with other drugs.

Preparations

Sargramostim injection containing EDTA has been withdrawn from the US market because of reports of increased adverse effects associated with its use. (See Cautions.) Clinicians are advised to immediately stop using any remaining stock of EDTA-containing sargramostim injection and return unused vials to the manufacturer. The manufacturer has reformulated commercially available sargramostim injection without EDTA.

Excipients in commercially available drug preparations may have clinically important effects in some individuals; consult specific product labeling for details.

Sargramostim (Recombinant DNA Origin)

Parenteral		
For injection	250 mcg (1.4×10^6 units)	**Leukine®**, Bayer
Injection	500 mcg/mL (2.8×10^6 units/mL)	**Leukine®**, Bayer

†Use is not currently included in the labeling approved by the US Food and Drug Administration

Selected Revisions December 2008,

Table 1. Factor Xa (Recombinant), Inactivated-zhzo Dosage Based on Apixaban or Rivaroxaban Dose and Timing

Factor Xa Inhibitor	Factor Xa Inhibitor Last Dose	Timing of Last Dose of Factor Xa Inhibitor	
		<8 Hours or Unknown	≥8 Hours
Apixaban	≤5 mg	Low dose	Low dose
	>5 mg or unknown	High dose	Low dose
Rivaroxaban	≤10 mg	Low dose	Low dose
	>10 mg or unknown	High dose	Low dose

Patients receiving therapy with a factor Xa inhibitor have underlying disease states that predispose them to thromboembolic events, and reversing the effects of factor Xa inhibitor therapy increases the risk of thromboembolic events. (See Thromboembolic Risks, Ischemic Risks, Cardiac Arrest, and Sudden Death under Warnings/Precautions: Warnings, in Cautions.) To reduce thromboembolic risk, anticoagulant therapy should be resumed as soon as medically appropriate following treatment with factor Xa (recombinant), inactivated-zhzo.

■ **Special Populations** The manufacturer makes no recommendations regarding dosage of factor Xa (recombinant), inactivated-zhzo in patients with hepatic or renal impairment.

Cautions

■ **Contraindications** The manufacturer states that there are no contraindications to the use of factor Xa (recombinant), inactivated-zhzo.

■ **Warnings/Precautions** ***Warnings*** **Thromboembolic Risks, Ischemic Risks, Cardiac Arrest, and Sudden Death.** Life-threatening thromboembolic and ischemic complications, including sudden death, have been reported following administration of factor Xa (recombinant), inactivated-zhzo. In the ANNEXA-4 study, factor Xa inhibitor (recombinant), inactivated-zhzo was administered to patients with an acute major bleeding episode who were taking factor Xa inhibitors as anticoagulation treatment for atrial fibrillation or venous thromboembolism. In an interim analysis of this study, approximately 18% of patients had experienced at least one of the following events: deep-vein thrombosis (DVT), ischemic stroke, acute myocardial infarction (MI), pulmonary embolism (PE), cardiogenic shock, sudden death, congestive heart failure, acute respiratory failure, cardiac arrest, cardiac thrombus, embolic stroke, iliac artery thrombosis, and/or nonsustained ventricular tachycardia. Of the 86 safety-evaluable patients in the interim analysis who had received factor Xa (recombinant), inactivated-zhzo (generation 1 product) and had anticoagulation reinitiated, 12.7% experienced a thromboembolic event, ischemic event, cardiac event, or death; the median time to the first thromboembolic event was 6 days. No thromboembolic events were observed in the ANNEXA-A or ANNEXA-R trials involving healthy individuals who received factor Xa (recombinant), inactivated-zhzo.

Safety of factor Xa (recombinant), inactivated-zhzo has not been established in patients who experienced a thromboembolic event or disseminated intravascular coagulation (DIC) within 2 weeks prior to the life-threatening bleeding event requiring treatment with the drug. Safety of factor Xa (recombinant), inactivated-zhzo also has not been established in patients who received prothrombin complex concentrates (PCC), recombinant factor VIIa, or whole blood products within 7 days prior to the bleeding event.

Patients receiving factor Xa (recombinant), inactivated-zhzo should be monitored for manifestations of arterial and venous thromboembolic events, ischemic events, and cardiac arrest. Patients should be treated as medically appropriate if manifestations of cardiac arrest occur. Anticoagulation should be initiated when medically appropriate.

Other Warnings and Precautions **Re-elevation or Incomplete Reversal of Anti-factor Xa Activity.** A rapid and substantial decrease in anti-factor Xa activity corresponding to a direct IV ("bolus") dose of factor Xa (recombinant), inactivated-zhzo was observed in clinical trials conducted in healthy individuals. This decrease was sustained throughout the continuous infusion of the drug; anti-factor Xa activity returned to the placebo concentrations approximately 2 hours after completion of a direct IV injection or continuous infusion of the drug. Thereafter, the anti-factor Xa activity decreased at a rate similar to the expected clearance of the factor Xa inhibitor. Tissue factor pathway inhibitor (TFPI) activity in plasma returned to the pretreatment level approximately 96 hours following factor Xa (recombinant), inactivated-zhzo administration.

Factor Xa (recombinant), inactivated-zhzo has a relatively short half-life, whereas a factor Xa inhibitor may have a prolonged half-life in the elderly or those with renal impairment. These differences in half-life may result in transient or incomplete reversal of the anticoagulant effects of the factor Xa inhibitor.

In an interim analysis of the ANNEXA-4 study, the median decrease in anti-factor Xa activity from baseline to nadir (the smallest value measured within 5 minutes after the end of the continuous infusion of factor Xa [recombinant], inactivated-zhzo) was 93 or 90% for those who had been receiving apixaban or rivaroxaban, respectively. The safety and efficacy of repeat doses of factor Xa (recombinant), inactivated-zhzo have not been established.

Immunogenicity. As with all therapeutic proteins, there is a potential for immunogenicity with factor Xa (recombinant), inactivated-zhzo. Low titers of anti-factor Xa (recombinant), inactivated-zhzo antibodies have been observed in patients receiving the drug (generation 1 product). None of these anti-factor Xa (recombinant), inactivated-zhzo antibodies were neutralizing. The development of antibodies cross-reacting with factor X or factor Xa has not been observed.

Specific Populations **Pregnancy.** There are no adequate and well-controlled studies of factor Xa (recombinant), inactivated-zhzo in pregnant women. Animal reproductive studies conducted with factor Xa (recombinant), inactivated-zhzo are lacking. Safety and efficacy of the drug during labor and delivery have not been established.

Lactation. It is not known whether factor Xa (recombinant), inactivated-zhzo is distributed into human milk. The benefits of breast-feeding and the clinical need for factor Xa (recombinant), inactivated-zhzo in the woman should be considered along with any potential adverse effects on the breast-fed infant from the drug or from the underlying maternal condition.

Pediatric Use. Safety and efficacy of factor Xa (recombinant), inactivated-zhzo have not been established in pediatric patients.

Geriatric Use. Clinical experience has not revealed age-related differences in safety or efficacy; however, the possibility that some older patients may exhibit increased sensitivity to factor Xa (recombinant), inactivated-zhzo cannot be ruled out. No differences in the pharmacokinetics of factor Xa (recombinant), inactivated-zhzo were observed in patients 65 years of age and older compared with younger patients (18–45 years of age).

■ **Common Adverse Effects** Adverse effects reported in at least 5% of patients receiving factor Xa (recombinant), inactivated-zhzo in clinical trials were urinary tract infections and pneumonia. Adverse effects reported in at least 3% of healthy individuals receiving factor Xa (recombinant), inactivated-zhzo were infusion-related reactions (e.g., flushing, feeling hot, cough, dysgeusia, dyspnea).

Drug Interactions

■ **Factor Xa Inhibitors** The pharmacokinetics of factor Xa (recombinant), inactivated-zhzo were not affected by concomitant therapy with apixaban (5 mg twice daily for 6 days) or rivaroxaban (20 mg once daily for 6 days).

Description

Factor Xa (recombinant), inactivated-zhzo (also known as andexanet alfa), a recombinant modified human factor Xa protein, is a specific reversal agent for the anticoagulant effects of apixaban or rivaroxaban. Factor Xa (recombinant), inactivated-zhzo is a decoy protein that binds to and sequesters factor Xa inhibitors (e.g., apixaban, rivaroxaban) with high affinity in a stoichiometric ratio of 1:1, thereby restoring the activity of native factor Xa. Factor Xa (recombinant), inactivated-zhzo differs from native factor Xa by substitution of alanine for serine at position 419 and deletion of the membrane-binding carboxyglutamic acid domain. These modifications allow the drug to have a similar affinity for factor Xa inhibitors as native factor Xa without having intrinsic anticoagulant or procoagulant activity; the drug is unable to cleave and activate prothrombin and cannot assemble into the prothrombinase complex. Factor Xa (recombinant), inactivated-zhzo also binds to and inhibits the activity of tissue factor pathway inhibitor (TFPI), a protein that normally binds to native factor Xa. Inhibition of TFPI activity can increase tissue factor-initiated thrombin generation.

Factor Xa (recombinant), inactivated-zhzo is prepared from cultures of genetically modified mammalian (Chinese hamster ovary) cells using recombinant DNA technology. To accommodate accelerated clinical development, manufacturing process modifications were made to increase drug production resulting in a generation 1 and generation 2 drug product. These products are produced from the same cell line, and the FDA has determined the 2 products to be bioequivalent.

Factor Xa (recombinant), inactivated-zhzo dose-dependently reverses the anti-factor Xa effects of apixaban and rivaroxaban. Factor Xa (recombinant), inactivated-zhzo also exhibits dose-dependent pharmacokinetics. The half-life (geometric mean) of the generation 1 or generation 2 factor Xa (recombinant), inactivated-zhzo product is 4.3 (range: 3.3–11.9) hours or 3.3 (range: 2.3–4) hours, respectively, when administered using the low-dose regimen. When administered using the high-dose regimen, the half-life (geometric mean) of the generation 1 or generation 2 factor Xa (recombinant), inactivated-zhzo product is 4 (range: 2–5.7) hours or 2.7 (range: 1.9–3.4) hours, respectively.

Advice to Patients

Importance of informing patients that reversing the effects of factor Xa inhibitor therapy increases the risk of thromboembolic events; arterial and venous thromboembolic events, including ischemic events, cardiac events, and sudden death, have been observed within 30 days following administration of factor Xa (recombinant), inactivated-zhzo.

Importance of women informing clinicians if they are or plan to become pregnant or plan to breast-feed.

Importance of informing clinicians of existing or contemplated concomitant therapy, including prescription and OTC drugs, as well as any concomitant illnesses.

Importance of informing patients of other important precautionary information. (See Cautions.)

Overview® (see Users Guide). For additional information on this drug until a more detailed monograph is developed and published, the manufacturer's labeling should be consulted. It is *essential* that the manufacturer's labeling be consulted for more detailed information on usual cautions, precautions, contraindications, potential drug interactions, laboratory test interferences, and acute toxicity.

Antihemorrhagic Agents, Miscellaneous 20:28.92

Factor Xa (Recombinant), Inactivated-zhzo

Andexanet Alfa

■ Factor Xa (recombinant), inactivated-zhzo (also known as andexanet alfa), a recombinant modified human factor Xa protein, is a specific reversal agent for the anticoagulant effects of apixaban or rivaroxaban.

Uses

■ **Reversal of Apixaban or Rivaroxaban Anticoagulation** Factor Xa (recombinant), inactivated-zhzo is used to reverse the anticoagulant effects of apixaban or rivaroxaban in patients receiving one of these drugs who have life-threatening or uncontrolled bleeding; factor Xa (recombinant), inactivated-zhzo has been designated an orphan drug by the US Food and Drug Administration (FDA) for this use. The accelerated approval of factor Xa (recombinant), inactivated-zhzo for this indication is based on the change from baseline in anti-factor Xa activity following administration in healthy individuals; an improvement in hemostasis has not been established. Because the concentration of factor Xa inhibitor has been shown to correlate with its anticoagulant action, the reduction of anti-factor Xa activity by factor Xa (recombinant), inactivated-zhzo was used to predict clinical benefit. Continued FDA approval of factor Xa (recombinant), inactivated-zhzo for this indication may be contingent on the results of studies demonstrating an improvement in hemostasis in patients receiving the drug.

Data from clinical trials indicate that factor Xa (recombinant), inactivated-zhzo is effective in rapidly reversing the anticoagulant effects of apixaban or rivaroxaban (as measured by anti-factor Xa activity, unbound anticoagulant concentration, and thrombin generation). Based on its mechanism of action (see Description), factor Xa (recombinant), inactivated-zhzo is expected to reduce the anti-factor Xa activity of all direct (apixaban, betrixaban, edoxaban, and rivaroxaban) and indirect (enoxaparin and fondaparinux) factor Xa inhibitors. However, data regarding reversal of the anticoagulant effect of factor Xa inhibitors other than apixaban and rivaroxaban are lacking, and the manufacturer states that factor Xa (recombinant), inactivated-zhzo is *not* indicated for the treatment of bleeding related to any factor Xa inhibitor other than apixaban or rivaroxaban.

Management of apixaban- or rivaroxaban-induced bleeding complications should be individualized according to the severity and location of hemorrhage; treatment with apixaban or rivaroxaban should be discontinued in patients with active pathological hemorrhage. While experts state that factor Xa (recombinant), inactivated-zhzo can be effective in reversing the anticoagulant effects of apixaban or rivaroxaban in patients with life-threatening or uncontrolled bleeding, obtaining and administering the reversal agent must not delay resuscitation and local hemostatic measures. The manufacturers of apixaban and rivaroxaban state that clotting tests such as prothrombin time (PT), international normalized ratio (INR), and activated partial thromboplastin time (aPTT) are not useful in monitoring the anticoagulant effects of these drugs. A chromogenic anti-factor Xa assay may be useful for assessing the anticoagulant activity of apixaban or rivaroxaban.

For further information regarding clinical manifestations, risk factors, and treatment of apixaban- or rivaroxaban-related bleeding, see Bleeding under Warnings/Precautions: Other Warnings and Precautions, in Cautions in Apixaban 20:12.04.14 and in Rivaroxaban 20:12.04.14.

To accommodate accelerated clinical development, manufacturing process modifications were made to increase factor Xa (recombinant), inactivated-zhzo production resulting in a generation 1 and generation 2 drug product; the same cell line was used for both generation 1 and 2 manufacturing processes. Both generations of drug product have been used in clinical trials; the generation 2 product is the currently commercially available product. The manufacturer has conducted comparability studies to demonstrate that the drug used during clinical trials is representative of the currently marketed product.

The current indication for factor Xa (recombinant), inactivated-zhzo for reversal of apixaban- or rivaroxaban-induced anticoagulation is based principally on the results of 2 randomized, placebo-controlled, double-blind, parallel trials in healthy older adults (ANNEXA-A and ANNEXA-R). In these trials, healthy adults 50–73 years of age (median age: 57 years) who had been given 5 mg of apixaban twice daily (ANNEXA-A) or 20 mg of rivaroxaban once daily (ANNEXA-R) for 3.5–4 days achieved rapid reversal (within 2–5 minutes) of the anticoagulant effects of these drugs (as determined principally by anti-factor Xa activity) following administration of factor Xa (recombinant), inactivated-zhzo on day 4 after steady-state plasma concentrations of apixaban or rivaroxaban had been achieved.

In the ANNEXA-A trial, individuals receiving apixaban were given 400 mg of factor Xa (recombinant), inactivated-zhzo by direct IV ("bolus") injection followed by 480 mg of the drug given by continuous IV infusion (4 mg/minute for 120 minutes). In the ANNEXA-R trial, individuals receiving rivaroxaban were given 800 mg of factor Xa (recombinant), inactivated-zhzo by direct IV injection followed by 960 mg of the drug by continuous IV infusion (8 mg/minute for 120 minutes). The dosages of factor Xa (recombinant), inactivated-zhzo used in these trials were based upon the findings of a phase 2 trial that determined the stoichiometric ratio needed for reversal of each anticoagulant's effects. The primary efficacy end point in both trials (mean percent change in anti-factor Xa activity) was measured using a validated chromogenic assay of factor Xa enzymatic activity. Administration of factor Xa (recombinant), inactivated-zhzo resulted in at least an 80% reversal of anti-factor Xa activity in all but one patient who did not receive the full dose of the drug. In both trials, anti-factor Xa activity was reduced to a greater extent with factor Xa (recombinant), inactivated-zhzo than with placebo (mean reduction of approximately 92–97 versus 33–45%, respectively). In placebo recipients, anti-factor Xa activity decreased in accordance with the expected rate for clearance of either apixaban or rivaroxaban. Administration of factor Xa (recombinant), inactivated-zhzo also was associated with a substantial reduction in the mean concentration of unbound apixaban or rivaroxaban. In all individuals receiving the full dose of factor Xa (recombinant), inactivated-zhzo, thrombin generation increased above the lower limit of the normal range within 2–10 minutes after administration of the direct IV injection. The extent and duration of factor Xa inhibitor reversal that is required to achieve hemostasis in patients has not been established. No serious or severe adverse events, including thrombotic events, were reported in the ANNEXA-A or ANNEXA-R trial.

A decrease in anti-factor Xa activity has been observed in patients receiving factor Xa (recombinant), inactivated-zhzo for the treatment of acute major bleeding (i.e., potentially life-threatening acute overt bleeding with manifestations of hemodynamic compromise, acute overt bleeding associated with a decrease in hemoglobin of at least 2 g/dL, hemoglobin of 8 g/dL or less, or acute symptomatic bleeding in a critical area or organ [retroperitoneal, intra-articular, pericardial, intracranial, or intramuscular with compartment syndrome]) associated with a factor Xa inhibitor. In an interim analysis of the ANNEXA-4 study in 185 patients (of a planned enrollment of 350 patients) who had acute major bleeding (e.g., intracranial hemorrhage, GI bleed) associated with a factor Xa inhibitor (e.g., apixaban, rivaroxaban), a median decrease of 90–93% in anti-factor Xa activity from baseline to nadir (the lowest value measured within five minutes after the end of the continuous infusion of the drug) was observed following administration of factor Xa (recombinant), inactivated-zhzo. Thromboembolic events, ischemic events, cardiac arrest, or sudden death occurred in 17.8% of patients receiving factor Xa (recombinant), inactivated-zhzo during the 30-day follow-up period, and 33% of these patients had been reinitated on anithrombotic therapy prior to the event. In the analysis of the completed study, factor Xa (recombinant), inactivated-zhzo substantially reduced anti-factor Xa activity and approximately 82% of patients who received the drug had excellent or good hemostatic efficacy, as assessed by an independent adjudication committee, 12 hours after the factor Xa (recombinant), inactivated-zhzo infusion.

Dosage and Administration

■ **Reconstitution and Administration** Factor Xa (recombinant), inactivated-zhzo is administered by direct IV ("bolus") injection (target rate of 30 mg/minute) from a prepared IV infusion bag, followed by a continuous IV infusion. The continuous infusion should be initiated within 2 minutes after direct IV injection of the drug and should be continued for up to 120 minutes.

Unopened vials of factor Xa (recombinant), inactivated-zhzo lyophilized powder for injection should be stored refrigerated at 2–8°C. Lyophilized factor Xa (recombinant), inactivated-zhzo for injection must be reconstituted prior to administration as directed by the manufacturer. The drug is reconstituted, using a 20-mL (or larger) syringe and a 20-gauge (or higher) needle, by adding 10 or 20 mL of sterile water for injection to a vial labeled as containing 100 or 200 mg of factor Xa (recombinant), inactivated-zhzo, respectively; the resultant solution contains 10 mg/mL of factor Xa (recombinant), inactivated-zhzo. The vial should be gently swirled (not shaken) to aid reconstitution (typical dissolution time for each vial is 3–5 minutes) and inspected for any evidence of particulate matter. The reconstituted solution should be clear, colorless to slightly yellow, and free from visible particles. The appropriate number of vials needed for the required dose should be reconstituted in succession to reduce the total reconstitution time. To prepare the direct IV injection dose, the appropriate amount of solution should be transferred from the reconstituted vial(s) using a 60-mL (or larger) syringe with a 20-gauge (or higher) needle into an empty polyolefin or PVC IV bag (250 mL or less). Similarly, to prepare the continuous infusion, the appropriate amount of reconstituted solution should be transferred to an empty polyolefin or PVC IV bag (250 mL or less); more than one 40- to 60-mL syringe, or an equivalent 100-mL syringe, may be used to transfer the reconstituted solution to the empty IV bag. An inline 0.2- or 0.22-μm polyethersulfone or equivalent low protein-binding filter should be used during IV administration.

Reconstituted vials of factor Xa (recombinant), inactivated-zhzo are stable at room temperature for up to 8 hours or may be stored refrigerated (2–8°C) for up to 24 hours. Reconstituted factor Xa (recombinant), inactivated-zhzo in an IV bag is stable at room temperature for up to 8 hours.

■ **Dosage** The recommended dosage of factor Xa (recombinant), inactivated-zhzo is based upon the specific factor Xa inhibitor, dosage of the factor Xa inhibitor, and the time since the patient's last dose of the factor Xa inhibitor. (See Table 1.) There are 2 recommended dosage regimens for factor Xa (recombinant), inactivated-zhzo: a low-dose and a high-dose regimen. The low-dose regimen consists of an initial direct IV injection of 400 mg administered at a target rate of 30 mg/minute followed by a continuous IV infusion of 4 mg/minute for up to 120 minutes (480 mg). The high-dose regimen consists of an initial direct IV injection dose of 800 mg administered at a target rate of 30 mg/minute followed by a continuous IV infusion of 8 mg/minute for up to 120 minutes (960 mg). The safety and efficacy of additional doses of factor Xa (recombinant), inactivated-zhzo have not been established.

Preparations

Excipients in commercially available drug preparations may have clinically important effects in some individuals; consult specific product labeling for details.

Factor Xa (Recombinant), Inactivated-zhzo

Parenteral		
For injection, for IV use only	100 mg	Andexxa®, Portola
	200 mg	Andexxa®, Portola

idaruCIZUmab

■ Idarucizumab, a recombinant humanized monoclonal antibody fragment, is a specific reversal agent for the anticoagulant effects of dabigatran etexilate mesylate (Pradaxa®).

Uses

■ **Urgent Reversal of Dabigatran Anticoagulation** Idarucizumab is used to reverse the anticoagulant effects of dabigatran in patients receiving the drug who have life-threatening or uncontrolled bleeding or a need for emergency surgery/urgent procedures; idarucizumab has been designated an orphan drug by the US Food and Drug Administration (FDA) for this use. The accelerated approval of idarucizumab for this indication is based on demonstration of a reduction in unbound plasma dabigatran and normalization of coagulation parameters with idarucizumab treatment in healthy individuals; continued FDA approval for this indication may be contingent on the results of an ongoing cohort case series study. Idarucizumab reverses dabigatran-induced anticoagulation with no impact on the effects of other anticoagulant or antithrombotic therapies. Some experts state that reversal agents such as idarucizumab should be used sparingly and generally should be reserved for patients with severe and life-threatening bleeding or those who must undergo an urgent procedure that requires immediate reversal of anticoagulation.

Management of dabigatran-induced bleeding complications should be individualized according to the severity and location of hemorrhage; treatment with dabigatran should be discontinued and the source of bleeding investigated. Data from clinical trials indicate that idarucizumab has no intrinsic procoagulant or prothrombotic activity and is effective in rapidly and completely reversing the anticoagulant effects of dabigatran. When necessary, ecarin clotting time (ECT) or activated partial thromboplastin time (aPTT) may be used to assess the degree of anticoagulation with dabigatran therapy. Idarucizumab can be used in conjunction with supportive measures (e.g., maintenance of adequate diuresis, mechanical compression, surgical hemostasis, volume replacement, blood products), which should be considered as medically appropriate. Obtaining and administering the reversal agent must not delay resuscitation and local hemostatic measures.

For further information regarding clinical manifestations, risk factors, and treatment of dabigatran-related bleeding, see Bleeding under Warnings/Precautions: Other Warnings and Precautions, in Cautions in Dabigatran Etexilate Mesylate 20:12.04.12.

The current indication for idarucizumab for reversal of dabigatran-induced anticoagulation is based principally on the results of 3 randomized, placebo-controlled, double-blind phase 1 trials in healthy individuals and interim analysis of an open-label, single-cohort, case series trial (Reversal Effects of Idarucizumab on Active Dabigatran [RE-VERSE AD]). In a phase 1 trial evaluating the safety, tolerability, and efficacy of various doses of idarucizumab in healthy men (mean age 29.9–31.9 years among dosing groups, range 18–45 years) receiving dabigatran, idarucizumab effectively reversed dabigatran-induced anticoagulation in a dose-dependent manner as measured by its effect on various coagulation parameters (diluted thrombin time [dTT], ECT, aPTT, thrombin time [TT], and activated clotting time [ACT]). In this trial, individuals received dabigatran 220 mg orally twice daily for 7 doses, followed by idarucizumab (a single 1-, 2-, or 4-g dose IV over 5 minutes, or 5 g IV over 5 minutes followed 1 hour later by an additional 2.5-g IV dose) or placebo approximately 2 hours after the last dose of dabigatran. Administration of at least 2 g of idarucizumab resulted in immediate, complete, and sustained reversal of dabigatran anticoagulant effects; reversal of anticoagulation was not maintained for the entire 72-hour observation period with the 1-g dose of idarucizumab. Idarucizumab was safe and well tolerated at all administered doses and there was no evidence of procoagulant activity with idarucizumab (as determined by no change in endogenous thrombin potential 15 minutes after idarucizumab administration). In another similar phase 1 trial in 80 healthy Japanese men 20–45 years of age, complete reversal of dabigatran anticoagulant effects was observed following IV administration of 4 or 5 g of idarucizumab in individuals receiving dabigatran 220 mg twice daily. In a third randomized, placebo-controlled phase 1 trial in healthy men and women 45–80 years of age and individuals with mild (creatinine clearance 60–89 mL/minute) or moderate (creatinine clearance 30–59 mL/minute) renal impairment, administration of idarucizumab 5 g IV resulted in almost complete reversal of dabigatran-induced anticoagulation regardless of the degree of renal impairment or age. In this trial, dabigatran was administered orally twice daily at a dosage of 220 mg (in those with normal renal function) or 150 mg (in those with mild or moderate renal impairment); idarucizumab was given IV over 5 minutes in doses of 1, 2.5, or 5 g (as a single dose or as two 2.5-g doses approximately 1 hour apart) approximately 2 hours after the last dose of dabigatran.

In the RE-VERSE AD trial, idarucizumab was administered to patients (median age 76.5 years, range 48–93 years) who required urgent reversal of dabigatran-induced anticoagulation because of uncontrolled or life-threatening bleeding (e.g., intracranial hemorrhage, GI bleeding, trauma) or the need for hemostasis required for emergency surgery or other urgent invasive procedures that could not be delayed for at least 8 hours. All patients received idarucizumab 5 g administered as 2 consecutive (2.5 g each) rapid IV ("bolus") infusions, administered no more than 15 minutes apart. The primary efficacy end point was the maximum percentage reversal of the anticoagulant effect of dabigatran as determined at any point from the end of the first idarucizumab infusion to 4 hours after the second infusion, with the percentage reversal assessed on the basis of dTT or ETC. Secondary end points were clinical outcomes (e.g., extent of bleeding and hemodynamic stability, hemostasis during surgical intervention) and were assessed by the treating physician.

Results of an interim analysis of data from 90 patients (of a planned enrollment of 300 patients for this trial) demonstrated a median maximum reversal of the anticoagulant effect of dabigatran (as measured by ECT or dTT) of 100% in the first 4 hours after IV administration of 5 g of idarucizumab, with most patients (at least 89%) achieving complete reversal of anticoagulant effect. Approximately 63–67% of patients had been treated with dabigatran 110 mg orally twice daily. The median time since the last dose of dabigatran as reported by patients was 15.4 hours. Reversal of the anticoagulant effects of dabigatran was evident immediately after the end of the first infusion of idarucizumab. In patients with uncontrolled or life-threatening bleeding who had received a bleeding assessment at baseline and in whom time to cessation of bleeding could be ascertained, median investigator-reported time to cessation of bleeding was 11.4 hours. Normal hemostasis was reported in more than 90% of patients who underwent procedures after the administration of idarucizumab. In this interim analysis, there were 18 deaths overall; 10 deaths were related to vascular causes, including 5 fatal bleeding events. Death within 96 hours after idarucizumab treatment appeared to be related to the index event, whereas all later deaths appeared to be associated with coexisting conditions.

Data are lacking on whether idarucizumab can be safely used to reverse dabigatran-induced anticoagulation before administration of thrombolytic therapy to patients with acute ischemic stroke. Further studies are needed to determine in which conditions or situations idarucizumab can improve clinical outcomes.

Dosage and Administration

■ **Administration** Idarucizumab is administered by IV infusion or by rapid IV ("bolus") injection; the injection should be administered undiluted. Once idarucizumab has been withdrawn from the vial, administration should begin promptly or within 1 hour. The manufacturer states that when administered by IV infusion, idarucizumab should be given as 2 consecutive doses (as rapidly as clinically feasible), with each dose administered directly from a 50-mL vial after spiking the vial with an infusion set. When administered by rapid IV injection, idarucizumab should be given as 2 separate, consecutive doses via syringe (as rapidly as clinically feasible). Some clinicians state that administration of each vial should take no longer than 5–10 minutes.

Idarucizumab injection is commercially available in single-use vials containing 2.5 g of the drug per 50 mL. The drug may be administered through an existing IV line; however, the line must be flushed with 0.9% sodium chloride injection prior to and upon completion of the idarucizumab infusion. Idarucizumab should not be admixed with any other drug, nor should any other drug be administered simultaneously in the same IV line with idarucizumab.

Idarucizumab should be stored at 2–8°C and should not be frozen. Prior to use, the unopened vial may be kept at room temperature (25°C) for up to 48 hours if stored in the original package and protected from light, or for up to 6 hours when exposed to light.

■ **Dosage** For urgent reversal of dabigatran-induced anticoagulation in patients with life-threatening or uncontrolled bleeding or in those undergoing emergency surgery/urgent procedures, the recommended dose of idarucizumab is 5 g administered in 2 divided consecutive doses (2.5 g each) by IV infusion or rapid IV injection. If clinically relevant bleeding recurs and coagulation parameters are elevated after the initial idarucizumab dose, administration of an additional 5-g dose may be considered. Similarly, patients who have elevated coagulation parameters and require a second emergency surgery/urgent procedure may be given an additional 5-g dose of idarucizumab. The safety and efficacy of repeat treatment with idarucizumab have not been established.

Dabigatran therapy can be reinitiated 24 hours after administration of idarucizumab; resumption of anticoagulant therapy should be considered as soon as medically appropriate. (See Thromboembolic Complications under Cautions: Warnings/Precautions.)

Specific Populations **Renal Impairment** No dosage adjustment is required for patients with renal impairment.

Hepatic Impairment Safety and efficacy of idarucizumab have not been established in patients with hepatic impairment.

Cautions

■ **Contraindications** The manufacturer states that there are no contraindications to the use of idarucizumab.

■ **Warnings/Precautions** ***Thromboembolic Complications*** Patients receiving therapy with dabigatran usually have underlying conditions that predispose them to thromboembolism; thus, reversal of anticoagulation by idarucizumab exposes these patients to their underlying thrombotic risk. Resumption of anticoagulant therapy should be considered as soon as medically appropriate to reduce the risk of thrombosis. In the interim analysis of the RE-VERSE AD trial, 5 of 123 patients reported thrombotic events; however, these patients were not receiving antithrombotic therapy at the time of the event and all of the thrombotic events could be attributed to the patient's underlying medical condition.

Hereditary Fructose Intolerance The recommended 5-g dose of idarucizumab contains 4 g of sorbitol as an excipient. The combined daily metabolic load of sorbitol/fructose from all sources, including idarucizumab and other drugs containing sorbitol, should be considered when prescribing idarucizumab to patients with hereditary fructose intolerance. Serious adverse reactions, including death, have been reported in patients with hereditary fructose intolerance who have received sorbitol parenterally. The minimum amount of IV sorbitol at which serious adverse reactions may occur in patients with hereditary fructose intolerance is not known. Other reactions in these patients have included hypoglycemia, hypophosphatemia, metabolic acidosis, increase in uric acid, and acute liver failure with breakdown of hepatic excretory and synthetic function.

Immunogenicity As with all therapeutic proteins, there is a potential for immunogenicity with idarucizumab therapy. Preexisting antibodies with cross-reactivity to idarucizumab were detected in some patients in clinical trials; no impact on the pharmacokinetics or reversal effect of idarucizumab and no hypersensitivity reactions were observed in these patients. Treatment-emergent, possibly persisting anti-idarucizumab antibodies with low titers were observed in approximately 4% of patients treated with idarucizumab.

Sensitivity Reactions **Hypersensitivity.** The manufacturer states that there is insufficient clinical experience to evaluate the risk of hypersensitivity to idarucizumab. Adverse events possibly indicative of hypersensitivity reactions (e.g., pyrexia, bronchospasm, rash, pruritus) where a possible relationship could not be excluded have been reported. The risk of hypersensitivity should be carefully weighed against the anticipated benefits of idarucizumab in patients with known hypersensitivity (e.g., anaphylactoid reaction) to idarucizumab or other ingredients in the formulation. If anaphylaxis or any severe hypersensitivity reaction occurs, idarucizumab should be discontinued immediately and appropriate therapy initiated as indicated.

Specific Populations **Pregnancy.** There are no adequate and well-controlled studies of idarucizumab in pregnant women. Data from animal reproductive and developmental studies with idarucizumab are lacking. It is not known whether idarucizumab can cause fetal harm when administered to a pregnant woman or if the drug can affect reproductive capacity. Idarucizumab should be used during pregnancy only when clearly needed. Safety and efficacy of the drug during labor and delivery have not been established.

Lactation. It is not known whether idarucizumab is distributed into human milk. Because many drugs are distributed into milk, the drug should be used with caution in nursing women.

Pediatric Use. Safety and efficacy of idarucizumab have not been established in pediatric patients.

Geriatric Use. In the interim analysis of the RE-VERSE AD trial, 90% of patients were 65 years of age or older. While clinical experience has not revealed age-related differences in safety or efficacy, the possibility that some older patients may exhibit increased sensitivity to the drug cannot be ruled out.

Renal Impairment. Renal impairment does not affect the dabigatran anticoagulation reversal effect of idarucizumab.

Hepatic Impairment. Data are lacking on the pharmacokinetics of idarucizumab in patients with hepatic impairment.

■ **Common Adverse Effects** Adverse effects reported in at least 5% of patients receiving idarucizumab in the RE-VERSE AD trial (at the interim analysis) were hypokalemia, delirium, constipation, pyrexia, and pneumonia. In phase 1 clinical trials, headache was reported in at least 5% of healthy individuals who received idarucizumab.

Drug Interactions

■ **Coagulation Factor Concentrates** In vitro data suggest that inhibition of dabigatran by idarucizumab is not affected by concomitant use of coagulation factor concentrates (3- or 4-factor prothrombin complex concentrates [PCC], activated PCC, or recombinant factor VIIa).

■ **Volume-replacement Preparations** Studies in animals (swine) suggest that neutralization of dabigatran anticoagulant activity is not influenced by 50% hemodilution with routinely used volume-replacement therapies (e.g., crystalloids, colloids).

Description

Idarucizumab is a recombinant humanized immunoglobulin G_1 (IgG_1) monoclonal antibody fragment that binds specifically to unbound and thrombin-bound dabigatran and its acylglucuronide metabolites, rapidly forming stable and essentially irreversible complexes. The drug is prepared from cultures of genetically modified mammalian (Chinese hamster ovary) cells using recombinant DNA technology. The affinity of idarucizumab for dabigatran is approximately 350-fold greater than that of dabigatran for thrombin. Because of the high affinity of idarucizumab for dabigatran, thrombin is no longer inhibited by dabigatran after idarucizumab administration and can regain its ability to trigger clotting. Idarucizumab has been shown to reverse the anticoagulant effects of dabigatran within minutes after administration. Idarucizumab is found mainly in plasma after administration whereas dabigatran is capable of moving freely between the blood and extravascular compartments. The concentration of unbound dabigatran (i.e., dabigatran and its conjugates that are not bound to plasma proteins or to idarucizumab) decreases when idarucizumab binds dabigatran in plasma. Any residual unbound dabigatran reestablishes equilibrium by moving from the extravascular compartment into plasma where it is bound by idarucizumab, provided that idarucizumab is administered in excess. This process continues until all of the dabigatran is bound and its anticoagulant activity is neutralized. Increases in plasma dabigatran concentrations as well as elevated coagulation parameters (e.g., activated partial thromboplastin time [aPTT], ecarin clotting time [ECT]) were seen in a limited number of patients in the RE-VERSE AD trial 12–24 hours after administration of idarucizumab; this finding is most likely attributable to redistribution of extravascular dabigatran into the intravascular compartment. Idarucizumab has many structural similarities to thrombin; however, it lacks thrombin-like enzymatic activity and does not bind thrombin substrates. In animal and human studies, idarucizumab did not promote or attenuate thrombin generation, suggesting that it has no intrinsic anticoagulant or procoagulant effects. The drug had no effect in stimulating platelet aggregation during in vitro studies. Idarucizumab does not affect the activity of factor Xa inhibitors (apixaban, edoxaban, rivaroxaban), direct thrombin inhibitors (argatroban, hirudin), vitamin K antagonists (warfarin), or heparin.

Idarucizumab exhibits multiphasic disposition kinetics and limited extravascular distribution. In clinical trials, no substantial differences in plasma concentration-time profiles of idarucizumab were evident following administration of the drug alone or after pretreatment with dabigatran. Idarucizumab has an initial half-life of 47 minutes and a terminal half-life of 10.3 hours. Idarucizumab is thought to be metabolized via biodegradation into smaller molecules (i.e., small peptides or amino acids), which are then reabsorbed and incorporated into general protein synthesis. Approximately 32% of a 5-g IV dose of idarucizumab is eliminated in urine within 6 hours followed by less than 1% of the dose during the following 18 hours; the remaining portion of drug is thought to be eliminated via protein catabolism, principally in the kidney.

Advice to Patients

Importance of informing patients of signs and symptoms of allergic hypersensitivity reactions (e.g., anaphylaxis) that may occur during or after injection of idarucizumab.

Importance of informing patients that reversing the effects of dabigatran therapy exposes them to the thromboembolic risk of their underlying disease. Clinicians should consider resuming anticoagulant therapy as soon as the patient is sufficiently stable.

Importance of advising patients to seek immediate medical attention for any signs or symptoms of bleeding.

Importance of informing patients with hereditary fructose intolerance that idarucizumab injection contains sorbitol. Importance of informing patients that parenteral administration of sorbitol in patients who have hereditary fructose intolerance has been associated with reports of hypoglycemia, metabolic acidosis, increase in uric acid, acute liver failure with breakdown of hepatic excretory and synthetic function, and death, which may occur during or after injection of idarucizumab.

Importance of women informing clinicians if they are or plan to become pregnant or plan to breast-feed.

Importance of informing clinicians of existing or contemplated concomitant therapy, including prescription and OTC drugs, as well as any concomitant illnesses.

Importance of informing patients of other important precautionary information. (See Cautions.)

Overview® (see Users Guide). For additional information on this drug until a more detailed monograph is developed and published, the manufacturer's labeling should be consulted. It is *essential* that the manufacturer's labeling be consulted for more detailed information on usual cautions, precautions, contraindications, potential drug interactions, laboratory test interferences, and acute toxicity.

Preparations

Excipients in commercially available drug preparations may have clinically important effects in some individuals; consult specific product labeling for details.

idaruCIZUmab

Parenteral		
Injection, for IV use	50 mg/mL (2.5 g)	**Praxbind®**, Boehringer Ingelheim

Selected Revisions October 2019,

24:00 Cardiovascular Drugs*

§ Omitted from the print version of *AHFS Drug Information*® because of space limitations. This monograph is available on the *AHFS Drug Information*® website, http://ahfsdruginformation.com. Username: ahfs2020; Password: ASHP94498.

* Please see the full *AHFS Pharmacologic-Therapeutic Classification*© on p. viii. Not all classes are used in the printed edition.

CARDIAC DRUGS 24:04
ANTIARRHYTHMIC AGENTS 24:04.04
CLASS IA ANTIARRHYTHMICS 24:04.04.04

Procainamide Hydrochloride

Procaine Amide Hydrochloride

■ Procainamide hydrochloride is a class Ia antiarrhythmic agent.

Uses

■ **Ventricular Arrhythmias** Procainamide hydrochloride is used for the treatment of ventricular arrhythmias (e.g., sustained ventricular tachycardia) that in the judgment of the physician are life-threatening, but the drug usually is not the antiarrhythmic of first choice. Because of the drug's arrhythmogenic potential, the lack of evidence for improved survival for class I antiarrhythmic agents, and the risk of serious (occurring in about 0.5% of patients), potentially fatal adverse hematologic effects (see Cautions: Hematologic Effects), particularly leukopenia or agranulocytosis, use of procainamide for less severe arrhythmias is not recommended by the manufacturer. Findings from the National Heart, Lung, and Blood Institute (NHLBI)'s Cardiac Arrhythmia Suppression Trial (CAST) study after an average of 10 months of follow-up have indicated that the rate of total mortality and nonfatal cardiac arrest in patients with recent myocardial infarction, mild-to-moderate left ventricular dysfunction, and asymptomatic or mildly symptomatic ventricular arrhythmias (principally frequent ventricular premature complexes [VPCs, PVCs]) who received encainide or flecainide increased substantially compared with placebo. (See Cautions in Flecainide 24:04.04.12.). Therefore, therapy with selected antiarrhythmic agents (e.g., procainamide) should be reserved for the suppression and prevention of documented life-threatening ventricular arrhythmias and treatment of patients with asymptomatic VPCs should be avoided. The manufacturers state that procainamide therapy should be initiated only in a hospital setting.

Procainamide has been used to suppress and prevent the recurrence of less severe but *symptomatic* ventricular arrhythmias†, including uniform, multiform, and/or coupled VPCs† and nonsustained ventricular tachycardia, and asymptomatic ventricular arrhythmias†; however, the arrhythmogenic potential of the drug and findings of the CAST study with other class I antiarrhythmic agents have called into question the safety of using such agents in arrhythmias that were not life-threatening. Therefore, procainamide therapy should be reserved for *life-threatening* ventricular arrhythmias in carefully selected patients in whom the benefits of procainamide therapy outweigh the possible risks.

Life-Threatening Ventricular Arrhythmias and Advanced Cardiovascular Life Support Antiarrhythmic drugs are used during cardiac arrest to facilitate the restoration and maintenance of a spontaneous perfusing rhythm in patients with refractory (i.e., persisting or recurring after at least one shock) ventricular fibrillation or pulseless ventricular tachycardia; however, there is no evidence that these drugs increase survival to hospital discharge when given routinely during cardiac arrest. High-quality cardiopulmonary resuscitation (CPR) and defibrillation are integral components of advanced cardiovascular life support (ACLS) and the only proven interventions to increase survival to hospital discharge. Other resuscitative efforts, including drug therapy, are considered secondary and should be performed without compromising the quality and timely delivery of chest compressions and defibrillation. The principal goal of pharmacologic therapy during cardiac arrest is to facilitate return of spontaneous circulation (ROSC), and epinephrine is considered the drug of choice for this use. (See Uses: Advanced Cardiovascular Life Support and Cardiac Arrhythmias, in Epinephrine 12:12.12.) Antiarrhythmic drugs may be considered for the treatment of refractory ventricular fibrillation or pulseless ventricular tachycardia during cardiac resuscitation; however, experts generally recommend the use of amiodarone (or lidocaine). Procainamide may be used for the management of regular wide-complex tachycardias during the periarrest period and is included as a recommended antiarrhythmic agent in current ACLS guidelines for adult and pediatric tachycardia.

Monomorphic and Polymorphic Ventricular Tachycardia Procainamide is one of several antiarrhythmic agents that may be used in the treatment of sustained, stable monomorphic ventricular tachycardia not associated with angina, pulmonary edema, or hypotension (blood pressure less than 90 mm Hg) in patients with preserved ventricular function. Drug regimens including amiodarone or procainamide may be used initially for the treatment of patients with episodes of sustained ventricular tachycardia that are somewhat better tolerated hemodynamically. If IV antiarrhythmic therapy is used for ventricular fibrillation or tachycardia, it probably should be discontinued (at least temporarily) after 6–24 hours so that the patient's ongoing need for antiarrhythmic drugs can be reassessed.

Although rare, episodes of drug-refractory sustained polymorphic ventricular tachycardia ("electrical storm") have been reported in cases of acute myocardial infarction. Some experts state that these episodes usually are treated with an IV β-adrenergic blocking agent, IV amiodarone, left stellate ganglion blockade, intra-aortic balloon counterpulsation (IABP), or emergency revascularization; IV magnesium also may be used. However, other experts recommend revascularization and β-blockade followed by IV antiarrhythmic drugs, such as procainamide or amiodarone, for patients with recurrent or incessant polymorphic ventricular tachycardia due to acute myocardial ischemia.

Ventricular Premature Complexes Procainamide decreases the frequency of VPCs associated with acute myocardial infarction, but IV lidocaine is considered the drug of choice because normal doses of lidocaine do not decrease cardiac contractility or peripheral resistance or slow AV conduction to the degree produced by procainamide. Like other antiarrhythmic drugs, procainamide has not been shown to decrease mortality rate in patients with VPCs associated with acute myocardial infarction. The use of procainamide in the treatment of asymptomatic VPCs should be avoided. Procainamide generally is not used to treat cardiac glycoside-induced ventricular arrhythmias. (See Cautions: Precautions and Contraindications.)

■ **Supraventricular Tachyarrhythmias** Procainamide has been used for the treatment of various supraventricular tachycardias (SVTs)†; because of a higher risk of toxicity and proarrhythmic effects, antiarrhythmic agents generally should be reserved for patients who do not respond to or cannot be treated with AV nodal blocking agents (β-adrenergic blocking agents and nondihydropyridine calcium-channel blocking agents). Some experts state that procainamide may be useful for restoring sinus rhythm or slowing ventricular rate in patients with preexcited atrial fibrillation and rapid ventricular response associated with Wolff-Parkinson-White syndrome† since AV nodal blocking agents are contraindicated in such patients; however, direct-current cardioversion is the treatment of choice in hemodynamically compromised patients. Procainamide also has been used in the management of junctional tachycardia†, but the drug has a more limited role in this arrhythmia and is usually considered only when IV β-adrenergic blocking agents are ineffective.

■ **Other Uses** IV procainamide has been used effectively in the treatment of malignant hyperthermia†. Procainamide is also used parenterally (preferably IM) in the treatment of arrhythmias that occur during surgery and anesthesia.

Dosage and Administration

■ **Administration** Procainamide hydrochloride may be administered by IM or IV injection or by IV infusion. ECG and blood pressure should be continuously monitored during IV administration of procainamide. IV administration may produce transient high plasma levels of the drug, which can cause severe hypotension.

Procainamide may be administered by intraosseous (IO) injection† in the setting of pediatric advanced cardiovascular life support (PALS); onset of action and systemic concentrations are comparable to those achieved with venous administration. The drug also has been administered orally; however, an oral dosage form no longer is commercially available in the US.

■ **Dosage** Dosage of procainamide must be carefully adjusted according to individual requirements and response, age, renal function, and the general condition and cardiovascular status of the patient. ECG monitoring of cardiac function and monitoring of renal function (i.e. creatinine clearance) is recommended during procainamide therapy, especially when the drug is given IV or when it is given in patients with increased risk of adverse reactions to procainamide, such as patients older than 50 years of age and patients with severe heart disease, hypotension, or hepatic or renal disease. Dosage should be reduced in patients with renal insufficiency and/or congestive heart failure and in critically ill patients; plasma concentrations of procainamide and its major metabolite *N*-acetyl procainamide (NAPA) should be determined and dosage should be adjusted to maintain desired concentrations.

Adult Dosage **Ventricular and Supraventricular Arrhythmias.** The usual initial adult IM dosage of procainamide hydrochloride is 50 mg/kg given in divided doses (every 3–6 hours). For the treatment of arrhythmias that occur during surgery and anesthesia, 100–500 mg of procainamide hydrochloride may be administered parenterally (preferably IM) in adults.

To facilitate control of the rate of administration, it is recommended that commercially available injections of procainamide hydrochloride be diluted prior to direct IV injection. Administration of the drug by IV injection should be done slowly at a rate not exceeding 50 mg/minute. If procainamide hydrochloride is administered by IV infusion, the drug should be diluted with a suitable IV infusion fluid (usually 5% dextrose injection) to a concentration of 20 mg/mL (for initial loading infusion) or 2 or 4 mg/mL (for maintenance infusion). *Blood pressure and ECG should be monitored continuously and the rate of administration adjusted accordingly.* If a fall in blood pressure of more than 15 mm Hg occurs, or if excessive widening of the QRS complex (greater than 50%) or prolongation of the PR interval occurs, or if severe adverse effects appear, the drug should be temporarily discontinued.

For initial control of arrhythmias in adults, IV doses of 100 mg of procainamide hydrochloride may be given every 5 minutes until the arrhythmia is controlled, adverse effects occur, or until a total of 500 mg has been administered, after which it may be advisable to wait 10 minutes or longer to allow for distribution of the drug before additional doses are given. Alternatively, a loading-dose IV infusion of 500–600 mg may be administered at a constant rate over a period of 25–30 minutes. Although it is unusual to require more than 600 mg to initially control an arrhythmia, the maximum recommended total dose given by either method of IV administration is 1 g. To maintain therapeutic plasma concentrations subsequently, a continuous IV infusion of 2–6 mg/minute may be administered. Alternatively, some clinicians have recommended a maintenance IV infusion of 0.02–0.08 mg/kg per minute.

If used in adults with cardiac arrest, some experts recommend an IV infusion of 20 mg/minute up to a total maximum dose of 17 mg/kg.

Malignant Hyperthermia. Various dosages of procainamide hydrochloride have been given in the treatment of malignant hyperthermia†. The IV dosage has ranged from 200–900 mg and has generally been followed by a maintenance infusion.

Pediatric Dosage **Ventricular and Supraventricular Arrhythmias.** The manufacturers have not established pediatric dosage recommendations for procainamide hydrochloride.

Pediatric parenteral dosage recommendations are variable, and clinicians should consult specialized references for specific information. Some clinicians recommend a pediatric IV dose of 2–6 mg/kg (not to exceed 100 mg) as a loading dose administered over 5 minutes, repeated as necessary at intervals of 5–10 minutes (not to exceed a total loading dose of 15 mg/kg or 500 mg in a 30-minute period). Also, some experts recommend a maintenance IV infusion dose of 0.02–0.08 mg (20–80 mcg)/kg per minute, up to a total maintenance infusion dose of 2 g in 24 hours. For pediatric resuscitation, some experts recommend an IV or IO† dose of 15 mg/kg given over 30–60 minutes with discontinuance of the drug if widening of the QRS complex (greater than 50%) from baseline occurs or hypotension develops. If the drug is administered IM, some clinicians recommend a pediatric dosage of 20–30 mg/kg daily (not to exceed 4 g in 24 hours), given in divided doses (every 4–6 hours).

Cautions

Procainamide has numerous adverse effects which may necessitate cessation of therapy in many patients.

■ **Sensitivity Reactions** Prolonged use of procainamide often results in the development of positive antinuclear antibody (ANA) titers. ANA titers are found in at least 50% of patients receiving long-term procainamide therapy (usually within 2–18 months after starting therapy); the induction of ANA by the drug appears to be independent of the dosage. Patients with procainamide-induced increases in ANA titers may develop a syndrome resembling systemic lupus erythematosus (SLE), characterized by polyarthralgia, arthritis, pleurisy, pleural effusion, dyspnea, fever, chills, myalgia, skin lesions (including urticaria, erythema multiforme, and morbilliform eruptions), headache, fatigue, weakness, abdominal pain, nausea, vomiting, pericarditis, pericardial effusion, pericardial tamponade, acute hepatomegaly, splenomegaly, lymphadenopathy, acute pancreatitis, and the presence of LE cells in the blood. Patients with procainamide-induced SLE may have a positive direct antiglobulin (Coombs') test. Thrombocytopenia, Coombs' positive hemolytic anemia, increased serum concentrations of AST (SGOT), ALT (SGPT), and amylase rarely have been associated with procainamide-induced SLE. Procainamide-induced SLE syndrome probably represents a hypersensitivity reaction in which procainamide anti-DNA antibodies are formed.

If a positive ANA titer develops during procainamide therapy, the relative benefits and risks of continued therapy with the drug should be assessed. Procainamide should be discontinued in patients who develop symptoms of SLE and/or who have rising ANA titer, unless the benefit of antiarrhythmic therapy with the drug outweighs the potential risk. If procainamide-induced SLE develops in a patient with a life-threatening arrhythmia uncontrolled by other antiarrhythmic drugs, the manufacturers state that corticosteroid therapy may be used concomitantly with procainamide. Signs and symptoms of SLE usually regress when the drug is discontinued, but long-term treatment with corticosteroids may be necessary if symptoms do not regress. If arthralgia, fever, rash, malaise, or other unexplained symptoms occur, laboratory studies such as LE cell preparations and ANA titer determinations should be performed.

■ **Hematologic Effects** Serious adverse hematologic effects, including agranulocytosis, leukopenia, bone marrow depression, hypoplastic anemia, and thrombocytopenia, have been reported in 0.5% of patients receiving procainamide. Pure red cell aplasia also has been reported. In most reported cases, such effects occurred with usual recommended dosages of procainamide during the first 12 weeks of therapy. The drug should be discontinued if any of these adverse hematologic effects occurs. Although blood cell counts usually return to normal within 1 month after discontinuance of procainamide, adverse hematologic effects have been fatal in some cases (e.g., in about 20–25% of patients who developed agranulocytosis). Because of the risk of these effects, careful monitoring of hematologic status is necessary during procainamide therapy (see Cautions: Precautions and Contraindications), and use of the drug should be limited to patients in whom the potential benefits clearly outweigh the possible risks (see Uses).

Leukopenia, hemolytic anemia, and eosinophilia also have occurred rarely in patients receiving procainamide. In at least one case, pancytopenia with generalized ecchymoses has been reported. Adverse hematologic effects also have been associated with a procainamide-induced syndrome resembling systemic lupus erythematosus. (See Cautions: Sensitivity Reactions.)

■ **GI Effects** GI disturbances such as anorexia, bitter taste, abdominal pain, nausea, vomiting, and diarrhea may occur in patients receiving procainamide and are most common with dosages of 4 g or more daily.

■ **Nervous System Effects** Adverse nervous system effects of procainamide are rare and have included dizziness, giddiness, seizures, mental depression, confusion, and psychosis with hallucinations.

■ **Dermatologic Effects** Urticaria, pruritus, and maculopapular rash have occurred occasionally in patients receiving procainamide. An urticarial vasculitis also has occurred.

■ **Cardiovascular Effects** Paradoxically, an extremely rapid ventricular rate may occur when procainamide is used in the treatment of atrial fibrillation or flutter, because of a reduction in the degree of AV nodal block to a 1:1 ratio. Patients with atrial flutter or fibrillation should be cardioverted or digitalized prior to procainamide administration to avoid enhanced AV conduction, which may result in ventricular rate acceleration beyond tolerable limits. The anticholinergic action of the drug on the AV node may also increase the heart rate. Procainamide-induced ventricular tachycardia may be prevented by prior digitalization; however, in atrial flutter or fibrillation, adequate digitalization reduces but does not eliminate the possibility of sudden increase in ventricular rate as the atrial rate is slowed by procainamide. If cessation of atrial fibrillation is accompanied by depression of the normal pacemaker, an idioventricular rhythm (including ventricular tachycardia and fibrillation) may result. Procainamide-induced ventricular tachycardia is particularly hazardous in patients with extensive myocardial injury. Conversion of atrial fibrillation also may be associated with embolism. Therefore, anticoagulant therapy may be necessary before procainamide conversion of atrial fibrillation to normal sinus rhythm. (See Uses: Supraventricular Tachyarrhythmias.) The arrhythmogenic effect of procainamide may result in atypical ventricular tachycardia (torsades de pointes). (See Cautions: Precautions and Contraindications.)

Procainamide cardiotoxicity is evidenced by conduction defects (50% widening of the QRS complex), ventricular tachycardia, frequent ventricular premature complexes, and complete AV block. When these ECG signs appear, procainamide should be discontinued and the patient should be monitored closely. Less frequently, ECG signs of toxicity may include prolongation of the PR and QT intervals and decreases in voltage of the QRS complexes and T waves. Adverse cardiac effects occur most commonly when procainamide is administered IV. The hazard of ventricular fibrillation increases with increasing dosage of procainamide and may be accompanied by ECG signs of toxicity. Large IV doses of the drug may cause heart block and asystole, and death has occurred rarely.

The manufacturers state that phenylephrine or norepinephrine should be available to treat severe hypotension caused by IV procainamide.

■ **Other Adverse Effects** Other adverse effects of procainamide include fever, flushing, angioedema, hypergammaglobulinemia, and, rarely, generalized or digital vasculitis, proximal myopathy, and Sjögren's syndrome. Hepatomegaly with increased serum aminotransferase concentrations has been reported after a single oral dose of the drug. Liver aminotransferase concentrations have been elevated, with or without elevations in alkaline phosphatase and bilirubin concentrations, in patients receiving oral procainamide. Abnormal liver function test results in some patients were accompanied by malaise, right upper-quadrant pain, liver failure, and death secondary to liver failure.

■ **Precautions and Contraindications** Findings from the postmarketing Cardiac Arrhythmia Suppression Trial (CAST), a long-term, multicenter, randomized, double-blind study in patients with asymptomatic non-life-threatening ventricular arrhythmias who had had myocardial infarctions more than 6 days but less than 2 years previously, indicate that the rate of total mortality and nonfatal cardiac arrest was increased in patients treated with encainide or flecainide compared with that seen in patients who received placebo. The applicability of these results to other populations (e.g., those without recent myocardial infarction) is uncertain. The manufacturers state that because of the drug's arrhythmogenic potential, the lack of evidence for improved survival for class I antiarrhythmic agents, and the risk of serious (occurring in about 0.5% of patients), potentially fatal adverse hematologic effects (see Cautions: Hematologic Effects), use of procainamide hydrochloride in patients with ventricular arrhythmias should be limited to those with *life-threatening* arrhythmias in carefully selected patients in whom benefits of procainamide therapy outweigh the possible risks, taking into account possible alternative antiarrhythmic therapy. Use of procainamide in less severe arrhythmias currently is not recommended and treatment of asymptomatic VPCs should be avoided.

Since procainamide, like other antiarrhythmic agents, has been associated with the development or exacerbation of arrhythmias in some patients, clinical and ECG evaluations are essential prior to and during procainamide therapy to monitor for the appearance of arrhythmias and to determine the need for continued therapy. Procainamide should be used with extreme caution, if at all, in patients with marked disturbances of AV conduction, such as second- or third-degree heart block, bundle-branch block, or severe cardiac glycoside intoxication because procainamide may cause additional depression of conduction, resulting in ventricular asystole or fibrillation. The drug is contraindicated in patients with complete AV heart block and in patients with second- or third-degree AV nodal block unless an electrical pacemaker is operative. The dosage should be reduced in patients who exhibit or develop first-degree heart block with procainamide; if the block persists despite dosage reduction, risk versus benefit of continued therapy with increased heart block must be carefully evaluated. Procainamide should be administered with caution (especially parenterally) in the treatment of ventricular arrhythmias in patients with severe organic heart disease, since these patients may have undiagnosed complete heart block; if the ventricular rate is slowed by procainamide and normal AV conduction does not occur, the drug should be discontinued and the patient reevaluated, since asystole may result. Procainamide also is contraindicated in patients with atypical ventricular tachycardia (torsades de pointes), since class IA antiarrhythmic agents may aggravate this ventricular arrhythmia. The possibility that potentially serious cardiac arrhythmias, including torsades de pointes, could occur if procainamide were used concomitantly with other drugs that prolong the QT_c interval also should be considered and such combined use should be avoided. Procainamide should be used with extreme caution in the treatment of ventricular tachycardia occurring during coronary occlusion. Hypokalemia, hypoxia, and disorders of acid-base balance must be eliminated as potentiating factors in patients who require large doses of antiarrhythmic agents to control ventricular arrhythmias. Procainamide should be used with caution in patients with congestive heart failure, acute ischemic heart disease, or cardiomyopathy, since even slight depression of contractility may further decrease cardiac output. Procainamide should be used with caution in patients with renal and hepatic disease, since accumulation of the drug may cause symptoms of overdosage, such as ventricular tachycardia and severe hypotension.

Commercially available formulations of procainamide hydrochloride injection may contain sulfites, which can cause allergic-type reactions, including anaphylaxis and life-threatening or less severe asthmatic episodes, in certain susceptible individuals. The overall prevalence of sulfite sensitivity in the general population is unknown but probably low; such sensitivity appears to occur more frequently in asthmatic than in nonasthmatic individuals.

Procainamide should be used with caution in patients with preexisting bone marrow depression or cytopenia of any type. Because of the risk of potentially severe, sometimes fatal adverse hematologic effects, the manufacturers recommend that complete blood cell counts, including differential leukocyte counts and platelet counts, optimally be performed at weekly intervals during the first 3 months of therapy and periodically thereafter. If a serious adverse hematologic effect is identified, the drug should be discontinued. Patients should be instructed to promptly report to their physician any sign of infection (e.g., sore mouth, throat, or gums; unexplained fever; chills), unusual bleeding or bruising, rash, arthralgia, myalgia, dark urine or icterus, wheezing, muscular weakness, chest or abdominal pain, palpitation, nausea, vomiting, anorexia, diarrhea, hallucinations, dizziness, or mental depression associated with procainamide therapy. If any of these signs and/or symptoms occur and granulocytopenia is present, the drug should be discontinued and appropriate treatment (e.g., measures to prevent infection) should be instituted immediately. Laboratory tests for detection of procainamide-induced SLE such as ANA titer determinations should be performed before and periodically during maintenance or prolonged procainamide therapy, even in asymptomatic patients. Procainamide is contraindicated in patients with an established diagnosis of SLE, since symptomatic aggravation is likely.

Procainamide is contraindicated in patients who are hypersensitive to the drug, and the possibility of cross-sensitivity to procaine and chemically related drugs (e.g., ester-type local anesthetics) must be considered, although cross-sensitivity is unlikely. Procainamide should not be used if it causes acute allergic dermatitis, asthma, or anaphylactic symptoms. Since procainamide has been reported to increase muscle weakness in patients with myasthenia gravis, the drug may be contraindicated in these patients. (See Drug Interactions: Anticholinesterase and Anticholinergic Agents.)

■ Pediatric Precautions Safety and efficacy of procainamide in pediatric patients have not been established. However, some experts state that procainamide may be considered in children with supraventricular tachycardia unresponsive to adenosine, vagal maneuvers, or electric cardioversion. Procainamide also has been used during pediatric resuscitation; expert consultation prior to use in a hemodynamically stable patient is strongly recommended. In addition, the drug should not be used in combination with another agent that prolongs the QT interval (e.g., amiodarone) without expert consultation.

■ Geriatric Precautions Clinical studies of procainamide did not include sufficient numbers of patients 65 years of age and older to determine whether geriatric patients respond differently than younger patients. Because the drug is known to be substantially excreted by the kidney, patients with renal impairment may be at increased risk of procainamide-induced toxicity. In general, dosage should be titrated carefully in geriatric patients, usually initiating therapy at the low end of the dosage range. (See Dosage and Administration: Dosage.) The greater frequency of decreased hepatic, renal, and/or cardiac function and of concomitant disease and drug therapy observed in the elderly also should be considered.

■ Mutagenicity and Carcinogenicity Studies to determine the mutagenic and carcinogenic potentials of procainamide have not been performed to date.

■ Pregnancy and Lactation Animal reproduction studies have not been performed with procainamide. It is not known whether procainamide can cause fetal harm when administered to pregnant women or can affect reproduction capacity. Procainamide does cross the placenta, but the extent to which it does so has not been well characterized. Procainamide should be used during pregnancy only when clearly needed.

Procainamide and NAPA are distributed into milk and can be absorbed by a nursing infant. Because of the potential for serious adverse reactions to procainamide in nursing infants, a decision should be made whether to discontinue nursing or the drug, taking into account the importance of the drug to the woman.

Drug Interactions

■ Histamine H_2-Receptor Antagonists Concomitant administration of procainamide and cimetidine may result in increased plasma procainamide and NAPA concentrations and subsequent toxicity. This interaction may be more marked in geriatric patients and patients with renal impairment since such patients eliminate procainamide, NAPA, and cimetidine more slowly. Cimetidine decreases the renal clearance of procainamide and NAPA; however, additional mechanisms also may contribute to this interaction. Limited evidence suggests that ranitidine also may increase plasma concentrations of procainamide and NAPA, but to a lesser extent than cimetidine; the precise mechanisms for this interaction are complex and are not fully understood. Evidence to date suggests that famotidine does not substantially interact with procainamide. Caution should be exercised when either cimetidine or ranitidine is administered concomitantly with procainamide, particularly in geriatric patients and patients with renal impairment; the patient and plasma procainamide concentrations should be monitored closely and procainamide dosage adjusted accordingly.

■ Neuromuscular Blocking Agents Procainamide may enhance the effects of skeletal muscle relaxants. The drug may potentiate the effects of both nondepolarizing and depolarizing skeletal muscle relaxants, such as gallamine triethiodide (no longer commercially available in the US), metocurine iodide (no longer commercially available in the US), pancuronium bromide, succinylcholine chloride, and tubocurarine chloride. Although the clinical significance of this interaction has not been established, procainamide should be used with caution in conjunction with neuromuscular blocking agents.

■ Anticholinesterase and Anticholinergic Agents Procainamide should be used with caution, if at all, in patients with myasthenia gravis and the dose of anticholinesterase drugs such as neostigmine and pyridostigmine may have to be increased. Theoretically, the anticholinergic effect of procainamide may be additive with anticholinergic drugs or procainamide may enhance the effects of anticholinergic agents.

■ Cardiovascular Drugs Since procainamide may reduce blood pressure, patients receiving hypotensive drugs and procainamide parenterally or in high oral doses should be observed for possible additive hypotensive effects. β-adrenergic blocking agents may increase plasma procainamide concentrations.

Concomitant use of procainamide with drugs that prolong the QT_c interval may result in potentially serious cardiac arrhythmias, including torsades de pointes.

Concurrent use of procainamide with class IA antiarrhythmics (e.g., disopyramide, quinidine) may enhance conduction prolongation, contractility depression, and hypotension, especially in patients with cardiac decompensation; combined use should be reserved for serious arrhythmias unresponsive to monotherapy and only if close observation is possible. When procainamide is administered with other antiarrhythmic drugs such as lidocaine, phenytoin, propranolol, or quinidine, the cardiac effects may be additive or antagonistic and toxic effects may be additive.

Concomitant use of procainamide and amiodarone may result in increased plasma procainamide and *N*-acetylprocainamide (NAPA) concentrations and subsequent toxicity. In a limited number of patients receiving 2–6 g of procainamide hydrochloride daily, initiation of amiodarone hydrochloride (1200 mg daily for 5–7 days and then 600 mg daily) increased plasma procainamide and NAPA concentrations by about 55 and 33%, respectively, during the first week of amiodarone therapy. The exact mechanism(s) has not been elucidated, but it has been suggested that amiodarone may decrease the renal clearance of procainamide or NAPA and/or inhibit the hepatic metabolism of procainamide. In addition to a pharmacokinetic interaction, additive electrophysiologic effects, including increased QT_c and QRS intervals, occur during concomitant use; adverse electrophysiologic effects (e.g., acceleration of ventricular tachycardia) may also occur. Pending further accumulation of data, it is recommended that procainamide dosage be reduced by 20–33% when amiodarone therapy is initiated in patients currently receiving procainamide or that procainamide therapy be discontinued.

■ Other Drugs Concomitant administration of procainamide and trimethoprim may result in increased plasma procainamide and NAPA concentrations.

Because alcohol appears to enhance acetylation of procainamide to NAPA, alcohol consumption may reduce the half-life of procainamide.

Ofloxacin may decrease the renal clearance of procainamide, which may result in an increase in the area under the serum concentration-time curve (AUC) and peak concentration of procainamide by 20–25%.

Para-aminobenzoic acid may decrease the renal clearance of NAPA, which may result in an increase in the plasma concentration and half-life of NAPA.

Acute Toxicity

■ Manifestations Overdosage of procainamide has produced hypotension, widening of the QRS complex, prolongation of PR and QT intervals, lowering of R and T waves, increasing AV block, ventricular extrasystole, ventricular tachycardia or fibrillation, junctional tachycardia, intraventricular conduction delay, oliguria, lethargy, confusion, nausea, and vomiting.

■ Treatment Management of procainamide overdosage generally involves symptomatic and supportive care with ECG and blood pressure monitoring. There is no known antidote to procainamide. If ingestion of the drug is recent, gastric lavage or emesis may reduce absorption. Procainamide toxicity can usually be treated, if necessary, by administering vasopressors after adequate fluid volume replacement. IV infusion of ⅙ *M* sodium lactate injection reportedly reduces the cardiotoxic effects of procainamide. If procainamide toxicity causes severe hypotension and renal insufficiency, urinary elimination of procainamide and NAPA is decreased and hemodialysis may be necessary.

Peritoneal dialysis is not effective. One patient who ingested approximately 7 g of procainamide hydrochloride recovered after treatment consisting of IV norepinephrine, IV furosemide, attempted volume expansion with albumin, and hemodialysis. Another patient recovered after ingestion of 19 g of procainamide hydrochloride; this patient was treated with IV isoproterenol and IV epinephrine.

Pharmacology

■ **Antiarrhythmic and Electrophysiologic Effects** Procainamide is an antiarrhythmic agent whose cardiac actions appear to be similar to those of quinidine. Procainamide is regarded as a myocardial depressant because it decreases myocardial excitability and conduction velocity, and may depress myocardial contractility. Procainamide, like disopyramide and quinidine, also possesses anticholinergic properties which may modify the direct myocardial effects of the drug.

The exact mechanism of antiarrhythmic action of procainamide has not been established, but the drug is considered a class I (membrane-stabilizing) antiarrhythmic agent. Like other class I antiarrhythmic agents, procainamide is believed to combine with fast sodium channels in their inactive state and thereby inhibit recovery after repolarization in a time- and voltage-dependent manner which is associated with subsequent dissociation of the drug from the sodium channels. Procainamide exhibits electrophysiologic effects characteristic of class IA antiarrhythmic agents. The electrophysiologic characteristics of the subgroups of class I antiarrhythmic agents may be related to quantitative differences in their rates of attachment to and dissociation from transmembrane sodium channels, with class IA agents exhibiting intermediate rates of attachment and dissociation. *N*-Acetylprocainamide (NAPA), a metabolite of procainamide, exhibits class III antiarrhythmic activity.

Like lidocaine and quinidine, procainamide suppresses automaticity in the His-Purkinje system. In usual doses, procainamide may decrease the automaticity of ectopic pacemakers, but the extent of this effect also depends upon the anticholinergic effect of the drug on the sinoatrial (SA) node, atria, and atrioventricular (AV) node. Extremely high concentrations of procainamide may increase myocardial automaticity. The drug decreases conduction velocity in the atria, ventricles, and His-Purkinje system, and may decrease or cause no change in conduction velocity through the AV node. Procainamide probably suppresses atrial fibrillation or flutter by prolonging the effective refractory period (ERP) and increasing the action potential duration in atrial and ventricular muscle and in the His-Purkinje system. Because prolongation of the ERP is greater than the increase in the duration of the action potential, the cardiac tissue remains refractory even after restoration of the resting membrane potential. Procainamide shortens the ERP of the AV node, and the anticholinergic action of the drug may also increase the conductivity of the AV node. The effects of procainamide on refractoriness and the action potential duration of atrial fibers may be modified by the anticholinergic effects of the drug. Procainamide decreases cardiac excitability both in diastole and in the relative refractory period by increasing the threshold potential for electrical excitation. In therapeutic plasma concentrations, procainamide causes prolongation of the PR and QT intervals, but the QRS complex is usually not prolonged beyond the normal range.

■ **Cardiovascular Effects** The effect of procainamide on heart rate is unpredictable, but generally the drug causes no change or slightly increases heart rate. Procainamide may have a direct negative inotropic effect, but therapeutic plasma concentrations of the drug do not usually depress contractility in the normal heart. Cardiac output is not usually decreased, except in the presence of myocardial damage. Procainamide may reduce peripheral resistance and blood pressure as a result of peripheral vasodilation. Decreased blood pressure is most likely to occur with high plasma concentrations of the drug. IV procainamide may decrease pulmonary arterial pressure. At high plasma concentrations, procainamide may produce sinus tachycardia because of reflex sympathetic response to its hypotensive effect.

■ **Other Effects** Procainamide has local anesthetic properties equal to but more sustained than those of procaine. Procainamide produces less CNS stimulation than does procaine.

Pharmacokinetics

■ **Absorption** Plasma procainamide concentrations of approximately 4–10 mcg/mL are required to suppress ventricular arrhythmias. Plasma procainamide concentrations exceeding 10 mcg/mL are increasingly associated with toxic findings, which are observed occasionally in the 10–12 mcg/mL range, more often in the 12–15 mcg/mL range, and commonly in patients with plasma concentrations greater than 15 mcg/mL; however, some clinicians state that plasma procainamide concentrations of 15–20 mcg/mL may be appropriate in selected patients with careful monitoring. With fixed dosage, there are large interindividual variations in the plasma concentrations of procainamide. Plasma concentrations of procainamide are approximately 25% higher than blood concentrations. *N*-Acetylprocainamide (NAPA), a metabolite of procainamide, has antiarrhythmic activity, and plasma concentrations of this metabolite may represent more than 50% of the total drug in the plasma. If renal excretion of procainamide is prolonged and conversion to NAPA is rapid, plasma concentrations of NAPA exceed procainamide concentrations at steady-state. The suggested therapeutic range for combined procainamide and NAPA concentrations is 5–30 mcg/mL.

Absorption of procainamide after IM administration is rapid, and the drug appears in the plasma in 2 minutes. Peak plasma procainamide concentrations after IM administration of the drug average 30% higher than after oral administration of the same dose. In one study in healthy individuals, peak plasma procainamide concentrations of 5–8.5 mcg/mL were attained in 15–60 minutes and plasma concentrations of 2–3 mcg/mL persisted for 6 hours after a single 1-g IM dose. The onset of action after IM administration of a single dose of the drug occurs within 10–30 minutes. In one study in patients with atherosclerotic heart disease, plasma concentrations of the drug ranged from 5.8–16 mcg/mL at the end of an IV infusion of 500 mg of procainamide hydrochloride at a rate of 50 mg/minute.

■ **Distribution** Procainamide is rapidly distributed into the CSF, liver, spleen, kidneys, lungs, muscles, brain, and heart. The apparent volume of distribution of the drug at steady state is approximately 2 L/kg. The apparent volume of distribution of procainamide is decreased in patients with heart failure. Studies using radiolabeled procainamide indicate that 14–23% of the drug is bound to plasma proteins at therapeutic plasma concentrations. Procainamide crosses the placenta, but the extent to which it does has not been well characterized. Procainamide and NAPA are distributed into milk and can be absorbed by a nursing infant.

■ **Elimination** After IV administration, procainamide has an initial half-life of 4–5 minutes and a terminal half-life of 2.5–4.7 hours in individuals with normal renal function. The elimination half-life of procainamide may be increased in patients with renal impairment and in geriatric patients. The half-life of NAPA is 6–7 hours in patients with normal renal function. In patients with congestive heart failure and/or renal insufficiency, plasma concentrations of procainamide are higher and decrease more gradually.

Procainamide is acetylated, presumably in the liver, to form NAPA. Acetylation of procainamide is related to genetic acetylator phenotype. The rate of acetylation is genetically determined and varies among individuals; however, it is constant for each person.

The total amount of unchanged procainamide excreted in urine varies from 40–70% of a dose due to differences in acetylator phenotype and in renal excretion. NAPA and 2 unidentified metabolites are also excreted in urine. Less than 0.2% of the dose is excreted in urine as either *p*-acetamidobenzoic acid or aminobenzoic acid. Procainamide and NAPA are excreted by active tubular secretion and glomerular filtration. The rate of renal excretion of procainamide and NAPA is not affected by changes in urine pH nor by acetylator phenotype. Rapid and slow acetylators excrete approximately the same amount of procainamide as unchanged drug, but rapid acetylators excrete more of a dose as NAPA. In patients with renal insufficiency, excretion of procainamide and NAPA is decreased. Procainamide and NAPA are removed by hemodialysis but not by peritoneal dialysis. NAPA also is removed by arteriovenous hemofiltration and by arteriovenous hemodiafiltration.

Chemistry and Stability

■ **Chemistry** Procainamide hydrochloride is an antiarrhythmic agent. The drug differs structurally from procaine in the replacement of the ester group of procaine with an amide group. Procainamide hydrochloride occurs as a white to tan, hygroscopic, crystalline powder and is very soluble in water and soluble in alcohol. The drug has a pK_a of 9.23.

Procainamide hydrochloride injection is a sterile solution of the drug in water for injection and is colorless or has not more than a slight yellow color. Hydrochloric acid and/or sodium hydroxide is used to adjust the pH of the commercially available injection to 4–6. At the time of manufacture, the air in the vials of procainamide hydrochloride injection is replaced with nitrogen. Sodium metabisulfite is present in the injection principally to prevent discoloration caused by oxidation of *p*-aminobenzoic acid (a procainamide degradation product) rather than to maintain product potency. Sodium metabisulfite is present in the injection principally to prevent discoloration caused by oxidation of *p*-aminobenzoic acid (a procainamide degradation product) rather than to maintain product potency.

■ **Stability** Procainamide hydrochloride injections are colorless or may turn slightly yellow on standing; injection of air into vials of the drug causes darkening of the solution. Solutions of procainamide that are darker than light amber or are otherwise discolored should not be used. Although procainamide hydrochloride injection may be stored at room temperature (10–27°C), refrigeration retards oxidation and associated development of color.

When procainamide hydrochloride injection is diluted with 0.9% sodium chloride injection or sterile water for injection, solutions containing 2–4 mg/mL are stable for 24 hours at room temperature or for 7 days at 2–8°C. While solutions diluted in 5% dextrose have been described as being less stable than this secondary to possible formation of an association complex between the drug and dextrose,/ and such complexation may not be readily reversible, at least in vitro, this phenomenon has *only* been observed in vitro to date and its clinical importance, if any, remains unclear. There is in vitro evidence indicating that complexation is pH dependent and that its rate and extent can be minimized by adjusting the pH of procainamide hydrochloride in 5% dextrose solutions to 7.5 with sodium bicarbonate. However, because this complexation has not been observed in vivo and its clinical importance has not been established, the need for such precautions remains questionable. Therefore, the manufacturer currently states that procainamide hydrochloride that has been diluted to a final concentration of 2–4 mg/mL in 5% dextrose can be considered stable for at least 24 hours at room temperature or for 7 days when refrigerated. In addition, because use of IV procainamide hydrochloride generally is limited to clinical situations in which ECG and blood pressure are monitored continuously, any potential alterations in clinical bioavailability resulting from such dilutions probably would be readily apparent. Procainamide hydrochloride injection has been reported to be physically incompatible with some drugs, but the compatibility depends on several factors (e.g., concentrations of the drugs, specific diluents used, resulting pH, temperature). Specialized references should be consulted for specific compatibility information.

Preparations

Excipients in commercially available drug preparations may have clinically important effects in some individuals; consult specific product labeling for details.

Procainamide Hydrochloride

Parenteral		
Injection	100 mg/mL*	**Procainamide Hydrochloride Injection**
	500 mg/mL*	**Procainamide Hydrochloride Injection**

*available from one or more manufacturer, distributor, and/or repackager by generic (nonproprietary) name

†Use is not currently included in the labeling approved by the US Food and Drug Administration

quiNIDine Gluconate
quiNIDine Sulfate

■ Quinidine is a class Ia antiarrhythmic agent that exhibits antimalarial activity.

Uses

■ **Arrhythmias** Quinidine is used to convert and prevent recurrence of atrial fibrillation or atrial flutter. The drug also has been used in the management of other supraventricular and ventricular arrhythmias such as paroxysmal atrial fibrillation, paroxysmal atrial tachycardia, paroxysmal AV junctional rhythm, paroxysmal ventricular tachycardia, and atrial or ventricular premature contractions. However, pooled analysis of data from several randomized controlled studies in patients with atrial flutter and fibrillation indicates that quinidine appears to be associated with a mortality rate more than 3 times higher compared with that associated with placebo. In addition, pooled analysis of data from several other randomized controlled studies in patients with non-life-threatening ventricular arrhythmias indicates that mortality rate associated with quinidine was consistently higher than that associated with other antiarrhythmic drugs (e.g., flecainide, mexiletine, propafenone, tocainide); the risk of mortality appeared to be increased in patients with structural heart disease, particularly those with left ventricular dysfunction.

Supraventricular Tachyarrhythmias **Atrial Fibrillation or Flutter.** Quinidine is used to convert atrial fibrillation or atrial flutter to normal sinus rhythm in patients whose symptoms are not adequately controlled by measures to reduce ventricular rate; the drug also is used to prevent recurrence of these arrhythmias following conversion. Quinidine was one of the first antiarrhythmic agents available for the treatment of atrial fibrillation and flutter; however, the drug is now infrequently used because of its propensity for adverse effects (e.g., QT-interval prolongation, torsades de pointes) and association with increased mortality. Experts currently consider quinidine an alternative agent for the treatment of atrial fibrillation when other antiarrhythmic drugs cannot be used.

The use of quinidine to prevent recurrence of atrial fibrillation or flutter is controversial. Although the drug may maintain normal sinus rhythm for long periods in patients with recent onset of atrial fibrillation or flutter without congestive heart failure, atrial enlargement, or left ventricular hypertrophy, patients who have had long-standing atrial fibrillation are likely to have recurrence of fibrillation even with quinidine maintenance therapy. Generally, quinidine should not be used prophylactically for atrial fibrillation unless the ventricular rate is inadequately controlled by alternative measures.

If quinidine is used for conversion of atrial fibrillation/flutter, appropriate measures should be taken to ensure that the patient is adequately anticoagulated since conversion to normal sinus rhythm may be associated with embolism, particularly when the arrhythmia has been present for more than 48 hours. (See Uses: Cardioversion of Atrial Fibrillation/Flutter, in Heparin 20:12.04.16.) The possibility of additive hypoprothrombinemic effects should be considered if oral anticoagulants and quinidine are administered concomitantly. (See Drug Interactions: Coumarin Anticoagulants.)

Paroxysmal Atrial Tachycardia and AV Junctional Rhythm. Quinidine has been used in the treatment of paroxysmal atrial tachycardia or paroxysmal AV junctional rhythm. If treatment of paroxysmal atrial tachycardia is necessary, however, measures to increase vagal tone (such as carotid sinus massage or Valsalva maneuver) and/or IV adenosine are the treatments of choice. Paroxysmal AV junctional rhythm is rarely treated unless there is an extremely rapid ventricular rate; if treatment is necessary, measures to increase vagal tone, IV adenosine, IV amiodarone, calcium-channel blocking agents (e.g., diltiazem, verapamil), β-adrenergic blockers, or electrical cardioversion are used.

Atrial Premature Complexes Although quinidine can be used for the treatment of atrial premature complexes, these arrhythmias are usually treated with a cardiac glycoside.

Ventricular Arrhythmias Quinidine is used to suppress and prevent the recurrence of ventricular arrhythmias (e.g., sustained ventricular tachycardia) that in the judgment of the physician are life-threatening. The manufacturers and many clinicians state that because of the drug's arrhythmogenic potential and the lack of evidence for improved survival for class I antiarrhythmic agents, use of quinidine for less severe ventricular arrhythmias is not recommended and treatment of patients with asymptomatic ventricular premature contractions (VPCs) should be avoided.

Parenteral lidocaine is the drug of choice for treatment of VPCs; although quinidine decreases the frequency of VPCs associated with acute myocardial infarction, usual doses may decrease myocardial contractility in these patients. Like other antiarrhythmic drugs, quinidine has not been shown to decrease mortality rate in patients with VPCs associated with acute myocardial infarction. Quinidine generally is not used to treat cardiac glycoside-induced ventricular arrhythmias. (See Cautions: Precautions and Contraindications.)

■ **Malaria** ***Treatment of Severe Malaria*** IV quinidine gluconate is used for initial treatment of severe, life-threatening malaria caused by *Plasmodium falciparum* or other *Plasmodium* species†. Severe malaria usually is caused by *P. falciparum*; *P. knowlesi* also can cause severe malaria, but other species (*P. ovale*, *P. malariae*, *P. vivax*) are less likely to cause severe disease.

Severe malaria can be a rapidly progressive, fatal illness. Because most deaths occur within the first 24–48 hours of illness, initial aggressive treatment with a parenteral antimalarial regimen is indicated as soon as possible after a diagnosis has been made (regardless of *Plasmodium* species involved) and whenever severe malaria is suspected based on possible exposure and symptoms. Manifestations of severe malaria include impaired consciousness/coma, severe normocytic anemia (hemoglobin less than 7 g/dL), renal failure, pulmonary edema, acute respiratory distress syndrome, hypotension, circulatory shock, disseminated intravascular coagulation, spontaneous bleeding, acidosis, hemoglobinuria, jaundice, repeated generalized seizures, and/or parasite density (parasitemia) greater than 5%.

For treatment of severe malaria in adults or children, the US Centers for Disease Control and Prevention (CDC) recommends an initial regimen of IV quinidine gluconate in conjunction with doxycycline, tetracycline, or clindamycin (oral or IV as tolerated). After at least 24 hours of continuous IV infusion of quinidine gluconate (or 3 intermittent IV doses) and when parasitemia is reduced to less than 1% and the patient can tolerate oral therapy, IV quinidine gluconate can be discontinued and oral quinine sulfate therapy initiated to complete 7 or 3 days of total quinidine and quinine therapy as determined by the geographic origin of the infecting parasite (7 days if malaria was acquired in Southeast Asia or 3 days if malaria was acquired elsewhere). Oral antimalarials are *not* recommended for initial treatment of severe malaria.

Although CDC previously recommended that exchange transfusions be considered an adjunct procedure for treatment of severe malaria in certain severely ill patients, CDC no longer recommends use of such transfusions in patients with severe malaria. Exchange transfusions have been used in treatment of severe malaria because they were thought to provide beneficial effects through removal of infected erythrocytes, improvement in blood rheology, and reduction of toxic factors (e.g., parasite-derived toxins, harmful metabolites, cytokines). However, clinical benefits have not been documented by a randomized clinical trial and survival benefits were not demonstrated in an analysis done by CDC involving cases of severe malaria treated with exchange transfusions. In addition, the risks of exchange transfusions include fluid overload, febrile and allergic reactions, metabolic disturbances (e.g., hypocalcemia), erythrocyte alloantibody sensitization, transmissible infection, and line sepsis.

In the past, IV quinine hydrochloride was considered the drug of choice for treatment of severe malaria, but was available in the US only from the Parasitic Diseases Drug Service of CDC and delivery of emergency supplies for specific patient needs was problematic. Evidence of the clinical efficacy and toxicity of IV quinidine gluconate over a 2-year period in the US and experience of an expert panel convened by the World Health Organization (WHO) supported a recommendation for use of quinidine gluconate for treatment of severe *P. falciparum* malaria. On an equimolar basis, quinidine is more active than quinine against *P. falciparum* and has been shown to be highly effective clinically; in addition, slow IV infusion of quinidine gluconate generally is well-tolerated, even in critically ill patients, patients with underlying cardiac disease, and children. For these reasons, IV quinine dihydrochloride is *no longer available* for use in the US, either commercially or from CDC, and IV quinidine gluconate has been the only parenteral cinchona alkaloid antimalarial agent commercially available in the US since 1991.

There have been several reports of fatal cases of *P. falciparum* malaria in the US and Canada in which delays in obtaining IV quinidine gluconate appeared to contribute to the deaths. As newer antiarrhythmics have replaced quinidine for many cardiac uses, some health-care facilities no longer have IV quinidine gluconate readily available for use. In addition, the number of clinicians with experience in using IV quinidine has decreased. Although most patients with malaria in the US respond to oral antimalarial agents and recover fully, a small number of fatal cases continue to occur each year, often in association with substantial delays in seeking medical attention and/or in initiating appropriate treatment.

Because of the potentially fatal consequences of delays in initiating appropriate therapy in patients with severe malaria, CDC, the US Food and Drug Administration (FDA), the manufacturer of parenteral quinidine gluconate, and other experts have alerted institutional pharmacy services regarding the essential role that ready availability of IV quinidine gluconate plays in treatment of severe and complicated malaria, and that this be weighed in any formulary decision that might affect availability of the drug. CDC and other experts encourage institutions within close geographic proximity to coordinate their respective formulary decisions so that IV quinidine gluconate remains readily available within the area (either by keeping IV quinidine gluconate on their formulary or knowing which neighboring hospitals or other health-care facilities maintain the drug on their formulary). In hospitals where IV quinidine gluconate is not maintained on formulary, health-care professionals (e.g., pharmacists) who require the drug for patients with severe *P. falciparum* malaria should contact local or regional distributors of the drug or the manufacturer.

If IV quinidine gluconate is unavailable locally and cannot be obtained quickly or cannot be used because of adverse effects or contraindications or if parasitemia is high and has not responded to quinidine gluconate, IV artesunate is available from CDC under an investigational new drug (IND) protocol for initial treatment of severe malaria. WHO recommends artesunate as the drug of choice for treatment of severe malaria.

Clinicians who desire assistance with the diagnosis or treatment of malaria or assistance obtaining IV quinidine gluconate or IV artesunate for treatment of severe malaria should contact the CDC Malaria Hotline at 770-488-7788 or 855-856-4713 from 9:00 a.m. to 5:00 p.m. Eastern Standard Time or CDC Emergency Operation Center at 770-488-7100 after hours and on weekends and holidays.

Treatment of Uncomplicated Malaria Oral quinidine sulfate has been used for treatment of uncomplicated *P. falciparum* malaria† in Thailand where this organism generally is resistant to chloroquine and/or the fixed combination of sulfadoxine and pyrimethamine (no longer commercially available in the US). Although quinidine appears to be more active than quinine in vitro on a weight basis against *P. falciparum* and it has been suggested that oral quinidine may be more effective than oral quinine for treatment of *P. falciparum* malaria, CDC and other experts recommend oral quinine sulfate (not oral quinidine sulfate) for treatment of uncomplicated *P. falciparum* malaria. Oral quinidine sulfate is not included in CDC recommendations for treatment of uncomplicated or severe malaria.

■ **Pseudobulbar Affect** Quinidine sulfate is used orally in fixed combination with dextromethorphan hydrobromide (Nuedexta®) in the treatment of pseudobulbar affect (PBA). Quinidine, a specific inhibitor of the hepatic cytochrome P-450 (CYP) isoenzyme 2D6, is used in the fixed combination to increase the systemic bioavailability of dextromethorphan. (See Dextromethorphan Hydrobromide and Quinidine Sulfate 28:92.)

Dosage and Administration

■ **Administration** Quinidine gluconate and quinidine sulfate are administered orally. Quinidine gluconate also is administered by IV infusion; IM administration is *not* recommended because absorption kinetics of the drug may vary depending on the patient's peripheral perfusion.

Oral Administration Quinidine gluconate is administered orally as extended-release tablets.

Quinidine sulfate is administered orally as conventional or extended-release tablets.

In the management of arrhythmias, extended-release tablets of quinidine are used primarily for maintenance therapy. If necessary, extended-release tablets of quinidine may be broken in half in order to titrate dosage; however, extended-release tablets should not be chewed or crushed.

Adverse GI effects of quinidine may be minimized by administering oral doses of the drug with food or antacids; however, the possibility that food and antacids may delay absorption and that antacids which increase urine pH may decrease quinidine excretion should be considered.

Because grapefruit juice may delay the absorption and inhibit the metabolism of quinidine to 3-hydroxyquinidine in the gut, grapefruit juice should be avoided in patients receiving quinidine. If grapefruit juice is ingested concomitantly, the patient should be monitored for evidence of the interaction. (See Cautions: Precautions and Contraindications.)

To determine possible idiosyncrasy to quinidine, a test dose of 200 mg of quinidine sulfate should be administered orally several hours before full dosage is begun. For children, the test dose for idiosyncrasy to quinidine is 2 mg/kg (up to 200 mg) of quinidine sulfate orally.

IV Administration For the treatment of arrhythmias, quinidine gluconate is administered by IV infusion.

For the treatment of severe *Plasmodium falciparum* malaria, quinidine gluconate is administered by continuous or intermittent IV infusion.

■ **Dosage** Dosage of quinidine gluconate or quinidine sulfate for the treatment of arrhythmias usually is expressed in terms of the salt. Dosage of quinidine gluconate for the treatment of malaria is expressed in terms of the base or salt.

On a molar basis, approximately 267 mg of quinidine gluconate is equivalent to 200 mg of quinidine sulfate.

Dosage of quinidine must be carefully adjusted according to individual requirements and response, and the general condition and cardiovascular status of the patient.

Quinidine therapy should be initiated or quinidine dosage adjusted in a setting where facilities and personnel for patient monitoring and resuscitation are continuously available, especially if the drug is used in patients with known structural heart disease or other risk factors for toxicity.

ECG monitoring of cardiac function and determination of plasma quinidine concentrations are recommended during quinidine therapy, especially when the drug is given IV or when more than 2 g of oral quinidine sulfate is administered daily, and in patients with an increased risk of adverse reactions to quinidine, such as patients with severe heart disease, hypotension, or hepatic or renal disease.

Quinidine should be used for conversion of atrial fibrillation/flutter only after alternative measures (e.g., use of other drugs to control ventricular rate) have been inadequate. Quinidine should be discontinued if sinus rhythm is not restored within a reasonable amount of time.

Quinidine should be discontinued if QRS complex widens to 130% of its pretreatment duration, QT_c interval widens to 130% of its pretreatment duration and is greater than 500 milliseconds, P waves disappear, or the patient develops clinically important tachycardia, symptomatic bradycardia, or hypotension.

Arrhythmias **Oral Quinidine Sulfate.** If oral quinidine sulfate (conventional tablets) is used for conversion of atrial fibrillation/flutter in adults, the manufacturers recommend that 400 mg of quinidine sulfate (332 mg of quinidine) be given every 6 hours initially. The dose may be cautiously increased if conversion is not attained after 4 or 5 doses.

Alternatively, if oral quinidine sulfate (extended-release tablets) is used for conversion of atrial fibrillation/flutter in adults, the manufacturer recommends that 300 mg of quinidine sulfate (249 mg of quinidine) be given every 8–12 hours initially. The dose may be cautiously increased if conversion is not attained, quinidine serum concentrations are within the therapeutic range, and the drug is well tolerated.

If successful conversion of atrial fibrillation does not occur when quinidine serum concentrations are in the therapeutic range, further increases in dosage are generally unsuccessful and increase the possibility of toxicity.

For reduction in frequency of relapse into atrial fibrillation/flutter, the initial adult dosage of oral quinidine sulfate (conventional tablets) recommended by the manufacturers is 200 mg of quinidine sulfate (166 mg of quinidine) every 6 hours. The dose may be cautiously increased if the drug is well tolerated, serum quinidine concentrations are within the therapeutic range, and the average time between arrhythmic episodes has not been satisfactorily increased.

Alternatively, if oral quinidine sulfate (extended-release tablets) is used for reduction in frequency of relapse into atrial fibrillation/flutter, the initial dosage recommended by the manufacturer is 300 mg of quinidine sulfate (249 mg of quinidine) every 8–12 hours. The dose may be cautiously increased if the drug is well tolerated, serum quinidine concentrations are within the therapeutic range, and average time between arrhythmic episodes has not been satisfactorily increased.

Quinidine sulfate (conventional or extended-release tablets) should be used for reduction in frequency of relapse into atrial fibrillation/flutter only if alternative measures have been inadequate and if potential benefits of such prophylaxis outweigh risks; the mortality risk should be considered.

The manufacturers of oral quinidine sulfate (conventional and extended-release tablets) state that dosage regimens for suppression of life-threatening ventricular arrhythmias have not been adequately studied, but regimens similar to those used in the management of atrial fibrillation/flutter have been described. Whenever possible, such therapy should be guided by results of programmed electrical stimulation and/or Holter monitoring with exercise.

Oral Quinidine Gluconate. If oral quinidine gluconate (extended-release tablets) is used for conversion of atrial fibrillation/flutter in adults, the manufacturers recommend an initial dosage of 648 mg of quinidine gluconate (403 mg of quinidine) every 8 hours. The dose may be cautiously increased if conversion is not attained after 3 or 4 doses. Alternatively, the manufacturers state that adults can receive an oral regimen of 324 mg of quinidine gluconate (202 mg of quinidine) every 8 hours for 2 days, then 648 mg of quinidine gluconate (403 mg of quinidine) every 12 hours for 2 days, and then 648 mg of quinidine gluconate (403 mg of quinidine) every 8 hours for up to 4 days. If the 648-mg dose is not tolerated, a lower dosage can be continued for the last 4 days.

If oral quinidine gluconate (extended-release tablets) is used for reduction in frequency of relapse into atrial fibrillation/flutter, the manufacturers recommend that adults receive an initial dosage of 324 mg of quinidine gluconate (202 mg of quinidine) every 8 or 12 hours. The dose may be cautiously increased if the drug is well tolerated, serum quinidine concentrations are within the therapeutic range, and the average time between arrhythmic episodes has not been satisfactorily increased. Quinidine gluconate should be used for such prophylaxis only if alternative measures have been inadequate and if potential benefits outweigh risks; the mortality risk should be considered.

The manufacturers of oral quinidine gluconate (extended-release tablets) state that dosage regimens for suppression of life-threatening ventricular arrhythmias have not been adequately studied, but regimens similar to those used in the management of atrial fibrillation/flutter have been described. Whenever possible, such therapy should be guided by results of programmed electrical stimulation and/or Holter monitoring with exercise.

IV Quinidine Gluconate. For IV treatment of symptomatic atrial fibrillation/flutter in adults, 800 mg of quinidine gluconate (10 mL of the commercially available injection containing 80 mg/mL) is diluted in 40 mL of 5% dextrose injection to provide a solution containing 16 mg/mL. The 16 mg/mL solution is infused at an initial rate of up to 0.25 mg/kg per minute (i.e., 1 mL/kg per hour).

Blood pressure and ECG should be monitored continuously during IV infusion and the rate of administration adjusted so the arrhythmia is abolished without disturbing the normal mechanism of the heart beat. If the QRS complex widens to 130% of its pretreatment duration, the QT_c interval widens to 130% of its pretreatment duration and is longer than 500 milliseconds, if disappearance of the P wave, severe hypotension, substantial tachycardia, or symptomatic bradycardia occurs, or if normal sinus rhythm is restored or severe adverse effects appear, IV administration of the drug should be discontinued.

Generally, the total IV dosage in the treatment of atrial fibrillation/flutter is less than 5 mg/kg, although 10 mg/kg may be required in some patients. If conversion to sinus rhythm has not occurred after infusion of quinidine gluconate 10 mg/kg, the infusion should be discontinued and other means of cardioversion should be considered.

While dosing regimens using IV quinidine gluconate for the management of life-threatening ventricular arrhythmias have not been systematically evaluated, regimens similar to that used in the management of atrial fibrillation/flutter have been described.

Malaria **Oral Quinidine Sulfate.** For treatment of uncomplicated *Plasmodium falciparum* malaria† in adults, 300–600 mg or 10 mg/kg of quinidine sulfate has been administered orally every 8 hours for 5–7 days.

Oral quinidine sulfate is not included in US Centers for Disease Control and Prevention (CDC) recommendations for treatment of uncomplicated or severe malaria. (See Uses: Malaria.)

IV Quinidine Gluconate. For treatment of severe malaria caused by *P. falciparum* or other *Plasmodium* species†, CDC states that IV quinidine gluconate in conjunction with doxycycline, tetracycline, or clindamycin (oral or IV as tolerated) should be initiated as soon as possible after a diagnosis of severe malaria has been made (regardless of *Plasmodium* species involved) and whenever severe malaria is suspected based on possible exposure and symptoms. Several dosage regimens (intermittent or continuous IV infusion) of quinidine gluconate have been employed for treatment of severe *P. falciparum* malaria. Because most deaths from severe malaria occur within the first 24–48 hours of illness, an initial loading dose of IV quinidine gluconate usually is used to rapidly provide therapeutic plasma concentrations of the drug.

When a continuous IV infusion regimen is used, an initial loading dose of 6.25 mg/kg of quinidine (10 mg/kg of quinidine gluconate) diluted in approximately 5 mL/kg of 0.9% sodium chloride injection should be given by IV infusion over 1–2 hours, followed by a continuous maintenance infusion of 12.5 mcg/kg of quinidine per minute (20 mcg/kg of quinidine gluconate per minute) given for at least 24 hours and until parasitemia is reduced to less than 1% and oral quinine sulfate can be substituted.

Alternatively, if an intermittent IV infusion regimen is used, an initial loading dose of 15 mg/kg of quinidine (24 mg/kg of quinidine gluconate) should be diluted in 250 mL of 0.9% sodium chloride injection and infused over 4 hours, followed 4 hours later (i.e., 8 hours after the beginning of the loading-dose infusion) by maintenance doses of 7.5 mg/kg of quinidine (12 mg/kg of quinidine gluconate) given by IV infusion over 4 hours at 8-hour intervals until 3 maintenance doses have been administered and parasitemia is reduced to less than 1% and oral quinine sulfate can be substituted.

The IV infusion rate should be decreased or the flow interrupted if corrected QT interval exceeds 0.6 seconds, corrected QT interval exceeds baseline by more than 25%, QRS widening exceeds 50% of baseline, or clinically important hypotension unresponsive to fluid expansion develops. Some clinicians state that the initial loading dose of quinidine gluconate should not exceed 375 mg of quinidine (600 mg of quinidine gluconate) when administered by a continuous IV infusion regimen.

Blood pressure and ECG should be continuously monitored and blood glucose periodically monitored in patients receiving quinidine for the treatment of malaria, and dosage adjusted accordingly. Clinicians should also consider that the risk of serious ventricular arrhythmias associated with quinidine is increased by bradycardia, hypokalemia, and hypomagnesemia. When deciding whether a patient should receive an initial loading dose of quinidine gluconate, clinicians should consider whether the patient has been receiving drugs that can prolong the QT interval (e.g., halofantrine [an antimalarial drug not commercially available in the US], mefloquine, quinine). A loading dose of quinidine gluconate should *not* be administered if the patient has received more than 40 mg/kg of quinine in the previous 48 hours or has received mefloquine in the previous 12 hours. Because clinical experience on which to base therapeutic decisions regarding quinidine gluconate is limited, these recommendations for administration of an initial loading dose are based on clinical experience with the use of initial loading doses of quinine. Both loading dose and infusion rate should be calculated carefully to prevent acute cardiac events. Consultation with a cardiologist and a clinician with experience using quinidine gluconate for treatment of severe malaria is advised.

After at least 24 hours of continuous IV quinidine gluconate infusion (or 3 intermittent doses) and if parasitemia is reduced to less than 1% and the patient can tolerate oral therapy, IV quinidine gluconate therapy can be discontinued and oral quinine sulfate therapy initiated to complete a total of 7 or 3 days of total quinidine and quinine therapy as determined by the geographic origin of the infecting parasite (7 days if acquired in Southeast Asia or 3 days if acquired elsewhere).

The initial IV quinidine gluconate regimen followed by oral quinine sulfate is used in conjunction with a 7-day regimen of doxycycline, tetracycline, or clindamycin administered IV or orally as tolerated. Adults intolerant of oral therapy may receive IV therapy with doxycycline hyclate (100 mg every 12 hours) or clindamycin (10 mg/kg loading dose followed by 5 mg/kg every 8 hours) until they can be switched to oral therapy. Rapid IV administration of doxycycline hyclate or clindamycin should be avoided. Adults who tolerate oral therapy may receive a 7-day course of therapy with doxycycline (100 mg every 12 hours), tetracycline (250 mg every 6 hours), or clindamycin (20 mg/kg daily given in 3 equal doses).

Additional information on the management of malaria can be obtained by contacting the CDC Malaria Hotline at 770-488-7788 or 855-856-4713 from 9:00 a.m. to 5:00 p.m. Eastern Standard Time or the CDC Emergency Operation Center at 770-488-7100 after hours and on weekends and holidays.

■ **Pediatric Dosage** ***Arrhythmias*** **Oral Quinidine Sulfate.** Although safety and efficacy for use as an antiarrhythmic agent in children have not been established in well-controlled clinical trials, some clinicians recommend that children with arrhythmias† receive oral quinidine sulfate in a dosage of 15–60 mg/kg daily given in divided doses every 6 hours. Other clinicians recommend that children with arrhythmias receive 30 mg/kg daily or 900 mg/m² daily, given in 5 divided doses.

Oral Quinidine Gluconate. Although safety and efficacy for use as an antiarrhythmic agent in children have not been established in well-controlled clinical trials, some clinicians recommend that children with arrhythmias† receive oral quinidine gluconate in a dosage of 20–60 mg/kg daily given in divided doses every 8 hours.

IV Quinidine Gluconate. Although safety and efficacy for use as an antiarrhythmic agent in children have not been established in well-controlled clinical trials, some clinicians have recommended parenteral quinidine gluconate dosages of 30 mg/kg daily or 900 mg/m² daily, given in 5 divided doses.

Malaria **IV Quinidine Gluconate.** For treatment of severe malaria caused by *P. falciparum* or other *Plasmodium* species† in pediatric patients†, CDC and other clinicians recommend that quinidine gluconate be given in the same dosage regimen recommended for adults. (See IV Quinidine Gluconate under Dosage: Malaria, in Dosage and Administration.) In addition, the appropriate pediatric dosages of oral quinine sulfate and IV or oral doxycycline, tetracycline, or clindamycin should be used in conjunction with IV quinidine gluconate. (See the dosage sections in Doxycycline and Tetracycline Hydrochloride in 8:12.24 and the dosage section in Clindamycin in 8:12.28.20.)

■ **Dosage in Renal Impairment** For the treatment of severe malaria, the initial loading dose and continuous IV infusion rate of quinidine gluconate do not need to be reduced in patients with renal failure. If renal failure persists or clinical improvement does not occur in such patients, the maintenance infusion rate should be reduced by one-third to one-half on the third day of the quinidine gluconate infusion.

Cautions

Quinidine has numerous adverse effects which may necessitate cessation of therapy in many patients.

■ **GI Effects** Adverse GI effects such as diarrhea, anorexia, abdominal pain and cramps, colic, nausea, bitter taste, esophagitis, and vomiting occur commonly with quinidine therapy and are the most frequent reasons for discontinuance of the drug. Adverse GI effects may be less severe with extended-release preparations than with other oral dosage forms, but there are no well-controlled clinical trials to date comparing adverse effects of quinidine salts after administration of doses that produce similar plasma concentrations.

■ **Dermatologic and Sensitivity Reactions** Idiosyncratic and hypersensitivity reactions to quinidine may occur, and the reaction of the patient to a test dose or the first dose of the drug should be observed carefully. (See Dosage and Administration: Administration.) Observation of the patient for hypersensitivity should be continued for the first weeks of therapy. Symptoms of cinchonism such as tinnitus, headache, vertigo, fever, dizziness, lightheadedness, tremor, nausea, and disturbed vision may occur in sensitive patients after a single dose of quinidine. Dosage should be decreased if signs of cinchonism appear.

Other hypersensitivity reactions to quinidine include fever, thrombocytopenic purpura, hypoprothrombinemia, hemorrhage, acute hemolytic anemia, agranulocytosis, aplastic anemia, leukopenia, acute asthmatic episode, angioedema, vascular collapse, respiratory arrest, and anaphylactic shock. Quinidine may cause hemolysis in patients with glucose-6-phosphate dehydrogenase (G-6-PD) deficiency.

Skin reactions to quinidine are rare and include morbilliform and scarlatiniform eruptions, urticaria, rash, pruritus, exfoliative dermatitis, eczema, severe exacerbation of psoriasis, lichenoid reactions, flushing, pigmentary abnormalities, photodermatitis (photosensitivity), and contact dermatitis.

Quinidine has produced a systemic lupus erythematosus-like syndrome characterized by polyarthritis, fever, pleuritic chest pain, lupus nephritis, and the presence of antinuclear antibodies (ANA) in the blood.

Hepatotoxicity, including granulomatous hepatitis, increased serum AST (SGOT) and alkaline phosphatase concentrations, and jaundice, has been reported with quinidine. Quinidine-induced hepatotoxicity appears to be the result of hypersensitivity to the drug. The possibility of quinidine-induced hepatotoxicity should be considered in any patient who develops unexplained fever and/or elevation of hepatic enzymes, particularly during the initial stages of therapy.

■ **Cardiovascular Effects** Paradoxically, an extremely rapid ventricular rate may occur when quinidine is used in the treatment of atrial flutter or fibrillation, due to a reduction in the degree of AV nodal block to a 1:1 ratio. The anticholinergic action of the drug on the AV node may also increase the heart rate. This tachycardia may be prevented by prior digitalization. If cessation of atrial fibrillation or flutter is accompanied by depression of the normal pacemaker, an idioventricular rhythm (including ventricular tachycardia and fibrillation) may result. Conversion of atrial fibrillation also may be associated with embolism. Therefore, anticoagulant therapy may be necessary before administration of quinidine for conversion of atrial fibrillation to normal sinus rhythm. (See Atrial Fibrillation or Flutter under Arrhythmias: Supraventricular Tachyarrhythmias, in Uses and see Drug Interactions: Coumarin Anticoagulants.)

The risk of fibrillation increases with increasing dosage and may be accompanied by ECG signs of toxicity. Quinidine-induced cardiotoxicity is evidenced by conduction defects (50% widening of the QRS complex), ventricular tachycardia or flutter, frequent ventricular premature contractions, and complete AV block. When these ECG signs appear, quinidine should be discontinued and the patient should be monitored closely. Lidocaine may be effective in treating quinidine-induced ventricular premature contractions, tachycardia, or fibrillation. Adverse cardiac effects occur most commonly when quinidine is administered IV. Large IV doses of the drug may cause heart block and asystole, and death has occurred during IV administration of quinidine in seriously ill patients.

In usual doses, quinidine may cause syncope, probably due to ventricular tachycardia or fibrillation. These syncopal episodes may subside spontaneously, but occasionally they are fatal. If quinidine-induced syncope occurs, the drug should be discontinued. Quinidine also may cause bradycardia.

Severe hypotension may occur following IV administration or oral overdosage of quinidine. Vascular collapse, respiratory distress, and respiratory arrest may occur. Quinidine-induced hypotension is reportedly related to the dose and rate of administration of the drug. Rapid IV injection of as little as 200 mg of quinidine reportedly may cause a decrease in blood pressure of 40–50 mm Hg. Norepinephrine or metaraminol may be used if necessary to treat vascular collapse; artificial respiration and other supportive measures may be required.

While substantial cardiovascular toxicity generally has not occurred, ECG changes, including prolonged QT interval, widened QRS complex, and flattened T waves (without dysrhythmia), have occurred frequently and hypotension and ventricular tachycardia have occurred occasionally in patients receiving IV quinidine gluconate for the treatment of *Plasmodium falciparum* malaria.

■ **Other Adverse Effects** Adverse nervous system effects of quinidine include headache, vertigo, faintness, apprehension, excitement, confusion, dementia, cold sweat, delirium, ataxia, and mental depression. Hearing disturbances such as tinnitus, decreased auditory acuity, and transitory deafness have occurred. Vision disturbances have included mydriasis, blurred vision, disturbed color perception, photophobia, diplopia, night blindness, reduced visual fields, scotomata, and optic neuritis. Increased serum skeletal muscle creatine kinase (CK, creatine phosphokinase, CPK), myalgia, and arthralgia also have been reported. Quinidine can decrease blood glucose concentrations, possibly by inducing insulin secretion, and has been associated with severe hypoglycemia in at least one patient with cerebral malaria and acute renal failure.

■ **Precautions and Contraindications** Quinidine is contraindicated in patients with an AV junctional or idioventricular pacemaker, including those in complete AV block. The drug is contraindicated in patients with a history of quinidine- or quinine-associated thrombocytopenic purpura and in patients with myasthenia gravis or other conditions that might be adversely affected by anticholinergic effects. Quinidine also is contraindicated in patients with known hypersensitivity to the drug.

Since pooled analysis of data from several randomized, controlled studies in patients with non-life-threatening ventricular arrhythmias indicates that the mortality rate associated with quinidine therapy was consistently higher than that associated with various other antiarrhythmic agents (e.g., flecainide, mexiletine, propafenone, tocainide), quinidine should only be used for life-threatening ventricular arrhythmias. Use of the drug for less severe ventricular arrhythmias is not recommended and treatment of patients with asymptomatic ventricular premature contractions should be avoided. In addition, pooled analysis of data from several randomized, controlled studies in patients with atrial flutter and fibrillation indicates that quinidine therapy may be associated with a mortality rate more than 3 times higher compared with that associated with placebo. The mortality risk should be considered when initiating quinidine therapy. Quinidine should be used with extreme caution, if at all, in patients with incomplete AV nodal block, since complete heart block and asystole may result. Parenteral quinidine is especially hazardous in the presence of AV block, in the absence of atrial activity, and in patients with extensive myocardial injury. The possibility that potentially serious cardiac arrhythmias, including torsades de pointes, could occur if quinidine were used concomitantly with other drugs that prolong the QT_c interval also should be considered. Hypokalemia, hypoxia, and disorders of acid-base balance must be eliminated as potentiating factors in patients who require large doses of antiarrhythmic agents to control ventricular arrhythmias.

Quinidine should be used with extreme caution in patients with cardiac glycoside intoxication, since cardiac glycoside intoxication may cause serious impairment of cardiac conduction and produce arrhythmias which may contraindicate use of quinidine. Conversely, quinidine may cause unpredictable, abnormal rhythms and decrease contractility in the presence of cardiac glycoside intoxication.

Since quinidine-induced decreases in cardiac contractility and blood pressure may aggravate congestive heart failure or preexisting hypotension, the drug should be used cautiously, if at all, in patients with these conditions.

Rapid IV infusion of quinidine gluconate may cause peripheral vascular collapse and severe hypotension. (See Dosage and Administration.) If hypotension or congestive heart failure is caused or aggravated by an arrhythmia treatable with quinidine, the drug may be useful, but the potential risks and benefits must be considered.

Concomitantly administered grapefruit juice may delay absorption of quinidine and inhibit metabolism of the drug to 3-hydroxyquinidine by cytochrome P-450 (CYP) isoenzyme 3A4 in the gut; in one study, the delay in quinidine absorption tended to delay the effects of the drug on the QT_c interval. Although the clinical importance of this interaction is unknown, the manufacturers of extended-release tablets recommend avoiding concomitant ingestion of grapefruit juice and quinidine. Some experts state that the clinical significance of resultant pharmacokinetic interactions appears to be limited and that no specific action other than being alert for evidence of the interaction is indicated.

Quinidine should be used with caution in patients with preexisting asthma, muscle weakness, or infection with fever, since hypersensitivity reactions to the drug may be masked. The drug should also be used with caution in patients with hepatic and/or renal (particularly if renal tubular acidosis is present) insufficiency, since systemic accumulation of quinidine potentially may result.

Patients receiving chronic quinidine therapy should be instructed to notify their physician if rash, fever, unusual bleeding or bruising, ringing in the ears, or visual disturbance occurs. During long-term administration of quinidine, complete blood counts (CBCs) and liver (particularly during the initial 4–8 weeks of therapy) and renal function tests should be performed periodically. The drug should be discontinued if blood dyscrasias or signs of hepatic or renal dysfunction occur.

Since prolongation of the QT interval, ventricular arrhythmias, hypotension, and hypoglycemia may occur when quinidine is administered parenterally for the treatment of severe *P. falciparum* malaria, therapy preferably should be undertaken in an intensive care facility where central hemodynamic and ECG monitoring is available. In addition, careful monitoring of hydration status, blood glucose, and parasitemia is required.

■ **Pediatric Precautions** Safety and efficacy of quinidine as an antiarrhythmic agent in children have not been determined. Quinidine has been used in children with arrhythmias†.

Study and experience in children with malaria suggest that safety and efficacy of IV quinidine gluconate are similar to those in adults.

■ **Geriatric Precautions** Safety and efficacy of quinidine have not been systematically studied in geriatric patients, and clinical studies did not include sufficient numbers of patients 65 years of age or older to determine whether they respond differently than younger adults. Other reported clinical experience has not identified differences in responses between geriatric adults and younger patients.

When used in geriatric patients, quinidine dosage should be selected with caution, usually initiating therapy at the low end of the dosage range and taking into consideration the greater frequency of decreased hepatic, renal, and/or cardiac function and concomitant disease and drug therapy in this age group.

■ **Mutagenicity and Carcinogenicity** Animal studies to determine the carcinogenic or mutagenic potential of quinidine have not been performed to date.

■ **Pregnancy, Fertility, and Lactation** Animal reproduction studies have not been performed to date with quinidine. It is not known whether quinidine can cause fetal harm when administered to pregnant women. Another cinchona alkaloid, *quinine*, has caused fetal blindness and has been implicated in congenital deafness. Quinidine should be used during pregnancy only when clearly needed. The safety of quinidine during labor and delivery is not known, but the drug exhibits oxytocic properties; the clinical importance remains to be established.

There is no evidence to date of quinidine-induced impairment of fertility.

Since quinidine is distributed into milk, the drug should be avoided, if possible, in nursing women.

Drug Interactions

■ **Drugs or Foods Affecting or Metabolized by Hepatic Microsomal Enzymes** Quinidine is metabolized by cytochrome P-450 (CYP) isoenzyme 3A4 and pharmacokinetic interactions with drugs that are inhibitors, inducers, or substrates of CYP3A4 are possible.

Quinidine inhibits CYP2D6 and therapeutic serum quinidine concentrations may effectively convert CYP2D6 extensive metabolizers into CYP2D6 poor metabolizers. Quinidine should be used with caution concomitantly with drugs that are metabolized by CYP2D6 (e.g., mexiletine, some phenothiazines, polycyclic antidepressants). Reduced dosage of such drugs may be necessary to obtain clinical benefit without toxicity. Quinidine is used in fixed combination with dextromethorphan (Nuedexta®) to inhibit the CYP2D6-mediated metabolism of dextromethorphan and thereby increase its systemic bioavailability in patients with pseudobulbar affect (PBA). (See Dextromethorphan Hydrobromide and Quinidine Sulfate 28:92.) If quinidine is used concomitantly with some prodrugs that require CYP2D6 for conversion to an active metabolite (e.g., codeine, hydrocodone), it may not be possible to achieve the desired clinical benefits of the drugs.

■ **Alkalinizing Agents** Quinidine toxicity may result when the drug is administered with agents which increase urine pH; therefore, patients receiving quinidine should be monitored closely during initiation of therapy with drugs such as carbonic anhydrase inhibitors (e.g., acetazolamide), thiazide diuretics, some antacids, or sodium bicarbonate.

■ **Anticonvulsants** Anticonvulsants such as phenytoin and phenobarbital may increase the rate of metabolism and decrease the elimination half-life of quinidine, and caution should be used when therapy with these anticonvulsants is initiated or discontinued in patients receiving quinidine.

■ **Cardiovascular Drugs** ***Cardiac Glycosides*** Concomitant administration of quinidine and digoxin produces increased plasma concentrations of digoxin (in 90% or more of patients) which may result in GI and cardiac toxicity. Although variability exists in the magnitude of the increase, plasma digoxin concentrations usually increase twofold to threefold when quinidine therapy is initiated in patients digitalized with digoxin. Plasma digoxin concentrations may begin to increase within a few hours after initiation of quinidine therapy, but at least 5–7 days are usually required to achieve a new steady-state plasma digoxin concentration. The magnitude of the effect appears to depend on the serum quinidine concentration. Both the clearance (principally renal clearance) and volume of distribution of digoxin are generally decreased, but serum half-life of the drug may be unaffected. When quinidine therapy is initiated in a patient receiving digoxin, serum digoxin concentrations should be carefully monitored and digoxin dosage reduced as needed; the patient should be observed closely for signs of toxicity. Many clinicians recommend that digoxin dosage be reduced by one-half when quinidine therapy is initiated; however, because of the variability in magnitude of the interaction, additional dosage adjustments are likely to be necessary. If severe toxicity occurs or if digoxin dosage adjustment is difficult, an alternative antiarrhythmic agent (if possible, one that does not interact with digoxin) should be used instead of quinidine (e.g., procainamide). If digoxin therapy is initiated in a patient receiving quinidine, lower than usual dosages of digoxin may be sufficient to produce desired plasma concentrations of the cardiac glycoside. If quinidine is discontinued in a patient stabilized on therapy with both drugs, the patient should be observed for signs of decreased response to digoxin and dosage of the cardiac glycoside adjusted as necessary.

Calcium-Channel Blocking Agents A substantial hypotensive effect has occurred when verapamil was used concomitantly with quinidine in patients with arrhythmia or hypertrophic cardiomyopathy. Pending further accumulation of data on the safety of combined therapy, concomitant use of verapamil and quinidine in such patients should probably be avoided. For additional information, see Drug Interactions: Antiarrhythmic Agents, in Verapamil Hydrochloride 24:28.92.

Nifedipine may decrease serum quinidine concentrations in some patients. Reductions or increases in serum quinidine concentrations occasionally have been observed following initiation or discontinuance, respectively, of nifedipine. Such changes can be substantial and may manifest as therapeutic resistance to usual quinidine dosages during concomitant therapy and/or altered ECGs (e.g., prolongation in corrected QT interval following discontinuance of nifedipine). While it had been postulated that alterations in quinidine pharmacokinetics during concomitant nifedipine therapy may have resulted from changes in hemodynamics induced by the latter drug (e.g., reduced peripheral vascular resistance with resultantly increased quinidine volume of distribution) in some patients (e.g., those with left ventricular dysfunction), subsequent study failed to confirm left ventricular dysfunction as a predictor of this interaction. Therefore, the mechanism of this interaction remains to be established, and possible identification of patients at risk requires further study. The possibility of this interaction should be considered in any patient exhibiting unpredictably low serum quinidine concentrations during concomitant nifedipine therapy. Serum quinidine concentrations should be monitored whenever nifedipine is initiated or discontinued in patients maintained on the antiarrhythmic, and quinidine dosage adjusted accordingly.

Amiodarone Serum quinidine concentrations may increase following initiation of amiodarone therapy in patients currently receiving quinidine, with subsequent toxicity occurring in some patients. Administration of amiodarone hydrochloride (1200 mg daily for 5–7 days then reduced to 600 mg daily) to a limited number of patients receiving quinidine gluconate or sulfate (average dose of about 3 g daily) resulted in an increase in serum quinidine concentrations of about 33%. Serum quinidine concentrations may begin to increase within a couple days after initiation of amiodarone therapy. The mechanism of the interaction is not fully established, but it has been suggested that amiodarone may inhibit hepatic clearance or decrease renal clearance of quinidine and/or displace quinidine from tissue- and/or protein-binding sites. Although not clearly established, combination therapy with amiodarone and quinidine may also cause marked QT prolongation, predisposing patients to atypical ventricular tachycardia (torsades de pointes). It is generally recommended that quinidine dosage be reduced by 33–50% when amiodarone therapy is initiated in patients currently receiving quinidine or that quinidine therapy be discontinued. Serum quinidine concentrations should be monitored carefully and quinidine dosage reduced as necessary in patients receiving concomitant quinidine and amiodarone therapy; patients should be observed closely for signs of toxicity, including QT prolongation.

Other Antiarrhythmic Agents When quinidine is administered with other antiarrhythmic drugs such as lidocaine, phenytoin, procainamide, or propranolol, cardiac effects may be additive or antagonistic and toxic effects may be additive. Quinidine also may increase plasma procainamide and *N*-acetylprocainamide (NAPA) concentrations, possibly via competition for renal excretory mechanisms (e.g., tubular secretion). The pharmacologic effects of quinidine may be additive with those of quinine.

■ **Cholinergic and Anticholinergic Agents** Quinidine should be used with caution, if at all, in patients with myasthenia gravis and the dose of anticholinesterase drugs such as neostigmine and pyridostigmine may have to be increased. Since quinidine antagonizes the effect of vagal excitation on the atria and AV node, the administration of cholinergic drugs or any other procedures to enhance vagal activity may fail to terminate paroxysmal supraventricular tachycardia in patients receiving quinidine. The anticholinergic effects of quinidine may be additive with those of anticholinergic drugs.

■ **Cimetidine** Administration of cimetidine with quinidine may increase serum quinidine concentrations; however, the mechanism of this interaction has not been elucidated, and the clinical importance remains to be established.

■ **Clarithromycin** Torsades de pointes has been reported rarely in patients receiving quinidine and clarithromycin concomitantly. If quinidine and clarithromycin are used concomitantly, ECGs and serum quinidine concentrations should be monitored.

■ **Coumarin Anticoagulants** Patients who receive quinidine and coumarin anticoagulants should be closely observed for additive hypoprothrombinemic effects, since hypoprothrombinemic hemorrhage has reportedly occurred in patients receiving quinidine and chronic anticoagulant therapy.

■ **Hypotensive Agents** Since quinidine may reduce blood pressure, patients receiving antihypertensive drugs and quinidine parenterally or in high oral doses should be observed for possible additive hypotensive effects. Additive cardiac depressant effects are possible when quinidine and phenothiazines or reserpine are administered concomitantly.

■ **Ketoconazole** Concomitant use of ketoconazole results in increased plasma concentrations of quinidine.

■ **Neuromuscular Blocking Agents** Quinidine may potentiate the effects of both nondepolarizing and depolarizing skeletal muscle relaxants such as pancuronium bromide, succinylcholine chloride, and tubocurarine chloride. Neostigmine methylsulfate does not appear to reverse these effects. The use of quinidine should be avoided immediately after surgery when the effects of neuromuscular blocking agents may be present. If quinidine must be used, respiratory support may be needed.

Acute Toxicity

■ **Manifestations** Overdosage of quinidine has produced ataxia, respiratory depression or distress, apnea, vomiting, diarrhea, severe hypotension, syncope, anuria, absence of P waves, broadening of the QRS complex, PR and QT intervals, ventricular arrhythmias, extrasystoles, heart block, heart failure, coma, death, irritability, lethargy, thrashing, twitching, hallucinations, paresthesia, and generalized seizures. Signs of cinchonism may also occur. (See Cautions: Dermatologic and Sensitivity Reactions.)

■ **Treatment** Management of quinidine overdosage includes symptomatic treatment, ECG and blood pressure monitoring, and cardiac pacing if indicated. Administration of drugs that delay elimination of quinidine (e.g., cimetidine, carbonic anhydrase inhibitors, thiazide diuretics) should be avoided, unless absolutely necessary. If ingestion of the drug is recent, gastric lavage, emesis, and/or administration of activated charcoal may reduce absorption. Artificial respiration and other supportive measures may be required.

IV infusion of ⅙ *M* sodium lactate injection reportedly reduces the cardiotoxic effects of quinidine. Since marked CNS depression may occur even in the presence of seizures, CNS depressants should not be administered. Hypotension may be treated, if necessary, with metaraminol or norepinephrine after adequate fluid volume replacement. Tachyarrhythmias may be treated with phenytoin or lidocaine. Hemodialysis or forced diuresis may be effective in the treatment of quinidine overdosage in adults and children, but is rarely warranted. Peritoneal dialysis is not effective.

Pharmacology

■ **Antiarrhythmic and Electrophysiologic Effects** Quinidine is an antiarrhythmic agent whose cardiac actions appear to be similar to those of procainamide. Quinidine is regarded as a myocardial depressant because it decreases myocardial excitability and conduction velocity, and may depress myocardial contractility. Quinidine, like disopyramide and procainamide, also possesses anticholinergic properties that may modify the direct myocardial effects of the drug.

Like other class I antiarrhythmic agents, quinidine is believed to combine with fast sodium channels in their inactive state and thereby inhibit recovery after repolarization in a time- and voltage-dependent manner, which is associated with subsequent dissociation of the drug from the sodium channels. Quinidine exhibits electrophysiologic effects characteristic of class IA antiarrhythmic agents. The electrophysiologic characteristics of the subgroups of class I antiarrhythmic agents may be related to quantitative differences in their rates of attachment to and dissociation from transmembrane sodium channels, with class IA agents exhibiting intermediate rates of attachment and dissociation.

Like lidocaine and procainamide, quinidine suppresses automaticity in the His-Purkinje system. In usual doses, quinidine may decrease the automaticity of ectopic pacemakers, but the extent of this effect also depends upon the anticholinergic effect of the drug on the sinoatrial (SA) node, atria, and atrioventricular (AV) node. Extremely high concentrations of quinidine may increase myocardial automaticity. The drug decreases conduction velocity in the atria, ventricles, and His-Purkinje system, and may decrease or cause no change in conduction velocity through the AV node. Quinidine probably suppresses atrial fibrillation or flutter by prolonging the effective refractory period (ERP) and increasing the action potential duration in atrial and ventricular muscle and in the His-Purkinje system. Because prolongation of the ERP is greater than the increase in the duration of the action potential, the cardiac tissue remains refractory even after restoration of the resting membrane potential. Quinidine shortens the ERP of the AV node, and the anticholinergic action of the drug may also increase the conductivity of the AV node. The effects of quinidine on refractoriness and the action potential duration of atrial fibers may be modified by the anticholinergic effects of the drug. Quinidine decreases cardiac excitability, both in diastole and in the relative refractory period, by increasing the threshold potential for electrical excitation. At therapeutic plasma concentrations, quinidine causes prolongation of the QRS complex and QT interval.

■ **Cardiovascular Effects** In therapeutic doses, quinidine may produce sinus tachycardia via its anticholinergic effects. Quinidine has a direct negative inotropic effect, but therapeutic plasma concentrations of the drug do not usually depress contractility in the normal heart. Quinidine may reduce peripheral resistance and blood pressure by blockade of α-adrenergic receptors and by its effects on myocardial contractility; decreased blood pressure is most likely to occur with high plasma concentrations of the drug. At high plasma concentrations, quinidine may produce sinus tachycardia because of reflex sympathetic response to the drug's hypotensive effect.

■ **Other Effects** Like quinine, quinidine has antimalarial activity. In patients with malaria, quinidine acts principally as an intraerythrocytic schizonticide; the drug has little effect on sporozoites or preerythrocytic parasites. Quinidine is gametocidal against *Plasmodium vivax* and *P. malariae*, but not *P. falciparum*. In vitro on a weight basis, quinidine appears to be more active than quinine against *Plasmodium falciparum*.

Quinidine also exhibits some antipyretic and oxytocic properties. Quinidine has a very weak curare-like action on the myoneural junction and also causes depression of skeletal muscle action potential.

Pharmacokinetics

■ **Absorption** Quinidine salts are almost completely absorbed from the GI tract. The amount of quinidine that reaches the circulation after oral administration is variable and depends on the amount of drug metabolized on the first pass through the liver. Extended-release formulations of quinidine gluconate and quinidine sulfate are absorbed more slowly than conventional tablets of quinidine sulfate.

Following oral administration of quinidine sulfate conventional tablets, absolute bioavailability is about 70% (range 45–100%) and peak serum concentrations are attained in about 2 hours.

Following oral administration of quinidine gluconate extended-release tablets or quinidine sulfate extended-release tablets, absolute bioavailability is 70–80% and peak serum concentrations are attained within 3–6 hours.

In patients with congestive heart failure, the rate and extent of quinidine absorption is reduced but these patients have higher plasma concentrations of quinidine due to a decreased volume of distribution.

In healthy fasting individuals, mean peak plasma quinidine concentrations of 0.43–1.14 mcg/mL are attained 1–2 hours following oral administration of a single 200-mg dose of quinidine sulfate. Plasma concentrations of quinidine generally reach steady-state after oral administration of 4–6 doses (200–300 mg) of quinidine sulfate at 2-hour intervals. If higher plasma concentrations are necessary after this time, the size of the individual dose must be increased.

Immediately following IV infusion over 4 hours of a single 24-mg/kg dose of quinidine gluconate in patients with *Plasmodium falciparum* malaria, plasma quinidine concentrations average 9.4 mcg/mL.

Plasma quinidine concentrations necessary to produce a therapeutic cardiovascular effect depend on the type of cardiac arrhythmia, the severity and duration of the arrhythmia, and the sensitivity of the patient to the drug. In the past when nonspecific assay methods were used to determine plasma quinidine concentrations, therapeutic plasma concentrations of quinidine were reportedly approximately 2–7 mcg/mL. Toxicity was generally associated with plasma quinidine concentrations greater than 5 mcg/mL. However, more specific assay methods are currently available and plasma quinidine concentrations are lower when these methods are used. Therefore, clinicians interpreting plasma quinidine concentrations should be aware of the method of analysis used. Therapeutic plasma concentrations of quinidine when these more specific assays are used have not been definitely established, but effective reduction of ventricular premature contractions has been reported with plasma quinidine concentrations less than 1 mcg/mL. After oral administration of 400–600 mg of quinidine sulfate, the onset of cardiovascular effects usually occurs in 1–3 hours and therapeutic cardiovascular effects persist for 6–8 hours.

Concomitant administration of antacids may delay oral absorption of quinidine. However, concomitant administration of oral quinidine gluconate and an aluminum hydroxide antacid does not have a clinically important effect on the rate and extent of absorption of quinidine.

When quinidine sulfate conventional tablets are administered with food, the rate of absorption is decreased but the extent of absorption is not affected. When quinidine gluconate extended-release tablets are administered with food, the rate of absorption is increased 27% and the extent of absorption is increased 17%.

■ **Distribution** Quinidine is rapidly distributed into all body tissues except the brain. The volume of distribution of the drug reportedly averages 2 L/kg in healthy adults and 0.9–1.8 L/kg in patients with malaria.

Quinidine is concentrated in heart, liver, kidneys, and skeletal muscle. Quinidine also is distributed into erythrocytes, where it is bound to hemoglobin. In one study in patients with cerebral *P. falciparum* malaria who received IV quinidine gluconate, CSF concentrations of quinidine were 7–17% of plasma concentrations.

Quinidine is about 80–88% bound to plasma proteins in adults and older children. Protein binding is lower in pregnant women, infants, and neonates, and may be as low as 50–70% in neonates and infants.

Quinidine crosses the placenta and is distributed into milk.

■ **Elimination** Quinidine generally has a plasma half-life of 6–8 hours in healthy individuals, but half-life may range from 3–16 hours or longer. In children, the elimination half-life of quinidine is 3–4 hours. In one study in patients with *P. falciparum* malaria, the elimination half-life of the drug averaged 12.8 hours (range: 6.6–24.8 hours).

Quinidine is metabolized by cytochrome P-450 (CYP) isoenzyme 3A4. Quinidine is metabolized in the liver, principally via hydroxylation to 3-hydroxyquinidine and 2-quinidinone. Some metabolites have antiarrhythmic activity. Animal studies indicate that the major metabolite, 3-hydroxyquinidine, has at least half of the antiarrhythmic activity of quinidine.

Approximately 10–50% of a dose is excreted in urine (probably by glomerular filtration) as unchanged drug within 24 hours. The rate of renal excretion of quinidine increases when the pH of urine is 6 or less; the rate of excretion decreases and plasma quinidine concentrations increase when urine is alkaline. Less than 5% of the orally administered drug is excreted in feces. Small amounts of quinidine are removed by hemodialysis; the drug is not removed by peritoneal dialysis.

Chemistry and Stability

■ **Chemistry** Quinidine is an alkaloid obtained from various species of *Cinchona* or their hybrids, from *Remijia pedunculata*, or prepared from quinine. Quinidine is the dextrorotatory isomer of quinine and contains 2 basic nitrogen atoms with pK_a values of 4 and 8.6. Commercially available quinidine salts contain not more than 20% of the respective dihydroquinidine salt, 1% of the respective quinine salt, and 1% of the respective dihydroquinine salt as impurities. The gluconate and sulfate derivatives of quinidine are used as antiarrhythmic agents.

Quinidine gluconate occurs as a white powder and is freely soluble in water and slightly soluble in alcohol. Commercially available quinidine gluconate injection has a pH of 5.5–7. Quinidine sulfate occurs as fine, needle-like, white crystals that frequently cohere in masses or as a fine, white powder and is slightly soluble in water and soluble in alcohol. The gluconate and sulfate derivatives of quinidine have a very bitter taste.

■ **Stability** Quinidine gluconate extended-release tablets should be stored at 20–25°C in tight, light-resistant containers.

Quinidine sulfate conventional or extended-release tablets should be stored at 20–25°C in tight containers. The tablets should be protected from light and moisture.

Quinidine gluconate injection should be stored at 25°C, but may be exposed to temperatures ranging from 15–30°C. When diluted to a concentration of 16 mg/mL with 5% dextrose injection, quinidine gluconate injection is stable for 24 hours at room temperature and up to 48 hours when refrigerated at 4°C.

Quinidine gluconate and quinidine sulfate darken on exposure to light. Solutions of quinidine salts slowly acquire a brownish tint on exposure to light. Only colorless, clear solutions of quinidine gluconate injection should be used.

Quinidine gluconate injection has been reported to be physically incompatible with some drugs, but the compatibility depends on several factors (e.g., concentrations of the drugs, specific diluents used, resulting pH, temperature). Specialized references should be consulted for specific compatibility information.

Preparations

Excipients in commercially available drug preparations may have clinically important effects in some individuals; consult specific product labeling for details.

quiNIDine Gluconate

Oral		
Tablets, extended-release	324 mg (equivalent to quinidine 202 mg)*	**quiNIDine Gluconate Extended-release Tablets**
Parenteral		
Injection	80 mg (equivalent to quinidine 50 mg) per mL*	**quiNIDine Gluconate Injection**

*available from one or more manufacturer, distributor, and/or repackager by generic (nonproprietary) name

quiNIDine Sulfate

Oral		
Tablets	200 mg (equivalent to quinidine 166 mg)*	**quiNIDine Sulfate Tablets**
	300 mg (equivalent to quinidine 249 mg)*	**quiNIDine Sulfate Tablets**
Tablets, extended-release	300 mg (equivalent to quinidine 249 mg)*	**quiNIDine Sulfate Extended-release Tablets**

*available from one or more manufacturer, distributor, and/or repackager by generic (nonproprietary) name

†Use is not currently included in the labeling approved by the US Food and Drug Administration

CLASS IB ANTIARRHYTHMICS 24:04.04.08

Lidocaine Hydrochloride

Lignocaine Hydrochloride

■ Lidocaine hydrochloride is an amide-type local anesthetic that is also used as a class Ib antiarrhythmic agent.

Uses

■ **Ventricular Arrhythmias** ***Ventricular Arrhythmias Associated with Myocardial Infarction or Cardiac Manipulation*** Lidocaine hydrochloride is used parenterally as an alternative to other antiarrhythmic drugs (e.g., amiodarone, procainamide, sotalol) for the acute treatment of life-threatening ventricular arrhythmias such as those that occur following myocardial infarction (MI) or during cardiac manipulative procedures such as cardiac surgery. Lidocaine previously was recommended for the prevention of ventricular arrhythmias associated with acute myocardial ischemia or infarction. Such use was supported largely by animal studies and extrapolation from historical use of the drug to suppress premature ventricular contractions (PVCs) and prevent ventricular fibrillation and potentially, sudden death, following acute MI. However, although pooled analysis of randomized controlled trials of prophylaxis with lidocaine demonstrated a reduction of approximately 33% in primary ventricular fibrillation following acute MI, this benefit was offset by a trend toward *increased* mortality, probably as a result of fatal episodes of bradycardia and asystole. Therefore, experts no longer recommend routine *prophylactic* use of lidocaine during acute MI, and such use has largely been abandoned.

Shock-Resistant Ventricular Fibrillation or Pulseless Ventricular Tachycardia Lidocaine is used as adjunctive therapy for the management of ventricular fibrillation or pulseless ventricular tachycardia resistant to cardiopulmonary resuscitation (CPR), defibrillation, and a vasopressor (e.g., epinephrine).

Antiarrhythmic drugs are used during cardiac arrest to facilitate the restoration and maintenance of a spontaneous perfusing rhythm in patients with refractory (i.e., persisting or recurring after at least one shock) ventricular fibrillation or pulseless ventricular tachycardia; however, there is no evidence that these drugs increase survival to hospital discharge when given routinely during cardiac arrest. High-quality CPR and defibrillation are integral components of ACLS and the only proven interventions to increase survival to hospital discharge. Other resuscitative efforts, including drug therapy, are considered secondary and should be performed without compromising the quality and timely delivery of chest compressions and defibrillation. The principal goal of pharmacologic therapy during cardiac arrest is to facilitate return of spontaneous circulation (ROSC), and epinephrine is the drug of choice for this use. (See Uses: Advanced Cardiovascular Life Support and Cardiac Arrhythmias, in Epinephrine 12:12.12.) If an antiarrhythmic agent is needed for the treatment of refractory ventricular fibrillation or pulseless ventricular tachycardia during adult cardiac arrest, AHA recommends amiodarone as the first-line drug of choice because of its proven benefits in improving rates of ROSC and hospital admission; lidocaine may be used as an alternative. Results of several studies suggest that amiodarone is more effective than lidocaine in improving rates of ROSC and hospital admission in patients with shock-refractory ventricular fibrillation or pulseless ventricular tachycardia. In pediatric advanced life support (PALS), current evidence supports the use of either amiodarone or lidocaine for these arrhythmias.

In a randomized, double-blind, comparative study, approximately 23% of patients with out-of-hospital cardiac arrest due to defibrillation-refractory ventricular arrhythmias (i.e., ventricular fibrillation, pulseless ventricular tachycardia) who received IV amiodarone hydrochloride (5 mg/kg) or lidocaine-placebo survived to hospital admission compared with 12% of those who received IV lidocaine hydrochloride (1.5 mg/kg) or amiodarone-placebo following at least 3 precordial electrical shocks, IV epinephrine, and an additional precordial shock. Among patients for whom the time from dispatch of the ambulance to the administration of the drug was equal to or less than the median time (24 minutes), approximately 28% of those given amiodarone and 15% of those given lidocaine survived to hospital admission. Despite these results, only about 6 or 4% of patients receiving IV amiodarone or IV lidocaine, respectively, who survived to hospital admission lived to be discharged from the hospital. Evidence supporting the use of amiodarone and lidocaine in pediatric cardiac arrest is more limited and principally based on extrapolation of data from the adult population. In a retrospective cohort study that included data from 889 pediatric patients with in-hospital cardiac arrest, improved ROSC was observed with lidocaine compared with amiodarone. Neither drug was associated with improved survival to hospital discharge.

Monomorphic Ventricular Tachycardia Lidocaine may be considered as an alternative to other antiarrhythmic agents or synchronized cardioversion for the treatment of hemodynamically stable monomorphic ventricular tachycardia; however, other agents are preferred. Available evidence suggests that lidocaine is less effective in treating ventricular tachycardia than either procainamide, sotalol, or amiodarone.

■ **Status Epilepticus** IV lidocaine has been used as a last resort for the treatment of status epilepticus†.

■ **Local Anesthesia** For the use of lidocaine hydrochloride as a local anesthetic, see 72:00.

Dosage and Administration

■ **Administration** ***Parenteral Administration*** Lidocaine hydrochloride is administered IV for the treatment of ventricular arrhythmias. The drug also has been administered by IM injection, but an IM formulation no longer is commercially available in the US. Lidocaine hydrochloride also has been administered by intraosseous (IO) injection† in the setting of advanced cardiovascular life support (ACLS) when IV administration is not possible; onset of action and systemic concentrations of the drug are comparable to those achieved with venous administration. *Lidocaine solutions that contain epinephrine must not be used to treat arrhythmias.*

Lidocaine hydrochloride also is available as solutions of the drug in 5% dextrose. Contents of lidocaine hydrochloride in dextrose injections should be inspected visually for discoloration and/or particulate matter prior to administration whenever solution and container permit. Additives should not be introduced into the solution container. Lidocaine hydrochloride in dextrose injection should not be used in series connections with other plastic containers, since such use could result in air embolism from residual air being drawn from the primary container before administration of fluid from the secondary container is complete. Commercially available solutions of the drug in 5% dextrose should not be administered unless the solution is clear and the container and seals are undamaged. When the commercially available IV infusion solution of lidocaine hydrochloride and 5% dextrose is used, the accompanying labeling should be consulted for proper methods of administration and other associated precautions.

Endotracheal Administration Lidocaine hydrochloride may be administered via the endotracheal route† if vascular (IV or IO) access cannot be established during cardiac arrest; however, IV or IO administration is preferred whenever possible because of more predictable drug delivery and pharmacologic effect. (See Pharmacokinetics: Absorption.) For endotracheal administration in adults, the dose should be diluted in 5–10 mL of 0.9% sodium chloride or sterile water and administered directly into the endotracheal tube. In pediatric patients, the endotracheal dose should be followed with a flush of at least 5 mL of 0.9% sodium chloride injection. Absorption of lidocaine, when administered via an endotracheal tube, may be increased by diluting the drug in sterile water instead of 0.9% sodium chloride.

■ **Dosage** Dosage of lidocaine hydrochloride must be carefully adjusted according to individual requirements and response.

Ventricular Arrhythmias **Adult Dosage.** For the initial treatment of ventricular arrhythmias, lidocaine hydrochloride usually is administered as a rapid (i.e., bolus) IV injection. The manufacturer states that the usual adult dose of lidocaine hydrochloride is 50–100 mg administered at a rate of approximately 25–50 mg/minute by direct IV injection. If the desired response is not achieved, a second dose may be administered 5 minutes after completion of the first injection. The manufacturer states that *no more than 200–300 mg should be administered during a 1-hour period.* Patients with congestive heart failure or cardiogenic shock may require smaller loading doses.

For the treatment of hemodynamically stable monomorphic ventricular tachycardia, the American Heart Association (AHA) recommends an initial adult dose of 1–1.5 mg/kg IV; additional doses of 0.5–0.75 mg/kg may be administered every 5–10 minutes as necessary, up to a maximum total dose of 3 mg/kg.

For the treatment of shock-resistant ventricular fibrillation or pulseless ventricular tachycardia during cardiac resuscitation, the initial adult loading dose of lidocaine hydrochloride is 1–1.5 mg/kg by IV or IO† injection, followed by 0.5–0.75 mg/kg repeated at 5- to 10-minute intervals as necessary, up to a maximum total dose of 3 mg/kg.

If IV or IO† access cannot be established during cardiac arrest, lidocaine may be administered via the endotracheal† route. Although the optimum endotracheal dose of lidocaine hydrochloride remains to be established, some experts state that typical doses should be 2–2.5 times those administered IV, and generally should be diluted in 5–10 mL of 0.9% sodium chloride or sterile water.

A maintenance infusion of lidocaine hydrochloride may be required to maintain normal sinus rhythm if oral antiarrhythmic therapy is not feasible.

Following initial administration with direct IV injections, an IV infusion of lidocaine hydrochloride may be initiated at a rate of 1–4 mg/minute (14–57 mcg/kg per minute). Some clinicians recommend maintaining the infusion rate below 30 mcg/kg per minute in patients with congestive heart failure. In patients with liver disease, dosing must be carefully individualized.

Major differences in lidocaine pharmacokinetics may exist for different types of liver disease (e.g., cirrhosis, hepatitis) and no consistent correlation has been established between clearance of the drug and severity of liver disease (as determined by liver function tests). No dosing modification appears to be necessary in patients with renal failure.

When arrhythmias reappear during a constant infusion of lidocaine hydrochloride, a small bolus dose (e.g., 0.5 mg/kg) may be given to rapidly increase plasma concentrations of the drug; the infusion rate is maintained or increased simultaneously. If the infusion rate alone is increased, a plateau or peak concentration of lidocaine may not be reached for 3–4 half-lives (5–8 hours).

The infusion should be terminated as soon as the patient's basic cardiac rhythm appears to be stable or at the earliest sign of toxicity. If signs of excessive cardiac depression, such as prolongation of the PR interval and QRS complex or the appearance or aggravation of arrhythmias occur, the infusion should be stopped immediately. The manufacturers state that it should rarely be necessary to continue the infusion for longer than 24 hours. Clinical studies have reported continuation of lidocaine infusions for several days; however, there are data which indicate that the half-life of lidocaine may be increased to 3 hours or longer following infusions lasting longer than 24 hours, and dosage may need to be reduced accordingly (e.g., by 50%) to avoid accumulation of the drug and potential toxicity. If maintenance therapy is necessary, therapy should be changed to an oral antiarrhythmic agent.

Pediatric Dosage. Controlled clinical studies to establish pediatric dosing schedules of lidocaine hydrochloride have not been performed. Some clinicians have suggested that infants and children may be given an initial rapid IV injection (i.e., bolus) of 0.5–1 mg/kg; this dose may be repeated according to the response of the patient, but the total dose should not exceed 3–5 mg/kg. A maintenance IV infusion of 10–50 mcg/kg per minute may be given via an infusion pump.

For the treatment of shock-refractory ventricular fibrillation or pulseless ventricular tachycardia during pediatric resuscitation, the recommended dosage of lidocaine hydrochloride is an initial rapid IV or IO† injection (i.e., bolus) of 1 mg/kg, followed by a maintenance infusion of 20–50 mcg/kg per minute. A repeat IV injection should be given if there is more than a 15-minute delay from the time of the initial rapid IV injection dose to the onset of the infusion.

If IV or IO† access cannot be established, lidocaine may be administered via the endotracheal† route. Although the optimum endotracheal dose of lidocaine hydrochloride remains to be established, some experts state that typical doses should be 2–2.5 times those administered IV. If cardiopulmonary resuscitation (CPR) is in progress, chest compressions should be interrupted briefly to administer lidocaine. Following administration, the endotracheal tube should be flushed with 5 mL of 0.9% sodium chloride injection and followed by 5 consecutive positive-pressure ventilations.

Status Epilepticus For the treatment of status epilepticus†, some clinicians have suggested an initial IV lidocaine hydrochloride bolus dose of 1 mg/kg. If the seizure is not terminated, 0.5 mg/kg may be given 2 minutes after completion of the first injection. A maintenance IV infusion of 30 mcg/kg per minute has been given to prevent recurrence of seizures.

Cautions

Serious adverse reactions to lidocaine are uncommon. Adverse effects of the drug mainly involve the CNS, are usually of short duration, and are dose related.

If severe reactions occur, lidocaine administration should be discontinued; emergency resuscitative procedures and other supportive measures should be instituted. Maintenance of adequate ventilation and a patent airway are of primary importance. For the treatment of severe seizures, small IV doses of diazepam or an ultrashort-acting barbiturate (e.g., thiopental, thiamylal) may be given or, if these are not available, pentobarbital or secobarbital may be administered. If the patient is anesthetized, a short-acting neuromuscular blocking agent (e.g., succinylcholine) may be given IV. If circulatory depression occurs, IV fluids and vasopressors such as ephedrine or metaraminol may be used if necessary.

■ **Nervous System Effects** Adverse CNS reactions may be manifested by drowsiness; dizziness; disorientation; confusion; lightheadedness; tremulousness; psychosis; nervousness; apprehension; agitation; euphoria; tinnitus; visual disturbances including blurred or double vision; nausea; vomiting; paresthesia; sensations of heat, cold, or numbness; difficulty swallowing; dyspnea; and slurred speech. Muscle twitching or tremors, seizures, unconsciousness or altered consciousness, coma, and respiratory depression and arrest may also occur.

■ **Dermatologic and Sensitivity Reactions** Hypersensitivity to lidocaine is rare and may be characterized by skin lesions, urticaria, edema, and anaphylactoid reactions.

■ **Cardiovascular Effects** Although usual doses of lidocaine generally produce no adverse cardiovascular effects, patients with high plasma concentrations of the drug or myocardial conduction defects may develop hypotension, arrhythmias, heart block, cardiovascular collapse, and bradycardia which may lead to cardiac arrest. However, cardiac arrest caused by lidocaine is usually secondary to respiratory arrest. In anesthetized patients, CNS toxicity and seizures may not occur; cardiovascular depression may be the first manifestation of toxicity in these patients.

■ **Administration Effects** Local thrombophlebitis may occur in patients receiving prolonged IV infusions of lidocaine. Pain at the site of IM injection (no longer commercially available in the US) has been reported occasionally, and IM injection of lidocaine increases serum creatine kinase (CK, creatine phosphokinase, CPK) concentrations. (See Laboratory Test Interferences.)

■ **Precautions and Contraindications** Constant ECG monitoring is necessary during IV administration of lidocaine. ECG changes such as prolongation of the PR interval and QRS complex or the appearance or aggravation of arrhythmias necessitates prompt cessation of lidocaine infusion. Resuscitative equipment and drugs should be immediately available for the management of severe, adverse cardiovascular, respiratory, or CNS effects. If severe reactions occur, lidocaine should be discontinued and appropriate therapy instituted. Severe reactions are often preceded by somnolence and paresthesia, and these symptoms should *not* be ignored.

Although the manufacturers state that lidocaine should be used with caution in patients with severe renal disease, the drug has been used safely in these patients. Lidocaine should be administered with caution to patients with liver disease, congestive heart failure, marked hypoxia, severe respiratory depression, hypovolemia, or shock. Caution should be used when administering lidocaine to patients with sinus bradycardia or incomplete heart block for the treatment of ventricular premature contractions without prior acceleration of heart rate, since more frequent and serious ventricular arrhythmias or heart block may result. In addition, use of the drug in patients with symptomatic bradycardia may result in potentially life-threatening adverse effects (e.g., death), particularly if the bradycardia is a ventricular escape rhythm that is mistaken for preventricular contractions or slow ventricular tachycardia. Lidocaine may increase ventricular rate when it is administered to patients with atrial fibrillation. Hypokalemia, hypoxia, and disorders of acid-base balance must be eliminated as potentiating factors in patients who require large doses of antiarrhythmic agents to control ventricular irritability.

Lidocaine is contraindicated in patients with a known hypersensitivity to the amide-type local anesthetics. There have been no reports of cross-sensitivity reactions between lidocaine and procainamide or quinidine. Lidocaine should be used with caution in patients with any form of heart block and is contraindicated in patients with Adams-Stokes syndrome or with severe degrees of SA, AV, or intraventricular heart block in the absence of an artificial pacemaker. Although some manufacturers state that lidocaine is contraindicated in patients with Wolff-Parkinson-White syndrome, some clinicians have used the drug for the treatment of tachyarrhythmias in patients with this syndrome.

■ **Pediatric Precautions** Safety and efficacy of lidocaine in the management of ventricular arrhythmias in children have not been established by controlled clinical studies. However, lidocaine has been used for the treatment of ventricular arrhythmias in infants and children. Some experts state that use of the drug may be considered during pediatric resuscitation for the treatment of ventricular fibrillation or pulseless ventricular tachycardia that is resistant to cardiopulmonary resuscitation (CPR), cardioversion (i.e., defibrillation), and epinephrine.

■ **Mutagenicity and Carcinogenicity** Studies have not been performed to date to evaluate the mutagenic or carcinogenic potential of lidocaine.

■ **Pregnancy and Lactation** Safe use of lidocaine during pregnancy (prior to labor) has not been established. The drug should be used during pregnancy only when clearly needed.

Since lidocaine is distributed into milk, the drug should be used with caution in nursing women. Limited data suggest that the amount of drug that potentially would be ingested by a breast-fed infant is small.

Drug Interactions

■ **Succinylcholine** In anesthetized individuals, the neuromuscular blocking effect of succinylcholine has been reported to be increased by IV administration of lidocaine prior to or following succinylcholine administration; however, this effect appears to be important only following administration of lidocaine in doses higher than those usually used clinically.

■ **Antiarrhythmic Agents** When lidocaine is administered with other antiarrhythmic drugs such as phenytoin, procainamide, propranolol, or quinidine, the cardiac effects may be additive or antagonistic and toxic effects may be additive. Phenytoin may stimulate the hepatic metabolism of lidocaine, but the clinical importance of this effect is not known.

■ **Other Drugs** Concurrent use of lidocaine with cimetidine or propranolol may result in increased serum concentrations of lidocaine with resultant toxicity. Cimetidine and propranolol substantially reduce the systemic clearance of lidocaine, apparently by reducing hepatic blood flow and hepatic extraction of the drug; other mechanisms (e.g., altered distribution or metabolism of lidocaine) may also be involved. If lidocaine and cimetidine or propranolol are used concurrently, the patient should be closely observed for signs of lidocaine toxicity, and serum lidocaine concentrations should be carefully monitored; reduction of lidocaine dosage may be necessary.

Laboratory Test Interferences

Because IM injection of lidocaine (no longer commercially available in the US) may increase serum CK (CPK) concentrations, isoenzyme separation is necessary when CK determinations are used in the diagnosis of acute myocardial infarction in patients receiving the drug IM.

Pharmacology

The cardiac actions of lidocaine appear to be similar to those of phenytoin. Lidocaine is considered a class I (membrane-stabilizing) antiarrhythmic agent. Like other class I antiarrhythmic agents, lidocaine is believed to combine with fast sodium channels in their inactive state and thereby inhibit recovery after repolarization in a time- and voltage-dependent manner which is associated with subsequent dissociation of the drug from the sodium channels. Lidocaine exhibits electrophysiologic effects characteristic of class IB antiarrhythmic agents. The electrophysiologic characteristics of the subgroups of class I antiarrhythmic agents may be related to quantitative differences in their rates of attachment to and dissociation from transmembrane sodium channels, with class IB agents exhibiting rapid rates of attachment and dissociation.

Lidocaine controls ventricular arrhythmias by suppressing automaticity in the His-Purkinje system and by suppressing spontaneous depolarization of the ventricles during diastole. These effects occur at lidocaine concentrations that do not suppress automaticity of the sinoatrial (SA) node. At therapeutic plasma concentrations, lidocaine has little effect on atrioventricular (AV) node conduction and His-Purkinje conduction in the normal heart. Specialized conducting tissues of the atria are less sensitive to the effects of lidocaine than are those of ventricular tissues. Lidocaine has a variable effect on the effective refractory period (ERP) of the AV node; the drug shortens the ERP and the action potential duration of the His-Purkinje system. Lidocaine does not appear to affect excitability of normal cardiac tissue.

Unlike quinidine and procainamide, lidocaine has little effect on autonomic tone and generally does not produce a substantial fall in blood pressure, decreased myocardial contractility, or diminished cardiac output in usual doses. Although lidocaine usually has little effect on heart rate, patients with a diseased or abnormal sinus node may be especially sensitive to the cardiac depressant effects of the drug. Lidocaine may increase coronary blood flow in patients with recent myocardial infarction.

Lidocaine is a CNS depressant and produces sedative, analgesic, and anticonvulsant effects. With high doses, seizures may result from depression of inhibitory influences on motor pathways; severe overdosage may cause respiratory arrest because of motor nerve paralysis and/or inadequate medullary blood flow. Lidocaine also suppresses the cough and gag reflexes.

Pharmacokinetics

■ Absorption Although lidocaine hydrochloride is absorbed from the GI tract, it passes into the hepatic portal circulation and only about 35% of an oral dose reaches systemic circulation unchanged. One study showed that therapeutic plasma concentrations are not achieved after oral administration of 250 or 500 mg of the drug, but toxic effects appear, perhaps because of high concentrations of toxic metabolites.

Plasma lidocaine concentrations of approximately 1–5 mcg/mL are required to suppress ventricular arrhythmias. Toxicity has been associated with plasma lidocaine concentrations greater than 5 mcg/mL. Following IV administration of a bolus dose of 50–100 mg of lidocaine hydrochloride, the drug has an onset of action within 45–90 seconds and a duration of action of 10–20 minutes. If an IV infusion is initiated without an initial bolus dose, the attainment of therapeutic plasma concentrations is relatively slow. For example, therapeutic plasma concentrations are achieved in 30–60 minutes after the start of a continuous infusion of 60–70 mcg/kg per minute when no loading dose is given. Plasma concentrations of 1.5–5.5 mcg/mL have been reported to be maintained with an initial IV bolus of 1.5 mg/kg followed by infusion of 50 mcg/kg per minute in patients with heart disease.

Lidocaine hydrochloride is absorbed in the trachea; when the drug is administered endotracheally, plasma concentrations generally are lower than those achieved with vascular administration. A biphasic pattern of absorption is observed following endotracheal administration of lidocaine (initial instantaneous absorption of a small fraction of the dose, followed by a late, delayed absorption phase). Absorption may be increased by diluting the drug in sterile water instead of 0.9% sodium chloride injection.

After intradeltoid injection (an IM formulation no longer is commercially available in the US) of lidocaine hydrochloride 4.5 mg/kg in one study in patients with ventricular premature contractions, peak blood concentrations of 2.9 mcg/mL were achieved in 10 minutes and blood concentrations of 2.2 mcg/mL persisted for 60 minutes. Intradeltoid injection produces higher blood concentrations and more rapid development of peak blood concentrations than do injections into the gluteus maximus or vastus lateralis.

■ Distribution Lidocaine is widely distributed into body tissues. After an IV bolus, there is an early, rapid decline in plasma concentrations of the drug, principally associated with distribution into highly perfused tissues such as the kidneys, lungs, liver, and heart, followed by a slower elimination phase in which metabolism and redistribution into skeletal muscle and adipose tissue occur. Lidocaine has a high affinity for fat and adipose tissue. As plasma concentrations of the drug fall, the diffusion gradient from tissue to blood increases and the lidocaine that initially entered the highly perfused tissues and fat diffuses back into the blood. The volume of distribution is decreased in patients with congestive heart failure and increased in patients with liver disease.

Binding of lidocaine to plasma proteins is variable and concentration dependent. At concentrations of 1–4 mcg/mL, the drug is approximately 60–80% bound to plasma proteins. Lidocaine is partially bound to α_1-acid glycoprotein (α_1-AGP), and the extent of binding to α_1-AGP depends on the plasma concentration of the protein. In patients with myocardial infarction, increases in plasma α_1-AGP concentration are associated with increased lidocaine binding and increased total plasma concentrations of the drug, but only small increases in plasma concentration of free drug; these changes in α_1-AGP concentration and lidocaine binding are believed to account in part for accumulation of the drug observed in patients with myocardial infarction receiving prolonged infusions.

Lidocaine readily crosses the blood-brain barrier and the placenta. Lidocaine also is distributed into milk; in one lactating woman, milk lidocaine concentration was approximately 40% of the serum concentration (from a sample obtained 2 hours earlier).

■ Elimination Lidocaine has an initial half-life of 7–30 minutes and a terminal half-life of 1.5–2 hours. In healthy individuals, the elimination half-lives of the active metabolites, monoethylglycinexylidide (MEGX) and glycinexylidide (GX) are 2 hours and 10 hours, respectively. In patients with myocardial infarction (with or without cardiac failure), the half-lives of lidocaine and MEGX have been reported to be prolonged; the half-life of GX is reportedly prolonged in patients with cardiac failure secondary to myocardial infarction. The half-life of lidocaine is reportedly also prolonged in patients with congestive heart failure or liver disease and may be prolonged following continuous IV infusions lasting longer than 24 hours. MEGX elimination may also be decreased in patients with congestive heart failure.

Approximately 90% of a parenteral dose of lidocaine is rapidly metabolized in the liver by de-ethylation to form MEGX and GX followed by cleavage of the amide bond to form xylidine and 4-hydroxyxylidine which are excreted in urine. Less than 10% of a dose is excreted unchanged in urine. MEGX and GX are pharmacologically active and may also cause CNS toxicity in some patients. The rate of metabolism of lidocaine appears to be limited by hepatic blood flow which may be reduced in patients after acute myocardial infarction and/or with congestive heart failure. Patients with congestive heart failure excrete more of a dose of lidocaine as unchanged drug and MEGX and less as GX and 4-hydroxyxylidine than do those without congestive heart failure. The rate of lidocaine metabolism may also be decreased in patients with liver disease, possibly because of altered perfusion in the liver or hepatic tissue necrosis. Distribution and elimination of lidocaine and MEGX appear to remain normal in patients with renal failure, but GX may accumulate in these patients when lidocaine is administered IV for several days.

Chemistry and Stability

■ Chemistry Lidocaine hydrochloride is an amide-type local anesthetic that is also used as an antiarrhythmic agent. The drug occurs as a white, crystalline powder having a slightly bitter taste and is very soluble in water and in alcohol. The pK_a of the drug is 7.86. Sodium hydroxide and/or hydrochloric acid are used to adjust the pH of the commercially available injections to 5–7. Commercially available lidocaine hydrochloride in 5% dextrose injections are sterile, nonpyrogenic solutions of the drug; sodium hydroxide may have been added to adjust pH to 4 (range: 3–7). Commercially available 0.4 or 0.8% solutions of lidocaine hydrochloride in 5% dextrose have osmolarities of 280–282, or 305–311 mOsm/L, respectively. Potency of lidocaine hydrochloride is calculated on the anhydrous basis.

■ Stability Lidocaine hydrochloride injections and commercially available solutions of the drug in 5% dextrose should be stored at 25°C but may be exposed to temperatures up to 40°C; the injection and solutions should not be frozen, and the solutions should be protected from excessive heat. Commercially available solutions of lidocaine hydrochloride in 5% dextrose usually are stable for 18 months after the date of manufacture. Commercially available solutions of lidocaine hydrochloride in 5% dextrose may be provided in plastic containers. The amount of water that can permeate from the container into the overwrap is insufficient to significantly affect the injection. Solutions in contact with the plastic can leach out some of the chemical components in very small amounts; however, safety of the plastic has been confirmed in tests in animals according to USP biological tests for plastic containers.

At concentrations of 1–4 mg/mL in 5% dextrose injection, extemporaneously prepared lidocaine hydrochloride solutions appear to be stable at room temperature for at least 24 hours.

Lidocaine hydrochloride injection is compatible with most commercially available IV infusion fluids, but the pH of the drug may adversely affect additives such as dopamine, epinephrine, norepinephrine, or isoproterenol that require low pH for stability. If such admixtures are prepared, they should be administered shortly after preparation. Specialized references should be consulted for specific compatibility information. The manufacturers state that the commercially available solutions of lidocaine hydrochloride in 5% dextrose should not be mixed with other drugs.

Preparations

Excipients in commercially available drug preparations may have clinically important effects in some individuals; consult specific product labeling for details.

Lidocaine Hydrochloride

Parenteral		
Injection, for direct IV injection	10 mg/mL*	Lidocaine Hydrochloride Injection for Cardiac Arrhythmias
	20 mg/mL*	Lidocaine Hydrochloride Injection for Cardiac Arrhythmias

*available from one or more manufacturer, distributor, and/or repackager by generic (nonproprietary) name

Lidocaine Hydrochloride in Dextrose

Parenteral		
Injection, for IV infusion	4 mg/mL (1 or 2 g) Lidocaine Hydrochloride in 5% Dextrose	0.4% Lidocaine Hydrochloride and 5% Dextrose Injection
	8 mg/mL (2 or 4 g) Lidocaine Hydrochloride in 5% Dextrose	0.8% Lidocaine Hydrochloride and 5% Dextrose Injection

†Use is not currently included in the labeling approved by the US Food and Drug Administration

CLASS IC ANTIARRHYTHMICS 24:04.04.12

Flecainide Acetate

■ Flecainide acetate is a local anesthetic-type class Ic antiarrhythmic agent.

Uses

■ **Ventricular Arrhythmias** Flecainide acetate is used to suppress and prevent the recurrence of documented *life-threatening* ventricular arrhythmias (e.g., sustained ventricular tachycardia). Based on information from the National Heart, Lung, and Blood Institute (NHLBI) describing interim results of the Cardiac Arrhythmia Suppression Trial (CAST) (see the opening discussion in Cautions), flecainide therapy should be *reserved* for the suppression and prevention of documented ventricular arrhythmias that, in the clinician's judgment, are considered *life-threatening*.

Because of the drug's arrhythmogenic potential and associated risk of death identified in CAST, use of flecainide for less severe arrhythmias (e.g., nonsustained ventricular tachycardia†, frequent premature ventricular complexes† [PVCs]), even when the patient is symptomatic, is not recommended. The findings of CAST involved a select patient population with recent myocardial infarction (MI), mild-to-moderate left ventricular dysfunction (e.g., mean baseline ejection fraction of 0.4), and asymptomatic or mildly symptomatic ventricular arrhythmias† (mean baseline PVCs of 127/hour as evidenced via ambulatory ECG [Holter] monitoring during at least 18 hours of analyzable time, with about 20% of patients exhibiting at least one run of nonsustained ventricular tachycardia during such monitoring); such patients also had demonstrated drug-induced suppressibility of PVCs during the initial phase of the open trial. It currently is not known whether the findings of CAST can be extrapolated to other patient populations with non-life-threatening ventricular arrhythmias (e.g., patients with arrhythmias in the absence of ventricular dysfunction, myocardial ischemia, or recent MI). CAST principally involved suppression and prevention of PVCs, with only about 10% of patients exhibiting more than a single run of tachycardia at baseline. Some clinicians also question whether the results of CAST even can be extrapolated to patients with recurrent nonsustained ventricular tachycardia and ventricular dysfunction, since these patients are known to be at high risk of sudden death if untreated, and since CAST did not include sufficient numbers of such patients to clearly determine the benefit-to-risk ratio. However, despite the limitations of the CAST findings, the manufacturer, FDA, and other experts consider the potential risks of flecainide therapy substantial and currently do not recommend use of the drug in any patient with non-life-threatening ventricular arrhythmias in the absence of substantial evidence of safety and efficacy. The manufacturer states that it is prudent to consider the risks of class Ic antiarrhythmic agents and current lack of evidence of improved survival *unacceptable* in patients *without* life-threatening ventricular arrhythmias, even in patients experiencing unpleasant, but non-life-threatening signs and symptoms. However, some clinicians, while recognizing the strong evidence of risk in the patient population studied in CAST and the substantial limitations of current evidence on safety and efficacy in other patient populations, question such an extreme limitation of usage.

Life-threatening Ventricular Arrhythmias The optimum role of flecainide in the suppression and prevention of ventricular arrhythmias remains to be clearly determined.

In addition, it remains to be determined whether antiarrhythmic agents, including flecainide, have a beneficial effect on mortality or sudden death. Although flecainide has been effective in suppressing and preventing ventricular arrhythmias in carefully selected patients, further studies are needed to evaluate the long-term efficacy and safety and the relative role of the drug. Therefore, it is recommended that flecainide generally be reserved for patients who have an insufficient therapeutic response to, or who do not tolerate, conventional orally administered antiarrhythmic agents (e.g., class Ia agents). In addition, because of flecainide's arrhythmogenic potential, some clinicians avoid use of the drug as a first-line agent in patients with life-threatening ventricular arrhythmias who also have congestive heart failure or substantial ventricular dysfunction. While it currently is not known whether the findings of the CAST study apply to class Ic antiarrhythmic agents other than flecainide and encainide (no longer commercially available in the US), some experts state that, in the absence of specific evidence of safety and efficacy, other class Ic drugs should be considered to share these risks.

There is relatively limited experience with the use of flecainide for suppression and prevention of recurrent life-threatening ventricular arrhythmias. In the management of severe refractory arrhythmias, the efficacy of flecainide appears to be comparable to that of other first-line antiarrhythmic agents, with the drug being effective in up to about 40% of patients. Younger patients and patients without coronary heart disease and/or substantial ventricular dysfunction appear to have a greater likelihood of responding to flecainide. Further studies, including comparative studies with other antiarrhythmic agents, are needed to evaluate the use of flecainide in the management of life-threatening ventricular arrhythmias.

Limited information is available on the use of flecainide in conjunction with other antiarrhythmic agents for the management of severe refractory ventricular arrhythmias. (See Drug Interactions: Antiarrhythmic Agents.) In a limited number of patients, flecainide has been combined with amiodarone, with good results in selected patients; however, use of these two agents in combination requires extreme caution and is generally reserved for patients with life-threatening ventricular arrhythmias inadequately controlled by single-agent therapy with amiodarone or another antiarrhythmic agent. Combination antiarrhythmic therapy for severe refractory ventricular arrhythmias is generally empiric and must be individualized.

Other Ventricular Arrhythmias Controlled and uncontrolled clinical studies in patients with chronic stable ventricular arrhythmias† have shown that flecainide is highly effective in suppressing and preventing nonsustained ventricular tachycardia and frequent PVCs, including complex PVCs. In short-term clinical studies, flecainide therapy produced at least 80–90% suppression of PVCs in about 80–90% of patients; in many patients, essentially complete suppression of uniform and multiform PVCs, complex PVCs, and/or nonsustained ventricular tachycardia may occur. However, despite such documented evidence of efficacy in suppressing and preventing these arrhythmias, there currently is no evidence of beneficial effect on mortality, and in at least one patient population (those with mild-to-moderate ventricular dysfunction and recent MI) with such arrhythmias, there was evidence of substantial risk (including mortality and nonfatal cardiac arrest) associated with flecainide or encainide therapy. (See the opening discussion of Cautions.) Therefore, use of flecainide in nonlife-threatening ventricular arrhythmias currently is *not* recommended by the manufacturer, FDA, and other experts.

■ **Supraventricular Tachyarrhythmias** Flecainide is used for the prevention of paroxysmal supraventricular tachycardia (PSVT), including atrioventricular (AV) nodal reentrant tachycardia and AV reentrant tachycardia (e.g., Wolff-Parkinson-White syndrome); other symptomatic, disabling supraventricular tachycardias of unspecified mechanisms; and symptomatic, disabling paroxysmal atrial fibrillation/flutter (PAF) in patients without structural heart disease. Controlled and uncontrolled clinical studies have shown that flecainide may prevent or delay recurrence of PSVT and PAF episodes or may increase the interval between episodes of PSVT and PAF in 31–81% of patients, depending on the type of arrhythmia; suppression of arrhythmias refractory to other antiarrhythmic agents also has occurred. In some patients with atrial fibrillation or flutter associated with ventricular preexcitation and Wolff-Parkinson-White syndrome, flecainide may slow the ventricular rate or possibly restore and maintain normal sinus rhythm. Because of the risk of proarrhythmia, flecainide should not be used in patients with structural heart disease or ischemic heart disease.

Based on findings from the CAST study demonstrating substantial flecainide-associated risk in certain patients with ventricular arrhythmias, some experts currently caution that use of flecainide in supraventricular arrhythmias be limited to the management of symptomatic, disabling supraventricular arrhythmias (PAF, AV junctional tachycardias) in patients *without* structural heart disease. However, some clinicians state that even these patients may be at risk of developing drug-induced arrhythmogenic effects (e.g., during exercise testing). The risks versus benefits of flecainide for the management of such arrhythmias in patients *with* structural heart defects remains to be elucidated, and assessment of the possible risks and potential benefits in such patients must be individualized.

Paroxysmal Supraventricular Tachycardia For acute conversion of PSVT, vagal maneuvers, IV adenosine, AV nodal blocking agents (e.g., calcium-channel blocking agents, β-adrenergic blocking agents), and/or synchronized cardioversion are the treatments of choice. Flecainide is one of several drugs that may be used for the ongoing management of PSVT (to prevent recurrences of these arrhythmias) in patients without structural or ischemic heart disease; because of the risk of adverse effects, however, use of flecainide generally is reserved for patients in whom other therapies are ineffective or contraindicated. In a randomized, placebo-controlled, crossover study in 34 patients with symptomatic PSVT, episodes of PSVT occurred in 85% of patients receiving placebo but in only about 21% of patients receiving flecainide acetate in a median dosage of 300 mg daily (range: 100–400 mg daily in 2 divided doses) during the 16-week study period. The median time before initial recurrence of PSVT exceeded 55 days in patients receiving flecainide compared with 11 days in those receiving placebo, while median intervals between episodes of PSVT exceeded 55 days in patients receiving flecainide compared with 12 days in those receiving placebo.

Paroxysmal Atrial Fibrillation and Flutter In another randomized, crossover placebo-controlled study in 48 patients with PAF, episodes of PAF occurred in 92% of patients receiving placebo versus 69% of patients who received flecainide acetate in a median dosage of 300 mg daily (range: 100–600 mg daily in 2 divided doses) during the 8-week study period. The median time before initial recurrence of PAF was approximately 15 days in patients receiving flecainide versus 3 days in those receiving placebo, while the median interval between episodes of PAF was 27 days in patients receiving flecainide and approximately 6 days in patients receiving placebo.

Self-administration for Conversion of Paroxysmal Atrial Fibrillation. Limited evidence suggests that out-of-hospital *self-administration* of a single oral loading dose† of flecainide or propafenone ("pill-in-the-pocket" approach) is safe and effective for terminating recent-onset PAF† and can reduce hospitalizations and emergency room visits in carefully selected patients who have mild or no heart disease. Experts state that an initial conversion trial in a monitored setting is recommended before this approach is undertaken in an unmonitored setting outside of the hospital. In-hospital administration of flecainide or propafenone (as immediate-release tablets) as a single oral dose for terminating acute atrial fibrillation† has been shown to be effective with a low incidence of adverse effects in several randomized, controlled studies; however, the safety of such treatment without initial evaluation in a hospital setting or in patients with substantial structural heart disease has not been established. In addition, additional study and experience are required to assess the possible need for concomitant antithrombotic (e.g., warfarin) therapy and potential for adverse drug interactions (e.g., with warfarin or digoxin) in patients self-administering antiarrhythmic agents for recent-onset paroxysmal atrial fibrillation on an out-of-hospital basis.

In a prospective, uncontrolled study, 268 patients (18–75 years of age) with mild or no heart disease who had hemodynamically well-tolerated atrial fibrillation of recent (less than 48 hours) onset were treated in-hospital (i.e., in the emergency room or cardiology ward) with a single oral dose of flecainide or immediate-release propafenone (according to clinician preference) to restore normal sinus rhythm. Patients weighing 70 kg or more received 300 mg of flecainide acetate or 600 mg of propafenone hydrochloride and those weighing less than 70 kg received 200 mg of flecainide acetate or 450 mg of propafenone hydrochloride. In-hospital treatment was considered effective if conversion of atrial fibrillation to sinus rhythm occurred within 6 hours of administration of the antiarrhythmic agent without clinically important adverse effects (i.e., symptomatic hypotension, symptomatic bradycardia after restoration of sinus rhythm, dyspnea, presyncope, syncope, conversion to atrial flutter or atrial tachycardia, or episodes of sustained or unsustained ventricular tachycardia). The time to conversion to sinus rhythm following in-hospital treatment with flecainide or propafenone in these patients averaged 135 minutes (median: 120 minutes). Patients in whom inpatient administration of these antiarrhythmics was effective and who were not excluded during subsequent examination were discharged and given flecainide or propafenone for treatment of subsequent episodes of palpitations (presumed recurrent atrial fibrillation) on an outpatient basis. These patients were instructed to take a single oral dose of the assigned antiarrhythmic drug 5 minutes after noting the onset of palpitations (self-assessed) and then to assume a resting state (e.g., a supine or sitting position) until resolution of the palpitations or for at least four hours.

Analysis of data from 2 of the study sites indicated that 12% of patients presenting to the emergency room for recent-onset atrial fibrillation were candidates for out-of-hospital treatment with propafenone or flecainide. During a mean follow-up period of 15 months (range: 7–19 months), 79% of patients included in the out-of-hospital phase of the study experienced episodes of palpitations (presumed atrial fibrillation); patients self-administered propafenone hydrochloride (mean dose: 555 mg) or flecainide acetate (mean dose: 263 mg) within a mean of 36 minutes (median: 10 minutes) after the onset of symptoms in 92% of such episodes. Each antiarrhythmic agent was effective in interrupting 94% of episodes of palpitations (a primary end point); time to resolution of symptoms after drug administration averaged 113 minutes (median: 98 minutes). In patients who had multiple recurrences of palpitations during the follow-up period, self-administration of flecainide or propafenone terminated all such episodes in 84% of patients. Self-administration of oral flecainide or propafenone also was associated with reductions in emergency room visits and hospital admissions (secondary end points); calls for emergency room intervention during the study averaged 4.9 per month compared with 45.6 per month during the year prior to the study, while the number of hospitalizations averaged 1.6 per month during the study compared with 15 per month during the prior year.

Atrial Fibrillation and Flutter Flecainide is considered a drug of choice for pharmacologic cardioversion of atrial fibrillation or atrial flutter†. Conversion of atrial fibrillation or flutter to normal sinus rhythm may be associated with embolism, particularly when the arrhythmia has been present for more than 48 hours, unless the patient is adequately anticoagulated. (See Uses: Cardioversion of Atrial Fibrillation/Flutter, in Heparin 20:12.04.16.)

Limited data suggest that flecainide may also improve control of ventricular rate at rest and during exercise in digitalized patients with atrial fibrillation† in whom cardiac glycosides alone may not provide adequate control.

Some clinicians do not recommend the use of antiarrhythmic agents in patients with atrial fibrillation or flutter because increased mortality has been reported in patients receiving antiarrhythmic therapy after conversion of atrial fibrillation to normal sinus rhythm.

Other Supraventricular Tachycardias Flecainide may be used for the ongoing management of focal atrial tachycardia† or junctional tachycardia† in patients without structural or ischemic heart disease. Limited data suggest that flecainide may be effective in suppressing and preventing recurrent atrial tachycardia†.

Dosage and Administration

■ **Administration** Flecainide acetate is administered orally. Flecainide also has been administered IV†, but a parenteral dosage form of the drug is currently not commercially available in the US.

Flecainide acetate is administered orally, usually in 2 equally divided doses daily at 12-hour intervals; however, in patients in whom arrhythmias are not adequately controlled or the drug is not well tolerated with twice-daily dosing, the drug may be given in 3 divided doses daily at 8-hour intervals. The elimination half-life of flecainide suggests that once-daily oral dosing may be possible in some patients, but once-daily dosing regimens of the drug have not been evaluated to date.

Absorption of flecainide is not affected by food or antacids; however, milk may inhibit absorption in infants. Dosage reduction of flecainide acetate may be necessary when milk is removed from the diet in infants.

Because of the risk of proarrhythmia, initiation of therapy in a hospital setting is recommended in patients with sustained ventricular tachycardia, regardless of their cardiac status. Some clinicians recommend that withdrawal of therapy should also occur in a hospital setting under continuous ECG monitoring.

■ **Dosage** Dosage of flecainide acetate should be carefully adjusted according to individual patient response and tolerance. Clinical and ECG monitoring of cardiac function is recommended during therapy with the drug. When feasible, plasma trough flecainide concentrations should be monitored; monitoring is required in patients with severe renal or hepatic impairment, and is recommended in other patients in whom elimination of the drug may be impaired (e.g., those with moderate renal impairment or congestive heart failure, or those receiving concomitant amiodarone therapy). Dosage should be adjusted to maintain trough plasma flecainide concentrations at less than 0.7–1 mcg/mL since concentrations above this range have been associated with a higher rate of adverse cardiac effects, especially when the trough concentration exceeds 1 mcg/mL. Since steady-state plasma concentrations of flecainide and the optimum therapeutic effect may not be attained for 3–5 days (or longer in some patients) at a given dosage in patients with normal renal and hepatic function, increases in flecainide dosage should be made at intervals of not less than 4 days. Once adequate control of arrhythmias has been attained, dosage reduction to minimize adverse effects or effects on cardiac conduction may be possible in some patients; however, efficacy of the drug at the lower dosage should be evaluated. If congestive heart failure, myocardial dysfunction, or renal or hepatic failure develops in patients receiving flecainide, dosage reduction may be necessary. Many clinicians recommend the use of low initial dosages in geriatric patients.

Any use of flecainide in children should be supervised directly by a cardiologist experienced in the treatment of arrhythmias in this age group. (See Cautions: Pediatric Precautions.) In pediatric patients, flecainide should be initiated in a hospital setting with facilities available for cardiac rhythm monitoring. Because of the evolving nature of flecainide use in children, specialized references should be consulted for the most recent information. The manufacturer states that the initial flecainide acetate dosage in infants younger than 6 months of age is approximately 50 mg/m^2 daily, divided into 2 or 3 equally spaced doses. For older children, an initial dosage of 100 mg/m^2 daily may be given. The maximum dosage recommended by the manufacturer for pediatric patients is 200 mg/m^2 daily, which should not be exceeded. Plasma trough flecainide concentrations (less than 1 hour before dosing) and ECGs should be obtained at presumed steady state (after at least 5 doses) after initiation of therapy or after any change in dosing, whether the dosage was increased for lack of effectiveness or for increased growth of the child. In some children receiving higher dosages, plasma drug concentrations are labile; while receiving the same dosage, plasma flecainide concentrations have increased rapidly to far above therapeutic concentrations, despite previously low plasma concentrations. Small changes in dosage also may lead to disproportionate increases in plasma drug concentrations. For the first year of flecainide treatment whenever the pediatric patient is seen for clinical follow-up, a 12-lead ECG and plasma trough flecainide concentrations are suggested. The usual therapeutic concentration of flecainide in children is 200–500 ng/mL, although concentrations up to 800 ng/mL may be required for adequate control in some children.

Since initial flecainide acetate dosages higher than those recommended and dosage adjustments at shorter intervals than recommended have resulted in an increased risk of arrhythmogenicity and congestive heart failure in patients with sustained ventricular tachycardia, especially during the first few days of flecainide therapy, a loading dose of the drug is *not* recommended; however, single oral loading doses (e.g., 200–300 mg) have been used for conversion of recent-onset atrial fibrillation to normal sinus rhythm† in selected patients ("pill-in-the-pocket" approach). IV lidocaine has occasionally been used concomitantly and without any apparent adverse interaction until the therapeutic effect of oral flecainide therapy was attained; however, studies have not been performed to determine the value of this regimen.

Based on theoretical considerations, it is recommended that, when transferring patients from therapy with another antiarrhythmic agent to flecainide, at least 2–4 plasma half-lives of the agent being discontinued be allowed to elapse before therapy with flecainide is initiated at the usual dosage. When withdrawal of another antiarrhythmic agent is likely to result in life-threatening arrhythmias, initiation of flecainide therapy in a hospital setting should be considered.

Life-threatening Ventricular Arrhythmias For the prevention of life-threatening ventricular arrhythmias (e.g., sustained ventricular tachycardia), the recommended initial adult dosage of flecainide acetate is 100 mg every 12 hours. Some clinicians suggest an initial dosage of 50 mg twice daily in these patients. Dosage may be increased in increments of 50 mg twice daily every 4 days until an effective response is attained. Most patients do not require dosages greater than 150 mg every 12 hours or 300 mg daily. The maximum recommended dosage of flecainide acetate in most patients with sustained ventricular tachycardia is 400 mg daily.

Supraventricular Tachyarrhythmias For the prevention of paroxysmal supraventricular tachycardias (PSVT), including atrioventricular nodal reentrant tachycardia, atrioventricular reentrant tachycardia, and other disabling supraventricular tachycardias of unspecified mechanism, and disabling paroxysmal atrial fibrillation/flutter (PAF), the recommended initial adult dosage of flecainide acetate is 50 mg every 12 hours. Dosage may be increased in increments of 50 mg twice daily every 4 days until an effective response is attained. In patients with PAF who do not attain the desired response, the manufacturer states that increasing flecainide acetate dosage to 100 mg twice daily can increase effective response without increasing the incidence of adverse effects (which might lead to discontinuance of flecainide therapy). The maximum recommended dosage of flecainide in patients with paroxysmal supraventricular arrhythmias is 300 mg daily.

Self-administration for Conversion of Paroxysmal Atrial Fibrillation. For *self-administration*† on an outpatient basis for termination of atrial fibrillation of recent onset in carefully selected patients with mild or no heart disease ("pill-in-the-pocket" approach), flecainide acetate has been given as a single oral loading dose of 300 mg in patients weighing 70 kg or more or 200 mg in patients weighing less than 70 kg.

Some clinicians suggest that flecainide be taken 5 minutes after noting the onset of palpitations and that patients remain in a supine or sitting position until resolution of palpitations or for a period of at least 4 hours following the dose. Patients should seek medical advice if palpitations do not resolve within 6–8 hours, if previously unexperienced symptoms (e.g., dyspnea, presyncope, syncope) occur, or if a marked increase in heart rate occurs after taking the antiarrhythmic drug. Patients should not take more than a single oral dose of flecainide during a 24-hour period.

■ **Dosage in Renal and Hepatic Impairment** In patients with renal impairment, dosage of flecainide acetate must be carefully adjusted based on the degree of renal impairment. The recommended initial oral dosage of flecainide acetate in patients with severe renal impairment (creatinine clearance of 35 mL/minute per 1.73 m^2 or less) is 100 mg once daily (or 50 mg twice daily). In patients with less severe renal impairment, an initial dosage of 100 mg every 12 hours is recommended. Since the elimination half-life of the drug may be prolonged in patients with renal impairment, steady-state plasma concentrations with a given dosage may not be attained for longer than 4 days. Consequently, increases in dosage should be made with caution and at intervals of longer than 4 days, with the patient closely monitored for signs of adverse cardiac effects or other toxicity. Plasma trough flecainide concentrations should be monitored in patients with severe renal impairment and also may be useful in patients with moderate renal impairment.

Since flecainide is extensively metabolized, probably in the liver, elimination may be markedly prolonged in patients with substantial hepatic impairment, and therefore the drug should not be used in such patients unless the potential benefits are considered to clearly outweigh the risks. If flecainide is used in patients with hepatic impairment, plasma flecainide concentrations should be monitored closely to guide dosage, and dosage should be increased cautiously at intervals of longer than 4 days.

Cautions

While clinical studies have indicated that adverse reactions to flecainide occur frequently but are usually mild to moderate in severity and transient, and the drug is generally well tolerated in most patients, concerns about the long-term safety and efficacy of the drug in patients with nonlife-threatening arrhythmias have been raised by findings of the Cardiac Arrhythmia Suppression Trial (CAST). Findings from the CAST study after an average of 10 months of follow-up indicate that the rate of total mortality and nonfatal cardiac arrest in patients with recent myocardial infarction (MI), mild-to-moderate left ventricular dysfunction, and asymptomatic or mildly symptomatic ventricular arrhythmias (principally frequent premature ventricular complexes [PVCs]) who received flecainide was increased substantially.

The CAST study, which began in 1987, was designed to evaluate the efficacy (in terms of reduced sudden cardiac death and total mortality) and safety of flecainide, encainide, and moricizine for the suppression and prevention of PVCs following recent MI (more than 6 days but less than 2 years previously) in patients with asymptomatic or mildly symptomatic ventricular arrhythmias. Findings from this large, multicenter, double-blind, placebo-controlled study, sponsored by the National Heart, Lung, and Blood Institute (NHLBI), indicate that the rates of total mortality (from arrhythmia, cardiac arrest, other cardiac causes, or noncardiac or unclassified causes) and nonfatal cardiac arrest combined in such patients receiving flecainide was increased substantially to 2.2 times that observed in patients receiving placebo. These findings were consistent across a variety of patient subgroups, and the degree of undesirable effects associated with flecainide or encainide was similar. When the effects of flecainide or encainide were considered together, the rate of total mortality and nonfatal cardiac arrest was 2.5 times that observed with placebo, and the rate of death secondary to arrhythmia or cardiac arrest for these drugs was 3.6 times that observed with placebo. Because there was evidence suggesting a potential harmful effect and no evidence of substantial benefit in the type of patient studied, flecainide and encainide were removed from the CAST study in early 1989. The relevance of the findings of the CAST study to patients with ventricular arrhythmias associated with a high risk of death currently is not known, and the manufacturers and FDA state that current evidence does *not* require discontinuance of flecainide in patients being treated for *life-threatening* arrhythmias.

The frequency of flecainide-induced adverse effects tends to decrease with time, and adverse effects tend to occur intermittently. Flecainide-induced adverse effects are often alleviated by dosage reduction, occasionally disappear despite continued treatment and without dosage reduction, and are usually reversible following discontinuance of the drug. The risk of adverse effects, particularly adverse cardiac effects, may increase when trough plasma flecainide concentrations increase above 0.7–1 mcg/mL, especially when the trough concentration exceeds 1 mcg/mL.

The most common adverse effects of flecainide are dizziness and visual disturbances, which are dose related, often occur concomitantly, and are also the most common adverse reactions requiring discontinuance of the drug. Adverse extracardiac effects requiring discontinuance of flecainide therapy occur in about 5–15% of patients. The need to discontinue flecainide results most often from multiple adverse effects rather than a single adverse effect, and adverse effects requiring discontinuance of the drug are most likely to occur during the first 2–4 weeks of therapy.

■ **Nervous System Effects** Dizziness (including dizziness, lightheadedness, faintness, unsteadiness, near syncope), which is dose related and often accompanied by visual disturbances, occurs in about 11–13% of patients receiving flecainide acetate dosages of 200–400 mg daily. Dizziness has required discontinuance of therapy in about 4–6% of patients. Flecainide-induced dizziness may also be associated with other adverse nervous system effects (e.g., nervousness) and probably results from an effect of the drug on the CNS.

Headache, which appears to be dose related, occurs in about 5–9% of patients receiving flecainide acetate dosages of 200–400 mg daily. Headache has required discontinuance of therapy in less than 1% of patients.

Fatigue has occurred in about 3–8% of patients receiving flecainide and required discontinuance in about 1% of patients. Tremor or nervousness has occurred in about 3–5% of patients and required discontinuance in less than 1% of patients. Hypoesthesia and paresthesia, which tend to occur in the perioral region or the extremities, occur in about 1–3% of patients receiving flecainide. Other adverse nervous system effects occurring in about 1–3% of patients receiving the drug include paresis, ataxia, vertigo, syncope, somnolence, tinnitus, anxiety, insomnia, and depression. Twitching, weakness, change in taste perception, dry mouth, speech disorder, stupor, seizures, amnesia, confusion, neuropathy, hallucinations, depersonalization, euphoria, morbid dreams, and apathy have been reported in less than 1% of patients.

■ **Ocular Effects** Visual disturbances (including blurred vision, difficulty in focusing, spots before eyes), which are dose related and often associated with dizziness, occur in about 5–20% of patients receiving flecainide acetate dosages of 200–400 mg daily and about 18–30% of patients receiving 400–600 mg daily. Visual disturbances have required discontinuance of therapy in about 2–3% of patients. The most common visual disturbance is blurred vision on lateral gaze and/or turning the head to the side. Diplopia has occurred in about 1–3% of patients receiving flecainide, and photophobia, nystagmus, and ocular pain or irritation have occurred in less than 1% of patients.

Flecainide-induced visual disturbances tend to be mild to moderate in severity and transient; persistent disturbances often respond to dosage reduction. Visual disturbances occur intermittently, usually last only for a few seconds, and occur most often during the time of expected peak plasma concentrations following an individual dose. The mechanism(s) of flecainide-induced visual disturbances is not known, but blurred vision may result from difficulty in accommodation caused by a local anesthetic effect of the drug on the ciliary muscle, from an effect on vestibulo-ocular reflexes, or from an effect on the CNS.

■ **Arrhythmogenic Effects** Like other antiarrhythmic agents, flecainide can worsen existing arrhythmias or cause new arrhythmias, and the arrhythmogenic potential is the most serious risk associated with the drug. Arrhythmogenic effects associated with flecainide range from an increased frequency of PVCs to the development of new and/or more severe and potentially fatal ventricular tachyarrhythmias. About 75% of the arrhythmogenic effects associated with the drug have been new or worsened ventricular tachyarrhythmias (e.g., new occurrence of sustained or nonsustained ventricular tachycardia, including exercise-induced or spontaneous wide QRS complex tachycardia, or progression of ventricular tachycardia to ventricular fibrillation), with the remainder consisting of increased frequency of PVCs or new or worsened supraventricular arrhythmias. In some patients, principally those with factors predisposing them to the risk of arrhythmogenic effects, flecainide therapy has been associated with episodes of ventricular tachycardia or fibrillation that required prolonged or unusual resuscitative measures or that resulted in death despite resuscitative measures.

The risk of flecainide-induced arrhythmogenic effects appears to be directly related to dosage and underlying cardiac disease, including severity of the preexisting ventricular arrhythmia and myocardial dysfunction. Patients with atherosclerosis, cardiac disease, previous MI, congestive heart failure, or nonsustained ventricular tachycardia appear to have approximately twice the risk of arrhythmogenic effects during flecainide therapy as those without these conditions. Patients with a history of sustained ventricular tachycardia appear to have about a 10-fold overall increased risk, and patients with both a history of sustained ventricular tachycardia and structural heart disease appear to have about a 14-fold increased risk compared with those with structural heart disease and only PVCs. When flecainide is given according to currently recommended dosage regimens and precautions, the risk of arrhythmogenic effects appears to be comparable to that associated with other antiarrhythmic agents.

Because of difficulties in distinguishing spontaneous and drug-related variations in an underlying arrhythmia disorder in patients with complex arrhythmias, reported occurrence rates must be considered approximations. In clinical studies, new or worsened arrhythmias occurred with an overall frequency of about 1–7%. In patients with sustained ventricular tachycardia who also often had heart failure, a low left ventricular ejection fraction, a history of MI, and/or an episode of cardiac arrest, the incidence of arrhythmogenic effects during flecainide therapy was 13% when dosage was initiated at 200 mg daily, was titrated upward slowly, and did not exceed 300 mg daily in most patients. In early clinical studies in patients with sustained ventricular tachycardia who received an initial flecainide acetate dosage of 400 mg daily (twice the currently recommended initial dosage), the incidence of arrhythmogenic effects was 26%, and arrhythmogenic effects resulted in death in about 10% of patients receiving the drug despite immediate medical attention. With lower initial dosages in these patients, the incidence of arrhythmogenic effects resulting in death has decreased to about 0.5% of patients. In patients with less severe arrhythmias (chronic PVCs, nonsustained ventricular tachycardia) receiving flecainide, the overall incidence of arrhythmogenic effects appears to be approximately 3–4%. It is not known whether the incidence of arrhythmogenic effects is increased in patients with chronic atrial fibrillation, high ventricular rate, and/or exercise. Wide complex tachycardia and ventricular fibrillation have been reported in about 17% of patients with chronic atrial fibrillation who were undergoing maximal exercise tolerance testing.

In patients with supraventricular arrhythmias including paroxysmal atrial fibrillation (PAF), the incidence of arrhythmogenic effects during flecainide therapy was about 4%; proarrhythmic events resulted in one fatal case of ventricular tachycardia/ventricular fibrillation and one case of wide complex ventricular tachycardia.

Flecainide-induced arrhythmogenic effects appear to be directly related to dosage and the rate of dosage escalation, particularly in patients with sustained ventricular tachycardia. A relationship with plasma concentrations of the drug has not been established; however, some data suggest that arrhythmogenicity may be associated with plasma concentrations higher than 1 mcg/mL. Arrhythmogenic effects appear to be most likely to occur within 1–4 weeks of initiation of flecainide therapy and/or within 1 week of an increase in dosage. In patients with sustained ventricular tachycardia, 80% of the arrhythmogenic effects occur within 14 days of initiation of flecainide therapy. The exact role is not clear, but concomitant use of other antiarrhythmic agents may increase the risk of arrhythmogenic effects during flecainide therapy. When transferring patients from another antiarrhythmic drug to flecainide, a transition period is recommended to allow the effects of the previous antiarrhythmic to dissipate prior to initiating flecainide. (See Dosage and Administration: Dosage.) Because of the risk of arrhythmogenic effects, initiation of flecainide therapy in a hospital setting is recommended for patients with sustained ventricular tachycardia and should be considered for other patients in whom withdrawal of a previous antiarrhythmic agent is likely to produce life-threatening arrhythmia. (See Cautions: Precautions and Contraindications.)

■ **Cardiovascular Effects** Because of its mild to moderate negative inotropic effect, flecainide may cause or worsen congestive heart failure, particularly in patients with cardiomyopathy, preexisting severe heart failure (New York Heart Association [NYHA] class III or IV), or low left ventricular ejection fractions (less than 30%). New or worsened congestive heart failure associated with flecainide has occurred in about 6% of patients with PVCs, non-sustained or sustained ventricular tachycardia. Worsened congestive heart failure associated with flecainide therapy occurred with a frequency of about 26% in patients with a history of congestive heart failure and sustained ventricular tachycardia. New or worsened congestive heart failure occurred in about 0.4% of patients with supraventricular arrhythmias.

Exacerbation of preexisting congestive heart failure during flecainide therapy has occurred most frequently in patients with advanced stages of failure (i.e., NYHA class III or IV). When congestive heart failure has developed or worsened, the onset has occurred within hours to several months after initiation of therapy; the risk appears to be greatest during the first 1–4 weeks of treatment. Some patients who develop signs and/or symptoms of congestive heart failure during flecainide therapy can continue to receive the drug at the same dosage with adjustment of concomitant cardiac glycoside and/or diuretic therapy; however, others may require a reduction in flecainide dosage or discontinuance of the drug.

Palpitation has occurred in about 6%, chest pain in about 5%, and edema in about 3% of patients receiving flecainide. Tachycardia and flushing have occurred in about 1–3% of patients, and bradycardia, angina pectoris, hypertension, and hypotension have occurred in less than 1% of patients receiving the drug.

■ **Effects on Cardiac Conduction** Clinically important conduction disturbances occur infrequently during flecainide therapy in patients without preexisting conduction abnormalities; however, the risk of adverse cardiac effects appears to increase as plasma flecainide concentrations increase above 0.7–1 mcg/mL. Sinus bradycardia, pause, and arrest have occurred collectively in about 1.2% of patients. First-degree AV block occurs in about 30–40% of patients receiving flecainide. Second-degree AV block occurs in about 0.5% of patients and third-degree AV block in about 0.4% of patients. New bundle-branch block may develop rarely. Some patients with atrial flutter may develop 1:1 AV conduction with flecainide due to slowing of the atrial rate. Paradoxically, an increase in ventricular rate also may occur when flecainide is used in patients with atrial fibrillation. Discontinuance of the drug may be necessary in some patients unless a temporary or permanent artificial pacemaker is in place. (See Cautions: Precautions and Contraindications.) Syncope also has occurred rarely as a result of sinus node dysfunction. Torsades de pointes-type arrhythmia associated with flecainide therapy also has been reported rarely.

Flecainide-induced increases in PR and QRS intervals are usually not clinically important. The degree of lengthening of PR and QRS intervals does not allow prediction of therapeutic efficacy or the development of adverse cardiac effects, although some data suggest that absolute increases in PR and QRS intervals (at least 40 ms) may be associated with adverse cardiac effects. Although prolongation of PR and QRS intervals is to be expected during therapy with the drug and is usually not clinically important, substantial increases require caution and consideration of dosage reduction. (See Cautions: Precautions and Contraindications.) Rarely, substantial prolongation of QT_c may occur and also require caution and dosage reduction.

■ **GI Effects** Nausea occurs in about 9–10% of patients receiving flecainide and has required discontinuance of the drug in about 1% of patients. Dyspepsia, anorexia, vomiting, constipation, and diarrhea have occurred in about 1–4% of patients and flatulence in less than 1% of patients.

■ **Dermatologic Effects** Rash occurs in about 1–3% of patients receiving flecainide. Urticaria, pruritus, and exfoliative dermatitis have occurred in less than 1% of patients.

■ **Other Adverse Effects** Dyspnea has occurred in about 5–10% of patients receiving flecainide. Malaise, fever, and increased sweating have occurred in about 1–3% of patients receiving the drug. Decreased libido, impotence, polyuria, urinary retention, arthralgia, myalgia, bronchospasm, and swelling of the lips, tongue, and mouth have been reported in less than 1% of patients.

There have been rare reports of asymptomatic, isolated increases in serum alkaline phosphatase or aminotransferase concentrations in patients receiving long-term flecainide therapy; however, a causal relationship to the drug has not been established. There have also been rare reports of hepatic dysfunction, including cholestasis and hepatic failure, and extremely rare reports of blood dyscrasias (leukopenia, thrombocytopenia) in patients receiving flecainide, but these effects have not been directly attributed to the drug. (See Cautions: Precautions and Contraindications.) However, in one patient who developed granulocytopenia, there was evidence of a specific IgG antibody directed against a flecainide (hapten)-neutrophil complex.

■ **Precautions and Contraindications** Findings from the CAST study indicate that use of flecainide and other class I antiarrhythmic agents (e.g., disopyramide, quinidine, procainamide) may be associated with substantial risk in certain patients with ventricular arrhythmias. Therefore, the manufacturer, FDA, and some experts currently recommend that use of flecainide and other class I agents in patients with ventricular arrhythmias be limited to those with *life-threatening* arrhythmias. (See Uses.) Use in less severe ventricular arrhythmias, even when symptomatic, currently is not recommended. In addition, it has been recommended that use of these drugs in patients with supraventricular arrhythmias be limited to those with symptomatic disabling arrhythmias. It is essential that patients not alter their antiarrhythmic therapy without first consulting their physician. The decision to discontinue therapy with flecainide must be made by the physician, and physicians have been advised by FDA and the manufacturers to contact their patients receiving the drug and determine whether alternative therapy is indicated, reserving therapy with flecainide only for arrhythmias considered *life-threatening*. Some experts state that discontinuance of therapy in patients with symptomatic sustained ventricular arrhythmias that have been treated effectively for prolonged periods seems unwarranted and is potentially dangerous. However, if withdrawal of therapy with flecainide is contemplated in these or other patients with sustained arrhythmias, it is recommended that it be performed in a hospital setting under continuous ECG monitoring. It also has been suggested that the need for hospitalization and ECG monitoring be considered when withdrawing therapy with these drugs in patients with nonsustained arrhythmias.

Since flecainide, like other antiarrhythmic agents, can worsen existing arrhythmias or cause new arrhythmias in some patients, clinical and ECG evaluations are essential prior to and during flecainide therapy to monitor for the appearance of arrhythmias and to determine the need for continued therapy. To minimize the risk of arrhythmogenic effects, the recommended flecainide dosage schedule should be closely followed, plasma drug concentrations should be monitored and concentrations higher than 1 mcg/mL avoided, ECG monitoring should be carefully evaluated before each dosage adjustment, and, if possible, concomitant use of other antiarrhythmic agents should be avoided. If flecainide is suspected or determined to be causing an increased frequency of PVCs despite adequate dosage or to be causing an increased frequency of complex PVCs or new and/or more serious arrhythmias, alternative therapy should be substituted. There is some evidence that exercise (e.g., treadmill) testing may be useful for detecting arrhythmogenic potential in some patients (e.g., those with preexisting sustained or nonsustained ventricular tachycardia and/or ventricular dysfunction), but additional study and experience are necessary.

Because of the relatively high incidence of arrhythmogenic effects in patients with sustained ventricular tachycardia and serious underlying heart disease and the need for careful dosage titration and monitoring, flecainide therapy should be initiated in a hospital setting with ECG monitoring in patients with sustained ventricular tachycardia, regardless of their cardiac status. Initiation of flecainide therapy in a hospital setting should also be considered for other patients with underlying structural heart disease, particularly those with serious disease, and for patients transferring from therapy with another antiarrhythmic agent in whom discontinuance of the current antiarrhythmic agent is likely to result in life-threatening arrhythmias. In patients with less severe and/or stable ventricular arrhythmias (frequent PVCs, nonsustained ventricular tachycardia), flecainide therapy may be initiated in an ambulatory setting with careful clinical and ECG monitoring.

Because of flecainide's mild to moderate negative inotropic effect, as well as an increased risk of arrhythmogenic effects, the drug should be used with caution in patients with a history of congestive heart failure or myocardial dysfunction, particularly those with advanced failure or dysfunction. Patients with a history of congestive heart failure or myocardial dysfunction who receive flecainide must be carefully monitored, and the recommended initial dosage in these patients should not be exceeded. When feasible, plasma flecainide concentrations should be monitored and dosage adjusted to maintain trough concentrations less than 0.7–1 mcg/mL. Particular attention should be given to maintenance of cardiac function, including optimum management with cardiac glycoside, diuretic, and/or other therapy. If myocardial dysfunction occurs, the patient may be managed with a reduction in flecainide dosage, discontinuance of therapy, or an adjustment in other drug therapy (e.g., diuretics, digoxin).

If the PR interval increases to 300 ms or greater, QRS duration increases to 180 ms or greater, or QT_c interval increases substantially during flecainide therapy, caution is necessary and dosage reduction should be considered. To minimize effects on cardiac conduction, an attempt should be made to manage patients on the lowest possible effective dosage. If second- or third-degree AV block or bifascicular block (right bundle-branch block associated with left hemiblock) occurs during flecainide therapy, the drug should be discontinued unless a temporary or implanted artificial ventricular pacemaker is in place to ensure an adequate ventricular rate.

Because its effects on sinus node function may be marked, flecainide should be used with particular caution in patients with preexisting sinus node dysfunction. Flecainide should be used only with extreme caution, if at all, in patients with sick sinus syndrome (including bradycardia-tachycardia syndrome), since the drug may cause sinus bradycardia, pause, or arrest in such patients.

Flecainide can increase acute and chronic endocardial pacing thresholds and may suppress ventricular escape rhythms; these effects are reversible following discontinuance of the drug. Flecainide should be used with particular caution in patients with permanent artificial pacemakers or temporary pacing electrodes and should not be administered to patients with existing poor thresholds or nonprogrammable artificial pacemakers unless suitable pacing rescue is available. In patients with pacemakers, the pacing threshold should be determined before and 1 week after initiating therapy with the drug and at regular intervals thereafter. Flecainide-induced changes in pacing threshold are generally within the range of multiprogrammable pacemakers and, when such changes occur, doubling of voltage or pulse width is usually sufficient to regain capture.

Since hypokalemia or hyperkalemia may alter the effects of class I antiarrhythmic agents, the possibility of a potassium imbalance should be evaluated and, if present, corrected before administration of flecainide.

Since elimination of flecainide may be impaired, the drug should be used with caution and dosage adjusted carefully in patients with renal impairment, particularly severe impairment. Because the urinary excretion of flecainide can be markedly affected by extremes of urinary pH, the potential effects of dietary regimens (e.g., very alkaline pH in strict vegetarians), disease states or conditions (e.g., renal tubular acidosis or metabolic alkalosis or acidosis), or concomitant drugs that may affect urinary pH should be kept in mind. Since flecainide is extensively metabolized, probably in the liver, elimination may be markedly prolonged in patients with substantial hepatic impairment, and therefore the drug should not be used in such patients unless the potential benefits are considered to clearly outweigh the risks. If flecainide is used in patients with severe renal or hepatic impairment, periodic monitoring of plasma concentrations of the drug is necessary.

Flecainide therapy should be discontinued in patients who develop unexplained jaundice, signs of hepatic dysfunction, or a blood dyscrasia to rule out the drug as a possible cause.

Use of flecainide in chronic atrial fibrillation is not recommended. Flecainide should not be used in patients with recent MI. In the absence of a pacemaker, flecainide is contraindicated in patients with preexisting second- or third-degree AV block or bifascicular block (right bundle-branch block associated with left hemiblock). Flecainide also is contraindicated in patients with cardiogenic shock or known hypersensitivity to the drug.

■ **Pediatric Precautions** The manufacturer states that safety and efficacy of flecainide in infants or children have not been established in randomized controlled studies. Limited data suggest that the drug may be useful in children for the management of refractory supraventricular tachycardias. The proarrhythmic effects of flecainide observed in adults also may occur in children. In pediatric patients with structural heart disease, flecainide has been associated with cardiac arrest and sudden death. Because of these risks, flecainide generally is not a preferred antiarrhythmic drug in pediatric patients; if use is necessary, therapy should be initiated in a hospital setting equipped with ECG monitoring and supervised directly by a cardiologist experienced in the treatment of arrhythmias in children.

■ **Mutagenicity and Carcinogenicity** No evidence of flecainide-induced mutagenicity was seen with in vitro microbial (Ames test) or mammalian (mouse lymphoma) test systems, or with in vivo cytogenetic tests in rats receiving dosages up to 180 mg/kg daily for 5 days.

No evidence of carcinogenesis was seen in mice and rats receiving oral flecainide acetate dosages up to 60 mg/kg daily for 18 and 24 months, respectively.

■ **Pregnancy, Fertility, and Lactation** Reproduction studies in rats and mice using oral flecainide acetate dosages up to 50 and 80 mg/kg daily, respectively, have not revealed evidence of fetal malformation; however, delayed sternebral and vertebral ossification were observed in rats receiving the highest dosages. Club paws, sternebral and vertebral abnormalities, pale hearts with contracted ventricular septum, and increased fetal resorptions were observed in one breed of rabbits (New Zealand white rabbits) receiving dosages of 30 and 35 mg/kg daily; reproduction studies in Dutch Belted rabbits using similar dosages did not reveal evidence of teratogenicity or embryotoxicity. There are no adequate and controlled studies to date using oral flecainide acetate in pregnant women, and the drug should be used during pregnancy only when the potential benefits justify the possible risks to the fetus. It is not known whether use of the drug during labor or delivery could have any immediate or delayed adverse effects on the mother or fetus, affect the duration of labor, or increase the likelihood of forceps delivery or other obstetrical intervention.

The effect of flecainide on fertility in humans is not known. In vitro, the drug inhibits sperm motility. Reproduction studies in male and female rats using flecainide acetate dosages up to 50 mg/kg daily (7 times the usual human dosage) have not revealed evidence of impaired fertility.

Limited data suggest that flecainide is distributed into milk in humans. In one study in postpartum women receiving multiple doses of flecainide, milk flecainide concentration averaged 2.5 times (sometimes as high as 4 times) that of maternal plasma concentrations. It is estimated that less than 3 mg of the drug would be ingested by a nursing infant (receiving about 700 mL of milk) over a 24-hour period assuming a maternal plasma flecainide concentration of 1 mcg/mL, which is considered at the top of the therapeutic range.

Drug Interactions

■ **Drugs Affecting or Metabolized by Hepatic Microsomal Enzymes** Metabolism of flecainide is mediated by the cytochrome P-450 (CYP) isoenzyme 2D6, and concurrent use of flecainide with CYP2D6 inhibitors (e.g., quinidine) could result in increased plasma flecainide concentrations.

Limited data indicate that the rate of flecainide elimination is increased by 30% in patients receiving flecainide concurrently with enzyme inducers (e.g., carbamazepine, phenytoin, phenobarbital).

■ **Protein-bound Drugs** Flecainide is not extensively bound to plasma proteins. Concomitant use of flecainide with other drugs that are highly protein-bound (e.g., oral anticoagulants) is not expected to result in an interaction.

■ **Antiarrhythmic Agents** There is limited information on the use of flecainide in conjunction with other antiarrhythmic agents for the management of severe refractory ventricular or supraventricular† arrhythmias. Combination antiarrhythmic therapy for severe refractory arrhythmias is generally empiric and must be individualized. Since the cardiac effects of multiple antiarrhythmic agents may be additive, synergistic, or antagonistic and adverse effects may be additive, combination therapy must be used with particular caution and careful monitoring. Because concomitant administration may increase the risk of arrhythmogenic effects, it is generally recommended that concomitant use of flecainide with other antiarrhythmic agents be avoided, if possible; however, combination therapy may be useful in carefully selected and managed patients with severe refractory arrhythmias. When transitioning from another antiarrhythmic drug to flecainide, sufficient time should elapse (at least 2–4 half-lives of the discontinued antiarrhythmic agent) before initiating flecainide therapy. (See Dosage and Administration: Dosage.)

Flecainide has been used in combination with amiodarone, with good results in selected patients, for the management of severe refractory ventricular arrhythmias or refractory atrial fibrillation†. Combined therapy may allow the use of lower dosages of flecainide and/or amiodarone and thereby potentially reduce the risk of toxicity. Plasma flecainide concentrations adjusted for daily dosage increased by an average of 60% (range: 5–190%) when amiodarone therapy was initiated in a limited number of patients receiving flecainide. Although the mechanism(s) of this interaction is not known, it has been suggested that amiodarone may inhibit the hepatic metabolism and/or decrease the renal clearance of flecainide. Pending further accumulation of data, it is recommended that dosage of flecainide be reduced by 30–50% several days after initiation of amiodarone therapy; subsequently, the patient and plasma flecainide concentrations should be monitored closely and flecainide dosage adjusted as necessary.

The effects of concomitant administration of flecainide and disopyramide have not been evaluated and experience with combined use of the drugs is limited. Because both drugs have negative inotropic effects, there appears to be little rationale for their combined use and the manufacturer cautions that they not be used concomitantly unless the potential benefits are considered to outweigh the risks.

■ **Cardiac Glycosides** Studies in healthy individuals indicate that plasma digoxin concentrations may be increased by an average of about 13–25% when flecainide and digoxin are administered concomitantly. The increase in plasma digoxin concentration may occur within a few days of initiating flecainide therapy in patients receiving digoxin and may result from a decrease in the volume of distribution of digoxin. Although the PR interval was substantially prolonged in most healthy individuals during concomitant administration of flecainide and digoxin, it was not determined whether this resulted from an additive effect of the drugs or mainly from flecainide. Flecainide has been administered concomitantly with cardiac glycosides without adverse effects. Additional studies to determine the potential importance of an interaction in patients with congestive heart failure are needed. Flecainide-induced increases in plasma digoxin concentration generally appear to be of a small magnitude and are unlikely to be clinically important in most cases; however, patients with AV nodal dysfunction, plasma digoxin concentrations in the upper end of the therapeutic range, and/or high plasma flecainide concentrations may be at increased risk of digoxin toxicity. Pending further accumulation of data, patients receiving flecainide and digoxin should be monitored for signs of digoxin toxicity.

■ **β-Adrenergic Blocking Agents** In healthy individuals, plasma flecainide concentrations are increased by about 20% and plasma propranolol concentrations are increased by about 30% when the drugs are administered concomitantly compared with administration of each drug alone. The mechanism(s) of this interaction is not known, but the elimination half-lives of both drugs are apparently unchanged. The negative inotropic effects of flecainide and propranolol are additive in healthy individuals, but the increases in PR interval produced by the drugs are less than additive. Flecainide has been administered concomitantly with β-adrenergic blocking agents in patients with ventricular arrhythmias without unusual adverse effects or an increased incidence of adverse effects; however, if flecainide and a β-adrenergic blocking agent are administered concomitantly, the possibility of additive negative inotropic effects should be considered.

■ **Calcium-Channel Blocking Agents** The effects of concomitant administration of flecainide and calcium-channel blocking agents have not been evaluated, and experience with combined use of the drugs is limited. Because verapamil also has a negative inotropic effect and decreases AV nodal conduction, the manufacturer cautions that flecainide and verapamil not be used concomitantly unless the potential benefits are considered to outweigh the risk. The manufacturer also cautions that there is insufficient experience with concomitant administration of flecainide and diltiazem or nifedipine to recommend such combined use.

■ **Acidifying and Alkalinizing Agents** The urinary excretion and systemic elimination of flecainide may be substantially affected by extremes of urinary pH, with urinary excretion of the drug decreased and elimination half-life increased in the presence of very alkaline urine and vice versa in the presence of very acidic urine. (See Pharmacokinetics: Elimination.) When drugs that can markedly affect urinary acidity (e.g., ammonium chloride) or alkalinity (e.g., high-dose antacids, carbonic anhydrase inhibitors, sodium bicarbonate) are administered concomitantly with flecainide, the potential effect on elimination of the antiarrhythmic agent and need for appropriate flecainide dosage adjustment should be kept in mind.

■ **Diuretics** Flecainide has been used concomitantly with diuretics in a large number of patients without any apparent drug interaction.

■ **Cimetidine** Plasma flecainide concentrations and half-life reportedly increased by approximately 30 and 10%, respectively, in a study in healthy individuals receiving flecainide in conjunction with cimetidine (1 g daily for 1 week). Further study of this potential interaction is needed, but these data suggest that reduction of flecainide dosage might be necessary in patients receiving cimetidine concomitantly.

Acute Toxicity

Limited information is available on the acute toxicity of flecainide.

■ **Pathogenesis** The acute lethal dose of flecainide acetate in humans is not known. The oral and IV LD_{50}s of the drug in mice were 190 and 24 mg/kg, respectively. Following IV, intraperitoneal, or oral administration of single large doses of flecainide acetate (up to 500 mg/kg) in animals, vomiting, ataxia, dyspnea, seizures, and death were observed; death appeared to result from respiratory depression and arrest. Surviving animals recovered within several hours after administration of flecainide with no apparent residual effects.

■ **Manifestations** In general, overdosage of flecainide may be expected to produce effects that are extensions of pharmacologic effects, particularly those involving cardiac conduction and function. Animal studies and case reports in humans indicate that possible effects may include increases in PR, QRS, and QT intervals; conduction disturbances; hypotension; asystole; or cardiac arrest and death. In one adult who reportedly intentionally ingested 2.5 g of flecainide acetate, somnolence, tremor, and sweating resulted. Plasma flecainide concentrations 3 and 4.5 hours after ingestion of the drug were 1.9 and 3 mcg/mL, respectively, with an AV nodal escape rhythm and substantial prolongation of QRS and QT intervals occurring in association with the higher of these concentrations. The patient recovered following symptomatic and supportive treatment, as well as the use of charcoal hemoperfusion and forced diuresis to enhance elimination of the drug. Other ECG abnormalities associated with flecainide intoxication have included regular ventricular tachycardia with right bundle-branch block that progressed to polymorphous tachycardia (possibly torsades de pointes); substantial prolongation of the PR and JT intervals; broadened P waves; and inverted T waves. Regular or polymorphous ventricular tachycardia may progress to ventricular fibrillation and sudden death.

■ **Treatment** Treatment of flecainide overdosage generally involves symptomatic and supportive care, with ECG, blood pressure, and respiratory monitoring. There is no specific antidote for flecainide intoxication.

Supportive treatment may include IV administration of inotropic agents or cardiac stimulants (e.g., dopamine, dobutamine, isoproterenol), circulatory assistance (e.g., intra-aortic balloon counterpulsation), mechanically assisted respiration, and transvenous pacing. Because of the long elimination half-life of flecainide and the possibility of markedly nonlinear pharmacokinetics at very high doses, treatment for an extended period of time may be necessary. Hemodialysis is not an effective means for enhancing elimination of flecainide. Specific data are not available, but acidification of the urine may be potentially useful for enhancing elimination of flecainide, particularly if the urine is very alkaline; however, the potential effects of acidification on serum electrolyte concentrations (e.g., potassium) would have to be considered. The value of forced diuresis is not known.

Pharmacology

■ **Antiarrhythmic and Electrophysiologic Effects** Flecainide acetate is a local anesthetic-type antiarrhythmic agent. Studies in animals have shown that flecainide is at least as effective and more potent on a weight basis than most currently available antiarrhythmic agents in preventing and/or suppressing experimentally induced arrhythmias.

The exact mechanism of antiarrhythmic action of flecainide has not been conclusively determined, but the drug is considered a class I (membrane-stabilizing) antiarrhythmic agent. The principal effect of flecainide on cardiac tissue appears to be a concentration-dependent inhibition of the transmembrane influx of extracellular sodium ions via fast sodium channels, as indicated by a decrease in the maximal rate of depolarization of phase 0 of the action potential and a shift of the membrane-responsiveness curve in the hyperpolarizing direction. Like other class I antiarrhythmic agents, flecainide is believed to combine with fast sodium channels in their inactive state and thereby inhibit recovery after repolarization in a time- and voltage-dependent manner which is associated with subsequent dissociation of the drug from the sodium channels. Flecainide also appears to have a slight inhibitory effect on the transmembrane influx of extracellular calcium ions via slow calcium channels, but generally only at high drug concentrations. Flecainide has no vagomimetic, vagolytic, or β-adrenergic blocking activity and does not antagonize the positive inotropic effect of calcium on cardiac muscle.

Flecainide exhibits electrophysiologic effects characteristic of class Ic antiarrhythmic agents. The electrophysiologic characteristics of the subgroups of class I antiarrhythmic agents may be related to quantitative differences in their rates of attachment to and dissociation from transmembrane sodium channels, with class Ic agents exhibiting slow rates of attachment and dissociation. Flecainide decreases the amplitude and maximal rate of rise of the action potential in a concentration-dependent manner and has little or no effect on resting potential. Like other class Ic antiarrhythmic agents, flecainide slows intracardiac conduction at low concentrations, has relatively small effects on refractoriness, and generally has little effect on repolarization and action potential duration (APD). The drug produces a slight increase in APD in atrial and ventricular muscle and a decrease in APD in Purkinje fibers. The electrophysiologic effects of flecainide generally appear to be comparable following multiple oral or single IV doses of the drug.

Effects on Cardiac Conduction and Refractoriness Flecainide produces a dose-related decrease in intracardiac conduction throughout the heart, with the most marked effect on conduction within the His-Purkinje system. The effect of the drug on intra-atrial and atrioventricular (AV) conduction is less pronounced than its effect on intraventricular conduction. Flecainide may also prolong refractoriness in most parts of the heart, with the most marked effect on the ventricles; however, the effects of the drug on refractoriness are less pronounced than its effects on intracardiac conduction.

The effects of flecainide on intracardiac conduction are manifested by dose-related increases in PR, QRS, and, to a lesser degree, QT intervals. Increases in PR and QRS intervals average about 25% (40 and 20 ms, respectively) at dosages of 400 mg or more daily but may be as large as approximately 118 and 150%, respectively, in some patients. About 30–40% of patients may develop first-degree AV block during flecainide therapy, and many patients develop a QRS interval of 120 ms or longer; however, PR intervals usually do not increase to 300 ms or longer and QRS intervals usually do not increase to 180 ms or longer. Flecainide generally increases QT interval by about 8%, but about 60–90% of this increase is secondary to the increase in QRS interval. Consequently, the JT interval (QT minus QRS) increases by an average of about 4%. Substantial prolongation of the JT interval occurs in less than 2% of patients. The QT interval corrected for rate (QT_c) may be unchanged or slightly increased. AH and HV intervals are prolonged. The atrial effective refractory period (ERP) may be unchanged or slightly increased, and ventricular ERP may be increased by about 5–15%. The AV nodal ERP may be unchanged or slightly increased.

Effects on Sinus Node Flecainide generally has minimal effects on normal sinus node function. Spontaneous sinus rate may be unchanged or decreased, and corrected sinus node recovery time following pacing and spontaneous cycle lengths is somewhat increased. Sinoatrial conduction time may be slightly increased. In contrast to its effects on normal sinus node function, flecainide may have a marked depressive effect on sinus node function in individuals with preexisting sinus node dysfunction; corrected sinus node recovery time and sinoatrial conduction time may be substantially increased in some individuals.

Effects on Dual AV Nodal and Anomalous AV Pathways The relatively selective effects of flecainide on retrograde pathways of dual AV nodal and anomalous AV conduction are responsible for the drug's ability to effectively terminate paroxysmal reentrant supraventricular tachycardias in many patients. In patients with dual AV pathways, flecainide decreases conduction, markedly increases refractoriness of the retrograde fast pathway, and increases or has little effect on refractoriness of the anterograde fast pathway or the anterograde and retrograde slow pathways; complete block of the retrograde fast pathway and, rarely, the anterograde fast pathway may result. In patients with Wolff-Parkinson-White syndrome or concealed accessory AV pathways, flecainide decreases conduction and increases the refractoriness of anterograde and retrograde accessory pathways, with the effects more pronounced on the retrograde pathway. In addition, the effects of flecainide may be greater on accessory pathways that have a long pretreatment refractory period. Complete block of the retrograde pathway and, sometimes, the anterograde pathway may result.

Effects on Endocardial Pacing Threshold Flecainide can increase acute and chronic endocardial pacing thresholds and may suppress ventricular escape rhythms; these effects are reversible following discontinuance of the drug. (See Cautions: Precautions and Contraindications.) Increases in endocardial pacing threshold as large as 200% have occurred. Flecainide-induced increases in endocardial pacing threshold appear to be correlated with plasma concentrations of the drug. Flecainide appears to have a greater effect on endocardial pacing threshold than most other class I antiarrhythmic agents.

■ **Arrhythmogenic Effects** Like other antiarrhythmic agents, flecainide can worsen existing arrhythmias or cause new arrhythmias. (See Cautions: Arrhythmogenic Effects.) The arrhythmogenic effects of the drug may range from an increased frequency of premature ventricular complexes (PVCs) to the development of more severe and potentially fatal ventricular tachyarrhythmias. The exact mechanism(s) by which various antiarrhythmic agents, including flecainide, produce arrhythmogenic effects has not been fully determined, but the arrhythmogenic potential of flecainide may be related to its effects on conduction and possibly myocardial contractility.

■ **Cardiovascular Effects** Flecainide generally exhibits minimal cardiovascular effects following oral or IV administration. The cardiovascular effects of the drug appear to be more pronounced following IV than oral administration, but evaluations have been more extensive following IV administration.

Flecainide exhibits a mild to moderate negative inotropic effect. The negative inotropic effect and other cardiovascular effects may be more pronounced and clinically important in patients with coronary heart disease, acute myocardial infarction (MI), congestive heart failure, or myocardial dysfunction. (See Cautions: Cardiovascular Effects.) The exact mechanism of flecainide's negative inotropic effect has not been determined, but it may be related in part to its effect on slow calcium channels. The myocardial depressant effect of flecainide appears to be less than that of disopyramide, but further evaluation is needed.

Heart rate is usually unchanged following oral or IV administration of flecainide, but slight increases may occur; occasionally, bradycardia or tachycardia has been reported. Similarly, blood pressure is usually unchanged following oral or IV administration of the drug, but small increases in mean systolic and/or diastolic blood pressure have been observed.

Following IV administration of flecainide in patients with coronary heart disease, acute MI, congestive heart failure, or myocardial dysfunction, cardiac output and left ventricular ejection fraction are generally decreased, pulmonary artery and/or wedge pressures are generally increased, and systemic vascular resistance may be unchanged or increased. The negative inotropic and other cardiovascular effects of IV flecainide are generally transient, being most marked during and immediately following administration of the drug, and are generally more pronounced in patients with preexisting ventricular dysfunction. Following chronic oral administration of flecainide, left ventricular ejection fraction generally appears to be unchanged or only slightly decreased, although both increases and decreases have been observed in patients receiving usual dosages of the drug. The drug can worsen or cause congestive heart failure, particularly in patients with a history of congestive heart failure and/or a preexisting ejection fraction of 30% or less. (See Cautions: Cardiovascular Effects.)

■ **Other Effects** Flecainide exhibits a local anesthetic action that is more potent and sustained than that of procaine (no longer commercially available in the US) in vitro. In animals, flecainide also exhibits anticonvulsant activity at doses higher than those required for antiarrhythmic action.

Pharmacokinetics

■ **Absorption** Flecainide acetate is rapidly and almost completely absorbed from the GI tract following oral administration. The absolute bioavailability of the commercially available flecainide acetate tablets averages approximately 85–90%. The rate of absorption may be slightly decreased by the presence of food, but the extent of absorption is not affected. The rate and extent of absorption are not affected by concomitant ingestion of an aluminum hydroxide antacid. Flecainide does not undergo any substantial first-pass metabolism.

Peak plasma flecainide concentrations usually occur within approximately 3 hours (range: 1–6 hours) after oral administration. Following oral administration of a single 200-mg dose of flecainide acetate in fasting, healthy adults, peak plasma flecainide concentrations of approximately 0.19–0.34 mcg/mL are attained. The pharmacokinetic profile of flecainide is apparently not substantially affected by dose or plasma concentrations at usual dosages, but does deviate somewhat from linearity. Within the usual dosage range, plasma concentrations of the drug are approximately proportional to dosage, with average concentrations increasing from direct proportionality by about 10–15% per 100-mg increment in dosage. Although plasma flecainide concentrations are relatively linearly related and approximately proportional to dosage, there is considerable interindividual and intraindividual variation in plasma concentrations attained with a given dosage. Following single oral doses, total plasma concentrations of flecainide metabolites (free and conjugated) are generally 1–2 times higher than those of unchanged flecainide; however, free plasma concentrations of the 2 major metabolites, *m-O*-dealkylated flecainide and the *m-O*-dealkylated lactam derivative, are very low (less than 0.05 mcg/mL), even after multiple dosing. (See Pharmacokinetics: Elimination.)

In patients with premature ventricular complexes (PVCs), flecainide-induced decreases in single and multiple PVCs are related to dosage and plasma concentrations of the drug. The dose-related increases in PR, QRS, and, to a lesser degree, QT intervals also appear to be related to plasma concentrations of the drug. Based on greater than 90% suppression of PVCs, plasma flecainide concentrations of approximately 0.2–1 mcg/mL (mean of about 0.5–0.6 mcg/mL) appear to be necessary for optimum therapeutic effect, with minimum therapeutic concentrations ranging from about 0.2–0.4 mcg/mL. Plasma flecainide concentrations necessary to suppress serious ventricular arrhythmias are not clearly established, but trough plasma concentrations of the drug in patients effectively treated for recurrent ventricular tachycardia have also ranged from about 0.2–1 mcg/mL. The risk of adverse cardiac effects (e.g., conduction defects, bradycardia) increases as plasma flecainide concentrations increase above 0.7–1 mcg/mL, particularly when concentrations exceed 1 mcg/mL. A relationship between plasma flecainide concentrations and arrhythmogenic effects has not been established, but some data suggest that adverse cardiac effects may be associated with plasma concentrations higher than 1 mcg/mL. In clinical studies of patients with ventricular tachycardia, reduction of flecainide dosage (i.e., use of a lower initial dosage with slow upward titration) appeared to be associated with a decreased frequency and severity of arrhythmogenic effects.

■ **Distribution** Distribution of flecainide acetate into human body tissues and fluids has not been fully characterized. Following IV administration in rats, flecainide and/or its metabolites are distributed extensively into many tissues, including the heart, but only minimally into the CNS. Studies in animals also indicate that the drug and/or its metabolites are distributed into and may accumulate in pigmented ocular tissues; however, chronic toxicity studies in animals and clinical experience to date in humans have not revealed evidence of specific flecainide-induced ocular toxicity. Following IV administration in humans, flecainide is rapidly and apparently widely distributed. The apparent volume of distribution of the drug in healthy adults reportedly averages 5.5–8.7 L/kg (range: 5–13.4 L/kg) following a single IV dose and about 10 L/kg following a single oral dose.

In vitro, flecainide is approximately 40–50% bound to plasma proteins, mainly α_1-acid glycoprotein (α_1-AGP). At in vitro plasma flecainide concentrations of 0.015–10 mcg/mL, binding is independent of the plasma concentration of the drug. Following acute myocardial infarction, protein binding of flecainide may be increased to an average of approximately 60% for about 24 hours, but this effect is not likely to be clinically important in most circumstances.

It is not known whether flecainide crosses the placenta in humans, but the drug and/or its metabolites cross the placenta in rats. A multiple-dose study conducted in mothers soon after delivery indicated that flecainide is distributed into human milk in concentrations as high as 4 times (with average concentrations about 2.5 times) corresponding plasma concentrations; assuming a high maternal plasma concentration of 1 mcg/mL, the calculated daily dose to a nursing infant (assuming about 700 mL of breast milk over 24 hours) would be less than 3 mg.

■ **Elimination** Plasma concentrations of flecainide acetate appear to decline in a biphasic manner. Following a single IV dose in healthy adults, the half-life of flecainide in the initial distribution phase ($t_{1/2\alpha}$) is about 3–6 minutes and the half-life in the terminal elimination phase ($t_{1/2\beta}$) has been reported to average 11–14 hours (range: 7–19 hours). Following single or multiple oral doses in healthy adults, the elimination half-life has averaged 11.5–16 hours (range: 7–25 hours), but the half-life tends to be slightly more prolonged following multiple rather than single doses. The elimination half-life of flecainide following multiple oral doses in patients with PVCs is slightly longer than in healthy individuals, averaging 19–22 hours (range: 12–30 hours). The elimination half-life tends to increase with age in patients with PVCs. Although data are limited in infants younger than 1 year of age, currently available data suggest that half-life of flecainide at birth may be as long as 29 hours, decreasing to 11–12 hours by 3 months of age, and to 6 hours by 1 year of age. In children 1–12 years of age, the half-life of flecainide is approximately 8 hours. In adolescents 12–15 years of age, the plasma elimination half-life is approximately 11–12 hours. Following a single oral dose in patients with congestive heart failure, the elimination half-life is also slightly longer than in healthy individuals but similar to that in patients with PVCs, averaging 19 hours (range: 14–26 hours). Steady-state plasma concentrations are reached in 3–5 days; once at steady state, no additional accumulation of drug is expected during chronic therapy. Over the usual therapeutic range, plasma concentrations of flecainide increase in an approximately dose-proportional manner.

The elimination half-life of flecainide is prolonged in patients with renal impairment, particularly in those with severe renal impairment. Following a single oral dose, the elimination half-life reportedly averaged 17 hours (range: 12–26 hours) and 26 hours (range: 9–58 hours) in patients with creatinine clearances of 4–41 and 0–2 mL/minute per m^2, respectively. The elimination half-lives of flecainide metabolites have not been determined to date, but their elimination appears to occur somewhat more slowly than that of unchanged flecainide and free plasma concentrations of *m-O*-dealkylated flecainide appear to persist in some patients with severe renal impairment. Extremes of urinary pH can markedly affect the elimination half-life of flecainide, prolonging it when very alkaline (pH 7.2–8.3) and reducing it when very acidic (pH 4.4–5.8).

Flecainide is extensively metabolized, probably in the liver, to 2 major metabolites and to at least 3 unidentified minor metabolites. In vitro metabolic studies indicate that the cytochrome P-450 (CYP) isoenzyme 2D6 is involved in the drug's metabolism. The 2 major metabolites, *m-O*-dealkylated flecainide and the *m-O*-dealkylated lactam derivative, are formed by preferential *O*-dealkylation at the *meta* position of the benzamide ring and by subsequent oxidation of the piperidine ring of *m-O*-dealkylated flecainide, respectively. Both metabolites undergo extensive conjugation at the *m-O*-dealkylated position with glucuronic or sulfuric acid. Studies in animals indicate that, on a weight basis, *m-O*-dealkylated flecainide has up to 20–50% of the antiarrhythmic and electrophysiologic activity of flecainide and the *m-O*-dealkylated lactam derivative has less than 10% of the electrophysiologic activity of flecainide. Because free plasma concentrations of the major metabolites are so low following multiple oral doses, it is unlikely that these metabolites would contribute to the therapeutic or toxic effects of the parent drug under most clinical circumstances; however, further studies are needed to evaluate their potential contribution, if any, in the presence of conditions that might affect their formation and/or elimination (e.g., severe hepatic or renal impairment). The minor metabolites remain to be identified, but some data suggest that they may result from amide hydrolysis. Some data also suggest that cigarette smoking may induce metabolism of flecainide.

Following oral administration, flecainide and its metabolites are excreted almost completely in urine; only small amounts of the drug and/or its metabolites are excreted in feces. Flecainide appears to be excreted in urine mainly by glomerular filtration, but some tubular secretion may also occur. Following a single oral dose of flecainide in healthy individuals, about 80–90% of the dose is excreted in urine and about 5% in feces within 6 days; most excretion occurs within 24 hours, and excretion is almost complete within 72 hours. In healthy individuals, about 30% (range: 10–50%) of a single oral dose is excreted in urine as unchanged drug, 10–20% as *m-O*-dealkylated flecainide and its conjugates, 10–15% as the *m-O*-dealkylated lactam derivative and its conjugates, and 3% or less as 3 unidentified minor metabolites. The major metabolites of the drug are excreted in urine principally as conjugates.

The fraction of flecainide excreted in urine as unchanged drug decreases with decreasing renal function and is markedly reduced in patients with severe renal impairment. Following a single oral dose in patients with creatinine clearances of 4–41 and 0–2 mL/minute per m^2, the fraction excreted in urine within 72 hours as unchanged drug averaged approximately 15% (range: 5–30%) and 1% (range: 0–3%), respectively. The fraction of flecainide excreted in urine as unchanged drug is also inversely related to urinary pH, increasing with decreasing urinary pH and vice versa. Although usual variations in urinary pH would generally be expected to have minimal effects, extremes of urinary pH may substantially affect the fraction of unchanged flecainide excreted in urine, approximately doubling it when very acidic (pH 4.4–5.8) and decreasing it by half when very alkaline (pH 7.2–8.3).

Following oral administration in healthy individuals, total apparent plasma clearance of flecainide averages approximately 10 mL/minute per kg (range: 4–20 mL/minute per kg); renal clearance of the drug is about 25–40% of the total plasma clearance. In healthy geriatric individuals, total apparent plasma clearance decreases following multiple oral doses, apparently as a result of decreased nonrenal clearance of the drug. Total apparent plasma clearance is decreased in patients with PVCs compared with healthy individuals, averaging 6.2 mL/minute per kg (range: 3.1–12.6 mL/minute per kg) in a small group of patients. Total apparent plasma clearance of flecainide is somewhat decreased in patients with congestive heart failure compared with healthy individuals, averaging 8.1 mL/minute per kg (range: 3.1–13.4 mL/minute per kg) in a small group of patients; renal clearance is also decreased in these patients, but still accounts for about 25% of total plasma clearance. It appears that an increase in nonrenal clearance can, to some extent, compensate for decreased renal clearance in some patients. Renal clearance of flecainide is inversely related to urinary pH, increasing with decreasing urinary pH and vice versa. Extremes of urinary pH may substantially affect renal clearance of the drug. The manufacturer states that elimination of flecainide from plasma may be markedly prolonged in patients with substantial hepatic impairment.

Only about 1% of an oral dose of flecainide is removed by hemodialysis as unchanged drug; however, about 10% of a dose is removed by hemodialysis as *m-O*-dealkylated flecainide and its conjugates. It is not known if flecainide and/or its metabolites are removed by peritoneal dialysis. There is some evidence that flecainide may be removed by charcoal hemoperfusion.

Chemistry and Stability

■ **Chemistry** Flecainide acetate is a local anesthetic-type antiarrhythmic agent. Flecainide is an amide-type local anesthetic and is structurally related to procainamide in that the drug is a benzamide derivative. The antiarrhythmic potency of flecainide is associated with the presence and positions of the trifluoroethoxy groups on the benzamide ring, which enhance lipophilicity, and with the presence of the nonsubstituted piperidylmethyl group in the amide side chain.

Flecainide acetate occurs as a white to slightly off-white crystalline powder and has a solubility of 48.4 mg/mL in water and 300 mg/mL in alcohol at 37°C. The drug has a pK_a of 9.3.

■ **Stability** Flecainide acetate tablets should be stored in tight, light-resistant containers at 20–25°C. However, USP states that the tablets can be stored in well-closed containers.

Preparations

Excipients in commercially available drug preparations may have clinically important effects in some individuals; consult specific product labeling for details.

Flecainide Acetate

Oral		
Tablets	50 mg*	Flecainide Acetate Tablets
	100 mg*	Flecainide Acetate Tablets
	150 mg*	Flecainide Acetate Tablets

*available from one or more manufacturer, distributor, and/or repackager by generic (nonproprietary) name

†Use is not currently included in the labeling approved by the US Food and Drug Administration

Propafenone Hydrochloride

■ Propafenone hydrochloride is a local anesthetic-type class Ic antiarrhythmic agent. The drug is commercially available as immediate-release tablets and extended-release capsules.

Uses

■ **Supraventricular Tachyarrhythmias** When given as *immediate-release tablets*, propafenone hydrochloride is used to prolong the time to recurrence of symptomatic, disabling paroxysmal supraventricular tachycardia (PSVT) (e.g., atrioventricular [AV] nodal reentrant tachycardia or AV reentrant tachycardia [Wolff-Parkinson-White, WPW, syndrome]) and symptomatic, disabling paroxysmal atrial fibrillation/flutter (PAF) in patients without structural heart disease. While comparative studies are limited, propafenone appears to be comparable to other antiarrhythmic agents (e.g., quinidine, disopyramide, flecainide, procainamide, sotalol) in preventing recurrences of PAF and maintaining sinus rhythm following successful cardioversion of atrial fibrillation.

When given as *extended-release capsules*, propafenone is used to prolong the time to recurrence of symptomatic paroxysmal atrial fibrillation in patients without structural heart disease. The safety and efficacy of propafenone as extended-release capsules have not been established in patients with exclusively PSVT or atrial flutter.

Propafenone also has been used for termination of supraventricular tachycardias; analysis of combined data from controlled and uncontrolled clinical studies in patients receiving oral (immediate-release tablets) or IV (IV dosage form not commercially available in the US) propafenone therapy has demonstrated termination of PAF, PSVT, or tachycardia associated with WPW syndrome in 73, 57, or 45%, respectively, of patients. However, vagal maneuvers, IV adenosine, AV nodal blocking agents (e.g., calcium-channel blocking agents, β-adrenergic blocking agents) and/or synchronized cardioversion are the treatments of choice for acute conversion of PSVT.

The safety and efficacy of propafenone hydrochloride as immediate-release tablets or extended-release capsules have not been established in patients with chronic atrial fibrillation, and the manufacturer states that the drug should not be used to control ventricular rate in patients with atrial fibrillation.

Because of the risk of proarrhythmia, propafenone should not be used in patients with structural heart disease or ischemic heart disease.

Paroxysmal Atrial Fibrillation/Flutter and Paroxysmal Supraventricular Tachyarrhythmias **Immediate-release Propafenone Hydrochloride.** Controlled and uncontrolled clinical studies have shown that propafenone (immediate-release tablets) may prevent or delay recurrence of PAF or increase the interval between recurrences of PAF in 39–64% of patients monitored for 6–18 months. Preliminary analysis of combined data from clinical studies indicates that propafenone prevented or delayed recurrence of PAF in 51 or 33% of patients monitored for 1 or 2 years, respectively, and prevented or delayed recurrence of PSVT or AV reentrant tachycardia (WPW syndrome) syndrome in 63 or 83%, respectively, of patients treated during a 10-month period. Long-term therapy with oral propafenone also has been effective in some patients for suppression and prevention of atrial fibrillation refractory to other antiarrhythmic agents. It has been suggested that propafenone may be more effective than flecainide in patients with adrenergically mediated atrial fibrillation or flutter, possibly because of its β-adrenergic blocking activity.

Control of ventricular rate should be the first therapeutic step in most patients with hemodynamically stable, acute atrial fibrillation. The goal of therapy should be a reduction of ventricular rate to less than 80–90 beats/minute and prevention of inappropriately high ventricular rates during activity. The use of propafenone in patients with chronic atrial fibrillation has not been adequately evaluated to date, and the manufacturer states that the drug should not be used to control ventricular rate in patients with atrial fibrillation. However, some experts and clinicians suggest that propafenone may be useful in controlling ventricular response rate in patients with stable but rapid atrial fibrillation/flutter and ventricular preexcitation via an accessory pathway (e.g., WPW syndrome).

In a randomized, crossover clinical trial of approximately 2–3 months' duration, the median time to arrhythmia recurrence was greater than 98 days in patients with PAF or PSVT receiving propafenone and 8 or 12 days in patients with PAF or PSVT, respectively, receiving placebo. Recurrences of PAF or PSVT were completely prevented in 53 or 47%, respectively, of patients receiving propafenone and in 13 or 16%, respectively, of those receiving placebo. In another randomized, crossover clinical trial of 2–3 months' duration, the median time to arrhythmia recurrence in patients with PAF or PSVT was 62 or 31 days, respectively, with propafenone therapy and 5 or 8 days, respectively, with placebo. Recurrences of PAF or PSVT were completely prevented in 67 or 38%, respectively, of patients receiving propafenone and in 22 or 7%, respectively, of those receiving placebo. Patients enrolled in these 2 trials had a mean age of 57.3 years; 50% of patients were male, and 80% received a daily propafenone hydrochloride dosage of 600 mg. Patients with PSVT or PAF were equally represented in the 2 studies.

Propafenone has been used orally for the long-term management of AV nodal reentrant tachycardia; however, the drug is generally reserved for patients in whom other therapies (e.g., catheter ablation, β-adrenergic blocking agents, diltiazem, verapamil) are ineffective or contraindicated.

In a randomized crossover study, the rate of recurrence of tachycardia with propafenone therapy was approximately one-fifth that with placebo. Propafenone may be particularly effective and may be considered first-line therapy in patients with atrial fibrillation/flutter associated with ventricular preexcitation and WPW syndrome; in these patients, the drug may slow the ventricular rate and possibly restore and maintain normal sinus rhythm. However, in patients with WPW syndrome whose condition is unstable (e.g., those with hypotension or heart failure), immediate cardioversion may be required. In studies in patients with recurrent episodes of supraventricular tachyarrhythmia associated with WPW syndrome, administration of oral propafenone hydrochloride (300–1200 mg daily prevented arrhythmia recurrence in 38–100% of patients during 7–36 months of follow-up. Propafenone therapy also has been effective for arrhythmias associated with WPW syndrome and a short anterograde refractory period of the accessory pathway, although radiofrequency catheter ablation of the accessory pathway may be preferred for the long-term management of this condition.

Based on findings from the Cardiac Arrhythmia Suppression (CAST) study of substantial risk associated with flecainide or encainide therapy in certain patients with ventricular arrhythmias, some experts currently caution that use of class Ic antiarrhythmic agents in supraventricular arrhythmias be limited to the management of symptomatic, disabling supraventricular arrhythmias (paroxysmal atrial fibrillation, AV junctional tachycardias) in patients *without* structural heart disease. However, some clinicians state that even these patients may be at risk of developing drug-induced arrhythmogenic effects (e.g., during exercise testing). The risks versus benefits of propafenone for the management of such arrhythmias in patients *with* structural heart disease remain to be elucidated, and assessment of the possible risks and potential benefits in such patients must be individualized. Current evidence indicates that initiation of antiarrhythmic therapy in patients with atrial fibrillation is associated with a notable risk for adverse cardiac events, particularly in geriatric patients or those with structural heart disease (e.g., heart failure); initiation of antiarrhythmic therapy in such patients should be performed in a hospital setting with ECG monitoring for the initial 24–48 hours. Some clinicians do not recommend the use of antiarrhythmic agents in patients with atrial fibrillation or flutter because increased mortality has been reported in patients receiving antiarrhythmic therapy after conversion of atrial fibrillation to normal sinus rhythm.

Extended-release Propafenone Hydrochloride. The FDA-labeled indication for *extended-release* propafenone hydrochloride in prolonging the time to first recurrence of symptomatic paroxysmal atrial fibrillation is based principally on the results of 2 multicenter, randomized, double-blind, placebo-controlled trials in patients with a history of ECG-documented recurrent episodes of this arrhythmia. Patients had a median duration of paroxysmal atrial fibrillation of 13 months and ECG-documented symptomatic atrial fibrillation within 12 months in one trial, and a median duration of paroxysmal atrial fibrillation of 39.6 months and ECG-documented symptomatic atrial fibrillation within 28 days in the second trial. In the first trial, the median time to first recurrence of atrial fibrillation from day 1 of randomization (primary efficacy variable) was 112, 291, or 41 days in patients receiving extended-release propafenone hydrochloride 225 or 325 mg twice daily or placebo, respectively, for up to 39 weeks. Additional analysis indicated that extended-release propafenone hydrochloride 425 mg twice daily also increased the interval to first recurrence of symptomatic atrial fibrillation. A dose-response relationship was observed with respect to time to first recurrence of ECG-documented symptomatic atrial fibrillation. The time to first recurrence of atrial fibrillation from day 5 of randomization (primary efficacy variable) also was increased in patients receiving extended-release propafenone hydrochloride (325 or 425 mg twice daily) for 91 days in the second trial.

IV† Propafenone Hydrochloride. Propafenone has been administered IV† with some success in the acute treatment of supraventricular reentrant tachycardias. In a randomized, crossover, placebo-controlled study in patients with AV nodal reentrant tachycardia, intraatrial orthodromic reentrant tachycardia, or tachycardia associated with WPW syndrome, conversion to normal sinus rhythm occurred in 75% of patients receiving 1 or 2 rapid IV injections† of propafenone hydrochloride (2 mg/kg) and in no patients receiving placebo. However, an IV dosage form is not commercially available in the US and other therapies (e.g., vagal maneuvers, IV adenosine, calcium-channel blocking agents, β-adrenergic blocking agents, synchronized cardioversion) are recommended for acute conversion of PSVT.

Conversion of Atrial Fibrillation or Flutter to Normal Sinus Rhythm Propafenone has been used for pharmacologic cardioversion of atrial fibrillation or flutter†. Both oral (immediate-release tablets) and IV propafenone (IV dosage form currently not commercially available in the US) have been effective for conversion of recent-onset atrial fibrillation, including atrial fibrillation occurring after open-heart surgery, to normal sinus rhythm†, and some clinicians suggest that propafenone may be considered first-line therapy for this use. Conversion rates are inversely related to both duration of atrial fibrillation, number of previous drug treatment failures, and degree of atrial enlargement. Some patients with atrial flutter receiving propafenone (immediate-release tablets) may develop 1:1 AV conduction and a rapid ventricular response; therefore, concomitant therapy with drugs that prolong the functional AV refractory period (e.g., cardiac glycoside, β-adrenergic blocking agent) is recommended in such patients.

In acute, hemodynamically stable atrial fibrillation of less than 48 hours' duration, antiarrhythmic drug therapy may result in conversion to sinus rhythm in about 60–90% of patients; however, such therapy is effective in only 15–30% or less of patients with atrial fibrillation of longer duration. Conversion of atrial fibrillation or flutter to normal sinus rhythm may be associated with embolism, particularly when the arrhythmia has been present for more than 48 hours, unless the patient is adequately anticoagulated. (See Uses: Cardioversion of Atrial Fibrillation/Flutter, in Heparin 20:12.04.16.)

Propafenone hydrochloride also has been administered orally (150–600 mg as immediate-release tablets) or IV (2 mg/kg over 10 minutes) as a single dose for restoration of sinus rhythm† in patients with infrequent episodes of paroxysmal atrial fibrillation when it is desirable to avoid potential adverse effects of long-term antiarrhythmic drug therapy. Limited data suggest that oral propafenone therapy (immediate-release tablets) initiated 48 hours prior to electrical cardioversion of patients with chronic atrial fibrillation† may decrease the recurrence rate of this arrhythmia without an untoward effect on defibrillation threshold or electrical cardioversion rates.

Self-administration for Conversion of Paroxysmal Atrial Fibrillation. Limited evidence suggests that out-of-hospital *self-administration*† ("pill-in-the-pocket" approach) of a single oral loading dose of propafenone hydrochloride (immediate-release tablets) or flecainide is safe and effective for terminating recent-onset paroxysmal atrial fibrillation† and can reduce hospitalizations and emergency room visits in carefully selected patients who have mild or no heart disease. *In-hospital administration* of propafenone hydrochloride (immediate-release tablets) or flecainide as a single oral dose for terminating acute atrial fibrillation† has been shown to be effective with a low incidence of adverse effects in several randomized, controlled studies; however, the safety of such treatment without initial evaluation in a hospital setting or in patients with substantial structural heart disease has not been established. In addition, additional study and experience are required to assess the possible need for concomitant antithrombotic (e.g., warfarin) therapy and potential for adverse drug interactions (e.g., with warfarin or digoxin) in patients self-administering antiarrhythmic agents for recent-onset paroxysmal atrial fibrillation on an out-of-hospital basis.

In a prospective, uncontrolled study, 268 patients (18–75 years of age) with mild or no heart disease who had hemodynamically well-tolerated atrial fibrillation of recent (less than 48 hours) onset were treated in-hospital (i.e., in the emergency room or cardiology ward) with a single oral dose of propafenone hydrochloride (immediate-release tablets) or flecainide (according to clinician preference) to restore normal sinus rhythm. Patients weighing 70 kg or more received 600 mg of propafenone hydrochloride (immediate-release tablets) or 300 mg of flecainide acetate and those weighing less than 70 kg received 450 mg of propafenone hydrochloride (immediate-release tablets) or 200 mg of flecainide acetate. In-hospital treatment was considered effective if conversion of atrial fibrillation to sinus rhythm occurred within 6 hours of administration of the antiarrhythmic agent without clinically important adverse effects (i.e., symptomatic hypotension, symptomatic bradycardia after restoration of sinus rhythm, dyspnea, presyncope, syncope, conversion to atrial flutter or atrial tachycardia, or episodes of sustained or unsustained ventricular tachycardia). The time to conversion to sinus rhythm following in-hospital treatment with propafenone hydrochloride (immediate-release tablets) or flecainide in these patients averaged 135 minutes (median: 120 minutes). Patients in whom inpatient administration of these antiarrhythmics was effective and who were not excluded during subsequent examination were discharged and given propafenone hydrochloride (immediate-release tablets) or flecainide for treatment of subsequent episodes of palpitations (presumed recurrent atrial fibrillation) on an outpatient basis. These patients were instructed to take a single oral dose of the assigned antiarrhythmic drug 5 minutes after noting the onset of palpitations (self-assessed) and then to assume a resting state (e.g., a supine or sitting position) until resolution of the palpitations or for a period of at least four hours.

Analysis of data from 2 of the study sites indicated that 12% of patients presenting to the emergency room for recent-onset atrial fibrillation were candidates for out-of-hospital treatment with propafenone hydrochloride or flecainide. During a mean follow-up period of 15 months (range: 7–19 months), 79% of patients included in the out-of-hospital phase of the study experienced episodes of palpitations (presumed atrial fibrillation); patients self-administered propafenone hydrochloride (immediate-release tablets) (mean dose: 555 mg) or flecainide acetate (mean dose: 263 mg) within a mean of 36 minutes (median: 10 minutes) after the onset of symptoms in 92% of such episodes. Each antiarrhythmic agent was effective in interrupting 94% of episodes of palpitations (a primary end point); time to resolution of symptoms after drug administration averaged 113 minutes (median: 98 minutes). In patients who had multiple recurrences of palpitations during the follow-up period, self-administration of propafenone or flecainide hydrochloride terminated all such episodes in 84% of patients. Self-administration of oral propafenone (immediate-release tablets) or flecainide also was associated with reductions in emergency room visits and hospital admissions (secondary end points); calls for emergency room intervention during the study averaged 4.9 per month compared with 45.6 per month during the year prior to the study, while the number of hospitalizations averaged 1.6 per month during the study compared with 15 per month during the prior year.

Other Atrial Tachycardias Propafenone is one of several drugs that may be used for the ongoing management of focal atrial tachycardia† or junctional tachycardia† in patients without structural or ischemic heart disease.

Supraventricular Tachyarrhythmias in Children Although controlled studies generally are lacking, oral (immediate-release tablets) or IV propafenone (IV dosage form currently not commercially available in the US) has been used successfully for the management of supraventricular tachyarrhythmias (e.g., PSVT, postoperative or congenital junctional ectopic tachycardia, atrial ectopic tachycardia, chaotic atrial tachycardia, atrial fibrillation or flutter) in children†. Oral propafenone (immediate-release tablets) reportedly has been effective in treating refractory atrial flutter in children†; however, experience is limited and the drug cannot currently be recommended as first-line therapy for this use.

■ **Ventricular Arrhythmias** Propafenone hydrochloride (immediate-release tablets) is used orally to suppress and prevent the recurrence of documented *life-threatening* ventricular arrhythmias (e.g., sustained ventricular tachycardia, ventricular fibrillation). Based on the results of the Cardiac Arrhythmia Suppression Trial (CAST) (see the opening discussion in Cautions in Flecainide Acetate 24:04.04.12), FDA, the manufacturer, and many clinicians recommend that therapy with antiarrhythmic agents, including propafenone, be *reserved* for the suppression and prevention of documented ventricular tachyarrhythmias that, in the clinician's judgment, are considered *life-threatening*.

Because of propafenone's arrhythmogenic potential and the associated risk of death identified with other class Ic antiarrhythmic drugs (encainide, flecainide) in CAST, use of propafenone for less severe ventricular arrhythmias (e.g., asymptomatic ventricular premature complexes† [VPCs]), is *not* recommended. The findings of CAST involved a select patient population with recent myocardial infarction, mild to moderate left ventricular dysfunction (e.g., mean baseline ejection fraction of 40%), and asymptomatic or mildly symptomatic ventricular arrhythmias (mean baseline VPCs of 127/hour as evidenced by ambulatory ECG [Holter] monitoring during at least 18 hours of analyzable time, with about 20% of patients exhibiting at least one run of nonsustained ventricular tachycardia during such monitoring); such patients also had demonstrated drug-induced suppressibility of VPCs during the initial phase of the open trial.

It currently is not known whether the findings of CAST can be extrapolated to other patient populations with non-life-threatening ventricular arrhythmias (e.g., patients with arrhythmias in the absence of ventricular dysfunction, myocardial ischemia, or recent myocardial infarction) or to other antiarrhythmic drugs (e.g., propafenone). CAST principally involved suppression and prevention of VPCs, with only about 10% of patients exhibiting more than a single run of tachycardia at baseline. Some clinicians also question whether the results of CAST even can be extrapolated to patients with recurrent nonsustained ventricular tachycardia and ventricular dysfunction, since these patients are known to be at high risk of sudden death if untreated, and since CAST did not include sufficient numbers of such patients to clearly determine the benefit-to-risk ratio. However, despite the limitations of the CAST findings, the manufacturer, FDA, and other experts consider the potential risks of antiarrhythmic therapy substantial and currently do not recommend use of propafenone in any patient with non-life-threatening ventricular arrhythmias in the absence of substantial evidence of safety and efficacy. They state that it is prudent to consider the risks of class Ic antiarrhythmic agents and current lack of evidence of improved survival *unacceptable* in patients *without* life-threatening ventricular arrhythmias, even in patients experiencing unpleasant but non-life-threatening manifestations. However, some clinicians, while recognizing the strong evidence of risk in the patient population studied in CAST and the substantial limitations of current evidence on safety and efficacy in other patient populations, question such an extreme limitation of usage.

Life-threatening Ventricular Arrhythmias **Monotherapy.** The optimum role of propafenone (immediate-release tablets) in the suppression and prevention of ventricular arrhythmias remains to be clearly determined. In addition, it remains to be determined whether antiarrhythmic agents, including propafenone, have a beneficial effect on mortality or sudden death. Although propafenone (immediate-release tablets) has been used for chronic suppression and prevention of ventricular arrhythmias in carefully selected patients, further study is needed to evaluate the long-term efficacy and safety and the relative role of the drug in such patients. Therefore, it is recommended that propafenone (immediate-release tablets) generally be reserved for patients who have an insufficient therapeutic response to, or who do not tolerate, conventional orally administered antiarrhythmic agents (e.g., class IA agents). In addition, because of propafenone's negative inotropic potential, some clinicians would avoid use of the drug as a first-line agent in patients with life-threatening ventricular arrhythmias who also have congestive heart failure and/or substantial ventricular dysfunction (e.g., left ventricular ejection fraction less than 30%). While it currently is not known whether the findings of the CAST study apply to class Ic antiarrhythmic agents other than flecainide and encainide, some experts state that, in the absence of specific evidence of safety and efficacy, other class Ic drugs should be considered to share the risks of flecainide and encainide.

Available data suggest that the efficacy of propafenone (immediate-release tablets) for suppression and prevention of recurrent, life-threatening ventricular arrhythmias is comparable to that of other antiarrhythmic agents (e.g., quinidine, procainamide, disopyramide), with propafenone considered effective in approximately 22–50% of patients. The decision to use propafenone therapy (immediate-release tablets) should be based on an analysis of each patient's risk profile, including consideration of the type and prognosis of the specific arrhythmia, presence of underlying heart disease, degree of ventricular dysfunction, and any other serious comorbidities (e.g., hepatic or renal impairment, conduction abnormalities). Additional studies, including comparative studies with other antiarrhythmic agents, are needed to evaluate the use of propafenone (immediate-release tablets) in the management of life-threatening ventricular arrhythmias.

In a cohort study, oral propafenone hydrochloride (750–900 mg daily) (immediate-release tablets) was effective in rendering arrhythmias noninducible in 26% of patients with documented sustained ventricular arrhythmias and/or ventricular fibrillation as determined by programmed ventricular stimulation. An analysis of 27 studies in a combined total of 684 patients with malignant ventricular arrhythmias receiving propafenone yielded overall efficacy rates of 61 and 71% as determined by invasive and noninvasive testing methods, respectively. In the invasive method efficacy studies, propafenone therapy (immediate-release tablets) was considered effective in 25% of patients whose arrhythmias became noninducible, 32% of patients whose arrhythmias remained inducible but who developed improved hemodynamic tolerance and prolongation of ventricular tachycardia cycle length (100 msec or greater), and 4% of patients whose inducible sustained ventricular tachycardia was improved to inducible nonsustained ventricular tachycardia. In the noninvasive method efficacy studies, short-term propafenone therapy (1–5 days) (immediate-release tablets) was considered effective in 53–92% (mean: 71%) of patients as determined by the complete elimination of ventricular tachycardia, greater than 90% reduction in frequency of ventricular coupled beats, or greater than 50% reduction in the total number of VPCs compared with baseline arrhythmia frequency. Overall long-term efficacy, defined as the absence of symptomatic recurrence of the baseline arrhythmia, was determined by evaluation of the 90% of patients who had a positive initial response to therapy (measured by invasive or noninvasive efficacy criteria) and who continued propafenone therapy (immediate-release tablets) after hospital discharge. Long-term propafenone therapy (immediate-release tablets) (mean duration of follow-up: 14 months; range: 1–57 months) was considered effective in 67% of patients discharged on the drug and in 36% of the combined total of patients enrolled in the studies.

Combination Therapy. Limited information is available on the use of propafenone (immediate-release tablets) in conjunction with other antiarrhythmic agents for the management of severe, refractory ventricular arrhythmias. In a limited number of patients, propafenone (immediate-release tablets) has been combined with procainamide, quinidine, or mexiletine with good results in selected patients. (See Drug Interactions: Antiarrhythmic Agents.)

Concomitant use of 2 or more antiarrhythmic drugs requires extreme caution and generally is reserved for patients with life-threatening ventricular arrhythmias inadequately controlled by single-agent therapy with propafenone (immediate-release tablets) or another antiarrhythmic agent. Combination antiarrhythmic therapy for severe refractory ventricular arrhythmias generally is empiric and must be individualized.

Other Ventricular Arrhythmias Controlled and uncontrolled clinical studies in patients with chronic stable ventricular arrhythmias† have shown that propafenone (immediate-release tablets) is highly effective in suppressing and preventing nonsustained ventricular tachycardia and frequent VPCs, including complex VPCs. In short-term clinical studies, propafenone therapy (immediate-release tablets) produced approximately 66–98% suppression of VPCs in about 90% of patients; in approximately 75% of patients, ventricular tachycardia was abolished and ventricular couplets suppressed. However, despite such documented evidence of efficacy in suppressing and preventing these arrhythmias, there currently is no evidence of a beneficial effect on mortality, and in at least one patient population (those with mild-to-moderate ventricular dysfunction and recent myocardial infarction) with such arrhythmias treated with other class Ic antiarrhythmic drugs (i.e., flecainide, encainide), there was evidence of substantial risk (including mortality and nonfatal cardiac arrest) associated with therapy. (For additional information, see the opening discussion of Cautions in Flecainide Acetate 24:04.04.12.) Therefore, use of propafenone in non-life-threatening ventricular arrhythmias currently is *not* recommended by the manufacturer, FDA, and other experts.

Although controlled studies generally are lacking, both oral (immediate-release tablets) and IV propafenone (IV dosage form currently not commercially available in the US) have been used successfully in the management of ventricular arrhythmias (e.g., VPCs, coupled VPCs, nonsustained ventricular tachycardia) in children†.

Dosage and Administration

■ **Administration** Propafenone hydrochloride is administered orally. Propafenone hydrochloride is commercially available as conventional (immediate-release) tablets and extended-release capsules. The drug also has been administered IV†, but a parenteral dosage form of propafenone hydrochloride currently is not commercially available in the US.

Propafenone hydrochloride (immediate-release tablets) usually is administered orally in 3 equally divided doses daily at 8-hour intervals. Administration of single doses of propafenone hydrochloride (immediate-release tablets) with food has increased the rate and extent of drug absorption in healthy individuals with the extensive-metabolizer phenotype, and limited data indicate that this effect also may occur in those with the poor-metabolizer phenotype. Therefore, while appreciable alterations in propafenone bioavailability have not been documented during multiple-dose administrations of immediate-release tablets with food, patients should be advised of the importance of taking propafenone hydrochloride (immediate-release tablets) in a consistent manner relative to food intake to ensure consistent bioavailability and clinical effect.

Extended-release capsules of propafenone hydrochloride usually are administered orally in equally divided doses every 12 hours. The extended-release capsules should be swallowed intact and should *not* be crushed; extended-release capsules of the drug may be taken without regard to food.

Concomitant oral administration of grapefruit juice with drugs that undergo hepatic oxidation by cytochrome P-450 isoenzymes (e.g., cyclosporine, midazolam, felodipine, nifedipine) has been reported to increase bioavailability of these drugs, resulting in increased plasma concentrations of the unchanged drugs and potential adverse effects. The possibility that a similar interaction could occur between grapefruit juice and propafenone should be considered since the reported increase in bioavailability appears to result from inhibition, probably prehepatic, of the cytochrome P-450 enzyme system. Therefore, pending further accumulation of data, clinicians should be aware of this potential interaction and should discourage patients from ingesting grapefruit juice concomitantly with propafenone. For additional information on drug interactions with grapefruit juice, see Grapefruit Juice, under Drug Interactions: Drugs and Foods Affecting Hepatic Microsomal Enzymes, in the Antihistamines General Statement 4:00.

■ **Dosage** Dosage of propafenone hydrochloride must be adjusted carefully according to individual requirements and response, patient tolerance, and the general condition and cardiovascular status of the patient. The manufacturer recommends that propafenone therapy (immediate-release tablets) for life-threatening ventricular arrhythmias be initiated in a hospital setting. Clinical and ECG monitoring of cardiac function, including appropriate ambulatory ECG monitoring (e.g., Holter monitoring), is recommended during therapy with the drug. However, ECG determination of propafenone's effect on the QT interval may be confounded by drug-induced prolongation of the QRS interval. (See Effects on Cardiac Conduction under Cautions.) Because of considerable interindividual variation in plasma concentrations of propafenone and its metabolites with a given dosage and their variable contribution to clinical response, the value of monitoring plasma concentrations of the drug and its metabolites has not been established.

At a given dosage, the relative proportion of propafenone in plasma is substantially higher in poor metabolizers than in extensive metabolizers. (See Pharmacokinetics: Absorption.) However, these differences in plasma propafenone concentrations are smaller at higher dosages of the drug and the pharmacologic effects of the drug in poor metabolizers are attenuated by the lack of the active 5-OHP metabolite; in addition, steady state is achieved after 4–5 days of dosing in all patients. Therefore, based on pharmacokinetic considerations and clinical experience, the recommended oral dosage regimens for propafenone are appropriate for initial dosing regardless of the patient's genetically determined ability to metabolize the drug. Reduction of the initial dosage of immediate-release tablets should be considered in patients weighing less than 70 kg.

The manufacturer and some clinicians state that oral loading doses of propafenone hydrochloride (immediate-release tablets) may lead to acute toxicity and are not recommended; however, oral loading doses (e.g., 450–750 mg as immediate-release tablets have been used with apparent safety for conversion of recent-onset atrial fibrillation to normal sinus rhythm† in individuals without heart failure. (See Conversion of Atrial Fibrillation or Flutter to Normal Sinus Rhythm, under Uses: Supraventricular Tachyarrhythmias.)

Since steady-state plasma concentrations of propafenone and the optimum therapeutic effect may not be attained for 1–3 days at a given dosage (immediate-release tablets) in patients with normal renal and hepatic function, increases in propafenone hydrochloride (immediate-release tablets) dosage should be made at intervals of not less than 3–4 days. More gradual dosage escalation should be performed in geriatric patients and patients with marked previous myocardial damage during initiation of propafenone therapy (immediate-release tablets). Increases in propafenone hydrochloride dosage as (extended-release capsules) should be made at intervals of not less than 5 days. Dosage reduction also should be considered in patients who develop excessive prolongation of the PR interval, excessive QRS widening, or second- or third-degree AV block during propafenone therapy. While it has been suggested that a reduction in propafenone hydrochloride dosage (immediate-release tablets) from initial levels may be needed because of a decrease in propafenone metabolism with long-term therapy, other limited data suggest that a partial tolerance to the antiarrhythmic effects of the drug may develop with continued therapy. (See Pharmacokinetics: Absorption.)

Supraventricular Arrhythmias For the prevention of paroxysmal supraventricular tachycardia (PSVT) associated with disabling symptoms and for disabling paroxysmal atrial fibrillation/flutter (PAF), the recommended initial adult dosage of propafenone hydrochloride (immediate-release tablets) is 150 mg every 8 hours. Dosage (immediate-release tablets) may be increased after 3–4 days to 225 mg 3 times daily if necessary. If the desired therapeutic response is not attained after an additional 3–4 days, dosage (immediate-release tablets) may be increased again to 300 mg 3 times daily. The safety and efficacy of propafenone hydrochloride dosages (immediate-release tablets) exceeding 900 mg daily have not been established.

Some clinicians suggest a maximum daily propafenone hydrochloride dosage (immediate-release tablets) of 600 mg/m^2 in children.

When propafenone hydrochloride is given as *extended-release capsules* for the prevention of symptomatic atrial fibrillation, the recommended initial adult dosage is 225 mg every 12 hours. Dosage may be increased after at least 5 days to 325 mg every 12 hours if necessary. If the desired therapeutic response is not attained after an additional 5 days, dosage may be increased again to 425 mg every 12 hours. If a dose of propafenone hydrochloride as extended-release capsules is missed, the patient should take only the next scheduled dose (i.e., the next dose should *not* be doubled to make up for the missed dose).

During relative bioavailability studies, a higher daily dosage of propafenone hydrochloride as extended-release capsules was required to obtain similar exposure to propafenone compared with that following immediate-release tablets. Because of decreased saturation of hepatic metabolic pathways and increased first-pass hepatic metabolism associated with the extended-release formulation compared with the immediate-release formulation, the bioavailability of propafenone hydrochloride 325 mg given every 12 hours as extended-release capsules is similar to that following 150 mg of the drug given every 8 hours as immediate-release tablets. Therefore, when switching therapy in a patient who currently is receiving the immediate-release dosage form to the extended-release dosage form, the dosage conversion ratio is *not* a 1:1 substitution (e.g., a patient who currently is receiving 150 mg every 8 hours of propafenone hydrochloride immediate-release tablets may be switched to 325 mg of extended-release capsules every 12 hours).

Self-administration for Conversion of Paroxysmal Atrial Fibrillation. For *self-administration* on an outpatient basis for termination of atrial fibrillation of recent onset in carefully selected patients with mild or no heart disease†, propafenone hydrochloride (immediate-release tablets) has been given as a single oral loading dose of 600 mg in patients weighing 70 kg or more and 450 mg in patients weighing less than 70 kg. Some clinicians suggest that propafenone hydrochloride (immediate-release tablets) be taken 5 minutes after noting the onset of palpitations and that patients remain in a supine or sitting position until resolution of palpitations or for a period of at least four hours following the dose. Patients should seek medical advice if palpitations do not resolve within 6–8 hours, if previously unexperienced symptoms (e.g., dyspnea, presyncope, syncope) occur, or if a marked increase in heart rate occurs after taking the antiarrhythmic drug. Patients should not take more than a single oral dose of propafenone hydrochloride (immediate-release tablets) during a 24-hour period.

Life-threatening Ventricular Arrhythmias For the suppression and prevention of life-threatening ventricular arrhythmias (e.g., sustained ventricular tachycardia), the recommended initial adult dosage of propafenone hydrochloride (immediate-release tablets) is 150 mg every 8 hours. Dosage (immediate-release tablets) may be increased after 3–4 days to 225 mg 3 times daily if necessary. If the desired therapeutic response is not attained after an additional 3–4 days, dosage (immediate-release tablets) may be increased again to 300 mg 3 times daily. The safety and efficacy of propafenone hydrochloride dosages (immediate-release tablets) exceeding 900 mg daily have not been established.

Some clinicians suggest a maximum daily propafenone hydrochloride dosage (immediate-release tablets) of 600 mg/m^2 in children.

■ **Dosage in Renal and Hepatic Impairment** Propafenone should be used with caution in patients with renal impairment since a considerable proportion of the dose (approximately 20–40%) administered as the immediate-release formulation is excreted in urine as active metabolites over a 48-hour period. The amount of the extended-release formulation excreted in urine has not been determined. The manufacturer states that data currently are insufficient to recommend a propafenone hydrochloride dosage for patients with renal impairment; however, such patients should be monitored closely for manifestations of toxicity, including hypotension, somnolence, bradycardia, conduction disturbances (intra-atrial and intraventricular), seizures, and serious ventricular arrhythmias.

Elimination of propafenone may be decreased in patients with hepatic impairment, including cirrhosis and alcoholic liver disease; the terminal elimination half-life of propafenone (immediate-release tablets) of the drug is increased to approximately 9 hours in such patients. (See Pharmacokinetics: Elimination.) In addition, the bioavailability of propafenone (immediate-release tablets) is increased to approximately 70% in patients with substantial hepatic impairment compared with a range of 3–40% in patients with normal hepatic function; absolute bioavailability of propafenone as the extended-release formulation has not been determined. When propafenone (immediate-release tablets) is used in patients with hepatic impairment, the initial dosage of the drug should be approximately 20–30% of the dosage given to patients with normal hepatic function (i.e., a 70–80% reduction in dosage), and these patients should be monitored for signs of toxicity, including hypotension, somnolence, bradycardia, conduction disturbances (intra-atrial and intraventricular), seizures, and/or ventricular arrhythmias.

Cautions

The most common adverse effects of propafenone involve the GI, cardiovascular, and central nervous systems and generally are dose related. Discontinuance of propafenone therapy was required in about 20% of patients receiving the drug in clinical trials. Drug discontinuance in patients treated for ventricular arrhythmias was required most frequently (i.e., in greater than 1% of patients) for proarrhythmia (4.7%), nausea and/or vomiting (3.4%), dizziness (2.4%), dyspnea (1.6%), congestive heart failure (1.4%), and ventricular tachycardia (1.2%). In patients treated for supraventricular arrhythmias in clinical trials, discontinuance of therapy was required most frequently (i.e., in greater than 1% of patients) for nausea and/or vomiting (2.9%), wide-complex tachycardia (1.9%), dizziness (1.7%), fatigue (1.5%), unusual taste (1.3%), and weakness (1.3%).

Propafenone-induced adverse effects tend to decrease with time and may be attenuated by dosage reduction and/or adjustment of dosage interval. Patients with the poor-metabolizer phenotype (see Pharmacokinetics: Elimination) and geriatric patients may be at increased risk of adverse effects because of increased plasma propafenone concentrations. In a multicenter, randomized study in patients with paroxysmal atrial fibrillation or paroxysmal supraventricular tachycardia (PSVT) who had no evidence of ischemic heart disease, the safety and tolerability (i.e., the incidence of adverse effects, including proarrhythmic events) of propafenone hydrochloride (450–900 mg daily, mean daily dosage: 569 mg) was comparable to that of flecainide acetate (100–300 mg daily, mean daily dosage: 167 mg) during a 12-month period of follow-up. In another multicenter, randomized study in patients with paroxysmal atrial fibrillation (more than 90% who were New York Heart Association [NYHA] functional class I) receiving extended-release capsules of propafenone hydrochloride (225 mg, 325 mg, or 425 mg twice daily) for up to 39 weeks, the most common adverse events included dizziness, chest pain, palpitations, taste disturbance, dyspnea, nausea, constipation, anxiety, fatigue, upper respiratory tract infection, influenza, first-degree heart block, and vomiting. The incidence of adverse effects in patients treated with extended-release propafenone hydrochloride capsules in this study was similar regardless of age or gender.

■ **Nervous System Effects** Adverse nervous system effects reported in US clinical trials in patients receiving propafenone for the treatment of ventricular arrhythmias included dizziness and/or lightheadedness in 13% of patients, fatigue/lethargy in 6%, and headache in 5%. Weakness, ataxia, insomnia, or anxiety was reported in 2%, and tremor or drowsiness in 1% of patients receiving propafenone for ventricular arrhythmias. Pain or loss of balance also has been reported with propafenone therapy in patients with ventricular arrhythmias.

In US clinical trials in patients with supraventricular arrhythmias, adverse nervous system effects reported with propafenone therapy included dizziness in 9% of patients, headache or fatigue in 6%, weakness in 3%, and tremor or ataxia in 2%. Abnormal dreams, abnormal speech, agitation, delusions, disorientation, coma, confusion, decreased libido, depression, memory loss, paranoia, paresthesia/numbness, psychosis/mania, seizures, unusual smell sensation, or vertigo has been reported in less than 1% of patients receiving propafenone in clinical trials or during postmarketing experience.

Transient global amnesia, which resolved within hours after drug discontinuance, has been reported in at least one patient receiving propafenone. Peripheral neuropathy, which was characterized by episodic jabbing and crushing pain in the hands and feet and hyperesthesia of the extremities and resolved following discontinuance of the drug, has been reported rarely with propafenone therapy.

■ **GI Effects** The most common adverse GI effect of propafenone therapy is nausea and/or vomiting, which was reported in 11% of patients receiving the drug for ventricular arrhythmias in US clinical trials. Propafenone is secreted by the salivary glands, and unusual (e.g., metallic or salty) taste (dysgeusia) was reported in 9% of patients treated for ventricular arrhythmias. Constipation occurred in 7%; dyspepsia and/or diarrhea in 3%; dry mouth, anorexia, and/or abdominal pain/cramps in 2%; and flatulence in 1% of patients receiving the drug for ventricular arrhythmias. Esophagitis and gastroenteritis also have been reported in clinical trials or during postmarketing experience in patients treated with propafenone for ventricular arrhythmias.

Unusual taste or nausea and/or vomiting was reported in 14 or 11%, respectively, of patients receiving propafenone for supraventricular arrhythmias in US clinical trials. Constipation occurred in 8% and anorexia or diarrhea in 2% of patients with supraventricular arrhythmias.

■ **Arrhythmogenic Effects** Like other antiarrhythmic agents, propafenone can worsen existing arrhythmias or cause new arrhythmias; the arrhythmogenic potential is the most serious risk associated with the drug. Arrhythmogenic effects associated with propafenone range from an increased frequency of ventricular premature complexes (VPCs) to the development of new and/or more severe and potentially fatal ventricular tachyarrhythmias. Because of difficulties in distinguishing between spontaneous and drug-related variations in an underlying arrhythmia disorder in patients with complex arrhythmias, reported occurrence rates must be considered approximations.

Arrhythmogenic events associated with propafenone therapy in clinical trials reportedly have occurred with an overall frequency of about 5%. In patients with malignant ventricular arrhythmias monitored by invasive and noninvasive methods, the incidence of arrhythmogenic effects during propafenone therapy was 8–19%. About 82–85% of the arrhythmogenic effects associated with the drug have been new or worsened ventricular tachyarrhythmias (e.g., new occurrence of sustained or nonsustained ventricular tachycardia, including spontaneous wide-QRS complex tachycardia, torsades de pointes, progression of ventricular tachycardia to ventricular fibrillation), with the remainder consisting of increased frequency of VPCs. VPCs were reported in 2% of patients receiving propafenone for treatment of ventricular arrhythmias in US clinical trials.

An increased incidence of arrhythmogenic events also has been reported during propafenone therapy in patients with supraventricular tachyarrhythmias. Wide-QRS complex tachycardia was reported in 2% of patients receiving propafenone for supraventricular arrhythmias in overall US clinical trials. In a long-term multicenter trial in patients with symptomatic supraventricular tachycardia, ventricular tachycardia or ventricular fibrillation developed in 9 of 474 patients (1.9 %) receiving propafenone therapy. Ventricular tachycardia or ventricular fibrillation developed within the first 14 days of therapy in 6 of 9 patients; ventricular tachycardia appeared to be of atrial origin in 4 of these 9 patients. Approximately 2.3% of patients in this trial may have experienced an arrhythmogenic event manifested as a recurrence of supraventricular tachycardia. Increased VPCs, ventricular tachycardia, ventricular fibrillation, and death have been reported in patients with atrial fibrillation/flutter receiving propafenone therapy. The overall annual mortality rate based on data from 8 clinical studies was 2.5 or 4% per year in patients receiving propafenone (extended-release or immediate-release formulation) or placebo, respectively.

Although the occurrence of propafenone-induced arrhythmias generally is unpredictable, the risk of arrhythmogenic effects generally appears to be related to dosage and underlying cardiac disease, including severity of the preexisting ventricular arrhythmia and myocardial dysfunction (e.g., low left ventricular ejection fraction, congestive heart failure (New York Heart Association [NYHA] functional class III or IV), myocardial ischemia). Of patients in clinical trials who had worsening of ventricular tachycardia while receiving propafenone, 92% had a history of ventricular tachycardia and/or ventricular fibrillation, 71% had coronary artery disease, and 68% had a history of myocardial infarction. During long-term (mean: 14.4 months) therapy in patients with symptomatic atrial fibrillation, atrial flutter, or supraventricular tachycardia, propafenone therapy was associated with a 20% incidence of adverse cardiovascular effects (e.g., arrhythmogenicity, congestive heart failure, conduction disturbance) in patients with structural heart disease compared with a 13% incidence in those without structural heart disease. While the overall incidence of adverse reactions was similar for patients with or without structural heart disease, the incidence was directly related to dosage and age. The incidence of proarrhythmia in patients receiving propafenone for less serious or benign arrhythmias, including an increased frequency of VPCs, was 1.6%.

Although most proarrhythmic events occurred during the first week of therapy in clinical trials with propafenone, such events also occurred later in therapy, and results of the CAST study suggest that an increased risk of proarrhythmic events is present throughout treatment with antiarrhythmic agents. When propafenone is administered according to currently recommended dosage regimens and precautions, the risk of arrhythmogenic effects appears to be comparable to or less than that associated with other antiarrhythmic agents (e.g., encainide, flecainide).

■ **Effects on Cardiac Conduction** Clinically important conduction disturbances may occur during propafenone therapy in patients without preexisting conduction abnormalities; however, the risk of adverse cardiac effects probably increases progressively as plasma propafenone concentrations increase. There is a correlation between propafenone dosage, plasma concentration, and the degree of lengthening of PR and QRS intervals.

First-, second-, or third-degree AV block occurred in about 2.5, 0.6, or 0.2%, respectively, of patients with ventricular arrhythmias receiving propafenone (immediate-release tablets) in clinical trials. First-degree AV block occurred in approximately 2–3% of patients with symptomatic paroxysmal atrial fibrillation receiving the extended-release formulation of propafenone hydrochloride in a clinical trial. There were no cases of sinus rhythm with Mobitz type I (Wenckenbach) second-degree AV block, sinus rhythm with Mobitz Type II second-degree AV block, third-degree AV block, or increased sinus bradycardia in a clinical trial of patients with symptomatic paroxysmal atrial fibrillation receiving the extended-release formulation of the drug. Dosage reduction or discontinuance of the drug may be necessary in patients who develop second- or third-degree AV block. (See Cautions: Precautions and Contraindications.) Bundle branch block, intraventricular conduction delay/increased QRS duration, or bradycardia occurred in about 1–2% of patients with ventricular arrhythmias in clinical trials. Bradycardia was reported in 2% of patients receiving propafenone therapy for supraventricular arrhythmias in clinical trials. A paradoxical increase in ventricular rate also has occurred with propafenone therapy in patients with atrial flutter or fibrillation because of a reduction in the degree of AV nodal block or enhanced conduction through an accessory bypass tract (e.g., in patients with Wolff-Parkinson-White [WPW] syndrome). (See Cautions: Precautions and Contraindications.)

■ **Cardiovascular Effects** The manufacturer states that clinically important decreases in left ventricular ejection fraction with oral propafenone therapy did not occur in clinical trials in patients with depressed baseline ejection fraction (mean ejection fraction: 33.5%). However, because of propafenone's dose-related β-adrenergic blocking and negative inotropic effects, the drug may cause or worsen congestive heart failure, particularly in patients with preexisting heart failure or decreased left ventricular ejection fraction (less than 30%). New or worsened congestive heart failure occurred in about 1–4% of patients treated for ventricular arrhythmias in clinical trials. In patients in whom these adverse effects were considered probably or definitely related to propafenone therapy (about 1%), 80% had preexisting heart failure and 85% had coronary artery disease. Patients with no prior history of congestive heart failure receiving propafenone rarely (less than 0.2%) developed congestive heart failure. Congestive heart failure or palpitations occurred in about 2% of patients receiving propafenone therapy for supraventricular arrhythmias (PAF or PSVT) in clinical trials.

Chest pain or angina, palpitations, or syncope/near syncope occurred in about 2–5% of patients receiving propafenone in clinical trials for treatment of ventricular arrhythmias. Atrial fibrillation or edema has occurred in about 1% of patients receiving propafenone therapy for ventricular arrhythmias. Atrial flutter, AV dissociation, cardiac arrest, flushing, hot flashes, sick sinus syndrome, sinus pause, sinus arrest, or supraventricular tachycardia has been reported in less than 1% of patients receiving propafenone.

■ **Hepatic Effects** Propafenone is extensively metabolized in the liver and should be administered with caution to patients with impaired hepatic function. (See Cautions: Precautions and Contraindications.) There have been postmarketing reports of hepatic dysfunction, including hepatocellular, cholestatic, and mixed hepatotoxicity in patients receiving the drug. In at least one case, hepatotoxicity recurred upon rechallenge with propafenone. Cholestasis, hepatitis, and increases in serum aminotransferase (AST [SGOT], ALT [SGPT]) and alkaline phosphatase concentrations have been reported in patients receiving the drug. In toxicology studies, fatty degenerative liver changes were observed in rats following long-term (6 months) administration of oral propafenone hydrochloride at a dosage of 270 mg/kg daily (about 3 times the maximum recommended human daily dosage based on body surface area) but not at 90 mg/kg daily (equivalent to the maximum recommended human daily dosage based on body surface area).

■ **Dermatologic and Sensitivity Reactions** Rash has been reported in 3% of patients with ventricular arrhythmias receiving propafenone in clinical trials, and diaphoresis has been reported in 1% of such patients. Pruritus also have been reported in patients receiving the drug. Possible propafenone-associated drug fever has been reported in at least one patient receiving oral propafenone therapy for sustained ventricular tachycardia. Fever and an erythematous, papular rash developed 10 days after initiation of propafenone therapy and resolved following drug discontinuance; fever recurred upon rechallenge with the drug but resolved completely upon termination of therapy.

Alopecia also has been reported with propafenone therapy.

■ **Hematologic Effects** Granulocytopenia, leukopenia, lymphopenia, leukocytosis, thrombocytosis, thrombocytopenia, purpura, anemia, bruising, and increased bleeding time have been reported in less than 1% of patients receiving propafenone. Agranulocytosis (fever, chills, weakness, and neutropenia) also has been reported with propafenone therapy, generally within 8 weeks after initiation of therapy. The leukocyte count generally returned to normal within 14 days after discontinuance of therapy. The possibility of agranulocytosis should be considered in any patient receiving propafenone who develops unexplained fever and/or decreases in leukocyte count, particularly during the 3 months following initiation of therapy. (See Cautions: Precautions and Contraindications.)

■ **Musculoskeletal Effects** Joint pain occurred in about 1% of patients receiving propafenone for ventricular arrhythmias in clinical trials. Arthritis, arthralgia, gout, muscle pain, muscle weakness, or muscle cramps were reported in less than 1% of such patients. Lupus erythematosus has been reported in less than 1% of patients receiving propafenone therapy in clinical trials or during postmarketing experience; in at least one patient, propafenone-induced lupus erythematosus recurred following rechallenge with the drug but resolved completely upon discontinuance of therapy. Positive antinuclear antibody (ANA) titers have been reported with propafenone therapy; these abnormalities generally were not associated with clinical manifestations and resolved upon discontinuance of the drug or even with continued therapy. In a randomized, controlled trial, positive ANA titers were found in about 24% of patients who had negative ANA titers before initiation of propafenone therapy.

Exacerbation of myasthenia gravis, which was evident within a few hours after initiation of propafenone hydrochloride (450 mg daily) in a patient with ocular myasthenia gravis and resolved upon drug discontinuance, has been reported with propafenone therapy.

■ **Other Adverse Effects** Blurred vision occurred in 4% of patients receiving propafenone therapy for ventricular arrhythmias in clinical trials; abnormal vision also has been reported. Asthma, increased serum glucose concentration, diabetes mellitus, hypochloremia, hyponatremia, syndrome of inappropriate antidiuretic hormone (SIADH) secretion, nephrotic syndrome, renal failure, nasal congestion, ocular irritation, tinnitus,pneumonia, respiratory failure, pain, increased urinary frequency or urgency, impotence, or prostatitis occurred in less than 1% of patients receiving propafenone for treatment of ventricular arrhythmias in clinical trials.

Blurred vision was reported in 3% and dyspnea in 2% of patients receiving propafenone therapy for supraventricular arrhythmias in clinical trials.

Both inflammatory and noninflammatory lesions in the renal tubules, with accompanying interstitial nephritis, have been observed in rats following administration of oral propafenone hydrochloride for 6 months at dosages of 180 and 360 mg/kg daily (2 or 4 times the maximum recommended human daily dosage based on body surface area) but not at 90 mg/kg daily (equivalent to the maximum recommended human daily dosage based on body surface area). However, these lesions appeared reversible as they were not found 6 weeks after discontinuance of the drug.

■ **Precautions and Contraindications** Findings from the postmarketing Cardiac Arrhythmia Suppression Trial (CAST), a long-term, multicenter, randomized, double-blind study in patients with asymptomatic, non-life-threatening ventricular arrhythmias who had had a myocardial infarction more than 6 days but less than 2 years previously, indicate that the rate of total mortality and nonfatal cardiac arrest in patients treated with encainide or flecainide (7.7%) was increased compared with that seen in patients who received placebo (3%). The applicability of these results to other populations (e.g., those without recent myocardial infarction) or to other antiarrhythmic drugs is uncertain; however, the manufacturer of propafenone states that use of any class Ic antiarrhythmic drug in patients with structural heart disease may be associated with substantial risk. In addition, the manufacturer, FDA, and some experts currently recommend that use of propafenone or other class I agents in patients with ventricular arrhythmias be limited to those with *life-threatening* arrhythmias. (See Uses.) Use in less severe ventricular arrhythmias, including even those with unpleasant manifestations, currently is not recommended, and treatment of asymptomatic VPCs should be avoided. In addition, current evidence indicates that initiation of antiarrhythmic therapy in patients with atrial fibrillation is associated with a notable risk for adverse cardiac events, particularly in geriatric patients or those with structural heart disease.

Since propafenone, like other antiarrhythmic agents, can worsen existing arrhythmias or cause new arrhythmias in some patients, clinical and ECG evaluations are essential prior to and during propafenone therapy to monitor for the appearance of arrhythmias and to determine the need for continued therapy. Use of propafenone in patients with atrial flutter has resulted in an increase in AV conduction (1:1 ratio) and the development of very rapid ventricular rates. (See Cautions: Effects on Cardiac Conduction.) Risk of this tachycardia may be reduced by concomitant administration of a cardiac glycoside or a β-adrenergic blocking agent. Patients with permanent artificial pacemakers should be monitored and, if necessary, have their pacemakers reprogrammed since propafenone may affect endocardial pacing and sensing thresholds (e.g., increased stimulation threshold) of these devices.

The patient's medication history should be carefully screened prior to and during propafenone therapy, including obtaining information on all OTC, prescription, and herbal/natural preparations with emphasis on those that may affect the pharmacodynamics or pharmacokinetics of propafenone. (See Drug Interactions.) Patients should be advised to inform their health-care providers of any change in the use of medications (OTC, prescription) and supplements. Patients should be advised to inform their health-care providers that they are receiving propafenone when hospitalized or prescribed a new medication for any condition. Patients should be advised to immediately inform their health care providers if they experience symptoms associated with electrolyte imbalance (e.g., excessive or prolonged diarrhea, sweating, vomiting, loss of appetite or thirst).

Because of propafenone's mild to moderate negative inotropic and β-adrenergic blocking effects, as well as an increased risk of arrhythmogenic effects, the immediate-release formulation of the drug should be used with caution in patients with a history of congestive heart failure or myocardial dysfunction; the manufacturer of the extended-release formulation of propafenone states that the drug should not be used in patients with congestive heart failure. Congestive heart failure should be fully compensated before propafenone therapy with the immediate-release formulation is initiated. If cardiovascular manifestations increase, therapy should be discontinued (unless congestive heart failure is caused by the cardiac arrhythmia) and adequate cardiac compensation reestablished before resuming propafenone therapy, if indicated, at a lower dosage of the immediate-release formulation.

Propafenone slows AV conduction and may cause AV block. A correlation exists between dosage and plasma concentrations of propafenone hydrochloride and the degree of lengthening of PR and QRS intervals. Some clinicians have suggested limiting QRS interval increases to 25% or less in patients receiving propafenone. If second- or third-degree AV block occurs during propafenone therapy, the dosage should be reduced or the drug discontinued.

Because reversible granulocytopenia and agranulocytosis have occurred rarely with propafenone therapy, patients receiving the drug should be advised to promptly report fever, sore throat, chills, or any other manifestations of infection.

Positive antinuclear antibody (ANA) titers have been reported in patients receiving propafenone therapy. (See Cautions: Musculoskeletal Effects.) Patients who develop an abnormal ANA test following initiation of propafenone therapy should be monitored carefully and, if titers remain elevated or increase further, drug discontinuance should be considered.

Propafenone is extensively metabolized in the liver, and dosage should be reduced substantially in patients with impaired hepatic function. The drug also should be used with caution in patients with renal dysfunction since a considerable portion of the dose is excreted in urine as active metabolites. (See Dosage and Administration: Dosage in Renal and Hepatic Impairment.)

Reversible disorders of spermatogenesis have been demonstrated in animals following high-dose IV administration of propafenone. Transient, reversible decreases (within the normal range) in sperm count have been reported in healthy men receiving short-term propafenone therapy but subsequent evaluations in patients receiving long-term therapy have suggested no effect of the drug on sperm count. (See Cautions: Pregnancy, Fertility, and Lactation.)

Pending further accumulation of data, patients should be discouraged from ingesting grapefruit juice concomitantly with propafenone because of the potential for increased propafenone bioavailability and possible adverse effects associated with such concomitant administration. (See Dosage and Administration: Administration.)

Propafenone, like other agents with nonselective β-adrenergic blocking activity, generally should *not* be used in patients with asthma/bronchospastic disease or nonallergic bronchospastic disease (e.g., chronic bronchitis, emphysema) since the drugs may inhibit bronchodilation produced by endogenous catecholamines.

Propafenone has been reported to exacerbate myasthenia gravis, and it has been suggested that use of the drug be avoided in patients with this condition.

Propafenone (immediate-release formulation) is contraindicated in patients with uncontrolled congestive heart failure; the extended-release formulation of the drug is contraindicated in patients with congestive heart failure. Propafenone is contraindicated in patients with cardiogenic shock, atrioventricular or intraventricular disorders of impulse generation and/or conduction (e.g., sick sinus node syndrome, atrioventricular block) unless an artificial pacemaker is present, bradycardia, severe hypotension, marked electrolyte imbalance, or known hypersensitivity to the drug.

The manufacturer of ritonavir states that concomitant use of ritonavir with propafenone is contraindicated because such use is likely to produce substantially increased plasma concentrations of propafenone and associated serious toxicity. (See Drug Interactions: Ritonavir.)

■ **Pediatric Precautions** Safety and efficacy of propafenone in patients younger than 18 years of age have not been established. However, the drug has been used successfully and without unusual adverse effects in a limited number of infants and children for the management of various refractory supraventricular (e.g., PSVT, junctional ectopic tachycardia, atrial fibrillation or flutter) and ventricular (e.g., VPCs, ventricular tachycardia) arrhythmias. (See Uses.)

■ **Geriatric Precautions** Data from clinical studies with propafenone (immediate-release tablets) in patients 65 years of age or older is insufficient to determine whether geriatric patients respond differently than younger adults. Dosage of propafenone (immediate-release tablets) should be selected with caution and generally initiated at the lower end of the recommended range since geriatric patients are more likely to have impaired renal, hepatic, and/or cardiac function and concomitant disease and drug therapy. Data from clinical studies indicate that safety and efficacy of propafenone as extended-release capsules are similar in geriatric patients and younger adults. Nevertheless, the manufacturer states that the possibility that some older patients may exhibit increased sensitivity to the drug as extended-release capsules cannot be ruled out.

■ **Mutagenicity and Carcinogenicity** No evidence of propafenone-induced mutagenicity was seen with in vitro microbial (Ames test), dominant lethal tests in mice, mammalian mutagenicity assays using Chinese hamster spermatogonoia and bone marrow cells, rat bone marrow, and Chinese hamster micronucleus test.

No evidence of carcinogenesis was seen in mice and rats receiving oral propafenone hydrochloride dosages up to 360 mg/kg (about 2 times the maximum recommended human daily dosage based on body surface area) and 270 mg/kg daily (about 3 times the maximum recommended human daily dosage based on body surface area), respectively.

■ **Pregnancy, Fertility, and Lactation** ***Pregnancy*** Propafenone has been shown to be embryotoxic, but not teratogenic, in rabbits and rats when given at a dosage 3 (150 mg/kg daily) and 6 times (600 mg/kg daily), respectively, the maximum recommended human daily dose based on body surface area. Embryotoxic effects were not observed in rats given propafenone hydrochloride dosages up to 270 mg/kg daily (about 3 times the maximum recommended human daily dose based on body surface area); however, dose-dependent increases in post-implantation loss were observed in rabbits given propafenone hydrochloride dosages as low as 15 mg/kg daily (about 33% of the maximum recommended human daily dose based on body surface area). Increased maternal death was observed in rats receiving oral propafenone hydrochloride dosages as low as 90 mg/kg daily (equivalent to the maximum recommended human daily dosage) from mid-gestation through weaning. Decreases in neonatal survival, weight gain, and physiologic development were observed in rats receiving oral propafenone hydrochloride dosages of 360 mg/kg or more daily (4 or more times the maximum recommended human daily dosage) from mid-gestation through weaning. Unchanged propafenone and its metabolite, 5-hydroxypropafenone (5-OHP), have been reported to cross the placenta in humans. However, there are no adequate and controlled studies to date using propafenone in pregnant women, and the drug should be used during pregnancy only when the potential benefits justify the possible risks to the fetus. It is not known whether use of the drug during labor or delivery could have any immediate or delayed adverse effects on the mother or fetus, affect the duration of labor, or increase the likelihood of forceps delivery or other obstetrical intervention.

Fertility The effect of propafenone on fertility in humans is not known. Temporary decreases in sperm count have been observed in healthy men receiving short-term, oral propafenone therapy; this effect was reversible following discontinuance of the drug and did not persist during long-term propafenone therapy. Administration of large IV doses of propafenone in monkeys, dogs, and rabbits has caused transient, reversible decreases in spermatogenesis; this effect was observed only at lethal or sublethal dosages and was not seen in rats receiving oral or IV propafenone. Reproduction studies in male rabbits using an oral propafenone hydrochloride dosage of 120 mg/kg daily (about 2.4 times the maximum recommended human daily dosage based on body surface area) or an IV dosage of 3.5 mg/kg daily (a dosage associated with impairment of spermatogenesis) have not revealed evidence of impaired fertility. In addition, reproduction studies in male and female rats using oral propafenone hydrochloride dosages up to 270 mg/kg daily (about 3 times the maximum recommended human daily dosage based on body surface area) have not revealed evidence of impaired fertility.

Lactation Since propafenone is distributed in milk, caution is advised if the drug is administered in nursing women. (See Pharmacokinetics: Distribution.) Because of the potential for serious adverse reactions to propafenone in nursing infants, a decision should be made whether to discontinue nursing or the drug, taking into account the importance of the drug to the woman.

Drug Interactions

■ **Drugs Affecting or Metabolized by Hepatic Microsomal Enzymes** Metabolism of propafenone is mediated by the cytochrome P-450 (CYP) isoenzyme system, including CYP2D6 (major metabolic pathway), CYP1A2 and CYP3A4; patients should be monitored and dosage of propafenone hydrochloride should be reduced accordingly when the drug is used concurrently with inhibitors of CYP2D6 (e.g., desipramine, paroxetine, quinidine, ritonavir, sertraline), CYP1A2 (e.g., amiodarone), or CYP3A4 (e.g., erythromycin, ketoconazole, ritonavir, saquinavir), because plasma propafenone concentrations may increase. In addition, propafenone inhibits CYP2D6 and caution is advised if the drug is used concurrently with substrates of CYP2D6 (e.g., desipramine, haloperidol, imipramine, metoprolol, propranolol, venlafaxine) since increased plasma concentrations of these drugs may occur, and consideration should be given to reduction of dosage for drugs that are substrates of CYP2D6 when such drugs are used concurrently with propafenone.

■ **Drugs Metabolized by P-glycoprotein Transporter** The effect, if any, of propafenone on the *p*-glycoprotein transport system has not been systematically evaluated.

■ **Digoxin** Concomitant administration of propafenone and oral or IV digoxin has resulted in increased serum or plasma digoxin concentrations, associated in some cases with enhanced effects of digoxin (e.g., decreased heart rate, shortened QT interval) and at least one case of digoxin toxicity.In some studies, increases in serum digoxin concentrations with propafenone hydrochloride dosages of 450 or 900 mg daily averaged about 35 or 85%, respectively; such increases in digoxin concentrations have been maintained over a period of up to 16 months of concomitant therapy with the drugs. Changes in digoxin concentrations in patients receiving concomitant propafenone therapy have exhibited wide interindividual and intraindividual variation, with a relationship to propafenone and/or digoxin dosage or plasma propafenone concentration being reported in some studies.

Although the exact mechanism of this interaction has not been established, some evidence suggests that propafenone may reduce the renal clearance of digoxin by inhibiting renal tubular transport of the drug. Other data suggest no alterations in digoxin renal clearance, but decreases in total body and/or nonrenal clearance or volume of distribution of digoxin have been reported.

Digoxin dosage generally should be reduced in patients in whom propafenone therapy is initiated, especially in those who have relatively high digoxin dosages or serum concentrations. Careful monitoring of serum digoxin concentrations and appropriate adjustments in digoxin dosage should be performed in patients receiving concomitant propafenone and digoxin therapy.

■ **β-Adrenergic Blocking Agents** In healthy individuals, concomitant administration of propafenone and propranolol or metoprolol has resulted in substantial increases in plasma concentrations and terminal elimination half-lives of the β-adrenergic blocking agents; plasma propafenone concentrations were unchanged. These increases in plasma concentration and half-life apparently are the result of propafenone's inhibition of the hydroxylation pathway responsible for metabolism of the β-adrenergic blocking agents. Increases in plasma metoprolol concentrations may result in loss of the drug's relative cardioselectivity and an increase in adverse effects. Although pharmacokinetics of propafenone were not affected and concomitant use of β-adrenergic blocking agents was not associated with an increased incidence of adverse effects in clinical trials of propafenone, an increase in the manifestations of acute metoprolol-induced brain syndrome (e.g., delirium, fatigue, lassitude) has been reported in a patient receiving concomitant metoprolol and propafenone. Patients receiving propafenone and β-adrenergic blocking agents concomitantly may require a reduction in the dosage of the β-adrenergic blocking agent.

■ **Antiarrhythmic Agents** There is limited information on the use of propafenone in conjunction with other antiarrhythmic agents for the management of severe, refractory ventricular or supraventricular arrhythmias. (See Combination Therapy under Ventricular Arrhythmias: Life-threatening Ventricular Arrhythmias, in Uses.) Combination antiarrhythmic therapy for severe refractory arrhythmias generally is empiric and must be individualized. Since the cardiac effects of multiple antiarrhythmic agents may be additive, synergistic, or antagonistic and adverse effects may be additive, combination therapy must be used only when the increased risk is justified and with careful monitoring.

The manufacturer of propafenone states that the extended-release formulation of the drug should *not* be used concomitantly with class Ia or III antiarrhythmic agents (including quinidine or amiodarone) and that class Ia or III antiarrhythmic agents should be withheld for at least 5 half-lives prior to administration of extended-release propafenone. Experience is limited with the concomitant use of propafenone and class Ib or other class Ic antiarrhythmic agents.

Quinidine Quinidine, even at small doses, completely inhibits the CYP2D6 hydroxylation pathway responsible for propafenone's metabolism; therefore, patients receiving concomitant quinidine and propafenone effectively are rendered poor metabolizers. Propafenone clearance decreased by 60%, plasma steady-state propafenone concentrations increased twofold, and 5-hydroxypropafenone (5-OHP) concentrations were reduced by approximately 50%, in patients with the extensive-metabolizer phenotype who received concomitant quinidine (50 mg 3 times daily) and propafenone as the immediate-release formulation (150 mg every 8 hours); steady-state plasma propafenone concentrations increased threefold in such patients who received concomitant quinidine at a dosage of 100 mg every 8 hours. Poor metabolizers receiving the 2 drugs concomitantly did not exhibit changes in plasma concentrations of propafenone or 5-OHP.

In a limited number of patients with ventricular arrhythmias refractory to procainamide or quinidine monotherapy, combined therapy with propafenone and quinidine or procainamide resulted in a substantial reduction in the frequency of ventricular premature complexes (VPCs) compared with drug-free baseline VPC frequencies. VPC frequency was reduced from a baseline geometric mean of 406/hour before treatment to 33/hour in patients receiving concomitant propafenone/quinidine therapy and from a baseline geometric mean of 211/hour to 27/hour in patients receiving concomitant propafenone/procainamide.

The manufacturer states that the concomitant use of propafenone and quinidine is not recommended; however, some clinicians have suggested that such combined therapy may be useful in selected patients.

Mexiletine Combined therapy with propafenone and mexiletine was effective in preventing the induction of ventricular tachycardia by programmed electrical stimulation in 3 of 16 patients with refractory sustained ventricular tachycardia; however, ventricular tachycardia with hemodynamic deterioration requiring defibrillation occurred in 5 patients (31%) receiving propafenone alone and 2 patients (13%) receiving propafenone and mexiletine. Additional data are needed to determine whether the observed benefit from combined therapy is attributable to potential synergism of the electrophysiologic effects of the 2 drugs or to alterations in hepatic metabolism of the drug(s), resulting in increased plasma concentrations of one or both drugs and decreased plasma concentrations of drug metabolites.

Lidocaine In patients with ventricular arrhythmias who received propafenone and lidocaine concomitantly by IV infusion, the negative inotropic effect of propafenone was increased and the effect of propafenone in prolonging atrial and ventricular refractoriness was attenuated. Although propafenone and lidocaine have been used concomitantly without notable effect on the pharmacokinetics of either drug, an increased risk of lidocaine-related adverse effects involving the central nervous system has been reported in patients receiving such concomitant therapy.

Other Antiarrhythmic Agents Sotalol or amiodarone reportedly may enhance the antiarrhythmic effect of propafenone. However, prolongation of the QT interval and atypical ventricular tachycardia (torsades de pointes) have been reported rarely in patients receiving concomitant propafenone and amiodarone therapy. Concomitant use of propafenone and amiodarone may affect cardiac conduction and repolarization. The manufacturer of propafenone states that concomitant use of propafenone and amiodarone is not recommended.

■ **Other Drugs That Prolong QT Interval** Although specific pharmacokinetic drug interaction studies are not available, the manufacturer of propafenone states that the drug should *not* be used concomitantly with other drugs that prolong the QT interval, including certain phenothiazines, cisapride, bepridil (not currently commercially available in the US), tricyclic antidepressant agents, or macrolides.

■ **Ritonavir** Although specific pharmacokinetic drug interaction studies are not available, the manufacturer of ritonavir states that ritonavir should *not* be used concomitantly with certain cardiovascular agents, including propafenone, because of the potential for substantially increased plasma concentrations of these cardiovascular drugs and potentially serious and/or life-threatening adverse effects. (See Cautions: Precautions and Contraindications, in Ritonavir 8:18.08.08.) This pharmacokinetic interaction may occur because ritonavir has high affinity for several cytochrome P-450 (CYP) isoenzymes (e.g., CYP3A, CYP2D6, CYP1A2) involved in propafenone metabolism. (See Drug Interactions in Ritonavir 8:18.08.08.)

■ **Local Anesthetic Agents** The manufacturer states that concomitant use of propafenone and local anesthetic agents (i.e., during pacemaker implantation, surgery, or dental procedures) may increase the risk of adverse nervous system effects.

■ **Warfarin** Concomitant administration of propafenone and warfarin results in increased plasma warfarin concentrations and corresponding increases in prothrombin times (PTs), possibly because of competition for a common metabolic pathway. Steady-state plasma warfarin concentrations and PTs increased an average of 39 and 25%, respectively, in a limited number of healthy individuals receiving concomitant propafenone and warfarin therapy. PTs or international normalized ratios (INRs) should be monitored closely and, if required, adjustments in warfarin dosage should be made in patients receiving concurrent propafenone and warfarin therapy.

■ **Cimetidine** In a limited number of healthy individuals receiving concomitant propafenone and cimetidine therapy, steady-state plasma propafenone concentrations averaged 20% higher than those with propafenone therapy alone.

■ **Theophylline** Increased serum theophylline concentrations have been reported in patients receiving theophylline concomitantly with propafenone and some clinicians suggest that serum theophylline concentrations and ECGs be monitored closely in patients receiving such combined therapy.

■ **Rifampin** Rifampin may increase the metabolism of concomitant propafenone; reductions in plasma propafenone concentrations and decreased antiarrhythmic efficacy have been reported in patients receiving these drugs concomitantly. Plasma propafenone concentrations decreased 67%, 5-OHP concentrations were reduced by 65%, and *N*-depropylpropafenone (NDPP) concentrations were increased by 35% in patients with the extensive-metabolizer phenotype who received concomitant propafenone and rifampin. Plasma propafenone concentrations decreased 50%, NDPP exposure and peak plasma concentration increased by 74 and 20%, respectively, and urinary excretion of propafenone, 5-OHP, and NDPP was reduced in patients with the poor-metabolizer phenotype who received such concomitant therapy. Propafenone exposure and peak plasma concentration both decreased by 84% and 5-OHP exposure and peak plasma concentration decreased by 69 and 57% in elderly patients with the poor-metabolizer phenotype who received concomitant propafenone and rifampin.

■ **Phenobarbital** Concomitant therapy with phenobarbital and propafenone reportedly may increase the clearance of propafenone, resulting in decreased plasma propafenone concentrations.

■ **Fluoxetine** Concomitant therapy with fluoxetine and propafenone in patients with the extensive-metabolizer phenotype increased the peak plasma concentrations and area under the plasma concentration-time curve (AUC) of the *S*-enantiomer by 39 and 59%, respectively, and the peak plasma concentrations and AUC of the *R*-enantiomer by 71 and 50%, respectively.

■ **Orlistat** Orlistat may limit absorption of propafenone during concomitant therapy with the drugs. There have been postmarketing reports of severe adverse effects, including seizures, atrioventricular block, and acute circulatory failure that occurred following abrupt discontinuance of orlistat in patients receiving chronic propafenone therapy.

■ **Other Drugs** Increases in blood cyclosporine or serum desipramine concentrations have been reported during concomitant administration of propafenone.

The manufacturer states that clinical experience in patients receiving propafenone concomitantly with calcium-channel blocking agents or diuretics has not revealed evidence of clinically important adverse interactions.

Acute Toxicity

Limited information is available on the acute toxicity of propafenone.

■ **Manifestations** In general, overdosage of propafenone may be expected to produce effects that are extensions of the drug's pharmacologic effects, particularly those involving cardiac conduction and function and the CNS. Overdosage of propafenone may result in nausea and/or vomiting, hypotension, somnolence, intra-atrial and intraventricular conduction disturbances, and high-grade ventricular arrhythmias; fatalities also have occurred. Cardiac manifestations may occur within 30–120 minutes after ingestion. Manifestations of overdosage generally are most severe during the 3 hours following the overdose. Nausea generally is the first manifestation of toxicity and may occur within 30 minutes of ingestion of the drug.

■ **Treatment** Effective management of propafenone overdosage requires early diagnosis and prompt detoxification, since no specific antidote is available and resuscitative measures (e.g., external cardiac massage, assisted mechanical ventilation) and supportive measures (e.g., pacemaker placement, cardiopulmonary bypass) may be of limited benefit. Some clinicians state that any adult or pediatric patient who has ingested a propafenone hydrochloride dose exceeding 1 g or exceeding 600 mg/m^2, respectively, should be admitted to intensive care and monitored closely for 24 hours. If ingestion of the drug is recent, emesis or gastric lavage with at least 30 g of activated charcoal may reduce absorption. Some experts recommend insertion of a transvenous pacemaker prior to gastric lavage, since vagal stimulation associated with such lavage may induce bradycardia. Defibrillation and IV infusion of dopamine and isoproterenol have been used successfully to restore normal cardiac rhythm and blood pressure, while IV diazepam has been used to control seizures. Limited data suggest that alkalinization with IV sodium lactate and potassium chloride may be of benefit in propafenone overdosage. IV infusion of small amounts of a concentrated (20%) sodium chloride injection reportedly has been used successfully in a patient with propafenone overdosage unresponsive to hemoperfusion.

Hemodialysis is probably of no value in enhancing elimination of propafenone hydrochloride since the drug is highly bound to plasma proteins and has a large volume of distribution.

Pharmacology

■ **Antiarrhythmic and Electrophysiologic Effects** Propafenone hydrochloride is a local anesthetic-type antiarrhythmic agent. Studies in animals have demonstrated the effectiveness of propafenone in preventing and/or suppressing experimentally induced arrhythmias.

Propafenone is considered a class I (membrane stabilizing) antiarrhythmic agent, although the antiarrhythmic and electrophysiologic actions of the drug are complex in that it also has demonstrated some β-adrenergic blocking and calcium-channel blocking activity. Like encainide and flecainide, the principal effect of propafenone on cardiac tissue appears to be a concentration-dependent inhibition of the transmembrane influx of extracellular sodium ions via fast sodium channels, as indicated by a decrease in the maximal rate of depolarization of phase 0 of the action potential and a shift of the membrane-responsiveness curve in the hyperpolarizing direction. Since this effect is greater at higher stimulation frequencies and less negative membrane potentials, the drug's sodium blockade is enhanced in ischemic cardiac tissue. Studies in cardiac tissue in animals indicate that propafenone binds to fast sodium channels in both their active and inactive states; the drug thereby inhibits recovery after repolarization in a time- and voltage-dependent manner, which is associated with subsequent dissociation of the drug from the sodium channels. Propafenone induces phasic (frequency-dependent) sodium channel blockade faster than encainide or flecainide, while recovery is similar to flecainide and faster than encainide. Propafenone also appears to have a slight inhibitory effect (approximately 1/75 the potency of verapamil) on the transmembrane influx of extracellular calcium ions via slow calcium channels (calcium-channel blocking effect), but this effect generally occurs only at high drug concentrations and probably does not contribute to antiarrhythmic efficacy. Propafenone has no vagomimetic or vagolytic effect on cardiac muscle.

Propafenone exhibits electrophysiologic effects characteristic of class Ic antiarrhythmic agents, with local anesthetic effects and a direct stabilizing action on myocardial membranes. The electrophysiologic characteristics of the subgroups of class I antiarrhythmic agents may be related to quantitative differences in their rates of attachment to and dissociation from transmembrane sodium channels, with class Ic agents exhibiting slow rates of attachment and dissociation. Propafenone decreases the amplitude and maximal rate of rise (phase 0) of the action potential in a concentration-dependent manner and has little or no effect on resting potential. Like other class Ic antiarrhythmic agents, propafenone slows intracardiac conduction at low concentrations, has relatively minimal effects on refractoriness, and generally has little effect on repolarization. The drug increases action potential duration (APD) in the sinus node and ventricular myocytes and decreases APD in Purkinje fibers. Propafenone decreases cardiac excitability in diastole by increasing the threshold potential for electrical excitation and prolonging the effective refractory period in the atria, AV node, and, to a lesser extent, the ventricles. The effective refractory period in accessory pathways also is prolonged, and both anterograde and retrograde conduction are decreased by the drug. The electrophysiologic effects of propafenone in ischemic cardiac tissue are qualitatively similar to those in healthy cardiac tissue but are more marked; increases in action potential amplitude and refractoriness and decreases in conduction velocity have been attributed to the voltage-dependent sodium channel blockade produced by the drug. This differential activity in ischemic versus healthy cardiac tissue may contribute to propafenone's antiarrhythmic action in ischemic heart disease.

The antiarrhythmic and electrophysiologic effects of propafenone result from the parent drug and its 2 major metabolites, 5-hydroxypropafenone (5-OHP) and *N*-depropylpropafenone (NDPP). (See Pharmacokinetics.) Concentrations and relative proportions of propafenone and its metabolites attained in plasma vary considerably depending on the patient's genetically determined ability to metabolize the drug, dosage, and duration of drug administration. Consequently, the observed effects of propafenone are a somewhat complex aggregate that depends on the relative proportions and serum concentrations of parent drug and metabolites. Following acute IV administration (IV dosage form currently not commercially available in the US), antiarrhythmic and electrophysiologic effects appear to result principally from propafenone regardless of the patient's metabolizer phenotype; however, following long-term oral administration, these effects appear to result principally from propafenone and 5-OHP in patients with the extensive-metabolizer phenotype and principally from propafenone in patients with the poor-metabolizer phenotype.

Effects on Cardiac Conduction and Refractoriness Propafenone and its metabolites produce a dose-related decrease in intracardiac conduction within the His-Purkinje system, atrioventricular (AV) node, and intraventricular pathways. The effects of the drug on conduction are manifested by dose-related increases in PR, QRS, AH, and HV intervals; at higher workload and heart rates, dose-related increases in QT interval also occur. PR interval increased about 11–28% with oral propafenone hydrochloride dosages of 450–1200 mg daily (immediate-release tablets), while QRS duration was prolonged from 8–32% after 1 or 2 IV doses of 1–2 mg/kg or oral dosages of 450–1200 mg daily (immediate-release tablets). Increases in mean PR interval of 9–21 msec, mean QRS duration of 4–6 msec, and the mean QT interval corrected for rate (QT_c) of 2–6 msec were observed with oral propafenone hydrochloride dosages of 500–850 mg daily as extended-release capsules. The range of maximum increases in the QT_c observed were greater than 20, 10–20, or 10% or less compared to baseline in 1–5, 16–26, or 72–83%, respectively, of patients receiving oral propafenone hydrochloride dosages of 500–850 mg daily as extended-release capsules. Effects on PR and QRS intervals (prolongation) were maintained for up to 2 years in patients receiving propafenone hydrochloride 600–900 mg daily (immediate-release tablets). Increases in AH and HV intervals of about 16–32% and up to 67% or less, respectively, were observed with dosages of 900–1200 mg daily (immediate-release tablets). Conduction slowing was greatest in patients with prolonged baseline HV intervals. 5-OHP further prolongs QRS duration and, to a lesser degree, PR interval.

Propafenone also prolongs atrial and ventricular refractoriness. Increases of approximately 17% in ventricular effective refractory period (ERP) during ventricular pacing have been reported with a propafenone hydrochloride dosage of 900 mg daily. In patients with recurrent ventricular tachycardia receiving 2 mg/kg of propafenone hydrochloride IV, atrial and AV nodal ERP were prolonged. Ventricular repolarization as determined by the QT interval corrected for rate (QT_c) has been reported to be increased by 7–15% or unaffected. The JT_c interval (QT_c-QRS interval) does not appear to be affected by propafenone.

Effects on Sinus Node Propafenone appears to have minimal effects on normal sinus node function, although some depression of function may occur. Sinus node recovery time, sinus cycle length, sinus node automaticity, and sinoatrial conduction time may increase or remain unaffected. Sinus cycle length generally is unchanged by propafenone; however, an 8% decrease in sinus cycle length was observed in children with recurrent paroxysmal supraventricular tachycardia (PSVT) receiving propafenone hydrochloride 1.5 mg/kg IV over 3 minutes. In patients with ventricular tachycardia, propafenone may have a depressant effect on sinus node function; sinus node recovery time increased by approximately 0.2 seconds in such patients receiving usual dosages of the drug.

Effects on Dual AV Nodal and Anomalous AV Pathways In patients with Wolff-Parkinson-White (WPW) syndrome or dual AV nodal pathways, propafenone decreases conduction and increases the refractoriness of anterograde and retrograde accessory pathways; complete block of the anterograde accessory pathway may result.

■ **Arrhythmogenic Effects** Like other antiarrhythmic agents, propafenone can worsen existing arrhythmias or cause new arrhythmias. (See Cautions: Arrhythmogenic Effects.) The arrhythmogenic effects of the drug may range from an increased frequency of ventricular premature complexes (VPCs) to the development of more severe and potentially fatal ventricular tachyarrhythmias. The exact mechanism(s) by which various antiarrhythmic agents, including propafenone, produce arrhythmogenic effects has not been fully determined, but the arrhythmogenic potential of propafenone may be related to its effects on conduction. The risk of arrhythmogenesis during propafenone therapy appears to correlate directly with the severity of the presenting arrhythmia and the degree of ventricular dysfunction, if present.

■ **Cardiovascular Effects** ***Inotropic Effects*** Propafenone exhibits a dose-dependent negative inotropic effect. The exact mechanism of the drug's negative inotropic effect has not been determined but may involve blockade of sodium channels as well as β-adrenergic receptors and/or, at high concentrations, calcium-channel blockade. Both propafenone and 5-OHP exhibit negative inotropic effects at high concentrations in vitro and, in large doses, have depressed left ventricular function in animals. The negative inotropic effect and other cardiovascular effects of propafenone may be more pronounced and clinically important in patients with coronary artery disease, acute myocardial infarction, congestive heart failure, or myocardial dysfunction. (See Cautions: Cardiovascular Effects.) However, conflicting data have been reported regarding the depressant effects of propafenone on left ventricular function, and reductions in left ventricular ejection fraction (LVEF) with oral propafenone therapy may be less than that with flecainide or disopyramide. No appreciable effects of propafenone on LVEF were observed in a study in patients with ventricular arrhythmias who had baseline LVEFs less than 40%. However, in another study, patients with baseline LVEFs less than 50% had reductions of 20–26% in LVEF with propafenone therapy compared with reductions of only 4–8% in patients who had no preexisting impairment in LVEF. Reductions in left ventricular function as measured by peak flow velocity have been observed in patients with ventricular arrhythmias receiving propafenone, but left ventricular ejection time was not affected. Increases in left ventricular end-systolic and end-diastolic diameter have been reported in patients with impaired left ventricular function receiving the drug. Increases in intracardiac pressure (assessed by measurement of right atrial, pulmonary artery, and pulmonary capillary wedge pressure) manifested as a depression of cardiac index have been reported in some patients receiving IV propafenone but not in others.

β-Adrenergic Blocking Effects Propafenone has β-adrenergic blocking activity in humans about 1–5% that of propranolol on a molar basis. While the clinical importance of propafenone's β-adrenergic blocking activity has not been fully elucidated, clinically important β-adrenergic blocking effects potentially could occur at usual dosages of the drug since long-term therapy may result in steady-state plasma propafenone concentrations 10–50 times greater than those of propranolol. Because plasma propafenone concentrations are high relative to those of propranolol, the functional relative β-adrenergic blocking activity of propafenone may be up to one-fourth the potency of propranolol.

β-Adrenergic blockade associated with propafenone is evidenced by inhibition of the positive inotropic effects of isoproterenol and attenuation of isoproterenol-induced increases in left ventricular pressure, contractile index, heart rate, and carotid arterial pressure. In addition, up-regulation of β_2-adrenergic receptors similar to that observed with nonselective β-adrenergic blocking agents has been reported in patients with symptomatic VPCs receiving 450–900 mg of propafenone hydrochloride daily. The extent of propafenone's β-adrenergic blocking activity may vary with a patient's genetically determined metabolizer phenotype and the differing ratios of parent drug to metabolites. The 2 principal metabolites of propafenone, 5-hydroxypropafenone (5-OHP) and *N*-depropylpropafenone (NDPP), have no clinically relevant β-adrenergic blocking effects at concentrations achieved with usual therapeutic dosages of propafenone. Therefore, in patients whose ability to metabolize the drug into 5-OHP is impaired (i.e., poor metabolizers), plasma concentrations of propafenone are increased, and β-adrenergic blocking effects are more evident, than those in whom the drug is rapidly and extensively metabolized (i.e., extensive metabolizers). Patients with poor-metabolizer phenotypes receiving 450–900 mg of propafenone hydrochloride daily had increased plasma propafenone concentrations and greater attenuation of exercise- and isoproterenol-induced tachycardia than patients with the extensive-metabolizer phenotype.

The β-adrenergic blocking effect of propafenone appears to be stereoselective. The *S*-enantiomer of propafenone possesses 50–100 times greater affinity for β-adrenergic receptors than the *R*-enantiomer and has a dissociation constant (K*i* value) for these receptors about 140 times less than that of the *R*-enantiomer. Although conflicting data exist regarding the effects of propafenone on heart rate and blood pressure, decreases of 4–5% in systolic blood pressure consistent with a negative inotropic or a peripheral vasodilatory effect have been reported in healthy individuals after oral or IV administration of *S*-propafenone or a racemic mixture of the drug, but not with the *R*-enantiomer.

Chronotropic Effects Following oral or IV administration of propafenone, heart rate may be reduced or unchanged. Propafenone's effect on heart rate varies at least in part according to evaluative conditions; sinus rate generally is unaffected at usual dosages in patients with arrhythmias, but decreases in heart rate have been reported in patients receiving such dosages during exercise. Propafenone-induced decreases in diurnal and nocturnal heart rate of 14–31 and 6.3–8.3%, respectively, have been reported; however, the normal circadian variation in heart rate was not affected. Propafenone-induced bradycardia is associated with high plasma drug concentrations and may be related to the patient's metabolizer phenotype; patients with the poor-metabolizer phenotype develop bradycardia more frequently than those with the extensive-metabolizer phenotype. The bradycardic effect appears to be attributable only to the parent drug.

■ **Local Anesthetic Effects** Propafenone exhibits a local anesthetic action approximately equal to that of procaine (no longer commercially available in the US).

Pharmacokinetics

■ **Absorption** Propafenone hydrochloride (immediate-release tablets) is rapidly and almost completely absorbed from the GI tract following oral administration. The absolute bioavailability averages approximately 5–50% for propafenone immediate-release tablets and has not been determined for extended-release capsules. The absolute bioavailability of propafenone depends principally on a patient's genetically determined ability to metabolize the drug. (See Pharmacokinetics: Elimination.) In most patients (those with the extensive-metabolizer phenotype), propafenone is metabolized extensively and undergoes first-pass metabolism in the liver, producing the 2 major, active metabolites 5-hydroxypropafenone (5-OHP) and *N*-depropylpropafenone (NDPP). In these patients, the absolute bioavailability of propafenone is dependent on dosage and dosage form; 150- and 300-mg immediate-release tablets of propafenone hydrochloride had absolute bioavailabilities of 3.4 and 10.6%, respectively, while a more rapidly absorbed solution of propafenone hydrochloride 3.5 mg/mL had an absolute bioavailability of 21.4%. In patients with the extensive-metabolizer phenotype, the drug exhibits nonlinear pharmacokinetics: a threefold increase in propafenone hydrochloride dosage (300 versus 900 mg as immediate-release tablets) results in a 10-fold increase in steady-state plasma concentration, while in a small fraction of patients (those with the poor-metabolizer phenotype or those receiving concurrent quinidine) (see Antiarrhythmic Agents: Quinidine, in Drug Interactions) propafenone exhibits linear pharmacokinetics, and 5-OHP is not formed or only minimally formed because the drug undergoes little or no first-pass metabolism. The nonlinear pharmacokinetics observed in patients with the extensive-metabolizer phenotype has been attributed to the saturation of the hydroxylation pathway.

Although the rate and extent of propafenone absorption were increased (bioavailability was increased by an average of 147%) when the drug was administered with food in a single-dose study in healthy individuals, the manufacturer states that bioavailability of the drug is not appreciably affected by food during multiple-dose administration of immediate-release tablets. Propafenone exposure was increased 4-fold when a single 425-mg extended-release capsule was administered with food in healthy individuals; however, the bioavailability of the drug is not appreciably affected by food during multiple-dose administration (425-mg extended-release capsules twice daily).

Bioavailability of propafenone is increased in patients with hepatic impairment (e.g., cirrhosis) and is inversely proportional to indocyanine green clearance. Bioavailability of immediate-release propafenone averages approximately 60–70% in patients with marked hepatic impairment (indocyanine green clearance of 7 mL/minute or less) and 3–40% in patients with normal hepatic function; the relative bioavailability of the extended-release formulation has not been determined.

Peak plasma propafenone concentrations generally occur approximately 2–3.5 hours after oral administration of immediate-release tablets in most individuals. Peak plasma concentration of propafenone after a single 300-mg oral dose of propafenone hydrochloride immediate-release tablets in patients with ventricular arrhythmias averaged 416 ng/mL; peak drug concentrations were 1198 and 1213 ng/mL with a dosage of 900 mg (immediate-release tablets) daily for 1 and 3 months, respectively. Increases in area under the plasma concentration-time curve (AUC) in these patients were similar following single- or multiple-dose drug administration of immediate-release tablets. Following single-dose administration of propafenone immediate-release tablets, the ratio of the AUCs of parent drug to 5-OHP was 0.43; with multiple dosing for 1 or 3 months, the ratio was 0.24 or 0.25, respectively. Peak plasma propafenone concentrations generally occur approximately 3–8 hours after oral administration of extended-release capsules in most individuals.

In healthy individuals, administration of propafenone hydrochloride as a single oral (300- or 450-mg immediate-release tablet) or IV (35–50 mg) dose produced similar peak plasma concentrations of the parent drug (278 versus 295 ng/mL, respectively). However, neither 5-OHP nor NDPP was detectable in plasma after IV administration in these individuals. Since 5-OHP and NDPP has clinically important antiarrhythmic activity, propafenone's effect may differ with oral versus IV administration. Considerable interindividual variation exists in plasma concentrations of propafenone and its metabolites with a given dosage. Peak plasma concentrations of 5-OHP and NDPP average 101–288 and 8–40 ng/mL, respectively, in healthy individuals after administration of a single oral dose (300–450 mg) of propafenone hydrochloride immediate-release tablets. Propafenone, 5-OHP, and NDPP exhibit nonlinear pharmacokinetics in patients with the extensive-metabolizer phenotype, although the pharmacokinetics of 5-OHP and NDPP deviate from linearity only to a small extent. The pharmacokinetic profiles of propafenone, 5-OHP, and NDPP apparently are not affected substantially by age or gender.

The considerable degree of interindividual variability observed in the pharmacokinetics of propafenone in individuals with the extensive-metabolizer phenotype is principally attributable to first-pass hepatic metabolism and non-linear pharmacokinetics. The degree of interindividual variability in propafenone pharmacokinetic parameters is increased following single and multiple dose administration of propafenone hydrochloride extended-release capsules. The fact that interindividual variability in the pharmacokinetics of propafenone appears to be substantially less in individuals with the poor-metabolizer phenotype than in those with the extensive-metabolizer phenotype suggests that such variability may be due to CYP2D6 polymorphism rather than to the formulation.

The pattern of plasma concentrations of propafenone and its metabolites observed in an individual patient with long-term oral propafenone therapy depends principally on the genetically determined metabolizer phenotype and, to a lesser extent, on hepatic blood flow and enzyme function. (See Pharmacokinetics: Elimination.) Following oral administration of propafenone (immediate-release tablets), steady-state plasma concentrations of the parent drug and its metabolites are attained within 4–5 days in individuals with normal hepatic and renal function. Plasma concentrations of 5-OHP and NDPP generally average less than 20% those of propafenone. Poor metabolizers achieve plasma propafenone concentrations 1.5–2 times higher than those of extensive metabolizers at propafenone hydrochloride dosages of 675–900 mg (immediate-release tablets) daily; at lower dosages, poor metabolizers may attain plasma propafenone concentrations more than fivefold higher than those of extensive metabolizers.

In patients with ventricular arrhythmias and the extensive-metabolizer phenotype receiving 337.5, 450, 675, or 900 mg of propafenone hydrochloride daily (immediate-release tablets), the proportions of 5-OHP to propafenone in plasma were 45, 40, 24, or 19%, respectively, while a subset of patients with the poor-metabolizer phenotype had higher relative plasma concentrations of the parent drug at each dosage and no detectable 5-OHP. Ratios of NDPP to propafenone are similar in extensive and poor metabolizers (approximately 10 and 6%, respectively). In poor metabolizers, NDPP is the principal metabolite and 5-OHP may not be detectable. Following oral administration of propafenone hydrochloride 300 mg (immediate-release tablets) every 8 hours for 14 days, plasma propafenone, 5-OHP, and NDPP concentrations averaged 1010, 174, and 179 ng/mL, respectively, in healthy individuals with the extensive-metabolizer phenotype. In an individual presumed to have the poor-metabolizer phenotype, plasma concentrations of propafenone, 5-OHP, and NDPP concentrations were 1048, undetectable, and 219 ng/mL, respectively, following oral administration of immediate-release tablets. Following administration of extended-release capsules of propafenone hydrochloride, plasma concentrations of 5-OHP and NDPP are generally less than 40 and 10% of plasma propafenone concentrations, respectively.

In extensive metabolizers, propafenone bioavailability following administration of extended-release capsules is less than that following administration of the immediate-release tablets; the more gradual release of propafenone from the extended-release formulation results in an increase in the extent of first-pass hepatic metabolism. During relative bioavailability studies, higher daily dosages of propafenone administered as extended-release capsules compared with immediate-release tablets were required to obtain similar exposure to propafenone. The bioavailability of propafenone following 325-mg extended-release capsules given twice daily is similar to 150-mg immediate-release tablets given 3 times daily. Following administration of extended-release capsules, the mean exposure to 5-OHP was approximately 20-25% higher compared with such exposure following immediate-release tablets.

Because propafenone, 5-OHP, and NDPP are pharmacologically active and plasma concentrations of the parent drug and these metabolites vary considerably depending on the patient's metabolizer phenotype, duration of drug administration, and dosage formulation relationships between plasma concentrations of propafenone and/or its metabolites and antiarrhythmic and electrophysiologic effects are complex. (See Pharmacology: Antiarrhythmic and Electrophysiologic Effects.) Limited data suggest that in patients with the extensive-metabolizer phenotype, the antiarrhythmic and electrophysiologic effects are correlated principally with plasma concentrations of unchanged propafenone and 5-OHP. In patients with the poor-metabolizer phenotype, the antiarrhythmic and electrophysiologic effects appear to be correlated with plasma concentrations of unchanged propafenone. In a study in patients with chronic ventricular arrhythmias, plasma propafenone concentrations of 250–490 ng/mL were associated with at least 90% suppression of ventricular premature complexes (VPCs), ventricular coupled beats, and nonsustained ventricular tachycardia in 47, 70, and 78% of patients, respectively; propafenone concentrations of 1500 ng/mL or higher produced at least 90% suppression of VPCs, ventricular coupled beats, and nonsustained ventricular tachycardia in 67, 83, and 100% of patients, respectively.

Following long-term administration of 850 mg of propafenone hydrochloride daily as extended-release capsules, plasma concentrations of propafenone in individuals with the poor-metabolizer phenotype was approximately twice that observed in individuals with the extensive-metabolizer phenotype. Following lower daily dosages of propafenone hydrochloride as extended-release capsules, the difference in plasma concentrations of propafenone is larger between the metabolizer phenotypes; plasma concentrations of propafenone in individuals with the poor-metabolizer phenotype are approximately 3–4 times higher than those observed in individuals with the extensive-metabolizer phenotype. Following saturation of the hydroxylation pathway (CYP2D6) in individuals with the extensive-metabolizer phenotypes, plasma propafenone concentrations increase at a greater-than-linear rate after administration of extended-release capsules of propafenone hydrochloride. In individuals with the poor-metabolizer phenotype, propafenone exhibits linear pharmacokinetics.

Despite the complex nature of the contribution of propafenone and its metabolites to clinical response in individual patients, clinical response generally is related to dosage and the usually effective dosages in patients with the poor- or extensive-metabolizer phenotype are comparable. (See Dosage and Administration: Dosage.) This recommendation is based on consideration of propafenone pharmacokinetics including the fact that differences in pharmacokinetics between metabolizer phenotypes decrease as dosage is increased, mitigation by the lack of the active 5-OHP metabolite in individuals with the poor-metabolizer phenotype, and the fact that steady-state occurs following 4–5 days of therapy in all patients. However, plasma concentrations of the drug may increase disproportionately during dosage titration in patients with the poor-metabolizer phenotype, resulting in an increased occurrence of adverse effects, especially CNS effects (e.g., dizziness, blurred vision, taste disturbances).

Limited data suggest that a partial tolerance to the antiarrhythmic effects of propafenone may develop during long-term therapy so that higher plasma concentrations are required to produce equivalent effects.

A relationship between plasma concentrations of propafenone or its metabolites and arrhythmogenic effects has not been established. (See Cautions: Arrhythmogenic Effects.)

■ Distribution Distribution of propafenone and its metabolites into human body tissues and fluids has not been fully characterized. Propafenone is highly lipophilic and rapidly distributed into lung, liver, and heart tissue. The apparent volume of distribution of propafenone averages 3 L/kg (range: 2.5–4 L/kg). In patients receiving propafenone who underwent heart surgery, 5-OHP was detected in higher concentrations in right atrial tissue than in plasma, and ratios of parent drug to metabolites were lower in plasma than in atrial tissue (1.7 versus 3.9, respectively).

The degree of protein binding of propafenone is concentration dependent. In healthy individuals, 81–97% of propafenone is bound in vitro to plasma proteins at plasma propafenone concentrations of 0.25–100 mcg/mL, while protein binding averages 96% at plasma propafenone concentrations of 0.5–2 mcg/mL. Most propafenone in plasma is bound to α_1-acid glycoprotein and a lesser extent to albumin.

In patients with severe hepatic dysfunction, approximately 88% of propafenone is bound in vitro to plasma proteins.

Propafenone and 5-OHP cross the placenta and are distributed into milk. (See Cautions: Pregnancy, Fertility, and Lactation.)

■ Elimination There are two principal patterns of propafenone metabolism. These patterns are genetically determined by an individual's ability to metabolize the drug via a hepatic oxidation pathway. The ability to oxidatively metabolize propafenone is dependent on an individual's ability to metabolize debrisoquin (debrisoquin phenotype). The debrisoquin phenotype or the observed pattern of propafenone metabolites may be used to determine an individual's metabolic phenotype for propafenone. Individuals who extensively metabolize propafenone via the oxidation pathway exhibit the extensive-metabolizer phenotype, while those who have an impaired ability to metabolize the drug by this pathway exhibit the poor-metabolizer phenotype. Approximately 90–95% of Caucasians exhibit the extensive-metabolizer phenotype, with the remainder being poor metabolizers. Propafenone metabolism in patients with the poor-metabolizer phenotype is characterized by a linear dose-concentration relationship and a relatively long terminal elimination half-life; these individuals have increased plasma propafenone concentrations relative to individuals with the extensive-metabolizer phenotype and are more likely to experience β-adrenergic blocking and adverse effects of the drug.

Following single or multiple oral doses of immediate-release tablets in adults with the extensive-metabolizer phenotype and normal renal and hepatic function, the elimination half-life of propafenone averages about 1–3 hours (range: 2–10 hours). The half-life of propafenone averages approximately 8–13 hours (range: 6–36 hours) in adults with the poor-metabolizer phenotype. Following a single oral dose of 300 mg of propafenone hydrochloride as immediate-release tablets, a half-life of 3.5 hours was reported; after administration of 300 mg of propafenone hydrochloride daily for 1 and 3 months, the reported half-lives were 6.7 and 5.8 hours, respectively. Steady-state plasma elimination half-life of propafenone is prolonged in poor metabolizers, averaging 17.2 hours (range: 10–32 hours) compared with 5.5 hours (range: 2–10 hours) in extensive metabolizers.

In individuals with the extensive-metabolizer phenotype, propafenone is metabolized in the liver to 2 active metabolites and at least 9 additional metabolites. The 2 active metabolites, 5-hydroxypropafenone (5-OHP) and *N*-depropylpropafenone (NDPP), are formed through hydroxylation and dealkylation of the parent drug. Propafenone hydroxylation via cytochrome CYP2D6, a cytochrome P-450 isoenzyme under genetic control, produces 5-OHP. Formation of NDPP is catalyzed by different isoenzymes, cytochrome CYP1A2 and CYP3A4. Differences in metabolism between *R*- and *S*-propafenone related to stereoselective interaction with the CYP2D6 isoenzyme have been observed in animals and humans receiving single enantiomers of the drug. Following a 250-mg oral dose of *R*- or *S*-propafenone hydrochloride administered to adults with the extensive-metabolizer phenotype, the mean values for elimination half-life, clearance, and volume of distribution for *R*-propafenone were smaller than those for *S*-propafenone, while AUC was larger; however, these stereospecific effects were not observed in an adult with the poor-metabolizer phenotype who received the separate drug enantiomers. In vitro and in vivo studies indicate that the *R*-enantiomer is cleared faster than the *S*-enantiomer via the 5-hydroxylation pathway (CYP2D6). This results in a higher ratio of the *S*-enantiomer to *R*-enantiomer at steady state. Although the enantiomers have equivalent sodium-channel blocking potency, the *S*-enantiomer is a more potent β-adrenergic antagonist than the *R*-enantiomer. Following administration of propafenone hydrochloride (immediate-release tablets or extended-release capsules), the observed ratio of *S*-enantiomer to *R*-enantiomer (*S/R* ratio) for AUC was approximately 1.7. The *S/R* ratios after administration of 225-, 325-, or 425-mg extended-release capsules were independent of dose. In addition, similar *S/R* ratios were observed among metabolizer genotypes and following long-term administration.

When racemic propafenone is administered, some data indicate that metabolic inhibition between the enantiomers appears to result in reversal of these enantiomer-dependent pharmacokinetic differences. In patients with extensive or poor metabolizer phenotypes receiving propafenone hydrochloride 450 mg daily (immediate-release tablets), the clearance of *R*-propafenone was approximately 1.7 times that of the *S*-enantiomer, and the AUC was smaller for *R*-propafenone regardless of metabolizer phenotype. In adults with the poor-metabolizer phenotype, the clearance of both enantiomers is reduced; however, the clearance of the *R*-enantiomer still exceeds that of the *S*-enantiomer.

Although conflicting data exist, clearance of propafenone appears to be reduced during long-term administration, presumably as a result of reduced hepatic metabolism. Increases in steady-state bioavailability, elimination half-life, and peak plasma concentration have been reported following oral administration of propafenone hydrochloride (150–300 mg as immediate-release tablets 3 times daily) for 5–30 days compared with these values after single-dose administration, suggesting a reduction in propafenone clearance during chronic dosing. However, the minimum plasma propafenone concentration required for antiarrhythmic efficacy also has been reported to increase with long-term therapy, suggesting the development of partial tolerance to the drug. (See Pharmacokinetics: Absorption.)

Propafenone clearance directly correlates with hepatic function as indicated by indocyanine green clearance, prothrombin time, and serum concentrations of albumin, total bilirubin, and AST (SGOT). The drug's terminal elimination half-life is increased to approximately 9 hours in patients with moderate to severe hepatic impairment (e.g., cirrhosis).

The volume of distribution, clearance, and elimination half-life of propafenone were similar in healthy individuals, patients undergoing hemodialysis, and those with moderate renal impairment (mean creatinine clearance: about 40 mL/minute per 1.73 m^2) receiving a single IV dose of the drug. Propafenone is not removed by hemodialysis.

Limited data indicate that mean interdose plasma propafenone concentrations in patients with the extensive-metabolizer phenotype and renal impairment receiving maintenance therapy with oral propafenone hydrochloride 450 mg daily (immediate-release tablets) may be decreased slightly compared with those in healthy individuals with normal renal function. However, steady-state concentrations of 5-OHP were decreased, and those of NDDP were increased, in patients with the extensive-metabolizer phenotype and renal impairment compared with those concentrations in healthy individuals with normal renal function. In another study, impaired renal function did not alter plasma concentrations of propafenone or 5-OHP at steady state in patients receiving 600 mg of propafenone hydrochloride (immediate-release tablets) daily for 4 days. The disposition of propafenone hydrochloride after administration of a single IV dose (70 mg) was similar in a limited number of patients with renal impairment (mean creatinine clearance: 0.66 mL/minute per 1.73 m^2) or renal failure compared with those with normal renal function (mean creatinine clearance: 1.43 mL/minute per 1.73 m^2). More data from long-term studies are needed to determine the effect of decreased renal function on the pharmacokinetics of propafenone.

Less than 1% of a dose of propafenone is excreted unchanged in urine or feces following oral administration of the drug; metabolites are mainly excreted in feces via biliary elimination. Urinary excretion of propafenone and its metabolites in patients with the extensive-metabolizer phenotype and cirrhosis generally is similar to that in healthy individuals with the same metabolizer phenotype, although the fraction of the dose excreted as unchanged drug is increased substantially and some NDDP also is excreted.

Chemistry and Stability

■ **Chemistry** Propafenone hydrochloride is a local anesthetic-type antiarrhythmic agent. Propafenone is structurally related to other class Ic antiarrhythmic drugs and also to β-adrenergic blocking agents (e.g., propranolol); both propafenone and β-adrenergic blocking agents contain an aromatic ring joined by a methylenenoxy bridge to the asymmetric carbon atom of *N*-substituted hydroxyethylamine.

Propafenone hydrochloride is commercially available as a racemic mixture. While limited data suggest that the *R*- and *S*-enantiomers of the drug have similar antiarrhythmic activity, only the *S*-isomer exerts a β-adrenergic blocking effect. (See Pharmacology.)

Propafenone hydrochloride occurs as a white crystalline powder or as colorless crystals and is slightly soluble in water and alcohol, having solubilities of 5 mg/mL in water and 11 mg/mL in alcohol. The drug has a pK_a of 9.

■ **Stability** Commercially available propafenone hydrochloride immediate-release tablets and extended-release capsules should be stored in tight containers at a controlled room temperature of 25°C, but may be exposed to temperatures ranging from 15–30°C. Propafenone hydrochloride immediate-release tablets should be stored in light-resistant containers. When stored under such conditions, the commercially available immediate-release tablets have an expiration date of 3 years following the date of manufacture.

Preparations

Excipients in commercially available drug preparations may have clinically important effects in some individuals; consult specific product labeling for details.

Propafenone Hydrochloride

Oral		
Capsules, extended-release	225 mg	**Rythmol®SR**, Reliant
	325 mg	**Rythmol®SR**, Reliant
	425 mg	**Rythmol®SR**, Reliant
Tablets, film-coated	150 mg*	**Propafenone Hydrochloride Tablets**
		Rythmol® (scored), Reliant
	225 mg*	**Propafenone Hydrochloride Tablets**
		Rythmol® (scored), Reliant
	300 mg*	**Propafenone Hydrochloride Tablets**
		Rythmol® (scored), Reliant

*available from one or more manufacturer, distributor, and/or repackager by generic (nonproprietary) name

†Use is not currently included in the labeling approved by the US Food and Drug Administration

Selected Revisions November 2016,

CLASS III ANTIARRHYTHMICS 24:04.04.20

Amiodarone Hydrochloride

■ Amiodarone hydrochloride is considered to be predominantly a class III antiarrhythmic agent, but the drug also appears to exhibit activity in each of the 4 Vaughn-Williams antiarrhythmic classes, including some class I (membrane-stabilizing) antiarrhythmic action.

Uses

Amiodarone appears to be effective in the management of a wide variety of ventricular as well as supraventricular arrhythmias†. Because of amiodarone's potentially life-threatening adverse effects and the management difficulties associated with its use, the drug previously was not considered a first-line antiarrhythmic but generally was reserved for use in life-threatening ventricular arrhythmias. The drug also was used infrequently for the suppression or prevention of any type of arrhythmia and only when conventional antiarrhythmic therapy was considered ineffective or was not tolerated. However, amiodarone generally appears to exhibit greater efficacy and a lower incidence of proarrhythmic effects than class I or other class III antiarrhythmic drugs and therefore has become a mainstay in the management of various tachyarrhythmias, including expert recommendations for advanced cardiovascular life support (ACLS), despite labeling that continues to recommend more limited use. In addition, although no antiarrhythmic agent given routinely during cardiac arrest has been shown to increase survival to hospital discharge, amiodarone has been shown to increase short-term survival to hospital admission relative to lidocaine or placebo. Amiodarone should be used only by clinicians who are familiar with and have access to, either directly or through referral, the use of all currently available modalities for the management of recurrent life-threatening ventricular arrhythmias and who have access to appropriate evaluative and monitoring procedures, including continuous ECG monitoring and electrophysiologic techniques for evaluating the patient in both ambulatory and hospital settings.

■ **Ventricular Arrhythmias** Amiodarone is used orally or IV to suppress and prevent the recurrence of documented life-threatening ventricular arrhythmias (recurrent ventricular fibrillation and recurrent, hemodynamically unstable ventricular tachycardia) that do not respond to documented adequate dosages of other currently available antiarrhythmic agents or when alternative antiarrhythmic agents are not tolerated. Amiodarone is designated an orphan drug by the FDA for use in this condition. Amiodarone may be used IV to treat patients with ventricular tachycardia or fibrillation in whom oral amiodarone therapy is indicated, but who are unable to take oral medication.

It is difficult to assess the overall efficacy of amiodarone since response to the drug depends on many factors, including the specific cardiac arrhythmia being treated, the criteria used to evaluate efficacy, the presence of underlying cardiac disease in the patient, the number of antiarrhythmic agents used prior to amiodarone, the duration of follow-up, and the concomitant use of other antiarrhythmic agents. In addition, overall arrhythmia recurrence rates (fatal and nonfatal) appear to be highly variable and depend on many factors, including response to programmed electrical stimulation (PES) or other measures, and whether patients who do not appear to respond initially are included. When considering only those patients who responded well enough to amiodarone to be placed on long-term treatment, ventricular arrhythmia recurrence rates have ranged from 20–40% in most studies having an average follow-up period of 1 year or longer.

Life-Threatening Ventricular Arrhythmias and Advanced Cardiovascular Life Support There is relatively limited experience from controlled studies with the use of amiodarone for suppression and prevention of recurrent life-threatening ventricular arrhythmias. Although comparative data are lacking, the efficacy of amiodarone in the management of severe refractory arrhythmias generally is considered to be at least comparable to and probably better than that of other antiarrhythmic agents (e.g., quinidine, procainamide). Data from most clinical studies indicate that the drug is effective in approximately 50–80% of patients with life-threatening ventricular arrhythmias, including those refractory to other antiarrhythmic agents. Previously, the potential severity of the drug's adverse effects generally had precluded amiodarone from being considered a first-line† agent in the management of life-threatening ventricular arrhythmias, and use of the drug generally was reserved for patients in whom other antiarrhythmic agents were ineffective or not tolerated. Currently, however, amiodarone is considered a preferred† or alternative agent for the management of various life-threatening ventricular arrhythmias, in part because of comparable or better efficacy and its apparent reduced risk of proarrhythmic activity.

Shock-Resistant Ventricular Fibrillation or Pulseless Ventricular Tachycardia. Amiodarone is used as adjunctive therapy for the treatment of ventricular fibrillation or pulseless ventricular tachycardia resistant to cardiopulmonary resuscitation (CPR), defibrillation, and a vasopressor (e.g., epinephrine).

Antiarrhythmic drugs are used during cardiac arrest to facilitate the restoration and maintenance of a spontaneous perfusing rhythm in patients with refractory (i.e., persisting or recurring after at least one shock) ventricular fibrillation or pulseless ventricular tachycardia; however, there is no evidence that these drugs increase survival to hospital discharge when given routinely during cardiac arrest. High-quality CPR and defibrillation are integral components of ACLS and the only proven interventions to increase survival to hospital discharge. Other resuscitative efforts, including drug therapy, are considered secondary and should be performed without compromising the quality and timely delivery of chest compressions and defibrillation. The principal goal of pharmacologic therapy during cardiac arrest is to facilitate return of spontaneous circulation (ROSC), and epinephrine is the drug of choice for this use. (See Uses: Advanced Cardiovascular Life Support and Cardiac Arrhythmias, in Epinephrine 12:12.12.) If an antiarrhythmic agent is needed for the treatment of refractory ventricular fibrillation or pulseless ventricular tachycardia during adult cardiac arrest, the American Heart Association (AHA) recommends amiodarone as the first-line drug of choice because of its proven benefits in improving rates of ROSC and hospital admission; lidocaine may be used as an alternative. Results of several studies suggest that amiodarone is more effective than lidocaine in improving rates of ROSC and hospital admission in patients with shock-refractory ventricular fibrillation or pulseless ventricular tachycardia. In pediatric advanced life support (PALS), current evidence supports the use of either amiodarone or lidocaine for these arrhythmias.

Results of a randomized, double-blind, placebo-controlled study in patients with out-of-hospital cardiac arrest due to defibrillation-refractory ventricular arrhythmias (i.e., ventricular fibrillation, pulseless ventricular tachycardia) who received a single 300-mg dose of IV amiodarone hydrochloride (after at least 3 precordial electrical shocks were administered) indicate that the drug improved the rate of survival to hospital admission by 29%. In a randomized, double-blind, comparative study with lidocaine, approximately 23% of patients with out-of-hospital cardiac arrest due to defibrillation-refractory ventricular arrhythmias who received IV amiodarone hydrochloride (5 mg/kg) or its matching placebo survived to hospital admission compared with 12% of those who received IV lidocaine (1.5 mg/kg) or its matching placebo following at least 3 precordial electrical shocks, IV epinephrine, and an additional precordial electrical shock. Among patients for whom the time from dispatch of the ambulance to the administration of the drug was equal to or less than the median time (24 minutes), approximately 28% of those given amiodarone and 15% of those given lidocaine survived to hospital admission. Despite these results, only about 5% of patients receiving IV amiodarone who survived to hospital admission lived to be discharged from the hospital compared with about 3% of those receiving IV lidocaine. Evidence supporting the use of amiodarone and lidocaine in pediatric cardiac arrest is more limited and principally based on extrapolation of data from the adult population. In a retrospective cohort study that included data from 889 pediatric patients with in-hospital cardiac arrest, improved ROSC was observed with lidocaine compared with amiodarone. Neither drug was associated with improved survival to hospital discharge.

IV amiodarone also may be used for the treatment of regular wide-complex tachycardias during the periarrest period and is included as a recommended antiarrhythmic agent in current ACLS guidelines for both adult and pediatric tachycardia.

Monomorphic and Polymorphic Ventricular Tachycardia. Some experts recommend that sustained monomorphic ventricular tachycardia not associated with angina, pulmonary edema, or hypotension (blood pressure less than 90 mm Hg)† be treated with amiodarone or synchronized electrical cardioversion. Other experts recommend amiodarone for control of hemodynamically stable monomorphic ventricular tachycardia†. Drug regimens including amiodarone or procainamide may be used initially† for the treatment of patients with episodes of sustained ventricular tachycardia that are associated with myocardial infarction and somewhat better tolerated hemodynamically. If IV antiarrhythmic therapy is used for ventricular fibrillation or tachycardia, it probably should be discontinued (at least temporarily) after 6–24 hours so that the patient's ongoing need for antiarrhythmic drugs can be reassessed.

Amiodarone also may be used for the treatment of polymorphic (irregular) ventricular tachycardia† associated with myocardial ischemia in the absence of QT interval prolongation. Although rare, episodes of drug-refractory sustained polymorphic ventricular tachycardia (electrical storm) have been reported in cases of acute myocardial infarction. Some experts state that these episodes should be managed by aggressive attempts at reducing myocardial ischemia†, including therapies such as an IV β-adrenergic blocking agent, IV amiodarone, left stellate ganglion blockade, intra-aortic balloon counterpulsation (IABP), or emergency revascularization (percutaneous transluminal coronary angioplasty [PTCA], coronary artery bypass graft [CABG] surgery); IV magnesium also may be used. Polymorphic ventricular tachycardia associated with QT interval prolongation usually is treated with IV magnesium sulfate.

Prevention of Ventricular Arrhythmias and Death Associated with Cardiac Arrest **Primary Prevention.** Oral amiodarone has been used for primary prevention† of sustained ventricular tachycardia (i.e., ventricular tachycardia lasting greater than 30 seconds and/or associated with hemodynamic compromise), ventricular fibrillation, or sudden cardiac death in patients with nonsustained ventricular arrhythmia following myocardial infarction. Such use of the drug was once thought to prevent sudden cardiac death because ventricular premature complexes (VPCs) were believed to be harbingers of more serious ventricular arrhythmias (e.g. ventricular fibrillation or tachycardia). However, conflicting results have been reported in studies evaluating the efficacy of antiarrhythmic agents on the risk of sudden death from cardiac causes in post-myocardial infarction patients.

Results of 2 multicenter, randomized, placebo-controlled studies in patients with frequent or repetitive ventricular premature complexes (Canadian Amiodarone Myocardial Infarction Arrhythmia Trial [CAMIAT]) or with left ventricular dysfunction (European Myocardial Infarct Amiodarone Trial [EMIAT]) indicate that therapy with oral amiodarone in patients who had survived a recent myocardial infarction appeared to reduce resuscitated cardiac arrest or ventricular fibrillation or arrhythmic death but was *not* associated with reduction of total mortality after 1–2 years of follow-up. These data are consistent with results of pooled analysis of small controlled trials in patients with structural heart disease, including post-myocardial infarction patients. However, in a smaller study (Basel Antiarrhythmic Study of Infarct Survival [BASIS]) comparing amiodarone with usual care in patients with persisting asymptomatic complex arrhythmias (multiform or repetitive ventricular arrhythmias [Lown class 3 or 4b]) after acute myocardial infarction, long-term therapy with amiodarone was associated with a reduction in mortality at 1 year compared with no antiarrhythmic therapy, possibly as a result of a decreased incidence of sudden death from ventricular tachycardia and fibrillation. In addition, analysis of pooled data from several other randomized studies in patients at risk of sudden cardiac death (e.g., those with congestive heart failure or left ventricular dysfunction, recent myocardial infarction, prior cardiac arrest) suggested that amiodarone therapy may reduce total mortality by 10–19%, and such risk reduction associated with the drug may be similar in the mentioned patient populations.

Findings from the National Heart, Lung, and Blood Institute (NHLBI)'s Cardiac Arrhythmia Suppression Trial (CAST) study indicated a substantially increased rate of total mortality and nonfatal cardiac arrest in patients with recent myocardial infarction, mild to moderate left ventricular dysfunction, and asymptomatic or mildly symptomatic ventricular arrhythmias (principally frequent VPC) who received encainide or flecainide (class I antiarrhythmic drugs) compared with placebo after an average of 10 months of follow-up, which resulted in considerably modified clinicians' use of not only class IC antiarrhythmics, but also class I antiarrhythmic agents in general, in post-myocardial infarction patients. (See Cautions in Flecainide 24:04.04.12.) Although it has been suggested that the applicability of the CAST results to other populations (e.g., those without recent myocardial infarction) or to predominantly class III antiarrhythmic agents such as amiodarone (a drug that has some characteristics of class IA and IC antiarrhythmic agents) is uncertain, the American College of Cardiology (ACC) and AHA state that β-adrenergic blocking agents are preferred over amiodarone for general prophylaxis. In addition, results of prospective, randomized clinical studies indicate improved survival following use of implantable cardioverter defibrillator (ICD) therapy compared with conventional drug therapy, including amiodarone, in patients with nonsustained ventricular tachycardia, reduced ejection fraction (less than 40%), and/or a history of myocardial infarction. However, preliminary reports suggest that only a small proportion of patients with a previous myocardial infarction would benefit from ICD therapy and it remains unclear whether routinely screening patients with impaired left ventricular function for prophylactic ICD therapy is clinically feasible and cost-effective.

Secondary Prevention. Amiodarone hydrochloride is used orally or IV to suppress or prevent the recurrence of documented life-threatening ventricular arrhythmias (e.g., recurrent ventricular fibrillation and recurrent, hemodynamically unstable ventricular tachycardia) that do not respond to documented adequate dosages of other currently available antiarrhythmic agents or when alternative antiarrhythmic agents cannot be tolerated. The effectiveness of IV amiodarone in suppressing recurrent ventricular fibrillation or hemodynamically unstable (destabilizing) ventricular tachycardia is supported by 2 randomized, parallel, dose-response studies of approximately 300 patients each. In patients with recurrent ventricular fibrillation or destabilizing ventricular tachycardia that was refractory to first-line (e.g., lidocaine) therapy, amiodarone produced a dose-dependent decrease in arrhythmia recurrence, although not in mortality. Patients with at least 2 episodes of ventricular fibrillation or hemodynamically unstable ventricular tachycardia within the preceding 24 hours were randomly assigned to receive IV amiodarone hydrochloride doses of 125 mg or 1 g over 24 hours; one study also evaluated a dose of 500 mg. After 48 hours, patients were eligible to receive open access to any treatment deemed necessary (including IV amiodarone) to control their arrhythmias. Amiodarone was administered in a 3-phase sequence, with an initial rapid loading infusion, followed by a slower 6-hour loading infusion, and a subsequent 18-hour maintenance infusion. Maintenance infusion was continued up through hour 48. Additional supplemental 10-minute infusions of 150 mg were administered for breakthrough arrhythmias; these occurred more frequently in patients receiving the 125-mg dosage regimen. Fewer patients receiving the 1-g IV amiodarone hydrochloride regimen required supplemental infusions. During treatment with IV amiodarone, median episodes of ventricular tachycardia or ventricular fibrillation were 0.02/hour in the group receiving the 1-g dosage regimen and 0.07/hour in the group receiving the 125-mg dosage regimen, or approximately 0.5 versus 1.7 episodes daily in patients receiving the 1-g versus 125-mg dosage regimen, respectively. In one study, the time to first episode of ventricular tachycardia or ventricular fibrillation was approximately 10 or 14 hours in patients receiving the 125- or 1000-mg amiodarone hydrochloride dosage regimens, respectively. Mortality rate was not affected by treatment in either of these studies.

Because there has been no evidence of improved survival with use of antiarrhythmic agents, including amiodarone and β-adrenergic blocking agents, whereas such evidence does exist for ICD therapy, ICDs have increasingly been used in the secondary prevention of life-threatening ventricular arrhythmias. In comparative studies, ICD therapy has been shown to be superior to antiarrhythmic drugs, principally amiodarone, for increasing overall survival of patients who had been resuscitated from near-fatal ventricular fibrillation or sustained ventricular tachycardia. Analysis of pooled data indicates that ICD therapy prolongs life by 2.1 or 4.4 months compared with amiodarone after a follow-up period of 3 or 6 years, respectively. Subgroup analysis of patients enrolled in the Antiarrhythmics Versus Implantable Defibrillators (AVID) study indicates that patients with an isolated episode of ventricular fibrillation in the absence of cerebrovascular disease or history of prior arrhythmia who have undergone revascularization or who have moderately preserved left ventricular function (i.e., left ventricular ejection fraction greater than 27%) are not likely to benefit from ICD therapy compared with amiodarone therapy. However, results of this analysis must be considered speculative because the specific criteria used in defining the subgroups were not planned prior to collection of data, and additional studies are needed to verify these findings.

Prediction of the efficacy of any antiarrhythmic agent in the long-term prevention of recurrent ventricular tachycardia and ventricular fibrillation is difficult and controversial. Many authorities currently recommend the use of ambulatory ECG monitoring, programmed electrical stimulation (PES), or a combination of both to assess patient response to amiodarone. There is no consensus on many aspects of how best to assess patient response to the drug; however, there is reasonable agreement on some aspects. If a patient with a prior history of cardiac arrest does not manifest a hemodynamically unstable arrhythmia during ECG monitoring prior to treatment, some provocative approach such as exercise or PES is required to assess the efficacy of amiodarone. The need for provocation in patients who do manifest life-threatening arrhythmias spontaneously remains to be established, although there are reasons to consider PES or other means of provocation in such patients. In patients whose PES-induced arrhythmia is made noninducible by amiodarone, the prognosis is almost uniformly excellent, with very low rates of arrhythmia recurrence or sudden death. The meaning of continued inducibility during therapy with the drug is controversial. Although not clearly established, increased difficulty of arrhythmia induction by PES and/or the ability to tolerate the induced ventricular tachycardia without severe symptoms may be useful criteria for identifying patients who may benefit from amiodarone therapy despite continued inducibility of the arrhythmia during therapy with the drug. Generally, easier inducibility or poorer tolerance of the induced arrhythmia should suggest consideration of the need to revise treatment. Other criteria for predicting the efficacy of amiodarone therapy, including complete suppression of nonsustained ventricular tachycardia determined by ambulatory ECG monitoring and the documentation of very low rates of VPCs, also have been suggested. These issues remain unsettled for amiodarone as well as for other antiarrhythmic agents. Specialized references should be consulted for additional information.

Combination Antiarrhythmic Regimens Amiodarone has been used in combination with numerous other antiarrhythmic agents for the management of severe refractory ventricular arrhythmias; however, such combination therapy has not been evaluated in well-controlled studies and is associated with an increased risk of adverse cardiovascular effects. (See Drug Interactions: Antiarrhythmic Agents.)

Other Ventricular Arrhythmias Amiodarone has been used with good results in a limited number of patients experiencing life-threatening ventricular arrhythmias associated with post-infarction aneurysm† or with chronic myocarditis induced by Chagas' disease.† IV amiodarone has been used with some success in a limited number of patients for the management of ventricular tachycardia and ventricular fibrillation associated with cardiac glycoside intoxication†.

■ **Supraventricular Tachyarrhythmias** Amiodarone appears to be effective in the suppression and prevention of various supraventricular tachycardias (SVTs)†; because of a higher risk of toxicity and proarrhythmic effects, antiarrhythmic agents generally should be reserved for patients who do not respond to or cannot be treated with AV nodal blocking agents (β-adrenergic blocking agents and nondihydropyridine calcium-channel blocking agents). Some experts state that amiodarone may be useful in situations where ventricular rate control is needed but AV nodal blocking agents are contraindicated, such as in patients with preexcited atrial arrhythmias associated with an accessory pathway†. However, IV amiodarone is potentially harmful when used for the acute treatment of patients with preexcited atrial fibrillation since it has the potential to accelerate the ventricular response and precipitate fatal arrhythmias.

Atrial Fibrillation and Flutter Amiodarone has been used orally and IV in the management of atrial fibrillation† or flutter†.

Amiodarone is one of several antiarrhythmic agents that may be used to maintain sinus rhythm in patients with atrial fibrillation or flutter. Long-term therapy with oral amiodarone alone or in combination with other antiarrhythmic agents has been effective for suppression and prevention of refractory atrial fibrillation†. Limited data indicate that long-term amiodarone therapy may be effective in about 70% (range: 35–95%) of patients with atrial fibrillation†, including those whose arrhythmia is refractory to conventional therapy. Although not clearly established, the efficacy of amiodarone in the suppression of atrial fibrillation† may result from the drug's ability to maintain normal sinus rhythm (probably by increasing atrial refractoriness), suppress atrial premature complexes (which may precipitate atrial fibrillation), and control ventricular rate. There is some evidence that amiodarone may be substantially more effective than sotalol or propafenone for long-term prevention of recurrent atrial fibrillation. Whether maintaining sinus rhythm in patients with recurrent atrial fibrillation will result in improved survival or a reduction in the risk of thromboembolic complications remains to be established.

Oral or IV† amiodarone may be effective for conversion of atrial fibrillation† to normal sinus rhythm (i.e., rhythm control). In current expert guidelines, amiodarone is considered a reasonable option for pharmacological conversion of atrial fibrillation; however, other antiarrhythmic agents (e.g., flecainide, dofetilide, propafenone, ibutilide) are preferred. IV amiodarone may be harmful, and therefore should not be used, in patients with Wolff-Parkinson-White (WPW) syndrome who have preexcited atrial fibrillation because the drug can accelerate ventricular rate and potentially cause life-threatening ventricular arrhythmias. Conversion of atrial fibrillation to normal sinus rhythm may be associated with embolism, particularly when atrial fibrillation has been present for more than 48 hours, unless the patient is adequately anticoagulated. (See Uses: Cardioversion of Atrial Fibrillation/Flutter, in Heparin 20:12.04.16.)

Further studies are needed to evaluate the comparative efficacy and safety of oral amiodarone, other antiarrhythmic agents, and cardioversion (direct-current countershock). Although cardioversion has been used safely and effectively following oral or IV amiodarone administration, decreased efficacy of cardioversion in patients receiving the drug has also been reported. Further studies are needed to evaluate the effect of amiodarone therapy on the efficacy of cardioversion.

Paroxysmal Supraventricular Tachycardia Limited data suggest that IV amiodarone is effective in terminating paroxysmal supraventricular tachycardia (PSVT)†, including atrioventricular nodal reentrant tachycardia (AVNRT) and atrioventricular reentrant tachycardia (AVRT) (e.g., WPW syndrome). Some experts state that IV amiodarone may be considered for the acute treatment of hemodynamically stable patients with AVNRT when other therapies are ineffective or contraindicated. However, IV use of amiodarone can be potentially harmful in patients with preexcited atrial fibrillation because the drug may accelerate ventricular rate and cause life-threatening ventricular arrhythmias.

Long-term oral amiodarone therapy appears to be particularly effective in the suppression and prevention of paroxysmal reentrant supraventricular tachycardias† (AVNRT and AVRT [e.g., WPW syndrome]) including those refractory to other antiarrhythmic agents. Some experts state that oral amiodarone may be reasonable for ongoing management of AVNRT or AVRT in patients who are not candidates for, or prefer not to undergo, catheter ablation and in whom first-line drugs (e.g., β-adrenergic blocking agents, diltiazem, verapamil) are not effective or contraindicated. Oral amiodarone also has been effective in some patients for the suppression and prevention of atrial fibrillation or flutter associated with WPW syndrome†. Although amiodarone also has been used IV in such patients, IV use of the drug has resulted in acceleration of ventricular rate. (See Cautions: Arrhythmogenic Effects.)

Atrial Tachycardia IV amiodarone may be used for the acute treatment of patients with hemodynamically stable focal atrial tachycardia† (i.e., regular SVT arising from a localized atrial site), and oral amiodarone may be reasonable for the ongoing management of such patients.

While evidence is more limited, amiodarone also has been used in patients with multifocal atrial tachycardia† (i.e., rapid, irregular rhythm with at least 3 distinct P-wave morphologies). However, such arrhythmia is commonly associated with an underlying condition (e.g., pulmonary, coronary, or valvular heart disease) and is generally not responsive to antiarrhythmic therapy. Antiarrhythmic drug therapy usually is reserved for patients who do not respond to initial attempts at correcting or managing potential precipitating factors (e.g., exacerbation of chronic obstructive pulmonary disease or congestive heart failure, electrolyte and/or ventilatory disturbances, infection, theophylline toxicity).

Junctional Tachycardia Amiodarone may be used for the treatment of junctional tachycardia† (i.e., nonreentrant SVT originating from the AV junction), a rapid, occasionally irregular, narrow-complex tachycardia; however, efficacy data is available only for pediatric patients. *β*-Adrenergic blocking agents generally are considered the drugs of choice for terminating and/or reducing the incidence of junctional tachycardia.

Bradycardia-Tachycardia Syndrome Amiodarone has been effective in the prevention of supraventricular arrhythmias associated with bradycardia-tachycardia syndrome† in a limited number of patients; however, the drug should be used with caution in such patients, since it may depress sinoatrial node function, possibly resulting in marked bradycardia. Some clinicians recommend insertion of a temporary or permanent artificial pacemaker prior to initiation of amiodarone therapy in patients with bradycardia-tachycardia syndrome†.

■ **Angina** Amiodarone has been used in a limited number of patients for the management of chronic stable angina pectoris†. Limited data suggest that amiodarone is as effective as diltiazem and more effective than sublingual nitroglycerin in increasing exercise tolerance and decreasing ST-segment depression in patients with chronic stable angina pectoris†. Amiodarone also has been used with good results in some patients with Prinzmetal variant angina†. Because of the potential toxicity associated with amiodarone, the drug generally is not considered a first-line agent for the management of chronic stable angina pectoris† or Prinzmetal variant angina† but may have a beneficial antianginal effect in patients receiving the drug for the management of arrhythmias.

■ **Hypertrophic Cardiomyopathy** Amiodarone has been used with good results in some patients for the management of ventricular and supraventricular arrhythmias associated with hypertrophic cardiomyopathy†. In addition to its antiarrhythmic effects, the drug may also relieve symptoms and increase exercise capacity in some patients, including those whose arrhythmias are refractory to conventional treatment. Pending further accumulation of data, some clinicians recommend that treatment with amiodarone be considered only in patients with refractory hypertrophic cardiomyopathy†.

Dosage and Administration

■ **Reconstitution and Administration** Amiodarone hydrochloride is administered orally or by IV infusion. Amiodarone also has been administered by intraosseous (IO) injection† in the setting of advanced cardiovascular life support (ACLS); however, there is limited experience with the drug given by this route.

For the management of life-threatening ventricular arrhythmias, oral amiodarone hydrochloride usually is administered once daily. When dosages of 1 g or more daily are administered (e.g., during the loading-dose phase of therapy) or when intolerable adverse GI effects occur with once-daily dosing, it is recommended that the drug be given in divided doses (e.g., twice daily) with meals. Because food can increase the rate and extent of absorption of amiodarone, the drug should be administered in a consistent manner relative to food intake.

Patients should be advised not to stop taking amiodarone without their clinician's knowledge, even if they feel better, as their condition may worsen. If a patient misses an oral dose of amiodarone, a double dose should not be taken to make up for the missed dose; instead, the next dose should be taken at the regularly scheduled time. If additional oral doses of amiodarone are ingested, patients should seek medical attention urgently by contacting their clinician or immediately proceeding to the nearest hospital emergency department.

IV Infusion Commercially available amiodarone hydrochloride concentrate for injection containing 50 mg of the drug per mL *must* be diluted prior to administration. To produce the solution required for the first rapid loading infusion or for supplemental amiodarone infusions, 3 mL of amiodarone hydrochloride concentrate should be added to 100 mL of 5% dextrose, resulting in a final concentration of 1.5 mg/mL. To produce the solution for slow infusion and the maintenance infusion, 18 mL of amiodarone hydrochloride concentrate should be added to 500 mL of 5% dextrose, resulting in a final amiodarone concentration of 1.8 mg/mL. For subsequent maintenance infusions, solutions containing a final amiodarone hydrochloride concentration of 1–6 mg/mL may be used. Parenteral amiodarone hydrochloride solutions should be inspected visually for particulate matter whenever solution and container permit.

For IV infusion, the recommended dose of the diluted amiodarone hydrochloride solution is administered in a 3-phase sequence: a rapid loading phase, a slow loading phase, and a maintenance infusion phase. Parenteral amiodarone therapy should be used for acute antiarrhythmic therapy until the patient's cardiac rhythm is stabilized and oral therapy can be initiated. The manufacturer states that most patients will require IV therapy for 48–96 hours, but that parenteral therapy may be administered safely for longer periods of time.

Solutions containing an amiodarone hydrochloride concentration of 2 mg/mL or more should be administered via a central venous catheter, although the manufacturer states that parenteral amiodarone solutions should be administered via a central venous catheter dedicated to administration of the drug whenever possible. An in-line filter also should be used for administration of IV amiodarone hydrochloride solutions. Amiodarone hydrochloride infusions that will exceed 2 hours must be administered in glass or polyolefin bottles. (See Chemistry and Stability: Stability.) Although amiodarone hydrochloride adsorbs to polyvinyl chloride (PVC), the drug dosages used in clinical trials were designed to take this factor into account; therefore, the manufacturer recommends that solutions containing amiodarone hydrochloride injection be administered through PVC tubing. Polysorbate (Tween®) 80, a component of IV amiodarone, can cause leaching of diethylhexylphthalate (DEHP) from IV tubing, including PVC tubing. Leaching of DEHP increases at lower than recommended flow rates and at higher than recommended infusion concentrations. Therefore, the manufacturer's dosage recommendations should be followed closely.

The surface properties of solutions containing amiodarone hydrochloride injection are altered such that the drop size may be reduced. This reduction may lead to underdosage of the patient by up to 30% if drop counter infusion sets are used. Therefore, the manufacturer states that solutions containing amiodarone hydrochloride injection must be administered by a volumetric infusion pump.

■ **Dosage** A uniform and optimal dosage schedule for amiodarone hydrochloride has not been established. *Amiodarone is a highly toxic drug, and the lowest effective dosage should be used to minimize the risk and occurrence of adverse effects.* Dosage of amiodarone hydrochloride must be carefully adjusted according to individual requirements and response, patient tolerance, and the general condition and cardiovascular status of the patient. Clinical and ECG monitoring of cardiac function, including appropriate ambulatory ECG monitoring (e.g., Holter monitoring) and/or programmed electrical stimulation (PES), as appropriate, is recommended during therapy with the drug. When dosage adjustment is necessary, the patient should be monitored closely for an extended period of time because of the long and variable elimination half-life of amiodarone and the difficulty in predicting the length of time required to attain a new steady-state plasma concentration of the drug. When feasible, monitoring of plasma amiodarone concentrations may be helpful in evaluating patients who are not responding to the drug or who experience unexpectedly severe toxicity. Monitoring of plasma amiodarone concentrations may also be useful in identifying patients whose concentrations are unusually low and who might benefit from an increase in dosage or those whose concentrations are unusually high in whom dosage reduction might minimize the risk of adverse effects.

Patients should be advised not to double the next dose if a dose is missed.

Although amiodarone dosage requirements generally appear to be similar in geriatric and younger adults, relatively high dosages should be used with caution in geriatric patients since they may be more susceptible to bradycardia and conduction disturbances induced by the drug. In addition, some manufacturers state that dosage in general for geriatric patients should be selected carefully, usually starting at the low end of the dosage range, because these individuals frequently have decreased hepatic, renal, and/or cardiac function and concomitant disease and drug therapy.

Life-threatening Ventricular Arrhythmias in Adults **Oral Dosage.** For the management of life-threatening ventricular arrhythmias, loading doses of amiodarone hydrochloride are required to ensure an antiarrhythmic effect without waiting several months. The loading-dose phase of therapy should be performed in a hospital setting. Close monitoring of patients is necessary, especially until the risk of recurrent ventricular tachycardia or fibrillation has abated. Upon initiating amiodarone therapy in patients receiving other antiarrhythmic agents, an attempt should be made to gradually discontinue the other antiarrhythmic agents. (See Drug Interactions: Antiarrhythmic Agents.)

In adults, oral amiodarone hydrochloride loading dosages of 800–1600 mg daily generally are required for 1–3 weeks (and occasionally for longer periods of time) until an initial therapeutic response occurs. Some clinicians have used oral loading dosages exceeding 1600 mg daily or IV† loading-dose regimens. Clinicians should consult published protocols for specific information on oral loading-dose regimens using dosages greater than 1600 mg daily or on IV loading-dose regimens. If an IV loading-dose regimen is used, oral therapy should be initiated as soon as possible after an adequate response is obtained and IV amiodarone therapy gradually eliminated. If adverse effects become excessive during the loading-dose phase of therapy, a reduction in dosage is recommended. Elimination of recurrent ventricular tachycardia and recurrent ventricular fibrillation as well as reduction in VPCs and total ventricular ectopic beats usually occur within about 1–3 weeks.

When adequate control of ventricular arrhythmias is achieved or adverse effects become prominent, the dosage of amiodarone hydrochloride should be reduced to 600–800 mg daily for about 1 month and then reduced again to the lowest effective maintenance dosage, usually 400 mg daily. Further cautious reductions in maintenance dosage (e.g., to 200 mg daily) may be possible in some patients. Adequate maintenance dosages generally range from less than 400 mg daily up to 600 mg daily. Because absorption and elimination of amiodarone are variable, adjustment of maintenance dosage is difficult, and it is not unusual to require dosage reductions or temporary withdrawal or discontinuance of the drug.

Parenteral Dosage. For the management of life-threatening ventricular arrhythmias, the recommended starting dose of IV amiodarone hydrochloride over the first 24 hours is approximately 1000 mg. The amiodarone hydrochloride dose for the first rapid loading infusion is 150 mg administered at a rate of 15 mg/minute (i.e., over 10 minutes); the initial infusion rate should not exceed 30 mg/minute. The slow loading phase of the infusion is 360 mg of amiodarone hydrochloride administered at a rate of 1 mg/minute (i.e., over 6 hours). The first maintenance phase of the infusion is 540 mg of amiodarone hydrochloride administered at a rate of 0.5 mg/minute (i.e., over 18 hours). The first 24-hour dose of amiodarone hydrochloride may be individualized for each patient; however, in controlled clinical trials, mean daily dosages exceeding 2.1 g were associated with an increased risk of hypotension.

After the first 24 hours, the maintenance infusion rate of 0.5 mg/minute (i.e., 720 mg over 24 hours) should be continued; however, the rate of the maintenance infusion may be increased to achieve effective arrhythmia suppression. In the event of breakthrough episodes of ventricular fibrillation or hemodynamically unstable ventricular tachycardia, supplemental amiodarone hydrochloride infusions of 150 mg administered at a rate of 15 mg/minute (i.e., over 10 minutes) may be given. Based on experience from clinical trials of IV amiodarone hydrochloride, a maintenance infusion of up to 0.5 mg/minute can be administered with caution for 2–3 weeks, regardless of the patient's age, renal function, or left ventricular function. The manufacturer states that there is limited experience in patients receiving parenteral amiodarone hydrochloride for longer than 3 weeks.

For cardiac arrest secondary to pulseless ventricular tachycardia or ventricular fibrillation, experts recommend an initial adult loading dose of amiodarone hydrochloride of 300 mg, given by rapid IV or IO† injection; an additional dose of 150 mg may be considered.

Supraventricular Arrhythmias in Adults For acute treatment of supraventricular tachycardia (SVT) in adults, an IV amiodarone hydrochloride loading dose of 150 mg over 10 minutes is recommended. The drug should then be administered at a rate of 1 mg/minute for 6 hours, then 0.5 mg/minute for the remaining 18 hours or until oral dosing is initiated. For ongoing management of SVT, some experts recommend an oral amiodarone hydrochloride loading dosage of 400–600 mg daily (in divided doses) in adults for approximately 2–4 weeks, followed by a maintenance dosage of 100–200 mg daily. Clinicians should consult published protocols for specific information on oral loading-dose regimens using higher dosages.

When used for rate control of atrial fibrillation, some experts recommend an initial IV amiodarone hydrochloride dose of 300 mg over 1 hour, followed by 10–50 mg/hr over 24 hours; the usual oral maintenance dose is 100–200 mg daily.

For the long-term management of recurrent atrial fibrillation† in adults, an oral dosage regimen that includes an initial amiodarone hydrochloride loading dose of 10 mg/kg daily for 14 days, followed by 300 mg daily for 4 weeks, and then by a maintenance dosage of 200 mg daily has been used effectively to prevent recurrences.

Pediatric Dosage **Oral Dosage.** Pediatric dosage of oral amiodarone hydrochloride has not been established, and dosage may vary considerably. For the management of ventricular and supraventricular arrhythmias in children†, some clinicians have recommended oral amiodarone hydrochloride loading dosages of 10–15 mg/kg daily or 600–800 mg/1.73 m^2 daily for approximately 4–14 days and/or until adequate control of cardiac arrhythmias is achieved or adverse effects become prominent. Dosage of the drug is then reduced to 5 mg/kg daily or 200–400 mg/1.73 m^2 for several weeks. If possible, dosage is then reduced gradually to the lowest effective level. Children younger than 1 year of age appear to require higher loading and maintenance dosages of amiodarone hydrochloride than older children when dosage of the drug is calculated on the basis of body weight, but not on the basis of body surface area.

Parenteral Dosage. The manufacturer states that pediatric dosage of IV amiodarone hydrochloride has not been established. For the management of refractory ventricular fibrillation or pulseless ventricular tachycardia† during pediatric resuscitation, the recommended amiodarone hydrochloride IV or IO† dose is 5 mg/kg as a rapid bolus injection. Some experts recommend that if adequate control of cardiac arrhythmia is not achieved, the dose may be repeated twice (maximum single dose of 300 mg) up to a total dosage of 15 mg/kg. If used for the management of wide-complex tachycardias or SVT in pediatric patients who are not in cardiac arrest, an IV amiodarone hydrochloride dose of 5 mg/kg is recommended (infused slowly over 20–60 minutes depending on the urgency). Alternative methods of dosing IV amiodarone hydrochloride (e.g., loading dose of 5 mg/kg given in 5 divided doses of 1 mg/kg, with each incremental dose infused over 5–10 minutes) may be considered in order to minimize pediatric exposure to the plasticizer DEHP. (See Cautions: Pediatric Precautions).

Conversion from IV to Oral Dosage Patients whose arrhythmias have been controlled successfully with IV amiodarone hydrochloride may be switched to oral therapy. The manufacturer states that since there are some differences in the safety and efficacy profiles of the oral and IV preparations of amiodarone, clinicians should review the prescribing information for oral amiodarone when switching from IV to oral therapy. The optimal dose of oral amiodarone hydrochloride will depend on the dose and duration of IV therapy, as well as the bioavailability of the oral drug. The manufacturer suggests that for patients receiving a daily dose of 720 mg of amiodarone hydrochloride IV (assuming an infusion rate of 0.5 mg/minute) for less than 1 week, 1–3 weeks, or longer than 3 weeks, the initial daily oral amiodarone hydrochloride dose should be 800–1600, 600–800, or 400 mg of the drug, respectively. These recommendations are made on the basis of a comparable total body amount of amiodarone hydrochloride delivered by IV and oral routes, taking into consideration the drug's oral bioavailability of 50%. When switching from IV to oral amiodarone hydrochloride therapy, clinical monitoring is recommended, particularly for geriatric patients.

■ **Dosage in Renal and Hepatic Impairment** Routine reduction of amiodarone hydrochloride dosage in patients with renal impairment does not appear to be necessary, although the risk of excessive accumulation of iodine and possible resultant thyroid effects should be considered.

The effects of hepatic impairment on the elimination of amiodarone have not been evaluated. Because the drug is extensively metabolized, probably in the liver, some clinicians caution that dosage reduction is probably warranted in patients with substantial hepatic impairment. Dosage reduction or discontinuance of amiodarone may be necessary in patients who develop evidence of hepatotoxicity during therapy with the drug. (See Cautions: Precautions and Contraindications.)

Cautions

Amiodarone is a highly toxic drug and exhibits several potentially fatal toxicities, notably pulmonary toxicity. Adverse reactions to amiodarone are common in nearly all patients receiving the drug for the treatment of ventricular arrhythmias. With relatively large dosages of amiodarone hydrochloride (400 mg or more daily), adverse reactions occur in about 75% of patients and require discontinuance of the drug in about 5–20% of patients.

The most severe reactions to oral amiodarone are pulmonary toxicity, arrhythmogenic effects, and rare, but potentially serious, liver injury; however, numerous other adverse reactions to the drug also may be clinically important. Amiodarone-induced adverse effects are often reversible following dosage reduction and nearly always reversible following discontinuance of the drug, although adverse effects may persist for weeks or months after discontinuance of therapy because of the drug's prolonged elimination. The most common adverse reactions requiring discontinuance of oral amiodarone are pulmonary infiltrates or fibrosis, paroxysmal ventricular tachycardia, congestive heart failure, and elevations of serum hepatic enzyme concentrations. The likelihood of most adverse reactions appears to increase after the first 6 months of therapy with the drug and then remains relatively constant beyond 1 year of therapy. The most common adverse effect observed with IV amiodarone therapy in clinical trials was hypotension, which resulted in discontinuation of therapy in less than 2% of patients. Additional experience with amiodarone is needed to more fully characterize the adverse effect profile of the drug, particularly in relation to duration of therapy and dosage.

■ **Pulmonary Effects** Pulmonary toxicity, which is potentially fatal, is the most severe adverse effect associated with oral amiodarone therapy with or without initial IV therapy. Acute-onset (days to weeks) pulmonary toxicity has been reported during postmarketing experience; manifestations include radiographic evidence of pulmonary infiltrates and/or mass, pulmonary alveolar hemorrhage, pleural effusion, bronchospasm, wheezing, fever, dyspnea, cough, hemoptysis, hypoxia, or adult respiratory distress syndrome (ARDS), sometimes leading to respiratory failure and/or death.

Amiodarone-induced pulmonary toxicity may result from pulmonary interstitial pneumonitis (or alveolitis) or from hypersensitivity pneumonitis (e.g., eosinophilic pneumonia). Clinically apparent interstitial pneumonitis (or alveolitis), hypersensitivity pneumonitis, and pulmonary fibrosis have occurred in up to 10–17% of patients with ventricular arrhythmias receiving amiodarone hydrochloride therapy at oral dosages of about 400 mg daily, and an abnormal diffusion capacity without symptoms occurs in a much higher percentage of patients. Only one patient in clinical trials of IV amiodarone therapy developed pulmonary fibrosis; in this patient, the condition was diagnosed 3 months after IV therapy, during which time the patient had begun treatment with oral amiodarone. Amiodarone-induced pulmonary toxicity has been fatal in about 10% of cases. Rarely, amiodarone has been associated with exacerbation of bronchial asthma, possibly because of its antiadrenergic effects. Hemoptysis has been reported during postmarketing experience.

Amiodarone pneumonitis is a clinical syndrome consisting of progressive dyspnea and cough accompanied by functional, radiographic, scintigraphic, and pathological data consistent with pulmonary toxicity. The clinical course of pulmonary toxicity appears to be quite variable. Although a slow, progressive course is often described, an abrupt onset of febrile illness resembling infectious illness (e.g., pneumonia) also may occur. Early symptoms may include dyspnea (particularly with exertion), cough (generally without sputum production), fever or chills, chest pain (generally pleuritic), malaise, weakness, fatigue, myalgia, myopathy, nausea, anorexia, and/or weight loss. Bronchiolitis obliterans organizing pneumonia (that may be fatal) and pleuritis have been reported during postmarketing experience.

The overall incidence of amiodarone-induced pulmonary toxicity has generally been reported to range from about 2–7%, but some studies indicate that pulmonary toxicity may occur in about 10–17% of patients receiving the drug orally. Adult respiratory distress syndrome (ARDS) and lung edema were reported in 2% and less than 2%, respectively, of patients receiving IV amiodarone therapy. Limited evidence suggests that the incidence may increase with duration of therapy, total daily dose, age of the patient, and cumulative dose. However, pulmonary toxicity has been reported during postmarketing experience in patients receiving low dosages. Although not clearly established, limited data suggest that patients with evidence of pulmonary disease prior to amiodarone therapy may have an increased risk of amiodarone-induced pulmonary toxicity, although there may be a bias toward detection in such patients.

Some clinicians state, however, that preexisting pulmonary disease does not appear to increase the risk of amiodarone-induced pulmonary toxicity; however, these patients have a poorer prognosis than patients without preexisting pulmonary disease if toxicity develops. The syndrome is usually reversible following discontinuance of the drug (with or without corticosteroid therapy), but pulmonary toxicity may be fatal in some patients.

Hypersensitivity pneumonitis has been reported in about one-third of patients with amiodarone-induced pulmonary toxicity, and may occur earlier during amiodarone therapy than interstitial pneumonitis. Hypersensitivity pneumonitis does not appear to be dose related and may be characterized by acute onset of symptoms (e.g., fever). Alveolar infiltrates appear to be the most common radiographic findings in patients with amiodarone-induced hypersensitivity pneumonitis; increased suppressor/cytotoxic ($CD8^+$, $T8^+$) T cells and neutrophils often are found in the bronchoalveolar lavage of these patients. It is not known whether fatalities secondary to amiodarone-induced hypersensitivity pneumonitis occur more frequently than fatalities secondary to other pulmonary toxicity induced the drug. The precise mechanism of amiodarone-induced hypersensitivity pneumonitis, including the possible role of immunoglobulins, complement deposition, and cytokines in the development of pulmonary toxicity, remains to be more fully elucidated.

Physical findings in patients with amiodarone interstitial pneumonitis (alveolitis) may include rales, decreased breath sounds, and/or a pleuritic friction rub. Laboratory abnormalities may include hypoxemia, hypercarbia, leukocytosis, and elevated erythrocyte sedimentation rate. Diffuse interstitial infiltrates appear to be the most common radiographic finding in patients with amiodarone-induced pulmonary toxicity; however, airspace opacities (particularly patchy, peripheral alveolar infiltrates), well-localized infiltrates, and mixed interstitial and airspace disease patterns have also been reported.

Microscopic tissue changes in patients with amiodarone pneumonitis appear to be nonspecific but generally are consistent. Pathologic changes may include accumulation of foamy macrophages in alveolar spaces (the presence of lamellated cytoplasmic inclusions probably causes their foamy appearance), hyperplasia of type II pneumocytes, and thickening of the alveolar septal membrane by connective tissue. Although lamellated cytoplasmic inclusions appear to occur predominantly in macrophages, they may also occur in epithelial cells of respiratory bronchioles, type II pneumocytes, endothelial cells, and interstitial cells. Interstitial thickening secondary to an infiltrate of lymphocytes, histiocytes, and occasional plasma cells may also occur. Because foamy alveolar macrophages and lamellated cytoplasmic inclusions have been reported in approximately 50% of patients receiving amiodarone without clinical evidence of pulmonary toxicity, these pathologic changes alone should not be relied on in the diagnosis of amiodarone pneumonitis.

Pulmonary function tests most commonly reveal impairment of diffusion capacity, but reductions of total lung capacity (TLC) and forced vital capacity (FVC) may also occur. Limited data suggest that pulmonary function testing is neither sensitive nor specific enough to be the only method employed in monitoring for amiodarone-induced pulmonary toxicity.

Patients receiving amiodarone should be carefully monitored for the development of pulmonary toxicity. (See Cautions: Precautions and Contraindications.) If hypersensitivity pneumonitis occurs, corticosteroid therapy should be initiated and amiodarone discontinued. Rechallenge with the drug in patients with hypersensitivity pneumonitis results in more rapid and more severe adverse effects. If interstitial pneumonitis (alveolitis) occurs, dosage reduction and preferably discontinuance of the drug is necessary, especially in patients in whom other acceptable antiarrhythmic therapies are available. Following dosage reduction or discontinuance of amiodarone in patients with interstitial pneumonitis, clinical improvement usually is evident within the first week and is maximal after 2 or 3 weeks; radiographic abnormalities usually resolve within 2–4 months. In some patients with interstitial pneumonitis, rechallenge with a lower dosage of amiodarone has not resulted in recurrence of pulmonary toxicity; however, in some patients (e.g., those with severe alveolar damage), pulmonary lesions have been irreversible. Treatment of amiodarone pneumonitis is mainly supportive and may include mechanical ventilation, if necessary. Although data from uncontrolled studies suggest that corticosteroid therapy is of some benefit, controlled studies are needed to fully evaluate the safety and efficacy of corticosteroids in the management of amiodarone-induced pulmonary toxicity. Some patients have received prednisone dosages of 40–60 mg daily, which were tapered in small decrements during several weeks, depending on the patient's condition.

Adult respiratory distress syndrome (ARDS) has occurred occasionally following cardiothoracic or other surgery in patients with or without preexisting amiodarone-induced pulmonary toxicity. A causal relationship between ARDS and amiodarone has not been clearly established, and other factors (e.g., prolonged pump-oxygenator time, oxygen toxicity, anesthetic agents) may have contributed to the development of the syndrome. Although patients usually have responded to vigorous respiratory therapy, fatalities have occurred rarely. Some manufacturers state that forced inspiratory oxygen (FiO_2) and determinants of tissue oxygenation (e.g., arterial oxygen saturation [SaO_2], arterial oxygen pressure [PaO_2]) should be monitored closely.

■ Hepatic Effects Abnormalities of liver function test results have generally been reported in about 3–20% of patients receiving amiodarone, although the incidence has been as high as 40–55% in some studies. Nonspecific hepatic disorders have occurred in about 1–3% of patients.

Amiodarone-induced elevations in serum AST (SGOT), ALT (SGPT), γ-glutamyltransferase (GGT, γ-glutamyltranspeptidase, GGTP), and alkaline phosphatase concentrations usually are minor, not accompanied by clinical symptoms, and generally return to normal following dosage reduction or discontinuance of the drug. Rarely, severe hepatic injury (i.e., clinical hepatitis, cholestatic hepatitis, hepatocellular necrosis, cirrhosis), which has been fatal in some patients (including at least one child), has occurred. Signs and symptoms of amiodarone-induced hepatotoxicity may include hepatomegaly, ascites, abdominal pain, nausea, vomiting, anorexia, and weight loss. Hypoalbuminemia, hyperbilirubinemia, and hyperammonemia have also been reported.

Liver biopsies performed in a limited number of patients with amiodarone-induced hepatic dysfunction have revealed histologic changes resembling alcoholic hepatitis or cirrhosis. Microscopic tissue changes may include Mallory bodies within hepatocytes, mixed inflammatory infiltrates, collagen deposits and/or fibrosis, steatosis, hepatocyte destruction, and/or cholangitis. Electron microscopic studies have revealed the presence of phospholipid-laden lysosomal inclusions within hepatocytes, bile duct epithelium, Kupffer cells, and endothelial cells, even in the absence of clinically apparent hepatic disease. Although the exact mechanism of amiodarone-induced hepatic injury has not been determined, limited evidence suggests that the drug may form amiodarone-phospholipid complexes within lysosomes, resulting in phospholipidosis. Acute centrolobular confluent hepatocellular necrosis, leading to hepatic coma, acute renal failure, and death, has been associated with administration of IV amiodarone at a much higher loading dose concentration and more rapid infusion rate than recommended. (See Precautions and Contraindications.)

Serum hepatic enzyme concentrations should be monitored in patients receiving amiodarone. (See Cautions: Precautions and Contraindications.) Persistent elevations in enzyme concentrations or the development of hepatomegaly may necessitate dosage reduction or discontinuance of the drug.

■ Arrhythmogenic Effects Like other antiarrhythmic agents, amiodarone can worsen existing arrhythmias or cause new arrhythmias. Arrhythmogenic effects associated with amiodarone have occurred in approximately 2–5% of patients and have included progression of ventricular tachycardia to ventricular fibrillation, sustained ventricular tachycardia, increased resistance to cardioversion, atrial fibrillation, nodal arrhythmia, and atypical ventricular tachycardia (torsades de pointes). Transient exacerbation of preexisting cardiac arrhythmias with subsequent control during continued therapy has also been reported. Prolongation of the QT interval was reported in less than 2% of patients receiving IV amiodarone. Acceleration of ventricular rate was reported in a patient receiving IV amiodarone for the treatment of atrial fibrillation associated with Wolff-Parkinson-White syndrome. In most cases, amiodarone-induced arrhythmogenic effects should be manageable in the proper clinical setting.

Arrhythmogenic effects do not appear to occur more frequently with amiodarone than with other antiarrhythmic agents; however, such effects may be prolonged if they occur. Concomitant use of cardiac glycosides and/or other antiarrhythmic agents may increase the risk of arrhythmogenic effects during amiodarone therapy. Limited data suggest that hypokalemia may increase the risk of amiodarone-induced atypical ventricular tachycardia.

Chronic administration of antiarrhythmic drugs (e.g., amiodarone) in patients with an implanted cardiac device (e.g., defibrillator, pacemaker) may affect pacing and/or defibrillating thresholds. Therefore, the manufacturer recommends that pacing and defibrillation thresholds should be assessed at the inception of and during amiodarone therapy.

■ Nervous System Effects Adverse nervous system effects occur in approximately 20–40% of patients receiving oral amiodarone. Amiodarone-induced nervous system effects may be alleviated by dosage reduction and rarely require discontinuance of the drug.

Malaise and fatigue, tremor and/or involuntary movements, lack of coordination, abnormal gait and/or ataxia, dizziness, and paresthesia occur in about 4–9% of patients. Other adverse nervous system effects occurring in about 1–3% of patients receiving the drug include abnormal smell, insomnia, sleep disturbances, headache, and decreased libido. Adverse nervous system effects occurring less frequently include difficulty in handwriting, postural instability, dyskinetic movements, decreased ability to concentrate, confusion, memory loss, and mood lability. Delirium, hallucination, confusional state, disorientation, and parkinsonian symptoms (e.g., akinesia, bradykinesia) have been reported during postmarketing experience.

Peripheral neuropathy, demyelinating polyneuropathy, and proximal myopathy have been reported rarely in patients receiving amiodarone. Although not fully established, these adverse effects may be dose related. Amiodarone-induced peripheral neuropathy, which occurs rarely during chronic oral administration of the drug, is usually symmetrical and involves all four limbs; the neurologic deficit is usually more marked in the lower limbs than in the upper limbs. Signs and symptoms may include distal sensory loss, sensory ataxia, loss of vibratory sensation, paresthesia, and/or decreased tendon reflexes. Proximal muscle weakness also may be present. Nerve biopsies in patients with amiodarone-induced peripheral neuropathy have demonstrated complete loss of large myelinated fibers, marked reduction of small myelinated and unmyelinated axons, and evidence of lysosomal inclusion bodies within Schwann cells. Nerve conduction studies have demonstrated normal or reduced nerve conduction velocities. Although the mechanism(s) of amiodarone-induced peripheral neuropathy has not been fully determined, the mechanism may involve formation of drug-phospholipid complexes within neurons. Peripheral neuropathy and proximal myopathy generally are slowly reversible following dosage reduction or discontinuance of the drug, although resolution of peripheral neuropathy has been incomplete.

Amiodarone-induced tremor generally presents as a fine hand tremor that is clinically indistinguishable from essential tremor; the tremor may be more prominent on one side of the body than the other. Amiodarone has also reportedly exacerbated preexisting tremor or parkinsonian tremor in some patients. Although limited data suggest that cautious use of propranolol may be of some benefit in the management of amiodarone-induced tremor, further study is needed.

Pseudotumor cerebri (with papilledema) has been reported rarely during postmarketing experience in patients receiving amiodarone. Although a causal relationship has not been established, chronic anxiety reactions have also occurred during therapy with the drug.

■ Thyroid Effects Thyroid nodules or thyroid cancer, sometimes accompanied by hyperthyroidism, has been reported during postmarketing experience.

Amiodarone alters thyroid function test results in many patients and thyroid function in some patients. Because amiodarone appears to partially inhibit the peripheral conversion of thyroxine (T_4) to triiodothyronine (T_3), serum T_4 and reverse triiodothyronine (reverse T_3, rT_3) concentrations may be increased and serum T_3 concentrations may be decreased. Most patients remain clinically euthyroid despite these changes in serum thyroid hormone concentrations; however, clinical hypothyroidism or hyperthyroidism may occur, and thyroid function should therefore be monitored in patients receiving amiodarone. (See Cautions: Precautions and Contraindications.) Geriatric patients and/or patients with a history of thyroid dysfunction (e.g., goiter, hypothyroidism, hyperthyroidism, thyroid nodules) may be more likely to develop adverse thyroid effects while receiving the drug. Because of the slow elimination of amiodarone and its metabolites from the body, increased plasma iodide concentration, alterations in thyroid function, and/or abnormal thyroid function test results may persist for several weeks or months following discontinuance of the drug.

Amiodarone-induced increases in serum T_4 and rT_3 concentrations with normal or decreased serum T_3 concentrations often occur in patients receiving amiodarone and generally are not accompanied by clinical evidence of thyroid dysfunction. Such changes may be referred to as "euthyroid hyperthyroxinemia" and generally do not require specific treatment. Periodic monitoring of thyroid function tests, including serum T_3, T_4, and thyrotropin (thyroid-stimulating hormone, TSH) concentrations, is recommended in these patients.

Amiodarone-induced hypothyroidism has been reported in about 2–4% of patients receiving oral drug therapy in most clinical studies, although this effect has occurred more frequently (8–10%) in some patient series. Although not clearly established, limited data suggest that hypothyroidism may be more likely to occur in females and in patients with a prior history of thyroid dysfunction. The clinical manifestations of hypothyroidism associated with amiodarone appear to be the same as those occurring in primary idiopathic hypothyroidism. Amiodarone-induced hypothyroidism is probably best detected by monitoring for the signs and symptoms of hypothyroidism and for an elevation in serum thyrotropin concentration, a decrease in serum T_3 concentration, and/or a decrease or no change in free serum T_4 concentration compared with baseline values.

Hypothyroidism induced by amiodarone may be managed by reduction in amiodarone dosage and/or careful supplementation with thyroid agents (e.g., levothyroxine sodium) if necessary. Some clinicians have recommended cautious titration of levothyroxine sodium until serum T_4 concentrations, but not serum thyrotropin concentrations, are within the normal range. Thyroid agents must be administered with extreme caution, however, in patients with angina pectoris or cardiovascular disease; if chest pain or aggravation of cardiovascular disease occurs, dosage of the thyroid agent should be reduced or the thyroid agent discontinued. Amiodarone-induced hypothyroidism may require discontinuance of the drug in some patients and appears to regress slowly once the drug is discontinued, usually over a period of 2–3 months.

Amiodarone-induced hyperthyroidism occurs in approximately 2% of patients receiving the drug orally and may require dosage reduction or discontinuance of amiodarone therapy. Hyperthyroidism may occur more frequently in geographic areas where iodine intake is relatively low. Hyperthyroidism may occur 3 or more months following discontinuance of amiodarone therapy. Hyperthyroidism associated with amiodarone therapy generally is more difficult to diagnose and manage and more poorly tolerated than hypothyroidism. Amiodarone-associated hyperthyroidism can be fatal. The clinical manifestations of amiodarone-induced hyperthyroidism may include weight loss, anxiety, tremor, heat intolerance, thyrotoxicosis, and breakthrough arrhythmias or exacerbation of cardiac arrhythmias. Patients receiving the drug should contact their physician if exacerbation of angina or recurrence of cardiac arrhythmias occurs after an initial apparent response to therapy, even several months after discontinuing the drug, since these signs may suggest the presence of amiodarone-induced hyperthyroidism. Hyperthyroidism is probably best detected by monitoring for signs and symptoms associated with hyperthyroidism and by monitoring for elevations in serum T_3 concentrations, elevations in serum T_4 concentrations, or subnormal serum thyrotropin concentrations. A thyrotropin-releasing hormone (protirelin) stimulation test may be performed in patients with suspected hyperthyroidism to confirm diagnosis in equivocal cases, although the availability of sensitive assays for serum thyrotropin concentrations has virtually eliminated the need for such a test. Secretion of thyrotropin, induced by exogenous administration of synthetic thyrotropin-releasing hormone (protirelin), is flat or blunted in such patients.

Because clinical manifestations of hyperthyroidism (i.e., cardiac arrhythmias) may be potentially serious in patients receiving amiodarone, aggressive therapy is indicated including dosage reduction or discontinuance of amiodarone, if necessary. Conventional antithyroid agents (e.g., methimazole, propylthiouracil) have been recommended for the management of amiodarone-induced hyperthyroidism; however, these agents appear to be of limited benefit when used alone, since the intrathyroidal thyroglobulin stores generally are fully iodinated in patients receiving long-term amiodarone therapy. High intrathyroidal iodine stores antagonize the inhibitory effects of antithyroid drugs on thyroidal iodine utilization. Combination therapy with methimazole and potassium perchlorate has been used with good results in a limited number of patients with hyperthyroidism and evidence of goiter. The use of β-adrenergic blocking agents (e.g., propranolol) and/or corticosteroids may be of some benefit in the management of hyperthyroidism associated with amiodarone therapy. Radioactive iodine therapy is contraindicated in patients with amiodarone-associated hyperthyroidism because of the low radioiodine uptake due to the high concentrations of circulating iodine from amiodarone therapy and the large intrathyroidal iodine load. In patients in whom aggressive treatment of thyrotoxicosis has failed or amiodarone cannot be discontinued because it is the only drug effective against the resistant arrhythmia, surgical management may be an option. Experience with thyroidectomy as a treatment for amiodarone-induced thyrotoxicosis is limited and could induce thyroid storm. Therefore, careful surgical and anesthetic management is required. Transient hypothyroidism occasionally may occur following resolution of amiodarone-induced hyperthyroidism. Further studies are needed to determine the optimum management of hyperthyroidism in patients receiving amiodarone.

■ GI Effects Adverse GI effects, principally nausea, vomiting, constipation, and anorexia, occur in about 25% of patients receiving amiodarone orally but only rarely necessitate discontinuance of the drug. Amiodarone-induced GI disturbances occur most commonly during administration of relatively large oral dosages of the drug (e.g., loading doses) and usually are alleviated by dosage reduction or administration in divided doses with meals.

Nausea and vomiting occur in about 10–33% of patients receiving oral amiodarone; nausea and vomiting occur in approximately 4% and less than 2% of patients receiving IV amiodarone, respectively. Constipation and anorexia have occurred in about 4–9% of patients, and abdominal pain, abnormal salivation, and abnormal taste have occurred in about 1–3% of patients. Epigastric burning or fullness and diarrhea have been reported rarely in patients receiving oral amiodarone; however, a causal relationship to the drug has not been established. Diarrhea has been reported in less than 2% of patients receiving the drug IV. Pancreatitis has been reported during postmarketing experience.

■ Ocular Effects Asymptomatic corneal microdeposits are present in practically all adults who receive oral amiodarone for longer than 6 months. These corneal deposits generally are detectable only by slit-lamp ophthalmologic examination and usually are not associated with visual disturbances; however, subjective visual disturbances including halo vision (particularly at night and/or while looking at bright objects), blurred vision, photophobia, and dry eyes may occur in up to 10% of patients receiving the drug.

The development of amiodarone-induced corneal deposits appears to be related to both dosage and duration of therapy. Limited data suggest that more extensive deposits occur in patients receiving amiodarone hydrochloride dosages of 400–1400 mg daily than in patients receiving dosages of 100–200 mg daily. The corneal deposits generally develop within 1–4 months but have occurred as soon as a few weeks after beginning therapy with the drug. Amiodarone keratopathy appears to occur rarely in pediatric patients, possibly because of greater lacrimal secretion and more rapid lacrimal circulation in children than in adults.

Corneal microdeposits generally occur bilaterally and symmetrically. Slit-lamp examination during the early stage of amiodarone keratopathy usually demonstrates fine, punctate, gray to golden brown opacities in a horizontal, linear pattern in the inferior cornea; these deposits then progress gradually into a characteristic, whorl-like pattern with continued therapy. Although the mechanism of amiodarone-induced keratopathy is not known, the presence of complex lipid deposits within lysosome-like intracytoplasmic inclusions suggests possible deposition of amiodarone-phospholipid complexes or lipofuscin within corneal epithelium as well as other epithelial structures of the eye. Corneal microdeposits and visual disturbances are reversible following dosage reduction or discontinuance of amiodarone, usually within about 3 months (range: 2–7 months). Methylcellulose ophthalmic solutions have been used in patients receiving amiodarone in an attempt to decrease the severity of existing microdeposits and progression of the keratopathy, but the efficacy of such therapy has not been established. The presence of asymptomatic corneal microdeposits does *not* necessitate dosage reduction or withdrawal of amiodarone. If severe and/or persistent visual disturbances occur, they may subside with dosage reduction if continued amiodarone therapy is considered necessary.

Optic neuropathy and/or optic neuritis, which may occur at any time following initiation of amiodarone therapy and usually results in visual impairment, has been reported in patients receiving amiodarone. In some patients, such visual impairment has progressed to permanent blindness. Diplopia, nystagmus, and itching of the eyes have been reported rarely. In addition, papilledema, corneal degeneration, scotoma, lens opacities, ocular discomfort, and macular degeneration have been reported in patients receiving amiodarone therapy. Visual disturbances infrequently impair visual acuity to a substantial degree and rarely require discontinuance of the drug.

■ Local, Dermatologic, and Sensitivity Reactions Local injection-site reactions (i.e., pain, erythema, edema, pigment changes, phlebitis, cellulitis, necrosis, skin sloughing) have been reported during postmarketing experience in patients receiving IV injection of amiodarone in recommended dosages.

Adverse dermatologic reactions occur in about 15% of patients receiving oral amiodarone. The most common adverse dermatologic effect associated with amiodarone is photosensitivity, which occurs in about 10% of patients but usually does not require discontinuance of the drug. When photosensitivity occurs, it generally begins within 2 hours of exposure to sunlight, and symptoms may consist of a burning or tingling sensation followed by erythema; blistering occurs infrequently. Swelling of sunlight-exposed areas has been reported rarely. Amiodarone-induced photosensitivity reactions generally last for 1–3 days, but may last as long as a week in severe cases. Photosensitivity reactions may occur up to 4 months following discontinuance of the drug. Enhanced tanning ability has also been reported in some patients receiving the drug.

Since exposure to visible light (wavelengths longer than 400 nm) and/or ultraviolet (UV) wavelengths near the visible spectrum (longer than 320 nm) has resulted in photosensitivity reactions in patients receiving amiodarone, both sunlight and light transmitted through window glass may potentially induce photosensitivity reactions in patients receiving the drug. Sunscreen agents may help to at least partially prevent amiodarone-induced photosensitivity reactions, particularly opaque physical sunscreens (i.e., agents containing zinc oxide, titanium dioxide) and chemical sunscreens that absorb longer UV light wavelengths (i.e., dioxybenzone, oxybenzone). Protective clothing and avoidance of exposure to sunlight are also recommended to at least partially prevent photosensitivity reactions. Although administration of pyridoxine hydrochloride has been recommended for the prevention of photosensitivity in patients receiving amiodarone, in vitro data and data from clinical use suggest that pyridoxine does not prevent and possibly may worsen amiodarone-induced photosensitivity reactions. Reduction in amiodarone dosage may partially alleviate photosensitivity reactions in some patients.

Long-term administration of amiodarone is associated with pigment deposition resulting in a blue-gray discoloration of the skin. The manufacturer states that blue-gray skin pigmentation occurred in less than 1% of patients who had received the drug for an average of about 440 days (range: 2–1515 days); however, in clinical studies, blue-gray skin pigmentation was reported in approximately 2–5% of patients. The incidence appears to be related to both the cumulative dosage and duration of therapy. Pigmentary changes of the skin generally are restricted to exposed areas of the body, particularly the face and hands, and may be mistaken for cyanosis. Exposure to sunlight or visible light and fairness of complexion appear to be risk factors. Although not clearly established, limited data suggest that photosensitivity reactions may predispose to the development of blue-gray pigmentation. The mechanism(s) of amiodarone-induced blue-gray discoloration is not known; however, histologic examination in a limited number of patients has revealed lysosomal, membrane-bound bodies containing amiodarone, *N*-desethylamiodarone, lipids, and possibly lipofuscin. Blue-gray pigmentation is of cosmetic importance only. The pigmentation usually is slowly reversible following discontinuance of the drug, although this may require up to a year in some cases. Occasionally, the pigmentation may not be completely reversible. Skin cancer has been reported during postmarketing experience with amiodarone.

Rash and hair loss have been reported in less than 1% of patients receiving oral amiodarone. Toxic epidermal necrolysis (sometimes fatal) and generalized pustular psoriasis also have been reported in patients receiving amiodarone. Exfoliative dermatitis and erythema multiforme also have been reported. Stevens-Johnson syndrome has been reported in less than 2% of patients receiving the drug IV and also has been reported during postmarketing experience with amiodarone. Pruritus has been reported during postmarketing experience with amiodarone.

Angioedema, urticaria, eczema, or bronchospasm has been reported during postmarketing experience with amiodarone therapy; anaphylactic/anaphylactoid reactions, including shock, also have been reported during postmarketing experience in patients receiving amiodarone.

Granuloma has been reported through postmarketing experience in patients receiving amiodarone.

■ Cardiovascular Effects New or worsened heart failure reportedly occurs in about 3% or about 2% of patients receiving oral or IV amiodarone therapy, respectively; however, it is often difficult to distinguish between spontaneous and amiodarone-induced depression of left ventricular function. Congestive heart failure rarely requires discontinuance of the drug.

Hypotension was the most frequent adverse effect observed in clinical trials of IV amiodarone, occurring in approximately 16% of patients. Hypotension has occurred in less than 1% of patients receiving oral amiodarone. Hypotension refractory to treatment and resulting in death has been reported during postmarketing experience with IV amiodarone. The relationship to amiodarone is not known, but hypotension (probably resulting from decreased cardiac output and/or decreased peripheral vascular resistance) has occurred rarely during open-heart surgery (during and/or following cardiopulmonary bypass) in patients receiving the drug. (See Cautions: Precautions and Contraindications.) An interaction between amiodarone and various anesthetic agents has been suggested but not clearly established. Some manufacturers and clinicians state that close perioperative monitoring is recommended in amiodarone-treated patients undergoing general anesthesia, since amiodarone may sensitize patients to the myocardial depressant and conduction effects of halogenated hydrocarbon general anesthetics.

Flushing and edema have occurred in about 1–3% of patients receiving oral amiodarone. In patients receiving IV amiodarone, cardiac arrest and shock have been reported in 2.9% and less than 2% of patients, respectively; asystole also has been reported. Venous thrombosis and thrombophlebitis have been reported with IV amiodarone during postmarketing experience.

■ Effects on Cardiac Conduction and Sinus Node Function Clinically important conduction disturbances, mainly AV and intraventricular block, occur infrequently in patients receiving amiodarone and are reversible following discontinuance of the drug. Sinoatrial block has also been reported. Rarely, amiodarone-induced QT prolongation has been associated with arrhythmogenicity.

Amiodarone generally depresses sinus node function. SA node dysfunction, including symptomatic sinus bradycardia or sinus arrest with suppression of escape foci, has occurred in approximately 1–5% of patients. Concomitant administration of a cardiac glycoside, β-adrenergic blocking agent, and/or calcium-channel blocking agent may increase the risk of sinus bradyarrhythmias. The relationship to amiodarone is not known, but atropine-resistant sinus bradycardia, sinus arrest, and/or AV block have also occurred in some amiodarone-treated patients undergoing general anesthesia, mainly for open-heart surgery. (See Cautions: Precautions and Contraindications.) Patients with preexisting sinus bradycardia or sinus node disease may have an increased risk of amiodarone-induced sinus bradyarrhythmias. Sinus bradycardia induced by amiodarone generally is not fully responsive to atropine.Bradycardia usually responds to dosage reduction, but administration of a β-adrenergic agonist (e.g., isoproterenol) and/or insertion of an artificial ventricular pacemaker may be necessary in patients with severe amiodarone-induced sinus bradyarrhythmias; amiodarone has been discontinued in several patients because of bradycardia.

■ Hematologic Effects Coagulation abnormalities have occurred in about 1–3% of patients receiving oral amiodarone, and spontaneous ecchymosis has occurred in less than 1% of patients receiving the drug. Severe thrombocytopenia, resulting in ecchymoses and petechiae, has occurred in a few patients receiving the drug. Following discontinuance of amiodarone and initiation of corticosteroid therapy, platelet counts gradually increased to normal values over a period of 12–16 days; subsequent administration of the drug resulted in recurrence of thrombocytopenia. Thrombocytopenia has been reported in less than 2% of patients receiving IV amiodarone. Although not clearly established, positive lymphocyte stimulation test results suggest that a delayed hypersensitivity reaction may be responsible for the thrombocytopenia. Hemolytic anemia, aplastic anemia, pancytopenia, agranulocytosis, and neutropenia have been reported during postmarketing experience in patients receiving amiodarone.

■ Other Adverse Effects Noninfectious epididymitis or epididymo-orchitis and/or scrotal pain have occurred in some patients receiving high oral dosages of amiodarone and/or long-term therapy with the drug. In patients who developed epididymitis, epididymal enlargement initially occurred unilaterally but later progressed bilaterally. Epididymitis subsided in some patients with reduction of amiodarone dosage but resolved in other patients despite continued therapy without dosage adjustment. Abnormal kidney function has been reported in less than 2% of patients receiving the drug IV. Renal insufficiency/impairment or acute renal failure has been reported with IV amiodarone during postmarketing experience. Impotence also has been reported during postmarketing experience with amiodarone therapy.

Gynecomastia, which was reversible following withdrawal of amiodarone but recurred upon rechallenge, has been reported. Hyperglycemia, symptomatic hypoglycemia, and vasculitis have been reported rarely. Myopathy, rhabdomyolysis, and muscle weakness have been reported during postmarketing experience in patients receiving amiodarone. (See HMG-CoA Reductase Inhibitors (Statins), under Drug Interactions: Drugs, Foods, and Dietary or Herbal Supplements Affecting Hepatic Microsomal Enzymes.) Syndrome of inappropriate antidiuretic hormone secretion (SIADH) has been reported during postmarketing experience in patients receiving amiodarone therapy.

Symptomatic bradycardia, sometimes requiring pacemaker intervention, has been reported in patients receiving amiodarone concomitantly with a hepatitis C virus (HCV) treatment regimen containing sofosbuvir in conjunction with another HCV direct-acting antiviral (DAA), including ledipasvir, simeprevir, or daclatasvir. Fatal cardiac arrest was reported in a patient receiving amiodarone concomitantly with the fixed combination containing ledipasvir and sofosbuvir (ledipasvir/sofosbuvir). In most reported cases, bradycardia occurred within hours to days after HCV treatment containing sofosbuvir with another DAA was initiated in patients receiving amiodarone, but has been observed up to 2 weeks after initiation of such HCV treatment regimens in patients receiving amiodarone. Bradycardia generally resolved after the HCV treatment regimen was discontinued. The mechanism for this adverse cardiovascular effect is unknown. Patients who may be at increased risk for symptomatic bradycardia if amiodarone is used concomitantly with an HCV treatment regimen containing sofosbuvir and another DAA include those also receiving a β-adrenergic blocking agent, those with underlying cardiac comorbidities, and/or those with advanced liver disease. Because of these reports of symptomatic bradycardia, concomitant use of amiodarone with an HCV treatment regimen containing sofosbuvir with another DAA (e.g., ledipasvir, simeprevir, daclatasvir) is not recommended. (See Drug Interactions: HCV Antivirals.)

■ Precautions and Contraindications Patients should be instructed to read the medication guide provided by the manufacturer before initiating therapy with amiodarone and each time the prescription is refilled, since new information may be available.

Amiodarone is a highly toxic drug and exhibits several potentially fatal toxicities, notably pulmonary toxicity. Because of its pharmacokinetic properties, difficult dosing schedule, and severity of adverse effects in patients who are improperly monitored, amiodarone should be administered only by clinicians who are experienced in the management of life-threatening arrhythmias, who are thoroughly familiar with the risks and benefits associated with amiodarone therapy, and who have access to laboratory facilities necessary to adequately monitor the efficacy and adverse effects of the drug, including continuous ECG monitoring and electrophysiologic techniques for evaluating the patient in both ambulatory and hospital settings. Because of the risks of substantial toxicity, amiodarone therapy currently is reserved principally for the management of documented life-threatening ventricular arrhythmias. Even in patients at high risk of death from arrhythmia, in whom the risks of toxicity are acceptable, use of amiodarone poses major management difficulties that could be life-threatening in a patient population at risk of sudden death, and maximum efforts should be made to utilize alternative antiarrhythmic agents initially.

Because of the life-threatening nature of the arrhythmias treated, lack of a predictable time course of antiarrhythmic effect, and the risks of arrhythmogenic effects and potential interactions with previous drug therapy, the loading-dose phase of oral amiodarone therapy should be performed in a hospital setting. Close monitoring of patients during the loading-dose phase of therapy is necessary, especially until the risk of recurrent ventricular tachycardia or fibrillation has abated. The difficulties associated with using amiodarone effectively and safely pose substantial risks to the patient. Even with an oral loading-dose regimen, a response to orally administered drug generally requires at least 1 week and usually 2 or more weeks of therapy. Because absorption and elimination of amiodarone are variable, adjustment of maintenance dosage is difficult, it is not unusual to require dosage reduction or temporary withdrawal or discontinuance of the drug. Patients who experience serious adverse effects during therapy with amiodarone should immediately contact their clinician or seek medical attention; in addition, patients should contact their clinician before discontinuance of the drug.

The time at which a previously controlled life-threatening arrhythmia will recur after reduction of amiodarone dosage or discontinuance of the drug is unpredictable, ranging from weeks to months. During this period, the patient is at great risk and may need prolonged hospitalization or intensive ambulatory monitoring (e.g., via telemetric ECG), possibly with periodic determination of plasma concentrations of the drug. Attempts to substitute other antiarrhythmic agents when amiodarone must be discontinued because of inefficacy or intolerance are difficult because of the gradually, but unpredictably, changing body burden of the drug, the drug's residual effects, and its potential interactions with subsequent treatment.

Because amiodarone may cause pulmonary toxicity that is potentially fatal, baseline pulmonary function tests, including diffusion capacity, should be performed prior to initiation of oral amiodarone therapy, and periodic chest radiographs and clinical evaluation should be performed every 3–6 months during therapy with the drug. Periodic pulmonary function testing also should be considered. Preoperative pulmonary function tests are recommended for patients undergoing cardiothoracic surgery since ARDS may develop postoperatively in patients receiving the drug. Until further studies have been performed, some manufacturers recommend that FiO_2 and tissue oxygenation (as determined by SaO_2 or PaO_2) be closely monitored in patients receiving amiodarone. (See Cautions: Pulmonary Effects.) Amiodarone should be used with caution, if at all, in patients with preexisting pulmonary disease, including chronic obstructive disease, or reduced pulmonary diffusion capacity. Patients should inform their clinician of preexisting lung or breathing disorders prior to initiation of amiodarone therapy. The possibility of amiodarone-induced pulmonary toxicity should be considered in any patient developing a new respiratory symptom during therapy with the drug. Patients should contact their clinician if dyspnea, wheezing, coughing, chest pain, hemoptysis, or any other breathing disorders occur during therapy with amiodarone. Clinical and radiographic evaluation, as well as scintigraphic and pulmonary function testing (including diffusion capacity), if necessary, are recommended in such patients. Respiratory symptoms should be carefully assessed and other causes of respiratory impairment (e.g., congestive heart failure, pulmonary embolism, malignancy) should be ruled out before discontinuance of the drug. Measurement of pulmonary capillary wedge pressure may help exclude congestive heart failure as a cause of symptoms or radiographic findings. Since amiodarone-induced pulmonary toxicity may mimic infection, possible infectious causes should be excluded; bronchoalveolar lavage, transbronchial lung biopsy, and/or open lung biopsy may aid in the diagnosis, especially in patients in whom alternative antiarrhythmic therapy is not available. The manufacturer states that the presence of suppressor/cytotoxic ($CD8^+$, $T8^+$) T-cell lymphocytosis in bronchoalveolar lavage specimens should be considered confirmatory of hypersensitivity pneumonitis. If hypersensitivity pneumonitis occurs, corticosteroid therapy should be initiated and amiodarone should be discontinued. If evidence of interstitial pneumonitis (alveolitis) is present, dosage of amiodarone should be reduced and, preferably, therapy with the drug withdrawn in an attempt to determine whether the toxicity is reversible; however, amiodarone should be discontinued with caution in patients with life-threatening arrhythmias, since sudden cardiac death is common in these patients.

Because amiodarone can alter results of thyroid function tests and/or cause clinical hypothyroidism or hyperthyroidism, thyroid function tests should be performed prior to initiating amiodarone therapy and at periodic intervals (approximately every 3–6 months) thereafter, particularly in geriatric patients and/or in patients with a prior history of thyroid nodules, goiter, or other thyroid dysfunction. Patients should inform their clinician if they have thyroid dysfunction or a history of such dysfunction prior to initiation of therapy. In addition, patients receiving amiodarone should be instructed to report episodes of chest pain, weight loss or gain, weakness, heat or cold intolerance, hair thinning, diaphoresis, menstrual cycle changes, swelling in the neck (e.g., goiter), nervousness, irritability, restlessness, decreased concentration, depression in geriatric patients, tremor, or aggravation of cardiovascular disease to their clinician, since such manifestations may indicate amiodarone-induced thyroid dysfunction. If any new signs of cardiac arrhythmias appear, the possibility of hyperthyroidism should be considered. The risks and benefits of amiodarone therapy in patients with thyroid dysfunction should be carefully considered because of the potential for arrhythmia breakthrough or exacerbation of arrhythmias, which may result in death, in such patients.

Because amiodarone may cause elevations in serum hepatic enzyme concentrations and may rarely cause severe, potentially fatal, hepatic injury, serum hepatic enzyme concentrations should be monitored at regular intervals in patients receiving the drug, particularly those receiving relatively high maintenance dosages. Patients should inform their clinician of preexisting liver dysfunction prior to initiation of amiodarone therapy. Patients should contact their clinician if nausea or vomiting, dark urine, fatigue, jaundice, or stomach pain occurs during amiodarone therapy. In patients with life-threatening arrhythmias, the potential risk of hepatic injury should be weighed against the potential benefit of IV amiodarone therapy. If serum hepatic enzyme concentrations increase to more than 3 times normal values in patients with normal pretreatment values or twice baseline pretreatment values in patients with elevated values prior to amiodarone therapy, or if hepatomegaly or progressive hepatic injury occurs, a reduction in oral amiodarone dosage, a decrease in the infusion rate during parenteral amiodarone therapy, or discontinuance of the drug should be considered. Because the risk of hepatic necrosis during IV amiodarone therapy may be related to the use of rapid infusion rates and excessive drug concentrations in the initial loading dose, the initial amiodarone concentration and IV infusion rate should be monitored closely and should not exceed those recommended by the manufacturer. Liver biopsy with ultrastructural study by electron microscopy may aid in the diagnosis of amiodarone-induced hepatic toxicity.

Because amiodarone causes corneal microdeposits in almost all patients and optic neuropathy occasionally may result in visual disturbances, the manufacturer and some clinicians recommend that a baseline ophthalmologic examination (e.g., a slit-lamp evaluation) be performed before initiating therapy with the drug and then possibly at periodic intervals during long-term therapy (e.g., after the first 6 months and then annually and/or as necessary). Patients experiencing visual disturbances or those receiving long-term therapy should be monitored carefully. Patients experiencing visual disturbances (e.g., blurred vision, visual halos, ocular photosensitivity) should contact their clinician. The presence of nonprogressive, asymptomatic corneal microdeposits does *not* necessitate dosage reduction or discontinuance of amiodarone. In addition, optic neuropathy and/or optic neuritis (usually resulting in visual impairment, which sometimes may progress to permanent blindness) has been reported in patients receiving amiodarone and although a causal relationship to the drug has not been clearly established, some manufacturers state that if visual impairment occurs (e.g., changes in visual acuity, decreases in peripheral vision), a prompt ophthalmologic examination should be performed. If optic neuropathy and/or optic neuritis has developed, amiodarone therapy should be reevaluated and the described risks and complications should be weighed against the possible benefits of antiarrhythmic therapy. Routine ophthalmologic examinations, including slit-lamp and funduscopic tests, should performed in patients receiving amiodarone therapy. Most manufacturers of corneal refractive laser surgery devices consider the procedure to be contraindicated in patients receiving amiodarone.

The use of sunscreen agents and protective clothing and avoidance of excessive exposure to sunlight are recommended to help prevent photosensitivity reactions associated with amiodarone therapy. Patients with fair complexions or excessive exposure to sunlight or those who have received prolonged amiodarone therapy and/or relatively large cumulative doses appear to be more susceptible to amiodarone-induced blue-gray skin discoloration.

Hypotension has been reported during open-heart surgery (during and/or following cardiopulmonary bypass) in amiodarone-treated patients. Patients should inform their clinician of blood pressure abnormalities prior to initiating amiodarone therapy. Atropine-resistant sinus bradycardia, sinus arrest, and/or AV block also have occurred in some amiodarone-treated patients undergoing general anesthesia for major surgery. The relationship of these effects to amiodarone is not known. An interaction between the antiarrhythmic agent and various anesthetic agents has been suggested but not clearly established. The hypotension may be severe in some patients and require larger than usual dosages of sympathomimetic agents and/or intra-aortic balloon counterpulsation. Sinus bradyarrhythmias and/or AV block may require insertion of an artificial pacemaker. Pending further evaluation, the anesthesiologist should be aware of potential complications in patients undergoing general anesthesia who are currently receiving amiodarone or who have previously received the drug within the past 1–2 months. In addition, close perioperative monitoring is recommended in patients undergoing general anesthesia while receiving amiodarone, since amiodarone may sensitize patients to the myocardial depressant and conduction effects of halogenated hydrocarbon general anesthetics.

Because IV amiodarone therapy is associated with bradycardia, patients with a known predisposition to bradycardia or AV block should be treated with IV amiodarone in a setting where a temporary pacemaker is available. Patients should contact their clinician if they experience heart pounding, irregular heart beat, very fast or slow heartbeat, lightheadedness, or faintness during amiodarone therapy. Also, because of the risk of proarrhythmia during parenteral amiodarone therapy, patients should be monitored for QT_c prolongation during infusion of amiodarone. The need to coadminister amiodarone with other drugs that are known to prolong the QT_c interval must be based on a careful assessment of the potential risks and benefits in individual patients. (See Drugs Affecting the QT Interval, under Drug Interactions.)

Since antiarrhythmic agents, including amiodarone, may be less effective and/or more arrhythmogenic in patients with hypokalemia or hypomagnesemia, the possibility of a potassium or magnesium deficiency should be evaluated and, if present, corrected prior to initiation of amiodarone therapy. Special attention should be given to electrolyte and acid-base balance in patients experiencing severe or prolonged diarrhea or in patients receiving concomitant diuretics.

Because of the possibility of clinically important interactions when amiodarone is used concomitantly with other drugs, patients should inform their clinicians of their use of other drugs, including prescription and nonprescription drugs, or of dietary and herbal supplements such as St. John's wort. (See Drug Interactions.) Grapefruit juice is known to inhibit cytochrome P-450 (CYP) 3A4-mediated metabolism of oral amiodarone, resulting in increased plasma concentrations of the drug; therefore, patients should be instructed not to consume grapefruit juice during treatment with oral amiodarone. (See Grapefruit Juice under Drug Interactions: Drugs, Foods, and Dietary or Herbal Supplements Affecting Hepatic Microsomal Enzymes.)

Amiodarone is contraindicated in patients with cardiogenic shock, in patients with severe sinus node dysfunction resulting in marked sinus bradycardia, in patients with second- or third-degree AV block, and in patients with episodes of bradycardia that have caused syncope, except when used concomitantly with an artificial pacemaker. Amiodarone also is contraindicated in patients with known hypersensitivity to the drug or any ingredient in the formulation, including iodine; IV amiodarone is contraindicated in patients with known hypersensitivity to any components of the parenteral formulation, including iodine.

■ **Pediatric Precautions** Safety and efficacy of amiodarone in children† have not been established. In a clinical trial in pediatric patients 30 days to 15 years of age, hypotension (36%), bradycardia (20%), and atrioventricular block (15%) were common dose-related adverse effects, and in some cases were severe or life-threatening. In this trial, injection-site reactions were observed in 5 of 20 patients receiving IV amiodarone through a peripheral vein. Limited data suggest that the drug may be useful in carefully selected cases for the management of refractory supraventricular or ventricular tachycardias in children, and current guidelines for pediatric advanced life support (PALS) recommend the use of amiodarone or lidocaine for the treatment of shock-refractory ventricular fibrillation or pulseless ventricular tachycardia. This recommendation is based principally on extrapolation of data from adult studies as well as an observational study in pediatric patients suggesting improved return of spontaneous circulation (ROSC) with lidocaine compared with amiodarone.

Each mL of the commercially available amiodarone hydrochloride IV injection contains 20.2 mg of benzyl alcohol as a preservative. Although a causal relationship has not been established, administration of injections preserved with benzyl alcohol has been associated with toxicity in neonates. Toxicity appears to have resulted from administration of large amounts (i.e., 100–400 mg/kg daily) of benzyl alcohol in these neonates. Although use of drugs preserved with benzyl alcohol should be avoided in neonates whenever possible, the American Academy of Pediatrics states that the presence of small amounts of the preservative in a commercially available injection should not proscribe its use when indicated in neonates.

In addition, the commercially available amiodarone hydrochloride IV injection has been found to leach diethylhexyl phthalate (DEHP) plasticizer from IV tubing (e.g., PVC tubing). Leaching of DEHP is increased when IV amiodarone hydrochloride is infused at higher concentrations and slower infusion rates than those recommended by the manufacturer. After reviewing data from animal studies and limited experience in humans, an expert panel of the National Toxicology Program Center for the Evaluation of Risks to Human Reproduction (NTP-CERHR) concluded that exposure to DEHP may adversely affect male reproductive tract development during fetal, infant, and toddler stages of development if the exposure at these stages is severalfold higher than that in adults, a situation that might be associated with intensive medical procedures such as those performed in critically ill infants. In studies in sexually mature rats, an oral amiodarone hydrochloride dosage of 3.7–14 mg/kg daily was associated with no observable adverse effects; however, in rats at the postnatal stage, a dosage level associated with no observable adverse effects was not identified. The maximum anticipated exposure to DEHP following IV administration of amiodarone hydrochloride in pediatric patients has been calculated to be about 1.9 mg/kg daily for a 3-kg infant, which provides about a 2- to 7-fold margin of safety. In pediatric patients requiring therapy with IV amiodarone hydrochloride, dosing methods that may reduce potential exposure to DEHP (e.g., IV loading dose of 5 mg/kg given in 5 divided doses of 1 mg/kg, with each incremental dose infused over 5–10 minutes) may be considered.

■ **Geriatric Precautions** While clinical experience to date has not revealed age-related differences in response to amiodarone, clinical studies evaluating the drug have not included sufficient numbers of adults 65 years of age and older to determine whether geriatric patients respond differently than younger adults. The manufacturers state that dosage in general for geriatric patients should be selected carefully, usually starting at the low end of the dosage range, because these individuals frequently have decreased hepatic, renal, and/or cardiac function and concomitant disease and drug therapy. In addition, geriatric patients may be more susceptible to bradycardia and conduction disturbances induced by the drug.

■ **Mutagenicity and Carcinogenicity** No evidence of amiodarone-induced mutagenicity was seen with an in vitro microbial test system (Ames test). Amiodarone also was not mutagenic in the micronucleus or lysogenic test.

Long-term studies in rats indicated that oral amiodarone caused a substantial, dose-related increase in thyroid tumors (follicular adenoma and/or carcinoma), with an increase in tumors occurring even at dosages as low as 5 mg/kg daily (approximately 0.08 times the maximum recommended human maintenance dosage of 600 mg for a 50-kg patient [calculated on the basis of body surface area]). No carcinogenicity studies were conducted with IV amiodarone.

■ **Pregnancy, Fertility, and Lactation** ***Pregnancy*** Reproduction studies in pregnant rats or rabbits receiving oral amiodarone hydrochloride dosages of 25 mg/kg daily (approximately 0.4 and 0.9 times, respectively, the maximum recommended human maintenance dosage of 600 mg for a 50-kg patient [calculated on the basis of body surface area]) revealed no evidence of harm to the fetus. However, in pregnant rabbits receiving oral amiodarone hydrochloride dosages of 75 mg/kg daily (approximately 2.7 times the maximum recommended human maintenance dosage of 600 mg for a 50-kg patient [calculated on the basis of body surface area]), abortions occurred in more than 90% of these rabbits. Slight displacement of the testes and an increased incidence of incomplete ossification of some skull and digital bones were reported in pregnant rats receiving oral amiodarone hydrochloride dosages of 50 mg/kg daily (approximately 0.8 times the maximum recommended human maintenance dosage of 600 mg for a 50-kg patient [calculated on the basis of body surface area]) or more. In addition, in rats receiving oral amiodarone hydrochloride dosages of 100 mg/kg daily (approximately 1.6 times the maximum recommended human maintenance dosage of 600 mg for a 50-kg patient [calculated on the basis of body surface area] or more, or 200 mg/kg daily (approximately 1.6 or 3.2 times the maximum recommended human maintenance dosage of 600 mg for a 50-kg patient [calculated on the basis of body surface area]), reduced fetal body weight or increased incidence of fetal resorptions, respectively, were observed. Adverse effects on fetal growth and survival also were reported in 1 of 2 strains of mice receiving oral amiodarone hydrochloride dosages of 5 mg/kg daily (approximately 0.04 times the maximum recommended human maintenance dosage of 600 mg for a 50-kg patient [calculated on the basis of body surface area]).

In a reproductive study in which amiodarone was administered IV to rabbits at dosages of 5, 10, or 25 mg/kg daily (approximately 0.1, 0.3, or 0.7 times the recommended maximum human dose on the basis of body surface area, respectively), maternal deaths occurred in all groups, including controls. Embryotoxicity, as manifested by fewer full-term fetuses and increased resorptions with concomitantly lower litter weights, occurred at dosages of 10 mg/kg and greater. No evidence of embryotoxicity was observed at the 5 mg/kg dosage and no teratogenicity was observed at any dosage level tested. In a teratology study in which amiodarone was administered by continuous IV infusion to rats at dosages of 25, 50, or 100 mg/kg daily (approximately 0.4, 0.7, or 1.4 times the recommended maximum human dose on the basis of body surface area, respectively), maternal toxicity (as evidenced by reduced weight gain and food consumption) and embryotoxicity (as evidenced by increased resorptions, decreased live litter size, reduced body weights, and retarded sternum and metacarpal ossification) were observed in the group receiving 100 mg/kg daily.

Amiodarone and *N*-desethylamiodarone cross the placenta to a limited extent. QT prolongation and transient sinus bradycardia have been observed in neonates of a limited number of pregnant women who received the drug during the second and/or third trimester. Specific data are not available, but there are concerns that amiodarone potentially could adversely affect fetal thyroid function and overall development. Congenital goiter/hypothyroidism and hyperthyroidism have been observed in a limited number of neonates born to women who received amiodarone during pregnancy. Amiodarone should be used during pregnancy only when the potential benefits justify the possible risks to the fetus. Women should inform their clinicians if they are or plan to become pregnant or plan to breast-feed. If amiodarone is used during pregnancy or if the patient becomes pregnant while receiving the drug, the patient should be apprised of the potential hazard to the fetus. Women of childbearing potential should avoid becoming pregnant during amiodarone therapy. The prolonged elimination of amiodarone from the body after discontinuance of the drug should be considered when a woman of childbearing potential receiving amiodarone plans to become pregnant. It is not known whether use of amiodarone during labor and delivery could have any immediate or delayed adverse effects on the mother or fetus. Studies in rodents have not shown any effect of the drug on duration of gestation or on parturition.

Fertility Reproduction studies in male and female rats using oral amiodarone hydrochloride dosages of 90 mg/kg daily (approximately 1.4 times the maximum recommended human maintenance dosage of 600 mg for a 50-kg patient [calculated on the basis of body surface area]) and initiated 9 weeks prior to mating, have revealed evidence of reduced fertility. Amiodarone and *N*-desethylamiodarone are distributed in high concentrations into human testes and semen. No fertility studies were conducted with IV amiodarone.

Lactation Amiodarone and, to a lesser extent, *N*-desethylamiodarone are distributed into milk in concentrations substantially higher than concurrent maternal plasma concentrations. Nursing offspring of lactating rats receiving amiodarone have been shown to be less viable and to have reduced bodyweight gains. Because nursing may expose the infant to a substantial dose of amiodarone and its metabolite, it is recommended that nursing be discontinued during amiodarone therapy. The slow elimination of amiodarone from the body after discontinuance of the drug should also be considered.

Drug Interactions

While only a limited number of drug interactions with amiodarone have been investigated, most drugs studied to date have been shown to interact with amiodarone. Few data are available on drug interactions with parenteral amiodarone therapy; most of the information on drug interactions with amiodarone comes from experience with *oral* administration of the drug. The possibility of interactions with any concomitantly administered drug and amiodarone should be anticipated, particularly for drugs with potentially serious toxic effects such as other antiarrhythmic agents. If such drugs are needed, their dosage should be carefully reassessed and adjusted as necessary, and plasma concentrations of such drugs should be measured, if appropriate.

Because of the long and variable elimination half-life of amiodarone, the potential for interactions exists not only with concomitantly administered drugs but also with drugs administered after discontinuance of amiodarone therapy.

■ **Drugs Affecting the QT Interval** Amiodarone prolongs the QT_c interval, and clinicians should consider the possibility that potentially serious cardiac arrhythmias, including torsades de pointes, could occur if amiodarone were used concomitantly with other drugs that prolong the QT_c interval (e.g., cisapride [no longer commercially available in the US], halofantrine [no longer commercially available in the US], dolasetron, pimozide, disopyramide, fluoroquinolones, loratadine, macrolide antibiotics, trazodone, ziprasidone, azole antifungal agents). Use of amiodarone with any other agent known to prolong the QT_c interval must be based on a careful assessment of the potential risks and benefits of such combination therapy. Some manufacturers state that such combined use should be avoided or is contraindicated. If dolasetron and amiodarone are used concomitantly, caution should be exercised and cardiac function should be monitored.

■ **Drugs with P-Glycoprotein-mediated Clearance** Amiodarone inhibits the P-glycoprotein transport system, which may result in unexpectedly high plasma concentrations of drugs that are substrates for this transport system.

■ **Drugs, Foods, and Dietary or Herbal Supplements Affecting Hepatic Microsomal Enzymes** Amiodarone is metabolized by the cytochrome P-450 (CYP) microsomal enzyme system, principally the isoenzymes CYP3A4 and CYP2C8. Therefore, amiodarone has the potential for interactions with drugs or substances that may be substrates, inhibitors, or inducers of CYP3A4 and CYP2C8. Amiodarone also inhibits CYP2D6, CYP1A2, CYP2C9, and CYP3A4 isoenzymes. Inhibition of these isoenzymes by amiodarone may result in unexpectedly high plasma concentrations of other drugs which are metabolized by these isoenzymes. (See Cyclosporine and see HMG-CoA Reductase Inhibitors (Statins) under Drug Interactions: Drugs, Food, and Dietary or Herbal Supplements Affecting Hepatic Microsomal Enzymes.)

Antiarrhythmic Agents The use of amiodarone in conjunction with other antiarrhythmic agents generally should be reserved for patients with life-threatening arrhythmias who do not respond completely to either a single antiarrhythmic agent or amiodarone alone. When combination therapy with amiodarone is employed, it is generally recommended that dosage of the currently administered antiarrhythmic agent(s) be reduced by 30–50% several days after initiation of amiodarone therapy, since the onset of amiodarone's antiarrhythmic effect may be delayed. The necessity of continuing the other antiarrhythmic agent(s) should be assessed after the antiarrhythmic effect of amiodarone has been established, and discontinuance of the other antiarrhythmic agent(s) usually should be attempted. If combination therapy with the other antiarrhythmic agent(s) is continued, patients should be monitored with particular care for possible adverse effects, especially conduction disturbances and exacerbation of tachyarrhythmias. In patients already receiving amiodarone, the initial dosage of other antiarrhythmic agents should be reduced to approximately 50% of their usual recommended initial dosages.

Atypical ventricular tachycardia (torsades de pointes) has been reported rarely when amiodarone was administered concomitantly with various antiarrhythmic agents, including disopyramide, mexiletine, propafenone, and quinidine. Pending further accumulation of data, amiodarone should be used with caution when administered concomitantly with other antiarrhythmic agents, particularly class IA antiarrhythmic agents.

Flecainide. Plasma flecainide concentrations adjusted for daily dosage increased by an average of about 60% (range: 5–190%) when amiodarone therapy was initiated in a limited number of patients receiving flecainide. Although the mechanism(s) of this interaction is not known, it has been suggested that amiodarone may inhibit the hepatic metabolism and/or decrease the renal clearance of flecainide. Pending further accumulation of data, it is recommended that the dosage of flecainide be reduced by 30–50% several days after initiation of amiodarone therapy; subsequently, the patient and plasma flecainide concentrations should be monitored closely and flecainide dosage adjusted as necessary.

Procainamide. Concomitant use of amiodarone and procainamide may result in increased plasma procainamide and *N*-acetylprocainamide (NAPA) concentrations and subsequent toxicity. In a limited number of patients receiving 2–6 g of procainamide hydrochloride daily, initiation of amiodarone hydrochloride (1200 mg daily for 5–7 days and then 600 mg daily) increased plasma procainamide and NAPA concentrations by about 55 and 33%, respectively, during the first week of amiodarone therapy. The exact mechanism(s) has not been elucidated, but it has been suggested that amiodarone may decrease the renal clearance of procainamide or NAPA and/or inhibit the hepatic metabolism of procainamide. In addition to a pharmacokinetic interaction, additive electrophysiologic effects, including increased QT_c and QRS intervals, occur during concomitant use; adverse electrophysiologic effects (e.g., acceleration of ventricular tachycardia) may also occur. Pending further accumulation of data, it is recommended that procainamide dosage be reduced by 20–33% when amiodarone therapy is initiated in patients currently receiving procainamide or that procainamide therapy be discontinued.

Quinidine. Serum quinidine concentrations may increase following initiation of amiodarone therapy in patients currently receiving quinidine, with subsequent toxicity occurring in some patients. Administration of amiodarone hydrochloride (1200 mg daily for 5–7 days then reduced to 600 mg daily) to a limited number of patients receiving quinidine gluconate or sulfate (average dose of about 3 g daily) resulted in an increase in serum quinidine concentrations of about 33%. Serum quinidine concentrations may begin to increase within a couple days after initiation of amiodarone therapy. The mechanism of the interaction is not fully established, but it has been suggested that amiodarone may inhibit hepatic clearance or decrease renal clearance of quinidine and/or displace quinidine from tissue- and/or protein-binding sites. Although not clearly established, combination therapy with amiodarone and quinidine may also cause marked QT prolongation, predisposing patients to atypical ventricular tachycardia (torsades de pointes). It is generally recommended that quinidine dosage be reduced by 33–50% when amiodarone therapy is initiated in patients currently receiving quinidine or that quinidine therapy be discontinued. Serum quinidine concentrations should be monitored carefully and quinidine dosage reduced as necessary in patients receiving concomitant amiodarone and quinidine therapy; patients should be observed closely for signs of toxicity, including QT prolongation.

Lidocaine. Sinus bradycardia was observed in a patient receiving oral amiodarone who was given lidocaine for local anesthesia. Seizures associated with increased lidocaine concentrations were observed in one patient receiving concomitant IV amiodarone therapy.

HIV Protease Inhibitors HIV protease inhibitors inhibit CYP3A4 to varying degrees, which may result in a decrease in the metabolism of amiodarone. Concomitant use of amiodarone and an HIV protease inhibitor used with low-dose ritonavir (*ritonavir-boosted*) or without low-dose ritonavir (unboosted) may result in increased plasma concentrations of amiodarone and the HIV protease inhibitor.

Concomitant use of amiodarone and *ritonavir-boosted* saquinavir or *ritonavir-boosted* tipranavir is not recommended. If amiodarone is used concomitantly with other *ritonavir-boosted* HIV protease inhibitors or with unboosted HIV protease inhibitors, some experts recommend caution and state that the patient should be monitored for amiodarone toxicity and consideration given to monitoring ECG and amiodarone plasma concentrations.

Histamine H_2-Receptor Antagonists Cimetidine inhibits CYP3A4 and can increase plasma amiodarone concentrations.

Histamine H_1-Receptor Antagonists Use of amiodarone with loratadine may result in a decrease in the metabolism of loratadine, a substrate of CYP3A4. QT-interval prolongation and torsades de pointes have been reported with concomitant use of amiodarone and loratadine.

Cyclosporine Amiodarone inhibits CYP3A4, which may result in a decrease in the metabolism of cyclosporine, a substrate of CYP3A4. Concomitant use of amiodarone and cyclosporine has been reported to produce persistently elevated plasma concentrations of cyclosporine, resulting in elevated serum creatinine concentrations despite reduction in the dose of cyclosporine.

HMG-CoA Reductase Inhibitors (Statins) Potent inhibitors of CYP3A4 can increase plasma concentrations of HMG-CoA reductase inhibitory activity and increase the risk of myopathy. Because the risk of myopathy/rhabdomyolysis is increased following concomitant use of amiodarone with higher dosages of certain HMG-CoA reductase inhibitors (e.g., simvastatin dosages exceeding 20 mg daily), the daily dosage of lovastatin or simvastatin should not exceed 40 or 20 mg, respectively, during concomitant therapy with amiodarone. (See Amiodarone under Drugs and Foods Affecting Hepatic Microsomal Enzymes: Cardiac Drugs, in Drug Interactions in the HMG CoA Reductase Inhibitors General Statement 24:06.08.)

Rifampin Concomitant administration of amiodarone and rifampin has been associated with decreases in plasma concentrations of amiodarone and desethylamiodarone because of induction of CYP3A4 by rifampin.

St. John's Wort (Hypericum perforatum) St. John's wort is an extract of hypericum and contains at least 7 different components that may contribute to its pharmacologic effects, including hypericin, pseudohypericin, and hyperforin. There is evidence that hypericum extracts can induce several different CYP isoenzymes, including CYP3A4 and CYP1A2. Since amiodarone is a substrate for CYP3A4, concomitant use of amiodarone and St. John's wort has the potential to result in decreased plasma concentrations of amiodarone.

Other Drugs Affecting Hepatic Microsomal Enzymes Concomitant administration of fentanyl and amiodarone may result in hypotension, bradycardia, and decreased cardiac output. Prolonged (exceeding 2 weeks) administration of oral amiodarone impairs the metabolism of dextromethorphan, phenytoin, and methotrexate.

Use of amiodarone concurrently with trazodone may result in a decrease in the metabolism of trazodone, a substrate of CYP3A4. QT-interval prolongation and torsades de pointes have been reported with concomitant use of amiodarone and trazodone.

Clopidogrel undergoes biotransformation through the CYP3A4 isoenzyme, and concomitant use with amiodarone may decrease the biotransformation of clopidogrel to the active form. Ineffective inhibition of platelet aggregation has been reported during concomitant use of clopidogrel and amiodarone.

Grapefruit Juice Grapefruit juice inhibits CYP3A4-mediated metabolism of oral amiodarone in intestinal mucosa, resulting in increased plasma concentrations of amiodarone. In healthy individuals receiving grapefruit juice and oral amiodarone concurrently, the area under the plasma concentration-time curve (AUC) and peak plasma concentration of amiodarone increased by 50 and 84%, respectively, and desethylamiodarone plasma concentrations decreased to below the detection limits of the assay. Therefore, grapefruit juice should not be consumed during treatment with oral amiodarone. This interaction should be considered when switching from IV to oral amiodarone therapy.

Phenytoin Concomitant use of amiodarone and phenytoin has resulted in a twofold to threefold increase in steady-state serum concentrations of phenytoin and subsequent signs of phenytoin toxicity (e.g., nystagmus, ataxia, lethargy) in a limited number of patients. The increase in serum phenytoin concentrations occurred within 3–4 weeks of initiating amiodarone therapy. Although the exact mechanism(s) has not been clearly established, amiodarone may inhibit hepatic metabolism of phenytoin. Patients receiving phenytoin should be monitored closely for signs of phenytoin toxicity when amiodarone is administered concomitantly; serum phenytoin concentrations also should be monitored and dosage of phenytoin reduced as necessary.

Phenytoin has been reported to decrease plasma amiodarone concentrations.

■ **Anticoagulants** An increase in prothrombin time (PT) appears to occur in almost all patients treated with amiodarone and a coumarin or indandione anticoagulant concomitantly and can result in serious or fatal hemorrhage. The increase in PT usually begins within 3–4 days, although onset of the effect may be delayed for 1–3 weeks in some patients. Bleeding episodes generally have been reported to occur 1–4 weeks following initiation of amiodarone therapy. The magnitude of the increase in PT appears to average 100%. Because of amiodarone's long elimination half-life, the PT may not return to normal for 1–4 months following discontinuance of the antiarrhythmic agent. The exact mechanism is not fully established, but amiodarone appears to decrease the hepatic clearance of warfarin. If amiodarone therapy is initiated in patients receiving warfarin or another coumarin or indandione anticoagulant, a reduction in anticoagulant dosage of 33–50% is recommended. In patients receiving amiodarone and an oral anticoagulant concomitantly, the PT should be determined frequently and patients should be observed closely for adverse effects; dosage of the anticoagulant should be adjusted as necessary.

■ **Cardiac Glycosides** Concomitant use of amiodarone and digoxin regularly results in increased serum digoxin concentrations, which may reach toxic levels with subsequent digoxin toxicity. Serum digoxin concentrations generally increase by an average of 70–100% in adults, but substantial variability exists in the magnitude of the increase. Limited data suggest that the magnitude of the increase may be much greater in children than in adults (i.e., 70–800%).

The amiodarone-induced increase in serum digoxin concentrations usually begins within 1–7 days and progresses gradually over a period of several weeks or even months. The exact mechanism(s) of this interaction appears to be complex and remains to be fully established, but data indicate that amiodarone may decrease the renal and/or nonrenal clearance of digoxin. It has also been suggested that amiodarone may increase the oral bioavailability of digoxin or displace digoxin from tissue binding sites. When initiating amiodarone therapy in patients receiving digoxin, the need for continued cardiac glycoside therapy should be reassessed, and digoxin discontinued if appropriate; if concomitant therapy is considered necessary in patients receiving digoxin, a 50% reduction in digoxin dosage is recommended when amiodarone therapy is begun. Serum digoxin concentrations should be monitored carefully and digoxin dosage reduced as necessary in patients receiving amiodarone and digoxin concomitantly; patients should be observed closely for signs of cardiac glycoside toxicity. In addition, thyroid function should be monitored carefully in patients receiving concurrent amiodarone and digoxin therapy, since amiodarone-induced changes in thyroid function may increase or decrease serum digoxin concentrations or alter sensitivity to the therapeutic and toxic effects of the cardiac glycoside.

■ **Other Cardiovascular Drugs** Amiodarone should be used with caution in patients receiving calcium-channel blocking agents (e.g., diltiazem, verapamil) and/or β-adrenergic blocking agents (e.g. propranolol), since possible potentiation of sinus bradycardia, sinus arrest, and AV block may occur. If amiodarone therapy is considered necessary, the drug may continue to be used in patients with severe sinus bradycardia or sinus arrest following insertion of an artificial pacemaker and institution of cardiac monitoring.

■ **General Anesthetics** The effects of concomitant administration of amiodarone and anesthetic agents have not been fully evaluated. However, potentially serious adverse cardiovascular and cardiac effects have occurred in some amiodarone-treated patients undergoing general anesthesia, suggesting the possibility of an interaction between the antiarrhythmic agent and various anesthetic agents. (See Cautions: Precautions and Contraindications.) In addition, close perioperative monitoring is recommended in patients undergoing general anesthesia while receiving amiodarone, since amiodarone may sensitize patients to the myocardial depressant and conduction effects of halogenated hydrocarbon general anesthetics.

■ **HCV Antivirals** Concomitant use of amiodarone and a hepatitis C virus (HCV) treatment regimen containing sofosbuvir with another HCV direct-acting antiviral (DAA), including ledipasvir, simeprevir, or daclatasvir, may result in serious symptomatic bradycardia and is not recommended. The mechanism for this adverse cardiovascular effect is unknown; the effect of concomitant use of amiodarone with these HCV treatment regimens on plasma concentrations of the drugs is unknown. If there are no alternative HCV treatment options and a regimen of sofosbuvir with another DAA (e.g., ledipasvir, simeprevir, daclatasvir) must be used in a patient receiving amiodarone, the patient should be advised about the risk of serious symptomatic bradycardia before HCV treatment is initiated. Cardiac monitoring should be performed in an inpatient setting during the first 48 hours of concomitant use of amiodarone and a regimen containing sofosbuvir with another DAA; heart rate monitoring should then be performed daily (outpatient or self-monitoring) through at least the first 2 weeks of concomitant use. Similar cardiac monitoring is recommended in patients who discontinued amiodarone just prior to initiation of a regimen that includes sofosbuvir with another DAA or if an alternative antiarrhythmic agent cannot be used and amiodarone must be initiated in a patient already receiving such sofosbuvir regimens. Patients receiving amiodarone concomitantly with a regimen containing sofosbuvir with another DAA should be advised about the risk of serious symptomatic bradycardia and the importance of immediately contacting a clinician if signs or symptoms of bradycardia (e.g., near-fainting or fainting, dizziness, lightheadedness, malaise, weakness, excessive tiredness, shortness of breath, chest pain, confusion, memory problems) occur.

Concomitant use of oral amiodarone and simeprevir is expected to result in modestly increased amiodarone concentrations due to intestinal CYP3A4 inhibition by simeprevir. If amiodarone is used concomitantly with a simeprevir-containing HCV treatment regimen that does *not* include sofosbuvir, caution is warranted and therapeutic drug monitoring of the antiarrhythmic agent, if available, is recommended.

Concomitant use of amiodarone and the fixed combination of ombitasvir, paritaprevir, and ritonavir (ombitasvir/paritaprevir/ritonavir) with dasabuvir is expected to increase plasma concentrations of amiodarone. If amiodarone is used concomitantly with ombitasvir/paritaprevir/ritonavir with dasabuvir, caution is warranted and therapeutic drug monitoring of the antiarrhythmic agent, if available, is recommended.

■ **Cholestyramine Resin** Limited data indicate that administration of cholestyramine resin following a single oral dose of amiodarone may decrease the elimination half-life and plasma concentrations of amiodarone, possibly by interfering with enterohepatic circulation of the antiarrhythmic agent. Further evaluation of this potential interaction is needed.

■ **Agalsidase Beta** Some clinicians state that because of a theoretical risk of inhibited intracellular α-galactosidase activity with amiodarone, it should not be administered concurrently with agalsidase beta, a biosynthetic form of α-galactosidase.

Acute Toxicity

Limited information is available on the acute toxicity of amiodarone. However, cases of amiodarone overdosage, sometimes fatal, have been reported. If an overdosage occurs, patients should contact their clinician or proceed immediately to a hospital emergency room.

■ **Pathogenesis** The acute lethal dose of amiodarone hydrochloride in humans is not known. The oral LD_{50} of the drug in rats, mice, and dogs is greater than 3 g/kg. Following oral administration of single large doses of amiodarone hydrochloride (up to 3 g/kg) in dogs, emesis, tremors, and hindlimb paresis were observed.

■ **Manifestations** In general, overdosage of amiodarone may be expected to produce effects that are extensions of pharmacologic effects, including sinus bradycardia and/or heart block, hypotension, and QT prolongation. The most likely effects of an inadvertent overdosage of IV amiodarone are hypotension, cardiogenic shock, bradycardia, AV block, and hepatotoxicity. Nausea is likely to occur with ingestions of greater than 1 g of the drug. Slight, asymptomatic bradycardia and QT prolongation occurred about 1–3 days following acute ingestion of 2.6–8 g of amiodarone hydrochloride in 3 patients.

In an adult who reportedly intentionally ingested 8 g of amiodarone hydrochloride and an unknown amount of diazepam and lorazepam, profuse perspiration occurred within 12 hours and slight bradycardia and QT prolongation (to about 500 ms) occurred 2–3 days after ingestion. In another adult who had received 200 mg of amiodarone hydrochloride daily for 1 week and then intentionally ingested 2.6 g of the drug, no ECG changes were apparent 6 hours after ingestion, but QT prolongation, T-wave inversion, and transient disappearance of precordial R waves occurred the day following ingestion. No symptoms were reported, and the patient's heart rate remained normal; repolarization returned to baseline about 10 days after ingestion. No deaths or permanent sequelae occurred in these patients.

■ **Treatment** Management of amiodarone overdosage generally involves symptomatic and supportive care, with ECG and blood pressure monitoring. In case of hypotension or cardiogenic shock in patients receiving amiodarone IV, the infusion rate should be decreased. There is no specific antidote for amiodarone intoxication.

Following recent acute ingestion of amiodarone, the stomach should be emptied immediately by inducing emesis or by gastric lavage. If the patient is comatose, having seizures, or lacks the gag reflex, gastric lavage may be performed if an endotracheal tube with cuff inflated is in place to prevent aspiration of gastric contents. Administration of activated charcoal after emesis or gastric lavage may be useful in minimizing absorption of amiodarone, although specific data are not available. Because the onset of toxicity may be delayed, ECG monitoring may be necessary for several days following acute ingestion of the drug. For bradycardia, IV administration of a β-adrenergic agonist (e.g., isoproterenol) or use of a transvenous cardiac pacemaker is recommended; amiodarone-induced bradycardia generally is not fully responsive to atropine. For AV block, the use of a transvenous cardiac pacemaker may be necessary. Administration of IV fluids and placement of the patient in Trendelenburg's position is recommended for the initial treatment of hypotension. An inotropic agent or vasopressor (e.g., dopamine, norepinephrine) should be given for hypotension accompanied by signs of inadequate tissue perfusion. Hepatic enzymes also should be monitored closely in the case of IV amiodarone overdosage. Hemodialysis or peritoneal dialysis is not useful for enhancing elimination of amiodarone or *N*-desethylamiodarone in acute overdosage.

Pharmacology

■ **Antiarrhythmic and Electrophysiologic Effects** The antiarrhythmic and electrophysiologic actions of amiodarone hydrochloride are complex and differ from those of other currently available antiarrhythmic agents. Studies in animals have shown that amiodarone is effective in preventing and/or suppressing experimentally induced arrhythmias.

The exact mechanism(s) of antiarrhythmic action of amiodarone has not been conclusively determined. Amiodarone is considered to be predominantly a class III antiarrhythmic agent, but the drug also appears to exhibit activity in each of the four Vaughn-Williams antiarrhythmic classes, including some class I (membrane-stabilizing) antiarrhythmic action. The principal effect of amiodarone on cardiac tissue is to delay repolarization by prolonging the action potential duration (APD) and effective refractory period (ERP). The drug also appears to inhibit transmembrane influx of extracellular sodium ions via fast sodium channels, as indicated by a decrease in the maximal rate of depolarization of phase 0 of the action potential. Like class I antiarrhythmic agents, amiodarone is believed to combine with fast sodium channels in their inactive state and thereby inhibit recovery after repolarization in a time- and voltage-dependent manner, which is associated with subsequent dissociation of the drug from the sodium channels. Amiodarone appears to have little affinity for activated fast sodium channels. Amiodarone also produces a noncompetitive inhibition of α- and β-adrenergic activity that may contribute to the drug's antiarrhythmic activity. Limited data suggest that the drug may possess some vagolytic and/or calcium-channel blocking activity, and that recovery from calcium-channel blockade may be substantially more rapid than that with diltiazem or verapamil, but additional study is needed. Amiodarone does not appear to have vagomimetic or local anesthetic activity.

Amiodarone predominantly exhibits electrophysiologic effects characteristic of class III antiarrhythmic agents (i.e., prolonged repolarization and refractoriness), but the drug also appears to exhibit activity in each of the four Vaughn-Williams antiarrhythmic classes, including some electrophysiologic effects characteristic of class I (particularly class IA or IC) antiarrhythmic agents. The drug prolongs APD in atrial and ventricular muscle, the sinus node, the atrioventricular (AV) node, and the His-Purkinje system without substantially altering resting membrane potential or action potential height, except in automatic cells (e.g., those in the sinus node or His-Purkinje system) in which it reduces the slope of diastolic depolarization and thereby generally reduces automaticity. Although several investigators have suggested that the myocardial effects observed during chronic amiodarone therapy are comparable to those associated with hypothyroidism and may be related to competitive inhibition of sodium-potassium-activated adenosine triphosphatase (Na^+-K^+-ATPase) activity, other data suggest that amiodarone's effects on thyroid function contribute minimally, if at all, to the overall electrophysiologic effects of the drug.

Effects on Cardiac Conduction and Refractoriness Amiodarone appears to prolong refractoriness throughout the myocardium including the atria, ventricles, His-Purkinje system, sinus node, and AV node, as well as in accessory pathways, if present. The effect of amiodarone on cardiac conduction is less well defined, but the drug appears to decrease AV conduction following a single IV dose or chronic oral administration; the decrease appears to be heart-rate dependent, with substantially larger reductions in AV conduction at high rates. Amiodarone may also partially impair conduction within the His-Purkinje system. When administered IV, amiodarone prolongs intranodal conduction and AV node refractoriness, but has little to no effect on sinus cycle length, refractoriness of the right atrium or right ventricle, repolarization, intraventricular conduction, or intranodal conduction. At higher than usual IV doses (e.g., greater than 10 mg/kg), amiodarone prolongation of right ventricular refractoriness and modest prolongation of the QRS complex have been observed. Differences in the effect between parenterally versus orally administered amiodarone are seen predominantly in effects on AV nodal conduction; IV amiodarone causes an intranodal conduction delay and increased nodal refractoriness secondary to slow-channel blockade (class IV activity) and noncompetitive adrenergic antagonism (class II activity). The effects of amiodarone on intracardiac conduction may result from its class I antiarrhythmic activity; the drug's effects on slow calcium channels also may be involved. Further studies are needed to fully determine the effects of the drug on intracardiac conduction.

The effects of amiodarone on refractoriness and intracardiac conduction are manifested by increases in PR and QT intervals. Following chronic oral administration of the drug, increases in PR interval and QT interval corrected for rate (QT_c) average about 10–17% and 10–23%, respectively. Limited data suggest that amiodarone-induced QT prolongation may constitute an antiarrhythmic mechanism, although additional study is necessary. Rarely, QT prolongation induced by the drug is associated with arrhythmogenicity. QRS intervals may be unchanged or increased. Amiodarone generally increases the AH interval but has a variable effect on the HV interval, which may be unchanged or prolonged following chronic oral administration of the drug. Changes in T-wave contour, such as widening, bifurcation, or reduction in amplitude, and the development of prominent U waves may also occur during amiodarone therapy.

The antiarrhythmic and electrophysiologic effects of amiodarone following single IV doses appear to differ substantially from those observed during chronic oral administration of the drug. Following a single IV dose, the major effect of the drug is on the AV node with lengthening of ERP and prolongation of intranodal conduction time, whereas during chronic oral therapy, prolongation of APD and ERP in the atria, ventricles, and AV nodal tissue occurs. At a constant oral dosage, the electrophysiologic effects of amiodarone, including increases in APD and refractoriness, appear to develop as a function of time.

Effects on Sinus Node Amiodarone generally depresses sinus node function. Following chronic oral administration of amiodarone, sinus rate is reduced by about 10–20%; however, changes in sinus rate following single IV doses of the drug do not appear to be substantial. Marked sinus bradycardia or sinus arrest and heart block may occur in some patients. Amiodarone appears to depress sinus node automaticity. Data are conflicting, but amiodarone may in part reduce automaticity by increasing the APD and depressing the slope of diastolic depolarization in the sinus node. Administration of propranolol or atropine does not appear to substantially influence these changes, but a low calcium concentration enhances the drug's negative chronotropic effect. Following chronic administration of amiodarone, spontaneous cycle lengths are increased. The effects of amiodarone on sinus node recovery time (SNRT) and sinoatrial conduction time (SACT) have not been fully established; however, prolongation of both SNRT and SACT has occurred in some patients receiving long-term therapy with the drug.

Effects on His-Purkinje System In addition to prolonging repolarization and refractoriness, amiodarone reduces the maximum rate of phase 0 depolarization in Purkinje fibers in a use-dependent manner (i.e., the magnitude of depression of the maximum rate of phase 0 depolarization increases at faster stimulation rates). Clinical experience indicates that chronic oral therapy with the drug may result in prolongation of intraventricular conduction as manifested by lengthening of the HV interval. However, amiodarone's effect on the HV interval appears to be variable; data from clinical studies indicate that the HV interval may either be unchanged or prolonged by up to about 15–30% during chronic administration of the drug. In addition, amiodarone therapy reportedly has exacerbated preexisting His-Purkinje delay in some patients.

Effects on Accessory AV Pathways and Reentry Mechanisms The electrophysiologic effects of amiodarone on accessory pathways, the AV node, the His-Purkinje system, and/or atrial and ventricular myocardium may contribute to the drug's efficacy in terminating and preventing paroxysmal reentrant supraventricular tachycardias. In patients with Wolff-Parkinson-White syndrome or concealed accessory AV pathways, amiodarone generally increases refractoriness of the anterograde and retrograde accessory pathways, but the effect on refractoriness of the retrograde accessory pathway appears to be somewhat more variable and less pronounced. Limited data indicate that the effects of amiodarone may be greater on anterograde accessory pathways that have relatively long pretreatment refractory periods. In addition to its effects on accessory pathways, amiodarone may increase refractoriness in atrial and ventricular tissue, the AV node, and the His-Purkinje system, resulting in possible prevention or interruption of reentrant tachyarrhythmias. Amiodarone may also decrease the occurrence of atrial premature complexes (APCs) and ventricular premature complexes (VPCs) responsible for initiation of reentrant tachyarrhythmias.

■ **Antiadrenergic Effects** Amiodarone noncompetitively inhibits α- and β-adrenergic responses to sympathetic stimulation and catecholamine administration. In vitro and in vivo data indicate that the drug noncompetitively antagonizes cardiovascular effects (e.g., tachycardia, hypertension, increase in myocardial oxygen consumption) induced by epinephrine, norepinephrine, and/or isoproterenol. The precise mechanism of adrenergic inhibition is unclear. Some data suggest that amiodarone does not bind directly to the catecholamine-recognition site on β-adrenergic receptors but instead may reduce β-adrenergic activity by decreasing the number of β-adrenergic receptors. Although conflicting results have been reported, limited data suggest that amiodarone may also inhibit the release of neurotransmitter from presynaptic adrenergic neurons. Although not clearly established, the antiadrenergic activity of amiodarone may contribute to its antiarrhythmic and antianginal efficacy.

■ **Arrhythmogenic Effects** Like other antiarrhythmic agents, amiodarone can worsen existing arrhythmias or cause new arrhythmias. (See Cautions: Arrhythmogenic Effects.) The arrhythmogenic effects of the drug have included ventricular fibrillation, sustained ventricular tachycardia, increased resistance to cardioversion, and atypical ventricular tachycardia (torsades de pointes).

■ **Cardiovascular Effects** Amiodarone generally exhibits minimal cardiovascular effects following oral administration. The cardiovascular effects of the drug appear to be more pronounced following IV than oral administration, but evaluations have been more extensive following IV administration. In addition, some cardiovascular effects observed following IV administration may be related to the solvent, polysorbate (Tween®) 80, used in the parenteral dosage form of the drug.

Long-term oral administration of amiodarone generally depresses sinus node function, and heart rate is reduced by an average of about 10–20%. Following a single IV dose of amiodarone, heart rate may be increased, decreased, or unchanged; however, changes in heart rate after IV administration, if present, generally are minimal and transient. Amiodarone generally does not appear to have a substantial negative inotropic effect following long-term oral administration, even in patients with depressed left ventricular ejection fraction (LVEF); however, a mild negative inotropic effect (possibly related to the rate of injection) may occur following IV administration of the drug.

Amiodarone generally relaxes cardiac and vascular smooth muscle, thereby dilating both systemic and coronary arteries. Following IV administration of 5 mg/kg of amiodarone hydrochloride, systemic blood pressure, systemic vascular resistance, coronary vascular resistance, and left ventricular end-diastolic pressure (LVEDP) are generally decreased, while coronary sinus flow may increase transiently and cardiac index may increase slightly. Studies in humans and animals indicate that IV amiodarone may produce a transient, dose-related increase in coronary artery blood flow, mainly as a result of a direct relaxant effect on coronary arteries, but reductions in contractility and LVEF may also be involved. Although not clearly established, limited data suggest that the transient reduction in coronary and systemic vascular resistance observed following IV administration may at least partially result from the vasodilatory effects of polysorbate 80 present as a solvent in the injection. Studies in humans and animals also suggest that amiodarone reduces myocardial oxygen consumption, resulting in a protective effect on ischemic myocardium. Although not clearly established, decreased myocardial oxygen consumption appears to result from a reduction in heart rate, systemic vascular resistance, and possibly myocardial contractility.

Long-term oral administration of amiodarone generally does not appear to produce substantial changes in LVEF, even in patients with left ventricular dysfunction. The drug, however, has been associated with new or worsened heart failure in some patients receiving chronic oral therapy. (See Cautions: Cardiovascular Effects.) IV administration of amiodarone may transiently depress left ventricular function, probably as a result of the drug's negative inotropic effect, particularly in patients with preexisting left ventricular dysfunction or at high doses. Although decreases in left ventricular function following IV administration of the drug are generally transient and well tolerated, severe hypotension has occurred rarely in patients with severe heart failure.

■ **Thyroid Effects** Amiodarone has variable and complex effects on thyroid function. The drug's principal effect appears to be inhibition of extrathyroidal deiodinases, resulting in decreased peripheral conversion of thyroxine (T_4) to triiodothyronine (T_3) and a subsequent increase in serum T_4 and inactive reverse triiodothyronine (reverse T_3, rT_3) concentrations and decrease in serum T_3 concentrations. Serum concentrations of thyrotropin (thyroid-stimulating hormone, TSH) usually increase initially but return to baseline or slightly below baseline values within a few months to a year despite continued therapy. In addition, the thyrotropin response to protirelin initially may be accentuated in patients receiving amiodarone; normal or depressed responses may occur during long-term therapy.

Despite the changes in serum thyroid hormone concentrations, most patients receiving amiodarone remain clinically euthyroid; however, clinical hypothyroidism or hyperthyroidism may occur. (See Cautions: Thyroid Effects.) The mechanism(s) of amiodarone-induced hypothyroidism or hyperthyroidism has not been fully elucidated, but may be related to the iodine content of amiodarone (See Chemistry and Stability: Chemistry.) and/or involve a direct effect of the drug or its major metabolite on thyroid function. It has also been proposed that amiodarone may alter the sensitivity of the pituitary gland and peripheral organs to the actions of thyroid hormones; however, additional study is needed.

■ **Other Effects** Amiodarone inhibits phospholipase (including phospholipase A_1, A_2, and C) activity in vitro. In patients receiving the drug, histologic examination has revealed the presence of phospholipid-laden lysosomal inclusions within pulmonary cells, liver cells, Schwann cells, leukocytes, epithelial cells in skin, and possibly within epithelial cells in the eye. The exact mechanism(s) of amiodarone-induced injury to various body organs remains to be clearly established; however, the production of amiodarone-phospholipid complexes within certain organs may play a role in the development of many of the adverse effects associated with the drug. It also has been suggested that accumulation of phospholipids within pulmonary cells also may result from increased phospholipid synthesis. In addition, amiodarone-induced pulmonary toxicity may be related to surfactant ingestion by macrophages, release of free oxygen radicals, increased iodide content, and/or altered cellular function secondary to the amphophilic nature of the drug. Although pulmonary toxicity appears to result from a hypersensitivity reaction in some patients, and there was evidence of an IgG-mediated immune response initiated against an amiodarone/native pulmonary protein complex (hapten-protein complex) in at least one patient, the mechanism of amiodarone-induced hypersensitivity, including the possible role of immunoglobulins, complement deposition, and cytokines in this reaction remains to be more fully elucidated. In patients developing amiodarone-induced hypersensitivity pneumonitis, suppressor/cytotoxic ($CD8^+$, $T8^+$) T-cell lymphocytosis often is present in bronchoalveolar lavage specimens.

Amiodarone theoretically can inhibit intracellular α-galactosidase activity. (See Drug Interactions: Agalsidase Beta.)

The effects of amiodarone on serum lipid concentrations have not been clearly established. Serum cholesterol and triglyceride concentrations in patients receiving the drug have variably been reported to be increased or decreased.

Pharmacokinetics

■ **Absorption** Amiodarone hydrochloride is slowly and variably absorbed from the GI tract following oral administration. The absolute bioavailability of commercially available amiodarone hydrochloride tablets averages approximately 50%, but varies considerably, ranging from 22–86%. The sometimes low and often variable bioavailability of amiodarone may possibly result from *N*-dealkylation or other metabolism in the intestinal lumen and/or GI mucosa, from first-pass metabolism in the liver, and/or from poor dissolution characteristics of the drug. Food increases the rate and extent of absorption of amiodarone. Results of a study in healthy adults indicate that administration of a single 600-mg oral dose of amiodarone hydrochloride after a high-fat meal increases the area under the plasma concentration-time curve (AUC) and the peak plasma concentration of amiodarone by 2.3 (range: 1.7–3.6) and 3.8 (range: 2.7–4.4) times, respectively, compared with administration in the fasting state. Food also increases the rate of absorption of amiodarone; when administered with food, the time to achieve peak plasma concentration of unchanged drug is decreased by about 37% to 4.5 hours. The mean AUC and mean peak plasma concentrations of *N*-desethylamiodarone (the major metabolite) increase by about 55 and 32%, respectively; however, the time to peak plasma concentration of this metabolite remains unchanged in the presence of food. Limited data suggest that the drug may undergo enterohepatic circulation.

Following oral administration, peak plasma amiodarone concentrations usually occur within 3–7 hours (range: 2–12 hours). Following oral administration of a single 400-mg dose of amiodarone hydrochloride in fasting, healthy adults, peak plasma amiodarone concentrations of approximately 0.15–0.7 mcg/mL are attained. Within the oral dosage range of 100–600 mg daily, steady-state plasma concentrations of the drug are approximately proportional to dosage, increasing by an average of 0.5 mcg/mL per 100-mg increment in dosage; however, there is considerable interindividual variation in plasma concentrations attained with a given dosage. Following continuous oral administration of the drug in the absence of an initial loading-dose regimen, steady-state plasma amiodarone concentrations would not be attained for at least 1 month and generally not for up to 5 months or longer. Following chronic oral administration of amiodarone, plasma concentrations of *N*-desethylamiodarone, the major metabolite of the drug, are approximately 0.5–2 times those of unchanged drug.

In a study of single-dose IV amiodarone hydrochloride (5 mg/kg over 15 minutes) in healthy individuals, peak drug concentration ranged from 5–41mcg/mL. Following 10-minute IV infusions of amiodarone hydrochloride at a dose of 150 mg in patients with ventricular fibrillation or hemodynamically unstable ventricular tachycardia, peak drug concentration ranged from 7–26 mcg/mL. Because of a rapid distribution phase, the concentration of amiodarone declines to 10% of peak values within 30–45 minutes after the end of the infusion. In clinical trials after 48 hours of continuous IV infusions (125, 500, or 1000 mg daily) plus supplemental infusions (150 mg) as needed for recurrent arrhythmias, mean plasma concentrations of amiodarone ranged from 0.7–1.4 mcg/mL.Following administration of a single IV dose of amiodarone in patients with cirrhosis, lower peak and mean plasma concentrations of *N*-desethylamiodarone are observed; mean amiodarone concentration remains unchanged.

Following oral administration of amiodarone, the onset of antiarrhythmic activity is highly variable. A therapeutic response may begin within 2–3 days in some patients but generally is not evident until 1–3 weeks after beginning therapy with the drug, even when loading doses are administered. Limited data suggest that the onset of action occurs earlier in patients receiving loading doses of the drug and in pediatric patients. Although not clearly established, the time of maximal antiarrhythmic effect usually occurs within 1–5 months after initiating oral amiodarone therapy. Antiarrhythmic effects generally persist for 10–150 days following withdrawal of long-term amiodarone therapy; however, duration of antiarrhythmic activity is variable and unpredictable and appears to depend on the length of therapy as well as the type of cardiac arrhythmia being treated. In general, when amiodarone therapy is resumed after prior discontinuance of the drug and subsequent recurrence of the arrhythmia, control of the arrhythmia occurs relatively rapidly compared to the initial response, presumably because tissues are not fully depleted of the drug at the time therapy is resumed.

There is considerable interindividual variation in the relationship between plasma amiodarone concentrations and antiarrhythmic effects. Limited data suggest that prolongation of the QT_c interval is correlated with plasma amiodarone concentrations. Based on suppression of arrhythmias, plasma amiodarone concentrations of approximately 1–2.5 mcg/mL are usually necessary for optimum therapeutic effect, although therapeutic response may be apparent at lower concentrations in some patients; plasma concentrations higher than 2.5 mcg/mL are generally not necessary. There is no established relationship between drug concentration and therapeutic response for short-term IV amiodarone therapy. Although considerable overlap exists between therapeutic and toxic plasma concentrations, certain adverse reactions including adverse hepatic, ocular, and neuromuscular effects appear to occur more frequently when plasma amiodarone concentrations exceed 2.5 mcg/mL.

■ **Distribution** Distribution of amiodarone into human body tissues and fluids has not been fully characterized. Following IV administration in rats, amiodarone is distributed extensively into many tissues, including adipose tissue, liver, kidneys, heart, and, to a lesser extent, the CNS. Following chronic oral administration of the drug in humans, amiodarone and *N*-desethylamiodarone are distributed extensively into many body tissues and fluids, including adipose tissue, liver, lung, spleen, skeletal muscle, bone marrow, adrenal glands, kidneys, pancreas, testes, semen, saliva, lymph nodes, myocardium, thyroid gland, skin, and brain. Amiodarone is also distributed into bile. Limited data indicate that peak biliary concentrations of the drug may be approximately 50 times greater than peak plasma concentrations. Tissue concentrations of amiodarone generally exceed concurrent plasma concentrations of the drug. *N*-Desethylamiodarone appears to accumulate in the same body tissues as amiodarone; however, after long-term therapy, concentrations of the metabolite are usually substantially higher than concentrations of unchanged drug in almost all tissues, except adipose tissue, which mainly contains amiodarone. *N*-Desethylamiodarone and, to a lesser extent, amiodarone also distribute into erythrocytes. Ratios of erythrocyte-to-plasma concentrations of amiodarone and *N*-desethylamiodarone were 0.33 and 0.67, respectively, after a single oral dose of amiodarone and 0.38–0.48 and 1.3–1.76, respectively, after long-term oral therapy with the drug. Following a single IV dose, the mean blood-to-plasma ratio for amiodarone is 0.73.

Following IV administration, amiodarone is rapidly and widely distributed. The apparent volume of distribution of the drug or its major metabolite, *N*-desethylamiodarone, in healthy adults reportedly averages 65.8 L/kg (range: 18.3–147.7 L/kg) or ranges from 68–168 L/kg, respectively, following a single IV dose.

In vitro, amiodarone is approximately 96% bound to plasma proteins, mainly to albumin and, to a lesser extent, a high-density lipoprotein that is probably β-lipoprotein.

Amiodarone and *N*-desethylamiodarone cross the placenta to a limited extent. In pregnant women receiving amiodarone, ratios of umbilical venous to maternal venous plasma concentrations of amiodarone and *N*-desethylamiodarone were 0.1–0.28 and 0.25–0.55, respectively. Amiodarone and its major metabolite are distributed into milk in concentrations substantially higher than concurrent maternal plasma concentrations. Limited data in a lactating woman indicate amiodarone and *N*-desethylamiodarone milk-to-plasma ratios ranging from 2.3–9.1 and 0.8–3.8, respectively.

■ **Elimination** Plasma concentrations of amiodarone appear to decline in at least a biphasic manner, although more complex, multicompartmental pharmacokinetics have been described. Following a single IV dose in healthy adults, the half-life of the drug in the terminal elimination phase ($t_{1/2\beta}$) has been reported to average 25 days (range: 9–47 days). The elimination half-life of the major metabolite, *N*-desethylamiodarone, is equal to or longer than that of the parent drug. Following single-dose administration of amiodarone in a limited number of healthy individuals, amiodarone exhibits multicompartmental pharmacokinetics; the mean apparent terminal plasma elimination half-life of amiodarone and *N*-desethylamiodarone were 58 (range: 15–142) and 36 (range: 14–75) days, respectively. The half-life of amiodarone appears to be substantially more prolonged following multiple rather than single doses. It has been suggested that differences in reported elimination half-lives may result in part from misinterpretation of slow distribution phases as elimination phases following IV administration of the drug. Following chronic oral administration of amiodarone hydrochloride in patients with cardiac arrhythmias (200–600 mg daily for 2–52 months), the drug appears to be eliminated in a biphasic manner with an initial elimination half-life of about 2.5–10 days, which is followed by a terminal elimination half-life averaging 53 days (range: 26–107 days), with most patients exhibiting a terminal elimination half-life in the range of 40–55 days. The elimination half-life of the major metabolite, *N*-desethylamiodarone, averages 57–61 days (range: 20–118 days) following long-term oral administration of amiodarone. The elimination profile of amiodarone probably reflects an initial elimination of the drug from well-perfused tissues followed by prolonged elimination from poorly perfused tissues such as adipose tissue.

In a study of single-dose amiodarone hydrochloride (5 mg/kg over 15 minutes) in healthy individuals, clearance of the drug and its major active metabolite, *N*-desethylamiodarone, ranged from 90–158 and 197–290 mL/hour per kg, respectively. In clinical studies lasting 2–7 days, clearance of IV amiodarone in patients with ventricular fibrillation or ventricular tachycardia ranged from 220–440 mL/hour per kg. Clearance of the drug in healthy geriatric individuals (i.e., older than 65 years of age) was decreased to approximately 100 mL/hour per kg, as compared with clearance of approximately 150 mL/hour per kg in younger individuals; in addition, the elimination half-life of the drug was increased in these geriatric individuals to 47 days, as compared with 20 days in younger individuals.

The exact metabolic fate of amiodarone has not been fully elucidated, but the drug appears to be extensively metabolized, probably in the liver and possibly in the intestinal lumen and/or GI mucosa, to at least one major metabolite. The major metabolite, *N*-desethylamiodarone, is formed by *N*-deethylation. Although not clearly established, limited data in animals indicate that the desethyl metabolite possesses substantial electrophysiologic and antiarrhythmic activity similar to amiodarone's. Following IV administration of a single dose of *N*-desethylamiodarone in animals, the metabolite prolonged atrial and ventricular refractoriness and decreased conduction within the AV node; however, further studies are needed to determine the effects of the desethyl metabolite following chronic administration. The precise role of *N*-desethylamiodarone in the antiarrhythmic activity of amiodarone has not been clearly established. The development of maximal ventricular class III antiarrhythmic effects after oral amiodarone administration in humans correlates more closely with *N*-desethylamiodarone accumulation over time than with amiodarone accumulation. A minor metabolite of amiodarone, di-*N*-desethylamiodarone, has been identified in animals following chronic administration of the drug. Amiodarone and *N*-desethylamiodarone may undergo deiodination to form deiodoamiodarone and deiodo-*N*-desethylamiodarone, respectively; iodine (in the form of iodide); and possibly other iodine-containing metabolites. It is not known whether deiodinated metabolites are pharmacologically active.

The excretory patterns of amiodarone and its metabolite have not been well characterized. Following oral or IV administration, amiodarone appears to be excreted almost completely in feces as unchanged drug and *N*-desethylamiodarone, presumably via biliary elimination. Although not clearly established, limited data suggest that amiodarone may undergo enterohepatic circulation. Renal excretion of amiodarone and *N*-desethylamiodarone appears to be negligible.

Following IV administration of amiodarone in healthy individuals, total plasma clearance of the drug averages approximately 1.9 mL/minute per kg (range: 1.4–2.5 mL/minute per kg). Although not clearly established, total apparent plasma clearance of the drug appears to decrease with time. Clinical experience suggests that clearance of amiodarone may be more rapid in pediatric patients; however, further studies are needed to fully determine the effects of age on clearance of the drug. Factors of age, gender, or renal or hepatic disease appear to have no effect on the disposition of amiodarone or its major metabolite, *N*-desethylamiodarone.

In patients with severe left ventricular dysfunction, the pharmacokinetics of amiodarone are not significantly altered; however, the terminal elimination half-life of *N*-desethylamiodarone is prolonged in these patients.

Amiodarone and *N*-desethylamiodarone are not appreciably removed by hemodialysis or peritoneal dialysis.

Chemistry and Stability

■ **Chemistry** Amiodarone hydrochloride is an iodinated benzofuran-derivative antiarrhythmic agent. The drug differs structurally and pharmacologically from other currently available antiarrhythmic agents.

Amiodarone hydrochloride occurs as a white to cream-colored, crystalline powder and has solubilities of approximately 0.72 mg/mL in water and 12.8 mg/mL in alcohol at 25°C. The drug is highly lipophilic. Amiodarone hydrochloride contains 37.3% iodine; each 200-mg tablet of the drug or each mL of the commercially available injection contains approximately 75 or 18.7 mg of iodine, respectively. The commercially available injection contains benzyl alcohol as a preservative. Amiodarone has a pK_a of approximately 6.6.

■ **Stability** Amiodarone hydrochloride tablets should be protected from light and stored in tight containers at 20–25°C. The manufacturer of one commercially available amiodarone hydrochloride tablet preparation (Pacerone®) states that the tablets may be exposed to temperatures ranging from 15–30°C. Commercially available amiodarone tablets have an expiration date of 3 years following the date of manufacture.

Commercially available amiodarone hydrochloride injection concentrate should be stored at 20–25°C and protected from light and excessive heat. Ampuls containing the injection concentrate should be stored in the carton to protect the solution from light until used. Diluted solutions of amiodarone hydrochloride injection do not need to be protected from light during administration.

Although amiodarone hydrochloride adsorbs to polyvinyl chloride (PVC) tubing, the parenteral drug doses and administration schedule studied in clinical trials were designed to take this fact into account. Therefore, the manufacturer recommends using PVC tubing and closely following the suggested infusion regimen when administering amiodarone hydrochloride by IV infusion. Leaching of diethylhexyl phthalate (DEHP) from IV tubing may occur. (See IV Infusion under Dosage and Administration: Reconstitution and Administration.)

Following dilution of amiodarone hydrochloride injection concentrate to a concentration of 1–6 mg/mL in 5% dextrose in a PVC container, there is physical compatibility, with a loss of less than 10% of drug at 2 hours at room temperature. Following dilution of amiodarone hydrochloride injection concentrate to a concentration of 1–6 mg/mL in 5% dextrose in a glass or polyolefin container, there is physical compatibility, with no loss of drug at 24 hours at room temperature. Therefore, the manufacturer states that amiodarone hydrochloride infusions exceeding 2 hours should be administered in 5% dextrose in a glass or polyolefin containers. However, evacuated glass containers should not be used since incompatibility with a buffer in the container may cause precipitation.

When admixed in 5% dextrose, amiodarone hydrochloride injection is incompatible with aminophylline, cefamandole nafate, cefazolin sodium, mezlocillin sodium, heparin sodium, or sodium bicarbonate. Specialized references should be consulted for specific compatibility information.

Clinicians should provide information to patients regarding proper techniques for storage and disposal of out-of-date amiodarone tablets.

Preparations

Excipients in commercially available drug preparations may have clinically important effects in some individuals; consult specific product labeling for details.

Amiodarone Hydrochloride

Oral		
Tablets	100 mg	**Pacerone®**, Upsher-Smith
	200 mg*	**Amiodarone Hydrochloride Tablets**
		Cordarone® (scored), Wyeth
		Pacerone® (scored), Upsher-Smith
	400 mg*	**Amiodarone Hydrochloride Tablets**
		Pacerone® (scored), Upsher-Smith
Parenteral		
Concentrate for injection, for IV infusion	50 mg/mL*	**Amiodarone Hydrochloride Injection**

*available from one or more manufacturer, distributor, and/or repackager by generic (nonproprietary) name

†Use is not currently included in the labeling approved by the US Food and Drug Administration

Dofetilide

■ Dofetilide is a class III antiarrhythmic agent.

REMS

FDA approved a REMS for dofetilide to ensure that the benefits outweigh the risks. However, FDA later rescinded REMS requirements. See the FDA REMS page (https://www.accessdata.fda.gov/scripts/cder/rems/index.cfm).

Uses

■ **Supraventricular Tachyarrhythmias** Dofetilide is used for the maintenance of normal sinus rhythm in patients with atrial fibrillation/ atrial flutter of more than 1 week duration who have been converted to normal sinus rhythm. Because dofetilide can cause life-threatening ventricular arrhythmias, it should be reserved for patients in whom atrial fibrillation/ atrial flutter is highly symptomatic. Dofetilide also is used for the conversion of atrial fibrillation and atrial flutter to normal sinus rhythm. Dofetilide has not been shown to be effective in patients with paroxysmal atrial fibrillation.

In 2 randomized, double-blind, dose-response studies, about 30% of patients with atrial fibrillation/ atrial flutter who received 500 mcg of dofetilide twice daily were successfully converted to normal sinus rhythm compared with about 10 or 6% of those receiving 250 or 125 mcg twice daily and 1% of those who received placebo. Approximately 70% of the patients who successfully achieved normal sinus rhythm did so within 24–36 hours of beginning dofetilide therapy. After 12 months of therapy, the probabilities of remaining in normal sinus rhythm were 58–66 or 25–21% in patients who had converted to normal sinus rhythm and were still receiving dofetilide (500 mcg twice daily) or placebo, respectively. In one of these studies, dofetilide also was more effective than sotalol (80 mg orally twice daily) in converting atrial fibrillation to normal sinus rhythm or maintaining normal sinus rhythm for up to 12 months. In a third study, dofetilide was effective in converting and preventing the recurrence of atrial fibrillation without affecting mortality in patients with congestive heart failure and reduced left ventricular function.

Dosage and Administration

■ **Administration** Dofetilide is administered orally twice daily without regard to meals.

Restricted Distribution Program Commercially available dofetilide must be obtained through a restricted distribution program. Clinicians and pharmacies in institutions must confirm their participation in a designated Tikosyn® educational program before prescribing or ordering the drug; the drug is not available through community pharmacies. The status of clinicians who have participated in these programs may be verified on the internet (www.tikosynlist.com); for information regarding such educational programs, contact the manufacturer at 877-845-6796.

■ **Dosage** The recommended adult dosage of dofetilide is 500 mcg twice daily, which is modified according to creatinine clearance and QT_c interval. The risk of torsades de pointes is related to the dosage of dofetilide, and clinicians may elect to initiate therapy with lower dosages. Dosages exceeding 500 mcg twice daily have been associated with an increased incidence of torsades de pointes.

Because of the arrhythmogenic potential of dofetilide, the manufacturer recommends that both initiation of therapy with the drug and any subsequent increases in dosage be performed in a hospital setting where creatinine clearance calculations, continuous ECG monitoring, and cardiac resuscitation can be performed and where the patient can be monitored by personnel trained in the management of serious ventricular arrhythmias. Prior to initiation of dofetilide, the creatinine clearance must be calculated and QT_c interval (or QT interval if the heart rate is less than 60 beats/minute) must be determined using an average of 5–10 beats. If the QT_c interval exceeds 440 msec (500 msec in patients with ventricular conduction abnormalities), dofetilide is contraindicated. If creatinine clearance is less than 60 mL/minute, the initial dosage of dofetilide must be reduced. (See Dosage and Administration: Special Populations.) Serum potassium should be within the normal range (above 3.6–4 mEq/L) before initiation of dofetilide therapy and maintained in that range during therapy. Within 2–3 hours of administering the first dose of dofetilide, determine the QT_c interval. If QT_c interval has increased by more than 15% or exceeds 500 msec (550 msec in patients with ventricular conduction abnormalities), adjust subsequent dosages as indicated in Table 1.

Table 1.

Initial Dosage (Based on Creatinine Clearance)	Adjusted Dosage (for QT_c Prolongation)
500 mcg twice daily	250 mcg twice daily
250 mcg twice daily	125 mcg twice daily
125 mcg twice daily	125 mcg once daily

Within 2–3 hours after each subsequent dose of dofetilide (for in-hospital doses 2–5), determine the QT_c interval. No further downward titration of dofetilide based on QT_c is recommended. However, if at any time after the second dose of dofetilide is given the QT_c exceeds 500 msec (550 msec in patients with ventricular conduction abnormalities), discontinue dofetilide. Continuous ECG monitoring should be performed for a minimum of 3 days or for a minimum of 12 hours after electrical or pharmacologic conversion to normal sinus rhythm, whichever is greater.

Reevaluate renal function and QT_c interval every 3 months or as medically warranted. If QT_c exceeds 500 msec (550 msec in patients with ventricular conduction abnormalities), discontinue dofetilide and carefully monitor the patient until QT_c returns to baseline levels. If renal function deteriorates, adjust dosage as described in Dosage and Administration: Special Populations.

The manufacturer recommends that patients be hospitalized and closely monitored for 3 days (until steady-state plasma concentrations are obtained) whenever treatment is initiated or reinitiated or when dofetilide dosage is increased. Previously successful use of such dosages of dofetilide does not eliminate the need for rehospitalization when the dosage is increased.

■ **Special Populations** In patients with impaired renal function, dosage of dofetilide must be modified according to the degree of impairment. *Because increase in QT interval and the risk of ventricular arrhythmias are directly related to plasma dofetilide concentrations, dosage adjustment based on calculated creatinine clearance is essential.* The patient's creatinine clearance (Ccr) can be estimated by using the following formulas:

$$Ccr\ male = \frac{(140 - age) \times weight}{72 \times serum\ creatinine}$$

$$Ccr\ female = 0.85 \times Ccr\ male$$

where age is in years, weight is in kg, and serum creatinine is in mg/dL.

The manufacturer recommends that patients receive the following dosage based on calculated creatinine clearance (see Table 2).

Table 2.

Calculated Creatinine Clearance (mL/minute)	Dosage
>60	500 mcg twice daily
40–60	250 mcg twice daily
20 to <40	125 mcg twice daily
<20	Dofetilide is contraindicated

No dosage adjustment is required in patients with mild to moderate hepatic impairment (Child-Pugh class A or B). The pharmacokinetics of the drug have not been studied in patients with severe hepatic insufficiency (Child-Pugh class C) and such patients should be treated cautiously.

Cautions

■ **Contraindications** Congenital or acquired long QT syndromes; baseline QT or QT_c interval exceeding 440 msec (500 msec in patients with ventricular conduction abnormalities). Severe renal impairment (calculated creatinine clearance below 20 mL/minute). Concomitant use of verapamil or cation transport system inhibitors (e.g., cimetidine, ketoconazole, megestrol, prochlorperazine, trimethoprim [alone or in combination with sulfamethoxazole]). Concomitant use of hydrochlorothiazide (alone or in combination with triamterene). (See Drug Interactions.) Known hypersensitivity to dofetilide.

■ **Warnings/Precautions** ***Warnings*** **Arrhythmogenic Effects.** Dofetilide may cause serious ventricular arrhythmias, principally polymorphic ventricular tachycardia associated with QT interval prolongation (i.e., torsades de pointes). The risk of torsades de pointes can be reduced by controlling the plasma concentration (e.g., adjustment of initial dofetilide dosage according to creatinine clearance, avoiding certain drug interactions) and monitoring the ECG for excessive increases in the QT interval. In clinical trials, the overall incidence of torsades de pointes was 0.8% and was dose-related in patients with supraventricular arrhythmias. Most episodes of torsades de pointes occurred within the first 3 days of dofetilide therapy, and the risk was threefold greater in women than in men.

Drug Interactions. Because there is a linear relationship between plasma dofetilide concentration and QT_c, drug interactions that increase plasma dofetilide concentrations either through decreased renal excretion (e.g., inhibitors of cationic renal secretion) or decreased metabolism (e.g., inhibitors of cytochrome P-450 [CYP] isoenzyme 3A4) may increase the risk of torsades de pointes. Use of dofetilide with other drugs that prolong the QT interval has not been studied, and concomitant use of dofetilide with such drugs is not recommended. Carefully screen patients' medication history, including all over-the-counter, prescription, and herbal/natural preparations with emphasis on those that may affect dofetilide pharmacokinetics. If dofetilide must be discontinued to permit administration of potentially interacting drug(s), allow a washout period of at least 2 days. (See Drug Interactions.)

General Precautions **Effects on Cardiac Conduction.** Animal and human studies have not shown any adverse effects of dofetilide on conduction velocity. No effect on AV nodal conduction following dofetilide treatment was noted in normal volunteers or in patients with first degree heart block. Dofetilide has been used safely in conjunction with pacemakers.

Drug Transfer. The manufacturer recommends a transition period for patients being transferred from another antiarrhythmic agent to dofetilide. Class I and class III antiarrhythmic agents should be withheld for at least 3 half-lives prior to initiating dofetilide. Amiodarone should be withheld for at least 3 months or until serum amiodarone concentration is less than 0.3 mcg/mL prior to administering dofetilide. (See Drug Interactions.)

Anticoagulants. Patients with atrial fibrillation should receive appropriate anticoagulant therapy. (See Uses: Embolism Associated with Mitral Valve Disease and/or Atrial Fibrillation in Warfarin 20:12.04.08.)

Electrolyte Imbalance. Hypokalemia or hypomagnesemia may increase the risk of torsades de pointes in patients receiving dofetilide. Patients experiencing prolonged or excessive diarrhea, sweating, vomiting, loss of appetite, or thirst or receiving concomitant therapy with drugs that may increase the risk of such electrolyte imbalance (e.g., diuretics) should be closely monitored. Hypokalemia should be corrected before initiation of dofetilide. (See Drug Interactions.)

Specific Populations **Pregnancy.** Category C. (See Users' Guide.)

Lactation. Not known whether dofetilide is distributed in milk. Patients should not breast-feed while receiving dofetilide.

Pediatric Use. Safety and efficacy not established in children younger than 18 years of age.

Geriatric Use. No substantial differences in safety and efficacy relative to younger adults. Because geriatric patients may have decreased renal function, cautious dosage selection is advised.

Renal Impairment. Safety and efficacy not established in patients with creatinine clearance less than 20 mL/minute. (See Dosage and Administration: Special Populations.)

Hepatic Impairment. No dosage adjustment necessary in mild to moderate hepatic impairment. Use with caution in patients with severe hepatic impairment. (See Dosage and Administration: Special Populations.)

■ **Common Adverse Effects** Adverse effects occurring in 2% or more of patients receiving dofetilide and more frequently than placebo include headache, chest pain, dizziness, respiratory tract infection, dyspnea, nausea, flu syndrome, insomnia, accidental injury, back pain, medical, surgical, or other health service procedure, diarrhea, rash, and abdominal pain.

Drug Interactions

■ **Drugs Inhibiting Renal Tubular Cationic Transport** Pharmacokinetic interaction (decreased dofetilide excretion) when dofetilide is used with drugs inhibiting renal tubular cationic transport (e.g., cimetidine, ketoconazole, megestrol, prochlorperazine, trimethoprim [with or without sulfamethoxazole]). (See Cautions: Contraindications.)

■ **Drugs Secreted by Renal Tubular Cationic Transport** Potential pharmacokinetic interaction (decreased dofetilide excretion and increased plasma concentration) when dofetilide is used with drugs secreted by renal tubular cationic transport (e.g., amiloride, metformin, triamterene). (See Cautions: Contraindications.)

■ **Verapamil** Pharmacokinetic interaction (increased dofetilide concentrations). (See Cautions: Contraindications.)

■ **Drugs Affecting Hepatic Microsomal Enzymes** Potential pharmacokinetic interaction (decreased dofetilide metabolism and possible increased systemic exposure to dofetilide) with inhibitors of cytochrome P-450 (CYP) 3A4 isoenzyme (e.g., macrolide antibiotics, azole antifungal agents, protease inhibitors, serotonin reuptake inhibitors, amiodarone, cannabinoids, diltiazem, grapefruit juice, nefazodone, norfloxacin, quinine, zafirlukast).

■ **Drugs that Prolong QT Interval** Potential pharmacodynamic interaction (increased toxicity) when dofetilide is used with drugs that prolong QT interval (e.g., class I or III antiarrhythmic agents, bepridil, cisapride, phenothiazines, tricyclic antidepressants, certain oral macrolides, hydrochlorothiazide-containing preparations).

■ **Warfarin** Pharmacodynamic or pharmacokinetic interaction unlikely.

■ **Potassium-depleting Diuretics** Potential pharmacodynamic interaction (increased dofetilide toxicity). Concomitant use with hydrochlorothiazide alone or in combination (e.g., with triamterene) is contraindicated.

Description

Dofetilide, a class III antiarrhythmic agent, is a methanesulfonamide derivative that is structurally related to sotalol. Dofetilide exhibits electrophysiologic effects characteristic of class III antiarrhythmic agents (e.g., prolongs repolarization and refractoriness without affecting cardiac conduction velocity and sinus node function). However, unlike ibutilide and sotalol, dofetilide has no effect on sodium channels (associated with class I antiarrhythmic agents) or β-adrenergic receptors at clinically relevant concentrations.

Dofetilide prolongs the action potential duration and effective refractory period in both atrial and ventricular cardiac tissue, principally due to delayed repolarization. The antiarrhythmic action of dofetilide results from selective inhibition of the rapidly activating component of the potassium channel involved in repolarization of cardiac cells (i.e., the rapidly activated component of the delayed rectifier potassium current I_{Kr}). Like other class III antiarrhythmics, effects on cardiac repolarization induced by the drug can result in proarrhythmic effects (principally torsades de pointes).

Dofetilide, like ibutilide, appears to be more selective in its cellular actions than some other currently available class III antiarrhythmic agents (e.g., amiodarone, sotalol) and therefore has been referred to as a "pure" class III antiarrhythmic. Dofetilide has negligible effects on heart rate or blood pressure and may slightly improve cardiac contractility.

Advice to Patients

Importance of reading the manufacturer's patient information prior to beginning therapy and rereading it each time the prescription is refilled in case status has changed. (See REMS.)

Importance of informing clinician immediately if new rapid heartbeats, lightheadedness, or fainting occur; if clinician cannot be contacted, go to nearest hospital emergency room.

Importance of adherence to dosage and medical appointment schedule. Take drug at same time each day and omit any missed doses.

Importance of informing clinicians of existing or contemplated concomitant therapy, including prescription and OTC drugs, as well as concomitant illnesses. Importance of women informing clinicians if they are or plan to become pregnant or breast-feed.

Overview (see Users Guide). For additional information until a more detailed monograph is developed and published, the manufacturer's labeling should be consulted. It is *essential* that the manufacturer's labeling be consulted for more detailed information on usual cautions, precautions, contraindications, potential drug interactions, laboratory test interferences, and acute toxicity.

Preparations

Distribution of dofetilide is restricted. (See Restricted Distribution under Dosage and Administration: Administration.)

Excipients in commercially available drug preparations may have clinically important effects in some individuals; consult specific product labeling for details.

Dofetilide

Oral		
Capsules	0.125 mg	**Tikosyn®**, Pfizer
	0.25 mg	**Tikosyn®**, Pfizer
	0.5 mg	**Tikosyn®**, Pfizer

Dronedarone Hydrochloride

■ Dronedarone hydrochloride is considered to be predominantly a class III antiarrhythmic agent, but the drug appears to exhibit activity in each of the 4 Vaughan-Williams antiarrhythmic classes.

REMS

FDA approved a REMS for dronedarone hydrochloride to ensure that the benefits outweigh the risks. However, FDA later rescinded REMS requirements. See the FDA REMS page (https://www.accessdata.fda.gov/scripts/cder/rems/index.cfm).

Uses

■ **Supraventricular Tachyarrhythmias** Dronedarone hydrochloride is used to reduce the risk of hospitalization for atrial fibrillation in patients in sinus rhythm who have a history of paroxysmal or persistent atrial fibrillation. Current evidence from a comparative trial suggests that dronedarone is less effective than amiodarone in preventing recurrence of atrial fibrillation but has an improved safety profile (based on short-term follow-up) with regard to certain serious adverse effects (e.g., thyroid, neurologic) and potential for drug interactions (e.g., with warfarin). However, long-term data and experience are needed to fully elucidate the relative safety and tolerability of dronedarone versus amiodarone because some adverse effects of amiodarone (e.g., pulmonary toxicity) have been reported to occur up to 2–3 years after initiation of therapy.

Dronedarone should *not* be used in patients with *permanent* atrial fibrillation (i.e., patients in whom normal sinus rhythm will not or cannot be restored); results of a clinical trial indicate an increased risk of cardiovascular events and death in such patients. (See Cardiovascular Death and Heart Failure in Patients with Permanent Atrial Fibrillation under Warnings/Precautions: Warnings, in Cautions.)

The efficacy of retreatment with dronedarone in patients who relapse after initial successful treatment or in those who fail therapy with amiodarone remains to be determined. Some clinicians suggest that based on current data, dronedarone should be considered alternative (e.g., second- or third-line) therapy in selected patients in whom control of ventricular rate alone is not feasible or successful and who do not have advanced (i.e., New York Heart Association [NYHA] class IV or recently decompensated class II or III) heart failure and are not receiving drugs that prolong QT interval or strongly inhibit cytochrome P-450 (CYP) isoenzyme 3A4 (CYP3A4). (See Cautions: Contraindications.) Treatment of atrial fibrillation/flutter should be individualized, with consideration given to the relative benefits and risks of various therapies (e.g., rhythm versus rate control, nondrug therapies such as ablation and pacemaker implantation), patient age, as well as patient preference and tolerance of the arrhythmia.

In a multicenter, placebo-controlled, double-blind, parallel-arm trial to assess the efficacy of dronedarone for the prevention of hospitalization for cardiovascular events or death from any cause in patients with atrial fibrillation/flutter (ATHENA study), the incidence of the combined primary outcome (first hospitalization due to cardiovascular events or death from any cause) was reduced with dronedarone compared with placebo. In this study, 4628 patients with a recent history of paroxysmal or persistent atrial fibrillation/flutter were randomized to receive dronedarone (400 mg twice daily) or placebo in addition to conventional therapy for cardiovascular diseases (i.e., β-adrenergic blocking agents, angiotensin-converting enzyme [ACE] inhibitors, angiotensin II receptor antagonists, digoxin, calcium-channel blocking agents, HMG-CoA reductase inhibitors, oral anticoagulants, aspirin, other maintenance antiplatelet therapy, and diuretics). Eligible patients included those who were at least 75 years of age or those at least 70 years of age who had one or more risk factors (i.e., hypertension, diabetes, prior cerebrovascular accident, left atrial diameter of 50 mm or greater, left ventricular ejection fraction of 40% or less) and who were in sinus rhythm or were to undergo cardioversion to sinus rhythm. Patients ineligible for participation in the study included, but were not limited to, patients with NYHA class IV heart failure. The median duration of follow-up was 22 months (range: 12–30 months).

In the ATHENA study, the combined primary outcome of first hospitalization due to cardiovascular events or death from any cause occurred in 31.9% of patients who received dronedarone (individual event rates of 29.3 and 2.6% were reported for cardiovascular hospitalization and death from any cause, respectively) compared with 39.4% of patients who received placebo (individual event rates of 36.9 and 2.5% were reported for cardiovascular hospitalizations and death from any cause, respectively). The reduction in the rate of the combined primary outcome with dronedarone was mainly attributable to a reduction in the rate of first hospitalization due to cardiovascular events, principally hospitalization related to atrial fibrillation; the incidence of death from any cause was not substantially reduced. The numbers of first hospitalizations for congestive heart failure (CHF), ventricular arrhythmia, nonfatal cardiac arrest, or syncope were similar for patients who received dronedarone or placebo; however, there were fewer first hospitalizations for acute coronary syndromes in the dronedarone group.

In 2 other multicenter, double-blind, placebo-controlled trials in outpatients with atrial fibrillation/flutter receiving dronedarone for the maintenance of sinus rhythm (the EURIDIS study in 12 European countries and the ADONIS study in the US, Canada, Australia, South Africa, and Argentina), patients who received dronedarone had a longer median time to first recurrence of atrial fibrillation/flutter (116 versus 53 days) and a lower rate of recurrence at 12 months (64.1 versus 75.2%) than those who received placebo. In these studies, a total of 1237 patients 21 years of age or older who had at least one episode of atrial fibrillation/flutter (as documented by electrocardiogram [ECG]) during the previous 3 months and were in sinus rhythm for at least 1 hour were randomized to receive dronedarone (400 mg twice daily) or placebo, in addition to conventional therapy, for 12 months. Patients ineligible for participation in the studies included, but were not limited to, patients with NYHA class III or IV congestive heart failure. The primary outcome was time from randomization to first documented recurrence of atrial fibrillation/flutter, which was defined as an episode lasting for at least 10 minutes and confirmed by 2 consecutive ECG or transtelephonic recordings taken 10 minutes apart.

In another double-blind, placebo-controlled trial of dronedarone therapy in patients with moderate to severe CHF (ANDROMEDA study), the study was terminated prematurely (after enrollment of 627 of 1000 planned patients and a median follow-up of 63 days) because of excess mortality, mainly as a result of worsening heart failure, in the dronedarone group (8.1%) compared with the placebo group (3.8%). However, at study termination, the combined primary end point of death from any cause or hospitalization for worsening heart failure was not significantly different between patients who received dronedarone or placebo (crude estimate: 17.1 versus 12.6%). After an additional 6 months of follow-up without study treatment, the rate of mortality and the percentage of patients who had reached the combined primary end point were not significantly different between the 2 groups.

In the ANDROMEDA study, patients 18 years of age or older who were hospitalized with new or worsening heart failure and who had at least one episode of shortness of breath on minimal exertion or at rest (NYHA class III or IV heart failure) or paroxysmal nocturnal dyspnea within the previous month and a wall-motion index of 1.2 or less (ejection fraction of about 35% or less) were randomized to receive dronedarone (400 mg twice daily) or placebo. Outcomes were assessed up to the day active treatment was discontinued, 1 month after the date of cessation of the active-treatment phase, and at the end of a 6-month follow-up phase following completion of the study. The study was originally scheduled to last for 2 years and each patient was to be treated for a minimum of 12 months; however, 7 months after the first patient was assigned to a study group, enrollment and treatment were discontinued for safety reasons on the recommendation of the data and safety monitoring board. Dronedarone is contraindicated in patients with NYHA class IV heart failure or heart failure with recent decompensation requiring hospitalization. (See Cautions: Contraindications and also see Cardiovascular Death in Decompensated Heart Failure under Warnings/Precautions: Warnings, in Cautions.)

Dronedarone appears to be less effective than amiodarone in preventing recurrence of atrial fibrillation but may be less likely to cause serious adverse effects, at least in the short term. In a randomized, double-blind study (DIONYSOS) in 504 amiodarone-naive patients (mean age: 64 years) with persistent atrial fibrillation, the primary composite (efficacy/safety) end point (time to first ECG-documented recurrence of atrial fibrillation or premature discontinuance of the study drug due to lack of efficacy or intolerance) was reached in 75.1% of patients receiving dronedarone (400 mg twice daily) compared with 58.8% of those receiving amiodarone (600 mg daily for 28 days, then 200 mg daily) at 12 months; the median duration of treatment was 7 months (maximum treatment duration of 13.8 months in both groups).

Patients enrolled in the DIONYSOS study had documented atrial fibrillation of more than 72 hours' duration, and almost all (95.6%) were receiving concomitant oral anticoagulant therapy. Recurrence of atrial fibrillation (including documented atrial fibrillation after successful conversion, unsuccessful electrical cardioversion, and no spontaneous conversion and no electrical cardioversion on days 10–28) accounted for the largest component of the composite primary end point (63.5 or 42% for dronedarone or amiodarone, respectively) compared with the premature drug discontinuance component (10.4 or 13.3% for dronedarone or amiodarone, respectively). Recurrence of atrial fibrillation after successful conversion was more frequent with dronedarone than with amiodarone (36.5 versus 24.3%, respectively). The incidence of the predefined main safety end point, which included thyroid, hepatic, pulmonary, neurologic, skin, ocular, and GI adverse effects as well as premature drug discontinuance, was similar for dronedarone and amiodarone at 12 months. Bradycardia and QT_c (QT interval corrected for rate, Bazett's formula) prolongation, thyroid and neurologic events, and premature drug discontinuance due to adverse effects were less frequent with dronedarone; however, GI events, none of which were serious (mainly diarrhea), occurred at a higher incidence in the dronedarone group. However, when GI events were excluded, the relative risk of the main safety end point was reduced by 39% with dronedarone. In addition, the proportion of patients with supratherapeutic INR levels (exceeding 4.5) was smaller and the incidence of hemorrhagic events was reduced with dronedarone compared with amiodarone therapy.

In the PALLAS study, patients with permanent atrial fibrillation (defined as the presence of atrial fibrillation or atrial flutter for at least 6 months prior to randomization and patient and clinician decision not to make further efforts to restore sinus rhythm) and additional cardiovascular risk factors who received dronedarone had a higher incidence of heart failure, stroke, and cardiovascular death than those receiving placebo, and the study was terminated early for safety reasons. In this study, patients received dronedarone (400 mg twice daily) or placebo in addition to standard therapy (e.g., drugs to control heart rate, digoxin, anticoagulation with a vitamin K antagonist [e.g., warfarin]). Patients were at least 65 years of age and considered at high risk for vascular events because of the presence of at least one of the following risk factors:

coronary artery disease, previous stroke or transient ischemic attack (TIA); symptomatic heart failure, left ventricular ejection fraction of 40% or less; peripheral arterial disease; or the combination of age exceeding 75 years, hypertension, and diabetes. Dronedarone therapy was associated with a more-than-twofold increase in the rate of the first coprimary outcome (stroke, myocardial infarction, systemic embolism, or cardiovascular death) and a near-doubling of the second coprimary outcome (unplanned hospitalization for cardiovascular causes or death). Dronedarone is contraindicated in patients with *permanent* atrial fibrillation. (See Cautions: Contraindications and see Cardiovascular Death and Heart Failure in Patients with Permanent Atrial Fibrillation under Warnings/Precautions: Warnings, in Cautions.)

Dosage and Administration

■ **Administration** Dronedarone hydrochloride is administered orally twice daily with the morning and evening meals (to enhance bioavailability). (See Description.)

■ **Dosage** Dosage of dronedarone hydrochloride is expressed in terms of dronedarone.

Supraventricular Tachyarrhythmias The recommended dosage of dronedarone to reduce the risk of hospitalization for atrial fibrillation in selected patients in sinus rhythm who have a history of paroxysmal or persistent atrial fibrillation (See Uses: Supraventricular Tachyarrhythmias) is 400 mg twice daily with the morning and evening meals.

In a small dose-response study, patients with recurrent atrial fibrillation received dronedarone dosages of 400, 600, or 800 mg twice a day; dosages above 400 mg twice daily were not more effective and were less well tolerated.

Treatment with class I or III antiarrhythmic agents or drugs that are potent inhibitors of the cytochrome P-450 (CYP) 3A isoenzyme must be discontinued prior to initiating dronedarone therapy. (See Cautions: Contraindications and also see Drug Interactions.)

■ **Special Populations** No dosage adjustment is required in patients with moderate hepatic impairment. However, dronedarone is contraindicated in patients with severe hepatic impairment. (See Hepatic Impairment under Warnings/Precautions: Specific Populations, in Cautions.)

No dosage adjustment is required in patients with renal impairment. (See Renal Impairment under Warnings/Precautions: Specific Populations, in Cautions.)

The manufacturer states that no dosage of dronedarone other than 400 mg twice daily is recommended for any population at this time.

Cautions

■ **Contraindications** Permanent atrial fibrillation (patients in whom normal sinus rhythm will not or cannot be restored).

Symptomatic heart failure with NYHA Class IV symptoms or recent decompensation requiring hospitalization.

Second- or third-degree atrioventricular (AV) block or sick sinus syndrome (except in patients with a functioning pacemaker).

Bradycardia (less than 50 beats/minute).

QT interval corrected for rate (Bazett's formula, QT_c) of 500 milliseconds or greater or PR interval exceeding 280 milliseconds. (See Other Warnings and Precautions: Prolongation of QT Interval, under Cautions: Warnings/Precautions.)

Concomitant use of potent inhibitors of the cytochrome P-450 (CYP) 3A isoenzyme (e.g., clarithromycin, cyclosporine, itraconazole, ketoconazole, nefazodone, ritonavir, telithromycin, voriconazole). (See Drug Interactions: Drugs Affecting Hepatic Microsomal Enzymes and also see Drug Interactions: Drugs Metabolized by Hepatic Microsomal Enzymes.)

Concomitant use with drugs or herbal supplements that prolong the QT interval and may increase the risk of torsades de pointes (e.g., class I or III antiarrhythmic agents, phenothiazine antipsychotics, tricyclic antidepressants, certain oral macrolides [e.g., erythromycin]). (See Drug Interactions: Drugs that Prolong the QT Interval.)

Liver toxicity related to previous use of amiodarone. (See Other Warnings and Precautions: Severe Hepatic Injury, under Warnings/Precautions, in Cautions.)

Severe hepatic impairment. (See Hepatic Impairment under Warnings/Precautions: Specific Populations.)

Women who are or may become pregnant. (See Other Warnings and Precautions: Fetal/Neonatal Morbidity and Mortality under Cautions: Warnings/Precautions.)

Nursing women.

■ **Warnings/Precautions** ***Warnings*** **Cardiovascular Death in Decompensated Heart Failure.** Dronedarone should not be used in patients with NYHA Class IV heart failure or symptomatic heart failure and recent decompensation requiring hospitalization because of a twofold increase in cardiovascular death in such patients receiving the drug. (See Cautions: Contraindications.)

Cardiovascular Death and Heart Failure in Patients with Permanent Atrial Fibrillation. Dronedarone doubles the risk of cardiovascular death (principally due to arrhythmia) and heart failure in patients with *permanent* atrial fibrillation (i.e., those who cannot or will not be converted to normal sinus rhythm); the drug offers no benefit and is contraindicated in such patients.

Patients receiving dronedarone should have heart rate monitored by electrocardiogram (ECG) at least every 3 months. Patients who have atrial fibrillation should have dronedarone therapy discontinued or, if clinically indicated, should undergo cardioversion.

Increased Risk of Stroke in Patients with Permanent Atrial Fibrillation. Dronedarone should only be initiated in patients in sinus rhythm who are receiving appropriate antithrombotic therapy. In a placebo-controlled study in patients with permanent atrial fibrillation, dronedarone therapy was associated with an increased risk of stroke, particularly during the first 2 weeks of therapy.

Other Warnings and Precautions **New-Onset or Worsening Heart Failure.** New-onset or worsening heart failure has been reported in patients receiving dronedarone during postmarketing experience. In a placebo-controlled study in patients with permanent atrial fibrillation, increased rates of heart failure were observed in patients with normal left ventricular function and no history of symptomatic heart failure, and also in those with a history of heart failure or left ventricular dysfunction. If heart failure develops or worsens, dronedarone therapy should be discontinued. In addition, the manufacturer states that dronedarone is contraindicated in patients with NYHA class IV heart failure or heart failure with recent decompensation requiring hospitalization. (See Cautions: Contraindications.)

Severe Hepatic Injury. Severe hepatocellular injury, including acute hepatic failure requiring liver transplantation, has been reported during postmarketing experience in patients receiving dronedarone. Hepatic failure requiring transplantation was reported in 2 women 4.5 and 6 months, respectively, after initiation of dronedarone therapy. No alternative etiologies for hepatic failure were identified in either case; in both cases, the explanted liver showed evidence of extensive hepatocellular necrosis. A causal relationship between dronedarone exposure and hepatic failure has not been established because these events were reported voluntarily from a population of unknown size.

Patients should be advised to contact a clinician immediately if they experience manifestations of hepatic injury (e.g., anorexia, nausea, vomiting, fever, malaise, fatigue, right upper quadrant pain, jaundice, dark urine, itching) while taking dronedarone. Clinicians should consider periodic monitoring of serum hepatic enzymes in patients receiving dronedarone, especially during the first 6 months of therapy; it is not known whether routine periodic monitoring of hepatic enzymes will prevent development of severe hepatic injury. If hepatic injury is suspected, dronedarone therapy should be discontinued promptly and serum hepatic enzymes (AST, ALT, and alkaline phosphatase) and bilirubin assessed. Appropriate therapy should be initiated if hepatic injury is found, and the probable cause of such injury should be investigated. Dronedarone should not be reinitiated in patients who experience hepatic injury without another explanation for such injury.

Hypokalemia and Hypomagnesemia. Hypokalemia or hypomagnesemia may occur in patients receiving dronedarone concomitantly with potassium-depleting diuretics. Serum potassium and magnesium concentrations should be within the normal range prior to initiation of dronedarone therapy and maintained within the normal range during dronedarone therapy.

Prolongation of QT Interval. Dronedarone prolongs the QT_c interval by an average of about 10 milliseconds; however, much greater prolongation of the QT_c interval has been observed. If the QT_c interval is 500 milliseconds or greater, dronedarone should be discontinued. (See Cautions: Contraindications.)

Increased Serum Creatinine Concentrations. Small increases in serum creatinine concentrations (about 0.1 mg/dL) following initiation of dronedarone therapy have been reported to result from inhibition of the tubular secretion of creatinine by dronedarone.

Larger increases in serum creatinine after dronedarone initiation have been reported during postmarketing experience. In clinical studies, a 10–15% increase in serum creatinine concentration has been observed in healthy individuals and patients receiving dronedarone without any clinical or laboratory evidence of structural renal damage. The increase in serum creatinine concentration associated with dronedarone has a rapid onset, reaches a plateau after 7 days, and is reversible following discontinuance of the drug. In some cases, increases in BUN were also reported. These effects generally appear to be reversible upon drug discontinuance. Renal function should be monitored periodically in patients receiving dronedarone.

Fetal/Neonatal Morbidity and Mortality. Dronedarone may cause fetal harm; teratogenicity has been demonstrated in animals at dosages equivalent to human dosages. Pregnancy should be avoided during therapy. Women of childbearing potential (i.e., premenopausal women who have not undergone hysterectomy or oophorectomy) should be counseled regarding appropriate contraceptive choices and must use effective contraception while receiving dronedarone. If dronedarone is used during pregnancy or if the patient becomes pregnant while receiving the drug, the patient should be apprised of the potential hazard to the fetus. (See Advice to Patients.) Dronedarone is contraindicated in women who are or may become pregnant.

Specific Populations **Pregnancy.** Category X. (See Cautions: Contraindications and also see Fetal/Neonatal Morbidity and Mortality under Cautions: Warnings/Precautions.)

Lactation. Dronedarone and its metabolites are distributed into milk in rats. It is not known whether dronedarone is distributed into human milk. Because of the potential for serious adverse reactions to dronedarone in nursing infants, a decision should be made whether to discontinue nursing or the drug, taking into account the importance of the drug to the woman. Dronedarone is contraindicated in nursing women.

Pediatric Use. Safety and efficacy have not been established in children or adolescents younger than 18 years of age.

Geriatric Use. No substantial differences in safety and efficacy have been observed in geriatric patients compared with younger adults. In clinical studies, exposure to dronedarone was increased by 23% in patients 65 years of age or older compared with younger adults.

Hepatic Impairment. Dronedarone has not been studied in patients with severe hepatic impairment and limited clinical experience is available in patients with moderate hepatic impairment. Dronedarone is contraindicated in patients with severe hepatic impairment.

Severe liver injury has been reported rarely with dronedarone therapy. (See Severe Hepatic Injury under Warnings/Precautions, in Cautions.)

In patients with moderate hepatic impairment, the mean exposure to dronedarone increased by 1.3-fold compared with that in individuals with normal hepatic function, and the mean exposure to the *N*-debutyl metabolite decreased by about 50%. The pharmacokinetics of dronedarone have not been studied in patients with severe hepatic impairment.

Renal Impairment. Because dronedarone undergoes minimal renal excretion, the manufacturer states that dosage adjustment in patients with renal impairment is not necessary.

No apparent differences in the pharmacokinetics of dronedarone have been observed in individuals with mild or moderate renal impairment versus those with normal renal function or in patients with atrial fibrillation with mild to severe renal impairment versus those with normal renal function. (See Dosage and Administration: Special Populations.)

■ **Common Adverse Effects** Adverse effects reported in at least 1% of patients receiving dronedarone and more frequently than with placebo include early increases in serum creatinine (at least 10% increase), prolonged QT interval corrected for rate (QT_c, Bazett's formula), diarrhea, asthenic conditions, nausea, skin reactions (e.g., rash [generalized, macular, maculopapular, erythematous], pruritus, eczema, dermatitis, allergic dermatitis), abdominal pain, bradycardia, vomiting, and dyspeptic manifestations. (See Cautions: Contraindications and also see Other Warnings and Precautions: Prolongation of QT Interval and Other Warnings and Precautions: Increased Serum Creatinine Concentrations under Cautions: Warnings/Precautions.)

Drug Interactions

Dronedarone is metabolized mainly by the cytochrome P-450 (CYP) 3A isoenzyme.

Dronedarone is a moderate inhibitor of CYP 3A and 2D6; however, the drug does not appear to substantially inhibit CYP 1A2, 2C9, 2C19, 2C8, or 2B6. Dronedarone may potentially inhibit the P-glycoprotein transport system. Dronedarone or its metabolites are weak inhibitors of organic cation transporter (OCT1), organic anion transporting polypeptide (OATP1B1, OATP1B3), and organic anion transporter (OAT3) in vitro.

■ **Drugs Affecting Hepatic Microsomal Enzymes** Potent inhibitors of CYP3A (e.g., clarithromycin, cyclosporine, itraconazole, ketoconazole, nefazodone, ritonavir, telithromycin, voriconazole): Pharmacokinetic interaction (increased peak plasma concentrations of and exposure to dronedarone). Concomitant use is contraindicated.

Moderate inhibitors of CYP3A (e.g., diltiazem, verapamil): Potential pharmacokinetic interaction (increased exposure to dronedarone). Initiate calcium-channel blocking agents at a low dosage and increase dosage only after ECG verification of good tolerability.

Inducers of CYP3A (e.g., carbamazepine, phenobarbital, phenytoin, rifampin, St. John's wort [*Hypericum perforatum*]): Potential pharmacokinetic interaction (substantially decreased exposure to dronedarone). Concomitant use should be avoided.

■ **Drugs Metabolized by Hepatic Microsomal Enzymes** Substrates of CYP3A: Potential pharmacokinetic interaction (possible increased plasma concentrations of the CYP3A substrate). Initiation of dronedarone therapy in one patient receiving sirolimus following kidney transplantation resulted in a threefold increase in trough sirolimus concentrations compared with the patient's baseline trough concentration. The manufacturer states that plasma concentrations of sirolimus, tacrolimus, and other CYP3A substrates with a narrow therapeutic index when administered orally should be monitored and dosage of these drugs should be adjusted appropriately when used concomitantly with dronedarone. Some clinicians state that dronedarone should be used with caution in patients receiving drugs with a narrow therapeutic index that are metabolized by CYP3A4. Due to the potential for sirolimus toxicity and excessive immunosuppression, some clinicians recommend that concurrent use of sirolimus and dronedarone be avoided when possible. However, if concurrent administration cannot be avoided, these clinicians suggest a 50–75% reduction in sirolimus dosage prior to dronedarone initiation and regular monitoring (possibly even daily) of trough sirolimus concentrations during the titration phase.

Substrates of CYP2D6 (e.g., β-adrenergic blocking agents, selective serotonin-reuptake inhibitors [SSRIs], tricyclic antidepressants): Potential pharmacokinetic interaction (possible increased exposure to the CYP2D6 substrate).

■ **Drugs that Prolong the QT Interval** Pharmacologic interaction (potential risk of torsades de pointes-type ventricular tachycardia). Concomitant use of dronedarone with drugs that prolong the QT interval (e.g., class I or III antiarrhythmic agents such as amiodarone, disopyramide, dofetilide, flecainide, propafenone, quinidine, sotalol; tricyclic antidepressants; certain phenothiazines; certain oral macrolides) is contraindicated.

■ **Drugs Affected by the P-glycoprotein Transport System** Potential pharmacokinetic interaction; increased exposure to substrates of the P-glycoprotein transport system (e.g., dabigatran, digoxin) is expected when such drugs are used concomitantly with dronedarone. Some clinicians state that dronedarone should be used with caution in patients receiving drugs with a narrow therapeutic index that are metabolized by the P-glycoprotein transport system.

■ **β-Adrenergic Blocking Agents** Potential pharmacologic and pharmacokinetic interactions. In clinical studies, bradycardia was observed more frequently when dronedarone was given concomitantly with β-adrenergic blocking agents. Dronedarone increases exposure to propranolol and metoprolol.

If dronedarone is used concomitantly with a β-adrenergic blocking agent, a lower initial dosage of the β-adrenergic blocking agent is recommended and the dosage should be increased only if well tolerated as documented by electrocardiogram (ECG). (Also see Drug Interactions: Drugs Metabolized by Hepatic Microsomal Enzymes.)

■ **Calcium-channel Blocking Agents** Potential pharmacologic and pharmacokinetic interactions. Calcium-channel blocking agents associated with depressant effects on the sinus and AV nodes may potentiate the myocardial conduction effects of dronedarone. In addition, dronedarone may increase exposure to calcium-channel blocking agents (diltiazem, nifedipine, verapamil). Initiate calcium-channel blocking agents at a low dosage and increase dosage only after ECG verification of good tolerability.

In addition, verapamil and diltiazem (moderate CYP3A inhibitors) may increase exposure to dronedarone. (See Drug Interactions: Drugs Affecting Hepatic Microsomal Enzymes.)

■ **Clopidogrel** Concomitant administration of dronedarone does not require dosage adjustment of clopidogrel.

■ **Dabigatran** Potential pharmacokinetic interaction. Concomitant administration of dronedarone may increase systemic exposure to dabigatran. (See Drug Interactions: Drugs Affected by the P-glycoprotein Transport System.)

■ **Digoxin** Potential pharmacologic and pharmacokinetic interactions. Digoxin may potentiate the electrophysiologic effects of dronedarone (e.g., decreased AV node conduction). In clinical studies, increased serum digoxin concentrations and an increased incidence of GI disorders were reported with concomitant use of dronedarone and digoxin. When dronedarone therapy is initiated in patients receiving digoxin, the need for continued digoxin therapy should be reassessed and digoxin discontinued if appropriate; if digoxin therapy is continued, a 50% reduction in digoxin dosage is recommended when dronedarone therapy is initiated. In addition, serum digoxin concentrations should be monitored carefully and patients should be observed closely for signs of digoxin toxicity if dronedarone and digoxin are used concomitantly. (See Drug Interactions: Drugs Affected by the P-glycoprotein Transport System.)

■ **Grapefruit Juice** Potential pharmacokinetic interaction (grapefruit juice increases exposure to dronedarone by threefold); use of grapefruit juice during dronedarone therapy should be avoided.

■ **HMG-CoA Reductase Inhibitors (Statins)** Simvastatin: Potential pharmacokinetic interaction; dronedarone increases exposure to simvastatin and simvastatin acid by fourfold and twofold, respectively. Simvastatin dosages exceeding 10 mg once daily should be avoided.

Other statins (e.g., atorvastatin, rosuvastatin): The manufacturer's labeling for the respective statin should be consulted for specific recommendations regarding concomitant use with CYP3A or P-glycoprotein transport system inhibitors, such as dronedarone. Concomitant administration of dronedarone does not require adjustment of atorvastatin or rosuvastatin dosage.

■ **Ketoconazole** Pharmacokinetic interaction; concomitant administration of ketoconazole, a potent CYP3A inhibitor, results in substantially increased exposure to dronedarone. Concomitant use of ketoconazole and dronedarone is contraindicated.

■ **Losartan** No losartan dosage adjustment required with concomitant administration of dronedarone and losartan.

■ **Metformin** No dosage adjustment to metformin hydrochloride required with concomitant dronedarone.

■ **Oral Contraceptives** No dosage adjustments to ethinyl estradiol or levonorgestrel required with concomitant dronedarone.

■ **Omeprazole** No dosage adjustment to omeprazole required with concomitant dronedarone.

■ **Pantoprazole** Pantoprazole does not necessitate dosage adjustment of concomitant dronedarone.

■ **Potassium-depleting Diuretics** Potential pharmacologic interaction (possible risk of hypokalemia or hypomagnesemia) with concomitant use of dronedarone and potassium-depleting diuretics. (See Other Warnings and Precautions: Hypokalemia and Hypomagnesemia under Cautions: Warnings/Precautions.)

■ **Rifampin** Potential pharmacokinetic interaction (rifampin substantially decreases exposure to dronedarone); concomitant use of dronedarone and rifampin should be avoided.

■ **Theophylline** No adjustment of theophylline dosage is required with concomitant dronedarone.

■ **Warfarin** Concomitant administration of dronedarone and warfarin resulted in slightly increased exposure to *S*-warfarin; however, there was no clinically important increase in the international normalized ratio (INR). In the ATHENA study, more patients experienced clinically important increases in INR (INR ≥5) usually within 1 week after adding dronedarone to warfarin therapy compared with placebo, but an excess risk of bleeding was not observed in such patients. However, cases of increased INR with or without bleeding events have been reported during postmarketing experience in warfarin-treated patients who received dronedarone. The INR should be monitored after initiation of dronedarone therapy in patients taking warfarin.

Description

Dronedarone hydrochloride is considered to be predominantly a class III antiarrhythmic agent, but the drug also appears to exhibit activity in each of the 4 Vaughan-Williams antiarrhythmic classes. The exact mechanism of antiarrhythmic action has not been fully elucidated, and the exact contribution of each of these activities to the clinical effect of dronedarone is unknown. Dronedarone is a benzofuran derivative that is structurally related to amiodarone, but with structural modifications that include removal of the iodine moiety and addition of a methane-sulfonyl group. The removal of the iodine group was intended to reduce the risk of non-target organ (e.g., thyroid, pulmonary) adverse effects associated with amiodarone, while the addition of the methane-sulfonyl group was aimed at reducing lipophilicity and thus decreasing the risk of neurotoxic adverse effects and shortening the half-life of dronedarone. Dronedarone also has an electrophysiologic profile similar to that of amiodarone, but with different relative effects on individual ion channels. Dronedarone prolongs the action potential duration (APD), principally due to inhibition of potassium channels including transmembrane delayed rectifier, ultrarapid delayed rectifier, inward rectifier, and transient outward potassium currents. Dronedarone also appears to inhibit sodium currents (at rapid pacing rates), calcium channels and slow L-type calcium currents, and demonstrates noncompetitive, antiadrenergic (α- and β-blocking) activity. Dronedarone prolongs the PR interval and slows the sinus rate by prolonging the atrial and ventricular refractory periods. Similar to amiodarone, dronedarone produces a dose-dependent increase in the PR interval, as well as moderate prolongation of the QT interval corrected for rate (QT_c, Bazett's formula). The drug also prolongs the RR and QT intervals.

Because dronedarone undergoes first-pass metabolism, the drug has low systemic bioavailability; the absolute bioavailability is about 4% when administered without food. Bioavailability is increased when the drug is given with meals and is approximately 15% when administered with a high-fat meal. Peak plasma concentrations of dronedarone and its main circulating *N*-debutyl metabolite are reached within 3–6 hours following oral administration with food. Steady-state concentrations are achieved within 4–8 days following repeated oral administration of dronedarone 400 mg twice daily. Dronedarone and its *N*-debutyl metabolite are greater than 98% bound to plasma proteins, mainly albumin; plasma protein binding does not appear to be saturable. Dronedarone is extensively metabolized, mainly by the cytochrome P-450 (CYP) 3A isoenzyme. The initial metabolic pathway includes *N*-debutylation to form the active *N*-debutyl metabolite, oxidative deamination to form the inactive propanoic acid metabolite, and direct oxidation. Monoamine oxidases contribute partially to the metabolism of the active metabolite of dronedarone. The metabolites undergo further metabolism to yield over 30 uncharacterized metabolites. The *N*-debutyl metabolite exhibits pharmacodynamic activity, but is only up to one-third as potent as dronedarone. Approximately 6 and 84% of an oral dose is excreted in urine and feces, respectively, mainly as metabolites; no unchanged drug is excreted in urine. The elimination half-life of dronedarone ranges from 13–19 hours following IV administration.

Advice to Patients

Importance of instructing patients to carefully read the manufacturer's patient information (medication guide) before initiating therapy and each time the prescription is refilled. (See REMS.)

Importance of patients not taking dronedarone if they have signs and symptoms of heart failure that recently worsened or required hospitalization, or if they have severe heart failure, because of an increased risk of dying. Importance of informing clinicians if signs or symptoms of heart failure (e.g., weight gain, dependent edema, increasing shortness of breath) occur during dronedarone treatment.

May cause hepatic injury, including life-threatening hepatic failure. Importance of patients not taking dronedarone if they have severe hepatic injury or had hepatic injury after using amiodarone. Importance of advising patients receiving dronedarone to immediately report symptoms suggesting hepatic injury (e.g., anorexia, nausea, vomiting, fever, malaise, fatigue, right upper quadrant pain or discomfort, jaundice, dark urine, itching).

Importance of patients not taking dronedarone if they have permanent atrial fibrillation. Importance of patients informing clinicians immediately if they notice an irregular pulse (a sign of atrial fibrillation) during treatment with dronedarone.

Importance of advising patients to avoid grapefruit juice while taking dronedarone. (See Drug Interactions: Grapefruit Juice.)

Importance of women informing clinicians immediately if they are or plan to become pregnant or plan to breast-feed; necessity of clinicians advising women to avoid pregnancy and breast-feeding during dronedarone therapy. Necessity of advising women of childbearing potential to use an effective method of contraception while receiving therapy and importance of advising these patients regarding appropriate contraceptive choices (taking into consideration their underlying medical conditions and lifestyle preferences). If pregnancy occurs, advise patient of risk to the fetus.

Importance of informing clinicians of existing or contemplated concomitant therapy, including prescription and OTC drugs and herbal supplements (e.g., St. John's wort) (see Drug Interactions), as well as any concomitant illnesses (e.g., heart failure, rhythm disturbance other than atrial fibrillation/flutter, uncorrected hypokalemia).

Importance of taking dronedarone exactly as prescribed (e.g., with meals). Importance of advising patients that if a dose of dronedarone is missed, the next dose should be taken at the regularly scheduled time; the dose should not be doubled.

Importance of informing patients of other important precautionary information. (See Cautions.)

Overview® (See Users Guide). For additional information on this drug until a more detailed monograph is developed and published, the manufacturer's labeling should be consulted. It is *essential* that the manufacturer's labeling be consulted for more detailed information on usual cautions, precautions, contraindications, potential drug interactions, laboratory test interferences, and acute toxicity.

Preparations

Excipients in commercially available drug preparations may have clinically important effects in some individuals; consult specific product labeling for details.

Dronedarone Hydrochloride

Oral

Tablets, film-coated	400 mg (of dronedarone)	**Multaq®**, Sanofi-Aventis

Ibutilide Fumarate

■ Ibutilide fumarate is a class III antiarrhythmic agent.

Uses

■ **Supraventricular Tachyarrhythmias** Ibutilide fumarate is used IV for the rapid conversion of recent-onset atrial fibrillation or atrial flutter to sinus rhythm. Ibutilide is considered a drug of choice for pharmacologic cardioversion of atrial fibrillation or flutter. Some experts also state that ibutilide may be useful for restoring sinus rhythm or slowing ventricular rate in hemodynamically stable patients with preexcited atrial fibrillation and rapid ventricular response (e.g., Wolff-Parkinson-White syndrome)†, although direct-current (DC) cardioversion is the intervention of choice for this indication when the patient is hemodynamically compromised. In addition, IV ibutilide may be considered for the treatment of focal atrial tachycardia†, usually after failure of other preferred therapies (e.g., diltiazem, verapamil, β-adrenergic blocking agents). Atrial arrhythmias that are not of recent onset are less likely to respond to the drug, and ibutilide's effectiveness has not been determined in atrial arrhythmias of more than 90 days' duration.

Ibutilide may cause potentially fatal arrhythmias, particularly sustained polymorphic ventricular tachycardia, usually associated with QT prolongation (i.e., torsades de pointes), but occasionally without documented QT interval prolongation; such ventricular arrhythmias that were severe enough to require treatment with DC cardioversion occurred during or within a few hours of ibutilide fumarate administration in 1.7% of patients in clinical trials. The risk of torsades de pointes may be increased in patients with bradycardia, varying heart rate, or hypokalemia. In addition, patients with a history of congestive heart failure or low ventricular ejection fraction appear to have a higher incidence of sustained polymorphic ventricular tachycardia. Therefore, it is essential that the drug be administered in a setting of continuous ECG monitoring and by personnel trained in the identification and treatment of acute ventricular arrhythmias, especially polymorphic ventricular tachycardia. In addition, the manufacturer states that patients with atrial fibrillation of more than 2 to 3 days' duration must be adequately anticoagulated, generally for at least 2 weeks before administration of ibutilide. Conversion of atrial fibrillation or flutter to normal sinus rhythm may be associated with embolism, particularly when the arrhythmia has been present for more than 48 hours, unless the patient is adequately anticoagulated. (See Uses: Cardioversion of Atrial Fibrillation/Flutter, in Heparin 20:12.04.16.) Ibutilide is *not* recommended for use in patients with a history of polymorphic ventricular tachycardia (e.g., torsades de pointes).

Chronic atrial fibrillation that has been converted by treatment such as ibutilide to sinus rhythm has a strong tendency to revert, and therapy required to maintain sinus rhythm is associated with risks. Therefore, patients for whom parenteral ibutilide therapy is considered should be selected carefully such that the expected benefits of conversion to sinus rhythm and continuous treatment to maintain it outweigh the immediate risks associated with use of ibutilide and the risks of maintenance therapy, and that they are likely to offer an advantage compared with alternative management methods for atrial flutter or fibrillation.

Because of their potential to prolong refractoriness, class Ia (e.g., disopyramide, quinidine, procainamide) or III (e.g., amiodarone, sotalol) antiarrhythmic agents should *not* be administered concomitantly with, or within 4 hours after completion of, ibutilide administration. In clinical trials, class I or III agents were withheld for at least 5 half-lives prior to, and 4 hours after completion of, ibutilide infusion, but thereafter were permitted at the clinician's discretion. The possibility that drugs that prolong the QT interval (e.g., certain antihistamines such as terfenadine [no longer commercially available in the US] and astemizole [no longer commercially available in the US], phenothiazines, tricyclic or tetracyclic antidepressants) may potentiate the proarrhythmic effects of ibutilide should be considered.

Current evidence of safety and efficacy of ibutilide in the acute termination of recent-onset atrial arrhythmias is based on several placebo-controlled studies that included hundreds of patients with atrial flutter and/or fibrillation of 3 hours' to 90 days' duration and in one active treatment (i.e., sotalol)-controlled study that included 319 patients with such arrhythmias of 3 hours' to 45 days' duration. In one study comparing single doses of ibutilide and sotalol, conversion to sinus rhythm reportedly occurred in 53 or 70% of patients with atrial flutter, and in 22 or 43% of patients with atrial fibrillation receiving a 1 or 2 mg of ibutilide fumarate IV, respectively; conversion to sinus rhythm occurred in 18% of those with atrial flutter, and 10% of patients with atrial fibrillation receiving 1.5 mg/kg of sotalol hydrochloride, respectively. In another placebo-controlled study, 14, 30, 58, or 55 % of patients with atrial flutter, and 10, 35, 32, or 40% of those with atrial fibrillation reportedly experienced conversion to sinus rhythm after receiving a single IV ibutilide fumarate dose of 0.005, 0.01, 0.015, or 0.025 mg/kg, respectively. In the other placebo-controlled study in which patients received up to 2 doses of ibutilide (i.e., an initial IV ibutilide fumarate dose of 1 mg followed by a second IV dose of either 0.5 or 1 mg), 48 or 63% of eligible patients with atrial flutter and 38 or 25% of those with atrial fibrillation receiving a total dose of 1.5 or 2 mg, respectively, converted to sinus rhythm.

In a double-blind, placebo-controlled, dose-ranging study in patients with atrial flutter or fibrillation of 1 hour's to 3 days' duration that developed 1–7 days after coronary bypass graft or valvular surgery, 56, 61, or 78% of patients with atrial flutter and 28, 42, or 44% of those with atrial fibrillation treated with two 10-minute IV ibutilide fumarate infusions (10 minutes apart) of 0.25, 0.5, or 1 mg (each), respectively, reportedly experienced conversion to sinus rhythm at 90 minutes. Four or 20% of patients with atrial flutter or atrial fibrillation, respectively, reportedly experienced conversion to sinus rhythm after receiving two 10-minute infusions of placebo. The mean time to conversion to sinus rhythm decreased as the dose of ibutilide fumarate was increased. In addition, 53 or 72% of patients who experienced conversion to sinus rhythm after receiving 10-minute IV ibutilide fumarate infusions of 0.5 or 1 mg (each), respectively, remained in sinus rhythm for 24 hours without the use of additional antiarrhythmic agents.

Direct-current (DC) cardioversion often is the treatment of choice for patients with atrial flutter and/or fibrillation, and up to 70–95% of such arrhythmias may initially be converted to sinus rhythm by DC cardioversion. However, while ibutilide also can effectively convert such arrhythmias in many patients, the role of the drug, particularly in light of its proarrhythmic potential, relative to DC cardioversion for acute conversion of atrial flutter or fibrillation to sinus rhythm remains to be established.

Dosage and Administration

■ **Administration** Ibutilide fumarate is administered by IV infusion. The commercially available injection containing 0.1 mg (100 mcg) of the drug per mL may be administered undiluted. Alternatively, ibutilide fumarate injection may be diluted prior to administration by adding the contents of a 10-mL vial of the drug to 50 mL of 0.9% sodium chloride or 5% dextrose injection, resulting in a final ibutilide fumarate concentration of about 0.017 mg/mL (17 mcg/mL). Undiluted or diluted infusion solutions of ibutilide should be administered IV over 10 minutes.

■ **Dosage** Dosage of ibutilide fumarate is expressed in terms of the hemifumarate salt. Safety and efficacy of the drug in children younger than 18 years of age have not been established.

Proarrhythmic effects of ibutilide must be anticipated, and the drug should be administered only by skilled personnel in a setting in which proper equipment (e.g., cardiac monitors, intracardiac pacing, cardioverter/defibrillator) and therapy for sustained ventricular tachycardia such as polymorphic ventricular tachycardia are available during and after administration of ibutilide. In clinical trials, many initial episodes of such proarrhythmic effects were observed after completion of the ibutilide infusion but no later than 40 minutes after initiation of the infusion. However, instances of recurrent polymorphic ventricular tachycardia occurring about 3 hours after the initial infusion also were observed in these trials. Therefore, patients should be observed with continuous ECG monitoring for at least 4–6 hours after completion of ibutilide administration or until the corrected QT interval (QT_c) has returned to baseline. Longer monitoring may be required if any arrhythmic activity is noted. Most cases of ventricular tachycardia observed in clinical trials responded to cardiac pacing and magnesium sulfate infusions, although degeneration to ventricular fibrillation requiring immediate defibrillation also can occur. If polymorphic ventricular tachycardia occurs in patients receiving ibutilide, the manufacturer recommends that the drug be discontinued and that electrolyte abnormalities (especially potassium and magnesium) be corrected and overdrive cardiac pacing, electrical cardioversion, and/or defibrillation be undertaken as necessary. Treatment with antiarrhythmic drugs generally should be avoided, although pharmacologic intervention with magnesium sulfate infusions may prove beneficial.

Supraventricular Tachyarrhythmias For the acute management of recent-onset atrial flutter or fibrillation in adults weighing 60 kg or more, 1 mg of ibutilide fumarate should be given initially; for adults weighing less than 60 kg, an initial dose of 0.01 mg/kg (10 mcg/kg) is recommended. If the arrhythmia does not terminate within 10 minutes after completion of the initial infusion, the initial dose may be repeated 10 minutes after completion of such infusion. In a clinical study comparing ibutilide with sotalol, 2 mg of ibutilide fumarate administered as a single infusion to patients weighing more than 60 kg also was effective in terminating atrial flutter or fibrillation. Results of a clinical study in patients who developed atrial flutter and/or fibrillation after undergoing coronary bypass graft or valvular surgery indicate that lower doses (i.e., 1 or 2 infusions of 0.5 mg each [0.005 mg/kg per dose for patients weighing less than 60 kg]) was effective in producing conversion to sinus rhythm in these patients. The value and patient tolerance of additional doses of the drug have not been established and currently are not recommended by the manufacturer.

Clinical studies of ibutilide did not include sufficient numbers of patients younger than 65 years of age to determine whether they respond differently than older patients. While other clinical experience has not revealed age-related differences in response, dosage of ibutilide should be selected with caution for geriatric patients, usually initiating therapy at the low end of the dosing range. The greater frequency of decreased hepatic, renal, and/or cardiac function and of concomitant disease or other drug therapy observed in geriatric patients also should be considered.

■ **Dosage in Renal and Hepatic Impairment** The safety, efficacy, and pharmacokinetics of ibutilide fumarate in patients with renal and/or hepatic impairment have not been established. The manufacturer states that it is unlikely that dosing adjustments based on renal or hepatic function are necessary. Nonetheless, because the drug undergoes substantial hepatic clearance, the manufacturer recommends that patients with abnormal liver function undergo continuous ECG monitoring that extends beyond the usual 4-hour period recommended for other patients.

Description

Ibutilide fumarate is a class III antiarrhythmic agent. Like sotalol, ibutilide is a methanesulfonanilide derivative, and exhibits electrophysiologic effects characteristic of class III antiarrhythmic agents (e.g., prolongs repolarization and refractoriness without affecting conduction). However, unlike sotalol, ibutilide lacks β-adrenergic blocking activity.

Ibutilide fumarate prolongs repolarization of cardiac tissue by prolonging the action potential duration (APD) and effective refractory period (ERP) in both atrial and ventricular cardiac tissue. In vitro studies of its electrophysiologic effects suggest that the antiarrhythmic action of ibutilide may result at least in part from activation of a slow, predominantly sodium, inward current at very low (i.e., less than nanomolar) concentrations, and/or from inhibition of the rapidly activating component of the potassium channel involved in repolarization of cardiac cells (i.e., the rapidly activated component of the delayed rectifier potassium current I_{Kr}) at higher (100-fold) concentrations. However, the exact mechanism of action of the drug remains to be more fully elucidated. Like other class III antiarrhythmics, effects on cardiac repolarization induced by the drug can result in proarrhythmic effects (principally torsades de pointes). (See Uses.)

Ibutilide appears to be more selective in its cellular actions than some other currently available class III antiarrhythmic agents (e.g., amiodarone, sotalol), and therefore has been referred to as a "pure" class III antiarrhythmic. Ibutilide has negligible effects on heart rate, cardiac contractility, or blood pressure.

SumMon® (see Users Guide). For additional information on this drug until a more detailed monograph is developed and published, the manufacturer's labeling should be consulted. It is *essential* that the labeling be consulted for detailed information on the usual cautions, precautions, and contraindications.

Preparations

Excipients in commercially available drug preparations may have clinically important effects in some individuals; consult specific product labeling for details.

Ibutilide Fumarate

Parenteral		
Injection, for IV infusion	1 mg (0.1 mg/mL)*	**Corvert®**, Pfizer
		Ibutilide Fumarate Injection

*available from one or more manufacturer, distributor, and/or repackager by generic (nonproprietary) name

†Use is not currently included in the labeling approved by the US Food and Drug Administration

CLASS IV ANTIARRHYTHMICS 24:04.04.24

Adenosine

Adenocard, Adenoscan

■ Adenosine, an endogenous nucleoside present in all cells of the body, is an antiarrhythmic and pharmacologic stress test agent.

Uses

■ **Treatment of Supraventricular Tachyarrhythmias** Adenosine is used as initial drug therapy for termination of paroxysmal supraventricular tachycardia (PSVT), including that associated with accessory bypass tracts (e.g., Wolff-Parkinson-White [WPW] syndrome). Adenosine is considered a drug of choice for terminating stable, regular narrow-complex tachycardias, the most common of which are reentry supraventricular tachycardias (SVTs) such as PSVT due to AV nodal reentrant tachycardia (AVNRT) and AV reentrant tachycardia (AVRT). In addition, the American Heart Association (AHA) states that a trial of adenosine may be considered in selected patients with unstable, narrow-complex tachycardia before cardioversion†. There also is evidence suggesting that adenosine may be useful for both diagnosis and treatment of stable, regular monomorphic wide-complex tachycardias† if the etiology of the rhythm cannot be determined. Appropriate vagal maneuvers (e.g., Valsalva maneuver, carotid sinus massage) should be attempted prior to adenosine administration when clinically indicated.

In controlled clinical studies, the cumulative percentage of patients with PSVT that converted to sinus rhythm within 1 minute after administration of 6 or 12 mg of adenosine by rapid IV injection was 60 or 92%, respectively; the conversion rate following 1–4 injections of placebo was 7–16%. Response to adenosine was not influenced by factors such as concomitant digoxin therapy, presence of WPW syndrome, gender, or race (black, white, Hispanic).

Adenosine is not effective in terminating arrhythmias that are not due to reentry involving the AV or sinus node; these arrhythmias include atrial flutter, atrial fibrillation, and ventricular tachycardia. Although a transient AV block with modest slowing of ventricular response may occur immediately following administration of adenosine in patients with atrial fibrillation or flutter, which may help clarify the type of arrhythmia present, serious arrhythmias and/or hypotension has occurred in some patients with preexcited arrhythmias who received the drug. (See Cardiovascular and Cerebrovascular Effects under Cautions: Warnings/Precautions.) Some clinicians state that adenosine is contraindicated in patients with atrial fibrillation or atrial flutter associated with WPW syndrome because of the risk of dramatically accelerating ventricular rate.

In pediatric patients, adenosine is considered the drug of choice for conversion of supraventricular tachycardia (SVT) when pharmacologic therapy is indicated. If IV or intraosseous (IO) access is readily available, adenosine should be administered; synchronized cardioversion is recommended if IV/IO access is not available, the patient is hemodynamically unstable, or adenosine is not effective. Some experts also state that adenosine may be useful for diagnosis and treatment of wide-complex tachycardias of supraventricular origin in pediatric patients if the rhythm is regular and monomorphic. Synchronized cardioversion is the treatment of choice in hemodynamically unstable patients. (See Cardiovascular and Cerebrovascular Effects under Cautions: Warnings/Precautions.)

■ **Adjunct to Thallium Stress Test** Adenosine is used as an adjunct to thallous (thallium) chloride TI 201 myocardial perfusion scintigraphy (thallium stress test) in patients unable to exercise adequately.

Adenosine substantially increases blood flow in normal coronary arteries while producing little or no increase in blood flow in stenotic arteries. Because myocardial uptake of thallous chloride TI 201 is directly proportional to coronary blood flow, relatively less thallous chloride TI 201 uptake as well as slower washout occurs in myocardium perfused by stenotic versus normal coronary arteries and the differences in blood flow between areas served by stenotic versus normal arteries are enhanced during thallium testing with adenosine infusion. Intracoronary Doppler flow catheter studies showed maximum coronary artery hyperemia (relative to intracoronary papaverine) in about 95% of cases within 2–3 minutes following initiation of an adenosine infusion at 140 mcg/kg per minute. Coronary artery blood flow velocity returns to baseline within 1–2 minutes after discontinuing the infusion.

In crossover, comparative studies in 319 individuals who could exercise, including 213 patients known or suspected to have coronary artery disease and 106 healthy individuals, thallium images obtained after IV infusion of adenosine or after a treadmill exercise test yielded comparable findings by blind assessment. Agreement regarding the presence of perfusion defects between thallium images obtained after adenosine and after exercise was 85.5% by global analysis and up to 93% when considered by coronary vascular territory. The sensitivity and specificity of thallium imaging using adenosine versus exercise in the detection of angiographically significant coronary artery disease (i.e., more than 50% reduction in the luminal diameter of at least one coronary artery) were determined by comparing results of thallium imaging with those of recent coronary arteriography in 193 patients. The sensitivity (true positive thallium stress tests divided by number of patients with positive [abnormal] angiograms) was 64% with use of either adenosine or exercise, while the specificity (true negative thallium stress tests divided by the number of patients with negative angiograms) was 54 or 65% with use of adenosine or exercise, respectively. The 95% confidence intervals for the sensitivity and specificity of adenosine were 56–78% and 37–71%, respectively.

■ **Diagnosis of Supraventricular Tachycardias** Adenosine has been used to aid diagnosis of stable, regular narrow-complex SVTs†. A transient AV block may occur following administration of the drug, which can unmask atrial activity in certain arrhythmias such as atrial tachycardia and atrial flutter. Adenosine also has been used diagnostically in patients with stable, regular wide-complex tachycardias; if the tachycardia is a result of SVT with aberrancy, adenosine will likely be effective in slowing or converting the arrhythmia to normal sinus rhythm. Some clinicians discourage overuse of adenosine for diagnostic purposes and recommend that the drug be used only when an arrhythmia of supraventricular origin is strongly suspected. (See Cardiovascular and Cerebrovascular Effects under Cautions: Warnings/Precautions.) Appropriate resuscitative equipment should be readily available during use of the drug.

Dosage and Administration

■ **Administration** ***Supraventricular Tachyarrhythmias*** For termination of paroxysmal supraventricular tachycardia (PSVT), adenosine is administered by rapid (over 1–2 seconds) IV ("bolus") injection into a peripheral vein. The drug also has been administered via a central vein† or by intraosseous (IO) injection† in pediatric patients without reliable/immediate IV access.

To ensure that the drug reaches the systemic circulation, the solution should be administered either directly into a vein or an IV line at a site as close to the patient as possible, followed by a rapid flush of 0.9% sodium chloride injection (e.g., flush with 5 mL or more for pediatric patients and 20 mL for adults).

Adjunct to Thallium Stress Testing For use as an adjunct to thallium stress testing, adenosine is administered by continuous IV infusion into a peripheral vein; the drug should be infused over a period of 6 minutes.

Safety and efficacy of intracoronary administration of adenosine as an adjunct to thallium stress testing has not been established.

■ **Dosage** ***Supraventricular Tachyarrhythmias*** When used for the treatment of PSVT in children weighing less than 50 kg, the manufacturer recommends an initial adenosine dose of 0.05–0.1 mg/kg by rapid IV (bolus) injection. If conversion does not occur within 1–2 minutes, subsequent doses should be increased by 0.05–0.1 mg/kg until sinus rhythm is established or a maximum single dose of 0.3 mg/kg (not exceeding 12 mg) has been given. When used for the treatment of PSVT in children weighing 50 kg or more, the manufacturer recommends an initial dose of 6 mg by rapid IV (bolus) injection. If conversion does not occur within 1–2 minutes, a 12-mg dose should be administered and repeated once, if necessary. The manufacturer states that doses greater than 12 mg are not recommended. Some experts recommend a maximum single dose of 6 mg for the initial injection in pediatric patients.

When used for the treatment of PSVT in adults, an initial adenosine dose of 6 mg by rapid IV (bolus) injection (over 1–3 seconds) is recommended. If conversion does not occur within 1–2 minutes, a 12-mg dose should be administered and repeated once, if necessary. Patients receiving methylxanthines (e.g., theophylline) may require higher adenosine doses because of decreased sensitivity to the effects of adenosine, but experience with such doses is limited and the manufacturer does not recommend doses exceeding 12 mg. (See Drug Interactions: Methylxanthines.) Some experts state that recurrences of PSVT may be treated with additional doses of adenosine or a longer-acting AV nodal blocking agent (e.g., diltiazem, β-adrenergic blocking agent). If adenosine fails to convert PSVT, rate control may be attempted with a nondihydropyridine calcium-channel blocking agent (e.g., diltiazem, verapamil) or a β-adrenergic blocking agent.

The manufacturer-recommended dosage regimen for adenosine in the treatment of PSVT is based on clinical studies of the drug administered by peripheral IV injection. However, the manufacturer and some clinicians suggest that a lower initial dose of adenosine (3 mg for adults or 50% of the usual recommended initial dose for children) may be effective if the drug is given via a central vein because the rhythm effects of adenosine are concentration dependent. In addition, the drug is metabolized by an enzyme on the surface of erythrocytes and more of the dose will be metabolized before reaching the heart when given by peripheral versus central IV injection.

Adjunct to Thallium Stress Testing When used as an adjunct to thallium stress testing, adenosine is administered by continuous IV infusion at a rate of 0.14 mg/kg per minute for 6 minutes (total dose of 0.84 mg/kg). The appropriate rate of infusion corrected for total body weight may be determined using the following formula:

$$\text{infusion rate (mL/minute)} = \frac{0.14\ \text{mg/kg per minute} \times \text{total body weight (kg)}}{\text{adenosine concentration (3 mg/mL)}}$$

The required dose of thallous (thallium) chloride TI 201 should be administered at the midpoint (i.e., after the first 3 minutes) of the adenosine infusion.

Adenosine and thallous chloride TI 201 are physically compatible, allowing direct injection of thallous chloride TI 201 into the infusion set containing adenosine. Thallous chloride TI 201 should be injected as close as possible to the venous access site to prevent an inadvertent increase in the dose of adenosine (the contents of the IV tubing) being administered.

■ **Special Populations** Adenosine should be administered with caution to cardiac transplant recipients because of cardiac denervation-related hypersensitivity to the drug. (See Cardiovascular and Cerebrovascular Effects under Cautions: Warnings/Precautions.)

Cautions

■ Contraindications

Known hypersensitivity to adenosine.

Second- or third-degree AV block (except in patients with a functioning artificial pacemaker).

Sinus node disease, such as sick sinus syndrome or symptomatic bradycardia (except in patients with a functioning artificial pacemaker).

Known or suspected bronchoconstrictive or bronchospastic lung disease (e.g., asthma).

■ Warnings/Precautions

Cardiovascular and Cerebrovascular Effects Serious cardiovascular and cerebrovascular events, including myocardial ischemic events, rhythm and conduction abnormalities, hypotension, hypertension, and stroke, have been reported rarely in patients receiving adenosine. Cardiac resuscitation equipment and trained staff should be available prior to administration of the drug.

Myocardial Ischemic Events. Fatal or nonfatal cardiac arrest, sustained ventricular arrhythmias (e.g., ventricular tachycardia), and myocardial infarction, have occurred in patients receiving adenosine as a cardiac stress test agent during myocardial perfusion imaging. At least 6 cases of myocardial infarction and 27 deaths associated with the use of adenosine (as Adenoscan®) have been reported to the FDA Adverse Event Reporting System since the date of initial marketing of the drug. A similar risk has been observed with regadenoson, another pharmacologic stress test agent used in myocardial perfusion imaging. (See Myocardial Ischemic Events under Warnings/Precautions: Cardiovascular and Cerebrovascular Effects, in Cautions in Regadenoson 36:18.) Available data indicate that these adverse cardiovascular events tended to occur within 6 hours following administration of adenosine (as Adenoscan®). Fatal outcomes with adenosine (as Adenoscan®) were most often associated with cardiorespiratory arrest, dyspnea, cardiac arrest, respiratory arrest, and ventricular tachycardia. A few cases of myocardial infarction also have been reported in the medical literature in patients receiving adenosine or regadenoson as a pharmacologic stress test agent. Published studies generally do not suggest a difference in the incidence of cardiovascular events between adenosine and regadenoson. However, many factors, including differences in patient exposure, underlying cardiac risk factors that may influence choice of drug, and longer time on the market for adenosine, may complicate analysis of the true incidence of such adverse events with these drugs.

Prior to performing a cardiac stress test with adenosine, clinicians should assess the suitability of patients to receive the drug. Because patients with signs or symptoms of acute myocardial ischemia (e.g., unstable angina, cardiovascular instability) may be at increased risk of serious cardiovascular events with adenosine, the drug should not be used in such patients.

Rhythm and Conduction Abnormalities. When adenosine is used for termination of paroxysmal supraventricular tachycardia (PSVT), new arrhythmias (ventricular premature complexes [VPCs], atrial premature complexes, atrial fibrillation, sinus bradycardia, sinus tachycardia, skipped beats, and varying degrees of AV nodal block) may appear at the time of conversion to normal sinus rhythm. These arrhythmias generally last only a few seconds and resolve without intervention. However, transient or prolonged episodes of asystole, sometimes fatal, have been reported with IV injection of adenosine. Ventricular fibrillation has been reported rarely with IV injection of the drug, including both resuscitated and fatal events. In most cases, these adverse effects occurred in patients receiving concomitant therapy with digoxin or, less frequently, digoxin and verapamil, although a causal relationship has not been established. (See Drug Interactions: Digoxin or Digoxin/Verapamil.) Atrial fibrillation also has been reported in patients receiving continuous IV infusion of adenosine (as Adenoscan®) as a pharmacologic stress test agent; the abnormal rhythm generally occurred shortly (1.5–3 minutes) after administration, was not persistent (lasting only 15 seconds to 6 hours), and converted to normal sinus rhythm spontaneously. Some clinicians state that adenosine should not be used in patients with wide-complex tachycardias of unknown origin because of the risk of inducing potentially serious arrhythmias, including atrial fibrillation with a rapid ventricular rate or prolonged asystole with severe hypotension in preexcited tachycardias (e.g., atrial flutter); the drug also may induce ventricular fibrillation in patients with severe coronary artery disease.

Because of adenosine's depressant effects on the SA and AV nodes, sinus bradycardia, varying degrees of AV block (asymptomatic and transient), and (rarely) sinus pauses may occur following IV administration of the drug; however, these effects generally are transient due to the short half-life of the drug. Cardiac denervation in patients who have undergone cardiac transplantation reportedly may enhance sensitivity to the bradycardic effects of adenosine. Adenosine should not be used in patients with sinus node dysfunction or high-grade AV block unless the patient has a functioning artificial pacemaker (see Cautions: Contraindications); caution is advised if the drug is used in patients with preexisting first-degree AV block or bundle branch block. If persistent or symptomatic high-grade AV block occurs during therapy, adenosine should be discontinued.

Hemodynamic and Associated Effects. Adenosine may decrease or increase blood pressure. Marked hypotension is possible due to the potent peripheral vasodilating effects of adenosine, and the risk of serious hypotension may be increased in patients with autonomic dysfunction, stenotic valvular heart disease, pericarditis or pericardial effusions, stenotic carotid artery disease with cerebrovascular insufficiency, or hypovolemia. Adenosine should be discontinued in any patient who develops persistent or symptomatic hypotension. Clinically important *increases* in systolic and diastolic blood pressure also have occurred in patients receiving adenosine; these effects generally are transient but reportedly have lasted for several hours in some cases.

Cerebrovascular events, including hemorrhagic and ischemic stroke, have occurred in patients receiving adenosine, and may be associated with the drug's effects on blood pressure.

Respiratory Effects Adenosine is a respiratory stimulant and adverse respiratory effects, including dyspnea, bronchospasm, bronchoconstriction, and respiratory compromise, have occurred in patients receiving the drug. Dyspnea was reported in approximately 28 or 12% of patients receiving adenosine for pharmacologic stress testing or conversion of PSVT, respectively, in clinical trials. In addition, respiratory compromise has occurred during adenosine infusion in patients with obstructive pulmonary disease. Other respiratory effects reported during postmarketing experience with the drug include bronchospasm, respiratory arrest, and throat tightness.

Adenosine should not be used in patients with bronchoconstriction or bronchospasm (e.g., asthma) since the drug may exacerbate respiratory symptoms in such patients; caution is advised if adenosine is used in patients with obstructive pulmonary disease not associated with bronchoconstriction (e.g., emphysema, bronchitis). (See Cautions: Contraindications.) Appropriate resuscitative measures should be available prior to administration of the drug. Adenosine should be discontinued in any patient who develops severe respiratory difficulties.

CNS Effects New-onset or recurrent seizures, including tonic-clonic (grand mal) seizures, have been reported following administration of adenosine. In some cases, seizure activity was prolonged and required emergency management. Concomitant use of aminophylline may increase the risk of seizures. (See Drug Interactions: Methylxanthines.)

Sensitivity Reactions **Hypersensitivity.** Hypersensitivity reactions may occur following administration of adenosine, possibly requiring resuscitative measures; reported manifestations have included dyspnea, throat tightness, flushing, erythema, and chest discomfort. Prior to administration of adenosine, clinicians should ensure that appropriate personnel and resuscitative equipment are available. (See Cautions: Contraindications.)

Specific Populations **Pregnancy.** Category C. Some clinicians suggest that because of its rapid onset and brief duration of action, adenosine may have advantages over other antiarrhythmic agents (e.g., verapamil, digoxin) in the acute treatment of PSVT in pregnant women in whom vagal maneuvers have failed. However, caution is advised because hypotension may compromise placental (fetal) blood flow.

Lactation. It is not known whether adenosine is distributed into human milk. Because of the potential for serious adverse reactions from adenosine in nursing infants, a decision should be made whether to discontinue nursing or the drug, taking into account the importance of the drug to the woman. Some clinicians suggest that use of adenosine during lactation may be possible because of the drug's short half-life.

Pediatric Use. Although the manufacturer states that controlled studies establishing the safety and efficacy of adenosine for treatment of PSVT in pediatric patients are lacking, the drug has been used for the treatment of PSVT in neonates, infants, children, and adolescents, and some clinicians consider it a drug of choice for SVT in pediatric patients.

Safety and efficacy as an adjunct to thallium stress testing not established in children 18 years of age or younger.

Geriatric Use. Insufficient experience in patients 65 years of age or older to determine whether geriatric patients respond differently than younger adults. However, use with caution because increased sensitivity cannot be ruled out; some geriatric patients may have diminished cardiac function, nodal dysfunction, or concomitant disease or drug therapy that may alter hemodynamic function and result in severe bradycardia or AV block.

Hepatic Impairment. Adenosine does not require hepatic function for therapeutic effect or inactivation; therefore, hepatic dysfunction would not be expected to alter the drug's effectiveness or tolerability.

Renal Impairment. Adenosine does not require renal function for therapeutic effect or inactivation; therefore, renal dysfunction would not be expected to alter the drug's effectiveness or tolerability.

■ Common Adverse Effects

Adverse effects reported in at least 1% of patients receiving adenosine for the treatment of PSVT in controlled clinical trials include facial flushing, shortness of breath/dyspnea, chest pressure, nausea, headache, lightheadedness, dizziness, numbness, and tingling in the arms.

Adverse effects reported in at least 1% of patients receiving adenosine as an adjunct to thallium stress testing in controlled and uncontrolled clinical trials include facial flushing; chest discomfort; dyspnea or urge to breathe deeply; headache; discomfort in the throat, neck, or jaw; GI discomfort; lightheadedness/dizziness; upper extremity discomfort; ST-segment depression; first-degree AV block; second-degree AV block; paresthesia; hypotension; nervousness; and arrhythmias.

Drug Interactions

When possible, drugs that may augment or inhibit adenosine effects should be withheld for 5 half-lives prior to adenosine administration.

■ **ACE Inhibitors** Potential pharmacodynamic interaction (additive or synergistic depressant effects on SA and AV nodes); the drugs should be used concomitantly with caution.

■ **β-Adrenergic Blocking Agents** Potential pharmacodynamic interaction (additive or synergistic depressant effects on SA and AV nodes); the drugs should be used concomitantly with caution.

■ **Calcium-channel Blocking Agents** Potential pharmacodynamic interaction (additive or synergistic depressant effects on SA and AV nodes); the drugs should be used concomitantly with caution.

■ **Carbamazepine** Potential pharmacodynamic interaction (higher degrees of heart block).

■ **Digoxin or Digoxin/Verapamil** Potential pharmacodynamic interaction (additive or synergistic depressant effects on SA and AV nodes); serious and/or life-threatening effects (asystole, ventricular fibrillation) have been reported rarely. (See Cardiovascular and Cerebrovascular Effects under Cautions: Warnings/Precautions.) The drugs should be used concomitantly with caution and with appropriate resuscitative measures available.

■ **Dipyridamole** Potential pharmacodynamic interaction (potentiation of vasoactive effects of adenosine). caution should be exercised.

The manufacturer of adenosine (Adenoscan®) states that safety and efficacy of the drug in the presence of dipyridamole have not been established. In general, administration of drugs that may inhibit or augment the pharmacologic effects of adenosine should be withheld for at least 5 half-lives prior to administration of adenosine.

■ **Methylxanthines** Potential pharmacodynamic interaction (inhibition of vasoactive effects of adenosine) with methylxanthines such as caffeine, aminophylline, or theophylline; larger doses of adenosine may be required or the drug may not be effective during such concomitant therapy. (See Advice to Patients.) The manufacturer of adenosine (Adenoscan®) states that safety and efficacy of the drug in the presence of methylxanthines have not been established. In general, administration of drugs that may inhibit or augment the pharmacologic effects of adenosine should be withheld for at least 5 half-lives prior to administration of adenosine.

Methylxanthines are competitive adenosine receptor antagonists, and theophylline has been used effectively to terminate persistent adverse effects of adenosine. However, the manufacturer states that aminophylline may increase the risk of seizures associated with adenosine and that methylxanthines should not be used in patients who experience adenosine-induced seizures. (See CNS Effects under Cautions: Warnings/Precautions.)

■ **Quinidine** Potential pharmacodynamic interaction (additive or synergistic depressant effects on SA and AV nodes); the drugs should be used concomitantly with caution.

Description

Adenosine is an endogenous nucleoside present in all cells of the body. Adenosine may exert its pharmacologic effects by activation of purine (cell-surface A_1 and A_2 adenosine) receptors; relaxation of vascular smooth muscle may be mediated by reduction in calcium uptake through inhibition of slow inward calcium current and activation of adenylate cyclase in smooth muscle cells. Adenosine may reduce vascular tone by modulation of sympathetic neurotransmission.

Adenosine has negative chronotropic, dromotropic, and inotropic effects on the heart. The drug slows conduction time through the AV node and can interrupt AV nodal reentry pathways, leading to restoration of normal sinus rhythm in patients with paroxysmal supraventricular tachycardia (PSVT), including that associated with Wolff-Parkinson-White syndrome.

Adenosine is a potent vasodilator in most vascular beds; however, vasoconstriction is produced in renal afferent arterioles and hepatic veins. The drug typically produces a net mild to moderate reduction in systolic, diastolic, and mean arterial blood pressure and a reflex increase in heart rate. Adenosine increases blood flow in normal coronary arteries with little or no increase in stenotic arteries, resulting in a relative difference in thallous (thallium) chloride TI 201 uptake in myocardium supplied by normal versus stenotic coronary arteries.

Adenosine is a respiratory stimulant, probably because of activation of carotid body chemoreceptors; IV administration produces an increase in minute ventilation and a reduction in arterial PCO_2, resulting in respiratory alkalosis.

Adenosine is rapidly metabolized intracellularly to the inactive metabolites adenosine monophosphate and inosine; the plasma half-life of adenosine is less than 10 seconds. The drug is cleared by cellular uptake, principally by erythrocytes and vascular endothelial cells, via a specific transmembrane nucleoside transport system.

Advice to Patients

Importance of informing patients about serious adverse effects associated with adenosine, such as myocardial infarction, arrhythmias, cardiac arrest, heart block, substantial changes in blood pressure, bronchoconstriction, hypersensitivity reactions, seizures, and stroke.

Importance of patient informing clinicians of existing or contemplated concomitant therapy, including prescription and OTC drugs (e.g., aminophylline, theophylline), caffeine-containing foods or beverages, as well as any concomitant illnesses (e.g., asthma, chronic obstructive pulmonary disease [COPD]).

Importance of women informing clinicians if they are or plan to become pregnant or plan to breast-feed.

Importance of informing patients of other important precautionary information. (See Cautions.)

Overview® (see Users Guide). For additional information on this drug until a more detailed monograph is developed and published, the manufacturer's labeling should be consulted. It is *essential* that the manufacturer's labeling be consulted for more detailed information on usual cautions, precautions, contraindications, potential drug interactions, laboratory test interferences, and acute toxicity.

Preparations

Excipients in commercially available drug preparations may have clinically important effects in some individuals; consult specific product labeling for details.

Adenosine

Parenteral

Injection, for rapid IV injection only	3 mg/mL*	**Adenocard®**, Astellas
		Adenosine Injection
Injection, for IV infusion only	3 mg/mL	**Adenoscan®**, Astellas

*available from one or more manufacturer, distributor, and/or repackager by generic (nonproprietary) name

†Use is not currently included in the labeling approved by the US Food and Drug Administration

CARDIOTONIC AGENTS 24:04.08

Digoxin

Cardiac glycoside

■ Digoxin is a cardiac glycoside with positive inotropic and antiarrhythmic effects.

Uses

Digoxin is a cardiac glycoside that is used principally in the management of heart failure and atrial fibrillation. Cardiac glycosides are a class of drugs that increase force and velocity of myocardial systolic contraction (positive inotropic action) and also decrease conduction velocity through the atrioventricular (AV) node. Although several cardiac glycoside preparations were previously available for medicinal use (see Chemistry and Stability: Chemistry), digoxin is currently the only commercially available cardiac glycoside in the US.

■ **Heart Failure** Digoxin is used in conjunction with other agents in the management of mild to moderate (New York Heart Association [NYHA] class II-III) heart failure associated with left ventricular systolic dysfunction. Although digoxin has been used extensively in the management of heart failure, current use is generally limited because of the lack of demonstrated survival benefit, potential for serious adverse effects, and availability of other drugs that have been shown to substantially reduce morbidity and mortality.

Current guidelines for the management of heart failure in adults generally recommend inhibition of the renin-angiotensin-aldosterone system with a combination of drug therapies, including neurohormonal antagonists (e.g., angiotensin-converting enzyme [ACE] inhibitors, angiotensin II receptor antagonists, angiotensin receptor-neprilysin inhibitors [ARNIs], β-adrenergic blocking agents [β-blockers], aldosterone receptor antagonists) to inhibit the detrimental compensatory mechanisms in heart failure and reduce morbidity and mortality. (See Uses: Heart Failure, in Enalaprilat/Enalapril 24:32.04 and in Sacubitril and Valsartan 24:32.92.) Additional agents (e.g., digoxin, diuretics, sinoatrial modulators [i.e., ivabradine]) added to a heart failure treatment regimen in selected patients have been associated with symptomatic improvement of heart failure and/or reduction in heart failure-related hospitalizations. Experts state that digoxin therapy may be initiated in severely symptomatic patients with heart failure and reduced left ventricular ejection fraction who have started, but not yet responded to, an ACE inhibitor or a β-blocker. Alternatively, digoxin may be withheld until the patient's symptomatic response to the ACE inhibitor or β-blocker has been defined and then used only in those patients who remain symptomatic while receiving ACE inhibitor or β-blocker therapy. In patients with heart failure who are receiving digoxin without an ACE inhibitor or β-blocker, digoxin should not be withdrawn, but appropriate therapy with an ACE inhibitor and/or a β-blocker should be added. The beneficial effects of digoxin have been shown to be additive with those of ACE inhibitors and/or diuretics; symptomatic and functional deterioration can occur when digoxin is withdrawn from patients whose heart failure was stabilized on a regimen of combined therapy.

In patients with heart failure, digoxin may alleviate symptoms and decrease heart failure-related hospitalizations. Although data demonstrating an overall survival benefit of digoxin are lacking, a large, controlled study (the Digitalis

Investigation Group [DIG] study) showed reductions in hospitalization rates, both overall and for worsening heart failure, as well as a reduction in the combined incidence of death from worsening heart failure and hospitalization for such worsening, when digoxin was added to a regimen of ACE inhibitors and/or diuretics in patients with normal sinus rhythm and chronic left ventricular heart failure (principally mild to moderate). The decision to use digoxin in patients with symptomatic heart failure caused by systolic left ventricular dysfunction should be based not on an anticipated improvement in survival but on potential benefits of less deterioration of the condition and associated improvement in hospitalization rates as well as of improved symptomatic and functional status.

Digoxin increases left ventricular ejection fraction and improves symptoms of heart failure (as evidenced by exercise capacity, heart failure-related hospitalizations and emergency care), while having no apparent effect on overall mortality. The acute and sustained hemodynamic efficacy of digoxin is well established, at least in patients with symptomatic heart failure caused by predominant systolic ventricular dysfunction. Digoxin is less effective in the management of high-output heart failure caused by bronchopulmonary insufficiency, infection, hyperthyroidism, anemia, fever, arteriovenous fistula, thiamine deficiency, Paget's disease, cor pulmonale, acute glomerulonephritis, or toxic or infectious myocarditis (e.g., diphtheria, acute rheumatic fever). Heart failure resulting from hypermetabolic or hyperdynamic states (e.g., hyperthyroidism, hypoxia, AV shunt) is best treated by addressing the underlying condition rather than by using digoxin. In addition, digoxin is of limited value in the management of heart failure caused by mechanical disturbances such as constrictive pericarditis, pericardial tamponade, mitral stenosis with normal sinus rhythm, and pure valvular aortic stenosis. Patients with idiopathic hypertrophic subaortic stenosis receiving digoxin may have a worsening of outflow obstruction as a result of the inotropic effects of the drug.

■ **Supraventricular Tachyarrhythmias** ***Atrial Fibrillation*** Digoxin is used for controlling rapid ventricular rate in patients with chronic atrial fibrillation; however, the drug is not considered first-line therapy for this use, in part because of its slow onset of action. In addition, concerns have been raised regarding possible increased mortality in patients with atrial fibrillation receiving digoxin, particularly when used for long-term therapy. In the AFFIRM (AF Follow-up Investigation of Rhythm Management) study, use of digoxin was associated with a 41% increase in mortality in patients with atrial fibrillation; however, additional post-hoc analyses have reported conflicting results.

Experts recommend the use of β-blockers or nondihydropyridine calcium-channel blocking agents (e.g., diltiazem, verapamil) as the preferred drugs for ventricular rate control in patients with atrial fibrillation. Digoxin may be used in combination with one of these agents to improve heart rate control during exercise and also may be useful in patients with concomitant heart failure. (See Uses: Heart Failure.) Choice of therapy should be individualized based on the clinical situation and patient-related factors. Digoxin should not be used in patients with preexcited atrial fibrillation because the drug may increase ventricular response and result in ventricular fibrillation.

Other Supraventricular Tachycardias Digoxin also is used in the management of paroxysmal supraventricular tachycardia (PSVT) due to AV nodal reentry tachycardia (AVNRT) or AV reentry tachycardia (AVRT)†. Some experts state that oral digoxin may be reasonable for ongoing management of PSVT in patients who are not candidates for, or prefer not to undergo, catheter ablation. Because of the potential for adverse effects, digoxin generally is reserved as a third-line agent for patients who are not responsive to, or are not candidates for, the preferred therapies (e.g., β-blockers, nondihydropyridine calcium-channel blocking agents, flecainide, propafenone). If acute treatment of PSVT is necessary, however, measures to increase vagal tone (such as carotid sinus massage and Valsalva maneuver) or administration of adenosine are the treatments of choice.

Digoxin has been used in the management of regular supraventricular (reciprocating) tachycardia associated with Wolff-Parkinson-White (WPW) syndrome†, but the drug may be potentially harmful if used in patients with WPW syndrome and preexcited atrial fibrillation because acceleration of the ventricular rate may occur. Digoxin should therefore not be administered to patients with WPW syndrome and preexcited atrial fibrillation. The preferred treatment of choice in hemodynamically compromised patients with WPW syndrome usually is prompt direct-current cardioversion.

■ **Myocardial Infarction** Use of digoxin in acute myocardial infarction (MI) is controversial. (See Cautions: Precautions and Contraindications.) Because the drug can increase myocardial oxygen demand and exacerbate ongoing ischemia, it is generally not recommended during acute MI. However, digoxin may be used in selected patients with left ventricular systolic dysfunction after acute MI. (See Uses: Heart Failure.)

Dosage and Administration

■ **Administration** Digoxin usually is administered orally. When oral therapy is not feasible or when rapid therapeutic effect is necessary, the drug may be administered parenterally. Although digoxin may be given IM or IV, the IV route of administration is preferred because IM injection can cause severe local irritation and pain at the site of injection. If the drug must be administered by the IM route, injections should be made deep into the muscle followed by massage of the injection site, and no more than 2 mL of the drug should be injected at a single site.

Oral Administration Digoxin is administered orally as tablets or oral solution. The manufacturers recommend once-daily dosing in adults and children older than 10 years of age; divided daily dosing is recommended in infants and children younger than 10 years of age.

The manufacturer recommends that the oral solution be used to obtain the appropriate dose in infants, young children, or patients with very low body weights. The calibrated dosing syringe supplied by the manufacturer should be used to measure doses of the oral digoxin solution; a separate measuring device should be used to accurately measure doses less than 0.1 mL.

IV Administration For IV administration, digoxin injection may be given undiluted or may be diluted with a fourfold or greater volume of sterile water for injection, 5% dextrose injection, or 0.9% sodium chloride injection; use of less than a fourfold volume of diluent may cause precipitation of the drug. Diluted IV solutions of digoxin should be used immediately.

Digoxin should be administered by slow IV infusion (over at least 5 minutes); rapid IV (i.e., bolus) administration may cause systemic and coronary vasoconstriction and should be avoided.

Mixing of digoxin injection with other drugs in the same container or simultaneous administration in the same IV line is not recommended.

■ **Dosage** ***General Considerations*** Digoxin has a narrow therapeutic index; therefore, cautious dosage determination is essential and dosage must be carefully individualized based on clinical assessment and therapeutic drug monitoring. Dosage guidelines provided are based upon average patient response and substantial patient variation can be expected. When selecting an appropriate dosage, the patient's renal function, body weight, age, concomitant disease states, concurrent drugs, and other factors likely to alter serum concentrations of digoxin should be considered. Because the drug is largely distributed into tissues, lean body weight should be used for dosage calculations. Serum digoxin concentrations can be used to guide dosing, but should always be interpreted in the overall clinical context.

Digoxin dosage may be initiated with or without a loading dose depending on whether rapid titration or a more gradual titration is desired; the different approaches vary in dosage and frequency of administration but achieve the same total amount of digoxin accumulated in the body. Loading doses may be used to reach adequate and effective drug concentrations for control of ventricular response in patients with atrial fibrillation. However, in patients with heart failure, experts state there is no reason to use loading doses and maintenance dosing can be initiated immediately.

Loading doses of digoxin are administered in divided doses, with about 50% of the total dose given as the first (i.e., initial) dose and additional fractions (usually 25%) usually administered every 6–8 hours with careful assessment of the patient's clinical response (including possible toxicity) before each additional dose. If a change from the calculated loading dose is required, then the maintenance dosage should be calculated based upon the amount (i.e., total loading dose) actually administered.

More gradual attainment of digoxin concentrations can be achieved by initiating therapy with a maintenance dosage without a loading dose. Steady-state serum digoxin concentrations will be achieved in about 5 half-lives of the drug for the individual patient; depending on the patient's renal function, this may take approximately 1–3 weeks.

Differences in the bioavailability of parenteral and oral preparations of digoxin should be considered when patients are switched from one dosage form to another. Because the absolute bioavailability of digoxin tablets and solution are similar, equivalent dosages may be used. (See Pharmacokinetics: Absorption.) When switching from oral to IV therapy, dosage of digoxin should be reduced by about 20–25%.

Since daily maintenance digoxin dosage is a replacement of daily digoxin loss from the body, an alternative dosing method has been used where the maintenance dosage for a particular patient is *estimated* by multiplying the daily percentage loss (see Pharmacokinetics: Elimination) by the peak body stores (i.e., loading dose) that produced a satisfactory response. The percentage of digoxin eliminated from the body daily can be *estimated* by the following equation:

$$\text{daily \% loss} = 14 + \frac{\text{creatinine clearance (in mL/minute)}}{5}$$

Heart Failure in Adults Loading doses are generally not required in patients with heart failure. If a loading dose is to be given, the manufacturers recommend an oral loading dose of 10–15 mcg/kg or an IV loading dose of 8–12 mcg/kg in adults, administered in divided doses. (See General Considerations under Dosage and Administration: Dosage.)

Experts state that digoxin is commonly initiated and maintained at a dosage of 125–250 mcg (0.125–0.25 mg) daily for the management of heart failure in adults. The manufacturers recommend an initial oral digoxin maintenance dosage of 3.4–5.1 mcg/kg once daily as tablets or 3–4.5 mcg/kg once daily as the oral solution in adults with normal renal function; dosage may be increased every 2 weeks according to clinical response, serum digoxin concentrations, and toxicity. If IV administration is necessary, the manufacturer recommends an initial IV maintenance dosage of 2.4–3.6 mcg/kg once daily in adults with normal renal function; dosage may be increased every 2 weeks according to clinical response, serum digoxin concentrations, and toxicity. The manufacturer's prescribing information should be consulted for recommended maintenance oral and IV dosages based on renal function.

Atrial Fibrillation in Adults If a loading dose is to be given for rate control in patients with atrial fibrillation, the manufacturers recommend an oral loading dose of 10–15 mcg/kg or an IV loading dose of 8–12 mcg/kg in adults, administered in divided doses. (See General Considerations under Dosage and Administration: Dosage.) Some experts recommend an initial IV dose of 250 mcg (0.25 mg) with repeat dosing to a maximum of 1500 mcg (1.5 mg) over 24 hours. These experts state that the usual oral maintenance dosage of digoxin for ventricular rate control in adults with atrial fibrillation is 125–250 mcg (0.125–0.25 mg) daily.

Heart Failure in Pediatric Patients Dosage should be carefully titrated in neonates, especially in premature infants, because renal clearance of digoxin is reduced in such patients. Infants and young children (up to 10 years of age) generally require proportionally larger doses than children older than 10 years of age and adults when calculated on the basis of lean body weight or body surface area. Children older than 10 years of age require adult dosages in proportion to the child's body weight.

Loading doses and maintenance dosages recommended by the manufacturers for the treatment of heart failure in pediatric patients are given in the tables that follow based on the dosage form administered. (See General Considerations under Dosage and Administration: Dosage.)

Table 1. Usual Pediatric Loading Doses and Maintenance Dosages for Digoxin Tablets (normal renal function, based on lean body weight)

Age	Oral Loading Dose[a]	Initial Oral Maintenance Dosage
5–10 years	20–45 mcg/kg	3.2–6.4 mcg/kg twice daily
>10 years	10–15 mcg/kg	3.4–5.1 mcg/kg once daily

[a] Loading doses are administered in divided doses, with about 50% of the total dose given as the first (i.e., initial) dose; additional 25% fractions are administered every 6–8 hours

Table 2. Usual Pediatric Loading Doses and Maintenance Dosages for Digoxin Solution (normal renal function, based on lean body weight)

Age	Oral Loading Dose[a]	Initial Oral Maintenance Dosage
Premature neonates	20–30 mcg/kg	2.3–3.9 mcg/kg twice daily
Full-term neonates	25–35 mcg/kg	3.8–5.6 mcg/kg twice daily
1–24 months	35–60 mcg/kg	5.6–9.4 mcg/kg twice daily
2–5 years	30–45 mcg/kg	4.7–6.6 mcg/kg twice daily
5–10 years	20–35 mcg/kg	2.8–5.6 mcg/kg twice daily
>10 years	10–15 mcg/kg	3–4.5 mcg/kg once daily

[a] Loading doses are administered in divided doses, with about 50% of the total dose given as the first (i.e., initial) dose; additional fractions may be administered every 4–8 hours

Table 3. Usual Pediatric Loading Doses and Maintenance Dosages for IV Digoxin (normal renal function, based on lean body weight)

Age	IV Loading Dose[a]	Initial IV Maintenance Dosage
Premature neonates	15–25 mcg/kg	1.9–3.1 mcg/kg twice daily
Full-term neonates	20–30 mcg/kg	3–4.5 mcg/kg twice daily
1–24 months	30–50 mcg/kg	4.5–7.5 mcg/kg twice daily
2–5 years	25–35 mcg/kg	3.8–5.3 mcg/kg twice daily
5–10 years	15–30 mcg/kg	2.3–4.5 mcg/kg twice daily
>10 years	8–12 mcg/kg	2.4–3.6 mcg/kg once daily

[a] Loading doses are administered in divided doses, with 50% of the total dose given as the first (i.e., initial) dose; additional 25% fractions are administered every 6–8 hours

Geriatric Dosage Dosage of digoxin should be selected carefully in geriatric patients since they are more likely to have impaired renal function. (See Dosage in Renal Impairment under Dosage and Administration: Dosage.) Lower dosages (125 mcg [0.125 mg] daily or every other day) are recommended for the management of heart failure in geriatric patients older than 70 years of age.

Dosage in Hepatic Impairment No dosage adjustment is necessary in patients with hepatic impairment; however, serum digoxin concentrations may be used to guide dosing in such patients.

Dosage in Renal Impairment Renal function should be considered during dosage selection. Digoxin is principally excreted by the kidneys and impaired renal function may predispose patients to digoxin toxicity. Dosage should be reduced and titrated carefully in patients with renal impairment based on clinical response and serum digoxin concentrations as appropriate.

Cautions

In addition to toxicity (see Acute Toxicity and also see Chronic Toxicity), other adverse effects may occur in patients receiving digoxin.

■ **Adverse Effects** GI effects, including nausea, vomiting, abdominal pain, and intestinal ischemia and hemorrhagic necrosis, have occurred in patients receiving digoxin. CNS effects associated with digoxin include headache, weakness, dizziness, apathy, confusion, and mental disturbances (e.g., anxiety, depression, delirium, hallucinations).

Estrogen-like effects may occur with chronic administration of cardiac glycosides, especially in geriatric men and women whose endogenous concentrations of sex hormones are low. Cardiac glycosides increase plasma estrogen and decrease serum luteinizing hormone in men and postmenopausal women and decrease plasma testosterone in men. Gynecomastia and enlargement of the mammary glands in women have been reported after chronic therapy with digoxin and were reversible when the drug was withdrawn. Digoxin also may produce vaginal cornification in postmenopausal women and result in the incorrect diagnosis of endometrial carcinoma. The estrogen-like effects of cardiac glycosides also cause reduced excretion of pituitary gonadotropin in postmenopausal women. Digoxin may cause an increase in urinary 17-hydroxycorticosteroids.

Hypersensitivity reactions to cardiac glycosides are rare but may occur, usually within 6–10 days after initiating therapy. Skin reactions may be erythematous, scarlatiniform, papular, vesicular, or bullous. Rashes usually are accompanied by eosinophilia; eosinophilia also may occur without skin reactions. Urticaria; fever; pruritus; facial, angioneurotic, or laryngeal edema; alopecia of the scalp; shedding of finger and toe nails; and desquamation have been reported. Rarely, thrombocytopenic purpura has been reported to occur during administration of cardiac glycosides.

■ **Precautions and Contraindications** The possibility that use of digoxin in patients with acute myocardial infarction (MI) may increase oxygen demand and associated ischemia should be considered. Patients with idiopathic hypertrophic subaortic stenosis may experience worsening of their condition because of the inotropic effects of digoxin. Patients with certain disorders involving heart failure associated with preserved left ventricular ejection fraction (e.g., restrictive cardiomyopathy, constrictive pericarditis, amyloid heart disease, acute cor pulmonale) may experience decreased cardiac output with digoxin. Digoxin should not be administered to patients with substantial sinus or atrioventricular (AV) block, unless the conduction block has been addressed with a permanent pacemaker. Digoxin should be used cautiously with other drugs that can depress sinus or AV nodal function.

Digoxin should be used with caution in patients with Wolff-Parkinson-White (WPW) syndrome and atrial fibrillation since the drug may enhance conduction via the accessory pathway and result in extremely rapid ventricular rates and ventricular fibrillation. (See Other Supraventricular Tachycardias under Uses: Supraventricular Tachyarrhythmias.) Carotid sinus massage has caused ventricular fibrillation in patients receiving cardiac glycosides.

Since digoxin can induce ventricular arrhythmias, it is recommended that dosage of the drug be reduced or therapy discontinued for 1–2 days before elective cardioversion in patients with atrial fibrillation; however, clinicians should consider the consequences of increasing the ventricular response if digoxin is decreased or withdrawn. Elective cardioversion should be postponed in patients with signs and symptoms of cardiac glycoside toxicity. If it is not possible to delay cardioversion, the lowest possible energy level should be used to avoid provoking ventricular arrhythmias.

Digoxin is contraindicated in patients with ventricular fibrillation.

Digoxin is contraindicated in patients who have demonstrated hypersensitivity to the drug or to other forms of digitalis.

■ **Pediatric Precautions** Safety and efficacy of digoxin in controlling ventricular rate have not been established in pediatric patients with atrial fibrillation.

The manufacturer states that safety and efficacy of digoxin in pediatric patients with heart failure have not been established in adequate and well-controlled studies; however, improvements in hemodynamics and clinical manifestations have been reported in pediatric patients with heart failure of various etiologies in the published literature.

Neonates exhibit considerable variability in their tolerance to digoxin. Premature and immature infants are particularly sensitive to the drug, and dosage must be reduced and individualized according to maturity. The adverse effect profile of digoxin differs in infants and children, particularly in regard to initial signs of toxicity. Cardiac arrhythmias, including sinus bradycardia, usually occur earliest and most frequently. In children, any arrhythmia can occur. Therefore, any arrhythmia or alteration in cardiac conduction in a child should be considered a sign of toxicity.

■ **Pregnancy and Lactation** Available data from retrospective clinical studies and case reports have not identified a drug-associated risk of major birth defects, miscarriage, or adverse maternal and fetal effects with digoxin. However, the underlying maternal condition (e.g., heart failure, atrial fibrillation) may increase the risk of adverse pregnancy outcomes during digoxin therapy. Animal reproduction studies have not been conducted with the drug.

Dosage requirements for digoxin may increase during pregnancy and decrease during the postpartum period; serum digoxin concentrations should be monitored.

Because digoxin crosses the placenta and is found in amniotic fluid, neonates should be monitored for signs and symptoms of digoxin toxicity (e.g., vomiting, cardiac arrhythmias).

Although digoxin is distributed into milk, the quantities present are unlikely to be clinically important. The effects of digoxin on the breast-fed infant or on milk production are not known.

Drug Interactions

Because digoxin has a narrow therapeutic window, increased monitoring of serum digoxin concentrations and for possible clinical manifestations of digoxin toxicity is necessary when initiating, adjusting, or discontinuing therapy with any drugs that may interact with digoxin. Clinicians should also consult the prescribing information for any drugs that are concurrently administered with digoxin for potential drug interaction information.

Concomitant use of certain drugs may increase serum concentrations of digoxin by interfering with absorption of the cardiac glycoside via P-glycoprotein (P-gp) interaction or other mechanisms. Drugs that have been shown to increase serum digoxin concentrations by more than 50% include amiodarone, captopril, clarithromycin, dronedarone, gentamicin, erythromycin, itraconazole, lapatinib, propafenone, quinidine, ranolazine, ritonavir, tetracycline, and verapamil. Serum digoxin concentrations should be measured prior to initiating these drugs and dosage of digoxin should be adjusted by either decreasing the dose by approximately 30–50% or modifying the dosing frequency and continuing monitoring.

Drugs that have been shown to increase digoxin concentrations by less than 50% include atorvastatin, carvedilol, conivaptan, diltiazem, indomethacin, mirabegron, nefazodone, nifedipine, propantheline, quinine, rabeprazole, saquinavir, spironolactone, telmisartan, ticagrelor, tolvaptan, and trimethoprim. Serum digoxin concentrations should be measured prior to initiating these drugs and dosage of digoxin should be adjusted by either decreasing the dose by approximately 15–30% or modifying the dosing frequency and continuing monitoring.

Drugs that have been shown to increase serum digoxin concentrations with unclear magnitude include alprazolam, azithromycin, cyclosporine, diclofenac, diphenoxylate, epoprostenol, esomeprazole, ibuprofen, ketoconazole, lansoprazole, metformin, and omeprazole. Serum digoxin concentrations should be measured prior to initiating these drugs; monitoring should be continued and dosage of digoxin should be reduced as necessary.

Drugs or therapies that have been shown to decrease serum digoxin concentrations include acarbose, albuterol, antacids, certain cancer chemotherapy or radiation therapy, cholestyramine, colestipol, exenatide, kaolin-pectin, metoclopramide, miglitol, neomycin, penicillamine, phenytoin, rifampin, St. John's wort (*Hypericum perforatum*), sucralfate, and sulfasalazine. Serum digoxin concentrations should be measured prior to initiating these drugs or therapies; monitoring should be continued and dosage of digoxin should be increased by approximately 20–40% as necessary.

■ **Drugs Affecting P-glycoprotein Transport** Digoxin is a substrate of the P-gp transport protein at the level of intestinal absorption, renal tubular secretion, and biliary-intestinal secretion. Clinically important interactions may occur when digoxin is used concomitantly with drugs that induce (e.g., rifampin, neomycin, penicillamine) or inhibit (e.g., amiodarone, dronedarone, verapamil, propafenone, quinidine, cyclosporine, atorvastatin, simvastatin, darunavir, saquinavir, ritonavir) P-gp.

■ **Drugs Affecting GI Absorption of Digoxin** A number of drugs are capable of binding digoxin and/or inhibiting the absorption of the cardiac glycoside from the GI tract, which may result in low serum concentrations of the glycoside.

Single-dose studies indicate that aluminum hydroxide, magnesium hydroxide, magnesium trisilicate, kaolin-pectin, aminosalicylic acid, metoclopramide, and sulfasalazine reduce GI absorption of digoxin (resulting in low serum digoxin concentrations), especially when these drugs are administered at the same time as digoxin; therefore, doses of these drugs should be spaced as far apart as possible from doses of digoxin.

Orally administered neomycin may cause malabsorption of digoxin, which may result in low serum digoxin concentrations, but administration of neomycin to digitalized patients apparently does not affect the terminal half-life of digoxin.

Macrolide antibiotics (e.g., clarithromycin, erythromycin) may increase oral bioavailability of digoxin by altering the GI flora that metabolize digoxin, possibly resulting in increased serum concentrations of digoxin and risk of digoxin toxicity. (See Drug Interactions: Anti-infective Agents.)

GI absorption of oral digoxin tablets may be substantially reduced in patients receiving radiation therapy, certain antineoplastic agents, or various combination chemotherapy regimens, possibly as a result of temporary damage to intestinal mucosa caused by the radiation or cytotoxic agents. Colestipol and cholestyramine may bind digoxin in the GI tract and impair its absorption (resulting in low serum digoxin concentrations), particularly if the glycoside and colestipol or cholestyramine are administered simultaneously or close together. Digoxin should be given at least 1.5–2 hours before cholestyramine or colestipol. Drugs that alter GI transit time and/or motility of the GI tract, such as antimuscarinics and diphenoxylate, may alter the rate of absorption of digoxin. Patients receiving an antimuscarinic and digoxin should be closely observed for signs of digitalis toxicity.

■ **Drugs Affecting Electrolyte Balance** In patients receiving digoxin, electrolyte disturbances produced by diuretics such as ethacrynic acid, furosemide, and thiazides (primarily hypokalemia but also hypomagnesemia and, with the thiazides, hypercalcemia) predispose the patient to digoxin toxicity. Fatal cardiac arrhythmias may result. Periodic electrolyte determinations must be performed in patients concurrently receiving digoxin and a diuretic, and corrective measures undertaken if warranted. Other drugs that deplete body potassium (e.g., amphotericin B, corticosteroids, corticotropin, edetate disodium, laxatives, sodium polystyrene sulfonate) or that reduce extracellular potassium (e.g., glucagon, large doses of dextrose, dextrose-insulin infusions) also may predispose digitalized patients to toxicity.

■ **Drugs Affecting Renal Function** Drugs that affect renal function (e.g., angiotensin-converting enzyme [ACE] inhibitors, angiotensin II receptor antagonists, nonsteroidal anti-inflammatory agents [NSAIAs]) may impair elimination of digoxin, and thus predispose patients to digoxin toxicity.

■ **Calcium Salts** The inotropic and toxic effects of digoxin and calcium are synergistic and arrhythmias may occur if these drugs are given together (particularly when calcium is administered rapidly IV). IV administration of calcium should be avoided in patients receiving digoxin; if necessary, calcium should be given slowly in small amounts.

■ **Antiarrhythmic Agents** Although quinidine, procainamide, disopyramide, phenytoin, propranolol, and lidocaine have been used effectively in conjunction with digoxin to treat arrhythmias and also alone to treat cardiac glycoside-induced arrhythmias, these antiarrhythmic agents may have negative inotropic effects with larger than usual doses, especially in patients with cardiac glycoside toxicity (propranolol has negative inotropic effects with usual doses).

Amiodarone Concomitant administration of digoxin and amiodarone may result in increased serum digoxin concentrations and subsequent digoxin toxicity. Serum digoxin concentrations generally increase by an average of 70–100% in adults, but substantial variability exists in the magnitude of the increase. Limited data suggest that the magnitude of the increase may be much greater in children than in adults (i.e., 70–800%).

The amiodarone-induced increase in serum digoxin concentrations usually begins within 1–7 days and progresses gradually over a period of several weeks or even months. The exact mechanism(s) of this interaction appears to be complex and remains to be fully established, but data indicate that amiodarone may decrease the renal and/or nonrenal clearance of digoxin. It also has been suggested that amiodarone may increase the oral bioavailability of digoxin or displace digoxin from tissue binding sites. When initiating amiodarone therapy in patients receiving digoxin, the need for continued digoxin therapy should be reassessed, and digoxin discontinued if appropriate; if concomitant therapy is considered necessary, serum digoxin concentrations should be measured prior to initiating amiodarone and dosage of digoxin adjusted by either decreasing the dose by approximately 30–50% or modifying the dosing frequency. Patients should be observed closely for signs of cardiac glycoside toxicity. In addition, thyroid function should be monitored carefully in patients receiving concurrent amiodarone and digoxin therapy, since amiodarone-induced changes in thyroid function may increase or decrease serum digoxin concentrations or alter sensitivity to the therapeutic and toxic effects of the cardiac glycoside.

Dofetilide Concomitant use of dofetilide and digoxin was associated with an increased risk of torsades de pointes. Dosage of digoxin should be individualized when used concomitantly with dofetilide.

Dronedarone Concomitant use of digoxin and dronedarone (a P-gp inhibitor) may result in a substantial increase (150%) in systemic exposure to digoxin; possible digoxin toxicity may occur. In clinical studies, baseline use of digoxin was associated with an increased risk of arrhythmic or sudden death in patients receiving dronedarone. Because digoxin can potentiate the electrophysiologic effects of dronedarone and dronedarone can increase exposure to digoxin, concomitant use of these drugs is not recommended. If concomitant use of dronedarone is necessary in a patient receiving digoxin, serum digoxin concentrations should be determined prior to initiating dronedarone and dosage of digoxin should be reduced by decreasing the dose by approximately 30–50% or modifying the dosing frequency.

Flecainide Studies in healthy individuals indicate that serum digoxin concentrations may be increased by an average of about 15–25% when flecainide and digoxin are administered concomitantly. The increase in serum digoxin concentration may occur within a few days of initiating flecainide therapy in patients receiving digoxin and may result from a decrease in the volume of distribution of digoxin. Although the PR interval was substantially prolonged in most healthy individuals during concomitant administration of flecainide and digoxin, it was not determined whether this resulted from an additive effect of the drugs or mainly from flecainide. Flecainide has been administered concomitantly with cardiac glycosides in patients with ventricular arrhythmias without unusual adverse effects. Additional studies to determine the potential importance of an interaction in patients with heart failure are needed. Flecainide-induced increases in serum digoxin concentration generally appear to be of a small magnitude and are unlikely to be clinically important in most cases; however, patients with AV nodal dysfunction, serum digoxin concentrations in the upper end of the therapeutic range, and/or high plasma flecainide concentrations may be at increased risk of digoxin toxicity. Pending further accumulation of data, patients receiving flecainide and digoxin should be monitored for signs of digoxin toxicity.

Quinidine Concomitant administration of quinidine and digoxin increases serum concentrations of digoxin (in 90% or more of patients), which may result in digoxin toxicity. Although variability exists in the magnitude of the increase, serum digoxin concentrations usually increase twofold to threefold when quinidine therapy is initiated in patients digitalized with digoxin. Serum digoxin concentrations may begin to increase within a few hours after initiating quinidine therapy, but at least 5–7 days are usually required to achieve a new steady-state serum digoxin concentration. The magnitude of the increase appears to depend on the serum quinidine concentration. Both the clearance (principally renal clearance) and volume of distribution of digoxin generally are decreased, but serum half-life of the drug may be unaffected.

When quinidine therapy is initiated in a patient receiving digoxin, serum digoxin concentrations should be carefully monitored and digoxin dosage reduced (by decreasing dose by approximately 30–50% or modifying dosing frequency) as needed; the patient should be observed closely for signs of toxicity. Because of the variability in magnitude of the interaction, additional dosage adjustments are likely to be necessary. If digoxin therapy is initiated in a patient receiving quinidine, lower than usual dosages of digoxin may be sufficient to produce desired serum concentrations of the cardiac glycoside. If quinidine is discontinued in a patient stabilized on therapy with both drugs, the patient should be observed for signs of decreased response to digoxin and dosage of the cardiac glycoside adjusted as necessary.

Sotalol In clinical studies, proarrhythmic events were more common in patients receiving sotalol and digoxin concomitantly than when either drug was used alone. It is not known if this represents an adverse drug interaction or is related to the presence of heart failure, which is a known risk factor for proarrhythmia, in patients receiving digoxin. Dosage of digoxin should be individualized when used concomitantly with sotalol.

■ **β-Adrenergic Blocking Agents** Concomitant use of digoxin and β-adrenergic blocking agents (β-blockers) can have additive negative effects on AV conduction, which can result in complete heart block. Although such combined therapy may be useful in controlling ventricular rate in patient with atrial fibrillation and/or flutter, digoxin dosage in patients receiving such therapy should be carefully individualized given the considerable variability of these interactions.

■ **Calcium-channel Blocking Agents** Although combination therapy with digoxin and calcium-channel blocking agents may be useful in controlling atrial fibrillation, such concomitant use can have negative effects on AV conduction, which can result in complete heart block. Digoxin dosage should be carefully individualized when used in conjunction with calcium-channel blocking agents because of the considerable variability of these interactions.

Diltiazem There are conflicting reports on whether diltiazem substantially affects the pharmacokinetics of digoxin when the drugs are administered concomitantly. In some studies, diltiazem reportedly increased average steady-state serum digoxin concentrations by about 20–50%, possibly by decreasing the renal and nonrenal clearance of the glycoside; however, in other studies, diltiazem did not substantially alter serum digoxin concentrations. Despite conflicting reports, serum digoxin concentrations should be carefully monitored and the patient observed closely for signs of digoxin toxicity when diltiazem and digoxin are administered concomitantly, especially in geriatric patients, patients with unstable renal function, or those with serum digoxin concentrations in the upper therapeutic range before diltiazem is administered. Dosage of digoxin should be reduced by either decreasing the dose by approximately 15–30% or modifying the dosing frequency. Digoxin does not appear to affect the pharmacokinetics of diltiazem.

Nifedipine Most evidence indicates that nifedipine does not substantially affect the pharmacokinetics of digoxin when the drugs are administered concomitantly; however, some data suggest that serum digoxin concentrations may increase by about 15–45% during concomitant therapy. Further evaluation of this potential interaction is needed. Patients receiving the drugs concomitantly should be monitored for signs and symptoms of digoxin toxicity. Serum digoxin concentrations should be determined prior to initiating nifedipine and dosage of digoxin should be reduced by either decreasing the dose by approximately 15–30% or modifying the dosing frequency.

Verapamil Verapamil, a potent P-gp inhibitor, may increase serum digoxin concentrations by 50–75% during the first week of verapamil therapy. This effect may be more substantial in patients with underlying hepatic disease (e.g., cirrhosis). When verapamil is administered to a patient receiving digoxin, serum digoxin concentrations should be measured and dosage of digoxin adjusted by either decreasing the dose by approximately 30–50% or modifying the dosing frequency. The patient should be monitored closely for clinical response and digoxin toxicity. Combined therapy with the drugs (e.g., for control of ventricular rate in patients with atrial fibrillation and/or flutter) usually is well tolerated if dosage of digoxin is properly adjusted.

■ **Other Cardiovascular Drugs** Sympathomimetics (e.g., dopamine, epinephrine, norepinephrine) should be used with caution in patients receiving digoxin, since the risk of arrhythmias may be increased in patients receiving these drugs concomitantly.

Altered responses to digoxin therapy have occurred in patients receiving digoxin and amiloride concomitantly. In healthy individuals in one study, amiloride increased the renal clearance but decreased the extrarenal clearance of digoxin, resulting in slight increases in serum digoxin concentration. Inhibition of the positive inotropic effect of digoxin has also been observed in healthy individuals receiving amiloride. Patients receiving amiloride and digoxin concurrently should be carefully observed for altered responses to digoxin therapy. Further studies are needed to determine the clinical importance of the potential drug interaction between amiloride and digoxin.

Concomitant use of captopril and digoxin has been reported to increase serum concentrations and systemic exposure to digoxin by about 58 and 39%, respectively. Such increases may result from decreased renal clearance (probably both glomerular filtration and tubular secretion) of digoxin and, possibly, displacement of the glycoside from tissue-binding sites by captopril-induced increases in serum potassium. Captopril has been administered concomitantly with digoxin in patients with congestive heart failure *without* unusual adverse effects or apparent increased risk of cardiac glycoside toxicity. It has been postulated that captopril-induced increases in serum potassium may offset the potential toxic effects of increased serum digoxin concentrations. If captopril is initiated in a patient receiving digoxin, serum digoxin concentrations should be measured prior to initiating captopril and dosage of digoxin should be adjusted by either decreasing the dose by approximately 30–50% or modifying the dosing frequency.

■ **Anti-infective Agents** Data suggest that, in about 10% of patients receiving digoxin, substantial amounts of the drug are metabolized by bacteria within the lumen of the large intestine to cardioinactive compounds (reduced metabolites) following oral and possibly parenteral administration. The extent of such metabolism following oral administration appears to vary inversely with the bioavailability of the preparation. In patients who form substantial amounts of reduced metabolites, alteration of enteric bacterial flora by some anti-infective agents (e.g., oral erythromycin or tetracycline hydrochloride) may result in an increase in the bioavailability of active drug and as much as a twofold increase in serum digoxin concentrations. When concomitant therapy with a systemic anti-infective agent is administered in patients receiving digoxin, the possibility that serum digoxin concentrations may increase should be considered and dosage of the cardiac glycoside should be reduced if necessary.

Concomitant administration of digoxin and itraconazole may result in increased serum digoxin concentrations (by 80%); digoxin toxicity may occur. If itraconazole is initiated in a patient receiving digoxin, serum digoxin concentrations should be measured prior to initiating itraconazole and dosage of digoxin should be adjusted by either decreasing the dose by approximately 30–50% or modifying the dosing frequency. Such patients should be observed for clinical manifestations of digoxin toxicity.

■ **Other Drugs** Succinylcholine appears to potentiate the effects of digoxin on conduction and ventricular irritability. Cardiac arrhythmias have occurred in patients receiving these drugs concomitantly and, therefore, succinylcholine should be administered with caution in patients receiving digoxin. Dosage of digoxin should be individualized when used concomitantly with neuromuscular blocking agents such as succinylcholine.

Teriparatide can transiently increase serum calcium concentrations, which may predispose patients to digoxin toxicity.

Thyroid supplements may increase dosage requirements of digoxin.

Indomethacin may prolong the elimination half-life and increase serum concentrations of digoxin; the mechanism of this interaction requires further elucidation. (See Drug Interactions: Digoxin, in Indomethacin 28:08.04.92.) Serum digoxin concentrations should be monitored carefully in patients receiving the drugs concomitantly. The manufacturer states that dosage of digoxin should be reduced by either decreasing the dose by approximately 15–30% or modifying the dosing frequency.

Laboratory Test Interferences

Digoxin may cause false-positive ST-T changes during exercise testing.

Acute Toxicity

The widespread use of digoxin and the very narrow margin between effective therapeutic and toxic dosages contribute to the high incidence of toxicity and the relatively high associated mortality rate.

Toxic effects of digoxin are mainly GI, CNS, biochemical, and cardiac in origin. The minimum toxic and lethal doses of digoxin are not well established. Based on both accidental and suicidal ingestions, the single oral lethal dose in otherwise healthy individuals is approximately 20–50 times the usual daily maintenance dose. However, patients with predisposing factors (e.g., preexisting heart disease) and patients receiving chronic digoxin therapy may tolerate lesser amounts. Infants and children appear to be more tolerant to the therapeutic and toxic actions of digoxin; children without underlying cardiac problems can usually tolerate an acute dose of several milligrams of the drug without potentially life-threatening cardiac toxicity.

Serum digoxin concentrations are useful in confirming the diagnosis of intoxication; however, clinical diagnosis and management should not be based on serum concentrations alone but should always be interpreted in the overall clinical context with all other relevant information. At least 6–10 hours usually are necessary for digoxin to equilibrate between plasma and tissue; plasma specimens drawn prior to this time may show digoxin concentrations greater than those present after equilibration. Many factors, including adequacy of tissue oxygenation, electrolyte and acid-base balance, thyroid function, autonomic nervous system tone, age of the patient, renal function, other concurrently administered drugs, and the nature and severity of the underlying cardiac disease, influence whether a patient manifests toxicity with a given dosage or serum concentration. There is some concern that therapeutic serum concentrations of digoxin (e.g., less than 2 ng/mL) may exert deleterious cardiovascular effects in the long term, although such concentrations appear to be well tolerated in the short term.

■ **Manifestations** Overdosage of digoxin is manifested by a wide variety of signs and symptoms that are difficult to distinguish from effects associated with cardiac disease (e.g., adverse GI effects, arrhythmias). Before additional doses of the drug are administered, attempts should be made to determine whether the patient's manifestations are glycoside induced. However, this may be difficult since signs of intoxication do not occur in regular sequence, and subjective signs of toxicity are frequently less easily recognized in infants and children than in adults.

Extracardiac Effects The extracardiac manifestations of digoxin intoxication are similar in both acute and chronic intoxication. However, GI effects and, to a lesser extent, CNS and visual disturbances may be more pronounced following acute overdosage. Acute toxicity may cause hyperkalemia, whereas patients with chronic toxicity may be hypokalemic or normokalemic. In addition, patients receiving chronic digoxin therapy may be hyperkalemic, normokalemic, or hypokalemic if acute intoxication occurs. In pediatric patients, drowsiness and vomiting are often the most prominent extracardiac effects. However, life-threatening cardiac arrhythmias have developed suddenly in children without evidence of any extracardiac signs of intoxication.

Anorexia, nausea, and vomiting are common early signs of toxicity and may precede or follow evidence of cardiotoxicity. Clinical evaluation of the cause of these symptoms should be attempted before further administration of digoxin; determination of serum digoxin concentrations may aid in deciding whether or not toxicity is present. GI effects probably are at least partially mediated by the area postrema of the medulla since they occur following administration by all routes. Large doses of cardiac glycosides may also produce emesis by direct GI irritation. Episodes of nausea and vomiting may start and stop abruptly. Other GI effects include salivation, epigastric or abdominal pain, abdominal distention, diarrhea, constipation, and weight loss. Acute hemorrhage and intestinal, esophageal, and gastric necrosis have occurred rarely in patients receiving cardiac glycosides.

Headache, fatigue, malaise, drowsiness, and generalized muscle weakness are common nervous system signs of cardiac glycoside toxicity. Dizziness, vertigo, syncope, apathy, lethargy, excitement, euphoria, insomnia, irritability, agitation, hiccups, restlessness, nervousness, seizures, opisthotonos, stupor, and coma also have occurred.

Severe facial pain, simulating trigeminal neuralgia and usually involving the lower third of the face, has occurred in some patients. The pain usually is characterized by aching of the teeth and lower jaw and sharp stabbing pain throughout the mandible and maxilla. Neuralgic pain also has occurred in the upper extremities and lumbar area; paresthesias and tremors have accompanied the pain.

Visual disturbances induced by toxic doses of digoxin probably result from a direct effect on the retina (cones are affected more than rods). Transient retrobulbar neuritis has been reported to cause visual changes in digoxin intoxication; however, it is likely that most visual disturbances result from functional changes of the retina in the presence of high concentrations of the drug. Color vision is commonly affected and objects may appear yellow or green or, less commonly, brown, red, blue, or white. Blurred vision, flashes or flickering of light, photophobia, halos or borders on objects (often are white and appear on dark objects), diplopia, macropsia, and micropsia may occur. Transient or permanent amblyopia and scotoma, including teichopsia, also have occurred. Visual disorders generally are reversible after withdrawal of digoxin therapy; transient or total blindness is rare.

Patients with digoxin toxicity are often hypokalemic or normokalemic. However, severe intoxication may cause hyperkalemia, presumably secondary to inhibition of the Na^+-K^+-ATPase pump. Hyperkalemia may develop rapidly and can result in life-threatening cardiac manifestations, such as AV block and asystole. Presence of hyperkalemia during the early stages of intoxication appears to be a poor prognostic indicator; data from clinical studies indicate that mortality correlates better with the severity of initial hyperkalemia than with the dosage of digoxin ingested, initial serum glycoside concentration, or initial ECG changes in patients treated with conventional supportive and symptomatic measures that do not include digoxin immune Fab therapy.

Cardiac Effects The most well defined and most dangerous toxic actions of digoxin are those affecting the heart. Cardiac signs of glycoside toxicity may occur with or without other signs of toxicity and often precede other toxic effects. Digoxin has caused almost every kind of cardiac arrhythmia, and various combinations of arrhythmias may occur in the same patient. In addition, arrhythmias associated with digoxin intoxication may result in worsening of heart failure.

Since most of the toxic cardiac effects of digoxin also can occur as manifestations of heart disease, it is often difficult to determine whether toxic cardiac effects are caused by an underlying heart disease or the glycoside. The type of arrhythmia, presence or absence of other manifestations of toxicity, serum concentrations of the drug, and the patient's age, disease state, renal function, and serum potassium concentration should be considered.

Cardiac effects occurring in acute overdosage in otherwise healthy individuals often differ from those in patients with underlying heart disease who are receiving chronic digoxin therapy. Otherwise healthy individuals with acute toxicity frequently present with atrioventricular (AV) conduction disturbances and supraventricular arrhythmias, such as sinus bradycardia. Ventricular arrhythmias are uncommon in these individuals; however, when present, they are associated with severe toxicity and high mortality.

Pediatric patients with healthy hearts often present with sinus bradycardia and conduction disturbances; ventricular arrhythmias also occur but are less common than in adults. In neonates, premonitory signs of toxicity may include sinus bradycardia, sinoatrial (SA) arrest, or prolongation of the PR interval. Multifocal premature ventricular complexes (PVCs), including bigeminy and trigeminy, and, less commonly, unifocal PVCs are common arrhythmias in adults with digoxin toxicity, especially in the presence of heart disease. Patients with glycoside-induced ventricular tachycardia have a high mortality rate, since ventricular fibrillation or asystole may result. Bidirectional ventricular tachycardia may occur in severe digoxin toxicity.

First-degree AV block is common in patients receiving digoxin and generally indicates a therapeutic rather than a toxic effect. However, AV block may progressively increase in patients with toxicity. Mobitz type I (Wenckebach) second-degree AV block and AV junctional exit block are relatively common AV conduction disorders associated with digoxin toxicity; complete (third-degree) AV block may occur in advanced intoxication.

Paroxysmal and nonparoxysmal AV junctional rhythms, especially nonparoxysmal AV junctional tachycardia, AV dissociation (with or without some degree of AV block), and paroxysmal atrial tachycardia with variable AV block, are common in both adults and children and somewhat characteristic of digoxin toxicity.

Digoxin toxicity also may cause various atrial and SA nodal arrhythmias and conduction disorders, including atrial tachycardia, atrial fibrillation, atrial flutter, atrial premature complexes, wandering atrial pacemaker, sinus bradycardia, SA arrest, SA exit block, and sinus tachycardia. Junctional premature complexes also may occur. Sinus bradycardia may be a sign of impending digoxin intoxication, especially in infants and children.

Electrolyte imbalances, especially hypokalemia and, to a lesser extent, hypomagnesemia or hypercalcemia, may predispose patients to the cardiotoxic effects of digoxin. Potassium depletion sensitizes the myocardium to digoxin, and calcium has effects similar to digoxin on contractility and excitability of the heart. Conversely, hypocalcemia may cause resistance to the effects of digoxin on the AV node, and digoxin may be ineffective until serum calcium is restored to normal.

■ Treatment

If signs of toxicity appear, digoxin should be discontinued immediately and serum digoxin concentrations obtained; the patient should be placed on a cardiac monitor while possible contributing factors (e.g., electrolyte and thyroid abnormalities, concomitant drugs) are addressed.

Measures to Reduce Absorption or Enhance Elimination of Digoxin Activated charcoal may be administered if acute ingestion (intentionally or accidently) of a potentially toxic amount of digoxin occurs. Administration of activated charcoal appears to be useful in preventing further absorption of the glycoside. Although activated charcoal is most effective when administered soon after ingestion, doses given later also appear to be effective, presumably because of the prolonged absorption and/or enterohepatic circulation of the drug. Multiple oral doses of activated charcoal have been used to enhance the elimination of digoxin, especially in patients with substantial renal impairment, since the drug undergoes enterohepatic circulation. Adults have been given 20–60 g of activated charcoal every 4–12 hours until objective evidence and clinical observations indicated that serum glycoside concentration had declined to the subtoxic range.

An anion-exchange resin such as cholestyramine or colestipol administered soon after ingestion of digoxin may reduce initial absorption of the glycoside. When administered after onset of toxicity, these resins also may reduce the duration of toxicity by binding digoxin in the GI tract during enterohepatic circulation. These agents probably do not have substantial value in the treatment of advanced digoxin toxicity.

Although these measures may be used to reduce the absorption or enhance elimination of digoxin, severe digoxin toxicity generally should be treated with digoxin-specific antibody fragments (digoxin immune Fab).

Therapeutic Measures Supportive and symptomatic treatment should be initiated depending on the type of cardiotoxicity; continuous ECG monitoring is recommended to monitor for signs of arrhythmias and hyperkalemia. Serum electrolytes, especially potassium, and serum digoxin concentrations should be monitored carefully. Hypoxia and acid-base and fluid and electrolyte imbalances should be corrected, when necessary.

Milder forms of cardiotoxicity, such as occasional PVCs, AV junctional rhythm with a slow rate, and possibly atrial fibrillation with a slow ventricular rate, usually are treated by temporary withdrawal of digoxin and, if necessary, careful correction of hypokalemia and subsequent adjustment of dosage to prevent recurrence. However, cardiac irregularities that impair cardiac output because of substantial bradycardia or tachycardia should be treated. Ventricular tachycardia, bidirectional ventricular tachycardia, nonparoxysmal AV junctional rhythm with rapid rate or with exit block, and frequent multifocal PVCs generally should be treated since these arrhythmias may be forerunners of ventricular fibrillation. In hypokalemic patients, some clinicians believe these ventricular arrhythmias should be treated initially with potassium supplements and/or IV phenytoin. In patients with ventricular arrhythmias who are normokalemic or hyperkalemic or in whom potassium is ineffective or contraindicated, phenytoin and/or lidocaine may be used. Phenytoin appears to be particularly useful in the treatment of ventricular arrhythmias, especially in the presence of AV block, because the drug improves conduction through the AV node. Limited data suggest that phenytoin is also occasionally useful in the treatment of supraventricular arrhythmias.

Although propranolol is effective in the treatment of cardiac glycoside-induced ventricular and supraventricular arrhythmias, the drug should be used with caution because it may compromise conduction through the AV node and also may cause bradycardia. Refractory ventricular or junctional tachycardia has been treated with ventricular overdrive pacing, but temporary ventricular pacing has been associated with decreased fibrillatory threshold of the ventricle and with mechanical damage to the heart in rare instances. Therefore, use of digoxin immune Fab, if available, generally is preferable in the management of ventricular or junctional tachyarrhythmias unresponsive to conventional therapy.

In adults with severe sinus bradycardia, SA arrest, or second- or third-degree AV block, 0.6–2 mg of atropine sulfate administered IV or IM may be effective, especially in those without heart disease. In pediatric patients, recommended dosages of atropine sulfate range from 0.01–0.03 mg/kg per dose. If atropine is ineffective, administration of digoxin immune Fab, if available, may reverse severe sinus bradycardia and advanced AV block. Insertion of a transvenous bipolar electrode catheter may be necessary if sinus bradyarrhythmias and/or AV block result in hemodynamic compromise.

Cardioversion is used only as a last resort for refractory supraventricular or ventricular tachycardia or for ventricular fibrillation caused by cardiac glycosides. Cardioversion is potentially hazardous in the treatment of ectopic rhythms induced by glycoside toxicity because it may cause ventricular tachycardia or fibrillation that is resistant to further cardioversion. If cardioversion is mandatory, initial shocks should be at low energy levels (e.g., 5, 20, then 40 watt-seconds) and gradually increased in successive shocks until the arrhythmia is terminated or evidence of worsened electrophysiologic instability emerges. Many clinicians recommend administration of phenytoin or lidocaine prophylactically before cardioversion and to suppress PVCs if they occur after cardioversion.

In patients with hypokalemia, potassium supplementation should be given to maintain serum concentrations between 4 and 5.5 mEq/L. Potassium generally should not be administered to patients with second- or third-degree AV block caused by cardiac glycosides since excess potassium may further impair AV conduction. Caution should be exercised when using potassium in acute digoxin intoxication since potentially life-threatening hyperkalemia may develop rapidly in advanced toxicity. Close ECG monitoring for evidence of hyperkalemia (e.g., tall peaked T-waves) is recommended.

Hypomagnesemia also should be corrected. Rarely, magnesium sulfate has been used slowly IV as an antiarrhythmic (e.g., to control ventricular arrhythmias unresponsive to other antiarrhythmics) and to correct demonstrated magnesium deficiency in patients with cardiac glycoside toxicity.

Digoxin immune Fab (ovine) is a specific antidote that can be used in the treatment of life-threatening or potentially life-threatening acute or chronic digoxin toxicity. Specific antigen-binding fragments present in the immune Fab bind to free (unbound) digoxin intravascularly and in extracellular fluid, thereby preventing and reversing the pharmacologic and toxic effects of the glycoside and enhancing its elimination as the bound, inactivated glycoside-Fab fragment complex. In cases of potentially life-threatening cardiotoxicity or hyperkalemia, digoxin immune Fab should be administered. Clinical trials with the immune Fab have been promising, with complete reversal of toxicity occurring in most cases. Massive glycoside overdosage may cause hyperkalemia, which can be refractory to conventional therapy. Prognosis appears to correlate with serum potassium concentration (i.e., the greater the serum potassium concentration, the worse the prognosis) in patients treated by conventional symptomatic and supportive measures that do not include digoxin immune Fab. Severe hyperkalemia refractory to standard measures is an indication for digoxin immune Fab. For further information on the immune Fab, see Digoxin Immune Fab 80:04. If digoxin immune Fab is not readily available, emergency measures for the treatment of hyperkalemia have included IV administration of glucose and insulin, sodium bicarbonate, peritoneal dialysis or hemodialysis, and/or use of exchange resins; however, these treatments have not been shown to reduce mortality. Use of calcium infusions in the treatment of hyperkalemia traditionally has been avoided because calcium may worsen cardiac irregularities.

Forced diuresis does not accelerate the renal elimination of cardiac glycosides and may worsen electrolyte imbalances. Because of the large volume of distribution and extensive protein binding of digoxin, hemodialysis and peritoneal dialysis are ineffective in removing the glycoside from the body and potentially may worsen toxicity because of a reduction in body potassium. Hemoperfusion using charcoal or extracorporeal resins or hemofiltration may result in limited removal of digoxin from the body. However, because of the risks involved in these procedures, their use cannot be routinely recommended.

Chronic Toxicity

Most cases of digoxin toxicity occur following multiple doses and result, at least in part, from the cumulative effects of the drug. Administration of digoxin in conjunction with diuretics (see Drug Interactions: Drugs Affecting Electrolyte Balance) is a frequent cause of chronic digoxin toxicity. Failure to individualize dosage is another contributing factor in many cases of toxicity.

Patients with chronic digoxin toxicity commonly present with ventricular arrhythmias, such as PVCs or ventricular tachycardia. AV conduction disturbances also are frequent in chronic toxicity. The extracardiac manifestations of digoxin intoxication are similar in both acute and chronic intoxication. Neuropsychiatric disturbances are especially likely to develop in geriatric patients with atherosclerotic disease and are easily overlooked in patients receiving chronic digoxin therapy. These effects include disorientation, confusion, depression, memory impairment, amnesia, aphasia, bad dreams, delirium, delusions, illusions, and hallucinations.

The initial treatment of chronic overdosage is the same as in an acute overdosage situation. (See Acute Toxicity.) If signs of toxicity appear, digoxin should be discontinued immediately and serum digoxin concentrations obtained; the patient should be placed on a cardiac monitor while possible contributing factors (e.g., electrolyte and thyroid abnormalities, concomitant drugs) are addressed. In patients with hypokalemia, potassium supplementation should be given to maintain serum concentrations between 4 and 5.5 mEq/L.

Pharmacology

The main pharmacologic property of cardiac glycosides is their ability to increase the force and velocity of myocardial systolic contraction (positive inotropic action) by a direct action on the myocardium both in patients with nonfailing hearts and in those with failing hearts. When the force of contraction is increased in patients with failing hearts, cardiac output is increased, systolic emptying is more complete, and diastolic heart size is decreased. Elevated ventricular end-diastolic pressure also is reduced and, consequently, pulmonary and systemic venous pressures are decreased. However, in normal subjects, cardiac output is unchanged or slightly decreased, and total peripheral resistance is increased by direct constriction of vascular smooth muscle and by CNS-mediated increase in sympathetic tone. In patients with heart failure, cardiac glycosides cause reflex reduction in peripheral resistance by increasing myocardial contractility; this compensates for the direct vasoconstrictor action of the drugs and, therefore, total peripheral resistance usually is reduced.

Digoxin inhibits the activity of sodium-potassium-activated adenosine triphosphatase (Na^+-K^+-ATPase), an enzyme required for active transport of sodium across myocardial cell membranes. Inhibition of this enzyme in cardiac cells results in an increase in the contractile state of the heart. Toxic doses of digoxin cause efflux of potassium from the myocardium and concurrent influx of sodium. Toxicity results in part from loss of intracellular potassium associated with inhibition of Na^+-K^+-ATPase. With therapeutic doses, augmentation of calcium influx to the contractile proteins with resultant enhancement of excitation-contraction coupling is involved in the positive inotropic action of cardiac glycosides; the role of Na^+-K^+-ATPase in this effect is controversial.

In patients with heart failure, increased myocardial contractility and cardiac output reflexly reduce sympathetic tone, thus slowing increased heart rate and causing diuresis in edematous patients. In patients without heart failure, increased myocardial contractility produced by cardiac glycosides is accompanied by increased myocardial oxygen consumption. In patients with heart failure, reduced ventricular end-diastolic pressure and increased myocardial contractility produce a net decrease or no change in myocardial oxygen consumption. Cardiac glycosides do not decrease coronary blood flow, and in patients with heart failure the restoration of efficient heart action may improve coronary circulation. Cardiac glycosides have a minor inotropic effect on skeletal muscle.

Digoxin decreases conduction velocity through the atrioventricular (AV) node and prolongs the effective refractory period (ERP) of the AV node by increasing vagal activity, by a direct effect on the AV node, and by a sympatholytic effect. The effects of the drug on the AV node are not apparent clinically when the atrial rate is slow enough to allow time for the AV node to recover between each beat, but in patients with supraventricular tachyarrhythmias such as atrial flutter or atrial fibrillation, the number of waves of depolarization reaching the ventricles is decreased. With usual doses, conduction velocity and refractoriness of the His-Purkinje system are not directly affected. Digoxin shortens the ERP of the atria and increases conduction velocity by a reflex increase in vagal tone and by a direct effect on the atria. With therapeutic doses, digoxin may cause prolongation of the PR interval and ST segment depression, but these ECG effects are not indicative of toxicity.

Digoxin-induced slowing of heart rate in patients without heart failure is negligible and is primarily due to vagal (cholinergic) and sympatholytic effects on the sinoatrial (SA) node, but with toxic doses is due to direct depression of SA node automaticity. Therapeutic doses of digoxin apparently have minimal direct effects and do not have cholinergic or sympatholytic effects on the ventricles. Low concentrations of digoxin produce little effect on the action potential, but toxic concentrations cause progressive loss of resting membrane potential, decreased rate of rise of the action potential, and increased rate of spontaneous diastolic depolarization producing increased automaticity and ectopic impulse activity, especially in the ventricles. Therefore, toxic doses of digoxin increase the automaticity (increased spontaneous diastolic depolarization) of all areas of the heart except the SA node.

Anorexia, nausea, and vomiting caused by cardiac glycosides are probably mediated by chemoreceptors located in the area postrema of the medulla.

Pharmacokinetics

■ **Absorption** Absorption of digoxin is mainly from the small intestine, presumably by a passive, nonsaturable process. The presence of food in the GI tract may slow the rate, but not extent, of absorption of orally administered digoxin from the tablet formulation. Decreased absorption may occur if the drug is administered with a high fiber meal. Gastric pH apparently does not affect the degree of digoxin absorption. Intestinal absorption of the drug may be impaired in patients with certain malabsorption states (e.g., short bowel syndrome, celiac sprue, jejunoileal bypass). Digoxin is a substrate of P-glycoprotein (P-gp), a transport protein involved in absorption of the drug.

There are interindividual variations in plasma concentrations of digoxin with a specific dose and in plasma concentrations of the drug that produce therapeutic and toxic effects. A specific plasma concentration may be therapeutic or toxic in an individual patient depending on factors other than dosage (e.g., serum electrolytes, acid-base balance, concurrently administered drugs, thyroid status, underlying disease states). Plasma concentrations of digoxin are the same as its serum concentrations. If plasma concentrations of digoxin are to be determined, blood samples should be obtained at least 6–8 hours after the daily dose and preferably just prior to the next scheduled daily dose. Therapeutic plasma concentrations of digoxin in adults generally are 0.5–2 ng/mL. Some experts suggest that plasma concentrations of 0.5–0.9 ng/mL are sufficient for the treatment of heart failure in adults; however, limited data are available. In adults, toxicity is usually, but not always, associated with steady-state plasma digoxin concentrations exceeding 2 ng/mL. Toxicity may also occur with lower digoxin levels, especially if hypokalemia, hypomagnesemia, or hypothyroidism coexists. Although neonates and infants appear to tolerate higher plasma concentrations of digoxin than do adults, evidence suggests that plasma concentrations greater than those in the generally accepted therapeutic ranges for adults are associated with little, if any, additional therapeutic benefit in these patients. *Serum concentrations of digoxin should be interpreted in the overall clinical context; thus, an isolated serum concentration measurement should not be used alone as the basis for adjusting dosage.*

Following oral administration of a single dose of digoxin, onset of action occurs in 0.5–2 hours and maximal effects occur in 2–6 hours. After IV administration of a single dose of digoxin, the onset of action occurs in 5–30 minutes depending on the rate of infusion and maximal effects occur in 1–4 hours.

The absolute bioavailability of digoxin tablets is 60–80% and the absolute bioavailability of the oral solution is 70–85%; when switching from IV to oral dosage forms, the differences in bioavailability should be considered.

■ **Distribution** Cardiac glycosides are widely distributed in body tissues; highest concentrations are found in the heart, kidneys, intestine, stomach, liver, and skeletal muscle. Lowest concentrations are in the plasma and brain. In the myocardium, cardiac glycosides are found in the sarcolemma-T system bound to a receptor (probably Na^+-K^+-ATPase). Only small amounts of digoxin are distributed into fat. Digoxin crosses the placenta and, in pregnant women receiving digoxin, fetal and maternal plasma concentrations are equal. Maternal concentrations of digoxin in plasma and milk are similar.

With therapeutic plasma concentrations, about 20–30% of digoxin in the blood is bound to plasma proteins.

■ **Elimination** In patients with normal renal function, the elimination half-life ($t_{1/2}$) of digoxin is 36 hours. The elimination $t_{1/2}$ of digoxin is increased in patients with impaired renal function. In undigitalized patients, institution of fixed daily maintenance doses of digoxin without an initial loading dose results in steady-state plasma concentrations after 4–5 elimination $t_{1/2}$s.

Digoxin is not metabolized appreciably (only about 13%) prior to excretion. Metabolism includes stepwise cleavage of the sugar molecules, hydroxylation, epimerization, and formation of glucuronide and sulfate conjugates. The cytochrome P-450 (CYP) system is not involved in the metabolism of digoxin. Digoxin is also apparently metabolized by bacteria within the lumen of the large intestine following oral administration and possibly after biliary elimination following parenteral administration.

Digoxin is excreted primarily by the kidneys mainly as unchanged drug. In healthy individuals, about 50–70% of an IV dose of digoxin is excreted unchanged in urine. Digoxin is eliminated from the body by first-order kinetics, with a fixed proportion of the residual drug in the body being eliminated each day. Renal excretion of digoxin is proportional to creatinine clearance and is largely independent of urine flow. Orally administered activated charcoal has been shown to enhance total body clearance and elimination of digoxin, probably by adsorbing the cardiac glycoside in the GI tract with subsequent excretion in feces. Digoxin is not appreciably removed by hemodialysis or peritoneal dialysis. Similarly, only minor amounts of the drug are removed during cardiopulmonary bypass or exchange transfusion.

Chemistry and Stability

■ **Chemistry** Digoxin is a cardiac glycoside, a class of drugs with common specific effects on the myocardium. Glycosides with positive inotropic actions on the diseased heart occur widely in nature and/or can be prepared synthetically. Cardiac glycosides of medicinal importance have been obtained from *Digitalis purpurea* Linné (Fam. *Scrophulariaceae*) (digitoxin, digitalis, gitalin), *Digitalis lanata* Ehrhart (Fam. *Scrophulariaceae*) (digoxin, digitoxin, lanatoside C, deslanoside, acetyldigitoxin), *Strophanthus gratus* (ouabain), and *Acokanthera schimperi* (ouabain). The term "digitalis" is sometimes used to designate the entire class of cardiac glycosides. Currently, digoxin is the only cardiac glycoside commercially available in the US.

Cardiac glycosides have a characteristic ring structure known as an aglycone (or genin) coupled with one or more types of sugars. The aglycone portion of the glycoside consists of a steroid nucleus (cyclopentanoperhydrophenanthrene nucleus) and an α,β-unsaturated 5- or 6-membered lactone ring at the C 17 position of the steroid nucleus. A β-oriented hydroxyl substitution usually is present at the C 3 and C 14 positions. Increasing the number of hydroxyl groups on the aglycone increases polarity and decreases lipid solubility; additional sugars also may increase polarity. The sugar portion of the glycoside is attached to the steroid nucleus, usually through a hydroxyl group at the C 3 position. The sugar moiety affects in part the activity of the cardiac glycoside by influencing solubility, absorption, distribution, and toxicity.

Digoxin has an hydroxyl group at the C 12 position and a tridigitoxose at the C 3 position.

Digoxin occurs as clear to white crystals or as a white, crystalline powder and has a bitter taste. Digoxin is practically insoluble in water, slightly soluble in diluted alcohol, and very slightly soluble in 40% propylene glycol. The pH of commercially available digoxin injection is 6.8–7.2.

■ **Stability** Digoxin preparations should be protected from light and stored at 20–25°C.

Digoxin injection is compatible with most commercially available IV infusion fluids. Before IV administration, digoxin injection may be diluted with a fourfold or greater volume of sterile water for injection, 5% dextrose injection, or 0.9% sodium chloride injection; use of less than a fourfold volume of diluent may cause precipitation of digoxin. Diluted solutions of digoxin should be used immediately.

Solutions of digoxin have been reported to be physically incompatible with other drugs, but the compatibility depends on several factors (e.g., concentrations of the drugs, specific diluents used, resulting pH, temperature). Specialized references should be consulted for specific compatibility information.

Preparations

Excipients in commercially available drug preparations may have clinically important effects in some individuals; consult specific product labeling for details.

Digoxin

Oral		
Solution	50 mcg/mL*	**Digoxin Oral Solution**
Tablets	62.5 mcg	**Lanoxin®**, Concordia
	125 mcg*	**Digitek®**, Mylan
		Digoxin Tablets
		Lanoxin® (scored), Concordia
	187.5 mcg	**Lanoxin®**, Concordia
	250 mcg*	**Digitek®**, Mylan
		Digoxin Tablets
		Lanoxin® (scored), Concordia
Parenteral		
Injection	100 mcg/mL	**Lanoxin® Injection Pediatric**, Covis
	250 mcg/mL*	**Digoxin Injection**
		Lanoxin®, Covis

*available from one or more manufacturer, distributor, and/or repackager by generic (nonproprietary) name

†Use is not currently included in the labeling approved by the US Food and Drug Administration

CARDIAC DRUGS, MISCELLANEOUS 24:04.92

Ivabradine Hydrochloride

■ Ivabradine hydrochloride, a hyperpolarization activated cyclic nucleotide-gated (HCN) channel (funny-channel [f-channel]) blocking agent, is a sinoatrial modulator.

Uses

■ **Heart Failure** Ivabradine is used to reduce the risk of hospitalization for worsening heart failure in patients with stable, symptomatic, mild to severe chronic heart failure (New York Heart Association [NYHA] class II–IV) with reduced ejection fraction (left ventricular ejection fraction [LVEF] of 35% or less), who are in sinus rhythm with a resting heart rate of 70 beats/minute or more and are either on maximally tolerated dosages of a β-adrenergic blocking agent (β-blocker) or have a contraindication to β-blocker use.

Current guidelines for the management of heart failure in adults generally recommend a combination of drug therapies to reduce morbidity and mortality, including neurohormonal antagonists (e.g., angiotensin-converting enzyme [ACE] inhibitors, angiotensin II receptor antagonists, angiotensin receptor-neprilysin inhibitors [ARNIs], β-blockers, aldosterone receptor antagonists) that inhibit the detrimental compensatory mechanisms in heart failure. (See Uses: Heart Failure, in Enalapril 24:32.04 and in Sacubitril and Valsartan 24:32.92.) Additional agents (e.g., cardiac glycosides, diuretics, sinoatrial modulators [i.e., ivabradine]) added to a heart failure treatment regimen in selected patients have been associated with symptomatic improvement and/or reduction in heart-failure related hospitalizations. Experts recommend that all *asymptomatic* patients with reduced LVEF (i.e., American College of Cardiology Foundation [ACCF]/American Heart Association [AHA] stage B heart failure) receive therapy with an ACE inhibitor and a β-blocker to prevent symptomatic heart failure and to reduce morbidity and mortality. In patients *with prior or current symptoms* of chronic heart failure with reduced LVEF (ACCF/AHA stage C heart failure), ACCF, AHA, and the Heart Failure Society of America (HFSA) recommend inhibition of the renin-angiotensin-aldosterone (RAA) system with an ACE inhibitor, angiotensin II receptor antagonist, or ARNI in conjunction with a β-blocker, and an aldosterone antagonist in selected patients, to reduce morbidity and mortality. If a patient cannot tolerate a β-blocker or if increasing the dosage of the β-blocker is ineffective, experts suggest that ivabradine be considered in symptomatic patients as an alternative or additional treatment option to reduce heart failure-related hospitalizations. Unlike β-blockers, ivabradine selectively reduces heart rate without any adverse effects on myocardial contractility, left ventricular relaxation, and coronary tone. Ivabradine also has a use-dependent mechanism of action, in which the reduction in heart rate is greater at higher heart rates than at lower heart rates, minimizing the risk of severe bradycardia. (See Description.) Unlike β-blockers, ivabradine has not been shown to reduce cardiovascular mortality. Given the well-established mortality benefits of β-blocker therapy, it remains important to initiate and titrate the dosage of β-blockers upwards to optimal level, as tolerated, before assessing the resting heart rate for consideration of ivabradine therapy.

Efficacy and safety of ivabradine as an adjunct to or a substitute for therapy with a β-blocker in the management of chronic heart failure has been established principally by the results of a randomized, double-blind, placebo-controlled trial (SHIFT) in patients with chronic heart failure receiving standard-of-care therapy at baseline, which included a β-blocker if tolerated. In this trial, ivabradine reduced the risk of the combined end point of hospitalization for worsening heart failure or cardiovascular death by 18% when added to guideline- and evidence-based treatment within 3 months. The trial was conducted in 6558 adults with stable NYHA class II–IV chronic heart failure with an LVEF of 35% or less, who were in sinus rhythm with a resting heart rate of 70 beats/minute or more and had been admitted to the hospital for worsening of heart failure within the previous 12 months. Patients received ivabradine or placebo in addition to standard-of-care therapy that included maximally tolerated dosages of β-blockers. Approximately 89% of enrolled patients received a β-blocker; 26% of patients were receiving guideline-defined target daily dosages of these drugs. The predominant reasons for patients not achieving target dosages of β-blockers were hypotension, fatigue, dyspnea, dizziness, cardiac decompensation, and excessive bradycardia. Approximately 11% of patients did not receive a β-blocker, principally because of chronic obstructive pulmonary disease (COPD), asthma, or hypotension. Most patients' baseline treatment regimens included an ACE inhibitor or angiotensin II receptor antagonist (91% of patients), diuretic (83%), and aldosterone antagonist (60%). The initial dosage of ivabradine was 5 mg twice daily. After a 14-day titration period, the dosage was increased to 7.5 mg twice daily unless the resting heart rate was 60 beats/minute or less. The dosage of ivabradine was adjusted throughout the trial (range: 2.5–7.5 mg twice daily) as tolerated to maintain a resting heart rate of 50–60 beats/minute. The primary end point of the trial was the composite of cardiovascular death or hospital admission for worsening heart failure.

The benefit of ivabradine in the SHIFT trial was attributable mainly to a reduction in the risk of hospitalization for worsening heart failure with ivabradine compared with placebo (15.6 versus 20.2%, respectively). Ivabradine did not have a favorable effect on the mortality component of the primary end point and did not substantially reduce cardiovascular death in the overall treatment population. The beneficial effect of ivabradine on the primary end point appeared to diminish as the dosage of β-blockers increased, with negligible benefit seen in patients taking guideline-defined target dosages of β-blockers. The composite end point of hospitalization for worsening heart failure or cardiovascular death was not substantially reduced by ivabradine in the subgroup of patients receiving at least 50% of the evidence-based target daily dosage of a β-blocker. Ivabradine therapy was associated with an average reduction in heart rate of 15 beats/minute (baseline value 80 beats/minute), which was generally maintained throughout the course of the trial. Patients with heart rates higher than the median were at increased risk of an end point event and exhibited greater event-reducing benefit from ivabradine than those with lower heart rates. A diminishing benefit of ivabradine was also seen in patients with lower baseline heart rates (less than 77 beats/minute). It has been suggested that this diminished benefit may be due to the lower risk of all end points in patients with lower heart rates and/or ivabradine's use-dependent mechanism of action, which may limit the heart rate reduction in patients with lower baseline heart rates. Whether ivabradine can improve patient outcomes when added to optimally managed heart failure therapies has not been established.

■ **Angina** Ivabradine also has been used for the treatment of chronic stable angina pectoris† in patients with normal sinus rhythm as an adjunct to, or a substitute for, β-blockers in patients whose symptoms are inadequately controlled by β-blockers or in those who have a contraindication or intolerance to the drugs. In some clinical trials in patients with chronic stable angina, ivabradine has reduced heart rate, improved exercise capacity, and decreased the number of anginal attacks. Evidence from randomized controlled trials using standard stress testing indicates that ivabradine may be as effective as atenolol or amlodipine in patients with stable coronary artery disease and that adding ivabradine to atenolol therapy may provide better control of heart rate and anginal symptoms. However, clinical trials (e.g., BEAUTIFUL, SIGNIFY) have not demonstrated any benefit of ivabradine in terms of cardiovascular outcomes (e.g., myocardial infarction [MI], cardiovascular death) among patients who have stable coronary artery disease with or without stable heart failure and are receiving guideline-based therapy for angina (e.g., including aspirin, statins, ACE inhibitors, β-blockers). Some clinical trial data suggest that ivabradine should be used with caution in patients with more severe forms of angina due to the possibility of an increased risk of death due to cardiovascular causes or nonfatal MI; however, further study and experience are needed to confirm these findings. Since ivabradine therapy has not been associated with a reduction in cardiovascular mortality, it is important to ensure that dosages of β-blockers (which do reduce cardiovascular mortality) are adjusted to clinically optimal levels before initiating ivabradine therapy.

The BEAUTIFUL trial was a randomized, double-blind placebo-controlled trial evaluating the use of ivabradine in approximately 11,000 patients with coronary artery disease, LVEF less than 40%, and a heart rate of at least 60 beats/minute. Eligible patients had heart failure and/or angina with stable symptoms for at least 3 months and were receiving conventional drug therapy for these conditions at stable dosages for at least 1 month. Patients who received ivabradine were given an initial dosage of 5 mg twice daily, which was increased to 7.5 mg twice daily depending on resting heart rate and tolerability. The primary end point was the composite of time to cardiovascular death, hospitalization for acute MI, or hospitalization for new-onset or worsening heart failure. After a median follow-up of 19 months, the primary composite end point was not reduced with ivabradine therapy. However, in a post hoc analysis of a subgroup of patients with activity-limiting anginal symptoms (e.g., pain, fatigue, palpitations, dyspnea) and a heart rate of at least 70 beats/minute at the time of randomization, ivabradine therapy was associated with reductions in the primary composite end point of cardiovascular death or hospitalization for fatal and nonfatal MI or heart failure and in coronary revascularization; these reductions were observed despite almost all patients in the subgroup receiving concomitant β-blocker therapy.

The findings of the post hoc subgroup analysis in the BEAUTIFUL trial, which were generally considered hypothesis generating, were further evaluated in the SIGNIFY trial in which approximately 19,000 patients with stable coronary artery disease, no clinical heart failure (NYHA class I), and a heart rate of at least 70 beats/minute received ivabradine or placebo in addition to standard therapy. After a median follow-up of 24.1 months, ivabradine did not substantially affect the primary end point (first occurrence of either cardiovascular death or MI). However, in the prespecified subgroup of patients with angina of Canadian Cardiovascular Society (CCS) class II or higher in the SIGNIFY trial, ivabradine increased the absolute risk of the primary composite end point of death from cardiovascular causes or nonfatal MI (7.6 versus 6.5%) compared with placebo, despite improving angina symptoms. The use of β-blockers was not required for inclusion in the SIGNIFY trial, but approximately 83% of patients in the ivabradine and placebo groups received a β-blocker as a part of their therapy. Approximately 12,000 patients in the trial had activity-limiting (CSS Class II or greater) angina. Ivabradine was initiated at a dosage of 7.5 mg twice daily, which could be increased to 10 mg twice daily or decreased to 5 mg twice daily to achieve a target heart rate of 55–60 beats/minute. Further study is needed to evaluate the adverse effects seen in the subgroup analysis of SIGNIFY as these effects may be attributable to the high dosages of ivabradine (10 mg twice daily) used in the trial and potentially exacerbated by concurrent use of drugs that increase ivabradine plasma concentrations and have negative chronotropic actions (e.g., verapamil, diltiazem). However, some experts currently suggest that ivabradine not be used in patients with activity-limiting angina who do not have clinical heart failure.

Dosage and Administration

■ **General** Dosage of ivabradine should be individualized according to the patient's heart rate response and tolerance to a target resting heart rate of 50–60 beats/minute.

■ **Administration** Ivabradine is administered orally twice daily with meals. If a dose is missed, the next dose should be taken at the usual time; the dose should not be doubled to make up for the missed dose. (See Advice to Patients.)

■ **Dosage** Dosage of ivabradine hydrochloride is expressed in terms of ivabradine.

Heart Failure For the management of chronic symptomatic heart failure, the initial dosage of ivabradine is 5 mg twice daily. In patients with a history of conduction defects, or other patients in whom bradycardia could lead to hemodynamic compromise, therapy should be initiated at a dosage of 2.5 mg twice daily. Patients should be assessed 2 weeks after initiation of therapy and the dosage adjusted to achieve a resting heart rate of 50–60 beats/minute. After the initial adjustment period, the dosage may be adjusted as needed based on resting heart rate and tolerability. If the heart rate exceeds 60 beats/minute, the dosage should be increased by 2.5 mg (given twice daily) up to a maximum of 7.5 mg twice daily. If the heart rate is less than 50 beats/minute or if the patient is experiencing signs and symptoms of bradycardia, the dosage should be decreased by 2.5 mg (given twice daily). If a patient is receiving ivabradine 2.5 mg twice daily and their heart rate is less than 50 beats/minute or they are experiencing signs and symptoms of bradycardia, ivabradine therapy should be discontinued.

Angina For the treatment of chronic stable angina†, ivabradine dosages of 2.5–10 mg twice daily have been used. In 2 large clinical trials in patients with stable angina with or without heart failure, ivabradine was initiated at dosages of 5 or 7.5 mg twice daily and titrated after 2–4 weeks to a target heart rate of 50–60 beats/minute. In the BEAUTIFUL trial, if the patient's resting heart rate was less than 50 beats/minute or if signs or symptoms of bradycardia were present, the dosage was titrated downward. In clinical trials, ivabradine was discontinued if the resting heart rate was less than 50 beats/minute or if signs or symptoms related to bradycardia were present despite reduction of ivabradine dosage.

Specific Populations **Hepatic Impairment** No dosage adjustment is required in patients with mild or moderate hepatic impairment. Ivabradine is contraindicated in patients with severe hepatic impairment (Child-Pugh class C) as safety and efficacy have not been established in this population and an increase in systemic exposure is expected. (See Cautions: Contraindications.)

Renal Impairment No dosage adjustment is required in patients with creatinine clearance 15–60 mL/minute. Data are lacking on use of ivabradine in patients with creatinine clearance less than 15 mL/minute.

Cautions

■ **Contraindications** Acute decompensated heart failure.

Blood pressure less than 90/50 mm Hg.

Heart rate less than 60 beats/minute prior to treatment.

Severe hepatic impairment. (See Hepatic Impairment under Warnings/Precautions: Specific Populations, in Cautions.)

Pacemaker dependence (heart rate maintained exclusively by the pacemaker).

Concomitant use of potent cytochrome P-450 (CYP) isoenzyme 3A4 inhibitors. (See Drug Interactions: Drugs and Foods Affecting Hepatic Microsomal Enzymes.)

Sick sinus syndrome, sinoatrial (SA) block, or third-degree atrioventricular (AV) block (unless a functioning demand pacemaker is present).

■ **Warnings/Precautions** ***Fetal Toxicity*** Based on findings in animal studies, ivabradine may cause fetal toxicity and teratogenicity when administered to pregnant women. Embryofetal toxicity and cardiac teratogenic effects (abnormal shape of the heart, interventricular septal defect, complex anomalies of primary arteries) were observed in fetuses of pregnant rats treated with ivabradine during organogenesis at exposures 1–3 times the human exposures at the maximum recommended human dose. Reduced fetal and placental weights and teratogenic effects (ectrodactylia) were observed in pregnant rabbits treated with ivabradine during organogenesis at exposures 15 times the human exposures at the maximum recommended human dose.

Women of childbearing potential should be advised to use effective contraception while taking ivabradine. (See Advice to Patients.)

Atrial Fibrillation Ivabradine increases the risk of atrial fibrillation. In the SHIFT trial, the rate of atrial fibrillation was 5 versus 3.9% per patient-year in patients treated with ivabradine or placebo, respectively. Results of a meta-analysis evaluating clinical trial data from 11 studies indicated a 15% increase in the relative risk of atrial fibrillation with ivabradine therapy. Patients receiving ivabradine should receive regular cardiac rhythm monitoring and the drug should be discontinued if atrial fibrillation occurs.

Bradycardia and Conduction Disturbances Bradycardia, sinus arrest, and heart block have occurred with ivabradine therapy. The rate of bradycardia was 6% per patient-year with ivabradine (2.7% symptomatic; 3.4% asymptomatic) and 1.3% per patient-year with placebo. Risk factors for bradycardia include sinus node dysfunction, conduction defects (e.g., first or second degree AV block, bundle branch block), ventricular dyssynchrony, and the use of other negative chronotropes (e.g., digoxin, diltiazem, verapamil, amiodarone). Concurrent use of verapamil or diltiazem can increase ivabradine exposure, may contribute to heart rate lowering, and should be avoided. (See Drug Interactions: Calcium-channel Blocking Agents.)

Ivabradine should be avoided in patients with second degree AV block, unless a functioning demand pacemaker is present. (See Cautions: Contraindications.) Patients with demand pacemakers set to a rate of 60 beats/minute or more cannot achieve a target heart rate less than 60 beats/minute, and these patients were excluded from clinical trials. The use of ivabradine is not recommended in patients with demand pacemakers set to rates of 60 beats/minute or higher.

Sensitivity Reactions **Hypersensitivity.** Hypersensitivity reactions (e.g., angioedema, erythema, rash, pruritus, urticaria) have been reported during postmarketing experience in patients receiving ivabradine.

Specific Populations **Pregnancy.** There are no adequate and well-controlled studies of ivabradine in pregnant women. Studies in rats and rabbits indicate that ivabradine can cause fetal harm when administered to pregnant women. (See Fetal Toxicity under Cautions: Warnings/Precautions.) Increased postnatal mortality was associated with the teratogenic effects seen in rats. In pregnant rabbits, increased postimplantation loss was observed at an exposure 5 times the human exposure at the maximum recommended human dose. Pregnant women receiving ivabradine should be informed of the potential risk to the fetus.

Stroke volume and heart rate increase during pregnancy, which increases cardiac output, especially during the first trimester. Pregnant patients with left ventricular ejection fraction (LVEF) less than 35% on maximally tolerated dosages of β-adrenergic blocking agents (β-blockers) may be particularly dependent on increases in heart rate for augmentation of cardiac output. Therefore, pregnant patients taking ivabradine, especially during the first trimester, should be closely monitored for destabilization of their heart failure that could result from heart rate slowing. Pregnant women with chronic heart failure in their third trimester of pregnancy should be monitored for preterm birth.

Lactation. Ivabradine is distributed into milk in rats; it is not known whether ivabradine is distributed into human milk. Because of the potential risk to breast-fed infants from exposure to ivabradine, breast-feeding is not recommended.

Pediatric Use. Safety and efficacy have not been established in patients younger than 18 years of age.

Geriatric Use. No pharmacokinetic differences with ivabradine have been observed in patients 65 years of age or older compared with the overall population. However, there is limited experience with ivabradine in patients 75 years of age or older.

Renal Impairment. Renal impairment (creatinine clearance 15–60 mL/minute) has minimal effect on the pharmacokinetics of ivabradine. Data are lacking on use of ivabradine in patients with creatinine clearance less than 15 mL/minute.

Hepatic Impairment. In patients with mild or moderate hepatic impairment, the pharmacokinetics of ivabradine were similar to that in patients with normal hepatic function. Safety and efficacy have not been established in patients with severe hepatic impairment (Child-Pugh class C); use is contraindicated in these patients as increased systemic exposure is anticipated. (See Cautions: Contraindications.)

■ **Common Adverse Effects** Adverse effects reported in more than 1% of patients receiving ivabradine in the SHIFT trial and occurring at least 1% more frequently with ivabradine than with placebo include bradycardia, hypertension, atrial fibrillation, and phosphenes/visual brightness. Phosphenes are described as a transiently enhanced brightness in a limited area of the visual field, or as halos, image decomposition (stroboscopic or kaleidoscopic effects), colored bright lights, or multiple images (retinal persistency). Phosphenes generally are triggered by sudden changes in light intensity. Phosphenes generally become apparent within the first 2 months of treatment, after which they may occur repeatedly. This phenomenon generally has been of mild to moderate intensity and usually has resolved during or after ivabradine treatment.

Drug Interactions

■ **Drugs and Foods Affecting Hepatic Microsomal Enzymes** Ivabradine is metabolized principally by cytochrome P-450 (CYP) isoenzyme 3A4. The major metabolite of ivabradine is the *N*-desmethylated derivative (S 18982), which is also metabolized by CYP3A4. Drugs that inhibit or induce CYP3A4 can increase or decrease, respectively, ivabradine plasma concentrations; increased concentrations may exacerbate bradycardia and conduction disturbances. Concomitant use of potent CYP3A4 inhibitors such as azole antifungal agents, macrolide antibiotics, HIV protease inhibitors, and nefazodone is contraindicated. (See Cautions: Contraindications.) The concomitant use of moderate CYP3A4 inhibitors such as diltiazem, verapamil, and grapefruit juice should be avoided. Inducers of CYP3A4 such as St. John's wort (*Hypericum perforatum*), rifampin, barbiturates, and phenytoin also should be avoided during ivabradine therapy.

■ **Azole Antifungal Agents** Concomitant use of ivabradine and potent CYP3A4 inhibitors such as azole antifungal agents (e.g., itraconazole, ketoconazole) increases the plasma concentrations of ivabradine and is contraindicated. (See Cautions: Contraindications.)

■ **Calcium-channel Blocking Agents** Concomitant use of ivabradine and moderate CYP3A4 inhibitors such as diltiazem and verapamil increases plasma ivabradine concentrations and should be avoided. Calcium-channel blocking agents such as diltiazem and verapamil that act as negative chronotropes also may increase the risk of bradycardia. Heart rate should be monitored in patients taking ivabradine with other negative chronotropes.

■ **HIV Protease Inhibitors** Concomitant use of ivabradine and potent CYP3A4 inhibitors such as HIV protease inhibitors (e.g., nelfinavir) increases plasma concentrations of ivabradine and is contraindicated. (See Cautions: Contraindications.)

■ **Macrolide Antibiotics** Concomitant use of ivabradine and potent CYP3A4 inhibitors such as macrolide antibiotics (e.g., clarithromycin, telithromycin) increases plasma concentrations of ivabradine and is contraindicated. (See Cautions: Contraindications.)

■ **Metformin** Ivabradine (10 mg twice daily dosed to steady state) did not affect the pharmacokinetics of concomitantly administered metformin, an organic cation transporter (OCT2) sensitive substrate. No dosage adjustment is required for metformin when administered with ivabradine.

■ **Nefazodone** Concomitant use of ivabradine and potent CYP3A4 inhibitors such as nefazodone increases plasma concentrations of ivabradine and is contraindicated. (See Cautions: Contraindications.)

■ **Negative Chronotropes** The risk of bradycardia increases with concomitant administration of drugs that slow heart rate (e.g., digoxin, amiodarone, β-adrenergic blocking agents [β-blockers]). Heart rate should be monitored in patients taking ivabradine with other negative chronotropes. Digoxin exposure did not change when used concomitantly with ivabradine.

■ **Proton-pump Inhibitors** Concomitant administration of lansoprazole (60 mg daily) or omeprazole (40 mg daily) did not have a clinically important effect on the pharmacokinetics of ivabradine; no dosage adjustment is required.

■ **Sildenafil** Sildenafil (100 mg) did not have a clinically important effect on the pharmacokinetics of ivabradine; no dosage adjustment is required.

■ **Simvastatin** Simvastatin (20 mg daily) did not have a clinically important effect on the pharmacokinetics of ivabradine; no dosage adjustment is required.

■ **Warfarin** Warfarin (1–5 mg daily) did not have a clinically important effect on the pharmacokinetics of ivabradine; no dosage adjustment is required.

Description

Ivabradine is a hyperpolarization-activated cyclic nucleotide-gated (HCN) channel (funny-channel [f-channel]) blocking agent that reduces the spontaneous pacemaker activity of the sinoatrial (SA) node by selectively inhibiting the funny-current (I_f) in pacemaker cells, resulting in heart rate reduction with no effect on ventricular repolarization or myocardial contractility.

The f-channels are part of the HCN channel family, which is comprised of many distinct isoforms (HCN 1–4), and are expressed in the heart and nervous system. The HCN4 channel is found in the heart and is active in the pacemaker cells of the SA node. The f-channels, unlike other voltage-gated ion channels, open with hyperpolarization rather than depolarization and have a mixed permeability to sodium and potassium ions. These channels open and close in response to ambient voltage and local intracellular cyclic adenosine monophosphate (cAMP) concentrations. Adrenergic agonists activate adenylate cyclase, which causes an increase in intracellular cAMP, whereas cholinergic transmitters decrease local cAMP by inhibiting adenylate cyclase. Intracellular cAMP acts as a second messenger and favors f-channel opening by direct binding to the c-terminus of the channel, which induces a depolarizing shift of the activation curve, leading to an increase in the number of open f-channels. The I_f current, which is a mixed sodium-potassium current, is able to move across open f-channels; this causes a deeper slope of diastolic depolarization and a reduction in diastolic duration, leading to an elevation in heart rate.

Ivabradine has a unique mechanism of action in that it displays state-dependent, use-dependent, and current-dependent properties. Ivabradine enters cardiac pacemaker cells and blocks the f-channel from the cytoplasmic side of the membrane preferentially when the channel is in an open state (state-dependence) and is more efficient at depolarized than hyperpolarized voltages. Therefore, the interaction between ivabradine and the f-channel binding site is dependent upon the rate of opening and closing of the channels in response to repolarization and depolarization (i.e., related to heart rate). As a result of this use-dependent inhibition, the reduction in pacemaker activity by ivabradine is more pronounced at higher firing rates in the SA node. Ivabradine also displays a current-dependence property by which ivabradine is drawn to the binding site of the f-channel by the electrostatic forces generated by the depolarization process and dissociates from the binding site in response to the inward current generated from the repolarization process. The blockade of f-channels by ivabradine inhibits the I_f current, which leads to a reduction in the slow diastolic depolarization phase of the SA node action potential, thereby reducing heart rate. The selective binding of ivabradine to f-channels makes it a pure heart-rate-reducing agent. Reduction in heart rate with ivabradine decreases myocardial oxygen consumption and increases oxygen supply due to prolongation of diastolic perfusion time.

The adverse effects of ivabradine on vision are due to interaction of ivabradine with retinal ion channels (I_h current), which closely resemble the I_f channels in the SA node. The I_h current is involved in curtailing retinal responses to bright light stimuli. Under circumstances that trigger these I_h channels (e.g., rapid changes in luminosity), partial inhibition of the I_h current by ivabradine may cause the luminous phenomena experienced by some patients. (See Cautions: Common Adverse Effects.)

Following oral administration, peak plasma concentrations of ivabradine are reached in approximately 1 hour under fasting conditions. Food delays absorption by approximately 1 hour and increases plasma ivabradine exposure by 20–40%; therefore, it is recommended that the drug be taken with meals to reduce individual variability in systemic exposure. (See Dosage and Administration: Administration.) The absolute oral bioavailability of ivabradine is approximately 40% due to first-pass elimination in gut and liver via cytochrome P-450 (CYP) isoenzyme 3A4-mediated oxidation. The major metabolite of ivabradine is the *N*-desmethylated derivative (S 18982), which is equipotent to ivabradine and circulates at concentrations approximately 40% that of ivabradine and is also metabolized by CYP3A4. Ivabradine has a low affinity for CYP3A4 and does not modify CYP3A4 substrate metabolism or plasma concentrations. Conversely, potent inhibitors and inducers may substantially affect ivabradine's bioavailability and plasma concentrations. (See Drug Interactions: Drugs and Foods Affecting Hepatic Microsomal Enzymes.) Ivabradine is approximately 70% bound to plasma proteins. Ivabradine plasma concentrations decline with a distribution half-life of 2 hours and an effective half-life of approximately 6 hours.

Advice to Patients

Importance of advising patients to read the FDA-approved patient labeling (medication guide).

Importance of women informing clinicians if they are or plan to become pregnant or plan to breast-feed. Importance of advising females of reproductive potential to use effective contraception and to notify their healthcare provider about a known or suspected pregnancy. Importance of informing pregnant women about the potential risks to the fetus.

Importance of advising patients to report substantial decreases in heart rate or symptoms such as dizziness, fatigue, or hypotension.

Importance of advising patients to report symptoms of atrial fibrillation, such as heart palpitations or racing pulse, chest pressure, or worsened shortness of breath. Importance of patients receiving regular cardiac rhythm monitoring.

Importance of advising patients about the possible occurrence of luminous phenomena (phosphenes) in the field of vision. Importance of advising patients to use caution if they are driving or using machines in situations where sudden changes in light intensity could occur, especially when driving at night. Importance of informing patients that phosphenes may subside spontaneously during continued treatment with ivabradine.

Importance of informing clinician of existing or contemplated concomitant therapy, including prescription and OTC drugs, as well as any concomitant diseases. Importance of advising patients to avoid ingestion of grapefruit juice or St. John's wort.

Importance of advising patients to take ivabradine twice daily with meals. If a dose is missed, the next dose should be taken at the usual time; the dose should not be doubled to make up for the missed dose.

Importance of informing patients of other important precautionary information. (See Cautions.)

Overview® (see Users Guide). For additional information on this drug until a more detailed monograph is developed and published, the manufacturer's labeling should be consulted. It is *essential* that the manufacturer's labeling be consulted for more detailed information on usual cautions, precautions, contraindications, potential drug interactions, laboratory test interferences, and acute toxicity.

Preparations

Excipients in commercially available drug preparations may have clinically important effects in some individuals; consult specific product labeling for details.

Ivabradine Hydrochloride

Oral		
Tablets (film-coated)	5 mg (of ivabradine)	Corlanor®, Amgen
	7.5 mg (of ivabradine)	Corlanor®, Amgen

†Use is not currently included in the labeling approved by the US Food and Drug Administration

ANTILIPEMIC AGENTS 24:06

CHOLESTEROL ABSORPTION INHIBITORS 24:06.05

Ezetimibe

■ Ezetimibe, a cholesterol absorption inhibitor, is an antilipemic agent.

Uses

■ **Dyslipidemias** Ezetimibe is used alone or in combination with other antilipemic agents (i.e., a hydroxymethylglutaryl-coenzyme A [HMG-CoA] reductase inhibitor [statin], fenofibrate) as an adjunct to dietary therapy in the treatment of primary hyperlipidemia and mixed dyslipidemia, homozygous familial hypercholesterolemia, and/or homozygous familial sitosterolemia. Efficacy of ezetimibe, alone or in fixed combination with simvastatin, in patients with Fredrickson type I, III, IV, or V dyslipidemias has not been established.

Effects of ezetimibe on cardiovascular morbidity and mortality have not been established.

The American College of Cardiology (ACC)/American Heart Association (AHA) guideline for management of blood cholesterol to reduce atherosclerotic cardiovascular risk in adults states that nondrug therapies (i.e., lifestyle modifications), which include adherence to a heart-healthy diet, regular exercise, avoidance of tobacco products, and maintenance of a healthy weight, are the foundation of atherosclerotic cardiovascular disease (ASCVD) prevention. Drug therapy is not a substitute for but an adjunct to these nondrug therapies and measures, which should be continued when drug therapy is initiated. For additional details on lifestyle modifications, consult the most recent AHA/ACC Guideline on Lifestyle Management to Reduce Cardiovascular Risk (available at http://www.cardiosource.org or http://my.americanheart.org).

The ACC/AHA cholesterol management guideline states that nonstatin therapies (e.g., ezetimibe) do not provide acceptable ASCVD risk reduction benefits compared to their potential for adverse effects in the routine prevention of ASCVD. However, nonstatin drugs may be useful as adjuncts to statin therapy in high-risk patients (e.g., patients with ASCVD, low-density lipoprotein [LDL]-cholesterol concentrations of at least 190 mg/dL, or diabetes mellitus) who have a less-than-anticipated response to statins, are unable to tolerate a less-than-recommended intensity of a statin, or are completely intolerant to statin therapy, particularly when there is evidence from randomized controlled studies suggesting that the nonstatin drug further reduces ASCVD events when added to statin therapy. When a nonstatin drug is required, selection of the nonstatin drug should be based on a favorable benefit-risk ratio (i.e., demonstrated benefit of ASCVD risk reduction outweighs risks of adverse effects and drug interactions) and patient preferences. For additional details on prevention of ASCVD, see the HMG-CoA Reductase Inhibitors General Statement 24:06.08 and also consult the most recent ACC/AHA Guideline on the Treatment of Blood Cholesterol to Reduce Atherosclerotic Cardiovascular Risk in Adults (available at http://www.cardiosource.org or http://my.americanheart.org).

Primary Hyperlipidemia and Mixed Dyslipidemia Ezetimibe is used alone or in combination with a statin as an adjunct to dietary therapy to decrease elevated serum total cholesterol, LDL-cholesterol, apolipoprotein B (apo B), and non-high-density lipoprotein (non-HDL)-cholesterol concentrations in the treatment of primary (heterozygous familial and nonfamilial) hyperlipidemia. Ezetimibe in fixed combination with simvastatin (Vytorin®) is used as an adjunct to dietary therapy to decrease elevated serum total cholesterol, LDL-cholesterol, apo B, triglyceride, and non-HDL-cholesterol concentrations, and to increase HDL-cholesterol concentrations in the treatment of primary hyperlipidemia or mixed dyslipidemia. Ezetimibe also is used in combination with fenofibrate as an adjunct to dietary therapy to decrease elevated serum total cholesterol, LDL-cholesterol, apo B, and non-HDL-cholesterol concentrations in the treatment of mixed dyslipidemia.

Efficacy and safety of ezetimibe monotherapy in the management of primary hyperlipidemia were established in 2 multicenter, randomized, double-blind, placebo-controlled studies of 12 weeks' duration in approximately 1700 patients with primary hyperlipidemia. In these studies, patients who received ezetimibe (10 mg daily) had mean reductions of approximately 12–13% in total cholesterol, 18% in LDL-cholesterol, 15–16% in apo B, 16% in non-HDL-cholesterol, and 7–9% in triglyceride concentrations; increases in high-density lipoprotein (HDL)-cholesterol concentrations in patients receiving ezetimibe were negligible (1%). In most patients with primary hyperlipidemia, maximal or near-maximal reductions in serum lipoprotein and apolipoprotein concentrations are achieved within 2 weeks and maintained during continued therapy. Reductions in LDL-cholesterol concentrations appear to be consistent across age, gender, and baseline LDL-cholesterol concentrations.

Data from several multicenter, randomized, double-blind, placebo-controlled studies indicate that concomitant therapy with ezetimibe and a statin may produce additive antilipemic effects. In a study in patients with primary hyperlipidemia and either multiple cardiovascular risk factors or documented coronary heart disease (CHD) who had not achieved their target LDL-cholesterol goal with diet and statin monotherapy, addition of ezetimibe (10 mg daily) to existing statin therapy reduced total cholesterol, LDL-cholesterol, apo B, non-HDL-cholesterol, and triglyceride concentrations by an additional 17, 25, 19, 23, and 14%, respectively, at 8 weeks and increased HDL-cholesterol concentrations by an additional 3% compared with statin monotherapy. For patients whose LDL-cholesterol levels were above the target levels recommended by the Second Report of the National Cholesterol Education Program (NCEP) (Adult Treatment Panel [ATP] II), approximately 72% of patients receiving combination therapy achieved their target LDL-cholesterol goal compared with 19% of those receiving statin monotherapy. In 4 multicenter, randomized, double-blind, placebo-controlled studies in hyperlipidemic patients, combination therapy with ezetimibe (10 mg daily) and a statin (i.e., atorvastatin 10–80 mg daily, lovastatin 10–40 mg daily, pravastatin 10–40 mg daily, or simvastatin 10–80 mg daily), initiated concurrently and continued for 12 weeks, reduced total cholesterol, LDL-cholesterol, apo B, non-HDL-cholesterol, and triglyceride concentrations and, except for the combination of ezetimibe and pravastatin, increased HDL-cholesterol concentrations compared with monotherapy with the corresponding statin. Following combination therapy with ezetimibe and either atorvastatin, simvastatin, pravastatin, or lovastatin, total reductions in LDL-cholesterol concentrations averaged 53–61, 46–58%, 34–42, or 34–46, respectively, compared with reductions of 37–54, 27–45, 21–31, or 20–30% with atorvastatin, simvastatin, pravastatin, or lovastatin monotherapy, respectively. Results of one study in patients with known CHD or CHD risk equivalents indicated that reductions in LDL-cholesterol concentrations achieved with the combination of ezetimibe 10 mg and simvastatin 10 mg (47%) were greater than those achieved with simvastatin 20 mg alone (38%).

Similar additive antilipemic effects were observed following therapy with the fixed-combination preparation containing ezetimibe and simvastatin. Data from several randomized, double-blind studies in patients with primary hyperlipidemia indicated that reductions in LDL-cholesterol concentrations achieved with pooled doses of the fixed-combination preparation were greater than those achieved with pooled doses of atorvastatin, rosuvastatin, or simvastatin monotherapy. In one study, LDL-cholesterol concentrations were reduced by 47–59% following therapy with the fixed-combination preparation containing ezetimibe (10 mg) and simvastatin (10–80 mg) and by 36–53% following monotherapy with atorvastatin (10–80 mg daily). In another study, LDL-cholesterol concentrations were reduced by 52–61% following therapy with the fixed-combination preparation containing ezetimibe (10 mg) and simvastatin (20–80 mg) and by 46–57% following monotherapy with rosuvastatin (10–40 mg daily). In the third study, LDL-cholesterol concentrations were reduced by 45–60% following therapy with the fixed-combination preparation containing ezetimibe (10 mg) and simvastatin (10–80 mg) and by 33–49% following monotherapy with simvastatin (10–80 mg daily).

Despite its additive effects on LDL-cholesterol reduction, early findings from a randomized, double-blind, active-controlled study (Ezetimibe and Simvastatin in Hypercholesterolemia Enhances Atherosclerosis Regression [ENHANCE]) in patients with heterozygous familial hypercholesterolemia indicated that the fixed-combination preparation containing ezetimibe and simvastatin (10 and 80 mg daily, respectively) was *not* superior to simvastatin monotherapy (80 mg daily) in reducing carotid intimal-medial wall thickness (cIMT). In this study, treatment with the fixed-combination preparation for 2 years resulted in a change in cIMT (increase of 0.011 mm) that was not statistically different from the change in cIMT observed with simvastatin monotherapy (increase of 0.006 mm). However, reductions in LDL-cholesterol concentrations achieved with the fixed-combination preparation (56%) were substantially greater than those achieved with simvastatin monotherapy (39%). Although the greater reductions in LDL-cholesterol concentrations did not translate into substantial improvement in cIMT in the ENHANCE study, the cardiovascular benefits of reducing LDL-cholesterol concentrations are well established and have been demonstrated in other studies.

The addition of ezetimibe to simvastatin therapy resulted in further LDL-cholesterol lowering and improved cardiovascular outcomes in the Improved Reduction of Outcomes: Vytorin® Efficacy International (IMPROVE-IT) study. IMPROVE-IT was a large randomized, double-blind study in 18,144 patients who had been hospitalized for an acute coronary syndrome in the preceding 10 days and had baseline LDL-cholesterol concentrations of 50–125 mg/dL (or 50–100 mg/dL if they were receiving lipid-lowering therapy). Patients were randomized to receive the fixed-combination preparation containing ezetimibe and simvastatin (10 and 40 mg daily, respectively) or simvastatin monotherapy (40 mg daily). After a median duration of follow-up of 6 years, the fixed-combination preparation produced a 24% further reduction in mean LDL-cholesterol concentration and also reduced the rate of the primary end point (composite of cardiovascular death, nonfatal myocardial infarction [MI], unstable angina requiring hospitalization, coronary revascularization, or nonfatal stroke) compared with simvastatin monotherapy; the absolute risk reduction for the primary composite outcome was 2% over 7 years. The treatment benefit of combined simvastatin/ezetimibe therapy began to emerge after 1 year and appeared to be particularly pronounced in patients with diabetes mellitus and geriatric patients (75 years of age or older).

The combination of ezetimibe and fenofibrate has been shown to reduce total and LDL-cholesterol, apo B, and non-HDL-cholesterol concentrations in patients with mixed dyslipidemia. In a randomized, double-blind, placebo-controlled study in patients with mixed dyslipidemia, combination therapy with ezetimibe and fenofibrate (160 mg daily) was superior to fenofibrate monotherapy in reducing total cholesterol (22 versus 11%), LDL-cholesterol (20 versus 6%), apo B (26 versus 15%), and non-HDL-cholesterol (30 versus 16%) concentrations at 12 weeks. Effects on triglyceride and HDL-cholesterol concentrations in patients receiving combination therapy were comparable to those in patients receiving fenofibrate monotherapy. Following an additional 48 weeks of combination therapy or monotherapy, changes in lipoprotein concentrations were consistent with those observed at 12 weeks of therapy. The manufacturer states that efficacy and safety of ezetimibe in combination with a fibric acid derivative other than fenofibrate have not been studied and currently is not recommended. (See Fibric Acid Derivatives under Drug Interactions: Antilipemic Agents.)

Patients with Chronic Kidney Disease In the Study of Heart and Renal Protection (SHARP), the fixed-combination preparation containing ezetimibe and simvastatin was shown to reduce the risk of major vascular and atherosclerotic events in patients with chronic kidney disease, a population known to be at increased risk of cardiovascular disease. More than 9000 patients with moderate to severe chronic kidney disease (33% receiving dialysis) and no known history of MI or coronary revascularization were initially randomized in a 4:4:1 ratio to receive the fixed-combination preparation containing ezetimibe and simvastatin (10 and 20 mg daily, respectively), placebo, or simvastatin alone (20 mg daily) for 1 year to assess the safety of adding ezetimibe to simvastatin; patients in the simvastatin monotherapy group were then re-randomized to the fixed-combination preparation or placebo. After a median duration of follow up of 4.9 years, the risk of a major vascular event (nonfatal MI or cardiac death, stroke, or revascularization excluding dialysis access procedures) was reduced by 16% (based on the primary intent-to-treat analysis in patients initially randomized to the fixed-combination preparation or placebo groups) and the risk of a major atherosclerotic event (nonfatal MI or cardiac death, nonhemorrhagic stroke, or arterial revascularization excluding dialysis access procedures) was reduced by 17% (based on the total number of patients randomized at any time to the fixed-combination preparation or placebo groups) with the fixed-combination preparation compared with placebo. The treatment effect was largely driven by a substantial reduction in ischemic strokes and arterial revascularization procedures. The subgroup of patients receiving dialysis at baseline experienced a smaller risk reduction benefit compared with those not receiving dialysis. In addition, therapy with the fixed-combination preparation did not appear to slow the progression to end-stage renal disease.

Homozygous Familial Hypercholesterolemia Ezetimibe may be used in combination with atorvastatin or simvastatin to decrease elevated serum total and LDL-cholesterol concentrations in patients with homozygous familial hypercholesterolemia as an adjunct to other lipid-lowering therapies (e.g., plasma LDL apheresis) or when such therapies are not available.

Efficacy and safety of ezetimibe combined with atorvastatin or simvastatin for the management of homozygous familial hypercholesterolemia were established in a randomized, double-blind study of 12 weeks' duration in a limited number of patients with a clinical and/or genotypic diagnosis of homozygous familial hypercholesterolemia who were already receiving atorvastatin (40 mg daily) or simvastatin (40 mg daily), with or without concomitant LDL apheresis. In this study, patients were randomized to receive 1 of 3 regimens: atorvastatin (80 mg daily) or simvastatin (80 mg daily) monotherapy; ezetimibe (10 mg daily) with either atorvastatin (40 mg daily) or simvastatin (40 mg daily); or ezetimibe (10 mg daily) with either atorvastatin (80 mg daily) or simvastatin (80 mg daily). The addition of ezetimibe (10 mg daily) to therapy with atorvastatin (40 or 80 mg daily) or simvastatin (40 or 80 mg daily) was more effective in reducing LDL-cholesterol concentrations (21% additional reduction based on pooled data from 40-mg and 80-mg groups) than increasing the dosage of atorvastatin or simvastatin monotherapy from 40 to 80 mg daily (7% additional reduction based on pooled data from 40-mg and 80-mg groups).

In the entire group of patients receiving higher dosages (80 mg daily) of either atorvastatin or simvastatin in combination with ezetimibe (10 mg daily), LDL-cholesterol concentrations were reduced by approximately 27% compared with a 7% reduction with statin monotherapy. Comparable reductions in LDL-cholesterol concentrations were observed in the subgroup of patients with genotype-confirmed homozygous familial hypercholesterolemia.

Beneficial effects of ezetimibe combined with atorvastatin or simvastatin in patients with homozygous familial hypercholesterolemia who currently are undergoing LDL apheresis compared with effects in patients not undergoing the procedure have not been established. Effects on clinical outcome and modification of other disease parameters (e.g., xanthoma formation, regression of atherosclerosis) also have not been established.

Homozygous Familial Sitosterolemia (Phytosterolemia) Ezetimibe is used as an adjunct to dietary therapy to decrease elevated serum sitosterol and campesterol concentrations in patients with homozygous familial sitosterolemia.

Efficacy and safety of ezetimibe in the management of homozygous sitosterolemia were established in a randomized, double-blind study of 8 weeks' duration in a limited number of patients with homozygous sitosterolemia who had plasma sitosterol concentrations exceeding 5 mg/dL and were already receiving standard antilipemic therapy (dietary therapy, bile acid sequestrants, statins, ileal bypass surgery, and/or LDL apheresis). In this study, treatment with ezetimibe (10 mg daily) reduced plasma sitosterol and campesterol concentrations by 21 and 24%, respectively, compared with increases of 4 and 3% in placebo-treated patients. Reductions in sitosterol and campesterol concentrations were consistent between patients receiving ezetimibe with or without bile acid sequestrants. The effect of reducing plasma concentrations of sitosterol and campesterol on cardiovascular morbidity and mortality has not been established.

For additional information on the role of antilipemic therapy in the treatment of lipoprotein disorders, prevention of cardiovascular events, and other conditions, see General Principles of Antilipemic Therapy in the HMG-CoA Reductase Inhibitors General Statement 24:06.08.

Dosage and Administration

■ Administration Ezetimibe is administered orally without regard to meals. Ezetimibe in fixed combination with simvastatin (Vytorin®) is administered orally in the evening without regard to meals. Patients should be placed on a standard cholesterol-lowering diet before initiation of ezetimibe therapy and should remain on this diet during treatment with the drug. For recommendations on dietary and other nondrug therapies (i.e., lifestyle modifications), consult the most recent American Heart Association (AHA)/American College of Cardiology (ACC) Guideline on Lifestyle Management to Reduce Cardiovascular Risk (available at http://www.cardiosource.org or http://my.americanheart.org).

When used in combination with a hydroxymethylglutaryl-coenzyme A [HMG-CoA] reductase inhibitor (statin) or fenofibrate for additive antilipemic effects, ezetimibe may be administered at the same time as the statin or fenofibrate, in accordance with the recommended dosing schedule for these drugs. When used in combination with a bile acid sequestrant, ezetimibe should be administered at least 2 hours before or at least 4 hours after administration of the bile acid sequestrant. The manufacturer states that pending further accumulation of data, use of ezetimibe in combination with a fibric acid derivative other than fenofibrate is not recommended. (See Drug Interactions: Antilipemic Agents.)

■ Dosage For the management of primary hyperlipidemia, mixed dyslipidemia, homozygous familial hypercholesterolemia, or homozygous familial sitosterolemia in adults and children 10 years of age and older, the recommended dosage of ezetimibe (alone or in combination with a statin or fenofibrate) is 10 mg once daily without regard to meals.

Ezetimibe/Simvastatin Combination Therapy The recommended initial dosage of the commercially available fixed-combination preparation (Vytorin®) for the management of primary hyperlipidemia or mixed dyslipidemia in adults is 10 mg of ezetimibe and 10 or 20 mg of simvastatin once daily in the evening. Patients requiring reductions in LDL-cholesterol concentration of more than 55% to achieve their goal may receive an initial dosage of 10 mg of ezetimibe and 40 mg of simvastatin once daily in the absence of moderate to severe renal impairment (estimated glomerular filtration rate [GFR] less than 60 mL/minute per 1.73 m²). Serum lipoprotein concentrations should be determined 2 or more weeks after initiation or titration of therapy, and dosage adjusted as needed. The usual maintenance dosage of ezetimibe in fixed combination with simvastatin is 10 mg of ezetimibe and 10–40 mg of simvastatin once daily. Because higher simvastatin dosages (e.g., 80 mg daily) have been associated with a greater risk of myopathy, including rhabdomyolysis, particularly during the first year of treatment, the manufacturer states that patients who are unable to achieve their LDL-cholesterol target goal with the fixed-combination preparation containing 10 mg of ezetimibe and 40 mg of simvastatin should *not* be titrated to the dosage containing 10 mg of ezetimibe and 80 mg of simvastatin but should be switched to alternative antilipemic agents that provide greater LDL-cholesterol reduction. The manufacturer also states that use of the fixed-combination preparation containing 10 mg of ezetimibe and 80 mg of simvastatin should be restricted to patients who have been receiving long-term therapy (e.g., 12 months or longer) at this dosage without evidence of muscle toxicity. (See Cautions.) Patients currently tolerating the fixed-combination preparation containing 10 mg of ezetimibe and 80 mg of simvastatin who require therapy with an interacting drug (i.e., a drug with which concomitant use is contraindicated or is associated with a dose limit for simvastatin) should be switched to an alternative statin or statin-based regimen with less drug interaction potential.

The recommended dosage of ezetimibe in fixed combination with simvastatin for the management of homozygous familial hypercholesterolemia in adults is 10 mg of ezetimibe and 40 mg of simvastatin once daily in the evening. Ezetimibe in fixed combination with simvastatin should be used as an adjunct to other lipid-lowering treatments (e.g., LDL apheresis) in these patients or as an alternative if such therapy is unavailable.

The risk of myopathy appears to be increased among Chinese patients versus non-Chinese patients receiving simvastatin 40 mg daily (alone or in combination with ezetimibe 10 mg daily) concomitantly with preparations containing antilipemic dosages (1 g daily or higher) of niacin. The cause of the increased risk of myopathy is not known, and it is not known whether these findings apply to patients of other Asian ancestries. Because of such increased risk, caution is advised when Chinese patients receive fixed-combination dosages exceeding 10 mg of ezetimibe and 20 mg of simvastatin daily concomitantly with preparations containing antilipemic dosages of niacin. Because the risk of myopathy is dose related, patients of Chinese descent should avoid concomitant use of the fixed-combination preparation containing 10 mg of ezetimibe and 80 mg of simvastatin with preparations containing antilipemic dosages of niacin.

■ Special Populations No dosage adjustment is necessary in geriatric patients (65 years of age or older), in patients with mild hepatic impairment, or in patients with renal impairment. However, the manufacturer states that ezetimibe should not be used in patients with moderate or severe hepatic impairment. (See Specific Populations under Cautions: Warnings/Precautions.)

In patients receiving ezetimibe in fixed combination with simvastatin, the manufacturer states that no dosage adjustment is necessary in geriatric patients or in patients with mild renal impairment (estimated GFR of 60 mL/minute per 1.73 m² or greater). However, in patients with chronic kidney disease and an estimated GFR of less than 60 mL/minute per 1.73 m², the dosage of the fixed-combination preparation is 10 mg of ezetimibe and 20 mg of simvastatin once daily in the evening; in such patients, higher dosages should be used with caution and close monitoring. (See Specific Populations under Cautions: Warnings/Precautions.)

Cautions

■ Contraindications Known hypersensitivity to ezetimibe or any ingredient in the formulation.

Ezetimibe, in combination with a hydroxymethylglutaryl-coenzyme A (HMG-CoA) reductase inhibitor (statin), is contraindicated in patients with active liver disease or unexplained, persistent increases in serum aminotransferase (transaminase) concentrations.

All statins are contraindicated in pregnant or nursing women. If ezetimibe is used in combination with a statin in a woman of childbearing age, the prescribing information for the statin should be consulted for detailed information on contraindications of the drug.

Concomitant use of the fixed combination of ezetimibe and simvastatin with potent inhibitors of cytochrome P-450 (CYP) isoenzyme 3A4, cyclosporine, danazol, or gemfibrozil is contraindicated.

■ Warnings/Precautions ***Sensitivity Reactions*** Anaphylaxis, angioedema, rash, and urticaria have been reported.

Major Toxicities **Hepatic Effects.** Consecutive elevations in serum aminotransferase (transaminase) concentrations (i.e., AST, ALT) exceeding 3 times the upper limit of normal were reported in approximately 0.5% of patients receiving ezetimibe and in 0.3% of those receiving placebo in clinical studies. In studies in which ezetimibe was initiated concurrently with a statin, these elevations were reported in 1.3% of patients receiving combination therapy and in 0.4% of those receiving statin monotherapy. Consecutive elevations in serum transaminase concentrations exceeding 3 times the upper limit of normal were reported in approximately 1.7–1.8% of patients receiving the fixed-combination preparation containing ezetimibe and simvastatin; these elevations appeared to be dose related and occurred in 2.6–3.6% of patients receiving the fixed combination containing 10 mg of ezetimibe and 80 mg of simvastatin. In a study in which ezetimibe was used in combination with fenofibrate, consecutive elevations in serum transaminase concentrations exceeding 3 times the upper limit of normal were reported in 2.7% of patients receiving combination therapy and in 4.5% of those receiving fenofibrate monotherapy. Increases in transaminase concentrations generally were asymptomatic and not associated with cholestasis; transaminase concentrations usually returned to pretreatment values during continued therapy or following discontinuance of ezetimibe. Hepatitis has been reported during postmarketing surveillance; however, a causal relationship to the drug has not been established.

The American College of Cardiology (ACC)/American Heart Association (AHA) cholesterol management guideline states that it is reasonable to obtain baseline hepatic aminotransferase concentrations before initiating ezetimibe. When ezetimibe is used in combination with a statin, liver function tests should be performed at initiation of therapy and in accordance with the recommended monitoring schedule for the specific statin and as clinically indicated. If ALT or AST concentrations increase to 3 or more times the upper limit of normal (ULN) and are persistent, discontinuance of ezetimibe and/or the statin should be considered.

Musculoskeletal Effects. Marked (exceeding 10 times the upper limit of normal) elevations of serum creatine kinase (CK, creatine phosphokinase, CPK) were reported in 0.2% of patients receiving ezetimibe and in 0.1% of patients receiving placebo in clinical studies. In clinical studies evaluating safety and efficacy of ezetimibe in combination with a statin, these elevations were reported in 0.1% of patients receiving combination therapy and in 0.4% of those receiving statin monotherapy.

In clinical studies, the incidence of myopathy (manifested as unexplained muscle pain, tenderness, or weakness and increases in serum CK concentration exceeding 10 times the upper limit of normal) or rhabdomyolysis appears to be similar among patients receiving ezetimibe, statin monotherapy, or placebo. Myalgia, myopathy, and/or rhabdomyolysis have been reported during postmarketing surveillance in patients receiving ezetimibe alone or in combination with other antilipemic agents. Most reported cases of rhabdomyolysis have occurred in patients who were receiving statin therapy prior to initiating ezetimibe. However, rhabdomyolysis also has been reported following ezetimibe monotherapy or following addition of ezetimibe to therapy with agents known to be associated with increased risk of rhabdomyolysis (e.g., fibric acid derivatives).

Predisposing factors for the development of myopathy and/or rhabdomyolysis include increased dosages of statins, age exceeding 65 years, uncontrolled hypothyroidism, renal impairment, and potential statin-drug interactions. Patients initiating therapy with ezetimibe should be advised of the risk of myopathy and instructed to promptly report any unexplained muscle pain, tenderness, or weakness, particularly if accompanied by malaise or fever or if such manifestations persist after discontinuance of therapy. If myopathy is diagnosed or suspected, ezetimibe and other concomitant antilipemic agents (e.g., statin, fibric acid derivative) should be discontinued immediately.

General Precautions **Combination Therapy with Statins or Fenofibrate.** When ezetimibe is used in combination with a statin or fenofibrate, the prescribing information for the specific statin or for fenofibrate also should be consulted for detailed information on the usual cautions, precautions, and contraindications for these drugs.

Risk of Cancer. The fixed combination of ezetimibe and simvastatin was reported in the Simvastatin and Ezetimibe in Aortic Stenosis (SEAS) study to be possibly associated with an increased risk of cancer; these findings prompted the FDA to issue an early communication in 2008 about this potential safety risk. Results of this study in 1873 patients with mild to moderate asymptomatic aortic stenosis revealed a higher incidence of cancer and cancer-related deaths (11.1 and 4.1%, respectively) in patients receiving the fixed-combination preparation compared with those receiving placebo (7.5 and 2.5%, respectively). However, results of 2 subsequent large randomized studies (the Study of Heart and Renal Protection [SHARP] and the Improved Reduction of Outcomes: Vytorin® Efficacy International Trial [IMPROVE-IT]) involving a combined study population of 27,414 patients with chronic kidney disease or acute coronary syndrome found no consistent pattern of increased cancer risk among patients receiving the fixed-combination preparation of ezetimibe and simvastatin. In the SHARP study, cancer or cancer-related mortality occurred in 9.4 or 2.8%, respectively, of patients receiving the fixed-combination preparation, and these rates were similar to those reported in placebo recipients. In the IMPROVE-IT study, cancer or cancer-related mortality occurred in 10.2 or 3.8%, respectively, of patients receiving the fixed combination of ezetimibe and simvastatin and these rates were similar to those reported in patients who received simvastatin monotherapy. Based on the currently available evidence, FDA has concluded that neither ezetimibe nor the fixed-combination preparation of ezetimibe and simvastatin is likely to increase the risk of cancer or cancer-related deaths.

Specific Populations **Pregnancy.** Category C. (See Users Guide.) Category X for fixed combination of ezetimibe and simvastatin (due to simvastatin component). (See Users Guide.)

Lactation. Ezetimibe is distributed into milk in rats. It is not known whether ezetimibe is distributed into milk in humans. Because many drugs are distributed into human milk, caution should be used if ezetimibe is used in nursing women; the drug should not be used in nursing women unless the potential benefits justify the possible risks to the infant.

Pediatric Use. There are no differences in the pharmacokinetics of ezetimibe between adolescents and adults. Pharmacokinetic data are not available for pediatric patients younger than 10 years of age.

Use of ezetimibe in combination with simvastatin has been evaluated in a limited number of adolescent boys and girls with heterozygous familial hypercholesterolemia. In a randomized, double-blind, controlled study in boys and postmenarchal girls 10–17 years of age with heterozygous familial hypercholesterolemia, discontinuance of therapy because of adverse effects occurred in more patients receiving ezetimibe in combination with simvastatin (10–40 mg daily) (6%) than in those receiving simvastatin monotherapy (2%); in addition, increases in aminotransferase or CK concentrations also occurred more frequently in patients receiving combination therapy (3 or 2%, respectively) than in those receiving simvastatin monotherapy (2 or 0%, respectively). There were no detectable adverse effects on growth or sexual maturation in adolescent boys or girls or on duration of menstrual cycle in girls. Use of ezetimibe in combination with simvastatin dosages exceeding 40 mg daily has not been evaluated in adolescents; safety and efficacy of ezetimibe, alone or in fixed combination with simvastatin, have not been evaluated in prepubertal girls or in children younger than 10 years of age.

Geriatric Use. In clinical studies in patients receiving ezetimibe, 28% of patients were 65 years of age or older, and 5% of patients were 75 years of age or older. Following administration of ezetimibe (10 mg daily for 10 days), plasma concentrations of the drug were approximately twofold higher in geriatric individuals (65 years of age or older) than in younger adults; however, no overall differences in safety and efficacy of ezetimibe have been observed in geriatric patients relative to younger adults. Nevertheless, the manufacturer states that the possibility that some older patients may exhibit increased sensitivity to the drug cannot be ruled out.

In clinical studies in patients receiving ezetimibe in fixed combination with simvastatin, 32% of patients were 65 years of age or older, and 8% of patients were 75 years of age or older. No substantial differences in safety or efficacy of the fixed-combination preparation were observed in geriatric patients relative to younger patients; however, greater sensitivity in some older patients cannot be ruled out. Because advanced age (65 years of age or older) is a risk factor for myopathy, including rhabdomyolysis, ezetimibe in fixed combination with simvastatin should be used with caution in geriatric patients.

Hepatic Impairment. Following a single 10-mg dose of ezetimibe, the mean area under the plasma concentration-time curve (AUC) of total ezetimibe was increased by approximately 1.7 fold in individuals with mild hepatic impairment (Child-Pugh score 5–6). In individuals with moderate (Child-Pugh score 7–9) or severe (Child-Pugh score 10–15) hepatic impairment, the mean AUC of total ezetimibe was increased by approximately threefold to fourfold and that of ezetimibe was increased by approximately fivefold to sixfold. In a multiple-dose study, administration of ezetimibe (10 mg daily) for 14 days resulted in fourfold increases in the AUCs of total ezetimibe and ezetimibe on days 1 and 14 in patients with moderate hepatic impairment compared with healthy individuals. Because the effects of increased exposure to ezetimibe in patients with moderate or severe hepatic impairment currently is not known, the manufacturer states that the drug is not recommended in such patients.

Renal Impairment. Following a single 10-mg dose of ezetimibe, the mean AUC of ezetimibe was increased by approximately 1.5-fold in individuals with severe renal impairment (mean creatinine clearance of 30 mL/minute per 1.73 m^2 or less) compared with healthy individuals. When ezetimibe is used as monotherapy, no dosage adjustment is necessary in patients with renal impairment. (See Dosage and Administration: Special Populations.)

In the SHARP study in patients with moderate to severe renal impairment, the incidence of serious adverse effects, adverse effects leading to discontinuance of therapy, or adverse effects of special interest (adverse musculoskeletal effects, liver enzyme abnormalities, incident cancer) was similar in patients receiving the fixed combination of ezetimibe 10 mg and simvastatin 20 mg compared with those receiving placebo following a median of 4.9 years. However, because renal impairment is a risk factor for statin-associated myopathy, dosages of the fixed-combination preparation exceeding ezetimibe 10 mg and simvastatin 20 mg daily should be used with caution and close monitoring in patients with moderate to severe renal impairment. (See Dosage and Administration: Special Populations.)

■ **Common Adverse Effects** Adverse effects occurring in 2% or more of patients receiving ezetimibe and more frequently with the drug than with placebo include upper respiratory tract infection, diarrhea, arthralgia, sinusitis, pain in extremity, fatigue, and influenza.

Adverse effects occurring in 2% or more of patients receiving ezetimibe in combination with statins and more frequently with the drug than with placebo include nasopharyngitis, myalgia, upper respiratory tract infection, arthralgia, diarrhea, back pain, influenza, headache, and pain in extremity. Adverse effects occurring in patients receiving ezetimibe in combination with statins generally were similar to those reported in patients receiving statin therapy alone. However, the incidence of increased transaminase concentrations was higher in patients receiving combination therapy (1.3%) than in those who received statin monotherapy (0.4%). (See Hepatic Effects under Warnings/Precautions: Major Toxicities, in Cautions.)

Drug Interactions

When using the fixed-combination preparation containing ezetimibe and simvastatin, the drug interactions associated with simvastatin should be considered. No formal drug interaction studies have been performed to date with the fixed-combination preparation other than that with extended-release niacin. (See Niacin under Drug Interactions: Antilipemic Agents.)

■ **Drugs Affecting Hepatic Microsomal Enzymes** Based on results of a study evaluating possible interactions with caffeine, dextromethorphan, tolbutamide, and IV midazolam in a limited number of healthy men, the potential for drug interactions mediated by hepatic cytochrome P-450 (CYP) with ezetimibe is low.

■ **Antacids** Concomitant use of ezetimibe (10 mg) and an aluminum and magnesium hydroxides-containing antacid decreased AUC and peak plasma concentration of total ezetimibe by 4 and 30%, respectively.

■ **Antilipemic Agents** ***Bile Acid Sequestrants*** Concomitant administration of cholestyramine (4 g twice daily for 14 days) and ezetimibe (10 mg) decreased the AUC and peak plasma concentration of total ezetimibe by 55 and 4%, respectively. Reduced LDL-cholesterol lowering effect may occur as a result of this interaction. Ezetimibe should be administered at least 2 hours before or at least 4 hours after administration of the bile acid sequestrant.

Fibric Acid Derivatives Concomitant use of fenofibrate (200 mg daily for 14 days) and ezetimibe (10 mg) increased AUC and peak plasma concentration of total ezetimibe by 48 and 64%, respectively. Concomitant use of fenofibrate (200 mg daily for 14 days) and ezetimibe (10 mg daily for 14 days) increased AUC and peak plasma concentration of fenofibrate by 11 and 7%, respectively.

Concomitant use of gemfibrozil (600 mg twice daily for 7 days) and ezetimibe (10 mg) increased AUC and peak plasma concentration of total ezetimibe by 64 and 91%, respectively. Concomitant use of gemfibrozil (600 mg twice daily for 7 days) and ezetimibe (10 mg daily for 7 days) decreased AUC and peak plasma concentration of gemfibrozil by 1 and 11%, respectively.

Fibric acid derivatives may increase cholesterol excretion into bile, leading to cholelithiasis, and ezetimibe has been shown to increase cholesterol in the gall bladder bile in animals. In clinical studies, cholecystectomy has been reported in 1.7% of patients receiving ezetimibe concomitantly with fenofibrate and in 0.6% of those receiving fenofibrate monotherapy.

The efficacy and safety of concomitant use of ezetimibe with a fibric acid derivative other than fenofibrate have not been established. Such concomitant use currently is *not* recommended pending further accumulation of data from adequate study in humans. Concomitant use of the fixed combination of ezetimibe and simvastatin with gemfibrozil is contraindicated. (See Ezetimibe/Simvastatin Combination Therapy under Dosage and Administration: Dosage.) If cholelithiasis is suspected in a patient receiving ezetimibe with fenofibrate, gallbladder studies should be performed, and alternative antilipemic therapy should be considered.

Hydroxymethylglutaryl-Coenzyme A (HMG-CoA) Reductase Inhibitors (Statins) Concomitant use of atorvastatin (10 mg daily for 14 days) and ezetimibe (10 mg) decreased AUC of total ezetimibe by 2% and increased peak plasma concentration of total ezetimibe by 12%. Concomitant use of atorvastatin (10 mg daily for 14 days) and ezetimibe (10 mg daily for 14 days) decreased AUC of atorvastatin by 4% and increased peak plasma concentration of atorvastatin by 7%.

Concomitant use of fluvastatin (20 mg daily for 14 days) and ezetimibe (10 mg) decreased AUC of total ezetimibe by 19% and increased peak plasma concentration of total ezetimibe by 7%. Concomitant use of fluvastatin (20 mg daily for 14 days) and ezetimibe (10 mg daily for 14 days) decreased AUC and peak plasma concentration of fluvastatin by 39 and 27%, respectively.

Concomitant use of lovastatin (20 mg daily for 7 days) and ezetimibe (10 mg) increased AUC and peak plasma concentration of total ezetimibe by 9 and 3%, respectively. Concomitant use of lovastatin (20 mg daily for 7 days) and ezetimibe (10 mg daily for 7 days) increased AUC and peak plasma concentration of lovastatin by 19 and 3%, respectively.

Concomitant use of pravastatin (20 mg daily for 14 days) and ezetimibe (10 mg) increased AUC and peak plasma concentration of total ezetimibe by 7 and 23%, respectively. Concomitant use of pravastatin (20 mg daily for 14 days) and ezetimibe (10 mg daily for 14 days) decreased AUC and peak plasma concentration of pravastatin by 20 and 24%, respectively.

Concomitant use of rosuvastatin (10 mg daily for 14 days) and ezetimibe (10 mg) increased AUC and peak plasma concentration of total ezetimibe by 13 and 18%, respectively. Concomitant use of rosuvastatin (10 mg daily for 14 days) and ezetimibe (10 mg daily for 14 days) increased AUC and peak plasma concentration of rosuvastatin by 19 and 17%, respectively.

Mipomersen No clinically relevant pharmacokinetic interactions were observed when ezetimibe was used concomitantly with mipomersen. Therefore, dosage adjustment of ezetimibe and mipomersen is not necessary during such concomitant use.

Niacin Following concomitant use of the fixed combination of ezetimibe and simvastatin (10 mg of ezetimibe and 20 mg of simvastatin administered daily for 7 days) with extended-release niacin (Niaspan® 1 g administered daily for 2 days, then 2 g administered daily for 5 days), mean peak plasma concentrations or AUC of niacin were increased by 9 or 22%, respectively; mean peak plasma concentrations or AUC of nicotinuric acid were increased by 10 or 19%, respectively; mean peak plasma concentrations of simvastatin acid were increased by 18%; and mean AUC of total ezetimibe, simvastatin, or simvastatin acid were increased by 26, 20, or 35%, respectively. (See Ezetimibe/Simvastatin Combination Therapy under Dosage and Administration: Dosage.)

■ **Cimetidine** Concomitant use of cimetidine (400 mg twice daily for 7 days) and ezetimibe (10 mg) increased AUC and peak plasma concentration of total ezetimibe by 6 and 22%, respectively.

■ **Cyclosporine** Concomitant use of cyclosporine (75–150 mg twice daily) and ezetimibe (10 mg) in renal transplant recipients with normal renal function or mild renal impairment increased AUC and peak plasma concentration of total ezetimibe by 3.4- and 3.9-fold, respectively. Exposure to ezetimibe may be greater in patients with severe renal insufficiency. In a renal transplant patient with severe renal impairment (creatinine clearance 13.2 mL/minute per 1.73 m^2) receiving multiple medications in addition to cyclosporine and ezetimibe, a 12-fold increase in total ezetimibe exposure occurred.

Concomitant use of cyclosporine (single 100-dose on day 7) and ezetimibe (20 mg daily for 8 days) increased AUC and peak plasma concentration of cyclosporine by 15 and 10%, respectively.

Because of increased exposure to ezetimibe and cyclosporine, caution should be exercised with concomitant use and cyclosporine concentrations should be monitored. The potential benefits versus risks of such concomitant therapy should be considered.

■ **Digoxin** Concomitant use of digoxin (single 0.5-mg dose) and ezetimibe (10 mg daily for 8 days) increased AUC of digoxin by 2% and decreased peak plasma concentration of digoxin by 7%.

■ **Fat-soluble Vitamins** Pharmacokinetic interactions with vitamins A, D, and E are unlikely.

■ **Glipizide** Concomitant use of glipizide (single 10-mg dose) and ezetimibe (10 mg) increased AUC of total ezetimibe by 4% and decreased peak plasma concentration of total ezetimibe by 8%. Concomitant use of glipizide (10 mg on days 1 and 9) and ezetimibe (10 mg daily on days 2–9) decreased AUC and peak plasma concentration of glipizide by 3 and 5%, respectively.

■ **Oral Contraceptives** Concomitant use of an oral contraceptive containing ethinyl estradiol and levonorgestrel (daily for 21 days) and ezetimibe (10 mg daily on days 8–14) decreased the peak plasma concentrations of ethinyl estradiol and levonorgestrel by 9 and 5%, respectively; AUCs of both components remained unchanged.

■ **Warfarin** Pharmacokinetic or pharmacodynamic interaction with ezetimibe is unlikely based on one small study. Concomitant use of warfarin (single 25-mg dose on day 7) and ezetimibe (10 mg daily for 11 days) decreased the AUCs of *R*- and *S*-warfarin by 2 and 4%, respectively, and increased peak plasma concentrations of *R*- and *S*-warfarin by 3 and 1%, respectively.

Increased international normalized ratio (INR) with concomitant use of ezetimibe and warfarin has been reported during postmarketing experience; however, most patients also were receiving other drugs. If ezetimibe is initiated in a patient receiving warfarin, the INR should be monitored.

Description

Ezetimibe, a cholesterol absorption inhibitor, is an antilipemic agent that differs chemically and pharmacologically from other currently available antilipemic agents. Following absorption, the drug localizes at the brush border of the small intestine and inhibits absorption of cholesterol through the sterol transporter, Niemann-Pick C1-Like 1 (NPC1L1), resulting in decreased delivery of intestinal cholesterol to the liver. This causes a reduction in hepatic cholesterol stores, a compensatory increase in hepatic uptake of cholesterol from systemic circulation, and consequently, an increase in systemic clearance of cholesterol. Ezetimibe does not appear to inhibit hepatic cholesterol synthesis or increase bile acid excretion.

Intestinal absorption of cholesterol reportedly was reduced by approximately 54% in a limited number of patients with hypercholesterolemia who received ezetimibe (10 mg daily) for 2 weeks. The cholesterol-lowering effects of ezetimibe and hydroxymethylglutaryl-coenzyme A (HMG-CoA) reductase inhibitors (statins) or of ezetimibe and fenofibrate are additive. In addition to reducing lipoprotein concentrations, ezetimibe also has been shown to reduce concentrations of noncholesterol sterols, including sitosterol and campesterol. Effects of ezetimibe on cardiovascular morbidity and mortality have not been established.

Ezetimibe does not appear to inhibit the absorption of triglycerides, fatty acids, bile acids, progesterone, or ethinyl estradiol. In 2 separate studies in more than 100 patients each, ezetimibe exhibited no clinically relevant effects on plasma concentrations of fat-soluble vitamins A, D, or E and did not appear to impair adrenocortical steroid production.

Following oral administration, approximately 93% of a radiolabeled dose of ezetimibe is absorbed systemically (as ezetimibe and ezetimibe glucuronide). Food does not appear to affect the extent of absorption of ezetimibe; however, concomitant administration of the drug with a high-fat meal resulted in a 38% increase in peak plasma concentrations of the drug. Following absorption, ezetimibe is rapidly and extensively metabolized in the small intestine and liver to a pharmacologically active phenolic glucuronide metabolite, ezetimibe glucuronide; the drug or its glucuronide metabolite constitutes 10–20 or 80–90%, respectively, of the total absorbed drug in plasma. Ezetimibe and ezetimibe glucuronide are more than 90% bound to human plasma proteins. The preparation containing ezetimibe in fixed combination with simvastatin is bioequivalent to corresponding dosages of the individual components.

Ezetimibe and ezetimibe glucuronide are each slowly eliminated from plasma with a half-life of approximately 22 hours. Plasma concentration-time profiles of ezetimibe exhibit multiple peaks, suggesting that the drug and its active metabolite may undergo enterohepatic recycling. Following oral administration of 20 mg of ^{14}C-ezetimibe, approximately 78 or 11% of the radioactivity was excreted in feces or urine, respectively, in 10 days; ezetimibe was the major component in feces, while ezetimibe glucuronide was the major component in urine.

Based on a meta-analysis of multiple-dose pharmacokinetic studies, there were no differences in pharmacokinetic parameters between blacks and Caucasians. Studies in Asian individuals indicated that the pharmacokinetics of ezetimibe were similar to those seen in Caucasian individuals.

Advice to Patients

Importance of adherence to prescribed directions for use, particularly when used concomitantly with other antilipemic agents.

Importance of adherence to a standard cholesterol-lowering diet.

Risk of myopathy and/or rhabdomyolysis; risk is increased when used concomitantly with certain other drugs or grapefruit juice. Importance of promptly informing clinicians of any unexplained muscle pain, tenderness, or weakness, particularly if accompanied by malaise or fever or if such manifestations persist after discontinuance of therapy.

Risk of adverse hepatic effects. Importance of monitoring liver function tests at initiation of ezetimibe if used in combination with a statin and thereafter in accordance with the recommendation of the statin. Importance of promptly reporting any symptoms suggestive of liver injury (e.g., fatigue, anorexia, right upper abdominal discomfort, dark urine, jaundice) when ezetimibe is used in combination with simvastatin.

Importance of women informing clinicians if they are or plan to become pregnant. Importance of advising women and adolescent girls to avoid pregnancy (i.e., using effective and appropriate contraceptive methods) and informing pregnant women of the risk to the fetus when using ezetimibe in combination with statin therapy.

Importance of avoiding breast-feeding when using ezetimibe in combination with statin therapy. If the patient has a lipid disorder and is breast-feeding, importance of contacting a clinician to discuss other antilipemic treatment options.

Importance of informing clinicians of existing or contemplated concomitant therapy, including prescription and OTC drugs, as well as concomitant illnesses.

Importance of informing patients of other important precautionary information. (See Cautions.)

Overview® (see Users Guide). For additional information on this drug until a more detailed monograph is developed and published, the manufacturer's labeling should be consulted. It is *essential* that the manufacturer's labeling be consulted for more detailed information on usual cautions, precautions, contraindications, potential drug interactions, laboratory test interferences, and acute toxicity.

Preparations

Excipients in commercially available drug preparations may have clinically important effects in some individuals; consult specific product labeling for details.

Ezetimibe

Oral		
Tablets	10 mg*	**Ezetimibe Tablets**
		Zetia®, Merck/Schering-Plough

*available from one or more manufacturer, distributor, and/or repackager by generic (nonproprietary) name

Ezetimibe Combinations

Oral		
Tablets	10 mg with Simvastatin 10 mg	**Vytorin®**, Merck
	10 mg with Simvastatin 20 mg	**Vytorin®**, Merck
	10 mg with Simvastatin 40 mg	**Vytorin®**, Merck
	10 mg with Simvastatin 80 mg	**Vytorin®**, Merck

HMG-CoA Reductase Inhibitors 24:06.08

HMG-CoA Reductase Inhibitors General Statement

■ Hydroxymethylglutaryl-coenzyme A (HMG-CoA) reductase inhibitors (statins) are antilipemic agents that competitively inhibit HMG-CoA reductase, the enzyme that catalyzes the conversion of HMG-CoA to mevalonic acid, an early precursor of cholesterol.

General Principles of Antilipemic Therapy

■ **Rationale for Intervention** Results of numerous epidemiologic studies indicate that elevated serum cholesterol, especially the low-density lipoprotein (LDL)-cholesterol fraction, is a major cause of clinical atherosclerotic cardiovascular disease (ASCVD), including coronary heart disease (CHD), stroke, and peripheral arterial disease. Clinical, epidemiologic, and angiographic evidence from primary and secondary prevention studies involving various HMG-CoA reductase inhibitors (statins) indicates that decreasing elevated serum cholesterol concentrations (specifically, LDL-cholesterol) can reduce the incidence of ASCVD events and/or the progression of atherosclerosis and result in a decrease in associated morbidity and mortality. It has been estimated that each 1% reduction in LDL-cholesterol concentration may result in a 1% decrease in the incidence of CHD. An analysis of pooled data from primary and secondary prevention studies found that treatment with a statin for a median duration of 5.4 years was associated with 31 and 21% reductions in the risk of major coronary events (i.e., coronary death, fatal or nonfatal myocardial infarction [MI], unstable angina, sudden cardiac death) and total mortality, respectively. This represents an absolute risk reduction of 36 major coronary events and 16 deaths from all causes per 1000 patients. The risk reduction in major coronary events was similar among men (31%), women (29%), and geriatric (65 years of age and older) patients (32%). Data from secondary prevention studies involving various statins (e.g., atorvastatin, pravastatin, simvastatin) indicate that decreasing elevated serum cholesterol concentrations reduces the risk of fatal and nonfatal cerebrovascular events (e.g., stroke, transient ischemic attack [TIA]). An analysis of pooled data from clinical trials of statins indicates that patients receiving statin therapy had a 29% reduction in the risk of stroke and a 22% reduction in total mortality, which was attributable to a 28% reduction in CHD death. In a prospective meta-analysis conducted by the Cholesterol Treatment Trialists' (CTT) Collaboration, which included data from approximately 90,000 patients in 14 randomized studies of statins, the risk of major coronary events, revascularization, and stroke was found to be reduced by about one-fifth for each 1 mmol/L (38.7 mg/dL) reduction in LDL cholesterol achieved. Results of this and other studies showed that further reduction in LDL cholesterol concentrations (e.g., more intensive statin therapy) produced greater cardiovascular risk reduction benefits. Clinical studies with statin therapy have not identified substantial adverse effects from LDL-cholesterol lowering per se; therefore, the decision to achieve very low LDL-cholesterol concentrations in very high risk patients should be based on evidence of benefit and recognition that there appears to be only a remote possibility of adverse effects from LDL-cholesterol lowering.

Data from observational epidemiologic studies have indicated a strong inverse relationship between high-density lipoprotein (HDL)-cholesterol and the incidence of CHD; a lower HDL-cholesterol concentration correlates with higher CHD risk across levels of LDL-cholesterol of 100–200 mg/dL. It has been estimated that each 4-mg/dL reduction in HDL-cholesterol concentration may result in a 10% increase in the incidence of CHD. It is not clear whether increasing HDL-cholesterol concentration reduces the risk of cardiovascular events; however, data from large randomized studies in patients with established cardiovascular disease indicate that addition of niacin to existing statin-based therapy did not further reduce the incidence of major cardiovascular events compared with statin-based therapy alone. (See Secondary Prevention under Uses: Prevention of Cardiovascular Events.)

■ **Initial Evaluation** The Third Report of the National Cholesterol Education Program (NCEP) (Adult Treatment Panel [ATP] III) and the more recent American College of Cardiology (ACC)/American Heart Association (AHA) guideline for management of blood cholesterol to reduce atherosclerotic cardiovascular risk in adults state that patients with and without clinical ASCVD should receive an initial evaluation that consists of a fasting lipoprotein profile, ALT concentration, and creatine kinase (CK, creatine phosphokinase, CPK) concentration (if indicated) prior to initiation of antilipemic therapy; baseline hemoglobin A_{1c} (HbA_{1c}) also should be obtained in patients without clinical ASCVD in whom diabetes status is unknown.

Patients with LDL-cholesterol concentrations of 190 mg/dL or greater or triglyceride concentrations of 500 mg/dL or greater should be evaluated to rule out secondary causes of hyperlipidemia. Secondary causes of elevated LDL-cholesterol concentrations include high intake of saturated or trans fats, weight gain, anorexia, current therapy with drugs that increase LDL-cholesterol concentration (e.g., diuretics, cyclosporine, glucocorticoids, amiodarone), biliary obstruction, nephrotic syndrome, hypothyroidism, obesity, and pregnancy. Secondary causes of elevated triglyceride concentrations include weight gain, very low-fat diets, high intake of refined carbohydrates, excessive alcohol intake, current therapy with drugs that increase triglyceride concentration (e.g., oral estrogens, glucocorticoids, bile acid sequestrants, protease inhibitors, retinoic acid, anabolic steroids, sirolimus, raloxifene, tamoxifen, β-adrenergic blocking agents [except carvedilol], thiazides), nephrotic syndrome, chronic renal failure, lipodystrophies, poorly controlled diabetes mellitus, hypothyroidism, obesity, and pregnancy. Patients with unexplained elevations in ALT concentrations of more than 3 times the upper limit of normal also should receive appropriate evaluation and treatment prior to initiating antilipemic therapy.

■ **Risk Assessment** Following initial evaluation, the patient's risk status should be determined in order to guide intensity of antilipemic therapy; the most intensive therapy should be reserved for patients in the highest risk category.

ATP III previously identified 4 categories of risk: *High risk* (CHD or CHD risk equivalents [e.g., abdominal aortic aneurysm, diabetes mellitus, peripheral arterial disease, renal artery disease, symptomatic carotid artery disease] with a 10-year CHD risk exceeding 20%), *moderately high risk* (2 or more major risk factors with a 10-year CHD risk of 10–20%), *moderate risk* (2 or more major risk factors with a 10-year CHD risk of less than 10%), and *lower risk* (one or no major risk factors). Major risk factors in adults and children include current cigarette smoking, hypertension (blood pressure of 140/90 mm Hg or greater) or use of antihypertensive therapy, low HDL-cholesterol concentrations (less than 40 mg/dL in adults and less than 35 mg/dL in children), family history of premature CHD (before 55 years of age in a male first-degree relative or before 65 years of age in a female first-degree relative), and age (men 45 years of age or older and women 55 years of age or older); HDL-cholesterol concentrations of 60 mg/dL or greater constitute a *negative* risk factor for CHD. The 10-year CHD risk is estimated using Framingham scoring; an electronic 10-year risk calculator is available at http://www.nhlbi.nih.gov/health-pro/guidelines/.

In the more recent ACC/AHA cholesterol management guideline, which is narrower in scope and focuses specifically on antilipemic therapies proven to reduce ASCVD risk (i.e., statins), the cholesterol expert panel identified 4 categories of risk (i.e., statin benefit groups): Patients with *clinical ASCVD* (i.e., acute coronary syndromes, history of MI, stable or unstable angina, coronary or other arterial revascularization, stroke, TIA, peripheral arterial disease presumed to be of atherosclerotic origin); patients with *primary, severe elevations in LDL-cholesterol concentration (190 mg/dL or greater)*; patients 40–75 years of age with *type 1 or 2 diabetes mellitus*; and patients without clinical ASCVD or diabetes mellitus who have LDL-cholesterol concentrations of 70–189 mg/dL and an *estimated 10-year ASCVD risk of 7.5% or higher*. In assessing risk, the ACC/AHA cholesterol management guideline does not require specific risk factor counting; instead, a global ASCVD risk assessment is used to guide initiation of statin therapy. The 10-year ASCVD risk (defined as first occurrence of nonfatal MI, CHD death, or nonfatal and fatal stroke) is estimated using the Pooled Cohort Equations, which were developed using data from 5 longitudinal, population-based studies in geographically diverse patient populations (i.e., African American and non-Hispanic white men and women); the Pooled Cohort Equations estimate ASCVD risk on the basis of age, gender, race, smoking status, total cholesterol concentration, HDL-cholesterol concentration, systolic blood pressure, use of antihypertensive therapy, and diabetes mellitus. A downloadable spreadsheet is available at http://my.americanheart.org, and a web-based calculator is available at http://www.cardiosource.org/science-and-quality/clinical-tools. The ASCVD risk-assessment calculator estimates 10-year ASCVD risk in patients 40–79 years of age. In patients 40–75 years of age without clinical ASCVD or diabetes mellitus who have LDL-cholesterol concentrations of 70–189 mg/dL and are not receiving antilipemic therapy, the ACC/AHA cholesterol management guideline recommends that an estimated 10-year risk of ASCVD be assessed every 4–6 years.

The ASCVD risk-assessment calculator adopted by the ACC/AHA cholesterol management guideline is controversial and has not been widely implemented. Despite its strength of incorporating the Pooled Cohort Equations, which currently are considered by some clinicians to be the best available method for estimating 10-year ASCVD risk (because the equations provide gender- and race-specific estimates and include stroke as an outcome), the ASCVD risk-assessment calculator has been shown by other clinicians to overestimate ASCVD risk, which may result in overtreatment in some patients, particularly in primary prevention.

In an analysis comparing the predicted 10-year risk (using the ASCVD risk-assessment calculator) with observed event rates in 3 large-scale primary prevention cohorts (the Women's Health Study, the Physicians' Health Study, and the Women's Health Initiative Observational Study), investigators found that the ASCVD risk-assessment calculator systematically overestimated observed risk by 75–150%, roughly doubling the actual observed risk; these investigators estimated that as many as 40–50% of middle-aged patients who qualify for statin therapy under the new ACC/AHA cholesterol management guideline do not actually have risk thresholds that exceed the 7.5% threshold suggested for treatment. (See Primary Prevention in Patients with Elevated ASCVD Risk under Treatment Recommendations: Adults, in General Principles of Antilipemic Therapy.) The cholesterol expert panel states that while some overestimation has been observed with the calculator, the 75–150% overestimation reported in the comparative analysis may not be reliable because the investigators used cohorts that were not representative of the US population, and that these cohorts probably had lower risk due to high rates of statin use during the follow-up period. The expert panel also states that modest overestimation of ASCVD risk generally does not affect most decisions to recommend therapy in adults with a 10-year ASCVD risk of 7.5% or higher because clinical data indicate that the benefit of statin therapy (i.e., reduction of ASCVD risk) outweighs the risk of adverse effects even in patients with a 10-year ASCVD risk of 5%. Nevertheless, some clinicians state that miscalibration of the risk calculator should be reconciled and addressed in additional external validation cohorts before the calculator can be widely implemented.

■ Determination of LDL-cholesterol Concentrations and Target Goals

Adults ATP III recommended that a fasting lipoprotein profile (total cholesterol, LDL-cholesterol, HDL-cholesterol, and triglycerides) be obtained at least once every year in patients with CHD or CHD risk equivalents, at least once every 2 years in patients with 2 or more major risk factors or those with one or no major risk factors who have LDL-cholesterol concentrations of 130–159 mg/dL, and once every 5 years in low-risk adults (i.e., those with one or no major risk factors) 20 years of age and older. Because ATP III recommended a treat-to-target approach, regular measurements of lipoprotein concentrations were required (i.e., at baseline to determine whether therapy was necessary, and periodically following initiation of therapy to ensure that target goals were achieved). LDL-cholesterol concentrations at which to initiate therapy and target goals varied depending on risk. (See Table 1 under General Principles of Antilipemic Therapy: Treatment Recommendations.)

The ACC/AHA cholesterol management guideline recommends that a fasting lipoprotein profile be obtained in adults prior to initiation of antilipemic (i.e., statin) therapy, 4–12 weeks after initiation of antilipemic therapy (to determine the patient's response to therapy and adherence), and every 3–12 months thereafter as clinically indicated. The guideline makes no recommendations for or against the treat-to-target approach but recommends that clinicians focus on *intensity* of statin therapy rather than LDL-cholesterol or non-HDL-cholesterol (calculated as total cholesterol minus HDL-cholesterol) targets. This new recommendation is based on the finding that the majority of studies used fixed-dose statin therapy rather than titrating therapy to achieve a specific target LDL-cholesterol concentration, and that there were no studies comparing 2 target goals; the ACC/AHA cholesterol management guideline states that use of LDL-cholesterol targets may result in undertreatment with statin therapy (i.e., using a suboptimal dose of statin because the goal has been achieved, particularly in patients with lower baseline LDL-cholesterol concentrations) or overtreatment with nonstatin drugs that have not been shown to reduce ASCVD events (e.g., adding a nonstatin drug to further reduce LDL-cholesterol and/or non-HDL-cholesterol concentrations and subsequently reducing the dose of the statin for safety reasons). The guideline states that by eliminating target goals, a patient who is adhering to optimal lifestyle management and statin therapy can avoid additional, nonevidence-based therapy even if his/her LDL-cholesterol concentration is higher than an arbitrary cutpoint; the requirement to achieve target goals under ATP III could make some patients unnecessarily feel like a failure. Many clinicians agree with the cholesterol expert panel's decision, stating that eliminating target goals greatly simplifies therapy for clinicians and patients because of less frequent laboratory monitoring and fewer dosage adjustments. However, other clinicians state that reversal of prior practice can confuse healthcare professionals and the public; furthermore, lipoprotein measurements during follow-up can serve as a marker of therapeutic response, promote adherence, motivate lifestyle improvements, and guide discussions about add-on pharmacologic therapy in high-risk patients.

The American Diabetes Association (ADA) recommends that a lipoprotein profile be obtained in all adult patients with diabetes mellitus at least annually to determine lipoprotein status; more frequent monitoring is recommended in patients whose LDL-cholesterol concentrations exceed the target goal. In low-risk patients (i.e., LDL-cholesterol concentrations less than 100 mg/dL, HDL-cholesterol concentrations exceeding 50 mg/dL, and triglyceride concentrations less than 150 mg/dL), lipoprotein analysis may be obtained once every 2 years.

Pediatric Patients There is no clear consensus on screening pediatric patients for lipid disorders. According to the NCEP expert panel, the American Academy of Pediatrics (AAP), and the AHA, a lipoprotein profile (preferably under fasting conditions) should be performed once every 5 years in children older than 2 years of age at *high* risk of developing dyslipidemia as adults (i.e., family history of premature cardiovascular disease [including CHD, atherosclerosis, peripheral vascular disease, cerebrovascular disease, MI], family history of dyslipidemia, presence of major risk factors [including obesity, hypertension, cigarette smoking, diabetes mellitus]) or in those for whom a family history is unavailable. However, studies have shown that this targeted screening approach will miss 30–60% of pediatric patients with elevated cholesterol concentrations. Therefore, an expert panel on integrated guidelines for cardiovascular health and risk reduction in children and adolescents recommends universal screening (nonfasting lipoprotein profile with non-HDL-cholesterol concentrations) in all children 9–11 years of age and 17–21 years of age.

Thresholds for therapy considerations and target LDL-cholesterol goals vary among pediatric guidelines, and clinicians are encouraged to consult individual guidelines for additional information. According to the AAP Committee on Nutrition, the AHA, and the NCEP expert panel on blood cholesterol concentrations in children and adolescents, dietary measures should be considered in all adolescents and children 2 years of age and older who have LDL-cholesterol concentrations exceeding 110 mg/dL. The AHA, NCEP expert panel, and the expert panel on integrated guidelines for cardiovascular health and risk reduction in children and adolescents state that antilipemic drug therapy should be reserved for children 10 years of age and older who, despite strict dietary management, have a serum LDL-cholesterol concentration of 190 mg/dL or greater *or* a serum LDL-cholesterol concentration of 160 mg/dL or greater and either a family history of definite premature cardiovascular disease (e.g., CHD, cerebrovascular or occlusive peripheral vascular disease) or at least 2 other risk factors (i.e., cigarette smoking, hypertension, low serum HDL-cholesterol concentrations, diabetes mellitus, severe obesity [30% or more overweight], physical inactivity) despite an adequate trial (6–12 months) of dietary management. The AAP supports the above thresholds but states that antilipemic therapy may be initiated in children as young as 8 years of age. The AAP also states that antilipemic therapy may be considered in children 8 years of age and older who have diabetes mellitus and a serum LDL-cholesterol concentration of 130 mg/dL or greater; the AHA and the expert panel on integrated guidelines for cardiovascular health and risk reduction in children and adolescents state that antilipemic therapy may be considered in *selected* children younger than 10 years of age who have severe lipid abnormalities along with other risk factors and/or high-risk conditions (e.g., diabetes mellitus). Some clinicians recommend initiating antilipemic therapy in selected children 5 years of age or older who have a serum LDL-cholesterol concentration of 160 mg/dL or greater and a family history of definite premature cardiovascular disease. Although antilipemic therapy may be initiated at a younger age in selected children who have extremely high cholesterol concentrations, the NCEP expert panel states that only a small proportion of children and adolescents should be considered for drug therapy because of the adverse effects, expense, and the lack of definitive, prospective data on the effects of such treatment on coronary heart disease. (See Cautions: Pediatric Precautions.) The AHA and the NCEP expert panel state that the minimum goal of dietary or drug therapy in children 2 years of age and older and adolescents is to achieve an LDL-cholesterol concentration of less than 130 mg/dL or, if possible, less than 110 mg/dL. The AAP states that these target goals may be warranted in patients with a strong family history of cardiovascular disease or in those with multiple risk factors.

■ Treatment Recommendations

Adults The goal of antilipemic therapy is to reduce the risk of ASCVD in patients with or without clinical ASCVD (secondary or primary prevention, respectively). The intensity of therapy is guided by the initial risk status of the patient, with the most intensive approach reserved for those in the highest risk category.

ATP III and the ACC/AHA cholesterol management guideline state that nondrug therapies (i.e., lifestyle modifications) are the foundation of ASCVD prevention. Drug therapy is not a substitute for but an adjunct to these nondrug therapies and measures, which should be continued when drug therapy is initiated. Lifestyle modifications include adherence to a heart-healthy diet (i.e., intake of vegetables, fruits, and whole grains with an appropriate caloric requirement; restriction of saturated fat intake to 5–6% of total daily calories; reduction in the percent of calories from saturated and trans fat), regular exercise (i.e., aerobic physical activity 3–4 times per week), avoidance of tobacco products, and maintenance of a healthy weight.

ATP III previously recommended that the intensity of antilipemic drug therapy be guided by initial risk status and LDL-cholesterol concentrations (treat-to-target approach). (See Table 1.)

Table 1. ATP III LDL-cholesterol Goals and Cutpoints for Lifestyle Modifications and Drug Therapy in Different Risk Categories

Risk Category	LDL-cholesterol Goal (mg/dL)	LDL-cholesterol Concentration at Which to Initiate Lifestyle Modifications (mg/dL)	LDL-cholesterol Concentration at Which to Consider Drug Therapy (mg/dL)
High risk: CHD or CHD risk equivalents (10-year risk >20%)	<100 (optional goal: <70)	≥100	≥100 (<100: consider drug options)
Moderately high risk: 2+ risk factors (10-year risk 10–20%)	<130 (optional goal: <100)	≥130	≥130 (100–129: consider drug options)
Moderate risk: 2+ risk factors (10-year risk <10%)	<130	≥130	≥160
Lower risk: 0–1 risk factor	<160	≥160	≥190 (160–189: drug optional)

Adapted from Grundy SM, Cleeman JI, Bairey Merz CN et al. Implications of recent clinical trials for the National Cholesterol Education Program Adult Treatment Panel III guidelines. Circulation. *2004; 110: 227-39.*

The more recent ACC/AHA cholesterol management guideline states that statins are the drugs of choice for prevention of ASCVD in adults; nonstatin therapies do not provide acceptable ASCVD risk reduction benefits compared to their potential for adverse effects in the routine prevention of ASCVD. The ACC/AHA cholesterol management guideline recommends a fixed-dose approach (high-, moderate-, or low-intensity statin therapy). (See Table 2.) The guideline states that giving a maximally tolerated statin intensity should be emphasized over giving lower statin dosages and adding nonstatin drugs to address low HDL-cholesterol or high triglyceride concentrations, a strategy that has not yet been shown to reduce ASCVD risk. However, consideration may be given to adding a nonstatin drug to statin therapy in certain high-risk patients (i.e., patients with ASCVD, patients with LDL-cholesterol concentrations of 190 mg/dL or greater, patients with diabetes mellitus) who have a less-than-anticipated response to statins, are unable to tolerate even a less-than-recommended intensity of a statin, or are completely intolerant to statin therapy. When a nonstatin drug is required, selection of the nonstatin drug should be based on a favorable benefit-risk ratio (i.e., demonstrated benefit of ASCVD risk reduction outweighs risks of adverse effects and drug interactions) and patient preferences.

Table 2. ACC/AHA Cholesterol Management Guideline Recommendations for High-, Moderate-, and Low-Intensity Statin Therapy[a,b]

High-intensity Statin Therapy[c]	Moderate-intensity Statin Therapy[d]	Low-intensity Statin Therapy[e]
Atorvastatin (40[f])–80 mg daily	**Atorvastatin 10** *(20)* **mg daily**	*Fluvastatin 20–40 mg daily*
Rosuvastatin 20 *(40)* **mg daily**	**Fluvastatin 40 mg twice daily**	**Lovastatin 20 mg daily**
	Fluvastatin 80 mg daily (extended-release)	*Pitavastatin 1 mg daily*
	Lovastatin 40 mg daily	**Pravastatin 10–20 mg daily**
	Pitavastatin 2–4 mg daily	*Simvastatin 10 mg daily*
	Pravastatin 40 *(80)* **mg daily**	
	Rosuvastatin *(5)* **10 mg daily**	
	Simvastatin 20–40 mg daily[g]	

[a] Statins and dosages that have been evaluated in randomized controlled studies are noted in **bold** (all of these randomized controlled studies with ASCVD outcomes have demonstrated a reduction in major cardiovascular events). Entries that appear in *italics* are FDA labeled, but these statins and dosages were not evaluated in the randomized controlled studies reviewed by the ACC/AHA expert panel.

[b] Individual responses to statin therapy varied in randomized controlled studies and should be expected to vary in clinical practice. There might be a biologic basis for a less-than-average response.

[c] Daily dosage reduces LDL-cholesterol concentration by approximately 50% or greater

[d] Daily dosage reduces LDL-cholesterol concentration by approximately 30–49%

[e] Daily dosage reduces LDL-cholesterol concentration by less than 30%

[f] Evidence from 1 randomized controlled study only. If patients cannot tolerate atorvastatin 80 mg daily (as in IDEAL study), reduce dosage to 40 mg daily.

[g] Although simvastatin 80 mg daily was evaluated in randomized controlled studies, initiation of or titration to a simvastatin dosage of 80 mg daily is not recommended by FDA because of the increased risk of myopathy, including rhabdomyolysis.

Adapted from Stone NJ, Robinson JG, Lichtenstein AH et al. 2013 ACC/AHA guideline on the treatment of blood cholesterol to reduce atherosclerotic cardiovascular risk in adults: A report of the American College of Cardiology/American Heart Association Task Force on Practice Guidelines. Circulation. *2014; 129(25 Suppl 2): S1-S45.*

The ACC/AHA cholesterol management guideline states that treatment decisions for women and racial and ethnic subgroups should be based on estimated 10-year ASCVD risk. (See General Principles of Antilipemic Therapy: Risk Assessment.) Because of insufficient data, the guideline makes no recommendations regarding initiation or discontinuance of statin therapy in patients with New York Heart Association (NYHA) class II–IV heart failure or in patients undergoing hemodialysis; if statin therapy is considered in individuals with these conditions, the clinician must evaluate the potential for ASCVD risk reduction benefit, adverse effects, drug interactions, and other cautions and contraindications associated with statin therapy.

Primary Prevention in Adults with Primary, Severe Elevations in LDL-cholesterol Concentration (190 mg/dL or Greater). Adults 21 years of age and older with primary, severe elevations in LDL-cholesterol concentration (190 mg/dL or higher) have a high lifetime risk for ASCVD events because of their lifetime exposure to markedly elevated LDL-cholesterol concentrations arising from genetic causes (i.e., familial [heterozygous and homozygous] hypercholesterolemia, familial defective apolipoprotein B-100, polygenic hypercholesterolemia). Therefore, these patients require substantial reductions in LDL-cholesterol concentrations and intensive management of other risk factors to reduce ASCVD risk. Although there are no controlled studies involving *only* patients with LDL-cholesterol concentrations of 190 mg/dL or higher, many studies evaluating statin therapy did include these patients, and all of these studies consistently demonstrated a reduction in ASCVD events. In addition, data from a meta-analysis indicate that each 39-mg/dL reduction in LDL-cholesterol concentration with statin therapy reduced ASCVD events by 22%, and the relative reductions in ASCVD events were consistent across the range of LDL-cholesterol concentrations. Therefore, ATP III and the ACC/AHA cholesterol guideline state that all patients with markedly elevated LDL-cholesterol concentrations arising from genetic causes should receive intensive antilipemic therapy to reduce risk. Because the hypercholesterolemia in these high-risk individuals often is genetically determined, family screening is especially important in this group to identify additional family members who would benefit from assessment and early treatment.

ATP III previously recommended that lifestyle modifications be initiated in all patients with heterozygous familial hypercholesterolemia, familial defective apolipoprotein B-100, or polygenic hypercholesterolemia to achieve a target LDL-cholesterol goal of less than 100, 130, or 160 mg/dL depending on initial risk status. (See Table 1.) ATP III stated that therapy with antilipemic agents (e.g., statins) should be considered as soon as it is apparent that the LDL-cholesterol goal cannot be achieved with lifestyle modifications alone. Combination therapy containing a statin and a bile acid sequestrant, or addition or substitution of another antilipemic agent, was considered useful in patients with very high LDL-cholesterol concentrations in whom initial drug therapy did not provide an adequate response. In patients who require even greater reductions in serum lipid concentrations, ATP III recommended that triple-drug therapy with a statin, a bile acid sequestrant, and niacin be considered. However, concomitant use of statins and fibric acid derivatives or niacin (at lipid-modifying dosages [i.e., at least 1 g daily]) can greatly increase the risk of adverse muscular effects and should be undertaken with caution. (See Drug Interactions: Antilipemic Agents.) ATP III stated that combination therapy generally is required less often in patients with familial defective apolipoprotein B-100 or polygenic hypercholesterolemia than in those with heterozygous familial hypercholesterolemia. Patients with homozygous familial hypercholesterolemia have poorly functioning, few, or no LDL receptors and generally are much less responsive to antilipemic therapy than those who have the heterozygous form of the disease. ATP III stated that although dietary therapy generally does not appear to be effective, high dosages of certain antilipemic agents (i.e., niacin, statins) have been shown to produce mild to moderate cholesterol reductions in some patients. According to ATP III, acceptable therapy in patients with homozygous familial hypercholesterolemia consisted of modified forms of plasmapheresis that selectively remove VLDL- and LDL-cholesterol from the plasma, although other techniques (e.g., heparin-induced extracorporeal lipoprotein precipitation) also may be employed.

The ACC/AHA cholesterol management guideline classifies patients 21 years of age and older without clinical ASCVD who have primary, severe elevations in LDL-cholesterol concentration (190 mg/dL or greater) as a major statin benefit group and recommends that lifestyle modifications and statin therapy be initiated simultaneously in such patients. However, before initiating statin therapy, patients should be evaluated to rule out secondary causes of hyperlipidemia (see General Principles of Antilipemic Therapy: Initial Evaluation); in addition, it is reasonable for clinicians and patients to discuss the potential for ASCVD risk reduction benefits, adverse effects, and drug interactions, as well as patient preferences for treatment. The ACC/AHA cholesterol management guideline recommends that high-intensity statin therapy be initiated unless contraindicated; in patients who are unable to tolerate high-intensity statin therapy, the maximum tolerated statin intensity should be used. (See Table 2.) In general, it is reasonable to intensify statin therapy to achieve at least a 50% reduction in LDL-cholesterol concentrations.

Primary Prevention in Adults with Diabetes Mellitus. Diabetes mellitus has been found to be an independent risk factor for several forms of cardiovascular disease (e.g., atherosclerotic CHD, diabetic cardiomyopathy, cerebrovascular disease, peripheral vascular disease) in men and women. Because diabetes mellitus often is associated with hyperglycemia, atherogenic dyslipidemia (i.e., presence of elevated triglycerides, small dense LDL particles, and low HDL-cholesterol), and other lipid and nonlipid risk factors of the metabolic syndrome, the risk for major coronary events (MI and CHD death) in patients with diabetes mellitus has been found to be similar to that in nondiabetic patients with CHD. In addition, patients 40–75 years of age with diabetes mellitus have a substantially increased lifetime risk for ASCVD events and death, and such patients experience greater morbidity and worse survival following the onset of clinical ASCVD.

Because of the increased risk of cardiovascular morbidity and mortality, ATP III identified diabetes mellitus as a *CHD risk equivalent* and recommended that patients receive antilipemic therapy to achieve an LDL-cholesterol target goal of less than 100 mg/dL (or, alternatively, less than 70 mg/dL). (See Table 1.) The guideline stated that pharmacologic therapy should be initiated simultaneously with lifestyle modifications when LDL-cholesterol concentrations are 100 mg/dL or greater. A statin was considered the initial drug of choice for diabetic dyslipidemia, although a bile acid sequestrant also could be a useful alternative. ATP III stated that a fibric acid derivative or niacin (with or without a statin) could be considered in patients in whom initial therapy did not provide an adequate response. However, the ACC/AHA cholesterol management guideline states that use of a statin in combination with fenofibrate in patients with diabetes mellitus has not been shown to provide additional ASCVD risk reduction benefit beyond that already demonstrated with statin monotherapy. (See Patients with Diabetes Mellitus under Prevention of Cardiovascular Events: Primary Prevention, under Uses.) In patients with triglyceride concentrations of 200 mg/dL or greater, ATP III stated that non-HDL-cholesterol concentrations should be recognized as a secondary target of cholesterol-lowering therapy. (See Hypertriglyceridemia under Treatment Recommendations: Adults, in General Principles of Antilipemic Therapy.) Although ATP III provided no specific target concentration for triglycerides, some clinicians recommended a target serum triglyceride concentration of 200 mg/dL or less in diabetic patients without clinically evident CHD and 150 mg/dL or less in those with clinically evident CHD. According to ATP III, clinical judgment is required in deciding how intensively to apply treatment guidelines in geriatric patients (65 years of age and older) with diabetes mellitus; treatment in such patients should take into account factors such as the presence of concomitant disease (e.g., other CHD risk factors), general health status, and social issues.

The ACC/AHA cholesterol management guideline classifies patients 40–75 years of age with type 1 or 2 diabetes mellitus and LDL-cholesterol concentrations of 70–189 mg/dL as a major statin benefit group and recommends that lifestyle modifications and statin therapy be initiated simultaneously in such patients. However, before initiating statin therapy, it is reasonable for clinicians and patients to discuss the potential for ASCVD risk reduction benefits, adverse effects, and drug interactions, as well as patient preferences for treatment. The ACC/AHA cholesterol management guideline states that moderate-intensity statin therapy should be initiated or continued in patients 40–75 years of age with type 1 or 2 diabetes mellitus and LDL-cholesterol concentrations of 70–189 mg/dL; in those with an estimated 10-year ASCVD risk of 7.5% or higher, it is reasonable to consider high-intensity statin therapy. (See Table 2.) In patients with diabetes mellitus who are younger than 40 or older than 75 years of age, it is reasonable to evaluate the potential benefits, adverse effects, drug interactions, and patient preferences when deciding to initiate, continue, or intensify statin therapy.

ADA states that statin therapy should be considered (in addition to lifestyle modifications) in diabetic patients younger than 40 years of age without overt CHD who have LDL-cholesterol concentrations exceeding 100 mg/dL or multiple cardiovascular risk factors. In diabetic patients with overt CHD or in those without CHD who are older than 40 years of age and have one or more other CVD risk factors (e.g., family history of CHD, hypertension, smoking, dyslipidemia, albuminuria), ADA states that statin therapy should be added to lifestyle modifications regardless of baseline LDL-cholesterol concentrations. The target LDL-cholesterol goal for diabetic patients without overt CHD is less than 100 mg/dL; an optional goal of 70 mg/dL (with high-dose statin therapy) is suggested for those with overt CHD. The ADA states that a target triglyceride concentration of less than 150 mg/dL and an HDL-cholesterol concentration exceeding 40 mg/dL (in men) or 50 mg/dL (in women) also are desirable, but LDL-cholesterol concentration remains the preferred target of therapy. If target LDL-cholesterol goal cannot be achieved with the maximally tolerated statin intensity, a reduction in LDL-cholesterol concentration of 30–40% from baseline is an alternative therapeutic goal. ADA states that use of a statin in combination with a nonstatin drug has not been shown not to provide additional cardiovascular benefit beyond that already demonstrated with statin monotherapy and is generally not recommended.

The American College of Physicians (ACP) also recommends antilipemic therapy in patients with type 2 diabetes mellitus based on the presence of CHD and/or major risk factors. ACP recommends that statin therapy be initiated in all patients with type 2 diabetes mellitus who have clinically evident CHD; patients with low HDL- and LDL-cholesterol concentrations may benefit more from gemfibrozil than statin therapy. Statin therapy also should be initiated in all patients with type 2 diabetes mellitus who do not have established CHD but have other cardiovascular risk factors; there are no data supporting the use of statins in low-risk patients younger than 55 years of age who have type 2 diabetes mellitus and no other cardiovascular risk factors. If statin therapy is initiated in patients with type 2 diabetes mellitus, ACP recommends that at least moderate dosages of the drugs be used. Based on results of primary prevention trials, ACP states that it would be reasonable to use atorvastatin 20 mg daily, lovastatin 40 mg daily, pravastatin 40 mg daily, or simvastatin 40 mg daily in diabetic patients without clinical evidence of CHD. For secondary prevention in diabetic patients, the following statin regimens have been used in clinical trials: fluvastatin 80 mg daily, lovastatin 40–80 mg daily, pravastatin 40 mg daily, and simvastatin 20 or 40 mg daily.

Primary Prevention in Patients with Elevated ASCVD Risk. ATP III previously recommended that lifestyle modifications be initiated in all patients with LDL-cholesterol concentrations above the target goal. (See Table 1.) If the target LDL-cholesterol goal was not achieved after an appropriate trial of lifestyle modifications (approximately 3 months), drug therapy could be initiated and lifestyle modifications continued to maintain the LDL-cholesterol target goal. A statin was considered the initial drug of choice, although a bile acid sequestrant or niacin also could be a useful alternative. Niacin or a fibric acid derivative was recommended for patients with moderately elevated LDL-cholesterol concentrations who have low HDL-cholesterol or high triglyceride concentrations. In patients in whom initial drug therapy does not provide an adequate response, ATP III stated that dosage of the statin could be increased or combination therapy containing a statin and a bile acid sequestrant or niacin could be employed. (See Cautions: Precautions and Contraindications and also Drug Interactions: Antilipemic Agents.)

The ACC/AHA cholesterol management guideline classifies patients 40–75 years of age without clinical ASCVD or diabetes mellitus who have LDL-cholesterol concentrations of 70–189 mg/dL and an estimated 10-year ASCVD risk of 7.5% or higher as a major statin benefit group and recommends that lifestyle modifications and statin therapy be initiated simultaneously in such patients. However, before initiating statin therapy, it is reasonable for clinicians and patients to discuss the potential for ASCVD risk reduction benefits, adverse effects, and drug interactions, as well as patient preferences for treatment. When antilipemic drug therapy is considered, the ACC/AHA cholesterol management guideline states that moderate- to high-intensity statin therapy should be initiated or continued. (See Table 2.) In those with an estimated 10-year ASCVD risk of 5 to less than 7.5%, it is reasonable to offer treatment with moderate-intensity statin therapy. In adults with LDL-cholesterol concentrations less than 190 mg/dL who are not otherwise identified in a statin benefit group, or for whom a treatment decision is uncertain, additional factors (e.g., LDL-cholesterol concentration greater than 160 mg/dL, evidence of genetic hyperlipidemias, family history of premature ASCVD [before 55 years of age in a male first-degree relative or before 65 years of age in a female first-degree relative]) may be considered to guide therapy; the ACC/AHA cholesterol management guideline states that statin therapy may be considered in these patients after evaluating the potential benefits, adverse effects, drug interactions, and patient preferences for such treatment.

The ACC/AHA cholesterol management guideline's recommendations for primary prevention are controversial and have not been widely implemented. Some clinicians state that the lowering of the statin treatment threshold to a 10-year risk of 7.5% and the adoption of the ASCVD risk-assessment calculator, which has been shown to potentially overestimate risk (see General Principles of Antilipemic Therapy: Risk Assessment), may result in overtreatment of some patients, particularly in primary prevention. ATP III previously recommended that statin therapy be initiated in patients with a 10-year CHD risk of 10–20% or less than 10% only if baseline LDL-cholesterol concentrations exceed 130 or 160 mg/dL, respectively. However, the ACC/AHA cholesterol management guideline recommends statin therapy based on 10-year ASCVD risk without considering baseline LDL-cholesterol concentration; for example, a 65 year-old man without hypertension, diabetes mellitus, or a history of smoking would be considered to have a 10-year ASCVD risk greater than 7.5%, and, therefore, would receive statin therapy regardless of baseline LDL-cholesterol concentration. If the ACC/AHA cholesterol management recommendations are widely implemented, some clinicians predict that millions more adults will be eligible for statin therapy, and such overtreatment may result in an increased incidence of statin-related adverse effects (e.g., myositis, rhabdomyolysis), which would generate a remarkable clinical and economic burden. To manage potential limitations of the lower treatment threshold and potential overestimation of the ASCVD risk-assessment calculator recommended by the ACC/AHA cholesterol management guideline, some clinicians suggest increasing the statin treatment threshold for primary prevention from 7.5% to 10 or 15% and expanding the definition of lower risk from a range of 5 to less than 7.5% to a range of 5–15%.

The ACC/AHA cholesterol management guideline's adoption of a global risk assessment approach to determine therapy for primary prevention also has been questioned. Some clinicians state that no trial of statin therapy has ever used a global risk prediction score as an enrollment criterion. Furthermore, statins have been shown to be effective for primary prevention only in certain patients (i.e., those with elevated LDL-cholesterol concentrations, low HDL-cholesterol concentrations, elevated C-reactive protein concentrations, diabetes mellitus, or hypertension). Therefore, these clinicians state that statin therapy should be used only in patient populations in whom efficacy has been demonstrated; in addition, rather than initiating statin therapy to reduce global risk, therapy for primary prevention should focus on the patient's underlying clinical conditions, such as eliminating cigarette use in a smoker or initiating antihypertensive therapy to manage hypertension.

Secondary Prevention. ATP III recommended that patients with clinical evidence of CHD receive antilipemic therapy to achieve an LDL-cholesterol target goal of less than 100 mg/dL (or, alternatively, less than 70 mg/dL). (See Table 1.) The guideline stated that antilipemic drug therapy should be started simultaneously with lifestyle modifications. A statin was considered the initial drug of choice, although a bile acid sequestrant or niacin could be a useful alternative. If target LDL-cholesterol goal was not achieved, ATP III suggested increasing dosage of the statin or, alternatively, adding a fibric acid derivative or niacin. If the target LDL-cholesterol goal has been achieved, ATP III stated that management of other lipid and nonlipid risk factors (e.g., low HDL-cholesterol concentrations, hypertriglyceridemia) should be considered.

The ACC/AHA cholesterol management guideline classifies patients with clinical ASCVD as a major statin benefit group and recommends that lifestyle modifications and statin therapy be initiated simultaneously in such patients. For secondary prevention in patients 21–75 years of age with clinical ASCVD, the guideline recommends that high-intensity statin therapy be initiated or continued as first-line therapy unless contraindicated. In patients 21–75 years of age with clinical ASCVD who are at increased risk for developing statin-associated adverse effects or in whom high-intensity statin therapy is inappropriate or contraindicated, moderate-intensity statin therapy should be given if tolerated. In patients older than 75 years of age with clinical ASCVD, use of statin therapy should be individualized based on the potential benefits, adverse effects, drug interactions, and patient preferences; it is reasonable to consider initiating or continuing moderate-intensity statin therapy in such patients if tolerated.

Metabolic Syndrome. According to ATP III, a diagnosis of the metabolic syndrome is established when 3 or more of the following risk factors are present: abdominal obesity (waist circumference exceeding 102 cm [40 inches] in men or exceeding 88 cm [35 inches] in women), triglyceride concentration of 150 mg/dL or greater, HDL-cholesterol concentrations less than 40 mg/dL in men or less than 50 mg/dL in women, blood pressure of 130/85 mm Hg or higher, and fasting blood glucose of 110–125 mg/dL. ATP III recommended that the metabolic syndrome be recognized as a secondary target of risk-reduction therapy (after appropriate control of LDL-cholesterol) in patients with multiple life-style and emerging risk factors.

The principal goals of therapy in the management of the metabolic syndrome are treatment of the underlying causes (i.e., obesity, physical inactivity) and management of other associated lipid and nonlipid risk factors. Weight reduction and increased physical activity generally are considered first-line therapies for the management of the metabolic syndrome. These measures, which effectively reduce most lipid and nonlipid risk factors, should be emphasized after appropriate control of LDL-cholesterol. Weight reduction can enhance LDL-cholesterol lowering, while regular physical activity can reduce very-low-density lipoprotein (VLDL)-cholesterol (and, in some patients, LDL-cholesterol) concentrations, increase HDL-cholesterol concentrations, lower blood pressure, reduce insulin resistance, and favorably influence cardiovascular function.

Management of other associated lipid and nonlipid risk factors also should be considered in patients with clinical evidence of the metabolic syndrome. These measures include treatment of hypertension, use of aspirin in patients with CHD to reduce the prothrombotic state, and management of elevated triglycerides and low HDL-cholesterol concentrations.

Hypertriglyceridemia. Pooled analysis of data from prospective studies indicates that elevated serum triglycerides, particularly when coupled with low HDL-cholesterol and a predominance of small, dense LDL particles (i.e., the lipid triad) are an independent risk factor for CHD. Elevated serum triglycerides have been found to increase the risk of developing hypertension and insulin resistance and to promote atherogenesis by inducing a prothrombotic state (i.e., increased platelet aggregability, elevated fibrinogen concentrations, increased plasminogen activator inhibitors [PAI], increased factor VII, and increased factor X clotting activity). This lipid abnormality most often is observed in individuals with the metabolic syndrome.

The finding that elevated triglycerides are an independent risk factor for CHD suggests that some triglyceride-rich lipoproteins (i.e., remnant lipoproteins) may be atherogenic. Therefore, atherogenic remnant lipoproteins levels (as determined by measurement of VLDL-cholesterol concentrations) should be included in the initial assessment of risk and determination of target goals. ATP III considered non-HDL-cholesterol concentration as a *secondary* target of therapy in patients with triglyceride concentrations of 200–499 mg/dL. Because a VLDL-cholesterol concentration of 30 mg/dL or less is considered normal, the goal for non-HDL-cholesterol in patients with triglyceride concentrations of 200 mg/dL or greater generally can be set at 30 mg/dL higher than that for LDL-cholesterol concentrations. Table 3 summarizes ATP III guidelines for target LDL-cholesterol and non-HDL-cholesterol goals in patients in each risk category who have elevated triglycerides.

Table 3. ATP III LDL-cholesterol and Non-HDL-cholesterol Goals for 3 Risk Categories

Risk Category	LDL-cholesterol Goal (mg/dL)	Non-HDL-cholesterol Goal (mg/dL)
CHD or CHD risk equivalents (10-year risk >20%)	<100	<130
2+ Risk factors (10-year risk ≤20%)	<130	<160
0–1 Risk factor	<160	<190

Modified from Expert Panel on Detection, Evaluation, and Treatment of High Blood Cholesterol in Adults. Executive summary of the third report of the National Cholesterol Education Program (NCEP) Expert Panel on Detection, Evaluation, and Treatment of high Blood Cholesterol in Adults (Adult Treatment Panel III). JAMA. *2001; 285:2486-97.*

ATP III stated that initiation of therapy and target goals in the management of hypertriglyceridemia depend on initial risk status and preexisting triglyceride concentrations. In patients with borderline high (150–199 mg/dL) or high (200–499 mg/dL) triglyceride concentrations, LDL-cholesterol should be considered the principal target of therapy; in those with high triglyceride concentrations, non-HDL-cholesterol becomes a secondary target of therapy. The principal aim of therapy in patients with very high triglyceride concentrations (500 mg/dL or greater) is to prevent acute pancreatitis through triglyceride lowering; target LDL- and non-HDL-cholesterol concentrations similar to those used in patients with borderline high or high triglycerides may be considered in these patients when triglyceride concentrations are reduced to less than 500 mg/dL.

ATP III stated that nondrug therapies and measures (i.e., weight reduction, increased physical activity, smoking cessation, restriction of excessive alcohol use, avoidance of high-carbohydrate [more than 60% of calories] diets) are considered the initial treatments of choice in the management of patients with *borderline high* or *high* triglyceride concentrations. Drug therapy, in addition to nonpharmacologic measures, also may be considered (after LDL-lowering therapy) in patients with *high* triglyceride concentrations to achieve the non-HDL-cholesterol goal. In these patients, ATP III recommended one of several options: intensifying therapy with an LDL-lowering drug (i.e., statin), initiating therapy with a triglyceride-lowering drug (i.e., fibric acid derivative or niacin), or combining moderate doses of statins and triglyceride-lowering drugs. AHA states that although statins have consistently shown benefit in subgroups with or without high triglyceride concentrations, fibric acid derivatives have more commonly been shown to provide greater benefit in subgroups with increased triglyceride concentrations. Concomitant use with a fibric acid derivative (i.e., fenofibrate) requires reduction in the daily dosage of the statin and should be used with *extreme caution* to minimize the potential risk of myopathy and/or rhabdomyolysis. In addition, some clinicians state that such combined regimens generally should be avoided in geriatric patients, in patients with acute or serious chronic illnesses (especially chronic renal disease), in patients undergoing surgery, and in patients receiving certain interacting medications. (See Cautions: Precautions and Contraindications and see Drug Interactions: Antilipemic Agents.) In patients who require even greater reductions in serum lipid concentrations, some clinicians recommend that triple-drug therapy with a statin, niacin, and a bile acid sequestrant be considered.

Patients with *very high* triglyceride concentrations should be treated more intensively to prevent development of acute pancreatitis. However, before initiating antilipemic therapy, patients with triglyceride concentrations of 500 mg/dL or greater should be evaluated to rule out secondary causes of hyperlipidemia. (See General Principles of Antilipemic Therapy: Initial Evaluation.) ATP III recommended elimination of alcohol from diet and identification and, preferably, discontinuance of drugs that increase triglyceride concentrations. In addition, insulin or oral antidiabetic therapy may be initiated (or dosage increased) in patients with hyperglycemia. In patients with triglyceride concentrations exceeding 1000 mg/dL, a very low-fat diet (less than 15% of total daily calories as fat) should be initiated immediately to improve chylomicronemia that contributes to hypertriglyceridemia. Weight reduction and increased physical activity as components of lifestyle modifications should be emphasized. Pharmacologic therapy with triglyceride-lowering drugs (i.e., niacin or, preferably, a fibric acid derivative) usually is required in patients with very high triglyceride concentrations and often can prevent acute pancreatitis. Because niacin may worsen hyperglycemia (and thus increase triglyceride concentrations), high doses (exceeding 2 g daily) of the drug generally should be used with caution in patients with elevated serum glucose concentrations. For most patients with very high triglyceride concentrations, therapy is considered successful if triglyceride concentrations are reduced to less than 500 mg/dL; triglyceride concentrations often cannot be normalized in these patients. The principal aim of therapy is to prevent acute pancreatitis; efforts to modify CHD risk (by lowering LDL- and/or non-HDL-cholesterol concentrations) may be considered once triglyceride concentrations have been reduced to less than 500 mg/dL.

A fibric acid derivative or niacin generally is considered the initial drug of choice when drug therapy is indicated for the treatment of primary dysbetalipoproteinemia, although a statin may be a useful alternative. Both triglyceride-lowering drugs (i.e., fibric acid derivatives and niacin) and statins have been shown to effectively reduce β-VLDL (i.e., cholesterol- and triglyceride-rich remnant lipoprotein) concentrations in patients with primary dysbetalipoproteinemia.

Patients with very high triglyceride and chylomicron concentrations usually have a genetic form of the disease and generally are unresponsive to triglyceride-lowering drugs. Treatment for these patients includes very low-fat diets, which may be supplemented with medium-chain triglycerides to minimize production of chylomicrons.

Low HDL-Cholesterol. Because low HDL-cholesterol (less than 40 mg/dL) is a strong independent risk factor for CHD (see General Principles of Antilipemic Therapy: Rationale for Intervention), ATP III and some clinicians stated that therapeutic decisions should take into account the level of HDL-cholesterol, and the use of agents that raise HDL-cholesterol should be considered if antilipemic drug therapy is needed in a patient who has both high LDL-cholesterol and low HDL-cholesterol concentrations.

ATP III stated that the primary goal of therapy in patients with low HDL-cholesterol concentrations was reduction of LDL-cholesterol to target levels similar to those established for patients requiring primary and secondary prevention of CHD. Therefore, therapeutic approaches in patients with low HDL-cholesterol concentrations generally are similar to those used for primary or secondary prevention of CHD and include lifestyle modifications (e.g., dietary management, weight reduction, increased physical activity) and antilipemic therapy (i.e., statins) to lower LDL-cholesterol concentrations.

In patients with clinical signs of the metabolic syndrome, weight reduction and increased physical activity should be emphasized. (See Metabolic Syndrome under Treatment Recommendations: Adults, in General Principles of Antilipemic Therapy.) In those with low HDL-cholesterol associated with high triglycerides (200–499 mg/dL), ATP III stated that non-HDL-cholesterol should be recognized as a secondary target of therapy. (See Hypertriglyceridemia under Treatment Recommendations: Adults, in General Principles of Antilipemic Therapy.) Although drugs that raise HDL-cholesterol (i.e., niacin, fibric acid derivatives) generally may be considered in patients with isolated low HDL-cholesterol concentrations (i.e., in those with triglycerides less than 150 mg/dL), ATP III stated that such therapy should be reserved for those with CHD or CHD risk equivalents. It should be noted that the addition of niacin to existing statin-based therapy has not been shown to further reduce the incidence of major cardiovascular events in patients with established cardiovascular disease compared with statin-based therapy alone; therefore, it is not clear whether increasing HDL-cholesterol concentration reduces cardiovascular risk. (See Secondary Prevention under Uses: Prevention of Cardiovascular Events.)

Patients with HIV Infection. HIV infection has been associated with altered lipoprotein concentrations (e.g., elevated serum triglycerides, reduced total cholesterol). In addition, use of highly active antiretroviral therapy (HAART) containing protease inhibitors (PIs) has resulted in dyslipidemias (e.g., hypercholesterolemia, hypertriglyceridemia) and, possibly, carotid atherosclerosis and endothelial dysfunction. Data from several observational studies indicate that use of HAART, with or without an HIV PI, is associated with an increased risk of MI; however, conflicting data have been reported. Although specific effects of PI use and dyslipidemia on the risk of CHD remain to be elucidated, preliminary findings suggest that the risk of coronary events is increased in HIV-infected patients. These findings provide a strong rationale for initiating conventional risk-reducing interventions in patients who have the potential for long-term survival while receiving HAART, regardless of whether PIs are a component of the antiretroviral regimen.

The Infectious Disease Society of America (IDSA) and the Adult AIDS Clinical Trials Group currently recommend that all HIV-infected adults undergo evaluation and treatment on the basis of NCEP ATP III guidelines for dyslipidemia. A fasting lipoprotein profile should be obtained before initiation of antiretroviral therapy in such patients, within 3–6 months after initiation of antiretroviral therapy, and then yearly (unless abnormalities are detected or therapeutic interventions are initiated). For patients with elevated triglyceride concentrations (i.e., exceeding 200 mg/dL) at baseline, it may be preferable to obtain the lipoprotein profile sooner (e.g., within 1–2 months after initiating antiretroviral therapy). Risk assessment and identification of target LDL-cholesterol goals should be performed to determine the intensity of therapy. (See General Principles of Antilipemic Therapy: Risk Assessment.)

Nondrug therapies (i.e., lifestyle modifications) should be initiated in all patients with HIV infection who have LDL-cholesterol concentrations exceeding the target goal. Attention also must be given to other modifiable risk factors for CHD, such as cigarette smoking, diabetes mellitus, physical inactivity, obesity, and hypertension. In addition, it must be noted that interventions for advanced immunosuppression, opportunistic infections, malignancies, and HIV-associated wasting should take precedence during the initial stages of treatment.

Patients who fail to achieve the target LDL-cholesterol goal after an appropriate trial of nondrug therapy (i.e., lifestyle modifications) should be switched to alternative antiretroviral drugs *or* receive antilipemic drug therapy. Clinicians should weigh the risks of new treatment-related toxicities and the possibility of virologic relapse when switching antiretroviral drugs against the risks of potential drug interactions and new treatment-related toxicities from antilipemic agents that are added to existing regimens.

Switching to alternative antiretroviral drugs has the potential advantage of avoiding pharmacologic therapy for dyslipidemia. However, because of the multifactorial nature of dyslipidemia in HIV infection, abnormalities may not resolve simply by switching drugs. Replacing the HIV PI in the regimen with atazanavir or changing to a regimen that contains antiretrovirals with less propensity for causing hyperlipidemia may be indicated. Switching from an HIV PI to nevirapine or abacavir generally has resulted in an improvement in total cholesterol and triglyceride concentrations, whereas switching to efavirenz has produced less consistent results. Results of switching from stavudine to abacavir have been inconclusive. Based on available data, IDSA and the Adult AIDS Clinical Trials Group state that in patients with a favorable treatment history (i.e., no previous treatment with a nucleoside reverse transcriptase inhibitor [NRTI]-based regimen that was less than fully suppressive, no history of virologic rebound occurring while receiving treatment), switching from a potentially lipid level-increasing PI to nevirapine or abacavir may be preferable to pharmacologic therapy with antilipemic agents.

Antilipemic therapy may be considered in patients who fail to achieve the target LDL-cholesterol goal after an appropriate trial of nondrug therapy (i.e., lifestyle modifications) and in whom alternative antiretroviral therapy is not appropriate. In patients with elevated LDL-cholesterol concentrations *or* in those with elevated non-HDL-cholesterol concentrations and triglyceride concentrations of 200–500 mg/dL, IDSA and the Adult AIDS Clinical Trials Group recommend initiating therapy with a statin, preferably pravastatin (20–40 mg once daily initially) or atorvastatin (10 mg once daily initially); fluvastatin (20–40 mg once daily initially) is a reasonable alternative. The fact that pharmacokinetic interactions can occur between certain statins and HIV PIs and nonnucleoside reverse transcriptase inhibitors (NNRTIs) should be considered. (See Antiretroviral Agents under Drug Interactions: Drugs and Foods Affecting or Metabolized by Hepatic Microsomal Enzymes.) A fibric acid derivative, either gemfibrozil (600 mg twice daily) or micronized fenofibrate (54–160 mg once daily), is a reasonable alternative only when statins are not appropriate. Based on studies in individuals without HIV infection, the addition of a fibric acid derivative or niacin may be considered in patients who fail to respond adequately to full doses of a statin. (See Drug Interactions: Antilipemic Agents.) IDSA and the Adult AIDS Clinical Trials Group state that when used in combination with a fibric acid derivative, pravastatin or fluvastatin may be the preferred statins.

Patients with triglyceride concentrations exceeding 500 mg/dL who are candidates for antilipemic therapy may be treated with gemfibrozil (600 mg twice daily) or micronized fenofibrate (54–160 mg once daily); fish oils and niacin are reasonable alternatives. In patients who fail to respond adequately to fibric acid derivative therapy and maximal lifestyle changes, the *addition* of a fish oil supplement or niacin may be considered. Addition of a statin to a fibric acid derivative regimen when elevated triglyceride concentration is the predominant abnormality (e.g., when triglyceride concentrations exceed 500 mg/dL and LDL-cholesterol or non-HDL-cholesterol concentrations are at or near the target goal) generally is not recommended. (See Drug Interactions: Antilipemic Agents.)

Children and Adolescents For *primary prevention* in children 2 years of age or older and adolescents, lifestyle modifications, including dietary management (e.g., restriction of total and saturated fat and cholesterol intake), weight control, an appropriate program of physical activity, and management of potentially contributory disease, are the initial treatments of choice. The National Heart, Lung, and Blood Institute (NHLBI)-appointed expert panel on integrated guidelines for cardiovascular health and risk reduction in children and adolescents recommends that the Cardiovascular Health Integrated Lifestyle Diet (CHILD)-1 diet (intake of 25–30% of total calories from fat, with 8–10% of total calories from saturated fatty acids, and intake of less than 300 mg of cholesterol daily) be initiated in all children 2 years of age or older and adolescents who have LDL-cholesterol concentrations exceeding 130 mg/dL. A CHILD-2 diet (intake of 25–30% of total calories from fat, with 7% or less of total calories from saturated fatty acids, and intake of less than 200 mg of cholesterol daily) may be considered after 3 months in patients whose LDL-cholesterol concentrations remain at 130 mg/dL or greater. As part of lifestyle modifications, the AHA recommends addition of viscous (soluble) fiber to the diet. The recommended daily intake of soluble fiber is calculated as 5–10 g plus age (in years); the maximum recommended daily intake is 25 g daily. The expert panel on integrated guidelines for cardiovascular health and risk reduction in children and adolescents recommends a daily dietary fiber intake from food sources of at least 5 g plus age (in children 2–10 years of age) or up to 14 g per 1000 kcal (in children 11 years and older). For most patients without severe hypercholesterolemia, a 6- to 12-month trial of lifestyle modifications generally is recommended before considering pharmacologic measures.

The AAP, AHA, and the NCEP expert panel on blood cholesterol concentrations in children and adolescents state that pharmacologic therapy generally should be limited to patients who have serum LDL-cholesterol concentrations of 190 mg/dL or greater *or* those who have LDL-cholesterol concentrations of 160 mg/dL or greater and either a family history of premature cardiovascular disease or multiple risk factors despite an adequate trial of dietary management. The NHLBI expert panel on integrated guidelines for cardiovascular health and risk reduction in children and adolescents states that statin therapy should be considered in high-risk patients 10 years of age older only after a 6-month trial of dietary and lifestyle management (e.g., restriction of total and saturated fat and cholesterol intake, addition of plant stanols/sterols and viscous fiber to diet, an appropriate program of physical activity).

Recommendations for selection of antilipemic drug therapy vary among pediatric guidelines, and clinicians are encouraged to consult individual guidelines for additional information. Bile acid sequestrants (e.g., cholestyramine) previously were considered by NCEP as the initial drugs of choice for the management of hyperlipoproteinemia or primary prevention of CHD in children and adolescents. However, data from recent studies indicate that these agents are associated with a high incidence of adverse GI effects, poor palatability, and low compliance; furthermore, because of their limited effectiveness, bile acid sequestrants are unlikely to reduce LDL-cholesterol concentrations to target levels in children who meet the criteria for antilipemic therapy. In light of these findings, the AHA currently recommends statins as first-line therapy for the management of hyperlipoproteinemia or primary prevention of CHD in children and adolescents. Niacin may be effective in reducing LDL-cholesterol and triglyceride concentrations and increasing HDL-cholesterol concentrations; however, because of poor tolerance, potential for severe adverse effects (e.g., flushing, hepatic failure, myopathy, decreased glucose tolerance, hyperuricemia), and limited available data, the AAP and AHA state that niacin should not be recommended for routine use in the management of pediatric dyslipidemia but may be considered in selected patients. Fibric acid derivatives have not been extensively studied in children and, therefore, should be used cautiously and preferentially in children with severe elevations in triglyceride concentration who are at risk of developing pancreatitis. Cholesterol absorption inhibitors (i.e., ezetimibe) may potentially become an important treatment option; however, additional studies are needed to evaluate their use as monotherapy and their long-term effectiveness in pediatric patients.

For additional details on management of dyslipidemias in pediatric patients, consult the most recent Integrated Guidelines for Cardiovascular Health and Risk Reduction in Children and Adolescents (available at http://www.nhlbi.nih.gov).

Uses

■ **Overview** HMG-CoA reductase inhibitors (statins) are used as adjuncts to nondrug therapies (i.e., lifestyle modifications) to reduce the risk of a first major acute coronary event (e.g., coronary death, myocardial infarction [MI], unstable angina, stroke) and the risk of coronary revascularization procedures in patients *without* clinical evidence of coronary heart disease (CHD) (*primary prevention*). The drugs also are used to reduce the risk of recurrent acute coronary events (e.g., total mortality secondary to coronary death, MI, stroke, transient ischemic attack [TIA]) and the risk of coronary revascularization procedures in patients *with* clinical evidence of CHD (*secondary prevention*) who have normal or elevated cholesterol concentrations. The drugs also are used to slow the progression of atherosclerosis.

Statins are used as adjuncts to nondrug therapies (e.g., dietary management) in the management of specific dyslipidemias, including primary hypercholesterolemia or mixed dyslipidemia, homozygous familial hypercholesterolemia, primary dysbetalipoproteinemia, and hypertriglyceridemia.

Statins generally are considered first-line therapy for primary or secondary prevention of atherosclerotic cardiovascular disease (ASCVD) in patients with clinical ASCVD or in patients with elevated ASCVD risk. Reductions in LDL-cholesterol concentrations with statins generally exceed those attainable with recommended dosages of other antilipemic agents, including bile acid sequestrants, niacin, and fibric acid derivatives (e.g., gemfibrozil). Data from several placebo-controlled, comparative studies report greater reductions in total and LDL-cholesterol concentrations among patients who received statin therapy (23–36 and 30–40%, respectively) than in those treated with cholestyramine (18–23 and 15–32%, respectively), niacin (11 and 16%, respectively), or gemfibrozil (14–15 and 16–17%, respectively). (See Primary Hypercholesterolemia or Mixed Dyslipidemia under Uses: Dyslipidemias.) When given as monotherapy for primary or secondary prevention of CHD, statins have been shown to reduce the incidence of coronary events by approximately 24–37% and the risk of death from any cause by about 22–30%. Statin therapy also reduces the risk of angina pectoris, cerebrovascular accidents, and the need for coronary revascularization procedures (e.g., coronary artery bypass grafting [CABG], angioplasty).

Results of comparative clinical studies using recommended dosages of various statins indicate that these agents differ in lipid-lowering as well as non-lipid-lowering effects. Reductions in LDL-cholesterol concentrations averaging 27–60, 25–42, 17–36, 21–48, 31–45, 19–41, 45–63, and 26–51% have been reported with recommended daily dosages of atorvastatin, cerivastatin (no longer commercially available in the US), fluvastatin, lovastatin, pitavastatin, pravastatin, rosuvastatin, and simvastatin, respectively, in patients with various forms of dyslipidemia who received statin therapy for at least 6 weeks. While atorvastatin and rosuvastatin generally have produced greater reductions in total and LDL-cholesterol, apolipoprotein B (apo B), and triglycerides than equipotent dosages of other statins, the superiority of a given statin in terms of improvement in cardiovascular outcomes compared with other drugs in this class has not been clearly defined to date. However, pooled analysis of data from trials in which various statins were used for primary or secondary prevention of cardiovascular events or for reducing progression of atherosclerotic plaques indicate similar reductions in death and major cardiovascular events despite differences in the effects of these statins on cholesterol components. It has been suggested that these benefits may result from antilipemic as well as pleiotropic effects (e.g., inhibition of arterial smooth muscle cell proliferation, stabilization of atherosclerotic plaques) of statins. (See Pharmacology.) In addition, factors other than antilipemic potency, such as baseline LDL-cholesterol concentration, baseline CHD risk, time of assessment of clinical benefit (i.e., early angiographic improvement may not translate into clinical improvement for several years), or other characteristics of the study population also may affect outcome in clinical trials of patients receiving statin therapy. Further study is needed to determine the impact of differences in antilipemic and pleiotropic effects of statins on clinical outcomes.

Atorvastatin, lovastatin, and simvastatin are metabolized by the cytochrome P-450 isoenzyme 3A4 (CYP3A4) and are contraindicated, should be avoided, or used with extreme caution in patients receiving certain drugs or foods that inhibit CYP3A4 (e.g., cyclosporine, erythromycin, clarithromycin, telithromycin, delavirdine, efavirenz, itraconazole, ketoconazole, posaconazole, voriconazole, HIV protease inhibitors [PIs], nefazodone, cobicistat-containing preparations, grapefruit juice). Fluvastatin, pitavastatin, pravastatin, and rosuvastatin are not substantially metabolized by CYP3A4; however, some clinicians and the manufacturer recommend that rosuvastatin be used with caution in patients receiving certain HIV or hepatitis C virus (HCV) PIs (e.g., certain *ritonavir-boosted* HIV PIs, simeprevir). (See Drug Interactions: Drugs and Foods Affecting or Metabolized by Hepatic Microsomal Enzymes.)

■ **Prevention of Cardiovascular Events** ***Primary Prevention***
Statins are used as adjuncts to nondrug therapies (e.g., dietary management) to reduce the risk of a first major acute coronary event (e.g., MI, unstable angina, coronary revascularization procedure, coronary death, stroke) in patients *without* clinical evidence of CHD (*primary prevention*). For additional details regarding the use of specific statins, see the individual statin monographs in 24:06.08.

In a randomized, double-blind, placebo-controlled study (West of Scotland Coronary Prevention Study [WOSCOPS]) in men with moderate hypercholesterolemia and no history of MI, therapy with pravastatin (40 mg daily) for a median of 4.9 years lowered total and LDL-cholesterol by 20 and 26%, respectively, and reduced the incidence of MI and death from cardiovascular causes by approximately 31%; the risks of undergoing coronary angiography and myocardial revascularization procedures also were reduced by 31 and 37%, respectively. In another randomized, double-blind, placebo-controlled study (Air Force/Texas Coronary Atherosclerosis Prevention Study [AFCAPS/TexCAPS]) in men and women (45–73 years of age) with *average* or moderately elevated total and LDL-cholesterol and below-average HDL-cholesterol concentrations (i.e., 36–40 mg/dL), treatment with lovastatin (20–40 mg daily) for a median of 5.2 years reduced the incidence of first acute major coronary events (defined as fatal or nonfatal MI, unstable angina, or sudden cardiac death) by 37% and the need for revascularization procedures by 33%. Clinical benefit was achieved within 1 year of initiating therapy and continued throughout the remainder of the study.

Despite favorable findings from the WOSCOPS and AFCAPS/TexCAPS studies, clinical benefit (i.e., reduction in CHD-related morbidity or all-cause mortality) was not observed in a randomized, open-label study, the Lipid Lowering Trial (LLT), in a subset of patients from the Antihypertensive and Lipid Lowering Treatment to Prevent Heart Attack Trial (ALLHAT). In this study (ALLHAT-LLT) in patients 55 years of age or older with well-controlled hypertension and moderately elevated LDL-cholesterol concentrations, the incidence of all-cause mortality or CHD-related adverse events (i.e., CHD death, nonfatal MI, stroke, congestive heart failure) was similar among patients receiving pravastatin (40 mg daily) or usual care (i.e., moderate LDL-cholesterol lowering according to the discretion of the patient's primary care clinician) for a mean duration of 4.8 years. The lack of clinical benefit may be attributable to the modest difference in total and LDL-cholesterol reduction between pravastatin and usual care recipients (17 versus 8% reduction in total cholesterol and 28 versus 11% reduction in LDL-cholesterol) compared with the differences reported in other statin trials. This modest difference may have resulted from poor adherence to initially prescribed therapy; at year 6 of follow-up, only 70% of patients randomized to receive pravastatin were still taking the protocol-specified dosage (40 mg daily), while 28.5% of patients randomized to receive usual care were receiving antilipemic therapy (26.1% with a statin). Despite the reported lack of clinical benefit in this study, study results are consistent with previous findings indicating that lesser degrees of cholesterol lowering are associated with less clinical benefit. Adherence to treatment should be particularly emphasized when antilipemic therapy is implemented in routine clinical practice in order to achieve adequate reduction in LDL-cholesterol concentrations.

Results of a recent pooled analysis of randomized, controlled trials in patients (90% without clinical evidence of CHD) who are at moderate to moderately high risk of developing CHD indicate that treatment with a statin over a mean of 4.3 years substantially reduced the relative risk of major coronary events (including nonfatal MI) by 29.2%, major cerebrovascular events by 14.4%, and revascularization procedures by 33.8%, but not CHD or overall mortality, compared with placebo. Statin therapy did not appear to increase the risk of cancer or increase concentrations of aminotransferase or creatine kinase (CK, creatine phosphokinase, CPK), although the confidence intervals for these safety measures were very wide. Although the relative risk reductions observed in this study were similar to those reported in secondary prevention studies, the absolute benefit is substantially lower because of the lower risk in primary prevention patients. Some clinicians state that statins appear to be cost-effective for primary prevention in patients at high risk of developing CHD (10-year risk exceeding 20%) but cost-*in*effective in patients at low risk (10-year risk of less than 10%); further studies are needed to clarify the cost-effectiveness of statin therapy for primary prevention in patients at moderately high risk of developing CHD (10-year risk of 10–20%).

Patients with Diabetes Mellitus. Statins are used as adjuncts to nondrug therapies (e.g., dietary management) to decrease elevated serum total and LDL-cholesterol concentrations and to reduce the risk of initial or recurrent acute coronary events (primary or secondary prevention, respectively) in patients with or without clinical evidence of CHD and hypercholesterolemia associated with or exacerbated by diabetes mellitus (diabetic dyslipidemia).

Safety and efficacy of statins (e.g., atorvastatin) for the prevention of cardiovascular events in patients without clinical evidence of CHD, but with diabetes mellitus and other risk factors, have been established in at least one randomized, double-blind, placebo-controlled study. In the Collaborative Atorvastatin Diabetes Study (CARDS) in hypercholesterolemic patients (median total cholesterol concentration of 207 mg/dL, LDL-cholesterol concentration of 120 mg/dL, triglyceride concentration of 151 mg/dL) with type 2 diabetes mellitus (mean hemoglobin A_{1c} [HbA_{1c}] of 7.7%) *and* at least one other risk factor (e.g., smoking, hypertension, retinopathy, microalbuminuria, macroalbuminuria), therapy with atorvastatin (10 mg daily) for a median of 3.9 years reduced the risk of stroke by 48% and the risk of MI by 42% compared with placebo. Lipoprotein concentrations were lowered to levels similar to those observed with atorvastatin 10 mg daily in previous clinical studies. Treatment with atorvastatin did not reduce the risk of unstable angina, revascularization procedures, or acute CHD death.

Several subgroup analyses evaluating the benefits of statins in patients with established CHD and mildly elevated fasting glucose concentrations or diabetes mellitus have reported improvements in the risk of cardiovascular events, as evidenced by reductions in the risks of recurrent coronary events and revascularization procedures. In several subgroup analyses evaluating effects of statin therapy in CHD patients with elevated cholesterol concentrations and normal fasting glucose (defined as fasting plasma glucose concentrations less than

110 mg/dL [6 mmol/L]), impaired fasting glucose (defined as fasting plasma glucose concentrations between 110 and 126 mg/dL [6–7 mmol/L]), or diabetes mellitus (defined as fasting plasma glucose concentrations equal to or exceeding 126 mg/dL [7 mmol/L] with or without a clinical history of diabetes mellitus), treatment with pravastatin (40 mg daily) or simvastatin (40 mg daily) for at least 5 years was associated with reductions in the risk of major coronary events (23–32, 38, and 25–42% in patients with normal fasting glucose, impaired fasting glucose, and those with diabetes mellitus, respectively) and the risk of undergoing myocardial revascularization procedures (33, 43, and 32–48%, respectively). The risk of total mortality and coronary mortality was markedly reduced in patients with normal fasting glucose (28 and 42%, respectively) and impaired fasting glucose (43 and 55%, respectively) but was only modestly reduced in diabetic patients (21 and 28%, respectively).

The addition of fenofibrate to statin therapy has not been shown to provide an incremental benefit on cardiovascular morbidity and mortality beyond that already demonstrated with statin monotherapy. In the Action to Control Cardiovascular Risk in Diabetes (ACCORD Lipid) Study, the combination of fenofibrate (160 mg daily) and a statin (simvastatin at dosages up to 40 mg daily) was compared with statin therapy alone in patients with type 2 diabetes mellitus at high risk for cardiovascular disease. Despite a favorable effect on serum lipid concentrations (e.g., increased HDL-cholesterol, reduced triglycerides), the addition of fenofibrate to simvastatin therapy did not substantially reduce the rate of major adverse cardiovascular events (i.e., nonfatal MI, nonfatal stroke, death from cardiovascular causes) compared with statin monotherapy over a mean follow-up period of 4.7 years. In general, routine use of fenofibrate in combination with a statin to further reduce ASCVD risk is not recommended in patients with type 2 diabetes mellitus; while subgroup analyses indicate that such a combination may provide some benefit in certain groups of patients (e.g., those with type 2 diabetes mellitus and atherogenic dyslipidemia), further study is required to confirm these findings. The ACC/AHA cholesterol management guideline states that the combination of fenofibrate and low- or moderate-intensity statin therapy may be considered only if the benefits from ASCVD risk reduction or triglyceride lowering (when triglyceride concentrations exceed 500 mg/dL) outweigh the potential risk of adverse effects.

Secondary Prevention Statins are used as adjuncts to nondrug therapies (e.g., dietary management) in patients with clinical evidence of CHD (*secondary prevention*), including prior MI and angina pectoris, to reduce the risk of total mortality (by reducing coronary death), recurrent MI, stroke or transient ischemic attack (TIA), angina, or hospitalization for congestive heart failure (CHF), and to reduce the risk of undergoing myocardial revascularization procedures.

Several clinical trials designed to evaluate the benefits of statins in patients with established CHD, including prior MI and angina pectoris, have reported improvements in cardiovascular risk status, as evidenced by reductions in the risks of total mortality and nonfatal coronary events. In the Scandinavian Simvastatin Survival Study (4S), therapy with simvastatin (20–40 mg daily) in 4444 patients with hypercholesterolemia and angina pectoris or prior MI was associated with reductions in total mortality (30%), CHD mortality (42%), and hospital-verified nonfatal MI (37%) compared with placebo over a median of 5.4 years of follow-up; the risk of undergoing myocardial revascularization procedures also was reduced by 37%. In addition, simvastatin therapy reduced the risk of fatal and nonfatal cerebrovascular events (combined incidence of stroke and TIA) by 28%.

In the Heart Protection Study (HPS), therapy with simvastatin (40 mg daily) in over 20,000 patients with CHD, history of stroke, or other cerebrovascular disease, other occlusive arterial disease (e.g., peripheral arterial disease), hypertension, or diabetes mellitus reduced the risk of total mortality (13%), CHD mortality (18%), nonfatal MI (38%), ischemic stroke (25%), coronary revascularization procedures (30%), and peripheral and other noncoronary revascularization procedures (16%) compared with placebo over approximately 5 years of follow-up, irrespective of baseline lipoprotein concentrations.

In the Cholesterol and Recurrent Events (CARE) study, therapy with pravastatin (40 mg daily) in patients with prior MI and *average* cholesterol concentrations (baseline total, LDL-, and HDL-cholesterol concentrations averaging 209, 139, and 39 mg/dL, respectively) was associated with a 24% reduction in CHD mortality or nonfatal MI compared with placebo after an average follow-up period of approximately 5 years. Therapy with pravastatin also reduced the risk of undergoing myocardial revascularization procedures (e.g., coronary artery bypass grafting [CABG], percutaneous transluminal coronary angioplasty) by 27% and the risk of stroke or TIA by 26% (risk reduction of 31% for stroke alone). The reduction in combined coronary events was greater in women and in those with higher pretreatment LDL-cholesterol concentrations. In addition, risk reduction reported in the CARE trial also was observed in geriatric patients (65 years of age and older) and in patients who had undergone coronary revascularization.

In the Long-term Intervention with Pravastatin in Ischaemic Disease (LIPID) Study, therapy with pravastatin (40 mg daily) in patients with a history of MI or hospitalization for unstable angina and *normal* or elevated total cholesterol concentrations resulted in reductions in overall mortality (22%), CHD mortality (24%), MI (29%), stroke (19%), and coronary revascularization procedures (20%) compared with placebo after an average follow-up period of 6.1 years.

Certain statins have been shown to reduce the risk of recurrent stroke. In the Stroke Prevention by Aggressive Reduction in Cholesterol Levels (SPARCL) study in hypercholesterolemic patients (LDL-cholesterol concentrations of 100–190 mg/dL) who had a stroke or TIA within the past 1–6 months, therapy with high-dose atorvastatin (80 mg daily) for a median of 4.9 years reduced the risk of subsequent nonfatal or fatal stroke and of major cardiovascular events by approximately 16 and 20%, respectively, compared with placebo. However, atorvastatin therapy did not reduce overall mortality. In addition, hemorrhagic stroke and elevated aminotransferase (transaminase) concentrations were reported in more patients receiving atorvastatin than in those receiving placebo; patients with a history of hemorrhagic stroke at study entry appeared to be at increased risk of developing hemorrhagic stroke. Some clinicians state that the results of this study should be interpreted with caution due to the heterogeneity of enrolled patients (i.e., with respect to stroke etiology and vascular risk). Furthermore, because patients with atrial fibrillation or other cardiac sources of embolism were excluded from the study, it is not known whether the observed benefits of atorvastatin apply to ischemic strokes of cardioembolic origin.

Intensive Statin Therapy for Stable CHD. Intensive antilipemic therapy (i.e., with atorvastatin 80 mg daily) has been shown to be more effective than moderate antilipemic therapy (i.e., with atorvastatin 10 mg daily) in reducing the risk of cardiovascular events in patients with stable CHD. In a randomized, double-blind, active-controlled study (Treating to New Targets [TNT]) in approximately 10,000 patients with clinically evident CHD (i.e., history of MI, history of or current angina with objective evidence of atherosclerotic CHD, history of coronary revascularization) and LDL-cholesterol concentrations less than 130 mg/dL, treatment with atorvastatin 80 or 10 mg daily for a median of 4.9 years reduced LDL-cholesterol concentrations to a mean of 77 or 101 mg/dL, respectively. Compared with the 10-mg daily regimen, treatment with the 80-mg daily regimen resulted in a 22% relative reduction in the composite risk of primary end points (i.e., death from CHD, nonfatal non-procedure-related MI, resuscitated cardiac arrest, fatal or nonfatal stroke). Of the events that comprised the primary composite endpoint, treatment with the intensive regimen substantially reduced the rate of nonfatal non-procedure-related MI and fatal and nonfatal stroke, but not death from CHD or resuscitated cardiac arrest. Of the predefined secondary endpoints, treatment with the intensive regimen reduced the rate of coronary revascularization, angina, and hospitalization for CHF, but not peripheral vascular disease. The intensive regimen did not reduce overall mortality and was associated with a slightly (but not statistically significant) increased risk of death from noncardiovascular causes. In addition, severe adverse effects (e.g., elevations in concentrations of aminotransferase or creatine kinase [CK, creatine phosphokinase, CPK] to at least 3 or 10 times greater than the upper limit of normal, respectively) and discontinuance of therapy due to adverse effects occurred more frequently in patients receiving the 80-mg daily regimen compared with the 10-mg daily regimen. Although results of this study suggest that lowering LDL-cholesterol concentrations well below currently recommended levels may have some clinical benefit, previous National Cholesterol Education Program (NCEP) guidelines (Adult Treatment Panel III [ATP III]) recommended that the lower goal (i.e., 70 mg/dL) be considered only for patients at *very high risk.* Some clinicians state that further study is needed to evaluate the safety of high-dose statin therapy in patients with stable CHD before adopting a lower target LDL-cholesterol goal in these patients.

In a randomized, comparative study (Incremental Decrease in Endpoints through Aggressive Lipid Lowering [IDEAL]) in 8888 patients with a history of CHD and an average LDL-cholesterol concentration of approximately 122 mg/dL, treatment with atorvastatin (80 mg daily) or simvastatin (20–40 mg daily) for a median of 4.8 years resulted in similar reduction in the risk of the primary composite end point (i.e., fatal CHD, nonfatal MI, and resuscitated cardiac arrest). In addition, no difference in overall mortality was observed between atorvastatin- or simvastatin-treated patients, and the rates of death from cardiovascular or noncardiovascular causes were similar in both treatment groups.

Intensive Statin Therapy for CHD and the Metabolic Syndrome. Intensive antilipemic therapy (i.e., with atorvastatin 80 mg daily) has been shown to be more effective than moderate antilipemic therapy (i.e., with atorvastatin 10 mg daily) in reducing the risk of cardiovascular events in patients with CHD and the metabolic syndrome. In a post hoc analysis of the TNT study in 5584 patients with CHD and the metabolic syndrome, treatment with the intensive regimen was associated with a lower incidence of major cardiovascular events than treatment with the moderate regimen (9.5 versus 13%); this represented a 29% relative reduction in the risk of major cardiovascular events in favor of the intensive regimen. However, consistent with the overall population in the TNT study, the intensive regimen did not reduce overall mortality compared with the moderate regimen.

Early and Intensive Statin Therapy for Acute Coronary Syndrome. Intensive antilipemic therapy has been shown to be more effective than standard antilipemic therapy in reducing the risk of cardiovascular events in patients with an acute coronary syndrome (ACS). In a randomized, double-blind study (A to Z trial) in about 4500 patients with manifestations of ACS within the preceding 5 days, early initiation of intensive antilipemic therapy (simvastatin 40 mg daily for 1 month, then simvastatin 80 mg daily) for 6–24 months resulted in a 25% reduction in the risk of cardiovascular mortality compared with delayed initiation of a less aggressive antilipemic regimen (placebo for 4 months, then simvastatin 20 mg daily thereafter). There was a reduction (11%) in the rate of the primary end point (a composite of cardiovascular death, nonfatal MI, readmission for ACS, and stroke) for the entire study period (not statistically significant). Although no difference was evident between the intensive and less aggressive regimens during the first 4 months of therapy, the primary end point was substantially reduced (by 25%) from month 4 through the end of the study in patients receiving the intensive regimen. Intensive or less aggressive antilipemic therapy reduced LDL-cholesterol concentrations to a median of 63 or 77 mg/dL, respectively, at 8 months. While a favorable trend toward reduction of major cardiovascular events was observed in this study, it is possible that more intensive therapy is required immediately after the onset of ACS during the period of greatest clinical instability to achieve a more rapid clinical benefit. However, the possible adverse effects of high dosage of statins (e.g., myopathy) should be considered when contemplating early and intensive statin therapy.

In a randomized, double-blind, active-controlled study (Pravastatin or Atorvastatin Evaluation and Infection Therapy—Thrombolysis in Myocardial Infarction 22 [PROVE IT—TIMI 22]) in over 4000 patients hospitalized for ACS within the preceding 10 days, treatment with intensive antilipemic therapy (atorvastatin 80 mg daily) or standard antilipemic therapy (pravastatin 40 mg daily) for a mean of 2 years reduced LDL-cholesterol concentrations to a median of 62 or 95 mg/dL, respectively. Compared with the standard regimen, treatment with the intensive regimen resulted in a 16% reduction in the composite risk of primary end points, including a 14% reduction in the need for revascularization procedures and a 29% reduction in the risk of recurrent unstable angina. Atorvastatin therapy also was associated with reductions in the end points of death from any cause (28%) and of death or MI (18%) compared with pravastatin therapy, but these differences were not statistically significant. Results of this study suggest that among patients who have recently had an ACS, an intensive statin regimen provides greater protection against death or major cardiovascular events than does a standard regimen, and that patients benefit from early and continued lowering of LDL-cholesterol to levels substantially below currently recommended target levels. However, the possible adverse effects of high dosage of statins (e.g., myopathy) should be considered when contemplating early and intensive statin therapy.

Recent findings from a large prospective, observational study (involving review of a database of over 300,000 patients hospitalized for acute MI) indicate that initiation or continuation of statins within the first 24 hours of hospitalization for an acute MI is associated with a decreased risk of in-hospital mortality compared with no statin use (4 or 5.3% for initiation or continuation of statins, respectively, compared with 15.4% for no statin therapy); discontinuation of statin therapy after hospitalization was associated with a slightly *increased* risk of mortality (16.5%) compared with no statin therapy (15.4%). In this study, early statin use also was associated with a lower incidence of cardiogenic shock, cardiac arrest, cardiac rupture, and ventricular tachycardia/fibrillation, but not recurrent MI. While results of this study provide the strongest clinical evidence to date to support the hypothesis of early, direct cardioprotective effects of statins in acute MI, adequately powered, prospective randomized clinical trials are needed to confirm these findings.

In a Myocardial Ischemia Reduction with Aggressive Cholesterol Lowering (MIRACL) substudy in patients hospitalized for acute MI or unstable angina, initiation of high-dose atorvastatin therapy (80 mg daily) in the early phase of an acute coronary event (i.e., between 24 and 96 hours following hospital admission) reduced the risk of nonfatal stroke and fatal plus nonfatal stroke by approximately 50%; effects of lower dosages of the drug on the risk of stroke have not been established. Because of the short duration (16 weeks) of therapy and the small absolute number of cerebrovascular events (12 fatal or nonfatal strokes in the atorvastatin group and 24 in the placebo group), further study is needed to confirm the findings of this study.

Results of a recent pooled analysis of randomized, controlled trials in patients with ACS indicate that, compared with moderate antilipemic therapy or placebo, early (i.e., initiated within 14 days of hospitalization for ACS) and intensive statin therapy reduced the overall incidence of cardiovascular events and cardiovascular death. The overall cardiovascular benefit began to occur between 4–12 months of therapy and was maintained during the 2 years of follow-up. However, results of this analysis should be interpreted with caution because of several limitations (e.g., statistical heterogeneity, limited number of trials, data abstracted from literature and not from individual patient data); an additional pooled analysis using data from individual patients may be needed to confirm the results of this study.

Statin Therapy Following Percutaneous Coronary Intervention. Certain statins (i.e., fluvastatin) have been shown to reduce the risk of cardiovascular events in patients undergoing percutaneous coronary intervention (PCI). In a randomized, double-blind, placebo-controlled study (Lescol Intervention Prevention Study [LIPS]) in 1677 patients with stable or unstable angina or silent ischemia who had undergone a first percutaneous coronary intervention (PCI), therapy with fluvastatin (40 mg twice daily), initiated within a mean of 3 days following PCI and continued for a median of 3.9 years, resulted in a 22% reduction in the relative risk and a 5.3% reduction in the absolute risk of fatal or nonfatal major adverse cardiac events (e.g., cardiac death, nonfatal MI, PCI for a new lesion, or repeat PCI or coronary artery bypass grafting [CABG] procedure). Reduction in the risk of adverse cardiac events also was observed in geriatric patients (older than 65 years of age). Revascularization procedures (repeat PCI or CABG) involving the originally instrumented site comprised most of the initial recurrent adverse cardiac events; these procedures were performed in 143 or 171 patients receiving fluvastatin or placebo, respectively, within the first 6 months following the initial procedure. Treatment with fluvastatin also was associated with a 32% reduction in the risk of *late* revascularization procedures (i.e., PCI or CABG occurring at the original site more than 6 months following the initial procedure, or at another site).

Statins have been shown to reduce the rate of restenosis following coronary stent implantation. In a retrospective study in patients undergoing coronary stent implantation, statin therapy was associated with a substantial reduction in restenosis development (25.4% in statin-treated patients versus 38% in placebo-treated patients) during a follow-up period of 6 months. In addition, statin-treated patients also had a reduced incidence of MI and repeat revascularization procedures.

Statin Therapy in Patients with Heart Failure. Data from observational studies indicate that statins may have beneficial effects on clinical outcomes in patients with heart failure†. In one study, adult patients with heart failure who received statin therapy had a 24 or 21% lower relative risk of death or hospitalization for heart failure, respectively, compared with those who did not receive statin therapy. In another study, geriatric patients (65 years of age or older) with heart failurewho received statin therapy had a 20 or 18% reduction in mortality risk at 1 or 3 years, respectively, compared with those who did not receive statin therapy. However, randomized, controlled studies evaluating clinical outcomes (particularly in patients with nonischemic heart failure in whom antilipemic therapy is not otherwise recommended) are needed to clarify the roles of statins in the management of heart failure.

Reducing Progression of Coronary Atherosclerosis Statins are used to slow the progression of coronary atherosclerosis. For additional details regarding the use of specific statins, see the individual statin monographs in 24:06.08.

Statin therapy has been shown to slow the progression and/or induce regression of atherosclerosis in both coronary and carotid arteries by reducing intimal-medial wall thickness (IMT). (See Pharmacology: Antiatherogenic Effects.) In numerous double-blind, placebo-controlled studies in men and women with documented CHD (e.g., atherosclerosis, angina pectoris) and normal to moderately elevated lipoprotein concentrations, progression of atherosclerosis at 2–4 years (measured as the mean per-patient changes from baseline in mean and minimal coronary artery lumen diameters, diameter stenosis, and formation of new lesions) was reduced in patients who received recommended daily dosages of a statin compared with that in those receiving placebo.

Treatment with a statin also has been shown to reduce the rate of progression of atherosclerosis in the carotid arteries. In several double-blind, placebo-controlled studies, hypercholesterolemic patients with or without CHD who received recommended daily dosages of atorvastatin, lovastatin, pravastatin, or rosuvastatin for a median of 2–3 years showed less progression of atherosclerosis (as determined by B-mode ultrasound quantification of carotid artery IMT) compared with those receiving placebo.

Results from several atherosclerosis regression trials in patients with documented CHD, including atherosclerosis and angina pectoris, and mild to moderate hypercholesterolemia indicate that treatment with statins is associated with a reduction in the incidence of clinical events (i.e., death, MI, revascularization procedures) compared with that in patients receiving placebo.

Intensive antilipemic therapy with atorvastatin has been shown to slow the progression of coronary atherosclerosis† in patients with CHD. In a randomized, double-blind, active-control study (Reversal of Atherosclerosis with Aggressive Lipid Lowering [REVERSAL]) in 654 patients with CHD, treatment with intensive antilipemic therapy (atorvastatin 80 mg daily) or moderate antilipemic therapy (pravastatin 40 mg daily) for 18 months reduced LDL-cholesterol concentrations to a mean of 79 or 110 mg/dL, respectively. Treatment with the intensive regimen was associated with a substantially lower progression rate (measured by percent change in atheroma volume) compared with treatment with the moderate regimen. Compared with baseline values, patients treated with atorvastatin had no change in atheroma burden, whereas patients treated with pravastatin showed progression of coronary atherosclerosis. In addition, concentrations of C-reactive protein were reduced by 36.4% in atorvastatin-treated patients and by 5.2% in pravastatin-treated patients. It has been suggested that the differences in atherosclerosis progression between atorvastatin and pravastatin may be related to the greater reduction in atherogenic lipoproteins and C-reactive protein concentrations in patients treated with atorvastatin.

Combination Antilipemic Therapy The ACC/AHA cholesterol management guideline states that the addition of a nonstatin drug (e.g., ezetimibe, bile acid sequestrant, fibric acid derivative, niacin) to statin therapy may be considered in patients who require further reductions in LDL-cholesterol concentrations, have a less-than-anticipated response to statins, are unable to tolerate a less-than-recommended intensity of a statin, or are completely intolerant to statin therapy, especially if there is evidence from randomized controlled studies suggesting that addition of the nonstatin drug further reduces ASCVD events. Because there are no data supporting the routine use of statin therapy in combination with nonstatin drugs, the guideline states that adherence to lifestyle modifications and to statin therapy should be re-emphasized before considering combination therapy. If combination therapy is considered, selection of the nonstatin drug should be based on the risk and benefit profile (i.e., reduction in ASCVD risk outweighs the drug's potential for adverse effects and drug interactions) and patient preferences. If combination therapy with a fibric acid derivative is necessary, fenofibrate or fenofibric acid is preferred because of a reduced incidence of drug interactions compared with gemfibrozil. (See Fibric Acid Derivatives under Drug Interactions: Antilipemic Agents.)

The addition of niacin to statin-based therapy has not been shown to provide an incremental benefit in reducing cardiovascular morbidity and mortality beyond that already demonstrated with statin-based therapy. In the Impact on Global Health Outcomes (AIM-HIGH) study, the combination of extended-release niacin (1.5–2 g daily) and statin-based therapy (simvastatin 40–80 mg once daily, with or without ezetimibe 10 mg daily) was compared with statin-based therapy alone in patients with established cardiovascular disease (i.e., documented stable CHD, cerebrovascular or carotid disease, peripheral arterial disease). Despite a favorable effect on serum lipid concentrations (median HDL-cholesterol concentration increased from 35 to 42 mg/dL, triglyceride concentration decreased from 164 to 122 mg/dL, and LDL-cholesterol concentration decreased from 74 to 62 mg/dL), the addition of niacin to simvastatin-based therapy did not further reduce the incidence of the primary end point (i.e., composite of death from CHD, nonfatal MI, ischemic stroke, hospitalization for more than 23 hours for ACS, or symptom-driven coronary or cerebral revascularization) compared with simvastatin-based therapy alone over a follow-up period of 36 months. The addition of extended-release niacin to existing simvastatin-based therapy, however, did increase the risk of adverse effects (e.g., pruritus, flushing, adverse GI effects, increased blood glucose concentrations). The investigators of this study stated that whether such combination therapy provides incremental benefit in higher-risk patients or in those receiving suboptimal statin therapy remains to be established.

Data from another large randomized, double-blind, multicenter study involving 25,673 adults with cardiovascular disease confirmed findings of the AIM-HIGH study. In the Heart Protection Study 2–Treatment of HDL to Reduce the Incidence of Vascular Events (HPS2-THRIVE), the combination of extended-release niacin/laropiprant (2 g/40 mg daily) (no longer commercially available) and statin-based therapy (simvastatin 40 mg once daily, with or without ezetimibe 10 mg daily) was compared with statin-based therapy alone in patients with established cardiovascular disease (i.e., history of MI, cerebrovascular disease, peripheral arterial disease, diabetes mellitus with evidence of symptomatic coronary disease). Despite a favorable effect on serum lipid concentrations (additional 6-mg/dL increase in HDL-cholesterol concentration, 33-mg/dL reduction in triglyceride concentration, and 10-mg/dL reduction in LDL-cholesterol concentration), the addition of niacin/laropiprant to simvastatin-based therapy did not further reduce the incidence of major cardiovascular events (i.e., nonfatal MI, death from coronary causes, stroke of any type, coronary or noncoronary revascularization) compared with simvastatin-based therapy alone over a median follow-up of 3.9 years. The addition of niacin/laropiprant to existing simvastatin-based therapy, however, did increase the risk of severe adverse effects, including disturbances in glycemic control requiring hospitalization, development of diabetes mellitus, adverse GI effects, myopathy, gout, rash, skin ulceration, and, unexpectedly, infection and bleeding. In light of these findings, some clinicians state that niacin should be reserved as a fourth-line agent (after intensive lifestyle modifications, fibric acid derivatives, and omega-3-acid ethyl esters) for patients with severe hypertriglyceridemia in whom the primary goal of treatment is prevention of pancreatitis.

Early findings from a randomized controlled study (Ezetimibe and Simvastatin in Hypercholesterolemia Enhances Atherosclerosis Regression [ENHANCE]) indicated that the fixed-combination preparation containing simvastatin and ezetimibe was not superior to simvastatin monotherapy in reducing carotid intimal-medial wall thickness (cIMT) in patients with heterozygous familial hypercholesterolemia despite the observed additive effects of the combination regimen on LDL cholesterol. However, a more recent study (the Improved Reduction of Outcomes: Vytorin® Efficacy International trial [IMPROVE-IT]) in 18,144 post-ACS patients with baseline LDL-cholesterol concentrations of 50–125 mg/dL (or 50–100 mg/dL if they were receiving lipid-lowering therapy) demonstrated that the addition of ezetimibe (10 mg daily) to simvastatin (40 mg daily) not only achieved a 24% further reduction in LDL cholesterol concentrations, but also improved cardiovascular outcomes (a composite end point of cardiovascular death, nonfatal MI, unstable angina requiring hospitalization, coronary revascularization, or nonfatal stroke) compared with simvastatin (40 mg daily) monotherapy; the absolute risk reduction for the composite primary outcome was 2% over 7 years.

Patients with Chronic Kidney Disease Several clinical studies have evaluated the potential benefits of LDL-cholesterol lowering with statins in patients with chronic kidney disease, a population at high risk of cardiovascular disease. In the Deutsche Diabetes Dialyse Studie (4D) in which 1255 patients with type 2 diabetes mellitus on maintenance hemodialysis received atorvastatin 20 mg daily or placebo, atorvastatin had no substantial effect on the primary composite end point of cardiovascular death, nonfatal MI, and stroke after a median follow-up of 4 years. Although atorvastatin reduced the rate of all cardiac events, a secondary end point in the study, the difference between drug and placebo was only nominally significant. Similar findings were reported with rosuvastatin in the Study to Evaluate the Use of Rosuvastatin in Subjects on Regular Hemodialysis (AURORA), a randomized, double-blind study in 2776 patients undergoing hemodialysis. In this study, treatment with rosuvastatin 10 mg daily did not substantially reduce the primary composite end point of cardiovascular death, nonfatal MI, or nonfatal stroke compared with placebo. Results of another randomized, double-blind study (Assessment of Lescol in Renal Transplantation [ALERT]) in 2102 renal transplant patients showed no substantial effect of fluvastatin on the primary end point of major adverse cardiac events (defined as cardiac death, nonfatal MI, or coronary intervention procedure) compared with placebo at a mean duration of follow-up of 5.1 years, although fluvastatin appeared to reduced the risk of cardiac deaths and nonfatal MI.

In contrast to studies evaluating statin monotherapy, results of a large, randomized, double-blind study (Study of Heart and Renal Protection [SHARP]) in more than 9000 patients with moderate to severe chronic kidney disease and no known history of MI or coronary revascularization demonstrated that the fixed-combination preparation containing ezetimibe and simvastatin (10 and 20 mg daily, respectively) reduced major vascular and atherosclerotic events; at a median duration of follow up of 4.9 years, the risk of a major vascular event (nonfatal MI or cardiac death, stroke, or revascularization excluding dialysis access procedures) was reduced by 16% and the risk of a major atherosclerotic event (nonfatal MI or cardiac death, nonhemorrhagic stroke, or arterial revascularization excluding dialysis access procedures) was reduced by 17% in patients receiving the fixed-combination preparation compared with those receiving placebo. The treatment effect was largely driven by a substantial reduction in ischemic strokes and arterial revascularization procedures.

■ **Dyslipidemias** Statins are used as adjuncts to nondrug therapies (e.g., dietary management) to decrease elevated serum total and LDL-cholesterol, apolipoprotein B (apo B), and triglyceride concentrations, and to increase HDL-cholesterol concentrations in the treatment of specific dyslipidemias, including primary hypercholesterolemia or mixed dyslipidemia, homozygous familial hypercholesterolemia, primary dysbetalipoproteinemia, and hypertriglyceridemia. Statins have not been studied in conditions where the principal lipoprotein abnormality is elevated chylomicrons.

Primary Hypercholesterolemia or Mixed Dyslipidemia Statins are used as an adjunct to nondrug therapies (e.g., dietary management) in adults to decrease elevated serum total and LDL-cholesterol, apo B, and triglyceride concentrations, and to increase serum HDL-cholesterol concentrations in the management of primary hypercholesterolemia or mixed dyslipidemia, including heterozygous familial hypercholesterolemia and other causes of hypercholesterolemia (e.g., polygenic hypercholesterolemia). Statins also are used as adjuncts to dietary therapy and lifestyle modifications in the treatment of heterozygous familial hypercholesterolemia in children who, despite an adequate trial of dietary management, have a serum LDL-cholesterol concentration of 190 mg/dL or greater *or* a serum LDL-cholesterol concentration of 160 mg/dL or greater and either a family history of premature cardiovascular disease or 2 or more other risk factors. Statins also are used in combination with fenofibric acid to decrease triglyceride concentrations and increase HDL-cholesterol concentrations in patients with mixed dyslipidemia and CHD (or CHD risk equivalents) who are receiving optimal statin therapy; however, no additional benefit on cardiovascular morbidity and mortality has been demonstrated with such combination therapy beyond that already established with statin monotherapy. (See Patients with Diabetes Mellitus under Prevention of Cardiovascular Events: Primary Prevention, in Uses.)

Reductions in total and LDL-cholesterol concentrations produced by usual dosages of statins substantially exceed those achieved with placebo. Mean reductions of 16–46% in total cholesterol concentration, 21–63% in LDL-cholesterol concentration, 18–54% in apo B concentration, and 6–37% in triglyceride concentration have been reported in controlled and uncontrolled studies in patients with primary hypercholesterolemia who received recommended daily dosages of a statin for at least 6 weeks. Modest and variable increases in HDL-cholesterol concentrations (2–16%) also were observed in patients receiving statin therapy.

Data from comparative studies suggest that reductions in total and LDL-cholesterol concentrations produced by statins generally equal or exceed those produced by other antilipemic agents (e.g., bile acid sequestrants, niacin, fibric acid derivatives). Pooled data from several placebo-controlled studies comparing 12–24 weeks of statin therapy (40–80 mg of pravastatin or 20–40 mg of simvastatin daily) with that of cholestyramine (8–24 g daily in divided doses) in patients with primary hypercholesterolemia indicate that statins may be equally or more effective than cholestyramine in reducing total cholesterol (25–36% for pravastatin or simvastatin versus 15–23% for cholestyramine) and LDL-cholesterol concentrations (31–43 versus 21–32%). Statins also were found to be more effective than cholestyramine in improving triglyceride concentrations, as evidenced by 13–21% reductions in statin-treated patients versus 11–21% increases in cholestyramine-treated patients.

Statin therapy has been shown to be superior to niacin in reducing total and LDL-cholesterol concentrations but less effective in reducing triglyceride and increasing HDL-cholesterol concentrations. In a multicenter, randomized, placebo-controlled, comparative study in patients with primary types IIa and IIb hyperlipoproteinemia, treatment with pravastatin (40 mg daily) for 8 weeks was associated with 23 and 33% reductions in total and LDL-cholesterol concentrations, respectively, compared with 11 and 16% reductions, respectively, achieved with niacin therapy (0.5–1 g twice daily). Although results of this study indicate no substantial difference between pravastatin and niacin in improving triglyceride and HDL-cholesterol concentrations, evidence from a randomized, crossover, comparative trial in a limited number of patients with combined hyperlipidemia suggests that niacin may more effective than pravastatin in improving these lipid parameters. Treatment with niacin (1.5 g 3 times daily) for 8 weeks resulted in a 32% reduction in triglycerides and a 27% increase in HDL-cholesterol concentrations, while treatment with pravastatin (40 mg daily) produced only modest improvements in these lipid parameters (-4 and +3%, respectively).

Statins have been shown to be superior to fibric acid derivatives in lowering total and LDL-cholesterol concentrations but less effective in improving triglyceride and HDL-cholesterol concentrations. In 2 randomized studies comparing therapy with pravastatin (40 mg daily) with that of gemfibrozil (600 mg twice daily) for 12–24 weeks in patients with primary hypercholesterolemia, pravastatin was more effective in reducing total cholesterol (23–26% for pravastatin versus 14–15% for gemfibrozil) and LDL-cholesterol (30–34% versus 16–17%); however, the drug was less effective than gemfibrozil in reducing triglyceride (5–14% versus 37–42%) and raising HDL-cholesterol concentrations (5–6% versus 13–15%).

Combined use of a statin and other antilipemic agents (e.g., bile acid sequestrants, niacin, fibric acid derivatives, ezetimibe) produces additive antilipemic effects and, in some cases, can also result in additional cardiovascular benefits. (See Combination Antilipemic Therapy under Uses: Prevention of Cardiovascular Events.) The addition of a bile acid sequestrant to statin therapy further reduces LDL-cholesterol by an additional 3–20%. The addition of ezetimibe (10 mg daily) to statin therapy reduces LDL-cholesterol by an additional 25% compared with a 4% reduction following addition of placebo. Combining niacin (1–3 g daily) with various statins (e.g., fluvastatin, pravastatin) for 8–18 weeks in hypercholesterolemic patients with or without coronary artery disease further reduced total cholesterol, LDL-cholesterol, apo B, and triglyceride concentrations by an additional 9–12, 9–19, 11%, and 18–27%, respectively, and increased HDL-cholesterol and apo A concentrations by an additional 3–29 and 11%, respectively. Combining a fibric acid derivative (e.g., fenofibrate, gemfibrozil) with statin therapy (e.g., pravastatin, simvastatin) in patients with primary hypercholesterolemia further reduced triglyceride concentrations by an additional 28–32% and increased HDL-cholesterol concentrations by an additional 7–12%.

The benefits of combined use of a statin and other lipid-lowering drugs should be weighed against the potential risks of hepatotoxicity, myopathy, and rhabdomyolysis; it should be noted that the addition of fenofibrate or niacin to existing statin-based therapy has not been shown to further reduce the incidence of major cardiovascular events in patients with diabetes mellitus or established cardiovascular disease, respectively, compared with statin-based therapy alone. (See Uses: Prevention of Cardiovascular Events.)

Homozygous Familial Hypercholesterolemia Statins are used alone or in combination with other lipid-lowering treatments (e.g., LDL apheresis) to reduce total cholesterol, LDL-cholesterol, and apo B concentrations in patients with homozygous familial hypercholesterolemia. Patients with homozygous familial hypercholesterolemia usually respond poorly to combined dietary management and drug therapy, including regimens containing a statin, in part because these patients have poorly functioning, few, or no LDL receptors.

Data concerning the effectiveness of statins in the management of homozygous familial hypercholesterolemia are limited. In several small controlled and uncontrolled studies, 86–92% of patients with homozygous familial hypercholesterolemia who received atorvastatin (20–80 mg daily) or simvastatin (40–80 mg daily) had marked reductions in LDL-cholesterol concentrations (7–53%) while 8–14% of patients showed *increases* (7–24%) in this lipoprotein fraction. In an open-label study, reductions in LDL-cholesterol concentrations achieved with usual dosages of rosuvastatin (20–40 mg daily) reportedly averaged 22%. In a randomized placebo-controlled study in 14 children and adolescents 7 years of age or older with homozygous familial hypercholesterolemia, rosuvastatin (20 mg daily) reduced LDL-cholesterol concentrations by approximately 22%, total cholesterol by approximately 20%, non-HDL-cholesterol by approximately 23%, and apo B by approximately 17%. In another small, open-label study in patients with homozygous familial hypercholesterolemia undergoing plasma exchange or LDL-apheresis, treatment with atorvastatin (80 mg daily) for 8 weeks further reduced LDL-cholesterol concentrations by approximately 31% during pre- and post-apheresis. The addition of ezetimibe (10 mg daily) to atorvastatin or simvastatin therapy (40 or 80 mg daily) further reduced LDL-cholesterol concentrations by an additional 21%.

Primary Dysbetalipoproteinemia Statins are used as adjuncts to nondrug therapies (e.g., dietary management) for the treatment of primary dysbetalipoproteinemia in patients who do not respond adequately to diet.

In several small double-blind, crossover studies in a limited number of patients with primary dysbetalipoproteinemia who received recommended daily dosages of a statin (e.g., pravastatin, rosuvastatin, simvastatin), total cholesterol, triglyceride, and non-HDL-cholesterol concentrations decreased by 31–58, 12–53, and 36–64%, respectively.

Hypertriglyceridemia Statins are used as adjuncts to nondrug therapies (e.g., dietary management) in the treatment of elevated serum triglyceride concentrations.

Mean reductions in total cholesterol concentrations of 22–44%, LDL-cholesterol concentrations of 27–45%, VLDL-cholesterol concentrations of 25–62%, triglyceride concentrations of 21–52%, and non-HDL-cholesterol concentrations of 27–52% have been reported in patients with hypertriglyceridemia who received recommended daily dosages of a statin (e.g., atorvastatin, pravastatin, rosuvastatin, simvastatin). Modest increases in HDL-cholesterol concentrations (3–22%) also were observed in patients receiving statin therapy.

An analysis of pooled data from a number of studies in which statins were used suggests that these agents are effective in decreasing triglyceride concentrations principally in patients with hypertriglyceridemia (baseline concentrations exceeding 250 mg/dL); in this analysis, such benefit was not observed in those with baseline triglyceride concentrations below 150 mg/dL. In addition, limited evidence suggests that the relative potency of a statin in reducing triglyceride concentrations may be related to its efficacy in reducing LDL-cholesterol concentrations.

Secondary Dyslipidemias Some statins have been used to reduce total and LDL-cholesterol concentrations in a limited number of patients with hypercholesterolemia associated with chronic renal insufficiency†, cardiac† or renal† transplantation, or nephrotic syndrome†. Additional studies are necessary to determine the role, if any, of statins in patients with these disorders.

■ **Other Uses** Limited data indicate that use of statins may be associated with an increase in bone mass density†; however, results of epidemiologic studies evaluating the effect of statins on risk of fractures† have been conflicting. Results of an observational study indicate a lower prevalence of Alzheimer's disease† among patients who received certain statins (i.e., lovastatin, pravastatin). Further study is needed to establish the usefulness of statins in these conditions.

Dosage and Administration

■ **Administration** All statins are administered orally once daily. While the manufacturers of atorvastatin, pitavastatin, pravastatin, and rosuvastatin state that these drugs may be taken without regard to time of day, some evidence suggests that statins should be administered in the evening or at bedtime for optimal efficacy in lowering LDL-cholesterol since the rate of hepatic cholesterol synthesis is greatest at night. Most statins may be administered without regard to meals; however, the manufacturer of lovastatin states that the drug should be given with the evening meal for optimal absorption.

Patients should be placed on a standard cholesterol-lowering diet before initiation of statin therapy and should remain on this diet during treatment with these agents. The most recent American Heart Association/American College of Cardiology (AHA/ACC) Guideline on Lifestyle Management to Reduce Cardiovascular Risk (available at http://www.cardiosource.org or http://my.americanheart.org) should be consulted for details on dietary therapy and lifestyle modifications.

The ACC/AHA guideline for management of blood cholesterol to reduce atherosclerotic cardiovascular risk in adults states that lipoprotein concentrations should be determined within 4–12 weeks following initiation of statin therapy (to determine the patient's response to therapy and adherence) and monitored every 3–12 months thereafter as clinically indicated.

Adherence to lifestyle modifications and to statin therapy are required for atherosclerotic cardiovascular disease (ASCVD) risk reduction and, thus, should be reinforced periodically.

Concomitant administration of statins and bile acid sequestrants has been associated with additive or synergistic antilipemic effects in hypercholesterolemic patients. However, since bile acid sequestrants may bind and delay absorption of statins, some manufacturers recommend that statins be administered 1 hour or more before or at least 4 hours after the resin.

■ **Dosage** Dosage of statins must be carefully adjusted according to individual requirements and response. Because the risk of myopathy is dose related, ACC, AHA, and the National Heart, Lung and Blood Institute (NHLBI) clinical advisory panel on statins state that statin dosages generally should not exceed those required to attain the desired percent reduction in LDL-cholesterol concentration. The manufacturer of simvastatin states that the 80-mg dose of the drug should be restricted to patients who have been receiving long-term therapy (e.g., 12 months or longer) at this dosage without evidence of muscle toxicity. (See Dosage and Administration in Simvastatin 24:06.08.) Serum lipoprotein concentrations should be determined periodically during statin therapy. (See Cautions: Precautions and Contraindications.) Dosage should be increased at intervals of no less than 4 weeks until the desired effect on lipoprotein concentrations is observed; reduction of statin dosage can be considered in patients whose serum cholesterol concentrations fall below the desired target range.

Therapy with statins, in conjunction with dietary measures, should continue throughout the patient's lifetime pending further data defining a more appropriate treatment period.

Use of certain statins with potent inhibitors of cytochrome P-450 (CYP) isoenzyme 3A4, immunosuppressants (e.g., cyclosporine), fibric acid derivatives, antilipemic dosages (exceeding 1 g daily) of niacin, cobicistat-containing preparations, danazol, amlodipine, amiodarone, dronedarone, diltiazem, verapamil, colchicine, lomitapide, ranolazine, or grapefruit juice may be associated with an increased risk of myopathy or rhabdomyolysis. (See Cautions: Musculoskeletal Effects and also see Drug Interactions.) Use of such combinations with certain statins are contraindicated, should be avoided, should be employed with caution, or may require statin dosage adjustments or limitations (e.g., lower initial or maximum dosages). (See Dosage and Administration in the individual statin monographs in 24:06.08.)

■ **Dosage in Renal and Hepatic Impairment** Since most statins (e.g., atorvastatin, fluvastatin, lovastatin, rosuvastatin, simvastatin) do not undergo substantial renal excretion, the manufacturers state that modification of dosage should not be necessary in patients with mild renal impairment (creatinine clearance of 61–90 mL/minute per 1.73 m^2). However, pitavastatin and pravastatin undergo renal and hepatic elimination, with renal excretion reaching 15 and 20–47% of the administered dose, respectively. (See Pharmacokinetics: Elimination.) Because the possibility of accumulation of pravastatin and other statins cannot be ruled out, these drugs should be administered with caution in patients with moderate to severe renal impairment (creatinine clearance less than 60 mL/minute per 1.73 m^2), initiating therapy with the drug under close monitoring and at reduced daily dosages.

Since statins are partially metabolized in the liver and potentially may accumulate in the plasma of patients with hepatic impairment, these drugs should be used with caution in patients who consume substantial amounts of alcohol and/or who have a history of liver disease; such patients should be monitored closely while receiving statin therapy. Statins are *contraindicated* in patients with active liver disease or unexplained, persistent increases in serum aminotransferase concentrations.

Cautions

At usual dosages, statins usually are well tolerated and are associated with a low incidence of adverse effects. Adverse effects reported in the Cautions section include those reported in clinical trials and during postmarketing studies, and a causal relationship to statin therapy has not necessarily been established.

Adverse effects reported with statin therapy usually have been mild and transient and similar in incidence to placebo. The most common adverse effects observed with statin therapy in controlled studies were GI disturbances, fatigue, localized pain, and headache. In controlled clinical trials, 0.3–4.6% of patients receiving statins discontinued the drugs because of adverse effects. Adverse effects most frequently resulting in drug discontinuance in long-term clinical studies were rash, musculoskeletal pain, asymptomatic increases in serum aminotransferase concentrations, and mild, nonspecific GI disturbances. No overall differences in the adverse effect profile were observed between geriatric and younger patients.

■ **Hepatic Effects** Increases in serum aminotransferase (transaminase) concentrations (i.e., AST [SGOT], ALT [SGPT]), including to more than 3 times the upper limit of normal, have been reported in patients receiving statins. (See Cautions: Precautions and Contraindications.) Increases in serum aminotransferase concentrations generally are dose dependent, are not related to the LDL-cholesterol reduction, and have not been associated with jaundice or cholestasis, although at least one patient in clinical trials developed jaundice. Increases in ALT and/or AST to more than 3 times the upper limit of normal most often are transient and will resolve spontaneously in 70% of patients even if the statin and original dosage are continued unchanged; following reduction of dosage or interruption or discontinuance of statin therapy, serum aminotransferase concentrations usually return slowly to pretreatment values without adverse sequelae. Increases in serum aminotransferase concentrations usually do not recur following rechallenge with the same statin or selection of another statin. Cases of fatal and nonfatal hepatic failure have been reported rarely in patients receiving statins during postmarketing surveillance. Pancreatitis, hepatitis (including chronic active hepatitis), cholestatic jaundice, fatty liver changes, biliary pain, increased serum alkaline phosphatase concentrations, increased serum γ-glutamyltransferase (γ-glutamyltranspeptidase, GGT, GGTP) concentrations, increased serum bilirubin concentrations, cirrhosis, fulminant hepatic necrosis, and hepatoma also have been reported with statin therapy.

■ **Musculoskeletal Effects** Uncomplicated myalgia (characterized by muscle pain or weakness) is the most common adverse musculoskeletal effect of statins, occurring in approximately 1–6% of patients receiving the drugs in controlled clinical trials, Arthralgia occurred in about 1–5% of patients receiving statins in controlled clinical trials. Increased serum creatine kinase (CK, creatine phosphokinase, CPK) concentrations, muscle cramps, leg cramps, back pain, shoulder pain, arthritis, and myositis, also have been reported with statin therapy. Bursitis, tenosynovitis, arthropathy, myasthenia, tendinous contracture, tendon rupture, tendon disorder, and polymyositis also have been reported with some statins.

Myopathy (manifested as muscle pain, tenderness, soreness, weakness, and/or cramps plus serum CK concentration increases exceeding 10 times the upper limit of normal) occurred in less than 0.7% of patients receiving statins in clinical trials. Immune-mediated necrotizing myopathy (IMNM), an autoimmune myopathy, has been reported rarely in patients receiving statins. The risk of myopathy appears to be increased in patients receiving higher dosages of statins, patients with multisystem disease (e.g., renal [particularly with pravastatin] or hepatic impairment), patients with concurrent serious infections or uncontrolled hypothyroidism, geriatric patients (65 years of age and older), women, patients with small body frame and frailty, and patients undergoing surgery (i.e., during perioperative periods). The risk of myopathy and/or rhabdomyolysis also is increased with concomitant use of statins and certain drugs or foods (e.g., cyclosporine, niacin, fibric acid derivatives, macrolide antibiotics [e.g., erythromycin, clarithromycin, telithromycin], certain azole antifungals [i.e., itraconazole, ketoconazole, posaconazole, voriconazole], alcohol, HIV protease inhibitors, nefazodone, amiodarone, cobicistat-containing preparations, dronedarone, amlodipine, verapamil, diltiazem, danazol, colchicine, ranolazine, lomitapide, simeprevir, grapefruit juice). (See Drug Interactions.)

Rhabdomyolysis (characterized by muscle pain or weakness with marked increases [exceeding 10 times the upper limit of normal] in serum CK concentrations and increases in serum creatinine concentrations [usually accompanied by brown urine and urinary myoglobinuria]) with or without acute renal failure secondary to myoglobinuria has occurred rarely with all statins. Fatalities secondary to rhabdomyolysis also have been reported in patients receiving statin therapy. As of June 2001, fatal rhabdomyolysis was reported in 6, 31, 0, 19, 3, or 14 of patients receiving atorvastatin, cerivastatin (no longer commercially available in the US), fluvastatin, lovastatin, pravastatin, or simvastatin, respectively. Among the 31 cases of fatal rhabdomyolysis associated with cerivastatin, 12 occurred with concomitant gemfibrozil therapy (see Fibric Acid Derivatives under Drug Interactions), while another 12 occurred following administration of a higher initial dosage (0.8 mg daily) of the drug (as monotherapy); fatal rhabdomyolysis associated with cerivastatin also appears to occur more frequently in geriatric patients. (See Cautions: Geriatric Precautions.) Based on available data, the reporting rate (calculated as the number of reported cases divided by the total number of prescriptions dispensed since initial marketing of the drug to May 2001) of fatal rhabdomyolysis associated with atorvastatin, cerivastatin, fluvastatin, lovastatin, pravastatin, or simvastatin monotherapy is 0.04, 1.9, 0, 0.19, 0.04, or 0.12 per million prescriptions, respectively. In view of a substantially higher reporting rate of fatal rhabdomyolysis associated with cerivastatin (10–50 times higher than that for other statins), the manufacturer (Bayer) announced a voluntary withdrawal of the drug from the world market in August 2001.

FDA notes that the data on severe or fatal rhabdomyolysis represent reporting rates, *not* incidence rates, and that statistically rigorous comparisons between drugs are not recommended. However, the American College of Cardiology (ACC), the American Heart Association (AHA), and the National Heart, Lung and Blood Institute (NHLBI) clinical advisory panel on statins state that there appears to be no clinically important differences in the reporting rate of fatal rhabdomyolysis among atorvastatin, fluvastatin, lovastatin, pravastatin, and simvastatin, and that clinicians should consider the rates of severe myopathy equivalent among all of these statins. The risk of severe adverse musculoskeletal effects associated with rosuvastatin appears to be similar to that with other statins.

Any patient taking a statin with or without gemfibrozil who experiences muscle pain, tenderness (especially in the calves or lower back), or weakness; brown urine; flu-like symptoms; and malaise should consult a clinician immediately. (See Cautions: Precautions and Contraindications.) However, it should be noted that myopathy or rhabdomyolysis also has occurred in the absence of such manifestations of muscle injury. All serious adverse effects associated with use of statins should be reported to the FDA MedWatch Program by phone (800-FDA-1088), fax (800-FDA-0178), through the Internet (http://www.fda.gov/Safety/MedWatch), or by mail (MedWatch, HF-2, FDA, 5600 Fishers Lane, Rockville, MD 20852-9787).

■ **GI Effects** The most frequent adverse GI effects of statins are diarrhea, abdominal pain, flatulence, nausea and/or vomiting, constipation, dyspepsia, and heartburn, which occurred in approximately 1–7% of patients receiving a statin in controlled clinical trials. Anorexia also has been reported with statin therapy. Other adverse GI effects reported with at least one statin include increased or decreased appetite, dysphagia, cheilitis, dry mouth, stomatitis, mouth ulceration, gum hemorrhage, glossitis, tooth disorder esophagitis, eructation, acid regurgitation, gastritis, GI hemorrhage, gastroenteritis, stomach ulcer, enteritis, duodenal ulcer, colitis, rectal hemorrhage, tenesmus, and melena.

■ **Respiratory Effects** Upper respiratory tract infection occurred in about 1–16% of patients receiving statins in controlled clinical trials. Pharyngitis, rhinitis, sinusitis, bronchitis, and cough, occurred in approximately 3–13, 1–11 , 2–7, 2, and 1–2%, respectively, of patients receiving various statins in controlled clinical trials. Pneumonia, asthma, epistaxis, and interstitial lung disease also have been reported with some statins.

■ **Dermatologic and Sensitivity Reactions** Rash is the most common dermatologic reaction of statins, occurring in about 1–4% of patients receiving the drugs in controlled clinical trials. Alopecia, pruritus, and skin changes (e.g., nodules, discoloration, dry skin and mucous membranes, changes to hair and nails) also have been reported with statins. Sweating,acne, eczema, seborrhea, phlebitis, and skin ulcer have been reported with at least one statin.

Hypersensitivity reactions have occurred rarely with statin therapy during clinical trials or postmarketing surveillance. Such reactions may include anaphylaxis, angioedema, head/neck edema, contact dermatitis, lupus erythematosus-like syndrome, polymyalgia rheumatica, dermatomyositis, vasculitis, purpura, thrombocytopenia, leukopenia, hemolytic anemia, positive antinuclear antibody (ANA) titer, increased erythrocyte sedimentation rate, eosinophilia, arthritis, arthralgia, urticaria, asthenia, photosensitivity, fever, chills, flushing, malaise, dyspnea, toxic epidermal necrolysis, erythema multiforme, and Stevens-Johnson syndrome.

■ **Nervous System Effects** Headache is the most frequent adverse nervous system effect of statins, occurring in about 2–17% of patients receiving the drugs in controlled clinical trials. Asthenia, fatigue, and dizziness occurred in about 1–4% of patients receiving statin therapy in controlled clinical trials. Dysfunction of certain cranial nerves (including alteration of taste, impairment of extraocular movement, and facial paresis), tremor, hypertonia, vertigo, paresthesia, peripheral neuropathy, peripheral nerve palsy, anxiety, insomnia, somnolence, and depression also have been reported with statin therapy. Psychic disturbances, sleep disturbances, abnormal dreams, nightmares, torticollis, hypesthesia, hyperkinesia, incoordination, paralysis, neck rigidity, migraine, emotional lability, and amnesia have been reported with at least one statin.

Cognitive impairment (e.g., memory loss, forgetfulness, amnesia, memory impairment, confusion) has been reported rarely with all statins during postmarketing surveillance. This adverse CNS effect generally was nonserious and reversible, with variable times to symptom onset (1 day to years) and symptom resolution (median of 3 weeks following discontinuance of statin therapy). Following review of available data (i.e., from the Adverse Event Reporting System [AERS] database, randomized clinical trials, observational studies, case reports), FDA concluded that cases of cognitive impairment did not appear to be associated with fixed or progressive dementia (e.g., Alzheimer's disease) or result in clinically important cognitive decline. Development of cognitive impairment did not appear to be associated with any specific statin, age of the patient, statin dosage, or concomitant drug therapy. Therefore, FDA continues to believe that the cardiovascular benefits of statins outweigh this small increased risk of cognitive impairment. The National Lipid Association (NLA) statin safety assessment task force recommends that patients experiencing manifestations consistent with cognitive impairment be evaluated and managed appropriately. (See CNS Effects under Cautions: Precautions and Contraindications.)

Although peripheral neuropathy has been reported with statin therapy, the NLA statin safety assessment task force states that the potential risk of developing peripheral neuropathy during statin therapy is very small, if it exists at all. Nevertheless, the task force recommends that patients experiencing manifestations consistent with peripheral neuropathy be evaluated and managed appropriately. (See CNS Effects under Cautions: Precautions and Contraindications.)

■ Ocular Effects Because of experience with a previously studied inhibitor of cholesterol synthesis (i.e., triparanol, MER-29), the cataractogenic potential of statins has been closely monitored during clinical studies. Unlike triparanol, however, statins affect an earlier step in the cholesterol biosynthetic pathway that does not appear to result in accumulation of potentially toxic intermediate sterols (e.g., desmosterol). However, concern remains that statin-induced inhibition of cholesterol synthesis could potentially adversely affect the lens since the lens may be completely dependent on *de novo* cholesterol synthesis for ongoing membranal synthetic processes.

Progression of cataracts (including lens opacities) has been reported in patients receiving statins. However, data from several controlled studies in patients receiving lovastatin or simvastatin for up to 3 years indicate that the incidence of lens opacity is similar to that reported in placebo-treated patients and increases at a rate consistent with that expected as a result of normal aging. Ophthalmoplegia, blurred vision, visual disturbance (e.g., diplopia), ocular irritation, glaucoma, ocular hemorrhage, amblyopia, refraction disorder, and dry eyes have been reported with at least one statin.

■ Cardiovascular Effects Adverse cardiovascular effects reported in patients receiving statin therapy include chest pain, hypertension, and angina pectoris. Palpitation, vasodilation, syncope, postural hypotension, peripheral edema, and arrhythmia have been reported with at least one statin.

■ Genitourinary Effects Genitourinary system abnormalities reported in patients receiving statin therapy include change or loss of libido, sexual dysfunction, and erectile dysfunction. Impotence, epididymitis, abnormal ejaculation, vaginal hemorrhage, uterine hemorrhage, metrorrhagia, fibrocystic breast, urinary tract infection, urinary abnormality (e.g., dysuria, frequency, nocturia), cystitis, hematuria, proteinuria, renal calculus, nocturia, albuminuria, nephritis, urinary incontinence, urinary retention, and urinary urgency have been reported with at least one statin.

Dipstick-positive proteinuria and microscopic hematuria reportedly occurred more frequently in patients receiving rosuvastatin 40 mg compared with lower doses of rosuvastatin or comparator statins in clinical trials. In an analysis of available data, the FDA concluded that proteinuria in patients receiving statins is not associated with renal impairment or renal failure. Nevertheless, the NLA statin safety assessment task force recommends that patients experiencing adverse renal effects (including proteinuria) be evaluated and managed appropriately. (See Renal Effects under Cautions: Precautions and Contraindications.)

■ Endocrine Effects Increases in glycosylated hemoglobin (hemoglobin A_{1c} [HbA_{1c}]) and fasting serum glucose concentrations that in some cases may exceed the threshold for the diagnosis of diabetes mellitus have been reported in patients receiving statins. Data from clinical trials and meta-analyses indicate that statin therapy may increase the risk of developing diabetes mellitus. Despite these findings, FDA continues to believe that the cardiovascular benefits of statins outweigh these small increased risks. (See Endocrine Effects under Cautions: Precautions and Contraindications.)

■ Other Adverse Effects Other adverse effects reported in patients receiving statins include accidental injury, gynecomastia, and flu-like syndrome. Gout, weight gain, ecchymosis, anemia, lymphadenopathy, petechia, tinnitus, deafness, parosmia, taste loss, and taste perversion have been reported with at least one statin.

■ Precautions and Contraindications ***General Precautions and Contraindications*** Prior to institution of antilipemic therapy with statins, a vigorous attempt should be made to control serum cholesterol by appropriate dietary regimens, weight reduction, exercise, and treatment of any underlying disorder that might be the cause of lipid abnormality. (See General Principles of Antilipemic Therapy.) Serum lipoprotein concentrations should be determined prior to and regularly during (e.g., at intervals of not less than every 4 weeks until maximum drug effect has been established and periodically thereafter) statin therapy. Statin dosages generally should not exceed those required to attain the desired percent reduction in LDL-cholesterol concentration, and reduction in dosage should be considered in patients whose cholesterol concentrations fall below the desired target range.

Statins are contraindicated in patients with hypersensitivity to any component of the drug formulations. These drugs also are contraindicated in patients with active liver disease or unexplained persistent elevations of serum transaminases. Statins are contraindicated in pregnant or lactating women and in women of childbearing age, unless the latter are highly unlikely to conceive.

Hepatic Effects The manufacturers state that liver function tests should be performed prior to initiation of statin therapy and repeated as clinically indicated (e.g., presence of manifestations suggestive of liver damage). Although the manufacturers previously recommended more frequent monitoring of liver function, FDA concluded that serious statin-related liver injury is rare and unpredictable in individual patients, and that routine periodic monitoring of liver enzymes does not appear to be effective in detecting or preventing serious liver injury. The ACC/AHA cholesterol management guideline states that, during statin therapy, it is reasonable to obtain liver function tests in adults experiencing symptoms of hepatotoxicity (e.g., unusual fatigue or weakness, loss of appetite, abdominal pain, dark colored urine, yellowing of the skin or sclera). However, an NHLBI-appointed expert panel on integrated guidelines for cardiovascular health and risk reduction in children and adolescents states that routine monitoring of hepatic function is strongly recommended in children and adolescents receiving statin therapy.

If serious liver injury with clinical manifestations and/or hyperbilirubinemia or jaundice occurs, the manufacturers state that statin therapy should be promptly interrupted. If an alternate etiology is not found, statin therapy should not be restarted. Patients receiving statin therapy should be advised to promptly report any symptoms suggestive of liver injury (e.g., fatigue, anorexia, right upper abdominal discomfort, dark urine, jaundice).

Statins should be used with caution in patients who consume substantial amounts of alcohol or in patients who have a history of liver disease; such patients should be closely monitored. The NLA expert liver panel states that patients with chronic liver disease, nonalcoholic fatty liver disease, or nonalcoholic steatohepatitis may safely receive statin therapy. Statins are contraindicated in patients with active liver disease or unexplained, persistent increases in serum aminotransferase concentrations. (See Cautions: Hepatic Effects.)

Musculoskeletal Effects Severe or fatal rhabdomyolysis has occurred rarely with all statins. (See Cautions: Musculoskeletal Effects.) Therefore, some experts recommend that baseline serum CK concentrations be performed prior to initiation of statin therapy, particularly in patients at high risk of developing musculoskeletal toxicity (e.g., patients with personal or family history of statin intolerance or muscle disease, geriatric patients, black men, patients receiving concomitant therapy with myotoxic drugs) to aid in the diagnosis of myopathy in patients who later present with adverse musculoskeletal effects; however, routine laboratory monitoring of serum CK concentrations in the absence of clinical manifestations is not recommended. During statin therapy, it is reasonable to measure CK concentrations in adults experiencing muscle symptoms (e.g., pain, tenderness, stiffness, cramping, weakness, generalized fatigue).

An NHLBI-appointed expert panel on integrated guidelines for cardiovascular health and risk reduction in children and adolescents states that baseline CK concentrations should be obtained before initiating statin therapy in pediatric patients. In addition, routine monitoring for muscle toxicity is strongly recommended in children and adolescents receiving statin therapy.

Patients receiving statin therapy should be advised to report promptly any unexplained muscle pain, tenderness, weakness, or other symptoms suggestive of a possible myopathy, especially if these symptoms are accompanied by malaise or fever. The ACC, AHA, NLA statin safety assessment task force, and other experts recommend that serum CK concentrations be obtained and compared to baseline concentrations in any patient presenting with musculoskeletal symptoms suggestive of myopathy (e.g., pain, tenderness, stiffness, cramping, weakness, generalized fatigue). Because hypothyroidism may be a predisposing factor for the development of myopathy, thyrotropin (thyroid-stimulating hormone, TSH) concentrations also should be obtained in such patients. Prior to diagnosis of myopathy, common causes of musculoskeletal symptoms (e.g., exercise, strenuous work, trauma, falls, accidents, seizure, shaking chills, hypothyroidism, infections, carbon monoxide poisoning, polymyositis, dermatomyositis, alcohol abuse, drug [cocaine, amphetamines, heroin, or phencyclidine hydrochloride] abuse) should be ruled out; patients who experience musculoskeletal symptoms should be advised to minimize strenuous activities during combination therapy.

Myopathy should be considered in any patient receiving statin therapy who has diffuse myalgias, muscle tenderness or weakness, and/or marked (greater than 10 times the upper limit of normal) elevation of serum CK concentration. Statin therapy should be discontinued if serum CK concentrations become markedly elevated or if myopathy is diagnosed or suspected. The NLA statin safety assessment task force states that once musculoskeletal manifestations resolve, the same or different statin (at the same or lower dosage) may be restarted to determine the reproducibility of manifestations; recurrence of manifestations with multiple statins and dosages requires initiation of other antilipemic therapy. If myalgia (muscle pain, tenderness) is present with either no CK elevation or a moderate elevation (3–10 times the upper limit of normal), some experts recommend that patients be monitored weekly until manifestations improve; statin therapy should be discontinued if manifestations worsen. In patients with muscle discomfort and/or weakness in the presence of progressive elevations of CK concentrations on serial measurements, either a reduction in statin dosage or temporary discontinuance of therapy may be prudent; a decision can then be made whether or when to reinstitute statin therapy. Statin therapy should be withheld temporarily in any patient experiencing an acute or serious condition suggestive of myopathy or predisposing to the development of acute renal failure secondary to rhabdomyolysis (e.g., sepsis; hypotension; dehydration; major surgery; trauma; severe metabolic, endocrine, or electrolyte disorders; uncontrolled seizures). The NLA statin safety assessment task force states that IV hydration therapy in a hospital setting should be instituted if needed in patients experiencing rhabdomyolysis; once manifestations resolve, the risks and benefits of statin therapy should be carefully reconsidered.

Because the risk of myopathy appears to be increased in geriatric patients (65 years of age and older), women, patients with small body frame and frailty, and patients with multisystem disease (e.g., chronic renal insufficiency [especially secondary to diabetes mellitus], uncontrolled hypothyroidism), statin therapy should be used with caution in such patients.

The manufacturers state that concomitant use of statins and gemfibrozil is contraindicated or should be avoided, and caution is advised when statins are used concomitantly with other fibric acid derivatives (e.g., fenofibrate). The ACC/AHA cholesterol management guideline states that the combination of fenofibrate and low- or moderate-intensity statin therapy may be considered only if the benefits from atherosclerotic cardiovascular disease (ASCVD) risk reduction or triglyceride lowering (when triglyceride concentrations exceed 500 mg/dL) outweigh the potential risk of adverse effects. (See Fibric Acid Derivatives under Drug Interactions.)

Since statins may produce elevations in serum CK and aminotransferase concentrations, this should be considered in the differential diagnosis of patients receiving statin therapy who are being evaluated for chest pain. The manufacturer of cerivastatin (no longer commercially available in the US) states that degeneration of muscle fibers, hyperkeratosis in the non-glandular stomach, and liver lesions also have been observed in animals receiving high dosages of statins.

Endocrine Effects Increases in HbA_{1c} and fasting serum glucose concentrations have been reported in patients receiving statins. (See Cautions: Endocrine Effects.) The ACC/AHA cholesterol management guideline states that patients receiving statin therapy should be evaluated for new-onset diabetes mellitus according to current diabetes screening guidelines. If diabetes mellitus develops during statin therapy, patients should be encouraged to adhere to a heart-healthy diet, engage in physical activity, achieve and maintain a healthy body weight, cease tobacco use, and continue statin therapy to reduce the risk of ASCVD events.

Statins interfere with cholesterol synthesis and lower circulating cholesterol concentrations and therefore theoretically may blunt adrenal or gonadal steroid hormone production. However, clinical studies have shown that statins do not decrease basal plasma cortisol concentration or impair adrenal reserve. Certain statins (e.g., fluvastatin, pravastatin) have been shown to decrease plasma testosterone response to human chorionic gonadotropin. The effects of statins on spermatogenesis and fertility have not been studied in adequate numbers of patients. The effects on the pituitary-gonadal axis in premenopausal females, if any, are unknown.

The manufacturers recommend that patients receiving statins who exhibit clinical evidence of endocrine dysfunction be evaluated appropriately. Caution should be used when administering a statin or another agent used to lower cholesterol concentrations concomitantly to patients also receiving other drugs (e.g., spironolactone, cimetidine) that may decrease the concentrations or activity of endogenous steroid hormones.

Renal Effects The NLA statin safety assessment task force recommends that renal function tests be performed prior to initiating statin therapy; however, routine monitoring of serum creatinine concentrations and proteinuria for the purpose of identifying adverse renal effects is not necessary. If serum creatine concentration is elevated in the absence of rhabdomyolysis, the task force states that statin therapy may be continued; however, per labeling recommendations, dosage adjustment may be required for some statins. If unexpected proteinuria develops, the etiology should be determined; although statin therapy may be continued in patients who developed proteinuria, the task force states that dosage adjustment may be required per labeling recommendations. Although the clinical importance of proteinuria and hematuria associated with rosuvastatin is not known, the manufacturer of rosuvastatin states that dosage reduction should be considered in patients receiving the drug who have unexplained persistent proteinuria and/or hematuria during routine urinalysis testing. (See Cautions: Genitourinary Effects.) The task force states that chronic renal disease does not preclude the use of statins; however, the dosage of some statins should be adjusted in those with moderate or severe renal impairment. (See Dosage and Administration: Dosage in Renal and Hepatic Impairment.)

CNS Effects CNS vascular lesions, characterized by perivascular hemorrhage and edema, mononuclear cell infiltration of perivascular spaces, and perivascular fibrin deposits and necrosis of small vessels have been observed in animals receiving statins at various dosages (producing plasma drug concentrations approximately 14–59 times higher than the mean serum drug concentration in humans receiving recommended dosages).

The NLA statin safety assessment task force states that routine neurologic monitoring for the purpose of identifying peripheral neuropathy or impaired cognition is not recommended. Patients experiencing manifestations consistent with peripheral neuropathy should be evaluated to rule out secondary causes (e.g., diabetes mellitus, renal impairment, alcohol abuse, vitamin B_{12} deficiency, cancer, hypothyroidism, acquired immunodeficiency syndrome [AIDS], Lyme disease, heavy metal intoxication). If a secondary cause is not identified, the task force recommends that statin therapy be discontinued for 3–6 months. If neurologic manifestations improve over this period without statin therapy, a presumptive diagnosis of statin-induced peripheral neuropathy may be made; however, because of the proven benefit of statin therapy, reinitiation of statin therapy (i.e., with a different statin and dosage) should be considered. If neurologic manifestations do not improve during the period of discontinuance, statin therapy should be reinitiated, taking into consideration the risks and benefits of such therapy. The NLA task force states that patients experiencing manifestations consistent with impaired cognition should be evaluated and managed in a similar manner as those experiencing peripheral neuropathy. These patients should first be evaluated to rule out secondary causes. If a secondary cause is not identified, statin therapy should be discontinued for 1–3 months. If cognitive impairment is not improved during this period of discontinuance, statin therapy should be reinitiated, taking into consideration the risks and benefits of such therapy. FDA continues to believe that the cardiovascular benefits of statins outweigh the small increased risk of cognitive impairment. (See Cautions: Nervous System Effects.) The ACC/AHA cholesterol management guideline states that, in patients presenting with confusion or memory impairment, it is reasonable to evaluate the patient for statin as well as nonstatin causes (e.g., exposure to other drugs, systemic or neuropsychiatric causes).

Ocular Effects Dose-dependent increases in optic nerve degeneration were observed in animals receiving certain statins (e.g., lovastatin, simvastatin) at dosages which produced mean plasma drug concentrations approximately 12–30 times higher than the mean plasma drug concentrations observed in humans receiving the highest recommended dosages. Vestibulocochlear Wallerian-like degeneration and retinal ganglion cell chromatolysis also were observed in animals receiving certain statins (e.g., lovastatin, simvastatin) at dosages which produced mean plasma drug concentrations approximately 30 times higher than the mean plasma drug concentrations observed in humans receiving the highest recommended dosages.

Neuromuscular Effects Use of statins does not appear to increase the risk of developing amyotrophic lateral sclerosis (ALS, Lou Gehrig disease). According to FDA analysis of data from 41 long-term (6 months to 5 years) controlled clinical trials of 7 statins (atorvastatin, cerivastatin [no longer commercially available in the US], fluvastatin, lovastatin, pravastatin, rosuvastatin, and simvastatin), ALS was diagnosed in 9 of approximately 64,000 patients receiving statin therapy and in 10 of approximately 56,000 patients receiving placebo. The incidence of ALS was 4.2 cases per 100,000 patient-years in patients receiving statin therapy and 5 cases per 100,000 patient-years in those receiving placebo. Because of the extensive use of statins and the serious nature of ALS, FDA states that continued evaluation of the effects of statin therapy on ALS is warranted.

■ **Pediatric Precautions** Results of several randomized, double-blind, placebo-controlled studies in children 8 years of age and older receiving pravastatin (20–40 mg daily for 2 years) or 10 years of age and older (postmenarchal girls) receiving atorvastatin (10–20 mg daily for 26 weeks), lovastatin (10–40 mg daily for at least 24 weeks), rosuvastatin (5–20 mg daily for 12 weeks), or simvastatin (10–40 mg daily for up to 24 weeks) indicate that the adverse effect profile in children receiving these statins generally is similar to that with placebo. However, elevations in serum CK concentrations exceeding 10 times the upper limit of normal were observed more frequently in children receiving rosuvastatin compared with those receiving placebo. In open-label, uncontrolled studies of 2 years' duration in pediatric patients 9–16 years of age receiving fluvastatin, the most common adverse effects observed were influenza and infections. There were no detectable adverse effects on growth or sexual maturation in adolescent boys or on duration of menstrual cycle in girls who received atorvastatin, fluvastatin, lovastatin, or simvastatin. In children who received pravastatin, there were no detectable differences in height, weight, testicular volume, Tanner score, or endocrine parameters (i.e., corticotropin [ACTH], cortisol, dehydroepiandrosterone sulfate [DHEA-S], follicle-stimulating hormone [FSH], luteinizing hormone [LH], thyrotropin [TSH], estradiol [in girls], testosterone [in boys]) relative to placebo-treated children. In children 10–17 years of age who received rosuvastatin, there were no detectable adverse effects on growth, weight, body mass index (BMI), or sexual maturation. If therapy with a statin is considered, the manufacturers of atorvastatin, fluvastatin, lovastatin, pravastatin, rosuvastatin, and simvastatin state that adolescent girls should be advised to use effective and appropriate contraceptive methods during therapy to reduce the likelihood of unintended pregnancy. (See Cautions: Pregnancy, Fertility, and Lactation.) Pharmacologic therapy generally should be undertaken in consultation with a specialist in the treatment of pediatric dyslipidemia.

Controversy exists regarding the implementation of screening for elevated cholesterol concentrations and use of long-term cholesterol-lowering interventions in children and adolescents based on the anticipated and/or demonstrated effects of dietary modification on LDL-cholesterol concentrations, the delayed effect of cholesterol-lowering therapy on cardiovascular risk reduction, and the potential for adverse effects related to such cholesterol-lowering interventions. The long-term safety of statins for any age group has not been fully elucidated to date. Safety data from clinical trials in hypercholesterolemic adults receiving statins for 2–8 years suggest that these drugs are well tolerated with an adverse effect profile similar to that of placebo, but long-term data are limited and additional follow-up is needed. The uncertainty about potential long-term toxicity of statins is of particular concern in pediatric patients, since they might be most susceptible to any potential adverse effects resulting from chronic suppression of cholesterol biosynthesis. For additional details regarding the use of specific statins in pediatric patients, see Pediatric Precautions in the individual statin monographs in 24:06.08.

■ **Geriatric Precautions** Statins generally are well tolerated in geriatric patients; the adverse effect profile reported in patients older than 65 years of age is similar to that in younger adults. Although no overall differences in efficacy or safety were observed between geriatric and younger patients, and other clinical experience has not revealed age-related differences in response, the possibility that some geriatric patients may exhibit increased sensitivity to statins cannot be ruled out.

According to reports by the AHA and ATP III, evidence suggests that substantial benefit in coronary heart disease risk reduction for geriatric patients may occur with efforts to decrease serum cholesterol concentrations. However, because advanced age (65 years of age or older) is a predisposing factor for myopathy, statins should be used with caution in geriatric patients. (See Musculoskeletal Effects under Cautions: Precautions and Contraindications.) In addition, the greater frequency of decreased hepatic, renal, and/or cardiac function and of concomitant disease and drug therapy observed in geriatric individuals should be considered when assessing the potential benefit of antilipemic therapy.

The ACC/AHA cholesterol management guideline states that initiation of statin therapy for primary prevention of ASCVD in patients older than 75 years of age requires consideration of additional factors, including increasing comorbidities, safety considerations, and priorities of care. Therefore, the potential for an ASCVD risk reduction benefit, adverse effects, and drug interactions, along with patient preferences, must be considered before initiating statin therapy in patients older than 75 years of age.

■ **Mutagenicity and Carcinogenicity** Statins did not exhibit mutagenic potential in vitro with or without metabolic activation in microbial mutagen tests, forward mutation assays, chromosomal aberration tests, and gene conversion assays.

In rats and mice receiving oral dosages of statins that produced plasma concentrations or AUCs 1–50 times higher than plasma concentrations or AUCs in humans receiving usual dosages of statins for 2 years, there was an increased incidence of hepatocellular adenomas and carcinomas, forestomach squamous papillomas and carcinomas, thyroid follicular adenomas and carcinomas, lung adenomas, and adenomas of the Harderian gland.

While the number of cases of breast cancer in patients receiving pravastatin was higher than that with placebo in one clinical trial, the expected number of breast cancer cases in the placebo group was low compared with that in the general population for women of similar race and age, and data from another study (the Long-term Intervention with Pravastatin in Ischaemic Disease [LIPID] study) indicate a similar incidence of breast cancer among pravastatin- and placebo-treated patients. Long-term (median duration of 7.4 years) follow-up data from the Scandinavian Simvastatin Study (4S) demonstrated a slightly lower incidence of cancer deaths (not statistically significant) in patients treated with simvastatin than in placebo recipients. However, a recent meta-analysis of randomized, controlled statin trials with patient follow-up of at least 1 year in which cancer diagnosis or cancer deaths were reported showed no effect of statins on cancer incidence or cancer death.

While early animal studies raised concerns about the possible carcinogenic effects of simvastatin, a large body of evidence indicates that long-term statin therapy is not associated with an increased risk of cancer. However, the fixed combination of simvastatin and ezetimibe (Vytorin®) was reported in one study (the Simvastatin and Ezetimibe in Aortic Stenosis [SEAS] study) to be possibly associated with an increased risk of cancer. Results of this study in 1873 patients with mild to moderate asymptomatic aortic stenosis revealed a higher incidence of cancer and fatal cancer (11.1 and 4.1%, respectively) in patients receiving the fixed-combination preparation compared with those receiving placebo (7.5 and 2.5%, respectively). Findings from the SEAS study prompted FDA to issue an early communication in 2008 about this potential safety risk. However, results of 2 subsequent large randomized studies (the Study of Heart and Renal Protection [SHARP] and the Improved Reduction of Outcomes: Vytorin® Efficacy International Trial [IMPROVE-IT]) found no consistent pattern of increased cancer risk among patients receiving the fixed-combination preparation. Based on the currently available evidence, FDA has concluded that the fixed-combination preparation of ezetimibe and simvastatin (Vytorin®) is not likely to increase the risk of cancer.

■ **Pregnancy, Fertility, and Lactation** ***Pregnancy*** There are no adequate and well-controlled studies using statins in pregnant women; limited published data are insufficient to determine whether these drugs are associated with an increased risk of major congenital malformations or miscarriage. Since atherosclerosis is a chronic process, discontinuance of antilipemic agents during pregnancy generally should not have a substantial effect on the outcome of long-term therapy for primary hypercholesterolemia. There is no known clinical benefit for continued use during pregnancy. Currently, most experts recommend that dyslipidemias in pregnant women be managed with dietary measures; consultation with a lipid specialist is recommended for pregnant women with severe forms of dyslipidemia. If antilipemic drugs are necessary, however, bile acid sequestrants may be considered.

Cholesterol and other products of the cholesterol biosynthetic pathway are essential for fetal development, including synthesis of steroids and cell membranes. Because of the ability of statins to decrease the synthesis of cholesterol and possibly other products of the cholesterol biosynthetic pathway, these agents may cause fetal harm when administered to pregnant women. Rarely, congenital anomalies have been reported following intrauterine exposure to statins. Therefore, statins are *contraindicated* in women who are or may become pregnant. These agents should be administered to women of childbearing age only when such patients are highly unlikely to conceive and have been informed of the potential hazards. If the patient becomes pregnant while receiving the drug, the drug should be discontinued immediately and the patient informed of the potential fetal hazard and the lack of known clinical benefit with continued use during pregnancy.

Fertility Effects of statins on spermatogenesis and fertility have not been studied in adequate numbers of patients. In animals receiving statins, no adverse effects on fertility were observed. However, in male rats receiving certain statins (e.g., simvastatin) in dosages resulting in AUCs of 4 times the maximum human exposure level for 34 weeks, decreased fertility was observed. This effect was not reproduced during a subsequent study using the same drug and dosage for 11 weeks (the entire duration of the spermatogenesis cycle in rats, including epididymal maturation). Seminiferous tubule degeneration, testicular atrophy, decreased spermatogenesis, spermatocytic degeneration, and giant cell formation were observed. The clinical importance of these effects has not been established.

Lactation Fluvastatin and pravastatin are distributed into human milk; atorvastatin, pitavastatin, and rosuvastatin are distributed into milk in animals. Because of the potential for serious adverse reactions from these drugs in nursing infants, statins are contraindicated in nursing women; women who are taking these drugs should be advised not to breast-feed their infants.

Drug Interactions

■ **Drugs and Foods Affecting or Metabolized by Hepatic Microsomal Enzymes** Current evidence suggests that certain adverse effects of statins (i.e., myotoxicity) are more common in patients receiving concomitant therapy with drugs metabolized by the hepatic cytochrome P-450 (CYP) isoenzyme system. Metabolism of most statins is mediated by the CYP isoenzyme system (see Pharmacokinetics: Elimination), principally by CYP3A4 and 2C9; concomitant use of drugs that inhibit these isoenzymes may increase plasma concentrations of these statins and increase the risk of adverse effects. Conversely, drugs that induce CYP isoenzymes may reduce plasma concentrations of statins metabolized by these isoenzymes. The clinical importance of these CYP-mediated interactions is based on the degree of inhibition or induction of CYP enzymes and the pharmacokinetic profile of the individual statin. Simvastatin and lovastatin are substantially metabolized by CYP3A4 and, therefore, are subject to more drug interactions that will likely require intervention. Atorvastatin also undergoes CYP3A4 metabolism, but to a lesser extent. Fluvastatin, pitavastatin, and rosuvastatin are principally metabolized by CYP2C9, and pravastatin does not undergo CYP metabolism.

Antifungals Rhabdomyolysis has occurred in at least one patient receiving concomitant lovastatin and itraconazole therapy. Concomitant use of itraconazole with lovastatin or simvastatin has resulted in a 10- to 20-fold increase in plasma concentrations of the antilipemic agents and more than a 14.8- to 36-fold increase in the area under the plasma concentration-time curve (AUC) of lovastatin. Itraconazole increased peak plasma concentration and AUC of atorvastatin by approximately 20% and 3.3-fold, respectively; of pravastatin by approximately 17 and 11%, respectively; and of rosuvastatin by 1.2- to 1.4-fold and 1.3- to 1.4-fold, respectively. Itraconazole decreased peak plasma concentration and AUC of pitavastatin by 22 and 23%, respectively. Concomitant administration of itraconazole with fluvastatin did not result in clinically important alterations in the pharmacokinetic profile of either drug.

Other azole antifungals that inhibit CYP3A4 (e.g., fluconazole, ketoconazole, posaconazole, voriconazole) also may inhibit the metabolism of certain statins, resulting in increased statin concentrations and an increased risk of myopathy and/or rhabdomyolysis. There is some evidence that voriconazole is a less potent inhibitor of CYP3A4 than ketoconazole or itraconazole; however, voriconazole has been shown to inhibit lovastatin metabolism in vitro and is likely to increase plasma concentrations of lovastatin and other statins metabolized by CYP3A4.

The manufacturer of atorvastatin states that clinicians considering concomitant use of atorvastatin with azole antifungals should weigh the benefits and risks (e.g., myopathy, rhabdomyolysis) of such concomitant use and should carefully monitor patients for manifestations of muscle pain, tenderness, or weakness, particularly during the initial months of therapy and following an increase in dosage of either drug; in addition, if atorvastatin is used concomitantly with itraconazole, the lowest necessary dosage of atorvastatin should be employed, and dosage of atorvastatin should be limited.

If fluvastatin and fluconazole are used concomitantly, dosage of fluvastatin should be limited.

Because of an increased risk of myopathy and/or rhabdomyolysis, concomitant administration of lovastatin or simvastatin with itraconazole, ketoconazole, posaconazole, or voriconazole is *contraindicated*; if therapy with itraconazole, ketoconazole, posaconazole, or voriconazole is unavoidable, therapy with lovastatin or simvastatin must be suspended during the course of antifungal treatment.

The manufacturer of voriconazole states that if voriconazole must be used concomitantly with a statin, the patient should be monitored frequently for statin-associated adverse effects and toxicity, and dosage adjustment of the statin should be considered and may be needed to reduce the risk of myopathy, including rhabdomyolysis.

Antimycobacterials Concomitant use of atorvastatin with rifampin may result in variable reductions in plasma concentrations of atorvastatin; administration of rifampin followed by delayed administration of atorvastatin resulted in 40 and 80% decreases in atorvastatin peak plasma concentration and AUC, respectively, while *simultaneous* administration of the drugs resulted in 2.7-fold and 30% *increases* in atorvastatin peak plasma concentration and AUC, respectively. Concomitant use of pitavastatin and rifampin increased pitavastatin peak plasma concentration and AUC by twofold and 29%, respectively, and decreased rifampin peak plasma concentration and AUC by 18 and 15%, respectively. Following concomitant administration with rifampin, peak plasma concentration and AUC of fluvastatin decreased by 42 and 53%, respectively.

The manufacturer of atorvastatin states that if atorvastatin and rifampin are used concomitantly, these drugs should be administered simultaneously, as delayed administration of atorvastatin following administration of rifampin has been associated with substantial reductions in plasma concentrations of atorvastatin.

The manufacturer of pitavastatin states that if this statin and rifampin are used concomitantly, dosage of pitavastatin should be limited.

Antiretroviral Agents **HIV Protease Inhibitors.** Concomitant use of certain statins (e.g., atorvastatin, lovastatin, rosuvastatin, simvastatin) with HIV protease inhibitors (atazanavir, darunavir, indinavir, fosamprenavir, lopinavir, nelfinavir, ritonavir, saquinavir, tipranavir) increases plasma concentration and AUC of the antilipemic agent, resulting in increased effects and/or increased risk of toxicity (e.g., myopathy and/or rhabdomyolysis).

Concomitant use of HIV protease inhibitors with lovastatin or simvastatin is *contraindicated*.

The manufacturer of atorvastatin states that concomitant use of atorvastatin and *ritonavir-boosted* tipranavir should be *avoided*. In addition, the manufacturer states that the benefits of concomitant use of atorvastatin with fosamprenavir (with or without low-dose ritonavir), the fixed combination of lopinavir and ritonavir (lopinavir/ritonavir), *ritonavir-boosted* darunavir, or *ritonavir-boosted* saquinavir should be weighed against the possible risk of myopathy or rhabdomyolysis, and patients should be monitored carefully for manifestations of muscle pain, tenderness, or weakness, particularly during the initial months of therapy and following an increase in dosage of either drug. If atorvastatin is used concomitantly with fosamprenavir (with or without low-dose ritonavir), nelfinavir, *ritonavir-boosted* darunavir, or *ritonavir-boosted* saquinavir, caution is advised; the lowest necessary dosage of atorvastatin should be used, and dosage of atorvastatin should be limited. If atorvastatin is used concomitantly with lopinavir/ritonavir, caution is advised, and the lowest necessary dosage of atorvastatin should be used.

If rosuvastatin is used concomitantly with *ritonavir-boosted* HIV protease inhibitors, caution is advised because such concomitant use has differing effects on exposure to rosuvastatin; dosage of rosuvastatin should be limited during concomitant therapy with *ritonavir-boosted* atazanavir or lopinavir/ritonavir.

Alternatively, use of a statin that is not principally metabolized by CYP3A (e.g., fluvastatin, pitavastatin, pravastatin [except with *ritonavir-boosted* darunavir]) should be considered. Although FDA states that there are no dosage limitations when pravastatin is used concomitantly with *ritonavir-boosted* darunavir, some experts state that the lowest necessary dosage of pravastatin should be used and with careful monitoring because such concomitant therapy increased pravastatin peak plasma concentration and AUC by 63 and 81%, respectively. Some experts and FDA state that dosage adjustments are not necessary when pitavastatin is used concomitantly with atazanavir (with or without ritonavir), lopinavir/ritonavir, or *ritonavir-boosted* darunavir, or when pravastatin is used concomitantly with lopinavir/ritonavir or *ritonavir-boosted* saquinavir.

Nonnucleoside Reverse Transcriptase Inhibitors. Concomitant use of certain statins (e.g., atorvastatin, lovastatin, simvastatin) and certain nonnucleoside reverse transcriptase inhibitors (efavirenz, etravirine, nevirapine) may alter plasma concentrations of the antilipemic agent.

Concomitant use of efavirenz with atorvastatin, pravastatin, or simvastatin has resulted in decreased AUC of the antilipemic agent. If efavirenz is used in patients receiving atorvastatin, pravastatin, rosuvastatin, or simvastatin, dosage of the antilipemic agent should be adjusted according to lipid response (up to the maximum recommended dosage).

Etravirine has been shown to decrease atorvastatin AUC; the drug may increase fluvastatin concentrations and decrease lovastatin or simvastatin concentrations, but has no substantial effects on either pravastatin or rosuvastatin concentrations. If etravirine is used in patients receiving atorvastatin, lovastatin, or simvastatin, dosage of the antilipemic agent should be adjusted according to lipid response (up to the maximum recommended dosage); if etravirine is used with fluvastatin, dosage adjustments for fluvastatin may be necessary. If etravirine is used in patients receiving pravastatin or rosuvastatin, dosage adjustments are not needed.

Nevirapine may decrease lovastatin or simvastatin concentrations. If nevirapine is used in patients receiving lovastatin or simvastatin, dosage of the antilipemic agent should be adjusted according to lipid response (up to the maximum recommended dosage).

Rilpivirine has been shown to increase concentrations of atorvastatin metabolites but does not affect atorvastatin AUC; dosage adjustments are not needed. Data are not available regarding concomitant use of rilpivirine and other statins.

Data are not available regarding concomitant use of pitavastatin with efavirenz, etravirine, or nevirapine, or of rosuvastatin with efavirenz.

Cardiac Drugs **Amiodarone.** Amiodarone is metabolized by the CYP microsomal enzyme system, principally by the isoenzyme CYP3A4. In addition, amiodarone inhibits the activity of CYP3A4 and potentially may interact with drugs that also are metabolized by this enzyme. Concomitant use of simvastatin and amiodarone increased simvastatin peak plasma concentration and AUC by 1.79- and 1.76-fold, respectively.

Because the risk of myopathy or rhabdomyolysis is increased following concomitant use of amiodarone with certain statins (e.g., lovastatin, simvastatin), dosages of these statins should be limited during concomitant therapy. In addition, the benefits versus risks of such concomitant therapy should be considered.

Diltiazem. Concomitant use of atorvastatin with diltiazem did not alter atorvastatin peak plasma concentration, but atorvastatin AUC was increased by 51%; in addition, rhabdomyolysis with renal failure and acute hepatitis have been reported in at least one patient receiving these agents concomitantly.

Concomitant administration of various other statins (e.g., lovastatin, simvastatin) and diltiazem has resulted in marked increases (i.e., 257–333% and fourfold to fivefold, respectively) in plasma concentrations of the antilipemic agents. Because the risk of myopathy and/or rhabdomyolysis is increased in patients receiving lovastatin or simvastatin (particularly with higher dosages of the statin) concomitantly with diltiazem, dosage of lovastatin or simvastatin should be limited during concomitant therapy. In addition, the benefits versus risks of such concomitant therapy should be considered.

Concomitant use of pitavastatin and extended-release diltiazem increased pitavastatin peak plasma concentration and AUC by 15 and 10%, respectively, and decreased diltiazem peak plasma concentration and AUC by 7 and 2%, respectively.

Concomitant use of pravastatin and diltiazem increased pravastatin peak plasma concentration and AUC by 30 and 2.7%, respectively.

Dronedarone. The risk of myopathy, including rhabdomyolysis, is increased following concomitant use of dronedarone with certain statins (e.g., lovastatin, simvastatin).

Concomitant administration of dronedarone and simvastatin increased peak plasma concentration and AUC of simvastatin by 3.75- and 3.9-fold, respectively; peak plasma concentration and AUC of the active simvastatin acid metabolite were increased by 2.14- and 1.96-fold, respectively. While there are no specific studies evaluating the interaction potential between dronedarone and lovastatin, it is expected that dronedarone also may increase lovastatin exposure to the same degree as simvastatin. The manufacturers of lovastatin and simvastatin state that dosage of these statins should be limited if used concomitantly with dronedarone and the benefits versus risks of such concomitant therapy should be carefully considered.

Verapamil. Concomitant use of certain statins (e.g., lovastatin, simvastatin) with verapamil increases the risk of myopathy and/or rhabdomyolysis. In a randomized, double-blind, crossover study in healthy individuals, concomitant administration of verapamil with simvastatin resulted in a threefold to fivefold increase in simvastatin concentrations and a threefold increase in simvastatin acid concentrations. In addition, concomitant use of simvastatin and extended-release verapamil increased simvastatin and simvastatin acid peak plasma concentration (2.1- and 2.4-fold, respectively) and AUC (2.5- and 2.3-fold, respectively). Because of such risk, some clinicians state that concomitant use of simvastatin and verapamil generally should be avoided. However, if concomitant use with verapamil is necessary, dosages of lovastatin and simvastatin should be limited, and close monitoring for adverse effects (i.e., muscle tenderness, elevated CK concentrations) is advised. In addition, the benefits versus risks of such concomitant therapy should be considered.

It has been suggested that since fluvastatin and pravastatin are not substantially metabolized by the CYP3A4 isoenzyme, verapamil would not be expected to have a clinically important effect on the pharmacokinetics of these statins. However, concomitant use of pravastatin and verapamil (immediate- and extended-release) has been shown to increase pravastatin peak plasma concentration and AUC by 42 and 31%, respectively.

Cobicistat-containing Preparations Concomitant use of cobicistat-containing preparations and certain statins (e.g., lovastatin, simvastatin) can increase plasma concentrations of the antilipemic agent, and possibly increase the risk of myopathy and/or rhabdomyolysis. The manufacturers of lovastatin and simvastatin state that concomitant use of cobicistat-containing preparations with these statins is *contraindicated*.

Danazol Myositis with rhabdomyolysis has developed in at least one patient receiving lovastatin and danazol concomitantly. Although the mechanism of the interaction has not been fully elucidated, it has been suggested that this adverse effect probably resulted from danazol-induced inhibition of lovastatin metabolism (by CYP3A4). Because the risk of myopathy and/or rhabdomyolysis is increased in patients receiving danazol concomitantly with certain statins, the manufacturer states that dosage of lovastatin should be limited during concomitant therapy with danazol; in addition, the benefits versus risks of such concomitant therapy should be considered.

Concomitant use of simvastatin with danazol is *contraindicated*.

The risk of myositis with rhabdomyolysis in patients receiving danazol with other statins currently is not known.

Diclofenac Concomitant administration of diclofenac with fluvastatin has resulted in a 60 or 25% increase in peak plasma concentration or AUC, respectively, of diclofenac and an 80 or 50% increase in peak plasma concentration or AUC, respectively, of fluvastatin. Although the precise mechanism of this interaction has not been fully elucidated, it has been suggested that this interaction probably resulted from fluvastatin-induced inhibition of diclofenac metabolism (particularly first-pass metabolism) by the CYP2C9 isoenzyme. The clinical importance of this pharmacokinetic interaction is unclear.

Grapefruit Juice Grapefruit juice is a potent inhibitor of the CYP3A4 isoenzyme and can increase plasma concentrations of various statins metabolized by CYP3A4 (e.g., atorvastatin, lovastatin, simvastatin).

The extent of this interaction may be influenced by the quantity and timing of grapefruit juice consumption (relative to administration of the statin) and also may vary depending on the specific statin used. In several studies in healthy individuals, plasma concentrations of lovastatin or simvastatin were increased by approximately twofold following administration of regular-strength grapefruit juice (240 mL) with breakfast and a single dose of lovastatin (40 mg) or simvastatin (20 mg) in the evening. In several other studies in individuals who received repeated quantities of double-strength grapefruit juice concomitantly with a single dose of atorvastatin (40 mg), lovastatin (80 mg), or simvastatin (60 mg), plasma concentrations of the antilipemic agents were increased by approximately 3.3-, 15-, or 16-fold, respectively. In a crossover study in healthy individuals, concurrent administration of simvastatin (40 mg) with large amounts of grapefruit juice (200 mL double-strength 3 times daily for 3 days) increased peak plasma concentrations and AUC of simvastatin by 12- and 13.5-fold, respectively; however, the inhibitory effects of grapefruit juice were considerably decreased when simvastatin was taken 24 hours after ingestion of grapefruit juice. In a study evaluating the interaction potential of grapefruit juice and atorvastatin, concomitant administration of a single dose of atorvastatin (40 mg) with grapefruit juice (240 mL once daily) increased atorvastatin peak plasma concentration and AUC by 16 and 37%, respectively; more substantial increases in atorvastatin peak plasma concentration (up to 71%) and/or AUC (up to 2.5-fold) have been reported following ingestion of large quantities (750–1200 mL daily or more) of grapefruit juice.

Because the risk of myopathy may be increased with high plasma concentrations of statins, the manufacturers of lovastatin and simvastatin and some clinicians state that concomitant administration of these statins with grapefruit juice should be *avoided*. The manufacturer of atorvastatin states that the risk of myopathy may be increased with ingestion of large quantities (more than one liter daily) of grapefruit juice. However, there is some difference of opinion regarding the actual risk of this drug interaction versus the perceived risk based on studies that used unusually large volumes of grapefruit juice. Some clinicians suggest that a small amount of grapefruit juice (e.g., 240 mL regular-strength) may be acceptable and may even be used to therapeutic advantage, although consumption should be separated from statin administration (i.e., grapefruit juice given in the morning and statin in the evening) to minimize this potentially serious interaction. Because of interindividual variations in CYP3A4-mediated drug metabolism and other factors, some patients may be more susceptible to the interacting effects of grapefruit juice.

Concomitant administration of grapefruit juice does not appear to affect the pharmacokinetics of fluvastatin, pitavastatin, or pravastatin because CYP3A4 is either not involved or only minimally involved in the metabolism of these statins.

HCV Protease Inhibitors Concomitant use of rosuvastatin and simeprevir can increase plasma concentrations of the antilipemic agent and increase the risk of myopathy. Caution should be exercised and dosage of the statin should be reduced when the drugs are coadministered.

Immunosuppressive Agents Cyclosporine has been shown to increase AUC of statins. Concomitant administration of atorvastatin or lovastatin with cyclosporine resulted in an 8.7-fold increase in atorvastatin AUC and a fivefold to eightfold increase in lovastatin AUC. Cyclosporine increased pitavastatin peak plasma concentration and AUC by 6.6- and 4.6-fold, respectively; such effects are considered clinically important. In addition, myopathy and/or rhabdomyolysis has developed in some patients receiving cyclosporine concomitantly with certain statins (e.g., atorvastatin, lovastatin, simvastatin). Although the mechanism of the interaction has not been fully elucidated, it has been suggested that this adverse effect probably results from cyclosporine-induced inhibition of statin metabolism (by CYP3A4); cyclosporine-induced inhibition of organic anion transporter (OATP) 1B1 also may be responsible for increasing bioavailability of atorvastatin, pitavastatin, and simvastatin acid. Concomitant administration of cyclosporine with fluvastatin, pravastatin, or rosuvastatin has resulted in substantial increases in the peak plasma concentration (i.e., 30%, 327%, or 11-fold, respectively) or AUC (i.e., 90%, 282%, or sevenfold, respectively) of the antilipemic agent. However, neither myopathy nor substantial increases in CK concentrations have been observed in 3 reports involving 100 posttransplant patients (24 renal and 76 cardiac) receiving concomitant therapy with cyclosporine and pravastatin for up to 2 years.

The manufacturers of pitavastatin and simvastatin state that concomitant use of these statins with cyclosporine is *contraindicated*. The manufacturers of atorvastatin and lovastatin state that concomitant use of these statins with cyclosporine should be *avoided*. The manufacturers of fluvastatin, pravastatin, and rosuvastatin state that dosages of these statins should be limited during concomitant therapy with cyclosporine.

Although data are more limited with everolimus, sirolimus, and tacrolimus, the drug interaction potential of these other immunosuppressants is expected to be similar to that of cyclosporine because of similar metabolism. Some experts state that concomitant use of everolimus, tacrolimus, or sirolimus with lovastatin, pitavastatin, or simvastatin should be avoided. These experts state that if atorvastatin is used concomitantly with any of these immunosuppressants, dosage of the statin should be limited.

Macrolides Rhabdomyolysis with or without renal impairment has occurred in patients receiving erythromycin or clarithromycin concomitantly with certain statins (e.g., lovastatin). Certain macrolides, including erythromycin, clarithromycin, and telithromycin are inhibitors of the CYP3A4 isoenzyme. Concomitant administration of erythromycin with atorvastatin or simvastatin resulted in marked increases (i.e., 38%, or fourfold to sixfold, respectively) in plasma concentrations of the antilipemic agents. Concomitant administration of clarithromycin with atorvastatin or pravastatin resulted in increased peak plasma concentrations (i.e., 5.4-fold and 128%, respectively) and AUC (i.e., 4.4-fold and 110%, respectively) of the antilipemic agents. Erythromycin increased pitavastatin peak plasma concentration and AUC by 3.6- and 2.8-fold, respectively; such effects are considered clinically important. Concomitant use of erythromycin with rosuvastatin decreased rosuvastatin peak plasma concentration and AUC by 31 and 20%, respectively. No clinically important changes in the pharmacokinetic profile of fluvastatin or pravastatin were reported following concomitant administration with erythromycin. Concomitant administration of telithromycin and simvastatin has resulted in increased simvastatin concentrations and AUC.

The manufacturer of atorvastatin states that the benefits of concomitant use of atorvastatin with macrolide antibiotics (e.g., clarithromycin, erythromycin) should be weighed against the possible risk of myopathy or rhabdomyolysis, and patients should be monitored carefully for manifestations of muscle pain, tenderness, or weakness, particularly during the initial months of therapy and following an increase in dosage of either drug. If atorvastatin is used concomitantly with clarithromycin, caution is advised; the lowest necessary dosage of atorvastatin should be used, and dosage of atorvastatin should be limited. If atorvastatin is used concomitantly with other macrolide antibiotics (e.g., erythromycin), caution is advised and lower initial and maintenance dosages of atorvastatin should be considered.

Because of an increased risk of myopathy and/or rhabdomyolysis, concomitant use of lovastatin or simvastatin with clarithromycin, erythromycin, or telithromycin is *contraindicated*. If therapy with clarithromycin, erythromycin, or telithromycin is unavoidable, therapy with lovastatin or simvastatin must be suspended during the course of macrolide treatment.

If pitavastatin and erythromycin are used concomitantly, dosage of pitavastatin should be limited.

If pravastatin and clarithromycin are used concomitantly, dosage of pravastatin should be limited. Other macrolides (e.g., erythromycin, azithromycin) also may potentially increase exposure to pravastatin and should therefore be used concomitantly with caution.

Nefazodone Administration of single 40-mg doses of atorvastatin or simvastatin in healthy individuals who had received nefazodone (200 mg twice daily) for 6 days resulted in threefold to fourfold increases in plasma concentrations of atorvastatin and atorvastatin lactone and 20-fold increases in plasma concentrations of simvastatin and simvastatin acid. In addition, myositis or rhabdomyolysis has occurred in a few patients following concomitant therapy with nefazodone and various statins (e.g., lovastatin, simvastatin). Although the mechanism of the interaction has not been fully elucidated, it has been suggested that this adverse effect probably resulted from nefazodone-induced inhibition of statin metabolism and subsequent marked increases in plasma concentrations of the antilipemic agent. Concomitant administration of pravastatin with nefazodone has resulted in increased serum CK concentrations in at least one patient.

Because of the risk of rhabdomyolysis, the manufacturer of nefazodone suggests that concomitant administration of nefazodone and certain statins (e.g., atorvastatin, lovastatin, simvastatin) be used with caution and at reduced dosages. However, the manufacturers of lovastatin and simvastatin and some clinicians state that concomitant use of nefazodone with lovastatin or simvastatin is *contraindicated*.

Oral Antidiabetic Agents Concomitant oral administration of glyburide or tolbutamide with certain statins (e.g., fluvastatin, simvastatin) reportedly has resulted in increased bioavailability of the antidiabetic agents without altering oral glucose tolerance. It has been suggested that these interactions probably resulted from inhibition of the CYP microsomal enzyme system (e.g., CYP2C9) involved in the metabolism of both agents. Although concomitant administration of fluvastatin with glyburide did not substantially alter the hypoglycemic effects of the antidiabetic agent, the manufacturer of fluvastatin recommends that patients receiving concomitant therapy with fluvastatin and glyburide should continue to be monitored appropriately.

Pharmacokinetic interactions were not reported during concomitant use of lovastatin with chlorpropamide or glipizide in patients with type 2 (noninsulin-dependent) diabetes mellitus.

The effect of other statins on antidiabetic agents currently is unknown.

Phenytoin Concomitant administration of phenytoin (300 mg once daily) with fluvastatin (40 mg twice daily for 5 days) has resulted in a 27 or 40% increase in peak plasma concentrations or AUC, respectively, of fluvastatin and a 5 or 20% increase in the respective parameters of phenytoin. Although the precise mechanism of this interaction has not been fully elucidated, it has been suggested that this interaction probably resulted from inhibition of the CYP2C9 isoenzyme involved in the metabolism of both agents. It has been calculated that addition of 40 mg of fluvastatin daily to an existing phenytoin regimen may increase steady-state plasma concentrations of phenytoin by approximately 33%. The manufacturer of fluvastatin recommends that patients receiving phenytoin should continue to be monitored appropriately when fluvastatin therapy is initiated or dosage is adjusted.

■ **Acid-reducing Agents** Concomitant administration of fluvastatin with cimetidine, ranitidine, or omeprazole resulted in increased peak plasma concentrations (40, 50, or 37%, respectively) and AUC (30, 10, or 20%, respectively) of fluvastatin. Although the mechanism of the interaction has not been fully elucidated, this effect probably resulted from a reduction in acid-catalyzed degradation of the antilipemic agent. It has been suggested that cimetidine also may inhibit the CYP enzyme system, resulting in increased concentrations of fluvastatin. Concomitant administration of cimetidine with atorvastatin or pravastatin decreased atorvastatin peak plasma concentration and AUC by 11 and less than 1%, respectively, and increased pravastatin peak plasma concentration and AUC by 9.8 and 30%, respectively.

■ **Amlodipine** The risk of myopathy, including rhabdomyolysis, is increased following concomitant use of simvastatin with amlodipine. Concomitant use of simvastatin and amlodipine increased simvastatin peak plasma concentration and AUC by 1.47- and 1.77-fold, respectively. The manufacturer of simvastatin states that if this statin and amlodipine are used concomitantly, dosage of simvastatin should be limited, and the benefits versus risks of such concomitant therapy should be considered.

Concomitant use of atorvastatin and amlodipine decreased atorvastatin peak plasma concentration by 12%, while increasing atorvastatin AUC by 15%.

■ **Antacids** Concomitant administration of atorvastatin with an antacid containing aluminum hydroxide and magnesium hydroxide resulted in 34 and 33% decreases in atorvastatin peak plasma concentration and AUC, respectively.

Simultaneous administration of rosuvastatin and an antacid containing aluminum hydroxide and magnesium hydroxide decreased rosuvastatin peak plasma concentration and AUC by 50 and 54%, respectively; such effects were considered clinically important. In contrast, when rosuvastatin and the antacid were administered 2 hours apart, rosuvastatin peak plasma concentration and AUC were decreased by 16 and 22%, respectively. Antacids containing aluminum and magnesium hydroxides should be administered at least 2 hours after rosuvastatin.

■ **Antilipemic Agents** ***Bile Acid Sequestrants*** The cholesterol-lowering effects of statins and bile acid sequestrants (e.g., cholestyramine, colestipol) are additive or synergistic.

Concomitant use of atorvastatin and colestipol decreased atorvastatin peak plasma concentration by 26%.

When fluvastatin was administered 4 hours after cholestyramine and a meal, peak plasma concentration and AUC of fluvastatin were decreased by 83 and 51%, respectively.

When pravastatin (20 mg as a single dose) was administered with cholestyramine (4 g as a single dose) or colestipol (10 g as a single dose), peak plasma concentration and AUC of pravastatin decreased by 39–53 and 40–47%, respectively. However, when pravastatin was administered 1 hour prior to cholestyramine, peak plasma concentration and AUC of pravastatin increased by 30 and 12%, respectively; when pravastatin was administered 4 hours after cholestyramine, peak plasma concentration and AUC of pravastatin decreased by 6.8 and 12%, respectively. Concomitant use of pravastatin (5–20 mg twice daily for 8 weeks) and cholestyramine (24 g once daily for 4 weeks) decreased pravastatin AUC by 18–51% but produced variable effects on pravastatin peak plasma concentration.

Therefore, some statin manufacturers recommend that statins be administered either 1 hour or more before, or at least 4 hours after, a bile acid sequestrant when these agents are used concomitantly.

Fibric Acid Derivatives Since both drugs are independently associated with a risk of muscle toxicity, the risk of myopathy and rhabdomyolysis is increased in patients receiving statins concomitantly with fibric acid derivatives (e.g., gemfibrozil). Severe (with or without renal failure) and, rarely, fatal rhabdomyolysis has occurred in some patients receiving cerivastatin (no longer commercially available in the US) concomitantly with gemfibrozil. (See Cautions: Musculoskeletal Effects.) Muscle-related toxicity also has been reported with other statin-fibric acid derivative combinations. In controlled clinical trials in nearly 600 patients receiving such combinations, moderate increases (exceeding 3 times the upper limit of normal) in serum creatine kinase (CK, creatine phosphokinase, CPK) concentrations or discontinuance of therapy because of muscle pain/discomfort was reported in 1% of patients; the reporting rates of mild adverse musculoskeletal effects (e.g., muscle pain) is expected to be similar among statin-fibric acid derivative combinations containing atorvastatin, fluvastatin, lovastatin, pravastatin, or simvastatin. The precise mechanism of the interaction between statins and fibric acid derivatives has not been fully elucidated; however, it has been suggested that the increased risk of myopathy and/or rhabdomyolysis may have both pharmacokinetic (i.e., decreased statin metabolism) and pharmacodynamic origins.

The manufacturer of simvastatin states that concomitant use of this statin with gemfibrozil is *contraindicated*, and the manufacturers of atorvastatin, fluvastatin, lovastatin, pitavastatin, pravastatin, and rosuvastatin state that concomitant use of these statins with gemfibrozil should be *avoided*. The ACC/AHA cholesterol management guideline states that gemfibrozil should not be used in combination with statins because of the increased risk of muscle toxicity and rhabdomyolysis. In a more recent scientific statement, AHA states that some statin-gemfibrozil combinations (i.e., gemfibrozil with atorvastatin, pitavastatin, or rosuvastatin) may be considered if clinically indicated. If gemfibrozil must be used in combination with atorvastatin, pitavastatin, or rosuvastatin, dosage of the statin should be limited; AHA states that fluvastatin may be used in combination with gemfibrozil without any specific dose restrictions.

The manufacturers state that caution is advised if statins are used concomitantly with other fibric acid derivatives (e.g., fenofibrate). In addition, the manufacturers of atorvastatin, lovastatin, pravastatin, and simvastatin state that the benefits (e.g., further alterations in lipid levels) of concomitant use of these statins and fibric acid derivatives other than gemfibrozil (e.g., fenofibrate) should be carefully weighed against the possible risk of myopathy. The manufacturer of atorvastatin also states that lower initial and maintenance dosages of this statin should be considered during such concomitant therapy, and patients should be carefully monitored for manifestations of muscle pain, tenderness, or weakness, particularly during the initial months of therapy and following an increase in dosage of either drug. The ACC/AHA cholesterol management guideline states that the combination of fenofibrate and low- or moderate-intensity statin therapy may be considered only if the benefits from atherosclerotic cardiovascular disease (ASCVD) risk reduction or triglyceride lowering (when triglyceride concentrations exceed 500 mg/dL) outweigh the potential risk of adverse effects.

Lomitapide Concomitant use of certain statins (i.e., atorvastatin, lovastatin, rosuvastatin, simvastatin) with lomitapide has resulted in increased exposure to the statin. The manufacturer of lomitapide states that dosage of lomitapide should be limited to 30 mg daily when the drug is used concomitantly with atorvastatin. When lomitapide is used concomitantly with lovastatin, reduction in lovastatin dosage should be considered. When lomitapide is initiated in patients receiving simvastatin, dosage of simvastatin should be reduced by 50%; during concomitant use, dosage of simvastatin should not exceed 20 mg daily (or 40 mg daily in patients who have received the 80-mg daily dosage for at least 1 year without evidence of adverse muscular effects).

Mipomersen No clinically relevant pharmacokinetic interactions were reported when simvastatin was administered concomitantly with mipomersen. Therefore, dosage adjustment of simvastatin and mipomersen is not necessary during such concomitant use.

Niacin ATP III states that it is not known whether concomitant use of statins and niacin increases the risk of myopathy. However, the manufacturers state that concomitant use of statins and niacin (particularly at antilipemic dosages [exceeding 1 g daily]) increases the risk of myopathy and/or rhabdomyolysis. Severe myopathy or rhabdomyolysis has occurred in some patients receiving certain statins concomitantly with antilipemic dosages (exceeding 1 g daily) of niacin. Therefore, the manufacturers state that caution is advised if statins are used concomitantly with antilipemic dosages of niacin.

The manufacturer of atorvastatin states that lower initial and maintenance dosages of this statin should be considered during concomitant therapy with antilipemic dosages of niacin, and patients should be carefully monitored for manifestations of muscle pain, tenderness, or weakness, particularly during the initial months of therapy and following an increase in dosage of either drug.

The manufacturers of fluvastatin, pitavastatin, and pravastatin state that dosage reduction of these statins should be considered if used concomitantly with antilipemic dosages of niacin.

The manufacturer of simvastatin recommends that dosage of this statin be limited in Chinese patients receiving antilipemic dosages of niacin-containing preparations concomitantly, since risk of myopathy is dose related and interim results of an ongoing clinical trial (Heart Protection Study 2 [HPS2)]) found a higher incidence of myopathy in Chinese patients receiving concomitant therapy with simvastatin (40 mg daily) and a niacin-containing preparation (antilipemic dosages of 1 g daily or higher) compared with non-Chinese patients receiving this drug combination.

The manufacturers of atorvastatin, lovastatin, and simvastatin state that the benefits (e.g., further alterations in lipid concentrations) of concomitant use of these statins and antilipemic dosages of niacin should be carefully weighed against the possible risk of myopathy. According to ATP III and other experts, concomitant use of relatively *low* dosages of niacin with a statin produces an improvement in the lipoprotein profile comparable to that obtained with a statin-fibric acid combination, and probably with a lower risk of myopathy. However, the potential advantage of this combination may be offset by the inability of some patients to tolerate the adverse effects of niacin.

Omega-3-acid Ethyl Esters Concomitant use of certain statins (i.e., atorvastatin, rosuvastatin, simvastatin) with omega-3-acid ethyl esters for 14 days did not affect the rate or extent of exposure to these statins or their metabolites at steady state.

■ **Colchicine** Specific drug interaction studies have not been conducted with statins and colchicine to determine whether specific pharmacokinetic parameters are affected when the drugs are used concomitantly; however, myopathy, including rhabdomyolysis, has been reported in patients receiving various statins (e.g., atorvastatin, fluvastatin, lovastatin, pravastatin, rosuvastatin, simvastatin) concomitantly with colchicine. The manufacturers generally caution against the concomitant use of these statins with colchicine; however, other experts state that concomitant use of rosuvastatin, fluvastatin, lovastatin, pitavastatin, or pravastatin with colchicine is reasonable when clinically indicated, and concomitant use of atorvastatin or simvastatin with colchicine may be considered in appropriate patients. Dosage reduction for some of these statins should be considered to minimize the risk of potential interaction.

■ **Conivaptan** Cases of muscle-related toxicity have been reported in patients receiving concomitant therapy with conivaptan and simvastatin or lovastatin. Such combinations should be avoided. If concomitant use of a statin and conivaptan is required, some experts state that atorvastatin, pravastatin, fluvastatin, rosuvastatin, or pitavastatin may be considered.

■ **Digoxin** Concomitant administration of digoxin with various statins (e.g., atorvastatin, pitavastatin, pravastatin, rosuvastatin) has resulted in variable effects on plasma digoxin concentrations. Concomitant use of atorvastatin 80 mg and digoxin increased peak plasma concentration and AUC of digoxin by 20 and 15%, respectively; however, atorvastatin 10 mg did not alter the pharmacokinetics of digoxin. Concomitant use of lovastatin and digoxin in patients with hypercholesterolemia had no effect on plasma concentrations of digoxin. Concomitant use of fluvastatin and digoxin increased fluvastatin peak plasma concentration by 11% while not affecting fluvastatin AUC. Concomitant use of pitavastatin and digoxin decreased pitavastatin peak plasma concentration by 9% while increasing pitavastatin AUC by 4%. Concomitant use of pravastatin and digoxin increased pravastatin peak plasma concentration and AUC by 26 and 23%, respectively. Patients receiving digoxin should be monitored appropriately, particularly when statins are initiated.

■ **Estrogens/Progestins** Concomitant administration of atorvastatin or rosuvastatin with an oral contraceptive increased peak plasma concentrations and AUC of the oral contraceptive components (i.e., ethinyl estradiol, norethindrone, norgestrel). The manufacturer of atorvastatin states that this interaction should be considered when selecting oral contraceptives for patients receiving atorvastatin or other statins.

■ **Ranolazine** The risk of myopathy, including rhabdomyolysis, is increased following concomitant use of lovastatin or simvastatin with ranolazine. Concomitant use of simvastatin and ranolazine increased simvastatin or simvastatin acid peak plasma concentration by 1.75- or 2.28-fold, respectively, and AUC by 1.86- or 2.26-fold, respectively. The manufacturer of lovastatin states that dosage adjustment of lovastatin may be considered during concomitant therapy with ranolazine. The manufacturer of simvastatin states that dosage of simvastatin should be limited when used concomitantly with ranolazine, and the risks versus benefits of such concomitant therapy should be carefully considered.

■ **Sacubitril/Valsartan** Interactions mediated by the organic anion-transporting polyprotein (OATP) and the organic anion transporter (OAT) are possible when certain statins (e.g., atorvastatin, fluvastatin, pitavastatin, pravastatin, rosuvastatin, simvastatin) are administered concomitantly with sacubitril/valsartan. Some experts recommend that lower doses of these statins be considered during concomitant use.

■ **Ticagrelor** Concomitant use of atorvastatin and ticagrelor increased atorvastatin peak plasma concentration and AUC by 23 and 36%, respectively; however, these changes were not statistically significant. Ticagrelor increased peak plasma concentration and AUC of simvastatin by 81 and 56%, respectively, with some individuals experiencing even greater increases in simvastatin exposure. Some experts state that dosage of simvastatin or lovastatin should not exceed 40 mg daily when administered concomitantly with ticagrelor.

■ **Warfarin** Increased prothrombin time/international normalized ratio (PT/INR) and/or clinically evident bleeding has been reported in patients receiving warfarin concomitantly with various statins (e.g., fluvastatin, lovastatin, pravastatin, rosuvastatin, simvastatin). Such effects have not been observed in patients receiving atorvastatin or pitavastatin concomitantly with warfarin. While the mechanism of this interaction has not been established, it has been proposed that highly protein-bound statins (e.g., lovastatin) may displace warfarin from plasma protein binding sites. Some clinicians also suggest that certain statins (e.g., lovastatin) may inhibit warfarin metabolism. Since fluvastatin is principally metabolized by CYP2C9, it may be expected to inhibit the metabolism of *S*-warfarin and thereby increase the anticoagulant response.

Concomitant use of fluvastatin and warfarin increased fluvastatin peak plasma concentration and AUC by 67 and 30%, respectively; increased *S*-warfarin peak plasma concentration and AUC by 10 and 7%, respectively; and increased *R*-warfarin peak plasma concentration by 6%.

Concomitant use of pitavastatin and warfarin increased *R*-warfarin peak plasma concentration and AUC by 3 and 7%, respectively, and *S*-warfarin peak plasma concentration and AUC by 3 and 6%, respectively.

Concomitant use of pravastatin and warfarin increased pravastatin peak plasma concentration by 6.7%, decreased pravastatin AUC by 13%, and increased warfarin peak plasma concentration and AUC by 15 and 17%, respectively.

Concomitant use of rosuvastatin and warfarin increased *R*- and *S*-warfarin AUC by 4 and 6%, respectively; decreased *R*-warfarin peak plasma concentration by 1%; and did not alter *S*-warfarin peak plasma concentration. The manufacturer of rosuvastatin states that caution should be exercised when the drug is used concomitantly with anticoagulants.

The PT/INR should be monitored closely until stabilized when a statin is initiated or dosage of the drug is adjusted in patients receiving warfarin concomitantly.

Acute Toxicity

Limited information is available on the acute toxicity of statins.

■ **Manifestations** A few cases of accidental statin overdosage have been reported. Although accidental ingestion of single oral doses of lovastatin as high as 3–75 times the maximum recommended human oral daily dosage resulted in no toxic effect, various adverse GI effects and increases in serum transaminase concentrations were reported with a 2-week ingestion of 640 mg of fluvastatin daily as extended-release tablets (8 times the maximum recommended human oral daily dosage). Simvastatin dosages as high as 100 g/m^2 in dogs were associated with emesis and mucus in the stool.

■ **Treatment** If acute statin overdosage occurs, supportive and symptomatic treatment should be initiated and the patient observed closely. Pending additional experience, specific recommendations for the management of statin overdosage currently are not available. It is not known whether statins or their metabolites are removed by hemodialysis or peritoneal dialysis. Some manufacturers state that these procedures are not expected to substantially enhance clearance of statins, since these agents (other than pravastatin) are extensively bound to plasma proteins.

Pharmacology

Statins are antilipemic agents that competitively inhibit hydroxymethylglutaryl-coenzyme A (HMG-CoA) reductase, the enzyme that catalyzes the conversion of HMG-CoA to mevalonic acid, an early precursor of cholesterol. These agents are structurally similar to HMG-CoA and produce selective, reversible, competitive inhibition of HMG-CoA reductase. The high affinity of statins for HMG-CoA reductase may result from their binding to 2 separate sites on the enzyme.

■ **Antilipemic Effects** The antilipemic action of statins results from their inhibition of HMG-CoA reductase and subsequent reduction in hepatic cholesterol synthesis. In humans, biosynthesis of cholesterol from acetyl-CoA in the liver accounts for 60–70% of the total cholesterol pool. Thus, at usual therapeutic dosages, inhibition of HMG-CoA reductase (and subsequent mevalonic acid and cholesterol synthesis) by statins via this mechanism is incomplete, and adrenal and gonadal steroidogenesis are not affected substantially as evidenced by a lack of effect of statins on plasma cortisol concentrations.

Effects on Plasma Lipoprotein Concentrations Statins reduce serum concentrations of low-density lipoprotein (LDL)-cholesterol, very low-density lipoprotein (VLDL)-cholesterol, apolipoprotein B (apo B), and triglycerides. The precise mechanisms by which statins reduce plasma LDL-cholesterol concentrations have not been fully elucidated but appear to be complex. Normally, the cell synthesizes cholesterol *de novo* for use in cell-membrane and steroid-hormone synthesis or obtains it from circulating low-density lipoproteins (LDLs) via receptor-mediated endocytosis. Most cholesterol in human serum is contained within LDL particles. Cellular cholesterol content is regulated by a feedback mechanism involving both cholesterol synthesis and the uptake and clearance of LDLs by LDL receptors, principally in the liver. Inhibition of hepatic cholesterol biosynthesis by statins results in a compensatory increase in the production of LDL receptors by cells in the liver; these receptors bind circulating LDLs and remove them from serum. In addition to the increased production of LDL receptors, in vitro and animal studies indicate that a simultaneous compensatory increase in the amount of HMG-CoA reductase in the liver occurs as a result of increased synthesis and/or decreased degradation of this enzyme. Production of LDLs also may be decreased by statins as a result of decreased hepatic production of VLDLs or increased binding and catabolism of VLDL remnants (i.e., intermediate-density lipoproteins, IDLs) by the LDL receptor, since VLDLs and VLDL remnants normally are converted to LDLs. Thus, LDL receptors are involved both in enhancing clearance and inhibiting production of LDLs. Inhibition of hepatic synthesis of apolipoprotein B (apo B), and thus the secretion of the apo B-containing LDLs and VLDLs, also has been suggested to account for some of the cholesterol- and triglyceride-lowering effects of statins. Statins produce modest increases in HDL-cholesterol and apolipoprotein A (apo A) concentrations. The mechanism by which statins increase HDL-cholesterol concentrations has not been fully elucidated but may be related to an increased synthesis of apo A-I.

Statins also have been shown to reduce hepatic lipase activity, increase LDL-cholesterol buoyancy, and decrease cholesteryl ester transfer protein (CETP) activity, alterations that may favorably influence coronary artery disease regression. Effects of statins on lipoprotein(a) (Lp[a]), fibrinogen, and certain other independent biochemical risk factors for coronary heart disease (CHD) have not been fully elucidated.

In patients with primary hypercholesterolemia or mixed dyslipidemia who received recommended daily dosages of various statins for at least 6 weeks, serum total and LDL-cholesterol concentrations were reduced by an average of 16–46 and 21–63%, respectively. Dose-related reductions in apo B (18–54%) and triglyceride (6–37%) concentrations, and small, variable increases in HDL-cholesterol concentrations (2–16%) also were observed in these patients. Patients with homozygous familial hypercholesterolemia have poorly functioning, few, or no LDL receptors and generally are much less responsive to statin therapy than those who have the heterozygous form of the disease; however, reductions of 14–46% in LDL-cholesterol concentrations have been reported in patients with homozygous familial hypercholesterolemia who received atorvastatin, rosuvastatin, or simvastatin. Reductions of 22–58% in serum total cholesterol, 27–57% in LDL-cholesterol, and 12–53% in triglyceride concentrations have occurred during therapy with various statins in patients with other primary types of hypercholesterolemia (including primary dysbetalipoproteinemia and hypertriglyceridemia). In most patients with primary hypercholesterolemia, marked reductions in serum lipoprotein and apolipoprotein concentrations occur within 1–2 weeks of initiating statin therapy, and maximal changes usually are observed within 4–6 weeks. Serum lipoprotein concentrations usually return to baseline levels within the same time period after discontinuance of the drug.

Tolerance to Antilipemic Effects Development of clinically important tolerance to the cholesterol-lowering effects of statins does not appear to occur commonly, even in patients treated for several (e.g., 2–6) years with the drug. However, in some patients receiving monotherapy with a statin, small increases in serum total and LDL-cholesterol concentrations (compared with those observed early in therapy) have been noted after 1–2 years of therapy, and it has been suggested (in the absence of other identifiable causes such as changes in compliance with drug therapy or diet, other medical conditions) that compensatory increases in HMG-CoA reductase concentrations may be responsible for these minor increases.

Relative Potency Results from clinical studies indicate that statins are not equipotent (on a weight basis) in their LDL-cholesterol-lowering effects. On a mg/kg basis, cerivastatin (no longer commercially available in the US) appears to be the most potent statin based on in vitro enzyme inhibition assays. However, in clinical trials, the greatest reductions in LDL-cholesterol and triglyceride concentrations generally have been observed in patients receiving rosuvastatin. In a randomized, parallel-group study, rosuvastatin 10 mg produced LDL-cholesterol reductions that were similar to atorvastatin 20 or 40 mg and superior to atorvastatin 10 mg, pravastatin 40 mg, or simvastatin 40 mg. In another randomized, parallel-group study, atorvastatin 10 mg produced LDL-cholesterol reductions similar to or exceeding those produced by up to 40 mg of simvastatin, pravastatin, lovastatin, or fluvastatin. In several randomized studies, pitavastatin 1 mg produced LDL-cholesterol reductions that were superior to pravastatin 10 mg in geriatric patients; pitavastatin 2 mg produced LDL-cholesterol reductions that were noninferior to atorvastatin 10 mg, superior to simvastatin 20 mg, and superior to pravastatin 20 mg; pitavastatin 4 mg produced LDL-cholesterol reductions that were noninferior to atorvastatin 20 mg and simvastatin 40 mg, and superior to pravastatin 40 mg; pitavastatin 4 mg produced LDL-cholesterol reductions that were *not* noninferior to atorvastatin 20 mg in patients with type 2 diabetes. Some clinicians suggest that 20 mg of simvastatin is approximately equipotent to 40 mg of lovastatin or pravastatin or to 80 mg of fluvastatin. Others propose that simvastatin is approximately 3 times more potent than lovastatin or pravastatin and 8 times more potent than fluvastatin (i.e., with 5 mg of simvastatin being approximately equipotent to 15 mg of lovastatin or pravastatin or to 40 mg of fluvastatin). Limited data indicate that 20 mg of simvastatin produces greater LDL-cholesterol reductions than 0.2 mg of cerivastatin.

■ **Antiatherogenic Effects** Most statins have been shown to slow the progression and/or induce regression† of atherosclerosis in coronary and/or carotid arteries. (See Reducing Progression of Coronary Atherosclerosis under Uses: Prevention of Cardiovascular Events.) The precise mechanism by which statins slow the progression of and/or induce regression of atherosclerotic lesions in patients with dyslipidemia has not been fully elucidated; however, limited evidence suggests that some of these effects of statins may be independent of their antilipemic effects.

Limited data from in vitro studies indicate that most statins may reduce intimal-medial wall thickness by producing a concentration-dependent inhibition of aortic or femoral arterial smooth muscle cell proliferation and/or inducing apoptosis of vascular smooth muscle cells. Pravastatin does not appear to exert such inhibition because the lower lipophilicity of the drug impairs its passive diffusion into extrahepatic cells; the ability of the drug to inhibit cholesterol synthesis like other statins is explained by its active transport into hepatocytes. Limited data from experimental studies suggest that statins also may stabilize atherosclerotic plaques by preventing oxidation of LDL-cholesterol, inhibiting macrophage cholesterol ester accumulation, and impairing the release of proteolytic enzymes (i.e., metalloproteases) that may weaken the fibrous cap and predispose plaques to rupture.

■ **Vascular Effects** Statins have been reported to decrease blood pressure in patients with hypertension and primary hypercholesterolemia. In several small randomized, placebo-controlled studies, patients with moderate hypercholesterolemia and hypertension who received pravastatin (10–40 mg daily) or simvastatin (10–40 mg daily) for at least 12 weeks had mean reductions in systolic, diastolic, and pulse pressures of 7–8, 4–5, and 3 mm Hg, respectively, compared with those values in patients receiving placebo. The precise mechanism by which statins modulate blood pressure in hypercholesterolemic patients with hypertension has not been fully elucidated; however, some evidence suggests that these antihypertensive effects may be related to statin-induced restoration of endothelial dysfunction (i.e., increased arterial compliance), activation of endothelial nitric oxide synthase, and reduction of plasma aldosterone concentrations. Additional study is needed to determine the long-term antihypertensive effects, if any, of statins in patients with comorbid conditions, in patients with higher baseline blood pressure and cholesterol concentrations, and in patients receiving antihypertensive therapy.

Improvements in endothelium-dependent vasodilation, as evidenced by improved coronary blood flow, decreased peripheral resistance, increased myocardial perfusion, and increased cardiac output, have been reported in a limited number of normocholesterolemic or hypercholesterolemic patients who received statin therapy for at least 4 weeks. Although the mechanism of these vascular effects has not been fully elucidated, it has been suggested that such effects may result from increased expression of endothelial nitric oxide synthase (eNOS) and subsequently, release of nitric oxide, both of which may improve endothelial function in systemic and cerebral vasculatures.

■ **Antithrombotic Effects** Conflicting data have been reported regarding the effects of statins on hemostatic abnormalities (i.e., prothrombotic state) associated with hypercholesterolemia. While some statins appear to inhibit platelet aggregation and tissue factor expression, none has been shown consistently to produce beneficial changes in plasminogen activator inhibitor-1 (PAI-1, the principal inhibitor of the fibrinolytic system), fibrinogen concentrations, or whole blood viscosity. However, in a large, randomized, placebo-controlled study (Heart and Estrogen/Progestin Replacement Study [HERS]) evaluating the effect of estrogen/progestin replacement therapy on coronary events (nonfatal myocardial infarction and coronary death) in postmenopausal women with CHD, the risk of venous thromboembolic disease (deep-vein thrombosis and pulmonary embolism) was reduced in patients receiving statin therapy compared with placebo recipients.

■ **Anti-inflammatory Effects** Evidence from controlled and uncontrolled studies in hypercholesterolemic patients with or without documented CHD suggests that statins may possess anti-inflammatory activity. Data from retrospective and prospective studies in hypercholesterolemic patients with or without documented CHD indicate that statin therapy reduces plasma C-reactive protein (CRP) concentrations; CRP concentrations also were reduced among relatively normocholesterolemic patients with high baseline CRP levels. Effects on CRP concentrations do not appear to correlate with changes in LDL-cholesterol concentrations and are more pronounced in patients with high baseline C-reactive protein levels. Data from recent studies with statins indicate that lowering CRP concentrations may reduce the risk of recurrent MI or death from coronary causes in patients with acute coronary syndromes (ACS) or slow the progression of coronary atherosclerosis in patients with documented CHD.

Limited data indicate that statins also may exert neuroprotective effects by preventing induction of inducible nitric oxide synthase (iNOS) and attenuating inflammatory cytokine responses (e.g., interleukin-1 [IL-1], IL-6, tumor necrosis factor [TNF]-α), mechanisms that accompany tissue injury and cerebral ischemia.

Statins also have been shown to inhibit the growth of lymphocytes and other blood mononuclear cells; the clinical relevance of these effects has not been fully elucidated.

Effects on Bone Limited data indicate that use of statins may be associated with an increase in bone mineral density. (See Uses: Other Uses.) The mechanism of this effect has not been fully elucidated but may be indirectly related to a decreased production of intermediate metabolites responsible for prenylation of proteins that regulate osteoclast cell processes.

■ **Other Effects** Results of an observational study indicate a lower prevalence of Alzheimer's disease among patients who received certain statins (i.e., lovastatin, pravastatin); however, the mechanism of these effects currently is not known.

Pharmacokinetics

Plasma concentrations of statins have been measured using a radioenzymatic assay and, more recently, high-performance liquid chromatography (HPLC) or gas chromatography coupled with mass spectrometry (GC/MS) techniques. HPLC and GC/MS techniques, which directly measure plasma drug and metabolite concentrations, are more specific than the radioenzymatic assay, which reports concentrations of total active inhibitors by determining total HMG-CoA reductase inhibitory activity. It must be noted, however, that the antilipemic effects of statins correlate with dosage rather than with plasma concentrations of the drugs.

■ **Absorption** Statins appear to be rapidly absorbed following oral administration and undergo extensive first-pass metabolism in the liver. The extent of absorption following oral administration varies considerably among statins. In animals, approximately 30–98% of oral radiolabeled doses of the drugs reaches systemic circulation. Because of extensive hepatic extraction, the amount of drug reaching systemic circulation as active inhibitors following oral administration in animals or humans is low; the absolute bioavailabilities of atorvastatin, fluvastatin, lovastatin, pitavastatin, pravastatin, rosuvastatin, and simvastatin are 14, 24, 5, 51, 17, 20, and less than 5%, respectively. The mean relative bioavailability of the extended-release formulation of fluvastatin is approximately 29% compared with that of the immediate-release capsule administered under fasting conditions. The relative bioavailability of lovastatin following administration of the extended-release formulation is greater than that achieved with the immediate-release formulation; however, the bioavailability of total and active inhibitors of HMG-CoA reductase is similar between the 2 formulations.

Food appears to alter the systemic bioavailability of certain statins (e.g., atorvastatin, fluvastatin, lovastatin, pravastatin) following oral administration. While administration of atorvastatin, conventional (immediate-release) fluvastatin, extended-release lovastatin, or pravastatin with food generally results in a decreased rate and/or extent of absorption of these agents, such reductions are small and not associated with clinically important alterations in antilipemic effects. Optimal absorption of extended-release fluvastatin and lovastatin, however, occurs when the drugs are administered with food. Following oral administration of a single dose of conventional (immediate-release) lovastatin in the fasted state, the plasma concentration of active inhibitors averaged about two-thirds that achieved when the drug was administered after a meal. Bioavailability of extended-release fluvastatin also increased (by approximately 50%) following a high-fat meal; however, such increase was not associated with clinically important alterations in antilipemic effects of the drug.

Some evidence suggests that plasma concentrations following oral administration of some statins may be related to circadian rhythms; evening administration of atorvastatin and pravastatin was associated with a 30–60% decrease in peak plasma concentrations and areas under the plasma-concentration time curve (AUCs). Despite the decrease in systemic bioavailability, the antilipemic activity of these statins following evening administration remains unchanged and appears to be marginally superior to that achieved with morning administration.

Mean peak plasma concentrations of active inhibitors occur at 1–5 hours following oral administration of conventional formulations of various statins. A therapeutic response to statins usually is apparent within 1–2 weeks after initiating therapy, with maximal changes in lipoprotein and apolipoprotein concentrations occurring within 4–6 weeks.

Peak plasma concentrations of some statins (e.g., atorvastatin, fluvastatin, pitavastatin) appear to be slightly higher in women than in men; however, such variability does not appear to correlate with the antilipemic activity of these drugs. It has been suggested that such variability may result from body weight differences since adjusting for body weight decreases the magnitude of the observed variation.

Limited data indicate that plasma concentrations of most statins may be higher in geriatric individuals (65 years of age and older) than in younger adults. Nevertheless, such alterations do not appear to alter the antilipemic effects of these statins.

The pharmacokinetics of statins are not altered substantially in patients with mild renal impairment (creatinine clearance of 61–90 mL/minute per 1.73 m^2). However, increased plasma concentrations of lovastatin or rosuvastatin have been observed in patients with severe renal impairment (creatinine clearance of 10–30 mL/minute). The manufacturers of pravastatin and simvastatin state that patients with moderate to severe renal insufficiency may be predisposed to higher systemic exposure of these drugs and their metabolites. (See Cautions: Precautions and Contraindications.)

Some evidence indicates that certain statins may accumulate in the plasma of patients with hepatic impairment. (See Cautions: Hepatic Effects and see Precautions and Contraindications.) Mean peak plasma concentrations and AUCs of atorvastatin, fluvastatin, pitavastatin, pravastatin, and rosuvastatin are substantially higher and more variable in patients with hepatic insufficiency, chronic liver disease, or cirrhosis compared with those observed in healthy individuals.

■ **Distribution** Distribution of statins into body tissues and fluids has not been fully characterized. All statins are distributed mainly to the liver, although distribution into extrahepatic tissues (e.g., spleen, kidney, adrenal glands) also has been reported with certain statins (e.g., lovastatin, pravastatin). Pitavastatin undergoes carrier-mediated uptake into hepatocytes, principally via organic anionic transport polypeptide (OATP) 1B1 (OATP2) and, to a lesser extent, by OATP1B3 and OATP2B1. Data from in vivo assays indicate that atorvastatin (which has a mean volume of distribution of 381 L) also may distribute into the spleen and adrenal glands.

With the exception of pravastatin, which is approximately 50% bound to human plasma proteins, all statins are 88–99% bound to human plasma proteins, principally albumin.

Results of studies in animals and humans indicate that statins may cross the placenta and distribute into milk. (See Cautions: Pregnancy, Fertility, and Lactation.) Some statins (e.g., lovastatin and simvastatin, which are lactones) have been shown to cross the blood-brain barrier, while other less lipophilic statins (e.g., fluvastatin, pravastatin) do not substantially distribute into the CNS.

■ **Elimination** Statins appear to be extensively metabolized, principally in the liver. Atorvastatin, lovastatin, and simvastatin appear to be metabolized by the cytochrome P-450 (CYP) microsomal enzyme system, mainly by the isoenzyme 3A4 (CYP3A4). Fluvastatin is metabolized principally (approximately 75%) by the isoenzyme 2C9 (CYP2C9), although CYP2C8 and CYP3A4 also may be involved (approximately 5 and 20%, respectively). Pitavastatin is principally metabolized by uridine 5′-diphosphate (UDP) glucuronosyltransferase (i.e., UGT1A1, UGT1A3, UGT2B7); the drug is minimally metabolized by CYP2C9 and CYP2C8. Pravastatin undergoes enzymatic and nonenzymatic biotransformation independent of the CYP microsomal enzyme system. Rosuvastatin is not extensively metabolized; approximately 10% of the drug is metabolized in the liver, principally by CYP2C9. Atorvastatin, lovastatin, rosuvastatin, and simvastatin have active metabolites, while the principal metabolites of fluvastatin, pitavastatin, and pravastatin are pharmacologically inactive. With the exception of atorvastatin, pitavastatin, and rosuvastatin (which have plasma elimination half-lives of 14, 12, and 19 hours, respectively), most statins have relatively short half-lives (between 0.5–3 hours); the elimination half-life of fluvastatin given as extended-release tablets is 9 hours. Despite differences in the mean elimination half-lives among statins, there appears to be little, if any, correlation between this pharmacokinetic parameter and duration of therapeutic effect (which reportedly is at least 24 hours for all statins). There is no evidence of drug accumulation during repeated administration of most statins. However, systemic exposure to fluvastatin (administered as conventional capsules or extended-release tablets) appears to be increased following multiple oral doses of the drug. Because of its long plasma elimination half-life, atorvastatin may accumulate in plasma following administration of multiple oral doses.

Statins are excreted in urine and feces. Following oral administration of single radiolabeled doses of various statins, approximately 2–20% of the dose is excreted in urine and 60–90% in feces. Although renal excretion appears to be a minor route of elimination, the amount of drug eliminated via this route has been shown to reach 20% of the orally administered dose for pravastatin. Following IV administration of a radiolabeled dose of pravastatin in healthy individuals, approximately 47% of the drug was cleared from the blood by renal excretion and 53% was cleared by nonrenal mechanisms (e.g., biliary excretion, biotransformation). Statins do not appear to undergo enterohepatic recirculation.

Limited data indicate that urinary excretion of pravastatin may be lower in geriatric patients than in younger adults. In a single-dose pharmacokinetic study, mean cumulative urinary excretion of the drug in geriatric patients (65–78 years of age) was 18–19% lower compared with that reported in younger adults (18–38 years of age).

It is not known whether statins or their metabolites are removed by hemodialysis or peritoneal dialysis. Some manufacturers state that these procedures are not expected to substantially enhance clearance of statins, since these agents (other than pravastatin) are extensively bound to plasma proteins.

Chemistry and Stability

■ **Chemistry** Hydroxymethylglutaryl-coenzyme A (HMG-CoA) reductase inhibitors are antilipemic agents that competitively inhibit HMG-CoA reductase, the enzyme that catalyzes the conversion of HMG-CoA to mevalonic acid, an early precursor of cholesterol. Because of the similarity in their United States Adopted Names (USAN), HMG-CoA reductase inhibitors often are referred to as statins. This short-hand term also has been adopted by various experts (e.g., the National Institutes of Health, National Cholesterol Education Program, American College of Cardiology, American Heart Association) as a simplified means for referring to this class of antilipemic agents and is used throughout the HMG-CoA Reductase Inhibitors General Statement to simplify discussion.

Mevastatin (compactin, not commercially available) is the prototype of the statins, and all currently available statins were developed as structural derivatives of mevastatin. Statins are either fungus-derived (lovastatin, pravastatin, simvastatin) or are produced synthetically (atorvastatin, cerivastatin [no longer commercially available in the US], fluvastatin, pitavastatin, rosuvastatin). The fungus-derived compound lovastatin is a fermentation product of *Aspergillus terreus*, whereas pravastatin and simvastatin are produced by chemical modification of lovastatin. Fully synthetic statins exist either as racemic mixtures (fluvastatin) or as pure enantiomers (atorvastatin, cerivastatin).

All commercially available statins contain a nucleus that interacts with the coenzyme A recognition site of HMG-CoA reductase and a β,δ-dihydroxy acid side chain that competes with HMG-CoA for interaction with HMG-CoA reductase. The nucleus is structurally distinct among fungus-derived and synthetic statins and consists of a hexahydronaphthalene moiety or an indole/pyrrole/pyridine moiety, respectively. Structural modification of the nucleus alters the lipophilicity of individual statin compounds. Among fungus-derived statins, substitution of a hydroxyl group for the methyl group on the hexahydronaphthalene ring of lovastatin produces a compound (i.e., pravastatin) with lower lipophilicity, while addition of a methyl group on the butyryl ester side chain produces one (i.e., simvastatin) with a more than twofold increase in lipophilicity, resulting in a greater potential for the latter compound to cross the blood-brain barrier. However, limited evidence indicates that these differences in lipophilicity do not appear to be clinically important. The β,δ-dihydroxy acid side chain (which is structurally similar to HMG-CoA and necessary for catalytic activity of HMG-CoA reductase) exists either as an active dihydroxy acid salt or an inactive lactone. Compounds possessing the dihydroxy acid salt (e.g., atorvastatin, cerivastatin [no longer commercially available in the US], fluvastatin, pitavastatin, pravastatin, rosuvastatin) are orally active, while those with the lactone moiety (e.g., lovastatin, simvastatin) are prodrugs and have little, if any, antilipemic activity until hydrolyzed in vivo to the corresponding ring-opened, β,δ-dihydroxy acid form.

Lovastatin and simvastatin are practically insoluble in water; atorvastatin is very slightly soluble in water; rosuvastatin is sparingly soluble in water and methanol, and slightly soluble in ethanol; and cerivastatin, fluvastatin, and pravastatin are each soluble in water. The solubilities of atorvastatin, cerivastatin, fluvastatin, lovastatin, pravastatin, and simvastatin in water are 0.11, greater than 195, 2, 0.0013, 300, and 0.0014 mg/mL, respectively. Pitavastatin is slightly soluble in methanol and very slightly soluble in water or ethanol.

■ **Stability** Statins generally should be stored in well-closed, light-resistant containers at 5–30°C. When stored under these conditions, statins generally are stable for 24 months after the date of manufacture.

For additional information on chemistry and stability, uses, cautions, and dosage and administration of individual statins, see the individual monographs in 24:06.08.

†Use is not currently included in the labeling approved by the US Food and Drug Administration

Atorvastatin Calcium

■ Atorvastatin calcium, a hydroxymethylglutaryl-CoA (HMG-CoA) reductase inhibitor (i.e., statin), is an antilipemic agent.

Uses

Atorvastatin is used as an adjunct to nondrug therapies (i.e., lifestyle modifications) for prevention of cardiovascular events and for the management of dyslipidemias.

■ Prevention of Cardiovascular Events The American College of Cardiology (ACC)/American Heart Association (AHA) cholesterol management guideline recommends statins as first-line therapy for prevention of atherosclerotic cardiovascular disease (ASCVD) in adults. There is extensive evidence demonstrating that statins can substantially reduce ASCVD risk when used for secondary prevention or primary prevention (in high-risk patients). Because the relative reduction in ASCVD risk is correlated with the degree of low-density lipoprotein (LDL)-cholesterol lowering, the maximum tolerated statin intensity should be used to achieve optimum ASCVD benefits. According to the ACC/AHA guidelines, atorvastatin may be used for primary or secondary prevention in adults when moderate- or high-intensity statin therapy is indicated. (See Prevention of Cardiovascular Events under Dosage and Administration: Dosage.) Nonstatin therapies do not provide acceptable ASCVD risk reduction benefits compared to their potential for adverse effects in the routine prevention of ASCVD. For additional details on prevention of ASCVD, see the HMG-CoA Reductase Inhibitors General Statement 24:06.08 and also consult the most recent ACC/AHA Guideline on the Treatment of Blood Cholesterol to Reduce Atherosclerotic Cardiovascular Risk in Adults (available at http://www.cardiosource.org or http://my.americanheart.org).

Primary Prevention The ACC/AHA cholesterol management guideline states that, before initiating statin therapy for primary prevention in patients without clinical ASCVD or diabetes mellitus, it is reasonable for clinicians and patients to discuss the potential for ASCVD risk reduction benefits, adverse effects, and drug interactions, as well as patient preferences for treatment.

Patients without Clinical Evidence of CHD. Atorvastatin is used as an adjunct to nondrug therapies (i.e., lifestyle modifications) in patients *without* clinical evidence of coronary heart disease (CHD) who have multiple risk factors (e.g., age, smoking, hypertension, low high-density lipoprotein [HDL]-cholesterol concentrations, family history of early CHD) to reduce the risk of myocardial infarction (MI), stroke, or angina, and to reduce the risk of undergoing revascularization procedures. Atorvastatin in fixed combination with amlodipine is used in patients for whom treatment with both atorvastatin and a calcium-channel blocking agent (i.e., amlodipine) is appropriate.

The ACC/AHA cholesterol management guideline recommends statins as first-line therapy for primary prevention in patients 21 years of age and older without clinical ASCVD who have primary, severe elevations in LDL-cholesterol concentration (190 mg/dL or greater) and in patients 40–75 years of age with LDL-cholesterol concentrations of 70–189 mg/dL and an estimated 10-year ASCVD risk of 7.5% or higher.

Safety and efficacy of atorvastatin for primary prevention of cardiovascular disease have been established in several randomized, double-blind, placebo-controlled studies in patients without clinical evidence of CHD. In the Anglo-Scandinavian Cardiac Outcomes Trial (ASCOT) in 10,305 hypertensive, hypercholesterolemic (total cholesterol 251 mg/dL or less) patients with no history of MI who had multiple risk factors for CHD, therapy with atorvastatin (10 mg daily) for a median of 3.3 years reduced the risk of coronary events (i.e., fatal CHD or nonfatal MI) by 36% and the risk of undergoing revascularization procedures by 42%. Lipoprotein concentrations were lowered to levels similar to those observed with atorvastatin 10 mg daily in previous clinical studies. The risk of fatal and nonfatal stroke was reduced by 26%, although this was not statistically significant. Treatment with atorvastatin did not reduce the risk of death from cardiovascular or noncardiovascular causes.

In the Stroke Prevention by Aggressive Reduction in Cholesterol Levels (SPARCL) study in hypercholesterolemic patients (LDL-cholesterol concentrations of 100–190 mg/dL) who had a stroke or transient ischemic attack (TIA) within the past 1–6 months, therapy with high-dose atorvastatin (80 mg daily) for a median of 4.9 years reduced the risk of subsequent nonfatal or fatal stroke and of major cardiovascular events by approximately 16 and 20%, respectively, compared with placebo. However, atorvastatin therapy did not reduce overall mortality. In addition, hemorrhagic stroke and elevated aminotransferase (transaminase) concentrations (to at least 3 times the upper limit of normal) were reported in more patients receiving atorvastatin than in those receiving placebo. (See Use in Patients with Recent Stroke or Transient Ischemic Attack under Cautions: Precautions/Contraindications.) Some clinicians state that the results of this study should be interpreted with caution due to the heterogeneity of enrolled patients (i.e., with respect to stroke etiology and vascular risk). Furthermore, because patients with atrial fibrillation or other cardiac sources of embolism were excluded from the study, it is not known whether the observed benefits of atorvastatin apply to ischemic strokes of cardioembolic origin.

Patients with Diabetes Mellitus. Atorvastatin is used as an adjunct to nondrug therapies (i.e., lifestyle modifications) in patients *without* clinical evidence of CHD who have type 2 diabetes mellitus and multiple risk factors for CHD (e.g., retinopathy, albuminuria, smoking, hypertension) to reduce the risk of MI or stroke. Atorvastatin in fixed combination with amlodipine is used in patients for whom treatment with both atorvastatin and a calcium-channel blocking agent (i.e., amlodipine) is appropriate.

The ACC/AHA cholesterol management guideline recommends statins as first-line therapy for primary prevention in patients 40–75 years of age with type 1 or 2 diabetes mellitus. In patients with diabetes mellitus who are younger than 40 or older than 75 years of age, it is reasonable to evaluate the potential benefits, adverse effects, drug interactions, and patient preferences when deciding to initiate, continue, or intensify statin therapy.

Safety and efficacy of atorvastatin for prevention of cardiovascular disease in patients with type 2 diabetes mellitus have been established in a randomized, double-blind, placebo-controlled study. In the Collaborative Atorvastatin Diabetes Study (CARDS) in 2838 hypercholesterolemic patients (median total cholesterol concentration of 207 mg/dL, LDL-cholesterol concentration of 120 mg/dL, triglyceride concentration of 151 mg/dL) with type 2 diabetes mellitus (mean hemoglobin A_{1c} [HbA_{1c}] of 7.7%) *and* one or more other risk factors (e.g., smoking, hypertension, retinopathy, microalbuminuria, macroalbuminuria), therapy with atorvastatin (10 mg daily) for a median of 3.9 years reduced the risk of stroke by 48% and the risk of MI by 42% compared with placebo. Lipoprotein concentrations were lowered to levels similar to those observed with atorvastatin 10 mg daily in previous clinical studies. Treatment with atorvastatin did not reduce the risk of unstable angina, revascularization procedures, or acute CHD death.

The addition of fenofibrate to statin therapy has not been shown to provide an incremental ASCVD risk reduction benefit beyond that already established with statin monotherapy. In the Action to Control Cardiovascular Risk in Diabetes (ACCORD Lipid) study in patients with type 2 diabetes mellitus, addition of fenofibrate (160 mg once daily) to simvastatin therapy (up to 40 mg once daily) did not further reduce the rate of fatal cardiovascular events, nonfatal MI, or nonfatal stroke compared with simvastatin alone.

Secondary Prevention **Patients with Clinical Evidence of CHD.** Atorvastatin is used as an adjunct to nondrug therapies (i.e., lifestyle modifications) in patients *with* clinical evidence of CHD to reduce the risk of nonfatal MI, fatal and nonfatal stroke, angina, or hospitalization for congestive heart failure (CHF), and to reduce the risk of undergoing revascularization procedures. Atorvastatin in fixed combination with amlodipine is used in patients for whom treatment with both atorvastatin and a calcium-channel blocking agent (i.e., amlodipine) is appropriate.

The ACC/AHA cholesterol management guideline recommends statins as first-line therapy for secondary prevention in patients 21–75 years of age who have clinical ASCVD (i.e., acute coronary syndromes; history of MI, stable or unstable angina, coronary or other arterial revascularization, stroke, TIA, or peripheral arterial disease presumed to be of atherosclerotic origin) unless contraindicated.

Safety and efficacy of atorvastatin for secondary prevention of cardiovascular disease were established in several randomized studies in patients with clinically evident CHD. In one randomized, double-blind study (Treating to New Targets [TNT]) in 10,001 patients with clinically evident CHD (i.e., history of MI, history of or current angina with objective evidence of atherosclerotic CHD, history of coronary revascularization) and LDL-cholesterol concentrations less than 130 mg/dL, treatment with intensive antilipemic therapy (atorvastatin 80 mg daily) or moderate antilipemic therapy (atorvastatin 10 mg daily) for a median of 4.9 years reduced LDL-cholesterol concentrations to a mean of 77 or 101 mg/dL, respectively. Compared with the moderate regimen, treatment with the intensive regimen resulted in a 22% relative reduction in the risk of the primary composite end point (i.e., death from CHD, nonfatal non-procedure-related MI, resuscitated cardiac arrest, and fatal or nonfatal stroke). Of the events that comprised the primary composite end point, treatment with the intensive regimen substantially reduced the rate of nonfatal non-procedure-related MI and fatal and nonfatal stroke, but not death from CHD or resuscitated cardiac arrest. Of the predefined secondary end points, treatment with the intensive regimen reduced the rate of coronary revascularization, angina, and hospitalization for CHF, but not peripheral vascular disease. The intensive regimen did not reduce overall mortality and was associated with a slightly (but not statistically significant) increased risk of death from noncardiovascular causes. In addition, severe adverse effects (e.g., increases in concentrations of aminotransferase or creatine kinase [CK, creatine phosphokinase, CPK] to at least 3 or 10 times greater than the upper limit of normal, respectively) and discontinuance of therapy due to adverse effects were more common in patients receiving the intensive regimen compared with the moderate regimen. In a post hoc analysis in 5584 patients with CHD and the metabolic syndrome, treatment with the intensive regimen was associated with a lower incidence of major cardiovascular events than treatment with the moderate regimen (9.5 versus 13%); this represented a 29% relative reduction in the risk of major cardiovascular events in favor of the intensive regimen. However, consistent with the overall population, the intensive regimen did not reduce overall mortality compared with the moderate regimen.

In a randomized, comparative study (Incremental Decrease in Endpoints through Aggressive Lipid Lowering [IDEAL]) in 8888 patients with a history of CHD and an average LDL-cholesterol concentration of approximately 122 mg/dL, treatment with atorvastatin (80 mg daily) or simvastatin (20–40 mg daily) for a median of 4.8 years resulted in similar reduction in the risk of the primary composite end point (i.e., fatal CHD, nonfatal MI, and resuscitated cardiac arrest). In addition, no difference in overall mortality was observed between atorvastatin- or simvastatin-treated patients, and the rates of death from cardiovascular or noncardiovascular causes were similar in both treatment groups.

In a multicenter, randomized, open-label study comparing the incidence of ischemic events in CHD patients undergoing angioplasty or receiving aggressive lipid-lowering therapy with atorvastatin 80 mg daily (Atorvastatin Versus Revascularization Treatments [AVERT] trial), atorvastatin was as effective as angioplasty in reducing the incidence of ischemic events (defined as death from cardiac causes, resuscitation after cardiac arrest, nonfatal MI, cerebrovascular accident, coronary artery bypass grafting, angioplasty, or worsening angina with objective evidence resulting in hospitalization) and delaying the onset of the first ischemic event. However, atorvastatin-treated patients had smaller increases in quality of life scores and were more likely to report worsening of angina (12 versus 7%) compared with patients in the angioplasty group.

High-intensity Statin Therapy. Early and intensive antilipemic therapy with a high dosage of atorvastatin has been shown to be more effective than a moderate dosage of a statin in reducing the risk of cardiovascular events in patients with acute coronary syndrome (ACS).

In a randomized, double-blind, placebo-controlled study (Myocardial Ischemia Reduction with Aggressive Cholesterol Lowering [MIRACL]) in patients with unstable angina or non-ST-segment elevation (e.g., non-Q-wave) acute MI, therapy with atorvastatin (80 mg daily), initiated within 24–96 hours after admittance to the hospital, was associated with a lower incidence of recurrent ischemic events (particularly symptomatic ischemia requiring rehospitalization) in the subsequent 16 weeks; however, the validity of these results has been questioned due to the large number of atorvastatin-treated patients lost during follow-up.

In a randomized, double-blind, study (Pravastatin or Atorvastatin Evaluation and Infection Therapy [PROVE-IT]) in over 4000 patients hospitalized for ACS within the preceding 10 days, treatment with intensive antilipemic therapy (atorvastatin 80 mg daily) or moderate antilipemic therapy (pravastatin 40 mg daily) for 2 years reduced LDL-cholesterol concentrations to a median of 62 or 95 mg/dL, respectively. Compared with the moderate regimen, treatment with the intensive regimen resulted in a 16% reduction in the composite risk of primary endpoints, including a 14% reduction in the need for revascularization procedures and a 29% reduction in the risk of recurrent unstable angina. Atorvastatin therapy also was associated with reductions in the rates of death from any cause (28%) and of death or MI (18%) compared with pravastatin therapy, but these differences were not statistically significant. Results of this study suggest that, among patients who have recently had an acute coronary syndrome, an intensive antilipemic regimen provides greater protection against death or major cardiovascular events than does a standard regimen.

Reducing Progression of Coronary Atherosclerosis Intensive antilipemic therapy with atorvastatin has been shown to slow the progression of coronary atherosclerosis† in patients with CHD. In a randomized, double-blind, active-control study (Reversal of Atherosclerosis with Aggressive Lipid Lowering [REVERSAL]) in 654 patients with CHD, treatment with intensive antilipemic therapy (atorvastatin 80 mg daily) or moderate antilipemic therapy (pravastatin 40 mg daily) for 18 months reduced LDL-cholesterol concentrations to a mean of 79 or 110 mg/dL, respectively; concentrations of C-reactive protein were reduced by 36.4% in atorvastatin-treated patients and by 5.2% in pravastatin-treated patients. Treatment with the intensive regimen was associated with a substantially lower progression rate (measured by percent change in atheroma volume) compared with treatment with the moderate regimen. Compared with baseline values, patients treated with atorvastatin had no change in atheroma burden, whereas patients treated with pravastatin showed progression of coronary atherosclerosis. It has been suggested that the differences in atherosclerosis progression between atorvastatin and pravastatin may be related to the greater reduction in atherogenic lipoproteins and C-reactive protein concentrations in patients treated with atorvastatin.

Intensity of Statin Therapy The ACC/AHA cholesterol management guideline states that the appropriate intensity of a statin should be used to reduce the risk of ASCVD in patients most likely to benefit. Based on the average LDL-cholesterol response observed with specific statins and dosages used in the randomized controlled studies evaluated by the guideline expert panel, ACC/AHA considers atorvastatin 10–20 mg daily to be a moderate-intensity statin (producing approximate LDL-cholesterol reductions of 30% to less than 50%) and atorvastatin 40–80 mg daily to be a high-intensity statin (producing average LDL-cholesterol reductions of at least 50%). Individual patient response may vary in clinical practice.

Combination Antilipemic Therapy The ACC/AHA cholesterol management guideline states that nonstatin drugs may be useful adjuncts to statin therapy in certain high-risk patients (e.g., patients with ASCVD, LDL-cholesterol concentrations of at least 190 mg/dL, or diabetes mellitus) who have a less-than-anticipated response to statins, are unable to tolerate a less-than-recommended intensity of a statin, or are completely intolerant to statin therapy, particularly if there is evidence from randomized controlled studies suggesting that the addition of the nonstatin drug further reduces ASCVD events. If combination therapy is necessary, selection of the nonstatin drug should be based on the risk and benefit profile (i.e., reduction in ASCVD risk outweighs the drug's potential for adverse effects and drug interactions) and patient preferences.

Patients with Chronic Kidney Disease The potential benefits of atorvastatin in patients with chronic kidney disease, a population at high risk of cardiovascular disease, were evaluated in the Deutsche Diabetes Dialyse Studie (4D), a randomized, double-blind, placebo-controlled study in 1255 patients with type 2 diabetes mellitus on maintenance hemodialysis. After a median follow-up of 4 years, therapy with atorvastatin 20 mg daily had no substantial effect on the primary composite end point of cardiovascular death, nonfatal MI, and stroke compared with placebo. Although atorvastatin reduced the rate of all cardiac events (a secondary end point in the study) relative to placebo, the difference was only nominally significant.

■ **Dyslipidemias** Atorvastatin is used as an adjunct to nondrug therapies (e.g., dietary management) for the management of primary hypercholesterolemia or mixed dyslipidemia (Fredrickson type IIa or IIb), hypertriglyceridemia (Fredrickson type IV), primary dysbetalipoproteinemia (Fredrickson type III), and/or homozygous familial hypercholesterolemia. Atorvastatin has not been studied in conditions where the principal lipoprotein abnormality is elevated chylomicrons (Fredrickson types I and V). Atorvastatin in fixed combination with amlodipine is used in patients for whom treatment with both atorvastatin and a calcium-channel blocking agent (i.e., amlodipine) is appropriate.

Primary Hypercholesterolemia or Mixed Dyslipidemia **Adults.** Atorvastatin, alone or in combination with ezetimibe, is used as an adjunct to nondrug therapies (e.g., dietary management) in adults to decrease elevated serum total and LDL-cholesterol, apolipoprotein B (apo B), and triglyceride concentrations, and to increase HDL-cholesterol concentrations in the management of primary hypercholesterolemia (heterozygous familial and nonfamilial) or mixed dyslipidemia (Fredrickson type IIa or IIb). Statins such as atorvastatin also are used in combination with fenofibrate to decrease triglyceride concentrations and increase HDL-cholesterol concentrations in patients with mixed dyslipidemia and CHD (or CHD risk equivalents) who are receiving optimal statin therapy; however, no additional benefit on cardiovascular morbidity and mortality has been demonstrated with such combination therapy beyond that already established with statin monotherapy. (See Patients with Diabetes Mellitus under Prevention of Cardiovascular Events: Primary Prevention, under Uses.)

Reductions in total and LDL-cholesterol concentrations produced by usual dosages of atorvastatin substantially exceed those of placebo. Mean reductions of 29–45% in total cholesterol, 39–60% in LDL-cholesterol, 32–50% in apo B, and 19–37% in triglyceride concentrations, and increases of 5–9% in HDL-cholesterol concentrations have been reported in 2 controlled studies in 107 patients with primary hypercholesterolemia who received atorvastatin 10–80 mg daily for 6 weeks. Increases in HDL-cholesterol concentrations also have been observed in other studies in patients with primary hypercholesterolemia or mixed dyslipidemia; pooled data from 24 controlled studies indicate median increases of 5–9% in HDL-cholesterol concentrations in patients receiving atorvastatin 10–80 mg daily. Analysis of pooled data demonstrated consistent and substantial decreases in total cholesterol, LDL-cholesterol, triglyceride, total-cholesterol/HDL-cholesterol ratio, and LDL-cholesterol/HDL-cholesterol ratio in patients receiving atorvastatin. In patients with dyslipidemia and hypertension who received atorvastatin (10–80 mg daily) in combination with amlodipine (5–10 mg daily), LDL-cholesterol concentrations were reduced by 36–48% following 8 weeks of therapy.

Data from comparative studies indicate that therapy with atorvastatin may produce greater reductions in total and LDL-cholesterol concentrations than certain other statins. In 3 multicenter, double-blind, comparative studies, patients with hypercholesterolemia who received atorvastatin 10 mg daily for 16 weeks experienced greater reductions in total and LDL-cholesterol concentrations (25–29 and 35–37%, respectively) than those receiving lovastatin 20 mg daily (19 and 27%, respectively), pravastatin 20 mg daily (17 and 23%, respectively), or simvastatin 10 mg daily (24 and 30%, respectively). In other multicenter, randomized, open-label, comparative studies, patients with hypercholesterolemia who received atorvastatin 10–40 mg daily experienced greater reductions in total and LDL-cholesterol concentrations (25–40 and 35–51%, respectively) than those receiving fluvastatin 20–40 mg daily (13–19 and 17–23%, respectively), lovastatin 20–40 mg daily (21–23 and 29–31%, respectively), pravastatin 10–40 mg daily (13–24 and 19–34%, respectively), or simvastatin 10–40 mg daily (21–31 and 28–41%, respectively). The impact of differences in antilipemic effects between various statins on clinical outcomes is not known.

Compared with certain other statins, the effects of atorvastatin on HDL-cholesterol concentrations may be less pronounced, particularly with higher doses of atorvastatin. In several studies designed to evaluate the effects of atorvastatin (20–80 mg daily) and simvastatin (40–80 mg) on HDL-cholesterol and apolipoprotein (apo) A-I concentrations, increases in HDL-cholesterol and apo A-I concentrations were greater with simvastatin therapy (7–9 and 3–6%, respectively) than with atorvastatin (0–7 and 0–5%, respectively). The mechanisms of these effects have not been fully elucidated but may be related to differences in the 2 drugs' plasma elimination half-lives (approximately 20 and 2 hours for atorvastatin and simvastatin, respectively) and/or differential effects of the drugs on lipolytic enzymes (e.g., lipoprotein lipase, hepatic lipase).

Limited data from comparative studies suggest that reductions in total and LDL-cholesterol concentrations produced by atorvastatin may exceed those produced by fibric acid derivatives. In an open-label study in patients with mixed dyslipidemia, treatment with atorvastatin (10 mg daily) was associated with greater reductions in serum total and LDL-cholesterol concentrations compared with fenofibrate therapy (200 mg daily); however, fenofibrate-treated patients had greater reductions in triglyceride concentrations and larger increases of HDL-cholesterol and apo A-I concentrations than those who received atorvastatin.

The combination of atorvastatin and other antilipemic agents (e.g., bile acid sequestrants, ezetimibe) generally results in additive antilipemic effects; however, the risk of myopathy and rhabdomyolysis may be increased. (See Combination Antilipemic Therapy under Uses: Prevention of Cardiovascular Events.) The addition of a bile acid sequestrant (e.g., colestipol 20 g daily) to atorvastatin therapy (10 mg daily) further reduced LDL-cholesterol by 10%, resulting in an overall LDL-cholesterol reduction of 45% in patients receiving the combination; however, frequent adverse effects (e.g., GI effects such as constipation) reported with this combination regimen may discourage adherence to therapy. The addition of ezetimibe (10 mg daily) to atorvastatin therapy (10–80 mg daily) further reduced LDL-cholesterol by 7–16%, resulting in an overall LDL-cholesterol reduction of 53–61%. (See Primary Hypercholesterolemia and Mixed Dyslipidemia under Uses: Dyslipidemias, in Ezetimibe 24:06.05.)

Pediatric Patients. Atorvastatin is used as an adjunct to nondrug therapies (e.g., dietary management) to decrease elevated serum total cholesterol, LDL-cholesterol, and apo B concentrations in the management of heterozygous familial hypercholesterolemia in boys and postmenarchal girls 10–17 years of age who, despite an adequate trial of dietary management, have a serum LDL-cholesterol concentration of 190 mg/dL or greater *or* a serum LDL-cholesterol concentration of 160 mg/dL or greater and either a family history of premature cardiovascular disease or 2 or more other cardiovascular risk factors. The long-term effect of atorvastatin therapy in childhood on reducing cardiovascular morbidity and mortality in adulthood has not been established. For additional details on management of dyslipidemias in pediatric patients, see General Principles of Antilipemic Therapy in the HMG-CoA Reductase Inhibitors General Statement 24:06.08 and also consult the most recent Integrated Guideline for Cardiovascular Health and Risk Reduction in Children and Adolescents (available at http://www.nhlbi.nih.gov).

In a double-blind, placebo-controlled study (followed by an open-label phase), 187 boys and postmenarchal girls 10–17 years of age with heterozygous familial hypercholesterolemia or severe hypercholesterolemia (mean baseline LDL-cholesterol concentration of 219–230 mg/dL) were randomized to receive either atorvastatin (10 mg daily for the first 4 weeks, increased to 20 mg daily if LDL-cholesterol concentration exceeded 130 mg/dL) or placebo for 26 weeks; after 26 weeks of the double-blind phase, all patients entered an open-label phase and received atorvastatin for an additional 26 weeks. During the 26-week double-blind phase, treatment with atorvastatin 10–20 mg daily resulted in mean reductions of 31% in total cholesterol, 40% in LDL-cholesterol, 34% in apo B, and 12% in triglyceride concentrations, while concentrations of these lipoprotein fractions in placebo recipients changed minimally. HDL-cholesterol concentrations increased by 2.8% in atorvastatin-treated patients and decreased by 1.9% in placebo recipients. The mean LDL-cholesterol concentration achieved with atorvastatin therapy was 130.7 mg/dL compared with 228.5 mg/dL achieved with placebo during the 26-week double-blind phase.

Hypertriglyceridemia Atorvastatin is used as an adjunct to nondrug therapies (e.g., dietary management) in the treatment of elevated serum triglyceride concentrations (Fredrickson type IV). AHA states that although statins have consistently shown benefit in subgroups with or without high triglyceride concentrations, fibric acid derivatives have more commonly been shown to provide greater benefit in subgroups with increased triglyceride concentrations.

While statins are effective in reducing LDL-cholesterol concentrations, most statins generally have a limited effect on serum triglyceride concentrations. However, limited data suggest that triglyceride reductions produced by usual dosages of atorvastatin substantially exceed those of placebo and appear to be similar to those reported with usual dosages of fibrates or niacin. In several clinical studies in 64 patients with isolated hypertriglyceridemia, treatment with atorvastatin (10–80 mg daily) resulted in median reductions of 39–52% in triglyceride, 28–44% in total cholesterol, 27–41% in LDL-cholesterol, 45–62% in very low-density lipoprotein (VLDL)-cholesterol, and 33–52% in non-HDL-cholesterol concentrations, and a median increase of 8–14% in HDL-cholesterol concentrations; however, no patient achieved normal triglyceride concentrations as a result of treatment.

Atorvastatin 10 mg daily reportedly has produced greater reductions in LDL-cholesterol than niacin 3 g daily or fenofibrate 300 mg daily in patients with combined hyperlipidemia or isolated hypertriglyceridemia. However, reductions in triglyceride concentrations and increases in HDL-cholesterol concentrations were less than those reported with usual dosages of niacin or fenofibrate.

Primary Dysbetalipoproteinemia Atorvastatin is used as an adjunct to nondrug therapies (e.g., dietary management) for the treatment of primary dysbetalipoproteinemia (Fredrickson type III) in patients who do not respond adequately to diet.

In an open-label, crossover study in 16 patients with primary dysbetalipoproteinemia (genotypes 14 apo E2/E2 and 2 apo E3/E2), treatment with atorvastatin (10 or 80 mg daily) for at least 8 weeks resulted in substantial reductions in total cholesterol (37 or 58%, respectively), triglyceride (39 or 53%, respectively), combined intermediate-density lipoprotein (IDL)- and VLDL-cholesterol (32 or 63%, respectively), and non-HDL-cholesterol concentrations (43 or 64%, respectively).

Homozygous Familial Hypercholesterolemia Atorvastatin is used alone or in combination with ezetimibe to decrease elevated serum total and LDL-cholesterol concentrations in patients with homozygous familial hypercholesterolemia as an adjunct to other lipid-lowering therapies (e.g., plasma LDL-apheresis) or when such therapies are not available. Patients with homozygous familial hypercholesterolemia usually respond poorly to combined dietary management and drug therapy, including regimens containing a statin, in part because these patients have poorly functioning, few, or no LDL receptors. In an uncontrolled study in 29 patients 6–37 years of age with homozygous familial hypercholesterolemia, LDL-cholesterol concentrations were reduced by 7–53% (mean reduction of 20%) in 25 of 29 patients (86%) and *increased* by 7–24% in 4 of 29 patients (14%) who received atorvastatin dosages of 20–80 mg daily; 5 of the 29 patients had absent LDL-receptor function (of these, 2 patients also had a portacaval shunt and had no substantial reduction in LDL-cholesterol concentrations, and the remaining 3 receptor-negative patients had a mean LDL-cholesterol reduction of 22%). Similar reductions (17–28%) were observed in another open-label study in which patients received atorvastatin dosages of 40–80 mg daily for at least 4 weeks. In a limited number of patients undergoing plasma LDL-apheresis to lower cholesterol concentrations, addition of atorvastatin (80 mg daily) for 8 weeks reduced plasma total and LDL-cholesterol concentrations by an additional 29 and 31%, respectively. Limited evidence indicates that treatment with atorvastatin also may slow the progression of atherosclerosis in these patients.

In a randomized, double-blind study of 12 weeks' duration in a limited number of patients with a clinical and/or genotypic diagnosis of homozygous familial hypercholesterolemia, the addition of ezetimibe (10 mg daily) to atorvastatin or simvastatin therapy (40 or 80 mg daily) was more effective in reducing LDL-cholesterol concentrations (21% additional reduction based on pooled data from 40-mg and 80-mg statin groups) than increasing the dosage of atorvastatin or simvastatin monotherapy from 40 to 80 mg daily (7% additional reduction based on pooled data from 40-mg and 80-mg statin groups). In patients receiving ezetimibe (10 mg daily) in combination with higher dosages (80 mg daily) of atorvastatin or simvastatin, LDL-cholesterol concentrations were reduced by an additional 27% compared with LDL-cholesterol reductions achieved with the 40-mg daily statin dosage. (See Homozygous Familial Hypercholesterolemia under Uses: Dyslipidemias, in Ezetimibe 24:06.05.)

■ **Other Uses** Atorvastatin has reduced total and LDL-cholesterol concentrations in a few patients with renal transplantation†. In addition, the drug has reduced total and LDL-cholesterol concentrations in hypercholesterolemic patients on peritoneal dialysis†. Atorvastatin, alone or in combination with gemfibrozil, also has been shown to reduce cholesterol and triglyceride concentrations in patients with hypercholesterolemia associated with the use of protease inhibitors†.

For additional information on the role of atorvastatin or other statins in the treatment of lipoprotein disorders, prevention of cardiovascular events, or other uses, see General Principles of Antilipemic Therapy and see Uses in the HMG-CoA Reductase Inhibitors General Statement 24:06.08. For additional information on the use of amlodipine, see Uses in Amlodipine Besylate 24:28.08.

Dosage and Administration

■ **General** Patients should be placed on a standard cholesterol-lowering diet before initiation of atorvastatin therapy and should remain on this diet during treatment with the drug. In patients with coronary heart disease (CHD) or multiple risk factors for CHD, atorvastatin may be initiated simultaneously with dietary therapy. For recommendations on dietary and other nondrug therapies (i.e., lifestyle modifications), consult the most recent American Heart Association (AHA)/American College of Cardiology (ACC) Guideline on Lifestyle Management to Reduce Cardiovascular Risk (available at http://www.cardiosource.org or http://my.americanheart.org).

The manufacturer states that lipoprotein concentrations should be determined within 2–4 weeks following initiation and/or titration of atorvastatin, and that dosage should be adjusted accordingly. The ACC/AHA cholesterol management guideline states that lipoprotein concentrations should be determined within 4–12 weeks following initiation of statin therapy (to determine the patient's response to therapy and adherence) and monitored every 3–12 months thereafter as clinically indicated.

Adherence to lifestyle modifications and to statin therapy are required for atherosclerotic cardiovascular disease (ASCVD) risk reduction and, thus, should be reinforced periodically.

■ **Administration** Atorvastatin is administered orally once daily. While food can reduce the systemic bioavailability of atorvastatin, such reduction does not appear to affect the drug's antilipemic activity, and atorvastatin may be taken without regard to meals. Although the manufacturer suggests that atorvastatin can be administered without regard to the time of day, the drug was given in the evening or at bedtime in most studies, when maximum HMG-CoA reductase inhibition occurs.

■ **Dosage** Dosage of atorvastatin calcium is expressed in terms of atorvastatin and must be carefully adjusted according to individual requirements (i.e., percent reduction in low-density lipoprotein [LDL]-cholesterol concentrations) and response.

Prevention of Cardiovascular Events The ACC/AHA cholesterol management guideline states that the appropriate intensity of statin therapy should be used to reduce ASCVD risk in patients most likely to benefit. Giving a maximally tolerated statin intensity should be emphasized over giving lower statin dosages and adding nonstatin drugs to address low high-density lipoprotein (HDL)-cholesterol or high triglyceride concentrations, a strategy that has not yet been shown to reduce ASCVD risk. It should be noted that although 20 mg once daily is an FDA-labeled dosage of atorvastatin, this dosage was not evaluated in randomized controlled studies reviewed by the ACC/AHA expert panel.

Primary Prevention. For primary prevention of cardiovascular disease in patients 21 years of age and older without clinical ASCVD who have primary, severe elevations in LDL-cholesterol concentration (*190 mg/dL or greater*), the ACC/AHA cholesterol management guideline recommends that high-intensity statin therapy (e.g., atorvastatin 80 mg once daily, or, if not tolerated, atorvastatin 40 mg once daily) be initiated unless contraindicated. In patients who are unable to tolerate high-intensity statin therapy, the maximally tolerated statin intensity should be used. The ACC/AHA cholesterol management guideline states that it is reasonable to intensify statin therapy to achieve at least a 50% reduction in LDL-cholesterol concentrations. In patients currently receiving the maximum intensity of statin therapy, addition of a nonstatin drug may be considered to achieve further reductions in LDL-cholesterol concentrations; however, the potential benefits and risks (e.g., adverse effects, drug interactions) of such combined therapy, along with patient preferences, should be considered.

For primary prevention of cardiovascular disease in patients 40–75 years of age with *type 1 or 2 diabetes mellitus* and LDL-cholesterol concentrations of 70–189 mg/dL, the ACC/AHA cholesterol management guideline recommends that moderate-intensity statin therapy (e.g., atorvastatin 10–20 mg once daily) be initiated or continued. In those with an estimated 10-year ASCVD risk of 7.5% or higher, it is reasonable to consider high-intensity statin therapy (e.g., atorvastatin 80 mg once daily, or, if not tolerated, atorvastatin 40 mg once daily) unless contraindicated. In patients with diabetes mellitus who are younger than 40 or older than 75 years of age, it is reasonable to evaluate the potential benefits, adverse effects, drug interactions, and patient preferences when deciding to initiate, continue, or intensify statin therapy.

For primary prevention of cardiovascular disease in patients 40–75 years of age without clinical ASCVD or diabetes mellitus who have LDL-cholesterol concentrations of 70–189 mg/dL and an *estimated 10-year ASCVD risk of 7.5% or higher*, the ACC/AHA cholesterol management guideline recommends that moderate- (e.g., atorvastatin 10–20 mg once daily) to high-intensity statin therapy (e.g., atorvastatin 80 mg once daily, or, if not tolerated, atorvastatin 40 mg once daily) be initiated or continued. In those with an estimated 10-year ASCVD risk of 5 to less than 7.5%, it is reasonable to offer treatment with moderate-intensity statin therapy. Before initiating statin therapy for primary prevention of ASCVD in patients 40–75 years of age without clinical ASCVD or diabetes mellitus who have LDL-cholesterol concentrations of 70–189 mg/dL, it is reasonable for clinicians and patients to discuss the potential benefits, adverse effects, drug interactions, and patient preferences for such therapy.

Secondary Prevention. For secondary prevention of cardiovascular disease in patients 21–75 years of age with *clinical ASCVD*, the ACC/AHA cholesterol management guideline recommends that high-intensity statin therapy (e.g., atorvastatin 80 mg once daily, or, if not tolerated, atorvastatin 40 mg once daily) be initiated or continued unless contraindicated; in patients currently receiving atorvastatin 40 mg once daily, the decision to increase the dosage to 80 mg once daily should be based on the potential for an ASCVD risk reduction benefit, adverse effects, drug interactions, as well as patient preferences. In patients 21–75 years of age with clinical ASCVD who are at increased risk for developing statin-associated adverse effects or in whom high-intensity statin therapy is inappropriate or contraindicated, moderate-intensity statin therapy (e.g., atorvastatin 10–20 mg once daily) should be given if tolerated. In patients older than 75 years of age with clinical ASCVD, use of statin therapy should be individualized based on the potential benefits, adverse effects, drug interactions, and patient preferences; it is reasonable to consider initiating or continuing moderate-intensity statin therapy in such patients if tolerated.

Dyslipidemias **Primary Hypercholesterolemia (Heterozygous Familial and Nonfamilial) or Mixed Dyslipidemia.** The recommended initial oral dosage of atorvastatin in adults for the management of primary hypercholesterolemia (heterozygous familial or nonfamilial) or mixed dyslipidemia is 10 or 20 mg once daily. The manufacturer states that patients requiring reductions in LDL-cholesterol of more than 45% may be started on an atorvastatin dosage of 40 mg daily. The usual maintenance dosage of atorvastatin in adults is 10–80 mg once daily.

The recommended initial dosage of atorvastatin for the management of heterozygous familial hypercholesterolemia in boys and postmenarchal girls 10–17 years of age is 10 mg once daily. Dosage adjustments should be made at intervals of 4 weeks or longer. The maximum recommended dosage of atorvastatin is 20 mg daily. Safety and efficacy of atorvastatin dosages exceeding 20 mg daily have not been evaluated in controlled trials in this patient population.

Homozygous Familial Hypercholesterolemia. The usual oral dosage of atorvastatin for the management of homozygous familial hypercholesterolemia is 10–80 mg once daily; the drug should be used as an adjunct to other lipid-lowering therapies (e.g., plasma LDL-apheresis) or when such therapies are not available.

Atorvastatin/Amlodipine Combination Therapy. The fixed-combination preparation containing atorvastatin and amlodipine (Caduet®) may be used as a *substitute* for individually titrated drugs. In patients currently receiving atorvastatin and amlodipine, the initial dosage of the fixed-combination preparation should be the equivalent of titrated dosages of atorvastatin and amlodipine. Increased amounts of atorvastatin, amlodipine, or both components may be added for additional antilipemic, antianginal, or antihypertensive effects.

The fixed-combination preparation may be used to provide *additional therapy* for patients currently receiving one component of the preparation. The fixed-combination preparation also may be used to *initiate treatment* in patients with dyslipidemias *and* either hypertension or angina. Doses of amlodipine and atorvastatin should be selected independently. For dosage recommendations for amlodipine, see Dosage and Administration: Dosage, in Amlodipine 24:28.08. The maximum dosage of atorvastatin or amlodipine in the fixed-combination preparation is 80 or 10 mg daily, respectively.

Concomitant Drug Therapy. Atorvastatin may be used in combination with other antilipemic agents (e.g., bile acid sequestrants, certain fibric acid derivatives). For specific recommendations for concomitant use of atorvastatin with other antilipemic agents, see Drug Interactions.

Because concomitant use of atorvastatin with certain drugs (e.g., inhibitors or inducers of cytochrome P-450 [CYP] isoenzyme 3A4) may increase the risk of myopathy, such concomitant use should be avoided or employed with caution. For specific recommendations (including dosage recommendations) for such concomitant use, see Drug Interactions.

Dosage Modification The ACC/AHA cholesterol management guideline states that decreasing the statin dosage in adults may be considered when LDL-cholesterol concentrations are less than 40 mg/dL on 2 consecutive measurements; however, there are no data to suggest that LDL-cholesterol concentrations below 40 mg/dL would increase the risk of adverse effects.

■ **Special Populations** Atorvastatin is metabolized predominantly in the liver and potentially may accumulate in the plasma of patients with hepatic impairment; however, the manufacturer makes no specific recommendations for dosage adjustment in patients with hepatic impairment. (See Cautions: Contraindications and also see Hepatic Impairment under Warnings/Precautions: Specific Populations, in Cautions.)

Because renal impairment does not affect plasma concentrations or antilipemic effects of atorvastatin, the manufacturer states that dosage modification in patients with renal impairment is not necessary.

Although there are no specific dosage recommendations for geriatric patients, caution is recommended when atorvastatin is used in these patients. (See Geriatric Use under Warnings/Precautions: Specific Populations, in Cautions.)

Cautions

■ **Contraindications** Active liver disease, including unexplained, persistent elevations in hepatic aminotransferase (transaminase) concentrations.

Women who are or may become pregnant. (See Fetal/Neonatal Morbidity and Mortality under Cautions: Warnings/Precautions.)

Nursing women. (See Lactation under Warnings/Precautions: Specific Populations, in Cautions.)

Known hypersensitivity to atorvastatin or any ingredient in the formulation.

■ **Warnings/Precautions** ***Fetal/Neonatal Morbidity and Mortality*** Serum cholesterol and triglyceride concentrations increase during normal pregnancy, and cholesterol or cholesterol derivatives are essential for fetal development; therefore, suppression of cholesterol biosynthesis by atorvastatin during pregnancy may cause fetal harm. Atherosclerosis is a chronic process, and discontinuance of antilipemic drugs during pregnancy should have little impact on long-term outcomes of primary hypercholesterolemia therapy. There is no known clinical benefit for continued use of antilipemic drugs during pregnancy.

Congenital anomalies following intrauterine exposure to statins have been reported rarely.

Atorvastatin should be administered to women of childbearing age only when such patients are highly unlikely to conceive and have been informed of the potential hazards. (See Advice to Patients.) If the patient becomes pregnant while taking the drug, atorvastatin should be immediately discontinued and the patient apprised of the potential fetal hazard and the lack of known clinical benefit with continued use during pregnancy.

Musculoskeletal Effects Myopathy (defined as muscle aches or weakness in conjunction with increases in creatine kinase [CK, creatine phosphokinase, CPK] concentrations exceeding 10 times the upper limit of normal [ULN]) has been reported occasionally in patients receiving statins, including atorvastatin. Rhabdomyolysis with acute renal failure secondary to myoglobinuria also has been reported rarely in patients receiving statins, including atorvastatin.

The risk of myopathy or rhabdomyolysis is increased in geriatric patients (65 years of age or older) and in patients with uncontrolled hypothyroidism or renal impairment. Patients with renal impairment should be more closely monitored for adverse musculoskeletal effects. The risk of myopathy and/or rhabdomyolysis also is increased when atorvastatin is used concomitantly with cyclosporine, fibric acid derivatives, antilipemic dosages (1 g daily or higher) of niacin, or potent inhibitors of cytochrome P-450 (CYP) isoenzyme 3A4 (e.g., azole antifungals, certain macrolide antibiotics, certain HIV protease inhibitors or *ritonavir-boosted* protease inhibitor regimens, certain hepatitis C virus

[HCV] protease inhibitors). (See Drug Interactions.) Myopathy, including rhabdomyolysis, has been reported following concomitant use of atorvastatin and colchicine.

Although periodic monitoring of CK concentrations may be considered, there is no assurance that such monitoring will prevent the occurrence of severe myopathy. The American College of Cardiology (ACC)/American Heart Association (AHA) cholesterol management guideline does not recommend routine monitoring of CK concentrations in patients receiving statin therapy. However, the guideline states that it is reasonable to obtain baseline CK concentrations in adults at increased risk of developing adverse musculoskeletal effects (e.g., patients with personal or family history of statin intolerance or muscle disease, patients receiving concomitant therapy with myotoxic drugs) before initiating statin therapy. During statin therapy, it is reasonable to measure CK concentrations in adults experiencing muscle symptoms (e.g., pain, tenderness, stiffness, cramping, weakness, generalized fatigue).

The National Heart, Lung, and Blood Institute (NHLBI)-appointed expert panel on integrated guidelines for cardiovascular health and risk reduction in children and adolescents states that baseline CK concentrations should be obtained before initiating statin therapy in pediatric patients. In addition, routine monitoring for muscle toxicity is strongly recommended in children and adolescents receiving statin therapy.

Myopathy should be considered in any patient with diffuse myalgias, muscle tenderness or weakness, and/or marked increases in CK concentrations. Atorvastatin should be discontinued if CK concentrations become markedly elevated or if myopathy is diagnosed or suspected. Atorvastatin therapy should be temporarily withheld or discontinued in any patient experiencing an acute, serious condition suggestive of myopathy or predisposing to the development of renal failure secondary to rhabdomyolysis (e.g., severe acute infection; hypotension; major surgery; trauma; severe metabolic, endocrine, or electrolyte disorders; uncontrolled seizures). (See Advice to Patients.)

For additional details on management of musculoskeletal effects in adults and pediatric patients, see Musculoskeletal Effects under Cautions: Precautions and Contraindications in the HMG-CoA Reductase Inhibitors General Statement 24:06.08 and also consult the most recent ACC/AHA Guideline on the Treatment of Blood Cholesterol to Reduce Atherosclerotic Cardiovascular Risk in Adults (available at http://www.cardiosource.org or http://my.americanheart.org.) and the Integrated Guidelines for Cardiovascular Health and Risk Reduction in Children and Adolescents (available at http://www.nhlbi.nih.gov).

Hepatic Effects Increases in serum aminotransferase (i.e., AST, ALT) concentrations have been reported in patients receiving statins, including atorvastatin. Persistent increases (exceeding 3 times the ULN and occurring on 2 or more occasions) in serum aminotransferase concentrations occurred in 0.7% of patients receiving atorvastatin in clinical trials (including in 0.2% of those receiving atorvastatin 10 or 20 mg daily, 0.6% of those receiving 40 mg daily, and 2.3% of those receiving 80 mg daily). Although jaundice occurred in at least one patient in clinical trials, increases in aminotransferase concentrations were not associated with jaundice or other clinical manifestations. Upon dosage reduction or therapy interruption or discontinuance, aminotransferase concentrations returned to pretreatment or near-pretreatment levels without sequelae. Eighteen of 30 patients with persistent aminotransferase elevations continued therapy with a reduced dosage of atorvastatin.

Cases of fatal and nonfatal hepatic failure have been reported rarely in patients receiving statins, including atorvastatin, during postmarketing surveillance.

Liver function tests should be performed prior to initiation of atorvastatin therapy and repeated as clinically indicated (e.g., presence of manifestations suggestive of liver damage). Although the manufacturer previously recommended more frequent monitoring of liver function (i.e., at 12 weeks), FDA concluded that serious statin-related liver injury is rare and unpredictable in individual patients, and that routine periodic monitoring of liver enzymes does not appear to be effective in detecting or preventing serious liver injury. The ACC/AHA cholesterol management guideline states that, during statin therapy, it is reasonable to obtain liver function tests in adults experiencing symptoms of hepatotoxicity (e.g., unusual fatigue or weakness, loss of appetite, abdominal pain, dark colored urine, yellowing of the skin or sclera). However, the NHLBI expert panel on integrated guidelines for cardiovascular health and risk reduction in children and adolescents states that routine monitoring of hepatic function is strongly recommended in children and adolescents receiving statin therapy.

If serious liver injury with clinical manifestations and/or hyperbilirubinemia or jaundice occurs, atorvastatin therapy should be promptly interrupted. If an alternate etiology is not found, atorvastatin therapy should not be restarted.

Atorvastatin should be used with caution in patients who consume substantial amounts of alcohol and/or have a history of liver disease. The drug is *contraindicated* in patients with active liver disease or unexplained, persistent elevations in serum aminotransferase concentrations.

Endocrine Effects Increases in glycosylated hemoglobin (hemoglobin A_{1c} [HbA_{1c}]) and fasting serum glucose concentrations have been reported in patients receiving statins, including atorvastatin. Data from clinical trials and meta-analyses indicate that statin therapy may increase the risk of developing diabetes mellitus. Despite these findings, FDA continues to believe that the cardiovascular benefits of statins outweigh these small increased risks. The ACC/AHA cholesterol management guideline states that patients receiving statin therapy should be evaluated for new-onset diabetes mellitus according to current diabetes screening guidelines. If diabetes mellitus develops during statin therapy, patients should be encouraged to adhere to a heart-healthy diet, engage in physical activity, achieve and maintain a healthy body weight, cease tobacco use, and continue statin therapy to reduce the risk of atherosclerotic cardiovascular disease (ASCVD).

Statins interfere with cholesterol synthesis and theoretically may blunt adrenal and/or gonadal steroid production. Clinical studies have shown that atorvastatin does not reduce basal plasma cortisol concentration or impair adrenal reserve. Effects of statins on male fertility have not been studied in adequate numbers of patients. Effects of the drug, if any, on the pituitary-gonadal axis in premenopausal women are unknown. Caution should be exercised if a statin is used concomitantly with drugs that may decrease the concentrations or activity of endogenous steroid hormones (e.g., ketoconazole, spironolactone, cimetidine).

Cognitive Impairment Cognitive impairment (e.g., memory loss, forgetfulness, amnesia, memory impairment, confusion) has been reported rarely with all statins during postmarketing surveillance. This adverse CNS effect generally was nonserious and reversible, with variable times to symptom onset (1 day to years) and symptom resolution (median of 3 weeks following discontinuance of statin therapy). Following review of available data (i.e., from the Adverse Event Reporting System [AERS] database, randomized clinical trials, observational studies, case reports), FDA concluded that cases of cognitive impairment did not appear to be associated with fixed or progressive dementia (e.g., Alzheimer's disease) or result in clinically important cognitive decline. Development of cognitive impairment did not appear to be associated with any specific statin, age of the patient, statin dosage, or concomitant drug therapy. Therefore, FDA continues to believe that the cardiovascular benefits of statins outweigh this small increased risk of cognitive impairment. The National Lipid Association (NLA) statin safety assessment task force recommends that patients experiencing manifestations consistent with cognitive impairment be evaluated and managed appropriately. The ACC/AHA cholesterol management guideline states that, in patients presenting with confusion or memory impairment, it is reasonable to evaluate the patient for statin as well as nonstatin causes (e.g., exposure to other drugs, systemic or neuropsychiatric causes).

Use in Patients with Recent Stroke or Transient Ischemic Attack In a post-hoc analysis of the Stroke Prevention by Aggressive Reduction in Cholesterol Levels (SPARCL) study in hypercholesterolemic patients without clinically evident coronary heart disease (CHD) who had a stroke or transient ischemic attack (TIA) within the past 1–6 months, therapy with high-dose atorvastatin (80 mg daily) for a median of 4.9 years was associated with a higher incidence of hemorrhagic stroke (2.3%) compared with placebo (1.4%). The incidence of *fatal* hemorrhagic stroke was similar between atorvastatin and placebo, while the incidence of *nonfatal* hemorrhagic stroke was substantially higher with atorvastatin (1.6%) compared with placebo (0.7%). Among patients receiving atorvastatin, those with a history of hemorrhagic or lacunar stroke at study entry were at increased risk of developing hemorrhagic stroke.

Elevated aminotransferase concentrations (to 3 or more times the ULN) were reported more frequently in patients receiving high-dose atorvastatin (0.9%) compared with those receiving placebo (0.1%). Increases in CK concentrations (exceeding 10 times the ULN) were rare but were reported more frequently in patients receiving high-dose atorvastatin (0.1%) compared with those receiving placebo (0%). Diabetes was reported in 6.1% of patients receiving high-dose atorvastatin compared with 3.8% of patients receiving placebo.

Use of Fixed Combination When atorvastatin is used in fixed combination with amlodipine, the usual cautions, precautions, and contraindications associated with amlodipine must be considered in addition to those associated with atorvastatin.

Specific Populations **Pregnancy.** Category X. (See Users Guide.) (See Cautions: Contraindications and also see Fetal/Neonatal Morbidity and Mortality under Cautions: Warnings/Precautions.)

Lactation. Atorvastatin is distributed into milk in rats. It is not known whether atorvastatin is distributed into human milk; however, the drug is probably distributed into human milk because a small amount of another statin is distributed into human milk. Because of the potential for serious adverse reactions from atorvastatin in nursing infants, the drug is *contraindicated* in nursing women. Women who require atorvastatin therapy should not breast-feed their infants.

Pediatric Use. Safety and efficacy of atorvastatin have not been evaluated in prepubertal children or in children younger than 10 years of age with heterozygous familial hypercholesterolemia. In a randomized, double-blind, placebo-controlled study in boys and postmenarchal girls 10–17 years of age, the adverse effect profile of atorvastatin (10–20 mg daily for 26 weeks) generally was similar to that of placebo; dosages exceeding 20 mg daily have not been evaluated in this population. There were no substantial adverse effects on growth or sexual maturation in adolescent boys or on duration of menstrual cycle in girls. If therapy with atorvastatin is considered, the manufacturer states that adolescent girls should be advised to use effective and appropriate contraceptive methods during therapy to reduce the likelihood of unintended pregnancy.

The manufacturer states that atorvastatin dosages of up to 80 mg daily for 1 year have been evaluated in an uncontrolled study in 8 pediatric patients (6 years of age or older) with homozygous familial hypercholesterolemia.

Safety and efficacy of atorvastatin in fixed combination with amlodipine (Caduet®) have not been established in pediatric patients.

Geriatric Use. Of the 39,828 patients receiving atorvastatin in clinical studies, 40% were 65 years of age or older, and 7% were 75 years of age or older. Although no overall differences in efficacy or safety were observed between geriatric and younger patients, and other clinical experience has not revealed age-related differences in response, the possibility that some geriatric patients may exhibit increased sensitivity to the drug cannot be ruled out. Data from a pharmacokinetic study indicate that peak plasma concentration and area under the plasma concentration-time curve (AUC) of atorvastatin were 40 or 30% higher, respectively, in geriatric individuals (65 years of age or older) compared with younger adults. In addition, mean reductions in LDL-cholesterol concentrations appear to be higher in geriatric patients receiving any dose of atorvastatin compared with younger patients.

Because advanced age (65 years of age or older) is a predisposing factor for myopathy, atorvastatin should be used with caution in geriatric patients. The ACC/AHA cholesterol management guideline states that initiation of statin therapy for primary prevention of ASCVD in patients older than 75 years of age requires consideration of additional factors, including increasing comorbidities, safety considerations, and priorities of care. Therefore, the potential for an ASCVD risk reduction benefit, adverse effects, and drug interactions, along with patient preferences, must be considered before initiating statin therapy in patients older than 75 years of age.

Safety and efficacy of atorvastatin in fixed combination with amlodipine (Caduet®) have not been established in geriatric patients.

Hepatic Impairment. Plasma concentrations of atorvastatin are markedly increased in patients with chronic alcoholic liver disease. Peak plasma concentration and AUC of atorvastatin are increased by fourfold in patients with Child-Pugh class A disease and by approximately 16- and 11-fold, respectively, in patients with Child-Pugh class B disease.

Atorvastatin should be used with caution in patients who consume substantial amounts of alcohol and/or have a history of liver disease. Atorvastatin is *contraindicated* in patients with active liver disease, including unexplained, persistent elevations in hepatic aminotransferase concentrations.

Renal Impairment. Renal impairment does not affect plasma concentrations or antilipemic effects of atorvastatin; therefore, dosage modification in patients with renal impairment is not necessary. However, because history of renal impairment may be a risk factor for development of rhabdomyolysis, patients with renal impairment should be monitored more closely for adverse musculoskeletal effects.

Safety and efficacy of atorvastatin have not been established in patients with end-stage renal disease. However, hemodialysis is not expected to substantially enhance clearance of atorvastatin since the drug is extensively bound to plasma proteins.

■ **Common Adverse Effects** Adverse effects reported in 2% or more of patients receiving atorvastatin in clinical trials that occurred more frequently than with placebo include nasopharyngitis, arthralgia, diarrhea, pain in extremity, urinary tract infection, dyspepsia, nausea, musculoskeletal pain, muscle spasms, myalgia, insomnia, and pharyngolaryngeal pain.

Drug Interactions

Atorvastatin is metabolized by cytochrome P-450 (CYP) isoenzyme 3A4.

When atorvastatin is used in fixed combination with amlodipine, interactions associated with amlodipine should be considered. No formal drug interaction studies have been performed to date with the fixed-combination preparation containing atorvastatin and amlodipine.

■ **Drugs and Foods Affecting Hepatic Microsomal Enzymes** Concomitant use of atorvastatin with potent inhibitors of CYP3A4 (e.g., clarithromycin, itraconazole, HIV protease inhibitors, grapefruit juice) may result in increased plasma atorvastatin concentrations and increase the risk of myopathy or rhabdomyolysis. The extent of interaction and potentiation of effects depend on the extent of effect on CYP3A4.

Concomitant use of atorvastatin with inducers of CYP3A4 (e.g., efavirenz, rifampin) may result in variable reductions in plasma concentrations of atorvastatin.

■ **Drugs Transported by Organic Anion Transport Polypeptide 1B1** Atorvastatin and its metabolites are substrates of organic anion transport polypeptide (OATP) 1B1. Drugs that inhibit OATP1B1 (e.g., cyclosporine) can increase bioavailability of atorvastatin.

■ **Azole Antifungals** Concomitant use of atorvastatin and azole antifungals (e.g., itraconazole) increases the risk of myopathy or rhabdomyolysis. Following concomitant use of atorvastatin (40 mg as a single dose) and itraconazole (200 mg once daily for 4 days), atorvastatin peak plasma concentration and area under the plasma concentration-time curve (AUC) were increased by 20% and 3.3-fold, respectively.

Clinicians considering concomitant use of atorvastatin and itraconazole or other azole antifungals should weigh the benefits and risks of such concomitant therapy. During concomitant therapy with itraconazole, the lowest necessary dosage of atorvastatin should be employed, and dosage of atorvastatin should not exceed 20 mg daily. Patients receiving concomitant therapy with atorvastatin and azole antifungals should be monitored for manifestations of muscle pain, tenderness, or weakness, particularly during the initial months of therapy and following an increase in dosage of either drug.

■ **Bile Acid Sequestrants** The cholesterol-lowering effects of atorvastatin and bile acid sequestrants (e.g., cholestyramine) are additive. However, since bile acid sequestrants may decrease absorption of various drugs, some clinicians state that statins (e.g., atorvastatin) generally should be administered one hour before or 4 hours after the bile acid sequestrant.

■ **Colchicine** Myopathy, including rhabdomyolysis, has been reported in patients receiving atorvastatin concomitantly with colchicine. Caution is advised during such concomitant use.

■ **Cyclosporine** Concomitant use of atorvastatin and cyclosporine increases plasma atorvastatin concentrations, which may increase the risk of myopathy or rhabdomyolysis. Following concomitant use of atorvastatin (10 mg daily for 28 days) and cyclosporine (5.2 mg/kg daily), atorvastatin peak plasma concentration and AUC were increased by 10.7- and 8.7-fold, respectively. Concomitant use of atorvastatin and cyclosporine should be *avoided.*

■ **Digoxin** Concomitant use of atorvastatin (80 mg once daily for 14 days) and digoxin (0.25 mg once daily for 20 days) resulted in 20 and 15% increases in digoxin peak plasma concentration and AUC, respectively. Therefore, patients receiving such concomitant therapy should be monitored appropriately.

■ **Efavirenz** Concomitant use of atorvastatin with efavirenz may result in reductions in plasma concentrations of atorvastatin. Following concomitant use of atorvastatin (10 mg daily for 3 days) and efavirenz (600 mg once daily for 14 days), atorvastatin peak plasma concentration and AUC were decreased by 1 and 41%, respectively.

■ **Fibric Acid Derivatives** Concomitant use of atorvastatin and fibric acid derivatives (e.g., gemfibrozil, fenofibrate) increases the risk of myopathy. Following concomitant use of atorvastatin (40 mg as a single dose) and gemfibrozil (600 mg twice daily for 7 days), atorvastatin AUC was increased by 35%. Following concomitant use of atorvastatin (40 mg as a single dose) and fenofibrate (160 mg once daily for 7 days), atorvastatin peak plasma concentration and AUC were increased by 2 and 3%, respectively.

Concomitant use of atorvastatin and gemfibrozil should be *avoided.* The benefits of concomitant use of atorvastatin and other fibric acid derivatives (e.g., fenofibrate) should be weighed against the possible risk of myopathy. The manufacturer states that caution is advised if such concomitant therapy is employed; lower initial and maintenance dosages of atorvastatin should be considered during such concomitant therapy, and the patient should be carefully monitored for manifestations of muscle pain, tenderness, or weakness, particularly during the initial months of therapy and following an increase in dosage of either drug. The ACC/AHA cholesterol management guideline states that the combination of fenofibrate and low- or moderate-intensity statin therapy may be considered only if the benefits from atherosclerotic cardiovascular disease (ASCVD) risk reduction or triglyceride lowering (when triglyceride concentrations exceed 500 mg/dL) outweigh the potential risk of adverse effects.

■ **Grapefruit Juice** Because grapefruit juice contains one or more components that inhibit CYP3A4, ingestion of grapefruit juice may result in increased atorvastatin concentrations. Following concomitant use of atorvastatin (40 mg as a single dose) with grapefruit juice (240 mL once daily), atorvastatin peak plasma concentration and AUC were increased by 16 and 37%, respectively. More substantial increases in atorvastatin peak plasma concentration (up to 71%) and/or AUC (up to 2.5-fold) have been reported following ingestion of large quantities (750–1200 mL daily or more) of grapefruit juice. Ingestion of large quantities (more than one liter daily) of grapefruit juice may increase the risk of myopathy.

■ **HIV Protease Inhibitors** ***Darunavir*** Concomitant use of atorvastatin and *ritonavir-boosted* darunavir increases the risk of myopathy or rhabdomyolysis. Following concomitant use of atorvastatin (10 mg daily for 4 days) and *ritonavir-boosted* darunavir (darunavir 300 mg twice daily with ritonavir 100 mg twice daily for 9 days), atorvastatin peak plasma concentration and AUC were increased by 2.25- and 3.4-fold, respectively.

The benefits of concomitant use of atorvastatin and *ritonavir-boosted* darunavir should be weighed against the possible risk of myopathy or rhabdomyolysis. Caution is advised if such concomitant therapy is employed. During such concomitant therapy, the lowest necessary dosage of atorvastatin should be used, and dosage of atorvastatin should not exceed 20 mg daily. Patients should be carefully monitored for manifestations of muscle pain, tenderness, or weakness, particularly during the initial months of therapy and following an increase in dosage of either drug.

Fosamprenavir Concomitant use of atorvastatin and fosamprenavir (with or without low-dose ritonavir) increases the risk of myopathy or rhabdomyolysis. Following concomitant use of atorvastatin (10 mg daily for 4 days) and fosamprenavir (1.4 g twice daily for 14 days), atorvastatin peak plasma concentration and AUC were increased by 4.04- and 2.3-fold, respectively, while fosamprenavir peak plasma concentration and AUC were decreased by 18 and 27%, respectively. Following concomitant use of atorvastatin (10 mg daily for 4 days) and *ritonavir-boosted* fosamprenavir (fosamprenavir 700 mg twice daily with ritonavir 100 mg twice daily for 14 days), atorvastatin peak plasma concentration and AUC were increased by 2.84- and 2.53-fold, respectively, while fosamprenavir peak plasma concentration and AUC were unchanged.

The benefits of concomitant use of atorvastatin and fosamprenavir (with or without low-dose ritonavir) should be weighed against the possible risk of myopathy or rhabdomyolysis. Caution is advised if such concomitant therapy is employed. During such concomitant therapy, the lowest necessary dosage of atorvastatin should be used, and dosage of atorvastatin should not exceed 20 mg daily. Patients should be carefully monitored for manifestations of muscle pain, tenderness, or weakness, particularly during the initial months of therapy and following an increase in dosage of either drug.

Lopinavir Concomitant use of atorvastatin with the fixed combination of lopinavir and ritonavir (lopinavir/ritonavir) increases the risk of myopathy or rhabdomyolysis.

The benefits of concomitant use of atorvastatin and lopinavir/ritonavir should be weighed against the possible risk of myopathy or rhabdomyolysis. Caution is advised if such concomitant therapy is employed. During such concomitant therapy, the lowest necessary dosage of atorvastatin should be used. Patients should be carefully monitored for manifestations of muscle pain, tenderness, or weakness, particularly during the initial months of therapy and following an increase in dosage of either drug.

Nelfinavir Following concomitant use of atorvastatin (10 mg daily for 28 days) and nelfinavir (1.25 g twice daily for 14 days), atorvastatin peak plasma concentration and AUC were increased by 2.2-fold and 74%, respectively.

Patients receiving atorvastatin concomitantly with nelfinavir should be closely monitored. During such concomitant therapy, the lowest necessary dosage of atorvastatin should be employed, and dosage of atorvastatin should not exceed 40 mg daily.

Saquinavir Concomitant use of atorvastatin and *ritonavir-boosted* saquinavir increases the risk of myopathy or rhabdomyolysis.

The benefits of concomitant use of atorvastatin and *ritonavir-boosted* saquinavir should be weighed against the possible risk of myopathy or rhabdomyolysis. Caution is advised if such concomitant therapy is employed. During such concomitant therapy, the lowest necessary dosage of atorvastatin should be used, and dosage of atorvastatin should not exceed 20 mg daily. Patients should be carefully monitored for manifestations of muscle pain, tenderness, or weakness, particularly during the initial months of therapy and following an increase in dosage of either drug.

Tipranavir Concomitant use of atorvastatin and *ritonavir-boosted* tipranavir increases the risk of myopathy or rhabdomyolysis. Following concomitant use of atorvastatin (10 mg as a single dose) and *ritonavir-boosted* tipranavir (tipranavir 500 mg twice daily with ritonavir 200 mg twice daily for 7 days), atorvastatin peak plasma concentration and AUC were increased by 8.6- and 9.4-fold, respectively, while tipranavir peak plasma concentration and AUC were unchanged.

Concomitant use of atorvastatin and *ritonavir-boosted* tipranavir should be *avoided.*

■ **Lomitapide** Following concomitant use of atorvastatin (single 20-mg dose) with lomitapide (10 mg once daily for 7 days), peak plasma concentration and AUC of atorvastatin acid were increased by 19 and 11%, respectively. Following concomitant use of lomitapide (60 mg once daily for 7 days) with atorvastatin (single 20-mg dose), peak plasma concentration and AUC of atorvastatin acid were increased by 63 and 52%, respectively. When lomitapide is used concomitantly with atorvastatin, adjustment of atorvastatin dosage is not required; however, lomitapide dosage should not exceed 30 mg daily.

■ **Macrolide Antibiotics** Concomitant use of atorvastatin and macrolide antibiotics (e.g., clarithromycin, erythromycin) increases the risk of myopathy or rhabdomyolysis. Following concomitant use of atorvastatin (80 mg daily for 8 days) and clarithromycin (500 mg twice daily for 9 days), atorvastatin peak plasma concentration and AUC were increased by 5.4- and 4.4-fold, respectively. Following concomitant use of atorvastatin (10 mg as a single dose) and erythromycin (500 mg 4 times daily for 7 days), atorvastatin peak plasma concentration and AUC were increased by 38 and 33%, respectively.

The benefits of concomitant use of atorvastatin and macrolide antibiotics (e.g., clarithromycin, erythromycin) should be weighed against the possible risk of myopathy or rhabdomyolysis. Caution is advised if such concomitant therapy is employed. Lower initial and maintenance dosages of atorvastatin should be considered during such concomitant therapy. During concomitant therapy with clarithromycin, the lowest necessary dosage of atorvastatin should be used, and dosage of atorvastatin should not exceed 20 mg daily. Patients receiving atorvastatin concomitantly with macrolide antibiotics should be carefully monitored for manifestations of muscle pain, tenderness, or weakness, particularly during the initial months of therapy and following an increase in dosage of either drug.

■ **Niacin** Concomitant use of atorvastatin and antilipemic dosages (1 g daily or higher) of niacin increases the risk of myopathy. Data from several large randomized studies indicate that concomitant use of niacin (1.5–2 g daily) with another statin (i.e., simvastatin 40–80 mg once daily, with or without ezetimibe) resulted in an increased risk of severe adverse effects, including disturbances in glycemic control requiring hospitalization, development of diabetes mellitus, adverse GI effects, myopathy, gout, rash, skin ulceration, infection, and bleeding.

The benefits of concomitant use of atorvastatin and antilipemic dosages of niacin should be weighed against the possible risk of myopathy. If concomitant therapy is employed, caution is advised, and lower initial and maintenance dosages of atorvastatin should be considered; in addition, patients should be carefully monitored for manifestations of muscle pain, tenderness, or weakness, particularly during the initial months of therapy and following an increase in dosage of either drug.

■ **Omega-3-acid Ethyl Esters** Concomitant use of atorvastatin (80 mg daily) with omega-3-acid ethyl esters (4 g daily) for 14 days did not affect the rate or extent of exposure to atorvastatin, 2-hydroxyatorvastatin, or 4-hydroxyatorvastatin at steady state.

■ **Oral Contraceptives** Concomitant use of atorvastatin (40 mg once daily for 22 days) and an oral contraceptive (ethinyl estradiol 35 mcg with norethindrone 1 mg for 2 months) resulted in 30 and 19% increases in ethinyl estradiol peak plasma concentration and AUC, respectively, and 23 and 28% increases in norethindrone peak plasma concentration and AUC, respectively. This interaction should be considered when selecting oral contraceptives for patients receiving atorvastatin.

■ **Rifampin** Administration of rifampin (600 mg once daily for 5 days) followed by delayed administration of atorvastatin (40 mg as a single dose) resulted in 40 and 80% decreases in atorvastatin peak plasma concentration and AUC, respectively, while *simultaneous* administration of the drugs (rifampin 600 mg once daily for 7 days with atorvastatin 40 mg as a single dose) resulted in 2.7-fold and 30% *increases* in atorvastatin peak plasma concentration and AUC, respectively. Therefore, if atorvastatin and rifampin are used concomitantly, these drugs should be administered *simultaneously*.

■ **Warfarin** Atorvastatin had no clinically important effect on prothrombin time (PT) when administered to patients receiving long-term warfarin therapy. Some experts recommend closer monitoring of the international normalized ratio (INR) after initiation of a statin or a change in statin dosage.

Description

Atorvastatin calcium is a synthetic antilipemic agent. The drug is a selective, competitive inhibitor of 3-hydroxymethylglutaryl-CoA (HMG-CoA) reductase, an enzyme that catalyzes the conversion of HMG-CoA to mevalonate (an early and rate-limiting step in cholesterol biosynthesis). Inhibition of HMG-CoA reductase results in reduction of hepatic cholesterol biosynthesis, which leads to a compensatory increase in the expression of low-density lipoprotein (LDL) receptors on hepatic cell surfaces and, subsequently, increased hepatic uptake and clearance of LDL-cholesterol from blood. Atorvastatin reduces serum total cholesterol, LDL-cholesterol, apolipoprotein B (apo B), triglyceride, very low-density lipoprotein (VLDL)-cholesterol, intermediate-density lipoprotein (IDL)-cholesterol, and non-high-density lipoprotein (HDL) cholesterol concentrations, and increases serum HDL-cholesterol and apolipoprotein A-1 concentrations in patients with primary hypercholesterolemia, mixed dyslipidemia, hypertriglyceridemia, or primary dysbetalipoproteinemia.

Atorvastatin is distributed mainly to the liver, the primary site of action and principal site of cholesterol synthesis and LDL-cholesterol clearance. Drug dosage, rather than systemic drug concentration, correlates better with LDL-cholesterol reduction; therefore, individualization of drug dosage should be based on therapeutic response. Therapeutic response is observed within 2 weeks, and maximum response is usually achieved within 4 weeks and maintained during long-term therapy.

Atorvastatin is metabolized by cytochrome P-450 (CYP) isoenzyme 3A4 to active metabolites (i.e., *o*- and *p*-hydroxylated derivatives, various β-oxidation products). In vitro inhibition of HMG-CoA reductase by the active *o*- and *p*-hydroxylated metabolites is similar to that by atorvastatin. Approximately 70% of circulating inhibitory activity for HMG-CoA reductase is attributed to active metabolites. In animals, the *o*-hydroxy metabolite undergoes further glucuronidation. Atorvastatin and its metabolites are eliminated primarily in bile following hepatic and/or extrahepatic metabolism; however, the drug does not appear to undergo enterohepatic recirculation. The mean plasma elimination half-life of atorvastatin in humans is approximately 14 hours, but the half-life of inhibitory activity for HMG-CoA reductase is 20–30 hours due to the contribution of active metabolites. Less than 2% of an orally administered dose of atorvastatin is recovered in urine.

Advice to Patients

Importance of adhering to nondrug therapies and measures, including adherence to a heart-healthy diet, regular exercise, avoidance of tobacco products, and maintenance of a healthy weight.

Importance of periodic monitoring of lipoprotein profile to determine goal attainment.

Risk of myopathy and/or rhabdomyolysis; risk is increased with higher dosages or when used concomitantly with certain drugs. Importance of promptly reporting any unexplained and/or persistent muscle pain, tenderness, or weakness, particularly if accompanied by malaise or fever, or if manifestations persist after discontinuance of therapy.

Risk of adverse hepatic effects. Importance of promptly reporting any symptoms suggestive of liver injury (e.g., fatigue, anorexia, right upper abdominal discomfort, dark urine, jaundice).

Risk of nonserious, reversible cognitive impairment (e.g., memory loss, forgetfulness, amnesia, memory impairment, confusion).

Risk of increased glucose concentrations and development of type 2 diabetes mellitus; may need to monitor glucose concentrations following initiation of statin therapy.

Importance of advising women and adolescent girls to avoid pregnancy (i.e., using effective and appropriate contraceptive methods) during therapy and informing pregnant women of risk to fetus.

Importance of avoiding breast-feeding during therapy. If the patient has a lipid disorder and is breast-feeding, importance of contacting a clinician to discuss other antilipemic treatment options.

Importance of informing clinicians of existing or contemplated concomitant therapy, including prescription and OTC drugs, as well as any concomitant illnesses. Importance of informing other clinicians of current therapy with atorvastatin.

Importance of informing patients of other important precautionary information. (See Cautions.)

Overview® (see Users Guide). For additional information on this drug until a more detailed monograph is developed and published, the manufacturer's labeling should be consulted. It is *essential* that the manufacturer's labeling be consulted for more detailed information on usual cautions, precautions, contraindications, potential drug interactions, laboratory test interferences, and acute toxicity.

Preparations

Excipients in commercially available drug preparations may have clinically important effects in some individuals; consult specific product labeling for details.

Atorvastatin Calcium

Oral		
Tablets, film-coated	10 mg (of atorvastatin)*	**Atorvastatin Calcium Tablets**
		Lipitor®, Pfizer
	20 mg (of atorvastatin)*	**Atorvastatin Calcium Tablets**
		Lipitor®, Pfizer
	40 mg (of atorvastatin)*	**Atorvastatin Calcium Tablets**
		Lipitor®, Pfizer
	80 mg (of atorvastatin)*	**Atorvastatin Calcium Tablets**
		Lipitor®, Pfizer

*available from one or more manufacturer, distributor, and/or repackager by generic (nonproprietary) name

Atorvastatin Calcium Combinations

Oral		
Tablets, film-coated	10 mg (of atorvastatin) with Amlodipine Besylate 2.5 mg (of amlodipine)*	**Atorvastatin Calcium and Amlodipine Besylate Tablets**
		Caduet®, Pfizer
	10 mg (of atorvastatin) with Amlodipine Besylate 5 mg (of amlodipine)*	**Atorvastatin Calcium and Amlodipine Besylate Tablets**
		Caduet®, Pfizer
	10 mg (of atorvastatin) with Amlodipine Besylate 10 mg (of amlodipine)*	**Atorvastatin Calcium and Amlodipine Besylate Tablets**
		Caduet®, Pfizer
	20 mg (of atorvastatin) with Amlodipine Besylate 2.5 mg (of amlodipine)*	**Atorvastatin Calcium and Amlodipine Besylate Tablets**
		Caduet®, Pfizer
	20 mg (of atorvastatin) with Amlodipine Besylate 5 mg (of amlodipine)*	**Atorvastatin Calcium and Amlodipine Besylate Tablets**
		Caduet®, Pfizer
	20 mg (of atorvastatin) with Amlodipine Besylate 10 mg (of amlodipine)*	**Atorvastatin Calcium and Amlodipine Besylate Tablets**
		Caduet®, Pfizer
	40 mg (of atorvastatin) with Amlodipine Besylate 2.5 mg (of amlodipine)*	**Atorvastatin Calcium and Amlodipine Besylate Tablets**
		Caduet®, Pfizer
	40 mg (of atorvastatin) with Amlodipine Besylate 5 mg (of amlodipine)*	**Atorvastatin Calcium and Amlodipine Besylate Tablets**
		Caduet®, Pfizer
	40 mg (of atorvastatin) with Amlodipine Besylate 10 mg (of amlodipine)*	**Atorvastatin Calcium and Amlodipine Besylate Tablets**
		Caduet®, Pfizer
	80 mg (of atorvastatin) with Amlodipine Besylate 5 mg (of amlodipine)*	**Atorvastatin Calcium and Amlodipine Besylate Tablets**
		Caduet®, Pfizer
	80 mg (of atorvastatin) with Amlodipine Besylate 10 mg (of amlodipine)*	**Atorvastatin Calcium and Amlodipine Besylate Tablets**
		Caduet®, Pfizer

*available from one or more manufacturer, distributor, and/or repackager by generic (nonproprietary) name

†Use is not currently included in the labeling approved by the US Food and Drug Administration

Lovastatin

Mevinolin, Monacolin K

■ Lovastatin, a hydroxymethylglutaryl-CoA (HMG-CoA) reductase inhibitor (i.e., statin), is an antilipemic agent.

Uses

■ **Prevention of Cardiovascular Events** The American College of Cardiology (ACC)/American Heart Association (AHA) cholesterol management guideline recommends statins as first-line therapy for prevention of atherosclerotic cardiovascular disease (ASCVD) in adults. There is extensive evidence demonstrating that statins can substantially reduce ASCVD risk when used for secondary prevention or primary prevention (in high-risk patients). Because the relative reduction in ASCVD risk is correlated with the degree of low-density lipoprotein (LDL)-cholesterol lowering, the maximum tolerated statin intensity should be used to achieve optimum ASCVD benefits. According to the ACC/AHA guidelines, lovastatin may be used for primary or secondary† prevention in adults when moderate-intensity statin therapy is indicated. (See Prevention of Cardiovascular Events under Dosage and Administration: Dosage.) Nonstatin therapies do not provide acceptable ASCVD risk reduction benefits compared to their potential for adverse effects in the routine prevention of ASCVD. For additional details on prevention of ASCVD, see the HMG-CoA Reductase Inhibitors General Statement 24:06.08 and also consult the most recent ACC/AHA Guideline on the Treatment of Blood Cholesterol to Reduce Atherosclerotic Cardiovascular Risk in Adults (available at http://www.cardiosource.org or http://my.americanheart.org).

Primary Prevention Lovastatin is used as an adjunct to nondrug therapies (i.e., lifestyle modifications) in patients without symptomatic cardiovascular disease who have normal or moderate elevations of total and LDL-cholesterol and below-average high-density lipoprotein (HDL)-cholesterol concentrations to reduce the risk of myocardial infarction (MI) or unstable angina and to reduce the risk of undergoing coronary revascularization procedures.

The ACC/AHA cholesterol management guideline recommends statins as first-line therapy for primary prevention in patients 21 years of age and older without clinical ASCVD who have primary, severe elevations in LDL-cholesterol concentration (190 mg/dL or greater); patients 40–75 years of age with type 1 or 2 diabetes mellitus; and patients 40–75 years of age with LDL-cholesterol concentrations of 70–189 mg/dL and an estimated 10-year ASCVD risk of 7.5% or higher. Before initiating statin therapy for primary prevention in patients without clinical ASCVD or diabetes mellitus, it is reasonable for clinicians and patients to discuss the potential for ASCVD risk reduction benefits, adverse effects, and drug interactions, as well as patient preferences for treatment.

In a randomized, double-blind, placebo-controlled study (Air Force/Texas Coronary Atherosclerosis Prevention Study [AFCAPS/TexCAPS]) in patients who had total and LDL-cholesterol concentrations averaging 221 and 150 mg/dL, respectively, and HDL-cholesterol concentrations averaging 36 mg/dL (men) or 40 mg/dL (women), lovastatin therapy (20–40 mg daily) reduced the incidence of a first acute major event (i.e., primary end point defined as fatal or nonfatal MI, unstable angina, or sudden cardiac death) by 37% after an average follow-up period of 5.2 years. Lovastatin therapy also produced benefit in terms of secondary end points, including a 33% reduction in coronary revascularization procedures, a 32% reduction in unstable angina, a 40% reduction in the incidence of fatal or nonfatal MI, and a 25% reduction in cardiovascular (e.g., atherosclerotic) events.

Reducing Progression of Coronary Atherosclerosis Lovastatin is used as an adjunct to nondrug therapies (e.g., dietary management) in patients with coronary heart disease (CHD) to slow the progression of coronary atherosclerosis as part of a treatment strategy to lower total and LDL-cholesterol concentrations to target levels.

Lovastatin has been shown to slow the progression of atherosclerosis in both coronary and carotid arteries by reducing intimal-medial wall thickness. In several double-blind, placebo-controlled studies (e.g., Canadian Coronary Atherosclerosis Intervention Trial [CCAIT], Monitored Atherosclerosis Regression Study [MARS], Familial Atherosclerosis Treatment Study [FATS]) in men and women with or without documented CHD and elevated lipoprotein concentrations, progression of atherosclerosis at 2–3 years (measured as the mean per-patient changes from baseline in mean and minimal coronary artery lumen diameters, percent diameter stenosis, and formation of new lesions) was reduced in patients who received recommended daily dosages of lovastatin.

Treatment with lovastatin has been shown to reduce the rate of progression of atherosclerosis in the carotid arteries. In the MARS and the Asymptomatic Carotid Artery Progression Studies (ACAPS), hypercholesterolemic patients with or without CHD who received recommended daily dosages of lovastatin for a median of 2–4 years showed less progression of atherosclerosis (as determined by B-mode ultrasound quantification of carotid artery intimal-medial thickness [IMT]) compared with those receiving placebo. In addition, treatment with lovastatin also was associated with a reduction in the risk of major cardiovascular events and all-cause mortality.

Intensity of Statin Therapy The ACC/AHA cholesterol management guideline states that the appropriate intensity of a statin should be used to reduce the risk of ASCVD in patients most likely to benefit. Based on the average LDL-cholesterol response observed with specific statins and dosages used in the randomized controlled studies evaluated by the guideline expert panel, ACC/AHA considers lovastatin 20 mg daily to be a low-intensity statin (producing approximate LDL-cholesterol reductions of less than 30%) and lovastatin 40 mg daily to be a moderate-intensity statin (producing approximate LDL-cholesterol reductions of 30% to less than 50%). Individual patient response may vary in clinical practice.

Combination Antilipemic Therapy The ACC/AHA cholesterol management guideline states that nonstatin drugs may be useful adjuncts to statin therapy in certain high-risk patients (e.g., patients with ASCVD, LDL-cholesterol concentrations of at least 190 mg/dL, or diabetes mellitus) who have a less-than-anticipated response to statins, are unable to tolerate a less-than-recommended intensity of a statin, or are completely intolerant to statin therapy, particularly if there is evidence from randomized controlled studies suggesting that the addition of the nonstatin drug further reduces ASCVD events. If combination therapy is necessary, selection of the nonstatin drug should be based on the risk and benefit profile (i.e., reduction in ASCVD risk outweighs the drug's potential for adverse effects and drug interactions) and patient preferences.

■ **Dyslipidemias** ***Primary Hypercholesterolemia or Mixed Dyslipidemia*** Lovastatin is used as an adjunct to nondrug therapies (e.g., dietary management) in adults to decrease elevated serum total and LDL-cholesterol, apolipoprotein B (apo B), and triglyceride concentrations, and to increase HDL-cholesterol concentrations in the treatment of primary hypercholesterolemia, including heterozygous familial hypercholesterolemia and other primary causes of hypercholesterolemia (e.g., polygenic hypercholesterolemia). Lovastatin as conventional (immediate-release) tablets also is used as an adjunct to dietary therapy to reduce elevated serum total cholesterol, LDL-cholesterol, and apo B concentrations in the treatment of heterozygous familial hypercholesterolemia in boys and girls (who are at least 1 year postmenarchal) 10–17 years of age who, despite an adequate trial of dietary management, have a serum LDL-cholesterol concentration of 190 mg/dL or greater *or* a serum LDL-cholesterol concentration exceeding 160 mg/dL and either a family history of premature cardiovascular disease or 2 or more other cardiovascular risk factors. Statins such as lovastatin also are used in combination with fenofibrate to decrease triglyceride concentrations and increase HDL-cholesterol concentrations in patients with mixed dyslipidemia and CHD or CHD risk equivalents who are receiving optimal statin therapy; however, no additional benefit on cardiovascular morbidity and mortality has been demonstrated with such combination therapy beyond that already established with statin monotherapy.

Although lovastatin also has been used to reduce elevated LDL-cholesterol concentrations in patients with combined hypercholesterolemia and hypertriglyceridemia caused by genotypic familial combined hyperlipidemia, the drug has not been studied in conditions where the major abnormality is elevation of chylomicrons, very-low-density lipoproteins (VLDLs), or intermediate-density lipoproteins (IDLs).

Nondrug therapies and measures specific for the type of dyslipidemia (therapeutic lifestyle changes) are the initial treatments of choice, including dietary management (e.g., restriction of total and saturated fat and cholesterol intake, addition of plant stanols/sterols and viscous fiber to diet), weight control, an appropriate program of physical activity, and management of potentially contributory disease (e.g., hypothyroidism). Drug therapy is not a substitute for but an adjunct to these nondrug therapies and measures, which should be continued when drug therapy is initiated.

Reductions in total and LDL-cholesterol produced by usual dosages of lovastatin substantially exceed those of placebo and appear to be similar to or greater than those produced by monotherapy with usual dosages of certain other antilipemic agents. Mean reductions in total cholesterol concentrations of 13–34%, LDL-cholesterol concentrations of 17–48%, and triglyceride concentrations of 6–27% have been observed in controlled and uncontrolled studies in patients with heterozygous familial hypercholesterolemia or other forms of primary hypercholesterolemia who received 10–80 mg of lovastatin daily. Modest and variable increases in HDL-cholesterol concentrations (1–10%) also were observed in these patients. In 2 multicenter, placebo-controlled studies, 89% of patients with heterozygous familial hypercholesterolemia or 97% of patients with other forms of primary hypercholesterolemia who received lovastatin 40 mg twice daily and dietary management had reductions in LDL-cholesterol of at least 20%, while 61 or 51% of such patients had LDL-cholesterol reductions of at least 40%; reductions in LDL-cholesterol averaged 39% in both groups of patients.

Reductions in total and LDL-cholesterol concentrations produced by usual dosages of lovastatin generally appear to be similar to or greater than those produced by monotherapy with usual dosages of some statins (e.g., fluvastatin, pravastatin, simvastatin) but less than those produced by usual dosages of atorvastatin and rosuvastatin. In a randomized, multicenter, parallel-group study comparing the efficacy of various statins, patients with hypercholesterolemia who received lovastatin 20–80 mg daily experienced similar or greater reductions in total and LDL-cholesterol concentrations (21–36 and 29–48%, respectively) than those receiving fluvastatin 20–40 mg daily (13–19 and 17–23%, respectively), pravastatin 10–40 mg daily (13–24 and 19–34%, respectively), or simvastatin 10–40 mg daily (21–30 and 28–41%, respectively). However, atorvastatin dosages of 10–80 mg daily produced greater reductions in total and LDL-cholesterol concentrations (28–42 and 38–54%, respectively) than lovastatin. Maximum reductions in LDL-cholesterol concentrations with lovastatin reportedly average about 35–40% at maximum recommended dosages (80 mg daily in 1 or 2 divided doses). (See Intensity of Statin Therapy under Uses: Prevention of Cardiovascular Events.)

Limited data from comparative studies suggest that reductions in total and LDL-cholesterol concentrations produced by lovastatin are similar to or greater than those produced by certain other antilipemic agents (i.e., bile acid sequestrants, niacin, fibric acid derivatives). Lovastatin 40–80 mg daily reportedly has produced greater reductions in total cholesterol than cholestyramine 12–24 g daily. HDL-cholesterol increases produced by lovastatin are similar to or greater than those reported with usual cholestyramine dosages. Lovastatin appears to produce greater reductions in total and LDL-cholesterol than niacin or fibric acid derivatives (i.e., fenofibrate, gemfibrozil) in reducing total and LDL-cholesterol concentrations but is less effective than these agents in reducing triglycerides or increasing HDL-cholesterol concentrations. In several comparative studies in patients with primary hypercholesterolemia or familial combined hyperlipidemia, therapy with lovastatin (20–40 mg daily) reduced total and LDL-cholesterol concentrations by 17–23 and 21–28%, respectively, while total and LDL-cholesterol reductions averaged 6 and 5%, respectively, with niacin; 9 and 2%, respectively, with gemfibrozil; and 13 and 12%, respectively, with fenofibrate. Reductions in triglycerides and increases in HDL-cholesterol concentrations generally were less pronounced among patients treated with lovastatin (8–25% reduction and 6–13% increase) than in those receiving niacin (22% reduction and 18% increase), gemfibrozil (48% reduction and 18% decrease), or fenofibrate (42% reduction and 22% increase).

When lovastatin monotherapy combined with dietary management does not reduce LDL-cholesterol concentrations to optimal levels in patients with dyslipidemia, combination drug therapy may be required. Although combined therapy with lovastatin and another antilipemic agent generally results in cholesterol reductions exceeding those achieved with either therapy alone, the risk of myopathy and rhabdomyolysis may be increased with such concomitant use. Therapy with lovastatin (20–40 mg daily) in fixed combination with extended-release niacin (1–2 g daily) (no longer commercially available in the US) reduced LDL-cholesterol or triglyceride concentrations by 30–42 or 32–44%, respectively, and increased HDL-cholesterol concentrations by 20–30%. Limited data indicate that concomitant therapy with gemfibrozil and lovastatin may be superior to that with gemfibrozil and a bile acid sequestrant in patients with familial combined hyperlipidemia, in part because the bile acid sequestrant appears to lessen the favorable effects of gemfibrozil on HDL- and VLDL-cholesterol and total triglycerides. Lovastatin has been used concomitantly with the bile acid sequestrants colestipol or cholestyramine in a limited number of patients with heterozygous familial hypercholesterolemia or other forms of primary hypercholesterolemia. The addition of a bile acid sequestrant to lovastatin therapy further reduced LDL-cholesterol by 19–26%, resulting in overall LDL-cholesterol reductions of 46–60% in patients receiving lovastatin 40–80 mg daily and either colestipol hydrochloride 10–20 g daily or cholestyramine 4–24 g daily. Triple-drug therapy with lovastatin, niacin, and a bile acid sequestrant in patients with severe heterozygous familial hypercholesterolemia or other forms of severe primary hypercholesterolemia has produced further sustained reductions in LDL-cholesterol compared with those produced by combinations of any two of these drugs, and some clinicians have suggested that niacin may be more effective than a fibric acid derivative (e.g., gemfibrozil) in a three-drug regimen in patients whose cholesterol concentrations are controlled inadequately by the combination of a statin and a bile acid sequestrant. However, because of the increased risk of adverse muscular effects with combination therapy, some antilipemic drug combinations should be avoided or used with caution. (See Drug Interactions: Antilipemic Agents, in the HMG-CoA Reductase Inhibitors General Statement 24:06.08.)

■ **Other Uses** Lovastatin has reduced total and LDL-cholesterol concentrations in a few patients with familial dysbetalipoproteinemia or with hypercholesterolemia associated with or exacerbated by diabetes mellitus† (diabetic dyslipidemia), cardiac† or renal transplantation,† nephrotic syndrome† (nephrotic hyperlipidemia), or distal ileal bypass surgery†. The drug also has been used to lower total cholesterol, LDL-cholesterol, and/or apolipoprotein B in a limited number of patients with hypoalphalipoproteinemia† or in those with mild endogenous (primary) hypertriglyceridemia and borderline elevated total cholesterol, decreased HDL-cholesterol, and elevated apolipoprotein B† (type IV hyperlipoproteinemia with elevated total apo B). Additional studies are necessary to determine the role, if any, of lovastatin therapy in patients with these disorders.

For additional information on these and other uses of lovastatin or other statins, see General Principles of Antilipemic Therapy and see Uses in the HMG-CoA Reductase Inhibitors General Statement 24:06.08.

Dosage and Administration

■ **Administration** Lovastatin is administered orally in the evening or at bedtime. Lovastatin conventional tablets should be administered with the evening meal. Lovastatin extended-release tablets should be taken in the evening at bedtime.

Patients should be placed on a standard cholesterol-lowering diet before initiation of lovastatin therapy and should remain on this diet during treatment with the drug. For recommendations on dietary and other nondrug therapies (i.e., lifestyle modifications), consult the most recent American Heart Association (AHA)/American College of Cardiology (ACC) Guideline on Lifestyle Management to Reduce Cardiovascular Risk (available at http://www.cardiosource.org or http://my.americanheart.org).

Because administration of lovastatin with grapefruit juice has resulted in substantial increases in plasma concentrations of the antilipemic agent, the manufacturers and some clinicians recommend that concomitant administration of lovastatin with grapefruit juice should be avoided. However, the extent of this interaction may be influenced by the quantity and timing of grapefruit juice consumption, and other clinicians suggest that small amounts of grapefruit juice (e.g., 240 mL) may be acceptable and may even be used to therapeutic advantage. (See Drug Interactions: Drugs and Foods Affecting or Metabolized by Hepatic Microsomal Enzymes, in the HMG-CoA Reductase Inhibitors General Statement 24:06.08.)

■ Dosage

Dosage of lovastatin must be carefully adjusted according to individual requirements and response. Dosage should be increased at intervals of no less than 4 weeks until the desired effect on lipoprotein concentrations is observed; reduction of lovastatin dosage should be considered in patients whose serum cholesterol concentrations fall below the desired target range. The manufacturer recommends that serum lipoprotein concentrations be determined periodically during lovastatin therapy. The ACC/AHA cholesterol management guideline states that lipoprotein concentrations should be determined within 4–12 weeks following initiation of statin therapy (to determine the patient's response to therapy and adherence) and monitored every 3–12 months thereafter as clinically indicated.

Prevention of Cardiovascular Events

The ACC/AHA cholesterol management guideline states that the appropriate intensity of statin therapy should be used to reduce atherosclerotic cardiovascular disease (ASCVD) risk in patients most likely to benefit. Giving a maximally tolerated statin intensity should be emphasized over giving lower statin dosages and adding nonstatin drugs to address low high-density lipoprotein (HDL)-cholesterol or high triglyceride concentrations, a strategy that has not yet been shown to reduce ASCVD risk.

Primary Prevention. For primary prevention of cardiovascular disease in patients 21 years of age and older without clinical ASCVD who have primary, severe elevations in low-density lipoprotein (LDL)-cholesterol concentration (*190 mg/dL or greater*), the ACC/AHA cholesterol management guideline recommends that high-intensity statin therapy (i.e., with atorvastatin or rosuvastatin) be initiated unless contraindicated. (See Atorvastatin Calcium or Rosuvastatin Calcium 24:06.08.)

For primary prevention of cardiovascular disease in patients 40–75 years of age with *type 1 or 2 diabetes mellitus*† and LDL-cholesterol concentrations of 70–189 mg/dL, the ACC/AHA cholesterol management guideline recommends that moderate-intensity statin therapy (e.g., lovastatin 40 mg once daily) be initiated or continued. In those with an estimated 10-year ASCVD risk of 7.5% or higher, it is reasonable to consider high-intensity statin therapy (i.e., with atorvastatin or rosuvastatin) unless contraindicated. In patients with diabetes mellitus who are younger than 40 or older than 75 years of age, it is reasonable to evaluate the potential benefits, adverse effects, drug interactions, and patient preferences when deciding to initiate, continue, or intensify statin therapy.

For primary prevention of cardiovascular disease in patients 40–75 years of age without clinical ASCVD or diabetes mellitus who have LDL-cholesterol concentrations of 70–189 mg/dL and an *estimated 10-year ASCVD risk of 7.5% or higher*, the ACC/AHA cholesterol management guideline recommends that moderate- (e.g., lovastatin 40 mg once daily) to high-intensity statin therapy (i.e., with atorvastatin or rosuvastatin) be initiated or continued. In those with an estimated 10-year ASCVD risk of 5 to less than 7.5%, it is reasonable to offer treatment with moderate-intensity statin therapy. Before initiating statin therapy for primary prevention of ASCVD in patients 40–75 years of age without clinical ASCVD or diabetes mellitus who have LDL-cholesterol concentrations of 70–189 mg/dL, it is reasonable for clinicians and patients to discuss the potential benefits, adverse effects, drug interactions, and patient preferences for such therapy.

Secondary Prevention. For secondary prevention† of cardiovascular disease in patients 21–75 years of age with clinical ASCVD, the ACC/AHA cholesterol management guideline recommends that high-intensity statin therapy (i.e., with atorvastatin or rosuvastatin) be initiated or continued unless contraindicated. (See Atorvastatin Calcium or Rosuvastatin Calcium 24:06.08.) In patients 21–75 years of age with clinical ASCVD who are at increased risk for developing statin-associated adverse effects or in whom high-intensity statin therapy is inappropriate or contraindicated, moderate-intensity statin therapy (e.g., lovastatin 40 mg once daily) should be given if tolerated. In patients older than 75 years of age with clinical ASCVD, use of statin therapy should be individualized based on the potential benefits, adverse effects, drug interactions, and patient preferences; it is reasonable to consider initiating or continuing moderate-intensity statin therapy in such patients if tolerated.

Dyslipidemias

Immediate-Release Tablets. The usual initial dosage of lovastatin as conventional tablets in adults is 20 mg once daily given with the evening meal. The manufacturer states that patients requiring reductions in LDL-cholesterol of 20% or greater should receive an initial lovastatin dosage of 20 mg daily; a dosage of 10 mg daily may be considered for patients requiring smaller reductions in LDL-cholesterol concentration. The recommended dosage range of lovastatin as conventional tablets in adults is 10–80 mg daily given a single dose or in 2 divided doses. The maximum recommended dosage of lovastatin is 80 mg daily. Twice-daily dosing of lovastatin has been used in most clinical studies in patients with heterozygous familial hypercholesterolemia and appears to be slightly but consistently more effective than once-daily dosing; however, once-daily dosing may be acceptable for patients in whom dosing convenience is considered important for compliance, particularly if only moderate degrees of hypercholesterolemia are present. When given as a single daily dose, lovastatin appears to be more effective when administered in the evening, possibly because cholesterol synthesis occurs mainly at night.

The recommended dosage range of lovastatin as conventional tablets for the management of heterozygous familial hypercholesterolemia in children 10–17 years of age is 10–40 mg daily. The manufacturer states that patients requiring reductions in LDL-cholesterol of 20% or greater should receive an initial lovastatin dosage of 20 mg daily; a dosage of 10 mg daily may be considered for patients requiring smaller reductions in LDL-cholesterol concentration. The maximum recommended dosage of lovastatin in children 10–17 years of age is 40 mg daily.

Extended-Release Tablets. The recommended dosage of lovastatin as extended-release tablets in adults ranges from 20 to 60 mg once daily.

In geriatric patients (65 years of age or older), the usual initial dosage of lovastatin as extended-release tablets is 20 mg once daily at bedtime. Higher dosages should be used only after careful consideration of the potential risks and benefits. (See Cautions: Geriatric Precautions.)

Concomitant Therapy. Because of an increased risk of myopathy/rhabdomyolysis, concomitant use of lovastatin with potent inhibitors of cytochrome P-450 (CYP) isoenzyme 3A4 (CYP3A4) (e.g., clarithromycin, cobicistat-containing preparations, erythromycin, HIV protease inhibitors, itraconazole, ketoconazole, nefazodone, posaconazole, telithromycin, voriconazole) is *contraindicated.* Concomitant use of lovastatin with cyclosporine or gemfibrozil should be *avoided.* In patients receiving danazol, diltiazem, dronedarone, or verapamil concomitantly with lovastatin, dosage of lovastatin should be initiated at 10 mg daily and should not exceed 20 mg daily. In patients receiving amiodarone concomitantly with lovastatin, dosage of lovastatin should not exceed 40 mg daily. In patients receiving ranolazine concomitantly with lovastatin, dosage adjustment of lovastatin may be considered.

In clinical studies in a limited number of patients, lovastatin dosages of 40–80 mg daily combined with colestipol hydrochloride dosages of 10–20 g daily or cholestyramine dosages of 4–24 g daily have resulted in additive or synergistic effects in reducing serum total and/or LDL-cholesterol concentrations.

Dosage Modification

The ACC/AHA cholesterol management guideline states that decreasing the statin dosage in adults may be considered when LDL-cholesterol concentrations are less than 40 mg/dL on 2 consecutive measurements; however, there are no data to suggest that LDL-cholesterol concentrations below 40 mg/dL would increase the risk of adverse effects.

■ Dosage in Renal and Hepatic Impairment

Although lovastatin is only minimally excreted in urine, the manufacturer states that the drug should be used with caution in patients with severe renal impairment (creatinine clearance less than 30 mL/minute); dosage increases above 20 mg daily should be carefully considered and, if deemed necessary, implemented with extreme caution. The manufacturer of the extended-release lovastatin preparation states that dosage increases above 20 mg daily should only be considered in patients with severe renal impairment if the expected benefits exceed the increased risk of myopathy and rhabdomyolysis.

Because the pharmacokinetics of lovastatin have not been studied in patients with hepatic dysfunction, the drug should be used with caution in patients who consume substantial amounts of alcohol and/or have a history of liver disease. Use of lovastatin is *contraindicated* in patients with active liver disease or unexplained, persistent elevations in serum aminotransferase concentrations.

Cautions

Lovastatin shares the toxic potentials of other statins, and the usual cautions, precautions, and contraindications associated with these drugs should be observed. Patients should be fully advised about the risks, especially rhabdomyolysis, associated with statin therapy alone or combined with other drugs. (See Cautions and also see Drug Interactions in the HMG-CoA Reductase Inhibitors General Statement 24:06.08.)

■ Precautions and Contraindications

Lovastatin is *contraindicated* in patients with hypersensitivity to any component of the formulation; in patients with active liver disease or unexplained, persistent elevations of serum transaminases; in patients receiving concomitant therapy with potent inhibitors of cytochrome P-450 (CYP) isoenzyme 3A4 (CYP3A4) (e.g., clarithromycin, cobicistat-containing preparations, erythromycin, HIV protease inhibitors, itraconazole, ketoconazole, nefazodone, posaconazole, telithromycin, voriconazole); in pregnant or lactating women; and in women of childbearing age (unless these patients are unlikely to conceive).

■ Pediatric Precautions

In several randomized, double-blind, placebo-controlled studies in boys and postmenarchal girls 10–17 years of age with heterozygous familial hypercholesterolemia, the adverse effect profile of lovastatin (10–40 mg daily for at least 24 weeks) as conventional tablets generally was similar to that of placebo; dosages exceeding 40 mg daily have not been evaluated in this population. There were no detectable adverse effects on growth or sexual maturation in adolescent boys or on duration of menstrual cycle in girls. If therapy with lovastatin is considered, the manufacturer states that adolescent girls should be advised to use effective and appropriate contraceptive methods during therapy to reduce the likelihood of unintended pregnancy. (See Cautions: Pregnancy, Fertility, and Lactation.) Safety and efficacy of lovastatin have not been evaluated in prepubertal children or in children younger than 10 years of age.

Safety and efficacy of lovastatin as extended-release tablets have not been established in children or adolescents younger than 20 years of age. Therefore, the manufacturer states that this preparation should not be used in this population.

For additional information on the use of statins in pediatric patients, see Cautions: Pediatric Precautions in the HMG-CoA Reductase Inhibitors General Statement 24:06.08.

■ **Geriatric Precautions** Results of a pharmacokinetic study in a limited number of patients receiving lovastatin (80 mg daily) as conventional tablets indicate that mean plasma levels of HMG-CoA reductase inhibitory activity are approximately 45% higher in geriatric patients (70–78 years of age) than in younger adults (18–30 years of age). However, data from clinical studies and other reported clinical experience employing various preparations of lovastatin suggest that safety and efficacy of the drug in geriatric patients appear to be similar to those in younger adults. Although dosage adjustment based on age-related pharmacokinetic differences does not appear to be necessary for geriatric patients, greater sensitivity in some older patients cannot be ruled out. Because advanced age (65 years of age or older) is a predisposing factor for myopathy, including rhabdomyolysis, the manufacturer states that lovastatin should be prescribed with caution in this population. Lower initial dosages of extended-release lovastatin are recommended in geriatric patients. (See Extended-Release Tablets under Dosage: Dyslipidemias, in Dosage and Administration.)

The ACC/AHA cholesterol management guideline states that initiation of statin therapy for primary prevention of atherosclerotic cardiovascular disease (ASCVD) in patients older than 75 years of age requires consideration of additional factors, including increasing comorbidities, safety considerations, and priorities of care. Therefore, the potential for an ASCVD risk reduction benefit, adverse effects, and drug interactions, along with patient preferences, must be considered before initiating statin therapy in patients older than 75 years of age.

■ **Mutagenicity and Carcinogenicity** Lovastatin did not exhibit mutagenic potential in in vitro mammalian cell systems (rat or mouse hepatocytes, V-79 cell forward mutation study), in vitro (Chinese hamster ovary cell) or in vivo (mouse bone marrow) chromosomal aberration studies, or microbial (Ames test) systems with or without metabolic activation. There is some in vitro evidence, however, that inhibition of HMG-CoA reductase can inhibit DNA synthesis during the S phase of the cell life cycle; this inhibition appears to result from depletion of mevalonic acid and is independent of its conversion to cholesterol.

An increased incidence of hepatocellular carcinoma and adenoma was observed after 21 months in mice given oral lovastatin 500 mg/kg daily resulting in plasma concentrations up to 3–4 times the estimated human exposure; similar changes were not observed at oral dosages of 20 or 100 mg/kg daily resulting in plasma concentrations up to 0.3–2 times the estimated human exposure. An increased incidence of pulmonary adenomas also was observed in female mice receiving oral lovastatin 500 mg/kg daily (resulting in plasma concentrations up to 4 times the estimated human exposure), but the relationship of these adenomas to administration of the drug is not known since the incidence of these tumors was within the range of that found in untreated animals in studies of similar duration. Similar changes were not observed in female mice given oral dosages of 20 or 100 mg/kg daily or in male mice at any dosage.

In mice given oral lovastatin dosages of 100 or 500 mg/kg daily, an increase in the incidence of papilloma in the nonglandular mucosa of the stomach was observed. There is a strong association between the development of papilloma and hyperplasia of squamous epithelium (acanthosis) in this region of the stomach; such acanthosis in these rodents appears to be related to inhibition of HMG-CoA reductase in this nonglandular tissue. Since the glandular mucosa of the stomach in these rodents was not affected and the human stomach contains only glandular mucosa, the importance of this finding to humans is unclear. Also, although similar squamous epithelium is found in the esophagus and anorectal junction of the mouse and rat, no evidence of similar drug-induced hyperplasia was observed in these tissues in studies of up to 21 months in mice given oral lovastatin dosages up to 500 mg/kg daily or of up to 24 months in rats given 180 mg/kg daily (112 times the maximum recommended human dosage).

In a 24-month study in rats, hepatocellular carcinogenicity showed a positive relationship to lovastatin dosage in males, but the incidence of hepatocellular carcinogenicity in this study was similar to that observed spontaneously in this strain of rat.

An increased incidence of thyroid neoplasms has been observed in rats given statins, including lovastatin.

The relevance has not been established, but mevastatin (compactin, not commercially available) has been shown to enhance adhesion of metastatic melanoma cells to epithelial cells in vitro.

■ **Pregnancy, Fertility, and Lactation** ***Pregnancy*** Safety of lovastatin in pregnant women has not been established. Lovastatin should be discontinued as soon as pregnancy is recognized. Currently, most experts recommend that dyslipidemias in pregnant women be managed with dietary measures; consultation with a lipid specialist is recommended for pregnant women with severe forms of dyslipidemia.

Lovastatin has produced skeletal malformations in offspring of pregnant mice and rats receiving dosages of 80 mg/kg daily during gestation (7 times the human dose based on body surface area and 5 times the human exposure based on area under the plasma concentration-time curve [AUC], respectively). Administration of the active β,δ-dihydroxyacid form of lovastatin (mevinolinic acid) at 60 mg/kg daily produced similar skeletal malformations; these teratogenic effects were markedly or completely suppressed by concomitant administration of the inhibited product mevalonic acid but not by cholesterol coadministration. No evidence of malformations was observed when pregnant rabbits were given 5 mg/kg daily (equivalent to a human dose of 80 mg daily based on body surface area) or a maternally toxic dose of 15 mg/kg daily (3 times the human dose of 80 mg daily based on body surface area).

Cholesterol and other products of the cholesterol biosynthetic pathway are essential for fetal development, including synthesis of steroids and cell membranes. Because of the ability of statins such as lovastatin to decrease the synthesis of cholesterol and possibly other products of the cholesterol biosynthetic pathway, lovastatin may cause fetal harm when administered to pregnant women. Rarely, congenital anomalies have been reported clinically following intrauterine exposure to statins. In an analysis of more than 200 prospectively followed pregnancies exposed during the first trimester to lovastatin or another closely related statin, the incidence of congenital anomalies was comparable to that seen in the general population; this number of pregnancies was sufficient to exclude a threefold or greater increase in congenital anomalies over the background incidence.

Lovastatin is *contraindicated* in women who are or may become pregnant. The drug should be administered to women of childbearing age only when such patients are highly unlikely to conceive and have been informed of the potential hazard. If the patient becomes pregnant while receiving lovastatin, the drug should be discontinued immediately and the patient informed of the potential hazard to the fetus.

Fertility Although the manufacturer states that reproduction studies in rats receiving lovastatin have not revealed evidence of impaired fertility, an increase in the rate of spontaneous testicular degeneration (i.e., testicular atrophy, decreased spermatogenesis, spermatocytic degeneration, and giant cell formation) was observed in dogs given oral lovastatin 20 mg/kg daily (12.5 times the maximum recommended human dosage) in a 1-year study; however, this effect was poorly reproducible and appeared to be unrelated to dosage. In a study in patients with type II hyperlipoproteinemia receiving oral lovastatin 40 mg daily for 4 months, there was a small but statistically significant reduction in sperm motility compared with that observed during dietary management alone but not compared with neomycin therapy. No alterations in sperm morphology or testicular dimensions or of biochemical indices of gonadal function (serum concentrations of testosterone, luteinizing hormone, follicle-stimulating hormone, prolactin) have been found in patients receiving lovastatin in clinical studies. However, at least one case of hypospermia, which resolved following discontinuance of lovastatin, has been reported.

Lactation It is not known whether lovastatin is distributed into human milk; however, other statins are distributed into human milk. Because of the potential for serious adverse reactions from lovastatin in nursing infants, the drug is contraindicated in nursing women; women who require lovastatin therapy should not breast-feed their infants.

Chemistry and Stability

■ **Chemistry** Lovastatin is a mevinic acid-derivative antilipemic agent. Lovastatin is the δ-lactone of mevinolinic acid and is produced by fermentation of *Aspergillus terreus.* The drug also has been isolated as a fermentation metabolite of *Monascus ruber.* Lovastatin is a hydroxymethylglutaryl-CoA (HMG-CoA) reductase inhibitor (statin) that is pharmacologically related to other statins (e.g., atorvastatin, fluvastatin, pravastatin, simvastatin).

Lovastatin is a prodrug and has little, if any, antilipemic activity until hydrolyzed in vivo to mevinolinic acid (the corresponding ring-opened, β,δ-dihydroxyacid form). The ring-opened acid forms of lovastatin (i.e., mevinolinic acid) and other mevinic acid-derivative statins are similar structurally to HMG-CoA and compete with this compound for interaction with HMG-CoA reductase.

Lovastatin occurs as a white, nonhygroscopic crystalline powder and is insoluble in water and sparingly soluble in alcohol, having solubilities of 0.44 mcg/mL and 16 mg/mL, respectively, at approximately 25°C.

Lovastatin is commercially available as conventional (immediate-release) or extended-release tablets.

■ **Stability** Lovastatin immediate-release tablets should be protected from light and stored in well-closed, light-resistant containers at 5–25°C. When stored under these conditions, the tablets are stable for 24 months after the date of manufacture. Lovastatin is sensitive to light. Following exposure to extreme light conditions, the drug is stable for 24 hours or 1 month when exposed to ultraviolet (approximately 3230 lux) or fluorescent (approximately 10,764 lux) light, respectively, at 28°C in air.

Lovastatin extended-release tablets should be stored at 20–25°C but may be exposed to temperatures ranging from 15–30°C; exposure to excessive heat and humidity should be avoided.

For further information on chemistry and stability, pharmacokinetics, uses, cautions, drug interactions, laboratory test interferences, and dosage and administration of lovastatin, see the HMG-CoA Reductase Inhibitors General Statement 24:06.08.

Preparations

Excipients in commercially available drug preparations may have clinically important effects in some individuals; consult specific product labeling for details.

Lovastatin

Oral		
Tablets	10 mg*	Lovastatin Tablets
	20 mg*	Lovastatin Tablets
	40 mg*	Lovastatin Tablets
Tablets, extended-release	20 mg	Altoprev®, Covis
	40 mg	Altoprev®, Covis
	60 mg	Altoprev®, Covis

*available from one or more manufacturer, distributor, and/or repackager by generic (nonproprietary) name

†Use is not currently included in the labeling approved by the US Food and Drug Administration

Pravastatin Sodium

Eptastatin Sodium

■ Pravastatin sodium, a hydroxymethylglutaryl-CoA (HMG-CoA) reductase inhibitor (i.e., statin), is an antilipemic agent.

Uses

■ Prevention of Cardiovascular Events The American College of Cardiology (ACC)/American Heart Association (AHA) cholesterol management guideline recommends statins as first-line therapy for prevention of atherosclerotic cardiovascular disease (ASCVD) in adults. There is extensive evidence demonstrating that statins can substantially reduce ASCVD risk when used for secondary prevention or primary prevention (in high-risk patients). Because the relative reduction in ASCVD risk is correlated with the degree of low-density lipoprotein (LDL)-cholesterol lowering, the maximum tolerated statin intensity should be used to achieve optimum ASCVD benefits. According to the ACC/AHA guidelines, pravastatin may be used for primary or secondary prevention in adults when moderate-intensity statin therapy is indicated. (See Prevention of Cardiovascular Events under Dosage and Administration: Dosage.) Nonstatin therapies do not provide acceptable ASCVD risk reduction benefits compared to their potential for adverse effects in the routine prevention of ASCVD. For additional details on prevention of ASCVD, see the HMG-CoA Reductase Inhibitors General Statement 24:06.08 and also consult the most recent ACC/AHA Guideline on the Treatment of Blood Cholesterol to Reduce Atherosclerotic Cardiovascular Risk in Adults (available at http://www.cardiosource.org or http://my.americanheart.org).

Primary Prevention Pravastatin is used as an adjunct to nondrug therapies (i.e., lifestyle modifications) in patients with hypercholesterolemia *without* clinical evidence of coronary heart disease (CHD) to reduce the risk of myocardial infarction (MI), to reduce the risk of undergoing myocardial revascularization procedures, and to reduce the risk of cardiovascular mortality (with no increase in death from noncardiovascular causes).

The ACC/AHA cholesterol management guideline recommends statins as first-line therapy for primary prevention in patients 21 years of age and older without clinical ASCVD who have primary, severe elevations in LDL-cholesterol concentration (190 mg/dL or greater); patients 40–75 years of age with type 1 or 2 diabetes mellitus; and patients 40–75 years of age with LDL-cholesterol concentrations of 70–189 mg/dL and an estimated 10-year ASCVD risk of 7.5% or higher. Before initiating statin therapy for primary prevention in patients without clinical ASCVD or diabetes mellitus, it is reasonable for clinicians and patients to discuss the potential for ASCVD risk reduction benefits, adverse effects, and drug interactions, as well as patient preferences for treatment.

In a randomized, placebo-controlled study (West of Scotland Coronary Prevention Study [WOSCOPS]) in men with moderate hypercholesterolemia and no history of MI, therapy with pravastatin sodium (40 mg daily) for a median of 4.9 years lowered plasma total and LDL-cholesterol by 20 and 26%, respectively, and reduced the incidence of MI and death from cardiovascular causes by approximately 31%; the risk of undergoing myocardial revascularization procedures also was reduced by 37%. Unlike some prior studies of cholesterol-lowering therapy, an increased risk of death from noncardiovascular causes was not observed in patients receiving pravastatin therapy in this study.

Despite favorable findings from the WOSCOPS study, clinical benefit (i.e., reduction in CHD-related morbidity or all-cause mortality) was not observed in a randomized, open-label study, the lipid lowering trial (LLT), in a subset of patients from the Antihypertensive and Lipid Lowering Treatment to Prevent Heart Attack Trial (ALLHAT). In this study (ALLHAT-LLT) in patients 55 years of age or older with well-controlled hypertension and moderately elevated LDL-cholesterol concentrations, the incidence of all-cause mortality or CHD-related adverse events (i.e., CHD death, nonfatal MI, stroke, congestive heart failure) was similar among patients receiving pravastatin sodium (40 mg daily) or usual care (i.e., moderate LDL-cholesterol lowering according to the discretion of the patient's primary care physician) for a mean duration of 4.8 years. The lack of clinical benefit may be attributable to the modest difference in total and LDL-cholesterol reduction between pravastatin and usual care recipients (17 versus 8% reduction in total cholesterol and 28 versus 11% reduction in LDL-cholesterol, respectively) compared with the differences reported in other statin trials. This modest difference may have resulted from poor adherence to initially prescribed therapy; at year 6 of follow-up, only 70% of patients randomized to receive pravastatin sodium were still taking the protocol-specified dosage (40 mg daily), while 28.5% of patients randomized to receive usual care were receiving antilipemic therapy (26.1% with a statin). Despite the reported lack of clinical benefit, the study results are consistent with previous findings indicating that lesser degrees of cholesterol lowering are associated with less clinical benefit. Adherence to treatment should be particularly emphasized when antilipemic therapy is implemented in routine clinical practice in order to achieve adequate reductions in LDL-cholesterol concentrations.

Secondary Prevention Pravastatin is used as an adjunct to nondrug therapies (i.e., lifestyle modifications) in patients with clinical evidence of CHD to reduce the risk of total mortality by reducing coronary death, to reduce the risk of MI, to reduce the risk of undergoing myocardial revascularization procedures, and to reduce the risk of stroke or transient ischemic attack (TIA).

The ACC/AHA cholesterol management guideline recommends statins as first-line therapy for secondary prevention in patients 21–75 years of age who have clinical ASCVD (i.e., acute coronary syndromes, history of MI, stable or unstable angina, coronary or other arterial revascularization, stroke, TIA, peripheral arterial disease presumed to be of atherosclerotic origin) unless contraindicated.

Several clinical trials designed to evaluate the benefits of pravastatin for secondary prevention of cardiovascular disease in patients with established CHD, including prior MI and angina pectoris, have reported improvements in cardiovascular risk status, as evidenced by reductions in the risks of total mortality and nonfatal coronary events. In the Cholesterol and Recurrent Events (CARE) study, therapy with pravastatin sodium (40 mg daily) in patients with prior MI and *average* cholesterol concentrations (baseline total, LDL-, and high-density lipoprotein [HDL]-cholesterol concentrations averaging 209, 139, and 39 mg/dL, respectively), was associated with a 24% reduction in fatal or nonfatal coronary events (i.e., CHD death, nonfatal MI) compared with placebo after an average follow-up period of approximately 5 years. Therapy with pravastatin also reduced the risk of undergoing myocardial revascularization procedures (e.g., coronary artery bypass grafting, percutaneous transluminal coronary angioplasty) by 27% and the risk of stroke or TIA by 26% (risk reduction of 31% for stroke alone). The reduction in the incidence of combined coronary events (coronary death, nonfatal MI, revascularization procedures, stroke or TIA) reported in the CARE trial also was observed in women, in geriatric patients (65 years of age and older), in patients with diabetes mellitus, and in those who had undergone coronary revascularization. Treatment with pravastatin also was associated with a reduction in overall mortality when compared with placebo. In the Long-term Intervention with Pravastatin in Ischaemic Disease (LIPID) study, therapy with pravastatin sodium (40 mg daily) in patients with a history of MI or hospitalization for unstable angina and *normal* or elevated total cholesterol concentrations resulted in reductions in overall mortality (22%), CHD mortality (24%), MI (29%), stroke (19%), and coronary revascularization procedures (20%) compared with placebo after an average follow-up period of 6.1 years.

Recent findings indicate that intensive antilipemic therapy may be more effective than moderate antilipemic therapy in reducing the risk of cardiovascular events in patients with acute coronary syndrome. In a randomized, double-blind, active-control study (Pravastatin or Atorvastatin Evaluation and Infection Therapy [PROVE-IT]) in over 4000 patients hospitalized for an acute coronary syndrome within the preceding 10 days, treatment with intensive antilipemic therapy (atorvastatin 80 mg daily) or moderate antilipemic therapy (pravastatin sodium 40 mg daily) for 2 years reduced LDL-cholesterol concentrations to a median of 62 or 95 mg/dL, respectively. Compared with the moderate regimen, treatment with the intensive regimen resulted in a 16% reduction in the composite risk of primary endpoints, including a 14% reduction in the need for revascularization procedures and a 29% reduction in the risk of recurrent unstable angina. Atorvastatin therapy also was associated with reductions in the endpoints of death from any cause (28%) and of death or MI (18%) compared with pravastatin therapy, but these differences were not statistically significant. Results of this study suggest that among patients who have recently had an acute coronary syndrome, an intensive antilipemic regimen provides greater protection against death or major cardiovascular events than does a standard regimen, and patients benefit from early and continued lowering of LDL-cholesterol to levels substantially below currently recommended target levels.

Reducing Progression of Coronary Atherosclerosis Pravastatin is used as an adjunct to nondrug therapies (e.g., dietary management) in patients with clinical evidence of CHD to slow the progression of coronary atherosclerosis.

Pravastatin has been shown to slow the progression and/or induce regression† of atherosclerosis in both coronary and carotid arteries by reducing intimal-medial wall thickness. In several double-blind, placebo-controlled studies (i.e., the Pravastatin Limitation of Atherosclerosis in the Coronary Arteries [PLAC I] and the Regression Growth Evaluation Statin Study [REGRESS] in men and women with clinical evidence of CHD and/or angina pectoris and normal to moderately elevated lipoprotein concentrations), progression of atherosclerosis at 2–3 years (measured as the mean per-patient changes from baseline in mean and minimal coronary artery lumen diameters, percent diameter stenosis, and formation of new lesions) was reduced in patients who received pravastatin sodium (40 mg daily) compared with that in those receiving placebo.

Treatment with pravastatin also has been shown to reduce the rate of progression of atherosclerosis in the carotid arteries. In several randomized, placebo-controlled studies (the Pravastatin, Lipids, and Atherosclerosis in the Carotid Arteries [PLAC II], the Kuopio Atherosclerosis Prevention Study [KAPS], the REGRESS subgroup study), hypercholesterolemic patients with or without CHD who received pravastatin sodium (20–40 mg daily) for a median of 2–3 years had less progression of atherosclerosis (as determined by B-mode ultrasound quantification of carotid artery intimal-medial thickness [IMT]) compared with those receiving placebo. Limited data indicate that pravastatin also may slow progression of atherosclerosis in patients with clinical evidence of CHD who have normal cholesterol concentrations.

Recent findings indicate that intensive antilipemic therapy may be more effective than moderate antilipemic therapy in slowing the progression of coronary atherosclerosis in patients with CHD. In a randomized, double-blind, active-control study (Reversal of Atherosclerosis with Aggressive Lipid Lowering [REVERSAL]) in 654 patients with CHD, treatment with intensive antilipemic therapy (atorvastatin 80 mg daily) or moderate antilipemic therapy (pravastatin sodium 40 mg daily) for 18 months reduced LDL-cholesterol concentrations to a mean of 79 or 110 mg/dL, respectively; concentrations of C-reactive protein were reduced by 36.4% in atorvastatin-treated patients and by 5.2% in pravastatin-treated patients. Treatment with the intensive regimen was associated with a substantially lower progression rate (measured by percent change in atheroma volume) compared with treatment with the moderate regimen. Compared with baseline values, patients treated with atorvastatin had no change in atheroma burden, whereas patients treated with pravastatin showed progression of coronary atherosclerosis. It has been suggested that the differences in atherosclerosis progression between atorvastatin and pravastatin may be related to the greater reduction in atherogenic lipoproteins and C-reactive protein concentrations in patients treated with atorvastatin.

Pooled data from several atherosclerosis regression trials in patients with documented CHD, including atherosclerosis and angina pectoris, and mild to moderate hypercholesterolemia indicate that treatment with pravastatin is associated with a reduction in the incidence of clinical events (i.e., death, MI, revascularization procedures) compared with that in patients receiving placebo.

Intensity of Statin Therapy The ACC/AHA cholesterol management guideline states that the appropriate intensity of a statin should be used to reduce the risk of ASCVD in patients most likely to benefit. Based on the average LDL-cholesterol response observed with specific statins and dosages used in the randomized controlled studies evaluated by the guideline expert panel, ACC/AHA considers pravastatin 10–20 mg daily to be a low-intensity statin (producing approximate LDL-cholesterol reductions of less than 30%) and pravastatin 40–80 mg daily to be a moderate-intensity statin (producing approximate LDL-cholesterol reductions of 30% to less than 50%). Individual patient response may vary in clinical practice.

Combination Antilipemic Therapy The ACC/AHA cholesterol management guideline states that nonstatin drugs may be useful adjuncts to statin therapy in certain high-risk patients (e.g., patients with ASCVD, LDL-cholesterol concentrations of at least 190 mg/dL, or diabetes mellitus) who have a less-than-anticipated response to statins, are unable to tolerate a less-than-recommended intensity of a statin, or are completely intolerant to statin therapy, particularly if there is evidence from randomized controlled studies suggesting that the addition of the nonstatin drug further reduces ASCVD events. If combination therapy is necessary, selection of the nonstatin drug should be based on the risk and benefit profile (i.e., reduction in ASCVD risk outweighs the drug's potential for adverse effects and drug interactions) and patient preferences.

■ **Dyslipidemias** Pravastatin is used as an adjunct to nondrug therapies (e.g., dietary management) to decrease elevated serum total and LDL-cholesterol, apolipoprotein B (apo B), and triglyceride concentrations, and to increase HDL-cholesterol concentrations in the treatment of primary hypercholesterolemia and mixed dyslipidemia, primary dysbetalipoproteinemia, and/or hypertriglyceridemia. Patients with homozygous familial hypercholesterolemia usually respond poorly to combined dietary management and drug therapy, including regimens containing a statin, in part because these patients have poorly functioning, few, or no LDL receptors. The manufacturer states that efficacy of pravastatin remains to be established in patients with elevated chylomicrons as their primary lipid abnormality.

Nondrug therapies and measures specific for the type of dyslipidemia (therapeutic lifestyle changes) are the initial treatments of choice, including dietary management (e.g., restriction of total and saturated fat and cholesterol intake, addition of plant stanols/sterols and viscous fiber to diet), weight control, an appropriate program of physical activity, and management of potentially contributory disease. Drug therapy is not a substitute for but an adjunct to these nondrug therapies and measures, which should be continued when drug therapy is initiated.

Primary Hypercholesterolemia or Mixed Dyslipidemia Pravastatin is used as an adjunct to nondrug therapies (e.g., dietary management) in adults to decrease elevated serum total and LDL-cholesterol, apo B, and triglyceride concentrations, and to increase HDL-cholesterol concentrations in the treatment of primary hypercholesterolemia or mixed dyslipidemia (Fredrickson type IIa or IIb). Pravastatin also is used as an adjunct to dietary therapy and therapeutic lifestyle changes in the management of heterozygous familial hypercholesterolemia in children 8 years of age and older who, despite an adequate trial of dietary management, have a serum LDL-cholesterol concentration of 190 mg/dL or greater *or* a serum LDL-cholesterol concentration of 160 mg/dL or greater and either a family history of premature cardiovascular disease or 2 or more other cardiovascular risk factors. Statins such as pravastatin also are used in combination with fenofibrate to decrease triglyceride concentrations and increase HDL-cholesterol concentrations in patients with mixed dyslipidemia and CHD (or CHD risk equivalents) who are receiving optimal statin therapy; however, no additional benefit on cardiovascular morbidity and mortality has been demonstrated with such combination therapy beyond that already established with statin monotherapy.

Reductions in total and LDL-cholesterol produced by usual dosages of pravastatin sodium substantially exceed those of placebo and appear to be similar to or less than those produced by monotherapy with usual dosages of some other antilipemic agents. Mean reductions in total cholesterol concentrations of 13–27%, LDL-cholesterol concentrations of 21–37%, and triglyceride concentrations of 9–24% have been reported in controlled and uncontrolled studies in patients with primary hypercholesterolemia who received 5–80 mg of pravastatin daily for at least 6 weeks. Modest and variable increases in HDL-cholesterol concentrations (2–12%) also were observed in these patients. In long-term controlled and uncontrolled studies (at least 36 weeks), mean total and LDL-cholesterol reductions of 20–29 and 26–34%, respectively, were observed with 40 mg of pravastatin daily.

Reductions in total and LDL-cholesterol concentrations produced by usual dosages of pravastatin sodium appear to be similar to or less than those produced by monotherapy with most other statins (e.g., atorvastatin, lovastatin, rosuvastatin, simvastatin). In a randomized, multicenter, parallel-group study comparing the efficacy of various statins, patients with hypercholesterolemia who received pravastatin sodium 10–40 mg daily experienced similar or smaller reductions in plasma total and LDL-cholesterol concentrations (13–24 and 19–34%, respectively) than those who received atorvastatin 10–80 mg daily (28–4% and 38–54%, respectively), lovastatin 20–80 mg daily (21–36 and 29–48%, respectively), and simvastatin 10–40 mg daily (21–30 and 28–41%, respectively). However, patients receiving pravastatin sodium dosages of 10–40 mg daily had greater reductions in plasma total and LDL-cholesterol concentrations (13–24 and 19–34%, respectively) than those who received fluvastatin 20–40 mg daily (13–19 and 17–23%, respectively).

Limited data from comparative studies suggest that reductions in total and LDL-cholesterol concentrations produced by pravastatin may be similar to or greater than those of other antilipemic agents (i.e., bile acid sequestrants, niacin, fibric acid derivatives). In 2 placebo-controlled studies comparing 12–24 weeks of pravastatin sodium therapy (40–80 mg daily) with that of cholestyramine (24 g daily in 2 divided doses) in patients with primary hypercholesterolemia, total and LDL-cholesterol reductions with pravastatin (24–30 and 30–39%, respectively) were similar to those with cholestyramine (18–23 and 28–32%, respectively); effects on increasing HDL-cholesterol concentrations also were similar (5–8% for pravastatin versus 5% for cholestyramine). However, pravastatin was more effective than cholestyramine in improving triglyceride concentrations, as evidenced by 13–19% decreases in pravastatin-treated patients and 12–21% increases in cholestyramine-treated patients. Pravastatin appears to be more effective than niacin or gemfibrozil in reducing total and LDL-cholesterol concentrations but less effective than these agents in reducing triglycerides and increasing HDL-cholesterol concentrations. In several randomized, comparative studies in patients with primary types IIa and IIb hyperlipoproteinemia, therapy with pravastatin sodium 40 mg daily produced greater reductions in total and LDL-cholesterol concentrations (23–26 and 30–34%, respectively) than niacin 1–4 g daily in 2 or 3 divided doses (11 and 16%, respectively) or gemfibrozil 600 mg twice daily (14–15 and 16–17%, respectively); however, reductions in triglyceride (4–14%) and increases in HDL-cholesterol concentrations (3–6%) associated with pravastatin therapy were less pronounced than those reported with niacin (32% reduction and 27% increase) or gemfibrozil (37–42% reduction and 13–15% increase).

The combination of pravastatin and other antilipemic agents (e.g., bile acid sequestrants, niacin, fibric acid derivatives) generally results in additive antilipemic effects; however, the risk of myopathy and rhabdomyolysis may be increased. (See Combination Antilipemic Therapy under Uses: Prevention of Cardiovascular Events.) The addition of a bile acid sequestrant to pravastatin therapy further reduced LDL-cholesterol by 14–20%, resulting in overall LDL-cholesterol reductions of 45–51% in patients receiving pravastatin 40 mg daily and cholestyramine 24 g daily. Combining niacin (1–3 g daily in 2 or 3 divided doses) with pravastatin sodium (20–40 mg daily) for 8–18 weeks in hypercholesterolemic patients with or without documented CHD further reduced total cholesterol, LDL-cholesterol, apo B, and triglyceride concentrations by 9, 9–11, 11, and 20–27%, respectively, and increased HDL-cholesterol and apo A concentrations by 3–29 and 11%, respectively. Similar effects also were observed in diabetic patients with hyperlipidemia who received low-dose pravastatin sodium (20 mg daily) and niacin (500 mg 3 times daily) therapy for 4 weeks. Pravastatin (40 mg daily) in combination with gemfibrozil (600 mg twice daily) in patients with primary hypercholesterolemia further reduced triglyceride concentrations by 28% and increased HDL-cholesterol concentrations by 11%. The increased risk of adverse skeletal muscle effects should be considered when pravastatin is used in combination with some antilipemic agents (i.e., fibric acid derivatives, niacin at lipid-modifying dosages [at least 1 g daily]). (See Drug Interactions: Antilipemic Agents, in the HMG-CoA Reductase Inhibitors General Statement 24:06.08.)

Primary Dysbetalipoproteinemia Pravastatin is used as an adjunct to nondrug therapies (e.g., dietary management) for the treatment of primary dysbetalipoproteinemia (Fredrickson type III) in patients who do not respond adequately to diet.

Treatment with pravastatin has resulted in substantial reductions in total and LDL-cholesterol, VLDL-cholesterol, triglyceride, and non-HDL-cholesterol concentrations. In several small double-blind, crossover studies in a limited number of patients with primary dysbetalipoproteinemia who received pravastatin 40 mg daily, total cholesterol, LDL-cholesterol, VLDL-cholesterol, triglyceride, and non-HDL-cholesterol concentrations decreased by 31–33, 30–41, 36–44, 12–24, and 36–37%, respectively.

Hypertriglyceridemia Pravastatin is used as an adjunct to nondrug therapies (e.g., dietary management) in the treatment of elevated serum triglyceride concentrations (Fredrickson type IV). AHA states that although statins have consistently shown benefit in subgroups with or without high triglyceride concentrations, fibric acid derivatives have more commonly been shown to provide greater benefit in subgroups with increased triglyceride concentrations.

Mean reductions in total cholesterol concentrations of 22%, LDL-cholesterol concentrations of 32%, triglyceride concentrations of 21%, and non-HDL-cholesterol concentrations of 27% have been reported in a subgroup analysis of a double-blind, placebo-controlled study in patients with hypertriglyceridemia who received 40 mg of pravastatin daily for a median of 4.9 years. Modest increases in HDL-cholesterol concentrations (7%) also were observed in these patients.

■ **Other Uses** Pravastatin has been shown to slow the progression and/or induce regression of atherosclerosis in a few patients without clinical evidence of CHD† who had mild to moderate elevations of LDL-cholesterol.The drug also has reduced transient myocardial ischemia† in male patients with clinical evidence of CHD or unstable angina pectoris.

While some statins have been shown to reduce the rate of restenosis† following coronary stent implantation, pravastatin has not been shown to reduce the incidence of restenosis in patients undergoing coronary balloon angioplasty.

Pravastatin has reduced total and LDL-cholesterol concentrations in patients with hypercholesterolemia associated with or exacerbated by diabetes mellitus† (diabetic dyslipidemia), cardiac† or liver† transplantation, or nephrotic syndrome† (nephrotic hyperlipidemia).

For additional information on the role of pravastatin or other statins in the treatment of lipoprotein disorders, prevention of cardiovascular events, or other uses, see General Principles of Antilipemic Therapy and see Uses in the HMG-CoA Reductase Inhibitors General Statement 24:06.08.

Dosage and Administration

■ **Administration** Pravastatin sodium is administered orally. The drug may be taken without regard to meals or time of day.

Patients should be placed on a standard cholesterol-lowering diet before initiation of pravastatin therapy and should remain on this diet during treatment with the drug. For recommendations on dietary and other nondrug therapies (i.e., lifestyle modifications), consult the most recent American Heart Association (AHA)/American College of Cardiology (ACC) Guideline on Lifestyle Management to Reduce Cardiovascular Risk (available at http://www.cardiosource.org or http://my.americanheart.org).

Adherence to lifestyle modifications and to statin therapy are required for atherosclerotic cardiovascular disease (ASCVD) risk reduction and, thus, should be reinforced periodically.

■ **Dosage** Dosage of pravastatin sodium must be carefully adjusted according to individual requirements and response. Dosage should be increased at intervals of no less than 4 weeks until the desired effect on lipoprotein concentrations is observed. Serum lipoprotein concentrations should be determined periodically during pravastatin therapy. The ACC/AHA cholesterol management guideline states that lipoprotein concentrations should be determined within 4–12 weeks following initiation of statin therapy (to determine the patient's response to therapy and adherence) and monitored every 3–12 months thereafter as clinically indicated.

Prevention of Cardiovascular Events The ACC/AHA cholesterol management guideline states that the appropriate intensity of statin therapy should be used to reduce ASCVD risk in patients most likely to benefit. Giving a maximally tolerated statin intensity should be emphasized over giving lower statin dosages and adding nonstatin drugs to address low HDL-cholesterol or high triglyceride concentrations, a strategy that has not yet been shown to reduce ASCVD risk. It should be noted that although 80 mg once daily is an FDA-labeled dosage of pravastatin, this dosage was not evaluated in randomized controlled studies reviewed by the ACC/AHA expert panel.

Primary Prevention. For primary prevention of cardiovascular disease in patients 21 years of age and older without clinical ASCVD who have primary, severe elevations in low-density lipoprotein (LDL)-cholesterol concentration (*190 mg/dL or greater*), the ACC/AHA cholesterol management guideline recommends that high-intensity statin therapy (i.e., with atorvastatin or rosuvastatin) be initiated unless contraindicated. (See Atorvastatin Calcium or Rosuvastatin Calcium 24:06.08.)

For primary prevention of cardiovascular disease in patients 40–75 years of age with *type 1 or 2 diabetes mellitus*† and LDL-cholesterol concentrations of 70–189 mg/dL, the ACC/AHA cholesterol management guideline recommends that moderate-intensity statin therapy (e.g., pravastatin 40–80 mg once daily) be initiated or continued. In those with an estimated 10-year ASCVD risk of 7.5% or higher, it is reasonable to consider high-intensity statin therapy (i.e., with atorvastatin or rosuvastatin) unless contraindicated. In patients with diabetes mellitus who are younger than 40 or older than 75 years of age, it is reasonable to evaluate the potential benefits, adverse effects, drug interactions, and patient preferences when deciding to initiate, continue, or intensify statin therapy.

For primary prevention of cardiovascular disease in patients 40–75 years of age without clinical ASCVD or diabetes mellitus who have LDL-cholesterol concentrations of 70–189 mg/dL and an *estimated 10-year ASCVD risk of 7.5% or higher*, the ACC/AHA cholesterol management guideline recommends that moderate- (e.g., pravastatin 40–80 mg once daily) to high-intensity statin therapy (i.e., with atorvastatin or rosuvastatin) be initiated or continued. (See Atorvastatin Calcium or Rosuvastatin Calcium 24:06.08.) In those with an estimated 10-year ASCVD risk of 5 to less than 7.5%, it is reasonable to offer treatment with moderate-intensity statin therapy. Before initiating statin therapy for primary prevention of ASCVD in patients 40–75 years of age without clinical ASCVD or diabetes mellitus who have LDL-cholesterol concentrations of 70–189 mg/dL, it is reasonable for clinicians and patients to discuss the potential benefits, adverse effects, drug interactions, and patient preferences for such therapy.

Secondary Prevention. For secondary prevention of cardiovascular disease in patients 21–75 years of age with *clinical ASCVD*, the ACC/AHA cholesterol management guideline recommends that high-intensity statin therapy (i.e., with atorvastatin or rosuvastatin) be initiated or continued unless contraindicated. In patients 21–75 years of age with clinical ASCVD who are at increased risk for developing statin-associated adverse effects or in whom high-intensity statin therapy is inappropriate or contraindicated, moderate-intensity statin therapy (e.g., pravastatin 40–80 mg once daily) should be given if tolerated. In patients older than 75 years of age with clinical ASCVD, use of statin therapy should be individualized based on the potential benefits, adverse effects, drug interactions, and patient preferences; it is reasonable to consider initiating or continuing moderate-intensity statin therapy in such patients if tolerated.

Dyslipidemias The recommended initial dosage of pravastatin sodium in adults is 40 mg daily. If antilipemic response is inadequate with the initial dosage, the manufacturer states that dosage may be increased to 80 mg daily.

The recommended dosage of pravastatin sodium in children 8–13 or 14–18 years of age is 20 or 40 mg once daily, respectively. Safety and efficacy of dosages exceeding 20 or 40 mg daily in children 8–13 or 14–18 years of age, respectively, have not been evaluated. The manufacturer states that children and adolescents treated with pravastatin should be reevaluated in adulthood, and antilipemic therapy should then be modified appropriately.

The cholesterol-lowering effects of pravastatin sodium and bile acid sequestrants (e.g., cholestyramine) are additive or synergistic. However, since bile acid sequestrants may bind and delay absorption of pravastatin sodium, the manufacturer recommends that pravastatin sodium be administered 1 hour or more before and at least 4 hours after the bile acid sequestrant when these drugs are used concomitantly.

Because of an increased risk of myopathy during concomitant therapy, patients receiving immunosuppressive drugs such as cyclosporine concomitantly with pravastatin should receive an initial pravastatin sodium dosage of 10 mg daily at bedtime; titration to higher dosages should be done with caution. Most patients treated with this drug combination received a maximum pravastatin sodium dosage of 20 mg daily. The manufacturer states that in patients receiving cyclosporine, dosage of pravastatin sodium should not exceed 20 mg daily.

In patients receiving clarithromycin, dosage of pravastatin sodium should not exceed 40 mg daily.

Dosage Modification The ACC/AHA cholesterol management guideline states that decreasing the statin dosage in adults may be considered when LDL-cholesterol concentrations are less than 40 mg/dL on 2 consecutive measurements; however, there are no data to suggest that LDL-cholesterol concentrations below 40 mg/dL would increase the risk of adverse effects.

■ **Dosage in Renal and Hepatic Impairment** Patients with severe renal impairment should receive an initial pravastatin sodium dosage of 10 mg daily.

Pravastatin should be used with caution in patients who consume substantial amounts of alcohol, in patients who have a recent (less than 6 months) history of liver disease, and in those with manifestations of liver disease (e.g., unexplained increases in aminotransferase concentrations, jaundice). Pravastatin is *contraindicated* in patients with active liver disease or unexplained, persistent increases in serum aminotransferase concentrations.

Cautions

Pravastatin shares the toxic potentials of other statins, and the usual cautions, precautions, and contraindications associated with these drugs should be observed. Patients should be fully advised about the risks, especially rhabdomyolysis, associated with statin therapy alone or combined with other drugs. (See Cautions and also see Drug Interactions in the HMG-CoA Reductase Inhibitors General Statement 24:06.08.)

Data from controlled studies indicate that safety and tolerability of pravastatin at a dosage of 80 mg daily is similar to those at lower dosages. However, single instances of elevated serum creatine kinase (CK, creatine phosphokinase, CPK) concentrations exceeding 10 times the upper limit of normal occurred more frequently in patients receiving 80 mg daily (4 of 464 patients) than in those receiving 40 mg daily (none of 115 patients).

■ **Pediatric Precautions** In several randomized, double-blind, placebo-controlled studies in children 8 years of age and older, the adverse effect profile of pravastatin sodium (20–40 mg daily for 2 years) generally was similar to that of placebo; dosages exceeding 20 or 40 mg daily in children 8–13 or 14–18 years of age, respectively, have not been evaluated. There were no detectable differences in height, weight, testicular volume, or Tanner score in pravastatin-treated children compared with those who received placebo. There also were no detectable differences in endocrine parameters (i.e., corticotropin [ACTH], cortisol, dehydroepiandrosterone sulfate [DHEA-S], follicle stimulating hormone [FSH], luteinizing hormone [LH], thyrotropin [TSH], estradiol [in girls], testosterone [in boys]) relative to placebo. If therapy with pravastatin is considered, the manufacturer states that female children and adolescents of child-bearing potential should be advised to use effective and appropriate contraceptive methods during therapy to reduce the likelihood of unintended pregnancy. (See Cautions: Pregnancy, Fertility, and Lactation.) Safety and efficacy of pravastatin have not been evaluated in children younger than 8 years of age.

For additional information on the use of statins in pediatric patients, see Cautions: Pediatric Precautions in the HMG-CoA Reductase Inhibitors General Statement 24:06.08.

■ **Geriatric Precautions** Of the 6593 patients receiving pravastatin in 2 secondary prevention studies, 36.1% were 65 years of age or older, and 0.8% were 75 years of age or older. No overall differences in efficacy (i.e., reduction in cardiovascular events, modification of lipoprotein profiles) or safety were observed between geriatric and younger patients, and other clinical experience has not revealed age-related differences in response. Data from a pharmacokinetic study indicate that mean area under the plasma concentration-time curve (AUC) of pravastatin is 25–50% higher in geriatric individuals compared with younger adults. However, because mean peak plasma concentration, time to peak plasma concentration, and half-life are similar between geriatric and younger individuals, substantial accumulation of pravastatin would not be expected in geriatric patients.

Because advanced age (65 years of age or older) is a predisposing factor for myopathy, pravastatin should be used with caution in geriatric patients. The ACC/AHA cholesterol management guideline states that initiation of statin therapy for primary prevention of atherosclerotic cardiovascular disease (ASCVD) in patients older than 75 years of age requires consideration of additional factors, including increasing comorbidities, safety considerations, and priorities of care. Therefore, the potential for an ASCVD risk reduction benefit, adverse effects, and drug interactions, along with patient preferences, must be considered before initiating statin therapy in patients older than 75 years of age.

■ **Mutagenicity and Carcinogenicity** Pravastatin did not exhibit mutagenic potential in vitro with or without metabolic activation in microbial mutagen tests using mutant strains of *Salmonella typhimurium* or *Escherichia coli*, a forward mutation assay in L5178Y TK +/- mouse lymphoma cells, a chromosomal aberration test in hamster cells, and a gene conversion assay using *Saccharomyces cerevisiae*. The drug also did not exhibit mutagenic potential in vivo in a dominant lethal test in mice or a micronucleus test in mice.

In rats receiving oral pravastatin sodium dosages of 10, 30, or 100 mg/kg daily for 2 years, there was an increased incidence of hepatocellular carcinomas in males receiving the highest dosage. These effects in rats were observed at approximately 12 or 4 times the maximum human dosage (80 mg daily), based on body surface area (mg/m^2 or AUC, respectively.

In mice receiving oral pravastatin sodium dosages of 250 and 500 mg/kg for 2 years, there was an increased incidence of hepatocellular carcinomas in males and females receiving both dosages. There also was an increased incidence of lung adenomas in females receiving these dosages. Serum drug levels were 15 times (250 mg/kg daily) and 23 times (500 mg/kg daily) those observed in humans given 80 mg of pravastatin daily, based on AUC. In another study in mice receiving oral pravastatin sodium dosages up to 100 mg/kg daily (approximately 2 times the maximum human dosage of 80 mg daily based on AUC) for 2 years, no drug-induced tumors were reported.

■ **Pregnancy, Fertility, and Lactation** ***Pregnancy*** Safety of pravastatin has not been established in pregnant women; there are no known benefits of continued use of the drug during pregnancy. Limited published data are insufficient to determine whether pravastatin is associated with a risk of major congenital malformations or miscarriage. Since atherosclerosis is a chronic process, discontinuance of antilipemic agents during pregnancy generally should not have a substantial effect on the outcome of long-term therapy for primary hypercholesterolemia.

Pravastatin was not teratogenic in rats receiving dosages up to 1000 mg/kg daily (120 times the usual human exposure based on body surface area in mg/m^2) or in rabbits receiving dosages up to 50 mg/kg daily (10 times the usual human exposure based on body surface area in mg/m^2). However, another statin has produced skeletal malformations in rats and mice.

Cholesterol and other products of the cholesterol biosynthetic pathway are essential for fetal development, including synthesis of steroids and cell membranes. Because of the ability of statins such as pravastatin to decrease the synthesis of cholesterol and possibly other products of the cholesterol biosynthetic pathway, pravastatin may cause fetal harm when administered to pregnant women. Rarely, congenital anomalies have been reported following intrauterine exposure to other statins. Therefore, pravastatin is *contraindicated* in women who are or may become pregnant. The drug should be discontinued immediately if pregnancy is known or suspected. Women of childbearing potential should use effective contraception while receiving the drug. Pravastatin should be administered to women of childbearing age only when such patients are highly unlikely to conceive and have been informed of the potential hazards. If the patient becomes pregnant while receiving pravastatin, the drug should be discontinued immediately and the patient informed of the potential hazard to the fetus.

Fertility Effects of statins on spermatogenesis and fertility have not been studied in adequate numbers of patients. In rats receiving pravastatin sodium in dosages up to 500 mg/kg daily, no adverse effects on fertility or general reproductive performance were observed. However, decreased fertility (20%) with sperm abnormalities were observed in juvenile male rats receiving pravastatin sodium at a dosage producing an AUC of 90 times that achieved with a 40-mg dose in humans.

Lactation Pravastatin is distributed into human milk. Effects of the drug on breast-fed infants or milk production are not known. Because of the potential for serious adverse reactions from pravastatin in nursing infants, the drug is *contraindicated* in nursing women; women who require pravastatin therapy should not breast-feed their infants.

Chemistry and Stability

■ **Chemistry** Pravastatin sodium is a mevinic acid-derivative antilipemic agent. The drug is a hydroxymethylglutaryl-CoA (HMG-CoA) reductase inhibitor (statin) and is pharmacologically related to mevastatin (compactin, not commercially available) and other statins (e.g., atorvastatin, fluvastatin, lovastatin, simvastatin). Pravastatin is structurally related to lovastatin and simvastatin but differs from these agents by the substitution of a hydroxyl group for the methyl group on the hexahydronaphthalene ring. This structural modification increases the hydrophilicity of pravastatin, making it approximately 100-fold more soluble in water than lovastatin or simvastatin. The octanol/water (pH 7) partition coefficient (log P) for pravastatin is approximately 0.59; the octanol/water coefficient for pravastatin is lower than that for lovastatin or simvastatin (log P 50 or log P 115, respectively).

Unlike the lactone prodrugs lovastatin and simvastatin, pravastatin exists as an active hydroxy acid and does not require hydrolysis in vivo. Pravastatin is similar structurally to HMG-CoA and competes with this compound for interaction with HMG-CoA reductase.

Pravastatin sodium occurs as an odorless, white to off-white, fine or crystalline powder that is soluble in water and methanol, having solubilities of greater than 300 mg/mL. Pravastatin sodium is slightly soluble in isopropanol and practically insoluble in acetone, acetonitrile, chloroform, and ether.

■ **Stability** Pravastatin sodium tablets should be stored in well-closed, light-resistant containers at 25°C, but may be exposed to temperatures ranging from 15–30°C; the tablets should be protected from moisture. When stored under these conditions, the tablets are stable for 24 months after the date of manufacture.

For further information on chemistry and stability, pharmacology, pharmacokinetics, uses, cautions, drug interactions, laboratory test interferences, and dosage and administration of pravastatin, see the HMG-CoA Reductase Inhibitors General Statement 24:06.08.

Preparations

Excipients in commercially available drug preparations may have clinically important effects in some individuals; consult specific product labeling for details.

Pravastatin Sodium

Oral		
Tablets	10 mg*	**Pravastatin Sodium Tablets**
	20 mg*	**Pravachol®**, Bristol-Myers Squibb
		Pravastatin Sodium Tablets
	40 mg*	**Pravachol®**, Bristol-Myers Squibb
		Pravastatin Sodium Tablets
	80 mg*	**Pravachol®**, Bristol-Myers Squibb
		Pravastatin Sodium Tablets

*available from one or more manufacturer, distributor, and/or repackager by generic (nonproprietary) name

†Use is not currently included in the labeling approved by the US Food and Drug Administration

Rosuvastatin Calcium

■ Rosuvastatin calcium, a hydroxymethylglutaryl-CoA (HMG-CoA) reductase inhibitor (i.e., statin), is an antilipemic agent.

Uses

Rosuvastatin is used as an adjunct to nondrug therapies (i.e., lifestyle modifications) for prevention of cardiovascular events and for the management of dyslipidemias.

■ **Prevention of Cardiovascular Events** The American College of Cardiology (ACC)/American Heart Association (AHA) cholesterol management guideline recommends statins as first-line therapy for prevention of atherosclerotic cardiovascular disease (ASCVD) in adults. There is extensive evidence demonstrating that statins can substantially reduce ASCVD risk when used for secondary prevention or primary prevention (in high-risk patients). Because the relative reduction in ASCVD risk is correlated with the degree of low-density lipoprotein (LDL)-cholesterol lowering, the maximum tolerated statin intensity should be used to achieve optimum ASCVD benefits. According to the ACC/AHA guidelines, rosuvastatin may be used for primary or secondary† prevention in adults when moderate- or high-intensity statin therapy is indicated. (See Prevention of Cardiovascular Events under Dosage and Administration: Dosage.) Nonstatin therapies do not provide acceptable ASCVD risk reduction benefits compared to their potential for adverse effects in the routine prevention of ASCVD. For additional details on prevention of ASCVD, see the HMG-CoA Reductase Inhibitors General Statement 24:06.08 and also consult the most recent ACC/AHA Guideline on the Treatment of Blood Cholesterol to Reduce Atherosclerotic Cardiovascular Risk in Adults (available at http://www.cardiosource.org or http://my.americanheart.org).

Primary Prevention Rosuvastatin is used as an adjunct to nondrug therapies (i.e., lifestyle modifications) in patients *without* clinical evidence of coronary heart disease (CHD) who have an increased risk of cardiovascular disease based on age (men 50 years of age or older, women 60 years of age or older), high-sensitivity C-reactive protein (hsCRP) concentrations of 2 mg/L or greater, and at least one additional cardiovascular disease risk factor (e.g., hypertension, low high-density lipoprotein [HDL]-cholesterol concentrations, smoking, family history of premature CHD) to reduce the risk of stroke or myocardial infarction (MI) and to reduce the risk of undergoing arterial revascularization procedures.

The ACC/AHA cholesterol management guideline recommends statins as first-line therapy for primary prevention in patients 21 years of age and older without clinical ASCVD who have primary, severe elevations in LDL-cholesterol concentration (190 mg/dL or greater); patients 40–75 years of age with type 1 or 2 diabetes mellitus; and patients 40–75 years of age with LDL-cholesterol concentrations of 70–189 mg/dL and an estimated 10-year ASCVD risk of 7.5% or higher. Before initiating statin therapy for primary prevention in patients without clinical ASCVD or diabetes mellitus, it is reasonable for clinicians and patients to discuss the potential for ASCVD risk reduction benefits, adverse effects, and drug interactions, as well as patient preferences for treatment.

In the Justification for the Use of Statins in Prevention: an Intervention Trial Evaluating Rosuvastatin (JUPITER) study in 17,802 patients (men 50 years of age or older and women 60 years of age or older) without clinical evidence of cardiovascular disease who had LDL-cholesterol concentrations of less than 130 mg/dL and hsCRP concentrations of 2 mg/L or greater, therapy with rosuvastatin (20 mg daily) for a mean of 2 years reduced the risk of major cardiovascular events (i.e., composite of cardiovascular death, nonfatal MI, nonfatal stroke, and hospitalization for unstable angina or an arterial revascularization procedure) by 44% compared with placebo. Aside from reducing the risk of the primary composite end point, rosuvastatin also substantially reduced the risk of certain individual components of the primary end point (i.e., nonfatal MI, nonfatal stroke, arterial revascularization procedure), as well as the risk of *any* (fatal and nonfatal) MI and stroke. However, there were no treatment differences among the rosuvastatin and placebo groups for death secondary to cardiovascular causes or hospitalization for unstable angina. At one year, rosuvastatin increased HDL-cholesterol concentrations and reduced LDL-cholesterol, hsCRP, total cholesterol, and serum triglyceride concentrations compared with placebo. In a post hoc subgroup analysis of 1405 patients with hsCRP concentrations of 2 mg/L or greater and no other traditional risk factors (smoking, blood pressure of at least 140/90 mmHg or taking antihypertensives, low HDL-cholesterol concentrations) other than age, there was no substantial treatment benefit associated with rosuvastatin after adjustment for high HDL-cholesterol concentrations.

Reducing Progression of Coronary Atherosclerosis Rosuvastatin is used as an adjunct to dietary therapy to slow the progression of atherosclerosis as part of a treatment strategy to lower total and LDL-cholesterol concentrations to target levels.

In the Measuring Effects on Intima Media Thickness: an Evaluation of Rosuvastatin (METEOR) study in 984 patients with elevated LDL-cholesterol concentrations and subclinical atherosclerosis (as determined by carotid intimal-medial thickness [cIMT]) who were at low risk (Framingham risk less than 10% over 10 years) for symptomatic coronary artery disease, therapy with rosuvastatin (40 mg daily) for 2 years slowed progression of atherosclerosis (as determined by B-mode ultrasound of the rate of change in mean maximum cIMT) compared with placebo. However, rosuvastatin did not induce disease regression.

Intensity of Statin Therapy The ACC/AHA cholesterol management guideline states that the appropriate intensity of a statin should be used to reduce the risk of ASCVD in patients most likely to benefit. Based on the average LDL-cholesterol response observed with specific statins and dosages used in the randomized controlled studies evaluated by the guideline expert panel, ACC/AHA considers rosuvastatin 5–10 mg daily to be a moderate-intensity statin (producing approximate LDL-cholesterol reductions of 30% to less than 50%) and rosuvastatin 20–40 mg daily to be a high-intensity statin (producing average LDL-cholesterol reductions of at least 50%). However, individual response may vary in clinical practice.

Combination Antilipemic Therapy The ACC/AHA cholesterol management guideline states that nonstatin drugs may be useful adjuncts to statin therapy in certain high-risk patients (e.g., patients with ASCVD, LDL-cholesterol concentrations of at least 190 mg/dL, or diabetes mellitus) who have a less-than-anticipated response to statins, are unable to tolerate a less-than-recommended intensity of a statin, or are completely intolerant to statin therapy, particularly if there is evidence from randomized controlled studies suggesting that the addition of the nonstatin drug further reduces ASCVD events. If combination therapy is necessary, selection of the nonstatin drug should be based on the risk and benefit profile (i.e., reduction in ASCVD risk outweighs the drug's potential for adverse effects and drug interactions) and patient preferences.

Patients with Chronic Kidney Disease The potential benefits of rosuvastatin in patients with chronic kidney disease, a population at high risk of cardiovascular disease, were evaluated in the Study to Evaluate the Use of Rosuvastatin in Subjects on Regular Hemodialysis (AURORA), a randomized, double-blind study in 2776 patients undergoing hemodialysis. In this study, therapy with rosuvastatin 10 mg daily for a median duration of 3.8 years did not substantially reduce the primary composite end point of cardiovascular death, nonfatal MI, or nonfatal stroke compared with placebo.

■ **Dyslipidemias** Rosuvastatin is used as an adjunct to dietary therapy for the management of primary hyperlipidemia or mixed dyslipidemia, hypertriglyceridemia, primary dysbetalipoproteinemia, and/or homozygous familial hypercholesterolemia. Efficacy of rosuvastatin in patients with Fredrickson type I or V dyslipidemia has not been established.

Primary Hyperlipidemia or Mixed Dyslipidemia **Adults.** Rosuvastatin is used as an adjunct to nondrug therapies (e.g., dietary management) in adults to reduce elevated total cholesterol, LDL-cholesterol, apolipoprotein B (apo B), non-HDL-cholesterol, and triglyceride concentrations, and to increase HDL-cholesterol concentrations in the management of primary hyperlipidemia or mixed dyslipidemia. Efficacy of rosuvastatin in patients with hyperlipidemia or mixed dyslipidemia has been established in placebo-controlled studies and in comparative studies with other statins (e.g., atorvastatin, pravastatin, simvastatin). Statins such as rosuvastatin also are used in combination with fenofibrate to decrease triglyceride concentrations and increase HDL-cholesterol concentrations in patients with mixed dyslipidemia and CHD (or CHD risk equivalents) who are receiving optimal statin therapy; however, no additional benefit on cardiovascular morbidity and mortality has been demonstrated with such combination therapy beyond that already established with statin monotherapy.

Reductions in total cholesterol and LDL-cholesterol concentrations achieved with usual dosages of rosuvastatin substantially exceed those with placebo or compared with baseline values. In a dose-ranging study in patients with primary hyperlipidemia, mean reductions in total cholesterol averaged 33, 36, 40, or 46% with rosuvastatin dosages of 5, 10, 20, or 40 mg, respectively, compared with 5% with placebo; corresponding reductions in LDL-cholesterol concentrations were 45, 52, 55, or 63%, respectively, versus 7% with placebo, while increases in HDL-cholesterol averaged 13, 14, 8, or 10%, respectively, versus 3% with placebo.

In a 6-week comparative study in more than 2200 patients (approximately 50% were women and about 30% were 65 years of age or older) with primary hyperlipidemia, reductions in LDL-cholesterol concentrations in patients receiving rosuvastatin (10 mg daily) exceeded those with atorvastatin (10 mg daily), pravastatin (10, 20, or 40 mg daily), or simvastatin (10, 20, or 40 mg daily). LDL-cholesterol reductions from baseline averaged 46, 52, or 55% with rosuvastatin 10, 20, or 40 mg, respectively, daily in these patients.

Rosuvastatin alone or combined with extended-release niacin improves the atherogenic lipid profile in patients with mixed dyslipidemia and low HDL-cholesterol concentrations. In a 24-week, randomized, double-blind study, LDL-cholesterol reductions averaged 48, 0.1, 42, or 36% in patients receiving rosuvastatin 40 mg daily, extended-release niacin 2 g daily, rosuvastatin 40 mg plus extended-release niacin 1 g daily, or rosuvastatin 10 mg plus extended-release niacin 2 g daily, respectively; HDL-cholesterol concentrations with these regimens were increased by 11, 12, 17, or 24%, respectively. Reductions in triglyceride concentrations and increases in HDL-cholesterol concentrations were similar with the highest dosage of rosuvastatin (40 mg daily) or extended-release niacin (2 g daily) given as monotherapy. Patients receiving rosuvastatin had a lower incidence of treatment-related adverse effects than those receiving niacin-containing regimens. (See Musculoskeletal Effects under Cautions: Warnings/Precautions and also Drug Interactions: Niacin.)

Pediatric Patients. Rosuvastatin is used as an adjunct to nondrug therapies (e.g., dietary management) to decrease elevated serum total cholesterol, LDL-cholesterol, and apo B concentrations in the management of heterozygous familial hypercholesterolemia in children and adolescents 8–17 years of age who, despite an adequate trial of dietary management, have a serum LDL-cholesterol concentration exceeding 190 mg/dL *or* a serum LDL-cholesterol concentration exceeding 160 mg/dL and either a family history of premature cardiovascular disease or 2 or more other cardiovascular risk factors. The long-term effect of rosuvastatin therapy in childhood on reducing cardiovascular morbidity and mortality in adulthood has not been established. For additional details on management of dyslipidemias in pediatric patients, see the HMG-CoA Reductase Inhibitors General Statement 24:06.08 and also consult the most recent Integrated Guidelines for Cardiovascular Health and Risk Reduction in Children and Adolescents (available at http://www.nhlbi.nih.gov).

Efficacy and safety of rosuvastatin in pediatric patients with heterozygous familial hypercholesterolemia were evaluated in a double-blind, placebo-controlled study and an open-label uncontrolled study. In the controlled study (which was followed by a 40-week, open-label, dose-titration phase), 176 children and adolescents 10–17 years of age with heterozygous familial hypercholesterolemia (mean baseline LDL-cholesterol concentration of 233 mg/dL) were randomized to receive either rosuvastatin (5, 10, or 20 mg daily) or placebo for 12 weeks; after 12 weeks of the double-blind phase, all patients entered an open-label phase and received rosuvastatin for an additional 40 weeks. Treatment with rosuvastatin resulted in substantial reductions in concentrations of total cholesterol, LDL-cholesterol (primary end point), and apo B compared with placebo during the 12-week double-blind phase. Mean reductions in total cholesterol averaged 30, 34, or 39% with rosuvastatin dosages of 5, 10, or 20 mg, respectively, compared with 0% with placebo; corresponding reductions in LDL-cholesterol concentrations were 38, 45, or 50%, respectively, versus 1% with placebo, and in apo B concentrations were 32, 38, or 41%, respectively, versus 2% with placebo. Changes in concentrations of triglycerides and HDL-cholesterol were similar in patients receiving rosuvastatin and in those receiving placebo. At the end of the 12-week double-blind phase, 12, 41, or 41% of patients receiving rosuvastatin dosages of 5, 10, or 20 mg achieved the LDL-cholesterol goal of less than 110 mg/dL compared with 0% of those receiving placebo. During the 40-week open-label phase, 71% of patients were titrated to the maximum rosuvastatin dosage of 20 mg daily and 41% of the patients achieved the LDL-cholesterol goal of less than 110 mg/dL.

In the open-label study (Hypercholesterolaemia in Children and Adolescents taking Rosuvastatin Open Label [CHARON]), 175 children and adolescents 8–17 years of age with heterozygous familial hypercholesterolemia (defined as a documented genetic defect in the LDL receptor or in apo B) and a mean baseline LDL-cholesterol concentration of 236 mg/dL received rosuvastatin at an initial dosage of 5 mg once daily, titrated to a maximum tolerated dosage of 10 mg daily (in patients 8–9 years of age) or 20 mg daily (in patients 10–17 years of age). The observed reductions in LDL-cholesterol concentrations from baseline were consistent across age groups and consistent with previous experience in controlled trials of adults and pediatric patients. At 24 months, LDL-cholesterol concentrations were reduced from baseline by approximately 35-43%; 48, 46, or 32% of patients receiving rosuvastatin dosages of 5, 10, or 20 mg daily, respectively, achieved the LDL-cholesterol goal of less than 110 mg/dL.

Homozygous Familial Hypercholesterolemia **Adults.** Rosuvastatin is used as an adjunct to other lipid-lowering therapies (e.g., plasma LDL-apheresis) or alone, if such therapies are not available, to reduce elevated total cholesterol, LDL-cholesterol, and apo B concentrations in adults with homozygous familial hypercholesterolemia. In an open-label, forced-titration study in 40 patients with homozygous familial hypercholesterolemia, therapy with rosuvastatin (20–40 mg daily [titrated at a 6-week interval]) decreased LDL-cholesterol concentrations by a mean of 22%. Approximately 33% of patients achieved additional (at least 6%) LDL-cholesterol lowering with an increase in the rosuvastatin dosage from 20 to 40 mg daily. Among the 27 patients with LDL-cholesterol reductions of 15% or greater, the mean LDL-cholesterol reduction achieved was 30%; among the 13 patients with LDL-cholesterol reductions of less than 15%, 3 had no change or an increase in LDL-cholesterol concentrations. LDL-cholesterol reductions of 15% or greater were observed in 3 of 5 patients with known receptor-negative status.

Pediatric Patients. Rosuvastatin is used alone or in combination with other lipid-lowering therapies (e.g., LDL apheresis) to decrease elevated serum LDL-cholesterol, total cholesterol, non-HDL-cholesterol, and apo B concentrations in children and adolescents 7–17 years of age with homozygous familial hypercholesterolemia as an adjunct to nondrug therapies (e.g., dietary management). In a double-blind, placebo-controlled crossover study in 14 children and adolescents 6 years of age or older with homozygous familial hypercholesterolemia (mean baseline LDL-cholesterol concentration of 416 mg/dL, 50% receiving apheresis, 57% receiving ezetimibe), treatment with rosuvastatin 20 mg daily for 6 weeks resulted in substantial reductions in concentrations of LDL-cholesterol (22.3%), total cholesterol (20.1%), non-HDL-cholesterol (22.9%), and apo B (17.1%) compared with placebo.

Hypertriglyceridemia Rosuvastatin is used as an adjunct to nondrug therapies (e.g., dietary management) in the treatment of hypertriglyceridemia. In a 6-week, double-blind, placebo-controlled study in patients with primary hypertriglyceridemia (baseline triglyceride concentrations of 273–817 mg/dL), triglyceride concentrations were reduced by a median of 21, 37, 37, or 43% with rosuvastatin dosages of 5, 10, 20, or 40 mg daily, respectively, and increased by a median of 1% with placebo. AHA states that although statins have consistently shown benefit in subgroups with or without high triglyceride concentrations, fibric acid derivatives have more commonly been shown to provide greater benefit in subgroups with increased triglyceride concentrations.

Primary Dysbetalipoproteinemia Rosuvastatin is used as an adjunct to nondrug therapies (e.g., dietary management) for the treatment of primary dysbetalipoproteinemia (Fredrickson type III).

In a double-blind, crossover study in 32 patients with primary dysbetalipoproteinemia (genotypes 27 apo E2/E2 and 4 apo-E mutation [Arg145Cys]), treatment with rosuvastatin (10 or 20 mg daily) for 6 weeks resulted in reductions in concentrations of non-HDL-cholesterol (48 or 56%, respectively), total cholesterol (43 or 48%, respectively), triglycerides (40 or 43%, respectively), combined intermediate-density lipoprotein (IDL)- and very low-density lipoprotein (VLDL)-cholesterol (47 or 56%, respectively), and circulating remnant lipoproteins.

For additional information on the role of rosuvastatin or other statins in the treatment of lipoprotein disorders, prevention of cardiovascular events, or other uses, see General Principles of Antilipemic Therapy and also Uses in the HMG-CoA Reductase Inhibitors General Statement 24:06.08.

Dosage and Administration

■ General Patients should be placed on a standard cholesterol-lowering diet before receiving rosuvastatin and should continue on this diet during treatment. For recommendations on dietary and other nondrug therapies (i.e., lifestyle modifications), consult the most recent American Heart Association (AHA)/American College of Cardiology (ACC) Guideline on Lifestyle Management to Reduce Cardiovascular Risk (available at http://www.cardiosource.org or http://my.americanheart.org).

The manufacturer states that serum lipoprotein concentrations should be determined within 2–4 weeks following initiation and/or titration of rosuvastatin, and that dosage should be adjusted accordingly. The ACC/AHA cholesterol management guideline states that lipoprotein concentrations should be determined within 4–12 weeks following initiation of statin therapy (to determine the patient's response to therapy and adherence) and monitored every 3–12 months thereafter as clinically indicated.

Adherence to lifestyle modifications and to statin therapy are required for atherosclerotic cardiovascular disease (ASCVD) risk reduction and, thus, should be reinforced periodically.

■ Administration Rosuvastatin is administered orally as a single dose at any time of day, with or without food; the tablets should be swallowed whole. Two doses of rosuvastatin should not be taken within 12 hours of each other.

■ Dosage Dosage of rosuvastatin calcium is expressed in terms of rosuvastatin.

When initiating rosuvastatin therapy or switching from another statin, the appropriate initial dosage of rosuvastatin should be used; dosage may then be carefully adjusted according to individual requirements (i.e., percent reduction in low-density lipoprotein [LDL]-cholesterol concentration) and response.

Prevention of Cardiovascular Events The ACC/AHA cholesterol management guideline states that the appropriate intensity of statin therapy should be used to reduce ASCVD risk in patients most likely to benefit. Giving a maximally tolerated statin intensity should be emphasized over giving lower statin dosages and adding nonstatin drugs to address low HDL-cholesterol or high triglyceride concentrations, a strategy that has not yet been shown to reduce ASCVD risk. It should be noted that although dosages of 5 and 40 mg once daily are FDA-labeled dosages of rosuvastatin, these dosages were not evaluated in randomized controlled studies reviewed by the ACC/AHA expert panel.

Primary Prevention. For primary prevention of cardiovascular disease in patients 21 years of age and older without clinical ASCVD who have primary, severe elevations in LDL-cholesterol concentration (*190 mg/dL or greater*), the ACC/AHA cholesterol management guideline recommends that high-intensity statin therapy (e.g., rosuvastatin 20–40 mg once daily) be initiated. In patients who are unable to tolerate high-intensity statin therapy, the maximum tolerated statin intensity should be used. The ACC/AHA cholesterol management guideline states that it is reasonable to intensify statin therapy to achieve at least a 50% reduction in LDL-cholesterol concentrations. In patients currently receiving the maximum intensity of statin therapy, addition of a nonstatin drug may be considered to achieve further reductions in LDL-cholesterol concentrations; however, the potential benefits and risks (e.g., adverse effects, drug interactions) of such combined therapy, along with patient preferences, should be considered.

For primary prevention of cardiovascular disease in patients 40–75 years of age with *type 1 or 2 diabetes mellitus*† and LDL-cholesterol concentrations of 70–189 mg/dL, the ACC/AHA cholesterol management guideline recommends that moderate-intensity statin therapy (e.g., rosuvastatin 5–10 mg once daily) be initiated or continued. In those with an estimated 10-year ASCVD risk of 7.5% or higher, it is reasonable to consider high-intensity statin therapy (e.g., rosuvastatin 20–40 mg once daily) unless contraindicated. In patients with diabetes mellitus who are younger than 40 or older than 75 years of age, it is reasonable to evaluate the potential benefits, adverse effects, drug interactions, and patient preferences when deciding to initiate, continue, or intensify statin therapy.

For primary prevention of cardiovascular disease in patients 40–75 years of age without clinical ASCVD or diabetes mellitus who have LDL-cholesterol concentrations of 70–189 mg/dL and *an estimated 10-year ASCVD risk of 7.5% or higher*, the ACC/AHA cholesterol management guideline recommends that moderate- (e.g., rosuvastatin 5–10 mg once daily) to high-intensity statin therapy (e.g., rosuvastatin 20–40 mg once daily) be initiated or continued. In those with an estimated 10-year ASCVD risk of 5 to less than 7.5%, it is reasonable to offer treatment with moderate-intensity statin therapy. Before initiating statin therapy for primary prevention of ASCVD in patients 40–75 years of age without clinical ASCVD or diabetes mellitus who have LDL-cholesterol concentrations of 70–189 mg/dL, it is reasonable for clinicians and patients to discuss the potential benefits, adverse effects, drug interactions, and patient preferences for such therapy.

Secondary Prevention. For secondary prevention† of cardiovascular disease in patients 21–75 years of age with *clinical ASCVD*, the ACC/AHA cholesterol management guideline recommends that high-intensity statin therapy (e.g., rosuvastatin 20–40 mg once daily) be initiated or continued unless contraindicated. In patients 21–75 years of age with clinical ASCVD who are at increased risk for developing statin-associated adverse effects or in whom high-intensity statin therapy is inappropriate or contraindicated, moderate-intensity statin therapy (e.g., rosuvastatin 5–10 mg once daily) should be given if tolerated. In patients older than 75 years of age with clinical ASCVD, use of statin therapy should be individualized based on the potential benefits, adverse effects, drug interactions, and patient preferences; it is reasonable to consider initiating or continuing moderate-intensity statin therapy in such patients if tolerated.

Dyslipidemias **General Dosage.** The usual initial dosage of rosuvastatin in adults is 10–20 mg once daily. The dosage range of rosuvastatin in adults is 5–40 mg once daily. The maximum 40-mg daily dosage of rosuvastatin should be used only for those patients who have not achieved their LDL-cholesterol goal with the 20-mg daily dosage.

Following initiation and/or titration of rosuvastatin dosage, lipoprotein concentrations should be determined within 2–4 weeks and dosage adjusted accordingly.

Heterozygous Familial Hypercholesterolemia in Pediatric Patients. The recommended dosage range of rosuvastatin for the management of heterozygous familial hypercholesterolemia in children 8 to less than 10 years of age is 5–10 mg once daily.

The recommended dosage range of rosuvastatin for the management of heterozygous familial hypercholesterolemia in children and adolescents 10–17 years of age is 5–20 mg once daily.

The maximum dosage of rosuvastatin in pediatric patients is 20 mg daily.

Homozygous Familial Hypercholesterolemia. The usual initial dosage of rosuvastatin in adults with homozygous familial hypercholesterolemia is 20 mg once daily.

The recommended dosage of rosuvastatin in children and adolescents 7–17 years of age with homozygous familial hypercholesterolemia is 20 mg once daily.

Concomitant Drug Therapy. In patients receiving concomitant cyclosporine, dosage of rosuvastatin should be limited. (See Drug Interactions: Cyclosporine.)

Concomitant use of rosuvastatin and gemfibrozil should be *avoided*; if concomitant use cannot be avoided, dosage of rosuvastatin should be limited. (See Gemfibrozil under Drug Interactions: Fibric Acid Derivatives.)

Caution is advised if rosuvastatin is used concomitantly with *ritonavir-boosted* atazanavir or with the fixed combination of lopinavir and ritonavir (lopinavir/ritonavir). Dosage of rosuvastatin should be limited. (Drug Interactions: HIV Protease Inhibitors.)

Caution is advised if rosuvastatin is used concomitantly with simeprevir. Dosage of rosuvastatin should be limited. (See Simeprevir under Drug Interactions: HCV Protease Inhibitors.)

Dosage Modification The ACC/AHA cholesterol management guideline states that decreasing the statin dosage in adults may be considered when LDL-cholesterol concentrations are less than 40 mg/dL on 2 consecutive measurements; however, there are no data to suggest that LDL-cholesterol concentrations below 40 mg/dL would increase the risk of adverse effects.

■ **Special Populations** ***Asian Patients*** The manufacturer recommends that an initial rosuvastatin dosage of 5 mg once daily be considered in Asian patients. (See Asian Patients under Warnings/Precautions: Specific Populations, in Cautions.)

Renal Impairment In patients with severe renal impairment (creatinine clearance less than 30 mL/minute per 1.73 m²) who are not undergoing hemodialysis, rosuvastatin should be initiated at a dosage of 5 mg once daily, and dosage should not exceed 10 mg once daily. (See Renal Impairment under Warnings/Precautions: Specific Populations, in Cautions.)

Hepatic Impairment The manufacturer makes no specific dosage recommendations at this time for patients with hepatic impairment. (See Cautions: Contraindications and also Hepatic Impairment under Warnings/Precautions: Specific Populations, in Cautions.)

Geriatric Patients Although there are no specific dosage recommendations for geriatric patients, caution is recommended when rosuvastatin is used in these patients. (See Geriatric Use under Warnings/Precautions: Specific Populations, in Cautions.)

Cautions

■ **Contraindications** Active liver disease, including unexplained, persistent elevations in hepatic aminotransferase (transaminase) concentrations.

Pregnancy. (See Fetal/Neonatal Morbidity and Mortality under Cautions: Warnings/Precautions.)

Lactation. (See Lactation under Warnings/Precautions: Specific Populations, in Cautions.)

Known hypersensitivity to rosuvastatin or any ingredient in the formulation. (See Sensitivity Reactions under Cautions: Warnings/Precautions.)

■ **Warnings/Precautions** ***Fetal/Neonatal Morbidity and Mortality*** Serum cholesterol and triglyceride concentrations increase during normal pregnancy, and cholesterol products are essential for fetal development; therefore, suppression of cholesterol biosynthesis by rosuvastatin during pregnancy may cause fetal harm. Atherosclerosis is a chronic process, and discontinuance of antilipemic drugs during pregnancy should have little impact on long-term outcomes of primary hyperlipidemia therapy. There is no known clinical benefit for continued use of antilipemic drugs during pregnancy.

Limited human data available to date have not identified an increased risk of major congenital malformations or miscarriage with the use of rosuvastatin during pregnancy; however, congenital anomalies following intrauterine exposure to other statins have been reported rarely. In animal studies, there were no adverse developmental effects when rosuvastatin was administered to rats and rabbits during the period of organogenesis at systemic exposures equivalent to the maximum recommended human dosage of 40 mg daily; decreased pup survival occurred at doses equivalent to or higher than the maximum recommended human dose. (See Pregnancy under Warnings/Precautions: Specific Populations, in Cautions.)

Musculoskeletal Effects Myopathy and rhabdomyolysis with acute renal failure secondary to myoglobinuria have been reported in patients receiving statins, including rosuvastatin. These adverse effects can occur at any dosage, but the risk is increased with the highest dosage of rosuvastatin (40 mg daily).

Rosuvastatin should be used with caution in patients with predisposing factors for myopathy (e.g., advanced age [65 years or older], renal impairment, inadequately treated hypothyroidism). The risk of myopathy may be increased when rosuvastatin is used concomitantly with some other antilipemic agents (niacin or certain fibric-acid derivatives [i.e., gemfibrozil]), cyclosporine, *ritonavir-boosted* atazanavir, the fixed combination of lopinavir and ritonavir (lopinavir/ritonavir), or simeprevir. (See Drug Interactions.)

The American College of Cardiology (ACC)/American Heart Association (AHA) cholesterol management guideline does not recommend routine monitoring of CK concentrations in patients receiving statin therapy. However, the guideline states that it is reasonable to obtain baseline CK concentrations in adults at increased risk of developing adverse musculoskeletal effects (e.g., patients with personal or family history of statin intolerance or muscle disease, patients receiving concomitant therapy with myotoxic drugs) before initiating statin therapy. During statin therapy, it is reasonable to measure CK concentrations in adults experiencing muscle symptoms (e.g., pain, tenderness, stiffness, cramping, weakness, generalized fatigue).

The National Heart, Lung, and Blood Institute (NHLBI)-appointed expert panel on integrated guidelines for cardiovascular health and risk reduction in children and adolescents states that baseline CK concentrations should be obtained before initiating statin therapy in pediatric patients. In addition, routine monitoring for muscle toxicity is strongly recommended in children and adolescents receiving statin therapy.

Rosuvastatin should be discontinued if CK concentrations become markedly elevated or if myopathy is diagnosed or suspected. Rosuvastatin therapy should be temporarily withheld in any patient experiencing an acute, serious condition suggestive of myopathy or predisposing to the development of renal failure secondary to rhabdomyolysis (e.g., sepsis; hypotension; dehydration; major surgery; trauma; severe metabolic, endocrine, or electrolyte disorders; uncontrolled seizures). (See Advice to Patients.)

For additional details on management of musculoskeletal effects in adults and pediatric patients, see Musculoskeletal Effects under Cautions: Precautions and Contraindications in the HMG-CoA Reductase Inhibitors General Statement 24:06.08 and also consult the most recent ACC/AHA Guideline on the Treatment of Blood Cholesterol to Reduce Atherosclerotic Cardiovascular Risk in Adults (available at http://www.cardiosource.org or http://my.americanheart.org) and the Integrated Guidelines for Cardiovascular Health and Risk Reduction in Children and Adolescents (available at http://www.nhlbi.nih.gov).

Hepatic Effects Increases in serum aminotransferase (i.e., AST [SGOT], ALT [SGPT]) concentrations have been reported in patients receiving statins, including rosuvastatin. These increases usually were transient and resolved or improved with continued therapy or after temporary interruption of therapy. In a pooled analysis of placebo-controlled studies, increases in serum aminotransferase concentrations exceeding 3 times the upper limit of normal (ULN) occurred in 1.1% of patients receiving rosuvastatin compared with 0.5% of those receiving placebo. Jaundice has been reported in at least 2 patients but resolved following discontinuance of rosuvastatin therapy; a causal relationship to rosuvastatin has not been established. Although liver failure and irreversible liver disease have not been reported in clinical studies evaluating rosuvastatin, cases of fatal and nonfatal hepatic failure have been reported rarely in patients receiving statins, including rosuvastatin, during postmarketing surveillance.

Liver function tests should be performed prior to initiation of rosuvastatin therapy and repeated as clinically indicated (e.g., presence of manifestations suggestive of liver damage). Although the manufacturer previously recommended more frequent monitoring of liver function (i.e., at 12 weeks following initiation of therapy or any increase in dosage, then periodically [e.g., semi-annually] thereafter), FDA concluded that serious statin-related liver injury is rare and unpredictable in individual patients, and that routine periodic monitoring of liver enzymes does not appear to be effective in detecting or preventing serious statin-related liver injury. The ACC/AHA cholesterol management guideline states that, during statin therapy, it is reasonable to obtain liver function tests in adults experiencing symptoms of hepatotoxicity (e.g., unusual fatigue or weakness, loss of appetite, abdominal pain, dark colored urine, yellowing of the skin or sclera). However, the NHLBI expert panel on integrated guidelines for cardiovascular health and risk reduction in children and adolescents states that routine monitoring of hepatic function is strongly recommended in children and adolescents receiving statin therapy.

If serious liver injury with clinical manifestations and/or hyperbilirubinemia or jaundice occurs, rosuvastatin therapy should be promptly interrupted. If an alternate etiology is not found, rosuvastatin therapy should not be restarted.

Rosuvastatin should be used with caution in patients who consume substantial amounts of alcohol and/or have a history of chronic liver disease. The drug is *contraindicated* in patients with active liver disease, including unexplained, persistent elevations in serum aminotransferase concentrations.

Interactions with Coumarin-derivative Anticoagulants Because rosuvastatin may potentiate the anticoagulant effects of coumarin-derivative anticoagulants, caution should be exercised when these agents are used concomitantly. If rosuvastatin is used concomitantly with coumarin-derivative anticoagulants, international normalized ratio (INR) should be stable before initiating rosuvastatin and should be monitored frequently enough during early therapy (or following adjustment of rosuvastatin dosage) to ensure that no substantial alteration in INR occurs.

Proteinuria and Hematuria Transient dipstick-positive proteinuria and microscopic hematuria (not associated with worsening renal function) have been reported in patients receiving rosuvastatin. These findings occurred more frequently in patients receiving rosuvastatin 40 mg compared with lower doses of rosuvastatin or comparator statins in clinical trials. Although the clinical importance of this finding is not known, dosage reduction should be considered in patients receiving rosuvastatin who have unexplained persistent proteinuria and/or hematuria during routine urinalysis testing.

Endocrine Effects Increases in glycosylated hemoglobin (hemoglobin A_{1c} [HbA_{1c}]) and fasting serum glucose concentrations have been reported in patients receiving statins, including rosuvastatin. Data from clinical trials and meta-analyses indicate that statin therapy may increase the risk of developing diabetes mellitus. In the JUPITER study, a higher incidence of diabetes mellitus was reported in patients receiving rosuvastatin (2.8%) compared with those receiving placebo (2.3%). In addition, mean HbA_{1c} was increased by 0.1% in patients receiving rosuvastatin compared with those receiving placebo, and the number of patients with an HbA_{1c} greater than 6.5% also was substantially higher among those receiving rosuvastatin. Despite these findings, FDA continues to believe that the cardiovascular benefits of statins outweigh these small increased risks. The ACC/AHA cholesterol management guideline states that patients receiving statin therapy should be evaluated for new-onset diabetes mellitus according to current diabetes screening guidelines. If diabetes mellitus develops during statin therapy, patients should be encouraged to adhere to a heart-healthy diet, engage in physical activity, achieve and maintain a healthy body weight, cease tobacco use, and continue statin therapy to reduce the risk of atherosclerotic cardiovascular disease (ASCVD).

Although clinical studies have shown that rosuvastatin alone does not reduce basal plasma cortisol concentration or impair adrenal reserve, statins interfere with cholesterol synthesis and theoretically may blunt adrenal or gonadal steroid hormone production. Caution should be exercised if rosuvastatin is used concomitantly with drugs that may decrease the levels or activity of endogenous steroid hormones (e.g., ketoconazole, spironolactone, cimetidine).

Sensitivity Reactions Hypersensitivity reactions, including rash, pruritus, urticaria, and angioedema, have been reported in patients receiving rosuvastatin.

Cognitive Impairment Cognitive impairment (e.g., memory loss, forgetfulness, amnesia, memory impairment, confusion) has been reported rarely with all statins during postmarketing surveillance. This adverse CNS effect generally was nonserious and reversible, with variable times to symptom onset (1 day to years) and symptom resolution (median of 3 weeks following discontinuance of statin therapy). Following review of available data (i.e., from the Adverse Event Reporting System [AERS] database, randomized clinical trials, observational studies, case reports), FDA concluded that cases of cognitive impairment did not appear to be associated with fixed or progressive dementia (e.g., Alzheimer's disease) or result in clinically important cognitive decline. Development of cognitive impairment did not appear to be associated with any specific statin, age of the patient, statin dosage, or concomitant drug therapy. Therefore, FDA continues to believe that the cardiovascular benefits of statins outweigh this small increased risk of cognitive impairment. The National Lipid Association (NLA) statin safety assessment task force recommends that patients experiencing manifestations consistent with cognitive impairment be evaluated and managed appropriately. The ACC/AHA cholesterol management guideline states that, in patients presenting with confusion or memory impairment, it is reasonable to evaluate the patient for statin as well as nonstatin causes (e.g., exposure to other drugs, systemic or neuropsychiatric causes).

Specific Populations **Pregnancy.** Safety of rosuvastatin has not been established in pregnant women; there are no known benefits of therapy with the drug during pregnancy. (See Cautions: Contraindications and also see Fetal/Neonatal Morbidity and Mortality under Cautions: Warnings/Precautions.)

Rosuvastatin should be discontinued immediately if pregnancy is known or suspected. Women of childbearing potential should use effective contraception while receiving the drug. (See Advice to Patients.)

Lactation. Limited data indicate that rosuvastatin is distributed into human milk; however, the effects of the drug on breast-fed infants or milk production are not known. Because of the potential for serious adverse reactions from rosuvastatin in nursing infants, the drug is *contraindicated* in nursing women. Women who require rosuvastatin therapy should not breast-feed their infants.

Pediatric Use. Safety and efficacy of rosuvastatin have not been established in pediatric patients younger than 8 years of age.

In a randomized, double-blind, placebo-controlled study in children and adolescents 10–17 years of age (females were at least 1 year postmenarche) with heterozygous familial hypercholesterolemia, the adverse effect profile of rosuvastatin (5–20 mg daily for 12 weeks) generally was similar to that of placebo. However, elevations in serum CK concentrations exceeding 10 times the ULN were observed more frequently in children receiving rosuvastatin compared with those receiving placebo; 3% of children receiving rosuvastatin (2 receiving 10 mg daily and 2 receiving 20 mg daily) had increased CK concentrations exceeding 10 times the ULN compared with 0% of those receiving placebo. Although controlled clinical studies of rosuvastatin in children younger than 10 years of age with heterozygous familial hypercholesterolemia have not been conducted, the drug was evaluated in a 2-year, open-label study that included patients 8–17 years of age with heterozygous familial hypercholesterolemia; results of this study showed that safety and efficacy of rosuvastatin in this age group generally were similar to those observed in the adult population. In a population pharmacokinetic analysis of the 2 pediatric studies in patients with heterozygous familial hypercholesterolemia, rosuvastatin exposure appeared similar to or less than that observed in adults. In a 6-week double-blind, crossover study that was followed by 12 weeks of open-label treatment in children and adolescents 7–15 years of age with homozygous familial hypercholesterolemia, the safety profile of rosuvastatin (20 mg daily) was consistent with that in adults.

In studies evaluating rosuvastatin in the pediatric population, there were no detectable adverse effects on growth, weight, body mass index (BMI), or sexual maturation in children and adolescents.

If rosuvastatin therapy is considered, the manufacturer states that adolescent girls should be advised to use effective and appropriate contraceptive methods during therapy to reduce the likelihood of unintended pregnancy. (See Fetal/Neonatal Morbidity and Mortality under Cautions: Warnings/Precautions.)

Geriatric Use. Of the 10,275 patients receiving rosuvastatin in clinical studies, 31% were 65 years of age or older, and 6.8% were 75 years of age or older. Although no overall differences in efficacy or safety were observed between geriatric and younger patients, and other clinical experience has not revealed age-related differences in response, the possibility that some geriatric patients may exhibit increased sensitivity to the drug cannot be ruled out. Plasma concentrations of rosuvastatin were similar between geriatric (65 years of age or older) and younger patients.

Since geriatric patients (65 years of age and older) are at increased risk of myopathy, rosuvastatin should be used with caution in such patients. (See Musculoskeletal Effects under Cautions: Warnings/Precautions.) The ACC/AHA cholesterol management guideline states that initiation of statin therapy for primary prevention of ASCVD in patients older than 75 years of age requires consideration of additional factors, including increasing comorbidities, safety considerations, and priorities of care. Therefore, the potential for an ASCVD risk reduction benefit, adverse effects, and drug interactions, along with patient preferences, must be considered before initiating statin therapy in patients older than 75 years of age.

Hepatic Impairment. Plasma concentrations of rosuvastatin are modestly increased in patients with chronic alcoholic liver disease. Peak plasma concentrations and AUC of rosuvastatin are increased by 60 and 5%, respectively, in patients with Child-Pugh class A disease and by 100 and 21%, respectively, in patients with Child-Pugh class B disease compared with individuals with normal liver function.

Rosuvastatin should be used with caution in patients with a history of liver disease (e.g., chronic alcoholic liver disease) and/or in patients who consume substantial amounts of alcohol. Rosuvastatin is *contraindicated* in patients with active liver disease, including unexplained, persistent elevations in hepatic aminotransferase concentrations.

Renal Impairment. Exposure to rosuvastatin (i.e., plasma concentrations) does not appear to be influenced by mild or moderate renal impairment (creatinine clearance of 30 mL/minute per 1.73 m^2 or greater). However, plasma concentrations of rosuvastatin were increased to a clinically important extent (about threefold) in patients with severe renal impairment (creatinine clearance less than 30 mL/minute per 1.73 m^2) not undergoing hemodialysis compared with healthy individuals (creatinine clearance greater than 80 mL/minute per 1.73 m^2). Steady-state plasma concentrations of rosuvastatin in patients undergoing chronic hemodialysis are approximately 50% higher than those in healthy individuals with normal renal function.

Dosage adjustments are required in patients with severe renal impairment who are not undergoing hemodialysis. (See Renal Impairment under Dosage and Administration: Special Populations.)

Asian Patients. Pharmacokinetic studies, including a large study conducted in the US, show an approximate twofold elevation in median exposure to rosuvastatin (peak plasma concentration and AUC) in Asian patients compared with Caucasian patients. Dosage of rosuvastatin should be adjusted in Asian patients.

Increased systemic exposure should be taken into consideration in such patients not adequately controlled at rosuvastatin dosages up to 20 mg daily. (See Asian Patients under Dosage and Administration: Special Populations.)

■ **Common Adverse Effects** Adverse effects reported in at least 2% of patients receiving rosuvastatin in clinical studies include headache, nausea, myalgia, asthenia, constipation, and abdominal pain.

Drug Interactions

Rosuvastatin is minimally (approximately 10%) metabolized by cytochrome P-450 (CYP) isoenzyme 2C9. Clearance of rosuvastatin is not dependent on metabolism by CYP3A4 to a clinically important extent.

■ **Drugs Affecting Transport Systems** Rosuvastatin is a substrate for the organic anion transport protein (OATP) 1B1 and the breast cancer resistance protein (BCRP). Concomitant use of rosuvastatin with drugs that are inhibitors of these transport proteins (e.g., cyclosporine, certain HIV protease inhibitors) may potentially result in increased plasma concentrations of rosuvastatin and an increased risk of myopathy. Clinicians should consult the relevant prescribing information of such drugs when concomitant use with rosuvastatin is being considered.

■ **Antacids** In a pharmacokinetic study, *simultaneous* administration of rosuvastatin (40 mg as a single dose) and an antacid containing aluminum hydroxide and magnesium hydroxide decreased rosuvastatin peak plasma concentration and area under the plasma concentration-time curve (AUC) by 50%; such effects were considered clinically important. In contrast, when the antacid and rosuvastatin were administered 2 hours apart, rosuvastatin peak plasma concentration and AUC were decreased by 20%. Therefore, if rosuvastatin and an aluminum-magnesium hydroxide antacid are used concomitantly, the antacid should be administered at least 2 hours after rosuvastatin.

■ **Azole Antifungals** ***Fluconazole*** Concomitant use of rosuvastatin (80 mg as a single dose) and fluconazole (200 mg once daily for 11 days) increased rosuvastatin peak plasma concentration and AUC by 1.1-fold.

Itraconazole Concomitant use of rosuvastatin (10 mg as a single dose) and itraconazole (200 mg once daily for 5 days) increased rosuvastatin peak plasma concentration and AUC by 1.4-fold. Concomitant use of a higher dose of rosuvastatin (80 mg) and itraconazole (200 mg once daily for 5 days) increased rosuvastatin peak plasma concentration and AUC by 1.2- and 1.3-fold, respectively.

Ketoconazole Concomitant use of rosuvastatin (80 mg as a single dose) and ketoconazole (200 mg twice daily for 7 days) had no effect on rosuvastatin peak plasma concentration and AUC.

■ **Colchicine** Myopathy, including rhabdomyolysis, has been reported in patients receiving various statins, including rosuvastatin, concomitantly with colchicine. Caution is advised if rosuvastatin is used concomitantly with colchicine.

■ **Cyclosporine** Concomitant use of rosuvastatin and cyclosporine increases plasma rosuvastatin concentrations, which may increase the risk of myopathy. Following concomitant use of rosuvastatin (10 mg once daily for 10 days) and cyclosporine (at a stable dosage of 75–200 mg twice daily), rosuvastatin peak plasma concentration and AUC were increased by 11- and 7.1-fold, respectively; such effects were considered clinically important. If used concomitantly with cyclosporine, dosage of rosuvastatin should not exceed 5 mg once daily.

■ **Digoxin** Concomitant use of rosuvastatin (40 mg once daily for 12 days) and digoxin (0.5 mg as a single dose) increased both peak plasma concentration and AUC of digoxin by 4%.

■ **Dronedarone** Concomitant use of rosuvastatin (10 mg as a single dose) and dronedarone (400 mg twice daily) increased rosuvastatin AUC by 1.4-fold.

■ **Eltrombopag** Concomitant use of rosuvastatin (10 mg as a single dose) and eltrombopag (75 mg once daily for 5 days) increased rosuvastatin peak plasma concentration and AUC by 2- and 1.6-fold, respectively.

■ **Erythromycin** Concomitant use of rosuvastatin (80 mg as a single dose) and erythromycin (500 mg 4 times daily for 7 days) decreased rosuvastatin peak plasma concentration and AUC by 30 and 20%, respectively.

■ **Ezetimibe** Concomitant use of rosuvastatin (10 mg once daily for 14 days) and ezetimibe (10 mg once daily for 14 days) increased rosuvastatin peak plasma concentration and AUC by 1.2-fold.

■ **Fibric Acid Derivatives** ***Fenofibrate*** Concomitant use of rosuvastatin and fenofibrate may increase the risk of myopathy. Following concomitant use of rosuvastatin (10 mg as a single dose) and fenofibrate (67 mg three times daily for 7 days), rosuvastatin peak plasma concentration was increased by 1.2-fold and AUC was unchanged; such effects were not considered clinically important. However, the manufacturer states that caution is advised if rosuvastatin is used concomitantly with fenofibrate. The ACC/AHA cholesterol management guideline states that the combination of fenofibrate and low- or moderate-intensity statin therapy may be considered only if the benefits from atherosclerotic cardiovascular disease (ASCVD) risk reduction or triglyceride lowering (when triglyceride concentrations exceed 500 mg/dL) outweigh the potential risk of adverse effects.

Gemfibrozil Concomitant use of rosuvastatin and gemfibrozil increases the risk of myopathy and/or rhabdomyolysis. Following concomitant use of rosuvastatin (80 mg as a single dose) and gemfibrozil (600 mg twice daily for 7 days), rosuvastatin peak plasma concentration and AUC were increased by 2.2- and 1.9-fold, respectively; such effects were considered clinically important. Concomitant use of rosuvastatin and gemfibrozil should be *avoided*; if concomitant use cannot be avoided, rosuvastatin should be initiated at a dosage of 5 mg once daily and dosage of the statin should not exceed 10 mg once daily.

■ **HCV Protease Inhibitors** Concomitant use of rosuvastatin with certain protease inhibitors has differing effects on exposure to rosuvastatin; in some cases, rosuvastatin exposure may be increased by up to threefold. Caution is advised if these drugs are used concomitantly.

Simeprevir Concomitant use of rosuvastatin and simeprevir may increase the risk of myopathy. Following concomitant use of rosuvastatin (10 mg as a single dose) and simeprevir (150 mg once daily for 7 days), rosuvastatin peak plasma concentration and AUC were increased by 3.2- and 2.8-fold, respectively; such effects were considered clinically important. If used concomitantly with simeprevir, rosuvastatin should be initiated at a dosage of 5 mg once daily and dosage of the statin should not exceed 10 mg once daily.

■ **HIV Protease Inhibitors** Concomitant use of rosuvastatin with certain *ritonavir-boosted* HIV protease inhibitors has differing effects on exposure to rosuvastatin; in some cases, rosuvastatin exposure may be increased by up to threefold. Caution is advised if these drugs are used concomitantly.

Atazanavir Concomitant use of rosuvastatin and *ritonavir-boosted* atazanavir may increase the risk of myopathy. Following concomitant use of rosuvastatin (10 mg as a single dose) and *ritonavir-boosted* atazanavir (atazanavir 300 mg with ritonavir 100 mg once daily for 8 days), rosuvastatin peak plasma concentration and AUC were increased by 7- and 3.1-fold, respectively; such effects were considered clinically important. If used concomitantly with *ritonavir-boosted* atazanavir, rosuvastatin should be initiated at a dosage of 5 mg once daily and dosage of the statin should not exceed 10 mg once daily.

Darunavir Following concomitant use of rosuvastatin (10 mg once daily for 7 days) and *ritonavir-boosted* darunavir (darunavir 600 mg with ritonavir 100 mg twice daily for 7 days), rosuvastatin peak plasma concentration and AUC were increased by 2.4- and 1.5-fold, respectively.

Fosamprenavir Concomitant use of rosuvastatin and *ritonavir-boosted* fosamprenavir produces minimal to no change in exposure to rosuvastatin. Following concomitant use of rosuvastatin (10 mg as a single dose) and *ritonavir-boosted* fosamprenavir (fosamprenavir 700 mg with ritonavir 100 mg twice daily for 7 days), rosuvastatin peak plasma concentration and AUC were increased by 1.5- and 1.1-fold, respectively.

Lopinavir Concomitant use of rosuvastatin and the fixed combination of lopinavir and ritonavir (lopinavir/ritonavir) may increase the risk of myopathy. Following concomitant use of rosuvastatin (20 mg once daily for 7 days) and lopinavir/ritonavir (lopinavir 400 mg/ritonavir 100 mg twice daily for 17 days), rosuvastatin peak plasma concentration and AUC were increased by 5- and 2.1-fold, respectively; such effects were considered clinically important. If used concomitantly with lopinavir/ritonavir, rosuvastatin should be initiated at a dosage of 5 mg once daily and dosage of the statin should not exceed 10 mg once daily.

Tipranavir Concomitant use of rosuvastatin and *ritonavir-boosted* tipranavir produces minimal to no change in exposure to rosuvastatin. Following concomitant use of rosuvastatin (10 mg as a single dose) and *ritonavir-boosted* tipranavir (tipranavir 500 mg with ritonavir 200 mg twice daily for 11 days), rosuvastatin peak plasma concentration and AUC were increased by 2.2- and 1.4-fold, respectively.

■ **Lomitapide** Following concomitant use of rosuvastatin (20 mg as a single dose) and lomitapide (10 mg once daily for 7 days), peak plasma concentration and AUC of rosuvastatin were increased by 6 and 2%, respectively. Following concomitant use of rosuvastatin (20 mg as a single dose) and lomitapide (60 mg once daily for 7 days), peak plasma concentration and AUC of rosuvastatin were increased by 4 and 32%, respectively. Dosage adjustment of rosuvastatin is not required during concomitant use with lomitapide.

■ **Niacin** Concomitant use of rosuvastatin and antilipemic dosages (1 g daily or higher) of niacin may increase the risk of myopathy. Data from several large randomized studies indicate that concomitant use of niacin (1.5–2 g daily) with another statin (i.e., simvastatin 40–80 mg once daily, with or without ezetimibe) resulted in an increased risk of severe adverse effects, including disturbances in glycemic control requiring hospitalization, development of diabetes mellitus, adverse GI effects, myopathy, gout, rash, skin ulceration, infection, and bleeding.

Caution is advised if rosuvastatin is used concomitantly with antilipemic dosages of niacin.

■ **Omega-3-acid Ethyl Esters** Concomitant administration of rosuvastatin (40 mg daily) with omega-3-acid ethyl esters (4 g daily) for 14 days did not affect the rate or extent of exposure to rosuvastatin at steady state.

■ **Oral Contraceptives** Concomitant use of rosuvastatin (40 mg once daily for 28 days) and an oral contraceptive (ethinyl estradiol 0.035 mg with norgestrel 0.18, 0.215, and 0.25 mg once daily for 21 days) resulted in a 25 or 26% increase in ethinyl estradiol peak plasma concentration or AUC, respectively, and a 23 or 34% increase in norgestrel peak plasma concentration or AUC, respectively.

■ **Rifampin** Concomitant use of rosuvastatin (20 mg as a single dose) and rifampin (450 mg once daily for 7 days) did not affect rosuvastatin AUC.

■ **Warfarin** Rosuvastatin potentiates the effects of coumarin-derivative anticoagulants in prolonging prothrombin time (PT)/international normalized ratio (INR); the drug has been shown to substantially increase INR in patients receiving coumarin anticoagulants. Following concomitant use of rosuvastatin (40 mg once daily for 10 days) and warfarin sodium (25 mg as a single dose), AUC of *R*- or *S*-warfarin was increased by 4 or 6%, respectively, while peak plasma concentration of *R*- or *S*-warfarin was decreased by 1% or unchanged, respectively; such effects resulted in clinically important pharmacodynamic effects. Caution should be exercised when rosuvastatin is used concomitantly with anticoagulants. If rosuvastatin is used concomitantly with coumarin-derivative anticoagulants, INR should be stable prior to initiating rosuvastatin and should be monitored frequently enough during early therapy (or following adjustment of rosuvastatin dosage) to ensure that no substantial alteration in INR occurs.

Description

Rosuvastatin calcium is a synthetic heptenoic acid-derivative antilipemic agent. The drug is a selective, competitive inhibitor of 3-hydroxymethylglutaryl-CoA (HMG-CoA) reductase (i.e., statin), an enzyme that catalyzes the conversion of HMG-CoA to mevalonate (an early and rate-limiting step in cholesterol biosynthesis). Rosuvastatin reduces total and low-density lipoprotein (LDL)-cholesterol, apolipoprotein B (apo B), non-high-density lipoprotein (HDL)-cholesterol, and triglyceride concentrations, and increases HDL-cholesterol concentrations in patients with primary hyperlipidemia or mixed dyslipidemia. Rosuvastatin also reduces triglyceride concentrations in patients with primary hypertriglyceridemia.

Rosuvastatin is not extensively metabolized; approximately 10% of a radiolabeled dose is recovered as metabolite. The major metabolite is *N*-desmethyl rosuvastatin, which is formed principally by cytochrome P-450 (CYP) isoenzyme 2C9. Clearance of rosuvastatin is not dependent on metabolism by CYP3A4 to a clinically important extent. Based on in vitro studies, *N*-desmethyl rosuvastatin has approximately 17–50% of the HMG-CoA reductase inhibitory activity of the parent drug. The parent drug accounts for greater than 90% of the active plasma HMG-CoA reductase inhibitory activity. Rosuvastatin is a substrate for the organic anion transport protein (OATP) 1B1 and the breast cancer resistance protein (BCRP). Genetic polymorphism of the OATP1B1 gene may affect rosuvastatin exposure. Higher plasma rosuvastatin concentrations have been reported in a limited number of patients with 2 reduced-function variant OATP1B1 alleles. The frequency of this genotype (SLCO1B1 521 C/C) generally is less than 5% in most populations. The effect of this genetic variation on efficacy and safety of rosuvastatin has not been established. Rosuvastatin and its metabolites are mainly eliminated in feces (90%) following oral administration. The elimination half-life of rosuvastatin is approximately 19 hours. Following an IV dose, approximately 28% of total body clearance was via the renal route and 72% by the hepatic route.

Advice to Patients

Importance of advising patients to read the manufacturer's patient information.

Importance of adhering to nondrug therapies and measures, including adherence to a heart-healthy diet, regular exercise, avoidance of tobacco products, and maintenance of a healthy weight.

Importance of informing patients that 2 doses of rosuvastatin should not be taken within 12 hours of each other.

Risk of myopathy and/or rhabdomyolysis; risk is increased with higher dosages (i.e., 40 mg daily) or when used concomitantly with certain other drugs. Importance of promptly reporting any unexplained muscle pain, tenderness, or weakness, particularly if accompanied by malaise or fever, or if manifestations persist after discontinuance of therapy.

Risk of adverse hepatic effects. Importance of promptly reporting any symptoms suggestive of liver injury (e.g., fatigue, anorexia, right upper abdominal discomfort, dark urine, jaundice).

Risk of nonserious, reversible cognitive impairment (e.g., memory loss, forgetfulness, amnesia, memory impairment, confusion).

Risk of increased glucose concentrations and development of type 2 diabetes mellitus; may need to monitor glucose concentrations following initiation of statin therapy.

Importance of advising women and adolescent girls to avoid pregnancy (i.e., using effective and appropriate contraceptive methods) during therapy; if the patient becomes pregnant, importance of discontinuing rosuvastatin and contacting a clinician.

Importance of avoiding breast-feeding during therapy.

Importance of informing clinicians of existing or contemplated concomitant therapy, including prescription and OTC drugs, as well as any concomitant illnesses.

Importance of informing patients of other important precautionary information. (See Cautions.)

Overview® (see Users Guide). For additional information on this drug until a more detailed monograph is developed and published, the manufacturer's labeling should be consulted. It is *essential* that the manufacturer's labeling be consulted for more detailed information on usual cautions, precautions, contraindications, potential drug interactions, laboratory test interferences, and acute toxicity.

Preparations

Excipients in commercially available drug preparations may have clinically important effects in some individuals; consult specific product labeling for details.

Rosuvastatin Calcium

Oral		
Tablets	5 mg (of rosuvastatin)*	**Crestor®**, AstraZeneca
		Rosuvastatin Tablets
	10 mg (of rosuvastatin)*	**Crestor®**, AstraZeneca
		Rosuvastatin Tablets
	20 mg (of rosuvastatin)*	**Crestor®**, AstraZeneca
		Rosuvastatin Tablets
	40 mg (of rosuvastatin)*	**Crestor®**, AstraZeneca
		Rosuvastatin Tablets

*available from one or more manufacturer, distributor, and/or repackager by generic (nonproprietary) name

†Use is not currently included in the labeling approved by the US Food and Drug Administration

Simvastatin

Synvinolin

■ Simvastatin, a hydroxymethylglutaryl-CoA (HMG-CoA) reductase inhibitor (statin), is an antilipemic agent.

Uses

■ **Prevention of Cardiovascular Events** The American College of Cardiology (ACC)/American Heart Association (AHA) cholesterol management guideline recommends statins as first-line therapy for prevention of atherosclerotic cardiovascular disease (ASCVD) in adults. There is extensive evidence demonstrating that statins can substantially reduce ASCVD risk when used for secondary prevention or primary prevention (in high-risk patients). Because the relative reduction in ASCVD risk is correlated with the degree of low-density lipoprotein (LDL)-cholesterol lowering, the maximum tolerated statin intensity should be used to achieve optimum ASCVD benefits. According to the ACC/AHA guidelines, simvastatin may be used for primary† or secondary prevention in adults when moderate-intensity statin therapy is indicated. (See Prevention of Cardiovascular Events under Dosage and Administration: Dosage.) Nonstatin therapies do not provide acceptable ASCVD risk reduction benefits compared to their potential for adverse effects in the routine prevention of ASCVD. For additional details on prevention of ASCVD, see the HMG-CoA Reductase Inhibitors General Statement 24:06.08 and also consult the most recent ACC/AHA Guideline on the Treatment of Blood Cholesterol to Reduce Atherosclerotic Cardiovascular Risk in Adults (available at http://www.cardiosource.org or http://my.americanheart.org).

Secondary Prevention Simvastatin is used as an adjunct to nondrug therapies (e.g., lifestyle modification) in patients with coronary heart disease (CHD) or CHD risk equivalents (i.e., risk factors that confer a risk for major coronary events equal to that of established CHD, such as diabetes mellitus, peripheral arterial disease, history of stroke or other cerebrovascular disease) to reduce the risk of total mortality by reducing CHD deaths, to reduce the risk of nonfatal myocardial infarction (MI) and stroke, and to reduce the need for coronary and noncoronary revascularization procedures.

The ACC/AHA cholesterol management guideline recommends statins as first-line therapy for secondary prevention in patients 21–75 years of age who have clinical ASCVD (i.e., acute coronary syndromes [ACS]; history of MI, stable or unstable angina, coronary or other arterial revascularization, stroke, transient ischemic attack [TIA], or peripheral arterial disease presumed to be of atherosclerotic origin) unless contraindicated.

Several clinical trials designed to evaluate the benefits of simvastatin in patients with established CHD have reported improvements in the risk of cardiovascular events, as evidenced by reductions in the risks of total mortality and nonfatal coronary events. In the Scandinavian Simvastatin Survival Study (4S), therapy with simvastatin in 4444 patients with hypercholesterolemia and angina pectoris or prior MI was associated with reductions in total mortality (30%), CHD mortality (42%), and hospital-verified nonfatal MI (37%) compared with placebo over a median of 5.4 years of follow-up; the risk of undergoing myocardial revascularization procedures also was reduced by 37%. In addition, simvastatin therapy reduced the risk of fatal and nonfatal cerebrovascular events (combined incidence of stroke and TIA) by 28%. The reduction in the combined coronary events (nonfatal MI and revascularization procedures) reported in the 4S trial also was observed in women, geriatric patients (65 years of age and older), and in patients with diabetes mellitus. Unlike some prior studies of cholesterol-lowering therapy, an increased risk of death from noncardiovascular causes was not observed in patients receiving simvastatin therapy in this study.

In the Heart Protection Study (HPS), therapy with simvastatin (40 mg daily) in over 20,000 patients with CHD, history or stroke or other cerebrovascular disease, other occlusive arterial disease (e.g., peripheral arterial disease), hypertension or diabetes mellitus reduced the risk of total mortality (13%), CHD mortality (18%), nonfatal MI (38%), ischemic stroke (25%), coronary revascularization procedures (30%), and peripheral and other noncoronary revascularization procedures (16%) compared with placebo over approximately 5 years of follow-up, irrespective of baseline lipoprotein concentrations.

In another randomized, double-blind study (A to Z trial) in about 4500 patients who had manifestations of ACS within the preceding 5 days, treatment with intensive antilipemic therapy (simvastatin 40 mg daily for 1 month, then simvastatin 80 mg daily thereafter) for 6–24 months resulted in a 25% reduction in the risk of cardiovascular mortality compared with moderate antilipemic therapy (placebo for 4 months, then simvastatin 20 mg daily thereafter); there was a reduction (11%) in the rate of the primary endpoint (a composite of cardiovascular death, nonfatal MI, readmission for ACS, and stroke) for the entire study period but this difference failed to reach statistical significance. However, while no difference was evident between the intensive and moderate regimens during the first 4 months of therapy, from 4 months through the end of the study, the primary endpoint was substantially reduced (by 25%) in patients receiving the intensive regimen. Intensive or moderate antilipemic therapy reduced LDL-cholesterol concentrations to a median of 63 or 77 mg/dL, respectively, at 8 months. While a favorable trend toward reduction of major cardiovascular events was observed in this study, it is possible that more intensive therapy is required immediately after the onset of ACS during the period of greatest clinical instability to achieve a more rapid clinical benefit.

Simvastatin has been shown to slow the progression and/or induce regression of atherosclerosis in coronary arteries by reducing intimal-medial wall thickness. In the Multicenter Anti-Atheroma Study (MAAS) in hypercholesterolemic men and women with clinical evidence of CHD, progression of atherosclerosis at 2–4 years (measured as the mean per-patient changes from baseline in mean and minimal coronary artery lumen diameters, diameter stenosis, and formation of new lesions) was reduced in patients who received simvastatin (20 mg daily) compared with those receiving placebo.

Intensity of Statin Therapy The ACC/AHA cholesterol management guideline states that the appropriate intensity of a statin should be used to reduce the risk of ASCVD in patients most likely to benefit. Based on the average LDL-cholesterol response observed with specific statins and dosages used in the randomized controlled studies evaluated by the guideline expert panel, ACC/AHA considers simvastatin 10 mg daily to be a low-intensity statin (producing approximate LDL-cholesterol reductions of less than 30%) and simvastatin 20–40 mg daily to be a moderate-intensity statin (producing approximate LDL-cholesterol reductions of 30% to less than 50%). Individual patient response may vary in clinical practice.

Combination Antilipemic Therapy The ACC/AHA cholesterol management guideline states that nonstatin drugs may be useful adjuncts to statin therapy in certain high-risk patients (e.g., patients with ASCVD, LDL-cholesterol concentrations of at least 190 mg/dL, or diabetes mellitus) who have a less-than-anticipated response to statins, are unable to tolerate a less-than-recommended intensity of a statin, or are completely intolerant to statin therapy, particularly if there is evidence from randomized controlled studies suggesting that the addition of the nonstatin drug further reduces ASCVD events. If combination therapy is necessary, selection of the nonstatin drug should be based on the risk and benefit profile (i.e., reduction in ASCVD risk outweighs the drug's potential for adverse effects and drug interactions) and patient preferences.

Although early findings from the Ezetimibe and Simvastatin in Hypercholesterolemia Enhances Atherosclerosis Regression (ENHANCE) study demonstrated that combination therapy with simvastatin and ezetimibe was not superior to simvastatin monotherapy in reducing carotid intimal-medial wall thickness (cIMT), a more recent study (the Improved Reduction of Outcomes: Vytorin® Efficacy International [IMPROVE-IT]) in 18,144 post-ACS patients with baseline LDL-cholesterol concentrations of 50–125 mg/dL (or 50–100 mg/dL if they were receiving lipid-lowering therapy) showed that the addition of ezetimibe (10 mg daily) to simvastatin (40 mg daily) therapy not only produced a 24% further reduction in LDL-cholesterol concentrations, but also improved cardiovascular outcomes (a composite of cardiovascular death, nonfatal MI, unstable angina requiring hospitalization, coronary revascularization, or nonfatal stroke) compared with simvastatin (40 mg daily) monotherapy. Treatment with the simvastatin and ezetimibe combination resulted in an absolute risk reduction of 2% over 7 years for the primary composite end point.

The addition of niacin to statin-based therapy has not been shown to provide an incremental benefit in reducing cardiovascular morbidity and mortality beyond that already demonstrated with statin-based therapy. In the Impact on Global Health Outcomes (AIM-HIGH) study, the combination of extended-release niacin (1.5–2 g daily) and statin-based therapy (simvastatin 40–80 mg once daily, with or without ezetimibe 10 mg daily) was compared with statin-based therapy alone in patients with established cardiovascular disease (i.e., documented stable CHD, cerebrovascular or carotid disease, peripheral arterial disease). Despite a favorable effect on serum lipid concentrations (median high-density lipoprotein [HDL]-cholesterol concentration increased from 35 to 42 mg/dL, triglyceride concentration decreased from 164 to 122 mg/dL, and LDL-cholesterol concentration decreased from 74 to 62 mg/dL), the addition of niacin to simvastatin-based therapy did not further reduce the incidence of the primary end point (i.e., composite of death from CHD, nonfatal MI, ischemic stroke, hospitalization for more than 23 hours for ACS, or symptom-driven coronary or cerebral revascularization) compared with simvastatin-based therapy alone over a follow-up period of 36 months. The addition of extended-release niacin to existing simvastatin-based therapy, however, did increase the risk of adverse effects (e.g., pruritus, flushing, adverse GI effects, increased blood glucose concentrations). The investigators of this study stated that whether such combination therapy provides incremental benefit in higher-risk patients or in those receiving suboptimal statin therapy remains to be established.

Data from another large randomized, double-blind, multicenter study involving 25,673 adults with cardiovascular disease confirmed findings of the AIM-HIGH study. In the Heart Protection Study 2–Treatment of HDL to Reduce the Incidence of Vascular Events (HPS2-THRIVE), the combination of extended-release niacin/laropiprant (2 g/40 mg daily) (no longer commercially available) and statin-based therapy (simvastatin 40 mg once daily, with or without ezetimibe 10 mg daily) was compared with statin-based therapy alone in patients with established cardiovascular disease (i.e., history of MI, cerebrovascular disease, peripheral arterial disease, diabetes mellitus with evidence of symptomatic coronary disease). Despite a favorable effect on serum lipid concentrations (additional 6-mg/dL increase in HDL-cholesterol concentration, 33-mg/dL reduction in triglyceride concentration, and 10-mg/dL reduction in LDL-cholesterol concentration), the addition of niacin/laropiprant to simvastatin-based therapy did not further reduce the incidence of major cardiovascular events (i.e., nonfatal MI, death from coronary causes, stroke of any type, coronary or noncoronary revascularization) compared with simvastatin-based therapy alone over a median follow-up of 3.9 years. The addition of niacin/laropiprant to existing simvastatin-based therapy, however, did increase the risk of severe adverse effects, including disturbances in glycemic control requiring hospitalization, development of diabetes mellitus, adverse GI effects, myopathy, gout, rash, skin ulceration, and, unexpectedly, infection and bleeding.

Patients with Chronic Kidney Disease In the Study of Heart and Renal Protection (SHARP), the fixed-combination preparation containing ezetimibe and simvastatin was shown to reduce the risk of major vascular and atherosclerotic events in patients with chronic kidney disease, a population known to be at increased risk of cardiovascular disease. More than 9000 patients with moderate to severe chronic kidney disease (33% receiving dialysis) and no known history of MI or coronary revascularization were initially randomized in a 4:4:1 ratio to receive the fixed-combination preparation containing ezetimibe and simvastatin (10 and 20 mg daily, respectively), placebo, or simvastatin alone (20 mg daily) for 1 year to assess the safety of adding ezetimibe to simvastatin; patients in the simvastatin monotherapy group were then re-randomized to the fixed-combination preparation or placebo. After a median duration of follow-up of 4.9 years, the risk of a major vascular event (nonfatal MI or cardiac death, stroke, or revascularization excluding dialysis access procedures) was reduced by 16% (based on the primary intent-to-treat analysis in patients initially randomized to the fixed-combination preparation or placebo groups) and the risk of a major atherosclerotic event (nonfatal MI or cardiac death, nonhemorrhagic stroke, or arterial revascularization excluding dialysis access procedures) was reduced by 17% (based on all patients randomized at any time to the fixed-combination preparation or placebo groups) with the fixed-combination preparation compared with placebo. The treatment effect was largely driven by a substantial reduction in ischemic strokes and arterial revascularization procedures. The subgroup of patients receiving dialysis at baseline experienced a smaller risk reduction benefit compared with those not receiving dialysis. In addition, therapy with the fixed-combination preparation did not appear to slow the progression to end-stage renal disease.

■ **Dyslipidemias** Simvastatin is used as an adjunct to nondrug therapies (e.g., dietary management) to decrease elevated serum total cholesterol, LDL-cholesterol, apolipoprotein B (apo B), triglyceride, and very low-density lipoprotein (VLDL)-cholesterol concentrations, and to increase HDL-cholesterol concentrations in the management of primary hyperlipidemia of primary or mixed dyslipidemia, homozygous familial hypercholesterolemia, primary dysbetalipoproteinemia, and/or hypertriglyceridemia. The efficacy of simvastatin remains to be established in patients with elevated chylomicrons as their primary lipid abnormality (Fredrickson types I and V).

Nondrug therapies and measures specific for the type of dyslipidemia (therapeutic lifestyle changes) are the initial treatments of choice, including dietary management (e.g., restriction of total and saturated fat and cholesterol intake, addition of plant stanols/sterols and viscous fiber to diet), weight control, an appropriate program of physical activity, and management of potentially contributory disease. Drug therapy is not a substitute for but an adjunct to these nondrug therapies and measures, which should be continued when drug therapy is initiated.

Primary Hyperlipidemia or Mixed Dyslipidemia Simvastatin is used alone or in combination with ezetimibe as an adjunct to nondrug therapies (e.g., dietary management) in adults to decrease elevated serum total and LDL-cholesterol, apo B, and triglyceride concentrations, and to increase HDL-cholesterol concentrations in the treatment of primary hyperlipidemia (heterozygous familial and nonfamilial) or mixed dyslipidemia (Fredrickson type IIa or IIb). Simvastatin also is used to decrease elevated serum total cholesterol, LDL-cholesterol, and apo B concentrations in the treatment of heterozygous familial hypercholesterolemia in boys and girls (at least one year postmenarchal) 10–17 years of age who, despite an adequate trial of dietary management, have a serum LDL-cholesterol concentration of 190 mg/dL or greater *or* a serum LDL-cholesterol concentration of 160 mg/dL or greater and either a family history of premature cardiovascular disease or 2 or more other cardiovascular risk factors. The long-term effect of simvastatin therapy in childhood on reducing cardiovascular morbidity and mortality in adulthood has not been established. Statins such as simvastatin also are used in combination with fenofibrate to decrease triglyceride concentrations and increase HDL-cholesterol concentrations in patients with mixed dyslipidemia and CHD (or CHD risk equivalents) who are receiving optimal statin therapy; however, no additional benefit on cardiovascular morbidity and mortality has been established with such combination therapy beyond that already established with statin monotherapy.

Reductions in total and LDL-cholesterol produced by usual dosages of simvastatin substantially exceed those of placebo and appear to be similar to or greater than those produced by monotherapy with certain other antilipemic agents. Mean reductions in total cholesterol concentrations of 19–36%, LDL-cholesterol concentrations of 26–47%, apo B concentrations of 31–38%, and triglyceride concentrations of 12–33% have been reported in controlled studies in patients with primary hypercholesterolemia who received 5–80 mg of simvastatin daily for at least 6 weeks. Modest and variable increases in HDL-cholesterol concentrations (5–16%) also were observed in these patients.

Reductions in total and LDL-cholesterol concentrations produced by usual dosages of simvastatin appear to be similar to or greater than those produced by monotherapy with most other statins (e.g., fluvastatin, lovastatin, pravastatin). In several randomized, comparative studies with various statins, patients with hypercholesterolemia who received simvastatin 5–40 mg daily had greater reductions in plasma total and LDL-cholesterol concentrations (16–30 and 21–41%, respectively) than those who received fluvastatin 20–40 mg daily (12–19 and 16–23%, respectively), lovastatin 20–40 mg daily (21–23 and 29–31%, respectively), or pravastatin 10–40 mg daily (13–24 and 19–34%, respectively). However, patients treated with atorvastatin 10–40 mg daily had greater reductions in total and LDL-cholesterol concentrations (28–40 and 38–51%, respectively) than simvastatin-treated patients. Furthermore, atorvastatin (40 mg daily) appears to be more effective than simvastatin (40 mg daily) in the management of patients with severe hypercholesterolemia who require regular plasma LDL-apheresis. Limited data indicate that reductions in LDL-cholesterol concentrations may be similar among patients receiving high-dose simvastatin and atorvastatin (80 mg daily).

Increases in HDL-cholesterol concentrations appear to be greater among simvastatin- than atorvastatin-treated patients. In several studies designed to evaluate the effects of simvastatin (40–80 mg) and atorvastatin (20–80 mg daily) on HDL-cholesterol and apolipoprotein A-I (apo A-I) concentrations, increases in HDL-cholesterol and apo A-I concentrations were more pronounced in simvastatin-treated (7–9 and 3–6%, respectively) patients than in atorvastatin-treated (0–7 and 0–5%, respectively) patients. The mechanisms of these effects have not been fully elucidated but may be related to differences in plasma elimination half-lives (approximately 20 hours for atorvastatin and 2 hours for simvastatin) and differential effects on lipolytic enzymes (e.g., lipoprotein lipase, hepatic lipase).

Limited data from comparative studies suggest that reductions in total and LDL-cholesterol concentrations produced by simvastatin may be greater than those of some other antilipemic agents (i.e., bile acid sequestrants, fibric acid derivatives). In several controlled studies comparing 12 weeks of simvastatin therapy (20–40 mg daily) with that of cholestyramine (4–16 g in divided doses) in patients with familial and nonfamilial hypercholesterolemia, simvastatin was more effective than cholestyramine in reducing total and LDL-cholesterol concentrations (26–36 and 32–40% versus 23 and 15–21%, respectively). Simvastatin also was more effective than cholestyramine in improving triglyceride (21% reduction versus 11% increase) and HDL-cholesterol concentrations (16% versus 9% increase). Simvastatin appears to be more effective than fibric acid derivatives (e.g., gemfibrozil) in reducing total and LDL-cholesterol concentrations but less effective than these agents in reducing triglycerides and increasing HDL-cholesterol concentrations. In several randomized, comparative studies in patients with primary hypercholesterolemia, therapy with simvastatin (5–20 mg) produced greater reductions in total and LDL-cholesterol (14–27 and 22–34%, respectively) than treatment with gemfibrozil (600 mg twice daily) (5–14 and 17%, respectively); however, reductions in triglycerides and increases in HDL-cholesterol concentrations were less pronounced among patients treated with simvastatin (7–16% reduction and 6–13% increase) than in those receiving gemfibrozil (30–44% reduction and 16–26% increase). Similar results have been reported with other fibric acid derivatives (e.g., fenofibrate).

The combination of simvastatin and other antilipemic agents (e.g., bile acid sequestrants, fibric acid derivatives, ezetimibe) may produce additive antilipemic effects; however, the risk of myopathy and rhabdomyolysis may be increased with some combinations. (See Combination Antilipemic Therapy under Uses: Prevention of Cardiovascular Events.) The addition of a bile acid sequestrant to simvastatin therapy further reduced LDL-cholesterol by 11%, resulting in an overall LDL-cholesterol reduction of 54% in patients receiving simvastatin 20–40 mg daily and cholestyramine 8–16 g daily. Low-dose simvastatin (10 mg daily) in combination with fenofibrate (300 mg daily) in patients with combined hyperlipidemia further reduced triglyceride concentrations by 32% and increased HDL-cholesterol concentrations by an additional 7%. In a multicenter, double-blind study, the addition of ezetimibe (10 mg daily) to simvastatin therapy (10–80 mg daily) further reduced LDL-cholesterol by 10–19%, resulting in overall LDL-cholesterol reductions of 46–58% with combined therapy. Similar additive antilipemic effects were observed following therapy with the fixed-combination preparation containing simvastatin and ezetimibe; LDL-cholesterol was reduced by 45–60% following therapy with the fixed-combination preparation and by 33–49% following monotherapy with simvastatin (10–80 mg daily). In another multicenter, double-blind study, the fixed-combination preparation containing 10 mg of ezetimibe and 20 mg of simvastatin was substantially more effective than doubling the dose of simvastatin (e.g., from 20 to 40 mg).

The increased risk of adverse muscular effects should be considered when simvastatin is used in combination with certain antilipemic agents (e.g., fibric acid derivatives or niacin at lipid-modifying dosages [at least 1 g daily]). (See Drug Interactions: Antilipemic Agents, in the HMG-CoA Reductase Inhibitors General Statement 24:06.08.)

Homozygous Familial Hypercholesterolemia Simvastatin is used alone or in combination with ezetimibe to decrease elevated serum total and LDL-cholesterol concentrations in patients with homozygous familial hypercholesterolemia as an adjunct to other lipid-lowering therapies (e.g., plasma LDL-apheresis) or when such therapies are not available. Patients with homozygous familial hypercholesterolemia usually respond poorly to combined dietary management and drug therapy, including regimens containing a statin, in part because these patients have poorly functioning, few, or no LDL receptors. In several open-label clinical trials in a limited number of patients with homozygous familial hypercholesterolemia receiving simvastatin 40–80 mg daily, LDL-cholesterol concentrations were reduced by 8–46% in most patients; however, at least one patient with homozygous familial hypercholesterolemia experienced increases (15%) in LDL-cholesterol concentrations with simvastatin therapy.

In a randomized, double-blind study of 12 weeks' duration in a limited number of patients with a clinical and/or genotypic diagnosis of homozygous familial hypercholesterolemia, the addition of ezetimibe (10 mg daily) to simvastatin or atorvastatin therapy (40 or 80 mg daily) was more effective in reducing LDL-cholesterol concentrations (21% additional reduction based on pooled data from 40-mg and 80-mg statin groups) than increasing the dosage of simvastatin or atorvastatin monotherapy from 40 to 80 mg daily (7% additional reduction based on pooled data from 40-mg and 80-mg statin groups). In patients receiving ezetimibe (10 mg daily) in combination with higher dosages (80 mg daily) of simvastatin or atorvastatin, LDL-cholesterol concentrations were reduced by an additional 27% compared with LDL-cholesterol reductions achieved with the 40-mg daily statin dosage. (See Homozygous Familial Hypercholesterolemia under Uses: Dyslipidemias, in Ezetimibe 24:06.05.)

Primary Dysbetalipoproteinemia Simvastatin is used as an adjunct to nondrug therapies (e.g., dietary management) to decrease elevated serum triglyceride and VLDL-cholesterol concentrations in the treatment of primary dysbetalipoproteinemia (Fredrickson type III).

Treatment with simvastatin has resulted in substantial reductions in combined intermediate-density lipoprotein (IDL)- and VLDL-cholesterol, total cholesterol, triglyceride, and non-HDL-cholesterol concentrations. In several studies in a limited number of patients with primary dysbetalipoproteinemia who received simvastatin 20–80 mg daily for at least 6 weeks, combined IDL- and VLDL-cholesterol, total cholesterol, triglyceride, and non-HDL-cholesterol concentrations decreased by 50–60, 39–54, 32–55, and 32–59%, respectively. Simvastatin 20 mg daily reportedly has produced greater reductions in LDL-cholesterol than gemfibrozil 1200 mg daily in patients with primary dysbetalipoproteinemia. However, reductions in triglyceride concentrations and increases in HDL-cholesterol concentrations were less pronounced than those reported with usual dosages of gemfibrozil.

Hypertriglyceridemia Simvastatin is used as an adjunct to nondrug therapies (e.g., dietary management) to decrease elevated serum triglyceride concentrations in the treatment of hypertriglyceridemia (Fredrickson type IV). AHA states that although statins have consistently shown benefit in subgroups with or without high triglyceride concentrations, fibric acid derivatives have more commonly been shown to provide greater benefit in subgroups with increased triglyceride concentrations.

Median reductions in total cholesterol concentrations of 25–32%, LDL-cholesterol concentrations of 28–37%, VLDL-cholesterol concentrations of 37–41%, triglyceride concentrations of 29–34%, and non-HDL-cholesterol concentrations of 32–38% have been reported in a subgroup analysis in patients with hypertriglyceridemia who received 40–80 mg daily. Simvastatin 20 mg daily reportedly has produced greater reductions in total and LDL-cholesterol concentrations than gemfibrozil 600 mg twice daily in patients with borderline hypertriglyceridemia; however, reductions in triglyceride concentrations were less pronounced than those reported with usual dosages of gemfibrozil.

■ **Other Uses** Treatment with simvastatin preoperatively to control lipoprotein fractions has been shown to reduce the risk of postoperative thrombocytosis and thrombotic complications† following coronary artery bypass grafting (CABG) procedures. Postoperative thrombocytosis (platelet counts exceeding 400,000/ mm^3) and MI occurred less frequently in simvastatin-treated patients than in those who received placebo (3 and 0%, respectively, versus 81 and 14%, respectively).

Simvastatin has reduced total and LDL-cholesterol concentrations in a few patients with hypercholesterolemia associated with or exacerbated by diabetes mellitus† (diabetic dyslipidemia) (see Secondary Prevention under Uses: Prevention of Cardiovascular Events), cardiac† or renal† transplantation, or nephrotic syndrome†.

Simvastatin also has been shown to improve ejection fraction in cardiac transplant recipients. Improvement in renal cholesterol emboli syndrome† was reported in at least one patient who received simvastatin (10–40 mg daily) for 3 months. However, the relationship between simvastatin and these effects is unclear.

For additional information on the role of simvastatin or other statins in the treatment of lipoprotein disorders, prevention of cardiovascular events, or other uses, see General Principles of Antilipemic Therapy and see Uses in the HMG-CoA Reductase Inhibitors General Statement 24:06.08.

Dosage and Administration

■ **Administration** Simvastatin, alone or in fixed combination with ezetimibe, is administered orally in the evening without regard to meals. GI absorption of the drug does not appear to be affected substantially when simvastatin is administered immediately before a low-fat meal. Patients should be placed on a standard cholesterol-lowering diet before initiation of simvastatin therapy and should remain on this diet during treatment with the drug; in patients with coronary heart disease (CHD) or CHD risk equivalents, simvastatin may be initiated simultaneously with dietary management. For recommendations on dietary and other nondrug therapies (i.e., lifestyle modifications), consult the most recent American Heart Association (AHA)/American College of Cardiology (ACC) Guideline on Lifestyle Management to Reduce Cardiovascular Risk (available at http://www.cardiosource.org or http://my.americanheart.org).

Because administration of simvastatin with grapefruit juice has resulted in substantial increases in plasma concentrations of the antilipemic agent, the manufacturer and some clinicians recommend that concomitant administration of simvastatin with grapefruit juice should be avoided. Because the extent of this interaction may be influenced by the quantity and timing of grapefruit juice consumption, other clinicians suggest that small amounts (e.g., 240 mL) of grapefruit juice may be acceptable. (See Drug Interactions: Drugs and Foods Affecting or Metabolized by Hepatic Microsomal Enzymes in the HMG-CoA Reductase Inhibitors General Statement 24:06.08.)

Adherence to lifestyle modifications and to statin therapy are required for atherosclerotic cardiovascular disease (ASCVD) risk reduction and, thus, should be reinforced periodically.

■ **Dosage** Dosage of simvastatin must be carefully adjusted according to individual requirements and response. The manufacturers state that serum lipoprotein concentrations should be determined 4 weeks after initiation of simvastatin monotherapy or 2 or more weeks after initiation or titration of therapy with the fixed-combination preparation (Vytorin®), and then periodically thereafter. The ACC/AHA guideline for management of blood cholesterol to reduce atherosclerotic cardiovascular risk in adults states that lipoprotein concentrations should be determined within 4–12 weeks following initiation of statin therapy (to determine the patient's response to therapy and adherence) and monitored every 3–12 months thereafter as clinically indicated.

Prevention of Cardiovascular Events The ACC/AHA cholesterol management guideline states that the appropriate intensity of statin therapy should be used to reduce ASCVD risk in patients most likely to benefit. Giving a maximally tolerated statin intensity should be emphasized over giving lower statin dosages and adding nonstatin drugs to address low HDL-cholesterol or high triglyceride concentrations, a strategy that has not yet been shown to reduce ASCVD risk. It should be noted that although 10 mg once daily is an FDA-labeled dosage of simvastatin, this dosage was not evaluated in randomized controlled studies reviewed by the ACC/AHA expert panel.

Primary Prevention. For primary prevention† of cardiovascular disease in patients 21 years of age and older without clinical ASCVD who have primary, severe elevations in low-density lipoprotein (LDL)-cholesterol concentration (*190 mg/dL or greater*), the ACC/AHA cholesterol management guideline recommends that high-intensity statin therapy (i.e., with atorvastatin or rosuvastatin) be initiated unless contraindicated. (See Atorvastatin Calcium or Rosuvastatin Calcium 24:06.08.)

For primary prevention† of cardiovascular disease in patients 40–75 years of age with *type 1 or 2 diabetes mellitus* and LDL-cholesterol concentrations of 70–189 mg/dL, the ACC/AHA cholesterol management guideline recommends that moderate-intensity statin therapy (e.g., simvastatin 20–40 mg once daily) be initiated or continued. In those with an estimated 10-year ASCVD risk of 7.5% or higher, it is reasonable to consider high-intensity statin therapy (i.e., with atorvastatin or rosuvastatin) unless contraindicated. In patients with diabetes mellitus who are younger than 40 or older than 75 years of age, it is reasonable to evaluate the potential benefits, adverse effects, drug interactions, and patient preferences when deciding to initiate, continue, or intensify statin therapy.

For primary prevention† of cardiovascular disease in patients 40–75 years of age without clinical ASCVD or diabetes mellitus who have LDL-cholesterol concentrations of 70–189 mg/dL and an estimated 10-year ASCVD risk of 7.5% or higher, the ACC/AHA cholesterol management guideline recommends that moderate- (e.g., simvastatin 20–40 mg once daily) to high-intensity statin therapy (i.e., with atorvastatin or rosuvastatin) be initiated or continued. In those with an estimated 10-year ASCVD risk of 5 to less than 7.5%, it is reasonable to offer treatment with moderate-intensity statin therapy. Before initiating statin therapy for primary prevention† of ASCVD in patients 40–75 years of age without clinical ASCVD or diabetes mellitus who have LDL-cholesterol concentrations of 70–189 mg/dL, it is reasonable for clinicians and patients to discuss the potential benefits, adverse effects, drug interactions, and patient preferences for such therapy.

Secondary Prevention. For secondary prevention of cardiovascular disease in patients 21–75 years of age with clinical ASCVD, the ACC/AHA cholesterol management guideline recommends that high-intensity statin therapy (i.e., with atorvastatin or rosuvastatin) be initiated unless contraindicated. (See Atorvastatin Calcium or Rosuvastatin Calcium 24:06.08.) In patients 21–75 years of age with clinical ASCVD who are at increased risk for developing statin-associated adverse effects or in whom high-intensity statin therapy is inappropriate or contraindicated, moderate-intensity statin therapy (e.g., simvastatin 20–40 mg once daily) should be given if tolerated. In patients older than 75 years of age with clinical ASCVD, use of statin therapy should be individualized based on the potential benefits, adverse effects, drug interactions, and patient preferences; it is reasonable to consider initiating or continuing moderate-intensity statin therapy in such patients if tolerated.

Dyslipidemias The usual initial dosage of simvastatin in adults is 10 or 20 mg once daily in the evening. In patients with CHD or CHD risk equivalents (e.g., diabetes mellitus, peripheral arterial disease, history of stroke or other cerebrovascular disease), the recommended initial dosage of simvastatin is 40 mg daily. The usual maintenance dosage of simvastatin is 5–40 mg once daily in the evening; geriatric patients may respond to maintenance dosages of 20 mg or less daily. Because higher simvastatin dosages (e.g., 80 mg daily) have been associated with a greater risk of myopathy, including rhabdomyolysis, particularly during the first year of treatment, the manufacturer states that patients who are unable to achieve the desired percent reduction in LDL-cholesterol concentrations with the 40-mg daily dosage of simvastatin should *not* be titrated to the 80-mg daily dosage but should be switched to alternative antilipemic agents that provide greater LDL-cholesterol reduction. The manufacturer also states that use of the 80-mg daily dosage of simvastatin should be restricted to patients who have been receiving long-term therapy (e.g., 12 months or longer) at this dosage without evidence of adverse muscular effects. (See Cautions.) Patients currently tolerating the 80-mg daily dosage of simvastatin who require therapy with an interacting drug (i.e., a drug with which concomitant use is contraindicated or is associated with a dose limit for simvastatin) should be switched to an alternative statin with less drug interaction potential.

The recommended initial dosage of simvastatin for the treatment of heterozygous familial hypercholesterolemia in boys and postmenarchal girls 10–17 years of age is 10 mg once daily in the evening. The recommended dosage range of simvastatin is 10–40 mg daily. Dosage adjustments should be made at intervals of 4 weeks or longer. The maximum recommended dosage of simvastatin in children and adolescents 10–17 years of age is 40 mg daily. Safety and efficacy of simvastatin dosages exceeding 40 mg daily have not been evaluated in this patient population.

In patients with homozygous familial hypercholesterolemia, the recommended dosage of simvastatin is 40 mg daily in the evening. Simvastatin should be used as an adjunct to other lipid-lowering treatment (e.g., LDL apheresis) in these patients or as an alternative if such therapy is unavailable.

Because of an increased risk of myopathy, including rhabdomyolysis, during concomitant therapy, particularly at higher dosages of simvastatin, the manufacturer of simvastatin states that concomitant use of simvastatin with potent inhibitors of cytochrome P-450 isoenzyme 3A4 (CYP3A4) (e.g., itraconazole, ketoconazole, posaconazole, voriconazole, HIV protease inhibitors, clarithromycin, erythromycin, telithromycin, nefazodone, cobicistat-containing preparations), cyclosporine, danazol, or gemfibrozil is *contraindicated*. The manufacturer states that consumption of grapefruit juice should be avoided. In patients receiving diltiazem, dronedarone, or verapamil concomitantly with simvastatin, dosage of simvastatin should not exceed 10 mg daily. In patients receiving amiodarone, amlodipine, or ranolazine concomitantly with simvastatin, dosage of simvastatin should not exceed 20 mg daily. In patients with homozygous familial hypercholesterolemia receiving lomitapide, dosage of simvastatin should not exceed 20 mg daily (or 40 mg daily in patients who have been receiving the 80-mg daily dosage of simvastatin for at least 1 year without evidence of adverse muscular effects).

The risk of myopathy appears to be increased among Chinese patients versus non-Chinese patients receiving simvastatin 40 mg daily concomitantly with preparations containing antilipemic dosages (1 g daily or higher) of niacin. The cause of the increased risk of myopathy is not known, and it is not known whether these findings apply to patients of other Asian ancestries. Because of such increased risk, caution is advised when Chinese patients receive simvastatin dosages exceeding 20 mg daily with preparations containing antilipemic dosages of niacin. Because the risk of myopathy is dose related, patients of Chinese descent should avoid concomitant use of simvastatin 80 mg daily with preparations containing antilipemic dosages of niacin.

Combination Oral Therapy. The usual initial dosage of the commercially available fixed-combination preparation (Vytorin®) for the management of primary hyperlipidemia or mixed dyslipidemia is 10 or 20 mg of simvastatin and 10 mg of ezetimibe once daily in the evening. Patients requiring reductions in LDL-cholesterol concentrations of more than 55% may receive an initial dosage of 40 mg of simvastatin and 10 mg of ezetimibe once daily in the absence of moderate to severe renal impairment (estimated glomerular filtration rate [GFR] less than 60 mL/minute per 1.73 m^2). Serum lipoprotein concentrations should be determined 2 or more weeks after initiation or titration of therapy, and dosage adjusted as needed. The usual maintenance dosage of simvastatin in fixed combination with ezetimibe is 10–40 mg of simvastatin and 10 mg of ezetimibe daily. Because higher simvastatin dosages (e.g., 80 mg daily) have been associated with a greater risk of myopathy, including rhabdomyolysis, particularly during the first year of treatment, the manufacturer states that patients who have inadequate response to the fixed combination containing 40 mg of simvastatin and 10 mg of ezetimibe should *not* be titrated to the fixed combination containing 80 mg of simvastatin and 10 mg of ezetimibe but should be switched to alternative antilipemic agents that provide greater LDL-cholesterol reduction. The manufacturer also states that use of the fixed combination containing 80 mg of simvastatin and 10 mg of ezetimibe should be restricted to patients who have been receiving long-term therapy (e.g., 12 months or longer) at this dosage without evidence of adverse muscular effects. (See Cautions.) Patients currently tolerating the fixed combination containing 80 mg of simvastatin and 10 mg of ezetimibe who require therapy with an interacting drug (i.e., a drug with which concomitant use is contraindicated or is associated with a dose limit for simvastatin) should be switched to an alternative statin or statin-based regimen with less drug interaction potential.

The usual dosage of simvastatin in fixed combination with ezetimibe for the management of homozygous familial hypercholesterolemia is 40 mg of simvastatin and 10 mg of ezetimibe once daily in the evening. Simvastatin in fixed combination with ezetimibe should be used as an adjunct to other lipid-lowering treatment (e.g., LDL apheresis) in these patients or as an alternative if such therapy is unavailable.

Because of an increased risk of myopathy, including rhabdomyolysis, during concomitant therapy, particularly at higher dosages of simvastatin, the manufacturer of Vytorin® states that concomitant use of this fixed-combination preparation with potent inhibitors of CYP3A4 (e.g., itraconazole, ketoconazole, posaconazole, voriconazole, HIV protease inhibitors, clarithromycin, erythromycin, telithromycin, nefazodone, cobicistat-containing preparations), cyclosporine, danazol, or gemfibrozil is *contraindicated*. The manufacturer states that consumption of grapefruit juice should be avoided. In patients receiving diltiazem, dronedarone, or verapamil, dosage of the fixed-combination preparation should not exceed 10 mg of simvastatin and 10 mg of ezetimibe daily. In patients receiving amiodarone, amlodipine, or ranolazine, dosage of the fixed-combination preparation should not exceed 20 mg of simvastatin and 10 mg of ezetimibe daily. In patients with homozygous familial hypercholesterolemia receiving lomitapide, dosage of the fixed-combination preparation should not exceed 20 mg of simvastatin and 10 mg of ezetimibe daily (or 40 mg of simvastatin and 10 mg of ezetimibe daily in patients who have been receiving the 80-mg daily dosage of simvastatin for at least 1 year without evidence of adverse muscular effects).

The risk of myopathy appears to be increased among Chinese patients versus non-Chinese patients receiving simvastatin 40 mg daily (alone or in combination with ezetimibe 10 mg daily) concomitantly with preparations containing antilipemic dosages (1 g daily or higher) of niacin. The cause of the increased risk of myopathy is not known, and it is not known whether these findings apply to patients of other Asian ancestries. Because of such increased risk, caution is advised when Chinese patients receive fixed-combinations dosages exceeding 20 mg of simvastatin and 10 mg of ezetimibe daily with preparations containing antilipemic dosages of niacin. Because the risk of myopathy is dose related, patients of Chinese descent should avoid concomitant use of the fixed-combination preparation containing 80 mg of simvastatin and 10 mg of ezetimibe with preparations containing antilipemic dosages of niacin.

Dosage Modification The ACC/AHA cholesterol management guideline states that decreasing the statin dosage in adults may be considered when LDL-cholesterol concentrations are less than 40 mg/dL on 2 consecutive measurements; however, there are no data to suggest that LDL-cholesterol concentrations below 40 mg/dL would increase the risk of adverse effects.

■ **Dosage in Renal and Hepatic Impairment** Because simvastatin does not undergo substantial renal excretion, the manufacturer states that modifications of dosage should not be necessary in patients with mild to moderate renal impairment. However, simvastatin should be administered with caution in patients with severe renal impairment, initiating therapy with the drug under close monitoring at a dosage of 5 mg daily. In patients receiving simvastatin in fixed combination with ezetimibe, the manufacturer states that no dosage adjustment is necessary in patients with mild renal impairment (estimated GFR of 60 mL/minute per 1.73 m^2 or greater). However, in patients with chronic kidney disease and an estimated GFR of less than 60 mL/minute per 1.73 m^2, the dosage of the fixed-combination preparation is 20 mg of simvastatin and 10 mg of ezetimibe once daily in the evening; in such patients, higher dosages should be used with caution and close monitoring.

Because simvastatin is metabolized predominantly in the liver and potentially may accumulate in the plasma of patients with hepatic impairment, the drug should be used with caution in patients who consume substantial amounts of alcohol and/or have a history of liver disease. Simvastatin is *contraindicated* in patients with active liver disease or unexplained, persistent increases in serum aminotransferase concentrations.

Cautions

Simvastatin shares the toxic potentials of other statins, and the usual cautions, precautions, and contraindications associated with these drugs should be observed. Patients should be fully advised about the risks, especially myopathy and rhabdomyolysis, associated with statin therapy alone or combined with other drugs. (See Cautions in the HMG-CoA Reductase Inhibitors General Statement 24:06.08.)

Although myopathy, including rhabdomyolysis, is a known adverse effect of all statins, studies have shown that patients receiving higher dosages of simvastatin may be at greater risk of muscle injury than those receiving lower dosages of the drug and possibly other statins. In a clinical trial database of 41,413 patients receiving simvastatin, with approximately 60% of patients enrolled in studies with a median follow-up of at least 4 years, the incidence of myopathy was approximately 0.03 or 0.08% in patients receiving simvastatin 20 or 40 mg daily, respectively. The incidence of myopathy was disproportionately higher in patients receiving simvastatin 80 mg daily (0.61%). In a clinical study (Study of the Effectiveness of Additional Reductions in Cholesterol and Homocysteine [SEARCH]) in which over 12,064 patients with a history of myocardial infarction (MI) were randomized to receive either high- or low-dose simvastatin, the incidence of myopathy (defined as unexplained muscle weakness or pain with a serum creatine kinase [CK, creatine phosphokinase, CPK] concentration exceeding 10 times the upper limit of normal [ULN]), after a mean follow-up of 6.7 years, was approximately 0.9 or 0.02% in patients receiving simvastatin 80 or 20 mg daily, respectively. The incidence of rhabdomyolysis (defined as myopathy with a serum CK concentration exceeding 40 times the ULN) was approximately 0.4 or 0% in patients receiving simvastatin 80 or 20 mg daily, respectively. The incidence of myopathy, including rhabdomyolysis, was highest during the first year and notably decreased during subsequent years of treatment. The investigators of the SEARCH trial found a genetic variant (single-nucleotide polymorphism within the SLCOlBl gene on chromosome 12) that was strongly associated with the risk of developing statin-induced myopathy; more than 60% of the cases of myopathy could be attributed to the specific SLCOlBl genetic variant. The SLCO1B1 gene encodes organic anion transporter protein (OATP) 1B1, which has been shown to mediate hepatic uptake of statins.

Because the risk of myopathy, including rhabdomyolysis, is greater with simvastatin 80 mg daily compared with other statin therapies with similar or greater LDL-cholesterol lowering efficacy and compared with lower dosages of simvastatin, the manufacturer states that the 80-mg daily dosage of simvastatin should be restricted to patients who have been receiving long-term therapy (e.g., 12 months or longer) at this dosage without evidence of adverse muscular effects. (See Dosage and Administration: Dosage.) Patients should be advised of the increased risk of myopathy, including rhabdomyolysis, and to promptly report any unexplained muscle pain, tenderness or weakness, particularly if accompanied by malaise or fever or if adverse muscular effects persist after discontinuance of therapy. If markedly elevated CK concentrations occur or if myopathy is diagnosed or suspected, simvastatin should be discontinued immediately.

When simvastatin is used in fixed combination with ezetimibe, the usual cautions, precautions, and contraindications associated with ezetimibe must be considered in addition to those associated with simvastatin.

■ **Pediatric Precautions** Simvastatin has been administered to a limited number of hypercholesterolemic children and adolescents without apparent adverse effects. In a randomized, double-blind, placebo-controlled study in boys and postmenarchal girls 10–17 years of age, the adverse effect profile of simvastatin (10–40 mg daily) generally was similar to that of placebo; dosages exceeding 40 mg daily have not been evaluated in this population. There were no detectable adverse effects on growth or sexual maturation in adolescent boys or girls or on duration of menstrual cycle in girls. If therapy with simvastatin is considered, the manufacturer states that adolescent girls should be advised to use effective and appropriate contraceptive methods during therapy to reduce the likelihood of unintended pregnancy. (See Cautions: Pregnancy, Fertility, and Lactation.) Safety and efficacy of simvastatin have not been evaluated in prepubertal girls or in children younger than 10 years of age.For additional information on the use of statins in pediatric patients, see Cautions: Pediatric Precautions in the HMG-CoA Reductase Inhibitors General Statement 24:06.08.

Use of simvastatin in combination with ezetimibe has been evaluated in a limited number of adolescent boys and girls with heterozygous familial hypercholesterolemia. In a randomized, double-blind, controlled study in boys and postmenarchal girls 10–17 years of age with heterozygous familial hypercholesterolemia, discontinuance of therapy because of adverse effects occurred in more patients receiving simvastatin (10–40 mg daily) in combination with ezetimibe (6%) than in those receiving simvastatin monotherapy (2%); in addition, increases in aminotransferase or CK concentrations also occurred more frequently in patients receiving combination therapy (3 or 2%, respectively) than in those receiving simvastatin monotherapy (2 or 0%, respectively). There were no detectable adverse effects on growth or sexual maturation in adolescent boys or girls or on duration of menstrual cycle in girls. Use of simvastatin dosages exceeding 40 mg daily in combination with ezetimibe has not been evaluated in adolescents; safety and efficacy of simvastatin in fixed combination with ezetimibe have not been evaluated in prepubertal girls or in children younger than 10 years of age.

■ **Geriatric Precautions** Of the 2423 patients receiving simvastatin in phase 3 clinical studies and the 10,269 patients receiving the drug in the Heart Protection Study (HPS), 15 and 52%, respectively, were 65 years of age or older; in HPS, 6% of patients were 75 years of age or older. Although no overall differences in efficacy or safety were observed between geriatric and younger patients receiving simvastatin alone or in combination with ezetimibe, and other clinical experience has not revealed age-related differences in response, the possibility that some geriatric patients may exhibit increased sensitivity to the drug cannot be ruled out. Results of a pharmacokinetic study in a limited number of patients receiving simvastatin (40 mg daily) indicate that mean plasma levels of HMG-CoA reductase inhibitory activity are approximately 45% higher in geriatric patients (70–78 years of age) than in younger adults (18–30 years of age). In the Scandinavian Simvastatin Survival Study (4S) in which 23% of patients were 65 years of age or older, antilipemic effects of simvastatin in these patients were similar to those in younger patients, and simvastatin substantially reduced total mortality and CHD mortality in geriatric patients with a history of CHD; in this study, there were no overall differences in safety between the 2 groups. In HPS in which 52% of patients were 65 years of age or older, reduction in the risk of CHD death, nonfatal MI, stroke, or coronary or noncoronary revascularization procedures was similar in geriatric patients and in younger patients; of the 7 cases of myopathy/rhabdomyolysis reported among over 10,000 patients randomized to receive simvastatin, 4 occurred in patients 65 years of age or older.

In a clinical trial in which patients received higher dosages (i.e., 80 mg daily) of simvastatin, patients 65 years of age and older had an increased risk of myopathy, including rhabdomyolysis, compared with younger patients. Because advanced age (65 years and older) is a predisposing factor for myopathy, including rhabdomyolysis, simvastatin should be used with caution in geriatric patients. In addition, because geriatric patients frequently have decreased renal function (e.g., glomerular filtration), particular attention should be paid to evaluating renal function prior to initiation of simvastatin and subsequently thereafter in this age group. If evidence of severe renal impairment exists or develops, appropriate adjustments in dosage should be made and the patient closely monitored. (See Dosage and Administration: Dosage in Renal and Hepatic Impairment.)

The ACC/AHA cholesterol management guideline states that initiation of statin therapy for primary prevention of ASCVD in patients older than 75 years of age requires consideration of additional factors, including increasing comorbidities, safety considerations, and priorities of care. Therefore, the potential for an ASCVD risk reduction benefit, adverse effects, and drug interactions, along with patient preferences, must be considered before initiating statin therapy in patients older than 75 years of age.

■ Mutagenicity and Carcinogenicity Simvastatin did not exhibit mutagenic potential in vitro in microbial mutagen (Ames) tests with or without rat or mouse liver metabolic activation, the alkaline elution assay using rat hepatocytes, a V-79 mammalian cell forward mutation study, a chromosome aberration study in Chinese hamster ovary cells, or in vivo in a chromosomal aberration assay in mouse bone marrow.

In mice receiving simvastatin dosages of 25, 100, and 400 mg/kg daily (which produced mean plasma drug concentrations approximately equivalent to or 4 and 8 times higher, respectively, than the mean plasma drug concentration observed in humans with a simvastatin dose of 80 mg) for 72 weeks, there was an increased incidence of liver carcinomas in females receiving 400 mg/kg daily and in males receiving 100 and 400 mg/kg daily. The maximum incidence of liver carcinomas was 90% in male mice. An increased incidence of liver adenomas also was observed in female mice receiving 100 and 400 mg/kg daily. The incidence of lung adenomas also was increased in mice receiving 100 and 400 mg/kg daily, regardless of gender, and the incidence of adenomas of the Harderian gland (a gland of the rodent eye) was increased in mice receiving 400 mg/kg daily. A tumorigenic effect was not observed in mice receiving 25 mg/kg daily in this study. In a separate study, no evidence of a tumorigenic effect was observed in mice receiving simvastatin dosages up to 25 mg/kg daily (which produced mean plasma drug concentrations equivalent to those in humans receiving 80 mg daily) for 92 weeks.

An increased incidence of thyroid follicular adenomas was observed in female rats receiving simvastatin for 2 years at dosages that produced plasma drug exposure (as measured by AUC) approximately 11 times higher than that in humans receiving 80 mg daily. Hepatocellular adenomas and carcinomas were observed in female rats receiving simvastatin 50 mg/kg and 100 mg/kg daily (which produced plasma drug exposure [AUC] approximately 22 and 25 times, respectively, those in humans receiving 80 mg daily) and in male rats receiving 100 mg/kg daily (which produced plasma drug exposure approximately 15 times that in humans receiving 80 mg daily) for two years. Rats receiving both dosages also exhibited an increased incidence in thyroid follicular adenomas, regardless of gender, and female rats receiving 100 mg/kg daily exhibited an increased incidence of thyroid follicular cell carcinoma. In male rats, 50 mg/kg daily produced plasma drug exposure approximately 7 times that in humans receiving 80 mg daily.

While early animal studies raised concerns of possible carcinogenic properties of simvastatin, a large body of evidence indicates that long-term statin therapy is not associated with an increased risk of cancer. However, the fixed combination of ezetimibe and simvastatin was reported in one study (Simvastatin and Ezetimibe in Aortic Stenosis [SEAS]) to be possibly associated with an increased risk of cancer. Results of this study in 1873 patients with asymptomatic aortic stenosis revealed a higher incidence of cancer and cancer-related deaths (11.1 and 4.1%, respectively) in patients receiving the fixed-combination preparation compared with those receiving placebo (7.5 and 2.5%, respectively). Findings from the SEAS study prompted FDA to issue an early communication in 2008 about this potential safety risk. However, results of 2 subsequent large randomized studies (the Study of Heart and Renal Protection [SHARP] and the Improved Reduction of Outcomes: Vytorin® Efficacy International Trial [IMPROVE-IT]) found no consistent pattern of increased cancer risk among patients receiving the fixed-combination preparation. Based on the currently available evidence, FDA has concluded that the fixed-combination preparation of ezetimibe and simvastatin (Vytorin®) is not likely to increase the risk of cancer. (See Risk of Cancer under Cautions: General Precautions, in Ezetimibe 24:06.05.)

■ Pregnancy, Fertility, and Lactation ***Pregnancy*** Simvastatin was not teratogenic in rats receiving dosages of 25 mg/kg daily (3 times the usual human exposure based on mg/m^2) or in rabbits receiving dosages up to 10 mg/kg daily (3 times the usual human exposure based on mg/m^2). However, another structurally related statin has produced skeletal malformations in rats and mice.

There are no adequate and well-controlled studies using simvastatin in pregnant women; however, congenital anomalies have been reported rarely following intrauterine exposure to statins. In a review of approximately 100 prospectively followed pregnancies in women exposed to simvastatin or another structurally related statin, the incidences of congenital anomalies, spontaneous abortions, and fetal deaths/stillbirths did not exceed what would be expected in the general population. The number of cases is adequate only to exclude a three- to fourfold increase in congenital anomalies over the background incidence. In 89% of the prospectively followed pregnancies, drug treatment was initiated prior to pregnancy and was discontinued at some point in the first trimester when pregnancy was identified.

Cholesterol and cholesterol derivatives are essential for normal fetal development. Because statins (e.g., simvastatin) decrease the synthesis of cholesterol and possibly other products of the cholesterol biosynthetic pathway, simvastatin may cause fetal harm when administered to a pregnant woman; therefore, the drug is *contraindicated* in women who are or may become pregnant.

Since atherosclerosis is a chronic process, and discontinuance of antilipemic agents during pregnancy generally should not have a substantial effect on the outcome of long-term therapy for primary hypercholesterolemia, therapy with simvastatin should be immediately discontinued as soon as pregnancy is recognized, and the patient should be informed of the potential hazard to the fetus. Currently, most experts recommend that dyslipidemias in pregnant women be managed with dietary measures; consultation with a lipid specialist is recommended for pregnant women with severe forms of dyslipidemia.

Simvastatin should be administered to women of childbearing age only when such patients are highly unlikely to conceive; these women should be advised to use effective contraception. Women trying to conceive should consider discontinuing simvastatin therapy; if pregnancy occurs, simvastatin should be discontinued immediately, and the patient should be informed of the potential hazard to the fetus.

Fertility Decreased fertility was observed in male rats receiving simvastatin 25 mg/kg daily (4 times the maximum plasma drug exposure [based on AUC] in humans receiving 80 mg daily) for 34 weeks. This effect was not observed in a subsequent study using the same dosage for 11 weeks (the entire duration of the spermatogenesis cycle in rats, including epididymal maturation). No microscopic changes in the testes were observed in either study. At a simvastatin dosage of 180 mg/kg daily in rats (22 times the plasma drug exposure in humans receiving 80 mg daily on a mg/m^2 basis), seminiferous tubule degeneration was observed. Testicular atrophy, decreased spermatogenesis, spermatocytic degeneration, and giant cell formation in dogs were observed at a dosage of 10 mg/kg daily (which produced plasma drug exposure approximately 2 times that in humans receiving 80 mg daily). The clinical importance of these effects has not been established.

Lactation It is not known whether simvastatin is distributed into milk. However, a small amount of another statin is distributed into milk. Because of the potential for serious adverse reactions from simvastatin in nursing infants, the drug is contraindicated in nursing women; women who require simvastatin therapy should not breast-feed their infants. A decision should be made whether to discontinue nursing or the drug, taking into account the importance of the drug to the woman.

Chemistry and Stability

■ Chemistry Simvastatin is a semisynthetic mevinic acid-derivative antilipemic agent. The drug is a methyl analog of lovastatin and is produced by fermentation of *Aspergillus terreus*.

Simvastatin is a hydroxymethylglutaryl-CoA (HMG-CoA) reductase inhibitor (statin) and is pharmacologically related to mevastatin (compactin, not commercially available) and other statins (e.g., atorvastatin, fluvastatin, lovastatin, pravastatin). Simvastatin is a derivative of lovastatin and differs from this agent by the presence of an additional methyl group on the butyryl ester side chain. This structural modification enhances the in vitro HMG-CoA reductase-inhibitory activity of simvastatin acid by a factor of 2 compared with that of lovastatin; however, it also increases simvastatin's lipophilicity, resulting in a greater potential for the drug to cross the blood-brain barrier. The octanol/water partition coefficient (log P) for simvastatin is approximately 115 at 25°C; the octanol/water coefficient for simvastatin is higher than that for lovastatin or pravastatin (log P 50 or log P 0.59, respectively).

Simvastatin is a prodrug and has little, if any, antilipemic activity until hydrolyzed in vivo to mevinolinic acid (the corresponding ring-opened, β-hydroxyacid form), which is a potent inhibitor of HMG-CoA reductase.

Simvastatin occurs as a white to off-white, nonhygroscopic, crystalline powder that is practically insoluble in water, having a solubility of 0.0014 mg/mL at 23°C. The drug is freely soluble in chloroform, methanol, and ethanol.

■ **Stability** Simvastatin tablets should be stored at 5–30°C. When stored under these conditions, the tablets are stable for 24 months after the date of manufacture.

The fixed-combination preparation containing simvastatin and ezetimibe should be stored in well-closed containers at 20–25°C.

For further information on chemistry and stability, pharmacology, pharmacokinetics, uses, cautions, drug interactions, laboratory test interferences, and dosage and administration of simvastatin, see the HMG-CoA Reductase Inhibitors General Statement 24:06.08.

Preparations

Excipients in commercially available drug preparations may have clinically important effects in some individuals; consult specific product labeling for details.

Simvastatin

Oral		
Tablets, film-coated	5 mg*	Simvastatin Tablets Zocor®, Merck
	10 mg*	Simvastatin Tablets Zocor®, Merck
	20 mg*	Simvastatin Tablets Zocor®, Merck
	40 mg*	Simvastatin Tablets Zocor®, Merck
	80 mg*	Simvastatin Tablets Zocor®, Merck

*available from one or more manufacturer, distributor, and/or repackager by generic (nonproprietary) name

Simvastatin Combinations

Oral		
Tablets	10 mg with Ezetimibe 10 mg	Vytorin®, Merck
	20 mg with Ezetimibe 10 mg	Vytorin®, Merck
	40 mg with Ezetimibe 10 mg	Vytorin®, Merck
	80 mg with Ezetimibe 10 mg	Vytorin®, Merck

†Use is not currently included in the labeling approved by the US Food and Drug Administration

Selected Revisions June 2017,

Proprotein Convertase Subtilisin Kexin Type 9 (PCSK9) Inhibitors 24:06.24

Alirocumab

■ Alirocumab, a fully human IgG_1 monoclonal antibody that binds to proprotein convertase subtilisin kexin type 9 (PCSK9), is an antilipemic agent.

Uses

■ **Prevention of Cardiovascular Events** Alirocumab is used for secondary prevention to reduce the risk of myocardial infarction (MI), stroke, and unstable angina requiring hospitalization in patients with established cardiovascular disease.

Current guidelines from the American College of Cardiology/American Heart Association (ACC/AHA) and the National Lipid Association recommend that lifestyle modifications, which include adherence to a heart-healthy diet, regular exercise, avoidance of tobacco products, and maintenance of a healthy weight, be instituted in all patients with clinical atherosclerotic cardiovascular disease (ASCVD), defined as acute coronary syndrome (ACS), history of MI, stable or unstable angina, coronary or other arterial revascularization, stroke, transient ischemic attack (TIA), or peripheral arterial disease presumed to be of atherosclerotic origin. Drug therapy is not a substitute for but an adjunct to these nondrug therapies and measures, which should be continued when drug therapy is initiated. In addition to lifestyle modifications, pharmacologic therapy with a hydroxymethylglutaryl-coenzyme A (HMG-CoA) reductase inhibitor (i.e., statin) is recommended in all patients with clinical ASCVD to reduce the risk of cardiovascular events; the maximum appropriate and tolerated intensity of a statin should be used (e.g., atorvastatin or rosuvastatin titrated to dosages that produce low-density lipoprotein [LDL]-cholesterol reductions of at least 50% from baseline).

Despite optimal statin therapy, some patients may not achieve adequate reductions in LDL-cholesterol concentrations and may benefit from the addition of a nonstatin antilipemic agent. The ACC/AHA cholesterol management guideline states that the addition of a nonstatin drug may be considered in patients who have a less-than-anticipated response to statins, are unable to tolerate a less-than-recommended intensity of a statin, or are completely statin intolerant, particularly when there is evidence from randomized controlled studies suggesting that the nonstatin drug further reduces ASCVD events when added to statin therapy. An expert consensus panel was convened by ACC to provide further guidance on the role of nonstatin drugs in the management of ASCVD, specifically in regard to the specific patient populations and clinical situations in which these drugs may be considered. According to these experts, patients who may benefit from the addition of a nonstatin drug include those with clinical ASCVD with or without comorbidities (including severe elevations of baseline LDL-cholesterol concentrations greater than 190 mg/dL) who have not met certain thresholds of LDL-cholesterol reduction (e.g., at least 50% reduction in LDL-cholesterol, or an absolute LDL-cholesterol concentration of less than 70 mg/dL or non-high-density lipoprotein [non-HDL]-cholesterol concentration of less than 100 mg/dL) while receiving maximally tolerated statin therapy; nonstatin drugs that may be considered include ezetimibe or a proprotein convertase subtilisin kexin type 9 (PCSK9) inhibitor (or possibly both) depending on the specific situation. Selection of a nonstatin drug should be based on a favorable benefit-risk ratio (i.e., demonstrated benefit of ASCVD risk reduction outweighs risks of adverse effects and drug interactions) and patient preferences. Prior to initiation of nonstatin antilipemic drugs, it is critical that patients are treated first with maximally tolerated statin therapy and that lifestyle modifications are intensified/optimized. Because true statin intolerance is uncommon, patients should be systematically and rigorously evaluated for this condition to encourage adherence to evidence-based statin therapy. For additional details on prevention of ASCVD, see the HMG-CoA Reductase Inhibitors General Statement 24:06.08.

Efficacy of alirocumab in the prevention of cardiovascular events has been established in the ODYSSEY OUTCOMES study, which was a large, multicenter, randomized, double-blind, placebo-controlled study in 18,924 high-risk adults with recent ACS (i.e., in the preceding 1–12 months) and elevated levels of atherogenic lipoproteins inadequately controlled with intensive statin therapy or maximally tolerated statin therapy. Patients were included in the study if they had an LDL-cholesterol concentration of at least 70 mg/dL, a non-HDL-cholesterol concentration of at least 100 mg/dL, or an apolipoprotein B concentration of at least 80 mg/dL after receiving at least 2 weeks of stable treatment with atorvastatin (40 or 80 mg daily) or rosuvastatin (20 or 40 mg daily), or the maximum tolerated dosage of one of these statins, with or without other lipid-lowering therapy. Approximately 89% of the patients were receiving high-intensity statin therapy at the time of randomization. Prior to the index ACS event, 23% of the patients had coronary revascularization procedures and 19% had prior MI; additional risk factors included hypertension (65%), diabetes mellitus (25%), smoking (24%), and New York Heart Association (NYHA) class I or II heart failure (15%). Patients were randomized to receive add-on therapy with alirocumab (initial dosage of 75 mg every 2 weeks by subcutaneous injection) or matching placebo. A protocol-specified blinded dosage adjustment strategy was used in alirocumab-treated patients to target LDL-cholesterol concentrations of 25–50 mg/dL and to avoid very low concentrations of LDL cholesterol (i.e., less than 15 mg/dL). If additional LDL-cholesterol lowering was required after 2 months of therapy (i.e., LDL-cholesterol concentration of 50 mg/dL or greater), alirocumab dosage was increased to 150 mg every 2 weeks. Patients who experienced 2 consecutive LDL-cholesterol concentrations less than 25 mg/dL while receiving the increased dosage of alirocumab had their dosage decreased back to 75 mg every 2 weeks, and those who experienced 2 consecutive LDL-cholesterol concentrations less than 15 mg/dL were switched to placebo. The median baseline LDL-cholesterol concentration prior to the start of add-on therapy was 92 mg/dL. Alirocumab substantially reduced the risk for the primary composite end point of time to first occurrence of death from coronary heart disease (CHD), nonfatal MI, fatal or nonfatal ischemic stroke, or unstable angina requiring hospitalization (hazard ratio of 0.85). The absolute benefit of alirocumab with respect to the primary composite end point was greatest among the subgroup of patients who had baseline LDL-cholesterol concentrations of at least 100 mg/dL. The median duration of follow-up in the ODYSSEY OUTCOMES study was 33 months; longer-term efficacy and safety of alirocumab in the prevention of cardiovascular events remain to be established.

■ **Dyslipidemias** ***Primary Hyperlipidemia*** Alirocumab is used alone or in combination with other antilipemic agents (e.g., statins, ezetimibe) as an adjunct to diet in patients with primary hyperlipidemia (including heterozygous familial hypercholesterolemia) to reduce LDL-cholesterol concentrations.

Elevated serum cholesterol, especially the LDL-cholesterol fraction, is a major cause of clinical ASCVD; patients with heterozygous familial hypercholesterolemia in particular have excessive elevations in LDL-cholesterol concentrations that predispose them to a high risk of premature ASCVD. Therefore, the goal of antilipemic therapy in patients with hyperlipidemia is to reduce the risk of ASCVD. The ACC/AHA cholesterol management guideline states that lifestyle modifications, which include adherence to a heart-healthy diet, regular exercise, avoidance of tobacco products, and maintenance of a healthy weight, are the foundation of ASCVD risk reduction. If drug therapy is needed, statins are the first-line antilipemic agents of choice. A nonstatin drug may be considered in selected high-risk patients (e.g., those with known cardiovascular disease, markedly high LDL-cholesterol concentrations at baseline, or diabetes mellitus) who are not able to achieve adequate reductions in LDL-cholesterol concentration with diet and statins alone or who are completely intolerant of statin therapy. Clinical studies have demonstrated that alirocumab can further reduce LDL-cholesterol concentrations by approximately 40–60%, depending on dosage, when added to maximally tolerated statin therapy or when used as monotherapy and can also reduce the risk of cardiovascular events. (See Uses: Prevention of Cardiovascular Events.)

Efficacy and safety of alirocumab in the treatment of primary hyperlipidemia (including patients with heterozygous familial hypercholesterolemia) have been established in 9 multicenter, randomized, double-blind, placebo- or active-controlled studies; alirocumab was mainly evaluated as add-on therapy to maximally tolerated statin therapy in these studies, but was also evaluated as monotherapy or as an adjunct to apheresis.

The largest of these studies, the ODYSSEY LONG TERM study, included 2341 patients with heterozygous familial hypercholesterolemia or established CHD or CHD risk equivalents who had LDL-cholesterol concentrations of at least 70 mg/dL despite receiving maximally tolerated statin therapy. The mean LDL-cholesterol concentration at baseline was 122 mg/dL. Patients were randomized in a 2:1 ratio to receive alirocumab 150 mg or placebo every 2 weeks for 78 weeks. Alirocumab substantially reduced LDL-cholesterol concentrations from baseline compared with placebo; at 24 weeks, LDL-cholesterol concentrations were reduced by a mean of 58% with alirocumab, but were increased by a mean of 1% with placebo. In addition, 79% of patients in the alirocumab group achieved an LDL-cholesterol goal of less than 70 mg/dL at 24 weeks. Reductions in LDL cholesterol were observed at 4 weeks and sustained throughout the 78-week study. Post-hoc analysis of positively adjudicated major adverse cardiovascular events (i.e., CHD death, nonfatal MI, fatal or nonfatal ischemic stroke, or unstable angina requiring hospitalization) in the ODYSSEY LONG TERM study suggested some evidence of cardiovascular risk reduction with alirocumab therapy; however, the analysis was based on a relatively small number of events.

The ODYSSEY COMBO I study included 316 high-risk patients (i.e., established CHD or CHD risk equivalents) who had suboptimally controlled hypercholesterolemia despite receiving maximally tolerated statin therapy. The mean LDL-cholesterol concentration at baseline was 102 mg/dL. Patients were randomized in a 2:1 ratio to receive alirocumab (75 mg every 2 weeks initially, followed by an increase to 150 mg every 2 weeks at week 12 if additional LDL-cholesterol reduction was required based on prespecified criteria) or placebo for 52 weeks. Alirocumab substantially reduced LDL-cholesterol concentrations from baseline compared with placebo; at 24 weeks, LDL-cholesterol concentrations were reduced by a mean of 44% in patients receiving alirocumab compared with a reduction of 2% in those receiving placebo. In addition, 75% of patients in the alirocumab group achieved an LDL-cholesterol goal of less than 70 mg/dL at 24 weeks. Reductions in LDL cholesterol were observed as early as 4 weeks after beginning therapy and sustained throughout the 52-week study. Among patients who received alirocumab in this study, 17% required a dosage increase to 150 mg every 2 weeks.

The ODYSSEY FH I, FH II, HIGH FH, and ESCAPE studies were exclusively conducted in patients with heterozygous familial hypercholesterolemia (diagnosed by genotyping or clinical criteria). In the ODYSSEY FH I and II studies, a total of 735 patients with heterozygous familial hypercholesterolemia who had inadequately controlled LDL-cholesterol concentrations despite maximally tolerated statin therapy were randomized in a 2:1 ratio to receive alirocumab (75 mg every 2 weeks initially, followed by an increase to 150 mg every 2 weeks beginning at week 12 if additional LDL-cholesterol reduction was required based on prespecified criteria) or placebo; at baseline, the mean LDL-cholesterol concentration was 141 mg/dL. Combined results of the ODYSSEY FH I and II studies at 24 weeks demonstrated a 47% mean reduction in LDL-cholesterol concentration from baseline with alirocumab therapy compared with a mean increase of 7% with placebo. Longer-term data indicate that the reductions in LDL cholesterol achieved with alirocumab were maintained for up to 78 weeks. Among patients who received alirocumab in these studies, 42% required a dosage increase to 150 mg every 2 weeks. The ODYSSEY HIGH FH study evaluated patients with heterozygous familial hypercholesterolemia and a baseline LDL-cholesterol concentration of at least 160 mg/dL; a total of 107 patients were randomized in a 2:1 ratio to receive alirocumab 150 mg or placebo every 2 weeks. At baseline, patients had a mean LDL-cholesterol concentration of 198 mg/dL. At 24 weeks, LDL-cholesterol concentrations were reduced by a mean of 43% in patients receiving alirocumab compared with a reduction of 7% in those receiving placebo. In the ODYSSEY ESCAPE study, 62 patients with heterozygous familial hypercholesterolemia undergoing regular weekly or every-2-week lipoprotein apheresis and receiving a stable lipid-lowering regimen were randomized in a 2:1 ratio to receive alirocumab 150 mg or placebo every 2 weeks. Although all patients in the study were at high cardiovascular risk, a substantial portion were not receiving a statin or were not receiving the maximally tolerated dosage of a statin for various reasons. At baseline, patients had a mean pre-apheresis LDL-cholesterol concentration of 181 mg/dL. At 6 weeks, pre-apheresis LDL-cholesterol concentrations were reduced by a mean of 53% in patients receiving alirocumab compared with an increase of 1% in those patients receiving placebo.

The ODYSSEY CHOICE I study included 803 patients with primary hyperlipidemia and moderate to very high cardiovascular risk who were receiving maximally tolerated statin therapy or no statin therapy, with or without other lipid-lowering therapy. Patients were stratified by use of concomitant statin therapy and randomized in a 4:1:2 ratio to receive alirocumab 300 mg every 4 weeks, alirocumab 75 mg every 2 weeks, or placebo; dosage of alirocumab in both active treatment groups was adjusted to 150 mg every 2 weeks at week 12 if additional LDL-cholesterol reduction was required based on prespecified criteria. Patients who were not receiving statin therapy had a higher mean LDL-cholesterol concentration at baseline than those who were receiving a statin (142 versus 113 mg/dL, respectively). Alirocumab produced greater reductions in LDL-cholesterol concentrations than placebo regardless of statin use, and a similar treatment effect was demonstrated in both patients receiving and not receiving concomitant statin therapy. In the cohort of patients on concomitant statin therapy, LDL-cholesterol concentrations at 12 weeks were reduced by a mean of 54% with alirocumab 300 mg every 4 weeks and a mean of 44% with alirocumab 75 mg every 2 weeks, compared with placebo; at 24 weeks, the mean reduction in LDL-cholesterol concentration compared with placebo was 56% in patients initially assigned to receive alirocumab 300 mg every 4 weeks and 48% in those initially assigned to receive alirocumab 75 mg every 2 weeks.

The ODYSSEY MONO and COMBO II studies were active-controlled studies that compared efficacy of alirocumab and ezetimibe. ODYSSEY MONO was a 24-week study that evaluated alirocumab monotherapy in 103 patients with moderate cardiovascular risk and baseline LDL-cholesterol concentrations of 100–190 mg/dL who were not receiving statin therapy or other lipid-lowering therapy at baseline. Patients were randomized in a 1:1 ratio to receive monotherapy with alirocumab (75 mg every 2 weeks initially, followed by an increase to 150 mg every 2 weeks at week 12 if additional LDL-cholesterol reduction was required based on prespecified criteria) or ezetimibe 10 mg daily. The mean LDL-cholesterol concentration at baseline was 140 mg/dL. At 12 weeks, LDL-cholesterol concentrations were reduced by a mean of 48% in patients receiving alirocumab compared with a reduction of 19% in those receiving ezetimibe; at 24 weeks, LDL-cholesterol concentrations were reduced by a mean of 45% in patients receiving alirocumab compared with a reduction of 14% in those receiving ezetimibe. ODYSSEY COMBO II was a 104-week study that included 720 patients with high cardiovascular risk who required additional LDL-cholesterol reduction despite receiving maximally tolerated statin therapy. Patients were randomized in a 2:1 ratio to receive alirocumab (75 mg every 2 weeks initially, followed by an increase to 150 mg every 2 weeks at week 12 if additional LDL-cholesterol reduction was required based on prespecified criteria) or ezetimibe 10 mg daily. The mean LDL-cholesterol concentration at baseline was 107 mg/dL. At 12 weeks, LDL-cholesterol concentrations were reduced by a mean of 50% in patients receiving alirocumab compared with a reduction of 22% in those receiving ezetimibe; at 24 weeks, LDL-cholesterol concentrations were reduced by a mean of 48% in patients receiving alirocumab compared with a reduction of 20% in those receiving ezetimibe.

For additional information on general principles of antilipemic therapy, see the HMG-CoA Reductase Inhibitors General Statement 24:06.08.

Dosage and Administration

■ **General** Adherence to lifestyle modifications and to statin therapy are required for atherosclerotic cardiovascular disease (ASCVD) risk reduction and should be reinforced periodically.

Low-density lipoprotein (LDL)-cholesterol concentrations should be monitored to assess response to therapy and the need for dosage adjustments. For patients receiving the every-2-week regimen of alirocumab, LDL-cholesterol concentrations should be measured within 4–8 weeks of initiating therapy. For patients receiving the every-4-week (i.e., once-monthly) regimen, LDL-cholesterol concentrations should be measured just prior to the next scheduled dose since some patients may experience considerable variation in LDL-cholesterol concentrations during the monthly dosing interval. In all patients, LDL-cholesterol concentrations should be reassessed within 4–8 weeks of any dosage adjustment.

■ **Administration** Alirocumab is administered subcutaneously.

Patients and/or their caregivers should be trained on the proper techniques for preparation and administration of alirocumab using the prefilled injection pen provided by the manufacturer. (See Advice to Patients.) Prior to use, the prefilled pens should be stored at 2–8°C in their original carton to protect from light; the drug should not be frozen, shaken, or exposed to extreme heat or direct sunlight. Prior to administration, alirocumab prefilled pens should be allowed to warm to room temperature for 30–40 minutes; the drug should not be returned to the refrigerator after removal and should be used within 30 days or discarded.

Alirocumab injection should be inspected visually prior to administration and should not be used if the solution is discolored, cloudy, or contains any particulate matter (e.g., flakes, particles). Commercially available alirocumab injection contains no preservatives and is intended for single use only.

Subcutaneous injections of alirocumab should be administered into the thigh, abdomen (except for the 2-inch area around the navel), or upper arm; injection sites should be rotated. Injections should *not* be made into areas of active skin disease or injury (e.g., sunburns, rashes, inflammation, infections); areas that are tender, irritated, or erythematous; or areas that have visible veins, scars, or stretch marks. Injection of alirocumab may take up to 20 seconds to complete. Alirocumab should not be administered concomitantly with other drugs at the same injection site.

If a dose of alirocumab is missed, the dose should be administered as soon as possible within 7 days. If a missed dose is *not* administered within 7 days in a patient receiving the every-2-week regimen, the dose should be withheld and the next dose should be administered at the regularly scheduled time. If a missed dose is *not* administered within 7 days in a patient receiving the once-monthly regimen, the dose should be administered and a new dosing schedule should be initiated starting on that date.

■ **Dosage** ***Prevention of Cardiovascular Events*** The recommended initial dosage of alirocumab to reduce the risk of myocardial infarction (MI), stroke, and unstable angina requiring hospitalization in adults with established cardiovascular disease is 75 mg every 2 weeks; in clinical studies, most patients were able to achieve sufficient LDL-cholesterol reduction with this dosage. If response is inadequate based on LDL-cholesterol monitoring, dosage may be increased to a maximum of 150 mg every 2 weeks. (See Dosage and Administration: General.)

Alternatively, an initial dosage of 300 mg (administered as 2 consecutive 150-mg injections at 2 different injection sites) every 4 weeks (i.e., once monthly) may be used for patients who prefer less frequent dosing. If response is inadequate based on LDL-cholesterol monitoring, dosage may be adjusted to 150 mg every 2 weeks (with the first dose of the new regimen administered on the date of the next scheduled dose of the previous regimen). (See Dosage and Administration: General.)

Primary Hyperlipidemia (including Heterozygous Familial Hypercholesterolemia) The recommended initial dosage of alirocumab as an adjunct to diet alone or in combination with other lipid-lowering therapy (e.g., hydroxymethylglutaryl-coenzyme A [HMG-CoA] reductase inhibitor [i.e., statin], ezetimibe) in adults with primary hyperlipidemia (including heterozygous familial hypercholesterolemia) is 75 mg every 2 weeks; in clinical studies, most patients were able to achieve sufficient LDL-cholesterol reduction with this dosage. If response is inadequate based on LDL-cholesterol monitoring, dosage may be increased to a maximum of 150 mg every 2 weeks. (See Dosage and Administration: General.)

Alternatively, an initial dosage of 300 mg (administered as 2 consecutive 150-mg injections at 2 different injection sites) every 4 weeks (i.e., once monthly) may be used for patients who prefer less frequent dosing. If response is inadequate based on LDL-cholesterol monitoring, dosage may be adjusted to 150 mg every 2 weeks (with the first dose of the new regimen administered on the date of the next scheduled dose of the previous regimen). (See Dosage and Administration: General.)

In adults with heterozygous familial hypercholesterolemia undergoing LDL apheresis, the recommended dosage of alirocumab is 150 mg every 2 weeks. The drug may be administered without regard to timing of the procedure.

■ **Special Populations** No dosage adjustment is necessary in patients with mild or moderate hepatic impairment; data are lacking in patients with severe hepatic impairment.

No dosage adjustment is necessary in patients with mild or moderate renal impairment; data are lacking in patients with severe renal impairment.

No dosage adjustment is necessary based on age, weight, gender, or race.

Cautions

■ **Contraindications** Alirocumab is contraindicated in patients with a history of a serious hypersensitivity reaction to the drug. (See Sensitivity Reactions under Cautions: Warnings/Precautions.)

■ **Warnings/Precautions** ***Sensitivity Reactions*** **Hypersensitivity.** Serious hypersensitivity reactions including angioedema, vasculitis, nummular eczema, and hypersensitivity reactions requiring hospitalization have been reported in patients receiving alirocumab. (See Cautions: Contraindications.) Other less severe allergic reactions (e.g., pruritus, rash, urticaria) also have occurred.

If manifestations of serious hypersensitivity occur, alirocumab therapy should be discontinued and patients should be treated in accordance with the standard of care. Patients experiencing a hypersensitivity reaction should be monitored until signs and symptoms of the reaction resolve.

Immunogenicity As with all therapeutic proteins, there is a potential for immunogenicity with alirocumab therapy. In the ODYSSEY OUTCOMES study, antibodies to alirocumab were detected in 5.5% of patients receiving the drug and were persistent in 0.7% of such patients. In addition, 0.5% of alirocumab-treated patients developed neutralizing antibodies. The incidence of anti-alirocumab antibodies and neutralizing antibodies detected in other clinical studies generally was similar to that observed in the ODYSSEY OUTCOMES study. While efficacy of alirocumab based on LDL-cholesterol reduction was generally similar among patients who developed anti-alirocumab antibodies and those who did not, some patients with persistent or neutralizing antibodies experienced an attenuated response. In addition, patients who developed anti-alirocumab antibodies appeared to have a higher incidence of injection site reactions. The long-term effects of continued alirocumab therapy in patients with anti-alirocumab antibodies are not known.

Specific Populations **Pregnancy.** There are no adequate and well-controlled studies of alirocumab in pregnant women. The potential benefits of the drug should be weighed against the possible risks to the fetus when used during pregnancy.

In animal reproductive studies, no adverse embryofetal effects were observed in rats exposed to alirocumab during the period of organogenesis; however, in utero exposure to the drug appeared to suppress the humoral immune response in infant monkeys. Alirocumab was administered at dose exposures of 12–13 times the maximum recommended human dosage in these animal studies.

To monitor pregnancy outcomes in pregnant women exposed to alirocumab, a pregnancy registry has been established. Clinicians and patients are encouraged to call 877-311-8792 or visit https://mothertobaby.org/ongoing-study/praluent to obtain more information about the registry.

Lactation. It is not known whether alirocumab is distributed into human milk. Human IgG is distributed into human milk; however, published data suggest that IgG antibodies present in human milk are not substantially distributed into the circulation of neonates and infants. The potential adverse effects of alirocumab on the infant should be weighed against the known benefits of breastfeeding, taking into account the importance of the drug to the woman.

Pediatric Use. Safety and efficacy of alirocumab have not been established in pediatric patients.

Geriatric Use. Although no overall differences in safety or efficacy have been observed between geriatric patients and younger adults in controlled studies or in other clinical experience, the possibility of increased sensitivity to alirocumab in some geriatric patients cannot be ruled out.

Hepatic Impairment. Safety and efficacy of alirocumab in patients with severe hepatic impairment have not been established. In patients with mild or moderate hepatic impairment, pharmacokinetics of alirocumab following subcutaneous administration of a single 75-mg dose were similar to those observed in individuals with normal hepatic function. (See Dosage and Administration: Special Populations.)

Renal Impairment. Safety and efficacy of alirocumab in patients with severe renal impairment have not been established. However, renal function is not expected to alter the pharmacokinetics of alirocumab because monoclonal antibodies are not known to be eliminated through renal pathways. In a population pharmacokinetic analysis, creatinine clearance did not substantially affect alirocumab pharmacokinetics. (See Dosage and Administration: Special Populations.)

■ **Common Adverse Effects** Adverse effects reported in 2% or more of patients receiving alirocumab and occurring more frequently than with placebo in primary hyperlipidemia studies include nasopharyngitis, injection site reactions (e.g., erythema/redness, itching, swelling, pain/tenderness), influenza, urinary tract infection, diarrhea, bronchitis, myalgia, muscle spasms, sinusitis, cough, contusion, and musculoskeletal pain.

Adverse effects reported in more than 5% of patients receiving alirocumab and occurring more frequently than with placebo in the cardiovascular outcomes study (ODYSSEY OUTCOMES) include noncardiac chest pain, nasopharyngitis, and myalgia.

Findings from genetic studies and clinical and observational studies of lipid-lowering therapies have suggested an association between low LDL-cholesterol concentrations and an increased risk of new-onset diabetes mellitus. In pooled data from placebo- and active-controlled primary hyperlipidemia studies, 914 patients who received alirocumab had 2 consecutive LDL-cholesterol concentrations less than 25 mg/dL and 335 patients had 2 consecutive LDL-cholesterol concentrations less than 15 mg/dL Although most of these patients were receiving higher dosages of alirocumab (i.e., 150 mg every 2 weeks or 300 mg every 4 weeks), dosage modifications to either alirocumab or other background antilipemic drugs were not required. In the cardiovascular outcomes study, 4305 patients who received alirocumab had 2 consecutive LDL-cholesterol concentrations less than 25 mg/dL and 782 patients had 2 consecutive LDL-cholesterol concentrations less than 15 mg/dL. Because protocol-specified dosage adjustment or discontinuance of alirocumab was required for 2 consecutive LDL-cholesterol concentrations less than 15 mg/dL, the effects of prolonged very low LDL-cholesterol concentrations associated with alirocumab have not been established.

Drug Interactions

■ **Drugs Metabolized by Hepatic Microsomal Enzymes** Alirocumab is not expected to affect cytochrome P-450 (CYP) enzymes (e.g., CYP3A4, CYP2C9); therefore, pharmacokinetic interactions are unlikely with drugs that are substrates of these enzymes.

■ **Drugs Affected by Transport Systems** Alirocumab is not expected to affect transport proteins such as P-glycoprotein and organic anion transport protein (OATP); therefore, pharmacokinetic interactions are unlikely with drugs that are substrates of these transporters.

■ **Hydroxymethylglutaryl-Coenzyme A (HMG-CoA) Reductase Inhibitors (Statins)** Statins can stimulate the production of proprotein convertase subtilisin kexin type 9 (PCSK9), which may affect the duration of action of alirocumab. Concomitant use of alirocumab and a statin has been shown to decrease the median apparent half-life of alirocumab to 12 days; however, this effect is not considered to be clinically important and does not require dosage adjustments.

In clinical studies in which alirocumab was administered concomitantly with atorvastatin or rosuvastatin, no clinically important changes in the statin concentration were observed.

Description

Alirocumab, a fully human IgG_1 monoclonal antibody produced by recombinant DNA technology in Chinese hamster ovary cells, is an inhibitor of human proprotein convertase subtilisin kexin type 9 (PCSK9). PCSK9 is a serine protease that is produced principally in the liver. The major function of PCSK9 is to regulate the metabolism of low-density lipoprotein (LDL) cholesterol by promoting the degradation of LDL receptors, the primary receptors responsible for clearing circulating LDL cholesterol. PCSK9 binds to the LDL receptor on the surface of hepatocytes and directs it towards lysosomal degradation; this causes a reduction in the amount of LDL receptors available to bind and remove LDL particles from circulation, and consequently, increases plasma LDL-cholesterol concentrations. Alirocumab binds specifically and with high affinity to PCSK9, preventing the binding of PCSK9 to the LDL-cholesterol receptor and thereby increasing the number of receptors available to clear LDL cholesterol. Reductions in lipoprotein (a), apolipoprotein B, and other lipid fractions also have been demonstrated with alirocumab therapy.

Familial hypercholesterolemia is a group of inherited disorders characterized by excessive elevations in LDL-cholesterol concentrations and early atherosclerotic disease. In most cases, the condition is caused by mutations in the LDL-receptor gene, but mutations in other genes, including the gene encoding apolipoprotein B and PCSK9, also can cause the condition.

Alirocumab reduces circulating PCSK9 in a concentration-dependent manner. Following a single subcutaneous injection of the drug (75 or 150 mg), maximal suppression of free PCSK9 occurs within 4–8 hours and returns to baseline once drug concentrations fall below the limit of quantification. In healthy individuals who received a single subcutaneous injection of alirocumab 75 mg, maximal reduction of LDL-cholesterol concentration occurred 15 days after the dose. Alirocumab exhibits nonlinear pharmacokinetics with slightly greater than dose-proportional increases in plasma concentrations with increasing doses. Following subcutaneous administration, absolute bioavailability of alirocumab is approximately 85% and peak plasma concentrations are attained within 3–7 days. Monthly dose-normalized exposure of alirocumab was similar between patients receiving a dosage of 300 mg every 4 weeks and a dosage of 150 mg every 2 weeks. Steady-state concentrations are achieved after 2–3 doses with an accumulation ratio up to a maximum of approximately twofold. Although specific drug metabolism studies have not been conducted, alirocumab is expected to be degraded into small peptides and individual amino acids. Elimination of alirocumab is concentration-dependent; at low concentrations, elimination occurs principally through saturable binding to the PCSK9 target, while at higher concentrations, elimination occurs principally through a non-saturable proteolytic pathway. The median apparent half-life of alirocumab is 17–20 days.

Advice to Patients

Importance of patients reading the manufacturer's patient information and instructions for use prior to starting therapy and each time the prescription is refilled.

Importance of discontinuing alirocumab and promptly seeking medical attention if any signs or symptoms of serious hypersensitivity (e.g., severe pruritus, rash, or redness; swollen face; difficulty breathing) occur. (See Hypersensitivity under Warnings/Precautions: Sensitivity Reactions, in Cautions.)

Importance of instructing patients and/or caregivers regarding proper preparation and subcutaneous administration of alirocumab, including use of aseptic technique and safe disposal of the prefilled pens in a puncture-resistant container. Importance of informing patients that injection of alirocumab may take up to 20 seconds.

Importance of instructing patients on proper storage of the drug.

Importance of instructing patients not to reuse the prefilled pens.

Importance of informing clinicians of existing or contemplated concomitant therapy, including prescription and OTC drugs and dietary or herbal supplements, as well as any concomitant illnesses.

Importance of women informing clinicians if they are or plan to become pregnant or plan to breast-feed. Importance of encouraging women who become pregnant while receiving alirocumab to participate in the pregnancy registry. (See Pregnancy under Warnings/Precautions: Specific Populations, in Cautions.)

Importance of informing patients of other important precautionary information. (See Cautions.)

Overview® (see Users Guide). For additional information on this drug until a more detailed monograph is developed and published, the manufacturer's labeling should be consulted. It is *essential* that the manufacturer's labeling be consulted for more detailed information on usual cautions, precautions, contraindications, potential drug interactions, laboratory test interferences, and acute toxicity.

Preparations

Excipients in commercially available drug preparations may have clinically important effects in some individuals; consult specific product labeling for details.

Alirocumab

Parenteral		
Injection, for subcutaneous use	75 mg/mL	**Praluent®** (available as single-dose prefilled injection pens), Sanofi-Aventis and Regeneron
	150 mg/mL	**Praluent®** (available as single-dose prefilled injection pens), Sanofi-Aventis and Regeneron

Evolocumab

■ Evolocumab, a fully human IgG_2 monoclonal antibody that binds to proprotein convertase subtilisin kexin type 9 (PCSK9), is an antilipemic agent.

Uses

■ **Prevention of Cardiovascular Events** Evolocumab is used for secondary prevention to reduce the risk of myocardial infarction (MI), stroke, and coronary revascularization in patients with established cardiovascular disease.

Current guidelines from the American College of Cardiology/American Heart Association (ACC/AHA) and the National Lipid Association recommend that lifestyle modifications, which include adherence to a heart-healthy diet, regular exercise, avoidance of tobacco products, and maintenance of a healthy weight, be instituted in all patients with clinical atherosclerotic cardiovascular disease (ASCVD), defined as acute coronary syndrome (ACS), history of MI, stable or unstable angina, coronary or other arterial revascularization, stroke, transient ischemic attack (TIA), or peripheral arterial disease presumed to be of atherosclerotic origin. Drug therapy is not a substitute for but an adjunct to these nondrug therapies and measures, which should be continued when drug therapy is initiated. In addition to lifestyle modifications, pharmacologic therapy with a hydroxymethylglutaryl-coenzyme A (HMG-CoA) reductase inhibitor (i.e., statin) is recommended in all patients with clinical ASCVD to reduce the risk of cardiovascular events; the maximum appropriate and tolerated intensity of a statin should be used (e.g., atorvastatin or rosuvastatin titrated to dosages that produce low-density lipoprotein [LDL]-cholesterol reductions of at least 50% from baseline).

Despite optimal statin therapy, some patients may not achieve adequate reductions in LDL-cholesterol concentrations and may benefit from the addition of a nonstatin antilipemic agent. The ACC/AHA cholesterol management guideline states that the addition of a nonstatin drug may be considered in patients who have a less-than-anticipated response to statins, are unable to tolerate a less-than-recommended intensity of a statin, or are completely statin intolerant, particularly when there is evidence from randomized controlled studies suggesting that the nonstatin drug further reduces ASCVD events when added to statin therapy. An expert consensus panel was convened by ACC to provide further guidance on the role of nonstatin drugs in the management of ASCVD, specifically in regard to the specific patient populations and clinical situations in which these drugs may be considered. According to these experts, patients who may benefit from the addition of a nonstatin drug include those with clinical ASCVD with or without comorbidities (including severe elevations of baseline LDL-cholesterol concentrations greater than 190 mg/dL) who have not met certain thresholds of LDL-cholesterol reduction (e.g., at least 50% reduction in LDL-cholesterol, or an absolute LDL-cholesterol concentration of less than 70 mg/dL or non-high-density lipoprotein [non-HDL]-cholesterol concentration of less than 100 mg/dL) while receiving maximally tolerated statin therapy; nonstatin drugs that may be considered include ezetimibe or a proprotein convertase subtilisin kexin type 9 (PCSK9) inhibitor (or possibly both) depending on the specific situation. Selection of a nonstatin drug should be based on a favorable benefit-risk ratio (i.e., demonstrated benefit of ASCVD risk reduction outweighs risks of adverse effects and drug interactions) and patient preferences. Prior to initiation of nonstatin antilipemic drugs, it is critical that patients are treated first with maximally tolerated statin therapy and that lifestyle modifications are intensified/optimized. Because true statin intolerance is uncommon, patients should be systematically and rigorously evaluated for this condition to encourage adherence to evidence-based statin therapy. For additional details on prevention of ASCVD, see the HMG-CoA Reductase Inhibitors General Statement 24:06.08.

Efficacy of evolocumab in the prevention of cardiovascular events has been established in the FOURIER study, which was a large randomized, double-blind, placebo-controlled study in 27,564 high-risk adults with established cardiovascular disease (81% with prior MI, 19% with prior nonhemorrhagic stroke, 13% with symptomatic peripheral arterial disease) and additional risk factors (80% with hypertension, 36% with type 2 diabetes mellitus, 28% smokers, 23% with New York Heart Association [NYHA] class I or II heart failure). Patients were included in the study if they had a fasting LDL- or non-HDL-cholesterol concentration of at least 70 or 100 mg/dL, respectively, while receiving an optimized antilipemic regimen (preferably with a high-intensity statin, but at least a statin intensity equivalent to atorvastatin 20 mg daily, with or without ezetimibe). Approximately 70% of the patients were receiving high-intensity statin therapy. Patients were randomized to receive add-on therapy with evolocumab (140 mg every 2 weeks or 420 mg once monthly by subcutaneous injection) or matching placebo. The median baseline LDL-cholesterol concentration prior to the start of add-on therapy was 92 mg/dL. Evolocumab substantially reduced the rate of the primary composite end point (time to first occurrence of cardiovascular death, MI, stroke, unstable angina requiring hospitalization, or coronary revascularization) by 15% and also reduced the key secondary composite end point (time to first occurrence of cardiovascular death, MI, or stroke) by 20% compared with placebo. The benefits of evolocumab were largely consistent across major patient subgroups defined by baseline LDL-cholesterol concentrations, intensity of statin therapy, concomitant use of ezetimibe, and evolocumab dosing regimen. Evolocumab produced a 63 and 57% further reduction in mean LDL-cholesterol concentration from baseline at 12 and 72 weeks, respectively, that was sustained throughout the study.

Although the median duration of follow-up was initially planned to be approximately 4 years, the prespecified number of events occurred at a higher rate than anticipated, resulting in a shortened median duration of follow-up of 26 months. Because of this relatively short duration, long-term efficacy of evolocumab in the prevention of cardiovascular events remains to be established.

Findings from postmarketing reports, observational studies, and small randomized trials have suggested an association between LDL-lowering therapies including PCSK9 inhibitors (or the very low LDL-cholesterol concentrations that can result from their use) and impaired cognitive function or cognitive adverse effects. At week 48 of the FOURIER study, 47% of patients in the evolocumab group had an LDL-cholesterol concentration less than 25 mg/dL, and 76% of patients receiving the drug had at least one LDL-cholesterol concentration less than 25 mg/dL. Although not a controlled comparison, the safety profile of evolocumab appeared to be similar among patients whose LDL-cholesterol concentrations decreased to less than 25 mg/dL and those whose LDL-cholesterol concentrations remained at 40 mg/dL or greater. In the EBBINGHAUS study, which prospectively evaluated cognition in a subset of 1974 patients from the FOURIER study, no substantial differences were observed in cognitive function test scores (evaluating episodic and working memory, executive function, psychomotor speed, and attention) between patients receiving evolocumab and those receiving placebo over a median follow-up of 19 months.

■ **Dyslipidemias** ***Primary Hyperlipidemia*** Evolocumab is used alone or in combination with other antilipemic agents (e.g., statins, ezetimibe) as an adjunct to diet in patients with primary hyperlipidemia (including heterozygous familial hypercholesterolemia) to reduce LDL-cholesterol concentrations.

Elevated serum cholesterol, especially the LDL-cholesterol fraction, is a major cause of clinical ASCVD; patients with heterozygous familial hypercholesterolemia in particular have excessive elevations in LDL-cholesterol concentrations that predispose them to a high risk of premature ASCVD. Therefore, the goal of antilipemic therapy in patients with hyperlipidemia is to reduce the risk of ASCVD. The ACC/AHA cholesterol management guideline states that lifestyle modifications, which include adherence to a heart-healthy diet, regular exercise, avoidance of tobacco products, and maintenance of a healthy weight, are the foundation of ASCVD risk reduction. If drug therapy is needed, statins are the first-line antilipemic agents of choice. A nonstatin drug may be considered in selected high-risk patients (e.g., those with known cardiovascular disease, markedly high LDL-cholesterol concentrations at baseline, or diabetes mellitus) who are not able to achieve adequate reductions in LDL-cholesterol concentration with diet and statins alone or who are completely intolerant of statin therapy. Clinical studies have demonstrated that evolocumab can further reduce LDL-cholesterol concentrations by approximately 50–60% or more when used alone or added to maximally tolerated statin therapy and can also reduce the risk of cardiovascular events. (See Uses: Prevention of Cardiovascular Events.)

Efficacy and safety of evolocumab in the treatment of primary hyperlipidemia (including patients with heterozygous familial hypercholesterolemia) have been established in 4 multicenter, randomized, double-blind, controlled studies (LAPLACE-2, DESCARTES, MENDEL-2, and RUTHERFORD-2); in these studies, evolocumab demonstrated substantial reductions in LDL-cholesterol concentrations whether used alone or added to existing statin therapy with or without other antilipemic agents (e.g., ezetimibe).

The LAPLACE-2 study was a 12-week placebo- and active-controlled study that evaluated efficacy of evolocumab when added to moderate- or high-intensity statin therapy in 1896 adults with primary hyperlipidemia or mixed dyslipidemia. Patients initially received one of 5 open-label statin regimens (i.e., moderate-intensity statin [atorvastatin 10 mg, rosuvastatin 5 mg, or simvastatin 40 mg daily] or high-intensity statin [atorvastatin 80 mg or rosuvastatin 40 mg daily]) for 4 weeks. Following the 4-week lipid stabilization period, patients were then randomized to add-on therapy with evolocumab (140 mg every 2 weeks or evolocumab 420 mg once monthly) or matching placebo for 12 weeks; ezetimibe (10 mg daily) also was included as an active control in the atorvastatin group. The mean baseline LDL-cholesterol concentration prior to the start of add-on therapy was 77–127 mg/dL. At 12 weeks, LDL-cholesterol concentrations were reduced by a mean of 71 or 63% from baseline with evolocumab 140 mg every 2 weeks or evolocumab 420 mg once monthly, respectively, compared with placebo; LDL-cholesterol concentrations were reduced by a mean of 45 or 41% from baseline with evolocumab 140 mg every 2 weeks or evolocumab 420 mg once monthly, respectively, compared with ezetimibe.

The DESCARTES study was a 52-week placebo-controlled study that included 901 adults with hyperlipidemia. Following initial stabilization on the assigned open-label background antilipemic regimen (i.e., cholesterol-lowering diet alone or in combination with atorvastatin 10 or 80 mg daily, or cholesterol-lowering diet in combination with atorvastatin 80 mg daily and ezetimibe 10 mg daily), patients were randomized in a 2:1 ratio to receive add-on therapy with evolocumab 420 mg or matching placebo once monthly. The mean baseline LDL-cholesterol concentration prior to the start of add-on therapy was 90–117 mg/dL. At 52 weeks, LDL-cholesterol concentrations were reduced by a mean of 55% from baseline with evolocumab compared with placebo.

The RUTHERFORD-2 study evaluated efficacy and safety of evolocumab in 329 adults with heterozygous familial hypercholesterolemia (diagnosed by genotyping or clinical criteria) who were receiving stable dosages of a statin with or without other antilipemic agents (ezetimibe, resins, stanols, or niacin, but not fibric acid derivatives); patients were randomized to receive add-on therapy with evolocumab 140 mg every 2 weeks, evolocumab 420 mg once monthly, or matching placebo for 12 weeks. Approximately 38% of the patients had ASCVD and 76% were receiving high-intensity statin therapy; more than half of the patients were also receiving ezetimibe. The mean LDL-cholesterol concentration at baseline was 156 mg/dL. At 12 weeks, LDL-cholesterol concentrations were reduced by a mean of 61 or 60% in patients receiving evolocumab 140 mg every 2 weeks or evolocumab 420 mg once monthly, respectively, compared with placebo. Reductions in LDL-cholesterol concentration were observed at 2 weeks after beginning therapy and sustained throughout the 12-week study. In addition, approximately 66% of patients in the evolocumab group achieved an LDL-cholesterol goal of less than 70 mg/dL at 12 weeks. The study also demonstrated that LDL-cholesterol response in patients with heterozygous familial hypercholesterolemia was independent of the underlying LDL-receptor defect.

The MENDEL-2 study was a 12-week study that evaluated evolocumab monotherapy in 614 adults with hyperlipidemia who were not receiving any lipid-lowering therapy at baseline. Patients were randomized to receive evolocumab (140 mg every 2 weeks or 420 mg once monthly) or placebo; ezetimibe (10 mg daily) also was included as an active control. The mean baseline LDL-cholesterol concentration was 143 mg/dL. At 12 weeks, LDL-cholesterol concentrations were reduced by a mean of 55 or 57% from baseline with evolocumab 140 mg every 2 weeks or evolocumab 420 mg once monthly, respectively, compared with placebo; LDL-cholesterol concentrations were reduced by a mean of 37 or 38% from baseline with evolocumab 140 mg every 2 weeks or evolocumab 420 mg once monthly, respectively, compared with ezetimibe. The MENDEL-2 study did not specifically evaluate statin intolerance; however, other randomized controlled studies (GAUSS studies) have been conducted with evolocumab in patients who were unable to tolerate evidence-based dosages of statins because of muscle-related adverse effects. In these studies, use of evolocumab compared with ezetimibe resulted in substantially greater reductions in LDL-cholesterol concentrations; mean reductions in LDL-cholesterol concentrations with evolocumab were consistent with those demonstrated in other randomized controlled studies of the drug.

Long-term efficacy and safety of evolocumab were evaluated in 2 open-label extension studies (OSLER-1 and OSLER-2) that included patients who had previously participated in one of the short-term (8–12 weeks) phase 2 or 3 studies of the drug; a total of 4465 patients with varying degrees of cardiovascular risk were randomly assigned to receive evolocumab (140 mg every 2 weeks or 420 mg once monthly) plus standard therapy or standard therapy alone, and followed for a median duration of 11.1 months. Results in terms of LDL-cholesterol reductions were similar to those observed in the short-term trials, and the LDL-reducing effects of evolocumab were sustained through 48 weeks. In a prespecified exploratory analysis of prospectively adjudicated cardiovascular events (i.e., death, MI, unstable angina, coronary revascularization, cerebrovascular events, heart failure requiring hospitalization) in the OSLER studies, evolocumab-treated patients appeared to have a decreased rate of cardiovascular events compared with those in the standard therapy group; however, the analysis was based on a relatively small number of events.

Homozygous Familial Hypercholesterolemia Evolocumab is used as an adjunct to diet and other LDL-cholesterol lowering therapies (e.g., statins, ezetimibe, LDL apheresis) in patients with homozygous familial hypercholesterolemia who require additional lowering of LDL-cholesterol concentrations. Evolocumab has been designated an orphan drug by the FDA for use in this condition.

Homozygous familial hypercholesterolemia is a severe subtype of familial hypercholesterolemia characterized by extreme elevations of serum cholesterol concentrations typically in excess of 500 mg/dL. (See Description.) Such excessive elevations in cholesterol concentrations predispose patients to a high risk of premature atherosclerosis, cardiovascular disease, and death. Current treatments for patients with homozygous familial hypercholesterolemia include lifestyle modifications (e.g., low-fat diet, maintenance of a healthy body weight, smoking cessation), maximally tolerated dosages of statins, and, if necessary, combination therapy with other lipid-lowering medications (e.g., ezetimibe, bile acid sequestrants, niacin). Because there is some variability in the level of residual LDL-receptor activity in individuals with homozygous familial hypercholesterolemia and because statins rely on the upregulation of the LDL receptor to clear LDL particles, even maximally tolerated dosages of statins often do not result in sufficient reduction of LDL-cholesterol concentration in this population. Clinical studies have demonstrated that evolocumab can further reduce LDL-cholesterol concentrations by approximately 30% when used adjunctively with other antilipemic agents in patients with homozygous familial hypercholesterolemia.

Efficacy and safety of evolocumab in patients with homozygous familial hypercholesterolemia have been established in a multicenter, randomized, double-blind, placebo-controlled study (TESLA Part B) that showed substantial reductions in LDL-cholesterol concentrations when the drug was added to existing stable antilipemic therapy. The study included 49 patients 13 years of age or older with genetically or clinically diagnosed homozygous familial hypercholesterolemia who had LDL-cholesterol concentrations of approximately 130 mg/dL or greater despite treatment with a stable low-fat diet and an antilipemic regimen for at least 4 weeks; baseline antilipemic therapy consisted in most cases of intensive statin therapy (at least 40 mg of atorvastatin or 20 mg of rosuvastatin daily) with ezetimibe, but without lipid apheresis. Patients were randomized to receive evolocumab 420 mg or placebo once monthly for 12 weeks. The mean LDL-cholesterol concentration at baseline was 349 mg/dL. At 12 weeks, LDL-cholesterol concentrations were reduced by a mean of 22% in patients receiving evolocumab compared with an increase of 9% in those receiving placebo. Reductions in LDL-cholesterol concentrations were observed at 4 weeks and sustained throughout the 12-week study. Analysis of response according to LDL-receptor function revealed a greater treatment effect in patients with receptor-defective mutations in both alleles compared with those with one defective and one negative mutation; one patient in the study who had known receptor-negative mutations in both alleles (corresponding to little to no residual function) exhibited no response to evolocumab therapy. (See Description.)

For additional information on general principles of antilipemic therapy, see the HMG-CoA Reductase Inhibitors General Statement 24:06.08.

Dosage and Administration

■ General Adherence to lifestyle modifications and to statin therapy are required for atherosclerotic cardiovascular disease (ASCVD) risk reduction and should be reinforced periodically.

When monitoring low-density lipoprotein (LDL)-cholesterol concentrations in patients receiving evolocumab, it should be noted that some patients receiving the once-monthly dosage regimen may experience considerable variation in LDL-cholesterol concentrations during the monthly dosing interval.

■ Administration Evolocumab is administered subcutaneously. The drug is administered as an every-2-week or once-monthly dosing regimen.

Evolocumab is commercially available as a prefilled manual syringe, prefilled auto-injector, and single-use on-body infuser pump with prefilled cartridge. Patients and/or their caregivers should be trained on the proper techniques for preparation and administration of evolocumab using these devices. If the on-body infuser with prefilled cartridge is used in adolescents, adult supervision is necessary. A monthly evolocumab dose of 420 mg can be administered using the on-body infuser with prefilled cartridge or by consecutively administering three 140-mg subcutaneous injections within 30 minutes using the prefilled syringes or auto-injectors. Patient preference for dosing frequency and injection volume should be considered when determining the method of administration.

Prior to use, all commercially available dosage forms of evolocumab (prefilled syringes and auto-injectors, on-body infusers with prefilled cartridges) should be stored at 2–8°C in their original carton to protect from light; the drug should not be frozen or shaken. Alternatively, patients may store these products at room temperature at 20–25°C; however, the drug must be used within 30 days or otherwise discarded if stored under these conditions. Prior to administration, evolocumab prefilled syringes and auto-injectors should be allowed to warm to room temperature for at least 30 minutes, and the on-body infuser with prefilled cartridge should be allowed to warm to room temperature for at least 45 minutes.

Evolocumab injection should be inspected visually prior to administration and should not be used if the solution is discolored, cloudy, or contains particulate matter. Commercially available evolocumab injection contains no preservatives and is intended for single use only.

Evolocumab should be administered subcutaneously into the abdomen (except for the 2-inch area around the navel), thigh, or upper arm; injection sites should be rotated. Areas that are tender, bruised, red, or indurated, or that have scars or stretch marks should be avoided. The on-body infuser should be securely attached to a clean, firm and flat skin surface that is less likely to have body hair or on which the body hair can be trimmed; it should not be used on areas with wrinkles, skin folds, moles, or excessive hair. Injection of the drug using a prefilled syringe or auto-injector may take up to 15 seconds to complete; injection of the drug using the on-body infuser with prefilled cartridge takes about 9 minutes to complete. Evolocumab should not be administered with other drugs at the same injection site.

If a dose of evolocumab is missed, the missed dose should be administered as soon as possible within 7 days. If a dose of evolocumab is missed in a patient receiving the every-2-week regimen and the missed dose is *not* administered within 7 days, the dose should be withheld and the next dose should be administered at the regularly scheduled time. If a dose of evolocumab is missed in a patient receiving the once-monthly regimen and the missed dose is *not* administered within 7 days, the dose should be administered and a new dosing schedule should be initiated starting on that date.

■ Dosage ***Prevention of Cardiovascular Events*** The recommended dosage of evolocumab to reduce the risk of myocardial infarction (MI), stroke, and coronary revascularization in adults with established cardiovascular disease is 140 mg every 2 weeks or 420 mg once monthly (administered using the on-body infuser with prefilled cartridge or as 3 consecutive 140-mg injections within 30 minutes).

When switching between the every-2-week and once-monthly dosage regimens, the first dose of the new regimen should be administered on the date of the next scheduled dose of the previous regimen.

Primary Hyperlipidemia The recommended dosage of evolocumab as an adjunct to diet alone or in combination with other lipid-lowering therapy (e.g., hydroxymethylglutaryl-coenzyme A [HMG-CoA] reductase inhibitor [i.e., statin], ezetimibe) in adults with primary hyperlipidemia (including heterozygous familial hypercholesterolemia) is 140 mg every 2 weeks or 420 mg once monthly (administered using the on-body infuser with prefilled cartridge or as 3 consecutive 140-mg injections within 30 minutes).

Homozygous Familial Hypercholesterolemia The recommended dosage of evolocumab as an adjunct to diet and other LDL-lowering therapies in adults and adolescents 13 years of age or older with homozygous familial hypercholesterolemia is 420 mg once monthly (administered using the on-body infuser with prefilled cartridge or as 3 consecutive 140-mg injections within 30 minutes).

In patients with homozygous familial hypercholesterolemia, LDL-cholesterol concentrations should be measured 4–8 weeks after initiation of evolocumab since response to therapy is dependent upon the degree of residual LDL-receptor function.

■ Special Populations No dosage adjustment is necessary in patients with mild or moderate hepatic impairment (Child-Pugh class A or B); data are lacking in patients with severe hepatic impairment.

No dosage adjustment is necessary in patients with renal impairment.

Cautions

■ Contraindications Evolocumab is contraindicated in patients with a history of a serious hypersensitivity reaction to the drug. (See Hypersensitivity under Warnings/Precautions: Sensitivity Reactions, in Cautions.)

■ Warnings/Precautions ***Sensitivity Reactions*** **Hypersensitivity.** Hypersensitivity reactions (including angioedema), sometimes resulting in drug discontinuance, have been reported in patients receiving evolocumab. (See Cautions: Contraindications.) In placebo-controlled trials, allergic reactions occurred in 5.1 or 4.7% of patients receiving evolocumab or placebo, respectively. The most common manifestations were rash, eczema, erythema, and urticaria.

If signs or symptoms of serious hypersensitivity reactions occur, evolocumab therapy should be discontinued and patients should be treated according to the standard of care. Patients experiencing a hypersensitivity reaction should be monitored until symptoms resolve.

Latex Sensitivity. Some packaging components of evolocumab (e.g., needle covers of prefilled syringes and auto-injectors) contain natural latex proteins in the form of dry natural rubber (latex). Some individuals may be hypersensitive to such latex proteins found in a wide range of medical devices, including such packaging components, and the level of sensitivity may vary depending on the form of natural rubber present; rarely, hypersensitivity reactions to natural latex proteins have been fatal. The needle covers of the prefilled evolocumab syringes and the area within the needle caps of the prefilled auto-injectors contain dry natural rubber (latex), and should not be handled by individuals sensitive to latex.

Immunogenicity As with all therapeutic proteins, there is a potential for immunogenicity with evolocumab therapy. In a pooled analysis of randomized controlled studies that included both placebo- and active-controlled trials, antibodies to evolocumab were detected in 0.3% of the patients who received at least 1 dose of the drug; none of the patients tested positive for neutralizing antibodies. The long-term effects of continued evolocumab therapy in patients with persistent neutralizing antibodies to the drug are not known.

Specific Populations **Pregnancy.** There are no adequate and well-controlled studies of evolocumab in pregnant women. The potential benefits of the drug should be weighed against the possible risks to the fetus when used during pregnancy.

Adverse embryofetal or postnatal developmental effects have not been observed in monkeys exposed to evolocumab during the period of organogenesis through parturition at dose exposures up to 12 times the maximum recommended human dosage; however, studies with another proprotein convertase subtilisin kexin type 9 (PCSK9) inhibitor demonstrated some evidence of humoral immune suppression in infant monkeys exposed to the drug in utero.

To monitor pregnancy outcomes in pregnant women exposed to evolocumab, a pregnancy registry has been established. Clinicians and patients are encouraged to call 877-311-8792 or visit https://mothertobaby.org/ongoing-study/repatha to obtain more information about the registry.

Lactation. It is not known whether evolocumab is distributed into human milk. Human IgG is distributed into human milk; however, published data suggest that the IgG antibodies present in human milk are not substantially distributed into the circulation of neonates and infants.

The potential adverse effects of evolocumab on the infant should be weighed against the known benefits of breastfeeding, taking into account the importance of the drug to the woman.

Pediatric Use. Safety and efficacy of evolocumab have not been established in pediatric patients with primary hyperlipidemia or heterozygous familial hypercholesterolemia.

The principal efficacy study of evolocumab in patients with homozygous familial hypercholesterolemia included 7 adolescents 13–17 years of age who received the drug; safety and efficacy profiles among these adolescents were similar to those observed in adult patients. Safety and efficacy of evolocumab have not been established in pediatric patients younger than 13 years of age with homozygous familial hypercholesterolemia.

Geriatric Use. In clinical studies, 41% of patients who received evolocumab were 65 years of age or older and 8% were 75 years of age or older. Although no overall differences in safety or efficacy have been observed between geriatric patients and younger adults in controlled studies or in other clinical experience, the possibility of increased sensitivity to evolocumab in some geriatric patients cannot be ruled out.

Hepatic Impairment. Safety and efficacy of evolocumab in patients with severe hepatic impairment have not been established. In patients with mild or moderate hepatic impairment (Child-Pugh class A or B), peak plasma concentrations of and systemic exposure to evolocumab following a single subcutaneous dose of 140 mg were reduced by about 20–30 and 40–50%, respectively, compared with values achieved in healthy individuals; however, these differences are not considered to be clinically important. (See Dosage and Administration: Special Populations.)

Renal Impairment. In patients with severe renal impairment (i.e., estimated glomerular filtration rate [GFR] less than 30 mL/minute per 1.73 m^2) or end-stage renal disease (ESRD) receiving hemodialysis, exposure to evolocumab following a single subcutaneous dose of 140 mg was reduced compared with exposure to the drug in patients with normal renal function (i.e., estimated GFR of at least 90 mL/minute per 1.73 m^2); however, reductions in PCSK9 concentrations in patients with severe renal impairment or ESRD were similar to those in patients with normal renal function. Renal function is not expected to affect the pharmacokinetics of the drug because monoclonal antibodies are not known to be eliminated through renal pathways. (See Dosage and Administration: Special Populations.)

■ **Common Adverse Effects** Adverse effects reported in 3% or more of patients receiving evolocumab and occurring more frequently than with placebo in clinical studies of patients with primary hyperlipidemia (including heterozygous familial hypercholesterolemia) include nasopharyngitis, upper respiratory tract infection, influenza, back pain, injection site reactions (e.g., erythema, pain, bruising), cough, urinary tract infection, sinusitis, headache, myalgia, dizziness, musculoskeletal pain, hypertension, diarrhea, and gastroenteritis.

Adverse effects reported in more than 5% of patients receiving evolocumab and occurring more frequently than with placebo in the cardiovascular outcomes study (FOURIER) include diabetes mellitus, nasopharyngitis, and upper respiratory tract infection.

Drug Interactions

■ **Hydroxymethylglutaryl-Coenzyme A (HMG-CoA) Reductase Inhibitors (Statins)** Concomitant use of evolocumab and a high-intensity statin regimen decreased the peak plasma concentration and area under the concentration-time curve (AUC) of evolocumab by approximately 20%; however, this difference is not considered to be clinically important and does not require dosage adjustment.

Description

Evolocumab, a fully human IgG$_2$ monoclonal antibody produced in genetically engineered mammalian (Chinese hamster ovary) cells, is an inhibitor of human proprotein convertase subtilisin kexin type 9 (PCSK9). PCSK9 is a serine protease that is produced principally in the liver. The major function of PCSK9 is to regulate the metabolism of low-density lipoprotein (LDL) cholesterol by promoting the degradation of LDL receptors, the primary receptors responsible for clearing circulating LDL cholesterol. PCSK9 binds to the LDL receptor on the surface of hepatocytes and directs it towards lysosomal degradation; this causes a reduction in the amount of LDL receptors available to bind and remove LDL particles from circulation, and consequently increases plasma LDL-cholesterol concentrations. Evolocumab binds specifically and with high affinity to PCSK9, preventing the binding of PCSK9 to the LDL-cholesterol receptor, and thereby increasing the number of receptors available to clear LDL cholesterol. Reductions in lipoprotein (a), apolipoprotein B, and other lipid fractions also have been demonstrated with evolocumab therapy.

Familial hypercholesterolemia is a group of inherited disorders characterized by excessive elevations in LDL-cholesterol concentrations and early atherosclerotic disease. In most cases, the condition is caused by mutations in the LDL-receptor gene, but mutations in other genes, including the gene encoding apolipoprotein B and PCSK9, also can cause the condition. In the heterozygous form of familial hypercholesterolemia, LDL-receptor function is impaired by up to 50% and in the more serious but rare homozygous form, LDL-receptor function is reduced by 70–97%. In patients with homozygous familial hypercholesterolemia, the severity of the mutation and corresponding residual LDL-receptor activity affect response to evolocumab therapy. Patients with 2 receptor-defective mutations (corresponding to relatively functional LDL-receptor activity) appear to derive the greatest benefit from evolocumab therapy; patients with one negative (corresponding to very little or no LDL-receptor activity) and one defective mutation have a lesser response, and those with 2 receptor-negative mutations generally do not respond to therapy. (See Homozygous Familial Hypercholesterolemia under Uses: Dyslipidemias.)

After a single subcutaneous injection of evolocumab (140 or 420 mg), maximal suppression of free PCSK9 occurs within 4 hours and returns to baseline once drug concentrations fall below the limit of quantification. Evolocumab exhibits dose-dependent nonlinear pharmacokinetics. Following subcutaneous administration of a single 140- or 420-mg dose of the drug in healthy adults, the estimated absolute bioavailability was approximately 72% and peak plasma concentrations were attained in approximately 3–4 days. After multiple dosing, an accumulation ratio of approximately two- to threefold was observed, and serum trough concentrations approached steady state by 12 weeks. Elimination of evolocumab is concentration-dependent; at low concentrations, elimination occurs principally through saturable binding to the PCSK9 target, while at higher concentrations, elimination occurs principally through a non-saturable proteolytic pathway. The effective half-life of evolocumab is estimated to be 11–17 days.

Advice to Patients

Importance of patients reading the manufacturer's patient information and instructions for use prior to starting therapy and each time the prescription is refilled.

Importance of discontinuing evolocumab and promptly seeking medical attention if any signs or symptoms of serious hypersensitivity (e.g., severe pruritus, rash, or redness; swollen face; difficulty breathing) occur. (See Hypersensitivity under Warnings/Precautions: Sensitivity Reactions, in Cautions.)

Importance of instructing patients and/or caregivers regarding the preparation and subcutaneous administration of evolocumab, including use of the prefilled syringes and auto-injectors and on-body infusers with prefilled cartridges. Importance of informing patients that injection of evolocumab using the prefilled syringe or auto-injector may take up to 15 seconds to complete, and that injection of the drug using the on-body infuser with prefilled cartridge takes about 9 minutes to complete. Importance of informing patients that adult supervision is necessary if the on-body infuser is used in adolescent patients.

Importance of patients informing their clinician if they have an allergy to latex.

Importance of informing clinicians of existing or contemplated concomitant therapy, including prescription and OTC drugs and dietary or herbal supplements, as well as any concomitant illnesses.

Importance of women informing clinicians if they are or plan to become pregnant or plan to breast-feed. Importance of encouraging women who become pregnant while receiving evolocumab to participate in the pregnancy registry. (See Pregnancy under Warnings/Precautions: Specific Populations, in Cautions.)

Importance of informing patients of other important precautionary information. (See Cautions.)

Overview® (see Users Guide). For additional information on this drug until a more detailed monograph is developed and published, the manufacturer's labeling should be consulted. It is *essential* that the manufacturer's labeling be consulted for more detailed information on usual cautions, precautions, contraindications, potential drug interactions, laboratory test interferences, and acute toxicity.

Preparations

Excipients in commercially available drug preparations may have clinically important effects in some individuals; consult specific product labeling for details.

Evolocumab

Parenteral		
Injection, for subcutaneous use	140 mg/mL	Repatha® (available as single-use prefilled syringes and auto-injectors), Amgen
	420 mg/3.5 mL	Repatha® (available as single-use Pushtronex® system consisting of on-body infusor with prefilled cartridge), Amgen

Selected Revisions October 2019, © Copyright, June 2016, American Society of Health-System Pharmacists, Inc.

HYPOTENSIVE AGENTS 24:08

CENTRAL α-AGONISTS 24:08.16

cloNIDine
cloNIDine Hydrochloride

■ Clonidine hydrochloride, an imidazoline-derivative hypotensive agent, is a selective α_2-adrenergic agonist.

Uses

■ **Hypertension** Oral clonidine hydrochloride or transdermal clonidine is used alone or in combination with other classes of antihypertensive agents in the management of hypertension. However, because of established clinical benefits (e.g., reductions in overall mortality and in adverse cardiovascular, cerebrovascular, and renal outcomes), current evidence-based practice guidelines for the management of hypertension in adults generally recommend the use of drugs from 4 classes of antihypertensive agents (angiotensin-converting enzyme [ACE] inhibitors, angiotensin II receptor antagonists, calcium-channel blockers, and thiazide diuretics). Centrally acting agents such as clonidine may be considered as add-on therapy if goal blood pressure cannot be achieved with the recommended drugs. (See Uses: Hypertension in Adults, in the Thiazides General Statement 40:28.20.) Some experts state that centrally acting agents such as clonidine generally are reserved as a last-line treatment option because of the drugs' ability to cause substantial adverse CNS effects, especially in geriatric patients.

Clonidine may be more effective when used with a diuretic. Clonidine hydrochloride has been used in conjunction with thiazide diuretics, chlorthalidone, or furosemide, producing a greater reduction in blood pressure than is obtained with either drug alone. Use of a diuretic may aid in overcoming tolerance to clonidine and permit reduction of clonidine dosage.

Clonidine may be useful in some patients who are unable to tolerate other adrenergic blocking agents because of severe postural hypotension. Clonidine hydrochloride has been used with other hypotensive agents such as hydralazine, reserpine, or methyldopa, permitting a reduction in the dosage of each drug and, in some patients, minimizing adverse effects while maintaining blood pressure control. As when clonidine is used alone, satisfactory results are obtained in both supine and standing patients during combined drug therapy; marked fluctuations in blood pressure because of postural changes usually do not occur during combined therapy. As with other hypotensive agents, treatment with clonidine is not curative; upon withdrawal of the drug, blood pressure returns to pretreatment levels or greater. (See Cautions: Withdrawal Effects.)

Transdermal clonidine has been effective for the management of mild to moderate hypertension when used alone or in combination with an oral thiazide diuretic, and also has been substituted for oral clonidine hydrochloride in some patients with mild to moderate hypertension whose therapy included the oral form of the drug.

For additional information on overall principles and expert recommendations for treatment of hypertension, see Uses: Hypertension in Adults, and also see Uses: Hypertension in Pediatric Patients, in the Thiazides General Statement 40:28.20.

Hypertensive Crises Oral loading-dose regimens of clonidine hydrochloride have been effective in rapidly reducing blood pressure in patients with severe hypertension in whom reduction of blood pressure was considered urgent, but not requiring emergency treatment†. Hypertensive urgencies are those situations in which there is a severe elevation in blood pressure without progressive target organ damage. Hypertensive urgencies can be managed by intensification or reinstitution (e.g., following noncompliance) of the current antihypertensive regimen and treatment of anxiety if needed. Experts state that there is no need for rapid reduction of blood pressure in such patients in the emergency department and hospitalization also is unnecessary.

Some experts suggest that oral clonidine may be used for the initial treatment of acute severe hypertension in children and adolescents† who are able to tolerate oral therapy and who have not developed life-threatening symptoms.

■ **Pain** Clonidine hydrochloride administered by epidural infusion is used as adjunctive therapy in combination with opiates in the management of severe cancer pain that is not relieved by opiate analgesics alone. Epidural administration of analgesics should be considered only when maximum tolerated doses of opiate and adjunct analgesics administered by other routes (e.g., oral, transdermal, subcutaneous, IV) fail to relieve pain. (See Cautions: Precautions and Contraindications.) Consistent with the drug's mechanism of action, epidural clonidine is more likely to be effective in patients with neuropathic pain rather than somatic or visceral pain.

In a double-blind, placebo-controlled, randomized study, cancer patients with severe intractable pain below the cervical dermatomes not controlled by oral, epidural, or IV opiate analgesics received epidural morphine with either clonidine hydrochloride 30 mcg/hour by continuous epidural infusion or placebo for 14 days. Pain relief, measured by a decrease in use of epidural morphine or a decrease in visual analog pain score, was reported in 45 or 21% of patients receiving epidural clonidine or placebo, respectively. In this study, substantial analgesic effects of clonidine appeared to be restricted to patients with neuropathic pain, characterized as localized, burning, shooting, or electric-like pain in a dermatomal or peripheral nerve distribution.

■ **Pheochromocytoma** Clonidine is not indicated in patients with pheochromocytoma; however, unlike reserpine and guanethidine, it does not cause acute cardiovascular collapse in patients with this condition. Because of clonidine's ability to suppress plasma norepinephrine concentration in healthy individuals via stimulation of central α-adrenergic receptors, the drug has been used as an aid in the diagnosis of pheochromocytoma in hypertensive patients with suggestive symptoms and borderline catecholamine values†; in patients with pheochromocytoma, plasma norepinephrine concentration is generally unchanged following administration of a single oral dose of clonidine, while patients with sympathetic hyperactivity exhibit a decrease in plasma norepinephrine concentration.

■ **Vascular Headaches** Although clonidine has been used in the prophylaxis of migraine headaches†, the efficacy of the drug for this condition is questionable. Results of most studies using α-adrenergic agents (e.g., clonidine) for prevention of migraine headaches indicate that these drugs have limited or no efficacy in most patients, and therefore, some experts state that such use is not recommended. For further information on management and classification of migraine headache, see Vascular Headaches: General Principles in Migraine Therapy, under Uses in Sumatriptan 28:32.28.

■ **Dysmenorrhea** Because clonidine reduces the responsiveness of blood vessels to vasodilators or vasoconstrictors, the drug has been used for the treatment of severe dysmenorrhea†.

■ **Vasomotor Symptoms Associated with Menopause** Clonidine has been used orally and transdermally for the management of vasomotor symptoms† (e.g., hot flashes) associated with menopause. Although limited data indicate that the drug may improve the severity and frequency of vasomotor symptoms in some patients, albeit modestly, the required dosages (exceeding the equivalent of 0.1 mg daily administered orally) may result in increased and, sometimes, intolerable adverse effects. Therefore, some clinicians recommend the use of clonidine for management of vasomotor symptoms mainly in postmenopausal women in whom estrogen replacement therapy is contraindicated or in those with preexisting hypertension.

■ **Opiate Withdrawal** Clonidine hydrochloride has been used safely and effectively for symptomatic relief in the management of opiate withdrawal in opiate-dependent individuals†, in both inpatient and outpatient settings.

In patients with opiate dependence (i.e., opiate use disorder), opiate withdrawal management (also referred to as detoxification) generally involves short-term use of tapering dosages of buprenorphine (an opiate partial agonist) or methadone (a full opiate agonist) to reduce withdrawal symptoms. However, prescribing restrictions may limit use of these drugs, and α_2-adrenergic agonists (e.g., clonidine, lofexidine) also have been used for symptomatic relief of noradrenergic-mediated opiate withdrawal symptoms (e.g., lacrimation, sweating, shivering, rhinorrhea) in both inpatient and outpatient settings and may allow for withdrawal over a shorter period of time. The α_2-adrenergic agonists appear to be less effective than buprenorphine or methadone in the management of opiate withdrawal, and some experts suggest that α_2-adrenergic agonists may be most useful in withdrawal management as adjuncts to opiate agonists or partial agonists, to facilitate transition to opiate antagonist (naltrexone) treatment for relapse prevention, or in settings where therapy with opiate agonists or partial agonists is contraindicated, unacceptable, or unavailable. While α_2-adrenergic agonists relieve noradrenergic-mediated symptoms of opiate withdrawal, concomitant supportive therapy for other withdrawal symptoms (e.g., abdominal cramping, diarrhea, nausea and vomiting, muscle spasms, anxiety or restlessness, insomnia) may improve patient comfort, particularly in patients treated principally with an α_2-adrenergic agonist.

Although direct comparisons between lofexidine and clonidine are limited, results of several small comparative studies suggest that lofexidine and clonidine have similar efficacy in managing opiate withdrawal symptoms but lofexidine may be associated with less hypotension. However, the greater cost of lofexidine compared with off-label clonidine use also must be considered.

Because of the potential for hypotension and bradycardia, some experts state that α_2-adrenergic agonists are not drugs of choice for opiate withdrawal management in geriatric patients or patients with coronary insufficiency, ischemic heart disease, bradycardia, or cerebrovascular disease.

Withdrawal management alone does not provide adequate treatment for opiate use disorder; withdrawal management should be employed in patients with opiate use disorder only in conjunction with a comprehensive treatment program. Opiate withdrawal without subsequent maintenance treatment is associated with high rates of relapse in patients with opiate use disorder. For most patients with opioid use disorder, maintenance treatment with buprenorphine or methadone or treatment with naltrexone for relapse prevention is superior to opiate withdrawal management.

In patients receiving long-term opiate analgesia, withdrawal symptoms generally are managed by slow tapering of the opiate analgesic dosage.

■ **Alcohol Withdrawal** Clonidine also has been used in conjunction with benzodiazepines for the management of alcohol withdrawal†. Clonidine appears to be effective in reducing symptoms of the hyperadrenergic state associated with alcohol withdrawal, including elevated blood pressure, increased heart rate, tremor, sweating, and anxiety. However, clonidine has not been shown to prevent delirium or seizures, and the drug should be used only as an adjunct to benzodiazepines (*not* as monotherapy) for the treatment of alcohol withdrawal (see Uses: Alcohol Withdrawal in the Benzodiazepines General Statement 28:24.08). Some clinicians state that the use of clonidine may be particularly helpful in patients with certain coexisting conditions (e.g., opiate withdrawal).

■ **Smoking Cessation** Clonidine is used for the management of nicotine (tobacco) dependence†. Nicotine dependence is a chronic relapsing disorder that requires ongoing assessment and often repeated intervention. Because effective nicotine dependence therapies are available, every patient should be offered effective treatment, and those who are unwilling to attempt cessation should be provided at least brief interventions designed to increase their motivation to stop tobacco use. The US Public Health Service (USPHS) guideline for the treatment of tobacco use and dependence currently recommends clonidine as a second-line drug for use under the supervision of a clinician. Second-line pharmacotherapy (e.g., clonidine, nortriptyline) is of a more limited role than first-line pharmacotherapy (i.e., bupropion [as extended-release tablets], nicotine polacrilex gum or lozenge, transdermal nicotine, nicotine nasal spray, nicotine oral inhaler, varenicline) in part because of more concerns about potential adverse effects. The use of second-line pharmacotherapy should be considered after first-line therapies have been used without success or are contraindicated. For additional information on smoking cessation, see Guidelines under Uses: Smoking Cessation, in Nicotine 12:92, and also consult the most current USPHS Clinical Practice Guideline on Treating Tobacco Use and Dependence available at http://www.ahrq.gov/professionals/clinicians-providers/guidelines-recommendations/index.html.

■ **Other Uses** Because of its GI effects (see Pharmacology: Other Effects), clonidine hydrochloride has been used with some success in a limited number of patients for the management of diarrhea† of various etiologies (e.g., narcotic bowel syndrome, idiopathic diarrhea associated with diabetes).

Dosage and Administration

■ **Administration** Clonidine hydrochloride is administered orally or by epidural infusion, and clonidine is administered percutaneously by topical application of a transdermal system. To ensure overnight blood pressure control with oral administration, the last dose of the day should be administered immediately before retiring. If oral clonidine therapy is to be discontinued, dosage of the drug should be slowly reduced over a period of 2–4 days to avoid the possibility of precipitating a withdrawal syndrome. (See Cautions: Withdrawal Effects.)

Patients receiving transdermal clonidine therapy should be carefully instructed in the use of the transdermal system. To obtain optimum results, patients should also be given a copy of the patient instructions provided by the manufacturer. To expose the adhesive surface of the system, the clear plastic protective strip should be peeled and discarded prior to administration. The transdermal system is applied topically to a dry, hairless area of intact skin on the upper arm or chest by firmly pressing the system with the adhesive side touching the skin. If the system becomes loose during the period of use, an adhesive cover should be applied directly over the system to ensure good adhesion. If the patient develops isolated, mild localized skin irritation before completion of the intended period of use, the system may be removed and replaced with a new system at a different application site. To minimize and/or prevent potential skin irritation, each transdermal system should be applied at a different site (e.g., systems may be applied progressively across the arms and chest in one direction or the other).

Specialized techniques are required for continuous epidural administration of clonidine hydrochloride; the drug should be administered via this route only by qualified individuals familiar with the techniques of administration and patient management problems associated with this route of clonidine administration. Prior to the implantation of a permanent controlled infusion device, screening should be conducted to ensure adequate response to epidural therapy. Chronic epidural analgesia should only be used when adequate pain relief cannot be achieved with less invasive therapies.

The injection for epidural use concentrate containing 500 mcg/mL *must* be diluted prior to use in sodium chloride 0.9% injection to provide a final concentration of 100 mcg/mL.

For continuous epidural infusion of clonidine hydrochloride, a controlled-infusion device is used to administer the drug. Infusion of clonidine into the upper thoracic spinal segments may be associated with substantial decreases in blood pressure. (See Cautions: Cardiovascular Effects.) The manufacturer states that administration of epidural clonidine above the C4 dermatome is contraindicated because of inadequate safety data supporting such use. Careful monitoring of infusion pump function and inspection of catheter tubing for obstruction or dislodgement is recommended to reduce the risk of inadvertent abrupt withdrawal of epidural clonidine infusion. Clonidine hydrochloride injection for epidural infusion contains no preservatives, and partially used vials of the drug should be discarded. Parenteral drug products should be inspected visually for particulate matter and discoloration whenever solution and container permit.

■ **Dosage** To avoid the possibility of precipitating the withdrawal syndrome, clonidine therapy should *not* be discontinued abruptly. (See Cautions: Withdrawal Effects.)

Hypertension Dosage of clonidine and clonidine hydrochloride must be adjusted according to the patient's blood pressure response and tolerance. Adverse effects such as drowsiness and dry mouth may be minimized by increasing dosage gradually and/or by taking the larger portion of the daily dose at bedtime.

Tolerance to the hypotensive effect of clonidine or clonidine hydrochloride may develop in some patients necessitating increased dosage or concomitant administration of a diuretic to enhance the hypotensive response to the drug.

Oral Dosage. For the management of hypertension, the usual initial oral dosage of clonidine hydrochloride (as conventional tablets) in adults is 0.1 mg twice daily. Geriatric patients may benefit from a lower initial dosage of 0.05 mg twice daily. Dosage may be increased by 0.1 mg at weekly intervals until the desired response is achieved. In clinical studies, the most commonly used dosages have ranged from 0.2–0.6 mg daily, administered in divided doses. Some experts state that the usual dosage range for adults is 0.1–0.8 mg daily, administered in 2 divided doses. The maximum effective dosage in adults is 2.4 mg daily.

For information on overall principles and expert recommendations for treatment of hypertension in pediatric patients, see Uses: Hypertension in Pediatric Patients, in the Thiazides General Statement 40:28.20.

Smaller than usual dosages of clonidine hydrochloride may be adequate in patients who are also receiving diuretics or other hypotensive drugs.

Transdermal Dosage. When transdermal clonidine therapy is used for the management of hypertension in adults, transdermal therapy is initiated with one system delivering 0.1 mg/24 hours applied once every 7 days. Because of interpatient variability in transdermal absorption, it is recommended that this initial dosage be used in all patients, including those who had been receiving oral clonidine hydrochloride therapy, and that dosage subsequently be titrated according to individual requirements; the relationship between the effective dosage of oral clonidine hydrochloride and that of transdermal clonidine is not predictable.

If the desired reduction in blood pressure is not achieved after 1 or 2 weeks with the initial dosage, dosage may be increased by using 2 systems delivering 0.1 mg/24 hours or a larger dosage system. Subsequent dosage adjustments may be made at weekly intervals. Some experts state that the usual dosage range for transdermal clonidine is 0.1–0.3 mg/24 hours applied once every 7 days. Transdermal dosages exceeding 0.6 mg/24 hours (2 systems each delivering 0.3 mg/24 hours) are usually not associated with additional efficacy. In patients who develop localized skin irritation during the intended period of use (7 days), it may be necessary to move the transdermal system to a different site or replace it with another system at shorter intervals (e.g., every 3–5 days). Replacement of the transdermal system following a duration of less than 7 days may be required rarely to maintain blood pressure control.

When transdermal therapy is initiated in patients who have been receiving low dosages of oral clonidine hydrochloride, some clinicians recommend continuing the usual oral dosage the first day the initial transdermal system is applied. When transdermal clonidine therapy is administered to patients already receiving other hypotensive agents, dosage of the other hypotensive agents should be gradually reduced when transdermal therapy is initiated since the hypotensive effect of transdermal clonidine may not begin until 2–3 days after application of the initial system; the other hypotensive agents may have to be continued, particularly in patients with more severe hypertension.

Blood Pressure Monitoring and Treatment Goals. Blood pressure should be monitored regularly (i.e., monthly) during therapy and dosage of the antihypertensive drug adjusted until blood pressure is controlled. If an adequate blood pressure response is not achieved, the dosage may be increased or another antihypertensive agent with demonstrated benefit and preferably with a complementary mechanism of action (e.g., angiotensin-converting enzyme [ACE] inhibitor, angiotensin II receptor antagonist, calcium-channel blocker, thiazide diuretic) may be added; if target blood pressure is still not achieved with the use of 2 antihypertensive agents, a third drug may be added. (See Uses: Hypertension.) In patients who develop unacceptable adverse effects with clonidine, the drug should be discontinued and another antihypertensive agent from a different pharmacologic class should be initiated.

The goal of hypertension management and prevention is to achieve and maintain optimal control of blood pressure. However, the optimum blood pressure threshold for initiating antihypertensive drug therapy and specific treatment goals remain controversial. A 2017 multidisciplinary hypertension guideline from the American College of Cardiology (ACC), American Heart Association (AHA), and a number of other professional organizations generally recommends a blood pressure goal of less than 130/80 mm Hg in all adults, regardless of comorbidities or level of atherosclerotic cardiovascular disease (ASCVD) risk. Many patients will require at least 2 drugs from different pharmacologic classes to achieve this blood pressure goal; the potential benefits of hypertension management and drug cost, adverse effects, and risks associated with the use of multiple antihypertensive drugs also should be considered when deciding a patient's blood pressure treatment goal.

For additional information on target levels of blood pressure and on monitoring therapy in the management of hypertension, see Blood Pressure Monitoring and Treatment Goals under Dosage: Hypertension, in Dosage and Administration in the Thiazides General Statement 40:28.20.

Hypertensive Crises For rapid reduction of blood pressure in patients with hypertensive urgencies†, clonidine hydrochloride has been administered orally (as conventional tablets) in an initial dose of 0.1–0.2 mg, followed by hourly doses of 0.05–0.2 mg until a total dose of 0.5–0.7 mg has been given or diastolic blood pressure has been controlled. Oral loading doses of antihypertensive agents may have cumulative effects and may cause hypotension after a patient has been discharged from a hospital or clinic setting. Excessive falls in blood pressure should be avoided since they may precipitate renal, cerebral, or coronary ischemia. Maintenance dosage of clonidine hydrochloride should be adjusted according to the patient's response and tolerance.

For rapid reduction of blood pressure in children and adolescents with acute severe hypertension who can tolerate oral therapy and have not developed life-threatening symptoms†, some experts recommend an initial oral clonidine hydrochloride dose of 2–5 mcg/kg per dose (up to 10 mcg/kg per dose), which may be administered every 6–8 hours.

Pain **Adult Dosage.** When used for the relief of severe, intractable cancer pain that is unresponsive to epidural or spinal opiate analgesia or other more conventional methods of analgesia, the recommended initial epidural dosage of clonidine hydrochloride in adults is 30 mcg/hour, administered by continuous epidural infusion. The dosage may be adjusted based on clinical response and tolerance; however, clinical experience with infusion rates exceeding 40 mcg/hour is limited. Patients should be closely monitored, particularly during the first few days of epidural clonidine therapy.

Pediatric Dosage. The recommended initial dosage of epidural clonidine hydrochloride in pediatric patients is 0.5 mcg/kg of body weight per hour. The dosage of epidural clonidine in pediatric patients should be cautiously adjusted based on clinical response.

Pheochromocytoma As an aid in the diagnosis of pheochromocytoma†, clonidine hydrochloride has been administered orally as a single 0.3-mg dose (as conventional tablets). To conduct the test, patients should rest in the supine position for 30 minutes, after which time, 2 blood samples for baseline determination of catecholamine concentrations are drawn at 5-minute intervals. The 0.3-mg dose is then administered and blood samples for catecholamine determinations are drawn at hourly intervals for 3 hours. In patients with pheochromocytoma, plasma norepinephrine concentrations generally remain unchanged following administration of clonidine, whereas plasma norepinephrine concentrations generally decrease in patients without pheochromocytoma.

Vascular Headache The oral dosage of clonidine hydrochloride (as conventional tablets) used in the prophylaxis of migraine† is 0.025 mg 2–4 times a day or up to 0.15 mg daily in divided doses.

Dysmenorrhea For the treatment of dysmenorrhea†, 0.025 mg of clonidine hydrochloride has been administered orally twice daily (as conventional tablets) for 14 days before and during menses.

Vasomotor Symptoms Associated with Menopause **Oral Dosage.** Oral clonidine hydrochloride dosages of 0.025–0.2 mg twice daily (as conventional tablets) have been employed in the management of vasomotor symptoms (e.g., hot flashes) associated with menopause†.

Transdermal Dosage. While comparative efficacy of various transdermal clonidine dosages have not been established, patients in clinical studies have received one transdermal system delivering 0.1 mg/24 hours applied once every 7 days.

Opiate Withdrawal **Oral Dosage.** For symptomatic relief of opiate withdrawal in opiate-dependent individuals†, various dosage regimens of oral clonidine hydrochloride (as conventional tablets) have been used. Some experts state that the usual clonidine hydrochloride dosage for opiate withdrawal management is 0.1–0.3 mg every 6–8 hours, with dosage guided by withdrawal symptoms and adverse effects. Other experts recommend administration of an initial 0.1-mg test dose of clonidine hydrochloride; a 0.2-mg test dose may be considered for patients with severe manifestations of opiate withdrawal or for those weighing more than 200 pounds (91 kg). If blood pressure remains adequate (generally systolic and diastolic blood pressures of least 90 and 60 mm Hg, respectively) following the test dose, a clonidine hydrochloride dosage of 0.1–0.2 mg may be administered every 4–6 hours as needed; scheduled dosing may be considered in patients with severe withdrawal. Under this dosing method, the total dose administered during the initial 24 hours of treatment is tabulated to establish the patient's daily dosage requirement and is administered in 3 or 4 divided doses.

Doses of clonidine hydrochloride should be reduced, delayed, or omitted in individuals demonstrating greater sensitivity to the drug's adverse effects (e.g., hypotension, orthostasis, bradycardia). Individuals treated in the outpatient setting should be capable of performing self-monitoring for these adverse effects, and some experts suggest that lower dosages may be appropriate in this setting. As opiate withdrawal symptoms wane, clonidine hydrochloride dosage may be reduced gradually (e.g., by 0.1 mg per dose every 1–2 days). Other tapering schedules also have been used to discontinue therapy (e.g., dosage has been reduced by decrements of 50% per day for 3 days and then discontinued, or reduced by 0.1–0.2 mg daily). Clinicians should consult published protocols for more specific information.

Alcohol Withdrawal While dosages of clonidine hydrochloride in the management of alcohol withdrawal† have not been established, oral dosages of 0.5 mg 2 or 3 times daily (as conventional tablets) have been shown to reduce tremor, heart rate, and blood pressure in patients with alcohol withdrawal.

Smoking Cessation Optimum dosage of oral clonidine hydrochloride (as conventional tablets) or transdermal clonidine for smoking cessation† (nicotine [tobacco] dependence) has not been established, and various regimens have been employed.

Oral Dosage. For use in the cessation of smoking†, the initial adult oral dosage of clonidine hydrochloride is typically 0.1 mg twice daily (as conventional tablets). Therapy with the drug is initiated on the day set as the date of cessation of smoking or shortly before this date (e.g., up to 3 days prior). Dosage may be increased each week by 0.1 mg daily, if needed. In clinical studies, oral dosages varied from 0.15–0.75 mg daily without a clear relationship to achievement of cessation of smoking. The duration of oral therapy with clonidine hydrochloride also varied in these studies, ranging from 3–10 weeks.

Transdermal Dosage. When transdermal clonidine is used for the cessation of smoking†, therapy is initiated typically in adults with one system delivering 0.1 mg/24 hours applied once every 7 days. Therapy with the drug is initiated on the day set as the date of cessation of smoking or shortly before this date (e.g., up to 3 days prior). Dosage may be increased at weekly intervals by 0.1 mg/24 hours, if needed. In clinical studies, the transdermal dosage varied from 0.1–0.2 mg/24 hours without a clear relationship to achievement of cessation of smoking. The duration of transdermal clonidine therapy also varied in these studies, ranging from 3–10 weeks.

Dosage in Renal Impairment Smaller than usual dosages of clonidine or clonidine hydrochloride may be adequate in patients with renal impairment. Dosage should be adjusted according to the degree of renal impairment. Some clinicians suggest that adjustment of clonidine hydrochloride dosage is not necessary in patients with creatinine clearances of 10 mL/minute or greater, but those with lower clearances can receive 50–75% of the usual dosage. Supplemental doses after hemodialysis are not necessary.

Cautions

Adverse effects occurring most frequently during oral clonidine hydrochloride therapy are dry mouth, dizziness, drowsiness and sedation, and constipation; these adverse effects appear to be dose related. Headache, fatigue, and weakness also have been reported. Generally, these adverse effects are mild and tend to diminish with continued therapy or may be relieved by a reduction in dosage. Adverse effects occurring with transdermal clonidine generally appear to be similar to those occurring with oral therapy; however, systemic adverse effects with transdermal clonidine appear to be less severe and possibly may occur less frequently than with oral therapy. Most adverse systemic effects occurring during transdermal therapy have been mild and have tended to diminish with continued treatment. The most frequently occurring adverse effects during transdermal therapy have been dry mouth, drowsiness, and local adverse dermatologic effects. Adverse effects reported most frequently in patients with cancer receiving clonidine by epidural infusion in combination with epidural morphine in a controlled clinical trial included hypotension, postural hypotension, and dry mouth, which occurred in 45, 32, and 16% of patients, respectively.

■ Nervous System Effects Drowsiness has been reported in about 33, 13, or 12% of patients receiving oral, epidural, or transdermal clonidine, respectively. In addition to drowsiness, sedation, dizziness, headache, fatigue, and weakness, other adverse nervous system effects of clonidine include lethargy, vivid dreams, nightmares, insomnia, behavioral changes, nervousness, restlessness, anxiety, agitation, irritability, mental depression, visual and auditory hallucinations, delirium, localized numbness, and cerebrovascular accidents.

Depression, which occurs often in patients with cancer, may be exacerbated by the use of epidural clonidine. Therefore, the manufacturer recommends that patients be monitored for signs and symptoms of depression (especially those with a history of affective disorders). Sedation and ventilatory abnormalities, usually mild, have been reported in patients receiving bolus epidural doses of clonidine that were substantially higher than the infusion rate recommended for the treatment of cancer pain. Tolerance to these effects may occur with chronic administration of the drug.

■ GI Effects Dry mouth has been reported in about 40, 25, or 13% of patients receiving oral, transdermal, or epidural clonidine, respectively. Nausea and vomiting have occurred in about 5% of patients and anorexia and malaise in about 1% of patients receiving oral clonidine. In addition, parotid pain, parotitis, pseudo-obstruction, abdominal pain, and constipation have occurred rarely in patients receiving oral clonidine. Nausea and vomiting were reported in about 13 and 11%, respectively, of patients receiving clonidine by epidural infusion in combination with epidural morphine for the treatment of intractable cancer pain in a controlled clinical trial. Dry throat, constipation, nausea, dysgeusia, anorexia, and vomiting have been reported in patients receiving transdermal clonidine.

■ Cardiovascular Effects Orthostatic symptoms have occurred in about 3% of patients receiving oral clonidine; palpitation and tachycardia, and bradycardia have occurred in about 0.5% of patients receiving the oral drug. Rare cases of sinus bradycardia and atrioventricular block, with and without concomitant cardiac glycoside therapy, have been reported. Congestive heart failure, Raynaud's phenomenon, flushes, facial pallor, syncope, chest pain, increases in blood pressure, palpitations, and ECG abnormalities (e.g., arrhythmias, sick sinus syndrome disturbances, sinus node arrest, conduction disturbances such as AV block) also have been reported.

Hypotension occurred in about 45% of patients receiving clonidine by epidural infusion as adjunctive therapy with epidural morphine for the treatment of cancer pain. In a 14-day clinical trial, hypotension usually was reported within the first 4 days of epidural clonidine therapy; however, hypotension also occurred throughout the duration of the study. Hypotension, which can be severe, usually responds to treatment with IV fluids and, if necessary, parenteral ephedrine. Hypotension appears to occur more frequently in women, in patients with a lower body weight, and in patients with higher serum clonidine concentrations.

Decreased heart rate has been reported frequently in patients receiving epidural clonidine, while AV block greater than first degree in severity has been reported rarely. Atropine may be used to treat symptomatic bradycardia when necessary. Increases in heart rate associated with hypovolemia may be masked by clonidine therapy.

■ Metabolic and Endocrine Effects Weight gain has been reported in about 1% of patients receiving oral clonidine. Some patients gain weight during the first few days of oral clonidine therapy because of sodium and fluid retention. Sodium retention usually lasts only 3 or 4 days and may be avoided or relieved by administration of a diuretic. Gynecomastia has occurred in about 0.1% of patients receiving oral clonidine during clinical trials, and in up to 0.5% of patients during postmarketing experience with transdermal clonidine. Transient elevation of blood glucose concentration after single large doses of clonidine hydrochloride has been reported; however, no effects on glucose metabolism have been reported during long-term use of the drug, and diabetic patients have remained in control while taking clonidine hydrochloride. Rarely, transient elevation of serum creatine kinase (CK, creatine phosphokinase, CPK) concentrations have been associated with use of the drug.

■ Dermatologic Effects Rash has occurred in about 1% of patients; pruritus in about 0.7% of patients; angioedema and urticaria in about 0.5% of patients; and alopecia in about 0.2% of patients receiving oral clonidine.

Dermatologic effects were the most frequently occurring adverse effects in clinical trials of transdermal clonidine. In clinical studies, localized skin reactions (i.e., erythema, pruritus) occurred in up to 50% of patients receiving transdermal clonidine therapy. Localized skin reactions occur more commonly in patients who use an adhesive cover over the transdermal system for the entire 7-day application period. Localized skin reactions usually are readily reversible following removal of the transdermal system and have usually not required discontinuance of transdermal therapy. Allergic contact sensitization to clonidine has occurred in about 20% of patients with transdermal therapy, most frequently in white females and least frequently in black males; the dermatitis may require discontinuance of transdermal therapy. Although systemic anaphylactic reactions have not been reported to date, subsequent administration of oral clonidine (or continued administration of transdermal clonidine) to patients who experience allergic reactions with transdermal therapy may result in a recurrence of the reaction or development of a generalized rash, urticaria, or angioedema. (See Cautions: Precautions and Contraindications.) Localized vesiculation, hyperpigmentation (at the application site), edema, excoriation, burning, throbbing, blanching, generalized macular rash, urticaria, contact dermatitis, alopecia, and localized hypopigmentation or hyperpigmentation also have occurred in patients receiving transdermal clonidine.

■ **Genitourinary Effects** Decreased sexual activity, impotence, and loss of libido have occurred in about 3% of patients receiving oral clonidine. Nocturia has occurred in about 1% of patients, difficulty in micturition in about 0.2% of patients, and urinary retention in about 0.1% of patients receiving oral clonidine. Impotence/sexual dysfunction has been reported in about 2% of patients receiving transdermal clonidine, and loss of libido or decreased sexual activity and difficulty in micturition have been reported in up to 0.5% of patients receiving transdermal clonidine.

■ **Hepatic Effects** Mild, transient abnormalities in liver function test results have occurred in about 1% of patients during oral clonidine therapy. Hepatitis has been reported rarely; one case of hepatitis without icterus and hyperbilirubinemia occurred in a patient receiving clonidine hydrochloride, chlorthalidone, and papaverine, but a relationship to clonidine has not been established.

■ **Other Adverse Effects** Muscle or joint pain has occurred in about 0.6% of patients and leg cramps in about 0.3% of patients receiving oral clonidine. Dryness of the nasal mucosa; blurred vision; dryness and burning of the eyes; weakly positive Coombs' test results; fever, pallor, thrombocytopenia, and increased sensitivity to alcohol also have been reported in patients receiving oral clonidine.

Fever, malaise, pallor, muscle or joint pain, and leg cramps have been reported in up to 0.5% of patients during postmarketing experience with transdermal clonidine.

In several studies in albino rats receiving oral clonidine hydrochloride for 6 months or longer, the drug produced a dose-dependent increase in the frequency and severity of spontaneous retinal degeneration. Distribution studies in dogs and monkeys showed that clonidine is concentrated in the choroid of the eye. Ophthalmologic examinations performed prior to and periodically during oral clonidine hydrochloride therapy in humans (for 24 months or longer in some) revealed no evidence of drug-induced ophthalmologic abnormalities, except dry eyes, nor was there evidence of altered retinal function as determined by specialized tests such as electroretinography and macular dazzle. Blurred vision and burning and/or dryness of the eyes have been reported in up to 0.5% of patients during postmarketing experience with transdermal clonidine.

Implantable epidural catheters are associated with a risk of infection, including meningitis and/or epidural abscess. The incidence of catheter-related infections is about 5–20%, and depends on several factors, including the clinical status of the patient, type of catheter used, catheter placement technique, quality of catheter care, and duration of catheter placement. The possibility of catheter-related infection should be considered in patients receiving epidural clonidine who develop a fever.

■ **Withdrawal Effects** Abrupt withdrawal of clonidine therapy may result in a rapid increase of systolic and diastolic blood pressures with associated symptoms such as nervousness, agitation, confusion, restlessness, anxiety, insomnia, headache, sweating, palpitation, increased heart rate, tremor, hiccups, stomach pains, nausea, muscle pains, and increased salivation. The exact mechanism(s) of the withdrawal syndrome following discontinuance of α-adrenergic agonists has not been determined but may involve increased concentrations of circulating catecholamines, increased sensitivity of adrenergic receptors, enhanced renin-angiotensin system activity, decreased vagal function, failure of autoregulation of cerebral blood flow, and/or failure of central α_2-adrenergic receptor mechanisms that regulate sympathetic outflow from the CNS and modulate baroreflex function.

Withdrawal syndrome has been reported in about 1% of patients receiving oral clonidine. The clonidine withdrawal syndrome is more pronounced after abrupt cessation of long-term therapy than after short-term (1–2 months) therapy and has usually been associated with previous administration of high oral dosages (greater than 1.2 mg daily) and/or with continuation of concomitant β-adrenergic blocking therapy. In addition, the risk of adverse effects following abrupt discontinuance of clonidine therapy may be increased in patients with a history of hypertension and/or other underlying cardiovascular conditions. (See Cautions: Precautions and Contraindications.) When the drug is discontinued abruptly, symptoms such as restlessness and headache may begin to appear 2–3 hours after a dose is missed and blood pressure may increase substantially within 8–24 hours. In a few patients, blood pressure exceeded pretreatment levels. Rare cases of hypertensive encephalopathy, cerebrovascular accidents, and death occurring after abrupt cessation of clonidine therapy have been reported. It has been postulated that the risk of precipitating the withdrawal syndrome should be reduced substantially with use of transdermal clonidine because of the pharmacodynamics associated with this dosage form; however, withdrawal symptoms have been reported occasionally (in up to 0.5% of patients) following discontinuance of transdermal therapy or when absorption of the drug was impaired because of dermatologic changes (e.g., contact dermatitis) under the transdermal system. In one patient, withdrawal symptoms (severe rebound hypertension, tachycardia, headache, diaphoresis) appeared approximately 36–72 hours after discontinuance of transdermal therapy but responded to sublingual nifedipine and oral clonidine therapy. In a few geriatric patients, blood pressure has increased to levels exceeding baseline approximately 3–7 days after transdermal therapy was discontinued, although other signs of a hyperadrenergic state were not evident.

An excessive rise in blood pressure after oral or transdermal clonidine withdrawal can be reversed and symptoms relieved by resumption of oral clonidine or by combined administration of α- and β-adrenergic blocking agents (e.g., phentolamine or prazosin with atenolol, labetalol, or propranolol). Rebound hypertension may present a particular problem if oral clonidine therapy must be interrupted for surgery. It has been reported that when the drug was discontinued 8 hours or more prior to surgery, hypertension resulted during and after surgery; however, when clonidine was administered 4–6 hours preoperatively, only minor hypertension developed and hypotension requiring treatment did not occur.

The manufacturer of oral clonidine states that because children frequently experience vomiting associated with GI illnesses, they may be particularly susceptible to hypertensive episodes resulting from sudden inability to ingest the drug.

In a controlled clinical trial in cancer patients receiving epidural clonidine as an adjunct to epidural morphine for the treatment of pain, about 10% of patients receiving 720 mcg of clonidine hydrochloride daily experienced rebound hypertension following abrupt discontinuance of the drug; one patient subsequently suffered a cerebrovascular accident. Rebound hypertension following discontinuance of epidural clonidine can be reversed by administration of clonidine or IV phentolamine. In patients who are receiving concomitant therapy with a β-adrenergic blocking agent, the β-blocker should be discontinued several days prior to discontinuance of epidural clonidine (by gradual tapering).

■ **Precautions and Contraindications** Because of the risk of rebound hypertension, patients receiving clonidine preparations should be warned of the danger of missing doses or stopping the drug without consulting their clinician. (See Cautions: Withdrawal Effects.) When discontinuing clonidine therapy, a rapid rise in blood pressure may be minimized or prevented by tapered withdrawal of the drug over 2–4 days. Tapered withdrawal of transdermal clonidine or initiation of a tapered regimen of oral clonidine also is recommended by some clinicians when the transdermal dosage form is discontinued, particularly in geriatric patients. If clonidine therapy is to be discontinued in patients receiving clonidine and a β-adrenergic blocking agent concomitantly, the β-blocker should be discontinued several days before clonidine therapy is discontinued. It is recommended that clonidine therapy not be interrupted for surgery; transdermal therapy can be continued throughout the perioperative period and oral therapy should be continued to within 4 hours before surgery. Blood pressure should be carefully monitored during surgery and additional measures to control blood pressure should be available if necessary. If clonidine therapy must be interrupted for surgery, parenteral hypotensive therapy should be administered as necessary, and clonidine therapy should be resumed as soon as possible. If transdermal therapy is initiated during the perioperative period, it must be kept in mind that therapeutic plasma clonidine concentrations are not achieved until 2–3 days after initial application of the transdermal system.

Clonidine transdermal systems should be removed from the site(s) of application prior to attempting defibrillation or cardioversion since altered electrical conductivity and enhanced potential for electrical arcing may occur.

Patients receiving transdermal clonidine therapy should be advised that if the transdermal system begins to loosen from the skin after application, an adhesive cover should be applied directly over the system to ensure good adhesion over the period of application. Patients receiving transdermal therapy who develop moderate or severe localized erythema and/or localized vesicle formation at the application site or who develop a generalized rash should consult their physician promptly about the need to remove the transdermal system. If patients develop isolated, mild localized skin irritation before completion of the intended period of use (7 days), the system may be removed and replaced with a new system at a different application site. In patients who develop localized contact sensitization to clonidine with transdermal therapy, subsequent administration of oral clonidine hydrochloride (or continued administration of transdermal clonidine) may be associated with development of a generalized rash. In patients receiving transdermal therapy who develop an allergic reaction, subsequent administration of oral clonidine hydrochloride also may elicit an allergic reaction (e.g., generalized rash, urticaria, angioedema). Patients receiving transdermal clonidine therapy should be instructed to keep both used and unused transdermal systems out of the reach of children. In addition, these patients should be cautioned that even after use, the transdermal system contains active medication that may be harmful if accidentally applied or ingested by infants or children. (See Acute Toxicity: Manifestations.) Patients should be instructed to handle the used transdermal system carefully (e.g., fold the system in half with the sticky sides together) and to dispose of the system out of the reach of children.

In rare instances, loss of blood pressure control has been reported in patients using transdermal clonidine therapy according to the instructions for use.

Epidural clonidine should be used only in patients with severe cancer pain that has failed to respond to an adequate trial with opiate analgesics. The drug is *not* recommended for the management of obstetric, postpartum, or perioperative pain. Careful monitoring of infusion pump function and inspection of catheter tubing for obstruction or dislodgement is recommended to reduce the risk of accidental abrupt withdrawal of epidural clonidine. Patients should be instructed to notify their clinician immediately in case of inadvertent interruption of epidural clonidine administration. Specialized techniques are required for continuous epidural administration of clonidine hydrochloride; the drug should be administered via this route only by qualified individuals familiar with the techniques of administration and patient management problems associated with this route of clonidine administration. Epidural drug administration is contraindicated in patients receiving anticoagulant therapy, in those with a bleeding diathesis, and in the presence of an injection site infection. Administration of epidural clonidine also is not recommended in most patients with severe cardiovascular disease or in patients who are hemodynamically unstable. The manufacturer states that administration of epidural clonidine above the C4 dermatome is contraindicated because of inadequate safety data supporting such use.

Clonidine should be used with caution in patients with severe coronary insufficiency, recent myocardial infarction, conduction disturbances, cerebrovascular disease, chronic renal failure, Raynaud's disease, or thromboangiitis obliterans. Patients with a history of mental depression require careful supervision while receiving clonidine as they may be subject to further depressive episodes. Patients who engage in potentially hazardous activities such as operating machinery or driving should be warned of the possible sedative effect of the drug. In addition, patients should be informed that clonidine may be additive with, or may potentiate the action of, other CNS depressants such as opiate agonists or other analgesics, barbiturates or other sedatives, anesthetics, or alcohol.

The possibility that clonidine may lower blood pressure in patients receiving the drug for conditions other than hypertension (e.g., opiate withdrawal, smoking cessation, pain management) should be considered, and blood pressure should be monitored as appropriate. In addition, the possibility of rebound hypertension and other withdrawal effects should be considered when the drug is discontinued in such patients; abrupt discontinuance should be avoided.

Patients who wear contact lenses should be cautioned that clonidine may cause dryness of the eyes.

A dose-dependent increase in the incidence and severity of spontaneously occurring retinal degeneration was observed in albino rats receiving the drug for 6 months or longer, especially those receiving strong exposure to light. In 353 of 908 patients undergoing eye examinations over periods of at least 24 months in clinical trials, no drug-related ophthalmologic findings were recorded except for some dryness of the eyes, and retinal function as measured by specialized tests (e.g., electroretinography, macular dazzle) was unchanged.

Clonidine is contraindicated in patients with known hypersensitivity to the drug or to any ingredient or component in the formulation.

■ **Pediatric Precautions** Safety and efficacy of oral clonidine hydrochloride and clonidine transdermal system for the management of hypertension in children have not been established. Some experts have recommended oral dosages of clonidine for pediatric patients with hypertension or severe hypertension based on clinical experience. For information on overall principles and expert recommendations for treatment of hypertension in pediatric patients, see Uses: Hypertension in Pediatric Patients, in the Thiazides General Statement 40:28.20.

The safety and efficacy of clonidine hydrochloride epidural infusion have been established in pediatric patients who are old enough to tolerate placement and management of an epidural catheter, based on evidence from adequate, well-controlled studies in adults and experience with the use of clonidine in pediatric patients for other indications. Epidural clonidine should be used only in pediatric patients with severe, intractable cancer pain that is unresponsive to epidural or spinal opiates and to other conventional analgesic therapy.

Children may be more likely to experience CNS depression associated with clonidine overdosage than adults. In children, signs of toxicity have occurred with clonidine doses as low as 0.1 mg. Rare cases of clonidine toxicity (many involving children) associated with accidental or deliberate mouthing or ingestion of clonidine transdermal systems have been reported.

The manufacturer of oral clonidine states that because children frequently experience vomiting associated with GI illnesses, they may be particularly susceptible to hypertensive episodes resulting from sudden inability to ingest the drug.

■ **Mutagenicity and Carcinogenicity** There was no evidence of clonidine-induced mutagenesis in vitro in the Ames microbial mutagen test. Clonidine was not clastogenic in the mouse micronucleus test. Studies to determine the carcinogenic potential of clonidine were performed in rats receiving oral dosages up to 46 times the maximum recommended human dosage on a mg/kg basis for 132 weeks and in mice receiving up to 70 times the maximum recommended human dosage on a mg/kg basis for up to 78 weeks. These dosages were approximately 9 and 6 times the maximum recommended human daily dosage on a mg/m^2 basis in rats and mice, respectively.

■ **Pregnancy, Fertility, and Lactation** ***Pregnancy*** Reproduction studies in rabbits using oral clonidine hydrochloride dosages up to about 3 times the maximum recommended human dosage have not revealed evidence of teratogenicity or embryotoxicity. However, in female rats receiving the drug continuously for 2 months prior to mating, an increased incidence of fetal resorptions occurred with oral dosages as low as one-third the maximum recommended human dosage (1/15th the maximum recommended human dosage on a mg/m^2 basis); resorptions were not increased when these or higher dosages (up to 3 times the maximum recommended human dosage) were administered during days 6–15 of gestation. An increased incidence of fetal resorptions was observed when much higher dosages (40 times the maximum recommended human dosage on a mg/kg basis and 4–8 times the maximum recommended human dosage on a mg/m^2 basis) were administered to mice and rats during days 1–14 of gestation; the lowest dosage used in the study was 0.5 mg/kg. There are no adequate and controlled studies to date using clonidine in pregnant women, and the drug should be used during pregnancy only when clearly needed.

Fertility Reproduction studies in rats using oral clonidine hydrochloride dosages up to 0.15 mg/kg daily (about 3 times the maximum recommended human dosage) have not revealed evidence of impaired fertility; however, fertility in female rats was impaired at oral dosages ranging from 0.5–2 mg/kg daily (about 10–40 times the maximum recommended human oral dosage on a mg/kg basis [2–8 times the maximum recommended human dosage on a mg/m^2 basis]).

Lactation Since clonidine is distributed into milk, the drug should be used with caution in nursing women. The manufacturer of parenteral clonidine states that because of the potential for serious adverse reactions to clonidine in nursing infants, a decision should be made whether to discontinue nursing or the drug, taking into account the importance of the drug to the woman.

Drug Interactions

■ **CNS Depressants** Clonidine may be additive with, or may potentiate the action of, other CNS depressants such as opiates or other analgesics, barbiturates or other sedatives, anesthetics, or alcohol. Concomitant administration of opiate analgesics with clonidine also may potentiate the hypotensive effects of clonidine.

■ **Psychotherapeutic Agents** Tricyclic antidepressants (i.e., imipramine, desipramine) have reportedly inhibited the hypotensive effect of clonidine. The increase in blood pressure usually occurs during the second week of tricyclic antidepressant therapy, but occasionally may occur during the first several days of concomitant therapy. The possibility of this interaction should be considered in patients receiving clonidine and tricyclic antidepressants concomitantly; blood pressure should be closely monitored during the first several weeks of concurrent therapy, and dosage of clonidine should be increased to adequately control hypertension if necessary. Alternatively, other hypotensive agents that do not interact with tricyclic antidepressants may be substituted, but clonidine therapy should *not* be discontinued abruptly. If tricyclic antidepressant therapy is discontinued in patients receiving clonidine, the hypotensive effect of clonidine may increase; blood pressure should be monitored and dosage of clonidine reduced if necessary. In rats, concurrent administration of clonidine and amitriptyline has produced corneal lesions within 5 days. The effects of tricyclic antidepressants on the analgesic effect of epidural clonidine hydrochloride are not known.

Clonidine withdrawal may result in an excess of circulating catecholamines; therefore, caution should be exercised in concomitant use of drugs which affect the metabolism or tissue uptake of these amines (monoamine oxidase inhibitors or tricyclic antidepressants, respectively).

Acute delirium has been reported in at least one patient receiving fluphenazine concomitantly with oral clonidine. The symptoms resolved following discontinuance of clonidine and recurred upon rechallenge with the drug.

■ **Cardiovascular Drugs** When clonidine is administered with other hypotensive agents, including diuretics, the hypotensive effect of clonidine may be increased. This effect is usually used to therapeutic advantage in antihypertensive therapy; however, careful adjustment of dosage is necessary when these drugs are used concomitantly.

Because clonidine may produce bradycardia and atrioventricular (AV) block, the possibility of additive effects should be considered if it is given concomitantly with other drugs that affect sinus node function or AV nodal conduction (e.g., guanethidine), β-adrenergic blocking agents (e.g., propranolol), calcium-channel blocking agents, or cardiac glycosides.

Because β-blockers may exacerbate rebound hypertension that may occur following discontinuance of clonidine therapy, such drugs should be discontinued several days before gradual withdrawal of clonidine when clonidine therapy is to be discontinued. If clonidine therapy is to be replaced by a β-blocker, administration of the β-blocker should be delayed for several days after clonidine therapy has been discontinued.

■ **Other Drugs** Epidural clonidine may prolong the duration of the pharmacologic effects, including both sensory and motor blockade, of epidural local anesthetics.

Acute Toxicity

■ **Pathogenesis** The oral LD_{50} of clonidine hydrochloride is 206 and 465 mg/kg in mice and rats, respectively.

■ **Manifestations** Signs and symptoms of overdosage of clonidine include hypotension (which may be profound), transient hypertension, weakness, vomiting, irritability, diminished or absent reflexes, lethargy, somnolence, drowsiness, deep sedation, irritability, skin pallor, hypothermia, decreased or irregular heart rate, dryness of the mouth, constricted pupils with poor reaction to light, respiratory depression, and hypoventilation. Large overdoses may result in reversible cardiac conduction defects or dysrhythmias, apnea, coma, and seizures. Signs and symptoms of clonidine overdosage usually occur within 30–120 minutes after ingestion. Children may be more likely to experience CNS depression associated with clonidine overdosage. In children, signs of toxicity have occurred with oral clonidine doses as low as 0.1 mg. Rare cases of clonidine toxicity (many involving children) associated with accidental or deliberate mouthing or ingestion of clonidine transdermal systems have been reported. In one individual who reportedly ingested 100 mg of clonidine hydrochloride, plasma clonidine concentrations were 60, 90, 370, 120, and 120 ng/mL 1, 1.5, 2, 5.5, and 6.5 hours after ingestion. Signs and symptoms of overdosage in this patient included transient hypertension followed by hypotension, bradycardia, apnea, hallucinations, partial coma, and ventricular premature contractions; the patient recovered following intensive symptomatic and supportive treatment. In a 2-year old infant who apparently ingested clonidine from a used and discarded transdermal system, a serum clonidine concentration determined 24 hours after ingestion was approximately 8 ng/mL (therapeutic range: 0.5–4.5 ng/mL). In this infant, lethargy developed over several hours and was accompanied by bradycardia, hypotension, miosis, and gasping respirations; the patient was monitored in an intensive care unit and recovered over a period of 16 hours without specific treatment.

■ **Treatment** There is no known specific antidote for clonidine overdosage. If signs and symptoms of clonidine overdosage occur in patients receiving transdermal therapy, all transdermal systems should be removed. Following removal of the transdermal system(s), plasma concentrations of clonidine will persist for about 8 hours and then decline slowly over several days. Ipecac-induced emesis and gastric lavage would not be expected to remove significant amounts of clonidine following transdermal exposure. If the transdermal system has been ingested, whole bowel irrigation may be considered, and the administration of activated charcoal and/or cathartic agents may be beneficial.

In acute overdosage with oral clonidine, gastric lavage may be indicated following recent and/or large ingestions; administration of an activated charcoal slurry and/or cathartic agents may be beneficial. Because clonidine overdosage may result in the rapid development of CNS depression, induction of emesis using ipecac syrup is not recommended. If the patient is comatose, having seizures, or lacks the gag reflex, gastric lavage may be performed if an endotracheal tube with cuff inflated is in place to prevent aspiration of gastric contents. Supportive and symptomatic treatment should be initiated and an adequate airway established and maintained since respiratory depression or apnea may ensue. Supportive care may include atropine sulfate for symptomatic bradycardia, IV fluids and/or vasopressor agents for hypotension, and vasodilators for hypertension. Patients with hypotension also may be placed in Trendelenburg's position; IV infusion of dopamine may be useful for severe, persistent hypotension. The manufacturers state that administration of tolazoline has yielded inconsistent results and is not recommended as first-line therapy for clonidine overdosage. Hypertension has been managed with IV furosemide or diazoxide (parenteral formulation no longer commercially available in the US) or α-adrenergic blocking agents (e.g., phentolamine). Additional information on the efficacy of α-adrenergic blockers in the treatment of clonidine overdosage is necessary. Naloxone may be a useful adjunct for the management of respiratory depression, hypotension, and/or coma associated with clonidine overdosage; because paradoxical hypertension occasionally has been reported with the use of naloxone, blood pressure should be monitored. Seizures can be managed with IV administration of a benzodiazepine (e.g., diazepam). Although forced diuresis has been suggested to enhance the elimination of clonidine, there is no current evidence to support this procedure for clonidine overdosage; in addition, forced diuresis may potentiate clonidine-induced hypotension. Hemodialysis is of limited value in the treatment of clonidine overdosage, since a maximum of 5% of circulating drug is removed.

Pharmacology

■ **Cardiovascular Effects** Clonidine appears to stimulate α_2-adrenergic receptors in the CNS (mainly in the medulla oblongata), causing inhibition, but not blockade, of sympathetic vasomotor centers. Cardiovascular reflexes remain intact, and normal homeostatic mechanisms and hemodynamic responses to exercise are maintained. The central effects of the drug result in reduced peripheral sympathetic nervous system activity, reduced peripheral and renovascular resistance, reduction of systolic and diastolic blood pressure, and bradycardia. Peripheral venous pressure remains unchanged. It has been postulated that the hypotensive response to clonidine may result from reduced angiotensin II generation because of inhibition of renin release or from reduced stimulation of medullary vasomotor centers responsive to circulating angiotensin II; however, the exact relationship between the action of the drug in reducing renin activity and excretion of aldosterone and catecholamines and the hypotensive effect of the drug has not been fully elucidated.

Clonidine reduces blood pressure to essentially the same extent in both supine and standing patients; therefore, orthostatic effects are mild and infrequently encountered. However, the underlying hemodynamic effects differ with position of the patient. Administration of a single dose of clonidine hydrochloride to supine patients results in a reduction in cardiac output and decreased stroke volume. Total peripheral resistance remains unchanged. In patients in the standing position or at a 45° tilt, a smaller decrease in cardiac output occurs and total peripheral resistance is decreased, but stroke volume is maintained. Prolonged therapy results in circulatory adjustments, so that the hypotensive effect of the drug largely results from reduced peripheral resistance. Rapid IV, but not oral or IM, administration of clonidine produces direct stimulation of peripheral α_2-adrenergic receptors, resulting in transient vasoconstriction and a rise in systolic and diastolic blood pressure.

Urinary excretion of catecholamines is decreased during clonidine hydrochloride therapy; however, unlike reserpine, clonidine does not deplete catecholamines from the heart or other tissues. Abrupt withdrawal of clonidine following prolonged oral administration may cause increased urinary excretion of catecholamines and rebound of systolic and diastolic blood pressure.

Blood volume, as determined using iodinated I 131 serum albumin, is not substantially affected by clonidine. Circulation time is prolonged during use of the drug.

■ **Analgesic Effects** Epidurally administered α_2-agonists, including clonidine, produce analgesia by mimicking the activation of descending pain-suppressing pathways arising from supraspinal control centers (i.e., cortex, thalamus, and brainstem) and terminating in the dorsal horn of the spinal cord. Stimulation of spinal α_2-adrenergic receptors by clonidine inhibits sympathetically mediated ascending pain pathways that are activated by nociceptive stimuli and prevents transmission of pain signals to the brain. Activation of α_2-adrenergic receptors by α_2-adrenergic agonists also stimulates acetylcholine release and inhibits the release of substance P, an inflammatory neuropeptide. Clonidine-mediated analgesia is dose-dependent and is limited to regions of the body that are innervated by spinal segments containing analgesic concentrations of the drug. Analgesia resulting from clonidine therapy is not antagonized by opiate antagonists.

■ **Renal and Metabolic Effects** Acute or chronic administration of clonidine hydrochloride produces no substantial change in renal blood flow, renal plasma flow, or glomerular filtration rate. In standing patients, renal vascular resistance is substantially reduced. The moderate reduction in renal blood flow and glomerular filtration rate produced by head-up tilting are unchanged by administration of the drug. The increased renal vascular resistance which normally occurs after tilting does not occur in patients receiving clonidine.

Sodium and chloride excretion are markedly reduced after initial administration of clonidine hydrochloride; however, potassium excretion is not substantially changed. Sodium retention probably results from enhanced tubular reabsorption being stimulated by decreased renal perfusion pressure and generally persists for only 3–4 days after which natriuresis occurs. Renal vein plasma renin activity and aldosterone excretion rate are consistently reduced as a result of centrally mediated sympathetic inhibition.

■ **Other Effects** Acute administration of clonidine stimulates release of growth hormone in children and adults, but the drug does not produce sustained elevation of growth hormone during chronic administration.

The sedative effect of clonidine is thought to result from central α_2-agonist activity. The decrease in salivation induced by clonidine appears to result from both central and peripheral mechanisms, probably involving the drug's α_2-agonist activity. The peripheral mechanism of decreased salivation may involve inhibition of cholinergic transmission via stimulation of α_2-adrenergic receptors.

Clonidine has been shown to decrease GI motility and control diarrhea in animals, probably secondary to the drug's α_2-agonist activity. Clonidine has also been shown to increase intestinal absorption of sodium and chloride, with a secondary passive increase in water absorption.

IV or ocular administration of clonidine hydrochloride (ophthalmic preparation no longer commercially available in the US) in patients with glaucoma decreases intraocular pressure, reportedly by decreasing production of aqueous humor. It has been reported that when only one eye is treated topically with clonidine, ocular pressure in the untreated eye is also reduced.

Clonidine has been shown to reduce the signs and symptoms of opiate withdrawal in individuals physically dependent on opiates. Clonidine appears to reduce the severity of opiate withdrawal symptoms by stimulating central presynaptic α_2-adrenergic receptors; the stimulation results in attenuation in noradrenergic activity in the CNS, which may be responsible for the behavioral symptoms of opiate withdrawal.

Pharmacokinetics

■ **Absorption** Clonidine hydrochloride is well absorbed from the GI tract. The drug may also be absorbed when applied topically to the eye (ophthalmic preparation no longer commercially available in the US). Clonidine is well absorbed percutaneously following topical application of a transdermal system to the arm or chest. Plasma clonidine concentrations of 2 ng/mL have been detected 1 hour after administration of a single 0.39-mg oral dose of radiolabeled drug. Peak plasma concentrations following oral administration occur in approximately 3–5 hours.

Following initial application of a transdermal system of clonidine, the initial release of the drug saturates skin sites beneath the system; therapeutic plasma concentrations are attained within 2–3 days. To provide the concentration gradient necessary for controlled release and percutaneous absorption of drug, clonidine transdermal systems contain an excess amount of drug. Following removal of the systems in one study in healthy adults, analysis of residual concentration of drug in transdermal systems that initially contained 2.5 mg of clonidine per 3.5 cm² surface area indicated that release of clonidine averaged 48 and 65% after 7 and 11 days of wear, respectively, following topical application to the upper outer arm and averaged 70% after 11 days of wear following topical application to the chest. When given in dosages that produce comparable blood pressure reduction, steady-state plasma clonidine concentrations attained with the transdermal systems are generally similar to trough concentrations attained with twice-daily oral dosing regimens of the drug. Mean steady-state plasma clonidine concentrations of 0.39, 0.84, or 1.12 ng/mL have been reported following topical application of the 3.5-, 7-, or 10.5-cm² transdermal system (see Preparations), respectively, to the upper outer arm of healthy adults. Percutaneous absorption of the drug from the upper arm or chest is similar, but less drug is absorbed from the thigh. Replacement of the transdermal system at a different site at weekly intervals continuously maintains therapeutic plasma clonidine concentrations. Following discontinuance of transdermal therapy, therapeutic plasma drug concentrations persist for about 8 hours and then decline slowly over several days; over this time period, blood pressure returns gradually to pretreatment levels. If a transdermal system of clonidine is not removed after 7 days as recommended, absorption of the drug from the system may continue; if an additional system is then applied, higher plasma drug concentrations may result and, if an additional system is not applied, plasma drug concentrations may not decrease substantially for at least 2–4 more days while the system is still being worn.

Reduction in blood pressure is maximal at plasma clonidine concentrations less than 2 ng/mL. Blood pressure begins to decrease within 30–60 minutes after an oral dose of clonidine hydrochloride; the maximum decrease occurs in approximately 2–4 hours. The hypotensive effect lasts up to 8 hours. Following administration of clonidine by slow IV injection† in patients with acute hypertensive crisis, a hypotensive effect occurred within minutes, peaked in 30–60 minutes, and lasted more than 4 hours.

Following epidural administration of a single bolus dose of clonidine in healthy individuals and patients with cancer, clonidine is rapidly absorbed into the systemic circulation. A mean peak plasma clonidine concentration of 4.4 ng/mL (range: 3–5.8 ng/mL) was reported on average 19 minutes following epidural administration of 700 mcg of clonidine hydrochloride given over 5 minutes in healthy individuals. Mean peak plasma concentrations of clonidine were reported to be higher in women than in men. Following continuous epidural infusion of clonidine hydrochloride (30 mcg/hour for 14 days in addition to administration of morphine sulfate for patient-controlled analgesia [PCA]) in cancer patients, mean steady-state plasma concentrations were approximately 2.2 and 2.4–2.5 ng/mL on days 7 and 14 of dosing, respectively. Accumulation of clonidine does not appear to occur following continuous epidural infusion of the drug in adult cancer patients.

Following epidural administration of a single dose of clonidine hydrochloride, near maximal analgesia occurs within 30–60 minutes. Onset and duration of the analgesic effect of a single epidural dose of clonidine do not correlate with plasma drug concentrations; rather, analgesic effects appear to correlate with drug concentration in the CSF. Although the CSF is not the presumed site of action of clonidine-mediated analgesia, the drug appears to diffuse rapidly from the CSF to the dorsal horn. A lumbar CSF concentration of 130 ng/mL reportedly was associated with a 95% maximal analgesic effect in healthy individuals.

■ **Distribution** Animal studies indicate that clonidine is widely distributed into body tissues; tissue concentrations of the drug are higher than plasma concentrations. The mean volume of distribution of clonidine is reported to be 2.1 L/kg. After oral administration, highest concentrations of the drug are found in the kidneys, liver, spleen, and GI tract. High concentrations of the drug also appear in the lacrimal and parotid glands. Clonidine is concentrated in the choroid of the eye and is also distributed into the heart, lungs, testes, adrenal glands, fat, and muscle. The lowest concentration occurs in the brain. Clonidine is distributed into CSF. Following epidural infusion, clonidine is rapidly and extensively distributed into CSF and readily partitions into the plasma via epidural veins. In vitro, clonidine is approximately 20–40% bound to plasma proteins, mainly albumin. Clonidine crosses the placenta and is distributed into milk. In one lactating woman who received approximately 0.04 mg of oral clonidine hydrochloride twice daily and 25 mg of oral dihydralazine 3 times daily, clonidine concentrations were 0.33 ng/mL in a plasma sample obtained 1 hour after a dose and 0.6 ng/mL in a milk sample obtained 2.5 hours after a dose; the drug was not detected in the plasma of the infant 1 hour after nursing.

■ **Elimination** The plasma half-life of clonidine is 6–20 hours in patients with normal renal function. The half-life in patients with impaired renal function has been reported to range from 18–41 hours. The elimination half-life of the drug may be dose dependent, increasing with increasing dose.

Clonidine hydrochloride is metabolized in the liver. In humans, 4 metabolites have been detected but only one, the inactive *p*-hydroxyclonidine, has been identified.

In humans, 40–60% of an orally administered dose of clonidine hydrochloride (as conventional tablets) is excreted in urine as unchanged drug within 24 hours. Following IV administration of radiolabeled clonidine, 72% of the administered dose is excreted in urine within 96 hours; about 40–50% is excreted as unchanged drug. In humans, less than 10% of a dose usually is excreted as *p*-hydroxyclonidine. Approximately 20% of the dose is excreted in feces, probably via enterohepatic circulation. Approximately 85% of a single dose is excreted within 72 hours, and excretion is complete after 5 days. Following IV administration of clonidine, renal clearance of the drug averages 133 mL/minute. In patients undergoing hemodialysis, only 5% of a dose was removed into the dialysate. Following continuous epidural infusion of clonidine hydrochloride (30 mcg/hour for 14 days in addition to morphine sulfate administered for patient-controlled analgesia [PCA]) in cancer patients, mean total body clearance of the drug was approximately 279 and 272 mL/minute on days 7 and 14 of dosing, respectively.

Chemistry and Stability

■ **Chemistry** Clonidine hydrochloride, an imidazoline-derivative hypotensive agent, is a selective α_2-adrenergic agonist. Clonidine is commercially available as the base and as the hydrochloride salt. Clonidine hydrochloride occurs as a white, crystalline powder that has a bitter taste and is freely soluble in water and soluble in alcohol. Clonidine hydrochloride also is commercially available as a clear, colorless, preservative-free aqueous sterile injection. Sodium hydroxide and/or hydrochloric acid may be added during manufacture of the injection to adjust the pH to 5–7.

The commercially available transdermal system of clonidine consists of an outer layer of pigmented polyester film; a drug reservoir of clonidine, mineral oil, polyisobutylene, and colloidal silicon dioxide; a microporous polypropylene membrane that controls the rate of diffusion of the drug; and a final adhesive layer that provides an initial release of drug and contains those ingredients found in the reservoir. The adhesive layer is covered by a protective slit release liner which is removed prior to application.

■ **Stability** The commercially available transdermal system of clonidine should be stored at a temperature less than 30°C. Clonidine hydrochloride tablets should be stored in tight, light-resistant containers at a controlled room temperature of 25°C, but may be exposed to temperatures ranging from 15–30°C. Commercially available clonidine hydrochloride tablets have an expiration date of 42 months following the date of manufacture. Commercially available clonidine hydrochloride injection should be stored at controlled room temperature of 25°C, but may be exposed to temperatures ranging from 15–30°C. The injection contains no preservatives; any unused portion should be discarded.

Preparations

Excipients in commercially available drug preparations may have clinically important effects in some individuals; consult specific product labeling for details.

cloNIDine

Topical		
Transdermal System	0.1 mg/24 hours (2.5 mg/3.5 cm²)*	**Catapres-TTS**®, Boehringer Ingelheim
		Clonidine Transdermal System
	0.2 mg/24 hours (5 mg/7 cm²)*	**Catapres-TTS**®, Boehringer Ingelheim
		Clonidine Transdermal System
	0.3 mg/24 hours (7.5 mg/10.5 cm²)*	**Catapres-TTS**®, Boehringer Ingelheim
		Clonidine Transdermal System

*available from one or more manufacturer, distributor, and/or repackager by generic (nonproprietary) name

cloNIDine Hydrochloride

Oral		
Tablets	0.1 mg*	**Catapres**® (scored), Boehringer Ingelheim
		Clonidine Hydrochloride Tablets
	0.2 mg*	**Catapres**® (scored), Boehringer Ingelheim
		Clonidine Hydrochloride Tablets
	0.3 mg*	**Catapres**® (scored), Boehringer Ingelheim
		Clonidine Hydrochloride Tablets
Parenteral		
Injection, concentrate, for epidural use	500 mcg/mL*	**Clonidine Hydrochloride Injection**
		Duraclon®, Mylan
Injection, for epidural use	100 mcg/mL*	**Clonidine Hydrochloride Injection**
		Duraclon®, Mylan

*available from one or more manufacturer, distributor, and/or repackager by generic (nonproprietary) name

†Use is not currently included in the labeling approved by the US Food and Drug Administration

Methyldopa
Methyldopate Hydrochloride

■ Methyldopa is a centrally acting hypotensive agent.

Uses

■ **Hypertension** Methyldopa is used alone or in combination with other classes of antihypertensive agents in the management of hypertension. However, because of established clinical benefits (e.g., reductions in overall mortality and in adverse cardiovascular, cerebrovascular, and renal outcomes), current evidence-based practice guidelines for the management of hypertension in adults generally recommend the use of drugs from 4 classes of antihypertensive agents (angiotensin-converting enzyme [ACE] inhibitors, angiotensin II receptor antagonists, calcium-channel blockers, and thiazide diuretics). Centrally acting agents such as methyldopa may be considered as add-on therapy if goal blood pressure cannot be achieved with the recommended drugs. (See Uses: Hypertension in Adults, in the Thiazides General Statement 40:28.20.) Some experts state that centrally acting agents such as methyldopa generally are reserved as a last-line treatment option because of the drug's ability to cause substantial adverse CNS effects, especially in geriatric patients.

IV methyldopate hydrochloride may be used for the management of hypertension when parenteral hypotensive therapy is necessary.

Methyldopa generally is most effective when used with a diuretic. The use of a diuretic may prevent tolerance to methyldopa and permit reduction of methyldopa dosage. Diuretics may also prevent sodium retention and increased plasma volume that may occur after prolonged methyldopa therapy. (See Cautions: Cardiovascular Effects.) Methyldopa also has been used with other antihypertensive agents, permitting a reduction in the dosage of each drug and, in some patients, minimizing adverse effects while maintaining blood pressure control. (See Drug Interactions: Diuretics and Hypotensive Agents.) The possibility that geriatric patients may not tolerate the adverse cognitive effects of centrally acting hypotensive agents such as methyldopa should be considered. Methyldopa is generally considered to be safe for use in patients with renal failure.

For additional information on overall principles and expert recommendations for treatment of hypertension, see Uses: Hypertension in Adults and also see Uses: Hypertension in Pediatric Patients in the Thiazides General Statement 40:28.20.

Hypertension during Pregnancy Methyldopa has been used effectively for the management of hypertension in pregnant women without apparent substantial adverse effects on the fetus.

The goal of antihypertensive treatment in pregnant women with hypertension is to minimize the acute complications of maternal hypertension while avoiding therapy that would compromise fetal well-being. Antihypertensive therapy is recommended in pregnant women with chronic hypertension who have persistent, severely elevated levels of blood pressure (e.g., systolic blood pressure of 160 mm Hg or higher or diastolic blood pressure of 105 mm Hg or higher); it is less clear whether antihypertensive therapy should be initiated in women with mild to moderate chronic hypertension. The American College of Obstetricians and Gynecologists (ACOG) and other experts currently recommend use of one of several agents (labetalol, nifedipine, or methyldopa) when initiation of antihypertensive therapy is necessary in a pregnant woman. In women who are already receiving antihypertensive therapy prior to pregnancy, ACOG states there are insufficient data to make recommendations regarding the continuance or discontinuance of such therapy; treatment decisions should be individualized in these situations. Alternatively, other experts state that women with hypertension who become pregnant should be transitioned to methyldopa, nifedipine, and/or labetalol during pregnancy. Antihypertensive therapy can reduce the risk of severe hypertension but has not been shown to prevent the development of preeclampsia. Use of methyldopa in association with careful prenatal management during pregnancy appears to be safe for mother and fetus. (See Pregnancy under Cautions: Pregnancy, Fertility, and Lactation.)

Hypertensive Crises IV methyldopate hydrochloride has been used for the management of hypertensive emergencies; however, because of the slow onset of action of this drug, other agents (e.g., labetalol, esmolol, fenoldopam, nicardipine, sodium nitroprusside) are preferred.

Pheochromocytoma Methyldopa and methyldopate hydrochloride are not recommended for use in patients with pheochromocytoma.

Dosage and Administration

■ **Administration** Methyldopa is administered orally; methyldopate hydrochloride is administered by IV infusion. IM or subcutaneous administration of methyldopate hydrochloride is not recommended because of unpredictable absorption.

Methyldopate hydrochloride IV infusions are prepared by adding the required dose of the drug to 100 mL of 5% dextrose injection. Alternatively, the required dose may be administered in 5% dextrose injection in a concentration of 100 mg/10 mL. The IV infusion should be administered slowly over a period of 30–60 minutes. ADD-Vantage® vials labeled as containing 50 mg/mL of methyldopate hydrochloride should be diluted and administered according to the manufacturer's directions. Vials containing solutions of methyldopate hydrochloride for injection and reconstituted solutions of the drug should be inspected visually for particulate matter and discoloration prior to administration, whenever solution and container permit.

■ **Dosage** Dosage of methyldopa must be adjusted according to the patient's blood pressure response and tolerance. Adverse effects such as drowsiness may be minimized by starting dosage increases in the evening or by giving a larger dose at bedtime than in the morning. Geriatric patients may respond to smaller doses of methyldopa.

Hypertension **Monotherapy.** The usual initial oral dosage of methyldopa in adults is 250 mg 2 or 3 times daily for 2 days. Dosage may then be increased or decreased at intervals of at least 2 days until an adequate response is achieved. The usual maintenance dosage of methyldopa recommended by the manufacturers is 0.5–2 g daily given in 2–4 divided doses; dosages exceeding 3 g daily are not recommended by the manufacturers, although occasionally some patients have responded to such dosages. Some experts state that the usual dosage range is 0.25–1 g daily in 2 divided doses; it usually is preferable to add another antihypertensive agent to the regimen than to increase maximum methyldopa dosage beyond 1 g daily because of poor patient tolerance of increasing dosages of the drug. In some patients, administration of methyldopa as a single daily dose at bedtime may provide adequate blood pressure control during maintenance therapy.

In children, the usual initial oral dosage of methyldopa is 10 mg/kg daily, given in 2–4 divided doses. Dosage is adjusted until an adequate response is achieved. The maximum oral dosage in children is 65 mg/kg daily or 3 g daily, whichever is less.

Combination Oral Therapy. When methyldopa is administered with other hypotensive drugs, the initial oral dosage in adults should not exceed 500 mg daily in divided doses. Tolerance to methyldopa may occur between the second and third month of therapy and an increase in dosage or concomitant use of a thiazide diuretic may be required to restore effective blood pressure control.

When combination therapy is required, commercially available products containing methyldopa in fixed combination with a thiazide diuretic should not be used initially. Dosage should first be adjusted by administering each drug separately. If it is determined that the optimum maintenance dosage corresponds to the ratio in a commercially available fixed-combination preparation, such a product may be used. However, whenever dosage adjustment is necessary, the drugs should be administered separately. If combination therapy is initiated with the fixed-combination preparation, the initial dosage is 250 mg of methyldopa and 15 mg of hydrochlorothiazide given 2 or 3 times daily, or alternatively, 250 mg of methyldopa and 25 mg of hydrochlorothiazide given twice daily. Patients requiring higher dosages of the fixed-combination preparation may receive once-daily administration of 500 mg of methyldopa and 30 mg of hydrochlorothiazide, or alternatively, 500 mg of methyldopa and 50 mg of hydrochlorothiazide. When administered with another antihypertensive agent, dosages of hydrochlorothiazide should not exceed 50 mg daily.

IV Dosage. When parenteral drug therapy is indicated, the usual IV dosage of methyldopate hydrochloride in adults is 250–500 mg every 6 hours as required; the maximum dosage is 1 g every 6 hours.

The usual IV dosage of methyldopate hydrochloride in pediatric patients is 20–40 mg/kg per 24 hours, administered in equally divided doses at 6-hour intervals. The maximum IV dosage in children is 65 mg/kg daily or 3 g daily, whichever is less. When blood pressure is controlled, oral therapy should be substituted using the same dosage as the parenteral dosage.

Blood Pressure Monitoring and Treatment Goals. Blood pressure should be monitored regularly (i.e., monthly) during therapy and dosage of the antihypertensive drug adjusted until blood pressure is controlled. If an adequate blood pressure response is not achieved, the dosage may be increased or another antihypertensive agent with demonstrated benefit and preferably with a complementary mechanism of action (e.g., ACE inhibitor, angiotensin II receptor antagonist, calcium-channel blocker, thiazide diuretic) may be added; if target blood pressure is still not achieved with the use of 2 antihypertensive agents, a third drug may be added. (See Uses: Hypertension.) In patients who develop unacceptable adverse effects with methyldopa, the drug should be discontinued and another antihypertensive agent from a different pharmacologic class should be initiated.

The goal of hypertension management and prevention is to achieve and maintain optimal control of blood pressure. However, the optimum blood pressure threshold for initiating antihypertensive drug therapy and specific treatment goals remain controversial. A 2017 multidisciplinary hypertension guideline from the American College of Cardiology (ACC), American Heart Association (AHA), and a number of other professional organizations generally recommends a blood pressure goal of less than 130/80 mm Hg in all adults, regardless of comorbidities or level of atherosclerotic cardiovascular disease (ASCVD) risk. Many patients will require at least 2 drugs from different pharmacologic classes to achieve this blood pressure goal; the potential benefits of hypertension management and drug cost, adverse effects, and risks associated with the use of multiple antihypertensive drugs also should be considered when deciding a patient's blood pressure treatment goal.

For additional information on target levels of blood pressure and on monitoring therapy, see Blood Pressure Monitoring and Treatment Goals under Dosage: Hypertension, in Dosage and Administration in the Thiazides General Statement 40:28.20.

■ **Dosage in Renal Impairment** Patients with impaired renal function may respond to smaller doses of methyldopa.

Cautions

■ **Nervous System Effects** The most common adverse effect of methyldopa is drowsiness which occurs within the first 48–72 hours of therapy and may disappear with continued administration of the drug. Sedation commonly recurs when dosage is increased. A persistent decrease in mental acuity, including impaired ability to concentrate, lapses of memory, and difficulty in performing simple calculations, may occur and usually necessitates withdrawal of the drug. Other adverse nervous system effects which occur early in therapy include vertigo, headache, asthenia, and weakness.

Adverse CNS effects, which are less common than sedation and decreased mental acuity, include paresthesia, parkinsonism, and Bell's palsy. Involuntary choreoathetotic movements have been reported rarely in patients with severe bilateral cerebrovascular disease and are an indication for discontinuance of the drug. Psychic disturbances including nightmares and reversible mild psychoses or mental depression have also occurred.

■ **Cardiovascular Effects** Orthostatic hypotension with attendant dizziness, lightheadedness, and symptoms of cerebrovascular insufficiency may occur during methyldopa therapy and is an indication for dosage reduction. Orthostatic hypotension may be less pronounced with methyldopa than with guanethidine or ganglionic blocking agents but may be more severe than with reserpine, clonidine, hydralazine, propranolol, or thiazides. Syncope in older patients may be related to an increased sensitivity to methyldopa and advanced arteriosclerotic vascular disease and may be avoided by using lower dosages.

Bradycardia may occur occasionally in patients receiving methyldopa. Aggravation of angina pectoris, congestive heart failure, and prolonged carotid sinus hypersensitivity have also been reported. Following IV administration of methyldopate hydrochloride, a paradoxical pressor response has been reported. Rebound hypertension has occurred rarely following abrupt withdrawal of oral methyldopa.

Sodium retention resulting in edema and weight gain has been reported in patients receiving methyldopa and can usually be controlled by concomitant administration of a thiazide diuretic. If edema cannot be controlled by diuretics and becomes progressive or leads to congestive heart failure, methyldopa should be discontinued.

■ **Hematologic Effects** Positive direct antiglobulin (Coombs') test results have been reported in about 10–20% of patients receiving methyldopa, usually after 6–12 months of therapy. This phenomenon is dose related, with the lowest incidence in patients receiving 1 g or less of methyldopa daily. In most patients, a positive Coombs' test associated with methyldopa therapy is not clinically important. Reversal of the positive Coombs' test occurs within weeks to months after discontinuance of the drug and usually becomes negative within 6 months. Hemolytic anemia has only rarely occurred, although 2 deaths have been reported in patients with methyldopa-induced hemolytic anemia. If anemia or a positive Coombs' test occurs, appropriate laboratory studies should be performed to determine if hemolysis is present; if there is evidence of hemolytic anemia, the drug should be discontinued. (See Cautions: Precautions and Contraindications.) Discontinuance of the drug alone or initiation of corticosteroid therapy has produced remission of methyldopa-induced hemolytic anemia.

Reversible leukopenia (primarily granulocytopenia) and immune thrombocytopenia have occurred rarely during methyldopa therapy. Methyldopa may cause hemolysis in patients with glucose-6-phosphate dehydrogenase deficiency. Positive lupus and rheumatoid factor tests have been reported to result from methyldopa therapy.

■ **Sensitivity Reactions and Hepatic Effects** A major toxic effect of methyldopa is drug-induced fever, usually occurring within 3 weeks after initiation of treatment. In some patients, fever has been associated with an influenza-like illness (i.e., generalized malaise and anorexia). Fever may also be associated with eosinophilia or abnormal liver function test results, such as increased serum concentrations of alkaline phosphatase, aminotransferases, and bilirubin and abnormal prothrombin time. Rarely, reversible jaundice, with or without fever, has been reported, usually within the first 2–3 months of therapy, but occasionally after long-term therapy. In some patients, laboratory tests and liver biopsies have been consistent with cholestasis, hepatitis, hepatocellular injury, or cirrhosis. Hepatic necrosis, which may be fatal, is rare. Hepatic changes may represent hypersensitivity reactions. Methyldopa therapy should be stopped if unexplained fever or jaundice occurs or if liver function test results are abnormal. (See Cautions: Precautions and Contraindications.) If methyldopa is the causative agent, temperature and liver function generally return to normal within a few months after the drug is discontinued.

Eosinophilia, myocarditis, pericarditis, vasculitis, and lupus-like syndrome have been reported as hypersensitivity reactions to methyldopa. Three cases of sialadenitis accompanied by fever have been reported in patients receiving methyldopa; 2 of these patients also had nasal congestion and pharyngitis.

■ **GI Effects** Adverse GI effects including nausea, vomiting, diarrhea, dry mouth, distention, constipation, flatus, and sore or "black" tongue have been reported during methyldopa therapy. Pancreatitis has also occurred. At least one case of colitis associated with hepatitis has been reported.

■ **Dermatologic Effects** Adverse dermatologic effects associated with methyldopa include rash, urticaria, eczema, ulceration of the soles of the feet, hyperkeratosis, and lichenoid eruptions. At least one case of granulomatous nodular skin lesions associated with fever, arthralgia, and myalgia has been reported. Tongue ulcerations with features of lichen planus have occurred.

■ **Other Adverse Effects** Nasal congestion occurs commonly in patients receiving methyldopa. Decreased libido and impotence frequently occur in males during therapy with the drug. Breast enlargement, gynecomastia, hyperprolactinemia, lactation, and amenorrhea have been reported rarely in patients receiving the drug. At least one case of retroperitoneal fibrosis may have been caused by methyldopa. Blurred vision, nocturia, and increased BUN and serum amylase concentrations have been reported.

■ **Precautions and Contraindications** When methyldopa is used as a fixed-combination preparation that includes hydrochlorothiazide, the cautions, precautions, and contraindications associated with thiazide diuretics must be considered in addition to those associated with methyldopa.

When methyldopa therapy is started, hemoglobin, hematocrit, or a red blood cell count should be done and periodic blood counts should be performed during therapy to detect hemolytic anemia. Hepatic function should be determined periodically, especially during the first 6–12 weeks of therapy or whenever unexplained fever occurs. If the need for a blood transfusion occurs in patients receiving methyldopa, prior knowledge of a positive Coombs' reaction will aid in the evaluation of a cross match; therefore, a direct Coombs' test before methyldopa therapy and after 6 and 12 months of therapy may be useful. A positive direct Coombs' test prior to methyldopa therapy is not in itself a contraindication to use of the drug. Patients receiving methyldopa who need a transfusion should have both a direct and an indirect Coombs' test performed. In the absence of hemolytic anemia, usually only the direct Coombs' test will be positive; a positive direct Coombs' test alone will not interfere with typing or cross matching. If both the indirect and direct Coombs' tests are positive, problems with major cross matching may occur and the assistance of an expert in this area may be required.

If anemia or a positive Coombs' test occur during methyldopa therapy, appropriate laboratory studies should be performed to determine if hemolysis is present; if there is evidence of hemolytic anemia, the drug should be discontinued. The anemia usually remits promptly; if not, corticosteroids may be given and other causes of anemia should be considered and investigated. If the hemolytic anemia is related to methyldopa, therapy with the drug should not be reinstituted. Similarly, if unexplained fever, abnormal liver function test results, or jaundice occurs during methyldopa therapy, the drug should be discontinued; if these effects are caused by the drug, methyldopa therapy should not be reinstituted.

Patients who are receiving methyldopa and who undergo dialysis may occasionally become hypertensive after the dialysis, since the drug is dialyzable.

Patients should be warned that methyldopa may impair their ability to perform activities requiring mental alertness or physical coordination (e.g., operating machinery, driving a motor vehicle). Rarely, involuntary choreoathetotic movements have occurred during methyldopa therapy in patients with severe bilateral cerebrovascular disease; if these effects occur, the drug should be discontinued.

Commercially available formulations of methyldopate hydrochloride may contain sulfites, which can cause allergic-type reactions, including anaphylaxis and life-threatening or less severe asthmatic episodes, in certain susceptible individuals. The overall prevalence of sulfite sensitivity in the general population is unknown but probably low; such sensitivity appears to occur more frequently in asthmatic than in nonasthmatic individuals.

Methyldopa should be used with caution in patients with a history of previous liver disease or dysfunction and is not recommended for use in patients with pheochromocytoma. Methyldopa is contraindicated in patients with active hepatic disease, such as acute hepatitis and active cirrhosis, and in patients in whom previous methyldopa therapy was associated with liver abnormalities or direct Coombs' positive hemolytic anemia. Methyldopa is contraindicated in patients receiving monoamine oxidase (MAO) inhibitors. Methyldopa is also contraindicated in patients who are hypersensitive to the drug or any ingredient in its formulation.

■ **Pediatric Precautions** There have been no well-controlled studies to date using oral or IV preparations of methyldopa in pediatric patients. Dosage recommendations in children are based on published literature concerning use of methyldopa in hypertensive pediatric patients. The manufacturer states that safety and efficacy of preparations containing methyldopa in fixed combination with hydrochlorothiazide in pediatric patients have not been established. For information on overall principles and expert recommendations for treatment of hypertension in pediatric patients, see Uses: Hypertension in Pediatric Patients, in the Thiazides General Statement 40:28.20.

■ **Mutagenicity and Carcinogenicity** Methyldopa was not mutagenic in the Ames test and did not increase chromosomal aberration or sister chromatid exchanges in Chinese hamster ovary cells; the in vitro studies were performed both with and without metabolic activation.

In a 2-year study, there was no evidence of tumorigenic effect when methyldopa was given to mice at dosages up to 1800 mg/kg daily (30 or 2.5 times the maximum human daily dosage when compared on the basis of body weight or body surface area, respectively) or to rats at dosages up to 240 mg/kg daily (4 or 0.6 times the maximum human daily dosage when compared on the basis of the body weight or body surface area, respectively).

■ **Pregnancy, Fertility, and Lactation** *Pregnancy* Reproduction studies in mice, rabbits, and rats using oral methyldopa in dosages of 1000, 200, and 100 mg/kg, respectively, have not revealed evidence of harm to the fetus. These dosages are 16.6, 3.3, and 1.7 times, respectively, the maximum daily human dosage when compared on the basis of body weight and 1.4, 1.1, and 0.2 times, respectively, the maximum daily human dosage when compared on the basis of body surface area.

Methyldopa has been used for many years in the management of hypertension in pregnant women, and the drug is generally considered safe for mother and fetus when used in association with careful prenatal management. Uteroplacental blood flow and fetal hemodynamics have been reported to be stable during therapy with the drug. Although no teratogenic effects have been reported, the possibility that methyldopa may cause fetal injury (e.g., secondary to reduced placental blood flow or fetotoxicity) cannot be excluded.

In neonates born to women treated with methyldopa, systolic blood pressure may be decreased during the first 2–3 days after delivery; in some neonates, tremors have also been reported. Studies to date, including a long-term follow-up study, of children born to women who received methyldopa during pregnancy have not revealed evidence of substantial adverse effects of the drug on the offspring; however, in the longest follow-up study, treatment with methyldopa was associated with a smaller head circumference (without an apparent effect on intelligence quotient) in male offspring of those women whose therapy was initiated between 16 and 20 weeks' gestation. At 4 years of age, the developmental delay commonly seen in children born to hypertensive mothers was less evident in those whose mothers received methyldopa during pregnancy than in those whose mothers were untreated. Children born to mothers receiving methyldopa scored consistently higher on indices of intellectual and motor development than children born to untreated hypertensive mothers; however, these differences were not apparent by 7.5 years of age.

Methyldopa should be used during pregnancy only when clearly needed. In addition, excessive reduction in blood pressure should be avoided, and a conservative approach to treatment generally should be followed. (See Hypertension during Pregnancy under Uses: Hypertension.)

Fertility Reproduction studies in male and female rats using methyldopa dosages of 100 mg/kg daily (1.7 times or 0.2 times the maximum recommended daily human dosage when compared on the basis of body weight or body surface area, respectively) have not revealed evidence of impaired fertility. However, in male rats given 200 mg/kg daily (3.3 or 0.5 times the maximum daily human dosage when compared on the basis of body weight or body surface area, respectively) or 400 mg/kg daily (6.7 or 1 times the maximum daily human dosage on the basis of body weight or body surface area, respectively), there were decreases in sperm count, sperm motility, number of late spermatids, and male fertility index.

Lactation Since methyldopa is distributed into milk, the drug should be used with caution in nursing women; the possibility of adverse effects on a nursing infant cannot be excluded. The extent to which methyldopa distributes into milk has not been clearly established, but the amount of drug a nursing infant would ingest is believed to be too small to be clinically important; however, if a woman receiving methyldopa breastfeeds, the infant (particularly if preterm) should be monitored for potential systemic effects of the drug (e.g., decreased respiration, blood pressure, or alertness).

Drug Interactions

■ **Diuretics and Hypotensive Agents** When methyldopa is administered with diuretics or other hypotensive agents, the hypotensive effect of methyldopa may be increased. This effect is usually used to therapeutic advantage, but careful adjustment of dosage is necessary when these drugs are used concomitantly.

■ **Psychotherapeutic Agents** Patients receiving methyldopa and phenothiazines or tricyclic antidepressants should be monitored for a possible reduction in hypotensive effect. Although methyldopa has been used with haloperidol and chlorpromazine to treat patients with schizophrenic disorder, nonschizophrenic patients have developed symptoms such as psychomotor retardation, memory impairment, and inability to concentrate when haloperidol was added to methyldopa therapy; these symptoms disappeared when haloperidol was discontinued.

Methyldopa and monoamine oxidase inhibitors are not to be used concomitantly.

Patients receiving lithium carbonate have developed signs and symptoms of lithium toxicity when methyldopa was added to their therapy. Therefore, patients receiving the drugs concomitantly should be monitored for lithium toxicity and therapy with the drugs adjusted accordingly.

■ **Levodopa** Methyldopa should be used with caution in patients receiving levodopa, since an additive hypotensive effect may occur. In addition, methyldopa can cause toxic CNS effects such as psychosis if administered concomitantly with levodopa.

■ **Oral Iron Preparations** Results of one cross-over study in healthy adults indicate that concomitant administration of a single oral dose of ferrous sulfate (325 mg) or ferrous gluconate (600 mg) can decrease oral absorption of methyldopa (500 mg) by 61–73%. In addition, concomitant administration of these oral iron preparations appears to affect metabolism of methyldopa since there was a 79–88% decrease in urinary excretion of free methyldopa and an increase in urinary excretion of the sulfate conjugate of the drug. When oral ferrous sulfate therapy (325 mg every 8 hours) was initiated in a group of hypertensive patients receiving chronic methyldopa therapy (250 mg 1–3 times daily or 500 mg 3 times daily), there was an increase in blood pressure during concomitant therapy and a decrease in blood pressure when the oral iron preparation was discontinued. Therefore, at least one manufacturer states that concomitant administration of methyldopa with ferrous sulfate or ferrous gluconate is *not* recommended.

■ **Other Drugs** Patients receiving methyldopa may require reduced doses of general anesthetics; if hypotension occurs during anesthesia, the manufacturers state that vasopressor drugs are usually effective. In patients receiving methyldopa, norepinephrine should be administered cautiously, beginning with small doses, since the magnitude and duration of the pressor response to norepinephrine may be enhanced. Theoretically, the effect of ephedrine may be reduced in methyldopa-treated patients, since methyldopa reduces the quantity of norepinephrine in sympathetic nerve endings and ephedrine activity is due to an indirect effect resulting in release of norepinephrine. Clinically, methyldopa treatment has decreased the mydriasis produced by topical ephedrine. Theoretically, amphetamines may increase sympathetic activity and result in a decrease in the hypotensive effect of methyldopa.

Laboratory Test Interferences

Patients receiving methyldopa may develop positive direct antiglobulin (Coombs') tests. (See Cautions: Precautions and Contraindications.)

Methyldopa may interfere with measurement of creatinine by the alkaline picrate method and AST (SGOT) by colorimetric methods. Interference with spectrophotometric methods for AST analysis has not been reported. Although methyldopa has been reported to interfere with measurement of uric acid by the phosphotungstate method, a recent study indicated that interference occurs only with concentrations of the drug that are several times higher than therapeutic concentrations.

Methyldopa causes fluorescence in urine samples at the same wavelengths as catecholamines and, therefore, may cause a false report of elevated urinary catecholamines. The drug does not interfere with measurement of vanillylmandelic acid (VMA) by methods which convert VMA to vanillin.

In the modified Watson-Schwartz test for porphobilinogen, the urine of patients receiving methyldopa produces a characteristic equal distribution of a pink or red color between the aqueous and butanol layers. Rarely, when urine is exposed to air, it may darken because of breakdown of methyldopa or its metabolites. Alkaline urine containing iron and methyldopa or its metabolites has been reported to darken immediately on exposure to air.

Acute Toxicity

■ **Pathogenesis** The oral LD_{50} of methyldopa exceeds 1.5 g/kg in mice and rats. The IV LD_{50} of methyldopate hydrochloride in mice is 321 mg/kg.

■ **Manifestations** Overdosage with methyldopa may produce acute hypotension associated with excessive sedation, weakness, bradycardia, dizziness, lightheadedness, constipation, GI distention, flatus, diarrhea, nausea, and vomiting. A few patients have received 6 g of methyldopa daily without adverse effects.

■ **Treatment** Treatment of methyldopa overdosage generally involves symptomatic and supportive care. If ingestion of methyldopa is recent, gastric lavage or emesis may reduce absorption. Management of overdosage includes keeping the patient supine and symptomatic treatment with monitoring of the cardiac rate and output, blood volume, electrolyte balance, GI motility, renal function, and cerebral activity. Some experts suggest that keeping the patient supine and adequately hydrated with infusion of IV fluids should reverse most of the hypotension; if these measures are inadequate, norepinephrine or dopamine may be used with caution. (See Drug Interactions: Other Drugs.) Methyldopa is dialyzable. Infusion of IV fluids may promote urinary excretion of the drug.

Pharmacology

The mechanism of the hypotensive action of methyldopa has not been fully elucidated, but probably is predominantly due to an effect on the CNS. Methyldopa is decarboxylated to form α-methylnorepinephrine in the CNS, where it lowers arterial pressure by stimulation of central inhibitory α-adrenergic receptors. Reduction of plasma renin activity (PRA) may also contribute to the hypotensive effect of methyldopa. In one study, the drug decreased PRA and blood pressure in patients with moderate to severe hypertension and normal PRA, and in hypertensive patients with renal failure. In another study, blood pressure decreased but there was no effect on PRA in low or normal renin hypertensive patients receiving methyldopa.

Methyldopa inhibits the decarboxylation of dihydroxyphenylalanine (dopa)—the precursor of norepinephrine—and of 5-hydroxytryptophan (5-HTP)—the precursor of serotonin—in the CNS and in most peripheral tissues. Although the drug's major hypotensive effect is not attributed to decarboxylase inhibition nor to any other effect on peripheral sympathetic nerves or their mediators, some contribution by peripheral mechanisms cannot be ruled out.

Although reports are conflicting, the hypotensive effect of methyldopa is generally attributed to a decrease in total peripheral resistance with little change in cardiac output and heart rate. However, one study has shown that chronic oral administration of methyldopa reduces blood pressure mainly by decreasing cardiac output with little change in total peripheral resistance. Results of another study indicated that short-term oral administration of the drug in hypertensive patients with congestive heart failure may also decrease cardiac output. Although methyldopa has a somewhat greater hypotensive effect when the patient is standing, blood pressure is also significantly reduced in the supine position. The drug may cause postural hypotension. (See Cautions: Cardiovascular Effects.)

Renal blood flow and glomerular filtration rate are unchanged or increased in patients receiving methyldopa. Methyldopa causes sodium and water retention. Tolerance to the hypotensive effect develops during prolonged therapy, especially if a diuretic is not administered concurrently. Methyldopa increases serum prolactin concentrations.

Pharmacokinetics

■ **Absorption** Methyldopa is partially absorbed from the GI tract. The degree of absorption varies among individuals and in the same patient from day to day, but generally about 50% of an oral dose is absorbed. Plasma concentrations of methyldopa generally do not correlate with therapeutic effect. Following oral administration of methyldopa, peak plasma concentrations of the drug occur in approximately 3–6 hours. Mean plasma concentrations of the drug 3 hours after a 750-mg dose are approximately 3.4 mcg/mL. The maximum decrease in blood pressure occurs in 4–6 hours after oral administration of methyldopa. Once an adequate oral dosage level is attained, optimum blood pressure response occurs in 12–24 hours in most patients. After withdrawal of the drug, blood pressure usually returns to pretreatment levels within 24–48 hours.

Methyldopate hydrochloride is hydrolyzed in the body to form methyldopa; hydrolysis is somewhat delayed. The mean plasma concentration of methyldopa 60 minutes after IV administration of 250 mg of methyldopate hydrochloride is approximately 1.7 mcg/mL. After IV administration of methyldopate hydrochloride, the hypotensive effect begins in 4–6 hours and lasts 10–16 hours.

■ **Distribution** Methyldopa and its metabolites are weakly bound to plasma proteins.

Animal studies indicate that the drug crosses the blood-brain barrier. Methyldopa crosses the placenta in humans. Methyldopa is distributed into milk; peak milk concentrations of free methyldopa are approximately 20–35% of those in maternal plasma following an individual dose during continuous therapy. The extent of distribution of methyldopa into milk has not been clearly determined, but it is estimated that about 0.02% of a daily maternal dose of 1 g would be ingested by a nursing infant and that this amount is probably not clinically important.

■ **Elimination** Plasma concentrations of methyldopa decline in a biphasic manner; in patients with normal renal function, 95% of the drug is eliminated during the initial phase with a plasma half-life of 1.8 hours; the second phase is much slower. Renal clearance of the drug is decreased in patients with renal insufficiency. In patients with severely impaired renal function, about 50% of the drug is excreted during the initial phase with a half-life of 3.6 hours.

Methyldopa is extensively metabolized mainly to the conjugate, methyldopa mono-*O*-sulfate, probably in the GI tract and the liver. Conjugation occurs to a greater extent when the drug is given orally than when it is given IV. The sulfate conjugate of methyldopa may be therapeutically active. There is wide interindividual difference in the ratio of free to conjugated methyldopa in the plasma. The rate of conjugation of methyldopa is decreased in patients with renal insufficiency. Unchanged methyldopa and its conjugates are the major constituents found in plasma and urine, but small amounts of decarboxylated derivatives have also been identified.

Methyldopa is excreted in urine largely by glomerular filtration, primarily unchanged and as the mono-*O*-sulfate conjugate. Delayed excretion and accumulation of this metabolite occur in patients with renal insufficiency and may cause an increased hypotensive effect during methyldopa therapy. Unabsorbed methyldopa is excreted in the feces unchanged. Methyldopa is removed by hemodialysis and peritoneal dialysis.

Chemistry and Stability

■ **Chemistry** Methyldopa is a hypotensive agent that is structurally related to the catecholamines and their precursors. Methyldopa occurs as a white to yellowish white, fine powder that may contain friable lumps and is sparingly soluble in water and slightly soluble in alcohol.

Methyldopate hydrochloride, the ethyl ester of the hydrochloride salt of methyldopa, occurs as a white or practically white, odorless or practically odorless, crystalline powder and is freely soluble in water and in alcohol. Methyldopate hydrochloride injection is a sterile solution of the drug in water for injection. Sodium hydroxide is used to adjust the pH of the commercially available injection to 3–4.2. Methyldopate hydrochloride imparts some buffer capacity to IV solutions. When methyldopate hydrochloride injection is diluted with most IV infusion fluids, the resulting solutions generally have a pH of 7 or less, even when alkaline solutions are used.

■ **Stability** Methyldopa is decomposed by oxidizing agents. Methyldopa tablets should be stored in tight, light-resistant containers at 15–30°C unless otherwise directed by the manufacturer. Methyldopate hydrochloride injection should be stored at a temperature less than 30°C, preferably at 15–30°C; freezing should be avoided.

Methyldopate hydrochloride injection is stable at pH 3.5–6 for 24 hours in most IV infusion fluids. Exposure to air may accelerate decomposition. Methyldopate hydrochloride should be mixed cautiously with drugs that are poorly soluble in an acidic medium (e.g., sodium salts of barbiturates and sulfonamides) and with drugs that are acid labile. Methyldopate hydrochloride injection has been reported to be physically incompatible with other drugs, but compatibility depends on several factors (e.g., concentrations of the drugs, specific diluents used, resulting pH, temperature). Specialized references should be consulted for specific information.

Preparations

Excipients in commercially available drug preparations may have clinically important effects in some individuals; consult specific product labeling for details.

Methyldopa

Oral		
Tablets, film-coated	250 mg*	Methyldopa Tablets
	500 mg*	Methyldopa Tablets

*available from one or more manufacturer, distributor, and/or repackager by generic (nonproprietary) name

Methyldopa and Hydrochlorothiazide

Oral		
Tablets, film-coated	250 mg with Hydrochlorothiazide 15 mg*	Methyldopa and Hydrochlorothiazide Tablets
	250 mg with Hydrochlorothiazide 25 mg*	Methyldopa and Hydrochlorothiazide Tablets

*available from one or more manufacturer, distributor, and/or repackager by generic (nonproprietary) name

Methyldopate Hydrochloride

Parenteral		
Injection	50 mg/mL*	Methyldopate Hydrochloride Injection

*available from one or more manufacturer, distributor, and/or repackager by generic (nonproprietary) name

DIRECT VASODILATORS 24:08.20

hydrALAZINE Hydrochloride

Hydrallazine

■ Hydralazine hydrochloride is a vasodilating agent.

Uses

■ **Hypertension** Hydralazine is used in the management of moderate to severe hypertension. However, because of established clinical benefits (e.g., reductions in overall mortality and in adverse cardiovascular, cerebrovascular, and renal outcomes), current evidence-based practice guidelines for the management of hypertension in adults generally recommend the use of drugs from 4 classes of antihypertensive agents (angiotensin-converting enzyme [ACE] inhibitors, angiotensin II receptor antagonists, calcium-channel blockers, and thiazide diuretics). Some experts state that direct vasodilators such as hydralazine may be considered as add-on therapy if goal blood pressure cannot be achieved with the recommended drugs.

Hydralazine generally is used in conjunction with a diuretic and another hypotensive agent. The use of a diuretic may prevent tolerance to hydralazine and also the sodium retention and increased plasma volume that may occur after prolonged hydralazine therapy. Use of hydralazine in conjunction with other hypotensive agents also may permit a reduction in the dosage of each drug and minimizes adverse effects while maintaining blood pressure control. (See Drug Interactions: Diuretics and Hypotensive Agents.) Adverse effects such as tachycardia and precipitation of angina may be minimized by administering the drug in conjunction with a β-adrenergic blocking agent (β-blocker).

For additional information on overall principles and expert recommendations for treatment of hypertension, see Uses: Hypertension in Adults, in the Thiazides General Statement 40:28.20.

Hypertensive Crises Parenteral hydralazine may be used for the management of severe hypertension when the drug cannot be given orally or when blood pressure must be lowered immediately. Because hydralazine has a less predictable hypotensive effect and greater cardiac stimulating effects, other agents (e.g., labetalol, esmolol, fenoldopam, nicardipine, sodium nitroprusside) usually are preferred for the management of severe hypertension or hypertensive emergencies when a parenteral hypotensive agent is employed. In addition, because of potential adverse effects on cerebrovascular circulation, hydralazine generally is *not* recommended for the management of severe hypertension or hypertensive emergencies associated with cerebrovascular accidents or in patients with cerebral edema and encephalopathy. However, IV or IM hydralazine has been used effectively and historically has been considered the parenteral hypotensive agent of choice for the management of hypertensive emergencies associated with pregnancy (e.g., preeclampsia, eclampsia). (See Severe Hypertension During Pregnancy under Uses: Hypertension.) Excessive falls in blood pressure should be avoided in any hypertensive crisis since they may precipitate renal, cerebral, or coronary ischemia.

Severe Hypertension during Pregnancy Hydralazine has been used parenterally in the hospital setting for urgent lowering of blood pressure in severely hypertensive pregnant women, including those with preeclampsia†. Recommendations for the management of such patients are based principally on experience in women with preeclampsia or gestational hypertension in the third trimester. Delivery is the preferred method of management for women with severe preeclampsia; however, use of antihypertensive drugs is recommended in such women who have severely elevated blood pressures (sustained systolic blood pressure of at least 160 mm Hg or diastolic blood pressure of at least 110 mm Hg) to prevent potentially life-threatening cardiovascular, renal, and cerebrovascular complications. Results of several randomized clinical trials evaluating antihypertensive therapy in women with severe hypertension during pregnancy suggest that IV hydralazine, IV labetalol, or oral nifedipine are appropriate antihypertensives for urgently lowering blood pressure in such patients; choice of therapy should be based on clinician experience and preference as well as patient-specific-factors (e.g., concomitant medical conditions or therapies) and drug-related factors (e.g., route of administration, adverse effects, contraindications, local availability, cost). Although hydralazine historically has been considered the agent of choice for management of hypertensive emergencies associated with pregnancy, some clinicians now prefer IV labetalol for its more rapid onset, shorter duration of action, and more predictable hypotensive effect.

■ **Heart Failure** Hydralazine is used in fixed combination with isosorbide dinitrate (BiDil®) as an adjunct to standard therapy for the treatment of heart failure in self-identified black patients to improve survival, decrease rate of hospitalization for worsened heart failure, and improve patient-reported functional status. Current guidelines for the management of heart failure in adults generally recommend a combination of drug therapies to reduce morbidity and mortality, including neurohormonal antagonists (e.g., ACE inhibitors, angiotensin II receptor antagonists, angiotensin receptor-neprilysin inhibitors [ARNIs], β-blockers, aldosterone receptor antagonists) that inhibit the detrimental compensatory mechanisms in heart failure. (See Uses: Heart Failure in Carvedilol 24:24 and in Sacubitril and Valsartan 24:32.92.) The combination of hydralazine and isosorbide dinitrate is recommended by the American College of Cardiology Foundation (ACCF) and American Heart Association (AHA) for self-identified black patients with New York Heart Association (NYHA) functional class III or IV heart failure and reduced ejection fraction who are receiving optimal therapy with ACE inhibitors and β-blockers (unless contraindicated). The ACCF and AHA also state that combined therapy with hydralazine and isosorbide dinitrate may be considered in patients with current or prior symptomatic heart failure with reduced ejection fraction who cannot receive an ACE inhibitor or angiotensin II receptor antagonist† because of drug intolerance, hypotension, or renal insufficiency.

Efficacy of the hydralazine/isosorbide dinitrate fixed-combination preparation was evaluated in a multicenter, randomized, placebo-controlled, double-blind trial (the African-American Heart Failure Trial; A-HeFT trial) in 1050 self-identified black adults (mean age: 57 years) with stable moderate-to-severe heart failure (NYHA functional class III in over 95% of patients) secondary to left ventricular dysfunction (ejection fraction 35% or less). Patients were randomized to receive the fixed-combination preparation containing hydralazine and isosorbide dinitrate (initially, 37.5 mg of hydralazine hydrochloride and 20 mg of isosorbide dinitrate 3 times daily and titrated [as tolerated] to a target dosage of 75 mg of hydralazine hydrochloride and 40 mg of isosorbide dinitrate 3 times daily) or placebo for up to 18 months. Patients also received standard therapy (e.g., diuretics [mainly loop diuretics], β-blockers, ACE inhibitors, angiotensin II receptor antagonists, cardiac glycosides, and/or aldosterone antagonists).

The A-HeFT trial was terminated early (after a mean follow-up period of 10–12 months) primarily because of a significant reduction (43%) in all-cause mortality in patients receiving the fixed-combination preparation containing hydralazine and isosorbide dinitrate; mortality rate was about 10.2 or 6.2% in patients receiving placebo or the fixed combination, respectively.

The primary end point of the study (a mean primary composite score consisting of all-cause mortality, first hospitalization for worsening of heart failure, and improvement of quality of life [as assessed by responses to the Minnesota Living with Heart Failure questionnaire]) also showed substantial differences between drug therapy and placebo. Patients receiving the fixed combination containing hydralazine and isosorbide dinitrate experienced a significant reduction (33%) in the rate of first hospitalization for heart failure (16.4 or 24.4% for those receiving the drug or placebo, respectively) and a significant improvement in response to the Minnesota Living with Heart Failure questionnaire (a self-report of functional status). Factors of age, gender, baseline disease, or concomitant medications appeared to have no effect on survival or rate of hospitalization. The fixed combination containing hydralazine and isosorbide dinitrate had a slight but significant blood pressure-lowering effect; a mean decrease of 1.9 and 2.4 mm Hg from baseline in systolic and diastolic blood pressure, respectively, was observed in patients receiving the drugs, while an increase of 1.2 and 0.8 mm Hg from baseline in systolic and diastolic blood pressure, respectively, was observed in patients receiving placebo. However, the role of reduced blood pressure in the improved outcome of patients receiving the study medications has not been evaluated. The manufacturer states that there is no adequate clinical experience with hydralazine hydrochloride or isosorbide dinitrate as separate agents† or with dosages of the drugs other than those used in the A-HeFT trial for the treatment of heart failure.

In another randomized, placebo-controlled, comparative, long-term (median 2.3 years; range: 6–68 months) study (Vasodilator Heart Failure Trial [V-HeFT I]) in patients with chronic congestive heart failure (associated with ischemic or nonischemic cardiomyopathy) who were receiving conventional therapy (cardiac glycosides and diuretics, without an ACE inhibitor), addition of hydralazine hydrochloride (up to 300 mg daily) given concomitantly with isosorbide dinitrate (up to 160 mg daily) resulted in a 25–30% decrease in overall mortality rates after 2 years when compared with conventional therapy and placebo or prazosin (up to 20 mg daily). However, despite substantial increases in ejection fraction, the combination of the 2 vasodilators was not associated with decreased hospitalizations and many patients discontinued therapy during follow-up, although retrospective analysis of such data indicate that there was a trend favoring the administration of the 2 vasodilators, which was attributed to an effect observed in black patients.

In a subsequent randomized, comparative, long-term (median 2.5 years; range: 6–68 months) study (V-HeFT II) in patients with ischemic or nonischemic cardiomyopathy and mild to moderate heart failure (NYHA functional class II and III) who were receiving conventional therapy (cardiac glycosides and diuretics), addition of enalapril maleate (up to 20 mg daily) resulted in a 28% decrease in overall mortality rates after 2 years when compared with conventional therapy and concomitant use of hydralazine hydrochloride (up to 300 mg daily) with isosorbide dinitrate (up to 160 mg daily). Retrospective analysis of the data indicates that such decreases in mortality rates in patients receiving enalapril in conjunction with conventional therapy were not observed in black patients. In addition, concomitant therapy with the 2 vasodilators had more favorable effects on ventricular ejection fraction and exercise tolerance than those associated with enalapril.

■ **Pulmonary Hypertension** Hydralazine has produced hemodynamic and clinical improvement in some patients with unexplained pulmonary hypertension†; however, the drug does not produce consistent results and may cause serious adverse reactions (e.g., symptomatic hypotension, severe dyspnea) in patients with this condition. Further studies are needed to determine the safety, efficacy, and role of hydralazine in the treatment of unexplained pulmonary hypertension. The drug should be used for the treatment of this condition only with careful hemodynamic monitoring and clinical evaluation.

Dosage and Administration

■ **Administration** Hydralazine hydrochloride usually is administered orally. In patients who are unable to take the drug orally or when a rapid decrease in blood pressure is required, the drug may be given IM or IV. Oral therapy with hydralazine should replace parenteral therapy as soon as possible.

■ **Dosage** When hydralazine therapy is discontinued in patients with a marked reduction in blood pressure, withdrawal should be gradual to avoid a possible sudden increase in blood pressure. One study found 20–25 mg of IV hydralazine hydrochloride approximately equal to 75–100 mg of oral hydralazine hydrochloride.

Hypertension Dosage of hydralazine must be adjusted according to the patient's blood pressure response and tolerance. Generally, dosage of hydralazine required for satisfactory blood pressure control is higher in rapid acetylators than in slow acetylators.

Adult Dosage. For the management of hypertension, an initial adult oral dosage of hydralazine hydrochloride of 10 mg 4 times daily for 2–4 days has been suggested. Dosage then can be increased to 25 mg 4 times daily for the remainder of the week. If necessary, dosage can be increased for the second and subsequent weeks to 50 mg 4 times daily. In a few patients, 300–400 mg daily may be required. Generally, slow acetylators should not receive more than 200 mg daily of oral hydralazine hydrochloride. For maintenance therapy, dosage is adjusted to the lowest effective level. Studies have shown hydralazine may be administered twice daily in many patients for maintenance therapy. Some experts state that the usual dosage range is 100–200 mg daily, administered in 2 or 3 divided doses.

Pediatric Dosage. Although the manufacturers state that pediatric dosage recommendations have not been established in controlled clinical trials, there is experience with the use of hydralazine hydrochloride in pediatric patients. Based on such experience, an initial oral hydralazine hydrochloride dosage of 0.75 mg/kg daily given in 4 divided doses has been suggested for treatment of hypertension. If necessary, oral dosage may be increased gradually over a period of 3–4 weeks up to a maximum of 7.5 mg/kg (or 200 mg) daily. For information on overall principles and expert recommendations for treatment of hypertension in pediatric patients, see Uses: Hypertension in Pediatric Patients, in the Thiazides General Statement 40:28.20.

Blood Pressure Monitoring and Treatment Goals. Blood pressure should be monitored regularly (i.e., monthly) during therapy and dosage of the antihypertensive drug adjusted until blood pressure is controlled. If an adequate blood pressure response is not achieved, the dosage may be increased or another antihypertensive agent with demonstrated benefit and preferably with a complementary mechanism of action (e.g., ACE inhibitor, angiotensin II receptor antagonist, calcium-channel blocker, thiazide diuretic) may be added; if target blood pressure is still not achieved with the use of 2 antihypertensive agents, a third drug may be added. (See Uses: Hypertension.) In patients who develop unacceptable adverse effects with hydralazine, the drug should be discontinued and another antihypertensive agent from a different pharmacologic class should be initiated.

The goal of hypertension management and prevention is to achieve and maintain optimal control of blood pressure. However, the optimum blood pressure threshold for initiating antihypertensive drug therapy and specific treatment goals remain controversial. A 2017 multidisciplinary hypertension guideline from the American College of Cardiology (ACC), American Heart Association (AHA), and a number of other professional organizations generally recommends a blood pressure goal of less than 130/80 mm Hg in all adults, regardless of comorbidities or level of atherosclerotic cardiovascular disease (ASCVD) risk. Many patients will require at least 2 drugs from different pharmacologic classes to achieve this blood pressure goal; the potential benefits of hypertension management and drug cost, adverse effects, and risks associated with the use of multiple antihypertensive drugs also should be considered when deciding a patient's blood pressure treatment goal.

For additional information on target levels of blood pressure and on monitoring therapy in the management of hypertension, see Blood Pressure Monitoring and Treatment Goals under Dosage: Hypertension, in Dosage and Administration in the Thiazides General Statement 40:28.20.

Hypertensive Crises For the management of severe hypertension in hospitalized adults when there is an urgent need to lower blood pressure or when the drug cannot be given orally, the manufacturer states that the usual IM or IV dose of hydralazine hydrochloride is 20–40 mg, repeated as necessary; most patients can be transferred to oral therapy within 24–48 hours. Alternatively, some experts recommend an initial IV hydralazine hydrochloride dose of 10–20 mg, which may be repeated every 4–6 hours as needed, for the treatment of hypertensive emergencies in adults. However, such experts state that hydralazine's unpredictability of response and prolonged duration of action make it an undesirable first-line agent for acute treatment in most patients.

If IV hydralazine is used in the management of a hypertensive emergency in adults *with* a compelling indication (e.g., aortic dissection, pheochromocytoma hypertensive crisis, severe preeclampsia or eclampsia), some experts state that systolic blood pressure should be reduced to less than 140 mm Hg during the first hour or, in patients with acute aortic dissection, to less than 120 mm Hg within the first 20 minutes. If IV hydralazine is used in the management of a hypertensive emergency in adults *without* a compelling indication, such experts state that the initial goal of such therapy is to reduce mean systolic blood pressure by no more than 25% within the first hour, followed by further blood pressure reduction if stable to 160/110 or 160/100 mm Hg within the next 2–6 hours, avoiding excessive declines in pressure that could precipitate renal, cerebral, or coronary ischemia. If this blood pressure is well tolerated and the patient is clinically stable, further gradual reductions toward normal blood pressure can be implemented in the next 24–48 hours.

Although the manufacturers state that pediatric dosage recommendations for hydralazine hydrochloride have not been established in controlled clinical trials, there is experience with the use of the drug in pediatric patients. For the treatment of severe hypertension in pediatric patients when hydralazine hydrochloride cannot be administered orally or when urgent blood pressure reduction is needed, the manufacturer states that an IV or IM dosage of 1.7–3.5 mg/kg daily divided in 4–6 doses has been used. Alternatively, in pediatric patients with severe hypertension and life-threatening symptoms†, some experts have suggested an initial IV or IM hydralazine hydrochloride dose of 0.1–0.2 mg/kg per dose, which may be increased up to 0.4 mg/kg per dose; the drug may be given every 4 hours when administered by direct IV ("bolus") injection. Such experts suggest that blood pressure be reduced by no more than 25% of the planned blood pressure reduction over the first 8 hours, with the remainder of the planned reduction over the next 12–24 hours. For pediatric patients with severe hypertension and non-life-threatening symptoms†, an oral hydralazine dose of 0.25 mg/kg per dose (up to 25 mg per dose) every 6–8 hours has been recommended.

Severe Hypertension during Pregnancy For the urgent lowering of blood pressure in severely hypertensive pregnant women, the usual initial adult IV dose of hydralazine hydrochloride is 5 mg, followed by IV doses of 5–10 mg every 20–40 minutes as necessary to achieve an adequate reduction in blood pressure; a maximum total dose of 20 mg has been recommended. Alternatively, hydralazine hydrochloride has been infused IV at a rate of 0.5–10 mg/hour for the management of severe hypertension during pregnancy. Blood pressure should be closely monitored when parenteral hydralazine is employed.

Heart Failure For the adjunctive treatment of heart failure in self-identified black patients, the recommended initial dosage of the fixed-combination preparation is 37.5 mg of hydralazine hydrochloride and 20 mg of isosorbide dinitrate (1 tablet of BiDil®) 3 times daily. The dosage may be titrated to a maximum tolerated dosage, not to exceed 2 tablets (a total of 75 mg of hydralazine hydrochloride and 40 mg of isosorbide dinitrate) 3 times daily. Although rapid titration (over 3–5 days) of dosage can be undertaken, slower titration may be needed in some patients who experience adverse effects. In patients who experience intolerable adverse effects, the dosage may be decreased to as little as one-half of the fixed-combination tablet 3 times daily; however, an attempt should be made to titrate the dosage up once the adverse effects subside.

If the drugs are administered separately in the treatment of heart failure†, an initial dosage of hydralazine hydrochloride 25–50 mg 3 or 4 times daily, given concomitantly with isosorbide dinitrate 20–30 mg 3 or 4 times daily, is recommended by the American College of Cardiology Foundation (ACCF) and American Heart Association (AHA). Dosages of the drugs should be titrated to levels similar to those recommended for the fixed-combination preparation and administered at least 3 times daily. The maximum recommended dosages are hydralazine hydrochloride 300 mg daily and isosorbide dinitrate 120 mg daily.

■ **Dosage in Renal Impairment** Patients with severe renal failure may require a lower dosage of hydralazine.

Cautions

The most frequently occurring adverse effects of hydralazine are headache, palpitation, and tachycardia; these adverse effects can be minimized by starting with small doses and increasing dosage gradually to effective levels and by concomitant administration with other antihypertensive drugs such as propranolol. Patients should be instructed to consult a clinician if headache continues with repeated dosing. Generally, adverse effects of hydralazine are reversible when dosage is reduced, but in some cases it may be necessary to discontinue the drug.

■ **GI Effects** Adverse GI disturbances such as anorexia, nausea, vomiting, and diarrhea may occur, especially with large doses. Constipation and adynamic ileus also have been reported. Cholecystitis has been reported occasionally in patients receiving fixed-combination therapy with hydralazine and isosorbide dinitrate.

■ **Cardiovascular Effects** Hydralazine-induced tachycardia may precipitate angina pectoris and ECG effects characteristic of myocardial ischemia. The drug may accentuate specific cardiovascular abnormalities and has been implicated in the production of myocardial infarction. Orthostatic hypotension and dizziness may occur rarely, but are less pronounced with hydralazine than with guanethidine or ganglionic blockers. A paradoxical pressor response, edema, and palpitations also have been reported. IV administration of hydralazine in patients with preexisting increased intracranial pressure may produce increased cerebral ischemia.

Sodium retention resulting in edema and weight gain has been reported in patients receiving hydralazine and can usually be controlled by concomitant administration with a thiazide diuretic.

In clinical trials in patients receiving hydralazine hydrochloride (37.5 mg) in fixed combination with isosorbide dinitrate (20 mg), chest pain and ventricular tachycardia have been reported.

■ **Sensitivity Reactions** Hydralazine has produced a syndrome resembling systemic lupus erythematosus (SLE) or rheumatoid arthritis, characterized by fever, arthralgia, splenomegaly, glomerulonephritis, lymphadenopathy, asthenia, myalgia, malaise, pleuritic chest pain, edema, and the presence of antinuclear antibodies (ANA) and LE cells in the blood. Rash or maculopapular facial rash characteristic of SLE also has occurred. Patients with hydralazine-induced SLE may have a positive direct Coombs' test; Coombs'-positive hemolytic anemia without SLE has occurred rarely. One case of hydralazine-induced SLE associated with pericarditis and pericardial tamponade has been reported. Hydralazine-induced SLE syndrome probably represents a hypersensitivity reaction in which hydralazine antibodies and anti-DNA antibodies are formed. The incidence of hydralazine-induced SLE syndrome is greatest in patients receiving more than 200 mg of the drug daily for prolonged periods, but cases have occurred rarely in patients receiving 100 mg daily.

Other hypersensitivity reactions including urticaria, pruritus, chills, vascular collapse, and eosinophilia have occurred rarely. Hepatitis, including granulomatous hepatitis, has been reported rarely in patients receiving hydralazine. In clinical trials in patients receiving hydralazine hydrochloride (37.5 mg) in fixed combination with isosorbide dinitrate (20 mg), angioedema has been reported occasionally.

■ **Hematologic Effects** Blood dyscrasias consisting of reduction in hemoglobin concentration and erythrocyte count, leukopenia, agranulocytosis, lymphadenopathy, thrombocytopenia with or without purpura, and splenomegaly have been reported rarely; if these abnormalities occur, hydralazine should be discontinued.

■ **Nervous System Effects** Peripheral neuritis characterized by paresthesia, numbness, and tingling has been reported rarely. These symptoms of peripheral neuritis may be caused by pyridoxine deficiency, and pyridoxine should be administered concomitantly with hydralazine if these symptoms occur. Headache, dizziness, and tremors have been reported with hydralazine.

In clinical trials in patients receiving hydralazine hydrochloride (37.5 mg) in fixed combination with isosorbide dinitrate (20 mg), somnolence, malaise, and sweating have been reported.

■ **Other Adverse Effects** Nasal congestion, flushing, lacrimation, and conjunctivitis have occurred occasionally. Muscle cramps, weakness, asthenia, dyspnea, difficulty in micturition, and tremors also have been reported. In patients with severe hypertension and uremia, rapid increase in hydralazine dosage may produce a marked decrease in blood pressure, resulting in psychotic reactions such as anxiety, disorientation or depression, and coma. Impotence has been reported very rarely.

In clinical trials in patients receiving hydralazine and hydrochloride (37.5 mg) in fixed combination with isosorbide dinitrate (20 mg), bronchitis, sinusitis, rhinitis, hyperlipidemia, hypercholesterolemia, hyperglycemia, amblyopia, myalgia, tendon disorder, and alopecia have been reported.

■ **Precautions and Contraindications** When hydralazine is used in fixed combination with isosorbide dinitrate, the cautions, precautions, and contraindications associated with nitrates (see Cautions and Precautions and Contraindications in the Nitrates and Nitrites General Statement 24:12.08) should be considered in addition to those associated with hydralazine.

Hydralazine generally is considered to be safe for use in patients with renal impairment, but the manufacturers state the drug should be used with caution in patients with severe renal impairment.

Patients who are slow acetylators of hydralazine may have a higher risk of developing drug-induced SLE than rapid acetylators; decreased renal function also increases risk. Patients receiving hydralazine should be instructed to report abnormalities such as joint or chest pain or fever to their physicians. If arthralgia, fever, chest pain, continued malaise, or other unexplained signs and symptoms occur during hydralazine therapy, appropriate laboratory studies such as complete blood counts and ANA titer determinations should be performed. Hydralazine should be discontinued in patients who develop this syndrome unless the potential benefit of antihypertensive therapy with the drug outweighs the potential risk. Signs and symptoms of hydralazine-induced SLE usually regress when the drug is discontinued, but residual effects have been detected years later; long-term treatment with corticosteroids may be necessary if symptoms do not regress.

Complete blood counts and ANA titer determinations should be performed before and periodically during prolonged hydralazine therapy, even in asymptomatic patients. The manufacturers state that a positive ANA titer requires that the implications of the test result be weighed against the benefits from therapy with the drug, but some experts state that an increase in ANA titer requires immediate discontinuance of the drug.

Some commercially available formulations of hydralazine may contain sulfites that may cause allergic-type reactions, including anaphylaxis and life-threatening or less severe asthmatic episodes, in certain susceptible individuals. The overall prevalence of sulfite sensitivity in the general population is unknown but probably low; such sensitivity appears to occur more frequently in asthmatic than in nonasthmatic individuals.

Patients who engage in potentially hazardous activities such as operating machinery or driving motor vehicles should be warned about possible faintness, dizziness, or weakness.

Hydralazine should be used with caution in patients with cerebrovascular accidents or with severe renal damage. Because of the risk of orthostatic hypotension, preparations containing hydralazine should be used with caution in patients who may be volume depleted, those with preexisting hypotension, or those receiving other hypotensive agents. In addition, patients receiving hydralazine in fixed combination with isosorbide dinitrate should be advised that inadequate fluid intake or excessive fluid loss due to diarrhea, vomiting, or perspiration may result in excessive hypotension, possibly leading to lightheadedness or even syncope. If syncope occurs, the fixed-combination therapy with hydralazine and isosorbide dinitrate should be discontinued and the patient's clinician should be notified as soon as possible. Because of the risk of developing hypotension and tachycardia, careful clinical and hemodynamic monitoring is recommended when preparations containing hydralazine are used in patients with acute myocardial infarction. Patients receiving hydralazine in fixed-dose combination with isosorbide dinitrate should be cautioned against concomitant use of phosphodiesterase type 5 (PDE type 5) inhibitors (e.g., sildenafil [Viagra®, Revatio®], tadalafil [Cialis®]), vardenafil [Levitra®]. (See: Drug Interactions: Organic Nitrates and Nitrites, in Sildenafil 24:12.12.)

Hydralazine also should be used with caution, if at all, in patients with known or suspected coronary artery disease and is contraindicated in patients with mitral valve rheumatic heart disease or hypersensitivity to the drug.

■ Pediatric Precautions Safety and efficacy of hydralazine alone or in fixed combination with isosorbide dinitrate in children have not been established. However, there is some experience with use of hydralazine in children. For information on overall principles and expert recommendations for treatment of hypertension in pediatric patients, see Uses: Hypertension in Pediatric Patients, in the Thiazides General Statement 40:28.20.

■ Geriatric Precautions Clinical studies of hydralazine in fixed combination with isosorbide dinitrate did not include sufficient numbers of patients 65 years of age and older to determine whether geriatric patients respond differently than younger patients. Although other clinical experience has not revealed age-related differences in response or tolerance, drug dosage generally should be titrated carefully in geriatric patients, usually initiating therapy at the low end of the dosage range. The greater frequency of decreased hepatic and/or renal function and of concomitant disease and drug therapy observed in the elderly also should be considered. Hydralazine may be eliminated more slowly in geriatric patients.

■ Mutagenicity and Carcinogenicity Hydralazine has been shown to be mutagenic in bacterial systems. In addition, hydralazine was positive for mutagenicity in the in vitro rat and rabbit hepatocyte DNA repair assays. However, there was no evidence of mutagenicity or clastogenicity when hydralazine was tested with additional in vivo and in vitro studies, including mouse fibroblasts and lymphoma or germinal cells, Chinese hamster bone marrow cells, and human cell line fibroblasts.

In a lifetime study in Swiss albino mice, there was a statistically significant increase in the incidence of lung tumors (adenomas and adenocarcinomas) in female and male mice receiving hydralazine hydrochloride 250 mg/kg daily (approximately 6 or 80 times the maximum recommended human dosage daily, given as hydralazine hydrochloride in fixed combination with isosorbide dinitrate [on a body surface area basis] or alone, respectively). In addition, in a 2-year carcinogenicity study in rats that used hydralazine hydrochloride oral gavage dosages of 15, 30, and 60 mg/kg daily (up to 3 or 5–20 times, the maximum recommended human dosage daily, given as hydralazine hydrochloride in fixed combination with isosorbide dinitrate [on a body surface area basis] or alone, respectively), there was a small but statistically significant increase in benign neoplastic nodules in male (high-dosage group) and female (high- and intermediate-dosage groups) rats. A statistically significant increase in benign interstitial cell tumors of the testes also was observed in the high-dosage group.

The relevance of these findings to humans currently is not fully known. The manufacturer states that although long-term clinical observation has not suggested an association between carcinogenicity in humans and administration of hydralazine, there is insufficient experience from epidemiologic studies to draw definitive conclusions.

■ Pregnancy, Fertility, and Lactation Safe use of hydralazine in pregnancy has not been established. Hydralazine is teratogenic in mice and possibly in rabbits but not in rats. Teratogenic effects in animals have included cleft palate and malformation of facial and cranial bones.

A meta-analysis of randomized, controlled trials comparing hydralazine with other antihypertensive agents for the treatment of severe hypertension during pregnancy showed that hydralazine was associated with a higher incidence of maternal hypotension, placental abruption, cesarean sections, and oliguria, as well as a higher incidence of lower Apgar scores and adverse effects on fetal heart rate than the other hypotensive drugs. In one study in 13 pregnant women with long-standing hypertension during 15 pregnancies who received combination therapy with hydralazine and propranolol, 14 live births and one unexplained stillbirth were reported. The only neonatal complications observed were 2 cases of mild hypoglycemia. In patients receiving hydralazine during pregnancy, the drug and its metabolites have been detected in maternal and umbilical plasma using a nonselective assay. The manufacturers state that although clinical experience with the drug does *not* indicate any positive evidence of adverse effect on the human fetus to date, hydralazine should not be used during pregnancy unless the possible benefits outweigh the potential risks to the fetus.

It is not known whether hydralazine is distributed into breast milk. Because many drugs are distributed into milk, the drug should be used with caution in nursing women.

Drug Interactions

■ Diuretics and Hypotensive Agents When hydralazine is administered with diuretics or other hypotensive agents, the hypotensive effect of hydralazine may be increased. This effect is usually used to therapeutic advantage, but careful adjustment of dosage is necessary when these drugs are used concomitantly. When parenteral hydralazine and parenteral diazoxide (parenteral formulation no longer commercially available in the US) are used concomitantly, profound hypotensive episodes may occur. When other potent parenteral hypotensive agents are used in combination with hydralazine, patients should be continually observed for several hours for any excessive reduction in blood pressure.

■ Other Drugs The manufacturers state that monoamine oxidase (MAO) inhibitors should be used with caution in patients receiving hydralazine, since these drugs have a synergistic effect resulting in a marked decrease in blood pressure.

Hydralazine may reduce the pressor response to epinephrine.

The fixed-combination preparation containing hydralazine should not be used concomitantly with phosphodiesterase type 5 (PDE type 5) inhibitors (e.g., sildenafil, vardenafil, tadalafil). See Drug Interactions: Organic Nitrates and Nitrites, in Sildenafil 24:12.12.

Acute Toxicity

■ Manifestations Overdosage of hydralazine may produce hypotension, tachycardia, headache, and generalized skin flushing. Myocardial ischemia and cardiac arrhythmias may develop; profound shock can occur in severe overdosage.

■ Treatment There is no specific antidote for the treatment of hydralazine overdosage. Support of the cardiovascular system is most important for the treatment of hydralazine overdosage. Evacuation of gastric contents using adequate precautions to protect the airway and prevent aspiration should be done only after cardiovascular status has been stabilized, since this procedure may precipitate cardiac arrhythmias or increase the depth of shock. Activated charcoal may be instilled if the cardiovascular system is stable. Shock should be treated with plasma volume expanders without the use of vasopressor drugs if possible. If a vasopressor drug is necessary, a drug that is least likely to precipitate or aggravate cardiac arrhythmias (e.g., methoxamine or phenylephrine) should be used. Digitalization may be necessary. Renal function should be monitored and supported if necessary. Experience with hemodialysis or peritoneal dialysis has not been reported.

Pharmacology

Hydralazine reduces peripheral resistance and blood pressure as a result of a direct vasodilatory effect on vascular smooth muscle; the effect on arterioles is greater than on veins. It has been postulated that cyclic 3′,5′-adenosine monophosphate (cyclic AMP) mediates, at least partly, the relaxation of arterial smooth muscle by the drug probably by stimulation of a calcium-binding process. Diastolic blood pressure is usually decreased more than systolic pressure. The drug decreases blood pressure in both the supine and standing positions, and there is little orthostatic hypotension.

In hypertensive patients, the hydralazine-induced decrease in blood pressure is accompanied by increased heart rate, cardiac output, and stroke volume, probably because of a reflex response to decreased peripheral resistance. The drug has no direct effect on the heart. Changes in blood pressure do not correlate well with the degree of increase in cardiac output. Increased cardiac output partially offsets the hypotensive effect of arteriolar dilation and limits the antihypertensive effectiveness of the drug. Hydralazine may increase pulmonary arterial pressure. Coronary, splanchnic, cerebral, and renal blood flows usually increase. Glomerular filtration rate, renal tubular function, and urine volume are not consistently affected by the drug. Hydralazine causes sodium and water retention and expansion of plasma volume. Tolerance to the antihypertensive effect of the drug develops during prolonged therapy, especially if a diuretic is not administered concurrently. Hydralazine usually increases plasma renin activity. Parenteral administration of the drug usually causes respiratory stimulation.

In patients with heart failure, hydralazine markedly decreases systemic vascular resistance and increases cardiac output. Systemic blood pressure, pulmonary venous pressure, and right atrial pressure are slightly decreased or unchanged in these patients; pulmonary vascular resistance may be decreased and heart rate may be slightly increased or unchanged. Increased cardiac output may be accompanied by increased renal blood flow and decreased renal vascular resistance. In patients with heart failure precipitated or exacerbated by mitral or aortic regurgitation, hydralazine may increase cardiac output and decrease regurgitant volume.

In a small number of patients with heart failure, administration of single doses of hydralazine 75 mg with isosorbide dinitrate 20 mg resulted in a substantially greater decrease in pulmonary wedge pressure compared with that observed with hydralazine alone. However, the increase in cardiac output, renal blood flow, and limb blood flow associated with the combination was similar to that observed with hydralazine alone.

In some patients with unexplained pulmonary hypertension, hydralazine may decrease systemic and pulmonary vascular resistance and increase cardiac output, resulting in improved hemodynamic status; however, in other patients with this condition, only systemic vascular resistance may be decreased, and the drug may produce hazardous hemodynamic effects (e.g., symptomatic hypotension).

Although hydralazine has little effect on nonvascular smooth muscle, animal studies indicate that the drug decreases the frequency of uterine contractions and may decrease blood flow to the uterus in toxemia of pregnancy.

Pharmacokinetics

Because assay methods used in many published pharmacokinetic studies were nonspecific and measured inactive metabolites, the accuracy of the reported values for various pharmacokinetic parameters (e.g., bioavailability) of hydralazine has been questioned.

It is not known whether impaired renal or hepatic function has an effect on the pharmacokinetics of hydralazine.

■ **Absorption** Hydralazine hydrochloride is rapidly absorbed from the GI tract and is extensively metabolized in the GI mucosa during absorption and on first pass through the liver. Following oral administration of a single 50-mg dose of ^{14}C-hydralazine to patients with hypertension, about 66% of the dose was absorbed. With fixed dosage, there are large interindividual variations in the plasma concentrations of hydralazine; however, with a given dosage, plasma concentrations generally remain constant in individual patients. Acetylation phenotype is an important determinant of the plasma concentration of hydralazine; slow acetylators have been shown to have higher plasma concentrations of the drug than rapid acetylators when the same dose of hydralazine is administered orally. A mean absolute bioavailability of 10–26% has been reported in patients with heart failure receiving a single 75-mg oral hydralazine dose; the higher bioavailability values were observed in slow acetylators.

Following oral administration of 100 mg of ^{14}C-hydralazine to healthy adults in one study, peak plasma concentrations of the drug and metabolites occurred in 2 hours and plasma concentrations of the unchanged drug ranged from 1.6–3.2 mcg/mL. When escalating doses of hydralazine (75 mg to 1 g) were administered 3 times daily in patients with congestive heart failure, up to a ninefold increase in dose-normalized area under the plasma-concentration time curve (AUC) values was observed; this nonlinear pharmacokinetic pattern is likely to be associated with saturable first-pass metabolism. After oral administration of a single dose of hydralazine, the antihypertensive effect begins in 20–30 minutes and lasts 2–4 hours. In one study, plasma hydralazine concentrations were similar after IV administration in both slow and rapid acetylator phenotype adults; the plasma concentrations of hydralazine in these patients 3 hours after IV administration of 20–25 mg of the drug ranged from 0.11–0.33 mcg/mL. Following IV administration of hydralazine, the hypotensive effect begins within 5–20 minutes, is maximum in 10–80 minutes, and lasts 2–6 hours. After IM administration of 20 mg of the drug to healthy individuals, peak plasma concentrations of 0.16–0.61 mcg/mL occur within 1 hour. The hypotensive effect begins within 10–30 minutes and lasts 2–6 hours after IM administration.

Following oral administration of a single 75-mg dose of hydralazine hydrochloride given in fixed combination with 40 mg of isosorbide dinitrate (2 tablets of BiDil®) in 19 healthy adults, peak plasma hydralazine concentrations of 88 ng/mL per 65 kg were reached in 1 hour.

Administration of hydralazine with food has been reported to result in higher plasma concentrations of the drug. The effect of food on the bioavailability of hydralazine administered in fixed combination with isosorbide dinitrate is not known.

■ **Distribution** Animal studies indicate that hydralazine is widely distributed into body tissues. In rats, highest concentrations of the drug are found in the kidneys, plasma, and liver; lower concentrations are present in the brain, lungs, muscle, heart, and fat. Radioisotope studies indicate hydralazine has a high affinity for arterial walls. A steady-state volume of distribution of 2.2 L/kg has been reported in patients with congestive heart failure receiving a 0.3-mg/kg IV hydralazine dose.

Hydralazine appears to readily cross the placenta. In patients receiving hydralazine during pregnancy, the drug and its metabolites have been detected in maternal and umbilical plasma using a nonselective assay. The drug appears to be distributed into milk; limited data suggest that milk concentrations of the drug would be clinically unimportant.

Approximately 85–87% of hydralazine in the blood is bound to plasma proteins following administration of usual doses.

■ **Elimination** The plasma half-life of hydralazine generally is 2–4 hours, but may be up to 8 hours in some patients. Plasma concentrations are increased and possibly prolonged in patients with impaired renal function. In one study, the plasma half-life was the same in both rapid and slow acetylators.

Hydralazine is metabolized extensively in the GI mucosa during absorption and in the liver by acetylation, hydroxylation, and conjugation with glucuronic acid. Four metabolites have been identified, and they apparently have no therapeutic activity. A small amount of hydralazine is reportedly converted to a hydrazone, which may be responsible for some toxic effects. Following oral administration of the drug, the main circulating metabolites of hydralazine are hydralazine pyruvate hydrazone and methyltriazolophthalazine. First-pass acetylation in the GI mucosa and liver is related to genetic acetylator phenotype. The rate of acetylation is genetically determined and varies among individuals; however, it is constant for each person. Slow acetylation is an autosomal recessive trait and results from a relative deficiency of the hepatic enzyme *N*-acetyl transferase. About 50% of American blacks and whites and the majority of American Indians, Native Alaskans, and Asians are rapid acetylators of hydralazine. The metabolism of hydralazine appears to be similar in healthy individuals and in patients with systemic lupus erythematosus (SLE); however, patients with hydralazine-induced SLE are usually slow acetylators.

Hydralazine is rapidly excreted in urine, mainly as metabolites. The major identified metabolite of hydralazine present in the urine is acetylhydrazinophthalazinone. Negligible amounts of unchanged drug are excreted in the urine. Approximately 10% of an oral dose is excreted in feces. The rate of excretion of the drug is apparently unrelated to acetylator phenotype. It is not known whether hydralazine is dialyzable.

Chemistry and Stability

■ **Chemistry** Hydralazine hydrochloride is a phthalazine-derivative antihypertensive agent. Hydralazine hydrochloride occurs as a white to off-white, crystalline powder and has solubilities of approximately 40 mg/mL in water and 2 mg/mL in alcohol at 25°C. The drug has a pK_a of 7.3. Commercially available hydralazine hydrochloride injection has a pH of 3.4–4.

■ **Stability** Commercially available preparations of hydralazine hydrochloride should be stored at a temperature less than 40°C, preferably at 15–30°C; freezing of the injection should be avoided. Hydralazine hydrochloride tablets should be stored in tight, light-resistant containers. Commercially available fixed-combination tablets of hydralazine and isosorbide dinitrate should be stored in tight, light-resistant containers at a controlled room temperature of 25°C but may be exposed to temperatures ranging from 15–30°C.

When hydralazine hydrochloride injection is diluted with most IV infusion solutions, a color change develops. Generally, color changes over a period of 8–12 hours do not indicate loss of potency when the solution is stored at 30°C or lower. Hydralazine hydrochloride injection has been reported to be physically incompatible with some drugs. Specialized references should be consulted for specific compatibility information.

Preparations

Excipients in commercially available drug preparations may have clinically important effects in some individuals; consult specific product labeling for details.

hydrALAZINE Hydrochloride

Oral		
Tablets	10 mg*	**hydrALAZINE Hydrochloride Tablets**
	25 mg*	**hydrALAZINE Hydrochloride Tablets**
	50 mg*	**hydrALAZINE Hydrochloride Tablets**
	100 mg*	**hydrALAZINE Hydrochloride Tablets**
Parenteral		
Injection	20 mg/mL*	**hydrALAZINE Hydrochloride Injection**

*available from one or more manufacturer, distributor, and/or repackager by generic (nonproprietary) name

hydrALAZINE Hydrochloride Combinations

Oral		
Tablets, film-coated	37.5 mg with Isosorbide Dinitrate 20 mg	**BiDil®** (scored), Nitro-Med

†Use is not currently included in the labeling approved by the US Food and Drug Administration

Selected Revisions April 2019,

Sodium Nitroprusside

Sodium Nitroferricyanide

■ Sodium nitroprusside is a vasodilating and hypotensive agent.

Uses

■ **Hypertensive Crises** IV sodium nitroprusside is used in hypertensive crises for immediate reduction of blood pressure in patients in whom such reduction is considered an emergency (hypertensive emergencies). The drug is consistently effective in the management of hypertensive emergencies, irrespective of etiology; however, sodium nitroprusside is contraindicated in compensatory hypertension (e.g., arteriovenous shunt or coarctation of the aorta). Because of the potential for serious toxicity (see Cautions), sodium nitroprusside should be used for treatment of hypertensive emergencies in carefully selected patients.

Hypertensive emergencies are those rare situations requiring immediate blood pressure reduction (not necessarily to normal ranges) to prevent or limit target organ damage. Such emergencies may be associated with hypertensive encephalopathy, acute myocardial infarction (MI), unstable angina pectoris, acute left ventricular failure with pulmonary edema, acute renal failure, acute ischemic stroke, eclampsia, or aortic dissection. Some experts state that the use of sodium nitroprusside is contraindicated for the treatment of eclampsia or preeclampsia. (For additional information on the use of antihypertensive drugs in women with preeclampsia, see Uses: Hypertension, Severe Hypertension during Pregnancy, in Hydralazine 24:08.20.) Patients with hypertensive emergencies require hospitalization and are treated initially with an appropriate parenteral agent. Several antihypertensive drugs from various pharmacologic classes are available for the treatment of hypertensive emergencies; because of the lack of evidence to support the use of one antihypertensive drug over another, experts state that selection of an appropriate agent should be individualized based on the underlying cause of hypertension, degree of target organ damage, desired rate of blood pressure reduction, specific drug characteristics, and patient comorbidities. Excessive falls in blood pressure should be avoided in any hypertensive crisis since they may precipitate renal, cerebral, or coronary ischemia. Hypertensive urgencies (i.e., situations in which there is severe elevation in blood pressure without acute or impending target organ damage) generally can be managed with intensification or reinstitution (e.g., following noncompliance) of the current antihypertensive regimen; there is no indication that hospitalization and immediate reduction of blood pressure is required in these situations.

Almost any desired blood pressure can be maintained by varying the rate of IV sodium nitroprusside infusion. Blood pressure reduction by sodium nitroprusside is a temporary measure. Administration of other longer-acting hypotensive agents should be started as soon as possible while the blood pressure is being controlled by sodium nitroprusside to minimize the duration of sodium nitroprusside therapy. The IV infusion should be slowed or stopped as the other medication takes effect.

■ **Congestive Heart Failure** Sodium nitroprusside is used in the management of acute decompensated (e.g., congestive) heart failure. The precipitating cause of acute heart failure decompensation should be carefully assessed to inform appropriate treatment, optimize outcomes, and prevent future acute events in patients with heart failure. Current guidelines for the management of heart failure in adults generally recommend inhibition of the renin-angiotensin-aldosterone system with a combination of drug therapies, including neurohormonal antagonists (e.g., angiotensin-converting enzyme [ACE] inhibitors, angiotensin II receptor antagonists, angiotensin receptor-neprilysin inhibitors [ARNIs], β-adrenergic blocking agents [β-blockers], aldosterone receptor antagonists), to inhibit the detrimental compensatory mechanisms in heart failure and reduce morbidity and mortality. (See Uses: Heart Failure in Carvedilol 24:24 and in Sacubitril and Valsartan 24:32.92.) IV vasodilators have not been shown to improve outcomes in patients hospitalized for heart failure; however, in the absence of symptomatic hypotension, sodium nitroprusside may be considered as an adjunct to diuretic therapy for relief of dyspnea in patients hospitalized for acutely decompensated heart failure. Administration of the drug produces rapid hemodynamic and clinical improvement by inducing arteriolar dilatation with subsequent reduction in systemic vascular resistance, thereby increasing cardiac output; by producing vasodilation and thus decreasing left ventricular filling, ventricular filling pressures are reduced. In addition, sodium nitroprusside has been reported to be particularly useful in the management of severe heart failure caused by the regurgitant valvular lesions of aortic insufficiency and mitral regurgitation. Some experts state that sodium nitroprusside may also be potentially useful in the management of heart failure in patients with severe pulmonary congestion and hypertension.

■ **Controlled Hypotension during Surgery** Sodium nitroprusside also is used to produce controlled hypotension during anesthesia in order to reduce bleeding during surgical procedures when appropriate. Use of the drug is contraindicated in patients with inadequate cerebral circulation or in patients requiring emergency surgery who are near death.

■ **Acute Myocardial Infarction** Vasodilators such as sodium nitroprusside also have been used to improve cardiac output in patients with left ventricular failure and low cardiac output after acute MI†. An inotropic agent (e.g., dobutamine) should be used initially to improve myocardial contractility and cardiac output; if blood pressure permits, afterload-reducing agents may be added to decrease cardiac work and pulmonary congestion. Use of sodium nitroprusside may be limited by coronary steal, a phenomenon whereby altered myocardial blood flow distribution causes diversion of blood away from ischemic areas. Nitroglycerin is the preferred vasodilator in patients with acute MI because of its ability to relieve ischemia by reducing left ventricular preload and increasing coronary blood flow.

Dosage and Administration

■ **Administration** Sodium nitroprusside is administered by IV infusion only using a controlled-infusion device (i.e., infusion pump); *IV infusion devices regulated only by gravity or mechanical clamps should not be used.* The rate of administration should be adjusted to maintain the desired hypotensive effect, as determined by continuous monitoring of blood pressure, using either a continually reinflated sphygmomanometer or, preferably, an intra-arterial pressure sensor. Because of the potential for toxicity, the drug should be administered for the shortest possible duration. Prolonged infusions should not exceed a rate of 3 mcg/kg per minute to prevent thiocyanate (byproduct of sodium nitroprusside metabolism) concentrations from reaching neurotoxic levels; thiocyanate concentrations should be monitored daily if this rate is exceeded.

Commercially available sodium nitroprusside injection concentrate (25 mg/mL) *must be further diluted* prior to IV infusion. The contents of one vial containing 50 mg of the drug should be diluted in 250–1000 mL of 5% dextrose injection. Vials of the drug are for single use only. Nitroprusside solutions should be protected from light by promptly wrapping the containers in the supplied opaque sleeve, aluminum foil, or other opaque material; it is not necessary to cover the infusion drip chamber or IV tubing. If properly protected from light, diluted solutions of the drug are stable for 24 hours. (See Chemistry and Stability: Stability.) Parenteral solutions of the drug should be inspected visually for particulate matter and discoloration prior to administration. The freshly prepared infusion solution has a very faint brownish tint; if it is highly colored (e.g., blue, green, red) or contains particulate matter, it should be discarded. No other drug should be added to the infusion fluid for simultaneous administration with sodium nitroprusside.

■ **Dosage** ***Hypertensive Crises or Controlled Hypotension during Surgery*** In adults and pediatric patients receiving sodium nitroprusside for hypertensive crises or for controlled hypotension during surgery, the manufacturer states that the average effective IV dosage is about 3 mcg/kg per minute, with a range of 0.5–10 mcg/kg per minute; however, some patients will experience profound hypotension when receiving the drug at this rate. Therefore, the infusion should be started at a very low rate (e.g., 0.3 mcg/kg per minute) and gradually titrated upward every few minutes until adequate blood pressure control is achieved or the maximum recommended infusion rate of 10 mcg/kg per minute has been reached. Some experts state that for management of severe hypertension with life-threatening symptoms in children and adolescents, an initial infusion rate of 0–3 mcg/kg per minute should be used. These experts suggest that blood pressure be reduced by no more than 25% of the planned reduction over the first 8 hours, with the remainder of the planned reduction over the next 12–24 hours. For the management of a hypertensive emergency in adults, some experts recommend an initial dosage of 0.3–0.5 mcg/kg per minute, with increases in increments of 0.5 mcg/kg per minute, up to a maximum rate of 10 mcg/kg per minute, to achieve desired blood pressure control. The infusion duration should be as short as possible; if an adequate reduction in blood pressure is not obtained within 10 minutes at this maximum infusion rate, the infusion should be immediately discontinued. Because of the rapidity of sodium nitroprusside's hypotensive onset and dissipation of effect, small changes in infusion rate can lead to large, undesirable fluctuations in blood pressure. The manufacturer states that prior to increasing dosage, the drug's effects should be confirmed by measuring blood pressure 5 minutes after any change in infusion rate to achieve the desired blood pressure response.

Diastolic blood pressure usually is decreased and maintained about 30–40% below pretreatment levels with sodium nitroprusside dosages of 3 mcg/kg per minute. Smaller dosages of sodium nitroprusside are adequate in patients receiving other hypotensive agents and in geriatric patients.

In adults who have a hypertensive emergency *with* a compelling indication (i.e., aortic dissection, pheochromocytoma crisis), some experts recommend that systolic blood pressure be reduced to less than 140 mm Hg during the first hour and, in patients with acute aortic dissection, to less than 120 mm Hg within the first 20 minutes. In adults who have a hypertensive emergency *without* a compelling indication, systolic blood pressure should be reduced by no more than 25% over the first hour, followed by further blood pressure reduction *if stable* to 160/110 or 160/100 mm Hg within the next 2–6 hours; excessive declines in pressure that could precipitate renal, cerebral, or coronary ischemia should be avoided. If this blood pressure is well tolerated and the patient is clinically stable, further gradual reductions toward normal can be implemented in the next 24–48 hours.

Longer-acting hypotensive agents should be administered concomitantly with sodium nitroprusside to minimize the duration of sodium nitroprusside therapy.

Congestive Heart Failure When sodium nitroprusside is used in adults and pediatric patients with acute congestive heart failure, the manufacturer recommends that the infusion be initiated at a rate of 0.3 mcg/kg per minute. Dosage should be gradually titrated upward every few minutes until the desired effect is achieved or the maximum recommended infusion rate of 10 mcg/kg per minute has been reached. The manufacturer states that the average effective dosage is about 3 mcg/kg (range: 0.5–10 mcg/kg) per minute. Adjustment of the infusion rate must be guided by the results of invasive hemodynamic monitoring and monitoring of urine output. Titration of sodium nitroprusside dosage can be accomplished by increasing the infusion rate until cardiac output is no longer increasing, systemic blood pressure cannot be further reduced without compromising vital organ perfusion, or the maximum recommended infusion rate is reached, whichever occurs first. While specific hemodynamic goals must be tailored to the clinical situation, improvements in cardiac output and left ventricular filling pressure must not be achieved at the expense of undue hypotension and consequent hypoperfusion.

Cautions

The most clinically important adverse effects of sodium nitroprusside are profound hypotension and cyanide toxicity. Other adverse effects are less common and develop less rapidly.

■ **Hypotension** Sodium nitroprusside can produce precipitous decreases in blood pressure and profound hypotension when administered at transient, slightly excessive infusion rates; the subsequent hemodynamic changes can result in a variety of associated symptoms, or blood pressure may decrease to the point where perfusion of vital organs may be compromised. The hypotensive effect of the drug occurs rapidly and the possible sequelae of hypotension (e.g., irreversible ischemic injury, death) are serious. (See Cautions: Precautions and Contraindications.)

■ **Cyanogenic Effects** ***Manifestations*** Sodium nitroprusside infusions at rates exceeding 2 mcg/kg per minute generate cyanogen (cyanide radical) in amounts greater than can be effectively buffered by the methemoglobin normally present in the body; cyanide toxicity can result when this buffering system is exhausted. The capacity of this system is exceeded when more than 500 mcg/kg of sodium nitroprusside is given; this amount is produced in less than 1 hour when the drug is administered at a rate of 10 mcg/kg per minute. Most cases of cyanide toxicity have occurred when sodium nitroprusside is used for prolonged periods or at high dosages; however, elevated cyanide levels, metabolic acidosis, and marked clinical deterioration have been reported occasionally in patients receiving the drug at recommended rates of infusion for only a few hours, and in one case, for only 35 minutes. Infusions of sodium nitroprusside at the maximum recommended rate of 10 mcg/kg per minute should never last longer than 10 minutes; if blood pressure is not adequately controlled after 10 minutes, the infusion should be discontinued immediately.

The toxic effects of cyanide may be rapid, serious, and possibly fatal and may manifest as venous hyperoxemia (secondary to the inability of tissues to extract oxygen from erythrocytes, with resultant bright red venous blood), lactic acidosis, air hunger, confusion, and death. While acid-base balance and venous oxygen concentrations should be monitored and may indicate cyanide toxicity, these tests alone should not be relied upon to guide therapy. Cyanide toxicity resulting from causes other than sodium nitroprusside has been associated with angina and myocardial infarction, ataxia, seizures, stroke, and other diffuse ischemic damage.

Treatment Sodium thiosulfate has been administered concomitantly with sodium nitroprusside at infusion rates 5–10 times that of the sodium nitroprusside infusion to accelerate the metabolism of cyanide; however, coadministration of these agents has not been extensively researched and further study is necessary. Caution must be exercised to avoid prolonged or excessive dosages of sodium nitroprusside with sodium thiosulfate, since thiocyanate toxicity and/or hypovolemia may result. The same precautions and contraindications apply to this method of administration as to the administration of sodium nitroprusside alone.

■ **Methemoglobinemia** Infusions of sodium nitroprusside can result in the sequestration of hemoglobin as methemoglobin; cyanide combines with methemoglobin to form cyanmethemoglobin. Although the conversion of methemoglobin back to hemoglobin is normally rapid, clinically important methemoglobinemia (greater than 10%) rarely may occur. Even patients who are congenitally incapable of converting methemoglobin back to hemoglobin should demonstrate 10% methemoglobinemia only following a total sodium nitroprusside dose of 10 mg/kg (i.e., infusion at the maximum recommended rate of 10 mcg/kg per minute for greater than 16 hours). Methemoglobinemia should be suspected in patients who have received greater than 10 mg/kg of sodium nitroprusside and who exhibit signs of impaired oxygen delivery despite adequate cardiac output and arterial PaO_2.

■ **Thiocyanate Accumulation** Thiocyanate may accumulate in the blood of patients receiving sodium nitroprusside therapy, especially in those with impaired renal function, or in patients receiving prolonged infusions of sodium nitroprusside at infusion rates exceeding 3 mcg/kg per minute or receiving sodium thiosulfate concomitantly with sodium nitroprusside to accelerate the metabolism of cyanide. (See Cautions: Precautions and Contraindications, and Chronic Toxicity.) Thiocyanate is mildly neurotoxic (e.g., tinnitus, miosis, hyperreflexia) at serum concentrations of 60 mcg/mL and may be life-threatening at concentrations of 200 mcg/mL. (See Cautions: Precautions and Contraindications

Since thiocyanate inhibits both uptake and binding of iodine, symptoms of hypothyroidism may occur. Thiocyanate retention and hypothyroidism have been reported in one patient with severe hypertension and uremia who had received 3.9 g of sodium nitroprusside IV over a period of 21 days. Elevated plasma thiocyanate concentrations and signs of hypothyroidism diminished after peritoneal dialysis.

■ **Other Metabolic Effects** Cyanogen (cyanide radical) as well as thiocyanate may interfere with vitamin B_{12} distribution and metabolism. A fall in total plasma cobalamins has been reported during administration of sodium nitroprusside; however, a rise in plasma cyanocobalamin has been noted in patients receiving the drug for prolonged periods.

■ **Renal Effects** Increases in serum creatinine concentrations, which returned to normal after the infusion was stopped, have also occurred during sodium nitroprusside use.

■ **Other Adverse Effects** Other adverse effects resulting from IV administration of sodium nitroprusside are uncommon and are usually associated with a too-rapid reduction in blood pressure. Nausea, retching, diaphoresis, apprehension, headache, restlessness, muscle twitching, retrosternal discomfort, palpitation, dizziness, and abdominal pain or cramps have been reported during use of the drug. These symptoms may be relieved by slowing the rate of infusion or temporarily discontinuing the drug, or minimized by keeping the patient supine. In addition, bradycardia, tachycardia, ECG changes, rash, decreased platelet aggregation, ileus, increased intracranial pressure, flushing, venous streaking, and irritation at the site of injection have been reported.

■ **Precautions and Contraindications** Sodium nitroprusside injection concentrate is *not* suitable for direct injection; the drug *must* be further diluted in 5% dextrose injection before IV infusion. (See Dosage and Administration: Administration.)

Because sodium nitroprusside can produce precipitous decreases in blood pressure, the drug should be administered only when adequate facilities, equipment, and personnel are available for close monitoring of blood pressure. Hypotension generally is self-limiting within 1–10 minutes following the discontinuance of the infusion; during this time, patients may benefit from being placed in Trendelenburg's position to maximize venous return. If blood pressure does not normalize within a few minutes, sodium nitroprusside may not be the principal cause of the hypotension and another cause should be sought.

Except when used for short periods of time or at low infusion rates (e.g., 2 mcg/kg per minute or slower), therapy with sodium nitroprusside can result in the production of clinically important levels of cyanide, which can reach toxic or potentially lethal concentrations. If excessive dosages of sodium nitroprusside are used and/or sulfur (usually thiosulfate) stores become depleted, cyanogen toxicity may occur. (See Cautions: Cyanogenic Effects and see Chronic Toxicity.) Sodium nitroprusside infusions at the maximum recommended infusion rate of 10 mcg/kg per minute should never last longer than 10 minutes; if after 10 minutes the blood pressure has not been adequately controlled, the infusion should be immediately discontinued.

Sodium nitroprusside should be used with caution in patients with hepatic insufficiency, hypothyroidism, or hyponatremia. Thiocyanate may accumulate in patients with renal impairment or in patients receiving prolonged infusions of sodium nitroprusside at rates exceeding 3 mcg/kg per minute. To maintain the steady-state concentration of thiocyanate below 60 mcg/mL (the level at which mild neurotoxic effects have been observed), infusion rates of sodium nitroprusside should be maintained below 3 mcg/kg per minute in patients with normal renal function or 1 mcg/kg per minute in anuric patients. When prolonged infusions are more rapid than these, serum thiocyanate concentrations should be monitored daily. Some clinicians recommend that plasma cyanogen concentrations be monitored daily after 1 or 2 days in patients with impaired hepatic function. Peritoneal dialysis or hemodialysis may be required to remove excess thiocyanate and relieve the symptoms. (See Chronic Toxicity: Treatment.)

Because sodium nitroprusside may interfere with vitamin B_{12} distribution and metabolism, the drug should be used with caution in patients with low plasma vitamin B_{12} concentrations. Because hydroxocobalamin is an antidote for cyanogen (combining to form cyanocobalamin), its use may be advisable before and during sodium nitroprusside administration in these patients.

Frequent monitoring of acid-base balance is necessary in all patients, particularly if tolerance to the pharmacologic effects of sodium nitroprusside develops during therapy (manifested as the need for higher infusion rates to control blood pressure), since metabolic acidosis is one of the earliest and most reliable signs of cyanogen toxicity; however, laboratory tests alone should not be relied upon to guide therapy since acidosis may not be evident until more than 1 hour after the development of toxic cyanogen concentrations. If signs of metabolic acidosis or increased tolerance to the hypotensive effect of the drug occurs during sodium nitroprusside therapy, the drug should be discontinued and alternative treatment should be administered.

In patients with symptomatic methemoglobinemia (i.e., 10% or greater), 1–2 mg/kg of methylene blue should be administered IV slowly over several minutes. However, treatment of methemoglobinemia should be undertaken with extreme caution in patients who are likely to have substantial amounts of cyanide bound to methemoglobin as cyanmethemoglobin.

Young, healthy males may require higher than recommended dosages of sodium nitroprusside for hypotensive anesthetic procedures; however, the maximum infusion rate of 10 mcg/kg per minute should not be exceeded. (See Dosage and Administration: Dosage.) Deepening of anesthesia in these patients may produce adequate hypotension with administration of sodium nitroprusside in the recommended dosage range.

Sodium nitroprusside, like other vasodilating agents, can produce increases in intracranial pressure; therefore, the drug should be used only with extreme caution in patients with preexisting increased intracranial pressure.

When IV sodium nitroprusside is used for controlled hypotension during anesthesia, tolerance to loss of blood, anemia, and hypovolemia may be decreased. If possible, preexisting anemia and hypovolemia should be corrected prior to use of the drug. Hypotensive anesthetic techniques also may affect pulmonary ventilation perfusion ratio. In patients who cannot tolerate additional dead air space at normal oxygen partial pressure, higher oxygen partial pressure may be beneficial. Sodium nitroprusside IV infusion should be used with extreme caution in patients who are especially poor surgical risks.

The use of sodium nitroprusside to produce controlled hypotension during surgery is contraindicated in patients with inadequate cerebral circulation and is not intended for use during emergency surgery in patients near death. Sodium nitroprusside should not be used in the treatment of compensatory hypertension (e.g., arteriovenous shunt or coarctation of the aorta). Use of the drug also should be avoided in patients with congenital (Leber's) optic atrophy or tobacco amblyopia; these conditions, although rare, are associated with absent or deficient thiosulfate sulfurtransferase (rhodanase), and these patients have unusually high cyanogen to thiocyanate ratios. The manufacturer states that sodium nitroprusside should not be used in patients with acute heart failure associated with reduced peripheral vascular resistance, such as high-output heart failure that may accompany endotoxic sepsis. Concomitant use of sodium nitroprusside and phosphodiesterase (PDE) type 5 inhibitors (e.g., sildenafil) or soluble guanylate cyclase stimulators (e.g., riociguat) is contraindicated because of the potential for additive hypotensive effects.

■ **Pediatric Precautions** Sodium nitroprusside has been used to induce hypotension in a limited number of patients younger than 17 years of age; at least 50% of such patients were prepubertal, and about 50% of prepubertal patients were younger than 2 years of age, including 4 neonates. Efficacy of the drug in pediatric patients has been established in a parallel, dose-ranging study and a long-term infusion study in which sodium nitroprusside dosage was titrated according to blood pressure; the primary efficacy variable in these studies was mean arterial pressure (MAP). Both studies demonstrated the blood pressure-lowering effect of sodium nitroprusside. In the latter study, sodium nitroprusside reduced MAP below that of placebo control for at least 12 hours. Similar effects on MAP were observed in all age groups in these studies, and no novel safety issues were noted.

■ **Carcinogenicity** It is not known whether sodium nitroprusside is carcinogenic in animals or humans.

■ **Pregnancy, Fertility, and Lactation** Animal reproduction studies have not been performed with sodium nitroprusside. It is also not known whether the drug can cause fetal harm when administered to pregnant women. The manufacturer states that sodium nitroprusside should be used during pregnancy only when clearly needed; some experts state that the drug is contraindicated in women with preeclampsia or eclampsia.

The effects of sodium thiosulfate administration during pregnancy, either alone or in conjunction with sodium nitroprusside, are unknown.

It is not known whether sodium nitroprusside affects fertility in humans.

It is not known if sodium nitroprusside and its metabolites are distributed into human milk. Because many drugs are distributed into milk and because of the potential for serious adverse effects in nursing infants, a decision should be made whether to discontinue nursing or the drug, taking into account the importance of the drug to the woman.

Drug Interactions

■ **Hypotensive Agents** The hypotensive effects of sodium nitroprusside are additive when used concomitantly with ganglionic blocking agents, negative inotropic agents, general anesthetics (e.g., enflurane), and most other circulatory depressants.

■ **Phosphodiesterase Inhibitors** Additive hypotensive effects can occur if sodium nitroprusside is used concomitantly with phosphodiesterase (PDE) type 5 inhibitors (e.g., sildenafil). Concomitant use of these drugs is contraindicated.

■ **Soluble Guanylate Cyclase Stimulators** Additive hypotensive effects can occur if sodium nitroprusside is used concomitantly with soluble guanylate cyclase stimulators (e.g., riociguat). Concomitant use of these drugs is contraindicated.

Chronic Toxicity

■ **Pathogenesis** Following IV administration, sodium nitroprusside is rapidly metabolized to cyanogen (cyanide radical) and subsequently converted to thiocyanate by the enzyme rhodanase. The rate of conversion from cyanogen to thiocyanate depends on the availability of sulfur, usually thiosulfate; however, cyanide toxicity can occur if excessive dosages of sodium nitroprusside are used and/or sulfur stores become depleted.

The toxicity of sodium nitroprusside has been attributed to cyanogen; however, the role of cyanogen in sodium nitroprusside poisoning has been questioned and it has been postulated that some toxic effects may be caused by profound hypotension.

■ **Manifestations** The first signs of overdosage with sodium nitroprusside are those related to severe hypotension. Increasing tolerance to the hypotensive effects of the drug and metabolic acidosis are also early indications of overdosage with sodium nitroprusside and may be associated with or followed by dyspnea, headache, vomiting, dizziness, ataxia, or loss of consciousness. Frequent monitoring of acid-base balance is necessary in all patients receiving sodium nitroprusside, particularly in patients who develop tolerance to the drug's pharmacologic effects, since metabolic acidosis is the most reliable sign of cyanogen toxicity; however, laboratory tests alone should not be relied upon to guide therapy since acidosis may not be evident until more than 1 hour after the development of toxic cyanogen concentrations. Reasonable suspicion of cyanogen toxicity is adequate basis for initiation of treatment. If signs of metabolic acidosis or tolerance to the hypotensive effect of the drug occurs during sodium nitroprusside therapy, the drug should be discontinued and alternative treatment should be administered. Signs or symptoms of cyanogen toxicity may include coma, imperceptible pulse, absent reflexes, dilated pupils, pink coloration of the skin, distant heart sounds, or shallow breathing.

Deaths clearly caused by sodium nitroprusside are limited to cases in which large oral doses were taken in suicides. Autopsy showed all organs to be congested and some evidence of cyanogen poisoning was observed.

■ **Treatment** In the event of overdosage with sodium nitroprusside, nitrites should be administered to induce methemoglobin formation. Oxygen administration alone will not provide relief. Methemoglobin combines with cyanogen bound to cytochrome-c oxidase to yield cytochrome-c oxidase and cyanmethemoglobin, a nontoxic complex. Cyanogen gradually dissociates from cyanmethemoglobin and is converted to sodium thiocyanate by administration of thiosulfate in the presence of thiosulfate sulfurtransferase (rhodanase).

When overdosage with sodium nitroprusside occurs with signs of cyanogen toxicity, sodium nitroprusside should be discontinued; amyl nitrite inhalations may be administered until IV access can be established for sodium nitrite administration. A 3% sodium nitrite solution should then be administered IV at a dosage of 4–6 mg/kg (approximately 0.2 mL/kg of the 3% solution) injected over 2–4 minutes. This dose can be expected to convert about 10% of the patient's hemoglobin to methemoglobin; however, this degree of methemoglobinemia alone is not associated with any important hazard. Blood pressure should be carefully monitored during sodium nitrite administration since vasodilation and hypotension may occur; hypotension should be managed routinely. Following these steps, a 10 or 25% solution of sodium thiosulfate is administered IV in a dose of 150–200 mg/kg; a typical adult dose is 50 mL of the 25% solution. Injections of sodium nitrite and sodium thiosulfate may be repeated at one-half the initial recommended doses after 2 hours.

Thiosulfate treatment of acute cyanide toxicity will increase the serum concentration of thiocyanate; however, the increase should not pose any risk to the patient. Physiologic methods (e.g., altering urinary pH) have not been demonstrated to increase the elimination of thiocyanate. Although hemodialysis is ineffective for the removal of cyanide from circulation, most thiocyanate will be removed by this procedure; the clearance rate of thiocyanate can approach the blood flow rate of the dialyzer.

Pharmacology

Sodium nitroprusside is a potent direct arterial and venous dilator. When sodium nitroprusside is administered by IV infusion to hypertensive or normotensive patients, a marked lowering of arterial blood pressure is produced. Venous pressure is also lowered and a moderate reduction in total peripheral resistance occurs. The effects of the drug on blood pressure are more pronounced in hypertensive than in normotensive patients.

The hypotensive action of sodium nitroprusside results from peripheral vasodilation caused by a direct action on vascular smooth muscle. Animal tests performed *in situ* have demonstrated no relaxation of other smooth muscle tissue, such as the uterus or duodenum, by sodium nitroprusside. The drug has no direct effect on vasomotor centers, sympathetic nerves, or adrenergic receptors. The hypotensive effect of sodium nitroprusside is augmented by concomitant use of other hypotensive agents and is not blocked by adrenergic blocking agents or vagotomy. Pressor agents such as epinephrine which stimulate the myocardium directly are the only drugs that cause an increase in blood pressure during sodium nitroprusside therapy. Resistance to the drug's hypotensive effects is very rare.

The effects of sodium nitroprusside on cardiac performance appear to depend on preexisting performance. Changes in cardiac performance are attributed mainly to a reduction in left ventricular afterload resulting from vasodilation but may also be related to reduction in venous return to the heart resulting from peripheral vascular pooling of blood, decreased arteriolar resistance, and increased diastolic compliance. The drug may exert a direct coronary vasodilator effect. When sodium nitroprusside is administered to hypertensive patients, a slight increase in heart rate usually occurs and cardiac output is usually decreased slightly. Decreases in cardiac index and stroke index are common; however, these decreases do not occur consistently and increases have occurred in some patients. When sodium nitroprusside is administered to patients with refractory heart failure and/or acute myocardial infarction, substantial improvement in left ventricular performance results with cardiac output, cardiac index, and stroke volume being increased and left ventricular filling pressure being decreased. In patients with congestive heart failure, a slight but clinically important slowing of the heart rate results, as well as reduction or cessation of arrhythmias. A reduction in myocardial oxygen consumption during sodium nitroprusside use has been noted which could prove beneficial when infarcted areas of the heart are already short of oxygen. In patients with congestive heart failure, improvement in cardiac performance is accompanied by prompt diuresis, with urine volume and sodium excretion both being increased.

Moderate doses of sodium nitroprusside in hypertensive patients produce renal vasodilation without an appreciable increase in renal blood flow or a decrease in glomerular filtration. Mean renal arterial pressure and renal vascular resistance are slightly decreased. The acute reduction in mean arterial pressure is accompanied by an increase in renin activity of renal venous plasma.

Pharmacokinetics

■ **Absorption** IV infusion of sodium nitroprusside produces an almost immediate reduction in blood pressure. Blood pressure begins to rise immediately when the infusion is slowed or stopped and returns to pretreatment levels within 1–10 minutes.

■ **Distribution** Distribution of nitroprusside in the body as well as passage across the placenta, into milk, or across the blood-brain barrier has not been studied.

■ **Elimination** Sodium nitroprusside is rapidly metabolized, probably by interaction with sulfhydryl groups in the erythrocytes and tissues. Cyanogen (cyanide radical) is produced which is converted to thiocyanate in the liver by the enzyme thiosulfate sulfurtransferase (rhodanase). This mitochondrial enzyme normally is present in excess quantities such that the rate-limiting step in the conversion of cyanogen to thiocyanate usually is the availability of sulfur donors (e.g., thiosulfate, cystine, cysteine). A thiocyanate oxidase present in the erythrocytes may oxidize small quantities of thiocyanate back to cyanogen. Toxic symptoms begin to appear at plasma thiocyanate concentrations of 50–100 mcg/mL; fatalities have been reported at concentrations of 200 mcg/mL.

Sodium nitroprusside is excreted entirely as metabolites, principally thiocyanate. In animals, sodium nitroprusside metabolites are excreted mainly in urine, exhaled air, and probably in feces. The elimination half-life of thiocyanate is 2.7–7 days when renal function is normal but is longer in patients with impaired renal function or hyponatremia.

Chemistry and Stability

■ **Chemistry** Sodium nitroprusside is a hypotensive agent which is structurally unrelated to other available hypotensive agents. Sodium nitroprusside is commercially available as the dihydrate, and potency is expressed in terms of the hydrated drug. The drug occurs as reddish-brown, practically odorless, crystals or powder and is freely soluble in water and slightly soluble in alcohol.

■ **Stability** Sodium nitroprusside is sensitive to, and must be protected from, light, heat, and moisture. Sodium nitroprusside injection concentrate should be protected from light and stored at 20–25°C.

Exposure of sodium nitroprusside solutions to light causes deterioration which may be evidenced by a change from a brown to a blue color caused by reduction of the ferric ion to the ferrous ion. It has been reported that approximately 20% of sodium nitroprusside in solution in glass bottles undergoes degradation within 4 hours when exposed to fluorescent light. Solutions in Viaflex® bags exposed to fluorescent light are degraded even more rapidly. Specialized references should be consulted for specific stability information. Sodium nitroprusside solutions should be protected from light by wrapping the container with aluminum foil or other opaque material. If properly protected from light, diluted solutions of the drug are stable for 24 hours. Sodium nitroprusside solution is rapidly degraded by trace contaminants often forming highly colored products, usually blue, green, or red. If this occurs, the solution should be discarded. No other drug or preservative should be added to sodium nitroprusside infusions.

Preparations

Excipients in commercially available drug preparations may have clinically important effects in some individuals; consult specific product labeling for details.

Sodium Nitroprusside

Parenteral		
Injection concentrate, for IV infusion only	25 mg/mL*	**Nitropress®**, Hospira
		Sodium Nitroprusside Injection

*available from one or more manufacturer, distributor, and/or repackager by generic (nonproprietary) name

†Use is not currently included in the labeling approved by the US Food and Drug Administration

VASODILATING AGENTS 24:12

NITRATES AND NITRITES 24:12.08

Nitrates and Nitrites General Statement

■ Organic nitrates and nitrites are vasodilating agents.

Uses

■ **Chronic Stable Angina** Nitrates and nitrites are used for the acute symptomatic relief of angina pectoris secondary to coronary artery disease, for prophylactic management in situations likely to provoke angina attacks, and for long-term prophylactic management of chronic stable angina.

Conventional measures in the management of angina pectoris are aimed at reducing the frequency, duration, and severity of attacks, and include coronary risk reduction (e.g., discontinuance of smoking, weight control, antilipemic strategies) rest, avoidance of precipitating circumstances (e.g., eating heavy meals, getting emotionally upset, performing strenuous exercise, exposure to cold air) and, if possible, treatment of the underlying cause.

Since nitrites and individual nitrates have similar pharmacologic and therapeutic properties, the choice of a preparation depends mainly on the onset and duration of action required. Short-acting nitroglycerin preparations (e.g., sublingual nitroglycerin tablets or nitroglycerin spray) generally are used for the immediate relief of acute angina attacks, but also may be used prophylactically prior to anticipated angina provoked by physical or emotional stress. Sublingual nitroglycerin is considered the drug of choice for the acute relief of an attack of angina because it has a rapid onset of action, is inexpensive, and its efficacy is well established. Lingual nitroglycerin and other rapidly acting nitrates or nitrites (e.g., amyl nitrite inhalation) also may be useful. However, amyl nitrite is seldom, if ever, used for angina pectoris because it is expensive, inconvenient, has a high incidence of adverse effects (e.g., headache, orthostatic symptoms, tachycardia), and has an unpleasant odor.

β-Adrenergic blocking agents (β-blockers) generally are considered the initial antianginal drugs of choice for the long-term prophylactic management of chronic stable angina because of their proven benefits in reducing ischemic burden and threshold and in improving survival in patients with left ventricular dysfunction or prior myocardial infarction (MI). However, long-acting nitrates (i.e., oral preparations of isosorbide dinitrate or mononitrate and oral or topical nitroglycerin) also are effective antianginal agents and are recommended as second-line therapy in patients who do not tolerate or respond adequately to β-blocker therapy. Experts state that long-acting nitrate preparations may be considered for the prophylactic management of angina pectoris when β-blockers are contraindicated or associated with unacceptable adverse effects. Alternatively, long-acting nitrates may be added to β-blocker therapy if initial therapy with a β-blocker is not effective. Prolonged use of nitrates has been associated with the development of tolerance to the hemodynamic and antianginal effects of the drugs; therefore, a daily nitrate-free interval is recommended. (See Cautions: Tolerance and Dependence.) Physiologic changes (e.g., endothelial dysfunction from accumulation of oxygen free radicals) have occurred in patients receiving long-term nitrate therapy which may offset the short-term ischemic benefits of these drugs; however, further study is needed.

Nitrates and nitrites have been used effectively with β-blockers; since these drugs act by different mechanisms of action, greater antianginal and anti-ischemic effects may be achieved when these drugs are used in combination than when either is used alone, and each agent may counteract some of the undesirable cardiac effects of the other. Calcium-channel blocking agents and nitrates act by different mechanisms, and clinical experience suggests a beneficial antianginal and anti-ischemic interaction in patients with angina. Although concomitant therapy with a nitrate, calcium-channel blocking agent, and β-blocker may be beneficial in some patients, the safety and/or efficacy of such therapy have not been fully determined.

■ **Non-ST-Segment-Elevation Acute Coronary Syndromes** Nitrates are used in the management of non-ST-segment-elevation acute coronary syndromes (NSTE ACS). Patients with NSTE ACS have either unstable angina or non-ST-segment-elevation MI (NSTEMI); because these conditions are part of a continuum of acute myocardial ischemia and have indistinguishable clinical features upon presentation, the same initial treatment strategies are recommended. The American Heart Association/American College of Cardiology (AHA/ACC) guideline for the management of NSTE ACS recommends an early invasive strategy (angiographic evaluation with the intent to perform revascularization procedures such as percutaneous coronary intervention [PCI] with coronary artery stent implantation or coronary artery bypass grafting [CABG]) or an ischemia-guided strategy (initial medical management followed by catheterization and revascularization if indicated) in patients with definite or likely NSTE ACS; standard medical therapies for all patients should include a β-blocker, antiplatelet agents, anticoagulant agents, nitrates (e.g., nitroglycerin), and analgesic agents regardless of the initial management approach.

Sublingual nitroglycerin (0.3–0.4 mg every 5 minutes for up to 3 doses) is recommended in patients with NSTE ACS who have continuing ischemic pain; IV nitroglycerin may be used in patients with heart failure, hypertension, or persistent ischemia that is not relieved with sublingual nitroglycerin and administration of a β-blocker. Since prolonged use of nitrates has been associated with the development of tolerance to the hemodynamic and antianginal effects of the drugs, an intermittent dosage schedule may be required to maintain efficacy. (See Cautions: Tolerance and Dependence.) AHA and ACC state that topical or oral nitrates may be an acceptable alternative to IV therapy in patients who do not have refractory or recurrent ischemia. The use of nitrates in patients with NSTE ACS is principally based on extensive clinical experience, experimental studies, and the pathophysiologic effects of the drugs rather than from randomized controlled studies.

■ **Acute Myocardial Infarction** Nitroglycerin is used in the management of acute MI. The term MI is used when there is evidence of myocardial necrosis in the setting of acute myocardial ischemia. ST-segment-elevation MI (STEMI) is distinguished from NSTEMI based on the presence or absence of ST-segment elevation on ECG. Patients with STEMI typically have complete arterial occlusion; therefore, immediate reperfusion therapy (with primary PCI or thrombolytic agents) is the current standard of care for such patients. Because the clinical presentation of NSTEMI is similar to that of unstable angina, these conditions are considered together in current expert guidelines. (See Uses: Non-ST-Segment-Elevation Acute Coronary Syndromes.)

Sublingual nitroglycerin has been administered for the initial relief of ischemic discomfort in patients with acute MI. However, the manufacturer states that the benefits of sublingual nitroglycerin in patients with acute MI have not been established; if the drug is used in this setting, careful hemodynamic and clinical monitoring are essential because of the possibility of hypotension and tachycardia. IV nitroglycerin may be used in patients with acute MI who have ongoing chest pain, hypertension, or heart failure. Because of its onset of action, ease of titration, and opportunity for prompt termination if adverse effects occur, IV administration of the drug is preferred during the early stage of acute MI. In the years prior to the introduction and acceptance of reperfusion therapy, IV nitroglycerin was one of the principal initial therapies for reducing mortality and major cardiovascular mortality in patients with acute MI. In addition to potentially alleviating ischemic myocardial pain, beneficial hemodynamic effects of nitroglycerin include vasodilation of the coronary arteries (especially at or near the site of recent plaque disruption), peripheral arteries, and venous capacitance vessels. However, nitroglycerin generally does not reduce myocardial injury associated with epicardial coronary artery occlusion unless there is substantial vasospasm. Although studies conducted prior to the routine use of reperfusion therapy suggested a mortality benefit with nitrates in patients with acute MI, this benefit was not confirmed in 2 large randomized controlled studies. In addition, systemic hypotension with resultant worsening of myocardial ischemia is a potential complication of nitroglycerin therapy. Therefore, patients with preexisting hypotension or at risk of hypotension should not receive nitrates. Nitrates also should be avoided in patients with marked bradycardia (e.g., less than 50 bpm) or tachycardia (e.g., exceeding 100 bpm), and those with suspected right ventricular infarction. (See Cautions: Precautions and Contraindications.)

The American College of Cardiology Foundation/American Heart Association (ACCF/AHA) guideline for the management of STEMI states that IV nitroglycerin may be beneficial in patients with STEMI and heart failure or hypertension. When the drug is used in this setting, patients must be carefully monitored for hypotension. The benefits of oral nitroglycerin have not been established in patients with acute MI, and experts state there is no role for the routine use of oral nitroglycerin during the convalescent phase of STEMI.

■ **Heart Failure and Low-output Syndromes** ***Isosorbide Dinitrate and Hydralazine*** Isosorbide dinitrate is used in fixed combination with hydralazine (BiDil®) as an adjunct to standard therapy for the treatment of heart failure in self-identified black patients to improve survival, decrease rate of hospitalization for worsened heart failure, and improve patient-reported functional status. Current guidelines for the management of heart failure in adults generally recommend a combination of drug therapies to reduce morbidity and mortality, including neurohormonal antagonists (e.g., angiotensin-converting enzyme [ACE] inhibitors, angiotensin II receptor antagonists, angiotensin receptor-neprilysin inhibitors [ARNIs], β-blockers, aldosterone receptor antagonists) that inhibit the detrimental compensatory mechanisms in heart failure. Additional agents (e.g., cardiac glycosides, diuretics, sinoatrial modulators [i.e., ivabradine]) added to a heart failure treatment regimen in selected patients have been associated with symptomatic improvement and/or reduction in heart failure-related hospitalizations. The combination of isosorbide dinitrate and hydralazine is recommended by the American College of Cardiology Foundation (ACCF) and American Heart Association (AHA) for self-identified black patients with New York Heart Association (NYHA) functional class III or IV heart failure and reduced ejection fraction who are receiving optimal therapy with ACE inhibitors and β-blockers (unless contraindicated). The ACCF and AHA also state that combined therapy with isosorbide dinitrate and hydralazine can be useful in patients with current or prior symptomatic heart failure with reduced ejection fraction who cannot receive an ACE inhibitor or angiotensin II receptor antagonist† because of drug intolerance, hypotension, or renal insufficiency.

Efficacy of the isosorbide dinitrate/hydralazine fixed-combination preparation was evaluated in a multicenter, randomized, placebo-controlled, double-blind trial (the African-American Heart Failure Trial; A-HeFT trial) in 1050 self-identified black adults (mean age: 57 years) with stable moderate-to-severe heart failure (NYHA functional class III in over 95% of patients) secondary to left ventricular dysfunction (ejection fraction 35% or less). Patients were randomized to receive the fixed-combination preparation containing isosorbide dinitrate and hydralazine hydrochloride (initially, 20 mg of isosorbide dinitrate and 37.5 mg of hydralazine hydrochloride 3 times daily and titrated [as tolerated] to a dosage of 40 mg of isosorbide dinitrate and 75 mg of hydralazine hydrochloride 3 times daily) or placebo for up to 18 months. Patients also received standard therapy (e.g., diuretics [mainly loop diuretics], β-blockers, ACE inhibitors, angiotensin II receptor antagonists, cardiac glycosides, and/or aldosterone antagonists).

The A-HeFT trial was terminated early (after a mean follow-up period of 10–12 months) principally because of a substantial reduction (43%) in all-cause mortality in patients receiving the fixed-combination preparation containing hydralazine and isosorbide dinitrate; mortality rate was about 10.2 or 6.2% in patients receiving placebo or the fixed-dose combination drug, respectively.

The primary end point of the study (a mean primary composite score consisting of all-cause mortality, first hospitalization for worsening of heart failure, and improvement of quality of life [as assessed by responses to the Minnesota Living with Heart Failure questionnaire]) also showed significant differences between drug therapy and placebo. Patients receiving the fixed combination containing isosorbide dinitrate and hydralazine experienced a significant reduction (33%) in the rate of first hospitalization for heart failure (16.4 or 24.4% for those receiving the drug or placebo, respectively) and a significant improvement in response to the Minnesota Living with Heart Failure questionnaire (a self-report of functional status). Factors of age, gender, baseline disease, or concomitant medications appear to have no effect on survival or rate of hospitalization. The fixed combination containing isosorbide dinitrate and hydralazine had a slight but significant blood pressure-lowering effect at 6 months; a mean decrease of 1.9 and 2.4 mm Hg from baseline in systolic and diastolic blood pressure, respectively, was observed in patients receiving the drug, while an increase of 1.2 and 0.8 mm Hg from baseline in systolic and diastolic blood pressure, respectively, was observed in patients receiving placebo. However, the role of reduced blood pressure in the improved outcome of patients receiving the study drugs has not been evaluated. The manufacturer states that there is no adequate clinical experience with hydralazine hydrochloride or isosorbide dinitrate as separate agents† or dosages of the drugs other than those used in the A-HeFT trial for the treatment of congestive heart failure.

In another randomized, placebo-controlled, comparative, long-term (median 2.3 years; range: 6–68 months) study (Vasodilator Heart failure Trial [V-HeFT I]) in patients with chronic congestive heart failure associated with ischemic or nonischemic cardiomyopathy who were receiving conventional therapy (cardiac glycosides and diuretics, without an ACE inhibitor), addition of isosorbide dinitrate (up to 160 mg daily) given concomitantly with hydralazine hydrochloride (up to 300 mg daily) resulted in a 25–30% decrease in overall mortality rates after 2 years when compared with conventional therapy and placebo or prazosin (up to 20 mg daily). However, despite substantial increases in ejection fraction, the combination of the 2 vasodilators was not associated with decreased hospitalizations and many patients discontinued therapy during follow up, although retrospective analysis of such data indicate that there was a trend favoring the administration of the 2 vasodilators, which was attributed to an effect observed in black patients.

In a subsequent randomized comparative, long-term (median 2.5 years; range: 6–68 months) study (V-HeFT II) in patients with ischemic or nonischemic cardiomyopathy and mild to moderate heart failure (NYHA functional class II and III) who were receiving conventional therapy (cardiac glycosides and diuretics), addition of enalapril maleate (up to 20 mg daily) resulted in a 28% decrease in overall mortality rates after 2 years when compared with conventional therapy and concomitant use of hydralazine hydrochloride (up to 300 mg daily) with isosorbide dinitrate (up to 160 mg daily). Retrospective analysis of the data indicates that such decreases in mortality rates in patients receiving enalapril in conjunction with conventional therapy were not observed in black patients. Concomitant administration of the 2 vasodilators had more favorable effects on ventricular ejection fraction and exercise tolerance than those associated with enalapril.

Nitroglycerin IV nitroglycerin has been used effectively in the treatment of acutely decompensated (e.g., congestive) heart failure† or other low cardiac output states†. Experts recommend that the precipitating cause of acute heart failure decompensation be carefully assessed to inform appropriate treatment, optimize outcomes, and prevent future acute events in patients with heart failure. IV vasodilators have not been shown to improve outcomes in patients hospitalized for heart failure; however, in the absence of symptomatic hypotension, IV nitroglycerin may be considered as an adjunct to diuretic therapy for relief of dyspnea in patients hospitalized for acutely decompensated heart failure. IV nitroglycerin causes venodilation, which lowers preload and may help rapidly reduce pulmonary congestion. Patients with heart failure and hypertension, coronary ischemia, or substantial mitral regurgitation are often considered ideal candidates for the use of IV nitroglycerin. However, tachyphylaxis to nitroglycerin may develop rapidly (e.g., within 24 hours), and up to 20% of those with heart failure may have inadequate response to even high doses of the drug.

■ **Hypertension** IV nitroglycerin is used to control blood pressure in perioperative hypertension, especially hypertension associated with cardiovascular procedures; to control blood pressure in patients with severe hypertension† or in hypertensive crises† for the immediate reduction of blood pressure in patients in whom such reduction is considered an emergency (hypertensive emergencies), especially those associated with coronary complications (e.g., coronary ischemia, acute coronary insufficiency, acute left ventricular failure, postoperative hypertension [especially following coronary bypass surgery]) and/or acute pulmonary edema; and to produce controlled hypotension during surgical procedures. Elevated blood pressure alone, in the absence of manifestations or other evidence of target organ damage, rarely requires emergency therapy.

■ **Cocaine-induced Acute Coronary Syndrome** Nitroglycerin has been used adjunctively in the management of cocaine overdose† to reverse coronary vasoconstriction. Experts state that administration of nitroglycerin also may be beneficial for cocaine-induced hypertension or chest discomfort.

■ **Diffuse Esophageal Spasm** In a limited number of patients with diffuse esophageal spasm without gastroesophageal reflux†, long-term administration of oral isosorbide dinitrate or erythrityl tetranitrate (no longer commercially available in the US) has been effective in relieving pain, dysphagia, and spasm; sublingual nitroglycerin 0.4 mg also briefly relieved symptoms in these patients.

Dosage and Administration

■ **Administration** Nitrates, in appropriate dosage forms, may be administered orally, lingually, sublingually, intrabuccally, topically, or by IV infusion. With sublingual administration, tingling may occur at the point of tablet contact with the mucous membrane and, if objectionable, may be lessened by placing the tablet in the buccal pouch. Amyl nitrite is administered by nasal inhalation. Lingual, sublingual, or intrabuccal administration of a nitrate is preferred for the acute relief of angina pectoris.

Nitrates are administered lingually, sublingually, or intrabuccally for prophylactic management in situations likely to provoke angina attacks, such as climbing stairs, cold weather, walking uphill, or sexual activity. These patients should be instructed to take the nitrate shortly before an activity that is known to cause angina rather than waiting until an attack occurs. For long-term prophylactic management of angina pectoris, nitrates are given orally or applied topically. If acute attacks of angina occur in patients receiving long-term nitrate therapy, a short-acting preparation (e.g., sublingual nitroglycerin) should be administered for acute relief.

The possibility that lingual, sublingual, or intrabuccal nitrates may be inadequately absorbed, with resultant decreased efficacy, in patients with dry oral mucous membranes (e.g., xerostomia) should be considered. It has been suggested that wetting the mouth with water immediately before the administration of sublingual nitrate tablets may increase the rate of dissolution of these tablets. In one study in patients undergoing cardiac catheterization who had dry oral mucous membranes (due to fasting), wetting the mouth with water immediately before the administration of sublingual nitrate tablets consistently enhanced the hemodynamic effects (e.g., substantial decrease in aortic systolic blood pressure) of these tablets. Although improved relief of angina associated with nitrates as a result of wetting oral mucous membranes with water was not specifically studied, the time of hemodynamic changes reportedly coincided with the relief of angina.

■ **Dosage** Dosage of nitrates must be carefully adjusted according to the patient's requirements and response and the smallest effective dosage should be used. For increased exercise tolerance in patients with angina, nitrates generally decrease systolic blood pressure (in sitting position) at least 10 mm Hg and/or increase heart rate at least 10 bpm.

Cautions

■ **Adverse Effects** Serious adverse reactions to the organic nitrates and nitrites are uncommon and their adverse effects mainly involve the CNS and cardiovascular system. Adverse effects of IV nitroglycerin generally are dose-related.

■ **Nervous System Effects** Headache, the most frequent adverse effect, may be severe (persistent or transient) and is perceived as a pulsating, throbbing sensation; headache is especially common after inhalation of amyl nitrite. Headache is most frequent early in therapy, usually diminishes rapidly, and may disappear within several days to weeks if treatment is continued. Headache may be relieved by a temporary reduction in dosage or administration of an analgesic such as aspirin or acetaminophen. However, patients should be advised to resist altering their nitrate dosage or schedule on their own in an effort to avoid headaches since a loss in antianginal efficacy could result.

■ **Cardiovascular Effects** Postural hypotension may occur in patients receiving nitrates or nitrites and may cause dizziness, weakness, and other signs of cerebral ischemia, especially if the patient is in a warm environment or standing immobile. Severe hypotension may occur even with small doses of nitroglycerin, especially in patients with constrictive pericarditis, aortic or mitral stenosis, volume depletion, or existing hypotension. Syncope may result and may be confused with acute myocardial infarction (MI) because the patient may be transiently pulseless, cold, clammy, and profusely sweating. Some patients may have a marked sensitivity to the hypotensive effects of nitrates and nitrites and nausea, vomiting, weakness, restlessness, pallor, cold sweat, involuntary passing of urine and feces, tachycardia, syncope, increased angina pectoris, rebound hypertension, shock, and cardiovascular collapse may occur with usual therapeutic doses; consumption of alcohol may enhance these effects. (See Drug Interactions: Alcohol.) In addition, the drugs may aggravate angina caused by hypertrophic cardiomyopathy. After administration of a rapidly acting nitrate or nitrite, reflex tachycardia may be marked if the patient is in an upright position. Patients should be sitting immediately after administration of rapidly acting nitrates and nitrites (e.g., amyl nitrite, lingual or sublingual nitroglycerin). If syncope occurs, the patient should be placed in the recumbent position. Measures that facilitate venous return (e.g., head-low [Trendelenburg's] position, deep breathing, movements of the extremities) may increase recovery rate. The possibility that inadvertent systemic hypotension and associated reflex tachycardia may result in worsening of myocardial ischemia should be considered. Severe arterial hypotension with absolute or relative bradycardia has been reported in patients who received sublingual or IV nitroglycerin within the first 24 hours after MI; hypotension and bradycardia were reversed by discontinuing the drug and elevating the lower extremities.

Transient flushing may occur with nitrates, and inhalation of amyl nitrite commonly causes cutaneous flushing of the head, neck, and clavicular area. In patients with venous insufficiency or severe congestive heart failure receiving topical nitroglycerin, peripheral edema may occur or be exacerbated.

■ **Dermatologic and Sensitivity Reactions** Allergic contact dermatitis and fixed drug eruptions have occurred rarely with topical nitroglycerin. Rash and/or exfoliative dermatitis may occur occasionally and are most common with pentaerythritol tetranitrate (no longer commercially available in the US). If rash occurs, the nitrate should be discontinued. There have been a few reports of anaphylactoid reactions in patients receiving nitroglycerin. Cross-sensitivity among the drugs may occur.

In clinical trials in patients receiving isosorbide dinitrate (20 mg) in fixed combination with hydralazine hydrochloride (37.5 mg) alopecia has been reported occasionally.

■ **Hematologic Effects** Nitrate ions released during metabolism of nitroglycerin can oxidize hemoglobin to methemoglobin. In patients without cytochrome-b_5 reductase activity, about 1 mg/kg of nitroglycerin is required before patients manifest clinically important (at least 10%) methemoglobinemia; patients with normal cytochrome$_b$ reductase activity require even higher doses of nitroglycerin for methemoglobinemia to develop. Methemoglobinemia should be suspected in any patient who exhibits sign of impaired oxygen delivery (e.g., darkening of the blood) despite adequate cardiac output and adequate arterial pO_2. Methemoglobinemia also may occur in infants who receive large amounts of nitrite or nitrate; the infant's relatively high GI pH causes bacterial reduction of unabsorbed nitrate to nitrite ion. Methemoglobinemia is extremely rare with therapeutic doses of nitrates and nitrites. However, large doses of amyl nitrite may cause formation of excessive methemoglobin which is characterized by blue skin and mucous membranes, vomiting, shock, and coma.

■ **Local Effects** Nitrates may cause a burning or tingling sensation when administered sublingually.

■ **GI Effects** GI upset has been reported during nitrate therapy and may be controlled by temporarily reducing the dosage. In addition, dry mouth was reported in some patients; the drug should be discontinued if this symptom occurs.

Adverse GI effects reported in self-identified black patients receiving isosorbide dinitrate in fixed-dose combination with hydralazine for adjunctive treatment of congestive heart failure (CHF) include nausea and vomiting; cholecystitis also has been reported occasionally.

■ **Other Adverse Effects** These drugs may cause blurred vision and should be discontinued if this symptom occurs.

In clinical trials in patients receiving isosorbide dinitrate (20 mg) in fixed combination with hydralazine hydrochloride (37.5 mg) bronchitis, sinusitis, sweating, hyperlipidemia, hyperglycemia, hypercholesterolemia, amblyopia, myalgia, and tendon disorders have been reported.

■ **Tolerance and Dependence** Tolerance to the vascular and antianginal effects of nitrates and nitrites has been shown in clinical studies, by experience from occupational exposure, and in isolated in vitro tissue experiments; such tolerance is a principal factor limiting the efficacy of long-term nitrate therapy. Rapid development of tolerance has occurred with oral, IV, and topical nitrate therapy (i.e., transdermal systems or nitroglycerin ointment); however, tolerance to the pharmacologic effects is generally minor with intermittent use of sublingual nitrates. In some controlled clinical studies in patients with angina, the improvement in exercise time on stress testing was substantially less and of shorter duration during sustained therapy with some nitrate preparations than during acute therapy; exercise capacity and/or angina frequency in some patients receiving transdermal nitrate therapy was similar to that in placebo-treated patients 24 hours or less (e.g., as little as 2–6 hours) after application of the transdermal system. Tolerance to the hemodynamic benefits of nitrates also has been reported in some patients with congestive heart failure. However, nitrate tolerance does not develop to the same degree in all patients, and some evidence suggests that up to 50% of patients may receive benefit from continuous nitrate therapy. Therefore, careful individualization of therapy is necessary in patients receiving nitrates.

Some evidence suggests that the development of tolerance can be prevented or minimized by use of the lowest effective dose of nitrates and an intermittent dosing schedule with a nitrate-free interval of 10–14 hours (e.g., removal of a transdermal nitroglycerin system in the early evening and application of a new system the next morning; omission of the last daily dose of oral nitrate preparations or use of an asymmetric daily dosing regimen for isosorbide mononitrate). An intermittent dosing regimen also has been recommended for topical (ointment) nitrate preparations. However, the minimum nitrate-free interval necessary for restoration of full first-dose effects of nitrate therapy has not been determined. Further studies are needed to determine the optimum regimen for minimizing or preventing tolerance to nitrate therapy.

Cross-tolerance to the effects of sublingual nitroglycerin reportedly may occur during long-term administration of nitrates. However, cross-tolerance to the effects of sublingual nitroglycerin apparently does not occur with long-term administration of extended-release preparations of isosorbide dinitrate or topical nitroglycerin. Available evidence is insufficient to warrant avoiding concomitant administration of sublingual nitroglycerin and long-acting nitrates.

Nitrate dependence has occurred in persons who manufacture organic nitrates and are in daily contact (either respiratory or skin exposure) with the drugs. Initially, headache, dizziness, or postural hypotension occurs and then tolerance to these effects develops. Following withdrawal from exposure, nonexertional ischemic cardiac pain and peripheral ischemic pain have occurred in some individuals without demonstrable organic vascular disease. Acute MI and even sudden death have also occurred in some industrial workers during temporary withdrawal of nitroglycerin exposure. These adverse effects generally have not been reported following sudden cessation of oral nitrate therapy in patients who have been receiving these drugs for long-term prophylactic management of angina, but there have been reports of anginal attacks being more easily provoked and of rebound in the hemodynamic effects soon after nitrate withdrawal in angina patients. The relative importance of these reports to the routine clinical use of nitrates is not known. Although many clinicians do not gradually reduce the dosage when discontinuance of oral nitrates is planned, it appears prudent that dosage be gradually reduced (e.g., over a period of about 1–2 weeks). Supplementary doses of sublingual nitroglycerin should be given if necessary during dosage reduction.

■ Precautions and Contraindications Intermittent dosing of nitrates (e.g., use of a nitrate-free interval of 10–14 hours daily) has been recommended to minimize or prevent the development of tolerance to the hemodynamic and antianginal effects of the drugs. (See Cautions: Tolerance and Dependence.) However, controlled clinical studies suggest that such intermittent use is associated with decreased exercise tolerance compared with placebo during the latter part of the nitrate-free interval. The clinical relevance of this observation currently is unknown, but the possibility of an increased frequency or severity of angina during the nitrate-free interval should be considered. Because substantial tolerance does not occur in all patients receiving nitrate therapy and because of the potential risks associated with withdrawal of nitrates in patients with angina, careful individualization of nitrate therapy is necessary. In patients with moderate to severe angina, unstable angina, or frequent episodes of chest pain at rest in whom nitrate therapy is to be interrupted on a daily basis, use of concomitant antianginal therapy with another class of drugs (e.g., calcium-channel blocking agents, β-blockers) has been suggested.

When isosorbide dinitrate is used in fixed combination with hydralazine, the cautions, precautions, and contraindications associated with hydralazine (see Cautions in Hydralazine 24:08.20) must be considered in addition to those associated with isosorbide dinitrate.

Nitrates are contraindicated in patients with known hypersensitivity to the drugs or any ingredient in the formulations. Topical nitroglycerin (transdermal system) is contraindicated in patients who are allergic to the adhesives used in the system.

Some manufacturers state that nitrates and nitrites should be used with caution or are contraindicated in patients with angle-closure or open-angle glaucoma; however, intraocular pressure is at most increased only briefly and drainage of aqueous humor from the eye is not impeded. In addition, in several studies in patients with open-angle or angle-closure glaucoma, nitrates did not affect or slightly decreased intraocular pressure.

Extended-release oral nitrate preparations should not be used in patients with functional or organic GI hypermotility or malabsorption syndrome.

Nitrates and nitrites should be used with caution, if at all, in patients with increased intracranial pressure (e.g., head trauma, cerebral hemorrhage) and are contraindicated in patients with severe anemia or with a previous idiosyncratic or hypersensitivity reaction to these drugs.

Although some manufacturers state that the benefits of oral, sublingual, or topical nitrates have not been established in patients with acute MI, IV nitroglycerin has been used in such patients. (See Uses: Acute Myocardial Infarction.) The use of any dosage form of nitroglycerin during the initial days following an acute MI requires particular attention to monitoring the hemodynamic and clinical status of the patient in order to avoid possible hypotension and tachycardia. In general, long-acting dosage forms should be avoided in the early management of acute MI since the effects are difficult to terminate rapidly should excessive hypotension or tachycardia occur. Nitrates in the setting of suspected acute MI should be avoided in patients with marked bradycardia (e.g., less than 50 bpm) or tachycardia (e.g., exceeding 100 bpm), and should not be used in patients with suspected right ventricular infarction. Patients with right ventricular infarction are particularly dependent on adequate right ventricular preload, which is reduced by nitrates, to maintain cardiac output and can experience profound hypotension during administration of the drugs.

Nitrates should be used with caution in patients with diuretic-induced fluid depletion. Patients receiving isosorbide dinitrate in fixed-dose combination with hydralazine should be advised that inadequate fluid intake or excessive fluid loss due to diarrhea, vomiting, or perspiration may result in excessive hypotension, possibly leading to lightheadedness or even syncope. If syncope occurs, isosorbide dinitrate and hydralazine should be discontinued, and the patient's clinician should be notified as soon as possible. Isosorbide dinitrate is contraindicated in patients with shock or marked low blood pressure. In addition, IV nitroglycerin is contraindicated in patients with hypotension or uncorrected hypovolemia, since severe hypotension or shock could result, and in patients with constrictive pericarditis and pericardial tamponade. Nitrate-induced hypotension may produce paradoxical bradycardia and increased angina pectoris. The possibility that nitrates may aggravate angina associated with hypertrophic cardiomyopathy also should be considered.

IV administration of dilute solutions of nitroglycerin may cause fluid overload resulting in dilution of serum electrolytes, overhydration, congestive conditions, or pulmonary edema. The risk of dilutional conditions is inversely proportional to the electrolyte concentration administered, and the risk of solute overload and resultant congestive conditions with peripheral and/or pulmonary edema is directly proportional to the electrolyte concentration administered. Lower concentrations of IV nitroglycerin in 5% dextrose injection increases the potential precision of dosing, but such concentrations increase the total fluid volume, which is a consideration in patients with compromised cardiac, hepatic, and/or renal function.

Patients receiving lingual or sublingual nitroglycerin for relief of acute attacks of angina pectoris should be instructed that if pain persists after 3 doses (administered approximately every 5 minutes) they should seek prompt medical attention, because inability of these drugs to relieve chest pain may indicate acute MI.

Phosphodiesterase (PDE) type 5 inhibitors (e.g., sildenafil, tadalafil, vardenafil) are contraindicated in patients receiving organic nitrates or nitrites in any form (e.g., orally, sublingually, transmucosally, parenterally), given regularly or intermittently, or nitric oxide donors since severe, potentially fatal hypotensive episodes can occur. Experts state that coadministration of PDE type 5 inhibitors should be strictly avoided within 24 hours of nitrate administration. (See Drug Interactions: Selective Phosphodiesterase Inhibitors.) Clinicians unfamiliar with their patients' drug history, especially those involved in emergency care (e.g., for presumed MI or ischemia), should take a careful history so that concomitant use of organic nitrates or nitrites with selective PDE inhibitors can be avoided. All patients receiving organic nitrates or nitrites should be warned about the potential interaction between the drugs and selective PDE inhibitors, even if they currently are not receiving the drugs, since there is substantial potential for patients to receive the drugs from another clinician, from a friend, with little or no clinical intervention (e.g., via the Internet), or illicitly. Similarly, all patients taking either selective PDE inhibitors or organic nitrates or nitrites must be warned of the potential consequences of taking the drugs within close proximity (e.g., within 24 hours of sildenafil; possibly more prolonged periods of risk with longer-acting PDE inhibitors) of taking a nitrate- or nitrite-containing preparation. The use of nitrates (e.g., nitroglycerin) or nitrites (e.g., amyl nitrite) with a soluble guanylate cyclase (sGC) stimulator (e.g., riociguat) also is contraindicated because of the potential for additive hypotensive effects.

■ Pregnancy and Lactation Some experts state that use of nitroglycerin during pregnancy does not appear to present a risk to the fetus; however, experience with the drug in pregnant women is limited. Nitrates and nitrites generally should be used during pregnancy only when the potential benefits justify the possible risks to the fetus or only when clearly needed.

It is not known whether nitrates or nitrites are distributed into human milk. The low molecular weight of nitroglycerin suggests that some distribution into milk may occur. Some manufacturers state that caution is advised if nitroglycerin is used in nursing women.

Drug Interactions

■ Alcohol Concomitant use of nitrates or nitrites and alcohol may cause hypotension. Although the clinical importance of this interaction has not been established, nitrates or nitrites should be used with caution in conjunction with alcohol.

■ Aspirin Concomitant use of nitroglycerin and high-dose aspirin (1 g) may increase exposure to nitroglycerin and enhance its vasodilatory and hemodynamic effects.

■ Disopyramide Concomitant use of isosorbide dinitrate (as sublingual tablets) and disopyramide reportedly reduces the efficacy of isosorbide dinitrate. The antimuscarinic actions of disopyramide appear to decrease salivary secretions and thereby inhibit the dissolution of the sublingual tablets.

■ Ergot Alkaloids Dihydroergotamine may counteract the coronary vasodilatory effect of nitrates, including isosorbide dinitrate. Oral administration of nitroglycerin substantially decreases the first-pass metabolism of dihydroergotamine and subsequently increases its oral bioavailability. Since ergotamine is known to precipitate angina and has been used as a provocative test for angina, patients receiving nitroglycerin for antianginal therapy should not be receiving dihydroergotamine if possible. However, if nitrates are used concomitantly with ergotamine, patients should be monitored for enhanced ergotamine effects and dosages of the ergot alkaloid should be reduced as needed.

■ Heparin Because some, but not all, evidence indicates that IV nitroglycerin may antagonize the anticoagulant effect of heparin when these drugs are administered concomitantly, caution should be exercised. Although initial data suggested that the solvent propylene glycol, used in parenteral dosage forms of nitroglycerin was responsible for this effect, additional study indicates that this interaction also occurs when nitroglycerin preparations not containing the solvent are used. Patients receiving heparin and IV nitroglycerin concomitantly should be monitored (e.g., measurement of activated partial thromboplastin time) closely to avoid inadequate anticoagulation. If IV nitroglycerin therapy is discontinued in patients receiving heparin, reduction in heparin dosage may be necessary.

■ Selective Phosphodiesterase Inhibitors Sildenafil and other selective phosphodiesterase (PDE) type 5 inhibitors (e.g., avanafil, tadalafil, vardenafil) profoundly potentiate the vasodilatory effects (e.g., a greater than 25-mm Hg decrease in systolic blood pressure) of organic nitrates and nitrites (e.g., nitroglycerin, isosorbide dinitrate), and potentially life-threatening hypotension and/or hemodynamic compromise can result. Nitrates and nitrites promote the formation of cyclic guanosine monophosphate (cGMP) by stimulating guanylate cyclase, and sildenafil acts to decrease the degradation of cGMP via phosphodiesterase (PDE) type 5 by inhibiting this enzyme, resulting in increased accumulation of cGMP and more pronounced smooth muscle relaxation and vasodilation than with either sildenafil or nitrates/nitrites alone. This interaction probably occurs with any organic nitrate, nitrite, or nitric oxide donor (e.g., nitroprusside) regardless of their predominant hemodynamic site of action.

Selective PDE inhibitors also may potentiate the hypotensive effects of inhaled nitrites (e.g., amyl or butyl nitrite, sometimes referred to as "poppers"), which may be misused ("recreational use") during sexual activity for purported effects in enhancing the sexual experience. Because these agents are used recreationally, patients may be unaware of their pharmacologic effects and potential risks and may not report their use to clinicians. Concurrent use of selective PDE inhibitors with poppers, which dilate blood vessels with a rapid onset of action, could result in sudden and marked blood pressure reduction and potentially serious or even fatal effects. Interactions with organic nitrates and nitrites may be even more pronounced in patients who also are taking certain HIV protease inhibitors concomitantly. Homosexual males may be at particular risk because of the greater likelihood of recreational inhaled nitrite use and antiretroviral therapy in this population.

Because of the serious risk of concomitant use of organic nitrates or nitrites and selective PDE inhibitors, such combined use is contraindicated. At least 19 deaths have been reported in patients who may have taken sildenafil and who took or were given nitroglycerin or another nitrate/nitrite or who were found with nitroglycerin in their possession. The manufacturers of selective PDE type 5 inhibitors (e.g., sildenafil, tadalafil, vardenafil) state that the drugs are contraindicated in any patient receiving organic nitrates or nitrites, either regularly or intermittently and in any form (e.g., orally, sublingually, transmucosally, parenterally), or other nitric oxide donors. Although it is not known how much time must elapse between use of *sildenafil* and administration of a nitrate or nitrite, pharmacokinetic data suggest that these latter agents should *not* be given within 24 hours of *sildenafil* administration because an exaggerated hypotensive response is likely; plasma sildenafil concentrations 24 hours after a dose are substantially lower than peak concentrations. Pharmacodynamic data for tadalafil, a longer-acting PDE type 5 inhibitor, in healthy individuals (including geriatric individuals 70 years of age or older) indicate that the hypotensive effect of sublingual nitroglycerin (0.4 mg) was augmented by tadalafil when administered within 24 hours after administration of the last dose of tadalafil (20 mg once daily for 7 days) but not at 48, 72, or 96 hours after the dose. The potential interaction of nitrates or nitrites with vardenafil has not been well studied.

The point at which nitrates or nitrites can be given safely is unclear, and therefore the drugs should be avoided unless, in the view of the treating clinician, the benefits outweigh the risks. Some experts state that coadministration of PDE type 5 inhibitors with long-acting nitrates should be strictly avoided within 24 hours of nitrate administration. Nitrates should not be taken for 24 hours after use of sildenafil or 48 hours after tadalafil. If consideration is given to administering a nitrate or nitrite beyond 24 or 48 hours after *sildenafil* or *tadalafil* use, respectively, the response to the initial doses must be monitored carefully and proper facilities for fluid and vasopressor (e.g., α-adrenergic agonists) support must be readily available to prevent acute ischemic episodes. If severe hypotension occurs, some manufacturers state that it is reasonable to treat the situation as a nitrate overdosage and provide appropriate supportive care (e.g., elevation of the extremities and central volume expansion). No specific antagonist to the vasodilator effects of nitroglycerin is known. In patients in whom clearance of *sildenafil* and/or its metabolites may be prolonged (e.g., those with hepatic [e.g., cirrhosis] or severe renal impairment [e.g., creatinine clearance less than 30 mL/minute], those receiving a potent inhibitor of cytochrome P-450 [CYP] isoenzyme 3A4, geriatric patients older than 65 years of age), elapse of a more extended period of time between use of *sildenafil* and administration of a nitrate or nitrite may be necessary. In either case, a short-acting nitrate formulation that can be titrated readily (e.g., IV nitroglycerin) would be preferred and such use should be accompanied by close hemodynamic monitoring.

All patients receiving either an organic nitrate/nitrite or *sildenafil* should be warned about the contraindications and the potential consequences of taking *sildenafil* within 24 hours of nitrate or nitrite use, even sublingual nitroglycerin. Even more prolonged periods of risk are possible for longer-acting selective PDE inhibitors. Although sublingual nitroglycerin is relatively short-acting, any use during the previous 24 hours suggests that it may be needed again after *sildenafil*-enhanced sexual activity. In addition, the presence of even trace amounts of nitrates or nitrites may have unknown effects in combination with sildenafil.

Because selective PDE inhibitors may be obtained without the knowledge of the physician and/or pharmacist, including via the Internet or illicitly, all patients prescribed nitrates or nitrites should be warned of the potential consequences of combined use with these drugs (e.g., sildenafil, tadalafil, vardenafil). The possibility or recreational use of inhaled nitrites ("poppers") also should be considered whenever sildenafil is prescribed, particularly in homosexual males.

■ **Soluble Guanylate Cyclase Stimulators** Soluble guanylate cyclase (sGC) stimulators (e.g., riociguat) can potentiate the hypotensive effects of organic nitrates (e.g., nitroglycerin) and nitrites (e.g., amyl nitrite) when used concomitantly; such concomitant use is contraindicated. Because the time course and dose dependence of this interaction have not been established, use of these drugs within a few days of one another is not recommended. If severe hypotension occurs, some manufacturers state that it is reasonable to treat the situation as a nitrate overdosage and provide appropriate supportive care (e.g., elevation of the extremities and central volume expansion).

■ **Thrombolytic Agents** Concomitant administration of tissue-type plasminogen activator (t-PA) and IV nitroglycerin can reduce plasma levels of t-PA and its thrombolytic effect. Caution is advised if a patient is receiving such concomitant therapy.

■ **Other Drugs** Patients receiving antihypertensive drugs, calcium-channel blocking agents, β-blockers, or phenothiazines and nitrates or nitrites concomitantly should be observed for possible additive hypotensive effects. Dosage adjustment of either the nitrate/nitrite or the other agent with hypotensive activity may necessary to avoid orthostatic hypotension during concomitant use.

Laboratory Test Interferences

Nitrates and nitrites may interfere with the Zlatkis-Zak color reaction causing a false report of decreased serum cholesterol. Because of the propylene glycol content of IV nitroglycerin, serum triglyceride assays that rely on glycerol oxidase may yield falsely elevated serum triglyceride concentrations.

Acute Toxicity

■ **Manifestations** Adverse effects from nitrate and nitrite overdosage are extensions of the pharmacologic action of the drugs, namely the capacity to induce vasodilation, venous pooling, reduced cardiac output, and hypotension. Nitrate and nitrite overdosage may result in severe hypotension, tachycardia, bradycardia, heart-block, palpitation, death secondary to circulatory collapse, confusion, fever, syncope (especially in upright posture), persistent throbbing headache, visual disturbances, increased intracranial pressure, paralysis, and coma followed by seizures, flushing and diaphoresis, cold and clammy skin, nausea and vomiting, colic and diarrhea, dyspnea, and methemoglobinemia.

■ **Treatment** Laboratory determinations of serum drug concentrations are not widely available and do not have an established role in the management of nitrate and nitrite overdosage. Data are not available to suggest physiologic maneuvers to increase the excretion of nitrates and nitrites, such as altering the pH of the urine. It is not known whether hemodialysis would remove any of the parent drugs or active metabolites. No specific antagonist to the vasodilator effects of nitrates and nitrites is known and no intervention has been subject to controlled study as a therapy for overdosage; use of epinephrine or other arterial vasoconstrictors is not recommended by the manufacturer Hypotension from nitroglycerin overdosage results from venodilation and arterial hypovolemia, and its prudent management should be directed toward increasing central fluid volume; passive elevation of the patient's legs may be sufficient, although IV infusion of 0.9% sodium chloride injection or similar solution also may be necessary. If methemoglobinemia is present, IV administration of methylene blue (e.g., 1–2 mg/kg of body weight) may be required. Management of nitroglycerin overdosage in patients with renal disease or congestive heart failure may require invasive monitoring. Therapy that effects central volume expansion could be hazardous to such patients.

Pharmacology

All organic nitrates appear to have similar pharmacologic effects. The principal pharmacologic property of these drugs is relaxation of vascular smooth muscle, resulting in generalized vasodilation. Nitrates are metabolized to a free radical nitric oxide at or near the plasma membrane of vascular smooth muscle cells. Nitric oxide is an endothelium-derived relaxing factor (EDRF) that modulates vascular tone. Nitric oxide activates guanylate cyclase, resulting in an increase of guanosine-3′,5′monophosphate (cyclic GMP), which eventually leads to the dephosphorylation of the light chain of myosin, resulting in vasodilation. Nitrate administration provides an exogenous source of nitric oxide which replenishes or restores the actions of EDRF, which usually are impaired in patients with coronary artery disease.

■ **Vascular Effects** Peripheral venous resistance is decreased via a selective action on venous capacitance vessels and results in venous pooling of blood and decreased venous return to the heart. The vasodilatory effect of the drugs on arteriolar resistance is not as great as the action on the venous side. As a result of this combined action, both venous filling pressure (preload) and, to a lesser extent, arterial impedance (afterload) are reduced. Left ventricular end-diastolic pressure (LVEDP) and volume (LVEDV) are decreased resulting in reduction of ventricular size and wall tension, particularly in patients with occlusive coronary artery disease and especially after exercise, atrial pacing, or added fluid load. Although nitrates and nitrites reflexly increase heart rate and myocardial contractility which increase myocardial oxygen consumption, the reduction in both right and left ventricular preload that results from peripheral vasodilation, particularly in the splanchnic and mesenteric circulations, combined with afterload reduction from arterial vasodilation, results in decreased cardiac work and a net decrease in myocardial oxygen consumption. By decreasing myocardial oxygen consumption, nitrates and nitrites alter the imbalance of myocardial oxygen supply and consumption which is thought to cause angina pectoris. Because of their hemodynamic profile, nitrates and nitrites are particularly beneficial in patients with left ventricular systolic dysfunction or heart failure.

In addition, both direct vasodilatory effects of nitrates and nitrites on the coronary bed and drug-induced prevention of episodic coronary artery vasoconstriction increase total coronary blood flow. However, in patients with ischemic hearts in whom the coronary vessels may be occluded or maximally dilated secondary to regional hypoxia, these drugs may not increase total coronary blood flow, but instead may cause a beneficial redistribution of coronary blood flow resulting in decreased myocardial ischemia. Nitroglycerin has been shown to preferentially increase subendocardial blood flow without changing total coronary blood flow. Redistribution of coronary blood flow may occur because nitrates and nitrites preferentially dilate the large conductance vessels (e.g., epicardial coronary arteries) rather than the arteriolar resistance vessels with resultant shunting of blood to the ischemic myocardium or because collateral vessels which may develop secondary to myocardial ischemia may be dilated by these drugs. As a result of increased global and regional myocardial blood flow, nitrates and nitrites improve the subendocardial-to-epicardial blood flow ratio. Vasodilation in intact vascular smooth muscle contained in obstructive atherosclerotic lesions can increase the caliber of some stenoses, improving coronary flow. The drugs also have been shown to dilate coronary collateral vessels and reverse vasoconstriction of small coronary arteries distal to coronary obstruction.Although systemic and coronary vascular effects may vary slightly among these drugs (e.g., in animals, the coronary vasodilator activity of isosorbide-5-mononitrate and isosorbide-2-mononitrate are 1/100–1/30 and ¼–⅓ that of isosorbide dinitrate, respectively), both of these effects are probably responsible for the beneficial effect of nitrates and nitrites in the treatment of angina pectoris.

After therapeutic doses of nitrates and nitrites, cardiac output may increase transiently and then decrease. Systemic arterial pressure is usually decreased (systolic blood pressure more than diastolic) as a result of vasodilation, and the decrease may be marked in individuals kept in a static upright position. Some patients may be especially sensitive to these hypotensive effects, particularly when there is little compensatory tachycardia, and syncope may result. In doses that do not appreciably decrease blood pressure, inhalation of amyl nitrite causes intense cutaneous flush of the head, neck, and clavicular area; this effect is less marked with nitrates. The meningeal vessels are dilated and a pulsating headache may occur. Net splanchnic vasoconstriction and decreased renal blood flow may occur. Pulmonary vascular resistance and pulmonary arterial pressure are decreased in healthy individuals and in those with angina pectoris.

■ **Antiplatelet and Antithrombotic Effects** Results of in vitro and in vivo studies suggest that nitrates also may have antiplatelet and antithrombotic effects. Administration of IV nitroglycerin may inhibit platelet aggregation and adhesion. The free radical nitric oxide resultant of nitrate metabolism activates guanylate cyclase, resulting in an increase of cyclic GMP which leads to decreased fibrinogen binding to the glycoprotein IIb/IIIa receptors. The platelet inhibition by nitrates may suggest an additional mechanism to improve perfusion to ischemic myocardium.

■ **Other Effects** In addition to vascular smooth muscle, nitrates and nitrites relax bronchial, biliary (including the gallbladder, biliary ducts, and sphincter of Oddi), GI (including the esophagus), ureteral, and uterine smooth muscle. These drugs relax all smooth muscle irrespective of autonomic innervation and are functional antagonists of norepinephrine, acetylcholine, and histamine.

Nitroglycerin may cause a marked increase in urinary vanillylmandelic acid (VMA) and catecholamine excretion, possibly secondary to adrenergic response to the hypotensive effect of the drug.

Pharmacokinetics

■ **Absorption** Amyl nitrite is readily absorbed via the respiratory tract and probably is rapidly hydrolyzed to isoamyl alcohol and nitrite ion. In general, the organic nitrates are well absorbed from the oral mucosa following administration lingually, sublingually, intrabuccally, or as chewable tablets. The organic nitrates are also well absorbed from the GI tract but undergo first-pass metabolism in the liver. Nitroglycerin is well absorbed through intact skin when applied topically as an ointment or transdermal system.

Following nasal inhalation, amyl nitrite has a more rapid onset and a shorter duration of action than do sublingually administered organic nitrates. Sublingually administered nitroglycerin has the most rapid onset of antianginal and hemodynamic effects compared to the other organic nitrates. When administered lingually, sublingually, intrabuccally, or as chewable tablets, the organic nitrates have a more rapid onset of action than when they are given orally or topically. Amyl nitrite inhalation, sublingual or buccal nitroglycerin, or sublingual or chewable isosorbide dinitrate is rapidly acting. Generally, orally administered nitrates and topical nitroglycerin are relatively long acting, but rapid tolerance to the hemodynamic and antianginal effects of these dosage forms may occur with continuous therapy. (See Cautions: Tolerance and Dependence.)

■ **Distribution** Following IV administration, highly lipophilic nitrates (e.g., nitroglycerin, isosorbide dinitrate) are widely distributed into vascular and other peripheral tissues while less lipophilic nitrates (e.g., isosorbide mononitrate) are not as widely distributed in the body.

At plasma concentrations of 50–500 ng/mL, approximately 60, 60, or 30% of nitroglycerin, 1,2-dinitroglycerin, or 1,3-dinitroglycerin are bound to plasma proteins, respectively. In addition, isosorbide dinitrate and isosorbide mononitrate are approximately 28 and 4–5% bound to plasma proteins, respectively.

■ **Elimination** Animal studies indicate that the organic nitrates are rapidly denitrated in the liver by the glutathione-organic nitrate reductase system which is dependent on endogenous glutathione. In addition, nitrates are metabolized in the serum independent of glutathione. Hepatic biotransformation is initiated by a redox reaction and the therapeutically active lipid soluble parent ester is converted to less active soluble metabolites. Isosorbide mononitrate (isosorbide-5-mononitrate), the principal active metabolite of isosorbide dinitrate, also is prepared synthetically for formulation of commercially available preparations that share the uses of other nitrates and nitrites.

Studies using IV nitrates indicate that the active nitrate esters have a shorter plasma half-life than do the less active metabolites. The metabolites and, to a lesser extent, the active nitrate esters are excreted by the kidneys.

Chemistry and Stability

■ **Chemistry** The organic nitrates and nitrites are esters of nitrous or nitric acid and are used mainly for the acute relief and prophylactic management of angina pectoris. Amyl nitrite is the only commercially available organic nitrite and is a mixture of isomeric amyl nitrites, principally isoamyl nitrite. Structural variations in the organic nitrates result in differences in onset and duration of action and potency. Although the orientation of nitrate ester groups may affect potency, there is no relationship between the number of nitrate groups and the amount of activity. Isosorbide dinitrate is metabolized in the liver to 2 active metabolites, isosorbide-2-mononitrate and isosorbide-5-mononitrate; isosorbide-5-mononitrate, the principal active metabolite, also is commercially available and is referred to simply as isosorbide mononitrate.

■ **Stability** Amyl nitrite is very volatile and flammable. The organic nitrates (erythrityl tetranitrate [no longer commercially available in the US], isosorbide dinitrate, isosorbide mononitrate, nitroglycerin, and pentaerythritol tetranitrate [no longer commercially available in the US]) are rendered nonexplosive by the addition of an inert excipient such as lactose.

For specific dosages and additional information on nitrates and nitrites, see the individual monographs in 24:12.08.

†Use is not currently included in the labeling approved by the US Food and Drug Administration

Isosorbide Dinitrate
Isosorbide Mononitrate

ISD, ISDNIsosorbide-5-mononitrate, ISMN

■ Isosorbide dinitrate and isosorbide mononitrate, organic nitrates, are vasodilating agents.

Uses

■ **Angina** Isosorbide dinitrate and isosorbide mononitrate share the actions of the other nitrates and nitrites. The drugs are used for the acute relief of angina pectoris, for prophylactic management in situations likely to provoke angina attacks, and for long-term prophylactic management of angina pectoris. (For further information on the use of isosorbide dinitrate and isosorbide mononitrate in the management of stable and unstable angina, see Uses: Angina in the Nitrates and Nitrites General Statement 24:12.08.)

■ **Heart Failure** Isosorbide dinitrate is used in fixed combination with hydralazine (BiDil®) as an adjunct to standard therapy for the treatment of heart failure in self-identified black patients to improve survival, decrease rate of hospitalization for worsened heart failure, and improve patient-reported functional status. Current guidelines for the management of heart failure in adults generally recommend a combination of drug therapies to reduce morbidity and mortality, including neurohormonal antagonists (e.g., angiotensin-converting enzyme [ACE] inhibitors, angiotensin II receptor antagonists, angiotensin receptor-neprilysin inhibitors [ARNIs], β-adrenergic blocking agents [β-blockers], aldosterone receptor antagonists) that inhibit the detrimental compensatory mechanisms in heart failure. (See Uses: Heart Failure in Carvedilol 24:24 and in Sacubitril and Valsartan 24:32.92.) The combination of isosorbide dinitrate and hydralazine is recommended by the American College of Cardiology Foundation (ACCF) and American Heart Association (AHA) for self-identified black patients with New York Heart Association (NYHA) functional class III or IV heart failure and reduced ejection fraction who are receiving optimal therapy with ACE inhibitors and β-blockers (unless contraindicated). ACCF and AHA also state that combined therapy with isosorbide dinitrate and hydralazine may be considered in patients with current or prior symptomatic heart failure and reduced ejection fraction who cannot receive an ACE inhibitor or angiotensin II receptor antagonist† because of drug intolerance, hypotension, or renal insufficiency. For further information on the use of isosorbide dinitrate in the management of heart failure, see Uses: Heart Failure and Low-output Syndromes in the Nitrates and Nitrites General Statement 24:12.08.

■ **Diffuse Esophageal Spasm** In a limited number of patients with diffuse esophageal spasm without gastroesophageal reflux†, isosorbide dinitrate has been used effectively to relieve pain, dysphagia, and spasm.

Dosage and Administration

■ **Administration** *Isosorbide Dinitrate* Isosorbide dinitrate is administered sublingually, intrabuccally, or orally. The possibility that sublingual or intrabuccal nitrates may be inadequately absorbed, with resultant decreased efficacy, in patients with dry oral mucous membranes (e.g., xerostomia) should be considered. Chewable tablets (no longer commercially available in the US) should be chewed thoroughly before swallowing. Extended-release preparations should *not* be chewed. The patient should be sitting immediately after administration of isosorbide dinitrate sublingually or as a chewable tablet.

Isosorbide Mononitrate Isosorbide mononitrate is administered orally. Isosorbide mononitrate extended-release tablets can be administered as whole or halved tablets, but these should be swallowed intact and not chewed or crushed. In addition, isosorbide extended-release tablets should be administered with adequate amounts of fluid (e.g., 120 mL) on arising in the morning.

■ **Dosage** Dosage of isosorbide dinitrate and isosorbide mononitrate must be carefully adjusted according to the patient's requirements and response and the smallest effective dosage should be used.

When isosorbide dinitrate is used in fixed combination with hydralazine, the cautions, precautions, and contraindications associated with hydralazine must be considered in addition to those associated with isosorbide dinitrate (see Cautions and Precautions and Contraindications in the Nitrates and Nitrites General Statement 24:12.08).

Clinical studies of isosorbide dinitrate alone or in fixed combination with hydralazine did not include sufficient numbers of patients 65 years of age and older to determine whether geriatric patients respond differently than younger patients. Although other clinical experience has not revealed age-related differences in response or tolerance, drug dosage generally should be titrated carefully in geriatric patients, usually initiating therapy at the low end of the dosage range. The greater frequency of decreased hepatic, renal, and/or cardiac function and of concomitant disease and drug therapy observed in the elderly also should be considered. Elimination of isosorbide dinitrate and its metabolites may occur more slowly in geriatric patients than in younger adults.

Clinical studies of isosorbide mononitrate did not include sufficient numbers of patients 65 years of age and older to determine whether geriatric patients respond differently than younger patients. Other clinical experience has not identified any differences in responses between geriatric and younger patients. One manufacturer of isosorbide mononitrate states that if isosorbide mononitrate is used in geriatric patients, dosage of the drug should be selected with caution, usually initiating therapy at the low end of the dosage range, although age, renal, hepatic, and cardiovascular dysfunction do not appear to have a significant effect on the clearance of the drug.

Angina **Acute Symptomatic Relief and Prophylactic Management.** For the acute relief of angina pectoris or for prophylactic management in situations likely to provoke angina attacks in patients who fail to respond to nitroglycerin lingual or sublingual preparations, 2.5–5 mg of isosorbide dinitrate is administered sublingually, intrabuccally, or as a chewable tablet (no longer commercially available in the US). If relief is not attained after a single dose during an acute attack, additional doses may be given at 5- to 10-minute intervals; no more than 3 doses should be given in a 15- to 30- minute period.

For the prophylactic management in situations likely to provoke angina attacks in patients who fail to respond to sublingual nitroglycerin, 2.5–5 mg of isosorbide dinitrate should be placed under the tongue approximately 15 minutes prior to engaging in such activities.

Since the onset of action of extended-release preparations containing isosorbide dinitrate or any preparation containing isosorbide mononitrate is not sufficiently rapid to be efficacious in aborting an acute anginal episode, such preparations are not indicated for use in the management of acute relief of angina or in the prophylactic management in situations likely to provoke angina attacks.

Long-term Prophylactic Management. For long-term prophylactic management of angina pectoris, the usual initial dosage of oral isosorbide dinitrate conventional tablets (e. g., Isordil® Titradose®) is 5–20 mg administered 2 or 3 times daily. The usual recommended maintenance dosage is 10–40 mg 2 or 3 times daily, although some patients may require higher dosages. Some clinicians recommend that such dosages be administered at 7 a.m., 12 p.m., and 5 p.m. in most patients with chronic stable angina or at 7 a.m. and 12 p.m. in patients with less severe symptoms of angina in order to allow for a nitrate-free interval of 10–14 hours. Patients who arise earlier than 7 a.m. may need to adjust this schedule since early morning angina is common. There is some evidence that less frequent administration of isosorbide dinitrate in patients with angina pectoris may reduce the development of tolerance to the drug's antianginal effects (see Cautions: Tolerance and Dependence, in the Nitrates and Nitrites General Statement). In addition, the manufacturer of isosorbide dinitrate extended-release capsules (Dilatrate®-SR) states that results of the only multiple-dose study performed using an extended-release preparation of isosorbide dinitrate indicate that when these extended-release capsules were given twice daily (6 hours apart), the antianginal efficacy of the drug after 4 weeks of therapy was comparable to that of placebo. This manufacturer also states that an interdosing interval sufficient to avoid tolerance with these extended-release capsules is not known, but it must exceed 18 hours. The maximum daily dosages of Dilatrate® should not exceed 160 mg (4 capsules).

Alternatively, conventional or extended-release tablets of isosorbide mononitrate may be used for long-term prophylactic management of angina. The usual initial dosage of conventional isosorbide mononitrate tablets (e.g., Ismo®, Monoket®) is 20 mg twice daily, with the 2 doses administered 7 hours apart. Patients of particularly small stature may receive initial dosages of 5 mg (administered as one-half of a 10-mg tablet) twice daily, but since such a lower dosage is only effective (as determined by exercise tolerance) on the first day of therapy, the dosage should be increased to at least 10 mg twice daily by the second or third day of therapy. The recommended initial dosage of the extended-release isosorbide mononitrate tablets (e.g., Imdur®) is 30 (administered as a single 30-mg tablet or as one-half of a 60-mg tablet) or 60 mg (administered as a single 60-mg tablet) once daily. Dosage may be increased to 120 mg (administered as a single 120-mg tablet or as two 60-mg tablets) once daily after several days of therapy; dosages of 240 mg of these extended-release tablets are rarely needed.

Heart Failure For the adjunctive treatment of heart failure in self-identified black patients, the recommended initial dosage of the fixed-combination preparation is 20 mg of isosorbide dinitrate and 37.5 mg of hydralazine hydrochloride (1 tablet of BiDil®) 3 times daily. The dosage may be titrated to a maximum tolerated dosage, not to exceed 2 tablets (a total of 40 mg of isosorbide dinitrate and 75 mg of hydralazine hydrochloride) 3 times daily. Although rapid titration (over 3–5 days) of dosage can be undertaken, slower titration may be needed in some patients who experience adverse effects. In patients who experience intolerable adverse effects, the dosage may be decreased to as little as one-half of the fixed-combination tablet 3 times daily; however, an attempt should be made to titrate the dosage up once the adverse effects subside.

If the drugs are administered separately in the treatment of heart failure†, an initial dosage of isosorbide dinitrate 20–30 mg 3 or 4 times daily, given concomitantly with hydralazine hydrochloride 25–50 mg 3 or 4 times daily, is recommended by the American College of Cardiology Foundation (ACCF) and American Heart Association (AHA). Dosages of the drugs should be titrated to levels similar to those recommended for the fixed-combination preparation and administered at least 3 times daily. The maximum recommended dosages are isosorbide dinitrate 120 mg daily and hydralazine hydrochloride 300 mg daily.

Diffuse Esophageal Spasm In a limited number of patients with diffuse esophageal spasm without gastroesophageal reflux†, 10–30 mg of isosorbide dinitrate has been given orally 4 times daily.

Pharmacokinetics

■ **Absorption** Isosorbide dinitrate is readily (and almost completely) absorbed from the GI tract and oral mucosa, but considerable variations in the bioavailability of the drug (10–90%) have been reported as a result of extensive first-pass metabolism in the liver. The bioavailability of isosorbide dinitrate, as unchanged drug, following oral administration of conventional tablets (25%) generally appears to be about half that following sublingual administration (40–50%); however, in one study, systemic bioavailability of the drug was similar (about 29%) for both oral conventional tablets and sublingual tablets. It has been suggested that the reduced bioavailability of sublingual tablets of isosorbide dinitrate may result from swallowing a portion of the drug dissolved from such tablets, possibly because absorption of the drug is slow relative to the time that a sublingual dose might reasonably be retained in the mouth. Although multiple-dose studies of isosorbide dinitrate sublingual tablets have not been conducted, multiple-dose studies of isosorbide dinitrate oral conventional tablets indicate that progressive increases in bioavailability may occur during chronic therapy.

Although some evidence suggests that systemic bioavailability of isosorbide dinitrate from extended-release oral tablets is similar but slightly less than that from conventional oral tablets, other evidence suggests that considerable variability exists for various extended-release preparations and that some preparations may be substantially less bioavailable than conventional tablets. Because pharmacologic effects of the drug also depend on serum concentrations of active metabolites (e.g., isosorbide-5-mononitrate, isosorbide-2-mononitrate), comparisons should extend beyond systemic bioavailability of unchanged drug alone. Unfortunately, many studies do not specify or provide incomplete data on these metabolites. In addition, although most studies have employed single doses, the pharmacokinetics and/or bioavailability of the drug may be affected substantially during multiple dosing because the metabolites may decrease the metabolic clearance of isosorbide dinitrate; therefore, predictions based on single-dose studies are uncertain.

Although food may decrease substantially mean peak plasma concentrations of isosorbide dinitrate, total bioavailability of the drug does not seem to be affected.

Considerable interindividual variations (approximately 5- to 11-fold) in peak plasma concentrations attained have been reported with a specific oral dose of isosorbide dinitrate. Following administration of isosorbide dinitrate as sublingual or conventional oral tablets, peak plasma isosorbide dinitrate concentrations are reached in 10–15 or 60 minutes, respectively. Elevated blood concentrations of isosorbide dinitrate have been observed in patients with cirrhosis.

Isosorbide mononitrate also is readily absorbed from the GI tract. Because isosorbide mononitrate, unlike isosorbide dinitrate, does not undergo first-pass hepatic metabolism, the bioavailability of isosorbide mononitrate conventional or extended-release tablets is approximately 100 or 77–80%, respectively.

In general, food was found to delay the rate but not the extent of absorption (less than 10%) of conventional or extended-release isosorbide mononitrate tablets. Following oral administration of conventional or extended-release isosorbide mononitrate tablets, peak plasma concentrations of isosorbide mononitrate are achieved within 0.5–1 or about 3–4.5 hours, respectively. In one study, following oral administration of a 40-mg conventional isosorbide mononitrate tablet in fasted healthy individuals, mean peak plasma concentrations of about 930 ng/mL were achieved within about 1 hour. In addition, in another study, following oral administration of a 60- or 120-mg extended-release tablet of isosorbide mononitrate in healthy individuals, peak plasma concentrations of about 557 or 1151 ng/mL were achieved within about 3 hours, respectively.

Following oral administration of a single 40-mg dose of isosorbide dinitrate given in fixed combination with 75 mg of hydralazine hydrochloride (2 tablets of BiDil®) in a limited number of healthy adults, peak plasma isosorbide concentrations of 76 ng/mL per 65 kg were reached in 1 hour. The effect of food on the bioavailability of isosorbide dinitrate when administered in fixed combination with hydralazine hydrochloride is not known.

Although optimal therapeutic plasma concentrations have not been determined, it has been suggested that the therapeutic plasma concentration of isosorbide mononitrate (both for the management of angina and heart failure) is 100 ng/mL. In addition, evidence from clinical studies of isosorbide dinitrate and isosorbide mononitrate have shown that dosing regimens that result in plasma isosorbide mononitrate concentrations that fall below 100 ng/L prior to the administration of the next dose may be associated with a lower risk of developing tolerance.

The approximate onset and duration of action of various dosage forms of isosorbide dinitrate (ISDN) and isosorbide mononitrate (ISMN) are shown in Table 1 and Table 2.

Table 1. Antianginal Effects

Dosage Form	Onset	Duration
sublingual ISDN	within 3 min	2 h
chewable ISDN	within 3 min	2–2.5 h
oral ISDN	1 h	up to 8 h
oral ISMN	1 h	5–7 h
extended-release ISDN	1 h	8 h
extended-release ISMN	1 h	12 h

Table 2. Hemodynamic Effects

Dosage Form	Onset	Duration
sublingual ISDN	within 15–30 min	1.5–4 h
chewable ISDN	5 min	2–3 h
oral ISDN	within 20–60 min	4–6 h
oral ISMN	10–30 min	at least 6 h
extended-release ISDN	within 2 h	up to 12 h
extended-release ISMN	20–30 min	at least 6 h

The onset and duration of action following intrabuccal administration are probably similar to those after sublingual administration of isosorbide dinitrate; however, no studies are available.

■ **Distribution** Distribution of isosorbide dinitrate or isosorbide mononitrate into human body tissues and fluids has not been fully characterized. Once absorbed, isosorbide dinitrate is widely distributed into body tissues and fluids including smooth muscle cells of blood vessels with the apparent volume of distribution reported to be 2–4 L/kg in adults. Under steady-state conditions, substantial accumulation (relative to simultaneous plasma concentrations) of isosorbide dinitrate may occur in the pectoral muscle and saphenous vein walls. Following IV administration, isosorbide mononitrate is distributed into total body water in about 9 minutes with an apparent volume of distribution of approximately 0.6–0.7 L/kg in adults. Isosorbide mononitrate also is distributed into blood cells and saliva.

Isosorbide dinitrate and isosorbide mononitrate are approximately 28 and 4–5% bound to plasma proteins, respectively.

Although isosorbide dinitrate reportedly was detected in milk, it currently is not known if isosorbide dinitrate and isosorbide mononitrate are distributed into milk in humans.

■ **Elimination** The elimination half-life of isosorbide dinitrate is approximately 1 hour (although a longer half-life [about 2 hours] has been reported when administered in fixed combination with hydralazine hydrochloride). Isosorbide mononitrate has an elimination half-life of about 5 hours.

Isosorbide dinitrate is metabolized (denitrated) extensively; about 15–25 and 75–85% of a dose is metabolized to isosorbide-2-mononitrate and isosorbide-5-mononitrate (referred to simply as isosorbide mononitrate), respectively. Both metabolites are pharmacologically active, especially the isosorbide mononitrate.

Isosorbide mononitrate is metabolized principally in the liver, but unlike isosorbide dinitrate, it does not undergo first-pass metabolism. About 50% of a dose of isosorbide mononitrate undergoes denitration to form isosorbide, followed by partial dehydration to form sorbitol. Isosorbide mononitrate also appears to undergo glucuronidation to form the 5-mononitrate glucuronide. These metabolites apparently do not have pharmacologic activity.

After a single oral dose of isosorbide dinitrate, 80–100% of the amount is excreted in urine within 24 hours, chiefly as metabolites. Isosorbide mononitrate also is excreted mainly in the urine; compounds recovered in urine after isosorbide mononitrate administration have included isosorbide, sorbitol, and conjugates; only 2% of a dose is excreted as unchanged drug. About 96% of an administered dose of isosorbide mononitrate is excreted in urine and about 1% in feces within 5 days; most excretion (about 93%) occurs within 48 hours.

The plasma clearance of isosorbide dinitrate reportedly is 2–4 L/minute. Since plasma clearance exceeds hepatic blood flow, it appears that the drug also is metabolized at extrahepatic sites.

Renal clearance of isosorbide mononitrate accounts only for about 4% of total body clearance. Plasma clearance of isosorbide mononitrate does not appear to be affected by age, cardiac disease, or renal or hepatic impairment. Isosorbide mononitrate is substantially removed by hemodialysis.

Chemistry and Stability

■ **Chemistry** Isosorbide is commercially available as dinitrate and mononitrate organic salts. Organic nitrates (e.g., isosorbide dinitrate, isosorbide mononitrate) are powerful explosives that are rendered nonexplosive by the addition of an inert excipient such as lactose.

Isosorbide Dinitrate Isosorbide dinitrate occurs as a white to off-white, crystalline powder. Isosorbide dinitrate is sparingly soluble in water and freely soluble in alcohol. The drug is diluted with lactose, mannitol, or other suitable inert excipients to permit safe handling. Diluted isosorbide dinitrate occurs as an ivory-white, odorless powder.

Isosorbide dinitrate is commercially available as conventional tablets (e.g., Sorbitrate® and Isordil® Titradose®), extended-release capsules (e.g., Dilatrate®-SR), extended-release tablets, and sublingual-intrabuccal (e.g., Isordil®) tablets. The commercially available extended-release capsules of isosorbide dinitrate (Dilatrate-SR®) contain the drug in a microdialysis membrane delivery system that slowly releases the drug.

Isosorbide Mononitrate Isosorbide mononitrate is the major active metabolite of isosorbide dinitrate. Isosorbide mononitrate occurs as a white, crystalline, odorless powder, and is freely soluble in water and alcohol.

The drug is commercially available as conventional (e.g., Monoket®, Ismo®) or extended-release (e.g., Imdur®) tablets. The commercially available extended-release isosorbide mononitrate tablets contain the drug in an insoluble matrix designed for extended release. Isosorbide mononitrate also may be available as extended-release capsules (not commercially available in the US) that contain 30% of the drug in an immediate-release layer and the remaining 70% in controlled-release coated pellets.

■ **Stability** ***Isosorbide Dinitrate*** Isosorbide dinitrate tablets should be stored in tight, light-resistant containers at room temperature (25°C) and should not be exposed to extremes in temperature. Commercially available fixed-combination tablets of isosorbide dinitrate and hydralazine hydrochloride should be stored in tight, light-resistant containers at a controlled room temperature of 25°C but may be exposed to temperatures ranging from 15–30°C.

Isosorbide Mononitrate Some isosorbide mononitrate extended-release (Imdur®) and conventional tablets (Ismo®) should be stored in tight, light-resistant containers at 20–25°C; however, other conventional tablets of isosorbide mononitrate (e.g., Monoket®) should be stored in tight, light-resistant containers at 15–30°C.

For further information on chemistry and stability, pharmacology, pharmacokinetics, uses, cautions, drug interactions, laboratory test interferences, and dosage and administration of isosorbide dinitrate, see the Nitrates and Nitrites General Statement 24:12.08.

Preparations

Excipients in commercially available drug preparations may have clinically important effects in some individuals; consult specific product labeling for details.

Isosorbide Dinitrate

Oral		
Capsules, extended-release	40 mg	**Dilatrate®-SR,** Schwarz
Tablets	5 mg*	**Isordil® Titradose®** (scored), Biovail
		Isosorbide Dinitrate Tablets
	10 mg*	**Isosorbide Dinitrate Tablets**
	20 mg*	**Isosorbide Dinitrate Tablets**
	30 mg*	**Isosorbide Dinitrate Tablets**
	40 mg*	**Isordil® Titradose®** (scored), Biovail
Tablets, extended-release	40 mg*	**Isosorbide Dinitrate Tablets ER**
Sublingual (Intrabuccal)		
Tablets	2.5 mg*	**Isosorbide Dinitrate Tablets**
	5 mg*	**Isosorbide Dinitrate Tablets**

*available from one or more manufacturer, distributor, and/or repackager by generic (nonproprietary) name

Isosorbide Mononitrate

Oral		
Tablets	10 mg*	**Isosorbide Mononitrate Tablets**
		Monoket® (scored), Schwarz
	20 mg*	**Isosorbide Mononitrate Tablets**
		Monoket® (scored), Schwarz

Tablets, extended-release	30 mg*	**Imdur®** (scored), Schering-Plough
		Isosorbide Mononitrate Tablets ER
	60 mg*	**Imdur®** (scored), Schering-Plough
		Isosorbide Mononitrate Tablets ER
	120 mg*	**Imdur®**, Schering-Plough
		Isosorbide Mononitrate Tablets ER
Tablets, extended-release, film-coated	20 mg	**Ismo®**, ESP Pharma

*available from one or more manufacturer, distributor, and/or repackager by generic (nonproprietary) name

Isosorbide Dinitrate Combinations

Oral		
Tablets, film-coated	20 mg with Hydralazine Hydrochloride 37.5 mg	**BiDil®** (scored), NitroMed

†Use is not currently included in the labeling approved by the US Food and Drug Administration

Nitric Oxide

Nitrogen Oxide

■ Nitric oxide is a vasodilating agent.

Uses

■ **Neonatal Hypoxic Respiratory Failure** Nitric oxide gas is used in conjunction with ventilatory support and other appropriate therapy to improve oxygenation and reduce the need for extracorporeal membrane oxygenation (ECMO) in term or near-term (exceeding 34 weeks of age) neonates with hypoxic respiratory failure and clinical or ECG evidence of pulmonary hypertension. Results from 2 comparative clinical trials in term or near-term neonates who had hypoxic respiratory failure with or without pulmonary hypertension indicate that inhaled nitric oxide gas (20 ppm mixed with either 100% oxygen or nitrogen) improved the arterial partial pressure of oxygen (PaO_2) and decreased the need for extracorporeal membrane oxygenation at 30 or 120 days compared with ventilatory support and supplemental oxygen or nitrogen (placebo) gas alone. In these neonates, hypoxic respiratory failure was caused by idiopathic persistent pulmonary hypertension of the newborn (PPHN) or associated with a variety of other underlying conditions (e.g., meconium aspiration syndrome, pneumonia with or without sepsis, respiratory distress syndrome, pulmonary hypoplasia associated with congenital diaphragmatic hernia) and in many cases had not responded adequately to conventional therapy (e.g., vasodilators, IV fluids, bicarbonate therapy, mechanical ventilation). The need for extracorporeal membrane oxygenation was decreased from 55–57% with placebo or oxygen alone to 31–39% with inhaled nitric oxide. In addition, improvement in hypoxemia (as measured by an increase in PaO_2, a decrease in oxygenation index [mean airway pressure in cm of water × fraction of inspired oxygen concentration × 100/PaO_2 in mm Hg], or in the alveolar-arterial oxygen gradient) was greater in neonates receiving inhaled nitric oxide. Nitric oxide therapy reduced the combined incidence of death and/or need for extracorporeal membrane oxygenation in these studies but had no effect on mortality alone. Long-term follow-up data from one of these clinical trials indicate that neurodevelopmental, behavioral, or medical abnormalities were not increased in patients receiving inhaled nitric oxide at 18–24 months of age.

Similar beneficial effects (i.e., reduction in combined incidence of death and chronic lung disease) were observed in premature neonates† (less than 34 weeks' gestation) who were undergoing mechanical ventilation for respiratory distress syndrome in a randomized, double-blind, placebo-controlled study. However, the manufacturer states that the drug currently is not indicated in this age group. Nitric oxide therapy also decreased the incidence of severe intraventricular hemorrhage and periventricular leukomalacia, the principal cause of serious, long-term disability in this patient population.

Available data suggest that inhaled nitric oxide is most effective in patients with severe persistent pulmonary hypertension who have minimal underlying parenchymal lung disease (idiopathic persistent pulmonary hypertension) and least effective in neonates with pulmonary hypoplasia (e.g., congenital diaphragmatic hernia). In a large clinical trial, treatment failure (defined as no response to a dosage of 20 or 80 ppm of nitric oxide and/or an absolute decrease in oxygen saturation exceeding 10%) occurred in 34% of term or near-term neonates with respiratory failure and persistent pulmonary hypertension receiving nitric oxide (20 ppm).

Dosage and Administration

■ **General** The recommended initial inhalation dosage of nitric oxide gas in term or near-term neonates (those exceeding 34 weeks of age) for the treatment of hypoxic respiratory failure associated with pulmonary hypertension is 20 ppm given continuously for up to for 14 days or until the underlying oxygen desaturation has resolved and the patient is ready to be weaned from therapy. Inhaled nitric oxide should be used in conjunction with mechanical ventilation and other supportive therapy to maximize oxygen delivery. In clinical trials, the safety and efficacy of inhaled nitric oxide were established in neonates with respiratory failure receiving conventional treatment, such as vasodilators (e.g., tolazoline, sodium nitroprusside), IV fluids for volume support, bicarbonate therapy for induction of alkalosis, and mechanical ventilation. In neonates with collapsed alveoli, additional therapies to improve lung expansion have included pulmonary surfactant replacement and high-frequency oscillatory ventilation.

Precise monitoring of nitrogen dioxide, nitric oxide, and oxygen (PaO_2) concentrations should be performed in neonates receiving inhaled nitric oxide therapy, using a nitric oxide delivery system that does not cause generation of excessive nitrogen dioxide and with appropriate alarms. Monitoring of nitric oxide inhalation therapy also should include periodic measurement of methemoglobin and continuous monitoring of nitrogen dioxide, nitric oxide, and oxygen concentrations. (See Methemoglobinemia and also see Environmental Exposure to Nitrogen Dioxide and Nitric Oxide in General Precautions, under Warnings/Precautions in Cautions.)

In several clinical trials, the median duration of treatment with inhaled nitric oxide ranged from 5–60 hours (i.e., generally less than 5 days); however, therapy has been continued for up to 2 weeks in some studies. Following improvement in oxygenation with the initial dosage of nitric oxide, reduction in the dosage to smaller maintenance dosages (5–6 ppm) has been used. If the patient fails to respond to an initial inhaled dosage of 20 ppm of nitric oxide, higher than recommended dosages (e.g., 40–80 ppm) generally have not provided additional benefit but have been associated with an increased incidence of adverse effects, and the manufacturer states that dosages above 20 ppm ordinarily should not be used.

■ **Weaning and Discontinuance of Therapy** Weaning and discontinuance of nitric oxide therapy generally have been performed in neonates who had adequate oxygenation (as measured by a PaO_2 of greater than 50–60 mm Hg, an increase in PaO_2 from baseline exceeding 20 mm Hg, oxygen saturation exceeding 92%, lack of appreciable oxygen gradient through the ductus arteriosus or foramen ovale, requirement for an inspired oxygen concentration fraction [FiO_2] less than 0.60), and a mean airway pressure less than 10 cm of water. Nitric oxide therapy should not be discontinued abruptly since neonates may experience signs of withdrawal, such as an increase in pulmonary artery pressure, oxygen desaturation, and/or systemic hypotension. Several weaning regimens have been used to minimize withdrawal manifestations, including discontinuance of nitric oxide after successful maintenance of oxygenation at a reduced dosage (5– 6 ppm) and stepwise reduction in the dosage in increments as little as 1 ppm. In neonates with clinical deterioration during the weaning period, the nitric oxide dosage and/or FiO_2 have been increased transiently. In a clinical trial in neonates with deterioration after discontinuance of nitric oxide therapy, such therapy was reinstituted temporarily at the last dosage used. For information regarding management of inhaled nitric oxide withdrawal in neonates, see Drug Interactions: Nitric Oxide and Its Donors, in Sildenafil 24:12.12.

Cautions

■ **Contraindications** Neonates dependent on extrapulmonary right-to-left shunting of blood (e.g., ductal-dependent congenital heart disease). (See Uses: Ductus Arteriosus-dependent Congenital Heart Disease, in Alprostadil 24:12.92.)

■ **Warnings/Precautions** ***General Precautions*** **Withdrawal of Therapy.** Abrupt discontinuance of nitric oxide therapy can result in oxygen desaturation and a rebound increase in pulmonary artery pressure. Such manifestations also can occur in neonates who do not respond to inhaled nitric oxide therapy. Hypoxemia and hypotension during acute withdrawal from the drug have been reported during postmarketing experience. To minimize adverse effects associated with withdrawal of inhaled nitric oxide therapy, neonates should be weaned from therapy by a gradual reduction in dosage and should be monitored for evidence of deterioration during and after weaning. (See Dosage and Administration: General Dosage.) The nitric oxide delivery system should include a backup battery power supply to ensure continuous administration of the drug during a power failure.

Methemoglobinemia. Methemoglobin is an end product of nitric oxide disposition in the body, and blood methemoglobin concentrations are dose-dependent. Methemoglobinemia appears to occur infrequently with usual recommended dosages of nitric oxide (e.g., 20 ppm), but was observed in 35% of neonates in one study who received a higher dosage (80 ppm). Following dosage adjustment or discontinuance of nitric oxide in clinical studies, methemoglobin concentrations generally returned to baseline within several hours. Methemoglobin blood concentrations should be monitored periodically during inhaled nitric oxide therapy (e.g., within 4 hours of initiating therapy and daily thereafter). Methemoglobinemia that does not resolve after adjustment of nitric oxide dosage may be treated with IV vitamin C, IV methylene blue, or blood transfusion as clinically appropriate.

Environmental Exposure to Nitrogen Dioxide and Nitric Oxide. Nitrogen dioxide, formed from the combination of oxygen and nitric oxide, interacts with oxyhemoglobin to form methemoglobin; exposure to elevated nitrogen dioxide concentrations also can cause acute lung injury. In neonates receiving nitric oxide at recommended dosages (e.g., 20 ppm), only a small amount of nitrogen dioxide (less than 0.5 ppm) is formed; however, in a study in which a larger dosage of nitric oxide (80 ppm) was administered, the mean peak concentration of nitrogen dioxide was 2.6 ppm. In a study evaluating exposure of intensive-care unit staff to nitrogen oxides during administration of nitric oxide therapy (20 ppm) to pediatric patients, exposures to nitrogen dioxide were below the ceiling limit of 5 ppm for the entire work shift, and below the 15-minute exposure of 1 ppm established by the Occupational, Safety and Health Administration (OSHA) and the National Institute for Occupational Safety and Health (NIOSH), respectively. In clinical studies, nitrogen dioxide concentrations exceeding 3 ppm were treated by reduction in the dosage or discontinuance of nitric oxide.

Headaches associated with environmental exposure to nitric oxide have been reported by hospital staff during postmarketing experience. OSHA has set an exposure limit of 25 ppm for nitric oxide.

Specific Populations **Pregnancy.** Category C. (See Users Guide.) The manufacturer of INOmax® states that the drug is not intended for use in adults.

Lactation. Not known whether nitric oxide is distributed in milk; use not indicated in nursing women.

Pediatric Use. The manufacturer states that use in neonates older than 14 days or younger than 34 weeks of gestational age currently not indicated. However, there is evidence from a randomized, double-blind, placebo-controlled study of beneficial effects in premature neonates (younger than 34 weeks' gestation) with respiratory distress syndrome who received inhaled nitric oxide therapy while undergoing mechanical ventilation.

Adult Respiratory Distress Syndrome (ARDS). The manufacturer states that inhaled nitric oxide is not indicated in patients with ARDS.

■ **Common Adverse Effects** Adverse effects occurring in 5% or more of patients receiving nitric oxide include hypotension, withdrawal manifestations (e.g., increased pulmonary artery pressure, decreased partial pressure of arterial oxygen (PaO_2), increase in or return to right-to-left shunting of blood, atelectasis, hematuria, hyperglycemia, sepsis, infection, stridor, and cellulitis.

Drug Interactions

No formal drug interaction studies performed.

■ **Nitric Oxide Donor Compounds** Potential pharmacologic interaction (increased risk of methemoglobinemia) when nitric oxide is used with nitric oxide donor compounds (e.g., sodium nitroprusside, nitroglycerin).

■ **Prilocaine** Potential pharmacologic interaction (increased risk of methemoglobinemia) when nitric oxide is used with prilocaine (topical, parenteral formulations).

Description

Nitric oxide is a vasodilating agent. The commercially available gas for inhalation is a mixture of nitric oxide (100 or 800 ppm) and nitrogen.

Endogenous nitric oxide is produced by many cells of the body and relaxes smooth muscle by increasing intracellular levels of cyclic guanosine 3′,5′-monophosphate (cGMP), which lowers intracellular calcium concentrations and results in vasodilation. When inhaled as a gas, nitric oxide diffuses from the alveoli into vascular smooth muscle and causes selective pulmonary vasodilation.

Persistent pulmonary hypertension of the newborn (PPHN) is a developmental defect or acquired condition in which pulmonary vascular resistance is high, resulting in right-to-left shunting of blood through the patent ductus arteriosus and foramen ovale and subsequent hypoxemia. Exogenously administered nitric oxide gas appears to increase the partial pressure of arterial oxygen (PaO_2) by dilating pulmonary vessels in better ventilated areas of the lung, thereby redistributing pulmonary blood flow away from regions with poor gas exchange (as indicated by ventilation/perfusion ratios) toward regions with better gas exchange. When inhaled, nitric oxide is rapidly metabolized; thus, the inhaled drug does not affect systemic vascular resistance. The metabolic products of nitric oxide that reach systemic circulation are predominantly methemoglobin and nitrate. (See General Precautions: Methemoglobinemia, under Warnings/Precautions in Cautions.)

Overview® (see Users Guide). For additional information on this drug until a more detailed monograph is developed and published, the manufacturer's labeling should be consulted. It is *essential* that the manufacturer's labeling be consulted for more detailed information on usual cautions, precautions, contraindications, potential drug interactions, laboratory test interferences, and acute toxicity.

Preparations

Excipients in commercially available drug preparations may have clinically important effects in some individuals; consult specific product labeling for details.

Nitric Oxide

Oral Inhalation

Gas	100 ppm	**INOmax®**, INO Therapeutics
	800 ppm	**INOmax®**, INO Therapeutics

†Use is not currently included in the labeling approved by the US Food and Drug Administration

Nitroglycerin

Glyceryl Trinitrate, Nitroglycerol

■ Nitroglycerin, an organic nitrate, is a vasodilating agent.

Uses

■ **Chronic Stable Angina** Nitroglycerin shares the actions of other nitrates and nitrites and is used for the acute relief of angina pectoris secondary to coronary artery disease, for prophylactic management in situations likely to provoke angina attacks, and for long-term prophylactic management of chronic stable angina. Sublingual nitroglycerin is considered the drug of choice for the acute relief of angina pectoris, because it has a rapid onset of action, is inexpensive, and its efficacy is well established. (See Uses: Chronic Stable Angina, in the Nitrates and Nitrites General Statement 24:12.08).

■ **Hypertension** IV nitroglycerin is used to control blood pressure in perioperative hypertension, especially hypertension associated with cardiovascular procedures; to control blood pressure in patients with severe hypertension† or in hypertensive crises† for the immediate reduction of blood pressure in patients in whom such reduction is considered an emergency (hypertensive emergencies), especially those associated with coronary complications (e.g., coronary ischemia, acute coronary insufficiency, acute left ventricular failure, postoperative hypertension [especially following coronary bypass surgery]) and/or acute pulmonary edema; and to produce controlled hypotension during surgical procedures.

Hypertensive emergencies are those rare situations requiring immediate blood pressure reduction, although not necessarily to normal ranges, in order to prevent or limit target organ damage. Examples of such emergency situations include hypertensive encephalopathy, intracerebral hemorrhage, unstable angina pectoris, acute myocardial infarction (MI), acute left ventricular failure with pulmonary edema, dissecting aortic aneurysm, and eclampsia. Elevated blood pressure alone, in the absence of symptoms or new or progressive target organ damage, rarely is a hypertensive crisis requiring emergency therapy.

■ **Non-ST-Segment-Elevation Acute Coronary Syndromes** Nitroglycerin is used in the management of non-ST-segment-elevation acute coronary syndromes (NSTE ACS). Patients with NSTE ACS have either unstable angina or non-ST-segment-elevation MI (NSTEMI); because these conditions are part of a continuum of acute myocardial ischemia and have indistinguishable clinical features upon presentation, the same initial treatment strategies are recommended. The American Heart Association/American College of Cardiology (AHA/ACC) guideline for the management of patients with NSTE ACS recommends sublingual nitroglycerin (0.3–0.4 mg every 5 minutes for up to 3 doses) for the relief of ongoing ischemic pain in patients with NSTE ACS; IV nitroglycerin may be used in patients with persistent ischemia who do not respond to sublingual therapy and administration of a β-blocker or those with heart failure or hypertension. (See Uses: Non-ST-Segment-Elevation Acute Coronary Syndromes, in the Nitrates and Nitrites General Statement 24:12.08.)

■ **Acute Myocardial Infarction** Nitroglycerin is used in the management of acute MI, generally in patients with hypertension or heart failure. (See Uses: Acute Myocardial Infarction, in the Nitrates and Nitrites General Statement 24:12.08.) Sublingual nitroglycerin has been administered for the initial relief of ischemic discomfort in patients with acute MI. However, the manufacturer states that the benefits of sublingual nitroglycerin in patients with acute MI have not been established; if the drug is used in this setting, careful hemodynamic and clinical monitoring is essential because of the possibility of hypotension and tachycardia. IV nitroglycerin may be used in patients with acute MI who have ongoing chest pain, hypertension, or heart failure. In addition to potentially alleviating ischemic myocardial pain, beneficial hemodynamic effects of nitroglycerin include vasodilation of the coronary arteries (especially at or near the site of recent plaque disruption), peripheral arteries, and venous capacitance vessels; however, the drug generally does not reduce myocardial injury associated with epicardial coronary artery occlusion unless there is substantial vasospasm. Although studies conducted prior to the routine use of reperfusion therapy suggested a mortality benefit with nitrates in patients with acute MI, this benefit was not confirmed in 2 large randomized controlled studies.

The American College of Cardiology Foundation/American Heart Association (ACCF/AHA) guideline for the management of STEMI states that IV nitroglycerin may be beneficial in patients with STEMI and heart failure or hypertension. These experts state that there is no role for the routine use of oral nitrates during the convalescent phase of STEMI. For recommendations on the management of NSTEMI, see Uses: Non-ST-Segment-Elevation Acute Coronary Syndromes. For precautions associated with the use of nitroglycerin in patients with acute MI, see Uses: Acute Myocardial Infarction and also see Cautions: Precautions and Contraindications, in the Nitrates and Nitrites General Statement 24:12.08.

■ **Heart Failure and Low-output Syndromes** IV nitroglycerin has been used effectively for the treatment of acutely decompensated (e.g., congestive) heart failure† or other low cardiac output states†, including those associated with acute MI. The precipitating cause of acute heart failure decompensation should be carefully assessed to inform appropriate treatment, optimize outcomes, and prevent future acute events in patients with heart failure. Current guidelines for the management of heart failure in adults generally recommend inhibition of the renin-angiotensin-aldosterone system with a combination of drug therapies, including neurohormonal antagonists (e.g., angiotensin-converting enzyme [ACE] inhibitors, angiotensin II receptor antagonists, angiotensin receptor-neprilysin inhibitors [ARNIs], β-adrenergic blocking agents [β-blockers], aldosterone receptor antagonists), to inhibit the detrimental compensatory mechanisms in heart failure and reduce morbidity and mortality. (See Uses: Heart Failure in Carvedilol 24:24 and in Sacubitril and Valsartan 24:32.92.) IV vasodilators have not been shown to improve outcomes in patients hospitalized for heart failure; however, in the absence of symptomatic hypotension, IV nitroglycerin may be considered as an adjunct to diuretic therapy for relief of dyspnea in patients hospitalized for acutely decompensated heart failure. IV nitroglycerin causes venodilation, which lowers preload and may help to rapidly reduce pulmonary congestion. Patients with heart failure and hypertension, coronary ischemia, or substantial mitral regurgitation are often considered ideal candidates for the use of IV nitroglycerin. However, tachyphylaxis to nitroglycerin may develop within 24 hours, and up to 20% of those with heart failure may have inadequate response to even high doses. (See Uses: Heart Failure and Low-output Syndromes, in the Nitrates and Nitrites General Statement 24:12.08.)

■ **Chronic Anal Fissure** For topical (intra-anal) use of nitroglycerin 0.4% ointment in the treatment of chronic anal fissures, see Nitroglycerin 84:92.

Dosage and Administration

■ **Administration** Nitroglycerin is administered lingually, sublingually, intrabuccally, orally, topically, or by IV infusion. Intracoronary injection of nitroglycerin infusions has not been studied.

Nitroglycerin tablets for sublingual administration are dissolved under the tongue or in the buccal pouch and should not be swallowed. Nitroglycerin sublingual powder also should be allowed to dissolve under the tongue and not swallowed. Nitroglycerin lingual preparations (aerosol or solution in a spray pump) should be administered onto or under the tongue and not inhaled. The possibility that lingual, sublingual, or intrabuccal nitroglycerin may be inadequately absorbed, with resultant decreased efficacy, in patients with dry oral mucous membranes (e.g., xerostomia) should be considered. In addition, the patient should be sitting immediately after lingual, sublingual, or intrabuccal administration of nitroglycerin. The manufacturers' prescribing information should be consulted for additional details on administration of individual nitroglycerin preparations.

For IV infusion, nitroglycerin should be administered via a controlled-infusion device that maintains a constant infusion rate. The commercially available injection concentrate must be diluted in 5% dextrose or 0.9% sodium chloride injection before administration. Nitroglycerin also is commercially available as a premixed solution in 5% dextrose injection for IV administration. *Because nitroglycerin readily migrates into many plastics, the manufacturers' specific instructions for dilution, dosage, and administration must be carefully followed.* (See Chemistry and Stability: Stability.)

Nitroglycerin transdermal system is preferably applied at the same time each day to areas of clean, dry, hairless skin of the upper arm or body; the system should not be applied to the extremities below the knee or elbow. Skin areas with irritation, extensive scarring, or calluses should be avoided, and application sites should be rotated to avoid causing skin irritation. *Nitroglycerin transdermal systems should be removed from the site(s) of application prior to attempting defibrillation or cardioversion since altered electrical conductivity and enhanced potential for electrical arcing may occur.*

When applied topically as an ointment, the appropriate amount of nitroglycerin ointment should be squeezed onto the manufacturer-supplied applicator and placed ointment side down on the desired non-hairy area of skin (usually on the chest or back). The ointment is then spread on the skin area in a thin, uniform layer without massaging or rubbing and using the applicator to prevent absorption of the ointment through the fingers. Using the size of the applicator to measure the coverage area allows the ointment to be absorbed through a smaller area of skin than that used in clinical trials; the clinical importance of this difference is not known. The applicator should be taped into place after application. To protect clothing, plastic wrap held in place by an elastic bandage, hosiery, or tape may be used to cover the ointment applicator. Application of the ointment over the chest may provide an additional psychological effect. As with transdermal nitroglycerin systems, nitroglycerin ointment has been reported to alter electrical conductivity, and some clinicians suggest that areas of the chest where defibrillation paddles typically are placed not be used for application of the ointment if possible.

■ **Dosage** Dosage of nitroglycerin must be carefully adjusted according to the patient's requirements and response and the smallest effective dosage should be used. When nitroglycerin is administered IV, the type of IV administration set used, polyvinyl chloride (PVC) or non-PVC, must be considered in dosage estimations. *It should be noted that dosages commonly used in early published studies were based on the use of PVC administration sets and are too high when non-PVC administration sets are used.*

Continuous monitoring of blood pressure and heart rate, as well as other appropriate parameters (e.g., pulmonary capillary wedge pressure), must be performed in all patients. Adequate systemic blood pressure and coronary perfusion pressure must be maintained. Some patients with normal or low left ventricular filling pressures or pulmonary capillary wedge pressure may be extremely sensitive to the effects of IV nitroglycerin and may respond fully to dosages as low as 5 mcg/minute; these patients require particularly careful monitoring and dosage titration.

For dosage of topical (intra-anal) nitroglycerin 0.4% ointment in the treatment of chronic anal fissure, see Nitroglycerin 84:92.

Chronic Stable Angina **Lingual Dosage.** For the acute relief of angina pectoris or for prophylactic management in situations likely to provoke angina attacks, nitroglycerin may be administered onto or under the tongue using a metered-dose spray pump or aerosol container. The spray pump or aerosol container must be primed, but not shaken, prior to first use or after a period of nonuse (i.e., 6 weeks or more) according to the manufacturers' instructions.

Commercially available nitroglycerin lingual solution in a spray pump delivers about 60 or 200 metered sprays per 4.9- or 14.6-g bottle, respectively; when properly primed, each metered spray delivers 0.4 mg of nitroglycerin. Commercially available nitroglycerin lingual aerosol delivers about 90 or 230 metered sprays per 4.1- or 8.5-g bottle, respectively; when properly primed, each metered spray delivers 0.4 mg of nitroglycerin. To administer these preparations, the spray pump or aerosol container should be held upright with the valve head uppermost and the spray orifice as close to the opened mouth as possible. To release a spray, the valve head is pressed with the forefinger. The dose should be sprayed onto or under the tongue and then the mouth immediately closed; *the spray should not be inhaled.* In addition, the drug should not be expectorated nor the mouth rinsed for 5–10 minutes following administration of the drug.

For the acute relief of angina pectoris, 1 or 2 sprays (0.4 or 0.8 mg, respectively) of nitroglycerin as a lingual solution or aerosol may be administered. If relief is not attained after the initial spray(s), additional single sprays may be given at 5-minute intervals as necessary; no more than 3 sprays should be given in a 15-minute period. If pain persists after a total of 3 doses within a 15-minute period, prompt medical attention is recommended. Nitroglycerin lingual solution or aerosol also may be used prophylactically 5–10 minutes before situations likely to provoke angina attacks.

Sublingual Dosage. For the acute relief of angina pectoris, the manufacturer recommends 0.3–0.6 mg of nitroglycerin as sublingual tablets, placed under the tongue or in the buccal pouch and allowed to dissolve at the first sign of an acute attack. Most patients respond within 5 minutes of taking 1 or 2 doses. If relief is not attained after a single dose during an acute attack, additional doses may be given at 5-minute intervals. If chest pain persists after a total of 3 doses within a 15-minute period, or if the pain is different from the pain that is typically experienced, patients should be advised to seek prompt medical attention. For prophylactic management in situations likely to provoke angina attacks, nitroglycerin sublingual tablets may be administered 5–10 minutes prior to engaging in such activities.

If nitroglycerin sublingual powder is used for the acute relief of angina, the manufacturer recommends administering 1 or 2 packets (containing a dose of 0.4 or 0.8 mg of nitroglycerin, respectively) at the onset of an attack. To administer the sublingual powder, the contents of 1 or 2 packets should be placed under the tongue and not swallowed; patients should immediately close their mouth, breathe normally, and allow the powder to dissolve. The drug should not be expectorated nor the mouth rinsed for 5 minutes following administration of the drug. If relief is not attained after the initial dose, an additional packet (0.4 mg of nitroglycerin) may be given every 5 minutes as needed up to a total of 3 packets within a 15-minute period. If chest pain does not improve or worsens after administering a total of 3 packets, patients should be advised to seek immediate medical attention. For prophylactic management in situations likely to provoke angina attacks, nitroglycerin sublingual powder may be administered 5–10 minutes prior to engaging in such activities.

Oral Dosage. For long-term prophylactic management of angina pectoris, 2.5–6.5 mg of nitroglycerin as extended-release capsules has been administered 3–4 times daily as an initial dosage in clinical studies, with subsequent titration based on patient response and adverse effects. To minimize the occurrence of tolerance, a nitrate-free interval is recommended; however, the minimum nitrate-free interval necessary for restoration of the full effects of nitroglycerin extended-release capsules has not been determined. Studies with other nitroglycerin formulations suggest that 10–14 hours may be sufficient.

Because the onset of action of extended-release nitroglycerin formulations is not sufficiently rapid to abort acute attacks of angina, such formulations should *not* be used to treat acute attacks of angina.

Topical Dosage. When a nitroglycerin transdermal system is used for the long-term prophylactic management of angina pectoris, the usual initial adult dosage is one transdermal dosage system, delivering the smallest available dose of nitroglycerin in its dosage series, applied every 24 hours. To minimize the occurrence of tolerance to the effects of nitroglycerin, a nitrate-free interval of 10–14 hours has been recommended; however, the minimum nitrate-free interval necessary for restoration of full first-dose effects of nitrate therapy has not been determined. (See Cautions: Tolerance and Dependence, in the Nitrates and Nitrites General Statement 24:12.08.) Dosage may be adjusted by changing to the next larger dosage system in the series or by a combination of dosage systems in the series. The transdermal systems should *not* be used to treat acute attacks of angina.

When nitroglycerin is applied topically as an ointment, a suggested initial dosage is 0.5 inch (as squeezed from the tube) of the 2% ointment (i.e., approximately 7.5 mg) applied twice daily (once upon arising in the morning and repeated 6 hours later). When the dose to be applied is in multiples of whole inches, unit-dose preparations that provide the equivalent of 1 inch of the 2% ointment also may be used. The initial dose may be doubled (i.e., increased to

1 inch or approximately 15 mg) and subsequently doubled again (i.e., increased to 2 inches or approximately 30 mg) if tolerated in patients failing to respond adequately. Doses used in clinical trials have ranged from 0.5–2 inches (approximately 7.5–30 mg). Dosage should be titrated upward until angina is effectively controlled or adverse effects preclude further dosage increases.

The amount of nitroglycerin reaching the circulation varies directly with the size of the area of application and the amount of ointment applied. Coverage of an area approximately the size of the applicator (3.5 by 2.25 inches) should be sufficient to obtain the desired clinical effects, however, a larger area may be used. In clinical trials, the ointment generally has been spread over an area of 6 by 6 inches.

As with other nitroglycerin formulations, all regimens of nitroglycerin ointment should include a daily nitrate-free interval to avoid development of tolerance. (See Cautions: Tolerance and Dependence, in the Nitrates and Nitrites General Statement 24:12.08.) It is not known whether nitroglycerin ointment is effective in preventing exertional angina for longer than 7 hours after application of a dose. The efficacy of repeated applications of the ointment for the long-term management of angina pectoris has not been established.

The onset of action of topical nitroglycerin ointment is not sufficiently rapid to treat acute attacks of angina; therefore, the ointment should *not* be used for this purpose.

IV Dosage. For the treatment of angina in patients who have not responded to sublingual nitroglycerin and β-adrenergic blocking agents (β-blockers), the recommended initial adult IV dosage when non- PVC administration sets are used is 5 mcg/minute, with increases of 5 mcg/minute every 3–5 minutes until a blood pressure response is obtained or until the infusion rate is 20 mcg/minute. If no effect is obtained with 20 mcg/minute, dosage may be increased by increments of 10 mcg/minute and if later necessary, by increments of 20 mcg/minute. When PVC administration sets are used, higher dosages generally are required; the usual initial adult dosage when these sets are used is 25 mcg/minute. Dosage is then titrated according to the response and tolerance of the patient.

Non-ST-Segment-Elevation Acute Coronary Syndromes **Sublingual Dosage.** For the treatment of continuing ischemic pain in patients with non-ST-segment-elevation acute coronary syndromes (NSTE ACS), sublingual nitroglycerin 0.3–0.4 mg every 5 minutes for up to 3 doses is recommended.

IV Dosage. Following use of sublingual nitroglycerin, the need for IV nitroglycerin should be assessed, if not contraindicated; experts state that IV nitroglycerin may be useful in patients with heart failure, hypertension, or persistent ischemia not relieved with sublingual nitroglycerin and administration of a β-blocker.

The recommended initial adult IV dosage of nitroglycerin when a nonadsorptive (e.g., non-PVC) administration set is used is 5 mcg/minute, with increases of 5 mcg/minute every 3–5 minutes until a blood pressure response is obtained or until the infusion rate is 20 mcg/minute. If no effect is obtained with 20 mcg/minute, dosage may be increased by increments of 10 mcg/minute and, if necessary, by increments of 20 mcg/minute. When a PVC administration set is used, higher dosages generally are required; the usual initial adult dosage when these sets are used is 25 mcg/minute. Dosage should be titrated according to the patient's response. Blood pressure and heart rate should be continuously monitored during IV administration.

Hypertension **IV Dosage.** When nitroglycerin is used to control perioperative hypertension or for the induction of intraoperative hypotension, the manufacturer recommends an initial adult IV dosage (using a nonadsorptive [e.g., non-PVC] administration set) of 5 mcg/minute, with increases of 5 mcg/minute every 3–5 minutes until a blood pressure response is obtained or an infusion rate of 20 mcg/minute is reached. If no effect is obtained with 20 mcg/minute, dosage may be increased by increments of 10 mcg/minute and, if necessary, by increments of 20 mcg/minute. When a PVC administration set is used, higher dosages generally are required; an initial infusion rate of 25 mcg/minute or greater has been used in studies employing PVC tubing. Dosage should be titrated according to the patient's response and possible adverse effects. Blood pressure and heart rate should be continuously monitored during IV administration; in many cases, invasive monitoring of pulmonary capillary wedge pressure is indicated.

When nitroglycerin is used IV in hypertensive emergencies†, some experts recommend an initial adult dosage of 5 mcg/minute, with increases of 5 mcg/minute every 3–5 minutes up to a maximum of 20 mcg/minute. Adults with a hypertensive emergency *with* a compelling indication (e.g., eclampsia or severe preeclampsia or pheochromocytoma crisis) should have their systolic blood pressure reduced to less than 140 mm Hg during the first hour and, in patients with acute aortic dissection, to less than 120 mm Hg within the first 20 minutes.

The risks of overly aggressive therapy in any hypertensive crisis must always be considered. The initial goal of IV nitroglycerin therapy for a hypertensive emergency in adults *without* a compelling indication is to reduce systolic blood pressure by no more than 25% within the first hour, followed by further blood pressure reduction *if stable* to 160/110 or 160/100 mm Hg within the next 2–6 hours, avoiding excessive declines in pressure that could precipitate renal, cerebral, or coronary ischemia. If this blood pressure is well tolerated and the patient is clinically stable, further gradual reductions toward normal can be implemented in the next 24–48 hours.

Acute Myocardial Infarction **IV Dosage.** When IV nitroglycerin is used after acute MI, some experts recommend an initial continuous IV infusion rate of 10 mcg/minute, increasing the dosage as necessary according to hemodynamic and clinical response. Dosage will vary considerably among patients and should be adjusted based on individual requirements, blood pressure response, and adverse effects. The manufacturer states that the usual initial adult dosage of nitroglycerin when a nonadsorptive (e.g., non-PVC) administration set is used is 5 mcg/minute; the rate may be increased by 5 mcg/minute every 3–5 minutes until blood pressure response is obtained or the infusion rate is 20 mcg/minute. If no effect is obtained with 20 mcg/minute, dosage may be further increased by increments of 10 mcg/minute and, if necessary, by increments of 20 mcg/minute. When a PVC administration set is used, higher dosages generally are required; the usual initial adult dosage when these sets are used is 25 mcg/minute. Dosage should then be titrated according to the patient's response. Blood pressure and heart rate should be continuously monitored during IV administration.

Continuous IV infusions of nitroglycerin have been given for 12 hours with no attenuation of effect.

Pharmacokinetics

■ **Absorption** The approximate onset and duration of action of various dosage forms of nitroglycerin are as follows:

Table 1. Antianginal Effects

Dosage Form	Onset	Duration
sublingual	within 2 min	up to 30 min
ointment	30 min	3 h
oral extended-release	1 h	up to 12 h

Table 2. Hemodynamic Effects

Dosage Form	Onset	Duration
sublingual	2 min	up to 30 min
ointment	within 1 h	3–6 h

The onset of action of transdermal systems of nitroglycerin is delayed and the duration prolonged compared with other currently available dosage forms of the drug. Transdermal systems of the drug are designed to provide continuous, controlled release of nitroglycerin to the skin from which the drug undergoes percutaneous absorption. The rates of delivery and absorption of the drug vary depending on the specific preparation, and the individual manufacturers' information should be consulted for specific descriptions of these rates and other characteristics of the preparation. The rate of delivery is linearly dependent on the active surface area of the applied system. In general, each transdermal system contains a reservoir of excess nitroglycerin, which establishes a concentration gradient to promote delivery of the drug out of the system and into the skin, and not all of the drug is delivered from the system during normal use. The preparations currently are labeled in terms of the approximate rate of drug delivery per hour; previously, they were labeled in terms of the approximate rate of drug delivery per 24 hours.

Several studies suggest that percutaneous absorption of nitroglycerin ointment varies with the site of application, with application to the chest resulting in higher blood concentrations of the drug and greater hemodynamic effects than application to the extremities; however, there are conflicting data, and further studies are needed to more fully evaluate the effect of the application site on absorption and hemodynamic effects.

■ **Distribution** Nitroglycerin is widely distributed in the body. In adult males, nitroglycerin has an apparent volume of distribution of about 200 L. In one study in rats, ^{14}C-labeled nitroglycerin was distributed mainly to the liver and carcass, and to a lesser extent to the heart, lungs, kidneys, and spleen. It is not known if nitroglycerin is distributed into milk.

At plasma concentrations of 50–500 ng/mL, nitroglycerin is about 60% bound to plasma proteins while its metabolites, 1,3-glyceryl dinitrate and 1,2-glyceryl dinitrate, are approximately 60 and 30% bound, respectively.

■ **Elimination** The plasma half-life of nitroglycerin is about 1–4 minutes. Clearance of nitroglycerin occurs at a rate of about 1 L/kg per minute.

Nitroglycerin is metabolized to 1,3-glyceryl dinitrate, 1,2-glyceryl dinitrate, and glyceryl mononitrate. In animals, the vasodilator effects of nitroglycerin are 10–14 times greater than those of the dinitrate metabolites. Glyceryl mononitrate, which is inactive, is the principal metabolite. The dinitrate metabolites are metabolized further to inactive mononitrates and are metabolized ultimately to glycerol and carbon dioxide. Clearance of nitroglycerin exceeds hepatic blood flow. Extrahepatic sites of metabolism include red blood cells and vascular walls.

Chemistry and Stability

■ **Chemistry** Nitroglycerin, an organic nitrate, is a powerful explosive and the undiluted drug occurs as a volatile, white to pale yellow, thick, flammable, explosive liquid with a sweet, burning taste. The undiluted drug is slightly soluble in water and soluble in alcohol. Nitroglycerin that has been diluted with lactose, dextrose, alcohol, propylene glycol, or another suitable inert excipient usually contains about 10% nitroglycerin. Diluted nitroglycerin occurs as a white, odorless powder when diluted with lactose or as a clear, colorless or pale yellow liquid when diluted with alcohol or propylene glycol. Nitroglycerin sublingual tablets may produce a sweet, burning sensation when administered sublingually; however, the ability to produce a burning sensation should not be considered a reliable method for judging the potency of the tablets.

Nitroglycerin concentrate for injection is a sterile solution prepared from diluted nitroglycerin. The solvent of the concentrate for injection may contain alcohol, propylene glycol, and water for injection, and the concentrate for injection has a pH of 3–6.5 when determined according to USP specifications.

■ **Stability** Undiluted nitroglycerin should be handled cautiously since it is a powerful explosive that can be exploded by percussion or excessive heat. Nitroglycerin is diluted with lactose, dextrose, alcohol, propylene glycol, or another inert excipient to permit safe handling.

Nitroglycerin sublingual tablets should be stored in the original glass container at 20–25°C. Nitroglycerin can escape from the surface of one sublingual tablet and be adsorbed onto the surface of another tablet or packaging filler material in contact with tablets. To decrease intertablet nitroglycerin migration, some manufacturers have added stabilizing agents such as povidone and polyethylene glycol to decrease vapor pressure. Patients should be advised to keep the sublingual tablets in the original container and to close it tightly immediately after each use in order to prevent loss of potency. Nitroglycerin sublingual powder should be stored at 20–25°C but may be exposed to temperatures ranging from 5–40°C.

Nitroglycerin lingual spray pump and lingual aerosol should be stored at 25°C but may be exposed to temperatures ranging from 15–30°C. Because the contents of nitroglycerin lingual spray or lingual aerosol contain 20% alcohol or a highly flammable propellant (butane), respectively, the containers should *not* be forcefully opened, sprayed toward a flame, or placed into a fire or incinerator for disposal. Nitroglycerin ointment should be stored in tight containers at 20–25°C. Patients should be advised to tightly close multiple-dose containers of nitroglycerin ointment immediately after each use. Nitroglycerin extended-release capsules should be dispensed in a tight container and stored at 25°C but may be exposed to temperatures ranging from 15–30°C. Nitroglycerin transdermal systems should be stored in sealed, single-dose containers at 15–30°C; extremes of temperature and/or humidity should be avoided. Nitroglycerin concentrate for injection should be stored at 15–30°C; freezing should be avoided.

Since nitroglycerin readily migrates into many plastics, nitroglycerin IV solutions should be diluted and stored only in glass bottles; since some filters also absorb nitroglycerin, use of filters with IV solutions should be avoided. About 40–80% of the total amount of nitroglycerin in a diluted solution for IV infusion is absorbed by the polyvinyl chloride (PVC) tubing of the IV administration sets currently in general use. Special IV administration sets are now available which are of non-PVC plastic and cause minimal drug absorption; therefore, nearly all of the calculated dose of nitroglycerin is delivered to the patient when such sets are used. Nitroglycerin IV solutions should not be admixed with other drugs. Administration of IV nitroglycerin solutions through the same infusion set as blood can result in pseudoagglutination and hemolysis. Specialized references and the manufacturers' labeling should be consulted for specific stability and compatibility information.

For further information on chemistry and stability, pharmacology, pharmacokinetics, uses, cautions, drug interactions, laboratory test interferences, and dosage and administration of nitroglycerin, see the Nitrates and Nitrites General Statement 24:12.08.

Preparations

Excipients in commercially available drug preparations may have clinically important effects in some individuals; consult specific product labeling for details.

Nitroglycerin

Lingual		
Aerosol	0.4 mg/spray*	**Nitroglycerin Aerosol**
		NitroMist®, Mist
Solution	0.4 mg/spray*	**Nitroglycerin Spray**
		Nitrolingual® Pumpspray, Arbor
Oral		
Capsules, extended-release	2.5 mg*	**Nitroglycerin Capsules ER**
		Nitro-Time®, Time-Cap
	6.5 mg*	**Nitroglycerin Capsules ER**
		Nitro-Time®, Time-Cap
	9 mg*	**Nitroglycerin Capsules ER**
		Nitro-Time®, Time-Cap
Parenteral		
For injection concentrate, for IV infusion	5 mg/mL (50 mg)	**Nitroglycerin Injection**
Sublingual		
Powder	0.4 mg/packet	**GoNitro®**, Espero
Tablets	0.3 mg*	**Nitroglycerin Tablets**
		Nitrostat®, Pfizer
	0.4 mg*	**Nitroglycerin Tablets**
		Nitrostat®, Pfizer
	0.6 mg*	**Nitroglycerin Tablets**
		Nitrostat®, Pfizer
Topical		
Ointment	2%	**Nitro-Bid®**, Fougera
Transdermal System	0.1 mg/hour (total nitroglycerin content and transdermal system size may vary by manufacturer)*	**Minitran®**, Valeant
		Nitro-Dur®, Merck
		Nitroglycerin Transdermal System
	0.2 mg/hour (total nitroglycerin content and transdermal system size may vary by manufacturer)*	**Minitran®**, Valeant
		Nitro-Dur®, Merck
		Nitroglycerin Transdermal System
	0.3 mg/hour (60 mg/15 cm²)	**Nitro-Dur®**, Merck
	0.4 mg/hour (total nitroglycerin content and transdermal system size may vary by manufacturer)*	**Minitran®**, Valeant
		Nitro-Dur®, Merck
		Nitroglycerin Transdermal System
	0.6 mg/hour (total nitroglycerin content and transdermal system size may vary by manufacturer)*	**Minitran®**, Valeant
		Nitro-Dur®, Merck
		Nitroglycerin Transdermal System
	0.8 mg/hour (160 mg/40 cm²)	**Nitro-Dur®**, Merck

*available from one or more manufacturer, distributor, and/or repackager by generic (nonproprietary) name

Nitroglycerin in Dextrose

Parenteral		
Injection, for IV use only	100 mcg/mL (25 or 50 mg) Nitroglycerin in 5% Dextrose*	**Nitroglycerin in 5% Dextrose Injection**
	200 mcg/mL (50 mg) Nitroglycerin in 5% Dextrose*	**Nitroglycerin in 5% Dextrose Injection**
	400 mcg/mL (100 or 200 mg) Nitroglycerin in 5% Dextrose*	**Nitroglycerin in 5% Dextrose Injection**

*available from one or more manufacturer, distributor, and/or repackager by generic (nonproprietary) name

†Use is not currently included in the labeling approved by the US Food and Drug Administration

Vasodilating Agents, Miscellaneous 24:12.92

Alprostadil

■ Alprostadil, the naturally occurring prostaglandin E_1, is a vasodilating agent and a platelet-aggregation inhibitor.

Uses

■ **Erectile Dysfunction** *Treatment* Alprostadil is used as an intracavernosal injection or a urethral suppository to facilitate attainment of a sexually functional erection in males with erectile dysfunction (ED, impotence). Self-injection of alprostadil into a corpus cavernosum of the penis or administration of a urethral suppository (distributed into corpus spongiosum and corpus cavernosum of the penis) has been effective in patients with organic (neurogenic, vasculogenic) or psychogenic erectile dysfunction and in those whose erectile dysfunction was of mixed etiology. Intracavernosal or intraurethral administration of alprostadil can increase tumescence (in both cavernosa because of cross circulation) and produce erection probably secondary to drug-induced relaxation of trabecular smooth muscle and by dilation of cavernosal arteries and branches. Dilation of the cavernosal arteries is accompanied by increased arterial inflow velocity and increased venous outflow resistance resulting in penile blood engorgement and erection. (See Description.) The goal of such therapy is to provide an erection of adequate rigidity and duration to be sexually functional and that is satisfying to the patient and his partner, while avoiding prolonged erection or priapism in the patient.

Erection, which can be potentiated by sexual arousal (e.g., genital stimulation), usually occurs within 2–25 or 5–10 minutes after injection or intraurethral administration of the drug, respectively, and may persist for approximately one (which is optimal) to several hours or 0.5–1 hour, respectively; tolerance to the beneficial vascular effects of the drug does not appear to occur during long-term use. Following intracavernosal injection of alprostadil, prolonged erection (persisting for 4–6 hours) or priapism (erection persisting for longer than 6 hours) may occur occasionally, but alprostadil appears to cause a decreased incidence of priapism compared with combined phentolamine and papaverine or papaverine alone; the manufacturers state that prolonged erection or priapism occurred in about 4 or 0.4%, respectively, of patients receiving intracavernosal alprostadil in clinical trials. The manufacturer of alprostadil urethral suppositories states that although prolonged erection or priapism was reported very rarely in patients receiving the intraurethral preparation, occurring in 0.3 or less than 0.1% of patients, respectively, the possibility that overdosage of the intraurethral preparation may produce priapism should be considered. Patients should be instructed to contact their clinician immediately or, if unavailable, seek alternative immediate medical assistance for any erection persisting longer than 4 hours; priapism or prolonged erection should be treated according to established medical practice. (See Intracavernosal Dosage, under Dosage: Maintenance in Patients with Erectile Dysfunction, in the Dosage and Administration section.)

Therapeutic Options. Because of their convenience (e.g., ease of administration), patient and partner acceptance, and effectiveness in a broad range of patients, most experts (e.g., the American Urological Association [AUA]) currently recommend that selective phosphodiesterase (PDE) type 5 inhibitor therapy (sildenafil, tadalafil, vardenafil) be offered as first-line treatment of erectile dysfunction unless contraindicated. Intracavernosal or intraurethral vasoactive therapy generally is considered second-line, being reserved for patients who do not respond to psychotherapy/behavioral therapy, vacuum constriction devices, and/or selective PDE type 5 inhibitors and in whom attempts at identifying and modifying any drug-related (e.g., certain antihypertensive agents) or other potential reversible medical cause of erectile dysfunction have proved inadequate. Vasoactive therapy (e.g., alprostadil, selective PDE type 5 inhibitors) or vacuum constriction devices generally are considered or attempted before resorting to more invasive (e.g., surgical) therapies. Because selective PDE type 5 inhibitors are effective in most men with erectile dysfunction and are given orally, they are likely to be more acceptable than injections or mechanical devices and may be less expensive. Ultimately, the choice of therapy for erectile dysfunction should be individualized, taking into account differences in response, tolerability and safety, administration considerations, cost and patient reimbursement factors, experience and judgment of the clinician, and individual patient and partner preference, expectations, and satisfaction. In addition, it should be considered that selective PDE type 5 inhibitors, unlike intracavernosal or intraurethral vasoactive therapy or vacuum constriction devices, are *only* effective in the presence of adequate sexual stimulation. For additional information, see Erectile Dysfunction: Therapeutic Options under Uses, in Sildenafil Citrate 24:12.12.

Although not as effective, intraurethral alprostadil generally is preferred over intracavernosal vasoactive therapy because it is less invasive. Intraurethral alprostadil may be considered for patients who are not candidates for or who have failed selective PDE type 5 therapy. Intracavernosal vasoactive therapy (e.g., alprostadil, papaverine, papaverine and phentolamine, other combinations) is the most effective nonsurgical treatment for erectile dysfunction; however, it is invasive and associated with the highest risk of priapism. Clinician preference and experience often guide the initial treatment choice when intracavernosal therapy is indicated.

Although additional study of the long-term safety and efficacy of *intracavernosal* injection of vasoactive drugs for the treatment of erectile dysfunction is necessary and ongoing, particularly regarding the relative complications (e.g., penile scarring, penile fibrosis) and safety of each approach, some clinicians currently favor alprostadil, alone or combined with other agents, when intracavernosal treatment of erectile dysfunction is indicated because of possible improved efficacy and decreased adverse effects (e.g., priapism, fibrotic changes) compared with papaverine therapy. However, all currently popular forms of therapy for erectile dysfunction, including intracavernosal or intraurethral vasoactive therapy, have been associated with high dropout rates, often early in treatment (e.g., secondary to adverse effects, compromised sexual spontaneity, loss of motivation or partner, spontaneous return of function). The motivations and expectations of the patient and his partner, and the education, as well as inclusion in the treatment plan, of both partners are critical in facilitating efficacy and compliance. Provision of continued education and adequate follow-up support, including determination of reasons for unacceptable response and for discontinuance of therapy if this occurs as well as discussion of treatment options, also are important, although additional study is needed to identify optimal interventions that might improve compliance and decrease dropout. Patients should be instructed to visit their clinician regularly (e.g., at 3-month intervals) for assessment of therapeutic benefit, including the need for possible dosage adjustment, and of potential adverse effects of alprostadil therapy.

Because of the risk of priapism and other potential complications (e.g., adverse morphologic penile effects such as fibrosis) associated with intracavernosal vasoactive therapy, alprostadil is *not* recommended for simply enhancing erections in men who are not impotent†.

Clinical Experience. Efficacy of alprostadil is variable in patients with erectile dysfunction, in part depending on the underlying etiology and dose employed. The manufacturers of intracavernosal alprostadil state that about 70–90% of patients with erectile dysfunction of various etiologies experienced erections sufficient for sexual intercourse with alprostadil intracavernosal therapy at doses ranging up to 65 mcg in clinical trials. In some reports involving erectile dysfunction of various etiologies, response rates ranged from about 40–85% for alprostadil doses ranging from 10–20 mcg.

Results of a placebo-controlled multicenter study indicate that in the initial (dose titrating) phase about 66% of patients with erectile dysfunction of various etiologies experienced erections sufficient for sexual intercourse with alprostadil intraurethral therapy at doses ranging from 125–1000 mcg. In other studies in patients with erectile dysfunction, response rates ranged from 37–43% for intraurethral doses ranging from 125–1000 mcg.

Alprostadil has been effective in patients with organic (neurogenic and/or mild to moderate vasculogenic) erectile dysfunction or with psychogenic erectile dysfunction, but efficacy in those with a vasculogenic component of their erectile dysfunction may vary depending on the extent and type of vascular dysfunction. Generally, vasculogenic erectile dysfunction of arteriogenic origin is more responsive (both in terms of dose and rate) to alprostadil than that of venogenic origin. In addition, patients with neurogenic or psychogenic erectile dysfunction generally respond to lower doses than those with vasculogenic erectile dysfunction. Overall response rate generally is less in patients with erectile dysfunction of mixed etiology than in those with neurogenic or psychogenic erectile dysfunction and those with vasculogenic erectile dysfunction. In men with erectile dysfunction associated with diabetes mellitus, intracavernosal alprostadil was effective in producing satisfactory erections at doses ranging from 10–40 mcg; however, efficacy was less in men with long-standing diabetes (exceeding 10 years) and in those with long-standing erectile dysfunction (exceeding 5 years). In addition, lower response rates have been observed with intracavernosal alprostadil in older men, with or without diabetes, than in younger men, but dose escalation may increase efficacy in geriatric patients. Limited data indicate that response rates in patients using intraurethral alprostadil are independent of the etiology of erectile dysfunction.

The dose of alprostadil is adjusted by the clinician according to the patient's response toward a therapeutic goal of achieving an erection satisfactory for intercourse of 1-hour duration; erections persisting longer than 1-hour increase the risk of priapism. Most males with various etiologies of erectile dysfunction respond to initial single intracavernosal alprostadil doses of 5–20 mcg; some males, especially those with neurogenic or psychogenic erectile dysfunction, experience erections at doses as low as 0.5–5 mcg. In addition, while intracavernosal doses as high as 140 mcg have been used, almost all patients who respond do so at doses of 60 mcg or less, and doses exceeding 60–65 mcg generally are not recommended. Results of a multicenter placebo-controlled study in patients with erectile dysfunction of various organic etiologies using intraurethral alprostadil in the initial (dose titrating) phase indicate that about 19% of the patients experienced erection with 125- or 250-mcg doses while about another 47% of patients experienced erection with 500- or 1000-mcg doses of the drug. In addition, a correlation appears to exist between dose of intraurethral alprostadil and mean duration of response. In the home maintenance phase of the placebo-controlled multicenter study in patients receiving intraurethral alprostadil, at least one sexual intercourse occurred in about 65 or 19% of patients receiving alprostadil urethral suppositories or placebo, respectively, while orgasm (occurring at least once) was reported in about 64 or 24% of patients receiving the drug or placebo, respectively. In patients who responded to home maintenance therapy, 70% of administrations (7 out of 10) resulted in successful intercourse. In studies that evaluated sexual intercourse during the home maintenance phase, 66–87% of the men using intracavernosal alprostadil reported satisfactory intercourse per injection. However, efficacy of the intracavernosal injection in the home during intercourse may be reduced relative to office-based titration to adequate erection, possibly secondary to problems with injection technique, anxiety associated with sexual performance, and/or problems in partner acceptance; as a result, some patients may require an increase in the office-titrated dose once maintenance therapy is under way at home. In some cases, though, patients actually have a greater response to alprostadil in the home setting and may be able to decrease their dose.

Occasionally, it may be possible to discontinue alprostadil therapy because normal erectile function returns. In such cases, normal erectile functioning may result from decreased anxiety, improved self-confidence (e.g., in those with psychogenic erectile dysfunction), or improved penile circulation in those with vasculogenic erectile dysfunction.

While most males with erectile dysfunction respond to alprostadil therapy, treatment failures occur in about 20% (and up to 33% of geriatric men) or 35% of patients receiving intracavernosal or intraurethral therapy, respectively, during home maintenance. In addition, other males may not be able to complete the dose titration phase of therapy, and many patients, despite adequate response, eventually drop out from continued use for various reasons. Corporeal veno-occlusive dysfunction may hamper the effectiveness of the drug in the treatment of erectile dysfunction, but men with arteriogenic, psychogenic, and neurogenic impotence also have reported failure with alprostadil.

Several comparative studies have evaluated the efficacy of various formulations of alprostadil. Limited data indicate that intracavernosal alprostadil may be more effective than intraurethral alprostadil in the treatment of erectile dysfunction. In one comparative study using intracavernosal alprostadil (up to 20 mcg) or intraurethral alprostadil (up to 1000 mcg), complete rigid erections occurred in 48 or 10% of patients, respectively, while total responses (complete rigid erection or full tumescence with partial rigidity) were reported in 70 or 43% of patients, respectively. Substantially higher alprostadil doses are needed for treatment of erectile dysfunction when the intraurethral route is used compared with intracavernosal therapy, since the drug contained in the urethral suppository is distributed from the mucosal cells of the urethra into the corpus spongiosum and corpus cavernosum. Alprostadil may undergo some metabolism in the urogenital tract and in addition, some alprostadil may be distributed from the corpus spongiosum directly into the pelvic venous circulation bypassing the corpus cavernosum. It has been suggested that a new technique involving an adjustable external penile band used in conjunction with the urethral suppositories possibly may improve delivery of the drug into the corpus cavernosum and thus achieve efficacy with lower doses of the intraurethral drug. Results of a crossover study evaluating intracavernosal alprostadil with (Caverject® Impulse®) or without alfadex (α-cyclodextrin) (Caverject®) in a limited number of men with erectile dysfunction indicate that the safety and efficacy of the 2 formulations are comparable.

Although the manufacturers state that safety and efficacy of combined vasoactive therapy for erectile dysfunction that includes alprostadil have not been established by systematic study and therefore currently is not recommended, intracavernosal alprostadil has been used in combination with phentolamine and papaverine; phentolamine, atropine, and papaverine; calcitonin gene-related peptide; or papaverine in an attempt to increase response, decrease dosage of individual agents, and decrease the incidence of local pain, penile corporal fibrosis, fibrotic nodules, hypotension, and priapism. Combined therapy with *intraurethral* alprostadil and a vacuum constriction device or an oral selective PDE type 5 inhibitor has exhibited increased efficacy relative to alprostadil alone; combined therapy with *intracavernosal* alprostadil and a selective PDE type 5 inhibitor has not been adequately evaluated. Additional study is needed to elucidate the long-term safety and benefits of such combined therapy.

In a limited number of patients, intraurethral alprostadil has been used in combination with prazosin; increased response rates associated with the combination therapy were more pronounced in patients receiving the lower doses (i.e., 125 or 250 mcg) of alprostadil.

Alprostadil should *not* be used in patients who might have conditions predisposing to priapism (e.g., sickle cell anemia or trait, multiple myeloma, leukemia, thrombocythemia, polycythemia, propensity to develop venous thrombosis, hyperviscosity syndrome), in those with anatomic deformation of the penis (e.g., angulation, cavernosal fibrosis, Peyronie's disease), or in men for whom sexual activity is inadvisable or contraindicated. In addition, alprostadil should be discontinued in any patient who develops penile angulation, cavernosal fibrosis, or Peyronie's disease during therapy with the drug. The manufacturers also state that patients with penile implants should *not* be treated with intracavernosal alprostadil. Alprostadil urethral suppositories should not be used in patients with certain genitourinary tract disorders (e.g., urethral stricture or obstruction, balanitis, acute or chronic urethritis, severe hypospadias and curvature, anuria) or in those with an indwelling urethral catheter. Since alprostadil is embryotoxic in animals, patients using intraurethral alprostadil should not engage in sexual intercourse with a pregnant woman unless a condom is used.

Diagnosis Alprostadil also is used by intracavernosal injection as an adjunct in the differential diagnosis of erectile dysfunction and in evaluating the hemodynamic status of erectile tissue. The drug can be used alone (simply monitoring for erectile response after intracavernosal injection) or prior to other testing (e.g., penile angiography, duplex or Doppler ultrasonography, radioisotope penograms, cavernosography, radiolabeled-xenon penile clearance, cavernosometry) as an adjunct to facilitate visualization and assessment of the penile vasculature.

Pharmacologic test doses of intracavernosal alprostadil generally are used alone when simply assessing the adequacy of penile arterial and veno-occlusive function. The induction of a rigid or nearly rigid erection after intracavernosal alprostadil generally indicates that arterial inflow is adequate to occlude venous outflow drainage, and patients with such response generally are suitable candidates for intracavernosal vasoactive therapy. Genital stimulation may be used to increase the erectile response in such testing. Intracavernosal alprostadil testing also may be used as an aid in differentiating erectile dysfunction that is of vasculogenic versus neurogenic or psychogenic origin; a positive response, especially at low doses, may be indicative of neurogenic or psychogenic erectile dysfunction. If partial tumescence occurs, mild to moderate arterial or venous disease may be present, and an erection after alprostadil injection that is not sustained may be indicative of venous dysfunction.

Patients with an inadequate or negative response to intracavernosal alprostadil may benefit from further vascular testing; such additional testing may aid in differentiating between arteriogenic or venogenic erectile dysfunction. However, it should be recognized that failure to respond adequately may not indicate vascular insufficiency but rather could simply be secondary to patient anxiety or discomfort. In addition, the number of patients who may benefit from additional vascular testing is small but includes patients who are candidates for vascular surgery, such as young men with a history of perineal or pelvic trauma and resultant arterial blockage with or without neurologic deficit. Studies to further define vasculogenic disorders include duplex ultrasonography, dynamic infusion cavernosometry/cavernosography, radioisotope penogram, and pelvic-penile angiography; such testing can be performed alone or in conjunction with intracavernosal vasoactive agents such as alprostadil. Specialized references should be consulted for additional information on the performance and interpretation of tests of erectile function involving intracavernosal alprostadil, and consideration should be given to referral to clinicians with expertise and interest in evaluating the vascular aspects of erectile dysfunction, particularly when specialized tests such as ultrasonography, cavernosometry/cavernosography, or angiography are performed.

■ **Ductus Arteriosus-dependent Congenital Heart Disease** Alprostadil is used IV for palliative, not definitive, therapy in maintaining patency of the ductus arteriosus in neonates born with various ductal-dependent congenital heart defects such as pulmonary atresia, pulmonary stenosis, tricuspid atresia, tetralogy of Fallot, interruption of the aortic arch, coarctation of the aorta, and/or transposition of the great vessels with or without other defects. The drug is used to provide adequate circulation and oxygenation and prevent or correct resultant acidemia until corrective or palliative surgery can be performed. Alprostadil is only effective if initiated prior to complete anatomic closure of the ductus. Although alprostadil therapy is indicated principally as a short-term measure, more prolonged therapy (e.g., up to several months) with the drug occasionally may be indicated (e.g., when surgical risk to the neonate dictates delay of the procedure), but the possible risks of prolonged therapy with the drug (e.g., gastric outlet obstruction secondary to antral hyperplasia, cortical hyperostosis of long bones, morphologic changes in pulmonary arteries) should be weighed carefully against the potential benefits.

Because of the risk of respiratory depression and apnea, which is greatest during the first hour of drug infusion particularly in neonates weighing less than 2 kg at birth, the manufacturer of Prostin VR Pediatric® states that alprostadil therapy for maintaining ductal patency should be performed only by trained personnel in facilities providing pediatric intensive care where respiratory status can be monitored throughout treatment and facilities and equipment for assisted ventilation are readily available. However, some clinicians suggest that an alprostadil IV infusion can be initiated at the local neonatal unit prior to transport to a tertiary care center, provided adequate monitoring can be undertaken and respiratory support initiated if necessary.

Alprostadil should *not* be used in patients with neonatal respiratory distress syndrome. In such neonates, closure of the ductus arteriosus is necessary to prevent overload of the pulmonary circulation. Therefore, a differential diagnosis between neonatal respiratory distress syndrome (hyaline membrane disease) and cyanotic heart disease (restricted pulmonary blood flow) should be made prior to initiating alprostadil therapy. The manufacturer of Prostin VR Pediatric® states that if full diagnostic facilities are not readily available, cyanosis (evidenced by a PO_2 less than 40 mm Hg) and radiographic evidence of restricted pulmonary blood flow are appropriate indicators of congenital heart defects. Alprostadil also should *not* be used in premature neonates with patent ductus arteriosus since cardiopulmonary management of such neonates also depends on closure of the ductus. In addition, the risk to benefit of alprostadil therapy should be weighed carefully in neonates with bleeding disorders (because of the drug's platelet-aggregation inhibiting effects) and in those with conditions in which alprostadil-induced increases in pulmonary blood flow may precipitate pulmonary edema and/or congestive heart failure.

The ductus arteriosus is present during fetal life, connecting the pulmonary artery to the descending aorta and thus diverting from the lungs to the placenta (for gas exchange) most blood passing through this artery. The ductus arteriosus apparently is maintained in a dilated state by a low partial pressure of oxygen and by effects of prostaglandins, presumably of the E series, which are produced by the placenta and in the ductus itself. The ductus usually closes within 24–96 hours after birth, partly as a result of a loss of circulating prostaglandins, a decrease in sensitivity to prostaglandins, and an increase in pulmonary blood flow. In neonates with congenital heart defects that result in cyanosis either by restricting pulmonary blood flow (pulmonary atresia, pulmonary stenosis, tetralogy of Fallot, tricuspid atresia) or systemic arteriovenous mixing (transposition of the great arteries) or that result in restriction of systemic blood flow (interruption of the aortic arch, coarctation of the aorta), the ductus arteriosus functions to preserve blood oxygenation and lower body perfusion. The spontaneous closure of the ductus arteriosus after birth is associated with hypoxemia and metabolic acidosis in neonates with restricted pulmonary blood flow and with metabolic acidosis, poor systemic perfusion, oliguria, and severe heart failure in those with restricted systemic blood flow.

Dilation of the constricted ductus arteriosus with alprostadil in neonates with cyanotic congenital heart disease results in a temporary increase in arterial oxygen partial pressure (PaO_2) and oxygen saturation secondary to the increase in pulmonary blood flow and/or increased mixing between the systemic and pulmonary circulation. Efficacy of alprostadil in increasing PaO_2 or oxygen saturation has been established relative to pretreatment values in the same neonates; data from placebo-controlled or comparative trials are not available. The increase in pulmonary blood flow may result from combined maintenance of the patency of the ductus arteriosus and dilation of the pulmonary vascular bed induced by the drug.

Response to alprostadil therapy in cyanotic neonates is inversely related to pretreatment PO_2. Thus, while about half of cyanotic neonates respond to the drug with at least a 10- mm Hg (mm Hg) increase in blood PO_2, neonates having pretreatment values of 40 mm Hg or greater (e.g., those with a widely patent ductus) usually exhibit little response, and response increases to 77% in those with low pretreatment blood PO_2 (less than 20 mm Hg), with a narrowing of the ductus arteriosus, and who are 4 days old or younger. The age-dependent efficacy of alprostadil Prostin VR Pediatric® administration in cyanotic neonates suggests that anatomic closure progresses irreversibly or that permanent functional closure occurs secondary to decreased responsiveness of ductal tissue to prostaglandins.

Alprostadil has been used to increase arteriovenous mixing and pulmonary blood flow in neonates with transposition of the great arteries. However, the optimal timing of administration of the drug and the duration of therapy in conjunction with atrial septostomy or septectomy and arterial switching have not been established.

In neonates with restricted systemic blood flow, dilation of the ductus arteriosus with alprostadil can result in prevention or correction of acidemia, increased cardiac output accompanied by increased systemic blood pressure, increased femoral pulse volume, increased renal blood flow and function (urine production), decreased gradient of descending to ascending aortic blood pressures (in neonates with coarctation of the aorta), and/or decreased gradient of pulmonary artery to descending aortic pressures (in neonates with interruption of the aortic arch). Unlike cyanotic neonates, acyanotic neonates do not display as pronounced an age dependence for a positive effect, and efficacy does not depend on low pretreatment arterial partial pressure (PaO_2); acyanotic neonates may have normal or slightly reduced PaO_2. Alprostadil reportedly has increased arterial pH from pretreatment values of 6.8–7.22 to posttreatment values of 7.22–7.45 in acyanotic neonates; efficacy in reversing metabolic acidosis does not appear to be dose related. In addition, the need for alkalinizing agents generally is reduced or eliminated. Mean systolic and diastolic blood pressures in the descending aorta increased 48–52% and 21–25%, respectively, in neonates with coarctation of the aorta receiving alprostadil infusion. The mean pressure difference between the main pulmonary artery and the descending aorta decreased from 13–14 mm Hg to 2–3 mm Hg in neonates with interruption of the aorta receiving alprostadil therapy.

Dosage and Administration

■ **Administration** Alprostadil is administered by intracavernosal injection for the treatment and diagnosis of erectile dysfunction, by urethral suppository for the treatment of erectile dysfunction, or by continuous IV or intra-arterial infusion to maintain the patency of the ductus arteriosus in neonates.

Intracavernosal Administration Intracavernosal alprostadil therapy should be initiated in a medical setting (e.g., physician's office), with the initial injections being administered by medically trained personnel. Patients can begin intracavernosal self-injection of alprostadil only after they have received and reviewed a copy of the patient instructions provided by the manufacturer and have been instructed carefully and trained well about proper administration techniques, including aseptic techniques and precautions. Careful instruction about administration technique can minimize the likelihood of local adverse effects associated with faulty technique (e.g., hematoma, ecchymosis) and also can minimize patient frustration and treatment failure.

To improve compliance and potentially decrease treatment dropout, patients should be highly motivated and properly educated about intracavernosal therapy, and they and their partners should be provided long-term follow-up support to assist them in adjusting to this therapeutic intervention. Careful and continuous follow-up should include ongoing education and support in therapy, careful determination of reasons for discontinuing therapy if this occurs, and discussion of therapeutic options if alprostadil therapy is not tolerated or is unsuccessful. Adequate assessment of the motivations and expectations of the patient and partner prior to intracavernosal therapy also can aid in optimizing outcome. Follow-up is particularly important during the initial period of self-injections since dosage adjustment often is necessary during this period.

Patients also should be instructed that unreconstituted alprostadil sterile powder (Caverject®) may be stored for up to 3 months at 25°C or colder, while avoiding freezing. During travel, care should be taken to avoid exposure to freezing or temperatures exceeding 25°C; therefore, the powder should not be stored in checked airline baggage (storage in the passenger compartment is permitted) or in a closed automobile. The sterile lyophilized powder in an alfadex (α-cyclodextrin) inclusion complex (Edex®) should be stored at room temperature at 15–30°C. The sterile lyophilized powder with alfadex (Caverject® Impulse®) should be stored at 25°C but may be exposed to temperatures ranging from 15–30°C.

Prior to reconstitution, alprostadil sterile powder (Caverject®) should be warmed to room temperature under ambient conditions; use of a water bath to facilitate warming is *not* recommended. Commercially available alprostadil sterile powder (Caverject®) for intracavernosal use should be reconstituted just prior to administration by adding 1 mL of bacteriostatic water for injection or sterile water to a vial labeled as containing 11.9, 23.2, or 46.4 mcg of the drug to provide a solution containing 10.5, 20.5, or 41.1 mcg/mL, respectively. Although the resultant diluted solutions contain 10.5, 20.5, or 41.1 mcg/mL, the deliverable amount of alprostadil in these dilutions is 10, 20, or 40 mcg/mL, respectively, bacause approximately 0.5, 0.5, or 1.1 mcg, respectively, of the drug is adsorbed onto the vial and syringe.

Alternatively, the commercially available lyophilized powder of alprostadil in an alfadex inclusion complex (Edex®) for intracavernosal use should be reconstituted just prior to administration by adding 1.2 mL of bacteriostatic 0.9% sodium chloride injection (which is supplied by the manufacturer in a separate vial when the drug is contained in a kit) to a vial labeled as containing 12.45, 24.9, or 49.8 mcg of the drug, to deliver a solution containing 10, 20, or 40 mcg/mL, respectively. After adding the diluent but before removing the syringe from the vial, the contents of the vial may be swirled gently until a clear solution is obtained. The desired dose (determined by careful titration) of the reconstituted solution can then be withdrawn into the same syringe. If the reusable injection device containing alprostadil powder in an alfadex inclusion complex is used, the drug should be reconstituted immediately by placing the commercially available dual-chambered cartridge into the injection device and then turning the threaded plunger of the device to force the diluent (1.075 mL of 0.9% sodium chloride injection) into the lower chamber containing alprostadil powder and mixing the contents of the cartridge gently to dissolve the solid. The reconstituted solution of alprostadil in an alfadex inclusion complex may initially appear cloudy as a result of introduction of small air bubbles. The vial or cartridge containing alprostadil in an alfadex inclusion complex contains the drug in a cake approximately three-sixteenths or ⅜ inch in thickness, respectively. If the vial or cartridge is damaged or the cake is substantially smaller than the manufacturer's specifications, the vial or cartridge should not be used.

If the single-use, disposable dual-chambered syringe system containing alprostadil powder and alfadex (Caverject® Impulse®) is used, the drug should be reconstituted by turning the plunger rod clockwise until the rod meets resistance to force the diluent (sterile bacteriostatic water for injection) into the chamber containing alprostadil powder. The contents of the syringe should then be mixed thoroughly by turning the device upside down several times. The reconstituted solution of alprostadil should be clear. The dose to be delivered is set by slowly turning the end of the plunger rod clockwise until the number visible in the dose window matches the appropriate dose of the drug (in mcg). The delivery device labeled as containing 10 mcg of alprostadil can be set to deliver a dose of 2.5, 5, 7.5, or 10 mcg of the drug (solution volume of 0.125, 0.25, 0.375, or 0.5 mL, respectively), and the delivery device labeled as containing 20 mcg of alprostadil can be set to deliver a dose of 5, 10, 15, or 20 mcg (solution volume of 0.125, 0.25, 0.375, or 0.5 mL, respectively). The single-use delivery device and any remaining solution should be disposed of properly following use.

Reconstituted solutions of certain formulations of alprostadil for intracavernosal injection (Caverject®, Edex®) are intended for single-use only and should be used immediately. Reconstituted solutions of alprostadil (Caverject® Impulse®) prepared from the powder for injection are intended for single-use only and should be used within 24 hours when stored at or below 25°C. Reconstituted solutions of the drug should be inspected visually for particulate matter and discoloration prior to administration whenever solution and container permit.

For intracavernosal injection, the head (glans) of the penis (if uncircumcised, the foreskin should pulled back initially) is held between the thumb and forefinger and stretched lengthwise along the thigh while sitting upright or slightly reclined, and the needle of the syringe or injection device is then positioned so that the drug will be injected into a corpus cavernosum underneath the tunica albuginea along the dorsolateral aspect of the proximal third of the penis. Once positioned, the needle of the syringe or injection device provided by the manufacturer (a fixed-hub, ½-inch, 27-, 29- or 30-gauge needle) should be pushed straight into the site using a steady motion until the metal portion of the needle is almost entirely in the penis; the dose should then be injected slowly (over 5–10 seconds) into the chosen corpus cavernosum. If a syringe other than the one provided by the manufacturer is used, it is recommended that it be a ½-inch, 27- to 30-gauge needle. If the needle becomes severely bent at anytime during reconstitution or injection of alprostadil, the needle should be discarded and a new unused needle should be used for these procedures. Blood vessels, corpus spongiosum, subcutaneous tissue, urethra, and dorsal neural vascular structures should be avoided as injection sites. The syringe or injection device then should be withdrawn and pressure applied to the injection site with an alcohol swab for 5 minutes (or until bleeding stops) to avoid hematologic complications (e.g., intracorporeal hematoma, ecchymosis, hemorrhage at the site of injection), especially in patients receiving concomitant anticoagulant therapy. To minimize adverse effects related to repeated local injection, the side of the penis and the site of injection should be varied. Patients should be cautioned against reuse of syringes and needles and should be given instructions on the proper disposal in puncture-resistant containers. Unused reconstituted solutions of alprostadil should be discarded.

Patients should be advised of the potential for prolonged erections (priapism), particularly with intracavernosal therapy, and informed of the steps to take in the event that this potentially serious adverse effect occurs. (See Intracavernosal Dosage: Maintenance in Patients with Erectile Dysfunction, in Dosage and Administration.)

Patients should be advised that use of intracavernosal alprostadil provides no protection against sexually transmitted diseases, and they should be counseled regarding protective measures to guard against such transmission. In addition, they should be counseled about the potential increased risk of transmitting blood-borne diseases secondary to possible exposure of the sexual partner to the small amount of blood at the injection site.

IV and Intra-arterial Infusion To maintain patency of the ductus arteriosus, alprostadil (Prostin VR Pediatric®) preferably is administered by continuous IV infusion into a large vein (peripheral or central) via a controlled-infusion device (e.g., an electronic volumetric controller, volumetric IV infusion pump) or other apparatus to ensure precise control of the flow rate during infusion since inadvertent rapid administration could result in toxicity (e.g., apnea). Alternatively, alprostadil may be administered by controlled intra-arterial infusion through an umbilical or femoral artery catheter placed at the ductal level or main pulmonary artery; other sites of infusion (e.g., into the main pulmonary artery, descending aorta adjacent to the ductus arteriosus, atrium, vena cava) also have been studied. While it was expected on theoretical grounds that intra-aortic or intra-arterial infusion would be the optimal route, providing the greatest concentration to the ductus and allowing for rapid deactivation in the lungs (thus minimizing adverse effects), clinical studies have shown these routes to be no more effective than IV infusion, and the IV route actually has been better tolerated (e.g., flushing is more common with intra-arterial injection). Therefore, IV infusion currently is the preferred route of alprostadil administration for maintaining patency of the ductus arteriosus. If flushing occurs during intra-arterial infusion, the catheter should be repositioned or the route changed to IV since cutaneous vasodilation usually is a sign of improper placement (e.g., inadvertent placement into the left carotid or left subclavian artery); rapid reversal of cutaneous vasodilation generally occurs with repositioning. Because systemically administered alprostadil is metabolized rapidly with a substantial portion undergoing β- and ω-oxidation on first pass through the lungs, the drug must be infused continuously to maintain ductal patency.

Alprostadil for injection concentrate containing 500 mcg/mL must be diluted prior to infusion. For infusion, 1 mL of the concentrate labeled as containing 500 mcg of alprostadil is diluted in 0.9% sodium chloride or dextrose 5% injection to provide a solution containing 2–20 mcg/mL, depending on the controlled-infusion device employed and the needs of the neonate. When using a device with a volumetric infusion chamber, the appropriate volume of diluent should be added to the chamber first and then 1 mL of alprostadil concentrate for infusion should be added to the diluent. The following table lists sample alprostadil dilutions and infusion rates when a dosage of 0.1 mcg/kg of body weight per minute is employed. This dosage is commonly used for initiation of alprostadil therapy to maintain patency of the ductus arteriosus.

Dilutions and infusion rates to provide a dosage of 0.1 mcg/kg per minute

Add 500 mcg (1 mL) alprostadil (Prostin VR Pediatric®) to following diluent volumes:	Resultant approximate concentration (mcg/mL)	Infusion rate (mL/min per kg of body weight)
250 mL	2	0.05
100 mL	5	0.02
50 mL	10	0.01
25 mL	20	0.005

For example, to provide an alprostadil dosage of 0.1 mcg/kg of body weight per minute to an infant weighing 2.8 kg using 500 mcg of alprostadil concentrate in 100 mL of compatible diluent, the resultant infusion rate for this solution would be 0.056 mL/minute (i.e., 0.02 mL/minute per kg × 2.8 kg) or 3.36 mL/hour.

Alprostadil for injection concentrate should be stored at 2–8°C. The for injection concentrate and diluted solutions of the drug should be inspected visually for particulate matter and discoloration prior to administration whenever solution and container permit. During dilution, care should be taken to avoid direct contact of the concentrate with the wall of the plastic volumetric infusion chamber since the appearance of the chamber may change and a hazy solution may develop; if this occurs, the chamber and solution should be discarded. The manufacturer of Prostin VR Pediatric® recommends that diluted solutions of the drug be prepared freshly every 24 hours and that any remaining solution should be discarded.

Because of the risk of respiratory depression and apnea, respiratory status of the neonate should be monitored throughout alprostadil Prostin VR Pediatric® administration, and facilities and equipment for assisted ventilation should be readily available. (See Uses: Ductus Arteriosus-dependent Congenital Heart Disease.) Apnea is most likely to develop during the first hour of infusion, particularly in neonates weighing less than 2 kg at birth. In addition during infusion, arterial pressure should be monitored periodically via umbilical artery catheter, auscultation, or Doppler transducer and the rate of infusion decreased immediately if a clinically important decrease in arterial pressure occurs. The infusion rate also should be slowed if fever or hypotension (appropriate therapy also may be necessary) occurs since these may be signs of overdosage; once they subside, the rate can be increased cautiously if necessary. If apnea or bradycardia occurs, the infusion should be discontinued and appropriate treatment initiated; in some cases, the infusion can be reinitiated cautiously if continued therapy is considered necessary.

Intraurethral Administration Alprostadil is administered intraurethrally as a suppository. Therapy with intraurethral alprostadil should be initiated in a medical setting (e.g., physician's office). Patients should begin intraurethral self-administration of alprostadil only after they have received and reviewed a copy of the patient instructions (including a video) provided by the manufacturer and have been instructed carefully about proper administration techniques and precautions.

Patients should urinate immediately prior to insertion of the alprostadil urethral suppository and they should gently shake the penis to remove excess urine. The micro suppository (medicated pellet) is designed to dissolve in the small quantity of urine remaining in the urethra after urination. Alprostadil urethral suppository should be inserted with a urethral applicator according to the manufacturer's instructions. After the suppository has been inserted, the removed applicator should be visually inspected to confirm that the urethral suppository is no longer in the applicator tip. If some residual medication is left in the applicator, the insertion procedure should be repeated. Urination or dribbling immediately following intraurethral alprostadil may result in loss of drug from the urethral area.

After application of the medicated pellet (suppository), the penis should be held upright, stretched to its full length and rolled firmly between the hands for at least 10 seconds to ensure that the drug is adequately distributed along the walls of the urethra. If a burning sensation occurs, the penis may be rolled for an additional 30–60 seconds or until burning subsides. After administration, sitting, standing, or walking for 10 minutes will increase blood flow to the penis and enhance erection; lying down (especially on the back) immediately after administration of the suppository may reduce blood flow to the penis and reduce the development of erection. During sexual activity, erection may be better maintained in positions that favor blood flow into the penis.

Patients should be advised that use of intraurethral alprostadil provides no protection against sexually transmitted diseases, and they should be counseled regarding protective measures to guard against such transmission.

■ **Dosage** ***Initiation and Titration in Patients with Erectile Dysfunction*** **Intracavernosal Dosage.** Dosage of intracavernosal alprostadil must be individualized carefully according to the patient's erectile response. Initiation and titration of dosage should be undertaken in a medical setting, and the patient must remain in this setting during titration of each dose until complete detumescence occurs. If no response occurs with a given dose, upward titration should be attempted after about 1 hour; no more than 2 injections should be administered initially within a 24-hour period. If a response is observed, at least 24 hours should elapse before administering the next dose. Dosage should be titrated slowly to the lowest possible effective level in order to avoid priapism.

For the treatment of neurogenic impotence secondary to spinal cord injury, the usual adult intracavernosal dose of alprostadil ranges from 1.25–60 mcg. Generally, therapy is started with the smaller dosage and increased until the optimum dose (as determined by maintenance of an erection that is satisfactory for intercourse but persists no longer than 1 hour) is attained. For the treatment of pure neurogenic impotence (i.e., spinal cord injury), the manufacturers recommend an initial intracavernosal dose of 1.25 mcg of alprostadil administered in a medical setting. If no response is observed with the initial dose of alprostadil, the dose may be doubled to 2.5 mcg after about 1 hour; no more than 2 doses should be administered within a 24-hour period. If additional dosage titration is required, a dose of 5 mcg may be administered during the next 24 hours, followed by subsequent increases in 5-mcg increments, with each incremental increase separated by at least 24 hours, until optimum response is achieved. If the duration of the erection achieved exceeds 1 hour, the subsequent dose of alprostadil should be reduced.

For the treatment of vasculogenic erectile dysfunction, psychogenic erectile dysfunction, or erectile dysfunction of mixed etiology, the manufacturers recommend an initial intracavernosal test dose of alprostadil of 2.5 mcg. If a partial response is observed, the dose may be doubled to 5 mcg after about 1 hour. If no response to the initial test dose is observed, then the second dose may be increased to 7.5 mcg after about 1 hour. No more than 2 doses should be administered within a 24-hour period.If additional titration is required, dosage may be increased in increments of 5–10 mcg at intervals of at least 24 hours until optimum response is achieved.

In clinical trials, most patients with erectile dysfunction of various etiologies responded to initial intracavernosal alprostadil doses titrated to exceeding 5 but not exceeding 20 mcg, with the dose at the end of the titration phase averaging 17.8 mcg. Although doses ranging from 0.2–140 mcg have been reported, almost all patients who respond to alprostadil do so at doses of 60 mcg or less; therefore, doses exceeding 60–65 mcg generally are not recommended.

Intraurethral Dosage. Dosage of intraurethral alprostadil should be individualized according to the patient's erectile response. Since symptomatic hypotension and syncope occurred in 3 and 0.4% of patients, respectively, using intraurethral alprostadil during the initial (dose-titrating) phase, initiation and titration of dosage should be undertaken in a medical setting to monitor the patients for manifestations of such effects. Patients should inform their clinician if they have a history of syncope. It is recommended that therapy with intraurethral alprostadil be initiated with low doses (e.g., 125 or 250 mcg); dosage should be titrated (in separate visits) to the lowest possible effective level in order to avoid development of hypotension or syncope, which appear to be dose related. If no response occurs with these doses, subsequent doses may be increased in a stepwise manner to 500 or 1000 mcg, as needed. In clinical studies, 6–10, 17–20, 20–30 or 27–56% of patients achieved adequate penile response (erections sufficient for intercourse) at intraurethral alprostadil doses during the dosage-titration phase (to establish home maintenance dosage) of 125-, 250-, 500-, or 1000 mcg, respectively.

Maintenance in Patients with Erectile Dysfunction **Intracavernosal Dosage.** Intracavernosal alprostadil self-injection therapy for erectile dysfunction should be initiated at the dose that was determined as optimal during titration in a medical setting (e.g., physician's office); however, the first self-administered dose should be delayed for at least 1 day after completion of supervised dose titration but also should be administered in a medical setting. The optimal maintenance dose should result in an erection that is maintained for no longer than 1 hour. Adjustments to the initial office-titrated dose often are required to maintain response in the home, but should be attempted only after consultation with a clinician (not independently by the patient), following the same initial titration guidelines. The manufacturers recommend that patients self-administer intracavernosal alprostadil no more frequently than 3 times weekly with at least 1 day elapsing between each dose. Follow-up monitoring of patients should be performed every 3 months to determine safety (e.g., careful examination of the penis for fibrotic changes) and the possible need for additional dosage adjustment. Alprostadil therapy should be discontinued if penile angulation, cavernosal fibrosis, or Peyronie's disease develop. The manufacturer of Caverject® states that efficacy of long-term alprostadil therapy for erectile dysfunction has been established for up to 6 months by an uncontrolled, self-injection study; at 6 months, the optimal dose averaged 20.7 mcg. Doses exceeding 60–65 mcg generally are not recommended. (See Erectile Dysfunction: Treatment, in Uses.)

Prolonged erection (persisting 4–6 hours) or priapism (erection persisting

6 hours or longer) occurred in 4 or 0.4% of patients, respectively, receiving intracavernosal alprostadil in clinical studies. However, priapism is a medical emergency that could result in penile tissue damage and permanent loss of potency if not treated immediately, and therefore, patients should be advised to report promptly to their physician or, if unavailable, to seek alternative immediate medical attention if an erection that persists longer than 4 hours or that is extremely painful occurs. Management of priapism or prolonged erection should be according to established medical practice, and has included aspiration of cavernosal blood and/or intracavernosal injection of an α-adrenergic agonist (i.e., phenylephrine, epinephrine) or dopamine; priapism may be more likely during dose titration than during maintenance (home) therapy. Rarely, more radical therapy for priapism (e.g., cavernospongiosus or Winter's shunt) may be necessary, such as in patients with persistent priapism (e.g., for longer than 24 hours).

The most common adverse effect associated with intracavernosal alprostadil use is penile pain, which was reported at least once in 37% of patients in clinical studies of up to 18 months' duration. In most cases, such pain was described as mild to moderate in intensity, although 3% of patients discontinued therapy with the drug because of penile pain. Patients should be advised to report to their clinician penile pain that develops or intensifies during intracavernosal alprostadil therapy. Patients also should be vigilant for the development of nodules or hard areas in the penis and be instructed to report any sign of infection (e.g., penile erythema, swelling, tenderness, or unusual curvature).

Penile fibrosis, including Peyronie's disease, developed in 3% of patients receiving intracavernosal alprostadil in clinical studies; in one self-injection study in which the drug was administered for up to 18 months, the incidence of fibrosis was about 8%. Penile hematoma and ecchymosis occurred in 3 and 2% of patients, respectively; most cases were attributed to improper administration technique. The manufacturers' labeling should be consulted for other less common adverse effects associated with intracavernosal alprostadil and for additional information on usual precautions associated with such therapy.

Intraurethral Dosage. Intraurethral alprostadil therapy (in the home setting) should be administered at the dose that was determined as optimal during titration in a medical setting; no more than 2 urethral suppositories should be used within a 24-hour period. Erection that lasts longer than desired may be relieved by the application of an ice pack alternately to each inner thigh for a period not exceeding 10 minutes.

Prolonged erection (persisting 4–6 hours) or priapism (erection persisting 6 hours or longer) occurred in 0.3 and less than 0.1% of patients, respectively, receiving intarurethral alprostadil in clinical studies. Since priapism is a medical emergency that could result in penile tissue damage and permanent loss of potency if not treated immediately, patients should be advised to report promptly to their clinician or, if their clinician is unavailable, to seek alternative immediate medical attention if an erection occurs that persists longer than 4–6 hours or is extremely painful. (For further information on management of priapism, see: Intracavernosal Dosage under Dosage: Maintenance in Patients with Erectile Dysfunction, in the Dosage and Administration section.) The manufacturer of alprostadil urethral suppositories states that in patients who develop priapism or prolonged erection, dose should be decreased or, alternatively, discontinuance of intraurethral alprostadil therapy should be considered.

The most common adverse effect associated with intraurethral alprostadil is penile, urethral, or testicular pain, which was reported in 36, 13, or 5% of patients, respectively. In most cases, such pain was described as mild and transient, although about 7% of patients discontinued therapy with the drug because of such pain. Urethral bleeding and/or spotting and other minor urethral abrasions were reported in about 3% of patients. Adverse effects associated with intraurethral alprostadil that were reported in sexual partners included vaginal burning and/or itching; however, a causal relationship to the drug has not been established and it is not known if these effects were associated with resumption of sexual intercourse. Dizziness, symptomatic hypotension, or syncope was reported in 4, 3, or 0.4% of patients, respectively, using alprostadil urethral suppositories during the intial (dose-titrating) phase. Patients should be warned to avoid tasks requiring physical coordination (e.g., operating machinery, driving a motor vehicle) that could result in injury if hypotension or syncope were to occur following the use of such suppositories. In addition, patients should be advised to lie down and immediately raise their legs if they experience a light-headed feeling, dizziness, feeling of faintness, or rapid pulse and to promptly contact their clinician if symptoms persist.

Diagnostic Use. When used alone as a simple test for erectile dysfunction, patients usually have been given a single 10- to 20-mcg intracavernosal dose of alprostadil and then examined 5–15 minutes later; if only partial erection was present, the patient could be asked to perform manual genital stimulation short of ejaculation, with or without visual sexual stimulation, for up to 5 minutes and then reexamined. If adequate erection still could not be achieved, the dose could be titrated upward (e.g., up to 40 mcg, possibly administered on a subsequent day). A positive response generally was interpreted as a full erection maintained for at least 30 minutes. (See Erectile Dysfunction: Diagnosis, in Uses.) Alternatively, characterization of the onset, degree (e.g., soft, slight tumescence, full tumescence without rigidity, full rigidity), angle, and duration of erection with a given dose can be reported. Specialized references should be consulted for additional information on the performance and interpretation of tests of erectile function involving intracavernosal alprostadil.

When used as an adjunct to other vascular testing (e.g., duplex ultrasonography, cavernosometry/cavernosography, angiography, radioisotope penogram) as an aid in visualizing and assessing the penile vasculature in the diagnosis of erectile dysfunction, the manufacturer of Caverject® states that a single dose of intracavernosal alprostadil that produces an erection with firm rigidity is used. However, the clinical value of these invasive studies currently can be severely limited by factors such as lack of normative data, operator dependence, and variable interpretation of results. Therefore, such studies might best be performed in facilities with expertise and interest in the investigation of vascular aspects of erectile dysfunction. Additional study is needed to define further interpretive standards and associated diagnostic accuracy and predictability of treatment outcomes of these tests in patients with erectile dysfunction.

Ductus Arteriosus-dependent Congenital Heart Disease Alprostadil dosage for maintaining patency of the ductus arteriosus is adjusted according to therapeutic response and tolerance, using the lowest possible effective dosage for the shortest period necessary to provide desired effects. Therapy with the drug usually is continued until surgical repair is complete, usually within 24–48 hours after initiation, although the drug occasionally is continued postoperatively (e.g., to improve pulmonary blood flow in neonates with cyanotic congenital heart disease). If long-term alprostadil infusion is considered (e.g., when surgery is deferred in a poor-risk neonate), the risks of prolonged therapy should be weighed carefully against the anticipated benefits. Neonates receiving recommended dosages for longer than 120 hours should be monitored closely for evidence of antral hyperplasia and gastric outlet obstruction. Other potential risks of prolonged therapy include cortical hyperostosis of long bones and morphologic changes in the pulmonary arteries. In some infants (e.g., those with very small branch pulmonary arteries, those with severe cyanotic congenital heart disease), alprostadil therapy has been continued cautiously for several weeks to months.

In neonates with restricted pulmonary blood flow, monitoring for adequate response to alprostadil should include measures of improved blood oxygenation. For neonates with restricted systemic blood flow, such monitoring should include measures of improved systemic blood pressure and blood pH.

The usual initial neonatal dosage of alprostadil for maintaining patency of the ductus arteriosus is continuous infusion of 0.05–0.1 mcg/kg per minute. Based on experience from clinical studies, the manufacturer of Prostin VR Pediatric® recommends an initial dosage of 0.1 mcg/kg per minute; however, adequate clinical response has been reported with an initial dosage of 0.05 mcg/kg per minute, and some neonates may respond to lower initial dosages. If response to the initial dosage is inadequate, dosage can be increased gradually up to 0.4 mcg/kg per minute; however, dosages exceeding 0.1 mcg/kg per minute generally have not been shown to produce additional benefit. After a therapeutic response is achieved (increased PO_2 in infants with restricted pulmonary blood flow or increased systemic blood pressure and blood pH in infants with restricted systemic blood flow), the infusion rate should be reduced to provide the lowest possible dosage that maintains the response; such downward titration of dosage often is accomplished by progressively halving the alprostadil dose (e.g., from 0.1 down to 0.05 down to 0.025 mcg/kg per minute, etc) until the lowest effective dose is reached. If complications occur, a lower infusion rate or discontinuance of the drug may be considered. A maintenance infusion rate of 0.025–0.01 mcg/kg per minute may be adequate to maintain response. Lower maintenance infusion rates of 0.002–0.005 mcg/kg per minute also have been effective for maintenance in some neonates prior to surgery.

Description

Alprostadil, the naturally occurring prostaglandin E_1, is a vasodilating agent and a platelet-aggregation inhibitor and is prepared synthetically for commercial use. Parenteral alprostadil is commercially available as a sterile powder for injection with (Caverject® Impulse®) or without alfadex (α-cyclodextrin) (Caverject®), as an alcoholic solution (Prostin VR Pediatric®), and as a lyophilized powder with alfadex (Edex®). The inclusion complex enhances the water solubility of alprostadil. Alprostadil also is available as a urethral (micro) suppository, measuring 1.4 mm in diameter and 3 or 6 mm in length (Muse®). Prostaglandins of the E series occur naturally in the seminal vesicles and cavernous tissues of males and in the placenta and ductus arteriosus of the fetus. Alprostadil relaxes the smooth muscles of the corpus cavernosum and the ductus arteriosus. Alprostadil is absorbed through the urethral mucosa and then distributed to corpus spongiosum and corpus cavernosum when administered as a urethral suppository.

■ **Penile Effects** Alprostadil induces erection by relaxing trabecular smooth muscle and dilating cavernosal arteries and their branches (i.e., the helicine arterioles of the penis). As a result, the lacunar spaces expand and blood becomes entrapped secondary to compression of venules against the tunica albuginea (i.e., the corporal veno-occlusive mechanism). For sufficient tumescence and rigidity to occur, the tunica albuginea must be sufficiently stiff to compress the venules penetrating it and thus block venous outflow.

The precise mechanism(s) of action of alprostadil-induced cavernosal effects has not been established but appears to differ from that of papaverine. Although both agents appear to increase the intracellular concentrations of cyclic AMP, papaverine inhibits the inactivation of cyclic AMP via oxidative phosphorylation and interferes with calcium mobilization during muscle contraction, while alprostadil interacts with specific membrane-bound receptors that stimulate adenylate cyclase and elevate intracellular cyclic AMP, leading to activation of protein kinase and resultant smooth muscle relaxation. In addition, alprostadil may antagonize the vasoconstrictive actions of norepinephrine by preventing the neuronal release of this amine and may enhance the actions of nonadrenergic, noncholinergic vasodilatory neurotransmitters. Data from studies employing combination therapy suggest a possible additive effect between alprostadil and papaverine in promoting intracavernosal arterial smooth muscle relaxation, but additional study is necessary. In addition, the mechanisms of erection are complex, and the exact nature of neurotransmitters (e.g., acetylcholine, norepinephrine) involved as well as the various steps leading to relaxation of the vascular smooth muscles remain to be more fully elucidated; nitric oxide released from endothelial cells currently is hypothesized as being the principal nonadrenergic, noncholinergic neurotransmitter involved, but others (e.g., neuropeptide Y, calcitonin gene-related peptide, vasoactive intestinal polypeptide) also may be involved.

Alprostadil does not directly affect ejaculation or orgasm.

■ **Effects on the Ductus Arteriosus** In neonates with a closing ductus arteriosus, alprostadil markedly relaxes, and thus may reopen, the ductus. Thus in neonates with congenital cardiopulmonary defects that restrict pulmonary or systemic blood flow and who depend on a patent ductus arteriosus for blood oxygenation and lower body perfusion, the drug may improve cardiovascular status (e.g., blood flow and oxygenation) by maintaining ductal patency until corrective or palliative surgery can be performed. In those with restricted pulmonary blood flow, alprostadil increases blood oxygenation in a substantial proportion of such neonates, with the most marked improvement generally occurring in those with low pretreatment blood PO_2. In those with restricted systemic blood flow, the drug can increase systemic blood pressure, decrease the ratio of pulmonary artery to aortic pressures, and increase blood pH in those with acidosis. (See Uses: Ductus Arteriosus-Dependent Congenital Heart Disease.)

SumMon® (see Users Guide). For additional information on this drug until a more detailed monograph is developed and published, the manufacturer's labeling should be consulted. It is *essential* that the labeling be consulted for detailed information on the usual cautions, precautions, and contraindications.

Preparations

Excipients in commercially available drug preparations may have clinically important effects in some individuals; consult specific product labeling for details.

Alprostadil

Parenteral		
For injection concentrate, for IV infusion	500 mcg/mL*	Alprostadil Injection Prostin VR Pediatric®, Pfizer
For injection, for intracavernosal use	10 mcg	Caverject® (available as single-dose vials), Pfizer Caverject® Impulse® (available as disposable prefilled dual-chambered cartridges with bacteriostatic water for injection with benzyl alcohol 4.45 mcg diluent; needle and alcohol swabs), Pfizer Edex® (available in single-dose vials; kits with vial diluent; or cartridges [refill or starter packs] with one compartment of dual-chamber containing diluent [bacteriostatic 0.9% sodium chloride with benzyl alcohol 0.945% w/v] and with needles and alcohol swabs), Schwarz
	20 mcg	Caverject® (available as single-dose vials), Pfizer Caverject® Impulse® (available as disposable prefilled dual-chambered cartridges with bacteriostatic water for injection with benzyl alcohol 4.45 mcg diluent; needle and alcohol swabs), Pfizer Edex® (available in single-dose vials; kits with vial diluent; or cartridges [refill or starter packs] with one compartment of dual-chamber containing diluent [bacteriostatic 0.9% sodium chloride with benzyl alcohol 0.945% w/v] and with needles and alcohol swabs), Schwarz
	40 mcg	Caverject® (available as single-dose vials), Pfizer Edex® (available in single-dose vials; kits with vial diluent; or cartridges [refill or starter packs] with one compartment of dual-chamber containing diluent [bacteriostatic 0.9% sodium chloride with benzyl alcohol 0.945% w/v] and with needles and alcohol swabs), Schwarz

Urogenital		
Suppository	125 mcg	Muse® (with applicator), Vivus
	250 mcg	Muse® (with applicator), Vivus
	500 mcg	Muse® (with applicator), Vivus
	1 mg	Muse® (with applicator), Vivus

*available from one or more manufacturer, distributor, and/or repackager by generic (nonproprietary) name

†Use is not currently included in the labeling approved by the US Food and Drug Administration

Dipyridamole

■ Dipyridamole is a non-nitrate coronary vasodilator that also inhibits platelet aggregation.

Uses

■ **Prosthetic Heart Valves** Dipyridamole is used orally as an adjunct to coumarin anticoagulants (e.g., warfarin) in the prevention of postoperative thromboembolic complications of heart valve replacement. Because warfarin therapy alone may not completely prevent thrombosis in patients with mechanical prosthetic heart valves, dipyridamole has been used in conjunction with warfarin in an effort to reduce the risk of thrombosis in these patients. While some evidence suggests that dipyridamole used in conjunction with warfarin may be more effective in reducing postoperative thromboembolic events in patients with mechanical prosthetic heart valves than use of warfarin alone, the American College of Chest Physicians (ACCP) and other experts generally recommend the addition of low-dose aspirin (rather than dipyridamole) to warfarin therapy in such patients. (See Thrombosis: Prosthetic Heart Valves, under Uses, in Aspirin 28:08.04.24.) Dipyridamole should not be used alone, without warfarin, for the prevention of postoperative thromboembolic complications in patients undergoing placement of mechanical prosthetic heart valves since there is no evidence to date that dipyridamole (or other platelet-aggregation inhibitors) would be effective when used alone.

■ **Transient Ischemic Attacks and Completed Thrombotic Stroke** Extended-release dipyridamole in fixed combination with aspirin is used to reduce the risk of stroke in patients who have had transient ischemic attacks (TIAs) or completed thrombotic stroke (secondary prevention).

In a randomized, comparative, placebo-controlled study, patients who had experienced either an ischemic stroke or TIAs were assigned to receive treatment with aspirin (25 mg twice daily), extended-release dipyridamole (200 mg twice daily), aspirin plus extended-release dipyridamole (25 and 200 mg twice daily, respectively), or placebo. All active treatments reduced the risk of the primary end points of stroke (nonfatal or fatal) or stroke and/or death compared with placebo. Aspirin plus dipyridamole reduced the risk of stroke by about 23% compared with aspirin alone and by about 25% compared with dipyridamole alone at 2 years of follow-up; the effects of combined therapy on risk reductions with aspirin and dipyridamole were additive but not synergistic. Aspirin, dipyridamole, and the combination also reduced the incidence of TIAs and other vascular events in a manner consistent with these treatments' effects on the risk of stroke. None of the treatments had a statistically significant effect on the end point of death (i.e., no effect on survival). Headache and GI events were the most common adverse effects in this study, occurring more frequently in the dipyridamole-treated groups, while bleeding from the GI tract or from any site was more common in the aspirin-treated groups.

ACCP, the American Stroke Association (ASA), and the American Heart Association (AHA) recommend antiplatelet therapy for secondary prevention of ischemic atherothrombotic (noncardioembolic) stroke or TIAs in patients with prior TIAs or stroke. (See Transient Ischemic Attacks and Acute Ischemic Stroke under Uses: Thrombosis, in Aspirin 28:08.04.24.) These experts consider the combination of aspirin and dipyridamole (25 mg aspirin/200 mg extended-release dipyridamole twice daily) an acceptable antiplatelet option for the prevention of recurrent stroke or other cardiovascular events in such patients; other options include aspirin monotherapy, cilostazol, or clopidogrel. When selecting an appropriate antiplatelet regimen for the secondary prevention of noncardioembolic stroke, factors such as the patient's individual risk for recurrent stroke, tolerance, and cost of the different agents should be considered.

■ **Adjunct to Thallium Myocardial Perfusion Imaging** Dipyridamole is used IV as an adjunct to thallous (thallium) chloride Tl 201 myocardial stress perfusion imaging in patients unable to exercise adequately.

The sensitivity and specificity of dipyridamole-assisted thallium imaging versus coronary arteriography in the detection of coronary artery disease were determined by comparing the results of thallium imaging with those of coronary arteriography under blinded conditions. The sensitivity of dipyridamole-assisted thallium imaging (true positive thallium imaging divided by the number of patients with positive angiograms) was 85% and the specificity (true negative thallium imaging divided by the number of patients with negative angiograms) was about 50%. In a subset of patients who had exercise thallium imaging or dipyridamole-assisted thallium imaging, the sensitivity and specificity of the 2 tests were almost identical.

■ **Other Uses** Dipyridamole also has been used orally to decrease platelet aggregation in a number of other thromboembolic disorders†. ACCP suggests postoperative anticoagulant therapy with unfractionated heparin and antiplatelet therapy with aspirin and/or dipyridamole to reduce thromboembolic events in children with heart failure who require implantation of ventricular assist devices†. However, for most thromboembolic disorders, it has not been established whether the inclusion of dipyridamole in an antithrombotic regimen substantially enhances the potential benefit compared with that of the other antithrombotic agents (e.g., aspirin) alone, and some evidence suggests that in certain disorders, it may not (e.g., for prevention of thromboembolic complications in patients surviving a myocardial infarction (MI) or following PCI, coronary artery bypass graft [CABG] surgery, lower extremity vascular reconstruction).

ACCP recommends the use of dipyridamole in combination with aspirin as an option for long-term antiplatelet therapy in patients with symptomatic carotid stenosis†, including those who have undergone recent carotid endarterectomy.

There currently is no evidence that antiplatelet agents such as dipyridamole or ticlopidine have any advantage over aspirin for mortality reduction following an acute MI†.

Dipyridamole has been used in the long-term therapy of chronic angina pectoris† based on the premise that prolonged therapy with the drug may reduce the frequency of or eliminate anginal episodes, improve exercise tolerance, and reduce requirements for nitroglycerin. However, well-controlled clinical studies showed that long-term oral administration of dipyridamole does not prevent ECG signs of myocardial ischemia in patients with angina pectoris following exercise or decrease the frequency or severity of anginal attacks, and experts state that there is evidence and/or general agreement that dipyridamole is *not* useful or effective for the management of chronic angina pectoris. The drug also is *not* effective for the treatment of acute episodes of angina† and is *not* a substitute for appropriate medical programs for the treatment of angina pectoris†.

Dosage and Administration

■ **Administration** Dipyridamole is administered orally or IV. Capsules containing the fixed-combination of extended-release dipyridamole and aspirin should be swallowed whole and should not be chewed. The fixed-combination capsules containing extended-release dipyridamole and aspirin may be administered without regard to food.

Prior to IV administration, dipyridamole injection should be diluted in at least twice the injection volume with 0.45% sodium chloride injection, 0.9% sodium chloride injection, or 5% dextrose injection to a final volume of approximately 20–50 mL. Infusion of undiluted dipyridamole may cause local irritation.

■ **Dosage** The usual adult oral dosage of dipyridamole for adjunctive use with coumarin anticoagulant (e.g., warfarin) therapy in the prevention of postoperative thromboembolic complications of cardiac valve replacement is 75–100 mg 4 times daily.

For the prevention of thromboembolic complications in patients with various other thromboembolic disorders†, oral dosage of dipyridamole generally has ranged from 150–400 mg daily, in combination with another platelet-aggregation inhibitor (e.g., aspirin) or warfarin.

For reducing the risk of stroke in patients who have had transient ischemic attacks (TIAs) or completed stroke caused by thrombosis, the usual dosage of oral extended-release dipyridamole is 200 mg in fixed combination with aspirin 25 mg (1 capsule) twice daily in the morning and evening. If headaches become intolerable during initial treatment, the dosage of the dipyridamole/aspirin fixed combination should be reduced to 200 mg of dipyridamole and 25 mg of aspirin (1 capsule) once daily at bedtime and low-dose aspirin should be administered in the morning. Because no outcome data are available with this regimen and headaches diminish during continued treatment, patients should resume the usual regimen (200 mg of extended-release dipyridamole and 25 mg of aspirin twice daily) as soon as possible (usually within 1 week). The amount of aspirin in the fixed-combination preparation may not be adequate to prevent recurrent myocardial infarction (MI) or angina pectoris in patients with stroke or TIA.

When used as an adjunct to thallium myocardial imaging, dipyridamole usually is administered as a single IV dose of 0.57 mg/kg, infused at a rate of 0.142 mg/kg per minute for 4 minutes. Although the maximum tolerated IV dose of dipyridamole has not been determined, clinical experience suggests that a total dose exceeding 60 mg is not needed for any patient. Thallium-201 should be injected within 5 minutes following completion of the dipyridamole infusion.

Cautions

■ **Adverse Effects** Adverse effects associated with oral dipyridamole therapy are generally dose related and reversible and may include headache, dizziness, GI intolerance (e.g., abdominal distress), nausea, vomiting, diarrhea, peripheral vasodilation, flushing, weakness, syncope, rash, and pruritus. Headache is the most common adverse effect of dipyridamole and is most notable during the first month of treatment. (See Dosage and Administration: Dosage, for details on dosage adjustment for headache.) Rarely, angina pectoris or aggravation of angina pectoris has been reported, usually at the beginning of therapy. During postmarketing experience, hypersensitivity reactions (e.g., rash, urticaria, severe bronchospasm, angioedema), laryngeal edema, fatigue, myalgia, arthritis, nausea, dyspepsia, paresthesia, hepatitis, thrombocytopenia, alopecia, cholelithiasis, hypotension, palpitation, and tachycardia have been reported rarely. Most adverse effects of oral dipyridamole are transient and resolve during long-term therapy with the drug; rarely, adverse effects are persistent or intolerable but are reversible when the drug is discontinued. In a large randomized, comparative, placebo-controlled trial, there was no clear safety benefit of treatment with extended-release dipyridamole in fixed combination with aspirin compared with aspirin alone.

Liver dysfunction (e.g., elevations of hepatic enzymes, hepatic failure) have been reported rarely in association with oral dipyridamole.

IV dipyridamole has been associated with serious adverse effects, including acute myocardial ischemia or infarction, cardiac death, ventricular fibrillation, symptomatic ventricular tachycardia, stroke, transient cerebral ischemia, and seizures. Asystole, sinus node arrest, sinus node depression, and conduction block also have been reported with IV dipyridamole therapy. Patients with abnormalities of cardiac impulse formation and conduction or severe coronary artery disease (e.g., unstable angina) may be at increased risk for these events. Anaphylactoid reactions and bronchospasm also have been reported in patients with coronary artery disease undergoing IV dipyridamole-assisted thallium imaging. Patients with a history of asthma may be at greater risk for bronchospasm during IV dipyridamole use.

The most common adverse effects reported in a large clinical trial in which IV dipyridamole was used as an adjunct to thallium myocardial perfusion imaging were chest pain/angina pectoris, electrocardiographic changes (most commonly ST-T changes), headache, and dizziness. Other adverse effects occurring in greater than 1% of patients receiving IV dipyridamole were hypotension, nausea, flushing, dyspnea, unspecified pain, blood pressure lability, hypertension, paresthesia, and fatigue. Cardiovascular adverse effects occurring in 1% or less of patients receiving IV dipyridamole included unspecified ECG abnormalities, unspecified arrhythmia, palpitation, ventricular tachycardia, bradycardia, myocardial infarction (MI), atrioventricular block, syncope, orthostatic hypotension, atrial fibrillation, supraventricular tachycardia, ventricular arrhythmia unspecified, heart block unspecified, cardiomyopathy, intermittent claudication, and edema. Nervous system adverse effects occurring in 1% or less of patients receiving IV dipyridamole included hypoesthesia, hypertonia, nervousness/anxiety, tremor, abnormal coordination, somnolence, dysphonia, migraine, malaise, asthenia, depersonalization, and vertigo. GI system adverse effects occurring in 1% or less of patients receiving IV dipyridamole included dyspepsia, dry mouth, abdominal pain, flatulence, vomiting, eructation, dysphagia, tenesmus, dysgeusia, thirst, and increased appetite. Respiratory system adverse effects occurring in 1% or less of patients receiving IV dipyridamole included pharyngitis, bronchospasm, hyperventilation, rhinitis, coughing, and pleural pain. Musculoskeletal system adverse effects occurring in 1% or less of patients receiving IV dipyridamole included myalgia, back pain, arthralgia, rigor, and leg cramping. Other adverse effects occurring in 1% or less of patients receiving IV dipyridamole include unspecified injection site reaction, diaphoresis, injection site pain, earache, tinnitus, unspecified vision abnormalities, eye pain, renal pain, perineal pain, and breast pain. Allergic reactions including urticaria, pruritus, dermatitis, and rash have been reported rarely during postmarketing experience.

■ **Precautions and Contraindications** When dipyridamole is used orally in fixed combination with aspirin, the cautions, precautions, and contraindications associated with aspirin therapy must be considered in addition to those associated with dipyridamole.

Dipyridamole is contraindicated in patients with hypersensitivity to dipyridamole or any ingredient in the formulation.

Dipyridamole should be used cautiously in patients with hypotension or severe coronary artery disease (e.g., unstable angina or recently sustained MI) since it can cause peripheral vasodilation.

In considering the use of IV dipyridamole-assisted thallium imaging in patients with coronary artery disease, the important clinical information to be gained by the procedure should be weighed against the risk to the patient. The rate of false positive and false negative results of IV dipyridamole-assisted thallium imaging as compared with coronary arteriography should also be considered when choosing to use dipyridamole-assisted thallium imaging.

When thallium myocardial perfusion imaging is performed with IV dipyridamole, parenteral aminophylline (an adenosine receptor antagonist) should be readily available for relieving adverse effects such as bronchospasm or chest pain. Vital signs should be monitored during and for 10–15 minutes after IV infusion of dipyridamole, and an ECG should be obtained using at least 1 chest lead. Should severe chest pain or bronchospasm occur, parenteral aminophylline should be administered by slow IV injection (e.g., 50–100 mg over 30–60 seconds) in doses of 50–250 mg. Patients with severe hypotension should be placed in a supine position with the head tilted down, if necessary, before administration of parenteral aminophylline. If the highest recommended dosage of aminophylline (250 mg) does not relieve chest pain within a few minutes, sublingual nitroglycerin may be administered. If chest pain continues despite such combination therapy, the possibility of MI should be considered. If the clinical condition of the patient with an adverse event permits a 1-minute delay, thallium imaging may be performed during such a time period before reversal of the pharmacologic effects of dipyridamole.

Commercially available extended-release dipyridamole in fixed combination with aspirin is not interchangeable with the individual components of aspirin and conventional dipyridamole tablets (e.g., Persantine®).

For patients with stroke or TIA for whom aspirin is indicated to prevent recurrent MI or angina pectoris, the amount of aspirin in the commercially available fixed-combination product may not provide adequate treatment for these cardiac indications.

■ **Pediatric Precautions** Safety and efficacy of oral dipyridamole in pediatric patients younger than 12 years of age have not been established. Safety and efficacy of IV dipyridamole in children have not been established. The safety and efficacy of extended-release dipyridamole in fixed combination with aspirin in children have not been established. The manufacturer of Aggrenox® states that because of the aspirin component, this preparation should not be used in pediatric patients. (See Cautions: Pediatric Precautions, in the Salicylates General Statement 28:08.04.24.).

■ **Mutagenicity and Carcinogenicity** Studies using dipyridamole have not revealed evidence of mutagenicity. No evidence of significant carcinogenic effects was seen in mice or rats receiving 111 or 128–142 weeks, respectively, of oral dipyridamole in dosages not exceeding 75 mg/kg (1 or 2 times the maximum recommended daily human oral dosage in mice or rats, respectively, on a mg/m^2 basis). In vitro mutagenicity tests using dipyridamole in bacterial and mammalian cell systems also did not reveal evidence of mutagenicity.

■ **Pregnancy, Fertility, and Lactation** Safe use of dipyridamole during pregnancy has not been established. Reproduction studies in mice receiving dipyridamole dosages up to 125 mg/kg daily (1.5 times the maximum recommended daily human oral dosage on a mg/m^2 basis), rats receiving dosages not exceeding 1000 mg/kg daily (25 times the maximum recommended daily human oral dosage on a mg/m^2 basis), and rabbits receiving dosages not exceeding 40 mg/kg daily (2 times the maximum recommended daily human oral dosage on a mg/m^2 basis) have not revealed evidence of harm to the fetus. There are no adequate and controlled studies to date using dipyridamole in pregnant women, and the drug should be used during pregnancy only when clearly needed. Extended-release dipyridamole in fixed combination with aspirin should be avoided in the third trimester of pregnancy and during labor and delivery because of the aspirin component of this preparation; aspirin has been shown to be teratogenic in animals and to cause fetal harm when administered to a pregnant woman. If dipyridamole in fixed combination with aspirin is used during pregnancy or the patient becomes pregnant while taking the fixed combination, the patient should be apprised of the potential hazard to the fetus. (See Cautions: Pregnancy, Fertility, and Lactation, in the Salicylates General Statement 28:08.04.24.)

Reproduction studies in rats receiving dipyridamole dosages up to 12 times the maximum recommended daily human oral dosage on a mg/m^2 basis have not revealed evidence of impaired fertility. However, a substantial reduction in the number of corpora lutea with a subsequent reduction in the number of implantations and live fetuses was observed in rats receiving 30 times the maximum recommended daily human oral dosage of the drug on a mg/m^2 basis.

Because dipyridamole is distributed into milk, the drug should be used with caution in nursing women.

Drug Interactions

Since dipyridamole may inhibit platelet aggregation, heparin and dipyridamole should be used concomitantly with caution and patients should be monitored closely to prevent bleeding; however, the actual incidence of this reaction has not been established.

In a dosage of 400 mg daily, dipyridamole does not affect prothrombin time and can be administered with warfarin. Concomitant use of dipyridamole and warfarin does not appear to increase the frequency or severity of bleeding compared with use of warfarin alone. However, in rare instances, increased bleeding during or after surgery has been observed during such concurrent therapy. Some clinicians recommend maintenance of prothrombin time in the lower end of the therapeutic range during concomitant administration of these drugs to avoid possible bleeding.

Dipyridamole may increase the plasma concentrations and the cardiovascular effects of adenosine; adjustment of adenosine dosage may be necessary. Methylxanthines are competitive adenosine receptor antagonists, and aminophylline has been used effectively to terminate persistent adverse effects of dipyridamole. Use of other xanthine derivatives (e.g., caffeine) or maintenance dosages of oral theophylline may abolish the coronary vasodilation of dipyridamole and lead to false negative thallium imaging results. (See Pharmacology.)

In patients receiving an anticholinesterase agent for the treatment of myasthenia gravis, concomitant use of dipyridamole may counteract the anticholinesterase effects of such inhibitors and potentially aggravate myasthenia gravis.

Acute Toxicity

Limited information is available on the acute toxicity of dipyridamole in humans. The oral LD_{50} of the drug exceeds 6 g/kg in rats and approximately 400 mg/kg in dogs. Overdosage of dipyridamole is likely to produce symptoms that are mainly extensions of the usual pharmacologic effects of the drug. Based on the known hemodynamic effects of dipyridamole, symptoms such as warm feeling, flushes, sweating, restlessness, feelings of weakness, or dizziness may occur. Hypotension and tachycardia might also be observed. Overdosage with IV dipyridamole has not been reported.

In cases of overdosage, seek medical attention immediately; careful medical management is essential. Symptomatic treatment of overdosage is recommended and may include use of a vasopressor. Gastric lavage should be considered. Administration of a xanthine derivative (e.g., aminophylline) may reverse the hemodynamic effects of dipyridamole. Dialysis is not likely to be of benefit in the management of dipyridamole overdosage since the drug is highly protein bound.

Pharmacology

The coronary vasodilator effect of dipyridamole probably results from its ability to inhibit cellular reuptake of adenosine, thereby increasing extracellular concentrations of endogenous adenosine available for receptor binding and vascular vasodilation. The vasodilatory effects of dipyridamole are abolished by the adenosine receptor antagonists theophylline and aminophylline. (See Drug Interactions.) Dipyridamole also may cause vasodilation by delaying the hydrolysis of cyclic 3′,5′-adenosine monophosphate (cAMP) by inhibiting the enzyme phosphodiesterase.

The mechanism(s) by which dipyridamole inhibits platelet aggregation has not been fully elucidated. The mechanism(s) may be related to inhibition of platelet uptake and metabolism of adenosine (an inhibitor of platelet reactivity); inhibition of platelet phosphodiesterase, which leads to accumulation of cAMP within platelets; direct stimulation of the release of eicosanoids such as prostacyclin or prostaglandin D_2 from endothelial cells; and/or inhibition of thromboxane A_2 formation. Increased local concentrations of adenosine at the platelet surface act on the platelet A_2 receptor and stimulate platelet adenyl cyclase, thereby increasing platelet cAMP concentrations. Increased platelet cAMP concentrations affect platelet-activating factor, collagen, and adenosine diphosphate and inhibit mobilization of free calcium, which is involved in platelet activation. Therapeutic concentrations of dipyridamole inhibit platelet cyclic-3′,5′-guanosine monophosphate phosphodiesterase (cGMP-PDE), thereby augmenting the increase in platelet cGMP concentrations produced by nitric oxide. Increased cGMP platelet concentrations inhibit platelet activation and aggregation. Dipyridamole also stimulates prostacyclin synthesis and potentiates the antiplatelet effects of prostacyclin. Dipyridamole prolongs platelet survival time in patients with valvular heart disease in whom platelet survival is shortened.

The mechanism by which IV dipyridamole-induced vasodilation aids in thallium myocardial perfusion imaging has not been fully elucidated, but may be a result of a "coronary steal" phenomenon in which normal coronary arteries dilate and sustain increased blood flow while shunting blood away from stenotic arteries. Because myocardial uptake of thallous (thallium) chloride Tl 201 is directly proportional to coronary blood flow, relatively less thallous chloride Tl 201 uptake as well as slower washout occurs in myocardium perfused by stenotic versus normal coronary arteries and the differences in blood flow between areas served by stenotic versus normal arteries are enhanced during thallium testing with dipyridamole infusion. Myocardial oxygen consumption and cardiac work are not increased.

IV dipyridamole may decrease blood pressure and increase heart rate and cardiac output, because of dilation of systemic resistance vessels. However, usual oral doses of the drug generally produce no change in blood pressure or in blood flow in peripheral arteries.

Pharmacokinetics

Oral dipyridamole is incompletely absorbed from the GI tract; the extent of absorption exhibits interindividual variation. According to the manufacturer, the pharmacokinetics of dipyridamole and aspirin are not altered by concomitant administration in fixed combination. Following oral administration of a dose of dipyridamole as conventional tablets, peak plasma concentrations of the drug are attained in about 45–150 minutes (mean: 75 minutes). The mean serum concentration of dipyridamole 2 minutes following administration of an IV dose of dipyridamole (0.568 mg/kg infused over 4 minutes) was 4.6 mcg/mL. Following oral administration of 200 mg of extended-release dipyridamole in fixed combination with aspirin, oral bioavailability of dipyridamole averages 37–66% and peak plasma dipyridamole concentrations are achieved in about 2 hours (range: 1–6 hours) with twice-daily dosing. Steady-state peak and trough plasma concentrations of dipyridamole average 1.98 and 0.53 mcg/mL, respectively, following administration as the fixed-combination extended-release capsules. When dipyridamole in fixed combination with aspirin was administered with a high-fat meal, dipyridamole peak plasma concentrations and total absorption (area under the concentration-time curve [AUC]) decreased at steady state by 20–30% compared with administration in the fasted state; this effect does not appear to be clinically important.

Animal studies indicate that dipyridamole is widely distributed into body tissues and that small amounts of the drug cross the placenta. Dipyridamole does not cross the blood-brain barrier in animals. Dipyridamole is distributed into human milk. The apparent volume of distribution of IV dipyridamole at steady state is 1–2.5 L/kg, with an apparent central volume of 3–5 liters. The drug is highly bound to plasma proteins, principally to α_1-acid glycoprotein (α_1-AGP) but also to albumin; 91–99% of the drug reportedly is bound to protein.

Following oral administration, plasma concentrations of dipyridamole decline in a biphasic manner. Half-life of the drug in the initial phase ($t_{1/2\alpha}$) is approximately 40–80 minutes and half-life in the terminal elimination phase ($t_{1/2\beta}$) is approximately 10–12 hours.

Following IV administration, plasma concentrations of dipyridamole decline in a triphasic manner, with mean half-lives of 3–12 minutes, 33–62 minutes, and 11.6–15 hours.

Dipyridamole is metabolized in the liver and excreted in the bile, chiefly as the monoglucuronide and a small amount as the diglucuronide. Dipyridamole and its glucuronides may undergo enterohepatic circulation and are excreted mainly in feces. Small amounts are excreted in urine. The mean total body clearance is 2.3–3.5 mL/minute per kg.

Chemistry and Stability

Chemistry Dipyridamole is a non-nitrate coronary vasodilator. Dipyridamole occurs as an intensely yellow, crystalline powder or needles with a bitter taste. The drug is slightly soluble in water and very soluble in alcohol. Dipyridamole is commercially available as conventional tablets and in fixed combination with aspirin as a hard-gelatin capsule containing dipyridamole as extended-release pellets and aspirin as an immediate-release tablet. Dipyridamole injection is an odorless pale yellow liquid.

Stability Dipyridamole tablets should be stored in tight, light-resistant containers at a 25°C; excursions to 15–30°C are permitted. The fixed-combination preparation of extended-release dipyridamole with aspirin should be stored at a controlled room temperature of 25°C and protected from excessive moisture, but may be exposed to temperatures ranging from 15–30°C.

Dipyridamole injection should be stored at 20–25°C; freezing should be avoided, and the injection should be protected from light. Dipyridamole should not be mixed with other drugs in the same syringe or infusion container. Parenteral drugs should be inspected visually for particulate matter and discoloration prior to administration, whenever container and solution permit.

Preparations

Excipients in commercially available drug preparations may have clinically important effects in some individuals; consult specific product labeling for details.

Dipyridamole

Oral		
Tablets	25 mg*	**Dipyridamole Tablets**
		Persantine®, Boehringer Ingelheim
	50 mg*	**Dipyridamole Tablets**
		Persantine®, Boehringer Ingelheim
	75 mg*	**Dipyridamole Tablets**
		Persantine®, Boehringer Ingelheim
Parenteral		
Injection, for IV Use	5 mg/mL	**Dipyridamole Injection**

*available from one or more manufacturer, distributor, and/or repackager by generic (nonproprietary) name

Dypyridamole Combinations

Oral		
Capsules, extended-release (containing dipyridamole pellets and 25 mg immediate-release aspirin tablet)	200 mg with Aspirin 25 mg	**Aggrenox®**, Boehringer Ingelheim

†Use is not currently included in the labeling approved by the US Food and Drug Administration

α-ADRENERGIC BLOCKING AGENTS 24:20

Doxazosin Mesylate

Doxazosin mesylate is a quinazoline-derivative postsynaptic α_1-adrenergic blocking agent.

Uses

Hypertension Doxazosin mesylate is used alone or in combination with other classes of antihypertensive agents for the management of hypertension. However, because of established clinical benefits (e.g., reductions in overall mortality and in adverse cardiovascular, cerebrovascular, and renal outcomes), current evidence-based practice guidelines for the management of hypertension in adults generally recommend the use of drugs from 4 classes of antihypertensive agents (angiotensin-converting enzyme [ACE] inhibitors, angiotensin II receptor antagonists, calcium-channel blockers, and thiazide diuretics).

In a randomized, double-blind clinical study (the Antihypertensive and Lipid-Lowering Treatment to Prevent Heart Attack Trial [ALLHAT]), doxazosin, an α_1-blocker, was less effective in lowering mean systolic blood pressure (by about 2–3 mm Hg) than chlorthalidone, a thiazide-like diuretic. In order to achieve target blood pressure in hypertensive patients, use of doxazosin required additional hypotensive therapy more frequently than chlorthalidone. In addition, interim analysis (median follow-up: 3.3 years) of this study indicated that use of doxazosin in high-risk (at least 2 risk factors for coronary heart disease) hypertensive patients 55 years of age and older was associated with a higher risk of stroke and a higher incidence of combined cardiovascular disease events (including twice the risk of congestive heart failure) than use of chlorthalidone. Study investigators concluded that such increased risk of congestive heart failure could not have been caused by the relatively small difference in the mean target systolic blood pressure observed in patients receiving doxazosin compared with those receiving chlorthalidone. Therefore, based on these findings, the trial's Data Safety and Monitoring Board recommended that the doxazosin treatment arm be terminated prematurely. The remaining antihypertensive arms (e.g., calcium-channel blockers, ACE enzyme inhibitors, diuretics) and lipid-lowering (pravastatin vs usual care) components of the study subsequently were completed and reported.

Current antihypertensive and urology guidelines no longer recommend α_1-blockers as preferred *first-line* therapy for any patients with hypertension, principally because of negative findings observed in ALLHAT. However, α_1-blockers are effective antihypertensive drugs and many experts still consider their use appropriate for the management of resistant hypertension as a component of combination therapy. Therapy with an α_1-blocker is most effective when used in combination with a diuretic. Some experts state that an α_1-blocker may be a second-line agent in antihypertensive treatment regimens in men with coexisting benign prostatic hyperplasia (BPH); the American Urology Association (AUA) states that monotherapy with these drugs is not optimal in hypertensive patients with lower urinary tract symptoms (LUTS) or BPH and that such conditions should be managed separately.

The beneficial effects of α_1-blockers on blood glucose and lipid concentrations may mitigate some of the adverse metabolic effects of diuretics, and α_1-blockers may offer some advantage in patients with underlying lipoprotein disorders (e.g., hypercholesterolemia) or in those with lipoprotein abnormalities induced by other antihypertensive agents (e.g., thiazide diuretics). The possibility that geriatric patients may be more susceptible than younger patients to the postural hypotensive effects of α_1-blockers should be considered in the selection of therapy. Blood pressure response to α_1-blockers appears to be comparable in white and black patients.

For further information on overall principles and expert recommendations for treatment of hypertension, see Uses: Hypertension in Adults and also see Uses: Hypertension in Pediatric Patients, in the Thiazides General Statement 40:28.20.

Benign Prostatic Hyperplasia Doxazosin is used to reduce urinary obstruction and relieve associated manifestations in hypertensive or normotensive patients with symptomatic benign prostatic hyperplasia (BPH, benign prostatic hypertrophy). For patients who can tolerate the potential cardiovascular and other effects of α_1-adrenergic blockade, doxazosin can effectively relieve mild to moderate obstructive manifestations (e.g., hesitancy, terminal dribbling of urine, interrupted or weak stream, impaired size and force of stream, sensation of incomplete bladder emptying or straining) and improve urinary flow rates in a substantial proportion of patients and may be a useful alternative to surgery, particularly in those who are awaiting or are unwilling to undergo surgical correction of the hyperplasia (e.g., via transurethral resection of the prostate [TURP]) or who are not candidates for such surgery.

Therapy with α_1-blockers appears to be less effective in relieving irritative (e.g., nocturia, daytime frequency, urgency, dysuria) than obstructive symptomatology. In addition, therapy with the drugs generally can be expected to produce less subjective and objective improvement than prostatectomy, and periodic monitoring (e.g., performance of digital rectal examinations, serum creatinine determinations, serum prostate specific antigen [PSA] assays) is indicated in these patients to detect and manage other potential complications of or conditions associated with BPH (e.g., obstructive uropathy, prostatic carcinoma). While symptomatic improvement has been maintained for at least up to 2 years of doxazosin therapy in some patients, the long-term effects of α-blockers on the need for surgery and on the frequency of developing BPH-associated complications such as acute urinary obstruction remain to be established.

Although the etiology of benign prostatic hyperplasia currently is unclear, age-associated changes in circulating hormones (e.g., androgens, estrogens) appear to be involved; approximately 40% of men have been reported to have clinical evidence of BPH by age 70. Hyperplasia of the prostatic tissue encircling the urethra produces narrowing of the bladder neck and prostatic urethra, leading to both obstructive (e.g., urinary hesitancy, slow/weak stream, straining, incomplete voiding) and irritative (e.g., urinary frequency, urgency, nocturia) manifestations; progressive obstruction of urinary flow eventually may lead to urinary retention and subsequent complications (e.g., urinary tract infection, bladder calculi, hydronephrosis).

In addition to the mechanical component of urethral obstruction caused by the enlarged gland, a dynamic component of obstruction may be prominent in some patients; current evidence suggests that approximately 50% of prostate outflow obstruction is caused by reversible α-adrenergic (principally α_1) receptor-mediated contractions of smooth muscle in the prostatic capsule, prostatic adenoma, and bladder neck. While nonselective α-adrenergic blockers such as phenoxybenzamine have been used successfully to treat BPH, such nonselective blockade has been associated with adverse effects such as postural hypotension, dizziness, and tachycardia because blockade of α_2-adrenergic receptors interferes with the negative feedback mechanism controlling norepinephrine release from presynaptic nerve terminals. As a result, nonselective α-blocker therapy currently is not recommended for BPH; instead, therapy with selective α_1-blockers, which can relieve α_1-adrenergic-mediated bladder outflow obstruction, is recommended.

Patients with mildly symptomatic BPH and those with moderate to severe symptoms that are not bothersome (i.e., that do not interfere with daily activities of living) generally should simply be followed rather than actively treated. Active therapy (e.g., drug therapy; minimally invasive therapies such as transurethral microwave heat; surgery such as TURP) should be considered for patients with moderate to severe BPH that is bothersome; the potential benefits and possible risks of various therapeutic options, including watchful waiting, should be discussed with the patient. Although drug therapy usually is not as effective as surgical therapy, it may provide adequate symptomatic relief with fewer and less serious adverse effects compared with surgery. Most experts currently consider therapy with an α_1-adrenergic blocker such as doxazosin to be an appropriate option for symptomatic treatment of bothersome lower urinary tract symptoms in patients with BPH. With the exception of prazosin (for which there are insufficient data to compare), currently available α_1-adrenergic blockers are considered comparably effective. Therapy with an α_1-adrenergic blocker generally is more effective in relieving lower urinary tract symptoms than that with a 5α-reductase inhibitor (e.g., finasteride), and 5α-reductase inhibitors are ineffective in patients without prostatic enlargement.

Combination Therapy Although studies of up to 1 year in duration generally have found combination therapy with an α_1-blocker and 5α-reductase inhibitor (e.g., finasteride) to be no more effective than α_1-adrenergic blocker monotherapy in providing symptomatic relief of BPH, a long-term (mean follow-up: 4.5 years), double-blind study (Medical Therapy of Prostatic Symptoms [MTOPS]) found that combined therapy with doxazosin (4–8 mg daily) and finasteride (5 mg daily) was more effective than therapy with either drug alone in preventing symptom progression (defined as an increase from baseline of at least 4 points in the American Urological Association [AUA] symptom score, acute urinary retention, urinary incontinence, renal insufficiency, or recurrent urinary tract infection). The percent reduction in the risk of symptom progression (generally manifested as an increase in AUA symptom score) relative to placebo was 34% with finasteride, 39% with doxazosin, and 67% with combination therapy. The risks of long-term acute urinary retention and the need for invasive therapy were reduced by combination therapy and by finasteride monotherapy but not by doxazosin monotherapy. Combination therapy or doxazosin or finasteride monotherapy each were effective in providing improvement in symptom scores, with combination therapy providing greater improvement than either drug alone.

Most experts state that combined therapy with an α_1-adrenergic blocker and 5α-reductase inhibitor can be considered for men with bothersome moderate to severe BPH and demonstrable prostatic enlargement, weighing the benefit of preventing progression of BPH with the risks and cost of the combination. Men at risk for BPH progression are most likely to benefit from combination therapy. Although the benefit of combination therapy was not as substantial in men with low baseline prostate-specific antigen (PSA) levels compared with those with high baseline values in the MTOPS study, the potential benefit appears to be greatest in those in whom baseline risk of progression generally is high rather than specifically in those with larger prostates or higher PSA levels at baseline.

Adverse effects associated with combined α_1-adrenergic blocker and 5α-reductase inhibitor therapy generally reflect the combined toxicity profile of each drug alone, although certain adverse effects (e.g., effects on sexual function and libido, postural hypotension, peripheral edema, dizziness, asthenia, rhinitis) may be more common with combined therapy. For further information on adverse effects associated with combined doxazosin and finasteride therapy, see Cautions in Finasteride 92:08.

Dosage and Administration

■ **Administration** Doxazosin mesylate is administered orally.

The pharmacokinetics and safety were similar with morning or evening dosing of doxazosin conventional (immediate-release) tablets in a limited number of normotensive patients in one study; however, the area under the plasma concentration-time curve (AUC) was 11% less with morning dosing, and the time to peak concentration occurred later with evening dosing (5.6 versus 3.5 hours).

Peak plasma concentrations and oral bioavailability are increased by approximately 32 and 18%, respectively, when doxazosin mesylate extended-release tablets (Cardura® XL) are administered with food. Therefore, to provide more consistent systemic exposure to the drug, extended-release tablets should be administered with breakfast.

Doxazosin mesylate extended-release tablets should be swallowed intact and should *not* be chewed, crushed, or broken. Patients should be advised *not* to become alarmed if they notice a tablet-like substance in their stools; this is normal since the tablet is designed to release the drug slowly from a nonabsorbable shell during passage through the GI tract.

■ **Dosage** Dosage of doxazosin mesylate is expressed in terms of doxazosin and must be adjusted according to the patient's blood pressure response and tolerance.

Hypertension **Usual Dosage.** For the management of hypertension in adults, the usual initial dosage of doxazosin conventional (immediate-release) tablets is 1 mg once daily. Because of the risk of postural effects (see Cautions: Postural Effects), it is essential that therapy with the drug *not* be initiated with higher dosages. Patient response (standing blood pressure) should be assessed 2–6 and 24 hours after the initial dose and any subsequent dosage adjustments. Because postural effects are most likely to occur 2–6 hours after a dose, it is particularly important that the standing blood pressure response be assessed during this period after the first dose and any increases.

If blood pressure is not adequately controlled at a doxazosin dosage of 1 mg daily as conventional tablets, the dosage may be increased to 2 mg once daily in adults; subsequent dosage adjustments can be made by doubling the dose until the desired blood pressure control is achieved, the drug is not tolerated, or a maximum dosage of 16 mg once daily is reached. Some experts state that the usual adult dosage ranges from 1–16 mg once daily. The manufacturer recommends that dosage increases be made no more frequently than every 2 weeks. Doxazosin dosages exceeding 4 mg daily as conventional tablets are associated with an increased likelihood of excessive postural effects including syncope, dizziness, vertigo, and hypotension, and those exceeding 16 mg daily are *not* recommended because of the substantial risk of postural effects.

If doxazosin is used for the management of hypertension in children†, some experts have recommended an initial dosage of 1 mg once daily as conventional tablets; dosage may be increased as necessary to a maximum of 4 mg once daily. (See Cautions: Pediatric Precautions.) For information on overall principles and expert recommendations for treatment of hypertension in pediatric patients, see Uses: Hypertension in Pediatric Patients, in the Thiazides General Statement 40:28.20.

Extended-release doxazosin tablets (Cardura® XL) currently are not FDA-labeled for use in the management of hypertension.

Blood Pressure Monitoring and Treatment Goals. Blood pressure should be monitored regularly (i.e., monthly) during therapy and dosage adjusted until blood pressure is controlled. If an adequate blood pressure response is not achieved, the dosage may be increased or another antihypertensive agent with demonstrated benefit and preferably with a complementary mechanism of action (e.g., angiotensin-converting enzyme [ACE] inhibitor, angiotensin II receptor antagonist, calcium-channel blocker, thiazide diuretic) may be added; if target blood pressure is still not achieved with the use of 2 antihypertensive agents, a third drug may be added. (See Uses: Hypertension.) In patients who develop unacceptable adverse effects with doxazosin, the drug should be discontinued and another antihypertensive agent from a different pharmacologic class should be initiated.

The goal of hypertension management and prevention is to achieve and maintain optimal control of blood pressure. However, the optimum blood pressure threshold for initiating antihypertensive drug therapy and specific treatment goals remain controversial. A 2017 multidisciplinary hypertension guideline from the American College of Cardiology (ACC), American Heart Association (AHA), and a number of other professional organizations generally recommends a blood pressure goal of less than 130/80 mm Hg in all adults, regardless of comorbidities or level of atherosclerotic cardiovascular disease (ASCVD) risk. Many patients will require at least 2 drugs from different pharmacologic classes to achieve this blood pressure goal; the potential benefits of hypertension management and drug cost, adverse effects, and risks associated with the use of multiple antihypertensive drugs also should be considered when deciding a patient's blood pressure treatment goal.

For additional information on target levels of blood pressure and on monitoring therapy in the management of hypertension, see Blood Pressure Monitoring and Treatment Goals under Dosage: Hypertension, in Dosage and Administration in the Thiazides General Statement 40:28.20.

Benign Prostatic Hyperplasia For the management of benign prostatic hyperplasia (BPH), the usual initial adult dosage of doxazosin as conventional (immediate-release) tablets is 1 mg daily, given in the morning or in the evening. Some clinicians state that it is preferable to administer the drug at bedtime to minimize postural effects. Because of the risk of postural effects (see Cautions: Postural Effects), it is essential that therapy with the drug *not* be initiated with higher dosages.

To achieve the desired improvement in symptoms and urodynamics, subsequent doxazosin dosage as conventional tablets may be increased in a stepwise manner to 2, 4, and 8 mg daily as necessary; it is recommended that each doubling of dosage occur at intervals of not less than 1–2 weeks. Although higher dosages (e.g., 16 mg daily) have been used, maximally tolerable and effective dosages have not been established and the manufacturer and most experts recommend that the dosage for BPH not exceed 8 mg daily as conventional tablets. Blood pressure should be evaluated routinely in patients receiving doxazosin therapy, particularly with initiation of therapy and subsequent dosage adjustment (see Dosage: Hypertension).

In a study demonstrating the combined efficacy of an α_1-adrenergic blocker and 5α-reductase inhibitor, doxazosin therapy as conventional tablets was initiated at a dosage of 1 mg daily at bedtime for the first week and then doubled at 1-week intervals until a dosage of 8 mg daily was achieved. In patients who could not tolerate the 8-mg dose, dosage was reduced to 4 mg daily as conventional tablets; those unable to tolerate the 4-mg dose were counted as having discontinued the drug. Finasteride was administered concomitantly at a dosage of 5 mg daily at bedtime.

Alternatively, when extended-release tablets are used for the management of BPH, the usual initial dosage is 4 mg once daily with breakfast. This dosage also should be used initially in patients being switched from conventional tablets. Depending on patient response and tolerability, extended-release dosage may be increased to a maximum of 8 mg once daily with breakfast. If extended-release therapy is interrupted, it should be reinitiated at 4 mg once daily.

■ **Dosage in Renal and Hepatic Impairment** Clinically important alterations in the pharmacokinetics of doxazosin in patients with impaired renal function have not been observed to date, and the manufacturer makes no specific recommendations for modification of dosage in such patients.

The effect of hepatic impairment on the disposition of doxazosin has not been established in controlled clinical studies. However, administration of a single 2-mg dose of doxazosin as conventional tablets to patients with cirrhosis (Child-Pugh class A) resulted in a 40% increase in systemic exposure to the drug. Because doxazosin is eliminated almost entirely by metabolism in the liver, the manufacturer states that the drug should be administered cautiously in patients with hepatic impairment.

■ **Dosage in Geriatric Patients** While the manufacturer makes no specific recommendations for titration of doxazosin dosage in geriatric patients, patients in this age group generally are less tolerant of the postural hypotensive effects of α_1-adrenergic blocking agents because of impaired cardiovascular reflexes, and caution should be exercised. Therefore, dosage escalation in elderly hypertensive patients generally should be slower than in younger adults. Clinically important alterations in the pharmacokinetics of the drug in geriatric patients have not been observed to date.

Cautions

Adverse effects occurring most frequently during doxazosin mesylate therapy for hypertension include dizziness, headache, drowsiness, lack of energy (e.g, lethargy, fatigue), nausea, edema, and rhinitis. In patients receiving the drug for benign prostatic hyperplasia (BPH), the most frequent adverse effects are dizziness, headache, fatigue, edema, dyspnea, abdominal pain, and diarrhea. The frequency of adverse effects in controlled clinical trials generally has been lower in patients receiving doxazosin for BPH than in those receiving the drug for hypertension; however, dosages employed for this condition also generally have been lower than those for hypertension.

While adverse effects occur frequently in patients receiving the drug, most are mild to moderate in severity, and discontinuance of doxazosin secondary to adverse effects was required in only 7% of patients with hypertension during clinical trials. The principal reasons for discontinuance in patients with hypertension were postural effects in 2% of patients and edema, malaise/fatigue, and heart rate disturbance each in about 0.7% of patients. In controlled clinical trials in patients with hypertension, only dizziness (including postural effects), weight gain, somnolence, and malaise/fatigue occurred at rates significantly greater than those for placebo; postural effects and edema appeared to be dose related. Only dizziness, fatigue, hypotension, edema, and dyspnea occurred significantly more frequently with the drug than placebo in controlled clinical trials for BPH; dizziness and dyspnea appeared to be dose-related.

■ **Postural Effects** Doxazosin, like other α_1-adrenergic blocking agents, can cause marked hypotension, which may be accompanied by syncope and other postural effects. While syncope is the most severe orthostatic effect of the drug, other less severe symptoms, such as dizziness, lightheadedness, and vertigo, also can be associated with doxazosin-induced reductions in blood pressure. Syncope is uncommon when doxazosin dosage is initiated at low levels and titrated slowly, but dizziness and/or lightheadedness are frequent, occurring in about 20 or 16% of patients receiving the drug for hypertension or BPH, respectively, in controlled trials. Vertigo has been reported in 2%, syncope in 0.7%, and postural hypotension in 0.3% of hypertensive patients in controlled trials. In patients receiving the drug for BPH in controlled clinical trials, postural hypotension was reported in 0.3% and syncope in 0.5–0.7% of patients.

Doxazosin-induced postural effects are dose related, particularly likely in the upright position following an initial dose, and most likely to develop between 2–6 hours after administration. With continued therapy after careful dosage titration, adaptation of reflex mechanisms to α_1-blockade develop and the risk of postural effects generally subsides. However, marked hypotension also can occur with subsequent dosage increases or after therapy is interrupted for more than a few days. In clinical trials in patients with hypertension, postural effects occurred in 23% of patients receiving the drug and required discontinuance in 2% of patients. In clinical trials in patients with BPH receiving doxazosin dosages up to 8 mg daily, discontinuance of the drug for postural effects was required in 3.3% of patients. While the adverse effect profiles of doxazosin and prazosin generally appear to be similar, it has been suggested that postural effects may be less likely with doxazosin in part because of the drug's slower onset of action and reduced affinity for α_1-receptors; however, additional study and experience are needed to elucidate the relative risks of postural effects.

The risk of first-dose syncope with α_1-adrenergic blocking agents generally can be minimized by initiating therapy at low doses (i.e., 1 mg of doxazosin daily) and lessening the level of salt restriction and avoiding diuretics just prior to initiation of α_1-blocker therapy. It is essential that doxazosin therapy *not* be initiated at dosages exceeding 1 mg daily and that dosage escalation be slow with patient evaluations. In addition, it is important that standing blood pressure be evaluated 2 minutes after standing. If syncope develops, the patient should be placed in the recumbent position and treated supportively as necessary. Patients should be advised to lie or sit down if they develop any postural symptom (e.g., dizziness, vertigo) and to exercise caution upon standing from a sitting or supine position. Patients also should be cautioned to avoid situations, both during the day and through the night, that could result in injury if syncope were to occur. Other antihypertensive therapy should added cautiously in patients receiving doxazosin.

In an early dose-ranging study of the safety and tolerance of doxazosin in several normotensive individuals, two-thirds of these individuals could not tolerate dosages exceeding 2 mg daily because of symptomatic postural hypotension. In other studies in normotensive individuals, approximately 30% of individuals receiving initial doxazosin dosages of 2 mg daily experienced symptomatic hypotension 0.5–6 hours after the dose, and in subsequent trials in hypertensive patients in which doxazosin therapy was initiated at 1 mg daily, postural effects were observed following the initial dose in 4% of patients but were not associated with syncope. In multiple-dose clinical trials in hypertensive patients involving dosage initiation at 1 mg daily and titration every 1–2 weeks, syncope was reported in less than 1% of patients, occurring in no patients at a dosage of 1 mg daily but in 1.2% of those titrated to 16 mg daily. In dose titration trials, the frequency of orthostatic effects could be minimized by initiating therapy at 1 mg daily and titrating dosage no more frequently than every 2 weeks to a maximum of 2.4–8 mg daily. The frequency of orthostatic effects in these titration trials in hypertensive patients was about 12% in those receiving 16 mg of doxazosin once daily, 10% in those receiving 8 mg or more once daily, and 5% in those receiving 1–4 mg once daily. In controlled trials in patients with BPH, the frequency of orthostatic hypotension was not dose related at dosages up to 8 mg daily, titrated at intervals of 1–2 weeks.

■ **Nervous System Effects** Besides dizziness (see Cautions: Postural Effects), headache is the most common adverse nervous system effect associated with doxazosin therapy, occurring in about 14 or 10% of patients receiving the drug for hypertension or BPH, respectively. Somnolence occurs in 5 or 3% of such patients, respectively, and pain in 2% of patients. Nervousness occurs in about 2% of patients receiving doxazosin for hypertension, and insomnia and anxiety occur in 1.2 and 1.1%, respectively, of those receiving the drug for BPH; insomnia occurs in 1% of hypertensive patients. Adverse nervous system effects occurring in 0.5–1% of patients include paresthesia, kinetic disorders, ataxia, hypertonia, hypoesthesia, agitation, depression, and decreased libido. Paresis, tremor, twitching, confusion, migraine, paroniria, amnesia, emotional lability, impaired concentration, abnormal thinking, and depersonalization have been reported in less than 0.5% of patients, but a causal relationship to the drug has not been established.

■ **GI Effects** Nausea, diarrhea, and dry mouth are the most common adverse GI effects of doxazosin in hypertensive patients, occurring in 3, 2, and 2% of such patients, respectively, and abdominal pain, diarrhea, dyspepsia, nausea, and dry mouth are the most common in those with BPH, occurring in 2.4, 2.3, 1.7, 1.5, and 1.4% of such patients, respectively; dyspepsia occurs in 1% of hypertensive patients. Constipation and flatulence occur in 1% of patients receiving the drug for hypertension. Increased appetite, anorexia, fecal incontinence, and gastroenteritis have been reported in less than 0.5% of hypertensive patients but not directly attributed to the drug. Vomiting has been reported during postmarketing experience with doxazosin.

■ **Cardiovascular Effects** Besides postural effects of the drug (see Cautions: Postural Effects), other cardiovascular effects reported in patients receiving doxazosin for hypertension or BPH include edema in 4 or 2.7%, respectively, and palpitation and chest pain in 2 or 1.2% of such patients, respectively. Arrhythmia occurs in 1% of hypertensive patients, and tachycardia and angina pectoris occur in 0.9 and 0.6%, respectively, of patients with BPH. Tachycardia and peripheral ischemia have been reported in 0.3% of hypertensive patients. Hot flushes, ischemia, angina pectoris, myocardial infarction, and cerebral vascular accident have been reported in less that 0.5% of hypertensive patients, but a causal relationship has not been established. In addition, bradycardia has been reported with doxazosin during postmarketing experience.

An increased incidence of myocardial necrosis and fibrosis has been observed in Sprague-Dawley rats after 6 months of oral doxazosin dosages of 80 mg/kg daily, and after 12 months of oral dosages of 40 mg/kg daily (AUC exposure in rats was 8 times the human AUC exposure associated with a 12 mg daily dosage). Myocardial fibrosis also was observed in both rats and mice receiving an oral dosage of 40 mg/kg daily for 18 months (AUC exposure in rats was 8 times the human exposure and in mice was somewhat equivalent to the human exposure). No cardiotoxicity was associated with lower dosages (e.g., 10 or 20 mg/kg daily, depending on the study) in either species, and such effects also were not observed following 12 months of administration in dogs receiving maximum oral doxazosin dosages of 20 mg/kg daily nor in Wistar rats receiving maximum oral dosages of 100 mg/kg daily. While the clinical relevance of these findings to human is not known, the manufacturer states that there currently is no evidence that similar lesions occur in humans.

■ **Dermatologic Effects** Adverse dermatologic effects associated with doxazosin include rash, pruritus, and facial edema. In controlled clinical trials, these effects were reported in 1% of hypertensive patients. Pallor, alopecia, dry skin, and eczema have been reported in less than 0.5% of hypertensive patients receiving doxazosin, but a causal relationship to the drug has not been established.

■ **Musculoskeletal Effects** Arthralgia/arthritis, muscle weakness, myalgia, and muscle cramps have been reported in 1% of hypertensive patients receiving doxazosin. Back pain was reported in 1.8% or less than 0.5% of patients receiving the drug for BPH or hypertension, respectively.

■ **Respiratory Effects** Rhinitis occurs in 3% of hypertensive patients receiving doxazosin. Dyspnea occurs in 2.6 or 1% of patients with BPH or hypertension, respectively, and respiratory disorder occurs in 1.1% of those with BPH. Bronchospasm, sinusitis, cough, and pharyngitis have been reported in less than 0.5% of hypertensive patients but not directly attributed to the drug. In addition, aggravated bronchospasm has been reported with doxazosin during postmarketing experience.

■ **Genitourinary Effects** Polyuria occurs in 2% of hypertensive patients receiving doxazosin and urinary incontinence occurs in 1% of such patients. Sexual dysfunction occurred in 2% of hypertensive patients and impotence occurred in 1.1% of those with BPH receiving the drug. Urinary tract infection and dysuria were reported in 1.4 and 0.5%, respectively, of patients with BPH receiving doxazosin, but they occurred less frequently than with placebo. Renal calculus has been reported in less than 0.5% of hypertensive patients, but a causal relationship has not been established. Priapism (painful penile erection sustained for hours and unrelieved by sexual intercourse or masturbation) has been reported rarely (probably less frequently than 1 in several thousand patients) in patients receiving an α_1-adrenergic antagonist (e.g., doxazosin). Urinary frequency, nocturia, hematuria, and unspecified micturition disorder have been reported with doxazosin during postmarketing experience.

■ **Ocular and Otic Effects** Visual abnormalities occur in 2 or 1.4% of patients receiving doxazosin for hypertension of BPH, respectively, and conjunctivitis/ocular pain occurs in 1% of hypertensive patients. Tinnitus also occurs in 1% of patients receiving the drug. Photophobia, abnormal lacrimation, and earache have been reported in less than 0.5% of hypertensive patients, but these effects have not been directly attributed to the drug.

■ **Hematologic Effects** Adverse hematologic effects reported with doxazosin include decreased leukocyte and neutrophil counts. Mean reductions in these counts relative to placebo were 2.4 and 1%, respectively, in clinical trials in hypertensive patients. In clinical trials in patients with BPH, clinically important leukocyte abnormalities occurred in 0.4% of patients receiving doxazosin and in 0% of those receiving placebo, but the difference in incidence between these groups was not statistically different. Leukopenia and thrombocytopenia have been reported with doxazosin during postmarketing experience.

A search by the manufacturer of a database that included information on 2400 hypertensive patients and 665 with BPH revealed 4 cases in the hypertensive group and one case in the BPH group in which doxazosin-related neutropenia could not be ruled out. In 2 hypertensive patients, stable, nonprogressive neutropenia of about 1000/mm^3 was observed over periods of 20–40 weeks. In a patient with BPH, the leukocyte count decreased from 4800 to 2700/mm^3 at the end of the study, but there was no evidence of clinical impairment. In cases where follow-up was possible, leukocyte and neutrophil counts returned to normal after discontinuance of doxazosin; no cases of symptomatic reductions have been reported to date. Similar reductions in leukocyte and neutrophil counts have been observed with other α_1-adrenergic blocking agents.

■ **Other Adverse Effects** Sweating has been reported in 1.1 or 0.5–1% of patients receiving doxazosin for BPH or hypertension, respectively, and flu-like symptoms have been reported in 1.1 or less than 0.5% of such patients, respectively. Weight gain has been reported in 0.5–1% of hypertensive patients receiving the drug and thirst, gout, hypokalemia, lymphadenopathy, purpura, breast pain, taste perversion, parosmia, infection, fever/rigors, and weight loss have been reported in less than 0.5% of patients. In addition, gynecomastia, hepatitis, and cholestatic hepatitis have been reported with doxazosin during postmarketing experience.

■ **Precautions and Contraindications** Patients should be warned of the possibility of doxazosin-induced postural dizziness and measures to take if it develops (e.g., sitting, lying down). (See Cautions: Postural Effects.) During initiation of doxazosin therapy, the patient should be cautioned to avoid situations, both day and night, where injury could result if syncope occurs. If syncope occurs, the patient should be placed in the recumbent position and treated supportively as necessary. Patients who engage in potentially hazardous activities such as operating machinery or driving motor vehicles should be warned about possible drowsiness, dizziness, or lightheadedness.

Patients also should be advised that priapism has been reported rarely in patients receiving an α_1-adrenergic antagonist (e.g., doxazosin). Priapism is a medical emergency that could result in penile tissue damage and permanent loss of potency if not treated immediately; therefore, patients should be advised to report promptly to their clinician or, if their clinician is unavailable, to seek alternative immediate medical attention if an erection occurs that persists longer than several (e.g., 4–6) hours or is painful.

Experience to date with doxazosin under controlled conditions is limited to patients with normal liver function. However, because the drug is almost completely metabolized in the liver, particular caution should be exercised when using doxazosin in patients with impaired liver function or who are receiving other agents (e.g., cimetidine) that could influence hepatic clearance of the drug.

The possibility of carcinoma of the prostate and other conditions associated with manifestations that mimic those of BPH should be excluded in any patient for whom doxazosin therapy for presumed BPH is being considered. No evidence of an effect on plasma concentrations of prostate specific antigen (PSA) has been observed in patients treated with doxazosin for up to 3 years.

Doxazosin is contraindicated in patients with known sensitivity to the drug or any other quinazoline derivative (e.g., prazosin, terazosin).

■ **Pediatric Precautions** The manufacturer states that safety and efficacy of doxazosin in children and adolescents younger than 18 years of age have not been established. Some experts state that use of centrally acting antihypertensive agents (e.g., doxazosin) should be reserved for children who are not responsive to 2 or more of the preferred classes of antihypertensive agents (angiotensin-converting enzyme [ACE] inhibitors, angiotensin II receptor antagonists, long-acting calcium-channel blockers, or thiazide diuretics). For information on overall principles and expert recommendations for treatment of hypertension in pediatric patients, see Uses: Hypertension in Pediatric Patients, in the Thiazides General Statement 40:28.20.

■ **Geriatric Precautions** Geriatric patients may be particularly susceptible to postural effects of α_1-adrenergic blocking agents such as doxazosin. (See Dosage and Administration: Dosage.) The manufacturer states that certain pharmacokinetic parameters (i.e., plasma half-life, oral clearance) were similar for geriatric individuals 65 years of age or older compared with younger adults. In addition, safety and efficacy of the drug in patients with BPH were similar in those 65 years of age or older compared with younger patients. Clinical studies of doxazosin in patients with hypertension did not include sufficient numbers of patients 65 years of age and older to determine whether geriatric patients respond differently than younger patients. While other clinical experience has not revealed age-related differences in response, drug dosage generally should be titrated carefully in geriatric patients, usually initiating therapy at the low end of the dosage range. The greater frequency of decreased hepatic, renal, and/or cardiac function and of concomitant disease and drug therapy observed in the elderly also should be considered.

■ **Mutagenicity and Carcinogenicity** The manufacturer states that there was no evidence of mutagenicity associated with doxazosin or its metabolites at the chromosomal or subchromosomal level in mutagenicity studies.

No evidence of carcinogenicity was seen in rats receiving the maximally tolerated oral doxazosin dosage of 40 mg/kg daily (8 times the human AUC exposure) for up to 24 months. There also was no evidence of carcinogenicity in a similarly conducted study in mice receiving oral doxazosin for up to 18 months; however, the relevance, if any, of the findings of this study in mice is unclear since the maximally tolerated dosage was not employed.

■ **Pregnancy, Fertility, and Lactation** Reproduction studies in rabbits and rats using doxazosin dosages up to 41 and 20 mg/kg daily (plasma concentrations 10 and 4 times the peak plasma concentration and AUC exposures of humans receiving a dosage of 12 mg daily) have not revealed evidence of harm to the fetus. Postnatal development (weight gain, anatomical features, reflexes) was delayed in some offspring of rats given maternal oral doxazosin dosages of 40–50 mg/kg daily, and decreased fetal survival was associated with dosages of 82 mg/kg daily (in rabbits). There are no adequate and controlled studies to date using doxazosin in pregnant women, and the drug should be used during pregnancy only when clearly needed.

Reproduction studies in male rats using oral doxazosin dosages of 20 mg/kg daily demonstrated a reversible decrease in fertility; however, oral dosages of 10 mg/kg or less daily were not associated with impaired fertility. There have been no reports of adverse effects of the drug on fertility in men.

Since it is not known whether doxazosin is distributed into human milk, the drug should be used with caution in nursing women. Accumulation of the drug has been observed in the milk of lactating rats given a single 1-mg/kg oral dose; in these rats, concentrations of radiolabeled doxazosin in milk were about 20 times greater than those in maternal plasma.

Description

Doxazosin mesylate is a quinazoline-derivative postsynaptic α_1-adrenergic blocking agent. The drug is chemically and pharmacologically related to prazosin and terazosin. On a weight basis, the postsynaptic α_1-adrenergic blocking potency of doxazosin is half that of prazosin, and the α_1-receptor selectivity is one-fourth that of terazosin when tested in human prostate adenoma.

Doxazosin reduces peripheral vascular resistance and blood pressure as a result of its vasodilating effects; the drug produces both arterial and venous dilation. Doxazosin reduces blood pressure in both supine and standing patients; the effect is most pronounced on standing blood pressure, and postural hypotension can occur. Doxazosin generally causes no change in heart rate or cardiac output in the supine position. Cardiovascular responses to exercise (e.g., increased heart rate and cardiac output) are maintained during doxazosin therapy.

Effects of doxazosin on the cardiovascular system are mediated by the drug's activity at α_1-receptor sites on vascular smooth muscle. α_1-Adrenergic receptors also are located in nonvascular smooth muscle (e.g., bladder trigone and sphincters, GI tract and sphincters, prostate adenoma and capsule, ureters, uterus) and in nonmuscular tissues (e.g., CNS, liver, kidneys). Because of the prevalence of α-receptors on the prostate capsule, prostate adenoma, and the bladder trigone and the relative absence of these receptors on the bladder body, α-blockers decrease urinary outflow resistance in men.

Doxazosin may improve to a limited extent the serum lipid profile (e.g., small increases in high-density lipoprotein cholesterol concentrations [HDL] and HDL/total cholesterol ratio, small decreases in low-density lipoprotein cholesterol [LDL], total cholesterol, and triglyceride concentrations), and can reduce blood glucose and serum insulin concentrations. The drug does not appear to affect plasma renin activity appreciably.

Commercially available extended-release tablets of doxazosin mesylate (Cardura® XL) contain the drug in an oral osmotic delivery system formulation (elementary osmotic pump, GI therapeutic system [GITS]). The osmotic delivery system consists of an osmotically active core (comprised of a layer containing the drug and a layer containing osmotically active but pharmacologically inert components) that is surrounded by a semipermeable membrane with a laser-drilled delivery orifice and is designed to deliver the drug at an approximately constant rate over a 24-hour period (approximately zero-order delivery). The inert tablet ingredients remain intact and are eliminated in feces. Oral bioavailability from extended-release tablets at steady state with 4- or 8-mg doses is 54 or 59%, respectively, of that achieved with conventional (immediate-release) tablets. Food increases peak plasma concentrations and bioavailability achieved with extended-release tablets.

SumMon® (see Users Guide). For additional information on this drug until a more detailed monograph is developed and published, the manufacturer's labeling should be consulted. It is *essential* that the labeling be consulted for information on the usual cautions, precautions, and contraindications concerning potential drug interactions and/or laboratory test interferences and for information on acute toxicity.

Preparations

Excipients in commercially available drug preparations may have clinically important effects in some individuals; consult specific product labeling for details.

Doxazosin Mesylate

Oral		
Tablets	1 mg (of doxazosin)*	**Cardura®** (scored), Pfizer
		Doxazosin Mesylate Tablets
	2 mg (of doxazosin)*	**Cardura®** (scored), Pfizer
		Doxazosin Mesylate Tablets
	4 mg (of doxazosin)*	**Cardura®** (scored), Pfizer
		Doxazosin Mesylate Tablets
	8 mg (of doxazosin)*	**Cardura®** (scored), Pfizer
		Doxazosin Mesylate Tablets
Tablets, extended-release	4 mg (of doxazosin)	**Cardura® XL**, Pfizer
	8 mg (of doxazosin)	**Cardura® XL**, Pfizer

*available from one or more manufacturer, distributor, and/or repackager by generic (nonproprietary) name

†Use is not currently included in the labeling approved by the US Food and Drug Administration

Prazosin Hydrochloride

■ Prazosin hydrochloride is an α_1-adrenergic blocking agent.

Uses

■ Hypertension Prazosin hydrochloride is used alone or in combination with other classes of antihypertensive agents in the management of hypertension. However, because of established clinical benefits (e.g., reductions in overall mortality and in adverse cardiovascular, cerebrovascular, and renal outcomes), current evidence-based practice guidelines for the management of hypertension in adults generally recommend the use of drugs from 4 classes of antihypertensive agents (angiotensin-converting enzyme [ACE] inhibitors, angiotensin II receptor antagonists, calcium-channel blockers, and thiazide diuretics).

In a randomized, double-blind clinical study (the Antihypertensive and Lipid-Lowering Treatment to Prevent Heart Attack Trial [ALLHAT]), doxazosin, an α_1-blocker, was less effective in lowering mean systolic blood pressure (by about 2–3 mm Hg) than chlorthalidone, a thiazide-like diuretic. In order to achieve target blood pressure in hypertensive patients, use of doxazosin required additional hypotensive therapy more frequently than chlorthalidone. In addition, interim analysis (median follow-up: 3.3 years) of this study indicated that use of doxazosin in high-risk (at least 2 risk factors for coronary heart disease) hypertensive patients 55 years of age and older was associated with a higher risk of stroke and a higher incidence of combined cardiovascular disease events (including twice the risk of congestive heart failure than use of chlorthalidone. Study investigators concluded that such increased risk of congestive heart failure could not have been caused by the relatively small difference in the mean target systolic blood pressure observed in patients receiving doxazosin compared with those receiving chlorthalidone. Therefore, based on these findings, the trial's Data Safety and Monitoring Board recommended that the α-blocker treatment arm be terminated prematurely. The remaining antihypertensive arms (e.g., calcium-channel blocking agents, angiotensin-converting enzyme [ACE] inhibitors, diuretics) and lipid-lowering (pravastatin vs usual care) components of the study subsequently were completed and reported.

Current antihypertensive and urology guidelines no longer recommend α_1-blockers as preferred *first-line* therapy for any patients with hypertension, principally because of negative findings observed in ALLHAT. However, α_1-blockers are effective antihypertensive drugs and many experts still consider their use appropriate for the management of resistant hypertension as a component of combination therapy. Therapy with an α_1-blocker is most effective when used in combination with a diuretic. Some experts state that an α_1-blocker may be a second-line agent in antihypertensive treatment regimens in men with coexisting benign prostatic hyperplasia (BPH); the American Urology Association (AUA) states that monotherapy with these drugs is not optimal in hypertensive patients with lower urinary tract symptoms (LUTS) or BPH and that such conditions should be managed separately.

The beneficial effects of α_1-blockers on blood glucose and lipid concentrations may mitigate some of the adverse metabolic effects of diuretics, and α_1-blockers may offer some advantage in patients with underlying lipoprotein disorders (e.g., hypercholesterolemia) or in those with lipoprotein abnormalities induced by other antihypertensive agents (e.g., thiazide diuretics). The possibility that geriatric patients may be more susceptible than younger patients to the postural hypotensive effects of α_1-blockers should be considered in the selection of therapy. Blood pressure response to α_1-blockers appears to be comparable in white and black patients.

Prazosin generally is most effective when used with a diuretic. The use of a diuretic may permit reduction of prazosin dosage. Prazosin has also been used with other hypotensive drugs, permitting a reduction in the dosage of each drug and, in some patients, minimizing adverse effects while maintaining blood pressure control. (See Drug Interactions: Diuretics and Hypotensive Agents.)

For further information on overall principles and expert recommendations for treatment of hypertension, see Uses: Hypertension in Adults, in the Thiazides General Statement 40:28.20.

■ Benign Prostatic Hyperplasia Prazosin has been used to reduce urinary obstruction and relieve associated manifestations (e.g., urinary hesitancy and/or urgency, nocturia) in patients with symptomatic benign prostatic hyperplasia† (BPH, benign prostatic hypertrophy) but efficacy relative to other α_1-blockers remains to be established. For patients who can tolerate the potential cardiovascular and other effects of α_1-adrenergic blockade, the drug can effectively relieve mild to moderate obstructive manifestations in a substantial proportion of patients, at least in the short term, and may be a useful alternative to surgery, particularly in those who are awaiting or are unwilling to undergo surgical correction of the hyperplasia (e.g., via transurethral resection of the prostate [TURP]) or who are not candidates for such surgery.

Therapy with α_1-blockers appears to be less effective in relieving irritative than obstructive symptomatology. In addition, therapy with the drugs generally can be expected to produce less subjective and objective improvement than prostatectomy, and periodic monitoring (e.g., performance of digital rectal examination, serum creatinine determinations, serum prostate specific antigen [PSA] assays) is indicated in these patients to detect and manage other potential complications of or conditions associated with BPH (e.g., obstructive uropathy, prostatic carcinoma). While symptomatic improvement has been observed in the short term in some patients receiving prazosin therapy, the long-term effects of α_1-blockers on the need for surgery and on the frequency of developing BPH-associated complications such as acute urinary obstruction remain to be established. Currently available α_1-adrenergic blockers (with the exception of prazosin, for which there are insufficient data to compare) are considered comparably effective.

Current evidence from principally uncontrolled, short-term studies suggests that the α_1-selective adrenergic blocker prazosin produces beneficial effects in approximately 60–70% of treated patients without the degree of adverse effects associated with nonselective adrenergic blockers; alleviation of both obstructive and irritative manifestations of the hyperplasia has been reported in some patients with prazosin therapy. In a few placebo-controlled or comparative studies, therapy with prazosin in dosages of 1–9 mg daily (generally 2 mg twice daily) has improved urinary flow rates and reduced urinary frequency and nocturia in patients with BPH.

Combination therapy with an α_1-blocker and 5α-reductase inhibitor (e.g., finasteride) has been more effective than therapy with either drug alone in preventing long-term BPH symptom progression; combined therapy also can reduce the risks of long-term acute urinary retention and the need for invasive therapy compared with α_1-blocker monotherapy.

For additional information on the use of α_1-blockers in the management of BPH, see Uses: Benign Prostatic Hyperplasia, in Doxazosin 24:20.

■ Posttraumatic Stress Disorder Prazosin has been used in the management of posttraumatic stress disorder (PTSD)†, particularly in combat veterans and in patients experiencing nighttime PTSD symptoms (e.g., nightmares, sleep disturbances). Nightmares and other sleep disturbances reportedly occur in about 70–87% of patients with PTSD; such patients often have decreased sleep efficiency because of more frequent nocturnal awakenings, as well as a higher incidence of other parasomnias and sleep-related breathing disorders compared with patients who have idiopathic nightmares.

Although selective serotonin-reuptake inhibitors (SSRIs; e.g., paroxetine, sertraline) generally have been considered the drugs of choice for the pharmacologic treatment of PTSD, they usually have not been effective in treating nighttime PTSD symptoms, which can be very disturbing and substantially interfere with the patient's quality of life. Atypical antipsychotic agents also have been studied in the treatment of PTSD and have been shown to reduce nighttime PTSD symptoms and may help reduce accompanying psychotic and other symptoms (e.g., agitation, irritability) in some patients; however, routine and long-term use of these drugs is discouraged by some clinicians because of the risk of clinically important adverse effects, such as weight gain and diabetes mellitus.

Clinical experience with prazosin in PTSD to date, which is mainly from small case series, case reports, retrospective or open-label studies, and several small randomized placebo-controlled studies, indicates that the drug is effective in suppressing or eliminating the nighttime sleep-related symptoms associated with PTSD. In several open-label and retrospective studies, prazosin therapy substantially improved trauma-related nightmares and reduced the severity of PTSD (as assessed by the recurrent distressing dreams item of the Clinician-Administered PTSD Scale [CAPS] and/or the Clinical Global Impression of Change [CGI-C] Scale, a 7-point clinician-rated assessment measuring overall PTSD severity and function).

In 2 randomized, double-blind, placebo-controlled trials conducted in combat veterans with PTSD, prazosin was found to be superior to placebo in reducing trauma-related nightmares and sleep disturbances. In the first study, 10 Vietnam combat veterans (mean age: 53 years) with chronic PTSD and severe trauma-related nightmares were randomized to receive prazosin or placebo with crossover to the opposite treatment arm occurring midway through the 20-week study. Prazosin was found to be more effective than placebo in reducing nightmares and sleep disturbances (assessed by CAPS) as well as improving overall PTSD severity and functional status (assessed by the CGI-C Scale). The second study, which was 8 weeks in duration, was conducted in a larger group of patients (40 US combat veterans; mean age: 56 years) with chronic PTSD, distressing trauma nightmares, and sleep disturbances. Compared with placebo, patients receiving prazosin in this study experienced substantially greater improvements in each of the 3 primary outcome measures addressing frequency and intensity of trauma-related nightmares and sleep quality used in this study (the CAPS recurrent distressing dreams item, the Pittsburgh Sleep Quality Index, and the CGI-C).

In a double-blind, placebo-controlled study in 13 patients with civilian trauma-related PTSD, prazosin reduced trauma-related nightmares, distressed awakenings, and total PTSD Checklist-Civilian scores; improved Clinical Global Impression of Improvement scores; and changed the PTSD Dream Rating Scale toward normal dreaming compared with placebo; the drug also improved objective measures of sleep (total sleep time, total REM sleep time, mean REM period duration) without changing sleep onset latency. In a historical prospective cohort study using retrospective chart review, the short-term effectiveness of prazosin (62 patients) and quetiapine (175 patients) in treating nighttime PTSD symptoms in combat veterans was found to be similar. However, long-term effectiveness (3–6 years) of prazosin was better compared with quetiapine; the quetiapine-treated patients were found to be more likely to discontinue therapy because of adverse effects than the prazosin-treated patients (approximately 35 and 18%, respectively). Prazosin therapy was generally found to be well tolerated when used in the treatment of PTSD-associated nightmares and other symptoms.

Some clinicians recommend prazosin as either first-line or alternative therapy when treating PTSD patients with prominent nighttime symptoms (e.g., nightmares, insomnia, sleep disturbances), particularly in combat veterans. Prazosin therapy could potentially be beneficial in some older PTSD patients who have hypertension and/or benign prostatic hyperplasia, since these conditions also may respond to therapy with the drug. Although preliminary findings have been very encouraging, larger, well controlled studies are needed to more fully define the role and optimum dosing of prazosin in the pharmacologic management of PTSD. In addition, further studies are needed to determine the safety and efficacy of prazosin in civilians with noncombat trauma-related PTSD and in the treatment of daytime symptoms associated with PTSD. Several controlled studies, including comparative and augmentation trials, are planned or currently underway to further evaluate prazosin in patients with this disorder.

For additional information on management of PTSD, see Uses: Posttraumatic Stress Disorder, in Paroxetine 28:16.04.20.

■ **Other Uses** Prazosin has been effective in conjunction with cardiac glycosides and diuretics for the management of severe congestive heart failure†, often producing improvements in cardiac function indexes and exercise tolerance. Although partial or complete tolerance to the hemodynamic effects of prazosin has reportedly developed rapidly in some patients, the attenuated response may be transient and/or corrected by dosage adjustment, by temporarily withdrawing the drug, and/or by the addition of an aldosterone antagonist (e.g., spironolactone) to the treatment regimen; acute hemodynamic attenuation does not preclude a beneficial hemodynamic response, especially during exercise. Most studies evaluating the long-term effects of prazosin have suggested that beneficial clinical and hemodynamic effects are sustained; however, conflicting results have been reported. Further studies are needed to determine the efficacy and role of prazosin for the long-term treatment of severe congestive heart failure.

Prazosin has been used with good results alone or in combination with a β-blocker for the preoperative management of the signs and symptoms of pheochromocytoma† in a limited number of patients; however, these patients may be particularly susceptible to a marked hypotensive response to the initial dose of prazosin. Limited data also suggest that prazosin may be useful for the treatment of Raynaud's disease† or phenomenon† and ergotamine-induced peripheral ischemia†.

Dosage and Administration

■ **Administration** Prazosin hydrochloride is administered orally.

■ **Dosage** Dosage of prazosin hydrochloride is expressed in terms of prazosin and must be adjusted according to the patient's blood pressure response and tolerance.

Hypertension **Usual Dosage.** For the management of hypertension in adults, the usual initial dosage of prazosin is 1 mg given 2 or 3 times daily; higher doses should not be used for initial therapy, since initiation of therapy with doses in excess of 1 mg may cause syncope. (See Cautions: Postural Effects.) It has been suggested that syncopal episodes can be minimized by limiting the initial dose of the drug to 1 mg, by subsequently increasing dosage gradually, and by introducing other hypotensive agents into the patient's regimen cautiously. Dosage of prazosin may be gradually increased if necessary to a total dosage of 20 mg daily administered in divided doses. Higher dosages usually do not increase efficacy, but a few patients may benefit from up to 40 mg of prazosin daily in divided doses. The manufacturer states that the usual maintenance dosage is 6–15 mg daily given in divided doses. For maintenance therapy, prazosin may be administered twice daily in some patients. Some experts state that the usual dosage range is 2–20 mg daily, administered in 2 or 3 divided doses.

When other hypotensive agents or diuretics are added to existing prazosin therapy, the dosage of prazosin in adults should be reduced to 1 or 2 mg given 3 times daily and gradually increased according to the response and tolerance of the patient.

If prazosin is used for the management of hypertension in children†, some experts have recommended an initial dosage of 0.05–0.1 mg/kg daily given in 3 divided doses; dosage may be increased as necessary to a maximum of 0.5 mg/kg daily given in 3 divided doses. (See Cautions: Pediatric Precautions.) For information on overall principles and expert recommendations for treatment of hypertension in pediatric patients, see Uses: Hypertension in Pediatric Patients, in the Thiazides General Statement 40:28.20.

Blood Pressure Monitoring and Treatment Goals. Blood pressure should be monitored regularly (i.e., monthly) during therapy and dosage of the antihypertensive drug adjusted until blood pressure is controlled. If an adequate blood pressure response is not achieved, the dosage may be increased or another antihypertensive agent with demonstrated benefit and preferably with a complementary mechanism of action (e.g., angiotensin-converting enzyme [ACE] inhibitor, angiotensin II receptor antagonist, calcium-channel blocker, thiazide diuretic) may be added; if target blood pressure is still not achieved with the use of 2 antihypertensive agents, a third drug may be added. (See Uses: Hypertension.) In patients who develop unacceptable adverse effects with prazosin, the drug should be discontinued and another antihypertensive agent from a different pharmacologic class should be initiated.

The goal of hypertension management and prevention is to achieve and maintain optimal control of blood pressure. However, the optimum blood pressure threshold for initiating antihypertensive drug therapy and specific treatment goals remain controversial. A 2017 multidisciplinary hypertension guideline from the American College of Cardiology (ACC), American Heart Association (AHA), and a number of other professional organizations generally recommends a blood pressure goal of less than 130/80 mm Hg in all adults, regardless of comorbidities or level of atherosclerotic cardiovascular disease (ASCVD) risk. Many patients will require at least 2 drugs from different pharmacologic classes to achieve this blood pressure goal; the potential benefits of hypertension management and drug cost, adverse effects, and risks associated with the use of multiple antihypertensive drugs also should be considered when deciding a patient's blood pressure treatment goal.

For additional information on target levels of blood pressure and on monitoring therapy in the management of hypertension, see Blood Pressure Monitoring and Treatment Goals under Dosage: Hypertension, in Dosage and Administration in the Thiazides General Statement 40:28.20.

Benign Prostatic Hyperplasia In the treatment of benign prostatic hyperplasia†, prazosin generally has been used in a dosage of 2 mg twice daily; however, dosages ranging from 1–9 mg daily also have been used.

Posttraumatic Stress Disorder The optimum dosage regimen of prazosin for the management of posttraumatic stress disorder (PTSD)† in adults has not been fully established. However, in clinical studies, prazosin usually was initiated at a dosage of 1 mg given at bedtime; the dosage was gradually increased (i.e., in 1- or 2-mg increments every few days or week) until an effective (i.e., nighttime symptoms associated with PTSD, such as nightmares and sleep disturbances, were substantially reduced) and well tolerated dosage was reached. Some clinicians recommend monitoring patients receiving prazosin for PTSD for first-dose syncope and orthostatic hypotension, particularly early in therapy. (See Cautions: Postural Effects and also see Cautions: Precautions and Contraindications.) In the available clinical studies, maintenance dosages ranging from 1 to 25 mg daily have been used. Some experts recommend a target maintenance dosage of 1–10 mg daily, while others recommend a higher target maintenance dosage of 2–20 mg daily. Although prazosin usually has been given once daily at bedtime, particularly when lower daily dosages have been used, some clinicians recommend a twice-daily regimen to help control daytime PTSD symptoms; further trials are needed to determine the optimal timing of doses for symptom control. Symptom relief appears to occur within several days to 2 weeks after beginning therapy with the drug.

Although the optimal duration of therapy has not been established, PTSD is often a chronic disorder and requires long-term therapy (i.e., for at least 1 to 2 years). Some PTSD patients have received the drug for up to 6 years. Because a rapid return of symptoms following prazosin discontinuance has been reported, some patients may require therapy indefinitely.

■ **Dosage in Renal Impairment** For the management of hypertension in adults with renal failure, therapy with prazosin should be initiated with 1 mg twice daily. Patients with chronic renal failure may require only small doses of the drug.

Cautions

Adverse effects occurring most frequently during prazosin hydrochloride therapy include dizziness, lightheadedness, headache, drowsiness, lack of energy, weakness, palpitation, and nausea. These effects may diminish with continued therapy or may be relieved by a reduction in dosage.

■ **Postural Effects** Prazosin may cause syncope with sudden loss of consciousness. (See Cautions: Precautions and Contraindications.) Syncopal episodes occur unpredictably and have no relationship to plasma prazosin concentrations. The incidence of syncope is greatest in patients given an initial dose of 2 mg or more (approximately 1%) and may be minimized by administering 1 mg of the drug initially with subsequent gradual increases in dosage. Results of one study suggest that administration of prazosin with food may reduce the frequency of hypotension and dizziness in some patients. Syncope, which is self-limiting, may result from an excessive postural hypotensive effect; syncopal episodes occasionally have been preceded by tachycardia with heart rates of 120–160 beats/minute. Syncopal episodes usually have occurred within 30–90 minutes after the initial dose of prazosin and occasionally have been associated with rapid dosage increases or the introduction of another hypotensive drug to the regimen of patients taking high dosages of prazosin.

■ **Intraoperative Floppy Iris Syndrome** A condition named intraoperative floppy iris syndrome (IFIS) has been observed during cataract surgery in some patients treated with α_1-adrenergic blocking agents. IFIS is a variant of small pupil syndrome and is characterized by the combination of a flaccid iris that billows in response to intraoperative irrigation currents, progressive intraoperative miosis despite preoperative dilation with mydriatics, and potential prolapse of the iris toward the phacoemulsification incisions. Most reported cases of IFIS occurred in patients who continued α_1-blocker therapy at the time of cataract surgery. Some cases were reported in patients who had discontinued such therapy prior to surgery, generally 2 to 14 days prior to surgery, but occasionally 5 weeks to 9 months prior to surgery. (See Cautions: Precautions and Contraindications.)

■ **GI Effects** Nausea is the most common adverse GI effect of prazosin, occurring in about 5% of patients. Other adverse GI effects such as vomiting, diarrhea, constipation, and abdominal discomfort and/or pain have also been reported.

■ **Cardiovascular Effects** Palpitation is the most common adverse cardiovascular effect of prazosin, occurring in about 5% of patients. In addition to syncope, other adverse cardiovascular effects of the drug include edema, dyspnea, orthostatic hypotension, tachycardia, and angina. (See Cautions: Postural Effects.) Nonspecific chest pain also has been reported in a patient receiving prazosin for posttraumatic stress disorder.

■ **Nervous System Effects** Dizziness is the most common adverse effect of prazosin, occurring in about 10% of patients. Headache or drowsiness occur in about 8% of patients, and lack of energy or weakness occur in about 7% of patients. Other adverse nervous system effects of prazosin which occur rarely include nervousness, vertigo, depression, paresthesia, hallucinations, and insomnia.

Worsening of narcolepsy (e.g., exacerbation of associated cataplexy) has been associated with prazosin therapy in patients with a history of this disorder. Although the manufacturers state that a causal relationship to prazosin has not been established to date, the frequency of cataplectic attacks decreased when the drug was withdrawn and increased when it was resumed in at least 2 patients. In addition, prazosin has been shown to exacerbate canine narcolepsy-cataplexy, probably secondary to inhibition of a subtype of α_1-adrenergic receptor (e.g., α_{1b}) in the CNS. Therefore, some clinicians recommend that prazosin not be used in patients with a history of narcolepsy.

■ **Dermatologic Effects** Adverse dermatologic effects associated with prazosin include rash, pruritus, alopecia, and lichen planus.

■ **Other Adverse Effects** Other adverse effects reported to occur with prazosin include urinary frequency, incontinence, impotence, priapism, blurred vision, epistaxis, tinnitus, reddened sclera, dry mouth, nasal congestion, liver function test result abnormalities, pancreatitis, diaphoresis, fever, positive ANA titer, and arthralgia. A transient fall in leukocyte count and increased serum uric acid and BUN concentrations have also been reported during prazosin therapy. Single reports of pigmentary mottling and serous retinopathy, and a few cases of cataract development or disappearance have been reported, but these have not been directly attributable to the drug. In slit-lamp and funduscopic studies, no drug-related abnormal ophthalmologic findings have been reported.

■ **Precautions and Contraindications** Because syncope and orthostatic hypotension may occur in patients receiving prazosin, careful monitoring of blood pressure during initial titration or subsequent upward adjustment in dosage is recommended in patients receiving prazosin; patients also should be monitored for possible symptoms of orthostatic hypotension. Patients receiving prazosin should be warned of the possibility of prazosin-induced postural dizziness and advised of measures to take if it develops (e.g., lying down). During initiation of prazosin therapy, the patient should be cautioned to avoid situations where injury could result if syncope occurs. If syncope occurs, the patient should be placed in the recumbent position and treated supportively as necessary. Patients who engage in potentially hazardous activities such as operating machinery or driving motor vehicles should be warned about possible drowsiness, dizziness, or lightheadedness. (See Cautions: Postural Effects.)

Intraoperative floppy iris syndrome (IFIS) has been observed during cataract surgery in some patients treated with α_1-adrenergic blocking agents (see Cautions: Intraoperative Floppy Iris Syndrome). If a patient scheduled for cataract surgery has received such agents, the ophthalmologist should be prepared to modify the surgical technique (e.g., through use of iris hooks, iris dilator rings, or viscoelastic substances) to minimize complications of IFIS. There does not appear to be a benefit from discontinuing α_1-blocker therapy prior to cataract surgery.

The possibility of carcinoma of the prostate and other conditions associated with manifestations that mimic those of benign prostatic hyperplasia (BPH) should be excluded in any patient for whom prazosin therapy for presumed BPH is being considered.

Patients receiving prazosin for posttraumatic stress disorder (PTSD)† should be informed that prazosin may help reduce nightmares and improve their sleep and other symptoms, but that the drug does not cure PTSD and that their nightmares, anxiety, and other PTSD-related symptoms may return if the drug is stopped.

Caution should be used when adding prazosin to a preexisting antihypertensive regimen or when adding other hypotensive agents to a prazosin regimen in order to avoid a possible rapid fall in blood pressure. (See Drug Interactions: Diuretics and Hypotensive Agents.) Caution also should be used when administering prazosin to patients with chronic renal failure as they may require only small doses of the drug.

Prazosin is contraindicated in patients with known hypersensitivity to the drug, any other quinazoline derivative (e.g., alfuzosin, doxazosin, terazosin), or any ingredient in the commercially available formulation.

■ **Pediatric Precautions** The manufacturers state that safety and efficacy of prazosin in children have not been established. (See Dosage and Administration: Dosage.) Some experts state that use of centrally acting antihypertensive agents (e.g., prazosin) should be reserved for children who are not responsive to 2 or more of the preferred classes of antihypertensive agents (angiotensin-converting enzyme [ACE] inhibitors, angiotensin II receptor antagonists, calcium-channel blockers, or thiazide diuretics).

For information on overall principles and expert recommendations for treatment of hypertension in pediatric patients, see Uses: Hypertension in Pediatric Patients, in the Thiazides General Statement 40:28.20.

■ **Mutagenicity and Carcinogenicity** No evidence of prazosin-induced mutagenicity was seen with in vivo tests.

No evidence of carcinogenesis was seen in rats receiving prazosin hydrochloride dosages more than 225 times the usual maximum recommended human dosage for 18 months.

■ **Pregnancy, Fertility, and Lactation** Prazosin hydrochloride has been associated with decreased litter size at birth and at 1, 4, and 21 days of age in rats receiving more than 225 times the usual maximum recommended human dosage; no evidence of drug-related external, visceral, or skeletal fetal abnormalities was observed. No prazosin-related external, visceral, or skeletal abnormalities were observed in the offspring of pregnant rabbits and monkeys receiving dosages more than 225 and 12 times the usual maximum recommended human dosage, respectively. Prazosin has been used alone or in combination with other hypotensive agents for the management of severe hypertension in a limited number of pregnant women without apparent adverse effect on the fetus. There are no adequate and well-controlled studies to date using prazosin in pregnant women, however, and the drug should be used during pregnancy only when the potential benefits justify the possible risks to the fetus.

Decreased fertility has occurred in male and female rats receiving prazosin dosages of 75 mg/kg (225 times the usual maximum recommended human dosage) but did not occur in those receiving 25 mg/kg (75 times the usual maximum recommended human dosage). Testicular changes consisting of atrophy and necrosis have occurred in rats and dogs receiving prazosin dosages of 25 mg/kg daily for a year or longer but no such changes occurred in those receiving 10 mg/kg daily (30 times the usual maximum recommended human dosage). Because of the testicular changes observed in animals, a group of patients receiving long-term prazosin therapy was monitored for 17-ketosteroid excretion, but no changes indicating a drug effect were observed. In addition, a group of males receiving prazosin for up to 51 months did not exhibit changes in sperm morphology suggestive of a drug effect.

Since prazosin is distributed into milk in small amounts, the drug should be used with caution in nursing women.

Drug Interactions

■ **Analgesics and Antipyretics** Although clinical experience is limited, prazosin has been administered concomitantly with aspirin, indomethacin, phenylbutazone (no longer commercially available in the US), or propoxyphene (no longer commercially available in the US) without any apparent adverse interaction.

■ **Antiarrhythmic Agents** Although clinical experience to date is limited, prazosin has been administered concomitantly with procainamide, propranolol (see Drug Interactions: Diuretics and Hypotensive Agents), or quinidine without any apparent adverse drug interaction.

■ **Antidiabetic Agents** Although clinical experience to date is limited, prazosin has been administered concomitantly with insulin, chlorpropamide, phenformin (no longer commercially available in the US), tolazamide, and tolbutamide without any apparent adverse drug interaction.

■ **Antigout Agents** Although clinical experience is limited, prazosin has been administered concurrently with allopurinol, colchicine, or probenecid without any apparent adverse interaction.

■ **CNS Depressants** Although clinical experience is limited, prazosin has been administered concurrently with chlordiazepoxide, diazepam, or phenobarbital without any apparent adverse interaction.

■ **Digoxin** Although clinical experience is limited, prazosin has been administered concomitantly with digoxin without any apparent adverse interaction.

■ **Diuretics and Hypotensive Agents** When prazosin is administered with diuretics or other hypotensive agents, particularly β-adrenergic blocking agents (e.g., propranolol), the hypotensive effect of prazosin may be increased. This effect is usually used to therapeutic advantage, but careful adjustment of dosage is necessary when these drugs are used concomitantly. (See Dosage and Administration: Dosage.)

■ **Phosphodiesterase Type 5 Inhibitors** Concomitant administration of prazosin and a phosphodiesterase type 5 (PDE5) inhibitor (e.g., sildenafil, tadalafil, vardenafil) may result in additive hypotensive effects and symptomatic hypotension. Therefore, PDE5 inhibitor therapy should be initiated at the lowest possible dosage in patients receiving prazosin. (See Dosage and Administration: Dosage.)

For further information on this potential drug interaction, see Drug Interactions: Antihypertensive and Hypotensive Agents, in Sildenafil 24:12.12.

■ **Protein-bound Drugs** Since prazosin is highly bound to plasma proteins, the possibility that it may interact with other highly protein-bound drugs should be considered.

Acute Toxicity

■ **Manifestations** The manufacturers state that ingestion of at least 50 mg of prazosin by a 2-year-old child produced profound drowsiness and depressed reflexes. There was no decrease in blood pressure and recovery was uneventful. A 19-year-old man who ingested approximately 200 mg of prazosin had normal CNS responses and slightly decreased blood pressure. Treatment of overdosage consisted of induction of emesis and maintaining the patient in a supine position with the head of the bed lowered; recovery was uneventful.

■ **Treatment** If overdosage of prazosin causes hypotension, supportive therapy should be initiated. The patient should be kept in the supine position; if necessary, shock may be treated with plasma volume expanders and vasopressor drugs. Renal function should be monitored. The manufacturers state that laboratory data indicate prazosin is not dialyzable because it is highly protein bound.

Pharmacology

Prazosin reduces peripheral vascular resistance and blood pressure as a result of its vasodilating effects; the drug produces both arterial and venous dilation. Prazosin's effects appear to result principally from its selective, competitive inhibition of α_1-adrenergic receptors. Prazosin's effects were initially attributed to a direct effect on vascular smooth muscle, inhibition of phosphodiesterase, and/or inhibition of dopamine β-hydroxylase with a resultant reduction in neurotransmitter synthesis; however, it is unlikely that concentrations of the drug necessary for these effects are achieved when prazosin is administered in therapeutic doses. Animal studies indicate that prazosin does not have its antihypertensive effect in the CNS. Prazosin does not interfere with nerve impulse transmission across sympathetic ganglia nor does it cause adrenergic neuronal blockade.

Prazosin reduces blood pressure in both supine and standing patients; the effect is most pronounced on diastolic blood pressure. The drug may cause postural hypotension. (See Cautions: Postural Effects.) Tolerance to the hypotensive effect has not been observed during long-term prazosin therapy in hypertensive patients. Prazosin generally causes no change in heart rate or cardiac output in the supine position. Cardiovascular responses to exercise (e.g., increased heart rate and cardiac output) are maintained during prazosin therapy. Reports on the effect of the drug on glomerular filtration rate and renal plasma flow indicate that these parameters may increase or show no marked change. In patients with chronic renal failure, prazosin produces no clinically important change in renal function. In a limited number of patients treated with prazosin, plasma renin activity (PRA) decreased; however, no appreciable effect on PRA was demonstrated in other patients.

In patients with congestive heart failure, prazosin markedly decreases systemic and pulmonary venous pressures and right atrial pressure, and increases cardiac output. Systemic blood pressure and systemic vascular resistance are moderately decreased in these patients; pulmonary vascular resistance is decreased and heart rate may be slightly decreased or unchanged. In patients with congestive heart failure precipitated or exacerbated by mitral or aortic regurgitation, prazosin may increase cardiac output and decrease regurgitant volume.

The precise mechanism of action of prazosin in posttraumatic stress disorder (PTSD) has not been fully elucidated; however, preliminary studies suggest that norepinephrine and α_1-adrenergic receptors play an important role in the pathophysiology of PTSD-associated nightmares, arousal, selective attention, and vigilance. Norepinephrine concentrations in the cerebrospinal fluid appear to correlate with PTSD symptom severity. Hyperresponsiveness of postsynaptic α_1-adrenergic receptors occurs primarily at night and can disrupt certain stages of the sleep cycle (stage 1, stage 2, rapid eye movement [REM]) in which PTSD-associated nightmares are known to occur. In preclinical and clinical studies, prazosin has been shown to reduce the effects of α_1-adrenergic receptor hyperstimulation and to help normalize the sleep cycle. In a placebo-controlled trial of prazosin in civilian trauma-related PTSD, prazosin increased total sleep time, REM sleep time, and mean REM period duration compared with placebo without producing a sedative-like effect on sleep onset latency.

Pharmacokinetics

■ **Absorption** There is intraindividual and interindividual variation in the rate of absorption and plasma concentrations of prazosin. The absolute oral bioavailability of prazosin is also variable but is reported to average about 60% (range: 43–82%). Results of one study indicate that the presence of food may delay absorption of the drug in some patients, but does not affect the extent of absorption.

Following oral administration of prazosin hydrochloride, plasma concentrations of the drug reach a peak in 2–3 hours in most fasting patients. Plasma concentrations of prazosin generally do not correlate with therapeutic effect. One manufacturer reports that plasma concentrations of the drug after a single 5-mg dose range from 0.01–0.075 mcg/mL. Blood pressure begins to decrease within 2 hours after an oral dose; the maximum decrease occurs in 2–4 hours. The hypotensive effect of prazosin lasts less than 24 hours. At fixed dosage levels, 4–6 weeks of therapy are required before the full antihypertensive effect of the drug is achieved.

■ **Distribution** Animal studies indicate that prazosin is widely distributed in body tissues. After IV administration in dogs, highest concentrations of the drug are found in the lungs, coronary arteries, aorta, paw arteries and heart; the lowest concentrations are in the brain. During prazosin therapy, approximately 97% of the drug in plasma is bound to proteins. Prazosin crosses the blood-brain barrier. It is not known whether the drug crosses the placenta. Prazosin is distributed into milk in small amounts.

■ **Elimination** The plasma half-life of prazosin after oral administration has been reported to be 2–4 hours.

Animal studies show that prazosin hydrochloride is metabolized extensively in the liver, principally by demethylation and conjugation, and excreted as unchanged drug (5–11%) and metabolites. Four of the metabolites have been shown to possess 10–25% of the hypotensive activity of prazosin and they may contribute to the antihypertensive effect of the drug. Approximately 6–10% of a dose is excreted in urine and the remainder in feces via bile.

Chemistry and Stability

■ **Chemistry** Prazosin hydrochloride is a quinazoline-derivative postsynaptic α_1-adrenergic blocking agent. The drug is chemically and pharmacologically related to alfuzosin, doxazosin, and terazosin. Prazosin hydrochloride occurs as a white to tan powder, is slightly soluble in water and very slightly soluble in alcohol, and has a pK_a of 6.5 in 1:1 water and ethanol solution.

■ **Stability** Prazosin hydrochloride capsules should be stored in well-closed, light-resistant containers at 20-25°C.

Preparations

Excipients in commercially available drug preparations may have clinically important effects in some individuals; consult specific product labeling for details.

Prazosin Hydrochloride

Oral		
Capsules	1 mg (of prazosin)*	**Minipress®**, Pfizer
		Prazosin Hydrochloride Capsules
	2 mg (of prazosin)*	**Minipress®**, Pfizer
		Prazosin Hydrochloride Capsules
	5 mg (of prazosin)*	**Minipress®**, Pfizer
		Prazosin Hydrochloride Capsules

*available from one or more manufacturer, distributor, and/or repackager by generic (nonproprietary) name

†Use is not currently included in the labeling approved by the US Food and Drug Administration

Terazosin Hydrochloride

■ Terazosin hydrochloride is a α_1-adrenergic blocking agent.

Uses

■ **Hypertension** Terazosin hydrochloride is used alone or in combination with other classes of antihypertensive agents for the management of hypertension. However, because of established clinical benefits (e.g., reductions in overall mortality and in adverse cardiovascular, cerebrovascular, and renal outcomes), current evidence-based practice guidelines for the management of hypertension in adults generally recommend the use of drugs from 4 classes of antihypertensive agents (angiotensin-converting enzyme [ACE] inhibitors, angiotensin II receptor antagonists, calcium-channel blockers, and thiazide diuretics).

In a randomized, double-blind clinical study (the Antihypertensive and Lipid-Lowering Treatment to Prevent Heart Attack Trial; [ALLHAT]), doxazosin, an α_1-blocker, was less effective in lowering mean systolic blood pressure (by about 2–3 mm Hg) than chlorthalidone, a thiazide-like diuretic. In order to achieve target blood pressure in hypertensive patients, use of doxazosin required additional hypotensive therapy more frequently than chlorthalidone. In addition, interim analysis (median follow-up: 3.3 years) of this study indicated that use of doxazosin in high-risk (at least 2 risk factors for coronary heart disease) hypertensive patients 55 years of age and older was associated with a higher risk of stroke and a higher incidence of combined cardiovascular disease events (including twice the risk of congestive heart failure) than use of chlorthalidone. Study investigators concluded that such increased risk of congestive heart failure could not have been caused by the relatively small difference in the mean target systolic blood pressure observed in patients receiving doxazosin compared with those receiving chlorthalidone. Therefore, based on these findings, the trial's Data Safety and Monitoring Board recommended that the α-blocker treatment arm be terminated prematurely. The remaining antihypertensive arms (e.g., calcium-channel blockers, ACE inhibitors, diuretics) and lipid-lowering (pravastatin vs usual care) components of the study subsequently were completed and reported.

Current antihypertensive and urology guidelines no longer recommend α_1-blockers as preferred *first-line* therapy for any patients with hypertension, principally because of negative findings observed in ALLHAT. However, α_1-blockers are effective antihypertensive drugs and many experts still consider their use appropriate for the management of resistant hypertension as a component of combination therapy. Therapy with an α_1-blocker is most effective when used in combination with a diuretic. Some experts state that an α_1-blocker may be a second-line agent in antihypertensive treatment regimens in men with coexisting benign prostatic hyperplasia (BPH); the American Urology Association (AUA) states that monotherapy with these drugs is not optimal in hypertensive patients with lower urinary tract symptoms (LUTS) or BPH and that such conditions should be managed separately.

The beneficial effects of α_1-blockers on blood glucose and lipid concentrations may mitigate some of the adverse metabolic effects of diuretics, and α_1-blockers may offer some advantage in patients with underlying lipoprotein disorders (e.g., hypercholesterolemia) or in those with lipoprotein abnormalities induced by other antihypertensive agents (e.g., thiazide diuretics). The possibility that geriatric patients may be more susceptible than younger patients to the postural hypotensive effects of α_1-blockers should be considered in the selection of therapy. Blood pressure response to α_1-blockers appears to be comparable in white and black patients.

For further information on overall principles and expert recommendations for treatment of hypertension, see Uses: Hypertension in Adults and also see Uses: Hypertension in Pediatric Patients, in the Thiazides General Statement 40:28.20.

■ Benign Prostatic Hyperplasia Terazosin hydrochloride is used to reduce urinary obstruction and relieve associated manifestations in patients with symptomatic benign prostatic hyperplasia (BPH, benign prostatic hypertrophy). For patients who can tolerate the potential cardiovascular and other effects of α_1-adrenergic blockade, the drug can effectively relieve mild to moderate obstructive manifestations (e.g., hesitancy, terminal dribbling of urine, interrupted stream, impaired size and force of stream, sensation of incomplete bladder emptying or straining) and urinary flow rates in a substantial proportion of patients and may be a useful alternative to surgery, particularly in those who are awaiting or are unwilling to undergo surgical correction of the hyperplasia (e.g., via transurethral resection of the prostate [TURP]) or who are not candidates for such surgery.

Therapy with α_1-blockers appears to be less effective in relieving irritative (e.g., nocturia, daytime frequency, urgency, dysuria) than obstructive symptomatology. In addition, therapy with the drugs generally can be expected to produce less subjective and objective improvement than prostatectomy, and periodic monitoring (e.g., performance of digital rectal examinations, serum creatinine determinations, serum prostate specific antigen [PSA] assays) is indicated in these patients to detect and manage other potential complications of or conditions associated with BPH (e.g., obstructive uropathy, prostatic carcinoma). While symptomatic improvement has been maintained for at least up to 2 years of terazosin therapy in some patients, the long-term effects of the drug on the need for surgery and on the frequency of developing BPH-associated complications such as acute urinary obstruction remain to be established.

Combination therapy with an α_1-blocker and 5α-reductase inhibitor (e.g., finasteride) has been more effective than therapy with either drug alone in preventing long-term BPH symptom progression; combined therapy also can reduce the risks of long-term acute urinary retention and the need for invasive therapy compared with α-blocker monotherapy.

For additional information on the use of α_1-blockers in the management of BPH, see Uses: Benign Prostatic Hyperplasia, in Doxazosin 24:20.

Because many of the signs and symptoms of BPH can occur with carcinoma of the prostate and with certain genitourinary conditions, including prostatitis and neurologic disorders, the possibility of such conditions, particularly this carcinoma, should be ruled out in any patient for whom terazosin therapy for presumed hyperplasia is being considered.

Dosage and Administration

■ Administration Terazosin hydrochloride is administered orally. Food has little, if any, effect on the extent of absorption of terazosin but may delay achievement of peak plasma concentrations by about 1 hour.

■ Dosage Dosage of terazosin hydrochloride is expressed in terms of terazosin and must be individualized according to the patient's response and tolerance.

Hypertension **Usual Dosage.** For the management of hypertension, terazosin dosage should be adjusted according to blood pressure response and tolerance. The usual initial adult dosage of the drug is 1 mg once daily at bedtime. Because of the risk of postural effects (see Cautions: Postural Effects), it is essential that therapy with the drug *not* be initiated with higher dosages.

If blood pressure is not adequately controlled at a terazosin dosage of 1 mg daily, the dosage may be increased gradually up to 5 mg once daily in adults, but each incremental increase should be delayed until blood pressure has stabilized at a given dosage; some patients may benefit from further titration up to 20 mg daily. Maintenance doses of the drug can be administered in the morning rather than at bedtime. Blood pressure should be monitored at the end of the dosing interval to ensure maintenance of control, and additional measurements 2–3 hours after dosing may be helpful in determining whether peak and trough responses are similar and in assessing potential manifestations (e.g., dizziness, palpitation) of an excessive response. If blood pressure response is diminished substantially 24 hours after a dose, an increased dose may provide adequate control. If necessary for optimal blood pressure control, the daily dose can be divided and administered every 12 hours.

Some experts state the usual adult dosage of terazosin for the management of hypertension ranges from 1–20 mg daily administered as a single dose or in 2 divided doses daily. While higher dosages have been employed, those exceeding 20 mg daily do not appear to be associated with improved hypertensive control and those exceeding 40 mg daily have not been studied systematically. If terazosin is discontinued for several days or longer, therapy with drug should be reinstituted at 1 mg daily at bedtime and titrated as usual.

If terazosin is used for the management of hypertension in children†, some experts have recommended an initial dosage of 1 mg once daily; dosage may be increased as necessary to a maximum dosage of 20 mg once daily. (See Cautions: Pediatric Precautions.) For information on overall principles and expert recommendations for treatment of hypertension in pediatric patients, see Uses: Hypertension in Pediatric Patients, in the Thiazides General Statement 40:28.20.

Blood Pressure Monitoring and Treatment Goals. Blood pressure should be monitored regularly (i.e., monthly) during therapy and dosage of the antihypertensive drug adjusted until blood pressure is controlled. If an adequate blood pressure response is not achieved, the dosage may be increased or another antihypertensive agent with demonstrated benefit and preferably with a complementary mechanism of action (e.g., angiotensin-converting enzyme [ACE] inhibitor, angiotensin II receptor antagonist, calcium-channel blocker, thiazide diuretic) may be added; if target blood pressure is still not achieved with the use of 2 antihypertensive agents, a third drug may be added. (See Uses: Hypertension.) In patients who develop unacceptable adverse effects with terazosin, the drug should be discontinued and another antihypertensive agent from a different pharmacologic class should be initiated.

The goal of hypertension management and prevention is to achieve and maintain optimal control of blood pressure. However, the optimum blood pressure threshold for initiating antihypertensive drug therapy and specific treatment goals remain controversial. A 2017 multidisciplinary hypertension guideline from the American College of Cardiology (ACC), American Heart Association (AHA), and a number of other professional organizations generally recommends a blood pressure goal of less than 130/80 mm Hg in all adults, regardless of comorbidities or level of atherosclerotic cardiovascular disease (ASCVD) risk. Many patients will require at least 2 drugs from different pharmacologic classes to achieve this blood pressure goal; the potential benefits of hypertension management and drug cost, adverse effects, and risks associated with the use of multiple antihypertensive drugs also should be considered when deciding a patient's blood pressure treatment goal.

For additional information on target levels of blood pressure and on monitoring therapy in the management of hypertension, see Blood Pressure Monitoring and Treatment Goals under Dosage: Hypertension, in Dosage and Administration in the Thiazides General Statement 40:28.20.

Benign Prostatic Hyperplasia For the management of benign prostatic hyperplasia (BPH), the usual initial adult dosage of terazosin is 1 mg once daily at bedtime. Because of the risk of postural effects (see Cautions: Postural Effects), it is essential that therapy with the drug *not* be initiated with higher dosages. To achieve the desired improvement in symptoms and/or urinary flow rates, subsequent dosage may be increased in a stepwise manner to 2, 5, and 10 mg daily as necessary. Titration to a dosage of 10 mg once daily generally is required for adequate clinical response. A minimum of 4–6 weeks may be needed to adequately assess the response at this dosage, but some patients may not respond despite appropriate titration. While additional benefit occasionally may be observed by increasing the dosage to 20 mg daily, maximally tolerable and effective dosages have not been established and there currently is insufficient experience with this dosage in the management of BPH to draw definitive conclusions. In addition, there currently are insufficient data to support the use of dosages exceeding 20 mg daily in patients with an inadequate or no response at lower dosages. If terazosin therapy is discontinued for several days or longer, therapy should be restarted using the recommended initial dosage.

■ **Dosage in Renal and Hepatic Impairment** Clinically important alterations in the pharmacokinetics of terazosin in patients with impaired renal function have not been observed to date, and modification of dosage in such patients generally does not appear to be necessary. In addition, administration of supplemental doses of the drug following hemodialysis does not appear to be necessary.

The effects, if any, of hepatic impairment on the pharmacokinetics of terazosin have not been elucidated, and the manufacturer makes no specific recommendations for modification of terazosin dosage in patients with hepatic impairment.

■ **Dosage in Geriatric Patients** While the manufacturer makes no specific recommendations for titration of terazosin dosage in geriatric patients, patients in this age group generally are less tolerant of the postural hypotensive effects of α_1-adrenergic blocking agents because of impaired cardiovascular reflexes, and caution should be exercised. Therefore, dosage escalation in elderly patients generally should be slower than in younger adults. In addition, the elimination half-life may be prolonged and plasma clearance of the drug decreased in patients 70 years of age and older.

Cautions

Adverse effects occurring most frequently during terazosin hydrochloride therapy for hypertension include dizziness, headache, asthenia (weakness, tiredness, lassitude, fatigue), nasal congestion, peripheral edema, somnolence, nausea, and palpitation. In patients receiving the drug for benign prostatic hyperplasia (BPH), the most frequent adverse effects are dizziness, asthenia, headache, postural hypotension, and somnolence. The frequency of adverse effects in controlled clinical trials generally has been lower in patients receiving terazosin for BPH than in those receiving the drug for hypertension; however, dosages employed for this condition also generally have been lower than those for hypertension.

While adverse effects occur frequently in patients receiving terazosin, most are mild to moderate in severity, and discontinuance of the drug secondary to adverse effects was required in only 9% of patients with BPH and in only 13–21% of patients with hypertension during clinical trials. The principal reasons for discontinuance in patients with hypertension were postural effects (e.g., dizziness in about 3% of patients) and asthenia, palpitation, headache, and dyspnea each in about 1–2% of patients. In patients with BPH, the principal reasons for discontinuance were dizziness, headache, and blurred vision/amblyopia in 2, 1.1, and 0.6%, respectively, of patients and postural hypotension, syncope, vertigo, dyspnea, fever, nausea, and urinary tract infection each in 0.5% of patients. In controlled clinical trials in patients with hypertension, only dizziness (including postural effects), asthenia, blurred vision, nasal congestion, nausea, peripheral edema, palpitation, and somnolence occurred at rates significantly greater than those for placebo. Only asthenia, postural hypotension, dizziness, somnolence, nasal congestion/rhinitis, and impotence occurred significantly more frequently with the drug than with placebo in controlled clinical trials for BPH. The risk of postural hypotension and syncope appears to be higher in geriatric patients (i.e., those 65 years of age and older) than in younger patients. Asthenia and postural effects, including dizziness, appear to be dose related.

■ **Postural Effects** Terazosin, like other α_1-adrenergic blocking agents, can cause marked hypotension, which may be accompanied by syncope and other postural effects. While syncope is the most severe orthostatic effect of the drug, other less severe symptoms, such as dizziness, lightheadedness, tachycardia, palpitation, and vertigo, also can be associated with terazosin-induced reductions in blood pressure. Syncope is uncommon when terazosin dosage is initiated at low levels and titrated slowly, but dizziness is frequent, occurring in about 20 or 10% of patients receiving the drug for hypertension or BPH, respectively, in controlled trials. Palpitation has been reported in 4.3% of hypertensive patients receiving terazosin, and tachycardia (especially in the standing position) and postural hypotension have been reported in 1–2% of such patients. Postural hypotension, vertigo, and syncope have been reported in about 4, 1.4, and 0.6% of patients, respectively, receiving the drug for BPH; however, in several clinical trials in such patients, the frequency of postural hypotension ranged from 3.7–5.2%.

Terazosin-induced postural hypotension is dose related, particularly likely in the upright position following an initial dose, and most likely to develop shortly after dosing (e.g., within 90 minutes), particularly during the initial week of therapy. With continued therapy after careful dosage titration, adaptation of reflex mechanisms to α_1-blockade develops and the risk of postural effects generally subsides. However, marked hypotension also can occur with subsequent dosage increases or after therapy is interrupted for more than a few days. Occasionally, syncopal episodes have been preceded by episodes of severe supraventricular tachycardia with heart rates of 120–160 bpm. In addition, the possibility exists that hemodilution induced by the drug may contribute to postural hypotension. While the adverse effect profiles of terazosin and prazosin generally appear to be similar, it has been suggested that postural effects may be less likely with terazosin in part because of the drug's slower onset of action and reduced affinity for α_1-receptors; however, additional study and experience are needed to elucidate the relative risks of postural effects.

The risk of first-dose syncope with α_1-adrenergic blocking agents generally can be minimized by initiating therapy at low doses (i.e., 1 mg of terazosin daily), lessening the level of salt restriction and avoiding diuretics just prior to initiation of α_1-blocker therapy, and administering initial doses at bedtime. It is essential that terazosin therapy *not* be initiated at dosages exceeding 1 mg daily and that dosage escalation be slow. If syncope develops, the patient should be placed in the recumbent position and treated supportively as necessary. Patients should be advised to lie or sit down if they develop any postural symptom (e.g., dizziness, vertigo) and to exercise caution upon standing from a sitting or supine position. Patients also should be advised to contact their physician if dizziness, lightheadedness, or palpitations become bothersome since dosage adjustment may be necessary. Other antihypertensive therapy, especially verapamil (see Precautions and Contraindications), should be added cautiously in patients receiving terazosin.

In early trials in which increasing single terazosin doses up to 7.5 mg were administered at 3-day intervals, tolerance to the first-dose phenomenon did not necessarily develop, and first-dose postural effects were observed at all doses. In addition, syncope occurred in about 20% of patients at single-dose levels of 2.5, 5, or 7.5 mg, and a few patients developed severe orthostatic hypotension (blood pressure declining to 50/0 mm Hg) at these dosing levels. These effects occurred within 90 minutes of dosing in all cases.

■ **Nervous System Effects** Besides dizziness (see Cautions: Postural Effects), headache is the most common adverse nervous system effect associated with terazosin therapy, occurring in about 16 or 5% of patients receiving the drug for hypertension or BPH, respectively. Asthenia (weakness, tiredness, lassitude, fatigue) occurs in 11.3 or 7.4% of such patients, respectively, and somnolenceoccurs in 5.4 or 3.6%, respectively. Paresthesia and nervousness occur in 2–3% of patients receiving the drug for hypertension, and depression occurs in 0.3%. Anxiety and insomnia have been reported occasionally, but a causal relationship to the drug has not been established.

■ **GI Effects** Nausea is the most common adverse GI effect of terazosin, occurring in 4.4 or 1.7% of patients receiving the drug for hypertension or BPH, respectively. Constipation, diarrhea, dry mouth, dyspepsia, flatulence, abdominal pain, and vomiting have been reported occasionally, but these effects have not been directly attributed to the drug.

■ **Cardiovascular Effects** Besides postural effects of the drug (see Cautions: Postural Effects), other cardiovascular effects reported with terazosin include peripheral edema in about 6 or 1% of patients receiving the drug for hypertension or BPH, respectively, and tachycardia and nonperipheral edema in about 1–2% of those receiving the drug for hypertension. Arrhythmia, chest pain, and vasodilation have been reported occasionally, but a causal relationship has not been established. While clinically important nonpostural decreases in blood pressure generally are not observed in normotensive patients receiving the drug for BPH, some reduction may occur, and hypotension develops in less than 1% of patients. Atrial fibrillation has been reported during postmarketing surveillance in patients receiving terazosin.

■ **Dermatologic and Sensitivity Reactions** Adverse dermatologic effects have been reported occasionally in patients receiving terazosin, but a causal relationship to the drug has not been established. Such effects include facial edema, pruritus, and rash.

Allergic reactions, including anaphylaxis, have been reported rarely in patients receiving terazosin.

■ **Musculoskeletal Effects** Back pain or flu-like syndrome occurs in 2.4% of patients receiving terazosin for hypertension or BPH, respectively. These effects also have been reported in hypertensive patients, but a causal relationship to the drug could not be established. Other musculoskeletal effects for which a causal relationship has not been established include neck or shoulder pain, arthralgia, arthritis, joint disorder, and myalgia. Pain in the extremities also has been reported.

■ **Respiratory Effects** Nasal congestion/rhinitis occurs in about 6 or 2% of patients receiving terazosin for hypertension or BPH, respectively, and dyspnea occurs in about 3.1 and 1.7%, respectively. Sinusitis occurs in 2.6% of hypertensive patients receiving the drug. Occasionally, cold symptoms, bronchitis, epistaxis,cough, and pharyngitis have been reported, but these effects have not been directly attributed to the drug.

■ **Genitourinary Effects** Impotence is the most common adverse genitourinary effect of terazosin, occurring in 1.2 or 1.6% of patients receiving the drug for hypertension or BPH, respectively. Priapism (painful penile erection sustained for hours and unrelieved by sexual intercourse or masturbation) has been reported rarely (probably less frequently than 1 per several thousand patients) in patients receiving an α_1-adrenergic antagonist (e.g., terazosin). Urinary tract infection was reported in 1.3% of patients with BPH receiving the drug, but this frequency was less than that reported with placebo. Urinary tract infection also has been reported in hypertensive patients receiving terazosin but could not be directly attributed to the drug. Other adverse genitourinary effects for which a causal relationship has not been established include urinary frequency and urinary incontinence (principally in postmenopausal women).

■ **Ocular and Otic Effects** Blurred vision/amblyopia occurs in 1.6 or 1.3% of patients receiving terazosin for hypertension or BPH, respectively. Visual abnormalities, conjunctivitis, and tinnitus have been reported occasionally but have not been directly attributed to the drug.

■ **Hematologic Effects** Small decreases in hemoglobin concentration, hematocrit, leukocyte count, and total protein and albumin concentrations have been observed following administration of terazosin and were suggestive of hemodilution. Similar changes have been observed with other α_1-adrenergic blocking agents and attributed to hemodilution. Thrombocytopenia has been reported during postmarketing surveillance in patients receiving terazosin.

■ **Other Adverse Effects** Weight gain (in both males and females) occurs in 0.5% of patients receiving terazosin for hypertension or BPH, and decreased libido occurs in 0.6% of those receiving the drug for hypertension. Some evidence suggests that the likelihood of weight gain may increase with increasing dosage and/or duration of therapy in some patients. Other adverse effects have been reported occasionally with terazosin but have not been directly attributed to the drug. Such effects include fever, gout, and sweating.

■ **Precautions and Contraindications** Patients should be warned of the possibility of terazosin-induced postural dizziness and measures to take if it develops (e.g., sitting, lying down). (See Cautions: Postural Effects.) During initiation of terazosin therapy, the patient should be cautioned to avoid, for 12 hours after the first dose, subsequent dosage increases, and resumption of therapy, situations where injury could result (e.g., driving, hazardous tasks) if syncope were to occur. If syncope occurs, the patient should be placed in the recumbent position and treated supportively as necessary. Patients who engage in potentially hazardous activities such as operating machinery or driving motor vehicles should be warned about possible somnolence, drowsiness, or dizziness.

While the manufacturer questions the need for caution, some clinicians state that α_1-adrenergic blocking agents should be avoided in patients with micturition-associated syncope because of the risk of exaggerated postural effects.

Patients also should be advised that priapism has been reported rarely in patients receiving an α_1-adrenergic antagonist (e.g., terazosin). Priapism is a medical emergency that could result in penile tissue damage and permanent loss of potency if not treated immediately; therefore, patients should be advised to report promptly to their clinician or, if their clinician is unavailable, to seek alternative immediate medical attention if an erection occurs that persists longer than several (e.g., 4–6) hours or is painful.

The possibility of carcinoma of the prostate and other conditions associated with manifestations that mimic those of BPH should be excluded in any patient for whom terazosin therapy for presumed BPH is being considered.

Caution should be exercised when adding terazosin to a preexisting antihypertensive regimen or when adding other hypotensive agents to a terazosin regimen in order to avoid a possible rapid fall in blood pressure and exacerbation of postural effects. Dosage reduction and/or retitration of therapy may be necessary. Particular caution may be necessary when terazosin and verapamil are used concomitantly because of an added potential pharmacokinetic interaction (i.e., verapamil-induced increases in plasma terazosin concentrations).

Terazosin is contraindicated in patients with known sensitivity to the drug or any other quinazoline derivative (e.g., doxazosin, prazosin).

■ **Pediatric Precautions** The manufacturer states that safety and efficacy of terazosin in patients younger than 21 years of age have not been established. Some experts state that use of centrally acting antihypertensive agents (e.g., terazosin) should be reserved for children who are not responsive to 2 or more of the preferred classes of antihypertensive agents (angiotensin-converting enzyme [ACE] inhibitors, angiotensin II receptor antagonists, long-acting calcium-channel blockers, or thiazide diuretics). For information on overall principles and expert recommendations for treatment of hypertension in pediatric patients, see Uses: Hypertension in Pediatric Patients, in the Thiazides General Statement 40:28.20.

■ **Geriatric Precautions** Geriatric patients (e.g., those 65 years of age and older) may be particularly susceptible to postural as well as certain other adverse effects of terazosin. (See Dosage and Administration: Dosage.)

■ **Mutagenicity and Carcinogenicity** There was no evidence of terazosin-induced mutagenicity in in vitro and in vivo test systems (Ames test, in vivo cytogenetics, dominant lethal test in mice, in vivo Chinese hamster chromosome aberration test, V79 forward mutation assay).

Oral terazosin dosages of 250 mg/kg daily (695 times the maximum recommended human dosage of 20 mg daily adjusted for a 55-kg man) for 2 years were associated with an increase in benign adrenal medullary tumors in male rats; females were unaffected. The drug was not oncogenic in mice receiving oral dosages of 32 mg/kg daily for 2 years. The absence of mutagenicity in a battery of in vivo and in vitro tests, of tumorigenicity of any cell type in the mouse carcinogenicity assay, of increased total tumor incidence in rats or mice, and of proliferative adrenal lesions in female rats suggests that the observed increase in benign medullary tumors is a male-rat species-specific effect. In addition, numerous other drugs and chemicals have been associated with increased benign adrenal medullary tumors in male rats without evidence of carcinogenic effects in humans.

■ **Pregnancy, Fertility, and Lactation** Terazosin was not teratogenic in rats or rabbits at oral dosages up to 1330 or 165 times the maximum recommended human dosage, respectively. Fetal resorptions occurred in rats at an oral dosage of 480 mg/kg daily, which is approximately 1330 times the maximum recommended human dosage. Increased fetal resorptions, decreased fetal weight, and increased supernumerary ribs were observed in offspring of rabbits that received 165 times the maximum recommended human dosage. These fetal findings were most likely secondary to maternal toxicity. There are no adequate and controlled studies in pregnant women, and safety of terazosin during pregnancy has not been established. The drug should be used during pregnancy only when potential benefits justify the possible risks to the mother and fetus.

In a perinatal and postnatal development study in rats, there was an increased frequency of deaths in the offspring during the first 3 weeks postpartum at a maternal oral terazosin dosage of 120 mg/kg daily (more than 300 times the maximum recommended human dosage).

In reproduction studies in rats receiving oral terazosin dosages of 8, 30, or 120 mg/kg daily, failure to sire litters was observed in males receiving the latter 2 dosages, but testicular weight and morphology were unaffected. However, vaginal smears at these latter dosages appeared to contain less sperm than smears from control matings, and a positive correlation between sperm count and subsequent pregnancy was observed. An increase in testicular atrophy has been observed in rats receiving terazosin dosages of 40 or 250 mg/kg daily but not in those receiving 8 mg/kg daily (more than 20 times the maximum recommended human dosage). Testicular atrophy also was observed in dogs receiving 300 mg/kg daily (more than 800 times the maximum recommended human dosage) for 3 months but not with 1 year of administration at 20 mg/kg daily. Such atrophy also has been observed with prazosin.

Since it is not known whether terazosin is distributed into milk, the drug should be used with caution in nursing women.

Description

Terazosin hydrochloride is a quinazoline-derivative postsynaptic α_1-adrenergic blocking agent. The drug is chemically and pharmacologically related to prazosin and doxazosin. On a molar basis, the postsynaptic α_1-adrenergic receptor affinity of terazosin is one-third that of prazosin when tested in rat liver, and the α_1-receptor selectivity is 4 times that of doxazosin when tested in human prostate adenoma.

Terazosin reduces peripheral vascular resistance and blood pressure as a result of its vasodilating effects; the drug produces both arterial and venous dilation. Terazosin reduces blood pressure in both supine and standing patients; the effect is most pronounced on standing blood pressure, and postural hypotension can occur. Terazosin generally causes no change in heart rate or cardiac output in the supine position. Cardiovascular responses to exercise (e.g., increased heart rate and cardiac output) are maintained during terazosin therapy.

Effects of terazosin on the cardiovascular system are mediated by the drug's activity at α_1-receptor sites in vascular smooth muscle. α_1-Adrenergic receptors also are located in nonvascular smooth muscle (e.g., bladder trigone and sphincters, GI tract and sphincters, prostate adenoma and capsule, ureters, uterus) and in nonmuscular tissues (e.g., CNS, liver, kidneys). Because of the prevalence of α-receptors in the prostate capsule, prostate adenoma, and the bladder trigone and the relative absence of these receptors on the bladder body, α-blockers decrease urinary outflow resistance in men.

Terazosin may improve to a limited extent the serum lipid profile (e.g., small increases in high-density lipoprotein cholesterol concentrations [HDL]/total cholesterol ratio, small decreases in low-density lipoprotein [LDL] cholesterol, total cholesterol, and triglyceride concentrations). In addition, such potential effects of terazosin may counteract the negative effects of thiazide diuretics on serum lipoprotein concentrations.

SumMon® (see Users Guide). For additional information on this drug until a more detailed monograph is developed and published, the manufacturer's labeling should be consulted. It is *essential* that the labeling be consulted for information on the usual cautions, precautions, and contraindications concerning potential drug interactions and/or laboratory test interferences and for information on acute toxicity.

Preparations

Excipients in commercially available drug preparations may have clinically important effects in some individuals; consult specific product labeling for details.

Terazosin Hydrochloride

Oral		
Capsules	1 mg (of terazosin)*	**Terazosin Hydrochloride Capsules**
	2 mg (of terazosin)*	**Terazosin Hydrochloride Capsules**
	5 mg (of terazosin)*	**Terazosin Hydrochloride Capsules**
	10 mg (of terazosin)*	**Terazosin Hydrochloride Capsules**

*available from one or more manufacturer, distributor, and/or repackager by generic (nonproprietary) name

†Use is not currently included in the labeling approved by the US Food and Drug Administration

β-ADRENERGIC BLOCKING AGENTS 24:24

Atenolol

■ Atenolol is a β_1-selective adrenergic blocking agent (β-blocker).

Uses

Atenolol is used for the management of hypertension, angina, and acute myocardial infarction (MI). The drug also has been used for the management of supraventricular and ventricular tachyarrhythmias†, management of acute alcohol withdrawal (in conjunction with a benzodiazepine)†, and prophylaxis of migraine headache†.

The choice of a β-adrenergic blocking agent (β-blocker) depends on numerous factors, including pharmacologic properties (e.g., relative β-selectivity, intrinsic sympathomimetic activity, membrane-stabilizing activity, lipophilicity), pharmacokinetics, intended use, and adverse effect profile, as well as the patient's coexisting disease states or conditions, response, and tolerance. While specific pharmacologic properties and other factors may appropriately influence the choice of a β-blocker in individual patients, evidence of clinically important differences among the agents in terms of overall efficacy and/or safety is limited. Patients who do not respond to or cannot tolerate one β-blocker may be successfully treated with a different agent.

In the management of hypertension or chronic stable angina pectoris in patients with chronic obstructive pulmonary disease (COPD) or type 1 diabetes mellitus, many clinicians prefer to use low dosages of a β_1-selective adrenergic blocking agent (e.g., atenolol, metoprolol), rather than a nonselective agent (e.g., nadolol, pindolol, propranolol, timolol). However, selectivity of these agents is relative and dose dependent. Some clinicians also will recommend using a β_1-selective agent or an agent with intrinsic sympathomimetic activity (ISA) (e.g., pindolol), rather than a nonselective agent, for the management of hypertension or angina pectoris in patients with peripheral vascular disease, but there is no evidence that the choice of β-blocker substantially affects efficacy.

■ **Hypertension** Atenolol is used alone or in combination with other classes of antihypertensive agents in the management of hypertension. β-Blockers often are used concurrently with a diuretic because of their additive effects. β-Blockers also have been combined with vasodilators (e.g., hydralazine, minoxidil) to counteract the reflex tachycardia that occurs with vasodilators.

Current evidence-based practice guidelines for the management of hypertension in adults generally recommend the use of drugs from 4 classes of antihypertensive agents (angiotensin-converting enzyme [ACE] inhibitors, angiotensin II receptor antagonists, calcium-channel blockers, and thiazide diuretics). Most guidelines no longer recommend β-blockers as first-line therapy for hypertension because of the lack of established superiority over other recommended drug classes and evidence from at least one study (with atenolol) demonstrating that β-blockers may be less effective than angiotensin II receptor antagonists in preventing cardiovascular death, MI, or stroke. (See Uses: Hypertension in Adults, in the Thiazides General Statement 40:28.20.) However, therapy with a β-blocker may still be considered in hypertensive patients who have a compelling indication (e.g., prior MI, ischemic heart disease, heart failure) for their use or as add-on therapy in those who do not respond adequately to the preferred drug classes. (See Considerations for Drug Therapy in Patients with Underlying Cardiovascular and Other Risk Factors, under Uses: Hypertension.) Ultimately, choice of antihypertensive therapy should be individualized, considering the clinical characteristics of the patient (e.g., age, ethnicity/race, comorbid conditions, cardiovascular risk factors) as well as drug-related factors (e.g., ease of administration, availability, adverse effects, costs).

General Considerations for Initial and Maintenance Antihypertensive Therapy **Nonpharmacologic Therapy.** Nonpharmacologic measures (i.e., lifestyle/behavioral modifications) that are effective in lowering blood pressure include weight reduction (for those who are overweight or obese), dietary changes to include foods such as fruits, vegetables, whole grains, and low-fat dairy products that are rich in potassium, calcium, magnesium, and fiber (i.e., adoption of the Dietary Approaches to Stop Hypertension [DASH] eating plan), sodium reduction, increased physical activity, and moderation of alcohol intake. Such lifestyle/behavioral modifications, including smoking cessation, enhance antihypertensive drug efficacy and decrease cardiovascular risk and remain an indispensable part of the management of hypertension. Lifestyle/behavioral modifications without antihypertensive drug therapy are recommended for individuals classified by a 2017 multidisciplinary hypertension guideline of the American College of Cardiology (ACC), American Heart Association (AHA), and a number of other professional organizations as having elevated blood pressure (systolic blood pressure 120–129 mm Hg and diastolic blood pressure less than 80 mm Hg) and in those with stage 1 hypertension (systolic blood pressure 130–139 mm Hg or diastolic blood pressure 80–89 mm Hg) who do *not* have preexisting cardiovascular disease or an estimated 10-year atherosclerotic cardiovascular disease (ASCVD) risk of 10% or greater.

Initiation of Drug Therapy. Drug therapy in the management of hypertension must be individualized and adjusted based on the degree of blood pressure elevation while also considering cardiovascular risk factors. Drug therapy generally is reserved for patients who respond inadequately to nondrug therapy (i.e., lifestyle modifications such as diet [including sodium restriction and adequate potassium and calcium intake], regular aerobic physical activity, moderation of alcohol consumption, and weight reduction) or in whom the degree of blood pressure elevation or coexisting risk factors, especially increased cardiovascular risk, requires more prompt or aggressive therapy; however, the optimum blood pressure threshold for initiating antihypertensive drug therapy and specific treatment goals remain controversial.

The 2017 ACC/AHA hypertension guideline and many experts currently state that the treatment of hypertension should be based not only on blood pressure values but also on patients' cardiovascular risk factors. For *secondary prevention* of recurrent cardiovascular disease events in adults with clinical cardiovascular disease or for *primary prevention* in adults with an estimated 10-year ASCVD risk of 10% or higher, the 2017 ACC/AHA hypertension guideline recommends initiation of antihypertensive drug therapy in conjunction with lifestyle/behavioral modifications at an average systolic blood pressure of 130 mm Hg or an average diastolic blood pressure of 80 mm Hg or higher. For *primary prevention* of cardiovascular disease events in adults with a low (less than 10%) estimated 10-year risk of ASCVD, the 2017 ACC/AHA hypertension guideline recommends initiation of antihypertensive drug therapy in conjunction with lifestyle/behavioral modifications at a systolic blood pressure of 140 mm Hg or higher or a diastolic blood pressure of 90 mm Hg or higher. After initiation of antihypertensive drug therapy, regardless of the ASCVD risk, the 2017 ACC/AHA hypertension guideline generally recommends a blood pressure goal of less than 130/80 mm Hg in all adults. In addition, a systolic blood pressure goal of less than 130 mm Hg also is recommended for noninstitutionalized ambulatory patients 65 years of age or older. While these blood pressure goals are lower than those recommended for most patients in previous guidelines, they are based upon clinical studies demonstrating continuing reduction of cardiovascular risk at progressively lower levels of systolic blood pressure.

Most data indicate that patients with a higher cardiovascular risk will benefit the most from tighter blood pressure control; however, some experts state this treatment goal also may be beneficial in those at lower cardiovascular risk. Other clinicians believe that the benefits of such blood pressure lowering do not outweigh the risks in those patients considered to be at lower risk of cardiovascular disease and that reclassifying individuals formerly considered to have prehypertension as having hypertension may potentially lead to use of drug therapy in such patients without consideration of cardiovascular risk. Previous hypertension guidelines, such as those from the JNC 8 expert panel, generally have recommended initiation of antihypertensive treatment in patients with a systolic blood pressure of at least 140 mm Hg or diastolic blood pressure of at least 90 mm Hg, targeted a blood pressure goal of less than 140/90 mm Hg regardless of cardiovascular risk, and used higher systolic blood pressure thresholds and targets in geriatric patients. Some clinicians continue to support the target blood pressures recommended by the JNC 8 expert panel because of concerns that such recommendations in the 2017 ACC/AHA hypertension guideline are based on extrapolation of data from the high-risk population in the SPRINT study to a lower-risk population. Also, because more than 90% of patients in SPRINT were already receiving antihypertensive drugs at baseline, data are lacking on the effects of *initiating* drug therapy at a lower blood pressure threshold (130/80 mm Hg) in patients at high risk of cardiovascular disease. The potential benefits of hypertension management and drug cost, adverse effects, and risks associated with the use of multiple antihypertensive drugs should be considered when deciding a patient's treatment goal.

The 2017 ACC/AHA hypertension guideline recommends an ASCVD risk assessment for all adults with hypertension; however, experts state that it can be assumed that patients with hypertension and diabetes mellitus or chronic kidney disease (CKD) are at high risk for cardiovascular disease and that antihypertensive drug therapy should be initiated in these patients at a blood pressure of 130/80 mm Hg or higher. ACC/AHA also recommends a blood pressure goal of less than 130/80 mm Hg in patients with hypertension and diabetes mellitus or CKD. These recommendations are based on a systematic review of high-quality evidence from randomized controlled trials, meta-analyses, and post hoc analyses that have demonstrated substantial reductions in the risk of important clinical outcomes (e.g., cardiovascular events) regardless of comorbid conditions or age when systolic blood pressure is lowered to less than 130 mm Hg. However, some clinicians have questioned the generalizability of findings from some of the trials (e.g., SPRINT) used to support the 2017 ACC/AHA hypertension guideline. For example, SPRINT included adults (mean age: 68 years) *without* diabetes mellitus who were at high risk of cardiovascular disease. While benefits of intensive blood pressure control were observed in this patient population, some clinicians have questioned whether these findings apply to younger patients who have a low risk of cardiovascular disease. In patients with CKD in the SPRINT trial, intensive blood pressure management (achieving a mean systolic blood pressure of approximately 122 mm Hg compared with 136 mm Hg with standard treatment) provided a similar beneficial reduction in the composite cardiovascular disease primary outcome and all-cause mortality as in the full patient cohort. Because most patients with CKD die from cardiovascular complications, the findings of this study further support a lower blood pressure target of less than 130/80 mm Hg. Data are lacking to determine the ideal blood pressure goal in patients with hypertension and diabetes mellitus; also, studies evaluating the benefits of intensive blood pressure control in patients with diabetes mellitus have provided conflicting results.

Clinical studies reviewed for the 2017 ACC/AHA hypertension guideline have shown similar quantitative benefits from blood pressure lowering in hypertensive patients with or without diabetes mellitus. In a randomized, controlled study (ACCORD-BP) that compared a higher (systolic blood pressure less than 140 mm Hg) versus lower (systolic blood pressure less than 120 mm Hg) blood pressure goal in patients with diabetes mellitus, there was no difference in the incidence of cardiovascular outcomes (e.g., composite outcome of cardiovascular death, nonfatal MI, and nonfatal stroke). However, some experts state that this study was underpowered to detect a difference between the 2 treatment groups and that the factorial design of the study complicated interpretation of the results. Although SPRINT did not include patients with diabetes mellitus, patients in this study with prediabetes demonstrated a similar cardiovascular benefit from intensive treatment of blood pressure as normoglycemic patients. A meta-analysis of data from ACCORD and SPRINT suggests that the findings of both studies are consistent and that patients with diabetes mellitus benefit from more intensive blood pressure control. These data support the 2017 ACC/AHA hypertension guideline recommendation of a blood pressure treatment goal of less than 130/80 mm Hg in patients with hypertension and diabetes mellitus. Alternatively, the American Diabetes Association (ADA) recommends a blood pressure goal of less than 140/90 mm Hg in patients with diabetes mellitus. The ADA states that a lower blood pressure goal (e.g., less than 130/80 mm Hg) may be appropriate for patients with a high risk of cardiovascular disease and diabetes mellitus if it can be achieved without undue treatment burden.

Further study is needed to more clearly define optimum blood pressure goals in patients with hypertension, particularly in high-risk groups (e.g., patients with diabetes mellitus, cardiovascular disease, or cerebrovascular disease; black patients); when determining appropriate blood pressure goals, individual risks and benefits should be considered in addition to the evidence from clinical studies.

Experts state that in patients with stage 1 hypertension (especially the elderly, those with a history of hypotension, or those who have experienced adverse drug effects), it is reasonable to initiate drug therapy using the stepped-care approach in which one drug is initiated and titrated and other drugs are added sequentially to achieve the target blood pressure. However, although some patients can begin treatment with a single antihypertensive agent, the 2017 ACC/AHA hypertension guideline recommends initiation of antihypertensive therapy with 2 drugs from different pharmacologic classes (either as separate agents or in a fixed-dose combination) in patients with stage 2 hypertension and an average blood pressure more than 20/10 mm Hg above their target blood pressure. Such combined therapy may increase the likelihood of achieving goal blood pressure in a more timely fashion, but also may increase the risk of adverse effects (e.g., orthostatic hypotension) in some patients (e.g., elderly). Drug regimens with complementary activity, where a second antihypertensive agent is used to block compensatory responses to the first agent or affect a different pressor mechanism, can result in additive blood pressure lowering and are preferred. Drug combinations that have similar mechanisms of action or clinical effects (e.g., the combination of an ACE inhibitor and an angiotensin II receptor antagonist) generally should be avoided. Many patients who begin therapy with a single antihypertensive agent will subsequently require at least 2 drugs from different pharmacologic classes to achieve their blood pressure goal. Experts state that other patient-specific factors, such as age, concurrent medications, drug adherence, drug interactions, the overall treatment regimen, cost, and comorbidities, also should be considered when deciding on an antihypertensive drug regimen. For any stage of hypertension, antihypertensive drug dosages should be adjusted and/or other agents substituted or added until goal blood pressure is achieved. (See Follow-up and Maintenance Drug Therapy under Hypertension: General Considerations for Initial and Maintenance Antihypertensive Therapy, in Uses.)

Follow-up and Maintenance Drug Therapy. Several strategies are used for the titration and combination of antihypertensive drugs; these strategies, which are generally based on those used in randomized controlled studies, include maximizing the dosage of the first drug before adding a second drug, adding a second drug before achieving maximum dosage of the initial drug, or initiating therapy with 2 drugs simultaneously (either as separate preparations or as a fixed-dose combination). Combined use of an ACE inhibitor and angiotensin II receptor antagonist should be avoided because of the potential risk of adverse renal effects. After initiating a new or adjusted antihypertensive drug regimen, patients should have their blood pressure reevaluated monthly until adequate blood pressure control is achieved. Effective blood pressure control can be achieved in most hypertensive patients, but many will ultimately require therapy with 2 or more antihypertensive drugs. In addition to measuring blood pressure, clinicians should evaluate patients for orthostatic hypotension, adverse drug effects, adherence to drug therapy and lifestyle modifications, and the need for drug dosage adjustments. Laboratory testing such as electrolytes and renal function status and other assessments of target organ damage also should be performed.

Considerations for Drug Therapy in Patients with Underlying Cardiovascular and Other Risk Factors Drug therapy in patients with hypertension and underlying cardiovascular or other risk factors should be carefully individualized based on the underlying disease(s), concomitant drugs, tolerance to drug-induced adverse effects, and blood pressure goal. (See Table 2 on Compelling Indications for Drug Classes based on Comorbid Conditions, under Uses: Hypertension in Adults, in the Thiazides General Statement 40:28.20.)

Ischemic Heart Disease. The selection of an appropriate antihypertensive agent in patients with ischemic heart disease should be based on individual patient characteristics and may include a β-blocker, with the addition of other drugs (e.g., ACE inhibitors, thiazide diuretics, calcium-channel blockers) as necessary to achieve blood pressure goals. Because of the demonstrated mortality benefit of β-blockers following MI, these drugs should be administered in all patients who have survived an MI. The 2017 ACC/AHA hypertension guideline states that β-blockers used for ischemic heart disease/angina that are also effective in lowering blood pressure include bisoprolol, carvedilol, metoprolol succinate, metoprolol tartrate, nadolol, propranolol, and timolol. However, ACC/AHA state that the use of atenolol for the management of hypertension in patients with stable ischemic heart disease should be *avoided* because the drug has been shown to be less effective than placebo in reducing cardiovascular events and is not as effective in treating hypertension as other antihypertensive agents.

Heart Failure. While β-blockers as single therapies are not superior to other antihypertensive agents in the reduction of all cardiovascular outcomes, certain β-blockers (bisoprolol, carvedilol, extended-release metoprolol succinate) have been shown to be effective in reducing the incidence of heart failure† and associated morbidity and mortality. (See Uses: Heart Failure, in Carvedilol 24:24.)

Other Special Considerations for Antihypertensive Drug Therapy

Race. Most patients with hypertension, especially black patients, will require at least 2 antihypertensive drugs to achieve adequate blood pressure control. In general, black hypertensive patients tend to respond better to monotherapy with thiazide diuretics or calcium-channel blocking agents than to monotherapy with β-blockers, ACE inhibitors, or angiotensin II receptor antagonists. However, such diminished response to a β-blocker is largely eliminated when the drug is administered concomitantly with a thiazide diuretic. In addition, some experts state that when use of β-blockers is indicated in hypertensive patients with underlying cardiovascular or other risk factors, these indications should be applied equally to black hypertensive patients.

For information on overall principles and expert recommendations for treatment of hypertension, see Uses: Hypertension in Adults, in the Thiazides General Statement 40:28.20.

■ **Chronic Stable Angina** Atenolol is used for the management of chronic stable angina pectoris. β-Blockers are recommended as the anti-ischemic drugs of choice in most patients with chronic stable angina; despite differences in cardioselectivity, intrinsic sympathomimetic activity, and other clinical factors, all β-blockers appear to be equally effective for this indication. Long-term use of β-blockers in patients with chronic stable angina pectoris has been shown to reduce the frequency of anginal attacks, allow a reduction in nitroglycerin dosage, and increase exercise tolerance.

Combination therapy with a β-blocker and a nitrate appears to be more effective than either drug alone because β-blockers attenuate the increased sympathetic tone and reflex tachycardia associated with nitrate therapy while nitrate therapy (e.g., nitroglycerin) counteracts the potential increase in left-ventricular wall tension associated with a decrease in heart rate. Combined therapy with a β-blocker and a dihydropyridine calcium-channel blocker also may be useful because the tendency to develop tachycardia with the calcium-channel blocker is counteracted by the β-blocker. However, caution should be exercised in the concomitant use of β-blockers and the nondihydropyridine calcium-channel blockers verapamil or diltiazem because of the potential for excessive fatigue, bradycardia, or atrioventricular (AV) block. (See Drug Interactions: Cardiovascular Drugs.)

■ **Non-ST-Segment-Elevation Acute Coronary Syndromes** β-Blockers are used as part of the standard therapeutic measures for managing non-ST-segment-elevation acute coronary syndromes (NSTE ACS). Patients with NSTE ACS have either unstable angina or non-ST-segment-elevation MI (NSTEMI); because these conditions are part of a continuum of acute myocardial ischemia and have indistinguishable clinical features upon presentation, the same initial treatment strategies are recommended. The American Heart Association/American College of Cardiology (AHA/ACC) guideline for the management of patients with NSTE ACS recommends an early invasive strategy (angiographic evaluation with the intent to perform revascularization procedures such as percutaneous coronary intervention [PCI] with coronary artery stent implantation or coronary artery bypass grafting [CABG]) or an ischemia-guided strategy (initial medical management followed by cardiac catheterization and revascularization if indicated) in patients with definite or likely NSTE ACS; standard medical therapies for all patients should include a β-blocker, antiplatelet agents (aspirin and/or a P2Y12-receptor antagonist), anticoagulant agents (e.g., low molecular weight or unfractionated heparin), nitrates (e.g., nitroglycerin), and analgesic agents regardless of the initial management approach. The guideline states that oral β-blocker therapy should be initiated within the first 24 hours in patients who do not have manifestations of heart failure, evidence of a low-output state, increased risk of cardiogenic shock, or any other contraindications to β-blocker therapy; use of IV β-blockers is potentially harmful in patients with risk factors for cardiogenic shock. Continued therapy with a β-blocker proven to reduce mortality (bisoprolol, carvedilol, or metoprolol succinate) is recommended in patients with stabilized heart failure and reduced systolic function. (See Uses: Heart Failure, in Carvedilol 24:24.)

■ **Acute Myocardial Infarction** Atenolol is used to reduce the risk of cardiovascular mortality in hemodynamically stable patients with definite or suspected acute MI. The term MI is used when there is evidence of myocardial necrosis in the setting of acute myocardial ischemia. ST-segment-elevation MI (STEMI) is distinguished from NSTEMI based on the presence or absence of ST-segment elevation on ECG. Patients with STEMI typically have complete arterial occlusion; therefore, immediate reperfusion therapy (with primary PCI or thrombolytic agents) is the current standard of care for such patients. Because the clinical presentation of NSTEMI is similar to that of unstable angina, these conditions are considered together in current expert guidelines. (See Uses: Non-ST-Segment-Elevation Acute Coronary Syndromes.) During the early stage of a definite or suspected MI, atenolol has been initiated with IV doses (no longer commercially available in the US), followed by continued oral dosing; however, experts currently recommend that early IV use of β-blockers be limited to selected patients.

Because β-blockers can reduce myocardial oxygen demand during the first few hours of an acute MI by reducing heart rate, arterial blood pressure, and myocardial contractility, and also have been shown to reduce mortality, early IV therapy with these drugs was routinely recommended following acute MI. Evidence supporting this recommendation was generally based on studies conducted prior to the reperfusion era demonstrating a reduction in mortality and other clinical benefits (i.e., reduced infarct size, incidence of ventricular arrhythmias, chest pain, and cardiac enzyme elevations) with early use of β-blockers during MI. In one such study (the First International Study of Infarct Survival; ISIS-1), therapy with atenolol (initiated IV within the first 12 hours of symptom onset and continued orally for 7 days) was shown to reduce cardiovascular mortality by approximately 15% during the first few days of therapy, but did not substantially reduce cardiovascular mortality beyond this initial period. The difference in vascular mortality rate between those receiving atenolol or placebo was evident almost entirely during the first 2 days of therapy. Analysis of data from a subset of patients who died during early treatment in ISIS-1 suggested that the principal mechanism of early mortality reduction associated with atenolol therapy was prevention of cardiac rupture and of cardiac electromechanical dissociation. However, the relevance of these study findings to current clinical practice has been questioned since patients did not receive reperfusion therapy and only 5% received an antiplatelet agent.

Studies conducted after the widespread use of reperfusion therapy generally have demonstrated more attenuated benefits with early β-blocker therapy in patients with acute MI; while β-blockers may still confer benefits (e.g., reduction in the risk of reinfarction and ventricular arrhythmias), there is less certainty regarding the drugs' effects on mortality in patients receiving contemporary revascularization and pharmacologic therapies (antiplatelet agents, ACE inhibitors, and lipid-lowering therapies). In addition, early use of β-blockers (particularly when administered IV) has been associated with an increased risk of cardiogenic shock. (See Uses: Acute Myocardial Infarction in Metoprolol 24:24.) Based on the currently available evidence, the American College of Cardiology Foundation/American Heart Association (ACCF/AHA) guideline for the management of STEMI recommends oral β-blocker therapy in all patients who do not have manifestations of heart failure, evidence of a low-output state, increased risk of cardiogenic shock, or any other contraindications to β-blocker therapy. Such therapy should be initiated within the first 24 hours following acute MI and continued during and after hospitalization. Because of conflicting evidence of benefit and the potential for harm, the guidelines recommend limiting use of IV β-blockers to patients with refractory hypertension or ongoing ischemia.

Although the efficacy of atenolol in reducing cardiovascular mortality has been established only during the first 7 days after an acute MI, the benefits of long-term β-blocker therapy for secondary prevention have been well established in numerous clinical studies. Patients with MI complicated by heart failure, left ventricular dysfunction, or ventricular arrhythmias appear to derive the most benefit from long-term β-blocker therapy. Data from studies using other β-blockers suggest that optimum benefit may be achieved if treatment with these agents is continued for at least 1–3 years if not indefinitely after infarction unless contraindicated. Several large, randomized studies have demonstrated that prolonged oral therapy with a β-blocker can reduce the rates of reinfarction and mortality (e.g., sudden and nonsudden cardiac death) following acute MI. It is estimated that such therapy could result in a relative reduction in mortality of about 25% annually for years 1–3 after infarction, with high-risk patients exhibiting the greatest potential benefit; the benefit of continued therapy may persist for at least several years beyond this period, although less substantially. Therefore, atenolol, like other β-blockers, can be used for secondary prevention following acute MI to reduce the risk of reinfarction and mortality. The AHA/ACCF secondary prevention guideline recommends β-blocker therapy in all patients with left ventricular systolic dysfunction (ejection fraction of 40% or less) and a prior MI; use of a β-blocker with proven mortality benefit (bisoprolol, carvedilol, or metoprolol succinate) is recommended. (See Uses: Heart Failure, in Carvedilol 24:24.) Although the benefits of long-term β-blockade in post-MI patients with normal left ventricular function are less well established, the guideline recommends continued β-blocker therapy for at least 3 years in such patients. Further studies are needed to establish the optimal duration of β-blocker therapy for secondary prevention of MI.

■ Supraventricular Arrhythmias β-Blockers, including atenolol, have been used to slow ventricular rate in patients with supraventricular tachycardia (SVT)†. The American College of Cardiology/American Heart Association/Heart Rhythm Society (ACC/AHA/HRS) guideline for the management of adult patients with supraventricular tachycardia recommends the use of β-adrenergic blocking agents in the treatment of various SVTs (e.g., atrial flutter, junctional tachycardia, focal atrial tachycardia, atrioventricular nodal reentrant tachycardia [AVNRT]); in general, an IV β-blocker is recommended for acute treatment, while an oral preparation is recommended for ongoing management of these arrhythmias. Vagal maneuvers and/or IV adenosine are considered first-line interventions for the acute treatment of patients with SVT and should be attempted prior to other therapies when clinically indicated; if such measures are ineffective or not feasible, an IV β-blocker may be considered in hemodynamically stable patients. Although evidence of efficacy is limited, experts state that the overall safety of β-adrenergic blockers warrants their use in patients with SVT. Patients should be closely monitored for hypotension and bradycardia during administration of these drugs.

Atrial Fibrillation and Flutter β-Blockers are recommended as one of several drug therapy options for ventricular rate control in patients with nonpreexcited atrial fibrillation or flutter†. For acute treatment of atrial fibrillation or flutter, an IV β-adrenergic blocking agent (e.g., esmolol, propranolol, metoprolol) may be used for ventricular rate control in patients without preexcitation; an oral β-blocker such as atenolol may be used for ongoing rate control in such patients. Choice of a specific β-blocker should be individualized based on the patient's clinical condition.

Atrial Tachycardia IV β-blockers may be used for the treatment of patients with hemodynamically stable focal atrial tachycardia† (i.e., regular SVT arising from a localized atrial site), and an oral β-blocker may be used for ongoing management. Multifocal atrial tachycardia, characterized by a rapid, irregular rhythm with at least 3 distinct P-wave morphologies, is commonly associated with an underlying condition (e.g., pulmonary, coronary, or valvular heart disease) and is generally not responsive to antiarrhythmic drug therapy. Antiarrhythmic drug therapy usually is reserved for patients who do not respond to initial attempts at correcting or managing potential precipitating factors (e.g., exacerbation of chronic obstructive pulmonary disease or congestive heart failure, hypoxemia, anemia) or in whom a precipitating factor cannot be identified.

Paroxysmal Supraventricular Tachycardia IV β-blockers may be used for the acute treatment of hemodynamically stable patients with paroxysmal supraventricular tachycardia (PSVT), including AVNRT†, that is uncontrolled or unconverted by vagal maneuvers and adenosine; an oral β-blocker may be used for the ongoing management of such patients who are not candidates for, or prefer not to undergo, catheter ablation.

Junctional Tachycardia β-Blockers are considered one of several drug therapy options that may be used for the treatment of junctional tachycardia† (i.e., nonreentrant SVT originating from the AV junction), a rapid, occasionally irregular, narrow-complex tachycardia. While evidence is limited, there is some data indicating that β-blockers (specifically propranolol) are modestly effective in terminating and/or reducing the incidence of junctional tachycardia.

■ Ventricular Arrhythmias β-Blockers also have been used in patients with cardiac arrest precipitated by ventricular fibrillation or pulseless ventricular tachycardia†. However, AHA states that routine administration of β-blockers after cardiac arrest is potentially harmful (e.g., may worsen hemodynamic instability, exacerbate heart failure, or cause bradyarrhythmias) and is therefore not recommended.

β-Blockers may be useful in the management of certain forms of polymorphic ventricular tachycardia† (e.g., associated with acute ischemia).

■ Vascular Headache ***Migraine*** Atenolol has been used for the prophylaxis of migraine headache†. When used prophylactically, atenolol can prevent migraine or reduce the number of attacks in some patients. However, the US Headache Consortium states that the quality of evidence for atenolol is not as compelling as it is for propranolol for this indication. Atenolol is not recommended for the treatment of a migraine attack that has already started. For further information on management and classification of migraine headache, see Vascular Headaches: General Principles in Migraine Therapy, under Uses in Sumatriptan 28:32.28.

■ Alcohol Withdrawal Atenolol has been used in conjunction with a benzodiazepine in the management of acute alcohol withdrawal†. β-Blockers such as atenolol appear to be effective in reducing manifestations of the hyperadrenergic state associated with alcohol withdrawal, including elevated blood pressure, increased heart rate, and anxiety. However, β-blockers have not been shown to prevent delirium or seizures, and such drugs should be used only as adjuncts to benzodiazepines (not as monotherapy) for the treatment of alcohol withdrawal. (See Uses: Alcohol Withdrawal, in the Benzodiazepines General Statement 28:24.08.) Some clinicians state that the use of β-blockers may be particularly helpful in patients with certain coexisting conditions (e.g., coronary artery disease).

Dosage and Administration

■ Administration Atenolol is administered orally; the drug also has been administered by IV injection, however a parenteral preparation no longer is commercially available in the US.

Oral administration of atenolol more frequently than once daily for the management of hypertension usually is not necessary. If atenolol is used in patients with bronchospastic disorders, therapy should be initiated cautiously; concomitant administration of a β_2-adrenergic agonist and twice-daily dosing of atenolol may minimize the risk of bronchospasm in some patients.

■ Dosage Dosage of atenolol must be individualized and adjusted according to the patient's response and tolerance. If atenolol therapy is to be discontinued, dosage of the drug should be reduced gradually over a period of about 2 weeks. (See Cautions: Precautions and Contraindications.)

Hypertension **Atenolol Therapy.** The manufacturer recommends an initial adult atenolol dosage of 50 mg once daily, either alone or in combination with diuretic therapy; the full antihypertensive effect may not be evident for 1–2 weeks. If response is inadequate after a sufficient trial at the initial dosage, the manufacturer states that dosage should be increased to 100 mg once daily. Some experts state that the usual adult dosage range for treatment of hypertension is 25–100 mg daily administered in 2 divided doses. Dosages exceeding 100 mg daily usually do not result in further improvement in blood pressure control.

If atenolol is used for the management of hypertension in children†, some experts have recommended an initial oral dosage of 0.5–1 mg/kg daily given as a single dose or in 2 divided doses. Such experts have suggested that dosage may be increased as necessary to a maximum dosage of 2 mg/kg (up to 100 mg) daily given as a single dose or in 2 divided doses. For information on overall principles and expert recommendations for treatment of hypertension in pediatric patients, see Uses: Hypertension in Pediatric Patients, in the Thiazides General Statement 40:28.20.

Atenolol/Chlorthalidone Fixed-combination Therapy. When combination therapy is required, commercially available preparations containing atenolol in combination with chlorthalidone should not be used initially. Dosage should first be adjusted by administering each drug separately. If it is determined that the optimum maintenance dosage corresponds to the ratio in the commercial combination preparation, such a preparation may be used. If the fixed-combination preparation is used, the manufacturer recommends an initial dosage of 50 mg of atenolol and 25 mg of chlorthalidone once daily. If an optimal response is not achieved, the fixed-combination preparation containing 100 mg of atenolol and 25 mg of chlorthalidone may be used once daily.

Blood Pressure Monitoring and Treatment Goals. Blood pressure should be monitored regularly (i.e., monthly) during therapy and dosage of the antihypertensive drug adjusted until blood pressure is controlled. If an adequate blood pressure response is not achieved, the dosage may be increased or another antihypertensive agent with demonstrated benefit and preferably with a complementary mechanism of action (e.g., angiotensin-converting enzyme [ACE] inhibitor, angiotensin II receptor antagonist, calcium-channel blocker, thiazide diuretic) may be added; if target blood pressure is still not achieved with the use of 2 antihypertensive agents, a third drug may be added. (See Uses: Hypertension.) In patients who develop unacceptable adverse effects with atenolol, the drug should be discontinued and another antihypertensive agent from a different pharmacologic class should be initiated.

The goal of hypertension management and prevention is to achieve and maintain optimal control of blood pressure. However, the optimum blood pressure threshold for initiating antihypertensive drug therapy and specific treatment goals remain controversial. While other hypertension guidelines have based target blood pressure goals on age and comorbidities, the 2017 American College of Cardiology/American Heart Association (ACC/AHA) hypertension guideline incorporates underlying cardiovascular risk into decision making regarding treatment and generally recommends the same target blood pressure (i.e., less than 130/80 mm Hg) for all adults. Many patients will require at least 2 drugs from different pharmacologic classes to achieve this blood pressure goal; the potential benefits of hypertension management and drug cost, adverse effects, and risks associated with the use of multiple antihypertensive drugs also should be considered when deciding a patient's blood pressure treatment goal. (See General Considerations for Initial and Maintenance Antihypertensive Therapy under Uses: Hypertension.)

For additional information on target levels of blood pressure and on monitoring therapy in the management of hypertension, see Blood Pressure Monitoring and Treatment Goals under Dosage: Hypertension, in Dosage and Administration in the Thiazides General Statement 40:28.20.

Chronic Stable Angina For the management of chronic stable angina pectoris, the initial adult oral dosage of atenolol is 50 mg once daily. If an optimum response is not achieved within one week, oral dosage should be increased to 100 mg once daily. Some patients may require an oral atenolol dosage of 200 mg once daily for optimum effect. Dosage of β-blockers in angina pectoris usually is adjusted according to clinical response and to maintain a resting heart rate of 55–60 beats/minute. Control of angina pectoris over a 24-hour period with once-daily dosing of atenolol is achieved by the use of doses larger than those necessary to achieve an immediate maximum effect. The maximum early effect on exercise tolerance occurs with oral atenolol doses of 50–100 mg, but the effect at 24 hours is attenuated at these doses, averaging about 50–75% of that observed with once-daily oral doses of 200 mg.

Acute Myocardial Infarction **Early Treatment.** Atenolol therapy may be initiated as soon as possible after an acute myocardial infarction (MI) when the patient's hemodynamic condition has stabilized. During the early stage of a definite or suspected MI, atenolol has been initiated with IV doses, followed by continued oral dosing; however, a parenteral preparation of atenolol is no longer commercially available in the US. When IV dosing is excluded, atenolol can be administered orally at a dosage of 50 mg twice daily or 100 mg once daily for at least 7 days.

The American College of Cardiology Foundation (ACCF)/AHA guideline for the management of ST-segment-elevation MI (STEMI) recommends initiation of oral β-blocker therapy within the first 24 hours of an acute MI in all patients who do not have manifestations of heart failure, evidence of a low-output state, increased risk of cardiogenic shock, or any other contraindications to β-blocker therapy.

Long-term Secondary Prevention. The optimal duration of β-blocker therapy following MI remains to be clearly established. Experts generally recommend that such therapy be continued long-term in post-MI patients with left ventricular systolic dysfunction, and for at least 3 years in those with normal left ventricular function.

Supraventricular Arrhythmias For the ongoing treatment of various supraventricular tachycardias (SVTs)† (e.g., atrial flutter†, atrial tachycardia†, junctional tachycardia†) or atrial fibrillation† after initial IV therapy in adults, some experts recommend an initial oral atenolol dose of 25–50 mg daily and usual maintenance dosage of 25–100 mg daily.

Vascular Headaches **Migraine.** Although oral dosage of atenolol for the prophylaxis of migraine† in adults has not been established, the usual effective dosage of the drug in clinical studies was 100 mg daily.

■ **Dosage in Renal Impairment** In patients with impaired renal function, doses and/or frequency of administration of atenolol must be modified in response to the degree of renal impairment. Because decreased renal function is a physiologic consequence of aging, the possibility that modification of atenolol dosage may be necessary in geriatric patients should be considered. Initiation of oral atenolol therapy at 25 mg daily may be necessary in some renally impaired or geriatric patients being treated for hypertension; if this dosage is employed, measurement of blood pressure just prior to a dose is recommended to ensure persistence of adequate blood pressure reduction. Although similar, low-dose initial therapy may be warranted for other conditions, data currently are not available.

A maximum oral atenolol dosage of 50 mg daily is recommended for patients with creatinine clearances of 15–35 mL/minute per 1.73 m²; 25 mg daily or 50 mg every other day is recommended when creatinine clearance is less than 15 mL/minute per 1.73 m². In patients undergoing hemodialysis, a 25- or 50-mg oral dose of atenolol may be administered after each dialysis; since marked reductions in blood pressure may occur, it is recommended that the supplemental dose be given under careful supervision.

Cautions

Atenolol shares the toxic potentials of β-adrenergic blocking agents (β-blockers). In therapeutic dosage, atenolol usually is well tolerated and has a low incidence of adverse effects. The incidence and severity of adverse reactions may occasionally be obviated by a reduction in dosage. Abrupt withdrawal of the drug should be avoided, especially in patients with coronary artery disease, since it may exacerbate angina or precipitate myocardial infarction (MI).

■ **Cardiovascular Effects** Potentially serious adverse cardiovascular effects of atenolol include bradycardia, which occurs in 3% of patients; profound hypotension; second- or third-degree atrioventricular (AV) block; and precipitation of severe heart failure, which is more likely to occur in patients with preexisting left ventricular dysfunction. Sick sinus syndrome has been reported during postmarketing experience in patients receiving atenolol-containing therapy. Atenolol-containing therapy is not recommended for use in patients with untreated pheochromocytoma. Bradycardia and hypotension usually can be reversed with an antimuscarinic agent like IV atropine. Isoproterenol or a transvenous cardiac pacemaker may be required for AV block. Other adverse cardiovascular effects include coldness of the extremities, reportedly occurring in 0–12% of patients; postural hypotension (which may be associated with syncope), in 2–4% of patients; and leg pain, in 0–3% of patients. When IV and oral atenolol were used in the early post-MI infarction period (for up to 10 days after onset of symptoms) in clinical trials, the principal adverse effects were bradycardia and hypotension, which occurred in up to 25% of patients receiving the drug (often combined with other therapy) and required reduction in dosage or discontinuance of atenolol in many patients. In addition, analysis of data from a subset of patients who died during early treatment in the First International Study of Infarct Survival (ISIS-1) revealed evidence of a small but not statistically significant increase in early death secondary to bradycardia and shock associated with atenolol therapy, but this potential adverse effect was outweighed substantially by beneficial effects of the drug on reduction of mortality from other causes. Atenolol may aggravate peripheral arterial circulatory disorders.

■ **CNS Effects** Adverse CNS effects of atenolol include dizziness, fatigue, and mental depression. Lethargy, drowsiness, unusual dreams, lightheadedness, and vertigo usually occur in less than 3% of patients. Headache and hallucinations also have been reported in patients receiving atenolol. Adverse CNS effects seen with other β-blockers that may occur with atenolol include visual disturbances, disorientation, short-term memory impairment, emotional lability, psychoses, catatonia, and impaired performance on neuropsychometric tests.

■ **GI Effects** Adverse GI reactions include diarrhea and nausea, which reportedly occur in 2–4% of patients receiving atenolol. A few cases of mesenteric arterial thrombosis and ischemic colitis have been reported in patients receiving other β-blockers. Dry mouth also has been reported in patients receiving atenolol.

■ **Endocrine Effects** Results of a large prospective cohort study of nondiabetic adults 45–64 years of age indicate that use of β-blockers in hypertensive patients is associated with increased risk (about 28%) of developing type 2 diabetes mellitus compared with hypertensive patients who were not receiving hypotensive therapy. In this study, the number of new cases of diabetes per 1000 person-years was 33.6 or 26.3 in patients receiving a β-blocker or no drug therapy, respectively. The association between the risk of developing diabetes mellitus and use of β-blockers reportedly was not confounded by weight gain, hyperinsulinemia, or differences in heart rate. It is not known if the risk of developing type 2 diabetes is affected by β-receptor selectivity. Further studies are needed to determine whether concomitant use of ACE inhibitors (which may improve insulin sensitivity) would abrogate β-blocker-induced adverse effects related to glucose intolerance. Therefore, until results of such studies are available, the proven benefits of β-blockers in reducing cardiovascular events in hypertensive patients must be weighed carefully against the possible risks of developing type 2 diabetes mellitus.

Hypoglycemia, which may result in loss of consciousness, also may occur in nondiabetic patients receiving β-blockers. Patients most at risk for the development of β-blocker-induced hypoglycemia are those undergoing dialysis, prolonged fasting, or severe exercise regimens.

β-Blockers may mask signs and symptoms of hypoglycemia (e.g., palpitation, tachycardia, tremor) and potentiate insulin-induced hypoglycemia. Although it has been suggested that nonselective β-blockers are more likely to induce hypoglycemia than selective β-blockers, such an adverse effect also has been reported with selective β-blocking agents (e.g., atenolol). In addition, selective β-blockers are less likely to mask symptoms of hypoglycemia or delay recovery from insulin-induced hypoglycemia than nonselective β-blockers because of their vascular sparing effects; however, selective β-blockers can decrease insulin sensitivity by approximately 15–30%, which may result in increased insulin requirements.

■ Other Adverse Effects Wheezing and dyspnea have occurred in patients receiving atenolol and are more likely to occur when dosage of the drug exceeds 100 mg daily. Rashes (which may be psoriasiform), exacerbation of psoriasis, lupus syndrome, drying of the eyes, visual disturbances, reversible alopecia, Peyronie's disease, antinuclear antibodies (ANA), impotence, elevated serum concentrations of hepatic enzymes and bilirubin, purpura, and thrombocytopenia also have been reported with atenolol.

The possibility that other adverse effects associated with other β-blockers may occur during atenolol therapy should be considered. These include hematologic reactions (e.g., agranulocytosis, nonthrombocytopenic or thrombocytopenic purpura); allergic reactions characterized by fever, sore throat, laryngospasm, and respiratory distress; Raynaud's phenomenon; conjunctivitis sicca; otitis; sclerosing serositis; and erythematous rash.

■ Precautions and Contraindications Atenolol shares the toxic potentials of β-blockers, and the usual precautions of these agents should be observed. When atenolol is used as a fixed-combination preparation that includes chlorthalidone, the cautions, precautions, and contraindications associated with thiazide diuretics must be considered in addition to those associated with atenolol.

In patients with heart failure, sympathetic stimulation is vital for the support of circulatory function. Atenolol should be used with caution in patients with inadequate cardiac function, since heart failure may be precipitated by blockade of β-adrenergic stimulation when atenolol therapy is administered. In addition, in patients with latent cardiac insufficiency, prolonged β-adrenergic blockade may lead to cardiac failure. Although β-blockers should be avoided in patients with overt heart failure, atenolol may be administered cautiously, if necessary, to patients with well-compensated heart failure (e.g., those controlled with cardiac glycosides and/or diuretics). Patients receiving atenolol therapy should be instructed to consult their physician at the first sign or symptom of impending cardiac failure and should be adequately treated (e.g., with a cardiac glycoside and/or diuretic) and observed closely; if cardiac failure continues, atenolol should be discontinued, gradually if possible. In patients with acute MI, use of atenolol is contraindicated in those whose congestive heart failure cannot be controlled promptly and effectively with a parenteral loop diuretic or comparable therapy. In addition, good clinical judgment suggests that patients whose cardiac output and/or blood pressure depends on sympathetic stimulation are not good candidates for β-adrenergic blocker therapy for acute MI, and such use is not recommended for patients whose systolic blood pressure or heart rate persistently is less than 100 mm Hg or 50–60 beats/minute, respectively.

Since β-blockers may inhibit bronchodilation produced by endogenous catecholamines, the drugs generally should not be used in patients with bronchospastic disease; however, because of its relative β_1-selective adrenergic blocking activity, atenolol may be used with caution in patients with bronchospastic disease who do not respond to or cannot tolerate other hypotensive agents. If atenolol is used in such patients, the initial dosage should be 50 mg daily and the smallest effective dosage should be used. In patients who develop symptoms of bronchospasm, atenolol dosage should be reduced or the drug discontinued (gradually if possible), and supportive treatment administered. In patients with bronchospastic disease, concomitant administration of a β_2-adrenergic agonist and/or twice-daily dosing of the drug may minimize the risk of bronchospasm.

Abrupt withdrawal of atenolol may exacerbate angina symptoms and/or precipitate MI and ventricular arrhythmias in patients with coronary artery disease, or may precipitate thyroid storm in patients with thyrotoxicosis. Therefore, patients receiving atenolol (especially those with ischemic heart disease) should be warned not to interrupt or discontinue therapy without consulting their physician. Because coronary artery disease is common and may be undiagnosed, abrupt withdrawal also should be avoided in patients receiving atenolol for other conditions (e.g., hypertension). When atenolol is discontinued in patients with coronary artery disease or suspected thyrotoxicosis, the patients should be observed carefully; patients with coronary artery disease should be advised to temporarily limit their physical activity. If exacerbation of angina occurs or acute coronary insufficiency develops after atenolol therapy is interrupted or discontinued, treatment with the drug should be reinstituted, at least temporarily.

Patients who have a history of anaphylactic reactions to a variety of allergens reportedly may be more reactive to repeated accidental, diagnostic, or therapeutic challenges with such allergens while taking β-blockers. These patients may be unresponsive to usual doses of epinephrine or may develop a paradoxical response to epinephrine when used to treat anaphylactic reactions.

Atenolol should be used with caution in patients undergoing major surgery involving general anesthesia. The necessity of withdrawing β-adrenergic blocking therapy prior to major surgery is controversial. Severe, protracted hypotension and difficulty in restarting or maintaining a heart beat have occurred during surgery in some patients who have received β-blockers. As with other β-blockers, the effects of atenolol can be reversed by administration of β-agonists (e.g., dobutamine, isoproterenol). If atenolol is discontinued, this should be done 2 days before surgery. If patients continue to receive atenolol prior to or during surgery in which anesthetics with negative inotropic activity are used, the patients should be observed for signs and symptoms of heart failure; if vagal stimulation occurs, atropine may be administered.

Atenolol should be used with caution in patients with hyperthyroidism since the drug may mask the tachycardia associated with hyperthyroidism. In addition, it is recommended that atenolol be used with caution in patients with diabetes mellitus since β-blockers may mask the tachycardia associated with hypoglycemia (a few cases have been reported in patients with type 2 diabetes mellitus), and β-blockers, especially nonselective ones, may potentially precipitate severe, acute hyperglycemia. (See Cautions: Endocrine Effects.) However, many clinicians state that patients with diabetes mellitus may be particularly likely to experience a reduction in morbidity and mortality with the use of these drugs. β-Blockers usually will not mask dizziness and sweating seen with hypoglycemia.

Atenolol should be used with caution and in reduced dosage in patients with impaired renal function, especially when creatinine clearance is less than 35 mL/minute per 1.73 m^2. The manufacturers recommend that patients receiving atenolol after hemodialysis be administered the drug under close supervision in a hospital setting, since marked hypotension may occur.

Atenolol is contraindicated in patients with sinus bradycardia, AV block greater than first degree, cardiogenic shock, known hypersensitivity to any component of the drug formulations, and overt or decompensated cardiac failure. Atenolol-containing therapy is not recommended for use in patients with untreated pheochromocytoma.

■ Pediatric Precautions Safety and efficacy of atenolol in pediatric patients have not been established; however, some experts have suggested dosages for hypertension based on clinical experience.

■ Geriatric Precautions Clinical studies of atenolol (used for angina pectoris associated with coronary atherosclerosis or hypertension) and of atenolol in fixed combination with chlorthalidone (used for hypertension) did not include sufficient numbers of patients 65 years of age and older to determine whether geriatric patients respond differently than younger adults. In addition, in a large clinical study (ISIS-1) evaluating atenolol in 8037 patients for the management of suspected acute MI, 2644 patients (about 33%) were 65 years of age or older, and there were no overall differences in safety or efficacy observed between geriatric individuals and younger adults; however, geriatric patients with systolic blood pressure below 120 mmHg seemed less likely to benefit from atenolol therapy. Although other clinical experience has not revealed age-related differences in response to the drug, care should be taken in dosage selection of atenolol. Because of greater frequency of decreased hepatic, renal, and/or cardiac function and of concomitant disease and drug therapy in geriatric patients, the manufacturers suggest that patients in this age group receive initial dosages of the drug in the low end of the usual range.

The manufacturers state that evaluation of geriatric patients with hypertension or MI always should include assessment of renal function.

■ Mutagenicity and Carcinogenicity No evidence of atenolol-induced mutagenicity was seen with an in vitro microbial test system (Ames test) with or without metabolic activation. Atenolol also was not mutagenic in in vivo cytogenicity tests in Chinese hamsters or the dominant lethal assay in mice.

No evidence of carcinogenicity was observed following administration of atenolol at dosages up to 300 mg/kg daily (up to 150 times the maximum recommended human antihypertensive dosage) for 18 months in mice or 18 or 24 months in rats. However, an increased incidence of benign adrenal medullary tumors in males and females, mammary fibroadenomas in females, and anterior pituitary adenomas and thyroid parafollicular cell carcinomas in males was observed at 24 months in rats receiving 500–1500 mg/kg of atenolol daily (250–750 times the maximum recommended human antihypertensive dosage).

■ Pregnancy, Fertility, and Lactation Atenolol has been shown to cause a dose-related increase in embryonal and fetal resorptions in rats when given at dosages 25 or more times the maximum human antihypertensive dosage; similar effects were not observed in rabbits receiving atenolol dosages up to 12.5 times the maximum human antihypertensive dosage. Atenolol crosses the placenta and has been detected in cord blood. Atenolol can cause fetal harm when administered to pregnant women. There are no studies on use of the drug during the first trimester of pregnancy and the possibility of fetal injury cannot be excluded. Atenolol therapy initiated in the second trimester of pregnancy has been associated with birth of infants who were small for gestational age. Atenolol has been used effectively under close supervision for the management of hypertension during the third trimester in a limited number of women and was well tolerated, and apparently did not adversely affect the fetus. However, use of the drug for longer periods of time for the management of mild to moderate hypertension in pregnant women has been associated with intrauterine growth retardation. Neonates born to mothers who receive atenolol at parturition may be at risk for developing hypoglycemia and bradycardia. Caution is recommended when atenolol is administered during pregnancy. If atenolol is administered during pregnancy or if the patient becomes pregnant while receiving the drug, the patient should be informed of the potential hazard to the fetus.

Reproduction studies in male and female rats using atenolol dosages up to 200 mg/kg daily (100 times the maximum recommended human antihypertensive dosage) have not revealed evidence of impaired fertility.

Atenolol is distributed into milk. The drug distributes into milk in concentrations 1.5–6.8 times those in maternal serum. In at least one infant, potentially toxic serum atenolol concentrations (2 mcg/mL) have been reported 48 hours after discontinuance of breast-feeding. Neonates of mothers who receive atenolol during breast-feeding may be at risk of developing hypoglycemia and adverse β-adrenergic effects (e.g., bradycardia). Therefore, the manufacturers state that atenolol should be used cautiously in nursing women. Because clearance of the drug may be substantially impaired, premature neonates, and infants with impaired renal function, may be at increased risk of developing adverse effects from ingested atenolol during breast-feeding. If a woman receiving atenolol breast-feeds, the infant should be monitored closely for potential systemic effects of the drug. Alternatively, β-blockers that distribute less extensively into milk (e.g., propranolol) can be considered, although caution still must be exercised.

Drug Interactions

■ **Cardiovascular Drugs** Concomitant administration of atenolol with reserpine may increase the incidence of hypotension and bradycardia as compared with atenolol alone, because of reserpine's catecholamine-depleting activity. Atenolol also is additive with and may potentiate the hypotensive actions of other hypotensive agents (e.g., calcium-channel blockers, hydralazine, methyldopa). This effect usually is used to therapeutic advantage, but dosage should be carefully adjusted when these drugs are used concurrently. Because β-blockers may exacerbate rebound hypertension that may occur following discontinuance of clonidine therapy, atenolol should be discontinued several days before clonidine when clonidine therapy is to be discontinued in patients receiving atenolol and clonidine concurrently.

Patients currently receiving another β-blocker must be evaluated carefully prior to initiating atenolol therapy. Depending on clinical findings (e.g., blood pressure, pulse), initial and subsequent atenolol dosage can be adjusted downward.

Slowing or complete suppression of SA node activity with development of slow ventricular rates (e.g., 30–40 bpm), often misdiagnosed as complete AV block, has been reported in patients receiving the nondihydropyridine calcium-channel blocking agent mibefradil (no longer commercially available in the US), principally in geriatric patients and in association with concomitant β-adrenergic blocker therapy.

Parenteral atenolol should be used with caution in patients who recently have received another drug that also may have a negative inotropic effect on the myocardium. Concomitant therapy with a β-blocker and verapamil can result in potentially serious adverse reactions, particularly in patients with severe cardiomyopathy, heart failure, or recent myocardial infarction (MI). (See Drug Interactions: β-Adrenergic Blocking Agents, in Verapamil Hydrochloride 24:28.92.)

■ **Nonsteroidal Anti-inflammatory Agents** Concurrent use of cyclooxygenase (prostaglandin synthase) inhibitors (e.g., indomethacin) may decrease the hypotensive effects of β-blockers. However, information on concomitant use of atenolol and aspirin is limited. Evidence from several studies (e.g., Thrombolysis in Myocardial Infarction Phase II [TIMI-II], Second International Study of Infarct Survival [ISIS-2]) suggests a lack of any clinically important adverse interaction and that the drugs can be used safely and effectively together in patients with MI.

Acute Toxicity

■ **Manifestations** Limited information is available on atenolol overdosage. In one woman who reportedly ingested 1.2 g of the drug, no unusual effects occurred and the patient's recovery was uncomplicated, and adults have survived acute doses up to 5 g; however, in a woman 15 years of age who reportedly ingested a single 500-mg dose of atenolol, severe sinus bradycardia, hypotension, and marked hypoglycemia occurred, and death occurred in a man who may have ingested up to 10 g acutely. In general, overdosage of atenolol may be expected to produce effects that are mainly extensions of pharmacologic effects, including symptomatic bradycardia, hypotension, bronchospasm, and acute cardiac failure; hypoglycemia, impaired conduction, decreased cardiac contractility, heart block, shock, and cardiac arrest may also occur.

■ **Treatment** In acute atenolol overdose, the stomach should be emptied immediately by gastric lavage. Supportive and symptomatic treatment should be initiated. For symptomatic bradycardia, IV atropine sulfate may be given and for second- or third-degree AV block, IV isoproterenol hydrochloride or a transvenous cardiac pacemaker may be used. A vasopressor (e.g., dobutamine, dopamine, epinephrine, norepinephrine) may be given for severe hypotension; IV glucagon may be useful if hypotension is refractory to vasopressors. For heart failure, a cardiac glycoside, diuretic, and oxygen should be used; IV glucagon also may be useful. Hypoglycemia should be treated with IV dextrose. Hemodialysis may be useful in enhancing elimination of atenolol in patients with severe overdosage.

Pharmacology

Atenolol has pharmacologic actions similar to those of other β-blockers. The principal physiologic action of atenolol is to competitively block adrenergic stimulation of β-adrenergic receptors within the myocardium and within vascular smooth muscle. Like metoprolol, low doses of atenolol selectively inhibit cardiac and lipolytic β_1-adrenergic receptors while having little effect on the β_2-adrenergic receptors of bronchial and vascular smooth muscle. At high doses (e.g., greater than 100 mg daily), this selectivity of atenolol for β_1-adrenergic receptors usually diminishes, and the drug will competitively block β_1- and β_2-adrenergic receptors. Atenolol does not exhibit the intrinsic sympathomimetic activity seen with pindolol or the membrane-stabilizing activity possessed by propranolol or pindolol.

By inhibiting myocardial β_1-adrenergic receptors, atenolol produces negative chronotropic and inotropic activity. The negative chronotropic action of atenolol on the sinoatrial (SA) node results in a decrease in the rate of SA node discharge and an increase in recovery time, thereby decreasing resting and exercise-stimulated heart rate and reflex orthostatic tachycardia by about 25–35%. High doses of the drug may produce sinus arrest, especially in patients with SA node disease (e.g., sick sinus syndrome). Atenolol also slows conduction in the atrioventricular (AV) node. Although stroke index may be increased moderately by about 10%, atenolol usually reduces cardiac output by about 20%, probably secondary to its effect on heart rate. The decrease in myocardial contractility and heart rate, as well as the reduction in blood pressure, produced by atenolol generally lead to a reduction in myocardial oxygen consumption which accounts for the effectiveness of the drug in chronic stable angina pectoris; however, atenolol can increase oxygen requirements by increasing left ventricular fiber length and end-diastolic pressure, particularly in patients with cardiac failure.

Atenolol suppresses plasma renin activity and suppresses the renin-aldosterone-angiotensin system. The renin-lowering effect of β-blockers may lead to a minimal reduction in glomerular filtration rate and occasionally may reduce renal blood flow; however, other mechanisms (e.g., decreased cardiac output, unopposed α-mediated renal vasoconstriction) also probably contribute to these effects. Because of the suppression of aldosterone production, β-blockers usually produce no measurable increases in plasma volume or sodium and water retention.

The precise mechanism of atenolol's hypotensive effect has not been determined. Single doses of atenolol may increase peripheral vascular resistance at rest and with exercise. It has been postulated that β-blockers reduce blood pressure by blocking peripheral (especially cardiac) adrenergic receptors (decreasing cardiac output), by decreasing sympathetic outflow from the CNS, and/or by suppressing renal renin release.

Because of its β_1-receptor selectivity, low doses (100 mg or less) of atenolol usually have little effect on bronchial airway resistance. Higher doses of atenolol may result in an increase in airway resistance (as measured by decreasing forced expiratory volume in 1 second), especially in patients with asthma and/or chronic obstructive pulmonary disease (COPD).

Low doses of atenolol produce no changes in serum insulin concentrations or in time to recover from insulin-induced hypoglycemia, and little change in free fatty acid response to hypoglycemia. The drug reduces serum free fatty acid concentrations and slightly increases serum triglyceride concentrations.

Pharmacokinetics

■ **Absorption** Atenolol is rapidly but incompletely absorbed from the GI tract. Only about 50–60% of an oral dose of atenolol is absorbed. In healthy adults, peak plasma concentrations of 1–2 mcg/mL are achieved 2–4 hours after oral administration of a single 200-mg dose of atenolol. An approximately fourfold interindividual variation in plasma concentrations attained has been reported with a specific oral dose of atenolol. In geriatric patients, plasma concentrations are increased. Peak plasma atenolol concentrations are achieved within 5 minutes following direct IV injection of the drug, and decline rapidly during an initial distribution phase; after the first 7 hours, plasma concentrations reportedly decline with an elimination half-life similar to that of orally administered drug.

The effect of atenolol on heart rate usually has an onset of 1 hour, peaks at 2–4 hours, and persists for 24 hours following oral administration of the drug. Following IV administration of a single 10-mg dose, the effect on heart rate usually peaks within 5 minutes and generally is negligible by 12 hours after the dose. The antihypertensive and β-adrenergic blocking effect of a single 50- to 100-mg oral dose usually persists for 24 hours. Atenolol's effect on heart rate, but not on blood pressure, correlates linearly with plasma atenolol concentrations of 0.02–200 mcg/mL.

■ **Distribution** In animals, atenolol is well distributed into most tissues and fluids except brain and CSF. Unlike propranolol, only a small portion of atenolol is apparently distributed into the CNS.

Approximately 6–16% of atenolol is bound to plasma protein.

Atenolol readily crosses the placenta and has been detected in cord blood. During continuous administration, fetal serum concentrations of the drug are probably equivalent to those in maternal serum. Atenolol is distributed into milk; peak milk concentrations of the drug are higher than peak serum concentrations after an individual dose, and the area under the milk concentration-time curve (AUC) is substantially greater than that of the serum AUC in lactating women receiving the drug continuously. (See Cautions: Pregnancy, Fertility, and Lactation.)

■ **Elimination** In patients with normal renal function, atenolol has a plasma half-life ($t_{1/2}$) of 6–7 hours. Children with normal renal function may exhibit a shorter elimination half-life. In one study in children 5–16 (mean:

8.9) years of age with arrhythmias and normal renal and hepatic function, the terminal elimination half-life averaged 4.6 hours. The plasma half-life($t_{1/2}$) of atenolol is markedly prolonged in geriatric patients compared with that in younger patients. Plasma $t_{1/2}$ of the drug increases to 16–27 hours in patients with creatinine clearances of 15–35 mL/minute per 1.73 m^2 and exceeds 27 hours with progressive renal impairment. Little or no metabolism of atenolol occurs in the liver. Approximately 40–50% of an oral dose of the drug is excreted in urine unchanged. The remainder is excreted unchanged in feces, principally as unabsorbed drug. About 1–12% of atenolol is reportedly removed by hemodialysis.

In geriatric patients, total plasma clearance of atenolol is reduced by about 50% compared with that in younger patients, resulting in higher plasma concentrations of the drug. The decreased clearance in geriatric adults may be related to decreased renal function in this age group.

Chemistry and Stability

■ Chemistry Atenolol is a β_1-selective adrenergic blocking agent. The drug occurs as a white, crystalline powder and has a solubility of 26.5 mg/mL in water at 37°C.

■ Stability Atenolol tablets alone or in fixed combination with chlorthalidone should be protected from heat, light, and moisture and stored in well-closed, light-resistant containers at 20–25°C.

Preparations

Excipients in commercially available drug preparations may have clinically important effects in some individuals; consult specific product labeling for details.

Atenolol

Oral		
Tablets	25 mg*	**Atenolol Tablets**
		Tenormin®, AstraZeneca
	50 mg*	**Atenolol Tablets**
		Tenormin® (scored), AstraZeneca
	100 mg*	**Atenolol Tablets**
		Tenormin®, AstraZeneca

*available from one or more manufacturer, distributor, and/or repackager by generic (nonproprietary) name

Atenolol Combinations

Oral		
Tablets	50 mg with Chlorthalidone 25 mg*	**Atenolol and Chlorthalidone Tablets**
		Tenoretic® (scored), AstraZeneca
	100 mg with Chlorthalidone 25 mg*	**Atenolol and Chlorthalidone Tablets**
		Tenoretic® (scored), AstraZeneca

*available from one or more manufacturer, distributor, and/or repackager by generic (nonproprietary) name

†Use is not currently included in the labeling approved by the US Food and Drug Administration

Selected Revisions October 2018,

Carvedilol

■ Carvedilol is a nonselective β-adrenergic blocking agent (β-blocker) with selective α_1-adrenergic blocking activity.

Uses

Carvedilol is used for the management of hypertension and heart failure. Carvedilol also is used to reduce the risk of cardiovascular mortality in clinically stable patients with left ventricular dysfunction (manifested as a left ventricular ejection fraction [LVEF] of 40% or less) with or without symptomatic heart failure following an acute myocardial infarction (MI).

The choice of a β-adrenergic blocking agent (β-blocker) depends on numerous factors, including intended use, pharmacologic properties (e.g., relative β-selectivity, intrinsic sympathomimetic activity, membrane-stabilizing activity, lipophilicity), pharmacokinetics, and adverse effect profile, as well as the patient's coexisting disease states or conditions, response, and tolerance. While specific pharmacologic properties and other factors may appropriately influence the choice of a β-blocker in individual patients, evidence of clinically important differences among the agents in terms of overall efficacy and/or safety is limited. Patients who do not respond to or cannot tolerate a given β-blocker may be successfully treated with a different one.

■ Hypertension Carvedilol is used alone or in combination with other classes of antihypertensive agents in the management of hypertension.

Current evidence-based practice guidelines for the management of hypertension in adults generally recommend the use of drugs from 4 classes of antihypertensive agents (angiotensin-converting enzyme [ACE] inhibitors, angiotensin II receptor antagonists, calcium-channel blockers, and thiazide diuretics). Most guidelines no longer recommend β-blockers as first-line therapy for hypertension because of the lack of established superiority over other recommended drug classes and evidence from at least one study demonstrating that β-blockers may be less effective than angiotensin II receptor antagonists in preventing cardiovascular death, MI, or stroke. However, therapy with a β-blocker may still be considered in hypertensive patients who have a compelling indication (e.g., prior MI, ischemic heart disease, heart failure) for their use or as add-on therapy in those who do not respond adequately to the preferred drug classes. (See Considerations for Drug Therapy in Patients with Underlying Cardiovascular and Other Risk Factors under Uses: Hypertension, in Atenolol 24:24 and in Metoprolol 24:24.) Ultimately, choice of antihypertensive therapy should be individualized, considering the clinical characteristics of the patient (e.g., age, ethnicity/race, comorbid conditions, cardiovascular risk factors) as well as drug-related factors (e.g., ease of administration, availability, adverse effects, costs).

A 2017 multidisciplinary hypertension guideline of the American College of Cardiology (ACC), American Heart Association (AHA), and a number of other professional organizations generally recommends a target blood pressure goal (i.e., blood pressure to achieve with drug therapy and/or nonpharmacologic intervention) of less than 130/80 mm Hg in all adults regardless of comorbidities or level of atherosclerotic cardiovascular disease (ASCVD) risk. In addition, a systolic blood pressure goal of less than 130 mm Hg generally is recommended for noninstitutionalized ambulatory patients 65 years of age or older with an average systolic blood pressure of at least 130 mm Hg. These blood pressure goals are based upon clinical studies demonstrating continuing reduction of cardiovascular risk at progressively lower levels of systolic blood pressure. Previous hypertension guidelines, such as those from an expert panel of the Eighth Joint National Committee on the Prevention, Detection, Evaluation, and Treatment of High Blood Pressure (JNC 8), generally have recommended initiation of antihypertensive treatment in patients with a systolic blood pressure of at least 140 mm Hg or diastolic blood pressure of at least 90 mm Hg, targeted a blood pressure goal of less than 140/90 mm Hg regardless of cardiovascular risk, and used higher systolic blood pressure thresholds and targets in geriatric patients compared with those recommended by the 2017 ACC/AHA hypertension guideline. The blood pressure thresholds used to define hypertension, the optimum blood pressure threshold at which to initiate antihypertensive drug therapy, and the ideal target blood pressure values remain controversial.

Most patients with hypertension, especially black patients, will require at least 2 antihypertensive drugs to achieve adequate blood pressure control. In general, black hypertensive patients tend to respond better to monotherapy with thiazide diuretics or calcium-channel blocking agents than to monotherapy with β-blockers. Although β-blockers have lowered blood pressure in all races studied, monotherapy with these agents has produced a smaller reduction in blood pressure in black hypertensive patients; however, this population difference in response does not appear to occur during combined therapy with a β-blocker and a thiazide diuretic. (See Race under Hypertension: Other Special Considerations for Antihypertensive Therapy, in Uses in Atenolol 24:24 and in Metoprolol 24:24.)

For additional information on the role of β-blockers in the management of hypertension, see Uses: Hypertension, in Atenolol 24:24 and in Metoprolol 24:24. For information on overall principles and expert recommendations for treatment of hypertension, see Uses: Hypertension in Adults, in the Thiazides General Statement 40:28.20. For information on overall principles and expert recommendations for treatment of hypertension in pediatric patients, see Uses: Hypertension in Pediatric Patients, in the Thiazides General Statement 40:28.20.

■ Heart Failure Carvedilol is used (usually in conjunction with other heart failure therapies) in the management of mild to severe (New York Heart Association [NYHA] class II–IV) heart failure of ischemic or cardiomyopathic origin to increase survival and to reduce the risk of hospitalization. Current guidelines for the management of heart failure in adults generally recommend a combination of drug therapies to reduce morbidity and mortality, including neurohormonal antagonists (e.g., ACE inhibitors, angiotensin II receptor antagonists, angiotensin receptor-neprilysin inhibitors [ARNIs], β-blockers, aldosterone receptor antagonists), that inhibit the detrimental compensatory mechanisms in heart failure. Additional agents (e.g., cardiac glycosides, diuretics, sinoatrial modulators [i.e., ivabradine]) added to a heart failure treatment regimen in selected patients have been associated with symptomatic improvement of heart failure and/or reduction in heart failure-related hospitalizations. Experts recommend that all asymptomatic patients with reduced LVEF (American College of Cardiology Foundation [ACCF]/American Heart Association [AHA] stage B heart failure) receive therapy with an ACE inhibitor and a β-blocker to prevent symptomatic heart failure and reduce morbidity and mortality. In patients with prior or current symptoms of chronic heart failure and reduced LVEF (ACCF/AHA stage C heart failure), ACCF, AHA, and the Heart Failure Society of America (HFSA) recommend inhibition of the renin-angiotensin-aldosterone (RAA) system with an ACE inhibitor, angiotensin II receptor antagonist, or ARNI in conjunction with a β-blocker, and an aldosterone antagonist in selected patients, to reduce morbidity and mortality. While ACE inhibitors have been the preferred drugs for inhibition of the RAA system because of their established benefits in patients with heart failure and reduced ejection fraction, some evidence indicates that therapy with an ARNI (sacubitril/valsartan) may be more effective than ACE inhibitor therapy (enalapril) in reducing cardiovascular death and heart failure-related hospitalization in such patients. ACCF, AHA, and HFSA recommend that patients with chronic symptomatic heart failure and reduced LVEF (NYHA class II or III) who are able to tolerate an ACE inhibitor or angiotensin II receptor antagonist be switched to therapy containing an ARNI to further reduce morbidity and mortality.

Because of favorable effects on survival and disease progression, therapy with a clinical trial-proven β-blocker (bisoprolol, carvedilol, extended-release metoprolol succinate) should be initiated as soon as the patient is diagnosed with heart failure and reduced LVEF. While bisoprolol, carvedilol, and extended-release metoprolol have been effective in reducing the risk of death in patients with chronic heart failure, these positive findings should not be considered indicative of a β-blocker class effect. Even when symptoms are mild or improve with other therapies, β-blocker therapy should not be delayed until symptoms return or the disease progresses. Despite concerns about β-blockade potentially masking some signs of hypoglycemia, patients with diabetes mellitus may be particularly likely to experience a reduction in morbidity and mortality with the use of β-blockers. If a patient cannot tolerate a β-blocker or if increasing the β-blocker dosage to optimal levels is ineffective, ivabradine should be considered an alternative or additional treatment option. Some evidence suggests that ivabradine is effective in reducing hospitalizations related to heart failure, but unlike β-blockers, ivabradine has not been shown to reduce cardiovascular mortality. (See Uses: Heart Failure, in Ivabradine 24:04.92.)

In individualizing the decision to use a β-blocker, clinicians should consider that clinical studies establishing the effects of these drugs on morbidity and mortality excluded patients who were hospitalized or had unstable symptoms and enrolled few patients with current or recent NYHA class IV symptoms. The efficacy of β-blockers in such patients is not known, and they may be at particular risk of deterioration following initiation of therapy with β-blockers. In the Carvedilol Prospective Randomized Cumulative Survival Trial (COPERNICUS) evaluating such patients with severe but stable heart failure (patients with marked fluid retention or severe pulmonary disease or requiring intensive care, IV vasodilators, or positive inotropic agents were excluded), carvedilol decreased the rate of death and the combined risk of death and hospitalization for any reason compared with placebo.

The beneficial effects of β-blockers in the management of heart failure are thought to result principally from inhibition of the effects of the sympathetic nervous system. (See Description.) Although the specific effects on the heart and circulation that are responsible for progression of heart failure remain to be established, sympathetic activity can increase ventricular volumes and pressure secondary to peripheral vasoconstriction and by impairing sodium excretion by the kidneys. Other sympathetic effects (e.g., induction of cardiac hypertrophy, arrhythmogenic activity) also may be involved. The beneficial effect of carvedilol in patients with severe heart failure may be the result of other effects (α-adrenergic blockade, antioxidant activity, antiendothelin effects) in addition to β-adrenergic blockade. Collective experience indicates that long-term therapy with β-blockers, like that with ACE inhibitors, can reduce heart failure symptoms and improve clinical status in patients with chronic heart failure and also can decrease the risk of death as well as the combined risk of death and hospitalization. These beneficial effects were demonstrated in patients already receiving an ACE inhibitor, suggesting that combined inhibition of the renin-angiotensin system and sympathetic nervous system can produce additive effects.

β-Blockers should not be used in patients with acutely decompensated heart failure requiring IV inotropic therapy and those with substantial fluid retention requiring intensive diuresis. In the absence of hemodynamic instability or contraindications, it has been recommended that patients with heart failure and a reduced ejection fraction who are hospitalized for a symptomatic exacerbation continue to receive maintenance treatment with standard oral therapy for heart failure (e.g., β-blocker, ACE inhibitor). Withholding of or reduction in β-blocker therapy should be considered only in patients hospitalized after recent initiation or increase in β-blocker therapy or in those with marked volume overload or low/marginal cardiac output. Initiation of β-blocker therapy in hospitalized patients is recommended once the patient's condition is stabilized (i.e., after optimization of volume status and successful discontinuance of IV diuretics, vasodilators, and inotropic agents). Caution should be used when initiating β-blockers in patients who have required inotrope therapy during hospitalization.

Carvedilol has been shown in controlled studies to improve left ventricular function, symptoms, and submaximal exercise tolerance (although not in all studies) in patients with wide-ranging severity of manifestations. Change in NYHA classification was a secondary endpoint in all of the studies, and a trend toward improvement in NYHA class was reported in all studies. Subjective quality-of-life determined by a standard questionnaire was not improved in patients receiving carvedilol compared with those receiving placebo; however, global assessments by patients and clinicians supported an improvement in such assessments in patients receiving carvedilol.

■ **Left Ventricular Dysfunction After Acute Myocardial Infarction** Carvedilol is used to reduce the risk of cardiovascular mortality following the acute phase of MI in clinically stable patients with left ventricular dysfunction (manifested as an ejection fraction of 40% or less) with or without symptomatic heart failure. In these patients, when compared with those receiving placebo, carvedilol therapy initiated within 21 days after an acute MI reduced mortality from any cause by about 23%; all-cause mortality or cardiovascular hospitalization was reduced by 8%, which was not statistically significant. In addition, a 40% reduction in fatal and nonfatal MI was observed in patients receiving carvedilol. This evidence of efficacy was obtained from a large, double-blind, placebo-controlled, multicenter long-term (about 16 months) study (Carvedilol Post-Infarct Survival Control in Left Ventricular Dysfunction Study; CAPRICORN). For information on the use of β-blockers during the acute phase of MI, see Uses in Metoprolol 24:24.

The benefits of long-term β-blocker therapy for secondary prevention of MI have been well established in numerous clinical studies. Patients with MI complicated by heart failure, left ventricular dysfunction, or ventricular arrhythmias appear to derive the most benefit from long-term β-blocker therapy. AHA/ACCF secondary prevention guideline recommends β-blocker therapy in all patients with left ventricular systolic dysfunction (ejection fraction of 40% or less) and a prior MI; use of a β-blocker with proven mortality benefit (bisoprolol, carvedilol, or metoprolol succinate) is recommended. (See Uses: Heart Failure.)

For additional information on the use of β-blockers in the management of MI, see Uses in Metoprolol 24:24.

Dosage and Administration

■ **Administration** Carvedilol and carvedilol phosphate are administered orally. Food has little, if any, effect on the oral bioavailability of carvedilol immediate-release tablets but may decrease the rate of absorption, resulting in reduced and delayed peak plasma concentrations. Therefore, to potentially decrease the risk of orthostatic hypotension, it is recommended that carvedilol be administered with food. In addition, the manufacturer suggests that manifestations of vasodilation in patients receiving concomitant therapy with an angiotensin-converting enzyme (ACE) inhibitor may be reduced by administering carvedilol 2 hours prior to the latter drug.

Food increases the bioavailability of carvedilol phosphate extended-release capsules and the manufacturer states that the extended-release capsules should be taken with food. Carvedilol extended-release capsules should be taken once daily in the morning and should be swallowed whole; the capsule and/or its contents should not be crushed, chewed, or taken in divided doses. However, carvedilol extended-release capsules may be opened carefully and the entire contents sprinkled over a spoonful of applesauce, immediately prior to administration. The applesauce should not be warm, and the drug and applesauce mixture should be consumed in entirety. The drug and applesauce mixture should not be stored for future use. The absorption of the beads sprinkled on foods other than applesauce has not been studied.

■ **Dosage** Patients whose conditions are controlled with immediate-release carvedilol tablets alone or in combination with other drugs may be switched to carvedilol phosphate extended-release capsules. Patients who are receiving a daily carvedilol dosage of 6.25 (3.125 mg twice daily), 12.5 (6.25 mg twice daily), 25 (12.5 mg twice daily), or 50 mg (25 mg twice daily) as immediate-release tablets may be switched to a dosage of 10, 20, 40, or 80 mg once daily, respectively, as carvedilol phosphate extended-release capsules. Subsequent titration to higher or lower dosages may be necessary and should be guided by the patient's clinical response.

Hypertension Dosage of carvedilol must be individualized and adjusted according to the patient's blood pressure response and tolerance.

In hypertensive patients with left ventricular dysfunction, including those with heart failure who already are receiving a cardiac glycoside, diuretic, and/or an ACE inhibitor, the manufacturer states that the usual carvedilol dosages and instructions recommended for the treatment of heart failure should be followed instead of those for hypertension, since such patients generally depend, at least in part, on β-adrenergic stimulation for maintaining cardiovascular compensation. (See Heart Failure under Dosage and Administration: Dosage.)

Usual Dosage. For the management of hypertension in adults, the usual initial dosage of carvedilol (as immediate-release tablets) is 6.25 mg twice daily. The manufacturer recommends that patient response and tolerance to the initial dosage and subsequent dosage adjustments be evaluated by measurement of standing systolic blood pressure 1 hour after administration of carvedilol (trough blood pressure). In patients whose blood pressure is not controlled adequately with the initial carvedilol dosage, dosage can be increased gradually (usually increasing dosage every 7–14 days), as tolerated up to a maximum of 50 mg daily. For patients who received an initial dosage of 6.25 mg twice daily, the dosage may be increased to 12.5 mg twice daily and, if needed, to 25 mg twice daily. Some experts state the usual dosage range is 12.5–50 mg daily, administered in 2 divided doses.

For the management of hypertension in adults, the usual initial dosage of carvedilol phosphate extended-release capsules is 20 mg once daily. The manufacturer recommends that patient tolerance to the initial dosage and subsequent dosage adjustments be evaluated by measurement of standing systolic blood pressure 1 hour after administration of carvedilol phosphate extended-release capsules. In patients whose blood pressure is not controlled adequately with the initial carvedilol phosphate dosage (given as extended-release capsules), dosage can be increased gradually (usually increasing dosage every 7–14 days) up to a maximum of 80 mg once daily (given as carvedilol phosphate extended-release capsules). Some experts state the usual dosage range is 20–80 mg once daily administered as extended-release capsules.

Addition of a diuretic to carvedilol therapy or of carvedilol to diuretic therapy can be expected to produce additive effects. When carvedilol and a thiazide diuretic are used concomitantly, an additive hypotensive response, including an increased risk of orthostatic hypotension, can be expected.

Blood Pressure Monitoring and Treatment Goals. Blood pressure should be monitored regularly (i.e., monthly) during therapy and dosage of the antihypertensive drug adjusted until blood pressure is controlled. If an adequate blood pressure response is not achieved, the dosage may be increased or another antihypertensive agent with demonstrated benefit and preferably with a complementary mechanism of action (e.g., ACE inhibitor, angiotensin II receptor antagonist, calcium-channel blocker, thiazide diuretic) may be added; if target blood pressure is still not achieved with the use of 2 antihypertensive agents, a third drug may be added. (See Uses: Hypertension.) In patients who develop unacceptable adverse effects with carvedilol, the drug should be discontinued and another antihypertensive agent from a different pharmacologic class should be initiated.

The goal of hypertension management and prevention is to achieve and maintain optimal control of blood pressure. However, the optimum blood pressure threshold for initiating antihypertensive drug therapy and specific treatment goals remain controversial. While previous hypertension guidelines have based target blood pressure goals on age and comorbidities, the 2017 American College of Cardiology/American Heart Association (ACC/AHA) hypertension guideline incorporates underlying cardiovascular risk into decision making regarding treatment and generally recommends the same target blood pressure (i.e., less than 130/80 mm Hg) for all adults. Many patients will require at least 2 drugs from different pharmacologic classes to achieve this blood pressure goal; the potential benefits of hypertension management and drug cost, adverse effects, and risks associated with the use of multiple antihypertensive drugs also should be considered when deciding a patient's blood pressure treatment goal.

For additional information on target levels of blood pressure and on monitoring therapy in the management of hypertension, see Blood Pressure Monitoring and Treatment Goals under Dosage: Hypertension, in Dosage and Administration in the Thiazides General Statement 40:28.20.

Heart Failure Prior to initiation of carvedilol therapy for heart failure, fluid retention should be minimized, and patients who are receiving treatment that includes a cardiac glycoside, diuretic, and/or ACE inhibitor should be stabilized with respect to the dosage of these drugs. Initiation of carvedilol therapy for heart failure and subsequent dosage adjustments should occur under very close medical supervision, since the risk of cardiac decompensation and/or severe hypotension is highest during the initial 30 days of therapy.

For the management of mild to severe (NYHA class II–IV) heart failure, carvedilol often is administered in conjunction with other agents such as a cardiac glycoside, ACE inhibitor, and/or diuretic. Treatment with carvedilol should be initiated at a very low dosage. The usual initial carvedilol dosage as immediate-release tablets for the management of heart failure in adults is 3.125 mg twice daily for 2 weeks. The usual initial dosage of carvedilol phosphate extended-release capsules for the management of heart failure in adults is 10 mg once daily for 2 weeks. Prior to dosage increases, the patient's response and tolerance to carvedilol therapy should be determined in a clinical setting and should include an assessment of manifestations of declining cardiovascular status, vasodilation (e.g., dizziness, lightheadedness, symptomatic hypotension), and bradycardia.

If the patient experiences increases in manifestations of heart failure such as edema during the initiation and titration phases of carvedilol therapy, further increases in carvedilol dosage should be delayed until the patient regains clinical stability; such manifestations may require an increase in diuretic dosage. If increased manifestations of heart failure do not resolve in response to an increase in diuretic dosage, consideration should be given to decreasing the carvedilol dosage or temporarily discontinuing the drug. The occurrence of increased manifestations of heart failure during initiation of carvedilol therapy or dosage titration that require dosage decreases or discontinuance of the drug should not prevent future consideration of resuming therapy with or increasing dosage of carvedilol. If the patient develops manifestations of vasodilation, consideration should be given to decreasing the patient's dosage of diuretic or ACE inhibitor; however, if these dosage reductions do not result in improved circulatory status, carvedilol dosage may be decreased. Separating the time of dosing of carvedilol from that of the ACE inhibitor also may reduce vasodilatory symptoms. If the patient becomes bradycardic (heart rate less than 55 beats/minute), carvedilol dosage should be reduced. If the patient develops manifestations of worsening heart failure or vasodilation, carvedilol dosage should not be increased until the patient's cardiovascular status is stable.

If the patient tolerates the initial dosage, carvedilol dosage may be increased to 6.25 mg twice daily as the immediate-release tablets or to 20 mg once daily as carvedilol phosphate extended-release capsules for 2 weeks. When increases in dosage are considered, the patient should be observed in a clinical setting for manifestations of hypotension (e.g., dizziness, light-headedness) for 1 hour after administration of the initial dose at the increased dosage. Dosage of carvedilol as the immediate-release tablets and carvedilol phosphate as extended-release capsules can be doubled every 2 weeks if necessary (with strict adherence to the monitoring regimen described above) to the highest tolerated dosage that does not exceed the maximum recommended dosage of 50 mg daily (in patients weighing less than 85 kg) and 100 mg daily (in those weighing more than 85 kg) as carvedilol immediate-release tablets and of 80 mg once daily as carvedilol phosphate extended-release capsules.

Left Ventricular Dysfunction After Acute Myocardial Infarction Prior to initiation of carvedilol therapy for left ventricular dysfunction following acute myocardial infarction (MI), fluid retention should be minimized, and patients should be hemodynamically stable. Initiation of carvedilol therapy and subsequent dosage adjustments should occur under very close medical supervision, since the risk of cardiac decompensation and/or severe hypotension is highest during the initial 30 days of therapy. Therapy may be initiated on an inpatient or outpatient basis after the patient is hemodynamically stable and fluid retention is minimized.

To decrease the likelihood of syncope or excessive hypotension, treatment with carvedilol should be initiated at a low dosage of 6.25 mg twice daily as the immediate-release tablets or 20 mg of carvedilol phosphate once daily as the extended-release capsules. If the patient tolerates the initial dosage, carvedilol dosage may be increased after 3–10 days to 12.5 mg twice daily as the immediate-release tablets or 40 mg once daily as carvedilol phosphate extended-release capsules, and then to the target dosage of 25 mg twice daily as the immediate-release tablets or 80 mg of carvedilol phosphate once daily as the extended-release capsules. A lower initial dosage of 3.125 mg twice daily as the immediate-release tablets or 10 mg of carvedilol phosphate once daily as the extended-release capsules and/or a slower rate of dosage titration may be used when clinically indicated (e.g., low blood pressure or heart rate, fluid retention). Alteration of the recommended dosage regimen is not necessary in patients who received IV or oral treatment with a β-blocker during the acute phase of MI.

Although the optimal duration of β-blocker therapy following MI remains to be clearly established, experts generally recommend that such therapy be continued long-term in post-MI patients with left ventricular systolic dysfunction.

■ Special Populations

Use of carvedilol is not recommended in patients with clinical manifestations of hepatic impairment or with otherwise severe impairment. (See Contraindications.)

Although the manufacturer makes no specific recommendations for dosage adjustments in patients with renal impairment, plasma concentrations of carvedilol based on comparison of mean plasma concentration-time curves (AUC) reportedly are 40–50% higher in patients with hypertension and moderate to severe renal impairment compared with patients with hypertension and normal renal function receiving carvedilol therapy as the immediate-release tablets. Although the ranges of AUC values were similar for both groups, mean peak plasma concentrations were approximately 12–26% higher in patients with impaired renal function compared with those in patients with no such impairment. Carvedilol does not appear to be removed by hemodialysis.

If a deterioration in renal function is detected in patients with heart failure, dosage of carvedilol should be decreased or the drug should be discontinued.

Some clinicians suggest using a reduced initial carvedilol dosage in geriatric patients, since such patients are at increased risk of developing orthostatic hypotension and experience is limited regarding the use of the drug in patients 75 years of age or older.

Cautions

■ Contraindications

Bronchial asthma or related bronchospastic conditions.

Second or third degree AV block.

Sick sinus syndrome or severe bradycardia (unless permanent pacemaker is in place).

Cardiogenic shock or decompensated heart failure requiring IV inotropic therapy; initiate carvedilol only after the patient is weaned from IV therapy.

Clinically apparent or otherwise severe hepatic impairment.

History of serious hypersensitivity reaction (e.g., Stevens-Johnson syndrome, anaphylactic reaction, angioedema) to carvedilol or any ingredient in the formulation.

■ Warnings/Precautions

Warnings **Abrupt Withdrawal of Therapy.** Abrupt withdrawal of carvedilol may exacerbate angina symptoms and/or precipitate myocardial infarction (MI) and ventricular arrhythmias in patients with coronary artery disease or may precipitate thyroid storm in patients with thyrotoxicosis. Therefore, patients receiving carvedilol (especially those with ischemic heart disease) should be warned not to interrupt or discontinue therapy without consulting their clinician. Because coronary artery disease is common and may be undiagnosed, abrupt withdrawal also should be avoided in patients receiving carvedilol for other conditions (e.g., hypertension). When carvedilol is discontinued in patients with coronary artery disease or suspected thyrotoxicosis, the patient should be observed carefully; patients with coronary artery disease should be advised to temporarily limit their physical activity. If exacerbation of angina occurs or acute coronary insufficiency develops after carvedilol therapy is interrupted or discontinued, treatment with the drug should be reinstituted, at least temporarily.

If carvedilol therapy, alone or combined with another antihypertensive agent (e.g., a thiazide diuretic), is to be discontinued, dosage should be reduced gradually in a deliberate and progressive manner, if possible. When such cessation of therapy is planned, the manufacturer recommends that therapy with the drug be withdrawn gradually over approximately 1–2 weeks. Patients should be monitored closely during this period and, if manifestations of withdrawal (e.g., angina, exacerbation of hypertension) develop, dosage should be increased or the drug reinstituted, at least temporarily.

Peripheral Vascular Disease. Possible precipitation or aggravation of arterial insufficiency in patients with peripheral vascular disease. Use with caution.

Anesthesia and Major Surgery. If carvedilol therapy is continued perioperatively, use particular caution when anesthetic agents that depress myocardial function (e.g., ether, cyclopropane, trichloroethylene) are used. (See Drug Interactions.)

Diabetes and Hypoglycemia. β-Adrenergic blocking agents (β-blockers) may mask some of the manifestations of hypoglycemia (e.g., tachycardia). Non-selective β-blockers (e.g., carvedilol) are more likely to potentiate insulin-induced hypoglycemia and delay recovery of serum glucose concentrations.

In patients with heart failure and diabetes mellitus, blood glucose should be monitored when carvedilol therapy is initiated or discontinued or the dosage adjusted, since carvedilol therapy may worsen hyperglycemia.

Thyrotoxicosis. β-Adrenergic blockade may mask clinical signs of hyperthyroidism (e.g., tachycardia). Abrupt withdrawal of β-blockade may be followed by an exacerbation of symptoms of hyperthyroidism or may precipitate thyroid storm.

General Precautions Carvedilol shares the toxic potentials of β-adrenergic and α_1-adrenergic blocking agents; observe the usual precautions recommended with these agents.

Bradycardia. May cause bradycardia; dosage should be reduced if heart rate is less than 55 beats/minute.

Hypotension. May cause hypotension, postural hypotension, or syncope. Risk is highest in first 30 days of therapy in patients with heart failure. To decrease risk of orthostatic hypotension, administer with food and strictly adhere to the usual starting dose and titration recommendations. (See Dosage and Administration.)

Pheochromocytoma. In patients with pheochromocytoma, an α-adrenergic blocking agent should be administered before using a β-blocker. Although carvedilol has both α- and β-blocking pharmacologic activities, there has been no experience with its use in this condition; use with caution.

Prinzmetal's Variant Angina. Nonselective β-blockers may provoke chest pain in patients with Prinzmetal's variant angina; use with caution.

History of Anaphylactic Reactions. Possible increased reactivity to a variety of allergens; patients may be unresponsive to usual doses of epinephrine used to treat anaphylactic reactions.

Bronchospastic Disease. Bronchospasm reported rarely; deaths secondary to status asthmaticus have been reported following single doses of carvedilol. Patients with bronchospastic disease (e.g., chronic bronchitis, emphysema) generally should not receive β-blockers. Carvedilol should be used in patients with bronchospastic disease only when they are nonresponsive or intolerant of other antihypertensive agents; if used in such patients, the drug should be administered with caution and at the lowest dosage that achieves the desired clinical effect to minimize the drug's inhibition of endogenous or exogenous β-adrenergic agonists. (See Contraindications under Cautions.) If bronchospasm occurs, dosage should be reduced.

The manufacturer recommends that carvedilol be used with caution and strict adherence to recommendations regarding dosage titration in patients with heart failure and bronchospastic disease. If any evidence of bronchospasm occurs during initiation and/or titration of carvedilol, the dosage should be reduced.

Specific Populations **Pregnancy.** Category C. (See Users Guide.) Crosses the placenta in rats. Perinatal and neonatal distress have been reported with other α- and β-blockers.

Lactation. Distributed into milk in rats; not known whether distributed into human milk. Because of the risk of adverse effects in the infant, discontinue nursing or the drug, taking into account the importance of the drug to the woman.

Pediatric Use. Safety and efficacy not established in children younger than 18 years of age.

In a clinical trial in pediatric patients (mean age 6 years, range 2 months to 17 years) with chronic heart failure (NYHA class II–IV), carvedilol resulted in β-blockade activity as demonstrated by a placebo-corrected heart rate reduction of 4–6 beats/minute; however, no clinically important effect on treatment outcome was observed after 8 months of follow-up. Common adverse effects included chest pain, dizziness, and dyspnea.

Geriatric Use. No substantial differences in safety or efficacy relative to younger adults, but possibility exists of increased sensitivity to carvedilol in some individuals. Some clinicians suggest using a reduced initial carvedilol dosage in geriatric patients, since such patients are at increased risk of developing orthostatic hypotension and experience is limited regarding the use of the drug in patients 75 years of age or older. Plasma concentrations of carvedilol are about 50% higher in geriatric individuals than in younger individuals.

Hepatic Impairment. Not recommended for use in patients with manifestations of hepatic impairment or severe hepatic impairment. (See Contraindications under Cautions.)

Patients with hepatic cirrhosis developed plasma drug concentrations approximately 4–7 times higher than those in healthy individuals after a single dose of immediate-release carvedilol tablets.

Renal Impairment. Deterioration of renal function has been reported in patients receiving carvedilol.

Patients at risk appear to be those with low blood pressure (systolic blood pressure less than 100 mm Hg), ischemic heart disease and diffuse vascular disease, and/or underlying renal insufficiency. Renal function should be monitored in these patients during the dosage titration period; the drug should be discontinued or dosage reduced if worsening of renal function occurs.

■ **Common Adverse Effects** Adverse effects reported in 5% or more of patients with heart failure receiving immediate-release carvedilol tablets include dizziness, headache, fatigue, asthenia, arthralgia, hypotension, bradycardia, generalized edema, diarrhea, nausea, vomiting, hyperglycemia, weight gain, increased BUN, increased nonprotein nitrogen (NPN), increased cough, and abnormal vision.

Adverse effects reported in patients with left ventricular dysfunction following MI receiving immediate-release carvedilol tablets generally were similar to those in patients receiving the drug for the treatment of heart failure. Additional adverse effects reported in 3% or more of such patients include anemia, dyspnea, and pulmonary edema.

Adverse effects reported in 2% or more of patients receiving immediate-release carvedilol tablets for the treatment of hypertension include dizziness, bradycardia, diarrhea, insomnia, and postural hypotension.

Adverse effects reported in 2% or more of patients receiving extended-release carvedilol phosphate capsules for the treatment of hypertension include nasopharyngitis, dizziness, nausea, and peripheral edema.

Drug Interactions

Metabolized by cytochrome P-450 (CYP) isoenzymes, principally CYP2D6 and CYP2C9; also metabolized to a lesser extent by CYP3A4, CYP2C19, CYP1A2, CYP2E1.

■ **Drugs Affecting Hepatic Microsomal Enzymes** Potent inhibitors of CYP2D6 (e.g., fluoxetine, paroxetine, propafenone, quinidine): potential pharmacokinetic interaction (increased plasma concentrations of *R*(+)-carvedilol); however interactions with carvedilol have not been studied.

■ **Antidiabetic Agents (Oral and Parenteral [Insulin])** Possible increased hypoglycemic effect. Blood glucose concentrations should be monitored regularly.

■ **Calcium-channel Blocking Agents** Possible conduction disturbance, rarely with hemodynamic compromise. Blood pressure and ECG should be monitored during concomitant use with diltiazem or verapamil.

■ **Cardiac Glycosides** Potential pharmacokinetic and pharmacodynamic interaction. Digoxin concentrations are increased by about 15% in patients receiving concomitant therapy with digoxin and carvedilol. Both cardiac glycosides and carvedilol slow AV conduction and decrease heart rate; concomitant use may increase risk of bradycardia. Digoxin therapy should be carefully monitored when carvedilol dosage is initiated, adjusted, or discontinued.

■ **Catecholamine-depleting Agents (e.g., reserpine, MAO inhibitors)** Potential additive effects (e.g., hypotension, bradycardia). Patients should be monitored closely for symptoms (e.g., vertigo, syncope, postural hypotension).

■ **Cimetidine** Potential decreased carvedilol metabolism and increased (by 30%) bioavailability (area under the plasma concentration-time curve [AUC]) of carvedilol. No apparent change in peak plasma concentration of carvedilol.

■ **Clonidine** Potential additive effects (e.g., hypotension, bradycardia). If carvedilol is used concomitantly with clonidine, caution should be exercised, particularly when discontinuing therapy; carvedilol generally should be discontinued first, and clonidine continued for several days thereafter with gradual downward dosage titration.

■ **Cyclosporine** Possible increased cyclosporine concentrations. Cyclosporine concentrations should be closely monitored during carvedilol dosage titration; adjust cyclosporine dosage as necessary.

■ **Fluoxetine** Potential pharmacokinetic and pharmacodynamic interaction; potential for increased plasma concentrations of *R*(+)-carvedilol that may result in increased α-adrenergic blockade effects (vasodilation).

■ **Glyburide** Pharmacokinetic interaction unlikely.

■ **Hydrochlorothiazide** Pharmacokinetic interaction unlikely.

■ **Myocardial Depressant General Anesthetics (ether, cyclopropane, trichloroethylene)** Potential for increased risk of hypotension and heart failure. Use with caution.

■ **Pantoprazole** No clinically important increases in AUC and peak plasma concentrations of carvedilol reported with concomitant administration of carvedilol and pantoprazole.

■ **Paroxetine** Potential pharmacokinetic and pharmacodynamic interaction; potential for increased plasma concentrations of *R*(+)-carvedilol that may result in increased α-adrenergic blockade effects (vasodilation).

■ **Propafenone** Potential pharmacokinetic interaction; potential for increased plasma concentrations of *R*(+)-carvedilol that may result in increased α-adrenergic blockade effects (vasodilation).

■ **Quinidine** Potential pharmacokinetic interaction: potential for increased plasma concentrations of *R*(+)-carvedilol that may result in increased α-adrenergic blockade effects (vasodilation).

■ **Rifampin** In a pharmacokinetic study, rifampin decreased peak plasma concentration (by 70%) and AUC (by 70%) of carvedilol.

■ **Torsemide** Pharmacokinetic interaction unlikely.

■ **Warfarin** No effect on steady-state prothrombin times or warfarin pharmacokinetics.

Description

Carvedilol is a nonselective β-adrenergic blocking agent (β-blocker) with selective α_1-adrenergic blocking activity. The principal physiologic action of carvedilol is to competitively block adrenergic stimulation of β-receptors within the myocardium (β_1-receptors) and within bronchial and vascular smooth muscle (β_2-receptors), and to a lesser extent α_1-receptors within vascular smooth muscle. The β_1-antagonist activity of carvedilol is similar to that of propranolol and greater than that of labetalol, and the duration of carvedilol's effect is longer than those of labetalol and propranolol. Studies in animals indicate that the drug may exert an antioxidant effect on the myocardium and an antiproliferative effect on intimal tissue. The commercially available drug is a racemic mixture of the 2 enantiomers, (*R*)[+] and (*S*)[−], and both enantiomers have equal α_1-adrenergic blocking activity; however, only the S(-)-enantiomer of carvedilol has β-adrenergic blocking activity. Carvedilol does not exhibit intrinsic sympathomimetic (β_1-agonist) activity and possesses only weak membrane-stabilizing (local anesthetic) activity.

Vasodilation resulting in reduced total peripheral resistance mediated through carvedilol's α_1-adrenergic blockade and reduced sympathetic tone appear to play a major role in the drug's hypotensive effect. Carvedilol causes reductions in cardiac output, exercise-induced tachycardia, isoproterenol-induced tachycardia, and reflex orthostatic tachycardia. Clinically important β-adrenergic blocking activity of carvedilol usually is evident within 1 hour of oral administration, and the drug's hypotensive effect is similar to that of metoprolol. Carvedilol's α_1-adrenergic blocking effects, which contribute to the drug's hypotensive effects, generally are evident within 30 minutes of oral administration and include reductions in phenylephrine-induced pressor effects, vasodilation, and decreased peripheral vascular resistance. The dose-dependent hypotensive effect of carvedilol results in blood pressure (systolic and diastolic) reductions of 5–46% with little, if any, reflex tachycardia. This hypotensive effect occurs approximately 30 minutes after oral administration and has a maximum effect 1.5–7 hours after oral administration.

Carvedilol reduces peripheral vascular resistance and blood pressure as a result of its vasodilating effects; the drug produces both arterial and venous dilation. Carvedilol reduces blood pressure in both supine and standing patients; as a result of α_1-blockade, the effect is most pronounced on standing blood pressure, and orthostatic hypotension can occur. The manufacturer states that the frequency and severity of orthostatic hypotension may be decreased by administering the drug with food and by strictly adhering to the usual starting dose and titration recommendations. (See Dosage and Administration.)

The precise mechanism of the beneficial effects of carvedilol in the treatment of heart failure has not been fully elucidated. β-Adrenergic blockade and vasodilation generally are associated with reflex tachycardia and peripheral vasoconstriction in therapeutic agents in which one of these pharmacologic effects predominates, but the combined effects of carvedilol appear to attenuate these two major untoward responses by balancing the potential adverse effects associated with adrenergic blockade and vasodilation. The drug's vasodilatory action appears to enable the patient to tolerate the negative inotropic effect of carvedilol during the initiation and titration of therapy in the treatment of compensated heart failure. Chronic adrenergic stimulation and resultant activation of the renin-angiotensin system associated with compensated chronic heart failure result in sodium retention and vasoconstriction that, in turn, can induce further increases in preload and afterload that decrease cardiac output and stimulate additional sympathetic output. Some evidence suggests that the combined adrenergic effects of carvedilol, especially vasodilation, may ameliorate the negative inotropic effects that could otherwise lead to myocardial dysfunction in the compensating heart failure patient.

In patients with chronic heart failure and left ventricular dysfunction, carvedilol is associated with improvements in myocardial function through reduction in afterload as evidenced by improved left ventricular ejection fraction, reduced left ventricular volumes, and prevention of progression of left ventricular dilatation. Reductions in systemic blood pressure, pulmonary artery pressure, pulmonary capillary wedge pressure, and heart rate were observed in patients with heart failure (New York Heart Association [NYHA] functional class II–IV) receiving angiotensin-converting enzyme (ACE) inhibitors, cardiac glycosides, and/or diuretics after initiating concurrent carvedilol therapy. During initial therapy with carvedilol, small and variable responses in cardiac output, stroke volume index, and systemic vascular resistance occur. Chronic carvedilol therapy (12 –14 weeks) is associated with reductions in systemic blood pressure, pulmonary artery pressure, right atrial pressure, systemic vascular resistance, and heart rate, and increased stroke volume index. Increases (7%) in left ventricular ejection fraction (LVEF) were observed in patients with heart failure (NYHA class II-III) receiving carvedilol at a target dosage of 25–50 mg twice daily for 26–52 weeks. The effect of carvedilol on LVEF was dose-related, with increases of 5, 6, and 8% reported with twice-daily doses of 6.25 mg, 12.5 mg, and 25 mg, respectively.

The precise mechanism of the beneficial effects of carvedilol in the treatment of left ventricular dysfunction following myocardial infarction (MI) has not been fully elucidated.

Carvedilol is rapidly and extensively absorbed following oral administration. Food decreases the rate of the drug's absorption (i.e., increases time to peak plasma concentration), but not the extent (i.e., no effect on bioavailability) of absorption. Administration with food may decrease the risk of orthostatic hypotension. Carvedilol is substantially distributed into extravascular tissues. The half-life of carvedilol is 7–10 hours; 5–9 hours for *R*(+)-carvedilol, and 7–11 hours for *S*(−)-carvedilol. The drug is more than 98% bound to plasma proteins. Carvedilol is extensively metabolized; phenol ring demethylation and hydroxylation produce 3 metabolites with β-adrenergic blocking activity and (weak) vasodilating activity. Plasma concentrations of active metabolites are about 10% those of carvedilol. The 4′-hydroxyphenyl metabolite is 13 times more potent than carvedilol in β-adrenergic blocking activity. Carvedilol is excreted principally in feces as metabolites; less than 2% is excreted in urine unchanged.

Advice to Patients

Importance of taking carvedilol exactly as prescribed. Importance of taking with food.

Importance of advising patients receiving carvedilol phosphate extended-release capsules not to crush or chew the capsules.

Importance of not interrupting or discontinuing therapy without consulting clinician. When discontinuing therapy, importance of advising patients to temporarily limit physical activity.

Importance of advising patients to sit or lie down and avoid hazardous tasks (e.g., driving) if dizziness or fatigue occur. Importance of informing clinician if dizziness or faintness from decreased blood pressure occurs; dosage adjustment may be necessary.

Importance of diabetic patients informing clinician if changes in blood glucose concentrations occur. Importance of warning patients receiving insulin or oral hypoglycemic agents or those subject to spontaneous hypoglycemia about these potential effects.

Importance of immediately informing clinician at the first sign or symptom (e.g., weight gain, shortness of breath) of heart failure.

Importance of informing contact lens wearers that they may experience decreased lacrimation.

Importance of advising patients undergoing major surgery to inform anesthesiologist or dentist that they are receiving the drug.

Importance of informing clinicians of existing or contemplated therapy, including prescription and OTC drugs.

Importance of women informing clinicians if they are or plan to become pregnant or plan to breast-feed.

Importance of informing patient of other important precautionary information. (See Cautions.)

Overview® (see Users Guide). For additional information on this drug until a more detailed monograph is developed and published, the manufacturer's labeling should be consulted. It is *essential* that the manufacturer's labeling be consulted for more detailed information on usual cautions, precautions, contraindications, potential drug interactions, laboratory test interferences, and acute toxicity.

Preparations

Excipients in commercially available drug preparations may have clinically important effects in some individuals; consult specific product labeling for details.

Carvedilol

Oral		
Tablets, film-coated	3.125 mg*	**Carvedilol Tablets**
		Coreg®, GlaxoSmithKline
	6.25 mg*	**Carvedilol Tablets**
		Coreg® Tiltabs®, GlaxoSmithKline
	12.5 mg*	**Carvedilol Tablets**
		Coreg® Tiltabs®, GlaxoSmithKline
	25 mg*	**Carvedilol Tablets**
		Coreg® Tiltabs®, GlaxoSmithKline

*available from one or more manufacturer, distributor, and/or repackager by generic (nonproprietary) name

Carvedilol Phosphate

Oral		
Capsules, extended-release	10 mg (with 12.5% immediate-release and 87.5% extended-release)	**Coreg CR®**, GlaxoSmithKline
	20 mg (with 12.5% immediate-release and 87.5% extended-release)	**Coreg CR®**, GlaxoSmithKline
	40 mg (with 12.5% immediate-release and 87.5% extended-release)	**Coreg CR®**, GlaxoSmithKline
	80 mg (with 12.5% immediate-release and 87.5% extended-release)	**Coreg CR®**, GlaxoSmithKline

Labetalol Hydrochloride

Ibidomide Hydrochloride

■ Labetalol hydrochloride is an α- and β-adrenergic blocking agent.

Uses

Labetalol is used for the management of hypertension. The drug is used for hypertension associated with angina or pheochromocytoma and during pregnancy. IV labetalol is used for hypertension associated with myocardial infarction (MI) and to control blood pressure in patients with severe hypertension or in hypertensive crises.

In addition, IV labetalol has been used to produce controlled hypotension during anesthesia† and to control blood pressure in eclampsia† or preeclampsia†. The drug also has been used in the management of sympathetic overactivity syndrome with severe tetanus† and in angina†.

The choice of a β-adrenergic blocking agent (β-blocker) depends on numerous factors, including pharmacologic properties (e.g., relative β-selectivity, intrinsic sympathomimetic activity, membrane-stabilizing activity, lipophilicity), pharmacokinetics, intended use, and adverse effect profile, as well as the patient's coexisting disease states or conditions, response, and tolerance. While specific pharmacologic properties and other factors may appropriately influence the choice of a β-blocker in individual patients, evidence of clinically important differences among the agents in terms of overall efficacy and/or safety is limited. Patients who do not respond to or cannot tolerate one β-blocker may be successfully treated with a different agent.

■ **Hypertension** Labetalol hydrochloride is used alone or in combination with other classes of antihypertensive agents in the management of hypertension.

Current evidence-based practice guidelines for the management of hypertension in adults generally recommend the use of drugs from 4 classes of antihypertensive agents (angiotensin-converting enzyme [ACE] inhibitors, angiotensin II receptor antagonists, calcium-channel blockers, and thiazide diuretics). Most guidelines no longer recommend β-blockers as first-line therapy for hypertension because of the lack of established superiority over other recommended drug classes and evidence from at least one study demonstrating that β-blockers may be less effective than angiotensin II receptor antagonists in preventing cardiovascular death, MI, or stroke. However, therapy with a β-blocker may still be considered in hypertensive patients who have a compelling indication (e.g., prior MI, ischemic heart disease, heart failure) for their use or as add-on therapy in those who do not respond adequately to the preferred drug classes. (See Considerations for Drug Therapy in Patients with Underlying Cardiovascular and Other Risk Factors under Uses: Hypertension, in Atenolol 24:24 and in Metoprolol 24:24.) Ultimately, choice of antihypertensive therapy should be individualized, considering the clinical characteristics of the patient (e.g., age, ethnicity/race, comorbid conditions, cardiovascular risk factors) as well as drug-related factors (e.g., ease of administration, availability, adverse effects, costs).

A 2017 multidisciplinary hypertension guideline of the American College of Cardiology (ACC), American Heart Association (AHA), and a number of other professional organizations generally recommends a target blood pressure goal (i.e., blood pressure to achieve with drug therapy and/or nonpharmacologic intervention) of less than 130/80 mm Hg in all adults regardless of comorbidities or level of atherosclerotic cardiovascular disease (ASCVD) risk. In addition, a systolic blood pressure goal of less than 130 mm Hg generally is recommended for noninstitutionalized ambulatory patients 65 years of age or older. These blood pressure goals are based upon clinical studies demonstrating continuing reduction of cardiovascular risk at progressively lower levels of systolic blood pressure. Previous hypertension guidelines, such as those from an expert panel of the Eighth Joint National Committee on the Prevention, Detection, Evaluation, and Treatment of High Blood Pressure (JNC 8), generally have recommended initiation of antihypertensive treatment in patients with a systolic blood pressure of at least 140 mm Hg or diastolic blood pressure of at least 90 mm Hg, targeted a blood pressure goal of less than 140/90 mm Hg regardless of cardiovascular risk, and used higher systolic blood pressure thresholds and targets in geriatric patients compared with those recommended by the 2017 ACC/AHA hypertension guideline. The blood pressure thresholds used to define hypertension, the optimum blood pressure threshold at which to initiate antihypertensive drug therapy, and the ideal target blood pressure values remain controversial.

Most patients with hypertension, especially black patients, will require at least 2 antihypertensive drugs to achieve adequate blood pressure control. In general, black hypertensive patients tend to respond better to monotherapy with thiazide diuretics or calcium-channel blocking agents than to monotherapy with β-blockers. Although β-blockers have lowered blood pressure in all races studied, monotherapy with these agents has produced a smaller reduction in blood pressure in black hypertensive patients; however, this population difference in response does not appear to occur during combined therapy with a β-blocker and a thiazide diuretic. (See Race under Hypertension: Other Special Considerations for Antihypertensive Drug Therapy, in Uses in Atenolol 24:24 and in Metoprolol 24:24.)

For additional information on the role of β-blockers in the management of hypertension, see Uses: Hypertension, in Atenolol 24:24 and in Metoprolol 24:24. For information on overall principles and expert recommendations for treatment of hypertension, see Uses: Hypertension, in Adults, in the Thiazides General Statement 40:28.20.

Hypertension Associated with Angina or Myocardial Infarction Oral labetalol has been used effectively for the management of hypertension in patients with coexisting angina pectoris, and IV labetalol has been used effectively for the management of hypertension associated with acute myocardial infarction. In patients with hypertension and ischemic heart disease, oral labetalol therapy reduced blood pressure and heart rate and was associated with elimination or reduction of anginal pain, improvement in exercise tolerance, and decreased consumption of nitroglycerin. In the management of hypertension associated with acute myocardial infarction, IV infusions of labetalol decreased blood pressure and heart rate and generally decreased cardiac index and pulmonary artery wedge pressure, without producing adverse hemodynamic effects.

Hypertension during Pregnancy Labetalol has been used for the management of hypertension in pregnant women. The drug has been effective in controlling blood pressure in pregnant women with moderate to severe hypertension, in those with severe pregnancy-induced hypertension, and in those with hypertension and superimposed pregnancy-induced hypertension. In addition, in hypertensive pregnant women with proteinuria, labetalol therapy has resulted in substantially less proteinuria.

The goal of antihypertensive treatment in pregnant women with hypertension is to minimize the acute complications of maternal hypertension while avoiding therapy that would compromise fetal well-being. Antihypertensive therapy is recommended in pregnant women with chronic hypertension who have persistent, severely elevated blood pressure (e.g., systolic blood pressure of 160 mm Hg or higher or diastolic blood pressure of 105 mm Hg or higher); it is less clear whether antihypertensive therapy should be initiated in women with mild to moderate chronic hypertension. If initiation of antihypertensive therapy is considered necessary in a pregnant woman, use of labetalol, nifedipine, or methyldopa is recommended by the American College of Obstetricians and Gynecologists (ACOG) and other experts. In women who are already receiving antihypertensive therapy prior to pregnancy, ACOG states that data are insufficient to make recommendations regarding the continuance or discontinuance of such therapy; treatment decisions should be individualized in these situations. Some other experts state that women with hypertension who become pregnant or who are planning to become pregnant should have their antihypertensive therapy transitioned to methyldopa, nifedipine, and/or labetalol during pregnancy. Antihypertensive therapy can reduce the risk of severe hypertension but has not been shown to prevent the development of preeclampsia. Use of labetalol in association with careful prenatal management during pregnancy does not appear to adversely affect the fetus. (See Cautions: Pregnancy, Fertility, and Lactation.)

Labetalol also has been used parenterally in the hospital setting for urgent lowering of blood pressure in severely hypertensive pregnant women, including those with preeclampsia† or eclampsia†. Recommendations for the management of such patients are based principally on experience in women with preeclampsia or gestational hypertension in the third trimester. Delivery is the preferred method of management for women with severe preeclampsia; however, use of antihypertensive drugs is recommended in such women who have severely elevated blood pressures (sustained systolic blood pressure of at least 160 mm Hg or diastolic blood pressure of at least 110 mm Hg) to prevent potentially life-threatening cardiovascular, renal, and cerebrovascular complications. Results of several randomized clinical trials evaluating antihypertensive therapy in women with severe hypertension during pregnancy suggest that IV labetalol, IV hydralazine, or oral nifedipine are appropriate antihypertensives for urgently lowering blood pressure in such patients; choice of therapy should be based on clinician experience and preference as well as patient-specific factors (e.g., concomitant medical conditions or therapies) and drug-related factors (e.g., route of administration, adverse effects, contraindications, local availability, cost). Although hydralazine historically has been considered the agent of choice for management of hypertensive emergencies associated with pregnancy, some clinicians now prefer IV labetalol for its more rapid onset and shorter duration of action and its more predictable hypotensive effect.

Hypertension Associated with Pheochromocytoma Because of labetalol's α- and β-adrenergic blocking activity, the drug has been used alone to control hypertension and symptoms resulting from excessive β-receptor stimulation in patients with pheochromocytoma. Labetalol generally appears to be effective in these patients; some evidence suggests that the drug may be more effective in patients whose tumors predominantly secrete epinephrine rather than norepinephrine and in patients with sustained rather than paroxysmal hypertension. Since there have been reports that oral labetalol may induce a paradoxical hypertensive crisis in some patients with pheochromocytoma (possibly because the drug's predominant β-adrenergic blockade leaves α-adrenergic stimulation relatively unopposed), the manufacturers recommend that the drug be used with caution in patients with this tumor. Although labetalol has some α-adrenergic blocking activity, some clinicians caution that the drug, like other β-adrenergic blocking agents, should not be used in patients with pheochromocytoma unless they have received pretreatment with an α-adrenergic blocking agent (e.g., IV phentolamine). If labetalol is used in patients with known or suspected pheochromocytoma, appropriate methods for determining urinary catecholamines should be employed. (See Laboratory Test Interferences: Urinary Catecholamines.)

Severe Hypertension and Hypertensive Crises IV labetalol hydrochloride is used to control blood pressure in patients with severe hypertension or in hypertensive crises for the immediate reduction in blood pressure in patients in whom such reduction is considered an emergency (hypertensive emergencies). Hypertensive emergencies are those rare situations requiring immediate blood pressure reduction (not necessarily to normal ranges) to prevent or limit target organ damage. Such emergency situations include hypertensive encephalopathy, acute MI, intracerebral hemorrhage, acute left ventricular failure with pulmonary edema, eclampsia, dissecting aortic aneurysm, unstable angina pectoris, acute ischemic stroke, and acute renal failure, and labetalol generally is suitable for most hypertensive emergencies (e.g., acute aortic dissection, acute coronary syndromes) except when acute cardiac failure is present. Patients with hypertensive emergencies require hospitalization and are treated with an appropriate parenteral agent. Elevated blood pressure alone, in the absence of manifestations or other evidence of target organ damage, rarely requires emergency therapy. The risks of overly aggressive therapy in any hypertensive crisis must always be considered. Excessive falls in blood pressure should be avoided in any hypertensive crisis since they may precipitate renal, cerebral, or coronary ischemia.

Labetalol usually produces a prompt, but gradual reduction of blood pressure without substantial changes in heart rate or cardiac output. IV labetalol appears to adequately reduce blood pressure in about 80–90% of patients with severe hypertension or hypertensive emergencies, irrespective of etiology, and may be useful even when other drugs have failed. The exact effects of previous antihypertensive therapy on the efficacy of IV labetalol have not been fully determined. IV labetalol generally appears to be effective regardless of whether patients have received other hypotensive drugs, including β-blockers; however, in some studies, the drug was reported to be ineffective, usually in patients who received a single IV injection and who were receiving other hypotensive drugs, including β-blockers. The possibility of a diminished response to IV labetalol should be considered in patients receiving α- or β-blockers.

The comparative efficacy and safety of IV labetalol and other currently available parenteral hypotensive agents in the management of severe hypertension and hypertensive emergencies have not been fully evaluated, but IV labetalol is considered one of several parenteral drugs of choice for the management of these forms of hypertension. IV labetalol appears to be as effective as IV diazoxide (parenteral formulation no longer commercially available in the US), but may be less likely to induce excessive hypotension and adverse neurologic or cardiovascular sequelae. Because of its usual lack of substantial changes in heart rate or cardiac output, IV labetalol may be particularly useful in severely hypertensive patients with ischemic heart disease. In addition, IV labetalol has an advantage over most other parenteral hypotensive agents in that oral therapy with the drug may be continued after parenteral therapy when long-term control of blood pressure is necessary. IV labetalol also has been used effectively to control blood pressure and the rate of left ventricular pressure rise (dp/dt) in a few patients with acute dissection of the aorta; the drug produced a gradual reduction in blood pressure without a concomitant increase in heart rate.

Hypertensive urgencies are those situations in which there is a severe elevation in blood pressure without progressive target organ damage. Hypertensive urgencies generally can be managed by intensification or reinstitution (e.g., following noncompliance) of the current antihypertensive regimen and treatment of anxiety if needed. Experts state that there is no need for rapid reduction of blood pressure in the emergency department in such patients and hospitalization also is unnecessary.

IV labetalol has been used effectively in a small number of patients for the management of hypertensive crises following discontinuance of clonidine†, and oral labetalol has been used effectively in a small number of patients to prevent such crises during withdrawal from clonidine therapy†. However, since severe rebound hypertension reportedly has occurred in at least one patient during gradual withdrawal of clonidine and concurrent oral administration of labetalol, some clinicians caution that labetalol not be used in such patients unless they have received pretreatment with an α-blocker (e.g., IV phentolamine).

■ **Controlled Hypotension during Anesthesia** IV labetalol hydrochloride has been used effectively to produce controlled hypotension during anesthesia† in order to reduce bleeding resulting from surgical procedures. When labetalol and halothane are used concomitantly, a synergistic hypotensive effect results, which may be used to therapeutic advantage. (See Drug Interactions: Halothane.) Labetalol has also been effective in the management of uncontrolled hypertension before anesthesia and during surgery†, and for the management and/or prevention of acute hypertensive responses during laryngoscopy†.

■ **Chronic Stable Angina** Labetalol has been used in a limited number of patients for the long-term management of chronic stable angina pectoris†. Use of the drug has been associated with a reduction in the frequency and severity of anginal attacks, a decrease in nitrate dosage, and an increase in exercise tolerance. β-Blockers are recommended as the anti-ischemic drugs of choice in most patients with chronic stable angina; despite differences in cardioselectivity, intrinsic sympathomimetic activity, and other clinical factors, all β-blockers appear to be equally effective for this indication. For additional information on the role of β-blockers in the management of chronic stable angina, see Uses: Chronic Stable Angina, in Metoprolol 24:24.

■ **Tetanus** Labetalol has been used with good results for the management of the sympathetic overactivity syndrome associated with severe tetanus†. The drug generally has been effective in stabilizing the cardiovascular disturbances, including hypertension, tachycardia, and increased systemic arteriolar resistance, that occur in patients with severe tetanus.

Dosage and Administration

■ **Administration** Labetalol hydrochloride is usually administered orally, but may be administered by slow, direct IV injection or by slow, continuous IV infusion.

Oral Administration Labetalol hydrochloride is usually administered orally in 2 divided doses daily; however, if adverse effects (e.g., nausea, dizziness) occur and are intolerable (particularly with dosages of 1.2 g daily or higher), administration of the drug in 3 divided doses daily may improve patient tolerance and/or facilitate dosage titration.

IV Administration To control blood pressure in patients with severe hypertension or hypertensive emergencies, repeated doses of labetalol hydrochloride may be given by slow, direct IV injection over a 2-minute period at intervals of 10 minutes, or a diluted solution of the drug may be administered by slow, continuous IV infusion. For IV infusion, labetalol hydrochloride solutions are prepared by diluting the injection to an appropriate concentration in a compatible IV infusion solution. (See Chemistry and Stability: Stability.) For example, 200 mg of the drug may be added to 160 mL of 5% dextrose injection to provide a solution containing 1 mg/mL. To facilitate a desired rate of infusion, diluted solutions of the drug can be administered via a controlled-infusion device. Labetalol hydrochloride injection and diluted solutions of the drug should be inspected visually for particulate matter and discoloration prior to administration whenever solution and container permit. Prefilled syringes of the drug should be destroyed and discarded if damaged in any manner; if the cannula is bent, no attempt should be made to straighten it.

Patients receiving IV labetalol must be kept in a supine position during administration of the drug; a substantial fall in blood pressure on standing should be expected in these patients. Since symptomatic orthostatic hypotension is likely to occur if these patients are tilted upward or allowed to assume an upright position within 3 hours after administration of the drug, they should remain in a supine position during this time period. The patient's ability to tolerate an upright position must be established before any ambulation is permitted. (See Cautions: Precautions and Contraindications.) Blood pressure must be closely monitored during and after completion of IV administration of labetalol. Rapid or excessive reductions in systolic or diastolic blood pressure during IV therapy with the drug should be avoided. In patients with excessive systolic hypertension, the decrease in systolic pressure, as well as the decrease in diastolic pressure, should be used to assess response to the drug. When labetalol is administered by direct IV injection, blood pressure should be monitored before and at 5-minute intervals after each injection; the maximum hypotensive effect usually occurs within 5–15 minutes after each injection. When the drug is administered by continuous IV infusion, the rate of infusion may be adjusted according to the supine blood pressure response. After the desired supine blood pressure is attained or the maximum recommended cumulative dose has been given, IV administration of labetalol should be discontinued. Following discontinuance of IV labetalol, blood pressure is usually monitored at 5-minute intervals for 30 minutes, then at 30-minute intervals for 2 hours, then hourly for about 6 hours, and as necessary thereafter. Oral therapy with the drug may be initiated when it has been established that the supine diastolic blood pressure has begun to increase (usually determined by an increase of 10 mm Hg).

■ **Dosage** ***Hypertension*** Dosage of oral labetalol hydrochloride should be adjusted according to standing blood pressure. Some adverse effects (e.g., nausea, dizziness) of the drug may be minimized or avoided and patient tolerance improved if dosage is adjusted more gradually (e.g., every 2–4 weeks) over a period of 4–12 weeks. The maximum, steady-state blood pressure response with twice-daily dosing occurs within 1–3 days and, with continued dosing, blood pressure can be measured approximately 12 hours after a dose to determine if further dosage titration is necessary. Since the maximum hypotensive effect of the drug is usually evident within 1–4 hours, lack of an excessive hypotensive response to the initial dose or a dose increment can usually be established in an ambulatory clinical setting.

If long-term labetalol therapy is to be discontinued, dosage of the drug should be reduced gradually over a period of 1–2 weeks. (See Cautions: Precautions and Contraindications.)

Usual Dosage. For the management of hypertension in adults, the recommended initial oral dosage of labetalol hydrochloride is 100 mg twice daily, given alone or in combination with a diuretic. Dosage may be adjusted in increments of 100 mg twice daily every 2 or 3 days until the optimum blood pressure response is achieved.

The usual oral maintenance dosage of labetalol hydrochloride recommended by the manufacturers for adults is 200–400 mg twice daily. Some experts recommend a lower usual dosage range of 100–400 mg twice daily; the rationale for this reduced dosage is that it usually is preferable to add another antihypertensive agent to the regimen than to continue increasing labetalol hydrochloride dosage since the patient may not tolerate such continued increases. Because some geriatric individuals eliminate labetalol more slowly than younger adults, a lower maintenance dosage than that recommended for the general population may be adequate to control blood pressure in these older patients. Some manufacturers suggest that a maintenance dosage of 100–200 mg twice daily may be adequate for most geriatric patients. The manufacturers state that some adults with severe hypertension may require labetalol hydrochloride dosages of up to 2.4 g daily given in 2 divided doses, administered alone or in combination with a diuretic; in these patients, dosage titration increments should not exceed 200 mg twice daily.

When diuretic therapy is initiated in a patient already receiving labetalol hydrochloride, adjustment of labetalol dosage may be necessary. Optimum maintenance dosage of oral labetalol hydrochloride is usually lower in patients also receiving a diuretic.

When patients are transferred from therapy with other antihypertensive agents, oral therapy with labetalol hydrochloride should be initiated in the usual initial dosage and dosage of the existing regimen gradually decreased.

If labetalol hydrochloride is used for the management of hypertension in children†, some experts have recommended an initial oral dosage of 1–3 mg/kg daily given in 2 divided doses. Such experts have suggested that dosage may be increased as necessary to a maximum dosage of 10–12 mg/kg (up to 1.2 g) daily given in 2 divided doses. For information on overall principles and expert recommendations for treatment of hypertension in pediatric patients, see Uses: Hypertension in Pediatric Patients, in the Thiazides General Statement 40:28.20.

Blood Pressure Monitoring and Treatment Goals. Blood pressure should be monitored regularly (i.e., monthly) during therapy and dosage of the antihypertensive drug adjusted until blood pressure is controlled. If an adequate blood pressure response is not achieved, the dosage may be increased or another antihypertensive agent with demonstrated benefit and preferably with a complementary mechanism of action (e.g., angiotensin-converting enzyme [ACE] inhibitor, angiotensin II receptor antagonist, calcium-channel blocker, thiazide diuretic) may be added; if target blood pressure is still not achieved with the use of 2 antihypertensive agents, a third drug may be added. (See Uses: Hypertension.) In patients who develop unacceptable adverse effects with labetalol, the drug should be discontinued and another antihypertensive agent from a different pharmacologic class should be initiated.

The goal of hypertension management and prevention is to achieve and maintain optimal control of blood pressure. However, the optimum blood pressure threshold for initiating antihypertensive drug therapy and specific treatment goals remain controversial. While previous hypertension guidelines have based target blood pressure goals on age and comorbidities, the 2017 American College of Cardiology/American Heart Association (ACC/AHA) hypertension guideline incorporates underlying cardiovascular risk into decision making regarding treatment and generally recommends the same target blood pressure (i.e., less than 130/80 mm Hg) for all adults. Many patients will require at least 2 drugs from different pharmacologic classes to achieve this blood pressure goal; the potential benefits of hypertension management and drug cost, adverse effects, and risks associated with the use of multiple antihypertensive drugs also should be considered when deciding a patient's blood pressure treatment goal.

For additional information on target levels of blood pressure and on monitoring therapy in the management of hypertension, see Blood Pressure Monitoring and Treatment Goals under Dosage: Hypertension, in Dosage and Administration in the Thiazides General Statement 40:28.20.

Severe Hypertension and Hypertensive Crises Dosage of labetalol hydrochloride must be adjusted according to the severity of hypertension and the patient's blood pressure response and tolerance. IV dosage of labetalol hydrochloride should be adjusted according to supine blood pressure. When IV labetalol hydrochloride is used in the management of a hypertensive emergency in adults *without* a compelling indication, the initial goal of such therapy is to reduce systolic blood pressure by no more than 25% within the first hour, followed by further blood pressure reduction *if stable* to 160/110 or 160/100 mm Hg within the next 2–6 hours, avoiding excessive declines in pressure that could precipitate renal, cerebral, or coronary ischemia. If this blood pressure is well tolerated and the patient is clinically stable, further gradual reductions toward normal can be implemented in the next 24–48 hours. Adults who have hypertensive crisis *with* a compelling indication (e.g., aortic dissection, severe preeclampsia or eclampsia, pheochromocytoma crisis) should have their systolic blood pressure reduced to less than 140 mm Hg during the first hour, and, in patients with aortic dissection, to less than 120 mm Hg within the first 20 minutes.

To control blood pressure in adults with severe hypertension or hypertensive emergencies, the manufacturer recommends that IV labetalol hydrochloride be given in an initial dose of 20 mg by slow (over 2 minutes), direct IV injection. Alternatively, some experts recommend an initial IV labetalol dosage of 0.3–1 mg/kg (maximum 20 mg) administered by slow, direct IV injection every 10 minutes. Higher initial doses (e.g., 1–2 mg/kg) have been administered by direct IV injection, but the 20-mg dose is recommended to minimize adverse effects (e.g., nausea, excessive hypotension) and the risks associated with too rapid reduction in blood pressure. Additional labetalol doses of 40 or 80 mg may be given at 10-minute intervals until the desired supine blood pressure is achieved or a total cumulative dose of 300 mg has been administered; IV labetalol should then be discontinued and oral therapy with the drug (administered as tablets) may be initiated when the supine diastolic blood pressure begins to increase.

As an alternative to direct IV injections, the manufacturer states that labetalol hydrochloride may be given by continuous IV infusion at an initial rate of 2 mg/minute, with the rate of infusion adjusted according to the blood pressure response. Some experts recommend an initial IV infusion rate of 0.4–1 mg/kg per hour and increasing the rate as needed up to 3 mg/kg per hour. The usual effective cumulative dose administered by IV infusion is 50–200 mg, although up to 300 mg may be required in some patients. A total cumulative dose of 300 mg has been recommended by some experts. Because of the elimination half-life of labetalol, steady-state plasma concentrations of the drug are not attained during the usual infusion period. The infusion should be continued until an adequate response is obtained (or the maximum recommended cumulative dose has been given) and then discontinued, and oral therapy with the drug initiated when the supine diastolic blood pressure begins to increase. Some clinicians have used a progressive, incremental IV infusion regimen† (i.e., infusing 20, 40, 80, and 160 mg/hour for 1 hour at each dose level, or until the desired blood pressure is achieved) and believe this method may result in a more gradual reduction of blood pressure and minimize adverse effects compared with repeated IV injections of the drug; however, controlled comparisons of the various methods of IV administration are not available. Some clinicians have also used oral regimens† for urgent reduction of blood pressure in severely hypertensive patients.

For rapid reduction of blood pressure in children and adolescents with acute severe hypertension† and life-threatening symptoms, some experts recommend administration of labetalol hydrochloride as a direct IV injection of 0.2–1 mg/kg per dose, up to 40 mg per dose. As an alternative to direct IV injections, labetalol hydrochloride may be given by continuous IV infusion at a rate of 0.25–3 mg/kg per hour. These experts suggest that blood pressure should be reduced by no more than 25% of the planned reduction over the first 8 hours. For information on overall principles and expert recommendations for treatment of hypertension in pediatric patients, see Uses: Hypertension in Pediatric Patients, in the Thiazides General Statement 40:28.20.

When oral labetalol therapy is initiated following IV therapy with the drug, the recommended initial oral dose in adults is 200 mg, followed in 6–12 hours by an additional oral dose of 200 or 400 mg, depending on the blood pressure response. Thereafter, while the patient is hospitalized, oral dosage may be increased in usual increments at 1-day intervals (dosage range: 400–2400 mg daily administered in 2 or 3 divided doses), if necessary, to achieve the desired blood pressure control; for subsequent outpatient dosage titration or maintenance dosing, the usual oral dosage recommendations should be followed.

Severe Hypertension During Pregnancy. To control acute severe hypertension in pregnant women, including preeclampsia†, some experts recommend an initial IV labetalol hydrochloride dose of 10–20 mg administered by direct IV injection, followed by 20–80 mg every 20–30 minutes as needed up to a maximum cumulative dose of 300 mg. Alternatively, the drug may be administered by continuous IV infusion at a rate of 1–2 mg/minute. Antihypertensive therapy is recommended for women with preeclampsia who have persistent systolic blood pressures of 160 mm Hg or higher or diastolic blood pressures of 110 mm Hg or higher.

Controlled Hypotension during Anesthesia To produce controlled hypotension during halothane anesthesia† in adults, IV labetalol hydrochloride has been given in an initial dose of 20 mg (range: 10–25 mg) following induction of anesthesia; if necessary, additional doses of 5–10 mg (range: 2.5–15 mg) were given. When IV labetalol hydrochloride and halothane anesthesia are used concomitantly, the degree and duration of the synergistic hypotensive response can be controlled by adjusting the inspired halothane concentration. (See Drug Interactions: Halothane.) To produce controlled hypotension during anesthesia with other anesthetic agents† in adults, IV labetalol hydrochloride has been given in an initial dose of 30 mg, with additional doses of 5–10 mg given if necessary.

■ Dosage in Renal and Hepatic Impairment Modification of labetalol hydrochloride dosage does not appear to be necessary in patients with mild to moderate renal impairment. In patients with severe renal impairment (i.e., creatinine clearance less than 10 mL/minute) undergoing dialysis, adequate blood pressure control may be possible with once-daily dosing of the drug.

Although specific data are currently not available, dosage reduction may be necessary in patients with impaired hepatic function since metabolism of the drug may be decreased in these patients.

Cautions

Labetalol hydrochloride shares the toxic potentials of β-adrenergic and postsynaptic α_1-adrenergic blocking agents. Most adverse reactions to labetalol are mild, transient, and occur early in the course of treatment. Adverse effects of labetalol can generally be divided into 3 groups (in decreasing order of frequency): nonspecific effects, effects related to the α-adrenergic blocking activity of the drug, and effects related to its β-adrenergic blocking activity. During controlled clinical studies in patients receiving oral labetalol for 3–4 months, adverse reactions requiring discontinuance of the drug occurred in about 7% of patients; in these same comparative studies, adverse reactions requiring discontinuance of therapy occurred in 8–10% of patients receiving pure β-adrenergic blocking agents (i.e., metoprolol, propranolol) and in 30% of patients receiving a centrally acting adrenergic inhibitor (i.e., methyldopa). Evidence from clinical studies in patients receiving oral labetalol hydrochloride dosages of 200 mg to 2.4 g daily suggests that some adverse effects, including dizziness, fatigue, nausea, vomiting, dyspepsia, paresthesia, nasal congestion, failure to ejaculate, impotence, and edema, are dose related. The incidence and/or severity of some labetalol-induced adverse reactions may occasionally be obviated by slow, upward titration of dosage over 4–12 weeks.

■ Cardiovascular Effects The most frequent adverse cardiovascular effect of labetalol is symptomatic orthostatic hypotension, which occurs in about 1–5% or 60% of patients following oral or IV administration of the drug, respectively. Orthostatic hypotension has been associated with loss of consciousness occasionally following IV administration and rarely following oral administration. Symptomatic orthostatic hypotension is likely to occur if supine patients are tilted upward or allowed to assume the upright position within 3 hours following IV administration of labetalol. (See Cautions: Precautions and Contraindications.) Moderate hypotension occurs in about 1% of patients in the supine position who are receiving the drug IV. Following oral administration, orthostatic hypotension appears to occur more frequently during initiation of therapy, in patients receiving concomitant administration of a diuretic, and in those receiving higher dosages of the drug.

Development or exacerbation of heart failure has occurred in some patients receiving labetalol, although the drug appears to be less likely to precipitate heart failure than pure β-adrenergic blocking agents. At the first sign or symptom of impending cardiac failure during labetalol therapy, patients should receive adequate treatment (e.g., cardiac glycoside, diuretic) and should be observed closely; if cardiac failure continues, labetalol should be discontinued, gradually if possible.

Ventricular arrhythmia (including ventricular premature contractions), edema or fluid retention, bradycardia, hypotension, syncope, chest pain, atrioventricular (AV) conduction delay, and AV block have occurred during therapy with labetalol.

■ **Nervous System Effects** Adverse nervous system effects occur with variable frequency with labetalol and most of these effects appear to be dose related. At the usual labetalol hydrochloride dosage of 200–400 mg twice daily, most adverse nervous system effects occur in 5% or less of patients. Adverse nervous system effects of the drug include drowsiness or tiredness, dizziness or lightheadedness (often posture related), headache, fatigue, lethargy, and nightmares or vivid dreams. Paresthesia, usually mild, transient tingling of the scalp or skin, may also occur following oral or IV administration of the drug, usually at the beginning of therapy. Hypoesthesia or numbness and circumoral paresthesia have also occurred. Mental depression, paroniria, vertigo, somnolence, yawning, tremor, asthenia, and insomnia have also been reported. Some adverse nervous system effects such as fatigue, mental depression, and sleep disorders may occur less frequently with labetalol than with pure β-adrenergic blocking agents. Adverse nervous system effects of labetalol may be obviated by a reduction in dosage or alteration of dosage schedule.

■ **GI Effects** The most frequent adverse GI effects associated with labetalol therapy are nausea, dyspepsia, and vomiting. Alteration or distortion in taste, abdominal pain, constipation, diarrhea, and flatulence have also been reported.

■ **Hepatic Effects** Elevated liver function test results, including reversible increases in serum aminotransferase concentrations; jaundice (including cholestatic jaundice); and hepatitis have been reported in patients receiving labetalol. Severe hepatocellular injury, which has recurred during rechallenge, has occurred rarely during labetalol therapy; hepatocellular injury may be accompanied by clinical symptoms of hepatotoxicity, including pruritus, dark urine, persistent anorexia, jaundice, flu-like syndrome, and/or right upper quadrant tenderness. Hepatocellular injury is usually reversible; however, hepatic necrosis and death have been reported. Hepatic injury may occur after short- or long-term labetalol therapy. Similar severe adverse hepatic effects, including at least 2 fatalities, have been reported with dilevalol hydrochloride; dilevalol is one of the 4 stereoisomers that make up the racemic mixture labetalol. (See Chemistry and Stability: Chemistry.)

■ **Respiratory Effects** Adverse respiratory effects of labetalol, including dyspnea, wheezing, bronchospasm, and nasal congestion, occur occasionally. Rhinorrhea and rhinitis also have been reported.

■ **Genitourinary Effects** Ejaculatory failure, impotence, difficult or painful micturition, and acute urinary retention have occurred occasionally in patients receiving labetalol alone or in fixed combination with hydrochlorothiazide. Peyronie's disease and priapism have been reported rarely. Urinary frequency, nocturia, and polyuria have been reported when the drug was used in fixed combination with hydrochlorothiazide.

■ **Dermatologic and Sensitivity Reactions** Rashes, including maculopapular, lichenoid, urticarial, and psoriasiform lesions, have developed in some patients during labetalol therapy (alone or in fixed combination with hydrochlorothiazide). Pruritus, bullous lichen planus, facial erythema, and reversible alopecia have also occurred. Hypersensitivity (e.g., rash, urticaria, pruritus, angioedema, dyspnea) and anaphylactoid reactions have been reported rarely in patients receiving labetalol.

■ **Endocrine Effects** Results of a large prospective cohort study of nondiabetic adults 45–64 years of age indicate that use of β-adrenergic blocking agents in hypertensive patients is associated with increased risk (about 28%) of developing type 2 diabetes mellitus compared with hypertensive patients who were not receiving hypotensive therapy. In this study, the number of new cases of diabetes per 1000 person-years was 33.6 or 26.3 in patients receiving a β-adrenergic blocking agents or no drug therapy, respectively. The association between the risk of developing type 2 diabetes mellitus and use of β-adrenergic blocking agents reportedly was not confounded by weight gain, hyperinsulinemia, or differences in heart rate. It is not known if the risk of developing diabetes is affected by β-receptor selectivity. Further studies are needed to determine whether concomitant use of ACE inhibitors (which may improve insulin sensitivity) would abrogate β-blocker-induced adverse effects related to glucose intolerance. Therefore, until results of such studies are available, the proven benefits of β-adrenergic blocking agents in reducing cardiovascular events in hypertensive patients must be weighed carefully against the possible risks of developing type 2 diabetes mellitus.

Hypoglycemia, which may result in loss of consciousness, also may occur in nondiabetic patients receiving β-adrenergic blocking agents. Patients most at risk for the development of β-blocker-induced hypoglycemia are those undergoing dialysis, prolonged fasting, or severe exercise regimens.

β-Adrenergic blocking agents may mask signs and symptoms of hypoglycemia (e.g., palpitation, tachycardia, tremor) and potentiate insulin-induced hypoglycemia. Although it has been suggested that nonselective β-adrenergic blocking agents are more likely to induce hypoglycemia than selective β-blockers agents, such an adverse effect also has been reported with selective β-blocking agents (e.g., atenolol). In addition, selective β-adrenergic blocking agents are less likely to mask symptoms of hypoglycemia or delay recovery from insulin-induced hypoglycemia than nonselective β-adrenergic blocking agents because of their vascular sparing effects; however, selective β-blockers can decrease insulin sensitivity by approximately 15–30%, which may result in increased insulin requirements.

■ **Other Adverse Effects** Lupus erythematosus-like illness, positive antinuclear antibody (ANA) titer, mild hyperglycemia, leukopenia, and development of positive antimitochondrial antibodies have occurred in patients receiving labetalol. Transient increases in BUN and serum creatinine concentrations associated with decreases in blood pressure have also occurred, usually in patients with renal insufficiency. Flushing or a feeling of warmth, fever, rigors, increased sweating, dry mouth or eyes, blurred vision, visual disturbances, pallor, shivering, decreased libido, muscle cramps, toxic myopathy, claudication, Raynaud's phenomenon, burning sensation of the groin, and pain at the injection site have been reported. In addition, leg cramps, pain, gout, increased appetite, hypokalemia, and increased serum creatine kinase (CK, creatine phosphokinase, CPK) concentrations have been reported when the drug was used in fixed combination with hydrochlorothiazide.

The possibility that other adverse effects associated with other β-adrenergic blocking agents may occur during labetalol therapy should be considered. These include, but may not be limited to, hematologic reactions (e.g., agranulocytosis, nonthrombocytopenic or thrombocytopenic purpura); allergic reactions characterized by fever, sore throat, laryngospasm, and respiratory distress; GI reactions including mesenteric thrombosis or ischemic colitis; and CNS reactions including reversible mental depression progressing to catatonia, short-term memory loss, decreased performance on neuropsychometric tests, and oculomucocutaneous syndrome.

■ **Precautions and Contraindications** Labetalol shares the toxic potentials of β-adrenergic and postsynaptic α_1-adrenergic blocking agents, and the usual precautions of these agents should be observed.

In patients with heart failure, sympathetic stimulation is vital for the support of circulatory function. Labetalol should be used with caution in patients with inadequate cardiac function, since heart failure may be precipitated by blockade of β-adrenergic stimulation when labetalol therapy is administered. In addition, in patients with latent cardiac insufficiency, prolonged β-adrenergic blockade may lead to cardiac failure. Although β-adrenergic blocking agents should be avoided in patients with overt heart failure, labetalol may be administered cautiously, if necessary, to patients with well-compensated heart failure (e.g., those controlled with cardiac glycosides and/or diuretics). Patients receiving labetalol therapy should be instructed to consult their clinician at the first sign or symptom of impending cardiac failure and should be adequately treated (e.g., with a cardiac glycoside and/or diuretic) and observed closely; if cardiac failure continues, labetalol should be discontinued, gradually if possible.

Further experience is necessary, but labetalol may be less likely than pure β-adrenergic blocking agents to produce adverse cardiovascular withdrawal reactions (e.g., angina, rebound hypertension) following abrupt withdrawal. Although angina pectoris has *not* been reported to date following discontinuance of labetalol therapy, exacerbation of angina pectoris and precipitation of myocardial infarction have occurred following abrupt cessation of therapy with some β-adrenergic blocking agents in patients with coronary artery disease. Therefore, patients receiving labetalol (especially those with ischemic heart disease) should be warned not to interrupt or discontinue therapy without consulting their clinician. When discontinuance of long-term labetalol therapy is planned, particularly in patients with ischemic heart disease, dosage of the drug should be gradually reduced over a period of 1–2 weeks. When labetalol therapy is discontinued, patients should be carefully monitored and advised to temporarily limit their physical activity. If exacerbation of angina occurs or acute coronary insufficiency develops after labetalol therapy is interrupted or discontinued, treatment with the drug should be reinstituted promptly, at least temporarily, and appropriate measures for the management of unstable angina pectoris should be initiated. Because coronary artery disease is common and may be unrecognized, the manufacturers caution that it may be prudent not to discontinue labetalol therapy abruptly, even in patients being treated only for hypertension.

Since β-adrenergic blocking agents may inhibit bronchodilation produced by endogenous catecholamines, the drugs generally should not be used in patients with bronchospastic disease; however, oral labetalol may be used with caution in patients with nonallergic bronchospasm (e.g., chronic bronchitis, emphysema) who do not respond to or cannot tolerate other hypotensive agents. (See Pharmacology: Respiratory Effects.) If oral labetalol is administered to such patients, the smallest effective dose should be used so that inhibition of endogenous or exogenous β-adrenergic agonist activity is minimized. Because IV labetalol at the usual therapeutic doses has not been studied in patients with nonallergic bronchospasm, the manufacturers state that it should not be used in these patients.

Although labetalol has been used effectively in the management of hypertension and relief of symptoms associated with pheochromocytoma, the drug should be used with caution in patients with this tumor since paradoxical hypertensive responses have been reported in a few patients. (See Hypertension Associated with Pheochromocytoma under Uses: Hypertension.)

It is recommended that labetalol be used with caution in patients with diabetes mellitus receiving hypoglycemic agents, especially those with labile disease or those prone to hypoglycemia since the drug may mask the signs and symptoms associated with acute hypoglycemia (e.g., tachycardia and blood pressure changes but not sweating). β-Adrenergic blocking agents also may impair glucose tolerance; delay the rate of recovery of blood glucose concentration following drug-induced hypoglycemia; alter the hemodynamic response to hypoglycemia, possibly resulting in an exaggerated hypertensive response; and possibly impair peripheral circulation. (See Cautions: Endocrine Effects.) However, many clinicians state that patients with diabetes mellitus may be particularly likely to experience a reduction in morbidity and mortality with the use of β-adrenergic blocking agents. (See Uses: Heart Failure, in Metoprolol 24:24.) If labetalol is used in diabetic patients receiving hypoglycemic agents, it may be necessary to adjust the dosage of the hypoglycemic agent.

The necessity of withdrawing β-adrenergic blocking therapy prior to major surgery is controversial. Severe, protracted hypotension and difficulty in restarting or maintaining a heart beat have occurred during surgery in some patients who have received β-adrenergic blocking agents. The effect of labetalol's α-adrenergic activity in patients undergoing major surgery has not been evaluated. However, several deaths have been reported in patients in whom labetalol hydrochloride injection was used during surgery, including those receiving the drug to control bleeding. In addition, a synergistic hypotensive response occurs in patients receiving IV labetalol and halothane anesthesia concomitantly. (See Drug Interactions: Halothane.) If labetalol therapy is continued in a patient undergoing major surgery, the anesthesiologist should be informed that the patient is receiving the drug.

Caution must be employed when reducing severely elevated blood pressure. The manufacturers state that IV labetalol is intended for use in hospitalized patients. When IV labetalol is used in patients with severely elevated blood pressure, the desired blood pressure reduction should be achieved over as long a period of time as is compatible with the patient's clinical status. Serious adverse effects, including cerebral infarction, optic nerve infarction, angina, and ischemic changes in the ECG, have been reported with other hypotensive agents when severely elevated blood pressure was reduced over periods ranging from several hours to as long as 1 or 2 days. Rapid or excessive reductions in systolic or diastolic blood pressure should be avoided; while these effects are unlikely with the recommended dosage schedules of IV labetalol, they can occasionally occur. Transient hypotension occurring with IV labetalol is usually readily managed by placing the patient in Trendelenburg's position, administering IV fluids, and/or temporarily discontinuing administration of the drug. Patients should remain supine during and for up to 3 hours after IV administration of the drug, since symptomatic orthostatic hypotension is likely to occur if they are tilted upward or allowed to assume an upright position during this period. The patient's ability to tolerate an upright position should be established before any ambulation (e.g., use of toilet facilities) is permitted; the patient should be advised on how to proceed gradually to become ambulatory and should be observed at the time of initial ambulation.

Labetalol should be used with caution in patients with impaired hepatic function, since metabolism of the drug may be decreased in such patients. Since labetalol has been rarely associated with the development of jaundice, hepatitis, severe hepatocellular injury, and elevated liver function test results, the manufacturers recommend that the drug be discontinued immediately if jaundice or laboratory evidence of hepatic injury occurs. Jaundice and hepatic dysfunction usually are reversible following discontinuance of the drug. Liver function tests should be performed at the first signs or symptoms of liver dysfunction (e.g., pruritus, dark urine, persistent anorexia, jaundice, right upper quadrant tenderness, flu-like syndrome).

Routine laboratory tests are usually not required before or after IV administration of labetalol, but the manufacturers recommend that laboratory parameters be monitored at regular intervals in patients receiving long-term oral therapy with the drug. In patients with concomitant illnesses (e.g., impaired renal function), appropriate tests should be performed to monitor these conditions.

Patients should be advised that transient scalp tingling may occur, usually during initiation of labetalol therapy.

Patients with a history of atopy or severe anaphylactic reactions to a variety of allergens may be more reactive to repeated, accidental, diagnostic, or therapeutic challenge with such allergens while receiving a β-adrenergic blocking agent. These patients may be less responsive than other patients to usual dosages of epinephrine or may develop a paradoxical response to epinephrine when that drug is used to treat anaphylactic reactions.

Labetalol is contraindicated in patients with a history of obstructive airway disease (e.g., bronchial asthma), overt cardiac failure, heart block of severity greater than first degree, cardiogenic shock, severe bradycardia, and/or other conditions associated with severe and prolonged hypotension. The drug also is contraindicated in patients with a history of hypersensitivity to any component of the formulation.

Because of similarity in spelling between labetalol hydrochloride and Lamictal® (the trade name for lamotrigine, an anticonvulsant agent), several dispensing errors have been reported to the manufacturer of Lamictal® (GlaxoSmithKline). These medication errors may be associated with serious adverse events either due to lack of appropriate therapy for seizures (e.g., in patients not receiving the prescribed anticonvulsant, lamotrigine, which may lead to status epilepticus) or, alternatively, to the risk of developing adverse effects (e.g., serious rash) associated with the use of lamotrigine in patients for whom the drug was not prescribed and consequently was not properly titrated. Therefore, the manufacturer of Lamictal® cautions that extra care should be exercised in ensuring the accuracy of both oral and written prescriptions for Lamictal® and labetalol. The manufacturer also recommends that when appropriate, clinicians might consider including the intended use of the particular drug on the prescription in addition to alerting patients to carefully check the drug they receive and promptly bring any question or concern to the attention of the dispensing pharmacist. The manufacturer also recommends that pharmacists assess the measures of avoiding dispensing errors and implement them as appropriate (e.g., placing drugs with similar names apart from one another in product storage areas, patient counseling).

■ **Pediatric Precautions** Although safety and efficacy remain to be fully established in children, some experts have recommended pediatric dosages for hypertension based on clinical experience. For information on overall principles and expert recommendations for treatment of hypertension in pediatric patients, see Uses: Hypertension in Pediatric Patients, in the Thiazides General Statement 40:28.20.

■ **Geriatric Precautions** Orthostatic hypotension, dizziness, or lightheadedness, similar to that reported in younger adults, have been reported in geriatric patients (i.e., those 60 years of age or older) receiving labetalol. Geriatric individuals are generally more likely than younger adults to experience orthostatic symptoms and these individuals should be cautioned about the possibility of these adverse effects during therapy with the drug. Because elimination of labetalol may be decreased in some geriatric patients, usual maintenance dosage of the drug is slightly lower in geriatric individuals than in younger adults. (See Dosage and Administration: Dosage.)

■ **Mutagenicity and Carcinogenicity** It is not known if labetalol is mutagenic or carcinogenic in humans. No evidence of labetalol-induced mutagenesis was seen with the modified Ames test or in studies in mice and rats using dominant lethal assays.

No evidence of carcinogenesis was seen in mice receiving oral labetalol hydrochloride dosages up to 200 mg/kg daily for 18 months or in rats receiving oral dosages up to 225 mg/kg daily for up to 113 weeks in females and up to 116 weeks in males.

■ **Pregnancy, Fertility, and Lactation** Reproduction studies in rats and rabbits using oral labetalol hydrochloride dosages up to about 6 and 4 times the maximum recommended human dosage, respectively, have not revealed reproducible evidence of fetal malformation; however, oral dosages approximating the maximum recommended human dosage were associated with an increased incidence of fetal resorption in both species. There was no evidence of drug-related fetotoxicity in rabbits receiving IV dosages of the drug up to 1.7 times the maximum recommended human dosage.In rats, oral administration of labetalol hydrochloride at dosages 2–4 times the maximum recommended human dosage during the period of late gestation through weaning was associated with decreased neonatal survival. Reproduction studies in rats or rabbits using combined oral labetalol hydrochloride and hydrochlorothiazide dosages up to about 15 and 80 times the maximum recommended human dosage, respectively, have not revealed evidence of teratogenicity, although combined oral dosages 3.5 and 20 times the maximum recommended human dosage, respectively, were maternotoxic with resultant fetotoxicity in rabbits. The combination appeared to be more toxic than either drug alone in rabbits.

Labetalol has been used orally for the management of hypertension in pregnant women and IV to control blood pressure in severely hypertensive pregnant women requiring urgent blood pressure reduction. (See Hypertension during Pregnancy under Uses: Hypertension.) Labetalol has been effective for the management of hypertension associated with pregnancy, and is one of several preferred agents for such use. Infants of mothers who received labetalol for the management of hypertension during pregnancy have not appeared to be adversely affected by the drug; however, transient hypotension (including slight decreases in systolic blood pressure during the first 24 hours after delivery), bradycardia, respiratory depression, and hypoglycemia have been reported rarely in neonates. Maternal labetalol therapy reportedly has been associated with a beneficial effect on development of fetal pulmonary maturity. Use of labetalol in pregnant women with hypertension does not appear to affect the usual course of labor and delivery, and the drug has been used IV to treat severe hypertension during labor. Following a single IV dose of the drug in pregnant women with preeclampsia, maternal blood pressure was reduced but placental and fetal blood flow were not affected. The manufacturers state that there are no adequate and controlled studies to date using labetalol in pregnant women, and the drug should be used during pregnancy only when the potential benefits justify the possible risks to the fetus.

The effects of labetalol on fertility in humans have not been fully determined. Ejaculatory failure and impotence in males and decreased libido have been reported in patients receiving labetalol.

Since small amounts (about 0.004% of the maternal dose) of labetalol are distributed into milk, the drug should be used with caution in nursing women.

Drug Interactions

Since IV labetalol hydrochloride may be administered to patients receiving other drugs, including other hypotensive agents, careful monitoring of these patients is necessary to detect and promptly treat any adverse effect resulting from concomitant administration.

■ Diuretics and Cardiovascular Drugs When labetalol is administered with diuretics or other hypotensive drugs, the hypotensive effect may be increased. This effect is usually used to therapeutic advantage, but careful adjustment of dosage is necessary to avoid excessive hypotension when these drugs are used concomitantly. When β-adrenergic blocking agents are administered with calcium-channel blocking agents, therapeutic as well as adverse effects may be additive. Slowing or complete suppression of SA node activity with development of slow ventricular rates (e.g., 30–40 bpm), often misdiagnosed as complete AV block, has been reported in patients receiving the nondihydropyridine calcium-channel blocking agent mibefradil (no longer commercially available in the US), principally in geriatric patients and in association with concomitant β-adrenergic blocker therapy. The manufacturers of labetalol and some clinicians state that labetalol and a calcium-channel blocking agent (e.g., verapamil, diltiazem) should be used concomitantly with caution.

■ Halothane Concomitant administration of IV labetalol and halothane anesthesia results in a synergistic hypotensive effect, the degree and duration of which may be controlled by adjusting the halothane concentration; however, excessive hypotension can result in a large reduction in cardiac output and an increase in central venous pressure. To minimize the risk of excessive hypotension during controlled hypotensive anesthesia with IV labetalol and halothane, inspired halothane concentrations of 3% or higher should *not* be used. If labetalol therapy is continued in a patient undergoing major surgery, the anesthesiologist should be informed that the patient is receiving the drug.

■ Cimetidine Concomitant administration of oral cimetidine has been shown to substantially increase the absolute bioavailability of oral labetalol, possibly via enhanced absorption or decreased first-pass hepatic metabolism of labetalol. If labetalol and cimetidine are administered concomitantly, dosage of labetalol required for optimal control of blood pressure should be carefully adjusted.

■ Glutethimide Concomitant administration of oral glutethimide (no longer commercially available in the US) has been shown to substantially decrease the absolute bioavailability of oral labetalol, possibly by increasing first-pass hepatic metabolism (glucuronidation) of labetalol. If labetalol and glutethimide are administered concomitantly, dosage of labetalol required for optimal control of blood pressure should be carefully adjusted.

■ Other Drugs Labetalol, like other drugs with β-adrenergic blocking activity, can antagonize the bronchodilation produced by β-adrenergic agonists in patients with bronchospasm, and greater than usual dosages of β-adrenergic agonist bronchodilators may be required in patients receiving labetalol.

Labetalol antagonizes the reflex tachycardia produced by nitroglycerin without preventing the hypotensive effect of the nitrate. If labetalol is used concurrently with nitroglycerin, an additive hypotensive effect may occur.

An increased incidence of tremor has been reported in patients receiving labetalol and tricyclic antidepressants concomitantly compared with those receiving labetalol alone. Although the contribution of each drug to this adverse reaction is not known, the possibility of a drug interaction cannot be excluded.

Laboratory Test Interferences

■ Urinary Catecholamines The presence of labetalol metabolites in urine may result in false-positive elevations of urinary free and total catecholamines, metanephrine, normetanephrine, and 3-methoxy-4-hydroxymandelic acid (vanillylmandelic acid, VMA) measured by fluorometric or photometric methods. When screening labetalol-treated patients suspected of having pheochromocytoma or when evaluating labetalol-treated patients with the tumor, specific assay methods such as high-performance liquid chromatography (HPLC) with solid phase extraction should be used to determine concentrations of catecholamines or their metabolites.

Acute Toxicity

■ Pathogenesis The acute lethal dose of labetalol in humans is not known. The oral LD_{50} of labetalol hydrochloride is approximately 0.6, greater than 2, and greater than 1 g/kg in mice, rats, and dogs, respectively; the IV LD_{50} in these species is about 50–60 mg/kg.

■ Manifestations In general, overdosage of labetalol may be expected to produce effects that are extensions of pharmacologic effects, particularly those involving the cardiovascular system; hypotension (which is posture dependent and may be severe), bradycardia (which may be severe), cardiac failure, and bronchospasm may occur. Common, dose-related adverse effects (e.g., nausea, vomiting, headache) might also occur. In one adult who was reported to have intentionally ingested labetalol hydrochloride 7.2 g, acebutolol hydrochloride 9.6 g, and trimipramine 625 mg, loss of consciousness, bradycardia, and profound hypotension resulted.

■ Treatment Treatment of labetalol overdosage generally involves symptomatic and supportive care. Following acute ingestion of the drug, the stomach should be emptied immediately by inducing emesis or by gastric lavage. If the patient is comatose, having seizures, or lacks the gag reflex, gastric lavage may be performed if an endotracheal tube with cuff inflated is in place to prevent aspiration of gastric contents. Administration of activated charcoal after emesis or gastric lavage may be useful in preventing absorption of labetalol, although specific data are not available. Patients should be placed in a supine position and their legs elevated if necessary to improve blood supply to the brain. For symptomatic bradycardia, atropine or epinephrine may be given. A vasopressor (e.g., norepinephrine, dopamine) may be given for severe hypotension. For heart failure, a cardiac glycoside and diuretic may be used; dopamine or dobutamine may also be useful. Glucagon may also be useful for the management of myocardial depression and hypotension. A β_2-adrenergic agonist and/or a theophylline derivative may be used for bronchospasm. For seizures, diazepam may be used. Labetalol is not appreciably removed (less than 1% of a dose) by hemodialysis or peritoneal dialysis.

Pharmacology

Labetalol is a nonselective β-adrenergic blocking agent and a selective α_1-adrenergic blocking agent. The pharmacology of labetalol is complex and in some ways resembles that of other β-adrenergic blocking agents and that of postsynaptic α_1-adrenergic blocking agents such as prazosin; however, the overall pharmacologic profile of labetalol differs from that of these other drugs. The β-adrenergic blocking activity of labetalol is approximately 3 or 7 times greater than the α-adrenergic blocking activity following oral or IV administration, respectively; it has not been clearly established whether the ratio changes with dosage of the drug or following long-term administration.

The principal physiologic action of labetalol is to competitively block adrenergic stimulation of β-receptors within the myocardium (β_1-receptors) and within bronchial and vascular smooth muscle (β_2-receptors) and α_1-receptors within vascular smooth muscle. In addition to inhibiting access of endogenous or exogenous catecholamines to β-adrenergic receptors, labetalol has been shown to exhibit some intrinsic β_2-agonist activity in animals; however, the drug exerts little, if any, intrinsic β_1-agonist activity. Labetalol does not exhibit intrinsic α-adrenergic agonist activity. There is some evidence from animal studies suggesting that the drug may have a vasodilating effect, possibly resulting from a direct or β_2-agonist action. In animals, at doses greater than those required for α- or β-adrenergic blockade, labetalol also has a membrane-stabilizing effect on the heartwhich is similar to that of quinidine; however, this effect is unlikely to be clinically important since it occurs only at doses higher than those required for α- or β-adrenergic blockade.

■ Cardiovascular Effects The hemodynamic effects of labetalol are variable following oral or IV administration. Labetalol, unlike pure β-adrenergic blocking agents, produces a dose-dependent (at usual doses) decrease in systemic arterial blood pressure and systemic vascular resistance without a substantial reduction in resting heart rate, cardiac output, or stroke volume, apparently because of its combined α- and β-adrenergic blocking activity. Labetalol effectively reduces blood pressure in the standing or supine position, but because of the drug's α_1-adrenergic blocking activity, the effect on blood pressure is position dependent; labetalol-induced decreases in blood pressure are greater in the standing than in the supine position, and orthostatic hypotension can occur. (See Cautions: Cardiovascular Effects.) The blunting of exercise-induced increases in blood pressure by oral or IV labetalol is generally greater than that produced by pure β-adrenergic blocking agents (e.g., propranolol), but the blunting of exercise-induced tachycardia produced by labetalol is generally less than that produced by pure β-adrenergic blocking agents.

Following oral administration of labetalol hydrochloride dosages of 200 mg to 2.4 g daily for 1 week to 20 months in clinical studies in patients with hypertension, blood pressure and heart rate were reduced at rest or during exercise and in the supine or standing position. During oral labetalol therapy, cardiac output is generally decreased or unchanged and stroke volume is generally increased or unchanged; however, unlike most pure β-adrenergic blocking agents, oral labetalol usually decreases systemic vascular resistance. Following IV administration of single labetalol doses in patients with hypertension, the drug decreases blood pressure and systemic vascular resistance in the supine position without substantially reducing cardiac output or stroke volume. Although substantial changes in heart rate usually do not occur in the supine position following IV administration, heart rate and cardiac output generally are reduced in an upright or tilted upright position or during exercise. In one study in patients with severe hypertension, an initial 0.25-mg/kg IV dose of the drug decreased supine blood pressure by an average of 11/7 mm Hg; additional 0.5-mg/kg IV doses administered at 15-minute intervals up to a total cumulative dose of 1.75 mg/kg caused further dose-related decreases in blood pressure in these patients. Similar results in patients with severe hypertension have also been produced with an initial 20-mg IV dose followed by IV doses of 40 or 80 mg at 10-minute intervals until blood pressure was adequately controlled or a total cumulative dose of 300 mg was administered. Following continuous IV infusion of a mean labetalol hydrochloride dose of 136 mg (range: 27–300 mg) over 2–3 hours in patients with severe hypertension, blood pressure was reportedly decreased by an average of 60/35 mm Hg. IV administration of a single labetalol dose does not appear to produce a clinically important reduction in cerebral blood flow following rapid reduction of blood pressure in severely hypertensive patients, and long-term oral administration of the drug also does not appear to affect cerebral blood flow.

Following IV administration of labetalol in normotensive patients with coronary artery disease, blood pressure, heart rate, systemic vascular resistance, and coronary vascular resistance are generally decreased; cardiac index, left ventricular end-diastolic pressure (LVEDP), and pulmonary artery wedge pressure are generally unchanged; and coronary sinus blood flow may be increased. In patients with hypertension associated with acute myocardial infarction, IV labetalol decreases blood pressure and heart rate and generally decreases cardiac index and pulmonary artery wedge pressure. In normotensive patients with acute myocardial infarction, IV labetalol may decrease blood pressure, heart rate, and cardiac index without affecting systemic vascular resistance.

The electrophysiologic effects of labetalol are variable and appear to be mediated via the drug's myocardial β_1-adrenergic blocking activity. Labetalol may decrease conduction velocity through the atrioventricular (AV) node and increase the atrial effective refractory period (ERP), but the drug appears to have inconsistent effects on sinoatrial (SA) conduction time and the AV nodal refractory period; the decrease in AV nodal conduction velocity produced by labetalol is less than that produced by pure β-adrenergic blocking agents. In healthy individuals and in patients with cardiac disease (e.g., coronary artery disease), labetalol generally has little effect on sinus rate, intraventricular conduction, the His-Purkinje system, or duration of the QRS complex. In one study in hypertensive patients, oral labetalol therapy was associated with a substantial reduction in ventricular premature contractions, and in another study in hypertensive patients, IV labetalol rapidly restored sinus rhythm in some patients with supraventricular or ventricular arrhythmias. Further studies are needed to adequately evaluate the drug's antiarrhythmic activity.

■ **Renal Effects** Unlike therapy with some pure β-adrenergic blocking agents (e.g., propranolol), labetalol therapy does not appear to be associated with a reduction in glomerular filtration rate or renal plasma flow following short- or long-term administration in patients with hypertension and normal renal function. Labetalol's apparent lack of effect on renal hemodynamics may be related to the drug's α-adrenergic blocking action on renal vasculature or its minimal effect on cardiac output. Use of the drug in patients with hypertension and chronic renal failure has generally not been associated with any deterioration in renal function. Although not consistently found, increases in plasma volume have been reported in some patients with hypertension receiving oral labetalol alone, and edema and/or fluid retention have been reported in some patients during therapy with the drug.

In several studies in patients with hypertension and elevated plasma renin activity (PRA), long-term oral administration of labetalol hydrochloride (150 mg to 2.4 g daily) has been reported to suppress PRA at rest and during exercise, and in the supine and standing positions; in most of the studies, the net suppressive effect on renin was generally proportional to basal PRA. In other studies, labetalol has been reported to have an inconsistent overall effect on resting PRA, but there was considerable interindividual variation in PRA in these studies. Following acute IV administration, labetalol has been reported to produce substantial reductions in plasma angiotensin II concentration, particularly in patients with high basal values. Although labetalol has been reported to have little, if any, effect on plasma aldosterone concentration following long-term oral administration in several studies, there is some evidence that the drug may decrease plasma aldosterone concentration following oral or IV administration. Labetalol has also been reported to decrease urinary aldosterone excretion following oral administration in patients with hypertension.

■ **Endocrine and Metabolic Effects** The exact mechanism is unknown and the effect has not been clinically important, but labetalol may increase plasma glucose concentration. Serum cholesterol and triglyceride concentrations have generally been unchanged or very slightly decreased during labetalol therapy; although data currently are limited, long-term administration of the drug does not appear to be associated with any clinically important adverse effects on plasma lipid concentrations. Labetalol does not appear to substantially alter serum concentrations of insulin, C-peptide, free fatty acids, growth hormone, or prolactin; however, following IV administration in one preliminary study, labetalol caused a substantial increase in serum prolactin concentration which was more marked in females than in males. Although subsequent studies have not demonstrated an effect on serum prolactin concentration following oral administration of the drug, IV administration appears to be associated with hyperprolactinemia, apparently resulting from a drug-induced CNS effect; the clinical importance of this finding is not known.

■ **Respiratory Effects** Through its β_2-adrenergic blocking action in the respiratory tract, labetalol may increase airway resistance, especially in patients with asthma or chronic obstructive pulmonary disease; however, since α-adrenergic receptors in the respiratory tract may be involved in the pathogenesis of bronchoconstriction, it is possible that the α-adrenergic blocking action of labetalol may attenuate some of the potential adverse respiratory effects resulting from the drug's β-adrenergic blocking action. In addition, labetalol's apparent β_2-adrenergic agonist activity may contribute to attenuation of the drug's potential adverse respiratory effects. Although an increase in airway resistance as measured by forced expiratory volume in 1 second (FEV_1) or by resting and post-exercise peak expiratory flow rates was not observed in many studies in healthy individuals or patients with asthma or chronic obstructive pulmonary disease (COPD) who received labetalol, evidence of increased airway resistance has occurred in some studies in healthy individuals or in patients with or without COPD who received the drug. Labetalol's effect on airway resistance generally appears to be less than that of nonselective β-adrenergic blocking agents (e.g., propranolol), but generally comparable to that of β_1-selective agents (e.g., atenolol). Labetalol has been used without evidence of a substantial increase in airway resistance in a limited number of hypertensive patients with bronchial asthma in whom propranolol had increased airway resistance.

Pharmacokinetics

■ **Absorption** Labetalol hydrochloride is rapidly and approximately 90–100% absorbed from the GI tract following oral administration, but the drug undergoes extensive first-pass metabolism in the liver and/or GI mucosa. Only about 25% of an oral dose reaches systemic circulation unchanged in fasted adults. Although absolute bioavailability in one study reportedly ranged from 11–86% (mean: 33%) following oral administration of a single 100-mg dose in fasted adults, the considerable interindividual variability in this study may have resulted from use of a relatively insensitive spectrofluorometric assay. Food delays GI absorption of labetalol hydrochloride but increases absolute bioavailability of the drug, possibly by decreasing first-pass metabolism and/or hepatic blood flow. Following oral administration of a single 200-mg dose in healthy adults in one study, absolute bioavailability of the drug averaged 26 and 36% in the fasted and nonfasted state, respectively. First-pass metabolism may also be reduced and bioavailability substantially increased in geriatric patients and in patients with hepatic dysfunction. However, in one study in patients with hepatosplenic schistosomiasis, mean absolute bioavailability of the drug was reportedly decreased when compared with healthy individuals. Oral cimetidine increases, and glutethimide decreases, the bioavailability of labetalol. (See Drug Interactions.) Concomitant oral administration of labetalol hydrochloride and hydrochlorothiazide does not affect the bioavailability of either drug.

Following multiple-dose oral administration of labetalol hydrochloride, peak plasma concentrations are generally achieved within 40 minutes to 2 hours. Peak plasma concentrations reportedly increase proportionately with oral dosage at dosages ranging from 100 mg to 3 g daily. In one study in hypertensive patients, peak plasma labetalol concentration following oral administration of 200 mg 3 times daily or 300 mg twice daily averaged 323 or 430 ng/mL, respectively, and the steady-state plasma drug concentration averaged 149 or 145 ng/mL, respectively; based on pharmacokinetic and pharmacodynamic (i.e., blood pressure response) evaluation, these dosage regimens were considered equivalent. Following IV injection over 1 minute of a 1.5-mg/kg dose of labetalol hydrochloride in one study, a mean peak plasma concentration of about 5.7 mcg/mL occurred 2 minutes after injection and plasma concentration had declined to an average of 575 ng/mL at 10.5 minutes after injection.

The relationship between plasma labetalol concentration and pharmacologic effects of the drug has not been clearly established. Relationships between pharmacologic effects (e.g., blood pressure response, response of exercise-induced tachycardia) and dose, logarithm of plasma labetalol concentration, and/or area under the plasma concentration-time curve (AUC) have been reported in some studies, but such relationships were not found in other studies. In general, there appears to be a correlation between plasma labetalol concentration and blood pressure reduction, particularly in the upright position, but there is wide interindividual variation.

Following oral administration of labetalol hydrochloride, the hypotensive effect of the drug is generally apparent within 20 minutes to 2 hours, maximal within 1–4 hours, and persists in a dose-dependent manner for about 8–12 or 12–24 hours after a single 200- or 300-mg dose, respectively. The maximum, steady-state blood pressure response with twice-daily dosing occurs within 1–3 days. Following slow, direct IV injection of the drug, the hypotensive effect is apparent within 2–5 minutes, is usually maximal within 5–15 minutes, and generally persists for about 2–4 hours, although a longer duration of effect (i.e., up to 24 hours) has been reported in some patients.

■ **Distribution** Following IV administration, labetalol is rapidly and widely distributed into the extravascular space. The drug has an apparent volume of distribution of 3.2–15.7 L/kg. In one study in healthy adults, the volume of distribution in the central compartment (V_c) and at steady state (V_{ss}) averaged 1.1 and 9.4 L/kg, respectively. The apparent volume of distribution is reportedly decreased in patients with impaired hepatic function but is similar to that of healthy individuals in patients with impaired renal function or in pregnant women. In animals, the drug distributes in highest concentrations into the lungs, liver, and kidneys; only minimal amounts cross the blood-brain barrier.

In vitro, labetalol is approximately 50% bound to plasma proteins at plasma labetalol concentrations of 0.1–50 mcg/mL.

Labetalol crosses the placenta. In one study in several pregnant women receiving the drug orally (200 mg 3 times daily) for about 7 days, the median ratio of fetal cord to maternal plasma concentration at parturition was 0.5. Small amounts of unchanged labetalol have been shown to distribute into the fetal uveal tract following administration of radiolabeled drug in pregnant animals; the drug bound reversibly to melanin in the uveal tract but was not oculotoxic. Small amounts of labetalol and its metabolites are distributed into milk, principally as unbound labetalol.

■ **Elimination** Plasma concentrations of labetalol appear to decline in a biphasic or possibly triphasic manner. In healthy adults and adults with hypertension, the half-life in the distribution phase ($t_{1/2\alpha}$) has been reported to average 6–44 minutes and the half-life in the terminal elimination phase ($t_{1/2\beta}$) has been reported to average 2.5–8 hours. The variability in reported mean half-lives for the drug may have resulted in part from use of a relatively insensitive spectrofluorometric assay in some studies. The manufacturers state that the drug has a plasma elimination half-life of 5.5 or 6–8 hours following IV or oral administration, respectively. The elimination half-life of the drug appears to be unchanged in individuals with renal or hepatic impairment, but may be increased in patients with severe renal impairment (i.e., creatinine clearance less than 10 mL/minute) undergoing dialysis. Results of some studies indicate that elimination of labetalol may be reduced in geriatric individuals; elimination half-life of the drug reportedly may be slightly increased (but within the reported range) in some geriatric individuals. Total body clearance of labetalol from plasma has been reported to average 19–33 mL/minute per kg in individuals with normal renal and hepatic function. Plasma clearance appears to be unaffected by renal impairment but may be decreased in patients with hepatic impairment.

Labetalol is extensively metabolized in the liver and possibly in the GI mucosa following oral administration, principally by conjugation with glucuronic acid. The major metabolite is the *O*-alkylglucuronide, with smaller amounts of the *O*-phenylglucuronide and *N*-glucuronide being formed. Following oral administration, labetalol undergoes extensive first-pass metabolism in the liver and/or GI mucosa. (See Pharmacokinetics: Absorption.)

Labetalol and its metabolites are excreted in feces via biliary elimination and in urine. About 55–60% of a dose is excreted in urine, mainly as glucuronide conjugates, within 24 hours, and about 30% is excreted in feces within 4 days. Less than 5% of a dose is excreted unchanged in urine. Labetalol is not appreciably removed (less than 1% of a dose) by hemodialysis or peritoneal dialysis.

Chemistry and Stability

■ **Chemistry** Labetalol hydrochloride is an α- and β-adrenergic blocking agent. The drug is commercially available as a racemic mixture of its 4 stereoisomers. The *RR*-isomer, dilevalol, makes up 25% of the racemic mixture. Dilevalol has about 2–4 times the β-adrenergic blocking activity of the racemic mixture but has only minimal α_1-adrenergic blocking activity; dilevalol also appears to possess some β_2-agonist activity. Most of the α_1-adrenergic blocking activity of labetalol hydrochloride is attributable to the *SR*-isomer.

Labetalol hydrochloride occurs as a white or off-white crystalline powder and is sparingly soluble in water (approximately 20 mg/mL) and freely soluble to soluble in alcohol (at least 100 mg/mL). Labetalol is less lipophilic than propranolol but more lipophilic than most other currently available β-adrenergic blocking agents. The drug has a pK_a of 9.3. Labetalol hydrochloride injection is a sterile, isotonic solution of the drug in water for injection. The injection occurs as a clear, colorless to light yellow solution and has a pH of 3–4. The injection also contains parabens as preservatives, dextrose, and edetate sodium; citric acid and sodium hydroxide may be added during manufacture of the injection to adjust pH.

■ **Stability** Labetalol hydrochloride tablets should be stored in well-closed containers at 2–30°C; tablets in unit-dose packages should be protected from excessive moisture. Labetalol hydrochloride injection should be stored at 2–30°C and protected from light and freezing. Labetalol hydrochloride tablets and injection have an expiration date of 3 and 2 years, respectively, after the date of manufacture.

Labetalol hydrochloride is most stable in solutions having a pH of 2–4. The drug is physically and chemically compatible with the following IV solutions: 5% dextrose; 0.9% sodium chloride; 2.5% dextrose and 0.45% sodium chloride; 5% dextrose and 0.2, 0.33, or 0.9% sodium chloride; 5% dextrose and lactated Ringer's or Ringer's; lactated Ringer's; or Ringer's. Following dilution of labetalol hydrochloride injection with one of these IV solutions, solutions containing 1.25–3.75 mg/mL are stable for at least 24 hours when refrigerated or stored at room temperature. In one study, these solutions were stable for at least 72 hours at 4 or 25°C. Appreciable changes in pH or osmolarity of these IV solutions did not occur following admixture of labetalol hydrochloride injection. The drug is physically and/or chemically incompatible with 5% sodium bicarbonate injection; labetalol hydrochloride solutions containing 1.25–3.75 mg/mL in 5% sodium bicarbonate have a pH of 7.6–8 and form a white precipitate, probably the free base, within 6 hours after admixture. A white precipitate also has been observed following concomitant infusion of other alkaline drugs (e.g., furosemide) and labetalol hydrochloride injection; therefore, labetalol hydrochloride injection should not be given in the same infusion line with other alkaline solutions.

Preparations

Excipients in commercially available drug preparations may have clinically important effects in some individuals; consult specific product labeling for details.

Labetalol Hydrochloride

Oral		
Tablets, film-coated	100 mg*	**Labetalol Hydrochloride Tablets**
	200 mg*	**Labetalol Hydrochloride Tablets**
	300 mg*	**Labetalol Hydrochloride Tablets**
Parenteral		
Injection, for IV use	5 mg/mL*	**Labetalol Hydrochloride Injection**

*available from one or more manufacturer, distributor, and/or repackager by generic (nonproprietary) name

†Use is not currently included in the labeling approved by the US Food and Drug Administration

Metoprolol Succinate
Metoprolol Tartrate

■ Metoprolol is a β_1-selective adrenergic blocking agent (β-blocker).

Uses

Metoprolol is used for the management of hypertension, angina, acute myocardial infarction (MI), and heart failure. The drug also has been used for supraventricular and ventricular tachyarrhythmias† and prophylaxis of migraine headache†.

The choice of a β-adrenergic blocking agent (β-blocker) depends on numerous factors, including pharmacologic properties (e.g., relative β-selectivity, intrinsic sympathomimetic activity, membrane-stabilizing activity, lipophilicity), pharmacokinetics, intended use, and adverse effect profile, as well as the patient's coexisting disease states or conditions, response, and tolerance. While specific pharmacologic properties and other factors may appropriately influence the choice of a β-blocker in individual patients, evidence of clinically important differences among the agents in terms of overall efficacy and/or safety is limited. Patients who do not respond to or cannot tolerate one β-blocker may be successfully treated with a different agent.

In the management of hypertension or chronic stable angina pectoris in patients with chronic obstructive pulmonary disease (COPD) or type 1 diabetes mellitus, many clinicians prefer to use low dosages of a β_1-selective adrenergic blocking agent (e.g., atenolol, metoprolol), rather than a nonselective agent (e.g., nadolol, pindolol, propranolol, timolol). However, selectivity of these agents is relative and dose dependent. Some clinicians also will recommend using a β_1-selective agent or an agent with intrinsic sympathomimetic activity (ISA) (e.g., pindolol), rather than a nonselective agent, for the management of hypertension or angina pectoris in patients with peripheral vascular disease, but there is no evidence that the choice of β-blocker substantially affects efficacy.

■ **Hypertension** Metoprolol is used alone or in combination with other classes of antihypertensive agents in the management of hypertension. β-Blockers often are used concurrently with a diuretic because of their additive effects. β-Blockers also have been combined with vasodilators (e.g., hydralazine, minoxidil) to counteract the reflex tachycardia that occurs with vasodilators.

Metoprolol's efficacy in the management of hypertension is similar to that of other β-blockers; however, metoprolol may be preferred over a nonselective β-blocker, like propranolol, in hypertensive patients with certain concomitant disease states. Metoprolol may be associated with less risk of bronchospasm than propranolol in patients with bronchitis. Metoprolol's relative cardioselectivity may be advantageous in hypertensive patients with concomitant heart failure controlled by diuretics and cardiac glycosides; however, it remains to be established whether metoprolol is less likely to cause heart failure in these patients than is propranolol. In patients with catecholamine excess (e.g., pheochromocytoma, drug-induced hypoglycemia, or acute withdrawal of adrenergic blocking agents), metoprolol reportedly is less likely to produce impairment of peripheral circulation, heart failure, and hypertensive reactions than is propranolol. Because metoprolol may cause less inhibition of glycogenolysis than does propranolol, metoprolol may be preferred in patients with diabetes mellitus who are receiving insulin or oral antidiabetic agents (e.g., sulfonylurea drugs); however, additional study is required.

In contrast to many other antihypertensive agents, metoprolol lowers blood pressure equally well in the upright or supine position. The drug appears to be safe and effective in the management of hypertension in patients with renal damage. Although metoprolol is apparently more effective in reducing blood pressure in patients with normal or elevated plasma renin concentrations, the drug also lowers blood pressure in patients with low renin hypertension. Tolerance to the antihypertensive effect of metoprolol apparently does not occur during long-term administration.

Current evidence-based practice guidelines for the management of hypertension in adults generally recommend the use of drugs from 4 classes of antihypertensive agents (angiotensin-converting enzyme [ACE] inhibitors, angiotensin II receptor antagonists, calcium-channel blockers, and thiazide diuretics). Most guidelines no longer recommend β-blockers as first-line therapy for hypertension because of the lack of established superiority over other recommended drug classes and evidence from at least one study demonstrating that β-blockers may be less effective than angiotensin II receptor antagonists in preventing cardiovascular death, MI, or stroke. However, therapy with a β-blocker may still be considered in hypertensive patients who have a compelling indication (e.g., prior MI, ischemic heart disease, heart failure) for their use or as add-on therapy in those who do not respond adequately to the preferred drug classes. (See Considerations for Drug Therapy in Patients with Underlying Cardiovascular and Other Risk Factors, under Uses: Hypertension.) Ultimately, choice of antihypertensive therapy should be individualized, considering the clinical characteristics of the patient (e.g., age, ethnicity/race, comorbid conditions, cardiovascular risk factors) as well as drug-related factors (e.g., ease of administration, availability, adverse effects, costs).

General Considerations for Initial and Maintenance Antihypertensive Therapy **Nonpharmacologic Therapy.** Nonpharmacologic measures (i.e., lifestyle/behavioral modifications) that are effective in lowering blood pressure include weight reduction (for those who are overweight or obese), dietary changes to include foods such as fruits, vegetables, whole grains, and low-fat dairy products that are rich in potassium, calcium, magnesium, and fiber (i.e., adoption of the Dietary Approaches to Stop Hypertension [DASH] eating plan), sodium reduction, increased physical activity, and moderation of alcohol intake. Such lifestyle/behavioral modifications, including smoking cessation, enhance antihypertensive drug efficacy and decrease cardiovascular risk and remain an indispensable part of the management of hypertension. Lifestyle/behavioral modifications without antihypertensive drug therapy are recommended for individuals classified by a 2017 multidisciplinary hypertension guideline of the American College of Cardiology (ACC), American Heart Association (AHA), and a number of other professional organizations as having elevated blood pressure (systolic blood pressure 120–129 mm Hg and diastolic blood pressure less than 80 mm Hg) and in those with stage 1 hypertension (systolic blood pressure 130–139 mm Hg or diastolic blood pressure 80–89 mm Hg) who do *not* have preexisting cardiovascular disease or an estimated 10-year atherosclerotic cardiovascular disease (ASCVD) risk of 10% or greater.

Initiation of Drug Therapy. Drug therapy in the management of hypertension must be individualized and adjusted based on the degree of blood pressure elevation while also considering cardiovascular risk factors. Drug therapy generally is reserved for patients who respond inadequately to nondrug therapy (i.e., lifestyle modifications such as diet [including sodium restriction and adequate potassium and calcium intake], regular aerobic physical activity, moderation of alcohol consumption, and weight reduction) or in whom the degree of blood pressure elevation or coexisting risk factors requires more prompt or aggressive therapy; however, the optimum blood pressure threshold for initiating antihypertensive drug therapy and specific treatment goals remain controversial.

The 2017 ACC/AHA hypertension guideline and many experts currently state that the treatment of hypertension should be based not only on blood pressure values but also on patients' cardiovascular risk factors. For *secondary prevention* of recurrent cardiovascular disease events in adults with clinical cardiovascular disease or for *primary prevention* in adults with an estimated 10-year ASCVD risk of 10% or higher, the 2017 ACC/AHA hypertension guideline recommends initiation of antihypertensive drug therapy in conjunction with lifestyle/behavioral modifications at an average systolic blood pressure of 130 mm Hg or an average diastolic blood pressure of 80 mm Hg or higher. For *primary prevention* of cardiovascular disease events in adults with a low (less than 10%) estimated 10-year risk of ASCVD, the 2017 ACC/AHA hypertension guideline recommends initiation of antihypertensive drug therapy in conjunction with lifestyle/behavioral modifications at a systolic blood pressure of 140 mm Hg or higher or a diastolic blood pressure of 90 mm Hg or higher. After initiation of antihypertensive drug therapy, regardless of the ASCVD risk, the 2017 ACC/AHA hypertension guideline generally recommends a blood pressure goal of less than 130/80 mm Hg in all adults. In addition, a systolic blood pressure goal of less than 130 mm Hg also is recommended for noninstitutionalized ambulatory patients 65 years of age or older with an average systolic blood pressure of at least 130 mm Hg. While these blood pressure goals are lower than those recommended for most patients in previous guidelines, they are based upon clinical studies demonstrating continuing reduction of cardiovascular risk at progressively lower levels of systolic blood pressure.

Most data indicate that patients with a higher cardiovascular risk will benefit the most from tighter blood pressure control; however, some experts state this treatment goal also may be beneficial in those at lower cardiovascular risk. Other clinicians believe that the benefits of such blood pressure lowering do not outweigh the risks in those patients considered to be at lower risk of cardiovascular disease and that reclassifying individuals formerly considered to have prehypertension as having hypertension may potentially lead to use of drug therapy in such patients without consideration of cardiovascular risk. Previous hypertension guidelines, such as those from the JNC 8 expert panel, generally have recommended initiation of antihypertensive treatment in patients with a systolic blood pressure of at least 140 mm Hg or a diastolic blood pressure of at least 90 mm Hg, targeted a blood pressure goal of less than 140/90 mm Hg regardless of cardiovascular risk, and used higher systolic blood pressure thresholds and targets in geriatric patients. Some clinicians continue to support the target blood pressures recommended by the JNC 8 expert panel because of concerns that such recommendations in the 2017 ACC/AHA hypertension guideline are based on extrapolation of data from the high-risk population in the SPRINT study to a lower-risk population. Also, because more than 90% of patients in SPRINT were already receiving antihypertensive drugs at baseline, data are lacking on the effects of *initiating* drug therapy at a lower blood pressure threshold (130/80 mm Hg) in patients at high risk of cardiovascular disease. The potential benefits of hypertension management and drug cost, adverse effects, and risks associated with the use of multiple antihypertensive drugs should be considered when deciding a patient's treatment goal.

The 2017 ACC/AHA hypertension guideline recommends an ASCVD risk assessment for all adults with hypertension; however, experts state that it can be assumed that patients with hypertension and diabetes mellitus or chronic kidney disease (CKD) are at high risk for cardiovascular disease and that antihypertensive drug therapy should be initiated in these patients at a blood pressure of 130/80 mm Hg or higher. ACC/AHA also recommends a blood pressure goal of less than 130/80 mm Hg in patients with hypertension and diabetes mellitus or CKD. These recommendations are based on a systematic review of high-quality evidence from randomized controlled trials, meta-analyses, and post hoc analyses that have demonstrated substantial reductions in the risk of important clinical outcomes (e.g., cardiovascular events) regardless of comorbid conditions or age when systolic blood pressure is lowered to less than 130 mm Hg. However, some clinicians have questioned the generalizability of findings from some of the trials (e.g., SPRINT) used to support the 2017 ACC/AHA hypertension guideline. For example, SPRINT included adults (mean age: 68 years) *without* diabetes mellitus who were at high risk of cardiovascular disease. While benefits of intensive blood pressure control were observed in this patient population, some clinicians have questioned whether these findings apply to younger patients who have a low risk of cardiovascular disease. In patients with CKD in the SPRINT trial, intensive blood pressure management (achieving a mean systolic blood pressure of approximately 122 mm Hg compared with 136 mm Hg with standard treatment) provided a similar beneficial reduction in the composite cardiovascular disease primary outcome and all-cause mortality as in the full patient cohort. Because most patients with CKD die from cardiovascular complications, the findings of this study further support a lower blood pressure target of less than 130/80 mm Hg. Data are lacking to determine the ideal blood pressure goal in patients with hypertension and diabetes mellitus; also, studies evaluating the benefits of intensive blood pressure control in patients with diabetes mellitus have provided conflicting results.

Clinical studies reviewed for the 2017 ACC/AHA hypertension guideline have shown similar quantitative benefits from blood pressure lowering in hypertensive patients with or without diabetes mellitus. In a randomized, controlled study (ACCORD-BP) that compared a higher (systolic blood pressure less than 140 mm Hg) versus lower (systolic blood pressure less than 120 mm Hg) blood pressure goal in patients with diabetes mellitus, there was no difference in the incidence of cardiovascular outcomes (e.g., composite outcome of cardiovascular death, nonfatal MI, and nonfatal stroke). However, some experts state that this study was underpowered to detect a difference between the 2 treatment groups and that the factorial design of the study complicated interpretation of the results. Although SPRINT did not include patients with diabetes mellitus, patients in this study with prediabetes demonstrated a similar cardiovascular benefit from intensive treatment of blood pressure as normoglycemic patients. A meta-analysis of data from ACCORD and SPRINT suggests that the findings of both studies are consistent and that patients with diabetes mellitus benefit from more intensive blood pressure control. These data support the 2017 ACC/AHA hypertension guideline recommendation of a blood pressure treatment goal of less than 130/80 mm Hg in patients with hypertension and diabetes mellitus. Alternatively, the American Diabetes Association (ADA) recommends a blood pressure goal of less than 140/90 mm Hg in patients with diabetes mellitus. The ADA states that a lower blood pressure goal (e.g., less than 130/80 mm Hg) may be appropriate for patients with a high risk of cardiovascular disease and diabetes mellitus if it can be achieved without undue treatment burden.

Further study is needed to more clearly define optimum blood pressure goals in patients with hypertension, particularly in high-risk groups (e.g., patients with diabetes mellitus, cardiovascular disease, or cerebrovascular disease; black patients); when determining appropriate blood pressure goals, individual risks and benefits should be considered in addition to the evidence from clinical studies.

Experts state that in patients with stage 1 hypertension (especially the elderly, those with a history of hypotension, or those who have experienced adverse drug effects), it is reasonable to initiate drug therapy using the stepped-care approach in which one drug is initiated and titrated and other drugs are added sequentially to achieve the target blood pressure. However, although some patients can begin treatment with a single antihypertensive agent, the 2017 ACC/AHA hypertension guideline recommends initiation of antihypertensive therapy with 2 drugs from different pharmacologic classes (either as separate agents or in a fixed-dose combination) in patients with stage 2 hypertension and an average blood pressure more than 20/10 mm Hg above their target blood pressure. Such combined therapy may increase the likelihood of achieving goal blood pressure in a more timely fashion, but also may increase the risk of adverse effects (e.g., orthostatic hypotension) in some patients (e.g., elderly). Drug regimens with complementary activity, where a second antihypertensive agent is used to block compensatory responses to the first agent or affect a different pressor mechanism, can result in additive blood pressure lowering and are preferred. Drug combinations that have similar mechanisms of action or clinical effects (e.g., the combination of an ACE inhibitor and an angiotensin II receptor antagonist) generally should be avoided. Many patients who begin therapy with a single antihypertensive agent will subsequently require at least 2 drugs from different pharmacologic classes to achieve their blood pressure goal. Experts state that other patient-specific factors, such as age, concurrent medications, drug adherence, drug interactions, the overall treatment regimen, cost, and comorbidities, also should be considered when deciding on an antihypertensive drug regimen. For any stage of hypertension, antihypertensive drug dosages should be adjusted and/or other agents substituted or added until goal blood pressure is achieved. (See Follow-up and Maintenance Drug Therapy under Hypertension: General Considerations for Initial and Maintenance Antihypertensive Therapy, in Uses.)

Follow-up and Maintenance Drug Therapy. Several strategies are used for the titration and combination of antihypertensive drugs; these strategies, which are generally based on those used in randomized controlled studies, include maximizing the dosage of the first drug before adding a second drug, adding a second drug before achieving maximum dosage of the initial drug, or initiating therapy with 2 drugs simultaneously (either as separate preparations or as a fixed-dose combination). Combined use of an ACE inhibitor and angiotensin II receptor antagonist should be avoided because of the potential risk of adverse renal effects. After initiating a new or adjusted antihypertensive drug regimen, patients should have their blood pressure reevaluated monthly until adequate blood pressure control is achieved. Effective blood pressure control can be achieved in most hypertensive patients, but many will ultimately require therapy with 2 or more antihypertensive drugs. In addition to measuring blood pressure, clinicians should evaluate patients for orthostatic hypotension, adverse drug effects, adherence to drug therapy and lifestyle modifications, and the need for drug dosage adjustments. Laboratory testing such as electrolytes and renal function status and other assessments of target organ damage also should be performed.

Considerations for Drug Therapy in Patients with Underlying Cardiovascular and Other Risk Factors Drug therapy in patients with hypertension and underlying cardiovascular or other risk factors should be carefully individualized based on the underlying disease(s), concomitant drugs, tolerance to drug-induced adverse effects, and blood pressure goal. (See Table 2 on Compelling Indications for Drug Classes based on Comorbid Conditions, under Uses: Hypertension in Adults, in the Thiazides General Statement 40:28.20.)

Ischemic Heart Disease. The selection of an appropriate antihypertensive agent in patients with ischemic heart disease should be based on individual patient characteristics, and may include a β-blocker, with the addition of other drugs (e.g., ACE inhibitors, thiazide diuretics, calcium-channel blockers) as necessary to achieve blood pressure goals. Because of the demonstrated mortality benefit of β-blockers following MI, these drugs should be administered in all patients who have survived an MI. The 2017 ACC/AHA hypertension guideline states that β-blockers used for ischemic heart disease/angina that are also effective in lowering blood pressure include bisoprolol, carvedilol, metoprolol succinate, metoprolol tartrate, nadolol, propranolol, and timolol.

Heart Failure. While β-blockers as single therapies are not superior to other antihypertensive agents in the reduction of all cardiovascular outcomes, certain β-blockers (bisoprolol, carvedilol, extended-release metoprolol succinate) have been shown to be effective in reducing the incidence of heart failure and associated morbidity and mortality. (See Uses: Heart Failure.)

Other Special Considerations for Antihypertensive Drug Therapy

Race. Most patients with hypertension, especially black patients, will require at least 2 antihypertensive drugs to achieve adequate blood pressure control. In general, black hypertensive patients tend to respond better to monotherapy with thiazide diuretics or calcium-channel blockers than to monotherapy with β-blockers, ACE inhibitors, or angiotensin II receptor antagonists. However, such diminished response to a β-blocker is largely eliminated when the drug is administered concomitantly with a thiazide diuretic. In addition, some experts state that when use of β-blockers is indicated in hypertensive patients with underlying cardiovascular or other risk factors, these indications should be applied equally to black hypertensive patients.

For information on overall principles and expert recommendations for treatment of hypertension, see Uses: Hypertension in Adults, in the Thiazides General Statement 40:28.20.

■ Chronic Stable Angina

Metoprolol is used for the management of chronic stable angina pectoris. β-Blockers are recommended as the anti-ischemic drugs of choice in most patients with chronic stable angina; despite differences in cardioselectivity, intrinsic sympathomimetic activity, and other clinical factors, all β-blockers appear to be equally effective for this indication. In placebo-controlled studies, metoprolol reduced the frequency of anginal attacks, reduced nitroglycerin consumption, and increased exercise tolerance.

Combination therapy with a β-blocker and a nitrate appears to be more effective than either drug alone because β-blockers attenuate the increased sympathetic tone and reflex tachycardia associated with nitrate therapy while nitrate therapy (e.g., nitroglycerin) counteracts the potential increase in left-ventricular wall tension associated with a decrease in heart rate. Combined therapy with a β-blocker and a dihydropyridine calcium-channel blocker also may be useful because the tendency to develop tachycardia with the calcium-channel blocker is counteracted by the β-blocker. However, caution should be exercised in the concomitant use of β-blockers and the nondihydropyridine calcium-channel blockers verapamil or diltiazem because of the potential for excessive fatigue, bradycardia, or atrioventricular (AV) block. Concomitant use of metoprolol with cardiac glycosides may be beneficial in patients with angina pectoris, especially in those with cardiomegaly, because both drugs reduce myocardial oxygen consumption; however, the potential effect of combined therapy on AV conduction should be considered. (See Drug Interactions: Cardiovascular Drugs.)

■ Non-ST-Segment-Elevation Acute Coronary Syndromes

β-Blockers are used as part of the standard therapeutic measures for managing non-ST-segment-elevation acute coronary syndromes (NSTE ACS). Patients with NSTE ACS have either unstable angina or non-ST-segment-elevation MI (NSTEMI); because these conditions are part of a continuum of acute myocardial ischemia and have indistinguishable clinical features upon presentation, the same initial treatment strategies are recommended. The American Heart Association/American College of Cardiology (AHA/ACC) guideline for the management of patients with NSTE ACS recommends an early invasive strategy (angiographic evaluation with the intent to perform revascularization procedures such as percutaneous coronary intervention [PCI] with coronary artery stent implantation or coronary artery bypass grafting [CABG]) or an ischemia-guided strategy (initial medical management followed by cardiac catheterization and revascularization if indicated) in patients with definite or likely NSTE ACS; standard medical therapies for all patients should include a β-blocker, antiplatelet agents (aspirin and/or a P2Y12-receptor antagonist), anticoagulant agents (e.g., low-molecular weight or unfractionated heparin), nitrates (e.g., nitroglycerin), and analgesic agents regardless of the initial management approach. The guideline states that oral β-blocker therapy should be initiated within the first 24 hours in patients who do not have manifestations of heart failure, evidence of a low-output state, increased risk of cardiogenic shock, or any other contraindications to β-blocker therapy; use of IV β-blockers is potentially harmful in patients with risk factors for cardiogenic shock. Continued therapy with a β-blocker proven to reduce mortality (bisoprolol, carvedilol, or metoprolol succinate) is recommended in patients with stabilized heart failure and reduced systolic function. (See Uses: Heart Failure, in Carvedilol 24:24.)

■ Acute Myocardial Infarction

Metoprolol tartrate is used orally and IV to reduce the risk of cardiovascular mortality in hemodynamically stable patients with definite or suspected acute MI. The term MI is used when there is evidence of myocardial necrosis in the setting of acute myocardial ischemia. ST-segment-elevation MI (STEMI) is distinguished from NSTEMI based on the presence or absence of ST-segment elevation on ECG. Patients with STEMI typically have complete arterial occlusion; therefore, immediate reperfusion therapy (with primary PCI or thrombolytic agents) is the current standard of care for such patients. Because the clinical presentation of NSTEMI is similar to that of unstable angina, these conditions are considered together in current expert guidelines. (See Uses: Non-ST-Segment Elevation Acute Coronary Syndromes.) During the early stage of a definite or suspected MI, metoprolol has been initiated with IV doses, followed by continued oral dosing; however, experts currently recommend that early IV use of β-blockers be limited to selected patients.

Because β-blockers can reduce myocardial oxygen demand during the first few hours of an acute MI by reducing heart rate, arterial blood pressure, and/or myocardial contractility, and also have been shown to reduce mortality, early IV therapy with these drugs was routinely recommended following acute MI. Evidence supporting this recommendation was generally based on studies conducted prior to the reperfusion era demonstrating a reduction in mortality and other clinical benefits (i.e., reduced infarct size, incidence of ventricular arrhythmias, chest pain, and cardiac enzyme elevations) with early use of β-blockers during MI. In one double-blind, placebo-controlled study in patients with definite or suspected acute MI, therapy with metoprolol tartrate (initiated IV as soon as possible after arrival to the hospital and continued orally for 3 months) was associated with a 36% reduction in mortality. The mortality benefit of metoprolol was similar between patients who were treated early (no more than 8 hours from the onset of symptoms) and those who initiated treatment at a later time. Patients receiving metoprolol also had substantial reductions in ventricular fibrillation and chest pain. (See Uses: Acute Myocardial Infarction, in Atenolol 24:24.)

Studies conducted after the widespread use of reperfusion therapy generally have demonstrated more attenuated benefits with early β-blocker therapy in patients with acute MI; while β-blockers may still confer benefits (e.g., reduction in the risk of reinfarction and ventricular arrhythmias), there is less certainty regarding the drugs' effects on mortality in patients receiving contemporary revascularization and pharmacologic therapies (antiplatelet agents, ACE inhibitors, and lipid-lowering therapies). In addition, early use of β-blockers (particularly when administered IV) has been associated with an increased risk of cardiogenic shock. In the Clopidogrel and Metoprolol in Myocardial Infarction Trial (COMMIT), there was no difference in mortality or the combined end point of death, reinfarction, or cardiac arrest between patients receiving early metoprolol therapy (initiated IV for up to 3 doses and continued orally) and those receiving placebo. Although patients who received metoprolol had a lower risk of reinfarction and ventricular fibrillation, these benefits were accompanied by a substantially higher risk of cardiogenic shock, particularly within the first day of treatment. Based on the currently available evidence, the American College of Cardiology Foundation/American Heart Association (ACCF/AHA) guideline for the management of STEMI recommends oral β-blocker therapy in all patients who do not have manifestations of heart failure, evidence of a low-output state, increased risk of cardiogenic shock, or any other contraindications to β-blocker therapy. Such therapy should be initiated within the first 24 hours following acute MI and continued during and after hospitalization. Because of conflicting evidence of benefit and the potential for harm, the guidelines recommend limiting use of IV β-blockers to patients with refractory hypertension or ongoing ischemia.

Although the efficacy of metoprolol tartrate following administration of the drug for longer than 3 months has not been conclusively established, the benefits of long-term β-blocker therapy for secondary prevention have been well established in numerous clinical studies. Patients with MI complicated by heart failure, left ventricular dysfunction, or ventricular arrhythmias appear to derive the most benefit from long-term β-blocker therapy. Data from studies using other β-blockers suggest that treatment should be continued for at least 1–3 years if not indefinitely after infarction unless contraindicated. Several large, randomized studies have demonstrated that long-term therapy with a β-blocker can reduce the rates of reinfarction and mortality (e.g., sudden or nonsudden cardiac death) following acute MI. It is estimated that such therapy could result in a relative reduction in mortality of about 25% annually for years 1–3 after infarction, with high-risk patients exhibiting the greatest potential benefit; the benefit of continued therapy may persist for at least several years beyond this period, although less substantially. Therefore, metoprolol, like other β-blockers, can be used for secondary prevention following acute MI to reduce the risk of reinfarction and mortality. The AHA/ACCF secondary prevention guideline recommends β-blocker therapy in all patients with left ventricular systolic dysfunction (ejection fraction of 40% or less) and a prior MI; use of a β-blocker with proven mortality benefit (bisoprolol, carvedilol, or metoprolol succinate) is recommended. (See Uses: Heart Failure, in Carvedilol 24:24.) Although the benefits of long-term β-blockade in post-MI patients with normal left ventricular function are less well established, the guideline recommends continued β-blocker therapy for at least 3 years in such patients. Further studies are needed to establish the optimal duration of β-blocker therapy for secondary prevention of MI.

■ **Supraventricular Arrhythmias** β-Blockers, including metoprolol, have been used to slow ventricular rate in patients with supraventricular tachycardia† (SVT). The American College of Cardiology/American Heart Association/Heart Rhythm Society (ACC/AHA/HRS) guideline for the management of adult patients with supraventricular tachycardia recommends the use of β-blockers in the treatment of various SVTs (e.g., atrial flutter, junctional tachycardia, focal atrial tachycardia, AV nodal reentrant tachycardia [AVNRT]); in general, an IV β-blocker is recommended for acute treatment, while an oral β-blocker is recommended for ongoing management of these arrhythmias. Vagal maneuvers and/or IV adenosine are considered first-line interventions for the acute treatment of SVT and should be attempted prior to other therapies when clinically indicated; if such measures are ineffective or not feasible, an IV β-blocker may be considered in hemodynamically stable patients. Although evidence of efficacy is limited, experts state that the overall safety of β-adrenergic blockers warrants their use in patients with SVT. Patients should be closely monitored for hypotension and bradycardia during administration of these drugs.

Atrial Fibrillation and Flutter β-Blockers, including metoprolol, have been used to slow rapid ventricular response in patients with atrial fibrillation† or atrial flutter†. IV β-blockers (e.g., esmolol, propranolol, metoprolol) are recommended as one of several drug therapy options for ventricular rate control in patients with nonpreexcited atrial fibrillation or flutter; an oral β-blocker may be used for ongoing rate control in such patients. Choice of a specific β-blocker should be individualized based on the patient's clinical condition.

Atrial Tachycardia IV β-blockers may be used for the acute treatment of patients with hemodynamically stable focal atrial tachycardia† (i.e., regular SVT arising from a localized atrial site), and an oral β-blocker may be used for ongoing management.

While evidence is more limited, IV metoprolol also has been used in patients with multifocal atrial tachycardia† (rapid, irregular rhythm with at least 3 distinct P-wave morphologies) to control ventricular rate and convert to normal sinus rhythm.Multifocal atrial tachycardia is commonly associated with an underlying condition (e.g., pulmonary, coronary, or valvular heart disease) and is generally not responsive to antiarrhythmic drug therapy. Antiarrhythmic drug therapy usually is reserved for patients who do not respond to initial attempts at correcting or managing potential precipitating factors (e.g., exacerbation of COPD or congestive heart failure, electrolyte and/or ventilatory disturbances, infection, theophylline toxicity) or in whom a precipitating factor cannot be identified. Therapy with IV metoprolol has been associated with slowing of atrial and ventricular rates and conversion to sinus rhythm in many patients with this arrhythmia; therefore, some experts state that IV metoprolol may be useful for the acute treatment of patients with multifocal atrial tachycardia who do not have respiratory decompensation, sinus node dysfunction, or AV block. Metoprolol also may be useful orally for chronic suppression of symptomatic multifocal atrial tachycardia.

Paroxysmal Supraventricular Tachycardia IV β-blockers may be used for the acute treatment of hemodynamically stable patients with paroxysmal supraventricular tachycardia (PSVT), including AVNRT†, that is uncontrolled or unconverted by vagal maneuvers and adenosine; an oral β-blocker may be used for the ongoing management of such patients who are not candidates for, or prefer not to undergo, catheter ablation.

Junctional Tachycardia β-Blockers are considered one of several drug therapy options for the treatment of junctional tachycardia† (i.e., nonreentrant SVT originating from the AV junction), a rapid, occasionally irregular, narrow-complex tachycardia. While evidence is limited, there is some data indicating that β-blocking agents (specifically propranolol) are modestly effective in terminating and/or reducing the incidence of junctional tachycardia.

■ **Ventricular Arrhythmias** ***Ventricular Fibrillation*** β-Blockers have been used in patients with cardiac arrest precipitated by ventricular fibrillation or pulseless ventricular tachycardia†. However, AHA states that routine administration of β-adrenergic blocking agents after cardiac arrest is potentially harmful (e.g., may worsen hemodynamic instability, exacerbate heart failure, or cause bradyarrhythmias) and is therefore not recommended.

Polymorphic Ventricular Tachycardia β-Blockers may be useful in the management of certain forms of polymorphic ventricular tachycardia† (e.g., associated with acute ischemia).

■ **Heart Failure** Metoprolol is used (usually in conjunction with other heart failure therapies) in the management of mild to moderately severe (New York Heart Association [NYHA] class II or III) heart failure of ischemic, hypertensive, or cardiomyopathic origin. In clinical studies, metoprolol (as extended-release metoprolol succinate) increased survival and reduced the risk of hospitalization in patients with chronic heart failure. Current guidelines for the management of heart failure in adults generally recommend a combination of drug therapies to reduce morbidity and mortality, including neurohormonal antagonists (e.g., ACE inhibitors, angiotensin II receptor antagonists, angiotensin receptor-neprilysin inhibitors [ARNIs], β-blockers, aldosterone receptor antagonists) that inhibit the detrimental compensatory mechanisms in heart failure. Additional agents (e.g., cardiac glycosides, diuretics, sinoatrial modulators [i.e., ivabradine]) added to a heart failure treatment regimen in selected patients have been associated with symptomatic improvement and/or reduction in heart-failure related hospitalizations. Experts recommend that all asymptomatic patients with reduced left ventricular ejection fraction (LVEF) (ACCF/AHA stage B heart failure) receive therapy with an ACE inhibitor and a β-blocker to prevent symptomatic heart failure and to reduce morbidity and mortality. In patients with prior or current symptoms of heart failure and reduced LVEF (ACCF/AHA stage C heart failure), ACCF, AHA, and the Heart Failure Society of America (HFSA) recommend inhibition of the renin-angiotensin-aldosterone (RAA) system with an ACE inhibitor, angiotensin II receptor antagonist, or ARNI in conjunction with a β-blocker, and an aldosterone antagonist in selected patients, to reduce morbidity and mortality. While ACE inhibitors have been the preferred drugs for inhibition of the RAA system because of their established benefits in patients with heart failure and reduced ejection fraction, some evidence indicates that therapy with an ARNI may be more effective than ACE inhibitor therapy in reducing cardiovascular death and heart failure-related hospitalization in such patients. ACCF, AHA, and HFSA recommend that patients with chronic symptomatic heart failure with reduced LVEF (NYHA class II or III) who are able to tolerate an ACE inhibitor or angiotensin II receptor antagonist be switched to therapy containing an ARNI to further reduce morbidity and mortality.

Because of favorable effects on survival and disease progression, therapy with a clinical trial-proven β-blocker (bisoprolol, carvedilol, extended-release metoprolol succinate) should be initiated as soon as the patient is diagnosed with heart failure and reduced LVEF. While bisoprolol, carvedilol, and extended-release metoprolol have been effective in reducing the risk of death in patients with chronic heart failure, these positive findings should not be considered indicative of a β-blocker class effect. Even when symptoms are mild or improve with other therapies, β-blocker therapy should not be delayed until symptoms return or the disease progresses. Despite concerns about β-blockade potentially masking some signs of hypoglycemia, patients with diabetes mellitus may be particularly likely to experience a reduction in morbidity and mortality with the use of β-blockers. If a patient cannot tolerate a β-blocker or if increasing the β-blocker dosage is ineffective, ivabradine should be considered an alternative or additional treatment option. Some evidence suggests that ivabradine is effective in reducing hospitalizations related to heart failure, but unlike β-blockers, ivabradine has not been shown to reduce cardiovascular mortality. (See Uses: Heart Failure, in Ivabradine 24:04.92.)

In individualizing the decision to use a β-blocker, clinicians should consider that clinical studies establishing the effects of these drugs on morbidity and mortality excluded patients who were hospitalized or had unstable symptoms and enrolled few patients with current or recent NYHA class IV symptoms. The efficacy of β-blockers in such patients is not known, and they may be at particular risk of deterioration following initiation of therapy with β-blockers.

In a large, randomized, double-blind, placebo-controlled study (Metoprolol CR/XL Randomized Intervention Trial in Congestive Heart Failure [MERIT-HF]) in patients with mild to severe (NYHA class II–IV) heart failure and a left ventricular ejection fraction of 0.4 or less, therapy with metoprolol succinate (as extended-release tablets) 12.5–25 mg daily as the tartrate (initial dosage depending on NYHA class, with dosage increased over 8 weeks to a target daily dosage of 200 mg daily) in addition to optimal standard therapy (principally ACE inhibitors and diuretics) was associated with a reduction in all-cause mortality of 34% (mortality rates of 7.2 and 11% with metoprolol and placebo, respectively). The MERIT-HF trial was terminated early because of the favorable effects of metoprolol on overall mortality; the mean follow-up period was 1 year. Sudden deaths and deaths from worsening heart failure also were reduced with metoprolol therapy. In addition to improved survival, metoprolol therapy improved NYHA class, reduced hospitalizations due to worsening heart failure, and resulted in beneficial effects on patient well-being (as determined by quality-of-life measurements); the composite end point of overall mortality and hospitalization for any cause was reduced by 19%. Metoprolol therapy appeared to be well tolerated, with 64% of patients achieving the target dosage of 200 mg daily and 87% tolerating a daily dosage of 100 mg; the mean daily dosage of metoprolol as the tartrate was 159 mg.

The beneficial effects of β-blockers in the management of heart failure are thought to result principally from inhibition of the effects of the sympathetic nervous system. Although the specific effects on the heart and circulation that are responsible for progression of heart failure remain to be established, sympathetic activity can increase ventricular volumes and pressure secondary to peripheral vasoconstriction and by impairing sodium excretion by the kidneys. Other sympathetic effects (e.g., induction of cardiac hypertrophy, arrhythmogenic activity) also may be involved. Collective experience indicates that long-term therapy with β-blockers, like that with ACE inhibitors, can reduce heart failure symptoms and improve clinical status in patients with chronic heart failure and also can decrease the risk of death as well as the combined risk of death and hospitalization. These beneficial effects were demonstrated in patients already receiving an ACE inhibitor, suggesting that combined inhibition of the renin-angiotensin system and sympathetic nervous system can produce additive effects.

β-Blockers should not be used in patients with acutely decompensated heart failure requiring IV inotropic therapy (see Cautions: Precautions and Contraindications) and those with substantial fluid retention requiring intensive diuresis. In the absence of hemodynamic instability or contraindications, it has been recommended that patients with heart failure and a reduced ejection fraction who are hospitalized for a symptomatic exacerbation continue to receive maintenance treatment with standard oral therapy (e.g., β-blocker, ACE inhibitor). Withholding of, or reduction in, β-blocker therapy may be considered in patients hospitalized after recent initiation or increase in β-blocker therapy. Initiation of β-blocker therapy in hospitalized patients is recommended once the patient's condition is stabilized (i.e., after optimization of volume status and successful discontinuance of IV diuretics, vasodilators, and inotropic agents). Caution should be used when initiating β-blockers in patients who have required inotrope therapy during their hospitalization.

■ **Vascular Headache** ***Migraine*** Metoprolol has been used for the prophylaxis of migraine headache†. When used prophylactically, metoprolol can prevent migraine or reduce the number of attacks in some patients. Results of comparative studies suggest that metoprolol may be comparable to propranolol for this indication. However, the US Headache Consortium states that the quality of evidence for metoprolol is not as compelling as it is for propranolol for this indication. Metoprolol is not recommended for the treatment of a migraine attack that has already started. For further information on management and classification of migraine headache, see Vascular Headaches: General Principles in Migraine Therapy, under Uses in Sumatriptan 28:32.28.

Dosage and Administration

■ **Administration** Metoprolol tartrate and metoprolol succinate are administered orally. Metoprolol tartrate also may be administered IV.

Absorption of metoprolol tartrate may be enhanced by administration with food. The manufacturer recommends that metoprolol tartrate be administered with or immediately following meals. Although administration with meals is not required, metoprolol tartrate should be given in a standardized relation to meals to minimize variance in effect. Food does not appear to affect the bioavailability of metoprolol succinate extended-release tablets.

Metoprolol tartrate may be administered daily as a single dose or in divided doses; metoprolol succinate extended-release tablets should be administered daily as a single dose. If a dose is missed, the patient should take only the next scheduled dose (i.e., the next dose should not be doubled). Metoprolol succinate extended-release tablets are scored and can be divided; however, the tablet or half tablet should be swallowed whole and should not be chewed or crushed.

Dispensing and Administration Precautions Because of similarity in spelling between Toprol-XL® (a trade name for metoprolol succinate) and Topamax® (the trade name for topiramate, an anticonvulsant and antimigraine agent), the potential exists for dispensing or prescribing errors involving these drugs. In addition, there is a potential for dispensing errors involving confusion between Toprol-XL® and Tegretol® or Tegretol®-XR (trade names for carbamazepine, an anticonvulsant that also is used for relief of pain associated with trigeminal neuralgia, as well as for various psychiatric disorders). According to medication error reports, the overlapping tablet strengths between Toprol-XL® and Topamax® (25, 50, 100, and 200 mg) and between Toprol-XL® and Tegretol® or Tegretol®-XR (100 and 200 mg) and the fact that these drugs were stored closely together in pharmacies also may have been contributing factors in causing these errors. Another contributing factor to dispensing errors associated with Toprol-XL® and Topamax® may be the use of mnemonic abbreviations in computerized listings incorporating the first 3 letters and dose strength (e.g., "TOP25"). Extra care should be exercised to ensure the accuracy of both oral and written prescriptions for these drugs. The manufacturers of Toprol-XL® and Topamax® also recommend that pharmacists assess various measures of avoiding dispensing errors and implement them as appropriate (e.g., by verifying all orders for these drugs by citing both the trade and generic names to prescribers, attaching reminders to pharmacy shelves, separating the drugs on pharmacy shelves, counseling patients). (See Cautions: Precautions and Contraindications.)

■ **Dosage** Dosages of metoprolol tartrate and metoprolol succinate are expressed in terms of the tartrate. Since there is no consistent interpatient correlation between the dosage of metoprolol and therapeutic response, dosage must be individualized according to the response of the patient. Blood pressure should be measured near the end of a dosing interval to determine whether satisfactory control is being maintained throughout the day. When patients receiving metoprolol tartrate conventional tablets are switched to metoprolol succinate extended-release tablets, the same daily dosage should be used. If long-term metoprolol therapy is to be discontinued, dosage of the drug should be gradually reduced over a period of 1–2 weeks. (See Cautions: Precautions and Contraindications.)

Hypertension **Metoprolol Therapy.** The manufacturers state that the usual initial adult oral dosage of metoprolol tartrate conventional tablets, given alone or in combination with a diuretic, is 100 mg daily given in single or divided doses. When administered as metoprolol succinate extended-release tablets, the manufacturers state that the recommended initial dosage in terms of metoprolol tartrate is 25–100 mg administered once daily. Some clinicians recommend an initial dosage of at least 50 mg 3 times daily as metoprolol tartrate conventional tablets, for better control. Dosage may be increased at weekly (or longer) intervals until optimum hypotensive effect is achieved. In general, the maximum effect of any given dosage will be apparent within 1 week. The manufacturers state that oral dosages in terms of metoprolol tartrate should not exceed 450 mg daily as conventional tablets or 400 mg daily as extended-release tablets; dosages of the respective formulations exceeding these have not been studied.

Some experts state the usual dosage range is 100–200 mg daily, given in 2 divided doses daily as conventional tablets or 50–200 mg once daily given as extended-release tablets.

The fact that β_1-adrenergic blocking selectivity of metoprolol diminishes as dosage is increased should be considered.

Patients with severe hypertension may require more uniform plasma concentrations for adequate control and in some hypertensive patients, especially when lower dosages (e.g., 100 mg daily) are used, blood pressure increases slightly toward the end of the dosing interval with once- or twice-daily administration. If a satisfactory response is not maintained throughout the day, larger doses, more frequent administration, or use of extended-release tablets may achieve better control.

If metoprolol tartrate is used for the management of hypertension in children 1–17 years of age†, some experts have recommended an initial oral dosage of 1–2 mg/kg daily given in 2 divided doses. Such experts have suggested that dosage may be increased as necessary to a maximum dosage of 6 mg/kg (up to 200 mg) daily given in 2 divided doses. The manufacturer states that if extended-release metoprolol succinate is used for hypertension in children 6 years of age or older, an initial oral dosage of 1 mg/kg (up to 50 mg) daily in terms of metoprolol tartrate is recommended. The dosage should be adjusted according to blood pressure response. The safety and efficacy of dosages exceeding 2 mg/kg (or 200 mg) once daily have not been established in pediatric patients. For information on overall principles and expert recommendations for treatment of hypertension in pediatric patients, see Uses: Hypertension in Pediatric Patients, in the Thiazides General Statement 40:28.20.

Metoprolol/Hydrochlorothiazide Fixed-combination Therapy. When combination therapy is required, the manufacturer recommends that commercially available preparations containing metoprolol tartrate in fixed combination with a thiazide diuretic should not be used initially. Dosage should first be adjusted by administering each drug separately. If it is determined that the optimum maintenance dosage corresponds to the ratio in the commercial combination preparation, the fixed combination may be used. Dosage regimens using fixed-combination preparations that exceed 50 mg of hydrochlorothiazide daily are not recommended.

Blood Pressure Monitoring and Treatment Goals. Blood pressure should be monitored regularly (i.e., monthly) during therapy and dosage of the antihypertensive drug adjusted until blood pressure is controlled. If an adequate blood pressure response is not achieved, the dosage may be increased or another antihypertensive agent with demonstrated benefit and preferably with a complementary mechanism of action (e.g., angiotensin-converting enzyme [ACE] inhibitor, angiotensin II receptor antagonist, calcium-channel blocker, thiazide diuretic) may be added; if target blood pressure is still not achieved with the use of 2 antihypertensive agents, a third drug may be added. (See Uses: Hypertension.) In patients who develop unacceptable adverse effects with metoprolol, the drug should be discontinued and another antihypertensive agent from a different pharmacologic class should be initiated.

The goal of hypertension management and prevention is to achieve and maintain optimal control of blood pressure. However, the optimum blood pressure threshold for initiating antihypertensive drug therapy and specific treatment goals remain controversial. While previous hypertension guidelines have based target blood pressure goals on age and comorbidities, the 2017 American College of Cardiology/American Heart Association (ACC/AHA) hypertension guideline incorporates underlying cardiovascular risk into decision making regarding treatment and generally recommends the same target blood pressure (i.e., less than 130/80 mm Hg) for all adults. Many patients will require at least 2 drugs from different pharmacologic classes to achieve this blood pressure goal; the potential benefits of hypertension management and drug cost, adverse effects, and risks associated with the use of multiple antihypertensive drugs also should be considered when deciding a patient's blood pressure treatment goal.

For additional information on target levels of blood pressure and on monitoring therapy in the management of hypertension, see Blood Pressure Monitoring and Treatment Goals under Dosage: Hypertension, in Dosage and Administration in the Thiazides General Statement 40:28.20.

Chronic Stable Angina For the long-term management of angina pectoris, the initial adult dosage of metoprolol tartrate (conventional tablets) or metoprolol succinate (extended-release tablets) is 100 mg as the tartrate daily given in 2 divided doses or in a single dose, respectively. Dosage may be increased at weekly intervals until optimum control of angina is obtained or there is pronounced slowing of the heart rate. The usual maintenance dosage of metoprolol tartrate (conventional tablets) or metoprolol succinate (extended-release tablets) is 100–400 mg (expressed in terms of metoprolol tartrate) daily. Oral dosages exceeding 400 mg daily (given as metoprolol tartrate conventional tablets or as metoprolol succinate extended-release tablets) have not been studied. When discontinuance of metoprolol therapy is planned, dosage of the drug should be gradually reduced over a period of about 1–2 weeks. (See Cautions: Precautions and Contraindications.)

Acute Myocardial Infarction **Early Treatment.** The manufacturer states that metoprolol therapy may be initiated as soon as possible after an acute myocardial infarction (MI) when the patient's hemodynamic condition has stabilized. During the early stage of a definite or suspected MI, the manufacturer recommends that treatment with metoprolol tartrate be initiated with the administration of three 5-mg rapid IV injections given at approximately 2-minute intervals as tolerated. Heart rate, blood pressure, and ECG should be monitored during IV administration, and the drug should be titrated to response. In patients who tolerate the full IV dose (15 mg), the manufacturer states that oral administration of metoprolol tartrate should be initiated 15 minutes after the last IV dose at a dosage of 50 mg every 6 hours for 48 hours. Thereafter, an oral maintenance dosage of 100 mg twice daily should be used. Patients who appear not to tolerate the usual total IV dose should initially receive an oral metoprolol tartrate dosage of 25 or 50 mg (depending on the degree of intolerance) every 6 hours beginning 15 minutes after the last IV dose or as soon as their clinical condition allows. In patients with severe intolerance, metoprolol should be discontinued.

The American College of Cardiology Foundation/American Heart Association (ACCF/AHA) guideline for the management of ST-segment-elevation MI (STEMI) recommends initiation of oral β-blocker therapy within the first 24 hours in patients who do not have manifestations of heart failure, evidence of a low-output state, increased risk of cardiogenic shock, or any other contraindications to β-blocker therapy. The recommended oral dosage of metoprolol tartrate is 25–50 mg every 6–12 hours; patients should be transitioned over the following 2–3 days to twice-daily dosing (using metoprolol tartrate) or daily dosing (using metoprolol succinate). Dosage should be titrated up to a total daily dose of 200 mg as tolerated. Because IV β-blockers can be potentially harmful in patients with risk factors for cardiogenic shock, these experts recommend that IV use be limited to patients who have refractory hypertension or have ongoing ischemia at the time of presentation. If IV therapy is employed, the recommended IV dosage of metoprolol tartrate is 5 mg every 5 minutes as tolerated up to 3 doses.

Late Treatment and Long-term Secondary Prevention. In patients who have contraindications to metoprolol therapy during the early phase of definite or suspected acute MI, in patients who appear not to tolerate the full early treatment, or in patients in whom therapy is delayed for any other reason, the manufacturer recommends initiation of metoprolol therapy with an oral dosage of 100 mg twice daily as soon as their clinical condition allows. The manufacturer states that oral metoprolol therapy should be continued for at least 3 months; however, the optimal duration of β-blocker therapy following MI remains to be clearly established. Experts generally recommend that such therapy be continued long-term in post-MI patients with left ventricular systolic dysfunction, and for at least 3 years in those with normal left ventricular function.

Atrial Fibrillation To slow rapid ventricular response in adults with atrial fibrillation†, metoprolol tartrate has been administered IV in doses of 2.5–5 mg administered over 2 minutes, up to a total of 3 doses. Once adequate control of heart rate or conversion to normal sinus rhythm has been achieved with parenteral metoprolol therapy, some experts suggest an oral metoprolol tartrate dosage of 25–100 mg twice daily or extended-release metoprolol succinate at a dosage of 50–400 mg once daily for long-term rate control in patients with atrial fibrillation.

Other Supraventricular Arrhythmias For the acute treatment of supraventricular tachycardia (SVT) (e.g., atrial flutter†, junctional tachycardia†, paroxysmal supraventricular tachycardia [PSVT]†, atrial tachycardia†) in adults, some experts recommend an initial IV metoprolol tartrate dose of 2.5–5 mg administered over 2 minutes; additional doses may be given every 10 minutes up to a maximum of 3 doses. The usual oral maintenance dosage for ongoing treatment of SVT is 200 mg twice daily (as metoprolol tartrate tablets) or 400 mg once daily (as metoprolol succinate extended-release tablets).

Heart Failure Prior to initiation of therapy with a β-blocker in patients with heart failure, the dosage of any concomitant heart failure therapy should be stabilized. Because of the potential for severe adverse effects (e.g., hypotension, bradycardia, fluid retention, worsening of heart failure), initiation of β-blocker therapy for heart failure and subsequent dosage adjustments should occur under close medical supervision.

For the management of symptomatic heart failure, the manufacturer recommends an initial metoprolol succinate (extended-release tablets) dosage of 25 mg (expressed as the tartrate) once daily in adults with New York Heart Association (NYHA) class II heart failure; adults with more severe heart failure should receive an initial dosage of 12.5 mg once daily. The manufacturer recommends that the dosage be doubled every 2 weeks until a dosage of 200 mg once daily or the highest tolerated dosage is reached. Some experts recommend initiation of β-blocker therapy at a very low dosage (e.g., a metoprolol succinate dosage of 12.5–25 mg once daily [expressed as metoprolol tartrate] using the extended-release tablets) in patients with heart failure, with the dosage gradually titrated upward as tolerated (maximum dosage 200 mg once daily). If deterioration of heart failure (usually transient) becomes evident during titration of metoprolol therapy, the dosage of the concurrent diuretic should be increased and the dosage of metoprolol not escalated until symptoms of worsening heart failure (e.g., fluid retention) have stabilized; it may be necessary to decrease the dosage of metoprolol or temporarily discontinue the drug. Should patients with heart failure experience symptomatic bradycardia (e.g., dizziness) or second- or third-degree heart block, the dosage of metoprolol should be reduced. Initial difficulty in titrating metoprolol dosage should not preclude subsequent attempts to successfully titrate the dosage.

It should be recognized that symptomatic improvement may not be evident for 2–3 months after initiating therapy with β-blockers. However, β-blocker therapy may reduce the risk of disease progression even if symptomatic improvement is not evident. In clinical trials, metoprolol dosages were *not* adjusted according to response but instead were increased as tolerated to a prespecified target dose. Once titrated to the target or highest tolerated dosage, therapy generally can be maintained at this level long term. In clinical trials, dosages usually were titrated up to 150–200 mg daily.

Vascular Headaches **Migraine.** Although dosages of metoprolol tartrate or metoprolol succinate for the prophylaxis of migraine† in adults have not been established, oral dosages of 50–300 mg daily have been used in clinical studies. The usual effective dosage of the drug in these studies was 200 mg daily.

Cautions

Metoprolol shares the toxic potentials of β-adrenergic blocking agents (β-blockers). Most adverse effects of metoprolol are mild and transient and occur more frequently at the onset of therapy than during prolonged treatment. The most frequent adverse effects are dizziness, tiredness, insomnia, and gastric upset.

■ Cardiovascular and Cerebrovascular Effects The most common adverse cardiovascular effects of metoprolol are shortness of breath and bradycardia, occurring in about 3% of patients with hypertension or angina receiving metoprolol tartrate in clinical trials. Severe bradycardia should be treated with IM or IV administration of atropine sulfate. If there is an inadequate response to atropine, IV isoproterenol may be administered with caution. Cold extremities, arterial insufficiency (e.g., Raynaud's phenomenon), palpitations, congestive heart failure, peripheral edema, syncope, chest pain, or hypotension has been reported in about 1% of patients with hypertension or angina receiving metoprolol tartrate. Gangrene has been reported very rarely in patients with preexisting severe peripheral circulatory disorders receiving metoprolol tartrate. Claudication has been reported in patients with myocardial infarction (MI) receiving metoprolol tartrate, although a relationship to the drug is unclear. Raynaud's phenomenon may be treated by keeping the patient warm, stopping the drug, and, if necessary, administering a vasodilator. Adverse cardiovascular events occurring in greater than 1% of patients with heart failure receiving metoprolol succinate extended-release tablets but with a similar incidence (within 0.5%) in patients receiving placebo include MI, coronary artery disorder, cerebrovascular disorder, ventricular tachycardia, or aggravation of arrhythmia.

If hypotension (systolic blood pressure of 90 mm Hg or less) occurs in patients with MI, metoprolol should be discontinued and appropriate cardiovascular monitoring and therapy instituted as necessary. (See Cautions: Precautions and Contraindications.) In patients without a prior history of heart failure, prolonged depression of the myocardium by metoprolol occasionally has resulted in heart failure. Intensification of AV block has occurred with other β-blockers and is a potential adverse effect of metoprolol. AV dissociation, AV conduction delays, complete heart block or cardiac arrest also may occur, especially in patients with preexisting heart block caused by digitalis or other factors.

During surgery, some patients who have received β-blockers may experience severe, protracted hypotension and, occasionally, difficulty in restarting and maintaining heart beat. The untoward effects of metoprolol may be reversed during surgery by IV administration of β-adrenergic agonists (e.g., isoproterenol, dopamine, dobutamine).

■ Nervous System Effects Tiredness or dizziness has occurred in about 10% of patients with hypertension or angina receiving metoprolol tartrate in clinical trials; tiredness has been reported in about 1% of patients with MI receiving the drug. In addition, vertigo, sleep disturbances/insomnia, hallucinations, nightmares, headache, dizziness, visual disturbances, and confusion have been reported in patients with MI receiving the drug, although a causal relationship is unclear. Somnolence or increased dreaming also has been reported with metoprolol therapy; these effects may be alleviated by avoiding late-evening dosage. Rarely, impotence, nervousness, and general weakness have occurred. Depression has been reported in about 5% of patients receiving metoprolol tartrate for hypertension or angina. Reversible mental depression occurs less frequently with metoprolol than with propranolol but is a reason for withdrawal of the drugs, as it may progress to catatonia. An acute reversible syndrome characterized by disorientation to time and place, short-term memory loss, emotional lability, slightly clouded sensorium, and decreased performance on neuropsychometric tests has been reported with other β-blockers and should be considered a potential adverse effect of metoprolol. Lethargy and, rarely, fullheadedness have occurred.

■ GI Effects Diarrhea has occurred in about 5% of patients receiving metoprolol tartrate in clinical trials. Other GI symptoms such as nausea, gastric pain, constipation, flatulence, digestive tract disorders, heartburn, xerostomia, and hiccups also have been reported with oral metoprolol therapy. Nausea and abdominal pain have occurred in less than 1% of patients with MI receiving IV or oral metoprolol.

■ **Endocrine Effects** Unstable diabetes mellitus has been reported in patients with MI receiving metoprolol tartrate, although a relationship to the drug is unclear. Results of a large prospective cohort study of adults 45–64 years of age indicate that use of β-blockers in hypertensive patients is associated with increased risk (about 28%) of developing diabetes mellitus. In this study, the number of new cases of diabetes per 1000 person-years was 33.6 or 26.3 in patients receiving a β-blocker or no drug therapy, respectively. The association between the risk of developing diabetes mellitus and use of β-blockers reportedly was not confounded by weight gain, hyperinsulinemia, or differences in heart rate. It is not known if the risk of developing diabetes is affected by β-receptor selectivity. Further studies are needed to determine whether concomitant use of ACE inhibitors (which may improve insulin sensitivity) would abrogate β-blocker-induced adverse effects related to glucose intolerance. Therefore, until results of such studies are available, the proven benefits of β-blockers in reducing cardiovascular events in hypertensive patients must be weighed carefully against the possible risks of developing diabetes mellitus.

Hypoglycemia, which may result in loss of consciousness, also may occur in nondiabetic patients receiving β-adrenergic blocking agents. Patients most at risk for the development of β-blocker-induced hypoglycemia are those undergoing dialysis, prolonged fasting, or severe exercise regimens.

β-Blockers may mask signs and symptoms of hypoglycemia (e.g., palpitation, tachycardia, tremor) and potentiate insulin-induced hypoglycemia. Although it has been suggested that nonselective β-blockers are more likely to induce hypoglycemia than selective β-blockers, such an adverse effect also has been reported with selective β-blockers (e.g., atenolol). Selective β-blockers are less likely to mask symptoms of hypoglycemia or delay recovery from insulin-induced hypoglycemia than nonselective β-blockers; however, selective β-blockers can decrease insulin sensitivity by approximately 15–30%, which may result in increased insulin requirements.

■ **Other Adverse Effects** In spite of its relative β_1-blocking selectivity, β_2-adrenergic blockade leading to bronchoconstriction, dyspnea, and wheezing may occur with metoprolol dosages greater than 100 mg daily, particularly in patients with a history of asthma. Wheezing or dyspnea has been reported in about 1% of patients with hypertension or angina receiving metoprolol, and dyspnea of pulmonary origin has been reported in less than 1% of patients with MI receiving the drug. Rhinitis also has been reported in patients receiving metoprolol tartrate. In a large clinical trial, pneumonia was reported in greater than 1% of patients with heart failure receiving metoprolol succinate extended-release tablets but with a similar incidence (within 0.5%) in patients receiving placebo.

Peyronie's disease, tinnitus, restless legs, a polymyalgia-like syndrome, musculoskeletal pain, decreased libido, blurred vision, dry mucous membranes, and sweating have occurred rarely in patients receiving metoprolol. Fatigue was reported in greater than 1% of patients with heart failure receiving metoprolol succinate extended-release tablets in a large clinical trial but with a similar incidence (within 0.5%) in patients receiving placebo.

Pruritus, dry skin, worsening of psoriasis, and psoriasiform, maculopapular, and urticarial rash have occurred in some patients receiving metoprolol. Allergic reactions reported in patients receiving other β-blockers include erythematous rash, fever combined with aching and sore throat, laryngospasm, and respiratory distress. Reversible alopecia, agranulocytosis, thrombocytopenia, weight gain, arthritis, retroperitoneal fibrosis, and dry eyes have been reported rarely with metoprolol therapy. Discontinuance of the drug should be considered if any such reaction is not otherwise explicable. There have been some reported cases of increased antinuclear factor (ANF) levels during metoprolol therapy; however, other reports indicate decreased ANF levels, and no positive ANF findings have been associated with adverse effects of metoprolol involving the skin and eyes.

Potential hematologic effects of β-blockers include eosinophilia, agranulocytosis, and nonthrombocytopenic and thrombocytopenic purpura.

Other β-blockers may cause elevated BUN and serum creatinine concentrations in patients with severe heart disease, presumably because of decreased renal blood flow. Hepatitis, jaundice, or nonspecific hepatic dysfunction has been reported during postmarketing experience in patients receiving metoprolol. Subclinical hepatitis of unknown etiology occurred in one patient receiving metoprolol therapy for 6 months. Isolated instances of elevated serum transaminase, alkaline phosphatase, and lactate dehydrogenase concentrations also have been reported during postmarketing experience with metoprolol therapy. Metoprolol may increase serum uric acid concentration.

■ **Precautions and Contraindications** Metoprolol shares the toxic potentials of β-blockers, and the usual precautions of these agents should be observed. When metoprolol is used as a fixed-combination preparation that includes hydrochlorothiazide, the cautions, precautions, and contraindications associated with thiazide diuretics must be considered in addition to those associated with metoprolol.

In patients with heart failure, sympathetic stimulation is vital for the support of circulatory function. Metoprolol should be used with caution in patients with inadequate myocardial function, since heart failure may be precipitated by blockade of β-adrenergic stimulation when metoprolol therapy is administered. Exercise tolerance may decrease in patients with left ventricular dysfunction. In addition, in patients with latent cardiac insufficiency, prolonged β-adrenergic blockade may lead to cardiac failure. Although β-blockers should be avoided in patients with overt or decompensated heart failure, metoprolol may be administered cautiously to patients with well-compensated heart failure (e.g., those controlled with ACE inhibitors, diuretics, and/or cardiac glycosides). Patients receiving metoprolol therapy should be instructed to consult their physician at the first sign or symptom of impending cardiac failure (e.g., weight gain, increasing shortness of breath) and should be adequately treated (e.g., with a cardiac glycoside and/or diuretic) and observed closely; if cardiac failure continues, metoprolol should be discontinued, gradually if possible. Metoprolol should be administered with caution in patients with sinus node dysfunction, since the drug can depress SA node automaticity.

Abrupt withdrawal of β-blocker therapy may exacerbate angina symptoms or precipitate MI in patients with coronary artery disease. Therefore, patients receiving metoprolol (especially those with ischemic heart disease) should be warned not to interrupt or discontinue therapy without consulting their physician. When discontinuance of metoprolol therapy is planned, particularly in patients with ischemic heart disease, dosage of the drug should be gradually reduced over a period of about 1–2 weeks. When metoprolol therapy is discontinued, patients should be monitored carefully and advised to temporarily limit their physical activity. If exacerbation of angina occurs or acute coronary insufficiency develops after metoprolol therapy is interrupted, metoprolol therapy should be reinstituted promptly, at least temporarily, and appropriate measures for the management of unstable angina pectoris should be initiated. Because coronary artery disease is common and may be unrecognized, it may be prudent not to discontinue metoprolol therapy abruptly, even in patients receiving the drug for conditions other than angina.

In patients with MI, hemodynamic status should be carefully monitored during metoprolol therapy. If heart rate decreases to less than 40 beats/minute in patients receiving the drug, particularly if associated with evidence of decreased cardiac output, the manufacturer recommends that IV atropine be administered; if the bradycardia is refractory to atropine, the manufacturer recommends that metoprolol be discontinued and that cautious administration of isoproterenol or use of a cardiac pacemaker be considered. If heart block occurs in patients with MI during metoprolol therapy, the manufacturer recommends that the drug be discontinued and IV atropine be administered; if the heart block is refractory to atropine, the manufacturer recommends that cautious administration of isoproterenol or use of a cardiac pacemaker be considered. If hypotension (systolic blood pressure of 90 mm Hg or less) occurs in patients with MI, the manufacturer recommends that metoprolol be discontinued and the hemodynamic status of the patient and the extent of myocardial damage be carefully assessed. Invasive monitoring of central venous, pulmonary capillary wedge, and arterial pressures may be necessary; appropriate therapy with IV fluids and other treatment modalities should be instituted. If hypotension is associated with severe bradycardia or heart block, treatment should be directed at reversing these effects.

Metoprolol should be used with caution in patients undergoing major surgery involving general anesthesia, and the anesthetic used should be one that does not cause myocardial depression. (See Drug Interactions: Other Drugs.) The necessity of withdrawing β-adrenergic blocking therapy prior to major surgery is controversial. Metoprolol may impair the ability of the heart to respond to reflex β-adrenergic stimuli and may increase the risks associated with general anesthesia such as severe hypotension and maintenance of heart beat. As with other β-blockers, the effects of metoprolol can be reversed by administration of β-agonists (e.g., dobutamine, isoproterenol). If metoprolol is continued during major or dental surgery, the anesthesiologist or dentist should be informed that the patient is receiving the drug.

Since β-blockers may inhibit bronchodilation produced by endogenous catecholamines, the drugs generally should not be used in patients with bronchospastic disease; however, because of its relative β_1-selective adrenergic blocking activity, metoprolol may be used with caution in patients with bronchospastic disease who do not respond to or cannot tolerate other hypotensive agents. In such patients, the lowest effective dosage of metoprolol should be used in addition to maximal therapy with a β_2-adrenergic agonist (e.g., terbutaline); in addition, it would be prudent to initially administer metoprolol in lower dosage given in 3 divided doses daily to avoid the higher plasma concentrations of the drug associated with twice-daily dosing. Patients receiving metoprolol should contact their physician if any difficulty in breathing occurs. Bronchoconstriction is readily reversed with β_2-adrenergic agonists.

Although the oculomucocutaneous syndrome associated with practolol use has not occurred with metoprolol, some patients have experienced dry eyes and decreased tear production, minimal injection of conjunctivae and/or eyelids, punctate keratitis, keratoconjunctivitis or corneal ulceration; therefore, patients receiving metoprolol should be observed carefully for potential ocular adverse effects.

Signs of hyperthyroidism (e.g., tachycardia) may be masked by metoprolol, and patients having or suspected of developing thyrotoxicosis should be monitored carefully because abrupt withdrawal of β-adrenergic blockade might precipitate thyroid storm. In addition, it is recommended that metoprolol be used with caution in patients with diabetes mellitus (especially those with labile diabetes) since the drug also may mask signs and symptoms of hypoglycemia (e.g., tachycardia, palpitation, blood pressure changes, tremor, feelings of anxiety, but not sweating) and may potentiate insulin-induced hypoglycemia.(see Cautions: Endocrine Effects.) However, many clinicians state that patients with diabetes mellitus may be particularly likely to experience a reduction in morbidity and mortality with the use of β-blockers.

The manufacturer states that metoprolol should be used with caution in patients with impaired hepatic function.

Because of similarity in spelling between Toprol-XL® (metoprolol succinate) and Topamax® (the trade name for topiramate, an anticonvulsant and antimigraine agent), the potential exists for dispensing or prescribing errors involving these drugs. In addition, there is a potential for dispensing errors involving confusion between Toprol-XL® and Tegretol® or Tegretol®-XR (trade names for carbamazepine, an anticonvulsant that also is used for relief of pain associated with trigeminal neuralgia, as well as for various psychiatric disorders). These medication errors have been associated with serious adverse events sometimes requiring hospitalization as a result of either lack of the intended medication (e.g., seizure recurrence, return of hallucinations, suicide attempt, hypertension recurrence) or exposure to the wrong drug (e.g., bradycardia in a patient erroneously receiving metoprolol). Therefore, extra care should be exercised to ensure the accuracy of both oral and written prescriptions for these drugs. (See Dispensing and Administration Precautions, in Dosage and Administration: Administration.) Patients should be advised to carefully check their medications and to bring any questions or concerns to the attention of the dispensing pharmacist. Dispensing errors involving Toprol-XL® (metoprolol succinate) and Topamax® (topiramate) or Tegretol® or Tegretol®–XR (carbamazepine) should be reported to the manufacturers, the USP/ISMP (Institute for Safe Medication Practices) Medication Errors Reporting Program by phone (800-233-7767), or directly to the FDA MedWatch program by phone (800-FDA-1088), fax (800-FDA-0178), or internet (http://www.fda.gov/Safety/MedWatch).

Metoprolol should be used with caution, if at all, in patients with AV conduction defects. The drug should be used with extreme caution in patients with substantial cardiomegaly. Metoprolol is contraindicated in patients with hypertension or angina who have sinus bradycardia, heart block greater than first degree, cardiogenic shock, overt or decompensated cardiac failure, severe peripheral, arterial circulatory disorders, pheochromocytoma (unless administered after initiating treatment with an alpha-adrenergic blocking agent), or sick sinus syndrome (unless a permanent pacemaker is in place). The drug is contraindicated in patients with acute MI who have a heart rate less than 45–60 beats/minute, heart block greater than first degree, systolic blood pressure less than 100 mm Hg, or moderate to severe cardiac failure. Metoprolol also is contraindicated in patients with a known history of hypersensitivity to metoprolol or any component of the formulations and in patients with a known history of hypersensitivity to other β-blockers.

■ Pediatric Precautions Although safety and efficacy of metoprolol tartrate remain to be fully established in children, some experts have recommended pediatric dosages for hypertension based on currently limited clinical experience.

The safety and efficacy of extended-release metoprolol succinate in pediatric patients has been evaluated in a placebo-controlled study in hypertensive patients 6–16 years of age. In this study, patients received extended-release metoprolol succinate 0.2, 1, or 2 mg/kg orally once daily (dosage expressed in terms of metoprolol tartrate) or placebo and were followed for 4 weeks. Although the primary efficacy end point (dose response for reduction in systolic blood pressure) was not met, several prespecified secondary end points were achieved. Compared with placebo, extended-release metoprolol succinate substantially reduced systolic blood pressure at the 1- and 2-mg/kg once-daily dosages, reduced diastolic blood pressure at the 2-mg/kg once-daily dosage, and demonstrated a dose-response relationship for reductions in diastolic blood pressure. No substantial differences in safety relative to adults were observed. Safety and efficacy of metoprolol succinate has not been established in children younger than 6 years of age.

For information on overall principles and expert recommendations for treatment of hypertension in pediatric patients, see Uses: Hypertension in Pediatric Patients, in the Thiazides General Statement 40:28.20.

■ Geriatric Precautions Clinical trials of conventional metoprolol tartrate or extended-release metoprolol succinate tablets for hypertension did not include sufficient numbers of patients 65 years and older to determine whether they respond differently than younger adults. While clinical experience generally has not revealed age-related differences in response to the drug, care should be taken in dosage selection of metoprolol. Safety and efficacy of conventional metoprolol tartrate tablets are similar in geriatric adults with MI and younger adults. However, since the possibility of greater sensitivity of some older patients cannot be ruled out, initial dosage should be selected carefully in these patients. Safety and efficacy of extended-release metoprolol succinate are similar in geriatric adults with heart failure and in younger adults. Because of the greater frequency of decreased hepatic, renal, and/or cardiac function and of concomitant disease and drug therapy in geriatric patients, the manufacturer suggests that patients in this age group receive initial dosages of the drug in the lower end of the usual range.

■ Mutagenicity and Carcinogenicity There has been no evidence of mutagenic potential in tests performed to date with metoprolol. No evidence of metoprolol tartrate-induced mutagenicity was observed in dominant lethal tests in mice, chromosome tests in somatic cells, *Salmonella* mammalian microsome tests, or nucleus anomaly tests in somatic interphase nuclei. No evidence of mutagenicity was observed in the *Salmonella* mammalian microsome test using metoprolol succinate. In chronic toxicity studies, benign lung tumors (small adenomas) occurred more frequently in female Swiss albino mice receiving oral dosages of metoprolol tartrate up to 750 mg/kg daily (representing 18 times the daily dosage of 200 mg in a 60-kg patient on a mg/m^2basis) for 21 months than in untreated control animals, although there was no increase in malignant lung tumors or total (benign plus malignant) lung tumors. In CD-1 mice, however, no differences were observed between treated and control mice of either gender for any tumor. In a 2-year study in rats, there was no evidence of increased development of spontaneously occurring benign or malignant neoplasms at dosages of metoprolol tartrate up to 800 mg/kg daily. However, in these rats, histologic changes included an increased incidence of mild focal accumulation of foamy macrophages in alveolar spaces and slight increases of biliary hyperplasia.

■ Pregnancy, Fertility, and Lactation Distribution studies in mice have shown that the fetus is exposed to metoprolol when the drug is administered during pregnancy. Although there are no adequate and controlled studies to date in humans, metoprolol has been shown to increase postimplantation loss and to decrease neonatal survival in rats when given at metoprolol succinate dosages (expressed as the tartrate) up to 22 times a daily dosage of 200 mg in a 60-kg patient (on a mg/m^2 basis) or metoprolol tartrate dosages up to 55.5 times the maximum recommended human dosage of 450 mg daily. Metoprolol should be used during pregnancy only when clearly needed.

Reproduction studies in rats using metoprolol succinate dosages (expressed as the tartrate) up to 22 times a daily dosage of 200 mg in a 60-kg patient (on a mg/m^2 basis) or metoprolol tartrate dosages up to 55.5 times the maximum recommended human dosage of 450 mg have not revealed evidence of impaired fertility. Metoprolol has rarely caused Peyronie's disease in human males.

Since metoprolol is distributed into milk, the drug should be used with caution in nursing women. The extent to which metoprolol distributes into milk has not been clearly established, but the amount of drug a nursing infant would ingest (less than 1 mg/L of milk consumed daily) is believed to be too small to be clinically important; however, if a woman receiving metoprolol breast-feeds, the infant should be monitored for potential systemic effects of the drug.

Drug Interactions

■ Cardiovascular Drugs When metoprolol is administered with diuretics or other hypotensive drugs, the hypotensive effect of metoprolol may be increased. This effect is usually used to therapeutic advantage, but careful adjustment of dosage is necessary when these drugs are used concomitantly. An additive effect may be obtained when metoprolol is given to patients receiving catecholamine-depleting drugs, such as reserpine and monoamine oxidase inhibitors, resulting in hypotension and/or bradycardia. The β_1-adrenergic stimulating effects of sympathomimetic agents are antagonized by usual doses of metoprolol.

Concomitant use of β-adrenergic blocking agents (β-blockers) and certain other cardiovascular drugs (e.g., cardiac glycosides, nondihydropyridine calcium-channel blocking agents) can have additive negative effects on SA or AV nodal conduction. Caution should be exercised in the concomitant administration of β-blockers and other cardiovascular drugs (e.g., nondihydropyridine calcium-channel blocking agents). Slowing or complete suppression of SA node activity with development of slow ventricular rates (e.g., 30–40 bpm), often misdiagnosed as complete AV block, has been reported in patients receiving the nondihydropyridine calcium-channel blocking agent mibefradil (no longer commercially available in the US), principally in geriatric patients and in association with concomitant β-blocker therapy.

Because β-blockers may exacerbate rebound hypertension that may occur following discontinuance of clonidine therapy, β-blockers should be discontinued several days before gradual withdrawal of clonidine when clonidine therapy is to be discontinued in patients receiving a β-blocker and clonidine concurrently. If clonidine therapy is to be replaced by a β-blocker, administration of the β-blocker should be delayed for several days after clonidine therapy has been discontinued.

Verapamil may substantially increase the oral bioavailability of metoprolol, a lipophilic drug. Area under the plasma metoprolol concentration-time curve has increased up to 300% following initiation of verapamil therapy. Verapamil appears to increase oral bioavailability of metoprolol by decreasing its hepatic clearance, although the exact mechanism(s) has not been elucidated. A similar pharmacokinetic interaction does not appear to occur when atenolol, a hydrophilic drug, and verapamil are used concomitantly. Concomitant use of verapamil and metoprolol should be avoided if possible and another β-blocker with which verapamil does not interact pharmacokinetically (e.g., atenolol) preferably used when combined therapy is required. If verapamil and metoprolol are used concomitantly, dosage of metoprolol should be adjusted carefully and the patient monitored closely.

■ Drugs Affecting Hepatic Microsomal Enzymes Metabolism of certain β-blockers (e.g., metoprolol, timolol) is mediated by the cytochrome (CYP) P-450 isoenzyme 2D6 (CYP2D6), and concurrent use of metoprolol with drugs that inhibit CYP2D6 (e.g., bupropion, cimetidine, diphenhydramine, fluoxetine, hydroxychloroquine, paroxetine, propafenone, quinidine, ritonavir, terbinafine, thioridazine) may increase plasma metoprolol concentrations, resulting in decreased cardioselectivity of the drug. Pending further experience with combination therapy with paroxetine and metoprolol, caution should be exercised when paroxetine and metoprolol are used concomitantly. In healthy individuals with an extensive metabolizer phenotype, coadministration of quinidine (100 mg) and metoprolol conventional tablets (200 mg) doubled the half life of metoprolol and tripled the plasma concentration of the *S*-enantiomer. In a limited number of patients with cardiovascular disease, concurrent administration of propafenone (150 mg 3 times daily) with metoprolol conventional tablets (50 mg 3 times daily) resulted in a twofold to fivefold increase in the steady-state plasma concentration of metoprolol.

■ **Other Drugs** Use of myocardial depressant general anesthetics (e.g., diethyl ether) in patients receiving a β-blocker, such as metoprolol, leads to a risk of hypotension and heart failure.

Administration of a β-blocker with a vasodilator, such as hydralazine, in patients with uremia could cause pulmonary hypertension secondary to β-adrenergic blockade of the pulmonary vasculature and to the increased cardiac output caused by the vasodilator.

Acute Toxicity

■ **Pathogenesis** The acute lethal dose of metoprolol in humans is not known. The oral LD_{50} of the drug is 1158–2460 and 3090–4670 mg/kg in mice and rats, respectively.

■ **Manifestations** Limited information is available on acute metoprolol toxicity; several cases of overdosage with metoprolol tartrate or metoprolol succinate have been reported, some resulting in death. A 19-year-old man who ingested 10 g of metoprolol tartrate (160 mg/kg) was conscious with peripheral cyanosis, weak heart sounds, and no measurable blood pressure. Treatment consisted of gastric lavage, IV infusion of Ringer's injection, IV administration of sodium bicarbonate to correct acidosis, furosemide to relieve fluid retention, and glucagon and metaraminol to restore blood pressure. Within 12 hours after admission to the hospital, the patient exhibited no signs of cardiac depression. In general, overdosage of metoprolol may be expected to produce effects that are mainly extensions of pharmacologic effects, including symptomatic bradycardia, hypotension, bronchospasm, and acute cardiac failure; impaired conduction, decreased cardiac contractility, heart block, shock, and cardiac arrest also may occur. Other manifestations associated with overdosage of metoprolol succinate as extended-release tablets include atrioventricular block, cardiogenic shock, cardiac arrest, impairment of consciousness, nausea, vomiting, and cyanosis.

■ **Treatment** In acute metoprolol overdose, the stomach should be emptied immediately by gastric lavage. Supportive and symptomatic treatment should be initiated. For symptomatic bradycardia, IV atropine sulfate may be given; if bradycardia persists, IV isoproterenol hydrochloride may be administered cautiously. A vasopressor (e.g., dopamine, norepinephrine) may be given for severe hypotension; IV glucagon may be useful if hypotension is refractory to vasopressors. A β-adrenergic agonist (e.g., isoproterenol) and/or a theophylline derivative may be given for bronchospasm. For heart failure, a cardiac glycoside, diuretic, and oxygen should be used; IV glucagon also may be useful.

Pharmacology

At low doses, metoprolol is a selective inhibitor of β_1-adrenergic receptors. Like propranolol, metoprolol inhibits response to adrenergic stimuli by competitively blocking β_1-adrenergic receptors within the myocardium. Unlike propranolol, however, metoprolol blocks β_2-adrenergic receptors within bronchial and vascular smooth muscle only in high doses.

Through its myocardial β_1-adrenergic blocking action, metoprolol decreases resting heart rate and reflex orthostatic tachycardia, inhibits exercise-induced increases in heart rate, decreases myocardial contractility, and decreases cardiac output at rest and during exercise without a compensatory increase in peripheral resistance. The drug increases systolic ejection time and cardiac volume; stroke volume is unchanged. Metoprolol also decreases conduction velocity through the sinoatrial (SA) and atrioventricular (AV) nodes and decreases myocardial automaticity via β_1-adrenergic blockade. The drug has no intrinsic sympathomimetic activity and little or no membrane-stabilizing effect on the heart; membrane-stabilizing effects occur only at plasma concentrations much higher than those required for β-adrenergic blocking action.

The precise mechanism of metoprolol's hypotensive action has not been determined. It has been postulated that β-adrenergic blocking agents (β-blockers) reduce blood pressure by blocking peripheral (especially cardiac) adrenergic receptors (decreasing cardiac output), by decreasing sympathetic outflow from the CNS, and/or by suppressing renin release. Results of several studies suggest a reduction in peripheral resistance by inhibition of release of norepinephrine as a basis for metoprolol's hypotensive effect, but this requires further study. Like propranolol, metoprolol decreases blood pressure in both supine and standing positions.

In patients with normal or high concentrations of circulating renin, low doses of metoprolol are associated with a fall in plasma renin concentrations, possibly due, at least partly, to acute peripheral β_1-adrenergic blockade. Metoprolol also substantially reduces furosemide-induced renin release. Metoprolol and propranolol produce similar decreases in plasma renin activity (PRA) in patients with high PRA. The importance of these effects in decreasing blood pressure in hypertensive patients requires further investigation.

A small increase in serum potassium has been observed during metoprolol therapy and may be related to β_2-adrenergic blockade and reduced PRA and plasma aldosterone concentration.

The exact mechanism of action of metoprolol in patients with suspected or definite myocardial infarction (MI) has not been determined. In patients with MI, metoprolol reduces heart rate, systolic blood pressure, and cardiac output, but stroke volume, diastolic blood pressure, and pulmonary artery end diastolic pressure remain unchanged; the drug also appears to decrease the occurrence of ventricular fibrillation in these patients.

In the management of angina pectoris, the mechanism of action of metoprolol is thought to be blockade of catecholamine-induced increases in heart rate, velocity and extent of myocardial contraction, and blood pressure, which results in a net decrease in myocardial oxygen consumption. In some studies, metoprolol (given as extended-release tablets) has improved left ventricular ejection fraction and has been shown to delay increases in left ventricular end-systolic and end-diastolic volumes after 6 months of therapy.

Usual doses of metoprolol increase airway resistance and decrease ventilatory capacity in asthmatic patients but, because of its relatively selective β_1-adrenergic blocking activity, to a lesser degree than does an equivalent β_1-adrenergic receptor blocking dose of propranolol. Unlike propranolol, low dosages (up to 100 mg daily) of metoprolol tartrate do not appreciably inhibit isoproterenol-induced bronchodilation. Because of its relative β_1-adrenergic blocking selectivity, metoprolol causes little inhibition of glycogenolysis in skeletal and cardiac muscles. Metoprolol inhibits the increase in plasma glycerol caused by exercise. Metoprolol may cause less inhibition of insulin release than does propranolol and may therefore result in better glucose tolerance than does propranolol in patients with diabetes mellitus; however, results of studies of this effect are conflicting. Metoprolol does not appear to reduce free fatty acid concentrations in healthy individuals. Fasting triglyceride concentrations have been increased in some patients, while in others no consistent changes have occurred. Metoprolol may increase the peripheral platelet count by interfering with β-adrenergic receptors involved in platelet level regulation in the spleen.

Pharmacokinetics

■ **Absorption** Metoprolol tartrate is rapidly and almost completely absorbed from the GI tract; absorption of a single oral dose of 20–100 mg is complete in 2.5–3 hours. After an oral dose, about 50% of the drug administered as conventional tablets appears to undergo first-pass metabolism in the liver. Bioavailability of orally administered metoprolol tartrate increases with increased doses, indicating a possible saturable disposition process of low capacity such as tissue binding in the liver. Steady-state oral bioavailability of extended-release tablets of metoprolol succinate given once daily at dosages equivalent to 50–400 mg of metoprolol tartrate is about 77% of that of conventional tablets at corresponding dosages given once daily or in divided doses. Food does not appear to affect bioavailability of metoprolol succinate extended-release tablets. Following a single oral dose as conventional tablets, metoprolol appears in the plasma within 10 minutes and peak plasma concentrations are reached in about 90 minutes. When metoprolol tartrate conventional tablets are administered with food rather than on an empty stomach, peak plasma concentrations are higher and the extent of absorption of the drug is increased. Following oral administration of metoprolol succinate as extended-release tablets, peak plasma metoprolol concentrations are about 25–50% of those attained after administration of metoprolol tartrate conventional tablets given once daily or in divided doses. However, in patients with heart failure, peak plasma concentrations attained after administration of metoprolol succinate as extended-release tablets (200 mg [expressed as the tartrate] once daily) are similar to those attained with conventional metoprolol tartrate tablets (50 mg 3 times daily). Time to peak concentration is longer with extended-release tablets, with peak plasma concentrations being reached in about 7 hours following administration of such tablets.

Plasma concentrations attained 1 hour after an oral dose are linearly related to metoprolol tartrate doses ranging from 50–400 mg as conventional tablets. After an oral dose of metoprolol tartrate, plasma concentrations attained are quite variable among individuals (particularly in geriatric patients) and apparently do not correlate with hypotensive effects. However, oral doses ranging from 50–400 mg appear to cause dose-dependent reductions in systolic blood pressure and exercise-induced heart rate. In addition, a linear relationship between plasma concentration of the drug and reduction in exercise-induced heart rate appears to exist. In healthy adults, plasma metoprolol concentrations of 8–144 ng/mL are associated with an 8–23% reduction in exercised-induced tachycardia; plasma concentration-effect curves reach a plateau at about 53.5–80 ng/mL, and higher metoprolol plasma concentrations produce little additional β_1-adrenergic blocking effects. The relative β_1 selectivity of the drug diminishes at higher plasma metoprolol concentrations while β_2-blocking effects increase at higher plasma metoprolol concentrations. Such effects diminish at higher plasma metoprolol concentrations while β_2-adrenergic blocking effects increase at higher plasma metoprolol concentrations.

Following oral administration of dosages equivalent to 100–400 mg of metoprolol tartrate given once daily as metoprolol succinate extended-release tablets in healthy individuals, steady-state β-adrenergic blocking effects (as measured by blockade of exercise-induced increases in heart rate) over a 24-hour period were similar to those following administration of metoprolol tartrate conventional tablets given 1–4 times daily. However, β-adrenergic blocking effects over a 24-hour period were higher following oral administration of metoprolol succinate extended-release tablets given once daily in a dosage equivalent to 50 mg of metoprolol tartrate compared with those following administration of the same dosage given as metoprolol tartrate conventional tablets. Following oral administration of metoprolol succinate as extended-release tablets, reduction in exercise-induced heart rate is stable throughout the entire dosing interval, and oral doses (equivalent to the tartrate) ranging from 50–400 mg appear to cause dose-dependent reductions in exercise-induced heart rate while a larger peak effect on exercise-induced tachycardia occurs following administration of 50–100 mg once daily as conventional tablets; this effect is not observed 24 hours after dosing. To achieve a similar effect to that attained with metoprolol succinate extended-release tablets, a total daily dosage of 200–400 mg is given in 3 or 4 divided doses if administered as conventional metoprolol tartrate tablets. In a randomized, crossover trial in patients with heart failure who had prior chronic therapy with metoprolol, the reduction in the average or exercise-induced heart rate over 24 hours was greater during short-term therapy with metoprolol succinate 200 mg (expressed as the tartrate) daily as extended-release tablets than with metoprolol tartrate 50 mg 3 times daily as conventional tablets. The manufacturer of Toprol XL® states that the relationship between plasma metoprolol concentrations and reduction in exercise-induced heart rate is independent of the pharmaceutical formulation. In patients with angina pectoris, a relationship between metoprolol tartrate dose and exercise capacity and reductions in left ventricular ischemia appears to exist for oral doses ranging from 50–400 mg. Following oral administration of multiple doses of metoprolol tartrate (50–80 mg 3 times daily), peak plasma concentrations range from 20–340 ng/mL.

In hypertensive patients, a reduction in systolic blood pressure during exercise has been reported within 15 minutes after a single oral dose of 50–80 mg of metoprolol tartrate and the effect persisted for 6 hours. Dosages of 150–450 mg daily cause a dose-dependent decrease in systolic blood pressure which averages 20 mm Hg; the effect is usually maximal within 1 week in healthy or hypertensive patients at rest and during exercise. The same dosage causes a less rapid but appreciable reduction in diastolic blood pressure which averages 10–15 mm Hg. Metoprolol succinate extended-release tablets given once daily at dosages equivalent to 100–400 mg of metoprolol tartrate produce similar hypotensive effects as conventional metoprolol tartrate tablets at similar dosages given 2–4 times daily; the hypotensive effect of extended-release tablets may persist for 24 hours. Duration of the β-adrenergic blocking effect (as measured by blockade of exercise-induced increases in heart rate) is dose related, increasing with increasing doses. With chronic therapy, hypotensive effects may persist for up to 4 weeks after withdrawal of the drug, possibly as a result of tissue-bound drug.

Plasma metoprolol concentrations attained after IV administration of the drug are approximately 2 times those attained following oral administration. Following IV infusion of metoprolol over 10 minutes in healthy individuals, maximum β-adrenergic blocking activity occurred at 20 minutes. In healthy individuals, a maximum reduction in exercise-induced heart rate of approximately 10 and 15% occurs following IV administration of a single 5- and 15-mg metoprolol dose, respectively; the effect on exercise-induced heart rate decreased linearly with time at the same rate for both doses and persisted for approximately 5 and 8 hours for the 5- and 15-mg doses, respectively.

■ **Distribution** Metoprolol is widely distributed into body tissues. The concentration of the drug is greater in the heart, liver, lungs, and saliva than in the plasma. Metoprolol is 11–12% bound to serum proteins, apparently only to albumin. Following therapeutic doses, metoprolol concentrations in erythrocytes are about 20% greater than those in plasma, but the drug is available for elimination from these two sites at the same rate. Metoprolol crosses the placenta, and maternal and fetal blood concentrations are about equal. The drug crosses the blood-brain barrier; the concentration of metoprolol in CSF is about 78% of the simultaneous concentration in plasma. Metoprolol is distributed into milk in a concentration about 3–4 times that of maternal plasma concentrations, but the actual amount distributed into milk appears to be very small.

■ **Elimination** Elimination of metoprolol appears to follow first-order kinetics and occurs mainly in the liver; the time required for the process apparently is independent of dose and duration of therapy. In healthy individuals and hypertensive patients, the elimination half-life of both unchanged drug and metabolites is about 3–4 hours. In poor hydroxylators of the drug, the elimination half-life is prolonged to about 7.6 hours. There is more interindividual variation in elimination half-lives in geriatric patients than in young healthy individuals. The half-life of metoprolol does not increase appreciably with impaired renal function.

Metoprolol is metabolized by the cytochrome P-450 (CYP) microsomal enzyme system, predominantly by the 2D6 isoenzyme (CYP2D6). When administered orally, metoprolol exhibits stereoselective metabolism that is dependent on oxidation phenotype. The CYP2D6 isoenzyme is absent in about 8% of Caucasians (poor metabolizers) and about 2% of most other populations. Since CYP2D6 can be inhibited by other drugs, concomitant use of such drugs with metoprolol in poor metabolizers will lead to increases in plasma metoprolol concentrations and a decrease in the β_1-selectivity of the drug. Metoprolol does not inhibit or enhance its own metabolism. Three main metabolites of the drug are formed by oxidative deamination, *O*-dealkylation with subsequent oxidation, and aliphatic hydroxylation; these metabolites account for 85% of the total urinary excretion of metabolites. The metabolites apparently do not have appreciable pharmacologic activity. The rate of hydroxylation, resulting in α-hydroxymetoprolol, is genetically determined and is subject to considerable interindividual variation. Poor hydroxylators of metoprolol have increased areas under the plasma concentration-time curves (AUCs), prolonged elimination half-lives (about 7.6 hours), higher urinary concentrations of unchanged drug, and negligible urinary concentrations of α-hydroxymetoprolol compared with extensive hydroxylators. β-Adrenergic blockade of exercise-induced tachycardia persists for at least 24 hours after administration of a single 200-mg oral dose of metoprolol tartrate in poor hydroxylators.

Metoprolol and its metabolites are excreted in urine mainly via glomerular filtration, although tubular secretion and reabsorption may be involved. About 95% of a single oral dose is excreted in urine within 72 hours. Less than 5% and approximately 10% of a metoprolol dose is excreted unchanged in urine following oral and IV administration of the drug, respectively.

Chemistry and Stability

■ **Chemistry** Metoprolol is a β_1-selective adrenergic blocking agent. Metoprolol is commercially available as the tartrate salt in oral tablets and parenteral injection and as the succinate salt in oral extended-release tablets containing controlled-release coated pellets. Metoprolol tartrate is commercially available as a racemic mixture. Metoprolol tartrate occurs as a white, crystalline powder with a bitter taste and is very soluble in water and freely soluble in alcohol. The drug has a pK_a of 9.68. Metoprolol succinate occurs as a white, crystalline powder and is freely soluble in water and sparingly soluble in alcohol.

■ **Stability** Commercially available preparations of metoprolol tartrate should be protected from light. Metoprolol tartrate tablets should be protected from moisture and stored in tight, light-resistant containers at 25°C but may be exposed to temperatures ranging from 15–30°C. Metoprolol tartrate injection should be stored at a temperature of 25°C but may be exposed to temperatures ranging from 15–30°C; freezing of the injection should be avoided.

Preparations

Excipients in commercially available drug preparations may have clinically important effects in some individuals; consult specific product labeling for details.

Metoprolol Succinate

Oral		
Tablets, extended-release, film-coated	23.75 mg (equivalent to 25 mg of metoprolol tartrate)*	**Metoprolol Succinate Extended-release Tablets** **Toprol XL®** (scored), AstraZeneca
	47.5 mg (equivalent to 50 mg of metoprolol tartrate)*	**Metoprolol Succinate Extended-release Tablets** **Toprol XL®** (scored), AstraZeneca
	95 mg (equivalent to 100 mg of metoprolol tartrate)*	**Metoprolol Succinate Extended-release Tablets** **Toprol XL®** (scored), AstraZeneca
	190 mg (equivalent to 200 mg of metoprolol tartrate)*	**Metoprolol Succinate Extended-release Tablets** **Toprol XL®** (scored), AstraZeneca

*available from one or more manufacturer, distributor, and/or repackager by generic (nonproprietary) name

Metoprolol Tartrate

Oral		
Tablets	50 mg*	**Lopressor®** (scored), Validus **Metoprolol Tartrate Tablets**
	100 mg*	**Lopressor®** (scored), Validus **Metoprolol Tartrate Tablets**
Parenteral		
Injection	1 mg/mL*	**Lopressor®**, Novartis **Metoprolol Tartrate Injection**

*available from one or more manufacturer, distributor, and/or repackager by generic (nonproprietary) name

Metoprolol Tartrate and Hydrochlorothiazide

Oral		
Tablets	50 mg Metoprolol Tartrate and Hydrochlorothiazide 25 mg*	**Lopressor® HCT** (scored), Validus **Metoprolol Tartrate and Hydrochlorothiazide Tablets**
	100 mg Metoprolol Tartrate and Hydrochlorothiazide 25 mg*	**Lopressor® HCT** (scored), Validus **Metoprolol Tartrate and Hydrochlorothiazide Tablets**
	100 mg Metoprolol Tartrate and Hydrochlorothiazide 50 mg*	**Lopressor® HCT** (scored), Validus **Metoprolol Tartrate and Hydrochlorothiazide Tablets**

*available from one or more manufacturer, distributor, and/or repackager by generic (nonproprietary) name

†Use is not currently included in the labeling approved by the US Food and Drug Administration

Propranolol Hydrochloride

■ Propranolol hydrochloride is a nonselective β-adrenergic blocking agent (β-blocker).

Uses

Propranolol is used for the management of hypertension, angina, supraventricular and ventricular arrhythmias, acute myocardial infarction (MI), and essential tremor. Propranolol also is used for prophylaxis of migraine headache, management of hypertrophic subaortic stenosis, and as an adjunct in the management of pheochromocytoma. The drug also has been used in the management of thyrotoxicosis†.

The choice of a β-adrenergic blocking agent (β-blocker) depends on numerous factors, including pharmacologic properties (e.g., relative β-selectivity, intrinsic sympathomimetic activity, membrane-stabilizing activity, lipophilicity), pharmacokinetics, intended use, and adverse effect profile, as well as the patient's coexisting disease states or conditions, response, and tolerance. While specific pharmacologic properties and other factors may appropriately influence the choice of a β-blocker in individual patients, evidence of clinically important differences among the agents in terms of overall efficacy and/or safety is limited. Patients who do not respond to or cannot tolerate one β-blocker may be successfully treated with a different agent.

In the management of hypertension or chronic stable angina pectoris in patients with chronic obstructive pulmonary disease (COPD) or type 1 diabetes mellitus, many clinicians prefer to use low dosages of a β_1-selective adrenergic blocking agent (e.g., atenolol, metoprolol), rather than a nonselective agent (e.g., nadolol, pindolol, propranolol, timolol). However, selectivity of these agents is relative and dose dependent. Some clinicians also will recommend using a β_1-selective agent or an agent with intrinsic sympathomimetic activity (e.g., pindolol), rather than a nonselective agent, for the management of hypertension or angina pectoris in patients with peripheral vascular disease, but there is no evidence that the choice of β-blocker substantially affects efficacy. Nonselective β-blockers are preferred for the management of hypertension or angina pectoris in patients with coexisting essential tremor or vascular (e.g., migraine) headache. For further information on management and classification of migraine headache, see Vascular Headaches: General Principles in Migraine Therapy, under Uses in Sumatriptan 28:32.28.

■ **Hypertension** Propranolol is used alone or in combination with other classes of antihypertensive agents in the management of hypertension.

Current evidence-based practice guidelines for the management of hypertension in adults generally recommend the use of drugs from 4 classes of antihypertensive agents (angiotensin-converting enzyme [ACE] inhibitors, angiotensin II receptor antagonists, calcium-channel blockers, and thiazide diuretics). Most guidelines no longer recommend β-blockers as first-line therapy for hypertension because of the lack of established superiority over other recommended drug classes and evidence from at least one study demonstrating that β-blockers may be less effective than angiotensin II receptor antagonists in preventing cardiovascular death, MI, or stroke. However, therapy with a β-blocker may still be considered in hypertensive patients who have a compelling indication (e.g., prior MI, ischemic heart disease, heart failure) for their use or as add-on therapy in those who do not respond adequately to the preferred drug classes. (See Considerations for Drug Therapy in Patients with Underlying Cardiovascular and Other Risk Factors under Uses: Hypertension, in Atenolol 24:24 and in Metoprolol 24:24.) Ultimately, choice of antihypertensive therapy should be individualized, considering the clinical characteristics of the patient (e.g., age, ethnicity/race, comorbid conditions, cardiovascular risk factors) as well as drug-related factors (e.g., ease of administration, availability, adverse effects, costs).

A 2017 multidisciplinary hypertension guideline of the American College of Cardiology (ACC), American Heart Association (AHA), and a number of other professional organizations generally recommends a target blood pressure goal (i.e., blood pressure to achieve with drug therapy and/or nonpharmacologic intervention) of less than 130/80 mm Hg in all adults regardless of comorbidities or level of atherosclerotic cardiovascular disease (ASCVD) risk. In addition, a systolic blood pressure goal of less than 130 mm Hg generally is recommended for noninstitutionalized ambulatory patients 65 years of age or older with an average systolic blood pressure of at least 130 mm Hg. These blood pressure goals are based upon clinical studies demonstrating continuing reduction of cardiovascular risk at progressively lower levels of systolic blood pressure. Previous hypertension guidelines, such as those from an expert panel of the Eighth Joint National Committee on the Prevention, Detection, Evaluation, and Treatment of High Blood Pressure (JNC 8), generally have recommended initiation of antihypertensive treatment in patients with a systolic blood pressure of at least 140 mm Hg or diastolic blood pressure of at least 90 mm Hg, targeted a blood pressure goal of less than 140/90 mm Hg regardless of cardiovascular risk, and used higher systolic blood pressure thresholds and targets in geriatric patients compared with those recommended by the 2017 ACC/AHA hypertension guideline. The blood pressure thresholds used to define hypertension, the optimum blood pressure threshold at which to initiate antihypertensive drug therapy, and the ideal target blood pressure values remain controversial.

Most patients with hypertension, especially black patients, will require at least 2 antihypertensive drugs to achieve adequate blood pressure control. In general, black hypertensive patients tend to respond better to monotherapy with thiazide diuretics or calcium-channel blocking agents than to monotherapy with β-blockers. Although β-blockers have lowered blood pressure in all races studied, monotherapy with these agents has produced a smaller reduction in blood pressure in black hypertensive patients; however, this population difference in response does not appear to occur during combined therapy with a β-blocker and a thiazide diuretic. (See Race under Hypertension: Other Special Considerations for Antihypertensive Drug Therapy, in Uses in Atenolol 24:24 and in Metoprolol 24:24.)

Propranolol is *not* indicated for the treatment of hypertensive emergencies.

In contrast to many other antihypertensive agents, propranolol lowers blood pressure equally well in the upright or supine position. The drug appears to be safe and effective for the treatment of hypertension in patients with renal damage. Although it apparently is more effective in patients with normal or elevated plasma renin concentrations than in those with low plasma renin concentrations, propranolol does lower blood pressure in patients with low-renin hypertension.

For additional information on the role of β-blockers in the management of hypertension, see Uses: Hypertension, in Atenolol 24:24 and in Metoprolol 24:24. For information on overall principles and expert recommendations for treatment of hypertension, see Uses: Hypertension in Adults and also see Uses: Hypertension in Pediatric Patients, in the Thiazides General Statement 40:28.20.

■ **Chronic Stable Angina** Propranolol is used for the long-term management of chronic stable angina pectoris. β-Blockers are recommended as the anti-ischemic drugs of choice in most patients with chronic stable angina; despite differences in cardioselectivity, intrinsic sympathomimetic activity, and other clinical factors, all β-blockers appear to be equally effective for this indication. In a double-blind study in patients with stable angina, propranolol reduced the frequency of anginal attacks and increased exercise tolerance compared with placebo.

Combination therapy with a β-blocker and a nitrate appears to be more effective than either drug alone because β-blockers attenuate the increased sympathetic tone and reflex tachycardia associated with nitrate therapy while nitrate therapy (e.g., nitroglycerin) counteracts the potential increase in left-ventricular wall tension associated with a decrease in heart rate. Combined therapy with a β-blocker and a dihydropyridine calcium-channel blocker also may be useful because the tendency to develop tachycardia with the calcium-channel blocker is counteracted by the β-blocker. However, caution should be exercised in the concomitant use of β-blockers and the nondihydropyridine calcium-channel blockers verapamil or diltiazem because of the potential for excessive fatigue, bradycardia, or atrioventricular (AV) block. (See Drug Interactions: Diuretics and Cardiovascular Drugs.)

■ **Cardiac Arrhythmias** ***Supraventricular Arrhythmias*** β-Blockers, including propranolol, are used to slow ventricular rate in patients with supraventricular tachycardia (SVT). The American College of Cardiology/American Heart Association/Heart Rhythm Society (ACC/AHA/HRS) guideline for the management of adult patients with supraventricular tachycardia recommends the use of β-blockers in the treatment of various SVTs (e.g., atrial flutter, junctional tachycardia, focal atrial tachycardia, atrioventricular nodal reentrant tachycardia [AVNRT]); in general, an IV β-blocker is recommended for acute treatment, while an oral β-blocker is recommended for ongoing management of these arrhythmias. Vagal maneuvers and/or IV adenosine generally are considered first-line interventions for the acute treatment of SVT and should be attempted prior to other therapies when clinically indicated; if such measures are ineffective or not feasible, an IV β-blocker may be considered in hemodynamically stable patients. Although evidence of efficacy is limited, experts state that the overall safety of β-blockers warrants their use in patients with SVT. Patients should be closely monitored for hypotension and bradycardia during administration of these drugs.

IV β-blockers may be used for the acute treatment of patients with hemodynamically stable focal atrial tachycardia (i.e., regular SVT arising from a localized atrial site), and an oral β-blocker may be used for ongoing management. Multifocal atrial tachycardia, characterized by a rapid, irregular rhythm with at least 3 distinct P-wave morphologies, is commonly associated with an underlying condition (e.g., pulmonary, coronary, or valvular heart disease) and is generally not responsive to antiarrhythmic drug therapy.

Propranolol is used to slow ventricular rate in patients with atrial fibrillation or atrial flutter when ventricular rate cannot be controlled with standard measures. For acute treatment of atrial fibrillation or flutter, an IV β-blocker (e.g., esmolol, propranolol, metoprolol) may be used for ventricular rate control in patients without preexcitation; an oral β-blocker may be used for ongoing rate control in such patients. Choice of a specific β-blocker should be individualized based on the patient's clinical condition.

IV β-blockers may be used for the acute treatment of hemodynamically stable patients with paroxysmal supraventricular tachycardia (PSVT), including AVNRT, that is uncontrolled or unconverted by vagal maneuvers and adenosine; an oral β-blocker may be used for the ongoing management of such patients who are not candidates for, or prefer not to undergo, catheter ablation. Propranolol may be useful in the prophylactic management of refractory PSVT, especially when caused by catecholamines or cardiac glycosides or associated with Wolff-Parkinson-White syndrome.

β-Blockers are considered one of several drug therapy options for the treatment of junctional tachycardia (i.e., nonreentrant SVT originating from the AV junction), a rapid, occasionally irregular, narrow-complex tachycardia. While evidence is limited, there is some data indicating that β-blockers (specifically propranolol) are modestly effective in terminating and/or reducing the incidence of junctional tachycardia.

Ventricular Arrhythmias Although propranolol generally is less effective in the management of ventricular arrhythmias than supraventricular arrhythmias and is usually not the first drug of choice for ventricular arrhythmias, it may be considered when cardioversion or other drugs are not effective. Propranolol also may be used in the treatment of persistent premature ventricular complexes that impair the well-being of the patient and do not respond to conventional therapy.

β-Blockers may be useful in the management of certain forms of polymorphic ventricular tachycardia (e.g., associated with acute ischemia).

β-Blockers also have been used in patients with cardiac arrest precipitated by ventricular fibrillation† or pulseless ventricular tachycardia†. However, AHA states that routine administration of β-blockers after cardiac arrest is potentially harmful (e.g., may worsen hemodynamic instability, exacerbate heart failure, or cause bradyarrhythmias) and is therefore not recommended.

Tachyarrhythmias Associated with Cardiac Glycoside Intoxication When AV block is not present, propranolol may be useful in the management of supraventricular or ventricular tachyarrhythmias associated with cardiac glycoside toxicity; however, because of the risk of adverse cardiovascular effects, the drug has a limited role in the management of these arrhythmias and other drugs are usually preferred. Propranolol can compromise conduction through the SA and AV nodes (possibly resulting in sinus bradycardia or asystole) and decrease myocardial automaticity; in addition, β-adrenergic blockade may result in deterioration of hemodynamic status in patients whose myocardial contractility depends on increased sympathetic nervous system activity. Oral propranolol may be useful in some patients for the management of cardiac glycoside-induced tachyarrhythmias that persist following discontinuance of the glycoside and correction of electrolyte abnormalities. IV propranolol should be used only if arrhythmias caused by cardiac glycoside intoxication are life-threatening and other therapy is ineffective. Use of digoxin immune Fab, if available, may be preferable and should be considered for the management of life-threatening cardiac glycoside-induced tachyarrhythmias that are unresponsive to conventional therapy.

Resistant Tachyarrhythmias Associated with Catecholamine Excess During Anesthesia Propranolol may be used with extreme caution and constant ECG and central venous pressure monitoring in the management of resistant tachyarrhythmias associated with catecholamine excess during anesthesia; however, more effective and less hazardous therapy such as lessening the depth of anesthesia or improving ventilation is preferred. (See Cautions: Precautions and Contraindications.)

■ **Hypertrophic Subaortic Stenosis** Propranolol may be of benefit in the management of exertional or other stress-induced angina, vertigo, syncope, and palpitation in some patients with hypertrophic subaortic stenosis; however, clinical improvement may be only temporary.

■ **Pheochromocytoma** An α-adrenergic blocking agent (e.g., phenoxybenzamine or phentolamine) alone is usually sufficient for management of the signs and symptoms of pheochromocytoma. Propranolol, however, may be used as an adjunct to α-adrenergic blocking agents to control symptoms resulting from excessive β-receptor stimulation in patients with inoperable or metastatic pheochromocytoma, or to control tachycardia prior to or during surgery in patients with pheochromocytoma. To prevent severe hypertension caused by unopposed α-adrenergic stimulation, treatment with an α-adrenergic blocking agent must always be instituted prior to the use of propranolol and continued during propranolol therapy in patients with pheochromocytoma.

■ **Thyrotoxicosis** Propranolol, which will not alter thyroid function tests, may be used orally as short-term (2–4 weeks) adjunctive therapy in the treatment of tachycardia and supraventricular arrhythmias in patients with thyrotoxicosis when these symptoms are distressful or hazardous, or when immediate therapy is necessary. Propranolol has been used IV and orally to treat symptomatic hypercalcemia secondary to thyrotoxicosis†, but this use requires further study. Propranolol has also been used for the management of thyrotoxicosis in neonates†. Safety of long-term administration of the drug in patients with thyrotoxicosis has not been established. The drug does not affect the underlying disease, which must be treated with an antithyroid agent.

■ **Vascular Headache** ***Migraine*** Propranolol may be used for the prophylaxis of common migraine headache. When used prophylactically, the drug can prevent common migraine or reduce the number of attacks in some patients. The US Headache Consortium states that there is good evidence from multiple well-designed clinical trials that propranolol has medium to high efficacy for the prophylaxis of migraine headache. Propranolol is not recommended for the treatment of a migraine attack that has already started nor for the prevention or treatment of cluster headaches. For further information on management and classification of migraine headache, see Vascular Headaches: General Principles in Migraine Therapy, under Uses in Sumatriptan 28:32.28.

■ **Myocardial Infarction** Propranolol is used to reduce the risk of cardiovascular mortality in patients who have survived the acute phase of MI and are clinically stable. In these patients, long-term (up to 39 months) administration of propranolol (begun within 5–21 days following MI) reduced overall mortality, cardiovascular mortality, arteriosclerotic heart disease (ASHD) mortality, and sudden death mortality within the ASHD category. Evidence of efficacy was obtained from a double-blind, placebo-controlled, multicenter study (Beta-Blocker Heart Attack Trial; BHAT). The effect of propranolol on reinfarction remains to be fully evaluated. For information on the use of β-blockers during the acute phase of MI, see Uses in Metoprolol 24:24.

The benefits of long-term β-blocker therapy for secondary prevention of MI have been well established in numerous clinical studies. Patients with MI complicated by heart failure, left ventricular dysfunction, or ventricular arrhythmias appear to derive the most benefit from long-term β-blocker therapy. Several large, randomized studies have demonstrated that prolonged oral therapy with a β-blocker can reduce the long-term rates of reinfarction and mortality (e.g., sudden or nonsudden cardiac death) following acute MI. It is estimated that such therapy could result in a relative reduction in mortality of about 25% annually for years 1–3 after infarction, with high-risk patients exhibiting the greatest potential benefit; the benefit of continued therapy may persist for at least several years beyond this period, although less substantially. Therefore, propranolol, like other β-blockers, can be used for secondary prevention following acute MI to reduce the risk of reinfarction and mortality. The American Heart Association/American College of Cardiology Foundation (AHA/ACCF) secondary prevention guideline recommends β-blocker therapy in all patients with left ventricular systolic dysfunction (ejection fraction of 40% or less) and prior MI; use of a β-blocker with proven mortality benefit (e.g., bisoprolol, carvedilol, or metoprolol succinate) is recommended. (See Uses: Heart Failure, in Carvedilol 24:24.) Although the benefits of long-term β-blockade in post-MI patients with normal left ventricular function are less well established, the guideline recommends continued β-blocker therapy for at least 3 years in such patients.

■ **Essential Tremor** Propranolol is used for the management of essential (familial, hereditary) tremor. The tremor is a postural and action tremor manifested as involuntary, rhythmic, oscillatory movements, principally of the upper limbs and, less frequently, the head; other areas, including the voice, legs, jaw, eyelids, and mouth, also may be involved. Essential tremor occurs during active movement and when the limb is held in a fixed posture or position against gravity; the tremor usually is absent at rest, although, when it is of large amplitude, tremor occasionally may be evident at rest, particularly in geriatric patients.

Propranolol decreases the amplitude but not the frequency of essential tremor; complete suppression of the tremor rarely is achieved with treatment. Response to propranolol therapy is variable, but the drug appears to be most effective in the management of high-amplitude, low-frequency tremor. Clinical benefit often is most evident for tremor affecting the upper extremities, although benefit also has been observed for head and other tremors; voice tremor may be less responsive to therapy with the drug. Propranolol hydrochloride doses of 120–320 mg generally produce tremor amplitude reductions averaging about 4–50%; however, reductions averaging 25–75% have been reported. Therapy with the drug may improve functional ability (e.g., handwriting, eating, drinking, dressing) and provide some subjective improvement (e.g., reduced anxiety and embarrassment), but patients should be advised that complete relief rarely is achieved so that their expectations about potential therapeutic benefit are realistic. Although propranolol often is used for chronic suppressive therapy in essential tremor, single oral doses may be useful in some patients to prevent or minimize tremor that is considered bothersome during specific, planned activity or to manage an exacerbation of tremor during periods of stress (e.g., business meetings, examinations).

■ **Other Uses** Propranolol has been used in the management of cyanotic spells of Fallot's tetralogy†, acute exacerbations of schizophrenic disorder† and anxiety states†, recurrent GI bleeding in patients with cirrhosis†, and many other conditions. In addition to essential tremor (see Uses: Essential Tremor), propranolol also has been used in the management of other action tremors†, including those associated with lithium therapy (see Cautions: Nervous System and Neuromuscular Effects, in Lithium Salts 28:28), anxiety, and thyrotoxicosis.

Dosage and Administration

■ **Administration** Propranolol hydrochloride is usually administered orally. When administered orally in divided doses, the drug should be given before meals and at bedtime. When propranolol hydrochloride extended-release capsules are administered, the entire daily dose is given once daily. When propranolol hydrochloride oral concentrate solution is used, the dose should be diluted (e.g., with water, juice, carbonated beverages) or mixed with semisolid foods (e.g., applesauce, puddings) just prior to administration.

For the treatment of cardiac arrhythmias, propranolol has been given IV. Oral therapy should replace IV therapy as soon as possible.

■ **Dosage** Since there is no consistent interpatient correlation between the dosage of propranolol hydrochloride and therapeutic response, especially after oral administration, dosage must be carefully individualized according to the response of the patient. If patients are switched from the conventional tablets to the extended-release capsules, care should be taken to ensure that the desired therapeutic effect is maintained. The extended-release capsules should not be considered a simple substitute for the conventional tablets on a mg-for-mg basis, since the capsules produce lower blood concentrations. If patients are switched to the extended-release capsules, the need for dosage retitration should be considered, especially to maintain effectiveness at the end of the dosing interval.

The manufacturers of propranolol hydrochloride injection state that a reduction in the dosage of propranolol hydrochloride may be necessary in geriatric patients.

Hypertension **Propranolol Therapy.** For the management of hypertension in adults, the initial oral dosage of propranolol hydrochloride, administered either alone or in combination with a diuretic, is 40 mg twice daily as conventional tablets or oral solution or 80 mg once daily as extended-release capsules. The usual effective oral dosage is 120–240 mg daily as conventional tablets or oral solution or 120–160 mg once daily as extended-release capsules; some manufacturers state that some patients may require dosages up to 640 mg daily. However, the manufacturer of Innopran XL® states that dosage of the extended-release capsules may be increased, if needed, up to 120 mg once daily, since dosages exceeding 120 mg once daily did not provide additional hypotensive effects. Some experts state the usual dosage range is 80–160 mg daily given in 2 divided doses as conventional tablets or oral solution or 80–160 mg once daily as extended-release capsules. It usually is preferable to add another antihypertensive agent to the regimen than to continue increasing propranolol hydrochloride dosage since the patient may not tolerate such continued increases. The full hypotensive effect of the drug usually is evident within 2–3 weeks, but the timing is variable. While twice-daily dosing using the conventional tablets or oral solution is usually effective, some patients may require larger doses or 3 divided doses daily to maintain effective blood pressure control throughout the day.

Propranolol/Hydrochlorothiazide Fixed-combination Therapy. When combination therapy is required, the manufacturers recommend that commercially available preparations containing propranolol hydrochloride in fixed combination with a thiazide diuretic should not be used initially. Dosage should first be adjusted by administering each drug separately. If it is determined that the optimum maintenance dosage corresponds to the ratio in the commercial combination preparation, the fixed combination may be used. Therapy with propranolol hydrochloride in fixed combination with hydrochlorothiazide is administered twice daily for a total daily dosage of up to 160 mg of propranolol hydrochloride and 50 mg of hydrochlorothiazide; use of this combination formulation is not appropriate for propranolol hydrochloride dosages exceeding 160 mg daily since it would provide an excessive dosage of the thiazide component. When necessary, another antihypertensive agent may be added gradually using half of the usual initial dosage to avoid an excessive decrease in blood pressure.

Blood Pressure Monitoring and Treatment Goals. Blood pressure should be monitored regularly (i.e., monthly) during therapy and dosage of the antihypertensive drug adjusted until blood pressure is controlled. If an adequate blood pressure response is not achieved, the dosage may be increased or another antihypertensive agent with demonstrated benefit and preferably with a complementary mechanism of action (e.g., angiotensin-converting enzyme [ACE] inhibitor, angiotensin II receptor antagonist, calcium-channel blocker, thiazide diuretic) may be added; if target blood pressure is still not achieved with the use of 2 antihypertensive agents, a third drug may be added. (See Uses: Hypertension.) In patients who develop unacceptable adverse effects with propranolol, the drug should be discontinued and another antihypertensive agent from a different pharmacologic class should be initiated.

The goal of hypertension management and prevention is to achieve and maintain optimal control of blood pressure. However, the optimum blood pressure threshold for initiating antihypertensive drug therapy and specific treatment goals remain controversial. While previous hypertension guidelines have based target blood pressure goals on age and comorbidities, the 2017 American College of Cardiology/American Heart Association (ACC/AHA) hypertension guideline incorporates underlying cardiovascular risk into decision making regarding treatment and generally recommends the same target blood pressure (i.e., less than 130/80 mm Hg) for all adults. Many patients will require at least 2 drugs from different pharmacologic classes to achieve this blood pressure goal; the potential benefits of hypertension management and drug cost, adverse effects, and risks associated with the use of multiple antihypertensive drugs also should be considered when deciding a patient's blood pressure treatment goal.

For additional information on target levels of blood pressure and on monitoring therapy in the management of hypertension, see Blood Pressure Monitoring and Treatment Goals under Dosage: Hypertension, in Dosage and Administration in the Thiazides General Statement 40:28.20.

Chronic Stable Angina For the management of angina pectoris, the initial oral dosage of propranolol hydrochloride as extended-release capsules is 80 mg daily; dosage is gradually increased as needed to control symptoms, usually at 3- to 7-day intervals. Although optimum response usually occurs at a dosage of 160 mg daily, there is a wide variation in individual requirements.

When using conventional tablets or oral solutions, the usual dosage of propranolol hydrochloride is 80–320 mg daily (given in 2–4 divided doses). The value and safety of dosages greater than 320 mg daily have not been established, but some clinicians have stated that dosage may be increased further if there is only a partial response to usual dosage.

During long-term therapy, the patient should be periodically reevaluated to determine the need for dosage alteration or continued therapy. When propranolol hydrochloride is to be discontinued, dosage should be reduced slowly over a period of at least a few weeks (about 2). (See Cautions: Precautions and Contraindications.)

Cardiac Arrhythmias The usual adult oral dosage of propranolol hydrochloride for the treatment of arrhythmias is 10–30 mg 3 or 4 times daily as conventional tablets or oral solution. For arrhythmias in adults which are life-threatening or occur during anesthesia, the manufacturer states that 1–3 mg may be administered IV under careful monitoring (e.g., ECG, central venous pressure). If necessary, a second IV dose may be administered after 2 minutes. Additional IV doses may be administered at intervals of no less than 4 hours until the desired response is obtained.

For the acute treatment of supraventricular tachycardia (SVT) (e.g., atrial flutter, junctional tachycardia, paroxysmal supraventricular tachycardia [PSVT], atrial tachycardia) in adults, some experts recommend an initial IV propranolol hydrochloride dose of 1 mg administered over 1 minute; additional doses may be given every 2 minutes up to a total of 3 doses. The usual oral maintenance dosage for ongoing treatment of SVT is 40–160 mg daily in divided doses or single doses (with long-acting preparations). To slow ventricular response in adults with acute atrial fibrillation, experts recommend an initial IV propranolol hydrochloride dose of 1 mg administered over 1 minute; additional doses may be given at 2-minute intervals up to a total of 3 doses. The usual oral maintenance dosage for ongoing treatment of atrial fibrillation is 40–160 mg daily in divided doses.

Hypertrophic Subaortic Stenosis Hypertrophic subaortic stenosis in adults is usually treated with 20–40 mg of propranolol hydrochloride orally 3 or 4 times daily as conventional tablets or oral solution or 80–160 mg once daily as extended-release capsules.

Pheochromocytoma In adults with pheochromocytoma, 60 mg of oral propranolol hydrochloride may be administered daily in divided doses as conventional tablets or oral solution in conjunction with an α-adrenergic blocking agent for 3 days prior to surgery. As an adjunct to prolonged treatment of inoperable pheochromocytoma, 30 mg of propranolol hydrochloride daily in divided doses with an α-adrenergic blocker is usually sufficient.

Vascular Headaches **Migraine.** For prophylaxis of migraine in adults, the initial oral dosage of propranolol hydrochloride is 80 mg daily, given in divided doses as the conventional tablets or oral solution or once daily as the extended-release capsules. Dosage may be increased gradually to achieve optimum migraine prophylaxis. The usual effective dosage is 80–240 mg daily. If an adequate response is not obtained within 4–6 weeks after reaching the maximum dose, propranolol therapy should be discontinued; it may be advisable to withdraw the drug gradually over several weeks.

Myocardial Infarction When used for secondary prevention after the acute phase of myocardial infarction (MI), the recommended oral dosage of propranolol hydrochloride is 180–240 mg daily (in divided doses) as conventional tablets or oral solution. In the study demonstrating mortality benefit with propranolol, the drug was initiated 5–21 days following infarction. Although the drug was given in 3 or 4 divided doses daily in clinical studies, there are considerable clinical, pharmacologic, and pharmacokinetic data suggesting that a twice-daily dosing regimen would also be adequate. Safety and efficacy of propranolol hydrochloride dosages exceeding 240 mg daily for the prevention of cardiac mortality have not been established; however, higher dosages may be required for the treatment of coexisting conditions such as angina or hypertension. Although the optimal duration of β-blocker therapy following MI remains to be clearly established, experts generally recommend that such therapy be continued long-term in post-MI patients with left ventricular systolic dysfunction, and for at least 3 years in those with normal left ventricular function.

Essential Tremor The initial oral dosage of propranolol hydrochloride for the management of essential tremor in adults is 40 mg twice daily as conventional tablets. Response to the drug is variable and dosage must be individualized; optimum suppression of tremor usually is achieved with a dosage of 120–320 mg daily (administered in 3 divided doses when conventional tablets are used). In adjusting propranolol hydrochloride dosage, it should be remembered that complete suppression of essential tremor rarely is achieved. Some evidence suggests that dosages exceeding 320 mg daily do not provide substantial added benefit but are associated with an increased risk of adverse effects. Although currently not recommended by the manufacturer, usual dosages administered once daily each morning as extended-release capsules appear to be at least as effective as equivalent dosages administered in divided doses daily as conventional tablets. Some patients may benefit from intermittent rather than maintenance therapy; single 80- to 120-mg doses as conventional tablets have been administered 1–3 hours before planned activity or anticipated stress associated with tremor.

Pediatric Dosage **Hypertension.** For the management of hypertension in children†, some experts have recommended an initial oral propranolol hydrochloride dosage of 1–2 mg/kg daily given in 2 or 3 divided doses as an immediate-release formulation. Dosage may be increased as necessary to a maximum dosage of 4 mg/kg (up to 640 mg) daily given in 2 or 3 divided doses. The extended-release formulation may be administered once daily.

Cardiac Arrhythmias. Although parenteral propranolol hydrochloride currently is not recommended by the manufacturer for use in children†, an initial IV dose of 10–20 mcg/kg infused over 10 minutes has been recommended by some clinicians for the treatment of cardiac arrhythmias in children. Some clinicians state that pediatric oral dosages exceeding 4 mg/kg daily may be necessary for the management of supraventricular tachyarrhythmias. Oral propranolol hydrochloride therapy has been initiated at 1.5–2 mg/kg daily and titrated upward as necessary to control the arrhythmia, up to a maximum dosage of 16 mg/kg daily given in 4 divided doses.

Thyrotoxicosis. For the treatment of tachyarrhythmias in neonates with thyrotoxicosis†, an oral propranolol hydrochloride dosage of 2 mg/kg daily given in 2–4 divided doses has been used, although higher dosages occasionally may be needed.

■ **Dosage in Hepatic Impairment** The manufacturers of propranolol hydrochloride injection state that a reduction in the dosage of propranolol hydrochloride may be necessary in patients with hepatic impairment.

Cautions

The most common, serious adverse effects of propranolol hydrochloride are related to its β-adrenergic blocking activity. Adverse reactions are more frequent and may be more severe after IV administration than after oral administration. In one large study of hospitalized patients receiving propranolol, reactions were most common in azotemic patients and in those older than 60 years of age. The incidence of adverse reactions to oral propranolol was unrelated to the dose, and adverse reactions usually occurred soon after the initiation of therapy. The investigators concluded that many severe adverse reactions result from the inability of severely ill patients to withstand a decrease in normal β-adrenergic stimulation.

■ **Cardiovascular Effects** The most common adverse cardiovascular effect of propranolol is bradycardia, especially in patients with digitalis intoxication. Bradycardia is occasionally severe and may be accompanied by hypotension, syncope, shock, or angina pectoris. Severe bradycardia should be treated with IM or IV administration of atropine sulfate. (See Drug Interactions: Sympathomimetic Agents.) In patients with Wolff-Parkinson-White syndrome, propranolol has produced severe bradycardia requiring a demand pacemaker.

In patients with heart failure, sympathetic stimulation is vital for the support of circulatory function. In patients with inadequate cardiac function, heart failure may be precipitated as a result of removal of β-adrenergic stimulation when propranolol therapy is initiated. A decrease in exercise tolerance may be experienced by patients with left ventricular dysfunction. In patients without a prior history of heart failure, prolonged depression of the myocardium by propranolol has resulted in heart failure in rare instances. (See Cautions: Precautions and Contraindications.) Intensification of AV block, AV dissociation, AV conduction delays, complete heart block, or cardiac arrest may occur, especially in patients with preexisting partial heart block caused by a cardiac glycoside or other factors. Ventricular fibrillation has been reported in a patient with hypertrophic subaortic stenosis.

After sudden cessation of propranolol therapy in some patients treated for angina, increased frequency, duration, and severity of angina episodes have occurred, often within 24 hours. These episodes are unstable and are not relieved by nitroglycerin. Acute and sometimes fatal myocardial infarction and sudden death have also occurred after abrupt withdrawal of propranolol therapy in some patients treated for angina. In hypertensive patients, sudden cessation of propranolol has produced a syndrome similar to florid thyrotoxicosis, characterized by tenseness, anxiety, tachycardia, and excessive perspiration; these symptoms occurred within one week of cessation of the drug and were relieved by reinstituting propranolol therapy.

During surgery, some patients who have been receiving propranolol may experience severe, protracted hypotension and, occasionally, difficulty in restarting and maintaining heart beat. These adverse cardiovascular effects of propranolol may be reversed during surgery by IV administration of β-adrenergic agonists such as isoproterenol or norepinephrine.

Severe hypertension has been reported in a few patients with schizophrenic disorder who received only propranolol orally in rapidly increasing doses; the hypertension responded to treatment with IV phentolamine followed by oral phenoxybenzamine.

Fluid retention, pulmonary edema, and peripheral arterial insufficiency, usually of the Raynaud's type, may occur in patients receiving propranolol. When the drug is used alone, dietary sodium restriction may be necessary. Intermittent claudication has occurred in patients with previously asymptomatic peripheral arterial disease who received propranolol, although one study which used the drug for the treatment of intermittent claudication did not note any deterioration of occlusive peripheral arterial disease.

■ **Nervous System Effects** A number of adverse CNS effects, which are usually reversible after withdrawal of the drug, have been reported with propranolol. Adverse CNS effects usually occur after long-term treatment with high dosages of propranolol hydrochloride and range from lightheadedness, giddiness, ataxia, dizziness, irritability, sleepiness, hearing loss, and visual disturbances to vivid dreams, hallucinations, and confusion. Insomnia, lassitude, weakness, fatigue, and mental depression progressing to catatonia have been reported. Dosages exceeding 160 mg daily, when administered in divided doses exceeding 80 mg each, may be associated with an increased incidence of fatigue, lethargy, and vivid dreams. Organic brain syndrome, characterized by disorientation to time and place, short-term memory loss, emotional lability, slightly clouded sensorium, and decreased performance on neuropsychometric tests, has been reported rarely. Paresthesia of the hands, peripheral neuropathy, and precipitation of myotonia have been reported. Impotence has been reported rarely. Ptosis has been reported in at least 2 patients. A few patients receiving propranolol for hypertrophic obstructive cardiomyopathy have developed migraine in some cases associated with sensory disturbances and teichopsia.

■ **GI Effects** Adverse GI effects such as nausea, vomiting, diarrhea, epigastric distress, abdominal cramping, constipation, and flatulence may occur in patients receiving propranolol and occasionally necessitate reduction of dosage or withdrawal of the drug. Mesenteric arterial thrombosis and ischemic colitis have also occurred.

■ **Dermatologic and Sensitivity Reactions** Rarely, rashes have been reported during propranolol usage. Rashes are most commonly erythematous (maculopapular or acneiform), dry, scaly, pruritic, psoriasiform lesions which occur on the trunk, extremities, and scalp. Hyperkeratosis of the scalp, palms, and soles of the feet have been reported during treatment with propranolol; nail changes such as thickening, pitting, and discoloration have occurred. At least one case of exfoliative dermatitis has been reported. Dermatologic reactions disappear after the drug is withdrawn. Other allergic manifestations reported during propranolol therapy include fever accompanied by aching and sore throat, rhinitis, dry mouth, laryngospasm, respiratory distress, and pharyngitis. A lupus-like syndrome characterized by fever, pruritus, severe myalgia, and positive lupus erythematosus cell tests has been reported. Reversible alopecia, which recurred following readministration of the drug, also has been reported.

■ **Hematologic Effects** Adverse hematologic effects of propranolol include transient eosinophilia (a pharmacologic effect of β-adrenergic blockade) and idiosyncratic reactions including thrombocytopenic and nonthrombocytopenic purpura and, rarely, agranulocytosis.

■ **Endocrine Effects** Results of a large prospective cohort study of adults 45–64 years of age indicate that use of β-adrenergic blocking agents (β-blockers) in hypertensive patients is associated with increased risk (about 28%) of developing type 2 diabetes mellitus compared with hypertensive patients who were not receiving hypotensive therapy. In this study, the number of new cases of diabetes per 1000 person-years was 33.6 or 26.3 in patients receiving a β-blocker or no drug therapy, respectively. The association between the risk of developing diabetes mellitus and use of β-blockers reportedly was not confounded by weight gain, hyperinsulinemia, or differences in heart rate. It is not known if the risk of developing diabetes is affected by β-receptor selectivity. Further studies are needed to determine whether concomitant use of ACE inhibitors (which may improve insulin sensitivity) would abrogate β-blocker-induced adverse effects related to glucose intolerance. Therefore, until results of such studies are available, the proven benefits of β-blockers in reducing cardiovascular events in hypertensive patients must be weighed carefully against the possible risks of developing diabetes mellitus.

Hypoglycemia, which may result in loss of consciousness, also may occur in nondiabetic patients receiving β-blockers. Patients most at risk for the development of β-blocker-induced hypoglycemia are those undergoing dialysis, prolonged fasting, or severe exercise regimens.

β-Blockers may mask signs and symptoms of hypoglycemia (e.g., palpitation, tachycardia, tremor) and potentiate insulin-induced hypoglycemia. Acute increases in blood pressure have occurred after insulin-induced hypoglycemia in patients receiving propranolol. Although it has been suggested that nonselective β-blockers are more likely to induce hypoglycemia than selective β-blockers, such an adverse effect also has been reported with selective β-blockers (e.g., atenolol). In addition, selective β-blockers are less likely to mask symptoms of hypoglycemia or delay recovery from insulin-induced hypoglycemia than nonselective β-blockers because of their vascular sparing effects; however, selective β-blockers can decrease insulin sensitivity by approximately 15–30%, which may result in increased insulin requirements.

■ **Other Adverse Effects** Propranolol may cause elevated BUN in patients with severe heart disease, elevated serum creatinine, aminotransferase, alkaline phosphatase, or lactic dehydrogenase concentrations. In hypertensive patients, propranolol may cause small increases in serum potassium concentration. Peyronie's disease has been reported rarely. Generalized hyperemia of the conjunctivae with decreased tear production and a prickling sensation of the eyes, eye dryness, eye pain, discoloration of the tongue, and bad taste have been reported rarely.

■ **Precautions and Contraindications** Propranolol shares the toxic potentials of β-blockers, and the usual precautions of these agents should be observed. When propranolol is used as a fixed-combination preparation that includes hydrochlorothiazide, the cautions, precautions, and contraindications associated with thiazide diuretics must be considered in addition to those associated with propranolol.

In patients with heart failure, sympathetic stimulation is vital for the support of circulatory function. Propranolol should be used with caution in patients with inadequate cardiac function, since heart failure may be precipitated by blockade of β-adrenergic stimulation when propranolol therapy is administered. In addition, in patients with latent cardiac insufficiency, prolonged β-adrenergic blockade may lead to cardiac failure. Although β-blockers should be avoided in patients with overt heart failure, propranolol may be administered cautiously, if necessary, to patients with well-compensated heart failure (e.g., those controlled with cardiac glycosides and/or diuretics). Patients receiving propranolol therapy should be instructed to consult their physician at the first sign or symptom of impending cardiac failure and should be adequately treated (e.g., with a cardiac glycoside and/or diuretic) and observed closely; if cardiac failure continues, propranolol should be discontinued, gradually if possible.

Abrupt withdrawal of propranolol may exacerbate angina symptoms or precipitate myocardial infarction in patients with coronary artery disease. Abrupt withdrawal of the drug in patients treated for hypertension has also been associated with adverse effects. (See Cautions: Cardiovascular Effects.) Therefore, patients receiving propranolol (especially those with ischemic heart disease) should be warned not to interrupt or discontinue therapy without consulting their clinician. When discontinuance of propranolol therapy is planned, particularly in patients with ischemic heart disease, dosage of the drug should be gradually reduced over a period of at least a few (about 2) weeks. When propranolol therapy is discontinued, patients should be carefully monitored and their activity restricted. If exacerbation of angina occurs after propranolol therapy is interrupted, treatment with the drug should generally be reinstituted and appropriate measures taken for the management of unstable angina pectoris. Because coronary artery disease is common and may be unrecognized, the manufacturers caution that it may be prudent not to discontinue propranolol therapy abruptly, even in patients receiving the drug for conditions other than angina.

The necessity of withdrawing β-adrenergic blocking therapy prior to major surgery is controversial. Severe, protracted hypotension and difficulty in restarting or maintaining a heart beat have occurred during surgery in some patients who have received β-blockers. As with other β-blockers, the effects of propranolol can be reversed by administration of β-agonists (e.g., dobutamine, isoproterenol). If propranolol therapy is discontinued prior to major surgery, oral therapy with the drug may be restarted as soon after surgery as possible; patients who are unable to take oral drugs after surgery may be treated with IV propranolol if necessary.

Caution should be used when administering propranolol to patients with sinus node dysfunction, since the drug can cause marked depression of SA node automaticity. Propranolol should be used with extreme caution for the management of arrhythmias occurring during anesthesia with myocardial depressant anesthetics, since excessive myocardial depression, bradycardia, and hypotension may occur.

Signs of hyperthyroidism may be masked by propranolol, and patients with thyrotoxicosis who receive the drug should be monitored closely. In addition, the drug may alter thyroid function test results, increasing thyroxine (T_4) and reverse triiodothyronine (rT_3) and decreasing triiodothyronine (T_3) determinations.

It is recommended that propranolol be used with caution in patients with diabetes mellitus (especially those with labile diabetes or those prone to hypoglycemia) since the drug also may block the signs and symptoms of hypoglycemia (e.g., tachycardia and blood pressure changes but not sweating). However, many clinicians state that patients with diabetes mellitus may be particularly likely to experience a reduction in morbidity and mortality with the use of β-blockers. In addition, the drug occasionally causes hypoglycemia, even in nondiabetic patients, presumably by interfering with catecholamine-induced glycogenolysis. Propranolol may also inhibit the insulin-releasing mechanism of the pancreas and has been implicated in hyperglycemic reactions. Propranolol-induced alterations in glucose tolerance appear to occur only rarely. (See Cautions: Endocrine Effects.) Some sources state that hypertensive patients who are prone to hypoglycemia should not receive propranolol because the drug may cause a sharp rise in blood pressure.

Since β-blockers may inhibit bronchodilation produced by endogenous catecholamines, the drugs generally should not be used in patients with bronchospastic disease. Propranolol should be used with caution in patients with a history of nonallergic bronchospasm (e.g., chronic bronchitis, emphysema). β-adrenergic blockade may lead to an increase in airway resistance and bronchospasm, particularly in patients with a history of asthma. Bronchospasm may be treated with IV administration of aminophylline; isoproterenol may also be administered. (See Drug Interactions: Sympathomimetic Agents.) IV administration of atropine has been suggested if the patient fails to respond to the above or if bradycardia is present.

Since treatment with β-blockers (e.g., propranolol) may reduce intraocular pressure, patients should be advised that such therapy may interfere with glaucoma screening tests. Withdrawal of propranolol may lead to an increase in intraocular pressure.

Propranolol should be used with caution in patients with renal or hepatic impairment. Laboratory parameters should be monitored in patients receiving prolonged therapy with the drug.

Patients with a history of severe anaphylactic reactions to a variety of allergens may be more reactive to repeated, accidental, diagnostic, or therapeutic challenge with such allergens while receiving a β-blocker. These patients may be unresponsive to usual doses of epinephrine or may develop a paradoxical response to epinephrine when it is used to treat anaphylactic reactions.

Propranolol is contraindicated in patients with Raynaud's syndrome, bronchial asthma, sinus bradycardia and heart block greater than first degree, and overt and decompensated heart failure (unless the failure is secondary to a tachyarrhythmia treatable with propranolol). The drug is not indicated in the management of hypertensive emergencies. Although the manufacturers state that propranolol is contraindicated in patients with cardiogenic shock, results of some studies indicate that the drug may have a beneficial effect in patients with myocardial infarction with or without cardiogenic shock. (See Uses: Acute Myocardial Infarction.) Because propranolol has produced a myasthenic condition characterized by ptosis, weakness of limbs, and double vision in 2 patients, the drug may be contraindicated in patients with myasthenia gravis. In addition, since propranolol appears to impair metabolism of thioridazine which may result in increased plasma concentrations of thioridazine that may be associated with prolongation of the QT interval, the manufacturer of thioridazine states that concomitant use of thioridazine and propranolol is contraindicated. (See Drug Interactions: Phenothiazines and Other Psychotherapeutic Agents.)

■ Pediatric Precautions Although safety and efficacy of propranolol have not been as extensively or systematically studied in children as in adults, current information from the medical literature allows fair estimates, and specific dosing information has been reasonably studied. Cardiovascular diseases that are common to adults and children generally are as responsive to propranolol therapy in children as in adults, and adverse reactions also are similar. For information on overall principles and expert recommendations for treatment of hypertension in pediatric patients, see Uses: Hypertension in Pediatric Patients, in the Thiazides General Statement 40:28.20. One manufacturer states that the possibility that oral bioavailability of propranolol hydrochloride may be increased in children with Down's syndrome should be considered. Safety and efficacy of propranolol hydrochloride extended-release capsules, oral solution, and injection have not been established in children.

■ Geriatric Precautions Clinical studies of propranolol tablets, injections, and extended-release capsules did not include sufficient numbers of patients 65 years of age and older to determine whether geriatric patients respond differently than younger patients. If propranolol is used in geriatric patients, dosage of the drug should be selected with caution, usually initiating therapy at the low end of the dosage range since decreased hepatic, renal, or cardiac function and concomitant disease or other drug therapy are more common in this age group than in younger patients.

Decreased propranolol clearance and a prolonged elimination half-life have been reported in geriatric patients receiving propranolol hydrochloride injection, and the manufacturers recommend that dosage reduction be considered in these patients.

■ Carcinogenicity In long-term studies in animals, no evidence of propranolol-related tumorigenic effects was observed.

■ Pregnancy, Fertility, and Lactation There are no adequate and well-controlled studies to date using propranolol in pregnant women. Safe use of propranolol during pregnancy has not been established. Low birthweight infants with respiratory distress and hypoglycemia have been born to women who received propranolol throughout pregnancy. Bradycardia, hypoglycemia, and respiratory depression also have been reported in neonates whose mothers received propranolol at parturition; adequate facilities for monitoring such infants at birth should be available. The manufacturers state that the drug should be used during pregnancy only when the possible benefits outweigh the potential risks to the fetus.

Embryotoxicity (reduced litter size, increased resorption rates) and neonatal toxicity (deaths) have been reported in reproductive studies in rats receiving propranolol hydrochloride 150 mg/kg daily by gavage or in the diet throughout pregnancy and lactation; however, such effects were not observed in rats receiving 80 mg/kg daily (equivalent to the maximum recommended human dosage on a mg/m^2 basis). No evidence of embryotoxicity or neonatal toxicity was observed in rabbits receiving oral doses of propranolol hydrochloride of up to 150 mg/kg daily (about 5 times the maximum recommended oral human daily dose) throughout pregnancy and lactation.

Reproduction studies in animals using propranolol have not revealed evidence of impaired fertility.

Since propranolol is distributed into milk, the drug should be used with caution in nursing women.

Drug Interactions

■ Drugs Affecting or Metabolized by Hepatic Microsomal Enzymes Because metabolism of propranolol is mediated by cytochrome P-450 (CYP) isoenzymes 2D6, 1A2, and 2C19, drugs that induce or inhibit these isoenzymes may alter the metabolism of propranolol, which may result in clinically important drug interactions. Inhibitors or substrates of the isoenzymes 2D6 (e.g., amiodarone, cimetidine, delavirdine, fluoxetine, paroxetine, quinidine, ritonavir), 1A2 (e.g., cimetidine, ciprofloxacin, fluvoxamine, imipramine, isoniazid, ritonavir, rizatriptan, theophylline, zileuton, zolmitriptan), or 2C19 (e.g., cimetidine, fluconazole, fluoxetine, fluvoxamine, teniposide, tolbutamide) could decrease the metabolism and increase plasma concentrations of propranolol. Drugs that induce cytochrome P-450 activity (e.g., alcohol, rifampin) may increase the metabolism of propranolol and decrease its plasma concentrations; in current smokers, plasma propranolol concentrations also may be decreased because cigarette smoking may induce hepatic metabolism of the drug, increasing propranolol clearance up to 100%.

■ Phenothiazines and Other Psychotherapeutic Agents Phenothiazines and propranolol may have additive hypotensive activity, especially when phenothiazines are administered in large doses. Chlorpromazine has been shown to reduce the clearance of propranolol and increase plasma propranolol concentrations. Increased plasma concentrations of chlorpromazine also have been reported in patients receiving the drug concomitantly with propranolol. Hypotension and cardiac arrest have occurred during concomitant therapy with propranolol and haloperidol.

In addition, since propranolol may inhibit metabolism of thioridazine, concomitant use of propranolol hydrochloride (100–800 mg daily) and thioridazine, reportedly resulted in increased plasma concentrations of thioridazine and its metabolites by about 50–400 and 80–300%, respectively. Because such increased concentrations of thioridazine may enhance thioridazine-induced prolongation of the QT_c interval, and increase the risk of serious, potentially fatal cardiac arrhythmias (e.g., torsades de pointes), the manufacturer of thioridazine states that concomitant use of thioridazine and propranolol is contraindicated.

Complete heart block has been reported in a patient receiving fluoxetine concomitantly with propranolol. The mechanism of this interaction is not known; however, it has been postulated that fluoxetine may inhibit metabolism of lipophilic β-adrenergic blocking agents (β-blockers) (e.g., propranolol, metoprolol), increase their bioavailability, and increase their β-adrenergic blocking effects. Therefore, some clinicians recommend that fluoxetine be administered with caution in patients receiving β-blockers and in those with impaired cardiac conduction.

The hypotensive effects of monoamine oxidase (MAO) inhibitors or tricyclic antidepressants may be exacerbated in patients receiving β-blockers.

Decreased metabolism and increased plasma concentrations of diazepam and its metabolites have been reported in patients receiving the drug concomitantly with propranolol; propranolol does not appear to alter pharmacokinetics of other benzodiazepines (e.g., alprazolam, lorazepam, oxazepam, triazolam). Diazepam does not alter pharmacokinetics of propranolol.

■ **Sympathomimetic Agents** The β-adrenergic stimulating effects of sympathomimetic agents are antagonized by propranolol. This interaction is especially pronounced with isoproterenol, and very large doses of isoproterenol may be needed to overcome the β-adrenergic blocking effects of propranolol. The effects of propranolol also can be reversed by administration of dobutamine. In addition, propranolol may reduce sensitivity to dobutamine stress echocardiography in patients undergoing evaluation for myocardial ischemia. Patients receiving long-term propranolol therapy may experience uncontrolled hypertension upon administration of epinephrine as a result of unopposed α-receptor stimulation. In patients receiving propranolol, epinephrine should be administered with caution since a decrease in pulse rate with first- and second-degree heart block may occur.

■ **Antimuscarinic Agents and Drugs with Anticholinergic Effects** Antimuscarinic agents, such as atropine, may counteract the bradycardia caused by propranolol by reestablishing the balance between sympathetic and parasympathetic actions on the heart. Tricyclic antidepressants (e.g., amitriptyline) also have anticholinergic activity and may similarly antagonize the cardiac β-adrenergic blocking effects of propranolol, although not as intensely as do the antimuscarinics.

■ **Catecholamine-depleting Drugs** When propranolol and a catecholamine-depleting drug (e.g., reserpine) are administered concomitantly, the effects of the drugs may be additive. Excessive reduction of resting sympathetic nervous system activity, which may lead to hypotension, severe bradycardia, vertigo, syncope, or orthostatic hypotension, has been reported in patients receiving both drugs concurrently. Concomitant use of reserpine and propranolol also may potentiate depression.

■ **Selective Serotonin Agonists** Increased concentrations of zolmitriptan and rizatriptan have been reported in patients receiving concomitant propranolol therapy.

■ **Diuretics and Cardiovascular Drugs** When propranolol is administered with diuretics or other antihypertensive drugs, the hypotensive effect of propranolol may be increased. This effect is usually used to therapeutic advantage, but careful adjustment of dosage is necessary when these drugs are used concomitantly. In addition to its potentially additive hypotensive effect, reserpine theoretically may add to the β-adrenergic blocking activity of propranolol through its catecholamine-depleting activity. (See Drug Interactions: Catecholamine-depleting Drugs.)

Clonidine The antihypertensive effects of clonidine may be antagonized by β-blockers, including propranolol. Because β-blockers (e.g., propranolol) may exacerbate rebound hypertension that may occur following discontinuance of clonidine therapy, β-blockers should be discontinued several days before gradual withdrawal of clonidine when clonidine therapy is to be discontinued in patients receiving a β-blocker and clonidine concurrently.

Angiotensin-converting Enzyme Inhibitors Concomitant therapy with angiotensin-converting enzyme (ACE) inhibitors and β-blockers (e.g., propranolol) may result in hypotension, particularly in patients with acute myocardial infarction. Increased bronchial hyperreactivity has been reported in patients receiving ACE inhibitors concomitantly with propranolol.

α-Adrenergic Blocking Agents Prolonged hypotension associated with administration of a first prazosin dose has been reported in patients receiving β-blockers. In addition, postural hypotension has been reported in patients receiving β-blockers concomitantly with terazosin or doxazosin.

Other Cardiovascular Agents When propranolol is administered with antiarrhythmic drugs such as lidocaine, phenytoin, procainamide, quinidine, or verapamil (see Drug Interactions: β-Adrenergic Blocking Agents, in Verapamil 24:28.92), cardiac effects may be additive or antagonistic and toxic effects may be additive.

Concomitant use of β-blockers (e.g., propranolol) and certain other cardiovascular drugs (e.g., cardiac glycosides, lidocaine, nondihydropyridine calcium-channel blocking agents) can have additive negative effects on SA or AV nodal conduction. Slowing or complete suppression of SA node activity with development of slow ventricular rates (e.g., 30–40 bpm), often misdiagnosed as complete AV block, has been reported in patients receiving the nondihydropyridine calcium-channel blocking agent mibefradil (no longer commercially available in the US), principally in geriatric patients and in association with concomitant β-adrenergic blocker therapy. Concomitant therapy with an *IV* β-blocker and *IV* verapamil has resulted rarely in serious adverse reactions, especially in patients with severe cardiomyopathy, heart failure, or recent myocardial infarction. Severe bradycardia, heart failure, and cardiovascular collapse have been reported in patients receiving verapamil concomitantly with β-blockers.

Caution should be used in patients receiving propranolol concomitantly with a calcium-channel blocking agent with negative inotropic and/or chronotropic effects, since both drugs may depress myocardial contractility and AV conduction. Severe bradycardia, asystole, heart failure, and cardiovascular collapse have been reported in patients receiving propranolol concomitantly with disopyramide or verapamil. In addition, bradycardia, hypotension, high-degree heart block, and heart failure have been reported in patients with cardiac disease receiving concomitant therapy with propranolol and diltiazem. Concomitant use of propranolol with amiodarone also may result in additive negative chronotropic effects, while additive negative inotropic and β-adrenergic blocking effects may occur when propafenone and propranolol are used concomitantly. In patients currently receiving a cardiac glycoside, concomitant propranolol therapy may reduce the positive inotropic effect of the glycoside. (See Cautions: Precautions and Contraindications.)

Increased propafenone exposure has been reported in patients receiving the drug concomitantly with propranolol. Verapamil does not appear to affect pharmacokinetics of propranolol and propranolol does not affect pharmacokinetics of verapamil or norverapamil. Increased propranolol concentrations have been reported in patients receiving concomitant therapy with nisoldipine or nicardipine with propranolol; increased concentrations of nifedipine may occur in patients receiving the drug concomitantly with propranolol.

Administration of quinidine has been reported to cause decreased propranolol metabolism, resulting in increased propranolol plasma concentrations and increased β-blocking effects (and possible postural hypotension). Reduced lidocaine metabolism and clearance resulting in lidocaine toxicity have been reported in patients receiving the drug concomitantly with propranolol.

■ **Antilipemic Agents** Decreased propranolol plasma concentrations have been reported in patients receiving the drug concomitantly with cholestyramine or colestipol. Decreased plasma concentrations of lovastatin and pravastatin have been reported in patients receiving the drugs concomitantly with propranolol; however, the pharmacodynamics of the antilipemics were not altered.

■ **Warfarin** Increases in warfarin bioavailability and prothrombin time have been reported in patients receiving warfarin concomitantly with propranolol. Prothrombin time should be monitored in patients receiving warfarin concomitantly with propranolol.

■ **Neuromuscular Blocking Agents** High doses of propranolol may potentiate the effects of neuromuscular blocking agents such as tubocurarine chloride, possibly because of propranolol's interference with ionic permeability of the postjunctional membrane. Propranolol should be administered with caution to patients who are receiving neuromuscular blocking agents or who are recovering from their effects.

■ **Antidiabetic Agents** β-Blockers may impair glucose tolerance; increase the frequency or severity of hypoglycemia; block hypoglycemia-induced tachycardia but not hypoglycemic sweating, which may actually be increased; delay the rate of recovery of blood glucose concentration following drug-induced hypoglycemia; alter the hemodynamic response to hypoglycemia, possibly resulting in an exaggerated hypertensive response; and possibly impair peripheral circulation. Nonselective β-blockers (e.g., propranolol, nadolol) without intrinsic sympathomimetic activity are more likely to affect glucose metabolism than more selective β-blockers (e.g., metoprolol, atenolol) or those with intrinsic sympathomimetic activity (e.g., acebutolol, pindolol). Signs of hypoglycemia (e.g., tachycardia, blood pressure changes, tremor, feelings of anxiety) mediated by catecholamines may be masked by either nonselective or selective β-blockers. When an oral antidiabetic agent or insulin and a β-blocker are used concomitantly, the patient should be advised about and monitored closely for altered antidiabetic response.

■ **Ergot Alkaloids** One case of severe peripheral vasoconstriction with pain and cyanosis has been reported in a patient who received propranolol orally and high doses of ergotamine in a rectal suppository concurrently for the treatment of migraine; however, several patients have received these drugs concomitantly without adverse effects. Caution should be used during simultaneous administration of propranolol and high doses of ergot alkaloids because of the possibility of additive peripheral vasoconstriction.

■ **Cimetidine** Cimetidine can substantially reduce the clearance of propranolol (apparently by inhibiting the hepatic metabolism of propranolol), which results in increased propranolol concentrations. If propranolol and cimetidine are administered concomitantly, the patient should be monitored for signs and symptoms of increased β-adrenergic blocking activity.

■ **Antacids** Concomitant oral administration of an aluminum hydroxide antacid with propranolol may reduce the GI absorption of propranolol. In a study in healthy adults, oral administration of 30 mL of an aluminum hydroxide (1.2 g) suspension with a single, 80-mg dose of propranolol hydrochloride reduced the peak plasma propranolol concentration and bioavailability of the drug by about 60%. The mechanism of this potential interaction has not been elucidated, but propranolol adsorption to or complexation with aluminum hydroxide does not appear to be involved. In another study in healthy adults, however, concomitant oral administration of 30 mL of an aluminum hydroxide suspension with a single, 40-mg dose of propranolol hydrochloride did *not* substantially affect bioavailability of propranolol. The need to avoid concomitant use or stagger dosing of an aluminum hydroxide antacid and propranolol has not been fully elucidated, but increasing propranolol dosage may be considered if an interaction is suspected.

■ **Levodopa** Propranolol may antagonize the hypotensive and positive inotropic effects of levodopa. This interaction is not well documented; however, the possibility of its occurrence should be kept in mind.

■ **Nonsteroidal Anti-inflammatory Agents** The possibility that nonsteroidal anti-inflammatory agents (NSAIAs; e.g., indomethacin) may reduce the hypotensive effect of β-blockers such as propranolol should be considered. (See Drug Interactions, in Indomethacin 28:08.04.92.)

■ **Theophylline** Propranolol decreases the clearance of theophylline in a dose-dependent manner by inhibiting hepatic microsomal metabolism (principally demethylation). In addition, propranolol can antagonize theophylline-induced bronchodilation.

Acute Toxicity

■ **Manifestations** Limited information is available on the acute toxicity of propranolol hydrochloride. In adults who intentionally ingested the drug, estimates of the ingested doses have ranged from 0.8–6 g. The principal manifestations of overdosage were bradycardia and severe hypotension (which may result in peripheral cyanosis); loss of consciousness and seizures have also occurred. In most cases of acute propranolol overdosage, the patient recovered; however, in a few cases, toxicity was severe enough to result in death. Two small children who ingested a total of 150 mg of propranolol hydrochloride became drowsy, perspired, and experienced periods of SA node block; they were treated with IV and oral dextrose. Severe paradoxical rise in blood pressure has been reported in 8 patients with schizophrenic disorder who received propranolol hydrochloride in rapidly increasing doses (600 mg in the first 24 hours); these patients responded to IV phentolamine.

■ **Treatment** Treatment of propranolol hydrochloride overdosage generally involves symptomatic and supportive care. Following acute ingestion of the drug, the stomach should be emptied immediately by inducing emesis or by gastric lavage. If the patient is comatose, having seizures, or lacks the gag reflex, gastric lavage may be performed if an endotracheal tube with cuff inflated is in place to prevent aspiration of gastric contents. For symptomatic bradycardia, IV atropine may be given; if bradycardia persists, IV isoproterenol hydrochloride may be administered cautiously (large doses may be required), and in refractory cases, use of a transvenous cardiac pacemaker should be considered. A vasopressor (e.g., norepinephrine, dopamine) may be given for severe hypotension. For heart failure, a cardiac glycoside and diuretic may be used. Because of the possibility of uncontrolled hypertension secondary to unopposed α-receptor stimulation in patients receiving long-term propranolol therapy, epinephrine is not indicated for the treatment of propranolol overdosage. Glucagon also may be useful for the management of myocardial depression and hypotension. Phosphodiesterase inhibitors also may be useful in the management of propranolol overdosage. A β_2-adrenergic agonist and/or a theophylline derivative may be used for bronchospasm. IV diazepam may be useful for controlling seizures. Hemodialysis is probably not useful for enhancing elimination of propranolol in acute overdosage.

Pharmacology

Propranolol hydrochloride is a nonselective β-adrenergic blocking agent (β-blocker). Propranolol inhibits response to adrenergic stimuli by competitively blocking β-adrenergic receptors within the myocardium and within bronchial and vascular smooth muscle. Only the *l*-isomer of propranolol has substantial β-adrenergic blocking activity. Propranolol has no intrinsic sympathomimetic activity.

Through its myocardial β-adrenergic blocking action, propranolol decreases heart rate and prevents exercise-induced increases in heart rate, decreases myocardial contractility, decreases cardiac output, increases systolic ejection time, and increases cardiac volume. The drug also decreases conduction velocity through the sinoatrial (SA) and atrioventricular (AV) nodes and decreases myocardial automaticity via β-adrenergic blockade. At blood concentrations greater than those required for β-adrenergic blockade, propranolol has a membrane-stabilizing effect on the heart which is similar to that of quinidine. The clinical importance of this effect is not clear, but it appears to be less important than its β-adrenergic blocking activity.

β-Adrenergic blockade may also increase peripheral resistance initially, but peripheral resistance tends to decrease after chronic administration of the drug as a result of unopposed α-adrenergic vasoconstriction. The cardiac effects of β-adrenergic blockade cause an increase in sodium reabsorption because of alterations in renal hemodynamics; renal blood flow and glomerular filtration rate generally decrease during chronic therapy. Plasma volume may increase if dietary sodium is not restricted. Hepatic blood flow is decreased.

The precise mechanism of propranolol's hypotensive effect has not been determined. It has been postulated that β-blockers reduce blood pressure by blocking peripheral (especially cardiac) adrenergic receptors (decreasing cardiac output), by decreasing sympathetic outflow from the CNS, and/or by suppressing renin release. In patients with high concentrations of circulating renin, low doses of the drug are associated with a fall in both blood pressure and in plasma renin concentrations, probably because of acute peripheral β-adrenergic blockade. With higher doses of propranolol, the hypotensive effect is probably unrelated to plasma renin activity and may be caused by a delayed centrally mediated reduction of adrenergic outflow. However, there appears to be some overlap between these mechanisms, and both mechanisms seem to be operative with usual therapeutic doses. Propranolol decreases blood pressure in both the supine and standing positions.

Several effects of propranolol may contribute to its usefulness in the management of angina pectoris. The drug usually causes decreased myocardial oxygen consumption and, secondarily, a decrease in coronary blood flow. The drug may reduce the oxygen requirements of the heart because of its β-adrenergic blockade. Propranolol also appears to cause redistribution of 2,3-diphosphoglyceric acid in erythrocytes which results in a decrease in the affinity of hemoglobin for oxygen, enhancing oxygen delivery to the tissues. This action is unrelated to β-adrenergic blockade. Propranolol may also affect platelet aggregation through a nonspecific platelet membrane effect unrelated to β-adrenergic blockade and possibly because of interference with calcium flux. In one study of patients with angina, the drug restored previously elevated platelet aggregability to normal. Abrupt withdrawal of the drug in patients with angina may cause rebound platelet hyperaggregability.

When used prophylactically, propranolol can prevent common migraine or reduce the number of attacks in some patients. β-Adrenergic receptors have been shown to be present in the pial vessels of the brain; however, the exact mechanism of the antimigraine effect of propranolol is not known. Some evidence suggests that propranolol may prevent migraines through diminishing central catecholaminergic hyperactivity, possibly by inhibiting norepinephrine release, reducing neuronal activity and excitability, exerting membrane-stabilizing effects, and inhibiting nitric oxide production.

Through its β-adrenergic blocking action in other body systems, propranolol increases airway resistance (especially in asthmatic patients), inhibits glycogenolysis in the skeletal and cardiac muscles, blocks the release of free fatty acids and insulin by adrenergic stimulation, and increases the number of circulating eosinophils. Propranolol increases uterine activity, more in the nonpregnant than in the pregnant uterus.

Pharmacokinetics

■ **Absorption** Propranolol is almost completely absorbed from the GI tract; however, plasma concentrations attained are quite variable among individuals. There is no difference in the rate of absorption of the 2 isomers of propranolol. Propranolol appears in the plasma within 30 minutes, and peak plasma concentrations are reached about 60–90 minutes after oral administration of the conventional tablets. The time when peak plasma concentrations are reached may be delayed, but concentrations are not necessarily lowered, when the drug is administered with food. One manufacturer states that oral bioavailability of the drug may be increased in children with Down's syndrome; higher than expected plasma propranolol concentrations have been observed in such children. Bioavailability of a single 40-mg oral dose of propranolol hydrochloride as a conventional tablet or oral solution reportedly is equivalent in adults. Propranolol is slowly absorbed following administration of the drug as extended-release capsules, and peak blood concentrations are reached about 6 hours after administration. When measured at steady-state over a 24-hour period, the area under the plasma concentration-time curve (AUC) for the extended-release capsules is about 60–65% of the AUC for a comparable divided daily dose of the conventional tablets. The lower AUC is probably caused by the slower rate of absorption of the drug from the extended-release capsules with resultant greater hepatic metabolism. After administration of a single dose of propranolol hydrochloride as the extended-release capsules, blood concentrations of propranolol are fairly constant for about 12 hours and then decline exponentially during the following 12 hours.

Plasma propranolol concentrations attained after IV administration of the drug are relatively consistent among individuals. After administration of a 0.5-mg IV bolus of propranolol hydrochloride, peak plasma propranolol concentrations of 40 ng/mL are produced in 1 minute and the drug is undetectable in the plasma in 5 minutes. Following IV administration of propranolol, the onset of action is almost immediate. Animal studies indicate that propranolol is rapidly absorbed after IM administration.

After absorption from the GI tract, propranolol is bound by the liver through nonspecific tissue binding. There are large individual differences in hepatic extraction, probably because of differences in hepatic blood flow. Following oral administration, the drug does not reach the general circulation until hepatic binding sites are saturated. Once saturation occurs, hepatic binding no longer affects the passage of the drug into the blood. The amount of drug that reaches the circulation after oral administration also depends on the amount of drug metabolized on the first pass through the liver. Propranolol decreases its own rate of metabolism by decreasing hepatic blood flow. Studies indicate that hepatic extraction and possibly metabolism of propranolol are reduced following oral administration of the drug in patients with chronic renal disease, resulting in higher peak plasma concentrations of the drug after the first dose than are attained in patients with normal renal function.

There is considerable interpatient variation in the relationship of plasma propranolol concentrations and therapeutic effect, but therapeutic plasma concentrations of propranolol are usually 50–100 ng/mL. Concentrations of 100 ng/mL generally represent a high degree of β-adrenergic blockade. There are several possible metabolic explanations for the discrepancies between plasma concentrations and therapeutic effect. (See Pharmacokinetics: Elimination.) Individual differences in sympathetic tone may also contribute to interpatient differences in response.

■ **Distribution** Propranolol is widely distributed into body tissues including lungs, liver, kidneys, and heart. Propranolol readily crosses the blood-brain barrier and the placenta. The drug is distributed into milk.

The apparent volume of distribution of propranolol at steady-state varies widely in proportion to the fraction of unbound drug in whole blood. Propranolol is more than 90% bound to plasma proteins over a wide range of blood concentrations. Both free and protein-bound propranolol are metabolized. Increased plasma protein binding of the drug increases its metabolism and decreases its volume of distribution, resulting in a shorter terminal half-life.

■ **Elimination** Elimination of propranolol appears to follow first-order kinetics and seems to be independent of plasma concentration or the dose administered, at least with oral doses of 160–320 mg/day. The reported elimination half-life varies considerably among different studies. After IV administration of 10 mg of propranolol hydrochloride at a rate of 1.03 mg/minute in one study, plasma concentrations declined in a biphasic manner; the half-life during the initial phase ($t_{1/2}\alpha$) was 10 minutes and that during the terminal phase ($t_{1/2}\beta$) was 2.3 hours. Results from one study indicate that the half-life of the *l*-isomer is about 50% longer than that of the *d*-isomer. When usual therapeutic doses of propranolol hydrochloride are administered chronically, the half-life of propranolol ranges from 3.4–6 hours. Single-dose studies generally have shown a shorter half-life of 2–3 hours. This difference in half-life between chronic and single-dose studies may be the result of initial removal of the drug into a large extravascular space (especially hepatic binding sites) and also a saturation of systemic clearance (including drug metabolizing enzymes and excretion). The half-life of propranolol may decrease with decreasing renal function; however, there is insufficient evidence to indicate that any alteration in maintenance dosage is necessary in patients with impaired renal function.

During initial oral therapy (but not during IV or chronic oral therapy), an active metabolite, 4-hydroxypropranolol, is formed. 4-Hydroxypropranolol has about the same β-adrenergic blocking potency as does propranolol and may be present in plasma in amounts about equal to propranolol. This metabolite is eliminated more rapidly than propranolol and is virtually absent from the plasma 6 hours after oral administration of the drug. Results of one study indicate that after IV administration or chronic oral administration of propranolol, 4-hydroxypropranolol is not formed to a substantial extent, and β-adrenergic blocking activity is more closely reflected by propranolol concentrations. Individual variations in ability to hydroxylate propranolol to the active metabolite may also exist. In addition, some other metabolites of propranolol may possess antiarrhythmic activity without β-adrenergic blocking activity.

Propranolol is almost completely metabolized in the liver and at least 8 metabolites have been identified in urine. Only 1–4% of an oral or IV dose of the drug appears in feces as unchanged drug and metabolites. In patients with severely impaired renal function, a compensatory increase in fecal excretion of propranolol occurs. Reduced propranolol plasma clearance and increased peak plasma concentrations have been reported in patients with chronic renal failure compared with healthy individuals and patients receiving dialysis. Chronic renal failure may be associated with reduced drug metabolism secondary to downregulation of hepatic cytochrome P-450 (CYP) enzyme system activity. Propranolol is apparently not substantially removed by hemodialysis.

Decreased propranolol clearance and prolonged elimination half-life have been reported in geriatric patients compared with younger patients. In addition, reduced clearance, increased volume of distribution, decreased protein binding, and considerable variation in elimination half-life of propranolol have been reported in patients with chronic liver disease compared with individuals with normal liver function. Increased propranolol exposure and decreased clearance also have been reported in obese individuals compared with nonobese individuals.

Chemistry and Stability

■ **Chemistry** Propranolol hydrochloride is a nonselective β-adrenergic blocking agent (β-blocker). Propranolol hydrochloride occurs as a white or off-white, crystalline powder with a bitter taste and is soluble in water and in alcohol. The commercially available drug is a racemic mixture of the 2 optical isomers. Solutions of propranolol hydrochloride fluoresce at pH 4–5. The injection is adjusted to pH 2.8–3.5 with citric acid.

■ **Stability** Propranolol hydrochloride preparations should be protected from light and stored at room temperature (20–25°C). The manufacturer recommends that propranolol hydrochloride extended-release capsules be stored in tight, light-resistant containers and be protected from moisture, freezing, and excessive heat. Propranolol hydrochloride injection also should be protected from freezing and excessive heat. USP recommends that propranolol hydrochloride preparations be stored in well-closed containers. Solutions of the drug have maximum stability at pH 3 and decompose rapidly at alkaline pH. Decomposition in aqueous solution is accompanied by a lowered pH and discoloration. Propranolol hydrochloride injection is reportedly compatible with 0.9% sodium chloride injection; however, specialized references should be consulted for specific compatibility information.

Preparations

Excipients in commercially available drug preparations may have clinically important effects in some individuals; consult specific product labeling for details.

Propranolol Hydrochloride

Oral		
Capsules, extended-release	60 mg	**Inderal® LA,** Ani Pharms
	80 mg	**Inderal® LA,** Ani Pharms **Innopran® XL,** Ani Pharms
	120 mg	**Inderal® LA,** Ani Pharms **Innopran® XL,** Ani Pharms
	160 mg	**Inderal® LA,** Ani Pharms
Solution	20 mg/5 mL*	**Propranolol Hydrochloride Solution**
	40 mg/5 mL*	**Propranolol Hydrochloride Solution**
Tablets	10 mg*	**Propranolol Hydrochloride Tablets**
	20 mg*	**Propranolol Hydrochloride Tablets**
	40 mg*	**Propranolol Hydrochloride Tablets**
	60 mg*	**Propranolol Hydrochloride Tablets**
	80 mg*	**Propranolol Hydrochloride Tablets**
Parenteral		
Injection	1 mg/mL*	**Propranolol Hydrochloride Injection**

*available from one or more manufacturer, distributor, and/or repackager by generic (nonproprietary) name

Propranolol Hydrochloride and Hydrochlorothiazide

Oral		
Tablets	40 mg Propranolol Hydrochloride and Hydrochlorothiazide 25 mg*	**Propranolol Hydrochloride and hydroCHLOROthiazide Tablets**
	80 mg Propranolol Hydrochloride and Hydrochlorothiazide 25 mg*	**Propranolol Hydrochloride and hydroCHLOROthiazide Tablets**

*available from one or more manufacturer, distributor, and/or repackager by generic (nonproprietary) name

†Use is not currently included in the labeling approved by the US Food and Drug Administration

Sotalol Hydrochloride

■ Sotalol hydrochloride is a nonselective β-adrenergic blocking agent that exhibits antiarrhythmic activity characteristic of class II and class III antiarrhythmic agents.

Uses

Sotalol is used to suppress and prevent the recurrence of documented life-threatening ventricular arrhythmias (e.g., sustained ventricular tachycardia). The drug also is used to maintain normal sinus rhythm in patients with symptomatic atrial fibrillation or flutter who are currently in sinus rhythm. Sotalol also has been used in the management of other supraventricular arrhythmias such as paroxysmal supraventricular tachycardia (PSVT)†.

The choice of a β-adrenergic blocking agent depends on numerous factors, including pharmacologic properties (e.g., relative β-selectivity, intrinsic sympathomimetic activity, membrane-stabilizing activity, lipophilicity), pharmacokinetics, intended use, and adverse effect profile, as well as the patient's coexisting disease states or conditions, response, and tolerance. While specific pharmacologic properties and other factors may appropriately influence the choice of a β-blocker in individual patients, evidence of clinically important differences among the agents in terms of overall efficacy and/or safety is limited. Patients who do not respond to or cannot tolerate one β-blocker may be successfully treated with a different agent.

■ **Ventricular Arrhythmias** Sotalol is used to suppress and prevent the recurrence of documented life-threatening ventricular arrhythmias (e.g., sustained ventricular tachycardia) and has been designated an orphan drug by the FDA for such use.

Although antiarrhythmic agents, including sotalol, may suppress the recurrence of arrhythmias and improve symptoms, there is no evidence from randomized controlled studies indicating that these drugs have a beneficial effect on mortality or sudden death. Findings from the National Heart, Lung, and

Blood Institute (NHLBI)'s Cardiac Arrhythmia Suppression Trial (CAST) after an average of 10 months of follow-up have indicated that the rate of total mortality and nonfatal cardiac arrest in patients with recent myocardial infarction (MI), mild to moderate left ventricular dysfunction, and asymptomatic or mildly symptomatic ventricular arrhythmias (principally frequent premature ventricular complexes [PVCs]) who received encainide or flecainide (class I antiarrhythmic drugs) increased substantially compared with placebo. (See Cautions in Flecainide 24:04.04.12.) Like other antiarrhythmic agents, sotalol can worsen existing arrhythmias or cause new arrhythmias, including torsades de pointes. Because of the drug's arrhythmogenic potential, use of sotalol for less severe arrhythmias, even if symptomatic, is not recommended by the manufacturer, and treatment of asymptomatic PVCs should be avoided. (See Cautions: Arrhythmogenic Effects.)

Although comparative data are limited, sotalol generally is considered to be as effective as some other antiarrhythmic agents (e.g., procainamide, quinidine) for the management of severe refractory arrhythmias. Data from clinical studies indicate that the drug is effective in approximately 55–85% of patients with life-threatening ventricular arrhythmias, including those refractory to other antiarrhythmic agents, and also is effective in patients with less severe arrhythmias. Sotalol can reduce PVCs, paired PVCs, and nonsustained ventricular tachycardia in patients with frequent PVCs, and can also suppress the recurrence of ventricular tachyarrhythmias in patients with ventricular tachycardia and/or fibrillation. The drug also has suppressed Holter monitor evidence of sustained ventricular tachycardia and ventricular tachycardia induced by programmed electrical stimulation (PES). Although some studies have shown that sotalol may reduce the risk of death from any cause and from cardiac causes compared with several class I antiarrhythmics (e.g., mexiletine, procainamide, propafenone, quinidine) in patients with ventricular tachyarrhythmias, the effect of the drug on survival (e.g., relative to placebo) remains to be established.

Life-threatening Ventricular Arrhythmias During Cardiac Arrest Antiarrhythmic drugs are used during cardiac arrest to facilitate and maintain a spontaneous perfusing rhythm in patients with refractory (i.e., persisting or recurring after at least one shock) ventricular fibrillation or pulseless ventricular tachycardia; however, there is no evidence that these drugs increase survival to hospital discharge when given routinely during cardiac arrest. High-quality cardiopulmonary resuscitation (CPR) and defibrillation are integral components of advanced cardiovascular life support (ACLS) and the only proven interventions to increase survival to hospital discharge. Other resuscitative efforts, including drug therapy, are considered secondary and should be performed without compromising the quality and timely delivery of chest compressions and defibrillation. The principal goal of pharmacologic therapy during cardiac arrest is to facilitate return of spontaneous circulation (ROSC), and epinephrine is considered the drug of choice for this use. (See Uses: Advanced Cardiovascular Life Support and Cardiac Arrhythmias, in Epinephrine 12:12.12.) Antiarrhythmic drugs may be considered for the treatment of refractory ventricular fibrillation or pulseless ventricular tachycardia during cardiac resuscitation; however, experts generally recommend the use of amiodarone (or lidocaine). IV sotalol may be used for the management of hemodynamically stable sustained monomorphic ventricular tachycardia during the periarrest period and is included as a recommended antiarrhythmic agent in current ACLS guidelines for adult tachycardia.

■ **Supraventricular Arrhythmias** Sotalol appears to be effective in the suppression and prevention of various supraventricular tachycardias (SVTs), including atrial fibrillation or flutter and PSVT†. Because of a higher risk of toxicity and proarrhythmic effects, antiarrhythmic agents such as sotalol generally should be reserved for patients who are not candidates for catheter ablation and who do not respond to or cannot be treated with AV nodal blocking agents (i.e., β-adrenergic blocking agents, nondihydropyridine calcium-channel blocking agents).

Atrial Fibrillation and Flutter Sotalol is used to maintain normal sinus rhythm in patients with symptomatic atrial fibrillation or flutter who are currently in sinus rhythm. Because of the potential to cause life-threatening ventricular arrhythmias, the manufacturer states that sotalol should be reserved for the treatment of highly symptomatic atrial fibrillation/flutter. (See Cautions: Arrhythmogenic Effects.) In addition, patients with paroxysmal atrial fibrillation that is easily reversed (e.g., by the Valsalva maneuver) should *not* receive sotalol.

Available data suggest that the efficacy of oral sotalol for prevention of recurrences of atrial fibrillation or flutter is comparable to that of quinidine or propafenone and less than that of amiodarone. Maintenance of sinus rhythm with oral sotalol does not appear to be related to either duration of previous episodes of atrial fibrillation (e.g., paroxysmal or persistent atrial fibrillation) or the degree of atrial enlargement.

Other Supraventricular Tachycardias Sotalol also has been used in patients with other SVTs, including PSVT due to AV nodal reentry tachycardia (AVNRT) or AV reentry tachycardia (AVRT).† However, vagal maneuvers and IV adenosine generally are preferred for initial treatment of PSVT in patients without contraindications. Sotalol may be a reasonable choice of therapy for the ongoing management of symptomatic SVT in patients who are not candidates for, or prefer not to undergo, catheter ablation and in whom first-line drugs (e.g., β-adrenergic blocking agents, diltiazem, verapamil) are not effective or are contraindicated.

Dosage and Administration

■ **Administration** Sotalol hydrochloride is administered orally or by IV infusion when oral administration is not feasible.

Because of the arrhythmogenic potential of sotalol, initiation or reinitiation of therapy, or conversion from IV to oral therapy should be performed in a facility capable of providing cardiac resuscitation, continuous electrocardiogram (ECG) monitoring, and calculation of creatinine clearance; treatment should be initiated in the presence of personnel trained in the management of serious arrhythmias. Patients should be closely monitored for at least 3 days (or until steady-state plasma concentrations are achieved) whenever treatment is initiated or dosage is increased. Prior to initiating therapy, the patient's baseline QT interval and creatinine clearance should be determined; therapy should not be initiated if the QT interval corrected for rate (QT_c) exceeds 450 msec or creatinine clearance is less than 40 mL/minute. Because the potential for arrhythmogenic events increases with increasing dosage, patients should be monitored closely during the dose titration phase until steady-state concentrations are reached. When titrating dosage, QT interval should be determined 2–4 hours after each dose increase (if the drug is given orally) or after completion of each IV infusion; dose should be reduced, dosing interval increased, or therapy discontinued if prolongation of the QT interval to 500 msec or greater occurs.

Patients should be advised not to discontinue or interrupt sotalol therapy without consulting their clinician. Patients should be given an adequate supply of the drug upon hospital discharge to allow uninterrupted therapy until their outpatient prescription can be filled.

Patients with atrial fibrillation should be anticoagulated according to usual medical practice. (See Uses: Embolism Associated with Atrial Fibrillation in Warfarin 20:12.04.08.)

Oral Administration Sotalol hydrochloride is administered orally as tablets or oral solution.

If the drug is administered as an oral solution, the commercially available oral solution containing 25 mg/5 mL may be used or an oral solution may be extemporaneously prepared by adding five 120-mg tablets to a 180-mL polyethylene terephthalate (PET) prescription bottle containing 120 mL of simple syrup with 0.1% sodium benzoate (syrup NF); alternatively, the syrup may be added to the tablets. An oversized bottle is used to allow more effective shaking of the mixture. The tablets may be added intact to the syrup or crushed; if crushed, care should be taken to transfer the entire quantity of tablet powder to the syrup. The mixture should be shaken to wet the tablets and the tablets allowed to hydrate for at least 2 hours. The bottle should then be shaken intermittently over another 2 hours until dispersion of fine particles is obtained; alternatively, the tablets may be allowed to hydrate overnight to simplify the disintegration process. An appropriate measuring device (e.g., oral dosing syringe) should be used to administer oral solutions of sotalol; use of a teaspoon or tablespoon may result in dosing errors and is not recommended.

Administration of oral sotalol within 2 hours of administration of an aluminum oxide and magnesium hydroxide-containing antacid resulted in decreased absorption of sotalol as evidenced by 26 and 20% reductions in peak plasma concentrations and area under the plasma concentration-time curve (AUC), respectively, of the drug. Since such decreased absorption was associated with a 25% reduction in bradycardic effect, the manufacturer states that antacids should not be administered within 2 hours of administration of sotalol; however, when the antacid was administered 2 hours after sotalol, no effects on the pharmacokinetics or pharmacodynamics of sotalol were observed.

IV Administration Sotalol hydrochloride is administered by IV infusion over 5 hours using a volumetric pump to ensure that the drug is delivered at a constant rate.

The commercially available 15-mg/mL injection concentrate must be diluted with a suitable diluent (i.e., 0.9% sodium chloride injection, 5% dextrose injection, lactated Ringer's injection) prior to administration. The manufacturer recommends that the volume of injection concentrate used to prepare the infusion solution and the final infusion solution volume exceed those required for the intended dose to account for the volume loss in the dead space of the infusion set. Preparation of a final volume of 120 or 300 mL is recommended; however, the actual volume that should be infused is 100 or 250 mL, respectively. For a dose of 75 mg, the manufacturer recommends that 6 mL of the injection concentrate be diluted with 114 or 294 mL of diluent to prepare a final volume of 120 or 300 mL, respectively. For a dose of 112.5 mg, the manufacturer recommends that 9 mL of the injection concentrate be diluted with 111 or 291 mL of diluent to prepare a final volume of 120 or 300 mL, respectively. For a dose of 150 mg, the manufacturer recommends that 12 mL of injection concentrate be diluted with 108 or 288 mL of diluent to prepare a final volume of 120 or 300 mL, respectively.

■ **Dosage** Dosage of sotalol hydrochloride must be adjusted carefully according to individual requirements and response, patient tolerance, renal function, and QT interval.

Appropriate dosage adjustments should be made for patients with impaired renal function to minimize the risk of drug accumulation and arrhythmogenic events. (See Dosage and Administration: Dosage in Renal and Hepatic Impairment.) If a dose is missed, patients should be advised to take the next dose at the regularly scheduled time and to not take a double dose or increase the dosing frequency to compensate for the missed dose.

Adult Oral Dosage **Life-threatening Ventricular Arrhythmias.** For the management of life-threatening ventricular arrhythmias in adults with normal renal function (creatinine clearance exceeding 60 mL/minute), an initial oral sotalol hydrochloride dosage of 80 mg twice daily is recommended. Dosage may be increased every 3 days in increments of 80 mg daily provided QT_c does not exceed 500 msec. The usual oral maintenance dosage in adults is 160–320 mg daily, given in 2 or 3 divided doses; because of the long elimination half-life of the drug, dosing more than 2 times a day usually is not necessary. In patients with life-threatening refractory ventricular arrhythmias, oral sotalol hydrochloride dosages as high as 480–640 mg daily have been used; however, the risk of serious arrhythmias increases with higher dosages.

Atrial Fibrillation/Flutter. For maintenance of normal sinus rhythm in adults with atrial fibrillation or flutter who have normal renal function (creatinine clearance exceeding 60 mL/minute), an initial oral sotalol hydrochloride dosage of 80 mg twice daily is recommended. Dosage may be increased every 3 days in increments of 80 mg daily provided QT_c does not exceed 500 msec. In a dose-response study, the most effective dosage in preventing recurrence of atrial fibrillation or flutter was 120 mg once or twice daily. Some clinicians state that dosage may be increased up to a maximum of 160 mg twice daily (provided the drug is well tolerated without excessive QT interval prolongation) if patients continue to experience recurrences of symptomatic atrial fibrillation or flutter.

Adult Parenteral Dosage When oral therapy is not feasible, sotalol may be administered as an IV infusion. Because oral bioavailability of sotalol is 90–100%, equivalent IV doses are lower than oral doses. The manufacturer recommends the following dose equivalencies when converting between oral and IV dosing: 75 mg IV for an oral dose of 80 mg, 112.5 mg IV for an oral dose of 120 mg, and 150 mg IV for an oral dose of 160 mg.

Life-threatening Ventricular Arrhythmias. The recommended initial IV dosage of sotalol hydrochloride for the management of life-threatening ventricular arrhythmias in adults is 75 mg once or twice daily (depending on creatinine clearance) by IV infusion over 5 hours. (See Dosage and Administration: Dosage in Renal and Hepatic Impairment.) If the desired response has not been achieved and the drug is well tolerated without excessive QT interval prolongation, dosage may be increased to 112.5 mg once or twice daily (depending on creatinine clearance); the manufacturer recommends that dosage be increased in increments of 75 mg daily every 3 days. Based on experience with oral sotalol hydrochloride, the usual therapeutic effect should be observed with IV dosages of 75–150 mg once or twice daily; however, patients with life-threatening refractory ventricular arrhythmias have received higher dosages (e.g., oral dosages of 240–320 mg once or twice daily corresponding to IV dosages of 225–300 mg once or twice daily).

Atrial Fibrillation/Flutter. The recommended initial IV dosage of sotalol hydrochloride for the maintenance of normal sinus rhythm in adults with atrial fibrillation or flutter is 75 mg once or twice daily (depending on creatinine clearance) by IV infusion over 5 hours. (See Dosage and Administration: Dosage in Renal and Hepatic Impairment.) If the desired response has not been achieved and the drug is well tolerated without excessive QT interval prolongation, dosage may be increased after at least 3 days to 112.5 mg once or twice daily (depending on creatinine clearance). Based on experience with oral sotalol hydrochloride, the usual therapeutic effect should be observed with an IV dosage of 112.5 mg once or twice daily; however, the manufacturer states that IV dosage may be increased up to 150 mg once or twice daily if necessary provided the drug is well tolerated.

Pediatric Dosage Dosage of sotalol hydrochloride in pediatric patients is based on pharmacokinetic data. (See Cautions: Pediatric Precautions.) The usual precautions observed in adults should also be taken when initiating or reinitiating therapy in pediatric patients. Dosage increases should preferably be performed in an inpatient setting where patients can be closely monitored. Because sotalol has similar potency in children and adults, dosages used in pediatric patients should achieve plasma concentrations similar to those within the adult dosage range; however, dosage should be individualized based on clinical response, heart rate, and QT_c. There are no studies of IV sotalol hydrochloride in pediatric patients.

The recommended initial oral dosage of sotalol hydrochloride for the management of ventricular arrhythmias or atrial fibrillation/flutter in children about 2 years of age or older with normal renal function is 30 mg/m^2 3 times daily (total daily dose of 90 mg/m^2); dosage may be increased up to a maximum of 60 mg/m^2 3 times daily, allowing at least 36 hours to elapse between dosage escalations to achieve steady-state concentrations.

Dosage of sotalol hydrochloride in children about 2 years of age or younger should be reduced from the usual oral dosage for older children (i.e., 30 mg/m^2 3 times daily) by an age-dependent factor obtained from the manufacturer's prescribing information. The age-dependent factor is approximately 0.3 in neonates about 1 week old, 0.68 in infants 1 month of age, and 0.97 in infants 20 months of age. The calculated dose after multiplying the age-dependent factor by 30 mg/m^2 is 9 mg/m^2 in neonates about 1 week old, 20 mg/m^2 in infants 1 month of age, and 29.1 mg/m^2 in infants 20 months of age, administered 3 times daily.

Use of sotalol in pediatric patients with renal impairment has not been evaluated; in general, lower doses should be used or the dosing interval should be increased.

Conversion from other Antiarrhythmic Agents The manufacturer recommends a transition period when converting patients from another antiarrhythmic agent to sotalol therapy. In general, initiation of sotalol therapy should be delayed for a period of at least 2–3 elimination half-lives of the previously administered antiarrhythmic; the patient should be monitored carefully during the transition. Class I or Class III antiarrhythmic agents should be withheld for at least 3 half-lives prior to dosing with sotalol hydrochloride.

■ **Dosage in Renal and Hepatic Impairment** In patients with renal impairment, the dose or dosing frequency of sotalol hydrochloride should be reduced to minimize the risk of proarrhythmia; as in patients with normal renal function, QT interval and heart rate should be closely monitored. (See Cautions: Arrhythmogenic Effects.) Dosing interval should be modified according to the patient's estimated creatinine clearance. In general, the initial oral adult sotalol hydrochloride dose of 80 mg and subsequent doses should be administered twice daily in patients with a creatinine clearance greater than 60 mL/minute and once daily in patients with a creatinine clearance of 40–60 mL/minute. The drug is generally contraindicated in patients with creatinine clearance less than 40 mL/minute. In patients with ventricular arrhythmias, some manufacturers recommend a dosing interval of 36–48 hours in adults with creatinine clearance of 10–29 mL/minute and individualized dosing in those with creatinine clearance less than 10 mL/minute. Since terminal elimination half-life of the drug is prolonged in patients with renal impairment, dosage increases generally should be made after administration of at least 5 doses at appropriate intervals. Sotalol is partially removed by dialysis; however, the manufacturers make no dosing recommendations for patients undergoing dialysis. Dosage of sotalol hydrochloride in children with renal impairment has not been established; however, reduced doses and increased dosing intervals are recommended in patients of all age groups with renal impairment.

The manufacturer states that clearance of sotalol is not altered by impaired hepatic function.

Cautions

Sotalol shares the toxic potentials of nonselective β-adrenergic blocking agents and, in therapeutic dosage, generally is well tolerated during long-term therapy. However, as a class III antiarrhythmic agent (see Description), sotalol, unlike conventional β-blockers, can prolong the QT interval and precipitate torsades de pointes. Adverse effects associated with sotalol are generally dose related and typically result from the drug's class II (beta-blocking) and class III (cardiac action potential duration prolongation) effects.

The most serious adverse effect of sotalol is torsades de pointes, which occurred in almost 4 or 1% of patients with a history of sustained ventricular tachycardia or other less serious ventricular arrhythmias, respectively, who received the drug orally in clinical studies. The most frequent adverse effects of sotalol involve the cardiovascular and nervous systems and GI tract, and occasionally they may be severe enough to require discontinuance of the drug. The most common adverse effects resulting in discontinuance of the drug include effects usually associated with β-blockade. Fatigue caused discontinuance of sotalol in 4–5% of patients, bradycardia (heart rate less than 50 bpm) in 2–3%, dyspnea in 2–3%, arrhythmogenic effects in 1.5–3%, asthenia in 2%, and dizziness in 2% of patients receiving the drug in clinical trials. Overall, discontinuance of sotalol as a result of adverse effects occurred in 17% of patients receiving the drug in clinical trials and in 10% of those treated for at least 2 weeks. Abrupt withdrawal of sotalol should be avoided, especially in patients with coronary artery disease, since it may exacerbate angina or precipitate myocardial infarction (MI).

■ **Arrhythmogenic Effects** Like other antiarrhythmic agents, sotalol can worsen existing arrhythmias or cause new arrhythmias, including sustained ventricular tachycardia or ventricular fibrillation which potentially may be fatal; the arrhythmogenic potential is the most serious risk associated with the drug. Because sotalol prolongs the QT interval corrected for rate (QT_c), torsades de pointes, a polymorphic ventricular tachycardia with prolongation of the QT interval and a shifting electrical axis, is the most common arrhythmogenic effect of the drug, occurring in about 0.6 or 4% of patients with a history of supraventricular arrhythmias (i.e., atrial fibrillation or flutter) or ventricular arrhythmias (i.e., sustained ventricular tachycardia or ventricular fibrillation), respectively. The risk of torsades de pointes increases progressively with prolongation of the QT interval and is worsened by a reduction in heart rate and serum potassium concentration. (See Cautions: Precautions and Contraindications.)

In patients with a history of sustained ventricular tachycardia, the frequency of torsades de pointes was 4% and the frequency of worsened ventricular tachycardia was about 1%; in patients with other, less serious ventricular arrhythmias, the frequency of torsades de pointes was 1% and the frequency of new or worsened ventricular tachycardia was 0.7%.

In clinical trials of sotalol, the incidence of cardiac mortality was 3.8% overall and 5.9% in patients with sustained ventricular tachycardia or ventricular fibrillation. Overall, cardiac death was associated with low left ventricular ejection fraction, history of congestive heart failure and/or cardiomegaly, and increasing age; the risk of death in patients with a history of both cardiomegaly and congestive heart failure was more than 3 times that in patients with no history of either condition. In patients with sustained ventricular tachycardia or ventricular fibrillation, the risk of cardiac death was most strongly associated with a history of cardiomegaly and then with a history of congestive heart failure and low left ventricular ejection fraction. A clear relationship between sotalol dosage and the frequency of death has not been demonstrated to date.

Prolongation of the QT_c interval and the occurrence of torsades de pointes are dose related. In patients with sustained ventricular tachycardia or ventricular fibrillation, the incidence of torsades de pointes ranged from 0.5% at 160 mg daily to 1.6% at 320 mg daily but increased more abruptly at higher dosages, to about 4% at 480–640 mg daily and to almost 6% at higher dosages. The frequency of torsades de pointes in patients with ventricular arrhythmias was 1.6% when the change in QT_c interval was less than 65 msec but increased by about 1% with each additional increase of about 20–30 msec in the QT_c interval, with a frequency of 7.1% at QT_c interval increases exceeding 130 msec. In addition, the risk of sotalol-induced torsades de pointes was increased with female gender, reduced renal function, large doses of the drug, and a history of cardiomegaly or heart failure. Patients with sustained ventricular tachycardia and a history of heart failure appeared to be at greatest risk of a serious arrhythmogenic event, with an occurrence rate of 7%. Approximately two-thirds of patients experiencing sotalol-induced torsades de pointes reverted spontaneously to their baseline rhythm. The remaining patients required either cardioversion or overdrive pacing or treatment with other drugs. Although it is not possible to determine whether some sudden deaths resulted from episodes of torsades de pointes, some instances of sudden death did follow documented episodes. Most cases of torsades de pointes required discontinuance of sotalol therapy, but 17% of patients continued the drug at a lower dosage. Sotalol should be used with particular caution if the QT_c interval exceeds 500 msec during treatment, and dosage reduction or discontinuance of the drug should be seriously considered when the QT_c interval exceeds 500 msec. Regardless of the QT_c interval, caution should be exercised because of the multiple risk factors associated with torsades de pointes.

Sotalol-induced arrhythmogenic events can occur not only when initiating therapy, but with every upward dosage adjustment. About 75% of such serious events (e.g., torsades de pointes, worsened ventricular tachycardia) occur within 7 days of initiating therapy with the drug, and about 60% occur within 3 days of initiation of the drug or dosage adjustment. Initiation of sotalol therapy at low dosages with gradual upward titration and appropriate monitoring should reduce the risk of arrhythmogenic events. Because of the arrhythmogenic potential of the drug and the life-threatening nature of the arrhythmias against which the drug is being employed, the manufacturer recommends that both initiation and reinitiation of sotalol therapy and any subsequent upward dosage adjustments be performed in an institutional setting.

■ **Cardiovascular Effects** Sympathetic stimulation is necessary for supporting circulatory function in heart failure. Therefore, because of its β-adrenergic blocking effects, sotalol may cause or worsen heart failure, particularly in patients with preexisting heart failure (New York Heart Association [NYHA] class II–IV) or sustained ventricular tachycardia or ventricular fibrillation, and/or a history of cardiomegaly, cardiomyopathy, coronary artery disease, or myocardial infarction. The effect of these risk factors appears to be cumulative, with patients exhibiting more risk factors being at greater risk for precipitated or worsened heart failure during therapy with the drug.

New or worsened heart failure occurred in 3% of patients receiving sotalol in premarketing studies and required discontinuance of the drug in about 1% of patients. The frequency of new or worsened heart failure was 5% in patients with sustained ventricular tachycardia or ventricular fibrillation and 7% in patients with a history of heart failure. In patients with sustained ventricular tachycardia or ventricular fibrillation, the most reliable predictive risk factors were a history of congestive heart failure or cardiomegaly. The 1-year frequency of new or worsened heart failure was 3% in patients without a previous history and 10% in those with a previous history of heart failure. The risk of new or worsened heart failure was closely related to NYHA classification. The occurrence of heart failure was not related to dosage of sotalol, regardless of heart failure history. New or worsened heart failure occurred in 2.7% of patients with nonsustained ventricular tachycardia or premature ventricular complexes (PVCs) and in 2.3% of patients with supraventricular arrhythmias.

Chest pain and palpitation occurred in 16 and 14%, respectively, of patients with sustained ventricular tachycardia or ventricular fibrillation receiving sotalol in clinical trials, but each of these adverse effects required discontinuance of the drug in less than 1% of patients. In pooled data from several clinical trials in a limited number of patients with atrial fibrillation or flutter, angina pectoris occurred in 1.6–2% of patients receiving sotalol hydrochloride 160–320 mg daily. Nonanginal chest pain occurred in 2.5–4.6% of these patients. Edema was reported in 8%, abnormal ECG in 7%, and syncope in 5% of patients with a history of ventricular arrhythmias receiving sotalol, and each of these adverse effects required discontinuance of the drug in 1% of patients. Hypotension was reported in 6% of patients with a history of ventricular arrhythmias and required discontinuance in 2% of patients. Presyncope was reported in 4%; peripheral vascular disorder, cardiovascular disorder, vasodilation, or AICD discharge in 3%; and hypertension in 2% of patients with a history of ventricular arrhythmias receiving sotalol, and each of these adverse effects required discontinuance of the drug in less than 1% of patients.

■ **Effects on Cardiac Conduction** Sinus bradycardia (heart rate less than 50 bpm), which increases the risk of torsades de pointes, occurred in 13% of patients with sustained ventricular tachycardia or ventricular fibrillation receiving sotalol in clinical trials and required discontinuance of the drug in about 2.4% of patients. Pooled data from several clinical trials in patients with atrial fibrillation or flutter indicate that bradycardia occurred in 12–13% of patients receiving oral sotalol; discontinuance of therapy was required in 2.4% of these patients. Sinus pause, arrest, and nodal dysfunction occurred in less than 1% of patients, and second- or third-degree AV block occurred in about 1% of patients receiving sotalol.

QRS intervals are affected minimally by sotalol; however, at dosages of 160–640 mg daily, sotalol causes dose-related mean increases of 40–100 msec in the QT interval and 10–40 msec in the QT_c interval. Excessive prolongation of the QT interval (to greater than 550 msec) can promote serious arrhythmias and should be avoided during sotalol therapy. (See Cautions: Arrhythmogenic Effects.)

■ **Nervous System Effects** Fatigue, dizziness, and asthenia, which appear to be dose related, are the most common adverse nervous system effects of sotalol, occurring in 20% of patients with sustained ventricular tachycardia or ventricular fibrillation receiving the drug in clinical trials. Fatigue and dizziness also are the most common adverse nervous system effects of sotalol in patients with a history of atrial fibrillation or flutter, occurring in 18.9–19.6 or 13.1–16.3% of these patients, respectively. Fatigue resulted in discontinuance of sotalol in 4.6% of patients with a history of these supraventricular arrhythmias. Lightheadedness, dizziness, and syncope also are symptoms of torsades de pointes. Asthenia and lightheadedness were reported in 13 and 12%, respectively, of patients with a history of ventricular arrhythmias receiving sotalol in clinical trials. Weakness was reported in about 5% of patients with a history of atrial fibrillation or flutter receiving sotalol in clinical trials. Headache and sleep disturbances were reported in 8% of patients with ventricular arrhythmias receiving sotalol and required discontinuance in less than 1% of patients. Insomnia was reported in 2.6–4.1% of patients with a history of atrial fibrillation or flutter receiving sotalol in clinical trials. Perspiration was reported in 6% of patients; altered consciousness, depression, paresthesia, or anxiety in 4% of patients; and localized pain, mood change, or appetite disorder in 3% of patients with a history of ventricular arrhythmias receiving sotalol in clinical trials; each of these adverse effects required discontinuance of the drug in less than 1% of patients. Cold sensation was reported in 2–2.5% of patients with a history of atrial fibrillation or flutter receiving sotalol in clinical trials. Rarely, emotional lability, slightly clouded sensorium, incoordination, vertigo, and paralysis have been reported during postmarketing experience. One case of peripheral neuropathy, which resolved on discontinuance of sotalol therapy and recurred when the patient was rechallenged with the drug, also has been reported.

■ **Respiratory Effects** Dyspnea was reported in 21% of patients with sustained ventricular tachycardia or ventricular fibrillation receiving the drug in clinical trials but required discontinuance of therapy in only 2% of patients. Dyspnea also has been reported in 9.2–9.8% of patients with a history of atrial fibrillation or flutter receiving sotalol in clinical trials, requiring discontinuance of therapy in 2% of these patients. Pulmonary problems were reported in 8%, upper respiratory tract problems in 5%, and asthma in 2% of patients with ventricular arrhythmias receiving sotalol; each of these adverse effects required discontinuance of therapy in less than 1% of patients. Influenza or upper respiratory tract infection has been reported in 0.8–2 or 2.6–3.3%, respectively, of patients with a history of atrial fibrillation or flutter receiving sotalol in clinical trials. Cough or tracheobronchitis has been reported in 2.5–3.3 or 0.7–3.3%, respectively, of patients with a history of these supraventricular arrhythmias receiving sotalol in clinical trials. Rarely, pulmonary edema has been reported during postmarketing experience with the drug. As with other nonselective β-adrenergic blocking agents, sotalol can increase airway resistance by inhibiting bronchodilation mediated by endogenous or exogenous catecholamine stimulation of β_2-adrenergic receptors; such changes may be clinically important in patients with underlying airway disease. (See Cautions: Precautions and Contraindications.)

■ **GI Effects** Nausea and vomiting are the most frequent adverse GI effects of sotalol, occurring in 5.7–7.8 or 10% of patients with supraventricular (i.e., atrial fibrillation or flutter) or ventricular (i.e., sustained ventricular tachycardia or ventricular fibrillation) arrhythmias, respectively, receiving the drug in clinical trials and requiring discontinuance in up to 1% of patients. Other adverse GI effects each required discontinuance of sotalol in less than 1% of patients with ventricular arrhythmias. Diarrhea and dyspepsia were reported in 7 and 6%, respectively, of patients with ventricular arrhythmias receiving sotalol in clinical trials. Diarrhea or dyspepsia was reported in 5.2–5.7 or 2–2.5% of patients, respectively, with a history of atrial fibrillation or flutter receiving sotalol in controlled clinical trials. Abdominal pain and colon problems occurred in 3% of patients, and flatulence occurred in 2% of patients with ventricular arrhythmias. Abdominal pain or abdominal distension was reported in 2.5–3.9% or 0.7–2.5%, respectively, of patients with a history of atrial fibrillation or flutter receiving sotalol in controlled clinical trials.

■ **Hepatic Effects** Increased serum concentrations of hepatic enzymes have occurred occasionally with sotalol therapy, but a causal relationship to the drug has not been established.

■ **Genitourinary Effects** Genitourinary disorders and sexual dysfunction were reported in 3 and 2%, respectively, of patients with ventricular arrhythmias receiving sotalol in clinical trials and each required discontinuance of the drug in less than 1% of patients.

■ **Musculoskeletal Effects** Extremity pain and back pain were reported in 7 and 3%, respectively, of patients with ventricular arrhythmias receiving sotalol in clinical trials and each required discontinuance of the drug in less than 1% of patients. Rarely, myalgia has been reported during postmarketing experience with the drug. Musculoskeletal pain or musculoskeletal chest pain has been reported in 2.6–4.1 or 2–2.5%, respectively, of patients with a history of atrial fibrillation or flutter receiving sotalol in clinical trials.

■ Dermatologic Effects Rash was reported in 5% of patients with ventricular arrhythmias receiving sotalol in clinical trials and required discontinuance of the drug in less than 1% of patients. Rarely, photosensitivity reactions, pruritus, and alopecia have been reported during postmarketing experience with the drug. Hyperhidrosis has been reported in 4.9–5.2% of patients with a history of atrial fibrillation or flutter receiving sotalol in clinical trials.

■ Hematologic Effects Bleeding was reported in 2% of patients with ventricular arrhythmias receiving sotalol in clinical trials and required discontinuance of the drug in less than 1% of patients. Rarely, thrombocytopenia, leukopenia, and eosinophilia have been reported during postmarketing experience with the drug.

■ Ocular Effects Visual disorders were reported in 5% of patients with ventricular arrhythmias receiving sotalol in clinical trials and required discontinuance of the drug in less than 1% of patients. Visual disturbances were reported in 0.8–2.6% of patients with a history of atrial fibrillation or flutter receiving sotalol in clinical trials.

■ Other Adverse Effects Fever, infection, and abnormal laboratory test results were each reported in 4% of patients and weight change in 2% of patients with sustained ventricular tachycardia or ventricular fibrillation receiving sotalol in clinical trials, and each of these adverse effects required discontinuance of the drug in less than 1% of patients. Pooled data from several clinical trials in patients with a history of atrial fibrillation or flutter indicate that fever was reported in 0.7–3.3% of patients receiving sotalol. Increases in blood glucose concentration and insulin requirements can occur in patients with diabetes mellitus receiving sotalol. Rarely, hyperlipidemia has been reported during postmarketing experience with the drug.

■ Precautions and Contraindications Sotalol shares the toxic potentials of other nonselective β-adrenergic blocking agents, and the usual precautions of these agents should be observed. In addition, as a class III antiarrhythmic agent, sotalol, unlike conventional β-blockers, can precipitate torsades de pointes.

Sotalol, like other antiarrhythmics, has been associated with the development or exacerbation of arrhythmias in some patients. (See Cautions: Arrhythmogenic Effects.) Concerns about the long-term safety and efficacy of several antiarrhythmic agents (e.g., encainide, flecainide, moricizine) in patients with nonlife-threatening arrhythmias have been raised by the postmarketing Cardiac Arrhythmia Suppression Trial (CAST). Findings from the CAST study after an average of 10 months of follow-up indicated that the rate of total mortality and nonfatal cardiac arrest in patients with recent MI, mild-to-moderate left ventricular dysfunction, and asymptomatic or mildly symptomatic ventricular arrhythmias (principally frequent PVCs) who received encainide or flecainide was increased substantially. (For additional information on the CAST study, see Cautions, in Flecainide 24:04.04.12.)

While sotalol can be used safely and effectively in the chronic management of life-threatening ventricular arrhythmias following MI, experience with the drug in the management of arrhythmias during the early phase of recovery from an acute MI is limited and at least at high initial doses (i.e., nontitrated initial dosage of 320 mg daily or 320 mg twice daily) has not been reassuring. Sotalol is devoid of class I antiarrhythmic activity, and there was no evidence of excess mortality associated with sotalol hydrochloride dosages up to 320 mg daily in a large (1456 patients), double-blind, placebo-controlled secondary prevention trial in patients with recent MI (but not necessarily concurrent ventricular arrhythmias). However, in patients who received an initial (i.e., not titrated) dosage of 320 mg daily in the study and in high-risk postinfarction patients who received high dosages (320 mg twice daily) in another smaller study, there was some evidence of a possible excess in early (within 2 weeks) sudden deaths. Therefore, sotalol should be used cautiously and with careful titration of dosage if the drug is used during the first 2 weeks following an acute MI, particularly in patients with markedly impaired ventricular function. Although specific studies of sotalol in treating supraventricular arrhythmias after a recent MI have not been performed to date, the usual precautions regarding heart failure, avoidance of hypokalemia, bradycardia, or prolonged QT interval apply.

Since sotalol, like other antiarrhythmic agents, can worsen existing arrhythmias or cause new arrhythmias in some patients, clinical and ECG evaluations are essential prior to and during sotalol therapy to monitor for the appearance of arrhythmias and to determine the need for continued therapy or dosage adjustment. (See Cautions: Arrhythmogenic Effects.) Arrhythmogenic events must be anticipated not only when sotalol therapy is initiated, but also with each upward dosage titration. To minimize the risk of arrhythmogenic effects, the recommendations for initiation of sotalol therapy and dosage adjustments should be closely followed. (See Dosage and Administration.) In addition, excessive accumulation of the drug in patients with diminished renal function should be avoided with appropriate dosage adjustment. Because of the arrhythmogenic potential, the manufacturer recommends that patients be hospitalized for a minimum of 3 days (or until steady-state concentrations are achieved) for initiation or reinitiation of sotalol therapy in a facility capable of providing cardiac resuscitation and continuous ECG monitoring.

Sotalol increases QT_c interval in a dose-related fashion and thereby increases the risk of torsades de pointes. Therefore, the QT interval should be monitored during therapy and dosage adjusted accordingly. (See Dosage and Administration: Administration.) Sotalol should not be *initiated* in patients with a QT interval exceeding 450 msec. If the QT interval exceeds 500 msec, the dose should be reduced, the dosing interval increased, or the drug should be discontinued. Excessive prolongation of the QT interval (to greater than 500 msec) can promote serious arrhythmias and should be avoided during sotalol therapy. The possibility that the development of syncope and/or dizziness may be signs of undetected torsades de pointes should be considered. Because of the multiple risk factors associated with torsades de pointes, however, caution should be exercised regardless of the QT_c interval.

Sotalol should not be used in patients with hypokalemia or hypomagnesemia until these imbalances are corrected, since such electrolyte abnormalities can exaggerate the degree of QT prolongation and increase the risk of torsades de pointes. Special attention should be given to electrolyte and acid-base balance in patients with severe or prolonged diarrhea and in patients receiving diuretics concomitantly. Patients should be advised to report immediately to their clinician conditions, concomitant therapy (e.g., diuretics), and/or manifestations associated with altered electrolyte balance such as severe or prolonged diarrhea, unusual sweating, vomiting, loss of appetite, or thirst. Sotalol generally should not be used concomitantly with other drugs known to prolong the QT interval (e.g., class I or other class III antiarrhythmic agents, certain oral macrolides [e.g., azithromycin, clarithromycin], phenothiazines, tricyclic antidepressants, certain quinolones [e.g., ciprofloxacin, levofloxacin]). The manufacturers state that class Ia antiarrhythmic agents such as disopyramide, quinidine, and procainamide and class III antiarrhythmic agents such as amiodarone should not be used concomitantly with sotalol and should be discontinued for at least 3 half-lives prior to dosing with sotalol. In clinical trials in patients with a history of atrial fibrillation or flutter, sotalol was not administered in patients previously treated with oral amiodarone for longer than 1 month in the previous 3 months. There is only limited experience with concomitant use of class Ib or Ic antiarrhythmics and sotalol. The manufacturers state that additive class II effects should be anticipated with the use of other β-blocking agents concomitantly with sotalol.

Sotalol is contraindicated in patients with sinus bradycardia, second- or third-degree AV block, or sick sinus syndrome, unless a functioning pacemaker is present. The risk of torsades de pointes in patients with atrial fibrillation and sinus node dysfunction is increased, especially after cardioversion. Because sotalol has a greater effect in prolonging the QT interval and the action potential duration at lower heart rates (reverse rate dependence), bradycardia following cardioversion in such patients is associated with greater QT_c prolongation than observed at higher heart rates.

Sotalol should be used with caution in patients with inadequate cardiac function. Because sympathetic stimulation is necessary to support circulatory function in patients with heart failure, β-blockade with sotalol carries the potential risk of depressing myocardial contractility and precipitating more severe heart failure. However, the fact that sotalol and cardiac glycosides both slow AV conduction also should be considered.

Since β-adrenergic blocking agents may inhibit bronchodilation produced by endogenous catecholamines, the drugs generally should not be used in patients with bronchospastic diseases. Use of sotalol is not recommended in patients with nonallergic bronchospasm (e.g., chronic bronchitis, emphysema). If sotalol is administered, it is prudent to use the lowest effective dosage to minimize inhibition of bronchodilation produced by endogenous or exogenous catecholamine stimulation of β_2-adrenergic receptors.

It is recommended that sotalol be used with caution in patients with diabetes mellitus (especially those with labile diabetes or those prone to hypoglycemia) since the drug may mask certain signs and symptoms associated with acute hypoglycemia (e.g., tachycardia). Sotalol may increase blood glucose concentrations and insulin requirements in diabetic patients. The drug also should be used with caution in patients with a history of episodic spontaneous hypoglycemia. However, many clinicians state that patients with diabetes mellitus may be particularly likely to experience a reduction in morbidity and mortality with the use of β-adrenergic blocking agents.

There is some controversy regarding the perioperative use of β-adrenergic blocking agents. Severe, protracted hypotension, bradycardia, and stroke have occurred during surgery in some patients who have received β-adrenergic blocking agents; in addition, it is unclear whether such use confers any mortality benefit or risk. It is generally recommended that β-blockers be continued during surgery in patients who are already receiving these drugs for a chronic condition. However, the risks versus benefits should be carefully considered in individual patients.

While receiving β-blockers such as sotalol, patients with a history of anaphylactic reaction to a variety of allergens may have a more severe reaction on repeated accidental, diagnostic, or therapeutic challenge. These patients may be unresponsive to the usual doses of epinephrine used to treat the reaction.

Abrupt withdrawal of sotalol may exacerbate angina symptoms and/or precipitate MI in patients with ischemic heart disease, or may precipitate thyroid storm (since signs of hyperthyroidism such as tachycardia may be masked by the drug) in patients with thyroid disease. Therefore, patients receiving sotalol (especially those with ischemic heart disease) should be warned not to interrupt or discontinue therapy without consulting their clinician. If possible, sotalol hydrochloride dosage should be reduced gradually and with close monitoring over 1–2 weeks, especially in patients with ischemic heart disease. If exacerbation of angina occurs or acute coronary insufficiency develops after sotalol therapy is interrupted or discontinued, appropriate treatment (e.g., temporary use of another β-blocker) should be instituted.

Sotalol reduces systolic and diastolic blood pressures and may result in hypotension. Hemodynamic monitoring is recommended in patients with marginal cardiac compensation.

Sotalol is contraindicated in patients with bronchial asthma or related bronchospastic conditions, sinus bradycardia (less than 50 beats per minute during waking hours), second- or third-degree AV block (unless a functioning pacemaker is present), congenital or acquired long-QT syndromes, cardiogenic shock, decompensated heart failure, hypokalemia (serum potassium concentrations less than 4 mEq/L), or hypersensitivity to the drug. In addition, sotalol is contraindicated for the treatment of atrial fibrillation or flutter in patients with baseline QT interval exceeding 450 msec and in patients with creatinine clearance less than 40 mL/minute.

■ **Pediatric Precautions** Safety and efficacy of sotalol in children younger than 18 years of age have not been established. Sotalol has been used in a limited number of infants younger than 3 months of age and children younger than 18 years of age and was effective for the treatment of supraventricular arrhythmias and to a lesser degree for the treatment of ventricular arrhythmias. Mild sinus bradycardia occurred in most of the infants, and fatigue, which required discontinuance in a few patients, occurred in several of the children receiving the drug. The physiologic effects and pharmacokinetics of sotalol have been evaluated in infants and children 3 days to 12 years of age. Dosage recommendations in pediatric patients are based on pharmacokinetic data. Similar to adults, serious adverse events including death, torsades de pointes, other proarrhythmias, AV block, and bradycardia have been reported in infants and children; therefore, the usual precautions in adults should also be observed when sotalol is used in pediatric patients.

■ **Geriatric Precautions** Safety and efficacy of sotalol in geriatric patients have not been studied specifically to date; however, life-threatening ventricular arrhythmias such as sustained ventricular tachycardia, for which safety and efficacy have been established, occur in many patients older than 50 years of age and clinical trials of sotalol included many such patients. In sotalol clinical trials, the overall risk of cardiac death was associated with increasing age. Because geriatric patients may have decreased renal function and because patients with renal impairment may be at increased risk of sotalol-induced toxicity, patients in this age group should be monitored closely and dosage adjusted accordingly.

■ **Mutagenicity and Carcinogenicity** Specific assays to determine the mutagenic or clastogenic potential of sotalol have not been performed to date.

There was no evidence of carcinogenic potential in a 24-month study in rats receiving sotalol hydrochloride dosages of 137–275 mg/kg daily (approximately 30 times the maximum recommended human oral dosage on a mg/kg basis or 5 times the maximum recommended human oral dosage on a mg/m² basis). There also was no evidence of carcinogenic potential in a study in mice receiving sotalol hydrochloride dosages of 4141–7122 mg/kg daily (approximately 450–750 times the maximum recommended human oral dosage on a mg/kg basis or 36–63 times the maximum recommended human oral dosage on a mg/m² basis).

■ **Pregnancy, Fertility, and Lactation** Reproduction studies in rats and rabbits during organogenesis did not reveal any teratogenic potential at sotalol hydrochloride doses that were 100 and 22 times the maximum recommended human oral dose on a mg/kg basis (9 and 7 times the maximum recommended human oral dose on a mg/m² basis), respectively. However, higher sotalol hydrochloride dosages of 160 mg/kg daily (16 times the maximum recommended human oral dosage on a mg/kg basis or 6 times the maximum recommended human oral dosage on a mg/m² basis) in rabbits were associated with a slight increase in fetal death likely resulting from maternal toxicity. A sotalol hydrochloride dosage of 80 mg/kg daily (8 times the maximum recommended human oral dosage on a mg/kg basis or 3 times the maximum recommended human oral dosage on a mg/m² basis) did not produce this effect. An increase in the number of early resorptions was associated with a sotalol hydrochloride dosage of 1000 mg/kg daily in rats (100 times the maximum recommended human oral dosage on a mg/kg basis or 18 times the maximum recommended human oral dosage on a mg/m² basis), while no increase was observed at 14 times the maximum recommended human oral dosage on mg/kg basis (2.5 times the maximum recommended human oral dosage on a mg/m² basis). Animal data are not always indicative of human response. There are no adequate and well-controlled studies using sotalol in pregnant women, but the drug has been shown to cross the placenta and is found in amniotic fluid.

Sotalol is distributed into milk, apparently in concentrations approximately 2.5–5.5 times concurrent maternal serum concentrations. Because of the potential for adverse reactions to sotalol in nursing infants, a decision should be made whether to discontinue nursing or the drug, taking into account the importance of the drug to the woman.

Description

Sotalol hydrochloride (MJ 1999) is a nonselective β-adrenergic blocking agent. Like propranolol, sotalol inhibits response to adrenergic stimuli by competitively blocking β_1-adrenergic receptors within the myocardium and β_2-adrenergic receptors within bronchial and vascular smooth muscle. In addition, sotalol, like propranolol, exhibits antiarrhythmic activity characteristic of class II antiarrhythmic agents. However, unlike propranolol, sotalol does not exhibit membrane-stabilizing activity but, as a methanesulfonanilide derivative, does exhibit electrophysiologic effects characteristic of class III antiarrhythmic agents (e.g., prolongs repolarization and refractoriness without affecting conduction). Sotalol does not exhibit intrinsic sympathomimetic activity.

The electrophysiologic effects of sotalol, like other methanesulfonanilide derivatives, also differ from those of many other commonly used antiarrhythmics (e.g., class I agents). In vitro studies suggest that sotalol selectively inhibits the rapidly activating component of the potassium channel involved in repolarization of cardiac cells (i.e., the rapidly activated inward component of the delayed rectifier potassium current I_{Kr}). In addition, sotalol does not appear to block sodium channels at usual doses (although it may at relatively high doses), and pharmacologic differences of the drug at potassium and sodium channels compared with class I antiarrhythmic agents (e.g., mexiletine, procainamide, propafenone, quinidine) have been proposed as possibly contributing to potential clinical superiority of sotalol in the management of ventricular tachyarrhythmias. However, other factors also may be involved.

Commercially available sotalol is a racemic mixture of the 2 optical isomers. Both isomers exhibit class III antiarrhythmic activity, but only the *l*-isomer exhibits β-blocking activity.

SumMon® (see Users Guide). For additional information on this drug until a more detailed monograph is developed and published, the manufacturer's labeling should be consulted. It is *essential* that the labeling be consulted for information on the usual cautions, precautions, and contraindications concerning potential drug interactions and/or laboratory test interferences and for information on acute toxicity.

Preparations

Excipients in commercially available drug preparations may have clinically important effects in some individuals; consult specific product labeling for details.

Sotalol Hydrochloride

Oral		
Solution	25 mg/5 mL	**Sotylize®**, Arbor
Tablets	80 mg*	**Betapace®** (scored), Covis
		Betapace AF® (scored), Covis
		Sorine® (scored), Upsher-Smith
		Sotalol Hydrochloride Tablets (scored)
	120 mg*	**Betapace®** (scored), Covis
		Betapace AF® (scored), Covis
		Sorine® (scored), Upsher-Smith
		Sotalol Hydrochloride Tablets (scored)
	160 mg*	**Betapace®** (scored), Covis
		Betapace AF® (scored), Covis
		Sorine® (scored), Upsher-Smith
		Sotalol Hydrochloride Tablets (scored)
	240 mg*	**Sorine®** (scored), Upsher-Smith
		Sotalol Hydrochloride Tablets (scored)
Parenteral		
Injection concentrate, for IV infusion	15 mg/mL*	**Sotalol Hydrochloride Injection**

*available from one or more manufacturer, distributor, and/or repackager by generic (nonproprietary) name

†Use is not currently included in the labeling approved by the US Food and Drug Administration

Calcium-Channel Blocking Agents 24:28

Dihydropyridines 24:28.08

amLODIPine Besylate

■ Amlodipine is a 1,4-dihydropyridine-derivative calcium-channel blocking agent with an intrinsically long duration of action.

Uses

■ **Hypertension** Amlodipine is used alone or in combination with other classes of antihypertensive agents in the management of hypertension. Amlodipine in fixed combination with atorvastatin (Caduet®) is used in patients for whom treatment with both amlodipine and atorvastatin is appropriate.

Current evidence-based practice guidelines for the management of hypertension in adults generally recommend the use of drugs from 4 classes of antihypertensive agents (angiotensin-converting enzyme [ACE] inhibitors, angiotensin II receptor antagonists, calcium-channel blockers, and thiazide diuretics); data from clinical outcome trials indicate that lowering blood pressure with any of these drug classes can reduce the complications of hypertension and provide similar cardiovascular protection. However, recommendations for initial drug selection and use in specific patient populations may vary across these expert guidelines. This variability is due, in part, to differences in the guideline development process and the types of studies (e.g., randomized controlled studies only versus a range of studies with different study designs) included in the evidence reviews. Ultimately, choice of antihypertensive therapy should be individualized, considering the clinical characteristics of the patient (e.g., age, ethnicity/race, comorbid conditions, cardiovascular risk factors) as well as drug-related factors (e.g., ease of administration, availability, adverse effects, costs). Because many patients eventually will need drugs from 2 or more antihypertensive classes, experts generally state that the emphasis should be placed on achieving appropriate blood pressure control rather than on identifying a preferred drug to achieve that control.

Disease Overview Worldwide, hypertension is the most common modifiable risk factor for cardiovascular events and mortality. The lifetime risk of developing hypertension in the US exceeds 80%, with higher rates observed among African Americans and Hispanics compared with whites or Asians. The systolic blood pressure and diastolic blood pressure values defined as hypertension in adults (see Blood Pressure Classification under Uses: Hypertension) in a 2017 multidisciplinary guideline of the American College of Cardiology (ACC), American Heart Association (AHA), and a number of other professional organizations (subsequently referred to as the 2017 ACC/AHA hypertension guideline in this monograph) are lower than those defined in the Seventh Report of the Joint National Committee on Prevention, Detection, Evaluation, and Treatment of High Blood Pressure (JNC 7) guidelines, which results in an increase of approximately 14% in the prevalence of hypertension in the US. However, this change in definition results in only a 2% increase in the percentage of patients requiring antihypertensive drug therapy because nonpharmacologic treatment is recommended for most adults now classified by the 2017 ACC/AHA hypertension guideline as hypertensive who would *not* meet the JNC 7 definition of hypertension. Among US adults receiving antihypertensive drugs, approximately 53% have inadequately controlled blood pressure according to current ACC/AHA treatment goals.

Cardiovascular and Renal Sequelae. The principal goal of preventing and treating hypertension is to reduce the risk of cardiovascular and renal morbidity and mortality, including target organ damage. The relationship between blood pressure and cardiovascular disease is continuous, consistent, and independent of other risk factors. It is important that very high blood pressure be managed promptly to reduce the risk of target organ damage. The higher the blood pressure, the more likely the development of myocardial infarction (MI), heart failure, stroke, and renal disease. For adults 40–70 years of age, each 20-mm Hg increment in systolic blood pressure or 10-mm Hg increment in diastolic blood pressure doubles the risk of developing cardiovascular disease across the entire blood pressure range of 115/75 to 185/115 mm Hg. For those older than 50 years of age, systolic blood pressure is a much more important risk factor for developing cardiovascular disease than is diastolic blood pressure. The rapidity with which treatment is required depends on the patient's clinical presentation (presence of new or worsening target organ damage) and the presence or absence of cardiovascular complications; the 2017 ACC/AHA hypertension guideline states that treatment of very high blood pressure should be initiated within at least 1 week.

Blood Pressure Classification Accurate blood pressure measurement is essential for the proper diagnosis and management of hypertension. Error in measuring blood pressure is a major cause of inadequate blood pressure control and may lead to overtreatment. Because a patient's blood pressure may vary in an unpredictable fashion, a single blood pressure measurement is not sufficient for clinical decision-making. An average of 2 or 3 blood pressure measurements obtained on 2–3 separate occasions using proper technique should be used to minimize random error and provide a more accurate blood pressure reading. Out-of-office blood pressure measurements may be useful for confirming and managing hypertension. The 2017 ACC/AHA hypertension guideline document (available on the ACC and AHA websites) should be consulted for key steps on properly measuring blood pressure.

According to the 2017 ACC/AHA hypertension guideline, blood pressure in adults is classified into 4 categories: normal, elevated, stage 1 hypertension, and stage 2 hypertension. (See Table 1.) The 2017 ACC/AHA hypertension guideline lowers the blood pressure threshold used to define hypertension in the US; previous hypertension guidelines (JNC 7) considered adults with systolic blood pressure of 120–139 mm Hg or diastolic blood pressure of 80–89 mm Hg to have prehypertension, those with systolic blood pressure of 140–159 mm Hg or diastolic blood pressure of 90–99 mm Hg to have stage 1 hypertension, and those with systolic blood pressure of 160 mm Hg or higher or diastolic blood pressure of 100 mm Hg or higher to have stage 2 hypertension. The blood pressure definitions in the 2017 ACC/AHA hypertension guideline are based upon data from studies evaluating the association between systolic blood pressure/diastolic blood pressure and cardiovascular risk and the benefits of blood pressure reduction. Individuals with systolic blood pressure and diastolic blood pressure in 2 different categories should be designated as being in the higher blood pressure category.

Table 1. ACC/AHA Blood Pressure Classification in Adults[a,b]

Category	SBP[c] (mm Hg)		DBP[d] (mm Hg)
Normal	<120	and	<80
Elevated	120–129	and	<80
Hypertension, Stage 1	130–139	or	80–89
Hypertension, Stage 2	≥140	or	≥90

[a] Source: Whelton PK, Carey RM, Aronow WS et al. 2017 ACC/AHA/AAPA/ABC/ACPM/AGS/APhA/ASH/ASPC/NMA/PCNA guideline for the prevention, detection, evaluation, and management of high blood pressure in adults: a report of the American College of Cardiology/American Heart Association Task Force on Clinical Practice Guidelines. Hypertension. 2018;71:e13-115.

[b] Individuals with SBP and DBP in 2 different categories (e.g., elevated SBP and normal DBP) should be designated as being in the higher blood pressure category (i.e., elevated BP).

[c] Systolic blood pressure

[d] Diastolic blood pressure

The blood pressure thresholds used to define hypertension, when to initiate drug therapy, and the ideal target blood pressure values remain controversial. The 2017 ACC/AHA hypertension guideline recommends a blood pressure goal of less than 130/80 mm Hg in all adults who have confirmed hypertension and known cardiovascular disease or a 10-year atherosclerotic cardiovascular disease (ASCVD) event risk of 10% or higher; the ACC/AHA guideline also states that this blood pressure goal is reasonable to attempt to achieve in adults with confirmed hypertension who do *not* have increased cardiovascular risk. The lower blood pressure values used to define hypertension and the lower target blood pressure goals outlined in the 2017 ACC/AHA hypertension guideline are based on clinical studies demonstrating a substantial reduction in the composite end point of major cardiovascular disease events and the combination of fatal and nonfatal stroke when a lower systolic blood pressure/diastolic blood pressure value (i.e., 130/80 mm Hg) was used to define hypertension. These lower target blood pressure goals also are based upon clinical studies demonstrating continuing reduction of cardiovascular risk at progressively lower levels of systolic blood pressure. A linear relationship has been demonstrated between cardiovascular risk and blood pressure even at low systolic blood pressures (e.g., 120–124 mm Hg). The 2017 ACC/AHA hypertension guideline recommends estimating a patient's ASCVD risk using the ACC/AHA Pooled Cohort equations (available online at http://tools.acc.org/ASCVD-Risk-Estimator), which are based on a variety of factors including age, race, gender, cholesterol levels, statin use, blood pressure, treatment for hypertension, history of diabetes mellitus, smoking status, and aspirin use. While the 2017 ACC/AHA hypertension guideline has lowered the threshold for *diagnosing* hypertension in adults, the threshold for *initiating drug therapy* has only been lowered for those patients who are at high risk of cardiovascular disease. Clinicians who support the 2017 ACC/AHA hypertension guideline believe that these recommendations have the potential to increase hypertension awareness, encourage lifestyle modification, and focus antihypertensive drug initiation and intensification in those adults at high risk for cardiovascular disease.

The lower blood pressure goals advocated in the 2017 ACC/AHA hypertension guideline have been questioned by some clinicians who have concerns regarding the guideline's use of extrapolated observational data, the lack of generalizability of some of the randomized trials (e.g., SPRINT) used to support the guideline, the difficulty of establishing accurate representative blood pressure values in typical clinical practice settings, and the accuracy of the cardiovascular risk calculator used in the guideline. Some clinicians state the lower blood pressure threshold used to define hypertension in the 2017 ACC/AHA hypertension guideline is not fully supported by clinical data, and these clinicians have expressed concerns about the possible harms (e.g., adverse effects of antihypertensive therapy) associated with classifying more patients as being hypertensive. Some clinicians also state that using this guideline, a large number of young, low-risk patients would need to be treated in order to observe a clinical benefit, while other clinicians state that the estimated gains in life-expectancy attributable to long-term use of blood pressure-lowering drugs are correspondingly greater in this patient population.

Treatment Benefits In clinical trials, antihypertensive therapy has been found to reduce the risk of developing stroke by about 34–40%, MI by about 20–25%, and heart failure by more than 50%. In a randomized, controlled study (SPRINT) that included hypertensive patients without diabetes mellitus who had a high risk of cardiovascular disease, intensive systolic blood pressure lowering of approximately 15 mm Hg was associated with a 25% reduction in cardiovascular disease events and a 27% reduction in all-cause mortality. However, the exclusion of patients with diabetes mellitus, prior stroke, and those younger than 50 years of age may decrease the generalizability of these findings. Some experts estimate that if the systolic blood pressure goals of the 2017 ACC/AHA hypertension guideline are achieved, major cardiovascular disease events may be reduced by an additional 340,000 and total deaths by an additional 156,000 compared with implementation of the JNC 8 expert panel guideline goals but these benefits may be accompanied by an increase in the frequency of adverse events. While there was no overall difference in the occurrence of serious adverse events in patients receiving intensive therapy for blood pressure control (systolic blood pressure target of less than 120 mm Hg) compared with those receiving less intense control (systolic blood pressure target of less than 140 mm Hg) in the SPRINT study, hypotension, syncope, electrolyte abnormalities, and acute kidney injury or acute renal failure occurred in substantially more patients receiving intensive therapy.

In the Antihypertensive and Lipid-lowering Treatment to Prevent Heart Attack Trial (ALLHAT), the long-term cardiovascular morbidity and mortality benefit of a long-acting dihydropyridine calcium-channel blocker (amlodipine), a thiazide-like diuretic (chlorthalidone), and an ACE inhibitor (lisinopril) were compared in a broad population of patients with hypertension at risk for coronary heart disease. Although these antihypertensive agents were comparably effective in providing important cardiovascular benefit, apparent differences in certain secondary outcomes were observed. Patients receiving the ACE inhibitor experienced higher risks of stroke, combined cardiovascular disease, GI bleeding, and angioedema, while those receiving the calcium-channel blocker were at higher risk of developing heart failure. The ALLHAT investigators suggested that the observed differences in cardiovascular outcome may be attributable, at least in part, to the greater antihypertensive effect of the calcium-channel blocker compared with that of the ACE inhibitor, especially in women and black patients. (See Clinical Benefits of Thiazides in Hypertension under Hypertension in Adults: Treatment Benefits in Uses in the Thiazides General Statement 40:28.20.)

General Considerations for Initial and Maintenance Antihypertensive Therapy **Nonpharmacologic Therapy.** Nonpharmacologic measures (i.e., lifestyle/behavioral modifications) that are effective in lowering blood pressure include weight reduction (for those who are overweight or obese), dietary changes to include foods such as fruits, vegetables, whole grains, and low-fat dairy products that are rich in potassium, calcium, magnesium, and fiber (i.e., adoption of the Dietary Approaches to Stop Hypertension [DASH] eating plan), sodium reduction, increased physical activity, and moderation of alcohol intake. Such lifestyle/behavioral modifications, including smoking cessation, enhance antihypertensive drug efficacy and decrease cardiovascular risk and remain an indispensable part of the management of hypertension. Lifestyle/behavioral modifications without antihypertensive drug therapy are recommended for adults classified by the 2017 ACC/AHA hypertension guideline as having elevated blood pressure (systolic blood pressure 120–129 mm Hg and diastolic blood pressure less than 80 mm Hg) and in those with stage 1 hypertension (systolic blood pressure 130–139 mm Hg or diastolic blood pressure 80–89 mm Hg) who do *not* have preexisting cardiovascular disease or an estimated 10-year ASCVD risk of 10% or greater.

Initiation of Drug Therapy. Drug therapy in the management of hypertension must be individualized and adjusted based on the degree of blood pressure elevation while also considering cardiovascular risk factors. Drug therapy generally is reserved for patients who respond inadequately to nondrug therapy (i.e., lifestyle modifications such as diet [including sodium restriction and adequate potassium and calcium intake], regular aerobic physical activity, moderation of alcohol consumption, and weight reduction) or in whom the degree of blood pressure elevation or coexisting risk factors, especially increased cardiovascular risk, require more prompt or aggressive therapy; however, the optimum blood pressure threshold for initiating antihypertensive drug therapy and specific treatment goals remain controversial.

The 2017 ACC/AHA hypertension guideline and many experts currently state that the treatment of hypertension should be based not only on blood pressure values but also on patients' cardiovascular risk factors. For *secondary prevention* of recurrent cardiovascular disease events in adults with clinical cardiovascular disease or for *primary prevention* in adults with an estimated 10-year ASCVD risk of 10% or higher, the 2017 ACC/AHA hypertension guideline recommends initiation of antihypertensive drug therapy in conjunction with lifestyle/behavioral modifications at an average systolic blood pressure of 130 mm Hg or an average diastolic blood pressure of 80 mm Hg or higher. For *primary prevention* of cardiovascular disease events in adults with a low (less than 10%) estimated 10-year risk of ASCVD, the 2017 ACC/AHA hypertension guideline recommends initiation of antihypertensive drug therapy in conjunction with lifestyle/behavioral modifications at a systolic blood pressure of 140 mm Hg or higher or a diastolic blood pressure of 90 mm Hg or higher. After initiation of antihypertensive drug therapy, regardless of the ASCVD risk, the 2017 ACC/AHA hypertension guideline generally recommends a blood pressure goal of less than 130/80 mm Hg in all patients. In addition, a systolic blood pressure goal of less than 130 mm Hg also is recommended for noninstitutionalized ambulatory patients 65 years of age or older. While these blood pressure goals are lower than those recommended for most patients in previous guidelines, they are based upon clinical studies demonstrating continuing reduction of cardiovascular risk at progressively lower levels of systolic blood pressure.

Most data indicate that patients with a higher cardiovascular risk will benefit the most from tighter blood pressure control; however, some experts state this treatment goal also may be beneficial in those at lower cardiovascular risk. Other clinicians believe that the benefits of such blood pressure lowering do not outweigh the risks in those patients considered to be at lower risk of cardiovascular disease and that reclassifying individuals formerly considered to have prehypertension as having hypertension may potentially lead to use of drug therapy in such patients without consideration of cardiovascular risk. Previous hypertension guidelines, such as those from the JNC 8 expert panel, generally recommended initiation of antihypertensive treatment in patients with a systolic blood pressure of at least 140 mm Hg or diastolic blood pressure of at least 90 mm Hg, targeted a blood pressure goal of less than 140/90 mm Hg regardless of cardiovascular risk, and used higher systolic blood pressure thresholds and targets in geriatric patients. Some clinicians continue to support the target blood pressures recommended by the JNC 8 expert panel because of concerns that such recommendations in the 2017 ACC/AHA hypertension guideline are based on extrapolation of data from the high-risk population in the SPRINT study to a lower-risk population. Also, because more than 90% of patients in SPRINT were already receiving antihypertensive drugs at baseline, data are lacking on the effects of *initiating* drug therapy at a lower blood pressure threshold (130/80 mm Hg) in patients at high risk of cardiovascular disease. The potential benefits of hypertension management and drug cost, adverse effects, and risks associated with the use of multiple antihypertensive drugs should be considered when deciding a patient's blood pressure treatment goal.

The 2017 ACC/AHA hypertension guideline recommends an ASCVD risk assessment for all adults with hypertension; however, experts state that it can be assumed that patients with hypertension and diabetes mellitus or chronic kidney disease (CKD) are at high risk for cardiovascular disease and that antihypertensive drug therapy should be initiated in these patients at a blood pressure of 130/80 mm Hg or higher. The 2017 ACC/AHA hypertension guideline also recommends a blood pressure goal of less than 130/80 mm Hg in patients with hypertension and diabetes mellitus or CKD. These recommendations are based on a systematic review of high-quality evidence from randomized controlled trials, meta-analyses, and post hoc analyses that have demonstrated substantial reductions in the risk of important clinical outcomes (e.g., cardiovascular events) regardless of comorbid conditions or age when systolic blood pressure is lowered to less than 130 mm Hg. However, some clinicians have questioned the generalizability of findings from some of the trials (e.g., SPRINT) used to support the 2017 ACC/AHA hypertension guideline. For example, SPRINT included adults (mean age: 68 years) *without* diabetes mellitus who were at high risk of cardiovascular disease. While benefits of intensive blood pressure control were observed in this patient population, some clinicians have questioned whether these findings apply to younger patients who have a low risk of cardiovascular disease. In patients with CKD in the SPRINT trial, intensive blood pressure management (achieving a mean systolic blood pressure of approximately 122 mm Hg compared with 136 mm Hg with standard treatment) provided a similar beneficial reduction in the composite cardiovascular disease primary outcome and all-cause mortality as in the full patient cohort. Because most patients with CKD die from cardiovascular complications, the findings of this study further support a lower blood pressure target of less than 130/80 mm Hg.

Data are lacking to determine the ideal blood pressure goal in adult patients with hypertension and diabetes mellitus; also, studies evaluating the benefits of intensive blood pressure control in patients with diabetes mellitus have provided conflicting results. Clinical studies reviewed for the 2017 ACC/AHA hypertension guideline have shown similar quantitative benefits from blood pressure lowering in hypertensive patients with or without diabetes mellitus. In a randomized, controlled study (ACCORD-BP) that compared a higher (systolic blood pressure less than 140 mm Hg) versus lower (systolic blood pressure less than 120 mm Hg) blood pressure goal in patients with diabetes mellitus, there was no difference in the incidence of cardiovascular outcomes (e.g., composite outcome of cardiovascular death, nonfatal MI, and nonfatal stroke). However, some experts state that this study was underpowered to detect a difference between the 2 treatment groups and that the factorial design of the study complicated interpretation of the results. Although SPRINT did not include patients with diabetes mellitus, patients in this study with prediabetes demonstrated a similar cardiovascular benefit from intensive treatment of blood pressure as normoglycemic patients. A meta-analysis of data from the ACCORD and SPRINT studies suggests that the findings of both studies are consistent and that patients with diabetes mellitus benefit from more intensive blood pressure control. These data support the 2017 ACC/AHA hypertension guideline recommendation of a blood pressure treatment goal of less than 130/80 mm Hg in adult patients with hypertension and diabetes mellitus. Alternatively, the American Diabetes Association (ADA) recommends a blood pressure goal of less than 140/90 mm Hg in patients with diabetes mellitus. The ADA states that a lower blood pressure goal (e.g., less than 130/80 mm Hg) may be appropriate for patients with a high risk of cardiovascular disease and diabetes mellitus if it can be achieved without undue treatment burden.

Further study is needed to more clearly define optimum blood pressure goals in patients with hypertension, particularly in high-risk groups (e.g., patients with diabetes mellitus, cardiovascular disease, or cerebrovascular disease; black patients); when determining appropriate blood pressure goals, individual risks and benefits should be considered in addition to the evidence from clinical studies.

Choice of Initial Drug Therapy. In current hypertension management guidelines, calcium-channel blockers are recommended as one of several preferred drugs for the initial treatment of hypertension; other preferred options include ACE inhibitors, angiotensin II receptor antagonists, and thiazide diuretics. (See Hypertension: Treatment Benefits, in Uses.) The 2017 ACC/AHA adult hypertension guideline states that a calcium-channel blocker, ACE inhibitor, angiotensin II receptor antagonist, or thiazide or thiazide-like diuretic (preferably chlorthalidone) are all acceptable choices for initial antihypertensive drug therapy in the general population of nonblack patients, including those with diabetes mellitus; drugs from any of these classes generally produce similar benefits in terms of overall mortality and cardiovascular, cerebrovascular, and renal outcomes. Calcium-channel blockers may be particularly useful in the management of hypertension in black patients; these patients tend to have a greater blood pressure response to calcium-channel blockers and thiazide diuretics than to other antihypertensive drug classes (e.g., ACE inhibitors, angiotensin II receptor antagonists). (See Race under Hypertension: Other Special Considerations for Antihypertensive Therapy, in Uses.) In black patients, including those with diabetes mellitus, the initial drug choice should include a thiazide diuretic or calcium-channel blocker. Use of a calcium-channel blocker also may be beneficial in patients with certain coexisting conditions such as ischemic heart disease (e.g., angina) and in geriatric patients, including those with isolated systolic hypertension. (See Considerations for Drug Therapy in Patients with Underlying Cardiovascular and Other Risk Factors and also see Other Special Considerations for Antihypertensive Drug Therapy, under Uses: Hypertension in Adults, in the Thiazides General Statement 40:28.20.) Because many patients eventually will need more than one antihypertensive drug to achieve blood pressure control, any of the recommended drug classes may be considered for add-on therapy.

Experts state that in patients with stage 1 hypertension (especially the elderly, those with a history of hypotension, or those who have experienced adverse drug effects), it is reasonable to initiate drug therapy using the stepped-care approach in which one drug is initiated and titrated and other drugs are added sequentially to achieve the target blood pressure. Although some patients can begin treatment with a single antihypertensive agent, starting with 2 first-line drugs in different pharmacologic classes (either as separate agents or in a fixed-dose combination) is recommended in patients with stage 2 hypertension and an average blood pressure more than 20/10 mm Hg above their target blood pressure. Such combined therapy may increase the likelihood of achieving goal blood pressure in a more timely fashion, but also may increase the risk of adverse effects (e.g., orthostatic hypotension) in some patients (e.g., elderly). Drug regimens with complementary activity, where a second antihypertensive agent is used to block compensatory responses to the first agent or affect a different pressor mechanism, can result in additive blood pressure lowering and are preferred. Drug combinations that have similar mechanisms of action or clinical effects (e.g., the combination of an ACE inhibitor and an angiotensin II receptor antagonist) generally should be avoided. Many patients who begin therapy with a single antihypertensive agent will subsequently require at least 2 drugs from different pharmacologic classes to achieve their blood pressure goal. Experts state that other patient-specific factors, such as age, concurrent medications, drug adherence, drug interactions, the overall treatment regimen, cost, and comorbidities, also should be considered when deciding on an antihypertensive drug regimen. For any stage of hypertension, antihypertensive drug dosages should be adjusted and/or other agents substituted or added until goal blood pressure is achieved. (See Follow-up and Maintenance Drug Therapy under Hypertension: General Considerations for Initial and Maintenance Antihypertensive Therapy, in Uses.)

Follow-up and Maintenance Drug Therapy. Several strategies are used for the titration and combination of antihypertensive drugs; these strategies, which are generally based on those used in randomized controlled studies, include maximizing the dosage of the first drug before adding a second drug, adding a second drug before achieving maximum dosage of the initial drug, or initiating therapy with 2 drugs simultaneously (either as separate preparations or as a fixed-dose combination). Combined use of an ACE inhibitor and angiotensin II receptor antagonist should be avoided because of the potential risk of adverse renal effects. After initiating a new or adjusted antihypertensive drug regimen, patients should have their blood pressure reevaluated monthly until adequate blood pressure control is achieved. Effective blood pressure control can be achieved in most hypertensive patients, but many will ultimately require therapy with 2 or more antihypertensive drugs. In addition to measuring blood pressure, clinicians should evaluate patients for orthostatic hypotension, adverse drug effects, adherence to drug therapy and lifestyle modifications, and the need for drug dosage adjustments. Laboratory testing such as electrolytes and renal function status and other assessments of target organ damage also should be performed.

Considerations for Drug Therapy in Patients with Underlying Cardiovascular and Other Risk Factors Drug therapy in patients with hypertension and underlying cardiovascular or other risk factors should be carefully individualized based on the underlying disease(s), concomitant drugs, tolerance to drug-induced adverse effects, and blood pressure goal. (See Table 2: Compelling Indications for Drug Classes based on Comorbid Conditions, in Considerations for Drug Therapy in Patients with Underlying Cardiovascular and Other Risk Factors under Uses: Hypertension in Adults, in the Thiazides General Statement 40:28.20.)

Other Special Considerations for Antihypertensive Therapy

Race. Most patients with hypertension, especially black patients, will require at least 2 antihypertensive drugs to achieve adequate blood pressure control. Blood pressure response to calcium-channel blockers appears to be comparable in white and black patients. In general, black hypertensive patients tend to respond better to monotherapy with calcium-channel blockers or thiazide diuretics than to monotherapy with other drug classes (e.g., ACE inhibitors, angiotensin II receptor antagonists, β-blockers). In a prespecified subgroup analysis of the ALLHAT study, a calcium-channel blocker was more effective than an ACE inhibitor in lowering blood pressure and was associated with a substantially reduced rate of stroke in black patients. When compared with a thiazide diuretic, the calcium-channel blocker appeared to be less effective in preventing heart failure, but comparable with respect to other outcomes (e.g., cerebrovascular, cardiovascular, renal, mortality). (See Clinical Benefits of Thiazides in Hypertension under Hypertension in Adults: Treatment Benefits, in Uses in the Thiazides General Statement 40:28.20.) However, the combination of an ACE inhibitor or an angiotensin II receptor antagonist with a calcium-channel blocker or thiazide diuretic produces similar blood pressure lowering in black patients as in other racial groups. In addition, some experts state that when use of ACE inhibitors, angiotensin II receptor antagonists, or β-blockers is indicated in hypertensive patients with underlying cardiovascular or other risk factors, these indications should be applied equally to black hypertensive patients. (See Considerations for Drug Therapy in Patients with Underlying Cardiovascular and Other Risk Factors under Uses: Hypertension in Adults, in the Thiazides General Statement 40:28.20.)

Advanced Age. Antihypertensive drugs recommended for initial therapy in geriatric patients, including those with isolated systolic hypertension, generally are the same as those recommended for younger patients. Antihypertensive therapy initiated with a calcium-channel blocking agent has been shown to reduce cardiovascular morbidity and mortality in older patients with isolated systolic hypertension.

Although some experts state that calcium-channel blocking agents or diuretics may be preferred in geriatric patients, ACE inhibitors and angiotensin II receptor antagonists also have shown beneficial effects and may be considered in this population.

For further information on overall principles and expert recommendations for treatment of hypertension, see Uses: Hypertension in Adults, and also see Uses: Hypertension in Pediatric Patients, in the Thiazides General Statement 40:28.20.

Hypertensive Crises Because of the slow onset of hypotensive effect with amlodipine, this drug is *not* suitable for use as acute therapy in rapidly reducing blood pressure in patients with severe hypertension in whom reduction of blood pressure is considered urgent (i.e., hypertensive urgencies) nor in hypertensive emergencies.

For additional information on the role of dihydropyridine calcium-channel blocking agents in the management of hypertension and angina, see Uses in Nifedipine 24:28.08.

■ **Coronary Artery Disease** Amlodipine in fixed combination with atorvastatin (Caduet®) is used in patients for whom treatment with both amlodipine and atorvastatin is appropriate.

Angina Amlodipine is used for the management of Prinzmetal variant angina and chronic stable angina pectoris. The drug has been used alone or in combination with other antianginal agents.

Angiographically Documented Coronary Artery Disease Amlodipine is used in patients with recently documented coronary artery disease by angiography (without heart failure or an ejection fraction less than 40%), to reduce the risk of coronary revascularization procedure and hospitalization due to angina.

Dosage and Administration

■ **Administration** Amlodipine besylate is administered orally. Amlodipine generally can be given without regard to meals.

■ **Dosage** Dosage of amlodipine besylate is expressed in terms of amlodipine.

Hypertension **Amlodipine Therapy.** The manufacturers state that the usual initial adult dosage of amlodipine is 2.5–5 mg once daily as monotherapy. In geriatric patients and small or frail individuals, an initial dosage of 2.5 mg once daily is recommended. This reduced initial dosage also can be used in adults when amlodipine is added to an existing antihypertensive drug regimen. Subsequent dosage of amlodipine should be adjusted according to the patient's blood pressure response and tolerance and usually should not exceed 10 mg once daily. Generally, dosage is increased gradually at 7- to 14-day intervals until optimum control of blood pressure is maintained. However, more rapid titration of dosage can be undertaken when clinically warranted, provided response and tolerance are assessed frequently. The usual maintenance dosage of amlodipine for the management of hypertension in adults is 2.5–10 mg once daily.

The manufacturer states that the safety and efficacy of amlodipine have not been established in pediatric patients younger than 6 years of age; however, for the management of hypertension in children 1–5 years of age†, an initial dosage of 0.1 mg/kg once daily and a maximum dosage of 0.6 mg/kg daily (up to 5 mg daily) has been recommended by some experts. In children 6 years of age and older, some experts recommend an initial dosage of 2.5 mg once daily and a maximum dosage of 10 mg once daily. However, the manufacturer states that the safety and efficacy of dosages exceeding 5 mg daily have not been established in pediatric patients. The manufacturer states that the usual effective dosage of amlodipine in children 6 years of age and older is 2.5–5 mg once daily. Experts state that the drug should be initiated at the low end of the dosage range; the dosage may be increased every 2–4 weeks until blood pressure is controlled, the maximum dosage is reached, or adverse effects occur. For information on overall principles and expert recommendations for treatment of hypertension in pediatric patients, see Uses: Hypertension in Pediatric Patients, in the Thiazides General Statement 40:28.20.

Amlodipine/Benazepril Fixed-combination Therapy. Therapy with the commercially available preparations containing amlodipine in fixed combination with benazepril hydrochloride usually should be initiated only after an adequate response is not achieved with amlodipine (or another dihydropyridine-derivative calcium-channel blocker) or benazepril (or another ACE inhibitor) alone.

Alternatively, such fixed combinations may be used if amlodipine dosages necessary for adequate response have been associated with development of edema. The fixed combination containing amlodipine and benazepril also may be used as a substitute for the individually titrated drugs. The recommended initial dosage is amlodipine 2.5 mg in fixed combination with benazepril hydrochloride 10 mg once daily. Dosage of the fixed combination containing amlodipine and benazepril should be adjusted according to the patient's response. The antihypertensive effect of a given dosage is largely attained with 2 weeks; if necessary, dosage of the fixed combination may be increased up to a maximum dosage of 10 mg of amlodipine in fixed combination with 40 mg of benazepril hydrochloride once daily.

The addition of benazepril to amlodipine therapy usually does not provide additional antihypertensive effects in black patients; however, benazepril appears to reduce the development of amlodipine-associated edema regardless of race. The manufacturers state that when the fixed combinations containing 2.5–10 mg of amlodipine with 10–40 mg of benazepril hydrochloride have been used, the antihypertensive effects of these combinations have increased with increasing dosages of amlodipine in all patients; in addition, antihypertensive effects increased with increasing dosages of benazepril in nonblack patients.

Amlodipine/Olmesartan Fixed-combination Therapy. In patients who do not respond adequately to monotherapy with amlodipine (or another dihydropyridine-derivative calcium-channel blocker) or, alternatively, with olmesartan medoxomil (or another angiotensin II receptor antagonist), combined therapy with the drugs can be used to provide additional antihypertensive effects. The fixed-combination preparation containing amlodipine and olmesartan medoxomil also can be used as a substitute for the individually titrated drugs. The patient can be switched to the fixed-combination preparation containing the corresponding individual doses of amlodipine and olmesartan medoxomil; alternatively, the dosage of one or both components can be increased for additional antihypertensive effects. If needed, dosage of the fixed combination may be increased after 2 weeks. Dosage adjustments generally should involve one drug at a time, although dosages of both drugs can be increased to achieve more rapid blood pressure control. Daily dosages exceeding 10 mg of amlodipine given in fixed combination with 40 mg of olmesartan medoxomil are not recommended by the manufacturer.

Commercially available preparations containing amlodipine in fixed combination with olmesartan medoxomil may be used for initial treatment of hypertension in patients likely to require combined therapy with multiple antihypertensive drugs to achieve blood pressure control. In such patients, therapy with the fixed-combination preparation usually should be initiated at a dosage of 5 mg of amlodipine and 20 mg of olmesartan medoxomil once daily. If necessary, dosage of the fixed combination may be increased after 1–2 weeks for additional blood pressure control (but should not exceed a maximum dosage of 10 mg of amlodipine and 40 mg of olmesartan medoxomil once daily). In patients whose baseline blood pressure is 160/100 mm Hg, the estimated probability of achieving control of systolic blood pressure (defined as systolic blood pressure of less than 140 mm Hg) is 48, 46, or 68% and of achieving control of diastolic blood pressure (defined as diastolic blood pressure of less than 90 mm Hg) is 51, 60, or 85% with olmesartan medoxomil (40 mg daily) alone, amlodipine (10 mg daily) alone, or amlodipine combined with olmesartan medoxomil (at the same dosages), respectively.

Amlodipine/Olmesartan/Hydrochlorothiazide Fixed-combination Therapy. The fixed-combination preparation containing amlodipine, olmesartan, and hydrochlorothiazide may be used to provide additional blood pressure control in patients who do not respond adequately to combination therapy with any 2 of the following classes of antihypertensive agents given at maximally tolerated, labeled, or usual dosages: calcium-channel blockers, angiotensin II receptor antagonists, or diuretics. Patients who experience dose-limiting adverse effects of amlodipine, olmesartan, or hydrochlorothiazide while receiving any dual combination of these drugs may be switched to a lower dosage of that drug, given as a fixed-combination preparation containing all 3 of these drugs, to achieve similar blood pressure reductions. The fixed-combination preparation containing amlodipine, olmesartan, and hydrochlorothiazide also can be used as a substitute for the individually titrated drugs. If necessary, dosage of the fixed-combination preparation may be increased after 2 weeks for additional blood pressure control (but should not exceed a maximum dosage of 10 mg of amlodipine, 40 mg of olmesartan medoxomil, and 25 mg of hydrochlorothiazide once daily). The commercially available preparation containing amlodipine in fixed combination with olmesartan and hydrochlorothiazide should not be used for the initial management of hypertension.

Amlodipine/Perindopril Fixed-combination Therapy. The commercially available preparation containing amlodipine in fixed combination with perindopril arginine may be used in patients receiving amlodipine monotherapy when amlodipine dosages necessary for adequate response have been associated with development of edema. In addition, patients who do not respond adequately to monotherapy may be switched to therapy with the fixed combination of amlodipine and perindopril arginine. Dosage of the fixed-combination preparation should be adjusted according to the patient's response at intervals of 7–14 days.

Commercially available preparations containing amlodipine in fixed combination with perindopril may be used for initial treatment of hypertension in patients likely to require combined therapy with multiple antihypertensive drugs to achieve blood pressure control. In such patients, therapy with the fixed-combination preparation usually should be initiated at a dosage of 2.5 mg of amlodipine and 3.5 mg of perindopril arginine once daily. The decision to use the fixed combination of amlodipine and perindopril for initial management of hypertension should be based on assessment of potential benefits and risks of such therapy, including consideration of whether the patient is likely to tolerate the lowest available dosage of the combined drugs. Dosage may be adjusted as needed at intervals of 7–14 days to a maximum dosage of amlodipine 10 mg and perindopril arginine 14 mg once daily.

In patients whose baseline blood pressure is 170/105 mm Hg, the estimated probability of achieving control of systolic blood pressure (defined as systolic blood pressure of less than 140 mm Hg) is 26, 40, or 50% and of achieving control of diastolic blood pressure (defined as diastolic blood pressure of less than 90 mm Hg) is 31, 46, or 65% with perindopril erbumine (16 mg daily) alone, amlodipine (10 mg daily) alone, or amlodipine (10 mg daily) combined with perindopril arginine (14 mg daily), respectively.

In black patients and patients with diabetes mellitus, the addition of perindopril arginine (14 mg daily) to amlodipine (10 mg daily) did not provide additional antihypertensive effects beyond those achieved with amlodipine monotherapy.

Amlodipine/Telmisartan Fixed-combination Therapy. The fixed-combination preparation containing amlodipine and telmisartan can be used as a substitute for the individually administered drugs; patients may be switched to the fixed-combination preparation containing the corresponding individual doses of amlodipine and telmisartan or, alternatively, the dosage of one or both components can be increased for additional antihypertensive effects. In addition, the manufacturers state that patients who do not respond adequately to monotherapy with amlodipine (or another dihydropyridine-derivative calcium-channel blocker) or, alternatively, with telmisartan (or another angiotensin II receptor antagonist) may be switched to therapy with the fixed-combination preparation containing amlodipine and telmisartan. Patients who experience dose-limiting adverse effects (e.g., edema) during monotherapy with amlodipine 10 mg may be switched to the fixed combination containing amlodipine 5 mg and telmisartan 40 mg to achieve similar blood pressure control. If needed, dosage of the fixed-combination preparation may be increased to a maximum dosage of 10 mg of amlodipine and 80 mg of telmisartan given once daily; because most of the antihypertensive effect of a given dosage is achieved within 2 weeks, dosage may be adjusted after at least 2 weeks, if needed, to attain blood pressure control.

Commercially available preparations containing amlodipine in fixed combination with telmisartan may be used for initial treatment of hypertension in patients likely to require combined therapy with multiple antihypertensive drugs to achieve blood pressure control. In such patients, therapy with the fixed-combination preparation usually should be initiated at a dosage of 5 mg of amlodipine and 40 mg of telmisartan once daily. An initial dosage of 5 mg of amlodipine and 80 mg of telmisartan once daily may be used in patients requiring larger blood pressure reductions. The decision to use the fixed combination of amlodipine and telmisartan for initial management of hypertension should be based on assessment of potential benefits and risks of such therapy, including consideration of whether the patient is likely to tolerate the lowest available dosage of the combined drugs. In patients whose baseline blood pressure is 160/110 mm Hg, the estimated probability of achieving control of systolic blood pressure (defined as systolic blood pressure of less than 140 mm Hg) is 46, 69, or 79% and of achieving control of diastolic blood pressure (defined as diastolic blood pressure of less than 90 mm Hg) is 26, 22, or 55% with telmisartan (80 mg daily) alone, amlodipine (10 mg daily) alone, or amlodipine combined with telmisartan (at the same dosages), respectively.

Amlodipine/Valsartan Fixed-combination Therapy. Patients whose hypertension is adequately controlled with amlodipine and valsartan administered separately may be switched to the fixed-combination preparation containing the corresponding individual doses. Alternatively, the manufacturers state that patients who do not respond adequately to monotherapy with amlodipine (or another dihydropyridine-derivative calcium-channel blocker) or, alternatively, with valsartan (or another angiotensin II receptor antagonist) may be switched to therapy with the fixed-combination preparation containing amlodipine and valsartan. In addition, patients who experience dose-limiting adverse effects during monotherapy with amlodipine or valsartan can be switched to a lower dosage of that drug, given as a fixed-combination preparation containing amlodipine and valsartan, to achieve similar blood pressure control; dosage should be adjusted according to the patient's response after 3–4 weeks of therapy. If needed, dosage of the fixed-combination preparation may be increased to a maximum of 10 mg of amlodipine and 320 mg of valsartan given once daily; because most of the antihypertensive effect of a given dosage is achieved within 2 weeks, dosage may be adjusted after 1–2 weeks, if needed, to attain blood pressure control.

Commercially available preparations containing amlodipine in fixed combination with valsartan may be used for initial treatment of hypertension in patients likely to require combined therapy with multiple antihypertensive drugs to achieve blood pressure control. In such patients, therapy with the fixed-combination preparation should be initiated at a dosage of 5 mg of amlodipine and 160 mg of valsartan once daily in individuals without depletion of intravascular volume. The decision to use the fixed combination of amlodipine and valsartan for initial management of hypertension should be based on assessment of potential benefits and risks of such therapy, including consideration of whether the patient is likely to tolerate the lowest available dosage of the combined drugs. In patients whose baseline blood pressure is 160/100 mm Hg, the estimated probability of achieving control of systolic blood pressure (defined as systolic blood pressure of less than 140 mm Hg) is 47, 67, or 80% and of achieving control of diastolic blood pressure (defined as diastolic blood pressure of less than 90 mm Hg) is 62, 80, or 85% with valsartan (320 mg daily) alone, amlodipine (10 mg daily) alone, or amlodipine combined with valsartan (at the same dosages), respectively.

Amlodipine/Valsartan/Hydrochlorothiazide Fixed-combination Therapy. The fixed-combination preparation containing amlodipine, valsartan, and hydrochlorothiazide may be used to provide additional blood pressure control in patients who do not respond adequately to combination therapy with any 2 of the following classes of antihypertensive agents: calcium-channel blockers, angiotensin II receptor antagonists, or diuretics. Patients who experience dose-limiting adverse effects of amlodipine, valsartan, or hydrochlorothiazide while receiving any dual combination of these drugs may be switched to a lower dosage of that drug, given as a fixed-combination preparation containing all 3 of these drugs, to achieve similar blood pressure reductions. The fixed-combination preparation containing amlodipine, valsartan, and hydrochlorothiazide also can be used as a substitute for the individually titrated drugs. If necessary, dosage of the fixed-combination preparation may be increased after 2 weeks for additional blood pressure control (but should not exceed a maximum dosage of 10 mg of amlodipine, 320 mg of valsartan, and 25 mg of hydrochlorothiazide given once daily). The commercially available preparation containing amlodipine in fixed combination with valsartan and hydrochlorothiazide should not be used for the initial management of hypertension.

Amlodipine/Atorvastatin Fixed-combination Therapy. The fixed-combination preparation containing amlodipine and atorvastatin may be used as a *substitute* for individually titrated drugs. In patients currently receiving amlodipine and atorvastatin, the initial dosage of the fixed-combination preparation is the equivalent of titrated dosages of amlodipine and atorvastatin. Increased amounts of amlodipine, atorvastatin, or both components may be added for additional antihypertensive or antilipemic effects.

The fixed-combination preparation may be used to provide *additional therapy* for patients currently receiving one component of the preparation. The initial dosage of the fixed-combination preparation should be selected based on the dosage of the current component being used and the recommended initial dosage for the added monotherapy.

The fixed-combination preparation may be used to *initiate treatment* in patients with hypertension *and* dyslipidemias. The initial dosage of the fixed-combination preparation should be selected based on the recommended initial dosages of the individual components. For dosage recommendations for atorvastatin, see Dosage and Administration: Dosage, in Atorvastatin 24:06.08. The maximum dosage of amlodipine or atorvastatin in the fixed-combination preparation is 10 or 80 mg daily, respectively.

Blood Pressure Monitoring and Treatment Goals. Blood pressure monitoring using an out-of-office (home [self-monitored]) or ambulatory method (using a device that measures blood pressure over a 24-hour period) as an adjunct to in-office monitoring generally is recommended to provide a more reliable assessment of blood pressure; studies suggest that out-of-office blood pressure may be a better predictor of hypertension-induced organ damage and cardiovascular risk than office blood pressure. Periodic determination of blood pressure in both the morning and evening (before taking the morning or evening dose) is useful in monitoring daytime control and ensuring that the surge in blood pressure that occurs with arising has been modulated adequately. Occasionally, particularly in geriatric patients and those with orthostatic symptoms, monitoring should include blood pressure determinations in both the seated position and, to recognize possible postural hypotension, after standing quietly for 2–5 minutes.

Once antihypertensive drug therapy has been initiated, dosage generally is adjusted at approximately monthly intervals if blood pressure control is inadequate at a given dosage; additional drugs may need to be added to an antihypertensive drug regimen to achieve adequate blood pressure control. Once blood pressure has been stabilized, follow-up visits generally can be scheduled at 3- to 6-month intervals, depending on patient status.

Blood pressure should be monitored regularly (i.e., monthly) during therapy and dosage of the antihypertensive drug adjusted until blood pressure is controlled. In patients who develop unacceptable adverse effects with amlodipine, the drug should be discontinued and another antihypertensive agent from a different pharmacologic class should be initiated. If an adequate blood pressure response is not achieved with amlodipine monotherapy, another antihypertensive agent with demonstrated benefit and preferably a complementary mechanism of action (e.g., angiotensin-converting enzyme [ACE] inhibitor, angiotensin II receptor antagonist, thiazide diuretic) may be added; if goal blood pressure is still not achieved with the use of 2 antihypertensive agents, a third drug may be added. (See Uses: Hypertension.)

The goal of hypertension management and prevention is to achieve and maintain optimal control of blood pressure. However, the optimum blood pressure threshold for initiating antihypertensive drug therapy and specific treatment goals remain controversial. While other hypertension guidelines have based target blood pressure goals on age and comorbidities, the 2017 American College of Cardiology (ACC)/ American Heart Association (AHA) hypertension guideline incorporates underlying cardiovascular risk into decision making regarding treatment and generally recommends the same target blood pressure (i.e., less than 130/80 mm Hg) for all adults. Many patients will require at least 2 drugs from different pharmacologic classes to achieve this blood pressure goal; the potential benefits of hypertension management and drug cost, adverse effects, and risks associated with the use of multiple antihypertensive drugs also should be considered when deciding a patient's blood pressure treatment goal. (See General Considerations for Initial and Maintenance Antihypertensive Therapy under Uses: Hypertension.)

For additional information on target levels of blood pressure and on monitoring therapy in the management of hypertension, see Blood Pressure Monitoring and Treatment Goals under Dosage: Hypertension, in Dosage and Administration in the Thiazides General Statement 40:28.20.

In children with hypertension with or without diabetes mellitus, blood pressure should be reduced to less than the corresponding age-adjusted 90th percentile value and to less than 130/80 mm Hg in adolescents at least 13 years of age. In children and adolescents with hypertension and chronic kidney disease (CKD), the 24-hour mean arterial pressure (MAP) as determined by ambulatory blood pressure monitoring should be decreased to a value less than the 50th percentile.

Coronary Artery Disease **Angina.** For the management of Prinzmetal variant angina or chronic stable angina, the usual adult dosage of amlodipine is 5–10 mg once daily. The manufacturers state that adequate control of angina usually requires a maintenance dosage of 10 mg daily.

Amlodipine has been used concomitantly with other antihypertensive and antianginal drugs, including thiazide diuretics, angiotensin-converting enzyme inhibitors, β-adrenergic blocking agents, long-acting nitrates, and/or sublingual nitroglycerin.

Angiographically Documented Coronary Artery Disease. For the management of coronary artery disease, the recommended adult dosage of amlodipine is 5–10 mg once daily. In clinical studies the majority of patients required a dosage of 10 mg daily.

Amlodipine/Atorvastatin Combination Therapy in Coronary Artery Disease. The fixed-combination preparation containing amlodipine and atorvastatin may be used as a *substitute* for individually titrated drugs. In patients currently receiving amlodipine and atorvastatin, the initial dosage of the fixed-combination preparation is the equivalent of titrated dosages of amlodipine and atorvastatin. Increased amounts of amlodipine, atorvastatin, or both components may be added for additional antianginal or antilipemic effects.

The fixed-combination preparation may be used to provide *additional therapy* for patients currently receiving one component of the preparation. The initial dosage of the fixed-combination preparation should be selected based on the dosage of the current component being used and the recommended initial dosage for the added monotherapy.

The fixed-combination preparation may be used to *initiate treatment* in patients with angina *and* dyslipidemias. The initial dosage of the fixed-combination preparation should be selected based on the recommended initial dosages of the individual components. For dosage recommendations for atorvastatin, see Dosage and Administration: Dosage, in Atorvastatin 24:06.08. The maximum dosage of amlodipine or atorvastatin in the fixed-combination preparation is 10 or 80 mg daily, respectively.

■ Special Populations

Hepatic Impairment Since the elimination of amlodipine may be impaired substantially in patients with hepatic impairment, resulting in increased exposure to the drug (area under the plasma concentration-time curve [AUC] increases of 40–60%), a reduced initial amlodipine dosage may be required and subsequent dosage should be titrated slowly in such patients.

For the management of hypertension in adults with hepatic insufficiency, an initial amlodipine dosage of 2.5 mg once daily generally is recommended. Subsequent dosage should be adjusted according to patient response and tolerance but usually should not exceed 10 mg once daily. Commercially available preparations containing amlodipine in fixed combination with olmesartan medoxomil (with or without hydrochlorothiazide), telmisartan, or valsartan (with or without hydrochlorothiazide) exceed the recommended initial dosage of amlodipine (2.5 mg daily) for patients with hepatic insufficiency. The manufacturer states that preparations containing amlodipine in fixed combination with perindopril are not recommended in patients with hepatic impairment, as insufficient data are available to support dosage recommendations.

For the management of Prinzmetal variant angina or chronic stable angina in patients with hepatic insufficiency, an amlodipine dosage of 5 mg daily is recommended. The manufacturers state that adequate control of angina usually requires a maintenance dosage of 10 mg daily.

Renal Impairment Adjustment of amlodipine dosage generally is not necessary in patients with renal impairment since elimination of the drug is not altered substantially by such impairment. However, use of the commercially available preparation containing benazepril in fixed combination with amlodipine is not recommended for patients with severe renal impairment (creatinine clearance of 30 mL/minute or less). In addition, use of preparations containing amlodipine in fixed combination with olmesartan medoxomil and hydrochlorothiazide are not recommended in patients with severe renal impairment; a loop diuretic generally is preferred over a thiazide diuretic in such patients. The safety and efficacy of preparations containing amlodipine in fixed combination with valsartan (with or without hydrochlorothiazide) in patients with creatinine clearances less than 30 mL/minute have not been established. The manufacturer states that preparations containing amlodipine in fixed combination with perindopril are not recommended in patients with creatinine clearances of less than 60 mL/minute, as insufficient data are available to support dosage recommendations. Dosage of the fixed combination of amlodipine and telmisartan should be titrated slowly in patients with severe renal impairment.

Geriatric Patients Since the elimination of amlodipine may be impaired substantially in geriatric patients, resulting in increased exposure to the drug (AUC increases of 40–60%), a reduced initial amlodipine dosage should be considered in such patients. For management of hypertension, some manufacturers recommend an initial amlodipine dosage of 2.5 mg once daily for geriatric patients; other manufacturers recommend this reduced dosage for geriatric patients 75 years of age or older. For management of Prinzmetal variant angina or chronic stable angina in geriatric patients, an amlodipine dosage of 5 mg daily is recommended; the manufacturers state that adequate control of angina usually requires a maintenance dosage of 10 mg once daily. Commercially available preparations containing amlodipine in fixed combination with olmesartan medoxomil (with or without hydrochlorothiazide), telmisartan, or valsartan (with or without hydrochlorothiazide) exceed the recommended initial dosage of amlodipine (2.5 mg daily) for geriatric patients. The manufacturer states that preparations containing amlodipine in fixed combination with perindopril are not recommended in geriatric patients, as insufficient data are available to support dosage recommendations.

Heart Failure Patients with moderate to severe heart failure have an increased AUC for amlodipine similar to that of geriatric patients and those with hepatic impairment, but the manufacturers currently make no specific recommendations for dosage adjustment in patients with congestive heart failure. The manufacturer states that preparations containing amlodipine in fixed combination with perindopril are not recommended in patients with heart failure, as insufficient data are available to support dosage recommendations.

Cautions

■ **Contraindications** Amlodipine is contraindicated in patients with known hypersensitivity to the drug.

■ **Warnings/Precautions** ***Hypotension*** Symptomatic hypotension may occur in patients receiving amlodipine, particularly in individuals with severe aortic stenosis; however, acute hypotension is unlikely because of the gradual onset of action of the drug.

Increased Angina or Acute Myocardial Infarction Worsening of angina or acute myocardial infarction can occur, particularly in patients with severe obstructive coronary artery disease, upon initiation of amlodipine therapy or an increase in amlodipine dosage.

Use of Fixed Combinations When amlodipine is used in fixed combination with other drugs (e.g., other antihypertensive agents, atorvastatin), cautions, precautions, contraindications, and interactions associated with the concomitant agent(s) should be considered in addition to those associated with amlodipine. Cautionary information applicable to specific populations (e.g., pregnant or nursing women, individuals with hepatic or renal impairment, geriatric patients) also should be considered for each drug in the fixed combination.

Heart Failure Although some calcium-channel blockers have been shown to worsen the clinical status of patients with heart failure, no evidence of worsening heart failure (based on exercise tolerance, New York Heart Association [NYHA] class, symptoms, or left ventricular ejection fraction) and no adverse effects on overall survival and cardiac morbidity were observed in controlled studies of amlodipine in patients with heart failure. Cardiac morbidity and overall mortality rates in these studies were similar in patients receiving amlodipine and those receiving placebo.

In patients with moderate to severe heart failure, amlodipine clearance is decreased and area under the concentration-time curve (AUC) is increased by about 40–60%.

Specific Populations **Pregnancy.** Category C. (See Users Guide.)

Lactation. It is not known whether amlodipine is distributed into milk; the manufacturer recommends discontinuance of nursing if amlodipine is used.

Pediatric Use. Safety and efficacy of amlodipine in children younger than 6 years of age have not been established. Efficacy of amlodipine (2.5–5 mg daily) for the treatment of hypertension has been established in pediatric patients 6–17 years of age.

Safety and efficacy of amlodipine in fixed combination with atorvastatin, benazepril, olmesartan (with or without hydrochlorothiazide), perindopril, telmisartan, or valsartan (with or without hydrochlorothiazide) have not been established in children.

Geriatric Use. In geriatric patients, amlodipine clearance is decreased and AUC is increased by about 40–60%. Therefore, amlodipine dosage should be selected carefully, usually initiating therapy with dosages at the lower end of the recommended range. The greater frequency of decreased hepatic, renal, and/or cardiac function and of concomitant disease and drug therapy observed in the elderly also should be considered. (See Geriatric Patients under Dosage and Administration: Special Populations.)

Clinical studies of amlodipine did not include sufficient numbers of patients 65 years of age and older to determine whether geriatric patients respond differently than younger patients; however, other clinical experience has not revealed age-related differences in response or tolerance. No substantial differences in safety and efficacy relative to younger adults have been observed in geriatric patients receiving amlodipine in fixed combination with benazepril, olmesartan (with or without hydrochlorothiazide), telmisartan, or valsartan (with or without hydrochlorothiazide), but increased sensitivity cannot be ruled out.

The manufacturer states that use of amlodipine in fixed combination with perindopril in geriatric patients is not recommended, as insufficient data are available to support dosage recommendations.

The manufacturers state that safety and efficacy of amlodipine in fixed combination with atorvastatin have not been established in geriatric patients.

Hepatic Impairment. In patients with hepatic impairment, amlodipine clearance is decreased and AUC is increased by about 40–60%. A reduced initial dosage of the drug is recommended, and subsequent dosage should be titrated slowly. (See Hepatic Impairment under Dosage and Administration: Special Populations.)

■ **Common Adverse Effects** Adverse effects reported in 1% or more of patients receiving amlodipine include edema, dizziness, flushing, palpitations, fatigue, nausea, abdominal pain, and somnolence. Edema, flushing, palpitations, and somnolence may occur more commonly in women than in men. Edema is dose related and may be less frequent with concomitant use of an angiotensin-converting enzyme (ACE) inhibitor or angiotensin II receptor antagonist.

Drug Interactions

When amlodipine is used in fixed combination with other drugs, interactions associated with the concomitant agent(s) must be considered in addition to those associated with amlodipine.

■ **Drugs Affecting Hepatic Microsomal Enzymes** Concomitant use of amlodipine with moderate (e.g., diltiazem) or potent (e.g., clarithromycin, itraconazole) inhibitors of cytochrome P-450 (CYP) 3A isoenzymes (CYP3A) results in increased systemic exposure to amlodipine. Reduction of amlodipine dosage may be necessary; patients receiving concomitant therapy with CYP3A inhibitors should be monitored for symptoms of hypotension or edema, which may indicate a need for dosage adjustment.

Data on the effects of CYP3A inducers on amlodipine exposure are lacking; blood pressure should be closely monitored in patients receiving such concomitant therapy.

■ **Alcohol** Concomitant administration of alcohol with amlodipine did not alter systemic exposure to alcohol.

■ **Antacids** Concomitant administration of a magnesium- and aluminum hydroxide-containing antacid with amlodipine did not alter systemic exposure to amlodipine.

■ **Cimetidine** Concomitant administration of cimetidine with amlodipine did not alter systemic exposure to amlodipine.

■ **Digoxin** Concomitant administration of amlodipine with digoxin did not alter systemic exposure to digoxin.

■ **Diltiazem** Concomitant use of diltiazem hydrochloride (180 mg daily) with amlodipine (5 mg) in geriatric patients with hypertension resulted in a 60% increase in amlodipine exposure.

■ **Erythromycin** Concomitant administration of erythromycin with amlodipine did not substantially alter systemic exposure to amlodipine in healthy individuals.

■ **Grapefruit Juice** The manufacturer states that concomitant administration of grapefruit juice with amlodipine did not alter systemic exposure to amlodipine. Although there is some evidence from healthy individuals that concomitant administration with grapefruit juice may increase oral bioavailability of the drug compared with concomitant administration with water, there currently is no evidence of altered amlodipine pharmacodynamics by concurrent ingestion of grapefruit juice in healthy individuals. Concomitant oral administration of other 1,4-dihydropyridine-derivative calcium-channel blocking agents (e.g., felodipine, nifedipine, nisoldipine) with grapefruit juice has resulted in potentially clinically important increases in the hemodynamic effects of these drugs. (See Drug Interactions: Grapefruit Juice, in Nifedipine 24:28.08.)

■ **HMG-CoA Reductase Inhibitors** ***Atorvastatin*** Concomitant administration of amlodipine with atorvastatin did not alter systemic exposure to atorvastatin.

Simvastatin Concomitant administration of amlodipine (multiple 10-mg doses) with simvastatin (80 mg) resulted in a 77% increase in simvastatin exposure compared with simvastatin alone. In patients receiving amlodipine, simvastatin dosage should not exceed 20 mg daily.

■ **Immunosuppressants** ***Cyclosporine*** Concomitant use of cyclosporine and amlodipine may result in increased systemic exposure to cyclosporine. Concomitant use of amlodipine with cyclosporine in renal allograft recipients resulted in a 40% increase in trough concentrations of the immunosuppressant. If concomitant use is required, cyclosporine concentrations should be monitored frequently and cyclosporine dosage adjusted as needed.

Tacrolimus Concomitant use of tacrolimus and amlodipine may result in increased systemic exposure to tacrolimus. If concomitant use is required, tacrolimus concentrations should be monitored frequently and tacrolimus dosage adjusted as needed.

In healthy Chinese individuals who expressed the CYP3A5 isoenzyme, concomitant administration of amlodipine with tacrolimus resulted in a 2.5- to 4-fold increase in tacrolimus exposure compared with tacrolimus alone; this finding was not observed in individuals who did not express CYP3A5. However, in a renal transplant patient who did not express CYP3A5, a threefold increase in systemic exposure to tacrolimus was observed following initiation of amlodipine therapy for posttransplantation hypertension; reduction in tacrolimus dosage was required. Irrespective of CYP3A5 genotype, the possibility of an interaction between tacrolimus and amlodipine cannot be excluded.

■ **Protein-bound Drugs** In vitro data indicate that amlodipine does not alter plasma protein binding of digoxin, indomethacin, phenytoin, or warfarin.

■ **Sildenafil** Concomitant administration of sildenafil with amlodipine did not alter systemic exposure to amlodipine; however, additional reductions in blood pressure are possible with such concomitant use. Patients receiving sildenafil concomitantly with amlodipine should be monitored for hypotension.

■ **Warfarin** Concomitant administration of amlodipine with warfarin did not alter prothrombin time.

Description

Amlodipine is a 1,4-dihydropyridine-derivative calcium-channel blocking agent that is structurally related to felodipine, nifedipine, and nimodipine. Unlike other currently available agents in the dihydropyridine class, amlodipine has an intrinsically long duration of action.

Following oral administration of amlodipine besylate, peak plasma concentrations of the drug are attained within 6–12 hours. Absolute bioavailability ranges from 64–90%; food does not affect bioavailability of amlodipine. Amlodipine is approximately 93% bound to plasma proteins. The drug is extensively (approximately 90%) metabolized to inactive metabolites in the liver. Amlodipine is excreted in urine as metabolites (60%) and unchanged drug (10%). The terminal elimination half-life of amlodipine is 30–50 hours.

Advice to Patients

When amlodipine is used in fixed combination with other drugs, importance of informing patients of important cautionary information about the concomitant agent(s).

Importance of instructing patients not to remove tablets containing amlodipine in fixed combination with telmisartan from the blister package until immediately before administration.

Importance of informing clinicians of existing or contemplated concomitant therapy, including prescription and OTC drugs, as well as any concomitant illnesses.

Importance of women informing clinicians if they are or plan to become pregnant or plan to breast-feed.

Importance of advising patients of other important precautionary information. (See Cautions.)

Overview® (see Users Guide). For additional information on this drug until a more detailed monograph is developed and published, the manufacturer's labeling should be consulted. It is *essential* that the manufacturer's labeling be consulted for more detailed information on usual cautions, precautions, contraindications, potential drug interactions, laboratory test interferences, and acute toxicity.

Preparations

Excipients in commercially available drug preparations may have clinically important effects in some individuals; consult specific product labeling for details.

amLODIPine Besylate

Oral		
Tablets	2.5 mg (of amlodipine)*	**Amlodipine Besylate Tablets**
		Norvasc®, Pfizer
	5 mg (of amlodipine)*	**Amlodipine Besylate Tablets**
		Norvasc®, Pfizer
	10 mg (of amlodipine)*	**Amlodipine Besylate Tablets**
		Norvasc®, Pfizer

*available from one or more manufacturer, distributor, and/or repackager by generic (nonproprietary) name

amLODIPine Besylate Combinations

Oral		
Capsules	2.5 mg (of amlodipine) with Benazepril Hydrochloride 10 mg*	**Amlodipine Besylate and Benazepril Hydrochloride Capsules**
		Lotrel®, Novartis
	5 mg (of amlodipine) with Benazepril Hydrochloride 10 mg*	**Amlodipine Besylate and Benazepril Hydrochloride Capsules**
		Lotrel®, Novartis
	5 mg (of amlodipine) with Benazepril Hydrochloride 20 mg*	**Amlodipine Besylate and Benazepril Hydrochloride Capsules**
		Lotrel®, Novartis
	5 mg (of amlodipine) with Benazepril Hydrochloride 40 mg*	**Amlodipine Besylate and Benazepril Hydrochloride Capsules**
		Lotrel®, Novartis
	10 mg (of amlodipine) with Benazepril Hydrochloride 20 mg*	**Amlodipine Besylate and Benazepril Hydrochloride Capsules**
		Lotrel®, Novartis
	10 mg (of amlodipine) with Benazepril Hydrochloride 40 mg*	**Amlodipine Besylate and Benazepril Hydrochloride Capsules**
		Lotrel®, Novartis
Tablets	2.5 mg (of amlodipine) with Perindopril Arginine 3.5 mg	**Prestalia®**, Symplmed
	5 mg (of amlodipine) with Olmesartan Medoxomil 20 mg	**Azor®**, Daiichi-Sankyo
	5 mg (of amlodipine) with Olmesartan Medoxomil 40 mg	**Azor®**, Daiichi-Sankyo
	5 mg (of amlodipine) with Perindopril Arginine 7 mg	**Prestalia®**, Symplmed
	10 mg (of amlodipine) with Olmesartan Medoxomil 20 mg	**Azor®**, Daiichi-Sankyo
	10 mg (of amlodipine) with Olmesartan Medoxomil 40 mg	**Azor®**, Daiichi-Sankyo
	10 mg (of amlodipine) with Perindopril Arginine 14 mg	**Prestalia®**, Symplmed
Tablets, film-coated	2.5 mg (of amlodipine) with Atorvastatin Calcium 10 mg (of atorvastatin)*	**Amlodipine Besylate and Atorvastatin Calcium Tablets**
		Caduet®, Pfizer
	2.5 mg (of amlodipine) with Atorvastatin Calcium 20 mg (of atorvastatin)*	**Amlodipine Besylate and Atorvastatin Calcium Tablets**
		Caduet®, Pfizer
	2.5 mg (of amlodipine) with Atorvastatin Calcium 40 mg (of atorvastatin)*	**Amlodipine Besylate and Atorvastatin Calcium Tablets**
		Caduet®, Pfizer
	5 mg (of amlodipine) with Atorvastatin Calcium 10 mg (of atorvastatin)*	**Amlodipine Besylate and Atorvastatin Calcium Tablets**
		Caduet®, Pfizer
	5 mg (of amlodipine) with Atorvastatin Calcium 20 mg (of atorvastatin)*	**Amlodipine Besylate and Atorvastatin Calcium Tablets**
		Caduet®, Pfizer
	5 mg (of amlodipine) with Atorvastatin Calcium 40 mg (of atorvastatin)*	**Amlodipine Besylate and Atorvastatin Calcium Tablets**
		Caduet®, Pfizer
	5 mg (of amlodipine) with Atorvastatin Calcium 80 mg (of atorvastatin)*	**Amlodipine Besylate and Atorvastatin Calcium Tablets**
		Caduet®, Pfizer
	5 mg (of amlodipine) with Hydrochlorothiazide 12.5 mg and Olmesartan Medoxomil 20 mg	**Tribenzor®**, Daiichi Sankyo
	5 mg (of amlodipine) with Hydrochlorothiazide 12.5 mg and Olmesartan Medoxomil 40 mg	**Tribenzor®**, Daiichi Sankyo
	5 mg (of amlodipine) with Hydrochlorothiazide 12.5 mg and Valsartan 160 mg*	**Amlodipine Besylate, Valsartan, and Hydrochlorothiazide Tablets**
		Exforge HCT®, Novartis
	5 mg (of amlodipine) with Hydrochlorothiazide 25 mg and Olmesartan Medoxomil 40 mg	**Tribenzor®**, Daiichi Sankyo
	5 mg (of amlodipine) with Hydrochlorothiazide 25 mg and Valsartan 160 mg*	**Amlodipine Besylate, Valsartan, and Hydrochlorothiazide Tablets**
		Exforge HCT®, Novartis
	5 mg (of amlodipine) with Valsartan 160 mg*	**Amlodipine Besylate and Valsartan Tablets**
		Exforge®, Novartis
	5 mg (of amlodipine) with Valsartan 320 mg*	**Amlodipine Besylate and Valsartan Tablets**
		Exforge®, Novartis
	10 mg (of amlodipine) with Atorvastatin Calcium 10 mg (of atorvastatin)*	**Amlodipine Besylate and Atorvastatin Calcium Tablets**
		Caduet®, Pfizer
	10 mg (of amlodipine) with Atorvastatin Calcium 20 mg (of atorvastatin)*	**Amlodipine Besylate and Atorvastatin Calcium Tablets**
		Caduet®, Pfizer

	10 mg (of amlodipine) with Atorvastatin Calcium 40 mg (of atorvastatin)*	**Amlodipine Besylate and Atorvastatin Calcium Tablets**
		Caduet®, Pfizer
	10 mg (of amlodipine) with Atorvastatin Calcium 80 mg (of atorvastatin)*	**Amlodipine Besylate and Atorvastatin Calcium Tablets**
		Caduet®, Pfizer
	10 mg (of amlodipine) with Hydrochlorothiazide 12.5 mg and Olmesartan Medoxomil 40 mg	**Tribenzor®**, Daiichi Sankyo
	10 mg (of amlodipine) with Hydrochlorothiazide 12.5 mg and Valsartan 160 mg*	**Amlodipine Besylate, Valsartan, and Hydrochlorothiazide Tablets**
		Exforge HCT®, Novartis
	10 mg (of amlodipine) with Hydrochlorothiazide 25 mg and Olmesartan Medoxomil 40 mg	**Tribenzor®**, Daiichi Sankyo
	10 mg (of amlodipine) with Hydrochlorothiazide 25 mg and Valsartan 160 mg*	**Amlodipine Besylate, Valsartan, and Hydrochlorothiazide Tablets**
		Exforge HCT®, Novartis
	10 mg (of amlodipine) with Hydrochlorothiazide 25 mg and Valsartan 320 mg*	**Amlodipine Besylate, Valsartan, and Hydrochlorothiazide Tablets**
		Exforge HCT®, Novartis
	10 mg (of amlodipine) with Valsartan 160 mg*	**Amlodipine Besylate and Valsartan Tablets**
		Exforge®, Novartis
	10 mg (of amlodipine) with Valsartan 320 mg*	**Amlodipine Besylate and Valsartan Tablets**
		Exforge®, Novartis
Tablets, multilayer	5 mg (of amlodipine) with Telmisartan 40 mg*	**Telmisartan and Amlodipine Besylate Tablets**
		Twynsta®, Boehringer Ingelheim
	5 mg (of amlodipine) with Telmisartan 80 mg*	**Telmisartan and Amlodipine Besylate Tablets**
		Twynsta®, Boehringer Ingelheim
	10 mg (of amlodipine) with Telmisartan 40 mg*	**Telmisartan and Amlodipine Besylate Tablets**
		Twynsta®, Boehringer Ingelheim
	10 mg (of amlodipine) with Telmisartan 80 mg*	**Telmisartan and Amlodipine Besylate Tablets**
		Twynsta®, Boehringer Ingelheim

*available from one or more manufacturer, distributor, and/or repackager by generic (nonproprietary) name

†Use is not currently included in the labeling approved by the US Food and Drug Administration

NIFEdipine

■ Nifedipine is a 1,4-dihydropyridine-derivative calcium-channel blocking agent.

Uses

■ **Angina** Nifedipine is used in the management of Prinzmetal variant angina and chronic stable angina pectoris. Calcium-channel blocking agents (used alone or in combination with nitrates) are considered the drugs of choice for the management of Prinzmetal variant angina. β-Adrenergic blocking agents (β-blockers) are recommended as the anti-ischemic drugs of choice in most patients with chronic stable angina; however, calcium-channel blockers may be substituted or added in patients who do not tolerate or respond adequately to β-blockers. In controlled clinical studies of up to 8 weeks' duration in patients with chronic stable angina, nifedipine reduced the frequency of attacks, allowed a decrease in sublingual nitroglycerin dosage, and increased exercise tolerance. All classes of calcium-channel blockers appear to be equally effective in reducing anginal episodes; however, choice of a specific agent should be individualized since the pharmacologic properties of these drugs differ. The potential risks of *short-acting* (conventional, immediate-release) nifedipine should be considered. (See Cautions.)

Calcium-channel blockers also have been used for the relief of ongoing or recurrent ischemia in patients with unstable angina†; however, a nondihydropyridine calcium-channel blocker (e.g., diltiazem, verapamil) generally is recommended.

Concurrent use of nifedipine and a β-blocker may have beneficial effects in some patients with chronic stable angina (e.g., reduction of dihydropyridine-induced tachycardia through β-blockade).

■ **Hypertension** Nifedipine is used alone or in combination with other classes of antihypertensive agents in the management of hypertension. Because of concerns about potentially serious adverse cardiovascular effects and increased mortality associated with short-acting (conventional, immediate-release) nifedipine (see Cautions), only extended-release formulations of the drug are recommended for the management of hypertension.

Calcium-channel blockers (e.g., nifedipine) are considered one of several preferred antihypertensive drugs for the initial management of hypertension according to current evidence-based hypertension guidelines; other preferred options include angiotensin-converting enzyme (ACE) inhibitors, angiotensin II receptor antagonists, and thiazide diuretics. While there may be individual differences with respect to recommendations for initial drug selection and use in specific patient populations, current evidence indicates that these antihypertensive drug classes all generally produce comparable effects on overall mortality and cardiovascular, cerebrovascular, and renal outcomes. (See Uses: Hypertension, in Amlodipine 24:28.08.)

Most patients with hypertension, especially black patients, will require at least 2 antihypertensive drugs to achieve adequate blood pressure control. Calcium-channel blockers may be particularly useful in the management of hypertension in black patients; these patients tend to have greater blood pressure response to calcium-channel blockers and thiazide diuretics than to other antihypertensive drug classes (e.g., ACE inhibitors, angiotensin II receptor antagonists). However, the combination of an ACE inhibitor or an angiotensin II receptor antagonist with a calcium-channel blocker or thiazide diuretic produces similar blood pressure lowering in black patients as in other racial groups. (See Race under Hypertension: Other Special Considerations for Antihypertensive Therapy, in Uses in Amlodipine 24:28.08.) Use of a calcium-channel blocker also may be beneficial in patients with certain coexisting conditions such as ischemic heart disease (e.g., angina) and in geriatric patients, including those with isolated systolic hypertension. (See Uses: Hypertension, in Amlodipine 24:28.08.)

In the Antihypertensive and Lipid-lowering Treatment to Prevent Heart Attack Trial (ALLHAT), the long-term cardiovascular morbidity and mortality benefit of a long-acting dihydropyridine calcium-channel blocker (amlodipine), a thiazide-like diuretic (chlorthalidone), and an ACE inhibitor (lisinopril) were compared in a broad population of patients with hypertension at risk of coronary heart disease. Although these antihypertensive agents were comparably effective in providing important cardiovascular benefit, apparent differences in certain secondary outcomes were observed. Patients receiving the ACE inhibitor experienced higher risks of stroke, combined cardiovascular disease, GI bleeding, and angioedema, while those receiving the calcium-channel blocker were at higher risk of developing heart failure. The ALLHAT investigators suggested that the observed differences in cardiovascular outcome may be attributable, at least in part, to the greater antihypertensive effect of the calcium-channel blocker compared with that of the ACE inhibitor, especially in women and black patients. (See Clinical Benefits of Thiazides in Hypertension under Hypertension in Adults: Treatment Benefits, in Uses in the Thiazides General Statement 40:28.20.)

For more detailed information on the role of calcium-channel blockers in the management of hypertension, see Uses: Hypertension, in Amlodipine 24:28.08. For information on overall principles and expert recommendations for treatment of hypertension, see Uses: Hypertension in Adults, in the Thiazides General Statement 40:28.20.

Hypertensive Crises *In the past*, when oral therapy was considered preferable to parenteral therapy in selected patients, short-acting (conventional, immediate-release capsules) nifedipine had been used for rapidly reducing blood pressure in patients with hypertensive crises† in whom reduction of blood pressure was considered urgent (hypertensive urgencies) or an emergency (hypertensive emergencies); however, most clinicians and the manufacturers now question the safety of short-acting nifedipine for this use because of occasional reports of poorly tolerated severe hypotension and the potential adverse cardiovascular consequences (e.g., cerebrovascular ischemia, stroke, myocardial ischemia and infarction, death). As a result of these and other (see Cautions) concerns and absence of substantial evidence clearly establishing superiority (both in terms of safety and efficacy) of nifedipine for this use, it is recommended that short-acting nifedipine no longer be used for the management of any form of hypertension, including hypertensive crises.

Patients with hypertensive emergencies (i.e., those rare situations requiring immediate blood pressure reduction, although not necessarily to normal ranges, in order to prevent or limit target organ damage) require hospitalization and are treated with an appropriate parenteral antihypertensive agent (e.g., labetalol, esmolol, fenoldopam, nicardipine, sodium nitroprusside). Hypertensive urgencies (i.e., situations in which there is severe elevation in blood pressure without progressive target organ damage) generally can be managed by intensification or reinstitution (e.g., following noncompliance) of the current antihypertensive regimen and treatment of anxiety if needed. Experts state that there is no need for rapid reduction of blood pressure in such patients and hospitalization or referral to the emergency department also is unnecessary. Excessive falls in blood pressure should be avoided in any hypertensive crisis since they may precipitate renal, cerebral, or coronary ischemia.

Hypertension During Pregnancy Antihypertensive therapy is recommended in pregnant women with chronic hypertension who have persistent, severely elevated blood pressure (e.g., systolic blood pressure of 160 mm Hg or higher or diastolic blood pressure of 105 mm Hg or higher); it is less clear whether antihypertensive therapy should be initiated in women with mild to moderate chronic hypertension. If initiation of antihypertensive therapy is necessary in a pregnant woman, use of labetalol, nifedipine, or methyldopa is recommended by the American College of Obstetricians and Gynecologists (ACOG) and other experts. In women who are already receiving antihypertensive therapy prior to pregnancy, ACOG states there are insufficient data to make recommendations regarding the continuance or discontinuance of such therapy; treatment decisions should be individualized in these situations. Alternatively, other experts state that women with hypertension who became pregnant, or are planning to become pregnant, should have their antihypertensive therapy transitioned to methyldopa, nifedipine, and/or labetalol during pregnancy.

Nifedipine also has been used orally in the hospital setting for urgent lowering of blood pressure in severely hypertensive pregnant women, including those with preeclampsia†. However, short-acting (conventional) formulations of nifedipine are not labeled by the US Food and Drug Administration (FDA) for acute reduction of blood pressure; cases of profound hypotension and other serious adverse cardiovascular consequences have been reported with the use of these preparations. (For additional information on the use of antihypertensive drugs in women with preeclampsia, see Uses: Hypertension, in Hydralazine 24:08.20.)

■ **Raynaud's Phenomenon** Nifedipine has been used effectively in the management of Raynaud's phenomenon† and is considered a drug of choice for the management of this condition. The drug has reduced the frequency, duration, and severity of attacks in patients with this condition. However, not all patients with this condition respond to nifedipine, and intolerable adverse effects (e.g., headache, flushing, orthostatic hypotension) may limit the usefulness of the drug in some other patients. Although most experience with nifedipine in the management of Raynaud's phenomenon had been with short-acting (conventional, immediate-release) formulations of the drug, recent concerns (e.g., risks of serious hypotension and associated cardiovascular consequences) about the safety of short-acting (conventional) nifedipine have prompted the manufacturers to warn against use of this preparation in conditions for which safety and efficacy have not been fully established. (See Cautions.) Therefore, while not studied as extensively as short-acting nifedipine, extended-release nifedipine (e.g., 30–60 mg daily) preferably should be used when the drug is indicated for the management of Raynaud's phenomenon. The extended-release preparation of nifedipine appears to be tolerated better than the short-acting preparation in patients with this condition. The principal troublesome adverse effect during long-term therapy in these patients appears to be peripheral (ankle) edema.

■ **Preterm Labor** Nifedipine has been used in selected patients to inhibit uterine contractions in preterm labor† (tocolysis) and thus prolong gestation when such prolongation of intrauterine life was expected to benefit pregnancy outcome. Current ACOG guidelines for management of preterm labor state that there is no clear first-line tocolytic agent because of conflicting results regarding efficacy in comparative trials. In addition, concerns about the safety of short-acting (conventional) nifedipine (e.g., risks of serious hypotension and associated cardiovascular consequences) have prompted the manufacturers to warn against use of this preparation in conditions for which safety and efficacy have not been fully established. (See Cautions.) However, an analysis of pooled data from a number of randomized, controlled studies suggests that calcium-channel blockers (principally nifedipine) may be more effective than, and preferable to, other agents (e.g., magnesium sulfate, β-adrenergic agonists) when tocolysis is deemed necessary. Results of this pooled analysis suggest that calcium-channel blockers are more effective in reducing births within 7 days of initiation of tocolytic treatment and before 34 weeks' gestation and are associated with improved neonatal outcomes (e.g., less neonatal respiratory distress syndrome, intraventricular hemorrhage, necrotizing enterocolitis, jaundice) and a reduced frequency of maternal adverse effects leading to treatment discontinuance compared with other tocolytic agents. A number of different dosages and dosage forms of nifedipine were used in these studies, and an optimal dosage regimen for the drug as a tocolytic has not been determined.

The main benefit currently derived from tocolytic therapy may be to forestall labor and provide time for patients to receive corticosteroids to increase fetal lung maturation and/or to be transferred to other (e.g., tertiary-care) facilities; any other potential benefits of prolonging pregnancy are unclear. For additional information, see Uses: Preterm Labor in Magnesium Sulfate 28:12.92.

■ **Acute Myocardial Infarction** Calcium-channel blocking agents have been used in the early treatment and secondary prevention of acute myocardial infarction (MI)†; although these drugs are effective anti-ischemic agents, they have not demonstrated mortality benefits and therefore are generally used as an alternative to β-blockers. A review of 28 randomized controlled studies involving 19,000 patients found no benefit with regard to infarct size, rate of reinfarction, or death when calcium-channel blockers were used during the acute or convalescent phase of ST-segment-elevation MI (STEMI). Calcium-channel blockers generally are used for their anti-ischemic and blood pressure-reducing properties in the MI setting, and only when β-blockers (which have been shown to reduce mortality after MI) are ineffective, not tolerated, or contraindicated.

Current expert guidelines state that a calcium-channel blocker may be used to relieve ischemic symptoms, lower blood pressure, or control rapid ventricular response associated with atrial fibrillation in patients with STEMI who are intolerant to β-blockers. A nondihydropyridine calcium-channel blocker (e.g., verapamil or diltiazem) may be used as an alternative to β-blockers for the relief of ongoing or recurring ischemia when β-blocker therapy is inadequate, not tolerated, or contraindicated in patients with non-ST-segment-elevation MI (NSTEMI) who do not have clinically important left ventricular dysfunction, increased risk of cardiogenic shock, or AV block.

The use of short-acting (conventional, immediate-release) nifedipine is generally contraindicated in patients with MI because of its negative inotropic effects and the reflex sympathetic activation, tachycardia, and hypotension associated with its use. Short-acting nifedipine may be particularly detrimental in patients with hypotension and/or tachycardia since the drug may induce a reduction in coronary perfusion pressure, disproportionate dilatation of coronary arteries adjacent to ischemic areas ("steal" phenomenon), and/or reflex activation of the sympathetic nervous system, resulting in an increase in myocardial oxygen demands. These findings are based on numerous clinical trials, including the Nifedipine Angina Myocardial Infarction Trial (NAMIS), the Trial of Early Nifedipine Treatment in Acute Myocardial Infarction (TRENT), the Norwegian Nifedipine Multicenter Trial, and the Secondary Prevention Reinfarction Israeli Nifedipine Trial (SPRINT).

Dosage and Administration

■ **Administration** Nifedipine is administered orally. The drug also has been administered sublingually† or intrabuccally† (e.g., for rapid reduction of blood pressure). When nifedipine is administered sublingually or intrabuccally, the conventional liquid-filled capsule must be punctured, chewed, and/or squeezed to express the liquid into the mouth. However, based on pharmacokinetic considerations (see Pharmacokinetics: Absorption), some clinicians recommend that when a relatively rapid response is desired the drug preferably be administered as conventional liquid-filled capsules that are bitten and then swallowed.

Nifedipine extended-release tablets should be swallowed intact and should *not* be chewed, crushed, or broken. The manufacturer of Adalat® CC states that the extended-release nifedipine tablets should be taken on an empty stomach. Patients should be advised *not* to become alarmed if they notice a tablet-like substance in their stools; this is normal since the tablet containing the drug is designed to remain intact and slowly release the drug from a nonabsorbable shell during passage through the GI tract.

Whenever extended-release tablets of nifedipine are dispensed or administered, care should be taken to ensure that the extended-release dosage form actually was prescribed. The manufacturers recommend that dosage of extended-release nifedipine tablets should be decreased gradually with close clinical supervision when discontinuance of the drug is required.

The manufacturer of Adalat® CC states that two 30-mg Adalat® CC extended-release tablets may be interchanged with one 60-mg Adalat® CC extended-release tablet; however, three 30-mg Adalat® CC extended-release tablets should *not* be considered interchangeable with one 90-mg Adalat® CC extended-release tablet (see Pharmacokinetics: Absorption).

Concomitant oral administration of 1,4-dihydropyridine-derivative calcium-channel blocking agents (e.g., nifedipine) with grapefruit juice usually should be avoided since potentially clinically important increases in hemodynamic effects may result. (See Grapefruit Juice under Drug Interactions: Drugs and Foods Affecting Hepatic Microsomal Enzymes.)

■ **Dosage** ***Angina*** The National Heart, Lung, and Blood Institute (NHLBI) states that, pending further accumulation of data, it seems prudent that conventional liquid-filled (short-acting) capsules of nifedipine, especially at high doses, be used in the management of angina with great caution, if at all. (See Cautions.)

If short-acting nifedipine is used for the management of Prinzmetal variant angina or chronic stable angina pectoris, the usual initial adult dosage of the drug as conventional liquid-filled capsules that are swallowed intact is 10 mg 3 times daily. Alternatively, nifedipine antianginal therapy can be initiated with extended-release tablets at a dosage of 30 or 60 mg once daily. Generally, dosage is gradually increased at 7- to 14-day intervals until optimum control of angina is obtained. If symptoms so warrant and the patient's tolerance and response to therapy are assessed frequently, dosage may be increased more rapidly to 90 mg daily in increments of 30 mg/day over a 3-day period using conventional liquid-filled capsules or after steady state is achieved (usually achieved on the second day of therapy with a given dose) using extended-release tablets. In hospitalized patients who are closely monitored, nifedipine dosage may be increased in 10-mg increments using conventional liquid-filled capsules at 4- to 6-hour intervals, as necessary to control pain and arrhythmias caused by ischemia. Single doses usually should not exceed 30 mg.

The usual adult maintenance dosage of nifedipine as conventional liquid-filled capsules is 10–20 mg 3 times daily. In some patients, especially those with evidence of coronary artery spasm, higher dosages (using conventional liquid-filled capsules or extended-release tablets) and/or more frequent administration (using conventional liquid-filled capsules *only*) are necessary. In such patients, the usual maintenance dosage is 20–30 mg 3 or 4 times daily using conventional liquid-filled capsules; rarely, more than 120 mg daily is necessary. Experience with antianginal dosages exceeding 90 mg once daily using the extended-release tablets is limited; therefore, higher dosages using this dosage form should be employed with caution and only when clinically necessary.

Dosage generally should not exceed 180 mg daily as conventional liquid-filled capsules or 120 mg daily as extended-release tablets, since the safety and efficacy of higher dosages have not been established. After anginal symptoms are controlled, dosage should be gradually reduced to the lowest level that will maintain relief of symptoms.

In patients whose angina is controlled with conventional liquid-filled capsules of nifedipine alone or in combination with other antianginal agents, extended-release tablets of nifedipine can be substituted for the conventional capsules at the nearest equivalent total daily dose. Thus, patients who are receiving a nifedipine dosage of 30 mg 3 times daily as conventional liquid-filled capsules can be switched to a dosage of 90 mg once daily as extended-release tablets. When the total daily dose as conventional liquid-filled capsules does not correspond exactly to the strength of a commercially available extended-release tablet, the nearest equivalent daily dose can be substituted; the extended-release tablets should *not* be divided in an attempt to exactly match total daily doses of conventional capsules. Subsequent titration to higher or lower dosages may be necessary and should be guided by the patient's clinical response and tolerance.

Hypertension Dosage of nifedipine should be adjusted according to the patient's blood pressure response and tolerance.

Usual Dosage. For the management of hypertension in adults, the usual initial dosage of nifedipine as extended-release tablets is 30 or 60 mg once daily. Generally, dosage is increased gradually at 7- to 14-day intervals until optimum control of blood pressure is obtained. If symptoms so warrant and the patient's tolerance and response to therapy are assessed frequently, dosage may be increased more rapidly. Steady state usually is achieved during the second day of therapy with a given dose as extended-release tablets. The manufacturers state that dosages exceeding 90 mg once daily (Adalat® CC) or 120 mg once daily (Procardia XL®) as extended-release tablets are not recommended. Some experts recommend a usual dosage range of 30–90 mg once daily.

If nifedipine is used for the management of hypertension in children†, some experts recommend a usual initial dosage of 0.2–0.5 mg/kg daily, administered as extended-release tablets once daily or in 2 divided doses daily. Dosage may be increased as necessary to a maximum dosage of 3 mg/kg (up to 120 mg), given once daily or in 2 divided doses. Experts state that the drug should be initiated at the low end of the dosage range and the dosage may be increased every 2–4 weeks until blood pressure is controlled, the maximum dosage is reached, or adverse effects occur. For information on overall principles and expert recommendations for treatment of hypertension in pediatric patients, see Uses: Hypertension in Pediatric Patients, in the Thiazides General Statement 40:28.20.

Because of concerns about potential cardiovascular risks associated with conventional liquid-filled (short-acting) capsules of the drug, short-acting preparations of nifedipine are no longer recommended for use in the management of hypertension.

Blood Pressure Monitoring and Treatment Goals. Blood pressure should be monitored regularly (i.e., monthly) during therapy and dosage of the antihypertensive drug adjusted until blood pressure is controlled. If an adequate blood pressure response is not achieved with nifedipine monotherapy, another antihypertensive agent with demonstrated benefit and preferably a complementary mechanism of action (e.g., angiotensin-converting enzyme [ACE] inhibitor, angiotensin II receptor antagonist, thiazide diuretic) may be added; if goal blood pressure is still not achieved with the use of 2 antihypertensive agents, a third drug may be added. (See Uses: Hypertension in Adults, in the Thiazides General Statement 40:28.20.) In patients who develop unacceptable adverse effects with nifedipine, the drug should be discontinued and another antihypertensive agent from a different pharmacologic class should be initiated.

The goal of hypertension management and prevention is to achieve and maintain optimal control of blood pressure. However, the optimum blood pressure threshold for initiating antihypertensive drug therapy and specific treatment goals remain controversial. While other hypertension guidelines have based target blood pressure goals on age and comorbidities, the 2017 American College of Cardiology (ACC)/American Heart Association (AHA) hypertension guideline incorporates underlying cardiovascular risk into decision making regarding treatment and generally recommends the same target blood pressure (i.e., less than 130/80 mm Hg) in all adults. Many patients will require at least 2 drugs from different pharmacologic classes to achieve this blood pressure goal; the potential benefits of hypertension management and drug cost, adverse effects, and risks associated with the use of multiple antihypertensive drugs also should be considered when deciding a patient's blood pressure treatment goal.

For additional information on target levels of blood pressure and on monitoring therapy in the management of hypertension, see Blood Pressure Monitoring and Treatment Goals under Dosage: Hypertension, in Dosage and Administration in the Thiazides General Statement 40:28.20.

Cautions

While serious adverse reactions requiring discontinuance of nifedipine therapy or dosage adjustments are uncommon, concerns about safety and efficacy of calcium-channel blocking agents (mainly conventional [short-acting] preparations of dihydropyridine derivatives) have been raised by findings of several studies. Results of a case-control study indicate dose-dependent increases in the risk of myocardial infarction (MI) (by about 60%) in hypertensive patients (with or without diagnosed cardiovascular disease, but excluding MI or heart failure) receiving a short-acting calcium-channel blocking agent (e.g., nifedipine, diltiazem, verapamil) compared with those receiving a diuretic or a β-adrenergic blocking agent (β-blocker). In addition, findings of several pooled analyses of studies indicate an increased risk of mortality (by about 16%) and reinfarction (by about 19%) in patients who have had an MI or in those with stable or unstable angina who were receiving dihydropyridine-derivative calcium-channel blocking agents (mainly conventional [short-acting] preparations of nifedipine) compared with those receiving placebo. Results of a pooled analysis of 16 studies indicate that the nifedipine-associated mortality may be dose dependent, especially in patients receiving short-acting nifedipine dosages of 80 mg or more daily when compared with those receiving placebo.

The National Heart, Lung, and Blood Institute (NHLBI) concluded from the apparent concordance of findings from observational studies in hypertensive patients and from randomized studies principally in acute MI and unstable angina patients that it seems prudent and consistent with current evidence to recommend that *short-acting* nifedipine, especially at high doses, be used in the management of hypertension, angina, or MI with great caution, if at all. In arriving at this conclusion, the NHLBI recognized the potential biases of observational studies. The NHLBI and some clinicians also state that while other calcium-channel blocking agents (e.g., diltiazem, verapamil) also were associated with increased risk of MI in the described case-control study, results of previous well-designed clinical studies indicate that the use of calcium-channel blocking agents was not associated with an increased risk of death; therefore, the adverse effects associated with short-acting nifedipine may not necessarily apply to other calcium-channel blocking agents, including other short-acting dihydropyridines (e.g., isradipine), or to long-acting preparations of nifedipine. Findings from the Antihypertensive and Lipid-Lowering Treatment to Prevent Heart Attack Trial (ALLHAT), which compared long-term therapy with an ACE inhibitor (lisinopril) or dihydropyridine-derivative calcium-channel blocker (amlodipine) revealed no difference in the primary outcome of combined fatal coronary heart disease or nonfatal MI among these therapies.

The increased risk of MI and death in patients receiving short-acting calcium-channel blocking agents may be associated with the arrhythmogenic, proischemic, negative inotropic, and/or prohemorrhagic effects of these agents; proischemic effects may result from reflex increases in sympathetic activity or from a reduction of coronary perfusion pressure induced by short-acting calcium-channel blocking agents. However, some clinicians state that while current evidence indicates an increased relative risk of MI associated with calcium-channel blocking agents, the actual increased risk for an individual patient may be low. Therefore, patients should not discontinue such therapy independently, but instead should consult their clinician about possible alternatives based on full evaluation of their medical condition, since the known risks of uncontrolled hypertension may be far greater than the postulated but unproven hazards associated with calcium-channel blocking agents.

■ **Cardiovascular Effects** Serious adverse reactions requiring discontinuance of nifedipine therapy or dosage adjustment are relatively rare. An increase in the frequency, intensity, and duration of angina, possibly resulting from hypotension, has occurred rarely during initiation of nifedipine therapy. Additional serious adverse effects including MI, congestive heart failure or pulmonary edema, and ventricular arrhythmia or conduction defects have reportedly occurred in 4%, 2%, and less than 0.5% of patients receiving conventional nifedipine capsules, respectively, but these have not been directly attributed to the drug. For additional information on potential serious cardiovascular effects associated with nifedipine, see the introductory discussion in Cautions and see also Cautions: Precautions and Contraindications.

Chest pain (nonspecific) has been reported in less than 3% of patients receiving extended-release nifedipine tablets in clinical trials. Adverse cardiovascular effects reported in up to 1% of patients receiving extended-release nifedipine tablets include substernal chest pain, arrhythmia, atrial fibrillation, bradycardia, tachycardia, cardiac arrest, extrasystole, hypotension, postural hypotension, syncope, increased angina, phlebitis, and cutaneous angiectases.

Most of the common adverse reactions to nifedipine result from its vasodilating action on vascular smooth muscle and include dizziness, lightheadedness, giddiness, flushing or heat sensation, and headache, reportedly occurring in up to 25% of patients, and less frequently, hypotension (usually mild to moderate and well tolerated), weakness, peripheral edema, and palpitation. The incidence and severity of syncope, peripheral (ankle) edema, and hypotension generally are dose related and occasionally may be obviated by a reduction in dosage. In patients receiving conventional liquid-filled (short-acting) nifedipine capsules, transient hypotension occurred in about 2% of patients receiving less than 60 mg daily and in about 5% of patients receiving 120 mg or more daily. Nifedipine-induced peripheral edema of the lower extremities usually responds to diuretic therapy. The relatively common adverse effects reported with conventional liquid-filled (short-acting) nifedipine capsules are similar in nature to those reported with extended-release tablets of the drug. However, some evidence indicates that the risk of certain adverse effects may be increased with short-acting preparations of the drug, particularly at high doses. (See the introductory discussion in Cautions.)

Although the hypotensive effect of nifedipine is modest and well tolerated in most patients receiving the drug for angina, excessive and poorly tolerated hypotension occurs occasionally in such patients. Such excessive hypotension usually occurs during initial dosage titration or subsequent upward titration of dosage, and may be more likely in patients receiving a β-blocker concomitantly. Severe hypotension and/or increased fluid requirements also have been reported in patients who were receiving these drugs concomitantly and underwent coronary artery bypass surgery involving high-dose fentanyl anesthesia. (See Drug Interactions: Fentanyl.) Several cases of profound hypotension, cerebrovascular ischemia or stroke, myocardial ischemia or infarction, and/or death have been reported when conventional short-acting preparations of nifedipine were used for the management of hypertensive crises, and therefore, the manufacturers currently warn that short-acting preparations should not be used for acute reduction in blood pressure. (See Hypertensive Crises under Uses: Hypertension.) However, profound hypotension, myocardial ischemia or infarction, and/or death also have been reported occasionally in patients receiving conventional short-acting preparations of the drug for other uses (e.g., angina, pulmonary hypertension). The manufacturers also warn that short-acting preparations of nifedipine should not be used for the chronic management of hypertension.

The frequency of nifedipine-induced peripheral edema appears to be dose related and reportedly occurs in 10–30% of patients receiving the drug. The edema is localized and probably occurs secondary to vasodilation of dependent arterioles and small blood vessels rather than to left ventricular dysfunction or generalized fluid retention. Intolerable adverse effects associated with nifedipine-induced vasodilation (e.g., headache, flushing, orthostatic hypotension) may limit the usefulness of nifedipine in some patients receiving the drug for Raynaud's phenomenon. The extended-release preparations of nifedipine appear to be tolerated better than the short-acting preparation in patients with this condition. The principal troublesome adverse effect during long-term therapy in these patients appears to be peripheral (ankle) edema.

Erythromelalgia has been reported in about 0.5% of patients receiving nifedipine. Characteristic manifestations of erythromelalgia include burning pain, increased skin temperature, and erythema of the extremities, usually the feet and lower legs, and less commonly, the hands. Manifestations resolve following discontinuance of the drug.

■ **Nervous System Effects** In patients receiving conventional liquid-filled (short-acting) nifedipine capsules, weakness was reported in 12% of patients, while tremor, nervousness, and mood changes occurred in about 7–8% of patients; fever and chills were reported in up to 2% of patients, and shakiness, jitteriness, disturbed sleep, and difficulty with postural balance occurred occasionally; mental depression and paranoid syndrome were reported rarely. In patients receiving extended-release nifedipine tablets, fatigue and asthenia were reported in about 4–6% of patients, pain occurred in less than 3% of patients, and paresthesia, vertigo, asthenia, insomnia, nervousness, and somnolence were reported in up to 3% of patients, while migraine, anxiety, confusion, ataxia, depression, hypertonia, hypoesthesia, paroniria, fever, and tremor were reported in up to 1% of patients. Chills occurred in less than 1% of patients. For nervous system effects associated with the vasodilating effect of nifedipine, see Cautions: Cardiovascular Effects.

■ **GI Effects** In patients receiving conventional liquid-filled (short-acting) nifedipine capsules, nausea and heartburn occurred in 11% of patients, while diarrhea, constipation, cramps, and flatulence were reported occasionally, and gingival hyperplasia occurred rarely. In patients receiving extended-release nifedipine tablets, nausea and constipation were reported in about 2–3 and about 1–3%, respectively, while abdominal pain, diarrhea, dry mouth, dyspepsia, and flatulence occurred in less than 3% of patients, and dysphagia, eructation, gastroesophageal reflux, esophagitis, vomiting, melena, GI hemorrhage, gum hemorrhage, gum hyperplasia, gum disorder, unspecified GI disorder, and taste perversion were reported in up to 1% of patients. GI irritation and GI bleeding have been reported in less than 1% of patients receiving Procardia XL® extended-release nifedipine tablets in open-label trials and during postmarketing experience, although a causal relationship to the drug has not been established.

Symptoms of GI obstruction have occurred in several patients with a history of GI strictures who were receiving extended-release tablets of the drug. (See Cautions: Precautions and Contraindications.) GI obstruction also has occurred in at least one patient with no preexisting abnormality who was receiving conventional capsules of the drug concomitantly with diltiazem; it was suggested that obstruction in this patient may have resulted from a pharmacologic effect on intestinal smooth muscle.

■ **Dermatologic and Sensitivity Reactions** In patients receiving conventional liquid-filled (short-acting) nifedipine capsules, dermatitis, pruritus, urticaria, and sweating have been reported occasionally, while angioedema (principally oropharyngeal edema and occasionally breathing difficulty) occurred in less than 0.5% of patients. Exfoliative dermatitis, exfoliative or bullous skin reactions (including erythema multiforme, Stevens-Johnson syndrome, and toxic epidermal necrolysis), and photosensitivity reactions have been reported rarely.

In patients receiving extended-release nifedipine tablets, rash and pruritus have been reported in up to 3% of patients, while angioedema, allergic reaction, cellulitis, facial edema, periorbital edema, alopecia, sweating, urticaria, photosensitivity reactions, and petechial rash were reported in up to 1% of patients.

Anaphylactic reactions have been reported rarely in patients receiving nifedipine.

■ **Respiratory Effects** In patients receiving conventional liquid-filled (short-acting) nifedipine capsules, dyspnea, cough, wheezing, nasal congestion, and sore throat occurred in 6% of patients, while chest congestion and shortness of breath have been reported in up to 2% of patients.

In patients receiving extended-release nifedipine tablets, dyspnea, epistaxis, and rhinitis were reported in up to 3% of patients, while cough, pharyngitis, sinusitis, upper respiratory tract infection, respiratory disorder, rales, and stridor were reported in up to 1% of patients.

■ **Musculoskeletal Effects** In patients receiving conventional liquid-filled (short-acting) nifedipine capsules, muscle cramps occurred in 8% of patients, while musculoskeletal complaints of inflammation and joint stiffness have been reported occasionally, and myalgia and arthritis with increased antinuclear antibodies (ANA) have been reported rarely.

In patients receiving extended-release nifedipine tablets, arthralgia, leg pain, and leg cramps occurred in up to 3% of patients, while myalgia, arthritis, joint disorder, myasthenia, back pain, neck pain, and gout occurred in up to 1% of patients.

■ **Genitourinary Effects** In patients receiving conventional liquid-filled (short-acting) nifedipine capsules, sexual difficulty has been reported occasionally, while gynecomastia, nocturia, and polyuria have been reported rarely.

In patients receiving extended-release nifedipine tablets, impotence, polyuria, and urinary frequency have been reported in up to 3% of patients, while decreased libido, breast pain, pelvic pain, dysuria, hematuria, and nocturia occurred in up to 1% of patients, and renal calculi, urogenital disorder, and breast engorgement were reported in less than 1% of patients. Gynecomastia has been reported in less than 1% of patients receiving Procardia XL® extended-release nifedipine tablets in open-label trials and during postmarketing experience, although a causal relationship to the drug has not been established.

■ **Hepatic Effects** Abnormal laboratory test results including mild to moderately increased serum concentrations of alkaline phosphatase, LDH, creatine kinase (CK, creatine phosphokinase, CPK), AST (SGOT), and ALT (SGPT) have been reported rarely in patients receiving nifedipine. Although a definite causal relationship of these laboratory test results to the drug has not been established, the relationship has been considered probable in several cases. In most cases, the laboratory test abnormalities were not associated with clinical symptoms; however, cholestasis (with or without jaundice) has been reported. Small increases (about 5%) in mean alkaline phosphatase concentrations have been reported in patients receiving extended-release nifedipine tablets; however, these increases were clinically asymptomatic, isolated incidents that rarely resulted in values outside the normal range. Increased γ-glutamyltransferase (GGT, γ-glutamyltranspeptidase, GGTP) concentrations have been reported in less than 1% of patients receiving Adalat® CC extended-release nifedipine tablets. Allergic hepatitis has occurred rarely.

■ **Renal Effects** In patients with preexisting chronic renal insufficiency receiving nifedipine, reversible increases in blood urea nitrogen (BUN) and serum creatinine concentrations have been reported rarely. Although a definite causal relationship of these laboratory test results to the drug has not been established, the relationship has been considered probable in several cases.

■ **Ocular and Otic Effects** In patients receiving conventional liquid-filled (short-acting) nifedipine capsules, blurred vision has been reported occasionally, while transient blindness at peak serum nifedipine concentrations and transient unilateral loss of vision have been reported rarely.

In patients receiving extended-release nifedipine tablets, abnormal lacrimation and vision abnormalities have been reported in up to 1% of patients, while amblyopia, conjunctivitis, diplopia, eye disorder, and ocular hemorrhage have been reported in less than 1% of patients.

Tinnitus has been reported in up to 1% of patients receiving nifedipine.

■ **Hematologic Effects** In patients receiving conventional liquid-filled (short-acting) nifedipine capsules, thrombocytopenia, anemia, leukopenia, and purpura have been reported rarely. In patients receiving extended-release nifedipine tablets, purpura occurred in up to 1% of patients, and eosinophilia and lymphadenopathy occurred in less than 1% of patients. Positive antiglobulin (Coombs') test results, with or without hemolytic anemia, have been reported in patients receiving nifedipine, but a causal relationship to the drug has not been established.

Like other calcium-channel blocking agents, nifedipine decreases platelet aggregation in vitro. A moderate decrease in platelet aggregation and increases in bleeding time, believed to be related to inhibition of calcium transport across the platelet membrane, have been reported in patients receiving nifedipine in a limited number of clinical studies; however, these findings were not considered to be clinically important.

■ **Metabolic Effects** Weight gain has been reported in up to 1% of patients receiving Procardia XL® extended-release nifedipine tablets, while weight loss has been reported in less than 1% of patients receiving Adalat® CC extended-release nifedipine tablets.

■ **Other Adverse Effects** In patients receiving extended-release nifedipine tablets, hot flushes (flashes), rigors, and malaise were reported in up to 1% of patients in clinical trials.

■ **Precautions and Contraindications** Some findings concerning possible risks of calcium-channel blocking agents have raised concerns about the safety and efficacy of these agents (mainly conventional [short-acting] preparations of nifedipine). However, findings with amlodipine in the ALLHAT study have shown a beneficial effect of dihydropyridine-derivative calcium-channel blockers on fatal coronary heart disease and nonfatal MI in patients treated with the drug for hypertension.

Nifedipine shares the toxic potentials of the calcium-channel blocking agents, and the usual precautions of these agents should be observed.

Because nifedipine decreases peripheral vascular resistance and occasionally causes excessive and poorly tolerated hypotension, blood pressure should be monitored carefully, especially during initiation of therapy and titration or upward adjustment of dosage. In addition, the manufacturers warn that the frequency, duration, and severity of angina may increase during initiation of therapy or upward adjustment of dosage.

Nifedipine should be used with caution in patients with congestive heart failure or aortic stenosis, especially in those receiving concomitant β-blockers, because nifedipine may precipitate or worsen heart failure in these patients. Peripheral edema occurring during the course of nifedipine therapy should be investigated, especially in patients with congestive heart failure, since it may indicate deterioration in left ventricular function induced by the drug.

Patients with acute stroke or acute MI may be at particular risk for the negative cardiovascular effects (both direct and reflex) of rapid blood pressure reduction, and the manufacturers warn that short-acting nifedipine should not be used during the first 1–2 weeks after acute MI. Preexisting hypovolemia or recent antihypertensive therapy may increase the risk of severe hypotension as may repeated doses of nifedipine. In patients with coronary artery disease and/or myocardial ischemia, reflex sympathetic activity with resultant increases in myocardial contractility, heart rate, and workload may aggravate preexisting myocardial ischemia. The manufacturers warn that short-acting nifedipine should be avoided in patients with acute coronary syndrome when MI may be imminent. When nifedipine therapy is initiated in patients with angina, they should be warned that the drug may cause increased angina, especially if β-blocker therapy is withdrawn abruptly when nifedipine therapy is being initiated. (See Drug Interactions: β-Adrenergic Blocking Agents.)

As with other nondeformable material, extended-release nifedipine tablets should be used with caution in patients with underlying severe GI narrowing (pathologic or iatrogenic) since obstruction may occur.

Nifedipine is contraindicated in patients with known hypersensitivity to the drug.

■ Pediatric Precautions Although safety and efficacy remain to be fully established in children younger than 18 years of age, some experts have recommended pediatric dosages for hypertension based on clinical experience. For information on overall principles and expert recommendations for treatment of hypertension in pediatric patients, see Uses: Hypertension in Pediatric Patients, in the Thiazides General Statement 40:28.20.

■ Geriatric Precautions Although a prolonged elimination half-life and an increase in peak plasma concentration and area under the plasma concentration-time curve (AUC) have been observed in pharmacokinetic studies in small numbers of patients (see Pharmacokinetics: Elimination), clinical studies of nifedipine did not include sufficient numbers of patients 65 years of age and older to determine whether geriatric patients respond differently than younger adults. While other clinical experience generally has not revealed age-related differences in response or tolerance, drug dosage generally should be titrated carefully in geriatric patients, usually initiating therapy at the low end of the dosage range and adjusting dosage as necessary based on patient response. The greater frequency of decreased hepatic, renal, and/or cardiac function and of concomitant disease and drug therapy observed in the elderly also should be considered.

■ Mutagenicity and Carcinogenicity In vivo studies using nifedipine have not revealed evidence of mutagenicity. No evidence of carcinogenicity was observed in rats receiving oral nifedipine for 2 years.

■ Pregnancy, Fertility, and Lactation Nifedipine has been shown to be teratogenic in rats and rabbits. Digital anomalies similar to those reported with phenytoin also have been reported in the offspring of animals receiving nifedipine or other dihydropyridines; these anomalies may occur secondary to compromised uterine blood flow. Nifedipine administration in rats, mice, rabbits, and monkeys also has been associated with a variety of other embryotoxic, placentotoxic, and fetotoxic effects, including stunted fetuses (rats, mice, and rabbits), rib deformities (mice), cleft palate (mice), small placentas and underdeveloped chorionic villi (monkeys), embryonic and fetal deaths (rats, mice, and rabbits), and prolonged pregnancy/decreased neonatal survival (rats; not evaluated in other species). The dosages (on a mg/kg basis) of nifedipine associated with teratogenic, embryotoxic, or fetotoxic effects in animals were higher (3.5–42 times) than the maximum recommended human dosage (120 mg daily); however, such dosages were within one order of magnitude of the maximum recommended human dosage. The dosages of nifedipine associated with placentotoxic effects in monkeys were equivalent to or lower than the maximum recommended human dosage on a mg/m^2 basis. There are no adequate and well-controlled studies using nifedipine in pregnant women, and the drug should be used during pregnancy only when the potential benefits justify the possible risks to the fetus.

Nifedipine caused decreased fertility when given to rats prior to mating at a dosage approximately 30 times the maximum recommended human dosage. A reversible reduction in the ability of human sperm to bind to and fertilize an ovum in vitro has been reported in a limited number of infertile men who were receiving usual dosages of nifedipine when the sperm was obtained.

Nifedipine is distributed into milk. In one lactating woman who received 10, 20, and 30 mg of the drug every 8 hours as conventional capsules, peak milk concentrations of nifedipine occurred within 1 hour after a dose and ranged from about 13–53 ng/mL; the drug generally was not detectable during the hour prior to a dose. Because of the potential for serious adverse reactions to nifedipine in nursing infants, a decision should be made whether to discontinue nursing or the drug, taking into account the importance of the drug to the woman.

Drug Interactions

■ Drugs and Foods Affecting Hepatic Microsomal Enzymes Metabolism of nifedipine is mediated by the cytochrome P-450 (CYP) microsomal enzyme system (principally the 3A isoenzyme) and concomitant use of nifedipine with inhibitors or inducers of CYP3A4 may be associated with altered nifedipine exposure resulting in favorable or adverse effects. In addition, in vitro and in vivo data indicate that nifedipine may inhibit metabolism of drugs that are substrates of CYP3A, thereby increasing exposure of other drugs. Nifedipine does not appear to affect the metabolism of CYP2D6 substrates.

Quinidine Quinidine appears to be a substrate of the CYP isoenzyme system and has been shown to inhibit CYP3A in vitro. In a multiple-dose study in healthy individuals, concomitant use of quinidine sulfate (200 mg 3 times daily) and nifedipine (20 mg 3 times daily) increased the area under the plasma concentration-time curve (AUC) and peak plasma concentration values of nifedipine 2.3 and 1.37 times, respectively. Heart rate during the initial interval following drug administration increased by up to 17.9 beats per minute.Heart rate should be monitored and nifedipine dosage adjusted as needed in patients receiving concomitant therapy with quinidine and nifedipine.

Although exposure to quinidine was not substantially affected by nifedipine in the previous study, nifedipine may decrease serum quinidine concentrations in some patients. Reductions or increases in serum quinidine concentrations occasionally have been observed following initiation or discontinuance, respectively, of nifedipine. Such changes can be substantial and may manifest as therapeutic resistance to usual quinidine dosages during concomitant therapy and/or altered ECGs (e.g., prolongation in corrected QT interval following discontinuance of nifedipine). While it had been postulated that alterations in quinidine pharmacokinetics during concomitant nifedipine therapy may have resulted from changes in hemodynamics induced by the latter drug (e.g., reduced peripheral vascular resistance with resultantly increased quinidine volume of distribution) in some patients (e.g., those with left ventricular dysfunction), subsequent study failed to confirm left ventricular dysfunction as a predictor of this interaction. Therefore, the mechanism of this interaction remains to be established, and possible identification of patients at risk requires further study. The possibility of this interaction should be considered in any patient exhibiting unpredictably low serum quinidine concentrations during concomitant nifedipine therapy. Serum quinidine concentrations should be monitored whenever nifedipine is initiated or discontinued in patients maintained on the antiarrhythmic, and quinidine dosage adjusted accordingly.

Verapamil Verapamil, an inhibitor of the isoenzyme CYP3A, may inhibit the metabolism of nifedipine. In patients receiving concomitant therapy with verapamil and nifedipine, blood pressure should be monitored, and nifedipine dosage reduction should be considered.

Diltiazem Since metabolism of diltiazem also is mediated principally by the CYP3A isoenzyme, diltiazem may competitively inhibit CYP3A4-dependent metabolism of other drugs (e.g., nifedipine). Administration of diltiazem 30- or 90-mg doses 3 times daily followed by a single 20-mg dose of nifedipine in healthy individuals increased nifedipine AUC values by 2.2 or 3.1 times, respectively, and peak plasma nifedipine concentrations by 2 or 1.7 times, respectively.

Angiotensin II Receptor Antagonists Nifedipine has been shown to inhibit the formation of oxidized metabolites of irbesartan in vitro; however, concomitant nifedipine therapy had no effect on irbesartan pharmacokinetics in clinical studies.

In addition, since candesartan is not substantially metabolized by the CYP isoenzyme system, no substantial drug interaction has been reported in individuals receiving nifedipine concomitantly with candesartan.

Antifungal Agents Concomitant use of nifedipine with ketoconazole, itraconazole, or fluconazole may affect the pharmacokinetics of nifedipine, possibly secondary to the inhibition of the CYP3A isoenzyme, and increased exposure of nifedipine may occur. Blood pressure should be monitored, and a decrease in nifedipine dosage should be considered.

Antiretroviral Agents Concomitant use of nifedipine with antiretroviral agents (HIV protease inhibitors [e.g., amprenavir, atazanavir, fosamprenavir, indinavir, nelfinavir, ritonavir] and nonnucleoside reverse transcriptase inhibitors [e.g., delavirdine]) may affect the pharmacokinetics of nifedipine, possibly secondary to the inhibition of the CYP3A isoenzyme, and may result in decreased nifedipine metabolism and increased nifedipine exposure. Caution is advised if nifedipine is administered concomitantly with these antiretroviral agents; patients should be monitored carefully.

Antituberculosis Agents Rifamycin derivatives (e.g., rifampin, rifabutin) can induce certain cytochrome P-450 liver enzymes (e.g., CYP3A isoenzyme) responsible for the metabolism of nifedipine. Concomitant use of these rifamycin derivatives and nifedipine may result in decreased plasma concentrations of nifedipine. In healthy individuals, concomitant use of oral rifampin (600 mg daily) and oral nifedipine (20 mcg/kg) or IV nifedipine resulted in an 87 or 30% decrease in nifedipine exposure, respectively. Adjustment of nifedipine dosage may be needed in patients receiving nifedipine concomitantly with rifamycin derivatives.

Quinupristin and Dalfopristin Concomitant use of nifedipine with quinupristin and dalfopristin may affect the pharmacokinetics of nifedipine, possibly secondary to the inhibition of the isoenzyme CYP3A. In healthy individuals, concomitant administration of repeated oral doses of nifedipine with

IV quinupristin and dalfopristin increased the median peak plasma concentration and the AUC of nifedipine by 18 and 44%, respectively. In patients receiving nifedipine concomitantly with quinupristin and dalfopristin, blood pressure should be monitored and nifedipine dosage reduced if needed.

Erythromycin Concomitant use of erythromycin (an inhibitor of the CYP3A4 isoenzyme) and nifedipine may result in inhibition of the metabolism of nifedipine and increased nifedipine exposure. Blood pressure should be monitored and nifedipine dosage reduced if necessary in patients in whom erythromycin is used concomitantly with nifedipine.

Histamine H_2-Receptor Antagonists Concomitant use of nifedipine (single 10-mg doses and 40–60 mg daily) with cimetidine (up to 1 g daily) in healthy individuals increased peak plasma nifedipine concentrations by approximately 60–102% and AUC of nifedipine by approximately 52–101%; plasma clearance of nifedipine was decreased by approximately 40%. Increases in the effect of nifedipine on blood pressure also have been observed in hypertensive patients receiving concomitant therapy with cimetidine (1 g daily) and nifedipine (10 mg daily). Peak plasma concentrations and AUCs of nifedipine also have increased with concomitant nifedipine and ranitidine therapy, but to a lesser degree than with cimetidine. Although the precise mechanism of these interactions is not known, cimetidine-induced inhibition of the cytochrome P-450 mixed-function oxidase system (the enzyme system that is probably responsible for the first-pass metabolism of nifedipine) may play a role. Pending further accumulation of data, cautious dosage titration of nifedipine is recommended in patients receiving cimetidine; a reduction in nifedipine dosage may be necessary in some patients previously stabilized on the drug when cimetidine therapy is initiated.

Since ranitidine interacts with the hepatic cytochrome P-450 (microsomal) enzyme system differently than does cimetidine, ranitidine appears to only minimally inhibit hepatic metabolism of some drugs. Results of several studies indicate that concomitant use of ranitidine with nifedipine did not affect exposure of nifedipine and no effects on blood pressure or heart rate have been observed when these drugs were used concomitantly in healthy individuals or hypertensive patients.

Anticonvulsant Agents Concomitant use of phenytoin with nifedipine may affect the pharmacokinetics of nifedipine. Phenytoin is an inducer of the CYP3A4 isoenzyme and may cause decreased nifedipine exposure. Concomitant use of nifedipine (as a 10-mg capsule or a 60-mg extended-release tablet) with phenytoin decreased (by about 70%) the AUC and peak plasma concentrations of nifedipine. Phenytoin toxicity has occurred within 4 weeks after initiating nifedipine in a patient stabilized on phenytoin. Manifestations of phenytoin toxicity (e.g., headaches, nystagmus, tremors, slurred speech, ataxia, mental depression) resolved and plasma concentrations of the drug decreased within 2 weeks after discontinuance of nifedipine. While the mechanism of this interaction has not been elucidated, it was suggested that nifedipine may have reduced the metabolism of phenytoin.

Phenytoin toxicity also reportedly has occurred in at least one patient with subarachnoid hemorrhage receiving nimodipine, another 1,4-dihydropyridine calcium-channel blocker. Whether this effect represented an actual drug interaction between phenytoin and nimodipine has not been determined to date. However, most patients with subarachnoid hemorrhage receiving nimodipine also received concomitant therapy with phenytoin or barbiturates reportedly with no apparent evidence of drug interactions.

Pending further accumulation of data, patients and plasma phenytoin concentrations should be monitored carefully whenever therapy with a 1,4-dihydropyridine calcium-channel blocker is initiated or withdrawn from a patient receiving phenytoin. Blood pressure should be monitored and nifedipine dosage adjusted as needed in patients receiving concomitant nifedipine and phenytoin therapy.

Phenobarbital and carbamazepine also may decrease exposure to nifedipine by inducing the CYP3A isoenzyme. In patients receiving nifedipine concomitantly with phenobarbital or carbamazepine, adjustment of nifedipine dosage may be needed. Conversely, nifedipine exposure may be increased in patients receiving valproic acid concomitantly with nifedipine; blood pressure should be monitored, and a reduction in nifedipine dosage should be considered in these patients.

Immunosuppressive Agents Because nifedipine may inhibit metabolism of tacrolimus, a substrate of CYP3A4, concomitant use of nifedipine and tacrolimus may result in increased tacrolimus exposure. In patients who underwent transplantation and received such concomitant therapy, tacrolimus dosage reductions of 26–38% were required; tacrolimus blood concentrations should be monitored, and a reduction in tacrolimus dosage should be considered in these patients.

Although sirolimus is a substrate for the isoenzyme 3A4, no clinically important pharmacokinetic interactions were observed in patients receiving nifedipine (a single 60-mg dose) concomitantly with oral sirolimus (a single 10-mg dose).

Dolasetron Although hydrodolasetron (the main active metabolite of dolasetron) is extensively metabolized, principally via the CYP system, including the 2D6 and 3A4 isoenzymes, concomitant use of IV or oral dolasetron with nifedipine did not alter the clearance of the metabolite.

Other Drugs Affecting Hepatic Microsomal Enzymes Ethanol can increase the oral bioavailability of nifedipine, possibly via inhibition of hepatic cytochrome P-450 microsomal metabolism. In one study in healthy adults, concomitant administration of ethanol with a single 20-mg oral dose of nifedipine capsules resulted in a 54% increase in the AUC of nifedipine.

Nefazodone, an inhibitor of the CYP3A isoenzyme, may inhibit the metabolism of nifedipine and increase nifedipine exposure; blood pressure should be monitored, and a reduction of nifedipine dosage should be considered in patients receiving nefazodone concomitantly with nifedipine.

St. John's wort may decrease nifedipine exposure by inducing the CYP3A4 isoenzyme. Adjustment of nifedipine dosage may be necessary in patients receiving nifedipine concomitantly with St. John's wort.

Grapefruit Juice Concomitant oral administration of grapefruit juice with nifedipine has been reported to increase bioavailability of the drug. Peak plasma concentrations and AUC values of nifedipine have been reported to increase by approximately twofold (with no change in elimination half-life) when the drug is administered with grapefruit juice. The interaction between grapefruit juice and the oral bioavailability of some 1,4-dihydropyridine-derivative calcium-channel blocking agents appears to result from inhibition, probably prehepatic, of the cytochrome P-450 enzyme system by some constituent(s) in the juice. Following oral administration of nifedipine, such prehepatic inhibition of drug metabolism by grapefruit juice appears mainly to involve the CYP3A4 isoenzyme, principally within the wall of the small intestine (e.g., in the jejunum), thus increasing systemic availability of the drug. (See Grapefruit Juice under Drug Interactions: Drugs and Foods Affecting Hepatic Microsomal Enzymes, in Cyclosporine 92:44.) Concomitant oral administration of grapefruit juice and nifedipine should be avoided. Consumption of grapefruit juice should be discontinued at least 3 days prior to initiating nifedipine therapy.

■ **β-Adrenergic Blocking Agents** Although concomitant therapy usually is well tolerated, the risk of severe hypotension, exacerbation of angina, congestive heart failure, and arrhythmia may be increased when nifedipine is used concomitantly with a β-adrenergic blocking agent (β-blocker) (e.g., propranolol, timolol), as compared with nifedipine alone. One manufacturer states that clinical monitoring is recommended in patients receiving nifedipine concomitantly with a β-blocker, and adjustment of nifedipine dosage should be considered. Exacerbation of anginal pain also has been observed when β-blocker therapy was being withdrawn concurrently with initiation of nifedipine therapy; gradual reduction of β-blocker dosage instead of abrupt withdrawal may minimize the risk of this effect.

■ **Fentanyl** Severe hypotension has occurred during surgery in patients receiving nifedipine, a β-blocker, and fentanyl concomitantly. The manufacturers recommend temporarily withholding nifedipine for at least 36 hours before surgery in which use of high-dose fentanyl is contemplated, if the patient's condition permits.

■ **Digoxin** Most evidence indicates that nifedipine does not substantially affect the pharmacokinetics of digoxin when the drugs are administered concomitantly; however, some data suggest that serum digoxin concentrations may increase by about 15–45% during concomitant therapy. Further evaluation of this potential interaction is needed. Since there have been isolated reports of increased serum digoxin concentrations during concomitant administration, serum digoxin concentrations should be monitored when nifedipine therapy is initiated or discontinued or dosage of nifedipine is adjusted in patients receiving digoxin. Patients receiving the drugs concomitantly should be monitored for signs and symptoms of digoxin toxicity and dosage of the cardiac glycoside reduced if necessary.

■ **Antidiabetic Agents** Since nifedipine may produce hyperglycemia which may lead to loss of glycemic control, glucose concentrations should be carefully monitored and adjustment of nifedipine dosage should be considered in patients receiving concomitant therapy with nifedipine and acarbose.

Nifedipine appears to enhance absorption of metformin. In healthy individuals, concomitant use of nifedipine with metformin was associated with 20 and 9% increases in peak plasma concentrations and AUC of metformin, respectively.

■ **Omeprazole** Administration of omeprazole 20 mg daily for 8 days followed by a single 10-mg dose of nifedipine in healthy individuals increased AUC of nifedipine by 26% and decreased peak plasma concentrations of nifedipine by 13% when compared with placebo followed by a single 10-mg dose of nifedipine. Concomitant use of omeprazole and nifedipine did not alter the effects of nifedipine on blood pressure or heart rate. The effect of omeprazole on nifedipine pharmacokinetics is unlikely to be clinically important.

■ **Hypotensive Agents** Concomitant administration of nifedipine with hypotensive agents (e.g., methyldopa, hydralazine, captopril, doxazosin) may increase the incidence of severe hypotension. When nifedipine is added to an existing antihypertensive therapy regimen, the patient should be observed closely for severe hypotension, especially during initial titration or upward adjustment of nifedipine dosage.

Attenuation of the tachycardic effect of nifedipine has been observed in patients receiving concomitant benazepril.

■ **Anticoagulants** Increased prothrombin time has been reported rarely in patients receiving concomitant therapy with nifedipine and coumarin anticoagulants; however, a causal relationship to nifedipine has not been established.

■ **Platelet-aggregation Inhibitors** No clinically important interactions have been reported in patients receiving nifedipine concomitantly with clopidogrel or tirofiban.

■ **Other Drugs** The manufacturer of Adalat® CC extended-release nifedipine tablets states that clinical experience is insufficient to recommend concomitant use of nifedipine with flecainide.

Acute Toxicity

Experience with acute overdosage of nifedipine is limited. Generally, overdosage with the drug would be expected to produce toxic effects that are extensions of the usual adverse effects of the drug, including pronounced hypotension. If pronounced hypotension occurs, symptomatic and supportive care should be initiated, including active cardiovascular support that includes monitoring of cardiovascular and respiratory function, elevation of the extremities, and judicious use of parenteral calcium salts, vasopressors, and fluids. Other symptoms associated with severe nifedipine overdosage include loss of consciousness, heart rhythm disturbances, metabolic acidosis, hypoxia, and cardiogenic shock with pulmonary edema. Clearance of nifedipine would be expected to be prolonged in patients with impaired hepatic function, since the drug is metabolized in the liver. Because nifedipine is highly protein bound, hemodialysis is unlikely to promote elimination of the drug; however, plasmapheresis may prove beneficial.

In a young man who intentionally ingested 4.8 g of extended-release nifedipine tablets, the principal manifestations of overdosage initially were dizziness, palpitations, flushing, and nervousness. Nausea, vomiting, and generalized edema developed within several hours following ingestion of the drug; however, no substantial hypotension developed approximately 18 hours after ingestion. Mild, transient elevation of serum creatinine and modest elevations in serum LDH and creatine kinase (CK, creatine phosphokinase, CPK) were observed, but serum AST was normal. The patient's vital signs remained stable, no ECG abnormalities were observed, and renal function returned to normal within 24–48 hours with routine supportive measures only. No prolonged sequelae were observed.

In a patient with angina and a history of bundle branch block who was receiving tricyclic antidepressants and ingested a single 900-mg dose of nifedipine capsules, loss of consciousness (within 30 minutes of nifedipine ingestion) and profound hypotension (which responded to calcium infusion, pressor agents, and fluid replacement) were observed. Because ECG abnormalities (e.g., sinus bradycardia, varying degrees of AV block) developed, a temporary ventricular pacemaker was required; thereafter, ECG abnormalities resolved spontaneously. Substantial hyperglycemia also was observed but resolved rapidly without treatment.

Ingestion of a single 280-mg dose of nifedipine capsules in a young patient with hypertension and advanced renal failure resulted in marked hypotension which responded to calcium infusion and fluids. No AV conduction abnormalities, arrhythmias, pronounced change in heart rate, or further deterioration in renal function were observed.

Pharmacology

Nifedipine has pharmacologic actions similar to those of other dihydropyridine calcium-channel blocking agents (e.g., felodipine, nisoldipine). The principal physiologic action of nifedipine is to inhibit the transmembrane influx of extracellular calcium ions across the membranes of myocardial cells and vascular smooth muscle cells, without changing serum calcium concentrations.

Calcium plays important roles in the excitation-contraction coupling processes of the heart and vascular smooth muscle cells and in the electrical discharge of the specialized conduction cells of the heart. The membranes of these cells contain numerous channels that carry a slow inward current and that are selective for calcium. Activation of these slow calcium channels contributes to the plateau phase (phase 2) of the action potential of cardiac and vascular smooth muscle cells.

The exact mechanism whereby nifedipine inhibits calcium ion influx across the slow calcium channels is not known, but the drug is thought to inhibit ion-control gating mechanisms of the channel, deform the slow channel, and/or interfere with release of calcium from the sarcoplasmic reticulum.

By inhibiting calcium influx, nifedipine inhibits the contractile processes of cardiac and vascular smooth muscle, thereby dilating the main coronary and systemic arteries. In patients with Prinzmetal variant angina (vasospastic angina), inhibition of spontaneous and ergonovine-induced coronary artery spasm by nifedipine results in increased myocardial oxygen delivery. Dilation of systemic arteries by nifedipine results in a decrease in total peripheral resistance, a usually modest decrease in systemic blood pressure (e.g., a decrease of 5–10 mm Hg), a decrease in the afterload of the heart, a small reflex increase in heart rate, and an increase in the cardiac index. The reduction in afterload, seen at rest and with exercise, and its resultant decrease in myocardial oxygen consumption are thought to be responsible for the effects of nifedipine in patients with chronic stable angina pectoris.

In contrast to verapamil and diltiazem, nifedipine has little or no effect on sinoatrial (SA) and atrioventricular (AV) nodal conduction at therapeutic doses.

Although negative inotropic effects have been noted in vitro and in animal studies with nifedipine, they are rarely, if ever, seen clinically, probably because of reflex responses to the drug's vasodilating actions including a small increase in heart rate. Major increases in left ventricular end-diastolic pressure (LVEDP) or volume (LVEDV) or decreases in cardiac ejection fraction usually are not seen following nifedipine administration in patients with normal ventricular function. In patients with impaired ventricular function, some increase in ejection fraction and reduction in left ventricular filling pressure may be seen acutely.

Pharmacokinetics

■ **Absorption** Approximately 90% of an oral dose of nifedipine is rapidly absorbed from the GI tract following oral administration of the drug as conventional capsules. Only about 45–75% of an oral dose as conventional capsules reaches systemic circulation as unchanged drug since nifedipine is metabolized on first pass through the liver. Peak serum concentrations usually are reached within 0.5–2 hours after oral administration as conventional capsules. Food appears to decrease the rate but not the extent of absorption of nifedipine as conventional capsules.

The manufacturer states that relative oral bioavailability differs little if conventional nifedipine capsules are swallowed intact, bitten and swallowed, or bitten and held sublingually. However, some data indicate that the rate and extent of absorption of nifedipine following sublingual administration may be decreased substantially. In several studies, peak plasma concentrations of nifedipine appeared to be delayed and decreased following sublingual administration. In one crossover study in healthy adults in which a 10-mg conventional capsule of the drug was bitten and held sublingually for 20 minutes or bitten and swallowed, the bioavailability following sublingual administration was 17% (range: 7–28%) of that following oral administration of a bitten capsule; on average, 86% of the dose remained in the mouth at the end of the 20-minute sublingual retention period. In this study, peak serum nifedipine concentrations following sublingual or oral administration of a bitten capsule occurred within 50 (range: 20–99) or 30 (range: 15–49) minutes, respectively, and averaged 10 (range: 5–17) or 82 (range: 44–146) ng/mL, respectively. Oral bioavailability of nifedipine may be increased up to twofold in patients with liver cirrhosis.

The commercially available extended-release tablets of nifedipine (Procardia XL®) contain the drug in an oral osmotic delivery system formulation (elementary osmotic pump, gastrointestinal therapeutic system [GITS]). The osmotic delivery system consists of an osmotically active core (comprised of a layer containing the drug and a layer containing osmotically active but pharmacologically inert components) that is surrounded by a semipermeable membrane with a laser-drilled delivery orifice and is designed to deliver the drug at an approximately constant rate over a 24-hour period (approximately zero-order delivery). When exposed to water in the GI tract, water is drawn osmotically into the core at a controlled rate that is determined by the permeability of the outer membrane and the osmotic pressure of the core formulation; as water enters the formulation, a resulting suspension of the drug is pushed out the delivery orifice of the membrane into the GI tract. Delivery of nifedipine from the formulation depends on the existence of an osmotic gradient between the fluid in the GI tract and the osmotically active core of the tablet, with drug delivery remaining approximately constant as long as the gradient is maintained and then declining parabolically to zero as the concentration inside the tablet falls below saturation. The rate of nifedipine delivery in the GI tract is independent of pH over the range of 1.2–7.5 and probably GI motility. The inert tablet ingredients remain intact and are eliminated in feces.

Extended-release tablets (Procardia XL®) labeled as containing 30, 60, or 90 mg of nifedipine reportedly deliver the drug into the GI tract at an approximately constant rate of 1.7, 3.4, and 5.1 mg/hour, respectively, throughout the 24-hour dosing period. Following oral administration of a single dose of the drug as extended-release tablets, plasma nifedipine concentrations increase gradually, reaching a peak at approximately 6 hours, and bioavailability is approximately 55–65% of that achieved with the same doses administered orally as conventional capsules. Following multiple doses, oral bioavailability from the extended-release tablets increases to approximately 75–86% of that achieved with the same doses administered as conventional capsules. Administration of Procardia XL® nifedipine extended-release tablets with food can increase the early rate of GI absorption but reportedly does not affect overall bioavailability.

The commercially available extended-release tablets of nifedipine (Adalat® CC) are composed of a slow-release outer coat and an immediate-release core. The bioavailability of nifedipine as Adalat® CC extended-release tablets relative to conventional nifedipine capsules is about 84–89%. Following oral administration of Adalat® CC in fasting individuals, peak plasma concentrations occur within 2.5–5 hours, with a small second peak (or "shoulder") occurring within 6–12 hours. Following oral administration of Adalat® CC extended-release nifedipine 30-mg tablets over a dosage range of 30–90 mg, the area under the plasma-concentration time curve (AUC) was proportional to the dose administered; however, peak plasma concentrations of the 90-mg dose (three 30-mg tablets) were 29% greater than that predicted from the 30- and 60-mg doses. Once-daily dosing of Adalat® CC extended-release tablets, under fasting conditions, resulted in less fluctuation in plasma nifedipine concentrations when compared with 3-times-daily dosing with conventional nifedipine capsules. Following administration of a single Adalat® CC 90-mg extended-release tablet under fasting conditions, mean peak plasma nifedipine concentration of about 115 ng/mL were reported. Administration of Adalat® CC extended-release tablets immediately after a high-fat meal increases peak plasma nifedipine concentrations by 60% and delays the time to peak plasma concentrations; however, no substantial changes in AUC occur. Peak plasma concentrations of nifedipine following administration of Adalat® CC extended-release tablets after a high-fat meal are slightly lower compared with those occurring after administration of the same daily dosage given in 3 divided doses as the conventional nifedipine capsules; this difference may be attributed to the lower bioavailability of Adalat® CC extended-release tablets compared with that of conventional nifedipine capsules.

Following oral administration of Adalat® CC extended-release nifedipine tablets in healthy geriatric individuals (older than 60 years of age), the mean peak plasma concentrations and average plasma concentrations of nifedipine increased by 36 and 70%, respectively, compared with those observed in younger adults.

With another extended-release tablet formulation (Adalat L®, not commercially available in the US), both the rate and extent (over 12 hours) of absorption of a single dose of nifedipine were increased by administration with food. Because orally administered nifedipine undergoes extensive metabolism on first pass through the liver, bioavailability of the drug from extended-release tablets is increased substantially in patients with liver cirrhosis and may be particularly increased in those with portacaval shunts. Substantial reductions in GI retention time for prolonged periods (e.g., in patients with short-bowel syndrome) can result in decreased absorption of nifedipine from extended-release tablets.

■ **Distribution** Binding of nifedipine to plasma proteins is concentration dependent and ranges from 92–98%. Protein binding may be reduced in patients with renal or hepatic (e.g., liver cirrhosis) impairment.

■ **Elimination** In patients with normal renal and hepatic function, the plasma half-life of nifedipine is about 2 hours when administered as conventional capsules, and about 7 hours when administered as extended-release tablets (Adalat® CC). The drug is extensively metabolized in the liver (to highly water-soluble, inactive metabolites) by the cytochrome P-450 microsomal enzyme system, including CYP3A. Approximately 60–80% of an oral dose of nifedipine is excreted as metabolites in the urine, with only traces (less than 0.1%) of an oral dose being excreted in urine as unchanged drug. The remainder of a dose is excreted in the feces as metabolites, possibly via biliary elimination. Nifedipine appears to be negligibly removed by hemodialysis or hemoperfusion.

Adalat® CC extended-release tablets should be used with caution in patients with renal impairment because absorption of the drug may be altered in such patients. In patients with hepatic impairment, elimination of the drug may be altered. The elimination half-life of nifedipine has been reported to increase to 7 hours in patients with liver cirrhosis; oral bioavailability of the drug also is increased in such patients.

Following IV administration of nifedipine, body clearance of the drug is 519 and 348 mL/minute in young adults and geriatric individuals, respectively.

Chemistry and Stability

■ **Chemistry** Nifedipine is a 1,4-dihydropyridine-derivative calcium-channel blocking agent. The drug occurs as a yellow, crystalline powder and is practically insoluble in water and soluble in alcohol.

■ **Stability** Nifedipine liquid-filled capsules should be protected from light and moisture and stored in tight, light-resistant containers at a temperature of 15–25°C, and extended-release tablets of the drug should be protected from light and moisture and stored in tight, light-resistant containers at a temperature less than 30°C.

Preparations

Excipients in commercially available drug preparations may have clinically important effects in some individuals; consult specific product labeling for details.

NIFEdipine

Oral		
Capsules, liquid-filled	10 mg*	**NIFEdipine Capsules**
		Procardia®, Pfizer
	20 mg*	**NIFEdipine Capsules**
Tablets, extended-release, film-coated	30 mg*	**Adalat® CC**, Bayer
		Afeditab® CR, Watson
		Nifedical® XL, Teva
		NIFEdipine ER
		Procardia XL®, Pfizer
	60 mg*	**Adalat® CC**, Bayer
		Afeditab® CR, Watson
		Nifedical® XL, Teva
		NIFEdipine ER
		Procardia XL®, Pfizer
	90 mg*	**Adalat® CC**, Bayer
		NIFEdipine ER
		Procardia XL®, Pfizer

*available from one or more manufacturer, distributor, and/or repackager by generic (nonproprietary) name

†Use is not currently included in the labeling approved by the US Food and Drug Administration

Calcium-Channel Blocking Agents, Miscellaneous 24:28.92

dilTIAZem Hydrochloride

Latiazem Hydrochloride

■ Diltiazem is a nondihydropyridine calcium-channel blocking agent (calcium-channel blocker).

Uses

Diltiazem is used in the management of Prinzmetal variant angina, chronic stable angina pectoris, supraventricular tachycardias, and hypertension.

■ **Angina** Diltiazem is used in the management of angina, including chronic stable angina, Prinzmetal variant angina, and unstable angina†. Calcium-channel blockers (used alone or in combination with nitrates) are considered the drugs of choice for the management of Prinzmetal variant angina. β-Adrenergic blocking agents (β-blockers) are recommended as the anti-ischemic drugs of choice in most patients with chronic stable angina; however, calcium-channel blockers may be substituted or added in patients who do not tolerate or respond adequately to β-blockers. In short-term, controlled clinical studies in patients with chronic stable angina, oral diltiazem reduced the frequency of attacks, allowed a decrease in sublingual nitroglycerin dosage, and increased exercise tolerance. All classes of calcium-channel blockers appear to be equally effective in reducing anginal episodes; however, choice of a specific agent should be individualized since the pharmacologic properties of these drugs differ.

Diltiazem also may be beneficial in patients with unstable angina†; experts recommend the use of a nondihydropyridine calcium-channel blocker (e.g., diltiazem, verapamil) for the relief of ongoing or recurrent ischemia when β-blocker therapy is inadequate, not tolerated, or contraindicated in patients with unstable angina who do not have clinically important left ventricular dysfunction, increased risk of cardiogenic shock, or AV block.

Although concurrent use of some calcium-channel blockers and a β-blocker may have beneficial effects in some patients (e.g., reduction of dihydropyridine-induced tachycardia through β-blockade), combined use of diltiazem with a β-blocker generally should be avoided because of the potential adverse effects on AV nodal conduction, heart rate, and cardiac contractility. (See β-Adrenergic Blocking Agents under Drug Interactions: Drugs Known to Impair Cardiac Contractility and Conduction.)

■ **Hypertension** Oral diltiazem is used alone or in combination with other classes of antihypertensive agents in the management of hypertension. Only extended-release formulations of diltiazem are recommended for the management of hypertension.

Calcium-channel blockers (e.g., diltiazem) are considered one of several preferred antihypertensive drug classes for the initial management of hypertension according to current evidence-based hypertension guidelines; other preferred options include angiotensin-converting enzyme (ACE) inhibitors, angiotensin II receptor antagonists, and thiazide diuretics. While there may be individual differences with respect to recommendations for initial drug selection and use in specific patient populations, current evidence indicates that these antihypertensive drug classes all generally produce comparable effects on overall mortality and cardiovascular, cerebrovascular, and renal outcomes. (See Uses: Hypertension, in Amlodipine 24:28.08.)

Calcium-channel blockers may be particularly useful in the management of hypertension in patients with certain coexisting conditions such as ischemic heart disease (e.g., angina) and in geriatric patients, including those with isolated systolic hypertension. (See Uses: Hypertension, in Amlodipine 24:28.08.) In addition, nondihydropyridine calcium-channel blockers may be beneficial in hypertensive patients with coexisting atrial fibrillation and a rapid ventricular rate. However, some experts recommend against the use of nondihydropyridine calcium-channel blockers in patients who have heart failure with reduced ejection fraction because of the drugs' myocardial depressant activity and unfavorable outcomes in some clinical trials in patients with heart failure receiving the drugs.

In the Antihypertensive and Lipid-lowering Treatment to Prevent Heart Attack Trial (ALLHAT), the long-term cardiovascular morbidity and mortality benefit of a long-acting dihydropyridine calcium-channel blocker (amlodipine), a thiazide-like diuretic (chlorthalidone), and an ACE inhibitor (lisinopril) were compared in a broad population of patients with hypertension at risk for coronary heart disease. Although these antihypertensive agents were comparably effective in providing important cardiovascular benefit, apparent differences in certain secondary outcomes were observed. Patients receiving the ACE inhibitor experienced higher risks of stroke, combined cardiovascular disease, GI bleeding, and angioedema, while those receiving the calcium-channel blocker were at higher risk of developing heart failure. The ALLHAT investigators suggested that the observed differences in cardiovascular outcome may be attributable, at least in part, to the greater antihypertensive effect of the calcium-channel blocker compared with that of the ACE inhibitor, especially in women and black patients. (See Clinical Benefits of Thiazides in Hypertension under Hypertension in Adults: Treatment Benefits, in Uses in the Thiazides General Statement 40:28.20.)

Most patients with hypertension, especially black patients, will require at least 2 antihypertensive drugs to achieve adequate blood pressure control. Calcium-channel blockers may be particularly useful in the management of hypertension in black patients; these patients tend to have greater blood pressure response to calcium-channel blockers and thiazide diuretics than to other antihypertensive drug classes (e.g., ACE inhibitors, angiotensin II receptor antagonists). However, the combination of an ACE inhibitor or an angiotensin II receptor antagonist with a calcium-channel blocker or thiazide diuretic produces similar blood pressure lowering in black patients as in other racial groups. (See Race under Hypertension: Other Special Considerations for Antihypertensive Therapy, in Uses in Amlodipine 24:28.08.)

For additional information on the role of calcium-channel blockers in the management of hypertension, see Uses: Hypertension, in Amlodipine 24:28.08. For information on overall principles and expert recommendations for treatment of hypertension, see Uses: Hypertension in Adults, and also see Uses: Hypertension in Pediatric Patients, in the Thiazides General Statement 40:28.20.

■ **Supraventricular Arrhythmias** Diltiazem is used in the management of supraventricular tachycardias (SVTs), including rapid conversion to sinus rhythm of paroxysmal supraventricular tachycardia (PSVT) (e.g., tachycardia associated with Wolff-Parkinson-White or Lown-Ganong-Levine syndrome), and control of rapid ventricular rate in atrial flutter or fibrillation. The American College of Cardiology/American Heart Association/Heart Rhythm Society (ACC/AHA/HRS) guideline for the management of adults with supraventricular tachycardia recommends the use of diltiazem in the treatment of various SVTs (e.g., atrial flutter, junctional tachycardia, focal atrial tachycardia, atrioventricular nodal reentrant tachycardia [AVNRT]); in general, IV diltiazem is recommended for acute treatment while oral diltiazem is recommended for ongoing management of these arrhythmias. Vagal maneuvers and/or IV adenosine are considered first-line interventions for the acute treatment of patients with SVT and should be attempted prior to other therapies when clinically indicated; if such measures are ineffective or not feasible, a nondihydropyridine calcium-channel blocker (i.e., diltiazem or verapamil) may be considered. Diltiazem should only be used in hemodynamically stable patients who do not have impaired ventricular function.

Paroxysmal Supraventricular Tachycardia IV diltiazem is used for rapid conversion of PSVT that is uncontrolled or unconverted by vagal maneuvers and adenosine, including atrioventricular nodal reentrant tachycardias and PSVT associated with extranodal accessory pathways (e.g., Wolff-Parkinson-White or Lown-Ganong-Levine syndrome). In about 86–88% of patients with PSVT, IV diltiazem produces rapid conversion (usually within 2–3 minutes of the first or second dose) to sinus rhythm; conversion to sinus rhythm appears to be dose related. Limited data indicate that conversion to sinus rhythm may occur spontaneously in 25% of placebo-treated patients with PSVT. Transient ventricular premature complexes may be present following conversion of PSVT to sinus rhythm but appear to be benign and of little clinical importance. While comparative trials have not been performed with IV diltiazem and other calcium-channel blockers, the efficacy rate of IV diltiazem in converting PSVT to sinus rhythm appears to be similar to that of verapamil.

Oral diltiazem also has been used to prevent PSVT, but efficacy of the drug for this condition has not been established.

Atrial Fibrillation and Flutter Nondihydropyridine calcium-channel blockers (e.g., diltiazem, verapamil) are recommended as one of several drug therapy options for ventricular rate control in patients with nonpreexcited atrial fibrillation or flutter. Management of atrial fibrillation or flutter depends on the clinical situation and the patient's condition. For acute treatment of atrial fibrillation, IV diltiazem may be used. Cardioversion is indicated, however, in hemodynamically unstable patients. IV diltiazem should *not* be used when atrial flutter or fibrillation is associated with an accessory pathway that has a short refractory period (e.g., Wolff-Parkinson-White or Lown-Ganong-Levine syndrome) or with preexcited ventricular complexes or wide QRS complexes, since ventricular tachyarrhythmias, including ventricular fibrillation and cardiac arrest, may be precipitated. Although approximately 95% of patients with atrial flutter or fibrillation respond to direct IV injection of 1 or 2 doses with at least a 20% reduction in ventricular rate and this reduction in heart rate is maintained in at least 83% of patients with continuous IV infusion of the drug, IV diltiazem alone rarely (i.e., less than 10% of patients) converts atrial flutter or fibrillation to normal sinus rhythm; limited data indicate that conversion to sinus rhythm may be dose-related and is not usually seen with recommended doses. Conversion to sinus rhythm after drug therapy is more likely to occur in atrial flutter or atrial fibrillation that is of recent onset (i.e., within 24–48 hours) in patients without structural heart disease.

While comparative trials have not been performed with IV diltiazem and IV digoxin, pharmacokinetic data indicate that diltiazem has a faster onset of action than digoxin and may be more useful for slowing ventricular response in patients with atrial flutter or fibrillation. Calcium-channel blockers (i.e., diltiazem or verapamil) may be used for the management of atrial fibrillation associated with an acute myocardial infarction (MI) in patients with a β-blocker intolerance. (See Uses: Acute Myocardial Infarction.)

Oral diltiazem also has been used to reduce heart rate in patients with atrial fibrillation†, but efficacy of the drug for this condition has not been established.

Atrial Tachycardia IV diltiazem may be used for the acute treatment of patients with hemodynamically stable focal atrial tachycardia† (i.e., regular SVT arising from a localized atrial site), and oral diltiazem may be used for ongoing management.

IV diltiazem also may be used in patients with multifocal atrial tachycardia† (i.e., rapid, irregular rhythm with at least 3 distinct P-wave morphologies), although such arrhythmia is commonly associated with an underlying condition (e.g., pulmonary, coronary, or valvular heart disease) and is generally not responsive to antiarrhythmic drugs. Antiarrhythmic drug therapy usually is reserved for patients who do not respond to initial attempts at correcting or managing potential precipitating factors (e.g., exacerbation of chronic obstructive pulmonary disease or congestive heart failure, electrolyte and/or ventilatory disturbances, infection, theophylline toxicity) or in whom a precipitating factor cannot be identified. While specific studies have not been performed with IV diltiazem in patients with multifocal atrial tachycardia, the effects of the drug are expected to be similar to that of IV verapamil, which has been shown to have some efficacy in the acute treatment of this arrhythmia. Orally administered diltiazem may be a reasonable choice for chronic suppression of recurrent symptomatic multifocal atrial tachycardia.

Junctional Tachycardia Diltiazem may be used for the treatment of junctional tachycardia† (i.e., nonreentrant SVT originating from the AV junction), a rapid, occasionally irregular, narrow-complex tachycardia. β-Adrenergic blocking agents generally are used for acute termination and/or ongoing management of junctional tachycardia; limited evidence suggests there may be a role for diltiazem when β-blocking agents (particularly propranolol) are ineffective.

■ **Acute Myocardial Infarction** Calcium-channel blockers have been used in the early treatment and secondary prevention of acute MI†; although these drugs are effective anti-ischemic agents, they have not demonstrated mortality benefits and therefore are generally used as an alternative to β-blockers. A review of 28 randomized controlled studies involving 19,000 patients found no benefit with regard to infarct size, rate of reinfarction, or death when calcium-channel blockers were used during the acute or convalescent phase of ST-segment-elevation MI (STEMI). Although some studies demonstrated a reduced risk of reinfarction when verapamil or diltiazem was administered after MI in patients without left ventricular dysfunction, other studies have not confirmed this finding. Calcium-channel blockers generally are used for their anti-ischemic and blood pressure-reducing properties in the MI setting, and only when β-blockers (which have been shown to reduce mortality after MI) are ineffective, not tolerated, or contraindicated; because the nondihydropyridine calcium-channel blockers (verapamil and diltiazem) can cause substantial negative inotropic effects, their use should be limited to patients without left ventricular dysfunction.

Current expert guidelines state that a calcium-channel blocker may be used to relieve ischemic symptoms, lower blood pressure, or control rapid ventricular response associated with atrial fibrillation in patients with STEMI who are intolerant to β-blockers. A nondihydropyridine calcium-channel blocker (e.g., verapamil or diltiazem) may be used as an alternative to β-blockers for relief of ongoing or recurring ischemia when β-blocker therapy is inadequate, not tolerated, or contraindicated in patients with non-ST-segment-elevation MI (NSTEMI) who do not have clinically important left ventricular dysfunction, increased risk of cardiogenic shock, or AV block. The use of immediate-release nifedipine is generally contraindicated because of the potential for hypotension and reflex sympathetic activation.

■ **Other Uses** Diltiazem has been used with good results as an alternative to β-adrenergic blocking agents (e.g., propranolol) for short-term adjunctive therapy in the treatment of tachycardia and tachyarrhythmias in a limited number of patients with hyperthyroidism and/or thyrotoxicosis†. Diltiazem hydrochloride (160–480 mg daily in divided doses) has reduced heart rate, blood pressure, and ventricular and supraventricular premature complexes in patients with these conditions. Diltiazem does not affect the underlying disease, which must be treated with antithyroid therapy. While additional study and experience are necessary, diltiazem may be a useful alternative to β-adrenergic blocking agents in patients in whom therapy with these agents is contraindicated or not tolerated.

Dosage and Administration

■ **Administration** Diltiazem hydrochloride is administered by direct IV injection, continuous IV infusion, or orally.

Oral Administration Diltiazem hydrochloride is administered orally as conventional tablets, extended-release capsules, and extended-release tablets. Diltiazem also has been available as diltiazem malate alone or in combination with enalapril, but these preparations no longer are commercially available in the US.

Directions for administration (e.g., dosing frequency, whether to administer with or without food, potential for opening capsules and mixing with food) may vary by manufacturer and formulation; the manufacturer's information for a specific preparation should be consulted for detailed information.

Parenteral Administration Diltiazem hydrochloride is administered by direct IV injection or continuous IV infusion in the management of supraventricular tachyarrhythmias.

For direct IV injection or continuous IV infusion, diltiazem is given slowly under continuous ECG and blood pressure monitoring during the administration period. Solutions of the drug should be inspected visually for particulate matter or discoloration prior to IV administration whenever solution and container permit.

IV Injection. When administered by direct IV injection, diltiazem hydrochloride injection containing 5 mg/mL requires no further dilution.

IV Infusion. When administered as a continuous IV infusion, 25, 50, or 50 mL of diltiazem hydrochloride injection containing 5 mg/mL should be added to 100, 250, or 500 mL of a compatible infusion solution (i.e., 0.9% sodium chloride, 5% dextrose, or 5% dextrose and 0.45% sodium chloride) to produce a final diltiazem hydrochloride concentration of 1, 0.83, or 0.45 mg/mL, respectively. Alternatively, IV infusions with a final concentration of 1 mg/mL can be prepared using the single-dose 100-mg ADD-Vantage® vials of diltiazem hydrochloride.

■ Dosage

Potency of diltiazem hydrochloride preparations is expressed in terms of the hydrochloride. (See Chemistry and Stability: Chemistry.)

Dosage of diltiazem hydrochloride must be carefully adjusted according to individual requirements, tolerance, and response. The manufacturers state that dosage of diltiazem for geriatric patients should be selected carefully because these individuals frequently have decreased hepatic, renal, and/or cardiac function and concomitant disease and drug therapy.

Angina For the management of Prinzmetal variant angina or chronic stable angina pectoris, the usual initial adult dosage of diltiazem hydrochloride as conventional tablets is 30 mg 4 times daily. Generally, dosage is gradually increased at 1- to 2-day intervals until optimum control of angina is obtained. The average optimum adult dosage range for diltiazem hydrochloride tablets appears to be 180–360 mg daily given in 3 or 4 divided doses. Geriatric patients may respond to lower dosages. After anginal symptoms are controlled, dosage should be gradually reduced to the lowest level that will maintain relief of symptoms.

When diltiazem hydrochloride is administered as extended-release capsules (Tiazac®, Dilt-XR®, Taztia XT®) or extended-release tablets (Cardizem® LA, Matzim® LA) for the management of chronic stable angina, the usual initial adult dosage is 120 mg (Dilt-XR®), 120–180 mg (Tiazac®, Taztia XT®) or 180 mg (Cardizem® LA, Matzim® LA) once daily. When diltiazem hydrochloride is administered as Cardizem® CD or Cartia XT® extended-release capsules for the management of chronic stable angina and angina secondary to coronary artery spasm, the usual initial adult dosage is 120–180 mg once daily.

Dosage should be individualized based on response; when dosage increases are necessary, they should be titrated over 7–14 days. Some patients may respond to higher dosages of up to 360 mg (Cardizem® LA, Matzim® LA), 480 mg (Dilt-XR®, Cardizem CD®, Cartia XT®), or 540 mg (Tiazac®, Taztia XT®) once daily.

Hypertension **Usual Dosage.** For the management of hypertension in adults receiving diltiazem hydrochloride as monotherapy, the usual initial dosage as the extended-release capsules (Cardizem® CD, Cartia XT®, Dilt-XR®) or extended-release tablets (Cardizem® LA, Matzim® LA) is 180–240 mg once daily. When the extended-release capsules of diltiazem hydrochloride (Tiazac®, Taztia XT®) are used, the usual initial dosage is 120–240 mg once daily. Dosage of the drug should be adjusted according to the patient's blood pressure response. Some patients may respond to lower initial dosages; the manufacturer of Dilt-XR® states that patients 60 years of age or older may respond to an initial dosage of 120 mg daily. The maximum hypotensive effect associated with a given dosage level usually is observed within 14 days. Some manufacturers state that maintenance dosages usually range from 240–360 mg daily, although diltiazem hydrochloride extended-release capsules (Dilt-XR®) have been administered during clinical trials in dosages of 180–480 mg once daily, and the diltiazem hydrochloride extended-release capsules (Tiazac®, Taztia XT®,Dilt-XR®) and the extended-release tablets (Cardizem® LA, Matzim® LA) may be administered at dosages of 120–540 mg once daily. Some experts state that the usual maintenance dosage of extended-release diltiazem hydrochloride for the management of hypertension is 120–360 mg once daily.

The manufacturers of Cardizem® CD or Cartia XT® extended-release capsules or Cardizem® LA or Matzim® LA extended-release tablets state that patients whose blood pressure is adequately controlled with diltiazem therapy alone or in combination with another antihypertensive agent may be safely switched to Cardizem® CD, Cartia XT®, Cardizem® LA, or Matzim® LA at the nearest equivalent daily dosage. Subsequent titration of dosage may be necessary depending on the clinical response of the patient. The manufacturers of Cardizem® CD or Cartia XT® extended-release capsules and Cardizem® LA extended-release tablets also state that there is limited clinical experience with diltiazem doses exceeding 360 mg, but doses up to 540 mg have been used during clinical trials; the incidence of adverse effects (especially first-degree AV block, dizziness, sinus bradycardia) increases with increasing dosage. The manufacturer of Dilt-XR® states that although clinical experience is limited, Dilt-XR® extended-release capsules have been administered in 540-mg doses with little or no increased risk of adverse effects.

Blood Pressure Monitoring and Treatment Goals. Blood pressure should be monitored regularly (i.e., monthly) during therapy and dosage of the antihypertensive drug adjusted until blood pressure is controlled. If an adequate blood pressure response is not achieved with diltiazem monotherapy, another antihypertensive agent with demonstrated benefit and preferably with a complementary mechanism of action (e.g., angiotensin-converting enzyme [ACE] inhibitor, angiotensin II receptor antagonist, thiazide diuretic) may be added; if goal blood pressure is still not achieved with the use of 2 antihypertensive agents, a third drug may be added. (See Uses: Hypertension in Adults, in the Thiazides General Statement 40:28.20.) In patients who develop unacceptable adverse effects with diltiazem, the drug should be discontinued and another antihypertensive agent from a different pharmacologic class should be initiated.

The goal of hypertension management and prevention is to achieve and maintain optimal control of blood pressure. However, the optimum blood pressure threshold for initiating antihypertensive drug therapy and specific treatment goals remain controversial. While other hypertension guidelines have based target blood pressure goals on age and comorbidities, the 2017 American College of Cardiology (ACC)/ American Heart Association (AHA) hypertension guideline incorporates underlying cardiovascular risk into decision making regarding treatment and generally recommends the same target blood pressure (i.e., less than 130/80 mm Hg) in all adults. Many patients will require at least 2 drugs from different pharmacologic classes to achieve this blood pressure goal; the potential benefits of hypertension management and drug cost, adverse effects, and risks associated with the use of multiple antihypertensive drugs also should be considered when deciding a patient's blood pressure treatment goal.

For additional information on target levels of blood pressure and on monitoring therapy in the management of hypertension, see Blood Pressure Monitoring and Treatment Goals under Dosage: Hypertension, in Dosage and Administration in the Thiazides General Statement 40:28.20.

Supraventricular Arrhythmias **Paroxysmal Supraventricular Tachycardia.** For rapid conversion to normal sinus rhythm in patients with paroxysmal supraventricular tachycardia (PSVT) or for stable, narrow-complex, reentry mechanism tachycardias (reentry SVT), if the rhythm is unresponsive to (i.e., not controlled or converted by) vagal maneuvers or adenosine, the usual initial IV dose of diltiazem hydrochloride is 0.25 mg/kg based on actual body weight (20 mg is reasonable for the average adult) given by direct IV injection over 2 minutes; some patients may respond to an initial dose of 0.15 mg/kg, but duration of action may be shorter and clinical experience with this dose is limited. If the patient tolerates the dose but response is inadequate (i.e., conversion to normal sinus rhythm does not occur) and no hypotension is observed, a second dose of 0.35 mg/kg based on actual body weight (25 mg is reasonable for the average adult) may be given 15 minutes after the initial dose. Subsequent doses should be individualized for each patient. Some clinicians suggest that additional doses of diltiazem should be given at intervals of no less than 15 minutes to allow for the full effect of the drug on AV conduction to be observed. Greater than recommended dosages (e.g., 0.45 mg/kg)† do not appear to be more effective in terminating PSVT. Patients with low body weights should be dosed on a mg/kg basis. The usual adult IV maintenance infusion dose of diltiazem hydrochloride is 5–15 mg/hour.

Atrial Fibrillation and Flutter. For temporary control of rapid ventricular rates in adults with atrial flutter or atrial fibrillation, an IV diltiazem hydrochloride loading dose of 0.25 mg/kg based on actual body weight (20 mg is reasonable for the average adult) is administered by direct IV injection over 2 minutes; some patients may respond to an initial dose of 0.15 mg/kg, but clinical experience with this dose is limited. If the patient tolerates but does not respond adequately to the initial dose (i.e., does not experience the desired reduction in ventricular rate), a second dose of 0.35 mg/kg based on actual body weight (25 mg is reasonable for the average adult) may be given 15 minutes after the initial dose. Subsequent doses should be individualized for each patient. Some clinicians suggest that additional doses of diltiazem should be given at intervals of not less than 15 minutes to allow for the full effect of the drug on AV conduction to be observed. For continued reduction of ventricular rate in patients with atrial flutter or fibrillation who have responded to initial therapy with diltiazem, the rate and duration of the diltiazem maintenance infusion should be adjusted carefully according to the patient's tolerance (e.g., reduction in blood pressure) and response (i.e., reduction in heart rate); infusions may be maintained for up to 24 hours. An initial maintenance infusion at the rate of 10 mg/hour (range: 5–15 mg/hour) is recommended. The maintenance infusion rate may be increased in increments of 5 mg/hour up to, but not exceeding, 15 mg/hour, as needed, if further reduction in heart rate is required. Optimal response usually is achieved with diltiazem hydrochloride maintenance dosages of 10–15 mg/hour, but some patients (e.g., those with small body frame) may achieve adequate heart rate control with infusion rates as low as 5 mg/hour; maintenance dosage requirements may be lower in patients with liver disease or in geriatric patients. The safety and efficacy of maintenance infusion rates exceeding 15 mg/hour for longer than 24 hours have not been established, and use of such dosages is not recommended by the manufacturers.

Once adequate control of heart rate or conversion to normal sinus rhythm has been achieved with diltiazem therapy, therapy with antiarrhythmic agents may be necessary to maintain reduced heart rate in patients with atrial fibrillation or atrial flutter or to prevent the further occurrence of paroxysmal supraventricular tachycardia. Attempts to transfer the patient to alternative antiarrhythmic therapy (e.g., IV or oral digoxin, quinidine, procainamide, oral calcium-channel blockers, oral β-adrenergic blockers) should be made. In controlled clinical trials, transference of therapy occurred within 3–24 hours of administration of direct IV injection of diltiazem. Clinical experience with transferring therapy following maintenance infusion of diltiazem hydrochloride is limited. In determining the appropriateness of transferring therapy, characteristics and dosing guidelines for the alternative drug must be considered.

After an acute reduction of heart rate in patients with atrial fibrillation or flutter is obtained with diltiazem therapy, clinicians may consider cardioversion, anticoagulant therapy (e.g., warfarin) to decrease the risk of peripheral embolization, or oral long-term antiarrhythmic agents, depending on the duration of atrial fibrillation and presence of concurrent cardiac disease.

Other Supraventricular Arrhythmias. For the treatment of other supraventricular tachycardias (e.g., junctional tachycardia†, atrial tachycardia†) in adults, an initial diltiazem hydrochloride dose of 0.25 mg/kg has been administered by direct IV injection over 2 minutes, followed by a maintenance IV infusion of 5–10 mg/hour (up to 15 mg/hour).

■ Dosage in Renal and Hepatic Impairment Diltiazem is metabolized extensively by the liver and excreted in urine and bile. Although specific dosage recommendations for patients with impaired renal function are not available, dosage of diltiazem hydrochloride should be titrated cautiously in these patients. However, some evidence suggests that the pharmacokinetics and bioavailability of the oral drug and its major active metabolite deacetyldiltiazem may not be altered substantially in patients with renal failure.

Diltiazem should be used with caution in patients with hepatic impairment, since acute hepatic injury has been reported rarely. (See Cautions: Hepatic Effects.) In addition, systemic clearance and half-life of the drug are increased in patients with liver cirrhosis receiving oral diltiazem; however, the manufacturers make no specific recommendations for dosage adjustment in patients with impaired hepatic function.

Cautions

In therapeutic dosage, diltiazem usually is well tolerated. Serious adverse reactions requiring discontinuance of diltiazem therapy or dosage adjustment are rare; however, GI tract disturbances, skin eruptions, and bradycardia may result in discontinuance of the drug in about 1% of patients.

■ Cardiovascular Effects The most common adverse cardiovascular effect noted with IV diltiazem is symptomatic or asymptomatic hypotension, which occurred in 3.2 or 4.3%, respectively, of patients receiving the drug in clinical trials. Hypotension or postural hypotension also was noted in approximately 1% or less of patients receiving oral diltiazem. If symptomatic hypotension occurs, appropriate therapy (e.g., placement of the patients in the Trendelenburg's position, plasma volume expansion) should be initiated. Hypotension occurred secondary to the vasodilating action of diltiazem on vascular smooth muscle. Vasodilation or flushing occurred in 1.7% of patients receiving IV diltiazem and in approximately 1% or less of patients receiving oral diltiazem in clinical trials.

Adverse cardiovascular effects of diltiazem generally occurring in approximately 1% or less of patients include angina; arrhythmia (e.g., junctional rhythm or isorhythmic dissociation); bradycardia; atrial fibrillation or flutter; chest pain; heart murmur; tachycardia; pallor; phlebitis; asymptomatic asystole; bigeminal extrasystole, ventricular extrasystole; sinus pause; sinus node dysfunction; congestive heart failure; worsening of congestive heart failure (in patients with impaired ventricular function); first-, second-, or third-degree AV block; bundle-branch block; ECG abnormalities; ST elevation; ventricular premature complexes; ventricular tachycardia; ventricular fibrillation; syncope; and palpitation. Some of these effects (e.g., first-degree AV block, bradycardia, ECG abnormalities, flushing) have been reported more frequently (but less than 10%) in patients receiving the drug in placebo-controlled studies for the treatment of angina or hypertension. Swelling and/or edema have been reported in about 2.5–9% or less than 1% of patients receiving the drug orally or IV, respectively. Myocardial infarction (MI) or ischemia also has been reported rarely in patients receiving diltiazem; however, this adverse effect is not readily distinguishable from the natural history of the disease in these patients.

■ GI Effects Nausea occurs in up to 3% of patients receiving diltiazem. Anorexia, vomiting, diarrhea, abdominal pain, paralytic ileus, dyspepsia, dysgeusia, tooth disorder, eructation, colitis, flatulence, GI hemorrhage, gastric ulcers, thirst, and weight gain have occurred in less than 2% of patients receiving the drug. Constipation or dry mouth has been reported in less than 2% of patients receiving the drug orally and in less than 1% of patients receiving the drug IV.

■ Nervous System Effects Adverse nervous system effects of diltiazem generally occurring in about 1–5% of patients include headache, somnolence, insomnia, and abnormal dreams. Dizziness or asthenia occurs in 1–5% of patients receiving the drug orally and in less than 1% of patients receiving the drug IV. However, headache, dizziness, and asthenia reportedly occurred in 8–12, 6–7, and 3–5%, respectively, of patients receiving the drug for hypertension. Other adverse nervous system effects including amnesia, depression, gait abnormality, neuropathy, sweating,paresthesia, personality change, malaise, fever, tinnitus, tremor, vertigo, hypertonia, nervousness, abnormal thinking, and hallucinationshave been reported in less than 1% of patients receiving the drug. Extrapyramidal reactions have been reported rarely in patients receiving diltiazem.

■ Hepatic Effects Mild to marked elevations in liver function test results (e.g., serum AST [SGOT], ALT [SGPT], LDH, creatine kinase [CK, creatine phosphokinase, CPK], alkaline phosphatase, bilirubin) and hepatocellular injury have been reported rarely in patients receiving oral diltiazem, usually early in therapy (e.g., 1–8 weeks after initiation); although a causal relationship to the drug is uncertain in most cases, it is likely in some cases. Mild elevations usually were transient and frequently resolved despite continued oral diltiazem therapy. Elevations in some indices of liver function (i.e., AST [SGOT], alkaline phosphatase) also have been reported in less than 1% of patients receiving IV diltiazem. Adverse hepatic effects of oral diltiazem have been reversible following discontinuance of the drug.

High dosages of diltiazem hydrochloride have been associated with hepatic damage in dogs and rats during subacute and chronic toxicity studies. Histologic liver changes occurred in rats receiving oral doses of 125 mg/kg or greater, but the changes were reversible following discontinuance of the drug. Doses of 20 mg/kg have also been associated with hepatic effects in dogs; however, the effects were reversible despite continued administration of the drug.

■ Local and Dermatologic Effects and Sensitivity Reactions Pruritus or burning at the injection site was reported in 3.9% of patients receiving IV diltiazem in clinical trials.

Rash has been reported in about 1% of patients receiving diltiazem. A generalized rash characterized by leukocytoclastic vasculitis also has been reported, but a causal relationship to the drug has not been established. Photosensitivity reactions, petechiae, urticaria, contact dermatitis, and skin hypertrophy (nevus) have occurred in less than 1% of patients receiving the drug orally; other allergic reactions also have been reported. Pruritus has been reported in less than 1% of patients receiving the drug orally or IV in clinical trials. Diaphoresis was reported in less than 1% of patients receiving IV diltiazem in clinical trials. Alopecia has occurred infrequently, but a causal relationship to the drug has not been established. Adverse dermatologic effects (e.g., rash) associated with diltiazem may be transient and resolve despite continued therapy with the drug; however, skin eruptions infrequently have progressed to erythema multiforme, toxic epidermal neurolysis, Stevens-Johnson syndrome, and/or exfoliative dermatitis. Recurrence of exfoliative dermatitis with rechallenge also has been reported. (See Cautions: Precautions and Contraindications.) Angioedema (including facial or periorbital edema) has been reported infrequently in patients receiving diltiazem. In at least one patient, a diffuse pruritic erythematous rash was associated with generalized lymphadenopathy and appeared to be a hypersensitivity reaction, which resolved following discontinuance of the drug.

■ Other Adverse Effects Hyperuricemia was reported in less than 1% of patients receiving IV diltiazem in clinical trials. Other adverse effects of diltiazem include amblyopia, dyspnea, respiratory distress, epistaxis, rhinitis, pharyngitis, pharyngeal edema,sinusitis or sinus disorder, bronchitis, ocular irritation, ophthalmitis, ocular hemorrhage, otic pain, otitis media, hyperglycemia, nasal congestion, sinus congestion, cough increase, flu syndrome, infection, pain, ecchymosis, osteoarticular pain, respiratory disorder, nocturia, polyuria, albuminuria, crystalluria, cystitis, kidney stones, renal failure, pyelonephritis, urinary tract infection, dysmenorrhea, vaginitis, prostate disease, gout, bone pain, neck pain, neck rigidity, blurred vision, muscle cramps, myalgia, back pain, arthrosis, arthralgia, bursitis, fatigue, accidental injury, gynecomastia, and sexual difficulties (e.g., impotence). Gingival hyperplasia, leukopenia, hemolytic anemia, increased bleeding time, purpura, myopathy, retinopathy, thrombocytopenia, and lymphadenopathy also have been reported rarely; however, a definite causal relationship to the drug has not been established.

■ Precautions and Contraindications Some findings concerning possible risks of calcium-channel blockers raised concerns about the safety and efficacy of these agents (mainly conventional [short-acting] preparations of nifedipine). (See Cautions, in Nifedipine 24:28.08.) Findings of the Antihypertensive and Lipid-Lowering Treatment to Prevent Heart Attack Trial (ALLHAT), which compared long-term therapy with a dihydropyridine-derivative calcium-channel blocker, a thiazide-like diuretic, or an angiotensin-converting enzyme (ACE) inhibitor, however, have failed to support these findings. (See Clinical Benefits of Thiazides in Hypertension under Hypertension in Adults: Treatment Benefits, in Uses in the Thiazides General Statement 40:28.20.)

Diltiazem shares the toxic potentials of other nondihydropyridine calcium-channel blockers, and the usual precautions of these agents should be observed.

IV diltiazem initially should be used only in a setting where ECG and hemodynamic monitoring can be performed and where resuscitative therapy and equipment (e.g., direct-current cardioconverter) are readily available. Once a clinician becomes familiar with an individual patient's response to diltiazem, IV administration of the drug in an office setting may be acceptable. All patients receiving IV diltiazem should be monitored electocardiographically. Because diltiazem decreases peripheral vascular resistance and occasionally causes symptomatic hypotension, blood pressure should be monitored carefully, especially during initiation of therapy or upward adjustment of dosage. In addition, the frequency, duration, and severity of angina may rarely increase during initiation of therapy or upward adjustment of dosage.

Diltiazem should be used with caution in patients with congestive heart failure, especially in those receiving concomitant β-adrenergic blocking agents or digoxin, since diltiazem may precipitate or worsen heart failure in these patients secondary to possible negative inotropic effects. Although negative inotropic effects have been noted in vitro with diltiazem, hemodynamic studies in humans with normal ventricular function and in patients with a compromised myocardium, (e.g., severe congestive heart failure, acute MI, hypertrophic cardiomyopathy) have not shown a reduction in cardiac index nor consistent negative effects on contractility. While IV diltiazem has been used successfully in patients with atrial flutter or fibrillation and concurrent moderate to severe congestive heart failure, clinical experience with IV diltiazem in patients with impaired ventricular function is limited, and the manufacturers state that the drug should be used with caution in such patients. Peripheral edema occurring during the course of diltiazem therapy should always be investigated as it may indicate deterioration in left ventricular function induced by the drug.

The manufacturers warn that diltiazem rarely may cause second- or third-degree AV block. If high-degree AV block occurs in patients with sinus rhythm,

IV diltiazem should be discontinued and appropriate supportive measures instituted. Diltiazem has been administered IV to patients receiving chronic oral β-adrenergic blocking therapy and the combination generally is well tolerated. However, the possibility of detrimental effects on myocardial contractility, heart rate, or AV conduction with such concomitant therapy should be considered. (See β-Adrenergic Blocking Agents under Drug Interactions: Drugs Known to Impair Cardiac Contractility and Conduction.)

The possibility that diltiazem-induced skin eruptions may progress to severe dermatologic reactions (e.g., erythema multiforme, exfoliative dermatitis) should be considered. While these dermatologic effects have not yet been reported with IV diltiazem, they potentially could occur with such administration. If an adverse dermatologic effect persists during diltiazem therapy, the drug should be discontinued.

The manufacturer of diltiazem hydrochloride extended-release capsules (Dilt-XR®) states that although the drug is contained in a slowly disintegrating matrix instead of nondeformable material, such capsules should be used with caution in patients with preexisting GI narrowing. While obstructive symptoms have not been reported in patients receiving diltiazem extended-release preparations, there have been reports of obstructive symptoms in patients with known GI strictures who were receiving other preparations containing nondeformable materials.

Diltiazem is contraindicated in patients with known hypersensitivity to the drug, sick sinus syndrome (unless a functioning ventricular pacemaker is in place), second- or third-degree AV block (unless a functioning ventricular pacemaker is in place), or severe hypotension (systolic blood pressure less than 90 mm Hg) or cardiogenic shock. Oral diltiazem is contraindicated in patients with acute MI with radiographically documented pulmonary congestion. Diltiazem should not be administered IV concomitantly with or within a few hours of IV β-adrenergic blocking agents. Prompt cardioversion to normal sinus rhythm is usually necessary in those patients with supraventricular tachycardias and hemodynamic compromise. Diltiazem also should not be used in patients with ventricular tachycardia, since administration of the drug in patients with wide-complex ventricular tachycardia (i.e., QRS of 0.12 seconds or longer) can result in marked hemodynamic deterioration and ventricular fibrillation; proper diagnosis and differentiation from wide-complex supraventricular tachycardia is imperative when administration of diltiazem is considered. The drug should not be used for the management of atrial flutter or fibrillation in patients with an accessory pathway (e.g., those with Wolff-Parkinson-White or Lown-Ganong-Levine syndrome) since life-threatening adverse effects (e.g., ventricular fibrillation, cardiac arrest) may be precipitated secondary to accelerated AV conduction across aberrant pathways that bypass the AV node.

■ **Pediatric Precautions** Safety and efficacy of diltiazem in children have not been established. For information on overall principles and expert recommendations for treatment of hypertension in pediatric patients, see Uses: Hypertension in Pediatric Patients, in the Thiazides General Statement 40:28.20.

■ **Geriatric Precautions** Diltiazem should be used with caution in geriatric patients, since the plasma half-life of the drug may be prolonged in these patients. Since diltiazem is extensively metabolized in the liver and is excreted by the kidneys, renal and hepatic function should be monitored periodically and the drug should be used cautiously in patients with renal or hepatic impairment. Pending further accumulation of data regarding the long-term safety of diltiazem, the manufacturers recommend that laboratory determinations be made at regular intervals when the drug is used for prolonged periods. While clinical experience to date has not revealed age-related differences in response to diltiazem, clinical studies evaluating diltiazem have not included sufficient numbers of adults 65 years of age or older to determine whether geriatric patients respond differently than younger adults. The manufacturers of diltiazem state that dosage for geriatric patients should be selected carefully because these individuals frequently have decreased hepatic, renal, and/or cardiac function and concomitant disease and drug therapy.

■ **Mutagenicity and Carcinogenicity** In vitro bacterial studies using diltiazem have not shown evidence of mutagenicity. No evidence of carcinogenicity was observed in rats or mice receiving diltiazem dosages up to 100 or 30 mg/kg daily for 24 or 21 months, respectively.

■ **Pregnancy, Fertility, and Lactation** Diltiazem has produced embryocidal and fetocidal effects, skeletal abnormalities, and reductions in early individual pup weights and survival rates during reproduction studies in mice, rats, and rabbits when given in dosages 5–10 times the usual human daily dosage, and an increased incidence of stillbirths at dosages 20 times or more the usual human dosage. There are no adequate and controlled studies to date with diltiazem in pregnant women, and the drug should be used during pregnancy only when the potential benefits justify the possible risks to the fetus.

Reproduction studies in male and female rats using diltiazem dosages of up to 100 mg/kg daily have not revealed evidence of impaired fertility.

Because diltiazem is distributed into milk, the manufacturers state that women receiving the drug should not breastfeed their infants; an alternative method of infant feeding should be used if diltiazem therapy is considered necessary in nursing women.

Drug Interactions

In all drug interactions described in the Drug Interactions section, diltiazem hydrochloride was used.

Because of the potential for additive cardiovascular effects, the manufacturers recommend caution when diltiazem is administered concomitantly with other drugs that may decrease peripheral resistance or myocardial filling, contractility, or impulse conduction.

■ **Cardiac Glycosides** There are conflicting reports on whether diltiazem substantially affects the pharmacokinetics of digoxin when the drugs are administered concomitantly. In some studies, diltiazem reportedly increased average steady-state serum digoxin concentrations by about 20–50%, possibly by decreasing the renal and nonrenal clearance of the glycoside; however, in other studies, diltiazem did not substantially alter serum digoxin concentrations. Despite conflicting reports, serum digoxin concentrations should be carefully monitored and the patient observed closely for signs of digoxin toxicity when diltiazem and digoxin are administered concomitantly, especially in geriatric patients, patients with unstable renal function, or those with serum digoxin concentrations in the upper therapeutic range before diltiazem is administered; digoxin dosage should be reduced if necessary. Digoxin does not appear to affect the pharmacokinetics of diltiazem. Concomitant use of diltiazem and a cardiac glycoside may result in an additive effect on AV nodal conduction. Although concomitant therapy with the drugs generally has been well tolerated, patients should be monitored for excessive slowing of the heart rate and/or AV block.

■ **Drugs Affecting Hepatic Microsomal Enzymes** Metabolism of diltiazem is mediated principally by the cytochrome P-450 (CYP) isoenzyme 3A4. The possibility exists that drugs that induce, inhibit, or compete for this isoenzyme may alter metabolism of diltiazem and therefore, may alter the efficacy and adverse effect profile of diltiazem.

Diltiazem may competitively inhibit CYP3A4-dependent metabolism of other drugs, potentially altering oral bioavailability and/or clearance of these drugs. Diltiazem has been shown to inhibit metabolism of aminopyrine in vitro, and the drug has substantially reduced antipyrine clearance via apparent inhibition of oxidative metabolism in healthy adults.

Dosage of drugs metabolized via CYP3A4 may require adjustment when concomitant diltiazem therapy is initiated or discontinued in order to maintain optimum therapeutic concentrations of such drugs, particularly drugs with a low therapeutic index or in patients with renal and/or hepatic impairment.

H_2-Receptor Antagonists Concomitant administration of diltiazem and cimetidine may result in increased plasma diltiazem concentrations. Peak plasma diltiazem concentrations were increased by approximately 58% and area under the plasma concentration-time curve by approximately 50% in several healthy adults who received a single, 60-mg oral dose of diltiazem after 1 week of oral cimetidine therapy (1.2 g daily). Concomitant administration of ranitidine produced some but not substantial alterations in these pharmacokinetic parameters of diltiazem. Cimetidine and ranitidine increased peak plasma deacetyldiltiazem concentrations by about 65 and 60%, respectively. Although the precise mechanism of this interaction is not known, cimetidine-induced inhibition of the cytochrome P-450 system may play a role; other mechanisms for the decreased clearance of diltiazem and its deacetyl metabolite also may be involved. Although the clinical importance of this potential interaction has not been elucidated, the effects of diltiazem should be monitored carefully when cimetidine therapy is initiated or discontinued in patients receiving cimetidine; dosage adjustment of diltiazem may be necessary.

Cyclosporine Concomitant use of diltiazem and cyclosporine has resulted in increased blood cyclosporine concentrations and consequent cyclosporine-induced nephrotoxicity. Although further study is needed, it has been suggested that diltiazem may interfere with metabolism of cyclosporine via CYP3A4 inhibition. The possibility that diltiazem may increase serum cyclosporine concentrations and thereby increase its nephrotoxic potential should be considered if the drugs are used concomitantly. Concomitant administration of cyclosporine with diltiazem (especially when diltiazem therapy is initiated, adjusted, or discontinued) requires monitoring of the concentration of cyclosporine in biologic fluid with appropriate adjustment of cyclosporine dosage.

Carbamazepine Concomitant use of oral diltiazem and carbamazepine can result in increased serum or plasma carbamazepine concentrations and subsequent neurologic and sensory manifestations of carbamazepine toxicity (e.g., dizziness, diplopia, nausea, anorexia, ataxia, fatigue, listlessness, lethargy, nystagmus, dysmetria, headache, paresthesia, depression, speech disturbances, visual hallucinations, hyperacusis); carbamazepine concentrations may increase by 40–72%. Limited experience indicates that a similar interaction also may occur when verapamil, but not nifedipine, is administered concomitantly with carbamazepine. Although further study is needed, it has been suggested that diltiazem may inhibit hepatic metabolism of carbamazepine via CYP3A4. Because of the risk of carbamazepine toxicity and the possibility of reduced diltiazem effect, concurrent use of diltiazem and carbamazepine should be avoided, if possible. If the combination is used, patients should be monitored closely for manifestations of carbamazepine toxicity and alterations in the pharmacokinetics of the drug during concomitant therapy, adjusting carbamazepine dosage accordingly.

Benzodiazepines Concomitant use of diltiazem and certain benzodiazepines (e.g., midazolam, triazolam) may result in increased plasma concentrations and decreased plasma clearance of those benzodiazepines. Although the exact mechanism has not been elucidated, diltiazem appears to inhibit the CYP3A4 isoenzyme responsible for metabolism of midazolam and triazolam. Results of clinical studies indicate that concomitant use of diltiazem with midazolam or triazolam increases area under the plasma concentration-time curve (AUC), peak plasma concentrations, and elimination half-lives of these benzodiazepines by about 300–400, 200, and 150–250%, respectively (compared with placebo). This interaction may result in increased adverse effects (e.g., prolonged sedation, respiratory depression) associated with the benzodiazepines.

Buspirone Concomitant use of diltiazem with buspirone may result in increased mean AUC and peak plasma concentrations of buspirone. Results of a placebo-controlled clinical study indicate that concomitant use of diltiazem with buspirone increases the AUC and peak plasma concentration of buspirone by about 550 and 410%, respectively. The elimination half-life and time to peak plasma concentration of buspirone were not affected by diltiazem. This interaction may result in enhanced effects and increased adverse reactions associated with buspirone. In patients receiving buspirone concomitantly with diltiazem, dosage adjustment of buspirone may be necessary.

Lovastatin Concomitant use of diltiazem with lovastatin may result in increased mean AUCs and peak plasma concentrations of lovastatin and an increased risk of myopathy/rhabdomyolysis. This drug interaction was not observed when diltiazem was used concomitantly with pravastatin. Results of a study in a limited number of individuals indicate that administration of diltiazem dosages of 120 mg twice daily for 2 weeks increases the mean AUC and peak plasma concentration of lovastatin (single dose of 20 mg) by 3- to 4-fold. When concomitant use is required, lovastatin therapy should be initiated at a dosage of 10 mg once daily and may be increased up to a maximum of 20 mg once daily. When a statin is required in a patient receiving diltiazem, a non-CYP3A4-metabolized statin should be used if possible. Patients receiving concomitant lovastatin concomitantly with diltiazem should be monitored for evidence of lovastatin toxicity (e.g., rhabdomyolysis, myositis).

Quinidine Concomitant use of diltiazem with quinidine may result in increases in mean AUC and elimination half-life quinidine and a decrease in oral clearance of quinidine. Results of clinical studies indicate that concomitant use of diltiazem with quinidine increases the AUC and elimination half-life of quinidine by about 51 and 36%, respectively, and decreases quinidine oral clearance by about 33%. Patients receiving quinidine concomitantly with diltiazem should be monitored for evidence of quinidine toxicity and quinidine dosage should be adjusted as necessary.

Rifampin Rifampin reduces the bioavailability and increases the clearance of diltiazem after oral administration via induction of CYP3A enzymes responsible for the metabolism of diltiazem. In a clinical study, concomitant use of rifampin with diltiazem lowered the plasma diltiazem concentrations to undetectable levels. Concomitant use of diltiazem with rifampin (or any other known inducer of CYP3A4) should be avoided when possible and alternative therapy should be considered.

Simvastatin Concomitant use of simvastatin with diltiazem may result in increased systemic exposure to simvastatin and possible increased risk of myopathy and rhabdomyolysis. In a limited number of healthy individuals, administration of a single 20-mg dose of simvastatin in patients who had been receiving extended-release diltiazem 120 mg twice daily for 2 weeks resulted in a fivefold increase in mean simvastatin AUC. Based on computer simulations using these data, administration of diltiazem 480 mg once daily may be expected to result in an eightfold to ninefold increase in mean simvastatin AUC. When a statin is required in a patient receiving diltiazem, a non-CYP3A4-metabolized statin should be used if possible. When concomitant use is required, daily dosages of diltiazem and simvastatin should not exceed 240 and 10 mg, respectively. Patients receiving simvastatin concomitantly with diltiazem should be monitored for evidence of simvastatin toxicity (e.g., rhabdomyolysis, myositis).

Atazanavir Concomitant use of diltiazem and atazanavir sulfate may result in increased plasma concentrations and AUC of diltiazem and an additive effect on PR interval prolongation. Caution is advised if diltiazem and atazanavir are used concomitantly; a 50% reduction in diltiazem dosage and ECG monitoring also are recommended.

■ Drugs Known to Impair Cardiac Contractility and Conduction

Concomitant use of diltiazem with drugs known to affect cardiac conduction or contractility may increase the risk of bradycardia, AV block, and heart failure.

β-Adrenergic Blocking Agents Concomitant use of diltiazem or other nondihydropyridine calcium-channel blockers with β-adrenergic blocking agents (β-blockers) can have additive negative effects on myocardial contractility, heart rate, and AV conduction. Although controlled studies indicate that concomitant use of diltiazem and a β-blocker in patients with chronic stable angina may reduce the frequency of angina attacks and increase exercise tolerance and usually is well tolerated, the risk of excessive bradycardia, cardiac conduction abnormalities (AV block), and congestive heart failure may be increased compared with diltiazem alone. Reflex enhancement in autonomic tone secondary to peripheral hypotensive effects has been noted with diltiazem alone, and concomitant use of β-blockers may increase the sensitivity of the AV node to the direct depressant effects of diltiazem or other nondihydropyridine calcium-channel blocker. Slowing or complete suppression of SA node activity with development of slow ventricular rates (e.g., 30–40 bpm), often misdiagnosed as complete AV block, has been reported in patients receiving the nondihydropyridine calcium-channel blocker mibefradil (no longer commercially available in the US), principally in geriatric patients and in association with concomitant β-blocker therapy.

Diltiazem has been administered IV to patients maintained on oral β-blockers therapy, and the combination generally is well tolerated. However, the possibility of detrimental effects on myocardial contractility, heart rate, or AV conduction with such concomitant therapy should be considered. When IV propranolol is used concomitantly with IV diltiazem in patients with coronary artery disease, heart rate and cardiac output are decreased and the PR interval is prolonged. Because of the depressive effects of the drugs on myocardial contractility and AV conduction, IV diltiazem and IV β-blockers should not be administered within a few hours of each other.

Oral bioavailability of propranolol has been increased by approximately 50% when diltiazem was administered concomitantly in several healthy individuals. Diltiazem has been shown to increase the mean plasma concentrations, elimination half-lives, AUC, and maximum plasma concentrations of propranolol or metoprolol. However, the mean plasma concentration and the pharmacokinetics of atenolol were not affected by concomitant use with diltiazem. In vitro, propranolol appears to be displaced from its binding sites by diltiazem. Dosage adjustment of propranolol may be necessary when concomitant diltiazem therapy is initiated or discontinued.

General Anesthetics Depression of cardiac contractility, conductivity, and automaticity as well as vascular dilation associated with the use of general anesthetics may be potentiated by concomitant use of a calcium-channel blocker, including diltiazem. When used concomitantly, anesthetics and calcium-channel blockers should be titrated carefully.

Ivabradine Concomitant use of diltiazem and ivabradine increases the systemic exposure of ivabradine and may exacerbate bradycardia and conduction disturbances. Concomitant use of ivabradine and diltiazem should be avoided.

■ Nitrates The manufacturers of diltiazem state that sublingual nitroglycerin may be administered as required during diltiazem therapy for relief of acute angina pectoris. The manufacturers also state that concomitant prophylactic therapy with short- or long-acting nitrates may be administered safely during diltiazem therapy, but that controlled studies to evaluate concomitant use of the drugs have not been performed.

■ Other Drugs Sinus bradycardia resulting in hospitalization and pacemaker insertion has been reported in patients receiving diltiazem and clonidine concomitantly. Patients receiving such concomitant therapy should have their heart rate monitored.

Acute Toxicity

Limited information is available on the acute toxicity of diltiazem. Because of the extensive metabolism of diltiazem, blood concentrations of the drug may vary tenfold. Therefore, the usefulness of such concentrations as a guide in the management of acute overdosages of diltiazem is limited.

Acute overdosages of diltiazem (up to 18 g) have been reported. Fatalities as a result of these overdosages usually occurred in individuals who ingested diltiazem in combination with other drugs. Most patients with a known outcome recovered.

■ Pathogenesis The acute lethal dose of diltiazem in humans is not known, but blood concentrations greater than 800 ng/mL have not been associated with toxicity. The oral LD_{50} of diltiazem hydrochloride is 415–740 and 560–810 mg/kg in mice and rats, respectively, and the IV LD_{50} in these animals is 60 and 38 mg/kg, respectively. The oral LD_{50} of diltiazem is greater than 50 mg/kg in dogs, and doses of 360 mg/kg are lethal in monkeys.

■ Manifestations Overdosage of diltiazem may be expected to produce signs and symptoms that are mainly extensions of common adverse reactions. Adverse effects observed following overdosage of diltiazem included bradycardia, hypotension, heart block, and heart failure.

■ Treatment If diltiazem overdosage or an exaggerated response to the drug occurs, general supportive and symptomatic treatment should be initiated in addition to gastric lavage and administration of activated charcoal. If bradycardia or second- or third-degree AV block occurs, IV atropine sulfate (0.6–1 mg) should be administered. If bradycardia and AV block do not respond to vagal blockade, isoproterenol hydrochloride may be administered with caution. Fixed second- or third-degree AV block should be treated with cardiac pacing. Sympathomimetic agents (e.g., isoproterenol, dopamine, dobutamine) and diuretics may be administered to treat cardiac failure. Ventilatory support also may be needed in some patients. Hypotension may be treated with fluids and a vasopressor agent (e.g., dopamine, levarterenol bitartrate, norepinephrine). IV calcium salts also may be useful for the management of hypotension, and possibly some other cardiovascular disturbances; however, use of IV calcium salts in the treatment of diltiazem overdosage has yielded conflicting results. In a few reported cases of calcium-channel blocker overdosage, hypotension and bradycardia that initially were refractory to atropine became more responsive to atropine following IV administration of calcium. In some cases, IV calcium (1 g calcium chloride or 3 g calcium gluconate) has been administered over 5 minutes and repeated every 10–20 minutes as needed. In addition, calcium gluconate has been administered by continuous IV infusion, at a rate of 2 g/hour for 10 hours; calcium infusions lasting 24 hours or more may be required. Patients receiving IV calcium should be monitored for signs of hypercalcemia. It appears that diltiazem is not eliminated by hemodialysis or peritoneal dialysis. Charcoal hemoperfusion has been used effectively, as adjunctive therapy, in eliminating diltiazem. Limited data suggest that plasmapheresis may hasten diltiazem elimination following overdosage.

Pharmacology

Diltiazem has pharmacologic actions similar to those of other calcium-channel blockers (e.g., nifedipine, verapamil). The principal physiologic action of diltiazem is to inhibit the transmembrane influx of extracellular calcium ions across the membranes of myocardial cells and vascular smooth muscle cells, without changing serum calcium concentrations.

Calcium plays important roles in the excitation-contraction coupling processes of the heart and vascular smooth muscle cells and in the electrical discharge of the specialized conduction cells of the heart. The membranes of these cells contain numerous channels that carry a slow inward current and that are selective for calcium. Activation of these slow calcium channels contributes to the plateau phase (phase 2) of the action potential of cardiac and vascular smooth muscle cells.

The exact mechanism whereby diltiazem inhibits calcium ion influx across the slow calcium channels is not known, but the drug is thought to inhibit ion-control gating mechanisms of the channel, deform the slow channel, and/or interfere with the release of calcium from the sarcoplasmic reticulum.

By inhibiting calcium influx, diltiazem inhibits the contractile processes of cardiac and vascular smooth muscle, thereby dilating the main coronary and systemic arteries and decreasing myocardial contractility. In patients with Prinzmetal variant angina (vasospastic angina), inhibition of spontaneous and ergonovine-induced coronary artery spasm by diltiazem results in increased myocardial oxygen delivery. Dilation of systemic arteries by diltiazem results in a decrease in total peripheral resistance, a decrease in systemic blood pressure, a decrease in the afterload of the heart, and, at high doses (e.g., 210 mg), an increase in the cardiac index. Decreases in peripheral vascular resistance usually occur without orthostatic decreases in blood pressure or tachycardia; however, orthostatic hypotension has occurred occasionally when the upright position was assumed suddenly. The reduction in afterload, seen at rest and with exercise, and its resultant decrease in myocardial oxygen consumption, are thought to be responsible for the effects of diltiazem in patients with chronic stable angina pectoris. Diltiazem also appears to reduce left ventricular mass and wall thickness that are associated with hypertension.

In contrast to nifedipine, diltiazem has substantial inhibitory effects on the cardiac conduction system, acting principally at the atrioventricular (AV) node, with some effects at the sinus node. When administered IV, diltiazem prolongs intranodal AV conduction and refractoriness, thereby prolonging the atria-His bundle (AH) interval; the drug usually has little or no effect on the His-Purkinje conduction system or intra-atrial or intraventricular conduction. Diltiazem increases AV nodal refractoriness by binding to calcium channels; binding is enhanced during depolarization, and the drug tends to unbind in a time-dependent manner during repolarization. Therefore, when heart rate is increased (e.g., tachycardia), calcium channel-bound diltiazem reportedly increases as a result of a greater number of depolarizations (allowing drug binding) and shorter diastolic periods (limiting drug unbinding). This frequency-dependent effect of diltiazem on AV nodal conduction allows it to selectively decrease heart rate during tachyarrhythmias involving the AV node while having little or no effect on normal AV nodal conduction at normal heart rates. Although diltiazem rarely produces clinically important changes in the rate of sinoatrial (SA) node discharge or recovery time, in patients without SA node dysfunction, the drug may decrease heart rate and prolong sinus cycle length, and may produce sinus arrest or sinus block in patients with SA node disease (e.g., sick sinus syndrome). Diltiazem has little effect on the QT interval and does not affect the His-Purkinje conduction system. In patients with paroxysmal supraventricular tachycardia (PSVT), including AV nodal reentrant tachycardias and reciprocating tachycardias associated with extranodal accessory pathways (e.g., Wolff-Parkinson-White [WPW] syndrome, short PR syndrome), the drug's effect at the AV node results in an interruption of conduction along the reentrant pathway and restoration of normal sinus rhythm. Similarly, diltiazem's effect on the AV node reduces rapid ventricular response rate (generally 150 bpm) caused by atrial flutter or atrial fibrillation. However, the drug does not prolong the refractoriness of the accessory pathway in patients with atrial flutter or fibrillation associated with an accessory pathway (e.g., WPW syndrome, short PR syndrome); these patients may experience a potentially life-threatening increase in heart rate accompanied by hypotension.

Although negative inotropic effects have been noted in vitro and in animal studies with diltiazem, they are rarely seen clinically. Major increases in left ventricular end-diastolic pressure (LVEDP) or volume (LVEDV) or decreases in cardiac ejection fraction usually are not seen following diltiazem administration in patients with normal ventricular function. However, worsening of congestive heart failure has been reported in patients with impaired ventricular function.

Diltiazem does not appear to affect blood glucose, serum insulin, and plasma renin or aldosterone concentrations. Following oral administration of diltiazem in hypertensive patients, serum total cholesterol, high- (HDL) and low-density lipoprotein (LDL)-cholesterol, and triglyceride concentrations have generally been unchanged. In patients with hypertension, diltiazem generally does not change renal plasma flow or glomerular filtration rate while it decreases renal vascular resistance; the drug does not cause sodium or water retention.

Pharmacokinetics

Unless otherwise specified, in all studies described in the Pharmacokinetics section, diltiazem was administered as the hydrochloride salt. The pharmacokinetics of diltiazem are subject to considerable interindividual variation.

■ **Absorption** Approximately 80% of an oral dose of diltiazem hydrochloride is rapidly absorbed from the GI tract following oral administration of conventional tablets of the drug. Only about 40% of an oral dose reaches systemic circulation as unchanged drug since diltiazem undergoes extensive metabolism on first pass through the liver. Oral bioavailability and average plasma concentrations at steady state reportedly are equivalent following oral administration of diltiazem hydrochloride dosages of 120 mg twice daily as extended-release capsules or 60 mg 4 times daily as conventional tablets; however, peak plasma concentration at steady state is lower and the time to peak concentrations is longer with extended-release capsules. The oral bioavailability of diltiazem from Cardizem® CD extended-release capsules at steady state is about 95% when compared with that of conventional diltiazem hydrochloride tablets. Oral bioavailability of diltiazem hydrochloride increases disproportionately with increasing doses; as the dosage of extended-release capsules increases from 120 to 240 mg daily (60 to 120 mg twice daily), oral bioavailability of the drug approximately triples, as the dosage of conventional tablets or extended-release capsules increases from 240 to 360 mg daily, the oral bioavailability approximately doubles, and as the dosage of extended-release capsules increases from 120 to 540 mg daily, the oral bioavailability of the drug approximately increases sevenfold. As the dose of diltiazem extended-release tablets (Cardizem® LA) increases from 120 to 240 mg, the area under the plasma concentration-time curve (AUC) increases by 250%.

Food does not appear to affect the extent of absorption of the (Cardizem® CD, Cartia XT®) extended-release diltiazem hydrochloride capsules or the (Cardizem® LA) extended-release diltiazem hydrochloride tablets; however, rate of absorption may be increased if the extended-release capsules (Tiazac®, Taztia XT®) are taken with a high-fat meal. Food may affect extent of absorption of some extended-release diltiazem hydrochloride capsules (Dilt-XR®); AUC was increased by 13 or 19%, while peak plasma concentrations increased by 37 or 51%, when Dilt-XR® extended-release capsules were administered with a high-fat meal. In healthy geriatric individuals 65–77 years of age who received oral or IV diltiazem, mean AUC of the drug was increased by approximately 50% relative to that in younger adults; these increases were attributed to slower elimination in the geriatric individuals.

Peak serum concentrations usually are reached within 2–3 or 4–11 hours after oral administration of conventional tablets or extended-release capsules, respectively; peak serum concentrations usually are reached within 10–14 hours after oral administration of Cardizem® CD extended-release capsules. Peak serum concentrations usually are reached within 11–18 hours following oral administration of diltiazem extended-release tablets (Cardizem® LA). In healthy adults, direct IV injection over 3 minutes of a single 10- or 15-mg dose of diltiazem hydrochloride results in median plasma diltiazem concentrations of 104 or 492 ng/mL, respectively. Following continuous infusion of 10 or 15 mg/hour of diltiazem, peak plasma concentrations average 242 or 470 ng/mL, respectively, in patients with atrial flutter/fibrillation and 170 or 270 ng/mL in healthy adults, respectively. After continuous IV infusion at a rate of 10 mg/hour in healthy adults, steady-state plasma diltiazem concentrations average approximately 160 ng/mL.

Plasma concentrations of 50–200 ng/mL appear to be required for antianginal effect. The manufacturer of diltiazem extended-release capsules (Cardizem® CD) states that administration of the capsules once daily provides 24-hour blood pressure control. When diltiazem is administered as a continuous IV infusion, plasma diltiazem concentrations of approximately 80–300 ng/mL are required to lower heart rate by 20–40% in patients with atrial flutter or atrial fibrillation; reductions in heart rate tend to correlate with plasma concentrations in these patients but not in healthy adults. Following administration of 1 or 2 direct IV injections of diltiazem hydrochloride, reductions in heart rate usually occur within 3 minutes; maximal heart rate reduction generally occurs within 2–7 minutes and persists for 1–3 hours. Following direct IV injection of diltiazem hydrochloride over a 2-minute period, hemodynamic effects (e.g., decrease in blood pressure) generally occur by the end of the 2-minute period and reach a maximum within 2–11 minutes. Blood pressure reductions following direct IV injection of diltiazem, if they occur, generally are short-lived but may last 1–3 hours. Plasma diltiazem concentrations required to prolong the AH interval in patients with paroxysmal supraventricular tachycardia (PSVT) vary considerably, ranging from 65–260 ng/mL following initial direct IV injection; conversion to normal sinus rhythm usually occurs within a mean of 0.4–8 minutes. Increases in plasma diltiazem concentrations or dosage roughly correlate with prolongation of AV nodal conduction in healthy individuals and patients with PSVT; individual differences in the extent of protein binding, tissue distribution, and autonomic tone may account for variability in the dose-response relationship. After initiation of a continuous IV infusion of diltiazem, effects on the AV node generally occur within minutes and may persist for 0.5–10 hours postinfusion. No consistent relationship has been established between plasma diltiazem concentrations or dosage and overall blood pressure reduction in healthy adults.

■ **Distribution** Diltiazem has a large volume of distribution because of its lipophilicity and is rapidly and extensively distributed into body tissues. The extensive distribution also may be secondary to the relatively high unbound fraction in plasma. The mean apparent volume of distribution of diltiazem at steady state ranges from 360–391 L in healthy adults receiving an IV infusion of 4.8–13.2 mg/hour for 24 hours. About 70–85% of diltiazem is bound to plasma proteins, but only 30–40% is bound to albumin.

Diltiazem is distributed into milk, apparently in concentrations approximately equal to maternal serum concentrations.

■ **Elimination** Following oral administration in healthy individuals, diltiazem has a plasma half-life of 2–11 hours; however, plasma half-life of unidentified metabolites may be increased to about 20 hours. Half-life may be slightly prolonged after multiple oral dosing. Following a single IV injection of diltiazem in healthy adults, pharmacokinetics are dose proportional over a dosage range of 10.5–21 mg with a half-life of approximately 3.4 hours and a systemic clearance of approximately 65 L/hour. In patients with atrial flutter or fibrillation receiving a single IV injection of diltiazem hydrochloride 2.5–38.5 mg, the systemic clearance averages 36 L/hour. After continuous IV infusion (10 and 15 mg/hour) in healthy adults, the plasma elimination half-life increases to 4.1–5 hours and the systemic clearance decreases to 52–68 or 48 L/hour, respectively; pharmacokinetics are nonlinear after continuous IV infusion. In patients with atrial fibrillation or atrial flutter receiving 10 or 15 mg/hour of diltiazem via continuous IV infusion, the half-life increases to 6.8 or 6.9 hours and the systemic clearance decreases to 42 or 31 L/hour, respectively. Plasma half-life of the drug may be increased in geriatric patients, but is unchanged or only slightly increased in patients with renal impairment. Liver cirrhosis has been shown to reduce diltiazem's apparent oral clearance and to prolong its half-life.

Diltiazem is rapidly and almost completely metabolized in the liver via deacetylation, *N*-demethylation, and *O*-demethylation to several active and at least 5 inactive metabolites principally via the cytochrome P-450 (CYP) microsomal enzyme system and mainly by the isoenzyme 3A4 (CYP3A4); the drug and its metabolites also undergo glucuronide and/or sulfate conjugation. Plasma diltiazem concentrations are higher following multiple oral doses of the drug than after single oral doses, indicating saturation of hepatic microsomal enzyme systems. Following single diltiazem doses administered via direct IV injection, plasma concentrations of the principal metabolites, deacetyldiltiazem and *N*-monodesmethyldiltiazem, are low or undetectable; plasma concentrations of active metabolites are detectable generally within 30 minutes of initiation of continuous IV infusion and peak at 0.25–5 hours after infusion. About 10–35% of diltiazem is metabolized to deacetyldiltiazem, which exhibits 25–50% of the coronary vasodilating activity of diltiazem.

The contribution of deacetyldiltiazem and *N*-monodesmethyldiltiazem to the observed efficacy of diltiazem is unclear. In one study, the plasma concentrations of the active metabolites were low in patients with atrial flutter or fibrillation receiving diltiazem hydrochloride by a continuous IV infusion; the metabolites are thought to contribute little to clinical response. However, data from a study in healthy individuals indicate the presence of appreciable concentrations of active metabolites following continuous IV infusion of the drug. Other unidentified metabolites were noted in the plasma after short-term IV administration in healthy adults and appeared in higher concentrations than unchanged diltiazem; these metabolites were more slowly eliminated than the parent drug.

Approximately 2–4% of a dose of the drug is excreted in urine unchanged. The remainder of the drug is eliminated in urine and via bile, mainly as metabolites.

Chemistry and Stability

■ **Chemistry** Diltiazem is a benzothiazepine-derivative calcium-channel blocker. Because most currently available calcium-channel blockers are dihydropyridines, diltiazem, like verapamil and mibefradil (no longer commercially available in the US), has been referred to as a nondihydropyridine calcium-channel blocker. Diltiazem is commercially available as diltiazem hydrochloride oral extended-release capsules, extended-release tablets, conventional tablets, and parenteral injections and powder for injection. Diltiazem also has been commercially available as diltiazem malate extended-release tablets and diltiazem malate extended-release tablets in fixed combination with enalapril; however, these preparations are no longer commercially available in the US. Diltiazem hydrochloride occurs as a bitter-tasting, white to off-white crystalline powder that is soluble in water and alcohol. Diltiazem malate occurs as a white to off-white crystalline powder that is soluble in water and slightly soluble in alcohol.

USP temporarily stated that potency of diltiazem hydrochloride preparations should be expressed both in terms of the salt and the base ("active moiety"). However, USP recently reverted to its previous standard that potency be expressed *only* in terms of diltiazem hydrochloride. Dosage of diltiazem hydrochloride currently is expressed in terms of diltiazem hydrochloride. Therefore, care should be taken to avoid confusion between potencies that during a transitional period may be labeled as the salt and/or base and dosage of diltiazem hydrochloride.

Diltiazem hydrochloride injection is a clear, colorless, nonpyrogenic, sterile solution of the drug in sorbitol and water for injection. Hydrochloric acid or sodium hydroxide may be added to the solution during manufacture to adjust the pH to 3.7–4.1. Diltiazem hydrochloride powder for IV infusion in ADD-Vantage® vials contains mannitol.

Each extended-release diltiazem hydrochloride capsule (Dilt-XR®) consists of multiple 60-mg tablets contained in a swellable matrix core that slowly releases the drug over approximately 24 hours. The commercially available Cardizem® CD extended-release diltiazem capsules contain 2 types of beads of diltiazem hydrochloride; the beads differ in the thickness of their copolymer membranes that surround the beads. In Cardizem® CD extended-release capsules 40% of the beads (surrounded by the thinner copolymer membrane) release the drug within 12 hours of oral administration of the extended-release diltiazem hydrochloride capsules and 60% of the beads (surrounded by the thicker copolymer membrane) release the drug throughout the last 12 hours of a 24-hour period following oral administration of these extended-release capsules. The manufacturer states that Cardizem® CD extended-release capsules and Cardizem® LA extended-release tablets provide continuous therapeutic plasma concentrations of diltiazem over a 24-hour period.

■ **Stability** Unless otherwise specified by the manufacturer, diltiazem hydrochloride conventional tablets, extended-release capsules, and extended-release tablets should be stored in tight, light-resistant, containers at a controlled room temperature of 25°C but may be exposed to temperatures ranging from 15–30°C; excessive humidity should be avoided.

Diltiazem hydrochloride injection in vials should be refrigerated at 2–8°C; freezing of the injection should be avoided. Diltiazem hydrochloride injection may be stored at room temperature for up to 1 month; after that time, the injection should be discarded. Diltiazem hydrochloride powder for IV infusion in ADD-Vantage® vials should be stored at a room temperature of 20–25°C; freezing of the powder for IV infusion should be avoided.

In concentrations up to 1 mg/mL, diltiazem hydrochloride-containing solutions are stable for at least 24 hours at controlled room temperature (15–30°C) or under refrigeration at 2–8°C, when stored in glass or polyvinyl chloride (PVC) bags in the following IV infusions: 0.9% sodium chloride, 5% dextrose, or 5% dextrose and 0.45% sodium chloride injection. The manufacturers state that, for IV infusion, diltiazem hydrochloride injection should be diluted to a final concentration of 0.45, 0.83, or 1 mg/mL by adding 250, 250, or 125 mg of diltiazem hydrochloride to 500, 250, or 100 mL, respectively, of a compatible IV infusion solution; these IV infusion solutions should be stored at room temperature or under refrigeration until administration and used within 24 hours.

After the ADD-Vantage® vials containing diltiazem hydrochloride 100 mg have been connected to an appropriate diluent container (containing 100 mL of 0.9% sodium chloride or 5% dextrose injection) and activated for dilution, the resultant 1-mg/mL solution is stable for 24 hours at controlled room temperature (15–30°C) or under refrigeration at 2–8°C; these IV infusion solutions should be stored at room temperature or under refrigeration until administration and used within 24 hours.

Diltiazem hydrochloride is potentially physically incompatible with many drugs, including acetazolamide, acyclovir, aminophylline, ampicillin, ampicillin sodium in fixed combination with sulbactam sodium, cefamandole, cefoperazone, diazepam, furosemide, heparin, hydrocortisone sodium succinate, insulin (regular; 100 units/mL), methylprednisolone sodium succinate, mezlocillin, nafcillin, phenytoin, rifampin, and sodium bicarbonate. Specialized references should be consulted for specific compatibility information.

Preparations

Excipients in commercially available drug preparations may have clinically important effects in some individuals; consult specific product labeling for details.

dilTIAZem Hydrochloride

Oral

Capsules, extended-release	60 mg*	**Diltiazem Hydrochloride Capsules Extended-release** (12 hours)
	90 mg*	**Diltiazem Hydrochloride Capsules Extended-release** (12 hours)
	120 mg*	**Cardizem® CD** (24 hours), Valeant
		Cartia XT® (24 hours), Actavis
		Dilt-XR® (24 hours), Apotex
		Diltiazem Hydrochloride Capsules Extended-release (12 hours)
		Diltiazem Hydrochloride Capsules Extended-release (24 hours)
		Taztia® XT (24 hours), Actavis
		Tiazac® (24 hours), Valeant
	180 mg*	**Cardizem® CD** (24 hours), Valeant
		Cartia XT® (24 hours), Actavis
		Dilt-XR® (24 hours), Apotex
		Diltiazem Hydrochloride Capsules Extended-release (24 hours)
		Taztia® XT (24 hours), Actavis
		Tiazac® (24 hours), Valeant

	240 mg*	**Cardizem® CD** (24 hours), Valeant
		Cartia XT® (24 hours), Actavis
		Dilt-XR® (24 hours), Apotex
		Diltiazem Hydrochloride Capsules Extended-release (24 hours)
		Taztia® XT (24 hours), Actavis
		Tiazac® (24 hours), Valeant
	300 mg*	**Cardizem® CD** (24 hours), Valeant
		Cartia XT® (24 hours), Actavis
		Dilt XR® (24 hours), Apotex
		Diltiazem Hydrochloride Capsules Extended-release (24 hours)
		Taztia® XT (24 hours), Actavis
		Tiazac® (24 hours), Valeant
	360 mg*	**Cardizem®CD** (24 hours), Valeant
		Diltiazem Hydrochloride Capsules Extended-release (24 hours)
		Taztia® XT (24 hours), Actavis
		Tiazac® (24 hours), Valeant
	420 mg	**Tiazac®** (24 hours), Valeant
Tablets	30 mg*	**Cardizem®**, Valeant
		Diltiazem Hydrochloride Tablets
	60 mg*	**Cardizem®** (scored), Valeant
		Diltiazem Hydrochloride Tablets
	90 mg*	**Cardizem®** (scored), Valeant
		Diltiazem Hydrochloride Tablets
	120 mg*	**Cardizem®** (scored), Valeant
		Diltiazem Hydrochloride Tablets
Tablets, extended-release	120 mg*	**Cardizem® LA** (24 hours), Valeant
		Diltiazem Hydrochloride Tablets Extended-release (24 hours)
	180 mg*	**Cardizem® LA** (24 hours), Valeant
		Diltiazem Hydrochloride Tablets Extended-release (24 hours)
		Matzim® LA (24 hours), Actavis
	240 mg*	**Cardizem® LA** (24 hours), Valeant
		Diltiazem Hydrochloride Tablets Extended-release (24 hours)
		Matzim® LA (24 hours), Actavis
	300 mg*	**Cardizem® LA** (24 hours), Valeant
		Diltiazem Hydrochloride Tablets Extended-release (24 hours)
		Matzim® LA (24 hours), Actavis
	360 mg*	**Cardizem® LA** (24 hours), Valeant
		Diltiazem Hydrochloride Tablets Extended-release (24 hours)
		Matzim® LA (24 hours), Actavis
	420 mg*	**Cardizem® LA** (24 hours), Valeant
		Diltiazem Hydrochloride Tablets Extended-release (24 hours)
		Matzim® LA (24 hours), Actavis
Parenteral		
For injection, for IV infusion only	100 mg*	**Diltiazem Hydrochloride for Injection ADD-Vantage®**, Hospira
Injection	5 mg/mL (25, 50, and 125 mg)*	**Diltiazem Hydrochloride Injection**

*available from one or more manufacturer, distributor, and/or repackager by generic (nonproprietary) name

†Use is not currently included in the labeling approved by the US Food and Drug Administration

Verapamil Hydrochloride

Iproveratril Hydrochloride

■ Verapamil hydrochloride is a nondihydropyridine calcium-channel blocking agent (calcium-channel blocker).

Uses

Verapamil is used in the management of supraventricular tachycardias (SVTs). The drug also is used for the management of Prinzmetal variant angina and unstable and chronic stable angina pectoris, and for the management of hypertension.

■ **Supraventricular Arrhythmias** Verapamil is used for rapid conversion to sinus rhythm of paroxysmal supraventricular tachycardia (PSVT), including tachycardia associated with Wolff-Parkinson-White or Lown-Ganong-Levine syndrome; the drug also is used for control of rapid ventricular rate in nonpreexcited atrial flutter or fibrillation. The American College of Cardiology/American Heart Association/Heart Rhythm Society (ACC/AHA/HRS) guideline for the management of adult patients with supraventricular tachycardia recommends the use of verapamil in the treatment of various SVTs (e.g., atrial flutter, junctional tachycardia, focal atrial tachycardia, atrioventricular nodal reentrant tachycardia [AVNRT]); in general, IV verapamil is recommended for acute treatment, while oral verapamil is recommended for ongoing management of these arrhythmias. Vagal maneuvers and/or IV adenosine are considered first-line interventions for the acute treatment of patients with SVT and should be attempted prior to other therapies when clinically indicated; if such measures are ineffective or not feasible, a nondihydropyridine calcium-channel blocker (i.e., verapamil or diltiazem) may be considered. Verapamil should only be used in hemodynamically stable patients who do not have impaired ventricular function.

Paroxysmal Supraventricular Tachycardia IV verapamil is used for rapid conversion of PSVT that is uncontrolled or unconverted by vagal maneuvers and adenosine, including atrioventricular nodal reentrant tachycardias and PSVT associated with accessory bypass tracts (e.g., Wolff-Parkinson-White or Lown-Ganong-Levine syndrome). In 60–100% of patients with PSVT, rapid (usually within 10 minutes after administration) conversion to sinus rhythm is achieved with IV verapamil.

Verapamil is used orally to prevent recurrent PSVT and is considered a drug of choice for this arrhythmia. The drug appears to be more effective in preventing PSVT associated with AV nodal reentry than that associated with a concealed accessory pathway.

Atrial Fibrillation and Flutter Nondihydropyridine calcium-channel blockers (e.g., diltiazem, verapamil) are recommended as one of several drug therapy options for ventricular rate control in patients with nonpreexcited atrial fibrillation or flutter. Management of atrial fibrillation or flutter depends on the clinical situation and the patient's condition. For acute treatment of atrial fibrillation, IV verapamil may be used to temporarily control rapid ventricular rate, usually decreasing heart rate by at least 20%. Cardioversion is indicated, however, in hemodynamically unstable patients. Verapamil should not be used when atrial flutter or fibrillation (especially when preexcited ventricular complexes are present) is associated with an accessory bypass tract (e.g., Wolff-Parkinson-White or Lown-Ganong-Levine syndrome), since ventricular tachyarrythmias, including ventricular fibrillation, and cardiac arrest may be precipitated. (See Cautions: Cardiovascular Effects.) Although approximately 70% of patients with atrial flutter and/or fibrillation respond to IV verapamil with a reduction in ventricular rate, the drug alone rarely converts atrial flutter or fibrillation to normal sinus rhythm. Conversion is more likely to occur in atrial flutter or fibrillation that is of recent onset and/or associated with only mild or moderate left-atrial enlargement.

Calcium-channel blockers (i.e., verapamil or diltiazem) may be used for the management of atrial fibrillation associated with acute myocardial infarction (MI) in patients with a β-blocker intolerance. (See Uses: Acute Myocardial Infarction.)

Oral verapamil is used in conjunction with a cardiac glycoside (e.g., digoxin) to control ventricular rate at rest and during stress in patients with chronic atrial fibrillation and/or flutter. Verapamil has also been used alone† and in combination with quinidine† to control ventricular rate in these patients. The drug should not be used when these arrhythmias are associated with an accessory bypass tract. Unlike cardiac glycosides, verapamil may be particularly useful in controlling tachycardia induced by exercise and stress. Verapamil reduces heart rate at rest (e.g., by 15–30%) and increases exercise capacity in patients with chronic atrial fibrillation and/or flutter, and has been effective in patients who did not respond adequately to a cardiac glycoside alone. Improvement in maximal exercise capacity occurs with a concomitant decrease in heart rate, blood pressure, and double product (heart rate times systolic blood pressure) at maximal exertion during verapamil therapy. Combined therapy with verapamil and a cardiac glycoside appears to be somewhat more effective than verapamil or a cardiac glycoside alone. Cardioversion has been used safely and effectively following IV or oral verapamil administration.

Although controlled studies have not been conducted to date, IV verapamil also has been used successfully in the management of PSVT and atrial fibrillation or flutter in neonates and children. However, most experts state that verapamil should *not* be used in infants because it may cause refractory hypotension and cardiac arrest and should be used with caution in children because it may cause hypotension and myocardial depression. (see Cautions: Pediatric Precautions.)

Atrial Tachycardia IV verapamil may be used for the acute treatment of patients with hemodynamically stable focal atrial tachycardia† (i.e., regular SVT arising from a localized atrial site), and oral verapamil may be used for ongoing management.

While evidence is more limited, IV verapamil also has been used in patients with multifocal atrial tachycardia† (i.e., rapid, irregular rhythm with at least 3 distinct P-wave morphologies) to control ventricular rate and convert to normal sinus rhythm. However, such arrhythmia is commonly associated with an underlying condition (e.g., pulmonary, coronary, or valvular heart disease) and is generally not responsive to antiarrhythmic therapy. Antiarrhythmic drug therapy usually is reserved for patients who do not respond to initial attempts at correcting or managing potential precipitating factors (e.g., exacerbation of chronic obstructive pulmonary disease or congestive heart failure, electrolyte and/or ventilatory disturbances, infection, theophylline toxicity). Therapy with verapamil has been associated with slowing of atrial and ventricular rates and conversion to sinus rhythm in some patients with this arrhythmia. Therefore, some clinicians suggest that IV verapamil may be useful for the acute treatment of patients with multifocal atrial tachycardia who do not have ventricular dysfunction, sinus node dysfunction, or AV block. Verapamil also may be useful orally for chronic suppression of recurrent symptomatic multifocal atrial tachycardia.

Junctional Tachycardia Verapamil may be used for the treatment of junctional tachycardia† (i.e., nonreentrant SVT originating from the AV junction), a rapid, occasionally irregular, narrow-complex tachycardia. β-Adrenergic blocking agents generally are used for acute termination and/or ongoing management of junctional tachycardia; limited evidence suggest there may be a role for verapamil when β-blocking agents (particularly propranolol) are ineffective.

■ **Angina** Verapamil is used in the management of angina, including chronic stable angina, unstable angina, and Prinzmetal variant angina. Calcium-channel blockers (used alone or in combination with nitrates) are considered the drugs of choice for the management of Prinzmetal variant angina. β-Blockers are recommended as the anti-ischemic drugs of choice in most patients with chronic stable angina; however, calcium-channel blockers may be substituted or added in patients who do not tolerate or respond adequately to β-blockers. In patients with chronic stable angina, verapamil may reduce the frequency of attacks, allow a decrease in sublingual nitroglycerin dosage, and increase exercise tolerance. All classes of calcium-channel blockers appear to be equally effective in reducing anginal episodes; however, choice of a specific agent should be individualized since the pharmacologic properties of these drugs differ. Verapamil also may be beneficial in patients with unstable angina; experts recommend the use of a nondihydropyridine calcium-channel blocker (e.g., diltiazem, verapamil) for the relief of ongoing or recurring ischemia when β-blocker therapy is inadequate, not tolerated, or contraindicated in patients with unstable angina who do not have clinically important left ventricular dysfunction, increased risk of cardiogenic shock, or AV block.

Although concurrent use of some calcium-channel blockers and a β-blocker may have beneficial effects in some patients (e.g., reduction of dihydropyridine-induced tachycardia through β-blockade), combined use of verapamil with a β-blocker generally should be avoided because of the potential adverse effects on AV nodal conduction, heart rate, and cardiac contractility. (See Drug Interactions: β-Adrenergic Blocking Agents.)

■ **Hypertension** Verapamil is used alone or in combination with other classes of antihypertensive agents in the management of hypertension.

Calcium-channel blockers (e.g., verapamil) are considered one of several preferred antihypertensive drugs for the initial management of hypertension according to current evidence-based hypertension guidelines; other preferred options include angiotensin-converting enzyme (ACE) inhibitors, angiotensin II receptor antagonists, and thiazide diuretics. While there may be individual differences with respect to recommendations for initial drug selection and use in specific patient populations, current evidence indicates that these antihypertensive drug classes all generally produce comparable effects on overall mortality and cardiovascular, cerebrovascular, and renal outcomes. (See Uses: Hypertension, in Amlodipine 24:28.08.)

Calcium-channel blockers may be particularly useful in the management of hypertension in patients with certain coexisting conditions such as ischemic heart disease (e.g., angina) and in geriatric patients, including those with isolated systolic hypertension. (See Uses: Hypertension, in Amlodipine 24:28.08.) In addition, nondihydropyridine calcium-channel blockers (e.g., diltiazem, verapamil) may be beneficial in hypertensive patients with coexisting atrial fibrillation and a rapid ventricular rate. However, some experts recommend against the use of nondihydropyridine calcium-channel blockers in patients who have heart failure with reduced ejection fraction because of the drugs' myocardial depressant activity and unfavorable outcomes in some clinical trials in patients with heart failure receiving the drugs.

In the Antihypertensive and Lipid-lowering Treatment to Prevent Heart Attack Trial (ALLHAT), the long-term cardiovascular morbidity and mortality benefit of a long-acting dihydropyridine calcium-channel blocker (amlodipine), a thiazide-like diuretic (chlorthalidone), and an ACE inhibitor (lisinopril) were compared in a broad population of patients with hypertension at risk for coronary heart disease. Although these antihypertensive agents were comparably effective in providing important cardiovascular benefit, apparent differences in certain secondary outcomes were observed. Patients receiving the ACE inhibitor experienced higher risks of stroke, combined cardiovascular disease, GI bleeding, and angioedema, while those receiving the calcium-channel blocker were at higher risk of developing heart failure. The ALLHAT investigators suggested that the observed differences in cardiovascular outcome may be attributable, at least in part, to the greater antihypertensive effect of the calcium-channel blocker compared with that of the ACE inhibitor, especially in women and black patients. (See Clinical Benefits of Thiazides in Hypertension under Hypertension in Adults: Treatment Benefits, in Uses in the Thiazides General Statement 40:28.20.)

Most patients with hypertension, especially black patients, will require at least 2 antihypertensive drugs to achieve adequate blood pressure control. Calcium-channel blockers may be particularly useful in the management of hypertension in black patients; these patients tend to have greater blood pressure response to calcium-channel blockers and thiazide diuretics than to other antihypertensive drug classes (e.g., ACE inhibitors, angiotensin II receptor antagonists). However, the combination of an ACE inhibitor or an angiotensin II receptor antagonist with a calcium-channel blocker or thiazide diuretic produces similar blood pressure lowering in black patients as in other racial groups. (See Race under Hypertension: Other Special Considerations for Antihypertensive Therapy, in Uses in Amlodipine 24:28.08.)

For additional information on the role of calcium-channel blockers in the management of hypertension, see Uses: Hypertension, in Amlodipine 24:28.08. For information on overall principles and expert recommendations for treatment of hypertension, see Uses: Hypertension in Adults, in the Thiazides General Statement 40:28.20.

■ **Hypertrophic Cardiomyopathy** Verapamil has been used as adjunctive therapy in the management of hypertrophic cardiomyopathy†. The drug is used to relieve cardiac manifestations (e.g., angina, dyspnea) and improve exercise capacity and quality of life associated with cardiomyopathy-induced outflow tract obstruction and also may alleviate and suppress concomitant supraventricular tachyarrhythmias. Verapamil therapy also has produced clinical improvement in patients without evidence of outflow obstruction. The drug can reduce the outflow tract gradient in patients with obstruction and enhance left ventricular diastolic filling (e.g., rate) and relaxation; the drug also appears to reduce regional systolic and diastolic asynchrony. In addition, limited evidence suggests that verapamil may limit the extent of ischemic myocardial changes in some patients with hypertrophic cardiomyopathy; however, the drug may not alter the underlying hypertrophic process, which apparently can progress slowly despite clinical and cardiac functional improvements induced by the drug and evidence of an increase in the number of calcium-channel blocker receptors (1,4-dihydropyridine receptors) in the myocardium of patients with this condition.

While clinical improvement frequently occurs in patients with hypertrophic cardiomyopathy treated with verapamil, improvement in the extent of hypertrophy as evidenced by changes in intraventricular septum (IVS) and left ventricular posterior wall (LVPW) thickness and in left ventricular diameters appears to occur only occasionally. In one study, there was no change in these parameters overall in patients receiving verapamil, although 13% of these patients exhibited decreases in IVS and/or LVPW thickness. The clinical importance of such changes is not known, but some evidence suggests that decreases in LVPW thickness in patients with hypertrophic cardiomyopathy actually may result in left ventricular systolic dysfunction.

Despite evidence of a lack of substantial effect on the underlying hypertrophic process, functional cardiac changes induced by verapamil, particularly those involving left ventricular diastolic filling, relaxation, and asynchrony, can result in decreased ischemic manifestations, including symptomatic improvement and increased exercise tolerance. While the role of chronic drug therapy in *asymptomatic* patients with hypertrophic cardiomyopathy remains controversial, verapamil has improved reversible perfusion defects and exercise capacity in such patients, and some clinicians suggest that such therapy can be considered for relatively young patients with a family history of premature sudden death and those with marked ventricular hypertrophy or marked subaortic stenosis.

Verapamil appears to be more effective than propranolol as adjunctive therapy in the management of hypertrophic cardiomyopathy† and often is effective and can delay the need for surgery in patients who fail to respond to β-adrenergic blocker therapy. In one study, most such patients improved clinically following discontinuance of propranolol and initiation of verapamil, and in many of those in whom symptoms were considered severe enough to warrant surgery, improvement was sufficient to delay the need for surgery. In another comparative study, clinical and hemodynamic improvement was greater with verapamil than with propranolol. However, because response to drug therapy in patients with hypertrophic cardiomyopathy is variable, probably secondary to the complexity and relative contribution of various underlying pathophysiologic mechanisms in this condition, such therapy should be individualized.

Additional study and experience are necessary to determine whether the beneficial effects of verapamil in hypertrophic cardiomyopathy† persist during long-term therapy. Some evidence suggests that potential benefits may diminish with time. In addition, verapamil should be used for hypertrophic cardiomyopathy with extreme caution and only when other alternatives are not considered suitable in patients with elevated pulmonary venous pressures (particularly when combined with a baseline outflow obstruction), paroxysmal nocturnal dyspnea or orthopnea, or clinically important SA nodal or AV junctional conduction abnormalities (unless a functional artificial ventricular pacemaker is in place).

■ **Acute Myocardial Infarction** Calcium-channel blockers have been used in the early treatment and secondary prevention of acute MI†; although these drugs are effective anti-ischemic agents, they have not demonstrated mortality benefits and therefore are generally used as an alternative to β-blockers. A review of 28 randomized controlled studies involving 19,000 patients found no benefit with regard to infarct size, rate of reinfarction, or death when calcium-channel blockers were used during the acute or convalescent phase of ST-segment-elevation MI (STEMI). Although some studies demonstrated a reduced risk of reinfarction when verapamil or diltiazem was administered after MI in patients without left ventricular dysfunction, other studies have not confirmed this finding. Calcium-channel blockers generally are used for their anti-ischemic and blood pressure-reducing properties in the MI setting, and only when β-blockers (which have been shown to reduce mortality after MI) are ineffective, not tolerated, or contraindicated; because the nondihydropyridine calcium-channel blockers (verapamil and diltiazem) can cause substantial negative inotropic effects, their use should be limited to patients without left ventricular dysfunction.

Current expert guidelines state that a calcium-channel blocker may be used to relieve ischemic symptoms, lower blood pressure, or control rapid ventricular response associated with atrial fibrillation in patients with STEMI who are intolerant to β-blockers. A nondihydropyridine calcium-channel blocker (e.g., verapamil or diltiazem) may be used as an alternative to β-blockers for relief of ongoing or recurring ischemia when β-blocker therapy is inadequate, not tolerated, or contraindicated in patients with non-ST-segment-elevation MI (NSTEMI) who do not have clinically important left ventricular dysfunction, increased risk of cardiogenic shock, or AV block. The use of immediate-release nifedipine is generally contraindicated because of the potential for hypotension and reflex sympathetic activation.

■ **Other Uses** Verapamil has been used orally with some success in a limited number of patients for the management of manic manifestations of bipolar disorder†, but additional study is needed.

Dosage and Administration

■ **Administration** Verapamil hydrochloride is administered by direct IV injection or orally. The drug has also been administered by IV infusion†, but safety and efficacy of this method of administration have not been established.

For IV administration, verapamil hydrochloride is given *slowly* under continuous ECG and blood pressure monitoring as a direct injection over a period of not less than 2 minutes or, in geriatric patients, of not less than 3 minutes. Solutions of the drug should be inspected visually for particulate matter prior to IV administration whenever solution and container permit.

The manufacturers recommend that extended-release tablets of the drug be administered with food, since smaller differences between peak and trough serum verapamil concentrations occur with such administration. Oral bioavailability of the extended-release tablets is not affected by halving the tablets. Conventional tablets, extended-release capsules, and controlled extended-release capsules can be administered without regard to food.

The commercially available extended-release capsules containing pellets of verapamil hydrochloride (Verelan®) may be swallowed intact and should not be chewed. Alternatively, the entire contents of a capsule may be sprinkled on a small amount of applesauce immediately prior to administration; patients should drink a glass of cool water to ensure complete swallowing the pellets. In addition, the applesauce should not be hot, and should be soft enough to be swallowed without chewing. The mixture of applesauce and pellets should not be stored for future use; subdividing the contents of a capsule is not recommended. Studies to establish bioequivalence of controlled extended-release pellets (Verelan PM®) sprinkled on applesauce have not been conducted to date.

■ **Dosage** Potency of verapamil hydrochloride preparations is expressed in terms of the hydrochloride salt. (See Chemistry and Stability: Chemistry.)

Dosage of verapamil hydrochloride must be carefully titrated according to individual requirements and response. Safety and efficacy of adult oral verapamil hydrochloride dosages exceeding 480 mg daily have not been established.

Supraventricular Arrhythmias **Parenteral Dosage.** For the management of supraventricular tachycardia (SVT) in adults, the usual initial IV dose of verapamil hydrochloride recommended by the manufacturer is 5–10 mg (0.075–0.15 mg/kg). Slower infusion rates (over at least 3 minutes) should be used in geriatric patients in order to minimize the risk of adverse effects. If the patient tolerates but does not respond adequately to the initial IV dose, a second IV dose of 10 mg (0.15 mg/kg) may be given 30 minutes after the initial dose.

For the management of SVT in children younger than 1 year of age, the usual initial IV dose of verapamil hydrochloride recommended by the manufacturer is 0.75–2 mg (0.1–0.2 mg/kg) administered over at least 2 minutes under continuous ECG monitoring. In children 1–15 years of age, the usual initial IV dose is 2–5 mg (0.1–0.3 mg/kg), but should not exceed 5 mg. The initial pediatric dose may be repeated once after 30 minutes if an adequate response is not achieved. In children 1–15 years of age, the repeat dose should not exceed 10 mg.

Because severe adverse cardiovascular effects have been associated with IV administration of verapamil, most experts state that IV verapamil should *not* be used in infants and should be used with caution in children. (See Cautions: Pediatric Precautions.)

Oral Dosage. The usual oral dosage of verapamil hydrochloride for the prevention of recurrent paroxysmal supraventricular tachycardia (PSVT) in adults is 240–480 mg daily given in 3 or 4 divided doses as conventional tablets. To control ventricular rate in digitalized adults with chronic atrial flutter and/or fibrillation, the usual adult oral dosage of verapamil hydrochloride is 240–320 mg daily given in 3 or 4 divided doses as conventional tablets. Maximum antiarrhythmic effects are generally apparent within 48 hours after initiating a given verapamil dosage.

Angina For the management of Prinzmetal variant angina or unstable or chronic stable angina pectoris, the usual initial adult oral dosage of verapamil hydrochloride is 80 mg every 6–8 hours. Dosage of the drug may be gradually increased by 80-mg increments at weekly intervals or, in patients with unstable angina, at daily intervals until optimum control of angina is obtained. Lower dosages (e.g., 40 mg every 8 hours) may be necessary in geriatric or other patients who may have an increased response to the drug. Although maximum pharmacologic effects may occur 24–48 hours after dosage adjustment, maximum pharmacologic and therapeutic response may be delayed since the half-life of the drug increases during this period of time after dosage adjustment. The adult oral maintenance dosage ranges from 240–480 mg daily but usually is 320–480 mg daily, given in 3 or 4 divided doses.

Hypertension For the management of hypertension in adults, verapamil hydrochloride extended-release capsules, extended-release tablets, or controlled extended-release capsules may be preferred because of less frequent dosing and potentially smoother blood pressure control.

The hypotensive effect of verapamil is usually evident within the first week of therapy. The need for upward titration of dosage with the extended-release capsules or tablets should be based on efficacy and safety and blood pressure determinations evaluated weekly at approximately 24 hours after a dose. When verapamil hydrochloride is administered at bedtime as controlled extended-release capsules, blood pressure determinations the following morning or early afternoon are necessary to determine maximum effect.

Verapamil Therapy. For the management of hypertension in adults, the usual dosage of verapamil as extended-release capsules (e.g., Verelan®) is 240 mg once daily in the morning; when given as extended-release tablets (e.g., Calan® SR), the usual initial dosage is 180 mg once daily in the morning. In patients who may have an increased response to the drug, such as geriatric patients and those of small stature, it may be preferable to initially administer 120 mg once daily in the morning as extended-release capsules or tablets.

If an adequate response is not obtained with an initial dosage of 120 mg once daily in the morning (as extended-release capsules [e.g., Verelan®]), the dosage may be adjusted upward as follows according to the patient's blood pressure response:

Extended-release capsules (e.g., Verelan®).

- 180 mg once daily in the morning;
- 240 mg once daily in the morning;
- 360 mg once daily in the morning;
- 480 mg once daily in the morning.

If an adequate response is not obtained with an initial dosage of 180 mg once daily in the morning (as extended-release tablets [e.g., Calan® SR]), the dosage may be adjusted upward as follows according to the patient's blood pressure response:

Extended-release tablets (e.g., Calan® SR).

- 240 mg each morning;
- 180 mg each morning plus 180 mg each evening, OR 240 mg each morning plus 120 mg each evening;
- 240 mg every 12 hours.

Some experts recommend a usual dosage range of 120–360 mg given as a single dose or in 2 divided doses daily as the extended-release capsules or tablets.

The usual manufacturer-recommended initial adult dosage of verapamil hydrochloride controlled extended-release capsules (Verelan® PM) is 200 mg daily at bedtime. Dosage may be increased to 300 mg daily at bedtime; if an adequate response is not achieved, dosage of the controlled extended-release capsules may be further increased to 400 mg (two 200-mg capsules) daily at bedtime. In patients who may have an increased response to the drug (e.g., elderly, low weight, those with impaired renal or hepatic function), an initial dosage of 100 mg daily may be warranted in rare instances.

Some experts recommend a usual dosage range of 100–300 mg once daily administered in the evening for verapamil delayed-onset extended-release capsules.

Conventional Tablets (e.g., Calan®). If a conventional (immediate-release) preparation is used for the management of hypertension in adults, the usual initial oral dosage of verapamil hydrochloride as monotherapy is 40 or 80 mg 3 times daily. Initiation of therapy with dosages at the lower end of this range should be considered in patients who might respond to low dosages, such as geriatric patients and those of small stature. Oral dosages up to 480 mg daily have been used in some adults, but there is no evidence that dosages exceeding 360 mg daily as conventional tablets provide any additional benefit in the management of hypertension. Some experts recommend a usual dosage range of 120–360 mg daily (given in 3 divided doses) as conventional tablets.

When switching from conventional verapamil hydrochloride tablets to extended-release capsules or tablets, the total daily dose may remain the same.

Verapamil/Trandolapril Fixed-combination Therapy. When combination therapy is required for the management of hypertension, the commercially available preparations containing verapamil in fixed combination with trandolapril should not be used for initial therapy. Instead, dosage should first be adjusted by administering each drug separately. If it is determined that the optimum maintenance dosage corresponds to the ratio in a commercial combination preparation, the fixed combination may be used. For patients receiving verapamil hydrochloride (up to 240 mg) and trandolapril (up to 8 mg) in separate tablets once daily, replacement with the fixed combination can be attempted using tablets containing the same component doses. Clinical trials with the verapamil and trandolapril fixed combination have investigated only once-daily dosing.

The fixed-combination tablets contain verapamil hydrochloride in an extended-release component and trandolapril in an immediate-release component. The antihypertensive effect or the adverse effects of adding 4 mg once daily of trandolapril to extended-release verapamil hydrochloride (120 mg twice daily) have not been studied, nor have the effects of adding 180 mg of verapamil hydrochloride extended-release tablets daily to 1 mg of trandolapril twice daily been evaluated. Over the dosage range of extended-release verapamil hydrochloride of 120–240 mg once daily and trandolapril 0.5–8 mg once daily, the effects of the fixed combination increase with increasing doses of either component.

Blood Pressure Monitoring and Treatment Goals. Blood pressure should be monitored regularly (i.e., monthly) during therapy and dosage of the antihypertensive drug adjusted until blood pressure is controlled. If an adequate blood pressure response is not achieved with verapamil monotherapy, another antihypertensive agent with demonstrated benefit and preferably with a complementary mechanism of action (e.g., angiotensin-converting enzyme [ACE] inhibitor, angiotensin II receptor antagonist, thiazide diuretic) may be added; if goal blood pressure is still not achieved with the use of 2 antihypertensive agents, a third drug may be added. (See Uses: Hypertension in Adults, in the Thiazides General Statement 40:28.20.) In patients who develop unacceptable adverse effects with verapamil, the drug should be discontinued and another antihypertensive agent from a different pharmacologic class should be initiated.

The goal of hypertension management and prevention is to achieve and maintain optimal control of blood pressure. However, the optimum blood pressure threshold for initiating antihypertensive drug therapy and specific treatment goals remain controversial. While other hypertension guidelines have based target blood pressure goals on age and comorbidities, the 2017 ACC/AHA hypertension guideline incorporates underlying cardiovascular risk into decision making regarding treatment and generally recommends the same target blood pressure (i.e., less than 130/80 mm Hg) in all adults. Many patients will require at least 2 drugs from different pharmacologic classes to achieve this blood pressure goal; the potential benefits of hypertension management and drug cost, adverse effects, and risks associated with the use of multiple antihypertensive drugs also should be considered when deciding a patient's blood pressure treatment goal.

For additional information on target levels of blood pressure and on monitoring therapy in the management of hypertension, see Blood Pressure Monitoring and Treatment Goals under Dosage: Hypertension, in Dosage and Administration in the Thiazides General Statement 40:28.20.

■ Dosage in Hepatic and Renal Impairment

Patients with impaired hepatic and/or renal function should be monitored for prolongation of the PR interval on ECG, blood pressure changes, or other signs of overdosage during therapy with verapamil hydrochloride. Neither verapamil nor norverapamil appear to be removed appreciably by hemodialysis; therefore, supplemental doses in patients undergoing hemodialysis are not necessary.

Because approximately 70% of a dose of verapamil is excreted renally as metabolites (norverapamil, the principal metabolite, is pharmacologically active) in patients with normal renal function, the manufacturers recommend that the drug be used cautiously and with close monitoring in patients with impaired renal function pending further accumulation of data. Some evidence suggests that the pharmacokinetics of the drug may not be altered substantially in patients with impaired renal function; however, the manufacturer of the controlled extended-release capsules (Verelan®PM) states that an initial dosage of 100 mg daily at bedtime rarely may be necessary in patients with impaired renal function.

In adults with severe hepatic impairment, dose and/or frequency of administration of verapamil hydrochloride must be modified according to the degree of impairment and the tolerance and therapeutic response of the patient. Usual oral daily doses for adults may need to be reduced by up to 60–70% in adults with severe hepatic dysfunction. The manufacturer of the controlled extended-release capsules (Verelan®PM) states that an initial dosage of 100 mg daily at bedtime rarely may be necessary in patients with impaired hepatic function.

Cautions

Verapamil shares the toxic potentials of the calcium-channel blockers, and the usual precautions of these agents should be observed. In therapeutic dosage, verapamil usually is well tolerated. Serious adverse effects requiring dosage reduction occur in 6.3% of patients receiving the drug orally; adverse effects requiring discontinuance of oral verapamil occur in approximately 5.5% of patients. The incidence and severity of adverse effects are increased in patients receiving the drug IV; in patients with hypertrophic cardiomyopathy, moderate to severe congestive heart failure, or sick sinus syndrome; and in patients receiving β-adrenergic blocking agents or digoxin concurrently with verapamil.

■ Cardiovascular Effects

Serious adverse effects attributed to verapamil's action on the cardiac conduction system occurring in less than 2% of patients include bradycardia; first-, second-, and third-degree AV block; AV dissociation; and bundle-branch block. First-degree AV block may be asymptomatic. Prolongation of the PR interval is correlated with plasma verapamil concentrations, especially during initial titration of therapy with the drug, but this correlation may disappear during chronic therapy. When first-degree AV block and transient bradycardia, sometimes accompanied by nodal escape rhythms, occur with oral verapamil, they usually are associated with peaks in serum concentrations of the drug. In patients with hypertrophic cardiomyopathy receiving the drug orally, the incidence of these adverse effects may be increased; in one study, 11% of these patients had bradycardia, 4% had second-degree AV block, and 2% had sinus arrest. Cardiovascular collapse, which may be fatal, has occurred rarely in patients receiving verapamil for hypertrophic cardiomyopathy and may be related to electrophysiologic and/or hemodynamic effects of the drug. Asystole has occurred with IV verapamil but AV nodal or normal sinus rhythm usually has returned within a few seconds. Conduction disturbances, including marked first-degree block or progression to second- or third-degree block, generally respond to discontinuance of IV verapamil, reduction of oral verapamil dosage, or, in the case of increased ventricular response rate, to cardioversion; severe AV block may rarely require discontinuance of the drug and initiation of appropriate treatment (e.g., IV atropine, isoproterenol, calcium), depending on the clinical situation. During clinical trials, ventricular rates less than 50 bpm and asymptomatic hypotension occurred in 15 and 5%, respectively, of patients with atrial fibrillation or flutter receiving verapamil and cardiac glycoside therapy to control ventricular response.

In patients with atrial fibrillation and/or flutter and an accessory AV pathway (e.g., Wolff-Parkinson-White or Lown-Ganong-Levine syndrome), increased anterograde conduction across aberrant pathways that bypass the AV node may result in a verapamil-induced increase in ventricular response rate. Ventricular fibrillation with loss of consciousness and atrial fibrillation with markedly increased ventricular response rate and resultant profound hypotension and syncope have occurred within minutes after IV administration of verapamil in patients with an accessory AV pathway. The risk of these effects occurring when the drug is used orally in patients with atrial fibrillation and/or flutter and an accessory AV pathway has not been established, but a similar risk may be associated with oral use of the drug. Because of the risk of potentially fatal adverse effects, verapamil should not be used (parenterally or orally) in these patients. (See Cautions: Precautions and Contraindications.)

Congestive heart failure or pulmonary edema, resulting from verapamil's negative inotropic action, occurs in less than 2% of patients receiving the drug orally. Most patients who develop congestive heart failure or pulmonary edema require reduction of verapamil dosage or discontinuance of the drug.

Adverse effects attributed to the vasodilating action of verapamil on vascular smooth muscle include dizziness or symptomatic hypotension, which occur in less than 4% of patients receiving the drug. Systolic and diastolic blood pressures less than 90 and 60 mm Hg, respectively, occur in 5–10% of patients receiving IV verapamil. Hypotension rarely may require treatment with an IV calcium salt (e.g., 7–14 mEq of calcium in adults) or vasopressor (e.g., dopamine, isoproterenol, metaraminol, methoxamine, norepinephrine, phenylephrine). Pretreatment with IV calcium chloride may prevent the hemodynamic changes associated with IV verapamil. Decreases in blood pressure to lower than normal are unusual in hypertensive patients receiving the drug.

Peripheral edema occurs in about 2% of patients receiving the drug orally and flushing occurs occasionally. Myocardial infarction (MI) has occurred in 1% or less of patients receiving oral verapamil, principally in those being treated for unstable angina; however, it is difficult to conclude whether this effect is drug related or associated with the natural history of the underlying disease. Angina, chest pain, palpitation, syncope, and claudication have also been reported in 1% or less of patients receiving oral verapamil but has not been directly attributed to the drug.

■ GI Effects

The most common adverse effect of oral verapamil is constipation, occurring in less than 9% of patients. Nausea, dyspepsia, and abdominal discomfort occur in less than 3% of patients receiving the drug orally and in less than 1% receiving the drug IV. Dry mouth, gingival hyperplasia, GI distress, and diarrhea have been reported in 1% or less of patients receiving the drug orally but have not been directly attributed to the drug. Paralytic ileus, which was reversible following discontinuance of the drug, has been reported rarely in patients receiving verapamil.

■ Nervous System Effects

Dizziness occurs in about 4% of patients receiving verapamil orally and in less than 2% of patients receiving the drug IV. Headache, lethargy, and fatigue occur in about 5, 3, and less than 2% of patients receiving oral verapamil, respectively; headache has occurred in less than 2% of patients receiving the drug IV. Seizures have occurred occasionally following IV administration of the drug.

Confusion, sleep disturbances (e.g., insomnia), sleepiness, equilibrium disorders, muscle cramps, paresthesia, shakiness, cerebrovascular accident, and psychotic symptoms have been reported in patients receiving oral verapamil but many of these have not been directly attributed to the drug. Similarly, mental depression, sleepiness, muscle fatigue, and vertigo have been reported with, but not directly attributed to, IV verapamil. Vivid, disturbing dreams, which recurred with rechallenge, have been reported in several patients receiving the drug for migraine headache prophylaxis. Morbid dreams (paroniria) also have been reported in several other patients receiving the drug.

■ **Hepatic Effects** Transient increases in serum concentrations of AST (SGOT) and ALT (SGPT), with or without concomitant increases in alkaline phosphatase and bilirubin, have been reported rarely with oral verapamil. These increases are occasionally transient and may resolve despite continued verapamil therapy. However, hepatocellular injury, which recurred during rechallenge, has occurred in several patients and may be accompanied by clinical symptoms of hepatotoxicity, including malaise, fever, and/or right upper quadrant pain. Periodic monitoring of liver function is recommended during chronic verapamil therapy.

■ **Other Adverse Effects** Blurred vision, tinnitus, dyspnea, hair loss, rash and arthralgia, Stevens-Johnson syndrome, erythema multiforme, macular eruptions, ecchymosis, bruising, purpura (vasculitis), exanthema, urticaria, hyperkeratosis, gynecomastia, urinary frequency, impotence, and spotty menstruation have been reported in approximately 1% of patients receiving oral verapamil, but some of these have not been directly attributed to the drug; myalgia also have been reported. Diaphoresis has been reported occasionally in patients receiving the drug IV or orally, and rotary nystagmus has been reported in a few patients receiving the drug IV. Rarely, hypersensitivity to verapamil has been manifested as bronchospasm and/or laryngospasm accompanied by pruritus and urticaria. Hyperprolactinemia, with or without galactorrhea, has occurred occasionally in females receiving verapamil; these effects were not associated with amenorrhea and subsided following discontinuance of the drug.

■ **Precautions and Contraindications** Some findings concerning possible risks of calcium-channel blockers have raised concerns about the safety and efficacy of these agents (mainly conventional [short-acting] preparations of nifedipine). (See Cautions, in Nifedipine 24:28.08.) Findings of the Antihypertensive and Lipid-Lowering Treatment to Prevent Heart Attack Trial (ALLHAT), which compared long-term therapy with a dihydropyridine-derivative calcium-channel blocker, a thiazide-like diuretic, or an angiotensin-converting enzyme (ACE) inhibitor, however, have failed to support these findings. (See Clinical Benefits of Thiazides in Hypertension under Hypertension in Adults: Treatment Benefits, in Uses in the Thiazides General Statement 40:28.20.)

Verapamil shares the toxic potentials of other nondihydropyridine calcium-channel blockers, and the usual precautions of these agents should be observed.

IV verapamil initially should only be used in a hospital setting using ECG and hemodynamic monitoring and where resuscitative therapy and equipment (e.g., direct-current cardioverter) are readily available. Once the physician becomes familiar with an individual patient's response to verapamil, the drug may be administered IV in an office setting. All patients receiving IV verapamil should be monitored electrocardiographically.

Because verapamil decreases peripheral vascular resistance and occasionally causes symptomatic hypotension, blood pressure should be monitored carefully.

Verapamil should be used with caution or not at all in patients with moderately severe to severe ventricular dysfunction or heart failure since the drug may precipitate or worsen heart failure. Signs and symptoms of heart failure in these patients should be controlled with a cardiac glycoside (e.g., digoxin) (see Drug Interactions: Digoxin) and/or diuretics before initiating verapamil therapy. The drug should also be used with caution in patients with hypertrophic cardiomyopathy since serious and sometimes fatal adverse cardiovascular effects (e.g., pulmonary edema, hypotension, second-degree AV block, sinus arrest) have occurred in such patients during verapamil therapy.

Dosage should be reduced, verapamil discontinued, and/or appropriate therapy or resuscitative measures instituted if congestive heart failure or conduction disturbances occur. (See Cautions: Cardiovascular Effects.)

Verapamil should be used with caution in patients with hepatic or renal impairment. Some clinicians state that extended-release preparations of verapamil hydrochloride should be used with caution in patients with renal impairment, since serious adverse (e.g., cardiovascular, metabolic, hepatic) effects secondary to accumulation of the drug and/or its metabolites have been reported in some of these patients. When the drug is administered orally or when multiple IV doses are given to these patients, the usual dosage should generally be reduced and the patient should be carefully monitored for signs (e.g., prolongation of the PR interval) and symptoms of overdosage. Because of the apparent potential for verapamil-induced hepatocellular toxicity, liver function should be determined periodically during chronic verapamil therapy.

Although verapamil has been used in a limited number of patients with pseudohypertrophic (Duchenne type) muscular dystrophy†, only minimal ergometric benefit was apparent during therapy with the drug, and the manufacturers state that verapamil should be used with caution in patients with this condition since the drug can precipitate respiratory paralysis. Caution should also be exercised and appropriate monitoring performed when verapamil is used in patients with supratentorial tumors who are undergoing anesthesia induction, since increased intracranial pressure can occur.

Patients with sick sinus syndrome and patients with atrial flutter and/or fibrillation with an accessory bypass tract are at increased risk of developing conduction disturbances during verapamil therapy. The drug should not be used for the management of atrial flutter or fibrillation in patients with an accessory bypass tract (e.g., those with Wolff-Parkinson-White or Lown-Ganong-Levine syndrome) since life-threatening adverse effects (e.g., ventricular fibrillation, cardiac arrest) may be precipitated secondary to accelerated AV conduction. Verapamil also should not be used in patients with ventricular tachycardia, since administration of the drug in patients with wide-complex ventricular tachycardia (QRS of 0.12 seconds or longer) can result in marked hemodynamic deterioration and ventricular fibrillation; proper diagnosis and differentiation of wide-complex ventricular tachycardia from wide-complex supraventricular tachycardia is imperative when administration of verapamil is considered.

Verapamil generally should not be used in patients with severe left ventricular dysfunction (i.e., pulmonary wedge pressure greater than 20 mm Hg, left ventricular ejection fraction less than 20–30%), unless the heart failure is caused by a supraventricular tachycardia amenable to verapamil, nor should the drug be used in patients with moderate to severe symptoms of cardiac failure. The drug also should generally not be used in patients with ventricular dysfunction or AV conduction abnormalities if they are receiving a β-adrenergic blocking agent. Verapamil is contraindicated in patients with severe hypotension (systolic blood pressure less than 90 mm Hg) or cardiogenic shock and, unless a functioning artificial ventricular pacemaker is in place, in patients with second- or third-degree AV block or with sick sinus syndrome. Verapamil also is contraindicated in patients with known hypersensitivity to the drug. Some experts state that verapamil is contraindicated in patients with borderline hypotension associated with drug-induced hemodynamically significant tachycardia, because the drug may further lower blood pressure.

■ **Pediatric Precautions** Controlled studies with verapamil in children have not been performed to date, but experience using IV verapamil in more than 250 children (about 50% were younger than 12 months of age and 25% were neonates) indicates that the drug produces effects similar to those in adults. However, severe adverse cardiovascular effects (e.g., refractory hypotension, cardiac arrest) have occurred rarely following IV administration of verapamil in neonates and infants. Therefore, the manufacturer states that IV verapamil should be used with caution in neonates and infants. However, some experts state that IV verapamil should *not* be used in infants. These experts also state that IV verapamil should be used with caution in children because such use also may result in adverse cardiovascular effects (e.g., hypotension, myocardial depression). Safety and efficacy of oral verapamil in children younger than 18 years of age have not been established. For information on overall principles and expert recommendations for treatment of hypertension in pediatric patients, see Uses: Hypertension in Pediatric Patients, in the Thiazides General Statement 40:28.20.

■ **Mutagenicity and Carcinogenicity** At a concentration of 3 mg/plate, verapamil was not mutagenic in the Ames microbial mutagen test with or without metabolic activation.

Studies in rats using verapamil dosages of 6 times the recommended maximum human dosage for 18 months did not reveal evidence of carcinogenicity. There was also no evidence of carcinogenic potential in rats receiving oral verapamil hydrochloride dosages approximately 1, 3.5, and 12 times the recommended maximum human dosage for 2 years.

■ **Pregnancy, Fertility, and Lactation** Reproduction studies in rabbits and rats using oral verapamil dosages up to 1.5 (15 mg/kg daily) and 6 (60 mg/kg daily) times the usual human oral dosage, respectively, have not revealed evidence of teratogenicity. However, in rats, this dosage has been shown to be embryocidal and was associated with retarded fetal growth and development, probably as a result of adverse maternal effects as evidenced by reduced maternal weight gain; this dosage has been shown to cause hypotension in rats. There are no adequate and controlled studies to date using verapamil in pregnant women, and the drug should be used during pregnancy only when clearly needed. Although the effects of verapamil on the mother and fetus during labor and delivery have not been fully determined, the drug has been used short-term without prolonging the duration of labor or increasing the need for forceps delivery or other obstetric intervention and without apparent adverse fetal effect in women who received verapamil as therapy for adverse cardiac effects induced by β-adrenergic agonists that were used in the management of premature labor.

Reproduction studies in female rats using oral verapamil hydrochloride dosages up to 5.5 times the recommended maximum human dosage have not revealed evidence of impaired fertility. The effects of verapamil on male fertility have not been determined, but the drug has increased human sperm motility in vitro.

Verapamil is distributed into milk. Because of the potential for serious adverse effects of verapamil in nursing infants, the manufacturers recommend that nursing be discontinued during therapy with the drug.

Drug Interactions

■ **Protein-bound Drugs** Because verapamil is highly protein bound, it theoretically could be displaced from binding sites by, or could displace from binding sites, other protein-bound drugs such as oral anticoagulants, hydantoins, salicylates, sulfonamides, and sulfonylureas. Verapamil should be used with caution in patients receiving any highly protein-bound drug.

■ β-Adrenergic Blocking Agents Concomitant use of nondihydropyridine calcium-channel blockers (e.g., verapamil, diltiazem, mibefradil [no longer commercially available in the US]) and β-adrenergic blocking agents can have additive negative effects on myocardial contractility, heart rate, and AV conduction. The incidence of congestive heart failure (CHF), arrhythmia, and severe hypotension may be increased when verapamil is administered concurrently with a β-adrenergic blocking agent (e.g., propranolol), especially if high doses of the latter agent are used, if the drugs are administered IV, or if the patient has moderately severe or severe CHF (e.g., left ventricular ejection fraction less than 20–30%), severe cardiomyopathy, or recent myocardial infarction (MI). In several studies in patients with chronic stable angina whose symptoms were inadequately controlled by conventional therapy, concomitant administration of verapamil and a β-adrenergic blocking agent (i.e., propranolol) resulted in greater antianginal effect than either drug alone; patients studied were usually refractory to propranolol or intolerant of its adverse effects. When low or moderate dosages of propranolol (i.e., 320 mg or less daily) were used concomitantly with verapamil, substantial negative inotropic, chronotropic, or dromotropic effects generally were not produced by combined therapy in patients with preserved left ventricular function; however, such effects have occurred in some patients.

Slowing or complete suppression of SA node activity with development of slow ventricular rates (e.g., 30–40 bpm), often misdiagnosed as complete AV block, has been reported in patients receiving the nondihydropyridine calcium-channel blocker mibefradil, principally in geriatric patients and in association with concomitant β-adrenergic blocker therapy. The hypotensive effects of concomitant therapy with verapamil and a β-adrenergic blocking agent are usually additive; this effect has been used to therapeutic advantage in some hypertensive patients, but careful adjustment of dosage is necessary. However, excessive bradycardia and AV block, including complete heart block, occasionally have occurred in hypertensive patients receiving combined therapy with the drugs, and the risks of such combined hypotensive therapy may outweigh the benefits. Verapamil should be used cautiously with a β-adrenergic blocking agent for the management of hypertension and only with close monitoring.

Patients considered for combined therapy with verapamil and a β-adrenergic blocking agent must be carefully selected and monitored. Pending further accumulation of data, concomitant therapy with the drugs should generally be avoided or used with extreme caution after conventional therapy has failed in patients with any degree of left ventricular dysfunction, patients with AV conduction abnormalities, and patients receiving drugs with a negative inotropic effect. If verapamil is used with a β-adrenergic blocking agent, the possibility of detrimental interactions on myocardial contractility or AV conduction should be considered, dosage of both drugs may need to be reduced, the clinical status of the patient should be carefully monitored, and the need for concomitant therapy should be reassessed periodically. Because of the depressant effects of the drugs on myocardial contractility and AV conduction, IV verapamil and an IV β-adrenergic blocking agent should not be administered within a few hours of each other.

Severe bradycardia (e.g., 36 bpm), which was associated with a wandering atrial pacemaker in one patient, and transient asystole have been reported when oral verapamil and ophthalmic timolol were used concomitantly. A single IV dose of atropine was effective in managing serious bradycardia in at least one patient. Verapamil should be used with extreme caution in patients receiving ophthalmic timolol; when therapy with a calcium-channel blocker is indicated (e.g., for angina) in such patients, an agent with minimal effects on the sinoatrial node and cardiac conduction (e.g., nifedipine) should be used if possible.

Verapamil may substantially increase the oral bioavailability of metoprolol, a lipophilic drug. Area under the plasma metoprolol concentration-time curve has increased up to 300% following initiation of verapamil therapy. Verapamil appears to increase oral bioavailability of metoprolol by decreasing its hepatic clearance, although the exact mechanism(s) has not been elucidated. A similar pharmacokinetic interaction does not appear to occur when atenolol (a hydrophilic drug) and verapamil are used concomitantly, although long-term administration of verapamil may increase steady-state plasma concentrations of atenolol. Concomitant use of verapamil and metoprolol should be avoided if possible and another β-adrenergic blocker with which verapamil does not interact pharmacokinetically (e.g., atenolol) preferably used when combined therapy is required. If verapamil and metoprolol are used concomitantly, dosage of metoprolol should be adjusted carefully and the patient monitored closely. Verapamil also may decrease oral clearance of propranolol; minimal increases in plasma propranolol concentrations have been reported in some individuals receiving verapamil concomitantly.

■ Digoxin Oral verapamil may increase serum digoxin concentrations by 50–75% during the first week of verapamil therapy. This effect may be more substantial in patients with underlying hepatic disease (e.g., cirrhosis). When verapamil is administered to a patient receiving digoxin, dosage of the glycoside generally should be reduced and the patient monitored closely for clinical response and cardiac glycoside toxicity. Combined therapy with the drugs is usually well tolerated if dosages of digoxin are properly adjusted. Whenever cardiac glycoside toxicity is suspected, dosage of digoxin should be further reduced and/or temporarily withheld. If verapamil is discontinued in a patient stabilized on digoxin, the patient should be monitored closely and dosage of the glycoside increased as necessary to avoid underdigitalization. Because of the possibility of additive effects of verapamil and digoxin on AV nodal conduction, patients receiving the drugs concomitantly should undergo periodic ECG monitoring for AV block or severe bradycardia during chronic therapy.

■ Hypotensive Agents Verapamil may be additive with or potentiate the hypotensive actions of hypotensive agents (e.g., diuretics, angiotensin-converting enzyme inhibitors, vasodilators). This effect is usually used to therapeutic advantage in hypertensive patients, but careful adjustment of dosage is necessary when these drugs are used concomitantly. An excessive reduction in blood pressure may occur in patients receiving verapamil concomitantly with drugs that attenuate α-adrenergic response (e.g., methyldopa, prazosin). In healthy normotensive individuals, 160 mg of oral verapamil hydrochloride substantially enhanced the hypotensive effect of 1 mg of oral prazosin. Patients receiving verapamil for the management of hypertension concomitantly with a hypotensive agent that inhibits α-adrenergic activity should be monitored closely for an exaggerated hypotensive effect.

■ Antiarrhythmic Agents A substantial hypotensive effect has occurred in some patients with hypertrophic cardiomyopathy when verapamil was used concurrently with quinidine; pending further accumulation of data on the safety of combined therapy, concomitant use of verapamil and quinidine in such patients should probably be avoided. Excessive hypotension has also been reported following an IV dose of verapamil in several other patients who were receiving quinidine therapy concomitantly but did not have hypertrophic cardiomyopathy. There is in vitro evidence that verapamil and quinidine have additive adrenergic-blocking activity at α_1- and α_2-receptors. Verapamil and quinidine have reportedly been used effectively in combination in a limited number of patients for the treatment of atrial fibrillation; verapamil has counteracted the effects of quinidine on AV conduction. The drugs have been used concomitantly in these patients without serious adverse effects; however, controlled studies to determine the safety and efficacy of this combination have not been conducted to date and the drugs should be used concomitantly with caution. There is also evidence that verapamil may substantially increase plasma quinidine concentrations during concomitant use. In one patient, the elimination half-life and peak and steady-state plasma concentrations of quinidine increased and clearance and volume of distribution decreased during verapamil therapy, requiring a reduction in quinidine dosage; an increase in quinidine dosage was subsequently necessary when verapamil was discontinued after 5 months of combined therapy.

Disopyramide should not be administered concomitantly with IV or oral verapamil because of the possibility of additive effects and impairment of left ventricular function. Pending further accumulation of data on the safety of combined therapy, disopyramide should be discontinued 48 hours prior to initiating verapamil therapy and should not be reinstituted until 24 hours after verapamil has been discontinued.

■ Carbamazepine Concomitant use of verapamil and carbamazepine may result in increased plasma carbamazepine concentrations and subsequent toxicity. In several patients receiving 1–2 g of carbamazepine daily, initiation of 360 mg of verapamil hydrochloride daily resulted in development of neurologic manifestations (e.g., diplopia, dizziness, ataxia, nystagmus) of carbamazepine toxicity within 36–96 hours. Plasma total and unbound carbamazepine concentrations increased by a mean of 46 and 33%, respectively, but returned to baseline values within 1 week after discontinuance of verapamil; manifestations of toxicity also resolved during this period. The ratio of plasma carbamazepine 10,11-epoxide to unchanged drug decreased during verapamil therapy but returned toward pretreatment levels following discontinuance of verapamil. Limited experience suggests that a similar interaction may also occur when diltiazem, but not nifedipine, is administered concomitantly with carbamazepine. It appears that verapamil and possibly diltiazem inhibit hepatic metabolism of carbamazepine via the cytochrome P-450 microsomal enzyme system.

If verapamil is initiated in patients receiving carbamazepine, a 40–50% reduction in carbamazepine dosage may be necessary during concomitant therapy. Patients should be monitored closely for manifestations of carbamazepine toxicity and for alterations in the pharmacokinetics of carbamazepine during concomitant therapy, adjusting carbamazepine dosage accordingly. If verapamil is discontinued, dosage of carbamazepine should be increased to avoid loss of seizure control.

■ Rifampin Rifampin may substantially reduce the oral bioavailability of verapamil. In a patient receiving 600 mg of rifampin daily, the patient's arrhythmias were resistant to oral verapamil therapy, requiring a verapamil hydrochloride dosage of 1920 mg daily. Steady-state trough serum concentrations of verapamil were 123 ng/mL at this dosage during rifampin use; 9 days after discontinuance of rifampin, trough serum verapamil concentrations increased almost fourfold. Arrhythmias were subsequently controlled at a lower verapamil dosage. It appears that rifampin may decrease oral bioavailability of verapamil by increasing first-pass metabolism via induction of hepatic microsomal enzymes. Patients receiving verapamil should be monitored closely for reduced clinical efficacy or for toxicity whenever rifampin is initiated or discontinued, respectively, and dosage of verapamil should be adjusted accordingly; the effects of this interaction may persist for several days or longer following discontinuance of rifampin.

■ **Cimetidine** Several manufacturers state that the pharmacokinetics of IV verapamil are not affected by concomitant use of cimetidine. However, conflicting data regarding the effects of cimetidine on clearance of IV or oral verapamil and on bioavailability of oral verapamil have been reported. Studies to date have determined the effects of cimetidine on single IV or oral doses of verapamil and may not reflect the effects during multiple-dose verapamil therapy. Pending further accumulation of data from well-designed studies performed under steady-state conditions for verapamil, some clinicians recommend that patients receiving verapamil should be monitored closely for alterations in the drug's pharmacokinetics and therapeutic and toxic effects whenever cimetidine is added to or deleted from the drug regimen and that verapamil dosage should be reduced if necessary (e.g., if oral bioavailability is increased and/or clearance is decreased).

■ **Lithium** Serum lithium concentrations may decrease, increase, or remain unchanged during concomitant use of verapamil. In a patient with bipolar disorder whose lithium dosage had been stabilized for several years, manic symptoms emerged and serum lithium concentrations decreased to subtherapeutic levels within 1 month after initiating 320 mg of verapamil hydrochloride daily, requiring an increase in lithium carbonate dosage from 900–1200 mg daily to 1800–2100 mg daily. Serum lithium concentrations also decreased in another patient and urinary excretion of the cation increased. Although the mechanism of this interaction currently is not known, serum lithium concentrations and the patient should be monitored closely and lithium dosage adjusted accordingly when verapamil is initiated or discontinued in patients receiving lithium therapy.

There is also some evidence that verapamil may potentiate the neurotoxic effects of lithium. When 240 mg of verapamil hydrochloride daily was initiated as investigational antimanic therapy in a patient whose bipolar disorder was inadequately controlled with a therapeutic dosage of lithium, bipolar disorder was controlled within 1 week after initiating combined therapy, but manifestations of neurotoxicity occurred 2 days later despite therapeutic serum lithium concentrations. Neurotoxicity subsided within 2 days following discontinuance of verapamil but recurred when the patient was rechallenged with verapamil in an attempt to regain control of the bipolar disorder. Verapamil did not appear to affect the pharmacokinetics of lithium in this patient. The mechanism of this interaction is not known, but a similar interaction has been described in a patient receiving lithium and diltiazem concomitantly. Calcium-channel blockers appear to share some of the neuropharmacologic effects of lithium, and combined therapy with the drugs may potentiate neurotoxicity. Pending further accumulation of data, verapamil and possibly other calcium-channel blockers should be used concomitantly with lithium cautiously.

■ **Flecainide** Experience with combined use of verapamil and flecainide is limited. In a small number of healthy individuals, concomitant administration of verapamil and flecainide showed possible additive effects on myocardial contractility. Because flecainide also has a negative inotropic effect and decreases AV nodal conduction, the manufacturer of flecainide cautions that flecainide and verapamil not be used concomitantly unless the potential benefits are considered to outweigh the risk.

■ **Theophylline** Concomitant use of verapamil in individuals receiving theophylline has resulted in decreased clearance of theophylline, elevated serum theophylline concentrations, and a prolonged serum half-life of the bronchodilator. Patients receiving theophylline should be closely monitored for signs of theophylline toxicity when verapamil is administered concomitantly; serum theophylline concentrations should be monitored and dosage of the bronchodilator reduced if indicated.

■ **Alcohol** Verapamil may increase blood alcohol concentrations and prolong its effects. Following oral administration of a single oral dose of alcohol (e.g., 0.8 g/kg of body weight) to healthy men receiving verapamil (80 mg 3 times daily for 5 days) or placebo, mean peak blood alcohol concentrations increased by 17% and the area under the blood alcohol concentration-time curve (AUC_{0-12}) increased by 30%.

■ **Other Drugs** Verapamil can produce marked increases in blood cyclosporine concentrations. Therefore, the drugs should be used concomitantly with caution; patients should be monitored closely for possible cyclosporine toxicity, and dosage of the drug should be adjusted accordingly.

Verapamil and a neuromuscular blocking agent should be used concomitantly with caution since there is some evidence that verapamil may potentiate the neuromuscular blockade of these agents. Careful monitoring of neuromuscular function is necessary, and dosage of verapamil and/or the neuromuscular blocking agent should be decreased as necessary.

The manufacturers state that dosages of each agent should be titrated carefully when a calcium slow-channel blocker such as verapamil is used concomitantly with inhalation anesthetics that depress cardiovascular activity since potentiation of this depression may occur.

Phenobarbital can increase the clearance of total and unbound verapamil, possibly via induction of hepatic cytochrome P-450 microsomal metabolism. Combined therapy with the drugs may decrease oral bioavailability of verapamil secondary to increased first-pass metabolism in the liver. The possibility that verapamil dosage may need to be adjusted following initiation or discontinuance of barbiturate therapy should be considered.

The clinical relevance to humans is not known, but animal studies suggest that concomitant use of IV verapamil and IV dantrolene may result in cardiovascular collapse.

Acute Toxicity

■ **Manifestations** Overdosage of oral or IV verapamil produces symptoms that are mainly extensions of common adverse reactions. Hypotension, bradycardia, and conduction abnormalities (junctional rhythm with AV dissociation and high degree AV block [including asystole]) have been reported in patients with verapamil overdosage. Other symptoms secondary to hypoperfusion (e.g., metabolic acidosis, hyperglycemia, hyperkalemia, renal dysfunction, seizures) also may occur.

■ **Treatment** All overdosages of verapamil should be considered serious; patients should be observed for at least 48 hours (especially those who ingested extended-release preparations) and preferably in a hospital setting. Delayed pharmacologic effects may occur following ingestion of the delayed-release preparations. Verapamil may decrease GI transit time. Ingestion of an overdose of verapamil extended-release tablets has been associated occasionally with intestinal or stomach concretions that were not detected by abdominal radiograph. GI evacuation techniques have not proven effective in removing such concretions; endoscopy may be considered in cases of large overdoses when symptoms last for an unusually long time.

In verapamil overdosage, supportive and symptomatic treatment, including administration of IV fluids and placement of the patient in Trendelenburg's position, should be initiated. Except in patients with hypertrophic cardiomyopathy, β-adrenergic agonists and IV calcium salts may be useful since they may increase the flux of calcium ions across the slow calcium channel. Clinically important hypotension should be treated with an IV calcium salt or vasopressor agent (e.g., isoproterenol, norepinephrine); in patients with hypertrophic cardiomyopathy, α-adrenergic agents (e.g., metaraminol, methoxamine, phenylephrine) should be used to treat hypotension, and isoproterenol and norepinephrine should be avoided. Bradycardia or a fixed second- or third-degree AV block should be treated with IV atropine, isoproterenol, calcium salt, or norepinephrine or a temporary cardiac pacemaker. In patients with bradycardia initially refractory to atropine, response was enhanced after the addition of large doses of calcium chloride (about 1 g/hour IV for more than 24 hours).

In calcium-channel blocker toxicity, an IV dose of 20 mg/kg (0.2 mL/kg) of 10% calcium chloride over 5–10 minutes has been administered; if a beneficial effect was observed from this dose, an IV infusion of 20–50 mg/kg per hour has been administered. Asystole should be treated using the appropriate resuscitative measures (e.g., isoproterenol, other vasopressor agents, cardiopulmonary resuscitation). Rapid ventricular response rate secondary to anterograde conduction (e.g., in patients with Wolff-Parkinson-White or Lown-Ganong-Levine syndrome) can be managed with direct-current cardioversion, possibly requiring high energy, or with IV lidocaine or procainamide. Verapamil is not removed by hemodialysis.

IV glucagon, sodium bicarbonate, and/or an infusion of insulin and glucose also has been used in calcium-channel blocker toxicity. Some experts state that isoproterenol should be used with caution, if at all, for the treatment of shock or hypotension associated with calcium-channel blocker toxicity. Also, atropine and prophylactic transvenous pacing should be used with caution, if at all, for bradycardia associated with calcium-channel blocker toxicity; atropine is seldom helpful for drug-induced bradycardia except for cholinesterase inhibitor poisoning. The effectiveness of IV calcium salt administration in calcium-channel blocker toxicity is variable. Ionized calcium concentrations should be monitored to prevent hypercalcemia in patients receiving calcium salts.

Pharmacology

Verapamil has pharmacologic actions similar to those of other calcium-channel blockers (e.g., diltiazem, nifedipine). The principal physiologic action of verapamil is to inhibit the transmembrane influx of extracellular calcium ions across the membranes of myocardial cells and vascular smooth muscle cells, without changing serum calcium concentrations.

Calcium plays important roles in the excitation-contraction coupling process of the heart and vascular smooth muscle cells and in the electrical discharge of the specialized conduction cells of the heart. The membranes of these cells contain numerous channels that carry a slow inward current and that are selective for calcium. Activation of these slow calcium channels contributes to the plateau phase (phase 2) of the action potential of cardiac and vascular smooth muscle cells.

The exact mechanism whereby verapamil inhibits calcium ion influx across the slow calcium channels is not known, but the drug is thought to inhibit ion-control gating mechanisms of the channel, deform the slow channel, and/or interfere with the release of calcium from the sarcoplasmic reticulum.

By inhibiting calcium influx, verapamil inhibits the contractile processes of cardiac and vascular smooth muscle, thereby dilating the main coronary and systemic arteries. In patients with Prinzmetal variant angina (vasospastic angina), inhibition of spontaneous and ergonovine-induced coronary artery spasm by verapamil results in increased myocardial oxygen delivery. Dilation of systemic arteries by verapamil results in a decrease in total peripheral resistance, systemic blood pressure, and the afterload of the heart. Decreases in peripheral vascular resistance usually occur without orthostatic decreases in blood pressure or reflex tachycardia. The reduction in afterload, seen at rest and with exercise, and its resultant decrease in oxygen consumption are thought to be responsible for the effects of verapamil in patients with unstable and chronic stable angina pectoris.

In contrast to nifedipine, verapamil has substantial inhibitory effects on the cardiac conduction system and is considered a class IV antiarrhythmic agent. Although verapamil rarely produces clinically important changes in the rate of sinoatrial (SA) node discharge or recovery time, the drug may reduce the resting heart rate and produce sinus arrest or SA block in patients with SA node disease (e.g., sick sinus syndrome). Verapamil also slows conduction and prolongs refractoriness in the atrioventricular (AV) node, thereby prolonging the AH (atria-His bundle) interval. This usually also results in PR-interval prolongation on ECG, which is correlated with plasma verapamil concentrations (especially during initial titration of verapamil therapy), and may rarely cause second- or third-degree AV block (even in patients without preexisting conduction defects). The correlation between plasma drug concentrations and PR-interval prolongation may disappear during chronic therapy. Verapamil has little effect on the QT interval. In patients with paroxysmal supraventricular tachycardia, including that associated with accessory pathways, verapamil's effects at the AV node result in an interruption of the reentrant pathway and restoration of normal sinus rhythm. Similarly, the drug's effects on the AV node reduce rapid ventricular rate caused by atrial flutter and/or fibrillation. Verapamil has minimal or no effects on anterograde or retrograde conduction of accessory bypass pathways. The drug may depress velocity of depolarization and amplitude and prolong intra-atrial conduction times in diseased or depressed but not normal atrial tissue. The drug does not alter normal intraventricular conduction, but acceleration of ventricular rate and/or ventricular fibrillation can occur in patients with atrial flutter or fibrillation and a coexisting accessory AV pathway.

Verapamil reduces afterload and myocardial contractility. Although negative inotropic effects have been noted in vitro and in animal studies of verapamil, they are seldom seen clinically in patients with normal left ventricular function. Even in patients with cardiac disease, the negative inotropic effect of verapamil is offset by reduced afterload, and cardiac index usually is not reduced; however, in patients with moderately severe or severe heart failure (i.e., pulmonary wedge pressure greater than 20 mm Hg, left ventricular ejection fraction less than 20–30%), substantial increases in left ventricular end-diastolic pressure (LVEDP) or volume (LVEDV) and decreases in cardiac ejection fraction may occur.

Verapamil also exhibits local anesthetic action (about 1.6 times that of procaine), but the clinical importance of this effect has not been determined.

Pharmacokinetics

In all studies described in the Pharmacokinetics section, verapamil was administered as the hydrochloride salt.

■ **Absorption** Approximately 90% of an oral dose of verapamil hydrochloride is rapidly absorbed from the GI tract following oral administration of conventional tablets of the drug. Only about 20–35% of an oral dose reaches systemic circulation as unchanged drug following administration of conventional tablets since verapamil is metabolized on first pass through the liver. The manufacturers state that oral bioavailability of extended-release capsules or tablets of the drug is similar to that of the conventional tablets when the drug is administered under fasting conditions. Oral bioavailability of the drug may be substantially increased in patients with hepatic dysfunction (e.g., in those with hepatic cirrhosis).

Considerable interindividual and intraindividual variations in plasma concentrations attained with a specific oral dose of verapamil have been reported. In healthy adults, peak plasma concentrations are reached within 1–2 hours after oral administration of conventional tablets of the drug, within 7–9 or 4–8 hours after extended-release capsules or tablets, respectively, and within about 11 hours after extended-release core tablets or controlled extended-release capsules. Following oral administration of a single 240-mg extended-release capsule or tablet under fasting conditions, mean peak plasma verapamil concentrations of about 77 or 150–165 ng/mL, respectively, were achieved, but there was considerable interindividual variation. Food decreases the rate and extent of absorption of extended-release verapamil tablets but produces smaller differences between peak and trough plasma concentrations of the drug; food does not appear to substantially affect the absorption of conventional tablets, extended-release capsules, or controlled extended-release capsules. of the drug. Mean steady-state plasma concentrations of verapamil range from 125–400 ng/mL following long-term oral administration of 120 mg every 6 hours as conventional tablets in healthy adults. Peak plasma concentrations after a 10-mg IV dose of verapamil range from 10–1500 ng/mL. In a limited number of infants receiving 1–3 mg/kg of the drug orally every 8 hours, peak plasma verapamil concentrations were attained within 1–4 hours after a dose but varied considerably, ranging from about 30–150 ng/mL.

Plasma concentrations greater than 100 ng/mL usually are required for acute antiarrhythmic effect, and PR-interval prolongation linearly correlates with plasma verapamil concentrations ranging from 10–250 ng/mL during initial dose titration, but this correlation may disappear during chronic therapy. Hemodynamic effects of verapamil usually peak at about 2 hours and persist for 6–8 hours after a single oral dose of the drug as conventional tablets. After a single IV injection of verapamil, hemodynamic effects peak within 5 minutes and persist for 10–20 minutes; effects on the AV node occur within 1–2 minutes, peak at 10–15 minutes, and usually persist for 30–60 minutes, but may persist for as long as 6 hours. No relationship has been established between plasma verapamil concentrations and blood pressure reduction.

■ **Distribution** The steady-state volume of distribution of verapamil ranges from 4.5–7 L/kg in healthy adults. An apparent volume of distribution of 12 L/kg has been reported in patients with hepatic cirrhosis. Approximately 90% of verapamil is bound to plasma proteins. Verapamil and norverapamil distribute into the CNS. Following oral administration of 120 mg of the drug 4 times daily in several schizophrenic patients, mean CSF concentrations of verapamil and norverapamil were 6 and 4%, respectively, of mean plasma concentrations.

Verapamil crosses the placenta and is present in umbilical vein blood at delivery. The drug is distributed into milk, reaching concentrations in breast milk similar to those in maternal plasma in some women.

■ **Elimination** Plasma concentrations of verapamil appear to decline in a biphasic or triphasic manner following IV administration of the drug. After IV infusion or administration of a single oral dose, verapamil has a plasma half-life of 2–8 hours. After 1–2 days of oral administration of the drug, plasma half-life may increase to 4.5–12 hours, presumably because of saturation of hepatic enzymes. Plasma half-life of the drug also is increased to 14–16 hours in patients with hepatic cirrhosis. Plasma elimination half-life also appears to be increased and clearance is decreased in geriatric patients. An elimination half-life of 4.4–6.9 hours has been reported in several infants.

Verapamil is rapidly and almost completely metabolized in the liver to at least 12 dealkylated or demethylated metabolites; only norverapamil is present in plasma in more than trace amounts. The drug appears to undergo stereoselective first-pass metabolism, with the *l*-isomer being preferentially metabolized. Norverapamil, an active (approximately 20% of the cardiovascular activity of verapamil) metabolite, achieves plasma concentrations approximately equal to those of verapamil within 4–6 hours of administration. Food decreases the rate and extent of drug reaching systemic circulation as norverapamil following oral administration of extended-release verapamil tablets. Approximately 70 and 16% of an oral or IV dose are excreted as metabolites in urine and feces, respectively, within 5 days. Only 3–4% of a dose is excreted in urine as unchanged drug. Metabolism of verapamil may differ in infants; in several infants receiving the drug orally, plasma concentrations of norverapamil were only 50% those of unchanged drug, and concentrations of 2 inactive metabolites were similar to or exceeded those of unchanged drug. Neither verapamil nor norverapamil appear to be removed appreciably by hemodialysis.

Chemistry and Stability

■ **Chemistry** Verapamil hydrochloride is a phenylalkylamine-derivative calcium-channel blocker. Because most currently available calcium-channel blockers are dihydropyridines, verapamil, like diltiazem and mibefradil (no longer commercially available in the US), has been referred to as a nondihydropyridine calcium-channel blocker. Verapamil hydrochloride is commercially available as a racemic mixture. The *l*-isomer of verapamil has been shown to inhibit the adenosine triphosphate (ATP)-dependent calcium-transport properties of the sarcolemma and intrinsic calcium-sensitive adenosine triphosphatase (ATPase). The *l*-isomer appears to be principally responsible for the negative dromotropic effects of the drug on atrioventricular nodal conduction.

Verapamil hydrochloride occurs as a white or practically white, crystalline powder with a bitter taste and is soluble in water and sparingly soluble in alcohol. Verapamil hydrochloride injection is a sterile solution of the drug in water for injection. The injection has a pH of 4–6.5.

The commercially available controlled extended-release capsules of verapamil hydrochloride (Verelan® PM) contain the drug in an oral diffusion delivery system formulation that also is designed to initiate delivery of the drug 4–5 hours after ingestion. The diffusion delivery system consists of controlled-release coated pellets enclosed in a hard gelatin capsule. The nonenteric controlled-release coat contains water-soluble and water-insoluble polymers. When exposed to water in the GI tract, the soluble polymer on individual pellets slowly dissolves, allowing the drug to diffuse through the resultant pores, while the insoluble polymer continues to act as a barrier maintaining controlled release of the drug into the GI tract. The rate of verapamil delivery in the GI tract is independent of posture, pH, GI motility, and presence of food in the GI tract.

■ **Stability** Verapamil hydrochloride injection should be stored at 15–30°C and protected from light; freezing of the injection should be avoided. Verapamil hydrochloride conventional tablets usually should be stored in tight, light-resistant containers at 15–25°C. Verapamil hydrochloride extended-release tablets should be stored in tight, light-resistant containers at 15–25°C. Verapamil hydrochloride extended-release capsules (Verelan®) should be stored in tight, light-resistant containers at 20–25°C. Verapamil hydrochloride controlled extended-release capsules (Verelan® PM) should be stored in tight, light-resistant containers at a controlled room temperature of 25°C, but may be exposed to temperatures ranging from 15–30°C.

Verapamil hydrochloride injection is reportedly physically compatible with parenteral solutions having a pH of 3–6. The drug is physically and chemically stable for at least 24 hours at 25°C in most common infusion solutions when protected from light. Dilution of the drug in ⅙ *M* sodium lactate injection in PVC containers is not recommended. In solutions with a pH greater than 6, the drug will precipitate. Admixing the drug with albumin human, amphotericin B, hydralazine hydrochloride, or co-trimoxazole should be avoided.

Preparations

Excipients in commercially available drug preparations may have clinically important effects in some individuals; consult specific product labeling for details.

Verapamil Hydrochloride

Oral		
Capsules, controlled- and extended-release (containing pellets)	100 mg	**Verelan® PM**, Schwarz
	200 mg	**Verelan® PM**, Schwarz
	300 mg	**Verelan® PM**, Schwarz
Capsules, extended-release (containing pellets)	120 mg*	**Verapamil Hydrochloride Extended-Release Capsules**
		Verelan®, Schwarz
	180 mg	**Verapamil Hydrochloride Extended-Release Capsules**
		Verelan®, Schwarz
	240 mg	**Verapamil Hydrochloride Extended-Release Capsules**
		Verelan®, Schwarz
	360 mg	**Verelan®**, Schwarz
Tablets, extended-release, film-coated	120 mg*	**Calan® SR Caplets®**, Pfizer
	180 mg*	**Calan® SR Caplets®** (scored), Pfizer
	240 mg*	**Calan® SR Caplets®** (scored), Pfizer
Tablets, film-coated	40 mg*	**Calan®**, Pfizer
	80 mg*	**Calan®** (scored), Pfizer
	120 mg*	**Calan®** (scored), Pfizer
Parenteral		
Injection, for IV use	2.5 mg/mL*	**Verapamil Hydrochloride Injection**

*available from one or more manufacturer, distributor, and/or repackager by generic (nonproprietary) name

Verapamil Hydrochloride Combinations

Oral		
Tablets, extended-release core (containing verapamil hydrochloride 180 mg), film-coated	180 mg with Trandolapril 2 mg	**Tarka®**, Abbott
Tablets, extended-release core (containing verapamil hydrochloride 240 mg), film-coated	240 mg with Trandolapril 1 mg	**Tarka®**, Abbott
Tablets, extended-release core (containing verapamil hydrochloride 240 mg), film-coated	240 mg with Trandolapril 2 mg	**Tarka®**, Abbott
Tablets, extended-release core (containing verapamil hydrochloride 240 mg), film-coated	240 mg with Trandolapril 4 mg	**Tarka®**, Abbott

†Use is not currently included in the labeling approved by the US Food and Drug Administration

RENIN-ANGIOTENSIN-ALDOSTERONE SYSTEM INHIBITORS 24:32

ANGIOTENSIN-CONVERTING ENZYME INHIBITORS 24:32.04

Benazepril Hydrochloride

■ Benazepril is an angiotensin-converting enzyme (ACE) inhibitor.

Uses

Benazepril hydrochloride is used alone or in combination with other classes of antihypertensive agents (e.g., thiazide diuretics) in the management of hypertension.

■ **Hypertension** Benazepril is used alone or in combination with other classes of antihypertensive agents in the management of hypertension.

ACE inhibitors are considered one of several preferred antihypertensive drugs for the initial management of hypertension according to current evidence-based hypertension guidelines; other preferred options include angiotensin II receptor antagonists, calcium-channel blockers, and thiazide diuretics. While there may be individual differences with respect to recommendations for initial drug selection and use in specific patient populations, current evidence indicates that these antihypertensive drug classes all generally produce comparable effects on overall mortality and cardiovascular, cerebrovascular, and renal outcomes. (See Uses: Hypertension, in Captopril 24:32.04.)

ACE inhibitors may be particularly useful in the management of hypertension in patients with certain coexisting conditions such as heart failure, ischemic heart disease, diabetes mellitus, chronic kidney disease (CKD), or cerebrovascular disease or following myocardial infarction (MI). (See Uses: Hypertension in Captopril 24:32.04 and in Enalaprilat/Enalapril 24:32.04.)

In patients with hypertension and compelling indications (e.g., CKD with albuminuria [urine albumin 300 mg/day or greater, or urine albumin:creatinine ratio of 300 mg/g or equivalent in the first morning void]), angiotensin II receptor antagonists are usually considered an alternative for ACE inhibitor-intolerant patients. However, data indicate no difference in efficacy between ACE inhibitors and angiotensin II receptor antagonists with regard to blood pressure lowering and clinical outcomes (i.e., all-cause mortality, cardiovascular mortality, MI, heart failure, stroke, and end-stage renal disease). Adverse events (e.g., cough, angioedema) leading to drug discontinuance occur more frequently with ACE inhibitor therapy than with angiotensin II receptor antagonist therapy. Because of similar efficacy and a lower frequency of adverse effects, some experts believe that an angiotensin II receptor antagonist should be used instead of an ACE inhibitor for the treatment of hypertension or hypertension with certain compelling indications.

Most patients with hypertension, especially black patients, will require at least 2 antihypertensive drugs to achieve adequate blood pressure control. In general, black hypertensive patients tend to respond better to monotherapy with thiazide diuretics or calcium-channel blockers than to monotherapy with ACE inhibitors. Although ACE inhibitors have lowered blood pressure in all races studied, monotherapy with these agents has produced a smaller reduction in blood pressure in black hypertensive patients, a population associated with low renin hypertension. However, the combination of an ACE inhibitor or an angiotensin II receptor antagonist with a calcium-channel blocker or thiazide diuretic produces similar blood pressure lowering in black patients as in other racial groups. In addition, ACE inhibitors appear to produce a higher incidence of angioedema in black patients than in other races. (See Race under Hypertension: Other Special Considerations for Antihypertensive Drug Therapy, in Uses in Captopril 24:32.04 and in Enalaprilat/Enalapril 24:32.04.)

For additional information on the role of ACE inhibitors in the management of hypertension, see Uses in Captopril 24:32.04 and in Enalaprilat/Enalapril 24:32.04. For information on overall principles and expert recommendations for treatment of hypertension, see Uses: Hypertension in Adults and also see Uses: Hypertension in Pediatric Patients, in the Thiazides General Statement 40:28.20.

■ **Heart Failure** ACE inhibitors have been used in the management of heart failure†, usually in conjunction with other agents such as cardiac glycosides, diuretics, and β-adrenergic blocking agents (β-blockers).

Current guidelines for the management of heart failure in adults generally recommend a combination of drug therapies to reduce morbidity and mortality, including neurohormonal antagonists (e.g., ACE inhibitors, angiotensin II receptor antagonists, angiotensin receptor-neprilysin inhibitors [ARNIs], β-blockers, aldosterone receptor antagonists) that inhibit the detrimental compensatory mechanisms in heart failure. Additional agents (e.g., cardiac glycosides, diuretics, sinoatrial modulators [i.e., ivabradine]) added to a heart failure treatment regimen in selected patients have been associated with symptomatic improvement and/or reduction in heart failure-related hospitalizations. Experts recommend that all asymptomatic patients with reduced left ventricular ejection fraction (LVEF) (American College of Cardiology Foundation [ACCF]/American Heart Association [AHA] stage B heart failure) receive therapy with an ACE inhibitor and β-blocker to prevent symptomatic heart failure and to reduce morbidity and mortality. If ACE inhibitors are not tolerated, then an angiotensin II receptor antagonist is recommended as alternative therapy. In patients with prior or current symptoms of chronic heart failure with reduced LVEF (ACCF/AHA stage C heart failure), ACCF, AHA, and the Heart Failure Society of America (HFSA) recommend inhibition of the renin-angiotensin-aldosterone (RAA) system with an ACE inhibitor, angiotensin II receptor antagonist, or ARNI in conjunction with a β-blocker, and an aldosterone antagonist in selected patients, to reduce morbidity and mortality. While ACE inhibitors have been the preferred drugs for inhibition of the RAA system because of their established benefits in patients with heart failure and reduced ejection fraction, some evidence indicates that therapy with sacubitril/valsartan, an ARNI, may be more effective than ACE inhibitor therapy (enalapril) in reducing cardiovascular death and heart failure-related hospitalization in such patients. ACCF, AHA, and HFSA recommend that patients with chronic symptomatic heart failure and reduced LVEF (New York Heart Association [NYHA] class II or III) who are able to tolerate an ACE inhibitor or angiotensin II receptor antagonist be switched to therapy containing an ARNI to further reduce morbidity and mortality. However, in patients in whom an ARNI is not appropriate, continued use of an ACE inhibitor for all classes of heart failure with reduced ejection fraction remains strongly advised. In patients in whom an ARNI or ACE inhibitor is not appropriate, an angiotensin II receptor antagonist may be used. For additional information on the use of ACE inhibitors in the management of heart failure, see Uses: Heart Failure, in Captopril 24:32.04 and in Enalaprilat/Enalapril 24:32.04. For further information on the use of ARNIs in patients with heart failure, see Uses: Heart Failure, in Sacubitril and Valsartan 24:32.92.

■ Diabetic Nephropathy Both ACE inhibitors and angiotensin II receptor antagonists have been shown to slow the rate of progression of renal disease in patients with diabetes mellitus and persistent albuminuria†, and use of a drug from either class is recommended in such patients with modestly elevated (30–300 mg/24 hours) or higher (exceeding 300 mg/24 hours) levels of urinary albumin excretion. The usual precautions of ACE inhibitor or angiotensin II receptor antagonist therapy in patients with substantial renal impairment should be observed. For additional information on the use of ACE inhibitors in the treatment of diabetic nephropathy, see Diabetic Nephropathy under Uses: Nephropathy, in Captopril 24:32.04.

Dosage and Administration

■ Administration Benazepril hydrochloride is administered orally.

For adult or pediatric patients unable to swallow tablets or those children for whom the daily dose does not correspond exactly to the strength of commercially available tablets, benazepril hydrochloride may be administered orally as an extemporaneously prepared suspension.

An extemporaneous suspension containing benazepril hydrochloride 2 mg/mL can be prepared in the following manner. First, 75 mL of suspending vehicle (Ora-Plus®) is added to an amber polyethylene terephthalate (PET) bottle containing fifteen 20-mg tablets of benazepril hydrochloride, and the contents are shaken for at least 2 minutes. The concentrated suspension should be allowed to stand for at least 60 minutes following reconstitution, and then should be shaken for an additional minute. The concentrated suspension of benazepril hydrochloride should be diluted with 75 mL of syrup (Ora-Sweet®), and the container then shaken to disperse the ingredients. The suspension should be shaken before dispensing each dose. The extemporaneous suspension is stable for 30 days when stored at 2–8°C.

■ Dosage Dosage of benazepril hydrochloride must be adjusted according to patient tolerance and response. Because of the risk of inducing hypotension, initiation of benazepril therapy requires consideration of recent and current antihypertensive therapy, the extent of blood pressure elevation, sodium intake, fluid status, and other clinical circumstances. If blood pressure is not controlled adequately with the ACE inhibitor alone, a low dosage of a diuretic may be added.

Hypertension **Benazepril Therapy.** For the management of hypertension in adults *not* receiving a diuretic, the usual initial dosage of benazepril hydrochloride is 10 mg once daily. In patients currently receiving a diuretic, an initial benazepril hydrochloride dosage of 5 mg daily is recommended. The divided-dose regimen has been more effective in controlling trough (pre-dose) blood pressure than the same dose given once daily.

The manufacturer states that the usual maintenance dosage in adults is 20–40 mg daily, given as a single dose or in 2 divided doses daily. Some experts state that the usual dosage range is 10–40 mg daily, given as a single dose or in 2 divided doses. Higher dosages (i.e., 80 mg daily) reportedly have resulted in increased response; however, there is limited experience with such dosages. The safety and efficacy of dosages exceeding 80 mg daily have not been established. If blood pressure is not controlled with benazepril alone, a second antihypertensive agent (e.g., diuretic) may be added.

For the management of hypertension in children 6 years of age or older, the usual initial dosage of benazepril hydrochloride is 0.2 mg/kg (up to 10 mg) once daily. Dosage may be adjusted until the desired blood pressure goal is achieved. Experts state that the dosage should be increased every 2–4 weeks until blood pressure is controlled, the maximum dosage is reached, or adverse effects occur. The safety and efficacy of dosages exceeding 0.6 mg/kg or in excess of 40 mg daily have not been established in pediatric patients. For information on overall principles and expert recommendations for treatment of hypertension in pediatric patients, see Uses: Hypertension in Pediatric Patients, in the Thiazides General Statement 40:28.20.

Benazepril/Hydrochlorothiazide Fixed-combination Therapy. The manufacturers state that therapy with the commercially available preparations containing benazepril hydrochloride in fixed combination with hydrochlorothiazide should only be initiated in adults after an adequate response is not achieved with benazepril or hydrochlorothiazide monotherapy. Alternatively, the fixed combination containing benazepril with hydrochlorothiazide may be used in patients who had been receiving the drugs separately and in whom dosage of the individual drugs has been adjusted. Patients whose blood pressure is not adequately controlled with benazepril or hydrochlorothiazide monotherapy may receive the fixed combination containing 10 mg of benazepril hydrochloride and 12.5 mg of hydrochlorothiazide initially. The maximum recommended dosage of the fixed combination preparation is 20 mg of benazepril hydrochloride and 25 mg of hydrochlorothiazide once daily.

Benazepril/Amlodipine Fixed-combination Therapy. The manufacturer states that therapy with the commercially available preparations containing benazepril hydrochloride in fixed combination with amlodipine should only be initiated in adults in whom an adequate response has not been achieved with benazepril or amlodipine monotherapy. Alternatively, such fixed combinations may be used if amlodipine dosages necessary for adequate response have been associated with development of edema. The fixed combination containing benazepril hydrochloride with amlodipine also may be used in patients who have been receiving the drugs separately, provided that the optimum dosage corresponds to the ratio in the commercial fixed-combination preparation. Dosage of the fixed combination containing benazepril hydrochloride and amlodipine should be adjusted according to the patient's response. The manufacturer states that when the fixed combinations containing 10–40 mg of benazepril hydrochloride and 2.5–10 mg of amlodipine have been used, the antihypertensive effects of these combinations have increased with increasing dosages of amlodipine regardless of race; in addition, antihypertensive effects increased with increasing dosages of benazepril in nonblack patients. The addition of benazepril to amlodipine therapy usually does not provide additional antihypertensive effects in black patients. The maximum recommended dosage of the fixed combination of benazepril hydrochloride and amlodipine is 40 mg of benazepril hydrochloride and 10 mg of amlodipine daily.

Blood Pressure Monitoring and Treatment Goals. Blood pressure should be monitored regularly (i.e., monthly) during therapy and dosage of the antihypertensive drug adjusted until blood pressure is controlled. If an adequate blood pressure response is not achieved with ACE inhibitor monotherapy, the dosage may be increased or another antihypertensive agent with demonstrated benefit and preferably with a complementary mechanism of action (e.g., calcium-channel blocker, thiazide diuretic) may be added; if target blood pressure is still not achieved, a third drug may be added. (See Uses: Hypertension.) In patients who develop unacceptable adverse effects with benazepril, the drug should be discontinued and another antihypertensive agent from a different pharmacologic class should be initiated.

The goal of hypertension management and prevention is to achieve and maintain optimal control of blood pressure. However, the optimum blood pressure threshold for initiating antihypertensive drug therapy and specific treatment goals remain controversial. While other hypertension guidelines have based target blood pressure goals on age and comorbidities, a 2017 multidisciplinary hypertension guideline from the American College of Cardiology (ACC), American Heart Association (AHA), and a number of other professional organizations incorporates underlying cardiovascular risk into decision making regarding treatment and generally recommends the same target blood pressure (i.e., less than 130/80 mm Hg) in all adults. Many patients will require at least 2 drugs from different pharmacologic classes to achieve this blood pressure goal; the potential benefits of hypertension management and drug cost, adverse effects, and risks associated with the use of multiple antihypertensive drugs also should be considered when deciding a patient's blood pressure treatment goal.

For additional information on target levels of blood pressure and on monitoring therapy in the management of hypertension, see Blood Pressure Monitoring and Treatment Goals under Dosage: Hypertension, in Dosage and Administration in the Thiazides General Statement 40:28.20.

■ Special Populations If benazepril is used in patients with impaired renal function, dosage must be modified in response to the degree of renal impairment, and, as with other ACE inhibitors, the theoretical risk of neutropenia must be considered. In adults with creatinine clearances less than 30 mL/minute per 1.73 m² or serum creatinine concentrations exceeding 3 mg/dL, the recommended initial dosage of benazepril hydrochloride is 5 mg once daily. If an adequate response is not achieved, dosage may be increased gradually until blood pressure is controlled or a maximum benazepril hydrochloride dosage of 40 mg daily is reached. There are insufficient data to date to make recommendations regarding dosage of benazepril hydrochloride in children with creatinine clearances less than 30 mL/minute per 1.73 m², and the manufacturer recommends that benazepril therapy not be used in such patients. Safety and efficacy of the fixed combination containing benazepril and hydrochlorothiazide have not been established in patients with severe renal impairment. Use of the commercially available preparation containing benazepril in combination with amlodipine is not recommended for patients with severe renal impairment.

Because of the greater frequency of decreased renal function in geriatric patients, the manufacturer states that dosage selection should be made with care and that it may be useful to monitor renal function in such patients receiving benazepril.

Preparations containing benazepril hydrochloride in fixed combination with 5 or 10 mg of amlodipine exceed the recommended initial dosage of amlodipine (2.5 mg daily) in geriatric patients and patients with hepatic impairment.

Cautions

■ Contraindications

Benazepril is contraindicated in patients with known hypersensitivity to benazepril, other angiotensin-converting enzyme (ACE) inhibitors, or any ingredient in the formulation; those with a history of angioedema with or without prior ACE inhibitor therapy; and in patients with diabetes mellitus who are receiving aliskiren therapy. Benazepril also is contraindicated in combination with a neprilysin inhibitor (e.g., sacubitril) and should not be administered within 36 hours of switching to or from sacubitril/valsartan.

■ Warnings/Precautions

Warnings **Fetal/Neonatal Morbidity and Mortality.** Drugs that act directly on the renin-angiotensin system (e.g., ACE inhibitors, angiotensin II receptor antagonists) reduce fetal renal function and can cause fetal and neonatal morbidity and mortality when used during pregnancy. Such potential risks of these drugs occur throughout pregnancy, especially during the second and third trimesters. ACE inhibitors also have been reported to increase the risk of major congenital malformations when administered during the first trimester of pregnancy. Potential neonatal effects include skull hypoplasia, anuria, hypotension, renal failure, and death. Resulting oligohydramnios can be associated with fetal lung hypoplasia and skeletal deformations. ACE inhibitors (e.g., benazepril) should be discontinued as soon as possible when pregnancy is detected, unless continued use is considered lifesaving. Nearly all women can be transferred successfully to alternative therapy for the remainder of pregnancy. For additional information on the risk of ACE inhibitors during pregnancy, see Cautions: Pregnancy, Fertility, and Lactation, in Captopril 24:32.04 and in Enalaprilat/Enalapril 24:32.04.

Sensitivity Reactions Sensitivity reactions, including anaphylactoid reactions and angioedema (including laryngeal angioedema and tongue edema), are potentially fatal. Head and neck angioedema have occurred in patients receiving an ACE inhibitor and have been reported at a higher rate in black patients compared with patients of other races. Patients with a history of angioedema unrelated to ACE inhibitor therapy may be at increased risk of angioedema while receiving an ACE inhibitor. In addition, concomitant use of an ACE inhibitor and a mammalian target of rapamycin (mTOR) inhibitor (e.g., everolimus, sirolimus, temsirolimus) or a neprilysin inhibitor (e.g., sacubitril) may increase the risk of angioedema; patients should be monitored for signs of angioedema during such concomitant therapy. Head and neck angioedema involving the tongue, glottis, or larynx may cause airway obstruction, especially in those with a history of airway surgery. If laryngeal stridor or angioedema of the face, tongue, or glottis occurs, ACE inhibitors (e.g., benazepril) should be discontinued promptly and appropriate therapy (e.g., epinephrine) and monitoring initiated until complete and sustained resolution of manifestations of angioedema has occurred.

Intestinal angioedema (occasionally without a prior history of facial angioedema or elevated serum levels of complement 1 [C1] esterase inhibitor) also has been reported in patients receiving ACE inhibitors. Intestinal angioedema, which frequently presents as abdominal pain (with or without nausea or vomiting), usually is diagnosed by abdominal CT scan, ultrasound, or surgery; symptoms usually have resolved after discontinuance of the ACE inhibitor. Intestinal angioedema should be considered in the differential diagnosis of patients who develop abdominal pain during therapy with an ACE inhibitor.

Life-threatening anaphylactoid reactions have been reported in at least 2 patients receiving ACE inhibitors while undergoing desensitization treatment with hymenoptera venom. When ACE inhibitors were temporarily discontinued before desensitization with the venom, anaphylactoid reactions did not recur; however, such reactions recurred after inadvertent rechallenge. Anaphylactoid reactions also have been reported following initiation of hemodialysis that used a high-flux membrane in patients receiving an ACE inhibitor. In addition, anaphylactoid reactions have been reported in patients undergoing low-density lipoprotein (LDL) apheresis with dextran sulfate absorption. In such patients, dialysis must be stopped immediately, and aggressive treatment for anaphylactoid reactions must be initiated. Antihistamine treatment has been ineffective in the alleviation of symptoms in these situations. In these patients, consideration should be given to using a different type of dialysis membrane or a different class of antihypertensive drug.

Other Warnings and Precautions **Renal Effects.** Deterioration of renal function, including acute renal failure, may occur in patients receiving ACE inhibitor therapy. Patients whose renal function depends on the activity of the renin-angiotensin system, particularly those with unilateral or bilateral renal artery stenosis, chronic kidney disease (CKD), severe congestive heart failure, myocardial infarction (MI), or volume depletion, may be at particular risk of developing acute renal failure while receiving benazepril. Increases in BUN and serum creatinine concentrations have occurred in patients with unilateral or bilateral renal artery stenosis; such increases generally are reversible following discontinuance of benazepril and/or diuretic therapy. Renal function should be monitored periodically in patients receiving benazepril. Withholding or discontinuance of therapy should be considered in patients who develop clinically important decreases in renal function while receiving benazepril.

Cardiovascular Effects. Symptomatic hypotension may occur; patients at particular risk include those with heart failure with systolic blood pressure less than 100 mm Hg, ischemic heart disease, cerebrovascular disease, hyponatremia, high-dose diuretic therapy, renal dialysis, or severe volume and/or salt depletion of any etiology. Symptomatic hypotension also may occur in patients with severe aortic stenosis. Volume and/or salt depletion should be corrected before starting benazepril therapy.

Excessive hypotension may occur in patients with heart failure (with or without associated renal impairment), which may be associated with oliguria and/or progressive azotemia and, rarely, acute renal failure and/or death. In patients with heart failure, benazepril therapy should be started under close medical supervision and patients should be followed closely for at least 2 weeks after initiation of benazepril or diuretic therapy or dosage adjustment of either drug. (See Dosage and Administration: Dosage.) Benazepril therapy should be avoided in patients who have hemodynamic instability following MI.

If hypotension occurs, the patient should be placed in the supine position, and if necessary, an IV infusion of 0.9% sodium chloride injection to expand fluid volume may be administered. Benazepril therapy usually may be continued following restoration of blood pressure and volume.

Hypotension may occur in patients undergoing major surgery or during anesthesia with agents that produce hypotension due to ACE inhibitor blockade of angiotensin II formation secondary to compensatory renin release. Hypotension in such patients may be corrected by volume expansion.

Effects on Potassium. Hyperkalemia can develop in patients receiving drugs that inhibit the renin-angiotensin system, especially in those with renal impairment or diabetes mellitus and those receiving other drugs that can increase serum potassium concentration (e.g., potassium-sparing diuretics, potassium supplements, potassium-containing salt substitutes). Serum potassium concentrations should be monitored periodically in patients receiving benazepril.

Hepatic Effects. An ACE inhibitor-associated clinical syndrome manifested initially by cholestatic jaundice has occurred; the syndrome may progress to fulminant hepatic necrosis and is potentially fatal. Patients receiving an ACE inhibitor, including benazepril, who develop jaundice or marked elevations of hepatic enzymes should discontinue the drug and receive appropriate monitoring and medical follow-up.

Hematologic Effects. Neutropenia/agranulocytosis, particularly in patients with renal impairment (especially those with concomitant collagen vascular disease), have been reported with another ACE inhibitor (captopril). Data are insufficient to rule out a similar incidence of agranulocytosis with benazepril in patients without prior reactions to other ACE inhibitors. Monitoring of leukocyte counts in patients with collagen vascular disease, especially if renal impairment exists, should be considered.

Respiratory Effects. Persistent, nonproductive cough has been reported with all ACE inhibitors; this effect resolves after drug discontinuance. ACE inhibitor-induced cough should be considered in the differential diagnosis of patients who develop cough during benazepril therapy.

Use of Fixed Combinations. When hydrochlorothiazide, amlodipine, or other drugs are used in fixed combination with benazepril, the usual cautions, precautions, and contraindications associated with these other drugs must be considered in addition to those associated with benazepril. (See Cautions, in the Thiazides General Statement 40:28.20 and in Amlodipine Besylate 24:28.08.)

Specific Populations **Pregnancy.** Category D. (See Users Guide.) Benazepril can cause fetal and neonatal morbidity and mortality when administered to a pregnant woman. Benazepril should be discontinued as soon as possible when pregnancy is detected. (See Fetal/Neonatal Morbidity and Mortality under Warnings/Precautions: Warnings, in Cautions.)

Lactation. Benazepril and benazeprilat are distributed into human milk in minimal amounts. Because of the unknown effects of benazepril or benazeprilat in nursing infants, a decision should be made whether to discontinue nursing or benazepril, taking into account the importance of the drug(s) to the woman.

Pediatric Use. If oliguria or hypotension occurs in neonates with a history of in utero exposure to benazepril, blood pressure and renal function should be supported; exchange transfusions or dialysis may be required. (See Fetal/Neonatal Morbidity and Mortality under Warnings/Precautions: Warnings, in Cautions.) Benazepril, which crosses the placenta, can theoretically be removed from the neonatal circulation by these means. There are occasional reports of benefit from these maneuvers with another ACE inhibitor; however, experience is limited.

Safety and efficacy of benazepril have not been established in children younger than 6 years of age and in pediatric patients with creatinine clearances of less than 30 mL/minute. Safety and efficacy of benazepril in fixed combination with amlodipine or hydrochlorothiazide have not been established in children. The long-term effects of benazepril on growth and development in children have not been studied. Although the safety profile of benazepril in pediatric patients is similar to that in adults, because of the potential for adverse effects on kidney development, ACE inhibitors should not be administered to pediatric patients younger than 1 year of age. For information on overall principles and expert recommendations for treatment of hypertension in pediatric patients, see Uses: Hypertension in Pediatric Patients, in the Thiazides General Statement 40:28.20.

Geriatric Use. No substantial differences in safety and efficacy have been observed in geriatric patients relative to younger adults, but increased sensitivity cannot be ruled out.

Because geriatric patients are more likely to have decreased renal function, dosage should be selected cautiously; it may be useful to monitor renal function in such patients.

Renal Impairment. Renal function may decrease with ACE inhibitor therapy in susceptible patients. Benazepril should be used with caution in those with renal impairment.

Benazepril in fixed combination with amlodipine is not recommended in patients with severe renal impairment; the recommended daily dosage of benazepril hydrochloride in such patients is 5 mg, which is not available in this combination preparation. (See Dosage and Administration: Special Populations and also Renal Effects under Warnings/Precautions: Other Warnings and Precautions, in Cautions.)

Black Patients. ACE inhibitors are not as effective and are associated with a higher incidence of angioedema in black patients compared with patients of other races. (See Uses: Hypertension.)

■ **Common Adverse Effects** Adverse effects reported in at least 2% of patients receiving benazepril and at an incidence more than 1% greater than that with placebo include headache, dizziness, somnolence, and postural dizziness. Adverse effects reported in greater than 1% of patients receiving benazepril in fixed combination with hydrochlorothiazide and possibly or probably study drug-related include dizziness, fatigue, postural dizziness, headache, cough, hypertonia, vertigo, nausea, impotence, and somnolence. Adverse effects reported in greater than 1% of patients receiving benazepril in fixed combination with amlodipine and possibly or probably drug-related include cough, headache, dizziness, and edema.

Drug Interactions

■ **Antidiabetic Agents** Concomitant administration of benazepril and insulin or oral antidiabetic agents may increase the risk of hypoglycemia. Patients receiving these drugs concomitantly should be informed of the possibility of hypoglycemia and monitored appropriately; dosage of the antidiabetic drug may need to be altered.

■ **Antihypertensive Agents and Drugs that Block the Renin-Angiotensin System** Benazepril potentiates the antihypertensive effect of other antihypertensive agents and drugs that block the renin-angiotensin system (e.g., curare derivatives, guanethidine, methyldopa, β-adrenergic blocking agents, vasodilators, calcium-channel blocking agents, ACE inhibitors, angiotensin II receptor antagonists, direct renin inhibitors [DRIs]).

Dual blockade of the renin-angiotensin system with angiotensin II receptor antagonists, ACE inhibitors, or aliskiren is associated with increased risks of hypotension, hyperkalemia, and changes in renal function (including acute renal failure) compared with monotherapy. Most patients receiving the combination of 2 renin-angiotensin system blocking agents do not obtain additional benefit compared with monotherapy. Concomitant use of 2 renin-angiotensin system blocking agents generally should be avoided. Blood pressure, renal function, and electrolytes should be closely monitored in patients receiving benazepril with other agents that affect the renin-angiotensin system.

■ **Diuretics** Potential pharmacokinetic and pharmacologic interaction (hypotensive effect).

■ **Drugs Increasing Serum Potassium Concentration** Potential pharmacologic interaction (additive hyperkalemic effect). Includes potassium-sparing diuretics, potassium supplements, and other drugs that can cause hyperkalemia. (See Effects on Potassium under Warnings/Precautions: Cautions: Other Warnings and Precautions, in Cautions.)

■ **Gold** Nitritoid reactions (e.g., facial flushing, nausea, vomiting, hypotension) have been reported rarely in patients receiving concomitant therapy with injectable gold (sodium aurothiomalate) and an ACE inhibitor.

■ **Lithium** Potential pharmacokinetic interaction (increased lithium concentrations and clinical toxicity). Lithium toxicity usually is reversible following discontinuance of lithium or benazepril. Serum lithium concentrations should be monitored during such concomitant use.

■ **Mammalian Target of Rapamycin Inhibitors** Concomitant use of an ACE inhibitor and a mammalian target of rapamycin (mTOR) inhibitor (e.g., everolimus, sirolimus, temsirolimus) may increase the risk of angioedema. (See Sensitivity Reactions under Cautions: Warnings/Precautions.)

■ **Neprilysin Inhibitors** Concomitant use of benazepril and a neprilysin inhibitor (e.g., sacubitril) may increase the risk for angioedema. (See Sensitivity Reactions under Cautions: Warnings/Precautions.)

■ **Nonsteroidal Anti-inflammatory Agents** In geriatric patients, patients who are volume depleted (including those who are receiving diuretic therapy), or in patients with compromised renal function, concomitant use of nonsteroidal anti-inflammatory agents (NSAIAs), including cyclooxygenase-2 (COX-2) inhibitors, with ACE inhibitors may result in the deterioration of renal function, including possible renal failure. These effects are usually reversible. Renal function should be monitored periodically in patients receiving concomitant benazepril and NSAIA therapy.

Description

Benazepril is an angiotensin-converting enzyme (ACE, bradykininase, kininase II) inhibitor. Benazepril, the ethylester of benazeprilat, is a prodrug and has little pharmacologic activity until hydrolyzed in the liver to benazeprilat. Like enalapril, fosinopril, lisinopril, quinapril, and ramipril, but unlike captopril, benazepril does not contain a sulfhydryl group.

Advice to Patients

When benazepril is used in fixed combination with hydrochlorothiazide, amlodipine, or other drugs, importance of advising patients about important precautionary information regarding the concomitant agent.

Risk of angioedema (including laryngeal edema), anaphylactoid, and other sensitivity reactions. Importance of discontinuing drug and reporting manifestations suggestive of angioedema (e.g., edema of face, eyes, lips, or tongue; swallowing or breathing with difficulty) to a clinician.

Risk of symptomatic hypotension (e.g., lightheadedness, syncope), especially during initial therapy or with volume depletion secondary to excessive perspiration, vomiting, or diarrhea; importance of reporting such symptoms to clinician. Importance of discontinuing drug and contacting clinician if syncope occurs.

Importance of informing clinicians of existing or contemplated concomitant therapy, including prescription and OTC drugs. Risk of hyperkalemia and hypoglycemia. Importance of avoiding the use of potassium supplements or salt substitutes containing potassium without consulting a clinician. Importance of monitoring closely for hypoglycemia in patients receiving oral antidiabetic agents or insulin, especially during first month of combined use with benazepril.

Risks of use during pregnancy. Importance of women informing clinicians immediately if they are or plan to become pregnant or plan to breast-feed; importance of discussing other options for hypertension treatment if pregnancy occurs.

Importance of informing patients of other important precautionary information. (See Cautions.)

Overview® (see Users Guide). For additional information on this drug until a more detailed monograph is developed and published, the manufacturer's labeling should be consulted. It is *essential* that the manufacturer's labeling be consulted for more detailed information on usual cautions, precautions, contraindications, potential drug interactions, laboratory test interferences, and acute toxicity.

Preparations

Excipients in commercially available drug preparations may have clinically important effects in some individuals; consult specific product labeling for details.

Benazepril Hydrochloride

Oral		
Tablets, film-coated	5 mg*	**Benazepril Hydrochloride Tablets**
		Lotensin®, Validus
	10 mg*	**Benazepril Hydrochloride Tablets**
		Lotensin®, Validus
	20 mg*	**Benazepril Hydrochloride Tablets**
		Lotensin®, Validus
	40 mg*	**Benazepril Hydrochloride Tablets**
		Lotensin®, Validus

*available from one or more manufacturer, distributor, and/or repackager by generic (nonproprietary) name

Benazepril Hydrochloride Combinations

Oral		
Capsules	10 mg with Amlodipine Besylate 2.5 mg (of amlodipine)*	**Amlodipine Besylate and Benazepril Hydrochloride Capsules**
		Lotrel®, Novartis
	10 mg with Amlodipine Besylate 5 mg (of amlodipine)*	**Amlodipine Besylate and Benazepril Hydrochloride Capsules**
		Lotrel®, Novartis
	20 mg with Amlodipine Besylate 5 mg (of amlodipine)*	**Amlodipine Besylate and Benazepril Hydrochloride Capsules**
		Lotrel®, Novartis
	20 mg with Amlodipine Besylate 10 mg (of amlodipine)*	**Amlodipine Besylate and Benazepril Hydrochloride Capsules**
		Lotrel®, Novartis

	40 mg with Amlodipine Besylate 5 mg (of amlodipine)*	**Amlodipine Besylate and Benazepril Hydrochloride Capsules**
		Lotrel®, Novartis
	40 mg with Amlodipine Besylate 10 mg (of amlodipine)*	**Amlodipine Besylate and Benazepril Hydrochloride Capsules**
		Lotrel®, Novartis
Tablets, film-coated	5 mg with Hydrochlorothiazide 6.25 mg*	**Benazepril with Hydrochlorothiazide Tablets**
		Lotensin® HCT (scored), Validus
	10 mg with Hydrochlorothiazide 12.5 mg*	**Benazepril with Hydrochlorothiazide Tablets**
		Lotensin® HCT (scored), Validus
	20 mg with Hydrochlorothiazide 12.5 mg*	**Benazepril with Hydrochlorothiazide Tablets**
		Lotensin® HCT (scored), Validus
	20 mg with Hydrochlorothiazide 25 mg*	**Benazepril with Hydrochlorothiazide Tablets**
		Lotensin® HCT (scored), Validus

*available from one or more manufacturer, distributor, and/or repackager by generic (nonproprietary) name

†Use is not currently included in the labeling approved by the US Food and Drug Administration

Captopril

■ Captopril is an angiotensin-converting enzyme (ACE) inhibitor.

Uses

■ **Hypertension** Captopril is used alone or in combination with other classes of antihypertensive agents in the management of hypertension. Because captopril can cause serious adverse effects (e.g., neutropenia, agranulocytosis), particularly in patients with renal impairment (especially those with collagen vascular disease) or in patients receiving immunosuppressive therapy, the drug was previously reserved for hypertension (usually severe) that was not manageable with maximal therapeutic dosages of other hypotensive agents in combination regimens (e.g., usually a diuretic, a β-adrenergic blocking agent [β-blocker], and a vasodilator) or when such regimens produced intolerable adverse effects. However, clinical experience with low dosages (up to 150 mg daily) has shown captopril to have a favorable benefit-to-risk ratio in the management of mild to moderate hypertension and the drug may currently be used as initial therapy in patients with normal renal function, in whom the risk of adverse hematologic effects is relatively low. In patients with impaired renal function, especially those with collagen vascular disease, captopril should be reserved for patients in whom other antihypertensive agents produce intolerable adverse effects or who do not have an adequate response to combination regimens of antihypertensive agents.

Current evidence-based practice guidelines for the management of hypertension in adults generally recommend the use of drugs from 4 classes of antihypertensive agents (angiotensin-converting enzyme [ACE] inhibitors, angiotensin II receptor antagonists, calcium-channel blockers, and thiazide diuretics); data from clinical outcome trials indicate that lowering blood pressure with any of these drug classes can reduce the complications of hypertension and provide similar cardiovascular protection. However, recommendations for initial drug selection and use in specific patient populations may vary across these expert guidelines. This variability is due, in part, to differences in the guideline development process and the types of studies (e.g., randomized controlled studies only versus a range of studies with different study designs) included in the evidence reviews. Ultimately, choice of antihypertensive therapy should be individualized, considering the clinical characteristics of the patient (e.g., age, ethnicity/race, comorbid conditions, cardiovascular risk factors) as well as drug-related factors (e.g., ease of administration, availability, adverse effects, costs). Because many patients eventually will need drugs from 2 or more antihypertensive classes, experts generally state that the emphasis should be placed on achieving appropriate blood pressure control rather than on identifying a preferred drug to achieve that control.

Disease Overview Worldwide, hypertension is the most common modifiable risk factor for cardiovascular events and mortality. The lifetime risk of developing hypertension in the US exceeds 80%, with higher rates observed among African Americans and Hispanics compared with whites or Asians. The systolic blood pressure and diastolic blood pressure values defined as hypertension (see Blood Pressure Classification under Uses: Hypertension) in a 2017 multidisciplinary guideline of the American College of Cardiology (ACC), American Heart Association (AHA), and a number of other professional organizations (subsequently referred to as the 2017 ACC/AHA hypertension guideline in this monograph) are lower than those defined in the Seventh Report of the Joint National Committee on Prevention, Detection, Evaluation, and Treatment of High Blood Pressure (JNC 7) guidelines, which results in an increase of approximately 14% in the prevalence of hypertension in the US. However, this change in definition results in only a 2% increase in the percentage of patients requiring antihypertensive drug therapy because nonpharmacologic treatment is recommended for most adults now classified by the 2017 ACC/AHA hypertension guideline as hypertensive who would *not* meet the JNC 7 definition of hypertension. Among US adults receiving antihypertensive drugs, approximately 53% have inadequately controlled blood pressure according to current ACC/AHA treatment goals.

Cardiovascular and Renal Sequelae. The principal goal of preventing and treating hypertension is to reduce the risk of cardiovascular and renal morbidity and mortality, including target organ damage. The relationship between blood pressure and cardiovascular disease is continuous, consistent, and independent of other risk factors. It is important that very high blood pressure be managed promptly to reduce the risk of target organ damage. The higher the blood pressure, the more likely the development of myocardial infarction (MI), heart failure, stroke, and renal disease. For adults 40–70 years of age, each 20-mm Hg increment in systolic blood pressure or 10-mm Hg increment in diastolic blood pressure doubles the risk of developing cardiovascular disease across the entire blood pressure range of 115/75 to 185/115 mm Hg. For those older than 50 years of age, systolic blood pressure is a much more important risk factor for developing cardiovascular disease than is diastolic blood pressure. The rapidity with which treatment is required depends on the patient's clinical presentation (presence of new or worsening target organ damage) and the presence or absence of cardiovascular complications; the 2017 ACC/AHA hypertension guideline states that treatment of very high blood pressure should be initiated within 1 week.

Blood Pressure Classification Accurate blood pressure measurement is essential for the proper diagnosis and management of hypertension. Error in measuring blood pressure is a major cause of inadequate blood pressure control and may lead to overtreatment. Because a patient's blood pressure may vary in an unpredictable fashion, a single blood pressure measurement is not sufficient for clinical decision-making. An average of 2 or 3 blood pressure measurements obtained on 2–3 separate occasions using proper technique should be used to minimize random error and provide a more accurate blood pressure reading. Out-of-office blood pressure measurements may be useful for confirming and managing hypertension. The 2017 ACC/AHA hypertension guideline document (available on the ACC and AHA websites) should be consulted for key steps on properly measuring blood pressure.

According to the 2017 ACC/AHA hypertension guideline, blood pressure in adults is classified into 4 categories: normal, elevated, stage 1 hypertension, and stage 2 hypertension. (See Table 1.) The 2017 ACC/AHA hypertension guideline lowers the blood pressure threshold used to define hypertension in the US; previous hypertension guidelines (JNC 7) considered adults with systolic blood pressure of 120–139 mm Hg or diastolic blood pressure of 80–89 mm Hg to have prehypertension, those with systolic blood pressure of 140–159 mm Hg or diastolic blood pressure of 90–99 mm Hg to have stage 1 hypertension, and those with systolic blood pressure of 160 mm Hg or higher or diastolic blood pressure of 100 mm Hg or higher to have stage 2 hypertension. The blood pressure definitions in the 2017 ACC/AHA hypertension guideline are based upon data from studies evaluating the association between systolic blood pressure/diastolic blood pressure and cardiovascular risk and the benefits of blood pressure reduction. Individuals with systolic blood pressure and diastolic blood pressure in 2 different categories should be designated as being in the higher blood pressure category.

Table 1. ACC/AHA Blood Pressure Classification in Adults[a,b]

Category	SBP[c] (mm Hg)		DBP[d] (mm Hg)
Normal	<120	and	<80
Elevated	120–129	and	<80
Hypertension, Stage 1	130–139	or	80–89
Hypertension, Stage 2	≥140	or	≥90

[a] Source: Whelton PK, Carey RM, Aronow WS et al. 2017 ACC/AHA/AAPA/ABC/ACPM/AGS/APhA/ASH/ASPC/NMA/PCNA guideline for the prevention, detection, evaluation, and management of high blood pressure in adults: a report of the American College of Cardiology/American Heart Association Task Force on Clinical Practice Guidelines. *Hypertension.* 2018;71:e13-115.

[b] Individuals with SBP and DBP in 2 different categories (e.g., elevated SBP and normal DBP) should be designated as being in the higher blood pressure category (i.e., elevated BP).

[c] Systolic blood pressure

[d] Diastolic blood pressure

The blood pressure thresholds used to define hypertension, when to initiate drug therapy, and the ideal target blood pressure values remain controversial. The 2017 ACC/AHA hypertension guideline recommends a blood pressure goal of less than 130/80 mm Hg in all adults who have confirmed hypertension and known cardiovascular disease or a 10-year atherosclerotic cardiovascular disease (ASCVD) event risk of 10% or higher; the ACC/AHA guideline also states that this blood pressure goal is reasonable to attempt to achieve in adults with confirmed hypertension who do *not* have increased cardiovascular risk. The lower blood pressure values used to define hypertension and the lower target blood pressure goals outlined in the 2017 ACC/AHA hypertension guideline are based on clinical studies demonstrating a substantial reduction in the composite end point of major cardiovascular disease events and the combination of fatal and nonfatal stroke when a lower systolic blood pressure/diastolic blood pressure value (i.e., 130/80 mm Hg) was used to define hypertension. These lower target blood pressure goals also are based upon clinical studies demonstrating continuing reduction of cardiovascular risk at progressively lower levels of systolic blood pressure. A linear relationship has been demonstrated between cardiovascular risk and blood pressure even at low systolic blood pressures (e.g., 120–124 mm Hg). The 2017 ACC/AHA hypertension guideline recommends estimating a patient's ASCVD risk using the ACC/AHA Pooled Cohort equations (available online at http://tools.acc.org/ASCVD-Risk-Estimator), which are based on a variety of factors including age, race, gender, cholesterol levels, statin use, blood pressure, treatment for hypertension, history of diabetes mellitus, smoking status, and aspirin use. While the 2017 ACC/AHA hypertension guideline has lowered the threshold for *diagnosing* hypertension in adults, the threshold for *initiating drug therapy* has only been lowered for those patients who are at high risk of cardiovascular disease. Clinicians who support the 2017 ACC/AHA hypertension guideline believe that these recommendations have the potential to increase hypertension awareness, encourage lifestyle modification, and focus antihypertensive drug initiation and intensification in those adults at high risk for cardiovascular disease.

The lower blood pressure goals advocated in the 2017 ACC/AHA hypertension guideline have been questioned by some clinicians who have concerns regarding the guideline's use of extrapolated observational data, the lack of generalizability of some of the randomized trials (e.g., SPRINT) used to support the guideline, the difficulty of establishing accurate representative blood pressure values in typical clinical practice settings, and the accuracy of the cardiovascular risk calculator used in the guideline. Some clinicians state the lower blood pressure threshold used to define hypertension in the 2017 ACC/AHA hypertension guideline is not fully supported by clinical data, and these clinicians have expressed concerns about the possible harms (e.g., adverse effects of antihypertensive therapy) associated with classifying more patients as being hypertensive. Some clinicians also state that using this guideline, a large number of young, low-risk patients would need to be treated in order to observe a clinical benefit, while other clinicians state that the estimated gains in life expectancy attributable to long-term use of blood pressure-lowering drugs are correspondingly greater in this patient population.

Treatment Benefits In clinical trials, antihypertensive therapy has been found to reduce the risk of developing stroke by about 34–40%, MI by about 20–25%, and heart failure by more than 50%. In a randomized, controlled study (SPRINT) that included hypertensive patients without diabetes mellitus who had a high risk of cardiovascular disease, intensive systolic blood pressure lowering of approximately 15 mm Hg was associated with a 25% reduction in cardiovascular disease events and a 27% reduction in all-cause mortality. However, the exclusion of patients with diabetes mellitus, prior stroke, and those younger than 50 years of age may decrease the generalizability of these findings. Some experts estimate that if the systolic blood pressure goals of the 2017 ACC/AHA hypertension guideline are achieved, major cardiovascular disease events may be reduced by an additional 340,000 and total deaths by an additional 156,000 compared with implementation of the JNC 8 expert panel guideline goals but these benefits may be accompanied by an increase in the frequency of adverse events. While there was no overall difference in the occurrence of serious adverse events in patients receiving intensive therapy for blood pressure control (systolic blood pressure target of less than 120 mm Hg) compared with those receiving less intense control (systolic blood pressure target of less than 140 mm Hg) in the SPRINT study, hypotension, syncope, electrolyte abnormalities, and acute kidney injury or acute renal failure occurred in substantially more patients receiving intensive therapy.

In the Antihypertensive and Lipid-lowering Treatment to Prevent Heart Attack Trial (ALLHAT), the long-term cardiovascular morbidity and mortality benefit of a long-acting dihydropyridine calcium-channel blocker (amlodipine), a thiazide-like diuretic (chlorthalidone), and an ACE inhibitor (lisinopril) were compared in a broad population of patients with hypertension at risk for coronary heart disease. Although these antihypertensive agents were comparably effective in providing important cardiovascular benefit, apparent differences in certain secondary outcomes were observed. Patients receiving the ACE inhibitor experienced higher risks of stroke, combined cardiovascular disease, GI bleeding, and angioedema, while those receiving the calcium-channel blocker were at higher risk of developing heart failure. The ALLHAT investigators suggested that the favorable cardiovascular outcome may be attributable, at least in part, to the greater antihypertensive effect of the calcium-channel blocker compared with that of the ACE inhibitor, especially in women and black patients. (See Clinical Benefit of Thiazides in Hypertension under Hypertension in Adults: Treatment Benefits, in Uses in the Thiazides General Statement 40:28.20.)

General Considerations for Initial and Maintenance Antihypertensive Therapy **Nonpharmacologic Therapy.** Nonpharmacologic measures (i.e., lifestyle/behavioral modifications) that are effective in lowering blood pressure include weight reduction (for those who are overweight or obese), dietary changes to include foods such as fruits, vegetables, whole grains, and low-fat dairy products that are rich in potassium, calcium, magnesium, and fiber (i.e., adoption of the Dietary Approaches to Stop Hypertension [DASH] eating plan), sodium reduction, increased physical activity, and moderation of alcohol intake. Such lifestyle/behavioral modifications, including smoking cessation, enhance antihypertensive drug efficacy and decrease cardiovascular risk and remain an indispensable part of the management of hypertension. Lifestyle/behavioral modifications without antihypertensive drug therapy are recommended for individuals classified by the 2017 ACC/AHA hypertension guideline as having elevated blood pressure (systolic blood pressure 120–129 mm Hg and diastolic blood pressure less than 80 mm Hg) and in those with stage 1 hypertension (systolic blood pressure 130–139 mm Hg or diastolic blood pressure 80–89 mm Hg) who do *not* have preexisting cardiovascular disease or an estimated 10-year ASCVD risk of 10% or greater.

Initiation of Drug Therapy. Drug therapy in the management of hypertension must be individualized and adjusted based on the degree of blood pressure elevation while also considering cardiovascular risk factors. Drug therapy generally is reserved for patients who respond inadequately to nondrug therapies or in whom the degree of blood pressure elevation or coexisting risk factors, especially increased cardiovascular risk, require more prompt or aggressive therapy; however, the optimum blood pressure threshold for initiating antihypertensive drug therapy and specific treatment goals remain controversial. Recommendations generally are based on specific blood pressure levels shown in clinical studies to produce clinical benefits and can therefore vary depending on the studies selected for review.

The 2017 ACC/AHA hypertension guideline and many experts currently state that the treatment of hypertension should be based not only on blood pressure values but also on patients' cardiovascular risk factors. For *secondary prevention* of recurrent cardiovascular disease events in adults with clinical cardiovascular disease or for *primary prevention* in adults with an estimated 10-year ASCVD risk of 10% or higher, the 2017 ACC/AHA hypertension guideline recommends initiation of antihypertensive drug therapy in conjunction with lifestyle/behavioral modifications at an average systolic blood pressure of 130 mm Hg or an average diastolic blood pressure of 80 mm Hg or higher. For *primary prevention* of cardiovascular disease events in adults with a low (less than 10%) estimated 10-year risk of ASCVD, the 2017 ACC/AHA hypertension guideline recommends initiation of antihypertensive drug therapy in conjunction with lifestyle/behavioral modifications at a systolic blood pressure of 140 mm Hg or higher or a diastolic blood pressure of 90 mm Hg or higher. After initiation of antihypertensive drug therapy, regardless of the ASCVD risk, the 2017 ACC/AHA hypertension guideline generally recommends a blood pressure goal of less than 130/80 mm Hg in all adults. In addition, a systolic blood pressure goal of less than 130 mm Hg is also recommended for noninstitutionalized ambulatory patients 65 years of age or older. While these blood pressure goals are lower than those recommended for most patients in previous guidelines, they are based upon clinical studies demonstrating continuing reduction of cardiovascular risk at progressively lower levels of systolic blood pressure.

Most data indicate that patients with a higher cardiovascular risk will benefit the most from tighter blood pressure control; however, some experts state this treatment goal also may be beneficial in those at lower cardiovascular risk. Other clinicians believe that the benefits of such blood pressure lowering do not outweigh the risks in those patients considered to be at lower risk of cardiovascular disease and that reclassifying individuals formerly considered to have prehypertension as having hypertension may potentially lead to use of drug therapy in such patients without consideration of cardiovascular risk. Previous hypertension guidelines, such as those from the JNC 8 expert panel, generally recommended initiation of antihypertensive treatment in patients with a systolic blood pressure of at least 140 mm Hg or diastolic blood pressure of at least 90 mm Hg, targeted a blood pressure goal of less than 140/90 mm Hg regardless of cardiovascular risk, and used higher systolic blood pressure thresholds and targets in geriatric patients. Some clinicians continue to support the target blood pressures recommended by the JNC 8 expert panel because of concerns that such recommendations in the 2017 ACC/AHA hypertension guideline are based on extrapolation of data from the high-risk population in the SPRINT study to a lower-risk population. Also, because more than 90% of patients in SPRINT were already receiving antihypertensive drugs at baseline, data are lacking on the effects of *initiating* drug therapy at a lower blood pressure threshold (130/80 mm Hg) in patients at high risk of cardiovascular disease. The potential benefits of hypertension management and drug cost, adverse effects, and risks associated with the use of multiple antihypertensive drugs should be considered when deciding a patient's blood pressure treatment goal.

The 2017 ACC/AHA hypertension guideline recommends an ASCVD risk assessment for all adults with hypertension; however, experts state that it can be assumed that patients with hypertension and diabetes mellitus or chronic kidney disease (CKD) are at high risk for cardiovascular disease and that antihypertensive drug therapy should be initiated in these patients at a blood pressure of 130/80 mm Hg or higher. The 2017 ACC/AHA guideline also recommends a blood pressure goal of less than 130/80 mm Hg in patients with hypertension and diabetes mellitus or CKD. These recommendations are based on a systematic review of high-quality evidence from randomized controlled trials, meta-analyses, and post-hoc analyses that have demonstrated substantial reductions in the risk of important clinical outcomes (e.g., cardiovascular events) regardless of comorbid conditions or age when systolic blood pressure is lowered to less than 130 mm Hg. However, some clinicians have questioned the generalizability of findings from some of the trials (e.g., SPRINT) used to support the 2017 ACC/AHA hypertension guideline. For example, SPRINT included adults (mean age: 68 years) *without* diabetes mellitus who were at high risk of cardiovascular disease. While benefits of intensive blood pressure control were observed in this patient population, some clinicians have questioned whether these findings apply to younger patients who have a low risk of cardiovascular disease. In patients with CKD in the SPRINT trial, intensive blood pressure management (achieving a mean systolic blood pressure of approximately 122 mm Hg compared with 136 mm Hg with standard treatment) provided a similar beneficial reduction in the composite cardiovascular disease primary outcome and all-cause mortality as in the full patient cohort. Because most patients with CKD die from cardiovascular complications, the findings of this study further support a lower blood pressure target of less than 130/80 mm Hg.

Data are lacking to determine the ideal blood pressure goal in patients with hypertension and diabetes mellitus; also, studies evaluating the benefits of intensive blood pressure control in patients with diabetes mellitus have provided conflicting results. Clinical studies reviewed for the 2017 ACC/AHA hypertension guideline have shown similar quantitative benefits from blood pressure lowering in hypertensive patients with or without diabetes mellitus. In a randomized, controlled study (ACCORD-BP) that compared a higher (systolic blood pressure less than 140 mm Hg) versus lower (systolic blood pressure less than 120 mm Hg) blood pressure goal in patients with diabetes mellitus, there was no difference in the incidence of cardiovascular outcomes (e.g., composite outcome of cardiovascular death, nonfatal MI, and nonfatal stroke). However, some experts state that this study was underpowered to detect a difference between the 2 treatment groups and that the factorial design of the study complicated interpretation of the results. Although SPRINT did not include patients with diabetes mellitus, patients in this study with prediabetes demonstrated a similar cardiovascular benefit from intensive treatment of blood pressure as normoglycemic patients. A meta-analysis of data from ACCORD and SPRINT suggests that the findings of both studies are consistent and that patients with diabetes mellitus benefit from more intensive blood pressure control. These data support the 2017 ACC/AHA hypertension guideline recommendation of a blood pressure treatment goal of less than 130/80 mm Hg in patients with hypertension and diabetes mellitus. Alternatively, the American Diabetes Association (ADA) recommends a blood pressure goal of less than 140/90 mm Hg in patients with diabetes mellitus. The ADA states that a lower blood pressure goal (e.g., less than 130/80 mm Hg) may be appropriate for patients with a high risk of cardiovascular disease and diabetes mellitus if it can be achieved without undue treatment burden.

Further study is needed to more clearly define optimum blood pressure goals in patients with hypertension, particularly in high-risk groups (e.g., patients with diabetes mellitus, cardiovascular disease, or cerebrovascular disease; black patients); when determining appropriate blood pressure goals, individual risks and benefits should be considered in addition to the evidence from clinical studies.

Choice of Initial Drug Therapy. In current hypertension management guidelines, ACE inhibitors are recommended as one of several preferred drugs for the initial treatment of hypertension; other options include angiotensin II receptor antagonists, calcium-channel blockers, and thiazide diuretics. The 2017 ACC/AHA hypertension guideline states that an ACE inhibitor, angiotensin II receptor antagonist, calcium-channel blocker, or thiazide diuretic (preferably chlorthalidone) are all acceptable choices for initial antihypertensive drug therapy in the general population of nonblack patients, including those with diabetes mellitus; drugs from any of these classes generally produce similar benefits in terms of overall mortality and cardiovascular, cerebrovascular, and renal outcomes. ACE inhibitors may be particularly useful in the management of hypertension in patients with certain coexisting conditions such as heart failure, ischemic heart disease, diabetes mellitus, CKD, or cerebrovascular disease or following myocardial infarction (MI). (See Considerations for Drug Therapy in Patients with Underlying Cardiovascular and Other Risk Factors under Uses: Hypertension.)

In patients with hypertension and compelling indications (e.g., CKD with albuminuria [urine albumin 300 mg/day or greater, or urine albumin:creatinine ratio of 300 mg/g or equivalent in the first morning void]), angiotensin II receptor antagonists are usually considered an alternative for ACE inhibitor-intolerant patients. (See Chronic Kidney Disease under Hypertension: Considerations for Drug Therapy in Patients with Underlying Cardiovascular and Other Risk Factors, in Uses.) However, data indicate no difference in efficacy between ACE inhibitors and angiotensin II receptor antagonists with regard to blood pressure lowering and clinical outcomes (i.e., all-cause mortality, cardiovascular mortality, MI, heart failure, stroke, and end-stage renal disease). Adverse events (e.g., cough, angioedema) leading to drug discontinuance occur more frequently with ACE inhibitor therapy than with angiotensin II receptor antagonist therapy. Because of similar efficacy and a lower frequency of adverse effects, some experts believe that angiotensin II receptor antagonists should be used instead of an ACE inhibitor for the treatment of hypertension or hypertension with certain compelling indications.

Experts state that in patients with stage 1 hypertension (especially the elderly, those with a history of hypotension, or those who have experienced adverse drug effects), it is reasonable to initiate drug therapy using the stepped-care approach in which one drug is initiated and titrated and other drugs are added sequentially to achieve the target blood pressure. Although some patients can begin treatment with a single antihypertensive agent, starting with 2 drugs in different pharmacologic classes (either as separate agents or in a fixed-dose combination) is recommended in patients with stage 2 hypertension and an average blood pressure more than 20/10 mm Hg above their target blood pressure. Such combined therapy may increase the likelihood of achieving goal blood pressure in a more timely fashion, but also may increase the risk of adverse effects (e.g., orthostatic hypotension) in some patients (e.g., elderly). Drug regimens with complementary activity, where a second antihypertensive agent is used to block compensatory responses to the first agent or affect a different pressor mechanism, can result in additive blood pressure lowering and are preferred. Drug combinations that have similar mechanisms of action or clinical effects (e.g., the combination of an ACE inhibitor and an angiotensin II receptor antagonist) generally should be avoided. Many patients who begin therapy with a single antihypertensive agent will subsequently require at least 2 drugs from different pharmacologic classes to achieve their blood pressure goal. Experts state that other patient-specific factors, such as age, concurrent medications, drug adherence, drug interactions, the overall treatment regimen, cost, and comorbidities, also should be considered when deciding on an antihypertensive drug regimen. For any stage of hypertension, antihypertensive drug dosages should be adjusted and/or other agents substituted or added until goal blood pressure is achieved. (See Follow-up and Maintenance Drug Therapy under Hypertension: General Considerations for Initial and Maintenance Antihypertensive Therapy, in Uses.)

Follow-up and Maintenance Drug Therapy. Several strategies are used for the titration and combination of antihypertensive drugs; these strategies, which are generally based on those used in randomized controlled studies, include maximizing the dosage of the first drug before adding a second drug, adding a second drug before achieving maximum dosage of the initial drug, or initiating therapy with 2 drugs simultaneously (either as separate preparations or as a fixed-dose combination). Combined use of an ACE inhibitor and angiotensin II receptor antagonist should be avoided because of the potential risk of adverse renal effects. After initiating a new or adjusted antihypertensive drug regimen, patients should have their blood pressure reevaluated monthly until adequate blood pressure control is achieved. Effective blood pressure control can be achieved in most hypertensive patients, but many will ultimately require therapy with 2 or more antihypertensive drugs. In addition to measuring blood pressure, clinicians should evaluate patients for orthostatic hypotension, adverse drug effects, adherence to drug therapy and lifestyle modifications, and the need for drug dosage adjustments. Laboratory testing such as electrolytes and renal function status and other assessments of target organ damage also should be performed.

Captopril can be used for the management of hypertension as initial monotherapy or as a component of a multiple-drug regimen. When captopril is used alone but the patient's hypertension does not respond adequately, addition of a thiazide diuretic often adequately controls blood pressure. Such combined therapy generally produces additive reduction in blood pressure and may permit dosage reduction of either or both drugs and minimize adverse effects while maintaining blood pressure control.

Captopril may be effective in the management of hypertension resistant to other drugs. Although captopril occasionally may be effective alone in patients with severe hypertension, it is usually necessary to use it in conjunction with a diuretic. (See Drug Interactions: Hypotensive Agents and Diuretics.)

Tolerance to the hypotensive effect of captopril apparently does not occur during long-term administration, particularly if the drug is used with a diuretic. Abrupt withdrawal of captopril therapy results in a gradual return of hypertension; rapid increases in blood pressure have not been reported to date.

Considerations for Drug Therapy in Patients with Underlying Cardiovascular and Other Risk Factors Drug therapy in patients with hypertension and underlying cardiovascular or other risk factors should be carefully individualized based on the underlying disease(s), concomitant drugs, tolerance to drug-induced adverse effects, and blood pressure goal. See Table 2 on Compelling Indications for Drug Classes based on Comorbid Conditions, under Uses: Hypertension in Adults, in the Thiazides General Statement 40:28.20.

Ischemic Heart Disease. The selection of an appropriate antihypertensive agent in patients with ischemic heart disease should be based on individual patient characteristics and may include ACE inhibitors and/or β-blockers, with the addition of other drugs such as thiazide diuretics or calcium-channel blockers as necessary to achieve blood pressure goals. Many experts recommend the use of an ACE inhibitor (or an angiotensin II receptor antagonist) and/or a β-blocker in hypertensive patients with stable ischemic heart disease because of the cardioprotective benefits of these drugs; in addition, all patients who have survived an MI should be treated with a β-blocker because of the demonstrated mortality benefit of these agents.

Heart Failure. While ACE inhibitors as single therapies are not superior to other antihypertensive agents in the reduction of cardiovascular outcomes, ACE inhibitors, usually in conjunction with other agents such as cardiac glycosides, diuretics, and β-blockers, have been shown to reduce morbidity and mortality in patients with existing heart failure. (See Uses: Heart Failure.) ACE inhibitors also have been shown to prevent subsequent heart failure and reduce morbidity and mortality in patients with systolic dysfunction following an acute MI. (See Uses: Left Ventricular Dysfunction after Acute Myocardial Infarction.)

Diabetes Mellitus. Experts state that initial treatment of hypertension in adults with diabetes mellitus and hypertension should include any of the usual first-line agents (ACE inhibitors, angiotensin II receptor antagonist, calcium-channel blockers, thiazide diuretics). In adults with diabetes mellitus, hypertension, and albuminuria, treatment with an ACE inhibitor or angiotensin II receptor antagonist may be considered to reduce the progression of kidney disease. While there is evidence demonstrating the benefits of ACE inhibitors in reducing the development or progression of microvascular or macrovascular complications in hypertensive patients with type 1 or type 2 diabetes mellitus, in the absence of albuminuria, the risk of progressive kidney disease is low, and ACE inhibitors and angiotensin II receptor antagonists have not demonstrated superior cardioprotection when compared with other first-line agents. Results of several studies indicate that adequate control of blood pressure in patients with type 2 diabetes mellitus reduces the development or progression of complications of diabetes (e.g., death related to diabetes, stroke, heart failure, microvascular disease). Most patients with diabetes mellitus will require 2 or more antihypertensive agents to achieve blood pressure control.

Chronic Kidney Disease. Hypertensive patients with CKD (glomerular filtration rate [GFR] less than 60 mL/minute per 1.73 m^2 or kidney damage for 3 or more months) usually will require more than one antihypertensive agent to reach target blood pressure. Use of ACE inhibitors or angiotensin II receptor antagonists may be reasonable in patients with diabetic or nondiabetic CKD (stage 1 or 2 with albuminuria or stage 3 or higher); these drugs have been shown to slow the progression of kidney disease. Evidence of a renoprotective benefit is strongest in those with higher levels of albuminuria. Increases in serum creatinine (up to 30%) may be observed as a result of a decrease in intraglomerular pressure and concurrent reduction in GFR. The 2017 ACC/AHA hypertension guideline states that in patients with less severe kidney disease (i.e., stage 1 or 2 CKD without albuminuria), any of the first-line antihypertensive agents (e.g., ACE inhibitors, angiotensin II receptor antagonists, calcium-channel blockers, thiazide diuretics) can be used for the initial treatment of hypertension. Diuretics also may be useful in the management of CKD, and may potentiate the effects of ACE inhibitors, angiotensin II receptor antagonists, and other antihypertensive agents when used in combination.

Cerebrovascular Disease. Some experts recommend a blood pressure goal of less than 140/90 mm Hg in patients with ischemic stroke or transient ischemic attack (TIA), while others state that a blood pressure goal of less than 130/80 mm Hg may be reasonable. The 2017 ACC/AHA hypertension guideline states that adults not previously treated for hypertension who experience a stroke or TIA and who have an established blood pressure of 140/90 mm Hg or higher should receive antihypertensive therapy within a few days after the event to reduce the risk of recurrent stroke or other vascular events. In patients with a recent lacunar stroke, experts suggest that a systolic blood pressure goal of 130 mm Hg may be reasonable based on results of a randomized open-label study (the Secondary Prevention of Small Subcortical Strokes [SPS3] trial). Although experts state that the optimal choice of drug for the management of hypertension in patients with a previous TIA or ischemic stroke is uncertain, available data indicate that an ACE inhibitor, angiotensin II receptor antagonist, thiazide diuretic, or the combination of a thiazide diuretic and an ACE inhibitor may be effective. Administration of an ACE inhibitor in combination with a thiazide diuretic has been shown to lower rates of recurrent stroke.

Other Special Considerations for Antihypertensive Drug Therapy

Race. Most patients with hypertension, especially black patients, will require at least 2 antihypertensive drugs to achieve adequate blood pressure control. In general, black hypertensive patients tend to respond better to monotherapy with thiazide diuretics or calcium-channel blockers than to monotherapy with ACE inhibitors. In a prespecified subgroup analysis of the ALLHAT study, a thiazide-type diuretic was more effective than an ACE inhibitor in improving cerebrovascular and cardiovascular outcomes in black patients; when compared with a calcium-channel blocker, the ACE inhibitor was less effective in reducing blood pressure and was associated with a 51% higher rate of stroke. (See Clinical Benefit of Thiazides in Hypertension under Hypertension in Adults: Treatment Benefits, in Uses in the Thiazides General Statement 40:28.20.) However, the combination of an ACE inhibitor or an angiotensin II receptor antagonist with a calcium-channel blocker or thiazide diuretic produces similar blood pressure lowering in black patients as in other racial groups. In addition, some experts state that when use of ACE inhibitors is indicated in hypertensive patients with underlying cardiovascular or other risk factors, these indications should be applied equally to black hypertensive patients.

Although captopril has lowered blood pressure in all races studied, monotherapy with this agent has produced a smaller reduction in blood pressure in black hypertensive patients, a population associated with low renin hypertension; however, this population difference in response does not appear to occur during combined therapy with captopril and a thiazide diuretic. In addition, ACE inhibitors appear to produce a higher incidence of angioedema in black patients than in other races studied.

For further information on overall principles and expert recommendations for treatment of hypertension, see Uses: Hypertension in Adults and also see Uses: Hypertension in Pediatric Patients, in the Thiazides General Statement 40:28.20.

Renovascular or Malignant Hypertension Captopril also has been effective in the management of renovascular or malignant hypertension and, in some patients, in the management of hypertension associated with chronic renal failure.

Hypertensive Crises Captopril has been used orally for rapidly reducing blood pressure in patients with hypertensive crises† in whom reduction of blood pressure was considered urgent (hypertensive urgencies) or emergent (hypertensive emergencies). Because even oral therapy for hypertensive crises can result in profound hypotension and associated adverse cardiovascular effects (e.g., myocardial ischemia or infarction, cerebrovascular hypoperfusion or stroke), captopril should not be used indiscriminately, and the benefits versus risks of rapidly reducing blood pressure with the drug must be weighed carefully.

Hypertensive urgencies are those situations in which there is a severe elevation in blood pressure without progressive target organ damage. Hypertensive urgencies generally can be managed by intensification or reinstitution (e.g., following noncompliance) of the current antihypertensive regimen and treatment of anxiety if needed. Experts state that there is no need for rapid reduction of blood pressure in such patients and hospitalization or referral to the emergency department also is unnecessary.

Hypertensive emergencies are those rare situations requiring immediate blood pressure reduction (not necessarily to normal ranges) to prevent or limit target organ damage. Such emergencies include hypertensive encephalopathy, acute MI, intracerebral hemorrhage, acute left ventricular failure with pulmonary edema, eclampsia, dissecting aortic aneurysm, unstable angina pectoris, acute ischemic stroke, and acute renal failure. Although oral therapy with captopril has been used to rapidly reduce blood pressure in such emergencies, patients with hypertensive emergencies should be hospitalized and treated initially with appropriate parenteral antihypertensive therapy (e.g., labetalol, esmolol, fenoldopam, nicardipine, sodium nitroprusside).

■ **Nephropathy** Captopril may be used in patients with nephropathy, including diabetic nephropathy. Use of ACE inhibitors or angiotensin II receptor antagonists is recommended in the management of diabetic or nondiabetic† CKD to slow progression of the disease. ACE inhibitors have stabilized or improved effective renal blood flow and glomerular filtration rate and decreased proteinuria in hypertensive or normotensive patients with moderately impaired renal function, moderate to severe renal disease, or diabetic nephropathy. Short-term administration of captopril improved blood flow and glomerular filtration rate in some hypertensive patients with moderately impaired renal function; however, long-term captopril therapy has not maintained sustained improvement in renal blood flow and glomerular filtration rate. In general, captopril should be used with caution in patients with impaired renal function, especially those with bilateral renal-artery stenosis or renal-artery stenosis in a solitary kidney. (See Cautions: Renal Effects and see Cautions: Hematologic Effects, and also see Precautions and Contraindications.) Captopril appears to be ineffective in the management of hypertension in anephric patients. (See Pharmacology: Renal and Electrolyte Effects.)

Diabetic Nephropathy Captopril is used in the management of diabetic nephropathy manifested by proteinuria (urinary protein excretion exceeding 500 mg per 24 hours) in patients with type 1 diabetes mellitus and diabetic retinopathy.

Both ACE inhibitors and angiotensin II receptor antagonists have been shown to slow the rate of progression of renal disease in patients with diabetes mellitus and persistent albuminuria, and use of a drug from either class is recommended in such patients with modestly elevated (30–300 mg per 24 hours) or higher (exceeding 300 mg per 24 hours) levels of urinary albumin excretion. Comparative trials evaluating the efficacy of ACE inhibitors and angiotensin II receptor antagonists for improving renal outcomes in diabetic patients are lacking. Evidence supporting use of ACE inhibitors generally is based on studies in patients with type 1 diabetes mellitus, while evidence supporting use of angiotensin II receptor antagonists generally is based on studies in patients with type 2 diabetes mellitus. Findings from these studies indicate that both drug classes delay progression of increased urinary albumin excretion in patients with diabetes mellitus and also may slow the decline in renal function. Because the available data are consistent, some experts suggest that the effects of both drug classes in improving renal outcomes in patients with diabetes mellitus and proteinuria are likely to be similar. Drugs that inhibit the renin-angiotensin system (i.e., ACE inhibitors, angiotensin II receptor antagonists) have been shown to delay the onset of albuminuria in patients with type 2 diabetes mellitus and hypertension who have normal levels of urinary albumin excretion†; however, experts state that in the absence of albuminuria, the risk of progressive kidney disease is low. Combined therapy with ACE inhibitors and angiotensin II receptor antagonists provides no additional cardiovascular benefit and increases the risk of adverse effects (e.g., impaired renal function, hyperkalemia). The American Diabetes Association (ADA) states that the use of an ACE inhibitor or angiotensin II receptor antagonist is not recommended for the primary prevention of diabetic nephropathy in patients with diabetes mellitus who are normotensive, have normal levels of urinary protein excretion, and have a normal glomerular filtration rate.

In a multicenter, controlled study in hypertensive and normotensive individuals who had type 1 diabetes mellitus for at least 7 years, diabetic retinopathy, proteinuria, and a serum creatinine concentration of 2.5 mg/dL or less, deterioration in renal function was substantially less pronounced in patients receiving long-term captopril therapy (median: 3 years [range: 1.8–4.8 years]) than in those receiving placebo. Patients with hypertension received hypotensive agents (e.g., diuretics, β-blockers, α-adrenergic blocking agents, vasodilators) as needed. Overall, patients receiving captopril had a 48% reduction in the risk of doubling of serum creatinine concentration. Captopril therapy was especially useful in patients with more advanced renal disease (i.e., baseline serum creatinine exceeding 1.5 mg/dL). Captopril therapy was associated with a 30% reduction in urinary protein excretion within 3 months and was evident throughout the study. In addition, patients receiving captopril had a 50% reduction in the risk of death and need for dialysis or renal transplantation, particularly in those with more advanced renal disease. It has been suggested that captopril and other ACE inhibitors may slow the progression of renal nephropathy by a mechanism independent of its antihypertensive properties.

Captopril also has been shown to delay the onset of diabetic nephropathy in normotensive patients with diabetes mellitus and microalbuminuria†. In multicenter controlled studies in normotensive patients with type 1 diabetes mellitus, retinopathy, and microalbuminuria (20–200 mcg/minute), treatment with captopril (50 mg twice daily) for 2 years was associated with a substantial reduction in the risk of developing diabetic nephropathy (based on progression of microalbuminuria to proteinuria). In one study, albumin excretion rate increased from a mean baseline value of 52 to 76 mcg/minute at 2 years in patients receiving placebo, while rates determined at the same time points in patients receiving captopril decreased from 52 to 41 mcg/minute. While clinical studies indicate that treatment with captopril can postpone the development of diabetic nephropathy in normotensive type 1 diabetic patients with microalbuminuria, the long-term clinical benefit of reducing the progression of microalbuminuria to proteinuria has not been determined.

■ **Heart Failure** Captopril is used in the management of heart failure, usually in conjunction with other agents such as cardiac glycosides, diuretics, and β-blockers.

Current guidelines for the management of heart failure in adults generally recommend a combination of drug therapies to reduce morbidity and mortality, including neurohormonal antagonists (e.g., ACE inhibitors, angiotensin II receptor antagonists, angiotensin receptor-neprilysin inhibitors [ARNIs], β-blockers, aldosterone receptor antagonists) that inhibit the detrimental compensatory mechanisms in heart failure. Additional agents (e.g., cardiac glycosides, diuretics, sinoatrial modulators [i.e., ivabradine]) added to a heart failure treatment regimen in selected patients have been associated with symptomatic improvement and/or reduction in heart failure-related hospitalizations. Experts recommend that all asymptomatic patients with reduced left ventricular ejection fraction (LVEF) (American College of Cardiology Foundation [ACCF]/American Heart Association [AHA] stage B heart failure) receive therapy with an ACE inhibitor and β-blocker to prevent symptomatic heart failure and to reduce morbidity and mortality. In patients with prior or current symptoms of chronic heart failure with reduced LVEF, ACCF, AHA, and the Heart Failure Society of America (HFSA) recommend inhibition of the renin-angiotensin-aldosterone (RAA) system with an ACE inhibitor, angiotensin II receptor antagonist, or ARNI in conjunction with a β-blocker, and an aldosterone antagonist in selected patients, to reduce morbidity and mortality. While ACE inhibitors have been the preferred drugs for inhibition of the RAA system because of their established benefits in patients with heart failure and reduced ejection fraction, some evidence indicates that therapy with sacubitril/valsartan, an ARNI, may be more effective than ACE inhibitor therapy (enalapril) in reducing cardiovascular death and heart failure-related hospitalization in such patients. ACCF, AHA, and HFSA recommend that patients with chronic symptomatic heart failure and reduced LVEF (New York Heart Association [NYHA] class II or III) who are able to tolerate an ACE inhibitor or angiotensin II receptor antagonist be switched to therapy containing an ARNI to further reduce morbidity and mortality. However, in patients in whom an ARNI is not appropriate, continued use of an ACE inhibitor for all classes of heart failure with reduced ejection fraction remains strongly advised. In patients in whom an ARNI or ACE inhibitor is not appropriate, an angiotensin II receptor antagonist may be used. For further information on the use of ARNIs in patients with heart failure, see Uses: Heart Failure, in Sacubitril and Valsartan 24:32.92.

Some clinicians state that ACE inhibitors usually are prescribed in clinical practice at dosages lower than those determined as target dosages in clinical trials, although results of several studies suggest that high dosages are associated with greater hemodynamic, neurohormonal, symptomatic, and prognostic benefits than lower dosages. Results of a large, randomized, double-blind study (Assessment of Treatment with Lisinopril and Survival [ATLAS] study) in patients with heart failure (NYHA class II–IV) indicate that high lisinopril dosages (32.5–35 mg daily) were associated with a 12% lower risk of death or hospitalization for any cause and 24% fewer hospitalizations for heart failure than low dosages (2.5–5 mg) of the drug.

Once ACE inhibitor therapy is initiated for heart failure, it generally is continued indefinitely, if tolerated, since withdrawal of an ACE inhibitor may lead to clinical deterioration. Patients with NYHA class II or III heart failure who are tolerating therapy with an ACE inhibitor may be switched to therapy containing an ARNI to further reduce morbidity and mortality; however, the ARNI should not be administered concomitantly with an ACE inhibitor or within 36 hours of the last dose of an ACE inhibitor.

Diuretics are recommended in all patients with heart failure and reduced ejection fraction who have evidence of fluid retention, unless contraindicated, to improve symptoms. Digoxin may be beneficial to patients with heart failure with reduced ejection fraction to decrease hospitalization for heart failure, especially in those with persistent symptoms despite treatment with guideline-directed medical therapy. The manufacturer states that most experience from controlled studies has been with combined captopril, cardiac glycoside, and diuretic therapy; however, the manufacturer also states that the beneficial effect of captopril does not require concomitant cardiac glycoside therapy. The addition of a sinoatrial modulator (i.e., ivabradine) is recommended in selected patients with chronic heart failure and reduced LVEF who are already receiving guideline-directed medical therapy, to reduce heart failure-related hospitalizations. (See Uses: Heart Failure, in Ivabradine 24:04.92.)

Results of a randomized, multicenter, double-blind, placebo-controlled study (Randomized Aldactone Evaluation Study [RALES]) indicate that addition of low-dosage spironolactone (25–50 mg daily) to standard therapy (e.g., an ACE inhibitor and a loop diuretic with or without a cardiac glycoside) in patients with severe (NYHA class IV within 6 months before enrollment and NYHA class III or IV at the time of enrollment) heart failure and LVEF of 35% or less was associated with decreases in overall mortality and hospitalization (for worsening heart failure) rates of approximately 30 and 35%, respectively, compared with standard therapy and placebo. Based on results of RALES and other studies, ACCF and AHA recommend the addition of an aldosterone antagonist (i.e., spironolactone or eplerenone) in selected patients with heart failure (NYHA class II–IV) and reduced LVEF (35% or less) who are already receiving standard therapy to reduce morbidity and mortality. (See Uses: Heart Failure, in Spironolactone 24:32.20.)

Many patients with heart failure respond to captopril with improvement in cardiac function indexes, symptomatic relief, improved functional capacity, and increased exercise tolerance. In some studies, improvement in cardiac function indexes and exercise tolerance were sustained for up to 6 months. In some patients, beneficial effects have been sustained for up to 1 year or longer. Captopril also has been effective in conjunction with cardiac glycosides and diuretics in the management of heart failure resistant to or inadequately controlled by cardiac glycosides, diuretics, and vasodilators.

ACE inhibitors also are used to prevent symptomatic heart failure in patients with ACCF/AHA stage B heart failure (see Uses: Asymptomatic Left Ventricular Dysfunction) and have been shown to reduce mortality after MI or acute coronary syndrome. (See Uses: Left Ventricular Dysfunction after Acute Myocardial Infarction.)

In patients with heart failure in whom renal perfusion is severely compromised, the renin-angiotensin system appears to substantially contribute to preservation of glomerular filtration; therefore, therapy with an ACE inhibitor may adversely affect renal function in such patients. (See Cautions: Renal Effects.)

■ **Left Ventricular Dysfunction After Acute Myocardial Infarction** Captopril is used to improve survival following acute MI in clinically stable patients with left ventricular dysfunction (manifested as an ejection fraction of 40% or less) and to reduce the incidence of overt heart failure and subsequent hospitalizations for heart failure in these patients.

Studies with various ACE inhibitors have shown that these drugs reduce fatal and nonfatal cardiovascular events in patients with recent MI. The magnitude of benefit appears to be greatest in certain high-risk patients (e.g., those with an anterior infarct, ejection fraction of 40% or less, heart failure, prior infarction, or tachycardia). In addition to their effects on mortality, ACE inhibitors also are used to minimize or prevent the development of left ventricular dilatation and dysfunction (ventricular "remodeling") following acute MI. Evidence regarding the efficacy of such therapy has been somewhat conflicting, particularly when parenteral therapy was initiated early (within 24–48 hours) and included patients with no evidence of baseline dysfunction. (See Uses: Left Ventricular Dysfunction After Acute Myocardial Infarction, in Enalaprilat/Enalapril 24:32.04.) However, the preponderance of evidence has shown a benefit of early oral therapy with ACE inhibitors, even in patients with no baseline dysfunction. In a multicenter, controlled study involving captopril in which initiation of therapy with the drug was delayed until 3–16 days after acute MI and limited to patients with low ejection fractions (40% or less), long-term (mean: 42 months; range: 24–60 months) therapy with the drug was associated with a reduction in overall mortality as well as a reduction in morbidity and mortality secondary to cardiovascular causes. In several other studies in which captopril was initiated within 24 hours to 4 weeks after acute MI, a beneficial effect also was observed, at least in terms of effects on left ventricular volume and/or infarct expansion.

Current expert guidelines recommend the use of an oral ACE inhibitor within the first 24 hours of acute MI in patients with an anterior infarction, heart failure, or ejection fraction of 40% or less who do not have any contraindications (e.g., hypotension, shock, renal dysfunction). While early treatment within the first 24 hours of MI has been shown to be beneficial, ACE inhibitors should be used with caution (and with gradual upward titration) during the initial postinfarction period because of the possibility of hypotension or renal dysfunction. ACE inhibitor therapy generally should be continued indefinitely in all patients with left ventricular dysfunction or other compelling indications for use (e.g., hypertension, diabetes mellitus, CKD). The benefits of long-term ACE inhibitor therapy are less certain in low-risk patients who have undergone revascularization and are receiving aggressive antilipemic therapy.

■ **Asymptomatic Left Ventricular Dysfunction** ACE inhibitors have been used to attenuate left ventricular enlargement and prevent progression to symptomatic dysfunction in asymptomatic patients with heart failure† (ACCF/AHA stage B heart failure). Captopril has reduced the development of symptomatic heart failure and associated morbidity and mortality in such patients. The drug's beneficial effect in preventing the development of symptomatic heart failure in these patients may result either from relieving symptoms that otherwise would have become apparent or from slowing the progression of asymptomatic ventricular dysfunction to overt, symptomatic disease. (See Uses: Asymptomatic Left Ventricular Dysfunction, in Enalaprilat/Enalapril 24:32.04.) If an ACE inhibitor is not tolerated, then an angiotensin II receptor antagonist is recommended as alternative therapy.

■ **Other Uses** Captopril has been shown to increase digital circulation in one patient with Raynaud's phenomenon† and decrease the orthostatic sodium and water retention in several women with idiopathic edema†. Therefore, it has been suggested that the drug may be useful in the treatment of these conditions; however, additional evaluation is necessary.

ACE inhibitors have been used to reduce the risk of cardiovascular events in patients 55 years of age or older who are at high risk for cardiovascular events† (e.g., diabetes mellitus, history of cardiovascular disease, stroke, peripheral vascular disease, dyslipidemia, smoking, microalbuminuria, hypertension). (See Uses: Prevention of Cardiovascular Events, in Ramipril 24:32.04.)

Dosage and Administration

■ **Administration** Captopril is administered orally. The manufacturer recommends that the drug be taken 1 hour before meals to ensure maximum absorption. (See Pharmacokinetics: Absorption.)

■ **Dosage** Dosage of captopril must be adjusted according to the patient's tolerance and response.

Hypertension Because of the risk of inducing hypotension, initiation of captopril therapy requires consideration of recent antihypertensive therapy, the extent of blood pressure elevation, sodium intake, fluid status, and other clinical circumstances. Except in patients with severe hypertension, it is recommended that other antihypertensive therapy be discontinued, if possible, 1 week before initiating captopril to minimize the possibility of severe hypotension. If captopril therapy is initiated in patients already receiving a diuretic, treatment with the drug should be initiated under close supervision, following the usual dosage and titration recommendations.

Concomitant sodium restriction may be helpful when captopril is used alone.

Captopril Therapy. The manufacturer states that the usual initial adult dosage of captopril for the management of hypertension in adults with normal renal function is 25 mg 2 or 3 times daily. However, lower initial dosages (e.g., 6.25 mg twice daily to 12.5 mg 3 times daily) may be effective in some patients, particularly in those already receiving a diuretic. Because the reduction in blood pressure may be gradual, most clinicians do not increase dosage during the first 1–2 weeks of captopril therapy. If blood pressure is not adequately controlled after 1–2 weeks, dosage may be increased to 50 mg 2 or 3 times daily. Similar dosages generally have been used in the management of hypertension in geriatric patients, although dosages of 6.25–12.5 mg 1–4 times daily have occasionally been used. The manufacturer states that it usually is not necessary to exceed a captopril dosage of 150 mg daily; if blood pressure is not adequately controlled after 1–2 weeks at a dosage of 50 mg 3 times daily, a thiazide diuretic should also be administered in a low dosage (e.g., 15 mg of hydrochlorothiazide daily). Because the full effect of a combined dose of therapy with captopril and a diuretic may not be attained for 6–8 weeks, dosage of either drug in a combined regimen generally should be increased no more frequently than every 6 weeks, unless the clinical situation requires more rapid adjustment. Diuretic dosage may be increased until its maximum usual antihypertensive dose is reached. If further reduction of blood pressure is necessary, dosage of captopril may be increased to 100 mg 2 or 3 times daily and, if necessary, to 150 mg 2 or 3 times daily, while continuing diuretic therapy. Although a β-adrenergic blocking agent (β-blocker) may be used with captopril, the hypotensive effects are less than additive and this combination is rarely employed. (See Uses: Hypertension.) For further information on dosage of captopril used in combination therapy, see Captopril/Hydrochlorothiazide Fixed-combination Therapy under Dosage: Hypertension. The usual adult maintenance dosage of captopril recommended by the manufacturers is 25–150 mg 2 or 3 times daily, and the maximum dosage is 450 mg daily.

The need for divided (2 or 3 doses) daily dosing of captopril may deter patient compliance and adequate blood pressure control throughout the day; optimally, the antihypertensive drug or dosage form should provide 24-hour efficacy with once-daily dosing, with at least 50% of the peak antihypertensive effect remaining at the end of the dosing interval.

Clinical experience with captopril in pediatric patients is limited (see Cautions: Pediatric Precautions), and dosage must be carefully titrated. In general, dosage for children has been reduced in proportion to body weight. Some experts have recommended an initial captopril dosage in infants of 0.05 mg/kg 1–4 times daily and an initial dosage of 0.5 mg/kg 3 times daily in children. Some experts state that the drug should be initiated at the low end of the dosage range and the dosage may be increased every 2–4 weeks until blood pressure is controlled, the maximum dosage (6 mg/kg per day) is reached, or adverse effects occur. For information on overall principles and expert recommendations for treatment of hypertension in pediatric patients, see Uses: Hypertension in Pediatric Patients, in the Thiazides General Statement 40:28.20.

Captopril/Hydrochlorothiazide Fixed-combination Therapy. When combination therapy is required for the management of hypertension, dosage first can be adjusted by administering each drug separately. If it is determined that the optimum maintenance dosage corresponds to the ratio in a commercial combination preparation, the fixed combination may be used. Alternatively, certain fixed-combination preparations containing low doses of captopril and hydrochlorothiazide can be used initially, thereby potentiating the antihypertensive effect of either drug alone while minimizing the likelihood of dose-related adverse effects. If combination therapy is initiated with the fixed-combination preparation, the initial adult dosage is 25 mg of captopril and 15 mg of hydrochlorothiazide once daily. Subsequent dosage can be adjusted by administering each drug separately or by advancing the once-daily administered fixed-combination preparation to that containing captopril and hydrochlorothiazide 50 and 15 mg, respectively; 25 and 25 mg, respectively; or 50 and 25 mg, respectively. The manufacturer states that dosage adjustments generally should be made at 6-week intervals. It may be necessary to administer captopril separately in divided doses in order to maintain adequate trough (prior to a dose) blood pressure control. Generally, combined dosage of captopril and hydrochlorothiazide in adults should not exceed 150 and 50 mg daily, respectively.

Blood Pressure Monitoring and Treatment Goals. Blood pressure should be monitored regularly (i.e., monthly) during therapy and dosage of the antihypertensive drug adjusted until blood pressure is controlled. If an adequate blood pressure response is not achieved with ACE inhibitor monotherapy, the dosage may be increased or another antihypertensive agent with demonstrated benefit and preferably with a complementary mechanism of action (e.g., calcium-channel blocking agent, thiazide diuretic) may be added; if target blood pressure is still not achieved, a third drug may be added. (See Uses: Hypertension.) In patients who develop unacceptable adverse effects with captopril, the drug should be discontinued and another antihypertensive agent from a different pharmacologic class should be initiated.

The goal of hypertension management and prevention is to achieve and maintain optimal control of blood pressure. However, the optimum blood pressure threshold for initiating antihypertensive drug therapy and specific treatment goals remain controversial. While other hypertension guidelines have based target blood pressure goals on age and comorbidities, the 2017 American College of Cardiology/American Heart Association (ACC/AHA) hypertension guideline incorporates underlying cardiovascular risk into decision making regarding treatment and generally recommends the same target blood pressure (i.e., less than 130/80 mm Hg) in all adults. Many patients will require at least 2 drugs from different pharmacologic classes to achieve this blood pressure goal; the potential benefits of hypertension management and drug cost, adverse effects, and risks associated with the use of multiple antihypertensive drugs also should be considered when deciding a patient's blood pressure treatment goal. (See General Considerations for Initial and Maintenance Antihypertensive Therapy under Uses: Hypertension.)

For additional information on target levels of blood pressure and on monitoring therapy in the management of hypertension, see Blood Pressure Monitoring and Treatment Goals under Dosage: Hypertension, in Dosage and Administration in the Thiazides General Statement 40:28.20.

Hypertensive Crises. In adults with severe hypertension (e.g., accelerated or malignant hypertension) in whom prompt blood pressure reduction is indicated or in whom temporary discontinuance of current antihypertensive therapy is not practical or desirable, diuretic therapy should be continued, other hypotensive agents should be discontinued, and captopril should be initiated promptly at a dosage of 25 mg 2 or 3 times daily, under close supervision with frequent monitoring of the patient's blood pressure.

When necessary, dosage of captopril may be increased at intervals of 24 hours or less under continuous supervision until the optimum blood pressure response is attained or 450 mg daily is given; in this regimen, a diuretic such as furosemide may also be necessary. If adequate control of blood pressure is not attained initially with captopril alone or in combination with a diuretic, some clinicians believe that temporary, adjunctive therapy with other hypotensive agents may be necessary.

Although acute captopril therapy (e.g., 12.5–25 mg, repeated once or twice if necessary at intervals of 30–60 minutes or longer) has been used orally in adults with hypertensive crises†, including those with severe hypertension in whom reduction of blood pressure was considered urgent† (hypertensive urgencies) or an emergency† (hypertensive emergencies), other management methods generally are preferred for patients with these conditions. (See Hypertensive Crises under Uses: Hypertension.)

Diabetic Nephropathy The recommended dosage of captopril for the long-term treatment of diabetic nephropathy is 25 mg 3 times daily. If adequate control of blood pressure is not attained with captopril alone, additional hypotensive agents (e.g., diuretics, β-blockers, calcium-channel blocking agents) may be administered concomitantly.

Heart Failure For the management of symptomatic heart failure, captopril usually is administered in conjunction with other agents such as a cardiac glycoside, a diuretic, and a β-blocker. Captopril therapy must be initiated under very close medical supervision with consideration given to recent diuretic therapy and the possibility of severe sodium and/or fluid depletion. ACE inhibitor therapy should be initiated with caution in patients with very low systemic blood pressure (systolic blood pressure less than 80 mm Hg), markedly increased serum concentrations of creatinine (greater than 3 mg/dL), bilateral renal artery stenosis, or elevated concentrations of serum potassium (greater than 5 mEq/L). Experts recommend that renal function and serum potassium should be assessed within 1–2 weeks of initiation of therapy and periodically thereafter, especially in patients with preexisting hypotension, hyponatremia, diabetes mellitus, or azotemia, or in those taking potassium supplements.

It should be recognized that although symptoms of heart failure may improve within 48 hours after initiating ACE inhibitor therapy in some patients, such improvement usually is not evident for several weeks or months after initiating ACE inhibitor therapy. In addition, it should be considered that such therapy may reduce the risk of disease progression even if symptomatic improvement is not evident. Therefore, dosages generally should be titrated to a prespecified target (i.e., 150 mg of captopril daily) or highest tolerated dosage rather than according to response.

The usual initial adult dosage of captopril recommended by the manufacturer for the management of heart failure in patients with normal renal function is 25 mg 3 times daily. In patients with normal or low blood pressure who have been vigorously treated with diuretics and who may be hyponatremic and/or hypovolemic, an initial dosage of 6.25 or 12.5 mg 3 times daily may minimize the magnitude or duration of the hypotensive effect; titration to the usual daily dosage can then be made within the next several days. Dosage is increased gradually according to the patient's tolerance and response. After a dosage of 50 mg 3 times daily is reached, further increases in dosage should be delayed when possible for at least 2 weeks to determine if an adequate response occurs.

Alternatively, the American College of Cardiology (ACC) and American Heart Association (AHA) recommend that captopril be initiated at low dosage (i.e., 6.25 mg 3 times daily) and titrated gradually upward as tolerated to a maximum dosage of 50 mg 3 times daily. It has been recommended that therapy with ACE inhibitors be titrated upwards to dosages that have been shown to reduce the risk of cardiovascular events in clinical trials rather than titrating based on a patient's therapeutic response. Most patients have an adequate response with 50 or 100 mg 3 times daily. The manufacturer states that a maximum dosage of 450 mg daily should not be exceeded. Some experts suggest a maximum dosage of 50 mg 3 times daily in patients with chronic heart failure.

Alternatively, for the management of heart failure in geriatric patients, some clinicians have initiated captopril therapy at a dosage of 6.25 mg twice daily; if necessary, dosage was increased to 25 mg twice daily after 2 weeks and was subsequently increased if heart failure was not adequately controlled after 4 weeks of therapy at this dosage. The median dosage after 12 weeks of therapy in these geriatric patients was 75 mg daily in 2 divided doses.

Left Ventricular Dysfunction After Acute Myocardial Infarction

When used following acute myocardial infarction (MI) in adults with left ventricular dysfunction, the manufacturer states that captopril therapy may be initiated as early as 3 days following MI. When this approach is followed, an initial 6.25-mg dose of captopril should be given, followed by 12.5 mg 3 times daily. During the next several days, dosage should be increased to 25 mg 3 times daily and then, during the next several weeks as tolerated, dosage should be increased to 50 mg 3 times daily. Some clinicians recommend initiation of therapy within the first 24 hours following MI. The recommended maintenance dosage for long-term use following MI is 50 mg 3 times daily.

■ **Dosage in Renal Impairment** If captopril is used in patients with impaired renal function, doses and/or frequency of administration must be modified in response to the degree of renal impairment and the risk of neutropenia must be considered. (See Cautions: Precautions and Contraindications.) The initial dosage of captopril should be reduced in these patients (i.e., less than 75 mg daily), and dosage should be slowly increased in small increments at 1- to 2-week intervals. After the desired therapeutic effect has been attained, dosage should be slowly decreased to the minimum effective level. It has been suggested that, after the minimum effective daily dosage has been determined in patients with impaired renal function, the dosing interval may be increased with appropriate dose modification; however, criteria for dosage adjustment have not been clearly established. Some clinicians suggest that patients with creatinine clearances of 10–50 mL/minute can receive 75% of the usual captopril dosage or the usual dose can be administered every 12–18 hours, and that those with creatinine clearances less than 10 mL/minute can receive 50% of the usual dosage or the usual dose can be administered every 24 hours. Patients undergoing hemodialysis may require a supplemental dose after dialysis.

When combination therapy with captopril and hydrochlorothiazide is required for the management of hypertension in patients with impaired renal function, the risk of precipitating hypotension during initiation of combined therapy should be considered. (See Cautions: Cardiovascular Effects and see Precautions and Contraindications.) Dosages of the drugs should be titrated carefully by slowly increasing the dosage of each drug separately in small increments. After the desired therapeutic effect has been attained, the manufacturer recommends that the dosing interval be increased and/or the doses decreased until the minimal effective daily dosage has been achieved. If after careful titration of each drug separately it is determined that the optimum maintenance dosage corresponds to the ratio in commercial combination preparation, the fixed combination may be substituted but should be replaced with the individual drugs if subsequent dosage adjustment is necessary. If concomitant diuretic therapy is required in patients with severe renal impairment, a loop diuretic such as furosemide is preferred to a thiazide diuretic. Therefore, use of commercially available preparations containing captopril in fixed combination with hydrochlorothiazide is usually not recommended for patients with severe renal impairment.

Cautions

Captopril is generally well tolerated in most patients; however, serious adverse effects (e.g., neutropenia, agranulocytosis, proteinuria, aplastic anemia) have been reported rarely, mainly in patients with renal impairment (especially those with collagen vascular disease). Captopril-induced adverse effects are often alleviated by dosage reduction, occasionally disappear despite continued treatment and without dosage reduction, and are usually reversible following discontinuance of the drug. The most common adverse effects of captopril are rash and loss of taste perception. Adverse effects requiring discontinuance of captopril therapy occur in about 4–12% of patients.

■ **Hematologic Effects** Neutropenia (less than 1000 neutrophils/mm^3) and agranulocytosis, both associated with myeloid hypoplasia, have occurred rarely in patients receiving captopril. In addition to myeloid hypoplasia, erythroid hypoplasia and decreased numbers of megakaryocytes (e.g., hypoplastic bone marrow and pancytopenia) were frequently observed in patients with captopril-induced neutropenia; anemia and thrombocytopenia also occurred occasionally in these patients. Systemic or oral cavity infections or other effects associated with agranulocytosis occurred in about half of the patients who developed neutropenia.

Neutropenia has occurred within 3–12 weeks after beginning treatment with captopril. The risk of captopril-induced neutropenia appears to depend principally on the degree of renal impairment and the presence of collagen vascular disease (e.g., systemic lupus erythematosus, scleroderma). In clinical studies in patients with some degree of renal impairment (serum creatinine concentration of at least 1.6 mg/dL), neutropenia occurred in about 0.2% of patients, a frequency greater than 15 times that in patients with uncomplicated hypertension who have normal renal function. Most of the patients with renal impairment received relatively high dosages, particularly in relation to their renal function; in some reports, the neutropenia was associated with concomitant administration of allopurinol while in other reports this association was not apparent. In clinical studies, neutropenia has occurred in about 3.7% of patients with collagen vascular disease and renal impairment. Neutropenia has also occurred in some patients receiving captopril for the management of heart failure and the risk factors appear to be similar; about 50% of the patients developing neutropenia had impaired renal function and about 75% were receiving procainamide concomitantly.

Following discontinuance of captopril and other drugs, the neutrophil count generally returned to normal in about 2 weeks. Serious infections have been limited to patients with complex clinical conditions. Death has occurred in about 13% of patients who developed neutropenia, but almost all deaths occurred in patients with serious illness who had collagen vascular disease, renal failure, and/or heart failure and/or who were receiving immunosuppressive therapy. Although a few patients have been rechallenged with captopril (usually with lower dosages) without recurrence, others have reportedly experienced recurrence, even with lower dosages. Although a causal relationship to captopril has not been established, anemia (e.g., aplastic, hemolytic) has been reported in some patients receiving the drug.

■ **Renal Effects** Proteinuria (total urinary proteins exceeding 1 g/day) has occurred in about 0.7% of patients receiving captopril, and nephrotic syndrome occurred in about one-fifth of these patients. About 90% of patients who have developed proteinuria during captopril therapy had evidence of prior renal disease and/or received relatively high dosages of the drug (greater than 150 mg daily). If proteinuria develops, it usually occurs by the eighth month of treatment with captopril, consists mainly of albumin, and is rarely accompanied by increases in BUN or serum creatinine concentrations. Renal biopsies in some patients who developed proteinuria showed that membranous glomerulopathy was present; however, it was not definitely established that this effect was caused by the drug since these patients did not have pretreatment renal biopsies, and membranous glomerulopathy has occurred in hypertensive patients who did not receive the drug. Proteinuria usually subsides or clears within 6 months whether or not captopril therapy is continued; however, in some patients, it may persist.

Deterioration in renal function, manifested as transient increases in BUN and serum creatinine concentrations may occur following administration of captopril, especially in patients with impaired renal function, sodium depletion, or hypovolemia; patients with renovascular hypertension, particularly those with bilateral renal-artery stenosis or those with renal-artery stenosis in a solitary kidney; or patients with chronic or severe hypertension in whom the glomerular filtration rate may decrease transiently. This effect was usually reversible following discontinuance of captopril and/or diuretic therapy. Acute reversible renal failure also may occur. Renal function should be monitored closely during the first few weeks of therapy and periodically thereafter in patients with bilateral renal-artery stenosis or those with renal-artery stenosis in a solitary kidney. (See Cautions: Precautions and Contraindications.) About 5–15% or 15–30% of patients with mild to moderate or severe heart failure, respectively, treated with an angiotensin-converting enzyme (ACE) inhibitor develop substantial elevations of serum creatinine concentrations (e.g., exceeding 5 mg/dL) and BUN. Some patients with heart failure, including those with severe preexisting renal disease, may require discontinuance of ACE inhibitor therapy, including captopril, because of progressively increasing serum creatinine concentration. The rapidity of onset and magnitude of captopril-induced renal insufficiency in patients with heart failure may depend in part on the degree of sodium depletion.

Because the renin-angiotensin system appears to contribute substantially to maintenance of glomerular filtration in patients with heart failure in whom renal perfusion is severely compromised, renal function may deteriorate markedly during therapy with an ACE inhibitor in these patients. Such drug-induced deterioration is generally well tolerated, and does not usually necessitate discontinuance of effective therapy with the drug when symptomatic improvement of the heart failure occurs. In addition, the magnitude of deterioration in renal function can usually be ameliorated by reducing the dosage of concomitantly administered diuretics and/or by liberalizing dietary sodium intake, since concomitant diuretic therapy and/or sodium restriction potentially increase the role of angiotensin II in maintaining glomerular filtration in these patients. In patients in whom renal perfusion pressure is very low and is further reduced by ACE inhibitor therapy, however, deterioration in renal function may be clinically important. Patients with concomitant underlying diabetes mellitus may be at risk for developing renal insufficiency during ACE inhibitor therapy; however, ACE inhibitors, including captopril, have been beneficial in the management of diabetic nephropathy.

Although a definite causal relationship to captopril has not been established, renal insufficiency, polyuria, oliguria, and urinary frequency have been reported in about 0.1–0.2% of patients.

■ Dermatologic and Sensitivity Reactions The most common adverse effect of captopril is rash, which occurs in about 4–7% of patients (depending on renal function and dosage) and is usually maculopapular and rarely urticarial. Rash is often accompanied by pruritus and erythema and sometimes by fever, arthralgia, eosinophilia, and/or positive antinuclear antibody (ANA) titers. Eosinophilia and/or positive ANA titers have been reported in 7–10% of patients with captopril-induced rash. The rash occurs most frequently on the upper extremities and trunk but may occur at other sites. It generally occurs during the first 4 weeks of therapy and has occurred rarely within 30 minutes after the initial dose of the drug. The rash is usually mild and disappears within a few days after dosage reduction, short-term treatment with an oral antihistamine, and/or discontinuance of the drug. In some patients, the rash may disappear despite continued treatment and without dosage adjustment. Although the cause has not been clearly determined, it has been suggested that the rash may be a reaction mediated by kinins. Pruritus without rash occurs in about 2% of patients receiving captopril.

Photosensitivity has occurred, and captopril has been associated with reversible, pemphigoid lesions. Bullous pemphigoid also has been reported; however, a causal relationship to the drug has not been established.

Angioedema of the face, mucous membranes, lips, tongue, larynx, glottis, or extremities has occurred in about 0.1% of patients and may be reversible following discontinuance of therapy. (See Cautions: Precautions and Contraindications.) Intestinal angioedema (occasionally without a prior history of facial angioedema or elevated serum levels of complement 1 [C1] esterase inhibitor) also has been reported in patients receiving ACE inhibitors. Intestinal angioedema, which frequently presents as abdominal pain (with or without nausea or vomiting), usually is diagnosed by abdominal CT scan, ultrasound, or surgery; manifestations usually have resolved after discontinuance of the ACE inhibitor. Intestinal angioedema should be considered in the differential diagnosis of patients who develop abdominal pain during therapy with an ACE inhibitor.

Other hypersensitivity reactions have included vasculitis and hypersensitivity pneumonitis, which was associated with eosinophilia and pulmonary infiltrates. Rarely, a serum sickness type of reaction with rash or other dermatologic manifestations, fever, myalgia, arthralgia, interstitial nephritis, increased erythrocyte sedimentation rate (ESR), and/or difficulty in breathing has been reported in patients receiving captopril. Alopecia has occurred, but a causal relationship to the drug has not been established.

Severe, sudden anaphylactoid reactions, which can be fatal, have been reported following initiation of hemodialysis that utilized a high-flux polyacrylonitrile [PAN] membrane (e.g., AN 69®) in patients receiving an ACE inhibitor. Manifestations of these reactions included nausea, abdominal cramps, burning, angioedema, and shortness of breath; progression to severe hypotension can develop rapidly. Dialysis should be stopped immediately and aggressive supportive and symptomatic therapy should be initiated as indicated.Antihistamines do *not* appear to be effective in providing symptomatic relief. While it currently does not seem to be necessary to exclude the use of ACE inhibitors in patients undergoing hemodialysis that involves PAN membranes, caution should be exercised during concomitant use. The mechanism of this interaction has not been established, and the incidence and risk of its occurrence remain to be elucidated. In these patients, consideration should be given to using a different type of dialysis membrane or a drug other than an ACE inhibitor. In addition, anaphylactoid reactions also have been reported in patients undergoing low-density lipoprotein (LDL) apheresis with dextran sulfate absorption, a procedure utilizing devices not approved in the US. Manifestations of these reactions included flushing, dyspnea, bradycardia, and hypotension. It has been postulated that these reactions may be associated with accumulation of polypeptides (e.g., bradykinin) since endogenous concentration of such polypeptides may be increased by LDL-apheresis with dextran sulfate and their metabolism may be decreased by ACE inhibitors. To avoid these anaphylactoid reactions, some clinicians recommend withdrawal of ACE inhibitors 12–30 hours before apheresis, while others state that ACE inhibitors should not be used in patients treated with LDL apheresis.

Life-threatening anaphylactoid reactions have been reported in at least 2 patients receiving ACE inhibitors while undergoing desensitization treatment with hymenoptera venom. When ACE inhibitors were temporarily discontinued 24 hours before desensitization with the venom, anaphylactoid reactions did not recur; however, such reactions recurred after inadvertent rechallenge.

Onycholysis and dystrophic changes in the fingernails have occurred rarely in patients receiving captopril. In at least one patient, these changes were associated with other manifestations of zinc deficiency (e.g., alopecia, asteatosis, dysgeusia, cutaneous eruptions). Although serum zinc concentrations were within the normal range in this patient, manifestations of zinc deficiency showed some improvement when captopril dosage was reduced and then gradually resolved when supplemental zinc therapy was initiated. However, other manifestations of zinc deficiency have been absent and serum zinc concentrations normal in other patients with nail changes, and the relationship, if any, of these effects to captopril-induced zinc deficiency has not been established.

■ Effects on Taste Decrease in taste acuity, or alteration (persistent metallic or salty taste) or loss of taste perception is another common adverse effect of captopril, occurring in about 2–4% of patients (depending on renal function and dosage). Taste impairment usually occurs during the first 3 months of therapy; it is usually reversible within 2–3 months even when captopril therapy is continued. In some patients, taste impairment has been associated with subsequent weight loss. The mechanism of taste impairment has not been established. In patients not receiving captopril, alterations in taste perception have been associated with decreased plasma zinc concentrations, but normal plasma zinc concentrations have been reported in a few patients with captopril-induced taste impairment and these patients did not respond to oral zinc supplements.

■ Cardiovascular Effects Excessive hypotension occurs rarely in hypertensive patients receiving captopril. Transient decreases in mean blood pressure greater than 20% may occur in about half of patients with heart failure treated with captopril. Hypotension has required discontinuance of therapy in about 3–5% of patients with heart failure receiving captopril.

Captopril-induced hypotension may occasionally be alleviated by initial dosage reduction (i.e., 6.25 or 12.5 mg 3 times daily), but hypotension has also occurred after low doses (i.e., a single 6.25-mg dose) of the drug. Orthostatic hypotension appears to occur more frequently during initiation of therapy and in patients with sodium depletion, hypovolemia, markedly elevated plasma renin or angiotensin II concentration, or overdosage. Transient hypotension in patients with heart failure or with hypertension may occur after any of the first several doses and usually is well tolerated, producing no symptoms or occasionally associated with brief, mild lightheadedness or dizziness, blurred vision, syncope, and, rarely, bradycardia or conduction defects. One patient with congestive heart failure who had markedly elevated PRA developed fatal refractory ventricular fibrillation, associated with hypotension, following two 6.25-mg doses of captopril. Patients who are volume and/or sodium depleted such as those receiving diuretics, especially those in whom diuretic therapy was recently initiated (e.g., patients with severe congestive heart failure), those whose sodium intake is severely restricted, and those who are undergoing dialysis, may occasionally experience a precipitous reduction of blood pressure within the first 3 hours after the initial dose of captopril. Symptomatic hypotension that occurs later in a course of captopril therapy (e.g., after the first 48 hours) may indicate the presence of sodium depletion (e.g., secondary to restriction of sodium intake or increased diuretic dosage).

Enalapril, another ACE inhibitor, has produced severe hypotension in patients with severe heart failure with or without renal insufficiency, which was occasionally associated with oliguria and/or progressive azotemia and, rarely, with acute renal failure, myocardial ischemia, and/or death. Captopril, which has a shorter duration of action than enalapril, may have a decreased risk associated with these adverse effects. Because of the risk of developing severe hypotension and potential compromise of the patient's hemodynamic status, patients with heart failure should be monitored closely for 2 weeks after initiation of captopril therapy and whenever dosage of captopril and/or a concomitantly administered diuretic is increased.

The possibility of severe hypotension may be minimized by withholding diuretic therapy and/or increasing sodium intake approximately 3–7 days prior to initiating captopril therapy. If hypotension occurs in patients receiving captopril, the patient should be placed in the supine or Trendelenburg's position; if hypotension is severe, IV infusion of 0.9% sodium chloride injection to expand fluid volume should be considered. Transient hypotension is not a contraindication to additional doses of captopril, and therapy with the drug can be cautiously reinstated after blood pressure has been stabilized (e.g., with volume expansion). Asymptomatic hypotension often does not require specific therapy and may be well tolerated with continued captopril therapy; however, severe hypotension occasionally may require discontinuance of captopril therapy. In patients with heart failure, the reduction in blood pressure stabilizes within 1–2 weeks after starting captopril therapy, and blood pressure generally returns to pretreatment levels within 2 months without a decrease in therapeutic efficacy. Hypotension may also occur in captopril-treated patients during major surgery or during anesthesia with agents that produce hypotension. This hypotensive effect results from inhibition by captopril of the angiotensin II formation that occurs subsequent to compensatory renin release, and, if it is thought to be caused by captopril, can generally be corrected with fluid volume expansion.

Tachycardia, chest pain, and palpitations have each occurred in about 1% of patients receiving captopril. Flushing, pallor, angina pectoris, myocardial infarction (MI), Raynaud's phenomenon, and heart failure have been reported rarely. Captopril has also produced hyperkinetic circulation (tachycardia, greatly increased cardiac output, and decreased mean blood transit time) in at least one patient with congestive heart failure. Although a causal relationship has not been established, other adverse cardiovascular effects that have been reported in patients receiving captopril include cardiac arrest, cerebrovascular accident and/or insufficiency, rhythm disturbances, and syncope.

■ Effects on Potassium Although small increases in serum potassium concentration occur frequently in patients receiving captopril without a thiazide diuretic, hyperkalemia has occurred rarely. Patients with impaired renal function or heart failure and patients concomitantly receiving drugs that can increase serum potassium concentration (e.g., potassium-sparing diuretics, potassium supplements, potassium-containing salt substitutes) may be at increased risk of developing hyperkalemia during captopril therapy, especially those with diabetes mellitus; serum potassium concentration should be monitored carefully in these patients, and potassium intake should be controlled and therapy with drugs that can increase serum potassium modified or discontinued as necessary. In a clinical trial in patients with type 1 diabetes mellitus who were receiving captopril for proteinuria, the drug was discontinued in about 2% of patients secondary to hyperkalemia. However, hyperkalemia was not reported in another trial in normotensive patients with type 1 diabetes mellitus who were receiving captopril for microalbuminuria.

■ Respiratory Effects Cough has been reported in about 0.5–2% of patients receiving captopril. However, cough often is overlooked as a potential adverse effect of ACE inhibitors and may occur more frequently (in about 5–15% of patients). The cough generally is persistent and nonproductive and reversible following discontinuance of the drug. It has been suggested that accumulation of kinins in the respiratory tract secondary to ACE inhibition may in part be responsible for this cough. Concomitant therapy with a nonsteroidal anti-inflammatory agent (i.e., sulindac) appeared to minimize cough in a few patients, but additional study of the safety (e.g., effects on renal function) of such combined therapy is necessary. Dyspnea and bronchospasm have been reported rarely during captopril therapy. Angioedema has occurred in 0.1% of patients receiving captopril, and, if associated with laryngeal edema or angioedema of the tongue or glottis, airway obstruction may occur, and angioedema may be fatal. (See Cautions: Precautions and Contraindications.)

■ Hepatic Effects Hepatitis (including rare cases of hepatic necrosis), cholestasis, jaundice, and elevations in serum concentrations of hepatic enzymes, alkaline phosphatase, and bilirubin have been reported occasionally but have not been directly attributed to the drug, and rare cases of cholestatic jaundice and of hepatocellular injury (with or without secondary cholestasis) have been associated with captopril therapy.

A clinical syndrome that usually is manifested initially by cholestatic jaundice and may progress to fulminant hepatic necrosis (which occasionally may be fatal) has been reported rarely in patients receiving ACE inhibitors. The mechanism of this reaction is not known.

■ Other Adverse Effects Hyponatremia (which may be symptomatic) has been reported occasionally in patients receiving captopril; some of these patients had heart failure or were receiving a low-sodium diet or concomitant diuretics. In at least one patient, gynecomastia occurred while receiving captopril, which was reversible following discontinuance of the drug.

Although a causal relationship has not been established, other adverse effects that have occurred rarely in patients receiving captopril include dry mouth, aphthous ulcers, ulceration of the tongue, reversible lymphadenopathy, abdominal pain, nausea, vomiting, diarrhea, anorexia, constipation, dyspepsia, gastric irritation, peptic ulcer, pancreatitis, glossitis, headache, dizziness, paresthesia, malaise, asthenia, myalgia, myasthenia, ataxia, confusion, depression, nervousness, somnolence, blurred vision, impotence, and insomnia.

■ Precautions and Contraindications Captopril may cause serious adverse effects (e.g., neutropenia) and must be used under close supervision, particularly in patients with renal impairment (especially those with collagen vascular disease). When the drug is used, the risk of neutropenia and agranulocytosis must be considered. When captopril is used as a fixed combination that includes hydrochlorothiazide, the cautions, precautions, and contraindications associated with thiazide diuretics must be considered in addition to those associated with captopril.

Because cough has been associated with the use of many ACE inhibitors, including captopril, it should be considered in the differential diagnosis of patients who develop cough during captopril therapy.

The possibility that proteinuria can develop and may progress to nephrotic syndrome in patients receiving captopril should be considered, particularly in those with preexisting renal disease or receiving captopril dosages exceeding 150 mg daily. (See Cautions: Renal Effects.)

Renal function should be evaluated prior to initiation of captopril therapy, and the drug should be used with caution in patients with renal impairment, particularly those with known or suspected renovascular disease. Reduction of captopril dosage, reduction in dosage or discontinuance of diuretic therapy, and/or adequate sodium repletion may be necessary in some patients who develop impaired renal function during captopril therapy; it may be impossible to reduce blood pressure to normal levels and maintain adequate renal perfusion. Because of an increased risk of reducing renal perfusion to a critically low level, captopril should be used with caution and renal function monitored closely for the first few weeks of therapy in patients with bilateral renal-artery stenosis and in those with renal-artery stenosis in a solitary kidney. Serum creatinine and electrolyte concentrations should be evaluated prior to and 1 week following initiation of therapy with ACE inhibitors in patients with heart failure. In patients with heart failure who have some degree of renal impairment (baseline serum creatinine concentrations less than 2 mg/dL) or more severe renal impairment (baseline serum creatinine concentrations exceeding 2 mg/dL), an increase in serum creatinine concentration exceeding 0.5 or 1 mg/dL, respectively, should prompt consideration of discontinuing ACE inhibitor therapy while additional renal evaluation and corrective action is undertaken. The possibility that ACE inhibitors might precipitate severe, sudden, potentially life-threatening anaphylactoid reactions in patients undergoing hemodialysis involving a high-flux membrane should be considered. (See Cautions: Dermatologic and Hypersensitivity Reactions.)

In patients with collagen vascular disease (e.g., systemic lupus erythematosus, scleroderma) or in those receiving other drugs known to affect leukocytes or immune response, particularly those with coexisting impaired renal function, captopril should be used only after an assessment of the benefits and risks, and then with caution. If captopril is administered to patients with any of these conditions and/or with impaired renal function, complete and differential leukocyte counts should be performed prior to initiation of therapy, at approximately 2-week intervals for the first 3 months of therapy, and periodically thereafter. In other patients receiving captopril, complete leukocyte counts may be performed at approximately 2-week intervals for the first 3 months of therapy and periodically thereafter; differential leukocyte counts should be performed if the complete leukocyte count is less than 4000/mm^3 or half of the pretreatment count. If the neutrophil count is less than 1000/mm^3, captopril should be discontinued and the patient closely monitored. Patients should be instructed to notify their clinician if any signs or symptoms of infection such as fever or sore throat occur. If infection is suspected, blood cell counts should be performed immediately.

Because rare cases of cholestatic jaundice and fulminant hepatic necrosis (sometimes fatal) have occurred in patients receiving ACE inhibitors, including captopril, the drug should be discontinued and patients monitored appropriately if jaundice or marked elevations in hepatic enzymes occur during therapy. (See Cautions: Hepatic Effects.)

Captopril should be used with caution in patients with sodium depletion or hypovolemia, those receiving diuretics, and those undergoing dialysis since severe hypotension may occur. The drug should also be used with caution in patients in whom excessive hypotension may have serious consequences (e.g., patients with coronary or cerebrovascular insufficiency). ACE inhibitor therapy should be initiated with caution in patients with very low systemic blood pressure (systolic blood pressure less than 80 mm Hg), markedly increased serum concentrations of creatinine (greater than 3 mg/dL), bilateral renal artery stenosis, or elevated concentrations of serum potassium (greater than 5 mEq/L). Experts recommend that treatment with an ACE inhibitor be initiated at low doses and gradually titrated upward as tolerated. Patients with heart failure should be closely monitored for the first 2 weeks of therapy and whenever the dosage of captopril and/or the diuretic is increased. Patients receiving captopril therapy should be informed that vomiting, diarrhea, excessive perspiration, and dehydration may lead to an exaggerated decrease in blood pressure because of fluid volume reduction; patients should notify their clinician if any of these conditions occurs. The possibility that patients with aortic stenosis might be at risk of decreased coronary perfusion when treated with captopril should be considered.

Patients receiving captopril should be warned not to interrupt or discontinue therapy unless instructed by their clinician. Patients with heart failure receiving captopril should be cautioned against rapid increases in physical activity.

Although captopril and penicillamine are not pharmacologically related, many adverse effects (e.g., rash, taste impairment, proteinuria) of these drugs are similar. Because captopril and penicillamine contain sulfhydryl groups and are structurally related, it has been suggested that the common toxicities may in part result from the chemical and structural characteristics of the drugs; however, such a relationship has not been clearly determined. Since therapy with ACE inhibitors has been associated with development of a rare syndrome that usually is manifested initially by cholestatic jaundice that may progress to fulminant hepatic necrosis and occasionally may be fatal, patients receiving an ACE inhibitor, including captopril, who develop jaundice or marked elevations of hepatic enzymes should discontinue the drug and receive appropriate medical follow-up. (See Cautions: Hepatic Effects.)

Angioedema may occur in patients receiving an ACE inhibitor (e.g., captopril), and, if associated with laryngeal edema, may be fatal. If swelling is confined to the extremities, face, lips, and mucous membranes of the mouth, the condition usually responds without treatment. Swelling of the tongue, glottis, or larynx may cause airway obstruction, and appropriate therapy (e.g., epinephrine) should be initiated immediately. Patients should be informed that swelling of the face, eyes, lips, tongue, larynx, or extremities or difficulty in breathing or in swallowing may be signs and symptoms of angioedema, and that they should discontinue captopril and notify their clinician immediately if any of these conditions occurs. The possibility that patients with a history of angioedema unrelated to ACE inhibitors may be at increased risk of developing angioedema while receiving the drugs should be considered.

Captopril is contraindicated in patients with known hypersensitivity to the drug or to another ACE inhibitor (e.g., those who experienced angioedema during therapy with another ACE inhibitor).

■ Pediatric Precautions Although there is limited clinical experience with captopril in children, safety and efficacy of the drug in children have not been established; however, pediatric dosage was reported to be comparable or less than dosage used in adults when calculated on the basis of body weight. Infants, especially neonates, may have increased susceptibility to captopril-induced adverse hemodynamic effects. Excessive, prolonged, and unpredictable decreases in blood pressure and associated complications (e.g., oliguria, seizures) have been reported in children receiving the drug. The manufacturer states that captopril should be used in children only when other measures for controlling blood pressure have not been effective. For information on overall principles and expert recommendations for treatment of hypertension in pediatric patients, see Uses: Hypertension in Pediatric Patients, in the Thiazides General Statement 40:28.20.

■ Mutagenicity and Carcinogenicity Mutagenicity studies with captopril in fixed combination with hydrochlorothiazide (Capozide®) have not been conducted, but the effects of the individual components in a 2:1 ratio have been studied. Captopril/hydrochlorothiazide did not exhibit mutagenic or clastogenic potential in vitro with or without metabolic activation in a bacterial reverse mutation (Ames) assays using *Salmonella*, a forward mutation assay in *Saccharomyces pombe*, a gene conversion assay using *Saccharomyces cerevisiae*, and a sister chromatid exchange test in human lymphocytes. In a cytogenetics assay in human lymphocytes exposed to captopril/hydrochlorothiazide concentrations of 5, 25, and 50 µg/mL (total concentration of both drugs) with metabolic activation, chromosomal abnormalities were not observed consistently. When such aberrations were observed, no concentration response was noted. Captopril and hydrochlorothiazide in a 2:1 ratio were not genotoxic in the in vivo mouse micronucleus test at an oral dose of 2,500 mg/kg (total concentration of both drugs).

No evidence of carcinogenesis was observed in rats or mice receiving captopril dosages of 50–1350 mg/kg daily for 2 years.

While an excess rate of GI cancer relative to placebo has been observed in several large trials in patients receiving prolonged ACE-inhibitor therapy, a causal relationship to the drugs has not been established. Some evidence suggests that such a relationship is unlikely since the observed risk did not increase with increasing exposure to the drugs and because of the heterogeneity of the reported cancers (involving the rectum, cecum, colon, esophagus, stomach, gallbladder, pancreas, or liver). However, the possibility of a causal relationship cannot be excluded, and additional study to further elucidate any possible relationship between use of ACE inhibitors and these cancers is necessary.

■ **Pregnancy, Fertility, and Lactation** ***Pregnancy*** Fetal and neonatal morbidity and mortality have been reported in at least 50 women who were receiving ACE inhibitors during pregnancy. Very limited epidemiologic data indicate that the rate of fetal and neonatal morbidity resulting from exposure to ACE inhibitors during the second and third trimesters may be as high as 10–20%. Hypotension, reversible or irreversible renal failure, anuria, skull hypoplasia, and/or death were reported in neonates whose mothers had received ACE inhibitors during the second and third trimesters of pregnancy. Other adverse effects associated with such use included oligohydramnios, presumably due to decreased renal function in the fetus, prematurity, fetal death, and patent ductus arteriosus; however, it is not known if these effects were associated with ACE inhibition or underlying maternal disease. Oligohydramnios has been associated with contractures of the limbs, craniofacial deformities, hypoplasia of the lungs, and intrauterine growth retardation.

Although fetal exposure limited to the first trimester previously was considered not to be associated with substantial risk, data from an epidemiologic study have shown that infants whose mothers had taken an ACE inhibitor during the first trimester of pregnancy have an increased risk of major congenital malformations compared with infants who had not undergone first trimester exposure to ACE inhibitors. The risk of major congenital malformations, primarily affecting the cardiovascular and central nervous systems, was increased by about 2.7 times in infants whose mothers had taken an ACE inhibitor during the first trimester of pregnancy compared with infants who had not undergone such exposure. Every effort should be made to discontinue captopril therapy as soon as possible in any woman who becomes pregnant while receiving the drug, regardless of the period of gestation. In addition, all women of childbearing potential who are receiving an ACE inhibitor should be advised to report pregnancy to their clinician as soon as possible. Women of childbearing potential who are receiving an ACE inhibitor also should be advised to inform their clinician if they are planning to become pregnant or think they might be pregnant. Nearly all women can be transferred successfully to alternative therapy for the remainder of their pregnancy. Rarely (probably less frequently than once in every 1000 pregnancies), no adequate alternative can be identified; in such rare cases, the woman should be informed of the potential hazard to the fetus and serial ultrasound examinations should be performed to assess the intra-amniotic environment. If oligohydramnios is present, captopril therapy should be discontinued, unless use of the drug is considered life-saving for the woman. Contraction stress testing (CST), a nonstress test (NST), or biophysical profiling may be performed, if appropriate, depending on the period of gestation. However, both clinicians and patients should realize that oligohydramnios may not become apparent until after irreversible fetal injury already has occurred.

Infants exposed in utero to ACE inhibitors should be observed closely for hypotension, oliguria, and hyperkalemia. If oliguria occurs, supportive measures (e.g., administration of fluids and pressor agents) to correct hypotension and renal perfusion should be considered. Exchange transfusion or dialysis may be required to reverse hypotension and/or substitute for impaired renal function. Although captopril may be removed by hemodialysis in adults, it is not known if the drug is removed from circulation of neonates or older children by hemodialysis. Peritoneal dialysis is not effective in enhancing the elimination of captopril, and it is not known whether the drug may be removed by exchange transfusion.

Reproduction studies in hamsters and rats using 150 and 625 times the maximum human dosage, respectively, of captopril have not revealed evidence of teratogenic effects. However, the drug was associated with a low incidence of craniofacial malformations in rabbits when given at dosages 0.8–70 times the maximum human dosage. Reduction in neonatal survival occurred in the offspring of rats receiving captopril dosages 400 times the usual human dosage continuously during gestation and lactation, and an increased incidence of stillbirths has reportedly occurred in ewes.

Fertility Reproduction studies in rats using captopril have not revealed evidence of impaired fertility.

Lactation Captopril is distributed into milk in concentrations about 1% of those in maternal blood. Because of the potential for serious adverse reactions to captopril in nursing infants, a decision should be made whether to discontinue nursing or the drug, taking into account the importance of the drug to the woman.

Drug Interactions

■ **Hypotensive Agents and Diuretics** When captopril is administered with diuretics or other hypotensive drugs, the hypotensive effect of captopril is increased. The effect is usually used to therapeutic advantage, but careful adjustment of dosage is necessary when these drugs are used concomitantly.

Captopril and diuretics appear to have additive hypotensive effects; however, severe hypotension and reversible renal insufficiency may occasionally occur, especially in volume- and/or sodium-depleted patients. (See Cautions: Cardiovascular Effects.) In addition, the duration of hypotensive effect is extended by concomitant diuretic therapy. The hypotensive effects of captopril and β-adrenergic blocking agents (β-blockers) (e.g., propranolol) are less than additive. Hypotensive drugs that cause release of renin (e.g., diuretics) will increase the hypotensive effect of captopril. Reduction of captopril dosage and/or dosage reduction or discontinuance of diuretic therapy may be necessary. Patients should be monitored closely during initiation and dosage adjustment of concomitant therapy with captopril and a diuretic; in patients already receiving diuretics, the risk of these effects may be minimized by withholding diuretic therapy and/or increasing sodium intake for 3–7 days prior to initiating captopril therapy.

While captopril may have pharmacodynamic interactions in patients receiving diuretics, use of furosemide concurrently with captopril in patients with renal impairment and hypertension does not alter the pharmacokinetics of captopril.

Hypotensive drugs that affect sympathetic nervous system activity such as ganglionic blocking agents (e.g., trimethaphan camsylate [no longer commercially available in the US]) or adrenergic neuron blocking agents (e.g., guanethidine sulfate) should be used with caution in patients receiving captopril, since the sympathetic nervous system may be especially important in maintaining blood pressure in patients treated with captopril.

■ **Vasodilating Agents** Data on the effect of concomitant use of captopril and other vasodilators in the management of heart failure are not currently available. Pending accumulation of clinical data on such concomitant use, nitroglycerin or other nitrates or other drugs with vasodilating activity (e.g., hydralazine, prazosin) should be discontinued if possible before starting captopril; if such agents are resumed during captopril therapy, they should be administered with caution and possibly at lower dosage.

■ **Drugs Increasing Serum Potassium Concentration** Since captopril decreases aldosterone secretion, small increases in serum potassium concentration frequently occur, especially in patients with impaired renal function; hyperkalemia has occurred rarely. Potassium-sparing diuretics (e.g., amiloride, spironolactone, triamterene), potassium supplements, or potassium-containing salt substitutes should be used with caution in patients receiving captopril and only if hypokalemia is documented, since hyperkalemia may occur; serum potassium should be monitored carefully. Dosage of the potassium-sparing diuretic and/or potassium supplement should be reduced or the diuretic and/or supplement discontinued as necessary. Patients with renal impairment may be at increased risk of hyperkalemia. If the patient has received spironolactone at any time up to several months before captopril is administered, serum potassium concentration should be determined frequently when captopril is administered since the potassium-sparing effect of spironolactone may persist. However, angiotensin-converting enzyme (ACE) inhibitors have been administered with low-dosage spironolactone therapy and hyperkalemia was reported rarely. (See Uses: Heart Failure.)

■ **Cardiac Glycosides** A study in healthy men revealed no evidence of a pharmacokinetic interaction between captopril and digoxin. However, studies in patients with heart failure indicate that serum digoxin concentrations may increase by about 15–30% when captopril and digoxin are used concomitantly. Such increases may result from decreased renal clearance (probably both glomerular filtration and tubular secretion) of digoxin and, possibly, displacement of the glycoside from tissue-binding sites by captopril-induced increases in serum potassium. Captopril has been administered concomitantly with digoxin in patients with heart failure *without* unusual adverse effects or apparent increased risk of cardiac glycoside toxicity. It has been postulated that captopril-induced increases in serum potassium may offset the potential toxic effects of increased serum digoxin concentrations. Reduction in digoxin dosage does not appear to be necessary when captopril is initiated; however, serum digoxin concentrations should be monitored and the patient observed for signs of glycoside toxicity when the drugs are used concomitantly. Further studies are needed to determine the clinical importance of this potential interaction.

■ **Nonsteroidal Anti-inflammatory Agents** Because ACE inhibitors may promote kinin-mediated prostaglandin synthesis and/or release, concomitant administration of drugs that inhibit prostaglandin synthesis (e.g., aspirin, ibuprofen) may reduce the blood pressure response to ACE inhibitors, including captopril. Limited data indicate that concomitant administration of ACE inhibitors with nonsteroidal anti-inflammatory agents (NSAIAs) occasionally may result in acute reduction of renal function; however, the possibility cannot be ruled out that one drug alone may cause such an effect. Blood pressure should be monitored carefully when an NSAIA is initiated in patients receiving ACE inhibitor therapy; in addition, clinicians should be alert for evidence of impaired renal function. Some clinicians suggest that if a drug interaction between an ACE inhibitor and an NSAIA is suspected, the NSAIA should be discontinued, or a different hypotensive agent used or, alternatively, the dosage of the hypotensive agent should be modified.

Aspirin and other NSAIAs also can attenuate the hemodynamic actions of ACE inhibitors in patients with heart failure. Because ACE inhibitors share and enhance the effects of the compensatory hemodynamic mechanisms of heart failure, with aspirin and other NSAIAs interacting with the compensatory mechanisms rather than with a given ACE inhibitor per se, these desirable mechanisms are particularly susceptible to the interaction and a subsequent potential loss of clinical benefits. As a result, the more severe the heart failure and the more prominent the compensatory mechanisms, the more appreciable the interaction between NSAIAs and ACE inhibitors. Even if optimal dosage of an ACE inhibitor is used in the treatment of heart failure, the potential cardiovascular and survival benefit may not be seen if the patient is receiving an NSAIA concomitantly. In several multicenter studies, concomitant administration of a single 350-mg dose of aspirin in patients with heart failure inhibited favorable hemodynamic effects associated with ACE inhibitors, attenuating the favorable effects of these drugs on survival and cardiovascular morbidity. However, these findings have not been confirmed by other studies. In one retrospective analysis of pooled data, patients who received an ACE inhibitor concomitantly with aspirin (160–325 mg daily) during the acute phase following myocardial infarction (MI) had proportional reductions in 7- and 30-day mortality rates comparable to patients who received an ACE inhibitor alone. Some clinicians have questioned the results of this study because of methodologic concerns (e.g., unsubstantiated assumptions about aspirin therapy [dosage, time of initiation, duration]; disparate distribution of patients). Although it has been suggested that patients requiring long-term management of heart failure avoid the concomitant use of ACE inhibitors and aspirin (and perhaps substitute another platelet-aggregation inhibitor for aspirin [e.g., clopidogrel, ticlopidine]), many clinicians state that existing data are insufficient to recommend a change in the current prescribing practices of clinicians concerning the use of aspirin in patients receiving therapy with an ACE inhibitor.

■ **Antacids** Concomitant oral administration of captopril and antacids may decrease the rate and extent of GI absorption of captopril. Oral administration of a single, 50-mg dose of captopril 15 minutes after an oral dose of an antacid containing magnesium carbonate and aluminum and magnesium hydroxides resulted in a 40–45% decrease in captopril bioavailability, and a delay and decrease in peak serum concentrations of the drug. However, there is some evidence that this potential interaction may not be clinically important, but additional study is necessary.

■ **Probenecid** Concomitant administration of probenecid may increase blood concentrations of captopril and its metabolites, probably through decreased tubular secretion of captopril and subsequently increased metabolism of the drug (the latter effect probably occurring indirectly as a result of decreased renal clearance of the drug). Prolongation of ACE inhibition by captopril and possible subsequent potentiation of clinical and toxic effects of the drug may occur during concomitant therapy, but the potential for such interaction has not been fully elucidated.

■ **Other Drugs** Neuropathy reportedly developed in 2 patients receiving captopril and cimetidine; however, further documentation of this potential interaction is necessary.

Initiation of captopril therapy has been associated with unexplained hypoglycemia in several diabetic patients whose diabetes had been controlled with insulin or oral antidiabetic agents. Testing in these patients indicated that captopril may increase insulin sensitivity; the mechanism of this effect is not known. The risk of precipitating hypoglycemia should be considered when captopril therapy is initiated in diabetic patients.

Lithium and an ACE inhibitor (e.g., captopril) should be used concomitantly with caution and serum lithium concentrations should be monitored frequently since elevated serum lithium concentrations and lithium toxicity have occurred following concomitant therapy with the drugs. The risk of lithium toxicity in patients receiving captopril may be increased in patients who are also receiving diuretic therapy.

Laboratory Test Interferences

Captopril may cause false-positive results in urine acetone determinations using sodium nitroprusside reagent.

Acute Toxicity

■ **Pathogenesis** The oral LD_{50} of captopril ranged from 5.7–8.6 g/kg in mice and rats, and the IV LD_{50} was 1 g/kg in mice. In dogs and monkeys, single oral doses of 0.5 and 1.5 g/kg, respectively, produced emesis and decreased blood pressure.

■ **Treatment** The manufacturer states that treatment of captopril overdose mainly involves correction of hypotension. Hypotension can be corrected with fluid volume expansion (e.g., IV infusion of 0.9% sodium chloride injection). Elimination of captopril may be enhanced by hemodialysis.

Pharmacology

The mechanism(s) of action of captopril has not been fully elucidated. The drug appears to reduce blood pressure in hypertensive patients and produce beneficial hemodynamic effects in patients with heart failure mainly by suppressing the renin-angiotensin-aldosterone system.

■ **Effects on Renin-Angiotensin-Aldosterone System** Captopril prevents the conversion of angiotensin I to angiotensin II (a potent vasoconstrictor) by competing with the physiologic substrate (angiotensin I) for the active site of angiotensin-converting enzyme (ACE); the affinity of the drug for ACE is approximately 30,000 times greater than that of angiotensin I.

Inhibition of ACE results in decreased plasma angiotensin II concentrations and, consequently, blood pressure may be reduced in part through decreased vasoconstriction. Plasma renin activity (PRA) increases, possibly as a result of loss of feedback inhibition (mediated by angiotensin II) on the release of renin from the kidneys and/or stimulation of reflex mechanisms via baroreceptors (as a result of the decrease in blood pressure). It has been suggested that the hypotensive effect of ACE inhibitors may in part result from a local effect (e.g., in vascular wall). By decreasing local angiotensin II production, ACE inhibitors may decrease vascular tone by reducing direct angiotensin II-induced vasoconstriction and/or angiotensin II-induced increases in sympathetic activity. The hypotensive effect of captopril persists longer than inhibition of ACE in blood; it is not known whether ACE is inhibited longer in vascular endothelium than in blood.

Captopril alone is apparently more effective in reducing blood pressure in patients with high or normal renin hypertension. The drug also may lower blood pressure in patients with low renin hypertension, but these patients are unlikely to respond unless a diuretic is given in conjunction with captopril. A positive correlation between pretreatment PRA and short-term reduction in blood pressure with captopril has been reported and is particularly evident when data from a large number of patients are combined; the magnitude of the initial decrease in blood pressure appears to be proportional to the pretreatment PRA. Although some clinicians have reported a positive correlation between pretreatment PRA and long-term response to captopril, such a correlation has not been consistently found and remains to be clearly established. Some clinicians believe that an individual pretreatment PRA is not useful in predicting a response to captopril because of the wide interpatient variation in PRA values. Since captopril increases PRA, renin profiling should not be performed during captopril therapy.

Decreases in plasma angiotensin II concentrations lead to decreased aldosterone secretion from the adrenal cortex and, therefore, decreased plasma aldosterone concentrations and decreased urinary aldosterone excretion. However, there is increasing evidence to suggest that plasma aldosterone concentrations may not decrease during therapy with usual dosages of ACE inhibitors in some patients and may return to pretreatment levels in others during prolonged therapy. It has been suggested that the addition of spironolactone, a drug that competitively inhibits the physiologic effects of aldosterone, appears to augment the suppressive effect of ACE inhibitors on aldosterone. The hypotensive effect of captopril may result in part from decreased sodium and water retention as a result of the reduction in aldosterone secretion.

■ **Effects on Catecholamines and Autacoids** Circulating plasma norepinephrine concentration is not affected by captopril, and the drug does not inhibit the increase in plasma norepinephrine concentration that results from orthostatic reflexes. However, by inhibiting angiotensin II formation, ACE inhibitors may affect catecholamine release and reuptake by noradrenergic nerve endings and/or may decrease vascular sensitivity to vasopressors. There is some evidence that high doses of ACE inhibitors may inhibit presynaptic norepinephrine release and postsynaptic α_2-adrenoceptor activity, thereby interfering with sympathetic reflexes, but the clinical importance of this finding is not known since dosages tested in animals substantially exceed usual human hypotensive dosages.

Because ACE also degrades the vasodilator bradykinin, it has been suggested that inhibition of ACE by captopril may cause accumulation of bradykinin in plasma or tissues with resultant vasodilation. However, the effects of captopril on plasma bradykinin concentration have varied, possibly because of the difficulties in measuring bradykinin; the contribution of bradykinin-mediated effects to the hypotensive action of captopril remains to be clearly established. It has been suggested that prostaglandins also may mediate some of the pharmacologic effects of captopril, since there is some evidence that the drug may increase prostaglandin production or release; prostaglandin release may in part result from increased concentrations of bradykinin. Some clinicians have reported that captopril may control blood pressure in patients with renovascular hypertension without affecting urinary excretion of prostaglandin E_2. However, the effects of captopril on prostaglandins have been inconsistent, and further evaluation is necessary to determine the importance of any prostaglandin-mediated effects. (See Drug Interactions: Nonsteroidal Anti-Inflammatory Agents.)

■ **Cardiovascular Effects** In hypertensive patients, captopril reduces blood pressure by decreasing total peripheral resistance with no change or an increase in heart rate, stroke volume, or cardiac output; these effects are independent of pretreatment blood pressure or cardiac output. The drug causes arterial and possibly venous dilation. Captopril generally decreases systolic and diastolic blood pressure by 15–25%; blood pressure is decreased to about the same extent in both the supine and standing positions. Orthostatic hypotension and tachycardia occur infrequently but are more common in sodium-depleted or hypovolemic patients. (See Cautions: Cardiovascular Effects.) Plasma volume has been reported to be unchanged or slightly increased. Animal studies indicate that captopril does not have a direct effect on vascular smooth muscle. The drug appears to have no direct effect on baroreceptor sensitivity although reflex stimulation may occur during captopril therapy.

In patients with heart failure, captopril decreases total peripheral resistance, pulmonary vascular resistance, pulmonary capillary wedge pressure, and mean arterial and right atrial pressures. Cardiac index, cardiac output, stroke volume, and exercise tolerance are increased in these patients; heart rate decreases or is unchanged. The drug may also cause regional redistribution of blood flow, principally increasing renal blood flow with slight or no increase in flow in the forearm or hepatic vasculature, respectively.

■ **Renal and Electrolyte Effects** Renal blood flow may increase but glomerular filtration rate is usually unchanged during captopril therapy. In some patients, however, both BUN and serum creatinine concentrations have occasionally increased. Increased BUN and serum creatinine occur more frequently in patients with preexisting renal impairment, in those receiving concomitant therapy with a diuretic, and in those with heart failure. In patients with heart failure and renal perfusion pressures less than 70 mm Hg, changes in creatinine clearance induced by 1–3 months of captopril therapy have varied linearly and inversely with pretreatment PRA; however, creatinine clearance was not substantially affected by the drug in patients with renal perfusion pressures of 70 mm Hg or greater. Transient increases in BUN and serum creatinine concentrations are more frequent in patients with renovascular hypotension than in hypertensive patients with normal renal function. In addition, renal function can markedly deteriorate during therapy with an ACE inhibitor in patients with preexisting, severely compromised renal function. (See Cautions: Renal Effects.) Although anephric patients may respond to captopril immediately following hemodialysis (i.e., when hypovolemia exists), they apparently do not respond to the drug when fluid repleted.

Small increases in serum potassium concentration may occur secondary to captopril-induced decreases in aldosterone secretion, especially in patients with impaired renal function. Concomitant administration of thiazide diuretics generally offsets this increase. Captopril apparently does not cause sodium retention. Urinary sodium excretion may be increased during the first 2–3 days of captopril therapy.

■ **Other Effects** Serum prolactin concentration has been reported to increase during captopril therapy.

Pharmacokinetics

■ **Absorption** Approximately 60–75% of an oral dose of captopril is rapidly absorbed from the GI tract in fasting healthy individuals or hypertensive patients. Food may decrease absorption of captopril by up to 25–40%, although there is some evidence that this effect is not clinically important. Following oral administration of a single 100-mg dose of captopril in fasting healthy individuals in one study, average peak blood drug concentrations of 800 ng/mL were attained in 1 hour.

The hypotensive effect of a single dose of orally administered captopril may be apparent within 15 minutes and is usually maximal in 1–2 hours. The duration of action is generally 2–6 hours but appears to increase with increasing doses and has been prolonged up to 12 hours in some patients receiving high doses. The reduction in blood pressure may be gradual, and several weeks of therapy may be required before the full effect of the drug is achieved. The reduction in blood pressure observed with the initial dose of captopril has been reported by some clinicians to be positively correlated with the reduction in blood pressure achieved by long-term therapy with the drug. Some clinicians have observed a triphasic hypotensive effect during the first 1–2 weeks of therapy: the initial blood pressure reduction in the first few days is followed by a period lasting 3–9 days during which blood pressure increases toward pretreatment levels or remains stable, and then, a further reduction in blood pressure occurs. Because of the apparent resistance that may occur, increases in captopril dosage are usually avoided in the first 1–2 weeks of therapy since the eventual reduction in blood pressure does not reflect the response observed during this period. After withdrawal of the drug, blood pressure gradually returns to pretreatment levels within 1–7 days; rebound hypertension has not been reported to date.

■ **Distribution** Animal studies indicate that captopril is rapidly distributed into most body tissues, except the CNS. Captopril crosses the placenta in humans and is distributed into milk in concentrations about 1% of maternal blood concentrations.

Captopril is approximately 25–30% bound to plasma proteins, mainly albumin.

■ **Elimination** The elimination half-life of unchanged captopril appears to be less than 2 hours in patients with normal renal function. The elimination half-life of captopril and its metabolites is correlated with creatinine clearance and increases to about 20–40 hours in patients with creatinine clearances less than 20 mL/minute and as long as 6.5 days in anuric patients.

About half the absorbed dose of captopril is rapidly metabolized, mainly to captopril-cysteine disulfide and the disulfide dimer of captopril. In vitro studies suggest that captopril and its metabolites may undergo reversible interconversions. It has been suggested that the drug may be more extensively metabolized in patients with renal impairment than in patients with normal renal function.

Captopril and its metabolites are excreted in urine. Renal excretion of unchanged captopril occurs principally via tubular secretion. In patients with normal renal function, more than 95% of an absorbed dose is excreted in urine in 24 hours; about 40–50% of the drug excreted in urine is unchanged captopril and the remainder is mainly the disulfide dimer of captopril and captopril-cysteine disulfide. In one study in healthy individuals, about 20% of a single dose of captopril was recovered in feces in 5 days, apparently representing unabsorbed drug. Captopril is removed by hemodialysis.

Chemistry and Stability

■ **Chemistry** Captopril is an angiotensin-converting enzyme (ACE, bradykininase, kininase II) inhibitor. The drug occurs as a white to off-white, crystalline powder with a slight acid-sulfhydryl odor and is freely soluble in water and in alcohol. The apparent pK_as of captopril are 3.7 and 9.8. Commercially available captopril tablets may have a slight sulfurous odor.

■ **Stability** Captopril tablets and fixed-combination captopril and hydrochlorothiazide tablets should be stored in tight containers at a temperature not exceeding 30°C.

Preparations

Excipients in commercially available drug preparations may have clinically important effects in some individuals; consult specific product labeling for details.

Captopril

Oral		
Tablets	12.5 mg*	Captopril Tablets
	25 mg*	Captopril Tablets
	50 mg*	Captopril Tablets
	100 mg*	Captopril Tablets

*available from one or more manufacturer, distributor, and/or repackager by generic (nonproprietary) name

Captopril and Hydrochlorothiazide

Oral		
Tablets	25 mg Captopril and Hydrochlorothiazide 15 mg*	Captopril and Hydrochlorothiazide Tablets
	25 mg Captopril and Hydrochlorothiazide 25 mg*	Captopril and Hydrochlorothiazide Tablets
	50 mg Captopril and Hydrochlorothiazide 15 mg*	Captopril and Hydrochlorothiazide Tablets
	50 mg Captopril and Hydrochlorothiazide 25 mg*	Captopril and Hydrochlorothiazide Tablets

*available from one or more manufacturer, distributor, and/or repackager by generic (nonproprietary) name

†Use is not currently included in the labeling approved by the US Food and Drug Administration

Selected Revisions November 2018, © Copyright, March 1982, American Society of Health-System Pharmacists, Inc.

Enalaprilat
Enalapril Maleate

■ Enalaprilat and enalapril are angiotensin-converting enzyme (ACE) inhibitors; enalapril, the ethylester of enalaprilat, is a prodrug and has little pharmacologic activity until hydrolyzed in the liver to enalaprilat.

Uses

■ **Hypertension** Enalapril is used alone or in combination with other classes of antihypertensive agents in the management of hypertension. Enalaprilat is used in the management of hypertension when oral therapy is not practical. Because captopril, another angiotensin-converting enzyme (ACE) inhibitor, may cause serious adverse effects (e.g., neutropenia, agranulocytosis), particularly in patients with renal impairment (especially those with collagen vascular disease) or in patients receiving immunosuppressive therapy, the possibility that similar adverse effects may occur with enalapril or enalaprilat should be considered since current experience is insufficient to rule out such risk. Enalapril has occasionally been used without recurrence of adverse effect in patients who developed intolerable adverse effects (i.e., rash, taste disturbances) during captopril therapy. Further studies are needed to evaluate the possible risks associated with the long-term use of enalapril. The hypotensive efficacy of enalapril in hypertensive patients is similar to that of captopril or β-adrenergic blocking agents (β-blockers). Enalapril may have a greater effect on systolic blood pressure at rest (but not with exercise) than do β-blockers, but additional study is necessary to establish the comparative efficacy of enalapril and β-blockers.

Current evidence-based practice guidelines for the management of hypertension in adults generally recommend the use of drugs from 4 classes of antihypertensive agents (ACE inhibitors, angiotensin II receptor antagonists, calcium-channel blockers, and thiazide diuretics); data from clinical outcome trials indicate that lowering blood pressure with any of these drug classes can reduce the complications of hypertension and provide similar cardiovascular protection. However, recommendations for initial drug selection and use in specific patient populations may vary across these expert guidelines. This variability is due, in part, to differences in the guideline development process and the types of studies (e.g., randomized controlled studies only versus a range of studies with different study designs) included in the evidence reviews. Ultimately, choice of antihypertensive therapy should be individualized, considering the clinical characteristics of the patient (e.g., age, ethnicity/race, comorbid conditions, cardiovascular risk factors) as well as drug-related factors (e.g., ease of administration, availability, adverse effects, costs). Because many patients eventually will need drugs from 2 or more antihypertensive classes, experts generally state that the emphasis should be placed on achieving appropriate blood pressure control rather than on identifying a preferred drug to achieve that control.

Disease Overview Worldwide, hypertension is the most common modifiable risk factor for cardiovascular events and mortality. The lifetime risk of developing hypertension in the US exceeds 80%, with higher rates observed among African Americans and Hispanics compared with whites or Asians. The systolic blood pressure and diastolic blood pressure values defined as hypertension (see Blood Pressure Classification under Uses: Hypertension) in a 2017 multidisciplinary guideline of the American College of Cardiology (ACC), American Heart Association (AHA), and a number of other professional organizations (subsequently referred to as the 2017 ACC/AHA hypertension guidelines in this monograph) are lower than those defined in the Seventh Report of the Joint National Committee on Prevention, Detection, Evaluation, and Treatment of High Blood Pressure (JNC 7) guidelines, which results in an increase of approximately 14% in the prevalence of hypertension in the US. However, this change in definition results in only a 2% increase in the percentage of patients requiring antihypertensive drug therapy because nonpharmacologic treatment is recommended for most adults now classified by the 2017 ACC/AHA hypertension guideline as hypertensive who would *not* meet the JNC 7 definition of hypertension. Among US adults receiving antihypertensive drugs, approximately 53% have inadequately controlled blood pressure according to current ACC/AHA treatment goals.

Cardiovascular and Renal Sequelae. The principal goal of preventing and treating hypertension is to reduce the risk of cardiovascular and renal morbidity and mortality, including target organ damage. The relationship between blood pressure and cardiovascular disease is continuous, consistent, and independent of other risk factors. It is important that very high blood pressure be managed promptly to reduce the risk of target organ damage. The higher the blood pressure, the more likely the development of myocardial infarction (MI), heart failure, stroke, and renal disease. For adults 40–70 years of age, each 20-mm Hg increment in systolic blood pressure or 10-mm Hg increment in diastolic blood pressure doubles the risk of developing cardiovascular disease across the entire blood pressure range of 115/75 to 185/115 mm Hg. For those older than 50 years of age, systolic blood pressure is a much more important risk factor for developing cardiovascular disease than is diastolic blood pressure. The rapidity with which treatment is required depends on the patient's clinical presentation (presence of new or worsening target organ damage) and the presence or absence of cardiovascular complications; the 2017 ACC/AHA hypertension guideline states that treatment of very high blood pressure should be initiated within 1 week.

Blood Pressure Classification Accurate blood pressure measurement is essential for the proper diagnosis and management of hypertension. Error in measuring blood pressure is a major cause of inadequate blood pressure control and may lead to overtreatment. Because a patient's blood pressure may vary in an unpredictable fashion, a single blood pressure measurement is not sufficient for clinical decision-making. An average of 2 or 3 blood pressure measurements obtained on 2–3 separate occasions using proper technique should be used to minimize random error and provide a more accurate blood pressure reading. Out-of-office blood pressure measurements may be useful for confirming and managing hypertension. The 2017 ACC/AHA hypertension guideline document (available on the ACC and AHA websites) should be consulted for key steps on properly measuring blood pressure.

According to the 2017 ACC/AHA hypertension guideline, blood pressure in adults is classified into 4 categories: normal, elevated, stage 1 hypertension, and stage 2 hypertension. (See Table 1.) The 2017 ACC/AHA hypertension guideline lowers the blood pressure threshold used to define hypertension in the US; previous hypertension guidelines (JNC 7) considered adults with systolic blood pressure of 120–139 mm Hg or diastolic blood pressure of 80–89 mm Hg to have prehypertension, those with systolic blood pressure of 140–159 mm Hg or diastolic blood pressure of 90–99 mm Hg to have stage 1 hypertension, and those with systolic blood pressure of 160 mm Hg or higher or diastolic blood pressure of 100 mm Hg or higher to have stage 2 hypertension. The blood pressure definitions in the 2017 ACC/AHA hypertension guideline are based upon data from studies evaluating the association between systolic blood pressure/diastolic blood pressure and cardiovascular risk and the benefits of blood pressure reduction. Individuals with systolic blood pressure and diastolic blood pressure in 2 different categories should be designated as being in the higher blood pressure category.

Table 1. ACC/AHA Blood Pressure Classification in Adults[a,b]

Category	SBP[c] (mm Hg)		DBP[d] (mm Hg)
Normal	<120	and	<80
Elevated	120–129	and	<80
Hypertension, Stage 1	130–139	or	80–89
Hypertension, Stage 2	≥140	or	≥90

[a] Source: Whelton PK, Carey RM, Aronow WS et al. 2017 ACC/AHA/AAPA/ABC/ACPM/AGS/APhA/ASH/ASPC/NMA/PCNA guideline for the prevention, detection, evaluation, and management of high blood pressure in adults: a report of the American College of Cardiology/American Heart Association Task Force on Clinical Practice Guidelines. Hypertension. 2018;71:e13-115.

[b] Individuals with SBP and DBP in 2 different categories (e.g., elevated SBP and normal DBP) should be designated as being in the higher blood pressure category (i.e., elevated BP).

[c] Systolic blood pressure

[d] Diastolic blood pressure

The blood pressure thresholds used to define hypertension, when to initiate drug therapy, and the ideal target blood pressure values remain controversial. The 2017 ACC/AHA hypertension guideline recommends a blood pressure goal of less than 130/80 mm Hg in all adults who have confirmed hypertension and known cardiovascular disease or a 10-year atherosclerotic cardiovascular disease (ASCVD) event risk of 10% or higher; the ACC/AHA guideline also states that this blood pressure goal is reasonable to attempt to achieve in adults with confirmed hypertension who do *not* have increased cardiovascular risk. The lower blood pressure values used to define hypertension and the lower target blood pressure goals outlined in the 2017 ACC/AHA hypertension guideline are based on clinical studies demonstrating a substantial reduction in the composite end point of major cardiovascular disease events and the combination of fatal and nonfatal stroke when a lower systolic blood pressure/diastolic blood pressure value (i.e., 130/80 mm Hg) was used to define hypertension. These lower target blood pressure goals also are based upon clinical studies demonstrating continuing reduction of cardiovascular risk at progressively lower levels of systolic blood pressure. A linear relationship has been demonstrated between cardiovascular risk and blood pressure even at low systolic blood pressures (e.g, 120–124 mm Hg). The 2017 ACC/AHA hypertension guideline recommends estimating a patient's ASCVD risk using the ACC/AHA Pooled Cohort equations (available online at http://tools.acc.org/ASCVD-Risk-Estimator), which are based on a variety of factors including age, race, gender, cholesterol levels, statin use, blood pressure, treatment for hypertension, history of diabetes mellitus, smoking status, and aspirin use. While the 2017 ACC/AHA hypertension guideline has lowered the threshold for *diagnosing* hypertension in adults, the threshold for *initiating drug therapy* has only been lowered for those patients who are at high risk of cardiovascular disease. Clinicians who support the 2017 ACC/AHA hypertension guideline believe that these recommendations have the potential to increase hypertension awareness, encourage lifestyle modification, and focus antihypertensive drug initiation and intensification in those adults at high risk for cardiovascular disease.

The lower blood pressure goals advocated in the 2017 ACC/AHA hypertension guideline have been questioned by some clinicians who have concerns regarding the guideline's use of extrapolated observational data, the lack of generalizability of some of the randomized trials (e.g., SPRINT) used to support the guideline, the difficulty of establishing accurate representative blood pressure values in typical clinical practice settings, and the accuracy of the cardiovascular risk calculator used in the guideline. Some clinicians state the lower blood pressure threshold used to define hypertension in the 2017 ACC/AHA hypertension guideline is not fully supported by clinical data, and these clinicians have expressed concerns about the possible harms (e.g., adverse effects of antihypertensive therapy) associated with classifying more patients as being hypertensive. Some clinicians also state that using this guideline, a large number of young, low-risk patients would need to be treated in order to observe a clinical benefit, while other clinicians state that the estimated gains in life expectancy attributable to long-term use of blood pressure-lowering drugs are correspondingly greater in this patient population.

Treatment Benefits In clinical trials, antihypertensive therapy has been found to reduce the risk of developing stroke by about 34–40%, MI by about 20–25%, and heart failure by more than 50%. In a randomized, controlled study (SPRINT) that included hypertensive patients without diabetes mellitus who had a high risk of cardiovascular disease, intensive systolic blood pressure lowering of approximately 15 mm Hg was associated with a 25% reduction in cardiovascular disease events and a 27% reduction in all-cause mortality. However, the exclusion of patients with diabetes mellitus, prior stroke, and those younger than 50 years of age may decrease the generalizability of these findings. Some experts estimate that if the systolic blood pressure goals of the 2017 ACC/AHA hypertension guideline are achieved, major cardiovascular disease events may be reduced by an additional 340,000 and total deaths by an additional 156,000 compared with implementation of the JNC 8 expert panel guideline goals but these benefits may be accompanied by an increase in the frequency of adverse events. While there was no overall difference in the occurrence of serious adverse events in patients receiving intensive therapy for blood pressure control (systolic blood pressure target of less than 120 mm Hg) compared with those receiving less intense control (systolic blood pressure target of less than 140 mm Hg) in the SPRINT study, hypotension, syncope, electrolyte abnormalities, and acute kidney injury or acute renal failure occurred in substantially more patients receiving intensive therapy.

In the Antihypertensive and Lipid-lowering Treatment to Prevent Heart Attack Trial (ALLHAT), the long-term cardiovascular morbidity and mortality benefit of a long-acting dihydropyridine calcium-channel blocker (amlodipine), a thiazide-like diuretic (chlorthalidone), and an ACE inhibitor (lisinopril) were compared in a broad population of patients with hypertension at risk for coronary heart disease. Although these antihypertensive agents were comparably effective in providing important cardiovascular benefit, apparent differences in certain secondary outcomes were observed. Patients receiving the ACE inhibitor experienced higher risks of stroke, combined cardiovascular disease, GI bleeding, and angioedema, while those receiving the calcium-channel blocker were at higher risk of developing heart failure. The ALLHAT investigators suggested that the favorable cardiovascular outcome may be attributable, at least in part, to the greater antihypertensive effect of the calcium-channel blocker compared with that of the ACE inhibitor, especially in women and black patients. (See Clinical Benefit of Thiazides in Hypertension under Hypertension in Adults: Treatment Benefits, in Uses in the Thiazides General Statement 40:28.20.)

General Considerations for Initial and Maintenance Antihypertensive Therapy **Nonpharmacologic Therapy.** Nonpharmacologic measures (i.e., lifestyle/behavioral modifications) that are effective in lowering blood pressure include weight reduction (for those who are overweight or obese), dietary changes to include foods such as fruits, vegetables, whole grains, and low-fat dairy products that are rich in potassium, calcium, magnesium, and fiber (i.e., adoption of the Dietary Approaches to Stop Hypertension [DASH] eating plan), sodium reduction, increased physical activity, and moderation of alcohol intake. Such lifestyle/behavioral modifications, including smoking cessation, enhance antihypertensive drug efficacy and decrease cardiovascular risk and remain an indispensable part of the management of hypertension. Lifestyle/behavioral modifications without antihypertensive drug therapy are recommended for individuals classified by the 2017 ACC/AHA hypertension guideline as having elevated blood pressure (systolic blood pressure 120–129 mm Hg and diastolic blood pressure less than 80 mm Hg) and in those with stage 1 hypertension (systolic blood pressure 130–139 mm Hg or diastolic blood pressure 80–89 mm Hg) who do *not* have preexisting cardiovascular disease or an estimated 10-year ASCVD risk of 10% or greater.

Initiation of Drug Therapy. Drug therapy in the management of hypertension must be individualized and adjusted based on the degree of blood pressure elevation while also considering cardiovascular risk factors. Drug therapy generally is reserved for patients who respond inadequately to nondrug therapy (i.e., life-style modifications such as diet [including sodium restriction and adequate potassium and calcium intake], regular aerobic physical activity, moderation of alcohol consumption, and weight reduction) or in whom the degree of blood pressure elevation or coexisting risk factors, especially cardiovascular risk, require more prompt or aggressive therapy; however, the optimum blood pressure threshold for initiating antihypertensive drug therapy and specific treatment goals remain controversial. Recommendations generally are based on specific blood pressure levels shown in clinical studies to produce clinical benefits and can therefore vary depending on the studies selected for review.

The 2017 ACC/AHA hypertension guideline and many experts currently state that the treatment of hypertension should be based not only on blood pressure values but also on patients' cardiovascular risk factors. For *secondary prevention* of recurrent cardiovascular disease events in adults with clinical cardiovascular disease or for *primary prevention* in adults with an estimated 10-year ASCVD risk of 10% or higher, the 2017 ACC/AHA hypertension guideline recommends initiation of antihypertensive drug therapy in conjunction with lifestyle/behavioral modifications at an average systolic blood pressure of 130 mm Hg or an average diastolic blood pressure of 80 mm Hg or higher. For *primary prevention* of cardiovascular disease events in adults with a low (less than 10%) estimated 10-year risk of ASCVD, the 2017 ACC/AHA hypertension guideline recommends initiation of antihypertensive drug therapy in conjunction with lifestyle/behavioral modifications at a systolic blood pressure of 140 mm Hg or higher or a diastolic blood pressure of 90 mm Hg or higher. After initiation of antihypertensive drug therapy, regardless of the ASCVD risk, the 2017 ACC/AHA hypertension guideline generally recommends a blood pressure goal of less than 130/80 mm Hg in all adults. In addition, a systolic blood pressure goal of less than 130 mm Hg is also recommended for noninstitutionalized ambulatory patients 65 years of age or older. While these blood pressure goals are lower than those recommended for most patients in previous guidelines, they are based upon clinical studies demonstrating continuing reduction of cardiovascular risk at progressively lower levels of systolic blood pressure.

Most data indicate that patients with a higher cardiovascular risk will benefit the most from tighter blood pressure control; however, some experts state this treatment goal also may be beneficial in those at lower cardiovascular risk. Other clinicians believe that the benefits of such blood pressure lowering do not outweigh the risks in those patients considered to be at lower risk of cardiovascular disease and that reclassifying individuals formerly considered to have prehypertension as having hypertension may potentially lead to use of drug therapy in such patients without consideration of cardiovascular risk. Previous hypertension guidelines, such as those from the JNC 8 expert panel, generally recommended initiation of antihypertensive treatment in patients with a systolic blood pressure of at least 140 mm Hg or diastolic blood pressure of at least 90 mm Hg, targeted a blood pressure goal of less than 140/90 mm Hg regardless of cardiovascular risk, and used higher systolic blood pressure thresholds and targets in geriatric patients. Some clinicians continue to support the target blood pressures recommended by the JNC 8 expert panel because of concerns that such recommendations in the 2017 ACC/AHA hypertension guideline are based on extrapolation of data from the high-risk population in the SPRINT study to a lower-risk population. Also, because more than 90% of patients in SPRINT were already receiving antihypertensive drugs at baseline, data are lacking on the effects of *initiating* drug therapy at a lower blood pressure threshold (130/80 mm Hg) in patients at high risk of cardiovascular disease. The potential benefits of hypertension management and drug cost, adverse effects, and risks associated with the use of multiple antihypertensive drugs should be considered when deciding a patient's blood pressure treatment goal.

The 2017 ACC/AHA hypertension guideline recommends an ASCVD risk assessment for all adults with hypertension; however, experts state that it can be assumed that patients with hypertension and diabetes mellitus or chronic kidney disease (CKD) are at high risk for cardiovascular disease and that antihypertensive drug therapy should be initiated in these patients at a blood pressure of 130/80 mm Hg or higher. The 2017 ACC/AHA hypertension guideline also recommends a blood pressure goal of less than 130/80 mm Hg in patients with hypertension and diabetes mellitus or CKD. These recommendations are based on a systematic review of high-quality evidence from randomized controlled trials, meta-analyses, and post-hoc analyses that have demonstrated substantial reductions in the risk of important clinical outcomes (e.g., cardiovascular events) regardless of comorbid conditions or age when systolic blood pressure is lowered to less than 130 mm Hg. However, some clinicians have questioned the generalizability of findings from some of the trials (e.g., SPRINT) used to support the 2017 ACC/AHA hypertension guideline. For example, SPRINT included adults (mean age: 68 years) *without* diabetes mellitus who were at high risk of cardiovascular disease. While benefits of intensive blood pressure control were observed in this patient population, some clinicians have questioned whether these findings apply to younger patients who have a low risk of cardiovascular disease. In patients with CKD in the SPRINT trial, intensive blood pressure management (achieving a mean systolic blood pressure of approximately 122 mm Hg compared with 136 mm Hg with standard treatment) provided a similar beneficial reduction in the composite cardiovascular disease primary outcome and all-cause mortality as in the full patient cohort. Because most patients with CKD die from cardiovascular complications, the findings of this study further support a lower blood pressure target of less than 130/80 mm Hg.

Data are lacking to determine the ideal blood pressure goal in patients with hypertension and diabetes mellitus; also, studies evaluating the benefits of intensive blood pressure control in patients with diabetes mellitus have provided conflicting results. Clinical studies reviewed for the 2017 ACC/AHA hypertension guideline have shown similar quantitative benefits from blood pressure lowering in hypertensive patients with or without diabetes mellitus. In a randomized, controlled study (ACCORD-BP) that compared a higher (systolic blood pressure less than 140 mm Hg) versus lower (systolic blood pressure less than 120 mm Hg) blood pressure goal in patients with diabetes mellitus, there was no difference in the incidence of cardiovascular outcomes (e.g., composite outcome of cardiovascular death, nonfatal MI, and nonfatal stroke). However, some experts state that this study was underpowered to detect a difference between the 2 treatment groups and that the factorial design of the study complicated interpretation of the results. Although SPRINT did not include patients with diabetes mellitus, patients in this study with prediabetes demonstrated a similar cardiovascular benefit from intensive treatment of blood pressure as normoglycemic patients. A meta-analysis of data from ACCORD and SPRINT suggests that the findings of both studies are consistent and that patients with diabetes mellitus benefit from more intensive blood pressure control. These data support the 2017 ACC/AHA hypertension guideline recommendation of a blood pressure treatment goal of less than 130/80 mm Hg in patients with hypertension and diabetes mellitus. Alternatively, the American Diabetes Association (ADA) recommends a blood pressure goal of less than 140/90 mm Hg in patients with diabetes mellitus. The ADA states that a lower blood pressure goal (e.g., less than 130/80 mm Hg) may be appropriate for patients with a high risk of cardiovascular disease and diabetes mellitus if it can be achieved without undue treatment burden.

Further study is needed to more clearly define optimum blood pressure goals in patients with hypertension, particularly in high-risk groups (e.g., patients with diabetes mellitus, cardiovascular disease, or cerebrovascular disease; black patients); when determining appropriate blood pressure goals, individual risks and benefits should be considered in addition to the evidence from clinical studies.

Choice of Initial Drug Therapy. In current hypertension management guidelines, ACE inhibitors are recommended as one of several preferred drugs for the initial treatment of hypertension; other options include angiotensin II receptor antagonists, calcium-channel blockers, and thiazide diuretics. The 2017 ACC/AHA hypertension guideline states that an ACE inhibitor, angiotensin II receptor antagonist, calcium-channel blocker, or thiazide diuretic (preferably chlorthalidone) are all acceptable choices for initial antihypertensive drug therapy in the general population of nonblack patients, including those with diabetes mellitus; drugs from any of these classes generally produce similar benefits in terms of overall mortality and cardiovascular, cerebrovascular, and renal outcomes. ACE inhibitors may be particularly useful in the management of hypertension in patients with certain coexisting conditions such as heart failure, ischemic heart disease, diabetes mellitus, CKD, or cerebrovascular disease or following myocardial infarction (MI). (See Considerations for Drug Therapy in Patients with Underlying Cardiovascular and Other Risk Factors under Uses: Hypertension.)

In patients with hypertension and compelling indications (e.g., CKD with albuminuria [urine albumin 300 mg/day or greater, or urine albumin:creatinine ratio of 300 mg/g or equivalent in the first morning void]), angiotensin II receptor antagonists are usually considered an alternative for ACE inhibitor-intolerant patients. (See Chronic Kidney Disease under Hypertension: Considerations for Drug Therapy in Patients with Underlying Cardiovascular and Other Risk Factors, in Uses.) However, data indicate no difference in efficacy between ACE inhibitors and angiotensin II receptor antagonists with regard to blood pressure lowering and clinical outcomes (i.e., all-cause mortality, cardiovascular mortality, MI, heart failure, stroke, and end-stage renal disease). Adverse events (e.g., cough, angioedema) leading to drug discontinuance occur more frequently with ACE inhibitor therapy than with angiotensin II receptor antagonist therapy. Because of similar efficacy and a lower frequency of adverse effects, some experts believe that angiotensin II receptor antagonists should be used instead of an ACE inhibitor for the treatment of hypertension or hypertension with certain compelling indications.

Experts state that in patients with stage 1 hypertension (especially the elderly, those with a history of hypotension, or those who have experienced adverse drug effects), it is reasonable to initiate drug therapy using the stepped-care approach in which one drug is initiated and titrated and other drugs are added sequentially to achieve the target blood pressure. Although some patients can begin treatment with a single antihypertensive agent, starting with 2 drugs in different pharmacologic classes (either as separate agents or in a fixed-dose combination) is recommended in patients with stage 2 hypertension and an average blood pressure more than 20/10 mm Hg above their target blood pressure. Such combined therapy may increase the likelihood of achieving goal blood pressure in a more timely fashion, but also may increase the risk of adverse effects (e.g., orthostatic hypotension) in some patients (e.g., elderly). Drug regimens with complementary activity, where a second antihypertensive agent is used to block compensatory responses to the first agent or affect a different pressor mechanism, can result in additive blood pressure lowering and are preferred. Drug combinations that have similar mechanisms of action or clinical effects (e.g., the combination of an ACE inhibitor and an angiotensin II receptor antagonist) generally should be avoided. Many patients who begin therapy with a single antihypertensive agent will subsequently require at least 2 drugs from different pharmacologic classes to achieve their blood pressure goal. Experts state that other patient-specific factors, such as age, concurrent medications, drug adherence, drug interactions, the overall treatment regimen, cost, and comorbidities, also should be considered when deciding on an antihypertensive drug regimen. For any stage of hypertension, antihypertensive drug dosages should be adjusted and/or other agents substituted or added until goal blood pressure is achieved. (See Follow-up and Maintenance Drug Therapy under Hypertension: General Considerations for Initial and Maintenance Antihypertensive Therapy, in Uses.)

Follow-up and Maintenance Drug Therapy. Several strategies are used for the titration and combination of antihypertensive drugs; these strategies, which are generally based on those used in randomized controlled studies, include maximizing the dosage of the first drug before adding a second drug, adding a second drug before achieving maximum dosage of the initial drug, or initiating therapy with 2 drugs simultaneously (either as separate preparations or as a fixed-dose combination). Combined use of an ACE inhibitor and angiotensin II receptor antagonist should be avoided because of the potential risk of adverse renal effects. After initiating a new or adjusted antihypertensive drug regimen, patients should have their blood pressure reevaluated monthly until adequate blood pressure control is achieved. Effective blood pressure control can be achieved in most hypertensive patients, but many will ultimately require therapy with 2 or more antihypertensive drugs. In addition to measuring blood pressure, clinicians should evaluate patients for orthostatic hypotension, adverse drug effects, adherence to drug therapy and lifestyle modifications, and the need for drug dosage adjustments. Laboratory testing such as electrolytes and renal function status and other assessments of target organ damage also should be performed.

Enalapril can be used for the management of hypertension as initial monotherapy or as a component of a multiple-drug regimen. When enalapril alone is used but the patient's hypertension does not respond adequately, addition of a thiazide diuretic often adequately controls blood pressure. Such combined therapy generally produces additive reduction in blood pressure and may permit dosage reduction of either or both drugs and minimize adverse effects while maintaining blood pressure control.

Enalapril may be effective in the management of hypertension resistant to other drugs. Although enalapril occasionally may be effective alone in patients with severe hypertension, it is usually necessary to use the drug in conjunction with a diuretic. (See Drug Interactions: Hypotensive Agents and Diuretics.) Enalapril has been used in some diabetic hypertensive patients with no adverse effect on control or therapy of diabetes; however, hypoglycemia has occasionally occurred when the drug was used in patients whose diabetes had been controlled with insulin or oral hypoglycemic agents. (See Drug Interactions: Other Drugs.)

Tolerance to the hypotensive effect of enalapril apparently does not occur during long-term administration, particularly if the drug is used with a diuretic. Abrupt withdrawal of enalapril or enalaprilat therapy results in a gradual return of hypertension; rapid increases in blood pressure have not been reported to date.

IV enalaprilat may be used in the management of hypertension when oral therapy is not practical. Enalaprilat generally produces a prompt reduction in blood pressure, usually without an orthostatic response, and with a slight reduction in heart rate. Occasional hypotension, or symptomatic postural hypotension in volume-depleted patients, might be anticipated. Enalaprilat also has been used effectively to control blood pressure in adults with severe hypertension or hypertensive emergencies† (see Hypertensive Crises under Uses: Hypertension) and in a small number of neonates with severe hypertension†.

Considerations for Drug Therapy in Patients with Underlying Cardiovascular and Other Risk Factors Drug therapy in patients with hypertension and underlying cardiovascular or other risk factors should be carefully individualized based on the underlying disease(s), concomitant drugs, tolerance to drug-induced adverse effects, and blood pressure goal. See Table 2 on Compelling Indications for Drug Classes based on Comorbid Conditions under Uses: Hypertension in Adults, in the Thiazides General Statement 40:28.20.

Ischemic Heart Disease. The selection of an appropriate antihypertensive agent in patients with ischemic heart disease should be based on individual patient characteristics and may include ACE inhibitors and/or β-blockers, with the addition of other drugs such as thiazide diuretics or calcium-channel blockers as necessary to achieve blood pressure goals. Many experts recommend the use of an ACE inhibitor (or an angiotensin II receptor antagonist) and/or a β-blocker in hypertensive patients with stable ischemic heart disease because of the cardioprotective benefits of these drugs; all patients who have survived an MI should be treated with a β-blocker because of the demonstrated mortality benefit of these agents.

Heart Failure. While ACE inhibitors as single therapies are not superior to other antihypertensive agents in the reduction of cardiovascular outcomes, ACE inhibitors, usually in conjunction with other agents such as cardiac glycosides, diuretics, and β-blockers, have been shown to reduce morbidity and mortality in patients with existing heart failure. (See Uses: Heart Failure.) ACE inhibitors also have been used to prevent subsequent heart failure and reduce morbidity and mortality in patients with systolic dysfunction following acute MI†. (See Uses: Left Ventricular Dysfunction After Acute Myocardial Infarction.)

Diabetes Mellitus. Experts state that initial treatment of hypertension in adults with diabetes mellitus and hypertension should include any of the usual first-line agents (ACE inhibitors, angiotensin II receptor antagonists, calcium-channel blockers, thiazide diuretics). In adults with diabetes mellitus, hypertension, and albuminuria, treatment with an ACE inhibitor or angiotensin II receptor antagonist may be considered to reduce the progression of kidney disease. While there is evidence demonstrating the benefits of ACE inhibitors in reducing the development or progression of microvascular or macrovascular complications in hypertensive patients with type 1 or type 2 diabetes mellitus, in the absence of albuminuria, the risk of progressive kidney disease is low, and ACE inhibitors and angiotensin II receptor antagonists have not demonstrated superior cardioprotection when compared with other first-line agents. Results of several studies indicate that adequate control of blood pressure in patients with type 2 diabetes mellitus reduces the development or progression of complications of diabetes (e.g., death related to diabetes, stroke, heart failure, microvascular disease). Most patients with diabetes mellitus will require 2 or more antihypertensive agents to achieve blood pressure control.

Chronic Kidney Disease. Hypertensive patients with CKD (glomerular filtration rate [GFR] less than 60 mL/minute per 1.73 m^2 or kidney damage for 3 or more months) usually will require more than one antihypertensive agent to reach target blood pressure. Use of ACE inhibitors or angiotensin II receptor antagonists may be reasonable in patients with diabetic or nondiabetic CKD (stage 1 or 2 with albuminuria or stage 3 or higher); these drugs have been shown to slow the progression of kidney disease. Evidence of a renoprotective benefit is strongest in those with higher levels of albuminuria. Increases in serum creatinine (up to 30%) may be observed as a result of a decrease in intraglomerular pressure and concurrent reduction in GFR. The 2017 ACC/AHA hypertension guideline states that in patients with less severe kidney disease (i.e., stage 1 or 2 CKD without albuminuria), any of the first-line antihypertensive agents (e.g., ACE inhibitors, angiotensin II receptor antagonists, calcium-channel blockers, thiazide diuretics) can be used for the initial treatment of hypertension. Diuretics also may be useful in the management of CKD, and may potentiate the effects of ACE inhibitors, angiotensin II receptor antagonists, and other antihypertensive agents when used in combination. (See Diabetic Nephropathy under Uses: Nephropathy, in Captopril 24:32.04.)

Cerebrovascular Disease. Some experts recommend a blood pressure goal of less than 140/90 mm Hg in patients with ischemic stroke or transient ischemic attack (TIA), while others state that a blood pressure goal of less than 130/80 mm Hg may be reasonable. The 2017 ACC/AHA hypertension guideline states that adults not previously treated for hypertension who experience a stroke or TIA and who have an established blood pressure of 140/90 mm Hg should receive antihypertensive therapy within a few days after the event to reduce the risk of recurrent stroke or other vascular events. In patients with a recent lacunar stroke, experts suggest that a systolic blood pressure goal of 130 mm Hg may be reasonable based on results of a randomized open-label study (the Secondary Prevention of Small Subcortical Strokes [SPS3] trial). Although experts state that the optimal choice of drug for the management of hypertension in patients with a previous TIA or ischemic stroke is uncertain, available data indicate that an ACE inhibitor, angiotensin II receptor antagonist, thiazide diuretic, or the combination of a thiazide diuretic and an ACE inhibitor may be effective. Administration of an ACE inhibitor in combination with a thiazide diuretic has been shown to lower rates of recurrent stroke.

Hypertension Associated with Scleroderma Renal Crisis. Enalapril has been effective for the management of hypertension associated with scleroderma renal crisis† in a limited number of patients who were unable to tolerate captopril because of adverse effects. Maintenance therapy with enalapril (5–30 mg daily) controlled blood pressure in these patients and was accompanied by improvement in renal function. Some clinicians consider ACE inhibitors the drugs of choice for this condition.

Other Special Considerations for Antihypertensive Drug Therapy

Race. Most patients with hypertension, especially black patients, will require at least 2 antihypertensive drugs to achieve adequate blood pressure control. In general, black hypertensive patients tend to respond better to monotherapy with thiazide diuretics or calcium-channel blockers than to monotherapy with

ACE inhibitors. In a prespecified subgroup analysis of the ALLHAT study, a thiazide-type diuretic was more effective than an ACE inhibitor in improving cerebrovascular and cardiovascular outcomes in black patients; when compared with a calcium-channel blocker, the ACE inhibitor was less effective in reducing blood pressure and was associated with a 51% higher rate of stroke. (See Clinical Benefit of Thiazides in Hypertension under Hypertension in Adults: Treatment Benefits, in Uses in the Thiazides General Statement 40:28.20.) However, the combination of an ACE inhibitor or an angiotensin II receptor antagonist with a calcium-channel blocker or thiazide diuretic produces similar blood pressure lowering in black patients as in other racial groups. In addition, some experts state that when use of ACE inhibitors is indicated in hypertensive patients with underlying cardiovascular or other risk factors, these indications should be applied equally to black hypertensive patients.

Although enalapril has lowered blood pressure in all races studied, monotherapy with enalapril has produced a smaller reduction in blood pressure in black hypertensive patients, a population associated with low renin hypertension; however, this population difference in response does not appear to occur during combined therapy with enalapril and a thiazide diuretic. In addition, ACE inhibitors appear to produce a higher incidence of angioedema in black patients than in other races studied.

For further information on overall principles and expert recommendations for treatment of hypertension, see Uses: Hypertension in Adults and also see Uses: Hypertension in Pediatric Patients, in the Thiazides General Statement 40:28.20.)

Renovascular or Malignant Hypertension Enalapril also has been effective in the management of renovascular or malignant hypertension, renal hypertension secondary to renal-artery stenosis, and, in some patients, hypertension associated with chronic renal failure. In addition to the drugs' hypotensive effect, ACE inhibitors also have stabilized or improved effective renal blood flow and glomerular filtration rate and decreased proteinuria in some hypertensive patients with moderately impaired renal function, moderate to severe renal disease, or diabetic nephropathy. However, enalapril should be used with caution in patients with impaired renal function, especially those with bilateral renal-artery stenosis or with renal-artery stenosis in a solitary kidney. (See Cautions: Renal Effects and see Hematologic Effects and see Precautions and Contraindications.)

Hypertensive Crises Enalaprilat has been used effectively to reduce blood pressure in adults with severe hypertension or hypertensive emergencies†.

Hypertensive emergencies are those rare situations requiring immediate blood pressure reduction (not necessarily to normal ranges) to prevent or limit target organ damage. Such emergencies include hypertensive encephalopathy, acute MI, intracerebral hemorrhage, acute left ventricular failure with pulmonary edema, eclampsia, dissecting aortic aneurysm, unstable angina pectoris, acute ischemic stroke, and acute renal failure. Patients with hypertensive emergencies require hospitalization and are treated initially with an appropriate parenteral agent. Elevated blood pressure alone, in the absence of manifestations or other evidence of target organ damage, rarely requires emergency therapy.

Acute enalaprilat therapy (e.g., 1.25–5 mg IV, repeated every 6 hours as necessary) is one of several parenteral regimens currently recommended for rapidly reducing blood pressure in patients with hypertensive crises in whom reduction of blood pressure is considered an emergency. However, reduction of blood pressure in a prompt but controlled manner may be more easily achieved with short-acting antihypertensive agents administered by continuous IV infusion (e.g., labetalol, esmolol, fenoldopam, nicardipine, sodium nitroprusside), and some clinicians state that such agents generally are preferred.

The risks of overly aggressive therapy in any hypertensive crisis must always be considered, as excessive falls in blood pressure may precipitate renal, cerebral, or coronary ischemia.

■ **Heart Failure** Enalapril is used in the management of symptomatic heart failure, usually in conjunction with other agents such as cardiac glycosides, diuretics, and β-blockers.

Current guidelines for the management of heart failure in adults generally recommend a combination of drug therapies to reduce morbidity and mortality, including neurohormonal antagonists (e.g., ACE inhibitors, angiotensin II receptor antagonists, angiotensin receptor-neprilysin inhibitors [ARNIs], β-blockers, aldosterone receptor antagonists) that inhibit the detrimental compensatory mechanisms in heart failure. Additional agents (e.g., cardiac glycosides, diuretics, sinoatrial modulators [i.e., ivabradine]) added to a heart failure treatment regimen in selected patients have been associated with symptomatic improvement and/or reduction in heart failure-related hospitalizations. In patients with prior or current symptoms of chronic heart failure with reduced left ventricular ejection fraction (LVEF) (American College of Cardiology Foundation [ACCF]/AHA stage C heart failure), ACCF, AHA, and the Heart Failure Society of America (HFSA) recommend inhibition of the renin-angiotensin-aldosterone (RAA) system with an ACE inhibitor, angiotensin II receptor antagonist, or ARNI (e.g., sacubitril/valsartan) in conjunction with a β-blocker, and an aldosterone antagonist in selected patients, to reduce morbidity and mortality. While ACE inhibitors have been the preferred drugs for inhibition of the RAA system because of their established benefits in patients with heart failure and reduced ejection fraction, some evidence indicates that therapy with an ARNI (sacubitril/valsartan) may be more effective than ACE inhibitor therapy (enalapril) in reducing cardiovascular death and heart failure-related hospitalization in such patients. ACCF, AHA, and HFSA recommend that patients with chronic symptomatic heart failure with reduced LVEF (New York Heart Association [NYHA] class II or III) who are able to tolerate an ACE inhibitor or angiotensin II receptor antagonist be switched to therapy containing an ARNI to further reduce morbidity and mortality. However, in patients in whom an ARNI is not appropriate, continued use of an ACE inhibitor for all classes of heart failure with reduced ejection fraction remains strongly advised. In patients in whom an ARNI or ACE inhibitor is not appropriate, an angiotensin II receptor antagonist may be used. For further information on the use of ARNIs in patients with heart failure, see Uses: Heart Failure, in Sacubitril and Valsartan 24:32.92.

Some clinicians state that ACE inhibitors usually are prescribed in clinical practice at dosages lower than those determined as target dosages in clinical trials, although results of several studies suggest that high dosages are associated with greater hemodynamic, neurohormonal, symptomatic, and prognostic benefits than lower dosages. Results of a large, randomized, double-blind study (Assessment of Treatment with Lisinopril and Survival [ATLAS] study) in patients with heart failure (NYHA class II–IV) indicate that high lisinopril dosages (32.5–35 mg daily) were associated with a 12% lower risk of death or hospitalization for any cause and 24% fewer hospitalizations for heart failure than low dosages (2.5–5 mg) of the drug.

Once ACE inhibitor therapy is initiated for heart failure, it generally is continued indefinitely, if tolerated, since withdrawal of an ACE inhibitor may lead to clinical deterioration. Patients with NYHA class II or III heart failure who are tolerating therapy with an ACE inhibitor may be switched to therapy containing an ARNI to further reduce morbidity and mortality; however, the ARNI should not be administered concomitantly with an ACE inhibitor or within 36 hours of the last dose of an ACE inhibitor.

Current evidence supports the use of ACE inhibitors and β-blocker therapy to prevent development of left ventricular dilatation and dysfunction ("ventricular remodeling") in patients with heart failure. (See Uses: Asymptomatic Left Ventricular Dysfunction.) The addition of other agents such as diuretics, cardiac glycosides, aldosterone antagonists, and/or sinoatrial modulators in the management of heart failure should be individualized. Unless contraindicated, diuretics are recommended in all patients with heart failure and reduced ejection fraction who have evidence of fluid retention to improve symptoms. Digoxin may be beneficial to patients with heart failure with reduced ejection fraction to decrease hospitalization for heart failure, especially in those with persistent symptoms despite treatment with guideline-directed medical therapy. The addition of a sinoatrial modulator (i.e., ivabradine) is recommended in selected patients with chronic heart failure and reduced LVEF who are already receiving guideline-directed medical therapy, to reduce heart failure-related hospitalizations. (See Uses: Heart Failure, in Ivabradine 24:04.92.)

Results of a randomized, multicenter, double-blind, placebo-controlled study (Randomized Aldactone Evaluation Study [RALES]) indicate that addition of low-dosage spironolactone (25–50 mg daily) to standard therapy (e.g., an ACE inhibitor and a loop diuretic with or without a cardiac glycoside) in patients with severe (NYHA class IV within 6 months before enrollment and NYHA class III or IV at the time of enrollment) heart failure and an LVEF of 35% or less, was associated with decreases in overall mortality and hospitalization (for worsening heart failure) rates of approximately 30 and 35%, respectively, compared with standard therapy and placebo. Based on the results of RALES and other studies, ACCF and AHA recommend the addition of an aldosterone antagonist (i.e., spironolactone or eplerenone) in selected patients with heart failure (NYHA class II–IV) and reduced LVEF (35% or less) who are already receiving standard therapy to reduce morbidity and mortality. (See Uses: Heart Failure, in Spironolactone 24:32.20.)

Many patients with heart failure respond to enalapril with improvement in cardiac function indexes, symptomatic (e.g., dyspnea, fatigue) relief, improved functional capacity, and increased exercise tolerance. In some studies, improvement in cardiac function indexes and exercise tolerance were sustained for up to 4 months. In some patients, beneficial effects have been sustained for up to 2–21 months. Enalapril also has been effective in conjunction with cardiac glycosides and diuretics for the management of heart failure resistant to or inadequately controlled by cardiac glycosides, diuretics, and vasodilators. In a multicenter, placebo-controlled study in patients with severe heart failure (NYHA class IV), the addition of enalapril to the therapeutic regimen (which included cardiac glycosides, diuretics, and/or vasodilators) was associated with a 40% reduction in overall mortality at 6 months and a 31% reduction at 12 months compared with patients who did not receive an ACE inhibitor, although the incidence of sudden cardiac death did not differ. In addition, there was a substantial improvement in NYHA functional class for patients receiving enalapril in this study. Follow-up of surviving patients 2 years after completion of the blinded, placebo-controlled phase showed a carry-over effect of enalapril on mortality reduction despite the availability of enalapril therapy for all surviving patients (whether treated initially with the drug or not) and the poorer clinical condition of the initial enalapril-treated group at the outset of follow-up; during follow-up, the carry-over effect on mortality reduction of initial enalapril therapy persisted for 15 months.

In 2 multicenter, controlled studies, enalapril substantially reduced mortality in patients with mild to moderate heart failure (NYHA class I–III) when added to a conventional therapeutic regimen (most commonly cardiac glycosides and diuretics); in these patients, enalapril therapy also may substantially reduce the rate of hospitalization. In one of these studies, the reduction in mortality was substantially greater with enalapril than with combined hydralazine and isosorbide dinitrate, although the latter regimen produced substantially greater improvement in exercise performance and left ventricular function. The beneficial effects of enalapril on reduction in mortality may result from a delay in worsening of heart failure, although other mechanisms (e.g., on causes of sudden death) may be involved. Analysis of the results of these studies according to racial subgroup indicates that white patients had substantially greater reductions in blood pressure and the risk of hospitalization for heart failure than black patients receiving similar dosages of enalapril. (See Race under Hypertension: Other Special Considerations for Antihypertensive Therapy, in Uses.) However, the risk of death in either racial subgroup was not altered by enalapril therapy.

It has not been determined whether addition of a vasodilator (e.g., hydralazine) to an ACE inhibitor is more effective than an ACE inhibitor alone. The efficacy of enalapril appears to be similar to that of captopril. However, because of enalapril's relatively long duration of action compared with captopril, enalapril may produce more prolonged hypotensive effects, particularly at high dosages, which potentially could result in adverse cerebral and renal effects. In addition, because the renin-angiotensin system appears to substantially contribute to preservation of glomerular filtration in patients with heart failure in whom renal perfusion is severely compromised, therapy with an ACE inhibitor in such patients may adversely affect renal function. (See Cautions: Renal Effects.)

ACE inhibitors also are used in patients with ACCF/AHA stage B heart failure (see Uses: Asymptomatic Left Ventricular Dysfunction) to prevent symptomatic heart failure and have been shown to reduce mortality after MI or acute coronary syndrome (ACS). (See Uses: Left Ventricular Dysfunction After Acute Myocardial Infarction.)

■ **Asymptomatic Left Ventricular Dysfunction** Enalapril is used in clinically stable asymptomatic patients with left ventricular dysfunction (manifested as an ejection fraction of 35% or less) in an effort to decrease the rate of development of overt heart failure and subsequent hospitalizations for heart failure in these patients. Experts recommend that all asymptomatic patients with reduced LVEF (ACCF/AHA stage B heart failure) receive therapy with an ACE inhibitor and β-blocker to prevent symptomatic heart failure and to reduce morbidity and mortality. If ACE inhibitors are not tolerated, then an angiotensin II receptor antagonist is recommended as an alternative.

Enalapril's beneficial effect in preventing the development of symptomatic heart failure in patients with asymptomatic left ventricular dysfunction may result either from relieving symptoms that otherwise would have become apparent or from slowing the progression of asymptomatic ventricular dysfunction to overt, symptomatic disease. In a multicenter, placebo-controlled study in patients with left ventricular dysfunction who did not have symptomatic heart failure (NYHA class I and II) and were not being treated for such at initiation of ACE inhibitor therapy, enalapril reduced the incidence of heart failure and rate of related hospitalizations relative to those receiving placebo during an average of 37.4 months of follow-up. Patients with higher ejection fractions and black patients appeared to benefit less from enalapril therapy than those with lower fractions and white patients, respectively. The effect of enalapril in preventing the development of heart failure was evident within 3 months after initiation of the drug and continued to increase for the remaining study period (approximately 3 years). Mortality rates increased substantially in patients who developed overt heart failure, suggesting the possibility of a secondary benefit on prognosis from prevention of symptomatic progression. In a follow-up study, treatment with enalapril for 3–4 years led to a sustained improvement in survival (11–12 years) in patients with reduced LVEF, including those who were asymptomatic at baseline.

■ **Left Ventricular Dysfunction After Acute Myocardial Infarction** ACE inhibitors, including enalapril and enalaprilat, have been used to reduce mortality and prevent the development of left ventricular dilatation and dysfunction following acute MI†. Studies with various ACE inhibitors have shown that these drugs reduce fatal and nonfatal cardiovascular events in patients with recent MI. The magnitude of benefit appears to be greatest in certain high-risk patients (e.g., those with an anterior infarct, ejection fraction of 40% or less, heart failure, prior infarction, or tachycardia). Evidence regarding the efficacy of such therapy has been somewhat conflicting, particularly when parenteral therapy was initiated early (within 24–48 hours) and included patients with no evidence of baseline dysfunction. While the preponderance of evidence (including a large, multinational, multicenter study) has shown a benefit of early oral therapy involving other ACE inhibitors, even in patients with no baseline dysfunction, one large study involving parenteral and oral enalapril found little if any early (within several months) benefit, particularly in terms of survival, from such therapy. In this multicenter, controlled study, IV enalaprilat (followed by oral enalapril) was initiated within 24 hours of the onset of chest pain associated with acute MI and continued for up to approximately 6 months; there was no evidence of improved survival from enalapril therapy during the 6-month period after MI and, in some patients, an actual worsening of heart failure was observed. In addition, enalapril therapy was associated with a substantial risk of hypotensive episodes, and long-term mortality was higher among patients who experienced hypotension with the first dose of enalapril than among other patients receiving the drug or among those who experienced hypotension with placebo. The lack of survival benefit observed in this study applied overall as well as to subgroups of patients (e.g., those with Q-wave infarction, anterior infarction, previous infarction, or current infarction complicated by pulmonary edema or heart failure). The results of this study are in contrast to other studies involving other ACE inhibitors initiated within 24 hours to 4 weeks after acute MI in which a beneficial effect was observed, in terms of effects on left ventricular volume, infarct expansion, and/or survival.

The reason for the differences in potential benefit observed between studies involving enalapril and those involving other ACE inhibitors (e.g., captopril, lisinopril, ramipril) is unclear, but the lack of benefit in the enalapril study may have resulted in part from an early adverse effect of ACE inhibition (e.g., inhibition of angiotensin II-stimulated protein synthesis involved in healing) combined with a rapid decrease in blood pressure associated with the initial administration of enalaprilat and with an inadequate period of follow-up to detect a delayed beneficial effect. Current expert guidelines recommend the use of an oral ACE inhibitor within the first 24 hours of acute MI in patients with an anterior infarction, heart failure, or ejection fraction of 40% or less who do not have any contraindications (e.g., hypotension, shock, renal dysfunction). While early treatment within the first 24 hours of MI has been shown to be beneficial, ACE inhibitors should be used with caution (and with gradual upward titration) during the initial postinfarction period because of the possibility of hypotension or renal dysfunction. ACE inhibitor therapy generally should be continued indefinitely in patients with left ventricular dysfunction or other compelling indications for use (e.g., hypertension, diabetes mellitus, CKD). The benefits of long-term ACE inhibitor therapy are less certain in low-risk patients who have undergone revascularization and are receiving aggressive antilipemic therapy.

■ **Diabetic Nephropathy** Both ACE inhibitors and angiotensin II receptor antagonists have been shown to slow the rate of progression of renal disease in patients with diabetes mellitus and persistent albuminuria†, and use of a drug from either class is recommended in such patients with modestly elevated (30–300 mg/24 hours) or higher (exceeding 300 mg/24 hours) levels of urinary albumin excretion. The usual precautions of ACE inhibitor or angiotensin II receptor antagonist therapy in patients with substantial renal impairment should be observed. For additional information on the use of ACE inhibitors in the treatment of diabetic nephropathy, see Diabetic Nephropathy under Uses: Nephropathy, in Captopril 24:32.04.

Dosage and Administration

■ **Administration** ***Oral Administration*** Enalapril maleate alone or in fixed combination with hydrochlorothiazide is administered orally. For patients unable to swallow tablets, enalapril maleate may be administered orally as an extemporaneously prepared suspension. The drug can be given before, during, or after meals since food does not appear to substantially affect the rate or extent of absorption of enalapril.

An extemporaneous suspension containing enalapril maleate 1 mg/mL can be prepared in the following manner. First, 50 mL of sodium citrate dihydrate (Bicitra®) is added to a polyethylene terephthalate (PET) bottle containing ten 20-mg tablets of enalapril maleate, and the contents are shaken for at least 2 minutes. The concentrated suspension should be allowed to stand for 60 minutes following reconstitution, and then should be shaken for an additional minute. The concentrated suspension of enalapril maleate should be diluted with 150 mL of syrup (Ora-Sweet SF®), and the container then shaken to disperse the ingredients. The suspension should be shaken before dispensing of each dose.

IV Administration Enalaprilat is administered by slow IV infusion over a period of at least 5 minutes. The drug should not be administered by other parenteral routes of administration. Enalaprilat may be administered by slow, direct IV infusion, or the injection can be diluted in up to 50 mL of compatible IV infusion solution for administration. (See Chemistry and Stability: Stability.) Enalaprilat injection and diluted solutions of the drug should be inspected visually for particulate matter and discoloration prior to administration whenever solution and container permit.

■ **Dosage** Dosage of enalapril maleate and enalaprilat must be adjusted according to the patient's tolerance and response. *Since enalapril maleate is a prodrug of enalaprilat and is well absorbed following oral administration, dosage of the two drugs is not identical and clinicians must give careful attention to dosage when converting from oral to IV therapy or vice versa.*

Because of the risk of inducing hypotension, initiation of enalapril maleate or enalaprilat therapy requires consideration of recent antihypertensive therapy, the extent of blood pressure elevation, sodium intake, fluid status, and other clinical circumstances. If therapy is initiated in patients already receiving a diuretic, symptomatic hypotension may occur following the initial dose of the angiotensin-converting enzyme (ACE) inhibitor. The possibility of hypotension may be minimized by discontinuing the diuretic, reducing the diuretic dosage, or cautiously increasing salt intake prior to initiation of oral enalapril maleate or IV enalaprilat therapy. (See Cautions: Cardiovascular Effects.) For information on initiating oral enalapril maleate or IV enalaprilat therapy when diuretic therapy is not being withheld, see the disease-specific dosage sections in Dosage and Administration: Dosage.

Hypertension **Oral Dosage.** The manufacturer states that the usual initial adult dosage of enalapril maleate for the management of hypertension in patients *not* receiving a diuretic is 5 mg once daily. In patients who are receiving a diuretic, it is recommended that diuretic therapy be discontinued, if possible, 2–3 days before initiating therapy. (See Cautions: Precautions and Contraindications.) If blood pressure is not adequately controlled with the ACE inhibitor alone, diuretic therapy may be resumed cautiously. If diuretic therapy cannot be discontinued, an initial enalapril maleate dose of 2.5 mg should be administered under medical supervision for at least 2 hours and until blood pressure has stabilized for at least an additional hour.

The usual initial pediatric (1 month to 16 years of age) dosage of enalapril maleate is 0.08 mg/kg once daily, up to 5 mg. Some experts state that the dose may be administered as a single dose or in 2 divided doses daily. Such experts also state that the dosage may be increased every 2–4 weeks until blood pressure is controlled, the maximum dosage is reached, or adverse effects occur. The manufacturer states that dosages of enalapril maleate exceeding 0.58 mg/kg or in excess of 40 mg daily have not been studied in pediatric patients. (For information on overall principles and expert recommendations for treatment of hypertension in pediatric patients, see Uses: Hypertension in Pediatric Patients, in the Thiazides General Statement 40:28.20.)

Dosage of enalapril maleate should be adjusted according to the patient's blood pressure response. If the blood pressure response diminishes toward the end of the dosing interval during once-daily administration, increasing the dosage or giving the drug in 2 divided doses daily should be considered. Because the reduction in blood pressure may be gradual, some clinicians suggest that enalapril maleate dosage generally be titrated at 2- to 4-week intervals if necessary. The manufacturer states that the usual maintenance dosage of enalapril maleate in adults is 10–40 mg daily, given as a single dose or in 2 divided doses daily, although most patients can be maintained on once-daily dosing. Some experts state that the usual adult dosage is 5–40 mg daily, given as a single dose or in 2 divided doses daily. Optimum blood pressure reduction may require several weeks of therapy in some patients. If blood pressure is not adequately controlled with enalapril alone, a second antihypertensive agent (e.g., a diuretic) may be added.

When oral therapy is initiated following IV enalaprilat therapy in adults *not* receiving a diuretic, the recommended initial dosage of enalapril maleate is 5 mg once daily with subsequent dosage adjustment as necessary. When oral therapy is initiated following IV enalaprilat therapy in adults receiving a diuretic, the recommended initial dosage of enalapril maleate in those who responded to enalaprilat 0.625 mg every 6 hours is 2.5 mg once daily with subsequent dosage adjustment as necessary.

Enalapril/Hydrochlorothiazide Fixed-combination Oral Therapy. To minimize the likelihood of adverse effects, therapy with the commercially available preparations containing enalapril in fixed combination with hydrochlorothiazide should only be initiated in adults after an adequate response is not achieved with enalapril or hydrochlorothiazide monotherapy. Alternatively, the fixed combination containing enalapril with hydrochlorothiazide may be used in adults who had been receiving the drugs separately and in whom dosage of the individual drugs has been adjusted. The recommended initial adult dosage of the commercially available fixed-combination tablets is 5 mg of enalapril maleate and 12.5 mg of hydrochlorothiazide or 10 mg of enalapril maleate and 25 mg of hydrochlorothiazide once daily. Further increases of either or both drugs depend on clinical response; however, generally, dosage of hydrochlorothiazide should not be increased for about 2–3 weeks after initiation of therapy. Because the suggested maximum adult dosage of enalapril maleate and hydrochlorothiazide during combined antihypertensive therapy is 20 or 50 mg daily, respectively, the combined dosage of enalapril maleate and hydrochlorothiazide in the fixed combination should not exceed these respective levels.

Blood Pressure Monitoring and Treatment Goals. Blood pressure should be monitored regularly (i.e., monthly) during therapy and dosage of the antihypertensive drug adjusted until blood pressure is controlled. If an adequate blood pressure response is not achieved with ACE inhibitor monotherapy, the dosage may be increased or another antihypertensive agent with demonstrated benefit and preferably with a complementary mechanism of action (e.g., calcium-channel blocking agent, thiazide diuretic) may be added; if target blood pressure is still not achieved, a third drug may be added. (See Uses: Hypertension.) In patients who develop unacceptable adverse effects with enalapril, the drug should be discontinued and another antihypertensive agent from a different pharmacologic class should be initiated.

The goal of hypertension management and prevention is to achieve and maintain optimal control of blood pressure. However, the optimum blood pressure threshold for initiating antihypertensive drug therapy and specific treatment goals remain controversial. While other hypertension guidelines have based target blood pressure goals on age and comorbidities, the 2017 American College of Cardiology/American Heart Association (ACC/AHA) hypertension guideline incorporates underlying cardiovascular risk into decision making regarding treatment and generally recommends the same target blood pressure (i.e., less than 130/80 mm Hg) in all adults. Many patients will require at least 2 drugs from different pharmacologic classes to achieve this blood pressure goal; the potential benefits of hypertension management and drug cost, adverse effects, and risks associated with the use of multiple antihypertensive drugs also should be considered when deciding a patient's blood pressure treatment goal. (See General Considerations for Initial and Maintenance Antihypertensive Therapy under Uses: Hypertension.)

For additional information on target levels of blood pressure and on monitoring therapy in the management of hypertension, see Blood Pressure Monitoring and Treatment Goals under Dosage: Hypertension, in Dosage and Administration in the Thiazides General Statement 40:28.20.

IV Dosage. When oral therapy is not feasible, the recommended initial IV enalaprilat dosage in adults *not* receiving a diuretic or in those converting from enalapril maleate therapy (without concomitant diuretic therapy) is 1.25 mg every 6 hours. Reduction in blood pressure usually occurs within 15 minutes, but the maximal hypotensive response after the first dose may not occur for up to 4 hours after administration. The maximum effects of the second and subsequent doses may exceed those of the first dose. Although no regimen has been shown to be more effective than 1.25 mg every 6 hours, dosages as high as 5 mg every 6 hours were well tolerated for up to 36 hours in controlled clinical studies. Experience with dosages greater than 20 mg daily is insufficient. In studies of patients with hypertension, enalaprilat was not administered for longer than 48 hours, but in other studies it has been administered for as long as 7 days.

When oral therapy is not feasible in adults receiving a diuretic, the recommended initial IV enalaprilat dose is 0.625 mg. A reduction in blood pressure usually occurs within 15 minutes. Although most of the effect is usually apparent within the first hour, the maximal hypotensive response may not occur for up to 4 hours after the initial dose. If the blood pressure response after 1 hour is inadequate, another dose of 0.625 mg may be given. Additional doses of 1.25 mg may be administered at 6-hour intervals.

To reduce blood pressure rapidly in adults with a hypertensive emergency†, an IV enalaprilat dosage of 1.25–5 mg, repeated every 6 hours as necessary, has been recommended. If IV enalaprilat is used in the management of a hypertensive emergency in adults without a compelling condition, the initial goal of such therapy is to reduce systolic blood pressure by no more than 25% within 1 hour, followed by further reduction *if stable* toward 160/100 to 110 mm Hg within the next 2–6 hours, avoiding excessive declines in pressure that could precipitate renal, cerebral, or coronary ischemia. If this blood pressure is well tolerated and the patient is clinically stable, further gradual reductions toward normal can be implemented in the next 24–48 hours. Enalaprilat is most useful in hypertensive emergencies associated with high plasma renin activity.

For information on converting patients from IV to oral therapy, see Oral Dosage under Dosage: Hypertension, in Dosage and Administration.

Heart Failure Because of the risk of severe hypotension, enalapril maleate therapy for heart failure should be initiated under very close medical supervision (e.g., in a hospital setting) with consideration given to recent diuretic therapy and the possibility of severe sodium and/or fluid depletion. ACE inhibitor therapy should be initiated with caution in patients with very low systemic blood pressure (systolic blood pressure less than 80 mm Hg), markedly increased serum concentrations of creatinine (greater than 3 mg/dL), bilateral renal artery stenosis, or elevated concentrations of serum potassium (greater than 5 mEq/L). Experts recommend that renal function and serum potassium be assessed within 1–2 weeks of initiation of therapy and periodically thereafter in patients receiving an ACE inhibitor, especially in those with preexisting hypotension, hyponatremia, diabetes mellitus, or azotemia, or in those taking potassium supplements. Use of low initial enalapril maleate dosages and reduction of the dosage of concomitantly administered diuretics may decrease the initial risk of hypotension. However, the long-term hemodynamic benefit of low enalapril maleate dosages (e.g., 10–20 mg daily) in this condition has not been established.

It should be recognized that although symptoms of heart failure may improve within 48 hours after initiating ACE inhibitor therapy in some patients, such improvement usually is not evident for several weeks or months after initiating ACE inhibitor therapy. In addition, it should be considered that such therapy may reduce the risk of disease progression even if symptomatic improvement is not evident. Therefore, dosages generally should be titrated to a prespecified target (i.e., at least 20 mg of enalapril daily) or highest tolerated dosage rather than according to response.

For the management of symptomatic heart failure, enalapril maleate often is administered in conjunction with other agents such as a cardiac glycoside, a diuretic, and a β-blocker. Enalapril maleate dosage for heart failure should be initiated at low doses and titrated gradually upward if lower doses have been well tolerated. The usual initial enalapril maleate dosage for the management of heart failure in adults with normal renal function and serum sodium concentration is 2.5 mg twice daily. After the initial dose, the patient should be monitored closely for at least 2 hours and for at least one additional hour after blood pressure has stabilized. Hypotension occurring after the initial dose does not preclude the administration of subsequent doses of the drug, provided due caution is exercised and the hypotension has been managed effectively. To minimize the likelihood of hypotension, the dosage of any diuretic given concomitantly with enalapril should be reduced, if possible. The usual maintenance dosage of enalapril maleate for heart failure is 2.5–20 mg twice daily. The maximum recommended daily dosage of the drug is 40 mg, given in 2 divided doses.

Asymptomatic Left Ventricular Dysfunction When used in adults with asymptomatic left ventricular dysfunction, enalapril maleate therapy has been initiated using a dosage of 2.5 mg twice daily. Therapy is then titrated as tolerated to a target daily dosage of 20 mg given in divided doses. After the initial dose of enalapril, the patient should be closely observed for at least 2 hours and for at least one additional hour after blood pressure has stabilized. To minimize the likelihood of hypotension, the dosage of any concomitant diuretic should be reduced, if possible. The appearance of hypotension after the initial dose of enalapril does not preclude subsequent carefully titrated doses of the drug after the hypotension has been effectively managed.

■ **Dosage in Renal or Hepatic Impairment, Hyponatremia, Pediatric Patients, and Geriatric Patients** If enalapril maleate or enalaprilat is used in patients with impaired renal function, dosage must be modified in response to the degree of renal impairment, and the theoretical risk of neutropenia must be considered. (See Cautions: Hematologic Effects.)

The manufacturer states that hypertensive adults with moderate renal impairment (i.e., creatinine clearances greater than 30 mL/minute) may receive the usual dosage of enalapril maleate. In adults with severe renal impairment (i.e., creatinine clearances of 30 mL/minute or less), dosage of enalapril maleate should be initiated at 2.5 mg daily. If an adequate response is not achieved, dosage may then be gradually increased until blood pressure is controlled or a maximum dosage of 40 mg daily is reached. Alternatively, some clinicians suggest that patients with creatinine clearances of 10–50 mL/minute can receive 75–100% of the usual dosage and those with creatinine clearances less than 10 mL/minute can receive 50% of the usual dosage. Patients undergoing hemodialysis should receive a supplemental dose of the drug after dialysis. The manufacturer recommends that hemodialysis patients be given a dose of 2.5 mg on dialysis days; on days between dialysis periods, enalapril maleate dosage should be adjusted according to the patient's blood pressure response.

For hypertensive adults with moderate renal impairment (i.e., creatinine clearances greater than 30 mL/minute) in whom oral therapy is not feasible, the recommended dosage of IV enalaprilat is 1.25 mg every 6 hours. In adults with severe renal impairment (i.e., creatinine clearances of 30 mL/minute or less), the initial dose of IV enalaprilat should be 0.625 mg; if the blood pressure response is inadequate after 1 hour, another dose of 0.625 mg may be given. Additional doses of 1.25 mg may be administered at 6-hour intervals. For patients undergoing dialysis, the initial dosage of IV enalaprilat should be 0.625 mg every 6 hours. When oral therapy is initiated following IV enalaprilat therapy, the recommended initial dosage of enalapril maleate is 5 mg once daily in patients with creatinine clearances greater than 30 mL/minute and 2.5 mg once daily in patients with creatinine clearances of 30 mL/minute or less. Dosage is subsequently adjusted according to the patient's blood pressure response.

The manufacturer states that adults with heart failure and hyponatremia (serum sodium concentration less than 130 mEq/L) or serum creatinine concentration greater than 1.6 mg/dL should receive an initial enalapril maleate dosage of 2.5 mg daily under close monitoring (see Heart Failure under Dosage and Administration: Dosage). Subsequent dosage may be increased gradually as necessary, usually at intervals of 4 or more days, to 2.5 mg twice daily, then 5 mg twice daily, and then higher, provided excessive hypotension or deterioration of renal function is not present at the time of intended dosage adjustment; dosage should not exceed 40 mg daily.

If concomitant diuretic therapy is required in patients with severe renal impairment, a loop diuretic is preferred to a thiazide diuretic. Therefore, use of commercially available preparations containing enalapril maleate in fixed combination with hydrochlorothiazide is not recommended for patients with severe renal impairment. The manufacturers state that dosage adjustment of commercially available preparations containing enalapril maleate in fixed combination with hydrochlorothiazide is not needed in patients with renal impairment whose creatinine clearance exceeds 30 mL/minute per 1.73 m^2. (For information on dosage of hydrochlorothiazide in other special populations, see Dosage and Administration, in Hydrochlorothiazide 40:28.20.)

Enalapril maleate is *not* recommended for neonates or for pediatric patients who have a glomerular filtration rate of less than 30 mL/minute per 1.73 m^2, since no data are available in such patients.

Since it is not known whether geriatric patients 65 years of age or older respond the same to enalapril in fixed combination with hydrochlorothiazide as younger adults, the manufacturer suggests that patients in this age group receive initial dosages of the fixed combination in the lower end of the usual range.

Cautions

Adverse reactions to enalapril usually are mild and transient but have required discontinuance of therapy in about 3 or 6% of patients receiving the drug for the management of hypertension or heart failure, respectively. Enalaprilat usually is well tolerated. Since enalapril is metabolized to enalaprilat, administration of enalaprilat can be expected to produce adverse effects associated with enalapril therapy. Overall, the frequency of many adverse effects produced by enalapril appears to be similar to or less than that produced by captopril. However, unlike captopril, enalapril lacks the sulfhydryl group which has been associated with certain captopril-induced adverse effects (e.g., cutaneous reactions, taste disturbances, proteinuria), and the risk of these effects may be decreased during enalapril therapy. Additional experience to determine the relative safety of enalapril is necessary, and the possibility that the risk may be similar should be considered. Because of enalapril's long duration of action, the risk of some adverse effects (e.g., hypotension, deterioration in renal function) may be increased compared with short-acting ACE inhibitors, particularly in patients whose cardiovascular and renal systems have increased dependency on the renin-angiotensin system (e.g., those with severe heart failure).

Adverse nervous system effects (e.g., headache, dizziness, fatigue) occur most frequently during enalapril therapy for hypertension. Although adverse effects of enalapril generally are mild, discontinuance of the drug has been necessary in about 6% of patients, principally because of dizziness, headache, hypotension, or rash. The manufacturer states that the incidence of the most frequently reported adverse effects was similar in patients receiving enalapril or placebo in clinical trials. In patients with heart failure, symptomatic hypotension, deterioration in renal function, and increased serum potassium concentration appear to occur most frequently, particularly during initiation of enalapril therapy in volume- and/or sodium-depleted patients (e.g., those receiving concomitant diuretic therapy).

The frequency of some adverse reactions may be increased during therapy with enalapril in fixed combination with hydrochlorothiazide compared with either drug alone, but the manufacturer states that adverse reactions reported to date with the combination have been reported previously with the individual drugs. No reactions peculiar to the combination have been reported.

■ **Nervous System Effects** Headache and dizziness occur in about 5% of patients receiving enalapril alone for hypertension, requiring discontinuance in 0.4 and 0.3% of patients, respectively, and occur in about 6 and 9%, respectively, of hypertensive patients receiving the drug in fixed combination with hydrochlorothiazide. In patients receiving enalapril for heart failure, dizziness and headache occurred in approximately 8 and 2% of patients, respectively, and required discontinuance of the drug in 0.6 and 0.1%, respectively. Headache has been reported in about 3% of patients receiving enalaprilat. Fatigue has occurred in about 3% of patients receiving the drug alone for hypertension, requiring discontinuance in less than 0.1%, and has occurred in about 4% of hypertensive patients receiving the drug in fixed combination with hydrochlorothiazide. Fatigue, fever, and dizziness have been reported in 0.5–1% of patients receiving enalaprilat. Vertigo has occurred in about 2% of patients receiving enalapril for heart failure and required discontinuance in about 0.1% of patients. Insomnia, nervousness, peripheral neuropathy (e.g., paresthesia, dysesthesia, asthenia, and somnolence occur in about 0.5–2% of patients receiving enalapril alone or in fixed combination with hydrochlorothiazide. Hyperesthesia of the oral mucosa, CNS depression, malaise, nightmares, confusion, ataxia, and coldness of the extremities have been reported rarely.

■ **GI Effects** Diarrhea and nausea occur in about 1–2% of patients with hypertension receiving enalapril alone or in fixed combination with hydrochlorothiazide and in patients with heart failure receiving the drug, and have required discontinuance of the drug in 0.2% or less of patients. Nausea has been reported in about 1% of patients receiving enalaprilat. Abdominal pain, vomiting, stomatitis, and dyspepsia occur in 0.5–2% of patients receiving enalapril, and ulceration of the oral mucosa, ileus, melena, anorexia, glossitis, dry mouth, and flatulence have been reported rarely. Constipation has been reported in 0.5–1% of patients receiving enalaprilat.

■ **Hepatic Effects** A clinical syndrome that usually is manifested initially by cholestatic jaundice and may progress to fulminant hepatic necrosis (which occasionally may be fatal), has been reported rarely in patients receiving ACE inhibitors. The mechanism of this reaction is not known.

■ **Cardiovascular Effects** The most frequent adverse cardiovascular effect of enalapril or enalaprilat is hypotension (including postural hypotension and other orthostatic effects), which occurs in about 1–2% of patients with hypertension and in about 5–7% of those with heart failure, following an initial dose or during extended therapy. Syncope occurred in approximately 0.5 or 2% of patients with hypertension or heart failure, respectively. Hypotension or syncope has required discontinuance of therapy in about 0.1 or 2% of patients with hypertension or heart failure, respectively, receiving enalapril.

Hypotensive effects, including excessive and/or symptomatic hypotension, appear to occur more frequently in patients receiving enalapril for heart failure rather than for uncomplicated hypertension. Some reduction in blood pressure occurs in most patients receiving the drug for heart failure and generally is beneficial when secondary to afterload reduction; however, pronounced hypotension can occur and may adversely affect renal and myocardial perfusion (see later discussion in this section). Enalapril-induced hypotension may occasionally be alleviated by dosage reduction, but severe hypotension has also occurred after low doses (i.e., a single 2.5- or 5-mg dose) of the drug.

The value of initiating enalapril therapy at low doses to decrease the risk of hypotension has not been fully elucidated, but such dosing has been suggested, particularly for patients at risk (e.g., those with heart failure). Orthostatic hypotension appears to occur more frequently during initiation of therapy and in patients with sodium depletion or hypovolemia. Transient hypotension in patients with heart failure or with hypertension may occur after any of the first several doses (i.e., with the first 24–48 hours), and sometimes is associated with dizziness, blurred vision, nausea, syncope, and, rarely, bradycardia. Patients who are volume and/or sodium depleted such as those receiving diuretics, especially those in whom diuretic therapy was recently initiated (e.g., patients with severe congestive heart failure), those whose sodium intake is severely restricted, and those who are undergoing dialysis, may occasionally experience a precipitous reduction in blood pressure within the first 3–4 hours after a dose of enalapril. The risk of orthostatic hypotension associated with concomitant use of enalapril and a diuretic may be affected by the sequence of initiation of therapy with each drug; the risk may be higher when enalapril is added to diuretic therapy than when a diuretic is added to enalapril therapy. Symptomatic hypotension that occurs later in a course of enalapril therapy (e.g., after the first 48 hours) may indicate the presence of sodium depletion (e.g., secondary to restriction of sodium intake or increased diuretic dosage).

When enalapril was used in fixed combination with hydrochlorothiazide in clinical trials in hypertensive patients, hypotension, orthostatic hypotension, and other orthostatic effects occurred in 0.9, 1.5, and 2.3% of patients, respectively. Syncope occurred in 1.3% of patients receiving the fixed combination, but the frequency of this effect can be minimized by proper titration of each drug separately and substitution with the combination preparation only when the optimum dosages correspond to the fixed ratio in the preparation.

Severe enalapril-induced hypotension may be associated with oliguria and/or progressive azotemia and, rarely, with acute renal failure, myocardial ischemia, and/or death in patients with heart failure, hyponatremia, or severe sodium or volume depletion of any etiology; patients undergoing dialysis; and those receiving high-dose or recent intensive diuretic therapy or in whom the diuretic dosage was recently increased. In such patients, it may be advisable to discontinue diuretic therapy (except in patients with heart failure), reduce the diuretic dosage, or cautiously increase salt intake, if possible, prior to initiating therapy with enalapril. Patients at risk for excessive hypotension should be closely monitored after an initial dose of the drug, and should be followed closely for 2 weeks after initiation of enalapril therapy and whenever dosage of enalapril and/or a concomitantly administered diuretic is increased. Some experts state that patients with heart failure should be under very close medical supervision (e.g., in a hospital setting) when enalapril therapy is initiated, since severe hypotension could potentially compromise the patient's hemodynamic status. The risk of hypotension and potential detrimental hemodynamic and clinical effects in patients with severe heart failure appears to be higher during therapy with a long-acting ACE inhibitor such as enalapril than with a short-acting inhibitor.

If hypotension occurs in patients receiving enalapril, the patient should be placed in the supine or Trendelenburg's position; if hypotension is severe or prolonged, IV infusion of 0.9% sodium chloride injection to expand fluid volume should be considered. Transient hypotension is not a contraindication to additional doses of enalapril, and therapy with the drug can usually be cautiously reinitiated after blood pressure has been stabilized (e.g., with volume expansion); enalapril dosage reduction and/or dosage reduction or discontinuance of concomitantly administered diuretics may be necessary. Some clinicians state that asymptomatic hypotension often does not require specific therapy and may be well tolerated with continued enalapril therapy. However, severe hypotension occasionally may require discontinuance of enalapril therapy, and the possibility should be considered that hypotension may persist for prolonged periods (e.g., for a week or longer) after discontinuance because of the drug's long duration of action. Patients with heart failure or those undergoing dialysis may be at particular risk of prolonged hypotension. The possibility of severe hypotension may be minimized by withholding diuretic therapy and/or increasing sodium intake for 2–3 days prior to initiating enalapril therapy.

Hypotension also may occur in enalapril-treated patients during major surgery or during anesthesia with agents that produce hypotension. This hypotensive effect results from inhibition by enalapril of the angiotensin II formation that occurs subsequent to compensatory renin release, and, if it is thought to be caused by enalapril, can generally be corrected with fluid volume expansion.

Palpitation and chest pain occur in about 0.5–2% of patients with hypertension receiving enalapril alone or in fixed combination with hydrochlorothiazide. Tachycardia, bradycardia, and development or worsening of Raynaud's phenomenon have been reported rarely in patients receiving the drug. Cardiac arrest or cerebrovascular accident, possibly secondary to excessive hypotension in high-risk patients, pulmonary embolism and infarction, pulmonary edema, rhythm disturbances (including atrial tachycardia and bradycardia), flushing, and atrial fibrillation have been reported in about 0.5–1% of patients with hypertension or heart failure. Angina or myocardial infarction (MI) was reported in about 1–1.5% of patients receiving enalapril for heart failure in controlled and uncontrolled studies, and required discontinuance in about 0.1–0.3% of patients, but a similar incidence for these effects was reported in patients receiving placebo in controlled studies. MI was reported in 0.5–1% of patients receiving enalaprilat.

■ **Renal Effects** Deterioration in renal function, manifested as transient increases in BUN and serum creatinine concentrations, has occurred in about 20% of patients with renovascular hypertension, especially those with bilateral renal-artery stenosis or those with renal-artery stenosis in a solitary kidney. This effect was usually reversible following discontinuance of enalapril and/or diuretic therapy. Renal function should be monitored closely during the first few weeks of therapy in these patients. (See Cautions: Precautions and Contraindications.) Transient increases in BUN and serum creatinine concentrations have also occurred in about 0.2% of patients with hypertension, but without preexisting renal vascular disease, who were receiving enalapril alone. These effects occur more frequently in patients receiving concomitant diuretic therapy, in patients with heart failure, and in patients with some degree of preexisting renal dysfunction. Dosage reduction of enalapril and/or dosage reduction or discontinuance of diuretic therapy may be necessary. The rapidity of onset and magnitude of enalapril-induced renal insufficiency in patients with heart failure may depend in part on the degree of sodium depletion. About 5–15 or 15–30% of patients with mild to moderate or severe heart failure, respectively, treated with an ACE inhibitor develop substantial elevations of serum creatinine concentrations (e.g., greater than 5 mg/dL). Acute reversible renal failure, flank pain, oliguria, uremia, glycosuria, and proteinuria have been reported rarely in patients receiving enalapril. Urinary tract infection has been reported in about 1% of patients receiving enalapril for heart failure in controlled and uncontrolled studies, but this effect occurred in about 2% of patients receiving placebo in controlled studies.

Because the renin-angiotensin system appears to contribute substantially to maintenance of glomerular filtration in patients with heart failure in whom renal perfusion is severely compromised, renal function may deteriorate markedly during therapy with an ACE inhibitor in these patients. Such drug-induced deterioration is generally well tolerated, and does not usually necessitate discontinuance of effective therapy with the drug when symptomatic improvement of the heart failure occurs. In addition, the magnitude of deterioration in renal function can usually be ameliorated by reducing the dosage of concomitantly administered diuretics and/or by liberalizing dietary sodium intake, since concomitant diuretic therapy and/or sodium restriction potentially increase the role of angiotensin II in maintaining glomerular filtration in these patients. In patients in whom renal perfusion pressure is very low and is further reduced by ACE-inhibitor therapy, however, deterioration in renal function may be clinically important. Patients with concomitant underlying diabetes mellitus may be at particular risk for developing renal insufficiency during ACE-inhibitor therapy. In some patients with severe heart failure, with or without associated renal insufficiency, treatment with an ACE inhibitor, including enalapril, may be associated with oliguria and/or progressive azotemia, and rarely with acute renal failure and/or death. The risk of developing functional renal insufficiency appears to be higher during therapy with a long-acting ACE inhibitor such as enalapril than with a short-acting inhibitor.

■ **Dermatologic and Sensitivity Reactions** The most frequent adverse dermatologic effect of enalapril is rash, which occurs in about 1.5% of patients and is usually maculopapular and rarely urticarial. Rash may sometimes be accompanied by pruritus, erythema, or eosinophilia, and has required discontinuance of the drug in approximately 0.3% of patients. A patient who developed enalapril-induced rash was subsequently treated with captopril without recurrence. However, the frequency of enalapril-induced rash appears to be less than that of captopril, possibly because enalapril lacks the sulfhydryl group, and several patients who developed captopril-induced rash have subsequently been treated with enalapril without recurrence of rash. Rash has been reported in 0.5–1% of patients receiving enalaprilat.

Pruritus, without rash, and excessive sweating have been reported in 0.5–2% of patients receiving enalapril alone or in fixed combination with hydrochlorothiazide. Alopecia has been reported in 0.5–1% of patients receiving enalapril. A symptom complex, consisting of positive ANA titer, increased erythrocyte sedimentation rate (ESR), arthralgias and/or arthritis, myalgias, fever, serositis, vasculitis, leukocytosis, eosinophilia, photosensitivity, rash, and other dermatologic reactions has been reported in 0.5–1% of patients receiving enalapril therapy. Exfoliative dermatitis, toxic epidermal necrolysis, Stevens-Johnson syndrome, pemphigus, herpes zoster, and erythema multiforme have been reported rarely in patients receiving enalapril therapy.

Severe, sudden anaphylactoid reactions, which can be fatal, have been reported following initiation of hemodialysis that utilized a high-flux polyacrylonitrile [PAN] membrane (e.g., AN 69®) in patients receiving an ACE inhibitor. Manifestations of these reactions included nausea, abdominal cramps, burning, angioedema, and shortness of breath; progression to severe hypotension can develop rapidly. Dialysis should be stopped immediately and aggressive supportive and symptomatic therapy should be initiated as indicated. Antihistamines do *not* appear to be effective in providing symptomatic relief. While it currently does not seem to be necessary to exclude the use of ACE inhibitors in patients undergoing hemodialysis that involves PAN membranes, caution should be exercised during concomitant use. The mechanism of this interaction has not been established, and the incidence and risk of its occurrence remain to be elucidated. The possibility that ACE inhibitors may precipitate similar reactions in patients undergoing hemodialysis involving other membrane types (new or reprocessed) should be considered. In addition, anaphylactoid reactions also have been reported in patients undergoing low-density lipoprotein (LDL) apheresis with dextran sulfate absorption. Manifestations of these reactions included flushing, dyspnea, bradycardia, and hypotension. It has been postulated that these reactions may be associated with accumulation of polypeptides (e.g., bradykinin) since endogenous concentration of such polypeptides may be increased by LDL-apheresis with dextran sulfate and their metabolism may be decreased by ACE inhibitors. To avoid these anaphylactoid reactions, some clinicians recommend withdrawal of ACE inhibitors 12–30 hours before apheresis, while others state that ACE inhibitors should not be used in patients treated with LDL apheresis.

Life-threatening anaphylactoid reactions have been reported in at least 2 patients receiving ACE inhibitors while undergoing desensitization treatment with hymenoptera venom. When ACE inhibitors were temporarily discontinued 24 hours before desensitization with the venom, anaphylactoid reactions did not recur; however, such reactions recurred after inadvertent rechallenge.

Angioedema of the face, lips, tongue, larynx, glottis, or extremities has occurred in patients receiving ACE inhibitor therapy, including enalapril. (See Cautions: Precautions and Contraindications.) In addition, intestinal angioedema (occasionally without a prior history of facial angioedema or elevated serum levels of complement 1 [C1] esterase inhibitor) has been reported in patients receiving ACE inhibitors. Intestinal angioedema, which frequently presents as abdominal pain (with or without nausea or vomiting), usually is diagnosed by abdominal CT scan, ultrasound, or surgery; manifestations usually have resolved after discontinuance of the ACE inhibitor. Intestinal angioedema should be considered in the differential diagnosis of patients who develop abdominal pain during therapy with an ACE inhibitor.

■ **Hematologic Effects** Decreases in hemoglobin and hematocrit averaging approximately 0.3 g/dL and 1%, respectively, occur frequently in hypertensive patients receiving enalapril alone or in fixed combination with hydrochlorothiazide, but rarely are clinically important unless another cause of anemia also exists. Enalapril-induced anemia has required discontinuance of therapy in less than 0.1% of patients. Hemolytic anemia, including cases of hemolysis in a few patients with glucose-6-phosphate-dehydrogenase (G-6-PD) deficiency, has been reported in patients receiving enalapril maleate therapy; a causal relationship has not been established.

Neutropenia (less than 1000 neutrophils/mm^3) and agranulocytosis, both associated with myeloid hypoplasia, have occurred rarely in patients receiving captopril. (See Cautions: Hematologic Effects, in Captopril 24:32.04.) Several cases of neutropenia, agranulocytosis, or thrombocytopenia have been reported, and a causal relationship to enalapril cannot be excluded. Because of pharmacologic and structural similarities between captopril and enalapril and the current lack of sufficient data to establish the relative risk of these adverse hematologic effects in patients receiving enalapril, the possibility that bone marrow depression, neutropenia, and agranulocytosis could occur in patients receiving enalapril should be considered. Experience with captopril indicates that patients with renal impairment, especially those with collagen vascular disease, appear to be at increased risk of these adverse hematologic effects, and complete and differential leukocyte counts should be performed periodically during enalapril therapy in these patients. Enalapril lacks a sulfhydryl group, the structural feature suggested as being associated with this toxicity in patients receiving captopril; however, this structural relationship has not been established and the lack of this group in enalapril may not exclude the possibility of these effects in patients receiving the drug.

■ Effects on Taste Loss of taste perception and decrease in taste acuity have been reported infrequently during enalapril therapy. Hyperesthesia of the oral mucosa has occurred in at least one patient receiving enalapril but was reversible following discontinuance of the drug. Patients with intolerable captopril-induced taste disturbances may tolerate enalapril better.

■ Effects on Potassium Although small increases (i.e., by an average of 0.2 mEq/L) in serum potassium concentrations frequently occur in patients receiving enalapril without a thiazide diuretic, hyperkalemia (i.e., increases to greater than 5.7 mEq/L) occurs in approximately 1 or 4% of patients with hypertension or heart failure, respectively, receiving the drug. In most cases, these were isolated increases that resolved despite continued therapy with the drug; however, hyperkalemia required discontinuance of enalapril therapy in about 0.3% of patients receiving the drug for hypertension. Hyperkalemia is less frequent in patients receiving enalapril and hydrochlorothiazide concomitantly, occurring in about 0.1% of patients. Patients with diabetes mellitus, impaired renal function, or heart failure and patients concomitantly receiving drugs that can increase serum potassium concentration (e.g., potassium-sparing diuretics, potassium supplements, potassium-containing salt substitutes) may be at increased risk of developing hyperkalemia during enalapril therapy; serum potassium concentration should be monitored frequently in these patients, and potassium intake should be controlled and therapy with drugs that can increase serum potassium modified or discontinued as necessary. The manufacturer recommends that potassium-sparing diuretics generally *not* be used in patients receiving enalapril for heart failure.

■ Respiratory Effects Cough has been reported in 1.3 or 3.5% of patients receiving enalapril alone or in fixed combination with hydrochlorothiazide for hypertension, respectively, and in about 2% of those receiving the drug for heart failure; discontinuance of the drug was required in less than 0.5% of patients. Nonproductive cough, particularly at night, may occur more frequently, especially in patients with chronic obstructive pulmonary disease. Some clinicians state that cough often is overlooked as a potential adverse effect of ACE inhibitors and may occur more frequently (in about 5–15% of patients). The cough generally is persistent and nonproductive, is not associated with other respiratory symptoms, and is reversible following discontinuance of the drug. Nasal congestion also has been reported. It has been suggested that accumulation of kinins in the respiratory tract secondary to ACE inhibition may in part be responsible for cough and nasal congestion. Concomitant therapy with a nonsteroidal anti-inflammatory agent (i.e., sulindac) appeared to minimize cough in a few patients, but additional study of the safety (e.g., effects on renal function) of such combined therapy is necessary. If cough develops in a patient receiving enalapril, ACE inhibitor-induced cough should be considered as part of the differential diagnosis.

Dyspnea and wheezing, which may persist if therapy with the drug is continued, have been reported in about 1% or less of patients receiving enalapril. Pneumonia or bronchitis has been reported in about 1% of patients receiving enalapril for heart failure. Asthma, upper respiratory infection, bronchospasm, pulmonary infiltrates, eosinophilic pneumonitis, and rhinorrhea also have been reported in patients receiving enalapril maleate therapy. Angioedema has occurred in 0.2 or 0.6% of patients receiving enalapril alone or in fixed combination with hydrochlorothiazide, respectively, and, if associated with laryngeal edema, may be fatal. ACE inhibitors appear to produce a higher incidence of angioedema in black patients than in other races studied. (See Cautions: Precautions and Contraindications.)

■ Other Adverse Effects Muscle cramps, and impotence have been reported in 0.5–1% of patients receiving enalapril alone, and decreased libido has been reported rarely. These effects have occurred more frequently when the drug was administered in fixed combination with hydrochlorothiazide. Hearing loss, which was reversible following discontinuance of the drug, has been reported rarely; however, the mechanism of this adverse effect is not known. Pancreatitis, hepatitis or cholestatic jaundice, hepatic failure, sore throat, hoarseness, anosmia, conjunctivitis, dry eyes, tearing eyes, gynecomastia, and myalgia have been reported in patients receiving enalapril. Vulvovaginal pruritus, burning urination, and dysuria were reported in at least one patient receiving enalapril.

Although a definite causal relationship to enalapril has not been established, elevations of serum hepatic enzymes and/or bilirubin concentrations have been reported rarely when enalapril was administered alone or in fixed combination with hydrochlorothiazide.

■ Precautions and Contraindications Since enalapril is metabolized to enalaprilat, both drugs share the same cautions, precautions, and contraindications. Because captopril, another ACE inhibitor, can cause serious adverse effects (e.g., neutropenia, agranulocytosis), particularly in patients with renal impairment (especially those with collagen vascular disease), the possibility that similar adverse effects may occur with enalapril should be considered. Periodic monitoring of leukocyte counts should be considered in these patients. (See Cautions: Hematologic Effects.) Patients should be instructed to notify their clinician if any sign or symptom of infection such as fever or sore throat occurs. When enalapril is used in fixed combination with hydrochlorothiazide, the cautions, precautions, and contraindications associated with thiazide diuretics must be considered in addition to those associated with enalapril. To minimize dose-independent adverse effects, it is recommended that therapy with enalapril in fixed combination with hydrochlorothiazide only be initiated in patients in whom an adequate response is not achieved with enalapril or hydrochlorothiazide monotherapy.

Renal function should be evaluated prior to initiation of enalapril therapy, and the drug should be used with caution in patients with renal impairment, particularly those with known or suspected renovascular disease. Reduction of enalapril dosage, reduction in dosage or discontinuance of diuretic therapy, and/or adequate sodium repletion may be necessary in some patients who develop impaired renal function during enalapril therapy. Because of an increased risk of reducing renal perfusion to a critically low level, enalapril should be used with caution and renal function monitored closely for the first few weeks of therapy in patients with bilateral renal-artery stenosis and those with renal-artery stenosis in a solitary kidney. Serum creatinine and electrolyte concentrations should be evaluated prior to and 1 week following initiation of therapy with ACE inhibitors in patients with heart failure. In patients with heart failure who have some degree of renal impairment (baseline serum creatinine concentrations less than 2 mg/dL) or more severe renal impairment (baseline serum creatinine concentrations exceeding 2 mg/dL), an increase in serum creatinine concentration exceeding 0.5 or 1 mg/dL, respectively, should prompt consideration of discontinuing ACE inhibitor therapy while additional renal evaluation and corrective action is undertaken. The possibility that ACE inhibitors might precipitate severe, sudden, potentially life-threatening anaphylactoid reactions in patients undergoing hemodialysis involving a high-flux membrane should be considered. (See Cautions: Dermatologic and Sensitivity Reactions.)

Enalapril should be used with caution in patients with sodium depletion or hypovolemia, those receiving diuretics, and those undergoing dialysis since severe hypotension may occur. The drug should also be used with caution in patients in whom excessive hypotension may have serious consequences (e.g., patients with coronary or cerebrovascular insufficiency). Because of the potential decrease in blood pressure in patients with heart failure, enalapril therapy should be initiated under very close medical supervision in these patients. (See Cautions: Cardiovascular Effects.) Like all vasodilators, enalapril should be administered with caution in patients with obstruction in the outflow tract of the left ventricle (e.g., aortic stenosis, hypertrophic cardiomyopathy). Patients at risk for excessive hypotension should be monitored closely for the first 2 weeks of therapy and whenever the dosage of enalapril and/or a concomitantly administered diuretic is increased. Patients receiving enalapril therapy should be informed that vomiting, diarrhea, excessive perspiration, and dehydration may lead to an exaggerated decrease in blood pressure because of fluid volume reduction; patients should notify their clinician if any of these conditions occurs. Patients should also be warned to report light headedness, especially during the first few days of therapy; if actual syncope occurs, they should discontinue enalapril therapy and contact their clinician. Since therapy with ACE inhibitors has been associated with development of a rare syndrome that usually is manifested initially by cholestatic jaundice, which may progress to fulminant hepatic necrosis and occasionally may be fatal, patients receiving an ACE inhibitor, including enalapril, who develop jaundice or marked elevations of hepatic enzymes should discontinue the drug and receive appropriate medical follow-up. (See Cautions: Hepatic Effects.)

Angioedema may occur, especially following the first dose of enalapril, and, if associated with laryngeal edema, may be fatal. If laryngeal stridor or angioedema of the face, extremities, lips, tongue, or glottis occurs, enalapril should be discontinued and the patient carefully observed until swelling disappears. If swelling is confined to the face and lips, the condition generally responds without treatment; however, antihistamines may provide symptomatic relief. Swelling of the tongue, glottis, or larynx may cause airway obstruction, and appropriate therapy (e.g., epinephrine, maintenance of patent airway) should be initiated immediately. Patients should be informed that swelling of the face, eyes, lips, or tongue or difficulty in breathing may be signs and symptoms of angioedema, and that they should discontinue enalapril and notify their clinician immediately if any of these conditions occurs. The possibility that patients with a history of angioedema unrelated to ACE inhibitors may be at increased risk of developing angioedema while receiving the drugs should be considered. Enalapril is contraindicated in patients with a history of angioedema related to ACE inhibitor therapy and those with hereditary or idiopathic angioedema. Enalapril also is contraindicated in patients with known hypersensitivity to the drug or any ingredient in the formulation.

■ **Pediatric Precautions** Antihypertensive effects of enalapril maleate have been established in hypertensive pediatric patients 1 month to 16 years of age. Enalapril maleate is not recommended for neonates or for pediatric patients with a glomerular filtration rate of less than 30 mL/minute per 1.73 m^2, since no data are available. The adverse effect profile of enalapril maleate in pediatric patients is similar to that in adults. Safety and efficacy of enalaprilat injection or of enalapril in fixed combination with hydrochlorothiazide in children have not been established. For information on overall principles and expert recommendations for treatment of hypertension in pediatric patients, see Uses: Hypertension in Pediatric Patients, in the Thiazides General Statement 40:28.20.

■ **Geriatric Precautions** Clinical studies of enalapril in fixed combination with hydrochlorothiazide did not include sufficient numbers of patients 65 years of age and older to determine whether geriatric patients respond differently than younger patients. While other clinical experience has not revealed age-related differences in response, drug dosage generally should be titrated carefully in geriatric patients, usually initiating therapy at the low end of the dosage range. The greater frequency of decreased hepatic, renal, and/or cardiac function and of concomitant disease and drug therapy observed in the elderly also should be considered. Enalapril is substantially eliminated by the kidneys; because geriatric patients may have decreased renal function and because patients with renal impairment may be at increased risk of toxicity, renal function should be monitored and dosage should be selected carefully.

■ **Mutagenicity and Carcinogenicity** No evidence of enalapril- or enalaprilat-induced mutagenicity or of mutagenicity induced by concomitant testing of enalapril and hydrochlorothiazide was seen with an in vitro microbial test system (Ames test) with or without metabolic activation. Enalapril alone or combined with hydrochlorothiazide also was not mutagenic in several other in vitro test systems, including mammalian systems, and in in vivo cytogenetic tests using mouse bone marrow.

No evidence of carcinogenesis was seen in rats or in male and female mice receiving enalapril maleate dosages up to 90 or 90 and 180 mg/kg daily, respectively (about 26 or 13 times the maximum daily human dosage on a mg/m^2 basis, respectively), for 106 or 94 weeks, respectively. Carcinogenicity studies have not been performed with enalaprilat.

While an excess rate of GI cancer relative to placebo has been observed in several large trials in patients receiving prolonged ACE-inhibitor therapy, a causal relationship to the drugs has not been established. Some evidence suggests that such a relationship is unlikely since the observed risk did not increase with increasing exposure to the drugs and because of the heterogeneity of the reported cancers (involving the rectum, cecum, colon, esophagus, stomach, gallbladder, pancreas, or liver). However, the possibility of a causal relationship cannot be excluded, and additional study to further elucidate any possible relationship between use of ACE inhibitors and these cancers is necessary.

■ **Pregnancy, Fertility, and Lactation** ***Pregnancy*** Fetal and neonatal morbidity and mortality have been reported in at least 50 pregnant women who were receiving ACE inhibitors during pregnancy. Very limited epidemiologic data indicate that the rate of fetal and neonatal morbidity resulting from exposure to ACE inhibitors during the second and third trimesters may be as high as 10–20%. Hypotension, reversible or irreversible renal failure, anuria, skull hypoplasia (defective skull ossification in some cases), and/or death were reported in neonates whose mothers had received ACE inhibitors during the second and third trimesters of pregnancy. In one premature neonate (35 weeks' gestation) born with acute, reversible renal failure following exposure to enalapril for several weeks prior to delivery, plasma ACE activity was completely suppressed at birth, and plasma active and total renin concentrations and renin activity were substantially increased in the neonate; the renal failure was managed with peritoneal dialysis, which was discontinued after 10 days. Other adverse effects associated with such use included oligohydramnios, presumably due to decreased renal function in the fetus, prematurity, fetal death, and patent ductus arteriosus; however, it is not known whether these effects were associated with ACE inhibition or underlying maternal disease. Oligohydramnios has been associated with contractures of the limbs, craniofacial deformities, hypoplasia of the lungs, and intrauterine growth retardation.

Although fetal exposure limited to the first trimester previously was considered not to be associated with substantial risk, data from an epidemiologic study have shown that infants whose mothers had taken an ACE inhibitor during the first trimester of pregnancy have an increased risk of major congenital malformations compared with infants who had not undergone first trimester exposure to ACE inhibitors. The risk of major congenital malformations, primarily affecting the cardiovascular and central nervous systems, was increased by about 2.7 times in infants whose mothers had taken an ACE inhibitor during the first trimester of pregnancy compared with infants who had not undergone such exposure. Every effort should be made to discontinue enalapril or enalaprilat therapy as soon as possible in any woman who becomes pregnant while receiving either of the drugs, regardless of the period of gestation. In addition, all women of childbearing potential who are receiving an ACE inhibitor should be advised to report pregnancy to their clinician as soon as possible. Women of childbearing potential who are receiving an ACE inhibitor also should be advised to inform their clinician if they are planning to become pregnant or think they might be pregnant. Nearly all women can be transferred successfully to alternative therapy for the remainder of their pregnancy. Rarely (probably less frequently than once in every 1000 pregnancies), no adequate alternative can be identified; in such rare cases, the woman should be informed of the potential hazard to the fetus and serial ultrasound examinations should be performed to assess the intra-amniotic environment. If oligohydramnios is present, enalapril therapy should be discontinued, unless use of the drug is considered life-saving for the woman.Contraction stress testing (CST), a nonstress test (NST), or biophysical profiling may be performed, if appropriate depending on the period of gestation. However, both clinicians and patients should realize that oligohydramnios may not become apparent until after irreversible fetal injury already has occurred.

Infants exposed in utero to ACE inhibitors should be observed closely for hypotension, oliguria, and hyperkalemia. If oliguria occurs, supportive measures (e.g., administration of fluids and pressor agents) to correct hypotension and renal perfusion should be considered. Exchange transfusion or dialysis may be required to reverse hypotension and/or substitute for impaired renal function. Enalapril, which crosses the placenta, has been removed from neonatal circulation by peritoneal dialysis with some clinical benefit. The manufacturer states that the drug theoretically may be removed by exchange transfusion; however, this latter procedure has not been used to date.

Reproduction studies in rats using enalapril maleate dosages up to 200 mg/kg daily (about 333 times the maximum daily human dosage) have not revealed evidence of teratogenicity or fetotoxicity. Decreases in average fetal weight occurred in rats receiving enalapril maleate dosages of 1200 mg/kg daily, but fetotoxicity did not occur when rats received a diet supplemented with sodium chloride. Fetotoxicity (decreased fetal weight) has been observed in rats receiving oral dosages up to 90 mg/kg of enalapril maleate combined with 10 mg/kg of hydrochlorothiazide daily (representing 26 and 1.6 times the maximum recommended human daily dosage of enalapril maleate and hydrochlorothiazide, respectively, on a mg/m^2 basis) and in mice receiving combined oral therapy with up to 30 and 10 mg/kg daily of enalapril maleate and hydrochlorothiazide, respectively (representing 4.3 and 0.8 times the maximum recommended human daily dosage of enalapril maleate and hydrochlorothiazide, respectively, on a mg/m^2 basis), but did not occur when lower dosages of enalapril maleate (30 and 10 mg/kg daily, respectively) were combined with 10 mg/kg of hydrochlorothiazide daily in these animals. Reproduction studies in rabbits receiving enalapril maleate dosages up to 30 mg/kg daily during days 6–18 of gestation did not reveal evidence of teratogenicity, but maternotoxicity and fetotoxicity occurred in rabbits at dosages of 1 mg/kg daily. Fetotoxicity and maternotoxicity did not occur in rabbits receiving enalapril maleate dosages of 3–10 mg/kg daily when their diet was supplemented with sodium chloride, but did occur at dosages of 30 mg/kg daily even when the diet was supplemented.

Fertility Reproduction studies in male and female rats using enalapril maleate dosages of 10–90 mg/kg daily (representing up to 4.3 and 0.8 times the maximum recommended human daily dosage of enalapril maleate and hydrochlorothiazide, respectively, on a mg/m^2 basis) have not revealed adverse effects on reproductive performance. Impotence and decreased libido have been reported occasionally in patients receiving enalapril alone or in fixed combination with hydrochlorothiazide.

Lactation Because enalapril alone or thiazide diuretics alone are distributed into human milk and potentially may cause serious adverse reactions in nursing infants, a decision should be made whether to discontinue nursing or enalapril (either alone or in fixed combination with hydrochlorothiazide), taking into account the importance of the drug(s) to the woman.

Drug Interactions

In addition to the drug interactions described, the possibility that other drug interactions reported with other angiotensin-converting enzyme (ACE) inhibitors (e.g., captopril) might occur with enalapril should be considered.

■ **Hypotensive Agents and Diuretics** When enalapril is administered with diuretics or other hypotensive drugs, the hypotensive effect of enalapril is increased. The effect is usually used to therapeutic advantage, but careful adjustment of dosage is necessary when these drugs are used concomitantly.

Enalapril and diuretics appear to have additive hypotensive effects; however, severe hypotension and reversible renal insufficiency may occasionally occur, especially in volume- and/or sodium-depleted patients. (See Cautions: Cardiovascular Effects; and Renal Effects.) Hypotensive drugs that cause release of renin (e.g., diuretics) will increase the hypotensive effect of enalapril. Reduction of enalapril dosage and/or dosage reduction or discontinuance of diuretic therapy may be necessary. Patients should be monitored closely during initiation and dosage adjustment of concomitant therapy with enalapril and a diuretic; in patients already receiving diuretics, the risk of these effects may be minimized by withholding diuretic therapy and/or increasing sodium intake for 2–3 days prior to initiating enalapril therapy. If diuretic therapy cannot be withheld, the patient should be under medical supervision for at least 2 hours after the initial dose of enalapril and until blood pressure has stabilized for at least an additional hour.

■ **Drugs Increasing Serum Potassium Concentration** Potassium-sparing diuretics (e.g., amiloride, spironolactone, triamterene), potassium supplements, or potassium-containing salt substitutes should be used with caution and serum potassium should be determined frequently in patients receiving enalapril, since hyperkalemia may occur. Dosage of the potassium-sparing diuretic and/or potassium supplement should be reduced or the diuretic and/or supplement discontinued as necessary. The manufacturer recommends that potassium-sparing diuretics generally *not* be used in patients receiving enalapril for heart failure. However, ACE inhibitors have been administrated with low-dosage spironolactone therapy and hyperkalemia was reported rarely. (See Uses: Heart Failure.) Patients should be advised to not use potassium-containing salt substitutes unless otherwise instructed by their clinician. Patients with renal impairment may be at increased risk of hyperkalemia.

■ **Nonsteroidal Anti-inflammatory Agents** Because ACE inhibitors may promote kinin-mediated prostaglandin synthesis and/or release, concomitant administration of drugs that inhibit prostaglandin synthesis (e.g., aspirin, ibuprofen) may reduce the blood pressure response to ACE inhibitors, including enalapril. Limited data indicate that concomitant administration of ACE inhibitors with nonsteroidal anti-inflammatory agents (NSAIAs) occasionally may result in acute reduction of renal function; however, the possibility cannot be ruled out that one drug alone may cause such an effect. Blood pressure should be monitored carefully when an NSAIA is initiated in patients receiving ACE inhibitor therapy; in addition, clinicians should be alert for evidence of impaired renal function. Some clinicians suggest that if a drug interaction between an ACE inhibitor and an NSAIA is suspected, the NSAIA should be discontinued, or a different hypotensive agent used or, alternatively, the dosage of the hypotensive agent should be modified.

Aspirin and other NSAIAs also can attenuate the hemodynamic actions of ACE inhibitors in patients with heart failure. Because ACE inhibitors share and enhance the effects of the compensatory hemodynamic mechanisms of heart failure, with aspirin and other NSAIAs interacting with the compensatory mechanisms rather than with a given ACE inhibitor per se, these desirable mechanisms are particularly susceptible to the interaction and a subsequent potential loss of clinical benefits. As a result, the more severe the heart failure and the more prominent the compensatory mechanisms, the more appreciable the interaction between NSAIAs and ACE inhibitors. Even if optimal dosage of an ACE inhibitor is used in the treatment of heart failure, the potential cardiovascular and survival benefit may not be seen if the patient is receiving an NSAIA concomitantly. In several multicenter studies, concomitant administration of a NSAIA (i.e., a single 350-mg dose of aspirin) in patients with heart failure inhibited favorable hemodynamic effects associated with ACE inhibitors, attenuating the favorable effects of these drugs on survival and cardiovascular morbidity. However, these findings have not been confirmed by other studies. In one retrospective analysis of pooled data, patients who received an ACE inhibitor concomitantly with aspirin (160– 325 mg daily) during the acute phase following myocardial infarction (MI) had proportional reductions in 7- and 30-day mortality rates comparable to patients who received an ACE inhibitor alone. Some clinicians have questioned the results of this study because of methodologic concerns (e.g., unsubstantiated assumptions about aspirin therapy [dosage, time of initiation, duration]; disparate distribution of patients). Although it has been suggested that patients requiring long-term management of heart failure avoid the concomitant use of ACE inhibitors and aspirin (and perhaps substitute another platelet-aggregation inhibitor for aspirin [e.g., clopidogrel, ticlopidine]), some clinicians state that existing data are insufficient to recommend a change in the current prescribing practices of clinicians concerning the use of aspirin in patients receiving therapy with an ACE inhibitor.

■ **Lithium** Lithium toxicity has occurred following concomitant administration of enalapril and lithium carbonate and was reversible following discontinuance of both drugs. In one patient, the toxicity was associated with elevated plasma lithium concentration and was manifested as ataxia, dysarthria, tremor, confusion, and altered EEG; bradycardia and T-wave depression also occurred. Moderate renal insufficiency (serum creatinine of 2.2 mg/dL) or acute renal failure has also occurred in these patients. The exact mechanism of this interaction remains to be established, but it has been suggested that enalapril may decrease renal elimination of lithium, possibly by increasing sodium excretion secondary to decreased aldosterone secretion or by altering renal function secondary to ACE inhibition. Renal function has returned to baseline within 2–4 days after discontinuing enalapril, and plasma lithium concentrations have returned to within normal limits following discontinuance of enalapril and temporary withdrawal of lithium therapy. The manufacturer of enalapril recommends that serum lithium concentrations be monitored frequently when enalapril and lithium are administered concomitantly.

■ **Other Drugs** Enalapril may reduce fasting blood glucose concentrations in nondiabetic individuals and may produce hypoglycemia in diabetic patients whose diabetes has been controlled with insulin or oral antidiabetic agents. Further studies are needed to evaluate the hypoglycemic effect of enalapril; however, similar effects have been reported in patients receiving captopril, and the risk of precipitating hypoglycemia should be considered when therapy with an ACE inhibitor is initiated in diabetic patients.

Concomitant use of enalapril and some vasodilating agents (e.g., nitrates) or anesthetic agents may cause an exaggerated hypotensive response. Patients receiving enalapril concomitantly with nitrates or with anesthetic agents that produce hypotension should be observed for possible additive hypotensive effects. Fluid volume expansion can correct hypotension during surgery or anesthesia if it is thought to result from an enalapril-induced inhibition of the angiotensin II formation that occurs secondary to compensatory renin release.

Acute Toxicity

Limited information is available on the acute toxicity of enalapril in humans. Specific information on overdosage with the fixed combination of enalapril and hydrochlorothiazide currently is not available.

■ **Pathogenesis** The oral LD_{50} of enalapril maleate ranged from 2000–3500 mg/kg in mice and male rats and 2000–3000 mg/kg in female rats. The IV LD_{50} ranged from 700–950 mg/kg in female mice and male rats, and the subcutaneous LD_{50} was 1150, 1400, 1500, and 1750 mg/kg in male mice, female rats, female mice, and male rats, respectively. The IV LD_{50} of enalaprilat was 3740–5890 mg/kg in female mice. In clinical studies, some hypertensive patients received a maximum IV enalaprilat dose of 80 mg over a 15-minute period, but no adverse effects other than those associated with the recommended dosages were observed. In animals, sublethal doses of enalapril produced ptosis, decreased activity, and bradypnea. In dogs, a single 200-mg/kg dose was lethal, but a single 100-mg/kg dose was not toxic. In mice and rats, single oral doses exceeding 1000 mg/kg or at least 1775 mg/kg, respectively, were lethal.

■ **Manifestations** Overdosage of enalapril produces effects that are mainly extensions of the drug's pharmacologic effects as an ACE inhibitor. Plasma ACE activity was completely suppressed within 10–15 hours after acute ingestion of 300–440 mg of enalapril maleate in 2 patients. The most likely manifestation of enalapril overdosage is hypotension, which may be profound. Onset and duration of the hypotensive effect may be prolonged following acute overdosage.Hypotension may be accompanied by stupor. Renal dysfunction, including acute renal failure; hyperkalemia; and hyponatremia may also occur.

■ **Treatment** Management of enalapril overdosage is mainly supportive and symptomatic. Hypotension can be corrected with fluid volume expansion (e.g., IV infusion of 0.9% sodium chloride injection). Renal function also improves during supportive therapy with sodium chloride infusion. Because of the long ACE-inhibitory effect of enalapril, prolonged observation (e.g., for several weeks) and supportive treatment may be necessary following overdosage with the drug. Treatment of acute oral overdosage may also include gastric lavage and administration of activated charcoal to prevent further GI absorption of the drug. The active metabolite enalaprilat may be removed by hemodialysis. Management of overdosage with the fixed combination of enalapril and hydrochlorothiazide should also include measures for the management of thiazide overdosage.

Pharmacology

Enalapril maleate is a prodrug of enalaprilat and has little pharmacologic activity until hydrolyzed in vivo to enalaprilat. Pharmacologic effects described for enalapril generally apply to enalaprilat, although the latter drug is substantially more potent on a weight basis. The mechanism(s) of action of enalaprilat and enalapril have not been fully elucidated. The drugs appear to reduce blood pressure in normotensive individuals and hypertensive patients and to produce beneficial hemodynamic effects in patients with heart failure mainly by suppressing the renin-angiotensin-aldosterone system.

■ **Effects on Renin-Angiotensin-Aldosterone System** Enalapril prevents the conversion of angiotensin I to angiotensin II (a potent vasoconstrictor) through inhibition of angiotensin-converting enzyme (ACE). The drug competes with physiologic substrate (angiotensin I) for the active site of ACE; the affinity of enalaprilat for ACE is approximately 200,000 times greater than that of angiotensin I. In vitro on a molar basis, the affinity of enalaprilat for ACE is 300–1000 or 2–17 times that of enalapril or captopril, respectively. However, in vitro on a molar basis, the ACE-inhibitory effect of enalapril was shown to be similar to that of enalaprilat in rat plasma and kidneys, because these tissues extensively hydrolyze enalapril to form enalaprilat. The drug apparently does not inhibit brain ACE in animals.

Inhibition of ACE initially results in decreased plasma angiotensin II concentrations and, consequently, blood pressure may be reduced in part through decreased vasoconstriction. Plasma renin activity (PRA) increases, possibly as a result of loss of feedback inhibition (mediated by angiotensin II) on the release of renin from the kidneys and/or stimulation of reflex mechanisms via baroreceptors (as a result of the decrease in blood pressure). Enalapril-induced increases in PRA are greater in the upright than in the supine position, and the effects of the drug on PRA and plasma angiotensin II concentrations may be potentiated by restriction of sodium intake. The initial hypotensive effect of enalapril appears to be proportional to inhibition of ACE in blood, but the hypotensive effect of the drug appears to persist longer than decreased angiotensin II concentrations. It has been suggested that the hypotensive effect of ACE inhibitors may in part also result from a local effect (e.g., in vascular wall). By decreasing local angiotensin II production, ACE inhibitors may decrease vascular tone by reducing direct angiotensin II-induced vasoconstriction and/or angiotensin II-induced increases in sympathetic activity. During prolonged enalapril use, plasma angiotensin II concentrations may return toward pretreatment levels, and inhibition of the renin-angiotensin system in various tissues (e.g., arterial wall, kidneys) rather than in blood may be more important determinants of the hypotensive effect of the drug, particularly long term.

Enalapril alone may be more effective in reducing blood pressure in patients with high or normal renin hypertension, but the drug may also lower blood pressure in patients with low renin hypertension. Although enalapril has lowered blood pressure in all races studied, the drug was less effective in black hypertensive patients, a population associated with low renin hypertension. Correlation between pretreatment PRA and short-term reduction in blood pressure has varied. Some clinicians have reported no correlation between pretreatment PRA and short-term reduction in blood pressure, while others have reported initial decreases in blood pressure to be proportional to pretreatment PRA. Correlation between pretreatment PRA and long-term response to the drug has not been consistently found.

Initial decreases in plasma angiotensin II concentrations lead to decreased aldosterone secretion from the adrenal cortex and, therefore, to decreased plasma concentrations and urinary excretion of aldosterone. However, there is increasing evidence to suggest that plasma aldosterone concentrations may not decrease with usual dosages of ACE inhibitors in some patients and may return to pretreatment levels in others during prolonged therapy. In addition, plasma aldosterone concentrations may not accurately reflect changes in aldosterone secretion, and reductions in these concentrations are usually greater when measured during ambulation than during rest in the supine position. It has been suggested that the addition of spironolactone, a drug that competitively inhibits the physiologic effects of aldosterone, appears to augment the suppressive effect of ACE inhibitors on aldosterone. Enalapril has blunted secondary hyperaldosteronism in healthy individuals receiving diuretics; the drug corrected hypokalemia associated with thiazides and increased sodium excretion. The drug has also improved potassium balance, increased PRA, decreased aldosterone secretion, and reduced blood pressure in a limited number of patients with idiopathic hyperaldosteronism.

■ **Effects on Catecholamines and Autacoids** Circulating plasma norepinephrine concentration generally is not affected by enalapril, but the drug has reduced these concentrations in some patients with hypertension or heart failure. In addition, the drug has attenuated the increase in plasma norepinephrine concentration that results from orthostatic reflexes. By inhibiting angiotensin II formation, ACE inhibitors may affect catecholamine release and reuptake by noradrenergic nerve endings and/or may decrease vascular sensitivity to vasopressors. There is some evidence that high doses of ACE inhibitors may inhibit presynaptic norepinephrine release and postsynaptic α_2-adrenoceptor activity, thereby interfering with sympathetic reflexes, but the clinical importance of this finding is not known since dosages tested in animals substantially exceed usual human hypotensive dosages.

Because ACE also degrades the vasodilator bradykinin, it has been suggested that inhibition of ACE may cause accumulation of bradykinin in plasma or tissues with resultant vasodilation; however, plasma and/or urinary concentrations of bradykinin and/or its metabolites have been unchanged in enalapril-responsive patients. Plasma and urinary concentrations of bradykinin may not indicate tissue activity of the peptide, and its role, if any, in the therapeutic effects of enalapril remains to be elucidated. It has been suggested that prostaglandins also may mediate some of the pharmacologic effects of enalapril since there is some evidence that the drug may increase prostaglandin production or release; however, most available evidence currently indicates that enalapril does not substantially affect prostaglandins, and further evaluation is necessary to determine the importance of any prostaglandin-mediated effects. (See Drug Interactions: Nonsteroidal Anti-inflammatory Agents.) Urinary concentration of thromboxane and prostacyclin metabolites have been unchanged during enalapril therapy.

■ **Cardiovascular Effects** In hypertensive patients, enalapril reduces blood pressure by decreasing total peripheral resistance with a slight increase or no change in heart rate, stroke volume, or cardiac output. The drug causes arterial and possibly venous dilation. Enalapril generally decreases systolic and diastolic blood pressures by approximately 10–15%; blood pressure is decreased to about the same extent in both the supine and standing positions.Orthostatic hypotension and tachycardia occur infrequently but are more common in sodium-depleted or hypovolemic patients. (See Cautions: Cardiovascular Effects.) Plasma volume has been reported to be unchanged or slightly increased; erythrocyte volume, extracellular fluid volume, and total body water have been unchanged. The drug appears to have no direct effect on baroreceptor sensitivity in normotensive or hypertensive individuals on a normal sodium diet. However, slight potentiation of baroreceptor sensitivity has been reported in mildly sodium-depleted individuals.

In patients with heart failure, enalapril, usually in conjunction with cardiac glycosides and diuretics, decreases total peripheral resistance, pulmonary capillary wedge pressure, heart size, and mean arterial and right atrial pressures. Cardiac index, cardiac output, stroke volume, and exercise tolerance increase in these patients; mean ejection fraction increases or remains unchanged; and heart rate decreases slightly or is unchanged. The drug may also cause a regional redistribution of blood flow, principally increasing renal blood flow with slight or no increase in flow in the forearm or hepatic vasculature, respectively.

■ **Renal and Electrolyte Effects** Renal blood flow may increase, but glomerular filtration rate is usually unchanged during enalapril therapy. In some patients, however, both renal blood flow and glomerular filtration rate have increased. BUN and serum creatinine concentrations have occasionally increased during long-term enalapril therapy. Increased BUN and serum creatinine occur more frequently in patients with preexisting renal impairment, in those receiving concomitant therapy with a diuretic, and in those with heart failure. However, in some hypertensive patients with preexisting renal impairment, renal blood flow and glomerular filtration rate have increased, presumably secondary to enalapril-induced intrarenal effects. In patients with heart failure and renal perfusion pressures less than 70 mm Hg, changes in creatinine clearance induced by 1–3 months of enalapril therapy have varied linearly and inversely with pretreatment PRA; however, creatinine clearance was not substantially affected by the drug in patients with renal perfusion pressures of 70 mm Hg or greater. Enalapril's effects on renal blood flow and glomerular filtration in patients with renovascular hypertension appear to be similar to those in hypertensive patients with normal renal function; however, transient increases in BUN and serum creatinine concentrations are more frequent in patients with renovascular hypertension than in hypertensive patients with normal renal function. In addition, renal function can markedly deteriorate during therapy with an ACE inhibitor in patients with preexisting, severely compromised renal perfusion. (See Cautions: Renal Effects.)

Increases in serum potassium concentration may occur secondary to enalapril-induced decreases in aldosterone secretion, especially in patients with impaired renal function. Concomitant administration of thiazide diuretics generally offsets this increase. Urinary sodium excretion may be increased during the first 2–3 days of enalapril therapy and may persist for longer periods in some patients with normal sodium intake, probably secondary to reduced tubular reabsorption of the ion. The hypotensive effect of enalapril may also result in part from decreased sodium and water retention secondary to reduced aldosterone secretion; however, decreases in aldosterone secretion during enalapril therapy are generally small.

Pharmacokinetics

■ **Absorption** Enalapril maleate, unlike enalaprilat, is well absorbed following oral administration. Although enalaprilat is a more potent angiotensin-converting enzyme (ACE) inhibitor than enalapril, it is poorly absorbed from the GI tract because of its high polarity, with only about 3–12% of an orally administered dose being absorbed. Approximately 55–75% of an oral dose of enalapril maleate is rapidly absorbed from the GI tract in healthy individuals and hypertensive patients. Food does not appear to substantially affect the rate or extent of absorption of enalapril maleate. Following oral administration, enalapril maleate appears to undergo first-pass metabolism principally in the liver, being hydrolyzed to enalaprilat. Concomitant oral administration of enalapril maleate and hydrochlorothiazide has little, if any, effect on the bioavailability of either drug. Oral administration of the commercially available fixed combination containing the drugs reportedly is bioequivalent to concurrent administration of the drugs as individual preparations. (See Pharmacokinetics: Elimination.)

Peak serum enalapril concentrations of 40–80 ng/mL occur within about 0.5–1.5 hours following oral administration of a single 10-mg dose of enalapril maleate in healthy individuals or hypertensive patients. Peak serum enalaprilat concentrations reportedly increase proportionally with oral doses of enalapril maleate ranging from 2.5–40 mg. Following oral administration of a single 2.5-, 5-, 10-, 20-, or 40-mg dose of enalapril maleate in these patients, average peak serum enalaprilat concentrations of 6–8, 15–28, 37–50, 70–80, or 123–150 ng/mL, respectively, occur within about 3–4.5 hours. Steady-state serum concentrations of enalaprilat were reached within 30–60 hours in patients with normal renal function receiving oral enalapril maleate dosages of 10 mg daily for 8 days; appreciable accumulation of the metabolite did not occur.

The hypotensive effect of a single oral dose of enalapril maleate is usually apparent within 1 hour and maximal in 4–8 hours. The hypotensive effect of usual doses of the drug generally persists for 12–24 hours but may diminish toward the end of the dosing interval in some patients. The reduction in blood pressure may be gradual, and several weeks of therapy may be required before the full effect is achieved. Following IV administration of enalaprilat, the hypotensive effect is usually apparent within 5–15 minutes with maximal effect occurring within 1–4 hours; the duration of hypotensive effect appears to be dose related, but with the recommended doses, the duration of action in most patients is approximately 6 hours. Plasma ACE inhibition and reduction in blood pressure appear to be correlated to a plasma enalaprilat concentration of 10 ng/mL, a concentration at which maximal blockade of plasma ACE is achieved. After withdrawal of enalapril or enalaprilat, blood pressure gradually returns to pretreatment levels; rebound hypertension following abrupt withdrawal of the drug has not been reported to date.

The onset and duration of hemodynamic effects of enalapril maleate appear to be slower and more prolonged than those of captopril. In patients with heart failure, the hemodynamic effects of enalapril maleate are generally apparent within 2–4 hours and may persist for up to 24 hours after an oral dose.

■ **Distribution** Distribution of enalapril into human body tissues and fluids has not been fully characterized.

Approximately 50–60% of enalaprilat is bound to plasma proteins. Two binding sites have been identified, a low-affinity, high-capacity site and a high-affinity, low-capacity site. Drug bound to the latter site may represent enalaprilat bound to circulating serum ACE, possibly accounting for the prolonged terminal elimination of the drug.

Information on distribution into the CNS is limited, but enalapril appears to cross the blood-brain barrier poorly, if at all, and enalaprilat does not appear to distribute into the CNS. The drug did not accumulate in any tissue following multiple-dose administration in animals. The drug crosses the placenta. In a premature neonate (35 weeks' gestation) whose mother received 20 mg of enalapril maleate daily for 17 days prior to delivery, plasma enalaprilat concentration soon after birth in the neonate was 28 ng/mL. Enalapril and enalaprilat are distributed into milk in trace amounts.

■ **Elimination** Following oral administration, the half-life of unchanged enalapril appears to be less than 2 hours in healthy individuals and in patients with normal hepatic and renal functions, but may be increased in patients with heart failure. Following oral administration of a single 5- or 10-mg dose of enalapril maleate in patients with heart failure, the half-life of enalapril was 3.4 or 5.8 hours, respectively. Serum concentrations of enalaprilat, the active metabolite of enalapril, appear to decline in a multiphasic manner. Elimination of enalaprilat may also be prolonged in patients with heart failure or impaired hepatic function compared with healthy individuals and patients with hypertension. Observations of serum concentrations of enalaprilat over long periods following oral or IV administration suggest that enalaprilat has an average terminal half-life of about 35–38 hours (range: 30–87 hours). The observed prolonged terminal phase may actually reflect enalaprilat binding to the high-affinity, low-capacity binding site of circulating serum ACE. The effective half-life for accumulation of enalaprilat (determined from urinary recovery) has been reported to average about 11 or 14 hours in healthy adults with normal renal function or in hypertensive pediatric patients, respectively.

Peak and trough enalaprilat concentrations and areas under the serum concentration-time curves (AUCs) may increase, time to peak and steady-state serum concentration may be delayed, and the effective half-life for accumulation may be prolonged in patients with impaired renal function. In patients with creatinine clearances less than 30 mL/minute, the effective half-life for accumulation of enalaprilat following multiple doses of enalapril maleate is prolonged. In patients with moderate renal impairment (i.e., creatinine clearances of 30–60 mL/minute), this half-life is not substantially prolonged, and there appears to be a lack of correlation between AUCs and creatinine clearance. Decreased urinary excretion of enalapril may increase the extent of hydrolysis of enalapril to enalaprilat or may increase extrarenal elimination of the drug (e.g., via biliary excretion).

About 60% of an absorbed dose of enalapril is extensively hydrolyzed to enalaprilat, principally in the liver via esterases. About 20% appears to be hydrolyzed on first pass through the liver; this hydrolysis does not appear to occur in plasma in humans. Enalaprilat is a more potent ACE inhibitor than enalapril. There is no evidence of other metabolites of enalapril in humans, rats, or dogs. However, a despropyl metabolite of enalaprilat was identified in urine in rhesus monkeys, accounting for 13% of an oral dose of enalapril maleate. Hydrolysis of enalapril to enalaprilat may be delayed and/or impaired in patients with severe hepatic impairment, but the pharmacodynamic effects of the drug do not appear to be significantly altered.

Following oral administration, enalapril and enalaprilat are excreted in urine and feces. In healthy individuals, a mean of 60–78% (a mean of 43–56% as enalaprilat and the remainder as unchanged drug) of a 10-mg oral dose of enalapril maleate is excreted in urine within 24–48 hours after administration and approximately 33% (about 27% as enalaprilat and 6% as unchanged drug) is excreted in feces within 24–48 hours. In a multiple-dose study (10 mg daily) in healthy individuals with normal renal function, urinary excretion of enalaprilat and total drug increased during the first 4 days of therapy and then stabilized; urinary excretion of the metabolite averaged 45% of the cumulative dose and that of total drug averaged 62%. In a multiple-dose study (0.07–0.14 mg/kg of enalapril maleate daily) in hypertensive pediatric patients (2 months to 16 years), 67% (64–76% as enalaprilat and the remainder as unchanged drug) of the administered dose is recovered in urine within 24 hours. It is not known whether enalapril and enalaprilat excreted in feces represent unabsorbed drug or that excreted via biliary elimination. Biliary excretion of enalapril and enalaprilat occurs in animals; however, this route of elimination has not been demonstrated in humans.

Renal clearance of enalaprilat and enalapril are reported to be approximately 100–158 and 300 mL/minute, respectively, in adults with normal renal function. The higher renal clearance of enalapril compared with that of the metabolite may indicate some degree of active tubular secretion of unchanged drug. Renal clearance may be decreased in hypertensive patients. In geriatric individuals, renal clearance and/or volume of distribution may decrease.

Enalaprilat is removed by hemodialysis. The amount of drug removed during hemodialysis depends on several factors (e.g., type of coil used, dialysis flow rate); however, the hemodialysis clearance of enalaprilat is reportedly 62 mL/minute. Enalaprilat also appears to be removed by peritoneal dialysis.

Chemistry and Stability

■ **Chemistry** Enalaprilat and enalapril are angiotensin-converting enzyme (ACE, bradykininase, kininase II) inhibitors. Enalapril, the ethylester of enalaprilat, is a prodrug and has little pharmacologic activity until hydrolyzed in the liver to enalaprilat. Enalapril is commercially available as the maleate salt and differs structurally from enalaprilat by the presence of an ethoxycarbonyl group rather than a carboxy group at position 1 of l-alanyl-l-proline and by the presence of the maleate salt. These structural modifications result in increased GI absorption of enalapril compared with enalaprilat, which is poorly absorbed from the GI tract. Enalapril is structurally and pharmacologically similar to captopril but contains a disubstituted nitrogen rather than a sulfhydryl group at position 3 of 2-methyl-1-oxopropyl-l-proline. The lack of the sulfhydryl group in enalapril may result in decreased risk of certain adverse effects (e.g., cutaneous reactions, taste disturbances, proteinuria).

Enalaprilat occurs as a white to off-white crystalline powder and is slightly soluble in water and sparingly soluble in methanol. Commercially available enalaprilat injection is a sterile, clear, colorless solution of the drug. Sodium chloride is added during manufacture of the injection to adjust tonicity, and sodium hydroxide is added to adjust pH; the injection also contains 0.9% benzyl alcohol as a preservative. Enalapril maleate occurs as a white to off-white, crystalline powder and has solubilities of 25 mg/mL in water and 80 mg/mL in alcohol at room temperature. The apparent pK_as of enalapril are 3 and 5.4 at 25°C.

■ **Stability** Commercially available enalaprilat injection should be stored at a temperature less than 30°C. Following dilution of enalaprilat injection in 5% dextrose, 0.9% sodium chloride, 5% dextrose and 0.9% sodium chloride, 5% dextrose in lactated Ringer's, or Isolyte® E, solutions of the drug are stable for 24 hours at room temperature. Enalaprilat is physically incompatible with amphotericin B and phenytoin sodium. Specialized references should be consulted for specific compatibility information.

The manufacturer recommends that enalapril maleate tablets be stored in tight containers at a temperature less than 30°C and that transient exposure to temperatures warmer than 50°C be avoided. The tablets should be protected from moisture. The tablets have an expiration date of 30 months following the date of manufacture when stored at less than 30°C. The manufacturer states that extemporaneous preparation of oral solutions of enalapril maleate should be avoided since the drug is not sufficiently stable in solution.

An extemporaneous preparation of enalapril maleate tablets in syrup (Ora-Sweet SF®) and sodium citrate dihydrate (Bicitra®) containing enalapril maleate 1 mg/mL is stable for 30 days when stored at 2–8°C.

Preparations

Excipients in commercially available drug preparations may have clinically important effects in some individuals; consult specific product labeling for details.

Enalaprilat

Parenteral

Injection, for IV use only	equivalent to 1.25 mg of anhydrous enalaprilat per mL*	**Enalaprilat Injection**

*available from one or more manufacturer, distributor, and/or repackager by generic (nonproprietary) name

Enalapril Maleate

Oral

Tablets	2.5 mg*	**Enalapril Maleate Tablets**
		Vasotec® (scored), Valeant
	5 mg*	**Enalapril Maleate Tablets**
		Vasotec® (scored), Valeant
	10 mg*	**Enalapril Maleate Tablets**
		Vasotec® (scored), Valeant
	20 mg*	**Enalapril Maleate Tablets**
		Vasotec® (scored), Valeant

*available from one or more manufacturer, distributor, and/or repackager by generic (nonproprietary) name

Enalapril Maleate and Hydrochlorothiazide

Oral

Tablets	5 mg Enalapril Maleate and Hydrochlorothiazide 12.5 mg*	**Enalapril Maleate and Hydrochlorothiazide Tablets**
	10 mg Enalapril Maleate and Hydrochlorothiazide 25 mg*	**Enalapril Maleate and Hydrochlorothiazide Tablets**
		Vaseretic®, Valeant

*available from one or more manufacturer, distributor, and/or repackager by generic (nonproprietary) name

†Use is not currently included in the labeling approved by the US Food and Drug Administration

Lisinopril

■ Lisinopril is an angiotensin-converting enzyme (ACE) inhibitor.

Uses

Lisinopril is used alone or in combination with other classes of antihypertensive agents (e.g., thiazide diuretics) in the management of hypertension. Lisinopril also is used in conjunction with other agents such as β-adrenergic blocking agents (β-blockers), cardiac glycosides, and diuretics in the management of heart failure. In addition, lisinopril may be used in conjunction with thrombolytic agents, aspirin, and/or β-blockers to improve survival in patients with acute myocardial infarction (MI) who are hemodynamically stable.

Because captopril, another angiotensin-converting enzyme (ACE) inhibitor, may cause serious adverse effects, (e.g., neutropenia, agranulocytosis), particularly in patients with renal impairment (especially those with collagen vascular disease) or in patients receiving immunosuppressive therapy, the possibility that similar adverse effects may occur with lisinopril should be considered since current evidence is insufficient to rule out such risk. (See Cautions: Hematologic Effects, in Captopril 24:32.04.)

■ **Hypertension** Lisinopril is used alone or in combination with other classes of antihypertensive agents in the management of hypertension. ACE inhibitors are considered one of several preferred antihypertensive drugs for the initial management of hypertension according to current evidence-based hypertension guidelines; other preferred options include angiotensin II receptor antagonists, calcium-channel blockers, and thiazide diuretics. While there may be individual differences with respect to recommendations for initial drug selection and use in specific patient populations, current evidence indicates that these antihypertensive drug classes all generally produce comparable effects on overall mortality and cardiovascular, cerebrovascular, and renal outcomes. (See Uses: Hypertension, in Captopril 24:32.04.)

ACE inhibitors may be particularly useful in the management of hypertension in patients with certain coexisting conditions such as heart failure, ischemic heart disease, diabetes mellitus, chronic kidney disease (CKD), or cerebrovascular disease or following MI. (See Uses: Hypertension in Captopril 24:32.04 and in Enalaprilat/Enalapril 24:32.04.)

In patients with hypertension and compelling indications (e.g., CKD with albuminuria [urine albumin 300 mg/day or greater, or urine albumin:creatinine ratio of 300 mg/g or equivalent in the first morning void]), angiotensin II receptor antagonists are usually considered an alternative for ACE inhibitor-intolerant patients. However, data indicate no difference in efficacy between ACE inhibitors and angiotensin II receptor antagonists with regard to blood pressure lowering and clinical outcomes (i.e., all-cause mortality, cardiovascular mortality, MI, heart failure, stroke, and end-stage renal disease). Adverse events (e.g., cough, angioedema) leading to drug discontinuance occur more frequently with ACE inhibitor therapy than with angiotensin II receptor antagonist therapy. Because of similar efficacy and a lower frequency of adverse effects, some experts believe that an angiotensin II receptor antagonist should be used instead of an ACE inhibitor for the treatment of hypertension or hypertension with certain compelling indications.

Most patients with hypertension, especially black patients, will require at least 2 antihypertensive drugs to achieve adequate blood pressure control. In general, black hypertensive patients tend to respond better to monotherapy with thiazide diuretics or calcium-channel blockers than to monotherapy with ACE inhibitors. Although ACE inhibitors have lowered blood pressure in all races studied, monotherapy with an ACE inhibitor has produced a smaller reduction in blood pressure in black hypertensive patients, a population associated with low renin hypertension. However, the combination of an ACE inhibitor or an angiotensin II receptor antagonist with a calcium-channel blocker or thiazide diuretic produces similar blood pressure lowering in black patients as in other racial groups. In addition, ACE inhibitors appear to produce a higher incidence of angioedema in black patients than in other races studied. (See ALLHAT study below and also see Race under Hypertension: Other Special Considerations for Antihypertensive Drug Therapy, in Uses in Captopril 24:32.04 and in Enalaprilat/Enalapril 24:32.04.)

The ALLHAT study, a large (33,357 patients), multicenter, randomized, active-control study in hypertensive patients 55 years of age or older with at least one other coronary heart disease risk factor, compared the cardiovascular benefit of therapy with an ACE inhibitor (lisinopril 10–40 mg daily) or a dihydropyridine-derivative calcium-channel blocker (amlodipine 2.5–10 mg daily) relative to therapy with a thiazide diuretic (chlorthalidone 12.5–25 mg daily). After a mean follow-up of 4.9 years, an intent-to-treat analysis revealed no difference in the primary outcome of combined fatal coronary heart disease or nonfatal MI among the treatments.

Compared with chlorthalidone, the relative risks for the primary outcome were 0.99 for lisinopril and 0.98 for amlodipine. In addition, all-cause mortality, a secondary outcome, did not differ among the treatments. Although each drug decreased blood pressure substantially, the extent of reduction was not equivalent. Five-year systolic blood pressures were significantly higher in the lisinopril (2 mm Hg) and amlodipine (0.8 mm Hg) groups relative to that achieved with chlorthalidone, and 5-year diastolic blood pressure was significantly lower with amlodipine (0.8 mm Hg) relative to the thiazide. Control of hypertension (systolic and diastolic blood pressures less than 140 and 90 mm Hg, respectively) was achieved in approximately two-thirds of patients by 5 years of follow-up (61, 66, or 68% of patients treated with lisinopril, amlodipine, lisinopril, or chlorthalidone, respectively).

Subgroup analysis of the ALLHAT study for race-related effects revealed no difference in the primary outcome of combined fatal coronary heart disease or nonfatal MI among the treatments in both black and nonblack patients. However, substantial race-related effects were observed in the incidence of secondary outcomes (e.g., stroke, combined cardiovascular disease events, heart failure). Compared with chlorthalidone, the relative risk for lisinopril was 1.4 or 1 (in black or nonblack patients, respectively) for stroke and 1.19 or 1.06 (in black or nonblack patients, respectively) for combined cardiovascular disease events. When amlodipine was compared with chlorthalidone, the only race-related difference observed was in the incidence of heart failure; the relative risk was 1.46 or 1.32 (in black or nonblack patients, respectively). The relative risk for heart failure in black versus nonblack patients receiving lisinopril was not considered to be statistically significant, and the overall relative risk for both groups was 1.19. In addition, after 4 years, in each treatment group, blood pressure reductions were greater in nonblack than in black patients; about 68 or 60% of nonblack or black patients, respectively, achieved a systolic/diastolic blood pressure of less than 140/90 mmHg. In nonblack patients receiving chlorthalidone, amlodipine, or lisinopril 69, 69, or 67% achieved the mentioned blood pressure, respectively, while in black patients receiving chlorthalidone, amlodipine, or lisinopril 63, 60, or 54% achieved such blood pressure, respectively.

Although the ALLHAT study provides strong evidence that these classes of antihypertensive agents (ACE inhibitors, dihydropyridine-derivative calcium-channel blockers, thiazide diuretics) are comparably effective in providing important cardiovascular benefit, apparent differences in certain secondary outcomes were observed. Thiazide diuretic therapy was superior to ACE inhibitor therapy in preventing aggregate cardiovascular events, principally stroke, heart failure, angina, and the need for coronary revascularization. Thiazide therapy also was better tolerated than ACE inhibitor therapy (e.g., angioedema, which was more likely in blacks than nonblacks).

Post hoc analysis of the ALLHAT study directly comparing cardiovascular and other outcomes in patients receiving amlodipine or lisinopril revealed no difference in the primary outcome of combined fatal coronary heart disease or nonfatal MI between patients receiving the ACE inhibitor and those receiving the calcium-channel blocking agent. However, patients receiving lisinopril were at higher risk for stroke, combined cardiovascular disease, GI bleeding, and angioedema, while those receiving amlodipine were at higher risk of developing heart failure. ALLHAT investigators suggested that the observed differences in cardiovascular outcome may be attributable, at least in part, to the greater antihypertensive effect of amlodipine compared with that of lisinopril, especially in women and black patients.

For additional information on the role of ACE inhibitors in the management of hypertension, see Uses in Captopril 24:32.04 and in Enalaprilat/Enalapril 24:32.04. For information on overall principles and expert recommendations for treatment of hypertension, see Uses: Hypertension in Adults and also see Uses: Hypertension in Pediatric Patients, in the Thiazides General Statement 40:28.20.

■ **Heart Failure** Lisinopril is used as adjunctive therapy in the management of heart failure in patients who do not respond adequately to diuretics and a cardiac glycoside.

Current guidelines for the management of heart failure in adults generally recommend a combination of drug therapies to reduce morbidity and mortality, including neurohormonal antagonists (e.g., ACE inhibitors, angiotensin II receptor antagonists, angiotensin receptor-neprilysin inhibitors [ARNIs], β-blockers, aldosterone receptor antagonists) that inhibit the detrimental compensatory mechanisms in heart failure. Additional agents (e.g., cardiac glycosides, diuretics, sinoatrial modulators [i.e., ivabradine]) added to a heart failure treatment regimen in selected patients have been associated with symptomatic improvement and/or reduction in heart failure-related hospitalizations. Experts recommend that all asymptomatic patients with reduced left ventricular ejection fraction (LVEF) (American College of Cardiology Foundation [ACCF]/American Heart Association [AHA] stage B heart failure) receive therapy with an ACE inhibitor and β-blocker to prevent symptomatic heart failure and to reduce morbidity and mortality. If ACE inhibitors are not tolerated, then an angiotensin II receptor antagonist is recommended as alternative therapy. In patients with prior or current symptoms of chronic heart failure and reduced LVEF (ACCF/AHA stage C heart failure), ACCF, AHA, and the Heart Failure Society of America (HFSA) recommend inhibition of the renin-angiotensin-aldosterone (RAA) system with an ACE inhibitor, angiotensin II receptor antagonist, or ARNI in conjunction with a β-blocker, and an aldosterone antagonist in selected patients, to reduce morbidity and mortality. While ACE inhibitors have been the preferred drugs for inhibition of the RAA system because of their established benefits in patients with heart failure and reduced ejection fraction, some evidence indicates that therapy with sacubitril/valsartan, an ARNI, may be more effective than ACE inhibitor therapy (enalapril) in reducing cardiovascular death and heart failure-related hospitalization in such patients. ACCF, AHA, and HFSA recommend that patients with chronic symptomatic heart failure and reduced LVEF (New York Heart Association [NYHA] class II or III) who are able to tolerate an ACE inhibitor or angiotensin II receptor antagonist be switched to therapy containing an ARNI to further reduce morbidity and mortality. However, in patients in whom an ARNI is not appropriate, continued use of an ACE inhibitor for all classes of heart failure with reduced ejection fraction remains strongly advised. In patients in whom an ARNI or ACE inhibitor is not appropriate, an angiotensin II receptor antagonist may be used. For additional information on the use of ACE inhibitors in the management of heart failure, see Uses: Heart Failure, in Captopril 24:32.04 and in Enalaprilat/Enalapril 24:32.04 For further information on the use of ARNIs in patients with heart failure, see Uses: Heart Failure, in Sacubitril and Valsartan 24:32.92.

Some clinicians state that ACE inhibitors usually are prescribed in clinical practice at dosages lower than those determined as target dosages in clinical trials, although results of several studies suggest that high dosages are associated with greater hemodynamic, neurohormonal, symptomatic, and prognostic benefits than lower dosages. Results of a large, randomized, double blind study (Assessment of Treatment with Lisinopril and Survival [ATLAS] study) in patients with heart failure (NYHA class II–IV) indicate that high lisinopril dosages (32.5–35 mg daily) were associated with a 12% lower risk of death or hospitalization for any cause and 24% fewer hospitalizations for heart failure than low dosages (2.5–5 mg) of the drug.

Many patients with heart failure respond to lisinopril with improvement in cardiac function indexes, symptomatic (e.g., dyspnea, fatigue) relief, improved functional capacity, and increased exercise tolerance. In some studies, improvement in cardiac function indexes and exercise tolerance were sustained for up to 3 months. Although additional studies are needed to determine the specific role of lisinopril in the management of heart failure and its long-term efficacy, the efficacy of the drug appears to be similar to that of captopril and enalapril. However, like enalapril, lisinopril has a relatively long duration of action compared with captopril; therefore, the drug may produce more prolonged hypotensive effects, particularly at high doses, which potentially could result in adverse cerebral and renal effects. In addition, because the renin-angiotensin system appears to contribute substantially to preservation of glomerular filtration in patients with heart failure in whom renal function is severely compromised, therapy with an ACE inhibitor may adversely affect renal function. (See Cautions: Renal Effects in Captopril 24:32.04 and in Enalaprilat/Enalapril 24:32.04.)

■ Mortality Reduction After Acute Myocardial Infarction Lisinopril is used in conjunction with standard therapies (e.g., thrombolytic agents, aspirin, β-blockers) to improve survival in hemodynamically stable patients with acute MI. Results of a multicenter, controlled, randomized, clinical study indicate that patients who received lisinopril or lisinopril concomitantly with nitrates within 24 hours of MI in addition to conventional therapy (thrombolytic agents, aspirin, β-blockers) had an 11% lower risk of death (6 weeks after infarction) compared with patients receiving conventional therapy only; mortality rates were 6.4 or 7.2% in patients receiving lisinopril and conventional therapy or conventional therapy alone, respectively.

Studies with various ACE inhibitors have shown that these drugs reduce fatal and nonfatal cardiovascular events in patients with recent MI. The magnitude of benefit appears to be greatest in certain high-risk patients (e.g., those with an anterior infarct, ejection fraction of 40% or less, heart failure, prior infarction, or tachycardia). In addition to their effects on mortality, ACE inhibitors also are used to minimize or prevent the development of left ventricular dilatation and dysfunction (ventricular "remodeling") following acute MI. Evidence regarding the efficacy of such therapy has been somewhat conflicting, particularly when parenteral therapy was initiated early (within 24–48 hours) and included patients with no evidence of baseline dysfunction. (See Uses: Left Ventricular Dysfunction After Acute Myocardial Infarction, in Enalaprilat/Enalapril 24:32.04.) However, the preponderance of evidence has shown a benefit of early oral therapy with ACE inhibitors, even in patients with no baseline dysfunction.

Current expert guidelines recommend the use of an ACE inhibitor within the first 24 hours of acute MI in patients with an anterior infarction, heart failure, or ejection fraction of 40% or less who do not have any contraindications (e.g., hypotension, shock, renal dysfunction). While early treatment within the first 24 hours of MI has been shown to be beneficial, ACE inhibitors should be used with caution (and with gradual upward titration) during the initial postinfarction period because of the possibility of hypotension or renal dysfunction. ACE inhibitor therapy generally should be continued indefinitely in all patients with left ventricular dysfunction or other compelling indications for use (e.g., hypertension, diabetes mellitus, CKD). The benefits of long-term ACE inhibitor therapy are less certain in low-risk patients who have undergone revascularization and are receiving aggressive antilipemic therapy.

■ Diabetic Nephropathy Both ACE inhibitors and angiotensin II receptor antagonists have been shown to slow the rate of progression of renal disease in patients with diabetes mellitus and persistent albuminuria†, and use of a drug from either class is recommended in such patients with modestly elevated (30–300 mg/24 hours) or higher (exceeding 300 mg/24 hours) levels of urinary albumin excretion. The usual precautions of ACE inhibitor or angiotensin II receptor antagonist therapy in patients with substantial renal impairment should be observed. For additional information on the use of ACE inhibitors in the treatment of diabetic nephropathy, see Diabetic Nephropathy under Uses: Nephropathy, in Captopril 24:32.04.

Dosage and Administration

■ Administration Lisinopril is administered orally. The manufacturers state that the absorption of lisinopril is not affected by the presence of food in the GI tract.

For pediatric patients and patients unable to swallow tablets, lisinopril may be administered orally as an extemporaneously prepared suspension. An extemporaneous suspension containing lisinopril 1 mg/mL can be prepared in the following manner. First, 10 mL of purified water is added to a polyethylene terephthalate (PET) bottle containing ten 20-mg tablets of lisinopril, and the contents are shaken for at least 1 minute. The concentrated suspension of lisinopril should be diluted with 30 mL of sodium citrate dihydrate (Bicitra®) and 160 mL of syrup (Ora-Sweet®), and the container then shaken gently for several seconds to disperse the ingredients. The suspension should be shaken before dispensing of each dose. The extemporaneous suspension is stable for 4 weeks when stored at or below 25°C.

■ Dosage Dosage of lisinopril must be adjusted according to patient tolerance and response. Because of the risk of inducing hypotension, initiation of lisinopril therapy requires consideration of recent antihypertensive therapy, the extent of blood pressure elevation, sodium intake, fluid status, and other clinical circumstances. If therapy is initiated in a patient already receiving a diuretic, symptomatic hypotension may occur following the initial dose of the angiotensin-converting enzyme (ACE) inhibitor. The possibility of hypotension may be minimized by discontinuing the diuretic, reducing the diuretic dosage, or cautiously increasing salt intake prior to initiation of lisinopril therapy. If diuretic therapy cannot be discontinued, lisinopril should be initiated in adults at a dosage of 5 mg daily under close medical supervision until blood pressure has stabilized. (See Cardiovascular Effects under Warnings/Precautions: Warnings, in Cautions.) For additional information on initiating lisinopril in patients receiving diuretic therapy, see the disease-specific dosage sections in Dosage and Administration.

Hypertension **Lisinopril Therapy.** For the management of uncomplicated hypertension in adults *not* receiving a diuretic, the usual initial dosage of lisinopril is 10 mg once daily. In patients currently receiving diuretic therapy, it is recommended that the diuretic be discontinued, if possible, 2–3 days before initiating lisinopril. If blood pressure is not adequately controlled with the ACE inhibitor alone, diuretic therapy may be resumed cautiously. If diuretic therapy cannot be discontinued, lisinopril should be initiated in adults at a reduced dosage of 5 mg daily under close medical supervision for at least 2 hours and until blood pressure has stabilized for at least an additional hour.

Dosage of lisinopril should be adjusted according to blood pressure response. If the blood pressure response diminishes toward the end of the dosing interval during once-daily administration, which may be particularly likely with a dosage of 10 mg or less daily, consideration should be given to increasing the dosage. The manufacturer states that the usual maintenance dosage of lisinopril in adults is 20–40 mg daily, given as a single dose. Some experts state that the usual dosage range is 10–40 mg daily, given as a single dose. Dosages up to 80 mg daily have been used, but do not appear to give a greater effect.

For the management of hypertension in children 6 years of age and older, the usual initial dosage of lisinopril is 0.07 mg/kg (up to 5 mg) once daily. Some experts state that the dosage may be increased every 2–4 weeks until blood pressure is controlled, the maximum dosage is reached, or adverse effects occur. The safety and efficacy of doses exceeding 0.61 mg/kg or in excess of 40 mg have not been established. For information on overall principles and expert recommendations for treatment of hypertension in pediatric patients, see Uses: Hypertension in Pediatric Patients, in the Thiazides General Statement 40:28.20.

Lisinopril/Hydrochlorothiazide Fixed-combination Therapy. The manufacturer states that therapy with the commercially available preparations containing lisinopril in fixed combination with hydrochlorothiazide should only be initiated in adults after an adequate response is not achieved with lisinopril or hydrochlorothiazide monotherapy. Alternatively, the fixed combination containing lisinopril with hydrochlorothiazide may be used in patients who have been receiving the drugs separately and in whom dosage of the individual drugs has been adjusted to the ratio in a commercial combination preparation. Such fixed combinations also may be used to prevent hydrochlorothiazide-induced potassium loss. Volume and/or salt depletion should be corrected before initiating therapy with lisinopril in fixed combination with hydrochlorothiazide. Patients whose blood pressure is not adequately controlled with lisinopril or hydrochlorothiazide monotherapy may receive the fixed combination containing 10 mg of lisinopril and 12.5 mg of hydrochlorothiazide or, alternatively, the preparation containing 20 mg of lisinopril and 12.5 mg of hydrochlorothiazide. Further increases of either or both drugs depend on clinical response; however, dosage of hydrochlorothiazide generally should not be increased for about 2–3 weeks after initiation of therapy. Patients whose blood pressure has been adequately controlled with a hydrochlorothiazide dosage of 25 mg daily, but who experienced potassium loss, may achieve a similar response if they are switched to therapy with the fixed-combination preparation containing 10 mg of lisinopril and 12.5 mg of hydrochlorothiazide. The dosages of lisinopril and hydrochlorothiazide should not exceed 80 and 50 mg daily, respectively.

Blood Pressure Monitoring and Treatment Goals. Blood pressure should be monitored regularly (i.e., monthly) and dosage of the antihypertensive drug adjusted until blood pressure is controlled. If an adequate blood pressure response is not achieved with ACE inhibitor monotherapy, the dosage may be increased or another antihypertensive agent with demonstrated benefit and preferably with a complementary mechanism of action (e.g., calcium-channel blocker, thiazide diuretic) may be added; if target blood pressure is still not achieved, a third drug may be added. (See Uses: Hypertension.) In patients who develop unacceptable adverse effects with lisinopril, the drug should be discontinued and another antihypertensive agent from a different pharmacologic class should be initiated.

The goal of hypertension management and prevention is to achieve and maintain optimal control of blood pressure. However, the optimum blood pressure threshold for initiating antihypertensive drug therapy and specific treatment goals remain controversial. While other hypertension guidelines have based target blood pressure goals on age and comorbidities, a 2017 multidisciplinary hypertension guideline from the American College of Cardiology (ACC), American Heart Association (AHA), and a number of professional organizations incorporates underlying cardiovascular risk into decision making regarding treatment and generally recommends the same target blood pressure (i.e., less than 130/80 mm Hg) in all adults. Many patients will require at least 2 drugs from different pharmacologic classes to achieve this blood pressure goal; the potential benefits of hypertension management and drug cost, adverse effects, and risks associated with the use of multiple antihypertensive drugs also should be considered when deciding a patient's blood pressure treatment goal.

For additional information on target levels of blood pressure and on monitoring therapy in the management of hypertension, see Blood Pressure Monitoring and Treatment Goals under Dosage: Hypertension, in Dosage and Administration in the Thiazides General Statement 40:28.20.

Heart Failure Because of the risk of severe hypotension, lisinopril therapy for heart failure should be initiated under very close medical supervision (e.g., in a hospital setting), especially in patients with low blood pressure (i.e., systolic blood pressure less than 80–100 mm Hg), with consideration given to recent diuretic therapy and the possibility of severe sodium and/or fluid depletion. Experts suggest that ACE inhibitor therapy also be initiated with caution in patients with markedly increased serum concentrations of creatinine (exceeding 3 mg/dL), bilateral renal artery stenosis, or elevated concentrations of serum potassium (exceeding 5 mEq/L).

For the management of heart failure, the usual initial dosage of lisinopril in adults with normal renal function and serum sodium concentration is 2.5–5 mg once daily. The usual effective dosage of lisinopril in adults with heart failure is 5–40 mg once daily.

Lisinopril often is administered in conjunction with other agents such as a cardiac glycoside, a diuretic, and a β-adrenergic blocking agent (β-blocker). After the initial dose, the patient should be monitored closely (especially those with systolic blood pressure less than 100 mg Hg) until blood pressure has stabilized. The mean peak blood pressure lowering usually occurs 6–8 hours after administration of a dose. Hypotension occurring after the initial dose does not preclude the administration of subsequent doses of the drug, provided due caution is exercised and the hypotension has been managed effectively. Evidence from a large clinical trial in patients with heart failure suggests that hypotension with lisinopril is dose-related. To minimize the likelihood of hypotension, the dosage of any diuretic given concomitantly with lisinopril should be reduced, if possible.

It should be recognized that although symptoms of heart failure may improve within 48 hours after initiating ACE inhibitor therapy in some patients, such improvement usually is not evident for several weeks or months after initiating ACE inhibitor therapy. In addition, it should be considered that such therapy may reduce the risk of disease progression even if symptomatic improvement is not evident. Therefore, some experts recommend that dosages generally be titrated to a prespecified target (i.e., 20–40 mg of lisinopril daily) or highest tolerated dosage rather than according to response. However, one manufacturer states that dosage adjustment of lisinopril should be based on the clinical response of individual patients. Patients with severe heart failure, with or without renal impairment, should be monitored closely for the first 2 weeks of lisinopril therapy and periodically thereafter (e.g., whenever dosage of the drug and/or concomitantly administered diuretic is increased), especially those taking potassium supplements or those with preexisting hypotension, hyponatremia, diabetes mellitus, or azotemia.

Mortality Reduction After Acute Myocardial Infarction Because of the risk of persistent hypotension (i.e., systolic blood pressure of less than 90 mm Hg lasting for more that 1 hour), lisinopril therapy should *not* be initiated in patients with myocardial infarction (MI) who are at risk of further severe hemodynamic deterioration (i.e., systolic blood pressure of 100 mm Hg or less after receiving therapy with a vasodilator) or who are in cardiogenic shock. In addition, because severe hypotension in patients with MI may result in MI or cerebrovascular accident, lisinopril therapy should be initiated under very close medical supervision in such patients, with close monitoring for the first 2 weeks of therapy and whenever dosage of the drug and/or concomitantly administered diuretic is increased. (See Hypotension under Warnings/Precautions: Warnings, in Cautions.)

To improve survival after acute MI in hemodynamically stable patients, the manufacturers state a 5-mg dose of lisinopril should be given within 24 hours of onset of symptoms of MI followed by a 5- and 10-mg dose 24 and 48 hours later, respectively; the drug should be administered in conjunction with standard therapies such as thrombolytic agents, aspirin, and/or β-blockers as appropriate. Thereafter, a maintenance dosage of 10 mg daily of lisinopril should be used and continued for 6 weeks. Patients who have low blood pressure (i.e., systolic pressure of 120 mm Hg or less) when lisinopril therapy is initiated or during the first 3 days after MI should be given a lower dose (i.e., 2.5 mg) of lisinopril; in addition, if hypotension (i.e., systolic pressure less than 100 mm Hg) occurs, the maintenance dosage should be reduced to 5 mg daily, which may be temporarily reduced further to 2.5 mg daily if needed. If prolonged hypotension occurs (i.e., systolic pressure less than 90 mm Hg lasting for more than 1 hour), lisinopril should be discontinued. Alternatively, experts recommend an initial lisinopril dosage of 2.5–5 mg daily (initiated within 24 hours of MI) titrated upward to 10 mg daily or higher as tolerated in patients with MI. For patients who develop symptoms of heart failure, the dosage indicated for heart failure should be administered. (See Dosage and Administration: Heart Failure).

■ **Special Populations** The manufacturers state that modification of the usual initial dosage (10 mg once daily) of lisinopril is not necessary in hypertensive adults with creatinine clearances exceeding 30 mL/minute per 1.73 m^2. If the drug is used in hypertensive adults with more than mildly impaired renal function, dosage must be modified in response to the degree of renal impairment, and as with other ACE inhibitors, the theoretical risk of neutropenia must be considered. Hypertensive adults with creatinine clearances of 10–30 mL/minute can receive an initial lisinopril dosage of 5 mg once daily and those with creatinine clearances less than 10 mL/minute (usually on hemodialysis) can receive an initial dosage of 2.5 mg once daily. Subsequent dosage should be titrated according to individual tolerance and blood pressure response up to a maximum of 40 mg once daily. The manufacturers state that use of lisinopril in hypertensive pediatric patients with creatinine clearances less than 30 mL/minute per 1.73 m^2 is not recommended.

The manufacturers state that adults with heart failure and hyponatremia (serum sodium concentration less than 130 mEq/L) or moderate to severe renal impairment (i.e., creatinine clearance of 30 mL/minute or less or serum creatinine exceeding 3 mg/dL) should receive an initial lisinopril dosage of 2.5 mg daily under close monitoring. (See Dosage and Administration: Dosage.)

The manufacturers state that lisinopril should be initiated with caution in patients with MI and renal impairment (serum creatinine concentrations exceeding 2 mg/dL). The manufacturers also state that dosage adjustments in patients with MI and severe renal impairment have not been evaluated. If renal impairment (serum creatinine concentrations exceeding 3 mg/dL) develops or if baseline serum creatinine concentrations are increased by 100% during lisinopril therapy, discontinuance of the drug should be considered.

When combination therapy with lisinopril and hydrochlorothiazide is required for the management of hypertension in patients with impaired renal function, the risk of precipitating hypotension during initiation of combined therapy should be considered. Dosages of the drugs should be titrated carefully by increasing slowly the dosage of each drug separately in small increments and the patient should be monitored closely. After careful titration of each drug separately, a fixed combination preparation can be substituted. If concomitant diuretic therapy is required in patients with severe renal impairment, a loop diuretic such as furosemide is preferred to a thiazide diuretic. Therefore, use of commercially available preparations containing lisinopril in fixed combination with hydrochlorothiazide is not recommended for patients with severe renal impairment.

Cautions

■ **Contraindications** History of angioedema related to previous angiotensin-converting enzyme (ACE) inhibitor treatment or of hereditary or idiopathic angioedema.

Known hypersensitivity to lisinopril, other ACE inhibitors, or any ingredient in the formulation.

Concomitant use of lisinopril and aliskiren in patients with diabetes mellitus. (See Drug Interactions: Drugs that Block the Renin-Angiotensin System.)

■ **Warnings/Precautions** ***Warnings*** When hydrochlorothiazide is used in fixed combination with lisinopril, the usual cautions, precautions, and contraindications associated with hydrochlorothiazide must be considered in addition to those associated with lisinopril. (See Cautions, in the Thiazides General Statement 40:28.20.)

Hypotension. Symptomatic hypotension may occur, sometimes associated with oliguria and/or progressive azotemia and, rarely, acute renal failure and/or death. Patients at particular risk include those with heart failure with systolic blood pressure less than 100 mm Hg, hyponatremia, high-dose or recent intensive diuretic therapy, recent increase in diuretic dose, dialysis, or severe volume and/or salt depletion of any etiology. In such patients, it may be advisable to discontinue the diuretic (except in patients with heart failure), reduce the diuretic dosage, or cautiously increase salt intake, if possible, prior to initiating lisinopril therapy. Treatment with lisinopril must not be initiated in patients with acute myocardial infarction (MI) at risk of further serious hemodynamic deterioration following treatment with a vasodilator (e.g., systolic blood pressure of 100 mm Hg or lower) or in those with cardiogenic shock. Marked hypotension may result in MI or stroke in those with acute MI or ischemic cardiovascular or cerebrovascular disease.

Hematologic Effects. Neutropenia/agranulocytosis, particularly in patients with renal impairment (especially those with concomitant collagen vascular disease), reported with captopril. Data insufficient to rule out similar incidence of agranulocytosis with lisinopril in patients without prior reactions with other ACE inhibitors. Hemolytic anemia reported rarely; causal relationship to lisinopril cannot be ruled out. Myelosuppression, leukopenia/neutropenia, and thrombocytopenia reported rarely.

Hepatic Effects. Rare ACE inhibitor-associated clinical syndrome manifested initially by cholestatic jaundice or hepatitis; may progress to fulminant hepatic necrosis and is potentially fatal. Patients receiving an ACE inhibitor, including lisinopril, who develop jaundice or marked elevations in hepatic enzymes should discontinue the drug and receive appropriate monitoring.

Fetal/Neonatal Morbidity and Mortality. ACE inhibitors can cause fetal and neonatal morbidity and mortality when used in pregnancy during the second and third trimesters. ACE inhibitors also increase the risk of major congenital malformations when administered during the first trimester of pregnancy. Discontinue as soon as possible when pregnancy is detected, unless continued use is considered lifesaving. Nearly all women can be transferred successfully to alternative therapy for the remainder of their pregnancy. For additional information on the risk of ACE inhibitors during pregnancy, see Cautions: Pregnancy, Fertility, and Lactation, in Captopril 24:32.04 and Enalaprilat/Enalapril 24:32.04.

Sensitivity Reactions Sensitivity reactions, including anaphylactoid reactions and angioedema (including laryngeal edema, tongue edema), are potentially fatal. Patients with head and neck angioedema involving the tongue, glottis, or larynx are likely to experience airway obstruction, especially in those with a history of airway surgery. If laryngeal stridor or angioedema of the face, lips, tongue, or glottis occurs, lisinopril should be discontinued and appropriate therapy (e.g., epinephrine) should be initiated immediately. Antihistamines and corticosteroids may not provide sufficient relief of symptoms even in patients experiencing only swelling of the tongue; prolonged observation may be necessary. Caution in patients with history of angioedema unrelated to ACE inhibitor therapy.

Intestinal angioedema (occasionally without a prior history of facial angioedema or elevated serum levels of complement 1 [C1] esterase inhibitor) also has been reported in patients receiving ACE inhibitors. Intestinal angioedema, which frequently presents as abdominal pain (with or without nausea or vomiting), usually is diagnosed by abdominal CT scan, ultrasound, or surgery; manifestations usually have resolved after discontinuance of the ACE inhibitor. Intestinal angioedema should be considered in the differential diagnosis of patients who develop abdominal pain during therapy with an ACE inhibitor.

Life-threatening anaphylactoid reactions reported in at least 2 patients receiving ACE inhibitors while undergoing desensitization with hymenoptera venom. Such reactions did not occur when ACE inhibitors were temporarily discontinued before desensitization but did recur following inadvertent rechallenge. Sudden and potentially life-threatening anaphylactoid reactions also have been reported in patients receiving ACE inhibitors while undergoing hemodialysis using high-flux membranes. In such patients, dialysis should be discontinued immediately, and aggressive therapy for anaphylactic reactions should be initiated. Antihistamines have not been effective for relieving symptoms in these patients; use of a different type of dialysis membrane or a different class of antihypertensive agent should be considered. In addition, anaphylactoid reactions have been reported in patients undergoing low-density lipoprotein (LDL) apheresis with dextran sulfate absorption.

General Precautions **Aortic Stenosis/Hypertrophic Cardiomyopathy.** Like other vasodilators, lisinopril should be administered with caution in patients with obstruction in the outflow tract of the left ventricle (e.g., aortic stenosis, hypertrophic cardiomyopathy).

Renal Effects. Inhibition of the renin-angiotensin-aldosterone (RAA) system may cause renal impairment and rarely renal failure and/or death in susceptible patients (e.g., those whose renal function depends on the activity of the RAA system such as patients with severe heart failure).

Deterioration of renal function, usually reversible upon discontinuance of the drug, manifested as minor and transient increases in BUN and serum creatinine concentrations, may occur following administration of ACE inhibitor therapy, particularly in hypertensive patients with unilateral or bilateral renal artery stenosis, preexisting renal impairment, or concomitant diuretic therapy. Renal function should be monitored during the first few weeks of therapy in such patients; dosage reduction and/or discontinuance of lisinopril and/or the diuretic may be required.

Renal artery stenosis, preexisting renal impairment, and concomitant diuretic therapy also are risk factors for renal impairment during ACE inhibitor therapy. In patients with acute MI who have evidence of renal dysfunction (i.e., serum creatinine concentration exceeding 2 mg/dL), consider discontinuance of lisinopril if serum creatinine exceeds 3 mg/dL or doubles from pretreatment value.

Hyperkalemia. Hyperkalemia can develop, especially in those with renal impairment or diabetes mellitus and those receiving drugs that can increase serum potassium concentration (e.g., potassium-sparing diuretics, potassium supplements, potassium-containing salt substitutes). Hyperkalemia can result in serious, potentially fatal, cardiac arrhythmias.

Cough. Persistent and nonproductive cough reported with all ACE inhibitors; resolves after drug discontinuance.

Surgery/Anesthesia. Hypotension may occur in patients undergoing surgery or during anesthesia with agents that produce hypotension.

Specific Populations **Pregnancy.** Category C (first trimester); Category D (second and third trimesters). (See Users Guide.) (See: Fetal/Neonatal Morbidity and Mortality under Warnings/Precautions: Warnings, in Cautions.)

Lactation. Lisinopril is distributed into milk (as determined by presence of radioactivity following administration of radiolabeled drug) in rats; not known whether the drug is distributed into milk in humans. Hydrochlorothiazide is distributed into human milk. Because of the potential for serious adverse reactions to ACE inhibitors (e.g., lisinopril) in nursing infants, a decision should be made whether to discontinue nursing or lisinopril (either alone or in fixed combination with hydrochlorothiazide), taking into account the importance of the drug(s) to the woman.

Pediatric Use. Safety and efficacy not established in children less than 6 years of age and in pediatric patients with creatinine clearances less than 30 mL/minute per 1.73 m^2. For information on overall principles and expert recommendations for treatment of hypertension in pediatric patients, see Uses: Hypertension in Pediatric Patients, in the Thiazides General Statement 40:28.20.

Geriatric Use. Clinical studies of lisinopril alone or in fixed combination with hydrochlorothiazide did not include sufficient numbers of patients (with hypertension and heart failure) 65 years of age and older to determine whether geriatric patients respond differently than younger patients, but other clinical experience has not revealed age-related differences. In pharmacokinetic studies, peak plasma concentrations and area under the plasma concentration-time curve (AUC) of lisinopril were increased in geriatric individuals compared with younger individuals. Drug dosage generally should be titrated carefully in geriatric patients, usually initiating therapy at the low end of the dosage range. The greater frequency of decreased hepatic, renal, and/or cardiac function and of concomitant disease and drug therapy observed in the elderly also should be considered.

Renal Impairment. Renal function may decrease with ACE inhibitor therapy in susceptible patients. Use with caution in those with renal impairment. (See Dosage and Administration: Special Populations and also Renal Effects under Warnings/Precautions: General Precautions, in Cautions.)

Black Patients. ACE inhibitors not as effective for decreasing blood pressure. Increased incidence of angioedema. (See Uses: Hypertension.)

■ **Common Adverse Effects** Adverse effects reported in greater than 1% of patients receiving lisinopril or lisinopril in fixed combination with hydrochlorothiazide for the management of hypertension and more frequently than with placebo include headache, dizziness, cough, fatigue, diarrhea, upper respiratory tract infection, nausea, asthenia, rash, orthostatic effects, hypotension, vomiting, hyperkalemia, or minor increases in BUN and serum creatinine concentrations. Additional adverse effects reported in 1% or more of patients receiving lisinopril in fixed combination with hydrochlorothiazide include dyspepsia, muscle cramps, paresthesia, decreased libido, vertigo, nasal congestion, influenza, or impotence.

Adverse effects reported in greater than 1% of patients receiving lisinopril for the management of heart failure and more frequently than with placebo include dizziness, hypotension, headache, diarrhea, chest pain, nausea, abdominal pain, rash, and upper respiratory tract infection.

In a large trial in patients with acute MI, hypotension and renal dysfunction occurred more frequently in patients receiving lisinopril than in those not receiving the drug.

Drug Interactions

■ **Drugs that Block the Renin-Angiotensin System** Increased risk of hypotension, syncope, hyperkalemia, and changes in renal function (e.g., acute renal failure) with concomitant use of other drugs that block the renin-angiotensin system (e.g., aliskiren, angiotensin II receptor antagonists); when lisinopril is used concomitantly with such drugs, blood pressure, renal function, and serum electrolyte concentrations should be monitored closely. Concomitant use of lisinopril and aliskiren is contraindicated in patients with diabetes mellitus; in addition, such concomitant use should be avoided in patients with renal impairment (glomerular filtration rate [GFR] less than 60 mL/minute per 1.73 m^2). (See Cautions in Aliskiren Hemifumarate 24:32.40.)

■ **Drugs Increasing Serum Potassium Concentration** Potential pharmacologic interaction (additive hyperkalemic effect). Includes potassium-sparing diuretics, potassium supplements, and other drugs that can increase serum potassium. The manufacturer states that lisinopril should be used cautiously (with frequent monitoring of serum potassium), if at all, with potassium supplements or salt substitutes containing potassium.

■ **Antidiabetic Agents** Potential pharmacologic interaction (increased hypoglycemic effect), especially during initial weeks of combined treatment and in patients with renal impairment.

■ **Digoxin** Clinically important adverse interaction not observed.

■ **Diuretics** Potential pharmacokinetic and pharmacologic interaction (hypotensive effect).

■ **Gold Compounds** Rare reports of nitritoid reactions (manifested by facial flushing, nausea, vomiting, and hypotension) in patients receiving parenteral aurothioglucose and gold sodium thiomalate concomitantly with ACE inhibitors, including lisinopril.

■ **Lithium** Potential pharmacokinetic interaction (increased lithium concentrations and clinical toxicity).

■ **Nonsteroidal Anti-inflammatory Agents** Potential pharmacologic interaction (decreased antihypertensive effect) when lisinopril is used concomitantly concurrently with nonsteroidal anti-inflammatory agents (NSAIAs). Potential pharmacologic interaction (decreased renal function) when lisinopril is used concomitantly with NSAIAs in patients with impaired renal function. (See Drug Interactions in Captopril 24:32.04.)

■ **Propranolol** Clinically important pharmacokinetic interaction not observed.

Description

Lisinopril is an angiotensin-converting enzyme (ACE, bradykinase, kininase II) inhibitor. Like benazepril, enalapril, fosinopril, quinapril, and ramipril but unlike captopril, lisinopril does not contain a sulfhydryl group.

Unlike enalapril, quinapril, fosinopril, and ramipril but like captopril, lisinopril is *not* a prodrug but instead is active unchanged.

Advice to Patients

Risk of angioedema, anaphylactoid, and other sensitivity reactions and importance of discontinuing the drug and reporting suggestive manifestations (e.g., edema of face, eyes, lips, or tongue; swallowing or breathing with difficulty) to a clinician.

Risk of hypotension (e.g., lightheadedness, syncope), especially during initial therapy and with volume depletion secondary to excessive perspiration or dehydration, vomiting, or diarrhea. Importance of adequate fluid intake. Importance of discontinuing drug and contacting clinician if symptoms of syncope occur.

Importance of contacting a clinician promptly if manifestations of infection or neutropenia (e.g., sore throat, fever) develop.

Importance of informing clinicians of existing or contemplated concomitant therapy, including prescription and OTC drugs. Risk of hyperkalemia; importance of avoiding use of potassium supplements or salt substitutes containing potassium without consultation with a clinician.

Risk of hypoglycemia in patients receiving concomitant therapy with insulin or oral antidiabetic agents. Importance of closely monitoring blood glucose concentrations, especially during the first month of combined use.

Importance of women informing clinicians immediately if they are or plan to become pregnant or plan to breast-feed. Risk of use during first, second, and third trimesters of pregnancy.

Importance of informing patients of other important precautionary information. (See Cautions.)

Overview® (see Users Guide). For additional information on this drug until a more detailed monograph is developed and published, the manufacturer's labeling should be consulted. It is *essential* that the manufacturer's labeling be consulted for more detailed information on usual cautions, precautions, contraindications, laboratory test interferences, and acute toxicity.

Preparations

Excipients in commercially available drug preparations may have clinically important effects in some individuals; consult specific product labeling for details.

Lisinopril

Oral		
Tablets	2.5 mg*	Zestril®, AstraZeneca
	5 mg*	Prinivil®, Merck
		Zestril®, AstraZeneca
	10 mg*	Prinivil®, Merck
		Zestril®, AstraZeneca
	20 mg*	Prinivil®, Merck
		Zestril®, AstraZeneca
	30 mg*	Zestril®, AstraZeneca
	40 mg*	Zestril®, AstraZeneca

*available from one or more manufacturer, distributor, and/or repackager by generic (nonproprietary) name

Lisinopril Combinations

Oral		
Tablets	10 mg with Hydrochlorothiazide 12.5 mg*	Prinzide®, Merck
		Zestoretic®, AstraZeneca
	20 mg with Hydrochlorothiazide 12.5 mg*	Prinzide®, Merck
		Zestoretic®, AstraZeneca
	20 mg with Hydrochlorothiazide 25 mg*	Prinzide®, Merck
		Zestoretic®, AstraZeneca

*available from one or more manufacturer, distributor, and/or repackager by generic (nonproprietary) name

†Use is not currently included in the labeling approved by the US Food and Drug Administration

Ramipril

■ Ramipril is an angiotensin-converting enzyme (ACE) inhibitor.

Uses

Ramipril is used alone or in combination with other classes of antihypertensive agents (e.g., thiazide diuretics) in the management of hypertension. Ramipril also is used to reduce the risk of mortality (mainly cardiovascular mortality) following myocardial infarction (MI) in hemodynamically stable patients who have demonstrated clinical signs of heart failure within a few days following acute MI; ramipril therapy also may reduce rate of heart failure-associated hospitalization and progression to severe and/or resistant heart failure. In addition, ramipril has been shown to reduce the rate of death, MI, and stroke in patients at high risk for cardiovascular events†.

Because captopril, another angiotensin-converting enzyme (ACE) inhibitor, may cause serious adverse effects (e.g., neutropenia, agranulocytosis), particularly in patients with renal impairment (especially those with collagen vascular disease) or in patients receiving immunosuppressive therapy, the possibility that similar adverse effects may occur with ramipril should be considered since current evidence is insufficient to rule out such risk. (See Cautions: Hematologic Effects, in Captopril 24:32.04.)

■ **Hypertension** Ramipril is used alone or in combination with other classes of antihypertensive agents in the management of hypertension. ACE inhibitors are considered one of several preferred antihypertensive drugs for the initial management of hypertension according to current evidence-based hypertension guidelines; other preferred options include angiotensin II receptor antagonists, calcium-channel blockers, and thiazide diuretics. While there may be individual differences with respect to recommendations for initial drug selection and use in specific patient populations, current evidence indicates that these antihypertensive drug classes all generally produce comparable effects on overall mortality and cardiovascular, cerebrovascular, and renal outcomes. (See Uses: Hypertension, in Captopril 24:32.04.)

ACE inhibitors may be particularly useful in the management of hypertension in patients with certain coexisting conditions such as heart failure, ischemic heart disease, diabetes mellitus, chronic kidney disease (CKD), or cerebrovascular disease or following MI. (See Uses: Hypertension in Captopril 24:32.04 and in Enalaprilat/Enalapril 24:32.04.)

In patients with hypertension and compelling indications (e.g., CKD with albuminuria [urine albumin 300 mg/day or greater, or urine albumin:creatinine ratio of 300 mg/g or equivalent in the first morning void]), angiotensin II receptor antagonists are usually considered an alternative for ACE inhibitor-intolerant patients. However, data indicate no difference in efficacy between ACE inhibitors and angiotensin II receptor antagonists with regard to blood pressure lowering and clinical outcomes (i.e., all-cause mortality, cardiovascular mortality, MI, heart failure, stroke, and end-stage renal disease). Adverse events (e.g., cough, angioedema) leading to drug discontinuance occur more frequently with ACE inhibitor therapy than with angiotensin II receptor antagonist therapy. Because of similar efficacy and a lower frequency of adverse effects, some experts believe that an angiotensin II receptor antagonist should be used instead of an ACE inhibitor for the treatment of hypertension or hypertension with certain compelling indications.

Most patients with hypertension, especially black patients, will require at least 2 antihypertensive drugs to achieve adequate blood pressure control. In general, black hypertensive patients tend to respond better to monotherapy with diuretics or calcium-channel blockers than to monotherapy with ACE inhibitors. Although ACE inhibitors have lowered blood pressure in all races studied, monotherapy with these agents has produced a smaller reduction in blood pressure in black hypertensive patients, a population associated with low renin hypertension. However, the combination of an ACE inhibitor or an angiotensin II receptor antagonist with a calcium-channel blocker or thiazide diuretic produces similar blood pressure lowering in black patients as in other racial groups. In addition, ACE inhibitors appear to produce a higher incidence of angioedema in black patients than in other races studied. (See Race under Hypertension: Other Special Considerations for Antihypertensive Drug Therapy, in Uses in Captopril 24:32.04 and in Enalaprilat/Enalapril 24:32.04.)

For additional information on the role of ACE inhibitors in the management of hypertension, see Uses in Captopril 24:32.04 and in Enalaprilat/Enalapril 24:32.04. For information on overall principles and expert recommendations for treatment of hypertension, see Uses: Hypertension in Adults and also see Uses: Hypertension in Pediatric Patients, in the Thiazides General Statement 40:28.20.

■ **Heart Failure After Acute Myocardial Infarction** Ramipril is used to reduce the risk of mortality (mainly cardiovascular mortality) following MI in hemodynamically stable patients who have demonstrated clinical signs of heart failure within a few days following acute MI; ramipril therapy also may reduce the rate of heart failure-associated hospitalization and progression to severe and/or resistant heart failure. In these patients, when compared with those receiving placebo, ramipril therapy initiated on average 5 (range: 2–9) days after acute MI reduced risk of mortality from any cause by approximately 27% (90% of mortality was cardiovascular, mainly sudden death); risk of progression to severe heart failure and heart failure-associated hospitalization were reduced by 23 and 26%, respectively. In addition, ramipril reduced risk of mortality combined with other events (e.g., reinfarction, stroke, development of severe heart failure) by 19%. This evidence of efficacy was obtained from a large, controlled, long-term (average: 15 months; range: 6–46 months) study (the Acute Infarction Ramipril Efficacy; AIRE). Benefits of ramipril were observed by day 30 of drug therapy and were not affected by gender, exact timing of initiation of drug therapy, or by concomitant drugs (e.g., aspirin, nitrates, β-adrenergic blocking agents [β-blockers], thrombolytic agents, calcium-channel blocking agents, cardiac glycosides); however, such benefits appeared to be increased in patients 65 years and older and in those receiving diuretics. Ramipril did not appear to reduce the rates of reinfarction, although there was a trend to fewer such events when compared with placebo.

Studies with various ACE inhibitors have shown that these drugs reduce fatal and nonfatal cardiovascular events in patients with recent MI. The magnitude of benefit appears to be greatest in certain high-risk patients (e.g., those with an anterior infarct, ejection fraction of 40% or less, heart failure, prior infarction, or tachycardia). In addition to their effects on mortality, ACE inhibitors also are used to minimize or prevent the development of left ventricular dilatation and dysfunction (ventricular "remodeling") following acute MI. Evidence regarding the efficacy of such therapy has been somewhat conflicting, particularly when parenteral therapy was initiated early (within 24–48 hours) and included patients with no evidence of baseline left ventricular dysfunction. (See Uses: Left Ventricular Dysfunction After Acute Myocardial Infarction in Enalaprilat/Enalapril 24:32.04.) However, the preponderance of evidence has shown a benefit of early oral therapy with ACE inhibitors, even in patients with no baseline dysfunction.

Current expert guidelines recommend the use of an oral ACE inhibitor within the first 24 hours of acute MI in patients with an anterior infarction, heart failure, or ejection fraction of 40% or less who do not have any contraindications (e.g., hypotension, shock, renal dysfunction). While early treatment within the first 24 hours of MI has been shown to be beneficial, ACE inhibitors should be used with caution (and with gradual upward titration) during the initial postinfarction period because of the possibility of hypotension or renal dysfunction. ACE inhibitor therapy generally should be continued indefinitely in all patients with left ventricular dysfunction or other compelling indications for use (e.g., hypertension, diabetes mellitus, CKD). The benefits of long-term ACE inhibitor therapy are less certain in low-risk patients who have undergone revascularization and are receiving aggressive antilipemic therapy.

■ Prevention of Major Cardiovascular Events Ramipril may reduce the rate of death, MI, and stroke in patients 55 years of age and older who are at high risk for cardiovascular events (e.g., those with a history of coronary artery disease, stroke, peripheral vascular disease, or diabetes mellitus, in addition to at least one other cardiovascular risk factor, including hypertension, elevated serum total cholesterol and/or decreased high-density lipoprotein [HDL]-cholesterol concentrations, smoking, or documented microalbuminuria) and who are not known to have low left ventricular ejection fraction (LVEF) or heart failure. Ramipril may be used concomitantly with antihypertensive, antiplatelet, or antilipemic drugs. Results of a randomized, multicenter, double-blind, placebo-controlled study (Heart Outcomes Prevention Evaluation [HOPE]) of approximately 5 years' duration in more than 9000 patients 55 years of age or older with a history of coronary artery disease, stroke, peripheral vascular disease, and at least one other cardiovascular risk factor (see above) indicate that ramipril (10 mg daily after an initial dosage of 2.5 mg daily for 1 week followed by 5 mg daily for 3 weeks) reduced the risk of cardiovascular death, stroke, and MI by about 25, 32, and 20%, respectively, compared with placebo. When compared with placebo, the drug also reduced the risk of cardiac arrest and heart failure by approximately 34 and 21%, respectively, and the need for coronary revascularization procedures by 15%. The exact mechanism of the beneficial effects of ramipril in high-risk patients for cardiovascular events has not been fully elucidated, but it appears that ACE inhibitors may antagonize the direct effects of angiotensin II thereby preventing the proliferation of vascular smooth muscle cells and rupture of fibrous plaques. ACE inhibitors also may improve vascular endothelial function, reduce left ventricular hypertrophy, and enhance fibrinolysis.

In addition to these beneficial cardiovascular effects, a reduction in the incidence of diabetic complications was reported in 6.2% of patients receiving ramipril compared with 7.4% of those receiving placebo. New diagnosis of diabetes was reported in fewer patients receiving ramipril compared with those receiving placebo. Although the exact mechanism of the endocrine effects of ramipril is not known, it has been suggested that ACE inhibitors may prevent diabetic complications and new diagnosis of diabetes by improving insulin sensitivity and blood flow to the pancreas and by decreasing hepatic clearance of insulin. In addition, results of other studies indicate that in patients with type 2 diabetes mellitus, intensive control of blood pressure (e.g., an approximate target systolic pressure of less than 150 mm Hg and diastolic pressure of less than 85 mm Hg) using an ACE inhibitor (e.g., captopril) or a β-blocker (e.g., atenolol) resulted in a reduction of development or progression of complications of diabetes (e.g., death related to diabetes, stroke, heart failure, microvascular disease).

In the HOPE study, reduction of cardiovascular risk factors was observed within 1 year of initiation of ramipril therapy and continued throughout the study (approximately 5 years). Because interim analysis of this study after about 5 years revealed a clear evidence of a beneficial effect of ramipril, the study was discontinued.

■ Heart Failure ACE inhibitors have been used in the management of heart failure†, usually in conjunction with other agents such as cardiac glycosides, diuretics, and β-blockers.

Current guidelines for the management of heart failure in adults generally recommend a combination of drug therapies to reduce morbidity and mortality, including neurohormonal antagonists (e.g., ACE inhibitors, angiotensin II receptor antagonists, angiotensin receptor-neprilysin inhibitors [ARNIs], β-blockers, aldosterone receptor antagonists) that inhibit the detrimental compensatory mechanisms in heart failure. Additional agents (e.g., cardiac glycosides, diuretics, sinoatrial modulators [i.e., ivabradine]) added to a heart failure treatment regimen in selected patients have been associated with symptomatic improvement and/or reduction in heart failure-related hospitalizations. Experts recommend that all asymptomatic patients with reduced LVEF (American College of Cardiology Foundation [ACCF]/American Heart Association [AHA] stage B heart failure) receive therapy with an ACE inhibitor and β-blocker to prevent symptomatic heart failure and to reduce morbidity and mortality. In patients with prior or current symptoms of chronic heart failure and reduced LVEF (ACCF/AHA stage C heart failure), ACCF, AHA, and the Heart Failure Society of America (HFSA) recommend inhibition of the renin-angiotensin-aldosterone (RAA) system with an ACE inhibitor, angiotensin II receptor antagonist, or ARNI in conjunction with a β-blocker, and an aldosterone antagonist in selected patients, to reduce morbidity and mortality. While ACE inhibitors have been the preferred drugs for inhibition of the RAA system because of their established benefits in patients with heart failure and reduced ejection fraction, some evidence indicates that therapy with sacubitril/valsartan, an ARNI, may be more effective than ACE inhibitor therapy (enalapril) in reducing cardiovascular death and heart failure-related hospitalization in such patients. ACCF, AHA, and HFSA recommend that patients with chronic symptomatic heart failure and reduced LVEF (New York Heart Association [NYHA] class II or III) who are able to tolerate an ACE inhibitor or angiotensin II receptor antagonist be switched to therapy containing an ARNI to further reduce morbidity and mortality. However, in patients in whom an ARNI is not appropriate, continued use of an ACE inhibitor for all classes of heart failure with reduced ejection fraction remains strongly advised. In patients in whom an ARNI or ACE inhibitor is not appropriate, an angiotensin II receptor antagonist may be used. For additional information on the use of ACE inhibitors in the management of heart failure, see Uses: Heart Failure, in Captopril 24:32.04 and in Enalaprilat/Enalapril 24:32.04. For further information on the use of ARNIs in patients with heart failure, see Uses: Heart Failure, in Sacubitril and Valsartan 24:32.92.

■ Diabetic Nephropathy Both ACE inhibitors and angiotensin II receptor antagonists have been shown to slow the rate of progression of renal disease in patients with diabetes mellitus and persistent albuminuria†, and use of a drug from either class is recommended in such patients with modestly elevated (30–300 mg/24 hours) or higher (exceeding 300 mg/24 hours) levels of urinary albumin excretion. The usual precautions of ACE inhibitor or angiotensin II receptor antagonist therapy in patients with substantial renal impairment should be observed. For additional information on the use of ACE inhibitors in the treatment of diabetic nephropathy, see Diabetic Nephropathy under Uses: Nephropathy, in Captopril 24:32.04.

Dosage and Administration

■ Administration Ramipril is administered orally. The rate but not the extent of GI absorption of the drug may be reduced by administration with food. Ramipril capsules usually are swallowed whole. However, if needed such capsules also may be opened and contents sprinkled in a small amount (about 120 mL) of applesauce or mixed in 120 mL of water or apple juice. To ensure that no drug is lost, the entire mixture should be consumed. These mixtures are stable for 24 hours at room temperature and 48 hours when refrigerated. The manufacturers state that serum ramiprilat concentrations are not affected when contents of ramipril capsules are mixed in applesauce or dissolved in water or apple juice.

■ Dosage Dosage of ramipril must be adjusted according to patient tolerance and response. Because of the risk of inducing hypotension, initiation of ramipril therapy requires consideration of recent antihypertensive therapy, the extent of blood pressure elevation, sodium intake, fluid status, and other clinical circumstances. If therapy is initiated in a patient already receiving a diuretic, symptomatic hypotension may occur following the initial dose of the angiotensin-converting enzyme (ACE) inhibitor. To minimize the possibility of hypotension, especially in patients in whom diuretic therapy was recently initiated, it is recommended that diuretic therapy be discontinued, the diuretic dosage decreased, or salt intake increased, if possible, before initiating ramipril. If such changes are not possible, ramipril therapy should be initiated at a reduced dosage of 1.25 mg once daily. (See Cardiovascular Effects under Warnings/Precautions: Warnings, in Cautions.) For additional information on initiating ramipril in patients receiving diuretic therapy, see the disease-specific dosage sections in Dosage and Administration. Hypotension does not preclude the administration of subsequent doses of the drug, provided the hypotension has been managed effectively.

Hypertension **Usual Dosage.** For the management of hypertension in adults *not* receiving a diuretic, the manufacturer states that the usual initial dosage of ramipril is 2.5 mg once daily. In patients currently receiving a diuretic, an initial ramipril dosage of 1.25 mg once daily is recommended; however, discontinuance or dosage reduction of the diuretic or an increase in salt intake is preferred. (See the introductory discussion under Dosage and Administration: Dosage.) Subsequent dosage of ramipril should be adjusted according to the patient's blood pressure response. If the blood pressure response diminishes toward the end of the dosing interval during once-daily administration, increasing the dosage or giving the drug in 2 divided doses daily should be considered. The usual maintenance dosage recommended by the manufacturer and some experts in adults is 2.5–20 mg daily, given as a single dose or in 2 divided doses.

Blood Pressure Monitoring and Treatment Goals. Blood pressure should be monitored regularly (i.e., monthly) during therapy and dosage of the antihypertensive drug adjusted until blood pressure is controlled. If an adequate blood pressure response is not achieved with ACE inhibitor monotherapy, the dosage may be increased or another antihypertensive agent with demonstrated benefit and preferably with a complementary mechanism of action (e.g., calcium-channel blocker, thiazide diuretic) may be added; if target blood pressure is still not achieved, a third drug may be added. (See Uses: Hypertension.) In patients who develop unacceptable adverse effects with ramipril, the drug should be discontinued and another antihypertensive agent from a different pharmacologic class should be initiated.

The goal of hypertension management and prevention is to achieve and maintain optimal control of blood pressure. However, the optimum blood pressure threshold for initiating antihypertensive drug therapy and specific treatment goals remain controversial. While other hypertension guidelines have based target blood pressure goals on age and comorbidities, a 2017 multidisciplinary hypertension guideline from the American College of Cardiology (ACC), American Heart Association (AHA), and a number of other professional organizations incorporates underlying cardiovascular risk into decision making regarding treatment and generally recommends the same target blood pressure (i.e., less than 130/80 mm Hg) in all adults. Many patients will require at least 2 drugs from different pharmacologic classes to achieve this blood pressure goal; the potential benefits of hypertension management and drug cost, adverse effects, and risks associated with the use of multiple antihypertensive drugs also should be considered when deciding a patient's blood pressure treatment goal.

For additional information on target levels of blood pressure and on monitoring therapy in the management of hypertension, see Blood Pressure Monitoring and Treatment Goals under Dosage: Hypertension, in Dosage and Administration in the Thiazides General Statement 40:28.20.

Heart Failure After Acute Myocardial Infarction When used after myocardial infarction (MI) in adults with clinical signs of heart failure, the manufacturer recommends an initial ramipril dosage of 2.5 mg twice daily, but if hypotension occurs, dosage should be reduced to 1.25 mg twice daily. Some clinicians recommend initiation of therapy within the first 24 hours following MI. After one week at the initial dosage, therapy is then titrated as tolerated, at intervals of about 3 weeks, to a target daily dosage of 5 mg twice daily. After the initial dose of ramipril, the patient should be observed closely for at least 2 hours and for at least 1 additional hour after blood pressure has stabilized. To minimize the likelihood of hypotension, the dosage of any concomitant diuretic should be reduced, if possible. The appearance of hypotension after the initial dose of ramipril does not preclude subsequent carefully titrated doses of the drug after the hypotension has been effectively managed. Dosage should be adjusted carefully under close medical supervision in patients with heart failure because of the risk of hypotension; such patients should be followed closely for at least 2 weeks after initiation of ramipril therapy or any increase in ramipril or diuretic dosage.

Prevention of Major Cardiovascular Events For reduction in the risk of MI, stroke, and death from cardiovascular causes, the manufacturers recommend that patients receive 2.5 mg once daily for the first week of therapy and 5 mg once daily for the following 3 weeks; dosage then may be increased, as tolerated, to a maintenance dosage of 10 mg once daily. In patients with hypertension or those with recent MI, dosage of ramipril may be given in divided doses.

Heart Failure In patients with prior or current symptoms of chronic heart failure and reduced LVEF (American College of Cardiology Foundation [ACCF]/American Heart Association [AHA] stage C heart failure†), ACCF and AHA recommend an initial ramipril dosage of 1.25–2.5 mg once daily. The dosage should be slowly titrated upward as tolerated to dosages that have been shown to reduce the risk of cardiovascular events in clinical trials; if such target dosages cannot be achieved or are poorly tolerated, ACCF and AHA state that intermediate doses should be used. ACCF and AHA recommend a maximum ramipril dosage of 10 mg once daily for patients with ACCF/AHA stage C heart failure.

■ **Special Populations** If ramipril is used in patients with impaired renal function, dosage must be modified in response to the degree of renal impairment, and as with other ACE inhibitors, the theoretical risk of neutropenia must be considered. In adults with creatinine clearances less than 40 mL/minute, 25% of the usual doses are expected to induce full therapeutic concentrations of ramiprilat. For the management of hypertension in these patients, the usual initial dosage of ramipril is 1.25 mg once daily. Subsequent dosage should be titrated according to individual tolerance and blood pressure response, up to a maximum of 5 mg daily. In patients with heart failure following acute MI and who have creatinine clearances less than 40 mL/minute, the usual initial dosage of ramipril is 1.25 mg once daily; dosage may be increased to 1.25 mg twice daily. Subsequent dosage should be titrated according to individual clinical response and tolerance up to a maximum dosage of 2.5 mg twice daily.

Patients with known or suspected renal artery stenosis should receive an initial ramipril dosage of 1.25 mg once daily; subsequent dosage should be adjusted based on blood pressure response.

Since ramipril is primarily metabolized by hepatic esterases to ramiprilat (its active moiety), hepatic impairment may result in increased ramipril plasma concentrations. In addition, the renin-angiotensin-aldosterone (RAA) system (see Renal Effects under Warnings/Precautions: General Precautions, in Cautions) may be activated in hypertensive patients with severe hepatic impairment (e.g., severe liver cirrhosis and/or ascites). However, the manufacturers make no specific recommendations regarding dosage adjustment in patients with hepatic impairment.

For additional information on initiating and adjusting ramipril dosage in the management of hypertension, including recommendations for blood pressure monitoring, see Dosage: Hypertension, under Dosage and Administration, in Captopril 24:32.04 and in Enalaprilat/Enalapril 24:32.04.

Cautions

■ **Contraindications** History of angioedema related to previous angiotensin-converting enzyme (ACE) inhibitor treatment.

Known hypersensitivity to ramipril, other ACE inhibitors, or any ingredient in the formulation.

Concomitant use of ramipril and aliskiren in patients with diabetes mellitus. (See Drug Interactions: Drugs that Block the Renin-Angiotensin System.)

■ **Warnings/Precautions** ***Warnings*** **Hypotension.** Like other ACE inhibitors, ramipril rarely is associated with hypotension in patients with uncomplicated hypertension. Symptomatic hypotension may occur; patients at particular risk include those with severe volume and/or salt depletion secondary to prolonged diuretic therapy, dietary salt restriction, dialysis, diarrhea, or vomiting. Volume and/or salt depletion should be corrected before starting ramipril therapy.

Marked hypotension may occur in patients with heart failure (with or without associated renal impairment), which may be associated with oliguria and/or progressive azotemia and, rarely, acute renal failure and/or death. In patients with heart failure, ramipril therapy should be started under close medical supervision, and patients should be followed closely for at least 2 weeks after initiation of ramipril or diuretic therapy or dosage adjustment of either drug. (See Dosage and Administration: Dosage.)

If hypotension occurs, the patient should be placed in the supine position, and if necessary, an IV infusion of 0.9% sodium chloride injection to expand fluid volume should be administered. Ramipril therapy usually may be continued following restoration of blood pressure and volume.

Hematologic Effects. Neutropenia/agranulocytosis, anemia, leukopenia, thrombocytopenia, pancytopenia may occur in patients receiving ACE inhibitors, particularly in patients with renal impairment (especially those with concomitant collagen vascular disease [e.g., systemic lupus erythematosus, scleroderma]). Monitoring of leukocytes in patients with collagen vascular disease, especially if renal impairment exists, should be considered.

Fetal/Neonatal Morbidity and Mortality. ACE inhibitors can cause fetal and neonatal morbidity and mortality when used in pregnancy during the second and third trimesters. ACE inhibitors also increase the risk of major congenital malformations when administered during the first trimester of pregnancy. Discontinue as soon as possible when pregnancy is detected, unless continued use is considered lifesaving. Nearly all women can be transferred successfully to alternative therapy for the remainder of their pregnancy. For additional information on the risk of ACE inhibitors during pregnancy, see Cautions: Pregnancy, Fertility, and Lactation, in Captopril 24:32.04.

Hepatic Effects. Rare ACE inhibitor-associated clinical syndrome manifested initially by cholestatic jaundice may occur; may progress to fulminant hepatic necrosis and is potentially fatal. Patients receiving an ACE inhibitor, including ramipril, who develop jaundice or marked elevations in hepatic enzymes should discontinue the drug and receive appropriate monitoring.

Sensitivity Reactions Sensitivity reactions, including anaphylactic reactions and angioedema (including laryngeal or tongue edema) are potentially fatal. Head and neck angioedema involving the tongue, glottis, or larynx may cause airway obstruction. If laryngeal stridor or angioedema of the face, tongue, or glottis occurs, ramipril should be discontinued and appropriate therapy (e.g., epinephrine) should be initiated immediately.

Intestinal angioedema (occasionally without a prior history of facial angioedema or elevated serum levels of complement 1 [C1] esterase inhibitor) also has been reported in patients receiving ACE inhibitors. Intestinal angioedema, which frequently presents as abdominal pain (with or without nausea or vomiting), usually is diagnosed by abdominal CT scan, ultrasound, or surgery; symptoms usually have resolved after discontinuance of the ACE inhibitor. Intestinal angioedema should be considered in the differential diagnosis of patients who develop abdominal pain during therapy with an ACE inhibitor.

Patients receiving concomitant mammalian target of rapamycin (mTOR) inhibitors (e.g., temsirolimus) may be at increased risk for angioedema.

Life-threatening anaphylactoid reactions have been reported in at least 2 patients receiving ACE inhibitors while undergoing desensitization treatment with hymenoptera venom. When ACE inhibitors were temporarily discontinued before desensitization with the venom, anaphylactoid reactions did not recur; however, such reactions recurred after inadvertent rechallenge. Anaphylactoid reactions have been reported following initiation of hemodialysis that used a high-flux membrane in patients receiving an ACE inhibitor. In addition, anaphylactoid reactions have been reported in patients undergoing low-density lipoprotein (LDL) apheresis with dextran sulfate absorption.

General Precautions **Renal Effects.** Inhibition of the renin-angiotensin-aldosterone (RAA) system may cause renal impairment and rarely renal failure and/or death in susceptible patients (e.g., those whose renal function depends on the activity of the RAA system such as patients with severe heart failure).

Deterioration in renal function, manifested as transient increases in BUN and serum creatinine concentrations may occur following administration of ACE inhibitor therapy, particularly in hypertensive patients with unilateral or bilateral renal-artery stenosis, preexisting renal impairment, or concomitant diuretic therapy. This effect was usually reversible following discontinuance of ACE inhibitor and/or diuretic therapy. Renal function should be monitored closely during the first few weeks of therapy and periodically thereafter in such patients.

Effects on Potassium. Hyperkalemia can develop, especially in those with renal impairment or diabetes mellitus and those receiving drugs that can increase serum potassium concentration (e.g., potassium-sparing diuretics, potassium supplements, potassium-containing salt substitutes).

Cough. Persistent and nonproductive; resolves after drug discontinuance.

Surgery/Anesthesia. Hypotension may occur in patients undergoing surgery or during anesthesia with agents that produce hypotension. Hypotension in such patients may be corrected by volume expansion.

Specific Populations **Pregnancy.** Category C (first trimester); Category D (second and third trimesters). (See Users Guide.) (See Fetal/Neonatal Morbidity and Mortality under Warnings/Precautions: Warnings, in Cautions.)

Lactation. Ramipril and its metabolites were undetectable in breast milk following a single 10-mg oral dose of the drug in nursing women; however, milk concentrations resulting from multiple doses of the drug have not been determined. Because of the potential for serious adverse reactions from ramipril in nursing infants, the manufacturers state that women receiving the drug should not breast-feed.

Pediatric Use. The manufacturers state that safety and efficacy of ramipril in children younger than 18 years of age have not been established. For information on overall principles and expert recommendations for treatment of hypertension in pediatric patients, see Uses: Hypertension in Pediatric Patients, in the Thiazides General Statement 40:28.20.

Geriatric Use. No substantial differences in safety and efficacy relative to younger adults, but increased sensitivity cannot be ruled out. Increased ramiprilat plasma concentrations and area under the concentration-time curve (AUC) have been reported in some geriatric patients.

Renal Impairment. Renal function may decrease with ACE inhibitor therapy in susceptible patients. Use with caution in those with renal impairment. (See Dosage and Administration: Special Populations and also under Warnings/Precautions: General Precautions, Renal Effects, in Cautions.)

Hepatic Impairment. Use with caution. (See Dosage and Administration: Special Populations.)

Black Patients. ACE inhibitors not as effective. (See Uses: Hypertension.)

■ **Common Adverse Effects** Adverse effects reported in 1% or more of patients receiving ramipril and considered possibly or probably related to treatment include asthenia/fatigue, hypotension, postural hypotension, increased cough, dizziness, headache, angina pectoris, nausea, syncope, vomiting, vertigo, abnormal kidney function, and diarrhea.

Drug Interactions

■ **Drugs that Block the Renin-Angiotensin System** Increased risk of renal impairment, hyperkalemia, and hypotension with concomitant use of other drugs that block the renin-angiotensin system (e.g., aliskiren, angiotensin II receptor antagonists); when ramipril is used concomitantly with such drugs, blood pressure, renal function, and serum concentrations of electrolytes should be monitored closely. Concomitant use of ramipril and aliskiren is contraindicated in patients with diabetes mellitus; in addition, such concomitant use should be avoided in patients with renal impairment (glomerular filtration rate [GFR] less than 60 mL/minute per 1.73 m^2). (See Cautions in Aliskiren Hemifumarate 24:32.40.)

■ **Drugs Increasing Serum Potassium Concentration** Potential pharmacologic interaction (additive hyperkalemic effect). Includes potassium-sparing diuretics, potassium supplements, and other drugs that can cause hyperkalemia.

■ **Diuretics** Potential pharmacokinetic and pharmacologic interaction (hypotensive effect).

■ **Lithium** Potential pharmacokinetic interaction (increased lithium concentrations and clinical toxicity).

■ **mTOR Inhibitors** Patients receiving concomitant mammalian target of rapamycin (mTOR) inhibitors (e.g., temsirolimus) may be at increased risk for angioedema.

■ **Nonsteroidal Anti-inflammatory Agents** Potential pharmacologic interaction (decreased renal function and increased serum potassium concentrations). (See Drug Interactions in Captopril 24:32.04.)

Description

Ramipril is an angiotensin-converting enzyme (ACE, bradykininase, kininase II) inhibitor. Unlike captopril or lisinopril but similar to benazepril, enalapril, fosinopril, moexipril, perindopril, quinapril, and trandolapril, ramipril is a prodrug and has little pharmacologic activity until hydrolyzed in the liver to ramiprilat. Like benazepril, enalapril, fosinopril, lisinopril, moexipril, and quinapril but unlike captopril, ramipril does not contain a sulfhydryl group.

Advice to Patients

Risk of angioedema, anaphylactoid, and other sensitivity reactions; importance of discontinuing the drug and immediately reporting suggestive manifestation (e.g., edema of face, eyes, lips, or tongue; swallowing or breathing with difficulty) to a clinician.

Risk of hypotension (e.g., lightheadedness, syncope), especially during initial therapy or with volume depletion secondary to excessive perspiration, vomiting, or diarrhea. Importance of adequate fluid intake. Importance of discontinuing drug and contacting clinician if symptoms of syncope occur.

Importance of contacting a clinician promptly if manifestations of infection or neutropenia (e.g., sore throat, fever) develop.

Importance of informing clinicians of existing or contemplated concomitant therapy, including prescription and OTC drugs. Risk of hyperkalemia. Importance of avoiding the use of potassium supplements or salt substitutes containing potassium without consultation with a clinician.

Importance of women informing clinicians immediately if they are or plan to become pregnant or plan to breast-feed. Risk of use during first, second, and third trimesters of pregnancy.

Importance of informing patients of other important precautionary information. (See Cautions.)

Overview® (see Users Guide). For additional information on this drug until a more detailed monograph is developed and published, the manufacturers' labelings should be consulted. It is *essential* that the manufacturers' labelings be consulted for more detailed information on usual cautions, precautions, contraindications, potential drug interactions, laboratory test interferences, and acute toxicity.

Preparations

Excipients in commercially available drug preparations may have clinically important effects in some individuals; consult specific product labeling for details.

Ramipril

Oral		
Capsules	1.25 mg*	**Altace®**, Pfizer **Ramipril Capsules**
	2.5 mg*	**Altace®**, Pfizer **Ramipril Capsules**
	5 mg*	**Altace®**, Pfizer **Ramipril Capsules**
	10 mg*	**Altace®**, Pfizer **Ramipril Capsules**

*available from one or more manufacturer, distributor, and/or repackager by generic (nonproprietary) name

†Use is not currently included in the labeling approved by the US Food and Drug Administration

ANGIOTENSIN II RECEPTOR ANTAGONISTS 24:32.08

Candesartan Cilexetil

■ Candesartan cilexetil, a nonpeptide tetrazole derivative, is an angiotensin II receptor (AT_1) antagonist (also referred to as an angiotensin II receptor blocker [ARB]).

Uses

■ **Hypertension** Candesartan cilexetil is used alone or in combination with other classes of antihypertensive agents in the management of hypertension. Angiotensin II receptor antagonists, such as candesartan cilexetil, are considered one of several preferred antihypertensive drugs for the initial management of hypertension according to current evidence-based hypertension guidelines; other preferred options include angiotensin-converting enzyme (ACE) inhibitors, calcium-channel blockers, and thiazide diuretics. While there may be individual differences with respect to recommendations for initial drug selection and use in specific patient populations, current evidence indicates that these antihypertensive drug classes all generally produce comparable effects on overall mortality and cardiovascular, cerebrovascular, and renal outcomes. (See Uses: Hypertension, in Valsartan 24:32.08.)

Angiotensin II receptor antagonists or ACE inhibitors may be particularly useful in the management of hypertension in patients with certain coexisting conditions such as diabetes mellitus or chronic kidney disease (CKD); angiotensin II receptor antagonists also may be preferred, generally as an alternative to ACE inhibitors, in hypertensive patients with heart failure or ischemic heart disease and/or following myocardial infarction (MI). (See Uses: Hypertension in Valsartan 24:32.08.)

In patients with hypertension and compelling indications (e.g., CKD with albuminuria [urine albumin 300 mg/day or greater, or urine albumin:creatinine ratio of 300 mg/g or equivalent in the first morning void]), angiotensin II receptor antagonists are usually considered an alternative for ACE inhibitor-intolerant patients. However, data indicate no difference in efficacy between ACE inhibitors and angiotensin II receptor antagonists with regard to blood pressure lowering and clinical outcomes (i.e., all-cause mortality, cardiovascular mortality, MI, heart failure, stroke, and end-stage renal disease). Adverse events (e.g., cough, angioedema) leading to drug discontinuance occur more frequently with ACE inhibitor therapy than with angiotensin II receptor antagonist therapy. Because of similar efficacy and a lower frequency of adverse effects, some experts believe that angiotensin II receptor antagonists should be used instead of an ACE inhibitor for the treatment of hypertension or hypertension with certain compelling indications.

Efficacy of candesartan cilexetil in the treatment of hypertension in adults has been established in placebo-controlled studies of 4–12 weeks' duration in patients with hypertension of mild to moderate severity. In these patients, candesartan cilexetil dosages of 8–32 mg daily decreased systolic blood pressure by about 8–12 mm Hg and diastolic blood pressure by about 4–8 mm Hg 24 hours after dosing. After withdrawal of candesartan cilexetil, blood pressure gradually returns to pretreatment levels; rebound hypertension following abrupt withdrawal of the drug has not been reported.

The efficacy of candesartan cilexetil for long-term use (i.e., exceeding 12 weeks) has been established in 2 open label, prospective studies in which the drug was administered in dosages 4–16 mg once daily for 6 or 12 months without apparent loss of clinical effect. Clinical studies have shown that the hypotensive effect of candesartan cilexetil in patients with mild to moderate hypertension is greater than that of placebo and comparable to that of usual dosages of enalapril or amlodipine. Like ACE inhibitors, angiotensin II receptor antagonists such as candesartan may produce a smaller blood pressure response in hypertensive black patients compared with nonblack patients. (See Race under Hypertension: Other Special Considerations for Antihypertensive Drug Therapy, in Uses in Valsartan 24:32.08.)

Efficacy of candesartan has been established in hypertensive pediatric patients 1 to less than 6 years of age and 6 to less than 17 years of age in 2 randomized, double-blind, multicenter, 4-week dose-ranging studies. Dosages of candesartan cilexetil used in these studies were adjusted for body weight to mimic dosages established in adults. Results of these studies indicate that efficacy and tolerability of candesartan in pediatric patients is comparable to that reported in adults. Changes in systolic and diastolic blood pressures from baseline with candesartan therapy in these studies were dose related and similar between the 2 patient age groups; antihypertensive effects were apparent within 1–2 weeks and full effects were observed by week 4. The pharmacokinetics of candesartan in these groups was comparable to that reported in adults and supported once-daily dosing.

In one study, 93 patients 1 to less than 6 years of age (74% with renal disease) received 0.05, 0.2 or 0.4 mg/kg of candesartan cilexetil once daily as an extemporaneously prepared oral suspension. The primary end point in this study was change in trough systolic blood pressure from baseline to the end of the study (i.e., at 4 weeks). Because this study did not include a placebo arm, the change in blood pressure from baseline likely overestimates the true magnitude of candesartan's blood pressure effects. However, reductions from baseline of 6–12 and 5–11 mm Hg in trough systolic blood pressure and diastolic blood pressure, respectively, were observed across the 3 doses of candesartan, supporting the appropriateness of the dosing regimen used. Blood pressure response to candesartan was similar in children with or without renal disease.

In another study, 240 patients 6 to less than 17 years of age were randomly allocated (in a 1: 2: 2: 2 ratio) to receive either placebo or low, medium, or high doses of candesartan. Dosages of candesartan cilexetil were 2, 8, or 16 mg once daily for patients who weighed less than 50 kg and 4, 16, or 32 mg once daily for those who weighed 50 kg or more. Mean age of patients in the study was approximately 13 years; 47% of those enrolled were black and 29% were female. The primary efficacy variable in this study was the placebo-corrected change from baseline in trough sitting systolic blood pressure to the end of week 4 of the study (or the last observation carried forward). The overall placebo-corrected changes in trough sitting systolic blood pressure and sitting diastolic blood pressure ranged from 4.9–7.5 and from 3–6.2 mmHg, respectively, after 4 weeks.

Most patients with hypertension, especially black patients, will require at least 2 antihypertensive drugs to achieve adequate blood pressure control. In children 6 to less than 17 years of age receiving candesartan in clinical studies, there was a trend for a lesser blood pressure effect in blacks compared with patients of other races. There were too few individuals in the age group of 1 to less than 6 years to determine whether blacks respond differently than other patients to candesartan.

For additional information on the use of angiotensin II receptor antagonists in the management of hypertension, see Uses: Hypertension, in Valsartan 24:32.08. For information on overall principles and expert recommendations for treatment of hypertension, see Uses: Hypertension in Adults and also see Uses: Hypertension in Pediatric Patients, in the Thiazides General Statement 40:28.20.

■ **Heart Failure** Candesartan is used in the management of mild to severe (New York Heart Association [NYHA] class II–IV) heart failure secondary to left ventricular dysfunction (i.e., a left ventricular ejection fraction [LVEF] of 40% or less) to reduce cardiovascular death and heart failure-associated hospitalization.

Current guidelines for the management of heart failure in adults generally recommend a combination of drug therapies to reduce morbidity and mortality, including neurohormonal antagonists (e.g., ACE inhibitors, angiotensin II receptor antagonists, angiotensin receptor-neprilysin inhibitors [ARNIs], β-adrenergic blocking agents (β-blockers), aldosterone receptor antagonists) that inhibit the detrimental compensatory mechanisms in heart failure. Additional agents (e.g., cardiac glycosides, diuretics, sinoatrial modulators [i.e., ivabradine]) added to a heart failure treatment regimen in selected patients have been associated with symptomatic improvement and/or reduction in heart-failure related hospitalizations. Experts recommend that all asymptomatic patients with reduced LVEF (American College of Cardiology Foundation [ACCF]/ American Heart Association [AHA] stage B heart failure) receive therapy with an ACE inhibitor and β-blocker to prevent symptomatic heart failure and to reduce morbidity and mortality. In patients with prior or current symptoms of chronic heart failure with reduced LVEF (ACCF/AHA stage C heart failure), ACCF, AHA, and the Heart Failure Society of America (HFSA) recommend inhibition of the renin-angiotensin-aldosterone (RAA) system with an ACE inhibitor, angiotensin II receptor antagonist, or ARNI in conjunction with a β-blocker, and an aldosterone antagonist in selected patients, to reduce morbidity and mortality. While ACE inhibitors have been the preferred drugs for inhibition of the RAA system because of their established benefits in patients with heart failure and reduced ejection fraction, some evidence indicates that therapy with sacubitril/valsartan, an ARNI, may be more effective than ACE inhibitor therapy (enalapril) in reducing cardiovascular death and heart failure-related hospitalization. ACCF, AHA, and HFSA recommend that patients with chronic symptomatic heart failure with reduced LVEF (NYHA class II or III) who are able to tolerate an ACE inhibitor or angiotensin II receptor antagonist be switched to therapy containing an ARNI to further reduce morbidity and mortality. However, in patients in whom an ARNI is not appropriate, continued use of an ACE inhibitor for all classes of heart failure with reduced ejection fraction remains strongly advised. In patients in whom an ARNI or ACE inhibitor is not appropriate, an angiotensin II receptor antagonist may be used. For further information on the use of ARNIs in patients with heart failure, see Uses: Heart Failure, in Sacubitril and Valsartan 24:32.92.

While angiotensin II receptor antagonists are considered reasonable alternatives in patients who are unable to tolerate ACE inhibitors (e.g., because of cough or angioedema), sensitivity reactions (e.g., various anaphylactoid reactions and/or angioedema) have been reported with use of angiotensin II receptor antagonists, including candesartan. (See Warnings: Sensitivity Reactions, under Warnings/Precautions in Cautions.)

Efficacy of candesartan for the management of heart failure has been studied in a large (2028 patients), multicenter, double-blind, placebo-controlled, randomized study (Candesartan in Heart failure: Assessment of Reduction in Mortality and morbidity [CHARM]-Alternative) in patients (32% were female and the mean age of all patients was 67 years) with NYHA class II–IV heart failure and a mean LVEF of 30%, who were intolerant of ACE inhibitors. Addition of candesartan cilexetil 4–8 mg once daily (initial dosage, with dosage doubled every 2 weeks to a target dosage of 32 mg once daily [mean daily dosage about 23 mg]) to standard therapy (diuretics, digoxin, β-blockers, spironolactone) was associated with a 23% reduction (compared with placebo) in the primary end point of cardiovascular death or hospitalization for worsened heart failure at a median follow-up of 34 months.

Efficacy of candesartan for the management of heart failure has been studied in a second large (2548 patients), multicenter, double-blind, placebo-controlled, randomized study (CHARM–Added) in patients (21% were female and the mean age of all patients was 64 years) with NYHA class II–IV heart failure and a mean LVEF of 28%. Addition of candesartan cilexetil 4–8 mg once daily (initial dosage, with dosage doubled every 2 weeks to a target dosage of 32 mg once daily [mean daily dosage about 24 mg]) to standard therapy (ACE inhibitors, diuretics, digoxin, β-blockers, spironolactone) was associated with a 15% reduction (compared with placebo) in the primary end point of cardiovascular death or hospitalization for worsened heart failure at a median follow-up of 41 months. Patients receiving combination therapy with drugs that block the renin-angiotensin system (angiotensin II receptor antagonists, ACE inhibitors, aliskiren), should be closely monitored. (See Drug Interactions: Drugs that Block the Renin-Angiotensin System.)

A third large (3023 patients), multicenter, double-blind, placebo-controlled, randomized study (CHARM-Preserved) was conducted in patients (40% were female and the mean age of all patients was 67 years) with NYHA class II–IV heart failure and preserved LVEF (higher than 40%)†. Addition of candesartan cilexetil 4–8 mg once daily (initial dosage, with dosage doubled every 2 weeks to a target dosage of 32 mg once daily [mean daily dosage about 25 mg]) to standard therapy, including an ACE inhibitor in about 19% of patients, was associated with a moderate reduction in the number of patients hospitalized one or more times for heart failure but no difference in the number of cardiovascular deaths at a median follow-up of 36.6 months.

■ **Diabetic Nephropathy** Both angiotensin II receptor antagonists and ACE inhibitors have been shown to slow the rate of progression of renal disease in patients with diabetes mellitus and persistent albuminuria†, and use of a drug from either class is recommended in such patients with modestly elevated (30–300 mg/24 hours) or higher (exceeding 300 mg/24 hours) levels of urinary albumin excretion. The American Diabetes Association (ADA) states that the use of an ACE inhibitor or angiotensin II receptor antagonist is not recommended for the primary prevention of diabetic nephropathy in patients with diabetes mellitus who are normotensive, have normal levels of urinary protein excretion, and have a normal glomerular filtration rate (GFR). The usual precautions of angiotensin II receptor antagonist or ACE inhibitor therapy in patients with substantial renal impairment should be observed. (See Renal Effects under Warnings/Precautions: General Precautions, in Cautions). For additional information on the use of angiotensin II receptor antagonists in the treatment of diabetic nephropathy, see Uses: Diabetic Nephropathy, in Losartan 24:32.08 and in Irbesartan 24:32.08.

Dosage and Administration

■ **General** Candesartan cilexetil is administered orally, and can be taken without regard to meals.

Candesartan cilexetil oral suspension can be extemporaneously prepared in concentrations within the range of 0.1–2 mg/mL; a concentration of 1 mg/mL generally is suitable for administering most dosages. Any strength of candesartan cilexetil tablet can be used to prepare the suspension. To prepare a suspension that will yield 160 mL of a 1-mg/mL suspension, equal volumes (80 mL each) of Ora-Plus® and Ora-Sweet SF® or, alternatively, 160 mL of Ora-Blend SF® should be used. A small amount of the vehicle should be added to five 32-mg candesartan cilexetil tablets and the tablets subsequently ground into a smooth paste using a mortar and pestle. The paste should then be added to a container of suitable size. The mortar and pestle should be rinsed clean using the vehicle and the resulting vehicle mixture should then be added to the container; this step should be repeated as necessary. The final amount of suspension should be prepared by adding the remaining vehicle to the container and mixing the suspension thoroughly. The suspension should be dispensed into suitably sized amber polyethylene terephthalate (PET) bottles. Each bottle of candesartan suspension should be labeled with an expiration date of 100 days and marked with the following instructions: store at room temperature (below 30°C/86°F), use within 30 days after first opening, do not use after the expiration date on the bottle, do not freeze, and shake well before each use.

Hypertension Dosage of candesartan cilexetil must be individualized and adjusted according to blood pressure response.

Candesartan Therapy. The usual initial dosage of candesartan cilexetil as monotherapy is 16 mg once daily in adults without depletion of intravascular volume and the usual dosage range is 8–32 mg daily, given in 1 dose or 2 divided doses. Experience with dosages exceeding 32 mg daily is limited, and there is no evidence that higher dosages provide additional therapeutic benefit. The manufacturer states that the antihypertensive effect of candesartan cilexetil generally is evident within 2 weeks, with a maximum blood pressure reduction after 4–6 weeks.

In pediatric patients, candesartan cilexetil may be administered once daily or twice daily in equally divided doses. Dosage should be adjusted according to blood pressure response. In patients with possible depletion of intravascular volume (e.g., those treated with diuretics, particularly those with impaired renal function), candesartan cilexetil should be initiated under close medical supervision and administration of a lower dosage should be considered. In patients 1 to less than 6 years of age, the recommended initial dosage is 0.2 mg/kg (oral suspension) daily, with a dosage range of 0.05–0.4 mg/kg daily. In patients 6 to less than 17 years of age who weigh less than 50 kg, the recommended initial dosage is 4–8 mg daily, with a dosage range of 2–16 mg daily. For patients 6 to less than 17 years of age who weigh more than 50 kg, the recommended initial dosage is 8–16 mg daily, with a dosage range of 4–32 mg daily. Safety and efficacy of dosages exceeding 0.4 mg/kg daily (in patients 1 to less than 6 years of age) or 32 mg daily (in patients 6 to less than 17 years of age) have not been established in this patient population. An antihypertensive effect usually is present within 2 weeks following initiation of candesartan therapy, with full effects generally obtained within 4 weeks. Some experts state that the drug should be initiated at the low end of the dosage range and the dosage may be increased every 2–4 weeks until blood pressure is controlled, the maximum dosage is reached, or adverse effects occur. Children younger than 1 year of age must not receive candesartan for hypertension. (See Infant Morbidity under Warnings/Precautions: Other Warnings and Precautions, in Cautions.) Safety and efficacy of candesartan have not been established in pediatric patients with a glomerular filtration rate less than 30 mL/minute per 1.73 m^2, and such patients should not receive the drug. For children who cannot swallow tablets, candesartan may be administered as an oral suspension.

Candesartan/Hydrochlorothiazide Fixed-combination Therapy. In patients who do not respond adequately to monotherapy with candesartan cilexetil or, alternatively, with hydrochlorothiazide, combined therapy with the drugs can be used. When combination therapy is necessary, the manufacturer states that commercially available preparation containing candesartan cilexetil in fixed combination with hydrochlorothiazide should not be used initially. Dosage preferably should first be adjusted by titrating the dosage of each drug separately; if it is determined that the optimum maintenance dosage corresponds to the ratio in the commercial combination preparation, this product may be used. The manufacturer states that combined therapy with the commercially available fixed-combination preparation containing 16 mg of candesartan cilexetil and 12.5 mg of hydrochlorothiazide can be used in adults whose blood pressure is not adequately controlled by monotherapy with 25 mg of hydrochlorothiazide or in those in whom control of blood pressure is maintained but hypokalemia is problematic at this hydrochlorothiazide dosage. In patients whose blood pressure is not adequately controlled by monotherapy with candesartan cilexetil dosages of 32 mg daily, the commercially available fixed-combination containing 32 mg of candesartan cilexetil and 12.5 mg of hydrochlorothiazide, or alternatively, 32 mg of candesartan cilexetil and 25 mg of hydrochlorothiazide can be used.

Blood Pressure Monitoring and Treatment Goals. Blood pressure should be monitored regularly (i.e., monthly) during therapy and dosage of the antihypertensive drug adjusted until blood pressure is controlled. If an adequate blood pressure response is not achieved with angiotensin II receptor antagonist monotherapy, the dosage may be increased or another antihypertensive agent with demonstrated benefit and preferably with a complementary mechanism of action (e.g., calcium-channel blocker, thiazide diuretic) may be added; if target blood pressure is still not achieved, a third drug may be added. (See Uses: Hypertension.) In patients who develop unacceptable adverse effects with candesartan, the drug should be discontinued and another antihypertensive agent from a different pharmacologic class should be initiated.

The goal of hypertension management and prevention is to achieve and maintain optimal control of blood pressure. However, the optimum blood pressure threshold for initiating antihypertensive drug therapy and specific treatment goals remain controversial. While previous hypertension guidelines have based target blood pressure goals on age and comorbidities, the 2017 ACC/AHA hypertension guideline incorporates underlying cardiovascular risk into decision making regarding treatment and generally recommends the same target blood pressure (i.e., less than 130/80 mm Hg) in all adults. Many patients will require at least 2 drugs from different pharmacologic classes to achieve their blood pressure goal; the potential benefits of hypertension management and drug cost, adverse effects, and risks associated with the use of multiple antihypertensive drugs also should be considered when deciding a patient's blood pressure treatment goal.

For additional information on target levels of blood pressure and on monitoring therapy in the management of hypertension, see Blood Pressure Monitoring and Treatment Goals under Dosage: Hypertension, in Dosage and Administration in the Thiazides General Statement 40:28.20.

Heart Failure Caution should be observed when initiating candesartan cilexetil therapy in patients with heart failure. For the management of symptomatic heart failure (New York Heart Association [NYHA] class II–IV), the manufacturer recommends an initial candesartan cilexetil dosage of 4 mg once daily, while some experts recommend an initial dosage of 4–8 mg once daily. Dosage should be increased (by doubling the dosage at approximately 2-week intervals) as tolerated to a target dosage of 32 mg once daily. The American College of Cardiology Foundation (ACCF) and American Heart Association (AHA) recommend a maximum candesartan cilexetil dosage of 32 mg once daily in patients with heart failure.

■ **Special Populations** The manufacturer recommends that patients with depletion of intravascular volume (e.g., patients receiving treatment with a diuretic, particularly those with renal impairment) should have this condition corrected prior to initiation of candesartan cilexetil therapy or they should be monitored closely and consideration should be given to administering a lower initial dose of the drug. The manufacturer states that no adjustment in initial candesartan cilexetil dosage is necessary in geriatric patients or in those with mild renal or hepatic impairment. However, the area under the concentration-time curve and peak plasma concentration of candesartan are increased substantially in patients with moderate (Child-Pugh B) hepatic impairment, and the manufacturer states that consideration should be given to initiating candesartan cilexetil therapy at a reduced dosage (e.g., 8 mg once daily). Some clinicians recommend an initial 4- or 8-mg daily dosage of candesartan cilexetil in patients with severe hepatic or renal impairment.

The commercially available preparation containing candesartan cilexetil in fixed combination with hydrochlorothiazide is not recommended for patients with renal impairment whose creatinine clearance is less than 30 mL/minute, and such preparations should be used with caution in patients with hepatic impairment. If a lower initial (less than 8 mg once daily) candesartan cilexetil dosage is selected in patients with moderate hepatic impairment, the commercially available preparation containing candesartan cilexetil in fixed combination with hydrochlorothiazide is not recommended for initial titration, because the appropriate starting dose of candesartan cilexetil is not available as a fixed-ratio preparation. The fixed combination preparation should be individualized and adjusted carefully in patients with hepatic impairment.

Cautions

■ **Contraindications** Known hypersensitivity to candesartan or any ingredient in the formulation.

Concomitant use of candesartan and aliskiren in patients with diabetes mellitus. (See Drug Interactions: Drugs that Block the Renin-Angiotensin System.)

■ **Warnings/Precautions** ***Warnings*** **Fetal/Neonatal Morbidity and Mortality.** Drugs that act on the renin-angiotensin system (e.g., angiotensin-converting enzyme [ACE] inhibitors, angiotensin II receptor antagonists) reduce fetal renal function and increase fetal and neonatal morbidity and mortality when used during the second and third trimesters of pregnancy. Resulting oligohydramnios can be associated with fetal lung hypoplasia and skeletal deformations. Potential neonatal effects include skull hypoplasia, anuria, hypotension, renal failure, and death. Candesartan should be discontinued as soon as possible when pregnancy is detected, unless continued use is considered life-saving. Nearly all women can be transferred successfully to alternative therapy for the remainder of their pregnancy. Cases of fetal and neonatal toxicity in infants born to women who received candesartan cilexetil during pregnancy have been reported during postmarketing experience with the drug. For additional information on the risk of such drugs during pregnancy, see Cautions: Pregnancy, Fertility, and Lactation, in Captopril 24:32.04 and Enalaprilat/Enalapril 24:32.04.

Sensitivity Reactions Sensitivity reactions, including various anaphylactoid reactions and/or angioedema, have been reported with use of angiotensin II receptor antagonists, including candesartan. Candesartan is not recommended in patients with a history of angioedema associated with or unrelated to ACE or angiotensin II receptor antagonist therapy.

Other Warnings and Precautions **Effects on Potassium.** Hyperkalemia can develop, especially in patients receiving agents that can increase serum potassium concentration (e.g., potassium-sparing diuretics, potassium supplements, potassium-containing salt substitutes). (See Drug Interactions: Agents that Increase Serum Potassium.) Serum potassium concentrations should be monitored periodically.

Hypotension. Symptomatic hypotension may occur. Patients at particular risk include those with volume or salt depletion secondary to salt restriction, prolonged diuretic therapy, heart failure, or dialysis. Volume and/or salt depletion should be corrected before initiation of candesartan therapy or a lower initial dosage should be used. In patients with symptomatic hypotension, a temporary reduction in the dosage of candesartan cilexetil and/or of a diuretic may be needed, as well as volume repletion; blood pressure should be monitored during dosage escalation and periodically thereafter.

Malignancies. In July 2010, the US Food and Drug Administration (FDA) initiated a safety review of angiotensin II receptor antagonists after a published meta-analysis suggested a possible association between the use of these agents and an increased risk of cancer. The meta-analysis, which combined cancer-related findings from 5 randomized, controlled trials in over 60,000 patients, found a modest but significant increase in the risk of new cancer occurrence in patients receiving an angiotensin II receptor antagonist (mostly telmisartan) compared with those in control groups (7.2 versus 6%, respectively; risk ratio 1.08). However, because of several limitations of the study (e.g., trials included in the meta-analysis were not specifically designed to evaluate cancer outcomes, lack of individual patient data), the validity of these findings has been questioned.

Subsequent studies, including a larger, more comprehensive meta-analysis conducted by FDA, have not shown an increased risk of cancer in patients receiving angiotensin II receptor antagonists. FDA's meta-analysis, which included trial-level data from 31 randomized studies (total of approximately 156,000 patients), found no evidence of an increased risk of cancer in patients who received an angiotensin II receptor antagonist compared with those who received other treatments (placebo or active control). The overall rate of new cancer occurrence was essentially the same in both groups of patients (1.82 and 1.84 cases per 100 patient-years, respectively). In addition, there was no difference in the risk of cancer-related death, breast cancer, lung cancer, or prostate cancer between the groups. Based on these results and a review of all currently available data related to this potential safety concern, FDA has concluded that use of angiotensin II receptor antagonists is not associated with an increased risk of cancer.

Renal Effects. Because the renin-angiotensin-aldosterone (RAA) system appears to contribute substantially to maintenance of glomerular filtration in patients with heart failure in whom renal perfusion is severely compromised, renal function may deteriorate markedly (e.g., oliguria, progressive azotemia, renal failure, death) in these patients during therapy with an ACE inhibitor or an angiotensin II receptor antagonist (e.g., candesartan cilexetil). Increases in serum creatinine requiring discontinuance of the drug may occur in patients with heart failure receiving candesartan. Serum creatinine should be monitored during dosage escalation and periodically thereafter. Renal artery stenosis, preexisting renal impairment, and concomitant diuretic therapy also are risk factors for renal impairment during therapy with drugs that inhibit the RAA system. (See Cautions: Renal Effects, in Enalapril 24:32.04.)

Infant Morbidity. Patients younger than 1 year of age must not receive candesartan for hypertension; drugs that act directly on the renin-angiotensin system can have effects on the development of immature kidneys.

Surgery/Anesthesia. Hypotension may occur in patients undergoing major surgery and anesthesia who are receiving angiotensin II receptor antagonists, including candesartan, presumably secondary to blockade of the renin-angiotensin system. Rarely, hypotension may be severe enough to require volume expansion with IV fluids and/or use of vasopressors.

Fixed-combination Preparations. When candesartan cilexetil is used as a fixed combination that includes hydrochlorothiazide, the cautions, precautions, and contraindications associated with thiazide diuretics must be considered in addition to those associated with candesartan cilexetil.

Specific Populations **Pregnancy.** Category D. (See Users Guide.) Candesartan can cause fetal and neonatal morbidity and mortality when administered to a pregnant woman. Candesartan should be discontinued as soon as possible when pregnancy is detected. (See Fetal/Neonatal Morbidity and Mortality under Warnings/Precautions: Warnings, in Cautions.)

The effects of candesartan on labor and delivery in humans have not been established.

Lactation. It is not known whether candesartan cilexetil is distributed into breast milk. Because of the potential for serious adverse reactions to candesartan in nursing infants, a decision should be made whether to discontinue nursing or the drug.

Pediatric Use. If oliguria or hypotension occurs in neonates with a history of in utero exposure to candesartan, blood pressure and renal function should be supported; exchange transfusions or dialysis may be required. (See Fetal/Neonatal Morbidity and Mortality under Warnings/Precautions: Warnings, in Cautions.)

The antihypertensive effects and pharmacokinetics of candesartan have been evaluated in patients 1 to less than 17 years of age in randomized double-blind studies. (See Uses: Hypertension.)

The pharmacokinetics of candesartan in pediatric patients 1 to less than 17 years of age were not modified by age, sex, or body weight. Data are lacking on the pharmacokinetics of candesartan in patients younger than 1 year of age or in children with renal impairment.

Candesartan must not be administered to children younger than 1 year of age. (See Infant Morbidity under Warnings/Precautions: Other Warnings and Precautions, in Cautions.) For information on overall principles and expert recommendations for treatment of hypertension in pediatric patients, see Uses: Hypertension in Pediatric Patients, in the Thiazides General Statement 40:28.20.

Geriatric Use. No substantial differences in safety and efficacy for the treatment of hypertension have been observed in geriatric patients relative to younger adults, but increased sensitivity cannot be ruled out.

Increased incidence of candesartan-associated adverse effects (e.g., abnormal renal function, hypotension, hyperkalemia) and consequent discontinuance of candesartan have been reported in patients with heart failure who were 75 years of age or older when compared with younger patients.

Renal Impairment. Candesartan should be used with caution in patients with renal impairment. (See Dosage and Administration: Special Populations.)

Hepatic Impairment. Candesartan should be used with caution in patients with hepatic impairment. (See Dosage and Administration: Special Population.)

■ **Common Adverse Effects** Adverse effects occurring in 1% or more of patients receiving candesartan cilexetil in clinical trials included back pain, dizziness, upper respiratory tract infection, pharyngitis, and rhinitis. The incidence of adverse effects was not affected by age, gender, or race.

Drug Interactions

■ **Agents that Increase Serum Potassium** Concomitant use of candesartan with potassium-sparing diuretics, potassium supplements, potassium-containing salt substitutes, or other drugs that increase serum potassium concentrations may result in hyperkalemia. Serum potassium concentrations should be monitored in such patients.

■ **Drugs Affecting Hepatic Microsomal Enzymes** Inhibitors or inducers of cytochrome P-450 (CYP) system; pharmacokinetic interaction unlikely.

■ **Drugs that Block the Renin-Angiotensin System** Increased risk of hypotension, hyperkalemia, and changes in renal function (e.g., renal impairment) with concomitant use of other drugs that block the renin-angiotensin system (e.g., angiotensin-converting enzyme [ACE] inhibitors, angiotensin II receptor antagonists, aliskiren); when candesartan is used concomitantly with such drugs, blood pressure, renal function, and serum concentrations of electrolytes should be monitored closely. Concomitant use of candesartan with aliskiren is contraindicated in patients with diabetes mellitus; in addition, such concomitant use should be avoided in patients with renal impairment (glomerular filtration rate [GFR] less than 60 mL/minute per 1.73 m^2). (See Use in Combination with Angiotensin-converting Enzyme Inhibitors or Angiotensin II Receptor Antagonists under Warnings/Precautions: Other Warnings and Precautions, in Cautions in Aliskiren Hemifumarate 24:32.40.)

■ **Cardiac Drugs** Pharmacologic interactions unlikely when candesartan is used concomitantly with cardiac drugs (e.g., digoxin, nifedipine).

■ **Lithium** Pharmacokinetic interaction (increased serum lithium concentrations) when candesartan is used concomitantly with lithium. Monitoring of serum lithium concentrations is recommended during concomitant use.

■ **Warfarin** Pharmacologic interaction unlikely.

■ **Glyburide** Pharmacologic interaction unlikely.

■ **Nonsteroidal Anti-inflammatory Agents** Concomitant use of nonsteroidal anti-inflammatory agents (NSAIAs), including selective cyclooxygenase-2 (COX-2) inhibitors, and angiotensin II receptor antagonists may result in deterioration of renal function, including possible acute renal failure, in patients who are geriatric, volume-depleted (including those on diuretic therapy), or who have compromised renal function. These effects usually are reversible. Renal function should be periodically monitored in patients receiving candesartan and NSAIA therapy.

Potential pharmacologic interaction (attenuated antihypertensive effects) when angiotensin II receptor antagonists are used concomitantly with NSAIAs, including selective COX-2 inhibitors.

■ **Oral Contraceptives** Pharmacokinetic interaction unlikely.

Description

Candesartan cilexetil, a nonpeptide tetrazole derivative, is an angiotensin II receptor (AT_1) antagonist. Candesartan cilexetil is a prodrug and has little pharmacologic activity until hydrolyzed during absorption in the GI tract to candesartan. Formulation of the drug as the cilexetil salt increases the bioavailability of candesartan. For additional information on the pharmacology of angiotensin II receptor antagonists, see Description in Irbesartan 24:32.08 and Valsartan 24:32.08.

Although candesartan is principally eliminated unchanged in feces (through biliary excretion) and in urine, a small clinically unimportant amount of the drug is metabolized by the cytochrome P-450 (CYP) 2C9 isoenzyme to an inactive metabolite.

Advice to Patients

Importance of informing clinicians of existing or contemplated concomitant therapy, including prescription and OTC drugs.

Importance of women informing clinicians if they plan to become pregnant or to breast-feed. All women of childbearing potential should be advised to report pregnancy to their clinician as soon as possible. See Fetal/Neonatal Morbidity and Mortality under Warnings/Precautions: Warnings, in Cautions.

Overview® (see Users Guide). For additional information on this drug until a more detailed monograph is developed and published, the manufacturer's labeling should be consulted. It is *essential* that the manufacturer's labeling be consulted for more detailed information on usual cautions, precautions, contraindications, potential drug interactions, laboratory test interferences, and acute toxicity.

Preparations

Excipients in commercially available drug preparations may have clinically important effects in some individuals; consult specific product labeling for details.

Candesartan Cilexetil

Oral		
Tablets	4 mg	Atacand®, AstraZeneca
	8 mg	Atacand®, AstraZeneca
	16 mg	Atacand®, AstraZeneca
	32 mg	Atacand®, AstraZeneca

Candesartan Cilexetil Combinations

Oral		
Tablets	16 mg with Hydrochlorothiazide 12.5 mg	Atacand® HCT, AstraZeneca
	32 mg with Hydrochlorothiazide 12.5 mg	Atacand® HCT, AstraZeneca

†Use is not currently included in the labeling approved by the US Food and Drug Administration

Irbesartan

■ Irbesartan, a nonpeptide tetrazole derivative, is an angiotensin II type 1 (AT_1) receptor antagonist (also referred to as an angiotensin II receptor blocker [ARB]).

Uses

■ **Hypertension** Irbesartan is used alone or in combination with other classes of antihypertensive agents in the management of hypertension. Angiotensin II receptor antagonists, such as irbesartan, are considered one of several preferred antihypertensive drugs for the initial management of hypertension according to current evidence-based hypertension guidelines; other preferred options include angiotensin-converting enzyme (ACE) inhibitors, calcium-channel blockers, and thiazide diuretics. While there may be individual differences with respect to recommendations for initial drug selection and use in specific patient populations, current evidence indicates that these antihypertensive drug classes all generally produce comparable effects on overall mortality and cardiovascular, cerebrovascular, and renal outcomes. (See Uses: Hypertension, in Valsartan 24:32.08.)

Angiotensin II receptor antagonists or ACE inhibitors may be particularly useful in the management of hypertension in patients with certain coexisting conditions such as diabetes mellitus or chronic kidney disease (CKD); angiotensin II receptor antagonists also may be preferred, generally as an alternative to ACE inhibitors, in hypertensive patients with heart failure or ischemic heart disease and/or following myocardial infarction (MI). (See Uses: Hypertension, in Valsartan 24:32.08.)

In patients with hypertension and compelling indications (e.g., CKD with albuminuria [urine albumin 300 mg/day or greater, or urine albumin:creatinine ratio of 300 mg/g or equivalent in the first morning void]), angiotensin II receptor antagonists are usually considered an alternative for ACE inhibitor-intolerant patients. However, data indicate no difference in efficacy between ACE inhibitors and angiotensin II receptor antagonists with regard to blood pressure lowering and clinical outcomes (i.e., all-cause mortality, cardiovascular mortality, MI, heart failure, stroke, and end-stage renal disease). Adverse events (e.g., cough, angioedema) leading to drug discontinuance occur more frequently with ACE inhibitor therapy than with angiotensin II receptor antagonist therapy. Because of similar efficacy and a lower frequency of adverse effects, some experts believe that angiotensin II receptor antagonists should be used instead of an ACE inhibitor for the treatment of hypertension or hypertension with certain compelling indications.

Efficacy of irbesartan for the management of hypertension has been established by controlled studies of 8–12 weeks' duration in patients with hypertension of mild to moderate severity in outpatient settings. Clinical studies have shown that the hypotensive effect of usual dosages of irbesartan in patients with mild to moderate hypertension is greater than that of placebo and comparable to that of usual dosages of losartan, enalapril, or atenolol.

Most patients with hypertension, especially black patients, will require at least 2 antihypertensive drugs to achieve adequate blood pressure control. Like ACE inhibitors, angiotensin II receptor antagonists such as irbesartan may produce a smaller blood pressure response in hypertensive black patients compared with nonblack patients. (See Race under Hypertension: Other Special Considerations for Antihypertensive Drug Therapy, in Uses in Valsartan 24:32.08.)

For additional information on the management of hypertension, see Uses: Hypertension, in Valsartan 24:32.08. For information on overall principles and expert recommendations for treatment of hypertension, see Uses: Hypertension in Adults and also see Uses: Hypertension in Pediatric Patients, in the Thiazides General Statement 40:28.20.

■ **Diabetic Nephropathy** Irbesartan is used in the management of diabetic nephropathy manifested by elevated serum creatinine and proteinuria (urinary protein excretion exceeding 300 mg daily) in patients with type 2 diabetes mellitus and hypertension.

Both angiotensin II receptor antagonists and ACE inhibitors have been shown to slow the rate of progression of renal disease in patients with diabetes mellitus and persistent albuminuria, and use of a drug from either class is recommended in such patients with modestly elevated (30–300 mg/24 hours) or higher (exceeding 300 mg/24 hours) levels of urinary albumin excretion. Some evidence suggests that these drugs may slow the progression of nephropathy by a mechanism independent of their antihypertensive effects.

Comparative trials evaluating the efficacy of angiotensin II receptor antagonists and ACE inhibitors for improving renal outcomes in diabetic patients are lacking. Evidence supporting use of ACE inhibitors generally is based on studies in patients with type 1 diabetes mellitus, while evidence supporting use of angiotensin II receptor antagonists generally is based on studies in patients with type 2 diabetes mellitus. Findings from these studies indicate that both drug classes delay progression of increased urinary albumin excretion in patients with diabetes mellitus and may also slow the decline in renal function. Because the available data are consistent, some experts suggest that the effects of both drug classes in improving renal outcomes in patients with diabetes mellitus and proteinuria are likely to be similar.

Drugs that inhibit the renin-angiotensin system (i.e., angiotensin II receptor antagonists, ACE inhibitors) also have been shown to delay the onset of albuminuria in patients with type 2 diabetes mellitus and hypertension who have normal levels of urinary albumin excretion†; however, some experts state that in the absence of albuminuria, the risk of progressive kidney disease is low. The American Diabetes Association (ADA) states that the use of an ACE inhibitor or angiotensin II receptor antagonist is not recommended for the primary prevention of diabetic nephropathy in patients with diabetes mellitus who are normotensive, have normal levels of urinary protein excretion, and have a normal glomerular filtration rate (GFR).

Combined therapy with ACE inhibitors and angiotensin II receptor antagonists provides no additional cardiovascular benefit and increases the risk of adverse effects (e.g., impaired renal function, hyperkalemia). The usual precautions of angiotensin II receptor antagonist therapy in patients with substantial renal impairment should be observed.

The current labeled indication for irbesartan in hypertensive patients with type 2 diabetes mellitus and nephropathy (indicated by an elevated serum creatinine and proteinuria exceeding 300 mg/day) is based principally on the results of a long-term (mean duration of follow-up: 2.6 years), multicenter, comparative controlled trial, the Irbesartan Diabetic Nephropathy Trial (IDNT). In the IDNT, therapy with irbesartan (dosage titrated from 75 to 300 mg daily) reduced the risk of the primary composite end point, which was defined as a doubling of the baseline serum creatinine concentration, end-stage renal disease (i.e., initiation of dialysis, renal transplantation, or a serum creatinine concentration of at least 6 mg/dL), or death, by 23% compared with amlodipine therapy (dosage titrated from 2.5 to 10 mg daily) and by 20% compared with placebo. Additional antihypertensive agents (diuretics, β-adrenergic blocking agents [β-blockers], peripheral α-adrenergic blocking agents, or central α_2-adrenergic agonists) were used as needed in all treatment groups to achieve a trough blood pressure of 135/85 mm Hg or less in the sitting position or 10 mm Hg reduction in systolic blood pressure if higher than 160 mm Hg; ACE inhibitors, other angiotensin II receptor antagonists, and calcium-channel blocking agents could not be used. Most of the delay in time to occurrence of composite clinical events seen with irbesartan-containing therapy was the result of a reduction in the risk of doubling of serum creatinine concentration; irbesartan-containing therapy had no appreciable effect on overall mortality, onset of end-stage renal disease, or secondary composite cardiovascular end point (death from cardiovascular causes, nonfatal myocardial infarction, hospitalization for heart failure, stroke with permanent neurologic deficit, amputation) compared with other treatments. Mean blood pressure achieved with either irbesartan- or amlodipine-containing therapies was similar (142/77 or 142/76 mm Hg, respectively) and lower than that achieved with placebo plus other antihypertensive agents (145/79 mm Hg). Despite therapy with an average of 3 other nonstudy antihypertensive agents per patient in all treatment groups, none of the treatment groups achieved the target blood pressure goal.

■ **Heart Failure** Angiotensin II receptor antagonists have been used in the management of heart failure†.

Current guidelines for the management of heart failure in adults generally recommend a combination of drug therapies to reduce morbidity and mortality, including neurohormonal antagonists (e.g., ACE inhibitors, angiotensin II receptor antagonists, angiotensin receptor-neprilysin inhibitors [ARNIs], β-blockers, aldosterone receptor antagonists) that inhibit the detrimental compensatory mechanisms in heart failure. Additional agents (e.g., cardiac glycosides, diuretics, sinoatrial modulators [i.e., ivabradine]) added to a heart failure treatment regimen in selected patients have been associated with symptomatic improvement and/or reduction in heart failure-related hospitalizations. Experts recommend that all asymptomatic patients with reduced left ventricular ejection fraction (LVEF) (American College of Cardiology Foundation [ACCF]/American Heart Association [AHA] stage B heart failure) receive therapy with an ACE inhibitor and β-blocker to prevent symptomatic heart failure and reduce morbidity and mortality. In patients with prior or current symptoms of chronic heart failure with reduced LVEF (ACCF/AHA stage C heart failure), ACCF, AHA, and the Heart Failure Society of America (HFSA) recommend inhibition of the renin-angiotensin-aldosterone (RAA) system with an ACE inhibitor, angiotensin II receptor antagonist, or ARNI in conjunction with a β-

blocker, and an aldosterone antagonist in selected patients, to reduce morbidity and mortality. While ACE inhibitors have been the preferred drugs for inhibition of the RAA system because of their established benefits in patients with heart failure and reduced ejection fraction, some evidence indicates that therapy with sacubitril/valsartan, an ARNI, may be more effective than ACE inhibitor therapy (enalapril) in reducing cardiovascular death and heart failure-related hospitalization. ACCF, AHA, and HFSA recommend that patients with chronic symptomatic heart failure and reduced LVEF (New York Heart Association [NYHA] functional class II or III) who are able to tolerate an ACE inhibitor or angiotensin II receptor antagonist be switched to therapy containing an ARNI to further reduce morbidity and mortality. However, in patients in whom an ARNI is not appropriate, continued use of an ACE inhibitor for all classes of heart failure with reduced ejection fraction remains strongly advised. In patients in whom an ARNI or ACE inhibitor is not appropriate, an angiotensin II receptor antagonist may be used. For additional information on the use of angiotensin II receptor antagonists in the management of heart failure, see Uses: Heart Failure, in Valsartan 24:32.08 and in Candesartan 24:32.08. For further information on the use of ARNIs in patients with heart failure, see Uses: Heart Failure, in Sacubitril and Valsartan 24:32.92.

Several clinical trials in patients with heart failure have evaluated the use of angiotensin II receptor antagonists as add-on therapy to conventional regimens compared with an ACE inhibitor, as add-on therapy to conventional regimens including an ACE inhibitor, as combination therapy with an ACE inhibitor compared with therapy with either type of agent alone, or as an alternative therapy in patients intolerant of ACE inhibitors. Data from these and other long-term placebo-controlled clinical trials indicate that angiotensin II receptor antagonists produce hemodynamic and neurohormonal effects associated with their suppression of the renin-angiotensin system; reduced hospitalizations and mortality also have been demonstrated. However, in some studies, these drugs did not show consistent effects on cardiac symptoms or exercise tolerance.

While angiotensin II receptor antagonists are considered reasonable alternatives in patients who are unable to tolerate ACE inhibitors (e.g., because of cough or angioedema), urticaria and angioedema (e.g., swelling of the face, lips, pharynx, and/or tongue) have been reported rarely during postmarketing experience in patients receiving irbesartan. (See Sensitivity Reactions under Cautions: Warnings/Precautions.)

Dosage and Administration

■ **Administration** Irbesartan is administered orally. Since food does not affect the oral bioavailability of irbesartan, the manufacturer states that the drug can be taken without regard to meals.

■ **Dosage** ***Hypertension*** Dosage of irbesartan must be individualized and adjusted according to blood pressure response.

Irbesartan Therapy. The manufacturer states that the usual initial dosage of irbesartan in adults is 150 mg once daily in patients without depletion of intravascular volume; in adults with depletion of intravascular volume, the usual initial dosage is 75 mg once daily. If blood pressure response is inadequate with the initial dosage, dosage may be increased as tolerated to 300 mg daily or a diuretic may be added. Increasing irbesartan dosages beyond 300 mg daily or dividing the total daily dosage into 2 doses usually does not result in additional therapeutic effect. Some experts state that the usual dosage range is 150–300 mg once daily. Addition of a diuretic generally has a greater effect on blood pressure reduction than dosage increases of irbesartan beyond 300 mg daily. Irbesartan also can be used concomitantly with other antihypertensive agents.

The manufacturer states that some of the irbesartan dosages used in a clinical study did not effectively lower blood pressure in pediatric patients 6–16 years of age. (See Pediatric Use under Cautions: Specific Populations.) In children 6–12 years of age, experts recommend an initial irbesartan dosage of 75 mg once daily and a maximum dosage of 150 mg once daily. In children at least 13 years of age, experts recommend an initial irbesartan dosage of 150 mg once daily and a maximum dosage of 300 mg once daily. These experts state the dosage may be increased every 2–4 weeks until blood pressure is controlled, the maximum dosage is reached, or adverse effects occur. For information on overall principles and expert recommendations for treatment of hypertension in pediatric patients, see Uses: Hypertension in Pediatric Patients, in the Thiazides General Statement 40:28.20.

Irbesartan/Hydrochlorothiazide Fixed-combination Therapy. In patients who do not respond adequately to monotherapy with irbesartan or, alternatively, with hydrochlorothiazide, combined therapy with the drugs can be used. The manufacturer states that combined therapy with the commercially available fixed-combination preparation containing 150 mg of irbesartan and 12.5 mg of hydrochlorothiazide, 300 mg of irbesartan and 12.5 mg of hydrochlorothiazide, or 300 mg of irbesartan and 25 mg of hydrochlorothiazide (in order of increasing mean effect) can be used in patients whose blood pressure is not adequately controlled by monotherapy with irbesartan or hydrochlorothiazide. The maximum antihypertensive effect is attained about 2–4 weeks after a change in dosage. Dosage of the fixed-combination preparation should not exceed 300 mg of irbesartan and 25 mg of hydrochlorothiazide once daily.

Irbesartan in fixed combination with hydrochlorothiazide also can be used for initial treatment of hypertension in patients who are likely to need multiple drugs to achieve their blood pressure goals. The decision to use irbesartan in fixed combination with hydrochlorothiazide as initial therapy should be based on an assessment of potential benefits and risks. Patients with moderate to severe hypertension are at relatively high risk for cardiovascular events (e.g., stroke, myocardial infarction, heart failure), kidney failure, and vision problems; therefore, prompt treatment is clinically important. The decision to use combination therapy as initial treatment should be individualized taking into account baseline blood pressure, target goal, and incremental likelihood of achieving blood pressure goal with combination therapy compared with monotherapy. In patients receiving fixed-combination tablets as initial therapy, the usual starting dosage is irbesartan 150 mg and hydrochlorothiazide 12.5 mg once daily. Dosage may be increased after 1–2 weeks of therapy to a maximum of irbesartan 300 mg and hydrochlorothiazide 25 mg once daily.

Blood Pressure Monitoring and Treatment Goals. Blood pressure should be monitored regularly (i.e., monthly) during therapy and dosage of the antihypertensive drug adjusted until blood pressure is controlled. If an adequate blood pressure response is not achieved with angiotensin II receptor antagonist monotherapy, the dosage may be increased or another antihypertensive agent with demonstrated benefit and preferably with a complementary mechanism of action (e.g., calcium-channel blocker, thiazide diuretic) may be added; if target blood pressure is still not achieved, a third drug may be added. (See Uses: Hypertension.) In patients who develop unacceptable adverse effects with irbesartan, the drug should be discontinued and another antihypertensive agent from a different pharmacologic class should be initiated.

The goal of hypertension management and prevention is to achieve and maintain optimal control of blood pressure. However, the optimum blood pressure threshold for initiating antihypertensive drug therapy and specific treatment goals remain controversial. While previous hypertension guidelines have based target blood pressure goals on age and comorbidities, the 2017 ACC/AHA hypertension guideline incorporates underlying cardiovascular risk into decision making regarding treatment and generally recommends the same target blood pressure (i.e., less than 130/80 mm Hg) in all adults. Many patients will require at least 2 drugs from different pharmacologic classes to achieve their blood pressure goal; the potential benefits of hypertension management and drug cost, adverse effects, and risks associated with the use of multiple antihypertensive drugs also should be considered when deciding a patient's blood pressure treatment goal.

For additional information on target levels of blood pressure and on monitoring therapy in the management of hypertension, see Blood Pressure Monitoring and Treatment Goals under Dosage: Hypertension, in Dosage and Administration in the Thiazides General Statement 40:28.20.

Diabetic Nephropathy For the management of diabetic nephropathy in patients with type 2 diabetes mellitus, the recommended target maintenance dosage of irbesartan is 300 mg once daily. No data are available on the effects of lower dosages of irbesartan on diabetic nephropathy. In a large clinical trial, approximately 83% of patients had dosage titrated from 75 mg daily initially up to 300 mg daily and maintained that dosage for more than 50% of the study period.

■ **Special Populations** Volume and/or salt depletion should be corrected prior to initiation of therapy or, alternatively, therapy should be initiated using a lower initial dosage (75 mg once daily). Fixed-combination tablets containing irbesartan and hydrochlorothiazide are *not* recommended as initial therapy in patients with intravascular volume depletion.

The manufacturer states that dosage modification of irbesartan is not necessary for adults with renal impairment; however, irbesartan should be used with caution in patients with renal impairment and depletion of intravascular volume. If concomitant diuretic therapy is required in patients with severe renal impairment (i.e., creatinine clearance less than 30 mL/minute), a loop diuretic is preferred to a thiazide diuretic. Therefore, commercially available preparations containing irbesartan in fixed combination with hydrochlorothiazide usually are *not* recommended for patients with severe renal impairment. Irbesartan is not removed by hemodialysis.

The manufacturer states that dosage adjustment is not necessary in patients with hepatic impairment.

The manufacturer states that dosage modification of irbesartan because of age in geriatric adults is not necessary. Because of the greater frequency of decreased hepatic, renal, and/or cardiac function and of concomitant disease and/or drug therapy in geriatric patients, dosage of irbesartan in fixed combination with hydrochlorothiazide should be carefully selected in such patients. The manufacturer recommends that dosage of the fixed combination be initiated at the lower end of the usual range in geriatric patients.

Cautions

■ **Contraindications** Known hypersensitivity to irbesartan or any ingredient in the formulation.

Concomitant use of irbesartan and aliskiren in patients with diabetes mellitus. (See Drug Interactions: Drugs that Block the Renin-Angiotensin System.)

■ **Warnings/Precautions** ***Warnings*** **Fetal/Neonatal Morbidity and Mortality.** Drugs that act on the renin-angiotensin system (e.g., angiotensin-converting enzyme [ACE] inhibitors, angiotensin II receptor antagonists) reduce fetal renal function and increase fetal and neonatal morbidity and mortality when used in pregnancy during the second and third trimesters. Resulting oligohydramnios can be associated with fetal lung hypoplasia and skeletal deformations. Potential neonatal effects include skull hypoplasia, anuria, hypotension, renal failure, and death. Irbesartan should be discontinued as soon as possible when pregnancy is detected, unless continued use is considered life-saving. Nearly all women can be transferred successfully to alternative therapy for the remainder of their pregnancy. For additional information on the risk of such drugs during pregnancy, see Cautions: Pregnancy, Fertility, and Lactation, in Captopril 24:32.04 and Enalaprilat/Enalapril 24:32.04.

Sensitivity Reactions Sensitivity reactions, including various anaphylactoid reactions and/or angioedema, have been reported with use of angiotensin II receptor antagonists, including irbesartan. Irbesartan is not recommended in patients with a history of angioedema associated with or unrelated to ACE inhibitor or angiotensin II receptor antagonist therapy.

Other Warnings and Precautions **Hypotension.** Symptomatic hypotension has been reported in patients receiving irbesartan, especially in volume- and/or salt-depleted patients (e.g., those treated with diuretics or undergoing dialysis). Volume and/or salt depletion should be corrected before initiation of irbesartan therapy or a lower initial dosage should be used. (See Dosage and Administration: Special Populations.)

Transient hypotension is not a contraindication to additional doses; therapy may be reinstated cautiously after blood pressure is stabilized (e.g., with volume expansion).

Malignancies. In July 2010, the US Food and Drug Administration (FDA) initiated a safety review of angiotensin II receptor antagonists after a published meta-analysis suggested a possible association between the use of these agents and an increased risk of cancer. The meta-analysis, which combined cancer-related findings from 5 randomized, controlled trials in over 60,000 patients, found a modest but significant increase in the risk of new cancer occurrence in patients receiving an angiotensin II receptor antagonist (mostly telmisartan) compared with those in control groups (7.2 versus 6%, respectively; risk ratio 1.08). However, because of several limitations of the study (e.g., trials included in the meta-analysis were not specifically designed to evaluate cancer outcomes, lack of individual patient data), the validity of these findings has been questioned.

Subsequent studies, including a larger, more comprehensive meta-analysis conducted by FDA, have not shown an increased risk of cancer in patients receiving angiotensin II receptor antagonists. FDA's meta-analysis, which included trial-level data from 31 randomized studies (total of approximately 156,000 patients), found no evidence of an increased risk of cancer in patients who received an angiotensin II receptor antagonist compared with those who received other treatments (placebo or active control). The overall rate of new cancer occurrence was essentially the same in both groups of patients (1.82 and 1.84 cases per 100 patient-years, respectively). In addition, there was no difference in the risk of cancer-related death, breast cancer, lung cancer, or prostate cancer between the groups. Based on these results and a review of all currently available data related to this potential safety concern, FDA has concluded that use of angiotensin II receptor antagonists is not associated with an increased risk of cancer.

Renal Effects. Because the renin-angiotensin-aldosterone (RAA) system appears to contribute substantially to maintenance of glomerular filtration in patients with heart failure in whom renal perfusion is severely compromised, renal function may deteriorate markedly (e.g., oliguria, progressive azotemia, renal failure, death) in these patients during therapy with an ACE inhibitor or an angiotensin II receptor antagonist (e.g., irbesartan). Increases in BUN and serum creatinine also may occur in patients with renal artery stenosis, chronic kidney disease (CKD), or volume depletion. Renal function should be monitored periodically in these patients. The clinician should consider withholding or discontinuing irbesartan in patients who develop a clinically important reduction in renal function while receiving irbesartan. (See Cautions: Renal Effects, in Enalapril 24:32.04.)

Fixed-combination Preparations. When hydrochlorothiazide is used in fixed combination with irbesartan, the usual cautions, precautions, and contraindications associated with hydrochlorothiazide must be considered in addition to those associated with irbesartan. (See Cautions, in the Thiazides General Statement 40:28.20.)

Specific Populations **Pregnancy.** Category D. (See Users Guide)

Irbesartan can cause fetal and neonatal morbidity and mortality when administered to a pregnant woman. Irbesartan should be discontinued as soon as possible when pregnancy is detected. (See Fetal/Neonatal Morbidity and Mortality under Warnings/Precautions: Warnings, in Cautions.)

Lactation. Irbesartan is distributed into milk in rats; it is not known whether the drug is distributed into human milk. Because of the potential risk in nursing infants, a decision should be made whether to discontinue nursing or the drug.

Pediatric Use. If oliguria or hypotension occurs in neonates with a history of in utero exposure to irbesartan, blood pressure and renal function should be supported; exchange transfusions or dialysis may be required. (See Fetal/Neonatal Morbidity and Mortality under Warnings/Precautions: Warnings, in Cautions.)

Administration of irbesartan in dosages of up to 4.5 mg/kg once daily did not appear to effectively lower blood pressure in pediatric patients 6–16 years of age. Safety and efficacy of irbesartan in children younger than 6 years of age have not been established.

Safety and efficacy of the fixed-combination preparation containing irbesartan and hydrochlorothiazide in pediatric patients have not been established.

For information on overall principles and expert recommendations for treatment of hypertension in pediatric patients, see Uses: Hypertension in Pediatric Patients, in the Thiazides General Statement 40:28.20.

Geriatric Use. No substantial differences in safety or efficacy of irbesartan monotherapy or fixed-combination irbesartan/hydrochlorothiazide tablets have been observed in geriatric patients relative to younger adults, but increased sensitivity cannot be ruled out.

Renal Impairment. Irbesartan should be used with caution in patients with renal impairment.

Deterioration of renal function may occur in patients receiving irbesartan.

Use of irbesartan in fixed combination with hydrochlorothiazide is *not* recommended in patients with severe renal impairment.

Black Patients. Blood pressure reduction may be smaller in black patients compared with nonblack patients; clinicians should consider using irbesartan in combination with a diuretic or calcium-channel blocker.

■ **Common Adverse Effects** Adverse effects occurring in at least 1% of patients with hypertension receiving irbesartan and at a higher incidence than with placebo in clinical trials include diarrhea, dyspepsia/heartburn, and fatigue. In patients receiving irbesartan for the treatment of diabetic nephropathy, dizziness, orthostatic dizziness, and orthostatic hypotension occurred with an incidence of at least 5% and were reported more frequently than in those receiving placebo.

Drug Interactions

■ **Agents that Increase Serum Potassium** Concomitant administration of irbesartan with potassium-sparing diuretics, potassium supplements, potassium-containing salt substitutes, or other drugs that increase serum potassium concentrations may result in hyperkalemia. Serum potassium concentrations should be monitored in such patients.

■ **Drugs Affecting Hepatic Microsomal Enzymes** Metabolized principally by cytochrome P-450 (CYP) 2C9 isoenzyme. Does not substantially induce or inhibit CYP1A1, 1A2, 2A6, 2B6, 2D6, 2E1, or 3A4. Potential pharmacokinetic interaction (decreased irbesartan metabolism) with CYP2C9 inhibitors.

■ **Drugs that Block the Renin-Angiotensin System** Increased risk of hypotension, hyperkalemia, and changes in renal function (e.g., renal impairment) with concomitant use of other drugs that block the renin-angiotensin system (e.g., angiotensin-converting enzyme [ACE] inhibitors, angiotensin II receptor antagonists, aliskiren); when irbesartan is used concomitantly with such drugs, blood pressure, renal function, and serum electrolyte concentrations should be monitored closely. The manufacturer states that most patients do not derive additional benefit from combination therapy with 2 renin-angiotensin system inhibitors compared with monotherapy. Concomitant use of irbesartan and aliskiren is contraindicated in patients with diabetes mellitus; in addition, such concomitant use should be avoided in patients with renal impairment (glomerular filtration rate [GFR] less than 60 mL/minute). (See Use in Combination with Angiotensin-converting Enzyme Inhibitors or Angiotensin II Receptor Antagonists under Warnings/Precautions: Other Warnings and Precautions, in Cautions in Aliskiren Hemifumarate 24:32.40.)

■ **Digoxin** Pharmacologic and/or pharmacokinetic interactions unlikely when irbesartan is used concomitantly with digoxin.

■ **Hydrochlorothiazide** Pharmacokinetic interactions unlikely when irbesartan is used concomitantly with hydrochlorothiazide.

Additive hypotensive effects expected when irbesartan is used concomitantly with hydrochlorothiazide.

■ **Lithium** Elevations in lithium concentrations and lithium toxicity have been reported when irbesartan is used concomitantly with lithium. Serum lithium concentrations should be carefully monitored.

■ **Nifedipine** Decreased irbesartan metabolism in vitro observed with nifedipine; alteration of irbesartan pharmacokinetics not observed in vivo when irbesartan is used concomitantly with nifedipine.

■ **Nonsteroidal Anti-inflammatory Agents** Possible deterioration of renal function in geriatric, volume-depleted (including those receiving concomitant diuretic therapy), or renally impaired patients; renal function should be monitored periodically in patients receiving concomitant therapy with irbesartan and a nonsteroidal anti-inflammatory agent (NSAIA), including selective cyclooxygenase-2 (COX-2) inhibitors.

Potential pharmacologic interaction (attenuated hypotensive effects) when angiotensin II receptor antagonists are used concomitantly with NSAIAs, including selective COX-29 inhibitors.

■ **Tolbutamide** Possible decreased irbesartan metabolism when irbesartan is used concomitantly with tolbutamide.

■ **Warfarin** Pharmacologic and/or pharmacokinetic interaction unlikely when irbesartan is used concomitantly with warfarin.

Description

Irbesartan, a nonpeptide tetrazole derivative, is an angiotensin II type 1 (AT_1) receptor antagonist. Irbesartan has pharmacologic actions similar to those of losartan; however, unlike losartan, irbesartan is not a prodrug and its pharmacologic activity does not depend on hydrolysis in the liver.

Irbesartan blocks the physiologic actions of angiotensin II, including vasoconstrictor and aldosterone-secreting effects, by selectively inhibiting access of angiotensin II to AT_1 receptors within many tissues, including vascular smooth muscle and the adrenal gland. By comparison, angiotensin-converting enzyme (ACE, kininase II) inhibitors block the conversion of angiotensin I to angiotensin II; however, the blockade of angiotensin II production by ACE inhibitors is not complete since the vasopressor hormone can be formed via other enzymes that are not blocked by ACE inhibitors. Because irbesartan, unlike ACE inhibitors, does not inhibit ACE, the drug does not interfere with response to bradykinins and substance P; a beneficial consequence is the absence of certain ACE inhibitor-induced adverse effects (e.g., cough), but possible renal and/or cardioprotective effects may be sacrificed.

Advice to Patients

Importance of informing women of risks of use during pregnancy. Importance of women informing clinicians if they plan to become pregnant or plan to breast-feed. All women of childbearing potential should be advised to report pregnancy to their clinician as soon as possible. See Fetal/Neonatal Morbidity and Mortality under Warnings/Precautions: Warnings, in Cautions.

Importance of informing clinicians of existing or contemplated concomitant therapy, including prescription and OTC drugs.

Importance of informing patients of other important precautionary information. (See Cautions.)

Overview® (see Users Guide). For additional information on this drug until a more detailed monograph is developed and published, the manufacturer's labeling should be consulted. It is *essential* that the manufacturer's labeling be consulted for more detailed information on usual cautions, precautions, contraindications, potential drug interactions, laboratory test interferences, and acute toxicity.

Preparations

Excipients in commercially available drug preparations may have clinically important effects in some individuals; consult specific product labeling for details.

Irbesartan

Oral		
Tablets	75 mg	**Avapro®**, Sanofi-Aventis
	150 mg	**Avapro®**, Sanofi-Aventis
	300 mg	**Avapro®**, Sanofi-Aventis

Irbesartan Combinations

Oral		
Tablets	150 mg with Hydrochlorothiazide 12.5 mg	**Avalide®**, Sanofi-Aventis
	300 mg with Hydrochlorothiazide 12.5 mg	**Avalide®**, Sanofi-Aventis

†Use is not currently included in the labeling approved by the US Food and Drug Administration

Losartan Potassium

■ Losartan potassium, a nonpeptide tetrazole derivative, is an angiotensin II type 1 (AT_1) receptor antagonist (also referred to as an angiotensin II receptor blocker [ARB]).

Uses

■ Hypertension Losartan is used alone or in combination with other classes of antihypertensive agents, including diuretics, in the management of hypertension.

Angiotensin II receptor antagonists, such as losartan, are considered one of several preferred antihypertensive drugs for the initial management of hypertension according to current evidence-based hypertension guidelines; other preferred options include angiotensin-converting enzyme (ACE) inhibitors, calcium-channel blockers, and thiazide diuretics. While there may be individual differences with respect to recommendations for initial drug selection and use in specific patient populations, current evidence indicates that these antihypertensive drug classes all generally produce comparable effects on overall mortality and cardiovascular, cerebrovascular, and renal outcomes. (See Uses: Hypertension, in Valsartan 24:32.08.)

Angiotensin II receptor antagonists or ACE inhibitors may be particularly useful in the management of hypertension in patients with certain coexisting conditions such as diabetes mellitus or chronic kidney disease (CKD); angiotensin II receptor antagonists also may be preferred, generally as an alternative to ACE inhibitors, in hypertensive patients with heart failure or ischemic heart disease and/or following myocardial infarction (MI). (See Uses: Hypertension, in Valsartan 24:32.08.)

In patients with hypertension and compelling indications (e.g., CKD with albuminuria [urine albumin 300 mg/day or greater, or urine albumin:creatinine ratio of 300 mg/g or equivalent in the first morning void]), angiotensin II receptor antagonists are usually considered an alternative for ACE inhibitor-intolerant patients. However, data indicate no difference in efficacy between ACE inhibitors and angiotensin II receptor antagonists with regard to blood pressure lowering and clinical outcomes (i.e., all-cause mortality, cardiovascular mortality, MI, heart failure, stroke, and end-stage renal disease). Adverse events (e.g., cough, angioedema) leading to drug discontinuance occur more frequently with ACE inhibitor therapy than with angiotensin II receptor antagonist therapy. Because of similar efficacy and a lower frequency of adverse effects, some experts believe that angiotensin II receptor antagonists should be used instead of an ACE inhibitor for the treatment of hypertension or hypertension with certain compelling indications.

Efficacy of losartan in the treatment of hypertension was established in placebo-controlled studies of 6–12 weeks' duration in patients with hypertension (baseline diastolic blood pressure: 95–115 mm Hg). In these patients, losartan potassium dosages of 50–150 mg once daily were associated with mean decreases in systolic blood pressure of 5.5–10.5 mm Hg and diastolic blood pressure of 3.5–7.5 mm Hg. Daily dosages of 150 mg did not result in greater decreases in blood pressure compared with daily dosages of 50–100 mg. Larger decreases in trough blood pressures were observed with twice-daily dosing compared with once daily dosing in patients receiving daily dosages of 50–100 mg. Rebound hypertension following abrupt withdrawal of the drug has not been reported.

Most patients with hypertension, especially black patients, will require at least 2 antihypertensive drugs to achieve adequate blood pressure control. Like ACE inhibitors, angiotensin II receptor antagonists such as losartan may produce a smaller blood pressure response in hypertensive black patients compared with nonblack patients. However, the combination of an ACE inhibitor or an angiotensin II receptor antagonist with a calcium-channel blocker or thiazide diuretic produces similar blood pressure lowering in black patients as in other racial groups. (See Race under Hypertension: Other Special Considerations for Antihypertensive Drug Therapy, in Uses in Valsartan 24:32.08.)

For additional information on the management of hypertension, see Uses: Hypertension, in Valsartan 24:32.08. For information on overall principles and expert recommendations for treatment of hypertension, see Uses: Hypertension in Adults and also see Uses: Hypertension in Pediatric Patients, in the Thiazides General Statement 40:28.20.

■ Prevention of Cardiovascular Morbidity and Mortality Losartan is used alone or in combination with other antihypertensive agents (e.g., hydrochlorothiazide) to reduce the risk of stroke in patients with hypertension and left ventricular hypertrophy; however, there is evidence that the benefit associated with such losartan-based antihypertensive therapy does not apply to black patients. In a randomized, double-blind, comparative study (Losartan Intervention for Endpoint [LIFE] reduction in hypertension) of approximately 4 years' duration in more than 9000 patients, losartan-based antihypertensive therapy (e.g., losartan 50–100 mg with hydrochlorothiazide 12.5–25 mg daily) reduced the risk of the primary outcome of combined cardiovascular death, stroke, and myocardial infarction (relative risk reduction of about 13%, adjusted for Framingham risk score and baseline left ventricular hypertrophy) compared with atenolol-containing therapy (e.g., atenolol 50–100 mg with hydrochlorothiazide 12.5–25 mg daily) despite similar control of blood pressure with each regimen. In addition, the rate of drug-related adverse events and the incidence of new-onset diabetes mellitus was less in patients receiving losartan-based therapy. The study population consisted primarily of white patients 55–80 years of age with ECG evidence of left ventricular hypertrophy but who did not have low left-ventricular ejection fraction (40% or less) or heart failure. The results of the study provided no evidence that the benefits of losartan in reducing the risk of cardiovascular events in patients with hypertension and left ventricular hypertrophy apply to black patients. Among black patients in the study, the risk of experiencing the primary outcome of combined cardiovascular death, stroke, and myocardial infarction was lower in patients receiving atenolol (11%) than in patients receiving losartan (17%).

Subgroup analysis of the LIFE study (mean follow-up 4.7 years) suggests that aspirin therapy at baseline in patients receiving losartan reduced the risk of the primary outcome of combined cardiovascular death, stroke, and myocardial infarction (relative risk reduction of about 32%, adjusted for Framingham risk score and baseline left ventricular hypertrophy) compared with aspirin therapy at baseline in patients receiving atenolol, despite similar control of blood pressure with each regimen. Further studies are needed to determine whether these differences are associated with a pharmacologic interaction or a selection by aspirin use of patients more likely to respond to losartan therapy.

■ Diabetic Nephropathy Losartan is used in the management of diabetic nephropathy manifested by elevated serum creatinine and proteinuria (urinary albumin to creatinine ratio of 300 mg/g or greater) in patients with type 2 diabetes mellitus and hypertension.

Both angiotensin II receptor antagonists and ACE inhibitors have been shown to slow the rate of progression of renal disease in patients with diabetes mellitus and persistent albuminuria, and use of a drug from either class is recommended in such patients with modestly elevated (30–300 mg/24 hours) or higher (exceeding 300 mg/24 hours) levels of urinary albumin excretion. Some evidence suggests that these drugs may slow the progression of nephropathy by a mechanism independent of their antihypertensive effects.

Comparative trials evaluating the efficacy of angiotensin II receptor antagonists and ACE inhibitors for improving renal outcomes in diabetic patients are lacking. Evidence supporting use of ACE inhibitors generally is based on studies in patients with type 1 diabetes mellitus, while evidence supporting use of angiotensin II receptor antagonists generally is based on studies in patients with type 2 diabetes mellitus. Findings from these studies indicate that both drug classes delay progression of increased urinary albumin excretion in patients with diabetes mellitus and also may slow the decline in renal function. Because the available data are consistent, some experts suggest that the effects of both drug classes in improving renal outcomes in patients with diabetes mellitus and proteinuria are likely to be similar.

Drugs that inhibit the renin-angiotensin system (i.e., ACE inhibitors, angiotensin II receptor antagonists) also have been shown to delay the onset of albuminuria in patients with type 2 diabetes mellitus and hypertension who have normal levels of urinary albumin excretion†; however, some experts state that in the absence of albuminuria, the risk of progressive kidney disease is low. The American Diabetes Association (ADA) states that the use of an ACE inhibitor or angiotensin II receptor antagonist is not recommended for the primary prevention of diabetic nephropathy in patients with diabetes mellitus who are normotensive, have normal levels of urinary protein excretion, and have a normal glomerular filtration rate (GFR).

Combined therapy with ACE inhibitors and angiotensin II receptor antagonists provides no additional cardiovascular benefit and increases the risk of adverse effects (e.g., impaired renal function, hyperkalemia). The usual precautions of angiotensin II receptor antagonist therapy in patients with substantial renal impairment should be observed.

The current labeled indication for losartan in hypertensive patients with type 2 diabetes mellitus and nephropathy (indicated by an elevated serum creatinine and urinary albumin to creatinine ratio of 300 mg/g or greater) is based principally on the results of a long-term (mean duration of follow-up: 3.4 years), multicenter, placebo-controlled trial, the Reduction of Endpoints in NIDDM with the Angiotensin II Receptor Antagonist Losartan (RENAAL) study. In the RENAAL trial, therapy with losartan potassium (50 mg daily initially and titrated to 100 mg daily) reduced the risk of the primary composite clinical end point, which was defined as a doubling of the baseline serum creatinine concentration, end-stage renal disease (i.e., need for dialysis or renal transplantation), or death, by 16% compared with placebo. Additional antihypertensive agents (diuretics, calcium-channel blocking agents, α- or β-adrenergic blocking agents (β-blockers), and/or centrally acting agents) were used as needed in all treatment groups to achieve a trough blood pressure of less than 140/90 mm Hg in the sitting position; ACE inhibitors and other angiotensin II receptor antagonists could not be used. Most of the delay in time to occurrence of composite clinical events seen with losartan-containing therapy was the result of a reduction in the risk of doubling serum creatinine concentration and end-stage renal disease (25 and 28% reductions, respectively); losartan-containing therapy had no appreciable effect on overall mortality. Similar mean blood pressures were achieved with losartan or placebo plus conventional antihypertensive therapy.

■ **Heart Failure** Angiotensin II receptor antagonists have been used in the management of heart failure†.

Current guidelines for the management of heart failure in adults generally recommend a combination of drug therapies to reduce morbidity and mortality, including neurohormonal antagonists (e.g., ACE inhibitors, angiotensin II receptor antagonists, angiotensin receptor-neprilysin inhibitors [ARNIs], β-blockers, aldosterone receptor antagonists) that inhibit the detrimental compensatory mechanisms in heart failure. Additional agents (e.g., cardiac glycosides, diuretics, sinoatrial modulators [i.e., ivabradine]) added to a heart failure treatment regimen in selected patients have been associated with symptomatic improvement and/or reduction in heart failure-related hospitalizations. Experts recommend that all asymptomatic patients with reduced left ventricular ejection fraction (LVEF) (American College of Cardiology Foundation [ACCF]/American Heart Association [AHA] stage B heart failure) receive therapy with an ACE inhibitor and β-blocker to prevent symptomatic heart failure and reduce morbidity and mortality. In patients with prior or current symptoms of chronic heart failure with reduced LVEF (ACCF/AHA stage C heart failure), ACCF, AHA, and the Heart Failure Society of America (HFSA) recommend inhibition of the renin-angiotensin-aldosterone (RAA) system with an ACE inhibitor, angiotensin II receptor antagonist, or ARNI in conjunction with a β-blocker, and an aldosterone antagonist in selected patients, to reduce morbidity and mortality. While ACE inhibitors have been the preferred drugs for inhibition of the RAA system because of their established benefits in patients with heart failure and reduced ejection fraction, some evidence indicates that therapy with sacubitril/valsartan, an ARNI, may be more effective than ACE inhibitor therapy (enalapril) in reducing cardiovascular death and heart failure-related hospitalization. ACCF, AHA, and HFSA recommend that patients with chronic symptomatic heart failure and reduced LVEF (New York Heart Association [NYHA] functional class II or III) who are able to tolerate an ACE inhibitor or angiotensin II receptor antagonist be switched to therapy containing an ARNI to further reduce morbidity and mortality. However, in patients in whom an ARNI is not appropriate, continued use of an ACE inhibitor for all classes of heart failure with reduced ejection fraction remains strongly advised. In patients in whom an ARNI or ACE inhibitor is not appropriate, an angiotensin II receptor antagonist may be used. For additional information on the use of angiotensin II receptor antagonists in the management of heart failure, see Uses: Heart Failure, in Valsartan 24:32.08 and in Candesartan 24:32.08. For further information on the use of ARNIs in patients with heart failure, see Uses: Heart Failure, in Sacubitril and Valsartan 24:32.92.

Several clinical trials have evaluated the use of angiotensin II receptor antagonists as add-on therapy to conventional regimens including an ACE inhibitor, as add-on therapy to conventional regimens compared with an ACE inhibitor, as combination therapy with an ACE inhibitor compared with therapy with either type of agent alone, or as an alternative therapy in patients intolerant of ACE inhibitors. Data from these and other long-term placebo-controlled clinical trials indicate that angiotensin II receptor antagonists produce hemodynamic and neurohormonal effects associated with their suppression of the renin-angiotensin system; reduced hospitalizations and mortality also have been demonstrated. However, in some studies, these drugs did not show consistent effects on cardiac symptoms or exercise tolerance.

In one comparative study (Evaluation of Losartan in the Elderly [ELITE]) in geriatric patients 65 years of age and older who received losartan (up to 50 mg daily) or captopril (up to 150 mg daily) in addition to conventional therapy for 48 weeks, patients receiving losartan had a 46% lower risk of death and also experienced a lower incidence of adverse effects than those receiving captopril. However, after interim analysis of data, the difference in survival was no longer significant and no difference in morbidity and mortality or frequency in hospitalizations for heart failure was found between the 2 therapies. Results of a follow-up study (ELITE II), failed to confirm a survival benefit for losartan therapy compared with captopril. In this study, losartan did not provide a statistically significant difference in reduction of overall death, sudden cardiac death, and/or resuscitated cardiac arrest compared with captopril, although ELITE II was not designed to demonstrate equivalence between the 2 therapies. For additional details on the use of angiotensin II receptor antagonists in the management of heart failure, see Uses: Heart Failure, in Valsartan 24:32.08 and in Candesartan 24:32.08.

While angiotensin II receptor antagonists are considered reasonable alternatives in patients who are unable to tolerate ACE inhibitors (e.g., because of cough or angioedema), angioedema, including swelling of the larynx and glottis (causing airway obstruction) and/or swelling of the face, lips, pharynx, and/or tongue, has been reported rarely during postmarketing experience in patients receiving losartan. The manufacturer states that some of these patients had a history of angioedema associated with other drugs (e.g., ACE inhibitors). (See Sensitivity Reactions under Cautions: Warnings/Precautions.)

Dosage and Administration

■ **Administration** Losartan is administered orally. Although food may decrease the rate of absorption of losartan and peak concentrations achieved, the magnitude of effect is not clinically important; the manufacturer states that the drug can be given without regard to meals.

For pediatric patients or patients unable to swallow tablets, losartan may be administered orally as an extemporaneously prepared suspension. An extemporaneous suspension containing losartan potassium 2.5 mg/mL can be prepared in the following manner. First, 10 mL of purified water is added to a 240-mL amber polyethylene terephthalate (PET) bottle containing ten 50-mg tablets of losartan potassium, and the contents are shaken for at least 2 minutes. The concentrated suspension should be allowed to stand for 60 minutes following reconstitution, and then should be shaken for an additional minute. A mixture containing equal parts (by volume) of syrup (Ora-Sweet SF®) and suspending vehicle (Ora-Plus®) should be prepared separately. The concentrated suspension of losartan should be diluted with 190 mL of the Ora-Sweet SF® and Ora-Plus® mixture, and the container then shaken an additional minute to disperse the ingredients. The suspension should be shaken before dispensing of each dose. The extemporaneous suspension is stable for up to 4 weeks when stored at 2–8°C.

■ **Dosage** Available as losartan potassium; dosage expressed in terms of the salt.

Hypertension Dosage of losartan potassium must be individualized and adjusted according to blood pressure response. Substantial therapeutic response to losartan generally occurs within 1 week of treatment initiation, but in some studies the maximum therapeutic response occurred in 3–6 weeks.

Losartan Therapy. The manufacturer states that the usual initial dosage of losartan potassium in adults is 50 mg daily; lower initial dosages (e.g., 25 mg daily) may be used in patients with possible depletion of intravascular volume, including those receiving a diuretic, or with hepatic impairment. (See Dosage and Administration: Special Populations.) The manufacturer states that the usual maintenance dosage is 25–100 mg daily given in 1 dose or 2 divided doses. Some experts state that the usual dosage range is 50–100 mg daily, given in 1 dose or 2 divided doses.

The usual initial dosage of losartan potassium in children 6 years of age and older is 0.7 mg/kg (up to 50 mg) once daily. Some experts state that the dosage may be increased every 2–4 weeks until blood pressure is controlled, the maximum dosage is reached, or adverse effects occur. The safety and efficacy of dosages exceeding 1.4 mg/kg or in excess of 100 mg daily have not been established. For information on overall principles and expert recommendations for treatment of hypertension in pediatric patients, see Uses: Hypertension in Pediatric Patients, in the Thiazides General Statement 40:28.20.

Losartan/Hydrochlorothiazide Fixed-combination Therapy. In patients who do not respond adequately to monotherapy with losartan or, alternatively, with hydrochlorothiazide, combined therapy with the drugs can be used. When combination therapy is necessary, the commercially available preparation containing losartan in fixed combination with hydrochlorothiazide generally should not be used initially. Dosage preferably should first be adjusted by titrating the dosage of each drug separately; if it is determined that the optimum maintenance dosage corresponds to the ratio in the commercial combination preparation, this product may be used. Alternatively, the manufacturer states that combined therapy can be initiated with the commercially available preparation in patients whose blood pressure is not adequately controlled with losartan monotherapy or with 25 mg daily of hydrochlorothiazide alone, in those in whom control is maintained but hypokalemia is problematic at this hydrochlorothiazide dosage, or in those with severe hypertension in whom the potential benefit of achieving prompt blood pressure control outweighs the potential risk of initiating therapy with the commercially available fixed combination. In such patients, the manufacturer states that combination therapy can be initiated with 50 mg of losartan potassium and 12.5 mg of hydrochlorothiazide daily as the fixed combination. In patients whose blood pressure is not adequately controlled with losartan 100 mg monotherapy, combination therapy can be initiated with 100 mg of losartan potassium and 12.5 mg of hydrochlorothiazide once daily as the fixed combination. If blood pressure is not controlled after about 3 weeks (or after 2–4 weeks of therapy in those with severe hypertension), dosage may be increased to 100 mg of losartan potassium and 25 mg of hydrochlorothiazide daily (administered as 2 tablets of the fixed combination containing 50 mg of losartan potassium and 12.5 mg of hydrochlorothiazide, or, alternatively, as 1 tablet of the fixed combination containing 100 mg of losartan potassium and 25 mg of hydrochlorothiazide). Additional increases using the fixed combination are not recommended. The fixed combination is *not* recommended for use in patients with creatinine clearances of 30 mL/minute or less, those with hepatic impairment, or those with intravascular volume depletion (e.g., patients receiving diuretics). (See Dosage and Administration: Special Populations.)

Blood Pressure Monitoring and Treatment Goals. Blood pressure should be monitored regularly (i.e., monthly) during therapy and dosage of the antihypertensive drug adjusted until blood pressure is controlled. If an adequate blood pressure response is not achieved with angiotensin II receptor antagonist monotherapy, the dosage may be increased or another antihypertensive agent with demonstrated benefit and preferably with a complementary mechanism of action (e.g., calcium-channel blocker, thiazide diuretic) may be added; if target blood pressure is still not achieved, a third drug may be added. (See Uses: Hypertension.) In patients who develop unacceptable adverse effects with losartan, the drug should be discontinued and another antihypertensive agent from a different pharmacologic class should be initiated.

The goal of hypertension management and prevention is to achieve and maintain optimal control of blood pressure. However, the optimum blood pressure threshold for initiating antihypertensive drug therapy and specific treatment goals remain controversial. While previous hypertension guidelines have based target blood pressure goals on age and comorbidities, the 2017 ACC/AHA hypertension guideline incorporates underlying cardiovascular risk into decision making regarding treatment and generally recommends the same target blood pressure (i.e., less than 130/80 mm Hg) in all adults. Many patients will require at least 2 drugs from different pharmacologic classes to achieve their blood pressure goal; the potential benefits of hypertension management and drug cost, adverse effects, and risks associated with the use of multiple antihypertensive drugs also should be considered when deciding a patient's blood pressure treatment goal.

For additional information on target levels of blood pressure and on monitoring therapy in the management of hypertension, see Blood Pressure Monitoring and Treatment Goals under Dosage: Hypertension, in Dosage and Administration in the Thiazides General Statement 40:28.20.

Diabetic Nephropathy For the management of diabetic nephropathy in patients with type 2 diabetes mellitus, the usual initial adult dosage of losartan potassium is 50 mg once daily. Dosage of losartan potassium may be increased to 100 mg once daily based on blood pressure response. In a large clinical trial, approximately 72% of patients had dosage titrated from 50 mg daily initially up to 100 mg daily and maintained that dosage for more than 50% of the study period.

Prevention of Cardiovascular Morbidity and Mortality When losartan potassium is used to reduce the risk of stroke in high-risk patients with hypertension and left ventricular hypertrophy, the usual starting dose is 50 mg once daily. Treatment should be adjusted based on blood pressure response. Adjustment of therapy, when indicated, should include the addition of hydrochlorothiazide 12.5 mg daily and/or an increase in losartan potassium dosage to 100 mg daily; subsequently, the hydrochlorothiazide dosage may be increased to 25 mg once daily. Alternatively, the fixed combination containing losartan potassium and hydrochlorothiazide may be used at the appropriate dosage.

Heart Failure In patients with prior or current symptoms of heart failure† and reduced left ventricular ejection fraction (LVEF) (American College of Cardiology Foundation [ACCF]/American Heart Association [AHA] stage C heart failure), ACCF and AHA recommend an initial losartan potassium dosage of 25–50 mg once daily. Blood pressure (including postural blood pressure changes), renal function, and serum potassium concentrations should be reevaluated within 1–2 weeks after initiation of therapy, and these parameters should be monitored closely after changes in dosage. ACCF and AHA recommend a maximum losartan potassium dosage of 50–150 mg once daily for patients with ACCF/AHA stage C heart failure.

■ **Special Populations** The manufacturer recommends that patients with depletion of intravascular volume (e.g., patients receiving treatment with a diuretic) should have this condition corrected prior to initiation of losartan potassium therapy, or alternatively, therapy should be initiated using a lower initial dosage (25 mg once daily). The manufacturer states that modification of losartan potassium dosage is not necessary for geriatric patients nor for other adults with renal impairment, including those undergoing hemodialysis. In patients with hepatic impairment, the manufacturer recommends that therapy be initiated with a lower dosage of losartan potassium (25 mg once daily).

The commercially available preparation containing losartan in fixed combination with hydrochlorothiazide is not recommended for patients with renal impairment whose creatinine clearance is less than 30 mL/minute, and such preparations should be used with caution in patients with hepatic impairment. The commercially available preparation containing losartan potassium in fixed combination with hydrochlorothiazide is not recommended for initial titration in patients with hepatic impairment, because the appropriate starting dose of losartan potassium (25 mg once daily) is not available as a fixed-ratio preparation.

Cautions

■ **Contraindications** Known hypersensitivity to losartan or any ingredient in the formulation.

Concomitant therapy with aliskiren in patients with diabetes mellitus. (See Drug Interactions: Drugs that Block the Renin-Angiotensin System.)

■ **Warnings/Precautions** ***Warnings*** **Fetal/Neonatal Morbidity and Mortality.** Drugs that act on the renin-angiotensin system (e.g., angiotensin-converting enzyme [ACE] inhibitors, angiotensin II receptor antagonists, aliskiren) reduce fetal renal function and increase fetal and neonatal morbidity and mortality when administered during pregnancy during the second and third trimesters. Resulting oligohydramnios can be associated with fetal lung hypoplasia and skeletal deformations. Potential neonatal effects include skull hypoplasia, anuria, hypotension, renal failure, and death. Losartan should be discontinued as soon as possible when pregnancy is detected, unless continued use is considered life-saving. Nearly all women can be transferred successfully to alternative therapy for the remainder of their pregnancy. For additional information on the risk of such drugs (i.e., angiotensin II antagonists and ACE inhibitors) during pregnancy, see Cautions: Pregnancy, Fertility, and Lactation, in Captopril 24:32.04 and in Enalaprilat/Enalapril 24:32.04.

Sensitivity Reactions Sensitivity reactions, including anaphylactoid reactions and/or angioedema, have been reported with use of angiotensin II receptor antagonists, including losartan. Losartan is not recommended in patients with a history of angioedema associated with or unrelated to ACE inhibitor or angiotensin II receptor antagonist therapy.

Other Warnings and Precautions **Hypotension.** Symptomatic hypotension has been reported in patients receiving losartan, especially in volume- and/or salt-depleted patients (e.g., those receiving diuretics). (See Dosage and Administration: Special Populations.)

Malignancies. In July 2010, the US Food and Drug Administration (FDA) initiated a safety review of angiotensin II receptor antagonists after a published meta-analysis suggested a possible association between the use of these agents and an increased risk of cancer. The meta-analysis, which combined cancer-related findings from 5 randomized, controlled trials in over 60,000 patients, found a modest but significant increase in the risk of new cancer occurrence in patients receiving an angiotensin II receptor antagonist (mostly telmisartan) compared with those in control groups (7.2 versus 6%, respectively; risk ratio 1.08). However, because of several limitations of the study (e.g., trials included in the meta-analysis were not specifically designed to evaluate cancer outcomes, lack of individual patient data), the validity of these findings has been questioned.

Subsequent studies, including a larger, more comprehensive meta-analysis conducted by FDA, have not shown an increased risk of cancer in patients receiving angiotensin II receptor antagonists. FDA's meta-analysis, which included trial-level data from 31 randomized studies (total of approximately 156,000 patients), found no evidence of an increased risk of cancer in patients who received an angiotensin II receptor antagonist compared with those who received other treatments (placebo or active control). The overall rate of new cancer occurrence was essentially the same in both groups of patients (1.82 and 1.84 cases per 100 patient-years, respectively). In addition, there was no difference in the risk of cancer-related death, breast cancer, lung cancer, or prostate cancer between the groups. Based on these results and a review of all currently available data related to this potential safety concern, FDA has concluded that use of angiotensin II receptor antagonists is not associated with an increased risk of cancer.

Renal Effects. Because the renin-angiotensin-aldosterone (RAA) system appears to contribute substantially to maintenance of glomerular filtration in patients with heart failure in whom renal perfusion is severely compromised, renal function may deteriorate markedly (e.g., oliguria, progressive azotemia, renal failure, death) in these patients during therapy with an ACE inhibitor or an angiotensin II receptor antagonist (e.g., losartan). Increases in BUN and serum creatinine may occur in patients with unilateral or bilateral renal artery stenosis, chronic kidney disease (CKD), or volume depletion. The clinician should consider withholding or discontinuing losartan in patients who develop a clinically important reduction in renal function while receiving losartan. (See Cautions: Renal Effects, in Enalapril 24:32.04.)

Effects on Potassium. Hyperkalemia can develop, especially in patients receiving agents that can increase serum potassium concentration (e.g., potassium-sparing diuretics, potassium supplements, potassium-containing salt substitutes). (See Drug Interactions: Agents that Increase Serum Potassium.)

Fixed-combination Preparations. When losartan is used in fixed combination with hydrochlorothiazide, the cautions, precautions, and contraindications associated with thiazide diuretics must be considered in addition to those associated with losartan.

Specific Populations **Pregnancy.** Category D. (See Users Guide.)

Losartan can cause fetal and neonatal morbidity and mortality when administered to a pregnant woman. Losartan should be discontinued as soon as possible when pregnancy is detected. (See Fetal/Neonatal Morbidity and Mortality under Warnings/Precautions: Warnings, in Cautions.)

Lactation. Losartan is distributed into milk in rats; it is not known whether the drug is distributed into human breast milk. A decision should be made whether to discontinue nursing or the drug because of the potential risk in nursing infants.

Pediatric Use. If oliguria or hypotension occurs in neonates with a history of in utero exposure to losartan, blood pressure and renal function should be supported; exchange transfusions or dialysis may be required. (See Fetal/Neonatal Morbidity and Mortality under Warnings/Precautions: Warnings, in Cautions.)

Safety and efficacy of losartan in pediatric patients younger than 6 years of age and in pediatric patients with glomerular filtration rate less than 30 mL/minute per 1.73 m^2 have not been established.For information on overall principles and expert recommendations for treatment of hypertension in pediatric patients, see Uses: Hypertension in Pediatric Patients, in the Thiazides General Statement 40:28.20.

Geriatric Use. No overall differences in safety and efficacy of losartan for the treatment of hypertension have been observed in geriatric patients relative to younger adults, but increased sensitivity cannot be ruled out.

No overall differences in efficacy with the fixed combination preparation containing losartan and hydrochlorothiazide have been observed in patients 65 years of age or older compared with younger adults. Geriatric patients had a somewhat higher incidence of adverse effects than younger patients; dosage should be selected with caution.

Hepatic Impairment. Systemic exposure to losartan and its active metabolite may be increased in patients with hepatic impairment. Initial dosage adjustment is recommended. (See Losartan Therapy under Dosage: Hypertension, in Dosage and Administration.)

Use of losartan in fixed combination with hydrochlorothiazide is not recommended in patients with hepatic impairment because the dosage of losartan potassium in the fixed-combination tablets exceeds the recommended initial dosage.

Renal Impairment. Deterioration of renal function may occur in patients with renal impairment receiving losartan. (See Renal Effects under Warnings/Precautions: Other Warnings and Precautions, in Cautions.)

Use of losartan in fixed combination with hydrochlorothiazide is not recommended in patients with creatinine clearances of 30 mL/minute or less.

Black Patients. Blood pressure reduction may be smaller in black patients compared with nonblack patients; losartan should be used in combination with a diuretic or calcium-channel blocker in such patients.

There is no evidence that the benefits of therapy in reducing the risk of cardiovascular events in hypertensive patients with left ventricular hypertrophy apply to black patients.

■ **Common Adverse Effects** Adverse effects occurring in at least 1% of patients with hypertension receiving losartan and at a higher incidence than with placebo include upper respiratory infection, dizziness, nasal congestion, back pain, leg pain, muscle cramp, and sinusitis. The incidence of adverse effects was not affected by age, gender, or race. In patients receiving losartan for the treatment of diabetic nephropathy, urinary tract infection, diarrhea, anemia, asthenia/fatigue, hypoglycemia, back pain, chest pain, cough, bronchitis, diabetic vascular disease, influenza-like disease, cataracts, cellulitis, hyperkalemia, hypotension, muscular weakness, sinusitis, gastritis, hypoesthesia, infection, knee pain, and leg pain occurred with an incidence of at least 5% and were reported more frequently than in those receiving placebo.

Drug Interactions

■ **Agents that Increase Serum Potassium** Hyperkalemia may occur with concomitant administration of losartan and potassium-sparing diuretics, potassium supplements, potassium-containing salt substitutes, or other drugs that increase serum potassium concentrations. Serum potassium concentrations should be monitored in patients receiving such concomitant therapy.

■ **Drugs Affecting Hepatic Microsomal Enzymes** Formation of active metabolite appears to be mediated by cytochrome P-450 (CYP) 2C9 isoenzyme. CYP3A4 apparently contributes to formation of inactive metabolites.

Potential pharmacokinetic interaction (inhibition of the formation of losartan's active metabolite) with CYP2C9 inhibitors. Clinically important interactions unlikely with CYP3A4 inhibitors (possible increased concentration of losartan, but no effects on formation of active metabolite observed).

■ **Drugs that Block the Renin-Angiotensin System** Increased risk of hypotension, hyperkalemia, and changes in renal function (e.g., renal impairment) with concomitant use of other drugs that block the renin-angiotensin system (e.g., angiotensin-converting enzyme [ACE] inhibitors, angiotensin II receptor antagonists, aliskiren); when losartan is used concomitantly with such drugs, blood pressure, renal function, and serum concentrations of electrolytes should be monitored closely. The manufacturer states that most patients do not derive additional benefit from combination therapy with 2 renin-angiotensin system inhibitors compared with monotherapy. Concomitant use of losartan and aliskiren is contraindicated in patients with diabetes mellitus; in addition, such concomitant use should be avoided in patients with renal impairment (glomerular filtration rate [GFR] less than 60 mL/minute). (See Use in Combination with Angiotensin-converting Enzyme Inhibitors or Angiotensin II Receptor Antagonists under Warnings/Precautions: Other Warnings and Precautions, in Cautions in Aliskiren Hemifumarate 24:32.40.)

■ **Cimetidine** Pharmacokinetic interactions unlikely when losartan is used concomitantly with cimetidine.

■ **Digoxin** Pharmacokinetic interactions unlikely when losartan is used concomitantly with digoxin.

■ **Erythromycin** Clinically important pharmacokinetic interactions unlikely when losartan is used concomitantly with erythromycin.

■ **Fluconazole** Decreased plasma concentrations of losartan's active metabolite and increased plasma losartan concentrations have been reported when losartan is used concomitantly with fluconazole.

■ **Hydrochlorothiazide** Pharmacokinetic interactions unlikely when losartan is used concomitantly with hydrochlorothiazide.

Additive hypotensive effects observed when losartan is used concomitantly with hydrochlorothiazide, which is used for therapeutic advantage. (See Uses and see Dosage and Administration: Dosage).

■ **Ketoconazole** Conversion of losartan to its active metabolite unaffected when losartan is used concomitantly with ketoconazole.

■ **Lithium** Lithium excretion may be reduced. Serum lithium concentrations should be carefully monitored.

■ **Nonsteroidal Anti-inflammatory Agents** Potential pharmacologic interaction (attenuated hypotensive effects) when angiotensin II receptor antagonists are used concomitantly with nonsteroidal anti-inflammatory agents (NSAIAs), including selective cyclooxygenase-2 (COX-2) inhibitors.

Possible deterioration of renal function in geriatric, volume-depleted (including those receiving concomitant diuretic therapy), or renally impaired patients; renal function should be monitored periodically in patients receiving concomitant therapy with losartan and an NSAIA, including selective COX-2 inhibitors.

■ **Phenobarbital** Pharmacokinetic interactions unlikely when losartan is used concomitantly with phenobarbital.

■ **Rifampin** Decreased plasma concentrations of losartan and its active metabolite observed when losartan is used concomitantly with rifampin.

■ **Warfarin** Pharmacokinetic interactions unlikely when losartan is used concomitantly with warfarin.

Description

Losartan, a nonpeptide tetrazole derivative, is an angiotensin II receptor (type AT_1) antagonist. Losartan is a prodrug and requires activation in the liver to exert its pharmacologic activity. Losartan's active carboxylic acid metabolite is 10 to 40 times more potent by weight than losartan and appears to be a reversible, noncompetitive inhibitor of the AT_1 receptor.

Losartan blocks the physiologic actions of angiotensin II, including vasoconstrictor and aldosterone-secreting effects. Losartan does not interfere with response to bradykinins and does not share the angiotensin-converting enzyme (ACE) inhibitor common adverse effect of dry cough. For additional information on the pharmacology of angiotensin II receptor antagonists, see Description in Irbesartan 24:32.08.

Advice to Patients

Importance of advising patients not to use potassium supplements or salt substitutes containing potassium without consulting their clinician.

Importance of informing women of risks of use during pregnancy. Importance of women informing clinicians if they are or plan to become pregnant or to breast-feed. All women of childbearing potential should be advised to report pregnancy to their clinician as soon as possible. (See Fetal/Neonatal Morbidity and Mortality under Warnings/Precautions: Warnings, in Cautions.)

Importance of informing clinicians of existing or contemplated concomitant therapy, including prescription and OTC drugs (including salt substitutes containing potassium).

Importance of informing patients of other important precautionary information. (See Cautions.)

Overview® (see Users Guide). For additional information on this drug until a more detailed monograph is developed and published, the manufacturer's labeling should be consulted. It is *essential* that the manufacturer's labeling be consulted for more detailed information on usual cautions, precautions, contraindications, potential drug interactions, laboratory test interferences, and acute toxicity.

Preparations

Excipients in commercially available drug preparations may have clinically important effects in some individuals; consult specific product labeling for details.

Losartan Potassium

Oral		
Tablets, film-coated	25 mg	Cozaar®, Merck
	50 mg	Cozaar®, Merck
	100 mg	Cozaar®, Merck

Losartan Potassium Combinations

Oral		
Tablets, film-coated	50 mg with Hydrochlorothiazide 12.5 mg	Hyzaar®, Merck
	100 mg with Hydrochlorothiazide 12.5 mg	Hyzaar®, Merck
	100 mg with Hydrochlorothiazide 25 mg	Hyzaar®, Merck

†Use is not currently included in the labeling approved by the US Food and Drug Administration

Olmesartan Medoxomil

■ Olmesartan medoxomil is a nonpeptide, benzimidazole derivative angiotensin II type 1 (AT_1) receptor antagonist (also referred to as an angiotensin II receptor blocker [ARB]).

Uses

■ **Hypertension** Olmesartan medoxomil is used alone or in combination with other classes of antihypertensive agents in the management of hypertension.

Angiotensin II receptor antagonists, such as olmesartan medoxomil, are considered one of several preferred antihypertensive drugs for the initial management of hypertension according to current evidence-based hypertension guidelines; other preferred options include angiotensin-converting enzyme (ACE) inhibitors, calcium-channel blockers, and thiazide diuretics. While there may be individual differences with respect to recommendations for initial drug selection and use in specific patient populations, current evidence indicates that these antihypertensive drug classes all generally produce comparable effects on overall mortality and cardiovascular, cerebrovascular, and renal outcomes. (See Uses: Hypertension, in Valsartan 24:32.08.)

Angiotensin II receptor antagonists or ACE inhibitors may be particularly useful in the management of hypertension in patients with certain coexisting conditions such as diabetes mellitus or chronic kidney disease (CKD); angiotensin II receptor antagonists also may be preferred, generally as an alternative to ACE inhibitors, in hypertensive patients with heart failure or ischemic heart disease, and/or following myocardial infarction (MI). (See Uses: Hypertension, in Valsartan 24:32.08.)

In patients with hypertension and compelling indications (e.g., CKD with albuminuria [urine albumin 300 mg/day or greater, or urine albumin:creatinine ratio of 300 mg/g or equivalent in the first morning void]), angiotensin II receptor antagonists are usually considered an alternative for ACE inhibitor-intolerant patients. However, data indicate no difference in efficacy between ACE inhibitors and angiotensin II receptor antagonists with regard to blood pressure lowering and clinical outcomes (i.e., all-cause mortality, cardiovascular mortality, MI, heart failure, stroke, and end-stage renal disease). Adverse events (e.g., cough, angioedema) leading to drug discontinuance occur more frequently with ACE inhibitor therapy than with angiotensin II receptor antagonist therapy. Because of similar efficacy and a lower frequency of adverse effects, some experts believe that angiotensin II receptor antagonists should be used instead of an ACE inhibitor for the treatment of hypertension or hypertension with certain compelling indications.

Efficacy of olmesartan medoxomil in the treatment of hypertension has been established in several placebo-controlled studies of 6–12 weeks' duration in patients with mild to moderate hypertension. In these patients, usual dosages of olmesartan medoxomil (20–40 mg administered once daily) decreased placebo-corrected systolic blood pressure by about 10–12 mm Hg and diastolic blood pressure by about 6–7 mm Hg 24 hours after dosing. There was no evidence of tachyphylaxis during long-term (e.g., 1 year) olmesartan therapy, and rebound hypertension following abrupt withdrawal of the drug has not been reported. Clinical studies have shown that the hypotensive effect of olmesartan in patients with mild to moderate hypertension is greater than that of placebo and comparable to or greater than that of captopril, irbesartan, losartan, and valsartan. In addition, olmesartan appears to be as effective as atenolol when used in conjunction with hydrochlorothiazide in the treatment of patients with moderate to severe hypertension.

Most patients with hypertension, especially black patients, will require at least 2 antihypertensive drugs to achieve adequate blood pressure control. Like ACE inhibitors, angiotensin II receptor antagonists such as olmesartan may produce a smaller blood pressure response in hypertensive black patients compared with nonblack patients. (See Race under Hypertension: Other Special Considerations for Antihypertensive Drug Therapy, in Uses in Valsartan 24:32.08.)

For additional information on the management of hypertension, see Uses: Hypertension, in Valsartan 24:32.08. For information on overall principles and expert recommendations for treatment of hypertension, see Uses: Hypertension in Adults and also see Uses: Hypertension in Pediatric Patients, in the Thiazides General Statement 40:28.20.

■ **Diabetic Nephropathy** Both angiotensin II receptor antagonists and ACE inhibitors have been shown to slow the rate of progression of renal disease in patients with diabetes mellitus and persistent albuminuria†, and use of a drug from either class is recommended in such patients with modestly elevated (30–300 mg/24 hours) or higher (exceeding 300 mg/24 hours) levels of urinary albumin excretion. The usual precautions of angiotensin II receptor antagonist or ACE inhibitor therapy in patients with substantial renal impairment should be observed. (See Renal Effects under Warnings/Precautions: Other Warnings and Precautions, in Cautions.) For additional information on the use of angiotensin II receptor antagonists in the treatment of diabetic nephropathy, see Uses: Diabetic Nephropathy, in Losartan 24:32.08 and in Irbesartan 24:32.08.

■ **Heart Failure** Angiotensin II receptor antagonists have been used in the management of heart failure†.

Current guidelines for the management of heart failure in adults generally recommend a combination of drug therapies to reduce morbidity and mortality, including neurohormonal antagonists (e.g., ACE inhibitors, angiotensin II receptor antagonists, angiotensin receptor-neprilysin inhibitors [ARNIs], β-adrenergic blocking agents [β-blockers], aldosterone receptor antagonists) that inhibit the detrimental compensatory mechanisms in heart failure. Additional agents (e.g., cardiac glycosides, diuretics, sinoatrial modulators [i.e., ivabradine]) added to a heart failure treatment regimen in selected patients have been associated with symptomatic improvement and/or reduction in heart failure-related hospitalizations. Experts recommend that all asymptomatic patients with reduced left ventricular ejection fraction (LVEF) (American College of Cardiology Foundation [ACCF]/American Heart Association [AHA] stage B heart failure) receive therapy with an ACE inhibitor and β-blocker to prevent symptomatic heart failure and reduce morbidity and mortality. In patients with prior or current symptoms of chronic heart failure with reduced LVEF (ACCF/AHA stage C heart failure), ACCF, AHA, and the Heart Failure Society of America (HFSA) recommend inhibition of the renin-angiotensin-aldosterone (RAA) system with an ACE inhibitor, angiotensin II receptor antagonist, or ARNI in conjunction with a β-blocker, and an aldosterone antagonist in selected patients, to reduce morbidity and mortality. While ACE inhibitors have been the preferred drugs for inhibition of the RAA system because of their established benefits in patients with heart failure and reduced ejection fraction, some evidence indicates that therapy with sacubitril/valsartan, an ARNI, may be more effective than ACE inhibitor therapy (enalapril) in reducing cardiovascular death and heart failure-related hospitalization. ACCF, AHA, and HFSA recommend that patients with chronic symptomatic heart failure and reduced LVEF (New York Heart Association [NYHA] class II or III) who are able to tolerate an ACE inhibitor or angiotensin II receptor antagonist be switched to therapy containing an ARNI to further reduce morbidity and mortality. However, in patients in whom an ARNI is not appropriate, continued use of an ACE inhibitor for all classes of heart failure with reduced ejection fraction remains strongly advised. In patients in whom an ARNI or ACE inhibitor is not appropriate, an angiotensin II receptor antagonist may be used. For additional information on the use of angiotensin II receptor antagonists in the management of heart failure, see Uses: Heart Failure, in Valsartan 24:32.08 and in Candesartan 24:32.08. For further information on the use of ARNIs in patients with heart failure, see Uses: Heart Failure, in Sacubitril and Valsartan 24:32.92.

While angiotensin II receptor antagonists are considered reasonable alternatives in patients who are unable to tolerate ACE inhibitors (e.g., because of cough or angioedema), angioedema and anaphylactic reactions have been reported rarely during postmarketing experience in patients receiving olmesartan. (See Sensitivity Reactions under Cautions: Warnings/Precautions.)

Dosage and Administration

■ **Administration** Olmesartan medoxomil is administered orally without regard to meals. Twice-daily dosing offers no therapeutic advantage over the same total dose given once daily.

For pediatric patients unable to swallow tablets, olmesartan may be administered orally as an extemporaneously prepared suspension. An extemporaneous suspension containing olmesartan medoxomil 2 mg/mL can be prepared in the following manner. First, 50 mL of purified water is added to an amber polyethylene terephthalate (PET) bottle containing twenty 20-mg tablets of olmesartan medoxomil, and the contents allowed to stand for a minimum of 5 minutes. The container should then be shaken for at least 1 minute and allowed to stand for at least 1 minute; this step of alternating shaking and standing should be repeated 4 additional times. The concentrated suspension should then be diluted with 100 mL of syrup (Ora-Sweet®) and 50 mL of a suspending vehicle (Ora-Plus®) and the container shaken well for at least 1 minute to disperse the ingredients. The suspension should be shaken well before dispensing each dose. The extemporaneous suspension is stable for up to 4 weeks when stored at 2–8°C. Olmesartan medoxomil tablets and the extemporaneously prepared oral suspension of the drug are bioequivalent.

■ **Dosage** ***Hypertension*** Dosage of olmesartan medoxomil must be individualized and adjusted according to blood pressure response.

Olmesartan Therapy. The usual initial dosage of olmesartan medoxomil as monotherapy is 20 mg once daily in adults without depletion of intravascular volume. If blood pressure response is inadequate with the initial dosage, dosage may be increased as tolerated to 40 mg daily or a diuretic may be added. Some experts state that the usual dosage of olmesartan medoxomil in adults is 20–40 mg once daily. Olmesartan medoxomil dosages exceeding 40 mg daily do not appear to provide additional therapeutic benefit. The antihypertensive effect of olmesartan medoxomil generally is evident within 2 weeks, with a maximum reduction observed after 4 weeks.

Dosage of olmesartan medoxomil in pediatric patients is based on weight. For pediatric patients 6–16 years of age weighing 20 to less than 35 kg, the usual initial dosage of olmesartan medoxomil is 10 mg once daily; dosage may be increased to a maximum of 20 mg once daily after 2 weeks if further reduction in blood pressure is needed. For pediatric patients 6–16 years of age weighing 35 kg or more, the recommended initial dosage of olmesartan medoxomil is 20 mg once daily; if necessary, dosage may be increased to a maximum of 40 mg once daily after 2 weeks.

Olmesartan/Amlodipine Fixed-combination Therapy. In patients who do not respond adequately to monotherapy with olmesartan medoxomil (or another angiotensin II receptor antagonist) or, alternatively, with amlodipine (or another dihydropyridine-derivative calcium-channel blocker), combined therapy with the drugs can be used to provide additional antihypertensive effects. The fixed-combination preparation containing olmesartan medoxomil and amlodipine also can be used as a substitute for the individually titrated drugs. The patient can be switched to the fixed-combination preparation containing the corresponding individual doses of olmesartan medoxomil and amlodipine; alternatively, the dosage of one or both components can be increased for additional antihypertensive effects. If needed, dosage of the fixed combination may be increased after 2 weeks. Dosage adjustments generally should involve one drug at a time, although dosages of both drugs can be increased to achieve more rapid blood pressure control. Daily dosages exceeding 40 mg of olmesartan medoxomil given in fixed combination with 10 mg of amlodipine are not recommended by the manufacturer.

Commercially available preparations containing olmesartan medoxomil in fixed combination with amlodipine may be used for initial treatment of hypertension in patients likely to require combined therapy with multiple antihypertensive drugs to achieve blood pressure control. In such patients, therapy with the fixed-combination preparation usually should be initiated at a dosage of 20 mg of olmesartan medoxomil and 5 mg of amlodipine once daily. If necessary, dosage of the fixed combination may be increased after 1–2 weeks for additional blood pressure control (but should not exceed a maximum dosage of 40 mg of olmesartan medoxomil and 10 mg of amlodipine once daily). In patients whose baseline blood pressure is 160/100 mm Hg, the estimated probability of achieving control of systolic blood pressure (defined as systolic blood pressure of less than 140 mm Hg) is 48, 46, or 68% and of achieving control of diastolic blood pressure (defined as diastolic blood pressure of less than 90 mm Hg) is 51, 60, or 85% with olmesartan medoxomil (40 mg daily) alone, amlodipine (10 mg daily) alone, or amlodipine combined with olmesartan medoxomil (at the same dosages), respectively.

Olmesartan/Hydrochlorothiazide Fixed-combination Therapy. In patients who do not respond adequately to monotherapy with olmesartan medoxomil or, alternatively, with hydrochlorothiazide, combined therapy with the drugs can be used. When combination therapy is necessary, the commercially available preparation containing olmesartan medoxomil in fixed combination with hydrochlorothiazide generally should not be used initially. Dosage preferably should first be adjusted by titrating the dosage of each drug separately; if it is determined that the optimum maintenance dosage corresponds to the ratio in the commercial combination preparation, this product may be used. The manufacturer states that combined therapy with the commercially available fixed-combination preparation containing 20 mg of olmesartan medoxomil and 12.5 mg of hydrochlorothiazide can be used in patients whose blood pressure is not adequately controlled by monotherapy with olmesartan medoxomil or 25 mg daily of hydrochlorothiazide. If needed, dosage of the fixed combination may be increased up to a maximum of 40 mg of olmesartan medoxomil and 25 mg of hydrochlorothiazide daily after 2–4 weeks. Daily dosages exceeding 40 mg of olmesartan medoxomil and 25 mg of hydrochlorothiazide given in combination are not recommended by the manufacturer.

Olmesartan/Amlodipine/Hydrochlorothiazide Fixed-combination Therapy. The fixed-combination preparation containing olmesartan medoxomil, amlodipine, and hydrochlorothiazide may be used to provide additional blood pressure control in patients who do not respond adequately to combination therapy with any 2 of the following classes of antihypertensive agents given at maximally tolerated, labeled, or usual dosages: angiotensin II receptor antagonists, calcium-channel blockers, or diuretics. Patients who experience dose-limiting adverse effects of olmesartan medoxomil, amlodipine, or hydrochlorothiazide while receiving any dual combination of these drugs may be switched to a lower dosage of that drug, given as a fixed-combination preparation containing all 3 of these drugs, to achieve similar blood pressure reductions. The fixed-combination preparation containing olmesartan medoxomil, amlodipine, and hydrochlorothiazide also can be used as a substitute for the individually titrated drugs. If necessary, dosage of the fixed combination preparation may be increased after 2 weeks for additional blood pressure control (but should not exceed a maximum dosage of 40 mg of olmesartan medoxomil, 10 mg of amlodipine, and 25 mg of hydrochlorothiazide daily). The commercially available preparation containing olmesartan medoxomil in fixed combination with amlodipine and hydrochlorothiazide should not be used for the initial management of hypertension.

Blood Pressure Monitoring and Treatment Goals. Blood pressure should be monitored regularly (i.e., monthly) during therapy and dosage of the antihypertensive drug adjusted until blood pressure is controlled. If an adequate blood pressure response is not achieved with angiotensin II receptor antagonist monotherapy, the dosage may be increased or another antihypertensive agent with demonstrated benefit and preferably with a complementary mechanism of action (e.g., calcium-channel blocker, thiazide diuretic) may be added; if target blood pressure is still not achieved, a third drug may be added. (See Uses: Hypertension.) In patients who develop unacceptable adverse effects with olmesartan, the drug should be discontinued and another antihypertensive agent from a different pharmacologic class should be initiated.

The goal of hypertension management and prevention is to achieve and maintain optimal control of blood pressure. However, the optimum blood pressure threshold for initiating antihypertensive drug therapy and specific treatment goals remain controversial. While previous hypertension guidelines have based target blood pressure goals on age and comorbidities, the 2017 ACC/AHA hypertension guideline incorporates underlying cardiovascular risk into decision making regarding treatment and generally recommends the same target blood pressure (i.e., less than 130/80 mm Hg) in all adults. Many patients will require at least 2 drugs from different pharmacologic classes to achieve their blood pressure goal; the potential benefits of hypertension management and drug cost, adverse effects, and risks associated with the use of multiple antihypertensive drugs also should be considered when deciding a patient's blood pressure treatment goal.

For additional information on target levels of blood pressure and on monitoring therapy in the management of hypertension, see Blood Pressure Monitoring and Treatment Goals under Dosage: Hypertension, in Dosage and Administration in the Thiazides General Statement 40:28.20.

■ **Special Populations** The manufacturer recommends that patients with depletion of intravascular volume be monitored closely and consideration be given to administering a lower initial dose of the drug. The manufacturer states that no adjustment in initial olmesartan medoxomil dosage is necessary in geriatric patients or in those with moderate-to-severe hepatic or renal impairment (creatinine clearance less than 40 mL/minute). However, some clinicians state that consideration should be given to administering a lower initial dose of the drug in patients with severe renal impairment (creatinine clearance less than 20 mL/minute) and recommend a maximum dosage of 20 mg once daily in such patients. The appropriate dosage in patients with end-stage renal disease has not been determined.

If concomitant diuretic therapy is required in patients with severe renal impairment (i.e., creatinine clearance of 30 mL/minute or less), a loop diuretic is preferred to a thiazide diuretic. Therefore, commercially available preparations containing olmesartan medoxomil in fixed combination with hydrochlorothiazide usually are not recommended for patients with severe renal impairment.

The amount of amlodipine in fixed-combination preparations containing olmesartan medoxomil and amlodipine exceeds the recommended initial dosage of amlodipine (2.5 mg daily) in patients 75 years of age or older and in those with hepatic impairment.

Cautions

■ **Contraindications** Concomitant therapy with aliskiren in patients with diabetes mellitus. (See Drug Interactions: Drugs that Block the Renin-Angiotensin System.)

■ **Warnings/Precautions** ***Warnings*** **Fetal/Neonatal Morbidity and Mortality.** Drugs that act on the renin-angiotensin system (e.g., angiotensin-converting enzyme [ACE] inhibitors, angiotensin II receptor antagonists, aliskiren) can reduce fetal renal function and increase fetal and neonatal morbidity and mortality when used in pregnancy during the second and third trimesters. ACE inhibitors also may increase the risk of major congenital malformations when administered during the first trimester of pregnancy. Resulting oligohydramnios can be associated with fetal lung hypoplasia and skeletal deformations. Potential neonatal effects include skull hypoplasia, anuria, hypotension, renal failure, and death. Olmesartan should be discontinued as soon as possible when pregnancy is detected, unless continued use is considered life-saving. Nearly all women can be transferred successfully to alternative therapy for the remainder of their pregnancy. For additional information on the risk during pregnancy of drugs that act on the renin-angiotensin system, see Cautions: Pregnancy, Fertility, and Lactation, in Captopril 24:32.04 and in Enalaprilat/Enalapril 24:32.04.

Sensitivity Reactions Facial edema has occurred in patients receiving olmesartan. Sensitivity reactions, including various anaphylactoid reactions and/or angioedema have been reported in patients receiving angiotensin II receptor antagonists.

Extreme caution is advised in patients with history of angioedema associated with or unrelated to ACE inhibitor or angiotensin II receptor antagonist therapy.

Other Warnings and Precautions **Infant Morbidity.** Olmesartan must not be used for the treatment of hypertension in infants younger than 1 year of age because drugs that act on the renin-angiotensin-aldosterone (RAA) system can affect the development of immature kidneys. (See Pediatric Use under Warnings/Precautions: Specific Populations, in Cautions.)

Hypotension. Because symptomatic hypotension may occur in patients with an activated RAA system (e.g., patients with volume or salt depletion secondary to salt restriction or prolonged diuretic therapy), olmesartan should be initiated in such patients under close medical supervision and consideration should be given to administering a lower initial dose of the drug.

If hypotension occurs in patients receiving olmesartan, the patient should be placed in the supine position; if hypotension is severe, IV infusion of 0.9% sodium chloride injection to expand fluid volume should be considered. Transient hypotension is not a contraindication to additional doses of olmesartan, and therapy with the drug can be cautiously reinstated after blood pressure has been stabilized (e.g., with volume expansion).

Malignancies. In July 2010, FDA initiated a safety review of angiotensin II receptor antagonists after a published meta-analysis suggested a possible association between the use of these agents and an increased risk of cancer. The meta-analysis, which combined cancer-related findings from 5 randomized, controlled trials in over 60,000 patients, found a modest but significant increase in the risk of new cancer occurrence in patients receiving an angiotensin II receptor antagonist (mostly telmisartan) compared with those in control groups (7.2 versus 6%, respectively; risk ratio 1.08). However, because of several limitations of the study (e.g., trials included in the meta-analysis were not specifically designed to evaluate cancer outcomes, lack of individual patient data), the validity of these findings has been questioned.

Subsequent studies, including a larger, more comprehensive meta-analysis conducted by FDA, have not shown an increased risk of cancer in patients receiving angiotensin II receptor antagonists. FDA's meta-analysis, which included trial-level data from 31 randomized studies (total of approximately 156,000 patients), found no evidence of an increased risk of cancer in patients who received an angiotensin II receptor antagonist compared with those who received other treatments (placebo or active control). The overall rate of new cancer occurrence was essentially the same in both groups of patients (1.82 and 1.84 cases per 100 patient-years, respectively). In addition, there was no difference in the risk of cancer-related death, breast cancer, lung cancer, or prostate cancer between the groups. Based on these results and a review of all currently available data related to this potential safety concern, FDA has concluded that use of angiotensin II receptor antagonists is not associated with an increased risk of cancer.

Renal Effects. Because the RAA system appears to contribute substantially to maintenance of glomerular filtration in patients with heart failure in whom renal perfusion is severely compromised, renal function may deteriorate markedly (e.g., oliguria, progressive azotemia, renal failure, death) in these patients during therapy with an ACE inhibitor or an angiotensin II receptor antagonist (e.g., olmesartan). Renal artery stenosis also is a risk factor for renal impairment during therapy with drugs that inhibit the RAA system. Although reports received to date have involved patients treated with ACE inhibitors, this adverse effect also would be expected to occur when drugs with similar pharmacologic activity (e.g., angiotensin II receptor antagonists) are used in a similar manner. (See Cautions: Renal Effects, in Enalaprilat/Enalapril 24:32.04.)

Sprue-like Enteropathy. Sprue-like enteropathy, an intestinal condition characterized by severe chronic diarrhea with substantial weight loss, has been reported during postmarketing experience in patients receiving olmesartan; in some cases, intestinal biopsy revealed villous atrophy. At least 23 cases of sprue-like enteropathy were identified through the FDA Adverse Event Reporting System, and an additional 22 patients were described as having a similar condition in a published case series. Clinical manifestations developed months to years after initiation of olmesartan therapy and sometimes resulted in hospitalization. In all of the reported cases, clinical improvement occurred after the drug was discontinued, and a positive rechallenge was observed in some of the patients. Although the exact mechanism of this adverse effect is not known, certain findings suggest that it may be associated with a localized delayed hypersensitivity or cell-mediated immune response to the prodrug olmesartan medoxomil.

If symptoms of sprue-like enteropathy develop during olmesartan therapy, the possibility of other etiologies (e.g., celiac disease) should be excluded; if no other causative factor can be identified, discontinuance of the drug should be considered. Sprue-like enteropathy has not been associated with other angiotensin II receptor antagonists to date and is not considered to be a class effect of the drugs.

Increased Cardiovascular Risk in Patients with Diabetes. Findings from 2 long-term, randomized, double-blind, placebo-controlled trials (the Randomized Olmesartan and Diabetes Microalbuminuria Prevention Study [ROADMAP] and the Olmesartan Reducing Incidence of End-stage Renal Disease in Diabetic Nephropathy Trial [ORIENT]) prompted concerns that high-dose olmesartan may be associated with an increased risk of cardiovascular death in patients with diabetes mellitus. The trials were designed to evaluate the renoprotective effects of olmesartan in patients with type 2 diabetes mellitus over a period of about 4–5 years, but unexpectedly found an increased risk of cardiovascular deaths (e.g., fatal myocardial infarction, sudden cardiac death) associated with olmesartan therapy. However, in the ROADMAP trial, there was a trend toward a lower incidence of nonfatal myocardial infarction in the olmesartan group. The US Food and Drug Administration (FDA) has reviewed the results of these studies in addition to several other studies to further evaluate this safety concern; although some studies appeared to support the initial findings of the ROADMAP trial, results were inconsistent and, in some cases, not statistically significant. In one such study (an observational study conducted in a large [more than 300,000 patient-years of exposure] cohort of patients 65 years of age or older), an increased risk of death was observed in patients receiving olmesartan as compared with other angiotensin II receptor antagonists, but only in the subgroup of patients with diabetes mellitus who received the highest dosage of the drug (40 mg daily) for longer than 6 months; in nondiabetic patients, high-dose olmesartan was associated with a lower incidence of death as compared with other angiotensin II receptor antagonists. FDA has concluded after considering all of the available data that the collective evidence to date is insufficient to clearly demonstrate an association between olmesartan and increased cardiovascular risk in diabetic patients. FDA states that the benefits of olmesartan in hypertensive patients continue to outweigh its potential risks when used according to the manufacturer's labeling.

Fixed-combination Preparations. When olmesartan is used in fixed combination with hydrochlorothiazide and/or amlodipine, the cautions, precautions, and contraindications associated with the concomitant agent(s) must be considered in addition to those associated with olmesartan.

Specific Populations **Pregnancy.** Category D. (See Users Guide.)

Olmesartan may cause fetal and neonatal morbidity and mortality when administered to a pregnant woman. Olmesartan should be discontinued as soon as possible when pregnancy is detected. (See Fetal/Neonatal Morbidity and Mortality under Warnings/Precautions: Warnings, in Cautions.)

Lactation. Olmesartan is distributed into milk in rats; it is not known whether the drug is distributed into milk in humans. Because of the potential for serious adverse reactions to olmesartan in nursing infants, a decision should be made whether to discontinue nursing or the drug, taking into account the importance of the drug to the woman.

Pediatric Use. If oliguria or hypotension occurs in neonates with a history of in utero exposure to olmesartan, blood pressure and renal function should be supported; exchange transfusions or dialysis may be required. (See Fetal/Neonatal Morbidity and Mortality under Warnings/Precautions: Warnings, in Cautions.)

Safety and efficacy of olmesartan have been established in a randomized, double-blind, placebo-controlled trial in pediatric patients 6–16 years of age with hypertension. Patients in the study were enrolled into 1 of 2 cohorts (an all-black or mixed racial cohort, 18% of whom were black). In both groups, olmesartan (given in a weight-adjusted dosage) substantially reduced systolic and diastolic blood pressures from baseline in a dose-dependent manner; systolic and diastolic blood pressures were, on average, 3.2 and 2.8 mm Hg lower, respectively, in patients receiving olmesartan than in those receiving placebo. Similar to that observed in the adult population, smaller blood pressure reductions were observed in the black compared with the predominantly nonblack pediatric patient cohort. The same pediatric study also included 59 patients who were 1–5 years of age; treatment with olmesartan medoxomil (0.3 mg/kg once daily) in this age group did not result in a statistically significant reduction in blood pressure compared with placebo. Adverse effects reported in the pediatric patients evaluated in this study generally were similar to those observed in adults.

Pharmacokinetics of olmesartan have been evaluated in pediatric patients 1–16 years of age; clearance of the drug (adjusted for body weight) in these pediatric patients was similar to that observed in adults.

The manufacturer states that olmesartan has not been shown to be effective for hypertension in patients younger than 6 years of age.

Olmesartan has not been evaluated in infants younger than 1 year of age; because of the possibility of abnormal kidney development, the drug *must* not be used in this age group.

Safety and efficacy of olmesartan in fixed combination with hydrochlorothiazide and/or amlodipine in pediatric patients have not been established.

For information on overall principles and expert recommendations for treatment of hypertension in pediatric patients, see Uses: Hypertension in Pediatric Patients, in the Thiazides General Statement 40:28.20.

Geriatric Use. No overall differences in safety and efficacy of olmesartan have been observed in geriatric patients 65 years of age or older relative to younger adults, but increased sensitivity to the drug cannot be ruled out. In general, dosage should be selected with caution because of age-related decreases in hepatic, renal, and/or cardiac function and concomitant disease and drug therapy.

Hepatic Impairment. Systemic exposure to olmesartan may be increased in patients with moderate hepatic impairment compared with those with normal hepatic function; however, no initial dosage adjustment is required in patients with moderate or severe hepatic impairment.

Renal Impairment. Serum concentrations of olmesartan may be increased in patients with renal impairment compared with those with normal renal function; however, the manufacturer states that no initial dosage adjustment is required. (See Dosage and Administration: Special Populations.)

Deterioration of renal function may occur during therapy. (See Renal Effects under Warnings/Precautions: Other Warnings and Precautions, in Cautions.)

Black Patients. Blood pressure reduction with olmesartan may be smaller in black patients than in patients of other races.

■ **Common Adverse Effects** Adverse effects occurring in 1% or more of patients receiving olmesartan, but also occurring at about the same or greater incidence in patients receiving placebo, include back pain, bronchitis, diarrhea, headache, hematuria, hyperglycemia, hypertriglyceridemia, influenza-like symptoms, pharyngitis, rhinitis, sinusitis, and upper respiratory tract infection. In placebo-controlled studies, the only adverse effect that occurred in more than 1% of patients receiving olmesartan and at an incidence greater than with placebo was dizziness. The incidence of adverse effects was not affected by age, gender, or race.

Drug Interactions

■ **Drugs Affecting or Metabolized by Hepatic Microsomal Enzymes** Olmesartan is not metabolized by the cytochrome P-450 (CYP) isoenzyme system and does not alter activity of CYP isoenzymes; pharmacokinetic interactions are unlikely with inhibitors or inducers of CYP isoenzymes or with drugs that are metabolized by these isoenzymes.

■ **Drugs that Block the Renin-Angiotensin System** Increased risk of renal impairment, hyperkalemia, and hypotension with concomitant use of other drugs that block the renin-angiotensin system (e.g., angiotensin-converting enzyme [ACE] inhibitors, angiotensin II receptor antagonists, aliskiren); when olmesartan is used concomitantly with such drugs, blood pressure, renal function, and serum concentrations of electrolytes should be monitored closely. The manufacturer states that most patients do not derive additional benefit from combination therapy with 2 renin-angiotensin system inhibitors compared with monotherapy. Concomitant use of olmesartan and aliskiren is contraindicated in patients with diabetes mellitus; in addition, such concomitant use should be avoided in patients with renal impairment (glomerular filtration rate [GFR] less than 60 mL/minute). (See Use in Combination with Angiotensin-converting Enzyme Inhibitors or Angiotensin II Receptor Antagonists under Warnings/Precautions: Other Warnings and Precautions, in Cautions in Aliskiren Hemifumarate 24:32.40.)

■ **Antacids** Pharmacokinetic interactions unlikely.

■ **Colesevelam Hydrochloride** Pharmacokinetic interaction (decreased systemic exposure and peak plasma concentrations of olmesartan). Administration of olmesartan at least 4 hours prior to colesevelam decreases the extent of this interaction and should be considered.

■ **Digoxin** Pharmacokinetic interactions unlikely.

■ **Lithium** Increased serum lithium concentrations resulting in lithium toxicity have been reported when angiotensin II receptor antagonists are used concomitantly with lithium. Serum lithium concentrations should be carefully monitored.

■ **Nonsteroidal Anti-inflammatory Agents** Potential pharmacologic interaction (attenuated hypotensive effects) when angiotensin II receptor antagonists are used concomitantly with nonsteroidal anti-inflammatory agents (NSAIAs), including selective cyclooxygenase-2 (COX-2) inhibitors. Possible deterioration of renal function, including possible acute renal failure, in geriatric, volume-depleted (including those receiving concomitant diuretic therapy), or renally impaired patients; renal function should be monitored periodically in patients receiving concomitant therapy with olmesartan and an NSAIA, including selective COX-2 inhibitors.

■ **Warfarin** Pharmacokinetic and pharmacologic interactions unlikely.

Description

Olmesartan medoxomil is a nonpeptide, benzimidazole-derivative angiotensin II type 1 (AT_1) receptor antagonist. For additional information on the pharmacology of angiotensin II receptor antagonists, see Description in Irbesartan 24:32.08 and Valsartan 24:32.08.

Olmesartan medoxomil is a prodrug that has little, if any, pharmacologic activity until hydrolyzed during absorption in the GI tract to olmesartan. Following rapid and complete ester hydrolysis of olmesartan medoxomil to olmesartan, there is virtually no further metabolism of olmesartan. Approximately 35–50% of an absorbed dose is recovered in urine while the remainder is excreted in feces via the bile. Olmesartan is not metabolized by the cytochrome P-450 (CYP) microsomal enzyme system.

Advice to Patients

When olmesartan is used in fixed combination with amlodipine and/or hydrochlorothiazide, importance of advising patients of important precautionary information about the concomitant agent(s).

Importance of informing clinicians of existing or contemplated concomitant therapy, including prescription and OTC drugs.

Importance of women informing clinicians if they are or plan to become pregnant or plan to breast-feed. Importance of advising women of childbearing age about the potential risks to the fetus if the drug is used during pregnancy. All women of childbearing potential should be advised to report pregnancy to their clinician as soon as possible. (See Fetal/Neonatal Morbidity and Mortality under Warnings/Precautions: Warnings, in Cautions.)

Importance of informing patients of other important precautionary information. (See Cautions.)

Overview® (see Users Guide). For additional information on this drug until a more detailed monograph is developed and published, the manufacturer's labeling should be consulted. It is *essential* that the manufacturer's labeling be consulted for more detailed information on usual cautions, precautions, contraindications, potential drug interactions, laboratory test interferences, and acute toxicity.

Preparations

Excipients in commercially available drug preparations may have clinically important effects in some individuals; consult specific product labeling for details.

Olmesartan Medoxomil

Oral		
Tablets, film-coated	5 mg	**Benicar®**, Daiichi Sankyo
	20 mg	**Benicar®**, Daiichi Sankyo
	40 mg	**Benicar®**, Daiichi Sankyo

Olmesartan Medoxomil Combinations

Oral		
Tablets	20 mg with Amlodipine Besylate 5 mg (of amlodipine)	**Azor®**, Daiichi Sankyo
	20 mg with Amlodipine Besylate 10 mg (of amlodipine)	**Azor®**, Daiichi Sankyo
	40 mg with Amlodipine Besylate 5 mg (of amlodipine)	**Azor®**, Daiichi Sankyo
	40 mg with Amlodipine Besylate 10 mg (of amlodipine)	**Azor®**, Daiichi Sankyo
Tablets, film-coated	20 mg with Amlodipine Besylate 5 mg (of amlodipine) and Hydrochlorothiazide 12.5 mg	**Tribenzor®**, Daiichi Sankyo
	20 mg with Hydrochlorothiazide 12.5 mg	**Benicar® HCT**, Daiichi Sankyo
	40 mg with Amlodipine Besylate 5 mg (of amlodipine) and Hydrochlorothiazide 12.5 mg	**Tribenzor®**, Daiichi Sankyo
	40 mg with Amlodipine Besylate 5 mg (of amlodipine) and Hydrochlorothiazide 25 mg	**Tribenzor®**, Daiichi Sankyo
	40 mg with Amlodipine Besylate 10 mg (of amlodipine) and Hydrochlorothiazide 12.5 mg	**Tribenzor®**, Daiichi Sankyo
	40 mg with Amlodipine Besylate 10 mg (of amlodipine) and Hydrochlorothiazide 25 mg	**Tribenzor®**, Daiichi Sankyo
	40 mg with Hydrochlorothiazide 12.5 mg	**Benicar® HCT**, Daiichi Sankyo
	40 mg with Hydrochlorothiazide 25 mg	**Benicar® HCT**, Daiichi Sankyo

†Use is not currently included in the labeling approved by the US Food and Drug Administration

Valsartan

Sacubitril and Valsartan

■ Valsartan is an angiotensin II type 1 (AT_1) receptor antagonist (also referred to as an angiotensin II receptor blocker [ARB]). Valsartan also is commercially available in fixed combination with sacubitril, a neprilysin inhibitor. (See the monograph on Sacubitril and Valsartan in 24:32.92.)

Uses

■ **Hypertension** Valsartan is used alone or in combination with other classes of antihypertensive agents (e.g., thiazide diuretics) in the management of hypertension. Efficacy of valsartan for the management of hypertension has been established by controlled studies of 8–12 weeks' duration in patients with hypertension of mild to moderate severity in outpatient settings. The efficacy of valsartan for long-term use (i.e., exceeding 12 weeks) has been established in noncontrolled, follow-up studies in which the drug was used for up to 2 years without apparent loss of clinical effect. Clinical studies have shown that the hypotensive effect of usual dosages of valsartan in patients with mild to moderate hypertension is greater than that of placebo and comparable to that of usual dosages of amlodipine, enalapril, lisinopril, or hydrochlorothiazide.

Current evidence-based practice guidelines for the management of hypertension in adults generally recommend the use of drugs from 4 classes of antihypertensive agents (angiotensin-converting enzyme [ACE] inhibitors, angiotensin II receptor antagonists, calcium-channel blockers, and thiazide diuretics); data from clinical outcome trials indicate that lowering blood pressure with any of these drug classes can reduce the complications of hypertension and provide similar cardiovascular protection. However, recommendations for initial drug selection and use in specific patient populations may vary across these expert guidelines. This variability is due, in part, to differences in the guideline development process and the types of studies (e.g., randomized controlled studies only versus a range of studies with different study designs) included in the evidence reviews. Ultimately, choice of antihypertensive therapy should be individualized, considering the clinical characteristics of the patient (e.g., age, ethnicity/race, comorbid conditions, cardiovascular risk factors) as well as drug-related factors (e.g., ease of administration, availability, adverse effects, costs). Because many patients eventually will need drugs from 2 or more antihypertensive classes, experts generally state that the emphasis should be placed on achieving appropriate blood pressure control rather than on identifying a preferred drug to achieve that control.

Disease Overview Worldwide, hypertension is the most common modifiable risk factor for cardiovascular events and mortality. The lifetime risk of developing hypertension in the US exceeds 80%, with higher rates observed among African Americans and Hispanics compared with whites or Asians. The systolic blood pressure and diastolic blood pressure values defined as hypertension in adults (see Blood Pressure Classification under Uses: Hypertension) in a 2017 multidisciplinary guideline of the American College of Cardiology (ACC), American Heart Association (AHA), and a number of other professional organizations (subsequently referred to as the 2017 ACC/AHA hypertension guideline in this monograph) are lower than those defined in the Seventh Report of the Joint National Committee on Prevention, Detection, Evaluation, and Treatment of High Blood Pressure (JNC 7) guidelines, which results in an increase of approximately 14% in the prevalence of hypertension in the US. However, this change in definition results in only a 2% increase in the percentage of patients requiring antihypertensive drug therapy because nonpharmacologic treatment is recommended for most adults now classified by the 2017 ACC/AHA hypertension guideline as hypertensive who would *not* meet the JNC 7 definition of hypertension. Among US adults receiving antihypertensive drugs, approximately 53% have inadequately controlled blood pressure according to current ACC/AHA treatment goals.

Cardiovascular and Renal Sequelae. The principal goal of preventing and treating hypertension is to reduce the risk of cardiovascular and renal morbidity and mortality, including target organ damage. The relationship between blood pressure and cardiovascular disease is continuous, consistent, and independent of other risk factors. It is important that very high blood pressure be managed promptly to reduce the risk of target organ damage. The higher the blood pressure, the more likely the development of myocardial infarction (MI), heart failure, stroke, and renal disease. For adults 40–70 years of age, each 20-mm Hg increment in systolic blood pressure or 10-mm Hg increment in diastolic blood pressure doubles the risk of developing cardiovascular disease across the entire blood pressure range of 115/75 to 185/115 mm Hg. For those older than 50 years of age, systolic blood pressure is a much more important risk factor for developing cardiovascular disease than is diastolic blood pressure. The rapidity with which treatment is required depends on the patient's clinical presentation (presence of new or worsening target organ damage) and the presence or absence of cardiovascular complications; the 2017 ACC/AHA hypertension guideline states that treatment of very high blood pressure should be initiated within 1 week.

Blood Pressure Classification Accurate blood pressure measurement is essential for the proper diagnosis and management of hypertension. Error in measuring blood pressure is a major cause of inadequate blood pressure control and may lead to overtreatment. Because a patient's blood pressure may vary in an unpredictable fashion, a single blood pressure measurement is not sufficient for clinical decision-making. An average of 2 or 3 blood pressure measurements obtained on 2–3 separate occasions using proper technique should be used to minimize random error and provide a more accurate blood pressure reading. Out-of-office blood pressure measurements may be useful for confirming and managing hypertension. The 2017 ACC/AHA hypertension guideline document (available on the ACC and AHA websites) should be consulted for key steps on properly measuring blood pressure.

According to the 2017 ACC/AHA hypertension guideline, blood pressure in adults is classified into 4 categories: normal, elevated, stage 1 hypertension, and stage 2 hypertension. (See Table 1.) The 2017 ACC/AHA hypertension guideline lowers the blood pressure threshold used to define hypertension in the US; previous hypertension guidelines (JNC 7) considered adults with systolic blood pressure of 120–139 mm Hg or diastolic blood pressure of 80–89 mm Hg to have prehypertension, those with systolic blood pressure of 140–159 mm Hg or diastolic blood pressure of 90–99 mm Hg to have stage 1 hypertension, and those with systolic blood pressure of 160 mm Hg or higher or diastolic blood pressure of 100 mm Hg or higher to have stage 2 hypertension. The blood pressure definitions in the 2017 ACC/AHA hypertension guideline are based upon data from studies evaluating the association between systolic blood pressure/diastolic blood pressure and cardiovascular risk and the benefits of blood pressure reduction. Individuals with systolic blood pressure and diastolic blood pressure in 2 different categories should be designated as being in the higher blood pressure category.

Table 1. ACC/AHA Blood Pressure Classification in Adults[a][b]

Category	SBP[c] (mm Hg)		DBP[d] (mm Hg)
Normal	<120	and	<80
Elevated	120–129	and	<80
Hypertension, Stage 1	130–139	or	80–89
Hypertension, Stage 2	≥ 140	or	≥ 90

[a] Source: Whelton PK, Carey RM, Aronow WS et al. 2017 ACC/AHA/AAPA/ABC/ACPM/AGS/APhA/ASH/ASPC/NMA/PCNA guideline for the prevention, detection, evaluation, and management of high blood pressure in adults: a report of the American College of Cardiology/American Heart Association Task Force on Clinical Practice Guidelines. Hypertension. 2018;71:e13-115.

[b] Individuals with SBP and DBP in 2 different categories (e.g., elevated SBP and normal DBP) should be designated as being in the higher blood pressure category (i.e., elevated BP).

[c] Systolic blood pressure

[d] Diastolic blood pressure

The blood pressure thresholds used to define hypertension, when to initiate drug therapy, and the ideal target blood pressure values remain controversial. The 2017 ACC/AHA hypertension guideline recommends a blood pressure goal of less than 130/80 mm Hg in all adults who have confirmed hypertension and known cardiovascular disease or a 10-year atherosclerotic cardiovascular disease (ASCVD) event risk of 10% or higher; the ACC/AHA guideline also states that this blood pressure goal is reasonable to attempt to achieve in adults with confirmed hypertension who do *not* have increased cardiovascular risk. The lower blood pressure values used to define hypertension and the lower target blood pressure goals outlined in the 2017 ACC/AHA hypertension guideline are based on clinical studies demonstrating a substantial reduction in the composite end point of major cardiovascular disease events and the combination of fatal and nonfatal stroke when a lower systolic blood pressure/diastolic blood pressure value (i.e., 130/80 mm Hg) was used to define hypertension. These lower target blood pressure goals also are based upon clinical studies demonstrating continuing reduction of cardiovascular risk at progressively lower levels of systolic blood pressure. A linear relationship has been demonstrated between cardiovascular risk and blood pressure even at low systolic blood pressures (e.g., 120–124 mm Hg). The 2017 ACC/AHA hypertension guideline recommends estimating a patient's ASCVD risk using the ACC/AHA Pooled Cohort equations (available online at http://tools.acc.org/ASCVD-Risk-Estimator), which are based on a variety of factors including age, race, gender, cholesterol levels, statin use, blood pressure, treatment for hypertension, history of diabetes mellitus, smoking status, and aspirin use. While the 2017 ACC/AHA hypertension guideline has lowered the threshold for *diagnosing* hypertension in adults, the threshold for *initiating drug therapy* has only been lowered for those patients who are at high risk of cardiovascular disease. Clinicians who support the 2017 ACC/AHA hypertension guideline believe that these recommendations have the potential to increase hypertension awareness, encourage lifestyle modification, and focus antihypertensive drug initiation and intensification in those adults at high risk for cardiovascular disease.

The lower blood pressure goals advocated in the 2017 ACC/AHA hypertension guideline have been questioned by some clinicians who have concerns regarding the guideline's use of extrapolated observational data, the lack of generalizability of some of the randomized trials (e.g., SPRINT) used to support the guideline, the difficulty of establishing accurate representative blood pressure values in typical clinical practice settings, and the accuracy of the cardiovascular risk calculator used in the guideline. Some clinicians state the lower blood pressure threshold used to define hypertension in the 2017 ACC/AHA hypertension guideline is not fully supported by clinical data, and these clinicians have expressed concerns about the possible harms (e.g., adverse effects of antihypertensive therapy) associated with classifying more patients as being hypertensive. Some clinicians also state that using this guideline, a large number of young, low-risk patients would need to be treated in order to observe a clinical benefit, while other clinicians state that the estimated gains in life-expectancy attributable to long-term use of blood pressure-lowering drugs are correspondingly greater in this patient population.

Treatment Benefits In clinical trials, antihypertensive therapy has been found to reduce the risk of developing stroke by about 34–40%, MI by about 20–25%, and heart failure by more than 50%. In a randomized, controlled study (SPRINT) that included hypertensive patients without diabetes mellitus who had a high risk of cardiovascular disease, intensive systolic blood pressure lowering of approximately 15 mm Hg was associated with a 25% reduction in cardiovascular disease events and a 27% reduction in all-cause mortality. However, the exclusion of patients with diabetes mellitus, prior stroke, and those younger than 50 years of age may decrease the generalizability of these findings. Some experts estimate that if the systolic blood pressure goals of the 2017 ACC/AHA hypertension guideline are achieved, major cardiovascular disease events may be reduced by an additional 340,000 and total deaths by an additional 156,000 compared with implementation of the JNC 8 expert panel guideline goals but these benefits may be accompanied by an increase in the frequency of adverse events. While there was no overall difference in the occurrence of serious adverse events in patients receiving intensive therapy for blood pressure control (systolic blood pressure target of less than 120 mm Hg) compared with those receiving less intense control (systolic blood pressure target of less than 140 mm Hg) in the SPRINT study, hypotension, syncope, electrolyte abnormalities, and acute kidney injury or acute renal failure occurred in substantially more patients receiving intensive therapy.

In the Antihypertensive and Lipid-lowering Treatment to Prevent Heart Attack Trial (ALLHAT), the long-term cardiovascular morbidity and mortality benefit of a long-acting dihydropyridine calcium-channel blocker (amlodipine), a thiazide-like diuretic (chlorthalidone), and an ACE inhibitor (lisinopril) were compared in a broad population of patients with hypertension at risk for coronary heart disease. Although these antihypertensive agents were comparably effective in providing important cardiovascular benefit, apparent differences in certain secondary outcomes were observed. Patients receiving the ACE inhibitor experienced higher risks of stroke, combined cardiovascular disease, GI bleeding, and angioedema, while those receiving the calcium-channel blocker were at higher risk of developing heart failure. The ALLHAT investigators suggested that the observed differences in cardiovascular outcome may be attributable, at least in part, to the greater antihypertensive effect of the calcium-channel blocker compared with that of the ACE inhibitor, especially in women and black patients. (See Clinical Benefits of Thiazides in Hypertension under Hypertension in Adults: Treatment Benefits, in Uses in the Thiazides General Statement 40:28.20.)

General Considerations for Initial and Maintenance Antihypertensive Therapy **Nonpharmacologic Therapy.** Nonpharmacologic measures (i.e., lifestyle/behavioral modifications) that are effective in lowering blood pressure include weight reduction (for those who are overweight or obese), dietary changes to include foods such as fruits, vegetables, whole grains, and low-fat dairy products that are rich in potassium, calcium, magnesium, and fiber (i.e., adoption of the Dietary Approaches to Stop Hypertension [DASH] eating plan), sodium reduction, increased physical activity, and moderation of alcohol intake. Such lifestyle/behavioral modifications, including smoking cessation, enhance antihypertensive drug efficacy and decrease cardiovascular risk and remain an indispensable part of the management of hypertension. Lifestyle/behavioral modifications without antihypertensive drug therapy are recommended for individuals classified by the 2017 ACC/AHA hypertension guideline as having elevated blood pressure (systolic blood pressure 120–129 mm Hg and diastolic blood pressure less than 80 mm Hg) and in those with stage 1 hypertension (systolic blood pressure 130–139 mm Hg or diastolic blood pressure 80–89 mm Hg) who do *not* have preexisting cardiovascular disease or an estimated 10-year ASCVD risk of 10% or greater.

Initiation of Drug Therapy. Drug therapy in the management of hypertension must be individualized and adjusted based on the degree of blood pressure elevation while also considering cardiovascular risk factors. Drug therapy generally is reserved for patients who respond inadequately to nondrug therapy (i.e., lifestyle modifications such as diet [including sodium restriction and adequate potassium and calcium intake], regular aerobic physical activity, moderation of alcohol consumption, and weight reduction) or in whom the degree of blood pressure elevation or coexisting risk factors, especially increased cardiovascular risk, requires more prompt or aggressive therapy; however, the optimum blood pressure threshold for initiating antihypertensive drug therapy and specific treatment goals remain controversial. Recommendations generally are based on specific blood pressure levels shown in clinical studies to produce clinical benefits and can therefore vary depending on the studies selected for review.

The 2017 ACC/AHA hypertension guideline and many experts currently state that the treatment of hypertension should be based not only on blood pressure values but also on patients' cardiovascular risk factors. For *secondary prevention* of recurrent cardiovascular disease events in adults with clinical cardiovascular disease or for *primary prevention* in adults with an estimated 10-year ASCVD risk of 10% or higher, the 2017 ACC/AHA hypertension guideline recommends initiation of antihypertensive drug therapy in conjunction with lifestyle/behavioral modifications at an average systolic blood pressure of 130 mm Hg or an average diastolic blood pressure of 80 mm Hg or higher. For *primary prevention* of cardiovascular disease events in adults with a low (less than 10%) estimated 10-year risk of ASCVD, the 2017 ACC/AHA hypertension guideline recommends initiation of antihypertensive drug therapy in conjunction with lifestyle/behavioral modifications at a systolic blood pressure of 140 mm Hg or higher or a diastolic blood pressure of 90 mm Hg or higher. After initiation of antihypertensive drug therapy, regardless of the ASCVD risk, the 2017 ACC/AHA hypertension guideline generally recommends a blood pressure goal of less than 130/80 mm Hg in all patients. In addition, a systolic blood pressure goal of less than 130 mm Hg also is recommended for noninstitutionalized ambulatory patients 65 years of age or older. While these blood pressure goals are lower than those recommended for most patients in previous guidelines, they are based upon clinical studies demonstrating continuing reduction of cardiovascular risk at progressively lower levels of systolic blood pressure.

Most data indicate that patients with a higher cardiovascular risk will benefit the most from tighter blood pressure control; however, some experts state this treatment goal also may be beneficial in those at lower cardiovascular risk. Other clinicians believe that the benefits of such blood pressure lowering do not outweigh the risks in those patients considered to be at lower risk of cardiovascular disease and that reclassifying individuals formerly considered to have prehypertension as having hypertension may potentially lead to use of drug therapy in such patients without consideration of cardiovascular risk. Previous hypertension guidelines, such as those from the JNC 8 expert panel, generally recommended initiation of antihypertensive treatment in patients with a systolic blood pressure of at least 140 mm Hg or diastolic blood pressure of at least 90 mm Hg, targeted a blood pressure goal of less than 140/90 mm Hg regardless of cardiovascular risk, and used higher systolic blood pressure thresholds and targets in geriatric patients. Some clinicians continue to support the target blood pressures recommended by the JNC 8 expert panel because of concerns that such recommendations in the 2017 ACC/AHA hypertension guideline are based on extrapolation of data from the high-risk population in the SPRINT study to a lower-risk population. Also, because more than 90% of patients in SPRINT were already receiving antihypertensive drugs at baseline, data are lacking on the effects of *initiating* drug therapy at a lower blood pressure threshold (130/80 mm Hg) in patients at high risk of cardiovascular disease. The potential benefits of hypertension management and drug cost, adverse effects, and risks associated with the use of multiple antihypertensive drugs should be considered when deciding a patient's blood pressure treatment goal.

The 2017 ACC/AHA hypertension guideline recommends an ASCVD risk assessment for all adults with hypertension; however, experts state that it can be assumed that patients with hypertension and diabetes mellitus or chronic kidney disease (CKD) are at high risk for cardiovascular disease and that antihypertensive drug therapy should be initiated in these patients at a blood pressure of 130/80 mm Hg or higher. The 2017 ACC/AHA hypertension guideline also recommends a blood pressure goal of less than 130/80 mm Hg in patients with hypertension and diabetes mellitus or CKD. These recommendations are based on a systematic review of high-quality evidence from randomized controlled trials, meta-analyses, and post-hoc analyses that have demonstrated substantial reductions in the risk of important clinical outcomes (e.g., cardiovascular events) regardless of comorbid conditions or age when systolic blood pressure is lowered to less than 130 mm Hg. However, some clinicians have questioned the generalizability of findings from some of the trials (e.g., SPRINT) used to support the 2017 ACC/AHA hypertension guideline. For example, SPRINT included adults (mean age: 68 years) *without* diabetes mellitus who were at high risk of cardiovascular disease. While benefits of intensive blood pressure control were observed in this patient population, some clinicians have questioned whether these findings apply to younger patients who have a low risk of cardiovascular disease. In patients with CKD in the SPRINT trial, intensive blood pressure management (achieving a mean systolic blood pressure of approximately 122 mm Hg compared with 136 mm Hg with standard treatment) provided a similar beneficial reduction in the composite cardiovascular disease primary outcome and all-cause mortality as in the full patient cohort. Because most patients with CKD die from cardiovascular complications, the findings of this study further support a lower blood pressure target of less than 130/80 mm Hg.

Data are lacking to determine the ideal blood pressure goal in adult patients with hypertension and diabetes mellitus; also, studies evaluating the benefits of intensive blood pressure control in patients with diabetes mellitus have provided conflicting results. Clinical studies reviewed for the 2017 ACC/AHA hypertension guideline have shown similar quantitative benefits from blood pressure lowering in hypertensive patients with or without diabetes mellitus. In a randomized, controlled study (ACCORD-BP) that compared a higher (systolic blood pressure less than 140 mm Hg) versus lower (systolic blood pressure less than 120 mm Hg) blood pressure goal in patients with diabetes mellitus, there was no difference in the incidence of cardiovascular outcomes (e.g., composite outcome of cardiovascular death, nonfatal MI, and nonfatal stroke). However, some experts state that this study was underpowered to detect a difference between the 2 treatment groups and that the factorial design of the study complicated interpretation of the results. Although SPRINT did not include patients with diabetes mellitus, patients in this study with prediabetes demonstrated a similar cardiovascular benefit from intensive treatment of blood pressure as normoglycemic patients. A meta-analysis of data from the ACCORD and SPRINT studies suggests that the findings of both studies are consistent and that patients with diabetes mellitus benefit from more intensive blood pressure control. These data support the 2017 ACC/AHA hypertension guideline recommendation of a blood pressure treatment goal of less than 130/80 mm Hg in adult patients with hypertension and diabetes mellitus. Alternatively, the American Diabetes Association (ADA) recommends a blood pressure goal of less than 140/90 mm Hg in patients with diabetes mellitus. The ADA states that a lower blood pressure goal (e.g., less than 130/80 mm Hg) may be appropriate for patients with a high risk of cardiovascular disease and diabetes mellitus if it can be achieved without undue treatment burden.

Further study is needed to more clearly define optimum blood pressure goals in patients with hypertension, particularly in high-risk groups (e.g., patients with diabetes mellitus, cardiovascular disease, or cerebrovascular disease; black patients); when determining appropriate blood pressure goals, individual risks and benefits should be considered in addition to the evidence from clinical studies.

Choice of Initial Drug Therapy. In current hypertension management guidelines, angiotensin II receptor antagonists are recommended as one of several preferred drugs for the initial treatment of hypertension; other preferred options include ACE inhibitors, calcium-channel blockers, and thiazide diuretics. The 2017 ACC/AHA adult hypertension guideline states that an ACE inhibitor, angiotensin II receptor antagonist, calcium-channel blocker, or thiazide or thiazide-like diuretic (preferably chlorthalidone) are all acceptable choices for initial antihypertensive drug therapy in the general population of nonblack patients, including those with diabetes mellitus; drugs from any of these classes generally produce similar benefits in terms of overall mortality and cardiovascular, cerebrovascular, and renal outcomes. Angiotensin II receptor antagonists or ACE inhibitors may be particularly useful in the management of hypertension in patients with certain coexisting conditions such as diabetes mellitus or CKD; angiotensin II receptor antagonists also may be preferred, generally as an alternative to ACE inhibitors, in hypertensive patients with heart failure or ischemic heart disease and/or following MI. (See Considerations for Drug Therapy in Patients with Underlying Cardiovascular and Other Risk Factors under Uses: Hypertension.)

In patients with hypertension and compelling indications (e.g., CKD with albuminuria [urine albumin 300 mg/day or greater, or urine albumin:creatinine ratio of 300 mg/g or equivalent in the first morning void]), angiotensin II receptor antagonists are usually considered an alternative for ACE inhibitor-intolerant patients. (See Chronic Kidney Disease under Hypertension: Considerations for Drug Therapy in Patients with Underlying Cardiovascular and Other Risk Factors, in Uses.) However, data indicate no difference in efficacy between ACE inhibitors and angiotensin II receptor antagonists with regard to blood pressure lowering and clinical outcomes (i.e., all-cause mortality, cardiovascular mortality, MI, heart failure, stroke, and end-stage renal disease). Adverse events (e.g., cough, angioedema) leading to drug discontinuance occur more frequently with ACE inhibitor therapy than with angiotensin II receptor antagonist therapy. Because of similar efficacy and a lower frequency of adverse effects, some experts believe that angiotensin II receptor antagonists should be used instead of an ACE inhibitor for the treatment of hypertension or hypertension with certain compelling indications.

Experts state that in patients with stage 1 hypertension (especially the elderly, those with a history of hypotension, or those who have experienced adverse drug effects), it is reasonable to initiate drug therapy using the stepped-care approach in which one drug is initiated and titrated and other drugs are added sequentially to achieve the target blood pressure. Although some patients can begin treatment with a single antihypertensive agent, starting with 2 first-line drugs in different pharmacologic classes (either as separate agents or in a fixed-dose combination) is recommended in patients with stage 2 hypertension and an average blood pressure more than 20/10 mm Hg above their target blood pressure. Such combined therapy may increase the likelihood of achieving goal blood pressure in a more timely fashion, but also may increase the risk of adverse effects (e.g., orthostatic hypotension) in some patients (e.g., elderly). Drug regimens with complementary activity, where a second antihypertensive agent is used to block compensatory responses to the first agent or affect a different pressor mechanism, can result in additive blood pressure lowering and are preferred. Drug combinations that have similar mechanisms of action or clinical effects (e.g., the combination of an ACE inhibitor and an angiotensin II receptor antagonist) generally should be avoided. Many patients who begin therapy with a single antihypertensive agent will subsequently require at least 2 drugs from different pharmacologic classes to achieve their blood pressure goal. Experts state that other patient-specific factors, such as age, concurrent medications, drug adherence, drug interactions, the overall treatment regimen, cost, and comorbidities, also should be considered when deciding on an antihypertensive drug regimen. For any stage of hypertension, antihypertensive drug dosages should be adjusted and/or other agents substituted or added until goal blood pressure is achieved. (See Follow-up and Maintenance Drug Therapy under Hypertension: General Considerations for Initial and Maintenance Antihypertensive Therapy, in Uses.)

Follow-up and Maintenance Drug Therapy. Several strategies are used for the titration and combination of antihypertensive drugs; these strategies, which are generally based on those used in randomized controlled studies, include maximizing the dosage of the first drug before adding a second drug, adding a second drug before achieving maximum dosage of the initial drug, or initiating therapy with 2 drugs simultaneously (either as separate preparations or as a fixed-dose combination). Combined use of an ACE inhibitor and angiotensin II receptor antagonist should be avoided because of the potential risk of adverse renal effects. After initiating a new or adjusted antihypertensive drug regimen, patients should have their blood pressure reevaluated monthly until adequate blood pressure control is achieved. Effective blood pressure control can be achieved in most hypertensive patients, but many will ultimately require therapy with 2 or more antihypertensive drugs. In addition to measuring blood pressure, clinicians should evaluate patients for orthostatic hypotension, adverse drug effects, adherence to drug therapy and lifestyle modifications, and the need for drug dosage adjustments. Laboratory testing such as electrolytes and renal function status and other assessments of target organ damage also should be performed.

Considerations for Drug Therapy in Patients with Underlying Cardiovascular and Other Risk Factors Drug therapy in patients with hypertension and underlying cardiovascular or other risk factors should be carefully individualized based on the underlying disease(s), concomitant drugs, tolerance to drug-induced adverse effects, and blood pressure goal. (See Table 2 on Compelling Indications for Drug Classes based on Comorbid Conditions, in Considerations for Drug Therapy in Patients with Underlying Cardiovascular and Other Risk Factors under Uses: Hypertension in Adults, in the Thiazides General Statement 40:28.20.)

Ischemic Heart Disease. The selection of an appropriate antihypertensive agent in patients with ischemic heart disease should be based on individual patient characteristics but may include ACE inhibitors and/or β-blockers, with the addition of other drugs such as thiazide diuretics or calcium-channel blockers as necessary to achieve blood pressure goals. Many experts recommend the use of an ACE inhibitor (or an angiotensin II receptor antagonist if ACE inhibitors are not tolerated) and/or a β-blocker in hypertensive patients with stable ischemic heart disease because of the cardioprotective benefits of these drugs; all patients who have survived an MI should be treated with a β-blocker because of the demonstrated mortality benefit of these agents.

Heart Failure. While available evidence suggests that angiotensin II receptor antagonists as single therapies are not superior to other antihypertensive agents in the reduction of cardiovascular outcomes, angiotensin II receptor antagonists, usually in conjunction with other agents such as cardiac glycosides, diuretics, and β-blockers, have been shown to reduce morbidity and mortality in patients with existing heart failure. Because of the established benefits of ACE inhibitors in patients with heart failure, the American College of Cardiology Foundation (ACCF), AHA, and Heart Failure Society of America (HFSA) recommend the use of these drugs in all patients with symptomatic or asymptomatic (i.e., structural heart disease but no signs or symptoms) heart failure with reduced left ventricular ejection fraction (LVEF). Experts recommend an angiotensin II receptor antagonist as an alternative to therapy with an ACE inhibitor in patients with symptomatic or asymptomatic (i.e., structural heart disease but no signs or symptoms) heart failure with reduced LVEF. (See Uses: Heart Failure.)

Diabetes Mellitus. Experts state that initial treatment of hypertension in adults with diabetes mellitus and hypertension should include any of the usual first-line agents (ACE inhibitors, angiotensin II receptor antagonists, calcium-channel blockers, thiazide diuretics). In adults with diabetes mellitus, hypertension, and albuminuria, treatment with an ACE inhibitor or angiotensin II receptor antagonist may be considered to reduce the progression of kidney disease. While there is evidence demonstrating the benefits of angiotensin II receptor antagonists in reducing the development or progression of microvascular or macrovascular complications in hypertensive patients with type 1 or type 2 diabetes mellitus, in the absence of albuminuria, the risk of progressive kidney disease is low, and ACE inhibitors and angiotensin II receptor antagonists have not demonstrated superior cardioprotection when compared with other first-line agents. Results of several studies indicate that adequate control of blood pressure in patients with type 2 diabetes mellitus reduces the development or progression of complications of diabetes (e.g., death related to diabetes, stroke, heart failure, microvascular disease). Most patients with diabetes mellitus will require 2 or more antihypertensive agents to achieve blood pressure control.

Chronic Kidney Disease. Hypertensive patients with CKD (glomerular filtration rate [GFR] less than 60 mL/minute per 1.73 m^2 or kidney damage for 3 or more months) usually will require more than one antihypertensive agent to reach target blood pressure. Use of angiotensin II receptor antagonists or ACE inhibitors may be reasonable in patients with diabetic or nondiabetic CKD (Stage 1 or 2 with albuminuria or Stage 3 or higher); these drugs have been shown to slow the progression of kidney disease. Evidence of a renoprotective benefit is strongest in those with higher levels of albuminuria. Increases in serum creatinine (up to 30%) may be observed as a result of a decrease in intraglomerular pressure and concurrent reduction in GFR. The 2017 ACC/AHA hypertension guideline states that in patients with less severe kidney disease (i.e., stage 1 or 2 CKD without albuminuria), any of the first-line antihypertensive agents (e.g., ACE inhibitors, angiotensin II receptor antagonists, calcium-channel blockers, thiazide diuretics) can be used for the initial treatment of hypertension. Diuretics also may be useful in the management of CKD, and may potentiate the effects of angiotensin II receptor antagonists, ACE inhibitors, and other antihypertensive agents when used in combination.

Cerebrovascular Disease. Some experts recommend a blood pressure goal of less than 140/90 mm Hg in patients with ischemic stroke or transient ischemic attack (TIA), while others state that a blood pressure goal of less than 130/80 mm Hg may be reasonable. The 2017 ACC/AHA hypertension guideline states that adults not previously treated for hypertension who experience a stroke or TIA and who have an established blood pressure of 140/90 mm Hg or higher should receive antihypertensive therapy a few days after the event to reduce the risk of recurrent stroke or other vascular events. In patients with a recent lacunar stroke, experts suggest that a systolic blood pressure goal of 130 mm Hg may be reasonable based on results of a randomized open-label study (the Secondary Prevention of Small Subcortical Strokes [SPS3] trial). Although experts state that the optimal choice of drug for the management of hypertension in patients with a previous TIA or ischemic stroke is uncertain, available data indicate that an ACE inhibitor, angiotensin II receptor antagonist, thiazide diuretic, or the combination of a thiazide diuretic and an ACE inhibitor may be effective. Administration of an ACE inhibitor in combination with a thiazide diuretic has been shown to lower rates of recurrent stroke.

Other Special Considerations for Antihypertensive Drug Therapy

Race. Most patients with hypertension, especially black patients, will require at least 2 antihypertensive drugs to achieve adequate blood pressure control. Like ACE inhibitors, angiotensin II receptor antagonists may produce a smaller blood pressure response in hypertensive black patients compared with nonblack patients. In general, black patients tend to respond better to thiazide diuretics or calcium-channel blocking agents than to angiotensin II receptor antagonists. However, the combination of an ACE inhibitor or an angiotensin II receptor antagonist with a calcium-channel blocker or thiazide diuretic produces similar blood pressure lowering in black patients as in other racial groups. In addition, some experts state that when use of angiotensin II receptor antagonists is indicated in hypertensive patients with underlying cardiovascular or other risk factors, these indications should be applied equally to black hypertensive patients.

For further information on overall principles and expert recommendations for treatment of hypertension, see Uses: Hypertension in Adults and also see Uses: Hypertension in Pediatric Patients, in the Thiazides General Statement 40:28.20.

■ **Diabetic Nephropathy** Both angiotensin II receptor antagonists (e.g., valsartan) and ACE inhibitors have been shown to slow the rate of progression of renal disease in patients with diabetes mellitus and persistent albuminuria†, and use of a drug from either class is recommended in such patients with modestly elevated (30–300 mg/24 hours) or higher (exceeding 300 mg/24 hours) levels of urinary albumin excretion. The ADA states that the use of an ACE inhibitor or angiotensin II receptor antagonist is not recommended for the primary prevention of diabetic nephropathy in patients with diabetes mellitus who are normotensive, have normal levels of urinary protein excretion, and have a normal GFR. The usual precautions of angiotensin II receptor antagonist or ACE inhibitor therapy in patients with substantial renal impairment should be observed. (See Renal Effects under Warnings/Precautions: Other Warnings/Precautions, in Cautions.) For additional information on the use of angiotensin II receptor antagonists in the treatment of diabetic nephropathy, see Uses: Diabetic Nephropathy, in Losartan 24:32.08 and in Irbesartan 24:32.08.

■ **Heart Failure** Valsartan is used in the management of heart failure.

Current guidelines for the management of heart failure in adults generally recommend a combination of drug therapies to reduce morbidity and mortality, including neurohormonal antagonists (e.g., ACE inhibitors, angiotensin II receptor antagonists, angiotensin receptor-neprilysin inhibitors [ARNIs], β-blockers, aldosterone receptor antagonists) that inhibit the detrimental compensatory mechanisms in heart failure. Additional agents (e.g., cardiac glycosides, diuretics, sinoatrial modulators [i.e., ivabradine]) added to a heart failure treatment regimen in selected patients have been associated with symptomatic improvement and/or reduction in heart failure-related hospitalizations. Experts recommend that all asymptomatic patients with reduced LVEF (ACCF/AHA stage B heart failure) receive therapy with an ACE inhibitor and β-blocker to prevent symptomatic heart failure and to reduce morbidity and mortality. In patients with prior or current symptoms of chronic heart failure with reduced LVEF (ACCF/AHA stage C heart failure), ACCF, AHA, and HFSA recommend inhibition of the renin-angiotensin-aldosterone (RAA) system with an ACE inhibitor, angiotensin II receptor antagonist, or ARNI in conjunction with a β-blocker, and an aldosterone antagonist in selected patients, to reduce morbidity and mortality. While ACE inhibitors have been the preferred drugs for inhibition of the RAA system because of their established benefits in patients with heart failure and reduced ejection fraction, some evidence indicates that therapy with sacubitril/valsartan, an ARNI, may be more effective than ACE inhibitor therapy (enalapril) in reducing cardiovascular death and heart failure-related hospitalization in such patients. ACCF, AHA, and HFSA recommend that patients with chronic symptomatic heart failure and reduced LVEF (New York Heart Association [NYHA] class II or III) who are able to tolerate an ACE inhibitor or angiotensin II receptor antagonist be switched to therapy containing an ARNI to further reduce morbidity and mortality. However, in patients in whom an ARNI is not appropriate, continued use of an ACE inhibitor for all classes of heart failure with reduced ejection fraction remains strongly advised. In patients in whom an ARNI or ACE inhibitor is not appropriate, an angiotensin II receptor antagonist may be used. For further information on the use of ARNIs in patients with heart failure, see Uses: Heart Failure, in Sacubitril and Valsartan 24:32.92.

While angiotensin II receptor antagonists are considered reasonable alternatives in patients who are unable to tolerate ACE inhibitors (e.g., because of cough or angioedema), angioedema has been reported rarely with the use of valsartan during postmarketing experience. (See Sensitivity Reactions under Cautions: Warnings/Precautions.)

Several clinical trials have evaluated the use of angiotensin II receptor antagonists in patients with heart failure as add-on therapy to conventional regimens compared with an ACE inhibitor, as add-on therapy to conventional regimens including an ACE inhibitor, as combination therapy with an ACE inhibitor compared with therapy with either type of agent alone, or as an alternative therapy in patients intolerant of ACE inhibitors. In a large, double-blind, placebo-controlled study (Valsartan Heart Failure Trial [Val-HeFT]) in patients with mild to severe (NYHA class II–IV) heart failure and LVEF less than 40%, addition of valsartan 40 mg twice daily (initial dosage, with dosage doubled every 2 weeks to a target dosage of 160 mg twice daily) to standard therapy (principally ACE inhibitors, diuretics, digoxin, and β-blockers) was associated with a reduction in the composite end point of heart failure-related morbidity and mortality (defined as cardiac arrest with resuscitation, hospitalization for worsening heart failure, or administration of IV inotropic or vasodilator drugs for 4 or more hours without hospitalization) after an average of approximately 23 months. Valsartan therapy also improved secondary cardiovascular outcomes such as NYHA class, ejection fraction, and symptoms of heart failure (dyspnea, fatigue, edema, rales), and prevented deterioration of the patients' well-being (as determined by quality of life measurements). However, improvement in heart failure morbidity occurred principally in patients not receiving adjunctive therapy with an ACE inhibitor, and overall mortality was not affected by valsartan therapy. For additional details of studies on the use of angiotensin II receptor antagonists in the management of heart failure, see Uses: Heart Failure, in Losartan 24:32.08 and and Candesartan 24:32.08.

Data from other long-term placebo-controlled clinical trials indicate that angiotensin II receptor antagonists produce hemodynamic and neurohormonal effects associated with their suppression of the renin-angiotensin system; reduced hospitalizations and mortality also have been demonstrated. However, these drugs did not show consistent effects on cardiac symptoms or exercise tolerance in some studies. In one comparative (Evaluation of Losartan in the Elderly [ELITE]) study in geriatric patients 65 years of age and older who received losartan (up to 50 mg daily) or captopril (up to 150 mg daily) in addition to conventional therapy for 48 weeks, patients receiving losartan had a 46% lower risk of death and also experienced a lower incidence of adverse effects than those receiving captopril. However, after interim analysis of data, the difference in survival was no longer statistically significant and no difference in morbidity and mortality or frequency in hospitalizations for heart failure was found between the 2 therapies. Results of a follow-up study (ELITE II) failed to confirm a survival benefit for losartan therapy compared with captopril. In this study, losartan did not provide a statistically significant difference in reduction of overall death, sudden cardiac death, and/or resuscitated cardiac arrest compared with captopril, although ELITE II was not designed to demonstrate equivalence between the 2 therapies. In addition, results of another study (Randomized Evaluation of Strategies for Left Ventricular Dysfunction [RESOLVD]) in patients with ischemic or nonischemic dilated cardiomyopathy and mild to moderate heart failure showed no differences in exercise capacity or risk of cardiac events in patients receiving candesartan (up to 16 mg daily), enalapril (up to 20 mg daily), or a combination of candesartan and enalapril, in addition to conventional therapy.

■ **Heart Failure or Left Ventricular Dysfunction After Acute Myocardial Infarction** Valsartan is used to reduce the risk of cardiovascular mortality following acute MI in clinically stable patients with demonstrated clinical evidence of heart failure (signs, symptoms, radiologic evidence) or left ventricular systolic dysfunction (i.e., LVEF 40% or less). While ACE inhibitors generally are the preferred agents for this use because of their established benefits, angiotensin II receptor antagonists may be substituted in patients who are intolerant to ACE inhibitor therapy.

Efficacy of valsartan for reducing risk of mortality from any cause has been evaluated in a large, double-blind, randomized, long-term (median follow-up: 24.7 months) study (VALsartan In Acute myocardial iNfarcTion trial [VALIANT]) involving 14,703 patients with acute MI complicated by heart failure or left ventricular systolic dysfunction. The primary end point of this study was death from any cause, while secondary end points included time to cardiovascular mortality and time to the first occurrence of cardiovascular reinfarction or hospitalization for heart failure. A prespecified analysis was designed to demonstrate the noninferiority or equivalence of valsartan to captopril in the event that valsartan would not clearly be shown to be superior to the ACE inhibitor. Such analysis also was based on results from previous placebo-controlled studies, in which administration of ACE inhibitors has been associated with reduction in mortality.

Results of VALIANT indicate that when compared with those receiving captopril (titrated to 50 mg 3 times daily) or the combination of valsartan (titrated to 80 mg twice daily) and captopril (titrated to 50 mg 3 times daily), valsartan therapy (titrated to 160 mg twice daily) initiated 0.5–10 days after an acute MI was associated with a reduction of all-cause mortality similar to the reduction observed among those receiving captopril or the combination of valsartan and captopril. Nine hundred and seventy-nine (19.9%) patients receiving valsartan died (hazard ratio of 1; 97.5% confidence interval: 0.9–1.11) compared with 958 (19.5%) of those receiving captopril. In addition, 941 (19.3%) patients receiving valsartan in combination with captopril died (compared with 19.5% of those receiving captopril) (hazard ratio of 0.98; 97.5% confidence interval: 0.89–1.09). Valsartan therapy also was comparable to ACE inhibitor therapy in terms of the composite end point of fatal and nonfatal cardiovascular events (hospitalization for heart failure and recurrent nonfatal MI). Benefits associated with valsartan were not affected by age, gender, race, or baseline therapies. In this study, combined therapy with valsartan and captopril increased the rate of adverse effects without providing further benefit on survival. Although findings of this study provide evidence of comparable benefit, at least in high-risk patients, most experts continue to recommend that angiotensin II receptor antagonists be reserved for patients who do not tolerate ACE inhibitors since experience with ACE inhibitors is more extensive.

Dosage and Administration

■ **Administration** Valsartan is administered orally. Although food may decrease the rate and extent (e.g., by about 40%) of valsartan absorption, the manufacturers state that the drug can be administered without regard to meals.

Valsartan may be administered as an extemporaneously prepared oral suspension in pediatric patients who are unable to swallow tablets or in those for whom the calculated daily dosage does not correspond to the available tablet strengths. An extemporaneous suspension containing valsartan 4 mg/mL can be prepared in the following manner. First, 80 mL of suspending vehicle (e.g., Ora-Plus®) is added to an amber glass bottle containing eight 80-mg tablets of valsartan, and the contents are shaken for at least 2 minutes. The concentrated suspension should be allowed to stand for at least 1 hour following reconstitution and then should be shaken for at least an additional minute. The concentrated suspension of valsartan should be diluted with 80 mL of sweetening vehicle (e.g., Ora-Sweet SE®), and the container then shaken for at least 10 seconds to disperse the contents. The suspension should be shaken for at least 10 seconds before each dose is dispensed. When stored in an amber glass bottle with child-resistant screw-cap closure at a temperature of less than 30°C or at 2–8°C, the extemporaneous suspension is stable for up to 30 or up to 75 days, respectively.

■ **Dosage** ***Hypertension*** Dosage of valsartan must be individualized and adjusted according to blood pressure response.

Valsartan Therapy. The manufacturers state the usual initial dosage of valsartan as monotherapy in adults is 80 or 160 mg once daily in patients without depletion of intravascular volume; patients requiring greater reductions in blood pressure initially may be started at the higher dosage. If blood pressure response is inadequate with the initial dosage, dosage may be increased as tolerated up to a maximum of 320 mg daily or a diuretic may be added. The usual maintenance dosage of valsartan is 80–320 mg given once daily. However, addition of a diuretic generally has a greater effect on blood pressure reduction than dosage increases of valsartan as dosage exceeds 80 mg daily. Valsartan also can be used concomitantly with other antihypertensive agents.

The usual initial dosage of valsartan in children and adolescents 6–16 years of age with hypertension is 1.3 mg/kg (up to 40 mg) once daily. Dosage should be adjusted according to blood pressure response. Some experts state that the dosage may be increased every 2–4 weeks until blood pressure is controlled, the maximum dosage is reached, or adverse effects occur. Dosages exceeding 2.7 mg/kg (up to 160 mg) once daily have not been evaluated in pediatric patients. Because systemic exposure to valsartan is 1.6 times greater when the drug is administered as an extemporaneously prepared suspension compared with administration as the commercially available tablets, children being switched from the suspension to the oral tablets may require an increase in dosage of the drug. For information on overall principles and expert recommendations for treatment of hypertension in pediatric patients, see Uses: Hypertension in Pediatric Patients, in the Thiazides General Statement 40:28.20.

Valsartan/Hydrochlorothiazide Fixed-combination Therapy. Commercially available preparations containing valsartan in fixed combination with hydrochlorothiazide can be used as a substitute for the individually titrated drugs. Alternatively, in patients who do not respond adequately to monotherapy with valsartan (or another angiotensin II receptor antagonist) or, alternatively, with hydrochlorothiazide, combined therapy with the drugs can be used. The manufacturers state that patients who do not respond adequately to monotherapy with valsartan (or another angiotensin II receptor antagonist) or hydrochlorothiazide may be switched to therapy with the fixed-combination preparation at an initial dosage of valsartan 160 mg and hydrochlorothiazide 12.5 mg once daily. In addition, patients who experience dose-limiting adverse effects during monotherapy with valsartan or hydrochlorothiazide can be switched to a lower dosage of that drug, given as a fixed-combination preparation containing valsartan and hydrochlorothiazide, to achieve similar blood pressure control. If needed, dosage of the fixed combination may be increased up to a maximum of 320 mg of valsartan and 25 mg of hydrochlorothiazide (given once daily) after 3–4 weeks. The maximum antihypertensive effect is attained within 2–4 weeks after initiation of therapy or a change in dosage.

Commercially available preparations containing valsartan in fixed combination with hydrochlorothiazide may be used for initial treatment of hypertension in patients likely to require combined therapy with multiple antihypertensive drugs to achieve blood pressure control. In such patients, therapy with the fixed-combination preparation should be initiated at a dosage of 160 mg of valsartan and 12.5 mg of hydrochlorothiazide once daily. Dosage should be adjusted according to the patient's response after 1–2 weeks of therapy. The decision to use the fixed combination of valsartan and hydrochlorothiazide for initial treatment of hypertension should be based on assessment of potential benefits and risks of such therapy. The fixed combination of valsartan and hydrochlorothiazide is not recommended as initial therapy in patients with depletion of intravascular volume. In patients whose baseline blood pressure is 160/100 mm Hg, the estimated probability of achieving control of systolic blood pressure (defined as systolic blood pressure of less than 140 mm Hg) is 41, 50, or 84% and of achieving control of diastolic blood pressure (defined as diastolic blood pressure of less than 90 mm Hg) is 60, 57, or 80% with valsartan (320 mg daily) alone, hydrochlorothiazide (25 mg daily) alone, or valsartan combined with hydrochlorothiazide (at the same dosages), respectively.

Valsartan/Amlodipine Fixed-combination Therapy. Patients whose hypertension is adequately controlled with valsartan and amlodipine administered separately may be switched to the fixed-combination preparation containing the corresponding individual doses. Alternatively, the manufacturers state that patients who do not respond adequately to monotherapy with valsartan (or another angiotensin II receptor antagonist) or, alternatively, with amlodipine (or another dihydropyridine-derivative calcium-channel blocker) may be switched to therapy with the fixed-combination preparation containing valsartan and amlodipine. In addition, patients who experience dose-limiting adverse effects during monotherapy with valsartan or amlodipine can be switched to a lower dosage of that drug, given as a fixed-combination preparation containing valsartan and amlodipine, to achieve similar blood pressure control; dosage should be adjusted according to the patient's response after 3–4 weeks of therapy. If needed, dosage of the fixed-combination preparation may be increased up to a maximum of 320 mg of valsartan and 10 mg of amlodipine given once daily; because most of the antihypertensive effect of a given dosage is achieved within 2 weeks, dosage may be adjusted after 1–2 weeks, if needed, to attain blood pressure control.

Commercially available preparations containing valsartan in fixed combination with amlodipine may be used for initial treatment of hypertension in patients likely to require combined therapy with multiple antihypertensive drugs to achieve blood pressure control. In such patients, therapy with the fixed-combination preparation should be initiated at a dosage of 160 mg of valsartan and 5 mg of amlodipine once daily in individuals without depletion of intravascular volume. The decision to use the fixed combination of valsartan and amlodipine for initial management of hypertension should be based on assessment of potential benefits and risks of such therapy, including consideration of whether the patient is likely to tolerate the lowest available dosage of the combined drugs. In patients whose baseline blood pressure is 160/100 mm Hg, the estimated probability of achieving control of systolic blood pressure (defined as systolic blood pressure of less than 140 mm Hg) is 47, 67, or 80% and of achieving control of diastolic blood pressure (defined as diastolic blood pressure of less than 90 mm Hg) is 62, 80, or 85% with valsartan (320 mg daily) alone, amlodipine (10 mg daily) alone, or valsartan combined with amlodipine (at the same dosages), respectively.

Valsartan/Amlodipine/Hydrochlorothiazide Fixed-combination Therapy. The fixed-combination preparation containing valsartan, amlodipine, and hydrochlorothiazide may be used to provide additional blood pressure control in patients who do not respond adequately to combination therapy with any 2 of the following classes of antihypertensive agents: angiotensin II receptor antagonists, calcium-channel blockers, or diuretics. Patients who experience dose-limiting adverse effects of valsartan, amlodipine, or hydrochlorothiazide while receiving any dual combination of these drugs may be switched to a lower dosage of that drug, given as a fixed-combination preparation containing all 3 of these drugs, to achieve similar blood pressure reductions. The fixed-combination preparation containing valsartan, amlodipine, and hydrochlorothiazide also can be used as a substitute for the individually titrated drugs. If necessary, dosage of the fixed-combination preparation may be increased after 2 weeks for additional blood pressure control (but should not exceed a maximum dosage of 320 mg of valsartan, 10 mg of amlodipine, and 25 mg of hydrochlorothiazide once daily). The commercially available preparation containing valsartan in fixed combination with amlodipine and hydrochlorothiazide should not be used for the initial management of hypertension.

Blood Pressure Monitoring and Treatment Goals. Blood pressure should be monitored regularly (i.e., monthly) during therapy and dosage of the antihypertensive drug adjusted until blood pressure is controlled. If an adequate blood pressure response is not achieved with angiotensin II receptor antagonist monotherapy, the dosage may be increased or another antihypertensive agent with demonstrated benefit and preferably with a complementary mechanism of action (e.g., calcium-channel blocker, thiazide diuretic) may be added; if target blood pressure is still not achieved, a third drug may be added. (See Uses: Hypertension.) In patients who develop unacceptable adverse effects with valsartan, the drug should be discontinued and another antihypertensive agent from a different pharmacologic class should be initiated.

The goal of hypertension management and prevention is to achieve and maintain optimal control of blood pressure. However, the optimum blood pressure threshold for initiating antihypertensive drug therapy and specific treatment goals remain controversial. While previous hypertension guidelines have based target blood pressure goals on age and comorbidities, the 2017 ACC/AHA hypertension guideline incorporates underlying cardiovascular risk into decision making regarding treatment and generally recommends the same target blood pressure (i.e., less than 130/80 mm Hg) in all adults. Many patients will require at least 2 drugs from different pharmacologic classes to achieve their blood pressure goal; the potential benefits of hypertension management and drug cost, adverse effects, and risks associated with the use of multiple antihypertensive drugs also should be considered when deciding a patient's blood pressure treatment goal. (See General Considerations for Initial and Maintenance Antihypertensive Therapy under Uses: Hypertension.)

For additional information on target levels of blood pressure and on monitoring therapy in the management of hypertension, see Blood Pressure Monitoring and Treatment Goals under Dosage: Hypertension, in Dosage and Administration in the Thiazides General Statement 40:28.20.

Heart Failure For the management of heart failure (New York Heart Association [NYHA] class II–IV) in patients unable to tolerate therapy with angiotensin-converting enzyme (ACE) inhibitors, the manufacturers recommend an initial valsartan dosage of 40 mg twice daily; some experts recommend an initial dosage of 20–40 mg twice daily in patients with chronic heart failure and reduced left ventricular ejection fraction (LVEF) (American College of Cardiology Foundation [ACCF]/American Heart Association [AHA] stage C heart failure). Dosage of valsartan should be increased until a dosage of 160 mg twice daily (the maximum dosage used in clinical trials) or the highest tolerated dosage is reached. While patients with heart failure generally have some reduction in blood pressure with valsartan therapy, discontinuance of therapy usually is not necessary when dosage recommendations are followed. Consideration should be given to reducing the dosage of concurrent diuretic therapy.

Heart Failure or Left Ventricular Dysfunction after Acute Myocardial Infarction When used after myocardial infarction (MI) in adults with clinical signs of heart failure or left ventricular systolic dysfunction, valsartan therapy may be initiated as early as 12 hours after the MI. An initial dosage of 20 mg twice daily is recommended. Dosage may be increased within 7 days to 40 mg twice daily with subsequent titrations to a target maintenance dosage of 160 mg twice daily, as tolerated. If hypotension or renal dysfunction occurs, dosage reduction should be considered. While post-MI patients generally have some reduction in blood pressure with valsartan therapy, discontinuance of therapy usually is not necessary when dosage recommendations are followed. Valsartan may be given with other standard post-MI therapy (e.g., thrombolytics, aspirin, β-adrenergic blocking agents [β-blockers], hydroxymethylglutaryl-CoA [HMG-CoA] reductase inhibitors [statins]).

■ Special Populations The manufacturers state that modification of valsartan dosage is not necessary for patients with mild to moderate renal impairment; however, valsartan has not been studied in patients with creatinine clearances of less than 10 mL/minute and should be used with caution in adults with severe renal impairment. Valsartan is not removed by hemodialysis. Use of valsartan in pediatric patients with glomerular filtration rates of less than 30 mL/minute per 1.73 m^2 has not been studied. Safety and efficacy of commercially available preparations containing valsartan in fixed combination with hydrochlorothiazide have not been established in patients with severe renal impairment.

The manufacturers state that valsartan should be used with caution in patients with hepatic impairment. Although systemic exposure to valsartan (as measured by area under the serum concentration-time curve [AUC]) is increased approximately twofold in patients with mild to moderate chronic liver disease, the manufacturers state that modification of valsartan dosage is not necessary for these patients. The amount of amlodipine in fixed-combination preparations containing valsartan and amlodipine exceeds the recommended initial dosage of amlodipine (2.5 mg daily) for patients with hepatic impairment.

The manufacturers state that modification of valsartan dosage is not necessary for geriatric patients. However, the amount of amlodipine in fixed-combination preparations containing valsartan and amlodipine exceeds the recommended initial dosage of amlodipine (2.5 mg daily) for geriatric patients.

Cautions

■ Contraindications Known hypersensitivity to valsartan or any ingredient in the formulation.

Concomitant use of valsartan and aliskiren in patients with diabetes mellitus. (See Drug Interactions: Drugs that Block the Renin-Angiotensin System.)

■ Warnings/Precautions ***Warnings*** **Fetal/Neonatal Morbidity and Mortality.** Drugs that act directly on the renin-angiotensin system (e.g., angiotensin-converting enzyme [ACE] inhibitors, angiotensin II receptor antagonists) can cause fetal and neonatal morbidity and mortality when used in pregnancy during the second and third trimesters. Valsartan should be discontinued as soon as possible when pregnancy is detected, unless continued use is considered life-saving. Nearly all women can be transferred successfully to alternative therapy for the remainder of their pregnancy. For additional information on the risk of such drugs (i.e., angiotensin II antagonists and ACE inhibitors) during pregnancy, see Cautions: Pregnancy, Fertility, and Lactation, in Captopril 24:32.04 and in Enalaprilat/Enalapril 24:32.04.

Sensitivity Reactions Sensitivity reactions, including various anaphylactoid reactions and/or angioedema, have been reported in patients receiving angiotensin II receptor antagonists, including valsartan. These drugs should be used with extreme caution in patients with a history of angioedema associated with or unrelated to ACE inhibitor or angiotensin II receptor antagonist therapy. The manufacturer states that valsartan should not be readministered to patients with a history of angioedema.

Other Warnings/Precautions **Cardiovascular Effects.** Valsartan rarely is associated with severe hypotension in patients with uncomplicated hypertension. Symptomatic hypotension may occur in patients with an activated renin-angiotensin system (e.g., patients with volume or salt depletion secondary to salt restriction or high-dose diuretic therapy). Volume and/or salt depletion should be corrected before starting valsartan therapy, or therapy should be initiated under close medical supervision.

Patients with heart failure and those with clinical signs of left ventricular systolic dysfunction following acute myocardial infarction (MI) generally have some reduction in blood pressure with valsartan therapy, but drug discontinuance generally is not necessary when recommended dosages are used. Caution should be observed when initiating valsartan therapy in these patients.

If symptomatic hypotension occurs, the patient should be placed in the supine position; if hypotension is severe, IV infusion of 0.9% sodium chloride injection to expand fluid volume should be considered. Transient hypotension is not a contraindication to additional doses of valsartan, and therapy with the drug can be reinstated cautiously after blood pressure has been stabilized (e.g., with volume expansion).

Malignancies. In July 2010, the US Food and Drug Administration (FDA) initiated a safety review of angiotensin II receptor antagonists after a published meta-analysis suggested a possible association between the use of these agents and an increased risk of cancer. The meta-analysis, which combined cancer-related findings from 5 randomized, controlled trials in over 60,000 patients, found a modest but significant increase in the risk of new cancer occurrence in patients receiving an angiotensin II receptor antagonist (mostly telmisartan) compared with those in control groups (7.2 versus 6%, respectively; risk ratio 1.08). However, because of several limitations of the study (e.g., trials included in the meta-analysis were not specifically designed to evaluate cancer outcomes, lack of individual patient data), the validity of these findings has been questioned.

Subsequent studies, including a larger, more comprehensive meta-analysis conducted by FDA, have not shown an increased risk of cancer in patients receiving angiotensin II receptor antagonists. FDA's meta-analysis, which included trial-level data from 31 randomized studies (total of approximately 156,000 patients), found no evidence of an increased risk of cancer in patients who received an angiotensin II receptor antagonist compared with those who received other treatments (placebo or active control). The overall rate of new cancer occurrence was essentially the same in both groups of patients (1.82 and 1.84 cases per 100 patient-years, respectively). In addition, there was no difference in the risk of cancer-related death, breast cancer, lung cancer, or prostate cancer between the groups. Based on these results and a review of all currently available data related to this potential safety concern, FDA has concluded that use of angiotensin II receptor antagonists is not associated with an increased risk of cancer.

Renal Effects. Because the renin-angiotensin-aldosterone (RAA) system appears to contribute substantially to maintenance of glomerular filtration in patients with heart failure in whom renal perfusion is severely compromised, renal function may deteriorate markedly (e.g., renal failure) in these patients during therapy with an ACE inhibitor or an angiotensin II receptor antagonist (e.g., valsartan). Dosage reduction or discontinuance of valsartan or diuretic therapy may be required. Renal artery stenosis, preexisting renal impairment, and concomitant diuretic therapy also are risk factors for renal impairment during therapy with drugs that inhibit the RAA system. Although reports received to date have involved patients treated with ACE inhibitors, this adverse effect also would be expected to occur when drugs with similar pharmacologic activity (e.g., angiotensin II receptor antagonists) are used in a similar manner. (See Cautions: Renal Effects, in Enalapril 24:32.04.)

Hyperkalemia. Hyperkalemia may occur in patients receiving valsartan, especially in those with heart failure and preexisting renal impairment. Dosage reduction or discontinuance of valsartan therapy may be required.

Fixed-combination Preparations. When valsartan is used as a fixed combination that includes amlodipine and/or hydrochlorothiazide, the cautions, precautions, and contraindications associated with the concomitant agent(s) must be considered in addition to those associated with valsartan.

Specific Populations **Pregnancy.** Category D. (See Users Guide.) Valsartan can cause fetal and neonatal morbidity and mortality when administered to a pregnant woman. Valsartan should be discontinued as soon as possible when pregnancy is detected. (See Fetal/Neonatal Morbidity and Mortality under Warnings/Precautions: Warnings, in Cautions.)

Lactation. Valsartan is distributed into milk in rats. It is not known whether valsartan is distributed into human milk. A decision should be made whether to discontinue nursing or the drug because of the potential risk in nursing infants.

Pediatric Use. Safety and efficacy of valsartan have been established in a randomized, double-blind clinical trial in pediatric patients 6–16 years of age with hypertension; adverse effects of the drug in this age group were similar to those observed in adults. Although there was some evidence of efficacy in randomized, double-blind clinical trials in pediatric patients 6 months to 5 years of age with hypertension, 2 deaths and 3 cases of transaminase elevations were observed in a one-year open-label extension study in patients 1–5 years of age. A causal relationship to the drug has not been established; however, use of valsartan in pediatric patients younger than 6 years of age is not recommended. In pediatric patients with hypertension in whom underlying renal abnormalities may be more common, renal function and serum potassium should be carefully monitored. Pharmacokinetics of the drug have been studied in pediatric patients 1–16 years of age.

Safety and efficacy of valsartan in fixed combination with hydrochlorothiazide and/or amlodipine in pediatric patients have not been established.

Safety and efficacy of valsartan in pediatric patients with glomerular filtration rates of less than 30 mL/minute per 1.73 m^2 have not been established.

For information on overall principles and expert recommendations for treatment of hypertension in pediatric patients, see Uses: Hypertension in Pediatric Patients, in the Thiazides General Statement 40:28.20.

Geriatric Use. No substantial differences in safety and efficacy of valsartan in geriatric patients relative to younger adults have been observed, but increased sensitivity cannot be ruled out.

Hepatic Impairment. Valsartan should be used with caution in patients with obstructive biliary disease or hepatic impairment since the drug is eliminated primarily by biliary excretion and clearance of the drug may be reduced.

Renal Impairment. Valsartan should be used with caution in patients with severe renal impairment. (See Renal Effects and also see Hyperkalemia under Warning/Precautions: Other Warnings/Precautions, in Cautions.)

■ Common Adverse Effects Adverse effects occurring in 1% or more of adults with hypertension receiving valsartan and more frequently than with placebo include viral infection, fatigue, and abdominal pain; adverse effects in pediatric patients 6–16 years of age generally are similar to those in adults.

Adverse effects occurring in 2% or more of patients with heart failure receiving valsartan and more frequently than with placebo include dizziness, hypotension, diarrhea, arthralgia, fatigue, back pain, postural dizziness, hyperkalemia, and postural hypotension. In patients receiving valsartan following acute MI, the most common adverse effects resulting in discontinuance of the drug included hypotension, cough, and increased serum creatinine concentration.

Drug Interactions

■ **Drugs Affecting or Metabolized by Hepatic Microsomal Enzymes** In vitro studies suggest valsartan is minimally metabolized by cytochrome P-450 (CYP) microsomal isoenzyme 2C9 and does not inhibit CYP enzymes at therapeutic concentrations. Therefore, drug interactions mediated by CYP enzymes are considered unlikely with valsartan.

■ **Drugs That Inhibit Hepatic Transport Systems** In vitro data suggest that valsartan is a substrate of organic anion transporter protein (OATP) 1B1 (hepatic uptake transporter) and multidrug resistance protein MRP2 (hepatic efflux transporter). Use of valsartan concomitantly with inhibitors of OATP 1B1 (e.g., cyclosporine, rifampin) or MRP2 (e.g., ritonavir) may result in increased systemic exposure to valsartan.

■ **Drugs that Block the Renin-Angiotensin System** Concomitant use of valsartan with other drugs that block the renin-angiotensin system (e.g., angiotensin-converting enzyme [ACE] inhibitors, aliskiren) may increase the risk of renal impairment, hyperkalemia, and hypotension; when valsartan is used concomitantly with such drugs, blood pressure, renal function, and serum concentrations of electrolytes should be monitored closely. Concomitant use of valsartan with aliskiren is contraindicated in patients with diabetes mellitus; in addition, such concomitant use should be avoided in patients with renal impairment (glomerular filtration rate [GFR] less than 60 mL/minute per 1.73 m^2). (See Cautions in Aliskiren Hemifumarate 24:32.40.)

■ **Drugs or Foods That Increase Serum Potassium Concentration** Concomitant use of potassium-sparing diuretics (e.g., amiloride, spironolactone, triamterene), potassium supplements, potassium-containing salt substitutes, or other drugs that may increase serum potassium concentrations (e.g., heparin) with valsartan may result in increased hyperkalemic effects and, in patients with heart failure, increases in serum creatinine concentration. Monitoring of serum potassium concentrations is recommended during concomitant use.

■ **Atenolol** Antihypertensive effect of combined atenolol and valsartan therapy exceeds that of either drug alone, but the reduction in heart rate with the drugs in combination does not exceed that observed with atenolol alone. Pharmacokinetic interaction is unlikely.

■ **Hydrochlorothiazide** Hypotensive effects of valsartan and hydrochlorothiazide are additive; pharmacokinetic interaction is unlikely.

■ **Lithium** Increased lithium concentrations and clinical toxicity have been reported in patients receiving valsartan concomitantly with lithium. Monitoring of serum lithium concentrations is recommended during concomitant use.

■ **Nonsteroidal Anti-inflammatory Agents** Hypotensive effects of angiotensin II receptor antagonists may be attenuated when these agents are used concomitantly with nonsteroidal anti-inflammatory agents (NSAIAs), including selective cyclooxygenase-2 (COX-2) inhibitors.

Deterioration of renal function may occur when angiotensin II receptor antagonists are used concomitantly with NSAIAs, including selective COX-2 inhibitors, in geriatric patients, patients with volume depletion (including those receiving concomitant diuretic therapy), or patients with renal impairment; renal function should be monitored periodically in patients receiving concomitant therapy with valsartan and an NSAIA.

■ **Warfarin** Concurrent use of valsartan and warfarin did not affect the pharmacokinetics of valsartan or the anticoagulant effect of warfarin.

■ **Other Drugs** Pharmacokinetic interactions with amlodipine, cimetidine, digoxin, furosemide, glyburide, and indomethacin are unlikely.

Description

Valsartan, a nonpeptide tetrazole derivative, is an angiotensin II type 1 (AT_1) receptor antagonist. Valsartan has pharmacologic actions similar to those of losartan; however, unlike losartan, valsartan is not a prodrug and its pharmacologic activity does not depend on hydrolysis in the liver.

Valsartan blocks the physiologic actions of angiotensin II, including vasoconstrictor and aldosterone-secreting effects, by selectively inhibiting access of angiotensin II to AT_1 receptors within many tissues, including vascular smooth muscle and the adrenal gland. By comparison, angiotensin-converting enzyme (ACE, kininase II) inhibitors block the conversion of angiotensin I to angiotensin II; however, the blockade of angiotensin II production by ACE inhibitors is not complete since the vasopressor hormone can be formed via other enzymes that are not blocked by ACE inhibitors. Because valsartan, unlike ACE inhibitors, does not inhibit ACE, the drug does not interfere with response to bradykinins and substance P; a beneficial consequence is the absence of certain ACE inhibitor-induced adverse effects (e.g., cough), but possible renal and/or cardioprotective effects may be sacrificed. Valsartan also does not interfere with angiotensin II synthesis.

Valsartan is eliminated mainly by biliary excretion; following oral administration, about 83% of the administered dose is recovered in feces and 13% in urine. The drug is eliminated mainly as unchanged drug, with only about 20% of a dose recovered as metabolites. In vitro studies indicate that valsartan is minimally metabolized by cytochrome P-450 (CYP) microsomal isoenzyme 2C9.

Advice to Patients

When valsartan is used in fixed combination with hydrochlorothiazide and/or amlodipine, importance of advising patients of important precautionary information about the concomitant agent(s).

Importance of informing women of childbearing potential about the risks of use during pregnancy.

Importance of women informing clinicians if they are or plan to become pregnant or plan to breast-feed. All women of childbearing potential should be advised to report pregnancy to their clinician as soon as possible. (See Fetal/Neonatal Morbidity and Mortality under Warnings/Precautions: Warnings, in Cautions.)

Importance of contacting clinician if dizziness or faintness develops or if unexplained weight gain or swelling of the feet, ankles, or hands occurs.

Importance of informing clinicians of existing or contemplated concomitant therapy, including prescription and OTC drugs.

Importance of informing patients of other important precautionary information. (See Cautions.)

Overview® (see Users Guide). For additional information on this drug until a more detailed monograph is developed and published, the manufacturer's labeling should be consulted. It is *essential* that the manufacturer's labeling be consulted for more detailed information on usual cautions, precautions, contraindications, potential drug interactions, laboratory test interferences, and acute toxicity.

Preparations

Excipients in commercially available drug preparations may have clinically important effects in some individuals; consult specific product labeling for details.

Valsartan

Oral		
Tablets	40 mg*	Diovan® (scored), Novartis **Valsartan Tablets**
	80 mg*	**Diovan®**, Novartis **Valsartan Tablets**
	160 mg*	**Diovan®**, Novartis **Valsartan Tablets**
	320 mg*	**Diovan®**, Novartis **Valsartan Tablets**

*available from one or more manufacturer, distributor, and/or repackager by generic (nonproprietary) name

Valsartan Combinations

Oral		
Tablets, film-coated	80 mg with Hydrochlorothiazide 12.5 mg*	**Diovan® HCT**, Novartis **Valsartan and Hydrochlorothiazide Tablets**
	160 mg with Amlodipine Besylate 5 mg (of amlodipine)*	**Amlodipine Besylate and Valsartan Tablets** **Exforge®**, Novartis
	160 mg with Amlodipine Besylate 5 mg (of amlodipine) and Hydrochlorothiazide 12.5 mg*	**Amlodipine Besylate, Valsartan, and Hydrochlorothiazide Tablets** **Exforge HCT®**, Novartis
	160 mg with Amlodipine Besylate 5 mg (of amlodipine) and Hydrochlorothiazide 25 mg*	**Amlodipine Besylate, Valsartan, and Hydrochlorothiazide Tablets** **Exforge HCT®**, Novartis
	160 mg with Amlodipine Besylate 10 mg (of amlodipine)*	**Amlodipine Besylate and Valsartan Tablets** **Exforge®**, Novartis
	160 mg with Amlodipine Besylate 10 mg (of amlodipine) and Hydrochlorothiazide 12.5 mg*	**Amlodipine Besylate, Valsartan, and Hydrochlorothiazide Tablets** **Exforge HCT®**, Novartis
	160 mg with Amlodipine Besylate 10 mg (of amlodipine) and Hydrochlorothiazide 25 mg*	**Amlodipine Besylate, Valsartan, and Hydrochlorothiazide Tablets** **Exforge HCT®**, Novartis
	160 mg with Hydrochlorothiazide 12.5 mg*	**Diovan® HCT**, Novartis **Valsartan and Hydrochlorothiazide Tablets**
	160 mg with Hydrochlorothiazide 25 mg*	**Diovan® HCT**, Novartis **Valsartan and Hydrochlorothiazide Tablets**
	320 mg with Amlodipine Besylate 5 mg (of amlodipine)*	**Amlodipine Besylate and Valsartan Tablets** **Exforge®**, Novartis

320 mg with Amlodipine Besylate 10 mg (of amlodipine)*	**Amlodipine Besylate and Valsartan Tablets**
	Exforge®, Novartis
320 mg with Amlodipine Besylate 10 mg (of amlodipine) and Hydrochlorothiazide 25 mg*	**Amlodipine Besylate, Valsartan, and Hydrochlorothiazide Tablets**
	Exforge HCT®, Novartis
320 mg with Hydrochlorothiazide 12.5 mg*	**Diovan® HCT**, Novartis
	Valsartan and Hydrochlorothiazide Tablets
320 mg with Hydrochlorothiazide 25 mg*	**Diovan® HCT**, Novartis
	Valsartan and Hydrochlorothiazide Tablets

*available from one or more manufacturer, distributor, and/or repackager by generic (nonproprietary) name

†Use is not currently included in the labeling approved by the US Food and Drug Administration

MINERALOCORTICOID (ALDOSTERONE) RECEPTOR ANTAGONISTS 24:32.20

Eplerenone

■ Eplerenone is considered a relatively selective competitive mineralocorticoid (aldosterone) receptor antagonist.

Uses

■ **Heart Failure** ***Heart Failure After Myocardial Infarction*** Eplerenone is used to improve survival following acute myocardial infarction (MI) in clinically stable patients with left ventricular dysfunction (i.e., left ventricular ejection fraction [LVEF] 40% or less) who have demonstrated clinical evidence of heart failure. The American College of Cardiology Foundation (ACCF) and the American Heart Association (AHA) recommend therapy with an aldosterone antagonist (i.e., spironolactone, eplerenone) to reduce morbidity and mortality following acute MI in patients with reduced LVEF (40% or less) who develop symptoms of heart failure or who have a history of diabetes mellitus, unless contraindicated. Efficacy of eplerenone for improving survival has been evaluated in a multicenter, randomized, double-blind, placebo-controlled study (the Eplerenone Post-Acute Myocardial Infarction Heart Failure Efficacy and Survival Study; EPHESUS) involving 6632 patients with acute MI complicated by congestive heart failure and left-ventricular dysfunction. Results of this study indicate that the addition of eplerenone (25–50 mg daily; mean dosage: 43 mg daily) to standard therapy (e.g., aspirin, nitrates, angiotensin-converting enzyme [ACE] inhibitors, angiotensin II receptor antagonists, β-adrenergic blocking agents (β-blockers), hydroxymethylglutaryl-coenzyme A [HMG-CoA] reductase inhibitors, loop diuretics) 3–14 days (mean: 7 days) after acute MI reduced the risk of mortality from any cause, and of hospitalization or mortality from cardiovascular causes by 15 and 13%, respectively, compared with standard therapy and placebo. In addition, eplerenone reduced the risk of mortality or hospitalization from any cause by 8% and mortality from cardiovascular causes by 17%. Eplerenone did not appear to affect the rates of re-infarction.

Chronic Heart Failure Eplerenone has been used in the management of chronic heart failure† (New York Heart Association [NYHA] class II–IV) with reduced ejection fraction in conjunction with standard therapy for heart failure to increase survival and reduce heart failure-related hospitalizations.

Current guidelines for the management of heart failure in adults generally recommend a combination of drug therapies to reduce morbidity and mortality, including neurohormonal antagonists (e.g., ACE inhibitors, angiotensin II receptor antagonists, angiotensin receptor-neprilysin inhibitors [ARNIs], β-blockers, aldosterone receptor antagonists) that inhibit the detrimental compensatory mechanisms in heart failure. ACCF and AHA recommend the addition of an aldosterone antagonist (i.e., spironolactone or eplerenone) in selected patients with heart failure and reduced LVEF† who are already receiving a β-blocker and an agent to inhibit the renin-angiotensin-aldosterone (RAA) system (e.g., ACE inhibitor, angiotensin II receptor antagonist, ARNI); careful patient selection is required to minimize the risk of hyperkalemia and renal insufficiency.

Aldosterone receptor antagonists are also recommended, unless contraindicated, in conjunction with standard heart failure therapy to reduce morbidity and mortality following acute MI in patients with reduced LVEF who develop symptoms of heart failure or who have a history of diabetes mellitus†. ACCF and AHA state that there are limited data to support or refute whether spironolactone and eplerenone are interchangeable. The perceived difference between eplerenone and spironolactone is attributed to the selectivity of aldosterone receptor antagonism and not the effectiveness of mineralocorticoid-blocking activity. (See Description.)

In a randomized, double-blind study (Eplerenone in Mild Patients Hospitalization and Survival Study in Heart Failure [EMPHASIS-HF]), in patients with mild heart failure symptoms (NYHA class II), eplerenone (in addition to therapy with an ACE inhibitor and/or angiotensin II receptor antagonist and β-blocker) reduced the risk of death and heart failure-related hospitalization compared with placebo. Patients enrolled in the study were at least 55 years of age, had an ejection fraction of 30% or less (mean: 26%), and were receiving treatment with a β-blocker and an ACE inhibitor and/or an angiotensin II receptor antagonist at the recommended or maximally tolerated dosage. Approximately 50% of patients had been previously hospitalized for heart failure and had a history of MI. In patients with serum potassium concentration of 5 mEq/L or less, eplerenone was administered in a dosage of 25 mg once daily, which was increased after 4 weeks of therapy to 50 mg once daily; patients with decreased renal function (estimated glomerular filtration rate [eGFR] 30–49 mL/minute per 1.73 m^2) received an initial eplerenone dosage of 25 mg once every *other* day with an increase to 25 mg once daily after 4 weeks. Eplerenone substantially reduced the primary composite end point of death from cardiovascular causes or hospitalization for heart failure compared with placebo (18.3 versus 25.9%, respectively). Hyperkalemia (serum potassium exceeding 5.5 mEq/L) developed in approximately 12% of patients receiving eplerenone.

■ **Hypertension** Eplerenone is used orally alone or in combination with other classes of antihypertensive agents in the management of hypertension.

Because of established clinical benefits (e.g., reductions in overall mortality and in adverse cardiovascular, cerebrovascular, and renal outcomes), current evidence-based practice guidelines for the management of hypertension in adults generally recommend the use of drugs from 4 classes of antihypertensive agents (ACE inhibitors, angiotensin II receptor antagonists, calcium-channel blockers, and thiazide diuretics). However, aldosterone antagonists (e.g., eplerenone, spironolactone) may be considered as add-on therapy if goal blood pressure cannot be achieved with the recommended drugs, and are considered preferred add-on therapy by some experts for resistant hypertension and for hypertension associated with primary aldosteronism. Some experts also state that aldosterone antagonists such as eplerenone may be useful for the management of resistant hypertension in patients with type 2 diabetes mellitus when added to an existing treatment regimen consisting of a renin-angiotensin system inhibitor (e.g., ACE inhibitor, angiotensin II receptor antagonist), diuretic, and calcium-channel blocker. However, therapy with an ACE inhibitor or angiotensin II receptor antagonist in conjunction with an aldosterone antagonist may increase the risk of hyperkalemia. Additionally, aldosterone antagonists may be particularly useful in selected patients with heart failure or following MI. For information on antihypertensive therapy for patients with heart failure or following MI, see Heart Failure and also see Ischemic Heart Disease under Hypertension in Adults: Considerations for Drug Therapy in Patients with Underlying Cardiovascular and Other Risk Factors, in Uses in the Thiazides General Statement 40:28.20.

Safety and efficacy of eplerenone, given alone or in combination with other antihypertensive agents, in the treatment of hypertension have been evaluated in several placebo-controlled studies. In 2 studies of 8–12 weeks' duration, patients with baseline diastolic pressure of 95–114 mm Hg were randomized to receive eplerenone (25–400 mg daily, administered as a single dose or in 2 divided doses) monotherapy (611 patients) or placebo (140 patients). In these patients, eplerenone (50–400 mg daily) decreased placebo-corrected seated and standing trough systolic blood pressure (determined 4 hours before morning dose) by about 5–13 mm Hg and diastolic blood pressure by about 3–7 mm Hg. Antihypertensive effect of eplerenone was maintained through 8–24 weeks. Results of other studies indicate that in patients not receiving other antihypertensive drugs, blood pressure may return to pretreatment levels within 1 week following discontinuance of eplerenone. Although eplerenone has lowered blood pressure in all races studied, monotherapy with the drug has produced a smaller reduction in blood pressure during the initial dosage titration period in black hypertensive patients, a population associated with low-renin hypertension; however, this population difference in response does not appear to occur during continued therapy.

For information on overall principles and expert recommendations for the management of hypertension, see Uses: Hypertension in Adults, in the Thiazides General Statement 40:28.20.

Dosage and Administration

■ **General** Eplerenone is administered orally and may be given without regard to meals.

Heart Failure **Heart Failure after Myocardial Infarction.** When used following myocardial infarction (MI) in adults with clinical evidence of heart failure, an initial eplerenone dosage of 25 mg once daily is recommended. Therapy is then titrated upward in one increment of 25 mg as tolerated to a target dosage of 50 mg once daily, preferably within 4 weeks of initiation of therapy, in patients without hyperkalemia (defined as serum potassium concentrations of 5.5 mEq/L or greater).

The manufacturer states that serum potassium concentrations should be measured prior to initiation of therapy, within the first week, and at 1 month after initiation of therapy or dosage adjustment. Serum potassium concentrations should be monitored periodically thereafter during eplerenone therapy and dosage of the drug should be modified according to serum potassium concentrations. Some experts recommend that serum potassium concentrations and renal function be checked within 2–3 days and again 7 days after initiation of an aldosterone antagonist. Subsequent monitoring should be performed as needed based upon the stability of renal function and fluid status but should occur at least monthly for the first 3 months and then every 3 months thereafter. The manufacturer recommends that in patients in whom serum potassium concentrations increase to 5.5–5.9 mEq/L, eplerenone dosage should be decreased to 25 mg daily in patients receiving 50 mg daily and to 25 mg every *other* day in those receiving eplerenone 25 mg daily; the drug should be withheld in patients with such serum potassium concentration increases who are receiving eplerenone 25 mg every *other* day. In patients in whom serum potassium concentrations increase to 6 mEq/L or more, eplerenone therapy should be withheld until serum potassium concentrations decrease to less than 5.5 mEq/L. Therapy with eplerenone may then be reinitiated at a dosage of 25 mg every *other* day. If serum potassium concentrations decrease to less than 5 mEq/L, dosage should be increased gradually (in 25-mg increments) to the maximum tolerated therapeutic dosage (up to 50 mg daily). Alternatively, the American College of Cardiology Foundation (ACCF) and the American Heart Association (AHA) recommend withholding eplerenone if the patient's serum potassium concentration exceeds 5.5 mEq/L or if renal function worsens; therapy may be resumed at a reduced dosage after confirming resolution (for at least 72 hours) of hyperkalemia (serum potassium decreases to less than 5 mEq/L) and of renal insufficiency. ACCF and AHA state that patients should also be specifically instructed to stop taking an aldosterone receptor antagonist if they have diarrhea or are dehydrated or if therapy with a concomitant loop diuretic is interrupted.

Chronic Heart Failure. When used in patients with chronic heart failure† and reduced LVEF in conjunction with standard heart failure therapy, eplerenone has been administered at an initial dosage of 25 mg once daily, which may be increased after 4 weeks of therapy to 50 mg once daily in patients with a serum potassium concentration of 5 mEq/L or less and adequate renal function (estimated glomerular filtration rate [eGFR] at least 50 mL/minute per 1.73 m^2). ACCF and AHA recommend that serum potassium concentrations and renal function be checked within 2–3 days and again at 7 days after initiation of an aldosterone antagonist. Subsequent monitoring should be performed as needed based upon the stability of renal function and fluid status, but should occur at least monthly for the first 3 months and every 3 months thereafter. ACCF and AHA recommend withholding eplerenone if the patient's serum potassium concentration exceeds 5.5 mEq/L or if renal function worsens; therapy may be resumed at a reduced dosage after confirming resolution (for at least 72 hours) of hyperkalemia (i.e., serum potassium decreases to less than 5 mEq/L) and of renal insufficiency. ACCF and AHA state that patients should also be specifically instructed to stop taking an aldosterone receptor antagonist if they have diarrhea or are dehydrated or if therapy with a concomitant loop diuretic is interrupted.

Hypertension Dosage of eplerenone must be individualized and adjusted according to the blood pressure response. The usual initial dosage of eplerenone in adults is 50 mg once daily. Following oral administration of eplerenone, the hypotensive effect is usually apparent within 2 weeks with full hypotensive effect occurring within 4 weeks. If blood pressure response is inadequate with the initial dosage, dosage may be increased to 50 mg twice daily. Administration of higher than recommended dosages (i.e., exceeding 100 mg daily) does not appear to provide added benefit, and has been associated with an increased risk of hyperkalemia. Some experts state the usual dosage range is 50–100 mg daily, given as a single dose or in 2 divided doses.

In hypertensive patients currently receiving therapy with moderate inhibitors of the cytochrome P-450 (CYP) 3A4 isoenzyme (e.g., erythromycin, saquinavir, verapamil, fluconazole), the initial dosage of eplerenone should be reduced to 25 mg once daily.

Monitoring and Blood Pressure Treatment Goals. The patient's renal function and electrolytes should be assessed 2–4 weeks after initiation of diuretic therapy. Blood pressure should be monitored regularly (i.e., monthly) during therapy and dosage of the antihypertensive drug adjusted until blood pressure is controlled. If an adequate blood pressure response is not achieved, the dosage may be increased or another antihypertensive agent with demonstrated benefit and preferably with a complementary mechanism of action (e.g., angiotensin-converting enzyme [ACE] inhibitor, angiotensin II receptor antagonist, calcium-channel blocker, thiazide diuretic) may be added. (See Uses: Hypertension.) In patients who develop unacceptable adverse effects with eplerenone, the drug should be discontinued and another antihypertensive agent from a different pharmacologic class should be initiated.

The goal of hypertension management and prevention is to achieve and maintain optimal control of blood pressure. However, the optimum blood pressure threshold for initiating antihypertensive drug therapy and specific treatment goals remain controversial. A 2017 multidisciplinary hypertension guideline from the American College of Cardiology (ACC), American Heart Association (AHA), and a number of other professional organizations generally recommends a blood pressure goal of less than 130/80 mm Hg in all adults, regardless of comorbidities or level of atherosclerotic cardiovascular disease (ASCVD) risk. Many patients will require at least 2 drugs from different pharmacologic classes to achieve this blood pressure goal; the potential benefits of hypertension management and drug cost, adverse effects, and risks associated with the use of multiple antihypertensive drugs also should be considered when deciding a patient's blood pressure treatment goal.

For additional information on target levels of blood pressure and on monitoring therapy in the management of hypertension, see Blood Pressure Monitoring and Treatment Goals under Dosage: Hypertension, in Dosage and Administration in the Thiazides General Statement 40:28.20.

■ **Special Populations** ***Renal Impairment*** ACCF and AHA state that the dosage of eplerenone should be reduced in heart failure patients with marginal renal function (eGFR 30–49 mL/minute per 1.73 m^2); an initial dosage of 25 mg once every *other* day and a maintenance dosage of 25 mg once daily (after 4 weeks of therapy and if serum potassium is 5 mEq/L or less) has been recommended. These experts state that use of an aldosterone antagonist is potentially harmful in patients with an eGFR less than 30 mL/minute per 1.73 m^2 because of the potential for life-threatening hyperkalemia or renal insufficiency. (See Endocrine, Electrolyte, and Metabolic Effects under Warnings/Precautions: Warnings, in Cautions.)

Cautions

■ **Contraindications** Eplerenone is contraindicated in patients with serum potassium concentrations exceeding 5.5 mEq/L at initiation of therapy, in those with creatinine clearance of 30 mL/minute or less, and in those receiving concomitant therapy with potent inhibitors of cytochrome P-450 (CYP) isoenzyme 3A4 (e.g., ketoconazole, itraconazole, nefazodone, troleandomycin, clarithromycin, ritonavir, nelfinavir) or any agent described as a potent CYP3A4 inhibitor in its prescribing information.

In addition, when used for hypertension, the drug is contraindicated in patients with type 2 diabetes mellitus with microalbuminuria; serum creatinine concentrations exceeding 2 or 1.8 mg/dL in males or females, respectively; creatinine clearance less than 50 mL/minute; and in those receiving potassium supplements or potassium-sparing diuretics (e.g., amiloride, spironolactone, triamterene).

■ **Warnings/Precautions** ***Warnings*** **Endocrine, Electrolyte, and Metabolic Effects.** The most serious risk associated with eplerenone therapy is hyperkalemia (serum potassium exceeding 5.5 mEq/L), which may cause serious, sometimes fatal, cardiac arrhythmias. Patients with impaired renal function or diabetes mellitus and patients receiving concurrent agents affecting the renin-angiotensin-aldosterone system (e.g., angiotensin-converting enzyme [ACE] inhibitors, angiotensin II receptor antagonists) are at an increased risk for developing hyperkalemia. Eplerenone should be used with caution in patients with heart failure following an acute myocardial infarction (MI), who have renal impairment (i.e., serum creatinine concentrations exceeding 2 or 1.8 mg/dL in males or females, respectively, or creatinine clearance of 50 mL/minute or less) or those with diabetes mellitus (including those with proteinuria). Serum potassium concentrations should be monitored periodically in patients receiving eplerenone. (See Heart Failure after Myocardial Infarction under Dosage and Administration: Dosage.) Dosage reduction has been shown to decrease serum potassium concentrations.

Specific Populations **Pregnancy.** Category B. (See Users Guide.)

Lactation. Eplerenone is distributed into milk in rats; a decision should be made whether to discontinue nursing or the drug, taking into account the importance of the drug to the woman.

Pediatric Use. Safety and efficacy have not been established in children younger than 18 years of age. For information on overall principles and expert recommendations for treatment of hypertension in pediatric patients, see Uses: Hypertension in Pediatric Patients, in the Thiazides General Statement 40:28.20.

Geriatric Use. No substantial differences in safety and efficacy have been observed in geriatric patients relative to younger adults. Geriatric patients 75 years of age and older with congestive heart failure following an acute MI did not benefit from the addition of eplerenone to standard medical therapy. Because geriatric patients may have decreased renal function (reduced creatinine clearance), the incidence of hyperkalemia may be increased in geriatric patients (65 years of age and older). (See Endocrine, Electrolyte, and Metabolic Effects under Warnings/Precautions: Warnings, in Cautions.)

Hepatic Impairment. Safety and efficacy have not been established in patients with severe hepatic impairment. Serum potassium concentrations were not affected in patients with mild-to-moderate hepatic impairment.

Renal Impairment. Patients with renal impairment are at an increased risk for developing hyperkalemia. For precautionary information about use of eplerenone in patients with renal impairment, see Cautions: Contraindications and see Endocrine, Electrolyte, and Metabolic Effects under Warnings/Precautions: Warnings in Cautions.

■ **Common Adverse Effects** Adverse effects occurring in 2% or more of patients receiving eplerenone for the management of congestive heart failure following acute MI, but occurring at greater incidence in patients receiving the drug than in those receiving placebo, include hyperkalemia, increased serum creatinine concentrations, urinary tract disorders, adverse CNS effects, and adverse GI effects.

Adverse effects reported in 1% or more of patients receiving eplerenone for the management of hypertension are dizziness, fatigue, flu-like symptoms, cough, diarrhea, abdominal pain, hyperkalemia, decreased serum sodium concentrations, abnormal vaginal bleeding, gynecomastia, hypercholesterolemia, hypertriglyceridemia, mastodynia, or albuminuria.

Drug Interactions

■ **Drugs Affecting Hepatic Microsomal Enzymes** Since eplerenone is primarily metabolized in the liver by the cytochrome P-450 (CYP) 3A4 isoenzyme, concomitant use of drugs that affect CYP3A4 hepatic microsomal enzymes may alter the metabolism of eplerenone. Following administration of a single 100-mg dose of eplerenone in individuals receiving ketoconazole 200 mg twice daily, peak plasma concentrations and area under the concentration-time curve (AUC) of eplerenone were increased by 1.7-fold and 5.4-fold, respectively, compared with administration of eplerenone alone. Concomitant administration of eplerenone and moderate CYP3A inhibitors (e.g., erythromycin 500 mg twice daily, verapamil hydrochloride 240 mg once daily, saquinavir 1.2 g three times daily, fluconazole 200 mg once daily) resulted in increases of 40–60 % in peak plasma eplerenone concentrations and 100–190% increases in AUC. For further precautionary information about concurrent use of eplerenone with inhibitors of the CYP3A4 isoenzyme, see Cautions: Contraindications and see Hypertension under Dosage and Administration: Dosage.

Concomitant use of eplerenone and grapefruit juice may result in a small (about 25%) increase in eplerenone exposure.

Coadministration of eplerenone and St. John's wort (*Hypericum perforatum*), a CYP3A4 isoenzyme inducer, resulted in a 30% decrease in AUC of eplerenone.

Eplerenone is not an inhibitor or inducer of the CYP isoenzymes 1A2, 3A4, 2C19, 2C9, or 2D6, suggesting that the drug is unlikely to alter the pharmacokinetics of drugs metabolized by these enzymes. In in vitro pharmacokinetic studies, eplerenone did not inhibit the metabolism of amiodarone, amlodipine, astemizole, chlorzoxazone, cisapride, dexamethasone, dextromethorphan, diclofenac, ethinyl estradiol, fluoxetine, losartan, lovastatin, mephobarbital, methylphenidate, methylprednisolone, metoprolol, midazolam, nifedipine, phenacetin (no longer commercially available in the US), phenytoin, simvastatin, tolbutamide, triazolam, verapamil, or warfarin.

■ **Drugs Affecting or Affected by P-glycoprotein Transport** Eplerenone is not a substrate or an inhibitor of P-glycoprotein at clinically relevant dosages.

■ **Drugs that Block the Renin-Angiotensin System** Potential pharmacodynamic interaction (increased serum potassium concentrations, hyperkalemia) when eplerenone is used concomitantly with an angiotensin-converting enzyme (ACE) inhibitor or an angiotensin II receptor antagonist for the treatment of hypertension. In patients with heart failure following myocardial infarction (MI), who were receiving eplerenone, the rates of developing hyperkalemia were similar regardless of treatment with an ACE inhibitor or angiotensin II receptor antagonist.

■ **Lithium** Potential pharmacokinetic and pharmacologic interaction (increased serum lithium concentrations resulting in lithium toxicity). No formal drug interaction studies have been performed. However, concomitant administration of diuretics and/or ACE inhibitors with lithium resulted in lithium toxicity. The manufacturer of eplerenone recommends that serum lithium concentrations be monitored frequently when eplerenone and lithium are administered concurrently.

■ **Nonsteroidal Anti-inflammatory Agents** Potential pharmacologic effects (decreased antihypertensive effect and/or severe hyperkalemia in patients with impaired renal function). No formal drug interaction studies have been performed. However, concomitant administration of other potassium-sparing antihypertensive agents with nonsteroidal anti-inflammatory agents (NSAIAs) resulted in the mentioned effects. Patients should be monitored to determine whether the desired therapeutic response is achieved.

■ **Drugs Increasing Serum Potassium Concentrations** Potential pharmacodynamic interaction (increased risk of hyperkalemia) when the drug is used concurrently with other potassium-sparing agents or potassium supplements. For further precautionary information about concurrent use of eplerenone with other potassium-sparing agents, see Cautions: Contraindications.

■ **Other Drugs** Pharmacokinetic interactions are unlikely with aluminum or magnesium-containing antacids, digoxin, warfarin, midazolam, cisapride, cyclosporine, simvastatin, glyburide, or oral contraceptives containing ethinyl estradiol and norethindrone.

Description

Although eplerenone shares many of the pharmacologic effects of spironolactone, eplerenone is considered a relatively *selective* mineralocorticoid (aldosterone) receptor antagonist, whereas spironolactone is nonselective. Eplerenone binds selectively to mineralocorticoid receptors and has low (less than 1%) affinity for glucocorticoid, progesterone, and androgen receptors. The steroid-related adverse effects (e.g., gynecomastia, impotence, menstrual abnormalities) occur less frequently with eplerenone than with spironolactone.

Aldosterone binds to mineralocorticoid receptors in both epithelial (e.g., kidney, salivary glands, GI tract) and nonepithelial (e.g., heart, blood vessels, brain) tissues and increases blood pressure through induction of sodium reabsorption, vascular remodeling, endothelial dysfunction, and possibly other mechanisms. Limited data indicate that increased serum aldosterone concentrations within the physiologic range may predispose individuals to the development of hypertension. Eplerenone is a competitive antagonist of aldosterone at mineralocorticoid receptors in the kidney, myocardium, salivary gland, GI tract, brain, and vasculature and the drug has been shown to inhibit the physiologic effects of aldosterone in these organs. Some of the antihypertensive effects of eplerenone may be related to restoration of endothelial function by increasing the release of nitric oxide, which results in vasodilation. Eplerenone has been shown to produce sustained increases in plasma renin and serum aldosterone concentrations, reflecting the inhibition of the negative feedback of aldosterone on renin secretion. The resulting increased plasma renin activity and circulating aldosterone concentrations do not overcome the antihypertensive effects of eplerenone.

Eplerenone appears to have cardioprotective effects in patients with congestive heart failure and left ventricular dysfunction following myocardial infarction (MI). The exact mechanism of the cardioprotective action of eplerenone in such patients has not been fully elucidated, but it appears to be related more to the drug's ability to competitively inhibit the pathophysiologic effects of aldosterone on the myocardium than to its hypotensive effects. In animals, aldosterone stimulates coronary inflammation and causes myocardial and coronary perivascular fibrosis and ventricular hypertrophy or remodeling. Eplerenone reduces coronary vascular inflammation, the risk of subsequent development of interstitial myocardial and coronary perivascular fibrosis, cardiac hypertrophy, and/or ventricular remodeling.

Eplerenone is extensively metabolized in the liver, principally via the cytochrome P-450 (CYP) 3A4 isoenzyme to inactive metabolites. The absolute bioavailability of eplerenone is 69% after oral administration of a 100-mg tablet. Steady-state concentrations of the drug are attained within 2 days with repeat dosing. Less than 5% of an eplerenone dose is recovered unchanged in the urine and feces. Approximately 67 and 32% of an orally administered dose of eplerenone is excreted in urine and feces, respectively.

Advice to Patients

Importance of informing clinicians of existing or contemplated concomitant therapy, including prescription and OTC drugs. Importance of not using concomitant potassium supplements, salt substitutes containing potassium, potassium-sparing diuretics (amiloride, triamterene, spironolactone), or potent inhibitors of liver enzymes without consulting a clinician. (See Cautions: Contraindications and see Drug Interactions: Drugs Affecting Hepatic Microsomal Enzymes.)

Importance of women informing clinicians if they are or plan to become pregnant or plan to breast-feed.

Importance of informing patients of other important precautionary information. (See Cautions.)

Overview® (see Users Guide). For additional information on this drug until a more detailed monograph is developed and published, the manufacturer's labeling should be consulted. It is *essential* that the manufacturer's labeling be consulted for more detailed information on usual cautions, precautions, contraindications, potential drug interactions, laboratory test interferences, and acute toxicity.

Preparations

Excipients in commercially available drug preparations may have clinically important effects in some individuals; consult specific product labeling for details.

Eplerenone

Oral		
Tablets, film-coated	25 mg*	**Eplerenone Tablets**
		Inspra®, Pfizer
	50 mg*	**Eplerenone Tablets**
		Inspra®, Pfizer

*available from one or more manufacturer, distributor, and/or repackager by generic (nonproprietary) name

†Use is not currently included in the labeling approved by the US Food and Drug Administration

Spironolactone

■ Spironolactone is a mineralocorticoid (aldosterone) receptor antagonist (aldosterone antagonist) and a potassium-sparing diuretic.

Uses

■ **Edema** Spironolactone is used in the management of edema associated with excessive aldosterone excretion such as idiopathic edema and edema accompanying cirrhosis of the liver, nephrotic syndrome, and heart failure, usually in conjunction with other diuretics. Careful etiologic diagnosis should precede the use of any diuretic. Although thiazides and chlorthalidone are more rapidly acting and more effective diuretics, spironolactone does not cause potassium depletion as may result from thiazide or chlorthalidone therapy. In addition, spironolactone is a useful adjunct to thiazide therapy when diuresis is inadequate or reduction of potassium excretion is necessary. When used in conjunction with a thiazide diuretic in the treatment of edema associated with cirrhosis of the liver, spironolactone should be given for 2–3 days prior to administration of the thiazide diuretic in order to prevent potassium depletion and precipitation of hepatic coma.

■ **Hypertension** Spironolactone is used in the management of hypertension, usually in conjunction with other diuretics or hypotensive agents. Used alone, spironolactone produces a modest lowering of blood pressure in most patients with hypertension, and blood pressure returns to within normal limits in about 20% of patients.

Because of established clinical benefits (e.g., reductions in overall mortality and in adverse cardiovascular, cerebrovascular, and renal outcomes), current evidence-based practice guidelines for the management of hypertension in adults generally recommend the use of drugs from 4 classes of antihypertensive agents (angiotensin-converting enzyme [ACE] inhibitors, angiotensin II receptor antagonists, calcium-channel blockers, and thiazide diuretics). However, aldosterone antagonists (e.g., spironolactone, eplerenone) may be considered as add-on therapy if goal blood pressure cannot be achieved with the recommended drugs, and are considered preferred add-on therapy by some experts for resistant hypertension and for hypertension associated with primary aldosteronism. Some experts also state that aldosterone antagonists such as spironolactone may be useful for the management of resistant hypertension in patients with type 2 diabetes mellitus when added to an existing treatment regimen consisting of a renin-angiotensin system inhibitor (e.g., ACE inhibitor, angiotensin II receptor antagonist), diuretic, and calcium-channel blocker. However, therapy with an ACE inhibitor or angiotensin II receptor antagonist in conjunction with an aldosterone antagonist may increase the risk of hyperkalemia. Additionally, aldosterone antagonists may be particularly useful in selected patients with heart failure or following myocardial infarction (MI). For information on antihypertensive therapy for patients with heart failure or following MI, see Heart Failure and also see Ischemic Heart Disease under Hypertension in Adults: Considerations for Drug Therapy in Patients with Underlying Cardiovascular and Other Risk Factors, in Uses in the Thiazides General Statement 40:28.20.

Spironolactone may be useful to decrease the potassium loss caused by other diuretics and potentiate the hypotensive effects of those agents or other more potent hypotensive agents. In addition, the drug may be useful in hypertensive patients with gout or diabetes mellitus that may be aggravated by thiazide diuretics. Spironolactone should be avoided in patients with renal insufficiency and in those receiving potassium supplements or other potassium-sparing diuretics.

For additional information on the role of aldosterone antagonists in the management of hypertension in patients with underlying cardiovascular risk factors and information on overall principles and expert recommendations for treatment of hypertension, see Uses: Hypertension in Adults, in the Thiazides General Statement 40:28.20.

■ Heart Failure Spironolactone is used in the management of severe heart failure (New York Heart Association [NYHA] functional class III-IV) in conjunction with standard therapy for heart failure to increase survival and reduce heart failure-related hospitalizations.

Current guidelines for the management of heart failure in adults generally recommend a combination of drug therapies to reduce morbidity and mortality, including neurohormonal antagonists (e.g., ACE inhibitors, angiotensin II receptor antagonists, angiotensin receptor-neprilysin inhibitors [ARNIs], β-blockers, aldosterone receptor antagonists) that inhibit the detrimental compensatory mechanisms in heart failure. Additional agents (e.g., cardiac glycosides, diuretics, sinoatrial modulators [i.e., ivabradine]) added to a heart failure treatment regimen in selected patients have been associated with symptomatic improvement and/or reduction in heart failure-related hospitalizations. For additional information on the management of heart failure, see Uses: Heart Failure, in Carvedilol 24:24, Enalaprilat/Enalapril 24:32.04, and Sacubitril and Valsartan 24:32.92. The American College of Cardiology Foundation (ACCF) and American Heart Association (AHA) recommend the addition of an aldosterone antagonist (i.e., spironolactone or eplerenone) in selected patients with heart failure and reduced LVEF who are already receiving a β-blocker and an agent to inhibit the renin-angiotensin-aldosterone (RAA) system (e.g., ACE inhibitor, angiotensin II receptor antagonist, ARNI); careful patient selection is required to minimize the risk of hyperkalemia and renal insufficiency. (See Cautions: Electrolyte and Metabolic Effects.)

Aldosterone receptor antagonists are also recommended, unless contraindicated, in conjunction with other heart failure therapy to reduce morbidity and mortality following acute MI in patients with reduced LVEF who develop symptoms of heart failure or who have a history of diabetes mellitus†. ACCF and AHA state that there are limited data to support or refute whether spironolactone and eplerenone are interchangeable. The perceived difference between eplerenone and spironolactone is attributed to the selectivity of aldosterone receptor antagonism and not the effectiveness of mineralocorticoid-blocking activity. (See Pharmacology.)

The concomitant use of spironolactone and an ACE inhibitor had been considered relatively contraindicated because of the potential for developing severe hyperkalemia. In addition, it was believed that ACE inhibitors would inhibit formation of aldosterone, a hormone associated with the pathophysiology of heart failure, by suppressing the RAA system. However, results of several studies have indicated that ACE inhibitors only transiently inhibit the production of aldosterone, and the addition of spironolactone to ACE inhibitor therapy may augment the suppressive effect of ACE inhibitors on aldosterone. (See Pharmacology: Cardiovascular Effects.)

Results of a randomized, multicenter, controlled study (Randomized Aldactone Evaluation Study [RALES]) in 1663 patients with moderate or severe heart failure (NYHA functional class III or IV) and LVEF of 35% or less indicate that addition of low-dose (25–50 mg daily) spironolactone to standard therapy (e.g., an ACE inhibitor and a loop diuretic with or without a cardiac glycoside was associated with decreases in overall mortality and hospitalization (for worsening heart failure) rates of approximately 30 and 35%, respectively, compared with standard therapy and placebo. The reduction in mortality and hospitalization rates was observed within 2–3 months of initiation of combined therapy and continued throughout the study (mean follow-up: 24 months). The combined therapy also was associated with an improvement in NYHA functional class in about 41% of patients. Because interim analysis of this study after a mean follow-up of 24 months revealed that morbidity and death were reduced significantly in patients receiving spironolactone concomitantly with standard therapy compared with those receiving standard therapy and placebo, the study was discontinued.

Spironolactone also is used for the management of edema and sodium retention in patients with heart failure who do not respond adequately to or are intolerant of other therapeutic measures. (See Uses: Edema.)

■ Primary Hyperaldosteronism Spironolactone is used for the short-term preoperative treatment of primary hyperaldosteronism and for long-term maintenance therapy in patients with discrete aldosterone-producing adrenal adenomas who are not candidates for surgery (e.g., adrenalectomy). The drug also is used for long-term maintenance therapy for patients with bilateral micronodular or macronodular adrenal hyperplasia (idiopathic hyperaldosteronism).

■ Precocious Puberty Spironolactone is used for its antiandrogenic effects in combination with testolactone in the management of certain forms of gonadotropin releasing hormone (GnRH)-independent (peripheral) precocious puberty† (e.g., familial male precocious puberty [testotoxicosis]). Such therapy has effectively controlled acne, spontaneous erections, and aggressive behavior and slowed accelerated growth and skeletal maturation, at least in the short term (e.g., 2 years), in boys with familial precocious puberty†. Neither drug alone effectively controls pubertal characteristics nor the rate of growth and skeletal maturation in boys with this condition, although some benefit (e.g., on height velocity) with testolactone alone may be apparent. Testolactone generally prevents the gynecomastia that may be associated with spironolactone. Testolactone also has been used in combination with other antiandrogens (e.g., flutamide) in the management of this condition, but experience is less extensive. While spironolactone currently is the most widely used antiandrogenic drug in familial male precocious puberty, alternative antiandrogenic drugs (e.g., flutamide) that avoid some of the potentially serious adverse effects of spironolactone therapy (e.g., mineralocorticoid-antagonist effects) are being studied for this condition and congenital adrenal hyperplasia. However, concerns about potential hepatotoxic effects of flutamide may limit the use of this drug in such precocious puberty. A gradual escape from the beneficial effects of combined therapy with spironolactone and testolactone may occur during long-term therapy because of the development of secondary GnRH-dependent precocity or pubertal increases in gonadotropins. In such cases, a GnRH analog has been added to the regimen to restore effective control of puberty progression. Additional study and experience are needed to elucidate further the optimum regimens for the management of these forms of precocious puberty and the long-term effects of such therapy, and such patients should be managed in consultation with experts in the diagnosis and treatment of these conditions. Combinations of testolactone with flutamide or with spironolactone also have been studied as a component in the complex regimen of therapy for boys and girls with congenital adrenal hyperplasia caused by steroid 21-hydroxylase or 11-hydroxylase deficiency†; the rationale for the addition of such therapy to the therapeutic regimen was similar to that for familial male precocious puberty (i.e., to control androgenic effects and accelerated growth and skeletal maturation).

■ Other Uses Spironolactone has been used effectively in the treatment of hirsutism† in women with polycystic ovary syndrome or idiopathic hirsutism. In the treatment of hirsutism, spironolactone appears to exert its therapeutic effects by interfering with ovarian androgen secretion and peripheral androgen activity.

Spironolactone has also been used as an adjunct in the treatment of myasthenia gravis† and familial periodic paralysis†.

Dosage and Administration

■ Administration Spironolactone is administered orally. For administration in children, spironolactone tablets may be pulverized and administered as an oral suspension in cherry syrup.

Administration of spironolactone with food increases the bioavailability of the drug by approximately 90–100%. The manufacturers state that patients should establish a routine time for taking the drug with regard to meals.

The commercially available oral suspension (CaroSpir®) is *not therapeutically equivalent* to spironolactone oral tablets (e.g., Aldactone®). In patients who require a dose exceeding 100 mg, tablets should be used; doses of CaroSpir® suspension exceeding 100 mg may result in higher than expected serum spironolactone concentrations.

Although it has frequently been recommended that spironolactone tablets be administered in 3 or 4 doses daily, more recent information suggests that 1 or 2 doses daily may be adequate.

■ Dosage ***Edema*** **Spironolactone Therapy.** For the management of edema associated with hepatic cirrhosis or nephrotic syndrome in adults, the recommended initial adult dosage of spironolactone (as oral tablets) is 100 mg daily administered as a single dose or in divided doses, but initial dosage may range from 25–200 mg daily.

When the commercially available oral suspension (CaroSpir®) is used for the treatment of edema associated with hepatic cirrhosis, the recommended initial adult dosage is 75 mg daily administered in a single dose or divided doses.

The manufacturers state that spironolactone should be initiated in patients with cirrhosis in a hospital setting and dosage titrated slowly.

Experts state that diuretics should be administered at a dosage sufficient to achieve optimal volume status and relieve congestion without inducing an excessively rapid reduction in intravascular volume, which could result in hypotension, renal dysfunction, or both.

For the management of edema in children, a spironolactone dosage of 3.3 mg/kg daily (as oral tablets) administered as a single dose or in divided doses has been suggested. Alternatively, an initial pediatric dosage of 60 mg/m^2 daily (as oral tablets) administered in divided doses has been suggested.

When used alone for the management of edema, spironolactone should be administered in the usual initial dosage for at least 5 days. If a satisfactory response is obtained, dosage may be adjusted to the optimal therapeutic or maintenance dosage.

Spironolactone/Hydrochlorothiazide Fixed-combination Therapy. The manufacturer of the fixed combination of spironolactone and hydrochlorothiazide states that the optimal dosage should be established by individual titration of the drug components.

For the management of edema in adults, the usual maintenance dosage of the fixed combination of spironolactone and hydrochlorothiazide is 100 mg each of spironolactone and hydrochlorothiazide daily administered as a single dose or in divided doses. The effective dosage may range from 25–200 mg of each component daily depending on the response to the initial titration. In some instances, it may be beneficial to administer separate tablets of either spironolactone or hydrochlorothiazide in addition to the fixed combination of spironolactone and hydrochlorothiazide in order to provide optimal individual therapy.

Hypertension **Spironolactone Therapy.** For the management of hypertension in adults, the usual initial dosage of spironolactone (as oral tablets) is 25–100 mg daily administered as a single dose or in divided doses. The dosage may be titrated at 2-week intervals. Dosages exceeding 100 mg daily generally do not provide additional reductions in blood pressure.

When the commercially available oral suspension (CaroSpir®) is used for the treatment of hypertension in adults, the recommended initial dosage is 20–75 mg daily administered in a single dose or divided doses. The dosage may be titrated at 2-week intervals. Dosages exceeding 75 mg daily generally do not provide additional reductions in blood pressure.

For the management of hypertension in children†, some experts have recommended an initial spironolactone dosage of 1 mg/kg daily (as tablets) administered as a single dose or in 2 divided doses. Such experts have suggested that dosage may be increased as necessary to a maximum dosage of 3.3 mg/kg (up to 100 mg) daily (as tablets) given as a single dose or in 2 divided doses. For information on overall principles and expert recommendations for treatment of hypertension in pediatric patients, see Uses: Hypertension in Pediatric Patients, in the Thiazides General Statement 40:28.20.

Spironolactone should be administered for a minimum of 2 weeks in order to assess its effectiveness in the management of hypertension in a specific patient. Subsequent dosage should be determined by the response of the patient.

Spironolactone/Hydrochlorothiazide Fixed-combination Therapy. The manufacturer of the fixed combination of spironolactone and hydrochlorothiazide states that the optimal dosage should be established by individual titration of the drug components. When the fixed combination is used for the management of hypertension, the dosage will vary depending on the results of the titration of the individual drug components. Most patients will have an optimal response to 50–100 mg each of spironolactone and hydrochlorothiazide daily administered as a single dose or in divided doses.

Monitoring and Blood Pressure Treatment Goals. The patient's renal function and electrolytes should be assessed 2–4 weeks after initiation of diuretic therapy. Blood pressure should be monitored regularly (i.e., monthly) during therapy and dosage of the antihypertensive drug adjusted until blood pressure is controlled. If an adequate blood pressure response is not achieved, the dosage may be increased or another antihypertensive agent with demonstrated benefit and preferably with a complementary mechanism of action (e.g., angiotensin-converting enzyme [ACE] inhibitor, angiotensin II receptor antagonist, calcium-channel blocker, thiazide diuretic) may be added. (See Uses: Hypertension.) In patients who develop unacceptable adverse effects with spironolactone, the drug should be discontinued and another antihypertensive agent from a different pharmacologic class should be initiated.

The goal of hypertension management and prevention is to achieve and maintain optimal control of blood pressure. However, the optimum blood pressure threshold for initiating antihypertensive drug therapy and specific treatment goals remain controversial. A 2017 multidisciplinary hypertension guideline from the American College of Cardiology (ACC), American Heart Association (AHA), and a number of other professional organizations generally recommends a blood pressure goal of less than 130/80 mm Hg in all adults, regardless of comorbidities or level of atherosclerotic cardiovascular disease (ASCVD) risk. Many patients will require at least 2 drugs from different pharmacologic classes to achieve this blood pressure goal; the potential benefits of hypertension management and drug cost, adverse effects, and risks associated with the use of multiple antihypertensive drugs also should be considered when deciding a patient's blood pressure treatment goal.

For additional information on target levels of blood pressure and on monitoring therapy in the management of hypertension, see Blood Pressure Monitoring and Treatment Goals under Dosage: Hypertension, in Dosage and Administration in the Thiazides General Statement 40:28.20.

Heart Failure For the management of severe heart failure, the manufacturer recommends an initial spironolactone dosage of 25 mg once daily (as oral tablets) in adults who have a serum potassium concentration of 5 mEq/L or less and an estimated glomerular filtration rate (eGFR) exceeding 50 mL/minute per 1.73 m^2. In patients who tolerate this initial dosage, dosage may be increased to 50 mg once daily as clinically indicated; those who do not tolerate the initial dosage (i.e., develop hyperkalemia) may receive 25 mg once every *other* day. Alternatively, the American College of Cardiology Foundation (ACCF) and the American Heart Association (AHA) recommend an initial spironolactone dosage of 12.5–25 mg once daily and a maintenance dosage (after 4 weeks of therapy) of 25 mg once or twice daily (as tablets) in patients who have a serum potassium concentration of 5 mEq/L or less and adequate renal function (eGFR at least 50 mL/minute per 1.73 m^2).

For the management of edema associated with heart failure in adults, some experts recommend initiating spironolactone (oral tablets) at a low dosage (e.g., 12.5–25 mg once daily) and increasing the dosage (maximum of 50 mg daily; higher dosages may be used with close monitoring) until urine output increases and weight decreases, generally by 0.5–1 kg daily.

The manufacturer recommends that serum potassium and renal function be monitored 1 week after initiation and then regularly thereafter; more frequent monitoring may be necessary when spironolactone is given with other drugs that cause hyperkalemia or in patients with impaired renal function. ACCF and AHA recommend that serum potassium and renal function be checked within 2–3 days and again 7 days after initiation of an aldosterone antagonist. Subsequent monitoring should be performed as needed based upon the stability of renal function and fluid status but should occur at least monthly for the first 3 months and then every 3 months thereafter. If hyperkalemia occurs, the dosage of spironolactone should be decreased or the drug discontinued and hyperkalemia should be treated. ACCF and AHA recommend withholding therapy with an aldosterone receptor antagonist if the patient's serum potassium concentration exceeds 5.5 mEq/L or if renal function worsens; therapy may be resumed at a reduced dosage after confirming resolution (for at least 72 hours) of hyperkalemia (i.e., serum potassium concentration decreases to less than 5 mEq/L) and of renal insufficiency. ACCF and AHA state that patients should also be specifically instructed to stop taking an aldosterone receptor antagonist if they have diarrhea or are dehydrated or if therapy with a concomitant loop diuretic is interrupted.

When the commercially available oral suspension (CaroSpir®) is used for the management of heart failure, the manufacturer recommends an initial dosage of 20 mg once daily in adults who have a serum potassium concentration of 5 mEq/L or less and an eGFR exceeding 50 mL/minute per 1.73 m^2. In patients who tolerate this initial dosage, dosage may be increased to 37.5 mg once daily as clinically indicated; those who develop hyperkalemia on the initial dosage may have their dosage reduced to 20 mg once every *other* day.

Primary Hyperaldosteronism After the diagnosis of hyperaldosteronism has been established, 100–400 mg of spironolactone (as oral tablets) may be administered daily for short-term preoperative therapy. When spironolactone is used for the treatment of primary hyperaldosteronism in patients unable or unwilling to undergo surgery, spironolactone may be used as long-term maintenance therapy at the lowest effective dosage determined for the individual patient.

Other Uses For the treatment of hirsutism† in women with polycystic ovary syndrome or idiopathic hirsutism, the usual dosage of spironolactone is 50–200 mg daily (as oral tablets). Regression of hirsutism is generally evident within 2 months, maximal within 6 months, and has been maintained up to at least 16 months with continued treatment.

■ Dosage in Hepatic Impairment In patients with cirrhosis, spironolactone should be initiated with the lowest dose and titrated slowly; patients with cirrhosis and ascites should have therapy initiated in the hospital. (See Cautions: Precautions and Contraindications.)

■ Dosage in Renal Impairment The manufacturer states, for the treatment of heart failure in patients with an eGFR of 30–50 mL/minute per 1.73 m^2, initiation of spironolactone at a dosage of 25 mg every *other* day (as oral tablets) should be considered because of the risk of hyperkalemia. Alternatively, ACCF and AHA state that the dosage of spironolactone should be reduced in heart failure patients with marginal renal function (eGFR 30–49 mL/minute per 1.73 m^2); an initial dosage of 12.5 mg once daily or every *other* day and a maintenance dosage of 12.5–25 mg once daily as tablets (after 4 weeks of therapy and if serum potassium is 5 mEq/L or less) has been recommended. The manufacturer of the commercially available spironolactone oral suspension (CaroSpir®) states in patients with heart failure and an eGFR of 30–50 mL/minute per 1.73 m^2, a reduced initial dosage of 10 mg once daily (as the oral suspension) should be considered because of the risk of hyperkalemia. The use of an aldosterone antagonist may be harmful in patients with an eGFR less than 30 mL/minute per 1.73 m^2 because of potentially life-threatening hyperkalemia or renal insufficiency. (See Cautions: Electrolyte and Metabolic Effects.)

Cautions

In general, adverse effects with recommended dosage of spironolactone are mild and respond to withdrawal of the drug.

■ Electrolyte and Metabolic Effects Patients receiving spironolactone may develop hyperkalemia. The risk of developing hyperkalemia is increased by impaired renal function or concomitant potassium supplementation, potassium-containing salt substitutes, or drugs that increase serum potassium (e.g., angiotensin-converting enzyme [ACE] inhibitors, angiotensin II receptor antagonists). (See Drug Interactions.) Hyperkalemia can cause cardiac irregularities that may be fatal.

Reversible hyperchloremic metabolic acidosis, usually in association with hyperkalemia, has occurred in some patients with decompensated hepatic cirrhosis, even in the presence of normal renal function. Mild acidosis also has occurred during spironolactone therapy. Spironolactone also may cause hypochloremic alkalosis.

Dehydration and hyponatremia manifested by a low serum sodium concentration, dry mouth, thirst, drowsiness, and lethargy may occur during spironolactone therapy, especially when spironolactone is used concomitantly with other diuretics. In patients with severe cirrhosis, dehydration and hyponatremia may be followed by further hepatic decompensation and asterixis. Hyponatremia occurs most frequently in patients with advanced cirrhosis and may be prevented by restriction of water intake, administration of corticosteroids, or administration of mannitol.

Spironolactone may cause hypomagnesemia, hypocalcemia, and hyperglycemia. Asymptomatic hyperuricemia also may occur and gout may rarely be precipitated.

Sudden alterations of fluid and electrolyte balance may precipitate impaired neurologic function, worsening hepatic encephalopathy, and coma in patients with hepatic disease with cirrhosis and ascites.

■ GI Effects Anorexia, nausea, vomiting, diarrhea, abdominal cramping, gastritis, gastric bleeding, and ulceration have occurred during spironolactone therapy.

■ Nervous System Effects Headache, drowsiness, lethargy, ataxia, mental confusion, and fever have occurred during spironolactone therapy. In addition, severe fatigue and lassitude have been associated with the rapid and profound weight loss that occurs at the start of high-dose spironolactone therapy in patients with primary hyperaldosteronism.

■ Dermatologic and Sensitivity Reactions Maculopapular and erythematous rashes (sometimes accompanied by eosinophilia), anaphylactic reaction, vasculitis, and urticaria have been reported rarely in patients receiving spironolactone. Stevens-Johnson Syndrome (SJS), toxic epidermal necrolysis (TEN), drug rash with eosinophilia and systemic symptoms (DRESS), alopecia, pruritus, and chloasma have also been reported in patients receiving spironolactone therapy.

■ Endocrine Effects Adverse effects related to the steroid-like structure of spironolactone include painful gynecomastia, decreased libido, and relative impotence in males, and menstrual irregularities, amenorrhea, postmenopausal bleeding, and breast soreness in females. Gynecomastia appears to be related to both dosage and duration of therapy (onset varies from 1–2 months to more than a year) and is usually reversible following discontinuance of spironolactone; however, some breast enlargement may rarely persist. Spironolactone may be associated with a greater risk of gynecomastia than eplerenone. In the RALES study, approximately 9% of the male patients who received spironolactone (mean dosage: 26 mg once daily) developed gynecomastia. Carcinoma of the breast has been reported in patients receiving spironolactone; however, a causal relationship to the drug has not been established. Androgen-like adverse effects such as hirsutism and deepening of the voice have also been reported.

■ Renal Effects and Hypotension Excessive diuresis may cause symptomatic dehydration, hypotension, and worsening renal function, especially in patients who are salt-depleted or those taking an ACE inhibitor or angiotensin II receptor antagonist. Worsening of renal function also may occur when spironolactone is used in conjunction with nephrotoxic drugs (e.g., aminoglycosides, cisplatin, nonsteroidal anti-inflammatory agents [NSAIAs]).

■ Other Adverse Effects Leg cramps, leukopenia (including agranulocytosis), and thrombocytopenia have been reported during spironolactone therapy. Mixed cholestatic/hepatocellular toxicity, with at least one fatality, has been reported rarely with spironolactone administration.

■ Precautions and Contraindications When spironolactone is used as a fixed-combination preparation that includes hydrochlorothiazide, the cautions, precautions, and contraindications associated with thiazide diuretics must be considered in addition to those associated with spironolactone.

Unless spironolactone is given concomitantly with another diuretic and a corticosteroid, the concurrent use of potassium supplements should generally be avoided. Serum electrolyte, uric acid, and blood glucose concentrations should be monitored periodically in patients receiving spironolactone. The manufacturer states that serum potassium concentrations should be monitored within 1 week of initiating or titrating spironolactone therapy and regularly thereafter. More frequent monitoring may be necessary when spironolactone is administered with other drugs that cause hyperkalemia or in patients with renal impairment. Serum potassium concentrations should be checked when concomitant ACE inhibitor or angiotensin II receptor antagonist therapy is altered. The patient's volume status and renal function also should be monitored periodically while on spironolactone therapy. Patients should be warned to avoid excessive ingestion of potassium-rich foods or salt substitutes. If hyperkalemia, occurs, the dosage of spironolactone should be decreased or the drug discontinued and hyperkalemia should be treated.

Spironolactone should be used with caution in patients with impaired renal function or hepatic disease. Spironolactone is contraindicated in patients with hyperkalemia. Some clinicians consider spironolactone to be contraindicated in patients whose serum creatinine or BUN concentration is more than twice normal. Spironolactone is also contraindicated in patients with Addison's disease or with concomitant use of eplerenone.

■ Pediatric Precautions The manufacturer states that safety and efficacy of spironolactone have not been established in pediatric patients.

■ Mutagenicity and Carcinogenicity Canrenone, a major metabolite of spironolactone, and canrenoic acid are the major metabolites of potassium canrenoate. In tests using bacteria or yeast and in an in vivo mammalian system, neither spironolactone nor potassium canrenoate was mutagenic. In the presence of metabolic activation, spironolactone has been reported to produce negative results in some mammalian mutagenicity tests in vitro and inconclusive but slightly positive results in other tests. In the presence of metabolic activation, results of in vitro mammalian mutagenicity tests of potassium canrenoate have been positive, inconclusive, or negative.

Spironolactone has been shown to be tumorigenic in chronic toxicity studies in rats. In an 18-month study in rats using spironolactone dosages of 50–500 mg/kg per day, a substantial increase in benign adenomas of the thyroid and testes was observed. In male rats, a dose-related increase in proliferative changes in the liver (including hepatocytomegaly and hyperplastic nodules) also was observed. In a 24-month study in rats using spironolactone dosages of 10–150 mg/kg per day, hepatocellular carcinoma and testicular interstitial cell tumors were observed; an increase in thyroid follicular cell adenomas and carcinomas and benign uterine endometrial stromal polyps also was reported.

■ Pregnancy and Lactation The use of spironolactone during pregnancy may affect the sex differentiation of a male fetus during embryogenesis. Studies in rats indicate that spironolactone may cause feminization of male fetuses and endocrine dysfunction in female fetuses exposed to the drug in utero. Data from published case reports and case series have not demonstrated an association of major malformations or other adverse pregnancy outcomes with spironolactone use. Because of the potential risk to the male fetus due to the antiandrogenic properties of spironolactone, the drug should be avoided during pregnancy; pregnant women who receive spironolactone should be advised of the potential risk to a male fetus.

Spironolactone is not distributed into milk; however, the active metabolite, canrenone, is distributed into milk in low amounts that are expected to be clinically inconsequential. The developmental and health benefits of breastfeeding along with the mother's clinical need for spironolactone and any potential adverse effects on the breastfed child from spironolactone or from the underlying maternal condition should be considered.

Drug Interactions

■ Drugs that Block the Renin-Angiotensin System Concomitant administration of spironolactone and an angiotensin-converting enzyme (ACE) inhibitor or angiotensin II receptor antagonist may cause severe hyperkalemia. Serum potassium concentrations should be monitored closely in patients receiving concomitant therapy with an ACE inhibitor or angiotensin II receptor antagonist and spironolactone.

■ Drugs or Foods that Increase Serum Potassium Concentration Concomitant use of spironolactone, potassium supplements or other substances containing potassium (e.g., salt substitutes), or potassium-rich diets may increase the risk of severe hyperkalemia as compared with spironolactone therapy alone. In general, potassium supplementation should be discontinued in patients with heart failure who are initiating spironolactone.

Spironolactone should not be used concurrently with another potassium-sparing agent or aldosterone receptor antagonist (e.g., eplerenone) since concomitant therapy with these drugs may increase the risk of severe hyperkalemia as compared with spironolactone alone; concomitant use of spironolactone and eplerenone is contraindicated. Concomitant use of spironolactone and other drugs that are known to cause hyperkalemia, such as ACE inhibitors, angiotensin II receptor antagonists, nonsteroidal anti-inflammatory agents (NSAIAs), heparin or low molecular weight heparin, or trimethoprim, may cause severe hyperkalemia.

■ Aminoglycosides Worsening of renal function may occur with concomitant use; the patient's renal function and volume status should be monitored periodically.

■ Antihypertensive and Hypotensive Agents When used in conjunction with other diuretics or hypotensive agents, spironolactone may be additive with or may potentiate the action of these drugs. Therefore, dosage of these drugs, particularly ganglionic blocking agents, may need to be reduced by at least 50% when concomitant spironolactone therapy is instituted.

■ Cholestyramine Hyperkalemic metabolic acidosis has been reported in patients who received spironolactone concurrently with cholestyramine.

■ Cisplatin Worsening of renal function may occur with concomitant use; the patient's renal function and volume status should be monitored periodically.

■ **CNS Depressants** Concomitant use of spironolactone and CNS depressants, including alcohol, barbiturates, and opiate agonists, may potentiate orthostatic hypotension.

■ **Corticosteroids** Concomitant use of spironolactone and corticosteroids may intensify electrolyte depletion, particularly hypokalemia.

■ **Digoxin** Spironolactone and its metabolites interfere with radioimmunoassays for digoxin and increase the apparent exposure to digoxin. The extent, if any, to which spironolactone actually increases digoxin exposure is unknown. In patients receiving concomitant therapy with spironolactone and digoxin, an assay that does not interact with spironolactone should be used to measure serum digoxin concentrations.

■ **Lithium** Renal clearance of lithium is decreased in patients receiving diuretics, and lithium toxicity may result. Serum lithium concentrations should be monitored periodically during concomitant spironolactone and lithium use.

■ **Nondepolarizing Neuromuscular Blocking Agents** Concomitant use of spironolactone and nondepolarizing neuromuscular blocking agents may potentially increase the neuromuscular blockade.

■ **Nonsteroidal Anti-inflammatory Agents** Concomitant use of spironolactone and NSAIAs (e.g., indomethacin) may cause severe hyperkalemia. NSAIAs, including aspirin, can reduce the diuretic, natriuretic, and antihypertensive effect of diuretics. When these drugs are used concomitantly, the maintenance dosage of spironolactone may need to be increased and the patient should be monitored closely to determine if the desired therapeutic effect of spironolactone is being achieved. Worsening of renal function also may occur with concomitant use; the patient's renal function and volume status should be monitored periodically.

■ **Vasopressors** Spironolactone reportedly reduces vascular responsiveness to norepinephrine, and regional or general anesthesia should be used with caution in patients receiving spironolactone.

Laboratory Test Interferences

■ **Tests for Plasma and Urinary Steroids** Because spironolactone metabolites produce fluorescence, the drug may interfere with fluorometric determinations of plasma and urinary 17-hydroxycorticosteroids (cortisol). Spurious plasma and urine fluorescence may persist for several days after termination of spironolactone therapy. It has been reported that spironolactone administration may also interfere with determinations of urinary 17-hydroxycorticosteroids by the Porter-Silber technique, urinary 17-ketosteroids by the Klendshoj, Feldstein and Sprague technique, and possibly urinary 17-ketogenic steroids.

■ **Tests for Urinary Aldosterone** Most methods of determining urinary aldosterone appear to be unaffected by spironolactone metabolites, but one report indicates that the metabolites may interfere with aldosterone radioimmunoassay procedures.

■ **Tests for Serum Digoxin** Spironolactone may cause false elevations in measurements of serum digoxin concentrations when radioimmunoassay procedures are used.

Acute Toxicity

■ **Pathogenesis** The oral LD_{50} of spironolactone is greater than 1000 mg/kg in mice, rats, and rabbits.

■ **Manifestations** Overdosage of spironolactone would be expected to produce signs and symptoms that are mainly extensions of common adverse reactions such as drowsiness, mental confusion, maculopapular or erythematous rash, nausea, vomiting, dizziness, or diarrhea. Rarely, hyponatremia or hyperkalemia may occur, especially in patients with impaired renal function; hepatic coma may occur in patients with severe liver disease but a causal relationship of these effects to overdosage of spironolactone has not been established.

■ **Treatment** In the event of overdosage, spironolactone should be discontinued and the patient should be carefully monitored. There is no specific antidote for spironolactone overdosage. In acute overdosage, the stomach should be emptied by inducing emesis or by gastric lavage. Supportive and symptomatic treatment should be initiated to maintain hydration, electrolyte balance, and vital functions. If severe hyperkalemia occurs (i.e., serum potassium concentration greater than 6.5 mEq/L), specific measures such as IV administration of calcium chloride solution, sodium bicarbonate, and/or oral or parenteral administration of glucose with a rapid-acting insulin preparation should be instituted to reduce serum potassium concentrations. If necessary, a cation exchange resin (e.g., sodium polystyrene sulfonate) may be administered orally or as a retention enema. Patients with persistent hyperkalemia may require dialysis.

Pharmacology

Spironolactone is a nonselective mineralocorticoid (aldosterone) receptor antagonist (aldosterone antagonist), as well as an androgen and progesterone receptor antagonist. Spironolactone exhibits magnesium- and potassium-sparing, natriuretic, diuretic, and hypotensive effects by competitively inhibiting the physiologic effects of the adrenocortical hormone aldosterone on the distal renal tubules, myocardium, and vasculature.

■ **Renal Effects** Spironolactone competitively inhibits the physiologic effects of the adrenocortical hormone aldosterone on the distal renal tubules, thereby producing increased excretion of sodium chloride and water, and decreased excretion of potassium, magnesium, ammonium, titratable acid, and phosphate. Spironolactone is a potassium-sparing diuretic that has diuretic activity only in the presence of aldosterone, and its effects are most pronounced in patients with hyperaldosteronism. Spironolactone does not interfere with renal tubular transport mechanisms and does not inhibit carbonic anhydrase. Renal plasma flow and glomerular filtration rate usually are unaffected, but free water clearance may increase. Prolonged administration of spironolactone may cause increased aldosterone secretion; however, reports are conflicting. Because most sodium is reabsorbed in the proximal renal tubules, spironolactone is relatively ineffective when administered alone, and concomitant administration of a diuretic which blocks reabsorption of sodium proximal to the distal portion of the nephron, such as a thiazide or loop diuretic, is required for maximum diuretic effects. When administered with other diuretics, spironolactone produces an additive or synergistic diuretic response and decreases potassium excretion caused by the other diuretic.

■ **Cardiovascular Effects** Spironolactone reportedly has hypotensive activity when given to hypertensive patients. The precise mechanism of hypotensive action has not been determined, but it has been suggested that the drug may act by blocking the effect of aldosterone on arteriolar smooth muscle or by altering the extracellular-intracellular sodium gradient.

Spironolactone appears to have cardioprotective effects when given to patients with severe heart failure. The exact mechanism of the cardioprotective action of spironolactone in patients with heart failure has not been fully elucidated, but it appears to be related more to the drug's ability to competitively inhibit the physiologic effects of aldosterone on the myocardium than to its diuretic effect. In addition to promoting retention of sodium and excretion of magnesium and potassium, aldosterone causes sympathetic activation, parasympathetic inhibition, myocardial and vascular fibrosis, direct vascular damage, and baroreceptor dysfunction; aldosterone also impairs arterial compliance and apparently prevents uptake of norepinephrine by the myocardium. Spironolactone appears to benefit patients with heart failure by increasing myocardial norepinephrine uptake and preventing myocardial fibrosis, sodium retention, and potassium and/or magnesium excretion. In addition, preliminary studies in animals and humans suggest that spironolactone may restore baroreceptor sensitivity and modulate baroreflex function in patients with heart failure.

It generally has been believed that angiotensin-converting enzyme (ACE) inhibitors would inhibit formation of aldosterone by suppressing the renin-angiotensin-aldosterone system. However, there is increasing evidence to suggest that plasma aldosterone concentrations may not decrease during therapy with usual dosages of ACE inhibitors in some patients and may return to pretreatment levels in others during prolonged therapy. Results of several studies indicate that the addition of spironolactone to ACE inhibitor therapy appears to augment the suppressive effect of the ACE inhibitors on aldosterone. In addition, although it has been suggested that concomitant administration of an ACE inhibitor and spironolactone was relatively contraindicated because of the potential for developing severe hyperkalemia, a low incidence of severe hyperkalemia has been reported in clinical studies in patients with heart failure receiving such combined therapy.

■ **Antiandrogenic Effects** Spironolactone exhibits antiandrogenic effects in males and females. The mechanism of antiandrogenic activity of spironolactone is complex and appears to involve several effects of the drug. Spironolactone decreases testosterone biosynthesis by inhibiting steroid 17α-monooxygenase (17α-hydroxylase) activity, possibly secondary to destruction of microsomal cytochrome P-450 in tissues with high steroid 17α-monooxygenase activity (e.g., testes, adrenals). The drug also appears to competitively inhibit binding of dihydrotestosterone to its cytoplasmic receptor protein, thus decreasing androgenic actions at target tissues. Spironolactone-induced increases in serum estradiol concentration also may contribute to its antiandrogenic activity, although such increases may not occur consistently; such increases appear to result from increased conversion of testosterone to estradiol. Spironolactone may have variable effects on serum 17-hydroxyprogesterone concentrations, possibly decreasing its production by inhibiting steroid 17α-monooxygenase activity or decreasing its conversion (with resultant accumulation) to androstenedione by inhibiting cytochrome P450-dependent 17α-hydroxyprogesterone aldolase (17,20-desmolase) activity. Serum progesterone concentrations may increase with the drug secondary to decreased hydroxylation (via steroid 17α-monooxygenase) to 17-hydroxyprogesterone. In children, compensatory increases in lutropin (luteinizing hormone, LH) and follicle-stimulating hormone (FSH) secretion can occur, probably secondary to the drug's antiandrogenic effects (i.e., a feedback response to decreasing serum testosterone concentrations and/or peripheral androgenic activity).

Pharmacokinetics

■ **Absorption** Absorption of spironolactone from the GI tract depends on the formulation in which it is administered. When spironolactone is administered as oral tablets, peak plasma concentrations of spironolactone and its active metabolite canrenone are achieved 2.6 and 4.3 hours, respectively, after dosing in healthy individuals.

When spironolactone is administered as the oral suspension (CaroSpir®), peak plasma concentrations of spironolactone are achieved 0.5–1.5 hours after dosing in healthy individuals; peak plasma concentrations of the active metabolite canrenone are reached 2.5–5 hours after dosing. When spironolactone (tablets or oral suspension) is administered concomitantly with food, peak serum concentrations and areas under the serum concentration-time curves (AUCs) of the drug and, to a lesser degree, its principal metabolites are increased substantially compared with the fasting state. (See Dosage and Administration: Administration.) At equivalent doses, serum concentrations of spironolactone are 15–37% higher following administration of the oral suspension (CaroSpir®) than with the oral tablets (Aldactone®).

When administered alone, spironolactone has a gradual onset of diuretic action with the maximum effect being reached on the third day of therapy. The delay in onset may result from the time required for adequate concentrations of the drug or metabolites to accumulate. After withdrawal of spironolactone, diuresis persists for 2 or 3 days. When a thiazide diuretic is used concomitantly with spironolactone, diuresis usually occurs on the first day of therapy.

■ **Distribution** Spironolactone and canrenone, a major metabolite of the drug, are both more than 90% bound to plasma proteins.

Spironolactone or its metabolites may cross the placenta. Canrenone, a major metabolite of spironolactone, is distributed into milk.

■ **Elimination** Spironolactone is rapidly and extensively metabolized. Spironolactone undergoes deacetylation at its sulfur group to form 7α-thiospironolactone (7α-thiospirolactone), which then undergoes further metabolism. 7α-Thiospironolactone is dethiolated to form canrenone and subsequently other non-sulfur-containing metabolites. 7α-Thiospironolactone also undergoes thiomethylation to form 7α-thiomethylspironolactone (7α-thiomethylspirolactone), which undergoes 6β-hydroxylation and subsequent metabolism to other sulfur-containing metabolites. Spironolactone metabolites are excreted principally in urine, but also in feces via biliary elimination.

The half-life of spironolactone averages 1–2 hours, and the half-life of canrenone,7α-thiomethylspironolactone, 6-β-hydroxy-7α-thiomethylspironolactone ranges from 10–35 hours depending on the formulation.

Chemistry and Stability

■ **Chemistry** Spironolactone is a synthetic steroid mineralocorticoid (aldosterone) receptor antagonist (aldosterone antagonist) that exhibits potassium-sparing diuretic and probably cardioprotective effects. Spironolactone occurs as a light cream-colored to light tan, crystalline powder with a faint to mild mercaptan-like odor. The drug is practically insoluble in water and soluble in alcohol.

■ **Stability** Spironolactone tablets should be stored in tight, light-resistant containers at a temperature less than 25°C.

Oral suspensions of spironolactone prepared by pulverizing commercially available tablets of the drug and adding them to cherry syrup have been reported to be stable for one month at 2–8°C.

The commercially available oral suspension of spironolactone (CaroSpir®) should be stored at a controlled room temperature of 20–25°C but may be exposed to temperatures ranging from 15–30°C.

Preparations

Excipients in commercially available drug preparations may have clinically important effects in some individuals; consult specific product labeling for details.

Spironolactone

Oral		
Suspension	25 mg/5 mL	**CaroSpir®**, CMP
Tablets, film-coated	25 mg*	**Aldactone®**, Pfizer
		Spironolactone Tablets
	50 mg*	**Aldactone®** (scored), Pfizer
		Spironolactone Tablets
	100 mg*	**Aldactone®** (scored), Pfizer
		Spironolactone Tablets

*available from one or more manufacturer, distributor, and/or repackager by generic (nonproprietary) name

Spironolactone and Hydrochlorothiazide

Oral		
Tablets, film-coated	25 mg Spironolactone and Hydrochlorothiazide 25 mg*	**Aldactazide®**, Pfizer
		Spironolactone and Hydrochlorothiazide Tablets
	50 mg Spironolactone and Hydrochlorothiazide 50 mg	**Aldactazide®** (scored), Pfizer

*available from one or more manufacturer, distributor, and/or repackager by generic (nonproprietary) name

†Use is not currently included in the labeling approved by the US Food and Drug Administration

RENIN-ANGIOTENSIN-ALDOSTERONE SYSTEM INHIBITORS, MISCELLANEOUS 24:32.92

Sacubitril and Valsartan

Sacubitril/Valsartan

■ Sacubitril and valsartan (sacubitril/valsartan) is a fixed combination of sacubitril (a neprilysin [neutral endopeptidase] inhibitor) and valsartan (an angiotensin II type 1 [AT_1] receptor antagonist [i.e., angiotensin II receptor blocker, ARB]); such drug combinations have been referred to as angiotensin receptor-neprilysin inhibitors (ARNIs).

Uses

■ **Heart Failure** Sacubitril and valsartan in fixed combination (sacubitril/valsartan) is used to reduce the risk of cardiovascular death and hospitalization for patients with chronic heart failure (New York Heart Association [NYHA] class II–IV) and reduced ejection fraction. Sacubitril/valsartan is usually administered in conjunction with other heart failure therapies (e.g., β-adrenergic blocking agent [β-blocker], aldosterone antagonist, diuretic) as a substitute for therapy with an angiotensin-converting enzyme (ACE) inhibitor or other angiotensin II receptor antagonist. Current evidence indicates that sacubitril/valsartan results in improved outcomes compared with enalapril based on reductions in cardiovascular death and heart failure hospitalization in patients with chronic heart failure and reduced ejection fraction receiving optimal heart failure therapy.

Current guidelines for the management of heart failure in adults generally recommend a combination of drug therapies to reduce morbidity and mortality, including neurohormonal antagonists (e.g., ACE inhibitors, angiotensin II receptor antagonists, angiotensin receptor-neprilysin inhibitors [ARNIs], β-blockers, aldosterone receptor antagonists) that inhibit the detrimental compensatory mechanisms in heart failure. Sacubitril/valsartan achieves dual neurohormonal modulation of the renin-angiotensin-aldosterone (RAA) system and neprilysin enzyme; the beneficial effects of RAA inhibition by valsartan are augmented by enhanced natriuretic peptide activity due to sacubitril. Additional agents (e.g., cardiac glycosides, diuretics, sinoatrial modulators [i.e., ivabradine]) added to a heart failure treatment regimen in selected patients have been associated with symptomatic improvement and/or reduction in heart failure-related hospitalizations.

Experts recommend that all asymptomatic patients with reduced left ventricular ejection fraction (LVEF) (i.e., American College of Cardiology Foundation [ACCF]/American Heart Association [AHA] stage B heart failure) receive therapy with an ACE inhibitor and β-blocker to prevent symptomatic heart failure and to reduce morbidity and mortality. In patients with prior or current symptoms of chronic heart failure with reduced LVEF (ACCF/AHA stage C), ACCF, AHA, and the Heart Failure Society of America (HFSA) recommend inhibition of the RAA system with an ACE inhibitor, angiotensin II receptor antagonist, or ARNI in conjunction with a β-blocker, and an aldosterone antagonist in selected patients, to reduce morbidity and mortality. While ACE inhibitors have been the preferred drugs for inhibition of the RAA system because of their established benefits in patients with heart failure and reduced ejection fraction, some evidence indicates that therapy with an ARNI (sacubitril/valsartan) may be more effective than ACE inhibitor therapy (enalapril) in reducing cardiovascular death and heart failure-related hospitalization and that such ARNI therapy is cost-effective. ACCF, AHA, and HFSA recommend that patients with NYHA class II or III chronic symptomatic heart failure with reduced LVEF who are able to tolerate an ACE inhibitor or angiotensin II receptor antagonist be switched to therapy containing an ARNI to further reduce morbidity and mortality. However, in patients in whom an ARNI is not appropriate, ACCF, AHA, and HFSA strongly advise continued use of an ACE inhibitor for all classes of heart failure with reduced ejection fraction. In patients in whom therapy with an ARNI or ACE inhibitor is not appropriate, an angiotensin II receptor antagonist may be used. For additional information on the use of angiotensin II receptor antagonists in the management of heart failure, see Uses: Heart Failure, in Valsartan 24:32.08 and in Candesartan 24:32.08.

Efficacy and safety of sacubitril/valsartan in the management of heart failure have been established principally by the results of a randomized, double-blind trial (PARADIGM-HF) comparing the long-term efficacy and safety of sacubitril/valsartan with that of enalapril in addition to standard-of-care therapy in 8442 patients with symptomatic (NYHA class II–IV) chronic heart failure and reduced ejection fraction (LVEF of 40% or less). In this trial, sacubitril/valsartan was superior to enalapril in reducing the risk of death and hospitalization for heart failure in patients who were receiving these drugs in addition to the best available medical therapy; the benefit of sacubitril/valsartan was similar for both death and hospitalization and was consistent across subgroups. Benefits of sacubitril/valsartan were observed in comparison with optimal therapy with enalapril; the mean dosage of enalapril was similar to the well-established target dosages shown to reduce mortality in patients with chronic heart failure and reduced ejection fraction.

Patients enrolled in the PARADIGM-HF trial were receiving an ACE inhibitor or angiotensin II receptor antagonist at a dosage equivalent to at least 10 mg of enalapril daily for at least 4 weeks prior to trial screening in addition to maximally tolerated dosages of β-blockers. Most patients also received diuretics and mineralocorticoid receptor antagonists and had mild to moderate heart failure symptoms. Patients with a systolic blood pressure of less than 100 mm Hg at the time of screening were excluded from the trial. All enrolled patients discontinued their existing ACE inhibitor or angiotensin II receptor antagonist therapy and entered sequential single-blind run-in periods during which they received enalapril 10 mg twice daily (a dosage that has previously been shown to reduce mortality), followed by sacubitril 49 mg/valsartan 51 mg twice daily, increasing to a target maintenance dosage of sacubitril 97 mg/valsartan 103 mg twice daily. To minimize the potential for angioedema caused by overlapping ACE and neprilysin inhibition, enalapril was withheld a day before initiating sacubitril/valsartan, and sacubitril/valsartan was withheld a day before initiating randomized therapy. The most common reason for patients failing to successfully complete the enalapril and sacubitril/valsartan run-in period was an adverse event, often related to renal dysfunction, hyperkalemia, or hypotension. Patients who successfully completed the sequential run-in periods were randomized to receive either sacubitril 97 mg/valsartan 103 mg twice daily or enalapril 10 mg twice daily in addition to standard-of-care therapy. The primary end point was a composite of death from cardiovascular causes or first hospitalization for heart failure.

The PARADIGM-HF trial was terminated prematurely following the revelation of a substantially lower rate of the primary composite outcome of cardiovascular death or heart failure hospitalization in the sacubitril/valsartan treatment group at a prespecified interim analysis. After a median follow-up duration of 27 months, sacubitril/valsartan reduced the primary end point by approximately 20% compared with enalapril. The treatment effect of sacubitril/valsartan compared with that of enalapril reflected a reduction in both cardiovascular death (20% reduction; event rate 13.3 or 16.5%, respectively) and first hospitalization for worsening heart failure (21% reduction; event rate 12.8 or 15.6%, respectively). Therapy with sacubitril/valsartan reduced the likelihood of a first hospitalization as well as of multiple hospitalizations. Sacubitril/valsartan therapy also improved measures of nonfatal clinical deterioration, including the need for intensification of outpatient treatment, frequency of emergency department visits for worsening heart failure, the requirement for intensive care or IV inotropic support during hospitalization, and the incidence of progression to heart failure mechanical device implantation or cardiac transplantation. Sacubitril/valsartan also substantially improved overall survival evidenced by a 16% reduction in all-cause mortality, which was attributable principally to a lower incidence of cardiovascular mortality. Symptomatic hypotension occurred more frequently with sacubitril/valsartan therapy than with enalapril (14 or 9.2%, respectively) but was not associated with an increased rate of discontinuance of therapy due to hypotension-related adverse effects. There were numerically more cases of angioedema with sacubitril/valsartan than with enalapril therapy but the difference was not statistically significant. While it has been stated that the final adverse event rate for sacubitril/valsartan may not reflect clinical practice because of exclusion of patients with intolerance to the drug during the initial run-in period, the overall number of patients who were excluded during this period was small and was higher in the enalapril treatment group; therefore, it is considered unlikely that the implementation of a run-in period in this trial substantially affected the observed safety profile of sacubitril/valsartan.

Dosage and Administration

■ **General** Each fixed-combination tablet of sacubitril and valsartan (sacubitril/valsartan [Entresto®]) contains sacubitril 24 mg/valsartan 26 mg, sacubitril 49 mg/valsartan 51 mg, or sacubitril 97 mg/valsartan 103 mg.

Bioavailability of the valsartan component of sacubitril/valsartan tablets is 40–60% higher than that of valsartan in other commercially available tablet formulations; the valsartan dose of 26, 51, or 103 mg in the fixed combination of sacubitril/valsartan is equivalent to valsartan doses of 40, 80, or 160 mg, respectively, in other commercially available valsartan tablets.

When switching from an angiotensin-converting enzyme (ACE) inhibitor to sacubitril/valsartan, ACE inhibitor treatment should be stopped 36 hours prior to initiation of sacubitril/valsartan therapy. (See Contraindications under Cautions.) Therapy with an angiotensin II receptor antagonist also should be discontinued before initiation of sacubitril/valsartan therapy. (See Drug Interactions: Drugs that Block the Renin-Angiotensin System.)

■ **Administration** Sacubitril/valsartan is administered orally twice daily without regard to food.

■ **Dosage** ***Heart Failure*** Dosage of sacubitril/valsartan in fixed combination is expressed in terms of both sacubitril and valsartan components.

Initial Dosage. The recommended initial dosage of sacubitril/valsartan in patients with chronic heart failure switching from therapy with an ACE inhibitor or angiotensin II receptor antagonist is sacubitril 49 mg/valsartan 51 mg twice daily; sacubitril/valsartan therapy should begin *after discontinuance* of the angiotensin II receptor antagonist or *36 hours after discontinuance* of the ACE inhibitor. (See Cautions: Contraindications.)

The recommended initial dosage of sacubitril/valsartan in patients switching from low dosages of an ACE inhibitor (i.e., in a clinical trial, "low dosage" was considered to be enalapril 10 mg daily or less or an equivalent dosage of another ACE inhibitor) or angiotensin II receptor antagonist (i.e., in a clinical trial, "low dosage" was considered to be valsartan 160 mg daily or less or an equivalent dosage of another angiotensin II receptor antagonist) is sacubitril 24 mg/valsartan 26 mg twice daily. Sacubitril/valsartan therapy in such patients should begin *after discontinuance* of the angiotensin II receptor antagonist or *36 hours after discontinuance* of the ACE inhibitor. (See Cautions: Contraindications.)

The recommended initial dosage of sacubitril/valsartan in patients *not* currently taking an ACE inhibitor or an angiotensin II receptor antagonist is sacubitril 24 mg/valsartan 26 mg twice daily.

Maintenance Dosage. The dosage of sacubitril/valsartan should be doubled every 2–4 weeks, as tolerated, to a target maintenance dosage of sacubitril 97 mg/valsartan 103 mg twice daily.

■ **Special Populations** ***Hepatic Impairment*** No adjustment of sacubitril/valsartan dosage is necessary in patients with mild hepatic impairment (Child-Pugh class A). An initial dosage of sacubitril 24 mg/valsartan 26 mg twice daily is recommended for patients with moderate hepatic impairment (Child-Pugh class B). The dosage of sacubitril/valsartan should be doubled every 2–4 weeks, as tolerated, to a target maintenance dosage of sacubitril 97 mg/valsartan 103 mg twice daily. Sacubitril/valsartan is not recommended in patients with severe hepatic impairment (Child-Pugh class C). (See Hepatic Impairment under Warnings/Precautions: Specific Populations, in Cautions.)

Renal Impairment No adjustment of sacubitril/valsartan dosage is necessary in patients with mild or moderate renal impairment. An initial dosage of sacubitril 24 mg/valsartan 26 mg twice daily is recommended for patients with severe renal impairment (estimated glomerular filtration rate [GFR] less than 30 mL/minute per 1.73 m²). The dosage of sacubitril/valsartan should be doubled every 2–4 weeks, as tolerated, to a target maintenance dosage of sacubitril 97 mg/valsartan 103 mg twice daily. Safety and efficacy have not been established in patients undergoing dialysis. (See Renal Impairment under Warnings/Precautions: Specific Populations, in Cautions.)

Volume- and/or Salt-Depleted Patients Patients with volume and/or salt depletion should have these imbalances corrected prior to the initiation of sacubitril/valsartan therapy; alternatively, sacubitril/valsartan may be initiated at a lower dosage.

Cautions

■ **Contraindications** Known hypersensitivity to sacubitril, valsartan, or any ingredient in the formulation.

History of angioedema related to prior treatment with an angiotensin-converting enzyme (ACE) inhibitor or angiotensin II receptor antagonist.

Concomitant use of ACE inhibitors. Sacubitril/valsartan should *not* be administered within 36 hours of switching from or to an ACE inhibitor.

Concomitant use of aliskiren in patients with diabetes mellitus.

■ **Warnings/Precautions** ***Warnings*** **Fetal/Neonatal Morbidity and Mortality.** Drugs that act directly on the renin-angiotensin system (e.g., angiotensin-converting enzyme [ACE] inhibitors, angiotensin II receptor antagonists) can cause fetal and neonatal morbidity and mortality when used in pregnancy during the second and third trimesters. The fixed combination of sacubitril and valsartan (sacubitril/valsartan) should be discontinued as soon as possible when pregnancy is detected, unless continued use is considered lifesaving. For additional information on the risk of such drugs (i.e., angiotensin II antagonists and ACE inhibitors) during pregnancy, see Cautions: Pregnancy, Fertility, and Lactation, in Captopril 24:32.04 and in Enalaprilat/Enalapril 24:32.04.

Sensitivity Reactions Angioedema may occur with sacubitril/valsartan therapy, and if associated with laryngeal edema, may be fatal. In cases of confirmed angioedema where swelling has been confined to the face and lips, the condition generally resolves without treatment; however, antihistamines may provide symptomatic relief. Swelling of the tongue, glottis, or larynx may cause airway obstruction, and appropriate therapy (e.g., epinephrine, maintenance of patent airway) should be initiated. Sacubitril/valsartan should *not* be used in patients with a known history of angioedema related to previous ACE inhibitor or angiotensin II receptor antagonist therapy (see Cautions: Contraindications); black patients and those with a prior history of angioedema may be at an increased risk of angioedema with sacubitril/valsartan therapy.

Other Warnings/Precautions **Precautions Related to Use of Fixed Combinations.** *When the fixed combination of sacubitril/valsartan is used, the cautions, precautions, contraindications, and drug interactions associated with sacubitril and valsartan must be considered.* Cautionary information applicable to specific populations (e.g., pregnant or nursing women, individuals with hepatic or renal impairment, geriatric patients) should be considered for each drug. (For cautionary information specific to valsartan, see Cautions in Valsartan 24:32.08.)

Cardiovascular Effects. Sacubitril/valsartan lowers blood pressure and may cause symptomatic hypotension. Symptomatic hypotension may occur in patients with an activated renin-angiotensin-aldosterone (RAA) system (e.g., patients with volume or salt depletion secondary to salt restriction or high-dose diuretic therapy). (See Volume- and/or Salt-Depleted Patients under Dosage and Administration: Special Populations.)

If hypotension occurs, dosage adjustments of diuretics or concomitant antihypertensive drugs, and treatment of other causes of hypotension (e.g., hypovolemia) should be considered. If hypotension persists despite such measures, the dosage of sacubitril/valsartan should be reduced or the drug temporarily discontinued. Permanent discontinuance of therapy is usually not required.

Renal Effects. Because the RAA system appears to contribute substantially to maintenance of glomerular filtration in patients with heart failure in whom renal perfusion is severely compromised, renal function may deteriorate markedly (e.g., leading to oliguria, progressive azotemia, and rarely acute renal failure and death) in these patients during therapy with an ACE inhibitor or an angiotensin II receptor antagonist (e.g., valsartan). Dosage reduction or interruption of sacubitril/valsartan therapy may be required in patients who develop a clinically important decrease in renal function. As with all drugs that affect the RAA system, sacubitril/valsartan may increase blood urea and serum creatinine concentrations in patients with bilateral or unilateral renal artery stenosis; renal function should be monitored. (See Cautions: Renal Effects, in Enalaprilat/Enalapril 24:32.04.)

Hyperkalemia. Hyperkalemia may occur in patients receiving sacubitril/valsartan, especially in those with severe renal impairment, diabetes mellitus, hypoaldosteronism, or a potassium-rich diet. Serum potassium should be monitored periodically and elevated values treated appropriately. Dosage reduction or interruption of sacubitril/valsartan therapy may be required in some instances of hyperkalemia.

Specific Populations **Pregnancy.** Sacubitril/valsartan can cause fetal and neonatal morbidity and mortality when administered to a pregnant woman. Sacubitril/valsartan should be discontinued as soon as possible when pregnancy is detected, unless continued use is considered life-saving; in such cases, the woman should be advised of the risk to the fetus. (See Advice to Patients.) Reproduction studies in rats and rabbits using sacubitril/valsartan during organogenesis have demonstrated increased embryofetal death and teratogenic effects. (See Fetal/Neonatal Morbidity and Mortality under Warnings/Precautions: Warnings, in Cautions.)

Lactation. Sacubitril/valsartan is distributed into milk in rats. It is not known whether sacubitril/valsartan is distributed into human milk. Because of the potential for serious adverse reactions to sacubitril/valsartan in nursing infants, a decision should be made whether to discontinue nursing or the drug, taking into account the importance of the drug to the woman.

Pediatric Use. Safety and efficacy of sacubitril/valsartan in pediatric patients have not been established.

Geriatric Use. No clinically relevant pharmacokinetic differences have been observed in patients 65 years of age and older compared with the overall population.

Hepatic Impairment. Results of a pharmacokinetic study indicate that sacubitril/valsartan exposure is increased in patients with mild or moderate hepatic impairment (Child-Pugh class A or B). Dosage adjustments are not necessary for patients with mild hepatic impairment; a lower initial dosage is recommended in patients with moderate hepatic impairment. (See Hepatic Impairment under Dosage and Administration: Special Populations.)

Sacubitril/valsartan is not recommended in patients with severe hepatic impairment (Child-Pugh class C); safety and efficacy have not been established in this population.

Renal Impairment. Results of a pharmacokinetic study indicate that exposure to LBQ657 (the active metabolite of sacubitril) is increased by approximately twofold in patients with mild or moderate renal impairment (creatinine clearance 30–80 mL/minute) and 2.7-fold in patients with severe renal impairment (creatinine clearance less than 30 mL/minute). Exposure to sacubitril and valsartan was not substantially altered in patients with renal impairment.

In the PARADIGM-HF trial, there was no increase in adverse events associated with the increased exposure to LBQ657 in patients with mild or moderate renal impairment; dosage adjustments are not necessary in these patients.

Sacubitril/valsartan should be used with caution in patients with severe renal impairment. (See Renal Effects and also see Hyperkalemia under Warnings/Precautions: Other Warnings/Precautions, in Cautions.) In patients with severe renal impairment, no change to the target maintenance dosage is recommended; however, a lower initial dosage of sacubitril/valsartan should be used in these patients. (See Renal Impairment under Dosage and Administration: Special Populations.) A lower initial dosage and slower titration to the target maintenance dosage may reduce potential tolerability issues.

Safety and efficacy have not been established in patients undergoing dialysis. Sacubitril/valsartan is unlikely to be removed by hemodialysis due to high protein binding.

■ **Common Adverse Effects** Adverse effects occurring in at least 5% of patients with heart failure receiving sacubitril/valsartan in the double-blind phase of the PARADIGM-HF trial included hypotension, cough, dizziness, and renal failure or acute renal failure. Laboratory abnormalities occurring in at least 5% of patients receiving sacubitril/valsartan in the double-blind phase of the PARADIGM-HF trial included decreases in hemoglobin and hematocrit exceeding 20%, increases in serum creatinine concentration exceeding 50%, and serum potassium concentrations exceeding 5.5 mEq/L.

Drug Interactions

■ **Drugs Affecting Hepatic Microsomal Enzymes** Cytochrome P-450 (CYP) enzyme-mediated metabolism of sacubitril and valsartan (sacubitril/valsartan) is minimal; therefore, drugs that affect activity of CYP enzymes are not expected to affect the pharmacokinetics of sacubitril/valsartan.

■ **Drugs Affected by Hepatic Transport Systems** In vitro data suggest that sacubitril inhibits organic anion transporter protein (OATP) 1B1 and OATP1B3 (hepatic uptake transporters). Sacubitril may increase systemic exposure of OATP1B1 and OATP1B3 substrates (e.g., atorvastatin).

■ **Drugs that Block the Renin-Angiotensin System** Concomitant therapy with sacubitril/valsartan and an angiotensin-converting enzyme (ACE) inhibitor is contraindicated because of the increased risk of angioedema. Concomitant therapy with sacubitril/valsartan and an angiotensin II receptor antagonist should be avoided because the valsartan component of sacubitril/valsartan is an angiotensin II receptor antagonist. Concomitant therapy with sacubitril/valsartan and aliskiren, a direct renin inhibitor, is contraindicated in patients with diabetes mellitus; in addition, such concomitant therapy should be avoided in patients with renal impairment (glomerular filtration rate [GFR] less than 60 mL/minute per 1.73 m^2). (See Cautions in Aliskiren Hemifumarate 24:32.40.)

■ **Drugs or Foods that Increase Serum Potassium Concentration** Concomitant use of potassium-sparing diuretics (e.g., amiloride, spironolactone, triamterene), potassium supplements, or potassium-containing salt substitutes with valsartan may result in an increased risk of hyperkalemia. Serum potassium concentrations should be monitored periodically during such concomitant use.

■ **Amlodipine** No clinically relevant pharmacokinetic interaction was observed with coadministration of sacubitril/valsartan and amlodipine.

■ **Atorvastatin** Concomitant administration of sacubitril/valsartan and atorvastatin did not alter systemic exposure to sacubitril/valsartan to a clinically important degree; however, the area under the concentration-time curve (AUC) and peak plasma concentration of atorvastatin were increased.

■ **Cardiac Drugs** No clinically relevant pharmacokinetic interactions were observed when sacubitril/valsartan was coadministered with carvedilol or digoxin.

■ **Diuretics** Volume depletion may potentiate symptomatic hypotension in patients receiving concomitant therapy with diuretics and sacubitril/valsartan. No clinically relevant pharmacokinetic interactions were observed when sacubitril/valsartan was coadministered with hydrochlorothiazide or furosemide.

■ **Lithium** Increased serum lithium concentrations and lithium toxicity have been reported with concomitant use of angiotensin II receptor antagonists and lithium. Monitoring of serum lithium concentrations is recommended during such concomitant use.

■ **Metformin** No clinically relevant pharmacokinetic interaction was observed with coadministration of sacubitril/valsartan and metformin.

■ **Nonsteroidal Anti-inflammatory Agents** Deterioration of renal function, including possible acute renal failure, may occur when sacubitril/valsartan is used concomitantly with nonsteroidal anti-inflammatory agents (NSAIAs), including selective cyclooxygenase-2 (COX-2) inhibitors, in geriatric patients, patients with volume depletion (including those receiving concomitant diuretic therapy), or patients with renal impairment. These effects are usually reversible; renal function should be monitored periodically in such patients receiving concomitant therapy with sacubitril/valsartan and an NSAIA.

■ **Omeprazole** No clinically relevant pharmacokinetic interaction was observed with concomitant administration of sacubitril/valsartan and omeprazole.

■ **Oral Contraceptives** No clinically relevant pharmacokinetic interaction was observed with concomitant administration of sacubitril/valsartan and an oral contraceptive containing ethinyl estradiol and levonorgestrel.

■ **Sildenafil** No clinically relevant pharmacokinetic interaction was observed with concomitant administration of sacubitril/valsartan and sildenafil. Coadministration of a 50-mg single dose of sildenafil with sacubitril/valsartan at steady state (sacubitril 194 mg/valsartan 206 mg once daily for 5 days) in patients with hypertension was associated with additive reductions in blood pressure (approximately 5 or 4 mm Hg for systolic or diastolic blood pressure, respectively) compared with administration of sacubitril/valsartan alone. Patients should be advised about potential adverse effects due to blood pressure-lowering effects with concomitant use of sacubitril/valsartan and sildenafil.

■ **Warfarin** No clinically relevant pharmacokinetic interaction was observed with concomitant administration of sacubitril/valsartan and warfarin.

Description

Sacubitril and valsartan (sacubitril/valsartan) is a combination of a neprilysin inhibitor (sacubitril) and an angiotensin II type 1 (AT_1) receptor antagonist (valsartan). The dual mechanism of sacubitril/valsartan suppresses harmful compensatory mechanisms of heart failure that are mediated by the renin-angiotensin-aldosterone (RAA) system, while simultaneously enhancing the beneficial adaptive mechanisms of natriuretic peptides by inhibiting their degradation.

The natriuretic peptide system consists of 3 major peptides (atrial natriuretic peptide [ANP], B-type natriuretic peptide [BNP], and C-type natriuretic peptide [CNP]), which are involved in maintaining normal hemodynamics and plasma volume. Natriuretic peptides stimulate natriuresis and diuresis, promote vasodilation, and oppose acute effects of volume overload by inhibiting the RAA system and the sympathetic nervous system. Natriuretic peptides also have been shown to attenuate the development of cardiac hypertrophy and fibrosis and enhance endothelial function. The effects of natriuretic peptides are mediated through guanylyl cyclase receptors. Activation of these receptors increases intracellular cyclic guanosine monophosphate (cGMP), which is ultimately responsible for the physiologic effects of natriuretic peptides.

Natriuretic peptides are predominantly catabolized via enzymatic cleavage by the membrane-bound, zinc-dependent enzyme neprilysin (also known as neutral endopeptidase or membrane-metallo-endopeptidase). Other substrates of neprilysin include enkephalins, oxytocin, gastrin, angiotensin I and II, endothelin-1, substance P, and bradykinin. Degradation of these substrates is inhibited by sacubitril, which results in increased concentrations of natriuretic peptides and enhances their beneficial counterregulatory effects in heart failure patients. Sole inhibition of neprilysin results in increased ANP, BNP, and cGMP concentrations but at the expense of increased potent vasoconstrictors (angiotensin II and endothelin-1), which partly counteracts the benefits of increased natriuretic peptides. Augmentation of natriuretic peptide effects through neprilysin inhibition requires concomitant suppression of angiotensin II to yield a beneficial effect. Valsartan blocks the physiologic actions of angiotensin II, including vasoconstrictor and aldosterone-secreting effects, by selectively inhibiting access of angiotensin II to AT_1 receptors within many tissues, including vascular smooth muscle and the adrenal gland. For additional information on the pharmacology of angiotensin II receptor antagonists, see Description in Irbesartan 24:32.08 and Valsartan 24:32.08

Following oral administration, sacubitril/valsartan dissociates into sacubitril and valsartan. The absolute oral bioavailability of sacubitril is at least 60%, and the bioavailability of valsartan from sacubitril/valsartan is 40–60% higher than that of valsartan administered as a single agent. Sacubitril is a prodrug; its neprilysin-inhibitory activity is dependent upon conversion to the active metabolite (LBQ657) by deethylation via plasma esterases. LBQ657 is not further metabolized to a substantial extent and valsartan is minimally metabolized; approximately 20% of the dose of valsartan is recovered as metabolites. The primary metabolite of valsartan, accounting for less than 10% of the dose, is a hydroxyl metabolite formed by metabolism via the cytochrome P-450 (CYP) isoenzyme 2C9. Administration of sacubitril/valsartan with food has no clinically important effect on the systemic exposure of sacubitril, LBQ657, or valsartan. The peak plasma concentrations of sacubitril, LBQ657, and valsartan are reached in 0.5, 2 , and 1.5 hours, respectively. Sacubitril, LBQ657, and valsartan are 94–97% bound to plasma proteins. The average elimination half-lives of sacubitril, LBQ657, and valsartan are 1.4, 11.5, and 9.9 hours, respectively. Sacubitril (mainly as LBQ657) is excreted in urine (52–68%) and feces (37–48%). Valsartan and its metabolites are excreted in urine (approximately 13%) and feces (86%).

Advice to Patients

Importance of advising patients to read the manufacturer's patient information.

Importance of women informing clinicians if they are or plan to become pregnant or plan to breast-feed. Importance of advising women of childbearing age about the potential risks to the fetus if sacubitril/valsartan is used during pregnancy. All women of childbearing potential should be advised to report pregnancy to their clinician as soon as possible. (See Fetal/Neonatal Morbidity and Mortality under Warnings/Precautions: Warnings, in Cautions.)

Risk of angioedema. Importance of advising patients to discontinue use of any angiotensin-converting enzyme (ACE) inhibitor or angiotensin II receptor antagonist before taking sacubitril/valsartan. Importance of advising patients to allow a 36-hour wash-out period if switching from or to an ACE inhibitor. (See Cautions: Contraindications and also see Sensitivity Reactions under Cautions: Warnings/Precautions.)

Importance of informing clinicians of existing or contemplated concomitant therapy, including prescription and OTC drugs (including salt substitutes containing potassium), as well as any concomitant diseases.

Importance of informing patients of other important precautionary information. (See Cautions.)

Overview® (see Users Guide). For additional information on this drug until a more detailed monograph is developed and published, the manufacturer's labeling should be consulted. It is *essential* that the manufacturer's labeling be consulted for more detailed information on usual cautions, precautions, contraindications, potential drug interactions, laboratory test interferences, and acute toxicity.

Preparations

Excipients in commercially available drug preparations may have clinically important effects in some individuals; consult specific product labeling for details.

Sacubitril and Valsartan

Oral		
Tablets, film-coated	Sacubitril 24 mg and Valsartan 26 mg	**Entresto®**, Novartis
	Sacubitril 49 mg and Valsartan 51 mg	**Entresto®**, Novartis
	Sacubitril 97 mg and Valsartan 103 mg	**Entresto®**, Novartis

28:00 Central Nervous System Agents*

28:56 Vesicular Monoamine Transporter 2 (VMAT2) Inhibitors

28:92 Central Nervous System Agents, Miscellaneous

§ Omitted from the print version of *AHFS Drug Information*® because of space limitations. This monograph is available on the *AHFS Drug Information*® website, http://ahfsdruginformation.com. Username: ahfs2020; Password: ASHP94498.

*Please see the full AHFS Pharmacologic-Therapeutic Classification© on p. viii. Not all classes are used in the printed edition.

General Anesthetics 28:04

General Anesthetics, Miscellaneous 28:04.92

Etomidate

■ Etomidate is a sedative and hypnotic agent used for general anesthesia.

Uses

■ **Induction and Maintenance of Anesthesia** Etomidate is used IV for induction of general anesthesia. Etomidate may be particularly useful in patients with compromised cardiopulmonary function because of its minimal hemodynamic effects and decreased respiratory depressant effects relative to other IV anesthetics (e.g., barbiturates, propofol). However, the manufacturers state that the potential benefits of the drug's hemodynamic effects must be weighed carefully against the possible risk of involuntary skeletal muscle movements (e.g., myoclonus). (See Cautions: Common Adverse Effects.)

Etomidate also is used during maintenance of anesthesia to supplement subpotent anesthetic agents (e.g., nitrous oxide and oxygen) during short surgical procedures (e.g., dilatation and curettage, cervical conization). Use of the drug for longer procedures is not recommended due to an increased risk of prolonged adrenal suppression. (See Adrenal Suppression under Cautions: Warnings/Precautions.)

When used for induction of anesthesia, etomidate is administered IV by rapid (over 30–60 seconds) injection. Induction with IV etomidate is rapid and results in dose-related hypnotic effects (progressing from light sleep to unconsciousness); the drug also has some amnestic effects, but lacks analgesic properties. Following administration of a standard induction dose of 0.3 mg/kg, hypnosis occurs in less than 1 minute and is maintained for about 3–10 minutes.

For further information on induction and maintenance of anesthesia, see Uses: Induction and Maintenance of Anesthesia, in Propofol 28:04.92.

■ **Rapid Sequence Intubation** Because of its rapid onset and favorable hemodynamic profile, etomidate is commonly used (and often the preferred induction agent) for rapid sequence intubation. Rapid sequence intubation involves the administration of a potent sedative (induction agent) and a neuromuscular blocking agent virtually simultaneously to facilitate rapid tracheal intubation. However, the potential for etomidate to cause adrenal suppression may limit its use in critically ill patients (particularly those with sepsis). (See Adrenal Suppression under Cautions: Warnings/Precautions.)

■ **Procedural Sedation** Etomidate has been used for procedural sedation† in the emergency department and other outpatient settings (e.g., clinic). Because of its relatively short duration of action, the drug is best suited for procedures of short duration. Etomidate does not exhibit analgesic properties and generally is used concomitantly with an opiate agonist (e.g., fentanyl).

Procedural sedation is a technique in which sedative or dissociative agents are administered with or without analgesics to allow patients to tolerate painful or unpleasant medical procedures; a depressed state of consciousness is intentionally induced while cardiorespiratory function is maintained. Because sedation is a continuum ranging from minimal sedation to general anesthesia, airway reflexes and cardiorespiratory function may be impaired if a deeper than intended level of sedation is produced. The appropriate level of sedation should be individualized according to the specific procedure and needs of the patient.

In clinical studies conducted in both adults and pediatric patients, etomidate (in doses less than those used for anesthesia) produced adequate sedation and facilitated the successful completion of a short painful procedure (e.g., fracture reduction, laceration repair, shoulder relocation). Time to onset of sedation and recovery with etomidate are comparable to those achieved with propofol, but considerably shorter than with midazolam. Adverse effects that occur more frequently with etomidate than with other sedative agents include myoclonus and pain at the injection site. Although respiratory depression or apnea also has been reported to occur in some patients receiving etomidate, the incidence is generally the same or less than that with other sedative agents.

Dosage and Administration

■ **General** Etomidate should be administered only by clinicians experienced in the use of general anesthetic drugs and in the management of possible complications associated with their use (e.g., airway or respiratory compromise).

Common premedications such as benzodiazepines (to relieve anxiety and produce anterograde amnesia) and opiate agonists (to relieve pain) may be administered as appropriate.

■ **Administration** Etomidate is administered by IV injection over 30–60 seconds. The drug should be injected undiluted by direct IV injection. Some clinicians state that etomidate may be administered by intraosseous (IO) injection† in the setting of pediatric rapid sequence intubation. Although the drug has been administered as a continuous IV infusion†, this method of delivery is currently not recommended because of the risk of adrenal toxicity. (See Adrenal Suppression under Cautions: Warnings/Precautions.)

Etomidate injection should be inspected visually for particulate matter and discoloration prior to administration whenever solution and container permit. The injection should not be administered unless the solution is clear and the container is undamaged; unused portions should be discarded.

Limited data from clinical and animal studies indicate that inadvertent intra-arterial administration of etomidate injection does not appear to be associated with tissue necrosis distant from the injection site; however, intra-arterial use of the drug is not recommended. Pain at the injection site, which occurs frequently and usually is mild to moderate in severity (although occasionally may be severe), can be minimized if the larger, more proximal veins of the forearm, rather than the smaller, distal hand or wrist veins are used. To prevent needlestick injuries, needles should not be recapped, bent, or broken by hand.

Etomidate injection is compatible with commonly used premedicants administered prior to induction of anesthesia.

■ **Dosage** Dosage of etomidate should be adjusted according to individual requirements and response, age, physical and clinical status, underlying pathologic conditions (e.g., shock, intestinal obstruction, malnutrition, anemia, burns, advanced malignancy, ulcerative colitis, uremia, alcoholism), and the type and amount of premedication or concomitant medication(s). In addition, dosage of the drug should be titrated to clinical effect.

Induction and Maintenance of Anesthesia The usual dose of etomidate for induction of anesthesia in adults and children older than 10 years of age is 0.3 mg/kg (0.2–0.6 mg/kg), administered by IV injection over 30–60 seconds.

When etomidate is used during maintenance of anesthesia to supplement subpotent anesthetic agents during short surgical procedures, smaller increments of etomidate may be administered.

Rapid Sequence Intubation For rapid sequence intubation, etomidate is usually administered in a dose of 0.3 mg/kg IV. The manufacturers state that there are inadequate data to make dosage recommendations for pediatric patients younger than 10 years of age; however, in published reports, etomidate was used in pediatric patients as young as 18 days of age at an average dose of 0.3 mg/kg. Some clinicians recommend an etomidate dose of 0.3 mg/kg by IV or IO† injection for pediatric rapid sequence intubation.

Procedural Sedation Doses of etomidate used for procedural sedation† are usually less than those used for induction of anesthesia; in clinical studies, an initial IV etomidate dose of 0.1–0.2 mg/kg was usually administered, followed by additional doses of 0.05–0.1 mg/kg given as needed for adequate sedation (average total dose of up to 0.26 mg/kg per procedure) in adults and pediatric patients. Some studies have found that a dose of 0.2 mg/kg was the most effective initial dose for short pediatric procedures in the emergency department.

■ **Special Populations** Since clinical studies have revealed pharmacokinetic differences (decreased initial distribution volumes and total clearance, decreased serum protein binding to albumin) between geriatric and younger patients, geriatric patients may require lower dosages of etomidate than younger patients.

Cautions

■ **Contraindications** Known hypersensitivity to etomidate.

■ **Warnings/Precautions** ***Administration Precautions*** To minimize the risk of adverse effects, recommendations for administration and monitoring of etomidate therapy should be followed. (See Dosage and Administration.)

Adrenal Suppression Etomidate is known to cause adrenal suppression by inhibiting 11-β-hydroxylase activity, the enzyme responsible for production of cortisol and aldosterone. Decreased plasma concentrations of cortisol, which usually persist for 6–8 hours and are unresponsive to stimulation by corticotropin (ACTH), have been reported following IV administration of a single induction dose of etomidate (0.3 mg/kg). Because of the risk of prolonged suppression of endogenous cortisol and aldosterone secretion from the adrenal cortex, administration of etomidate as a continuous IV infusion is not recommended.

Although it is well established that etomidate can cause adrenal suppression, there is controversy regarding the clinical importance of this observed effect. Some evidence from a randomized controlled study suggested a possible link between the use of etomidate and increased mortality in critically ill patients (particularly those with sepsis); however, other studies have not found such an association. Studies comparing etomidate to other induction agents (e.g., midazolam, ketamine) for endotracheal intubation have not shown any strong evidence that etomidate increases mortality when compared with these other agents.

Specific Populations **Pregnancy.** There are no adequate and well controlled studies of etomidate in pregnant women; in animal reproduction studies, reduced pup survival and maternal toxicity have been observed.

Based on animal data, repeated or prolonged use of general anesthetics and sedation drugs, including etomidate, during the third trimester of pregnancy may result in adverse neurodevelopmental effects in the fetus. The clinical relevance of these animal findings to humans is not known; the potential risk of adverse neurodevelopmental effects should be considered and discussed with pregnant women undergoing procedures requiring general anesthetics and sedation drugs. (See Pediatric Use under Warnings/Precautions: Specific Populations, in Cautions.)

There are insufficient data to support the use of etomidate during labor and delivery; use is therefore not recommended in the obstetric setting, including in patients undergoing cesarean section.

Lactation. It is not known whether etomidate is distributed into milk in humans. Because many drugs are distributed into human milk, caution is advised if etomidate is used in nursing women.

Pediatric Use. The manufacturers state that safety and efficacy of etomidate for induction or maintenance of anesthesia have not been established in children younger than 10 years of age. However, the drug has been used for rapid sequence intubation in pediatric patients as young as 18 days of age. Etomidate also has been used in children of all ages for procedural sedation† in the emergency department.

FDA warns that repeated or prolonged use of general anesthetics and sedation drugs, including etomidate, in children younger than 3 years of age or during the third trimester of pregnancy may affect brain development. Animal studies in multiple species, including nonhuman primates, have demonstrated that use for longer than 3 hours of anesthetic and sedation drugs that block *N*-methyl-D-aspartic acid (NMDA) receptors and/or potentiate γ-aminobutyric acid (GABA) activity leads to widespread neuronal and oligodendrocyte cell loss and alterations in synaptic morphology and neurogenesis in the brain, resulting in long-term deficits in cognition and behavior. Across animal species, vulnerability to these neurodevelopmental changes occurs during the period of rapid brain growth or synaptogenesis; this period is thought to correlate with the third trimester of pregnancy through the first year of life in humans, but may extend to approximately 3 years of age. The clinical relevance of these animal findings to humans is not known.

While some published evidence suggests that similar deficits in cognition and behavior may occur in children following repeated or prolonged exposure to anesthesia early in life, other studies have found no association between pediatric anesthesia exposure and long-term adverse neurodevelopmental outcomes. Most studies to date have had substantial limitations, and it is not clear whether the adverse neurodevelopmental outcomes observed in children were related to the drug or to other factors (e.g., surgery, underlying illness). There is some clinical evidence that a single, relatively brief exposure to general anesthesia in generally healthy children is unlikely to cause clinically detectable deficits in global cognitive function or serious behavioral disorders; however, further research is needed to fully characterize the effects of exposure to general anesthetics in early life, particularly for prolonged or repeated exposures and in more vulnerable populations (e.g., less healthy children). For further information, see Cautions: Pediatric Precautions, in Propofol 28:04.92.

Anesthetic and sedation drugs are an essential component of care for children and pregnant women who require surgery or other procedures that cannot be delayed; no specific general anesthetic or sedation drug has been shown to be less likely to cause neurocognitive deficits than any other such drug. Pending further accumulation of data in humans from well-designed studies, decisions regarding the timing of elective procedures requiring anesthesia should take into consideration both the benefits of the procedure and the potential risks. When procedures requiring the use of general anesthetics or sedation drugs are considered for young children or pregnant women, clinicians should discuss with the patient, parent, or caregiver the benefits, risks (including potential risk of adverse neurodevelopmental effects), and appropriate timing and duration of the procedure. FDA states that procedures that are considered medically necessary should not be delayed or avoided.

Geriatric Use. Clinical data indicate that etomidate may be associated with cardiac depression (decreased heart rate and cardiac index) and decreased mean arterial blood pressure in geriatric patients, especially those with hypertension. Etomidate is substantially excreted by the kidneys and the risk of severe adverse reactions to the drug may be increased in patients with impaired renal function. Because geriatric patients may have decreased renal function, it may be useful to monitor renal function, and dosage should be selected with caution in such patients. (See Dosage and Administration: Special Populations.)

Hepatic Impairment. Etomidate is metabolized by the liver; patients with hepatic insufficiency may be at higher risk of adverse effects (e.g., adrenal insufficiency). In patients with cirrhosis, elimination half-life of etomidate is approximately double that seen in healthy individuals.

Renal Impairment. Because etomidate is substantially excreted renally, the risk of serious adverse effects is increased in patients with renal impairment.

■ **Common Adverse Effects** The most frequent adverse effects associated with IV use of etomidate are transient venous pain at the injection site and transient skeletal muscle movements (i.e., myoclonus), which occur in about 20% (range: 1–42%) and 32% (range: 23–63%) of patients, respectively. Although generally mild to moderate in severity, such adverse effects can occasionally be severe.

Most (74%) cases of transient skeletal muscle movements have been classified as myoclonic, but tonic movements (10%), ocular movements (9%), and averting movements (7%) also have been noted. Such movements are usually bilateral (of the arms, legs, shoulders, neck, chest wall, trunk, and/or all 4 extremities, with one or more muscle groups predominating), with an electroencephalogram (EEG) suggesting that they are manifestations of cortical disinhibition in the absence of evidence of seizure activity. Alternatively, muscle movements may be unilateral or predominate on one side (e.g., predominance of movement of the arm in which the IV was started), or a mixture of bilateral and unilateral types may occur. The incidence of skeletal muscle movements, particularly those considered disturbing, has been minimized with IV administration of fentanyl immediately before induction of anesthesia with etomidate.

Other adverse effects reported in patients receiving etomidate include hyperventilation, hypoventilation, apnea (duration: 5–90 seconds), laryngospasm, hiccups and snoring (may be associated with partial upper airway obstruction), hypertension, hypotension, arrhythmias (e.g., tachycardia, bradycardia), and postoperative nausea and vomiting.

Drug Interactions

■ **Neuromuscular Blocking Agents** Etomidate does not appear to alter usual dosage requirements of neuromuscular blocking agents used for endotracheal intubation or any other purpose.

■ **Opiate Agonists** Because of a potential additive pharmacologic effect when etomidate is used with an opiate agonist (e.g., fentanyl), dosage adjustments (i.e., decrease in etomidate dosage) may be necessary.

Description

Etomidate, a carboxylated imidazole, is a sedative and hypnotic agent used for general anesthesia. The drug is structurally unrelated to other currently available IV anesthetics.

Following IV injection, etomidate has a rapid onset of action and will produce loss of consciousness within 1 arm-brain circulation time (i.e., usually within about 60 seconds). Etomidate produces its anesthetic activity by enhancing the activity of γ-aminobutyric acid (GABA), the principal inhibitory neurotransmitter in the CNS, through modulation and direct activation of the $GABA_A$ receptor complex.

Etomidate is capable of producing all levels of CNS depression—from light sleep to deep coma—depending on the dosage; however, the drug has no analgesic activity. The degree of depression and duration of action depend on dosage, rate and route of administration, and pharmacokinetics of the drug. Substantial changes on the EEG appear to occur following induction doses of etomidate. The EEG changes are indicative of the various stages of anesthesia and appear to be similar to those occurring following induction of anesthesia with barbiturates. Etomidate may decrease cerebral blood flow and intracranial pressure, while cerebral perfusion pressure is increased or maintained during induction of anesthesia.

Etomidate causes minimal hemodynamic changes and is associated with a decreased incidence and severity of cardiovascular effects compared with other IV anesthetic agents. Minor increases in cardiac index and slight decreases in heart rate, systemic vascular resistance, and arterial blood pressure have been reported with use of etomidate. In addition, equivalent induction doses of etomidate cause less respiratory depression than propofol or barbiturates. Increases in carbon dioxide tension (P_{CO_2}) have been reported with administration of etomidate.

Some data suggest that etomidate usually reduces intraocular pressure (IOP).

The pharmacokinetic profile of etomidate is characterized by a rapid distribution from blood into CNS, rapid clearance from the brain, and substantial tissue uptake. Following the usual induction dose (0.3 mg/kg) of etomidate, duration of hypnosis is short (about 3–10 minutes) and dose dependent. The elimination half-life of etomidate is about 1.25–5 hours. The drug is rapidly metabolized in the liver, principally by hydrolysis, to form etomidate carboxylic acid, which appears to be pharmacologically inactive. About 75% of an administered dose is excreted in urine within 24 hours, mainly (about 80%) as the carboxylic acid metabolite, while 13 and 10% of a dose are excreted in feces and bile, respectively.

Advice to Patients

When procedures requiring general anesthetics or sedation drugs, including etomidate, are considered for young children or pregnant women, importance of discussing with the patient, parent, or caregiver the benefits, risks (including potential risk of adverse neurodevelopmental effects), and appropriate timing and duration of the procedure.

Importance of informing clinicians of existing or contemplated concomitant therapy, including prescription and OTC drugs.

Importance of women informing clinicians if they are or plan to become pregnant or are breast-feeding.

Importance of informing patients of other important precautionary information. (See Cautions.)

Overview® (see Users Guide). For additional information on this drug until a more detailed monograph is developed and published, the manufacturer's labeling should be consulted. It is *essential* that the manufacturer's labeling be consulted for more detailed information on usual cautions, precautions, contraindications, potential drug interactions, laboratory test interferences, and acute toxicity.

Preparations

Excipients in commercially available drug preparations may have clinically important effects in some individuals; consult specific product labeling for details.

Etomidate

Parenteral		
Injection, for IV use	2 mg/mL (20 and 40 mg)*	**Amidate®**, Hospira **Etomidate Injection**

*available from one or more manufacturer, distributor, and/or repackager by generic (nonproprietary) name

†Use is not currently included in the labeling approved by the US Food and Drug Administration

Ketamine Hydrochloride

■ Ketamine hydrochloride, an *N*-methyl-D-aspartate (NMDA) receptor antagonist, is a nonbarbiturate general anesthetic that also has analgesic and antidepressant properties.

Uses

Ketamine hydrochloride has historically been used as an anesthetic agent; however, the drug also can produce profound analgesia and other pharmacologic effects, and is therefore being used for a variety of other indications such as procedural sedation in the emergency department, pain management†, sedation and analgesia in the intensive care setting†, and some psychiatric indications, including treatment-resistant depression and suicidality†.

■ Induction and Maintenance of Anesthesia Ketamine is used IV or IM for induction of anesthesia prior to administration of other general anesthetic agents. Ketamine also is used as the sole anesthetic agent for diagnostic and surgical procedures that do not require skeletal muscle relaxation. Although the drug is best suited for brief procedures, additional (i.e., maintenance) doses may be administered for longer procedures. Ketamine also may be used to supplement low-potency agents (e.g., nitrous oxide). While ketamine currently is FDA-labeled for use in adults only, the drug has been used widely in pediatric patients†.

Induction of anesthesia with ketamine is rapid and results in a trance-like cataleptic state characterized by profound analgesia and amnesia, with retention of protective airway reflexes, spontaneous respirations, and cardiopulmonary stability. This anesthetic state, known as dissociative anesthesia, is markedly different from that of other general anesthetic agents (e.g., barbiturates, benzodiazepines, propofol, inhalation anesthetics).

Efficacy of ketamine as an anesthetic agent has been evaluated in over 12,000 operative and diagnostic procedures involving over 10,000 patients from 105 studies. In these studies, ketamine was administered as the sole anesthetic agent, as an induction agent for other general anesthetics, or to supplement low-potency anesthetic agents; the anesthesia produced by ketamine was rated by anesthesiologists and surgeons, respectively, as excellent or good (90 and 93%), fair (6 and 4%), or poor (4 and 3%). Using another evaluation method, anesthesia was rated as adequate in at least 90% or inadequate in 10% or less of procedures studied. Procedures for which ketamine has been used include debridement, dressing changes, and skin grafting in burn patients; neurodiagnostic procedures (e.g., pneumoencephalograms, ventriculograms, myelograms, lumbar punctures); diagnostic and operative procedures of the eye, ear, nose, and mouth, including dental extractions; diagnostic and operative procedures of the pharynx, larynx, or bronchial tree; colonoscopy and minor surgery of the anus and rectum; circumcision; short gynecologic procedures (e.g., dilatation and curettage); orthopedic procedures (e.g., fracture reductions, manipulations, femoral pinning, amputation, biopsies); emergency cardioversion; and cardiac catheterization.

Due to the risk of emergence reactions (see Emergence Reactions under Cautions: Nervous System Effects) and the availability of other anesthetic agents, current use of ketamine is generally limited to certain patient populations (e.g., those with hemodynamic instability) or settings (e.g., prehospital environments that lack appropriate monitoring and respiratory support) where the drug's unique pharmacologic properties may be advantageous. Because ketamine produces sympathomimetic effects, the drug may be particularly useful for induction of anesthesia in hemodynamically unstable patients (e.g., those with traumatic injury or septic shock) or in poor-risk patients with depressed vital functions. Because of its bronchodilating effects, ketamine is generally considered the induction agent of choice in patients with reactive airway disease (e.g., asthma) or active bronchospasm.

Ketamine is commonly used as an induction agent for rapid sequence intubation, particularly in patients with reactive airway disease or hemodynamic compromise; studies have shown that ketamine may produce similar outcomes to etomidate and may be used as an alternative.

■ Procedural Sedation Ketamine is used to provide dissociative sedation during short painful or emotionally disturbing procedures (e.g., fracture reduction, laceration repair, abscess drainage, emergency cardioversion, chest tube insertion, central line placement) in the emergency department. Administration of a single IV or IM dose can effectively produce a dissociative state for approximately 5–10 or 20–30 minutes, respectively, while maintaining cardiovascular stability, spontaneous respiration, and protective airway reflexes.

Ketamine is commonly used for procedural sedation in pediatric patients†. Although used less frequently in adults due to an increased risk of emergence delirium, current evidence also supports the use of ketamine for procedural sedation in the adult population. Ketamine has a well-established role in the care of burn patients undergoing painful procedures (e.g., dressing changes, debridement, grafts). The drug may be administered by the IM route in patients in whom IV administration may be difficult (e.g., severely agitated or combative patients, young children, patients with extensive burns).

Ketamine has been used in combination with propofol (combined therapy commonly referred to as "ketofol") for procedural sedation in the emergency department. The rationale for the combination is to counteract the adverse effects of the drugs (i.e., ketamine mitigating propofol-induced hypotension and propofol mitigating ketamine-induced vomiting and recovery agitation).

■ Pain Ketamine exhibits potent analgesic properties in low (i.e., subanesthetic or subdissociative) doses and has been used for a variety of acute and chronic pain conditions†. Such conditions include acute pain† in the emergency department and prehospital settings, postoperative pain†, and chronic pain† of various etiologies. In addition to its analgesic effects, ketamine also can prevent the development of central sensitization, hyperalgesia, and opiate tolerance, which may be particularly useful in patients who are opiate tolerant or opiate dependent.

Postoperative Pain Ketamine in low (i.e., subanesthetic or subdissociative) doses has been used for the management of postoperative pain† following a variety of surgical procedures in both adults and pediatric patients. The drug should be used as part of a multimodal regimen consisting of a combination of pharmacologic and nonpharmacologic methods targeting different pain mechanisms in the peripheral and central nervous systems.

Efficacy of low-dose ketamine in the postoperative setting is well established and supported by numerous studies demonstrating reduced opiate requirements and, in some cases, additional reductions in postoperative pain when the drug was used as a component of multimodal analgesia; although some studies reported discrepant results, the inconsistency may be due to differences in patient populations, dosage regimens, and concomitant analgesics used. Because ketamine appears to be most beneficial for procedures associated with severe pain, some experts state that subanesthetic ketamine infusions should be reserved for patients undergoing surgeries in which the postoperative pain is expected to be severe; such procedures include thoracic, abdominal (upper, lower, and intra-abdominal), and orthopedic (limb and spinal) surgeries. These experts state that patients undergoing procedures associated with only mild postoperative pain (e.g., tonsillectomy, head and neck surgery) have not been shown to benefit from perioperative ketamine. For these procedures, standard analgesia with low dosages of opiates, nonsteroidal anti-inflammatory agents (NSAIAs), and local anesthetics usually can provide adequate pain relief. However, management of post-tonsillectomy pain in children can be difficult and several studies have demonstrated that administration of a single IV dose of ketamine 0.5 mg/kg (alone or in combination with other analgesics) can provide effective postoperative pain control.

Ketamine may be particularly useful in the management of opiate-tolerant or opiate-dependent patients undergoing surgery. In a randomized controlled study in opiate-dependent patients undergoing spinal surgery, intraoperative use of ketamine was associated with reduced opiate consumption at 48 hours and reduced opiate usage at 6 weeks. Ketamine also may be considered as an adjunct to reduce postoperative opiate consumption in patients who have an increased risk of opiate-related respiratory depression (e.g., those with obstructive sleep apnea).

Acute Pain Ketamine (in subanesthetic doses) has been used alone or as an adjunct to other analgesics (e.g., opiates) for relief of acute pain† in the emergency department and prehospital settings (e.g., ambulance). Studies evaluating subanesthetic ketamine for analgesia in these settings have been conducted principally in the adult population. However, low or subanesthetic doses of ketamine also have been used for analgesia in pediatric patients 3 months of age or older presenting to the emergency department. When used as an adjunct to opiate analgesics in the emergency department or prehospital setting, ketamine has resulted in greater reduction in pain scores compared with opiate therapy alone, and/or decreased opiate requirements. When given as a single agent for acute pain in the emergency department, IV ketamine has been reported to provide comparable reductions in pain scores to IV morphine.

Although evidence is limited, ketamine may be useful in opiate-dependent patients with acute exacerbations of chronic pain conditions (e.g., sickle cell disease)†.

Chronic Pain Ketamine has been used as an adjunct analgesic for the management of chronic pain of various etiologies, including complex regional pain syndrome (CRPS)†, neuropathic pain associated with spinal cord injury†, phantom limb pain†, fibromyalgia†, ischemic pain†, cancer pain†, and migraine pain†, in adults and pediatric patients. Evidence of efficacy varies depending on the specific pain condition treated and generally is limited to small randomized controlled studies, observational studies, and case reports demonstrating short-term benefits of ketamine infusions during and for a short time following the infusion; however, ketamine dosages and administration protocols varied widely in these studies.

Ketamine has been evaluated most extensively in chronic pain conditions associated with a neuropathic component. With regard to specific conditions, some experts state that there is weak to moderate evidence that ketamine infusions are effective for reducing pain related to CRPS in adults and pediatric patients; the evidence to date includes mostly systematic reviews, case reports, and observational studies with only a few small randomized controlled studies. In one study in 19 patients with CRPS, reductions in pain were reported for up to 12 weeks with continuous IV infusion of ketamine (maximum rate of 0.35 mg/kg per hour over 4 hours daily for 10 days). There also is weak evidence supporting ketamine infusions for short-term improvements in neuropathic pain associated with spinal cord injury. Other chronic pain syndromes that have been investigated generally have not responded to or only minimally responded to ketamine therapy; experts state that the available evidence remains inconclusive for the efficacy of ketamine infusions for mixed neuropathic pain, phantom limb pain, postherpetic neuralgia, fibromyalgia, ischemic pain, migraine, and low-back pain.

Although data are limited regarding the use of ketamine as an adjuvant treatment of cancer pain, some experts state that oral or IV ketamine may be considered for the management of refractory cancer pain in adults. Evidence to date remains inconclusive for the efficacy of ketamine in chronic cancer pain and is mostly based on case reports and uncontrolled studies. While a few randomized controlled studies indicate that the drug may have some benefit as an adjunct analgesic in cancer-related pain, these studies generally were small and had short durations of follow-up relative to the chronic nature of the pain being treated. In a larger controlled clinical trial in 214 adults with cancer-related neuropathic pain inadequately treated with adjuvant analgesics, the addition of oral ketamine (up to 400 mg daily for 16 days) was no more effective than placebo in improving pain scores. In another controlled clinical trial in 185 adults in palliative care settings who had refractory cancer-related pain, adjunctive therapy with ketamine (administered as a subcutaneous infusion in escalating doses up to 500 mg every 24 hours over 5 days) also was no more effective than placebo in improving pain scores. Studies of IV and oral ketamine have been conduced in children with cancer pain; although these studies were mostly retrospective, there is some evidence suggesting that pain control can be achieved with ketamine in these patients.

Additional study is needed to establish the role of ketamine in patients with chronic pain and to determine optimum dosages, durability of response, and long-term benefits and risks of the drug. Some clinicians recommend that use of ketamine be restricted to patients with refractory pain who have failed to obtain adequate relief from standard analgesics and nonpharmacologic treatments.

■ **Treatment-resistant Depression and Suicidality** Ketamine has been used in low (i.e., subanesthetic) doses for the treatment of severe and treatment-resistant depression associated with major depressive disorder or bipolar disorder†. Although there are various definitions for treatment-resistant depression, the condition often has been defined as the failure of at least 2 trials of first-line antidepressants given in an adequate dosage for an adequate duration of therapy. In patients with refractory forms of depression, ketamine usually has been given in subanesthetic doses as an IV infusion.

Ketamine has demonstrated rapid and potent antidepressant effects when administered to depressed patients in controlled studies and case series, with improvement in depression reported within several hours to a day following a single IV infusion of the drug. In controlled studies, single, low-dose IV infusions of the drug have resulted in response rates of approximately 37–71% in patients with treatment-resistant depression.

Most depressed patients who respond to a single IV infusion of ketamine experience a relapse of depression within several days to a week or two following the initial infusion. Therefore, multiple-infusion regimens of ketamine (i.e., weekly, biweekly, 3 times weekly) have been studied in depressed patients in open-label as well as blinded studies with encouraging results suggesting that repeated infusions are more effective than a single infusion and can extend the duration of depressive symptom remission. However, the long-term efficacy and safety of repeated infusions of ketamine have not been fully determined to date and further studies are needed to evaluate relapse prevention therapy with the drug. There is some concern that multiple-infusion regimens of ketamine may cause long-term cognitive impairment or neurotoxicity, although no evidence of such impairment has been seen in preliminary studies conducted to date. Some clinicians have suggested that the optimal use of ketamine infusions may be short-term to produce rapid antidepressant and antisuicidal effects until a less invasive relapse prevention strategy for a patient can be implemented.

In addition to its antidepressant effects, randomized controlled studies suggest that ketamine may be helpful in the short-term treatment of suicidal ideation†. In a systematic review and individual participant data meta-analysis, suicidal ideation rapidly decreased (within 1 day) following a single IV infusion of ketamine and the effect lasted for up to 1 week even among patients whose depression did not fully respond to ketamine therapy, suggesting that the drug may have a partially independent antisuicidal effect.

Despite the increasingly widespread use of IV ketamine to treat patients with treatment-resistant depression and suicidality, including in outpatient ketamine infusion centers and psychiatric clinics, some clinicians currently recommend that the drug's use for these psychiatric indications be limited to controlled settings under the care of skilled clinicians. Clinicians and patients should consider enrollment in clinical studies evaluating ketamine's efficacy and safety so that further data can be collected and analyzed to improve clinical practice. (See Dosage and Administration: Administration and see also Cautions: Precautions and Contraindications.)

When considering the use of ketamine for treating mood disorders, the American Psychiatric Association's (APA's) Council of Research Task Force on Novel Biomarkers and Treatments recommends balancing the potential benefits of ketamine infusion therapy with the potential risks of long-term exposure to the drug, including neurotoxicity, cystitis, and abuse potential. (See Uses: Misuse and Abuse and see also Chronic Toxicity.) A thorough pretreatment evaluation process to determine the appropriateness of ketamine therapy is recommended in such cases. If ketamine is prescribed outside of a controlled setting, careful screening, monitoring during treatment, and follow-up of patients are necessary. (See Dosage and Administration: Administration and see also Cautions: Precautions and Contraindications.)

Since conventional oral antidepressants generally require several weeks or months to be effective, the addition of ketamine to oral antidepressant therapy has been suggested as one possible method to produce a more rapid antidepressant response in patients with depression. In a randomized, double-blind, placebo-controlled study, the efficacy and safety of single-infusion ketamine augmentation of oral escitalopram therapy (10 mg daily) were evaluated in 30 outpatients with severe major depressive disorder. Ketamine was given as a single IV infusion (0.5 mg/kg over 40 minutes) on day 1 of escitalopram therapy. At 4 weeks, response occurred in significantly more escitalopram plus ketamine-treated patients than in the escitalopram plus placebo-treated patients (approximately 92 and 57% of patients, respectively). In addition, the escitalopram plus ketamine-treated patients had a shorter mean time to response than the escitalopram plus placebo-treated patients (6 days compared with 27 days).

Some clinicians state that electroconvulsive therapy (ECT) should still be considered as a first-line therapy for patients with refractory depression, and have expressed concern that a trial of single- or multiple-dose ketamine therapy might delay patients from being referred for an ECT consultation. Preliminary experience with the adjunctive use of ketamine in the course of ECT for depression does not suggest improved efficacy or tolerability.

Preliminary evidence suggests that intranasal† ketamine given in 50-mg doses is effective in rapidly improving depressive symptoms in patients with major depressive disorder and generally is well tolerated; however, further study is needed to more clearly determine the efficacy, tolerability, and optimal dosing of this alternative route of administration. The APA's Council of Research Task Force on Novel Biomarkers and Treatments currently advises against the prescription of self-administration of ketamine at home and recommends medical supervision whenever the drug is used pending further accumulation of safety data from controlled settings.

For information on the intranasal use of esketamine hydrochloride, the *S*-enantiomer of racemic ketamine, for treatment-resistant depression, see Esketamine Hydrochloride 28:16.04.92.

■ **Sedation and Analgesia in Critical Care Settings** Ketamine has been used by continuous IV infusion to provide short-term (i.e., less than 24 hours) sedation in critically ill patients† in the intensive care unit (ICU) setting.

However, evidence supporting this use is generally lacking, and other sedative agents (e.g., propofol, midazolam, dexmedetomidine) are more commonly used.

Ketamine also has been used for the management of pain in critically ill patients† in the ICU. Although opiate analgesics generally are considered the first-line drugs of choice for non-neuropathic pain in this setting, some experts state that non-opiate analgesics such as IV ketamine may be used adjunctively to reduce opiate requirements and opiate-related adverse effects.

■ **Misuse and Abuse** Ketamine is a known drug of abuse and is subject to control under the Federal Controlled Substances Act of 1970 as a schedule III drug. The pharmacologic and behavioral effects of ketamine are similar to, but somewhat less intense and shorter in duration than those of phencyclidine (PCP). Ketamine is most commonly abused by nasal insufflation (i.e., snorting) of the powder (evaporated from the injectable liquid), although IV, IM, and oral routes also have been used. Reported desired effects of ketamine include feelings of dissociation and unreality, altered state of consciousness, enhanced sensory perception, hallucinations, intoxication, mild euphoria, and a sensation of floating. Most cases of ketamine abuse have been reported in the context of multidrug or polysubstance abuse. Surveys and studies examining the use pattern of ketamine indicate that abuse of the drug may be more prevalent in certain geographic regions (e.g., Hong Kong). The annual prevalence rate for ketamine use in adolescents (17–18 years of age) in the US was 1.5% in 2012.

Although brief exposure to ketamine in a hospital setting is not likely to cause addiction, the possibility of addiction exists and patients should be individually assessed for their risk. Abuse of ketamine can result in adverse urinary, CNS, and hepatobiliary effects. (See Chronic Toxicity.) The manufacturer states that ketamine should be prescribed and administered with caution because of the risk of abuse.

Dosage and Administration

■ **Administration** Ketamine hydrochloride usually is administered by slow (e.g., over 60 seconds) IV injection, IV infusion, or IM injection. Ketamine also has been administered by oral†, intranasal†, rectal†, subcutaneous†, and intraosseous (IO)† routes. Because of extensive first-pass metabolism, the bioavailability of ketamine following oral or rectal administration is limited (approximately 20–30%). Although ketamine has been administered epidurally† or intrathecally†, there have been concerns about potential neurotoxicity with these routes, and some experts state it may be prudent to avoid neuraxial administration of the drug (see Neurotoxicity under Cautions: Nervous System Effects).

Some experts state that IV administration of ketamine is preferred to IM administration when access can be obtained readily. IM administration is associated with a higher rate of vomiting and longer recovery times compared with IV administration. In addition, IV access can permit convenient administration of additional doses for longer procedures and allow for rapid treatment of adverse effects (e.g., IV benzodiazepines for emergence reactions). In certain patients (e.g., severely agitated or uncooperative patients, young children), IM administration may be preferred.

General Anesthesia When used for general anesthesia, ketamine should be administered by or under the supervision of clinicians experienced in the use of general anesthetic drugs and in the management of possible complications (e.g., airway or respiratory compromise). Appropriate monitoring and resuscitation facilities should be readily available. Because rapid induction of anesthesia occurs following IV injection, patients should be in a supported position during administration. Purposeless and tonic-clonic movements may occur during the course of ketamine anesthesia; however, such movements do not imply a light plane of consciousness and are not indicative of the need for additional doses.

Procedural Sedation When used for procedural sedation in the emergency department, ketamine should be administered by appropriately trained individuals who can safely administer the drug and manage any possible complications (e.g., airway or respiratory compromise). Experts recommend that 2 individuals be present during the procedure (one to perform the procedure and one to monitor the patient). Patients should be continuously observed by a dedicated healthcare professional until recovery is well established. Because ketamine dissociation occurs rapidly, the drug should be administered just prior to initiation of the procedure.

Vomiting Risk Ketamine may be administered in a patient whose stomach is not empty if the benefits outweigh the potential risks. Vomiting has been reported following administration of ketamine and aspiration of gastric contents may occur; although protective laryngeal and pharyngeal reflexes generally are preserved with ketamine, the risk of aspiration must be considered when the drug is administered with other anesthetics and muscle relaxants that may impair such reflexes.

Prophylactic use of antiemetics (e.g., ondansetron) may reduce the rate of ketamine-associated vomiting. (See Cautions: GI Effects.)

Adjunctive Benzodiazepine Therapy Concomitant administration of benzodiazepines (e.g., diazepam, midazolam) may reduce the incidence of psychotomimetic manifestations during emergence from ketamine anesthesia, and is recommended in adults; however, because such benefit has not been observed in children and because the incidence of emergence reactions is much lower in children than in adults, routine use of prophylactic benzodiazepines is not recommended in pediatric patients. Benzodiazepines may be used to terminate unpleasant psychotomimetic reactions, should they occur, in adults and children.

The manufacturer states that a reduced dosage of ketamine supplemented with diazepam may be used in conjunction with other agents (e.g., nitrous oxide, oxygen) to produce balanced anesthesia. However, if ketamine hydrochloride and diazepam are used concurrently, the drugs should be administered separately, and should *not* be admixed in the same syringe or infusion container. (See Chemistry and Stability: Stability.)

Adjunctive Anticholinergic Therapy Anticholinergic agents (e.g., atropine, glycopyrrolate) may be administered prior to or concomitantly with ketamine to reduce hypersalivation and risk of laryngospasm; however, evidence to support a clinically important benefit or harm from routine anticholinergic prophylaxis is lacking, and some experts recommend that such therapy be reserved for patients with clinically important hypersalivation or impaired ability to mobilize secretions.

Treatment-resistant Depression and Suicidality When ketamine is used by IV infusion for the treatment of severe and treatment-resistant depression and suicidality†, the drug should be administered by experienced clinicians in facilities in which adequate monitoring for possible adverse reactions (e.g., altered cardiovascular and respiratory function, acute dissociative and psychotomimetic effects) and management of such reactions are possible.

Dilution Ketamine hydrochloride is commercially available as an injection containing 10, 50, or 100 mg/mL of ketamine for IV or IM use. The 100-mg/mL concentration should *not* be administered IV without proper dilution; the commercially available injection concentrate must be diluted with an equal volume of sterile water for injection, 0.9% sodium chloride injection, or 5% dextrose injection prior to IV injection.

For IV infusion, a diluted solution containing 1 mg of ketamine per mL (1 mg/mL) may be prepared by adding 500 mg of ketamine (10 mL from a vial labeled as containing 50 mg/mL of ketamine or 5 mL from a vial labeled as containing 100 mg/mL of ketamine) to an infusion bag containing 500 mL of 0.9% sodium chloride injection or 5% dextrose injection. In patients requiring fluid restriction, a 2-mg/mL solution may be prepared by adding 500 mg of ketamine (10 mL from a vial labeled as containing 50 mg/mL of ketamine or 5 mL from a vial labeled as containing 100 mg/mL of ketamine) to an infusion bag containing 250 mL of 0.9% sodium chloride injection or 5% dextrose injection. The manufacturer states that the 10-mg/mL vial of ketamine hydrochloride is not recommended for dilution; however, some stability studies have used ketamine hydrochloride solutions prepared by diluting a 10-mg/mL solution of the drug with 0.9% sodium chloride injection.

Rate of Administration Because rapid IV administration can cause respiratory depression, IV injections of ketamine should be administered slowly (e.g., over 60 seconds).

For dissociative sedation in emergency department settings, IV administration over 30–60 seconds has been recommended.

When ketamine is administered in a regimen with diazepam for induction of anesthesia, the manufacturer states that the drug may be administered by IV injection at a rate of 0.5 mg/kg per minute; for maintenance of anesthesia, ketamine may be administered by IV infusion at a rate of 0.1–0.5 mg/minute.

When ketamine is used in subanesthetic doses for acute pain†, some clinicians have recommended that the drug be administered as a short IV infusion over 15 minutes.

When ketamine is administered in subanesthetic doses for the treatment of severe and treatment-resistant depression and/or suicidality†, the drug is usually given as an IV infusion over 40 minutes. Although shorter and longer infusion rates have been used in some patients, clinical experience is too limited to recommend an alternative infusion rate at this time.

■ **Dosage** Dosage of ketamine hydrochloride is expressed in terms of ketamine.

Dose-dependency of Effects Dosage of ketamine depends on the intended use and desired pharmacologic effect. At low doses, ketamine produces analgesia and sedation, and at higher doses, the drug produces a state of dissociative anesthesia. Ketamine has a dosing threshold at which dissociation occurs (see Anesthetic Effects under Pharmacology: CNS Effects); doses at or above the threshold are referred to as "dissociative" or "anesthetic," and doses below this threshold are referred to as "subdissociative" or "subanesthetic." Although specific dosing ranges have not been established, dissociation generally appears at an IV dose of approximately 1–1.5 mg/kg or an IM dose of approximately 3–5 mg/kg. Once the dissociative threshold has been reached, additional administration of ketamine will not enhance or deepen sedation.

Induction and Maintenance of Anesthesia As with other general anesthetics, individual response to ketamine is variable and can depend on factors such as dosage, route of administration, patient age, or concomitant drugs. Dosage should be individualized based on therapeutic response and the patient's anesthetic needs. In general, higher doses of ketamine correspond with longer times to complete recovery from anesthesia.

Adult Dosage. For induction of anesthesia in adults, the manufacturer recommends an initial IV ketamine dose of 1–4.5 mg/kg (administered by slow IV injection over 60 seconds) or an initial IM dose of 6.5–13 mg/kg. On average, an IV dose of 2 mg/kg will produce surgical anesthesia for 5–10 minutes and an IM dose of 10 mg/kg will produce surgical anesthesia for 12–25 minutes.

For maintenance of anesthesia in adults, additional IV doses of 0.5–4.5 mg/kg or IM doses of 3.25–13 mg/kg may be administered as needed. A continuous IV infusion of 1–6 mg/kg per hour also has been recommended for maintenance of anesthesia. The maintenance dosage should be adjusted based on the patient's anesthetic requirements and concomitant use of other anesthetic agents.

Alternatively, the manufacturer states that the incidence of psychologic manifestations during emergence, particularly dream-like observations and emergence delirium, may be reduced by using an induction regimen consisting of ketamine (1–2 mg/kg administered IV at a rate of 0.5 mg/kg per minute) augmented with diazepam (doses of 2–5 mg administered by IV injection over 60 seconds in a separate syringe). For maintenance of anesthesia using this augmented regimen, ketamine may be administered by IV infusion at a rate of 0.1–0.5 mg/minute and diazepam (2–5 mg) may be administered by IV injection in a separate syringe as needed. A total diazepam dosage of no more than 15 mg usually is sufficient for induction, and a total diazepam dosage of no more than 20 mg usually is sufficient for combined induction and maintenance; however, higher amounts may be required depending on factors such as the type and duration of the procedure or physical status of the patient.

Pediatric Dosage. In general, pediatric patients require higher doses of ketamine compared with adults, although there is considerable interpatient variability in dosing requirements.

Some experts recommend an initial IV ketamine dose of 1–3 mg/kg for induction of anesthesia in pediatric patients†; supplemental IV doses of 0.5–1 mg/kg may be given if clinically indicated. The recommended IM dose of ketamine for induction of anesthesia in pediatric patients is 5–10 mg/kg. Because of possible airway complications, some experts state that ketamine is contraindicated in infants younger than 3 months of age.

Procedural Sedation **Adult Dosage.** For dissociative sedation in adults undergoing short painful or emotionally disturbing procedures in the emergency department, the usual IV dose of ketamine is 1 mg/kg administered by IV injection over 30–60 seconds. Dissociative sedation is usually achieved with a single IV loading dose; however, if sedation is inadequate or a prolonged period of sedation is needed for longer procedures, additional IV doses of 0.5–1 mg/kg may be administered every 5–15 minutes as needed. Lower IV doses of ketamine (e.g., 0.2–0.75 mg/kg) also have been used to produce analgesia, particularly if a dissociative effect is not required for the procedure.

Although the IM route is not preferred in adults, some experts state that an IM dose of 4–5 mg/kg may be administered; additional doses of 2–5 mg/kg may be given after 5–10 minutes if initial sedation is inadequate or additional doses are needed for longer procedures. Lower IM doses of ketamine (e.g., 0.4–2 mg/kg) also have been used, particularly if a dissociative effect is not required for the procedure.

Pediatric Dosage. For dissociative sedation in pediatric patients† 3 months of age or older undergoing short painful or emotionally disturbing procedures in the emergency department, some experts state that the usual IV dose of ketamine is 1.5–2 mg/kg administered by IV injection over 30–60 seconds. Dissociative sedation is usually achieved with a single IV loading dose; however, if initial sedation is inadequate or prolonged sedation is necessary for longer procedures, additional incremental IV doses of 0.5–1 mg/kg may be administered every 5–15 minutes as needed. These experts state that the minimum IV dose that will reliably elicit the dissociative state in children is 1.5 mg/kg; however, lower IV doses (e.g., 0.25–1 mg/kg) also have been used successfully to provide adequate procedural sedation in pediatric patients, particularly if a dissociative effect is not required for the procedure.

The recommended IM dose of ketamine for dissociative sedation in pediatric patients† 3 months of age or older undergoing short painful or emotionally disturbing procedures in the emergency department is 4–5 mg/kg. Although dissociative sedation is usually achieved with a single IM dose, additional doses of 2–5 mg/kg may be administered after 5–10 minutes if initial sedation is inadequate or additional doses are needed for longer procedures. Although some experts state that the minimum IM dose that will reliably elicit the dissociative state in children is 4–5 mg/kg, lower IM doses (e.g., 1–2 mg/kg) also have been used successfully, particularly if a dissociative effect is not required for the procedure.

Sedation and Analgesia in Critical Care Settings For sedation and analgesia in critically ill adults† with severe pain unresponsive to conventional therapies, initial IV ketamine doses of 0.1–0.5 mg/kg followed by IV infusion of 0.05–0.4 mg/kg per hour (0.83–6.67 mcg/kg per minute) have been recommended by some experts as an adjunct to opiates; other dosage regimens also have been used. If additional pain control is needed, additional IV doses may be administered up to a maximum of 0.5 mg/kg; alternatively, the infusion rate may be titrated in increments of 0.06 mg/kg per hour (1 mcg/kg per minute) every 15 minutes up to a maximum of 1.2 mg/kg per hour (20 mcg/kg per minute) as tolerated.

Pain Ketamine is used in low (i.e., subanesthetic or subdissociative) dosages for the management of pain; however, a dosage range that is considered subanesthetic has not been consistently defined. Most acute pain studies used IV bolus doses less than 0.5 mg/kg and infusion rates of 0.5 mg/kg per hour or less; however, there is wide variability in the dosage ranges and routes of administration used.

Postoperative Pain. For the management of postoperative pain† in pediatric patients and adults, IV ketamine bolus doses ranging from 0.1–0.5 mg/kg with or without continuous IV infusion (at rates usually ranging from 0.1–0.6 mg/kg per hour [1.67–10 mcg/kg per minute]) have been commonly used in clinical studies; however, dosages and timing of administration in relation to the surgical procedure varied widely in these studies and the optimum dosage regimen is not known. Some experts state that there is moderate evidence supporting the use of IV ketamine bolus doses up to 0.35 mg/kg and IV infusions up to 1 mg/kg per hour (16.67 mcg/kg per minute) as an adjunct to opiates for perioperative analgesia. In several studies, administration of a single IV ketamine dose of 0.5 mg/kg (alone or in combination with other analgesics) was effective in achieving postoperative pain control in children undergoing tonsillectomy. Because of possible airway complications, some experts state that ketamine is contraindicated in infants younger than 3 months of age.

IM administration of analgesic agents for postoperative pain is not recommended because of unreliable absorption and substantial pain at the site of injection.

Acute Pain. For the management of acute pain† in the emergency department and prehospital settings, the usual IV dose of ketamine is 0.1–0.3 mg/kg administered as a slow IV injection or short IV infusion over 10–15 minutes based on studies conducted principally in adults; although longer infusions of ketamine are rare in this setting, continuous IV infusions of 0.1–0.3 mg/kg per hour (1.67–5 mcg/kg per minute) have been used. Non-weight-based IV ketamine doses ranging from 10–20 mg also have been used in clinical studies of ketamine for the treatment of acute pain in adults. When ketamine is used for acute pain in settings without intensive monitoring, some experts state that IV bolus doses should not exceed 0.35 mg/kg and infusion rates generally should not exceed 1 mg/kg per hour (16.67 mcg/kg per minute), but also acknowledge that higher or lower doses may be necessary due to interindividual differences in response.

Because of possible airway complications, some experts state that ketamine is contraindicated in infants younger than 3 months of age.

Ketamine may be administered IM for acute pain in the emergency department or prehospital settings; however, experts state that a dosage range has not been definitively established and analgesic effects are less predictable when the drug is administered by IM injection.

Chronic Pain. Although there is no consensus on dosages or administration protocols for ketamine in patients with chronic pain†, the drug generally is administered in subanesthetic doses by IV infusion. There is some evidence suggesting that administration of higher dosages over longer periods and more frequent infusions may provide more benefit. Some experts state that it is reasonable to initiate a single outpatient infusion of ketamine at a minimum dose of 80 mg for at least 2 hours and then reassess before initiating further treatments. In a study in children and adolescents 12–17 years of age with chronic pain conditions (e.g., chronic headache, fibromyalgia, complex regional pain syndrome), ketamine was administered by continuous IV infusion at a rate of 0.1–0.3 mg/kg per hour for 4–8 hours each day up to a maximum of 16 hours (in total, up to a maximum of 3 consecutive days). Children with severe cancer-related pain have been treated with IV infusions of ketamine at 0.1–1 mg/kg per hour. Based on limited evidence, IV ketamine bolus doses up to 0.35 mg/kg followed by IV infusions of 0.5–2 mg/kg per hour have been recommended by some experts for the management of chronic pain; however, higher (e.g., up to 7 mg/kg per hour for the treatment of refractory pain) or lower (e.g., 0.1–0.5 mg/kg per hour) infusion rates also have been used.

Treatment-resistant Depression and Suicidality For severe and treatment-resistant depression and suicidality† in adults, ketamine usually is given as a low-dose (i.e., subanesthetic dose) IV infusion of 0.5 mg/kg over 40 minutes. Obese patients (i.e., body mass index [BMI] of 30 or higher) appear to be at increased risk for ketamine-associated hypertension and other adverse hemodynamic effects and potentially may benefit from adjusting the ketamine dosage to their calculated ideal body weight rather than actual body weight; further clinical experience to determine optimal dosing in such patients is needed. There is limited evidence that higher ketamine infusion dosages (e.g., 0.75 mg/kg) may be necessary in certain chronically ill and/or severely treatment-resistant patients, but further study is needed to determine the efficacy and safety of such higher-dosage regimens.

There currently is limited clinical experience with longer-term (multiple-dose) ketamine infusion therapy for treatment-resistant depression and suicidality; however, IV infusions of ketamine have been given once, twice, or 3 times weekly for the first 2 weeks during the acute treatment phase in some patients and sometimes have been continued once or twice weekly for another 2–4 weeks during the continuation phase for a total of 4–6 weeks of therapy or gradually tapered. Patients who do not initially respond to several infusions of ketamine appear unlikely to respond to subsequent infusions. Discontinuance of ketamine therapy is recommended by some experts if the interval between infusions cannot be extended to one week or longer by the second month of treatment; these experts state that the goal should be to eventually taper and discontinue ketamine treatment until additional long-term safety data with the drug become available.

Cautions

Ketamine generally is well tolerated; however, the drug can cause adverse effects as a result of its actions on a variety of receptors (e.g., *N*-methyl-D-aspartic acid [NMDA], acetylcholine, opiate, monoaminergic, histaminic).

■ Nervous System Effects

Like phencyclidine (PCP), ketamine, a PCP derivative, may cause psychotomimetic effects. When given in low (subanesthetic) doses, ketamine can produce mild cognitive, psychotic, and mood disturbances that are usually transient and limited to the time of administration; symptoms that have been reported include feelings of inebriation, positive and negative schizophrenic symptoms, dissociative symptoms, mania, confusion, lowered inhibition, perceptual disturbances, and impairments in attention, learning, and memory. At higher doses, ketamine can produce more severe schizophrenic-like symptoms, vivid hallucinations, psychosis, feelings of an "out of body" experience, mental confusion, hyperexcitability, and catalepsy.

Long-term use of ketamine can cause persistent neuropsychiatric symptoms, cognitive impairment, and psychologic abnormalities.

When used for treatment-resistant depression and suicidality, acute dissociative and psychotomimetic effects (e.g., psychotic symptoms) have been reported with IV infusions of ketamine. Such effects generally occur only during and immediately following ketamine infusion and resolve within 2–4 hours following the end of the infusion, are generally mild in severity, and are well tolerated. Clinical experience to date suggests that dissociative symptoms occur more commonly than psychotomimetic effects when ketamine is used in patients with treatment-resistant depression. (See Cautions: Precautions and Contraindications.)

Increased intracranial pressure has been reported following administration of ketamine as a result of cerebral vasodilation; however, cerebral perfusion may be increased.

Emergence Reactions Emergence reactions have been reported during recovery in patients receiving ketamine anesthesia; the manufacturer reports an incidence of approximately 12% for such emergence reactions, although higher rates have been reported in the published literature. Emergence reactions occur more frequently in adults (approximately 30–50%) than in pediatric patients (approximately 5–15%). A reduced risk has been observed in geriatric patients (older than 65 years of age) relative to younger adults and in patients who have previously received the drug.

Emergence manifestations vary in severity from pleasant to unpleasant dream-like states, vivid imagery, hallucinations, alterations in mood and body image, floating sensations, extracorporeal (out-of-body) experiences, and emergence delirium; in some cases, these states have been accompanied by confusion, excitement, and irrational behavior, which some patients recall as an unpleasant experience. The duration of such reactions is generally no more than a few hours; however, recurrences have occurred up to 24 hours following anesthesia. The manufacturer states that no residual psychologic effects have been reported from ketamine use.

Emergence reactions may be less frequent when ketamine is given IM. (See Cautions: Precautions and Contraindications.)

Neurotoxicity Animal studies suggest that ketamine may be neurotoxic when given intrathecally; however, pathologic findings were not observed in studies in which the preservative was omitted from the ketamine preparation. Studies evaluating this potential adverse effect of ketamine are lacking in humans.

■ **Cardiovascular Effects** Adverse cardiovascular effects of ketamine generally are a result of the drug's sympathomimetic effects. Mild to moderate increases in blood pressure, heart rate, and cardiac output can occur following administration of anesthetic or subanesthetic doses. Palpitations also have been reported with the drug.

Elevated blood pressure and/or heart rate may occur during IV infusions of ketamine for treatment-resistant depression and suicidality; these hemodynamic effects usually are transient and subside following completion of the IV infusion. Transient but significantly elevated blood pressure occurred in nearly one-third of ketamine-treated patients in one study. Short-term antihypertensive therapy sometimes has been used to treat ketamine infusion-associated blood pressure elevations in this and other studies.

Hypotension, bradycardia, and arrhythmia have been reported infrequently with ketamine. Precipitation of angina also has been reported. (See Cautions: Precautions and Contraindications.)

■ **Respiratory Effects** Adverse respiratory effects are rare with ketamine. When given in anesthetic doses, clinically important respiratory depression usually does not occur. Respiration is frequently stimulated; however, transient respiratory depression and apnea have been reported following rapid IV administration of the drug.

Ketamine can cause excessive secretions through stimulation of central cholinergic receptors; such increased secretions may cause laryngospasm or other airway obstruction.

Airway or respiratory complications have been reported in about 3.9% of pediatric patients receiving ketamine for dissociative sedation in the emergency department; transient apnea and respiratory depression have been reported in about 0.8% and transient laryngospasm has been reported in about 0.3% of pediatric patients in this setting.

When used in subanesthetic doses for the treatment of depression in otherwise healthy individuals, ketamine usually does not cause clinically important adverse respiratory effects.

■ **Musculoskeletal Effects** Skeletal muscle hypertonicity is a common adverse effect of ketamine and may manifest as involuntary random, purposeless, and/or tonic-clonic movements resembling seizures.

Clonus, hiccups, and hyperreflexia also have been reported following ketamine administration.

■ **Genitourinary Effects** Lower urinary tract and bladder symptoms including dysuria, urinary frequency, urgency, urge incontinence, cystitis, hematuria, and postmicturition pain have been reported in patients receiving ketamine. Pathologic changes (e.g., epithelial damage) also have been observed. In most cases, urologic symptoms have been associated with chronic ketamine use or abuse. (See Chronic Toxicity.)

■ **GI Effects** Nausea and vomiting are reported frequently in patients receiving ketamine. Vomiting has been reported in approximately 8% of pediatric patients and 5–15% of adults receiving ketamine for dissociative sedation in emergency department settings. In children, a higher incidence of vomiting (up to 33% depending on the route of administration) has been reported in the postoperative setting. Vomiting generally occurs well into the recovery period when the patient is alert and can clear the airway without assistance, but also may occur after the patient is discharged. The incidence of vomiting is highest in early adolescent patients and also may be more frequent with IM compared with IV administration.

There is some evidence suggesting that prophylactic use of antiemetics (e.g., ondansetron) may reduce the risk of ketamine-associated vomiting in pediatric patients receiving ketamine for procedural sedation. However, the effect appears to be modest and has not been consistently demonstrated in clinical studies. One approach that has been recommended is to administer prophylactic antiemetics only in those patients at highest baseline risk for vomiting (i.e., early adolescents).

Ketamine increases salivary secretions, which can cause laryngospasm; however, clinically important hypersalivation resulting in airway complications has been reported rarely.

Anorexia also has been reported in patients receiving ketamine.

■ **Hepatobiliary Effects** Elevated hepatic enzyme concentrations may occur with anesthetic and subanesthetic doses of ketamine, particularly following prolonged infusion and/or repeated doses within a short time frame. Hepatotoxicity has been reported following longer-term use (e.g., more than 3–4 days). Increased hepatic enzyme concentrations have been reported in approximately 10% of patients receiving repetitive low doses or continuous high doses of ketamine infusions clinically. In a small study in patients receiving IV infusions of *S*-ketamine for chronic pain, hepatic enzyme elevations up to 3 times the upper limit of normal occurred following a second exposure to the drug. Hepatic enzyme concentrations generally return to baseline over several months. (See Chronic Toxicity.)

■ **Ocular Effects** Nystagmus and diplopia occur frequently following administration of ketamine. Elevation of intraocular pressure (IOP) also may occur. Blurred vision and pupillary dilation have been reported with subanesthetic doses of ketamine. Transient blindness also has been reported.

■ **Dermatologic and Sensitivity Reactions** Transient erythema and morbilliform rash have been reported in patients receiving ketamine. Anaphylaxis also has been reported.

■ **Local Effects** Injection-site reactions (e.g., pain, erythema, rash) have been reported infrequently in patients receiving ketamine.

■ **Precautions and Contraindications** Ketamine hydrochloride should be administered only by or under the supervision of individuals who are experienced with its use and potential complications.

When used in anesthetic doses that may render patients unresponsive, administration of ketamine should occur in a monitored setting in the presence of personnel trained in advanced airway management and cardiovascular life support; resuscitative equipment should be readily available. When used in subanesthetic doses in the emergency department, adverse effects generally are mild and self-limiting; therefore, some experts state that ketamine administration may follow the same procedures and policies used for other analgesics in the emergency department. However, local protocols should be consulted since expectations may differ by institution.

When used in subanesthetic doses for the short-term treatment of mood disorders, ketamine generally appears to be well tolerated; however, adverse cardiovascular and CNS effects may occur. Therefore, some experts recommend that ketamine infusions only be given for mood disorders in settings in which adequate monitoring for possible adverse effects (e.g., altered cardiovascular and respiratory function, acute dissociative and psychotomimetic effects) and management of such reactions are possible.

CNS Precautions Because ketamine can cause sedation and potentially impair cognitive function, patients should be cautioned not to operate hazardous machinery, including driving a motor vehicle, or engage in potentially dangerous activities for at least 24 hours after anesthesia, depending on the dosage of ketamine administered and consideration of other drugs used during the procedure. The duration of ketamine administration also should be considered, especially in cases where early discharge is possible. When repeated administration of ketamine is used in treating patients with mood disorders, some experts recommend that assessment of cognitive function be considered.

Ketamine can exacerbate schizophrenia, and generally should be avoided in patients with schizophrenia or active psychosis. Although data are limited, caution is advised when ketamine is used for procedural sedation or acute pain in patients with other psychiatric disorders, including substance abuse-induced psychosis.

Emergence Reactions Emergence reactions may occur during the recovery period in patients receiving ketamine anesthesia. The incidence of emergence reactions may be reduced if verbal and tactile stimulation of the patient is minimized during the recovery period; however, this should not preclude appropriate monitoring of vital signs. Prophylactic administration of benzodiazepines (e.g., diazepam, midazolam) may reduce the incidence of ketamine-induced psychotomimetic manifestations during emergence and the manufacturer suggests a regimen using a decreased dosage of ketamine in conjunction with a benzodiazepine (e.g., diazepam, midazolam) during induction and maintenance of anesthesia. (See Dosage and Administration.) Benzodiazepines also may be used to terminate severe or unpleasant emergence reactions.

Patients should be informed that they may experience psychologic manifestations as the effects of ketamine wear off, and that these effects may vary in severity and range from pleasant dream-like states to hallucinations, confusion, and unpleasant experiences.

When ketamine is used on an outpatient basis, patients should not be released until complete recovery from anesthesia occurs, after which patients should then be accompanied by a responsible adult.

Cardiovascular Precautions Because ketamine has a stimulating effect on the cardiovascular system, elevations in blood pressure and heart rate can occur. Ketamine should be used with caution or avoided in patients with known or suspected cardiac conditions that may be exacerbated by the sympathomimetic effects of the drug (e.g., unstable angina, coronary artery disease, myocardial infarction [MI], congestive heart failure, hypertension).

The manufacturer states that ketamine is contraindicated in patients in whom a substantial elevation of blood pressure would constitute a serious hazard, and that cardiac function should be continuously monitored in patients who experience hypertension or cardiac decompensation during ketamine anesthesia.

Because sympathomimetic effects may be increased in patients with porphyria or hyperthyroidism, or in those receiving thyroid replacement therapy, some experts state that ketamine should be used with caution or avoided in such patients.

Respiratory Precautions Although respiration is frequently stimulated, respiratory depression or apnea may occur following rapid IV administration or overdosage of ketamine. If respiratory depression occurs, respiratory support (e.g., mechanical ventilation) should be provided. IV injections of ketamine should be administered slowly (e.g., over 60 seconds).

Laryngospasm and other forms of airway obstruction may occur during ketamine administration; therefore, clinicians should be prepared to rapidly identify and manage such complications (e.g., with assisted ventilation, oxygen, and possible intubation). Major stimulation of the posterior pharynx (e.g., endoscopy) may increase the risk of laryngospasm; therefore, the manufacturer states that ketamine should not be used alone during surgery or diagnostic procedures of the pharynx, larynx, or bronchial tree. If the drug is used alone, mechanical stimulation of the pharynx should be avoided whenever possible. Muscle relaxants, with proper maintenance of respiration, may be required in these situations.

Although the risk of laryngospasm is low with minor oropharyngeal procedures typically performed in the emergency department, efforts should be made to avoid vigorous stimulation of the posterior pharynx and accumulation of secretions or blood during these procedures.

Some experts state that ketamine should be used with caution or avoided in patients with active pulmonary infection or disease (e.g., upper respiratory infection, asthma) because such conditions may increase the risk of laryngospasm (particularly in children).

Because of a potential increased risk of airway complications, ketamine should be used with caution or avoided in patients with a history of airway instability, tracheal surgery, or tracheal stenosis.

Hepatic Precautions Prolonged effects of ketamine may occur in patients with hepatic impairment. Some experts recommend that ketamine use should be avoided or limited in patients with severe hepatic disease or cirrhosis, and that the drug should be used with caution (e.g., with monitoring of liver function tests) in patients with moderate hepatic disease. Discontinuance of ketamine therapy is recommended if hepatotoxicity occurs.

Alcohol Precautions Ketamine should be used with caution or avoided in patients with chronic alcoholism or acute alcohol intoxication.

Visceral Pain Precautions If ketamine is used in patients undergoing surgical procedures involving visceral pain pathways, the drug should be supplemented with an agent that obtunds visceral pain.

Intracranial Pressure and Head Injury Precautions The manufacturer states that ketamine should be used with extreme caution in patients with elevated intracranial pressure and some experts state that the drug should be avoided in such patients. However, there is some controversy regarding the use of ketamine in patients with head trauma. Despite concerns of increased intracranial pressure, cerebral perfusion is maintained and there is evidence that ketamine can be safely and effectively used in patients with head injuries or risk of intracranial hypertension.

Studies suggest that intracranial pressure increases are minimal in patients with normal ventilation and are associated with concomitant elevations in cerebral perfusion. In a systematic review of data from studies using ketamine in mechanically ventilated patients with traumatic brain injury, ketamine was not associated with increased intracranial pressure; in some cases, intracranial pressure was decreased.

Because of concerns about increased intracranial pressure, some experts state that ketamine should be used with caution or avoided in patients with CNS masses, abnormalities, or hydrocephalus.

Ocular Precautions Because ketamine can increase intraocular pressure (IOP), some experts state that the drug should be used with caution or avoided in patients with elevated IOP (e.g., glaucoma, acute globe injury).

Genitourinary Precautions Because ketamine has been associated with disorders of the urinary tract (including cystitis), particularly with long-term use, interruption of ketamine therapy should be considered in patients experiencing urinary symptoms (e.g., urinary frequency, urge incontinence, dysuria, hematuria, lower abdominal pain) without evidence of infection, and the patient should be evaluated by a specialist. The manufacturer states that discontinuance of ketamine should be considered if genitourinary pain continues in the setting of other genitourinary symptoms.

Some experts advise that patients receiving long-term ketamine therapy for mood disorders be assessed for urinary symptoms such as discomfort during therapy.

Misuse and Abuse The manufacturer states that ketamine should be prescribed and administered with caution because of the risk of abuse. (See Uses: Misuse and Abuse.) Tolerance and dependence may develop following prolonged administration of the drug. Because of the risk of abuse or diversion, careful monitoring and supervision are recommended during ketamine use.

Sensitivity Reactions The manufacturer states that ketamine is contraindicated in patients with known hypersensitivity to the drug.

■ **Pediatric Precautions** Although the manufacturer states that safety and efficacy of ketamine have not been established in patients younger than 16 years of age, the drug has been used widely in pediatric patients† in a variety of clinical settings for anesthesia, procedural sedation and analgesia, postoperative analgesia, and chronic pain management. Ketamine frequently is used in children to facilitate painful procedures in the emergency department and is considered a drug of choice for this use. Ketamine may be particularly useful in pediatric patients because the drug may be administered IM.

Ketamine may be preferred for induction of anesthesia in children with congenital heart disease with right-to-left shunt† because of its sympathomimetic effects and hemodynamic stability.

Ketamine generally should *not* be used in infants younger than 3 months of age because of the potential increased risk of airway complications (e.g., airway obstruction, laryngospasm, apnea) thought to be due to age-specific differences in airway reactivity and anatomy.

Neurodevelopmental and Cognitive Effects Prolonged use of general anesthetics and sedation drugs, including ketamine, in children younger than 3 years of age or during the third trimester of pregnancy may affect brain development. Animal studies in multiple species, including nonhuman primates, have demonstrated that use for longer than 3 hours of anesthetic and sedation drugs that block *N*-methyl-D-aspartic acid (NMDA) receptors and/or potentiate γ-aminobutyric acid (GABA) activity leads to widespread neuronal and oligodendrocyte cell loss and alterations in synaptic morphology and neurogenesis in the developing brain, resulting in long-term deficits in cognition and behavior. Across animal species, vulnerability to these neurodevelopmental changes occurs during the period of rapid brain growth or synaptogenesis; this period is thought to correlate with the third trimester of pregnancy through the first year of life in humans, but may extend to approximately 3 years of age. The clinical relevance of these animal findings to humans is not known.

While some published evidence suggests that similar deficits in cognition and behavior may occur in children following repeated or prolonged exposure to anesthesia early in life, other studies have found no association between pediatric anesthesia exposure and long-term adverse neurodevelopmental outcomes. Most studies to date have had substantial limitations, and it is not clear whether the adverse neurodevelopmental outcomes observed in children were related to the drug or to other factors (e.g., surgery, underlying illness). There is some clinical evidence that a single, relatively brief exposure to general anesthesia in generally healthy children is unlikely to cause clinically detectable deficits in global cognitive function or serious behavioral disorders; however, further research is needed to fully characterize the effects of exposure to general anesthetics in early life, particularly for prolonged or repeated exposures and in more vulnerable populations (e.g., less healthy children).

Results from an observational study (the Pediatric Anesthesia Neurodevelopment Assessment [PANDA] study) and preliminary results from an ongoing multicenter, randomized trial (the General Anesthesia Compared to Spinal Anesthesia [GAS] trial) provide some evidence that a single, relatively brief exposure to general anesthesia in generally healthy children is unlikely to cause clinically detectable deficits in global cognitive function or serious behavioral disorders. The PANDA study compared global cognitive function (as measured by intelligence quotient [IQ] score) of children 8–15 years of age who had a single anesthesia exposure for elective inguinal hernia surgery before the age of 3 years with that of a biologically related sibling who had no anesthesia exposure before the age of 3 years. All of the children had a gestational age at birth of at least 36 weeks, and sibling pairs were within 3 years of being the same age. Children who underwent the elective procedure were mostly males (90%) and generally healthy. The mean duration of anesthesia was 84 minutes; 16% of those receiving anesthesia had exposures exceeding 2 hours. The study found no substantial difference in IQ score between children who had a single anesthesia exposure before the age of 3 years and their siblings who had not. The GAS trial was designed to compare neurodevelopmental outcomes in children who received general anesthesia with those in children who received awake regional (caudal and/or spinal) anesthesia for inguinal herniorrhaphy before they reached a postmenstrual age of 60 weeks (with a gestational age at birth of more than 26 weeks); the primary outcome was the Wechsler Preschool and Primary Scale of Intelligence Third Edition (WPPSI-III) Full Scale IQ at 5 years of age. In an interim analysis at the age of 2 years, no difference in composite cognitive score (as measured by the Bayley Scales of Infant and Toddler Development III) was detected between children who had received sevoflurane anesthesia of less than 1 hour's duration (median duration: 54 minutes) compared with those who had received awake regional anesthesia.

Anesthetic and sedation drugs are an essential component of care for children and pregnant women who require surgery or other procedures that cannot be delayed; no specific general anesthetic or sedation drug has been shown to be less likely to cause neurocognitive deficits than any other such drug. Pending further accumulation of data in humans from well-designed studies, decisions regarding the timing of elective procedures requiring anesthesia should take into consideration both the benefits of the procedure and the potential risks. When procedures requiring the use of general anesthetics or sedation drugs are considered for young children or pregnant women, clinicians should discuss with the patient, parent, or caregiver the benefits, risks (including potential risk of adverse neurodevelopmental effects), and appropriate timing and duration of the procedure. FDA states that procedures that are considered medically necessary should not be delayed or avoided.

■ **Geriatric Precautions** While reported clinical experience to date has not revealed age-related differences in response to ketamine when used as an anesthetic agent, clinical studies have not included sufficient numbers of adults 65 years of age or older to determine whether geriatric patients respond differently than younger adults. A reduced risk of emergence reactions has been observed in geriatric patients older than 65 years of age relative to younger adults. When ketamine is used as an anesthetic agent in geriatric patients, the dosage should be selected carefully, usually starting at the low end of the dosing range, because of the greater frequency of age-related decreases in hepatic, renal, and/or cardiac function, and of concomitant disease or other drug therapy.

■ **Mutagenicity and Carcinogenicity** Long-term animal studies have not been conducted to evaluate the carcinogenic potential of ketamine.

Data are insufficient to evaluate the genotoxic potential of ketamine. Ketamine was clastogenic in an in vitro chromosomal aberration assay. However, unpublished data using *S*-ketamine did not reveal any evidence of genotoxic effects.

■ **Pregnancy, Fertility, and Lactation** There are no adequate and well-controlled studies of ketamine in pregnant women. Although ketamine has been used for induction of anesthesia during vaginal delivery and caesarean sections, the manufacturer states that the drug is not recommended for use during pregnancy or delivery because safety has not been established. Some neonates exposed to ketamine at maternal IV doses of 1.5 mg/kg or higher during delivery have experienced respiratory depression and low Apgar scores requiring resuscitation. Marked increases in maternal blood pressure and uterine tone have been observed following administration of IV ketamine doses greater than 2 mg/kg.

In animal reproduction studies using IM ketamine doses approximately 0.3–0.6 times the usual human dose of 10 mg/kg (based on body surface area), developmental delays, skeletal hypoplasia, and increased fetal resorptions were observed.

Based on animal data, repeated or prolonged use of general anesthetics and sedation drugs, including ketamine, during the third trimester of pregnancy may result in adverse neurodevelopmental effects in the fetus. The clinical relevance of these animal findings to humans is not known; the potential risk of adverse neurodevelopmental effects should be considered and discussed with pregnant women undergoing procedures requiring general anesthetics and sedation drugs. (See Neurodevelopmental and Cognitive Effects under Cautions: Pediatric Precautions.)

Reproduction studies in female and male rats given IV ketamine doses of 10 mg/kg (approximately 0.8 times the average human ketamine induction dose of 2 mg/kg based on body surface area) prior to mating did not reveal any evidence of impaired fertility.

It is not known whether ketamine is distributed into milk. Because the drug should be undetectable in plasma approximately 11 hours after administration, nursing after this time period should not expose the infant to clinically relevant amounts of ketamine.

Drug Interactions

■ **Drugs and Foods Affecting Hepatic Microsomal Enzymes**

The biotransformation of ketamine and its norketamine metabolite is mediated by cytochrome P-450 (CYP) isoenzymes, principally by CYP3A4 with lesser involvement by CYP2B6 and CYP2C9. (See Pharmacokinetics: Elimination.) Therefore, drugs that inhibit or induce these CYP isoenzymes, particularly CYP3A4, may increase or decrease, respectively, the systemic exposure of ketamine or norketamine.

Grapefruit Juice In healthy individuals, concomitant administration of the CYP3A4 inhibitor grapefruit juice (200 mL 3 times daily for 5 days) and *S*-ketamine (single oral dose of 0.2 mg/kg) increased peak plasma concentrations and area under the concentration-time curve (AUC) of ketamine by twofold and threefold, respectively. This interaction may be clinically important if ketamine is taken orally.

Itraconazole Concomitant administration of the CYP3A inhibitor itraconazole (200 mg orally once daily) and *S*-ketamine (single oral dose of 0.2 mg/kg) in healthy individuals had no effect on the AUC of ketamine.

Macrolide Antibiotics Concomitant administration of the CYP3A4 inhibitor clarithromycin and *S*-ketamine (single oral dose of 0.2 mg/kg) in healthy individuals increased peak plasma concentration and AUC of ketamine by 3.6- and 2.6-fold, respectively, and decreased the ratio of norketamine to ketamine by 54%. In addition, self-reported pharmacologic effects of ketamine were increased when *S*-ketamine was administered following pretreatment with clarithromycin. Erythromycin, but not azithromycin, is expected to have similar effects on the pharmacokinetics of *S*-ketamine.

Rifampin Concomitant use of the potent CYP3A4 and CYP2B6 inducer rifampin (600 mg orally daily for 5 days) and *S*-ketamine (0.57–1.14 mg/kg by IV infusion over 2 hours) in healthy individuals decreased the AUC of *S*-ketamine and *S*-norketamine by 10 and 50%, respectively.

St. John's Wort In healthy individuals, concomitant administration of the CYP3A4 inducer St. John's wort (*Hypericum perforatum*) and *S*-ketamine (single oral dose of 0.3 mg/kg) decreased peak plasma concentration and AUC of *S*-ketamine by 66 and 58%, respectively, and of *S*-norketamine by 18 and 23%, respectively.

Ticlopidine Concomitant use of the CYP2B6 inhibitor ticlopidine (250 mg orally twice daily) and *S*-ketamine (single oral dose of 0.2 mg/kg) in healthy individuals increased the AUC of *S*-ketamine by 2.4-fold and decreased the ratio of norketamine to ketamine.

■ **Anesthetic Agents** Ketamine is clinically compatible with commonly used general and local anesthetic agents when adequate respiration is maintained.

■ **CNS Depressants** Concomitant use of ketamine with CNS depressants (e.g., alcohol, benzodiazepines, opiate agonists, skeletal muscle relaxants) may result in additive CNS depression and increased risk of respiratory depression. Concomitant use of barbiturates and/or opiate agonists with ketamine during anesthesia may prolong recovery time. However, decreased half-life and plasma concentrations of ketamine have been observed in patients receiving long-term therapy with barbiturates, likely due to hepatic enzyme induction. (See Drug Interactions: Drugs and Foods Affecting Hepatic Microsomal Enzymes.)

Benzodiazepines *Increased* half-life of ketamine has been reported in patients who were premedicated with diazepam rectally (as a single dose) prior to anesthesia; these patients required lower doses of ketamine. However, *decreased* ketamine half-life was observed in patients who had been receiving long-term therapy with oral diazepam.

Ketamine metabolism was not substantially altered in patients who received IV clorazepate prior to anesthesia.

Administration of lorazepam has been reported to diminish the antidepressant response to repeated ketamine infusions in a patient with severe depression associated with bipolar disorder. Based on limited clinical evidence and theoretic concerns based on proposed mechanisms of action that benzodiazepines may diminish the antidepressant effects of ketamine, some clinicians recommend avoiding benzodiazepine administration for 8–12 hours prior to ketamine infusions.

■ **Ergonovine** Concomitant use of ketamine and ergonovine may result in increased blood pressure.

■ **Lamotrigine** Limited data suggest that lamotrigine, which inhibits the release of glutamate, may antagonize some of the effects of ketamine. Attenuated effects of ketamine, including perceptual abnormalities, schizophrenia-like symptoms, and learning and memory impairment, have been observed in healthy individuals who were pretreated with lamotrigine (300 mg) prior to receiving ketamine (0.26 mg/kg by IV injection or 0.65 mg/kg per hour by IV infusion). Failure of ketamine anesthesia following administration of IV doses totaling approximately 3.125 mg/kg has been reported in a patient with lamotrigine overdosage.

Lamotrigine has been reported to reduce ketamine cravings in a patient with ketamine abuse disorder.

■ **Neuromuscular Blocking Agents** Ketamine may potentiate the neuromuscular blocking effects of atracurium, resulting in respiratory depression and apnea. It is not known whether ketamine affects the duration of neuromuscular blockade of other neuromuscular blocking agents.

■ **Theophyllines** Concomitant use of ketamine and aminophylline or theophylline may result in a clinically important reduction in the seizure threshold. Tonic seizures have been reported during ketamine anesthesia in patients receiving aminophylline or theophylline.

■ **Thyroid Agents** Patients receiving thyroid replacement therapy may have an increased risk of ketamine-induced hypertension and tachycardia.

Acute Toxicity

Ketamine has a wide margin of safety. Overdosage of ketamine can result in respiratory depression, in which case respiratory support (e.g., mechanical ventilation) should be provided. Several cases of accidental ketamine overdosage (with doses up to 10 or 100 times the intended dose in adults or children, respectively) resulted in prolonged sedation, but no other clinically important adverse effects or complications; ventilator support was required rarely. Death secondary to acute ketamine overdosage in the absence of multidrug intoxication is rare, although accidental deaths have been reported. A lethal dose of ketamine in humans has not been identified.

In animal studies, vacuolation in neuronal cells of the posterior cingulate and retrosplenial cortices was observed in adult rats following intraperitoneal administration of ketamine at doses greater than 40 mg/kg. Vacuolation appeared to be reversible and did not progress to degeneration or neuronal death at doses up to 80 mg/kg (1.2 times the human dose of 10 mg/kg based on body surface area). The period of vulnerability to these changes is thought to correlate with the onset of puberty through adulthood in humans. The clinical relevance of these animal findings to humans is not known.

Chronic Toxicity

Ketamine is a known drug of abuse. Although cases of abuse and dependence have been reported with ketamine, the abuse potential with the drug has not been clearly defined.

Tolerance to the drug's effects may develop following prolonged administration. A sevenfold increase in the dose required for a desired "high" has been reported after 2 months of continuous use in recreational users of ketamine.

Although reported rarely, dependence on ketamine is possible. Cases of ketamine abuse resulting in physical or psychologic dependence have been reported. Evidence of withdrawal symptoms following discontinuance of ketamine is lacking; however, a withdrawal syndrome with psychotic features has been described following cessation of long-term ketamine use.

Urinary tract complications have been reported in association with long-term ketamine use, generally in the setting of chronic drug abuse, but also with clinical use of the drug. Reported lower urinary tract and bladder symptoms include cystitis, hematuria, dysuria, increased urinary frequency, urgency, incontinence, and postmicturition pain; secondary renal damage also can occur in severe cases. The exact mechanism of urinary tract damage is not clear, but ketamine and/or its metabolites are thought to have a direct irritant effect on the urothelium or interstitial cells of the bladder. Decreased bladder capacity and compliance, bladder wall thickening, transmural inflammation, detrusor muscle dysfunction, vesicoureteric reflux, hydronephrosis, and papillary necrosis have been observed.

Hepatobiliary toxicity also has been associated with long-term use of ketamine for therapeutic purposes or in the setting of chronic drug abuse. Epigastric pain, bile duct dilatation, and abnormal liver function tests consistent with posthepatic obstruction have been observed in chronic ketamine abusers.

Long-term use of ketamine has been reported to cause neuropsychiatric effects including hallucinatory flashbacks, inability to concentrate, and other cognitive deficits, possibly resulting from long-term effects of *N*-methyl-D-aspartic acid (NMDA)-receptor blockade. Both short-term and long-term memory impairment have been reported in chronic ketamine users. Magnetic resonance imaging (MRI) studies in chronic ketamine abusers have found areas of degeneration in the superficial white matter as early as 1 year of ketamine abuse; cortical atrophy and substantially decreased thalamocortical connectivity in the brain also have been observed.

Pharmacology

■ Mechanism of Action Ketamine is a nonbarbiturate general anesthetic that also has analgesic, amnestic, anti-inflammatory, and antidepressant properties. The pharmacologic effects of ketamine are dose dependent and mediated principally by its actions on the *N*-methyl-D-aspartate (NMDA) receptor, with contributory effects from other receptor interactions.

The anesthetic, amnestic, analgesic, and psychotomimetic effects of ketamine have been attributed to the drug's noncompetitive antagonism of the NMDA receptor. The NMDA receptor is a ligand-gated channel complex that plays an important role in excitatory glutamate-mediated neurotransmission, which can affect cognition, chronic pain, opiate tolerance, and mood regulation. The receptor is blocked at resting state by extracellular magnesium. Upon neuronal depolarization, magnesium is released, resulting in ligand-induced channel opening and calcium influx. Ketamine binds to the phencyclidine (PCP) site of the NMDA receptor channel, decreasing the frequency of channel opening and duration of time in the open active state, thereby inhibiting receptor activation and excitatory glutamatergic neurotransmission.

The NMDA receptor is closely involved in the development of opiate tolerance, opiate-induced hyperalgesia, and central sensitization (a condition closely related to the development of chronic pain). Activation of the NMDA receptor enhances neuronal excitability that can lead to hyperalgesia and allodynia. In the development of opiate tolerance and opiate-induced hyperalgesia, repeated activation of opiate receptors causes phosphorylation and opening of the NMDA receptor channel, leading to downregulation of opiate receptors and a reduction in opiate responsiveness. In chronic pain states, prolonged nociceptive stimulation causes activation and upregulation of NMDA receptors at dorsal horn synapses, resulting in enhanced and amplified trafficking of pain signals to the brain (central sensitization). Therefore, antagonism of NMDA receptors by ketamine decreases amplification of the response to repeated opiate receptor stimulation and can also prevent or reduce central sensitization.

In addition to its effects on the NMDA receptor, ketamine also acts on a wide range of other targets, including opiate, α-amino-3-hydroxy-5-methyl-4-isoxazolepropionic acid (AMPA), γ-aminobutyric acid A ($GABA_A$), cholinergic, nicotinic, and muscarinic receptors; L-type voltage-dependent calcium channels, hyperpolarization-activated cyclic nucleotide (HCN) channels, voltage-gated sodium channels, and large-conductance potassium (BK) channels; and the monoaminergic system.

■ CNS Effects Ketamine produces dissociative anesthesia as a result of a functional and electrophysiologic dissociation between the thalamocortical and limbic systems. The drug appears to selectively depress sensory association areas in the cortex, limbic systems, and thalamus without substantially obtunding the more primitive pathways (reticular-activating and limbic systems). At anesthetic doses, ketamine disrupts frontal-to-posterior corticocortical connectivity while maintaining thalamocortical somatosensory pathways. Thus, sensory input may reach cortical receiving areas but fail to be observed in some of the association areas, effectively dissociating the CNS from outside stimuli. At subanesthetic doses, ketamine has been shown to alter functional connectivity between the subgenual anterior cingulate cortex and a network cluster involving the thalamus, hippocampus, and the retrosplenial cortex, without reported loss of consciousness.

Ketamine increases cerebral metabolism and cerebral blood flow, and can also potentially increase intracranial pressure.

Anesthetic Effects At anesthetic doses, ketamine produces a dissociative, cataleptic state characterized by profound analgesia, sedation, and amnesia. The anesthetic state produced by ketamine is distinct from that of other general anesthetic drugs (e.g., barbiturates, propofol, benzodiazepines, inhalation anesthetics). Dissociated patients are nonresponsive and unable to respond to external stimuli (including pain). Although there is some variability, ketamine dissociation usually occurs at a dosing threshold of approximately 1–1.5 mg/kg when given IV or 3–4 mg/kg when given IM. Plasma ketamine concentrations associated with dissociative anesthesia have been reported to range from approximately 1.2–3 mcg/mL; concentrations associated with hypnosis and amnesia during surgery range from 0.8–4 mcg/mL and awakening usually occurs at plasma concentrations of 0.5–1.1 mcg/mL. Unlike other anesthetic or sedative drugs, increasing the dose of ketamine beyond the dissociative threshold does not enhance or deepen sedation.

Analgesic Effects At doses and plasma concentrations lower than those used for anesthesia, ketamine produces analgesia and sedation. Although there is some variability, doses less than 1 mg/kg generally have been considered subanesthetic.

Following IV or IM administration, analgesic effects are associated with plasma ketamine concentrations ranging from 0.07–0.2 mcg/mL. Analgesic effects following oral administration occur at plasma ketamine concentrations of 0.04 mcg/mL, possibly due to a higher ratio of norketamine. (See Pharmacokinetics: Absorption.)

Antidepressant Effects The precise mechanism(s) of ketamine's antidepressant activity has not been clearly established. Considerable preclinical research suggests that the NMDA class of glutamate receptors plays a role in the pathophysiology of depression as well as in the mechanism of action of antidepressant treatments. In addition, NMDA receptor antagonists, including ketamine, have been shown to be effective in animal models of depression and in models that predict antidepressant activity in many studies. Preclinical and clinical data suggest that the antidepressant effects of ketamine may be mediated by an increase in glutamate, which leads to a cascade of events that results in synaptogenesis and reversal of the negative effects of chronic stress and depression, particularly in the prefrontal cortex.

Following IV infusion of 0.5 mg/kg of ketamine over 40 minutes in patients with treatment-resistant major depressive disorder, peak plasma ketamine concentrations of 0.07–0.2 mcg/mL are achieved. These concentrations usually are associated with antidepressant effects but not general anesthetic effects.

Psychotomimetic Effects Like PCP, ketamine may cause psychotomimetic effects as a result of NMDA-receptor antagonism; such effects can occur following anesthetic or subanesthetic doses. At higher ketamine doses used for anesthesia, psychotomimetic effects appear to be dose related; however, a dose-related effect has not been clearly established at subanesthetic doses. The analgesic properties of ketamine are closely related to its psychotomimetic effects.

Psychotomimetic effects of ketamine may occur at IV doses in the range of 0.1–1 mg/kg or IM doses in the range of 25–200 mg. The most common manifestations reported following single subanesthetic IV doses include distortions in visual, auditory, or somatosensory stimuli; alterations in the perception of self or time; conceptual disorganization; hallucinations; suspiciousness; unusual thought content; blunted affect; emotional withdrawal; and motor retardation.

Psychotomimetic manifestations appearing during awakening or emergence from ketamine-induced dissociative anesthesia have been described as disturbances in visual and audio perception, mood, body image, and time; feelings of unreality, floating, or depersonalization; conscious dreams; and hallucinations. Such effects may occur at plasma concentrations as low as 0.05 mcg/mL, with more severe effects (e.g., anxiety, paranoid feelings) occurring around plasma concentrations of 0.5 mcg/mL. A linear concentration-effect relationship has been observed in healthy individuals for plasma concentrations ranging from 0.05–0.2 mcg/mL.

Psychotomimetic effects of ketamine usually are reversible following discontinuance of the drug.

■ Respiratory Effects Respiratory function generally is preserved during administration of ketamine, although transient and minimal respiratory depression may occur occasionally. Arterial hypoxemia and respiratory depression have been reported following rapid IV administration of the drug. The drug may have a respiratory stimulating effect at low doses.

Upper airway reflexes remain intact and may be slightly exaggerated during ketamine administration. Ketamine also produces bronchodilation, likely through vagolytic and other centrally mediated mechanisms.

■ **Cardiovascular Effects** Ketamine inhibits the reuptake of catecholamines and has other direct and indirect sympathomimetic effects at subanesthetic and anesthetic doses. Typical cardiovascular effects include increases in heart rate, blood pressure, cardiac output, and myocardial oxygen consumption; however, hypotension and bradycardia also have been observed. Ketamine also causes direct relaxation of vascular smooth muscle; however, systemic vascular resistance usually is unaffected. The sympathomimetic effects of ketamine often are used to therapeutic advantage (e.g., in patients with severe hypotension, sepsis, or other hemodynamically compromised state).

When ketamine is administered IV in anesthetic doses, increased blood pressure usually occurs shortly after the IV injection, reaches a maximum within a few minutes, and returns to preanesthetic levels within 15 minutes. Systolic and diastolic blood pressure usually peaks at 10–50% over baseline values, but increases can be higher or last longer in some individuals. In healthy individuals receiving subanesthetic doses of ketamine (0.5 mg/kg by IV infusion over 40 minutes), increases in blood pressure were observed 10 minutes after the start of infusion; mean maximum increases in systolic and diastolic blood pressure of 13.38 and 12.65 mm Hg, respectively, occurred approximately 28 minutes after initiation of the infusion and returned to baseline levels within 2 hours. The mean maximum increase in heart rate in these individuals was 10.69 beats per minute.

Ketamine may have negative inotropic effects in some patients.

Pharmacokinetics

■ **Absorption** Ketamine has a rapid onset of anesthetic action when given IV or IM. Following IV administration of the usual induction dose of 2 mg/kg, onset of surgical anesthesia occurs within 30 seconds and the duration of anesthetic effect is 5–10 minutes. Following IM administration of doses ranging from 9–13 mg/kg, onset of surgical anesthesia occurs within 3–4 minutes and the duration of anesthetic effect is usually 12–25 minutes. Plasma ketamine concentrations are about 1.8–2 mcg/mL at 5 minutes following IV injection of a 2-mg/kg dose and about 1.7–2.2 mcg/mL at 15 minutes following IM injection of a 6-mg/kg dose. Following IV administration of a 2.5-mg/kg dose, ketamine has an initial distribution phase (α) lasting about 45 minutes and a half-life of 10–15 minutes, which is associated with the duration of anesthetic effect (about 20 minutes).

Norketamine, the main active metabolite of ketamine, appears in the blood 2–3 minutes following IV administration of the drug and reaches peak plasma concentration in approximately 30 minutes.

Peak plasma concentrations following oral administration of ketamine occur within 20–120 minutes.

Bioavailability of ketamine following IM administration is 93% in adults; lower IM bioavailability has been reported in children. Due to extensive first-pass metabolism, bioavailability following oral or rectal administration is low (16–30 or 11–30%, respectively), with relatively higher concentrations of norketamine.

Bioavailability of ketamine following intranasal administration has been reported to be up to 45–50%, but can vary substantially.

In children 4–10 years of age, plasma ketamine concentrations are similar to those observed in adults. Plasma concentrations of norketamine are higher in children than adults following equivalent weight-adjusted doses.

■ **Distribution** Ketamine is rapidly and widely distributed into highly perfused tissues, including the CNS, with a distribution half-life of 10–15 minutes. Animal studies have shown ketamine to be highly concentrated in body fat, liver, and lung. Because ketamine is lipophilic, it has a large volume of distribution.

Termination of the anesthetic effect of ketamine occurs partly via redistribution from the CNS to peripheral tissues and partly by hepatic biotransformation.

Ketamine crosses the placenta. Following an IM dose of 250 mg (approximately 4.2 mg/kg) in parturient patients, placental transfer rate of ketamine from maternal artery to umbilical vein was 47% at the time of delivery (average of 12 minutes from the time of injection to vaginal delivery).

It is not known whether ketamine is distributed into milk.

Ketamine is less than 50% bound to plasma proteins (α_1-acid glycoprotein or albumin).

■ **Elimination** Ketamine is metabolized extensively in the liver, principally undergoing *N*-demethylation to the active metabolite norketamine, which has approximately one-third the anesthetic activity of the parent drug. *N*-demethylation of ketamine to norketamine is mediated principally by cytochrome P-450 (CYP) isoenzyme 3A4 and, to a lesser extent, by CYP2B6 and CYP2C9. Norketamine is further metabolized to hydroxynorketamines and dehydronorketamine.

Other biotransformation pathways of ketamine include hydroxylation of the cyclohexone ring, conjugation with glucuronic acid, and dehydration of the hydroxylated metabolites to form a cyclohexene derivative.

About 90% of a parenteral dose of ketamine is excreted in the urine, mostly as conjugates of hydroxylated metabolites. Less than 5% of a dose is excreted unchanged in feces and urine. Because ketamine is extensively metabolized prior to excretion, the effect of renal function on the pharmacokinetics of ketamine and norketamine is minimal. Plasma concentrations of ketamine have been reported to be 20% higher in individuals with acute renal failure than in those with normal renal function.

Ketamine is not appreciably removed by hemodialysis or hemofiltration (10 or 4%, respectively).

The elimination half-life of ketamine is approximately 2–4 hours and is shorter in children (approximately 100 minutes) than in adults. The half-life of norketamine is 12 hours.

Chemistry and Stability

■ **Chemistry** Ketamine hydrochloride is an arylcycloalkylamine general anesthetic derived from phencyclidine (PCP). Ketamine is commercially available in the US as a racemic mixture containing equal amounts of the *R*- and *S*-enantiomers. *S*-Ketamine, which is commercially available as esketamine in the US and some other countries, has a higher binding affinity for *N*-methyl-D-aspartate (NMDA) receptors and has approximately 3–4 times greater anesthetic potency than *R*-ketamine. *S*-Ketamine also appears to be associated with more frequent psychotomimetic adverse effects compared with *R*-ketamine.

Ketamine is commercially available as the hydrochloride salt. Ketamine hydrochloride injection is a sterile solution of the drug that contains benzethonium chloride as a preservative; sodium chloride has been added to the injection containing 10 mg of ketamine per mL to provide an isotonic solution. The sterile solution has a pH of 3.5–5.5.

Ketamine hydrochloride is soluble in both water and lipids.

■ **Stability** Ketamine hydrochloride injection should be stored at controlled room temperature between 20–25°C and protected from light.

The commercially available 100-mg/mL ketamine injection (as the hydrochloride) must be diluted with an equal volume of sterile water for injection, 5% dextrose, or 0.9% sodium chloride injection prior to IV injection. For IV infusion, a solution containing 1 or 2 mg/mL may be prepared by diluting an appropriate volume of ketamine from the commercially available 50- or 100-mg/mL vial with 5% dextrose or 0.9% sodium chloride injection. (See Dilution under Dosage and Administration: Administration.)

The manufacturer states that ketamine hydrochloride injection is incompatible with barbiturates and diazepam, and should *not* be mixed in the same syringe or infusion solution with these drugs due to the risk of precipitate formation. Ketamine has been reported to be compatible with several drugs when administered as additives, simultaneously in the same syringe, or when a Y-type administration set is used; specialized references should be consulted for more specific information.

Preparations

Ketamine is subject to control under the Federal Controlled Substances Act of 1970 as a schedule III (C-III) drug.

Excipients in commercially available drug preparations may have clinically important effects in some individuals; consult specific product labeling for details.

Ketamine Hydrochloride

Parenteral		
Injection	10 mg (of ketamine) per mL*	Ketalar® (C-III), Par **Ketamine Hydrochloride Injection** (C-III)
	50 mg (of ketamine) per mL*	Ketalar® (C-III), Par **Ketamine Hydrochloride Injection** (C-III)
	100 mg (of ketamine) per mL*	Ketalar® (C-III), Par **Ketamine Hydrochloride Injection** (C-III)

*available from one or more manufacturer, distributor, and/or repackager by generic (nonproprietary) name

†Use is not currently included in the labeling approved by the US Food and Drug Administration

Propofol

■ Propofol is a sedative and hypnotic agent.

Uses

Propofol is used for IV induction and maintenance of anesthesia in adults and pediatric patients. Propofol also is used IV for initiation and maintenance of monitored anesthesia care (MAC) sedation in adults undergoing diagnostic procedures or in those undergoing surgical procedures who are receiving local or regional anesthesia. In addition, propofol is used IV for sedation in intubated and mechanically ventilated adults in a critical care setting (e.g., intensive care unit [ICU]).

■ **Induction and Maintenance of Anesthesia** *General Overview of Anesthesia* The IV anesthetic agents propofol, etomidate, methohexital, and thiopental (no longer commercially available in the US) are widely used for induction and maintenance of general anesthesia. General anesthesia may be defined as a global, but reversible depression of the CNS that results in the loss of response to and perception of all external stimuli. The intraoperative period of general anesthesia consists of 3 phases: induction, maintenance, and emergence. General anesthesia should provide hypnosis, amnesia, analgesia, and muscle relaxation; these effects usually are provided by a combination of drugs. When used for induction of anesthesia, IV administration of propofol, etomidate, methohexital, or thiopental usually results in unconsciousness. Once unconsciousness is induced, anesthesia is maintained with a combination of drugs that provide attenuation of autonomic responses to surgery (e.g., cardiovascular, respiratory, GI), immobility, anterograde amnesia, analgesia, and muscle relaxation. Balanced anesthesia (e.g., an IV hypnotic and/or inhalation anesthetic, analgesic, skeletal muscle relaxant) or total IV anesthesia (balanced anesthesia in which an IV anesthetic agent replaces the inhalation anesthetic) will provide the effects necessary for maintenance of anesthesia. The degree of each of these desired effects will determine the depth of anesthesia experienced by the patient.

When these IV anesthetic agents are given either by an intermittent rapid ("bolus") injection or a continuous infusion, the drugs can be titrated to maintain unconsciousness (e.g., loss of response to voice command) whereas a low-dose continuous IV infusion of these agents (e.g., propofol) can maintain sedation for MAC in patients receiving a local anesthetic agent while undergoing surgery. Ideally, recovery from general anesthesia should be rapid without associated adverse effects; residual analgesia, however, is beneficial. Recovery, including of psychomotor function, from propofol-induced anesthesia generally is more rapid and the associated adverse effects (e.g., drowsiness, nausea, vomiting) are less frequent than those associated with thiopental, methohexital, or etomidate.

Use of Propofol for Anesthesia Propofol is used IV for induction and/or maintenance of anesthesia as the sedative and hypnotic component of balanced anesthesia (benzodiazepines, anticholinergic agents, depolarizing and nondepolarizing skeletal muscle relaxants, opiate analgesics, inhalation and/or regional anesthetic) or total IV anesthesia (balanced anesthesia in which the IV anesthetic completely replaces the inhalation anesthetic) in adults and pediatric patients 3 years of age and older undergoing inpatient or outpatient surgery. Propofol also is used for maintenance anesthesia in pediatric patients older than 2 months of age undergoing inpatient or outpatient surgery. When used for total IV anesthesia, propofol is administered by a constant IV infusion to provide adequate depth of anesthesia. The manufacturers state that prior to administration of propofol, patients may receive premedication with other drugs including benzodiazepines (to relieve anxiety and produce anterograde amnesia) and barbiturates (to relieve anxiety and provide sedation). Anticholinergic agents (e.g., atropine, scopolamine) also have been used as premedication (to suppress vagal reflexes and decrease secretions). Induction anesthesia with IV propofol is rapid and results in dose-related hypnotic effects (progressing from light sleep to unconsciousness) and anterograde amnesia, but not analgesia. Following induction, anesthesia can be maintained IV either by continuous infusion or by intermittent rapid ("bolus") injections.

The current indications for propofol are based principally on the results of numerous comparative (with sedatives or inhalation and IV anesthetic agents) clinical trials in several thousand adults undergoing general anesthesia or MAC sedation. Indications for pediatric anesthesia are based on multiple trials in children up to 16 years of age.

Surgery. Propofol has produced adequate general anesthesia in patients undergoing various types of surgery, including neurosurgery (e.g., craniotomy, intracranial aneurysm), cardiovascular (e.g., coronary artery bypass graft [CABG]), abdominal, ocular, ear, nose and throat (ENT), orthopedic, and general surgery. Because propofol decreases cerebral blood flow, intracranial pressure, and cerebral metabolic requirements and is associated with fast recovery from anesthesia and thus allows rapid postoperative neurologic assessment, the drug may be useful in neurosurgery.

Propofol also has been used in patients undergoing cardiac surgery. Use of the drug has been studied extensively in patients with coronary artery disease, but experience in patients with hemodynamically significant valvular or congenital heart disease is limited. When propofol is used for induction of anesthesia, substantial decreases in arterial pressure (by about 30%; 30–40 mm Hg) may occur in patients with normal or impaired ventricular or cardiac function. When compared with other IV induction agents, propofol-induced decreases in blood pressure usually are more substantial (especially when the drug is used concomitantly with opiates). Results of several comparative studies indicate that hemodynamic parameters (e.g., heart rate, systemic blood pressure, systemic vascular resistance) associated with use of propofol for maintenance anesthesia are similar to those associated with other IV anesthetics. Therefore, some clinicians recommend that patients undergoing cardiac surgery receive induction anesthesia with combination of a benzodiazepine and an opiate while for maintenance anesthesia they should receive propofol, an inhalation anesthetic, and/or an opiate.

Because propofol is associated with substantial decreases in intraocular pressure (IOP), the drug is used to provide anesthesia in patients undergoing ocular surgery.

Outpatient Surgery. Many clinicians state that propofol is particularly useful in patients undergoing outpatient surgery while others consider propofol the hypnotic of choice for such surgery. When compared with other IV anesthetic agents (e.g., etomidate, methohexital, thiopental) or conventional combinations (e.g., an IV induction agent and an inhalation anesthetic), IV propofol usually is associated with similar or faster early (time to awakening and eye opening) recovery from anesthesia, a more rapid recovery of psychomotor performance and time to discharge, and less incidence of adverse effects (e.g., nausea, vomiting, cough, hiccups).

When propofol is compared with the inhalation anesthetic desflurane, early recovery usually is faster with the use of the inhalation anesthetic, while time to intermediate recovery (return to cognitive and psychomotor functions) and to discharge appear to be similar. Lower incidence of nausea is observed with propofol than with desflurane. Similar findings have been reported when propofol was compared with the inhalation anesthetic sevoflurane when used as a component of balanced anesthesia with nitrous oxide. Time to emergence after discontinuance of primary maintenance anesthetics (measured by spontaneous eye opening, response to verbal commands, extubation, cognitive functions, time to discharge) was similar in patients receiving propofol compared with those receiving sevoflurane. However, incidence of nausea prior to discharge was lower in patients receiving propofol than in those receiving sevoflurane.

Special Populations. Propofol has been used safely in patients with susceptibility to malignant hyperthermia and those with porphyria; however, further studies are needed.

Monitored Anesthesia Care Propofol is used alone or in combination with an opiate analgesic and/or a benzodiazepine for initiation and maintenance of MAC sedation in adults undergoing diagnostic procedures or in conjunction with local or regional anesthesia for surgical procedures. MAC is a specific anesthesia service performed by a qualified anesthesia provider that includes the administration of sedatives, analgesics, anesthetic agents, and hypnotics as needed for a diagnostic or therapeutic procedure, while vital functions (e.g., hemodynamic stability, airway management) are continuously supported. MAC sedation is distinguished from moderate sedation (also referred to as conscious sedation), which is a drug-induced depression of consciousness during which patients respond purposefully to verbal commands. MAC sedation with propofol has been used prior to and/or during dental, endoscopic (e.g., gastroscopy, bronchoscopy, colonoscopy), diagnostic, oral, or other procedures such as extracorporeal lithotripsy, transvaginal oocyte retrieval, central venous catheter placement, herniorrhaphy, and electrical cardioversion. Propofol also is used in conjunction with local or regional anesthesia for surgical procedures, including orthopedic (hip or knee arthroplasty), abdominal, or urologic surgery.

For MAC sedation, initial propofol dosages (100–150 mcg/kg per minute for 3–5 minutes) usually are associated with a rapid onset of action (within 1–3 minutes) and recovery. If a procedure is longer than expected and a deeper level of anesthesia is required, increasing the rate of propofol or administration of incremental rapid IV ("bolus") doses of the drug (titrated to effect) will result in an easy transition to general anesthesia.

When used for sedation in patients undergoing diagnostic procedures or minor surgical procedures (under local or regional anesthesia), propofol produces less postoperative sedation, drowsiness, confusion, clumsiness, and nausea and a more rapid recovery of psychomotor performance than IV midazolam; however, midazolam has been associated with less pain at the injection site, less frequent oxygen requirements for decreased oxygen saturation, and more effective intraoperative amnesia. The quality of intraoperative sedation and time to discharge appear to be similar when using propofol or IV midazolam.

■ **Sedation in Critical Care Settings** Propofol is used as a continuous IV infusion for sedation in intubated and mechanically ventilated adults (including medical, trauma, and surgery patients) in a critical care setting (e.g., ICU). Efficacy and safety of propofol for this indication are based principally on the results of several comparative (with benzodiazepines and/or opiates) clinical trials in adults. Propofol, alone or in combination with an opiate analgesic (e.g., morphine, fentanyl), has been effective in achieving a desired level of sedation using the standardized Ramsay or modified Glasgow sedation scale and providing adequate sedation in intubated and mechanically ventilated patients.

Sedative agents are administered in critically ill patients to reduce agitation and anxiety, and increase tolerance to invasive procedures (e.g., mechanical ventilation). The provision of adequate analgesia and other measures to ensure patient comfort is recommended before sedatives are administered. Common sedative agents used in the ICU include benzodiazepines (e.g., midazolam, lorazepam), propofol, and dexmedetomidine. These agents appear to be similarly effective in providing adequate sedation in critically ill, mechanically ventilated adults. However, modest benefits with respect to other clinical outcomes (e.g., reduced duration of mechanical ventilation, shorter time to extubation, reduced risk of delirium) have been observed with the nonbenzodiazepine sedatives (dexmedetomidine and propofol) compared with benzodiazepines. Because of the apparent advantages and an overall favorable benefit-to-risk profile, nonbenzodiazepine sedatives (propofol or dexmedetomidine) are generally preferred to benzodiazepines (midazolam or lorazepam) in mechanically ventilated, critically ill adults. This recommendation should be considered in the context of the specific clinical situation since benzodiazepines may still be preferred in certain situations (e.g., patients with anxiety, seizures, or alcohol or benzodiazepine withdrawal). When selecting an appropriate sedative agent, the patient's individual sedation goals should be considered in addition to specific drug-related (e.g., pharmacology, pharmacokinetics, adverse effects, availability, cost) and patient-related (e.g., comorbid conditions) factors.

Comparative studies have shown that propofol may have a less variable effect on recovery of consciousness and time to recovery of function after cessation of therapy than midazolam. However, propofol may be associated with less frequent amnestic effects and more frequent hypotension than midazolam. When receiving short-term (less than 24 hours), intermediate-term (1–3 days), or long-term (more than 3 days) sedation, time to spontaneous breathing (ability to wean from mechanical ventilation), recovery (awakening or response to voice command), or extubation is often shorter in patients (especially those awakened from deep sedation) receiving propofol than in those receiving midazolam. However, certain clinical outcomes (e.g., discharge from an ICU) may be similar when the drugs are used for short- or intermediate-term sedation. Because of its short duration of sedative effect, some experts state that propofol may be particularly useful in patients requiring frequent awakenings (e.g., for neurologic assessments) or undergoing daily sedation interruption protocols. Results of several studies suggest that when used for long-term sedation, propofol is associated with more reliable and rapid awakening than use of midazolam. However, long-term administration of propofol can lead to prolonged emergence. Prolonged use of propofol also may be associated with increased serum lipid concentrations (e.g., hypertriglyceridemia) secondary to the injectable emulsion formulation. Studies comparing propofol and dexmedetomidine for ICU sedation generally have not found any importance differences in clinical outcomes between the drugs.

■ Other Uses Propofol also has been used in the management of refractory status epilepticus†, refractory complex-partial seizures†, postoperative or cancer chemotherapy-induced nausea and vomiting†, and spinal opiate- or cholestasis-induced pruritus†.

Although propofol has been associated rarely with development of seizures or seizure-like activity, the drug has been used in patients with refractory status epilepticus†, usually administered IV by a rapid injection followed by a continuous infusion. (See Other Uses, under Dosage and Administration: Dosage.) In some patients with status epilepticus refractory to conventional anticonvulsants, termination of seizure activity and/or EEG burst suppression occurred within seconds after administration of propofol by rapid IV ("bolus") injection and was sustained during propofol infusion (lasting 2 hours to 12 days). In at least one patient, propofol also has been used in the management of refractory complex-partial seizures†.

Because propofol appears to possess direct antiemetic activity, the drug has been administered in subhypnotic doses (10–15 mg IV) for the management of postoperative nausea and vomiting†. In addition, propofol (usually administered with conventional antiemetics) has been used effectively IV for the prevention of nausea and vomiting associated with emetogenic cancer chemotherapy†.

Subhypnotic doses of propofol have been used effectively for relief of pruritus† associated with use of spinal opiates or cholestasis.

■ Misuse and Abuse Cases of propofol abuse and dependence, in some cases resulting in death (following repeated *self-administration* of propofol by health-care providers), have been reported. While most reported cases have involved health-care professionals (primarily anesthesiology personnel), cases of propofol abuse among lay persons also have been reported. (See Chronic Toxicity.)

Propofol currently is not subject to control under the Federal Controlled Substances Act of 1970; however, some clinicians have suggested that the drug should be subject to such control (or some other means of ensuring greater accountability). Data from a 2005-2006 survey sent to all (126) anesthesiology departments with residency programs in the US indicate that 18% (23 out of 126) of the departments had one or more individuals abusing propofol in the last 10 years and 2 departments had more than one incident. Seven individuals died, 6 of whom were residents and one was an anesthesia technician. Among all anesthesia-based providers who were found to be abusing propofol, the overall mortality rate was 28% (7 out of 25), while the mortality rate among residents was found to be 38% (6 out of 16). Results of the survey have shown that 71% of institutions (90 out of 126) did not regulate propofol. Among the 25 programs that had individuals who abused the drug, 3 programs had some pharmacy control of propofol at the time of abuse. Data regarding regulation of propofol by pharmacy departments in academic anesthesia programs indicate a greater prevalence of abuse and related deaths at locations where there was no established system to control or monitor propofol use. The manufacturers and some clinicians recommend that restriction of access and accounting procedures appropriate to the particular practice setting should be used to prevent diversion of propofol. Some clinicians also suggest routine testing of drug screenings for propofol in individuals considered to be at risk for abuse.

Dosage and Administration

■ Administration Propofol injectable emulsion is administered by IV infusion (using a controlled-infusion device [pump], preferably a volumetric pump) or by IV injection (administered in incremental doses). In patients undergoing magnetic resonance imaging (MRI) who are receiving IV infusion of propofol, metered controlled devices may be used when mechanical pumps are not suitable. Rarely, the drug also has been administered by continuous IV infusion using a patient-controlled infusion device† in individuals receiving monitored anesthesia care (MAC) sedation while undergoing diagnostic or surgical procedures.

Propofol, a potent sedative/hypnotic, should be administered slowly to minimize adverse effects (e.g., hypotension, respiratory depression). Cardiorespiratory depression is more likely to occur at higher blood propofol concentrations resulting from either too-rapid administration of the IV injection or increases in the rate of infusion. In addition, the drug should not be administered by rapid IV ("bolus") injection (single or repeated doses) in geriatric, debilitated, or American Society of Anesthesiologists (ASA) physical status III or IV patients since such administration may result in cardiorespiratory depression (e.g., hypotension, oxyhemoglobin desaturation, apnea, airway obstruction) during general anesthesia or MAC sedation.

When using a continuous IV infusion, depth of anesthesia is controlled by rate of infusion. In the absence of clinical signs indicating light anesthesia and until a mild response to surgical stimulation develops, propofol IV infusion rates always should be titrated downward to avoid drug administration at rates higher than clinically necessary. To optimize recovery times, adults usually should receive propofol at a rate of about 50–100 mcg/kg per minute.

The commercially available 1% (10 mg/mL) propofol injectable emulsion may be used without dilution. However, if dilution of the emulsion is necessary, the drug may be diluted with 5% dextrose injection to a concentration of not less than 0.2% (2 mg/mL) in order to maintain the emulsion. Propofol injectable emulsion should be discarded if there is evidence of separation of the emulsion. When diluted with 5% dextrose injection, propofol has been shown to be more stable in glass rather than in plastic containers. (See Chemistry and Stability: Stability.) Propofol injectable emulsion and dilutions of the drug should be inspected visually for particulate matter and discoloration prior to administration whenever the emulsion and container permit. The injectable emulsion should be shaken well just prior to administration. Although commercially available preparations of propofol injectable emulsion contain ingredients that inhibit the rate of growth of microorganisms (e.g., Diprivan® contains 0.005% of edetate disodium), strict aseptic technique must be observed when handling the drug, because the emulsion still may support growth of microorganisms. Propofol injectable emulsion should not be used if contamination is suspected.

To administer propofol emulsion, contents of a vial may be transferred into a sterile, single-use syringe immediately after the vial is opened and after cleaning the rubber stopper with 70% isopropyl alcohol; when withdrawing the drug from vials, a sterile venting spike should be used. Propofol injectable emulsion should be prepared for single patient use only. Syringes should be labeled with appropriate information, including the date and time the vial was opened.

Clinical experience with use of inline filters for propofol administration during general anesthesia, MAC, or critical care setting sedation is limited. An inline membrane filter may be used during administration of the drug; however, the mean pore diameter of the filter should not be less than 5 μm, unless it has been demonstrated that the filter does not restrict the flow and/or cause the breakdown of the emulsion. Filters should be used with caution and only when clinically appropriate. Continuous monitoring for restricted flow and breakdown of the emulsion is required.

When used for general anesthesia or MAC sedation, the manufacturers state that administration of propofol should be started promptly and be completed within 12 hours after vials have been opened. Propofol injectable emulsion should be prepared for use just prior to initiation of each individual anesthetic/sedative procedure. The manufacturers also state that any unused portion, reservoirs, dedicated administration tubing, and/or solutions containing propofol injectable emulsion should be discarded at the end of the anesthetic procedure or after 12 hours. However, because of recent reports of acute febrile reactions following administration of propofol (see Cautions: Infectious Complications), the FDA states that, when used for general anesthesia or procedural sedation, administration from a single vial or syringe must be completed within 6 hours of opening. The IV line should be flushed every 12 hours (one manufacturer has recommended flushing with 5% dextrose) and at the end of the procedure to remove residual propofol emulsion. When propofol is used for sedation in critical care settings, manipulations of IV lines should be minimized and administration should be started promptly and be completed within 12 hours after the vial has been spiked. A sterile vent spike and sterile tubing must be used for administration of propofol injectable emulsion. When used for sedation in critical care settings, any unused portion and IV tubing should be discarded at the end of the procedure or after 12 hours. (See Chemistry and Stability: Stability.)

Pain at the injection site can be minimized in adults and children if the larger veins of the forearm or antecubital fossa rather than hand veins are used and by administering IV lidocaine prior to administration of propofol. (See Cautions: Local Effects.) Because of the possibility that lidocaine may cause instability of the propofol emulsion, the manufacturers recommend that lidocaine be administered prior to propofol administration or that lidocaine be added to propofol immediately before administration in a quantity not exceeding 20 mg of lidocaine per 200 mg of propofol. (See Chemistry and Stability: Stability.)

■ Dosage Because individual response to propofol is variable, dosage (including the infusion rate or amount and frequency of incremental doses) of the drug should be adjusted according to individual requirements and response, age, weight, clinical status (e.g., ASA physical status, degree of debilitation), blood lipid profile, underlying pathologic conditions (e.g., shock, intestinal obstruction, malnutrition, anemia, burns, advanced malignancy, ulcerative colitis, uremia, alcoholism), and the type and amount of premedication or concomitant medication(s) used. To provide adequate anesthesia in patients undergoing minor surgical procedures (e.g., on the body surface), propofol may be administered concomitantly with 60–70% nitrous oxide, while for major (e.g., intra-abdominal) surgical procedures or if nitrous oxide is not available or appropriate, administration rates of propofol and/or opiates may be increased. In general, the smallest effective dose should be used.

Induction and Maintenance of General Anesthesia **Adult Patients (Younger Than 55 Years of Age).** For induction of anesthesia, the manufacturers recommend that patients with ASA Physical Status I or II who have not been premedicated or those who received premedication with oral benzodiazepines or IM opiate agonists usually should receive 40 mg (2–2.5 mg/kg) of propofol every 10 seconds according to the patient's response, until onset of induction.

For maintenance of anesthesia in patients undergoing general surgery, the usual initial IV infusion rate of propofol is 100–200 mcg/kg per minute (6–12 mg/kg per hour), administered concomitantly with inhaled 60–70% nitrous oxide and oxygen. Immediately following induction, higher IV infusion rates of 150–200 mcg/kg per minute generally may be required for the first 10–15 minutes, and then decreased by 30–50% during the first 30 minutes of maintenance anesthesia. The manufacturers state that IV infusion rates of 50–100 mcg/kg per minute usually are used to optimize recovery times.

Alternatively, for maintenance anesthesia, healthy adults may receive propofol doses of 20–50 mg by intermittent IV injection in combination with inhaled nitrous oxide. Additional IV doses of 25–50 mg may be given if necessary, as determined by changes in vital signs (increases in pulse rate, blood pressure, sweating and/or lacrimation) indicating a stress response to surgical stimulation or emergence from anesthesia.

Geriatric (55 Years of Age and Older) or Debilitated Patients. Geriatric, debilitated, or ASA III or IV physical status patients usually require lower induction dosages of propofol, because of possible reduced clearance and higher blood drug concentrations. For induction of anesthesia, such patients usually receive 20 mg (1–1.5 mg/kg) of propofol every 10 seconds, according to the individual patient's condition and response, until onset of induction. For maintenance of anesthesia, the usual IV infusion rate is 50–100 mcg/kg per minute (3–6 mg/kg per hour), administered concomitantly with inhaled 60–70% nitrous oxide and oxygen.

Pediatric Patients. In healthy (ASA I or II physical status) pediatric patients 3–16 years of age (who have not been premedicated or those who received premedication with oral benzodiazepines or IM opiate agonists), the usual suggested IV induction dosage of propofol is 2.5–3.5 mg/kg administered over 20–30 seconds. Within this dosage range, younger pediatric patients may require higher induction dosages than older pediatric patients. However, a lower dosage for induction of anesthesia is recommended for pediatric patients with ASA physical status of III or IV.

For maintenance of anesthesia in healthy (ASA I or II physical status) pediatric patients 2 months to 16 years of age, the usual initial infusion rate is 125–300 mcg/kg per minute (7.5–18 mg/kg per hour) administered concomitantly with inhaled 60–70% nitrous oxide and oxygen. Immediately following induction, higher IV infusion rates of 200–300 mcg/kg per minute generally may be required for the first 30 minutes, which may be decreased to 125–150 mcg/kg per minute (unless clinical signs of light anesthesia develop) by titration, according to the patient's response.

Patients Undergoing Cardiac Anesthesia. For induction of anesthesia, adults undergoing cardiac surgery usually receive 20 mg (0.5–1.5 mg/kg) of propofol every 10 seconds, administered by slow IV injection until the onset of induction. Propofol dosages of 25 mcg/kg per minute may be used for management of anxiolysis prior to induction.

When used as the primary agent for maintenance of anesthesia, propofol is administered as a continuous IV infusion at a rate of 100–150 mcg/kg per minute and is supplemented with a continuous infusion of an opiate agonist (e.g., alfentanil, fentanyl, sufentanil) administered to provide analgesia. Higher propofol dosages will reduce opiate analgesic dosage requirements. When an opiate agonist is used as the primary agent for maintenance of anesthesia in cardiac surgery, propofol is administered at a rate of at least 50 mcg/kg per minute; care should be taken to ensure adequate amnesia.

Patients Undergoing Neurosurgery. For induction of anesthesia, adults undergoing neurosurgery usually receive 20 mg (1–2 mg/kg) of propofol IV every 10 seconds until the onset of induction. For maintenance of anesthesia, the usual IV infusion rate is 100–200 mcg/kg per minute (6–12 mg/kg per hour).

Monitored Anesthesia Care Sedation **Adult Patients (Younger Than 55 Years of Age).** For initiation of monitored anesthesia care (MAC) sedation in healthy adults, a slow rate of a continuous IV infusion or direct IV injection is recommended in order to reduce the risk of apnea and hypotension. These patients usually receive an initial propofol infusion of 100–150 mcg/kg per minute (6–9 mg/kg per hour) for 3–5 minutes or a slow injection of 0.5 mg/kg over 3–5 minutes.

The manufacturers state that a variable infusion rate with the drug is preferred to intermittent bolus administration for maintenance of MAC sedation in healthy adults, because such administration may be associated with a reduced risk of hypotension. The usual initial IV maintenance dosage of propofol in this patient population is 25–75 mcg/kg per minute (1.5–4.5 mg/kg per hour) for the first 10–15 minutes and then it is decreased to a dosage of 25–50 mcg/kg per minute. When dosage is adjusted according to clinical effect, approximately 2 minutes should be allowed for onset of peak drug response. Alternatively, intermittent IV propofol injections of 10 or 20 mg may be administered; however, the possibility of developing respiratory depression or transient increases in sedation depth and/or prolongation of recovery should be considered.

Geriatric and Debilitated Patients. For initiation of MAC sedation in geriatric (55 years of age and older), debilitated, or ASA III or IV physical status patients, dosages similar to those for healthy adults are required for most such patients.

For maintenance of MAC sedation, the manufacturers recommend that the usual adult dosage of propofol be reduced by 20% in geriatric, debilitated, ASA III or IV physical status, or neurosurgical patients. Rapid IV injection is *not* recommended in this patient population because of an increased risk of developing adverse cardiorespiratory effects.

Sedation in Critical Care Settings Dosage of sedative agents should be titrated to the desired level of sedation; in most cases, a light rather than deep level of sedation is recommended in critically ill, mechanically ventilated adults because of improved clinical outcomes that have been demonstrated (e.g., shortened duration of mechanical ventilation, reduced ICU length of stay). The depth and quality of sedation should be assessed frequently using a validated and reliable assessment tool (e.g., Richmond Agitation-Sedation Scale [RASS], Sedation-Agitation Scale [SAS]).

For sedation in intubated and mechanically ventilated adults during treatment in critical care settings (e.g., an ICU), propofol is administered as a continuous IV infusion. In patients with residual effects from anesthetic or sedative drugs, propofol should be injected slowly initially, at an IV infusion rate of 5 mcg/kg per minute (0.3 mg/kg per hour) for at least 5 minutes to minimize the risk of hypotension or acute overdosage. This rate of infusion may then be increased slowly in increments of 5–10 mcg/kg per minute (0.3–0.6 mg/kg per hour) over 5–10 minutes, until desired sedation is achieved. For maintenance of sedation, adults usually receive propofol IV infusion dosages of 5–50 mcg/kg per minute (0.3–3 mg/kg per hour); higher maintenance infusion rates occasionally may be required in some patients. Rapid IV ("bolus") administration of 10- or 20-mg doses of propofol may be used to rapidly increase depth of sedation in patients in whom development of hypotension is unlikely. It should be considered that patients with impaired myocardial function, intravascular volume depletion, or abnormally low vascular tone (sepsis) may be more susceptible to hypotension. The lowest effective dosages should be used in patients with residual effects from anesthetic drugs or in those currently receiving other sedatives or opiates. Assessment of the level of sedation and CNS function should be performed at regular intervals (at least daily during maintenance sedation) and IV infusion rate adjusted accordingly to ensure adequate titration of the sedation level.

Because certain propofol injectable emulsion formulations (i.e., Diprivan®) contain edetate disodium, a heavy metal antagonist, patients receiving continuous IV infusions for sedation in critical care settings should not receive this formulation for longer than 5 days without a drug-free interval, to allow replacement of estimated or measured urinary zinc losses. (See Cautions: Precautions and Contraindications.)

During long-term therapy (exceeding 7 days), some tolerance to the sedative effects of the drug may occur and increasing the infusion rate may be necessary. It has been suggested, however, that such effects may be associated with changes in drug elimination or an improved health status of the patient.

Other Uses For the management of patients with refractory status epilepticus†, 1- to 2-mg/kg doses of propofol have been administered initially by IV injection, over 5 minutes, which were repeated when seizure activity was no longer adequately controlled. In these patients, the rate of the IV maintenance infusion was adjusted to 2–10 mg/kg per hour until the lowest rate of infusion needed to suppress epileptiform activity was achieved; dosage then was decreased gradually to prevent withdrawal seizures.

Propofol has been administered in subhypnotic (10- to 15-mg) doses for the management of postoperative nausea and vomiting†. In addition, propofol, administered as a continuous IV infusion at a rate of 1 mg/kg per hour, also has been used for the prevention of nausea and vomiting associated with emetogenic cancer chemotherapy†.

For relief of pruritus associated with use of spinal opiates or cholestasis†, subhypnotic propofol doses given by direct IV injection (10 or 15 mg, respectively) or by IV infusion (at a rate of 0.5–1 or 1–1.5 mg/kg per hour, respectively) have been used.

Cautions

Information on adverse effects of propofol has been obtained principally from controlled clinical trials and worldwide postmarketing experience with the drug. The studies were conducted using various premedications, other anesthetic or sedative agents, and a range of lengths of surgical or diagnostic procedures. Most adverse effects were mild and transient. In adults, the adverse effect profile in patients undergoing monitored anesthesia care (MAC) sedation was similar to that of patients undergoing anesthesia, although more severe adverse respiratory effects (e.g., cough, upper airway obstruction, apnea, hypoventilation, dyspnea) were reported in those undergoing MAC sedation. In addition, the adverse effect profile in pediatric patients 6 days to 16 years of age undergoing anesthesia was similar to that of adults receiving propofol for anesthesia, although apnea may occur more frequently in children than in adults.

■ **Cardiovascular Effects** Propofol is a cardiovascular depressant with effects similar to or greater than those associated with other IV anesthetic induction agents. The main adverse cardiovascular effect of propofol during induction anesthesia is hypotension, with 30% or more decreases in both systolic and diastolic blood pressure. Concomitant use of propofol with an opiate agonist appears to increase the risk of severe hypotension. Administration of additional fluids and a cautious rate of IV infusion may help to prevent propofol-induced hypotension. Severe hypotensive effects may be alleviated by medical intervention. (See Cautions: Precautions and Contraindications.)

In clinical trials in patients undergoing anesthesia or MAC sedation, hypotension or arrhythmias (e.g., bradycardia, tachycardia) were reported in 3–10 or 1–3% of adults, respectively, while hypotension, hypertension, or arrhythmias (e.g., tachycardia) were reported in 17, 8, or 1.2–1.6% of pediatric patients undergoing anesthesia, respectively. In less than 1% of adults, ECG abnormalities, bigeminy, atrial arrhythmias, atrial premature complexes (APCs, PACs), ventricular premature complexes (VPCs, PVCs), and syncope, possibly associated with use of propofol, have been reported. Although a causal relationship to propofol has not been established, atrial fibrillation, atrioventricular (AV) heart block, bundle branch block, cardiac arrest, edema, extrasystole, hypertension, myocardial infarction, myocardial ischemia, ST-segment depression, supraventricular tachycardia, and ventricular fibrillation were reported in clinical trials in less than 1% of adults receiving propofol for anesthesia or MAC sedation.

In clinical trials in intubated, mechanically ventilated patients undergoing sedation with propofol in a critical care setting (e.g., an ICU), hypotension, bradycardia, and decreased cardiac output were reported in 26, 1–3, and 1–3% of patients, respectively. Although a causal relationship to propofol has not been established, arrhythmias (e.g., ventricular tachycardia), atrial fibrillation, bigeminy, cardiac arrest, extrasystole, and right-sided heart failure have been reported in less than 1% of adults receiving propofol for sedation in a critical care setting.

■ Respiratory Effects Propofol can depress respiration, and induction anesthesia frequently is associated with apnea. In clinical trials in adults receiving propofol for induction of anesthesia, duration of apnea was less than 30, 30–60, and more than 60 seconds in 7, 24, and 12% of patients, respectively. In addition, in clinical trials in pediatric patients (neonates and children 16 years of age and younger) receiving 1- to 3.6-mg/kg doses of rapid IV propofol injections for induction of anesthesia, duration of apnea was less than 30, 30–60, and more than 60 seconds in 12, 10, and 5% of patients, respectively. Overall, apnea was reported in 1–3% of adult patients undergoing anesthesia or MAC sedation. The respiratory depressant effects of propofol appear to be similar to those of other IV induction anesthetics; however, the incidence and duration of apnea associated with propofol may be greater. During maintenance of general anesthesia, propofol causes a decrease in spontaneous minute ventilation, usually associated with increased carbon dioxide tension ($Paco_2$), the likelihood of which depends on the rate of administration of propofol and other concomitantly used drugs (e.g., opiates, sedatives).

In clinical trials, wheezing and cough, possibly associated with use of propofol, were reported in less than 1% of adults undergoing anesthesia or MAC sedation. Although a causal relationship to propofol has not been established, hypoxia, laryngospasm, bronchospasm, laryngismus, pulmonary edema, burning of the throat, dyspnea, hiccups, hyperventilation, hypoventilation, pharyngitis, sneezing, tachypnea, and upper airway obstruction were reported in less than 1% of adults receiving propofol for anesthesia or MAC sedation.

Although the respiratory depressant effects of propofol are not clinically important during mechanical ventilation, such effects may be important during the weaning process. Respiratory acidosis during weaning has been reported in 3–10% of adults undergoing sedation in a critical care setting. Decreased pulmonary function, possibly related to use of propofol, has been reported in less than 1% of adults undergoing sedation in a critical care setting, while hypoxia occurred in less than 1% of such adults; however, a causal relationship to the drug has not been established.

■ Infectious Complications Propofol is commercially available in a lipid-based formulation that has been found to support rapid microbial growth at room temperature. Although currently available formulations contain an agent to retard the growth of microorganisms, they are not considered antimicrobially preserved products by USP standards. Contamination of propofol even with very small numbers of microorganisms may result in clinical disease. Therefore, strict aseptic technique and strict adherence to the manufacturer's preparation and handling instructions are required. (See Dosage and Administration: Administration.) The manufacturers state that when proper aseptic technique has not been used in handling propofol injectable emulsion, microbial contamination of the injection and consequent development of fever, infection, sepsis, other life-threatening illness, or death has occurred.

Outbreaks of postoperative surgical site infections, sepsis, and acute febrile episodes were reported following the initial marketing of propofol. The outbreaks were determined to be caused by extrinsic microbial contamination of propofol secondary to improper handling and use. Several practices were identified that were thought to contribute to this contamination: preparation of multiple syringes of propofol at one time for use throughout the day; reuse of syringes and/or infusion-pump lines on different patients; use of propofol syringes that had been prepared up to 24 hours in advance; failure to wear gloves during preparation and administration of propofol; failure to disinfect the rubber stopper of propofol vials prior to use; and transfer of prepared syringes of propofol between operating rooms or facilities. The frequency of reports of infection declined substantially after an agent to retard microbial growth was added to propofol vials and after the professional prescribing information was revised to include warnings to use strict aseptic technique, adhere to requirements to use a vial or syringe for a single patient only, begin administration immediately after opening the vial or syringe, and discard unused product within specified time limits. Propofol formulations containing 0.005% disodium edetate or 0.25 mg/mL sodium metabisulfate have been found to inhibit microbial growth for up to 12 hours as demonstrated by test data for representative USP organisms; however, strict aseptic technique and adherence to handling guidelines still are necessary to avoid the risk of infection.

Several clusters of patients experiencing chills, fever, and body aches shortly after receiving propofol for sedation or general anesthesia have been reported. Symptoms have developed 6–18 hours after propofol administration and have lasted for up to 3 days. Several patients have been hospitalized, and one patient experienced seizures; in all cases, patients have recovered without apparent sequelae. Tests of propofol vials and lots used in patients experiencing these symptoms have not identified any vials contaminated with bacteria or endotoxins. Patients who develop these symptoms shortly after receiving propofol should be evaluated for bacterial sepsis, and such cases should be reported to the FDA MedWatch program. In addition, although infections associated with propofol principally have been traced to extrinsic contamination of the drug, recall of specific lots of propofol (Teva) because of the presence of elevated endotoxin levels has occurred.

■ Nervous System Effects Involuntary movement has been reported in 3–10% of adults receiving propofol for anesthesia or MAC sedation, while this effect occurred in 17% of pediatric patients undergoing anesthesia. Hypertonia and/or dystonia, paresthesia, anticholinergic syndrome, agitation, chills, delirium, dizziness, and somnolence, possibly related to the use of propofol, have been reported in less than 1% of adults undergoing anesthesia or MAC sedation; in addition, abnormal dreams, increased sexual mood, anxiety, bucking/jerking/thrashing, confusion, shivering, clonic and/or myoclonic movement, asthenia, combativeness, confusion, depression, emotional lability, excitement, euphoria, fatigue, hallucinations, headache, hysteria, insomnia, moaning, neuropathy, opisthotonos, rigidity, seizures, somnolence, tremor, and twitching were reported in less than 1% of such adults, but causal relationship to propofol has not been established.

In less than 1% of adults undergoing sedation in a critical care setting, agitation, possibly related to the use of propofol, has been reported. In addition, chills and/or shivering, intracranial hypertension, seizures, somnolence, and abnormal thinking have been reported in less than 1% of such patients, although a causal relationship to propofol has not been established.

■ Local Effects Pain at the injection site occurs frequently (in up to 70% of patients) following peripheral IV administration of propofol. Pain at the injection site can be minimized in adults and children if the larger veins of the forearm or antecubital fossa rather than hand veins are used and by administering 1 mL of a 1% solution of IV lidocaine prior (30–120 seconds) to IV administration of propofol. Because of the possibility that lidocaine may cause instability of the propofol emulsion, the manufacturers recommend that lidocaine be administered prior to propofol administration or that lidocaine be added to propofol immediately before administration in a quantity not exceeding 20 mg of lidocaine per 200 mg of propofol. (See Chemistry and Stability: Stability.) For prevention of pain at the propofol injection site, other methods, including prior administration of opiates or metoclopramide, prior application of a tourniquet, topical nitroglycerin or a local anesthetic cream, or administration of propofol at low temperatures (4–5°C) also have been used. Intra-arterial injection in animals did not result in adverse local tissue effects and while pain was reported in patients who received inadvertent intra-arterial injection of propofol, there was no evidence of major sequelae. In animals, injection of propofol into subcutaneous or perivascular tissues was associated with minimal tissue reaction. Local pain, swelling, blisters and/or tissue necrosis has been reported rarely following inadvertent extravasation in postmarketing surveillance of propofol. The manufacturers state that in clinical trials, burning, stinging, or pain at the injection site was reported in 17.6% of adults undergoing anesthesia or MAC sedation and in 10% of pediatric patients. Phlebitis, thrombosis, and pruritus, possibly related to use of propofol, were reported in less than 1% of adults, while urticaria and/or pruritus and redness/discoloration were reported in less than 1% of such adults, but a causal relationship to the drug has not been established.

■ Dermatologic and Sensitivity Reactions Propofol has been associated with fatal and life-threatening anaphylactic and anaphylactoid reactions. Anaphylactoid and/or anaphylactic reactions (manifested by angioedema, bronchospasm, erythema, and hypotension), and flushing, possibly related to use of propofol, were reported in less than 1% of adults undergoing anesthesia or MAC sedation. In addition, urticaria and diaphoresis have been reported in less than 1% of such patients, but a causal relationship to the drug has not been established. Rash and pruritus have been reported in 1–3% of adults undergoing anesthesia and MAC sedation and in 5 and 2% of pediatric patients undergoing anesthesia, respectively.

Rash has been reported in less than 1% of adults receiving propofol for sedation in a critical care setting, but a causal relationship to the drug has not been established.

■ Metabolic and Electrolyte Effects Propofol infusion syndrome, a potentially life-threatening constellation of metabolic derangements and organ system failure, has been reported in adult and pediatric patients receiving propofol for sedation in a critical care setting. The syndrome, characterized by severe metabolic acidosis, hyperkalemia, lipidemia, rhabdomyolysis, hepatomegaly, and cardiac, renal, or circulatory failure, has occurred most frequently in patients receiving prolonged, high-dose infusions (greater than 5 mg/kg per hour for more than 48 hours); however, the syndrome also has occurred following short-term, high-dose infusions during surgical anesthesia. The manufacturers state that alternate means of sedation should be considered in the setting of prolonged need for sedation, increasing propofol dosage requirements to maintain a constant level of sedation, or onset of metabolic acidosis during propofol infusion.

Hypomagnesemia, possibly related to the use of propofol, has been reported in less than 1% of adults receiving propofol for anesthesia or MAC sedation. In addition, hyperkalemia and hyperlipemia have been reported in less than 1% of such adults, but a causal relationship to the drug has not been established.

Hyperlipemia was reported in 3–10% of adults receiving propofol in a critical care setting. Because the commercially available formulations of propofol are 1% oil-in-water emulsions, patients receiving IV infusion of the drug for longer than 3 days tend to have increased serum lipid concentrations (e.g., triglycerides) while propofol IV infusions administered for 7 days or longer have resulted in serum triglyceride concentrations 3–4 times the normal values. (See Cautions: Precautions and Contraindications.)

Certain formulations of propofol injectable emulsion (Diprivan®) contain edetate disodium, which can chelate many divalent and trivalent metals. In clinical trials, mean urinary zinc loss was about 2.5–3 and 1.5–2 mg daily in adult and pediatric patients, respectively, receiving propofol injectable emulsion formulations containing edetate disodium 0.005%. (See Cautions: Precautions and Contraindications.)

■ Genitourinary and Renal Effects Cloudy urine, possibly related to the use of propofol, was reported in less than 1% of adults receiving the drug for anesthesia or MAC sedation. In addition, oliguria and urinary retention were reported in less than 1% of such adults, but a causal relationship to the drug has not been established.

Green urine, possibly related to the use of propofol, has been reported in less than 1% of adults receiving propofol for sedation in a critical care setting. In addition, increased BUN, serum creatinine concentrations, and renal failure have been reported in less than 1% of such adults, but a casual relationship to the drug has not been established.

■ GI Effects Results of randomized, controlled clinical trials indicate that postoperative nausea and vomiting is less likely to occur in propofol-treated patients than in those receiving other anesthetic agents. It should be considered, however, that the incidence of postoperative nausea and vomiting also is influenced by other factors (e.g., age, gender, type and duration of surgery, concomitant drugs).

Hypersalivation, nausea, and vomiting, possibly related to the use of propofol, were reported in less than 1% of adults receiving the drug for anesthesia or MAC sedation. In addition, cramping, diarrhea, dry mouth, taste perversion, parotid gland enlargement, difficulty in swallowing, and vomiting occurred in less than 1% of such adults, but a causal relationship to the drug has not been established.

Ileus has been reported in adults receiving propofol for sedation in a critical care setting, but a causal relationship to the drug has not been established.

■ Ocular and Otic Effects Amblyopia and abnormal vision, possibly related to the use of propofol, have been reported in less than 1% of adults receiving the drug for anesthesia or MAC sedation. In addition, diplopia, conjunctival hyperemia, ocular pain, nystagmus, otic pain, and tinnitus have been reported in less than 1% of such adults, but a causal relationship to propofol has not been established.

■ Musculoskeletal Effects Pain of the extremities, possibly related to the use of propofol, has been reported in less than 1% of adults receiving propofol for anesthesia or MAC sedation. In addition, myalgia, neck rigidity and/or stiffness, and trunk pain have been reported in less than 1% of such adults, but a causal relationship to the drug has not been established.

Rhabdomyolysis has been reported in association with propofol infusion syndrome (see Cautions: Metabolic and Electrolyte Effects).

■ Hematologic Effects Hemorrhage and leukocytosis, possibly related to the use of propofol, have been reported in less than 1% of adults receiving the drug for anesthesia or MAC sedation. In addition, coagulation disorders have been reported in less than 1% of such adults, but a causal relationship to the drug has not been established.

■ Pancreatitis Pancreatitis (sometimes requiring hospitalization) has been reported in adults undergoing induction anesthesia or prolonged sedation in a critical care setting who received propofol. Following resolution of pancreatitis in at least one patient, the disease recurred after inadvertent rechallenge with the drug and therefore a causal relationship to propofol was suggested. However, some clinicians state that a variety of confounding factors (e.g., concomitant drugs, presence or absence of hypertriglyceridemia) make it difficult to conclude with certainty the effects of propofol on the risk of developing pancreatitis. Many clinicians state that further controlled studies are needed to determine whether there is an association between pancreatitis and administration of propofol and they further state that clinicians should consider the possibility of pancreatitis in patients receiving propofol.

■ Hepatic Effects Abnormal liver function test results have been reported in adults receiving propofol for sedation in a critical care setting, but a causal relationship to the drug has not been established.

■ Other Effects Perinatal disorder and fever, possibly related to the use of propofol, have been reported in less than 1% of adults receiving propofol for anesthesia or MAC sedation. In addition, intraoperative awareness, increased drug effect, and chest pain were reported in less than 1% of such adults, but a causal relationship to the drug has not been established. Fever, sepsis, and whole-body weakness were reported in less than 1% of adults receiving propofol for sedation in a critical care setting.

■ Precautions and Contraindications When used in general anesthesia or MAC sedation, propofol should be administered by individuals experienced in the use of general anesthesia who are not involved in the conduct of the surgical and/or diagnostic procedures. Sedated patients should be constantly monitored and facilities necessary for intubation, assisted respiration, administration of oxygen, and cardiopulmonary resuscitation should be readily available whenever propofol is used. Because propofol may produce cardiovascular depression, patients receiving the drug should be monitored continuously for early signs of hypotension and bradycardia. Patients also should be monitored for adverse respiratory effects (e.g., apnea, airway obstruction, and/or oxygen desaturation), especially those undergoing MAC sedation. These cardiorespiratory effects are more likely to occur following administration of rapid IV ("bolus") injections, especially in patients with American Society of Anesthesiologists (ASA) physical status III or IV, and in geriatric or debilitated patients. Therefore, geriatric, debilitated, and ASA physical status III or IV patients should receive lower induction and slower maintenance doses than other patients. In patients undergoing cardiac surgery, slower rates of IV administration of propofol should be used in those who received premedication and in those with recent fluid imbalance or who are hemodynamically unstable. It is recommended that fluid depletion be corrected prior to administration of propofol. Management of hypotension may include discontinuance of propofol, increasing the rate of IV fluid administration (except in those in whom additional fluid therapy is contraindicated), elevation of the lower extremities, and/or use of vasopressors.

Although propofol has no vagolytic activity, cases of bradycardia, asystole, and rarely, cardiac arrest have been reported, especially in pediatric patients who received concomitant administration with fentanyl. Intervention with anticholinergic agents (e.g., atropine, glycopyrrolate) should be considered to modify potential increases in vagal tone associated with surgical stimuli or concomitant use of certain drugs, including succinylcholine. Apnea, which may persist for more than 60 seconds, occurs frequently during induction anesthesia and ventilatory support should be considered.

Propofol has been associated with fatal and life-threatening anaphylactic and anaphylactoid reactions. (See Cautions: Dermatologic and Sensitivity Reactions.)

Propofol infusion syndrome, a potentially life-threatening constellation of metabolic derangements and organ system failures, has been reported in adult and pediatric patients receiving propofol for sedation in a critical care setting (see Cautions: Metabolic and Electrolyte Effects). The syndrome, characterized by severe metabolic acidosis, hyperkalemia, lipidemia, rhabdomyolysis, hepatomegaly, cardiac and/or renal, and/or circulatory failure, has occurred most frequently in patients receiving prolonged, high-dose infusions (greater than 5 mg/kg per hour for more than 48 hours); however, the syndrome also has occurred following short-term, high-dose infusions during surgical anesthesia. Patients should be closely monitored for development of unexplained acidosis, rhabdomyolysis, and cardiac and/or renal failure. The manufacturers state that alternate means of sedation should be considered in the setting of prolonged need for sedation, increasing propofol dosage requirements to maintain a constant level of sedation, or onset of metabolic acidosis during propofol infusion.

Because commercially available propofol preparations are oil-in-water emulsions, the drug should be used with caution in patients with disorders of lipid metabolism (e.g., primary hyperlipoproteinemia, diabetic hyperlipemia, pancreatitis). Since prolonged administration of the drug may result in increased serum lipid concentrations (e.g., hypertriglyceridemia) (see Cautions: Metabolic and Electrolyte Effects), patients undergoing sedation in a critical care setting (e.g., an ICU) who are at risk of developing hyperlipidemia should be monitored for increases in serum triglyceride concentrations or serum turbidity. The manufacturers state that the quantity of concurrently administered lipids (e.g., fat emulsions for parenteral nutrition) in these patients should be reduced in order to compensate for the amount of lipids contained in the propofol emulsion formulation (1 mL of propofol injectable emulsion contains 0.1 g of fat [1.1 kcal]).

When used for sedation in critical care settings in intubated, mechanically ventilated patients, propofol should be administered by individuals qualified in the management of patients in intensive-care settings and trained in cardiovascular resuscitation and airway management. Since excessively high blood concentrations of propofol may occur in patients receiving the drug for prolonged periods, infusion rate of propofol should be reduced and titrated according to individual clinical response and sedation levels should be evaluated at least daily. Prior to weaning patients from mechanical ventilator assistance, neuromuscular blocking agents should be discontinued or neuromuscular blockade reversed, and opiate therapy should be discontinued or the dosage adjusted to optimize respiratory function and/or to maintain a light level of sedation. If respiratory depression does not develop, this level of sedation may be maintained during the weaning process since abrupt withdrawal of propofol has been associated with rapid awakening, accompanied by anxiety, agitation, and resistance to mechanical ventilation, thus making the weaning process difficult. Therefore, the manufacturers recommend that administration of propofol be continued until about 10–15 minutes prior to extubation.

Because certain formulations of propofol injectable emulsion (Diprivan®) contain 0.005% of edetate disodium, a heavy metal antagonist that can chelate many divalent and trivalent cations, patients receiving continuous infusions for sedation in critical care settings should not receive such formulations for longer than 5 days without a drug-free interval. This drug-free interval is intended to allow replacement of estimated or measured urinary zinc losses. In patients who are predisposed to zinc deficiency (e.g., those with burns, diarrhea, major sepsis), the need for supplemental zinc should be considered during prolonged therapy with edetate disodium-containing formulations of propofol. Although renal toxicity has been reported rarely in patients receiving high (2–3 g daily) dosages of edetate disodium, decreased renal function has not been observed in clinical studies conducted to date in patients with normal or impaired renal function receiving propofol (Diprivan®) injectable emulsion. However, the manufacturer of Diprivan® recommends that laboratory analysis of urine (including urine sediment) should be performed prior to and during (every other day) initiation of propofol therapy in patients at risk for developing renal impairment.

Long-term propofol therapy in patients with renal or hepatic impairment has not been evaluated to date.

Similar to other sedatives, there appears to be wide interpatient variation in propofol dosage requirements that may increase or decrease with time.

When propofol is used for anesthesia in patients with increased intracranial pressure or impaired cerebral circulation who are undergoing neurosurgery, substantial decreases in mean arterial pressure should be avoided because of the resultant decreases in cerebral perfusion pressure. To avoid substantial hypotension and decreases in cerebral perfusion pressure, propofol should be administered IV by an infusion or a slow injection. (See Dosage and Administration: Dosage.)

Propofol has been associated rarely with a period of postoperative unconsciousness (sometimes preceded by a brief period of wakefulness), which may be accompanied by increased muscle tone; recovery has been spontaneous.

Patients with a history of seizure disorders who are receiving propofol are at increased risk of developing seizures during the recovery phase of anesthesia.

Patients should be warned that propofol may impair their ability to perform activities requiring mental alertness (e.g., operating machinery, driving a motor vehicle, signing legal documents) for some time after undergoing general anesthesia or sedation.

Cases of propofol dependence and abuse, in some cases resulting in death (following repeated *self-administration* of propofol by health-care providers) have been reported. While most reported cases have involved health-care professionals (principally anesthesiology personnel), cases of propofol abuse among lay persons also have been reported. (See Chronic Toxicity.) The manufacturers and some clinicians recommend that restriction of access and accounting procedures appropriate to the particular practice setting should be used to prevent diversion of propofol.

Although commercially available preparations of propofol injectable emulsion contain ingredients that retard the rate of growth of microorganisms (e.g., Diprivan® contains 0.005% of edetate disodium), the manufacturers state that strict aseptic technique must be observed when handling the drug, because the emulsion still may support growth of microorganisms. Propofol injectable emulsion should not be used if contamination is suspected, and unused portions should be discarded within the required time limits as recommended by the manufacturers. (See Dosage and Administration: Administration.) The manufacturers also state that when proper aseptic technique in handling propofol injectable emulsion has not been used, microbial contamination of the injection and consequent development of fever, infection, sepsis, other life-threatening illness, or death has occurred. Patients who develop chills, fever, body aches, or other symptoms of acute febrile reactions shortly after receiving propofol should be evaluated for bacterial sepsis, and such cases should be reported to the FDA MedWatch program. (See Cautions: Infectious Complications and see Dosage and Administration: Administration.)

Some commercially available formulations of propofol contain a sulfite that may cause allergic-type reactions, including anaphylaxis and life-threatening or less severe asthmatic episodes, in certain susceptible individuals. The overall prevalence of sulfite sensitivity in the general population is unknown but probably low; such sensitivity appears to occur more frequently in asthmatic than in nonasthmatic individuals.

Propofol is contraindicated in patients with known hypersensitivity to the drug or any component of the respective formulation. Propofol also is contraindicated in patients with allergies to eggs, egg products, soybeans, or soy products.

■ **Pediatric Precautions** The manufacturers state that the safety and efficacy of propofol for the induction of general anesthesia have not been established in pediatric patients younger than 3 years of age. For maintenance of general anesthesia, the manufacturers state that safety and efficacy of the drug have not been established in pediatric patients younger than 2 months of age. In addition, the manufacturers state that propofol is not recommended for sedation in critical care settings, for use in combination with regional anesthesia, or for MAC sedation in pediatric patients younger than 16 years of age, because safety for these procedures in this patient population has not been established.

Propofol has been used in pediatric patients undergoing sedation in critical care settings. Although a causal relationship to propofol has not been definitely established, case reports describe a severe, progressive metabolic (e.g., lactic) acidosis syndrome (that may progress to death) in several ventilated pediatric patients (mainly with respiratory infections) receiving propofol for sedation in an ICU. In some of these children, increasing metabolic acidosis was accompanied or followed by hypocalcemia, hypoglycemia, high serum lipid concentrations (hypertriglyceridemia), elevated serum liver enzyme concentrations, enlarged liver, oliguria, myoglobinuria, fever, multisystem organ failure, cardiac failure, bradycardia, hypotension, AV block of varying degrees, bundle branch block, asystole, and death. The mechanism of this syndrome is not known and the possibility that causes other than administration of propofol may be involved has been suggested.

Results of a multicenter, comparative, clinical trial (conducted by one manufacturer, AstraZeneca) in pediatric patients undergoing sedation in critical care settings (excluding those with upper respiratory infection) indicate that the incidence of mortality was increased in those receiving propofol (9%) compared with that seen in those receiving standard sedative agents (4%). Although a causal relationship of such incidence of mortality to propofol has not been established, this manufacturer and the FDA state that there may be important safety concerns associated with the use of propofol injectable emulsion in pediatric patients undergoing sedation in critical care settings. Therefore, propofol is *not* labeled and should not be employed for such use in children 16 years of age or younger.

Propofol also has been used in pediatric patients undergoing MAC sedation for surgical, diagnostic, and other procedures (e.g., lumbar puncture with intrathecal chemotherapy, bone marrow aspiration and biopsy, central venous catheter placement, transesophageal echocardiogram, cardiac catheterization, radiologic examinations, orthopedic manipulations). However, the manufacturers state that propofol should not be used for MAC sedation in pediatric patients, because safety and efficacy for such use have not been established.

In pediatric patients receiving prolonged IV infusions of propofol, abrupt discontinuance of the drug may result in flushing of the hands and feet, agitation, tremulousness, hyperirritability, increased incidence of bradycardia, agitation, or jitteriness.

FDA warns that repeated or prolonged use of general anesthetics and sedation drugs, including propofol, in children younger than 3 years of age or during the third trimester of pregnancy may affect brain development. Animal studies in multiple species, including nonhuman primates, have demonstrated that use for longer than 3 hours of anesthetic and sedation drugs that block *N*-methyl-D-aspartic acid (NMDA) receptors and/or potentiate γ-aminobutyric acid (GABA) activity leads to widespread neuronal and oligodendrocyte cell loss and alterations in synaptic morphology and neurogenesis in the brain, resulting in long-term deficits in cognition and behavior. Across animal species, vulnerability to these neurodevelopmental changes occurs during the period of rapid brain growth or synaptogenesis; this period is thought to correlate with the third trimester of pregnancy through the first year of life in humans, but may extend to approximately 3 years of age. The clinical relevance of these animal findings to humans is not known.

While some published evidence suggests that similar deficits in cognition and behavior may occur in children following repeated or prolonged exposure to anesthesia early in life, other studies have found no association between pediatric anesthesia exposure and long-term adverse neurodevelopmental outcomes. Most studies to date have had substantial limitations, and it is not clear whether the adverse neurodevelopmental outcomes observed in children were related to the drug or to other factors (e.g., surgery, underlying illness). There is some clinical evidence that a single, relatively brief exposure to general anesthesia in generally healthy children is unlikely to cause clinically detectable deficits in global cognitive function or serious behavioral disorders; however, further research is needed to fully characterize the effects of exposure to general anesthetics in early life, particularly for prolonged or repeated exposures and in more vulnerable populations (e.g., less healthy children).

Results from an observational study (the Pediatric Anesthesia Neurodevelopment Assessment [PANDA] study) and preliminary results from an ongoing multicenter, randomized trial (the General Anesthesia Compared to Spinal Anesthesia [GAS] trial) provide some evidence that a single, relatively brief exposure to general anesthesia in generally healthy children is unlikely to cause clinically detectable deficits in global cognitive function or serious behavioral disorders. The PANDA study compared global cognitive function (as measured by intelligence quotient [IQ] score) of children 8–15 years of age who had a single anesthesia exposure for elective inguinal hernia surgery before the age of 3 years with that of a biologically related sibling who had no anesthesia exposure before the age of 3 years. All of the children had a gestational age at birth of at least 36 weeks, and sibling pairs were within 3 years of being the same age. Children who underwent the elective procedure were mostly males (90%) and generally healthy. The mean duration of anesthesia was 84 minutes; 16% of those receiving anesthesia had exposures exceeding 2 hours. The study found no substantial difference in IQ score between children who had a single anesthesia exposure before the age of 3 years and their siblings who had not. The GAS trial was designed to compare neurodevelopmental outcomes in children who received general anesthesia with those in children who received awake regional (caudal and/or spinal) anesthesia for inguinal herniorrhaphy before they reached a postmenstrual age of 60 weeks (with a gestational age at birth of more than 26 weeks); the primary outcome was the Wechsler Preschool and Primary Scale of Intelligence Third Edition (WPPSI-III) Full Scale IQ at 5 years of age. In an interim analysis at the age of 2 years, no difference in composite cognitive score (as measured by the Bayley Scales of Infant and Toddler Development III) was detected between children who had received sevoflurane anesthesia of less than 1 hour's duration (median duration: 54 minutes) compared with those who had received awake regional anesthesia.

Anesthetic and sedation drugs are an essential component of care for children and pregnant women who require surgery or other procedures that cannot be delayed; no specific general anesthetic or sedation drug has been shown to be less likely to cause neurocognitive deficits than any other such drug. Pending further accumulation of data in humans from well-designed studies, decisions regarding the timing of elective procedures requiring anesthesia should take into consideration both the benefits of the procedure and the potential risks. When procedures requiring the use of general anesthetics or sedation drugs are considered for young children or pregnant women, clinicians should discuss with the patient, parent, or caregiver the benefits, risks (including potential risk of adverse neurodevelopmental effects), and appropriate timing and duration of the procedure. FDA states that procedures that are considered medically necessary should not be delayed or avoided.

■ **Geriatric Precautions** Studies in geriatric patients have shown that these patients may require lower dosages of propofol for anesthesia and other indications. The manufacturers state that lower induction doses and a slower rate of maintenance IV infusion should be used in patients 55 years of age and older. In addition, to minimize the risk of adverse effects, including cardiorespiratory depression (e.g., hypotension), apnea, airway obstruction, and/or arterial oxygen desaturation, rapid (single or repeated) IV ("bolus") administration of propofol should not be used in geriatric patients during general anesthesia or MAC sedation. (See Dosage and Administration: Dosage.)

■ **Mutagenicity and Carcinogenicity** No evidence of mutagenicity was seen when propofol was evaluated in several in vitro and in vivo test systems. The drug was not mutagenic in the Ames microbial (*Salmonella*) mutagen test, *Saccharomyces cerevisiae* gene mutation and/or gene conversion assay, in vitro cytogenic studies in Chinese hamsters, and the mouse micronucleus test.

Long-term animal studies to evaluate the carcinogenic potential of propofol have not been performed to date.

■ **Pregnancy, Fertility, and Lactation** Reproduction studies in rats and rabbits using IV propofol dosages of 15 mg/kg daily (approximately equivalent to the human propofol induction dose on a mg/m^2 basis) did not reveal evidence of harm to the fetus. Propofol readily crosses the placenta and similar to other general anesthetics, administration of propofol may be associated with neonatal depression. Limited data indicate that the ratio of umbilical vein to maternal vein concentration at parturition is about 0.7 after rapid IV ("bolus") administration of 2.5 mg/kg of propofol to women undergoing cesarean section. In one study, mean propofol concentrations of 0.078 mcg/mL were detected 2 hours after delivery in neonates whose mothers had received an IV propofol infusion of 5 mg/kg per hour for about 26 minutes while undergoing cesarean section. Because there are no adequate and controlled studies to date using propofol in pregnant women and animal studies are not always predictive of human response, propofol should be used during pregnancy only when clearly needed. The manufacturers state that propofol is not recommended for obstetric surgery (e.g., cesarean section).

Based on animal data, repeated or prolonged use of general anesthetics and sedation drugs, including propofol, during the third trimester of pregnancy may result in adverse neurodevelopmental effects in the fetus. The clinical relevance of these animal findings to humans is not known; the potential risk of adverse neurodevelopmental effects should be considered and discussed with pregnant women undergoing procedures requiring general anesthetics and sedation drugs. (See Cautions: Pediatric Precautions.)

Reproduction studies in female rats receiving IV propofol dosages up to 15 mg/kg daily (approximately equivalent to the human propofol induction dose on a mg/m^2 basis) for 2 weeks before pregnancy up to day 7 of gestation did not reveal evidence of impaired fertility. Impairment of male fertility was not observed in a dominant lethal study in rats receiving propofol dosages up to 15 mg/kg daily for 5 days.

Propofol reportedly is distributed into human milk. The manufacturers state that the drug should not be used in nursing women because the effects of oral absorption of small amounts of propofol are not known. Some clinicians state that nursing women undergoing surgery may receive usual anesthetic induction doses of propofol; however, since trace amounts of the drug may be present in milk, drowsiness of the infants may occur on the day of the procedure. It should be considered that in reproduction studies in rats and rabbits, IV propofol dosages (15 mg/kg daily) administered to dams during lactating periods have been shown to cause maternal deaths and decreased pup survival. It has been suggested that the pharmacologic effect (anesthesia) of propofol on the dams probably is responsible for the adverse effects observed in the offspring.

Drug Interactions

■ **Drugs Affecting Hepatic Microsomal Enzymes** In vitro data indicate that propofol is metabolized mainly by cytochrome P-450 (CYP) isoenzyme 2B6 and to a lesser extent by 2C9. In addition, results of in vitro studies indicate that propofol is an inhibitor of the CYP isoenzymes 1A1, 1A2, 2B1, 2C9, 2D6, 2E1, and 3A4, and the possibility exists that propofol may alter the pharmacokinetics of drugs metabolized by these isoenzymes. However, it has been suggested that because of the increased value for hepatic extraction (50 μM) of propofol, there have been relatively few clinically important drug interactions with agents affecting or being affected by the cytochrome P-450 system

Concomitant use of propofol with alfentanil in healthy young men reportedly has resulted in increased (up to 22%) blood concentrations of propofol. Limited data indicate that concomitant use of propofol with opiate agonists (e.g., alfentanil, fentanyl, sufentanil) may result in increased (10–20%) blood concentrations of the opiates. These effects presumably occur via inhibition of CYP isoenzymes involved in the metabolism of propofol and the opiates. However, alfentanil also may reduce both distribution and clearance of propofol. Although these variations in blood concentrations of propofol and opiates are unlikely to be clinically important, concomitant use of propofol with opiates has resulted in greater sedation and analgesia than those associated with administration of each drug alone.

■ **CNS Depressants** Concomitant use of propofol with other CNS depressants including sedatives (e.g., benzodiazepines), hypnotics (e.g., opiates), and inhalation anesthetics (e.g., nitrous oxide, enflurane, isoflurane, halothane) may increase the sedative, anesthetic, and cardiorespiratory depressant effects of propofol. Increased serum concentrations of propofol have been reported with concomitant use of propofol and inhalation anesthetics (e.g., halothane, isoflurane), possibly associated with decreased hepatic blood flow that may result in decreased clearance of propofol. Therefore, the manufacturers state that the induction dose requirements of propofol may need to be reduced in patients receiving premedication with IV or IM opiates (e.g., meperidine, morphine, fentanyl) or in those receiving a combination of opiates with sedatives (e.g., benzodiazepines, barbiturates, chloral hydrate, droperidol). In addition, during maintenance of anesthesia or sedation, IV infusion rates of propofol may need to be reduced with concomitant use of CNS depressants.

Limited data suggest that IV propofol may act synergistically with IV midazolam to produce induction of anesthesia and sedation (e.g., in an ICU). It has been postulated that the synergism observed between propofol and midazolam is the result of a pharmacodynamic interaction occurring at the $GABA_A$ receptors in the brain. In addition, concomitant use of propofol and midazolam resulted in increased (by about 20%) mean free plasma concentration of midazolam, although mean free concentrations of propofol did not appear to be affected.

In pediatric patients, concomitant use of propofol with fentanyl may result in severe bradycardia.

■ **Neuromuscular Blocking Agents** Propofol does not appear to cause clinically important changes in the onset, intensity, or duration of action of commonly used neuromuscular blocking agents (e.g., succinylcholine, nondepolarizing skeletal muscle relaxants). However, bradycardia and asystole have occurred in patients receiving propofol with atracurium or suxamethonium, but a causal relationship to the concomitant use of these agents has not been established. It also should be considered that administration of propofol alone has been associated with such cardiac effects.

■ **Anticoagulants** Limited data indicate that IV administration of lipids (e.g., those contained in the propofol injectable emulsion) may decrease patient response to coumarin-derivative anticoagulants (e.g., warfarin) in patients with malabsorptive states secondary to disease (e.g., those with Crohn's disease). The mechanism of such an interaction has not been elucidated, but lipid emulsions may interfere pharmacodynamically with warfarin activity by increasing synthesis of functional blood coagulation factors, increasing platelet aggregation, or supplying vitamin K. It is recommended that until further studies are available to evaluate this interaction, heparin therapy should be administered for initial anticoagulation in patients with malabsorptive states receiving high-dose lipid emulsions who require reliable anticoagulation. If warfarin is given, international normalized ratio (INR) should be monitored daily in these patients.

■ **Other Drugs** Administration of the local anesthetic agents bupivacaine or lidocaine reduced propofol dosage requirements for sedation or hypnosis, while premedication with clonidine has been reported to reduce intraoperative dosage requirements of propofol.

In one study, concomitant use of droperidol with propofol was found to increase twofold the frequency of postoperative incidence of nausea and vomiting associated with administration of propofol alone, suggesting a potential interaction between the drugs.

Acute Toxicity

■ **Pathogenesis** Limited information is available on the acute toxicity of propofol in humans. The IV LD_{50} of propofol, administered as the emulsion formulation, averaged 53 and 42 mg/kg in mice and rats, respectively, while the oral LD_{50} of propofol, administered as a solution in soybean oil, was 1230 and 600 mg/kg in mice and rats, respectively.

■ **Manifestations** Overdosage of propofol would be expected to produce manifestations that principally are extensions of the drug's pharmacologic and adverse effects. At least 2 fatalities have been reported following intentional self-administration of a 400- or 1600-mg dose of propofol.

■ **Treatment** In the event of overdosage, therapy with propofol should be discontinued immediately, and appropriate symptomatic therapy initiated. Overdosage of propofol is likely to be associated with cardiorespiratory depression. If respiratory depression occurs, patients require administration of oxygen and institution of artificial ventilation. In addition, for cardiovascular depression, elevation of the lower extremities, increasing the rate of IV fluid administration, and/or use of vasopressors or anticholinergic agents are suggested.

Chronic Toxicity

Cases of propofol dependence and abuse, in some cases resulting in death, have been reported. While most reported cases have involved healthcare professionals (principally anesthesiology personnel), cases of propofol abuse among lay persons also have been reported. (See Uses: Misuse and Abuse.)

Death secondary to propofol abuse usually has been associated with the drug's cardiorespiratory effects. Since ventilatory support is absent in cases of self-administration, death secondary to apnea and subsequent respiratory depression can occur at therapeutic concentrations of the drug. In one case report involving a clinician with a history of chronic propofol abuse who died of cardiac sudden death, development of ST-segment elevation in right precordial leads on ECG was observed, possibly indicating that the development of such elevation may be the first warning sign of electrical instability and predictive of imminent sudden death. It was hypothesized that a rise in cardioinhibitory cytokines (TNF-α) may be interpreted as an adaptive response of jeopardized myocardium to the cardiac dysfunction resulting from elevated catecholamine concentrations secondary to chronic propofol abuse.

Psychological dependence, manifested by intense craving for the drug and loss of control over the amount and frequency of drug use, has been reported in cases of propofol abuse. In some cases, abuse of the drug continued despite negative consequences (e.g., job loss, criminal activity to obtain drug). Rarely, withdrawal symptoms (e.g., insomnia, anxiety, difficulty concentrating), suggesting physical dependence, have been observed; however, in most cases of propofol abuse, withdrawal symptoms have not been reported. Signs of tolerance, including increases in use to 100 injections or more daily, have been observed. Prior history of substance abuse has been present in some, but not all, cases of propofol abuse. One case of propofol abuse occurred in a lay person who initially had received propofol for the treatment of tension headache; the remaining cases have been reported in patients who have not received prior medical treatment with the drug.

The abuse potential and mechanisms of propofol have not been defined in detail. Like alcohol, barbiturates, and benzodiazepines, propofol enhances the chloride content of the $GABA_A$ receptor. In addition, propofol has been shown to increase dopamine concentrations in the nucleus accumbens, a core region of the brain's reward system. Propofol also has been reported to bind to dopamine D_2 and *N*-methyl-D-aspartic acid (NMDA) receptors. Effects of the drug in cases of abuse have been described as pleasant feelings, feelings of euphoria or relaxation, sedation, and unconsciousness. In addition, sexual hallucinations and sexual disinhibition have been reported upon recovery from propofol anesthesia. Results of a clinical trial in healthy individuals indicate that subanesthetic doses of propofol could be rewarding in some participants. Animal studies also have shown that propofol is self-administered by rats and primates at subanesthetic doses, indicating a reinforcing effect of the drug.

Pharmacology

■ **CNS Effects** Following IV injection, propofol has a rapid onset of action and will produce a loss of consciousness within 1 arm-brain circulation time (the time required for the drug to travel from the site of injection to the site of action in the brain) (i.e., usually within 40–60 seconds). The exact mechanism(s) by which propofol exerts its effect on the CNS has not been fully elucidated. However, it is believed that such effects are related, at least partially, to the drug's ability to enhance the activity of γ-aminobutyric acid (GABA), the principal inhibitory neurotransmitter in the CNS, by interacting with the $GABA_A$ receptor complex both at spinal and supraspinal synapses. There is evidence that the drug enhances GABA-mediated transmission at a site distinct from benzodiazepine receptors and such activity may vary depending on plasma propofol concentrations. In addition to the effects on the $GABA_A$ receptors, propofol also may interact with other neurotransmitter sites, including glycine, nicotinic, glutamate, and G-protein coupled receptors; the drug also may inhibit sodium channels.

Anesthetic Effects Propofol is capable of producing all levels of CNS depression—from light sleep to deep coma—depending on the dosage. The degree of depression and duration of action depend on dosage, rate of administration, and pharmacokinetics of the drug. In addition, the patient's age, weight, medical condition, type of surgical procedure, and/or concurrent use of other drugs may alter the response. Therefore, dosage of propofol should be titrated based on assessment of clinical effect. Clinical assessment of the depth of anesthesia is based on responses to verbal commands and surgical stimulation (e.g., changes in heart rate and blood pressure), EEG changes (measured by bispectral [BIS] index), autonomic signs (e.g., lacrimation, diaphoresis), eyelash reflex, and movement.

Effects on EEG Dose-related changes on the EEG appear to occur with propofol. Following administration of sedative doses of propofol, activation of the EEG (particularly in beta wave activity) occurs while anesthetic doses have been associated with increased slow wave activity in the delta frequency range. High dosages (e.g., IV infusion rates exceeding 9 mg/kg per hour [150 mcg/kg per minute]) of propofol may result in an EEG pattern with isoelectric periods (burst suppression), which may last up to 15 seconds or longer.

Propofol appears to be associated with both anticonvulsant activity and excitatory effects on the nervous system. Propofol has been used effectively in patients with refractory status epilepticus, and the drug may substantially decrease seizures associated with electroconvulsive therapy (ECT). However, propofol also has been associated with a variety of excitatory effects (e.g., seizures, myoclonus, opisthotonos) on the nervous system, possibly resulting from glycine antagonism at subcortical sites.

Cerebrovascular Effects When administered in anesthetic doses, propofol may increase cerebral vascular resistance and decrease cerebral blood flow and cerebral metabolic rate for oxygen ($CMRO_2$) and glucose. The drug may slightly decrease intracranial pressure in patients undergoing intracranial surgery or in those undergoing sedation in a critical care setting.

Analgesic, Amnesic, and Anxiolytic Effects The analgesic effects of propofol have not been conclusively determined. Limited data indicate that hypnotic doses of propofol may be associated with analgesic effects, while responses to subhypnotic doses of the drug may vary from analgesia to hyperalgesia. Propofol also may be associated with some level of amnesia; however, the drug has lesser amnesic effects than the benzodiazepines.

In addition, limited data indicate that subhypnotic doses of propofol may be associated with anxiolytic effects comparable to those of midazolam or methohexital.

■ **Cardiovascular Effects** Propofol has caused cardiovascular depression, and such an effect may be similar or greater than that associated with other IV induction agents (e.g., barbiturates). The hemodynamic effects of propofol during induction of anesthesia are variable. If spontaneous pulmonary ventilation is maintained, the most severe cardiovascular effect of propofol is arterial hypotension (sometimes greater than a 30% decrease), which is accompanied by little or no changes in heart rate or appreciable decreases in cardiac output. However, if respiration is maintained via mechanically assisted ventilation, the incidence and degree of decreases in cardiac output are increased. Many factors, including age, gender, physical status, type of procedure, concomitant medications (e.g., opiates, benzodiazepines, β-adrenergic blocking agents), and dose and rate of IV infusion, can influence the extent of cardiovascular depression. Although the exact mechanism of action has not been elucidated, hypotension may result from peripheral vasodilation, reduction in ventricular preload, sympathetic activity, or myocardial contractility.

Propofol is associated with bradycardia that may lead to asystole in adult and pediatric patients. The drug also reduces myocardial oxygen consumption; further studies are needed to determine the extent of this effect on the myocardium and the coronary vascular system.

■ **Respiratory Effects** Administration of anesthetic induction doses of propofol frequently depress respiration, which usually begins with a fall in tidal volume and progresses to apnea in both adults and pediatric patients. Apnea may persist for longer than 1 minute, depending on the dose of propofol administered. In addition, maintenance anesthesia with propofol results in dose-dependent decreases in pulmonary ventilation and increases in carbon dioxide tension (PCO_2). Propofol-induced respiratory depression is affected by the choice of premedication and dose and rate of injection; respiratory depression is increased when propofol is administered with opiate agonists or benzodiazepines. Propofol-induced adverse respiratory effects are similar to those of other induction agents (e.g., methohexital, thiopental [no longer commercially available in the US]); however, the incidence and duration of apnea are greater with propofol. In addition, equivalent anesthetic doses of etomidate appear to cause less respiratory depression than propofol or thiopental sodium.

Propofol has been shown to depress pharyngeal reflexes and provide appropriate jaw tone for intubation. Rapid IV injection or sedative doses of propofol are reported to cause bronchodilation in patients with chronic obstructive pulmonary disease, status asthmaticus, or hyperactive airways.

When compared with midazolam, effects of propofol on arterial blood gas or other pulmonary measurements appear to be similar to those occurring in intubated and mechanically ventilated adult patients undergoing treatment in a critical care setting (e.g., an ICU).

■ **Other Effects** In clinical studies, a substantial reduction (30–60%) in intraocular pressure (IOP) was reported in adult and geriatric patients undergoing ophthalmic surgery who were receiving anesthesia with propofol. Decreases in IOP usually occur immediately following induction, and IOP may remain below baseline levels during intubation. It has been suggested that such decreases in IOP may be associated with a reduction in the extraocular muscular tone or depression of the ocular center in the brain.

Results of several clinical studies indicate that patients receiving propofol for induction and maintenance of anesthesia have a lower incidence of postoperative nausea and vomiting than those associated with other anesthetic agents. It appears that propofol has direct antiemetic properties; however, the mechanism of antiemetic action of propofol remains to be established.

Because the commercially available formulations of propofol are 1% oil-in-water emulsions, patients receiving IV infusions of the drug for longer than 3 days tend to have increased serum lipid concentrations (e.g., triglycerides), while IV propofol infusions administered for 7 days or longer may result in serum triglyceride concentrations 3–4 times the normal values.

Results of animal and human studies indicate that propofol injectable emulsion does not appear to suppress adrenocortical response to stimulation by corticotropin (ACTH) or increase plasma histamine concentrations.

Results of animal studies have shown development of hemosiderin deposits in livers of dogs receiving certain formulations of propofol injectable emulsion (Diprivan®) containing 0.005% of edetate disodium for 2 weeks; however, the clinical importance of this effect is not known.

In vitro studies indicate that high doses of propofol may affect immune responses by inhibiting neutrophil polarization by more than 50%. Although the clinical importance of such effects in vivo are not known, some clinicians state that these effects should be considered in patients receiving prolonged IV infusions of the drug (e.g., those in an ICU).

Pharmacokinetics

The pharmacokinetics of propofol after IV administration are best described by a 3-compartment model and they appear to be linear. The pharmacokinetic profile of propofol is characterized by rapid distribution of the drug from blood into tissues, rapid metabolic clearance from blood, and slow redistribution of the drug from the peripheral compartment.

The pharmacokinetics of propofol have been studied in adults and in pediatric patients 3–12 years of age. Distribution and clearance of propofol in pediatric patients are similar to those reported in adults. There is no evidence of gender-related differences in the pharmacokinetics of the drug. Studies in adults indicate that the pharmacokinetics of propofol do not appear to be affected by chronic renal failure or chronic hepatic cirrhosis; however, the pharmacokinetics of propofol have not been studied in patients with acute renal or hepatic failure.

■ **Absorption** Following a single (e.g., 2.5 mg/kg) IV injection, propofol has a rapid onset because the drug is distributed rapidly from plasma to the CNS. The onset of action of propofol as determined by time to unconsciousness (i.e., loss of response to voice command) usually ranges from 15–30 seconds, and depends on the rate of administration. Following a single rapid IV injection, propofol blood concentrations decline so rapidly that peak plasma concentrations cannot be readily measured; duration of action of the drug usually is about 5–10 minutes.

Following IV administration of repeated rapid IV injections of propofol (e.g., an initial induction dose of 2.5 mg/kg followed in 3 minutes by several 1-mg/kg doses, administered at 6-minute intervals), peak and trough venous blood concentrations of the drug in samples obtained immediately before each rapid IV dose and 2 minutes afterwards were 4–10 and 1–2.5 mcg/mL, respectively. When propofol is used alone for induction anesthesia, plasma concentrations of the drug necessary to provide loss of eyelash reflex, loss of consciousness, and the possibility for initiation of surgery in 50% of patients (IC_{50}) are estimated to be 2.1, 2.7–3.4, and 15.2 mcg/mL, respectively.

To provide adequate maintenance anesthesia when propofol is used as a component of total IV anesthesia, initial plasma propofol concentrations of 2–7.5 mcg/mL followed by 2.5–5 mcg/mL have been suggested. To achieve such concentrations, some clinicians have used a pharmacokinetic computer model interfaced with a target-controlled infusion (TCI) device† (e.g., Diprifusor®, AstraZeneca; not currently commercially available in the US) to administer the appropriate amounts of propofol.

Following initiation of a continuous IV infusion of propofol, there is an initial rapid increase in blood concentrations of the drug, which is followed by a slower rate of increase, probably associated with a rapid distribution from the blood to tissues. In a limited number of patients undergoing sedation with propofol in an ICU and who received a 1- to 3-mg/kg rapid IV ("bolus") dose followed by a constant-rate IV infusion (3 mg/kg per hour) for 72 hours, peak blood concentrations of the drug in samples obtained over the 72-hour period ranged from 0.77–15.3 mcg/mL. Limited data indicate that plasma propofol concentrations necessary to provide sedation in 50% of such patients (IC_{50}) are estimated to be 0.47 mcg/mL for a sedation score exceeding 2 (when measured by the Ramsey scale) and 1.1 mcg/mL for a sedation score exceeding 4.

Since propofol is rapidly distributed from CNS to inactive storage sites, recovery from anesthesia is rapid. Following a single rapid IV injection of propofol, most patients will awaken as blood concentrations of the drug decline to approximately 1 mcg/mL, and improvement of psychomotor performance (as measured by patient response to verbal command) usually occurs at blood propofol concentrations of 0.5–0.6 mcg/mL.

Following daily titration of propofol to achieve only the minimum effective therapeutic concentration, rapid awakening within 10–15 minutes may occur even after long-term administration. However, if higher than necessary infusion rates have been maintained for a long time, redistribution of propofol from fat and muscle to the plasma may be substantial resulting in slow recovery.

Recovery from anesthesia may be more rapid following administration of propofol than barbiturates (e.g., thiopental [no longer commercially available in the US], methohexital) or possibly, etomidate. In a double-blind, comparative, crossover study in healthy adults receiving IV propofol (2.5 mg/kg initially, followed by 1 mg/kg 3 minutes later) or thiopental sodium (5 mg/kg initially, followed by 2 mg/kg 3 minutes later), improvement of psychomotor performance (as measured by patient response to verbal command) was faster in patients receiving propofol (mean time: 33 minutes) than in those receiving thiopental sodium (mean time: 62 minutes). In addition, psychomotor performance was impaired for up to 5 hours after IV administration of thiopental sodium and for 1 hour after propofol.

■ **Distribution** Propofol is highly lipophilic and is rapidly distributed from plasma into human body tissues, including the CNS. Following IV administration, the drug is widely distributed, initially to highly perfused tissues (e. g., brain), then to lean muscle tissue, and finally to fat tissue. In humans, equilibration of propofol between blood and CSF occurs within about 2–3 minutes. Following rapid IV injection of propofol, the volume of distribution of the drug during the initial, steady-state, or elimination phase reportedly ranged from 13–76, 171–771, or 159–1011 L, respectively. Following long-term continuous IV infusion (longer than 72 hours) in patients undergoing sedation in a critical care setting, the volume of distribution at steady-state was much higher than that reported following short-term IV infusions (shorter than 9 hours), 25.5 vs 1.8–5.3 L/kg, possibly because of increased peripheral distribution associated with the long-term infusion. Volume of distribution of propofol may be reduced in geriatric patients when compared with younger individuals, perhaps because of a reduction in the volume of highly perfused tissues relative to body mass or a reduction in perfusion of these tissues associated with decreased cardiac output.

Propofol is approximately 95–99% bound to plasma proteins, mainly albumin and hemoglobin. Protein binding appears to be independent of the plasma concentration of the drug.

Propofol readily crosses the placenta. Limited data indicate that the ratio of umbilical venous to maternal venous blood concentration at parturition is about 0.7 after rapid IV ("bolus") administration of 2.5 mg/kg of propofol to women undergoing cesarean section. In one study, mean propofol blood concentrations of 0.078 mcg/mL were detected 2 hours after delivery in neonates whose mothers had received a propofol infusion of 5 mg/kg per hour for about 26 minutes while undergoing cesarean section. Propofol reportedly is distributed into human milk in low concentrations.

■ **Elimination** Pharmacokinetic data indicate that plasma concentrations of propofol decline in a triphasic manner, with the drug undergoing a very rapid initial distribution. In adults receiving IV propofol either as a single rapid injection or a continuous infusion, in the initial (distribution) phase ($t_{1/2\alpha}$) reportedly averages 1.8–9.5 minutes, in the second (redistribution) phase ($t_{1/2\beta}$) averages 21–70 minutes, and in the terminal (elimination) phase ($t_{1/2\gamma}$) averages 1.5–31 hours. It has been suggested that the terminal plasma half-life may not affect clinical outcome as substantially as the distribution half-life, because once blood propofol concentrations decrease below the range required for hypnosis, rapid awakening from the anesthesia will occur.

Propofol is rapidly and extensively metabolized in the liver. Propofol mainly undergoes glucuronidation at the C1-hydroxyl position, but hydroxylation of the benzene ring also may occur to form 4-hydroxypropofol which is subsequently conjugated with sulfuric and/or glucuronic acid. Hydroxypropofol has been reported to have approximately ⅓ of the hypnotic activity of propofol. Hydroxylation of propofol is mediated by the cytochrome P-450 (CYP) isoenzyme 2B6 and to a lesser extent by the 2C9 isoenzyme.

Propofol is excreted mainly in the urine principally as sulfate and/or glucuronide conjugates; less than 0.3% of propofol is eliminated unchanged in the urine. Limited data indicate that less than 2% of a dose of propofol is eliminated in feces.

Following IV administration of propofol by rapid injections or by a continuous infusion in healthy adults or in critically ill patients undergoing sedation, total body clearance of the drug is high and ranges from about 1.3–3.5 L/minute. Total body clearance of propofol may be substantially lower in geriatric patients compared with younger adults, possibly because of decreased hepatic metabolism resulting from decreased hepatic blood flow. Since plasma clearance exceeds hepatic blood flow, it appears that the drug also is metabolized at extrahepatic sites. Mean total body clearance of propofol appears to be proportional to body weight; obese patients have a substantially higher body clearance than leaner individuals.

Chemistry and Stability

■ **Chemistry** Propofol, an alkyl phenol, is an IV anesthetic agent. The drug is structurally unrelated to other currently available IV anesthetics. Propofol, which occurs as a colorless to pale straw-colored, oily, liquid, is very slightly soluble in water and is very soluble in alcohol. The octanol/water (pH 6–8.5) partition coefficient for propofol is approximately 5012:1 to 6761:1. Propofol has a pK_a of 11 in water. Commercially available parenteral propofol preparations are sterile, nonpyrogenic, isotonic, white oil-in-water emulsions containing 10 mg of propofol, 100 mg of soybean oil, 2.5 mg of glycerin, and 12 mg of egg lecithin per mL. Diprivan® injectable emulsion also contains edetate disodium (0.005%) as a pharmaceutic aid (chelating agent), and sodium hydroxide to adjust pH to 7–8.5.

■ **Stability** Commercially available propofol injectable emulsions should be stored at 4–22°C and should be protected from freezing. Since propofol undergoes oxidative degradation in the presence of oxygen, the commercially available injectable emulsions are packaged under nitrogen to prevent such degradation.

The manufacturers state that the commercially available 1% (10 mg/mL) propofol injectable emulsion may be used without dilution. When the emulsion is administered directly from the original container, administration should be completed within 12 hours and unused portions should be discarded. If propofol injectable emulsion is transferred to another container, administration should begin promptly and be completed within 12 hours; unused portions also should be discarded. If dilution of propofol injectable emulsion is necessary, the drug may be diluted with 5% dextrose injection to a concentration of not less than 0.2% (2 mg/mL). It appears that stability of the diluted solutions is greater in glass than in plastic containers; potency of the diluted emulsions may decrease by about 5–8% after continuous IV infusion of propofol through a plastic (PVC) tubing for 2 hours. Potency may decrease even further (up to 35%) when the diluted solution is left stationary in a PVC tubing. It has been suggested that propofol injectable emulsion may adsorb to plastic IV tubing and such adsorption may be decreased by maintaining a constant flow of the solution.

The manufacturers state that propofol is compatible with several IV fluids (e.g., 5% dextrose, 5% dextrose and lactated Ringer's, lactated Ringer's, 5% dextrose and 0.2% or 0.45% sodium chloride) when a Y-type administration set is used. Propofol should *not* be administered through the same catheter as blood, serum, or plasma, because compatibility of the drug with these fluids has not been established. In vitro tests have shown that aggregates of the globular component of the vehicle containing propofol may form when the drug has been in contact with blood, serum, or plasma. The clinical importance of these effects is not known.

Addition of lidocaine to propofol in quantities greater than 20 mg of lidocaine per 200 mg of propofol may cause instability of the propofol emulsion, resulting in increases in globule sizes over time; reduction of anesthetic potency has been reported in rats. The manufacturers recommend that lidocaine be given prior to administration of propofol or, alternatively, that lidocaine be added to propofol immediately before administration, in a quantities not exceeding 20 mg lidocaine/200 mg propofol.

The manufacturers state that propofol should *not* be mixed with other therapeutic agents prior to administration. Propofol has been reported to be physically and/or chemically incompatible with several drugs, but the compatibility depends on several factors (e.g., concentration of the drugs, specific diluents used, resulting pH, temperature). Specialized references should be consulted for more specific information.

Results of several studies indicate that propofol is chemically and physically compatible with thiopental (no longer commercially available in the US) when admixed in syringes for at least 24 hours at room temperature. In addition, limited data suggest that thiopental may decrease the potential for microbial growth associated with use of propofol when the drugs are admixed.

Preparations

Excipients in commercially available drug preparations may have clinically important effects in some individuals; consult specific product labeling for details.

Propofol

Parenteral		
Injectable emulsion, for IV use	10 mg/mL*	**Diprivan® Emulsion** (available as ready-to-use single patient infusion vials), Fresenius Kabi
		Propofol Injectable Emulsion

*available from one or more manufacturer, distributor, and/or repackager by generic (nonproprietary) name

†Use is not currently included in the labeling approved by the US Food and Drug Administration

Analgesics and Antipyretics 28:08
Nonsteroidal Anti-inflammatory Agents 28:08.04
Cyclooxygenase-2 (COX-2) Inhibitors 28:08.04.08

Celecoxib

■ Celecoxib is a nonsteroidal anti-inflammatory agent (NSAIA) that is a selective inhibitor of cyclooxygenase-2 (COX-2).

Uses

Celecoxib is used in the management of osteoarthritis, rheumatoid arthritis, juvenile rheumatoid arthritis, pain, ankylosing spondylitis, and dysmenorrhea. There currently is no evidence establishing superiority of selective COX-2 inhibitors relative to prototypical NSAIAs in the management of these conditions, and the principal benefit of selective COX-2 inhibitors is a potential reduction in the incidence of certain adverse effects (e.g., GI toxicity). Both COX-2 inhibitors and prototypical NSAIAs have been associated with an increased risk of cardiovascular events. A decision to use a selective COX-2 inhibitor rather than a prototypical NSAIA usually is based on an individual assessment of the risk of ulcer complications from NSAIA therapy. There is some evidence that therapy with a COX-2 inhibitor may be no more effective in reducing the risk of NSAIA-induced GI complications than a combined regimen of a prototypical NSAIA and a proton-pump inhibitor. (See Uses: Osteoarthritis.) Additional study is planned or under way to establish more definitively the role of COX-2 inhibitors relative to prototypical NSAIAs.

Celecoxib also is used to reduce the number of adenomatous colorectal polyps in adults with familial adenomatous polyposis (FAP).

The potential benefits and risks of celecoxib therapy as well as alternative therapies should be considered prior to initiating therapy with the drug. The lowest possible effective dosage and shortest duration of therapy consistent with treatment goals of the patient should be employed.

■ **Osteoarthritis** Celecoxib is used for the management of the signs and symptoms of osteoarthritis in adults. Medical management of osteoarthritis of the hip or knee includes both pharmacologic therapy to reduce pain and nonpharmacologic therapy to maintain and/or improve joint mobility and limit functional impairment (e.g., patient education, weight loss when necessary, aerobic and muscle-strengthening exercise programs, physical therapy and range-of-motion exercises, assistive devices for ambulation and activities of daily living, patellar taping, appropriate footwear or bracing). Pain management is considered an adjunct to nonpharmacologic measures, and is most effective when combined with nonpharmacologic strategies.

A variety of drugs have been used for management of pain in patients with osteoarthritis, including oral agents (e.g., acetaminophen, NSAIAs, tramadol), intraarticular agents (e.g., glucocorticoids, sodium hyaluronate), and topical agents (e.g., capsaicin, methylsalicylate). Factors to consider when making treatment decisions for the management of pain in patients with osteoarthritis include the presence of risk factors for serious adverse GI effects or renal toxicity (which may affect decisions regarding use of NSAIAs), existing comorbidities and concomitant therapy, and the adverse effects profiles and costs of specific therapies.

Because there is evidence that acetaminophen can be effective and because of its relative safety and low cost, the American College of Rheumatology (ACR) and other clinicians recommended use of the drug as the initial analgesic for many osteoarthritis patients. Acetaminophen appears to be as effective as NSAIAs for relief of mild to moderate joint pain in many patients with osteoarthritis; however, the drug is not effective in all patients and may not provide adequate relief in those with moderate to severe pain or when joint inflammation is present. An NSAIA can be considered an alternative initial drug of choice for patients with osteoarthritis, especially for those who have moderate to severe pain and signs of joint inflammation, and also can be considered in patients who fail to obtain adequate symptomatic relief with acetaminophen. NSAIAs that are selective inhibitors of COX-2 (e.g., celecoxib) are associated with a lower incidence of adverse GI effects than prototypical NSAIAs. Both COX-2 inhibitors and prototypical NSAIAs have been associated with an increased risk of cardiovascular events. A decision to use a selective COX-2 inhibitor (e.g., celecoxib) rather than a prototypical NSAIA usually is based on an individual assessment of the risk for GI toxicity. If a prototypical NSAIA (e.g., diclofenac, diflunisal, fenoprofen, ibuprofen, indomethacin, ketoprofen, meclofenamate, naproxen, piroxicam, sulindac, tolmetin) is used in osteoarthritis patients at risk for GI complications, concomitant use of misoprostol or a proton-pump inhibitor (e.g., omeprazole) can be considered for preventive therapy. However, in a study comparing the efficacy of celecoxib (200 mg twice daily) versus diclofenac sodium (75 mg twice daily) plus omeprazole (20 mg daily) in preventing recurrent ulcer bleeding in *H. pylori*-negative arthritis (principally osteoarthritis) patients with a recent history of ulcer bleeding while receiving long-term NSAIA therapy, the protective efficacy was unexpectedly low for both regimens (recurrent ulcer bleeding probabilities of 4.9 versus 6.4%, respectively, during the 6-month study) and it appeared that neither could completely protect patients at high risk.

In several double-blind, placebo-controlled, or comparative studies of up to 12 weeks' duration, celecoxib was at least as effective as naproxen and more effective than placebo in the symptomatic management of osteoarthritis of the knee or hip in patients who experienced exacerbation of symptoms (e.g., pain, joint stiffness) following discontinuance of standard therapy with NSAIAs or other analgesics. While celecoxib and naproxen generally are comparably effective in the management of osteoarthritis, current data suggest that adverse GI effects occur less frequently with celecoxib. (See Cautions: GI Effects.)

In controlled clinical studies in adults with osteoarthritis, therapy with celecoxib (100 mg twice daily or 200 mg once daily) resulted in improvement in the Western Ontario and McMasters Universities (WOMAC) osteoarthritis index; WOMAC is a 24-item questionnaire that measures pain, stiffness, and functioning. Following initiation of celecoxib 100 or 200 mg twice daily in patients with joint pain as a result of symptomatic exacerbation of osteoarthritis, pain relief generally occurs within 24–48 hours and therapy with the drug is associated with greater reductions in joint pain than placebo. In placebo-controlled and comparative studies in patients with symptomatic exacerbation of osteoarthritis of the hip or knee, 31–36% of patients receiving celecoxib 100 mg twice daily for 12 weeks improved as measured by patient and physician assessment of the arthritic condition; improvement occurred in 29–36% of patients receiving celecoxib 200 mg twice daily, 29–37% of patients receiving naproxen 500 mg twice daily, and 17–24% of patients receiving placebo twice daily. Celecoxib dosages of 100 mg twice daily and 200 mg once daily were comparably effective in patients with osteoarthritis as measured by joint pain, disease activity, functionality, and health-related quality of life. Celecoxib dosages of 200 mg twice daily do not appear to provide additional benefit compared with dosages of 100 mg twice daily or 200 mg once daily in these patients.

■ **Rheumatoid Arthritis in Adults** Celecoxib is used for the management of the signs and symptoms of rheumatoid arthritis in adults. Although current data suggest that the efficacy of celecoxib is similar to that of prototypical NSAIAs but with a lower risk of adverse GI effects, both selective COX-2 inhibitors and prototypical NSAIAs have been associated with an increased risk of cardiovascular events. A decision to use a selective COX-2 inhibitor (e.g., celecoxib) rather than a prototypical NSAIA usually is based on an individual assessment of the risk for GI toxicity. There is some evidence that therapy with a COX-2 inhibitor may be no more effective in reducing the risk of NSAIA-induced GI complications than a combined regimen of a prototypical NSAIA and a proton-pump inhibitor. (See Uses: Osteoarthritis.)

In the management of rheumatoid arthritis in adults, NSAIAs may be useful for initial symptomatic treatment; however, NSAIAs do not alter the course of the disease or prevent joint destruction. Disease modifying antirheumatic drugs (DMARDs) (e.g., azathioprine, cyclosporine, etanercept, oral or injectable gold compounds, hydroxychloroquine, infliximab, leflunomide, methotrexate, minocycline, penicillamine, sulfasalazine) have the potential to reduce or prevent joint damage, preserve joint integrity and function, and reduce total health care costs, and all patients with rheumatoid arthritis are candidates for DMARD therapy. DMARDs should be initiated early in the disease course and should not be delayed beyond 3 months in patients with active disease (i.e., ongoing joint pain, substantial morning stiffness, fatigue, active synovitis, persistent elevation of erythrocyte sedimentation rate [ESR] or C-reactive protein [CRP], radiographic evidence of joint damage) despite an adequate regimen of NSAIAs. NSAIA therapy may be continued in conjunction with DMARD therapy or, depending on patient response, may be discontinued. (For further information on the treatment of rheumatoid arthritis, see Uses: Rheumatoid Arthritis, Methotrexate 10:00.)

In double-blind, placebo-controlled studies, therapy with celecoxib was associated with greater reduction in joint tenderness/pain and swelling than placebo. In addition, several double-blind, comparative studies of up to 24 weeks' duration have demonstrated that celecoxib is at least as effective as naproxen or diclofenac in the symptomatic treatment of rheumatoid arthritis but is less likely to cause adverse GI effects. (See Cautions: GI Effects.) Clinical studies of celecoxib generally have included adults receiving standard therapy for rheumatoid arthritis (i.e., NSAIAs with or without DMARDs and/or low-dose oral corticosteroids) who experienced symptomatic exacerbation (symptom "flare") within 2–14 days of discontinuing the NSAIA component of their regimen. Symptom flare was defined as a minimum of 6 *tender* joints *and* an increase of 20% in the number of tender or painful joints or involvement of at least 2 additional joints since discontinuing NSAIA therapy; a minimum of 3 *swollen* joints *and* an increase of 20% in the number of swollen joints or involvement of at least 2 additional joints since discontinuing NSAIA therapy; and either a minimum of 45 minutes of morning stiffness*and* an increase of at least 15 minutes in the duration of morning stiffness *or* an increase in patient-assessed arthritis pain since discontinuing NSAIA therapy.

The American College of Rheumatology criteria for a 20% improvement (ACR 20 response) in measures of disease activity were used as the principal measure of clinical response in studies evaluating the efficacy of celecoxib. An ACR 20 response is achieved if the patient experiences a 20% improvement in the number of tender and swollen joints and a 20% or greater improvement in at least 3 of the following 5 criteria: patient pain assessment; patient global assessment; physician global assessment; patient self-assessed disability; and laboratory measures of disease activity (i.e., ESR or C-reactive protein level). In placebo-controlled and comparative studies in adults with rheumatoid arthritis who had symptom flare, an ACR 20 response was achieved in 30–40% of patients who received celecoxib 100 mg twice daily for 12 weeks, 39–44% of patients who received celecoxib 200 mg twice daily for 12 weeks, 36–42% of patients who received naproxen 500 mg twice daily for 12 weeks, and 23–29% of placebo-treated patients. While celecoxib 100 mg twice daily generally was as effective as celecoxib 200 mg twice daily, some patients experienced additional benefit from the higher dosage. Dosages of 400 mg twice daily provided no additional benefit compared with dosages of 100–200 mg twice daily.

■ Juvenile Arthritis Celecoxib is used for the management of the signs and symptoms of juvenile rheumatoid arthritis in children 2 years of age or older. Efficacy of celecoxib was established in pediatric patients with pauciarticular course, polyarticular course, or systemic onset juvenile rheumatoid arthritis (active systemic disease not present at study entry) in a double-blind, active-controlled study of 12 weeks' duration; pediatric patients 2–17 years of age were randomized to receive celecoxib 3 mg/kg (up to a maximum dose of 150 mg) twice daily, celecoxib 6 mg/kg (up to a maximum dose of 300 mg) twice daily, or naproxen 7.5 mg/kg (up to a maximum dose of 500 mg) twice daily. Response was measured using the juvenile rheumatoid arthritis definition of improvement (i.e., a 30% or greater improvement in at least 3 of 6 and a 30% or greater deterioration in no more than 1 of 6 core set criteria that included physician and patient/parent global assessments, active joint count, limitation of motion, functional assessment, and erythrocyte sedimentation rate: JRA DOI 30). Results of this study indicate that celecoxib is as effective as naproxen in the management of juvenile rheumatoid arthritis. Evaluation at week 12 indicated that clinical response (JRA DOI 30) was achieved in 69, 80, or 67% of pediatric patients receiving celecoxib 3 mg/kg twice daily, celecoxib 6 mg/kg twice daily, or naproxen 7.5 mg/kg twice daily, respectively. The manufacturer states that safety and efficacy of celecoxib therapy beyond 6 months in pediatric patients with juvenile arthritis have not been established.

Clinical trials indicate that either celecoxib or a prototypical NSAIA is effective in the management of juvenile rheumatoid arthritis. Celecoxib may have a lower risk of adverse GI effects compared with prototypical NSAIAs and may be useful in children who have experienced adverse GI effects with prototypical NSAIAs. In addition, celecoxib may be useful in children who have experienced other adverse effects with prototypical NSAIAs (e.g., naproxen-induced pseudoporphyria). It remains to be determined whether long-term cardiovascular risks in children exposed to celecoxib are similar to those observed in adults receiving celecoxib or other NSAIAs. (See Cautions: Cardiovascular Effects.)

■ Ankylosing Spondylitis Celecoxib is used for the management of the signs and symptoms of ankylosing spondylitis in adults. Clinical trials indicate that either selective COX-2 inhibitors or prototypical NSAIAs are effective for initial symptomatic management of ankylosing spondylitis. Although celecoxib may have a lower risk of adverse GI effects compared with prototypical NSAIAs, both selective COX-2 inhibitors and prototypical NSAIAs have been associated with an increased risk of cardiovascular events. A decision to use a selective COX-2 inhibitor (e.g., celecoxib) rather than a prototypical NSAIA usually is based on an individual assessment of the risk for GI toxicity. There is some evidence that therapy with a COX-2 inhibitor may be no more effective in reducing the risk of NSAIA-induced GI complications than a combined regimen of a prototypical NSAIA and a proton-pump inhibitor. (See Uses: Osteoarthritis.)

In placebo- and active-controlled studies of 6- and 12-weeks' duration in patients with ankylosing spondylitis, celecoxib (100 mg twice daily, 200 mg once daily, or 400 mg once daily) was more effective than placebo, as assessed by global pain intensity and global disease activity (both rated using visual analog scales) and functional impairment (measured using the Bath Ankylosing Spondylitis Functional Index [BASFI]). In the 12-week study, there was no difference in the extent of improvement in those receiving celecoxib 400 mg daily relative to those receiving celecoxib 200 mg daily, but more patients receiving the 400-mg daily dose (53%) than the 200-mg daily dose (44%) were classified as responders (defined as achieving 20% or greater improvement in the Assessment in Ankylosing Spondylitis [ASAS] response criteria). There was no change in responder rates after 6 weeks.

■ Colorectal Polyps Celecoxib is used to reduce the number of adenomatous colorectal polyps in adults with familial adenomatous polyposis (FAP) as an adjunct to usual care (e.g., endoscopic surveillance, surgery). Patients with FAP have an inherited mutation in the adenomatous polyposis coli (APC) gene that results in hundreds of adenomatous polyps and an almost 100% risk of colon cancer. The clinical benefit of reducing the number of polyps in individuals with FAP remains to be determined. It is not known whether use of celecoxib in patients with FAP will reduce the risk of colorectal, duodenal, or other FAP-related cancers or whether use of the drug reduces the need for endoscopic surveillance and prophylactic colectomy or other FAP-related surgery. Therefore, FAP patients receiving celecoxib should continue to receive usual care.

Efficacy of celecoxib in reducing the extent of polyposis has been evaluated in a randomized, placebo-controlled study in adults with FAP. In this study, patients with FAP were randomized to receive a 6-month regimen of celecoxib 400 mg twice daily, celecoxib 100 mg twice daily, or placebo. Patients underwent endoscopy at the beginning and end of the study to determine the number and size of polyps in specified areas (one area of the rectum and up to 4 areas of the colon); response to treatment was expressed as the mean percent change in the number of polyps and in polyp burden (expressed as the sum of polyp diameters). The mean pretreatment number of polyps was 11.5–15.5 and the mean pretreatment polyp burden was 34.8–44.7 mm. At month 6, the mean reduction in the number of polyps was 28% in patients who received celecoxib 400 mg twice daily, 12% in those who received celecoxib 100 mg twice daily, and 5% in those who received placebo; the mean reduction in polyp burden was 30.7, 14.6, and 4.9%, respectively. While administration of celecoxib (400 mg twice daily) appears to be associated with a reduction in the number of colorectal polyps in patients with FAP, the clinical benefit of reducing the number of polyps in such individuals remains to be determined and it is unclear whether the effect of celecoxib in reducing the number of polyps persists after the drug is discontinued. The manufacturer states that safety and efficacy of celecoxib therapy for longer than 6 months in patients with FAP have not been studied.

Use of celecoxib for the prevention of adenomatous colorectal polyps (colorectal adenomas) in patients without a history of FAP† has been investigated in 2 long-term, National Institute of Health (NIH)-supported, multicenter studies (Adenoma Prevention with Celecoxib [APC]; Prevention of Colorectal Sporadic Adenomatous Polyps [PreSAP]). Patients included in these studies had undergone recent removal of colorectal adenomas and were at high risk of recurrent adenomas. Results of these studies indicate that administration of celecoxib (200 mg twice daily, 400 mg twice daily, or 400 mg once daily) reduces the risk of recurrent colorectal adenomas. The cumulative rate of adenoma detection during up to 3 years of treatment was 33.6–43.2% among patients receiving celecoxib compared with 49.3–60.7% among those receiving placebo. However, some clinicians state that routine use of celecoxib for the prevention of sporadic colorectal adenomas cannot be recommended because of the potential for serious cardiovascular events in celecoxib-treated patients. The studies did not evaluate whether celecoxib alters the risk of a first occurrence of colorectal adenoma or prevents the development of colorectal cancer.

■ Pain Celecoxib is used in the management of acute pain, including postoperative (dental, orthopedic) pain, in adults. In pain studies evaluating the efficacy of celecoxib, the drug was effective in the relief of postoperative dental pain and postoperative orthopedic pain that was described as moderate to severe. Following administration of single doses of celecoxib, the onset of analgesia was 60 minutes. In a single-dose study, celecoxib 100 or 400 mg reportedly was more effective than placebo and as effective as aspirin 650 mg for relief of pain following dental extraction. However, limited data indicate that celecoxib 100 or 200 mg as a single dose may be less effective than single doses of ibuprofen 400 mg or naproxen sodium 550 mg for the acute relief of postoperative dental pain.

■ **Dysmenorrhea** Celecoxib is used for the relief of primary dysmenorrhea in adults. In pain studies evaluating the efficacy of celecoxib, the drug was effective in the relief of moderate to severe pain associated with primary dysmenorrhea.

■ **Other Uses** Celecoxib has no effect on platelet function and is not a substitute for aspirin in the prevention of adverse cardiovascular events (e.g., primary or secondary prevention of myocardial infarction).

Results from a large, prospective, population-based cohort study in geriatric individuals indicate a lower prevalence of Alzheimer's disease† among patients who received an NSAIA for 2 years or longer. Similar findings have been reported from some other, but not all, observational studies.

Dosage and Administration

■ **Administration** The potential benefits and risks of celecoxib therapy as well as alternative therapies should be considered prior to initiating celecoxib therapy.

Celecoxib is administered orally as a single daily dose or in 2 equally divided doses daily. Once- and twice-daily regimens were equally effective in the management of osteoarthritis. The manufacturer recommends a twice-daily dosing schedule for the management of rheumatoid arthritis and juvenile arthritis. The manufacturer states that celecoxib dosages up to 200 mg twice daily may be administered without regard to meals; higher celecoxib dosages (i.e., 400 mg twice daily) should be administered with food to improve absorption.

For patients with difficulty swallowing capsules, the celecoxib capsule may be opened, the contents carefully emptied onto a level teaspoonful of applesauce at room temperature or cooler, and the mixture swallowed immediately with water. This mixture is stable for 6 hours when refrigerated.

Dispensing and Administration Precautions Because of similarity in spelling of Celebrex® (celecoxib), Celexa® (citalopram hydrobromide), and Cerebyx® (fosphenytoin sodium), extra care should be exercised in ensuring the accuracy of prescriptions for these drugs.

■ **Dosage** The lowest possible effective dosage and shortest duration of therapy consistent with treatment goals of the patient should be employed.

When celecoxib is used in the management of arthritis in adults, the dosage of celecoxib should be adjusted according to individual requirements and response, using the lowest possible effective dosage.

Although peak plasma concentrations and area under the plasma concentration-time curve (AUC) were increased 40 and 50%, respectively, in geriatric individuals older than 65 years of age compared with younger adults, dosage adjustment in geriatric adults based solely on age generally is not required. However, for geriatric patients weighing less than 50 kg, celecoxib therapy should be initiated at the lowest recommended dosage.

Osteoarthritis For the symptomatic treatment of osteoarthritis, the usual adult dosage of celecoxib is 200 mg daily given as a single dose or in 2 equally divided doses. Celecoxib dosages exceeding 200 mg daily (e.g., 200 mg twice daily) do not appear to provide additional therapeutic benefit.

Rheumatoid Arthritis in Adults For the symptomatic treatment of rheumatoid arthritis, the usual adult dosage of celecoxib is 100–200 mg twice daily. Although the overall efficacy of celecoxib was similar in patients receiving 100 or 200 mg twice daily, additional benefit was observed in some patients receiving the higher dosage. However, celecoxib dosages of 400 mg twice daily do not appear to provide additional therapeutic benefit compared with dosages of 100–200 mg twice daily.

Juvenile Arthritis For the symptomatic management of juvenile rheumatoid arthritis in children 2 years of age or older, the recommended dosage of celecoxib for children weighing 10–25 kg is 50 mg twice daily, and the recommended dosage for children weighing more than 25 kg is 100 mg twice daily.

Ankylosing Spondylitis For the symptomatic treatment of ankylosing spondylitis, the usual initial adult dosage of celecoxib is 200 mg daily given as a single dose or in 2 equally divided doses. If no response is observed after 6 weeks, the dosage may be increased to 400 mg daily. If no response is observed following administration of celecoxib 400 mg daily for 6 weeks, response is unlikely and alternative treatment options should be considered.

Colorectal Polyps To reduce the number of adenomatous colorectal polyps in adults with familial adenomatous polyposis (FAP) as an adjunct to usual care (e.g., endoscopic surveillance, surgery), celecoxib should be given in a dosage of 400 mg twice daily. The manufacturer states that safety and efficacy of celecoxib therapy for longer than 6 months in patients with FAP have not been studied.

Pain and Dysmenorrhea For the relief of acute pain or dysmenorrhea, the usual initial adult dosage of celecoxib is 400 mg given as a single dose, followed by an additional dose of 200 mg, if necessary, on the first day. For continued relief, 200 mg may be administered twice daily as needed.

■ **Dosage in Renal and Hepatic Impairment** Celecoxib has not been studied in patients with severe renal impairment, and is not recommended for use in such patients. However, if celecoxib therapy must be used in patients with severe renal impairment, close monitoring of renal function is recommended. The AUC of celecoxib was 40% lower in adults with chronic renal insufficiency (e.g., glomerular filtration rate [GFR] 35–60 mL/minute) than that reported in adults with normal renal function although no substantial relationship was found between GFR and clearance of the drug. The manufacturer makes no specific recommendations for dosage modification in patients with chronic renal insufficiency.

The pharmacokinetics of celecoxib have not been studied in patients with severe hepatic impairment, and the manufacturer states that the drug should not be used in such patients. In addition, the AUC of celecoxib was 40 or 180% higher in adults with mild or moderate hepatic impairment, respectively, compared with that reported in patients with normal hepatic function. In patients with moderate hepatic impairment (Child-Pugh Class B), the manufacturer recommends that celecoxib dosage be reduced approximately 50%.

Cautions

Information on the safety of celecoxib has been obtained principally from clinical studies in about 12,000 patients, including those with osteoarthritis, rheumatoid arthritis, or postoperative pain. About 50 or 30% of these patients received the drug for at least 6 months or at least 1 year, respectively; a limited number of patients have received celecoxib for 2 years or longer. Information on the safety of the drug also has been obtained from studies in pediatric patients 2–17 years of age with juvenile rheumatoid arthritis who received the drug for up to 24 weeks and from colorectal adenoma prevention and Alzheimer's disease prevention studies in adults.

At usual dosages, celecoxib generally is well tolerated. Adverse effects of celecoxib usually are mild and mainly involve the GI tract. During controlled clinical studies in adults receiving celecoxib dosages of 100–800 mg daily, the incidence of celecoxib-associated adverse effects generally was similar to that reported with prototypical nonsteroidal anti-inflammatory agents (NSAIAs) (e.g., diclofenac, ibuprofen, naproxen) or placebo; however, the incidence of endoscopically confirmed GI ulceration and clinically observed upper GI perforations, ulcers, and bleeding was higher in patients receiving a prototypical NSAIA than in those receiving placebo or celecoxib. The adverse effects profile of celecoxib reported in a clinical study in adults with familial adenomatous polyposis (FAP) and in clinical studies in patients with ankylosing spondylitis or acute pain, including postoperative (e.g., dental, orthopedic) pain and primary dysmenorrhea, was similar to that reported in clinical studies in patients with arthritis. About 7.1% of adults receiving celecoxib in clinical studies discontinued therapy because of adverse effects compared with 6.1% of those receiving placebo. The most frequent adverse effects requiring discontinuance of celecoxib include dyspepsia (in about 0.8 or 0.6% of patients receiving celecoxib or placebo, respectively) and abdominal pain (in about 0.7 or 0.6% of patients receiving celecoxib or placebo, respectively).

■ **Cardiovascular Effects** Peripheral edema has been reported in 2.1% of adults receiving celecoxib in premarketing clinical studies. Angina pectoris, chest pain, coronary artery disorder, hot flushes, myocardial infarction, palpitation, tachycardia, or aggravated hypertension has been reported in 0.1–1.9% of adults receiving the drug. Adverse cardiovascular effects reported in less than 0.1% of adults receiving celecoxib include syncope, congestive heart failure, ventricular fibrillation, pulmonary embolism, cerebrovascular accident, peripheral gangrene, thrombophlebitis, deep-vein thrombosis, and vasculitis.

Peripheral edema or hypertension occurred in 4.5 or 2.4%, respectively, of patients receiving celecoxib (400 mg twice daily) in the Celecoxib Long-term Arthritis Safety Study (CLASS). Peripheral edema and hypertension also have been described as evidence of adverse renal effects. (See Cautions: Renal, Electrolyte, and Genitourinary Effects.)

Thrombotic Events NSAIAs, including selective cyclooxygenase-2 (COX-2) inhibitors and prototypical NSAIAs, increase the risk of serious adverse cardiovascular thrombotic events, including myocardial infarction and stroke (which can be fatal), in patients with or without cardiovascular disease or risk factors for cardiovascular disease.

The association between cardiovascular complications and use of NSAIAs is an area of ongoing concern and study. Findings of an FDA review of published observational studies of NSAIAs, a meta-analysis of published and unpublished data from randomized controlled trials of these drugs, and other published information indicate that NSAIAs may increase the risk of serious adverse cardiovascular thrombotic events by 10–50% or more, depending on the drugs and dosages studied. Available data suggest that the increase in risk may occur early (within the first weeks) following initiation of therapy and may increase with higher dosages and longer durations of use. Although the relative increase in cardiovascular risk appears to be similar in patients with or without known underlying cardiovascular disease or risk factors for cardiovascular disease, the absolute incidence of serious NSAIA-associated cardiovascular thrombotic events is higher in those with cardiovascular disease or risk factors for cardiovascular disease because of their elevated baseline risk.

Findings from some systematic reviews of controlled observational studies and meta-analyses of data from randomized studies of NSAIAs suggest that naproxen may be associated with a lower risk of cardiovascular thrombotic events compared with other NSAIAs. However, limitations of these observational studies and the indirect comparisons used to assess cardiovascular risk of the prototypical NSAIAs (e.g., variability in patients' risk factors, comorbid conditions, concomitant drug therapy, drug interactions, dosage, and duration of therapy) affect the validity of the comparisons; in addition, these studies were not designed to demonstrate superior safety of one NSAIA compared with another. Therefore, FDA states that definitive conclusions regarding relative risks of NSAIAs are not possible at this time.

Rofecoxib Experience. In September 2004, one selective COX-2 inhibitor, rofecoxib, was voluntarily withdrawn from the world market based on data from a prospective, randomized, placebo-controlled study (Adenomatous Polyp Prevention on Vioxx; APPROVe). This study was designed to evaluate the efficacy of rofecoxib in preventing recurrence of colorectal polyps in patients with a history of colorectal adenomas. The primary efficacy end point was the incidence of colorectal adenoma; safety was monitored on a regular basis by an external board. In this study, there was an increased relative risk of confirmed thrombotic events (e.g., myocardial infarction, unstable angina, sudden death from cardiac causes, ischemic stroke, transient ischemic attack, peripheral arterial thrombosis, peripheral venous thrombosis, pulmonary embolism) in patients receiving rofecoxib compared with those receiving placebo. At study end point, 27 patients had experienced confirmed thrombotic events during 3327 patient-years of placebo use, and 47 had experienced confirmed thrombotic events during 3059 patient-years of rofecoxib use. The relative risk of a confirmed thrombotic event in patients receiving rofecoxib compared with those receiving placebo was 1.89 (95% confidence interval: 1.18–3.04). The difference between the 2 groups was related mainly to an increased number of myocardial infarctions and strokes in patients receiving rofecoxib. The relative risk of an Antiplatelet Trialists' Collaboration end point (death from cardiovascular, hemorrhagic, or unknown causes; nonfatal myocardial infarction; nonfatal ischemic or hemorrhagic stroke) was 2.12 (95% confidence interval: 1.2–3.74). No difference in overall mortality was observed between treatment groups.

Extended posttreatment follow-up data regarding cardiovascular events and mortality were available for approximately 84 and 95%, respectively, of patients in the APPROVe study. The median posttreatment follow-up was 550 or 538 days for rofecoxib-treated patients or placebo recipients, respectively. Over the treatment and extended follow-up periods combined, 59 rofecoxib-treated patients and 34 placebo recipients experienced an Antiplatelet Trialists' Collaboration event (hazard ratio of 1.79; 95% confidence interval: 1.17–2.73). During the first year following discontinuance of the study drug, such events occurred more frequently in patients who had received rofecoxib compared with those who had received placebo (23 versus 12 patients; hazard ratio of 1.95; 95% confidence interval: 0.97–3.93), but no difference was evident after the first posttreatment year.

In a study in adults with rheumatoid arthritis who were randomized to receive rofecoxib (50 mg daily) or naproxen (500 mg twice daily) (Vioxx Gastrointestinal Outcomes Research; VIGOR), the risk of developing a serious cardiovascular thrombotic event was substantially higher in those receiving rofecoxib than in those receiving naproxen; mortality secondary to cardiovascular events was similar in both groups. In addition, information from pooled analyses and database reviews of large populations indicate that use of rofecoxib is associated with an increased risk of major cardiovascular events (e.g., myocardial infarction) relative to use of celecoxib, prototypical NSAIAs, or no NSAIAs; some evidence indicates that rofecoxib dosages exceeding 25 mg daily are associated with a higher risk of major cardiovascular events than rofecoxib dosages of 25 mg daily or less.

Celecoxib Experience. Data from clinical trials comparing celecoxib with prototypical NSAIAs in patients with osteoarthritis or rheumatoid arthritis and from placebo-controlled trials evaluating use of celecoxib for the prevention of adenomatous polyps or Alzheimer's disease have provided varied estimates of the cardiovascular risk associated with celecoxib. Although data from some large, randomized studies (Prevention of Spontaneous Adenomatous Polyps [PreSAP], Alzheimer's Disease Anti-inflammatory Prevention Trial [ADAPT]) and database reviews of large populations have not shown an increased risk of cardiovascular events in patients receiving celecoxib, an increased incidence of cardiovascular events was observed in patients receiving celecoxib in a colorectal adenoma prevention study (Adenoma Prevention with Celecoxib [APC]).

In a study (CLASS) in adults with osteoarthritis or rheumatoid arthritis who were randomized to receive celecoxib (400 mg twice daily), ibuprofen (800 mg 3 times daily), or diclofenac sodium (75 mg twice daily), no difference in thrombotic events (myocardial infarction, pulmonary embolism, deep-vein thrombosis, unstable angina, transient ischemic attacks, ischemic cardiovascular accidents) was observed between celecoxib and the prototypical NSAIAs used in this study. Although findings from the CLASS study suggested that the risk of cardiovascular events in patients receiving celecoxib was similar to the risk in those receiving prototypical NSAIAs, the study was not designed to establish cardiovascular safety as a primary end point. There are noteworthy differences between the VIGOR and CLASS studies (patient selection relative to cardiac-related factors [e.g., use of low-dose aspirin], indication for use of the selective COX-2 inhibitor, and the active comparator agent), and conclusions regarding differences in risk of cardiovascular events between rofecoxib and celecoxib cannot be made from these studies.

Additional information on the relationship between use of celecoxib and cardiovascular risk is available from 2 long-term National Institutes of Health (NIH)-supported colorectal adenoma prevention trials and an NIH-supported Alzheimer's disease prevention trial. In one colorectal adenoma prevention trial (APC), an interim analysis of safety data revealed an increased risk of cardiovascular events in patients receiving celecoxib compared with those receiving placebo. The cumulative rates of serious cardiovascular thrombotic events began to differ between those receiving celecoxib and those receiving placebo after about 1 year of treatment. Based on these adverse cardiovascular findings, NIH suspended the study early. Final data for this study became available in 2006, and the findings of the updated safety analysis, which included data for all patients with up to 3 years of follow-up, were similar to those reported in the interim analysis. The final analysis indicated that the risk of serious cardiovascular events (cardiovascular death, myocardial infarction, or stroke) was increased in patients receiving celecoxib 200 mg twice daily (hazard ratio of 2.8; 95% confidence interval: 1.1–7.2) or celecoxib 400 mg twice daily (hazard ratio of 3.4; 95% confidence interval: 1.4–8.5), compared with that in patients receiving placebo; the increase in risk with celecoxib compared with placebo was related mainly to an increased incidence of myocardial infarction.

Findings from another colorectal adenoma prevention trial (PreSAP) did not show an increased incidence of adverse cardiovascular events (cardiovascular death, myocardial infarction, stroke) in patients receiving celecoxib 400 mg once daily compared with patients receiving placebo. Serious cardiovascular events (death from cardiovascular causes, myocardial infarction, stroke, or heart failure) occurred in 2.5% of patients receiving celecoxib and in 1.9% of patients receiving placebo (relative risk of 1.3; 95% confidence interval: 0.65–2.62). An analysis of pooled data from the APC and PreSAP studies demonstrated an increased risk for death from cardiovascular causes, myocardial infarction, stroke, or heart failure in celecoxib-treated patients.

Analysis of results from ADAPT did not show an increased risk for cardiovascular-related death, myocardial infarction, stroke, or transient ischemic attack, either individually or as composite end points, in patients receiving celecoxib (200 mg twice daily) relative to patients receiving placebo.

Data concerning the risk of cardiovascular events in patients receiving celecoxib continue to be collected and evaluated. Current evidence suggests that cardiovascular risk associated with celecoxib use may be dose related, with dosages exceeding 200 mg daily associated with greater risk. Meta-analyses of data from published and unpublished controlled clinical trials, systematic reviews, and large observational studies have yielded varied estimates of the cardiovascular risks associated with celecoxib use. A systematic review of controlled observational studies that included 11 studies of celecoxib suggested that celecoxib is not associated with an increased risk of cardiovascular events, but because only 3 of these studies provided dose-stratified risk estimates, there were insufficient data to provide stable estimates of the effect of dosage on risk. In an update of this systematic review that included 35 studies of celecoxib, both low (200 mg or less daily) and higher (exceeding 200 mg daily) dosages of celecoxib were associated with an increased risk of cardiovascular events (low dosage: relative risk of 1.26; 95% confidence interval: 1.09–1.47) (higher dosage: 1.69; 1.11–2.57); the increase in the risk estimate at higher dosages compared with lower dosages did not reach conventional levels of significance. In observational studies in patients with prior myocardial infarction, both low and higher dosages of celecoxib were associated with increased cardiovascular risk, but risk appeared to be greater at dosages exceeding 200 mg daily. A pooled analysis of data from 6 randomized placebo-controlled studies evaluating any of 3 higher-dosage regimens of celecoxib suggested that the risk of cardiovascular events was highest for a celecoxib dosage of 400 mg twice daily (hazard ratio of 3.1; 95% confidence interval: 1.5–6.1), intermediate for a dosage of 200 mg twice daily (1.8; 1.1–3.1), and lowest for a dosage of 400 mg once daily (1.1; 0.6–2).

Experience with Other COX-2 Inhibitors. Results of pooled analyses of randomized studies of valdecoxib (no longer commercially available in the US) in patients with rheumatoid arthritis or osteoarthritis and a systematic review of controlled observational studies that included limited data on valdecoxib suggested that such use is not associated with an increased risk of cardiovascular thrombotic events. However, administration of valdecoxib with or without parecoxib (a prodrug of valdecoxib; a parenteral formulation not commercially available in the US) immediately after surgery in patients undergoing coronary artery bypass grafting† (CABG) has been associated with an increase in cardiovascular events compared with CABG patients receiving standard care (e.g., opiate analgesics) for postoperative pain. Therefore, NSAIAs are contraindicated in the setting of CABG surgery.

Findings of pooled analyses and observational studies suggest that use of lumiracoxib or etoricoxib (neither drug commercially available in the US) is associated with an increased risk of major cardiovascular events. Of the 7 NSAIAs studied in one meta-analysis (including celecoxib, diclofenac, etoricoxib, ibuprofen, lumiracoxib, naproxen, and rofecoxib), etoricoxib and diclofenac were associated with the highest risk of cardiovascular death; rofecoxib was associated with the highest risk of myocardial infarction, followed by lumiracoxib; and ibuprofen was associated with the highest risk of stroke, followed by diclofenac, lumiracoxib, and etoricoxib. (See Experience with Prototypical NSAIAs under Cardiovascular Effects: Thrombotic Events, in Cautions.)

Data from long-term studies of lumiracoxib and etoricoxib also are available. In the Therapeutic COX-189 Arthritis Research and Gastrointestinal Event Trial (TARGET), the incidence of myocardial infarction, stroke, or cardiac death in patients receiving lumiracoxib was similar to that in patients receiving a prototypical NSAIA (naproxen or ibuprofen). The study was designed as 2 substudies, and substudy results suggested that lumiracoxib was associated with a slightly, but not significantly, increased risk for cardiovascular events compared with naproxen and a slightly, but not significantly, decreased risk compared with ibuprofen. In the Multinational Etoricoxib and Diclofenac Arthritis Long-term (MEDAL) study, a randomized controlled study designed to evaluate relative cardiovascular thrombotic risk with etoricoxib (60 or 90 mg daily) compared with diclofenac (75 mg twice daily), the risk of a serious cardiovascular event in patients receiving etoricoxib was similar to that in patients receiving diclofenac; the most common cardiovascular event was myocardial infarction.

Experience with Prototypical NSAIAs. Data concerning the risk of cardiovascular events in patients receiving prototypical NSAIAs continue to be collected and evaluated. In some studies (CLASS, MEDAL), the risk of cardiovascular events in patients receiving selective COX-2 inhibitors has been similar to that in patients receiving prototypical NSAIAs (diclofenac, ibuprofen). The risk of cardiovascular events associated with selective COX-2 inhibitors and individual prototypical NSAIAs has been evaluated in several systematic reviews of controlled observational studies and meta-analyses of published and unpublished data from randomized studies.

In one systematic review, 23 observational studies providing data on individual prototypical NSAIAs reported mainly on diclofenac, indomethacin, ibuprofen, naproxen, and piroxicam. A meta-analysis utilizing tabular data from studies found through searches conducted for the period of 1966 to early 2005 provided estimates of cardiovascular risk for 3 of these drugs (diclofenac, ibuprofen, and naproxen, generally at relatively high dosages). In the meta-analysis, the risks associated with these 3 drugs were estimated indirectly relative to placebo (i.e., from studies of prototypical NSAIAs versus selective COX-2 inhibitors and studies of selective COX-2 inhibitors versus placebo) because of insufficient data from randomized placebo-controlled trials of prototypical NSAIAs. Findings from these 2 analyses suggested that use of certain prototypical NSAIAs is associated with an increased risk of cardiovascular events. The findings suggested that use of naproxen does not alter the risk of cardiovascular events (summary relative risk of 0.99; 95% confidence interval: 0.89–1.09; based on data from 16 observational studies) (summary relative risk of 0.92; 95% confidence interval: 0.67–1.26; meta-analysis) but that the risk of cardiovascular events is increased with use of diclofenac (summary relative risk of 1.4; 95% confidence interval: 1.19–1.65; 10 observational studies) (summary relative risk of 1.63; 95% confidence interval: 1.12–2.37; meta-analysis) or indomethacin (summary relative risk of 1.36; 95% confidence interval: 1.15–1.61; 7 observational studies). The findings also suggested that use of ibuprofen may be associated with an increased risk of cardiovascular events, although the reported risk estimates from these 2 analyses did not reach conventional levels of significance (summary relative risk of 1.09; 95% confidence interval: 0.99–1.2; 17 observational studies) (summary relative risk of 1.51; 95% confidence interval: 0.96–2.37; meta-analysis). Few data were available for meloxicam or piroxicam. The available data suggested that use of meloxicam may be associated with an increased risk of cardiovascular events (summary relative risk of 1.24; 95% confidence interval: 1.06–1.45; 4 observational studies); however, the finding of increased risk was based largely on results from one study. The risk ratio reported for piroxicam does not suggest increased risk (summary relative risk of 1.16; 95% confidence interval: 0.86–1.56; 5 observational studies).

The systematic review was subsequently updated to provide updated risk estimates and to evaluate dose-response effects for certain NSAIAs. The updated review included data from 51 controlled observational studies and 43 unique data sets, and provided estimates of cardiovascular risk for 11 NSAIAs. Of the 6 NSAIAs that were evaluated in 10 or more studies (range: 14–41 studies), pooled estimates of overall cardiovascular risk were highest for rofecoxib (pooled relative risk of 1.45; 95% confidence interval: 1.33–1.59) and diclofenac (1.4; 1.27–1.55) and lowest for naproxen (1.09; 1.02–1.16); the pooled risk estimate for indomethacin (1.3; 1.19–1.41) was close to that for diclofenac, and pooled risk estimates for ibuprofen (1.18; 1.11–1.25) and celecoxib (1.17; 1.08–1.27) were somewhat lower. Dose-response data were available from a subset of studies, and analyses utilizing these data indicated that low dosages of rofecoxib (25 mg or less daily), celecoxib (200 mg or less daily), and diclofenac (defined in most studies as 100 mg or less daily) were associated with elevated risk; higher dosages of these drugs were associated with even greater risk, although the increase in risk at higher dosages did not reach conventional levels of significance for celecoxib. With ibuprofen, elevated risk was observed only at high dosages (defined in most studies as more than 1.2 g daily). In this data subset, neither low nor high dosages of naproxen were associated with increased risk. Fewer data were available for etoricoxib, etodolac, meloxicam, piroxicam, and valdecoxib; of these drugs, etoricoxib appeared to be associated with the highest risk of cardiovascular events, followed by etodolac and meloxicam. Pair-wise comparisons suggested that cardiovascular risk was lower with naproxen compared with ibuprofen and was higher with diclofenac compared with celecoxib, ibuprofen, or naproxen; with etoricoxib compared with ibuprofen or naproxen; with indomethacin compared with naproxen; and with meloxicam compared with naproxen. No substantial differences in risk were found for diclofenac compared with rofecoxib, for naproxen compared with celecoxib, or for etodolac compared with diclofenac, ibuprofen, or naproxen.

A meta-analysis from the Coxib and Traditional NSAIDs Trialists' (CNT) Collaboration that utilized data from randomized trials with results available prior to 2011 provided estimates of cardiovascular risk for diclofenac, ibuprofen, and naproxen. Data for individual participants, rather than aggregate tabular data, were utilized when available. The risks associated with diclofenac, ibuprofen, and naproxen relative to placebo were obtained by combining estimates made directly (i.e., from a small number of placebo-controlled trials) or indirectly (i.e., from studies of prototypical NSAIAs versus selective COX-2 inhibitors and studies of selective COX-2 inhibitors versus placebo). The findings suggested that vascular risks of high-dose diclofenac, and possibly those of high-dose ibuprofen, are similar to those of selective COX-2 inhibitors, but high-dose naproxen may be associated with less vascular risk. The prototypical NSAIA regimens all involved high dosages with minimal variations in dosage (diclofenac 150 mg daily, ibuprofen 2.4 g daily, naproxen 1 g daily). The findings suggested that the risk of major vascular events was increased by about one-third by diclofenac (rate ratio of 1.41; 95% confidence interval: 1.12–1.78) or a selective COX-2 inhibitor (1.37; 1.14–1.66), mainly because of an increase in major coronary events (diclofenac: 1.7; 1.19–2.41) (selective COX-2 inhibitors: 1.76; 1.31–2.37). The findings also suggested that ibuprofen increased major coronary events (2.22; 1.1–4.48) but not major vascular events (1.44; 0.89–2.33). Naproxen did not appear to increase major vascular events (0.93: 0.69–1.27) or major coronary events (0.84; 0.52–1.35). In this analysis, the risk of vascular death was increased by diclofenac (1.65; 0.95–2.85) and selective COX-2 inhibitors (1.58; 1–2.49), increased but not to conventional levels of significance by ibuprofen (1.9; 0.56–6.41), but not increased by naproxen (1.08; 0.48–2.47). The estimated excess risks for diclofenac and selective COX-2 inhibitors compared with placebo suggested that diclofenac or a selective COX-2 inhibitor could cause approximately 3 additional major vascular events, including 1 fatal event, per 1000 patients per year.

Another meta-analysis of data from 31 large randomized controlled studies provided estimates of cardiovascular risk for diclofenac, ibuprofen, naproxen, and 4 selective COX-2 inhibitors. The results supported those of other analyses indicating that both prototypical NSAIAs and selective COX-2 inhibitors increase the risk of cardiovascular events. The cardiovascular safety profiles of the individual NSAIAs compared with placebo varied depending on the specific outcome. Of the 7 NSAIAs studied, etoricoxib (rate ratio of 4.07; 95% credibility interval of 1.23–15.7) and diclofenac (3.98; 1.48–12.7) were associated with the highest risk of cardiovascular death; rofecoxib was associated with the highest risk of myocardial infarction (2.12; 1.26–3.56), followed by lumiracoxib (2; 0.71–6.21); and ibuprofen was associated with the highest risk of stroke (3.36; 1–11.6), followed by diclofenac (2.86; 1.09–8.36), lumiracoxib (2.81; 1.05–7.48), and etoricoxib (2.67; 0.82–8.72). Naproxen appeared to have the least harmful cardiovascular effects of the 7 NSAIAs.

Patients with Elevated Cardiovascular Risk. Several observational studies utilizing data from national registries of hospitalization and drug dispensing from pharmacies in Denmark have examined the cardiovascular risk associated with use of NSAIAs in patients with prior myocardial infarction. In these studies, approximately 84,000–99,000 patients who had been hospitalized for a first-time myocardial infarction during the 10 or 13-year study period were identified; approximately 42–44% of these patients subsequently claimed at least one prescription for an NSAIA. Results from these studies indicated that patients who received NSAIAs following a myocardial infarction were at increased risk of reinfarction, cardiovascular-related death, and all-cause mortality beginning in the first week of treatment. Patients who received NSAIAs following myocardial infarction had a higher 1-year mortality rate compared with those who did not receive NSAIAs (20 versus 12 deaths per 100 person-years). Although the absolute mortality rate declined somewhat after the first year following the myocardial infarction, the increased relative risk of death in patients who received NSAIAs persisted over at least the next 4 years of follow-up. Similar patterns were observed for the composite end point of coronary death or nonfatal recurrent myocardial infarction.

In these Danish registry studies, the most commonly used NSAIAs were ibuprofen and diclofenac, followed by celecoxib, rofecoxib, and naproxen. When analyzed separately, these NSAIAs were associated with increased risk of cardiovascular death and increased risk of coronary death and nonfatal myocardial infarction, but increased risk was evident for ibuprofen and naproxen only at higher dosages (exceeding 1.2 g or 500 mg daily, respectively). Estimated risks were elevated at low dosages of celecoxib (200 mg or less daily), diclofenac (100 mg or less daily), and rofecoxib (25 mg or less daily), but were increased further at higher dosages of these drugs.

In 2 large controlled clinical trials of a selective COX-2 inhibitor for the management of pain in the first 10–14 days following CABG surgery, the incidence of myocardial infarction and stroke was increased. (See Experience with Other COX-2 Inhibitors under Cardiovascular Effects: Thrombotic Events, in Cautions.)

Limited data are available regarding cardiovascular risks associated with use of NSAIAs in patients with stable atherothrombotic disease. A post hoc analysis of data from the International Verapamil Trandolapril Study (INVEST), which compared antihypertensive regimens in patients with stable coronary artery disease and hypertension, indicated an increased risk for the composite end point of death, nonfatal myocardial infarction, or nonfatal stroke in patients who reported long-term NSAIA use compared with patients who did not report long-term use (4.4 versus 3.7 events per 100 patient-years; hazard ratio of 1.47; 95% confidence interval: 1.19–1.82). An ongoing randomized controlled study is evaluating the cardiovascular safety of celecoxib compared with ibuprofen or naproxen in patients with high cardiovascular risk. (See Ongoing Research under Cardiovascular Effects: Cardiovascular Risk Considerations for COX-2 Inhibitors and Prototypical NSAIAs, in Cautions.)

Heart Failure Data from observational studies indicate that use of NSAIAs in patients with heart failure is associated with increased morbidity and mortality. Results from a retrospective study utilizing Danish national registry data indicated that use of selective COX-2 inhibitors or prototypical NSAIAs in patients with chronic heart failure was associated with a dose-dependent increase in the risk of death and an increased risk of hospitalization for myocardial infarction or heart failure. In addition, findings from a meta-analysis of published and unpublished data from randomized controlled trials of NSAIAs indicated that use of selective COX-2 inhibitors or prototypical NSAIAs was associated with an approximate twofold increase in the risk of hospitalization for heart failure. Fluid retention and edema also have been observed in some patients receiving NSAIAs.

In the retrospective study utilizing Danish national registry data, more than 100,000 patients who had survived a first hospitalization for heart failure were identified from the registry; about 34% of these patients claimed at least one prescription for an NSAIA after discharge. Risks associated with the 5 most commonly used NSAIAs were analyzed separately. Low dosages of celecoxib (200 mg or less daily), diclofenac (100 mg or less daily), and rofecoxib (25 mg or less daily) were associated with an increased risk of death; higher dosages of these drugs were associated with even higher levels of risk. With ibuprofen and naproxen, only higher dosages (exceeding 1.2 g or 500 mg daily, respectively) were associated with an increased risk of death. All 5 NSAIAs were associated with an increased risk of hospitalization for myocardial infarction or heart failure.

Cardiovascular Risk Considerations for COX-2 Inhibitors and Prototypical NSAIAs FDA reviewed the safety of NSAIAs in early 2005 and concluded that the 3 selective COX-2 inhibitors that previously had been marketed in the US or were on the market in the US at that time (celecoxib, rofecoxib, valdecoxib) were associated with an increased risk of serious adverse cardiovascular events compared with placebo. In addition, FDA noted that data from some long-term controlled studies that included both a selective COX-2 inhibitor and a prototypical NSAIA did not clearly demonstrate that use of a selective COX-2 inhibitor was associated with a greater risk of serious adverse cardiovascular events than use of prototypical NSAIAs. Long-term data from placebo-controlled clinical trials were not available to assess the potential for prototypical NSAIAs to increase the risk of serious cardiovascular events. FDA interpreted data on cardiovascular risk available in 2005 as being applicable to all NSAIAs, including selective COX-2 inhibitors and prototypical NSAIAs.

As a result of this analysis, FDA directed manufacturers of all NSAIAs (except aspirin) to add a boxed warning to the labeling of their products to alert clinicians to the increased risk of serious cardiovascular events and GI toxicity. In addition to the boxed warning and other information in the professional labeling, FDA recommended that a patient medication guide explaining the risks and benefits of these drugs be provided to the patient each time the drugs are dispensed.

At that time, short-term use of NSAIAs to relieve acute pain, especially at low dosages, did not appear to be associated with an increased risk of serious cardiovascular events (except immediately following CABG surgery). Therefore, in early 2005, FDA concluded that preparations of NSAIAs that currently were available without a prescription (OTC) had a favorable benefit-to-risk ratio when used according to labeled instructions and determined that these preparations should remain available without a prescription despite the addition of a boxed warning to the professional labeling of prescription-only NSAIA preparations. FDA directed manufacturers of nonprescription NSAIAs to revise the labeling of these preparations to include more specific information on the potential cardiovascular and GI risks and information to assist individuals in the safe use of these agents.

Following completion of additional studies and analyses of pooled study data, FDA again reviewed the cardiovascular risks associated with NSAIAs. Findings of this FDA review of published observational studies of NSAIAs, the CNT meta-analysis of published and unpublished data from randomized controlled trials of these drugs, and other published information indicate that NSAIAs may increase the risk of serious adverse cardiovascular thrombotic events by 10–50% or more, depending on the drugs and dosages studied. Available data now suggest that the increase in risk may occur early (within the first weeks) following initiation of therapy and may increase with higher dosages and longer durations of use. Published observational studies also indicate that use of NSAIAs in patients who have had a myocardial infarction increases the risk of reinfarction and death. Although the relative increase in cardiovascular risk appears to be similar in patients with or without known underlying cardiovascular disease or risk factors for cardiovascular disease, the absolute incidence of serious NSAIA-associated cardiovascular thrombotic events is higher in those with cardiovascular disease or risk factors for cardiovascular disease because of their elevated baseline risk. Therefore, in July 2015, FDA strengthened an existing warning in the labeling of NSAIAs regarding the increased risk of cardiovascular thrombotic events in patients receiving NSAIAs and an existing caution regarding risk in patients with heart failure. FDA directed manufacturers of prescription and nonprescription NSAIA preparations to revise the labeling of these preparations to include updated information regarding cardiovascular risk.

Concomitant Aspirin Therapy. There is no consistent evidence that use of low-dose aspirin mitigates the increased risk of serious cardiovascular events associated with NSAIAs. In several studies (APC, TARGET APPROVe), post hoc analyses or planned subset analyses suggested that the overall risk for cardiovascular events in patients receiving a COX-2 inhibitor versus placebo or a prototypical NSAIA was not influenced by use of low-dose aspirin.

Ongoing Research. Studies designed specifically to assess the relationship between NSAIAs, including selective COX-2 inhibitors and prototypical NSAIAs, and cardiovascular events are needed to determine the precise risk of cardiovascular events in patients receiving these agents. As part of ongoing research, the manufacturer of celecoxib is conducting a large randomized, double-blind, controlled clinical study (Prospective Randomized Evaluation of Celecoxib Integrated Safety versus Ibuprofen or Naproxen [PRECISION]) to evaluate the effects of celecoxib compared with ibuprofen or naproxen on cardiovascular and GI events in patients with osteoarthritis or rheumatoid arthritis and high cardiovascular risk, including a history of coronary artery disease, other occlusive arterial disease, diabetes mellitus, or at least 2 risk factors for atherosclerosis, but no history of myocardial infarction, stroke, CABG surgery, or unstable angina within the prior 3 months. Decisions regarding use of NSAIAs should take into account risks and benefits of such therapy. These agents should be used with caution and careful monitoring of outcomes and adverse effects.

■ **GI Effects** Dyspepsia, diarrhea, abdominal pain, nausea, or flatulence occurred in 8.8, 5.6, 4.1, 3.5, or 2.2%, respectively, of adults receiving usual dosages of celecoxib in clinical studies. Anorexia, constipation, diverticulitis, dry mouth, dysphagia, eructation, esophagitis, gastritis, gastroenteritis, gastroesophageal reflux, hemorrhoids, hiatal hernia, increased appetite, melena, stomatitis, taste perversion, tenesmus, tooth disorder, or vomiting has been reported in 0.1–1.9% of adults receiving celecoxib. Adverse GI effects reported in less than 0.1% of adults include intestinal obstruction, intestinal perforation,colitis with bleeding, esophageal perforation, pancreatitis, cholelithiasis, and ileus. GI bleeding also was reported, albeit rarely, in patients receiving celecoxib during postmarketing surveillance. Intestinal anastomotic ulceration was reported in a few patients with FAP who received celecoxib in a clinical study; these patients had prior intestinal surgery. Dry socket (alveolar osteitis) was reported in patients receiving celecoxib for postoperative dental pain in a clinical study. Abdominal pain, nausea, diarrhea, or vomiting has been reported in 3–8% of children receiving celecoxib in an active-controlled clinical study.

GI Risk Considerations for COX-2 Inhibitors and Prototypical NSAIAs Numerous short-term (12–24 weeks' duration), comparative, randomized, controlled studies using endoscopy have been performed in patients with osteoarthritis or rheumatoid arthritis to evaluate the incidence of celecoxib-associated upper GI ulceration relative to that associated with prototypical NSAIAs. In these studies, the incidence of endoscopically confirmed GI ulceration generally was lower in patients receiving celecoxib than in those receiving a prototypical NSAIA (e.g., diclofenac, ibuprofen, naproxen). Results of two 3-month studies showed that gastroduodenal ulcer occurred in 2.7–5.9% of patients receiving celecoxib (50–400 mg twice daily), 16.2–17.6% of patients receiving naproxen (500 mg twice daily), and 2–2.3% of patients receiving placebo. Celecoxib was associated with a lower incidence of endoscopic ulcers than diclofenac (4% versus 15%) in one 6-month study. No consistent relationship between celecoxib dosage and the incidence of GI ulcers has been established in these studies. The correlation between endoscopic findings and the incidence of clinically important upper GI events remains to be determined.

The incidence of severe adverse upper GI effects in patients receiving celecoxib relative to the incidence in those receiving prototypical NSAIAs has been evaluated in a double-blind, randomized controlled study in patients with osteoarthritis or rheumatoid arthritis (the Celecoxib Long-term Arthritis Safety Study [CLASS]). Patients were randomized to receive celecoxib (400 mg twice daily), ibuprofen (800 mg 3 times daily), or diclofenac (75 twice daily) for up to 65 weeks; patients were allowed to continue aspirin therapy (up to 325 mg daily) for cardiovascular prophylaxis. Published results of the first 6 months of the study indicated that therapy with celecoxib was associated with a lower incidence of symptomatic ulcers and ulcer complications combined than therapy with ibuprofen or diclofenac; the decrease in upper GI toxicity in patients receiving celecoxib generally was observed only in those not receiving concomitant low-dose aspirin. However, results for celecoxib therapy were less favorable at 12 months than at 6 months, since almost all of the ulcer complications reported during the second half of the study occurred in patients receiving celecoxib; however, a greater percentage of patients receiving a prototypical NSAIA (i.e., diclofenac) than patients receiving celecoxib withdrew from the study because of GI intolerance, potentially biasing GI event rates at 12 months. Overall, the incidence of complicated ulcers in patients receiving celecoxib was similar to the incidence in those receiving the comparator agents (i.e., ibuprofen or diclofenac). Patients receiving celecoxib and low-dose aspirin experienced a fourfold higher rate of complicated ulcers compared with those receiving celecoxib alone. The rate of complicated and symptomatic ulcers at 9 months was 0.78 or 2.19% in those receiving celecoxib alone or celecoxib and low-dose aspirin, respectively; the rate of these adverse GI effects was 0.47 or 1.26% in patients younger than 65 years of age or 1.4 or 3.06% in those 65 years of age and older receiving celecoxib alone or celecoxib and low-dose aspirin, respectively. In patients with a history of peptic ulcer disease, the rate of complicated and symptomatic ulcers at 48 weeks was 2.56 or 6.85% in those receiving celecoxib or celecoxib and low-dose aspirin, respectively. Low-dose aspirin did not have a clinically important effect on the rate of upper GI complications in patients receiving prototypical NSAIAs.

Serious adverse GI effects (e.g., bleeding, ulceration, perforation of the stomach, small intestine, or large intestine) can occur at any time in patients receiving NSAIA therapy, and such effects may *not* be preceded by warning signs or symptoms. Only 1 in 5 patients who develop a serious upper GI adverse event while receiving NSAIA therapy is symptomatic. Therefore, clinicians should remain alert to the possible development of serious adverse GI effects (e.g., bleeding, ulceration) in any patient receiving NSAIA therapy, and such patients should be followed on a long-term basis for the development of manifestations of such effects and advised of the importance of this follow-up. In addition, patients should be advised about the signs and/or symptoms of serious NSAIA-induced GI toxicity and what action to take if such toxicity occurs. Longer duration of therapy with an NSAIA increases the likelihood of a serious adverse GI event. However, short-term therapy is not without risk.

Studies have shown that patients with a history of peptic ulcer disease and/or GI bleeding who are receiving NSAIAs have a substantially higher risk of developing GI bleeding than patients without these risk factors. In addition to a history of ulcer disease, pharmacoepidemiologic studies have identified several comorbid conditions and concomitant therapies that may increase the risk for GI bleeding, including concomitant use of oral corticosteroids or anticoagulants, longer duration of NSAIA therapy, smoking, alcoholism, older age, and poor general health status. Patients with rheumatoid arthritis are more likely to experience serious GI complications from NSAIA therapy than are patients with osteoarthritis. In addition, most spontaneous reports of fatal GI effects have been in geriatric or debilitated patients.

For patients at high risk for complications from NSAIA-induced GI ulceration (e.g., bleeding, perforation), concomitant use of misoprostol can be considered for preventive therapy. (See Misoprostol 56:28.28.) Alternatively, some clinicians suggest that a proton-pump inhibitor (e.g., omeprazole) may be used concomitantly to decrease the incidence of serious GI toxicity associated with NSAIA therapy. In one study, therapy with high dosages of famotidine (40 mg twice daily) was more effective than placebo in preventing peptic ulcers in NSAIA-treated patients; however, the effect of the drug was modest. In addition, efficacy of usual dosages of H_2-receptor antagonists for the prevention of NSAIA-induced gastric and duodenal ulcers has not been established. Therefore, most clinicians do not recommend use of H_2-receptor antagonists for the prevention of NSAIA-associated ulcers. Another approach in high-risk patients who would benefit from NSAIA therapy is use of an NSAIA that is a selective inhibitor of cyclooxygenase-2 (COX-2) (e.g., celecoxib), since these agents are associated with a lower incidence of serious GI bleeding than are prototypical NSAIAs. However, while celecoxib (200 mg twice daily) was comparably effective to diclofenac sodium (75 mg twice daily) plus omeprazole (20 mg daily) in preventing recurrent ulcer bleeding (recurrent ulcer bleeding probabilities of 4.9 versus 6.4%, respectively, during the 6-month study) in *H. pylori*-negative arthritis (principally osteoarthritis) patients with a recent history of ulcer bleeding, the protective efficacy was unexpectedly low for both regimens and it appeared that neither could completely protect patients at high risk. Additional study is necessary to elucidate optimal therapy for preventing GI complications associated with NSAIA therapy in high-risk patients.

■ **Nervous System Effects** Headache has been reported in about 16% of adults receiving celecoxib in clinical studies, whereas dizziness or insomnia occurred in 2 or 2.3% of these patients, respectively. Anxiety, asthenia, depression, hypertonia, hypoesthesia, migraine, nervousness, neuralgia, neuropathy, paresthesia, somnolence, or vertigo has been reported in 0.1–1.9% of adults receiving celecoxib, and aseptic meningitis, ataxia, ageusia, anosmia, fatal intracranial hemorrhage, or suicide occurred in less than 0.1% of these patients. Headache occurred in 10–13% of children receiving celecoxib in an active-controlled clinical study.

■ **Respiratory Effects** Upper respiratory tract infection, sinusitis, pharyngitis, or rhinitis has occurred in 8.1, 5, 2.3, or 2%, respectively, of adults receiving usual dosages of celecoxib in clinical studies. Bronchitis, bronchospasm (including aggravated bronchospasm), coughing, dyspnea, laryngitis, or pneumonia has been reported in 0.1–1.9% of adults. Cough or nasopharyngitis has been reported in 5–7% of celecoxib-treated children.

■ **Dermatologic and Sensitivity Reactions** Rash occurred in 2.2% of adults receiving celecoxib in clinical studies. Adverse dermatologic effects occurring in 0.1–1.9% of adults receiving celecoxib include alopecia, dermatitis, dry skin, erythematous rash, maculopapular rash, nail disorder, photosensitivity reaction, pruritus, skin disorder, increased sweating, and urticaria. Cellulitis, contact dermatitis, injection site reaction, or skin nodule has occurred in 0.1–1.9% of patients following *topical* application of celecoxib.

Allergic reactions, aggravated allergy, bronchospasm, or generalized or facial edema has been reported in 0.1–1.9% of adults receiving celecoxib. Anaphylactoid reactions and angioedema have occurred in patients receiving celecoxib. As with other NSAIAs, anaphylactic reactions have been reported rarely in patients with no previous exposure to the drug. Erythema multiforme, exfoliative dermatitis, Sweet's syndrome, Stevens-Johnson syndrome, and toxic epidermal necrolysis have been reported rarely in patients receiving celecoxib.

■ **Hematologic Effects** Anemia has been reported in 0.6% of celecoxib-treated adults. Ecchymosis, epistaxis, or thrombocythemia has occurred in 0.1–1.9% of adults receiving celecoxib in clinical studies, and agranulocytosis, aplastic anemia, pancytopenia, leukopenia, and thrombocytopenia has occurred in less than 0.1% of these patients.

In contrast to prototypical NSAIAs, including aspirin, usual dosages of celecoxib generally do not appear to inhibit platelet aggregation, serum thromboxane B concentrations, or bleeding time. In addition, usual dosages of the drug do not affect platelet counts, prothrombin time (PT), or partial thromboplastin time (PTT). (See Pharmacology: Hematologic Effects.)

Although comparative studies are limited, therapy with celecoxib is expected to be associated with fewer and less severe episodes of bleeding than therapy with prototypical NSAIAs. However, bleeding events have been reported in postmarketing experience, predominantly in geriatric patients, in association with increased PTs in patients receiving celecoxib concomitantly with warfarin. (See Warfarin under Drug Interactions: Drugs Affecting Hepatic Microsomal Enzymes.)

Modest prolongation of the activated partial thromboplastin time (aPTT) with no change in PT has been reported in celecoxib-treated pediatric patients with systemic onset juvenile rheumatoid arthritis.

■ **Renal, Electrolyte, and Genitourinary Effects** Whether COX-2 selectivity affects renal function is unclear. (See Pharmacology: Renal Effects.) Like prototypical NSAIAs, celecoxib has been associated with adverse renal effects. In one study in arthritis (principally osteoarthritis) patients with a recent history of ulcer bleeding while receiving long-term NSAIA therapy, celecoxib therapy (200 mg twice daily) was associated with a 24.3% incidence of adverse renal effects; however, this study defined hypertension as an adverse renal effect, and this was the principal adverse renal effect reported (occurring in 13.9% of treated patients and accounting for 57% of reported renal effects). Peripheral edema also was defined as an adverse renal effect in this study, occurring in 4.9% of treated patients; when its incidence was combined with that of hypertension, these 2 effects accounted for 77% of reported renal effects. The incidence of adverse renal effects was increased in patients with preexisting renal impairment.

Albuminuria; increased BUN, nonprotein nitrogen (NPN), and serum creatinine concentration; cystitis; dysuria; hematuria; frequent micturition; renal calculus; urinary incontinence; urinary tract infection; dysmenorrhea; genital moniliasis; menstrual disorder; vaginal hemorrhage; vaginitis; or prostatic disorder has occurred in 0.1–1.9% of adults receiving celecoxib. Acute renal failure, interstitial nephritis, or hyponatremia has been reported in less than 0.1% of adults receiving the drug. In one study in arthritis (principally osteoarthritis) patients receiving celecoxib 200 mg daily, renal failure (a progressive rise in serum creatinine concentration to exceed 2.2 mg/dL) was reported in 5.6% of patients; 25.7% of all celecoxib-treated patients in this study had baseline serum creatinine concentrations exceeding 1.2 mg/dL when therapy with the drug was initiated.

Long-term administration of NSAIAs has resulted in renal papillary necrosis and other renal injury.

■ **Musculoskeletal Effects** Back pain has been reported in 2.8% of adults receiving celecoxib. Arthralgia, arthrosis, bone disorder, leg cramps, myalgia, neck stiffness, synovitis, tendinitis, or accidental fracture has occurred in 0.1–1.9% of adults receiving the drug. Arthralgia has been reported in 3–7% of children receiving celecoxib in an active-controlled clinical study.

■ **Ocular and Otic Effects** Adverse ocular and otic effects reported in 0.1–1.9% of adults receiving celecoxib include blurred vision, cataract, conjunctivitis, ocular pain, glaucoma, deafness, ear abnormality, earache, otitis media, and tinnitus.

■ **Hepatic Effects** In controlled clinical studies in adults, the incidence of borderline elevations in liver function test results was similar in patients receiving celecoxib or placebo, occurring in 6 or 5% of patients, respectively. Substantial increases in serum concentrations of AST (SGOT) or ALT (SGPT) occurred in 0.2 or 0.3% of patients receiving the drug or placebo, respectively.

Borderline elevations in one or more liver function test results may occur in up to 15% of patients treated with NSAIAs; meaningful (3 times the upper limit of normal) elevations in serum ALT (SGPT) or AST (SGOT) have occurred in approximately 1% of patients receiving NSAIAs in controlled clinical studies. These abnormalities may progress, may remain essentially unchanged, or may be transient with continued therapy. Hepatitis, jaundice, or liver failure has been reported in patients receiving celecoxib during postmarketing surveillance. Rare cases of severe hepatic reactions, including jaundice and fatal fulminant hepatitis, liver necrosis, and hepatic failure (sometimes fatal), have been reported in patients receiving NSAIAs, including celecoxib.

■ **Other Adverse Effects** Accidental injury has been reported in 2.9% of adults receiving celecoxib. Other adverse effects reported in 0.1–1.9% of celecoxib-treated adults include cysts (not otherwise specified), fatigue, fever, flu-like symptoms, bacterial infections, fungal infections (including moniliasis), viral infections (including herpes simplex or herpes zoster), pain, and peripheral pain. Diabetes mellitus, increases in serum concentrations of creatine kinase (CK, creatine phosphokinase, CPK) or alkaline phosphatase, hypercholesterolemia, hyperglycemia, hypokalemia, or weight gain also has been reported in 0.1–1.9% of adults receiving celecoxib. Sepsis and hypoglycemia have been reported in less than 0.1% of celecoxib-treated adults. Fever has occurred in 8–9% of children receiving the drug.

Soon after celecoxib became commercially available, the death of 10 adults receiving the drug was reported in the lay media. Review of the data indicated that the death of these adults was not attributable to the drug; 8 of these adults had substantial concomitant medical conditions, and 3 were receiving multiple drugs concomitantly. The cause of death was not known or clearly specified for the other 2 patients.

■ **Precautions and Contraindications** Patients should be advised that celecoxib, like other NSAIAs, is not free of potential adverse effects, including some that can cause discomfort, and that more serious effects (e.g., myocardial infarction, stroke, GI bleeding), which may require hospitalization and may even be fatal, also can occur.

Patients should be advised to read the medication guide for NSAIAs that is provided to the patient each time the drug is dispensed.

Cardiovascular Precautions NSAIAs, including selective COX-2 inhibitors and prototypical NSAIAs, increase the risk of serious adverse cardiovascular thrombotic events. (See Cautions: Cardiovascular Effects.) Although findings from some systematic reviews of controlled observational studies and meta-analyses of data from randomized studies of these drugs suggest that naproxen may be associated with a lower risk of cardiovascular thrombotic events compared with other NSAIAs, FDA states that definitive conclusions regarding relative risks of NSAIAs are not possible at this time. Until more data are available, decisions to use an NSAIA, including a selective COX-2 inhibitor (e.g., celecoxib), depend on individual assessment of risk for GI and cardiac toxicity and availability of alternative therapies. Some clinicians have suggested that use of a selective COX-2 inhibitor remains an appropriate choice for patients at low cardiovascular risk who have had serious GI events, especially while receiving a prototypical NSAIA. Some clinicians also suggest that it is prudent to avoid use of NSAIAs whenever possible in patients with cardiovascular disease. Celecoxib should be avoided in patients with recent myocardial infarction unless the benefits of therapy are expected to outweigh the risk of recurrent cardiovascular thrombotic events; if celecoxib is used in such patients, the patient should be monitored for cardiac ischemia. Additional studies, preferably randomized controlled trials, are required to more fully assess cardiovascular risks associated with individual NSAIAs in patients with established cardiovascular disease.

To minimize the potential risk of adverse cardiovascular events in patients receiving NSAIAs, the lowest effective dosage and shortest possible duration of therapy should be employed. Patients receiving NSAIAs (including those without previous symptoms of cardiovascular disease) should be monitored for the possible development of cardiovascular events throughout therapy. Patients should be informed about the signs and symptoms of serious cardiovascular toxicity (chest pain, dyspnea, weakness, slurring of speech) and instructed to seek immediate medical attention if such toxicity occurs.

There is no consistent evidence that concomitant use of low-dose aspirin mitigates the increased risk of serious cardiovascular events associated with NSAIAs. The overall risk for cardiovascular events in patients receiving a COX-2 inhibitor versus placebo or a prototypical NSAIA was not influenced by use of low-dose aspirin. Concomitant use of aspirin and celecoxib increases the risk for serious GI events.

Use of NSAIAs, including celecoxib, can result in the onset of hypertension or worsening of preexisting hypertension; either of these occurrences may contribute to the increased incidence of cardiovascular events. Patients receiving NSAIAs may have an impaired response to diuretics (i.e., thiazide or loop diuretics), angiotensin-converting enzyme (ACE) inhibitors, angiotensin II receptor antagonists, or β-adrenergic blocking agents. NSAIAs, including celecoxib, should be used with caution in patients with hypertension. Blood pressure should be monitored closely during initiation of celecoxib therapy and throughout therapy.

Because NSAIAs increase morbidity and mortality in patients with heart failure, the manufacturer states that celecoxib should be avoided in patients with severe heart failure unless the benefits of therapy are expected to outweigh the risk of worsening heart failure; if celecoxib is used in such patients, the patient should be monitored for worsening heart failure. Some experts state that use of NSAIAs should be avoided whenever possible in patients with reduced left ventricular ejection fraction and current or prior symptoms of heart failure. Patients receiving NSAIAs should be advised to inform their clinician if they experience symptoms of heart failure, including dyspnea, unexplained weight gain, and edema. Use of NSAIAs may diminish the cardiovascular effects of certain drugs used to treat heart failure and edema (e.g., diuretics, ACE inhibitors, angiotensin II receptor antagonists). (See Drug Interactions.)

Use of celecoxib for longer than 6 months in children has not been systematically studied. It remains to be determined whether long-term cardiovascular risks in children exposed to celecoxib are similar to those observed in adults receiving celecoxib or other NSAIAs.

GI Precautions The risk of potentially serious adverse GI effects should be considered in patients receiving celecoxib, particularly in patients receiving chronic therapy with the drug. (See Cautions: GI Effects.) Because peptic ulceration and/or GI bleeding have been reported in patients receiving the drug, patients should be advised to report promptly signs or symptoms of GI ulceration or bleeding to their clinician.

NSAIAs, including celecoxib, should be used with extreme caution and under close supervision in patients with a history of ulcer disease or GI bleeding. Special care should be exercised if the drug is administered to geriatric or debilitated patients because most spontaneous reports of fatal GI effects have been in such patients. To minimize the potential risk of adverse GI effects, the lowest effective dosage and shortest possible duration of therapy should be employed. For patients who are at high risk, alternative therapy other than a NSAIA should be considered.

Renal Precautions Renal toxicity has been observed in patients in whom renal prostaglandins have a compensatory role in maintaining renal perfusion. Administration of an NSAIA to such patients may cause a dose-dependent reduction in prostaglandin formation and thereby precipitate overt renal decompensation. Patients at greatest risk of this reaction are those with impaired renal function, heart failure, or hepatic dysfunction; those with extracellular fluid depletion (e.g., patients receiving diuretics); those taking an ACE inhibitor or angiotensin II antagonist concomitantly; and geriatric patients. Patients should be advised to consult their clinician promptly if unexplained weight gain or edema occurs. Recovery of renal function to pretreatment levels usually occurs following discontinuance of NSAIA therapy. Celecoxib should be discontinued if abnormal renal function test results persist or worsen. The manufacturer states that celecoxib-induced renal effects are similar to those reported with prototypical NSAIAs.

Celecoxib has not been evaluated in patients with severe renal impairment, and the manufacturer states that use of celecoxib is not recommended in patients with advanced renal disease. If celecoxib therapy must be used in patients with severe renal impairment, close monitoring of renal function is recommended.

Hepatic Precautions Patients who experience signs and/or symptoms suggestive of liver dysfunction or an abnormal liver function test result while receiving celecoxib should be evaluated for evidence of the development of a severe hepatic reaction. Severe reactions, including jaundice and fatal fulminant hepatitis, liver necrosis, and hepatic failure (sometimes fatal), have been reported rarely in patients receiving NSAIAs. Celecoxib should be discontinued if clinical signs and symptoms consistent with liver disease develop or if systemic manifestations (e.g., eosinophilia, rash) occur. In addition, celecoxib should be discontinued if abnormal liver function test results persist or worsen. (See Cautions: Hepatic Effects.) Patients receiving celecoxib should be instructed to report to their clinician any early signs or symptoms of possible hepatic dysfunction (e.g., fatigue, lethargy, nausea, pruritus, jaundice, right upper quadrant pain, flu-like symptoms). In addition, patients should be advised to discontinue celecoxib and contact their clinician immediately if any of these manifestations occur.

The manufacturer states that celecoxib has not been evaluated in patients with severe hepatic impairment, and use of the drug in such patients is not recommended. In patients with poor metabolizer phenotypes of the cytochrome P-450 (CYP) 2C9 isoenzyme, the metabolic clearance of celecoxib may be decreased and plasma concentrations may be increased. Therefore, the drug should be used with caution in patients who are known or suspected poor metabolizers of this isoenzyme, because higher than expected plasma concentrations of celecoxib may occur.

Other Precautions and Contraindications The possibility that the anti-inflammatory and, perhaps, antipyretic effects of NSAIAs may mask the usual signs and symptoms of infection should be considered.

Use of corticosteroids during NSAIA therapy may increase the risk of GI ulceration, and the drugs should be used concomitantly with caution. Celecoxib is not a substitute for corticosteroid therapy, and the drug is not effective in the management of adrenal insufficiency. Abrupt withdrawal of corticosteroids may exacerbate corticosteroid-responsive conditions. If corticosteroid therapy is to be discontinued after prolonged therapy, the dosage should be tapered gradually.

It is not known whether use of celecoxib in patients with familial adenomatous polyposis (FAP) will reduce the risk of colorectal, duodenal, or other FAP-related cancers or whether use of the drug reduces the need for endoscopic surveillance, prophylactic colectomy, or other FAP-related surgery. Therefore, FAP patients receiving celecoxib should continue to receive usual care; the frequency of routine endoscopic surveillance should not be decreased and prophylactic colectomy or other FAP-related surgery should not be delayed.

Because of similarity in spelling of Celexa® (citalopram hydrobromide), Celebrex® (celecoxib), and Cerebyx® (fosphenytoin sodium), extra care should be exercised in ensuring the accuracy of prescriptions for these drugs.

Anaphylactoid reactions have been reported in patients receiving celecoxib. Patients receiving celecoxib should be informed of the signs and symptoms of an anaphylactoid reaction (e.g., difficulty breathing, swelling of the face or throat) and advised to seek immediate medical attention if an anaphylactoid reaction develops.

Serious skin reactions (e.g., exfoliative dermatitis, Stevens-Johnson syndrome, toxic epidermal necrolysis) can occur in patients receiving celecoxib. These serious skin reactions can occur without warning and in patients without a history of sulfonamide sensitivity reactions; patients should be advised to consult their clinician if skin rash and blisters, fever, or other signs of hypersensitivity reaction (e.g., pruritus) occur. Celecoxib should be discontinued at the first appearance of rash or any other sign of hypersensitivity.

Patients receiving long-term NSAIA therapy should have a complete blood cell count and chemistry profile performed periodically.

Use of NSAIAs, including celecoxib, has been associated with modest prolongation of activated partial thromboplastin time (aPTT) in children with systemic onset juvenile rheumatoid arthritis. NSAIAs should be used with caution in these children because of the risk of disseminated intravascular coagulation. Children with systemic onset juvenile rheumatoid arthritis who are receiving celecoxib should be monitored with coagulation tests.

If signs and/or symptoms of anemia occur during therapy with celecoxib, hemoglobin concentration and hematocrit should be determined.

The manufacturer states that celecoxib is contraindicated in patients with known hypersensitivity to the drug. In addition, celecoxib should not be given to patients who have experienced allergic-type reactions to sulfonamides. NSAIAs, including celecoxib, generally are contraindicated in patients in whom asthma, urticaria, or other sensitivity reactions are precipitated by aspirin or other NSAIAs, because there is potential for cross-sensitivity between NSAIAs and aspirin, and severe, often fatal, anaphylactic reactions may occur in such patients. Because patients with asthma may have aspirin-sensitivity asthma, celecoxib should be used with caution in patients with asthma. In patients with asthma, aspirin sensitivity is manifested principally as bronchospasm and usually is associated with nasal polyps; the association of aspirin sensitivity, asthma, and nasal polyps is known as the aspirin triad. For a further discussion of cross-sensitivity of NSAIAs, see Cautions: Sensitivity Reactions, in the Salicylates General Statement 28:08.04.24.

Celecoxib is contraindicated in the setting of CABG surgery.

■ **Pediatric Precautions** Celecoxib is used for the management of the signs and symptoms of juvenile rheumatoid arthritis in children 2 years of age or older; safety and efficacy of celecoxib therapy beyond 6 months in pediatric patients with juvenile arthritis have not been established. Celecoxib has been evaluated in pediatric patients 2–17 years of age with pauciarticular course, polyarticular course, or systemic onset juvenile rheumatoid arthritis in one clinical study. Celecoxib has not been studied in pediatric patients younger than 2 years of age, those weighing less than 10 kg, or children with active systemic disease.

Recommended pediatric dosages of celecoxib should achieve plasma concentrations of the drug that are similar to those achieved in the clinical study that demonstrated efficacy.

In the clinical study in pediatric patients with pauciarticular course, polyarticular course, or systemic onset juvenile rheumatoid arthritis (active systemic disease not present at study entry), children with systemic onset juvenile rheumatoid arthritis appeared to be at risk for the development of abnormal coagulation test results. Use of NSAIAs, including celecoxib, has been associated with modest prolongation of activated partial thromboplastin time (aPTT) in children with systemic onset juvenile rheumatoid arthritis. NSAIAs should be used with caution in these children because of the risk of disseminated intravascular coagulation. Children with systemic onset juvenile rheumatoid arthritis who are receiving celecoxib should be monitored with coagulation tests.

It remains to be determined whether long-term cardiovascular risks in children exposed to celecoxib are similar to those observed in adults receiving celecoxib or other NSAIAs. (See Cautions: Cardiovascular Effects.)

■ **Geriatric Precautions** In clinical trials of celecoxib more than 3300 patients were 65–74 years of age and about 1300 were 75 years of age and older. No overall differences in efficacy of celecoxib were observed between geriatric and younger patients. Although results from clinical studies indicated that renal (i.e., glomerular filtration rate, blood urea nitrogen, creatinine) and platelet function (i.e., bleeding time, platelet aggregation) in geriatric individuals receiving celecoxib did not differ from those in younger individuals, more of the spontaneous reports of fatal adverse GI effects and acute renal failure have been in geriatric individuals than in younger individuals.

Peak plasma concentration and area under the plasma concentration-time curve (AUC) were increased 40 and 50%, respectively, in geriatric individuals (i.e., older than 65 years of age), but dosage adjustment in this age group based solely on age generally is not required. However, in geriatric patients weighing less than 50 kg, celecoxib therapy should be initiated at the lowest recommended dosage.

■ **Mutagenicity and Carcinogenicity** Celecoxib was not mutagenic when tested in vitro in an Ames test and in mutagenicity assays in Chinese hamster ovary (CHO) cells. In addition, the drug did not exhibit clastogenic potential in a chromosome aberration test in CHO cells and in vivo in the micronucleus test in rat bone marrow.

In a 2-year study, there was no evidence of carcinogenicity in male and female rats receiving oral celecoxib dosages of up to 200 and 10 mg/kg daily, respectively; exposure with such dosages is about twofold to fourfold that with the human dosage of 200 mg twice daily, expressed in terms of AUC (0–24 hours). In the same study, no evidence of carcinogenic potential was found in male and female mice receiving oral celecoxib dosages of up to 25 and 50 mg/kg daily, respectively, resulting in exposures approximately equivalent to the usual human daily dosage of 200 mg twice daily, expressed in terms of AUC (0–24 hours).

■ **Pregnancy, Fertility, and Lactation** An increased incidence of fetuses with ventricular septal defects, sternebral fusion, rib fusion, and sternebrae abnormality was observed in reproduction studies in rabbits receiving oral celecoxib dosages of 150 mg/kg daily or more throughout organogenesis (exposure approximately twice the usual human dosage of 200 mg twice daily, expressed in terms of AUC [0–24 hours]). A dose-dependent increase in diaphragmatic hernias was observed in rats receiving oral celecoxib dosages of 30 mg/kg or more daily throughout organogenesis (exposure approximately sixfold the usual human dosage of 200 mg twice daily, expressed in terms of AUC [0–24 hours]). Reproduction studies in rats using oral dosages up to 100 mg/kg daily (exposure approximately sevenfold the usual human dosage of 200 mg twice daily, expressed in terms of AUC [0–24 hours]) did not reveal evidence of delayed labor or parturition. There are no adequate and controlled studies to date using celecoxib in pregnant women or during labor and delivery, and the drug should be used during pregnancy only when the potential benefits justify the possible risks to the fetus. Although reproduction studies evaluating the effect of celecoxib on the closure of the ductus arteriosus in humans have not been conducted, the drug should not be used during the third trimester of pregnancy, since inhibitors of prostaglandin synthesis may have adverse effects on the fetal cardiovascular system (e.g., premature closure of the ductus arteriosus).

In rats receiving oral celecoxib dosages of 50 mg/kg or more daily (exposure approximately sixfold the usual human dosage of 200 mg twice daily, expressed in terms of AUC [0–24 hours]), postimplantation and preimplantation losses and reduced embryonic/fetal survival were observed. The manufacturer states that these adverse effects probably resulted from prostaglandin synthesis inhibition by the drug and were not associated with permanent alteration of the female reproductive function; these effects would not be expected to occur in women receiving recommended dosages of celecoxib. Studies in female and male rats using celecoxib dosages up to 600 mg/kg daily (exposure approximately 11-fold the usual human dosage of 200 mg twice daily, expressed in terms of AUC [0–24 hours]) have not revealed evidence of impaired fertility.

Celecoxib is distributed in the milk of lactating rats at concentrations similar to those in plasma. It is not known whether the drug is distributed in human milk. Because of the potential for serious adverse reactions to celecoxib in nursing infants, a decision should be made whether to discontinue nursing or the drug, taking into account the importance of the drug to the woman.

Drug Interactions

■ **Drugs Affecting Hepatic Microsomal Enzymes** Metabolism of celecoxib is mediated by the cytochrome P-450 (CYP) isoenzyme 2C9, and the possibility exists that drugs that inhibit this enzyme (e.g., fluconazole, fluvastatin, zafirlukast) may affect the pharmacokinetics of celecoxib. Therefore, celecoxib and drugs that inhibit the CYP2C9 isoenzyme should be administered concomitantly with caution. In addition, celecoxib inhibits CYP2D6, and the possibility exists that celecoxib may alter the pharmacokinetics of drugs metabolized by this isoenzyme, including various β-adrenergic blocking agents, many tricyclic and other antidepressants, various antipsychotic agents, and some antiarrhythmics (e.g., encainide, flecainide). Results of in vitro studies indicate that celecoxib is not a substrate for CYP2D6, and the drug does not inhibit the CYP2C9, CYP2C19, or CYP3A4 isoenzymes.

Fluconazole Results of clinical studies indicate that clinically important drug interactions may occur if celecoxib is administered with fluconazole. Concomitant administration of celecoxib with fluconazole can result in substantially increased plasma concentrations of celecoxib. This pharmacokinetic interaction appears to occur because fluconazole inhibits the CYP2C9 isoenzyme involved in celecoxib metabolism. In one study, concomitant administration of fluconazole (200 mg daily) and celecoxib (a single 200-mg dose) increased plasma concentrations of celecoxib twofold. The manufacturer of celecoxib states that celecoxib therapy should be initiated at the lowest recommended dosage in patients receiving fluconazole concomitantly.

Warfarin In one short-term (7-day) premarketing study in healthy individuals, celecoxib (200 mg twice daily) did not appear to alter the anticoagulant effect of warfarin (2–5 mg daily) as determined by the prothrombin time (PT). However, during postmarketing surveillance, bleeding complications associated with increases in PT were reported in some (mainly geriatric) patients receiving celecoxib concomitantly with warfarin. Therefore, patients receiving such concomitant therapy should be monitored appropriately for changes in anticoagulant activity (e.g., PT), particularly during the first few days after initiating or altering therapy, since these patients may be at increased risk of bleeding complications.

Other Drugs Affecting Hepatic Microsomal Enzymes In clinical studies, concomitant administration of celecoxib with ketoconazole, phenytoin, or tolbutamide did not alter the pharmacokinetics and/or pharmacodynamics of these drugs, and no clinically important interactions have been reported.

■ **Antacids** Administration of an antacid containing magnesium or aluminum with celecoxib decreased peak plasma concentrations of celecoxib by 37% and the area under the plasma concentration-time curve (AUC) by 10% in clinical studies. However, the manufacturer makes no specific recommendation for administration of the drug with regard to antacids because these effects are not considered clinically important.

■ **Angiotensin-converting Enzyme Inhibitors and Angiotensin II Receptor Antagonists** Experience with other nonsteroidal anti-inflammatory agents (NSAIAs) suggests that clinically important changes in blood pressure response may occur when celecoxib is administered concomitantly with an angiotensin-converting enzyme (ACE) inhibitor or angiotensin II receptor antagonist. There is some evidence that concomitant administration of NSAIAs, including celecoxib, may reduce the blood pressure response to ACE inhibitors or angiotensin II receptor antagonists. Therefore, blood pressure should be monitored carefully when a NSAIA, including celecoxib, is initiated in patients receiving one of these agents.

■ **Diuretics** NSAIAs may interfere with the natriuretic response to diuretics with activity that depends in part on prostaglandin-mediated alterations in renal blood flow (e.g., furosemide, thiazides). (See Cautions: Renal, Electrolyte, and Genitourinary Effects and also see Pharmacology: Renal Effects.)

■ **Glyburide** In clinical studies, concomitant administration of celecoxib with glyburide did not alter the pharmacokinetics and/or pharmacodynamics of glyburide, and no clinically important interactions have been reported.

■ **Lithium** Results of clinical studies indicate that clinically important drug interactions may occur if celecoxib is administered with lithium. Celecoxib and other NSAIAs can decrease renal clearance of lithium, which may lead to increased serum or plasma lithium concentrations. The mechanism involved in the reduction of lithium clearance by NSAIAs is not known, but has been attributed to inhibition of prostaglandin synthesis, which may interfere with the renal elimination of lithium by increasing sodium retention and thus lithium reabsorption; alternatively, inhibition of prostaglandin synthesis may reduce renal blood flow and glomerular filtration rate. In a study in healthy individuals, concomitant administration of celecoxib (200 mg daily) with lithium carbonate (450 mg twice daily) increased the mean steady-state plasma concentrations of lithium by about 17% compared with administration of lithium alone. Patients receiving lithium and celecoxib concomitantly should be monitored closely for signs of lithium toxicity and lithium dosage adjusted accordingly when celecoxib is initiated or discontinued.

■ **Methotrexate** In clinical studies, concomitant administration of celecoxib with methotrexate did not alter the pharmacokinetics and/or pharmacodynamics of methotrexate, and no clinically important interactions have been reported.

■ **Nonsteroidal Anti-inflammatory Agents** Although celecoxib may be used with low doses of aspirin, concomitant use of the 2 NSAIAs may increase the incidence of GI ulceration or other complications compared with that associated with celecoxib alone. (See Cautions: GI Effects.) Because celecoxib does not exhibit antiplatelet activity, the drug is not a substitute for aspirin for cardiovascular prophylaxis. However, there is no consistent evidence that use of low-dose aspirin mitigates the increased risk of serious cardiovascular events associated with COX-2 inhibitors.

Acute Toxicity

Limited information is available on the acute toxicity of celecoxib in humans. Serious toxicity was not observed in 12 individuals who received celecoxib 2.4 g daily for 10 days.

■ **Manifestations** Overdosage of NSAIAs can cause lethargy, drowsiness, nausea, vomiting, and epigastric pain; these manifestations generally are reversible with supportive care. GI bleeding also has been reported. Rarely, hypertension, acute renal failure, respiratory depression, and coma may occur. Anaphylactoid reactions have been reported with therapeutic use of NSAIAs and may occur following an overdosage.

■ **Treatment** Treatment of NSAIA overdosage involves symptomatic and supportive care; there is no specific antidote for NSAIA overdosage. During the first 4 hours after overdosage, emesis and/or administration of activated charcoal (60–100 g in adults or 1–2 g/kg in children) and/or an osmotic cathartic may be useful in symptomatic patients or in those who reportedly ingested a large overdosage. It is not known whether celecoxib is removed by hemodialysis, but the drug's extensive protein binding suggests that forced diuresis, alkalinization of urine, hemodialysis, or hemoperfusion is likely to be ineffective in removing substantial amounts of celecoxib from the body.

Pharmacology

■ **Mechanism of Action** Celecoxib is a selective inhibitor of the cyclooxygenase-2 (COX-2) isoform of prostaglandin endoperoxide synthase (prostaglandin G/H synthase, PGHS) and exhibits many of the pharmacologic actions of prototypical NSAIAs, including anti-inflammatory, analgesic, and antipyretic activity. NSAIAs appear to inhibit prostaglandin synthesis via inhibition of cyclooxygenase (COX); at least 2 isoenzymes, cyclooxygenase-1 (COX-1) and -2 (COX-2) (also referred to as PGHS-1 and -2, respectively), have been identified that catalyze the formation of prostaglandins in the arachidonic acid pathway. Although the exact mechanisms have not been clearly established, NSAIAs appear to exert anti-inflammatory, analgesic, and antipyretic activity principally through inhibition of the COX-2 isoenzyme; COX-1 inhibition presumably is responsible for the drugs' unwanted effects on GI mucosa. While prototypical NSAIAs are nonselective, inhibiting both COX-1 and COX-2 to varying degrees, celecoxib's highly selective inhibition of COX-2 potentially may be associated with a decreased risk of certain adverse effects (e.g., on GI mucosa); however, additional experience is needed to evaluate fully the adverse effect profile of the drug.

COX-1 is a constitutive enzyme that is expressed in most tissues, blood monocytes, and platelets; COX-1 is involved in thrombogenesis (e.g., promotion of platelet aggregation), maintenance of the gastric mucosal barrier, and renal function (e.g., maintenance of renal perfusion). COX-2 is an inducible enzyme that is found principally at sites of inflammation, although it also is expressed constitutively in the brain, kidney, and reproductive organs. COX-2 is expressed within 2–12 hours in response to cytokines and growth factors. At clinically relevant concentrations, celecoxib inhibits COX-2 in a slow, time-dependent manner involving formation of a tight enzyme-inhibitor complex that is noncovalent but only slowly dissociable. The celecoxib IC_{50}s (concentrations that inhibit enzyme activity by 50%) for COX-1 and COX-2 are 15 and 0.04 μM, respectively; the ED_{50} (dose that results in an effect in 50% of individuals tested) for COX-1 exceeds 200 mg/kg and, for COX-2, 0.2 mg/kg. The ratios of the IC_{50}s and ED_{50}s for COX-1 and COX-2 are 375 and greater than 1000, respectively, indicating that celecoxib is a highly selective COX-2 inhibitor. When celecoxib is administered in the management of osteoarthritis and rheumatoid arthritis, the principal physiologic action of the drug is inhibition of COX-2; celecoxib does not inhibit COX-1 when given in recommended dosages.

■ **Anti-inflammatory, Analgesic, and Antipyretic Effects** The anti-inflammatory, analgesic, and antipyretic effects of celecoxib and prototypical NSAIAs appear to result from inhibition of prostaglandin synthesis. While the precise mechanism of the anti-inflammatory and analgesic effects of NSAIAs continues to be investigated, these effects appear to be mediated principally through inhibition of the COX-2 isoenzyme at sites of inflammation with subsequent reduction in the synthesis of certain prostaglandins from their arachidonic acid precursors. Evidence supporting the role of COX-2 in inflammation includes up-regulation of COX-2 expression by mediators of inflammation, including cytokines and bacterial endotoxin. In addition, anti-inflammatory glucocorticoids can selectively inhibit cytokine and endotoxin induction of COX-2 while having no effect on expression of COX-1. Selective inhibitors of COX-2 block prostaglandin production and acute tissue inflammation in vivo, and studies in animals suggest that the anti-inflammatory and analgesic properties of selective COX-2 inhibitor NSAIAs are similar to those of prototypical NSAIAs that inhibit both COX-1 and COX-2. Clinical evidence also indicates that COX-2 has an important role in joint inflammation because highly selective COX-2 inhibitor NSAIAs are as effective as prototypical NSAIAs in the management of rheumatoid arthritis and osteoarthritis.

Studies in animals indicate that celecoxib exerts antipyretic activity at concentrations that inhibit COX-2 in vitro.

■ **Renal Effects** Prototypical NSAIAs have been associated with reductions in renal blood flow and glomerular filtration rate (GFR) and with sodium retention and hyperkalemia. These effects have been attributed to inhibition of renal prostaglandin synthesis in states of low renal reserve when prostaglandin-related physiologic mechanisms are needed to support renal function.

COX-1 is located in the arteries and arterioles, glomeruli, and collecting ducts of the kidney and is believed to be important in the maintenance of renal blood flow. The location and role of COX-2 in the human kidney remains to be determined, but results of animal studies indicate that COX-2 may be important in the regulation of sodium, volume, and blood pressure homeostasis, and in postnatal renal development. Although the effects of celecoxib on renal function were expected to differ from those of prototypical NSAIAs, results of renal pharmacodynamic and clinical studies indicate that the renal effects of selective inhibitors of COX-2 (e.g., celecoxib) are similar to those of prototypical NSAIAs with respect to renal regulation of sodium excretion, blood pressure, and GFR. In healthy geriatric adults (65–85 years of age), a group likely to have compromised renal function, and in patients with renal impairment (serum creatinine 1.3–3 mg/dL, GFR 40–60 mL/minute per 1.73 m^2), celecoxib had minimal effects on renal function.

Current evidence suggests that primary dysmenorrhea is mediated by prostaglandins. Substantially higher concentrations of prostaglandins have been found in the endometrium and menstrual fluid of women with primary dysmenorrhea (painful menses without demonstrable pelvic abnormality) compared with women without primary dysmenorrhea, and the amount of prostaglandin F_2 in menstrual fluid correlates with symptom severity (i.e., cramps, pain). Whether increased production of prostaglandins associated with primary dysmenorrhea is mediated by COX-1 or -2 remains to be determined. Prototypical NSAIAs that inhibit COX-1 and -2 and selective inhibitors of COX-2 (e.g., celecoxib) have been effective in relieving menstrual pain.

Limited evidence indicates that inhibition of COX-2 might interfere with ovulation.

■ **GI Effects** Therapy with prototypical NSAIAs has been associated with gastric mucosal damage; these effects have been attributed to inhibition of the synthesis of prostaglandins produced by COX-1. Other factors possibly involved in NSAIA-induced gastropathy include local irritation, promotion of acid back-diffusion into gastric mucosa, uncoupling of oxidative phosphorylation, and enterohepatic recirculation of the drugs. Because celecoxib is a selective inhibitor of COX-2, the drug is not expected to produce gastric mucosal damage typical of prototypical NSAIAs. Short-term administration of celecoxib has been associated with a lower incidence of adverse upper GI effects and endoscopically confirmed GI ulcer than prototypical NSAIAs. Whether long-term therapy with celecoxib is associated with a better GI safety profile than therapy with prototypical NSAIAs remains to be established. Limited evidence (e.g., from animal studies) indicates that COX-2 may contribute to healing of GI ulcers and that inhibition of COX-2 might interfere with epithelial cell proliferation, angiogenesis, and maturation of granular tissue at regions of ulcer repair and thus may delay healing of gastric ulcers.

The effect, if any, of selective COX-2 inhibitors in patients with inflammatory bowel disease remains to be established.

Epidemiologic and laboratory studies suggest that NSAIAs may reduce the risk of colon cancer. The exact mechanism by which NSAIAs may inhibit colon carcinogenesis has not been fully determined, and inhibition of COX-1 and/or COX-2 or inhibition of other cellular targets of NSAIAs may be involved. Several lines of evidence suggest that inhibition of COX-2 by NSAIAs may play an important role in this effect, although pathways that do not involve cyclooxygenase also may be involved. Overexpression of COX-2 has been observed in colon tumors in rodents and humans and there is evidence that COX-2 contributes to tumorigenesis. Although the specific cellular pathways responsible for the effects of COX-2 on tumorigenesis remain to be determined, the enzyme apparently mediates mitogenic growth factor signaling and down-regulates apoptosis, thus promoting tumor growth. Biopsy specimens from patients with colorectal cancer (adenocarcinomas) indicate that COX-2 is present in and around colorectal tumors and the degree of expression of COX-2 correlates positively with Duke's stage and tumor size; COX-2 was not present in control tissue from patients without colorectal cancer. The distribution of COX-2 in colorectal tumors suggests that inhibition of COX-2 has the potential to restore apoptosis and prevent proliferation of colon cancer cells. Induction of apoptosis by inhibition of COX-2 may be important in reducing the number of adenomatous colorectal polyps in patients with familial adenomatous polyposis (FAP), a disorder in which apoptosis is believed to be attenuated, and there is evidence that celecoxib and some other NSAIAs can reduce the size and number of colorectal polyps in patients with FAP. Studies using genetic and carcinogen-induced rodent models of colon cancer indicate that NSAIAs can decrease both the incidence and multiplicity of colon tumors and decrease the overall colon tumor burden and that celecoxib is more effective than prototypical NSAIAs (e.g., aspirin, ibuprofen, piroxicam, sulindac) in these models.

■ **Hematologic Effects** Unlike prototypical NSAIAs, celecoxib administered in single doses up to 800 mg and in multiple doses of 600 mg twice daily for up to 7 days does not appear to inhibit platelet aggregation or prolong bleeding time. In addition, usual dosages of the drug do not appear to affect platelet counts, prothrombin time (PT), or partial thromboplastin time (PTT). However, bleeding complications have been reported during postmarketing surveillance in some patients with elevated PTs receiving concomitant warfarin therapy. (See Warfarin under Drug Interactions: Drugs Affecting Hepatic Microsomal Enzymes.)

It has been postulated that selective COX-2 inhibitors may increase cardiovascular thrombotic risk because they block synthesis of prostacyclin (which is antithrombotic) but leave generation of thromboxane A_2 (which is prothrombotic) unaffected, thereby allowing platelet aggregation and hemostasis to occur unopposed; in contrast, prototypical NSAIAs suppress synthesis of both prostacyclin and thromboxane A_2. However, individual prototypical NSAIAs vary in degree of selectivity for COX-1 relative to COX-2, and both selective COX-2 inhibitors and prototypical NSAIAs have been associated with increased risk of cardiovascular events. Because NSAIAs differ in their selectivity for the COX-2 enzyme and their potency as inhibitors of COX-2, effects of individual NSAIAs on the balance between suppression of prostacyclin and thromboxane A_2 may differ. Rofecoxib is one of the most potent COX-2 inhibitors; rofecoxib also is one of the most selective COX-2 inhibitors in vitro. Celecoxib is less selective than rofecoxib or valdecoxib. The clinical relevance of differences in COX-2 selectivity and potency of individual NSAIAs with regard to cardiovascular thrombotic risk remains to be fully determined.

Pharmacokinetics

The pharmacokinetics of celecoxib have been studied principally in healthy adults and in adults with acute pain, rheumatoid arthritis, or osteoarthritis. Certain pharmacokinetic parameters of celecoxib (i.e., peak plasma concentration, area under the plasma concentration-time curve [AUC]) are approximately dose proportional when the drug is administered to fasting adults in dosages up to 200 mg twice daily. However, there is a less-than-proportional increase in peak plasma concentration and AUC when the drug is administered to fasting adults in dosages exceeding 200 mg twice daily; this effect has been attributed to the low aqueous solubility of celecoxib. Limited data indicate that the pharmacokinetics of celecoxib are affected by advanced age, renal and/or hepatic function, and race. (See Pharmacokinetics: Absorption.)

■ **Absorption** Celecoxib is well absorbed from the GI tract, and peak plasma concentrations of the drug generally are attained within 3 hours after dosing in fasting individuals. Absolute bioavailability of celecoxib has not been determined. Following oral administration of a single 200-mg dose of celecoxib in healthy, fasting adults 19–52 years of age, peak plasma concentrations of the drug averaged 705 ng/mL. Bioavailability (AUC) was increased 10–20% and time to reach peak plasma concentrations of celecoxib was delayed by 1–2 hours when the commercially available 200-mg capsules were administered with a high-fat meal (24 g fat) compared with administration with a medium-fat meal (8 g fat) or under fasting conditions. In addition, AUC and plasma concentration 12 hours after the dose were slightly (about 10%) higher when the drug was given in the evening versus the morning. When a celecoxib capsule is opened and the contents sprinkled over applesauce prior to administration, the pharmacokinetic profile of the drug (i.e., AUC, peak plasma concentration, time to peak plasma concentration, plasma elimination half-life) is similar to that following oral administration of the intact capsule. Following oral administration of celecoxib at recommended dosages (200–400 mg daily), steady-state plasma concentrations are achieved within 5 days. Drug accumulation has not been observed in individuals receiving celecoxib 400 mg twice daily.

Following oral administration of celecoxib at recommended dosages in geriatric individuals older than 65 years of age, peak plasma concentration and AUC were increased 40 and 50%, respectively, compared with younger adults. Peak plasma celecoxib concentration and AUC values were higher in geriatric women than geriatric men, predominantly because of the lower body weight of these women. Analysis of pooled pharmacokinetic data indicates that the AUC of celecoxib is about 40% higher in blacks compared with whites; the cause and clinical importance of this finding are not known.

Limited information is available on the pharmacokinetics of celecoxib in patients with mild to moderate hepatic and/or renal impairment. AUC of celecoxib at steady state reportedly was increased 40 or 180% in individuals with mild (Child-Pugh class A) or moderate (Child-Pugh class B) hepatic impairment, respectively, compared with that in healthy adults with normal hepatic function. In adults with chronic renal insufficiency (glomerular filtration rates of 35–60 mL/minute), AUC of celecoxib reportedly was 40% lower than that in adults with normal renal function.

■ **Distribution** Distribution of celecoxib into body tissues and fluids has not been fully characterized. The apparent volume of distribution of celecoxib at steady state is about 400 L (about 7.14 L/kg), suggesting extensive tissue distribution.

At therapeutic plasma concentrations, celecoxib is about 97% bound to plasma proteins, principally albumin and to a lesser extent, α_1-acid glycoprotein. Celecoxib is not preferentially bound to erythrocytes in blood.

It is not known whether celecoxib crosses the placenta in humans. Although it also is not known whether celecoxib is distributed into human milk, the drug is distributed into milk in rats in concentrations similar to those in plasma.

■ **Elimination** The plasma elimination half-life of celecoxib following oral administration of a single 200-mg dose under fasting conditions is about 11 hours, and the apparent plasma clearance of the drug is about 500 mL/minute; these parameters exhibit wide intraindividual variability, presumably because the low aqueous solubility of celecoxib prolongs absorption. The half-life of celecoxib is prolonged in patients with renal or hepatic impairment and has been reported to be 13.1 hours in patients with chronic renal insufficiency and 11 or 13.1 hours in patients with mild or moderate hepatic impairment, respectively.

The metabolic fate of celecoxib has not been fully determined, but the drug is metabolized in the liver to inactive metabolites principally by the cytochrome P-450 (CYP) isoenzyme 2C9. Metabolism of celecoxib involves hydroxylation of the 4-methyl group to form a primary alcohol (SC-60613), followed by oxidation of the primary alcohol to the corresponding carboxylic acid (SC-62807), the major metabolite. The carboxylic acid metabolite is conjugated with glucuronic acid to some extent, forming the 1-*O*-glucuronide. Metabolites of celecoxib do not have pharmacologic activity as cyclooxygenase-1 (COX-1) or COX-2 inhibitors. In patients with poor metabolizer phenotypes of the CYP2C9 isoenzyme, the metabolic clearance of celecoxib may be decreased and plasma concentrations may be increased. (See Cautions: Precautions and Contraindications.)

Oral clearance of celecoxib appears to increase in a less-than-proportional manner with increasing weight; pediatric patients with juvenile rheumatoid arthritis weighing 10 or 25 kg are predicted to have a 40 or 24% lower clearance, respectively, than a 70-kg adult with rheumatoid arthritis.

Celecoxib is excreted in urine and feces principally as metabolites; less than 3% of the dose is excreted unchanged. Following oral administration of a single 300-mg dose of radiolabeled celecoxib as an oral suspension (not commercially available in the US), approximately 27 and 57% of the dose was excreted in urine and feces, respectively. The principal metabolite in both urine and feces was the carboxylic acid metabolite (73% of the dose); small amounts of the glucuronide metabolite were present in urine.

Chemistry and Stability

■ **Chemistry** Celecoxib, a diaryl substituted pyrazole derivative containing a sulfonamide substituent, is a nonsteroidal anti-inflammatory agent (NSAIA). Celecoxib is a selective inhibitor of cyclooxygenase-2 (COX-2). Because the goal of selective inhibitors of COX-2 is to inhibit COX-2 but not COX-1, the drugs also have been referred to as COX-1-sparing NSAIAs. Celecoxib differs chemically and, to some extent, pharmacologically from prototypical NSAIAs, which inhibit cyclooxygenase-1 (COX-1) and -2 (COX-2).

Celecoxib consists of a central pyrazole ring, 2 substituted aromatic rings, and a benzenesulfonamide attached to one of the rings. Spatial orientation of the 2 aromatic rings relative to the central ring is important for cyclooxygenase inhibitory activity; the 2 aromatic rings must reside at adjacent positions on the central ring for COX-2 activity. Unlike most prototypical NSAIAs, celecoxib does not contain a carboxylate group; it has been postulated that absence of such a group may contribute to the drug's high COX-2 selectivity.

Although the overall structures of COX-1 and COX-2 are similar, a principal difference between the 2 isoforms of cyclooxygenase is the presence of a much larger NSAIA binding site on COX-2 compared with the NSAIA binding site on COX-1. The larger binding site on COX-2 results from the substitution of valine for isoleucine at position 523 in COX-2. It has been postulated that the smaller valine molecule, unlike the larger isoleucine molecule in COX-1, gives access to a side pocket that may be the binding site for many selective COX-2 inhibitors, including celecoxib. It appears that the benzenesulfonamide moiety of celecoxib binds to the side pocket, although diaryl heterocyclic compounds, including celecoxib, may have multiple modes of binding to cyclooxygenases.

Celecoxib occurs as an odorless, white to off-white crystalline powder. The aqueous solubility of celecoxib at a pH less than 9 is about 5 mcg/mL at 5–40°C. Solubility of the drug increases in strongly basic solutions; celecoxib has a solubility of 0.8 mg/mL in water at 40°C and pH 12. The drug has a solubility of 111 mg/mL in alcohol at room temperature.

■ **Stability** Commercially available celecoxib capsules should be stored at 25°C, but may be exposed to temperatures ranging from 15–30°C. When stored as directed, the capsules have an expiration date of 2 years following the date of manufacture.

When a celecoxib capsule is opened and the contents mixed with applesauce, the mixture is stable for 6 hours when refrigerated.

Preparations

Because of similarity in spelling of Celexa® (citalopram hydrobromide), Celebrex® (celecoxib), and Cerebyx® (fosphenytoin sodium), extra care should be exercised in ensuring the accuracy of prescriptions for these drugs.

Excipients in commercially available drug preparations may have clinically important effects in some individuals; consult specific product labeling for details.

Celecoxib

Oral		
Capsules	50 mg*	CeleBREX®, Pfizer Celecoxib Capsules
	100 mg*	CeleBREX®, Pfizer Celecoxib Capsules
	200 mg*	CeleBREX®, Pfizer Celecoxib Capsules
	400 mg*	CeleBREX®, Pfizer Celecoxib Capsules

*available from one or more manufacturer, distributor, and/or repackager by generic (nonproprietary) name

†Use is not currently included in the labeling approved by the US Food and Drug Administration

SALICYLATES 28:08.04.24

Salicylates General Statement

■ Salicylates (synthetic derivatives of salicylic acid) are nonsteroidal anti-inflammatory agents (NSAIAs); the pharmacologic actions (e.g., analgesia, anti-inflammatory effects) of salicylates appear to result principally from the salicylate moiety.

Uses

Salicylates are used principally in the symptomatic treatment of mild to moderate pain, fever, inflammatory diseases, and rheumatic fever. Aspirin, but not other currently available salicylates, is also used in the prevention of arterial thrombosis. (See Uses: Thrombosis, in Aspirin 28:08.04.24.)

Aspirin is the most extensively evaluated and utilized salicylate. Although there are relatively few controlled comparative studies of aspirin and other salicylates (e.g., salicylate salts), the analgesic, antipyretic, and anti-inflammatory effects of other salicylates are generally considered to be comparable to those of aspirin. However, many clinicians prefer aspirin in most patients, at least initially, when a salicylate is indicated. Other salicylates may be particularly useful in patients with GI intolerance to aspirin or in patients in whom interference with normal platelet function by aspirin or other NSAIAs is considered undesirable. Generally, other commercially available salicylates are used only in the symptomatic treatment of rheumatoid arthritis, osteoarthritis, or related inflammatory diseases.

■ **Pain** Salicylates are generally used to provide temporary analgesia in the treatment of mild to moderate pain, particularly pain associated with inflammation. Salicylates are most effective in relieving low-intensity pain of nonvisceral origin, such as headache, neuralgia, myalgia, and arthralgia; however, the drugs may relieve mild to moderate postoperative pain, postpartum pain, oral surgery and other dental pain, dysmenorrhea, or other visceral pain such as that associated with trauma or cancer. Salicylates have lower maximum analgesic effects than most opiate analgesics and are generally not useful in the treatment of severe acute pain of visceral origin.

In addition to systemic administration, salicylates (e.g., trolamine salicylate) have been applied topically alone or as an adjunct to systemic therapy in the treatment of mild muscle or joint pain, such as that associated with inflammatory disease (e.g., rheumatoid arthritis). A chewing gum formulation or gargle containing aspirin has also been used for topical treatment of sore throat pain. However, the evidence that topical salicylates are effective analgesics is inconclusive.

■ **Fever** Salicylates are often used to lower body temperature in febrile patients in whom fever may be deleterious or in whom considerable relief is obtained when fever is lowered. However, antipyretic therapy is generally nonspecific, does not influence the course of the underlying disease, and may obscure the course of the patient's illness. For information on salicylates and Reye's syndrome, see Cautions: Pediatric Precautions.

■ **Inflammatory Diseases** Salicylates are frequently used for anti-inflammatory and analgesic effects in the initial and/or long-term symptomatic treatment of rheumatoid arthritis, juvenile arthritis, and osteoarthritis. Salicylates may also be useful in the symptomatic treatment of other polyarthritic conditions (e.g., psoriatic arthritis, Reiter's syndrome, ankylosing spondylitis), systemic lupus erythematosus, and nonarticular inflammation; however, other NSAIAs may be preferred in the treatment of some of these conditions (e.g., ankylosing spondylitis). Salicylates appear to be only palliative in rheumatic conditions and have not been shown to permanently arrest or reverse the underlying disease process. Salicylates are not effective in the treatment of chronic iridocyclitis in patients with juvenile arthritis.

Rheumatoid Arthritis, Juvenile Arthritis, and Osteoarthritis When used in the treatment of rheumatoid arthritis or juvenile arthritis, salicylates have relieved pain and stiffness; reduced swelling, fever, tenderness, the duration of morning stiffness, and the number of joints involved; and improved mobility. In patients with rheumatoid arthritis, salicylates have also improved grip strength. When used in the treatment of osteoarthritis, salicylates have relieved pain and stiffness, reduced tenderness, and improved mobility. In the treatment of osteoarthritis, NSAIAs are used principally for their analgesic rather than anti-inflammatory effect, although inflammation may be part of the symptomatology.

Most clinical studies have shown that the anti-inflammatory and analgesic effects of usual dosages of salicylates in the treatment of rheumatoid arthritis, juvenile arthritis, or osteoarthritis are greater than those of placebo and about equal to those of usual dosages of other currently available NSAIAs. Patient response to NSAIAs is variable, however, and patients who do not respond to one agent may be successfully treated with a different agent.

In the management of rheumatoid arthritis in adults, NSAIAs may be useful for initial symptomatic treatment; however, NSAIAs do not alter the course of the disease or prevent joint destruction. Disease modifying antirheumatic drugs (DMARDs) (e.g., azathioprine, cyclosporine, etanercept, oral or injectable gold compounds, hydroxychloroquine, infliximab, leflunomide, methotrexate, minocycline, penicillamine, sulfasalazine) have the potential to reduce or prevent joint damage, preserve joint integrity and function, and reduce total health care costs, and all patients with rheumatoid arthritis are candidates for DMARD therapy. DMARDs should be initiated early in the disease course and should not be delayed beyond 3 months in patients with active disease (i.e., ongoing joint pain, substantial morning stiffness, fatigue, active synovitis, persistent elevation of erythrocyte sedimentation rate [ESR] or C-reactive protein [CRP], radiographic evidence of joint damage). (For further information on the treatment of rheumatoid arthritis, see Uses: Rheumatoid Arthritis, in Methotrexate 10:00.) NSAIA therapy may be continued in conjunction with DMARD therapy or, depending on patient response, may be discontinued.

Psoriatic Arthritis and Reiter's Syndrome Salicylate therapy may be effective in the treatment of some patients with psoriatic arthritis or Reiter's syndrome but usually only when the disease is mild. Salicylates are also seldom effective in the treatment of ankylosing spondylitis unless the disease is mild.

Systemic Lupus Erythematosus Some clinicians consider salicylates (particularly aspirin) to be the drugs of choice for the treatment of fever, arthritis, pleurisy, and pericarditis in patients with systemic lupus erythematosus. The anti-inflammatory and analgesic effects of salicylates may also be useful in the symptomatic treatment of nonarticular inflammation such as bursitis and/or tendinitis (e.g., acute painful shoulder) and fibrositis.

■ **Rheumatic Fever** Salicylates are considered to be the drugs of choice for the symptomatic treatment of patients with rheumatic fever who have only polyarthritis or those (with or without polyarthritis) who develop mild carditis without cardiomegaly or congestive heart failure. Most clinicians consider aspirin to be the salicylate of choice. Although salicylates suppress the acute exudative inflammatory process of rheumatic fever, progression or duration of the disease is usually not altered. Within 1–4 days after an adequate dosage of salicylate has been initiated, there is usually considerable or complete relief of pain, swelling, immobility, local heat, and erythema of the involved joints; fever and heart rate are also decreased.

Although it has not been clearly established by controlled studies, most clinicians prefer corticosteroid therapy to salicylates in the treatment of patients with rheumatic fever who develop carditis with cardiomegaly or congestive heart failure. Corticosteroids control acute manifestations of carditis more rapidly than salicylates and may be life-saving in critically ill patients. However, corticosteroids, like salicylates, cannot prevent valvular damage and are no better than salicylates for long-term treatment. Some clinicians initiate therapy with salicylates in patients with carditis and cardiomegaly; if the disease is not rapidly and adequately controlled, salicylate therapy is discontinued and steroid therapy started immediately. In patients with carditis who are treated with steroids, most clinicians initiate salicylate therapy as steroid therapy is gradually withdrawn, to minimize potential inflammatory rebound. Salicylate therapy is continued for several weeks after steroids are discontinued. Rebound of rheumatic activity after discontinuance of therapy usually subsides within 5–10 days without further treatment.

■ **Thrombosis** Because of its ability to inhibit platelet aggregation, aspirin is used in the prevention of arterial thrombosis. (See Uses: Thrombosis, in Aspirin 28:08.04.24.) Since other currently available salicylates do not inhibit platelet aggregation, they should not be substituted for aspirin in the prophylaxis of thrombosis.

■ **Kawasaki Disease** The American Academy of Pediatrics (AAP), the American Heart Association (AHA), and the American College of Chest Physicians (ACCP) recommend aspirin therapy used in conjunction with immune globulin IV (IGIV) for initial treatment of the acute phase of Kawasaki disease†. High-dose aspirin therapy (80–100 mg/kg daily for up to 14 days) combined with a single dose of IGIV (2 g/kg) initiated within 10 days of the onset of fever is more effective than aspirin therapy alone for preventing or reducing the occurrence of coronary artery abnormalities associated with Kawasaki disease; fever and other manifestations of inflammation also may resolve more rapidly with concomitant therapy. Aspirin then is continued alone in lower dosages (i.e., 1–5 mg/kg daily) for antiplatelet effects for 6–8 weeks in those without coronary artery changes or with only transient coronary artery ectasia or dilatation (disappearing within the initial 6–8 weeks of illness). For additional information on initial treatment of Kawasaki disease, see Uses: Kawasaki Disease and see Kawasaki Disease under Dosage and Administration: Dosage for Immune Globulin IV, in Immune Globulin 80:04

Coronary artery abnormalities develop in 15–25% of children with Kawasaki disease if they are not treated within 10 days of fever onset; 2–4% of patients develop coronary artery abnormalities despite prompt treatment with aspirin and IGIV. Long-term management of those who develop coronary abnormalities depends on the severity of coronary involvement and may include low-dose aspirin (with or without clopidogrel or dipyridamole), anticoagulant therapy with warfarin or low molecular weight heparin, or a combination of antiplatelet and anticoagulant therapy (usually low-dose aspirin and warfarin). If giant coronary aneurysms are present, AHA and ACCP suggest long-term low-dose aspirin therapy in conjunction with warfarin . Specialized references should be consulted for additional information on long-term management of Kawasaki disease in individuals with coronary abnormalities.

■ **Gout** Because salicylates have a uricosuric effect, they were once used in the treatment of gout. However, other more effective agents are currently available for the treatment of this disease. Indeed, salicylates are generally contraindicated in patients with gout since they may cause uric acid retention (at low to intermediate dosages) and may antagonize the activity of other uricosuric agents. (See Drug Interactions: Uricosuric Agents.)

Other Uses of Aspirin For information on other uses of aspirin, see Uses in Aspirin 28:08.04.24.

Dosage and Administration

■ **Administration** Salicylates are usually administered orally, preferably with food or a large quantity (240 mL) of water or milk to minimize gastric irritation. In patients unable to take or retain oral medication, aspirin suppositories may be administered rectally; however, rectal absorption may be slow and incomplete. (See Pharmacokinetics: Absorption.) If gastric irritation and/or symptomatic GI disturbances occur with uncoated oral solid-dosage preparations, these effects may be reduced with enteric-coated tablets, extended-release tablets, or an oral solution of salicylate.

■ **Dosage** Dosage of salicylates must be carefully adjusted according to individual requirements and response, using the lowest possible effective dosage.

Pain and Fever For analgesia or antipyresis, salicylates are usually administered in divided doses every 4–6 hours. If a rapid response is required, the more slowly absorbed dosage forms (i.e., enteric-coated tablets, extended-release tablets) should *not* be used.

Salicylates should not be used for *self-medication* of pain for longer than 10 days in adults or 5 days in children, unless directed by a clinician, since pain of such intensity and duration may indicate a pathologic condition requiring medical evaluation and supervised treatment.

Salicylates should not be used in adults or children for *self-medication* of marked fever (greater than 39.5°C), fever persisting longer than 3 days, or recurrent fever, unless directed by a clinician, since such fevers may indicate serious illness requiring prompt medical evaluation and treatment.

To minimize the risk of overdosage, no more than 5 doses of a salicylate preparation should be administered to children for analgesia or antipyresis in any 24-hour period, unless directed by a clinician.

Inflammatory Diseases For the symptomatic treatment of inflammatory diseases, salicylates are usually administered in 4–6 divided doses daily. If large single doses are tolerated, salicylates can probably be given in 2 or 3 divided doses daily (every 8–12 hours) in many patients during long-term therapy, since the elimination half-life of salicylate is prolonged when high dosages are administered. In some patients, a single daily dose may be effective. At least 5–7 days is generally required to attain steady-state serum salicylate concentrations with high dosages. Therefore, when necessary, dosage is usually increased no more frequently than at weekly intervals.

Dosage should be adjusted according to the patient's response, tolerance, and serum salicylate concentration. Serum salicylate concentrations of 150–300 mcg/mL are usually required for an anti-inflammatory effect. Measurement of serum salicylate concentration should be performed no sooner than 5–7 days after a specific dosage has been initiated (unless toxicity is suspected); blood specimens usually should be obtained approximately 1–3 hours after a dose. In patients with decreased serum albumin concentrations, therapeutic effects may be associated with lower than usual serum salicylate concentrations since the fraction of total drug in serum as free salicylate is increased in these patients; measurement of free salicylate concentration in serum may be useful to guide therapy in such patients.

In the symptomatic treatment of inflammatory diseases, duration of salicylate therapy depends on the specific disease and the patient's response and tolerance; several weeks to months may be required to obtain optimum therapeutic response. In the symptomatic treatment of rheumatoid arthritis, osteoarthritis, or other polyarthritic conditions, therapy is usually continued for as long as a satisfactory response is obtained and no severe or intolerable adverse effect occurs. In the symptomatic treatment of juvenile rheumatoid arthritis, therapy is usually continued for 4–12 months after patients have achieved a complete clinical remission.

Rheumatic Fever Dosage and duration of salicylate therapy in the symptomatic treatment of rheumatic fever are generally determined by severity and duration of acute manifestations; many clinicians believe that optimum therapeutic effects are associated with serum salicylate concentrations of 250–350 mcg/mL.

In patients with rheumatic fever who have only polyarthritis or those (with or without polyarthritis) who develop mild carditis without cardiomegaly or congestive heart failure, salicylates are usually administered for approximately 4–8 weeks or as long as necessary. Patients who have only polyarthritis are usually asymptomatic after 2–3 weeks of therapy. Some clinicians suggest that salicylate therapy be continued for at least 2 weeks after the patient is asymptomatic and evidence of active inflammation has disappeared.

Patients who have carditis with cardiomegaly or congestive heart failure are usually treated with corticosteroids, and salicylate therapy is initiated as steroid therapy is gradually withdrawn; salicylates are usually administered for approximately 2–4 weeks after steroids are discontinued. High dosages of salicylates should be used with extreme caution in patients with carditis since congestive heart failure or pulmonary edema may be precipitated.

When salicylate therapy is discontinued in patients with rheumatic fever, the drug is withdrawn gradually over 1–2 weeks to minimize the risk of rebound of rheumatic activity. Only extremely severe clinical rebounds of rheumatic activity require reinstitution of therapy, in which case salicylates are administered in the usual dosage for 3–4 additional weeks.

Cautions

■ **GI Effects** Adverse reactions to salicylates mainly involve the GI tract and include symptomatic GI disturbances, GI bleeding, and/or mucosal lesions (e.g., erosive gastritis, gastric ulcer). These reactions apparently occur more frequently with aspirin than with other currently available salicylates.

Symptomatic GI Disturbances Symptomatic GI disturbances are manifested most frequently as dyspepsia, heartburn, epigastric distress, or nausea, and less frequently as vomiting, anorexia, or abdominal pain; these disturbances appear to occur more frequently with aspirin than with some other NSAIAs. Symptomatic GI disturbances reportedly occur in about 2–10% of healthy individuals receiving usual analgesic or antipyretic dosages of salicylates, in about 10–30% of patients receiving high dosages (e.g., greater than 3.6 g of aspirin daily), and in about 30–90% of patients with preexisting peptic ulcer, hemorrhagic gastritis, or duodenitis. Symptomatic GI disturbances frequently occur in the first few days of treatment with high dosages; although these disturbances disappear when therapy is discontinued, they also often subside despite continued treatment and without dosage adjustment. Centrally induced nausea and vomiting occur most often when the plasma salicylate concentration exceeds 270 mcg/mL, but nausea and vomiting may occur at lower concentrations as a result of local gastric irritation.

Symptomatic GI disturbances may be minimized by administering salicylates immediately after meals or with food, antacids, or a large quantity (240 mL) of water or milk. Alternatively, if symptomatic GI disturbances occur with an uncoated tablet, an enteric-coated tablet, extended-release tablet, or an oral solution of salicylate may be better tolerated. If burning in the throat or an unpleasant taste or aftertaste occurs with an uncoated tablet, a film-coated or enteric-coated tablet may be better tolerated. It has not been established that buffered aspirin tablets cause fewer symptomatic GI disturbances than uncoated plain aspirin tablets.

GI Bleeding Occult GI bleeding, which occurs in most patients receiving salicylates (particularly aspirin), is usually painless and appears to be the result of a local action on GI mucosa. Occult GI blood loss with usual dosages of aspirin appears to be greater than that with usual dosages of most other NSAIAs. There appears to be no correlation between the incidence of salicylate-induced occult GI bleeding and symptomatic GI disturbances. Uncoated plain aspirin tablets in an oral dosage of 1–4.5 g daily produce a blood loss of 2–8 mL daily in about 70% of patients. However, about 10–15% of patients lose 10 mL or more of blood daily, which may result in iron deficiency anemia with long-term therapy; tolerance to salicylate-induced bleeding apparently does not occur. Unlike aspirin, usual oral dosages of salicylate salts or salsalate produce little or no GI blood loss.

The incidence and severity of GI bleeding are generally dose related. GI bleeding is not reduced by administration of salicylates with food. GI bleeding is less in patients with achlorhydria than in healthy individuals with normal gastric acid production, apparently because gastric acid is necessary to produce gastric mucosal injury. There is adequate evidence that sufficient buffering to decrease gastric acidity and increase the pH of gastric contents substantially reduces aspirin-induced GI blood loss; however, concomitant oral administration of high dosages of antacids is necessary to provide sufficient buffering capacity. (See Drug Interactions: Acidifying and Alkalinizing Agents.) It has not been established that the amounts of buffers contained in commercially available buffered aspirin tablets have any effect in reducing GI blood loss. However, GI blood loss is reduced with oral aqueous aspirin solutions. Although single oral doses of highly buffered aqueous aspirin solutions (e.g., Alka-Seltzer®) cause little or no GI blood loss, multiple doses for 2–3 days do cause some GI bleeding; these solutions are not recommended for long-term therapy because of their high buffer and sodium content. Aspirin-induced GI blood loss also may be reduced with enteric-coated tablets, extended-release tablets, or by concomitant oral administration of a histamine H_2-receptor antagonist (e.g., cimetidine hydrochloride).

The risk of GI bleeding is increased in geriatric patients 60 years of age or older and in patients with a history of GI ulcers or bleeding, those receiving an anticoagulant or corticosteroid or taking multiple NSAIAs concomitantly, those consuming 3 or more alcohol-containing beverages daily, and those receiving excessive dosages or prolonged therapy.

In an FDA review of 41 reports of serious bleeding events (site unspecified but severe enough to require hospitalization) associated with use of OTC preparations containing aspirin in fixed combination with antacids (e.g., buffered effervescent tablets administered as oral solutions), 88% of the events occurred in patients with risk factors for bleeding.

Rarely, major upper GI bleeding may occur in patients receiving salicylates (particularly aspirin), regardless of the specific dosage form. A definite relationship between occult GI bleeding and major upper GI bleeding with aspirin therapy has not been established. Patients with active peptic ulcer or those who have recently had major upper GI bleeding do not experience greater occult blood loss after small doses of aspirin than do healthy individuals; however, these patients do have an increased risk of recurrent major bleeding. Most clinicians believe that aspirin and other salicylates can potentiate GI bleeding in patients with GI lesions.

In patients who have undergone tonsillectomy, severe bleeding from tonsillar blood vessels has been reported following topical application of aspirin via gargles or chewing gum tablets.

Mucosal Lesions Salicylates (especially aspirin) can cause gastric mucosal damage with varying degrees of erythema, petechiae, submucosal bleeding, erosions, and/or ulceration, with or without bleeding, and even in the absence of GI symptoms. Aspirin and other salicylates may also reactivate latent gastric or duodenal ulcers. Although not clearly established, the incidence of gastric mucosal damage may be higher with aspirin than with other NSAIAs. The exact relationships between salicylate-induced gastric mucosal damage and occult GI bleeding or major upper GI bleeding remain to be clearly determined. Microscopic mucosal damage that accompanies endoscopically observed mucosal abnormalities usually resolves within several hours following a single oral dose of aspirin and can be reduced or prevented by concomitant oral administration of sodium bicarbonate (in amounts sufficient to buffer gastric contents) or a histamine $_2$-receptor antagonist (e.g., cimetidine). However, with long-term aspirin therapy, many patients develop persistent gastric erythema and erosions and gastric ulcer (often in the distal antrum). Several studies using endoscopy have indicated that the incidence of aspirin-induced gastric erosions and ulceration is lower with enteric-coated tablets than with buffered or uncoated plain tablets; buffered tablets appear to provide little or no protection against gastric mucosal damage.

Although long-term aspirin therapy has not been clearly associated with the occurrence of duodenal ulceration, duodenal erythema and erosions have been reported to occur frequently in patients receiving aspirin; the incidence of duodenal mucosal damage appears to be lower with enteric-coated tablets than with buffered or uncoated plain tablets.

In patients who develop gastric or duodenal ulcers during treatment with salicylates, salicylate therapy is generally discontinued because of an increased risk of bleeding and/or ulcer perforation; occasionally, another NSAIA is substituted for the salicylate in these patients. However, gastric or duodenal ulcers 1 cm or less in diameter, which are induced by salicylates or other NSAIAs, may heal despite continued treatment with these agents when an oral histamine H_2-receptor antagonist (e.g., cimetidine) and high-dose antacid therapy are administered concomitantly. Although such regimens generally appear to be safe and effective, ulcer perforation has occurred in patients receiving a NSAIA and cimetidine concomitantly; further evaluation of these regimens is necessary.

Uncoated plain aspirin tablets allowed to remain in contact with mucous membranes of the mouth and aspirin chewing gum tablets have produced mucosal erosions and ulcerations of the mouth. Rectally administered aspirin suppositories may rarely cause rectal mucosal irritation, burning pain, rectal bleeding, diarrhea, and tenesmus.

Other Adverse GI Effects Although a causal relationship has not been established, one case-control analysis suggests that NSAIAs may contribute to the formation of esophageal stricture in patients with gastroesophageal reflux.

Gastric accumulation of enteric-coated aspirin tablets, sometimes resulting in gastric ulceration or salicylate intoxication, has been reported in some patients with gastric outlet obstruction. Removal of accumulated enteric-coated aspirin tablets from the stomach by usual methods (e.g., emesis, gastric lavage) may be unsuccessful in these patients and surgery may be necessary. However, some clinicians have reported successful removal by gastric lavage using an isotonic sodium bicarbonate solution (containing 150 mEq/L) to dissolve the enteric coating and allow dissolution of the aspirin; 300 mL of the solution was instilled into the stomach via a nasogastric tube over 30 minutes and then removed by continuous nasogastric suction for 30 minutes, the regimen being repeated continuously for 24 hours.

■ **Otic Effects** Tinnitus and hearing loss may occur in patients receiving large dosages of salicylates and/or long-term therapy. These effects are often the initial manifestations of chronic salicylate intoxication in adults. (See Chronic Toxicity: Manifestations.) Tinnitus and hearing loss are rarely noted by young children or patients with preexisting hearing impairment and are therefore usually not useful as indicators of early chronic intoxication in these patients.

Tinnitus and hearing loss are dose related, usually completely reversible (even after administration of large dosages for many years), and are more likely caused by actions on the inner ear than on the CNS. Patients receiving high dosages should be monitored periodically for tinnitus and hearing loss. Tinnitus usually develops only when the serum salicylate concentration exceeds 200 mcg/mL and generally occurs at a concentration of about 300 mcg/mL; however, it may develop only at higher concentrations in some patients. Tinnitus occurs infrequently in patients with preexisting hearing impairment, even at high serum salicylate concentrations (e.g., greater than 400 mcg/mL). Since serum salicylate concentrations of 200–300 mcg/mL are consistent with those considered necessary for anti-inflammatory effects, the occurrence of tinnitus in adults with inflammatory disease can indicate attainment of adequate concentrations, but only in those patients with normal hearing. Because tinnitus can occur over a wide range of concentrations, determinations of serum salicylate concentration are preferred as a guide to adjusting dosage. Tinnitus subsides gradually with reduction of salicylate dosage or usually within 24–48 hours after discontinuance of therapy.

Salicylate-induced hearing impairment involves bilateral loss of pure tone sensitivity for all sound frequencies. Hearing losses generally range from 20–40 decibels, occur initially at a serum salicylate concentration of about 200 mcg/mL, and increase with increasing concentrations. Maximum hearing loss occurs most frequently at a serum salicylate concentration of about 400 mcg/mL. Hearing loss is usually completely reversible, subsiding within 24–72 hours after discontinuance of therapy; rarely, permanent hearing loss has been reported.

■ **Hepatic Effects** Salicylates occasionally cause acute, reversible hepatotoxicity, particularly in patients with juvenile arthritis, active systemic lupus erythematosus, rheumatic fever, or preexisting hepatic impairment. Therefore, hepatic function should be monitored in these patients. In addition, salicylate therapy has been associated in a few patients with hepatic injury consistent with chronic active hepatitis. Salicylate-induced hepatotoxicity is usually mild, but death or hepatic injury with encephalopathy has occurred in a few patients.

Hepatic injury usually consists of mild, focal, cellular necrosis, eosinophilic degeneration of hepatocytes, and portal inflammation; the exact mechanism is not known. Salicylate-induced hepatotoxicity is manifested principally as elevations in serum aminotransferase concentrations; elevations in serum alkaline phosphatase concentration occur occasionally. Rarely, serum bilirubin concentration may be elevated and/or serum prothrombin concentration may be decreased with a resultant increase in the PT. Although most patients are asymptomatic, some develop nausea, vomiting, anorexia, abdominal distress, loss of taste for cigarettes, liver tenderness, and/or hepatomegaly.

Hepatotoxicity has generally developed after 1–4 weeks of therapy and appears to be related to serum salicylate concentration, occurring principally at concentrations exceeding 200–250 mcg/mL; however, it may occur at lower concentrations. Elevated serum aminotransferase concentrations usually return to pretreatment values within 1–2 weeks after dosage reduction or discontinuance of salicylate therapy; however, they may be transient and return to pretreatment values despite continued therapy and without dosage adjustment.

It is usually not necessary to discontinue salicylate therapy in patients who develop hepatotoxicity, but dosage reduction may be advisable in patients who develop signs of hepatotoxicity and whose serum salicylate concentration exceeds 250 mcg/mL. Some clinicians recommend that the PT be measured periodically in patients with abnormal hepatic function test results and that salicylate therapy be discontinued if prolonged PT occurs.

■ **Renal Effects** In usual dosages, salicylates rarely cause clinically important adverse renal effects. In overdosage, the drugs may cause a marked reduction in creatinine clearance or acute tubular necrosis with renal failure.

Although the exact mechanism(s) is not known, salicylates cause transient urinary excretion of renal tubular epithelial cells. Albuminuria, proteinuria, and urinary excretion of leukocytes and erythrocytes may also occur. Urinary excretion of renal tubular epithelial cells usually increases markedly in the first several days of continuous therapy and then subsides or continues at a low level with prolonged treatment. Salicylates have also been shown to cause urinary excretion of *N*-acetyl-β-glucosaminidase 2–4 hours after single doses equivalent in salicylate content to at least 1.95 g of aspirin; the mechanism is not known.

In patients with impaired renal function or systemic lupus erythematosus, aspirin may cause reversible (sometimes marked) decreases in renal blood flow and glomerular filtration rate; as a result, minimal water, sodium, and potassium retention may occur. These effects may also occur in patients with conditions predisposing to sodium and water retention (e.g., congestive heart failure, decompensated hepatic cirrhosis). However, aspirin may have less severe adverse renal effects than other currently available NSAIAs. Renal effects are usually rapidly reversed following discontinuance of aspirin therapy, but they may also subside despite continued treatment. Although these effects on renal function have not been reported to date with salicylates other than aspirin, other salicylates may cause similar effects.

Long-term therapy with aspirin alone or in combination with other analgesic-antipyretic agents (e.g., phenacetin) has been associated with analgesic nephropathy (renal papillary necrosis with subsequent chronic interstitial nephritis); however, evidence to date concerning aspirin alone is conflicting and a causal relationship remains to be clearly established. Several studies indicate that long-term aspirin or salicylate therapy rarely, if ever, causes substantial renal disease; however, some clinicians have reported a high incidence of renal papillary necrosis at autopsy in patients with rheumatoid arthritis who received long-term aspirin therapy. The exact mechanism(s) of renal damage is not known but may include renal medullary ischemia caused by inhibition of renal prostaglandin synthesis and/or a direct cytotoxic effect of the drugs or their metabolites. Further studies are needed to fully evaluate the effects of long-term salicylate therapy on the kidney and renal function.

■ **Cardiovascular Effects** Salicylates may cause moderate to severe noncardiogenic pulmonary edema, principally with chronic or acute intoxication. Salicylate-induced pulmonary edema may also be precipitated or aggravated by forced alkaline diuresis during the treatment of salicylate overdosage, but fluid volume overload is not necessary for its occurrence. It has been suggested that salicylates cause pulmonary edema by increasing alveolar capillary membrane permeability. Salicylate-induced noncardiogenic pulmonary edema appears to occur most frequently when the serum salicylate concentration exceeds 400 mcg/mL. It is usually manifested as diffuse bilateral infiltrates on chest radiographs, tachypnea or dyspnea, and hypoxemia, and is often associated with proteinuria and adverse neurologic effects such as lethargy or confusion. Patients receiving long-term salicylate therapy or those with a history of smoking appear to have an increased risk of developing pulmonary edema. Treatment of salicylate-induced pulmonary edema is generally supportive and includes measures to increase the excretion of salicylate; an adequate airway should be maintained and assisted pulmonary ventilation may be required. Following treatment, pulmonary edema generally resolves within 1–7 days.

In patients with rheumatic fever who have carditis, congestive heart failure and pulmonary edema may be precipitated with high dosages of salicylates, apparently as a result of increased circulating plasma volume and cardiac workload.

In one placebo-controlled study in a small number of patients with variant angina, aspirin therapy (2 g twice daily) was associated with an increased frequency of angina and an increased risk of exercise-induced angina.

■ **Hematologic Effects** Although aspirin alters hemostasis through effects on platelet function and high dosages of salicylates can decrease hepatic synthesis of blood coagulation factors (see Pharmacology: Hematologic Effects), salicylates cause few hematologic reactions. Daily aspirin doses of 3–4 g may decrease the hematocrit and plasma iron concentration, and reduce erythrocyte life span. Since the effects of aspirin on platelets are irreversible, ingestion of aspirin or aspirin-containing preparations within 3–5 days of platelet donation generally precludes use of an individual donor as a sole source of platelet preparations for a thrombocytopenic recipient. However, ingestion of aspirin or aspirin-containing preparations does not preclude donation of whole blood. Since other currently available salicylates do not affect platelet aggregation, ingestion of these other salicylates does not preclude donation of platelets or whole blood.

Leukopenia, thrombocytopenia, pancytopenia, eosinopenia, agranulocytosis, aplastic anemia, purpura, eosinophilia associated with aspirin-induced hepatotoxicity, and disseminated intravascular coagulation have been reported rarely in patients receiving salicylates. Leukocytosis has occurred with salicylate overdosage. Increased perioperative and postoperative bleeding, hematomas, and ecchymoses have occurred in patients who ingested aspirin before and for several days after oral surgery. In addition, adverse hematologic effects have been reported in neonates whose mothers ingested aspirin before delivery. (See Cautions: Pregnancy, Fertility, and Lactation.)

Macrocytic anemia associated with folic acid deficiency has been reported in patients abusing analgesic-combination preparations containing aspirin and in patients with rheumatoid arthritis receiving high dosages of aspirin. In one patient, megaloblastic anemia was associated with long-term ingestion of a preparation containing aspirin, salicylamide, and caffeine.

In vitro, salicylates reduce adenosine triphosphate (ATP) concentrations and inhibit hexose-monophosphate shunt activity in erythrocytes of patients with pyruvate kinase deficiency. Although the clinical significance of these effects in vivo is not known, salicylates might cause or aggravate hemolysis in these patients.

Salicylates (especially aspirin) may cause or aggravate hemolysis in patients with glucose-6-phosphate dehydrogenase (G-6-PD) deficiency; however, this has not been clearly established. In a study in patients with G-6-PD deficiency, salicylate did not inhibit hexose-monophosphate shunt activity in erythrocytes from these patients in vitro, and oral doses of aspirin (50 mg/kg daily for 4 days) did not cause hemolysis; however, none of the patients in this study had chronic hemolysis. Some clinicians suggest that aspirin or other salicylates can probably be used safely in most patients with G-6-PD deficiency, but effects of the drugs in patients with rare variants of this enzyme deficiency remain to be fully evaluated.

■ **Dermatologic Effects** Skin eruptions of a pustular acneiform nature may occur but are usually observed only in patients who have received salicylates continually for longer than 1 week or with overdosage. Erythematous, scarlatiniform, pruritic, eczematoid, or desquamative lesions, which rarely may be bullous or purpuric, have also been reported. Hemorrhage from mucous membranes may occur rarely. Rarely, aspirin has been associated with Stevens-Johnson syndrome and toxic epidermal necrolysis.

■ **Sensitivity Reactions** Sensitivity reactions to aspirin may occur rarely; sensitivity reactions to other salicylates are extremely rare. Sensitivity reactions manifested principally as bronchospasm appear to be related mainly to inhibition of prostaglandin synthesis. The exact mechanism(s) of sensitivity reactions manifested principally as urticaria and/or angioedema has not been determined; although these reactions may be immune-mediated in some patients, IgE antibodies or specific antibodies have not been detected. If an aspirin (or salicylate) sensitivity reaction occurs, it usually develops within 3 hours of ingestion and is characterized as urticaria, angioedema, bronchospasm, severe rhinitis, or shock. Facial edema also has been reported with aspirin. Lacrimation, complete vasomotor collapse, and loss of consciousness may also occur. Although extremely rare, severe reactions resulting in death have occurred within minutes following ingestion of 325–650 mg of aspirin in individuals with known aspirin sensitivity. If a severe reaction occurs, the drug should be discontinued and the patient given appropriate treatment (e.g., epinephrine, corticosteroids, maintenance of an adequate airway, oxygen) as indicated.

Aspirin sensitivity appears to occur in about 0.3% of the general population, in about 20% of patients with chronic urticaria, in about 4% of patients with asthma, and in about 1.5% of patients with chronic rhinitis. Aspirin sensitivity also appears to occur more frequently in adults 30–60 years of age than in younger adults or children, and more frequently in females.

In patients with asthma, aspirin sensitivity is manifested principally as bronchospasm and is usually associated with the presence of nasal polyps; the association of aspirin sensitivity, asthma, and nasal polyps is known as the aspirin triad. In these patients, nasal symptoms usually precede asthma, and the onset of asthma may precede the development of aspirin sensitivity by many years. Mild to marked bronchospasm of variable duration may occur with oral doses of aspirin as small as 20–30 mg and usually develops within 15–30 minutes after ingestion of the drug.

In one study in patients with asthma, the capacity of aspirin and other NSAIAs to induce bronchospasm was directly correlated with the degree of in vitro inhibition of prostaglandin synthesis caused by the drugs. As an inhibitor of cyclooxygenase, aspirin may alter the synthesis of prostaglandin E (a bronchodilator) and prostaglandin $F_{2\alpha}$ (a bronchoconstrictor), resulting in a predominance of prostaglandin $F_{2\alpha}$ and bronchoconstriction. It has also been suggested that the inhibition of cyclooxygenase favors the formation of leukotrienes that contribute to bronchoconstriction. Patients with aspirin-induced bronchospasm are often cross-sensitive to other inhibitors of prostaglandin synthesis. *Cross-sensitivity in these patients appears to occur most frequently with indomethacin, followed by ibuprofen, mefenamic acid, phenylbutazone, and sodium benzoate; therefore, these drugs and any NSAIA are generally contraindicated in patients with aspirin sensitivity and vice versa.* Patients with aspirin-induced bronchospasm are usually not cross-sensitive to salicylate salts, salicylamide, or acetaminophen. Aspirin desensitization in aspirin-sensitive asthmatic patients has been reported; in some of these patients, cross-desensitization with indomethacin and other NSAIAs was demonstrated. However, continuous aspirin therapy appears to be necessary to maintain desensitization, which disappears gradually over several days when aspirin is withheld. Further evaluation is needed to determine the clinical implications of these findings.

In patients with chronic urticaria or chronic rhinitis, aspirin sensitivity is manifested principally as urticaria and/or angioedema, but bronchospasm and shock may also occur. Patients with aspirin sensitivity who generally have dermatologic reactions to the drug appear to have an increased risk of cross-sensitivity to salicylate salts or acetaminophen.

In general, about 10% of patients with aspirin sensitivity appear to be cross-sensitive to the dye tartrazine (FD&C yellow No. 5) and about 5% appear to be cross-sensitive to acetaminophen; since the incidence of cross-sensitivity to acetaminophen is low, some clinicians state that, if necessary, acetaminophen may be used instead of aspirin for analgesic-antipyretic effects in some patients with aspirin sensitivity.

The manufacturer of salsalate states that patients with aspirin sensitivity are not cross-sensitive to salsalate; although specific data are not available, the manufacturer suggests that patients who have sensitivity reactions to non-salicylate NSAIAs are probably not cross-sensitive to salsalate.

■ **Precautions and Contraindications** Salicylates (particularly aspirin) should be used with caution in patients with active GI lesions (e.g., erosive gastritis, peptic ulcer) or with a history of recurrent GI lesions, since the drugs may cause or aggravate GI bleeding and/or ulcerations. Patients with ulcers or persistent or recurring stomach disorders (e.g., heartburn, stomach pain, dyspepsia) should contact their clinician prior to initiating therapy with aspirin. If salicylates must be administered, these patients should be closely monitored for signs of GI bleeding or ulcer perforation. For additional information on precautions associated with the use of salicylates in these patients, see Cautions: GI Effects. Use of enteric-coated salicylate preparations in patients with known or suspected gastric outlet obstruction should generally be avoided. When aspirin is used in fixed combination with dipyridamole, the cautions, precautions, and contraindications associated with dipyridamole must be considered in addition to those associated with aspirin.

Patients should be informed that alcohol has a synergistic effect with aspirin in causing GI bleeding. The manufacturers caution that patients who generally consume 3 or more alcohol-containing drinks per day should ask their clinician whether to use salicylates (e.g., aspirin, choline salicylate, magnesium salicylate) or an alternative analgesic for *self-medication* since salicylates may increase the risk of GI bleeding. In addition, the manufacturers caution that patients who generally consume 3 or more alcohol-containing drinks per day should ask their clinician whether to use a salicylate (e.g., aspirin) in fixed combination with acetaminophen or an alternative analgesic for *self-medication* since aspirin in fixed combination with acetaminophen may increase the risk of GI bleeding and hepatotoxicity.

Despite current warnings on OTC product labels, serious bleeding events continue to occur in patients receiving aspirin in fixed combination with antacids (e.g., buffered effervescent tablets administered as oral solutions) for *self-medication*. FDA is evaluating whether additional actions are needed to address this safety concern.

Patients should discontinue aspirin and consult a clinician if they experience erythema or edema in the area being treated for pain or if new symptoms occur.

Because of an increased risk of bleeding, salicylates (particularly aspirin) should be used with extreme caution, if at all, in patients with preexisting hypoprothrombinemia, vitamin K deficiency, thrombocytopenia, thrombotic thrombocytopenic purpura, or severe hepatic impairment, or in patients receiving anticoagulants (see Drug Interactions: Anticoagulants and Thrombolytic Agents). Since salicylates may cause or aggravate hemolysis in patients with pyruvate kinase deficiency or in patients with rare variants of G-6-PD deficiency, the drugs should probably be avoided in these patients. Most clinicians recommend that aspirin therapy be discontinued 5–7 days before surgery to prevent or minimize excessive perioperative bleeding; however, it has not been clearly established that patients receiving aspirin have substantially increased perioperative blood loss. Therapy with salicylates that do not affect platelet aggregation need not be discontinued before surgery.

Because of an increased risk of bleeding, aspirin is contraindicated in patients with bleeding disorders such as hemophilia, von Willebrand's disease, or telangiectasia. If salicylate therapy is considered necessary in patients with bleeding disorders, some clinicians suggest that salicylates which do not inhibit platelet aggregation (e.g., salicylate salts) may be used. Patients with bleeding disorders should contact their clinician prior to initiating therapy with aspirin for *self-medication*.

Because of an increased risk of bleeding, chewing gum tablets or gargles that contain aspirin should be avoided for at least 1 week after tonsillectomy or oral surgery. In addition, tablets containing aspirin should not be chewed before swallowing for at least 1 week after tonsillectomy or oral surgery because of possible injury to oral tissues from prolonged contact with aspirin particles.

Salicylates should be used with caution in patients with impaired renal function and with extreme caution, if at all, in patients with advanced chronic renal insufficiency, since salicylate and its metabolites are excreted almost completely in the urine; in addition, these patients may have an increased risk of developing adverse renal effects.

Hematocrit and renal function should be monitored periodically in patients receiving prolonged salicylate therapy or high dosages since iron deficiency anemia or adverse renal effects may occur. Because of an increased risk of hepatotoxicity, hepatic function should also be monitored in patients with juvenile arthritis, active systemic lupus erythematosus, rheumatic fever, or preexisting hepatic impairment who are receiving high dosages of salicylates.

Because of the high sodium content, highly buffered aspirin solutions (e.g., Alka-Seltzer®) should be used with extreme caution, if at all, in patients with congestive heart failure or other conditions in which a high sodium intake would be harmful; in addition, highly buffered aspirin solutions can result in alkalinization of the urine and enhance urinary excretion of salicylate. Salicylate salts containing magnesium or sodium should be avoided in patients in whom excessive amounts of these electrolytes might be harmful. Patients on a sodium-restricted diet should consult a clinician prior to initiating therapy with aspirin for *self-medication*.

If corticosteroid dosage is decreased during salicylate therapy, it should be done gradually and patients should be observed for adverse effects, including adrenocortical insufficiency or symptomatic exacerbation of the inflammatory condition being treated. In addition, since corticosteroids may increase renal excretion of salicylate or induce its metabolism, reduction of salicylate dosage may be necessary when steroid therapy is discontinued. (See Drug Interactions: Corticosteroids.)

The possibility that the antipyretic and anti-inflammatory effects of NSAIAs may mask the usual signs and symptoms of infection or other diseases should be considered.

Some commercially available formulations of salicylates contain sodium bisulfite, a sulfite that may cause allergic-type reactions, including anaphylaxis and life-threatening or less severe asthmatic episodes, in certain susceptible individuals. The overall prevalence of sulfite sensitivity in the general population is unknown but probably low; such sensitivity appears to occur more frequently in asthmatic than in nonasthmatic individuals. Some commercially available formulations of salicylates contain the dye tartrazine (FD&C yellow No. 5), which may cause allergic reactions including bronchial asthma in certain susceptible individuals. Although the incidence of tartrazine sensitivity is low, it frequently occurs in individuals who are sensitive to aspirin.

A specific salicylate preparation is contraindicated in patients with known hypersensitivity to that preparation or any of the ingredients in the formulation and should be used with extreme caution, if at all, in patients with known hypersensitivity to salicylates. The commercially available preparation containing aspirin in fixed combination with extended-release dipyridamole is contraindicated in patients with hypersensitivity to dipyridamole, aspirin, or any other ingredient in the formulation. Aspirin generally is contraindicated in patients in whom sensitivity reactions (e.g., urticaria, angioedema, bronchospasm, severe rhinitis, shock) are precipitated by any NSAIA and vice-versa, although the drugs have occasionally been used in aspirin- or NSAIA-sensitive patients who have undergone desensitization. Patients with known aspirin sensitivity should be warned to avoid aspirin and aspirin-containing preparations. If an allergic reaction with aspirin occurs, a clinician should be contacted immediately. Patients with asthma should consult their clinician prior to initiating therapy with aspirin. (See Cautions: Sensitivity Reactions.)

■ Pediatric Precautions Salicylates should be used with caution in pediatric patients who are dehydrated, since these patients are especially susceptible to salicylate intoxication.

Safety and efficacy of magnesium salicylate in children younger than 12 years of age have not been established. Safety and efficacy of salsalate in children have not been established.

The safety and efficacy of the commercially available preparation containing aspirin in fixed combination with extended-release dipyridamole have not been established in children.

Reye's Syndrome Use of salicylates (almost exclusively aspirin) in children with varicella infection or influenza-like illnesses reportedly is *associated with* an increased risk of developing Reye's syndrome; however, a *causal relationship* has *not* been established. In several initial epidemiologic studies, children with varicella or influenza-like illnesses who developed Reye's syndrome appeared to receive salicylates more frequently during their antecedent illness than those who did not develop the syndrome; however, the methodology and results of some of these studies have been questioned. Subsequent epidemiologic studies designed and implemented by the US Public Health Service Reye Syndrome Task Force found a *strong association* between development of the syndrome and ingestion of salicylates (almost exclusively aspirin) during the antecedent illness. Most evidence to date, including a decline in the use of aspirin in children accompanied by a continuing decline in reported cases of Reye's syndrome, strongly supports such an association, but some data do not and some controversy still remains. Whether an increased risk of developing the syndrome is associated with aspirin only or with all salicylates has not been adequately evaluated.

The exact pathogenesis of Reye's syndrome and the potential role of aspirin and other salicylates in its pathogenesis remain to be determined. The syndrome has occurred in children who did not receive salicylates and in children who received other medications.

Because of the evidence to date, the US Surgeon General, the American Academy of Pediatrics Committee on Infectious Diseases, the US Food and Drug Administration (FDA), and other authorities currently advise that *salicylates not be used in children and teenagers with varicella or influenza, unless directed by a clinician.* Use of salicylates also generally should be avoided in children and teenagers with suspected varicella or influenza and during presumed outbreaks of influenza, since diagnosis of these diseases may be impossible to establish accurately during the prodromal period; similarly, salicylates should not be used in the management of viral infections in children or adolescents because of the possibility that the infection may be one associated with an increased risk of Reye's syndrome. If antipyretic medication is considered necessary in children or teenagers with known or suspected varicella or influenza or other viral illness, acetaminophen may be used. It is not known whether Reye's syndrome may occur in children who receive salicylates following vaccination with varicella virus vaccine live. (See Drug Interactions: Varicella Virus Vaccine Live.)

■ Geriatric Precautions Geriatric individuals receiving salicylates are more likely than younger individuals to experience adverse effects secondary to age-related decline in renal function and/or increased use of concomitant drug therapy. The risk of GI bleeding is increased in geriatric patients 60 years of age or older. (See Cautions: GI Effects.)

Salicylates are highly protein bound and can be displaced from binding sites by other protein-bound drugs. Because geriatric patients are more likely to be taking multiple drugs than younger patients, geriatric patients are at increased risk of drug interactions mediated by alterations in protein binding (i.e., decrease in protein binding of salicylate and increased concentrations of unbound salicylate). (See Drug Interactions: Protein-bound Drugs.)

■ Pregnancy, Fertility, and Lactation Although safe use of salicylates during pregnancy has not been established, there is evidence indicating that aspirin is the most frequently used drug during pregnancy either as a single entity or in combination with other drugs. Salicylates have been shown to be teratogenic and embryocidal in animals. In humans, a slight positive association between chronic maternal salicylate ingestion during pregnancy and congenital abnormalities has been reported in some studies, but other studies have found no association. In some studies, chronic maternal salicylate ingestion has also been associated with decreased fetal birth weight; an increased incidence of stillbirth, neonatal mortality, antepartum and postpartum maternal hemorrhage, and complicated deliveries; and prolongation of gestation and spontaneous labor. There have been several reports of adverse hematologic effects (e.g., subconjunctival hemorrhage, hematuria, purpura, petechiae, cephalhematoma) in neonates whose mothers had ingested aspirin before delivery, and at least 2 reports of neonatal salicylate intoxication secondary to salicylate accumulation in utero. In one study, maternal ingestion of aspirin during the week before delivery was associated with an increased incidence of intracranial hemorrhage in premature neonates. In addition, it has been suggested that premature closure of the ductus arteriosus secondary to maternal salicylate ingestion may be one cause of persistent pulmonary hypertension in some infants.

Maternal and fetal hemorrhagic complications observed with maternal ingestion of large doses (e.g., 12–15 g daily) of aspirin generally have not been observed in studies in which low doses (60–150 mg daily) of the drug were used for prevention of complications of pregnancy† (e.g., preeclampsia, recurrent spontaneous abortions, prematurity, intrauterine growth retardation, stillbirth, low birthweight), including those associated with autoimmune disorders such as antiphospholipid syndrome, poor paternal blocking antibody production, or systemic lupus erythematosus. (See Uses: Complications of Pregnancy, in Aspirin 28:08.04.24.) Although current evidence indicates that low dosages of aspirin can be used safely during pregnancy, the possibility of maternal and/or fetal complications (e.g., bleeding) should be considered. At least one case of fatal cerebral hemorrhage has been reported in a woman who was receiving prophylactic therapy with aspirin, heparin, and immune globulin despite no history of recurrent pregnancy loss nor antiphospholipid antibodies; this woman was found to have had a congenital arteriovenous malformation as a predisposing risk for hemorrhage.

Salicylates should be used during pregnancy only when the potential benefits justify the possible risks to the fetus. The drugs (particularly aspirin) generally should be avoided during the last 3 months (although *low* dosages have been useful in the prevention of preeclampsia during this period) of pregnancy (especially during the 1–2 weeks before delivery). Similarly, aspirin in fixed combination with extended-release dipyridamole should be avoided in the third trimester of pregnancy.

If maternal ingestion of aspirin occurs within 1–2 weeks of delivery, the neonate should be closely evaluated for the presence of bleeding.

In animals, aspirin has been shown to cause testicular atrophy and inhibit spermatogenesis. Although the effect on fertility is not known, aspirin has been shown to decrease seminal fluid concentrations of prostaglandins E and F in healthy men.

Since salicylates are distributed into milk in low concentrations, the drugs should be administered with caution to nursing women. However, maternal consumption of high salicylate dosages potentially may result in adverse effects (e.g., rash, platelet abnormalities, bleeding) in nursing infants. At least one case of salicylate toxicity in an infant has been attributed to breast-feeding; however, some experts consider it unlikely that ingestion of breast milk alone could have resulted in the serum salicylate concentration reported in the infant. In general, nursing should be discontinued during long-term salicylate therapy with high dosages; however, some clinicians state that occasional single doses of salicylates in nursing women appear to be of little risk to nursing infants.

Drug Interactions

Numerous drug interactions involving salicylates have been reported but few appear to be clinically important. The salicylate interactions that many clinicians consider to be the most important include those with anticoagulants and thrombolytic agents, uricosuric agents, sulfonylureas, corticosteroids, and methotrexate.

■ **Protein-bound Drugs** Because salicylate is highly protein bound, it could be displaced from binding sites by, or could displace from binding sites, other protein-bound drugs such as oral anticoagulants, sulfonylureas, hydantoins, penicillins, and sulfonamides; salicylates could also theoretically displace bilirubin in neonates, resulting in hyperbilirubinemia. Patients receiving salicylates with any of these drugs should be observed for adverse effects. The acetylation of albumin by aspirin could alter protein binding of other drugs; acetylated albumin has been shown to have a higher affinity for phenylbutazone.

■ **Anticoagulants** Salicylates may enhance the hypoprothrombinemic effect of warfarin and other oral anticoagulants and increase the risk of bleeding complications with these agents; several mechanisms may be involved. However, low-dose aspirin (e.g., 75–100 mg daily) may be used in combination with heparin or oral anticoagulants for therapeutic benefit (i.e., additive antithrombotic effects) in selected patients at high risk for thromboembolism (e.g., patients with prosthetic mechanical heart valves).

Although salicylates can cause a dose-dependent hypoprothrombinemia, clinical data are conflicting regarding salicylate enhancement of oral anticoagulant-induced hypoprothrombinemia. In several studies in patients receiving warfarin or other oral anticoagulants, the PT was not affected when aspirin was administered concurrently in dosages up to 3 g daily for 3–14 days. However, in one study in which either a lower or a higher aspirin dosage (1.95 or 3.9 g daily, respectively) was administered concurrently, the PT was substantially increased; patients receiving the higher aspirin dosage also had signs of bleeding. Therefore, it appears that high dosages of salicylates (e.g., greater than 3 g of aspirin daily) may enhance the hypoprothrombinemic effect of oral anticoagulants when administered concurrently. At lower dosages, salicylates may not affect oral anticoagulant-induced hypoprothrombinemia and occasional low doses of salicylates (other than aspirin) can probably be used with caution in patients receiving anticoagulants; however, salicylates should generally be avoided in these patients since they also cause GI bleeding. Patients with preexisting hepatic impairment may have an increased risk of bleeding if salicylates and oral anticoagulants are administered concomitantly. Since aspirin also inhibits platelet aggregation, it should be used with caution in patients receiving anticoagulants. Patients receiving anticoagulants should consult a clinician prior to initiating therapy with aspirin for *self-medication*. If salicylates are indicated for other than their antithrombotic effects in patients receiving anticoagulants, salicylates (e.g., salicylate salts) that do not affect platelet aggregation are preferred to aspirin. In addition, the lowest effective salicylate dosage should be used, the PT should be determined frequently and anticoagulant dosage adjusted accordingly, and patients should be observed closely for adverse effects.

Because aspirin inhibits platelet aggregation and causes GI bleeding, it should be used with caution in patients receiving heparin. Although further documentation is necessary, severe bleeding complications have been reported in some patients with hip fractures who received aspirin in conjunction with heparin as prophylaxis for deep-vein thrombosis.

■ **Thrombolytic Agents** Aspirin has been administered concomitantly with and/or after therapy with thrombolytic agents (e.g., streptokinase, alteplase) to prevent coronary artery reocclusion and/or reinfarction in patients with acute myocardial infarction. Concomitant administration of low dosages of aspirin with IV streptokinase therapy has been associated with additive reductions in mortality compared with those attributed to streptokinase therapy alone. Although concurrent therapy with aspirin and streptokinase was associated with an increased risk of major bleeding (including a slight increase in the incidence of confirmed intracranial hemorrhage during the first days of therapy) compared with placebo, such therapy appeared to be associated with only a slight increase in minor bleeding complications and no overall increase in serious bleeding episodes compared with streptokinase alone. Concomitant administration of low dosages of oral aspirin and IV heparin with IV alteplase therapy also has been associated with a substantial reduction in acute post-myocardial infarction mortality compared with placebo, but this regimen was accompanied by an apparent increased risk of bleeding complications, notably intracranial hemorrhage. Use after thrombolysis of drugs that affect platelet function should be individualized since these drugs may increase the risk of bleeding complications and have not been shown to be unequivocally effective to date. Further study is needed to elucidate the contribution of anticoagulant and/or platelet-aggregation inhibitor (e.g., aspirin) therapies to mortality reduction and the incidence of hemorrhagic complications observed in patients receiving these agents concomitantly with thrombolytic therapy.

■ **Uricosuric Agents** The uricosuric effects of salicylates and phenylbutazone, probenecid, or sulfinpyrazone are antagonistic; therefore, salicylates are generally contraindicated during uricosuric therapy. Although the exact mechanism(s) of the interaction has not been established, it appears to involve competition for active renal tubular transport; salicylates may also displace these agents from protein-binding sites. Salicylate-induced uricosuria is inhibited by usual doses of any of these agents. However, probenecid-induced uricosuria appears to be inhibited principally when the serum salicylate concentration exceeds 50 mcg/mL; therefore, occasional doses of salicylates for analgesia or antipyresis in patients receiving probenecid may be insufficient to produce a clinically important interaction. Although high single doses (e.g., greater than 3 g of sodium salicylate) of salicylates inhibit sulfinpyrazone-induced uricosuria, the effect of lower doses has not been determined. Frequent doses of salicylates for analgesia or antipyresis in patients receiving sulfinpyrazone as a uricosuric should probably be avoided. Patients receiving uricosuric agents should consult a clinician prior to initiating therapy with aspirin for *self-medication*. Sulfinpyrazone decreases the renal excretion of salicylate, apparently as a result of preferential tubular secretion of sulfinpyrazone.

■ **Antidiabetic Agents** The hypoglycemic effect of sulfonylureas (e.g., chlorpropamide, tolbutamide) may be enhanced by salicylates. Although this effect occurs principally with high salicylate dosages, it may occur with serum salicylate concentrations less than 100 mcg/mL. The exact mechanisms of the interaction are not known, but the ability of salicylates to decrease blood glucose concentration in diabetics may be involved. In vitro studies indicate that salicylates displace chlorpropamide and tolbutamide from protein-binding sites. In addition, salicylates may interfere with the renal tubular secretion of chlorpropamide, resulting in increased serum concentrations of the sulfonylurea. Further evaluation of the interaction between salicylates and sulfonylureas is needed. Patients receiving antidiabetic agents should consult a clinician prior to initiation of aspirin for *self-medication*.If salicylates and sulfonylureas are administered concurrently, caution should be exercised. Patients receiving both drugs should be observed closely for signs and symptoms of hypoglycemia and appropriate dosage reduction of either drug should be made accordingly. If reduction in sulfonylurea dosage is necessary when salicylate therapy is initiated, an increase in sulfonylurea dosage may be necessary when salicylate therapy is discontinued. It is not known whether salicylates have similar effects on insulin.

Although the exact mechanism(s) is not known, aspirin appears to inhibit the flush effect induced by alcohol in some patients receiving chlorpropamide.

■ **Corticosteroids** Serum salicylate concentrations may decrease when corticosteroids are administered concomitantly. Likewise, when corticosteroids are discontinued in patients receiving salicylates, serum salicylate concentration may increase; salicylate intoxication has been precipitated rarely. Several mechanisms may be involved in this interaction. In one study in healthy individuals and in patients with polyarthritis who received both drugs concomitantly, corticosteroids increased the renal clearance of salicylate, possibly by increasing glomerular filtration rate. Corticosteroids may also induce the metabolism of salicylate. Salicylates and corticosteroids should be used concurrently with caution. Patients with receiving antiarthritic agents should consult a clinician prior to initiating therapy with aspirin for *self-medication*.Patients receiving both drugs should be observed closely for adverse effects of either drug. It may be necessary to increase salicylate dosage when corticosteroids are administered concurrently or decrease salicylate dosage when corticosteroids are discontinued in patients receiving salicylates.

■ **Methotrexate** Limited clinical data indicate that concurrent administration of salicylates and methotrexate may result in increased serum concentrations of methotrexate and thereby increase the risk of methotrexate toxicity. Salicylates displace methotrexate from plasma protein binding sites and decrease renal excretion of methotrexate by competing with and inhibiting renal tubular secretion of the antineoplastic agent. Several patients receiving both drugs reportedly developed severe pancytopenia; a few of these patients died. Since methotrexate has a low therapeutic index and may produce serious adverse effects, salicylates should be used with extreme caution, if at all, in patients receiving the drug. Geriatric patients and patients with impaired renal function may be at particular risk. If the drugs are administered concurrently, patients should be carefully monitored for signs of adverse effects of methotrexate. Patients receiving methotrexate should be warned to avoid nonprescription preparations containing salicylates.

■ **Acidifying and Alkalinizing Agents** Since the urinary excretion of salicylate is markedly pH dependent (see Pharmacokinetics: Elimination), concurrent administration of drugs that increase or decrease urine pH may increase or decrease urinary excretion of salicylate, respectively.

In patients receiving high dosages of salicylates, urinary acidifying agents (e.g., ammonium chloride) may increase renal tubular reabsorption of salicylate and possibly increase serum salicylate concentrations. However, if urine is acidic before administration of an acidifying agent, the increase in serum salicylate concentration is likely to be minimal; a substantial increase is likely only in patients who have an initial urine pH greater than 6.5.

Concurrent administration of high dosages of antacids (e.g., 4 g of sodium bicarbonate or at least 60–120 mL of aluminum and magnesium hydroxides suspension daily), or highly buffered aspirin solutions (e.g., Alka-Seltzer®) may increase urine pH and decrease serum salicylate concentrations by decreasing renal tubular reabsorption of salicylate. Although substantial reductions in serum salicylate concentration caused by concomitant antacid therapy have occasionally been reported, a quantitative reduction in serum salicylate concentration cannot be routinely predicted. Patients receiving high dosages of salicylates should be monitored for alterations in serum salicylate concentration if antacid therapy is initiated or discontinued, and salicylate dosage adjusted accordingly when necessary. Except for highly buffered tablets for preparation of an oral solution (Alka-Seltzer®), the amounts of buffer contained in other commercially available solid dosage forms of salicylates are insufficient to alter urine pH.

Carbonic anhydrase inhibitors (e.g., acetazolamide) may also increase urine pH and should generally be avoided in patients receiving high dosages of salicylates. More importantly, however, carbonic anhydrase inhibitors may induce metabolic acidosis and thereby enhance salicylate penetration into the CNS and other tissues, possibly resulting in salicylate intoxication. Likewise, use of a carbonic anhydrase inhibitor to alkalinize the urine in patients with salicylate overdosage may precipitate metabolic acidosis and lead to severe complications. (See Acute Toxicity: Treatment.) There is evidence from pharmacokinetic studies that salicylates competitively inhibit protein binding of acetazolamide and substantially reduce plasma clearance of the drug, probably by competitively inhibiting renal tubular secretion of the carbonic anhydrase inhibitor. These results and well-documented case reports of toxicity during concomitant administration of acetazolamide and salicylates suggest that the observed toxicity potentially may result from either drug or both, and not necessarily just from the salicylate.

■ **Alcohol** Concomitant ingestion of salicylates (particularly aspirin) and alcohol generally should be avoided since alcohol increases the incidence and severity of salicylate-induced GI bleeding and increases the risk of gastric mucosal erosions and ulceration. In one study, alcohol reportedly enhanced aspirin-induced prolongation of bleeding time in healthy individuals when ingested concomitantly or within at least 36 hours after a single dose of aspirin; the aspirin-induced prolongation of bleeding time was not potentiated when alcohol was ingested 12 hours before the dose of aspirin, and alcohol did not potentiate the effects of aspirin on platelet aggregation. Although further documentation is necessary, some clinicians have suggested that use of aspirin within 8–10 hours of heavy alcohol ingestion should be avoided when possible. The manufacturers caution that patients who generally consume 3 or more alcohol-containing drinks per day should ask their clinician whether to use oral salicylates (e.g., aspirin, choline salicylate, magnesium salicylate) or an alternative analgesic for *self-medication* since salicylates may increase the risk of GI bleeding. In addition, the manufacturers caution that patients who generally consume 3 or more alcohol-containing drinks per day should ask their clinician whether to use a salicylate (e.g., aspirin) in fixed combination with acetaminophen or an alternative analgesic for *self-medication* since salicylates in fixed combination with acetaminophen may increase the risk of GI bleeding and hepatotoxicity.

■ **Nonsteroidal Anti-inflammatory Agents** Salicylates should be used cautiously with non-salicylate NSAIAs. Salicylates appear to have various pharmacokinetic interactions with many other NSAIAs; however, these interactions appear to have little or no clinical importance. Although most of the interactions with other NSAIAs have been studied or detected during concurrent administration of aspirin, the salicylate moiety is probably responsible for the interactions.

Concurrent administration of aspirin may decrease plasma concentrations of diflunisal, fenoprofen, ibuprofen, indomethacin, piroxicam, meclofenamate, and possibly naproxen and the active sulfide metabolite of sulindac; plasma concentrations of free tolmetin may be slightly increased. Aspirin appears to decrease plasma concentrations of indomethacin by decreasing the efficiency of its GI absorption and its renal clearance, and by increasing its biliary clearance. Aspirin apparently decreases GI absorption of meclofenamate sodium. Although the mechanisms of interaction with many of the other NSAIAs remain to be clearly established, salicylates may displace these agents from protein-binding sites, thereby increasing their metabolism and/or excretion. In general, salicylate pharmacokinetics are not affected by other NSAIAs.

Although the pharmacokinetic interactions appear to be of little or no clinical importance, many clinicians recommend that salicylates not be used in conjunction with other NSAIAs, since it has not been established that combination therapy is more efficacious than the individual agents alone and the potential for adverse effects (particularly GI and renal effects) may be increased.

Ibuprofen can antagonize the irreversible inhibition of platelet aggregation induced by aspirin and therefore may limit the cardioprotective effects of aspirin in patients with increased cardiovascular risk. Administration of 400 mg of ibuprofen 3 times daily in patients receiving aspirin 81 mg daily blocked the aspirin-induced inhibition of platelet cyclooxygenase-1 activity as well as the impairment of platelet aggregation achieved with aspirin during prolonged dosing. Administration of aspirin 2 hours before the morning dose of ibuprofen failed to circumvent the interaction with such multiple-dose administration, although such dose timing did effectively obviate the interaction when only single doses of each drug were administered.

The US Food and Drug Administration (FDA) recommends that patients taking a single dose of ibuprofen 400 mg for *self-medication* in conjunction with immediate-release, low-dose aspirin therapy be advised to administer the ibuprofen dose at least 8 hours before or at least 30 minutes after administration of aspirin. Data currently are insufficient to support recommendations regarding the timing of ibuprofen administration relative to that of enteric-coated, low-dose aspirin. The occasional use of ibuprofen is likely to be associated with minimal risk of attenuating the effects of low-dose aspirin. FDA states that other NSAIAs that are used for *self-medication* (e.g., ketoprofen, naproxen) should be viewed as having the potential to interfere with the antiplatelet effect of aspirin unless data are available that indicate otherwise. In one study, concomitant administration of naproxen (500 mg) and low-dose aspirin (100 mg) interfered with the antiplatelet effect of aspirin. Whether ketoprofen interferes with the antiplatelet effect of aspirin has not been investigated. Use of alternative analgesics that do not interfere with the antiplatelet effect of low-dose aspirin (e.g., acetaminophen, opiates) should be considered for patients at high risk of cardiovascular events. Labeling for prescription NSAIAs states that concomitant use of NSAIAs with aspirin is not recommended because of the potential for increased adverse effects. Limited data indicate that administration of diclofenac sodium delayed-release tablets (75 mg twice daily) does not inhibit the antiplatelet effect of aspirin (81 mg daily).

■ **Salicylates** Patients receiving long-term salicylate therapy should be warned to avoid nonprescription preparations containing salicylates to prevent salicylate accumulation and potential toxicity. Results of several studies suggest that repeated doses or maximum recommended dosages of bismuth subsalicylate-containing antidiarrheal preparations (e.g., Pepto-Bismol®) could potentially lead to salicylate intoxication in patients receiving concurrent salicylate therapy.

■ **Anticonvulsants** At high dosages, salicylate appears to displace phenytoin from protein-binding sites; however, it is unlikely that this interaction is clinically important since the increase in serum concentration of free phenytoin is apparently small and transient. However, because the fraction of total drug in serum as free phenytoin is increased, therapeutic effects of phenytoin may be associated with lower than usual total serum phenytoin concentrations in patients receiving both drugs.

Salicylates (particularly aspirin) and valproic acid should be administered concurrently with caution. When aspirin and valproic acid were administered concurrently in one study in children with epilepsy, salicylate apparently displaced valproic acid from serum albumin; the serum concentration and elimination half-life of both free and total valproic acid were increased. Salicylate also appeared to alter the metabolism of valproic acid. Although further evaluation of this interaction is needed, the results of this study suggest that concomitant use of salicylates and valproic acid might result in increased serum concentrations of free valproic acid and thereby increase the risk of adverse effects of the anticonvulsant. In addition to this potential interaction, both salicylates (particularly aspirin) and valproic acid may affect coagulation and their combined use may increase the risk of bleeding complications. If the drugs are administered concurrently, patients should be carefully monitored for adverse effects.

■ **Diuretics** Aspirin has been shown to slightly reduce the natriuretic effect of spironolactone in healthy individuals, possibly by reducing active renal tubular secretion of canrenone, the active metabolite of spironolactone; the antihypertensive effect of spironolactone and its effect on urinary potassium excretion in hypertensive patients are apparently not affected. Until more clinical data are available on this potential interaction, patients receiving both drugs should be monitored for signs and symptoms of decreased clinical response to spironolactone.

Although reports are conflicting, aspirin appears to attenuate the diuretic effect of furosemide, possibly by competing with and inhibiting renal tubular secretion of furosemide. The clinical importance of this potential interaction has not been established; further evaluation is necessary.

Tetracyclines Because tetracyclines readily chelate divalent and trivalent cations such as aluminum or magnesium, concurrent administration of buffered salicylate preparations containing such cations (e.g., Bufferin®), or concurrent administration of salicylate salts containing magnesium, may decrease absorption of oral tetracyclines. Therefore, such salicylate preparations should be given at least 1 hour before or after the tetracycline.

Angiotensin-converting Enzyme Inhibitors Because angiotensin-converting enzyme (ACE) inhibitors may promote kinin-mediated prostaglandin synthesis and/or release, concomitant use of drugs that inhibit prostaglandin synthesis and release, including salicylates, may reduce the blood pressure response to ACE inhibitors (e.g., captopril, enalapril). In addition, salicylates (e.g., aspirin) can attenuate the hemodynamic actions of ACE inhibitors in patients with congestive heart failure. Because ACE inhibitors share and enhance the effects of the compensatory hemodynamic mechanisms of heart failure, with aspirin interacting with the compensatory mechanisms rather than with a given ACE inhibitor per se, these desirable mechanisms are particularly susceptible to the interaction and a subsequent potential loss of clinical benefits. As a result, the more severe the heart failure and the more prominent the compensatory mechanisms, the more appreciable the interaction between aspirin and ACE inhibitors. Even if optimal dosage of an ACE inhibitor is used in the treatment of congestive heart failure, the potential cardiovascular and survival benefit may not be seen if the patient is receiving aspirin concomitantly.

In several multicenter studies, concomitant administration of a single 350-mg dose of aspirin in patients with congestive heart failure inhibited favorable hemodynamic effects associated with ACE inhibitors, attenuating the favorable effects of these drugs on survival and cardiovascular morbidity. However, these findings have not been confirmed by other studies. In one retrospective analysis of pooled data, patients who received an ACE inhibitor concomitantly with aspirin (160–325 mg daily) during the acute phase following myocardial infarction had proportional reductions in 7- and 30-day mortality rates comparable to patients who received an ACE inhibitor alone. Some clinicians have questioned the results of this study because of methodologic concerns (e.g., unsubstantiated assumptions about aspirin therapy [dosage, time of initiation, duration]; disparate distribution of patients).

Although it has been suggested that patients requiring long-term management of heart failure avoid the concomitant use of ACE inhibitors and aspirin (and perhaps substitute another platelet-aggregation inhibitor [e.g., clopidogrel, ticlopidine] for aspirin), many clinicians state that existing data are insufficient to recommend a change in the current prescribing practices of clinicians concerning the use of aspirin in patients receiving therapy with an ACE inhibitor.

Varicella Virus Vaccine Live Because of the association between Reye's syndrome, natural varicella infection, and salicylates (see Reye's Syndrome under Cautions: Pediatric Precautions), the manufacturer of varicella virus vaccine live recommends that individuals who receive the vaccine avoid use of salicylates for 6 weeks following vaccination. However, an association between Reye's syndrome, administration of varicella virus vaccine live, and use of salicylates has not been established and the syndrome has not been reported to date in recipients of the vaccine. For children who are receiving long-term salicylate therapy, the American Academy of Pediatrics (AAP) suggests that the theoretical risks associated with the vaccine be weighed against the known risks of the wild-type virus. The ACIP states that, since the risk for serious salicylate-associated complications is likely to be greater in children in whom natural varicella disease develops than in children who receive the vaccine containing attenuated virus, children who have rheumatoid arthritis or other conditions requiring therapeutic salicylate therapy probably should receive varicella virus vaccine live in conjunction with subsequent close monitoring.

Other Drugs Salicylates should be used cautiously, if at all, with other drugs that might potentiate the adverse GI effects.

Concurrent administration of salicylates and pyrazinamide may prevent or reduce hyperuricemia which usually occurs with pyrazinamide therapy.

Although there are apparently no published reports to date, the possibility that concurrent administration of salicylates and antiemetics (including antihistamines and phenothiazines) might mask the symptoms of salicylate-induced otic effects should be considered.

Laboratory Test Interferences

At dosages equivalent in salicylate content to 2.4 g or more of aspirin daily, salicylates may cause false-negative results in urinary glucose determinations using glucose oxidase reagent (e.g., Clinistix®, Tes-Tape®) and false-positive results in urinary glucose determinations using the cupric sulfate method (Benedict's solution, Clinitest®). Gentisic acid, a salicylate metabolite, may be responsible for false-negative results with glucose oxidase reagent since it is a potent reducing agent. Although salicylates are generally considered not to substantially affect glucose tolerance tests, some clinicians have reported that 3 g of aspirin daily results in a slightly increased oral glucose tolerance in healthy individuals and in patients with type 2 (non-insulin-dependent) diabetes mellitus.

Salicylates interfere with the Gerhardt test for acetoacetic acid by reacting with ferric chloride to produce a reddish color which, unlike the color produced by acetoacetic acid, persists after boiling.

Salicylates may produce falsely increased or decreased results in urinary vanillylmandelic acid (VMA) determinations, depending on the method used; with the Pisano method, urinary VMA may be falsely decreased. Salicylates should be avoided before and during urine collections for VMA determinations.

Aspirin has been shown to interfere with urinary 5-hydroxyindoleacetic acid (5-HIAA) determinations that use a fluorescent method.

Salicylates may decrease urinary excretion of phenolsulfonphthalein by competing for renal tubular secretion with the diagnostic agent. Therefore, the phenolsulfonphthalein excretion test should not be performed in patients receiving salicylates.

Although the evidence is somewhat conflicting, salicylates probably do not interfere with urinary 17-hydroxycorticosteroid determinations using the Porter-Silber method or with urinary 17-ketosteroid determinations using the Zimmerman color reaction. However, high dosages may cause false decreases in urinary 17-hydroxycorticosteroid determinations which utilize β-glucuronidase to hydrolyze the steroid glucuronides before extraction.

Concurrent administration of aspirin with xylose reportedly reduces urinary excretion of the sugar; the exact mechanism is not known.

At high dosages, salicylates competitively bind to thyroxine-binding globulin and thyroxine-binding prealbumin. As a result, serum protein-bound iodine is decreased; total serum concentrations of thyroxine and triiodothyronine are decreased while the unbound fractions of these hormones are increased. Secretion of thyrotropin, induced by exogenous administration of synthetic thyrotropin-releasing hormone (protirelin), is decreased in patients receiving salicylates, apparently as a result of the increased unbound fraction of thyroid hormones. Resin triiodothyronine uptake may be unchanged or slightly increased in patients receiving salicylates. Although reports are conflicting, 24-hour thyroid uptake of iodine 131 may be reduced following high dosages of salicylates.

Salicylates may falsely increase serum uric acid concentrations determined by colorimetric methods; serum uric acid concentrations determined by the uricase method are not affected.

Salicylates may completely interfere with or falsely decrease plasma theophylline concentrations determined by the Schack and Waxler method.

Acute Toxicity

Pathogenesis Acute salicylate overdosage results from ingestion of a single toxic dose. The acute lethal dose of salicylate varies with the specific preparation ingested. Death has occurred in adults who ingested single 10- to 30-g doses of aspirin or sodium salicylate, but one patient survived after ingestion of 130 g of aspirin. In salicylate overdosage resulting from acute ingestion, little or no toxicity generally occurs in individuals ingesting less than 150 mg/kg, mild to moderate toxicity in those ingesting 150–300 mg/kg, severe toxicity in those ingesting 300–500 mg/kg, and potentially lethal toxicity in those ingesting greater than 500 mg/kg.

The pathophysiology of salicylate overdosage is complex because of the variety of toxic effects produced and their resultant manifestations. The principal toxic effects are extensions of pharmacologic actions and include local GI irritation, direct CNS stimulation of respiration, uncoupling of oxidative phosphorylation, altered glucose metabolism through inhibition of Krebs cycle enzymes, stimulation of gluconeogenesis and lipid metabolism, increased tissue glycolysis, inhibition of amino acid metabolism, and interference with hemostatic mechanisms.

Manifestations Acute salicylate overdosage produces manifestations similar to those of chronic intoxication, but the effects are often more pronounced and occur in more rapid succession.

Ingestion may cause mild burning pain in the throat and stomach; vomiting, particularly in infants and children, usually begins within 1–8 hours. An asymptomatic interval of several hours may follow these initial manifestations.

In addition to manifestations of chronic intoxication, oliguria or acute renal failure, hyperthermia, restlessness, irritability, garrulity, incoherent speech, apprehension, vertigo, asterixis, tremor, diplopia, confusion, disorientation, delirium, mania, hallucinations, EEG abnormalities, generalized seizures, lethargy, and coma may occur; toxic encephalopathy resembling chorea may also occur. The mental disturbances, sometimes referred to as *salicylate jag,* resemble alcoholic intoxication without euphoria. Pulmonary edema, skin eruptions (see Cautions: Dermatologic Effects), and pancreatitis occur less frequently. Hemorrhagic complications (e.g., petechiae in skin and mucous membranes, GI bleeding, perforated peptic ulcer) or a syndrome resembling inappropriate secretion of antidiuretic hormone (SIADH) occurs rarely. As salicylate intoxication progresses, CNS stimulation is replaced by CNS depression manifested as stupor and coma; respiratory insufficiency and cardiovascular collapse follow, sometimes with asphyxial seizures. Death usually occurs during coma and results from respiratory failure or cardiovascular collapse.

The principal physiologic manifestations of salicylate overdosage are acid-base and electrolyte disturbances, dehydration, hyperpyrexia, and hyperglycemia or hypoglycemia. As with high dosages, single toxic doses of salicylate produce respiratory stimulation by peripheral and central mechanisms, resulting in hyperventilation, hypocapnea, and respiratory alkalosis; compensation for the respiratory alkalosis occurs rapidly. (See Pharmacology: Metabolic Effects.) Hyperventilation usually occurs when the serum salicylate concentration exceeds 350 mcg/mL and begins within 6–12 hours after ingestion of a single toxic dose. Marked hyperpnea usually occurs at a serum concentration of about 500 mcg/mL.

Metabolic acidosis usually follows compensation of respiratory alkalosis; occasionally, respiratory acidosis also occurs, usually only when intoxication progresses and respiration is centrally depressed or when a CNS depressant has been ingested concomitantly. Metabolic acidosis develops principally from accumulation of organic acids (pyruvic, lactic, acetoacetic, and amino acids) secondary to salicylate interference with carbohydrate and amino acid metabolism and increased lipid metabolism; inorganic phosphoric and sulfuric acids also accumulate secondary to salicylate-induced renal impairment. Depletion of buffer capacity as a result of the initial compensatory increase in renal excretion of bicarbonate also contributes to development of metabolic acidosis. Depending on the relative contributions of the metabolic effects, either alkalemia or acidemia and either alkaluria or aciduria may be observed. Early in the course of acute intoxication in most adults and with mild to moderate intoxication in older children, respiratory alkalosis alone or with alkaluria may be present. In adults, alkalemia occurs often and may persist, but a mixed acid-base disturbance (usually metabolic acidosis and respiratory alkalosis) appears to occur most frequently. With acute intoxication in children, metabolic acidosis and respiratory alkalosis are usually present, with acidosis and acidemia predominating. Until adequate salicylate removal from the GI tract has been accomplished, the likelihood of acidosis increases with time elapsed since the ingestion; severe acidosis may not occur for 12–24 hours after acute ingestion.

In general, severity of acidosis increases with decreasing age; metabolic acidosis apparently predominates in young children because they are more susceptible to development of ketosis. The severity of acidosis also generally increases with increasing severity of intoxication and vice versa. Acidosis and acidemia increase the severity of intoxication by enhancing salicylate penetration into the CNS and other tissues (see Pharmacokinetics: Distribution); increased CNS concentrations of salicylate appear to be directly related to CNS dysfunction and death. Therefore, the greater severity of intoxication observed in young children appears to be due in part to the increased frequency and severity of acidosis in these patients. In adults, severe acidosis is associated with impaired consciousness and a poor prognosis.

Toxic effects that result in acid-base disturbances also cause alterations of fluid and electrolyte balance. Increased metabolism and heat production increase cutaneous insensible losses, principally of water, but also of sodium as a result of sweating. During compensation of initial respiratory alkalosis, renal excretion of bicarbonate is accompanied by increased renal excretion of sodium, potassium, and water. As intoxication progresses and metabolic acidosis develops, organic aciduria increases the solute load excreted by the kidney and is also accompanied by increased renal excretion of sodium, potassium, and water. The resultant dehydration and electrolyte imbalance may be enhanced by decreased fluid intake and vomiting, and hyperventilation (increased pulmonary insensible water loss). Electrolyte losses lead to total body depletion of sodium and potassium. However, hypernatremia is usually observed due to dehydration; hyponatremia is uncommon and associated with inappropriate fluid retention (SIADH). Hypokalemia is also usually observed; even if serum potassium concentration is normal, total body potassium depletion is likely. In general, water loss may be as great as 2–3 L/m^2 with moderate intoxication and 4–6 L/m^2 with severe intoxication. Oliguria may occur as a result of severe dehydration. Anuria or acute renal failure usually accompanies severe shock, hemorrhage, or cardiovascular collapse.

Hyperthermia, sometimes with rectal temperature as high as 40.5–42.2°C, is secondary to impaired oxidative phosphorylation and the consequent increase in heat production by body tissues. In toxic doses, salicylates appear to decrease efficiency of normal body cooling mechanisms; dehydration enhances this effect. When hyperthermia is present, it contributes to dehydration.

Altered glucose metabolism may result in hyperglycemia or hypoglycemia. Hyperglycemia usually occurs early in the course of intoxication as a result of interference with tissue utilization of glucose. Blood glucose concentration usually does not exceed 200 mg/dL but glucosuria may occur; hyperglycemia may persist for a few hours to a few days. Salicylate-induced hyperglycemia associated with coma, ketoacidosis, dehydration, and hyperventilation closely simulates diabetic ketoacidosis. Eventually, hypoglycemia may occur as a result of glucose depletion. Hypoglycemia may be life-threatening and is most likely to occur in infants or late in the course of intoxication. CNS hypoglycemia may occur despite the absence of systemic hypoglycemia and should be considered in children with seizures, coma, or cardiovascular collapse.

■ Treatment

In the treatment of acute salicylate intoxication, intensive symptomatic and supportive therapy should be instituted immediately. Treatment consists principally of removal of salicylate from the GI tract and prevention of further absorption; correction of fluid, electrolyte, and acid-base disturbances; and measures to enhance salicylate elimination.

■ Assessment of Severity of Intoxication

In acute ingestions, severity of intoxication can be estimated by assessing the amount reported to be ingested, by evaluating the clinical condition of the patient, and by measuring serum salicylate concentration.

Since the apparent volume of distribution of salicylate appears to increase with increasing doses, a specific serum salicylate concentration following acute ingestion of large doses may reflect a higher amount of salicylate in the body than the same serum concentration attained following ingestion of smaller doses; therefore, toxic effects may be more severe than generally anticipated, depending upon the ingested dose. In acute ingestions, a serum salicylate concentration obtained 6 hours or longer after the ingestion may be used in conjunction with the Done nomogram (below) to estimate severity of intoxication and provide a guide to treatment; *the nomogram cannot be used to estimate severity of chronic salicylate intoxication.*

Because absorption and distribution of salicylate may continue in the first 6 hours after ingestion, a serum salicylate concentration obtained during this period should not be used in conjunction with the nomogram unless serial determinations indicate that a peak concentration has occurred. In overdosage with massive doses, serum salicylate concentration may continue to increase for up to 24 hours. In overdosage with enteric-coated or extended-release salicylate preparations, absorption may be delayed and serum salicylate concentration may continue to increase up to 72 hours after the ingestion; *in such ingestions, the nomogram cannot be used to estimate severity of intoxication.* In the event that a serum concentration cannot be obtained or a preliminary estimate is desired, a Phenistix® reagent strip (as used in the diagnosis of phenylketonuria) may be dipped into separated plasma or serum obtained from the intoxicated individual; the reagent strip generally gives a tan color with salicylate concentrations less than 400 mcg/mL, a darker brown color with concentrations of 400–900 mcg/mL, and a purple color with concentrations exceeding 900 mcg/mL.

■ Measures to Reduce Salicylate Absorption

In acute overdosage, the stomach should be emptied immediately, preferably by ipecac syrup-induced emesis if the patient is alert, or by gastric lavage. These procedures are generally effective up to 3–4 hours after an acute ingestion and may be effective for up to 10 hours following ingestion of massive doses. If the patient is comatose, having seizures, or has lost the gag reflex, gastric lavage may be performed if an endotracheal tube with cuff inflated is in place to prevent aspiration of vomitus. Activated charcoal should be administered since it is extremely effective in reducing salicylate absorption. Activated charcoal is usually administered as an aqueous suspension; adults are usually given 50–100 g and children 30–60 g or 0.5–1 g/kg. *Activated charcoal should not be administered before induction of emesis with ipecac syrup since the emetic is inactivated by activated charcoal.* Administration of a saline cathartic (e.g., magnesium citrate, sodium sulfate) is also usually recommended, with repeated administration until the activated charcoal has been passed rectally. However, the efficacy of saline catharsis in salicylate overdosage remains to be clearly determined. Results of several studies in healthy individuals suggest that saline catharsis in combination with activated charcoal does not further decrease GI absorption of salicylate compared to activated charcoal alone; however, studies in acutely intoxicated patients are needed.

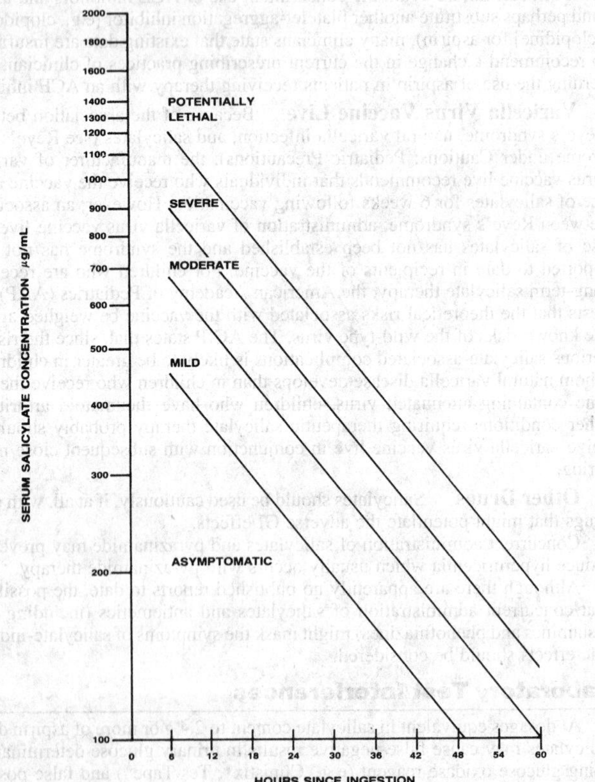

Nomogram relating serum salicylate concentration and estimated severity of intoxication at varying intervals following ingestion of a single toxic dose of salicylate. Modified from Done AK. Salicylate intoxication. Pediatrics. 1960; 26:800–7. © American Academy of Pediatrics 1960.

■ Fluid and Electrolyte Therapy

If hyperthermia and/or dehydration have developed, initial treatment should be directed to their correction and maintenance of normal renal function. Patients with a rectal temperature greater than 40°C should be cooled by cooling devices or by sponging with tepid water.

Appropriate fluid and electrolyte therapy should be administered promptly, based on evaluation of the patient's fluid, acid-base, and electrolyte status. Arterial pH and blood gases (Po_2, pCO_2, and total CO_2); serum sodium, potassium, chloride, bicarbonate, and creatinine concentrations; and blood glucose concentration and BUN should be determined immediately. Urinary output should be monitored hourly. The PT should also be monitored. Determinations of acid-base and electrolyte status and renal function should be performed frequently during treatment to guide therapy.

In patients with mild intoxication who have adequate urine output and do not vomit severely, fluids should be administered orally every hour up to a total of 100 mL/kg in the first 24 hours. In more severely intoxicated patients, IV fluid and electrolyte therapy is necessary; fluid requirements usually range from 2–6 L/m^2 in the first 24 hours. Patients are usually rehydrated initially with an IV solution containing 5–10% dextrose (to prevent hypoglycemia) with 75 mEq of sodium, 50 mEq of chloride, and 25 mEq of bicarbonate per liter; if metabolic acidosis is not present, the bicarbonate is replaced by chloride. This solution is usually administered at a rate of 10–20 mL/kg per hour for 1–2 hours; patients in shock may require more rapid fluid administration. Acidemia should be corrected as rapidly as possible to minimize entry of salicylate into the CNS and other tissues. Just as acidemia enhances intracellular movement of salicylate, correction of acidemia and/or maintenance of an alkaline serum pH facilitate movement of salicylate from intracellular sites to plasma and ultimately to urine. If acidosis is severe (serum pH less than 7.15), patients should receive additional IV sodium bicarbonate, 1–2 mEq/kg every 1–2 hours, as necessary. *Potassium is added to IV fluids to replace losses only after it has been determined that renal function is adequate;* potassium replacement may be necessary to accomplish alkalinization of the urine. Patients should be monitored by ECG and serum potassium determinations during potassium replacement. Subsequent hydration is usually performed with an IV solution containing 5–10% dextrose with 40 mEq of sodium, 35 mEq of potassium, 50 mEq of chloride, and 20 mEq of bicarbonate per liter; if acidosis persists, an additional 15 mEq of sodium bicarbonate is usually added to each liter. This solution is usually administered at a rate of 4–8 mL/kg per hour until the serum salicylate concentration is less than 300 mcg/mL, which may require several hours to several days. Thereafter, IV hydration is continued as necessary, usually with a solution containing 5% dextrose with 25 mEq each of sodium and chloride and 20 mEq each of potassium and bicarbonate per liter; this solution is usually administered at a rate of 2–3 mL/kg per hour.

■ **Other Supportive Therapies** If severe hypotension and/or manifestations of hemorrhagic complications (e.g., petechiae) are initially present, whole blood transfusions (10–15 mL/kg over 1 hour) may be necessary. Plasma transfusions may be beneficial, especially if shock develops. Although routine administration of vitamin K has been suggested in salicylate intoxication, the drug is usually administered only if hemorrhagic complications occur or if the PT is prolonged. Patients with respiratory depression may require assisted pulmonary ventilation and oxygen. CNS depressants (e.g., barbiturates, narcotics) should not be administered to counter salicylate-induced hyperventilation since they may lead to respiratory acidosis and coma. Seizures may usually be controlled by IV administration of a benzodiazepine (e.g., diazepam) or short-acting barbiturate; a short-acting skeletal muscle relaxant (e.g., succinylcholine), assisted pulmonary ventilation, and oxygen may occasionally be necessary.

■ **Measures to Enhance Salicylate Elimination** Although reduction of hyperthermia and appropriate IV fluid and electrolyte therapy constitute adequate treatment for many patients, therapeutic measures (e.g., forced alkaline diuresis, hemodialysis) to enhance salicylate elimination may also be useful and/or necessary, depending on severity of intoxication. Forced alkaline diuresis with IV sodium bicarbonate (and IV furosemide when necessary) may be employed since alkalinization of the urine to pH 7.5 or greater, with maintenance of sufficient urine flow, greatly enhances the rate of urinary salicylate excretion. (See Pharmacokinetics: Elimination.) Sodium bicarbonate should *not* be given orally since it might enhance absorption of salicylate. Forced alkaline diuresis is often employed when the serum salicylate concentration exceeds 500 mcg/mL 6 hours after the ingestion and the patient's condition indicates severe intoxication. However, dehydration must be corrected before the procedure is employed. Forced alkaline diuresis with sodium bicarbonate should be performed with caution, particularly in infants, or in older children and adults with respiratory alkalosis; hypernatremia, pulmonary edema, and severe alkalosis (possibly with tetany and/or hypokalemia) may occur. If forced alkaline diuresis is employed, sufficient urinary output must be maintained, urine and serum pH must be carefully monitored, and dosage of sodium bicarbonate adjusted accordingly; for optimum results, urine pH of 7.5 or greater and serum pH of 7.5 should be maintained. In most children, even high doses of sodium bicarbonate may not produce a sufficiently alkaline urine because the degree of inorganic acid production and resultant aciduria cannot be adequately compensated; in addition, alkalinization of the urine may not be accomplished until potassium depletion is corrected.

Following correction of acidemia with sodium bicarbonate, acetazolamide has been used as an adjunct to alkalinize the urine; *however, its use is dangerous and generally not recommended since it may precipitate metabolic acidosis and lead to severe complications.* (See Drug Interactions: Acidifying and Alkalinizing Agents.) Therefore, if acetazolamide is used at all, it should probably be used only in adults with respiratory alkalosis and only under the supervision of clinicians experienced in the use of the drug in salicylate overdosage. Some clinicians have also suggested that tromethamine may be useful in patients with severe, refractory metabolic acidosis or in patients in whom sodium restriction is necessary; *however, tromethamine should be used with extreme caution, if at all, since the drug produces intracellular as well as extracellular alkalinization and may therefore increase CNS and tissue concentrations of salicylate.*

The most effective measures for removal of salicylate from the body are hemodialysis or hemoperfusion in adults and older children, and peritoneal dialysis or exchange transfusions in young children and infants; however, these measures are rarely necessary. Most clinicians reserve these measures for patients with serum salicylate concentrations of 900–1300 mcg/mL or higher 6 hours after an ingestion, unresponsive acidosis (pH less than 7.1), impaired renal function or renal failure, pulmonary edema, persistent CNS manifestations (e.g., seizures, coma), progressive deterioration despite appropriate therapy, or preexisting disease that prohibits usual therapeutic measures. If any of these conditions occurs, hemodialysis may be useful regardless of serum salicylate concentration. Hemodialysis and hemoperfusion are considered to be equally effective in removing salicylate, but hemodialysis is preferred to hemoperfusion since acid-base and electrolyte disturbances are corrected more rapidly with hemodialysis. In patients with severe intoxication, peritoneal dialysis and exchange transfusions may be instituted while preparations for hemodialysis or hemoperfusion are undertaken. If peritoneal dialysis is employed, 50 g of albumin should be added to each liter of dialysate; binding of salicylate to albumin enhances the efficiency of peritoneal dialysis.

Chronic Toxicity

Since the pathophysiology, manifestations, and treatment of chronic salicylate intoxication are similar to those of acute salicylate intoxication, the Acute Toxicity section should be consulted for additional information.

■ **Pathogenesis** Chronic salicylate intoxication, also known as *salicylism,* results from high dosages or from prolonged therapy with high dosages. Some clinicians believe that chronic intoxication is generally associated with ingestion of dosages greater than 100 mg/kg daily for 2 days or longer. Severe chronic intoxication has often occurred in infants who were dehydrated as a result of fever and/or illness, and is best prevented by generally avoiding use of salicylates for antipyresis in infants or by limiting dosage in these patients.

■ **Manifestations** Chronic intoxication is manifested principally as tinnitus, hearing loss, dimness of vision, headache, dizziness, mental confusion, lassitude, drowsiness, sweating, thirst, hyperventilation, increased heart rate, nausea, vomiting, and occasionally diarrhea; however, if intoxication is severe, other manifestations associated with acute intoxication may occur. Chronic salicylate intoxication is sometimes not readily recognized since a preexisting disease or concomitant illness may produce signs and symptoms (e.g., nausea, vomiting, tachypnea, disorientation) that are similar to those of salicylate intoxication.

Tinnitus and hearing loss are the most frequent manifestations of chronic intoxication in adults. (See Cautions: Otic Effects.) In children, the most frequent manifestations are hyperventilation or CNS effects such as giddiness, drowsiness, or behavioral changes; these effects usually occur at serum salicylate concentrations greater than 300 mcg/mL.

The onset of hyperventilation is usually insidious. With chronic intoxication, metabolic acidosis and respiratory alkalosis are usually present, with acidosis and acidemia predominating. Acidosis is usually more severe with chronic intoxication than with ingestion of a single toxic dose. Hypoglycemia, which may be life-threatening, is also likely to occur.

■ **Treatment** Usually only evaluation of the clinical condition of patients with chronic intoxication is useful in determining the severity of intoxication. Serum salicylate concentrations may be determined but are not as useful in estimating the severity; severe symptomatology has been associated with concentrations as low as 150 mcg/mL. *The Done nomogram cannot be used to estimate severity of chronic salicylate intoxication.*

When chronic intoxication is mild, dosage reduction or discontinuance of salicylates, in conjunction with symptomatic and supportive therapy, usually constitutes adequate treatment. When intoxication is more severe, salicylates are discontinued and intensive symptomatic and supportive therapy, as in the treatment of acute salicylate intoxication, should be instituted immediately. Patients who experience hearing loss of tinnitus during aspirin therapy should discontinue therapy and consult a clinician. Hemodialysis may be particularly useful in chronically intoxicated patients with high serum salicylate concentrations. Regardless of serum salicylate concentration, hemodialysis may also be especially useful in those with unresponsive acidosis (pH less than 7.1), impaired renal function or renal failure, pulmonary edema, persistent CNS manifestations (e.g., seizures, coma), progressive deterioration despite appropriate therapy, or preexisting disease that prohibits usual therapeutic measures.

Pharmacology

Salicylates mainly exhibit analgesic, anti-inflammatory, and antipyretic activity. These effects appear to result principally from the salicylate moiety. Although aspirin hydrolyzes to salicylate and acetate, it does not require hydrolysis to produce its effects; in addition, aspirin appears to have some pharmacologic effects that are distinct from those of salicylate. The ability of aspirin to acetylate proteins results in some effects, such as inhibition of platelet aggregation, which other currently available salicylates do not exhibit. (See Pharmacology in Aspirin 28:08.04.24.)

The exact mechanisms have not been clearly established, but many actions (e.g., analgesic, anti-inflammatory) of salicylates appear to be associated principally with inhibition of prostaglandin synthesis. Aspirin inhibits the synthesis of prostaglandins in body tissues by irreversibly acetylating and inactivating cyclooxygenase; at least 2 isoenzymes, cyclooxygenase-1 (COX-1) and -2 (COX-2) (also referred to as prostaglandin G/H synthase-1 [PGHS-1] and -2 [PGHS-2], respectively), have been identified that catalyze the formation of prostaglandins in the arachidonic acid pathway. Salicylate only minimally inhibits cyclooxygenase in vitro but is as active as aspirin in vivo in decreasing prostaglandin synthesis. Salicylate may be a reversible inhibitor of cyclooxygenase, but this has not been clearly established. Inhibition of prostaglandin synthesis by aspirin and salicylate may also involve other mechanisms.

Although aspirin and other salicylates inhibit cyclooxygenase and thereby decrease production of prostaglandins, they apparently do not inhibit lipoxygenase, an enzyme involved in the formation of 12-hydroperoxyarachidonic acid (12-HPETE) and leukotrienes from arachidonic acid. Since cyclooxygenase and lipoxygenase appear to compete for the metabolism of arachidonic acid, the inhibition of cyclooxygenase by aspirin and other salicylates may actually result in increased formation of 12-HPETE and leukotrienes. In platelets, 12-HPETE increases lipoxygenase activity (thereby increasing its own formation) and inhibits cyclooxygenase. Therefore, in the presence of salicylate, increased formation of 12-HPETE via lipoxygenase may contribute to the inhibition of cyclooxygenase. In addition, high concentrations of aspirin or salicylate have been reported to reversibly inhibit the conversion of 12-HPETE to 12-hydroxyarachidonic acid (12-HETE) via peroxidase. By inhibiting this conversion, salicylates may also increase concentrations of 12-HPETE and thereby indirectly inhibit cyclooxygenase. However, further evaluation of these effects is needed.

■ **Analgesic Effect** The analgesic effect of salicylates may result from inhibition of prostaglandin synthesis. Prostaglandins appear to sensitize pain receptors to mechanical stimulation or to other chemical mediators (e.g., bradykinin, histamine). Since salicylates do not directly alter the pain threshold or prevent pain caused by exogenous or previously synthesized endogenous prostaglandins, the drugs may produce analgesia by inhibiting the formation of prostaglandins involved in pain. The analgesic effect of salicylates appears to result from mainly a peripheral action, but the drugs may also have similar activity and/or other mechanisms of action in the CNS, possibly in the hypothalamus. In addition, the anti-inflammatory effect of the drugs may contribute to their analgesic effect. There is no evidence that long-term therapy with salicylates results in tolerance to or physical dependence on the drugs.

■ **Anti-inflammatory Effect** Due in part to the complexity of the inflammatory response, the exact mechanisms of the anti-inflammatory effect of salicylates have not been fully elucidated. Since prostaglandins appear to mediate many inflammatory effects and have been shown to directly produce many of the signs and symptoms of inflammation, the anti-inflammatory effect of salicylates may be due in part to inhibition of prostaglandin synthesis and release during inflammation. The anti-inflammatory effect of salicylates and other NSAIAs generally appears to be positively correlated with their ability to inhibit prostaglandin synthesis; however, the relative contributions of this and other mechanisms of action remain to be determined.

Although aspirin and other salicylates inhibit cyclooxygenase and thereby decrease production of prostaglandins, they apparently do not inhibit the formation of leukotrienes. The exact roles of leukotrienes in inflammation have not been fully elucidated, but they may contribute to the inflammatory response. Inhibition of cyclooxygenase by aspirin and other salicylates, while reducing prostaglandin synthesis and release, may actually result in the increased formation of leukotrienes. However, the clinical importance of such an effect remains to be determined.

Although high concentrations of aspirin or salicylate have been reported to reversibly inhibit the conversion of 12-HPETE to 12-HETE, a compound that appears to be a chemotactic stimulus for polymorphonuclear leukocytes, it is not clear whether salicylates enhance or inhibit migration of leukocytes into inflamed tissue. Salicylates have been shown to stabilize lysosomal membranes in vitro; therefore, they may prevent the release of lysosomal substances which contribute to inflammation. The anti-inflammatory action of the drugs may also involve effects on other cellular and immunologic processes in mesenchymal and connective tissues. Salicylates may inhibit lymphocyte activation, and by inhibiting cyclooxygenase, salicylates and other NSAIAs may interfere with prostaglandin-mediated formation of autoantibodies that are involved in the inflammatory process. High serum concentrations of salicylates may also suppress antigen-antibody reactions, but the contribution of this effect to the anti-inflammatory action of salicylates has not been established. Although the mechanism is not known, salicylates have been shown to enhance monocyte-mediated cytotoxicity and thereby increase antigen removal. Salicylates may also alter the composition, synthesis, and metabolism of connective tissue mucopolysaccharides related to the ground substance that helps prevent spread of inflammation.

■ **Antipyretic Effect** Salicylates lower body temperature in patients with fever; the drugs rarely decrease body temperature in afebrile patients. Salicylates decrease body temperature principally by inhibiting the synthesis and release of prostaglandins that mediate the effect of endogenous pyrogen in the hypothalamus; however, other mechanisms may be involved. Although heat production is not directly inhibited by salicylates, centrally mediated dilation of peripheral blood vessels and sweating enhance dissipation of heat. Paradoxically, toxic doses of salicylates may increase body temperature by increasing oxygen consumption and metabolic rate, apparently as a result of salicylate-induced uncoupling of oxidative phosphorylation.

■ **Hematologic Effects** Aspirin, but not other currently available salicylates, inhibits platelet aggregation and prolongs bleeding time. (See Pharmacology: Hematologic Effects, in Aspirin 28:08.04.24.)

Salicylates alter the hepatic synthesis of blood coagulation factors VII, IX, and X, apparently by interfering with the action of vitamin K; this effect appears to be dose-dependent and occurs principally when serum salicylate concentration exceeds 300 mcg/mL. At usual dosages (e.g., 1.3–6 g of aspirin daily), the prothrombin time (PT) may rarely be increased by 2–3 seconds; larger increases in the PT may occur at higher dosages or in patients with fever or increased metabolic rate. The increased PT is due mainly to a deficiency in factor VII and can be reversed by administration of phytonadione (vitamin K_1) or discontinuance of salicylate therapy; in some patients, the PT may return to normal even if salicylate therapy is continued.

Although salicylates usually do not alter the leukocyte or erythrocyte count, the drugs may decrease leukocytosis and erythrocyte sedimentation rate in patients with rheumatic fever; the mechanisms of these effects are not known. Although reports are conflicting, salicylates also apparently increase fibrinolysis, possibly by enhancing the fibrinolytic action of leukocytes.

■ **Genitourinary and Renal Effects** Salicylates produce various effects on the uterus, apparently by inhibiting prostaglandin synthesis. Prostaglandins E_2 and $F_{2\alpha}$ increase the amplitude and frequency of uterine contractions in pregnant women; current evidence suggests that primary dysmenorrhea is also mediated by these prostaglandins. In some patients with primary dysmenorrhea, salicylate therapy has produced analgesic effects and has been associated with decreased synthesis of prostaglandin $F_{2\alpha}$. Administration of salicylates during late pregnancy may prolong gestation and labor by inhibiting the formation of prostaglandins involved in these processes.

Salicylates have dose-related effects on urinary excretion of uric acid. In large dosages (e.g., 1.3 g of aspirin 4 times daily), salicylates enhance urinary excretion of uric acid and decrease serum uric acid concentration by inhibiting reabsorption of uric acid in the proximal renal tubule. Intermediate dosages (e.g., 650 mg to 1 g of aspirin 3 times daily) inhibit secretion of uric acid in the distal renal tubule but only slightly inhibit its reabsorption; therefore, urinary uric acid excretion is usually not altered. Low dosages (e.g., 325 mg of aspirin 3 times daily or less) inhibit renal tubular secretion of uric acid and therefore may decrease urinary uric acid excretion and increase serum uric acid concentration. In general, serum uric acid concentrations are increased when plasma salicylate concentrations are less than 100 mcg/mL and decreased when plasma salicylate concentrations are greater than 100 mcg/mL. Salicylates antagonize the activity of other uricosuric agents. (See Drug Interactions: Uricosuric Agents.)

Although salicylates generally do not alter renal function in healthy individuals, aspirin has been reported to cause reversible (sometimes marked) decreases in renal blood flow and glomerular filtration rate (which may be accompanied by minimal water, sodium, and potassium retention) in sodium-restricted, otherwise healthy individuals and in patients with impaired renal function, systemic lupus erythematosus, or other conditions predisposing to sodium and water retention. (See Cautions: Renal Effects.) These effects appear to be associated with inhibition of renal synthesis of prostaglandins such as prostaglandin E_2 and prostacyclin (epoprostenol, PGI_2); these prostaglandins increase renal blood flow and help to maintain renal function. Aspirin-induced renal impairment has been directly correlated with decreased urinary excretion of immunoreactive prostaglandin E. In addition, aspirin has been associated with analgesic nephropathy. (See Cautions: Renal Effects.)

■ **GI Effects** Salicylates (especially aspirin) can cause gastric mucosal damage which may result in ulceration and/or bleeding. (See Cautions: GI Effects.) The damage is generally believed to be the result of a local action; however, IV administration of salicylates has also been reported to cause gastric mucosal lesions and bleeding.

The mechanism of salicylate-induced gastric mucosal damage is complex. Gastric mucosal effects have been attributed to inhibition of the synthesis of prostaglandins produced by COX-1. Salicylates appear to selectively increase permeability of the gastric mucosa to cations, and thus, enhance back diffusion of hydrogen ions; the increased entry of acid into the mucosa causes cellular damage. The resultant cellular damage leads to additional alterations in gastric mucosal permeability. Salicylates may also alter mucosal permeability by disrupting metabolism in gastric mucosal cells.

Salicylates cause nausea and vomiting as a result of local gastric irritation and/or by CNS stimulation.

■ **Cardiovascular Effects** Salicylates generally have no direct cardiovascular effects; however, large single doses (e.g., 2.4 g of aspirin) may result in dilation of peripheral blood vessels by a direct effect on smooth muscle. In patients receiving large dosages of salicylates, such as those with rheumatic fever, circulating plasma volume may increase by about 20% (with resultant hemodilution) and cardiac workload and output may also increase. The increase in plasma volume may be due to sodium and water retention secondary to salicylate-induced renal impairment. In overdosage, salicylates may directly suppress cardiac conduction and may cause circulatory depression and possibly collapse, both directly and through central vasomotor paralysis.

■ **Metabolic Effects** In high dosages (e.g., greater than 6 g of aspirin daily) or in the initial phase of overdosage, salicylates produce respiratory stimulation by peripheral and central mechanisms, with resultant changes in acid-base balance and electrolytes. Peripherally, salicylates uncouple oxidative phosphorylation, principally in skeletal muscle; the resultant increased production of carbon dioxide stimulates alveolar ventilation so that carbon dioxide tension is not changed. This increase in alveolar ventilation is characterized as an increase in depth of respiration and a slight increase in rate of respiration. As salicylates enter the CNS, the drugs directly stimulate the respiratory center in the medulla, resulting in marked hyperventilation that is characterized as an increase in depth of respiration and a pronounced increase in rate of respiration. Plasma carbon dioxide tension decreases, and intracellular and extracellular respiratory alkalosis develops. Compensation for respiratory alkalosis occurs rapidly and includes increased renal excretion of bicarbonate, sodium, potassium, and water; as a result, plasma bicarbonate concentration is decreased and blood pH returns toward normal. If substantial potassium depletion occurs, the kidneys retain potassium and excrete hydrogen ions instead, regardless of blood pH; therefore, a paradoxical aciduria can occur in the presence of salicylate-induced systemic alkalosis. These changes in acid-base balance and electrolytes are most often observed in adults receiving high dosages; more severe alterations in acid-base balance (e.g., metabolic acidosis) and electrolytes generally occur only in overdosage.

Salicylates produce a variety of other metabolic effects. The effects on carbohydrate metabolism are complex and involve numerous mechanisms, often with opposing results on blood glucose concentration. High dosages may cause hyperglycemia and glycosuria by interfering with tissue utilization of glucose; however, blood glucose concentration may be decreased in diabetics. It has been suggested that this effect in diabetics may result from increased uptake of glucose by muscle, increased rate of tissue glycolysis, and decreased synthesis of glucose from non-carbohydrate precursors, all of which may be due in part to uncoupling of oxidative phosphorylation. It has also been suggested that salicylates stimulate insulin secretion. In high dosages, or with long-term therapy or overdosage, salicylates eventually decrease aerobic metabolism of glucose and cause depletion of liver and muscle glycogen; hypoglycemia may occur. Depletion of liver glycogen may be caused by an increased rate of glycogenolysis and a decreased rate of glycogen synthesis; these effects may also be related to the uncoupling action of salicylates. In vitro studies have shown that salicylates also inhibit aldose reductase, the enzyme that catalyzes the formation of sorbitol. In overdosage, salicylates decrease synthesis and increase catabolism of proteins which results in a negative nitrogen balance characterized as aminoaciduria. Salicylates may also decrease fatty acid synthesis, increase metabolism of fatty acids and oxidation of ketone bodies, and decrease plasma concentrations of phospholipids and free fatty acids. With a dosage equivalent in salicylate content to at least 5 g of aspirin daily, plasma concentrations of cholesterol may be decreased.

Salicylates inhibit uptake of ascorbic acid by leukocytes and platelets. As a result, leukocyte and plasma concentrations of ascorbic acid are decreased to concentrations slightly higher than those associated with tissue depletion of the vitamin; however, there is no evidence to date that salicylate therapy precipitates ascorbic acid deficiency. Although concomitant administration of ascorbic acid supplements increases plasma ascorbic acid concentrations, leukocyte ascorbic acid concentrations are not increased and tissue stores of the vitamin may not be increased. Therefore, routine administration of ascorbic acid supplements to patients receiving salicylates is not warranted; however, patients receiving high dosages of salicylates who exhibit any signs or symptoms of ascorbic acid deficiency should be evaluated for such a deficiency.

Aspirin has been shown to inhibit osteolytic activity of human breast carcinoma in vitro, apparently by inhibiting the synthesis of prostaglandins that may mediate this activity. Supporting evidence for this effect and its mechanism has been obtained in patients with certain types of solid tumors (e.g., lung carcinoma) who developed hypercalcemia; in some of these patients, aspirin therapy has resulted in normalization of serum calcium concentrations and has been associated with a reduction in the urinary excretion of a metabolite of prostaglandin E.

Toxic doses of salicylates may stimulate corticosteroid secretion by the adrenal cortex through an effect on the hypothalamus and may transiently increase plasma concentrations of free corticosteroids by displacement from plasma proteins; however, the anti-inflammatory action of salicylates is not dependent on these effects.

Pharmacokinetics

■ **Absorption** In general, salicylates are rapidly and well absorbed from the GI tract following oral administration. Although some absorption occurs from the stomach, salicylates are absorbed primarily from the upper small intestine via passive diffusion of un-ionized molecules (e.g., salicylic acid).

The rate of absorption of an orally administered salicylate depends on many factors, including dosage form and its formulation characteristics, gastric and intestinal pH, gastric emptying time, and the presence of food in the GI tract. The rate of absorption is generally most rapid with effervescent and noneffervescent aqueous solutions, followed by uncoated tablets (plain or with buffers) or film-coated tablets, and capsules; however, clinically significant therapeutic differences between these dosage forms or specific preparations have not been established. The rate of absorption is slowest for enteric-coated tablets, followed by extended-release tablets.

Dissolution is usually the rate-limiting process in the absorption of tablets containing salicylate; however, the in vitro dissolution rate of a specific preparation does not necessarily reflect the in vivo absorption rate. Dissolution depends on several factors such as pH in the GI tract and formulation characteristics of the preparation. An increase in gastric pH (e.g., as a result of concomitant administration of an antacid) enhances dissolution by increasing solubility of salicylate, but it may also decrease gastric absorption by increasing the degree of ionization of salicylate and decreasing gastric emptying time. The buffers contained in buffered aspirin tablets may increase pH in the microenvironment of aspirin particles and thereby increase solubility of the drug in surrounding GI fluids; as a result, the dissolution rate of the tablets may be increased. (See Pharmacokinetics: Absorption, in Aspirin 28:08.04.24.) Although the increased pH in the small intestine also increases dissolution and degree of ionization of salicylate, the high degree of ionization does not appear to limit the absorption of salicylate from the small intestine, probably because of the large surface area of the small intestine.

Other formulation characteristics of tablets (e.g., particle size, compression pressure) may have varied effects on the rate of absorption. In general, the smaller the particle size, the faster the absorption rate since the resultant increase in surface area of dissolving drug enhances the rate of dissolution. Since enteric-coated tablets are formulated to resist dissolution in the stomach and thereby lessen gastric irritation, the rate of absorption from this dosage form is usually decreased compared to uncoated tablets. Absorption of aspirin from extended-release tablets is delayed and prolonged. Since salicylates are absorbed primarily from the upper small intestine, the rate of absorption is generally slower when gastric emptying time is increased, and faster when gastric emptying time is decreased (e.g., by metoclopramide or when gastric pH is increased by concomitant administration of an antacid). Gastric emptying time may be partially dependent on salicylate dosage; in overdosage, there is some evidence that salicylates may remain in the stomach for as long as 10 hours if not removed. Food delays absorption and decreases the rate, but not the extent, of absorption of orally administered salicylates.

In general, solid oral dosage forms of aspirin are 80–100% absorbed. Although well-designed bioavailability studies are generally lacking, solid oral dosage forms of most other salicylates also appear to be 80–100% absorbed. Oral aqueous solutions of aspirin or other salicylates appear to be completely absorbed. There is some evidence that absorption of salicylate following oral administration may be substantially impaired or is highly variable during the febrile phase of Kawasaki disease. Following rectal administration, salicylates are slowly and variably absorbed; the extent of absorption increases with increasing rectal retention time. Methyl salicylate, salicylic acid, and trolamine salicylate are rapidly and well absorbed percutaneously following topical application.

Salicylates are detected in serum within 5–30 minutes after oral administration of rapidly absorbed dosage forms (e.g., aqueous solutions, uncoated or film-coated tablets), and peak serum salicylate concentrations are usually attained within 0.25–2 hours, depending on dosage form and specific formulation. Although some rapidly absorbed dosage forms (e.g., aqueous solutions) may produce slightly higher peak serum salicylate concentrations than others (e.g., uncoated tablets), clinically significant therapeutic differences between such dosage forms or between specific preparations have not been established. However, if a rapid response is required (e.g., analgesic effect), the more slowly absorbed dosage forms (i.e., enteric-coated tablets, extended-release tablets) should not be used.

In general, analgesic and antipyretic effects of single oral doses of rapidly absorbed salicylates begin within 30 minutes, peak at 1–3 hours, and persist for 3–6 hours. Following rectal administration of aspirin as a suppository, the antipyretic effect generally begins within 1–2 hours, peaks at 4–5 hours, and may persist 7 or more hours. In patients with inflammatory diseases, the onset of anti-inflammatory effect generally occurs within 1–4 days of continuous oral salicylate therapy. The time required to achieve optimum anti-inflammatory effect depends principally on the attainment and maintenance of adequate serum salicylate concentrations; several weeks or longer may be required in some patients.

Onset, intensity, and duration of analgesic, antipyretic, and anti-inflammatory effects of single doses of salicylates do not directly coincide with the time course of serum salicylate concentrations; however, these effects appear to be related to total (protein-bound and free) serum salicylate concentration. The usual total serum salicylate concentration associated with analgesia and antipyresis is 30–100 mcg/mL. The usual total serum salicylate concentration required for anti-inflammatory effect is 150–300 mcg/mL; however, in the treatment of rheumatic fever, many clinicians believe a total serum salicylate concentration of 250–350 mcg/mL is associated with optimum therapeutic effects. Although many adverse effects are not well correlated with serum salicylate concentrations, most patients experience toxicity when the total serum salicylate concentration exceeds 300–350 mcg/mL. Because of large interindividual and intraindividual variations in the saliva to serum salicylate concentration ratio, salivary salicylate concentrations are generally not useful.

There is limited evidence from animal studies that the pharmacologic effects of salicylates are produced by free salicylate; however, serum concentrations of free salicylate are technically difficult to obtain and have not been clearly correlated with therapeutic effects. Measurements of serum free salicylate concentration may be useful in some patients with documented or suspected alterations in salicylate protein-binding (e.g., patients with extremely low serum albumin concentrations).

■ **Distribution** Salicylates are rapidly distributed throughout extracellular fluid and into most body tissues and fluids, with high concentrations in the liver and kidneys. During absorption from the stomach, salicylate concentrations in gastric mucosal cells may be 15–20 times higher than concentrations within the gastric lumen. Salicylate can be detected in synovial, peritoneal, and cerebrospinal fluids.

The apparent volume of distribution of salicylate is generally 0.15–0.2 L/kg at usual therapeutic concentrations but may be higher in neonates. The volume of distribution appears to increase with increasing doses and/or serum concentration of salicylate. This increase with increasing doses and/or serum concentration may be due in part to decreased binding of salicylate to serum proteins. The volume of distribution is decreased in patients with decreased serum albumin concentrations and is also affected by plasma and tissue pH.

Distribution of salicylate occurs principally by pH-dependent processes; studies in animals have shown that the tissue-to-plasma distribution ratio of salicylate is increased when plasma pH is greater than that of tissue and decreased when plasma pH is less than that of tissue. Since a large fraction of salicylate in blood is ionized at normal pH, it usually crosses the blood-brain barrier slowly. However, when blood pH is decreased from 7.4 to 7.2, the amount of un-ionized salicylate in blood increases about twofold. Since acidosis often occurs in salicylate overdosage, pH-dependent distribution of salicylate into the CNS and other tissues must be considered. Salicylate is actively transported out of CSF across the choroid plexus by a low-capacity, saturable process.

Salicylate is rapidly distributed into synovial fluid. The principal mechanism of distribution from blood into synovial fluid appears to be passive diffusion. Following single oral doses, salicylate concentrations attained in synovial fluid are about 50–75% of peak serum concentrations. At steady-state, free salicylate concentrations in synovial fluid and serum are approximately equal; however, the total salicylate concentration in synovial fluid is slightly less than in serum because of decreased protein binding of salicylate in synovial fluid.

Salicylate is variably bound to serum proteins, mainly albumin. The fraction bound to serum proteins depends on both the serum salicylate and serum albumin concentrations; even with comparable serum albumin concentrations at a specific serum salicylate concentration, there are interindividual differences in the amount of drug bound. In healthy individuals, salicylate is approximately 90–95% bound to serum proteins at serum salicylate concentrations up to 100 mcg/mL; approximately 70–85% bound to serum proteins at serum salicylate concentrations of 100–400 mcg/mL; and possibly as little as 25–60% bound to serum proteins at higher serum salicylate concentrations. As a result of decreased serum albumin concentrations, serum protein binding of salicylate is decreased and the free fraction is increased in pregnant women, neonates, anephric patients, patients with impaired renal function, and patients with inflammatory diseases. In pregnant women, anephric patients, and patients with impaired renal function, salicylate may be displaced from serum proteins by accumulating endogenous compounds. Protein binding of salicylate is lower in synovial fluid than in serum, possibly as a result of decreased concentrations of albumin in synovial fluid and/or decreased affinity of salicylate for binding sites on synovial fluid proteins.

Salicylate readily crosses the placenta and fetal serum salicylate concentrations may exceed maternal serum concentrations. During chronic oral administration, salicylate may be distributed throughout fetal tissues in concentrations higher than those in the mother.

Salicylate is distributed into milk; however, the extent of distribution into milk is not clearly established. In one study, peak concentrations of salicylate in milk were only 2–5% of peak maternal plasma concentrations. In another study, peak salicylate concentrations in milk were 170–480 mcg/mL at 5–8 hours following maternal ingestion of a single 650-mg dose of aspirin; concurrent maternal plasma concentrations were not reported.

■ **Elimination** Salicylate is metabolized principally in the liver by the microsomal enzyme system. Salicylate is predominantly conjugated with glycine to form salicyluric acid (salicylurate). Salicylate is also conjugated with glucuronic acid to form salicyl phenolic glucuronide and salicyl acyl glucuronide. In addition, small amounts of salicylate are hydroxylated to form 2,5-dihydroxybenzoic acid (gentisic acid), 2,3-dihydroxybenzoic acid, and 2,3,5-trihydroxybenzoic acid. Gentisuric acid, formed either by conjugation of gentisic acid with glycine or by hydroxylation of salicyluric acid, has also been identified as a minor metabolite. Of the salicylate metabolites, only gentisic acid appears to be active; although gentisic acid is a potent inhibitor of prostaglandin synthesis, its contribution to the clinical effects of salicylate is generally considered insignificant because only small amounts are formed. Salicyluric acid and salicyl phenolic glucuronide are formed by capacity-limited (saturable) processes which can be characterized by Michaelis-Menten kinetics. Other salicylate metabolites appear to be formed by first-order processes.

As a result of the capacity-limited processes, steady-state serum salicylate concentrations increase more than proportionally with increasing doses. The time required to attain steady-state concentrations also increases with increasing doses since the apparent serum half-life of salicylate increases with increasing serum salicylate concentration. With low doses (e.g., 325 mg of aspirin), elimination of salicylate is a first-order process and serum salicylate half-life is approximately 2–3 hours; however, with higher doses, elimination of salicylate is capacity limited and the apparent serum salicylate half-life may increase to 15–30 hours. Because of decreased serum protein binding, the effect of increasing doses is more pronounced on the free serum salicylate concentration than on the total serum salicylate concentration. However, in healthy adults, it has been shown that total serum salicylate clearance remains relatively constant at serum salicylate concentrations of 100–300 mcg/mL. The following pharmacokinetic parameters for adults, expressed in concentrations of salicylate and amounts of salicylate metabolized, have been reported for the Michaelis-Menten variables that characterize the capacity-limited metabolism of salicylate: the Michaelis-Menten constant (K_m) for salicyluric acid formation is approximately 5 mg/L; the maximum rate (V_{max}) of salicyluric acid formation is approximately 800–900 mcg/kg per hour (but may increase with long-term therapy, possibly as a result of enzyme induction); the Michaelis-Menten constant (K_m) for salicyl phenolic glucuronide formation is approximately 9 mg/L; and the maximum rate (V_{max}) of salicyl phenolic glucuronide formation is approximately 400 mcg/kg per hour. Specialized references should be consulted for more specific information on salicylate pharmacokinetics.

Genetically determined differences in salicylate metabolism have been reported. There is some evidence that salicylate may induce its own metabolism, as suggested by increased formation of salicyluric acid and decreased serum salicylate concentrations during long-term therapy. Although not clearly established, it has been reported that salicylate is eliminated more slowly by women. The elimination rate of salicylate is reduced in neonates compared to adults, apparently because neonatal metabolic and excretory pathways are incompletely developed; however, prolonged fetal exposure to salicylate resulting from chronic maternal ingestion of salicylate during pregnancy may increase the rate of development of fetal mechanisms of salicylate elimination.

Salicylate and its metabolites are rapidly and almost completely excreted in urine. Trace amounts of salicylate are also excreted in sweat, saliva, and feces. In patients with normal renal function, 80–100% of a single dose is excreted in the urine within 24–72 hours. The relative amounts of salicylate and its metabolites excreted in the urine are extremely variable, being dependent on the dose administered and urine pH. Following a single oral dose of salicylate of less than 10 mg/kg in patients with normal renal function, about 10% of the dose is excreted in urine as unchanged salicylate, 75% as salicyluric acid, 10% as salicyl phenolic glucuronide, 5% as salicyl acyl glucuronide, and less than 1% as gentisic acid and gentisuric acid. With higher single doses or long-term therapy, the proportions excreted in urine as unchanged salicylate, salicyl acyl glucuronide, and gentisic acid generally increase as a result of capacity-limited formation of salicyluric acid and salicyl phenolic glucuronide.

Unchanged salicylate and its metabolites are excreted in the urine via glomerular filtration and renal tubular secretion; since unchanged salicylate also undergoes renal tubular reabsorption, its urinary excretion is markedly pH dependent. As urine pH increases from 5 to 8, the urinary excretion rate of salicylate is greatly increased and the fraction of a single dose excreted in the urine as unchanged salicylate may increase from 5–10% to 85%. Therefore, concomitant administration of drugs that alter urine pH may have substantial effects on serum salicylate concentrations. (See Drug Interactions: Acidifying and Alkalinizing Agents.)

In patients with normal renal function, salicylate metabolites are excreted in the urine as rapidly as they are formed. Although anephric patients appear to eliminate small doses of salicylate (e.g., 650 mg of sodium salicylate) as rapidly as healthy individuals, the pharmacokinetics of salicylate in patients with severe renal impairment have not been clearly established and salicylates are usually avoided in these patients.

Salicylate and its metabolites are readily removed by hemodialysis and, to a lesser extent, by peritoneal dialysis.

Chemistry and Stability

■ **Chemistry** Salicylates are nonsteroidal anti-inflammatory agents (NSAIAs) that are synthetic derivatives of salicylic acid. The drugs hydrolyze or dissociate to salicylate (ionized salicylic acid) in vivo. Salicylic acid is not used systemically because of its severe irritating effect on GI mucosa and other tissues; therefore, better tolerated chemical derivatives have been prepared for systemic use.

The pharmacologic actions of salicylates appear to result principally from the salicylate moiety. The carboxyl group and an adjacent hydroxyl group on salicylic acid are necessary for activity; either or both groups may have substituents. The currently available salicylates are either esters of organic acids derived by substitution at the hydroxyl group of salicylic acid, or esters or salts of salicylic acid derived by substitution at the carboxyl group. Aspirin, the prototype of the salicylates, is the salicylate ester of acetic acid; the drug hydrolyzes to salicylate and acetate. Salsalate is the salicylate ester of salicylic acid; the drug hydrolyzes to 2 molecules of salicylate. Many commercially available salicylate preparations contain salts of salicylic acid (e.g., choline salicylate, magnesium salicylate, sodium salicylate, trolamine salicylate) which dissociate to form salicylate. Although related to the salicylates structurally and pharmacologically, diflunisal, salicylamide, and probably sodium thiosalicylate are not hydrolyzed to salicylate; therefore, these drugs are not considered true salicylates and are not included in this discussion.

Salicylic acid occurs as white crystals, usually in fine needles, or as a fluffy, white, crystalline powder. The drug has a sweetish taste and an acrid aftertaste and is slightly soluble in water and freely soluble in alcohol. The synthetic form is white and odorless; when prepared from natural methyl salicylate, the drug may have a slightly yellow or pink tint and a faint, mint-like odor. Salicylic acid has pK_as of 2.97 and 13.4. Most salicylates occur as white, crystalline powders and are practically insoluble to very soluble in water and soluble to freely soluble in alcohol.

■ **Stability** Aqueous solutions of salicylates slowly darken in color due to oxidation; however, the color change appears to have no effect on efficacy or toxicity. Darkening of solutions of salicylates is delayed by the presence of 0.1% of sodium bisulfite, sodium sulfite, sodium thiosulfate, or sodium hypophosphite, or 0.5% sodium citrate. Addition of mineral acids to aqueous solutions of salicylates results in precipitation of salicylic acid.

For specific dosages and additional information on chemistry and stability, pharmacology, pharmacokinetics, uses, and cautions, see the individual monographs on Aspirin, Salicylate Salts, and Salsalate in 28:08.04.24.

†Use is not currently included in the labeling approved by the US Food and Drug Administration

Aspirin

Acetylsalicylic Acid, ASA

■ Aspirin (the prototype of the salicylates) is a nonsteroidal anti-inflammatory agent (NSAIA) and also exhibits antithrombotic, analgesic, and antipyretic activity.

Uses

Aspirin is used extensively in the treatment of mild to moderate pain, fever, and inflammatory diseases. Aspirin is also used in the prevention of arterial and venous thrombosis. Aspirin, however, should be used with extreme caution, if at all, in patients in whom urticaria, angioedema, bronchospasm, severe rhinitis, or shock is precipitated by other salicylates or other NSAIAs. (See Cautions: Sensitivity Reactions in the Salicylates General Statement 28:08.04.24.)

■ **Pain** Aspirin is used to relieve headache, neuralgia, myalgia, arthralgia, and other low-intensity pain of nonvisceral origin, particularly pain associated with inflammation. Aspirin may also relieve mild to moderate postoperative pain, postpartum pain, oral surgery or other dental pain, dysmenorrhea, or other visceral pain such as that associated with trauma or cancer. Many studies have shown that the analgesic effects of aspirin are greater than those of placebo in the treatment of these types of pain. The drug, however, does not usually relieve severe acute pain of visceral origin. In addition, use of chewing gum tablets or gargles containing aspirin has not been shown to be effective in relieving sore throat pain.

The analgesic effect of aspirin appears to increase with increasing single oral doses up to at least 1.2 g; however, single oral doses of aspirin exceeding 650 mg apparently do not result in a greater incidence or degree of pain relief in most patients. Multiple oral doses of aspirin exceeding 650 mg each have not been shown to be more effective in relieving pain than multiple oral doses of 650 mg.

When used to relieve postoperative pain, 600-mg oral doses of aspirin appear to be as effective as 60-mg oral doses of codeine or 50-mg oral doses of pentazocine. When used to relieve oral surgery pain, 650-mg oral doses of aspirin appear to be more effective than 30-mg oral doses of codeine, as effective as 650-mg oral doses of acetaminophen, and less effective than 250-mg, 500-mg, or 1-g oral doses of diflunisal.

In the treatment of postpartum uterine pain, the analgesic effect of 650-mg oral doses of aspirin is about equal to that of 300- or 600-mg oral doses of naproxen or 275-mg oral doses of naproxen sodium and greater than that of 60-mg oral doses of codeine or codeine sulfate. When used to relieve episiotomy pain, several studies have shown that 600-mg to 1.2-g oral doses of aspirin are more effective than placebo; in one study, the analgesic effect of 900-mg oral doses of aspirin was about equal to that of 300- or 900-mg oral doses of ibuprofen. In another study, the analgesic effect of 600-mg oral doses of aspirin was less than that of 500-mg oral doses of diflunisal.

In the treatment of nonspecific pain associated with cancer, 650-mg oral doses of aspirin appear to be at least as effective as 650-mg oral doses of acetaminophen, 65-mg oral doses of codeine, 250-mg oral doses of mefenamic acid, or 50-mg oral doses of pentazocine, and more effective than 75-mg oral doses of ethoheptazine citrate or 65-mg oral doses of propoxyphene hydrochloride (no longer commercially available in the US). When used to relieve nonspecific pain associated with cancer, 650-mg oral doses of aspirin in combination with oral doses of codeine (65 mg), oxycodone (976 mcg), or pentazocine hydrochloride (25 mg) appear to be more effective than 650-mg oral doses of aspirin alone or in combination with oral doses of caffeine (65 mg), ethoheptazine citrate (75 mg), pentobarbital sodium (25 mg), promazine hydrochloride (25 mg), or propoxyphene napsylate (100 mg) (no longer commercially available in the US).

Results of studies comparing aspirin (500–650 mg 4 times daily) with placebo to relieve primary dysmenorrhea have been inconsistent. Although the effects of higher dosages of aspirin remain to be evaluated, most clinicians consider aspirin to be one of the *least* effective NSAIAs currently available for the treatment of primary dysmenorrhea.

In several double-blind placebo-controlled studies with small numbers of patients with migraine, prophylactic therapy with aspirin (650 mg twice daily) alone or aspirin (300 mg twice daily) with dipyridamole (25 mg 3 times daily) has reportedly been effective in reducing the frequency of headache; however, further evaluation is needed. In addition, aspirin in fixed combination with acetaminophen and caffeine (aspirin 500 mg, acetaminophen 500 mg, and caffeine 130 mg per dose) is used for the temporary relief of mild to moderate pain associated with migraine headache. Some experts state that an NSAIA (e.g., aspirin alone or in fixed combination with acetaminophen and caffeine) is a reasonable first-line therapy for mild to moderate migraine attacks or for severe attacks that have responded in the past to similar NSAIAs or non-opiate analgesics. The efficacy of oral aspirin in fixed combination with acetaminophen and caffeine for the management of mild to moderate pain associated with migraine headache was established by 3 double-blind, randomized, parallel-group, placebo-controlled studies (one of them a population-based study) in adults who had migraine with aura or migraine without aura as defined by criteria established by the International Headache Society (IHS). The efficacy of therapy for management of pain associated with migraine headache in these studies was evaluated in terms of a reduction in headache severity as rated by the patient (i.e., a reduction in pain from at least moderate to mild or to absent 2 hours after dosing using a 4-point scale). Pooled analysis of data from the 3 studies indicated that about 59% of patients receiving 500 mg of aspirin in fixed combination with acetaminophen 500 mg and caffeine 130 mg attained relief of pain associated with migraine headache (i.e., mild or no headache) within 2 hours compared with about 33% of placebo recipients; at 6 hours, about 79 and 52%, respectively, of drug- and placebo-treated patients had mild or no headache pain. In addition, about 21% of patients receiving the combination were pain-free 2 hours after dosing versus about 7% of those receiving placebo, while at 6 hours, 51% of drug-treated patients were pain-free versus 24% of those receiving placebo. It appears that this combination also may relieve manifestations of migraine other than headache, including nausea, vomiting, photophobia, and phonophobia. Patients in whom pain associated with migraine headache is not relieved by aspirin in fixed combination with acetaminophen and caffeine should consult their clinician about possible alternatives (e.g., use of prescription drugs including ergot alkaloids or vascular serotonin type 1-like receptor agonists) based on evaluation of their medical condition. In several double-blind controlled studies in patients with acute migraine headache, aspirin 900 or 1000 mg given as a single dose with or without metoclopramide 10 mg (as an antiemetic) was more effective than placebo and had efficacy generally similar to that of sumatriptan 50 or 100 mg for relief of pain and associated symptoms of migraine (nausea, vomiting, photophobia, phonophobia). For further information on management and classification of migraine headache, see General Principles in Migraine Therapy under Uses: Vascular Headaches, in Sumatriptan 28:32.28.

Aspirin has been used in the treatment of pain in various combinations with acetaminophen, caffeine, opiates, salicylamide, and/or other agents. However, combinations of aspirin with agents such as acetaminophen, caffeine, or salicylamide have not been clearly shown to have greater analgesic effect than an optimal dose of aspirin alone. In addition, there is little evidence that such combinations cause fewer adverse effects than higher doses of the individual agents alone. In one study, the simultaneous administration of 325- or 650-mg oral doses of acetaminophen with 650-mg oral doses of aspirin resulted in increased blood concentrations of unhydrolyzed aspirin compared with 650-mg oral doses of aspirin alone; however, the clinical importance of such an effect remains to be established. Aspirin (650-mg oral doses) in combination with oral doses of an opiate (e.g., codeine, oxycodone) produces greater analgesic effect than that produced by either aspirin or higher doses of the opiate alone. There is also some evidence that aspirin/opiate combinations may cause fewer adverse effects than equianalgesic doses of the individual drugs alone.

■ **Fever** Aspirin is used frequently to lower body temperature in febrile patients in whom fever may be deleterious or in whom considerable relief is obtained when fever is lowered. However, antipyretic therapy is generally nonspecific, does not influence the course of the underlying disease, and may obscure the course of the patient's illness. For information on salicylates and Reye's syndrome, see Cautions: Pediatric Precautions, in the Salicylates General Statement 28:08.04.24.

Aspirin and acetaminophen are equally effective as antipyretics. In one study in febrile children, the combination of oral doses of aspirin and acetaminophen was at least as effective in reducing fever as either drug alone, and the duration of fever reduction was longer with the combination than with the individual drugs. However, because of the study design, it could not be concluded that the combination had additive effects. Many clinicians use regimens of alternating doses of aspirin and acetaminophen; however, combined overdosage with both drugs has occurred with such a regimen and the efficacy and safety of these regimens remain to be established.

Several clinical studies have shown that the antipyretic effect of usual dosages of aspirin is about equal to that of usual dosages of mefenamic acid and naproxen, and less than that of usual dosages of indomethacin. However, efficacy of these other NSAIAs as antipyretics remains to be clearly established and they should not be used for routine treatment of fever because of their potential adverse effects.

■ **Inflammatory Diseases** Aspirin is used for anti-inflammatory and analgesic effects in the initial and/or long-term symptomatic treatment of rheumatoid arthritis, juvenile arthritis, and osteoarthritis. Aspirin may also be useful in the treatment of other polyarthritic conditions (e.g., psoriatic arthritis, Reiter's syndrome, ankylosing spondylitis), systemic lupus erythematous, and nonarticular inflammation; however, other NSAIAs may be preferred in the treatment of some of these conditions (e.g., ankylosing spondylitis).

Rheumatoid Arthritis, Juvenile Arthritis, and Osteoarthritis Most clinical studies have shown that the anti-inflammatory and analgesic effects of usual dosages of aspirin in the treatment of rheumatoid arthritis or osteoarthritis are greater than those of placebo and about equal to those of usual dosages of fenoprofen calcium, ibuprofen, indomethacin, meclofenamate sodium, naproxen, piroxicam, sulindac, and tolmetin sodium. In the treatment of juvenile arthritis, the anti-inflammatory and analgesic effects of usual dosages of aspirin are about equal to those of usual dosages of fenoprofen, naproxen, or tolmetin sodium. Patient response to NSAIAs is variable, however, and patients who do not respond to one agent may be successfully treated with a different agent.

Aspirin has been used in conjunction with other NSAIAs in the treatment of some patients with rheumatoid arthritis, but such combination therapy is generally not recommended because there is inadequate proof that such combination therapy is more efficacious than the individual agents alone and the potential for adverse reactions may be increased. In addition, there is evidence that aspirin alters plasma concentrations of some other NSAIAs.

Psoriatic Arthritis and Reiter's Syndrome Aspirin may be effective in the treatment of some patients with psoriatic arthritis or Reiter's syndrome but usually only when the disease is mild. Aspirin is seldom effective in the treatment of ankylosing spondylitis unless the disease is mild. In one study in patients with ankylosing spondylitis, the anti-inflammatory and analgesic effects of aspirin were less than those of indomethacin or phenylbutazone.

Systemic Lupus Erythematous Some clinicians consider aspirin to be a drug of first choice for the treatment of fever, arthritis, pleurisy, and pericarditis in patients with systemic lupus erythematous (SLE). In one study in patients with SLE, the anti-inflammatory and analgesic effects of aspirin were greater than those of ibuprofen. The anti-inflammatory and analgesic effects of aspirin may also be useful in the symptomatic treatment of nonarticular inflammation such as bursitis and/or tendinitis (e.g., acute painful shoulder) and fibrositis.

■ **Rheumatic Fever** Most clinicians consider aspirin to be the salicylate of choice when salicylate therapy is indicated in the treatment of rheumatic fever†. For information on salicylate therapy in the treatment of rheumatic fever, see Uses: Rheumatic Fever, in the Salicylates General Statement 28:08.04.24.

■ **Thrombosis** Generally accepted indications for prophylactic aspirin therapy include its use for reducing the risk of recurrent vascular events (e.g., recurrent stroke, death) in men and women who have had single or multiple transient ischemic attacks (TIAs)† or ischemic stroke†, for reducing the risk of vascular mortality in patients with suspected acute myocardial infarction† (MI), for reducing the risk of recurrent nonfatal MI and/or death in patients with previous MI or unstable angina†, for reducing the risk of MI and sudden death in patients with chronic stable angina pectoris†, and for reducing cardiovascular risks in patients undergoing percutaneous coronary intervention [PCI] or certain revascularization procedures (e.g., coronary artery bypass grafting [CABG]). Aspirin also has been used to prevent thrombosis in patients undergoing percutaneous transluminal angioplasty (PTA) of the lower extremities†, and for postoperative thromboprophylaxis in children undergoing surgery for placement of modified Blalock-Taussig shunts†, surgery for univentricular heart lesions (i.e., Fontan procedure†), surgery for placement of ventricular assist devices†, or surgery for hypoplastic left heart (i.e., Norwood procedure)†. Aspirin also has been used to prevent thromboembolism in patients with atrial fibrillation† or atrial flutter†, valvular heart disease† (e.g., mitral valve prolapse), chronic limb ischemia (e.g., intermittent claudication)†, or prosthetic heart valves†.

Transient Ischemic Attacks and Acute Ischemic Stroke Aspirin is used for *secondary prevention* of vascular events (e.g., recurrent stroke, death) in patients who have had an acute ischemic stroke or TIAs. The American College of Chest Physicians (ACCP), the American Stroke Association (ASA), the American Heart Association (AHA), and other clinicians recommend antiplatelet therapy over oral anticoagulation (e.g., warfarin) for *secondary prevention* of ischemic atherothrombotic (noncardioembolic) stroke or TIAs in patients with prior TIAs or ischemic stroke who do not have atrial fibrillation.

AHA and ASA recommend aspirin for *primary prevention* or *secondary prevention* of ischemic stroke in high-risk women (i.e., women with established coronary heart disease, cerebrovascular disease, peripheral arterial disease, abdominal aortic aneurysm, end-stage or chronic kidney disease, diabetes mellitus, or a 10-year Framingham risk exceeding 20%). AHA and ASA also suggest that low-dose aspirin therapy can be useful in women 65 years of age or older in whom the benefits for ischemic stroke and MI prevention are likely to outweigh the risk of GI bleeding and hemorrhagic stroke and may be reasonable to consider in women younger than 65 years of age in whom the benefits for ischemic stroke prevention are likely to outweigh the adverse effects of aspirin. Results of several trials suggest that use of aspirin therapy for *primary prevention* of stroke in men without a history of TIAs or stroke may be associated with a slightly increased risk of stroke, particularly hemorrhagic stroke, and aspirin is not recommended for *primary prevention* of ischemic stroke in men.

Restoring perfusion (e.g., with thrombolytic therapy) is the principal goal of acute stroke therapy, with the second goal being prevention of early recurrence of cerebrovascular events with anticoagulants and antiplatelet agents. Unless contraindicated or unless too much time (i.e., more than 3–4.5 hours†) has elapsed since the event, thrombolytic therapy generally is preferred for the acute treatment of ischemic stroke. (See Uses: Acute Ischemic Stroke, in Alteplase 20:12.20.) In patients with acute ischemic stroke or TIA in whom thrombolytic therapy is contraindicated or not appropriate, early aspirin therapy (160–325 mg initially, followed by 75–100 mg daily to reduce bleeding risk) is recommended. Aspirin should be initiated within 48 hours of stroke onset. The rationale for antithrombotic therapy such as aspirin in patients with acute ischemic stroke is to reduce the risk of stroke progression or recurrent cerebral thromboembolism and prevent thromboembolic complications. Current evidence indicates that aspirin therapy initiated within 48 hours of stroke onset is relatively safe and can produce a small but definite net benefit by reducing both stroke recurrence risk and mortality.

For *secondary prevention* of ischemic stroke in patients with cerebrovascular disease, including patients with a history of TIAs or previous ischemic stroke, aspirin is the most widely studied and used antiplatelet agent. Secondary prevention with aspirin has been shown to reduce the combined endpoint of stroke, MI, and/or vascular death by 13–25%. Data from numerous clinical studies have shown that aspirin reduces the risk of these cardiovascular events in a wide variety of patients at high risk for these atherosclerotic outcomes.

Because there is evidence from clinical studies to support the efficacy of low dosages of aspirin (e.g., 50–325 mg daily) in patients with a history of TIAs or cerebral ischemia and considerable evidence supporting the antithrombotic efficacy of such dosages in patients with MI, these dosages have supplanted the moderate- to high-dose regimens employed in the past. Further supporting this change in dosage recommendations is evidence that efficacy is not compromised with low-dosage regimens, but patient tolerance is improved. Although early evidence supporting the beneficial effects of aspirin in patients with TIAs came from studies that included mainly men, more recent studies have shown numerically similar results for men and women, and favorable trends generally have been seen in both genders. Current data suggest that an aspirin dosage of 75–81 mg daily may be sufficient for long-term cardiovascular prevention and is associated with less GI bleeding risk.

Aspirin in fixed combination with extended-release dipyridamole is used to reduce the risk of recurrent stroke in patients who have had TIAs or completed ischemic stroke caused by noncardioembolic thrombosis (e.g., atherothrombotic, lacunar, cryptogenic). In a randomized, comparative, placebo-controlled study, patients who had experienced either an ischemic stroke or TIAs were assigned to receive treatment with aspirin (25 mg twice daily), extended-release dipyridamole (200 mg twice daily), aspirin plus extended-release dipyridamole (25 and 200 mg twice daily, respectively), or placebo. All active treatments reduced the risk of the primary end points of stroke (nonfatal or fatal) or stroke and/or death compared with placebo. Aspirin plus dipyridamole reduced the risk of stroke by about 23% compared with aspirin alone and by about 25% compared with dipyridamole alone at 2 years of follow-up; the effects of combined therapy on risk reductions with aspirin and dipyridamole were additive but not synergistic. Aspirin, dipyridamole, and the combination also reduced the incidence of TIAs and other vascular events in a manner consistent with these treatments' effects on the risk of stroke. None of the treatments had a statistically significant effect on the end point of death (i.e., no effect on survival). Headache and GI events were the most common adverse effects in this study, occurring more frequently in the dipyridamole-treated groups, while bleeding from the GI tract or from any site was more common in the aspirin-treated groups.

In another randomized, placebo-controlled, open-label study (European/Australasian Stroke Prevention in Reversible ischemia Trial [ESPRIT]) in patients who had experienced a TIA or minor stroke within the previous 6 months, treatment with aspirin (median dosage 75 mg daily, range 30–325 mg daily) in combination with dipyridamole (200 mg twice daily) resulted in a reduction in the overall risk of the composite primary outcome (death from all vascular causes, nonfatal stroke, nonfatal MI, major bleeding complication) compared with that in patients receiving aspirin alone. Approximately 34% of patients discontinued treatment with the aspirin-dipyridamole combination during the study because of adverse effects, principally headache. Results from other trials evaluating combination therapy with aspirin (900 mg to 1.3 g daily) and dipyridamole (150–300 mg daily) also have been reported to reduce the risk of cerebral infarction in patients with TIAs or mild stroke. A meta-analysis of data from the ESPRIT and several prior studies comparing aspirin with or without dipyridamole in patients with cerebral ischemia of presumed arterial origin demonstrated an overall reduction of 18% in the incidence of primary outcome events with combined aspirin and dipyridamole treatment compared with aspirin alone.

ACCP, ASA, AHA, and other clinicians recommend long-term antiplatelet therapy for *secondary prevention* of ischemic atherothrombotic (noncardioembolic) stroke or TIAs in patients with prior TIAs or stroke. In such patients, ACCP states that aspirin, clopidogrel, the combination of aspirin and dipyridamole, or cilostazol are all acceptable options for long-term antithrombotic therapy. Based on a somewhat greater risk reduction for stroke, ACCP suggests that clopidogrel or the combination of aspirin and dipyridamole may be preferred over the other options for secondary prevention of noncardioembolic stroke. When selecting an appropriate antiplatelet regimen for the secondary prevention of noncardioembolic stroke, factors such as the patient's individual risk for recurrent stroke, tolerance, and cost of the different agents should be considered. Oral anticoagulation (e.g., warfarin) rather than antiplatelet therapy is recommended for the secondary prevention of cardioembolic stroke in patients with a history of ischemic stroke or TIA and concurrent atrial fibrillation; however, in patients who cannot take or choose not to take warfarin (e.g., those with difficulty maintaining stable international normalized ratios [INRs], compliance issues, dietary restrictions, cost limitations), dual antiplatelet therapy with aspirin and clopidogrel is recommended.

In children with acute arterial ischemic stroke†, aspirin is recommended as one of the options for initial antithrombotic therapy until cerebral arterial dissection and embolic causes have been excluded. Once dissection and cardioembolic causes have been excluded, secondary prevention with aspirin therapy (in prophylactic dosages for at least 2 years) is suggested. Children who experience recurrent arterial ischemic stroke or TIAs despite aspirin therapy may be switched to clopidogrel or anticoagulant therapy with a low molecular weight heparin or warfarin.

Coronary Artery Disease and Myocardial Infarction **ST-Segment-Elevation Myocardial Infarction.** The current standard of care in patients with ST-segment-elevation MI (STEMI) is timely reperfusion (with primary PCI or thrombolytic therapy). Adjunctive therapy with anticoagulant (e.g., heparin) and antiplatelet (e.g., aspirin and clopidogrel) agents should be used during and after successful coronary artery reperfusion for the prevention of early reocclusion and death, unless contraindicated. Aspirin reduces the risk of stroke, recurrent infarction, and death in adults with STEMI and should be administered in all such patients regardless of the reperfusion strategy. Aspirin in a dose of 162–325 mg, initiated as soon as possible after the clinical impression of an evolving acute STEMI is formed and continued indefinitely at a dosage of 81–325 mg daily, also is strongly recommended for the acute management of all patients (unless contraindicated) with suspected STEMI, regardless of whether thrombolytic therapy is to be given. Some experts prefer the use of a maintenance dosage of 81 mg daily because of a decreased risk of bleeding and lack of definitive evidence demonstrating that higher dosages confer greater benefit in this setting. A P2Y12 platelet adenosine diphosphate (ADP)-receptor antagonist (e.g., clopidogrel, prasugrel, ticagrelor) should be administered in conjunction with aspirin in patients with STEMI.

In a large, multicenter study (Second International Study of Infarct Survival; ISIS-2) of patients with an evolving STEMI allocated to treatment early (within 24 hours of symptom onset), therapy with aspirin 162.5 mg daily for 1 month was shown conclusively to be associated with a vascular mortality reduction at 5 weeks of 23% compared with placebo. In this study, a statistically significant difference in both vascular and all-cause mortality, which persisted for at least a median of 15 months after treatment, was observed. Patients receiving aspirin had fewer nonfatal reinfarctions and nonfatal strokes compared with those given placebo and, when given concomitantly with IV streptokinase therapy, aspirin appeared to prevent the increase in reinfarction observed with streptokinase treatment alone. Compared with placebo, aspirin treatment resulted in a small increase in the incidence of minor bleeding complications but no increase in major bleeding (e.g., intracranial hemorrhage). When aspirin is combined with thrombolytic therapy (streptokinase), the reduction in mortality associated with acute STEMI is even greater, being reported as a 42% reduction. Pooled analysis of clinical studies indicates that aspirin reduces coronary reocclusion and recurrent ischemic events after thrombolytic therapy with streptokinase or alteplase. At doses of at least 160 mg, aspirin produces a rapid clinical antithrombotic effect via immediate and near-total inhibition of thromboxane A_2. As a result, aspirin is an important therapy in the early management of suspected acute STEMI.

In patients with STEMI who have indications for anticoagulation (e.g., atrial fibrillation, left ventricular dysfunction, cerebral emboli, extensive wall-motion abnormality, mechanical heart valves), many experts recommend the addition of warfarin (INR 2–3) to antiplatelet therapy; in some cases, triple antithrombotic therapy (warfarin, low-dose aspirin, and clopidogrel) is suggested, such as in patients with an anterior STEMI and left ventricular thrombosis undergoing PCI with coronary artery stent implantation. However, triple-drug antithrombotic regimens are associated with an increased risk of bleeding. (See Uses: ST-Segment Elevation Myocardial Infarction, in Warfarin 20:12.04.08.)

Secondary Prevention of Cardiovascular Events. Unless contraindicated, therapy with low-dose aspirin currently is recommended by AHA and the American College of Cardiology Foundation (ACCF) for all patients with coronary artery disease in order to reduce the risk of vascular events (*secondary prevention*). ACCP recommends long-term, single-drug antiplatelet therapy with aspirin or clopidogrel in patients with established coronary artery disease (i.e., 1 year after ACS with prior revascularization, coronary stenosis greater than 50% by coronary angiogram, and/or evidence of cardiac ischemia on diagnostic testing). The efficacy of aspirin for secondary prevention of cardiovascular events does not appear to be influenced by gender or age. The American Diabetes Association (ADA) currently recommends low-dose aspirin (e.g., 75–162 mg daily) for secondary prevention of cardiovascular events (e.g., MI) in patients with diabetes mellitus and a history of atherosclerotic cardiovascular disease (ASCVD).

Primary Prevention of Ischemic Cardiac Events. The beneficial effects of aspirin for secondary prevention of cardiovascular disease are well established; however, use of aspirin for *primary prevention* of cardiovascular disease remains controversial. Low-dose aspirin (e.g., 75–162 mg daily) has been used to reduce the risk of a first cardiac event (*primary prevention*†) in patients with at least a moderate risk factor for a coronary event. However, recent evidence suggests that aspirin therapy should not be used routinely for *primary prevention* of cardiovascular disease because of a lack of net benefit.

Most clinical studies that demonstrated the beneficial effect of aspirin for primary prevention of cardiovascular disease (e.g., the US Physicians' Health Study [men 40–84 years of age without a history of ischemic heart disease], the British Doctors' Study [men younger than 60 up to 79 years of age without ischemic heart disease], the Medical Research Council's Thrombosis Prevention Trial [men 45–69 years of age with an increased risk of ischemic heart disease], the Hypertension Optimal Treatment [HOT] trial [men and women 50–80 years with hypertension], the Primary Prevention Project [PPP] [patients at least 50 years of age who had at least one major cardiovascular risk factor]) were conducted prior to modern preventative and therapeutic practices (i.e., emphasis on stricter blood pressure control, smoking cessation, and cholesterol reduction). While low-dose aspirin may still confer benefits in selected patients, there is less certainty regarding the drug's widespread use for primary prevention. In 3 recently conducted randomized, placebo-controlled primary prevention studies evaluating the use of low-dose aspirin regimens (100 mg once daily in all 3 studies) in various patient populations, there was no substantial net clinical benefit with low-dose aspirin therapy largely because of an increased risk of bleeding with aspirin use. In the ARRIVE (Aspirin to Reduce Risk of Initial Vascular Events) study, which included patients 55 years of age or older without diabetes mellitus and with a low to moderate cardiovascular risk, low-dose aspirin did not substantially reduce the combined outcome of first MI, stroke, cardiovascular death, unstable angina, or transient ischemic attack but was associated with an increased risk of GI bleeding. In the ASCEND (A Study of Cardiovascular Events In Diabetes) study, which included patients 40 years of age or older with type 1 or type 2 diabetes mellitus who did not have known cardiovascular disease, the use of low-dose aspirin for 7.4 years was associated with a 12% reduction in the rate of serious vascular events at the cost of a 29% increase in major bleeding. In this study, there was no substantial difference in all-cause mortality among patients who received aspirin therapy and those who did not. In the ASPREE (ASPirin in Reducing Events in the Elderly) study, which included healthy patients 65 years of age and older without cardiovascular disease, low-dose aspirin use resulted in a substantially higher risk of major hemorrhage (composite of hemorrhagic stroke, symptomatic intracranial bleeding, or clinically important extracranial bleeding) and did not substantially reduce the risk of cardiovascular disease.

Based on available evidence including the results of these recent clinical studies, experts from the American College of Cardiology and American Heart Association (ACC/AHA) recommend that low-dose aspirin (e.g., 75–100 mg daily) for *primary prevention* be reserved for adults 40–70 years of age who have a higher risk of cardiovascular disease without an increased risk of bleeding (e.g., patients with a history of previous GI bleed, peptic ulcer disease, thrombocytopenia, coagulopathy, chronic kidney disease, concomitant use of drugs that increase bleeding risk [e.g., nonsteroidal anti-inflammatory drugs, corticosteroids, direct oral anticoagulants, warfarin]). When determining a patient's risk for ASCVD, these experts state that the totality of patient risk factors should be considered (e.g., strong family history of premature MI; inability to achieve lipid, blood pressure, or blood glucose targets; substantial elevation in coronary artery calcium score) in conjunction with patient and clinician preferences. High-risk patients also include adults 40–70 years of age without diabetes mellitus who have a 10-year ASCVD risk of at least 20% and those with diabetes mellitus who have a 10-year ASCVD risk of at least 10%. Low-dose aspirin for *primary prevention* is not recommended for adults with a low ASCVD risk, and the routine use of aspirin for *primary prevention* is not recommended in patients younger than 40 years of age or older than 70 years of age. In addition, such experts state that it is unclear whether low-dose aspirin should be *continued* in patients already taking aspirin who turn 70 years of age. Additional studies are needed to clarify aspirin's role in the primary prevention of cardiovascular disease.

Based on a systematic review of evidence, the US Preventive Services Task Force (USPSTF) has concluded that the beneficial effects of aspirin for primary prevention of cardiovascular disease are modest and occur at daily dosages of 100 mg or less; subpopulation analyses suggest a greater relative benefit for MI prevention in older age groups.

The ADA states that the use of aspirin for *primary prevention* of cardiovascular disease should be carefully considered and generally may not be recommended. ADA states that *primary prevention* with low-dose aspirin may be considered in patients with type 1 or type 2 diabetes mellitus who are at high risk for cardiovascular events (i.e., familial history of premature ASCVD, smoking, hypertension, chronic kidney disease/albuminuria, elevated blood cholesterol or triglyceride concentrations) and have a low bleeding risk. ADA also states that aspirin use is not recommended for patients at low risk of ASCVD (e.g., men and women younger than 50 years of age with diabetes mellitus and no other major risk factors) as the risk of bleeding is likely to outweigh the small benefit. For patients older than 70 years of age (with or without diabetes mellitus), the risks associated with the use of low-dose aspirin appear to outweigh any potential benefits

Non-ST-Segment-Elevation Acute Coronary Syndromes. Aspirin is used to reduce the risk of death and/or nonfatal MI in patients with non-ST-segment-elevation acute coronary syndromes (NSTE ACS). Patients with NSTE ACS have either unstable angina or non-ST-segment-elevation MI (NSTEMI); because these conditions are part of a continuum of acute myocardial ischemia and have indistinguishable clinical features upon presentation, the same initial treatment strategies are recommended. The American Heart Association/American College of Cardiology (AHA/ACC) guideline for the management of patients with NSTE ACS recommends an early invasive strategy (angiographic evaluation with the intent to perform revascularization procedures such as PCI with coronary artery stent implantation or CABG) or an ischemia-guided strategy (initial medical management followed by cardiac catheterization and revascularization if indicated) in patients with definite or likely NSTE ACS; standard medical therapies for all patients should include a β-adrenergic blocking agent (β-blocker), antiplatelet agents, anticoagulant agents, nitrates, and analgesic agents regardless of the initial management approach. Aspirin is the mainstay of antiplatelet therapy in patients with NSTE ACS and should be administered in all such patients unless contraindicated; a loading dose of aspirin should be administered as soon as possible after diagnosis, followed by a maintenance dosage that should be continued indefinitely unless such therapy is not tolerated or contraindicated. A P2Y12-receptor antagonist (e.g., clopidogrel, ticagrelor) should be administered in conjunction with aspirin for up to 12 months unless contraindicated.

Aspirin therapy has been shown to substantially reduce the rates of total mortality or cardiac death and nonfatal MI in patients with NSTE ACS. Several randomized, placebo-controlled studies indicate that prophylactic aspirin therapy is associated with a reduction of at least 50% in the risk of death and/or nonfatal MI in men and women with NSTE ACS. In another randomized, controlled study in men with NSTE ACS who received 75 mg of aspirin daily, the risk of MI and death was reduced by 57–69% at least 5 days after initiation of therapy.

Chronic Stable Angina. In patients with chronic stable angina, low-dose aspirin is used to reduce the risk of MI and sudden death. Experts recommend that aspirin therapy (75–162 mg daily) be continued indefinitely in patients with stable ischemic heart disease who do not have contraindications. There is some evidence suggesting that an aspirin dosage not exceeding 75–81 mg daily may be sufficient for long-term cardiovascular prevention and is associated with less GI bleeding risk. Clopidogrel may be used as an alternative to aspirin in patients with symptomatic chronic stable angina who cannot tolerate aspirin.

Evidence from a large, randomized, placebo-controlled study in patients with stable chronic angina pectoris showed that aspirin (75 mg daily) combined with sotalol therapy is associated with 34% reduction in the primary endpoint of fatal or nonfatal MI and sudden death and a 22–32% reduction in secondary endpoints (vascular events, vascular death, all-cause mortality, stroke). There also was a reduction in nonfatal MI, the principal component of benefit of the primary end point. Although not significantly different from placebo, aspirin therapy also was associated with a favorable trend in decreasing vascular deaths and all-cause mortality when considered separately. Because all patients in this study received sotalol concomitantly, this study did not establish whether aspirin alone is effective in patients with chronic stable angina. However, the ability of aspirin to decrease the rate of thrombotic vascular events in various conditions has not depended on concomitant β-blocker therapy to date, and therefore it is likely that aspirin therapy would be beneficial in patients with chronic stable angina pectoris regardless of concomitant β-blocker therapy.

Percutaneous Coronary Intervention and Revascularization Procedures. Aspirin is used to reduce early ischemic complications in patients with ACS undergoing PCI (e.g., coronary angioplasty, coronary stent implantation). ACCF, AHA, and the Society for Cardiovascular Angiography and Interventions (SCAI) recommend pretreatment with aspirin (81–325 mg in those already receiving long-term aspirin therapy, otherwise 325 mg as non-enteric-coated aspirin) at least 2, and preferably 24, hours before the procedure. In addition to aspirin, a loading dose of a P2Y12-receptor antagonist (clopidogrel, prasugrel, or ticagrelor) is recommended in patients undergoing PCI with stent placement. Aspirin should be continued indefinitely after PCI, while a P2Y12-receptor antagonist generally should be continued for at least 12 months following stent placement.

In patients with anterior MI and left ventricular thrombus (or at high risk for left ventricular thrombus) who undergo stent placement, ACCP suggests the use of warfarin and clopidogrel in addition to aspirin therapy; the recommended duration of such triple antithrombotic therapy is dependent on whether the patient has a bare-metal or drug-eluting stent. However, such triple antithrombotic regimens are associated with an increased risk of bleeding.

An increased incidence of late stent thrombosis has been reported in patients with drug-eluting stents, often coincident with discontinuance of clopidogrel after initially recommended durations of dual-drug antiplatelet therapy. Stent thrombosis can be a catastrophic event leading to MI and/or death, and a broad range of experts currently recommend that dual-drug therapy with aspirin and a P2Y12-receptor antagonist (e.g., clopidogrel, prasugrel, ticagrelor) be continued for at least 12 months in patients with any type of coronary artery stent (drug-eluting or bare-metal) who are not at high risk of bleeding. Some evidence suggests that an even longer duration of dual antiplatelet therapy (more than 12 months) may be beneficial in some patients with drug-eluting stents, but such prolonged therapy may be associated with a higher risk of bleeding and other adverse effects. (See Uses: Prevention of Stent Thrombosis, in Clopidogrel 20:12.18.)

Aspirin is used to prevent reocclusion of the aortocoronary bypass graft in patients undergoing coronary revascularization procedures (e.g., CABG), and there is some evidence indicating that early (within 48 hours) administration of aspirin (75–325 mg daily) after CABG also is associated with a substantially reduced risk of both fatal and nonfatal (e.g., ischemic complications) outcomes in patients undergoing saphenous vein CABG. In a multicenter, prospective, longitudinal study, data on nonfatal and fatal outcomes (e.g., MI, heart failure, stroke, renal dysfunction or failure, GI ischemia or infarction) were recorded for patients with CHD who were refractory to medical therapy and who underwent CABG. Use of aspirin (total dose of 80–650 mg) within the first 48 hours following CABG was associated with a reduction in overall mortality during hospitalization of about 68% and reductions of 48, 50, 74, and 62% in the incidences of MI, stroke, renal failure, and bowel infarction, respectively. Duration of hospitalization also was shorter in patients receiving aspirin compared to those who did not (9.5 versus 11.5 days, respectively). Aspirin use was not associated with an increased risk of bleeding, gastritis, infection, or impaired wound healing. Subset analysis of data suggested that discontinuance of aspirin use prior to CABG and institution of hemostatic therapies (e.g., platelet transfusions, antifibrinolytic agents) during the perioperative period (i.e., during reperfusion following CABG) was associated with an increased risk of mortality and ischemic complications.

Some clinicians suggest that early administration of aspirin now be considered standard therapy in all patients undergoing CABG, including internal mammary artery bypass grafting, unless specifically contraindicated. AHA and ACCF recommend that aspirin therapy be initiated within 6 hours after CABG and continued for up to 1 year to reduce saphenous vein graft closure; aspirin dosages of 100–325 mg daily appear to be effective for this use. For long-term therapy after 1 year, ACCP recommends the use of low-dose aspirin in all patients with established coronary artery disease, including those with prior CABG. There are some data suggesting that an aspirin dosage not exceeding 75–81 mg daily may be sufficient for long-term cardiovascular prevention and is associated with less GI bleeding risk.

Aspirin has been used in combination with dipyridamole to prevent thrombosis in vein grafts in patients who undergo aortocoronary-artery bypass. However, dipyridamole does not appear to enhance the efficacy of aspirin, regardless of aspirin dosage, in patients receiving saphenous vein or internal mammary artery grafts.

Embolism Associated with Atrial Fibrillation Antiplatelet agents (e.g., aspirin) have been used as an alternative or adjunct to warfarin therapy to reduce the incidence of thromboembolic episodes in selected patients with chronic atrial fibrillation†. ACC, AHA, ACCP, ASA, and other experts currently recommend that antithrombotic therapy be administered to all patients with nonvalvular atrial fibrillation (i.e., atrial fibrillation in the absence of rheumatic mitral stenosis, a prosthetic heart valve, or mitral valve repair) who are considered to be at increased risk of stroke, unless such therapy is contraindicated.

Recommendations regarding choice of antithrombotic therapy in patients with atrial fibrillation are based on the patient's risk for stroke and bleeding. In general, oral anticoagulant therapy (traditionally warfarin) is recommended in patients with atrial fibrillation who have a high risk for stroke and acceptably low risk of bleeding, while aspirin or no antithrombotic therapy may be considered in patients at low risk of stroke. Although many risk stratification methods have been used, patients considered to be at increased risk of stroke generally include those with prior ischemic stroke or TIA, advanced age (e.g., 75 years or older), history of hypertension, diabetes mellitus, or congestive heart failure. In addition, population-based studies suggest that female sex is an important risk factor for stroke in patients with atrial fibrillation, particularly in patients 75 years of age or older, and AHA and ASA recommend the use of risk stratification tools that account for age- and sex-specific differences in stroke risk. One such tool is the CHA_2DS_2-VASc score, an extension of the $CHADS_2$ system (which considers the risk factors congestive heart failure, hypertension, age 75 years or older, diabetes mellitus, and prior stroke/TIA) that adds extra points for female sex (1 point); previous MI, peripheral arterial disease, or aortic plaque (1 point); and age 65–74 years (1 point) or 75 years or older (2 points). Pooled analyses of data from a number of comparative studies evaluating therapy with a coumarin derivative (e.g., warfarin) or aspirin suggest that warfarin therapy is more effective than aspirin in reducing thromboembolic complications (e.g., TIAs, ischemic stroke) in patients with atrial fibrillation. However, the anticipated greater benefit of warfarin compared with aspirin must be weighed against the greater risk of bleeding with warfarin. Because the net clinical benefit with warfarin relative to aspirin appears to be greatest in patients with a high (and possibly also intermediate) risk of stroke, ACCP and other experts recommend the use of warfarin (target INR 2–3) over aspirin in such patients. Some experts also suggest that a non-vitamin K antagonist oral anticoagulant (e.g., apixaban, dabigatran, rivaroxaban) may provide certain advantages over warfarin (e.g., rapid onset of action, predictable anticoagulant effect, no requirement for coagulation monitoring, less potential for drug-drug and drug-food interactions) and may be considered as alternative therapy to warfarin in selected patients. (See Uses: Embolism Associated with Atrial Fibrillation, in Apixaban 20:12.04.14.) For patients at low risk of stroke, the expected benefits of warfarin may not outweigh the risks of bleeding, and thus, aspirin is preferred.

Results of a study comparing dual antiplatelet therapy (clopidogrel and aspirin) with aspirin in patients with atrial fibrillation who had an increased risk of stroke but were unable to take warfarin showed that the combination of clopidogrel and aspirin was more effective than aspirin in reducing the risk of stroke; however, such dual antiplatelet therapy was associated with an increased risk of bleeding. Based on these findings, ACCP and other experts recommend the use of clopidogrel and aspirin rather than aspirin alone as an alternative to warfarin in patients with atrial fibrillation at increased risk of stroke who cannot take or choose not to take warfarin (e.g., those with difficulty maintaining stable INRs).

The risk of thromboembolism in patients with atrial flutter is not as well established as it is in those with atrial fibrillation. In addition, many patients with atrial flutter have alternating periods of atrial fibrillation. Experts state that antithrombotic therapy in patients with atrial flutter generally should be managed in the same manner as in patients with atrial fibrillation.

Peripheral Arterial Disease Aspirin also has been used for primary and secondary prophylaxis of cardiovascular events in patients with peripheral arterial disease, including those with intermittent claudication or carotid artery stenosis and those undergoing revascularization procedures (peripheral artery percutaneous transluminal angioplasty or peripheral arterial bypass graft surgery, carotid endarterectomy). ACCP recommendations for the use of aspirin in patients with peripheral arterial disease are largely similar to those in patients with coronary arterial disease. In general, aspirin is suggested in patients with asymptomatic disease (primary prevention) because of some evidence demonstrating a slight reduction in total mortality when the drug is taken over a period of 10 years. For patients with symptomatic peripheral arterial disease or those undergoing revascularization procedures, single-drug antiplatelet therapy with aspirin or clopidogrel is recommended; dual antiplatelet therapy with aspirin and clopidogrel generally is not suggested except in patients receiving below-the-knee prosthetic bypass grafts. AHA and ASA state that unless contraindicated, aspirin is recommended in patients who are to undergo carotid endarterectomy because aspirin was used in every trial that demonstrated the efficacy of this procedure. Aspirin or the combination of aspirin and dipyridamole also are recommended as 2 of several options for long-term antiplatelet therapy in patients with symptomatic carotid stenosis†, including those who have undergone recent carotid endarterectomy.

Although aspirin has generally been ineffective in preventing thrombosis after arterial catheterization, a single 600-mg oral dose the evening before surgery has been reported to reduce the incidence of thrombosis following radial-artery catheterization for surgery.

Valvular Heart Disease In selected patients with mitral valve prolapse and atrial fibrillation (i.e., those younger than 65 years of age who have no history of mitral valve regurgitation, hypertension, or heart failure), aspirin therapy (e.g., 75–325 mg daily) is recommended by ACC and AHA. Aspirin also is recommended for symptomatic patients with mitral valve prolapse who experience a TIA.

Prosthetic Heart Valves Aspirin is used for the prevention of thromboembolism in selected patients with prosthetic heart valves†. Warfarin generally is recommended in patients with *mechanical* heart valves because of the high risk of thromboembolism associated with these valves. In patients with a *bioprosthetic* heart valve in the aortic position who are in sinus rhythm and who have no other indications for warfarin, ACCP and ACC/AHA suggest the use of low-dose aspirin (50–100 mg daily) for initial (i.e., first 3 months after valve insertion) and long-term antithrombotic therapy. Warfarin therapy is suggested by ACCP in patients with bioprosthetic heart valves in the mitral position, at least for the first 3 months after valve insertion; after the first 3 months, aspirin may be substituted for warfarin therapy, provided the patient is in normal sinus rhythm.

Because warfarin therapy alone does not completely prevent thrombosis in patients with prosthetic mechanical heart valves†, aspirin has been used in conjunction with warfarin to reduce the incidence of thrombosis in these patients. The combination of aspirin and warfarin appears to be more effective than warfarin alone in patients with prosthetic mechanical valves, but the risk of bleeding complications may be increased. Pooled analysis of several randomized, controlled studies comparing combined therapy with an antiplatelet agent (aspirin or dipyridamole) and an oral anticoagulant (e.g., warfarin) versus oral anticoagulant monotherapy in patients who had received mechanical prosthetic heart valves showed that combined therapy substantially reduced systemic thromboembolism (principally manifested as stroke) and overall mortality compared with oral anticoagulant therapy alone; however, the risk of bleeding complications (e.g., hemorrhage, major GI hemorrhage) also was increased with combined therapy. In this analysis, it was estimated that for every 1.6 patients who had stroke prevented by combined therapy, there was an excess of one major GI bleeding episode, suggesting that the benefits derived from enhanced antithrombotic activity outweigh the risks resulting from enhanced bleeding potential. Subgroup analyses also showed that such benefits occur when only studies in which combined aspirin and oral anticoagulant therapy were considered, but that the increased risk of bleeding occurred mainly in patients receiving an oral anticoagulant combined with aspirin rather than with dipyridamole. Of 4 studies involving aspirin, 3 employed moderate (500 mg daily) or high (1 g daily) aspirin dosages, with the remaining one employing a low dosage of 100 mg daily.

Based on current evidence, ACCP and other experts recommend the addition of an antiplatelet agent such as low-dose aspirin to warfarin therapy in all patients with mechanical heart valves who are at low risk of bleeding. Combination therapy with aspirin and warfarin also is recommended by ACC/AHA in patients with bioprosthetic heart valves who have additional risk factors for thrombosis (e.g., atrial fibrillation, previous thromboembolism, left ventricular dysfunction, hypercoagulable condition).

In pregnant women with prosthetic heart valves, a low molecular weight heparin or unfractionated heparin is substituted for warfarin because of concerns about warfarin embryopathy. Based on extrapolation of data from nonpregnant patients with prosthetic heart valves, aspirin (75–100 mg daily) may be added to therapy with a low molecular weight heparin or unfractionated heparin in pregnant women with prosthetic heart valves who are at high risk for thrombosis.

In patients with a prosthetic heart valve receiving long-term oral antithrombotic therapy (warfarin and/or aspirin) who require surgical procedures, the risk of perioperative bleeding should be weighed against the increased risk of thromboembolism that may occur as a result of temporary discontinuance of oral antithrombotic therapy. Oral antithrombotic therapy generally should not be discontinued for procedures in which bleeding is unlikely or inconsequential, such as minor dental, dermatologic, or ophthalmologic procedures.

Thrombosis Associated with Heart Surgery in Children ACCP recommends aspirin (1–5 mg/kg daily) or unfractionated heparin followed by warfarin for the prevention of thromboembolic complications in children undergoing Fontan surgery† (the definitive palliative surgical treatment for most congenital univentricular heart lesions). However, despite even aggressive antithrombotic therapy in children who have undergone the Fontan procedure, thromboembolic events associated with the procedure result in a high mortality rate and respond to therapy in less than 50% of patients. There currently is no consensus on the optimal type or duration of antithrombotic therapy following Fontan surgery, and a wide variety of prophylactic regimens currently are in use.

Venous Thromboembolism **Thromboprophylaxis in Orthopedic Surgery.** Aspirin has been used for the prevention of venous thromboembolism in patients undergoing major orthopedic surgery (total-hip replacement†, total-knee replacement†, or hip-fracture surgery†). Although aspirin generally is not considered the drug of choice for this use, there is some evidence suggesting that aspirin may provide some benefit over placebo or no antithrombotic prophylaxis in patients undergoing major orthopedic surgery. (See Hip-Replacement, Knee-Replacement, or Hip-Fracture Surgery under Venous Thromboembolism: Prophylaxis, in Uses in Enoxaparin 20:12.04.16.) Results of a large, randomized placebo-controlled study (The Randomized Placebo-controlled Pulmonary Embolism Prevention [PEP] Trial) in patients undergoing hip-fracture surgery or elective arthroplasty showed that aspirin was associated with a modest reduction in the risk of symptomatic deep-vein thrombosis at the expense of a possible increased risk of major bleeding and nonfatal MI. Based on these findings, ACCP considers the use of aspirin to be an acceptable option for pharmacologic thromboprophylaxis in patients undergoing major orthopedic surgery. When selecting an appropriate thromboprophylaxis regimen, ACCP states that factors such as relative efficacy and bleeding risk as well as logistics and compliance issues should be considered. For additional information on the prevention of venous thromboembolism in patients undergoing major orthopedic surgery, consult the most recent ACCP Evidence-based Clinical Practice Guidelines on Antithrombotic Therapy and Prevention of Thrombosis available at http://www.chestnet.org.

Thromboprophylaxis in General Surgery. Aspirin also has been used for thromboprophylaxis in patients undergoing general (e.g., abdominal) surgery who are at high risk of venous thromboembolism. If pharmacologic prophylaxis is indicated in such patients undergoing general surgery, ACCP states that a low molecular weight heparin or low-dose unfractionated heparin is preferred, but when these agents are contraindicated or not available, aspirin or fondaparinux may be considered.

For additional information on the prevention of venous thromboembolism in patients undergoing surgery, consult the most recent ACCP Evidence-based Clinical Practice Guidelines on Antithrombotic Therapy and Prevention of Thrombosis available at http://www.chestnet.org.

Pericarditis In addition to its use for reducing the risk of death and/or nonfatal recurrent MI (secondary prevention) (see Coronary Artery Disease and Myocardial Infarction under Uses: Thrombosis), aspirin also is used for the treatment of pain associated with acute pericarditis that develops after an acute MI.

ACCF and AHA recommend that pericarditis be considered in the differential diagnosis of recurrent chest pain after STEMI. Pericarditis probably is not responsible for clinically important chest pain during the initial 24 hours after infarction and may not become evident for up to several weeks after an acute MI. Recurrent pain occurring during the initial 12 hours after onset of infarction usually is considered related to the original infarction itself. Pericarditis in acute MI occurs with extension of myocardial necrosis throughout the epicardial wall. The Multicenter Investigation of the Limitation of Infarct Size (MILIS) study found that pericarditis (defined as presence of pericardial friction rub) occurred in about 20% of patients following acute MI. In patients not treated with thrombolytic therapy, pericarditis occurs in about 25% of patients as evidenced by either typical symptoms or pericardial friction rub, but the incidence averages only 14% when the presence of a friction rub is required for diagnosis. Patients with pericarditis have larger infarcts, lower ejection fractions, and a higher incidence of congestive heart failure. Although anterior chest discomfort mimicking ischemia can occur with pericarditis, pericardial pain usually exhibits distinguishing characteristics, including pleural or positional discomfort; radiation to the left shoulder, scapula, or trapezius muscle; and a pericardial rub, ECG J-point elevation with concave upward ST-segment elevation, and PR depression. It is important to distinguish between pain caused by pericarditis and that caused by ischemia since management will differ. On occasion, pericarditis may be a clinical clue to the presence of subacute myocardial rupture. Although pericarditis is not an absolute contraindication to anticoagulation, ACCF and AHA state that anticoagulation therapy should be used with caution due to the potential for hemorrhagic conversion.

In one study, the effects of 2.6 g of oral aspirin daily were comparable to those of 100–200 mg of oral indomethacin daily, with either drug relieving symptoms within 48 hours. Although other NSAIAs (e.g., indomethacin, ibuprofen) or corticosteroids also can provide symptomatic relief, these drugs may be associated with adverse cardiac effects (e.g., increased coronary vascular resistance, thinning of the developing scar, myocardial rupture). The possibility that cardiac rupture, which occurs in about 1–4% of patients hospitalized for acute MI, may account for recurrent pain should be considered since use of NSAIAs may be a risk factor in its development. ACCF and AHA state the administration of acetaminophen, colchicine, or opiate analgesics may be reasonable if pain relief with aspirin therapy is ineffective.

Kawasaki Disease The American Academy of Pediatrics (AAP), AHA, and ACCP recommend aspirin therapy used in conjunction with immune globulin IV (IGIV) for initial treatment of the acute phase of Kawasaki disease†; aspirin also is used alone or in conjunction with other antiplatelet agents or anticoagulants for follow-up treatment.

High-dose aspirin therapy (80–100 mg/kg daily for up to 14 days) combined with a single dose of IGIV (2 g/kg) initiated within 10 days of the onset of fever is more effective than aspirin therapy alone for preventing or reducing the occurrence of coronary artery aneurysms associated with Kawasaki disease; fever and other manifestations of inflammation also may resolve more rapidly with concomitant therapy. Aspirin then is continued alone in lower dosages (i.e., 1–5 mg/kg daily) for antiplatelet effects for 6–8 weeks in those without coronary artery changes or with only transient coronary artery ectasia or dilatation (disappearing within the initial 6–8 weeks of illness). For additional information on initial treatment of Kawasaki disease, see Uses: Kawasaki Disease and see Kawasaki Disease under Dosage and Administration: Dosage for Immune Globulin IV, in Immune Globulin 80:04.

Coronary artery abnormalities develop in 15–25% of children with Kawasaki disease if they are not treated within 10 days of onset of fever; 2–4% of patients develop coronary artery abnormalities despite prompt treatment with aspirin and IGIV. Long-term management of those who develop coronary abnormalities depends on the severity of coronary involvement and may include low-dose aspirin (with or without clopidogrel or dipyridamole), anticoagulant therapy with warfarin or low molecular weight heparin, or a combination of antiplatelet and anticoagulant therapy (usually low-dose aspirin and warfarin). If giant coronary aneurysms are present, AHA and ACCP suggest long-term low-dose aspirin therapy in conjunction with warfarin for primary thromboprophylaxis. Specialized references should be consulted for additional information on long-term management of Kawasaki disease in individuals with coronary abnormalities.

Complications of Pregnancy Aspirin should be used during pregnancy only when clearly needed, weighing carefully the potential benefits versus the possible risks to the mother and fetus. (See Cautions: Pregnancy, Fertility, and Lactation, in the Salicylates General Statement 28:08.04.24.) Aspirin has been used alone or in combination with other drugs (e.g., unfractionated heparin, low molecular weight heparins, corticosteroids, immune globulin) for the prevention of complications of pregnancy† (e.g., preeclampsia, pregnancy loss in women with a history of antiphospholipid syndrome and recurrent fetal loss). Maternal and fetal hemorrhagic complications observed with maternal ingestion of large dosages (e.g., 12–15 g daily) of aspirin generally have not been observed in studies in which dosages of 50–150 mg daily of the drug were used during the second and third trimesters for prevention of complications of pregnancy (e.g., preeclampsia, recurrent spontaneous abortions, prematurity, intrauterine growth retardation, stillbirth, low birthweight), including those associated with autoimmune disorders such as antiphospholipid syndrome, poor paternal blocking antibody production, or systemic lupus erythematosus.

Results of several controlled studies suggest that low dosages of aspirin administered from preconception through delivery alone or in combination with heparin or corticosteroids in high-risk women may prevent the development of preeclampsia and fetal growth retardation and reduce perinatal death, possibly by suppressing thromboxane A_2-mediated vasospasm, ischemia, and thrombosis. The presence of maternal antiphospholipid antibodies is associated with an increased risk of thrombosis and pregnancy loss. Data from several small comparative studies indicate that combined prophylaxis with heparin and low dosages of aspirin may be more effective than aspirin alone or aspirin combined with a corticosteroid in preventing recurrent pregnancy loss (fetal death, miscarriage), preeclampsia, or premature delivery in women with antiphospholipid syndrome (Hughes syndrome). In at least one study in women with antiphospholipid antibodies and at least 2 prior pregnancy losses, combined aspirin (100 mg daily) and corticosteroid (prednisone 0.5–0.8 mg/kg daily) therapy was not effective in promoting live birth and was associated with an increased risk of prematurity. The beneficial effect of prophylactic therapy with aspirin and heparin may result from aspirin-induced suppression of thromboxane$_2$-mediated vasospasm, ischemia, and thrombosis in the placental vasculature and by heparin-induced anticoagulation combined with binding to phospholipid antibodies that protects the trophoblast from antibody attack and thus promotes successful implantation in early pregnancy.

Women with antiphospholipid syndrome and a history of multiple pregnancy losses are candidates for prophylactic therapy†, and most experts currently recommend combined prophylactic therapy with low dosages of aspirin and unfractionated heparin or low molecular weight heparin, followed by postpartum warfarin therapy. ACCP states that women with antiphospholipid antibody (APLA) syndrome and a history of multiple pregnancy losses (at least 3) should receive antepartum prophylaxis with low-dose aspirin in combination with subcutaneous unfractionated heparin or a low molecular weight heparin. (See Uses: Thromboembolism Occurring During Pregnancy, in Enoxaparin 20:12.04.16.)

Because of experience in women with antiphospholipid syndrome, aspirin and heparin (often combined with immune globulin) also have been used to prevent venous thromboembolism and early pregnancy loss in women who have undergone in vitro fertilization†. However, current evidence suggests that the overall absolute risk of symptomatic thrombosis appears to be low in women undergoing in vitro fertilization. Therefore, ACCP recommends against routine thromboprophylaxis in most women undergoing assisted reproduction.

Aspirin in low dosages throughout pregnancy also has been used to prevent preeclampsia† in pregnant women at high risk, including those with pregestational diabetes mellitus, obesity, age exceeding 40 years, chronic hypertension, nulliparity, multifetal gestations, preexisting vascular disease, collagen vascular disease, renal disease, and/or antiphospholipid syndrome (see preceding discussion), and those with a history of preeclampsia during prior pregnancy. The rationale for aspirin prophylaxis is that hypertension and coagulation abnormalities in preeclampsia are caused in part by an imbalance between vasodilating and vasoconstricting prostaglandins (prostacyclin and thromboxane A_2, respectively); by preferentially inhibiting thromboxane A_2 production at low doses, aspirin was postulated to provide some protection against the abnormalities associated with preeclampsia. Some clinicians have suggested that prophylaxis with low dosages of aspirin be considered in selected high-risk women (e.g., those with chronic hypertension, a history of early or recurrent preeclampsia, diabetes mellitus, underlying renal disease, high body mass index, those 35 years of age or older) who do not have thrombophilia.

Systematic reviews involving large numbers of patients have suggested beneficial effects of low-dose aspirin on preeclampsia and its complications. In a systematic review based on pooled data in more than 12,000 women with historical risk factors for preeclampsia, aspirin prophylaxis (generally 50–150 mg daily) was associated with a reduction of about 15% in the risk of preeclampsia and also some benefit on perinatal death, spontaneous preterm birth, and birth weight. Another systematic review in more than 30,000 women receiving prophylaxis with antiplatelet drugs (usually aspirin in a dosage of up to 75 mg daily) demonstrated similar findings. Neither of these reviews found evidence of a harmful effect of aspirin prophylaxis in these women. ACCP, AHA, and ASA recommend the use of low-dose aspirin during pregnancy (starting from the second trimester) in women who are at high risk for preeclampsia, including those with chronic primary or secondary hypertension or previous pregnancy-related hypertension.

Prevention of Cancer While data principally from observational studies suggest that aspirin or other NSAIAs may reduce the risk of various cancers† (e.g., colorectal, breast, gastric), results of several randomized, placebo-controlled studies generally have not confirmed these observations. A large, long-term randomized study (Women's Health Study) in women with no history of cancer or cardiovascular disease indicated *no* reduction in the risk of developing cancer overall or at specific sites, including breast, colorectal, or lung cancer, with use of low dosages of aspirin (100 mg every other day). In this study, approximately 40,000 predominantly middle-aged (mean age 54.6 years at study entry) women received aspirin or placebo in a 2 x 2 factorial design (patients also were randomized to receive vitamin E or placebo as part of the study; no effect of the vitamin E treatment arm was noted on the aspirin results); patients received aspirin for an average of 10 years. Aspirin use also was not associated with a reduction in overall cancer mortality, including deaths due to breast or colorectal cancer. However, a statistically significant reduction in lung cancer *mortality* and a trend toward a reduction in the risk of lung cancer were noted in patients taking aspirin. Given the variability of aspirin's effects on lung cancer reported in other trials, it has been suggested that the positive findings in this study may be due to chance; however, data from this study cannot rule out a protective effect of aspirin on lung cancer.

Observational studies and a few randomized, placebo-controlled trials in patients with a history of colorectal adenomas have shown a reduction in the risk of recurrent colorectal adenomas† with regular (e.g., daily) use of aspirin or other NSAIAs. However, evidence that aspirin and other NSAIAs prevent colorectal *cancer* itself currently is based principally on observational studies, and available data suggest that beneficial effects on cancer may only be evident following at least a decade of regular aspirin therapy. Almost all evidence indicates that the beneficial effects of NSAIAs in reducing colorectal cancer risk dissipate following discontinuance of NSAIA therapy. Current data suggest that the potential clinical benefits of aspirin for primary or secondary prevention of colorectal cancer may be small considering the efficacy of screening and removal of colorectal adenomas in preventing cancer and the risks of bleeding complications associated with long-term aspirin therapy in patients at average risk for colorectal cancer. Therefore, most clinicians state that such preventive therapy with aspirin currently is not recommended and, because randomized trials indicate that aspirin does not completely eliminate adenomas, it should not be considered a replacement for colorectal cancer screening and surveillance. Further studies are necessary to determine whether aspirin therapy can lessen the required intensity or frequency of such surveillance measures. Certain other NSAIAs, particularly selective inhibitors of cyclooxygenase-2 (COX-2) (e.g., celecoxib), currently are used as adjunctive therapy to reduce the number of colorectal polyps in patients with familial adenomatous polyposis; such patients are at particularly high risk for developing colorectal cancer. (See Uses: Colorectal Polyps, in Celecoxib 28:08.04.08.)

Epidemiologic studies have consistently demonstrated a 40–50% reduction in the risk of colorectal neoplasia with aspirin use that is not explained by differences in study design, study populations, patterns of aspirin use, or outcomes. The mechanism by which aspirin and other NSAIAs prevent the development of colorectal adenomas or neoplasms has not been fully elucidated, but some evidence suggests that NSAIAs may restore apoptosis in adenomatous colorectal polyps and/or inhibit angiogenesis, both through COX-2 inhibition and COX-independent mechanisms. (See Pharmacology: GI Effects, in Celecoxib 28:08.04.08.) Since most colorectal cancers arise from benign adenomas but have a long latency period (e.g., 5–10 years), prevention of adenomas has been used as a surrogate end point in clinical prevention trials of colorectal cancer. Several randomized, placebo-controlled trials involving patients with prior colorectal neoplasia have demonstrated reductions in the incidence of recurrent colorectal adenomas with regular use of aspirin.

Dosage and Administration

■ Administration Aspirin is usually administered orally, preferably with food or a large quantity (240 mL) of water (unless the patient is fluid restricted) or milk to minimize gastric irritation. In patients unable to take or retain oral medication, aspirin suppositories may be administered rectally; however, rectal absorption may be slow and incomplete. (See Pharmacokinetics: Absorption.) *Aspirin tablets should not be administered rectally, since they are likely to cause irritation and erosion of the rectal mucosa.* Aspirin preparations should not be used if a strong vinegar-like odor is present. (See Chemistry and Stability: Stability.)

If an unpleasant taste or aftertaste, burning in the throat, or difficulty in swallowing occurs with uncoated aspirin-containing tablets, these effects may be reduced with film-coated tablets. Although specific data are not available, these effects are also likely to be reduced with enteric-coated tablets. If gastric irritation and/or symptomatic GI disturbances occur with uncoated aspirin-containing tablets, these effects may be reduced with enteric-coated tablets or extended-release tablets. If a liquid dosage form of aspirin is desired for short-term treatment of pain, an oral solution may be prepared from commercially available effervescent tablets (e.g., Alka-Seltzer®) by dissolving tablets in 120 mL of water; ingest the entire solution to ensure adequate dosing.

In addition to potentially reducing adverse GI effects, some clinicians suggest that enteric-coated tablets may be swallowed more easily by children receiving chronic therapy with the drug and may therefore result in increased compliance.

Aspirin or buffered aspirin preparations should not be chewed before swallowing for at least 7 days following tonsillectomy or oral surgery because of possible injury to oral tissues from prolonged contact with aspirin particles. In addition, aspirin or buffered aspirin tablets should not be placed directly on a tooth or gum surface because of possible injury to tissues.

Capsules containing the fixed combination of aspirin and extended-release dipyridamole should be swallowed whole and should not be chewed.

Chewable aspirin tablets may be chewed, crushed, and/or dissolved in a liquid, or swallowed whole, followed by approximately 120 mL of water, milk, or fruit juice immediately after administration of the drug.

For information on the concomitant administration of aspirin with nonsteroidal anti-inflammatory agents (NSAIAs), see Drug Interactions: Nonsteroidal Anti-inflammatory Agents, in the Salicylates General Statement 28:08.04.24.

■ Dosage Dosage of aspirin must be carefully adjusted according to individual requirements and response, using the lowest possible effective dosage. When used at high (e.g., anti-inflammatory) dosages, the development of tinnitus can be used as a sign of elevated serum salicylate concentrations, except in patients with high-frequency hearing impairment.

When preparations containing aspirin in fixed combination with other drugs are used, the cautions, precautions, and contraindications applicable to each ingredient must be considered.

Pain and Fever Aspirin should not be used for *self-medication* of pain for longer than 10 days in adults or 5 days in children, unless directed by a physician, since pain of such intensity and duration may indicate a pathologic condition requiring medical evaluation and supervised treatment. Aspirin, including chewing gum pieces, should not be used for *self-medication* of sore throat pain for longer than 2 days in adults or children, unless directed by a physician, since prolonged use could cause mucosal erosions in the mouth. Patients should be warned that the risk of GI bleeding is increased in geriatric patients 60 years of age or older, in patients with a history of GI ulcers or bleeding, when recommended dosages and durations of *self-medication* are exceeded, when anticoagulants or corticosteroids are used concomitantly, in patients receiving more than one NSAIA, and in those consuming 3 or more alcohol-containing beverages daily. (See Cautions: GI Effects, in the Salicylates General Statement 28:08.04.24)

Aspirin should not be used in adults or children for *self-medication* of marked fever (exceeding 39.5°C), fever persisting longer than 3 days, or recurrent fever, unless directed by a physician, since such fevers may indicate serious illness requiring prompt medical evaluation.

Aspirin should not be used in adults or children for *self-medication* of sore throat for longer than 2 days, and should be discontinued and a clinician consulted if sore throat persists or is accompanied by fever, headache, rash, nausea, or vomiting.

To minimize the risk of overdosage, no more than 5 doses of aspirin should be administered to children for analgesia or antipyresis in any 24-hour period, unless directed by a physician.

For analgesia or antipyresis in adults or children older than 12 years of age, the usual oral or rectal dosage of aspirin is 324–650 mg every 4 hours as necessary, but should not exceed 3.9 g daily; higher single doses (e.g., 975 mg or 1 g) may be useful for analgesia in some patients. If a rapid response is required, the more slowly absorbed dosage forms (i.e., enteric-coated, extended-release tablets) should not be used. In children 2–11 years of age, the usual oral or rectal dosage for analgesia or antipyresis is 1.5 g/m^2 daily, administered in 4–6 divided doses; total daily rectal dosage should not exceed 2.5 g/m^2. Alternatively, children may receive the following *approximate* oral or rectal doses every 4 hours as necessary: children 11–12 years of age, 320–480 mg; children 9–11 years of age, 320–400 mg; children 6–7 years of age, 320–325 mg; children 4–6 years of age, 240 mg; and children 2–4 years of age, 160 mg. Dosage in children younger than 2 years of age must be individualized.

The usual dosage of aspirin (as chewing gum pieces) for analgesia and antipyresis in adults and children older than 12 years of age is 454 mg, repeated every 4 hours as necessary (maximum 3.632 g daily). The chewing gum pieces should be thoroughly chewed for about 15 minutes to ensure adequate dosing and then the gum should be expelled from the mouth and discarded. Children 6–12 years of age may be given 227–454 mg, repeated as necessary up to 4 times daily. Children 3–6 years of age may be given 227 mg, repeated as necessary up to 3 times daily. Aspirin chewing gum pieces should not be used in children younger than 3 years of age unless directed by a physician; dosage must be individualized.

The usual oral dosage of aspirin as a highly buffered effervescent solution (Alka-Seltzer® Original, Lemon-Lime) for analgesia in adults and children 12 years of age or older is 650 mg every 4 hours as necessary; total dosage in any 24-hour period should not exceed 2.6 g. Alternatively, in adults and children 12 years of age or older, the usual dosage of Alka-Seltzer Extra Strength is 1 g every 6 hours; total dosage in any 24-hour period should not exceed 3.5 g Because of the high sodium content of this preparation (approximately 24 mEq of sodium per 325 mg of aspirin), it should be used with extreme caution, if at all, in patients in whom excessive amounts of sodium may be harmful. The usual oral dosage of aspirin (Alka-Seltzer® lemon-Lime or Original) for patients 60 years of age or older is 650 mg every 4 hours as necessary, not to exceed 1.3 g in any 24-hour period. The usual dosage of aspirin (Alka-Seltzer® Extra Strength) for patients 60 years of age or older is 1 g every 6 hours; total dosage in any 24-hour period should not exceed 2 g. The manufacturer states that the preparation should not be used in children younger than 12 years of age unless directed by a physician. In addition, higher than usually recommended dosages of this preparation should not be used unless directed by a physician.

The usual oral dosage of aspirin (as 650-mg extended-release tablets) for analgesia in adults is 650 mg to 1.3 g every 8 hours as necessary, not to exceed 3.9 g daily. For patients who have difficulty swallowing the 650-mg tablets whole, the tablets may be gently broken or crumbled before administration (or in the mouth), but they must *not* be ground up if they are to retain the property of extended release. An 800-mg extended-release aspirin tablet is also commercially available but is indicated for use only in the symptomatic treatment of inflammatory disease; the 800-mg tablet *cannot* be broken or crumbled and must be swallowed whole. Most clinicians believe that extended-release aspirin tablets offer no therapeutic advantage over other types of aspirin tablets; this is particularly true at high dosages since the elimination half-life of salicylate is dose dependent and prolonged at high dosages. However, symptomatic GI disturbances and/or occult GI bleeding may be reduced with extended-release tablets.

For *self-medication* for the temporary relief of mild to moderate pain associated with migraine headache in adults, the recommended oral aspirin dosage is 500 mg (combined with 500 mg of acetaminophen and 130 mg of caffeine) as a single dose of an immediate-release (conventional) preparation taken with a full glass of water; no more than 500 mg of aspirin (in combination with 500 mg of acetaminophen and 130 mg of caffeine) should be taken in a 24-hour period unless directed by a clinician. Individuals younger than 18 years of age should consult their clinician before using this combination preparation. Patients receiving the combination for *self-medication* should be advised to discontinue the drug and consult a clinician if an allergic reaction occurs, if migraine headache pain worsens or persists after the first dose, or if new or unexpected symptoms, including tinnitus (ringing in the ears) or hearing loss, occur.

For temporary relief of acute migraine headache pain and associated symptoms (nausea, vomiting, photophobia, phonophobia) in adults, aspirin 900 or 1000 mg has been given as a single dose with or without metoclopramide 10 mg (as an antiemetic).

Inflammatory Diseases For the symptomatic treatment of rheumatoid arthritis, osteoarthritis, or other polyarthritic or inflammatory conditions (e.g., spondyloarthropathies, arthritis and pleurisy of systemic lupus erythematosus [SLE]), the usual initial adult dosage of aspirin is 2.4–3.6 g daily, administered in divided doses. When necessary, dosage is generally increased by 325 mg to 1.2 g daily at intervals of 1 week or more. The usual adult maintenance dosage is 3.6–5.4 g daily; however, higher dosages may be necessary. Dosage should be adjusted according to the patient's response, tolerance, and serum salicylate concentration. (See Dosage: Inflammatory Diseases under Dosage and Administration, in the Salicylates General Statement 28:08.04.24.)

For the symptomatic treatment of juvenile arthritis, the usual initial dosage is 60–130 mg/kg daily in children weighing 25 kg or less, or 2.4–3.6 g daily in children weighing more than 25 kg, administered in divided doses. Alternatively, some clinicians recommend an initial dosage of 1.5 g/m^2 daily, administered in divided doses. When necessary, dosage is generally increased by 10 mg/kg daily no more frequently than at weekly intervals. The usual maintenance dosage is 80–100 mg/kg daily; up to 130 mg/kg daily may be required in some children. Although some clinicians have reported a high incidence of chronic intoxication in children receiving 90–100 mg/kg daily, this has not been found by many others. However, it appears that dosages of at least 100 mg/kg daily should not be used in children weighing more than 25 kg. Based on body surface area, dosage should generally not exceed 3 g/m² daily. Dosage should be adjusted according to the patient's response, tolerance, and serum salicylate concentration. (See Dosage: Inflammatory Diseases under Dosage and Administration, in the Salicylates General Statement 28:08.04.24.)

Because of the prolonged elimination half-life of salicylate at high dosages, at least 5–7 days are generally required to achieve steady-state serum salicylate concentrations in the treatment of inflammatory diseases. Therefore, some clinicians have suggested that loading-dose regimens of aspirin may be useful to more rapidly attain serum concentrations associated with an anti-inflammatory effect. In one small study, healthy individuals were given oral dosages of 650 mg of aspirin every 4 hours for 4 days (conventional-dose regimen) or two 1.3-g doses 4 hours apart followed 2 hours later by initiation of a maintenance dosage of 650-mg oral doses every 4 hours through 4 days (loading-dose regimen). In this study, the time required to reach a serum salicylate concentration of 150 mcg/mL was approximately 15 hours with the loading-dose regimen and approximately 48 hours with the conventional-dose regimen; serum salicylate concentrations were higher during the first 36 hours with the loading-dose regimen. However, the actual clinical importance of any difference between these regimens in patients with inflammatory diseases is not known; further evaluation of loading-dose regimens in such patients is needed.

Rheumatic Fever For the symptomatic treatment of rheumatic fever†, dosage and duration of aspirin therapy are generally determined by the severity and duration of acute manifestations. For maximal suppression of acute inflammation, the usual initial dosage of aspirin is 4.9–7.8 g daily in adults and 90–130 mg/kg daily in children, administered in divided doses every 4–6 hours. Patients with only polyarthritis and fever usually respond to lower dosages. Subsequent dosage should be adjusted according to the patient's response, tolerance, and serum salicylate concentration. The initial dosage is generally administered for up to 1–2 weeks, then decreased to approximately 60–70 mg/kg daily for 1–6 weeks or as long as necessary, and then gradually withdrawn over 1–2 weeks. Various aspirin regimens have been suggested depending on the severity of acute manifestations, and the clinician should consult published protocols for more information on specific dosages and schedules of administration.

In patients with carditis and cardiomegaly or congestive heart failure who are treated with corticosteroids, aspirin therapy is usually initiated as steroid therapy is gradually withdrawn. In these patients, some clinicians recommend an aspirin dosage of 60 mg/kg daily, administered in divided doses. High dosages should be used with caution in patients with carditis since congestive heart failure or pulmonary edema may be precipitated. Aspirin is usually administered for approximately 2–4 weeks after steroids are discontinued. Only extremely severe clinical rebounds of rheumatic activity require reinstitution of therapy, in which case aspirin is administered in the usual dosage for 3–4 additional weeks.

Thrombosis **Transient Ischemic Attacks and Acute Ischemic Stroke.** For secondary prevention of vascular events (e.g., death, recurrent stroke) in patients with transient ischemic attacks (TIAs) or stroke, the usual oral dosage of aspirin in adults is 50–325 mg daily, continued long term. In patients with noncardioembolic ischemic stroke or TIA, the American College of Chest Physicians (ACCP) recommends an aspirin dosage of 75–100 mg daily, continued long term. While dosages up to 1.3 g daily, administered in 2 or 4 divided doses, have been recommended, there is little evidence supporting superiority of such dosages relative to currently recommended low dosages, and the risk of adverse effects (e.g., GI intolerance, bleeding) is increased with increasing dosage. Current data suggest that an aspirin dosage not exceeding 75–81 mg daily may be sufficient for long-term cardiovascular prevention and is associated with less GI bleeding risk.

For the acute treatment of ischemic stroke in patients who are not receiving a thrombolytic agent, the usual oral dosage of aspirin when given as monotherapy in adults is 150–325 mg initiated within 24–48 hours of stroke onset. In children with acute arterial ischemic stroke†, aspirin 1–5 mg/kg daily is recommended as an option for initial anticoagulation until dissection and embolic causes have been excluded. When cerebral arterial dissection and cardioembolic causes have been excluded, the usual suggested dosage of aspirin for secondary prevention in such children is 1–5 mg/kg daily for a minimum of 2 years. If aspirin is used in children with acute arterial ischemic stroke secondary to non-Moyamoya vasculopathy, ACCP recommends at least 3 months of therapy; ongoing antithrombotic therapy should be determined by repeat cerebrovascular imaging.

When aspirin is given in combination with dipyridamole to reduce the risk of stroke in patients who have had noncardioembolic stroke or TIAs, the usual dosage of aspirin in fixed combination with extended-release dipyridamole (200 mg) is 25 mg (1 capsule) twice daily in the morning and evening.

The American Heart Association (AHA) and American Stroke Association (ASA) state that unless contraindicated, an aspirin dosage of 75–325 mg daily is recommended for *secondary prevention* of ischemic stroke in high-risk women and is reasonable in selected women (e.g., those with diabetes mellitus) for *primary prevention* of ischemic stroke†. (See Transient Ischemic Attacks and Acute Ischemic Stroke under Uses: Thrombosis for definition of high risk.) If the benefit of aspirin for the prevention of ischemic stroke or myocardial infarction (MI) in women is considered to outweigh the risks of therapy, a dosage of 81 mg daily or 100 mg every *other* day has been suggested by AHA and ASA.

Coronary Artery Disease. For the secondary prevention of cardiovascular events in patients with coronary artery disease, a low dosage of aspirin (e.g., 75–162 mg daily) generally is recommended. ACCP recommends long-term, single-drug antiplatelet therapy with aspirin 75–100 mg daily in patients with established coronary artery disease (i.e., 1 year after ACS with prior revascularization, coronary stenosis greater than 50% by coronary angiogram, and/or evidence of cardiac ischemia on diagnostic testing).

ST-Segment-Elevation Myocardial Infarction. As an adjunct in the acute management of suspected acute ST-segment-elevation MI (STEMI), the usual initial adult oral dose of aspirin for prevention of early recurrence or extension of infarction and mortality reduction is 162–325 mg. Such acute aspirin therapy should be initiated as soon as possible after the clinical impression of an evolving acute STEMI is formed, preferably by chewing and/or swallowing a conventional tablet.

Aspirin therapy for the management of STEMI should be continued indefinitely at a dosage of 81–325 mg daily. Some experts prefer the use of a maintenance dosage of 81 mg daily because of a decreased risk of bleeding and lack of definitive evidence demonstrating that higher dosages confer greater benefit. Although higher dosages of aspirin have been used in patients surviving an MI (900 mg to 1.5 g daily in divided doses), lower-dosage regimens appear to be equally effective and may minimize adverse GI effects. Some data suggest that 75–81 mg of aspirin daily is sufficient for long-term cardiovascular disease prevention and is associated with less GI bleeding risk.

In patients with STEMI who have indications for anticoagulation (e.g., atrial fibrillation, left ventricular dysfunction, cerebral emboli, extensive wall-motion abnormality, mechanical heart valves), warfarin (INR 2–3) should be administered in addition to aspirin therapy; in some cases (e.g., patients with an anterior STEMI and left ventricular thrombosis undergoing percutaneous coronary intervention [PCI] with stenting), both warfarin (INR 2–3) and clopidogrel 75 mg daily may be added to aspirin therapy (triple antithrombotic therapy).

For primary prevention† to reduce the risk of atherosclerotic cardiovascular disease (ASCVD), including first STEMI in patients 40–70 years of age at increased risk for ASCVD but without an increased bleeding risk, the usual oral dosage of aspirin is 75–162 mg daily. The efficacy of dosages lower than 75 mg daily has not been established. An oral aspirin dosage of 325 mg every other day has been used but is no longer preferred.

Non-ST-Segment-Elevation Acute Coronary Syndromes. In patients with non-ST-segment-elevation acute coronary syndromes (NSTE ACS), the American College of Cardiology (ACC) and AHA recommend an initial aspirin dose of 162–325 mg as soon as possible after presentation, unless such therapy is contraindicated, followed by a maintenance dosage of 81–325 mg daily. Aspirin should be used in conjunction with a P2Y12-receptor antagonist (e.g., clopidogrel, ticagrelor) for up to 12 months. When used in conjunction with ticagrelor, aspirin should be administered in a maintenance dosage of 75–100 mg daily since aspirin dosages exceeding 100 mg daily have been associated with reduced efficacy of ticagrelor.

Percutaneous Coronary Intervention and Revascularization Procedures. To reduce the incidence of early ischemic complications in patients undergoing PCI (e.g., coronary angioplasty, coronary stent placement), ACCF, AHA, and the Society for Cardiovascular Angiography and Interventions (SCAI) recommend pretreatment with 81–325 mg of aspirin, initiated at least 2, and preferably 24, hours before the procedure. In patients not already receiving long-term aspirin therapy, an aspirin dose of 325 mg (as the non-enteric-coated formulation) initiated at least 2, and preferably 24, hours prior to PCI is recommended.

In addition to aspirin, a loading dose of a P2Y12-receptor antagonist (clopidogrel, prasugrel, or ticagrelor) should be administered in patients with ACS undergoing PCI with stent placement (bare-metal or drug-eluting). Aspirin should be continued indefinitely after PCI, while a P2Y12-receptor antagonist generally should be continued for at least 12 months following placement of an intracoronary stent.

In patients with anterior MI and left ventricular thrombus (or at high risk for left ventricular thrombus) undergoing stent placement, ACCP suggests the use of warfarin (INR 2–3) and clopidogrel 75 mg daily in addition to aspirin therapy; the recommended duration of such triple antithrombotic therapy is dependent on whether the patient has a bare-metal or drug-eluting stent.

When aspirin is used to prevent reocclusion in adults undergoing coronary artery bypass grafting (CABG), ACCF/AHA recommends a dosage of 100–325 mg daily; aspirin should be initiated within 6 hours after surgery and continued for up to 1 year. For long-term therapy after 1 year, ACCP recommends aspirin 75–100 mg daily. There are some data suggesting that an aspirin dosage not exceeding 75–81 mg daily may be sufficient for long-term cardiovascular prevention and is associated with less GI bleeding risk.

Managing Antiplatelet Therapy in Patients Undergoing Invasive Procedures. Temporary interruption of long-term aspirin therapy generally is not necessary for patients undergoing surgery or other invasive procedures. In patients receiving dual antiplatelet therapy (e.g., with aspirin and clopidogrel) who require surgery within 6 weeks of bare-metal stent implantation or within 6 months of drug-eluting stent implantation, ACCP suggests continuation of dual antiplatelet therapy during the periprocedural period. In patients receiving dual antiplatelet therapy (e.g., with aspirin and clopidogrel) who require CABG, interruption of clopidogrel therapy is recommended 5 days prior to surgery; however, aspirin may be continued around the time of surgery in such patients.

For additional information on the perioperative management of antithrombotic therapy, consult the most recent ACCP Evidence-based Clinical Practice Guidelines on Antithrombotic Therapy and Prevention of Thrombosis available at http://www.chestnet.org.

Embolism Associated with Atrial Fibrillation. When aspirin is used for the prevention of thromboembolism in patients with atrial fibrillation†, a dosage of 75–325 mg daily has been suggested.

Experts recommend that atrial flutter† generally be managed in the same manner as atrial fibrillation.

Valvular Heart Disease. Aspirin therapy at a dosage of 75–325 mg daily is recommended by ACC and AHA for selected patients with mitral valve prolapse† (i.e., symptomatic patients who experience a TIA or patients younger than 65 years of age with concurrent atrial fibrillation and no history of mitral valve regurgitation, hypertension, or heart failure).

Peripheral Arterial Disease. To reduce vascular morbidity and mortality in patients with asymptomatic peripheral arterial disease (*primary prevention*), ACCP suggests that aspirin be given a dosage of 75–100 mg daily.

For *secondary prevention* of cardiovascular events in patients with symptomatic peripheral arterial disease, ACCP recommends aspirin 75–100 mg daily. In patients with refractory intermittent claudication, ACCP suggests the use of cilostazol in addition to aspirin therapy.

Peripheral Artery Bypass Graft Surgery. To reduce graft occlusion in patients undergoing peripheral artery bypass graft surgery, aspirin 75–100 mg daily is recommended by ACCP; aspirin should be initiated preoperatively and continued long term. ACCP suggests the addition of clopidogrel 75 mg daily to aspirin therapy in patients undergoing below-the-knee prosthetic graft bypass surgery.

Prosthetic Heart Valves. In patients with a bioprosthetic heart valve† in the aortic position who are in sinus rhythm and who have no other indications for warfarin therapy, ACCP suggests aspirin 50–100 mg daily for initial (i.e., first 3 months after valve insertion) and long-term antithrombotic therapy. Aspirin 50–100 mg daily also may be used for long-term antithrombotic therapy after an initial 3 months of treatment with warfarin in patients with bioprosthetic heart valves in the mitral position. In all patients with a mechanical heart valve who are at low risk of bleeding, ACCP suggests the addition of low-dose aspirin (50–100 mg daily) to warfarin anticoagulation. Combination therapy with aspirin and warfarin also is recommended by ACC/AHA for patients with bioprosthetic heart valves with additional risk factors for thromboembolism.

In pregnant women with prosthetic heart valves who are at high risk for thromboembolism, aspirin (75–100 mg daily) may be added to therapy with a low molecular weight heparin or unfractionated heparin.

Thrombosis Associated with Heart Surgery in Children. Following the Fontan procedure† in children, aspirin in a dosage of 1–5 mg/kg daily is recommended by ACCP; the optimal duration of therapy in such patients is unknown.

Kawasaki Disease For initial treatment of the acute phase of Kawasaki disease†, the American Academy of Pediatrics (AAP), AHA, and ACCP recommend that aspirin therapy be initiated as soon as possible (optimally within 7–10 days of illness) and given in a dosage of 80–100 mg/kg daily in 4 equally divided doses for up to 14 days; a single dose (2 g/kg) of immune globulin IV (IGIV) also should be administered as soon as possible (optimally within 7–10 days of illness). Although absorption of aspirin may be impaired or is highly variable during the initial phase of the illness, AAP states that it is not necessary to monitor aspirin concentrations in most patients.

After the patient has been afebrile for 48 hours or longer (usually about day 14 of illness), the aspirin dosage should be decreased to 1–5 mg/kg once daily to provide antiplatelet effects for prevention of coronary aneurysm, thrombosis, and subsequent infarction. In patients without coronary artery changes or with only transient coronary artery ectasia or dilatation (disappearing within the initial 6–8 weeks of illness), low-dose aspirin therapy usually is discontinued at 6–8 weeks. In those with coronary abnormalities, long-term low-dose aspirin therapy (with or without anticoagulants) may be indicated. (See Uses: Kawasaki Disease.)

Complications of Pregnancy In women with antiphospholipid antibody (APLA) syndrome† and a history of multiple pregnancy losses (at least 3), ACCP recommends antepartum administration of aspirin (75–100 mg daily) plus prophylactic- or intermediate-dose subcutaneous unfractionated heparin or prophylactic-dose low molecular weight heparin.

In women at high risk for preeclampsia, including those with chronic primary or secondary hypertension or previous pregnancy-related hypertension, ACCP, AHA, and the American Stroke Association (ASA) recommend low-dose aspirin during pregnancy, starting from the second trimester.

Pharmacology

Aspirin exhibits analgesic, anti-inflammatory, and antipyretic activity. Although aspirin hydrolyzes to salicylate and acetate, the drug does not require hydrolysis to produce its effects and appears to have some pharmacologic effects that are distinct from those of salicylate. The ability of aspirin to acetylate proteins (e.g., platelet proteins, hormones, DNA, hemoglobin) results in some effects, such as inhibition of platelet aggregation, that other currently available salicylates do not exhibit.

Aspirin acetylates prostaglandin endoperoxide synthase (prostaglandin G/H-synthase) and irreversibly inhibits its cyclooxygenase (COX) activity. The enzyme catalyzes the conversion of arachidonic acid to PGH_2, the first committed step in prostanoid biosynthesis. Two isoforms of prostaglandin endoperoxide synthase exist, PGHS-1 and PGHS-2 (also referred to as COX-1 and COX-2, respectively). PGHS-1 (COX-1) is expressed constitutively in most cell types, including platelets. PGHS-2 (COX-2) is undetectable in most mammalian cells, but its expression can be induced rapidly in response to mitogenic and inflammatory stimuli. Aspirin is a relatively selective inhibitor of platelet PGHS-1 (cyclooxygenase-1, COX-1). The existence of 2 isoenzymes with different aspirin sensitivities, coupled with extremely different recovery rates of their cyclooxygenase (COX) activity following inactivation by aspirin, at least partially explains the different dosage requirements and durations of aspirin effects on platelet function versus the drug's analgesic and anti-inflammatory effects. Human platelets and vascular endothelial cells process PGH_2 to produce thromboxane A_2 and prostacyclin (epoprostenol, PGI_2), respectively. Thromboxane A_2 induces platelet aggregation and vasoconstriction, while prostacyclin inhibits platelet aggregation and induces vasodilation. Aspirin is antithrombotic in a wide range of doses inhibiting thromboxane A_2 and prostacyclin. (See Pharmacology: Antithrombotic Effects.)

■ Analgesic, Anti-inflammatory, and Antipyretic Effects

While unhydrolyzed aspirin has been shown to be more potent than sodium salicylate in relieving pain in animals, it remains to be clearly established that aspirin has greater analgesic effect than salicylate in humans. A direct correlation between onset, intensity, or duration of analgesia and the time course of serum aspirin (or salicylate) concentrations or peak serum aspirin (or salicylate) concentrations also remains to be established. There are relatively few controlled comparative studies of aspirin and other salicylates (e.g., salicylate salts), but the analgesic, anti-inflammatory, and antipyretic effects of aspirin and other salicylates are generally considered to be comparable. However, in terms of antipyretic activity, aspirin is approximately 1.6 times as potent as sodium salicylate on an equimolar basis.

For further information on analgesic, anti-inflammatory, antipyretic, and other effects of aspirin, see Pharmacology in the Salicylates General Statement 28:08.04.24.

■ Hematologic Effects

At usual dosages (e.g., 1.3–6 g daily), aspirin may rarely prolong the prothrombin time (usually only by 2–3 seconds) by inhibiting hepatic synthesis of blood coagulation factors VII, IX, and X.

Aspirin (but not other salicylates) inhibits platelet aggregation induced by epinephrine or low concentrations of collagen but not that induced by thrombin or high concentrations of collagen. Aspirin inhibits the second phase of platelet aggregation by preventing release of adenosine diphosphate (ADP) from platelets. The drug also prevents release of platelet factor 4 from platelets. Mean bleeding time may be prolonged by several minutes (approximately doubled) in healthy individuals and longer in children or in patients with bleeding disorders (e.g., hemophilia). In healthy individuals receiving a single 325-mg oral dose of aspirin, bleeding time may increase to a maximum within 12 hours and generally return to normal within 24 hours; any increase is usually of little clinical significance. Some clinicians have reported that mean bleeding time is progressively prolonged with increasing single doses of up to 1 g, but may be only slightly prolonged or unaffected by higher single doses; however, this has not been consistently found. The effect on bleeding time depends on the measurement method (e.g., Duke, Ivy, Mielke) used and technical variables (e.g., venostasis), and this may partially account for conflicting reports.

Like the analgesic and anti-inflammatory effects, the effects of aspirin on platelets appear to be mainly associated with inhibition of prostaglandin synthesis. Aspirin irreversibly acetylates and inactivates cyclooxygenase in circulating platelets and possibly in megakaryocytes. A single 325-mg oral dose of the drug results in about 90% inhibition of the enzyme in circulating platelets. This inactivation prevents platelet synthesis of prostaglandin endoperoxides and thromboxane A_2, compounds which induce platelet aggregation and constrict arterial smooth muscle. Since cyclooxygenase in platelets is not resynthesized, this effect of aspirin on platelet function persists for the life span of platelets (4–7 days). When approximately 20% of circulating platelets have not been exposed to aspirin (about 36 hours after the last dose), the hemostatic function of the platelet pool generally returns to normal; however, altered hemostasis has been reported to persist longer in some patients receiving long-term therapy.

■ Antithrombotic Effects

Because of its ability to inhibit platelet aggregation via platelet cyclooxygenase inhibition, aspirin has been extensively investigated for potential therapeutic effects in the prevention of thrombosis (particularly arterial thrombosis). (See Uses: Thrombosis.) Aspirin has also been found to inactivate cyclooxygenase in venous endothelium and thereby inhibit venous synthesis of prostacyclin (epoprostenol, PGI_2). Since prostacyclin inhibits platelet aggregation and causes vasodilation, it appears to oppose the effects of thromboxane A_2 (and prostaglandin endoperoxides) on hemostasis. Therefore, it has been suggested that the relative extent to which the formation of these compounds is inhibited by aspirin might result in an increased or decreased likelihood of thrombosis. It has not been established whether interruption of prostacyclin formation is a sufficient stimulus to initiate the thrombotic process, but studies in mice deficient in the gene that encodes the prostacyclin receptor support the importance of this prostanoid in the prevention of arterial thrombosis. Although prostacyclin is synthesized by arterial endothelium and in vitro studies suggest that arterial cyclooxygenase is less sensitive to inhibition by aspirin than venous cyclooxygenase, the actual effects of aspirin on arterial synthesis of prostacyclin in healthy or diseased human arteries remain to be established.

In some clinical studies that evaluated the effect of aspirin in preventing thrombosis, the dosages of aspirin (900 mg to 1.5 g daily in divided doses) probably inhibited the synthesis of prostacyclin as well as that of thromboxane A_2. Although concomitant inhibition of prostacyclin synthesis by aspirin may potentially decrease the antithrombotic efficacy of the drug, it is unlikely that this effect increases the risk of thrombosis since an increased risk has not been observed in these studies or in patients with rheumatoid arthritis receiving higher dosages of the drug. Cyclooxygenase in both platelets and venous endothelium has been found to be inhibited by single oral aspirin doses of 80–300 mg. However, at these doses, the duration of inhibition of thromboxane A_2 synthesis in platelets (about 48–96 hours) is longer than inhibition of prostacyclin synthesis in venous endothelium (about 24–48 hours), apparently because cyclooxygenase is resynthesized in venous endothelium but not in platelets. Since cyclooxygenase in platelets appears to be more sensitive to inactivation than cyclooxygenase in venous endothelium, it has been suggested that low dosages of aspirin might prevent thrombosis by selectively inhibiting prostaglandin endoperoxide and thromboxane A_2 synthesis. In addition, limited data indicate that modifying the absorption rate of aspirin to limit its systemic availability may result in such selective effects. Uncoated or film-coated, plain aspirin or buffered aspirin tablets or capsules have been used in most studies in which aspirin has been shown to prevent thrombosis, and limited data indicate that differences in the systemic availability of unhydrolyzed aspirin may be associated with different effects of the drug on thromboxane A_2 and prostacyclin synthesis, which might theoretically affect antithrombotic efficacy. In a comparative study in healthy men, administration of aspirin 75 mg daily as a controlled-release matrix formulation designed to release 10 mg of drug per hour produced essentially complete suppression of thromboxane A_2 formation (as determined by thromboxane B_2 concentrations) while having only modest effects on basal or bradykinin-stimulated prostacyclin synthesis. Suppression of thromboxane A_2 production and prolongation of template bleeding time in individuals receiving the controlled-release preparation daily for 28 days were comparable to those produced by immediate-release aspirin given as 162.5 mg daily or 325 mg every other day. Doses as low as 50–80 mg of enteric-coated aspirin have been shown to produce near-maximal inhibition of thromboxane A_2 synthesis, and some studies demonstrate that enteric-coated and controlled-release aspirin produce similar, although somewhat delayed, inhibition of cyclooxygenase activity and platelet aggregation compared with the same doses of plain or buffered aspirin. However, an optimum aspirin dose and administration schedule required to achieve these selective effects have not been clearly determined, and the actual clinical importance of such a selective inhibitory effect remains to be clearly established. In addition, salicylate appears to competitively inhibit the effect of aspirin on platelets; the relevance of this effect to the prevention of thrombosis is not known.

Pharmacokinetics

Since both unhydrolyzed aspirin and its metabolite, salicylate, are pharmacologically active, the pharmacokinetics of both compounds must be considered. For additional information on the distribution and elimination of *salicylate*, see Pharmacokinetics in the Salicylates General Statement 28:08.04.24.

■ **Absorption** Approximately 80–100% of an oral dose of aspirin is absorbed from the GI tract. However, the actual bioavailability of the drug as unhydrolyzed aspirin is lower since aspirin is partially hydrolyzed to salicylate in the GI mucosa during absorption and on first pass through the liver. There are relatively few studies of the bioavailability of unhydrolyzed aspirin. In one study in which aspirin was administered IV and as an oral aqueous solution, it was shown that the solution was completely absorbed but only about 70% reached the systemic circulation as unhydrolyzed aspirin. In another study in which aspirin was administered IV and orally as capsules, only about 50% of the oral dose reached the systemic circulation as unhydrolyzed aspirin. There is some evidence that the bioavailability of unhydrolyzed aspirin from slowly absorbed dosage forms (e.g., enteric-coated tablets) may be substantially decreased. Food does not appear to decrease the bioavailability of unhydrolyzed aspirin or salicylate; however, absorption is delayed and peak serum aspirin or salicylate concentration may be decreased. There is some evidence that absorption of salicylate following oral administration may be substantially impaired or is highly variable during the febrile phase of Kawasaki disease.

Most studies reported to date determined the bioavailability of aspirin preparations in terms of salicylate. Effervescent or noneffervescent oral aqueous solutions of aspirin appear to be completely absorbed. Oral buffered aspirin tablets, uncoated plain aspirin tablets, and methylcellulose film-coated (nonenteric) plain aspirin tablets are approximately 80–100% absorbed. Erratic and incomplete absorption of some enteric-coated aspirin tablets (particularly those with shellac coatings) has been reported, but recent studies indicate that the extent of absorption of currently available enteric-coated aspirin tablets is similar to that of buffered, uncoated plain, and film-coated plain aspirin tablets. Although well-designed studies are lacking, the extent of absorption of extended-release aspirin tablets appears to be similar to that of uncoated plain aspirin tablets. There are apparently no published studies on the bioavailability of aspirin capsules. Following rectal administration as a suppository, aspirin is slowly and variably absorbed; the extent of absorption increases with increasing rectal retention time. In general, 20–60% of the dose is absorbed if the suppository is retained for 2–4 hours and 70–100% is absorbed if the suppository is retained for at least 10 hours.

The rate of absorption of aspirin depends on the same factors that determine the rate of absorption of other salicylates and the relative rates of absorption from various oral aspirin dosage forms are generally the same as for oral dosage forms of other salicylates (e.g., aqueous solutions are the most rapidly absorbed). As with other salicylates, dissolution is usually the rate-limiting process in the absorption of tablets containing aspirin; however, the in vitro dissolution rate of a specific preparation does not necessarily reflect the in vivo absorption rate. According to the manufacturer, the in vitro dissolution of film-coated aspirin tablets does not differ from that of uncoated plain tablets; however, the film-coated tablet does not undergo dissolution in the mouth during administration.

Buffered Aspirin There has been controversy over the relative rates of absorption of buffered aspirin tablets and uncoated plain aspirin tablets and their relative potential for producing gastric irritation and analgesia.

The buffers contained in buffered aspirin tablets may increase the pH in the microenvironment of aspirin particles and thereby increase solubility of the drug in surrounding GI fluids; as a result, the dissolution rate of the tablets may be increased. However, it cannot be stated that *all* buffered aspirin tablets are dissolved and absorbed more rapidly than *all* uncoated plain aspirin tablets. The types and amounts of buffers affect dissolution rate, and claims for a specific preparation should be substantiated by appropriate data. Conflicting reports of the relative rates of absorption of buffered or uncoated plain aspirin tablets are most likely due to differences in the specific preparations studied. Some studies have shown that, like aqueous aspirin solutions, some buffered aspirin tablet preparations may be absorbed slightly more rapidly than some uncoated plain aspirin tablet preparations and may produce slightly higher peak serum salicylate concentrations; however, clinically important differences in the onset or intensity of analgesia produced by these dosage forms or specific preparations have not been established. Crossover studies directly comparing peak serum concentrations of unhydrolyzed aspirin attained with these dosage forms are lacking.

It has been suggested that buffered aspirin tablets cause less gastric irritation than uncoated plain aspirin tablets since the potentially more rapid dissolution of the former may reduce contact time between aspirin particles and gastric mucosa. However, several recent, well-designed studies indicate that buffered aspirin tablets do not cause less gastric irritation than uncoated plain aspirin tablets.

Rapidly Absorbed Dosage Forms Following oral administration of single doses of rapidly absorbed aspirin dosage forms, salicylate is detected in serum within 5–30 minutes, and peak serum salicylate concentrations are attained within 0.25–2 hours, depending on dosage form and specific formulation. Clinically important differences in the onset or intensity of analgesia produced by rapidly absorbed dosage forms or specific preparations have not been established.

Following oral administration of a single 650-mg dose of aspirin as an effervescent or noneffervescent aqueous solution in healthy adults, average peak plasma aspirin concentrations of about 13 mcg/mL are attained within 15–40 minutes and average peak plasma salicylate concentrations of about 40–55 mcg/mL are attained within 30–60 minutes. After a single 650-mg oral dose of aspirin (as two 325-mg uncoated plain tablets) in fasting healthy adults, average peak plasma aspirin concentrations of about 7–9 mcg/mL occur within 25–40 minutes and average peak plasma salicylate concentrations of about 35–50 mcg/mL occur within 1.5–2 hours. Following oral administration of a single 650-mg dose of buffered aspirin (as 2 tablets, each containing 325 mg of aspirin), average peak plasma salicylate concentrations of about 40–60 mcg/mL are attained within 45–60 minutes.

In one study in healthy fasting adults given a single 975-mg oral dose of aspirin (as three 325-mg uncoated plain tablets), peak serum salicylate concentrations averaged 60–75 mcg/mL and occurred within 2 hours. In another study in fasting rheumatoid arthritis patients given a single 1.95-g oral dose of aspirin (as six325-mg uncoated plain tablets), peak plasma aspirin concentrations of about 12–16 mcg/mL occurred within 1 hour and peak plasma salicylate concentrations of about 110–160 mcg/mL occurred within 4 hours. When these patients were given the same dose of buffered aspirin (as 6 tablets, each containing 325 mg of aspirin), peak plasma aspirin concentrations of about 14–18 mcg/mL occurred within 1–2 hours and peak plasma salicylate concentrations of about 140–160 mcg/mL occurred within 1–2 hours.

Enteric-Coated Aspirin There are few published studies reporting plasma aspirin or salicylate concentrations after single oral doses of enteric-coated aspirin tablets. In one crossover study, following single 975-mg oral doses (three 325-mg tablets) of 2 commercially available enteric-coated aspirin preparations in healthy adults, average peak serum salicylate concentrations of 48 mcg/mL occurred at 8 hours with one preparation, and average peak serum salicylate concentrations of 25 mcg/mL occurred at 14 hours with the other preparation. In one study in fasting rheumatoid arthritis patients given a single 1.92-g oral dose (as six 320-mg enteric-coated tablets), peak plasma aspirin concentrations of about 4–7 mcg/mL occurred within about 4 hours and average peak plasma salicylate concentrations of about 70 mcg/mL occurred within about 8 hours.

Extended-Release Aspirin There are few published studies reporting plasma aspirin or salicylate concentrations after single oral doses of extended-release aspirin tablets. Combining data from several small studies, some clinicians report that following a single 1.3-g oral dose of aspirin as two 650-mg extended-release tablets, an average peak serum aspirin concentration of about 3 mcg/mL was attained within 1 hour and peak serum salicylate concentrations of about 70–80 mcg/mL were attained within 4 hours; the serum aspirin concentration declined to less than 1 mcg/mL by 3 hours and the serum salicylate concentration was about 60 mcg/mL at 8 hours, 45 mcg/mL at 12 hours, and 25 mcg/mL at 16 hours. Following a single 1.6-g oral dose (as two 800-mg tablets) of one commercially available extended-release aspirin preparation in healthy adults in one crossover study, an average peak plasma aspirin concentration of about 1 mcg/mL was attained within 2 hours and average peak plasma salicylate concentrations of about 22 mcg/mL were attained within 8–12 hours; the plasma salicylate concentration declined to about 15 mcg/mL by 24 hours.

Suppositories In one study in children given a rectal dose of 150–300 mg of aspirin as a suppository, peak serum salicylate concentrations of 20–140 mcg/mL generally occurred within 3–4 hours.

■ **Distribution** Aspirin is rapidly and widely distributed, apparently into most body tissues and fluids. The volume of distribution of aspirin is approximately the same as that of salicylate and is generally 0.15–0.2 L/kg.

In one study in patients with rheumatic disease who received a single 650-mg oral dose of buffered aspirin, aspirin was detected in synovial fluid within 10–30 minutes and salicylate was detected in synovial fluid within 15–35 minutes. In this study, peak aspirin concentrations in synovial fluid occurred after an average of 1.3 hours and were about 75% of peak blood concentrations; peak salicylate concentrations in synovial fluid occurred after an average of 2.2 hours and were about 60% of peak blood concentrations.

Aspirin is poorly bound to plasma proteins; the unhydrolyzed drug is 33% bound at a serum salicylate concentration of 120 mcg/mL. However, aspirin acetylates serum albumin at the E-amino group of lysine; the acetylation may alter binding of other drugs (e.g., phenylbutazone) to the protein. Acetylation of serum albumin by aspirin is inhibited by salicylate.

■ **Elimination** The elimination half-life of aspirin in plasma is approximately 15–20 minutes. Unlike salicylate, unhydrolyzed aspirin does not undergo capacity-limited metabolism and does not accumulate in plasma following multiple doses.

Following oral administration, aspirin is partially hydrolyzed to salicylate during absorption by esterases in the GI mucosa. Following absorption, unhydrolyzed aspirin is rapidly and almost completely hydrolyzed by esterases principally in the liver but also in plasma, erythrocytes, and synovial fluid; hydrolysis occurs more slowly in synovial fluid apparently because the amounts of esterases in synovial fluid are lower. It has been reported that aspirin may be hydrolyzed more slowly in women because women apparently have lower amounts of plasma aspirin esterases.

Only about 1% of an oral dose of aspirin is excreted unhydrolyzed in urine. The remainder is excreted in urine as salicylate and its metabolites.

Chemistry and Stability

■ **Chemistry** Aspirin, the prototype of the salicylates, is a nonsteroidal anti-inflammatory agent (NSAIA). Aspirin is the salicylate ester of acetic acid. In vivo, the drug rapidly hydrolyzes to salicylate and acetate. Aspirin occurs as white crystals, which are usually tabular or needle-like, or as a white, crystalline powder. Aspirin is available in fixed combination with dipyridamole as a hard gelatin capsule containing dipyridamole as extended-release pellets and aspirin as an immediate-release tablet. The drug may have a faint odor, is slightly soluble in water and freely soluble in alcohol, and has a pK_a of 3.5. Each gram of aspirin contains approximately 760 mg of salicylate.

■ **Stability** Aspirin is stable in dry air. However, in moist air or in aqueous or hydroalcoholic solutions, the drug gradually hydrolyzes to salicylate and acetate and emits a strong vinegar-like odor; the rate of hydrolysis is increased by heat and is pH dependent.

In aqueous solutions, aspirin is most stable at a pH of 2–3, less stable at a pH of 4–8, and least stable at a pH less than 2 or exceeding 8. In a saturated aqueous solution at a pH of 5–7, aspirin is almost completely hydrolyzed within 1 week at 25°C. If a liquid dosage form of aspirin is desired for short-term treatment of pain, an oral solution may be prepared from commercially available buffered effervescent tablets (Alka-Seltzer®). Following dissolution of 1 Alka-Seltzer® tablet in approximately 90 mL of water, the solution has a pH of 6–7. In the resultant solution, aspirin is about 99% ionized and is at least 90% unhydrolyzed for approximately 10 hours at room temperature and about 90 hours at 5°C.

Chewable aspirin tablets containing 81 mg of the drug should be stored in child-resistant containers holding not more than 36 tablets each in order to limit the potential toxicity associated with accidental ingestion in children. Aspirin extra-strength (Anacin®) tablets should be stored at 20–25°C and protected from moisture. Aspirin (Bayer products, excluding Alka-Seltzer® products) tablets or caplets should be stored at room temperature; high humidity and excessive heat (40°C) should be avoided. Aspirin effervescent antacid and pain relief tablets (Alka-Seltzer® products) should be protected from excessive heat. Aspirin gum should be stored at 15–25°C and protected from excessive moisture. Aspirin suppositories should be stored at 2–15°C. The fixed-combination preparation of extended-release dipyridamole with aspirin should be stored at 25°C and protected from excessive moisture, but may be exposed to temperatures ranging from 15–30 degrees.

For further information on chemistry and stability, pharmacology, pharmacokinetics, uses, cautions, chronic toxicity, acute toxicity, drug interactions, laboratory test interferences, and dosage and administration of aspirin, see the Salicylates General Statement 28:08.04.24.

Preparations

Excipients in commercially available drug preparations may have clinically important effects in some individuals; consult specific product labeling for details.

Aspirin

Oral		
Pieces, chewing gum	227 mg	**Aspergum®**, Heritage, Schering Plough
Tablets	81 mg*	**Aspirin Tablets**
	325 mg*	**Aspirin Tablets**
		Norwich® Aspirin, Chattem
	500 mg*	**Aspirin Tablets**
		Norwich® Aspirin Maximum Strength, Chattem
	650 mg*	**Aspirin Tablets**
Tablets, chewable	81 mg*	**Aspirin Chewable Tablets**
		Bayer® Children's Chewable Aspirin, Bayer
		St. Joseph® Aspirin Adult Low Strength Chewable®, McNeil
Tablets, delayed-release (enteric-coated)	81 mg*	**Aspirin Delayed-release (Enteric-coated) Tablets**
		Bayer® Aspirin Regimen Adult Low Strength, Bayer
		Ecotrin® Adult Low Strength, GlaxoSmithKline
		Halfprin®, Kramer
		St. Joseph® Adult Low Strength Enteric Coated Tablets, McNeil
	162 mg	**Halfprin®**, Kramer
	325 mg*	**Aspirin Delayed-release (Enteric-coated) Tablets**
		Bayer® Aspirin Regimen Regular Strength Caplets®, Bayer
		Ecotrin® Regular Strength, GlaxoSmithKline
		Genacote®, Teva
	500 mg*	**Aspirin Delayed-release (Enteric-coated) Tablets**
		Ecotrin® Maximum Strength, GlaxoSmithKline
	650 mg*	**Aspirin Delayed-release (Enteric-coated) Tablets**
	975 mg	**Easprin®**, Harvest
Tablets, extended-release	800 mg	**ZORprin®**, Par
Tablets, film-coated	325 mg*	**Aspirin Film-coated Tablets**
		Bayer® Aspirin Caplets®, Bayer
		Genuine Bayer® Aspirin Tablets, Bayer
	500 mg	**Bayer® Aspirin Extra Strength Caplets®**, Bayer
		Bayer® Aspirin Extra Strength Gelcaplets®, Bayer
		Bayer® Aspirin Extra Strength Tablets, Bayer
Rectal		
Suppositories	60 mg*	**Aspirin Suppositories**
	120 mg*	**Aspirin Suppositories**
	200 mg*	**Aspirin Suppositories**
	300 mg*	**Aspirin Suppositories**
	600 mg*	**Aspirin Suppositories**

*available from one or more manufacturer, distributor, and/or repackager by generic (nonproprietary) name

Aspirin with Buffers

Oral		
Tablets	325 mg with buffers*	**Aspirin with Buffers Tablets**
Tablets, enteric-coated	81 mg with buffers*	**Aspirin with Buffers Enteric-coated Tablets**
	325 mg with buffers	**Ascriptin® Enteric Regular Strength,** Novartis

Tablets, film-coated	81 mg with buffers	**Bayer® Women's Aspirin Plus Calcium Caplets®**, Bayer
	325 mg with buffers	**Ascriptin® Regular Strength**, Novartis
		Ascriptin® Arthritis Pain Caplets®, Novartis
		Bufferin® Tablets, Novartis Consumer Health
	500 mg with buffers	**Ascriptin® Maximum Strength Caplets®**, Novartis
		Bayer® Aspirin Plus Buffered Extra Strength Caplets®, Bayer
		Bufferin® Arthritis Strength Caplets®, Bristol-Myers
		Bufferin® Extra Strength, Novartis Consumer Health
Tablets, for solution	325 mg	**Alka-Seltzer® Effervescent Pain Reliever and Antacid**, Bayer
		Alka-Seltzer® Lemon-Lime Effervescent Pain Reliever and Antacid, Bayer
	500 mg	**Alka-Seltzer® Extra Strength Effervescent Pain Reliever and Antacid**, Bayer

*available from one or more manufacturer, distributor, and/or repackager by generic (nonproprietary) name

Acetaminophen and Aspirin

Oral		
For solution	325 mg/packet Acetaminophen and Aspirin 500 mg/packet	**Goody's® Back & Body Pain Powder**, Prestige
Tablets, film-coated	250 mg Acetaminophen, Aspirin 250 mg, and buffer	**Excedrin® Back and Body Caplets**, Novartis

Acetaminophen, Aspirin, and Caffeine

Oral		
Capsules, gel-coated	250 mg Acetaminophen, Aspirin 250 mg, and Caffeine 65 mg*	**Acetaminophen, Aspirin, and Caffeine Gelcaps**
		Excedrin® Menstrual Complete Gelcaps, Novartis
For solution	260 mg/packet Acetaminophen, Aspirin 520 mg/packet, and Caffeine 32.5 mg/packet	**Goody's® Extra Strength Headache Powder**, Prestige
	325 mg/packet Acetaminophen, Aspirin 500 mg/packet, and Caffeine 65 mg/packet	**Goody's® Cool Orange Extra Strength Powder**, Prestige
Tablets, film-coated	194 mg Acetaminophen, Aspirin 227 mg, Caffeine 33 mg, and buffers	**Vanquish® Caplets**, Moberg
	250 mg Acetaminophen, Aspirin 250 mg, and Caffeine 65 mg	**Excedrin® Extra Strength Caplets**, Novartis
		Excedrin® Migraine Caplets, Novartis
		Goody's® Extra Strength Caplets, Prestige
		Pamprin® Max, Chattem

*available from one or more manufacturer, distributor, and/or repackager by generic (nonproprietary) name

Oxycodone and Aspirin

Oral		
Tablets	4.8355 mg Oxycodone Hydrochloride and Aspirin 325 mg*	**Endodan®** (C-II), Qualitest
		Oxycodone Hydrochloride and Aspirin Tablets (C-II)
		Percodan® (C-II; scored), Endo

*available from one or more manufacturer, distributor, and/or repackager by generic (nonproprietary) name

Other Aspirin Combinations

Oral		
Capsules	325 mg with Butalbital 50 mg and Caffeine 40 mg*	**Butalbital, Aspirin, and Caffeine Capsules** (C-III)
		Fiorinal® (C-III), Actavis
	325 mg with Butalbital 50 mg, Caffeine 40 mg, and Codeine Phosphate 30 mg*	**Butalbital, Aspirin, Caffeine, and Codeine Phosphate Capsules** (C-III)
		Fiorinal® with Codeine (C-III), Actavis
	356.4 mg with Caffeine 30 mg and Dihydrocodeine Bitartrate 16 mg	**Synalgos®-DC** (C-III), Leitner
Capsules, extended-release core (dipyridamole only)	25 mg with Dipyridamole 200 mg	**Aggrenox®**, Boehringer Ingelheim
For solution	845 mg/packet with Caffeine 65 mg/packet	**BC® Powder**, Prestige
		Stanback® Powder, Prestige
	1000 mg/packet with Caffeine 65 mg/packet	**BC® Powder Arthritis Strength**, Prestige
Tablets	325 mg with Butalbital 50 mg and Caffeine 40 mg*	**Butalbital, Aspirin, and Caffeine Tablets** (C-III)
		Fortabs® (C-III), United Research
	325 mg with Carisoprodol 200 mg*	**Carisoprodol and Aspirin Tablets** (C-IV)
		Soma® Compound (C-IV), Meda
	325 mg with Carisoprodol 200 mg and Codeine Phosphate 16 mg*	**Carisoprodol, Aspirin, and Codeine Phosphate Tablets** (C-III)
		Soma® Compound with Codeine (C-III), Meda
	325 mg with Meprobamate 200 mg	**Equagesic®** (C-IV; scored), Leitner
		Micrainin® (C-IV), Wallace
	385 mg with Caffeine 30 mg and Orphenadrine Citrate 25 mg*	**Norgesic®**, 3M
		Orphenadrine Citrate, Aspirin, and Caffeine Tablets
	400 mg with Caffeine 32 mg	**P-A-C® Analgesic**, Lee
	770 mg with Caffeine 60 mg and Orphenadrine Citrate 50 mg*	**Norgesic® Forte** (scored), 3M
		Orphenadrine Citrate, Aspirin, and Caffeine Tablets
Tablets, film-coated	400 mg with Caffeine 32 mg	**Anacin® Caplets®**, Wyeth
		Anacin® Tablets, Wyeth
	421 mg with Caffeine 32 mg and buffers	**Cope®**, Lee
	500 mg with Caffeine 32 mg	**Anacin® Maximum Strength**, Wyeth
	500 mg with Caffeine 32.5 mg	**Extra Strength Bayer® Back and Body Pain**, Bayer
Tablets, for solution	500 mg with Caffeine 65 mg	**Alka Seltzer® Morning Relief**, Bayer

Aspirin is also commercially available in combination with other drugs such as analgesics, antihistamines, antimuscarinics, antitussives, barbiturates, decongestants, and expectorants.

*available from one or more manufacturer, distributor, and/or repackager by generic (nonproprietary) name

†Use is not currently included in the labeling approved by the US Food and Drug Administration

OTHER NONSTEROIDAL ANTI-INFLAMMATORY AGENTS 28:08.04.92

Diclofenac

■ Diclofenac is a prototypical nonsteroidal anti-inflammatory agent (NSAIA) that also exhibits analgesic and antipyretic activity.

Uses

■ **Inflammatory Diseases** Diclofenac sodium and diclofenac potassium are used orally for anti-inflammatory and analgesic effects in the symptomatic treatment of acute and chronic rheumatoid arthritis, osteoarthritis, ankylosing spondylitis, and other inflammatory conditions.

Diclofenac sodium in fixed combination with misoprostol is used orally for anti-inflammatory activity and analgesic effects in the symptomatic treatment of rheumatoid arthritis and osteoarthritis in patients at high risk of developing NSAIA-induced gastric or duodenal ulcers and in patients at high risk of developing complications from these ulcers.

Diclofenac sodium 1% gel (Voltaren® gel) is used topically for the symptomatic treatment of osteoarthritis-related joint pain. The gel is used for joints amenable to topical therapy (e.g., hands, knees); the gel has not been evaluated for use on joints of the spine, hip, or shoulder.

The potential benefits and risks of diclofenac therapy as well as alternative therapies should be considered prior to initiating diclofenac therapy. The lowest possible effective dosage and shortest duration of therapy consistent with treatment goals of the patient should be employed.

Rheumatoid Arthritis and Osteoarthritis When used in the symptomatic treatment of rheumatoid arthritis, oral diclofenac has relieved pain and stiffness; reduced swelling, tenderness, and the number of joints involved; and improved mobility and grip strength. In the symptomatic treatment of osteoarthritis, diclofenac has relieved pain and stiffness, improved knee joint function, and increased range of motion and functional activity. Diclofenac appears to be only palliative in these conditions and has not been shown to permanently arrest or reverse the underlying disease process.

Most clinical studies have shown that the anti-inflammatory and analgesic effects of usual oral dosages of diclofenac sodium in the management of rheumatoid arthritis or osteoarthritis are greater than those of placebo and about equal to those of usual dosages of salicylates, diflunisal, ibuprofen, indomethacin, ketoprofen, mefenamic acid, naproxen, phenylbutazone (no longer commercially available in the US), piroxicam, or sulindac. In controlled clinical studies of 3 months' duration in patients with rheumatoid arthritis or osteoarthritis, diclofenac sodium dosages of 100–200 mg daily, given as delayed-release (enteric-coated) tablets, were as effective as 2.4–4.8 g of aspirin daily, 500 mg of naproxen daily, or 2.4 g of ibuprofen daily. Patient response to oral NSAIAs is variable; patients who do not respond to or cannot tolerate one NSAIA might be successfully treated with a different agent. However, NSAIAs are generally contraindicated in patients in whom sensitivity reactions (e.g., urticaria, bronchospasm, severe rhinitis) are precipitated by aspirin or other NSAIAs. (See Cautions: Precautions and Contraindications.)

In the management of rheumatoid arthritis in adults, NSAIAs may be useful for initial symptomatic treatment; however, NSAIAs do not alter the course of the disease or prevent joint destruction. Disease modifying antirheumatic drugs (DMARDs) (e.g., abatacept, adalimumab, anakinra, etanercept, hydroxychloroquine, infliximab, leflunomide, methotrexate, minocycline, rituximab, sulfasalazine) have the potential to reduce or prevent joint damage and to preserve joint integrity and function. DMARDs are used in conjunction with anti-inflammatory agents (i.e., NSAIAs, intra-articular and oral glucocorticoids) and physical and occupational therapies for the management of rheumatoid arthritis. DMARD therapy should be initiated early in the disease course to prevent irreversible joint damage. (For further information on the treatment of rheumatoid arthritis, including considerations in selecting a DMARD regimen, see Uses: Rheumatoid Arthritis, in Methotrexate 10:00.) Diclofenac has been used concomitantly with gold compounds, antimalarials, penicillamine, acetaminophen, and/or corticosteroids. Use of diclofenac with aspirin is not recommended, because the risk of serious adverse GI events may be increased and the pharmacokinetics of one or both of these drugs may be altered. (See Drug Interactions: Nonsteroidal Anti-inflammatory Agents.)

When used for the symptomatic treatment of osteoarthritis of the hand or knee, diclofenac sodium 1% gel has been more effective than vehicle (placebo) in relieving pain; however, results of clinical trials evaluating the formulation suggest that its analgesic effects may be modest.

Ankylosing Spondylitis In the symptomatic treatment of ankylosing spondylitis, oral diclofenac appears to provide relief of spinal pain, tenderness and/or spasm, morning stiffness, and pain at rest (including night pain) and to improve motion, posture, chest expansion, and spinal mobility. The anti-inflammatory and analgesic effects of usual dosages of diclofenac in the management of ankylosing spondylitis are about equal to those of usual dosages of indomethacin or sulindac. In a controlled clinical study in patients with ankylosing spondylitis, diclofenac sodium dosages of 75–125 mg daily, given as delayed-release (enteric-coated) tablets, were as effective as indomethacin 75–125 mg daily.

Juvenile Arthritis Diclofenac has been used orally with good results in a number of children for the management of juvenile rheumatoid arthritis†. Results of these studies suggest that usual dosages of the drug are more effective than placebo and at least as effective as usual dosages of salicylates, naproxen, or tolmetin in decreasing the number of painful, swollen, and tender joints. Further studies are needed to evaluate the efficacy and safety of diclofenac in the management of juvenile rheumatoid arthritis. (See Cautions: Pediatric Precautions.)

Other Inflammatory Conditions Oral diclofenac has been effective in a limited number of patients for the symptomatic relief of acute gouty arthritis†. The drug does not appear to correct hyperuricemia but has been used instead for its anti-inflammatory and analgesic effects to relieve pain, joint tenderness, and swelling associated with this condition.

Oral diclofenac also has been used for the symptomatic treatment of acute painful shoulder† (bursitis and/or tendinitis), sciatic pain†, backache†, myositis†, and radiohumeral bursitis† (radiohumeral epicondylitis, tennis elbow). The drug has been injected locally† (a parenteral dosage form currently is not commercially available in the US) for the relief of myofascial pain† in a limited number of patients with fibrositis, but additional study is necessary.

Oral or topical diclofenac has been used for the symptomatic treatment of infusion-related superficial thrombophlebitis†. In a controlled clinical trial in a limited number of patients, symptoms of thrombophlebitis improved in 60% of patients receiving diclofenac either orally (75 mg every 12 hours) or topically (as a gel applied to affected area every 8 hours) for 48 hours compared with 20% of those receiving placebo.

■ **Pain** Diclofenac potassium is used orally for symptomatic relief of postoperative pain (including that associated with orthopedic, gynecologic, and oral surgery) and orthopedic pain (including musculoskeletal sprains and traumatic joint distortions). Diclofenac epolamine transdermal system is used for symptomatic relief of acute pain due to minor strains, sprains, and contusions.

The potential benefits and risks of diclofenac therapy as well as alternative therapies should be considered prior to initiating diclofenac therapy. The lowest possible effective dosage and shortest duration of therapy consistent with treatment goals of the patient should be employed.

In patients with dental extraction or gynecologic surgery pain, single oral 50- and 100-mg doses of diclofenac potassium have been reported to be as effective as single 650-mg doses of aspirin; the duration of diclofenac potassium's analgesic effect appears to be longer than that of aspirin. When used to relieve postoperative orthopedic surgery pain, 50- or 100-mg doses of diclofenac potassium followed by 50 mg every 8 hours were as effective as 550 mg of naproxen sodium followed by 275 mg every 8 hours. When used to relieve orthopedic pain, 150 mg of diclofenac potassium daily was more effective than placebo and at least as effective as 1.2 g of ibuprofen daily or 20 mg of piroxicam daily.

Diclofenac sodium also has been used orally for symptomatic relief of postoperative (including that associated with dental surgery), postpartum, and orthopedic (including musculoskeletal strains or sprains) pain†, and visceral pain associated with cancer†. Because of the relatively slow onset of action of delayed-release (enteric-coated) or extended-release tablets of diclofenac sodium, other more rapid-acting NSAIAs (e.g., diclofenac potassium) may be preferred when prompt relief of acute pain is required. Diclofenac also has been used parenterally† (a parenteral dosage form is currently not commercially available in the US) for the relief of acute biliary or renal colic† , and for relief of postoperative pain† (including that associated with gynecologic and orthopedic surgery).

When used to relieve mild to moderate acute pain†, single oral diclofenac sodium doses of 50–150 mg have been more effective than placebo and at least as effective as usual analgesic doses of other NSAIAs or mild opiate analgesics. Diclofenac sodium dosages of 75–150 mg daily have been as effective as aspirin dosages of 0.9–2.7 g daily or ibuprofen dosages of 1.2 g daily. In patients with oral surgery pain†, 50-mg doses of diclofenac sodium have been reported to be as effective as 100-mg doses of pentazocine.

Efficacy of diclofenac epolamine transdermal system for the management of pain in patients with minor strains, sprains, and contusions has been demonstrated in 2 of 4 clinical studies. In one of these studies, diclofenac epolamine transdermal system (applied twice daily for 2 weeks) was more effective than a placebo transdermal system in relieving pain due to an acute minor sports injury.

■ **Dysmenorrhea** Diclofenac potassium is used orally in the management of primary dysmenorrhea. In patients with primary dysmenorrhea, NSAIAs may relieve pain and reduce the frequency and severity of uterine contractions, possibly as a result of inhibition of prostaglandin synthesis.

The potential benefits and risks of diclofenac therapy as well as alternative therapies should be considered prior to initiating diclofenac therapy. The lowest possible effective dosage and shortest duration of therapy consistent with treatment goals of the patient should be employed.

When used to relieve primary dysmenorrhea, 50- or 100-mg doses of diclofenac potassium followed by 50 mg every 8 hours were as effective as 550 mg of naproxen sodium followed by 275 mg every 8 hours.

Diclofenac sodium as delayed-release (enteric-coated) tablets also has been used for the symptomatic relief of dysmenorrhea†. When used to relieve dysmenorrhea, diclofenac sodium (delayed-release [enteric-coated]) dosages of 50–150 mg daily were more effective than placebo and as effective as naproxen dosages of 250–1250 mg daily.

■ **Other Uses** Oral diclofenac sodium has been used for its antipyretic effect in the management of fever†, usually associated with infection. In one study, the antipyretic effect of usual dosages of diclofenac sodium as delayed-release (enteric-coated) tablets was about equal to that of usual dosages of aspirin. The drug, however, should not be used routinely as an antipyretic because of its potential adverse effects.

Results from a large, prospective, population-based cohort study in geriatric individuals indicate a lower prevalence of Alzheimer's disease† among patients who received an NSAIA for 2 years or longer. Similar findings have been reported from some other, but not all, observational studies.

Diclofenac sodium also is used topically as an ophthalmic solution for the treatment of postoperative ocular inflammation in patients undergoing cataract extraction.

For use of diclofenac sodium in the topical treatment of actinic keratoses, see Diclofenac Sodium 84:92.

Dosage and Administration

■ **Administration** The potential benefits and risks of diclofenac therapy as well as alternative therapies should be considered prior to initiating diclofenac therapy.

Diclofenac sodium, diclofenac sodium in fixed combination with misoprostol, and diclofenac potassium are administered orally. The drug also has been administered rectally† and parenterally† (by IM injection), but commercially available dosage forms for the rectal and parenteral routes of administration currently are not available in the US.

Diclofenac sodium also is administered by topical application of a gel. Patients receiving diclofenac sodium 1% topical gel (Voltaren® gel) should be instructed in the use of the gel and given a copy of the patient instructions provided by the manufacturer. Diclofenac sodium 1% gel should be applied 4 times daily to the affected joint(s). To measure the appropriate dose using the dosing card provided by the manufacturer, gel is applied within the oblong area of the dosing card up to the appropriate (i.e., 2- or 4-g of gel) line; the dosing card can be used to apply the gel. The gel should be massaged gently into the skin, ensuring application to the entire joint (e.g., foot [including sole, top of foot, and toes], knee, ankle, hand [including palm, back of hand, and fingers], elbow, wrist). The patient should be advised to wait 10 minutes before covering the treated area with clothing and at least 60 minutes before bathing or showering. Hands should be washed after application of the gel unless the treated joint is in the hand. Diclofenac sodium gel should not be applied to open wounds, infected or inflamed areas of skin, or areas affected with exfoliative dermatitis; contact with eyes and mucous membranes should be avoided. The treated joint should not be exposed to external heat or to natural or artificial sunlight; use of occlusive dressings has not been evaluated and should be avoided. Other topical preparations (e.g., sunscreens, cosmetics, lotions, moisturizers, insect repellents) should not be applied to the treated joint; such use has not been evaluated.

Diclofenac epolamine is administered by topical application of a transdermal system. Patients receiving diclofenac epolamine transdermal system (Flector®) should be instructed in the use of the system and given a copy of the patient information provided by the manufacturer. The transdermal system should be applied to the most painful area twice daily. The system should be applied to intact skin only; application to damaged skin (e.g., wounds, burns, infected areas of skin, areas affected with eczema or exudative dermatitis) should be avoided. Hands should be washed after handling the system. Contact with the eyes and mucous membranes should be avoided. The transdermal system should not be worn while bathing or showering. If a system should begin to peel off during the period of use, the edges of the system may be taped to the skin.

■ Dosage

The lowest possible effective dosage and shortest duration of therapy consistent with treatment goals of the patient should be employed. Dosage of diclofenac must be carefully adjusted according to individual requirements and response, using the lowest possible effective dosage.

Based on safety reviews conducted to evaluate available data on cardiovascular risk of diclofenac, some authorities (e.g., Health Canada) now recommend that the dosage of systemically administered diclofenac not exceed 100 mg daily (except on the first day of treatment for dysmenorrhea when a total dose of 200 mg may be administered). (See Cautions: Cardiovascular Effects.)

Commercially available diclofenac sodium enteric-coated tablets (Voltaren®), diclofenac sodium extended-release tablets (Voltaren®-XR), and diclofenac potassium conventional tablets (Cataflam®) are not necessarily bioequivalent on a mg per mg basis.

Inflammatory Diseases

Based on safety reviews conducted to evaluate cardiovascular risk of diclofenac, some authorities (e.g., Health Canada) now recommend that systemic diclofenac dosage for inflammatory diseases not exceed 100 mg daily. (See Cautions: Cardiovascular Effects.)

Rheumatoid Arthritis and Osteoarthritis. For the symptomatic treatment of acute or chronic rheumatoid arthritis, the usual initial adult dosage of diclofenac sodium delayed-release (enteric-coated) tablets or diclofenac potassium conventional tablets is 150–200 mg daily, administered in divided doses of 75 mg (diclofenac sodium delayed-release [enteric-coated] tablets only) twice daily or 50 mg (diclofenac sodium delayed-release [enteric-coated] tablets or diclofenac potassium conventional tablets) 3 or 4 times daily. For the management of rheumatoid arthritis, the usual initial adult dosage of diclofenac sodium extended-release tablets is 100 mg daily. If dosage increase is necessary in patients receiving diclofenac sodium 100 mg daily as extended-release tablets, dosage can be increased to 100 mg twice daily.

When diclofenac is used in fixed combination with misoprostol for the symptomatic treatment of chronic rheumatoid arthritis, the usual dosage is 50 mg of diclofenac sodium 3 or 4 times daily. Dosage may be changed to 50 or 75 mg of diclofenac sodium twice daily in patients who do not tolerate the usual dosage; however, these dosages may be less effective in preventing NSAIA-induced ulcers. When therapy with diclofenac and misoprostol is required for the treatment of chronic rheumatoid arthritis, the commercially available combination of diclofenac in fixed combination with misoprostol should not be used for initial therapy. Instead, dosage should first be adjusted by administering each drug separately. If it is determined that the optimum maintenance dosage corresponds to the ratio in the commercial combination preparation, the fixed combination may be used. If clinically indicated, supplemental doses of misoprostol or diclofenac as the individual component can be administered with the fixed combination.

For the symptomatic treatment of osteoarthritis, the usual adult dosage of diclofenac sodium delayed-release (enteric-coated) tablets or diclofenac potassium conventional tablets is 100–150 mg daily, administered in divided doses of 75 mg (diclofenac sodium delayed-release [enteric-coated] tablets only) twice daily or 50 mg (diclofenac sodium delayed-release [enteric-coated] tablets or diclofenac potassium conventional tablets) 2 or 3 times daily. For the management of osteoarthritis, the recommended adult dosage of diclofenac sodium extended-release tablets is 100 mg daily.

When diclofenac is used in fixed combination with misoprostol for the symptomatic treatment of osteoarthritis, the usual dosage is 50 mg of diclofenac sodium 3 times daily. Dosage may be changed to 50 or 75 mg of diclofenac sodium twice daily in patients who do not tolerate the usual dosage; however, these dosages may be less effective in preventing NSAIA-induced ulcers. When therapy with diclofenac and misoprostol is required for the treatment of osteoarthritis, the commercially available combination of diclofenac in fixed combination with misoprostol should not be used for initial therapy. Instead, dosage should first be adjusted by administering each drug separately. If it is determined that the optimum maintenance dosage corresponds to the ratio in the commercial combination preparation, the fixed combination may be used. If clinically indicated, supplemental doses of misoprostol or diclofenac as the individual component can be administered with the fixed combination.

When diclofenac sodium 1% gel (Voltaren® gel) is used for the management of lower extremity (i.e., knees, ankles, feet) joint pain due to osteoarthritis, 4 g of gel is massaged into the affected joint 4 times daily. When the gel is used for the management of upper extremity (i.e., elbows, wrists, hands) joint pain, 2 g of gel is massaged into the affected joint 4 times daily. The total daily dose applied to all affected joints should *not* exceed 32 g of gel, with no more than 16 g of gel applied daily to any single lower extremity joint and no more than 8 g of gel applied daily to any single upper extremity joint.

Ankylosing Spondylitis. For the symptomatic treatment of ankylosing spondylitis, the usual adult dosage of diclofenac sodium delayed-release (enteric-coated) tablets is 100–125 mg daily, administered in divided doses of 25 mg 4 or 5 times daily. When diclofenac potassium is used for the management of ankylosing spondylitis, a dosage of 50 mg twice daily has been suggested by the manufacturers.

Pain and Dysmenorrhea

When diclofenac potassium conventional tablets are used for relief of pain or primary dysmenorrhea, an initial dose of 50 mg is recommended, followed by 50 mg every 8 hours as needed; some patients may benefit from an initial dose of 100 mg, followed by 50 mg every 8 hours as needed. Based on safety reviews conducted to evaluate available data on cardiovascular risk of diclofenac, some authorities (e.g., Health Canada) now recommend that the dosage of systemically administered diclofenac not exceed 100 mg daily (except on the first day of treatment for dysmenorrhea when a total dose of 200 mg may be administered). (See Cautions: Cardiovascular Effects.)

When diclofenac epolamine transdermal system (Flector®) is used for relief of acute pain due to strains, sprains, and contusions, one system is applied to the most painful area twice daily.

■ Dosage in Renal or Hepatic Impairment

Diclofenac dosage reductions do not appear to be necessary in patients with renal impairment. However, patients with substantially impaired renal function should be monitored closely during diclofenac therapy, because of potential risks of NSAIA therapy in such patients. (See Cautions: Renal, Electrolyte, and Genitourinary Effects.)

Reduction of oral diclofenac dosage may be necessary in patients with hepatic impairment.

Cautions

Adverse reactions to oral diclofenac are usually mild and transient and mainly involve the upper GI tract; however, adverse effects may be severe enough to require discontinuance of the drug in about 1.5–2% of patients. Most diclofenac-induced adverse effects occur during the first 3–6 months of treatment. The relationship of the frequency of adverse effects to dosage remains to be established. Overall, the frequency and nature of adverse effects produced by diclofenac sodium delayed-release (enteric-coated) tablets, diclofenac potassium conventional tablets, and ibuprofen appear to be similar. When diclofenac potassium was administered short-term (2 weeks or less), the incidence of adverse effects was about 10–50% of that associated with long-term administration of the drug.

■ Cardiovascular Effects

Fluid retention manifested principally as edema has occurred in up to 10% of patients receiving oral diclofenac. Adverse cardiovascular effects reported occasionally in diclofenac-treated patients include congestive heart failure, hypertension, tachycardia, and syncope. Arrhythmia, myocardial infarction, chest pain, palpitations, vasculitis, thrombophlebitis, hypotension, angina-like attack, and circulatory shock or distress have occurred rarely.

Nonsteroidal anti-inflammatory agents (NSAIAs), including selective cyclooxygenase-2 (COX-2) inhibitors and prototypical NSAIAs, increase the risk of serious adverse cardiovascular thrombotic events, including myocardial infarction and stroke (which can be fatal), in patients with or without cardiovascular disease or risk factors for cardiovascular disease. Use of NSAIAs also is associated with an increased risk of heart failure.

The association between cardiovascular complications and use of NSAIAs is an area of ongoing concern and study. Findings of an FDA review of published observational studies of NSAIAs, a meta-analysis of published and unpublished data from randomized controlled trials of these drugs, and other published information indicate that NSAIAs may increase the risk of serious adverse cardiovascular thrombotic events by 10–50% or more, depending on the drugs and dosages studied. Available data suggest that the increase in risk may occur early (within the first weeks) following initiation of therapy and may increase with higher dosages and longer durations of use. Although the relative increase in cardiovascular risk appears to be similar in patients with or without known underlying cardiovascular disease or risk factors for cardiovascular disease, the absolute incidence of serious NSAIA-associated cardiovascular thrombotic events is higher in those with cardiovascular disease or risk factors for cardiovascular disease because of their elevated baseline risk. (See Cautions: Cardiovascular Effects, in Celecoxib 28:08.04.08.)

Results from observational studies utilizing Danish national registry data indicated that patients receiving NSAIAs following a myocardial infarction were at increased risk of reinfarction, cardiovascular-related death, and all-cause mortality beginning in the first week of treatment. Patients who received NSAIAs following myocardial infarction had a higher 1-year mortality rate compared with those who did not receive NSAIAs (20 versus 12 deaths per 100 person-years). Although the absolute mortality rate declined somewhat after the first year following the myocardial infarction, the increased relative risk of death in patients who received NSAIAs persisted over at least the next 4 years of follow-up.

In 2 large controlled clinical trials of a selective COX-2 inhibitor for the management of pain in the first 10–14 days following coronary artery bypass graft (CABG) surgery, the incidence of myocardial infarction and stroke was increased. Therefore, NSAIAs are contraindicated in the setting of CABG surgery.

Findings from some systematic reviews of controlled observational studies and meta-analyses of data from randomized studies of NSAIAs suggest that naproxen may be associated with a lower risk of cardiovascular thrombotic events compared with other NSAIAs. However, limitations of these observational studies and the indirect comparisons used to assess cardiovascular risk of the prototypical NSAIAs (e.g., variability in patients' risk factors, comorbid conditions, concomitant drug therapy, drug interactions, dosage, and duration of therapy) affect the validity of the comparisons; in addition, these studies were not designed to demonstrate superior safety of one NSAIA compared with another. Therefore, FDA states that definitive conclusions regarding relative risks of NSAIAs are not possible at this time. (See Cautions: Cardiovascular Effects, in Celecoxib 28:08.04.08.)

Findings from some of these meta-analyses and systematic reviews also suggest that the cardiovascular risk associated with diclofenac, particularly at higher dosages (e.g., 150 mg or more daily), is similar to that observed with selective COX-2 inhibitors. (See Experience with Prototypical NSAIAs under Cautions: Cardiovascular Effects, in Celecoxib 28:08.04.08.) Some authorities (e.g., Health Canada) now recommend that the dosage of systemically administered diclofenac not exceed 100 mg daily (except for the first day of treatment for dysmenorrhea). (See Dosage and Administration: Dosage.)

Data from observational studies also indicate that use of NSAIAs in patients with heart failure is associated with increased morbidity and mortality. Results from a retrospective study utilizing Danish national registry data indicated that use of selective COX-2 inhibitors or prototypical NSAIAs in patients with chronic heart failure was associated with a dose-dependent increase in the risk of death and an increased risk of hospitalization for myocardial infarction or heart failure. In addition, findings from a meta-analysis of published and unpublished data from randomized controlled trials of NSAIAs indicated that use of selective COX-2 inhibitors or prototypical NSAIAs was associated with an approximate twofold increase in the risk of hospitalization for heart failure. Fluid retention and edema also have been observed in some patients receiving NSAIAs.

There is no consistent evidence that use of low-dose aspirin mitigates the increased risk of serious cardiovascular events associated with NSAIAs.

■ **GI Effects** Adverse GI effects, which mainly involve the upper GI tract, occur in up to 10% of patients receiving oral diclofenac. Adverse GI effects require discontinuance of the drug in about 3% of patients. Peptic ulcer, GI bleeding, and/or perforation have been reported in up to 10% of patients receiving oral diclofenac in controlled clinical studies. There is some evidence that the incidence of diclofenac-induced peptic ulcers and gastric lesions may be reduced with concomitant use of an appropriate ulcer preventive regimen. Nausea, diarrhea, constipation, abdominal pain or cramps, flatulence, vomiting, and dyspepsia occur in up to 10% of patients receiving oral diclofenac. Esophagitis, gastritis, glossitis, stomatitis, aphthous stomatitis, changes in appetite, dry mouth and mucous membranes, pancreatitis (with or without hepatitis), thirst, colitis, ulceration of the colon, and distress have occurred during diclofenac therapy. The incidence of abdominal pain, diarrhea, and other GI symptoms may be higher in patients receiving diclofenac in fixed combination with misoprostol than in patients receiving diclofenac without misoprostol. Nausea, altered taste, dyspepsia, or other adverse GI effects (including gastritis, vomiting, diarrhea, constipation, upper abdominal pain, and dry mouth) have occurred in 1–3% of patients receiving diclofenac epolamine transdermal system.

Usual oral dosages of diclofenac sodium reportedly produce fewer adverse GI effects than usual anti-inflammatory dosages of aspirin or naproxen. In healthy individuals, GI bleeding as determined by fecal blood loss was less in individuals receiving 150 mg of diclofenac sodium daily than in those receiving 3000, 750, or 150 mg of aspirin, naproxen, or indomethacin daily, respectively, for 3 weeks. In healthy adults, the frequency of GI mucosal lesions observed with endoscopic examination was lower with diclofenac than with naproxen. However, the clinical importance of these findings is not known since currently there is no evidence to indicate that diclofenac is less likely to produce serious GI lesions during chronic therapy than other prototypical NSAIAs.

Serious adverse GI effects (e.g., bleeding, ulceration, perforation) can occur at any time in patients receiving NSAIA therapy, and such effects may *not* be preceded by warning signs or symptoms. Only 1 in 5 patients who develop a serious upper GI adverse event while receiving NSAIA therapy is symptomatic. Minor upper GI effects (e.g., dyspepsia), which usually develop early, occur commonly during NSAIA therapy, but the absence of such early GI manifestations does not preclude the development of serious GI toxicity in patients receiving chronic NSAIA therapy. Therefore, clinicians should remain alert to the possible development of serious GI effects (e.g., bleeding, ulceration) in any patient receiving NSAIA therapy, and such patients should be followed chronically for the development of manifestations of such effects and advised of the importance of this follow-up. In addition, patients should be advised about the signs and symptoms of serious NSAIA-induced GI toxicity and what action to take if they occur. If signs and symptoms of a serious GI event develop, additional evaluation and treatment should be initiated promptly; the NSAIA should be discontinued until appropriate diagnostic studies have ruled out a serious GI event.

Results of studies to date are inconclusive concerning the relative risk of various prototypical NSAIAs in causing serious GI effects. In patients receiving NSAIAs and observed in clinical studies of several months' to 2 years' duration, symptomatic upper GI ulcers, gross bleeding, or perforation appeared to occur in approximately 1% of patients treated for 3–6 months and in about 2–4% of those treated for 1 year. Longer duration of therapy with an NSAIA increases the likelihood of a serious GI event. However, short-term therapy is not without risk. High dosages of any NSAIA probably are associated with increased risk of such effects, although controlled studies documenting this probable association are lacking for most NSAIAs. Therefore, whenever use of relatively high dosages (within the recommended dosage range) is considered, sufficient benefit to offset the potential increased risk of GI toxicity should be anticipated.

Studies have shown that patients with a history of peptic ulcer disease and/or GI bleeding who are receiving NSAIAs have a substantially higher risk of developing GI bleeding than patients without these risk factors. In addition to a history of ulcer disease, pharmacoepidemiologic studies have identified several comorbid conditions and concomitant therapies that may increase the risk for GI bleeding, including concomitant use of oral corticosteroids or anticoagulants, longer duration of NSAIA therapy, smoking, alcoholism, older age, and poor general health status. Patients with rheumatoid arthritis are more likely to experience serious GI complications from NSAIA therapy than are patients with osteoarthritis. In addition, geriatric or debilitated patients appear to tolerate GI ulceration and bleeding less well than other individuals, and most spontaneous reports of fatal GI effects have been in such patients.

For patients at high risk for complications from NSAIA-induced GI ulceration (e.g., bleeding, perforation), concomitant use of misoprostol can be considered for preventive therapy. (See Misoprostol 56:28.28.) Alternatively, some clinicians suggest that a proton-pump inhibitor (e.g., omeprazole) may be used concomitantly to decrease the incidence of serious GI toxicity associated with NSAIA therapy. In one study, therapy with high dosages of famotidine (40 mg twice daily) was more effective than placebo in preventing peptic ulcers in NSAIA-treated patients; however, the effect of the drug was modest. In addition, efficacy of usual dosages of H_2-receptor antagonists for the prevention of NSAIA-induced gastric and duodenal ulcers has not been established. Therefore, most clinicians do not recommend use of H_2-receptor antagonists for the prevention of NSAIA-associated ulcers. Another approach in high-risk patients who would benefit from NSAIA therapy is use of an NSAIA that is a selective inhibitor of COX-2 (e.g., celecoxib), since these agents are associated with a lower incidence of serious GI bleeding than prototypical NSAIAs. However, while celecoxib (200 mg twice daily) was comparably effective to diclofenac sodium (75 mg twice daily) plus omeprazole (20 mg daily) in preventing recurrent ulcer bleeding (recurrent ulcer bleeding probabilities of 4.9 versus 6.4%, respectively, during the 6-month study) in *H. pylori*-negative arthritis (principally osteoarthritis) patients with a recent history of ulcer bleeding, the protective efficacy was unexpectedly low for both regimens and it appeared that neither could completely protect patients at high risk. Additional study is necessary to elucidate optimal therapy for preventing GI complications associated with NSAIA therapy in high-risk patients.

■ **Nervous System Effects** Headache or dizziness has been reported in up to 10% of patients receiving oral diclofenac. Anxiety, asthenia, confusion, depression, abnormal dreams, drowsiness, insomnia, malaise, nervousness, paresthesia, somnolence, tremors, irritability, and vertigo have occurred occasionally in patients receiving the drug. Tingling sensation, dreams, myoclonus, and migraine have occurred rarely. Headache, paresthesia, somnolence, or other adverse nervous system effects (including hypoesthesia, dizziness, and hyperkinesias) have occurred in 1% of patients receiving diclofenac epolamine transdermal system. Although a causal relationship to diclofenac has not been established, seizures, coma, hallucinations, and meningitis have been reported during therapy with the drug.

■ **Renal, Electrolyte, and Genitourinary Effects** Diclofenac has caused impairment of renal function, resulting in acute renal failure, interstitial nephritis, nephrotic syndrome, increased BUN and serum creatinine concentrations, and renal papillary necrosis in patients receiving the drug. In at least one patient receiving oral diclofenac, acute renal failure became chronic. Cystitis, dysuria, hematuria, oliguria/polyuria, and proteinuria have been reported occasionally in patients receiving diclofenac. Urinary tract infection, renal calculi, and hyponatremia have occurred rarely.

■ **Hepatic Effects** Severe, sometimes fatal, hepatic reactions, including jaundice and fulminant hepatitis, liver necrosis, cholestasis, hepatic failure, asymptomatic hepatitis, acute hepatitis, and chronic active hepatitis, have been reported rarely in patients receiving diclofenac. Borderline (1.2–3 times the upper limit of normal) or greater elevations of one or more liver function test results have occurred in about 15% of patients treated with diclofenac. Liver function abnormalities associated with NSAIA therapy may progress, may remain essentially unchanged, or may be transient with continued therapy. Meaningful (more than 3 times the upper limit of normal) elevations of serum AST (SGOT) concentration have occurred in approximately 2% of patients at some time during therapy with diclofenac. In one large, open-label, controlled study, meaningful or marked (more than 8 times the upper limit of normal) elevations of serum AST and/or ALT (SGPT) concentrations occurred in 4 or 1% of patients, respectively, receiving diclofenac for 2–6 months. Increased serum concentrations of bilirubin have been reported rarely in patients receiving diclofenac therapy.

Misoprostol does not appear to exacerbate hepatic effects (e.g., increases in liver function test values) associated with diclofenac therapy.

Diclofenac should be discontinued if signs or symptoms of a severe hepatic reaction occur. (See Cautions: Precautions and Contraindications.)

■ Dermatologic and Sensitivity Reactions Rash or pruritus occurs in up to 10% of patients receiving oral diclofenac. Other adverse dermatologic reactions, including alopecia, photosensitivity, and excessive perspiration, have occurred occasionally. Bullous eruption, Stevens-Johnson syndrome, erythema multiforme, exfoliative dermatitis, toxic epidermal necrolysis, urticaria, and angioedema, have occurred rarely.

Sensitivity reactions, including anaphylaxis; swelling of the eyelids, tongue, lips, pharynx, or larynx; urticaria; asthma; bronchospasm; laryngeal edema; dyspnea; chest tightness; wheezing; anaphylactoid reactions; eosinophilic pneumonitis and angioedema, sometimes with concomitant, potentially severe hypotension, have been reported in patients receiving diclofenac.

In clinical studies that evaluated diclofenac sodium 1% gel, the most common adverse effect reported was dermatitis at the application site; this adverse effect has been reported in 4–11% of patients receiving the gel. Application site pruritus, erythema, paresthesia, dryness, vesicles, irritation, or papules also have occurred in patients receiving diclofenac gel.

Application site reactions (i.e., pruritus, dermatitis, burning, dryness, irritation, erythema, atrophy, discoloration, hyperhidrosis, vesicles) have been reported in 11% of patients receiving therapy with diclofenac epolamine transdermal system in clinical studies. Rash also has been reported in patients receiving diclofenac epolamine transdermal system. Skin infection developed in one individual after the diclofenac system that had been applied to the foot was subjected to prolonged exposure to wetness. Edema and abnormal sensation at the treated site and allergic skin reactions also have been reported.

■ Otic and Ocular Effects Tinnitus has occurred in up to 10% of patients receiving oral diclofenac.

Adverse ocular effects (including blurred vision and conjunctivitis) and hearing impairment have occurred in diclofenac-treated patients.

■ Hematologic Effects Anemia has been reported in up to 10% of patients receiving oral diclofenac. Leukopenia, thrombocytopenia, purpura, ecchymosis, eosinophilia, melena, and rectal bleeding have occurred occasionally in patients receiving diclofenac. Agranulocytosis, lymphadenopathy, hemolytic anemia, aplastic anemia, and pancytopenia have been reported rarely in diclofenac-treated patients. Bruising in the extremities and abdomen, spontaneous bleeding, and hematoma formation also have been reported rarely in patients receiving the drug. Diclofenac may inhibit platelet aggregation and prolong bleeding time. Diclofenac usually does not affect platelet count, prothrombin time, partial thromboplastin time, or thrombin time.

■ Respiratory Effects Asthma or dyspnea has been reported occasionally in patients receiving diclofenac. Respiratory tract infection (e.g., pneumonia, pharyngitis, bronchitis) or respiratory depression has been reported rarely.

■ Other Adverse Effects Fever, infection, and sepsis have occurred in patients receiving diclofenac. Back, leg, or joint pain and hyperglycemia have occurred rarely. Although a causal relationship to diclofenac has not been established, weight changes have occurred in patients receiving the drug.

■ Precautions and Contraindications Multiple diclofenac-containing preparations should not be used concomitantly. Concomitant use of diclofenac sodium 1% gel with oral NSAIAs may result in increased adverse effects.

When diclofenac sodium is used in fixed combination with misoprostol, the cautions, precautions, and contraindications associated with misoprostol must be considered in addition to those associated with diclofenac.

Patients should be advised that diclofenac, like other NSAIAs, is not free of potential adverse effects, including some that can cause discomfort, and that more serious effects (e.g., myocardial infarction, stroke, GI bleeding), which may require hospitalization and may even be fatal, also can occur. Patients also should be informed that, while NSAIAs may be commonly employed for conditions that are less serious, NSAIA therapy often is considered essential for the management of some diseases, and the drugs have a major role in the management of pain. Clinicians may wish to discuss with their patients the potential risks and likely benefits of NSAIA therapy, particularly when consideration is being given to use of these drugs in less serious conditions for which therapy without an NSAIA may represent an acceptable alternative to both the patient and clinician.

Patients should be advised to read the medication guide for NSAIAs that is provided to the patient each time the drug is dispensed.

NSAIAs increase the risk of serious adverse cardiovascular thrombotic events. (See Cautions: Cardiovascular Effects.) To minimize the potential risk of adverse cardiovascular events, the lowest effective dosage and shortest possible duration of therapy should be employed. Some clinicians suggest that it may be prudent to avoid use of NSAIAs whenever possible in patients with cardiovascular disease. Patients receiving NSAIAs (including those without previous symptoms of cardiovascular disease) should be monitored for the possible development of cardiovascular events throughout therapy. Patients should be informed about the signs and symptoms of serious cardiovascular toxicity (chest pain, dyspnea, weakness, slurring of speech) and instructed to seek immediate medical attention if such toxicity occurs. Diclofenac should be avoided in patients with recent myocardial infarction unless the benefits of therapy are expected to outweigh the risk of recurrent cardiovascular thrombotic events; if diclofenac is used in such patients, the patient should be monitored for cardiac ischemia.

There is no consistent evidence that concomitant use of low-dose aspirin mitigates the increased risk of serious cardiovascular events associated with NSAIAs. Concomitant use of aspirin and an NSAIA increases the risk for serious GI events. Because of the potential for increased adverse effects, patients receiving diclofenac should be advised not to take aspirin.

Use of NSAIAs can result in the onset of hypertension or worsening of preexisting hypertension; either of these occurrences may contribute to the increased incidence of cardiovascular events. Patients receiving NSAIAs may have an impaired response to diuretics (i.e., thiazide or loop diuretics), angiotensin-converting enzyme (ACE) inhibitors, angiotensin II receptor antagonists, or β-adrenergic blocking agents. NSAIAs should be used with caution in patients with hypertension. Blood pressure should be monitored closely during initiation of NSAIA therapy and throughout therapy.

Because NSAIAs increase morbidity and mortality in patients with heart failure, the manufacturer states that diclofenac should be avoided in patients with severe heart failure unless the benefits of therapy are expected to outweigh the risk of worsening heart failure; if diclofenac is used in such patients, the patient should be monitored for worsening heart failure. Some experts state that use of NSAIAs should be avoided whenever possible in patients with reduced left ventricular ejection fraction and current or prior symptoms of heart failure. Patients receiving NSAIAs should be advised to inform their clinician if they experience symptoms of heart failure, including dyspnea, unexplained weight gain, and edema. Use of NSAIAs may diminish the cardiovascular effects of certain drugs used to treat heart failure and edema (e.g., diuretics, ACE inhibitors, angiotensin II receptor antagonists). (See Drug Interactions.)

The risk of potentially serious adverse GI effects should be considered in patients receiving diclofenac, particularly in patients receiving chronic therapy with the drug. (See Cautions: GI Effects.) Diclofenac should be used with caution and under close supervision in patients with a history of GI disease. Because peptic ulceration and/or GI bleeding have been reported in patients receiving the drug, patients should be advised to promptly report signs or symptoms of GI ulceration or bleeding to their clinician.

Diclofenac should be used with extreme caution and under close supervision in patients with a history of GI bleeding or peptic ulceration, and such patients should receive an appropriate ulcer preventive regimen. All patients considered at increased risk of potentially serious adverse GI effects (e.g., geriatric patients, those receiving high therapeutic dosages of NSAIAs, those with a history of peptic ulcer disease, those receiving anticoagulants or corticosteroids concomitantly) should be monitored closely for signs and symptoms of ulcer perforation or GI bleeding.To minimize the potential risk of adverse GI effects, the lowest effective dosage and shortest possible duration of therapy should be employed. For patients who are at high risk, therapy other than an NSAIA should be considered.

Because severe hepatotoxic effects may develop without symptoms of liver dysfunction, serum transaminase values should be monitored periodically during long-term therapy with diclofenac. Serum transaminase values should be obtained 4–8 weeks after therapy with diclofenac is initiated. ALT (SGPT) is the recommended hepatic function marker for monitoring liver injury. Diclofenac should be discontinued if abnormal liver function test results persist or worsen, if clinical signs and symptoms consistent with liver disease develop, or if systemic manifestations occur (e.g., eosinophilia, rash). (See Cautions: Hepatic Effects.) Patients receiving diclofenac should be informed of the warning signs and symptoms of hepatotoxicity (e.g., nausea, anorexia, fatigue, lethargy, pruritus, jaundice, right upper quadrant tenderness, flu-like syndrome) and the appropriate actions to take if any of these manifestations develop.

Concomitant use of corticosteroids during NSAIA therapy may increase the risk of GI ulceration; therefore, NSAIAs should be used with caution when used concomitantly with corticosteroids.

Diclofenac should be used with caution in patients who may be adversely affected by a prolongation of bleeding time (e.g., patients receiving anticoagulant therapy), since the drug may inhibit platelet function. If signs and/or symptoms of anemia occur during therapy with diclofenac, hemoglobin concentration and hematocrit should be determined.

Renal toxicity has been observed in patients in whom renal prostaglandins have a compensatory role in maintaining renal perfusion. Administration of an NSAIA to such patients may cause a dose-dependent reduction in prostaglandin formation and thereby precipitate overt renal decompensation. Patients at greatest risk of this reaction are those with impaired renal function, heart failure, or hepatic dysfunction; those with extracellular fluid depletion (e.g., patients receiving diuretics); those taking an ACE inhibitor or angiotensin II receptor antagonist concomitantly; and geriatric patients. Patients should be advised to consult their clinician promptly if unexplained weight gain or edema occurs. Recovery of renal function to pretreatment levels usually occurs following discontinuance of NSAIA therapy.

Diclofenac has not been evaluated in patients with severe renal impairment, and the manufacturers state that use of the drug is not recommended in patients with advanced renal disease. If diclofenac is used in patients with severe renal impairment, close monitoring of renal function is recommended.

Anaphylactoid reactions have been reported in patients receiving diclofenac. Patients receiving diclofenac should be informed of the signs and symptoms of an anaphylactoid reaction (e.g., difficulty breathing, swelling of the face or throat) and advised to seek immediate medical attention if an anaphylactoid reaction develops.

Serious skin reactions (e.g., exfoliative dermatitis, Stevens-Johnson syndrome, toxic epidermal necrolysis) can occur in patients receiving diclofenac. These serious skin reactions may occur without warning; patients should be advised to consult their clinician if skin rash and blisters, fever, or other signs of hypersensitivity reaction (e.g., pruritus) occur. Diclofenac should be discontinued at the first appearance of rash or any other sign of hypersensitivity.

Patients receiving long-term NSAIA therapy should have a complete blood cell count and chemistry profile performed periodically.

Some clinicians state that NSAIAs should be used with caution in patients with systemic lupus erythematosus (SLE) since serious adverse CNS effects (e.g., aseptic meningitis) and possible activation of SLE occasionally have been observed in patients with SLE receiving NSAIAs.

Because NSAIAs have caused adverse ocular effects, patients who experience visual disturbances during diclofenac therapy should have an ophthalmologic examination.

The possibility that the antipyretic and anti-inflammatory effects of diclofenac sodium may mask the usual signs and symptoms of infection or other diseases should be considered.

Diclofenac is not a substitute for corticosteroid therapy, and the drug is not effective in the management of adrenal insufficiency. Abrupt withdrawal of corticosteroids may exacerbate corticosteroid-responsive conditions. If corticosteroid therapy is to be discontinued after prolonged therapy, the dosage should be tapered gradually.

When diclofenac sodium 1% gel or diclofenac epolamine transdermal system is used, patients should be advised to avoid contact with the eyes or mucous membranes. If the gel or transdermal system does come in contact with the eyes, the eyes should be thoroughly rinsed with water or saline. Patients should be advised to consult a clinician if ocular irritation persists for longer than one hour.

Patients should be advised to store and discard diclofenac epolamine transdermal systems in a manner that avoids accidental exposure or ingestion by children or pets.

Topical application of diclofenac gel formulations has resulted in early onset of ultraviolet (UV) light-related skin tumors in animal studies. When diclofenac sodium 1% gel is used, it may be prudent to minimize or avoid exposure of treated areas to natural or artificial sunlight. The potential effects of topical diclofenac gel on skin response to UV damage in humans are not known.

Patients receiving therapy with diclofenac epolamine transdermal system should be advised to bathe or shower after removing one system but before applying a new system; patients should not wear the system while bathing or showering.

The manufacturers state that diclofenac is contraindicated in patients with known hypersensitivity to the drug. In addition, NSAIAs, including diclofenac, generally are contraindicated in patients in whom asthma, urticaria, or other sensitivity reactions are precipitated by aspirin or other NSAIAs, since there is potential for cross-sensitivity between NSAIAs and aspirin, and severe, often fatal, anaphylactic reactions may occur in such patients. Although NSAIAs generally are contraindicated in these patients, the drugs have occasionally been used in NSAIA-sensitive patients who have undergone desensitization. Because patients with asthma may have aspirin-sensitivity asthma, diclofenac should be used with caution in patients with asthma. In patients with asthma, aspirin sensitivity is manifested principally as bronchospasm and usually is associated with nasal polyps; the association of aspirin sensitivity, asthma, and nasal polyps is known as the aspirin triad. For a further discussion of cross-sensitivity of NSAIAs, see Cautions: Sensitivity Reactions, in the Salicylates General Statement 28:08.04.24.

NSAIAs are contraindicated in the setting of CABG surgery.

■ **Pediatric Precautions** The manufacturer states that safety and efficacy of diclofenac in children have not been established. However, oral diclofenac has been used with good results for the management of juvenile rheumatoid arthritis† in a limited number of children 3–16 years of age. Further studies are needed to establish the optimum dosages and indications for use in children.

■ **Geriatric Precautions** Many of the spontaneous reports of fatal adverse GI effects in patients receiving NSAIAs involve geriatric individuals. NSAIAs, including diclofenac, should be used with caution in geriatric patients 65 years of age or older.

Of the total number of patients studied in clinical trials of diclofenac sodium 1% topical gel, 498 were 65 years of age or older. Although no overall differences in safety or efficacy were observed between geriatric individuals and younger adults in these studies, the possibility that some older patients may exhibit increased sensitivity to the drug cannot be ruled out.

Clinical trials of diclofenac epolamine transdermal system did not include sufficient numbers of patients 65 years of age and older to determine whether they respond differently than younger adults. Other clinical experience has not identified differences in response between geriatric and younger patients.

Diclofenac is substantially excreted by the kidneys, and the risk of toxicity may be greater in patients with renal impairment. Because geriatric patients are more likely to have decreased renal function, diclofenac should be used with caution; it may be useful to monitor renal function in such patients.

■ **Mutagenicity and Carcinogenicity** No evidence of diclofenac sodium-induced mutagenicity was seen with several in vitro test systems, including the microbial (Ames test) and mammalian (mouse lymphoma) test systems. Also, there was no evidence of mutagenicity when diclofenac sodium was tested with in vitro and in vivo mammalian tests, including dominant lethal and male germinal epithelial chromosomal tests in mice and nucleus anomaly and chromosome aberration tests in Chinese hamsters.

No evidence of carcinogenic potential was seen in rats receiving oral diclofenac sodium dosages up to 2 mg/kg daily (12 mg/m^2 daily; about the maximum recommended human dosage) for 2 years. In addition, no evidence of oncogenic potential was seen in male and female mice receiving diclofenac sodium dosages up to 0.3 (0.9 mg/m^2) and 1 mg/kg (3 mg/m^2) daily, respectively, for 2 years. There was an increase, however, in benign mammary fibroadenomas in female rats receiving oral diclofenac sodium dosages of 0.25–2 mg/kg for 2 years.

Animal photocarcinogenicity studies indicate a shortened time to skin tumor formation following application of diclofenac sodium gel in a concentration up to 0.035%.

■ **Pregnancy, Fertility, and Lactation** Reproduction studies in rabbits, rats, and mice receiving oral diclofenac sodium dosages up to 10, 10, and 20 mg/kg daily, respectively, have not revealed evidence of teratogenicity; however, these dosages produced maternal (e.g., dystocia, prolonged gestation) and fetal (e.g., reduced weight, growth, and survival) toxicity.

The effects of diclofenac on labor and delivery in humans currently are not known. There are no adequate and controlled studies to date using diclofenac in pregnant women. Diclofenac should be used during pregnancy only when the potential benefits justify the possible risks to the fetus. Diclofenac should not be used during late pregnancy, since inhibitors of prostaglandin synthesis may have adverse effects on the fetal cardiovascular system (e.g., premature closure of the ductus arteriosus).

Diclofenac sodium in fixed combination with misoprostol is contraindicated in women who are pregnant because misoprostol exhibits abortifacient activity and can cause serious fetal harm. In addition, it is recommended that diclofenac in fixed combination with misoprostol be used in women of childbearing potential *only* if they require NSAIA therapy and are considered at high risk of complications resulting from NSAIA-induced gastric or duodenal ulceration or at high risk of developing gastric or duodenal ulceration. (See Cautions: Pregnancy, Fertility, and Lactation, in Misoprostol 56:28.28.)

Reproduction studies in male and female rats using diclofenac sodium dosages up to 4 mg/kg (24 mg/m^2) daily have not revealed evidence of impaired fertility.

Because of the potential for serious adverse reactions to diclofenac in nursing infants, a decision should be made whether to discontinue nursing or the drug, taking into account the importance of the drug to the woman.

Drug Interactions

■ **Protein-bound Drugs** Because diclofenac is highly protein bound, it could be displaced from binding sites by, or it theoretically could displace from binding sites, other protein-bound drugs. In vitro studies suggest that diclofenac only minimally displaces from protein binding sites other highly protein-bound drugs (e.g., prednisolone, salicylates, tolbutamide, warfarin), although diclofenac may be displaced from binding sites by high doses of ionized protein-bound drugs (e.g., salicylates).

■ **Angiotensin-converting Enzyme Inhibitors and Angiotensin II Receptor Antagonists** There is some evidence that concomitant use of NSAIAs with angiotensin-converting enzyme (ACE) inhibitors or angiotensin II receptor antagonists may reduce the blood pressure response to the antihypertensive agent.

■ **Anticoagulants** The effects of warfarin and NSAIAs on GI bleeding are synergistic. Concomitant use of diclofenac and warfarin is associated with a higher risk of GI bleeding compared with use of either agent alone.

In short-term controlled studies in patients receiving maintenance doses of coumarin derivatives, diclofenac did not substantially alter the hypothrombinemic effect of these anticoagulants when the drugs were administered concomitantly. However, because diclofenac may cause GI bleeding, inhibit platelet aggregation, and prolong bleeding time, the drug should be used with caution and the patient carefully observed if the drug is used concomitantly with any anticoagulant (e.g., warfarin).

■ **Diuretics** Patients receiving diuretics may have an increased risk of developing renal failure secondary to decreased renal blood flow resulting from prostaglandin inhibition by NSAIAs, including diclofenac. (See Cautions: Precautions and Contraindications.) In addition, NSAIAs may interfere with the natriuretic response to diuretics with activity that depends in part on prostaglandin-mediated alterations in renal blood flow (e.g., furosemide, thiazides). In patients with hypertension, the antihypertensive effect of hydrochlorothiazide was attenuated by diclofenac. Patients receiving concomitant NSAIA and diuretic therapy should be monitored for signs of renal failure and for efficacy of the diuretic.

Concomitant use of diclofenac and potassium-sparing diuretics may be associated with increased serum potassium concentrations.

Concomitant administration of diclofenac and triamterene has resulted in reversible impairment of renal function. Similar adverse renal effects have been reported with concomitant use of triamterene and other NSAIAs (e.g., indomethacin), progressing to acute renal failure in some patients. Therefore, diclofenac and triamterene should be used concomitantly with caution. The mechanism of this interaction has not been determined, but it has been postulated that NSAIAs may inhibit triamterene-mediated renal vasoconstriction.

■ **Nonsteroidal Anti-inflammatory Agents** Concomitant use of aspirin and an NSAIA increases the risk for serious GI events. Because of the potential for increased adverse effects, patients receiving diclofenac should be advised not to take aspirin. There is no consistent evidence that use of low-dose aspirin mitigates the increased risk of serious cardiovascular events associated with NSAIAs.

While multiple-dose administration of ibuprofen may inhibit the cardioprotective effects of aspirin, limited data indicate that administration of diclofenac sodium delayed-release tablets (75 mg twice daily) does not inhibit the antiplatelet effect of aspirin (81 mg daily).

Following concomitant administration of diclofenac and aspirin in healthy individuals, protein binding of diclofenac is decreased, biliary excretion of diclofenac may be increased, and peak plasma concentrations and area under the plasma concentration-time curve (AUC) of diclofenac are reduced. Pretreatment with diclofenac for 14 days before administration of aspirin appeared to enhance renal elimination of salicylate. The clinical importance of these pharmacokinetic interactions remains to be determined.

■ **Methotrexate** Severe, sometimes fatal, toxicity has occurred following concomitant administration of diclofenac and methotrexate. The toxicity was associated with elevated serum concentrations of methotrexate. Patients at greatest risk of this reaction are those with renal impairment and those receiving relatively high (e.g., antineoplastic) dosages of methotrexate. Caution is advised if methotrexate and an NSAIA are administered concomitantly. (See Drug Interactions: Nonsteroidal Anti-inflammatory Agents, in Methotrexate 10:00.)

■ **Cyclosporine** Concomitant administration of diclofenac and cyclosporine may increase the nephrotoxic effects of cyclosporine; this interaction may be related to inhibition of renal prostaglandin (e.g., prostacyclin) synthesis. Diclofenac and cyclosporine should be used concomitantly with caution.

■ **Lithium** Diclofenac increases plasma lithium concentrations and reduces renal lithium clearance. The mechanism involved in the reduction of lithium clearance by NSAIAs (including diclofenac) is not known, but has been attributed to inhibition of prostaglandin synthesis, which may interfere with the renal elimination of lithium. In one study in healthy women, plasma lithium concentration was increased by 26% and renal clearance was reduced by 23%. In a patient receiving 1 g of lithium daily together with diclofenac sodium dosages of 75 mg daily, plasma lithium concentrations increased about fivefold; manifestations of lithium intoxication developed but resolved following discontinuance of both diclofenac and lithium. If diclofenac and lithium are administered concurrently, the patient should be closely observed for signs of lithium toxicity and plasma lithium concentrations should be monitored carefully during the initial stages of combined therapy or subsequent dosage adjustment. In addition, appropriate adjustment of lithium dosage may be required when therapy with diclofenac is discontinued.

■ **Quinolones** It has been suggested that concomitant use of ciprofloxacin and an NSAIA (e.g., diclofenac) could increase the risk of CNS stimulation (e.g., seizures), but additional study and experience are necessary.

■ **Antacids** Concomitant administration of diclofenac and an aluminum and magnesium hydroxides antacid may result in delayed diclofenac absorption; however, extent of absorption is not affected.

Because magnesium-containing antacids may increase the incidence of misoprostol-induced diarrhea, concomitant administration of diclofenac in fixed combination with misoprostol with a magnesium-containing antacid is not recommended. Antacids and food appear to decrease the oral bioavailability of misoprostol. (See Drug Interactions: Food and Antacids, in Misoprostol 56:28.28.)

■ **Other Drugs** Concomitant use of ulcerogenic drugs such as corticosteroids during NSAIA therapy may increase the risk of GI ulceration. Concomitant administration of more than one diclofenac-containing product should be avoided.

Acute Toxicity

Limited information is available on the acute toxicity of diclofenac.

■ **Pathogenesis** The acute lethal dose of diclofenac sodium in humans is not known. Individuals have survived reported ingestions of up to 4 g of the drug. The oral LD_{50} of diclofenac sodium is 55–240, 500, and 3200 mg/kg in rats, dogs, and monkeys, respectively. Hydroxylated metabolites of the drug have exhibited less toxic potential than did the unchanged drug in LD_{50} studies in rats.

■ **Manifestations** Acute diclofenac overdosage produces manifestations that are mainly extensions of adverse effects of the drug. Loss of consciousness, increased intracranial pressure, and aspiration pneumonitis were reported in a 17-year-old male, who died 2 days after ingesting 5 g of diclofenac. No signs or symptoms of toxicity were observed in a few patients who ingested 3.75–4 g of diclofenac. However, vomiting and drowsiness occurred in an adolescent who ingested 2.37 g of the drug. Several other adults who ingested overdosages of diclofenac along with other drugs, including CNS depressants, developed confusion, hypotonia, and loss of consciousness (requiring intubation and ventilation). In one of these patients, plasma diclofenac concentrations were 60.1 and 0.19 mcg/mL 7 and 15 hours after ingestion, respectively.

■ **Treatment** In acute diclofenac overdosage, general measures should include immediately emptying the stomach by inducing emesis or by gastric lavage, followed by initiation of symptomatic and supportive treatment. Administration of activated charcoal after emesis or gastric lavage may be useful in minimizing absorption of diclofenac and reabsorption of enterohepatically recirculated drug. Forced diuresis, alkalinization of urine, hemodialysis, or hemoperfusion may not be beneficial in enhancing elimination of diclofenac, because the drug is highly protein bound. If forced diuresis is used in an attempt to enhance urinary excretion of the drug, fluid and electrolyte balance should be monitored carefully, since potentially serious electrolyte disturbances and fluid retention may occur.

Pharmacology

Diclofenac has pharmacologic actions similar to those of other prototypical NSAIAs. The drug exhibits anti-inflammatory, analgesic, and antipyretic activity. The exact mechanisms have not been clearly established, but many of the actions appear to be associated principally with the inhibition of prostaglandin synthesis. Diclofenac inhibits the synthesis of prostaglandins in body tissues by inhibiting cyclooxygenase; at least 2 isoenzymes, cyclooxygenase-1 (COX-1) and -2 (COX-2) (also referred to as prostaglandin G/H synthase-1 [PGHS-1] and -2 [PGHS-2], respectively), have been identified that catalyze the formation of prostaglandins in the arachidonic acid pathway. Diclofenac, like other prototypical NSAIAs, inhibits both COX-1 and COX-2. Although the exact mechanisms have not been clearly established, NSAIAs appear to exert anti-inflammatory, analgesic, and antipyretic activity principally through inhibition of the COX-2 isoenzyme; COX-1 inhibition presumably is responsible for the drugs' unwanted effects on GI mucosa and platelet aggregation.

■ **Anti-inflammatory, Analgesic, and Antipyretic Effects** The anti-inflammatory, analgesic, and antipyretic effects of diclofenac and other NSAIAs, including selective inhibitors of COX-2 (e.g., celecoxib), appear to result from inhibition of prostaglandin synthesis. While the precise mechanism of the anti-inflammatory and analgesic effects of NSAIAs continues to be investigated, these effects appear to be mediated principally through inhibition of the COX-2 isoenzyme at sites of inflammation with subsequent reduction in the synthesis of certain prostaglandins from their arachidonic acid precursors.

High concentrations of diclofenac have been reported to inhibit formation of other arachidonic acid metabolites, including leukotrienes and 5- hydroxyeicosatetraenoic acid (5-HETE). Diclofenac may inhibit the migration of leukocytes, including polymorphonuclear leukocytes, into inflammatory sites. However, inhibition of leukotriene formation and migration of leukocytes do not appear to result from direct diclofenac-induced inhibition of lipoxygenase. Diclofenac also inhibits lysosomal enzyme release from polymorphonuclear leukocytes and may inhibit superoxide production and chemotaxis of polymorphonuclear leukocytes.

On a weight basis, the anti-inflammatory potency of diclofenac has been shown to be less than that of piroxicam, and to be about 2.5, 10, 24, 80, or 430 times that of indomethacin, naproxen, phenylbutazone, ibuprofen, or aspirin, respectively, as determined by inhibition of carrageenan-induced paw edema in rats. In adjuvant-induced arthritis in rats, the anti-inflammatory activity of diclofenac is similar to that of indomethacin, and about 30, 95, or 380 times that of naproxen, phenylbutazone, or ibuprofen, respectively. The anti-inflammatory activity of topically applied 4% diclofenac sodium is similar to that of topically applied 2–4% ibuprofen or indomethacin and 10% meclofenamic acid, mefenamic acid, or phenylbutazone, as determined by inhibition of UV light-induced erythema in animals.

On a weight basis, as determined by antagonism of phenylbenzoquinone-induced writhing in mice, the analgesic potency of diclofenac was similar to that of indomethacin and about 5, 10, 22, or 38 times that of naproxen, ibuprofen, phenylbutazone, or aspirin, respectively. On a weight basis in human studies, the analgesic effect of diclofenac was similar to that of codeine and about 3–8, 8–16, and 12–18 times that of naproxen, ibuprofen, and aspirin, respectively.

Tolerance to the analgesic effect of diclofenac apparently does not occur during long-term administration.

Diclofenac lowers body temperature in animals with antigen-induced fever. Although the mechanism of antipyretic effect of NSAIAs is not known, it has been suggested that suppression of prostaglandin synthesis in the CNS (probably in the hypothalamus) may be involved. In rats, the antipyretic activity of diclofenac 0.5 mg/kg was similar to that of 1.2, 24, 35, 55, or 185 mg/kg of indomethacin, ibuprofen, phenylbutazone, naproxen, or aspirin, respectively.

■ **Genitourinary and Renal Effects** Diclofenac has relieved symptoms associated with primary dysmenorrhea, probably by inhibiting the synthesis and/or actions of prostaglandins. Whether the increased production of prostaglandins associated with primary dysmenorrhea is mediated by COX-1 or COX-2 remains to be determined.

Diclofenac has been reported to adversely affect renal function. (See Cautions: Renal, Electrolyte, and Genitourinary Effects.) Although the exact mechanism of adverse renal effects of NSAIAs has not been determined, the effects may be related to inhibition of renal prostaglandin synthesis.

Diclofenac exhibited an antiproteinuric effect in a limited number of patients with glomerulonephritis and normal renal function. The mechanism(s) of this decreased proteinuria remains to be established.

Diclofenac does not appear to have uricosuric activity when administered in usual dosages.

■ **GI Effects** Diclofenac can cause gastric mucosal damage, which may result in ulceration and/or bleeding. These gastric effects have been attributed to inhibition of the synthesis of prostaglandins produced by COX-1. Other factors possibly involved in NSAIA-induced gastropathy include local irritation, promotion of acid back-diffusion into gastric mucosa, uncoupling of oxidative phosphorylation, and enterohepatic recirculation of the drugs.

Misoprostol, a synthetic prostaglandin E_1 analog, inhibits gastric acid secretion and protects the mucosa from irritant and/or other (e.g., pharmacologic) effects of certain drugs (e.g., nonsteroidal anti-inflammatory agents [NSAIAs]). (See Pharmacology, in Misoprostol 56:28.28.)

Epidemiologic and laboratory studies suggest that NSAIAs may reduce the risk of colon cancer. Although the exact mechanism by which NSAIAs may inhibit colon carcinogenesis remains to be determined, it has been suggested that inhibition of prostaglandin synthesis may be involved.

■ **Hematologic Effects** Diclofenac can inhibit platelet aggregation and may prolong bleeding time. Like other prototypical NSAIAs, these effects of diclofenac appear to be associated with inhibition of the synthesis of prostaglandins produced by COX-1. In a study in healthy individuals, the drug did not substantially affect collagen-induced platelet aggregation, platelet count, prothrombin time, or bleeding time. Reports of the effect of parenterally administered diclofenac on bleeding time have been equivocal. However, parenterally administered diclofenac has produced a dose-dependent increase in bleeding time in healthy adults when administered by IV infusion.

■ **Other Effects** Diclofenac may increase free fatty acid concentrations and plasma post-heparin lipoprotein lipase activity. In healthy men, diclofenac does not appear to alter substantially plasma concentrations of follicle-stimulating hormone, luteinizing hormone, or thyrotropin (thyroid-stimulating hormone, TSH) but has decreased plasma prolactin concentrations.

Like some other NSAIAs, diclofenac inhibits prostaglandin synthesis in the conjunctiva and uvea following topical application to the eye and thereby may prevent and/or decrease disruption of the blood-aqueous humor barrier.

Pharmacokinetics

■ **Absorption** Diclofenac sodium and diclofenac potassium are almost completely absorbed from the GI tract; however, the drugs undergo extensive first-pass metabolism in the liver, with only about 50–60% of a dose of diclofenac sodium or diclofenac potassium reaching systemic circulation as unchanged drug. Diclofenac also is absorbed into systemic circulation following rectal administration and percutaneously following topical application to the skin as a gel or transdermal system.

Measurable plasma concentrations of diclofenac have been observed in some fasting individuals within 10 minutes of receiving diclofenac potassium conventional tablets. Onset of absorption is delayed when diclofenac sodium is administered orally as delayed-release (enteric-coated) tablets, but the extent of absorption does not appear to be affected. Peak plasma concentrations of diclofenac generally occur within 1 hour (range: 0.33–2 hours) or 2–3 hours (range: 1–4 hours) after oral administration of diclofenac potassium conventional tablets or delayed-release (enteric-coated) diclofenac sodium tablets, respectively. Peak plasma concentrations occur within 10–30 minutes after administration of an oral solution of diclofenac sodium. Following oral administration of a single 25-, 50-, 75-, or 150-mg dose as delayed-release (enteric-coated) diclofenac sodium tablets in healthy adults, average peak plasma diclofenac concentrations of 0.5–1, 1–1.5, 2, and 2.5 mcg/mL, respectively, occur within about 1.5–3 hours. The area under the plasma concentration-time curve (AUC) increases linearly with single diclofenac sodium doses of 25–150 mg. There is considerable interindividual and intraindividual variation in plasma concentrations attained with a given dosage, and onset of absorption is variable secondary to differing dissolution of the enteric coating of diclofenac sodium delayed-release tablets. Following oral administration of a single 100-mg dose of diclofenac sodium as an extended-release tablet, mean peak plasma concentrations of 417 ng/mL generally occur within 5–6 hours. Following rectal administration of a single 25-, 50-, or 100-mg diclofenac sodium suppository in healthy adults, peak plasma diclofenac concentrations of approximately 0.6, 0.7, or 1.8 mcg/mL, respectively, occur within about 1 hour. The relationship between plasma diclofenac concentrations and therapeutic effect has not been established.

Food decreases the rate of absorption of conventional tablets of diclofenac potassium and of delayed-release (enteric-coated) tablets of diclofenac sodium, resulting in delayed and decreased peak plasma concentrations; however, the extent of absorption is not affected substantially. When diclofenac potassium conventional tablets are administered with food, time to achieve peak plasma concentrations of the drug is increased and peak plasma concentrations of the drug are decreased by approximately 30%. When single doses of diclofenac sodium delayed-release (enteric-coated) tablets are taken with food, the onset of absorption usually is delayed by 1–4.5 hours but may be delayed up to 12 hours in some patients. These food-induced alterations in GI absorption of the drug result from delayed transit of the delayed-release (enteric-coated) tablets to the small intestine, the site of dissolution. When diclofenac sodium extended-release tablets are taken with food, onset of absorption is delayed 1–2 hours and peak plasma concentrations are increased two-fold; however, extent of absorption is not substantially affected. Absorption of diclofenac does not appear to be affected substantially by the presence of food following continuous dosing of the drug. Antacids also may decrease the rate but not the extent of absorption of diclofenac.

Peak plasma diclofenac concentrations attained following administration of the drug may be reduced in patients with rheumatoid arthritis compared with those in healthy adults; however, AUCs appear to be similar. Peak plasma concentrations and AUCs of the drug in geriatric individuals may be increased up to about fourfold and twofold those, respectively, observed in younger individuals, although a lack of substantial age-related alterations also has been reported. No differences in pharmacokinetic values for diclofenac have been detected in patients with renal impairment relative to healthy adults.

Diclofenac is absorbed into systemic circulation following topical application, but plasma concentrations generally are very low compared with oral administration. Following application of a single diclofenac epolamine transdermal system to intact skin on the upper arm, peak plasma diclofenac concentrations of 0.7–6 ng/mL occur in 10–20 hours. Following application of a diclofenac transdermal system twice daily for 5 days, plasma diclofenac concentrations of 1.3–8.8 ng/mL have been reported. No difference in systemic absorption was observed between healthy individuals at rest and those engaging in moderate exercise.

Following topical application of 4 g of diclofenac sodium 1% gel 4 times daily to one knee, mean peak plasma diclofenac concentrations of 15 ng/mL occur in about 14 hours. Following application of the gel to both knees and both hands 4 times daily (48 g of gel), mean peak plasma diclofenac concentrations of 53.8 ng/mL occur in about 10 hours. Systemic exposure to the drug at these dosage levels (16 or 48 g of gel daily) is about 6 or 20%, respectively, of the systemic exposure attained when diclofenac sodium is administered orally at a dosage of 50 mg 3 times daily. Application of a heat patch for 15 minutes before application of the gel did not affect systemic absorption. It has not been established whether application of a heat patch following gel application affects systemic absorption of the drug. Moderate exercise did not affect systemic absorption of the drug.

■ **Distribution** Distribution of diclofenac into human body tissues and fluids has not been fully characterized. Following IV administration of diclofenac in rats, the drug is widely distributed, achieving highest concentrations in bile, liver, blood, heart, lungs, and kidneys and lower concentrations in adrenals, thyroid glands, salivary glands, pancreas, spleen, muscles, brain, and spinal cord.

Like other NSAIAs, diclofenac is distributed into synovial fluid, achieving peak synovial fluid concentrations about 60–70% of those attained in plasma following oral administration; however, synovial fluid concentrations of the drug and its metabolites substantially exceed those in plasma after 3–6 hours. Following oral administration of a single 75-mg dose of diclofenac sodium, peak synovial fluid concentrations of approximately 225 ng/mL occur within about 4 hours, but there is considerable interindividual variation in synovial concentrations attained with a given dosage of the drug. Diclofenac appears to be eliminated from synovial fluid less rapidly than from plasma.

The apparent total volume of distribution of diclofenac reportedly averages about 1.3–1.4 L/kg.

Diclofenac is extensively but reversibly bound to plasma proteins, mainly albumin. At plasma diclofenac concentrations of 0.15–105 mcg/mL, the drug is 99–99.8% protein bound in vitro. Two binding sites have been identified, a high-affinity, low capacity site and a low-affinity, high capacity site. In patients with rheumatoid arthritis, protein binding of diclofenac in synovial fluid appears to be lower than in plasma.

Diclofenac and its metabolites cross the placenta in mice and rats. While substantial distribution of the drug into the milk of lactating women does not appear to occur with oral diclofenac sodium dosages of 100 mg daily, milk diclofenac concentrations of approximately 100 ng/mL were achieved in at least one woman receiving 150 mg of the drug daily.

■ **Elimination** Plasma concentrations of diclofenac appear to decline in a triphasic manner. Following IV administration of diclofenac sodium in healthy adults, the half-life of diclofenac reportedly averages about 3 minutes in the initial distribution phase, about 16 minutes in the intermediate (redistribution) phase, and about 1–2 hours in the terminal (elimination) phase. Following oral administration of delayed-release (enteric-coated) diclofenac sodium tablets in healthy individuals or in patients with rheumatoid arthritis, the elimination half-life of the drug was approximately 1.2–2 hours. Following application of diclofenac epolamine transdermal system, the elimination half-life of diclofenac is approximately 12 hours. The elimination half-life of diclofenac in patients with moderate renal impairment appears to be similar to that in patients with normal renal function; however, half-life may be prolonged with severe renal impairment.

The exact metabolic fate of diclofenac has not been fully elucidated, but the drug is rapidly and extensively metabolized in the liver. Diclofenac undergoes extensive hydroxylation and subsequent conjugation with glucuronic acid, taurine amide, sulfuric acid, and other biogenic ligands. Conjugation of unchanged drug also may occur. Hydroxylation of the dichlorophenyl aromatic ring results in formation of 4′-hydroxydiclofenac (the principal metabolite of diclofenac) and 3′-hydroxydiclofenac, both of which subsequently undergo conjugation. Diclofenac also may undergo hydroxylation of the phenylacetic acid ring and subsequent conjugation to form conjugates of 5-hydroxydiclofenac and 4′,5-dihydroxydiclofenac. Conjugation with glucuronic acid and taurine usually occurs at the carboxyl group of the phenylacetic ring, while conjugation with sulfuric acid mainly occurs at the 4′ hydroxyl group of the dichlorophenyl aromatic ring; 3′- and/or 4′-hydroxydiclofenac may undergo further 4′-*O*-methylation to form 3′-hydroxy-4′-methoxydiclofenac.

Studies in animals indicate that on a weight basis, 4′-hydroxydiclofenac has about 3% of the anti-inflammatory potency of diclofenac and about 6 times the anti-inflammatory potency of aspirin. 3′-Hydroxydiclofenac also may have some anti-inflammatory activity, but other metabolites of the drug appear to be pharmacologically inactive.

Following oral or IV administration, diclofenac is excreted in urine and feces, with only minimal amounts being excreted unchanged. Fecal excretion of the drug occurs mainly via biliary elimination. Conjugates of unchanged diclofenac are excreted principally in bile, while hydroxylated metabolites are excreted in urine. Although there is evidence from animal studies that diclofenac undergoes enterohepatic circulation, such recirculation is minimal in humans.

Following oral or IV administration of diclofenac in healthy adults, about 50–70% of a dose is excreted in urine and about 30–35% is excreted in feces within 96 hours. About 20–30% of a dose is excreted in urine as conjugates of 4′-hydroxydiclofenac, 10–20% as conjugates of 5-, 3′-, and 4′,5-dihydroxydiclofenac, 5–10% as conjugates of unchanged diclofenac, 2% as unconjugated metabolites, 1.4% as an unidentified metabolite (with an elimination half-life of 80 hours), and less than 1% as unchanged drug.Approximately 10–20% of a dose is excreted in bile as conjugates of 4′-hydroxydiclofenac, 1–5% as conjugates of unchanged diclofenac, and about 5–6% total as conjugates of the other 3 major metabolites.

Following IV administration of diclofenac in healthy individuals, plasma clearance of the drug averages about 263–350 mL/minute. Plasma clearance of diclofenac does not appear to be affected by renal impairment, although clearance of metabolites may be decreased.

The degree of accumulation of metabolites of diclofenac in patients with renal failure has not been systematically evaluated. Metabolites of diclofenac may accumulate in patients with severe renal impairment. In these patients, steady-state plasma metabolite concentrations may be up to four times higher than those observed in healthy individuals.

It is not known whether diclofenac is removed from systemic circulation by hemodialysis, hemoperfusion, or peritoneal dialysis.

Chemistry and Stability

■ **Chemistry** Diclofenac, a phenylacetic acid derivative, is a prototypical nonsteroidal anti-inflammatory agent (NSAIA). The drug is structurally related to meclofenamate sodium and mefenamic acid, but unlike these anthranilic acid (2-aminobenzoic) acid derivatives, diclofenac is a 2-aminobenzeneacetic acid derivative.

Diclofenac is commercially available as diclofenac sodium delayed-release (enteric-coated) tablets, diclofenac sodium extended-release tablets, and as diclofenac potassium conventional tablets. Diclofenac also is commercially available as a fixed combination of diclofenac sodium in an enteric-coated core and misoprostol in an outer shell. Diclofenac sodium also is commercially available as a topical gel. Diclofenac epolamine is commercially available as a transdermal system. The transdermal system consists of an adhesive material containing diclofenac epolamine (13 mg of drug per g of adhesive) that is applied to a polyester felt backing and is covered with a polypropylene liner; the liner is removed prior to application to the skin. Each transdermal system measures 10 × 14 cm and contains 180 mg of diclofenac epolamine in an aqueous base.

Diclofenac sodium and diclofenac potassium occur as faintly yellowish white to light beige, practically odorless, slightly hygroscopic crystalline powders and, at 25°C, have a pK_a of approximately 4.

■ **Stability** Diclofenac sodium delayed-release (enteric-coated) tablets, diclofenac sodium extended-release tablets, and diclofenac potassium tablets should be protected from moisture and stored in tight containers at a temperature not exceeding 30°C. Commercially available diclofenac sodium and misoprostol tablets should be stored in a dry area at a temperature not exceeding 25°C. Commercially available diclofenac sodium delayed-release (enteric-coated) tablets have an expiration date of 2 years following the date of manufacture.

Diclofenac sodium 1% gel and diclofenac epolamine transdermal system should be stored at 25°C but may be exposed to temperatures ranging from 15–30°C. Diclofenac gel should not be frozen.

Preparations

Excipients in commercially available drug preparations may have clinically important effects in some individuals; consult specific product labeling for details.

Diclofenac Epolamine

Topical		
Transdermal System	1.3%	**Flector®**, King

Diclofenac Potassium

Oral		
Tablets	50 mg*	**Diclofenac Potassium Tablets**

*available from one or more manufacturer, distributor, and/or repackager by generic (nonproprietary) name

Diclofenac Sodium

Oral		
Tablets, delayed-release (enteric-coated)	25 mg*	**Diclofenac Sodium Delayed-release Tablets**
	50 mg*	**Diclofenac Sodium Delayed-release Tablets**
	75 mg*	**Diclofenac Sodium Delayed-release Tablets**
		Voltaren®, Novartis
Tablets, extended-release	100 mg*	**Diclofenac Sodium Extended Release Tablets**
		Voltaren®-XR, Novartis
Topical		
Gel	1%	**Voltaren®**, Novartis

*available from one or more manufacturer, distributor, and/or repackager by generic (nonproprietary) name

Diclofenac Sodium Combinations

Oral		
Tablets, delayed-release (enteric-coated core), film-coated	50 mg diclofenac sodium enteric-coated core, with 200 mcg of misoprostol outer layer*	**Arthrotec®**, Searle **Diclofenac Sodium and Misoprostol Delayed-release Tablets**
	75 mg diclofenac sodium enteric-coated core, with 200 mcg of misoprostol outer layer*	**Arthrotec®**, Searle **Diclofenac Sodium and Misoprostol Delayed-release Tablets**

*available from one or more manufacturer, distributor, and/or repackager by generic (nonproprietary) name

†Use is not currently included in the labeling approved by the US Food and Drug Administration

Ibuprofen
Ibuprofen Lysine

p-Isobutylhydratropic Acid

■ Ibuprofen is a prototypical nonsteroidal anti-inflammatory agent (NSAIA) that also exhibits analgesic and antipyretic activity.

Uses

Ibuprofen is used orally for anti-inflammatory and analgesic effects in the symptomatic treatment of rheumatoid arthritis, juvenile rheumatoid arthritis, and osteoarthritis. Ibuprofen also is used orally to relieve mild to moderate pain and for the management of primary dysmenorrhea.

Ibuprofen has been used orally in the management of pericarditis†.

Ibuprofen also may be used orally for *self-medication* for analgesic effects to provide temporary relief of *minor* aches and pains, including those of arthritis, and of dysmenorrhea and for its antipyretic effect to reduce fever.

Ibuprofen is used IV to relieve mild to moderate pain, to relieve moderate to severe pain (in conjunction with opiates), and to reduce fever.

Ibuprofen lysine is used IV in the treatment of patent ductus arteriosus (PDA) in premature neonates.

The potential benefits and risks of ibuprofen therapy as well as alternative therapies should be considered prior to initiating ibuprofen therapy. The lowest possible effective dosage and shortest duration of therapy consistent with treatment goals of the patient should be employed.

■ **Inflammatory Diseases** ***Rheumatoid Arthritis, Juvenile Arthritis, and Osteoarthritis*** Ibuprofen is used orally for anti-inflammatory and analgesic effects in the symptomatic treatment of acute and chronic rheumatoid arthritis and osteoarthritis. Ibuprofen is also used orally for anti-inflammatory and analgesic effects in the symptomatic treatment of nonarticular (e.g., muscular) inflammation.

When used in the treatment of rheumatoid arthritis, ibuprofen has relieved pain and stiffness, reduced swelling, and improved grip strength and joint flexion. The drug does not, however, alter the basic rheumatoid process. Most clinical studies have shown that the analgesic and anti-inflammatory effects of ibuprofen in the treatment of rheumatoid arthritis and/or osteoarthritis are greater than those of placebo, about equal to those of salicylates or indomethacin and less than those of phenylbutazone or prednisolone. Patient response to oral NSAIAs is variable; patients who do not respond to or cannot tolerate one NSAIA might be successfully treated with a different agent. However, NSAIAs generally are contraindicated in patients in whom sensitivity reactions (e.g., urticaria, bronchospasm, severe rhinitis) are precipitated by aspirin or other NSAIAs. (See Cautions: Precautions and Contraindications.)

In the management of rheumatoid arthritis in adults, NSAIAs may be useful for initial symptomatic treatment; however, NSAIAs do not alter the course of the disease or prevent joint destruction. Disease modifying antirheumatic drugs (DMARDs) (e.g., abatacept, adalimumab, anakinra, etanercept, hydroxychloroquine, infliximab, leflunomide, methotrexate, minocycline, rituximab, sulfasalazine) have the potential to reduce or prevent joint damage and to preserve joint integrity and function. DMARDs are used in conjunction with anti-inflammatory agents (i.e., NSAIAs, intra-articular and oral glucocorticoids) and physical and occupational therapies for the management of rheumatoid arthritis. DMARD therapy should be initiated early in the disease course to prevent irreversible joint damage. For further information on the treatment of rheumatoid arthritis, including considerations in selecting a DMARD regimen, see Uses: Rheumatoid Arthritis, in Methotrexate 10:00.

Ibuprofen is used orally in the symptomatic management of juvenile rheumatoid arthritis. In a very limited number of patients with juvenile rheumatoid arthritis receiving alternate-day corticosteroid therapy, ibuprofen relieved joint stiffness when administered on the corticosteroid "off" day.

Other Inflammatory Conditions Ibuprofen has been used with some success in other inflammatory diseases including ankylosing spondylitis†, gout†, and psoriatic arthritis†.

■ **Pericarditis** Ibuprofen has been used to reduce the pain, fever, and inflammation of pericarditis†; however, in the treatment of post-myocardial infarction pericarditis, NSAIAs are potentially harmful and aspirin is considered the treatment of choice. (See Cautions: Cardiovascular Effects and Cautions: Precautions and Contraindications.)

■ **Pain** Ibuprofen is used orally or IV for the relief of mild to moderate pain. Ibuprofen also may be used orally for *self-medication* for the temporary relief of minor aches and pains associated with the common cold, influenza, or sore throat; headache (including migraine); toothache; muscular aches; backache; and minor pain of arthritis.

Some experts state that an NSAIA (e.g., ibuprofen) is a reasonable first-line therapy for mild to moderate migraine attacks or for severe attacks that have responded in the past to similar NSAIAs or non-opiate analgesics. For further information on management and classification of migraine headache, see Vascular Headaches: General Principles in Migraine Therapy, under Uses in Sumatriptan 28:32.28.

Ibuprofen has been used to relieve postoperative pain (including that associated with dental or orthopedic surgery or episiotomy). In the relief of postoperative pain, ibuprofen has been shown to be more effective than placebo or propoxyphene and at least as effective as aspirin.

Ibuprofen has been used IV in conjunction with opiates to relieve pain following abdominal hysterectomy, other abdominal surgical procedures, or orthopedic surgery.

The fixed-combination preparation containing ibuprofen and hydrocodone bitartrate is used in the short-term (less than 10 days) treatment of acute pain.

The fixed-combination preparation containing ibuprofen and oxycodone hydrochloride is used in the short-term (no more than 7 days) treatment of acute moderate to severe pain.

■ **Dysmenorrhea** Ibuprofen is used orally for the relief of primary dysmenorrhea. Ibuprofen also may be used for *self-medication* for the relief of pain of menstrual cramps (dysmenorrhea). Ibuprofen has been used to relieve dysmenorrhea associated with insertion of an intrauterine contraceptive device†.

When used to relieve dysmenorrhea, ibuprofen has been reported to be as effective as mefenamic acid and more effective than placebo, aspirin, or propoxyphene. In patients with primary dysmenorrhea, ibuprofen has reduced resting and active intrauterine pressure and the frequency of uterine contractions, probably as a result of inhibition of prostaglandin synthesis.

■ **Fever** Ibuprofen is used orally or IV to reduce fever. Ibuprofen also may be used orally for *self-medication* to reduce fever.

When used to lower body temperature in febrile children (6 months–12 years of age) with viral infections and temperatures of 39°C or less, single ibuprofen doses of 10 mg/kg have been as effective as single ibuprofen doses of 5 mg/kg or single acetaminophen doses of 10–15 mg/kg; however, in children with temperatures exceeding 39°C, single 10-mg/kg doses of ibuprofen were most effective.

■ **Patent Ductus Arteriosus** Ibuprofen lysine is used IV in the treatment of patent ductus arteriosus (PDA) in premature neonates and is designated an orphan drug by the US Food and Drug Administration (FDA) for use in this condition. The drug is used IV to promote closure of a clinically important PDA in premature neonates weighing 500–1500 g who are no more than 32 weeks' gestational age when usual medical management (e.g., fluid restriction, diuretics, respiratory support) is ineffective. Ibuprofen lysine has been evaluated in premature neonates with echocardiographic evidence of PDA who were asymptomatic from their PDA at the time of study enrollment. Efficacy was determined by the need for rescue therapy (indomethacin, open-label ibuprofen, or surgery) for a hemodynamically important PDA through study day 14. Rescue therapy was indicated if the neonate developed a hemodynamically important PDA that was confirmed by echocardiograph. Rescue therapy was required by 25% of neonates receiving ibuprofen compared with 48% of those receiving placebo. Neonates enrolled in this study were followed for a short period of time (up to 8 weeks) following treatment; long-term consequences of such therapy have not been determined. Use of the drug should be reserved for neonates with clinically important PDA.

■ **Other Uses** Results from a large, prospective, population-based cohort study in geriatric individuals indicate a lower prevalence of Alzheimer's disease† among patients who received a NSAIA for 2 years or longer. Similar findings have been reported from some other, but not all, observational studies.

Dosage and Administration

■ **Administration** The potential benefits and risks of ibuprofen therapy as well as alternative therapies should be considered prior to initiating ibuprofen therapy.

Ibuprofen is administered orally or IV. Ibuprofen lysine is administered IV.

Ibuprofen is administered by IV infusion over a period of at least 30 minutes in adults and pediatric patients 17 years of age or older. All patients receiving IV ibuprofen should be well hydrated.

For *self-medication* in pediatric patients, ibuprofen is commercially available as oral drops, an oral suspension, chewable tablets, and film-coated tablets. The calibrated dosing device provided by the manufacturer should be used by parents or caregivers for measurement of the dose of oral drops; the calibrated dosage cup provided by the manufacturer should be used by parents or caregivers for measurement of the dose of pediatric oral suspension. Ibuprofen oral drops generally are used in infants 6–23 months of age, the oral suspension commonly is used in children 2 years of age and older, the 50-mg chewable tablets may be used in children 2 years of age and older, and the 100-mg chewable tablets or 100-mg film-coated tablets may be used in children 6 years of age and older.

If GI disturbances occur, ibuprofen should be administered with meals or with milk or dosage should be reduced.

For IV administration, ibuprofen injection concentrate containing 100 mg/mL must be diluted with a compatible IV solution (e.g., 0.9% sodium chloride injection, 5% dextrose injection, lactated Ringer's injection) to provide a solution containing 4 mg/mL (less-concentrated solutions are acceptable). Ibuprofen doses are administered over 30 minutes or longer. Parenteral solutions of ibuprofen should be inspected visually for particulate matter and/or discoloration prior to administration whenever solution and container permit. The solution should not be used if opaque particles, discoloration, or other foreign particulate matter is present.

For IV administration, ibuprofen lysine injection should be diluted with an appropriate volume of dextrose injection or sodium chloride injection and administered within 30 minutes of preparation. The drug should be administered using the IV port that is nearest to the IV insertion site. The dose should be infused over a period of 15 minutes. Care should be taken to avoid extravasation of the drug since it may be irritating to extravascular tissues. Ibuprofen lysine should not be infused simultaneously through the same IV line as parenteral nutrition solutions; if the same IV line must be used, infusion of the nutrition solution should be interrupted for 15 minutes before and after ibuprofen lysine administration, and patency of the IV line maintained by infusion of dextrose injection or sodium chloride injection. Parenteral solutions of ibuprofen lysine should be inspected visually for particulate matter and/or discoloration prior to administration whenever solution and container permit. Ibuprofen lysine injection contains no preservatives and is intended for single use only; any unused portion should be discarded.

■ **Dosage** The lowest possible effective dosage and shortest duration of therapy consistent with treatment goals of the patient should be employed. Dosage of ibuprofen must be carefully adjusted according to individual requirements and response, using the lowest possible effective dosage.

Patients receiving ibuprofen for *self-medication* should be advised to use the lowest effective dosage and not to exceed the recommended dosage or duration of therapy.

Dosage of ibuprofen lysine is expressed in terms of ibuprofen.

Patients should be warned that the risk of GI bleeding is increased when recommended durations of *self-medication* are exceeded and when more than one NSAIA are used concomitantly.

Inflammatory Diseases **Rheumatoid Arthritis, Juvenile Arthritis, and Osteoarthritis.** The usual adult oral dosage of ibuprofen in the symptomatic treatment of acute and chronic rheumatoid arthritis and osteoarthritis is 400–800 mg 3 or 4 times daily. Dosage should be adjusted according to the response and tolerance of the patient and should not exceed 3.2 g daily. Although well-controlled clinical studies did not show that the average response was greater with 3.2 g daily than with 2.4 g daily, some patients may have a better response with 3.2 g daily; in patients receiving 3.2 g daily, an adequate increase in clinical benefit should be evident to justify potential increased risks associated with this dosage. Optimum therapeutic response may occur within a few days to 1 week but usually occurs within 2 weeks after beginning ibuprofen therapy if the dosage is adequate. The manufacturers state that patients with rheumatoid arthritis usually require a higher dosage of ibuprofen than do patients with osteoarthritis. When a satisfactory response to ibuprofen therapy occurs, dosage of the drug should be reviewed and adjusted as required.

For the management of juvenile rheumatoid arthritis, the recommended ibuprofen oral dosage is 30–40 mg/kg daily divided into 3 or 4 doses. An ibuprofen dosage of 20 mg/kg daily in divided doses may be adequate for children with mild disease. Dosages exceeding 50 mg/kg daily are not recommended in children with juvenile arthritis, since such dosages have not been studied. In addition, dosages exceeding 40 mg/kg daily may increase the risk of drug-induced adverse effects. Optimum therapeutic response occurs from a few days to several weeks in children with juvenile rheumatoid arthritis.

Pain For relief of mild to moderate pain, the usual adult oral dosage of ibuprofen is 400 mg every 4–6 hours as necessary. Alternatively, for *self-medication* of mild to moderate pain, the usual initial adult dosage is 200 mg every 4–6 hours; dosage may be increased to 400 mg every 4–6 hours if pain does not respond to the lower dosage but should not exceed 1.2 g daily unless directed by a clinician. For *self-medication* of migraine pain, the usual adult dosage of ibuprofen liquid-filled capsules is 400 mg; unless directed by a clinician, dosage should not exceed 400 mg in a 24-hour period. *Self-medication* of pain should not exceed 10 days unless otherwise directed by a clinician. Doses greater than 400 mg have *not* provided a greater analgesic effect than the 400-mg dose.

For relief of mild to moderate pain in children 6 months to 12 years of age, the recommended ibuprofen oral dosage is 10 mg/kg every 6–8 hours; the maximum dosage of ibuprofen is 40 mg/kg daily. For *self-medication* of minor aches and pains in pediatric patients, ibuprofen dosages should be calculated based on body weight rather than age whenever possible. (See Cautions: Pediatric Precautions.) Infants 6–11 months of age or those weighing 12–17 pounds (approximately 5–8 kg) may receive 50 mg of ibuprofen, infants 12–23 months of age or those weighing 18–23 pounds (approximately 8–10 kg) may receive 75 mg, children 2–3 years of age or those weighing 24–35 pounds (approximately 11–16 kg) may receive 100 mg, children 4–5 years of age or those weighing 36–47 pounds (approximately 16–21 kg) may receive 150 mg, children 6–8 years of age or those weighing 48–59 pounds (approximately 22–27 kg) may receive 200 mg, children 9–10 years of age or those weighing 60–71 pounds (approximately 27–32 kg) may receive 250 mg, and children 11 years of age or those weighing 72–95 pounds (approximately 33–43 kg) may receive 300 mg; these doses may be administered every 6–8 hours and no more than 4 times daily. Parents and caregivers should be instructed to contact their clinician if minor aches and pain do not improve within 24 hours or if pain increases. *Self-medication* of pain in children should not exceed 3 days unless otherwise directed by a clinician.

For relief of pain, individuals 17 years of age or older may receive ibuprofen in a dosage of 400–800 mg IV every 6 hours as needed; ibuprofen dosage should not exceed 3.2 g in a 24-hour period.

When ibuprofen is used in fixed combination with hydrocodone bitartrate for short-term (generally less than 10 days) management of acute pain, the usual oral dosage is 200 mg of ibuprofen every 4–6 hours, as needed; ibuprofen dosage should not exceed 1 g in a 24-hour period.

When ibuprofen is used in fixed combination with oxycodone hydrochloride for short-term (not to exceed 7 days) management of acute pain, 400 mg of ibuprofen may be administered up to 4 times daily; ibuprofen dosage should not exceed 1.6 g in a 24-hour period.

Dysmenorrhea For the relief of primary dysmenorrhea, ibuprofen therapy should be started with the earliest onset of pain; the usual adult oral dosage in these patients is 400 mg every 4 hours as necessary for relief of pain. Alternatively, for *self-medication* of dysmenorrhea, the usual initial adult dosage is 200 mg every 4–6 hours; dosage may be increased to 400 mg every 4–6 hours if necessary but should not exceed 1.2 g daily unless otherwise directed by a clinician.

Fever For antipyresis in children 6 months to 12 years of age, the usual oral dosage of ibuprofen is 5 or 10 mg/kg for temperatures below or above 39°C, respectively. The maximum daily dosage of ibuprofen in febrile children is 40 mg/kg.

For *self-medication* of fever in pediatric patients, ibuprofen dosages should be calculated based on body weight rather than age whenever possible. (See Cautions: Pediatric Precautions.) Infants 6–11 months of age or those weighing 12–17 pounds (approximately 5–8 kg) may receive 50 mg of ibuprofen, infants 12–23 months of age or those weighing 18–23 pounds (approximately 8–10 kg) may receive 75 mg, children 2–3 years of age or those weighing 24–35 pounds (approximately 11–16 kg) may receive 100 mg, children 4–5 years of age or those weighing 36–47 pounds (approximately 16–21 kg) may receive 150 mg, children 6–8 years of age or those weighing 48–59 pounds (approximately 22–27 kg) may receive 200 mg, children 9–10 years of age or those weighing 60–71 pounds (approximately 27–32 kg) may receive 250 mg, and children 11 years of age or those weighing 72–95 pounds (approximately 33–43 kg) may receive 300 mg; these doses may be administered every 6–8 hours and no more than 4 times daily. Parents and caregivers should be instructed to contact their clinician if fever does not improve or worsens within 24 hours. *Self-medication* of fever in children should not exceed 3 days unless otherwise directed by a clinician.

For *self-medication* of fever, the usual initial adult dosage of ibuprofen is 200 mg every 4–6 hours; dosage may be increased to 400 mg every 4–6 hours if fever is not adequately reduced at the lower dosage but should not exceed 1.2 g daily unless otherwise directed by a clinician. In addition, limited data indicate that adequate antipyresis may be maintained in some patients in whom initial doses of ibuprofen were followed with lower doses of the drug. *Self-medication* of fever should not exceed 3 days unless otherwise directed by a clinician.

For reduction of fever, individuals 17 years of age or older may receive an initial dose of ibuprofen 400 mg IV followed by 400 mg IV every 4–6 hours or 100–200 mg IV every 4 hours. Ibuprofen dosage should not exceed 3.2 g in a 24-hour period.

Patent Ductus Arteriosus For the treatment of patent ductus arteriosus (PDA) in premature neonates, ibuprofen lysine is administered by IV infusion over 15 minutes. A course of therapy consists of 3 doses of ibuprofen lysine administered at 24-hour intervals. All doses are based on the neonate's birth weight. The first IV dose of ibuprofen in the course is 10 mg/kg; the second and third doses are 5 mg/kg each, administered 24 and 48 hours after the first dose. If anuria or oliguria (i.e., urine output less than 0.6 mL/kg per hour) is present at the time of the second or third dose, the dose should be withheld until laboratory determinations indicate that renal function has returned to normal. Subsequent doses are not necessary if the ductus arteriosus closes or is substantially constricted after completion of the first course of ibuprofen therapy. If the ductus fails to close or reopens, a second course of ibuprofen, alternative pharmacologic therapy, or surgery may be needed.

Cautions

■ **Cardiovascular Effects** Peripheral edema and fluid retention have been reported during ibuprofen therapy. Congestive heart failure has occurred in patients with marginal cardiac function. Increased blood pressure, hypotension, cerebrovascular accident, and palpitations also have been reported. Although a causal relationship has not been established, arrhythmias, including sinus tachycardia or bradycardia, have been reported during therapy with the drug.

Tachycardia, cardiac failure, and hypotension have occurred in premature neonates receiving ibuprofen for treatment of patent ductus arteriosus (PDA), although a causal relationship to the drug has not been established.

Nonsteroidal anti-inflammatory agents (NSAIAs), including selective cyclooxygenase-2 (COX-2) inhibitors and prototypical NSAIAs, increase the risk of serious adverse cardiovascular thrombotic events, including myocardial infarction and stroke (which can be fatal), in patients with or without cardiovascular disease or risk factors for cardiovascular disease. Use of NSAIAs also is associated with an increased risk of heart failure.

The association between cardiovascular complications and use of NSAIAs is an area of ongoing concern and study. Findings of an FDA review of published observational studies of NSAIAs, a meta-analysis of published and unpublished data from randomized controlled trials of these drugs, and other published information indicate that NSAIAs may increase the risk of serious adverse cardiovascular thrombotic events by 10–50% or more, depending on the drugs and dosages studied. Available data suggest that the increase in risk may occur early (within the first weeks) following initiation of therapy and may increase with higher dosages and longer durations of use. Although the relative increase in cardiovascular risk appears to be similar in patients with or without known underlying cardiovascular disease or risk factors for cardiovascular disease, the absolute incidence of serious NSAIA-associated cardiovascular thrombotic events is higher in those with cardiovascular disease or risk factors for cardiovascular disease because of their elevated baseline risk.

Results from observational studies utilizing Danish national registry data indicated that patients receiving NSAIAs following a myocardial infarction were at increased risk of reinfarction, cardiovascular-related death, and all-cause mortality beginning in the first week of treatment. Patients who received NSAIAs following myocardial infarction had a higher 1-year mortality rate compared with those who did not receive NSAIAs (20 versus 12 deaths per 100 person-years). Although the absolute mortality rate declined somewhat after the first year following the myocardial infarction, the increased relative risk of death in patients who received NSAIAs persisted over at least the next 4 years of follow-up.

In 2 large controlled clinical trials of a selective COX-2 inhibitor for the management of pain in the first 10–14 days following coronary artery bypass graft (CABG) surgery, the incidence of myocardial infarction and stroke was increased. Therefore, NSAIAs are contraindicated in the setting of CABG surgery.

Findings from some systematic reviews of controlled observational studies and meta-analyses of data from randomized studies of NSAIAs suggest that naproxen may be associated with a lower risk of cardiovascular thrombotic events compared with other NSAIAs. However, limitations of these observational studies and the indirect comparisons used to assess cardiovascular risk of the prototypical NSAIAs (e.g., variability in patients' risk factors, comorbid conditions, concomitant drug therapy, drug interactions, dosage, and duration of therapy) affect the validity of the comparisons; in addition, these studies were not designed to demonstrate superior safety of one NSAIA compared with another. Therefore, FDA states that definitive conclusions regarding relative risks of NSAIAs are not possible at this time. (See Cautions: Cardiovascular Effects, in Celecoxib 28:08.04.08.)

Data from observational studies also indicate that use of NSAIAs in patients with heart failure is associated with increased morbidity and mortality. Results from a retrospective study utilizing Danish national registry data indicated that use of selective COX-2 inhibitors or prototypical NSAIAs in patients with chronic heart failure was associated with a dose-dependent increase in the risk of death and an increased risk of hospitalization for myocardial infarction or heart failure. In addition, findings from a meta-analysis of published and unpublished data from randomized controlled trials of NSAIAs indicated that use of selective COX-2 inhibitors or prototypical NSAIAs was associated with an approximate twofold increase in the risk of hospitalization for heart failure. Fluid retention and edema also have been observed in some patients receiving NSAIAs.

There is no consistent evidence that use of low-dose aspirin mitigates the increased risk of serious cardiovascular events associated with NSAIAs.

■ **GI Effects** The most frequent adverse effects of ibuprofen involve the GI tract and have included dyspepsia, heartburn, nausea, vomiting, anorexia, diarrhea, constipation, stomatitis, flatulence, bloating, epigastric pain, and abdominal pain. Peptic ulcer and GI bleeding (including evidence of occult blood in stools), sometimes severe, have also been reported. Although a causal relationship has not been established, a few cases of GI ulceration with perforation and bleeding resulting in death have occurred.

Nonnecrotizing enterocolitis has occurred in premature neonates receiving ibuprofen for treatment of PDA. Gastroesophageal reflux, gastritis, ileus, GI perforation, and necrotizing enterocolitis also have occurred, although a causal relationship to the drug has not been established.

The frequency of mild adverse GI effects with usual dosages of ibuprofen is reported to be less than that with usual dosages of oral aspirin or indomethacin. It is not known whether ibuprofen causes less peptic ulceration than does aspirin. Usual dosages of ibuprofen generally have been associated with only minimal GI blood loss, and limited data indicate that the risk of GI bleeding and/or perforation with ibuprofen appears to be less than that with other prototypical NSAIAs (e.g., piroxicam, indomethacin, ketoprofen, naproxen, diclofenac).

The risk of GI bleeding is increased in geriatric patients older than 60 years of age and in patients with a history of GI ulcers or bleeding, those receiving an anticoagulant or taking multiple NSAIAs concomitantly, those consuming 3 or more alcohol-containing beverages daily, and those receiving prolonged therapy.

Adverse GI effects of orally administered ibuprofen may be minimized by administering the drug with meals or milk. Close supervision of ibuprofen therapy is necessary, particularly in patients with a history of upper GI disease.

Serious adverse GI effects (e.g., bleeding, ulceration, perforation) can occur at any time in patients receiving NSAIA therapy, and such effects may *not* be preceded by warning signs or symptoms. Only 1 in 5 patients who develop a serious upper GI adverse event while receiving NSAIA therapy is symptomatic. Therefore, clinicians should remain alert to the possible development of serious GI effects (e.g., bleeding, ulceration) in any patient receiving NSAIA therapy, and such patients should be followed chronically for the development of manifestations of such effects and advised of the importance of this follow-up. In addition, patients should be advised about the signs and symptoms of serious NSAIA-induced GI toxicity and what action to take if they occur. If signs and symptoms of a serious GI event develop, additional evaluation and treatment should be initiated promptly; the NSAIA should be discontinued until appropriate diagnostic studies have ruled out a serious GI event.

Results of studies to date are inconclusive concerning the relative risk of various prototypical NSAIAs in causing serious GI effects. In patients receiving NSAIAs and observed in clinical studies of several months' to 2 years' duration, symptomatic upper GI ulcers, gross bleeding, or perforation appeared to occur in approximately 1% of patients treated for 3–6 months and in about 2–4% of those treated for 1 year. Longer duration of therapy with an NSAIA increases the likelihood of a serious GI event. However, short-term therapy is not without risk. High dosages of any NSAIA probably are associated with increased risk of such effects, although controlled studies documenting this probable association are lacking for most NSAIAs. Therefore, whenever use of relatively high dosages (within the recommended dosage range) is considered, sufficient benefit to offset the potential increased risk of GI toxicity should be anticipated.

Studies have shown that patients with a history of peptic ulcer disease and/or GI bleeding who are receiving NSAIAs have a substantially higher risk of developing GI bleeding than patients without these risk factors. In addition to a history of ulcer disease, pharmacoepidemiologic studies have identified several comorbid conditions and concomitant therapies that may increase the risk for GI bleeding, including concomitant use of oral corticosteroids or anticoagulants, longer duration of NSAIA therapy, smoking, alcoholism, older age, and poor general health status. Patients with rheumatoid arthritis are more likely to experience serious GI complications from NSAIA therapy than are patients with osteoarthritis. In addition, geriatric or debilitated patients appear to tolerate GI ulceration and bleeding less well than other individuals, and most spontaneous reports of fatal GI effects have been in such patients.

For patients at high risk for complications from NSAIA-induced GI ulceration (e.g., bleeding, perforation), concomitant use of misoprostol can be considered for preventive therapy. (See Misoprostol 56:28.28.) Alternatively, some clinicians suggest that a proton-pump inhibitor (e.g., omeprazole) may be used concomitantly to decrease the incidence of serious GI toxicity associated with NSAIA therapy. In one study, therapy with high dosages of famotidine (40 mg twice daily) was more effective than placebo in preventing peptic ulcers in NSAIA-treated patients; however, the effect of the drug was modest. In addition, efficacy of usual dosages of H_2-receptor antagonists for the prevention of NSAIA-induced gastric and duodenal ulcers has not been established. Therefore, most clinicians do not recommend use of H_2-receptor antagonists for the prevention of NSAIA-associated ulcers. Another approach in high-risk patients who would benefit from NSAIA therapy is use of a NSAIA that is a selective inhibitor of COX-2 (e.g., celecoxib), since these agents are associated with a lower incidence of serious GI bleeding than are prototypical NSAIAs. However, while celecoxib (200 mg twice daily) was comparably effective to diclofenac sodium (75 mg twice daily) plus omeprazole (20 mg daily) in preventing recurrent ulcer bleeding (recurrent ulcer bleeding probabilities of 4.9 versus 6.4%, respectively, during the 6-month study) in *H. pylori*-negative arthritis (principally osteoarthritis) patients with a recent history of ulcer bleeding, the protective efficacy was unexpectedly low for both regimens and it appeared that neither could completely protect patients at high risk. Additional study is necessary to elucidate optimal therapy for preventing GI complications associated with NSAIA therapy in high-risk patients.

■ **Nervous System Effects** Adverse CNS effects of ibuprofen include dizziness, headache, and nervousness. Fatigue, drowsiness, malaise, lightheadedness, anxiety, confusion, mental depression, and emotional lability have also been reported. Although a causal relationship has not been established, paresthesia, hallucinations, dream abnormalities, and pseudotumor cerebri also have been reported.

Aseptic meningitis with fever and coma has occurred rarely in patients receiving ibuprofen, and has recurred upon rechallenge with the drug. Although meningitis probably is more likely to occur in patients with systemic lupus erythematosus or related connective tissue diseases, it has been reported in some patients without evidence of any underlying chronic disease. Other associated manifestations have included GI symptoms (e.g., nausea, vomiting, abdominal pain), transient conjunctivitis, CNS signs (e.g., confusion, combativeness, lethargy, headache), and hypotension. If signs and/or symptoms of meningitis develop in a patient receiving ibuprofen, the possibility that these effects may be associated with the drug should be considered.

Intraventricular (intracranial) hemorrhage has occurred in premature neonates receiving ibuprofen for treatment of PDA. Seizures also have occurred, although a causal relationship to the drug has not been established.

■ **Otic and Ocular Effects** Patients receiving ibuprofen have experienced tinnitus. Decreased hearing and amblyopia (blurred and/or decreased visual acuity, scotomata and/or changes in color vision) have also been reported. Vision generally has gradually improved when the drug was discontinued in patients with visual disturbances. Although a causal relationship has not been established, conjunctivitis, diplopia, optic neuritis, and cataracts have also been reported in patients receiving the drug. Ibuprofen should be discontinued and an ophthalmologic examination performed in patients who experience visual disturbances during therapy with the drug.

■ **Hepatic Effects** Severe hepatic reactions (sometimes fatal) including jaundice and hepatitis have occurred rarely during ibuprofen therapy. A transitory rise in serum AST (SGOT), ALT (SGPT), and serum alkaline phosphatase has occurred in a few patients during ibuprofen therapy.

Borderline elevations of one or more liver function test results may occur in up to 15% of patients treated with NSAIAs; meaningful (3 times the upper limit of normal) elevations of serum ALT or AST concentration have occurred in less than 1% of patients receiving NSAIAs in controlled clinical studies. These abnormalities may progress, may remain essentially unchanged, or may be transient with continued therapy. Ibuprofen should be discontinued if signs or symptoms of a severe hepatic reaction occur. (See Cautions: Precautions and Contraindications.)

Although a causal relationship to the drug has not been established, jaundice and cholestasis have occurred in premature neonates receiving ibuprofen for treatment of PDA.

■ **Dermatologic Effects** Urticarial, vesiculobullous, and erythematous macular rashes, erythema multiforme, exfoliative dermatitis, toxic epidermal necrolysis (Lyell's syndrome), and photosensitivity reactions have occurred occasionally during ibuprofen therapy. Pruritus without evidence of a rash has occurred in a few patients. Stevens-Johnson syndrome, flushes, alopecia, rectal itching, and acne have also been reported.

Skin lesion/irritation has occurred in premature neonates receiving ibuprofen for treatment of PDA.

■ **Hematologic Effects** Adverse hematologic effects of ibuprofen include neutropenia, agranulocytosis, aplastic anemia, hemolytic anemia (with or without positive direct antiglobulin test results), and thrombocytopenia (with or without purpura). Slight, dose-dependent reductions in serum hemoglobin concentrations and hematocrit have occurred in patients receiving ibuprofen dosages of 1.2–3.2 g daily, and the total decrease in hemoglobin may exceed 1 g in patients receiving 3.2 g or more of the drug. Data from clinical use indicate that a decrease in hemoglobin concentration of 1 g or more occurs in about 17% of patients receiving 1.6 g of ibuprofen daily and in about 23% of patients receiving 2.4 g of the drug daily. In the absence of clinical signs of bleeding, the decrease in hemoglobin probably is not clinically important. Although a causal relationship has not been established, bleeding episodes (e.g., epistaxis, menorrhagia, occult blood in the stool) have been reported during therapy with the drug. Ibuprofen can inhibit platelet aggregation and may prolong bleeding time. It appears that ibuprofen's inhibitory effect on platelet aggregation is of shorter duration and less pronounced than that of aspirin. Patients who may be adversely affected by a prolongation of bleeding time should be carefully observed during ibuprofen therapy.

Anemia and bleeding have occurred in premature neonates receiving ibuprofen for treatment of PDA. Neutropenia and thrombocytopenia also have occurred, although a causal relationship to the drug has not been established.

■ **Renal Effects** Acute renal failure has been reported in patients receiving ibuprofen and may be accompanied by acute tubular necrosis. Such acute deterioration in renal function may be evident soon (e.g., within several days) after initiation of ibuprofen therapy in certain patients at risk (e.g., those with preexisting renal impairment) (see Cautions: Precautions and Contraindications) and may be accompanied by hyperkalemia. Polyuria, azotemia, cystitis, hematuria, and decreased creatinine clearance also have been reported in patients receiving the drug. Elevations in serum creatinine concentrations and increases in BUN without other manifestation of renal failure also have occurred occasionally. In addition, acute interstitial nephritis accompanied by hematuria, proteinuria, and occasionally nephrotic syndrome has occurred. Recurrence of nephrotic syndrome has occurred in at least one patient during ibuprofen therapy. Increases in serum uric acid concentration, tubular necrosis, glomerulitis, and renal papillary necrosis also have been reported. Long-term studies in rats and monkeys have shown histologic evidence of ibuprofen-induced mild renal toxicity manifested as papillary edema and necrosis in some animals. An association between prolonged (e.g., daily for 1 year or longer) NSAIA use, including ibuprofen, and chronic renal failure also has been described in certain high-risk patients, but current evidence suggests that the potential risk, if any, is low overall in patients receiving the drug, and additional study and experience are necessary to confirm and elucidate these findings.

Renal insufficiency (including oliguria), increases in BUN (sometimes accompanied by hematuria), increases in serum creatinine concentration, and renal failure have been reported in ibuprofen-treated premature neonates. Reversible decreases in urine output have occurred in premature neonates receiving ibuprofen therapy for PDA. Urine output usually decreases during the first 2–6 days of life; this is followed by a compensatory increase in output by day 9.

■ **Other Adverse Effects** Hypersensitivity reactions manifested as a syndrome of abdominal pain, fever, chills, nausea, and vomiting have occasionally occurred during ibuprofen therapy. Anaphylaxis, anaphylactoid reactions, and bronchospasm have also occurred. Although a causal relationship has not been established, serum sickness, lupus erythematosus syndrome, Henoch-Schönlein vasculitis, and angioedema have also been reported during therapy with the drug.

Other adverse effects of ibuprofen include dry mouth, gingival ulceration, and rhinitis. Although a causal relationship has not been established, gynecomastia, hypoglycemic reactions, and acidosis have also been reported during therapy with the drug.

Infections (e.g., sepsis, respiratory infection, urinary tract infection), apnea, respiratory failure, atelectasis, edema, adrenal insufficiency, hypoglycemia, hypocalcemia, and hypernatremia have occurred in premature neonates receiving ibuprofen for treatment of PDA. Hyperglycemia, abdominal distension, feeding problems, inguinal hernia, and injection site reactions also have occurred, although a causal relationship to the drug has not been established.

■ **Precautions and Contraindications** Patients should be advised that ibuprofen, like other NSAIAs, is not free of potential adverse effects, including some that can cause discomfort, and that more serious effects (e.g., myocardial infarction, stroke, GI bleeding), which may require hospitalization and may even be fatal, also can occur. When preparations containing ibuprofen in combination with other drugs are used, the precautions and contraindications associated with each ingredient also must be considered. Patients also should be informed that, while NSAIAs may be commonly employed for conditions that are less serious, NSAIA therapy often is considered essential for the management of some diseases, and the drugs have a major role in the management of pain. Clinicians may wish to discuss with their patients the potential risks and likely benefits of NSAIA therapy, particularly when consideration is being given to use of these drugs in less serious conditions for which therapy without a NSAIA may represent an acceptable alternative to both the patient and clinician.

Patients should be advised to read the medication guide for NSAIAs that is provided to the patient each time the drug is dispensed.

NSAIAs increase the risk of serious adverse cardiovascular thrombotic events. (See Cautions: Cardiovascular Effects.) To minimize the potential risk of adverse cardiovascular events, the lowest effective dosage and shortest possible duration of therapy should be employed. Some clinicians suggest that it may be prudent to avoid use of NSAIAs whenever possible in patients with cardiovascular disease. Patients receiving NSAIAs (including those without previous symptoms of cardiovascular disease) should be monitored for the possible development of cardiovascular events throughout therapy. Patients should be informed about the signs and symptoms of serious cardiovascular toxicity (chest pain, dyspnea, weakness, slurring of speech) and instructed to seek immediate medical attention if such toxicity occurs. Ibuprofen should be avoided in patients with recent myocardial infarction unless the benefits of therapy are expected to outweigh the risk of recurrent cardiovascular thrombotic events; if ibuprofen is used in such patients, the patient should be monitored for cardiac ischemia.

There is no consistent evidence that concomitant use of low-dose aspirin mitigates the increased risk of serious cardiovascular events associated with NSAIAs. Concomitant use of aspirin and an NSAIA increases the risk for serious GI events. Because of the potential for increased adverse effects, patients receiving an NSAIA should be advised not to take aspirin.

Use of NSAIAs can result in the onset of hypertension or worsening of preexisting hypertension; either of these occurrences may contribute to the increased incidence of cardiovascular events. Patients receiving NSAIAs may have an impaired response to diuretics (i.e., thiazide or loop diuretics), angiotensin-converting enzyme (ACE) inhibitors, angiotensin II receptor antagonists, or β-adrenergic blocking agents. NSAIAs should be used with caution in patients with hypertension. Blood pressure should be monitored closely during initiation of NSAIA therapy and throughout therapy.

Because NSAIAs increase morbidity and mortality in patients with heart failure, the manufacturer states that ibuprofen should be avoided in patients with severe heart failure unless the benefits of therapy are expected to outweigh the risk of worsening heart failure; if ibuprofen is used in such patients, the patient should be monitored for worsening heart failure. Some experts state that use of NSAIAs should be avoided whenever possible in patients with reduced left ventricular ejection fraction and current or prior symptoms of heart failure. Patients receiving NSAIAs should be advised to inform their clinician if they experience symptoms of heart failure, including dyspnea, unexplained weight gain, and edema. Use of NSAIAs may diminish the cardiovascular effects of certain drugs used to treat heart failure and edema (e.g., diuretics, ACE inhibitors, angiotensin II receptor antagonists). (See Drug Interactions.)

Ibuprofen lysine is contraindicated in neonates with congenital heart disease when patency of the ductus arteriosus is necessary for adequate pulmonary or systemic blood flow (e.g., neonates with pulmonary atresia, severe tetralogy of Fallot, or severe coarctation of the aorta).

The risk of potentially serious adverse GI effects should be considered in patients receiving ibuprofen, particularly in patients receiving chronic therapy with the drug. Since peptic ulceration and/or GI bleeding have been reported in patients receiving the drug, patients should be advised to promptly report signs or symptoms of GI ulceration or bleeding to their clinician.

NSAIAs should be used with extreme caution and under close supervision in patients with a history of GI bleeding or peptic ulceration, and such patients should receive an appropriate ulcer preventive regimen. All patients considered at increased risk of potentially serious adverse GI effects (e.g., geriatric patients, those receiving high therapeutic dosages of NSAIAs, those with a history of peptic ulcer disease, those receiving anticoagulants or corticosteroids concomitantly) should be monitored closely for signs and symptoms of ulcer perforation or GI bleeding. To minimize the potential risk of adverse GI effects, the lowest effective dosage and shortest possible duration of therapy should be employed. For patients who are at high risk, therapy other than an NSAIA should be considered.

Ibuprofen lysine is contraindicated in premature neonates with suspected necrotizing enterocolitis.

Ibuprofen should be used with caution in patients with increased total bilirubin because of the potential for ibuprofen to displace bilirubin from albumin binding sites.

The possibility that the antipyretic and anti-inflammatory effects of ibuprofen may mask the usual signs and symptoms of infection or other diseases should be considered.

Ibuprofen lysine should be used with caution in premature neonates at risk for infection and in those with an existing infection that is adequately controlled. Clinicians should be alert to the masking effect of the drug in these neonates. The drug is contraindicated in neonates with proven or suspected, untreated infection.

Ibuprofen should be used with caution in patients who may be adversely affected by a prolongation of bleeding time (e.g., patients receiving anticoagulant therapy), since the drug may inhibit platelet function.

Premature neonates receiving ibuprofen lysine should be observed closely for bleeding tendencies. Ibuprofen lysine is contraindicated in neonates with active bleeding, such as those with intracranial hemorrhage or GI bleeding, and in neonates with thrombocytopenia or underlying coagulation defect.

Patients receiving ibuprofen for *self-medication* should be advised to use the lowest effective dosage and not to exceed the recommended dosage or duration of therapy. Unless otherwise directed by a clinician, patients receiving ibuprofen for *self-medication* should be advised to discontinue the drug and consult a clinician if pain persists for more than 10 days in adults or 3 days in children or fever persists for longer than 3 days. Patients should not use ibuprofen for *self-medication* immediately before or after cardiac surgery, or if they have experienced an allergic reaction to any analgesic or antipyretic. Patients receiving the drug for *self-medication* also should be advised to consult a clinician before initiating ibuprofen if they have experienced adverse effects associated with any analgesic or antipyretic; if they have a GI disorder, coagulation disorder, hypertension, cardiac disease, or renal disease; if they are receiving therapy with a diuretic; or if they are 60 years of age or older. Patients receiving the drug for *self-medication* should consult a clinician or pharmacist before initiating ibuprofen if they are under a clinician's care for any continuing serious medical condition; they are receiving an anticoagulant, a corticosteroid, or any other NSAIA-containing preparation; or they are taking any other drugs on a regular basis. They also should be advised to stop taking the drug and to report to their clinician symptoms of GI bleeding (faintness, vomiting blood, bloody or black stools); any new, unusual, or unexpected symptoms that occur during *self-medication* with the drug; if pain or fever gets worse during therapy; or if stomach pain intensifies or persists with use of the drug. Patients should be advised that the risk of GI bleeding is increased if they are 60 years of age or older, have a GI disorder (e.g., history of GI bleeding or peptic ulceration), are receiving an anticoagulant or corticosteroid, are receiving another NSAIA (including aspirin) concomitantly, if they generally consume 3 or more alcohol-containing drinks per day, or if they exceed the recommended dosage or duration of ibuprofen therapy. In addition, patients should be advised that NSAIAs may increase the risk of a cardiovascular event. For additional information on use of ibuprofen for *self-medication* in children, see Pediatric Precautions.

Individuals with phenylketonuria (i.e., homozygous genetic deficiency of phenylalanine hydroxylase) and other individuals who must restrict their intake of phenylalanine should be warned that Motrin® chewable tablets contain aspartame (NutraSweet®), which is metabolized in the GI tract to provide 3 or 6 mg of phenylalanine for each 50- or 100-mg tablet, respectively, following oral administration and that Advil® Children's chewable tablets and Advil® Junior Strength chewable tablets contain aspartame, which is metabolized to provide 2.1 and 4.2 mg of phenylalanine for each tablet, respectively. Diabetic patients should be warned that some commercially available preparations of ibuprofen may contain sucrose.

Because NSAIAs, including ibuprofen, have caused adverse ocular effects (e.g., blurred or diminished vision, scotoma, changes in color vision), patients who experience such visual disturbances during ibuprofen therapy should discontinue the drug and have an ophthalmologic examination, including testing of central visual fields and color vision.

Renal toxicity has been observed in patients in whom renal prostaglandins have a compensatory role in maintaining renal perfusion. Administration of an NSAIA to such patients may cause a dose-dependent reduction in prostaglandin formation and thereby precipitate overt renal decompensation. Patients at greatest risk of this reaction are those with impaired renal function, heart failure, or hepatic dysfunction; those with extracellular fluid depletion (e.g., patients receiving diuretics); those taking an ACE inhibitor or angiotensin II receptor antagonist concomitantly; and geriatric patients. Patients should be advised to consult their clinician promptly if unexplained weight gain or edema occurs. Recovery of renal function to pretreatment levels usually occurs following discontinuance of NSAIA therapy. Some clinicians recommend that renal function be monitored periodically in all patients receiving long-term NSAIA therapy, but other clinicians question the cost-effectiveness of this recommendation and instead recommend selective monitoring in patients considered at risk.

The manufacturers state that ibuprofen should be used with caution and close monitoring in patients with substantial renal impairment, since the drug and its metabolites are eliminated principally by the kidneys. To avoid excessive accumulation of the drug, the manufacturers recommend that decreased dosages of ibuprofen be considered in these patients. The safety of ibuprofen in patients with chronic renal failure has not been established.

Ibuprofen lysine is contraindicated in neonates with substantially impaired renal function.

Liver function should be monitored periodically during long-term ibuprofen therapy. Elevations in serum ALT may be the most sensitive indicator of NSAIA-induced liver dysfunction. Patients who experience signs and/or symptoms suggestive of liver dysfunction or an abnormal liver function test result while receiving ibuprofen should be evaluated for evidence of the development of a more severe hepatic reaction. Severe reactions, including jaundice and fatal fulminant hepatitis, liver necrosis, and hepatic failure (sometimes fatal), have been reported in patients receiving NSAIAs. Although such reactions are rare, ibuprofen should be discontinued if abnormal liver function test results persist or worsen, if clinical signs and symptoms consistent with liver disease develop, or if systemic manifestations occur (e.g., eosinophilia, rash).

Use of corticosteroids during NSAIA therapy may increase the risk of GI ulceration, and the drugs should be used concomitantly with caution. If corticosteroid dosage is decreased during ibuprofen therapy, it should be done gradually and patients should be observed for adverse effects, including adrenocortical insufficiency or symptomatic exacerbation of the inflammatory condition being treated.

Ibuprofen can interfere with the antiplatelet effect of low-dose aspirin. Patients receiving low-dose aspirin for its cardioprotective effects should be informed of this potential interaction and advised about appropriate timing of ibuprofen administration relative to aspirin administration in order to minimize the interaction. (See Drug Interactions: Nonsteroidal Anti-inflammatory Agents.)

Anaphylactoid reactions have been reported in patients receiving NSAIAs. Patients receiving NSAIAs should be informed of the signs and symptoms of an anaphylactoid reaction (e.g., difficulty breathing, swelling of the face or throat) and advised to seek immediate medical attention if an anaphylactoid reaction develops.

Serious skin reactions (e.g., exfoliative dermatitis, Stevens-Johnson syndrome, toxic epidermal necrolysis) can occur in patients receiving NSAIAs. These serious skin reactions may occur without warning; patients should be advised to consult their clinician if skin rash and blisters, fever, or other signs of hypersensitivity reaction (e.g., pruritus) occur. NSAIAs should be discontinued at the first appearance of rash or any other sign of hypersensitivity.

Ibuprofen is contraindicated in patients with known hypersensitivity to the drug. NSAIAs generally are contraindicated in patients in whom asthma, urticaria, or other sensitivity reactions are precipitated by aspirin or other NSAIAs, since there is potential for cross-sensitivity between NSAIAs and aspirin, and severe, often fatal, anaphylactic reactions may occur in such patients. Although NSAIAs generally are contraindicated in these patients, the drugs have occasionally been used in NSAIA-sensitive patients who have undergone desensitization. Because patients with asthma may have aspirin-sensitivity asthma, NSAIAs should be used with caution in patients with asthma. In patients with asthma, aspirin sensitivity is manifested principally as bronchospasm and usually is associated with nasal polyps; the association of aspirin sensitivity, asthma, and nasal polyps is known as the aspirin triad. Patients who are considering use of ibuprofen for *self-medication* should be advised that ibuprofen is contraindicated in patients who have experienced asthma, urticaria, or other sensitivity reaction to other analgesics or antipyretics. For further discussion of cross-sensitivity of NSAIAs, see Cautions: Sensitivity Reactions, in the Salicylates General Statement 28:08.04.24.

NSAIAs are contraindicated in the setting of CABG surgery.

■ Pediatric Precautions The manufacturers state that the safety and efficacy of oral ibuprofen in children younger than 6 months of age have not been established. Ibuprofen should not be used for *self-medication* in children younger than 6 months of age unless otherwise directed by a clinician. Ibuprofen should not be used for *self-medication* in children immediately before or after cardiac surgery or in children who have experienced an allergic reaction to any analgesic or antipyretic. Clinicians should be consulted before initiating ibuprofen for *self-medication* in children if the child has experienced adverse effects associated with any analgesic or antipyretic; if the child has a GI disorder, coagulation disorder, hypertension, cardiac disease, or renal disease or is receiving therapy with a diuretic; or if dehydration associated with vomiting, diarrhea, or lack of fluid intake has occurred. A clinician or pharmacist should be consulted before initiating ibuprofen for *self-medication* in children if the child is under a clinician's care for any continuing serious medical condition; is receiving an anticoagulant, a corticosteroid, or any other NSAIA-containing preparation; or is taking any other drugs on a regular basis. Ibuprofen *self-medication* should be discontinued and a clinician should be contacted if symptoms of GI bleeding (faintness, vomiting blood, bloody or black stools) develop; if any new, unusual, or unexpected symptoms occur during *self-medication* with the drug; if pain or fever gets worse during therapy or lasts more than 3 days; if no relief is observed within the first 24 hours of therapy; or if stomach pain intensifies or persists with use of the drug. In addition, a clinician should be contacted if the child experiences severe sore throat, if a sore throat of more than 2 days' duration occurs, or if sore throat is associated with fever, headache, rash, nausea, or vomiting. The risk of GI bleeding is increased if the child has a GI disorder (e.g., history of GI bleeding or peptic ulceration), is receiving an anticoagulant or corticosteroid, is receiving another NSAIA (including aspirin) concomitantly, or if the recommended dosage or duration of ibuprofen therapy is exceeded. Ibuprofen should not be used for *self-medication* in children for longer than 10 days unless directed by a clinician.

Results of a large (about 84,000 children) double-blind, randomized study indicate that risk of hospitalization for GI bleeding, renal failure, anaphylaxis, or Reye's syndrome in febrile children (6 months to 12 years of age) receiving ibuprofen doses of 5 or 10 mg/kg is similar to that in children receiving acetaminophen doses of 12 mg/kg. These data, however, provide no information on the risks of less severe adverse effects or the risks associated with prolonged use of ibuprofen in children.

Overdosage and toxicity (including death) have been reported in children younger than 2 years of age receiving nonprescription (over-the-counter, OTC) preparations containing antihistamines, cough suppressants, expectorants, and nasal decongestants alone or in combination for relief of symptoms of upper respiratory tract infection. Such preparations also may contain analgesics and antipyretics. There is limited evidence of efficacy for these preparations in this age group, and appropriate dosages (i.e., approved by the US Food and Drug Administration [FDA]) have not been established. Therefore, FDA stated that nonprescription cough and cold preparations should not be used in children younger than 2 years of age; the agency continues to assess safety and efficacy of these preparations in older children. Meanwhile, because children 2–3 years of age also are at increased risk of overdosage and toxicity, some manufacturers of oral nonprescription cough and cold preparations have agreed to voluntarily revise the product labeling to state that such preparations should not be used in children younger than 4 years of age. FDA recommends that parents and caregivers adhere to the dosage instructions and warnings on the product labeling that accompanies the preparation if administering to children and consult with their clinician about any concerns. Clinicians should ask caregivers about use of nonprescription cough and cold preparations to avoid overdosage. For additional information on precautions associated with the use of cough and cold preparations in pediatric patients, see Cautions: Pediatric Precautions in Pseudoephedrine 12:12.12.

Safety and efficacy of IV ibuprofen for relief of pain or reduction of fever have not been established in pediatric patients younger than 17 years of age.

Long-term follow-up (beyond a postconceptional age of 36 weeks) of premature neonates receiving ibuprofen lysine for patent ductus arteriosus (PDA) has not been conducted. The effects of ibuprofen on neurodevelopmental outcome, growth, and other complications of prematurity (e.g., retinopathy of prematurity, chronic lung disease) have not been assessed.

Ibuprofen lysine is contraindicated in neonates with substantially impaired renal function, thrombocytopenia, coagulation disorders, active bleeding (e.g., intracranial hemorrhage, GI bleeding), known or suspected necrotizing enterocolitis, or proven or suspected infection that is untreated. The drug also is contraindicated in neonates with congenital heart disease when patency of the ductus arteriosus is necessary for adequate pulmonary or systemic blood flow (e.g., neonates with pulmonary atresia, severe tetralogy of Fallot, or severe coarctation of the aorta).

■ Geriatric Precautions Geriatric individuals appear to tolerate GI ulceration and bleeding less well than other individuals, and many of the spontaneous reports of fatal adverse GI effects in patients receiving NSAIAs involve geriatric individuals.

Clinical studies of IV ibuprofen did not include sufficient numbers of patients 65 years of age or older to determine whether geriatric patients respond differently than younger adults. Dosage should be selected with caution, starting at the low end of the dosage range, because of the greater frequency of decreased hepatic, renal, and/or cardiac function and concomitant disease and drug therapy observed in the elderly.

■ Pregnancy and Lactation Although animal reproduction studies have not demonstrated any teratogenic effects, the safe use of ibuprofen during pregnancy has not been established. Ibuprofen inhibits prostaglandin synthesis and release, which may cause dystocia, interfere with labor, and delay parturition. Inhibitors of prostaglandin synthesis may have adverse effects on the fetal cardiovascular system (e.g., premature closure of the ductus arteriosus). Use of ibuprofen is not recommended during pregnancy (especially during the last trimester) or during labor and delivery.

Although ibuprofen has not been reported to distribute into milk in lactating women, the manufacturers state that use of the drug in nursing women is not recommended because of the potential risk of inhibitors of prostaglandin synthesis in neonates.

Drug Interactions

■ Anticoagulants and Thrombolytic Agents The effects of warfarin and NSAIAs on GI bleeding are synergistic. Concomitant use of an NSAIA and warfarin is associated with a higher risk of GI bleeding compared with use of either agent alone.

In several short-term, controlled studies, ibuprofen did not have a substantial effect on the prothrombin time of patients receiving oral anticoagulants; however, because ibuprofen may cause GI bleeding, inhibit platelet aggregation, and prolong bleeding time and because bleeding has occurred when ibuprofen and coumarin-derivative anticoagulants were administered concomitantly, the drug should be used with caution and the patient carefully observed if the drug is used concomitantly with any anticoagulant (e.g., warfarin) or thrombolytic agent (e.g., streptokinase).

■ Nonsteroidal Anti-inflammatory Agents In animal studies, blood concentrations of ibuprofen decreased when aspirin and ibuprofen were administered concomitantly. Although limited studies in humans have not shown decreased blood concentrations of ibuprofen when these drugs were administered concurrently, this possibility should be considered. In addition, concomitant administration of ibuprofen and salicylates, phenylbutazone, indomethacin, or other NSAIAs could potentiate the adverse GI effects of these drugs, and thus ibuprofen probably should not be administered with these agents.

Concomitant use of aspirin and an NSAIA increases the risk for serious GI events. Because of the potential for increased adverse effects, patients receiving an NSAIA should be advised not to take aspirin. There is no consistent evidence that use of low-dose aspirin mitigates the increased risk of serious cardiovascular events associated with NSAIAs.

Some NSAIAs (e.g., ibuprofen, naproxen) can interfere with the antiplatelet effect of low-dose aspirin. Ibuprofen can antagonize the irreversible inhibition of platelet aggregation induced by aspirin and therefore may limit the cardioprotective effects of aspirin in patients with increased cardiovascular risk. Administration of 400 mg of ibuprofen 3 times daily in patients receiving aspirin 81 mg daily blocked the aspirin-induced inhibition of platelet cyclooxygenase-1 activity as well as the impairment of platelet aggregation achieved with aspirin during prolonged dosing. Administration of aspirin 2 hours before the morning dose of ibuprofen failed to circumvent the interaction with such multiple-dose administration, although such dose timing did effectively obviate the interaction when only single doses of each drug were administered. The US Food and Drug Administration (FDA) recommends that patients taking a single dose of ibuprofen 400 mg for *self-medication* in conjunction with immediate-release, low-dose aspirin therapy be advised to administer the ibuprofen dose at least 8 hours before or at least 30 minutes after administration of aspirin. Data currently are insufficient to support recommendations regarding the timing of ibuprofen administration relative to that of enteric-coated, low-dose aspirin. The occasional use of ibuprofen is likely to be associated with minimal risk of attenuating the effects of low-dose aspirin. Use of alternative analgesics that do not interfere with the antiplatelet effect of low-dose aspirin (e.g., acetaminophen, opiates) should be considered for patients at high risk of cardiovascular events.

■ Lithium Ibuprofen has been reported to increase plasma or serum lithium concentrations by 12–67% and to reduce renal lithium clearance. The mechanism involved in the reduction of lithium clearance by NSAIAs (including ibuprofen) is not known, but has been attributed to inhibition of prostaglandin synthesis, which may interfere with the renal elimination of lithium. Some clinicians recommend that patients receiving lithium should not receive ibuprofen. However, if ibuprofen and lithium are used concurrently, the patient should be observed closely for signs of lithium toxicity, and plasma or serum lithium concentrations should be monitored carefully during the initial stages of combined therapy or subsequent dosage adjustment. Dosage of lithium may have to be reduced in some patients; appropriate adjustment of lithium dosage may be required when therapy with ibuprofen is discontinued.

■ Angiotensin-converting Enzyme Inhibitors and Angiotensin II Receptor Antagonists There is some evidence that concomitant use of drugs that inhibit prostaglandin synthesis, including ibuprofen, may reduce the blood pressure response to angiotensin-converting enzyme (ACE) inhibitors (e.g., captopril, enalapril) and angiotensin II receptor antagonists. Limited data indicate that concomitant use of NSAIAs with ACE inhibitors occasionally may result in acute reductions in renal function; however, the possibility cannot be ruled out that one of the drugs alone may cause such an effect. Blood pressure should be monitored carefully when an NSAIA is initiated in patients receiving an ACE inhibitor or angiotensin II receptor antagonist; in addition, clinicians should be alert for evidence of impaired renal function.

■ Diuretics NSAIAs may reduce the natriuretic effect of furosemide or thiazide diuretics. This effect may be related to inhibition of renal prostaglandin synthesis. Patients receiving concomitant NSAIA and diuretic therapy should be monitored for signs of renal failure and for efficacy of the diuretic.

■ Methotrexate Because of the possibility of enhanced toxicity of methotrexate, caution is advised if methotrexate and an NSAIA are administered concomitantly. (See Drug Interactions: Nonsteroidal Anti-inflammatory Agents, in Methotrexate 10:00.)

Acute Toxicity

■ Manifestations Limited information is available on the acute toxicity of ibuprofen. Adverse effects associated with overdosage of ibuprofen usually depend on the amount of drug ingested and time elapsed; however, because individual response may vary, each occurrence should be evaluated individually. Occasionally, overdosage of ibuprofen has been associated with severe toxicity, including death.

The most frequent manifestations of ibuprofen overdosage reportedly are abdominal pain, nausea, vomiting, lethargy, and drowsiness. In addition, other adverse effects, including headache, tinnitus, CNS depression, seizures, hypotension, bradycardia, tachycardia, and atrial fibrillation, may occur. Metabolic acidosis, coma, acute renal failure, hyperkalemia, apnea (mainly in young children), respiratory depression, and respiratory failure have been reported rarely. There appears to be little correlation between severity of manifestations associated with ibuprofen overdosage and plasma ibuprofen concentrations.

Drowsiness was the only adverse effect experienced by a child 1 year of age who ingested 1.2 g (120 mg/kg) of the drug even though the blood ibuprofen concentration 90 minutes after ingestion was 700 mcg/mL (nearly 10 times the highest concentration previously recorded in adults following a single oral 800-mg dose of the drug). Signs of acute intoxication or late sequelae also were not present following ingestion of a 120-mg/kg dose of the drug in another child. However, in a 12-kg child who ingested 2.8–4 g of the drug, apnea, cyanosis, and response only to painful stimuli were present about 1.5 hours after ingestion; respiration could be induced by painful stimuli. The blood ibuprofen concentration in this child was about 103 mcg/mL at about 8.5 hours after ingestion and the child appeared to have completely recovered at 12 hours following treatment with oxygen, sodium bicarbonate, and parenteral infusion of dextrose and 0.9% sodium chloride. Dizziness and nystagmus occurred in a 19-year-old who ingested 8 g of the drug over a period of a few hours.

■ Treatment Treatment of acute toxicity associated with ibuprofen overdosage mainly is supportive. When acute overdosage of ibuprofen occurs, the stomach should be emptied by inducing emesis with syrup of ipecac or by lavage, particularly if there is evidence that the drug has been ingested recently (within 30–60 minutes), and standard measures to maintain urine output should be instituted. Administration of activated charcoal may be useful in reducing absorption and reabsorption of ibuprofen. Since ibuprofen is acidic and is excreted in the urine, forced alkaline diuresis might be beneficial. Management of hypotension, GI bleeding, and acidosis also may be necessary.

In children, the estimated amount ingested per unit of body weight may be helpful in predicting the development of toxicity, but each case should be evaluated individually. One manufacturer and some clinicians state that toxicity is unlikely in children who have ingested less than 100 mg/kg of ibuprofen. In children who have ingested 100–200 mg/kg, the stomach should be emptied by inducing emesis and the child observed for at least 4 hours; in children who have ingested 200–400 mg/kg of the drug, the stomach should be emptied and the child observed in a health-care facility for at least 4 hours. Children who have ingested more than 400 mg/kg of ibuprofen require immediate medical referral, careful observation, and appropriate supportive therapy; syrup of ipecac is not recommended in these children because of risk of seizures and potential aspiration of gastric contents. In adults, the amount of ibuprofen ingested does not appear to predict toxicity; therefore, the need for referral and follow-up treatment should be assessed individually. Adults with symptomatic toxicity should be admitted to a health-care facility for observation.

Pharmacology

Ibuprofen has pharmacologic actions similar to those of other prototypical NSAIAs. Ibuprofen has shown anti-inflammatory, antipyretic, and analgesic activity in both animals and humans. The exact mechanisms of action of the drug have not been clearly established, but many of the actions appear to be associated principally with the inhibition of prostaglandin synthesis. Ibuprofen inhibits synthesis of prostaglandins in body tissues by inhibiting cyclooxygenase; at least 2 isoenzymes, cyclooxygenase-1 (COX-1) and -2 (COX-2) (also referred to as prostaglandin G/H synthase-1 [PGHS-1] and -2 [PGHS-2], respectively), have been identified that catalyze the formation of prostaglandins in the arachidonic acid pathway. Ibuprofen, like other prototypical NSAIAs, inhibits both COX-1 and COX-2. Although the exact mechanisms have not been clearly established, NSAIAs appear to exert anti-inflammatory, analgesic, and antipyretic activity principally through inhibition of the COX-2 isoenzyme; COX-1 inhibition presumably is responsible for the drugs' unwanted effects on GI mucosa and platelet aggregation.

■ **Anti-inflammatory, Analgesic, and Antipyretic Effects** The anti-inflammatory, analgesic, and antipyretic effects of ibuprofen and other NSAIAs, including selective inhibitors of COX-2 (e.g., celecoxib), appear to result from inhibition of prostaglandin synthesis. While the precise mechanism of the anti-inflammatory and analgesic effects of NSAIAs continues to be investigated, these effects appear to be mediated principally through inhibition of the COX-2 isoenzyme at sites of inflammation with subsequent reduction in the synthesis of certain prostaglandins from their arachidonic acid precursors.

Ibuprofen does not possess glucocorticoid or adrenocorticoid-stimulating properties. Higher doses usually are required for anti-inflammatory effects than for analgesia.

■ **Genitourinary and Renal Effects** Ibuprofen-induced inhibition of prostaglandin synthesis may result in decreased frequency and intensity of uterine contractility. Prostaglandins E_2 and $F_2\alpha$ increase the amplitude and frequency of uterine contractions in pregnant women; current evidence suggests that primary dysmenorrhea also is mediated by these prostaglandins. Whether the increased production of prostaglandins associated with primary dysmenorrhea is mediated by COX-1 or COX-2 remains to be determined. Therapy with ibuprofen has been effective in relieving menstrual pain probably by inhibiting the formation of these prostaglandins. Administration of ibuprofen during late pregnancy may prolong gestation by inhibiting uterine contractions.

Ibuprofen has been reported to adversely affect renal function. (See Cautions: Renal Effects.) The mechanisms of adverse renal effects of ibuprofen have not been determined, but may involve inhibition of renal synthesis of prostaglandins.

Ibuprofen does not appear to have uricosuric activity.

■ **GI Effects** Similar to other prototypical NSAIAs, ibuprofen can cause gastric mucosal damage, which may result in ulceration and/or bleeding. (See Cautions: GI Effects.) These gastric effects have been attributed to inhibition of the synthesis of prostaglandins produced by COX-1. Other factors possibly involved in NSAIA-induced gastropathy include local irritation, promotion of acid back-diffusion into gastric mucosa, uncoupling of oxidative phosphorylation, and enterohepatic recirculation of the drugs.

Limited data indicate that ibuprofen, in a dosage of 1.2 or 2.4 g daily, produced less severe gastric mucosal abnormalities (observed with endoscopic examination) than did aspirin in a dosage of 3.6 g daily. In addition, ibuprofen in a dosage of 1.2 g daily produces less severe gastric mucosal damage than indomethacin in a dosage of 100 mg daily.

Epidemiologic and laboratory studies suggest that NSAIAs may reduce the risk of colon cancer. Although the exact mechanism by which NSAIAs may inhibit colon carcinogenesis remains to determined, it has been suggested that inhibition of prostaglandin synthesis may be involved.

■ **Hematologic Effects** Ibuprofen inhibits platelet aggregation and prolongs bleeding time but does not affect prothrombin time or whole blood clotting time. Similar to aspirin and other prototypical NSAIAs, the effects of ibuprofen on platelets appear to be associated with inhibition of the synthesis of prostaglandins produced by COX-1.

■ **Cardiovascular Effects** In many premature neonates, administration of ibuprofen results in closure of the persistently patent ductus arteriosus. During fetal life, the ductus arteriosus apparently is maintained in a dilated state by prostaglandins, presumably of the E series, which are produced in the placenta and in the ductus itself. The ductus usually closes within 24 hours after birth, partly as a result of loss of placental prostaglandins and increased pulmonary blood flow. In premature neonates, however, the ductus may not close promptly, perhaps because of increased sensitivity of the immature ductus to prostaglandins; some of these neonates develop cardiopulmonary decompensation because of large left-to-right cardiac shunts. Ibuprofen appears to inhibit the synthesis of the prostaglandins, thereby permitting closure of the ductus. Other factors such as oxygenation and hydration status of the neonate also may contribute to successful ductus closure.

Pharmacokinetics

■ **Absorption** Approximately 80% of an oral dose of ibuprofen is absorbed from the GI tract. Absorption rate is slower and plasma concentrations are reduced when ibuprofen tablets, chewable tablets, or suspension are taken with food; however, the extent of absorption is not affected. When the drug is administered with food, peak plasma ibuprofen concentrations are reduced by 30–50% and time to achieve peak plasma concentrations is delayed by 30–60 minutes. Absorption of ibuprofen does not appear to be affected by concomitant administration of antacids containing aluminum hydroxide or magnesium hydroxide.

In adults, oral bioavailability of ibuprofen (measured by peak plasma concentrations and extent of absorption) is similar following administration of conventional tablets, chewable tablets, or suspension; however, time to reach peak plasma concentrations was reportedly about 120, 62, or 47 minutes following administration of each respective dosage form. Following oral administration of a single 200-mg dose of ibuprofen as chewable tablets, suspension, or conventional tablets in adults, peak plasma concentrations were 15, 19, or 20 mcg/mL, respectively. Following oral administration of ibuprofen in adults, the area under the serum concentration-time curves (AUCs) of total and free drug increase proportionally with single ibuprofen doses of 50–600 and up to 1200 mg, respectively. In febrile children, oral bioavailability (measured by peak plasma concentrations and extent of absorption) of ibuprofen also appears to be similar following administration of the respective dosage form; however, time to reach peak plasma concentrations was reportedly 86 or 58 minutes following administration of chewable tablets or suspension, respectively. Following oral administration of a 200-mg dose in adults or a 10-mg/kg dose in febrile children, peak plasma concentrations and plasma concentration-time curves (AUCs) of ibuprofen appear to be increased in children compared with those achieved in adults; these differences appear to result from age- or fever-related changes in the volume of distribution in children and also to the variability of doses (based on body weight) administered to pediatric patients. Peak plasma or serum ibuprofen concentrations of about 40–55 mcg/mL occur after about 1–1.5 hours in febrile children receiving a single 10-mg/kg dose of ibuprofen suspension or chewable tablets. Following oral administration of ibuprofen suspension in febrile children, AUCs increase with increasing single ibuprofen doses up to 10 mg/kg; it appears that pharmacokinetics of ibuprofen are not affected by age, in children 2 to 11 years of age.

In children, the antipyretic effect of ibuprofen suspension begins within 1 hour after oral administration and peaks within 2-4 hours. The antipyretic effect of single ibuprofen suspension doses of 5 or 10-mg/kg may last up to 6 or 8 hours, respectively. Following oral administration of ibuprofen chewable tablets, onset, peak, and duration of antipyretic effects reportedly are similar to that following oral administration of the suspension. The antipyretic effects of conventional ibuprofen tablets have not been studied in children. Plasma concentrations required for anti-inflammatory effect are not known. A few days to 2 weeks of therapy are required before therapeutic response occurs.

Following IV administration of 400 or 800 mg of ibuprofen in adults, peak plasma concentrations were 39.2 or 72.6 mcg/mL, respectively.

■ **Distribution** Animal studies indicate that ibuprofen distribution varies according to species; human distribution data have not been published. The volume of distribution reportedly is about 0.12 or 0.2 L/kg in adults or febrile children younger than 11 years of age, respectively, suggesting that the volume of distribution may be affected by age or fever; however, the clinical importance of this difference is not known. In one study in premature neonates receiving IV ibuprofen lysine, the volume of distribution of ibuprofen at birth averaged 0.32 L/kg. Approximately 90–99% of a dose is bound to plasma proteins; protein binding appears to be saturable, and at concentrations exceeding 20 mcg/mL, such binding is nonlinear. Ibuprofen and its metabolites cross the placenta in rats and rabbits. In preliminary studies, ibuprofen was not detected in the milk of nursing women.

■ **Elimination** Plasma concentrations of ibuprofen appear to decline in a biphasic manner. The terminal elimination half-life in children reportedly is similar to that in adults; however, total clearance may be affected by age or fever. It has been suggested that changes in total clearance may result from changes in the volume of distribution in febrile children. The plasma half-life of the drug has been reported to be 2–4 hours. Blood concentrations decline as rapidly after multiple doses as after single doses. In one study in premature neonates receiving IV ibuprofen lysine, clearance of ibuprofen at birth averaged 3 mL/kg per hour. Clearance increased rapidly (by an average of about 0.5 mL/kg per hour each day) as postnatal age increased, and interindividual variability (55%) in clearance was observed. The terminal elimination half-life is at least tenfold longer in premature neonates than in adults.

Ibuprofen is metabolized via oxidation to form 2 inactive metabolites, (+)-2[4′-(2-hydroxy-2-methylpropyl)phenyl]propionic acid (metabolite A) and (+)-2-[4′-(2-carboxypropyl)phenyl]propionic acid (metabolite B). About 50–60% of an oral dose is excreted in urine as metabolites A and B or their glucuronide conjugates within 24 hours. Less than 10% of the drug is excreted in urine unchanged; the remainder of the drug is eliminated in feces, both as metabolites and unabsorbed drug. Excretion of ibuprofen is essentially complete within 24 hours following oral administration. Some biliary excretion of the drug probably occurs in humans. Metabolism and excretion of ibuprofen in premature neonates have not been evaluated.

Chemistry and Stability

■ **Chemistry** Ibuprofen is a prototypical nonsteroidal anti-inflammatory agent (NSAIA). Ibuprofen is commercially available as the acid and as the potassium salt. Ibuprofen is a racemic mixture of 2 optical isomers. In vivo and in vitro studies indicate that only the *l*-isomer of ibuprofen has clinical activity. However, the *d*-isomer, which is considered clinically inactive, is slowly and incompletely (by about 60%) converted to the *l*-isomer in adults; the degree of such conversion is believed to be similar in children. It also has been suggested that the *d*-isomer serves as a circulating reservoir to maintain concentration of the active drug. Ibuprofen occurs as a white to off-white, crystalline powder having a slight, characteristic odor and is practically insoluble in water and very soluble in alcohol. The apparent pK_a of ibuprofen is about 4.4.

Commercially available ibuprofen lysine injection occurs as a clear sterile solution of the drug in water for injection. Sodium hydroxide or hydrochloric acid may be added during the manufacture of the injection to adjust the pH to 7.

■ **Stability** Oral preparations containing ibuprofen should be stored in well-closed, light-resistant containers at 20–25°C.

Ibuprofen injection concentrate should be stored at 20–25°C. The product contains no preservatives.

Ibuprofen lysine injection should be stored at 20–25°C; the injection should be stored in the manufacturer's carton until time of use and should be protected from light. The product contains no preservatives and is intended for single use only; any unused portions should be discarded.

Preparations

Excipients in commercially available drug preparations may have clinically important effects in some individuals; consult specific product labeling for details.

Ibuprofen

Oral		
Capsules, liquid-filled	200 mg	**Advil® Liqui-Gels®**, Wyeth
	equivalent to 200 mg ibuprofen (as free acid and ibuprofen potassium)	**Advil® Migraine®**, Wyeth
Suspension	40 mg/mL*	**Advil® Infants' Concentrated Drops**, Wyeth
		Ibuprofen Oral Suspension
		Motrin® Drops, McNeil
		Motrin® Infants' Concentrated Drops, McNeil
	100 mg/5 mL*	**Advil® Children's**, Wyeth
		Ibuprofen Oral Suspension
		Motrin® Children's, McNeil
Tablets	200 mg*	**Ibuprofen Tablets**
		Motrin® IB Gelcaps®, McNeil
	400 mg*	**Ibuprofen Tablets**
	600 mg*	**Ibuprofen Tablets**
	800 mg*	**Ibuprofen Tablets**
Tablets, chewable	50 mg	**Advil® Children's**, Wyeth
		Motrin® Children's, McNeil
	100 mg	**Advil® Junior Strength Chewable Tablets**, Wyeth
		Motrin® (scored), McNeil
		Motrin® Junior Strength, McNeil
Tablets, film-coated	100 mg	**Advil® Junior Strength Tablets**, Wyeth
		Motrin® Caplets® (scored), McNeil
		Motrin® Junior Strength Caplets®, McNeil
	200 mg*	**Advil® Caplets®**, Wyeth
		Advil® Gel Caplets, Wyeth
		Advil® Tablets, Wyeth
		Genpril® Caplets®, Teva
		Genpril® Tablets, Teva
		Haltran®, Lee
		Ibu-Tab®, Alra
		Ibuprofen Tablets
		Menadol® Captabs®, Watson
		Midol® Cramp, Bayer
		Motrin® IB Caplets®, McNeil
		Motrin® IB Tablets, McNeil
		Motrin® Migraine Pain Caplets®, McNeil
	400 mg*	**IBU®**, Par
		Ibu-Tab®, Alra
		Ibuprofen Tablets
		Motrin®, Pharmacia
	600 mg*	**IBU®**, Par
		Ibu-Tab®, Alra
		Ibuprofen Tablets
		Motrin®, Pharmacia
	800 mg*	**IBU®**, Par
		Ibuprofen Tablets
		Ibu-Tab®, Alra
		Motrin®, Pharmacia
Parenteral		
Injection concentrate, for IV use	100 mg/mL	**Caldolor®**, Cumberland

*available from one or more manufacturer, distributor, and/or repackager by generic (nonproprietary) name

Ibuprofen Combinations

Oral		
Suspension	100 mg with Pseudoephedrine Hydrochloride 15 mg/5 mL	**Motrin® Children's Cold**, McNeil
Tablets	200 mg with Pseudoephedrine Hydrochloride 30 mg	**Dristan® Sinus Caplets®**, Wyeth
Tablets, film-coated	200 mg with Hydrocodone Bitartrate 2.5 mg*	**Hydrocodone Bitartrate and Ibuprofen Film-coated Tablets** (C-II)
		Reprexain® (C-II), Gemini
	200 mg with Hydrocodone Bitartrate 5 mg*	**Hydrocodone Bitartrate and Ibuprofen Film-coated Tablets** (C-II)
		Reprexain® (C-II), Gemini
	200 mg with Hydrocodone Bitartrate 7.5 mg*	**Hydrocodone Bitartrate and Ibuprofen Film-coated Tablets** (C-II)
		Vicoprofen® (C-II), AbbVie
	200 mg with Hydrocodone Bitartrate 10 mg*	**Hydrocodone Bitartrate and Ibuprofen Film-coated Tablets** (C-II)
		Reprexain® (C-II), Gemini
	200 mg with Pseudoephedrine Hydrochloride 30 mg	**Advil® Cold & Sinus Caplets®**, Wyeth
		Advil® Cold & Sinus Tablets, Wyeth
		Advil® Flu & Body Ache Caplets®, Wyeth
		Motrin® Sinus Headache Caplets®, McNeil
	400 mg with Oxycodone Hydrochloride 5 mg*	**Oxycodone Hydrochloride and Ibuprofen Film-coated Tablets** (C-II)

*available from one or more manufacturer, distributor, and/or repackager by generic (nonproprietary) name

Ibuprofen Lysine

Parenteral		
For injection, for IV use only	10 mg/mL(of ibuprofen)	**NeoProfen®**, Lundbeck

†Use is not currently included in the labeling approved by the US Food and Drug Administration

Indomethacin
Indomethacin Sodium

Indometacin

■ Indomethacin is a prototypical nonsteroidal anti-inflammatory agent (NSAIA) that also exhibits analgesic and antipyretic activity.

Uses

Indomethacin is used orally or rectally for anti-inflammatory and analgesic effects in the symptomatic treatment of active stages of moderate to severe rheumatoid arthritis (including acute flares of chronic disease), osteoarthritis, and ankylosing spondylitis. Indomethacin is also used orally or rectally for symptomatic treatment of acute gouty arthritis and acute painful shoulder (bursitis and/or tendinitis). Extended-release capsules of indomethacin are *not* recommended for use in the treatment of acute gouty arthritis.

Indomethacin sodium is used IV in the treatment of patent ductus arteriosus in premature neonates.

The potential benefits and risks of indomethacin therapy as well as alternative therapies should be considered prior to initiating indomethacin therapy. The lowest possible effective dosage and shortest duration of therapy consistent with treatment goals of the patient should be employed.

■ **Inflammatory Diseases** ***Rheumatoid Arthritis and Osteoarthritis*** When used in the treatment of rheumatoid arthritis, indomethacin has relieved pain and stiffness; reduced swelling, fever, tenderness, and the number of joints involved; and improved mobility and grip strength. In the treatment of osteoarthritis, indomethacin has relieved pain and stiffness and improved mobility. In patients with rheumatoid arthritis or osteoarthritis, other NSAIAs (e.g., naproxen, fenoprofen) usually have been considered before indomethacin because of indomethacin's potential for adverse reactions, particularly at high dosages. However, because clinical experience indicates that indomethacin does not appear to be associated with a substantially greater risk of toxicity than most other NSAIAs, the drug may be considered for initial therapy. Indomethacin appears to be only palliative in these conditions and has not been shown to permanently arrest or reverse the underlying disease process.

Most clinical evaluations of indomethacin in the management of rheumatoid arthritis or osteoarthritis have shown that the anti-inflammatory and analgesic effects of usual dosages of indomethacin are greater than those of placebo and about equal to those of usual dosages of salicylates, phenylbutazone (no longer commercially available in the US), ibuprofen, and naproxen. Patient response to NSAIAs is variable; patients who do not respond to or cannot tolerate one drug might be successfully treated with a different agent. However, NSAIAs are generally contraindicated in patients in whom sensitivity reactions (e.g., urticaria, bronchospasm, severe rhinitis) are precipitated by aspirin or other NSAIAs. (See Cautions: Dermatologic and Sensitivity Reactions.)

In a controlled clinical study in patients with osteoarthritis, single daily doses of 75-mg extended-release capsules of indomethacin were as effective in relieving pain and stiffness and improving mobility as multiple daily doses of conventional 25-mg capsules of the drug administered 3 times daily.

In the management of rheumatoid arthritis in adults, NSAIAs may be useful for initial symptomatic treatment; however, NSAIAs do not alter the course of the disease or prevent joint destruction. Disease modifying antirheumatic drugs (DMARDs) (e.g., azathioprine, cyclosporine, etanercept, oral or injectable gold compounds, hydroxychloroquine, infliximab, leflunomide, methotrexate, minocycline, penicillamine, sulfasalazine) have the potential to reduce or prevent joint damage, preserve joint integrity and function, and reduce total health care costs, and all patients with rheumatoid arthritis are candidates for DMARD therapy. DMARDs should be initiated early in the disease course and should not be delayed beyond 3 months in patients with active disease (i.e., ongoing joint pain, substantial morning stiffness, fatigue, active synovitis, persistent elevation of erythrocyte sedimentation rate [ESR] or C-reactive protein [CRP], radiographic evidence of joint damage) despite an adequate regimen of NSAIAs. NSAIA therapy may be continued in conjunction with DMARD therapy or, depending on patient response, may be discontinued. (For further information on the treatment of rheumatoid arthritis, see Uses: Rheumatoid Arthritis, in Methotrexate 10:00.)

Indomethacin has been used in conjunction with corticosteroids in patients with rheumatoid arthritis; results of one study indicated that when indomethacin was used concomitantly with prednisolone in the treatment of rheumatoid arthritis, plasma concentrations of free prednisolone were increased (see Drug Interactions: Other Drugs).

Use of indomethacin with aspirin is not recommended. There is no proof that the combination is more efficacious than either drug alone, the potential for adverse reactions is increased, and there is some evidence that aspirin decreases plasma concentrations of indomethacin. (See Drug Interactions: Nonsteroidal Anti-inflammatory Agents.)

Gout Indomethacin is among the drugs of choice for relieving the pain, fever, redness, swelling, and tenderness of acute gouty arthritis. The drug does not correct hyperuricemia, but is used for its anti-inflammatory, antipyretic, and analgesic effects. Indomethacin is at least as effective as usual dosages of colchicine or phenylbutazone (no longer commercially available in the US) in relieving attacks of acute gouty arthritis and, for short-term use, indomethacin is better tolerated than usual dosages of colchicine. Extended-release capsules of indomethacin are *not* recommended for use in these patients.

For long-term prophylactic treatment of gouty arthritis, colchicine in usual dosages appears to be better tolerated and more effective than indomethacin. If probenecid is administered concurrently with indomethacin, a reduction in indomethacin dosage may be necessary. (See Drug Interactions: Probenecid.)

Ankylosing Spondylitis Many clinicians consider indomethacin a drug of choice in the management of ankylosing spondylitis. In one study, the anti-inflammatory and analgesic effects of indomethacin in the management of ankylosing spondylitis were greater than those of usual dosages of aspirin and about equal to those of usual dosages of phenylbutazone.

Pericarditis Indomethacin is used to reduce the pain, fever, and inflammation of pericarditis†, including that occurring during maintenance hemodialysis. However, in the treatment of post-myocardial infarction pericarditis, NSAIAs are potentially harmful and aspirin is considered the treatment of choice. (See Cautions: Cardiovascular Effects and Cautions: Precautions and Contraindications.)

Indomethacin has been used successfully in the treatment of idiopathic pericarditis† and postpericardiotomy pericarditis† in children (11–15 years of age).

Other Inflammatory Conditions In the management of Reiter's syndrome†, many clinicians consider indomethacin a drug of choice.

When used in the symptomatic treatment of acute painful shoulder (bursitis and/or tendinitis), the anti-inflammatory and analgesic effects of indomethacin are greater than those of placebo and about equal to those of naproxen sodium. Indomethacin has also been used for symptomatic treatment of traumatic synovitis†, tennis elbow†, athletic injuries†, psoriatic arthritis†, juvenile arthritis†, Paget's disease†, mild uveitis†, and acute pseudogout†.

Indomethacin also has been used to reduce the pain, fever, and inflammation of pleurisy† and pleuritic chest pain† of diverse origins.

■ **Patent Ductus Arteriosus** Indomethacin sodium is used IV in the treatment of patent ductus arteriosus (PDA) in premature neonates. The drug is believed to inhibit the synthesis of prostaglandins that maintain ductal patency. (See Pharmacology: Cardiovascular Effects.) The drug is used IV to promote closure of a hemodynamically significant PDA (i.e., a left-to-right shunt large enough to compromise cardiorespiratory status) in premature neonates weighing 500–1750 g when 36–48 hours of usual medical management (e.g., fluid restriction, diuretics, cardiac glycosides, respiratory support) is ineffective. Evidence of hemodynamically significant PDA includes the presence of a continuous murmur over the anterior thorax or a systolic murmur or, in the absence of a murmur, respiratory distress requiring prolonged ventilatory support (e.g., intermittent mandatory ventilation for 48 hours or longer or escalating need for respiratory support). In addition, other criteria for hemodynamically significant PDA may include one or more of the following: hyperactive precordium, increased pulse pressure or bounding pulses, tachycardia, tachypnea, hepatomegaly, the need for varying levels of respiratory support, echocardiographic abnormalities, and/or cardiomegaly with radiographic evidence of pulmonary plethora.

Although the reported rates for successful closure of the ductus have varied, experience with IV administration of the drug has shown that indomethacin is substantially more effective than usual medical management alone (placebo group) and that the rate of successful indomethacin-induced closure is 75–90%. In the National Collaborative Study on Patent Ductus Arteriosus (a large, multicenter, placebo-controlled study) in premature neonates with hemodynamically significant PDA who weighed 500–1750 g, IV indomethacin sodium trihydrate combined with usual medical management produced successful ductal closure within 48 hours in 79% of neonates versus a 28% 48-hour closure rate in neonates receiving only usual medical management (placebo group). Subsequent reopening of the ductus arteriosus occurred in 26 and 12% of the indomethacin-treated and placebo groups, respectively, but the ductus reclosed in 69 and 42% of these, respectively; final closure rates were 79% in indomethacin-treated neonates and 35% in the placebo group. Neonates who did not respond to indomethacin therapy required surgical ligation. In neonates who did not initially respond to usual medical management but were randomly selected to subsequently receive indomethacin, the final closure rate was 70% (54% within 48 hours after initiating indomethacin); the remainder required surgical ligation. In this study, closure rates were not significantly related to birthweight, gestational age, gender, race, or plasma indomethacin concentration, although the rates were lowest in neonates weighing less than 1 kg, in those with a gestational age less than 30 weeks, and in those younger than 5 days of age when therapy was initiated. Neonates weighing less than 1 kg who received indomethacin or only usual medical management prior to 5 days of age had a final closure rate of 54 or 26%, respectively. However, the ratio of the rate of indomethacin-induced ductal closure to that of only usual medical management was greatest among smaller neonates (less than 1 kg), those with a gestational age less than 29 weeks, and those initially treated after the fifth day of life. Following IV indomethacin therapy in another study in premature neonates with hemodynamically significant PDA, no correlations were found between the number of doses required for ductal closure (1–6 doses of 0.2 mg/kg) and birthweight, gestational age, or age at the time of the first dose. In this and another study, 50–60% of the responders achieved ductal closure within 48 hours of a single dose and about 90% of responders required 3 doses or fewer.

The relationship between plasma or serum indomethacin concentrations and successful closure of the ductus remains unclear. While substantial constriction of the ductus appears to be correlated with indomethacin concentrations 24 hours after a dose, generally appearing to be associated with concentrations exceeding 0.25 mcg/mL, current evidence indicates that exceeding this concentration may not be predictive of either successful initial or permanent closure of the ductus. In one study, however, the time of subsequent reopening of the ductus was related to the plasma concentration of the drug. Because serum indomethacin concentrations appear to be inversely related to postnatal age (see Pharmacokinetics: Elimination), age-dependent IV dosage schedules have been proposed. (See Dosage and Administration: Patent Ductus Arteriosus.)

IV indomethacin sodium trihydrate has been used prophylactically in premature neonates with subclinical PDA† and as routine prophylaxis† during the first day of life in low-birthweight premature neonates. In clinical studies, prophylactic IV administration of indomethacin in premature neonates less than 7 days of age and weighing less than 1 kg with subclinical PDA and routine prophylactic IV administration of indomethacin initiated soon after delivery in low-birthweight (500–1500 g) premature neonates have been shown to decrease the incidence of hemodynamically significant PDA (e.g., large ductal shunts) and the need for subsequent medical and surgical ductal closure in such neonates. In addition, routine prophylactic IV administration of indomethacin initiated soon after delivery in selected low-birthweight (500–1500 g) premature neonates substantially decreased the development of intraventricular or periventricular hemorrhage, particularly grade 3 or 4 intraventricular hemorrhage. However, despite these beneficial effects, results of one large randomized clinical study indicate that routine prophylactic IV administration of indomethacin (0.1 mg/kg once daily for 3 days) does not improve the rate of survival without neurosensory impairment (e.g., cerebral palsy, cognitive delay, deafness, blindness) at 18 months of age.

■ **Genitourinary and Renal Diseases** Indomethacin has been used occasionally to relieve severe primary dysmenorrhea†. Indomethacin in dosages of 25 mg 3 times daily is reported to be more effective than placebo or aspirin (500 mg 3 times daily) in relieving painful menstruation; however, because of potentially serious adverse effects of indomethacin, other NSAIAs (e.g., ibuprofen, mefenamic acid, naproxen sodium) have been studied more extensively and are preferred for treatment of primary dysmenorrhea.

Indomethacin has been used to inhibit uterine contractions during preterm labor† (tocolysis) and thus prolong gestation. However, safety and efficacy of indomethacin for tocolysis have not been established and such use is controversial since there have been reports of serious adverse fetal effects, including constriction of the fetal ductus arteriosus, neonatal primary pulmonary hypertension, and fetal deaths.(See Cautions: Pregnancy, Fertility, and Lactation.)

Indomethacin has been used for symptomatic treatment of Bartter's syndrome†. (See Pharmacology: Genitourinary and Renal Effects.) However, because of potentially serious adverse effects of indomethacin, the drug may not be suitable for the long-term therapy necessary to control the disease; use of other NSAIAs such as ibuprofen is being evaluated.

■ **Fever** Indomethacin has been used for its antipyretic effect in the management of fever† associated with infection in children and with neoplasms (e.g., Hodgkin's disease, hepatic metastases of solid tumors). The drug appears to be more effective in reducing fever associated with neoplasms than fever caused by infections. In adults with fever associated with various neoplasms, indomethacin has effectively controlled fever that had not responded to other antipyretics (e.g., aspirin, acetaminophen), antineoplastic agents, and/or anti-infective agents. Indomethacin has been reported to have a greater antipyretic effect than aspirin in children with infection. However, indomethacin should not be used routinely as an antipyretic because of potentially serious adverse effects.

■ **Orthostatic Hypotension** Indomethacin has been recommended by some clinicians to treat orthostatic hypotension associated with multiple system atrophy characterized by predominantly autonomic failure† (formerly known as Shy-Drager syndrome). It has been suggested, however, that at least some autonomic activity must be present for indomethacin therapy to be successful in this condition.

■ **Pulmonary Hypertension** Although indomethacin has been used in the treatment of primary pulmonary hypertension†, it appears that the drug provides little hemodynamic benefit in these patients and may adversely affect their hemodynamic status. (See Pharmacology: Cardiovascular Effects.)

■ **Cystoid Macular Edema** A 1% indomethacin suspension has been applied topically to the eye† for the prevention of postoperative cystoid macular edema† in patients undergoing cataract surgery or retinal surgery, but a commercially available ophthalmic preparation currently is not available in the US.

■ **Other Uses** Indomethacin has also been used for symptomatic treatment of postoperative pain†, biliary pain†, chronic erythema nodosum†, and certain types of headache† (e.g., cluster headache, exertional headache).

Results from a large, prospective, population-based cohort study in geriatric individuals indicate a lower prevalence of Alzheimer's disease† among patients who received a NSAIA for 2 years or longer. Similar findings have been reported from some other, but not all, observational studies.

Dosage and Administration

■ **Reconstitution and Administration** The potential benefits and risks of indomethacin therapy as well as alternative therapies should be considered prior to initiating indomethacin therapy.

Indomethacin is administered orally or rectally. Indomethacin sodium is administered by IV injection for the treatment of patent ductus arteriosus (PDA).

Oral and Rectal Administration Indomethacin conventional capsules, oral suspension, and rectal suppositories are administered in 2–4 divided doses daily. The extended-release capsules are administered once or twice daily. To reduce adverse GI effects of the drug, the conventional or extended-release capsules or oral suspension should be administered orally immediately after meals or with food or antacids. Extended-release capsules of indomethacin must be administered and swallowed intact. Extended-release capsules of indomethacin are *not* recommended for use in the symptomatic treatment of acute gouty arthritis. Once-daily administration of 75-mg extended-release capsules of indomethacin can be used as an alternative dosage form for thrice-daily administration of 25-mg conventional indomethacin capsules; twice-daily administration of 75-mg extended-release capsules of indomethacin can be substituted for thrice-daily administration of 50-mg conventional indomethacin capsules.

To ensure complete absorption of the drug, indomethacin suppositories should be retained in the rectum for at least 1 hour.

IV Administration For IV administration, indomethacin sodium trihydrate sterile powder should be reconstituted by adding 1 or 2 mL of sterile water for injection or 0.9% sodium chloride injection to the vial labeled as containing 1 mg of indomethacin to provide solutions containing approximately 1 or 0.5 mg/mL, respectively. *Preserved diluents (i.e., bacteriostatic water for injection or bacteriostatic sodium chloride injection) should not be used to reconstitute the drug.* Because reconstituted solutions of the drug contain no preservatives, solutions should be prepared just prior to administration of each dose and any unused portion should be discarded. Reconstituted indomethacin sodium solutions should *not* be further diluted in IV infusion solutions. (See Chemistry and Stability: Stability.) Solutions of the drug should be inspected visually for particulate matter and discoloration prior to administration whenever solution and container permit.

The manufacturer currently states that the optimal rate of injection has not been established, but some studies indicate that indomethacin sodium solutions may be injected IV over 20–30 minutes. Previously, indomethacin sodium was administered IV over 5–10 seconds. Limited data indicate that the slower administration rate (e.g., over 20–30 minutes) may produce some amelioration, albeit inconsistently, in the indomethacin-associated reduction in cerebral blood flow and cerebral blood-flow velocity in premature neonates with patent ductus arteriosus (PDA), effects that may result in cerebral ischemia in such neonates. Limited data indicate that fast (i.e., over 20 seconds or less) IV administration of indomethacin also may be associated with substantial decreases in mesenteric artery blood flow velocity in neonates with PDA, which presumably may contribute to the development of necrotizing enterocolitis. Indomethacin sodium also has been given by continuous infusion over 36 hours in a very limited number of premature neonates with PDA; cerebral blood flow or cerebral blood-flow velocity was not decreased in these neonates. Additional studies are needed to determine the optimum rate of IV administration of indomethacin in premature neonates with PDA, taking into consideration the drug's effects on cerebral ischemia or intraventricular hemorrhage.

Care should be taken to avoid extravasation of the drug since it may be irritating to extravascular tissues.

■ **Dosage** The lowest possible effective dosage and shortest duration of therapy consistent with treatment goals of the patient should be employed. Dosage of indomethacin must be carefully adjusted according to individual requirements and response, using the lowest possible effective dosage.

Dosage of indomethacin sodium, which is available as the trihydrate, is expressed in terms of anhydrous indomethacin.

Inflammatory Diseases Dosage of indomethacin must be carefully adjusted according to individual requirements and response, using the lowest possible effective dosage. Total dosages greater than 200 mg daily generally do not increase the effectiveness of the drug. If extended-release capsules of the drug are used for initiating or titrating dosage, the patient should be observed for possible signs and symptoms of intolerance to adverse effects.

Rheumatoid Arthritis, Osteoarthritis, and Ankylosing Spondylitis. For the symptomatic treatment of moderate to severe rheumatoid arthritis, osteoarthritis, or ankylosing spondylitis, the usual initial adult dosage of indomethacin is 25 mg 2 or 3 times daily. If this dosage is well tolerated, dosage may be increased by 25 or 50 mg daily at weekly intervals until a satisfactory response is obtained or a dosage of 150–200 mg daily is reached.

The usual initial adult dosage of extended-release capsules of indomethacin for the symptomatic treatment of these conditions is one 75-mg capsule daily, administered in the morning or at bedtime; if this dosage is well tolerated, dosage may be increased to 75 mg twice daily.

Symptomatic improvement may occur after 4–6 days of indomethacin therapy; some patients may require up to 1 month of therapy before benefit is apparent. In patients who have persistent night pain and/or morning stiffness, administration of a large portion (a maximum of 100 mg) of the total daily dose orally or rectally at bedtime may be helpful.

Acute Exacerbations of Chronic Rheumatoid Arthritis. For the symptomatic treatment of acute exacerbations of chronic rheumatoid arthritis, the usual initial dosage of indomethacin may be increased by 25 or 50 mg daily until a satisfactory response is obtained or until the total daily dose reaches 150–200 mg.

If minor adverse effects develop as indomethacin dosage is increased, the dosage should be rapidly reduced to a tolerated level while observing the patient closely. If serious adverse effects occur, indomethacin therapy should be discontinued.

After the acute phase of the disease is controlled, repeated attempts should be made to reduce the indomethacin dosage until the patient is receiving the smallest effective dosage or the drug has been discontinued.

Gout. Various dosages have been used in the symptomatic treatment of acute gouty arthritis. The manufacturers recommend 50 mg of indomethacin 3 times daily until the pain can be tolerated. When symptoms subside, dosage should be reduced rapidly until the drug is withdrawn. Relief of pain has been reported in 2–4 hours, tenderness and heat usually subside in 24–36 hours, and swelling gradually disappears in 3–5 days. Administration of extended-release capsules of indomethacin for acute gouty arthritis is not recommended.

Acute Painful Shoulder. For the symptomatic treatment of acute painful shoulder (bursitis and/or tendinitis), the usual initial adult dosage of indomethacin is 75–150 mg daily in 3 or 4 divided doses. After signs and symptoms of inflammation have been controlled for several days, indomethacin should be discontinued. The usual duration of treatment is 7–14 days.

Juvenile Arthritis. If the benefits are thought to outweigh the risks (see Cautions: Pediatric Precautions), children 2–14 years of age may receive an initial oral indomethacin dosage of 1–2 mg/kg daily in divided doses for the management of juvenile rheumatoid arthritis. Dosage may be increased until a satisfactory response is achieved or a maximum dosage of 3 mg/kg daily or 150–200 mg daily (whichever is less) in divided doses is reached; limited data support the use of a maximum dosage of 4 mg/kg daily or 150–200 mg daily (whichever is less) in divided doses. As symptoms subside, dosage should be reduced to the lowest effective level or, if possible, until the drug is discontinued.

Pericarditis. In children with idiopathic pericarditis† or postpericardiotomy pericarditis†, 50–100 mg of indomethacin daily in 2–4 divided doses has been administered.

Patent Ductus Arteriosus For the treatment of patent ductus arteriosus (PDA) in premature neonates, indomethacin sodium is administered by IV injection. Extemporaneously prepared oral or rectal suspensions or solutions of indomethacin have occasionally been used for the treatment of PDA†, but administration of such preparations may present problems in drug delivery and absorption in premature neonates. (See Pharmacokinetics: Absorption.)

For the treatment of PDA in premature neonates, each course of therapy consists of up to 3 doses of indomethacin sodium administered at 12- to 24-hour intervals. The manufacturer indicates that all 3 doses should be administered in the first course of therapy, but some clinicians state that subsequent doses occasionally may be omitted if there is evidence of complete closure (e.g., resolution of murmur and lack of need for respiratory support) after the first or second dose in the course.

The first IV dose of each course of indomethacin sodium trihydrate is 0.2 mg/kg of indomethacin, regardless of the neonate's age. Subsequent doses depend on the age of the neonate at the time of administration of the first dose in the first course. If anuria or oliguria (i.e., urine output less than 0.6 mL/kg per hour) is present at the time of a second or third dose, the dose should be withheld until laboratory determinations indicate that renal function has returned to normal. (See Cautions: Renal and Electrolyte Effects.) For neonates younger than 48 hours of age at the time of the first dose, second and third doses of 0.1 mg/kg each are used. Neonates 2–7 days of age at the time of the first dose should receive second and third doses of 0.2 mg/kg each, and those older than 7 days of age at the time of the first dose should receive second and third doses of 0.25 mg/kg each. If severe adverse effects occur during a course of therapy, the drug should be discontinued.

Subsequent doses are not necessary if the ductus arteriosus closes or is substantially constricted 48 hours or longer after completion of the first course of indomethacin sodium therapy. If the ductus reopens (i.e., evidence of recurrence of significant PDA), a second course of 1–3 doses, given at 12- to 24-hour intervals, may be administered; doses in the second course are the same as those used in the first course (i.e., determined by the age of the neonate at the time of the first dose in the first, not second, course). Surgical ligation of the ductus may be necessary if the ductus arteriosus is unresponsive to indomethacin therapy after 2 courses.

Indomethacin sodium trihydrate has also been administered prophylactically to premature neonates (less than age 7 days) with subclinical PDA† in an initial IV indomethacin dose of 0.2 mg/kg followed by two IV doses of 0.1 mg/kg at 12-hour intervals.

When indomethacin is administered shortly after birth, a long duration of action may be expected after a single dose; the risk of accumulation of the drug should be considered when more than one dose is required. (See Pharmacokinetics: Elimination.)

Genitourinary and Renal Diseases Although other NSAIAs are preferred in the management of primary dysmenorrhea†, 25 or 50 mg of indomethacin has been given 3 or 4 times daily in the management of severe primary dysmenorrhea until symptoms were relieved. Indomethacin has been reported to be most effective if therapy is initiated several days prior to menstruation.

When used in the management of Bartter's syndrome†, indomethacin has been administered to children in dosages of 0.5–2 mg/kg daily in divided doses; adults have received dosages of 150 mg daily in divided doses.

Cautions

Adverse effects have been estimated to occur in 30–60% of patients treated with indomethacin, and serious reactions requiring discontinuance of the drug occur in about 10% of patients. Most adverse reactions appear to be dose-related and mainly involve the CNS and GI tract. In controlled clinical studies, the frequency of indomethacin-induced adverse effects was similar in patients receiving equivalent daily dosages of extended-release or conventional capsules. Adverse reactions reported with conventional indomethacin capsules may also occur with rectal suppositories or the oral suspension of the drug. Although the relevance to premature neonates receiving indomethacin IV for the treatment of patent ductus arteriosus (PDA) is not known, the possibility that adverse reactions reported in adults receiving the drug orally may also occur in neonates receiving the drug IV should be considered.

Unless otherwise specified, the frequencies of adverse effects associated with indomethacin use for the treatment of PDA in premature neonates are derived from experience from clinical studies and anecdotal reports in which the drug was administered IV, rectally, or orally. Adverse reactions (especially psychotic episodes and GI effects) may be particularly likely to occur in geriatric patients. Careful instructions to, and observation of, patients taking indomethacin are essential to prevent serious and irreversible, possibly fatal, adverse reactions.

■ **Cardiovascular Effects** Adverse cardiovascular effects, including congestive heart failure, tachycardia, chest pain, arrhythmia, and palpitations, occur in less than 1% of patients receiving indomethacin. Indomethacin also may cause hypertension, pulmonary hypertension, and edema; reduce the actions of some hypotensive agents; and may enhance the hypertensive effect of sympathomimetic agents. (See Hypotensive Agents and Diuretics and also see Other Drugs, in Drug Interactions.) Hypotension has also occurred. Although a causal relationship has not been established, thrombophlebitis and bradycardia have been reported in patients receiving the drug. Intraventricular bleeding (see Cautions: Nervous System Effects) has been reported in 3–9% and bradycardia and pulmonary hypertension in 1–3% of premature neonates receiving the drug for PDA.

Nonsteroidal anti-inflammatory agents (NSAIAs), including selective cyclooxygenase-2 (COX-2) inhibitors and prototypical NSAIAs, increase the risk of serious adverse cardiovascular thrombotic events, including myocardial infarction and stroke (which can be fatal), in patients with or without cardiovascular disease or risk factors for cardiovascular disease. Use of NSAIAs also is associated with an increased risk of heart failure.

The association between cardiovascular complications and use of NSAIAs is an area of ongoing concern and study. Findings of an FDA review of published observational studies of NSAIAs, a meta-analysis of published and unpublished data from randomized controlled trials of these drugs, and other published information indicate that NSAIAs may increase the risk of serious adverse cardiovascular thrombotic events by 10–50% or more, depending on the drugs and dosages studied. Available data suggest that the increase in risk may occur early (within the first weeks) following initiation of therapy and may increase with higher dosages and longer durations of use. Although the relative increase in cardiovascular risk appears to be similar in patients with or without known underlying cardiovascular disease or risk factors for cardiovascular disease, the absolute incidence of serious NSAIA-associated cardiovascular thrombotic events is higher in those with cardiovascular disease or risk factors for cardiovascular disease because of their elevated baseline risk.

Results from observational studies utilizing Danish national registry data indicated that patients receiving NSAIAs following a myocardial infarction were at increased risk of reinfarction, cardiovascular-related death, and all-cause mortality beginning in the first week of treatment. Patients who received NSAIAs following myocardial infarction had a higher 1-year mortality rate compared with those who did not receive NSAIAs (20 versus 12 deaths per 100 person-years). Although the absolute mortality rate declined somewhat after the first year following the myocardial infarction, the increased relative risk of death in patients who received NSAIAs persisted over at least the next 4 years of follow-up.

In 2 large controlled clinical trials of a selective COX-2 inhibitor for the management of pain in the first 10–14 days following coronary artery bypass graft (CABG) surgery, the incidence of myocardial infarction and stroke was increased. Therefore, NSAIAs are contraindicated in the setting of CABG surgery.

Findings from some systematic reviews of controlled observational studies and meta-analyses of data from randomized studies of NSAIAs suggest that naproxen may be associated with a lower risk of cardiovascular thrombotic events compared with other NSAIAs. However, limitations of these observational studies and the indirect comparisons used to assess cardiovascular risk of the prototypical NSAIAs (e.g., variability in patients' risk factors, comorbid conditions, concomitant drug therapy, drug interactions, dosage, and duration of therapy) affect the validity of the comparisons; in addition, these studies were not designed to demonstrate superior safety of one NSAIA compared with another. Therefore, FDA states that definitive conclusions regarding relative risks of NSAIAs are not possible at this time. (See Cautions: Cardiovascular Effects, in Celecoxib 28:08.04.08.)

Data from observational studies also indicate that use of NSAIAs in patients with heart failure is associated with increased morbidity and mortality. Results from a retrospective study utilizing Danish national registry data indicated that use of selective COX-2 inhibitors or prototypical NSAIAs in patients with chronic heart failure was associated with a dose-dependent increase in the risk of death and an increased risk of hospitalization for myocardial infarction or heart failure. In addition, findings from a meta-analysis of published and unpublished data from randomized controlled trials of NSAIAs indicated that use of selective COX-2 inhibitors or prototypical NSAIAs was associated with an approximate twofold increase in the risk of hospitalization for heart failure. Fluid retention and edema also have been observed in some patients receiving NSAIAs.

There is no consistent evidence that use of low-dose aspirin mitigates the increased risk of serious cardiovascular events associated with NSAIAs.

■ **GI Effects** GI disturbances most frequently reported with indomethacin therapy include nausea, with or without vomiting, and dyspepsia (including indigestion, heartburn, and epigastric pain), which occur in 3–9% of patients. Diarrhea, abdominal distress or pain, or constipation occur in 1–3% of patients receiving the drug. Other adverse GI effects, occurring in less than 1% of patients, include anorexia, bloating (including distention), flatulence, gastroenteritis, rectal bleeding, proctitis, ulcerative stomatitis, intestinal strictures (diaphragms), and gingival ulcers.

Indomethacin may reactivate latent peptic or intestinal lesions. Single or multiple ulcerations of the esophagus, stomach, duodenum, or small and/or large intestine, occasionally resulting in death, have been reported in less than 1% of patients receiving indomethacin and may occur in patients with no previous history of ulcers; hemorrhage and perforation of such lesions have occurred. Rarely, ulceration has been associated with stenosis and obstruction. GI bleeding without obvious ulcer formation may occur. In one study, occult GI bleeding was reported to be less with indomethacin (200 mg daily) than with aspirin (3.9 g daily) and about the same as that occurring with tolmetin (1.2 g daily). In a study in healthy adults, gastroscopic evidence of mucosal abnormalities was greater in individuals receiving conventional oral capsules of the drug than in those receiving placebo or rectal suppositories. However, in a controlled clinical study in patients with rheumatoid arthritis, the incidence of adverse upper GI effects was similar in patients receiving rectal suppositories or conventional oral capsules, but the incidence of adverse lower GI effects was greater in patients receiving suppositories; gastroscopic findings also were similar following rectal suppositories or conventional oral capsules in a crossover study in patients with rheumatic diseases. Perforation of preexisting sigmoid lesions such as diverticula and carcinoma has been reported. Increased abdominal pain in patients with ulcerative colitis has been reported to occur rarely. The development of ulcerative colitis and regional ileitis also has occurred rarely.

GI bleeding has occurred in 3–9% of premature neonates receiving indomethacin for PDA. In a large, multicenter study, the frequency of major GI bleeding was similar for indomethacin-treated neonates and those not receiving the drug; however, minor GI bleeding, as evidenced by occult blood in feces, occurred more frequently in indomethacin-treated neonates. Vomiting, abdominal distention, and transient ileus have occurred in 1–3% of neonates. Necrotizing enterocolitis has occurred in premature neonates receiving the drug for PDA, but the frequency of this effect has been similar to that observed in premature neonates not receiving indomethacin and a causal relationship to the drug has not been established. Focal GI (gastric, jejunal, ileal, rectal) perforation has occurred in premature neonates who received the drug IV, orally via nasogastric tube, or rectally. Pathologic examination of resected specimens in several of these neonates revealed well-defined perforation that was surrounded by well-circumscribed, superficial, mucosal ulceration; histologic findings included moderate to marked mucosal hemorrhagic necrosis with some submucosal hemorrhage but without substantial inflammatory infiltration.

Although a causal relationship has not been directly determined, one case-control analysis suggests that NSAIAs may contribute to the formation of esophageal stricture in patients with gastroesophageal reflux.

Adverse GI effects of orally administered indomethacin may be minimized by administering the drug immediately after meals, with food, or with antacids. Because of the potential severity of adverse GI effects, clinicians must be alert to signs and symptoms of GI reactions in patients receiving indomethacin. Stools should be examined periodically for occult blood in patients receiving long-term indomethacin therapy. Therapy should be discontinued if GI bleeding occurs. If GI symptoms occur, the benefits of continued therapy with indomethacin should be weighed against the possible risks.

Serious adverse GI effects (e.g., bleeding, ulceration, perforation) can occur at any time in patients receiving NSAIA therapy, and such effects may *not* be preceded by warning signs or symptoms.Only 1 in 5 patients who develop a serious upper GI adverse event while receiving NSAIA therapy is symptomatic. Therefore, clinicians should remain alert to the possible development of serious GI effects (e.g., bleeding, ulceration) in any patient receiving NSAIA therapy, and such patients should be followed chronically for the development of manifestations of such effects and advised of the importance of this follow-up. In addition, patients should be advised about the signs and symptoms of serious NSAIA-induced GI toxicity and what action to take if they occur. If signs and symptoms of a serious GI event develop, additional evaluation and treatment should be initiated promptly; the NSAIA should be discontinued until appropriate diagnostic studies have ruled out a serious GI event.

Results of studies to date are inconclusive concerning the relative risk of various prototypical NSAIAs in causing serious GI effects. In patients receiving NSAIAs and observed in clinical studies of several months' to 2 years' duration, symptomatic upper GI ulcers, gross bleeding, or perforation appeared to occur in approximately 1% of patients treated for 3–6 months and in about 2–4% of those treated for 1 year. Longer duration of therapy with an NSAIA increases the likelihood of a serious GI event. However, short-term therapy is not without risk. High dosages of any NSAIA probably are associated with increased risk of such effects, although controlled studies documenting this probable association are lacking for most NSAIAs. Therefore, whenever use of relatively high dosages (within the recommended dosage range) is considered, sufficient benefit to offset the potential increased risk of GI toxicity should be anticipated.

Studies have shown that patients with a history of peptic ulcer disease and/or GI bleeding who are receiving NSAIAs have a substantially higher risk of developing GI bleeding than patients without these risk factors. In addition to a history of ulcer disease, pharmacoepidemiologic studies have identified several comorbid conditions and concomitant therapies that may increase the risk for GI bleeding, including concomitant use of oral corticosteroids or anticoagulants, longer duration of NSAIA therapy, smoking, alcoholism, older age, and poor general health status. Patients with rheumatoid arthritis are more likely to experience serious GI complications from NSAIA therapy than are patients with osteoarthritis. In addition, geriatric or debilitated patients appear to tolerate GI ulceration and bleeding less well than other individuals, and most spontaneous reports of fatal GI effects have been in such patients.

For patients at high risk for complications from NSAIA-induced GI ulceration (e.g., bleeding, perforation), concomitant use of misoprostol can be considered for preventive therapy. (See Misoprostol 56:28.28.) Alternatively, some clinicians suggest that a proton-pump inhibitor (e.g., omeprazole) may be used concomitantly to decrease the incidence of serious GI toxicity associated with NSAIA therapy. In one study, therapy with high dosages of famotidine (40 mg twice daily) was more effective than placebo in preventing peptic ulcers in NSAIA-treated patients; however, the effect of the drug was modest. In addition, efficacy of usual dosages of H_2-receptor antagonists for the prevention of NSAIA-induced gastric and duodenal ulcers has not been established. Therefore, most clinicians do not recommend use of H_2-receptor antagonists for the prevention of NSAIA-associated ulcers. Another approach in high-risk patients who would benefit from NSAIA therapy is use of a NSAIA that is a selective inhibitor of COX-2 (e.g., celecoxib), since these agents are associated with a lower incidence of GI bleeding than are prototypical NSAIAs. However, while celecoxib (200 mg twice daily) was comparably effective to diclofenac sodium (75 mg twice daily) plus omeprazole (20 mg daily) in preventing recurrent ulcer bleeding (recurrent ulcer bleeding probabilities of 4.9 versus 6.4%, respectively, during the 6-month study) in *H. pylori*-negative arthritis (principally osteoarthritis) patients with a recent history of ulcer bleeding, the protective efficacy was unexpectedly low for both regimens and it appeared that neither could completely protect patients at high risk. Additional study is necessary to elucidate optimal therapy for preventing GI complications associated with NSAIA therapy in high-risk patients.

■ **Nervous System Effects** Headache, which appears to be dose related, is the most frequent adverse effect, occurring in at least 10% (although some estimates range from 25–50%) of patients treated with indomethacin. Headache is more common and most severe in the morning and may be accompanied by frontal throbbing, apparent swelling of the temporal vessels, vomiting, tinnitus, ataxia, tremor, dizziness, insomnia, or vertigo. If headache persists despite reduction of dosage, indomethacin should be discontinued. In one study, adverse CNS effects (e.g., frontal headache and lightheadedness) appeared to increase when plasma indomethacin concentrations exceeded 6 mcg/mL. Dizziness also is common in patients receiving indomethacin, occurring in 3–9% of patients. Vertigo, somnolence, depression, and fatigue (including malaise and listlessness) occur in 1–3% of patients.

Less frequently reported adverse nervous system effects, occurring in less than 1% of patients receiving indomethacin, include lightheadedness, drowsiness, confusion, psychic disturbances (including psychotic episodes), hallucinations, nightmares, depersonalization, feelings of floating or unreality, insomnia, muzziness, anxiety (including nervousness), muscle weakness, involuntary muscle movements, ataxia, dysarthria, syncope, paresthesia, aggravation of epilepsy and parkinsonian syndrome, seizures, peripheral neuropathy, and coma.

Intraventricular (intracranial) hemorrhage has been reported in 3–9% of premature neonates receiving indomethacin for PDA; however, it appears that the frequency of this effect is similar for indomethacin-treated neonates and those not receiving the drug. Extension of intraventricular hemorrhage has also been reported in neonates receiving indomethacin for PDA, but this effect did not appear to be drug related. Although the risk, if any, remains to be clearly delineated, the possibility that indomethacin could potentially increase the risk of intraventricular hemorrhage in premature neonates should be considered since the drug can inhibit platelet aggregation and prolong bleeding time. (See Pharmacology: Hematologic Effects.) It should be remembered, however, that prematurity itself is associated with an increased risk of intraventricular hemorrhage. There is preliminary evidence that indomethacin may decrease cerebral blood flow in neonates and that prophylactic administration of the drug may have a beneficial effect in preventing the development of intraventricular hemorrhage, possibly by inhibiting prostaglandin-mediated cerebral blood flow and preventing germinal matrix capillary damage; however, in one study, a protective effect was not evident, and additional study is necessary to elucidate the effects of indomethacin on cerebral blood flow and whether such a protective effect occurs.

Pseudotumor cerebri occurred in one adult treated with indomethacin for Bartter's syndrome and was attributed to sodium and water retention induced by the drug. One suicide, possibly related to indomethacin-induced depression, has been reported.

If severe nervous system reactions occur, indomethacin should be discontinued.

■ **Hematologic Effects** Adverse hematologic effects of indomethacin occur in less than 1% of patients and include anemia secondary to GI bleeding, hemolytic anemia (including hemolytic anemia with positive antiglobulin [Coombs'] test results), bone marrow depression, aplastic anemia (sometimes fatal), agranulocytosis, leukopenia, thrombocytopenia, and thrombocytopenic purpura. Thrombocytopenia has also occurred in premature neonates receiving the drug for PDA. Iron deficiency anemia may develop secondary to GI bleeding in patients receiving indomethacin. There have been several reports of leukemia in patients who had received indomethacin, but a causal relationship to the drug has not been established. Disseminated intravascular coagulation also has been reported.

Indomethacin inhibits platelet aggregation, but this effect usually disappears within 24 hours after discontinuing the drug. Indomethacin may prolong bleeding time (but within the normal range) in healthy individuals; however, this effect may be exaggerated in patients with underlying hemostatic defects. Indomethacin therapy has been associated with platelet dysfunction and bleeding tendencies in premature neonates with PDA. In one study in premature neonates with PDA, a single oral dose of indomethacin (0.2–0.3 mg/kg by nasogastric tube) resulted in severe platelet dysfunction, with normal function returning only 9–10 days later. In another study in premature neonates with PDA who received indomethacin IV (0.2 mg/kg initially, followed by 0.1 mg/kg 12 and 24 hours later), bleeding time increased from a pretreatment mean of 3.6 minutes to means of 8.7 minutes 2 hours after the first dose and 8.9 and 5.3 minutes 2 and 48 hours, respectively, after the third dose; thrombocytopenia also occurred, but clinical signs of bleeding were minor. Intraventricular (intracranial) hemorrhage and GI bleeding have occurred in premature neonates receiving the drug for PDA. (See Cautions: Nervous System Effects and also GI Effects.) In a large, multicenter study in premature neonates with PDA, bleeding tendencies (e.g., gross macroscopic GI bleeding, oozing at the site of injection, pulmonary hemorrhage, disseminated intravascular coagulation), other than intraventricular hemorrhage, occurred more frequently in neonates receiving indomethacin than in those receiving usual medical management alone; however, life-threatening hemorrhage, other than intraventricular, did not occur.

Patients who may be adversely affected by a prolongation of bleeding time should be carefully observed during indomethacin therapy. Neonates should be carefully observed for bleeding.

■ Ocular and Otic Effects Corneal deposits and retinal disturbances, including those of the macula, have been reported in less than 1% of patients receiving prolonged indomethacin therapy; the drug should be discontinued if these effects occur. Other reported ocular effects occurring in less than 1% of patients include blurred vision, conjunctival pain, photophobia, diplopia, toxic amblyopia, nightblindness, mydriasis, and loss of vision. Patients who experience visual disturbances during indomethacin therapy should have an ophthalmologic examination.

The retinopathy of prematurity (retrolental fibroplasia) has developed in 3–9% of premature neonates who were treated with indomethacin for PDA; however, the frequency of this effect appears to be similar in indomethacin-treated neonates and in those not receiving the drug. In a large, multicenter study in premature neonates with PDA, indomethacin appeared to have a beneficial effect in reducing the development of severe (grade III–V), but not less severe, retinopathy; however, this possible beneficial effect was less evident after 1 year of follow-up and additional study is necessary to determine whether such an effect occurs. After 1 year of follow-up in this study, the frequency of strabismus was similar in indomethacin-treated neonates and in those not receiving the drug. After 3.5 years of follow-up in another study, the frequency of retinopathy, amblyopia, optic nerve atrophy, myopia, or hyperopia was similar in children who had received indomethacin for PDA as neonates and in those who had undergone surgical ligation of the ductus arteriosus.

Tinnitus occurs in 1–3% of patients receiving indomethacin. Hearing disturbances and deafness occur in less than 1% of patients. After 3.5 years of follow-up in one study, the frequency and severity of audiologic abnormalities were similar in children who had received indomethacin for PDA as neonates and in those who had undergone surgical ligation of the ductus arteriosus.

■ Renal and Electrolyte Effects Acute interstitial nephritis with hematuria, proteinuria, and, occasionally, nephrotic syndrome has occurred in less than 1% of patients receiving indomethacin. Reversible worsening of renal function, including renal failure, has been reported following indomethacin administration in patients with moderate to severe renal impairment or with sodium retention associated with hepatic disease or congestive heart failure. Abnormal laboratory findings may include increases in BUN and serum creatinine concentrations, proteinuria, hematuria, and albuminuria. Hematuria occurs in less than 1% of patients receiving indomethacin; transient occult hematuria has been reported in neonates receiving the drug. Acute renal failure has occurred in at least one patient who was not known to have prior renal dysfunction. As with other NSAIAs, long-term administration of indomethacin in animals has resulted in renal papillary necrosis and other pathologic renal abnormalities. Renal papillary necrosis occurred in 2 young adults who had received prolonged therapy with low dosages of indomethacin (37.5–100 mg daily for 12–17 years) in the treatment of juvenile rheumatoid arthritis. In addition, an association between prolonged (e.g., daily for 1 year or longer) NSAIA use, including indomethacin, and chronic renal failure also has been described in certain high-risk patients, but current evidence suggests that the overall potential risk, if any, is low in patients receiving the drug, and additional study and experience are necessary to confirm and elucidate these findings.

Increased serum potassium concentrations have occurred in 3–9% of premature neonates with PDA receiving indomethacin, and such increases, including hyperkalemia, have occurred in less than 1% of other patients receiving the drug, including some patients without renal impairment. Several patients with preexisting renal disease and at least one patient with no apparent renal disease developed severe hyperkalemia following indomethacin therapy. In one study in patients with baseline serum potassium concentrations of about 4–5 mEq/L who were receiving indomethacin for musculoskeletal pain, pericarditis, or fever, serum potassium concentrations increased in most patients during therapy with the drug. In some of these patients, serum potassium increased by more than 1 mEq/L and exceeded 5 mEq/L in most patients within 2–6 days of therapy. Patients most likely to experience increases in serum potassium during indomethacin therapy included those with preexisting mild to moderate renal dysfunction and geriatric patients. In patients with normal renal function, increases in serum potassium concentration during indomethacin therapy have been attributed to hyporeninemic hypoaldosteronism induced by the drug. Serum potassium concentrations have increased by about 0.5–0.8 mEq/L within 12–36 hours after administration of indomethacin in several studies in premature neonates but subsequently returned toward baseline (e.g., within 72 hours) following discontinuance of the drug.

Mild, transient renal insufficiency, usually manifested as a reversible decrease in urine output, occurs in about 40% of premature neonates during indomethacin therapy for PDA. Urine output usually decreases during the first 12 hours after indomethacin is administered and usually returns to pretreatment levels within 48 hours after the last dose of the drug (sometimes within 24 hours). Transient increases in serum potassium, BUN, and serum creatinine concentrations; transient decreases in urinary excretion of sodium, chloride, and potassium and in urinary osmolarity, free water clearance, and glomerular filtration rate; and transient and asymptomatic decreases in serum sodium concentrations have also occurred in these neonates. In a large, multicenter study, the frequency of transient oliguria and increased serum creatinine concentrations (1.8 mg/dL or greater) was higher in indomethacin-treated neonates than in those not receiving the drug. Weight gain secondary to fluid retention has occurred in 1–3% of premature neonates receiving the drug. Changes in acid-base balance, including acidosis and alkalosis, have also occurred in 1–3% of neonates; however, a causal relationship to the drug has not been established. Decreased urinary excretion of kallikrein and prostaglandins $F_{2\alpha}$, E-M, and 6-keto-$F_{1\alpha}$, and decreased plasma renin activity have also been reported in these neonates. There was no evidence of major delayed renal toxicity after 1 year of follow-up in one study in infants who had received indomethacin as neonates for PDA.

Fatal glomerulonephritis with nonthrombocytopenic purpura and urinary frequency has been reported but not definitely attributed to indomethacin.

Some clinicians recommend that renal function tests be performed every 3 months in patients receiving long-term indomethacin therapy. Renal function, including measurement of urine output and serum electrolytes, should be closely monitored in neonates receiving the drug. If a substantial reduction in urine output (i.e., less than 0.6 mL/kg per hour) occurs during indomethacin therapy in neonates, additional doses of the drug should be withheld until output returns toward normal.

■ Dermatologic and Sensitivity Reactions Adverse dermatologic effects of indomethacin occur in less than 1% of patients and include pruritus, urticaria, rash, macular and morbilliform eruptions, erythema nodosum, petechiae or ecchymosis, exfoliative dermatitis, loss of hair, Stevens-Johnson syndrome, erythema multiforme, and toxic epidermal necrolysis.

Acute anaphylaxis, asthma, angioedema, acute respiratory distress, dyspnea, purpura, angiitis, pulmonary edema, fever, and a rapid fall in blood pressure resembling shock have been reported as hypersensitivity reactions to indomethacin and occur in less than 1% of patients receiving the drug. The drug may precipitate asthma in aspirin-sensitive individuals who have had no previous exposure to indomethacin; it has been suggested that of the currently available NSAIAs, indomethacin may be most likely to induce signs and symptoms of a sensitivity reaction in individuals with aspirin-induced bronchospasm. Sensitivity reactions to the structurally different NSAIAs appear to be related mainly to inhibition of prostaglandin synthesis in patients with bronchospastic reactions; however, other mechanisms may be involved. For a further discussion of cross-sensitivity of NSAIAs, see Cautions: Sensitivity Reactions, in the Salicylates General Statement 28:08.04.24.

■ Hepatic Effects Jaundice and toxic hepatitis, possibly fatal, may occur rarely in patients receiving indomethacin. Increases in serum ALT (SGPT), AST (SGOT), alkaline phosphatase, and bilirubin concentrations and in cephalin flocculation and thymol turbidity values occurred in one case of fatal hepatitis. Green urine was reported in one patient with indomethacin-induced hepatitis with biliverdinemia. Histologic analysis of liver tissues from this patient revealed centrilobular degeneration, swelling, some fatty changes of parenchymal cells, regeneration of hepatic cells, and infiltration of both parenchyma and portal zone by neutrophils and mononuclear cells. The manufacturer of parenteral indomethacin sodium trihydrate states that displacement of bilirubin from albumin by indomethacin, as evidenced by an increased frequency of kernicterus, has not been observed in controlled studies in premature neonates receiving the drug for PDA. In vitro evidence suggests that indomethacin-induced displacement of bilirubin is unlikely at dosages used in these neonates.

Borderline elevations of one or more liver function test results may occur in up to 15% of patients treated with NSAIAs; meaningful (3 times the upper limit of normal) elevations of serum ALT (SGPT) or AST (SGOT) concentration have occurred in less than 1% of patients receiving NSAIAs in controlled clinical studies. These abnormalities may progress, may remain essentially unchanged, or may be transient with continued therapy. Patients, including neonates, who experience signs and/or symptoms suggestive of liver dysfunction or an abnormal liver function test result while receiving indomethacin should be evaluated for evidence of the development of a more severe hepatic reaction. Although such reactions are rare, indomethacin should be discontinued if abnormal liver function test results persist or worsen, if clinical signs and symptoms consistent with liver disease develop, or if systemic manifestations occur (e.g., eosinophilia, rash).

■ Respiratory Effects Apnea and exacerbation of pulmonary infection have occurred in 1–3% of premature neonates receiving indomethacin for PDA.

Bronchopulmonary dysplasia, hyaline membrane disease, and pulmonary insufficiency also have occurred in these neonates; however, the frequency of these effects in indomethacin-treated neonates appears to be similar to or less than that in neonates not receiving the drug. In addition, indomethacin-induced closure of the ductus arteriosus has been associated with a decreased need for ventilatory support in some studies. The frequency of pneumothorax in indomethacin-treated neonates has been similar to that in neonates not receiving the drug but less than that in neonates undergoing surgical ligation of the ductus.

■ Other Adverse Effects Fulminant necrotizing fasciitis, which may be fatal and usually is associated with group A β-hemolytic streptococcal infection, has been reported rarely in patients receiving nonsteroidal anti-inflammatory agents, including indomethacin. Vaginal bleeding, weight gain, flushing or sweating, epistaxis, and breast changes (including enlargement and tenderness) have occurred in less than 1% of patients receiving indomethacin. Acute pancreatitis with increased serum amylase concentration and urinary frequency have been reported, but a causal relationship to indomethacin has not been established.

Decreased plasma glucose concentrations, occasionally resulting in hypoglycemia, have been observed in 1–3% of premature neonates receiving indomethacin for PDA. Plasma glucose concentrations decreased from a pretreatment mean of about 95 mg/dL to means of about 70 mg/dL 24–72 hours after administration of the drug in one study in these neonates. Hyperglycemia and glucosuria have been reported in less than 1% of other patients receiving the drug.

■ Precautions and Contraindications Patients should be advised that indomethacin, like other NSAIAs, is not free of potential adverse effects, including some that can cause discomfort, and that more serious effects (e.g., myocardial infarction, stroke, GI bleeding), which may require hospitalization and may even be fatal, also can occur. Patients also should be informed that, while some NSAIAs may be commonly employed for conditions that are less serious, NSAIA therapy often is considered essential for the management of some diseases. Clinicians may wish to discuss with their patients the potential risks and likely benefits of NSAIA therapy, particularly when consideration is being given to use of these drugs in less serious conditions for which therapy without a NSAIA may represent an acceptable alternative to both the patient and clinician.

Patients should be advised to read the medication guide for NSAIAs that is provided to the patient each time the drug is dispensed.

NSAIAs increase the risk of serious adverse cardiovascular thrombotic events. (See Cautions: Cardiovascular Effects.) To minimize the potential risk of adverse cardiovascular events, the lowest effective dosage and shortest possible duration of therapy should be employed. Some clinicians suggest that it may be prudent to avoid use of NSAIAs whenever possible in patients with cardiovascular disease. Patients receiving NSAIAs (including those without previous symptoms of cardiovascular disease) should be monitored for the possible development of cardiovascular events throughout therapy. Patients should be informed about the signs and symptoms of serious cardiovascular toxicity (chest pain, dyspnea, weakness, slurring of speech) and instructed to seek immediate medical attention if such toxicity occurs. Indomethacin should be avoided in patients with recent myocardial infarction unless the benefits of therapy are expected to outweigh the risk of recurrent cardiovascular thrombotic events; if indomethacin is used in such patients, the patient should be monitored for cardiac ischemia.

There is no consistent evidence that concomitant use of low-dose aspirin mitigates the increased risk of serious cardiovascular events associated with NSAIAs. Concomitant use of aspirin and an NSAIA increases the risk for serious GI events. Because of the potential for increased adverse effects, patients receiving indomethacin should be advised not to take aspirin.

Use of NSAIAs, including indomethacin, can result in the onset of hypertension or worsening of preexisting hypertension; either of these occurrences may contribute to the increased incidence of cardiovascular events. Patients receiving NSAIAs may have an impaired response to diuretics (i.e., thiazide or loop diuretics), angiotensin-converting enzyme (ACE) inhibitors, angiotensin II receptor antagonists, or β-adrenergic blocking agents. NSAIAs, including indomethacin, should be used with caution in patients with hypertension. Blood pressure should be monitored closely during initiation of indomethacin therapy and throughout therapy.

Because NSAIAs increase morbidity and mortality in patients with heart failure, the manufacturer states that indomethacin should be avoided in patients with severe heart failure unless the benefits of therapy are expected to outweigh the risk of worsening heart failure; if indomethacin is used in such patients, the patient should be monitored for worsening heart failure. In patients with severe congestive heart failure, particularly those with hyponatremia, inhibition of prostaglandin synthesis induced by the drug may cause clinical deterioration of cardiovascular status by interfering with prostaglandin-mediated, circulatory homeostatic mechanisms. (See Pharmacology: Cardiovascular Effects.) Some experts state that use of NSAIAs should be avoided whenever possible in patients with reduced left ventricular ejection fraction and current or prior symptoms of heart failure. Patients receiving NSAIAs should be advised to inform their clinician if they experience symptoms of heart failure, including dyspnea, unexplained weight gain, and edema. Use of NSAIAs may diminish the cardiovascular effects of certain drugs used to treat heart failure and edema (e.g., diuretics, ACE inhibitors, angiotensin II receptor antagonists). (See Drug Interactions.)

Indomethacin is contraindicated in neonates with congenital heart disease when patency of the ductus arteriosus is necessary for adequate pulmonary or systemic blood flow (e.g., neonates with pulmonary atresia, severe tetralogy of Fallot, or severe coarctation of the aorta).

The risk of potentially serious adverse GI effects should be considered in patients receiving indomethacin, particularly in patients receiving chronic therapy with the drug. Indomethacin should be used with caution and under close supervision in patients with a history of GI disease. Since peptic ulceration and/or GI bleeding have been reported in patients receiving the drug, patients should be advised to promptly report signs or symptoms of GI ulceration or bleeding to their clinician.

Indomethacin should be used with extreme caution and under close supervision in patients with a history of GI bleeding or peptic ulcer disease, and such patients should receive an appropriate ulcer preventive regimen. All patients considered at increased risk of potentially serious adverse GI effects (e.g., geriatric patients, those receiving high therapeutic dosages of NSAIAs, those with a history of peptic ulcer disease, those receiving anticoagulants or corticosteroids concomitantly) should be monitored closely for signs of ulcer perforation or GI bleeding.To minimize the potential risk of adverse GI effects, the lowest effective dosage and shortest possible duration of therapy should be employed. For patients who are at high risk, therapy other than an NSAIA should be considered.

Indomethacin suppositories are contraindicated in patients with a history of proctitis or recent rectal bleeding. The possibility that adverse GI effects reported with oral or rectal administration of indomethacin in older children and adults also may occur with parenteral administration of the drug in premature neonates should be considered.

Indomethacin should not be used in premature neonates with active GI bleeding or known or suspected necrotizing enterocolitis. For additional information on adverse GI effects of indomethacin and associated precautions, see Cautions: GI Effects.

NSAIAs, including indomethacin, may mask the usual signs and symptoms of infection; the drug should be used with extreme caution in patients with an existing infection since fulminant necrotizing fasciitis, which may be fatal and usually is associated with group A β-hemolytic streptococcal infection, has been reported rarely in patients receiving nonsteroidal anti-inflammatory agents including indomethacin. In addition, deaths attributed to overwhelming sepsis have been reported very rarely in children with severe rheumatoid arthritis who received the drug; a direct causal relationship to indomethacin has not been established. Activation of latent infections including tuberculosis has been attributed to indomethacin. A severe reaction to a smallpox vaccination in one patient has also been attributed to indomethacin, although a causal relationship has not been established.

Indomethacin should be used with caution in premature neonates with an existing infection that is adequately controlled, and clinicians should be alert to the masking effect of the drug in these neonates. The drug is contraindicated in neonates with proven or suspected, untreated infection.

Renal toxicity has been observed in patients in whom renal prostaglandins have a compensatory role in maintaining renal perfusion. Administration of an NSAIA to such patients may cause a dose-dependent reduction in prostaglandin formation and thereby precipitate overt renal decompensation. Patients at greatest risk of this reaction include those with impaired renal function, heart failure, or hepatic dysfunction; those with extracellular fluid depletion (e.g., patients receiving diuretics); those taking an ACE inhibitor or angiotensin II antagonist; and geriatric patients. Patients should be advised to consult their clinician promptly if unexplained weight gain or edema occurs. Recovery of renal function to pretreatment levels usually occurs following discontinuance of NSAIA therapy.

Indomethacin has not been evaluated in patients with advanced renal disease, and the manufacturer states that use of indomethacin is not recommended in such patients. If indomethacin is used in patients with advanced renal disease, close monitoring of renal function is recommended.

Indomethacin also may precipitate renal insufficiency, including acute renal failure, in premature neonates with PDA, especially those with other conditions that might adversely affect renal function (e.g., those with extracellular fluid depletion, congestive heart failure, sepsis, or hepatic dysfunction and those receiving a nephrotoxic drug concomitantly). Renal function and serum electrolytes should be monitored closely in neonates receiving the drug. (See Caution: Renal and Electrolyte Effects.) The drug is contraindicated in neonates with substantially impaired renal function.

The risk of increased serum potassium concentration, including hyperkalemia, should be considered in any patient receiving indomethacin therapy, including those with normal renal function.

Indomethacin also should be used with extreme caution in patients with a history of mental depression or other psychiatric disorder, epilepsy, or parkinsonian syndrome because the drug may aggravate these conditions. If severe adverse nervous system effects occur during indomethacin therapy, the drug should be discontinued. The drug should also be discontinued in patients in whom indomethacin-induced headache persists despite a reduction in dosage. Patients should be warned that indomethacin may impair their ability to perform activities requiring mental alertness or physical coordination (e.g., operating machinery, driving a motor vehicle).

Patients who experience signs and/or symptoms suggestive of liver dysfunction or an abnormal liver function test result while receiving indomethacin should be evaluated for evidence of the development of a more severe hepatic reaction. Severe reactions, including jaundice and fatal fulminant hepatitis, liver necrosis, and hepatic failure (sometimes fatal), have been reported in patients receiving NSAIAs. Indomethacin should be discontinued if abnormal liver function test results persist or worsen, if clinical signs and symptoms consistent with liver disease develop, or if systemic manifestations occur (e.g., eosinophilia, rash).

Indomethacin can inhibit platelet aggregation and may prolong bleeding time. (See Cautions: Hematologic Effects.) The drug should be used with caution in patients who may be adversely affected by a prolongation of bleeding time (e.g., patients receiving anticoagulant therapy). If signs and/or symptoms of anemia occur during therapy with indomethacin, hemoglobin concentration and hematocrit should be determined. Premature neonates receiving the drug should be observed closely for bleeding tendencies. Indomethacin is contraindicated in neonates with active bleeding, such as those with intraventricular hemorrhage or GI bleeding, and in neonates with thrombocytopenia or underlying coagulation defect.

Because ocular changes may be asymptomatic, patients receiving prolonged indomethacin therapy should be given periodic ophthalmologic examinations at least once a year; a thorough examination is also indicated whenever blurred vision occurs. (See Cautions: Ocular and Otic Effects.)

Indomethacin is not a substitute for corticosteroid therapy. Use of corticosteroids during NSAIA therapy may increase the risk of GI ulceration, and the drugs should be used concomitantly with caution. If corticosteroid dosage is decreased during indomethacin therapy, it should be done gradually and patients should be observed for adverse effects, including adrenocortical insufficiency or symptomatic exacerbation of the inflammatory condition being treated.

Anaphylactoid reactions have been reported in patients receiving indomethacin. Patients receiving indomethacin should be informed of the signs and symptoms of an anaphylactoid reaction (e.g., difficulty breathing, swelling of the face or throat) and advised to seek immediate medical attention if an anaphylactoid reaction develops.

Serious skin reactions (e.g., exfoliative dermatitis, Stevens-Johnson syndrome, toxic epidermal necrolysis) can occur in patients receiving indomethacin. These serious skin reactions may occur without warning; patients should be advised to consult their clinician if skin rash and blisters, fever, or other signs of hypersensitivity reaction (e.g., pruritus) occur. Indomethacin should be discontinued at the first appearance of rash or any other sign of hypersensitivity.

Patients receiving long-term NSAIA therapy should have a complete blood cell count and chemistry profile performed periodically.

Indomethacin is contraindicated in patients with known hypersensitivity to the drug. In addition, NSAIAs, including indomethacin, generally are contraindicated in patients in whom asthma, urticaria, or other sensitivity reactions are precipitated by aspirin or other NSAIAs, since there is potential for cross-sensitivity between NSAIAs and aspirin, and severe, often fatal, anaphylactic reactions may occur in such patients. Although NSAIAs generally are contraindicated in these patients, the drugs have occasionally been used in NSAIA-sensitive patients who have undergone desensitization. Because patients with asthma may have aspirin-sensitivity asthma, indomethacin should be used with caution in patients with asthma. In patients with asthma, aspirin sensitivity is manifested principally as bronchospasm and usually is associated with nasal polyps; the association of aspirin sensitivity, asthma, and nasal polyps is known as the aspirin triad. For a further discussion of cross-sensitivity of NSAIAs, see Cautions: Sensitivity Reactions, in the Salicylates General Statement 28:08.04.24

Indomethacin is contraindicated in the setting of CABG surgery.

■ Pediatric Precautions Safety and efficacy of oral indomethacin have not been established in children 14 years of age and younger. Therefore, the drug should not be administered to children 2–14 years of age except under circumstances when inefficacy or toxicity associated with other drugs warrants the risk; such children should be monitored closely. The manufacturers state that experience with indomethacin in these children has been limited to use of conventional capsules of the drug. Adverse effects associated with use of conventional capsules of the drug in children 14 years of age and younger have been similar to those associated with use of this dosage form in adults. Hepatotoxicity (sometimes fatal) has occurred in children receiving the drug for juvenile rheumatoid arthritis. If the drug is used in children 2–14 years of age, liver function should be monitored periodically.

Indomethacin therapy has been associated with GI bleeding, necrotizing enterocolitis, intraventricular hemorrhage, and renal insufficiency in premature neonates receiving the drug for PDA. These effects have also been observed in neonates with PDA who did not receive the drug. (See Cautions: GI Effects, Nervous System Effects, and Renal and Electrolyte Effects.) The drug is generally contraindicated in neonates with substantially impaired renal function, thrombocytopenia, coagulation disorders, active bleeding from any cause, recent intracranial hemorrhage, known or suspected necrotizing enterocolitis, or proven or suspected, untreated infection. The drug also is contraindicated in neonates with congenital heart disease when patency of the ductus arteriosus is necessary for adequate pulmonary or systemic blood flow (e.g., neonates with pulmonary atresia, severe tetralogy of Fallot, or severe coarctation of the aorta). For additional information on precautions associated with indomethacin use in neonates, see Cautions: Precautions and Contraindications and other sections in Cautions.

■ Geriatric Precautions Indomethacin should be used with caution in geriatric individuals 65 years of age or older since increasing age may be associated with increased risk of adverse reactions. Geriatric individuals appear to tolerate GI ulceration or bleeding less well than other individuals, and many of the spontaneous reports of fatal adverse GI effects in patients receiving NSAIAs involve geriatric individuals. (See Cautions: GI Effects.) Indomethacin may cause confusion or, rarely, psychosis; clinicians should remain alert to the possibility of such adverse reactions in geriatric individuals.

Indomethacin is eliminated mainly by the kidneys and individuals with renal impairment may be at increased risk for toxic reactions to the drug. Because geriatric patients frequently have decreased renal function, particular attention should be paid to indomethacin dosage and it may be useful to monitor renal function in these patients.

■ Pregnancy, Fertility, and Lactation Although there are no adequate and controlled studies to date in humans, indomethacin has been shown to have various adverse effects in animals during reproduction studies. Dosages of 5–15 mg/kg daily have resulted in maternal toxicity and death, increased fetal resorptions, and fetal malformations in mice. Indomethacin inhibits prostaglandin synthesis which may result in prolongation of gestation and interference with labor if the drug is given late in pregnancy. When indomethacin was administered during the 27th–34th weeks of gestation to control premature uterine contractions in humans, adverse fetal reactions including constriction of the fetal ductus arteriosus, neonatal primary pulmonary hypertension, and fetal deaths have occurred. Other adverse effects associated with such use have included oligohydramnios (in the absence of premature rupture of the amniotic membrane) and neonatal edema (including hydrops), bleeding disorders, transient oliguric renal failure, and focal ileal perforation. Reduced number and excessive muscularity of pulmonary blood vessels have occurred in offspring of rats given 2–4 mg/kg daily during the last trimester of gestation; these findings are similar to those associated with the syndrome of persistent pulmonary hypertension of the newborn. Phocomelia and agenesis of the penis in one human neonate have tentatively been attributed to fetal exposure to indomethacin. Use of indomethacin during pregnancy is not recommended by the manufacturers, since safety of the drug in pregnant women has not been established and because of the drug's potential adverse effects on the fetus, including effects on the cardiovascular system (e.g., closure of the ductus arteriosus, degenerative myocardial changes), platelets (e.g., bleeding), renal function (e.g., renal failure with oligohydramnios), and GI system (e.g., bleeding, perforation) during the last trimester.

Indomethacin had no effect on fertility in rats or mice at dosages up to 0.5 mg/kg daily.

Indomethacin is distributed into milk. Seizures occurred in one breast-fed neonate (6 days of age) after the mother had taken approximately 200 mg of indomethacin daily for about 3 days. Indomethacin should not be used in nursing women.

Drug Interactions

■ Protein-bound Drugs Because indomethacin is highly protein bound, it theoretically could be displaced from binding sites by, or could displace from binding sites, other protein-bound drugs such as oral anticoagulants, hydantoins, salicylates, sulfonamides, and sulfonylureas. Patients receiving indomethacin with any of these drugs should be observed for adverse effects.

■ Anticoagulants and Thrombolytic Agents The effects of warfarin and NSAIAs on GI bleeding are synergistic. Concomitant use of indomethacin and warfarin is associated with a higher risk of GI bleeding compared with use of either agent alone.

It appears that indomethacin has little, if any, direct influence on the hypoprothrombinemic effect of warfarin or other oral anticoagulants when these drugs are administered concurrently. Because indomethacin may cause GI bleeding and may inhibit platelet aggregation, the drug should be used with caution in patients receiving any anticoagulant or thrombolytic agent (e.g., streptokinase).

■ Alcohol In one study in healthy adults, concomitant ingestion of a single dose of indomethacin (25 mg) and alcohol (50 g) resulted in a prompt prolongation of bleeding time compared with control values, although neither drug alone had any effect on bleeding time. The mechanism of this interaction was not determined.

■ Nonsteroidal Anti-inflammatory Agents Concomitant use of indomethacin and another NSAIA is not recommended because such use may increase the possibility of adverse GI effects with little or no increase in efficacy.

Administration of aspirin with indomethacin may decrease plasma indomethacin concentrations and diminish urinary excretion of indomethacin. Although the mechanism and clinical importance of this interaction have not been determined, it has been suggested that the efficiency of GI absorption of indomethacin is diminished and biliary clearance of the drug is increased during combined therapy. Fatal aplastic anemia has been reported in patients receiving indomethacin and aspirin, although indomethacin alone may produce this effect. Concomitant use of aspirin and an NSAIA increases the risk for serious GI events. Because of the potential for increased adverse effects, patients receiving indomethacin should be advised not to take aspirin. There is no consistent evidence that use of low-dose aspirin mitigates the increased risk of serious cardiovascular events associated with NSAIAs.

In healthy individuals, concomitant use of indomethacin and diflunisal resulted in decreased renal clearance and increased plasma concentrations of indomethacin. In addition, this combination has been associated with fatal GI hemorrhage in some patients. Indomethacin and diflunisal should therefore not be used concomitantly.

■ **Hypotensive Agents and Diuretics** Indomethacin may reduce the hypotensive effects of hydralazine, furosemide, β-adrenergic blocking agents (e.g., atenolol, propranolol), or thiazide diuretics. In at least one patient with severe congestive heart failure, administration of indomethacin appeared to antagonize the diuretic effects of furosemide and spironolactone, resulting in exacerbation of the clinical signs of cardiac failure. The mechanism(s) of these interactions is uncertain but has been attributed to indomethacin-induced inhibition of prostaglandin synthesis which may result in fluid retention and/or changes in vascular resistance. The clinical importance of these reactions has not been established; however, when indomethacin is added to the regimen of a patient receiving hydralazine, furosemide, thiazides, or a β-adrenergic blocking agent, or when one of these agents is added to a regimen of a patient receiving indomethacin, the patient should be closely observed to determine if the desired antihypertensive effect is obtained. When evaluating plasma renin activity in hypertensive patients, it should be kept in mind that indomethacin blocks the furosemide-induced increase in plasma renin activity.

It appears that concomitant furosemide therapy may have a beneficial effect on renal function in premature neonates with PDA who are receiving indomethacin. In one study in premature neonates with PDA who received indomethacin or combined therapy with indomethacin and furosemide, neonates who received combined therapy had higher urine output, urinary excretion of sodium and chloride, and glomerular filtration rate than those who received indomethacin alone.

Concomitant use of indomethacin and triamterene has adversely affected renal function. In one study, concomitant administration of indomethacin and triamterene to 4 healthy adults resulted in a 60–70% decrease in creatinine clearance in 2 individuals; renal function returned to normal within 2 weeks after both drugs were discontinued. When the drugs were given separately, triamterene caused no consistent change in renal function; indomethacin induced an average 10% decrease in creatinine clearance. Acute anuric renal failure occurred within 2 days after concomitant use of indomethacin and triamterene in a 79-year-old woman with compensated congestive heart failure. BUN and serum creatinine concentrations increased to 102 and 10.2 mg/dL, respectively, within several days of concomitant therapy in this woman, and subsequently returned toward normal over 2 months; anuria persisted for 11 days after discontinuance of the drugs. Although the mechanism of this interaction was not determined, it has been postulated that indomethacin may inhibit triamterene-stimulated synthesis of renal prostaglandins that mediate an adaptive mechanism for renal blood flow preservation in response to triamterene-mediated renal vasoconstriction. The manufacturers recommend that the combination of indomethacin and triamterene not be used.

There is some evidence that concomitant administration of drugs that inhibit prostaglandin synthesis, including indomethacin, may reduce the blood pressure response to angiotensin-converting enzyme (ACE) inhibitors (e.g., captopril, enalapril) or angiotensin II receptor antagonists (e.g., losartan). Limited data indicate that concomitant administration of NSAIAs with ACE inhibitors or angiotensin II receptor antagonists occasionally may result in acute reduction of renal function; however, the possibility cannot be ruled out that one drug alone may cause such an effect. Blood pressure should be monitored carefully when an NSAIA is initiated in patients receiving an ACE inhibitor or angiotensin II receptor antagonist, and clinicians should be alert for evidence of impaired renal function.

In healthy adults, indomethacin does not appear to influence the pharmacokinetics of hydrochlorothiazide.

■ **Digoxin** Therapy in premature neonates with PDA and associated heart failure often includes digoxin. Administration of indomethacin in premature neonates receiving digoxin may further prolong the half-life of digoxin in these neonates, as a result of an indomethacin-induced reduction in renal function. In one study in premature neonates with PDA receiving digoxin, initiation of indomethacin therapy (mean total dose of 0.32 mg/kg) resulted in a mean digoxin half-life of 97 hours and an increase in mean serum digoxin concentrations from 2.2 to 3.2 ng/mL; increased serum digoxin concentrations were correlated with decreased urine output in these neonates. When indomethacin and digoxin are used concomitantly in premature neonates, the neonate should be observed closely for signs of digoxin toxicity; frequent ECG monitoring and determinations of serum digoxin concentrations may be necessary to prevent or detect impending cardiac glycoside toxicity. Dosage reduction of digoxin should be considered when the glycoside is used concomitantly with indomethacin in neonates. Some clinicians have suggested that digoxin dosage be initially reduced by about 50% when indomethacin is initiated in these neonates, and that subsequent dosage be adjusted according to urine output and serum digoxin concentrations.

In adults, serum digoxin concentrations also may be increased and elimination half-life prolonged by concomitant indomethacin administration, but data are conflicting. In a study in healthy adults, indomethacin (150 mg orally daily) did not appear to alter substantially elimination half-life, systemic clearance, or distribution of digoxin. However, in a study in adults with congestive heart failure and normal renal and hepatic function who were maintained on digoxin, steady-state serum digoxin concentrations (obtained 12 hours after a dose) increased by a mean of about 40% (range: 0–100%) during concomitant administration of indomethacin (150 mg orally daily) and returned to pretreatment values following discontinuance of the NSAIA. In this study, concomitant administration of ibuprofen (1.8 g orally daily) had no apparent effect on serum digoxin concentrations. While the clinical importance and mechanism of this potential interaction require further elucidation, the manufacturers state that serum digoxin concentrations should be monitored closely when indomethacin is used concomitantly.

■ **Drugs Increasing Serum Potassium Concentrations** Because indomethacin may increase serum potassium concentrations, the drug should be used cautiously with other drugs that may increase serum potassium (e.g., potassium-sparing diuretics, angiotensin-converting enzyme inhibitors, potassium supplements). Patients most likely to experience indomethacin-induced increases in serum potassium concentration include those with preexisting mild to moderate renal dysfunction, geriatric patients, and premature neonates. The potential effects of indomethacin and other drugs that may increase serum potassium on renal function and potassium kinetics should be considered when the drugs are used concomitantly, and serum potassium concentrations should be monitored before and periodically during concomitant therapy.

■ **Lithium** In one study in psychiatric and healthy individuals with steady-state plasma lithium concentrations, indomethacin (150 mg daily) increased plasma lithium concentration by 30–60% and reduced renal lithium clearance. The mechanism involved in the reduction of lithium clearance by indomethacin is not known but has been attributed to inhibition of prostaglandin synthesis, possibly in the distal tubule. If indomethacin and lithium are administered concurrently, the patient should be closely observed for signs of lithium toxicity, and plasma lithium concentrations should be carefully monitored during the initial stages of combined therapy. In addition, appropriate adjustment in lithium dosage may be required when therapy with indomethacin is discontinued.

■ **Methotrexate** Severe, sometimes fatal, toxicity has occurred following administration of a NSAIA (e.g., indomethacin, ketoprofen) concomitantly with methotrexate (principally high-dose therapy) in patients with various malignant neoplasms or rheumatoid arthritis. The toxicity was associated with elevated and prolonged blood concentrations of methotrexate. The exact mechanism of the interaction remains to be established, but it has been suggested that NSAIAs may inhibit renal elimination of methotrexate, possibly by decreasing renal perfusion via inhibition of renal prostaglandin synthesis or by competing for renal elimination. Further studies are needed to evaluate the interaction between NSAIAs and methotrexate. Caution is advised if methotrexate and a NSAIA are administered concomitantly. (See Drug Interactions: Nonsteroidal Anti-inflammatory Agents, in Methotrexate 10:00.)

■ **Cyclosporine** Concomitant administration of a NSAIA and cyclosporine may increase the nephrotoxic effects of cyclosporine; this interaction may be related to inhibition of renal prostaglandin (e.g., prostacyclin) synthesis. NSAIAs and cyclosporine should be used concomitantly with caution and renal function should be closely monitored.

■ **Probenecid** When probenecid is administered concomitantly with indomethacin, plasma concentration, plasma half-life, and therapeutic effects of indomethacin have been reported to increase. The mechanisms of this interaction remain unknown but have been attributed to blockade of renal tubular secretion of indomethacin and to interference with the biliary clearance of indomethacin. Although the clinical importance of the interaction has not been established, the manufacturers suggest that a decreased total daily dose of indomethacin may produce a satisfactory therapeutic response when indomethacin and probenecid are used concurrently and that increases in indomethacin dosage, if necessary, should be made carefully and in small increments. Indomethacin does not interfere with the uricosuric action of probenecid.

■ **Other Drugs** Indomethacin has been reported to increase trough and peak serum aminoglycoside (e.g., amikacin, gentamicin) concentrations in premature neonates who were receiving the drugs concomitantly. Increases in serum aminoglycoside concentrations appeared to be related to indomethacin-induced decreases in urine output. Serum aminoglycoside concentrations and renal function should be closely monitored and aminoglycoside dosage adjusted accordingly when aminoglycosides are used concomitantly with indomethacin in premature neonates.

In one study in patients with rheumatoid arthritis, concomitant administration of indomethacin and prednisolone resulted in increased plasma concentrations of free prednisolone; total plasma prednisolone concentrations were unchanged.

Severe hypertension occurred in at least one patient when indomethacin was taken with phenylpropanolamine.

Indomethacin exacerbated phenylbutazone-related renal failure in one patient.

Acute renal failure was reported in 2 patients who received indomethacin with penicillin or nafcillin; however, a direct causal relationship has not been established.

Because indomethacin therapy may reduce renal function, reduction in dosage of any concurrently administered drug that depends on adequate renal function for elimination should be considered. Indomethacin should be used cautiously, if at all, with other drugs that might potentiate the adverse GI effects.

Laboratory Test Interferences

Indomethacin has been reported to augment the hypothalamic-pituitary-adrenal (HPA) axis response to the dexamethasone suppression test, potentially causing false normal results in patients with depression. In patients with depression who were given dexamethasone (1 mg orally) alone and with indomethacin (75 mg orally), indomethacin caused a further reduction in plasma cortisol concentrations compared with dexamethasone alone. Indomethacin alone did not affect plasma cortisol concentrations and the drug had no effect on plasma dexamethasone concentrations. Although the mechanism was not determined, it was suggested that indomethacin altered the suppressibility of the HPA axis at a site in the CNS.

Acute Toxicity

Limited information is available on the acute toxicity of indomethacin.

■ **Pathogenesis** The oral LD_{50} of indomethacin, based on 14-day mortality, is 50 and 12 mg/kg in mice and rats, respectively.

■ **Manifestations** Drowsiness, lethargy, mental confusion, nausea, vomiting, paresthesia, numbness, aggressive behavior, disorientation, and seizures have been reported following acute overdosage of the drug. The possibility of intense headache, dizziness, and GI bleeding should be considered. Cerebral edema, cardiac arrest, and death occurred in a child 2 days after ingestion of 30–40 capsules (strength unknown) of indomethacin.

■ **Treatment** In acute overdosage, the stomach should be emptied immediately by inducing emesis or by gastric lavage, followed by administration of activated charcoal. If the patient is comatose, having seizures, or lacks the gag reflex, gastric lavage may be performed if an endotracheal tube with cuff inflated is in place to prevent aspiration of gastric contents. Supportive and symptomatic treatment should be initiated. Close medical observation may be necessary depending on the condition of the patient. Because of the possibility of delayed GI ulceration and hemorrhage, the patient's progress should be monitored for several days. Administration of antacids may be useful. Hemodialysis appears to be of no value in enhancing elimination of indomethacin.

Pharmacology

Indomethacin has pharmacologic actions similar to those of other prototypical NSAIAs. The drug exhibits anti-inflammatory, analgesic, and antipyretic activity. The exact mechanisms have not been clearly established, but many actions appear to be associated principally with inhibition of prostaglandin synthesis. Indomethacin inhibits the synthesis of prostaglandins in body tissues by inhibiting cyclooxygenase; at least 2 isoenzymes, cyclooxygenase-1 (COX-1) and -2 (COX-2) (also referred to as prostaglandin G/H synthase-1 [PGHS-1] and -2 [PGHS-2], respectively), have been identified that catalyze the formation of prostaglandins in the arachidonic acid pathway. Indomethacin, like other prototypical NSAIAs, inhibits both COX-1 and COX-2. Although the exact mechanisms have not been clearly established, NSAIAs appear to exert anti-inflammatory, analgesic, and antipyretic activity principally through inhibition of the COX-2 isoenzyme; COX-1 inhibition presumably is responsible for the drugs' unwanted effects on GI mucosa and platelet aggregation.

■ **Anti-inflammatory, Analgesic, and Antipyretic Effects** The anti-inflammatory, analgesic, and antipyretic effects of indomethacin and other NSAIAs, including selective inhibitors of COX-2 (e.g., celecoxib), appear to result from inhibition of prostaglandin synthesis. While the precise mechanism of the anti-inflammatory and analgesic effects of NSAIAs continues to be investigated, these effects appear to be mediated principally through inhibition of the COX-2 isoenzyme at sites of inflammation with subsequent reduction in the synthesis of certain prostaglandins from their arachidonic acid precursors.

This effect may be related to inhibition of the synthesis of prostaglandins that are believed to play a role in modulating the rate and extent of leukocyte infiltration during inflammation. Indomethacin also inhibits lysosomal enzyme release from polymorphonuclear leukocytes. Although the mechanism has not been determined, this effect appears to depend on the nature of the stimulus and may not be related to inhibition of prostaglandin synthesis.

It has also been postulated that indomethacin, as an inhibitor of phosphodiesterase, may increase intracellular concentrations of cyclic adenosine monophosphate (AMP) which may play a role in the inflammatory response. In supratherapeutic concentrations, indomethacin depresses the synthesis of mucopolysaccharides through uncoupling of oxidative phosphorylation. By inhibiting cyclooxygenase, indomethacin and some other NSAIAs may also interfere with prostaglandin-mediated formation of autoantibodies that are involved in the inflammatory process.

Indomethacin does not possess glucocorticoid or adrenocorticoid-stimulating properties.

Indomethacin lowers body temperature in patients with fever. Although the mechanism of the antipyretic effect is not known, it has been suggested that suppression of prostaglandin synthesis in the CNS (probably in the hypothalamus) may be involved. It has been suggested that indomethacin's antipyretic effect in patients with neoplasm-associated fever results from inhibition (probably in the hypothalamus) of the synthesis of prostaglandins (e.g., PGE_1) that are involved in mediating the pyretic effect of tumor-induced endogenous pyrogen. The drug, however, should not be used routinely as an antipyretic because of potentially serious adverse effects. (See Cautions.)

■ **Genitourinary and Renal Effects** Indomethacin-induced inhibition of prostaglandin synthesis may result in decreased uterine tone and contractility. Prostaglandins E_2 and $F_{2\alpha}$ increase the amplitude and frequency of uterine contractions in pregnant women; current evidence suggests that primary dysmenorrhea is also mediated by these prostaglandins. Whether the increased production of prostaglandins associated with primary dysmenorrhea is mediated by COX-1 or COX-2 remains to be determined. In some patients with primary dysmenorrhea, indomethacin has produced an analgesic effect, probably by inhibiting the synthesis of prostaglandins. Administration of the drug during late pregnancy may prolong gestation by inhibiting uterine contractions.

Indomethacin has been reported to adversely affect renal function. (See Cautions: Renal and Electrolyte Effects.) The renal effects of indomethacin appear to be in part associated with inhibition of renal synthesis of prostaglandins. Indomethacin has decreased urinary sodium excretion and induced temporary sodium, potassium, and water retention in healthy adults and patients with impaired renal function. The drug has decreased effective renal plasma flow in patients with impaired renal function and has decreased glomerular filtration rate in some patients. In healthy adults and hypertensive patients, indomethacin causes a decrease in plasma renin activity which is associated with a marked decrease in urinary excretion of prostaglandins E and E_2; indomethacin also blunts the acute rise in plasma renin activity following furosemide administration in both groups of patients. In one study in premature neonates, indomethacin lowered urine output, fractional excretion of sodium and chloride, and urinary kallikrein excretion. In Bartter's syndrome, a condition associated with overproduction of renal prostaglandins, indomethacin has reduced urinary kallikrein excretion, urinary excretion of an immunoreactive prostaglandin E-like material, and plasma renin activity, while increasing sensitivity to intravenous angiotensin II and returning serum potassium concentration to within normal limits. The drug has also decreased plasma atrial natriuretic peptide (ANP) concentrations in patients with this syndrome, possibly via inhibition of a prostaglandin-mediated effect on ANP synthesis or release.

Indomethacin has no uricosuric activity.

■ **Cardiovascular Effects** In many premature neonates, administration of indomethacin results in closure of the persistently patent ductus arteriosus. During fetal life, the ductus arteriosus is apparently maintained in a dilated state by prostaglandins, presumably of the E series, which are produced in the placenta and in the ductus itself. The ductus usually closes within 24 hours after birth, partly as a result of loss of placental prostaglandins and increased pulmonary blood flow. In premature neonates, however, the ductus may not close promptly, perhaps because of increased sensitivity of the immature ductus to prostaglandins; some of these neonates develop cardiopulmonary decompensation because of large left-to-right cardiac shunts. Indomethacin appears to inhibit the synthesis of the prostaglandins, thereby permitting closure of the ductus. Other factors such as oxygenation and hydration status of the neonate may also contribute to successful ductus closure.

Some patients with orthostatic hypotension associated with multiple system atrophy characterized by predominantly autonomic failure (formerly known as Shy-Drager syndrome) have experienced increases in blood pressure following indomethacin therapy. The mechanism of this action has not been determined, but it has been associated with prostaglandin synthesis inhibition. The drug appears to augment the release of norepinephrine and restore vascular sensitivity to norepinephrine; therefore, it has been suggested that at least some autonomic activity must be present for indomethacin therapy to be successful in these patients. It is not clear whether indomethacin's effects on sodium and water retention contribute to an increase in blood pressure in these patients.

In one study, administration of large IV doses of indomethacin (0.5 mg/kg as the sodium salt) to patients with extensive coronary heart disease increased mean arterial pressure, myocardial arteriovenous oxygen difference, and coronary vascular resistance and decreased coronary blood flow. It is not known if these effects occur in patients with normal coronary arteries. In another study in patients with primary pulmonary hypertension, oral administration of indomethacin (50 mg, followed by 25 mg every 4 hours) had no effect on pulmonary artery pressure but increased pulmonary and systemic vascular resistances and reduced cardiac output and stroke volume. In a study in patients with severe, chronic, congestive heart failure (New York Heart Association class III or IV), indomethacin produced acute, substantial decreases in cardiac index and increases in pulmonary capillary wedge pressure and in systemic vascular resistance in patients with hyponatremia but not in those with normal serum sodium concentration, although some patients in the latter group also had increases in pulmonary capillary wedge pressure and in systemic vascular resistance. Although the mechanisms and sites of these cardiovascular effects have not been determined, it has been suggested that indomethacin blocks the synthesis of several vasoactive prostaglandins (e.g., prostacyclin, prostaglandins E_1 and $F_{2\alpha}$, thromboxane A_2) involved in the regulation of coronary, pulmonary, and systemic vascular tone. In patients with severe congestive heart failure, prostaglandins appear to increase in response to the degree of activation of neurohormonal vasoconstrictor systems (e.g., catecholamines, angiotensin, vasopressin); the vasoactive prostaglandins appear to contribute to circulatory homeostasis by limiting the magnitude of compensatory regional and systemic vasoconstriction that occurs when cardiac output decreases. Other mechanisms may also be involved.

Acute oral and IV administration of indomethacin have been reported to reduce basal and carbon dioxide-stimulated cerebral blood flow. In one study, following oral administration of indomethacin for 1 week, this effect on basal cerebral blood flow was no longer observed after 7 days of indomethacin therapy, probably because of tachyphylaxis. Following IV administration of indomethacin in premature neonates with patent ductus arteriosus, a transient decrease in cerebral blood flow velocity and in cerebral blood flow were observed; similar decreases in mesenteric blood flow and velocity have been observed. The clinical importance of these effects has not been established.

■ **Hematologic Effects** Indomethacin can inhibit platelet aggregation and may prolong bleeding time. Like aspirin and other prototypical NSAIAs, the effects of indomethacin on platelets appear to be associated with inhibition of the synthesis of prostaglandins produced by COX-1. In one study, the drug inhibited platelet response to collagen and, in a manner similar to that of aspirin, eliminated secondary aggregation induced by epinephrine; however, unlike the prolonged effects of aspirin, platelet aggregation following a single oral dose of indomethacin returned to normal within 24 hours. In the same study, bleeding time was prolonged in healthy individuals following multiple (but not single) doses of indomethacin.

■ **GI Effects** Indomethacin can cause gastric mucosal damage which may result in ulceration and/or bleeding. (See Cautions: GI Effects.) These gastric effects have been attributed to inhibition of the synthesis of prostaglandins produced by COX-1. Other factors possibly involved in NSAIA-induced gastropathy include local irritation, promotion of acid back-diffusion into gastric mucosa, uncoupling of oxidative phosphorylation, and enterohepatic recirculation of the drugs. In addition to local effects of indomethacin, the drug may have systemic GI effects; in one animal study, IV indomethacin decreased gastric blood flow and potentiated pentagastrin-stimulated (but not basal) acid output.

It has been suggested that indomethacin may inhibit prostaglandin synthesis in the gallbladder; the drug has relieved pain associated with cholelithiasis in the bile duct.

Epidemiologic and laboratory studies suggest that NSAIAs may reduce the risk of colon cancer. Although the exact mechanism by which NSAIAs may inhibit colon carcinogenesis remains to be determined, it has been suggested that inhibition of prostaglandin synthesis may be involved.

■ **Metabolic Effects** In premature neonates, decreased plasma glucose concentrations have been observed during indomethacin therapy for patent ductus arteriosus; the mechanism of this effect has not been established.

Indomethacin therapy has reduced elevated serum calcium concentrations in some patients with solid tumors associated with osteolytic activity (e.g., lung carcinoma). The drug has also been reported to reduce tumor growth and mean tumor weight, and enhance immune defenses. It has been suggested that indomethacin may inhibit the synthesis of prostaglandins that mediate osteolytic activity and that weaken the immune defense to endogenous mutagenic cells. However, other mechanisms independent of prostaglandins may be involved.

Pharmacokinetics

■ **Absorption** Indomethacin is rapidly and almost completely absorbed from the GI tract in healthy adults. Following oral administration, bioavailability is virtually 100%, with 90% of a single dose being absorbed within 4 hours. When administered orally with food, a single 50-mg dose of the oral suspension is reportedly bioequivalent to a single 50-mg conventional capsule. The extended-release capsules of indomethacin (designed to release 25 mg of the drug initially and the remaining 50 mg over an extended time period) are 90% absorbed within 12 hours. The rate of absorption following rectal administration of suppositories of the drug generally has been reported to be more rapid than that following oral administration of conventional capsules; however, in one study in healthy adults, the rate of absorption was slower following rectal administration of suppositories than following oral administration of conventional capsules. The bioavailability following rectal administration of suppositories of the drug has generally been reported to be comparable to or slightly less than that following oral administration of the drug. The manufacturer states that bioavailability following rectal administration of suppositories of the drug has been reported to be about 80–90% in controlled clinical studies; the decreased bioavailability compared with oral administration may have resulted from incomplete retention of the suppository (i.e., less than 1 hour) within the rectum. In one study following oral administration of a single 75-mg dose (as 25-mg conventional capsules) or rectal administration of a single 100-mg suppository in adults with normal renal, hepatic, and GI function, however, the dose-adjusted AUC was substantially smaller following rectal administration than following oral administration. Indomethacin is absorbed into the aqueous humor following topical application to the eye, but does not appear to achieve appreciable systemic concentrations. (See Pharmacokinetics: Distribution.)

In premature neonates, absorption of oral indomethacin appears to be poor and incomplete; bioavailability is reportedly only about 20%. It has been suggested that poor oral absorption of the drug in premature neonates may result from abnormal pH-dependent diffusion and gastric motility and from lower gastric acid secretion. In neonates, gastric emptying time and motility are increased and peristalsis is irregular and unpredictable. In addition, the lack of solubility of the capsule form of indomethacin in aqueous media (See Chemistry and Stability: Chemistry.) may present problems in drug delivery and absorption from extemporaneous preparations.

In one study in healthy fasting adults, peak plasma concentrations of indomethacin occurred in 0.5–2 hours and were about 0.8–2.5 mcg/mL following a 25-mg oral dose, and 2.5–4 mcg/mL following a 50-mg oral dose. When indomethacin was administered orally to healthy fasting individuals in 25-mg doses 3 times daily, mean steady-state plasma drug concentrations ranged from 0.39–0.63 mcg/mL.

When indomethacin is taken with food or an aluminum and magnesium hydroxides antacid, peak plasma concentrations of the drug may be slightly decreased or delayed; however, the clinical significance of this effect has not been established. Plasma concentrations of indomethacin fluctuate less and are more sustained following oral administration of a single 75-mg extended-release capsule (Indocin® SR) than following oral administration of 3 doses of 25-mg conventional capsules at 4- to 6-hour intervals.

In multiple-dose studies, the mean steady-state plasma concentration of indomethacin attained with daily administration of a 75-mg extended-release capsule was comparable to that following administration of conventional indomethacin capsules in a dosage of 25 mg 3 times daily (given at 6-hour intervals); however, there were differences in the plasma indomethacin concentrations achieved with the 2 regimens, especially after 12 hours. In one multiple-dose study, mean plasma indomethacin concentrations 11 and 16 hours after rectal administration of single daily doses as 100-mg suppositories or oral administration of single daily doses as four 25-mg conventional capsules were comparable. Although the relationship between plasma indomethacin concentrations and anti-inflammatory effect has not been precisely determined, a therapeutic range of 0.5–3 mcg/mL has been suggested.

The results of one study in healthy adults suggest that plasma concentrations following oral administration of indomethacin appear to be related to circadian rhythms; evening ingestion resulted in the smallest peak plasma drug concentration and longest time to peak. Further studies are necessary before recommendations based on this finding can be made.

In premature neonates, serum or plasma indomethacin concentrations appear to depend on postnatal age. In one study, neonates who received their first IV dose of indomethacin of 0.2 mg/kg at 48 hours of age or younger had mean serum indomethacin concentrations of approximately 0.6 mcg/mL at 12 hours after administration and those who received their first dose beyond 7 days of age had mean serum indomethacin concentrations of approximately 0.37 mcg/mL. In the same study, following multiple IV doses (0.2 mg/kg at 12-hour intervals), mean serum indomethacin concentrations 12 hours after the third dose were approximately 2.3 mcg/mL in the younger neonates and 0.75 mcg/mL in the older neonates. Limited pharmacokinetic data are available in premature neonates following oral administration of the drug. In one study, plasma indomethacin concentrations of 0.027–0.31 mcg/mL were attained 3–4 hours after oral doses of 0.1–0.3 mg/kg to premature neonates with gestational ages of 28–36 weeks and birthweights of 0.8–1.96 kg.

■ **Distribution** At therapeutic concentrations, indomethacin is approximately 99% bound to plasma proteins.

In healthy adults, the volume of distribution of indomethacin has been reported to range from 0.34–1.57 L/kg. In one study in premature neonates, the volume of distribution of indomethacin (calculated on the basis of birthweight) was about 0.287 L in neonates weighing greater than 1 kg and about 0.216 L in neonates weighing less than 1 kg.

Peak indomethacin concentrations in synovial fluid have been reported to occur 1.5 hours after peak serum drug concentrations and were approximately 20% of those in serum.

Following topical application of a 1% aqueous or oil suspension of indomethacin to the eye for 18–24 hours prior to cataract surgery, mean aqueous humor concentrations at the time of surgery were 198 or 429 ng/mL in patients receiving the aqueous or oil suspension, respectively. Indomethacin was not detected (lower limits of detection: 50 ng/mL) in aqueous humor at the time of surgery in patients who received 100 mg of the drug orally in divided doses during the 24-hour period prior to surgery (last dose was administered 2 hours prior to surgery); mean simultaneous plasma concentration of the drug in patients receiving oral indomethacin was 642 ng/mL.

Indomethacin crosses the blood-brain barrier in small amounts and appears to freely cross the placenta. The drug is distributed into milk; one breast-fed neonate (6 days of age) received an estimated 0.5–2 mg of indomethacin daily during maternal ingestion of 200 mg of the drug daily for 3 days. (See Cautions: Pregnancy, Fertility, and Lactation.)

■ **Elimination** In studies in healthy adults or patients with rheumatoid arthritis, the disappearance of indomethacin from plasma appears to be biphasic with a half-life of approximately 1 hour during the initial phase and 2.6–11.2 hours during the second phase; variations in terminal plasma half-life may be due to individual differences in enterohepatic circulation of the drug. There appears to be no difference between plasma half-life in healthy adults and in rheumatoid arthritis patients.

In premature neonates, the serum or plasma elimination half-life of indomethacin is inversely related to postnatal age. In a limited number of neonates, the mean plasma half-life of indomethacin has been reported to be about 20–28 hours in those receiving the drug during the first week of life, compared to about 12–19 hours in those receiving the drug after the first week. The elimination half-life in neonates may also be inversely related to body weight. In one study, the plasma indomethacin half-life showed considerable interindividual variation but averaged 21 hours in neonates weighing less than 1 kg and 15 hours in those weighing more than 1 kg. Total body clearance of indomethacin increases with increasing postnatal age. It was suggested that extensive enterohepatic circulation may commonly occur in premature neonates and may contribute to the relatively long half-life of elimination. Age-dependent IV dosage schedules have been proposed. (See Dosage and Administration: Patent Ductus Arteriosus.)

Geriatric patients have reportedly shown greater serum concentrations and longer plasma half-lives of indomethacin than younger adults; however, these findings need further documentation.

In one study in healthy adults and patients with arthritis, the half-life for disappearance of indomethacin from synovial fluid was 9 hours.

Indomethacin is metabolized in the liver to its glucuronide conjugate and to desmethyl, desbenzoyl, and desmethyl-desbenzoyl metabolites and their glucuronides. These metabolites do not appear to possess anti-inflammatory activity. A portion of the drug is also *N*-deacylated by a nonmicrosomal system.

Approximately 33% or more of a 25-mg oral dose of indomethacin is excreted in feces principally as demethylated metabolites in their unconjugated forms; 1.5% of fecal drug excretion occurs as indomethacin. Indomethacin and its conjugates undergo enterohepatic circulation.

About 60% of a 25-mg oral dose of indomethacin is excreted in urine in 48 hours; renal tubular secretion of indomethacin and/or its glucuronide derivative appears to occur. About 30% of urinary drug excretion occurs as indomethacin and its glucuronide, with the balance consisting of the metabolites and their glucuronides.

Chemistry and Stability

■ Chemistry Indomethacin, an indoleacetic acid derivative, is a prototypical nonsteroidal anti-inflammatory agent (NSAIA). Indomethacin is commercially available as the base and as the sodium trihydrate salt. The drug is structurally and pharmacologically related to sulindac.

Indomethacin occurs as a pale yellow to yellow-tan, crystalline powder with a slight odor and is practically insoluble in water and sparingly soluble in alcohol. Indomethacin sodium is available as the trihydrate; dosage and concentration are calculated on the dried basis in terms of anhydrous indomethacin. Commercially available sterile indomethacin sodium occurs as a lyophilized, white to yellow powder or plug and is soluble in water and in alcohol. When reconstituted as directed in sterile water for injection, indomethacin sodium solutions have a pH of 6–7.5. Indomethacin suppositories contain the drug in a glycerin, polyethylene glycol 4000 and 6000, sodium chloride, edetic acid, butylated hydroxyanisole, and butylated hydroxytoluene base. Indocin® oral suspension may contain sodium hydroxide or hydrochloric acid to adjust the pH to 4–5; Roxane's oral suspension has a pH of 2.9. Indomethacin has a pK_a of 4.5.

■ Stability Indomethacin is sensitive to light and is unstable in alkaline solution. Indomethacin capsules should be stored in well-closed containers at a controlled room temperature of 15–30°C. Indomethacin oral suspension should be stored in tight, light-resistant containers at a temperature less than 30°C; exposure to temperatures greater than 50°C should be avoided, and the suspension should be protected from freezing. Indomethacin suppositories should be stored at a temperature less than 30°C; exposure to temperatures greater than 40°C (even transiently) should be avoided.

Sterile indomethacin sodium trihydrate powder should be protected from light and stored at a temperature less than 30°C. The manufacturer states that following reconstitution of indomethacin sodium trihydrate with 0.9% sodium chloride injection, solutions containing 1 mg of indomethacin per mL appear to be chemically stable at room temperature for at least 16 days; however, the reconstituted solutions contain no preservatives or buffers and microbiologic contamination or precipitation of the drug may occur during prolonged storage. Because the solutions contain no preservatives, the manufacturer recommends that reconstituted solutions be prepared just prior to administration of the drug and used only if clear; any unused portion of the solution should be discarded. Further dilution of reconstituted solutions of the drug in IV infusion solutions is *not* recommended.

Preparations

Excipients in commercially available drug preparations may have clinically important effects in some individuals; consult specific product labeling for details.

Indomethacin

Oral		
Capsules	25 mg*	**Indomethacin Capsules**
	50 mg*	**Indomethacin Capsules**
Capsules, extended-release	75 mg*	**Indomethacin Extended-release Capsules**
Suspension	25 mg/5 mL	**Indocin®**, Iroko
Rectal		
Suppositories	50 mg*	**Indocin®**, Iroko
		Indomethacin Suppositories

*available from one or more manufacturer, distributor, and/or repackager by generic (nonproprietary) name

Indomethacin Sodium

Parenteral		
For injection, for IV use only	1 mg (of anhydrous indomethacin)*	**Indomethacin Sodium for Injection**

*available from one or more manufacturer, distributor, and/or repackager by generic (nonproprietary) name

†Use is not currently included in the labeling approved by the US Food and Drug Administration

Ketorolac Tromethamine

■ Ketorolac is a prototypical nonsteroidal anti-inflammatory agent (NSAIA) that also exhibits analgesic and antipyretic activity.

Uses

■ Pain Ketorolac tromethamine is used for the short-term (i.e., up to 5 days) management of moderately severe, acute pain. The manufacturer states that the drug is *not* indicated for use in minor or chronic painful conditions.

The potential benefits and risks of ketorolac therapy as well as alternative therapies should be considered prior to initiating ketorolac therapy. The lowest possible effective dosage and shortest duration of therapy consistent with treatment goals of the patient should be employed.

Ketorolac tromethamine has been used for the symptomatic relief of moderate to severe postoperative pain, including that associated with abdominal, gynecologic, oral, ophthalmologic, orthopedic, urologic, or otolaryngologic surgery. Ketorolac tromethamine should *not* be used in obstetric patients as a preoperative medication or for analgesia during labor since inhibitors of prostaglandin synthesis (e.g., ketorolac tromethamine) may affect uterine contractions and fetal circulation. In addition, ketorolac tromethamine should not be used as a preoperative medication for support of anesthesia, since the drug does not have sedative or anxiolytic effects but may inhibit platelet aggregation and prolong bleeding time. Ketorolac tromethamine also has been used for the relief of acute renal colic, pain associated with trauma, pain associated with vaso-occlusive crisis of sickle-cell disease, and visceral pain associated with cancer. IM ketorolac tromethamine generally produces analgesia comparable to that of moderate IM doses of opiate analgesics. However, unlike opiate agonists, ketorolac tromethamine does not appear to cause respiratory depression and there is no evidence that therapy with ketorolac tromethamine results in physical dependence on the drug.

When used to relieve moderate to severe pain in adults, a single 10-mg IM dose of ketorolac tromethamine has been reported to be more effective than placebo and at least as effective as a single 6-mg IM dose of morphine sulfate, a single 30-mg IM dose of pentazocine, or a single 50- or 100-mg IM dose of meperidine hydrochloride. A single 30-mg IM dose of ketorolac tromethamine has been reported to be more effective than placebo or a single 6-mg IM dose of morphine sulfate and at least as effective as a single 12-mg IM dose of morphine sulfate, a single 30-mg IM dose of pentazocine, or a single 50- to 100-mg IM dose of meperidine hydrochloride. The duration of analgesia produced by single IM doses of ketorolac tromethamine appears to be longer than that of single IM doses of morphine sulfate or meperidine hydrochloride.

In a short-term (up to 5 days) multiple-dose study in adults with moderate to severe postoperative pain, IM ketorolac tromethamine doses of 30 mg were more effective than IM morphine sulfate doses of 6 mg and as effective as IM morphine sulfate doses of 12 mg; the drugs were administered at an average frequency of every 5–6 hours. When used to relieve severe sciatic pain†, IM ketorolac tromethamine dosages of 30 mg 4 times daily have been at least as effective as IM ketoprofen dosages of 100 mg twice daily.

Use of ketorolac tromethamine in pediatric patients is supported by evidence from well-controlled studies in adults, data regarding the pharmacokinetics of ketorolac in children, and safety and efficacy data from studies in pediatric patients. In studies in children 2–16 years of age, a single dose of IV or IM ketorolac tromethamine has been effective in the management of moderately severe, acute pain; these studies usually have evaluated pain in the postoperative setting (e.g., pain following tonsillectomy). Limited data are available to support administration of more than one parenteral dose of ketorolac tromethamine in pediatric patients.

Parenteral ketorolac tromethamine has been used concomitantly with opiate agonist analgesics (e.g., meperidine, morphine) for the management of moderate to severe postoperative pain without apparent adverse drug interactions. Combined use of the drugs can result in reduced opiate analgesic requirements. Ketorolac tromethamine also has been administered concomitantly with nonopiate analgesics (e.g., aspirin, acetaminophen), but the manufacturer states that use of the drug with other NSAIAs is contraindicated because of the potential for additive adverse effects.

Ketorolac tromethamine also is used orally in adults for the symptomatic relief of moderate to severe pain such as postpartum, postoperative (including that associated with oral, orthopedic, or gynecologic surgery), orthopedic (including musculoskeletal strains or sprains), or sciatic pain and for visceral pain associated with cancer. When used to relieve moderate to severe pain in adults, a single 5-mg oral dose of ketorolac tromethamine has been reported to be more effective than placebo and as effective as a single 500-mg or 1-g oral dose of acetaminophen. A single 10-mg oral dose of ketorolac tromethamine has been reported to be more effective than placebo and at least as effective as single oral doses of acetaminophen 500 mg, 600 mg, or 1 g; aspirin 650 mg; pentazocine 100 mg; dihydrocodeine 30 mg; naproxen 550 mg; ibuprofen 400 mg; acetaminophen 600 mg or 1 g with codeine phosphate 60 mg; or propoxyphene napsylate 300 mg with aspirin 700 mg and antipyrine 300 mg. A single 20-mg oral dose of ketorolac tromethamine was more effective than placebo, a single 500- or 600-mg oral dose of acetaminophen, or a single 650-mg oral dose of aspirin and at least as effective as a single 1-g oral dose of acetaminophen, a single 400-mg oral dose of ibuprofen, a single 650-mg oral dose of aspirin with 60 mg of codeine phosphate, or a single 600-mg oral dose of acetaminophen with 60 mg of codeine phosphate.

Oral ketorolac tromethamine dosages of 5 or 10 mg 4 times daily have been as effective as oral diflunisal dosages of 500 mg twice daily. Oral ketorolac tromethamine dosages of 10 mg given up to 4 times daily have been as effective as oral pentazocine dosages of 100 mg given up to 4 times daily, oral dihydrocodeine dosages of 30 mg given up to 4 times daily, or oral acetaminophen dosages of 1 g with oral codeine phosphate dosages of 60 mg given up to 4 times daily. When used to relieve orthopedic (including musculoskeletal strains or sprains) pain, oral ketorolac tromethamine dosages of 10 mg 4 times daily have been at least as effective as oral diclofenac sodium dosages of 50 mg 3 times daily, oral ibuprofen dosages of 400 mg 4 times daily, oral diflunisal dosages of 500 mg twice daily, or oral acetaminophen dosages of 600 mg with oral codeine phosphate dosages of 60 mg 4 times daily.

Long-term† (e.g., up to 1 year) oral ketorolac tromethamine therapy at dosages of 10 mg given up to 4 times daily has been used in adults to relieve chronic pain, including that associated with osteoarthritis, fibromyopathies, fibromyalgias, or tension headaches, and was more effective than chronic aspirin therapy at dosages of 650 mg given up to 4 times daily. However, the manufacturer states that total combined duration of parenteral and oral ketorolac tromethamine therapy in adults should not exceed 5 days, and, therefore, the drug is not indicated for the management of chronic pain.

■ **Ophthalmic Uses** For ophthalmic uses of ketorolac tromethamine, see 52:08.20.

Dosage and Administration

■ **Administration** The potential benefits and risks of ketorolac therapy as well as alternative therapies should be considered prior to initiating ketorolac therapy.

Ketorolac tromethamine is administered by IM or IV injection in adults and children 2 years of age and older. The drug also is administered orally in adults. When ketorolac tromethamine is used in adults, the manufacturer states that therapy should be initiated with parenteral (i.e., IV or IM) ketorolac, with the oral formulation used as continuation therapy, as required. The manufacturer also states that the total combined duration of parenteral and oral ketorolac therapy in adults should *not* exceed 5 days. When ketorolac tromethamine is used in children 2–16 years of age, the manufacturer states that the drug should be administered as a single parenteral (i.e., IM or IV) dose. Patients should be switched to alternate analgesic therapy as soon as clinically possible.

IV administration of ketorolac tromethamine injection must be given over no less than 15 seconds. IM injection of ketorolac should be given slowly, via deep IM injection. While administration with food may delay and reduce peak plasma concentrations following oral administration, the extent of GI absorption of the drug is not affected. Concomitant administration of ketorolac tromethamine and antacids does not appear to affect oral absorption of the NSAIA.

Parenteral solutions of ketorolac tromethamine should be inspected visually for particulate matter and/or discoloration prior to administration whenever solution and container permit.

■ **Dosage** The lowest possible effective dosage and shortest duration of therapy consistent with treatment goals of the patient should be employed.

Current principles of pain management indicate that analgesics, including ketorolac tromethamine, preferably should be administered at regularly scheduled intervals, although the drug also has been administered on an as-needed basis (i.e., withholding subsequent doses until pain returns). The manufacturer states that clinicians should manage breakthrough pain in adults receiving ketorolac tromethamine therapy with supplemental low doses of opiate analgesics (unless contraindicated) as needed rather than considering higher or more frequent dosages of ketorolac tromethamine.

Because there is some evidence of dose-related adverse effects (e.g., GI bleeding), particularly in geriatric patients, the lowest possible effective ketorolac tromethamine dosage should be employed, and total combined duration of parenteral and oral therapy with the drug in adults should not exceed 5 days. Particular caution and reduced parenteral dosage should be employed in geriatric patients, adults weighing less than 50 kg, and those with renal impairment (see Dosage and Administration: Dosage in Renal and Hepatic Impairment). In addition, it is recommended that in these patients a lower first usual dose of ketorolac tromethamine should be used. Elimination of the drug generally is slower and sensitivity to adverse renal effects of NSAIAs generally is increased in geriatric patients.

For the short-term management of moderately severe, acute pain in adults, a single IM or IV ketorolac tromethamine dose of 60 or 30 mg, respectively, is recommended by the manufacturer. For geriatric patients (65 years of age or older) and adults weighing less than 50 kg, the manufacturer recommends a single IM or IV dose of 30 or 15 mg, respectively. Such single-dose parenteral ketorolac tromethamine may be followed by oral ketorolac therapy in adults. The manufacturer recommends that multiple-dose parenteral ketorolac tromethamine therapy be both initiated and continued with IM or IV dosages of 30 mg every 6 hours in adults; the maximum daily dose should not exceed 120 mg. For multiple-dose parenteral therapy in geriatric patients and adults weighing less than 50 kg, the manufacturer recommends 15 mg of ketorolac tromethamine every 6 hours; the maximum daily dose in these patients should not exceed 60 mg.

Adults receiving parenteral ketorolac tromethamine who have experienced pain relief without limiting adverse effects may be switched to oral ketorolac tromethamine therapy, if needed. The manufacturer states that oral ketorolac tromethamine should be used only as continuation therapy following parenteral ketorolac therapy. Adults whose last parenteral dose of single-dose IM or IV ketorolac tromethamine was 60 or 30 mg, respectively, or who were receiving multiple-dose IV or IM therapy of 30 mg every 6 hours, should receive a first oral dose of 20 mg, followed by 10 mg every 4–6 hours. Geriatric patients or adults who weigh less than 50 kg whose last parenteral dose of single-dose IM or IV ketorolac tromethamine was 30 or 15 mg, respectively, or who were receiving multiple-dose IV or IM therapy of 15 mg every 6 hours, should receive 10 mg of ketorolac tromethamine every 4–6 hours. The manufacturer states that the daily oral dosage in any patient should not exceed 40 mg/24 hours. Low supplemental doses of an opiate agonist may be administered concomitantly with ketorolac tromethamine if breakthrough pain occurs, unless administration of an opiate agonist is contraindicated.

For the management of moderately severe, acute pain in pediatric patients 2–16 years of age, a single IM or IV ketorolac tromethamine dose of 1 mg/kg (maximum dose 30 mg) or 0.5 mg/kg (maximum dose 15 mg), respectively, is recommended by the manufacturer.

The manufacturer recommends that only single doses of parenteral ketorolac be used in pediatric patients.

For the management of moderate to severe pain in adults, oral ketorolac tromethamine dosages of 10 mg up to 4 times daily (at 4- to 6-hour intervals) have been used as needed†, although higher oral doses also have been employed.

■ **Dosage in Renal and Hepatic Impairment** Since ketorolac and its metabolites are excreted mainly by the kidneys, dosage may need to be adjusted in geriatric patients and in other patients with reduced renal function. When ketorolac is used in adults with renal impairment the manufacturer recommends a single IM or IV ketorolac tromethamine dose of 30 or 15 mg, respectively. In these patients, multiple-dose parenteral ketorolac tromethamine therapy is administered at a dosage of 15 mg every 6 hours. Subsequent oral ketorolac tromethamine therapy should be administered at a dosage of 10 mg every 4–6 hours. The manufacturer states that the daily oral dosage in any patient should not exceed 40 mg/24 hours. The manufacturer also states that for breakthrough pain, supplemental doses of an opiate agonist may be administered concomitantly with these reduced doses of ketorolac tromethamine, unless opiate agonists are contraindicated. The safety of ketorolac tromethamine in patients with serum creatinine concentrations exceeding 5 mg/dL and/or undergoing dialysis has not been determined.

The need for ketorolac tromethamine dosage adjustment in patients with hepatic impairment has not been fully determined, but evidence from patients with liver cirrhosis suggests that modification may not be necessary. Pending further accumulation of data, caution should be exercised when the drug is used in patients with hepatic impairment.

Cautions

Ketorolac tromethamine shares the toxic potentials of nonsteroidal anti-inflammatory agents (NSAIAs); when NSAIAs are administered short-term, the incidence of adverse effects is about 10–50% of that associated with chronic administration. Adverse reactions to ketorolac tromethamine usually are mild, dose related, and reportedly occur in about 39% of patients. Ketorolac tromethamine usually is well tolerated. The most common adverse effects associated with short-term IM or oral therapy with the drug are nervous system and GI effects. Results of premarketing studies indicated that short-term IM ketorolac tromethamine therapy was associated with a lower incidence of adverse effects compared with short-term IM morphine therapy.

The manufacturer conducted a postmarketing, nonrandomized, observational study to examine the relative risks and benefits of ketorolac tromethamine and parenteral opiate agonists in a hospital setting. In this study, no attempt was made to assign the drug or dosage employed, and while patients included in the opiate group could not receive NSAIAs concomitantly, there was no limitation on concomitant opiate use by those receiving ketorolac. Interim analysis of data involving 6721 patients in the ketorolac group and 3943 patients in the opiate group revealed an association between mortality rate and age, increasing with age in both groups; the mortality rate was 0.9 and 1.7% for the respective drug groups. In addition, the frequency of GI bleeding, which ranged in severity from occult blood in stools to frank bleeding, also increased with age in both groups but was higher in the ketorolac than opiate group; about half of the reported GI effects involved occult blood in stools only, although death was attributed to GI bleeding in 2 patients (one in each drug group). Final analysis of data accumulated on approximately 10,000 patients revealed that the risk of clinically serious GI bleeding depended on the dose of ketorolac tromethamine; this appeared to be particularly important in geriatric patients who received an average daily dose greater than 60 mg. Serious adverse effects also were associated with long-term ketorolac therapy or therapy in patients with GI bleeding, renal impairment (without appropriate dose modification), or a history of sensitivity reactions to aspirin or other NSAIA-type agents. In addition, through December 4, 1992, the manufacturer had accumulated information on 73 spontaneously reported deaths in patients who received ketorolac.

■ **Cardiovascular Effects** Adverse cardiovascular effects occur in about 4% of patients receiving IM ketorolac tromethamine. Edema occurred in 1–3% of patients receiving the drug IM or orally. Hypertension has been reported in greater than 1% of patients receiving the drug. Vasodilation, pallor, hypotension, flushing, syncope, or palpitation has been reported in 1% or less of patients receiving the drug IM or orally.

NSAIAs, including selective cyclooxygenase-2 (COX-2) inhibitors and prototypical NSAIAs, increase the risk of serious adverse cardiovascular thrombotic events, including myocardial infarction and stroke (which can be fatal), in patients with or without cardiovascular disease or risk factors for cardiovascular disease. Use of NSAIAs also is associated with an increased risk of heart failure.

The association between cardiovascular complications and use of NSAIAs is an area of ongoing concern and study. Findings of an FDA review of published observational studies of NSAIAs, a meta-analysis of published and unpublished data from randomized controlled trials of these drugs, and other published information indicate that NSAIAs may increase the risk of serious adverse cardiovascular thrombotic events by 10–50% or more, depending on the drugs and dosages studied. Available data suggest that the increase in risk may occur early (within the first weeks) following initiation of therapy and may increase with higher dosages and longer durations of use. Although the relative increase in cardiovascular risk appears to be similar in patients with or without known underlying cardiovascular disease or risk factors for cardiovascular disease, the absolute incidence of serious NSAIA-associated cardiovascular thrombotic events is higher in those with cardiovascular disease or risk factors for cardiovascular disease because of their elevated baseline risk.

Results from observational studies utilizing Danish national registry data indicated that patients receiving NSAIAs following a myocardial infarction were at increased risk of reinfarction, cardiovascular-related death, and all-cause mortality beginning in the first week of treatment. Patients who received NSAIAs following myocardial infarction had a higher 1-year mortality rate compared with those who did not receive NSAIAs (20 versus 12 deaths per 100 person-years). Although the absolute mortality rate declined somewhat after the first year following the myocardial infarction, the increased relative risk of death in patients who received NSAIAs persisted over at least the next 4 years of follow-up.

In 2 large controlled clinical trials of a selective COX-2 inhibitor for the management of pain in the first 10–14 days following coronary artery bypass graft (CABG) surgery, the incidence of myocardial infarction and stroke was increased. Therefore, NSAIAs are contraindicated in the setting of CABG surgery.

Findings from some systematic reviews of controlled observational studies and meta-analyses of data from randomized studies of NSAIAs suggest that naproxen may be associated with a lower risk of cardiovascular thrombotic events compared with other NSAIAs. However, limitations of these observational studies and the indirect comparisons used to assess cardiovascular risk of the prototypical NSAIAs (e.g., variability in patients' risk factors, comorbid conditions, concomitant drug therapy, drug interactions, dosage, and duration of therapy) affect the validity of the comparisons; in addition, these studies were not designed to demonstrate superior safety of one NSAIA compared with another. Therefore, FDA states that definitive conclusions regarding relative risks of NSAIAs are not possible at this time. (See Cautions: Cardiovascular Effects, in Celecoxib 28:08.04.08.)

Data from observational studies also indicate that use of NSAIAs in patients with heart failure is associated with increased morbidity and mortality. Results from a retrospective study utilizing Danish national registry data indicated that use of selective COX-2 inhibitors or prototypical NSAIAs in patients with chronic heart failure was associated with a dose-dependent increase in the risk of death and an increased risk of hospitalization for myocardial infarction or heart failure. In addition, findings from a meta-analysis of published and unpublished data from randomized controlled trials of NSAIAs indicated that use of selective COX-2 inhibitors or prototypical NSAIAs was associated with an approximate twofold increase in the risk of hospitalization for heart failure. Fluid retention and edema also have been observed in some patients receiving NSAIAs.

There is no consistent evidence that use of low-dose aspirin mitigates the increased risk of serious cardiovascular events associated with NSAIAs.

■ **GI Effects** Adverse GI effects reportedly occur in about 13% of patients receiving IM ketorolac tromethamine. Dyspepsia, nausea, and GI pain are the most common adverse GI effects of ketorolac tromethamine, occurring in about 12–13% of patients receiving the drug. Diarrhea occurs in 3–9% of patients receiving ketorolac tromethamine. Constipation, flatulence, feeling of GI fullness, and vomiting occur in less than 3% of patients receiving ketorolac tromethamine. Melena, peptic ulcer, rectal bleeding, stomatitis, dysgeusia, gastritis, eructation, anorexia, increased appetite, GI bleeding, GI perforation, dry mouth, and excessive thirst occur in 1% or less of patients receiving the drug. GI ulceration has been reported rarely in patients receiving ketorolac tromethamine. Most of these adverse GI effects also have been reported in patients receiving the drug orally but may occur more frequently than in those receiving the drug IM, since the duration of oral therapy often exceeds that of IM therapy. Although a causal relationship to ketorolac tromethamine has not been established, acute pancreatitis has occurred during therapy with the drug.

Usual IM dosages of ketorolac tromethamine reportedly produce fewer adverse GI effects than usual analgesic dosages of aspirin. In healthy individuals, the frequency of GI mucosal lesions observed endoscopically was lower with usual dosages of IM ketorolac tromethamine than with usual analgesic dosages of aspirin; higher than usual dosages of ketorolac tromethamine (i.e., IM dosages of 90 mg 4 times daily) were associated with a frequency of GI mucosal lesions similar to that associated with usual analgesic dosages of aspirin. However, the frequency of adverse GI effects may be increased during long-term administration and, in chronic toxicity studies in animals, GI toxicity (irritation and/or ulceration) was observed with oral but not parenteral ketorolac administration. The incidence of GI ulceration and bleeding in patients receiving long-term oral therapy (10 mg 1–4 times daily for up to 1 year) with the drug occurs at a rate of 1.2–5.4% per year. In one short-term (5 days' duration) study, endoscopically evident ketorolac tromethamine-induced mucosal injury, including GI ulceration, was dose related and independent of the route of administration.

Serious adverse GI effects (e.g., bleeding, ulceration, perforation) can occur at any time in patients receiving NSAIA therapy, and such effects may *not* be preceded by warning signs or symptoms. Only 1 in 5 patients who develop a serious upper GI adverse event while receiving NSAIA therapy is symptomatic. Therefore, clinicians should remain alert to the possible development of serious GI effects (e.g., bleeding, ulceration) in any patient receiving NSAIA therapy, and such patients should be followed chronically for the development of manifestations of such effects and advised of the importance of this follow-up. In addition, patients should be advised about the signs and symptoms of serious NSAIA-induced GI toxicity and what action to take if they occur. If signs and symptoms of a serious GI event develop, additional evaluation and treatment should be initiated promptly; the NSAIA should be discontinued until appropriate diagnostic studies have ruled out a serious GI event.

Studies to date are inconclusive concerning the relative risk of various prototypical NSAIAs in causing serious GI effects. In patients receiving NSAIAs and observed in clinical studies of several months' to 2 years' duration, symptomatic upper GI ulcers, gross bleeding, or perforation appeared to occur in approximately 1% of patients treated for 3–6 months and in about 2–4% of those treated for 1 year. Longer duration of therapy with an NSAIA increases the likelihood of a serious GI event. However, short-term therapy is not without risk. High dosages of any NSAIA probably are associated with an increased risk of such effects, although controlled studies documenting this probable association are lacking for most NSAIAs. Therefore, whenever use of relatively high dosages (within the recommended dosage range) is considered, sufficient benefit to offset the potential increased risk of GI toxicity should be anticipated.

Studies have shown that patients with a history of peptic ulcer disease and/or GI bleeding who are receiving NSAIAs have a substantially higher risk for developing GI bleeding than patients without these risk factors. In addition to a history of ulcer disease, pharmacoepidemiologic studies have identified several comorbid conditions and concomitant therapies that may increase the risk for GI bleeding, including concomitant administration of oral corticosteroids or anticoagulants, longer duration of NSAIA therapy, smoking, alcoholism, older age, and poor general health status. Most spontaneous reports of fatal GI effects have been in geriatric or debilitated patients. In addition, geriatric or debilitated patients appear to tolerate ulceration and bleeding less well than other individuals, and most spontaneous reports of fatal GI effects have been in such patients. In addition, results of postmarketing studies suggest that geriatric patients receiving ketorolac tromethamine may be at increased risk of developing serious adverse GI effects (e.g., bleeding, ulceration, perforation).

For patients at high risk for complications from NSAIA-induced GI ulceration (e.g., bleeding, perforation), concomitant use of misoprostol can be considered for preventive therapy. (See Misoprostol 56:28.28.) Alternatively, some clinicians suggest that concomitant use of a proton-pump inhibitor (e.g., omeprazole) may be used to decrease the incidence of serious GI toxicity associated with NSAIA therapy.

■ **Nervous System Effects** Adverse nervous system effects reportedly occur in about 23% of patients receiving IM ketorolac tromethamine. Headache, somnolence or drowsiness, and dizziness have been reported in 17, 3–14, and 3–9%, respectively, of patients receiving ketorolac therapy. Nervousness, abnormal thinking, depression, euphoria, difficulty in concentration, insomnia, CNS stimulation, seizures, tremors, extrapyramidal manifestations, abnormal dreams, hallucinations, vertigo, asthenia, and paresthesia have been reported in 1% or less of patients receiving the drug. Psychosis also has been reported.

Nervousness, hyperkinesia, and asthenia/fatigue have been reported in 1–4% of patients receiving oral ketorolac tromethamine. Euphoria, stupor, and malaise have been reported rarely in patients receiving the drug orally.

■ **Local and Dermatologic Effects** IM administration of ketorolac tromethamine has produced pain at the injection site in about 2–4% of patients. Ecchymosis, bruising, hematoma or other signs of wound bleeding, and tingling at the injection site have been reported rarely. Adverse local effects may be minimized by applying pressure over the injection site for 15–30 seconds after administration. There has been no evidence (e.g., alterations in serum creatine kinase [CK, creatine phosphokinase, CPK] concentrations) of substantial adverse muscular tissue effects following single or multiple IM injections of ketorolac tromethamine.

Pruritus occurred in 3–9% of patients receiving ketorolac tromethamine therapy, and sweating has been reported in 1–3% of patients receiving IM ketorolac tromethamine. Rash (may be maculopapular), urticaria, toxic epidermal necrolysis (Lyell's syndrome), and exfoliative dermatitis have been reported in 1% or less of patients receiving the drug IM. These effects also have been reported in patients receiving ketorolac tromethamine orally.

■ **Sensitivity Reactions** Severe anaphylactoid reactions have been reported in patients receiving ketorolac tromethamine. Anaphylactoid reactions may occur in patients with known hypersensitivity to aspirin or other NSAIA, including ketorolac tromethamine; however, these reactions also have been reported in patients without a history of hypersensitivity or known previous exposure to these drugs. Patients should be questioned carefully before ketorolac tromethamine therapy is initiated about development of allergic reactions (e.g., asthma, nasal polyps, urticaria, hypotension) associated with administration of NSAIAs; if such manifestations occur during therapy, the drug should be discontinued. In premarketing studies in a limited number of patients previously exposed to ketorolac tromethamine but with no history of hypersensitivity to it, there was no evidence that the drug possessed an unusual propensity for causing hypersensitivity reactions. Anaphylaxis, bronchospasm, and laryngeal and/or lingual edema have been reported in 1% or less of patients receiving the drug. Angioedema and anaphylactoid reaction also have been reported.

■ **Renal, Electrolyte, and Genitourinary Effects** Chronic administration of oral ketorolac tromethamine occasionally has caused impairment of renal function, resulting in hematuria, proteinuria, and transiently increased BUN and serum creatinine concentrations. Increased BUN and serum creatinine concentrations have occurred in about 3 and 2% of patients, respectively, receiving the drug orally for 1 year. Oliguria, urinary frequency, urinary retention, hemolytic-uremic syndrome, acute renal failure, flank pain (with or without hematuria and/or azotemia), hyponatremia, and hyperkalemia have occurred in about 1% or less of patients receiving short-term, ketorolac tromethamine therapy. Glomerular nephritis, interstitial nephritis, renal papillary necrosis, and nephrotic syndrome have been reported in patients receiving ketorolac tromethamine; patients at greatest risk of adverse renal effects include those with impaired renal function and geriatric patients. Although a causal relationship to ketorolac tromethamine has not been established, polyuria has occurred during therapy with the drug. As with other NSAIAs, renal papillary necrosis and other evidence of renal toxicity have occurred following prolonged administration of the drug in animals.

■ **Hepatic Effects** Borderline elevations of one or more liver function test results may occur in up to 15% of patients treated with NSAIAs; meaningful (3 times the upper limit of normal) elevations of serum ALT (SGPT) or AST (SGOT) concentration have occurred in less than 1% of patients receiving oral ketorolac tromethamine in controlled clinical studies. In addition, liver function abnormalities have been reported in less than 1% of patients receiving short-term, IM therapy with the drug. Such abnormalities may progress, may remain essentially unchanged, or may be transient with continued therapy. Hepatitis, liver failure, and cholestatic jaundice have been reported in 1% or less of patients receiving ketorolac tromethamine.

■ **Hematologic Effects** Purpura has been reported in less than 3% of patients receiving IM ketorolac tromethamine. Ketorolac tromethamine may inhibit platelet adhesion and aggregation and prolong bleeding time (generally by approximately 3 minutes from baseline values). However, the drug has a transient effect on platelet function, and aggregation usually returns to normal within 24–48 hours after discontinuing ketorolac tromethamine. The drug usually does not affect prothrombin time, partial thromboplastin time, or kaolin-cephalin coagulation time. Platelet count may or may not be affected by ketorolac tromethamine; thrombocytopenia (which was not considered clinically important) has been reported rarely in patients receiving the drug IM. Patients who may be affected adversely by a prolongation of bleeding time should be observed carefully during ketorolac tromethamine therapy. (See Cautions: Precautions and Contraindications.)

Bleeding at the operative site (rarely requiring blood transfusions) has been reported in 1% or less of patients receiving parenteral ketorolac tromethamine therapy. Bleeding has occurred following tonsillectomy in pediatric patients receiving ketorolac tromethamine. In one retrospective analysis of patients undergoing tonsillectomy with or without adenoidectomy, the risk of bleeding was 10.1 or 2.2% in patients receiving ketorolac or an opiate agonist, respectively, for pain management. In pediatric patients 12 years of age or younger, postoperative hemorrhage occurred in 6.5% of those given ketorolac and in 3.3% of those who did not receive the drug. In a prospective study in children 3–9 years of age undergoing tonsillectomy with or without adenoidectomy, the overall incidence of bleeding in children receiving ketorolac (16.3%) was similar to the incidence in children receiving morphine (17%). However, the incidence of bleeding during the first 24 hours after surgery was higher in those receiving ketorolac (14.3%) than in those receiving morphine (4.2%).

Thrombocytopenia, epistaxis, and anemia have been reported in 1% or less of patients receiving the drug. Although a causal relationship to ketorolac tromethamine has not been established, leukopenia and eosinophilia have occurred during therapy with the drug.

■ **Ocular and Otic Effects** Visual disturbances (e.g., blurred vision) have occurred in 1% or less of patients receiving IM ketorolac tromethamine therapy and also have been reported in patients receiving the drug orally. Tinnitus and hearing loss have been reported in 1% or less of patients receiving the drug.

■ **Other Adverse Effects** Dyspnea, infection, pulmonary edema, and myalgia have been reported in 1% or less of patients receiving ketorolac tromethamine IM or orally. Chills occurred in at least one patient receiving the drug IM. Other adverse effects reported rarely in patients receiving oral ketorolac tromethamine include weight gain, generalized pain, and fever. Although a causal relationship to ketorolac tromethamine has not been established, aseptic meningitis, rhinitis, and cough have occurred during therapy with the drug.

■ **Precautions and Contraindications** Ketorolac tromethamine, like other NSAIAs, is not free of potential adverse effects, including some that can cause discomfort; more serious effects (e.g., myocardial infarction, stroke, GI bleeding), which may require hospitalization and may even be fatal, also can occur. The manufacturer warns that the total combined duration of parenteral and/or oral ketorolac therapy in adults is *not* to exceed 5 days because of an increased frequency and severity of adverse effects associated with more prolonged therapy; patients should be switched to alternative analgesic agents as soon as clinically possible.

Patients should be advised to read the medication guide for NSAIAs that is provided to the patient each time the drug is dispensed.

NSAIAs increase the risk of serious adverse cardiovascular thrombotic events. (See Cautions: Cardiovascular Effects.) To minimize the potential risk of adverse cardiovascular events, the lowest effective dosage and shortest possible duration of therapy should be employed. Some clinicians suggest that it may be prudent to avoid use of NSAIAs whenever possible in patients with cardiovascular disease. Patients receiving NSAIAs (including those without previous symptoms of cardiovascular disease) should be monitored for the possible development of cardiovascular events throughout therapy. Patients should be informed about the signs and symptoms of serious cardiovascular toxicity (chest pain, dyspnea, weakness, slurring of speech) and instructed to seek immediate medical attention if such toxicity occurs. Ketorolac tromethamine should be avoided in patients with recent myocardial infarction unless the benefits of therapy are expected to outweigh the risk of recurrent cardiovascular thrombotic events; if ketorolac tromethamine is used in such patients, the patient should be monitored for cardiac ischemia.

There is no consistent evidence that concomitant use of low-dose aspirin mitigates the increased risk of serious cardiovascular events associated with NSAIAs. Concomitant use of aspirin and an NSAIA increases the risk for serious GI events. Because of the potential for increased adverse effects, patients receiving ketorolac should be advised not to take aspirin.

Use of NSAIAs can result in the onset of hypertension or worsening of preexisting hypertension; either of these occurrences may contribute to the increased incidence of cardiovascular events. Patients receiving NSAIAs may have an impaired response to diuretics (i.e., thiazide or loop diuretics), angiotensin-converting enzyme (ACE) inhibitors, angiotensin II receptor antagonists, or β-adrenergic blocking agents. NSAIAs should be used with caution in patients with hypertension. Blood pressure should be monitored closely during initiation of NSAIA therapy and throughout therapy.

Because NSAIAs increase morbidity and mortality in patients with heart failure, the manufacturer states that ketorolac tromethamine should be avoided in patients with severe heart failure unless the benefits of therapy are expected to outweigh the risk of worsening heart failure; if ketorolac tromethamine is used in such patients, the patient should be monitored for worsening heart failure. Some experts state that use of NSAIAs should be avoided whenever possible in patients with reduced left ventricular ejection fraction and current or prior symptoms of heart failure. Patients receiving NSAIAs should be advised to inform their clinician if they experience symptoms of heart failure, including dyspnea, unexplained weight gain, and edema. Use of NSAIAs may diminish the cardiovascular effects of certain drugs used to treat heart failure and edema (e.g., diuretics, ACE inhibitors, angiotensin II receptor antagonists). (See Drug Interactions.)

Serious GI toxicity (e.g., bleeding, ulceration, perforation), with or without warning symptoms, can occur at any time during ketorolac tromethamine therapy. Studies to date have not identified any subset of patients who are not at risk of NSAIA-associated bleeding or peptic ulceration. Geriatric (i.e., 65 years of age or older) or debilitated patients appear to be more susceptible to such GI bleeding and ulceration and most spontaneous reports of fatal GI events during ketorolac therapy were in these populations. Postmarketing experience with parenterally administered ketorolac suggests that there may be a greater risk of GI ulcerations, bleeding, and perforation in geriatric patients. (See Geriatric Precautions.) The incidence and severity of adverse GI effects increase with increasing dose and duration of ketorolac tromethamine therapy. To minimize the potential risk of adverse GI effects, the lowest effective dosage and shortest duration of therapy should be employed. In a hospital-based, nonrandomized, observational postmarketing study comparing patients receiving parenteral ketorolac therapy with patients receiving parenteral opiate therapy, higher rates of clinically serious GI bleeding were observed in patients younger than 65 years of age who received an average total daily parenteral ketorolac tromethamine dose of greater than 90 mg. In this same study, patients with a history of peptic ulcer disease also appeared to be at increased risk of developing serious GI complications. The manufacturer states that clinicians should inform their patients of the potential risks of ketorolac tromethamine therapy prior to initiating treatment.

Patients receiving ketorolac tromethamine are at risk of developing adverse renal effects, including interstitial nephritis and acute renal failure. Renal toxicity has been observed in patients in whom renal prostaglandins have a compensatory role in maintaining renal perfusion. Administration of an NSAIA to such patients may cause a dose-dependent reduction in prostaglandin formation and thereby precipitate overt renal decompensation. Patients at greatest risk of this reaction include those with impaired renal function, heart failure, or hepatic dysfunction; those with extracellular fluid depletion (e.g., patients receiving diuretics, dehydrated patients); those taking an ACE inhibitor or angiotensin II receptor antagonist concomitantly; and geriatric patients. Recovery of renal function to pretreatment levels usually occurs following discontinuance of NSAIA therapy. The manufacturer recommends that hypovolemia be corrected prior to initiating therapy with ketorolac. Some clinicians recommend that renal function be monitored periodically in patients receiving long-term NSAIA therapy.

The manufacturer states that ketorolac tromethamine should be used with caution in patients with renal impairment or a history of kidney disease, since the drug and its metabolites are excreted principally by the kidneys. Such patients should be monitored closely during ketorolac therapy. Because patients with underlying renal insufficiency are at risk of developing acute renal failure, the risks and benefits of ketorolac therapy must be considered before instituting therapy with the drug in these patients. In patients with moderately elevated serum creatinine, the manufacturer recommends that the usual daily dose of parenteral ketorolac tromethamine be halved, and not exceed 60 mg daily in these patients. (See Dosage and Administration: Dosage in Renal and Hepatic Impairment.)

Elevations in serum ALT concentrations may be the most sensitive indicator of NSAIA-induced liver dysfunction. Patients who experience signs and/or symptoms suggestive of liver dysfunction or an abnormal liver function test result (especially those with a history of hepatic impairment) while receiving ketorolac tromethamine should be evaluated for evidence of the development of a more severe hepatic reaction; the manufacturer states that therapy with the drug should be discontinued in such patients. The manufacturer states that ketorolac tromethamine should be used with caution in patients with a history of hepatic impairment or with a history of liver disease.

Use of corticosteroids during NSAIA treatment may increase the risk of GI ulceration and the drugs should be used concomitantly with caution.

Ketorolac tromethamine should be used very cautiously and with careful monitoring in patients who may be adversely affected by prolongation of bleeding time (e.g., patients receiving anticoagulant therapy, patients with hemophilia, von Willebrand's disease, or platelet deficiency) and *only* when the potential benefits justify the possible risks to the patient, since the drug may inhibit platelet function and hemorrhage is possible. (See Drug Interactions: Anticoagulants and Thrombolytic Agents.) In patients who receive anticoagulants for any reason, there is an increased risk of intramuscular hematoma formation from administration of IM ketorolac tromethamine. In addition, since hematomas and other signs of wound bleeding have been reported in patients receiving ketorolac tromethamine perioperatively, the manufacturer states that postoperative administration of ketorolac tromethamine should be undertaken with caution in any patient in whom hemostasis is critical.

In adults who weigh less than 50 kg, the dosage of ketorolac tromethamine should be reduced. (See Dosage and Administration: Dosage.) Parenteral dosages of ketorolac tromethamine must not exceed 60 mg daily in these patients.

The possibility that the antipyretic and anti-inflammatory effects of ketorolac tromethamine may mask the usual signs and symptoms of infection or other diseases should be considered, although some evidence suggests that the likelihood of such an effect may be small.

Anaphylactoid reactions have been reported in patients receiving NSAIAs. Patients receiving ketorolac should be informed of the signs and symptoms of an anaphylactoid reaction (e.g., difficulty breathing, swelling of the face or throat) and advised to seek immediate medical attention if an anaphylactoid reaction develops.

Serious skin reactions (e.g., exfoliative dermatitis, Stevens-Johnson syndrome, toxic epidermal necrolysis) can occur in patients receiving ketorolac. These serious skin reactions may occur without warning; patients should be advised to consult their clinician if skin rash and blisters, fever, or other signs of hypersensitivity reaction (e.g., pruritus) occur. Ketorolac should be discontinued at the first appearance of rash or any other sign of hypersensitivity.

Ketorolac tromethamine therapy is contraindicated in patients with active peptic ulcer disease, recent GI bleeding or perforation, or a history of peptic ulcer disease or GI bleeding; in patients with advanced renal impairment or patients at risk of renal failure because of volume depletion; in patients with suspected or confirmed cerebrovascular bleeding, hemorrhagic diathesis, incomplete hemostasis, or patients at a high risk of bleeding; in patients receiving concomitant probenecid therapy; or in patients receiving concomitant aspirin or NSAIA therapy, because of the cumulative risk of serious NSAIA-related adverse effects. Use of ketorolac tromethamine as a prophylactic analgesic before any major surgery, or as an intraoperative analgesic during procedures where hemostasis is critical also is contraindicated. Because of the alcohol content of the parenteral formulations of the drug, epidural or intrathecal administration of ketorolac is contraindicated.

The manufacturers state that ketorolac is contraindicated in patients with known hypersensitivity to the drug. In addition, NSAIAs generally are contraindicated in patients in whom asthma, urticaria, or other sensitivity reactions are precipitated by aspirin or other NSAIAs, since there is potential for cross-sensitivity between NSAIAs and aspirin, and severe, often fatal, anaphylactic reactions may occur in such patients. Although NSAIAs generally are contraindicated in these patients, the drugs have occasionally been used in NSAIA-sensitive patients who have undergone desensitization. Because patients with asthma may have aspirin-sensitivity asthma, NSAIAs should be used with caution in patients with asthma. In patients with asthma, aspirin sensitivity is manifested principally as bronchospasm and usually is associated with nasal polyps; the association of aspirin sensitivity, asthma, and nasal polyps is known as the aspirin triad. For a further discussion of cross-sensitivity of NSAIAs, see Cautions: Sensitivity Reactions, in the Salicylates General Statement 28:08.04.24.

NSAIAs are contraindicated in the setting of CABG surgery.

■ **Pediatric Precautions** Safety and efficacy of parenteral (IM or IV) ketorolac tromethamine administered as a single dose have been established in children 2–16 years of age. Use of ketorolac tromethamine in pediatric patients is supported by evidence from well-controlled studies in adults, data regarding the pharmacokinetics of IV ketorolac in children, and safety and efficacy data from studies in pediatric patients. Since the safety and efficacy of ketorolac tromethamine in children younger than 2 years of age have not been established, the manufacturer recommends that the drug *not* be used in this age group. Limited data are available to support administration of more than one parenteral (IM or IV) dose of ketorolac tromethamine in pediatric patients. The manufacturer states that there are insufficient data available to support oral administration of ketorolac tromethamine in pediatric patients. In limited observational and double-blind, parallel-group studies of short-term ketorolac therapy for control of pain, including postoperative pain, or for antipyresis† in pediatric patients, the drug was generally effective and no unusual adverse effects were observed. In a randomized double-blind comparison of IV ketorolac versus rectal acetaminophen for post-tonsillectomy pain in pediatric patients aged 2–15 years, there was no difference in analgesic efficacy; however, hemostasis was more difficult to achieve in patients receiving ketorolac therapy.

Since ketorolac tromethamine appears to increase the risk of bleeding following tonsillectomy, clinicians should consider the increased risk of bleeding when prescribing the drug in children undergoing this operative procedure. The same contraindications and precautions that apply to adults receiving ketorolac tromethamine also apply to pediatric patients. (See Cautions: Precautions and Contraindications.)

■ **Geriatric Precautions** Geriatric individuals appear to tolerate GI ulcerations or bleeding less well than other individuals, and many of the spontaneous reports of fatal GI effects in patients receiving NSAIAs involve geriatric individuals. Because ketorolac tromethamine may be cleared more slowly in geriatric individuals (i.e., 65 years of age or older) and because this population may be more susceptible to the adverse effects of NSAIA-type drugs, ketorolac therapy must be instituted with caution and at reduced dosages in these patients. The incidence and severity of GI complications increases with increasing dose and duration of ketorolac therapy. The lower end of the parenteral ketorolac dosing range should be used in geriatric patients and the total daily dose of the drug should not exceed 60 mg. (See Dosage and Administration: Dosage.)

■ **Mutagenicity and Carcinogenicity** No evidence of ketorolac tromethamine-induced mutagenesis was seen in in vitro studies with *Salmonella typhimurium*, *Saccharomyces cerevisiae*, or *Escherichia coli*. There also was no evidence of mutagenicity when ketorolac tromethamine was tested for chromosome breaks in vivo in the micronucleus assay in mice. Ketorolac was not mutagenic in the Ames microbial mutagen test or in the forward mutation assay; there was no increase in DNA repair when ketorolac tromethamine was tested in an unscheduled DNA synthesis. Ketorolac tromethamine increased chromosomal aberrations in Chinese hamster ovarian cells when they were exposed to the drug at concentrations of 1.59 mg/mL (about 1000 times the average human plasma ketorolac concentrations).

No evidence of carcinogenic potential was seen in an 18-month study in mice receiving oral ketorolac tromethamine dosages up to 2 mg/kg daily (approximately equivalent to the maximum recommended human dosage of IM ketorolac tromethamine). There also was no evidence of carcinogenic potential in a 24-month study in rats receiving oral ketorolac tromethamine dosages up to 5 mg/kg daily (approximately 2.5 times the maximum recommended human dosage of IM ketorolac tromethamine).

■ **Pregnancy, Fertility, and Lactation** Reproduction studies in rabbits and rats receiving oral ketorolac tromethamine dosages of 3.6 and 10 mg/kg daily, respectively (about 1.8 and 5 times the maximum recommended human parenteral dosage, respectively), during the period of organogenesis have not revealed evidence of harm to the fetus; however, oral dosages exceeding the maximum recommended human parenteral dosage in rats produced delayed parturition and dystocia, probably secondary to inhibition of prostaglandin synthesis. There are no adequate and controlled studies to date using ketorolac tromethamine in pregnant women. The manufacturer states that ketorolac tromethamine is not recommended for use during pregnancy and should be used only when the potential benefits justify the possible risks to the fetus. Ketorolac tromethamine should *not* be used during late pregnancy or during labor or delivery, since inhibitors of prostaglandin synthesis may have adverse effects on the fetal cardiovascular system (e.g., premature closure of the ductus arteriosus) and on uterine contraction.

Reproduction studies in male and female rats using ketorolac tromethamine dosages of 9 or 16 mg/kg daily (about 4.5 or 8 times the maximum recommended human parenteral dosage, respectively) have not revealed evidence of impaired fertility.

Because ketorolac is distributed into milk (see Pharmacokinetics: Distribution), and because of the potential adverse effects of prostaglandin-inhibiting drugs in neonates, the drug should not be used in nursing women.

Drug Interactions

■ **Protein-bound Drugs** Because ketorolac tromethamine is highly protein bound, it could be displaced from binding sites by, or it could displace from binding sites, some other protein-bound drugs. However, the clinical importance of such potential drug interactions has not been established for ketorolac. In vitro studies indicate that salicylates may displace ketorolac from protein-binding sites. (See Drug Interactions: Nonsteroidal Anti-Inflammatory Agents.) In addition, in vitro studies indicate that ketorolac may displace warfarin slightly from protein-binding sites; however, it appears that the NSAIA does not displace digoxin from its protein-binding sites. Therapeutic plasma concentrations of digoxin, warfarin, ibuprofen, naproxen, acetaminophen, phenytoin, tolbutamide, or piroxicam do not appear to alter the protein binding of ketorolac.

■ **Angiotensin-converting Enzyme Inhibitors and Angiotensin II Receptor Antagonists** There is some evidence that concomitant use of NSAIAs with angiotensin-converting enzyme (ACE) inhibitors or angiotensin II receptor antagonists may reduce the blood pressure response to the antihypertensive agent.

The manufacturer states that the concomitant use of ketorolac and ACE inhibitor therapy may increase the risk of renal impairment, especially in patients who are hypovolemic.

■ **Nonsteroidal Anti-inflammatory Agents** In vitro studies indicate that therapeutic anti-inflammatory concentrations (e.g., 300 mcg/mL) of salicylates may displace ketorolac from protein binding sites, possibly resulting in elevated plasma concentrations of unbound ketorolac. Protein binding of ketorolac may be decreased from 99.2% to 97.5%, which would represent a potential two-fold increase in plasma concentrations of unbound drug. The manufacturer states that ketorolac tromethamine is contraindicated in patients receiving aspirin or other NSAIAs because of the potential for cumulative adverse effects.

Concomitant use of aspirin and an NSAIA increases the risk for serious GI events. Because of the potential for increased adverse effects, patients receiving ketorolac should be advised not to take aspirin. There is no consistent evidence that use of low-dose aspirin mitigates the increased risk of serious cardiovascular events associated with NSAIAs.

■ **Anticoagulants and Thrombolytic Agents** The effects of warfarin and NSAIAs on GI bleeding are synergistic. Concomitant use of NSAIAs and warfarin is associated with a higher risk of GI bleeding compared with use of either agent alone.

While in vitro studies indicate that protein binding of warfarin may be decreased slightly from 99.5 to 99.3% by ketorolac, a ketorolac dosage of 10 mg daily for 6 days did not substantially alter the pharmacokinetics or pharmacodynamics of a single dose of warfarin in one study in healthy adults. No drug interaction was observed in healthy adults following concomitant administration of heparin (5000 units) and ketorolac tromethamine. However, because ketorolac tromethamine can inhibit platelet function, the drug should be used with extreme caution and prothrombin time should be monitored carefully in patients who may be adversely affected by prolongation of bleeding time (e.g., patients receiving anticoagulant therapy, patients with hemophilia, von Willebrand's disease, or platelet deficiency). Patients receiving therapeutic doses of anticoagulants (e.g., heparin, warfarin) have an increased risk of bleeding complications if ketorolac is administered concomitantly; therefore, the manufacturer recommends that such concomitant therapy be undertaken with extreme caution. The concurrent use of ketorolac tromethamine and prophylactic low-dose heparin (2500–5000 units every 12 hours), warfarin, or dextrans has not been studied extensively, but also may be associated with an increased risk of bleeding. Until more data are available, the manufacturer recommends that such concomitant therapy be undertaken only very cautiously, and *only* when the potential benefits justify the possible risks to the patient.

■ **Diuretics** Patients receiving diuretics may have an increased risk of developing renal failure secondary to decreased renal blood flow resulting from prostaglandin inhibition by NSAIAs, including ketorolac tromethamine. (See Cautions: Precautions and Contraindications.) In addition, NSAIAs (including ketorolac tromethamine) can reduce the natriuretic effects of furosemide or thiazide diuretics. This effect may be related to inhibition of renal prostaglandin synthesis.

■ **Methotrexate** While the effect of ketorolac tromethamine on clearance of methotrexate has not been evaluated to date, severe, sometimes fatal, toxicity has occurred following administration of an NSAIA concomitantly with methotrexate (principally high-dose therapy) in patients with various malignant neoplasms or rheumatoid arthritis. The toxicity was associated with elevated and prolonged blood concentrations of methotrexate. The exact mechanism of the interaction remains to be established, but it has been suggested that NSAIAs may inhibit renal elimination of methotrexate, possibly by decreasing renal perfusion via inhibition of renal prostaglandin synthesis or by competing for renal elimination. Further studies are needed to evaluate the interaction between NSAIAs and methotrexate. Caution is advised if methotrexate and an NSAIA are administered concomitantly. (See Drug Interactions: Nonsteroidal Anti-inflammatory Agents, in Methotrexate 10:00.)

■ **Lithium** NSAIAs appear to decrease renal clearance of lithium, which may lead to an increase in serum or plasma lithium concentrations. Limited reports suggest that concomitant administration of ketorolac tromethamine and lithium results in increased lithium concentrations, with associated symptoms of lithium toxicity (e.g., nausea, vomiting, neurologic effects). Although such concomitant therapy is not recommended, if patients must receive concomitant ketorolac and lithium therapy, plasma lithium concentrations should be monitored closely, and the patient should be observed for signs and symptoms of lithium toxicity.

■ **Probenecid** Concomitant administration of ketorolac tromethamine and probenecid has reportedly decreased clearance and increased plasma concentration, total AUC (by approximately threefold), and half-life (by approximately twofold) of ketorolac. Therefore, the manufacturer states that ketorolac is contraindicated in patients receiving probenecid.

■ **Other Drugs** Ketorolac tromethamine has been administered concomitantly with morphine or meperidine for the management of postoperative pain without apparent adverse interaction. Seizures have been reported rarely in patients receiving concomitant ketorolac and anticonvulsant therapy (e.g., phenytoin, carbamazepine). Hallucinations have been reported in patients receiving therapy with ketorolac and psychoactive drugs (e.g., fluoxetine, thiothixene, alprazolam). No drug interactions were reported following concomitant administration of ketorolac with some anti-infective agents (e.g., cephalosporins, penicillins, aminoglycosides), antiemetic agents, laxatives, sedatives, anxiolytic agents, corticosteroids, bronchodilators, or hormones.Results of postmarketing studies indicate that ketorolac tromethamine may potentiate the effects of nondepolarizing skeletal muscle relaxants, resulting in apnea; however, the drug interaction potential of the drugs has not been specifically studied.

Evidence from animal or human drug interaction studies suggest that ketorolac is unlikely to interact with the metabolism of itself or other drugs via the hepatic microsomal enzyme system (cytochrome P-450 system).

Acute Toxicity

Limited information is available on the acute toxicity of ketorolac tromethamine. The acute lethal dose of ketorolac tromethamine in humans is not known. The oral LD_{50} of the drug is 200 mg/kg in mice.

Daily parenteral ketorolac tromethamine dosages of 360 mg (3 times the maximum daily recommended dose) for 5 days resulted in abdominal pain and peptic ulcers, which healed after drug discontinuance. Metabolic acidosis following intentional overdosage of ketorolac (amount of drug not specified) also has been reported. Dialysis does not appear to be effective in removing the drug from circulation. In rats, mice, and monkeys, single oral ketorolac tromethamine doses exceeding 100 mg/kg produced diarrhea, pallor, labored breathing, rales, vomiting, and decreased activity.

Chronic Toxicity

Tolerance, psychological dependence, or physical dependence does not appear to occur in patients receiving chronic (for 6 months) oral ketorolac tromethamine. There also was no evidence of manifestations of withdrawal following abrupt discontinuance of IM ketorolac tromethamine. The drug does not appear to affect opiate receptors and does not appear to exhibit opiate agonist or antagonist activity. The most frequent adverse effects observed during chronic toxicity studies in animals were GI irritation and/or ulceration, which at high dosages resulted occasionally in peritonitis, anemia, and death. Renal toxicity also was evident after prolonged therapy at relatively high dosages in animals.

Pharmacology

Ketorolac tromethamine has pharmacologic actions similar to those of other prototypical NSAIAs. The drug exhibits anti-inflammatory, analgesic, and antipyretic activity. The exact mechanisms have not been clearly established, but many of the actions appear to be associated principally with the inhibition of prostaglandin synthesis. Ketorolac tromethamine inhibits the synthesis of prostaglandins in body tissues by inhibiting cyclooxygenase; at least 2 isoenzymes, cyclooxygenase-1 (COX-1) and -2 (COX-2) (also referred to as prostaglandin G/H synthase-1 [PGHS-1] and -2 [PGHS-2], respectively), have been identified that catalyze the formation of prostaglandins in the arachidonic acid pathway. Ketorolac, like other prototypical NSAIAs, inhibits both COX-1 and COX-2. Although the exact mechanisms have not been clearly established, NSAIAs appear to exert anti-inflammatory, analgesic, and antipyretic activity principally through inhibition of the COX-2 isoenzyme; COX-1 inhibition presumably is responsible for the drugs' unwanted effects on GI mucosa and platelet aggregation.

■ **Analgesic Effect** The analgesic effect of ketorolac tromethamine appears to result from inhibition of prostaglandin synthesis. While the precise mechanism of the analgesic effect of NSAIAs continues to be investigated, these effects appear to be mediated principally through inhibition of the COX-2 isoenzyme at sites of inflammation with subsequent reduction in the synthesis of certain prostaglandins from their arachidonic acid precursors. Prostaglandins appear to sensitize pain receptors to mechanical stimulation and to other chemical mediators (e.g., bradykinin, histamine). Since many NSAIAs, including ketorolac tromethamine, do not directly alter the pain threshold or prevent pain caused by exogenous or previously synthesized prostaglandins, the drugs may produce analgesia by inhibiting the synthesis of prostaglandins peripherally and possibly centrally. Animal studies suggest that the analgesic activity of ketorolac tromethamine results principally from a peripheral action. In addition, the anti-inflammatory effect of NSAIAs may contribute to their analgesic effect. Ketorolac tromethamine does not appear to affect opiate receptors; however, in one animal study, naloxone decreased the analgesic activity of ketorolac tromethamine. There is no evidence that therapy with ketorolac tromethamine results in physical dependence on the drug.

On a weight basis, the analgesic potency of oral ketorolac tromethamine was about 3–6, 25–50, 180–350, or 180–350 times that of indomethacin, naproxen, aspirin, or phenylbutazone, respectively, as determined by antagonism of phenylbenzoquinone-induced writhing in mice. On a weight basis, as determined by the adjuvant-inflamed paw test in rats, the analgesic potency of oral ketorolac tromethamine was about 500–800 times that of aspirin. The analgesic potency of oral ketorolac tromethamine was similar to that of indomethacin and about 11–25, 30–90, or 100–200 times that of naproxen, phenylbutazone, or aspirin, respectively, as determined by the yeast-inflamed paw test in rats.

■ **Anti-inflammatory Effect** The anti-inflammatory effect of ketorolac tromethamine and other NSAIAs may result in part from inhibition of prostaglandin synthesis and release during inflammation. While the precise mechanism of the anti-inflammatory effect of NSAIAs continues to be investigated, these effects appear to be mediated principally through inhibition of the COX-2 isoenzyme at sites of inflammation with subsequent reduction in the synthesis of certain prostaglandins from their arachidonic acid precursors. It appears that ketorolac tromethamine does not suppress phagocytic activity of mononuclear macrophages. Ketorolac tromethamine does not possess glucocorticoid or mineralocorticoid activity.

On a weight basis, the anti-inflammatory potency of oral ketorolac tromethamine has been shown to be 2–3 times that of indomethacin or naproxen and about 36 times that of phenylbutazone, as determined by inhibition of carrageenan-induced paw edema in rats. However, when determined by inhibition of cotton pellet-induced granuloma in rats, the anti-inflammatory potency of ketorolac tromethamine was comparable to that of indomethacin. In adjuvant-induced arthritis in rats, the anti-inflammatory activity of oral ketorolac tromethamine was approximately twice that of naproxen. However, there is limited evidence from studies in patients with inflammatory diseases (e.g., rheumatoid arthritis) and in animals that the anti-inflammatory potency of ketorolac is less than the drug's analgesic potency.

■ **Antipyretic Effect** Ketorolac tromethamine lowers body temperature in animals with antigen-induced fever. Although the mechanism of antipyretic effect of NSAIAs is not known, it has been suggested that suppression of prostaglandin synthesis in the CNS (probably in the hypothalamus) may be involved. In rats, the antipyretic activity of a ketorolac tromethamine dose of 0.1–2.7 mg/kg was similar to that of an aspirin dose of 5–45 mg/kg. However, results of clinical studies on the antipyretic activity of ketorolac tromethamine in humans have been equivocal, and further studies are needed.

■ **Renal Effects** Ketorolac tromethamine has been reported to adversely affect renal function. (See Cautions: Renal, Electrolyte and Genitourinary Effects.) Although the exact mechanism of adverse renal effects of NSAIAs has not been determined, the effects may be related to inhibition of renal prostaglandin synthesis.

■ **GI Effects** Ketorolac tromethamine can cause gastric mucosal damage, which may result in ulceration and/or bleeding. (See Cautions: GI Effects.) These gastric effects have been attributed to inhibition of the synthesis of prostaglandins produced by COX-1. Other factors possibly involved in NSAIA-induced gastropathy include local irritation, promotion of acid back-diffusion into gastric mucosa, uncoupling of oxidative phosphorylation, and enterohepatic recirculation of the drugs.

Epidemiologic and laboratory studies suggest that NSAIAs may reduce the risk of colon cancer. Although the exact mechanism by which NSAIAs may inhibit colon carcinogenesis remains to be determined, it has been suggested that inhibition of prostaglandin synthesis may be involved.

■ **Hematologic Effects** Ketorolac tromethamine can inhibit collagen- and arachidonic acid-induced platelet aggregation and may prolong bleeding time. Information on the effect of the drug on ADP-induced platelet aggregation has been equivocal. It appears that ketorolac tromethamine does not affect thromboxane A_2-induced platelet aggregation, prothrombin time, or partial thromboplastin time; however, serum thromboxane B_2 concentrations are decreased by the drug. In vitro, ketorolac tromethamine is more potent than aspirin in inhibiting collagen-induced platelet aggregation.

Following IM administration of 30 mg of ketorolac tromethamine 4 times daily in healthy adults, bleeding time was prolonged from 4.9 minutes to 7.8 minutes; prolongation of bleeding time was more pronounced in men than in women. In controlled clinical studies, clinically important postoperative bleeding occurred in 0.4 or 0.2% of patients receiving ketorolac tromethamine or opiate analgesics, respectively. In healthy individuals, oral administration of single 2.5- to 200-mg doses of ketorolac tromethamine resulted in 75–100% inhibition of ADP-, collagen-, or arachidonic acid-induced platelet aggregation 3 hours after administration of the drug. Unlike the irreversible action of aspirin on platelets and the resultant prolonged effect on platelet aggregation, ketorolac tromethamine had a transient effect on platelet function, and aggregation returned to normal within 24–48 hours after discontinuance of the drug in individuals receiving oral doses up to 200 mg. Like other prototypical NSAIAs, these effects of ketorolac tromethamine appear to be associated with inhibition of synthesis of prostaglandins produced by COX-1. In healthy adults, ketorolac tromethamine does not produce excessive perioperative bleeding and it appears that prolongation of bleeding time is of little clinical importance in most patients. However, caution is necessary in some patients. (See Cautions: Precautions and Contraindications.)

■ **CNS Effects** In animals, high doses (up to 300 mg/kg) of ketorolac tromethamine did not appear to cause appreciable CNS effects (e.g., CNS depression, EEG disturbances). In mice, ketorolac tromethamine doses of 100 mg/kg did not potentiate barbiturate-induced sleep or protect against drug- or electroshock-induced seizures. Usual doses of ketorolac tromethamine did not appear to cause psychomotor effects in healthy individuals.

■ **Respiratory Effects** Unlike opiate agonists, ketorolac tromethamine does not appear to cause respiratory depression. In a limited number of patients undergoing surgery, postoperative increases in carbon dioxide tension (PCO_2) were less in patients receiving IM ketorolac tromethamine concomitantly with IM morphine than in patients receiving IM morphine with placebo, although the dose of morphine was higher in patients receiving morphine with placebo. In healthy adults, including some undergoing minor surgery, ketorolac tromethamine did not depress the ventilatory response to carbon dioxide. In patients with chronic obstructive pulmonary disease (COPD), ketorolac tromethamine did not produce substantial decreases in minute ventilation or inspiratory flow.

■ **Cardiovascular Effects** Usual doses of ketorolac tromethamine do not appear to cause appreciable cardiovascular effects. In healthy individuals, therapeutic doses of the drug did not affect mean arterial blood pressure, heart rate, stroke volume, left ventricular performance, or left ventricular stroke index. It appears that administration of parenteral ketorolac tromethamine does not alter the hemodynamics of anesthetized patients.

■ **Ocular Effects** Following topical application to the eye, ketorolac tromethamine may reduce some manifestations of ocular inflammation induced by ocular trauma (e.g., ocular surgery) or external agents and also may inhibit corneal neovascularization. The exact mechanism of the ocular effects of the drug has not been clearly established, but these actions appear to be associated principally with the inhibition of ocular prostaglandin synthesis. Topically applied ketorolac tromethamine does not appear to affect intraocular pressure (IOP) nor to worsen bacterial, fungal, or viral ocular infections.

■ **Other Effects** In a limited number of patients with diabetes mellitus receiving insulin or oral sulfonylurea antidiabetic agents, ketorolac tromethamine did not appear to affect glucose metabolism. Ketorolac tromethamine may exhibit weak anticholinergic and α-adrenergic blocking activity.

Pharmacokinetics

The pharmacokinetics of ketorolac after IM, IV, or oral administration are best described by a linear, two-compartment model with first-order absorption and elimination, and pharmacokinetics of the drug after IV administration are best described by a two- or three-compartment model.

■ **Absorption** Ketorolac tromethamine is rapidly and completely or almost completely absorbed following IM or oral administration, respectively. Bioavailability has been reported to range from 80–100% following oral administration. At physiologic pH, ketorolac tromethamine is present in dissociated form as ketorolac (anion) and tromethamine (cation). The rate of absorption appears to be slower following IM administration than following oral administration of the drug in fasting, healthy adults; however, the extent of absorption is similar following parenteral or oral routes of administration. Food decreases the rate, but not the extent, of absorption of orally administered ketorolac tromethamine. The rate of absorption from the GI tract also may be decreased in patients with hepatic or renal impairment and in geriatric individuals.

Following IV administration of 15- or 30-mg doses of ketorolac tromethamine injection in healthy adults, time to peak plasma concentration was about 1 or 3 minutes, respectively. Peak plasma concentration following single-dose IV administration of 15 or 30 mg of ketorolac in healthy adults was approximately 2.5 or 4.7 mcg/mL, respectively. Following IM administration of the drug in adults, plasma concentrations of the drug increase proportionally with increasing doses. Average peak plasma ketorolac concentrations of 0.7–1.4, 2.2–3, 4–4.6 or 6.9 mcg/mL occur within 30–60 minutes following IM administration of a single 10-, 30-, 60-, or 90-mg dose of ketorolac tromethamine, respectively, in healthy adults. Following IM administration of a single 30-, 60-, or 90-mg dose of ketorolac tromethamine in healthy adults, peak plasma *p*-hydroxyketorolac (the principal metabolite of ketorolac) concentrations of about 30, 63, or 102 ng/mL, respectively, occur at about 2 hours. Following oral administration of a single 10- or 30-mg dose of ketorolac tromethamine in healthy adults, average peak plasma ketorolac concentrations of 0.7–1.1 or 2.7 mcg/mL, respectively, occur at about 1 hour (range: 20–60 minutes). Peak plasma *p*-hydroxyketorolac concentrations of about 37 ng/mL occur in about 1 hour following oral administration of a single 30-mg dose of the drug in healthy adults. The area under the plasma concentration-time curves (AUCs) of ketorolac and *p*-hydroxyketorolac increase linearly with single IM ketorolac tromethamine doses of 30–90 mg. AUCs of ketorolac also increase proportionally with oral ketorolac tromethamine doses of 0.8–3.2 mg/kg, and may be increased in adults with renal impairment compared with those in healthy adults.

Following IV administration of a single ketorolac tromethamine dose of 0.6 mg/kg in children 3–18 years of age, peak plasma concentrations of about 4.3 mcg/mL were attained in 10.25 minutes.

In healthy adults, steady-state plasma concentrations of ketorolac generally are reached within 24 hours following multiple dosing and average approximately 0.6–0.8 (range: 0.2–1.7) or 1.3–1.5 (range: 0.3–3.5) mcg/mL with IM ketorolac tromethamine dosages of 15 or 30 mg, respectively, 4 times daily. In multiple-dose IV studies, peak plasma steady-state ketorolac concentration following administration of 15- or 30-mg doses 4 times daily in healthy adults was approximately 3.1 or 6.9 mcg/mL, respectively. Mean steady-state plasma concentration following IV ketorolac doses of 15 or 30 mg 4 times daily in healthy adults was approximately 1.1 or 2.2 mcg/mL, respectively. Mean steady-state plasma concentration following oral administration of 10 mg 4 times daily in adults was approximately 0.6 mcg/mL. Steady-state plasma concentrations of ketorolac also generally are reached within 24 hours following multiple dosing with oral ketorolac tromethamine dosages of 12.5 mg 3 times daily; appreciable accumulation of ketorolac does not appear to occur. However, accumulation of ketorolac in special populations (e.g., geriatric, renal failure, or hepatic disease patients) has not been studied.

Following IM administration of ketorolac tromethamine in adults, the onset of analgesic action usually is evident within 10 minutes, and peak analgesia occurs within 75–150 minutes; analgesia may be maintained for up to 6–8 hours. Following oral administration of the drug in adults, onset of analgesic action usually is evident within about 30–60 minutes, peak analgesia occurs within 1.5–4 hours, and analgesia usually is maintained up to 6–8 hours. Although the relationship between plasma ketorolac concentrations and therapeutic effect has not been precisely determined, an estimated therapeutic range of 0.3–5 mcg/mL has been suggested. In adults undergoing dental surgery, pain intensity was reduced by 50% at plasma concentrations of 0.1–0.3 mcg/mL, and adverse effects generally became frequent at concentrations exceeding 5 mcg/mL.

■ **Distribution** Distribution of ketorolac into human body tissues and fluids has not been fully characterized. Following oral administration in mice, ketorolac is distributed into the kidneys, liver, lungs, heart, muscle, gonads, and spleen, with an average tissue/plasma concentration ratio of about 1.5 for the kidney and less than 1 for the other tissues. However, following oral, IM, or IV administration of ketorolac tromethamine in humans, ketorolac does not appear to be distributed widely. The apparent volume of distribution of ketorolac during the terminal elimination phase in healthy adults is approximately 0.15–0.3 L/kg and the volume of distribution at steady state (V_{ss}) is about 0.11–0.33 L/kg following IV, IM, or oral administration. Following IV administration of a single dose of the drug in children 3–18 years of age, the apparent volume of distribution averaged 0.25–0.26 L/kg. Ketorolac appears to cross the blood-brain barrier poorly; CSF concentrations are reported to be about 0.2% of concurrent plasma concentrations. Following topical application of a ketorolac tromethamine gel to the knee, the drug is distributed into synovial fluid, achieving synovial fluid concentrations approximately 50% of those attained in plasma. Ketorolac is more than 99% bound to plasma proteins; the degree of protein binding appears to be independent of plasma concentration of the drug and constant over the therapeutic range of the drug.

Ketorolac crosses the placenta. In pregnant women receiving single 10-mg IM doses of ketorolac tromethamine during labor, cord blood concentrations averaged about 11.6% (range: 4–25%) of maternal plasma concentrations. Ketorolac is distributed into milk, but in relatively small amounts. Following oral administration of a single 10-mg dose of ketorolac tromethamine in nursing women, peak milk ketorolac concentrations of 7.3 ng/mL occurred within about 2 hours, and the milk-to-plasma ratio was about 0.04. Following oral administration of 10-mg of ketorolac tromethamine 4 times daily for 2 days in nursing women, peak milk ketorolac concentrations 2 hours after dosing on the first or second day were 5.2–7.9 ng/mL and the milk-to-plasma ratio ranged from 0.015–0.037.

■ **Elimination** Ketorolac tromethamine dissociates into ketorolac (anion) and tromethamine (cation) at physiologic pH. Following single oral, IM, or IV doses of ketorolac tromethamine in healthy adults, plasma concentrations of ketorolac appear to decline in a biphasic manner with a terminal elimination half-life of about 4–6 hours (range: 2.4–9.2 hours). In a limited number of pediatric patients receiving the drug IV, an elimination half-life of 3.8–6.1 hours has been reported. In geriatric individuals, the elimination half-life was reported to increase to an average of about 5–7 hours (range: 4.3–8.6 hours). The elimination half-life of ketorolac also is prolonged in patients with renal impairment to about 9–10 hours (range: 3.2–19 hours) following oral or IM administration of the drug; in patients undergoing dialysis, elimination half-life of ketorolac tromethamine was about 13.6 hours (range: 8–39.1 hours). There is poor correlation between creatinine clearance and total ketorolac tromethamine clearance in geriatric individuals and in patients with renal impairment. It appears that hepatic impairment (e.g., liver cirrhosis) does not affect substantially the elimination half-life of ketorolac. In patients with liver cirrhosis, elimination half-life of ketorolac was about 5.4 hours (range: 2.2–6.9 hours) and 4.5 hours (range: 1.6–7.6 hours) following IM and oral administration, respectively.

The exact metabolic fate of ketorolac is not clearly established, but the drug undergoes hydroxylation in the liver to form *p*-hydroxyketorolac. This hydroxy metabolite exhibits limited pharmacologic activity, having less than 20 or 1% of the anti-inflammatory or analgesic potency, respectively, of the parent drug. Ketorolac also undergoes conjugation with glucuronic acid. The drug also is metabolized to unidentified polar metabolites, which appear to be pharmacologically inactive probably because of their high polarity and rapid elimination.

Following oral, IM, or IV administration, ketorolac and its metabolites are excreted mainly in urine; only small amounts of the drug and its metabolites are excreted in feces, probably via biliary elimination. Following a single oral or IV dose of ketorolac tromethamine in healthy adults, about 91% of the dose is excreted in urine within 2 days and about 6% in feces within 3 days; most urinary excretion (about 75% of the dose) occurs within about 7 hours. In healthy adults, about 56–60% of a single oral or IV dose is excreted in urine as ketorolac, 20–26% as ketorolac glucuronide, 11–12% as *p*-hydroxyketorolac, and 6–7% as unidentified polar metabolites.

Following IM, IV, or oral administration of the drug in healthy adults, total plasma clearance of ketorolac averages approximately 0.42–0.55 (range: 0.21–0.83) mL/minute per kg. Following single IV doses of ketorolac tromethamine in children 3–18 years of age, plasma clearance of the drug reportedly averaged 0.7–1.13 mL/minute per kg. Total plasma clearance of ketorolac is decreased in patients with reduced renal function. Following IM or oral administration of ketorolac tromethamine in patients with serum creatinine concentrations of 1.9–5 mg/dL, total apparent plasma ketorolac clearance was reduced to about 0.27 (range: 0.1–0.87) mL/minute per kg. Total plasma clearance reportedly also is decreased in geriatric individuals. In geriatric individuals, total apparent plasma clearance of ketorolac averaged 0.32–0.4 (range: 0.22–0.57) mL/minute per kg. It appears that hepatic impairment does not affect total clearance of ketorolac. In a group of patients with liver cirrhosis, total apparent plasma clearance averaged about 0.5 (range: 0.22–1.1) mL/minute per kg.

The effect of hemodialysis and/or peritoneal dialysis on elimination of ketorolac is not known but probably is minimal secondary to the drug's high protein binding. Limited data indicate that following IM administration of the drug in patients undergoing dialysis total apparent plasma clearance of ketorolac averaged 0.27 (range: 0.05–0.6) mL/minute per kg.

Chemistry and Stability

■ **Chemistry** Ketorolac, a pyrrolizine carboxylic acid derivative, is a prototypical nonsteroidal anti-inflammatory agent (NSAIA). The drug is structurally and pharmacologically related to tolmetin, zomepirac, and indomethacin, but unlike these pyrrole acetic acid derivatives, ketorolac is a cyclic propionic acid derivative.

Ketorolac is commercially available as the tromethamine salt. The tromethamine moiety enhances the aqueous solubility of ketorolac. Ketorolac tromethamine is commercially available as a racemic mixture. The analgesic and anti-inflammatory activity of the drug results principally from the levorotatory (*l*) isomer, which has approximately twice the pharmacologic activity of the racemic mixture.

Ketorolac tromethamine occurs as an off-white crystalline powder and has solubilities of 3 mg/mL in alcohol and more than 500 mg/mL in water at 23°C. The pK_a of the drug in water is 3.54.

Ketorolac tromethamine injection is a sterile solution of the drug in alcohol and sterile water for injection. The commercially available injection occurs as a clear, slightly yellow solution; hydrochloric acid and/or sodium hydroxide may be added during manufacture to adjust the pH to 6.9–7.9. About 6.68 or 4.35 mg of sodium chloride is added to each mL of the injection containing 15 or 30 mg of ketorolac tromethamine per mL, respectively, to provide an isotonic solution.

■ **Stability** Ketorolac tromethamine injection and oral tablets should be stored at 15–30°C and protected from light. The tablets also should be stored in well-closed containers and protected from excessive humidity. Prolonged exposure of the injection to light may produce discoloration of the solution and also may promote precipitation of the 1-keto derivative (constituting more than 80% of the light-induced degradation products) and, to a lesser extent, the decarboxy and 1-hydroxy derivatives. In commercially available ketorolac tromethamine injections, air has been replaced with nitrogen; the injections have an expiration date of 24 months following the date of manufacture.

When stored at 15–30°C, ketorolac tromethamine solutions containing 0.6 mg/mL are chemically and physically compatible for at least 48 hours in the following IV solutions: 0.9% sodium chloride, 5% dextrose, 5% dextrose and 0.9% sodium chloride, Ringer's, lactated Ringer's, or Plasma-Lyte® A.

When admixed in the same syringe to produce the concentrations listed, ketorolac tromethamine (15 mg/mL) is incompatible with solutions of drugs such as opiate agonists (e.g., meperidine hydrochloride [50 mg/mL], morphine sulfate [7.5 mg/mL]), promethazine hydrochloride (25 mg/mL), or hydroxyzine hydrochloride (25 mg/mL) that result in a relatively low pH following admixture since precipitation of the NSAIA can occur. Therefore, ketorolac tromethamine should *not* be administered in the same syringe with any such drug solutions.

Preparations

Excipients in commercially available drug preparations may have clinically important effects in some individuals; consult specific product labeling for details.

Ketorolac Tromethamine

Oral		
Tablets, film-coated	10 mg*	**Ketorolac Tromethamine Tablets**
Parenteral		
Injection, for IM or IV use	15 mg/mL*	**Ketorolac Tromethamine Injection**
	30 mg/mL*	**Ketorolac Tromethamine Injection**
Injection, for IM use	30 mg/mL*	**Ketorolac Tromethamine Injection**

*available from one or more manufacturer, distributor, and/or repackager by generic (nonproprietary) name

†Use is not currently included in the labeling approved by the US Food and Drug Administration

Meloxicam

■ Meloxicam is a nonsteroidal anti-inflammatory agent (NSAIA) exhibiting analgesic, antipyretic, and anti-inflammatory actions that has been referred to as a "preferential" rather than "selective" COX-2 inhibitor.

Uses

Meloxicam is used for anti-inflammatory and analgesic effects in the symptomatic treatment of osteoarthritis or rheumatoid arthritis in adults and for the management of the signs and symptoms of pauciarticular or polyarticular course juvenile rheumatoid arthritis in children 2 years of age or older.

The potential benefits and risks of meloxicam therapy as well as alternative therapies should be considered prior to initiating meloxicam therapy. The lowest possible effective dosage and shortest duration of therapy consistent with treatment goals of the patient should be employed.

■ **Osteoarthritis** Meloxicam is used in the symptomatic treatment of osteoarthritis (OA) in adults. Efficacy for the management of the signs and symptoms of OA (e.g., pain, stiffness, quality of life) of the knee or hip has been established in controlled studies of 4 weeks' to 6 months' duration in adults. Efficacy of 7.5 or 15 mg once daily was comparable to that of piroxicam 20 mg daily or 100 mg daily of conventional or extended-release diclofenac. Meloxicam has not been compared with celecoxib in patients with osteoarthritis. For additional information on the management of osteoarthritis, see Uses: Osteoarthritis, in Celecoxib 28:08.04.08.

■ **Rheumatoid Arthritis in Adults** Meloxicam is used for the management of the signs and symptoms of rheumatoid arthritis in adults. In the management of rheumatoid arthritis in adults, NSAIAs may be useful for initial symptomatic treatment; however, NSAIAs do not alter the course of the disease or prevent joint destruction.

Efficacy of meloxicam for the management of rheumatoid arthritis was established in a placebo-controlled, double-blind study of 12 weeks' duration; the primary measure of clinical response in this study was the American College of Rheumatology criteria for a 20% improvement (ACR 20 response) in measures of disease activity. An ACR 20 response is achieved if the patient experiences a 20% improvement in the number of tender and swollen joints and a 20% or greater improvement in at least 3 of the following criteria: patient pain assessment, patient global assessment, physician global assessment, patient self-assessed disability, or laboratory measures of disease activity (i.e., erythrocyte sedimentation rate [ESR] or C-reactive protein [CRP] level). In this study, meloxicam 7.5 or 15 mg daily was substantially more effective than placebo as evaluated by ACR 20 response; the 22. 5-mg daily dosage provided no additional benefit compared with 15 mg daily.

For additional information on the management of rheumatoid arthritis, see Uses: Rheumatoid Arthritis in Adults, in Celecoxib 28:08.04.08.

■ **Juvenile Arthritis** Meloxicam is used for the management of the signs and symptoms of pauciarticular or polyarticular course juvenile rheumatoid arthritis in children 2 years of age or older. Efficacy of meloxicam was established in 2 double-blind, active-controlled studies of 12 weeks' duration; response rates were determined according to the American College of Rheumatology pediatric 30% improvement criteria (ACR pediatric 30; a composite of parent and investigator assessments, number of active joints, number of joints with limited range of motion, disability index, and ESR). Results of these studies indicate that meloxicam is as effective as naproxen in the treatment of juvenile rheumatoid arthritis. In one study, response rates (ACR pediatric 30 criteria) of 77, 76, or 74% were achieved at 12 months in children receiving meloxicam 0.125 mg/kg daily, meloxicam 0.25 mg/kg daily, or naproxen 10 mg/kg daily, respectively.

■ **Other Uses** Meloxicam also has been used in the management of ankylosing spondylitis†.

Dosage and Administration

■ **General** The potential benefits and risks of meloxicam therapy as well as alternative therapies should be considered prior to initiating meloxicam therapy.

■ **Administration** Meloxicam is administered orally once daily, without regard to meals or antacids. The manufacturer states that commercially available meloxicam tablets and oral suspension are bioequivalent. Meloxicam oral suspension should be shaken well prior to dispensing of each dose.

■ **Dosage** The lowest possible effective dosage and shortest duration of therapy consistent with treatment goals of the patient should be employed. Dosage of meloxicam must be carefully adjusted according to individual requirements and response, using the lowest possible effective dosage.

The initial and maintenance dosage of meloxicam for the management of osteoarthritis or rheumatoid arthritis in adults is 7.5 mg once daily. Titration to a maximum dosage of 15 mg once daily may provide additional benefit. Higher dosages (e.g., 22.5 mg daily or greater) were associated with increased adverse GI effects, and the manufacturer recommends that the dosage of meloxicam not exceed 15 mg daily.

For the symptomatic management of juvenile rheumatoid arthritis, the recommended dosage of meloxicam is 0.125 mg/kg (maximum 7.5 mg) once daily. Higher dosages evaluated in clinical studies were not associated with additional benefit.To improve dosing accuracy, meloxicam oral suspension preferably should be used in children who weigh less than 60 kg.

■ **Special Populations** No dosage adjustment is necessary in patients with mild-to-moderate hepatic or renal impairment. Use in patients with severe renal impairment is *not* recommended. Patients with severe hepatic impairment have not been studied.

Cautions

■ **Contraindications** Known hypersensitivity to meloxicam or any ingredient in the formulation. History of urticaria, angioedema, bronchospasm, severe rhinitis, or shock precipitated by aspirin or other nonsteroidal anti-inflammatory agents (NSAIAs). History of aspirin triad (aspirin sensitivity, asthma, and nasal polyps). In the setting of coronary artery bypass graft (CABG) surgery.

■ **Warnings/Precautions** ***Warnings*** **Cardiovascular Effects.** NSAIAs, including selective cyclooxygenase-2 (COX-2) inhibitors and prototypical NSAIAs, increase the risk of serious adverse cardiovascular thrombotic events, including myocardial infarction and stroke (which can be fatal), in patients with or without cardiovascular disease or risk factors for cardiovascular disease.

Findings of an FDA review of published observational studies of NSAIAs, a meta-analysis of published and unpublished data from randomized controlled trials of these drugs, and other published information indicate that NSAIAs may increase the risk of serious adverse cardiovascular thrombotic events by 10–50% or more, depending on the drugs and dosages studied. Available data suggest that the increase in risk may occur early (within the first weeks) following initiation of therapy and may increase with higher dosages and longer durations of use. Although the relative increase in cardiovascular risk appears to be similar in patients with or without known underlying cardiovascular disease or risk factors for cardiovascular disease, the absolute incidence of serious NSAIA-associated cardiovascular thrombotic events is higher in those with cardiovascular disease or risk factors for cardiovascular disease because of their elevated baseline risk.

Results from observational studies utilizing Danish national registry data indicated that patients receiving NSAIAs following a myocardial infarction were at increased risk of reinfarction, cardiovascular-related death, and all-cause mortality beginning in the first week of treatment. Patients who received NSAIAs following myocardial infarction had a higher 1-year mortality rate compared with those who did not receive NSAIAs (20 versus 12 deaths per 100 person-years). Although the absolute mortality rate declined somewhat after the first year following the myocardial infarction, the increased relative risk of death in patients who received NSAIAs persisted over at least the next 4 years of follow-up. Some clinicians suggest that it may be prudent to avoid use of NSAIAs whenever possible in patients with cardiovascular disease. Meloxicam should be avoided in patients with recent myocardial infarction unless the benefits of therapy are expected to outweigh the risk of recurrent cardiovascular thrombotic events; if meloxicam is used in such patients, the patient should be monitored for cardiac ischemia.

In 2 large controlled clinical trials of a selective COX-2 inhibitor for the management of pain in the first 10–14 days following CABG surgery, the incidence of myocardial infarction and stroke was increased. Therefore, NSAIAs are contraindicated in the setting of CABG surgery.

Findings from some systematic reviews of controlled observational studies and meta-analyses of data from randomized studies of NSAIAs suggest that naproxen may be associated with a lower risk of cardiovascular thrombotic events compared with other NSAIAs. However, limitations of these observational studies and the indirect comparisons used to assess cardiovascular risk of the prototypical NSAIAs (e.g., variability in patients' risk factors, comorbid conditions, concomitant drug therapy, drug interactions, dosage, and duration of therapy) affect the validity of the comparisons; in addition, these studies were not designed to demonstrate superior safety of one NSAIA compared with another. Therefore, FDA states that definitive conclusions regarding relative risks of NSAIAs are not possible at this time. (See Cautions: Cardiovascular Effects, in Celecoxib 28:08.04.08.)

To minimize the potential risk of adverse cardiovascular events, NSAIAs should be used at the lowest effective dosage and for the shortest possible duration of therapy. Patients receiving NSAIAs (including those without previous symptoms of cardiovascular disease) should be monitored for the possible development of cardiovascular events throughout therapy.

There is no consistent evidence that concomitant use of low-dose aspirin mitigates the increased risk of serious cardiovascular events associated with NSAIAs.

Hypertension. Use of NSAIAs, including meloxicam, can result in the onset of hypertension or worsening of preexisting hypertension; either of these occurrences may contribute to the increased incidence of cardiovascular events. Patients receiving NSAIAs may have an impaired response to diuretics (i.e., thiazide or loop diuretics), angiotensin-converting enzyme (ACE) inhibitors, angiotensin II receptor antagonists, or β-adrenergic blocking agents. NSAIAs, including meloxicam, should be used with caution in patients with hypertension. Blood pressure should be monitored closely during initiation of meloxicam therapy and throughout therapy.

Heart Failure and Edema. Data from observational studies indicate that use of NSAIAs in patients with heart failure is associated with increased morbidity and mortality. Results from a retrospective study utilizing Danish national registry data indicated that use of selective COX-2 inhibitors or prototypical NSAIAs in patients with chronic heart failure was associated with a dose-dependent increase in the risk of death and an increased risk of hospitalization for myocardial infarction or heart failure. In addition, findings from a meta-analysis of published and unpublished data from randomized controlled trials of NSAIAs indicated that use of selective COX-2 inhibitors or prototypical NSAIAs was associated with an approximate twofold increase in the risk of hospitalization for heart failure. Fluid retention and edema also have been observed in some patients receiving NSAIAs. Use of NSAIAs may diminish the cardiovascular effects of certain drugs used to treat these conditions (e.g., diuretics, ACE inhibitors, angiotensin II receptor antagonists). (See Drug Interactions.)

The manufacturer states that meloxicam should be avoided in patients with severe heart failure unless the benefits of therapy are expected to outweigh the risk of worsening heart failure; if meloxicam is used in such patients, the patient should be monitored for worsening heart failure. Some experts state that use of NSAIAs should be avoided whenever possible in patients with reduced left ventricular ejection fraction and current or prior symptoms of heart failure.

GI Effects. Risk of serious GI effects (e.g., bleeding, ulceration, perforation), which can occur at any time with or without warning signs or symptoms. Conditions or concomitant therapies that may increase risk include a history of GI bleeding or ulceration, longer duration of NSAIA therapy, treatment with anticoagulants or oral corticosteroids, smoking, alcohol dependence, poor general health, or older age (higher risk of fatal GI complications). Use with extreme caution in these patients. In some clinical studies, meloxicam was associated with a lower incidence of adverse GI effects compared with other NSAIAs (e.g., diclofenac, naproxen, piroxicam).

Renal Effects. Renal papillary necrosis or other renal medullary changes may occur with long-term administration of NSAIAs. Possibility of overt renal decompensation in patients dependent on renal prostaglandins for maintenance of renal perfusion. Patients at particular risk include those with heart failure, hepatic or renal dysfunction, or dehydration; those receiving a diuretic, ACE inhibitor, or angiotensin II antagonist; and geriatric patients. Recovery of renal function to pretreatment levels usually occurs following discontinuance of NSAIA therapy.

Sensitivity Reactions Sensitivity reactions, including anaphylactoid reactions, possible in patients without prior exposure to meloxicam. Immediate medical intervention and drug discontinuance required. Cross-sensitivity may exist with other NSAIAs. (See Cautions: Sensitivity Reactions, in the Salicylates General Statement 28:08.04.24.)

Serious skin reactions (e.g., exfoliative dermatitis, Stevens-Johnson syndrome, toxic epidermal necrolysis) can occur in patients receiving meloxicam. These serious skin reactions may occur without warning. Discontinue meloxicam at the first appearance of rash or any other sign of hypersensitivity.

General Precautions Provide the medication guide for NSAIAs to the patient each time the drug is dispensed.

Hepatic Effects. Borderline elevations of one or more liver function tests may occur in up to 15% of patients treated with NSAIAs, including meloxicam; meaningful (3 times the upper limit of normal) elevations of serum ALT (SGPT) or AST (SGOT) reported in approximately 1% of patients receiving other NSAIAs. Severe, sometimes fatal, reactions (e.g., jaundice, fulminant hepatitis, liver necrosis, hepatic failure) reported rarely in patients receiving NSAIAs. Discontinue use if clinical signs and symptoms occur.

Hematologic Effects. Anemia has been reported, principally in patients receiving long-term (e.g., 6 months' duration) therapy with meloxicam. Notable effects on platelets or bleeding times do not appear to occur.

Other Precautions. May mask certain signs of infection; cannot be used as a substitute for corticosteroid therapy nor used to treat adrenal insufficiency.

Specific Populations **Pregnancy.** Category C. (See Users Guide.) Avoid use in the third trimester because of possible premature closure of the ductus arteriosus.

Lactation. Meloxicam is distributed into milk in rats; discontinue nursing or drug because of potential risk in nursing infants.

Pediatric Use. Safety and efficacy not established in children younger than 2 years of age. Safety and efficacy of meloxicam have been established in pediatric patients 2–17 years of age with juvenile rheumatoid arthritis.

Geriatric Use. As with any NSAIA, use with caution.

Severe Renal Impairment. Use not recommended. If meloxicam must be used in patients with advanced renal disease, closely monitor renal function.

■ **Common Adverse Effects** Adverse effects occurring in 2% or more of adults receiving meloxicam include dyspepsia, headache, nausea, diarrhea, upper respiratory tract infection, abdominal pain, dizziness, edema, flatulence, influenza-like illness, musculoskeletal and connective tissue signs and symptoms (back pain, muscle spasms, musculoskeletal pain), and rash.

The most common adverse effects reported in pediatric patients include abdominal pain, vomiting, diarrhea, headache, and pyrexia.

Drug Interactions

■ **ACE Inhibitors and Angiotensin II Receptor Antagonists** Potential pharmacologic interaction (antagonized antihypertensive effects).

■ **Bile Acid Sequestrants** Pharmacokinetic interaction (increased meloxicam clearance; clinical importance not established) when meloxicam is used with bile acid sequestrants (e.g., cholestyramine).

■ **Cimetidine** Pharmacokinetic interaction unlikely.

■ **Digoxin** Pharmacokinetic interaction unlikely.

■ **Diuretics** Patients receiving diuretics may have an increased risk of developing renal failure secondary to decreased renal blood flow resulting from prostaglandin inhibition by NSAIAs. NSAIAs may reduce the natriuretic effects of furosemide and thiazides. Observe patient for signs of renal failure and for diuretic efficacy.

■ **Drugs Affecting Hepatic Microsomal Enzymes** Inhibitors or inducers of CYP2C9 or 3A4; interaction unlikely.

■ **Lithium** Pharmacokinetic interaction (increased plasma lithium concentration).

■ **Methotrexate** Potential pharmacokinetic interaction (enhanced toxicity of methotrexate resulting from inhibition of methotrexate renal elimination). (See Drug Interactions: Nonsteroidal Anti-inflammatory Agents, in Methotrexate 10:00.) No interaction was observed in a study of 12 adults with arthritis receiving concomitant methotrexate (weekly) and meloxicam; however, caution advised with concomitant use of NSAIAs and methotrexate.

■ **Aspirin** Concomitant use of aspirin increases serum meloxicam concentrations; clinical importance of this interaction is unknown. Concomitant use of aspirin and an NSAIA increases the risk for serious GI events. Because of the potential for increased adverse effects, concurrent use of meloxicam and aspirin generally is not recommended. Meloxicam is not a substitute for aspirin for cardioprophylaxis. There is no consistent evidence that use of low-dose aspirin mitigates the increased risk of serious cardiovascular events associated with NSAIAs.

■ **Warfarin** The effects of warfarin and NSAIAs on GI bleeding are synergistic. Concomitant use of an NSAIA and warfarin is associated with a higher risk of GI bleeding compared with use of either agent alone. Caution advised if meloxicam is used concomitantly with warfarin.

Potential pharmacologic interaction (increased adverse effects [e.g., bleeding], potential [though less likely] increased prothrombin time/INR).

Description

Meloxicam, an oxicam derivative that is structurally related to piroxicam, is a nonsteroidal anti-inflammatory agent (NSAIA) exhibiting analgesic, antipyretic, and anti-inflammatory actions. In vitro and in vivo studies indicate that meloxicam inhibits the cyclooxygenase-2 (COX-2) isoform of prostaglandin endoperoxide synthase (prostaglandin G/H synthase [PGHS]) to a greater extent than the COX-1 isoform. However, meloxicam's COX-2 selectivity is dose dependent and is diminished at higher dosages. Therefore meloxicam sometimes has been referred to as a "preferential" rather than "selective" COX-2 inhibitor. For additional information on COX-1 and COX-2, see Pharmacology: Mechanism of Action, in Celecoxib 28:08.04.08.

Meloxicam is extensively metabolized to inactive metabolites in the liver, principally via the cytochrome P-450 (CYP) 2C9 isoenzyme, with minor contribution by CYP3A4. The drug and its metabolites are excreted in urine and feces, and meloxicam undergoes substantial biliary secretion and enterohepatic recirculation.

Advice to Patients

Importance of reading the medication guide for NSAIAs that is provided to the patient each time the drug is dispensed.

Risk of serious cardiovascular toxicity (e.g., myocardial infarction, stroke). Importance of seeking immediate medical attention if signs and symptoms of serious cardiovascular toxicity (chest pain, dyspnea, weakness, slurring of speech) occur.

Risk of GI ulceration or bleeding; importance of reporting any signs or symptoms of GI ulceration or bleeding.

Importance of reporting signs or symptoms of hepatotoxicity, including nausea, fatigue, lethargy, pruritus, jaundice, right upper quadrant tenderness, or flu-like symptoms.

Risk of anaphylactoid and other sensitivity reactions. Importance of reporting signs of hypersensitivity reactions (e.g., skin rash and blisters, fever, pruritus).

Risk of heart failure or edema; importance of reporting dyspnea, unexplained weight gain, or edema.

Importance of informing clinicians of existing or contemplated concomitant therapy, including prescription and OTC drugs.

Importance of women informing clinicians if they are or plan to become pregnant or plan to breast-feed. Risk of use during late pregnancy.

Importance of informing patients of other important precautionary information. (See Cautions.)

Overview (see Users Guide). For additional information until a more detailed monograph is developed and published, the manufacturer's labeling should be consulted. It is *essential* that the manufacturer's labeling be consulted for more detailed information on usual cautions, precautions, contraindications, potential drug interactions, laboratory test interferences, and acute toxicity.

Preparations

Excipients in commercially available drug preparations may have clinically important effects in some individuals; consult specific product labeling for details.

Meloxicam

Oral		
Tablets	7.5 mg*	Meloxicam Tablets
		Mobic®, Boehringer Ingelheim (
	15 mg*	Meloxicam Tablets
		Mobic®, Boehringer Ingelheim (
Suspension	7.5 mg/5 mL	Mobic®, Boehringer Ingelheim

*available from one or more manufacturer, distributor, and/or repackager by generic (nonproprietary) name

†Use is not currently included in the labeling approved by the US Food and Drug Administration

Naproxen
Naproxen Sodium

■ Naproxen and naproxen sodium are prototypical anti-inflammatory agents (NSAIAs) that also exhibit analgesic and antipyretic activity.

Uses

Naproxen and naproxen sodium are used to relieve mild to moderately severe pain. Conventional (immediate-release) and delayed-release (enteric-coated) tablets and suspension formulations of naproxen or naproxen sodium are used for anti-inflammatory and analgesic effects in the symptomatic treatment of rheumatoid arthritis, osteoarthritis, juvenile rheumatoid arthritis, and ankylosing spondylitis. Conventional (immediate-release) tablets and suspension formulations of naproxen or naproxen sodium also are used for the symptomatic treatment of tendinitis, bursitis, acute gout, pain, and primary dysmenorrhea. Suspension formulations of naproxen are preferred for the management of juvenile arthritis since this formulation provides maximum dosage flexibility. Because of the delayed-release properties of enteric-coated naproxen tablets, this formulation is not recommended for the management of acute pain. Extended-release naproxen sodium tablets are used for the symptomatic treatment of rheumatoid arthritis, osteoarthritis, ankylosing spondylitis, tendinitis, bursitis, acute gout, mild to moderately severe pain, and primary dysmenorrhea. (Naproxen 250 mg is approximately equivalent to naproxen sodium 275 mg.) Naproxen sodium also may be used for *self-medication* for anti-inflammatory and analgesic effects to provide temporary relief of *minor* aches and pains, including those associated with arthritis, and of dysmenorrhea and for its antipyretic effect to reduce fever.

The potential benefits and risks of naproxen therapy as well as alternative therapies should be considered prior to initiating naproxen therapy. The lowest possible effective dosage and shortest duration of therapy consistent with treatment goals of the patient should be employed.

■ **Inflammatory Diseases** Naproxen and naproxen sodium are used for anti-inflammatory and analgesic effects in the symptomatic treatment of rheumatoid arthritis, osteoarthritis, juvenile rheumatoid arthritis, and ankylosing spondylitis. Naproxen also is used in fixed combination with esomeprazole magnesium for the symptomatic treatment of rheumatoid arthritis, osteoarthritis, and ankylosing spondylitis in patients at risk of developing gastric ulcers associated with NSAIA therapy. For information on the combined use of naproxen and esomeprazole, see Uses: Prevention of Nonsteroidal Anti-inflammatory Agent-induced Ulcers, in Esomeprazole 56:28.36.

Rheumatoid Arthritis, Juvenile Arthritis, and Osteoarthritis When used in the treatment of rheumatoid arthritis or juvenile rheumatoid arthritis, naproxen has relieved pain and stiffness, reduced swelling, and improved mobility and grip strength. In the treatment of osteoarthritis, naproxen has relieved pain and stiffness and improved knee joint function. Naproxen appears to be only palliative in these conditions and has not been shown to permanently arrest or reverse the underlying disease process. Naproxen sodium also may be used for *self-medication* to provide temporary relief of minor aches and pains associated with arthritis.

Most clinical evaluations of naproxen in the management of rheumatoid arthritis or osteoarthritis have shown that the anti-inflammatory and analgesic effects of usual dosages of naproxen are greater than those of placebo and about equal to those of usual dosages of salicylates, indomethacin, fenoprofen, or ibuprofen. The results of a study in patients with osteoarthritis suggested that naproxen (500 mg twice daily) was less effective than tolmetin (800 mg twice daily) in some measures of pain relief, although improvements in functional ability did not differ. In controlled studies in patients with juvenile rheumatoid arthritis, the anti-inflammatory and analgesic effects of usual dosages of naproxen were comparable to those of usual dosages of aspirin, indomethacin, or piroxicam. Patient response to oral NSAIAs is variable; patients who do not respond to or cannot tolerate one NSAIA might be successfully treated with a different agent. However, NSAIAs are generally contraindicated in patients in whom sensitivity reactions (e.g., urticaria, bronchospasm, severe rhinitis) are precipitated by aspirin or other NSAIAs. (See Cautions: Precautions and Contraindications.)

In the management of rheumatoid arthritis in adults, NSAIAs may be useful for initial symptomatic treatment; however, NSAIAs do not alter the course of the disease or prevent joint destruction. Disease modifying antirheumatic drugs (DMARDs) (e.g., azathioprine, cyclosporine, etanercept, oral or injectable gold compounds, hydroxychloroquine, infliximab, leflunomide, methotrexate, minocycline, penicillamine, sulfasalazine) have the potential to reduce or prevent joint damage, preserve joint integrity and function, and reduce total health care costs, and all patients with rheumatoid arthritis are candidates for DMARD therapy. DMARDs should be initiated early in the disease course and should not be delayed beyond 3 months in patients with active disease (i.e., ongoing joint pain, substantial morning stiffness, fatigue, active synovitis, persistent elevation of erythrocyte sedimentation rate [ESR] or C-reactive protein [CRP], radiographic evidence of joint damage) despite an adequate regimen of NSAIAs. NSAIA therapy may be continued in conjunction with DMARD therapy or, depending on patient response, may be discontinued. For further information on the treatment of rheumatoid arthritis, see Uses: Rheumatoid Arthritis in Methotrexate 10:00.

The manufacturers state that naproxen and its salt may be used safely in conjunction with gold compounds and/or corticosteroids in the treatment of rheumatoid arthritis. The manufacturers state that combined use of naproxen or its salt and corticosteroids has not resulted in greater improvement than with steroids alone, although addition of naproxen or its salt to a regimen of gold compounds has resulted in greater improvement than with gold salts alone.

Use of naproxen or its salt with aspirin is not recommended by the manufacturers. There is inadequate proof that the combination is more efficacious than either drug alone, and the potential for adverse reactions may be increased. (See Drug Interactions: Nonsteroidal Anti-inflammatory Agents.)

Ankylosing Spondylitis When used in patients with ankylosing spondylitis, naproxen has relieved night pain, morning stiffness, and pain at rest. In a limited number of controlled studies, the anti-inflammatory and analgesic effects of usual dosages of naproxen in the symptomatic treatment of ankylosing spondylitis were greater than those of placebo and comparable to those of usual dosages of aspirin or phenylbutazone (no longer commercially available in the US).

Other Inflammatory Conditions Naproxen has been used effectively to relieve pain, fever, redness, swelling, and tenderness in patients with acute gouty arthritis.

When used in the treatment of acute painful shoulder, the anti-inflammatory and analgesic effects of naproxen sodium are greater than those of placebo and about equal to those of indomethacin. When used in the treatment of tendinitis and bursitis, the anti-inflammatory and analgesic effects of usual dosages of naproxen sodium are comparable to those of usual dosages of oxyphenbutazone (no longer commercially available in the US).

■ **Pain** Naproxen and its salt are used to relieve postoperative pain (including that associated with dental surgery), postpartum pain, primary dysmenorrhea, pain following insertion of an intrauterine contraceptive device, orthopedic pain, headache (including migraine), and visceral pain associated with cancer. Naproxen sodium also may be used for *self-medication* to provide temporary relief of minor aches and pains associated with the common cold, headache, toothache, muscular aches, and backache.

There are few published studies comparing the effectiveness of naproxen and its salt with other analgesics in the relief of nonarthritic pain. In one study, a single 275-mg oral dose of naproxen sodium was as effective as a single 650-mg oral dose of aspirin in the relief of postpartum uterine pain. In another study, when used to relieve postoperative or orthopedic pain, 550 mg of oral naproxen sodium followed by 275 mg every 6 hours was at least as effective as 650 mg of acetaminophen orally every 6 hours or 50 mg of pentazocine orally every 6 hours; in this study, the onset of action appeared to be more rapid for naproxen sodium than for acetaminophen or pentazocine. In another study of patients with postoperative pain, the analgesic effects of 550 mg of oral naproxen sodium and 60 mg of oral codeine sulfate were additive (the combination was more effective than either drug alone).

Some experts state that an NSAIA (e.g., naproxen or its salt) is a reasonable first-line therapy for mild to moderate migraine attacks or for severe attacks that have responded in the past to similar NSAIAs or non-opiate analgesics. When used for prophylaxis† of migraine headache, naproxen and its salt appear to have a modest effect on headache frequency, intensity, and/or duration. For further information on management and classification of migraine headache and on efficacy of concomitant naproxen sodium and sumatriptan therapy, see Uses: Vascular Headaches, in Sumatriptan 28:32.28.

■ **Dysmenorrhea** When used to relieve dysmenorrhea, including that which develops after insertion of an intrauterine contraceptive device, an oral dosage of 500 mg of naproxen or 550 mg of naproxen sodium followed by 250 mg of naproxen or 275 mg of naproxen sodium every 6 hours, respectively, has been reported to be more effective than placebo or aspirin (650 mg 4 times daily). In a placebo-controlled study of women with primary menorrhagia† or menorrhagia associated with intrauterine contraceptive devices†, administration of naproxen (750 mg daily for the first 2 days of menstrual bleeding followed by 500 mg daily thereafter for up to 7 days) resulted in a reduction of blood loss.In one controlled study in patients with postpartum pain, a single oral dose of 550 mg of naproxen sodium appeared to provide greater pain relief after 4 and 5 hours than 500 mg of naproxen; however, there was no difference in onset of analgesia.

Naproxen sodium also may be used for *self-medication* to provide temporary relief of manifestations of dysmenorrhea (e.g., menstrual cramps).

■ **Other Uses** Naproxen sodium has been used in adults for *self-medication* as an antipyretic. The drug also has been used as an antipyretic in children; one study indicates that a single oral dose of naproxen (2.5 or 7.5 mg/kg) was at least as effective as a single oral dose of aspirin (15 mg/kg) in the reduction of fever in children. The results of one study suggested that the combination of naproxen sodium and ampicillin was more effective than ampicillin alone in alleviating fever, dyspnea, and coughing associated with acute respiratory infections in children†.

Naproxen has been used in the symptomatic management of osteitis deformans† (Paget's disease of bone) and Bartter's syndrome†.

Results from a large, prospective, population-based cohort study in geriatric individuals indicate a lower prevalence of Alzheimer's disease† among patients who received an NSAIA for 2 years or longer. Similar findings have been reported from some other, but not all, observational studies.

Dosage and Administration

■ **Administration** The potential benefits and risks of naproxen therapy as well as alternative therapies should be considered prior to initiating naproxen therapy.

Naproxen and naproxen sodium are administered orally. Enteric-coated tablets of naproxen should not be broken, crushed, or chewed, so that the delayed-release properties of this formulation are maintained. Adverse GI effects may be minimized by administering the drugs with meals, milk, or a magnesium and aluminum hydroxides antacid. When used for *self-medication*, the manufacturer recommends that each dose of naproxen sodium be taken with a full glass of water. Tablets containing naproxen sodium in fixed combination with sumatriptan succinate may be administered without regard to meals; the tablets should not be split, crushed, or chewed. Tablets containing delayed-release naproxen in fixed combination with immediate-release esomeprazole magnesium should be swallowed whole with liquid and administered at least 30 minutes before meals; the tablets should not be split, chewed, crushed, or dissolved. Because of the delayed-release properties of enteric-coated formulations, enteric-coated preparations of naproxen are not recommended for the management of acute pain. Also, the manufacturer states that because naproxen sodium is absorbed more rapidly than naproxen, the sodium salt conventional tablet formulation is recommended for the management of acute painful conditions when prompt onset of pain relief is desired.

■ **Dosage** The lowest possible effective dosage and shortest duration of therapy consistent with treatment goals of the patient should be employed. Dosage of naproxen must be carefully adjusted according to individual requirements and response, using the lowest possible effective dosage. Lower dosages of the drug should be considered in patients with renal or hepatic impairment or in geriatric patients. Use of naproxen or naproxen sodium in patients with moderate to severe renal impairment (creatinine clearance less than 30 mL/minute) is not recommended. The commercially available preparation containing naproxen in fixed combination with esomeprazole magnesium is not recommended for patients with severe hepatic impairment because the appropriate esomeprazole dosage is not available as a fixed-ratio preparation for twice-daily dosing. In addition, the commercially available preparation containing naproxen sodium in fixed combination with sumatriptan succinate should not be used in patients with hepatic impairment since sumatriptan dosage cannot be appropriately adjusted.

Patients receiving naproxen for *self-medication* should be advised to use the lowest effective dosage and not to exceed the recommended dosage or duration of therapy.

Patients should be warned that the risk of GI bleeding is increased when recommended durations of *self-medication* are exceeded and when more than one NSAIA are used concomitantly.

Each 220, 275, 412.5, or 550 mg of naproxen sodium is approximately equivalent to 200, 250, 375, or 500 mg of naproxen, respectively.

Different dose strengths and formulations are not necessarily bioequivalent, and this should be considered when changing from one strength to another or from one formulation to another.

Inflammatory Diseases **Rheumatoid Arthritis, Osteoarthritis, and Ankylosing Spondylitis.** For the symptomatic treatment of osteoarthritis, rheumatoid arthritis, or ankylosing spondylitis, but excluding acute gouty arthritis), the usual adult dosage of naproxen is 250–500 mg (275–550 mg of naproxen sodium) twice daily in the morning and evening. Alternatively, 250 mg of naproxen (275 mg of naproxen sodium) may be given in the morning, and 500 mg (550 mg of the sodium salt) may be given in the evening. It is not necessary to administer either drug more often than twice daily, and morning and evening doses do not have to be equal in size.

The usual adult dosage of extended-release naproxen tablets is 750 mg or 1 g (825 mg or 1.1 g of naproxen sodium) administered once daily. Patients receiving other naproxen dosage forms twice daily may be switched to the extended-release naproxen sodium tablets by replacing their total daily dosage with an equal dosage of the extended-release formulation and then administered once daily.

Subsequent dosage of naproxen or naproxen sodium should be adjusted according to the patient's response and tolerance. In patients who tolerate lower dosages well, the dosage of naproxen may be increased to 1.5 g (1.65 g of naproxen sodium) daily for limited periods of time (up to 6 months) when a greater level of anti-inflammatory and/or analgesic activity is necessary; when a dosage of 1.5 g (1.65 g of the sodium salt) daily is administered, an adequate increase in clinical benefit should be evident to justify potential increased risks associated with this dosage. Symptomatic improvement usually begins within 2 weeks after beginning therapy. If improvement does not occur within 2 weeks, an additional 2 weeks of therapy may be tried.

When naproxen is used in fixed combination with esomeprazole magnesium for the symptomatic relief of rheumatoid arthritis, osteoarthritis, or ankylosing spondylitis, the recommended adult dosage of naproxen is 375 or 500 mg twice daily.

For *self-medication* to provide temporary relief of pain associated with arthritis, adults 65 years of age and younger can receive 200 mg of naproxen (220 mg of naproxen sodium) every 8–12 hours or 400 mg (440 mg of the sodium salt) initially and 200 mg (220 mg of the sodium salt) 12 hours later; dosage should not exceed 600 mg of naproxen (660 mg of naproxen sodium) daily for *self-medication* in these adults unless otherwise directed by a clinician. In older adults, dosage for *self-medication* should not exceed 200 mg of naproxen (220 mg of naproxen sodium) every 12 hours unless otherwise directed by a clinician. Such *self-medication* should not exceed 10 days unless otherwise directed.

Juvenile Arthritis. For the symptomatic treatment of juvenile rheumatoid arthritis, the recommended dosage of naproxen is approximately 10 mg/kg daily given in 2 divided doses. Because naproxen and naproxen sodium tablets are not well suited for providing the calculated pediatric dosage of the drug, naproxen oral suspension preferably should be used in this age group. (See Cautions: Pediatric Precautions.)

Other Inflammatory Conditions. For the symptomatic treatment of acute gouty arthritis, the usual adult dosage of naproxen is 750 mg (825 mg of naproxen sodium) initially followed by 250 mg (275 mg of naproxen sodium) every 8 hours; therapy is continued until the attack subsides. Alternatively, in the management of acute gout, an initial dosage of 1–1.5 g of naproxen (using extended-release naproxen sodium tablets) may be used (as a single dose) on the first day, followed by 1 g given once daily until the attack subsides. The manufacturer states that delayed-release (enteric-coated) naproxen tablets are not recommended for treatment of acute gout because of the delayed absorption of the drug from this preparation. Relief of pain and tenderness and decreases in heat and swelling have been reported to occur within 24–48 hours.

For the relief of tendinitis or bursitis, the usual initial adult dose of naproxen is 500 mg (550 mg of naproxen sodium), followed by 500 mg (550 mg of the sodium salt) every 12 hours or 250 mg (275 mg of the sodium salt) every 6–8 hours as necessary. Total initial daily dose should not exceed 1.25 g of naproxen (1.375 g of naproxen sodium). Alternatively, the usual adult oral dosage of naproxen from extended-release tablets is 1 g (1.1 g of naproxen sodium) administered once daily. If adequate response does not occur, dosage of the extended-release tablets may be increased to 1.5 g of naproxen daily; however, such dosages should be used for a limited period only. Thereafter, the total daily dose should not exceed 1 g of naproxen (1.1 g of naproxen sodium).

Pain and Dysmenorrhea For relief of mild to moderate pain or dysmenorrhea, the usual initial adult dose of naproxen is 500 mg (550 mg of naproxen sodium), followed by 500 mg (550 mg of the sodium salt) every 12 hours or 250 mg (275 mg of the sodium salt) every 6–8 hours as necessary. Total initial daily dose should not exceed 1.25 g of naproxen (1.375 g of naproxen sodium). Alternatively, the usual adult oral dosage of naproxen from extended-release tablets is 1 g (1.1 g of naproxen sodium) administered once daily. If adequate response does not occur, dosage of the extended-release tablets may be increased to 1.5 g of naproxen daily; however, such dosages should be used for a limited period only. Thereafter, the total daily dose should not exceed 1 g of naproxen (1.1 g of naproxen sodium).

Alternatively, for *self-medication* of these conditions in adults 65 years of age and younger, a naproxen dosage of 200 mg (220 mg of naproxen sodium) every 8–12 hours can be used. Some patients may experience greater relief with an initial dose of 400 mg (440 mg of the sodium salt) and then 200 mg (220 mg of the sodium salt) 12 hours later. Regardless of the regimen employed, dosage for *self-medication* should not exceed 600 mg of naproxen (660 mg of naproxen sodium) daily unless otherwise directed by a clinician. For adults older than 65 years of age, dosage for *self-medication* should not exceed 200 mg (220 mg of the sodium salt) every 12 hours unless otherwise directed by a clinician. *Self-medication* of pain should not exceed 10 days unless otherwise directed.

When naproxen sodium is used in fixed combination with sumatriptan succinate for the acute management of migraine attacks in adults, the recommended dosage of naproxen sodium is 500 mg (given in fixed combination with sumatriptan 85 mg) as a single dose. Efficacy of more than 1 dose has not been established. If a second dose is administered, an interval of at least 2 hours should elapse between the first and second doses. No more than 2 doses (total sumatriptan dosage of 170 mg) should be administered in any 24-hour period. The safety of treating an average of more than 5 headaches per 30-day period has not been established.

Fever For *self-medication* of fever, the usual dosage recommended for *self-medication* of pain can be used. (See Dosage: Pain and Dysmenorrhea, in Dosage and Administration.) Antipyretic therapy with naproxen sodium should not exceed 3 days for *self-medication* unless otherwise directed by a clinician.

Cautions

■ Cardiovascular Effects Peripheral edema has occurred in patients receiving naproxen; congestive heart failure, palpitations, vasculitis, tachycardia, and dyspnea have occurred less frequently. Increases in blood pressure have been reported in patients receiving naproxen.

Nonsteroidal anti-inflammatory agents (NSAIAs), including selective cyclooxygenase-2 (COX-2) inhibitors and prototypical NSAIAs, increase the risk of serious adverse cardiovascular thrombotic events, including myocardial infarction and stroke (which can be fatal), in patients with or without cardiovascular disease or risk factors for cardiovascular disease. Use of NSAIAs also is associated with an increased risk of heart failure.

The association between cardiovascular complications and use of NSAIAs is an area of ongoing concern and study. Findings of an FDA review of published observational studies of NSAIAs, a meta-analysis of published and unpublished data from randomized controlled trials of these drugs, and other published information indicate that NSAIAs may increase the risk of serious adverse cardiovascular thrombotic events by 10–50% or more, depending on the drugs and dosages studied. Available data suggest that the increase in risk may occur early (within the first weeks) following initiation of therapy and may increase with higher dosages and longer durations of use. Although the relative increase in cardiovascular risk appears to be similar in patients with or without known underlying cardiovascular disease or risk factors for cardiovascular disease, the absolute incidence of serious NSAIA-associated cardiovascular thrombotic events is higher in those with cardiovascular disease or risk factors for cardiovascular disease because of their elevated baseline risk.

Results from observational studies utilizing Danish national registry data indicated that patients receiving NSAIAs following a myocardial infarction were at increased risk of reinfarction, cardiovascular-related death, and all-cause mortality beginning in the first week of treatment. Patients who received NSAIAs following myocardial infarction had a higher 1-year mortality rate compared with those who did not receive NSAIAs (20 versus 12 deaths per 100 person-years). Although the absolute mortality rate declined somewhat after the first year following the myocardial infarction, the increased relative risk of death in patients who received NSAIAs persisted over at least the next 4 years of follow-up.

In 2 large controlled clinical trials of a selective COX-2 inhibitor for the management of pain in the first 10–14 days following coronary artery bypass graft (CABG) surgery, the incidence of myocardial infarction and stroke was increased. Therefore, NSAIAs are contraindicated in the setting of CABG surgery.

Findings from some systematic reviews of controlled observational studies and meta-analyses of data from randomized studies of NSAIAs suggest that naproxen may be associated with a lower risk of cardiovascular thrombotic events compared with other NSAIAs. However, limitations of these observational studies and the indirect comparisons used to assess cardiovascular risk of the prototypical NSAIAs (e.g., variability in patients' risk factors, comorbid conditions, concomitant drug therapy, drug interactions, dosage, and duration of therapy) affect the validity of the comparisons; in addition, these studies were not designed to demonstrate superior safety of one NSAIA compared with another. Therefore, FDA states that definitive conclusions regarding relative risks of NSAIAs are not possible at this time. (See Cautions: Cardiovascular Effects, in Celecoxib 28:08.04.08.)

Data from observational studies also indicate that use of NSAIAs in patients with heart failure is associated with increased morbidity and mortality. Results from a retrospective study utilizing Danish national registry data indicated that use of selective COX-2 inhibitors or prototypical NSAIAs in patients with chronic heart failure was associated with a dose-dependent increase in the risk of death and an increased risk of hospitalization for myocardial infarction or heart failure. In addition, findings from a meta-analysis of published and unpublished data from randomized controlled trials of NSAIAs indicated that use of selective COX-2 inhibitors or prototypical NSAIAs was associated with an approximate twofold increase in the risk of hospitalization for heart failure. Fluid retention and edema also have been observed in some patients receiving NSAIAs.

There is no consistent evidence that use of low-dose aspirin mitigates the increased risk of serious cardiovascular events associated with NSAIAs.

■ GI Effects Adverse reactions to naproxen mainly involve the GI tract. Constipation, heartburn, abdominal pain, and nausea occur in about 3–9% of patients receiving the drug. Less frequently, dyspepsia, diarrhea, stomatitis, vomiting, anorexia, colitis, peptic ulcer, GI bleeding/perforation, hematemesis, and flatulence occur. In patients with rheumatoid arthritis, adverse GI effects appear to be more frequent and more severe at a naproxen dosage of 1.5 g (1.65 g of naproxen sodium) daily than at 750 mg (825 mg of naproxen sodium) daily. The frequency of adverse GI effects in children appears to be similar to that in adults. Adverse GI effects may be minimized by administering naproxen with meals, milk, or an aluminum and magnesium hydroxides antacid.

Naproxen may reactivate latent peptic ulcer and may cause peptic ulcers in patients with no previous history of ulcers. Hemorrhage and perforation of ulcers may occur, occasionally causing fatalities. Hematemesis, GI bleeding without obvious ulcer formation, and melena also have occurred. Prodromal symptoms do not always precede GI bleeding. Ulcerative stomatitis, esophagitis, and nonpeptic GI ulceration have been reported during postmarketing experience. Although a causal relationship has not been directly determined, one case-control analysis suggests that NSAIAs may contribute to the formation of esophageal stricture in patients with gastroesophageal reflux.

The risk of GI bleeding is increased in geriatric patients older than 60 years of age and in patients with a history of GI ulcers or bleeding, those receiving an anticoagulant or taking multiple NSAIAs concomitantly, those consuming 3 or more alcohol-containing beverages daily, and those receiving prolonged therapy.

Clinical studies of conventional versus delayed-release (enteric-coated) naproxen tablets demonstrated similar prevalence of minor GI complaints; however, individual patients may prefer one formulation over the other. In a dosage of 500 mg daily, naproxen has been reported to produce fewer adverse GI effects than 3.6–4.8 g of aspirin daily. In one study, a single dose of 550 mg of naproxen sodium produced fewer adverse GI effects than a single dose of 650 mg of aspirin. It is not known whether naproxen causes less peptic ulceration than does aspirin. In one study, the amount of GI bleeding as determined by fecal blood loss and gastroscopic evaluation in healthy adults was reported to be less with 1 g of naproxen or 1.1 g of naproxen sodium daily than with 3.25 g of aspirin daily. In another study in patients with rheumatoid arthritis, fecal blood loss following 750 mg of naproxen daily was less than that following 3.6 g of aspirin daily and no different than that during the control period. The frequency of adverse GI effects in patients receiving 500 mg of naproxen or 550 mg of naproxen sodium daily is reportedly similar to that in patients receiving 1.2 g of ibuprofen daily and less than that in patients receiving 100 mg of indomethacin daily or 2.4 g of fenoprofen daily.

Serious adverse GI effects (e.g., bleeding, ulceration, perforation) can occur at any time in patients receiving NSAIA therapy, and such effects may *not* be preceded by warning signs or symptoms. Only 1 in 5 patients who develop a serious upper GI adverse event while receiving an NSAIA is symptomatic. Therefore, clinicians should remain alert to the possible development of serious GI effects (e.g., bleeding, ulceration) in any patient receiving NSAIA therapy, and such patients should be followed chronically for the development of manifestations of such effects and advised of the importance of this follow-up. In addition, patients should be advised about the signs and symptoms of serious NSAIA-induced GI toxicity and what action to take if they occur. If signs and symptoms of a serious GI event develop, additional evaluation and treatment should be initiated promptly; the NSAIA should be discontinued until appropriate diagnostic studies have ruled out a serious GI event.

Results of studies to date are inconclusive concerning the relative risk of various prototypical NSAIAs in causing serious GI effects. In patients receiving NSAIAs and observed in clinical studies of several months' to 2 years' duration, symptomatic upper GI ulcers, gross bleeding, or perforation appeared to occur in approximately 1% of patients treated for 3–6 months and in about 2–4% of those treated for 1 year. Longer duration of therapy with an NSAIA increases the likelihood of a serious GI event. However, short-term therapy is not without risk. High dosages of any NSAIA probably are associated with increased risk of such effects, although controlled studies documenting this probable association are lacking for most NSAIAs. Therefore, whenever use of relatively high dosages (within the recommended dosage range) is considered, sufficient benefit to offset the potential increased risk of GI toxicity should be anticipated.

Studies have shown that patients with a history of peptic ulcer disease and/or GI bleeding who are receiving NSAIAs have a substantially higher risk of developing GI bleeding than patients without these risk factors. In addition to a history of ulcer disease, pharmacoepidemiologic studies have identified several comorbid conditions and concomitant therapies that may increase the risk for GI bleeding, including concomitant use of oral corticosteroids or anticoagulants, longer duration of NSAIA therapy, smoking, alcoholism, older age, and poor general health status. Patients with rheumatoid arthritis are more likely to experience serious GI complications from NSAIA therapy than are patients with osteoarthritis. In addition, geriatric or debilitated patients appear to tolerate GI ulceration and bleeding less well than other individuals, and most spontaneous reports of fatal GI effects have been in such patients.

For patients at high risk for complications from NSAIA-induced GI ulceration (e.g., bleeding, perforation), concomitant use of misoprostol can be considered for preventive therapy (See Misoprostol 56:28.28.) Alternatively, some clinicians suggest that a proton-pump inhibitor (e.g., esomeprazole, omeprazole) may be used concomitantly to decrease the incidence of serious GI toxicity associated with NSAIA therapy. (See Esomeprazole 56:28.36.) In one study, therapy with high dosages of famotidine (40 mg twice daily) was more effective than placebo in preventing peptic ulcers in NSAIA-treated patients; however, the effect of the drug was modest. In addition, efficacy of usual dosages of H_2-receptor antagonists for the prevention of NSAIA-induced gastric and duodenal ulcers has not been established. Therefore, most clinicians do not recommend use of H_2-receptor antagonists for the prevention of NSAIA-associated ulcers. Another approach in high-risk patients who would benefit from NSAIA therapy is use of an NSAIA that is a selective inhibitor of COX-2 (e.g., celecoxib), since these agents are associated with a lower incidence of serious GI bleeding than are prototypical NSAIAs. However, while celecoxib (200 mg twice daily) was comparably effective to diclofenac sodium (75 mg twice daily) plus omeprazole (20 mg daily) in preventing recurrent ulcer bleeding (recurrent ulcer bleeding probabilities of 4.9 versus 6.4%, respectively, during the 6-month study) in *H. pylori*-negative arthritis (principally osteoarthritis) patients with a recent history of ulcer bleeding, the protective efficacy was unexpectedly low for both regimens and it appeared that neither could completely protect patients at high risk. Additional study is necessary to elucidate optimal therapy for preventing GI complications associated with NSAIA therapy in high-risk patients.

■ Nervous System Effects Adverse nervous system effects of naproxen include headache, drowsiness, and dizziness, which occur in about 3–9% of patients. Vertigo, lightheadedness, inability to concentrate, mental depression, nervousness, irritability, fatigue, malaise, insomnia, sleep disorders, dream abnormalities, and aseptic meningitis may also occur. Although a causal relationship to naproxen has not been definitely established, reversible peripheral neuropathy, cognitive dysfunction, and seizures have occurred rarely in patients receiving the drug. The frequency of adverse nervous system effects in children appears to be similar to that in adults.

■ **Otic and Ocular Effects** Patients receiving naproxen have experienced tinnitus and, less frequently, other hearing or visual disturbances (e.g., hearing impairment). Corneal opacity, papillitis, papilledema, and retrobulbar optic neuritis have been reported during postmarketing experience.

■ **Hematologic Effects** Adverse hematologic effects of naproxen include thrombocytopenia, leukopenia, granulocytopenia, and eosinophilia. Although a causal relationship to naproxen has not been established, agranulocytosis, aplastic anemia, and hemolytic anemia have occurred in patients receiving the drug. Naproxen can inhibit platelet aggregation and may prolong bleeding time. The frequency of prolonged bleeding time may be greater in children than in adults.

■ **Renal and Electrolyte Effects** Renal disease, glomerulonephritis, interstitial nephritis, nephrotic syndrome, renal failure, renal papillary necrosis, dysuria, and hyperkalemia have been reported in patients receiving naproxen. Abnormal laboratory findings include hematuria and asymptomatic increases in BUN and serum creatinine. In one patient who developed increased serum creatinine concentration and decreased creatinine clearance during naproxen therapy, these measurements returned to pretreatment values following discontinuance of the drug and remained within normal limits after sulindac therapy was started. Chronic high doses of naproxen have caused nephritis and cortical and papillary necrosis in animals.

■ **Hepatic Effects** Jaundice (including cholestatic jaundice which cleared promptly when naproxen was discontinued) and fatal hepatitis have been reported rarely in patients receiving the drug. Abnormal liver function test results, including mild and generally transient increases in serum alkaline phosphatase, have occurred in some patients.

Borderline elevations of one or more liver function test results may occur in up to 15% of patients treated with NSAIAs; meaningful (3 times the upper limit of normal) elevations of serum ALT (SGPT) or AST (SGOT) concentration have occurred in less than 1% of patients receiving NSAIAs in controlled clinical studies. These abnormalities may progress, may remain essentially unchanged, or may be transient with continued therapy. Naproxen or naproxen sodium should be discontinued if signs or symptoms of a severe hepatic reaction occur. (See Cautions: Precautions and Contraindications.)

■ **Dermatologic Effects** Pruritus, skin eruptions or rashes, and ecchymoses occur frequently during naproxen administration. Sweating, photosensitive dermatitis, photosensitivity reactions resembling porphyria cutanea tarda and epidermolysis bullosa, and purpura have also occurred occasionally. The frequency of rash may be greater in children than in adults. Toxic epidermal necrolysis, erythema multiforme, Stevens-Johnson syndrome, urticaria, alopecia, erythema nodosum, fixed drug eruption, lichen planus, and pustular reaction have been reported during postmarketing experience.

■ **Other Adverse Effects** Thirst, myalgia, muscle weakness and cramps, pyrexia, sore throat, eosinophilic pneumonitis or colitis, anaphylactoid reactions, pancreatitis, and menstrual disturbances also have been reported during naproxen therapy. Hypoglycemia, hyperglycemia, angioedema, systemic lupus erythematosus, vasculitis, asthma, pulmonary edema, and female infertility have been reported during postmarketing experience. In a patient receiving naproxen in combination with aspirin, infective symptoms associated with an empyema appeared to be suppressed.

■ **Precautions and Contraindications** With the exception of precautions related to the sodium content of naproxen sodium, the cautions associated with naproxen sodium use are the same as those for naproxen use. Each 220-, 275-, 412.5, or 550-mg naproxen sodium tablet contains about 0.87, 1, 1.5, or 2 mEq of sodium, respectively, and each mL of the commercially available naproxen suspension contains about 0.3 mEq of sodium; this should be considered in patients whose sodium intake must be restricted. Multiple naproxen-containing preparations (e.g., naproxen conventional and delayed-release [enteric-coated] tablets, naproxen suspension, naproxen sodium conventional and extended-release tablets) should not be used concomitantly, as all of these products circulate in the plasma as naproxen anion and may result in naproxen toxicity.

When naproxen or naproxen sodium is used in fixed combination with other drugs (e.g., esomeprazole magnesium, sumatriptan succinate), the usual cautions, precautions, and contraindications associated with the concomitant agent must be considered in addition to those associated with naproxen.

Patients should be advised that naproxen, like other NSAIAs, is not free of potential adverse effects, including some that can cause discomfort, and that more serious effects (e.g., myocardial infarction, stroke, GI bleeding), which may require hospitalization and may even be fatal, can occur. Patients also should be informed that, while NSAIAs may be commonly employed for conditions that are less serious, NSAIA therapy often is considered essential for the management of some diseases, and the drugs have a major role in the management of pain. Clinicians may wish to discuss with their patients the potential risks and likely benefits of NSAIA therapy, particularly when consideration is being given to use of these drugs in less serious conditions for which therapy without an NSAIA may represent an acceptable alternative to both the patient and clinician.

Patients should be advised to read the medication guide for NSAIAs that is provided to the patient each time the drug is dispensed.

NSAIAs increase the risk of serious adverse cardiovascular thrombotic events. (See Cautions: Cardiovascular Effects.) To minimize the potential risk of adverse cardiovascular events, the lowest effective dosage and shortest possible duration of therapy should be employed. Some clinicians suggest that it may be prudent to avoid use of NSAIAs whenever possible in patients with cardiovascular disease. Patients receiving NSAIAs (including those without previous symptoms of cardiovascular disease) should be monitored for the possible development of cardiovascular events throughout therapy. Patients should be informed about the signs and symptoms of serious cardiovascular toxicity (chest pain, dyspnea, weakness, slurring of speech) and instructed to seek immediate medical attention if such toxicity occurs. Naproxen should be avoided in patients with recent myocardial infarction unless the benefits of therapy are expected to outweigh the risk of recurrent cardiovascular thrombotic events; if naproxen is used in such patients, the patient should be monitored for cardiac ischemia.

There is no consistent evidence that concomitant use of low-dose aspirin mitigates the increased risk of serious cardiovascular events associated with NSAIAs. Concomitant use of aspirin and an NSAIA increases the risk for serious GI events. Because of the potential for increased adverse effects, patients receiving an NSAIA should be advised not to take aspirin.

Use of NSAIAs can result in the onset of hypertension or worsening of preexisting hypertension; either of these occurrences may contribute to the increased incidence of cardiovascular events. Patients receiving NSAIAs may have an impaired response to diuretics (i.e., thiazide or loop diuretics), angiotensin-converting enzyme (ACE) inhibitors, angiotensin II receptor antagonists, or β-adrenergic blocking agents. NSAIAs should be used with caution in patients with hypertension. Blood pressure should be monitored closely during initiation of NSAIA therapy and throughout therapy.

Because NSAIAs increase morbidity and mortality in patients with heart failure, the manufacturer states that naproxen should be avoided in patients with severe heart failure unless the benefits of therapy are expected to outweigh the risk of worsening heart failure; if naproxen is used in such patients, the patient should be monitored for worsening heart failure. Some experts state that use of NSAIAs should be avoided whenever possible in patients with reduced left ventricular ejection fraction and current or prior symptoms of heart failure. Patients receiving NSAIAs should be advised to inform their clinician if they experience symptoms of heart failure, including dyspnea, unexplained weight gain, and edema. Use of NSAIAs may diminish the cardiovascular effects of certain drugs used to treat heart failure and edema (e.g., diuretics, ACE inhibitors, angiotensin II receptor antagonists). (See Drug Interactions.)

The risk of potentially serious adverse GI effects should be considered in patients receiving naproxen, particularly in patients receiving chronic therapy with the drug. (See Cautions: GI Effects.) Naproxen should be used with caution and under close supervision in patients with a history of GI disease. Since peptic ulceration and/or GI bleeding have been reported in patients receiving the drug, patients should be advised to promptly report signs or symptoms of GI ulceration or bleeding to their clinician.

Naproxen should be used with extreme caution and under close supervision in patients with a history of GI bleeding or peptic ulceration, and such patients should receive an appropriate ulcer preventive regimen. All patients considered at increased risk of potentially serious adverse GI effects (e.g., geriatric patients, those receiving high therapeutic dosages of NSAIAs, those with a history of peptic ulcer disease, those receiving anticoagulants or corticosteroids concomitantly) should be monitored closely for signs and symptoms of ulcer perforation or GI bleeding. To minimize the potential risk of adverse GI effects, the lowest effective dosage and shortest possible duration of therapy should be employed. For patients who are at high risk, therapy other than an NSAIA should be considered.

Elevations in serum ALT may be the most sensitive indicator of NSAIA-induced liver dysfunction. Patients who experience signs and/or symptoms suggestive of liver dysfunction or an abnormal liver function test result while receiving naproxen should be evaluated for evidence of the development of a severe hepatic reaction. Severe reactions, including jaundice and/or fatal hepatitis, have occurred during therapy with naproxen. Although such reactions are rare, naproxen should be discontinued if abnormal liver function test results persist or worsen, if clinical signs and symptoms consistent with liver disease develop, or if systemic manifestations occur (e.g., eosinophilia, rash).

Since naproxen can inhibit platelet aggregation, patients who may be adversely affected by a prolongation of bleeding time should be carefully observed during naproxen therapy. If signs and/or symptoms of anemia occur during therapy with naproxen, hemoglobin concentration and hematocrit should be determined.

Because renal prostaglandins may have a supportive role in maintaining renal perfusion in patients with prerenal conditions, administration of an NSAIA to such patients may cause a dose-dependent reduction in prostaglandin formation and thereby precipitate overt renal decompensation. Patients at greatest risk of this reaction include those with impaired renal function, heart failure, or hepatic dysfunction; those with extracellular fluid depletion (e.g., patients receiving diuretics); those taking an ACE inhibitor or angiotensin II receptor antagonist concomitantly; and geriatric patients. Patients should be advised to consult their clinician promptly if unexplained weight gain or edema occurs. Recovery of renal function to pretreatment levels usually occurs following discontinuance of NSAIA therapy. Some clinicians recommend that renal function be monitored periodically in patients receiving long-term NSAIA therapy.

Naproxen has not been evaluated in patients with renal impairment, and the manufacturer states that use of the drug is not recommended in patients with moderate to severe renal impairment (creatinine clearance less than 30 mL/minute). If NSAIAs are used in patients with advanced renal disease, close monitoring is recommended.

Lower dosages of naproxen should be considered in patients with renal or hepatic impairment and in geriatric patients.

Anaphylactoid reactions have been reported in patients receiving naproxen. Patients receiving naproxen should be informed of the signs and symptoms of an anaphylactoid reaction (e.g., difficulty breathing, swelling of the face or throat) and advised to seek immediate medical attention if an anaphylactoid reaction develops.

Serious skin reactions (e.g., exfoliative dermatitis, Stevens-Johnson syndrome, toxic epidermal necrolysis) can occur in patients receiving NSAIAs. These serious skin reactions may occur without warning; patients should be advised to consult their clinician if skin rash and blisters, fever, or other signs of hypersensitivity reaction (e.g., pruritus) occur. NSAIAs should be discontinued at the first appearance of rash or any other sign of hypersensitivity.

Patients receiving long-term NSAIA therapy should have a complete blood cell count and chemistry profile performed periodically.

Patients receiving naproxen for self-medication should be advised to use the lowest effective dosage and not to exceed the recommended dosage or duration of therapy. Unless otherwise directed by a clinician, patients receiving naproxen for *self-medication* should be advised to discontinue the drug and consult a clinician if pain persists for more than 10 days or fever persists for longer than 3 days. Patients should not use naproxen for *self-medication* immediately before or after cardiac surgery or if they have experienced an allergic reaction to any analgesic or antipyretic. Patients receiving the drug for *self-medication* also should be advised to consult a clinician before initiating naproxen if they have experienced adverse effects associated with any analgesic or antipyretic; if they have a GI disorder, coagulation disorder, hypertension, cardiac disease, or renal disease; if they are receiving therapy with a diuretic; or if they are 60 years of age or older. Patients receiving the drug for *self-medication* should consult a clinician or pharmacist before initiating naproxen if they are under a clinician's care for any continuing serious medical condition; they are receiving an anticoagulant, a corticosteroid, or any other NSAIA-containing preparation; or they are taking any other drugs on a regular basis. They also should be advised to stop taking the drug and to report to their clinician symptoms of GI bleeding (faintness, vomiting blood, bloody or black stools); any new, unusual, or unexpected symptoms that occur during *self-medication* with the drug; if pain or fever gets worse during therapy; or if stomach pain intensifies or persists with use of the drug. Patients should be advised that the risk of GI bleeding is increased if they are 60 years of age or older, have a GI disorder (e.g., history of GI bleeding or peptic ulceration), are receiving an anticoagulant or corticosteroid, are receiving another NSAIA (including aspirin) concomitantly, if they generally consume 3 or more alcohol-containing drinks per day, or if they exceed the recommended dosage or duration of naproxen therapy. In addition, patients should be advised that taking naproxen may increase the risk of a cardiovascular event.

Naproxen can interfere with the antiplatelet effect of low-dose aspirin. Patients receiving low-dose aspirin for its cardioprotective effects should be informed of this potential interaction. (See Drug Interactions: Nonsteroidal Anti-inflammatory Agents.)

Patients should be warned that naproxen may impair their ability to perform activities requiring mental alertness or physical coordination (e.g., operating machinery, driving a motor vehicle).

Because NSAIAs have caused adverse ocular effects, patients who experience visual disturbances or changes during naproxen therapy should have an ophthalmologic examination.

Naproxen is not a substitute for corticosteroids. If corticosteroid dosage is decreased during naproxen therapy, it should be done gradually and patients should be observed for adverse effects, including adrenocortical insufficiency or symptomatic exacerbation of the inflammatory condition being treated.

The possibility that the antipyretic and anti-inflammatory effects of NSAIAs may mask the usual signs and symptoms of infection or other diseases should be considered.

Naproxen is contraindicated in patients with known hypersensitivity to the drug. In addition, NSAIAs, including naproxen, generally are contraindicated in patients in whom asthma, urticaria, or other sensitivity reactions are precipitated by aspirin or other NSAIAs, since there is potential for cross-sensitivity between NSAIAs and aspirin, and severe, rarely fatal, anaphylactic reactions to NSAIAs have been reported in these patients. Although NSAIAs generally are contraindicated in these patients, the drugs have occasionally been used in NSAIA-sensitive patients who have undergone desensitization. Because patients with asthma may have aspirin-sensitivity asthma, naproxen should be used with caution in patients with asthma. In patients with asthma, aspirin sensitivity is manifested principally as bronchospasm and usually is associated with nasal polyps; the association of aspirin sensitivity, asthma, and nasal polyps is known as the aspirin triad. Patients who are considering use of naproxen for *self-medication* should be advised that naproxen is contraindicated in patients who have experienced asthma, urticaria, or other sensitivity reaction to other analgesics or antipyretics. For a further discussion of cross-sensitivity of NSAIAs, see Cautions: Sensitivity Reactions, in the Salicylates General Statement 28:08.04.24.

NSAIAs are contraindicated in the setting of CABG surgery.

■ Pediatric Precautions Safety and efficacy of naproxen in children younger than 2 years of age have not been established. Pediatric dosage recommendations for juvenile rheumatoid arthritis are based on well-controlled studies. There are no adequate efficacy or dose-response data for other pediatric conditions, but clinical experience in juvenile rheumatoid arthritis and other use experience indicate that single doses of 2.5–5 mg/kg with a total daily dose not exceeding 15 mg/kg are safe in children older than 2 years of age. The manufacturers of delayed-release naproxen tablets and extended-release naproxen sodium tablets state that studies using such tablets in pediatric patients have not been performed and therefore, the safety of these formulations in children has not been established. Naproxen sodium should not be used for *self-medication* in children younger than 12 years of age unless otherwise directed by a clinician.

Overdosage and toxicity (including death) have been reported in children younger than 2 years of age receiving nonprescription (over-the-counter, OTC) preparations containing antihistamines, cough suppressants, expectorants, and nasal decongestants alone or in combination for relief of symptoms of upper respiratory tract infection. Such preparations also may contain analgesics and antipyretics (e.g., naproxen). There is limited evidence of efficacy for these preparations in this age group, and appropriate dosages (i.e., approved by the US Food and Drug Administration [FDA]) have not been established. Therefore, FDA stated that nonprescription cough and cold preparations should not be used in children younger than 2 years of age; the agency continues to assess safety and efficacy of these preparations in older children. Meanwhile, because children 2–3 years of age also are at increased risk of overdosage and toxicity, some manufacturers of oral nonprescription cough and cold preparations recently have agreed to voluntarily revise the product labeling to state that such preparations should not be used in children younger than 4 years of age. FDA recommends that parents and caregivers adhere to the dosage instructions and warnings on the product labeling that accompanies the preparation if administering to children and consult with their clinician about any concerns. Clinicians should ask caregivers about use of nonprescription cough and cold preparations to avoid overdosage. For additional information on precautions associated with the use of cough and cold preparations in pediatric patients, see Cautions: Pediatric Precautions in Pseudoephedrine 12:12.12.

■ Geriatric Precautions Although the total plasma concentrations of naproxen in geriatric patients are similar to those attained in younger adults, the unbound plasma fraction of the drug is increased in geriatric patients when compared with that in younger adults. Therefore, consideration should be given for reduced dosage of naproxen or naproxen sodium in geriatric patients, and the lowest possible effective dose should be used. Naproxen and naproxen sodium should be used with caution in geriatric patients when high dosages are required and some adjustment of dosage may be needed. Geriatric individuals appear to tolerate GI ulceration and bleeding less well than other individuals, and many of the spontaneous reports of fatal adverse GI effects in patients receiving NSAIAs involve geriatric individuals. Naproxen is eliminated substantially by the kidneys, and individuals with renal impairment may be at increased risk of toxic reactions to the drug. Because geriatric patients frequently have decreased renal function, particular attention should be paid to naproxen dosage, and it may be useful to monitor renal function in these patients.

■ Carcinogenicity A 2-year study in rats was performed to evaluate the carcinogenic potential of naproxen at 8, 16, or 24 mg/kg daily (50, 100, or 150 mg/m^2, respectively); the maximum dose used was 0.28 times the human systemic exposure at the recommended dose. There was no evidence of carcinogenicity.

■ Pregnancy, Fertility, and Lactation Reproduction studies of naproxen in rats at 20 mg/kg daily (125 mg/m^2, 0.23 times the human systemic exposure), rabbits at 20 mg/kg daily (220 mg/m^2, 0.27 times the human systemic exposure), and mice at 170 mg/kg daily (510 mg/m^2, 0.28 times the human systemic exposure) have not revealed evidence of harm to the fetus. Naproxen inhibits prostaglandin synthesis which may result in prolongation of gestation and interference with labor if the drug is given late in pregnancy. Inhibitors of prostaglandin synthesis may have adverse effects on the fetal cardiovascular system (e.g., premature closure of the ductus arteriosus) and are associated with an increased risk of neonatal complications such as necrotizing enterocolitis or intracranial hemorrhage. Severe hypoxemia due to persistent pulmonary hypertension has occurred in infants whose mothers received naproxen to delay parturition. Neonatal death also has been reported when the drug was used to prevent preterm labor; autopsy of a neonate showed brain hemorrhage, multiple gastric ulcers, extensive GI bleeding, and an adverse cardiovascular effect known to be associated with use of NSAIAs. In addition, severe hyponatremia, water retention, cerebral irritation, and paralytic ileus was reported in a neonate whose mother ingested 5 g of naproxen 8 hours before delivery; it has been suggested that naproxen adversely affected renal function. Renal dysfunction and abnormal prostaglandin E concentrations in premature infants also have been reported. There are no adequate and controlled studies to date using naproxen in pregnant women. The drug should be used during the first and second trimesters of pregnancy only when the potential benefits justify the potential risks to the fetus; use of the drug in the third trimester should be avoided. Women who are pregnant or nursing should seek the advice of a health professional before using naproxen sodium for *self-medication*. It is especially important not to *self-administer* naproxen sodium during the last 3 months of pregnancy unless specifically directed to do so by a physician, because it may cause problems in the unborn child or complications during delivery.

Reproduction studies of naproxen in rats at 20 mg/kg daily (125 mg/m^2, 0.23 times the human systemic exposure), rabbits at 20 mg/kg daily (220 mg/m^2, 0.27 times the human systemic exposure), and mice at 170 mg/kg daily (510 mg/m^2, 0.28 times the human systemic exposure) have not revealed evidence of impaired fertility. Information on the effects of naproxen on fertility in humans is lacking. At least one human case was reported in which ejaculatory dysfunction occurred during naproxen therapy and was reversed upon discontinuing the drug; a definite causal relationship was not established.

Naproxen is distributed into milk. Because of the potential for adverse effects from naproxen or naproxen sodium in infants, use of the drug in nursing women should be avoided.

Drug Interactions

■ **Protein-bound Drugs** Because naproxen is highly protein bound, it theoretically could be displaced from binding sites by, or it could displace from binding sites, other protein-bound drugs such as oral anticoagulants, hydantoins, other nonsteroidal anti-inflammatory agents (NSAIAs; including aspirin), sulfonamides, and sulfonylureas. Patients receiving naproxen with any of these drugs should be observed for adverse effects.

■ **Angiotensin-converting Enzyme Inhibitors and Angiotensin II Receptor Antagonists** There is some evidence that concomitant use of NSAIAs with angiotensin-converting enzyme (ACE) inhibitors or angiotensin II receptor antagonists may reduce the blood pressure response to the antihypertensive agent.

■ **Anticoagulants and Thrombolytic Agents** The effects of warfarin and NSAIAs on GI bleeding are synergistic. Concomitant use of naproxen and warfarin is associated with a higher risk of GI bleeding compared with use of either agent alone.

Administration of naproxen with warfarin results in a slight increase in free warfarin in serum, but does not affect the hypoprothrombinemic effect of warfarin. Naproxen should be used with caution in patients receiving any anticoagulant or thrombolytic agent (e.g., streptokinase).

■ **Antidiabetic Agents** Results of a study in patients with diabetes mellitus showed no interference by naproxen on the effect of tolbutamide on plasma glucose concentrations.

■ **Diuretics** NSAIAs can reduce the natriuretic effects of furosemide or thiazide diuretics. This effect may be related to inhibition of renal prostaglandin synthesis. Patients receiving concomitant NSAIA and diuretic therapy should be monitored for signs of renal failure and efficacy of the diuretic.

■ **Nonsteroidal Anti-inflammatory Agents** Concomitant use of aspirin and an NSAIA increases the risk for serious GI events. Because of the potential for increased adverse effects, patients receiving naproxen should be advised not to take aspirin. There is no consistent evidence that use of low-dose aspirin mitigates the increased risk of serious cardiovascular events associated with NSAIAs.

Administration of aspirin with naproxen may decrease protein binding of naproxen, but clearance of free (unbound) naproxen does not appear to be altered. The clinical importance of this pharmacokinetic interaction has not been established.

Some NSAIAs (e.g., ibuprofen, naproxen) can interfere with the antiplatelet effect of low-dose aspirin. Ibuprofen can interfere with the antiplatelet effect of low-dose aspirin (81 mg daily; immediate-release preparation) when the drugs are administered concomitantly. The interaction can be minimized by appropriate timing of ibuprofen administration relative to that of immediate-release, low-dose aspirin. (See Drug Interactions: Nonsteroidal Anti-inflammatory Agents in Ibuprofen 28:08.04.92.) In one study, concomitant administration of naproxen (500 mg) and low-dose aspirin (100 mg) also interfered with the antiplatelet effect of aspirin.

■ **Probenecid** Administration of probenecid with naproxen substantially increases the plasma half-life of naproxen and plasma naproxen concentrations. In one study, the plasma half-life of naproxen increased to an average of 37 hours and plasma naproxen concentrations increased by an average of 50% when the drugs were administered concomitantly. It was suggested that probenecid interfered with the plasma clearance of naproxen by inhibiting the formation of glucuronide conjugates of naproxen, as well as inhibiting its renal clearance.

■ **Methotrexate** Severe, sometimes fatal, toxicity has occurred following administration of an NSAIA concomitantly with methotrexate (principally high-dose therapy) in patients with various malignant neoplasms or rheumatoid arthritis. The toxicity was associated with elevated and prolonged blood concentrations of methotrexate. The exact mechanism of the interaction remains to be established, but it has been suggested that NSAIAs may inhibit renal elimination of methotrexate, possibly by decreasing renal perfusion via inhibition of renal prostaglandin synthesis or by competing for renal elimination. Naproxen and methotrexate should be administered concomitantly with caution. (See Drug Interactions: Nonsteroidal Anti-inflammatory Agents, in Methotrexate 10:00.)

■ **Lithium** Naproxen may increase serum lithium concentrations and reduce renal lithium clearance. If naproxen and lithium are administered concurrently, the patient should be observed closely for signs of lithium toxicity, and serum lithium concentrations should be monitored carefully during the initial stages of combined therapy or subsequent dosage adjustment. In addition, appropriate adjustment of lithium dosage may be required when therapy with naproxen is discontinued.

■ **Drugs Affecting Gastric pH** Concomitant administration of naproxen and aluminum hydroxide or magnesium oxide antacids may result in delayed absorption of naproxen. Because delayed-release (enteric-coated) naproxen tablets are formulated to release the drug at relatively nonacidic pH (i.e., in the small intestine), concomitant use of this formulation with intensive antacid therapy or histamine H_2-receptor antagonists is not recommended.

In a controlled study in healthy adults, concomitant oral administration of naproxen and cimetidine did not appear to alter the pharmacokinetics of either drug and did not affect the inhibition of gastric acid output by cimetidine.

■ **Cholestyramine** Concomitant administration of naproxen and cholestyramine may result in delayed absorption of naproxen.

■ **Sucralfate** Concomitant administration of naproxen and sucralfate may result in delayed absorption of naproxen. Concomitant use of sucralfate with naproxen delayed-release tablets is not recommended.

■ **Other Drugs** Naproxen should be used cautiously, if at all, with other drugs that might potentiate the adverse GI effects.

Naproxen may interfere with the antihypertensive effects of β-adrenergic blocking agents, including propranolol.

Laboratory Test Interferences

Naproxen or its metabolites may cause falsely elevated urinary 17-ketogenic steroid concentrations by interfering with the *m*-dinitrobenzene reagent used in the test. Although 17-hydroxycorticosteroid measurements (Porter-Silber method) are not significantly altered, withdrawal of naproxen for 72 hours before testing has been recommended.

Naproxen may also interfere with some urinary assays of 5-hydroxyindoleacetic acid (5-HIAA).

Acute Toxicity

Limited information is available on the acute toxicity of naproxen or naproxen sodium.

■ **Pathogenesis** The acute dose of naproxen or naproxen sodium associated with life-threatening toxicity in humans is not known. The oral LD_{50} of naproxen is 4110, 1234, more than 1000, and 543 mg/kg in hamsters, mice, dogs, and rats, respectively.

■ **Manifestations** There have been several cases of naproxen overdosage in children which have resulted in acute toxicity. Acute renal failure and hyperkalemia were reported in a 2-year-old child with juvenile arthritis who received a naproxen sodium dosage of 20 mg/kg daily for 1 month. Death occurred in an 8-month-old child following administration of 110–440 mg of naproxen sodium for 5 days for fever and upper respiratory infection. A 2-year-old child recovered after ingesting up to 2 g of naproxen, hydrogen peroxide, and eucalyptus oil and who developed drowsiness, ataxia, and prolonged bleeding time. Another 2-year-old child developed dyspepsia after ingesting 625 mg of naproxen. In addition, seizures were reported in a 5-year-old child who ingested an unknown amount of naproxen sodium.

Most cases of naproxen overdosage have been reported in adults. Adverse GI effects (e.g., heartburn, vomiting) and seizures usually occur in these patients; drowsiness and prolongation of clotting time also may occur. The incidence of adverse effects in adults may differ from those in children since rash and prolonged bleeding time appear to occur more frequently in children while other reactions occur more frequently in adults; the incidence of adverse GI and CNS effects are similar.

One patient who ingested 25 g of naproxen experienced mild nausea and indigestion. Life-threatening adverse effects are uncommon; however, seizures, apnea, metabolic acidosis, and impaired renal function have been reported following overdosage of naproxen. One death due to CNS depression has been attributed to naproxen overdosage.

■ **Treatment** In acute naproxen overdosage, general measures should include immediately emptying the stomach by inducing emesis or by gastric lavage, followed by initiation of supportive and symptomatic treatment. If the patient is comatose, having seizures, or lacks the gag reflex, gastric lavage may be performed if an endotracheal tube with cuff inflated is in place to prevent aspiration of gastric contents. Hemodialysis appears to be of no value in enhancing elimination of naproxen.

Pharmacology

Naproxen has pharmacologic actions similar to those of other prototypical NSAIAs. The drug exhibits anti-inflammatory, analgesic, and antipyretic activity. The exact mechanisms have not been clearly established, but many of the actions appear to be associated principally with the inhibition of prostaglandin synthesis. Naproxen inhibits the synthesis of prostaglandins in body tissues by inhibiting cyclooxygenase; at least 2 isoenzymes, cyclooxygenase-1 (COX-1) and -2 (COX-2) (also referred to as prostaglandin G/H synthase-1 [PGHS-1] and -2 [PGHS-2], respectively), have been identified that catalyze the formation of prostaglandins in the arachidonic acid pathway. Naproxen, like other prototypical NSAIAs, inhibits both COX-1 and COX-2. Although the exact mechanisms have not been clearly established, NSAIAs appear to exert anti-inflammatory, analgesic, and antipyretic activity principally through inhibition of the COX-2 isoenzyme; COX-1 inhibition presumably is responsible for the drugs' unwanted effects on GI mucosa and platelet aggregation.

■ **Anti-inflammatory, Analgesic, and Antipyretic Effects** The anti-inflammatory, analgesic, and antipyretic effects of naproxen and other NSAIAs, including selective inhibitors of COX-2 (e.g., celecoxib, rofecoxib), appear to result from inhibition of prostaglandin synthesis. While the precise mechanism of the anti-inflammatory and analgesic effects of NSAIAs continues to be investigated, these effects appear to be mediated principally through inhibition of the COX-2 isoenzyme at sites of inflammation with subsequent reduction in the synthesis of certain prostaglandins from their arachidonic acid precursors.

Naproxen stabilizes lysosomal membranes and inhibits the response of neutrophils to chemotactic stimuli. The drug does not possess glucocorticoid or adrenocorticoid-stimulating properties.

There is no evidence that long-term therapy with naproxen results in tolerance to or physical dependence on the drug. The drug probably cannot suppress the abstinence syndrome in opiate-dependent patients.

Naproxen lowers body temperature in patients with fever. Although the mechanism of the antipyretic effect of NSAIAs is not known, it has been suggested that suppression of prostaglandin synthesis in the CNS (probably in the hypothalamus) may be involved.

■ **Genitourinary and Renal Effects** Naproxen-induced inhibition of prostaglandin synthesis may result in decreased frequency and intensity of uterine contractility. Prostaglandins E_2 and $F_{2\alpha}$ increase the amplitude and frequency of uterine contractions in pregnant women; current evidence suggests that primary dysmenorrhea is also mediated by these prostaglandins. Whether the increased production of prostaglandins associated with primary dysmenorrhea is mediated by COX-1 or COX-2 remains to be determined. Blood concentrations of a metabolite of prostaglandin $F_{2\alpha}$ have been found to decrease in women with dysmenorrhea who were receiving naproxen. Therapy with naproxen has been effective in relieving menstrual pain and has reduced blood loss in women with menorrhagia, probably by inhibiting the formation of these prostaglandins. Administration of naproxen during late pregnancy may prolong gestation by inhibiting uterine contractions.

Naproxen has been reported to adversely affect renal function. (See Cautions: Renal Effects.) The mechanisms of adverse renal effects of naproxen have not been determined, but may involve inhibition of renal synthesis of prostaglandins.

Naproxen does not appear to have uricosuric activity.

■ **GI Effects** Naproxen can cause gastric mucosal damage which may result in ulceration and/or bleeding. (See Cautions: GI Effects.) These gastric effects have been attributed to inhibition of the synthesis of prostaglandins produced by COX-1. Other factors possibly involved in NSAIA-induced gastropathy include local irritation, promotion of acid back-diffusion into gastric mucosa, uncoupling of oxidative phosphorylation, and enterohepatic recirculation of the drugs.

Epidemiologic and laboratory studies suggest that NSAIAs may reduce the risk of colon cancer. Although the exact mechanism by which NSAIAs may inhibit colon carcinogenesis remains to be determined, it has been suggested that inhibition of prostaglandin synthesis may be involved.

■ **Hematologic Effects** Although naproxen can inhibit platelet aggregation and may prolong bleeding time, it does not affect prothrombin or whole blood clotting time. (See Cautions: Hematologic Effects.) In one study, the drug inhibited the second phase of platelet aggregation induced by adenosine diphosphate or epinephrine. Like aspirin and other prototypical NSAIAs, the effects of naproxen on platelets appear to be associated with the inhibition of the synthesis of prostaglandins produced by COX-1.

Pharmacokinetics

Naproxen pharmacokinetics have not been determined in individuals with renal or hepatic impairment, nor in children younger than 5 years of age. Pharmacokinetics of the drug in the delayed-release (enteric-coated) formulation have not been determined in individuals younger than 18 years of age.

■ **Absorption** Preparations of naproxen differ in their pattern of absorption, owing to the chemical form of naproxen (i.e., the base or sodium salt) and the formulation used. When administered as the acid or the sodium salt, naproxen is completely absorbed from the GI tract; the sodium salt is absorbed more rapidly than the acid. Oral bioavailability of naproxen is 95%. There appears to be no difference in bioavailability between a single 500-mg conventional tablet and two 250-mg conventional tablets of naproxen. Commercially available formulations of naproxen (i.e., conventional tablets, delayed-release tablets, oral suspension) are bioequivalent in terms of extent of absorption (i.e., area under the curve [AUC]) and peak plasma concentrations; however, the rate of absorption varies depending on the formulation used. When naproxen (either as conventional or delayed-release tablets) or naproxen sodium (either as conventional or extended-release tablets) is taken with food, the rate but not the extent of absorption of the drug is decreased. Studies to date indicate that antacids may have variable, but probably clinically insignificant, effects on absorption of naproxen (either as conventional or delayed-release tablets) or naproxen sodium.

The manufacturers state that peak plasma concentrations of the drug occur in 2–4 hours following oral administration of naproxen as conventional tablets; peak plasma concentration occurs 1–4 hours following administration of the oral suspension. In several studies, following oral administration of a single 500-mg dose of naproxen (as one 500-mg or two 250-mg conventional tablets) to fasting, healthy adults, mean peak plasma concentrations of the drug ranged from 62–96 mcg/mL and occurred at 1.5–2 hours. The manufacturers state that peak plasma concentrations of the drug occur in 1–2 hours following oral administration of naproxen sodium as conventional tablets. Following oral administration of a single 550-mg dose of naproxen sodium as a conventional tablet (equivalent to 500 mg of naproxen) to a group of fasting, healthy adults, mean peak plasma concentrations of the drug were 70 mcg/mL and occurred at about 1 hour. In children 5–16 years of age, plasma naproxen concentrations following a single 5- to 10-mg/kg dose of the suspension are similar to those attained in healthy adults following a 500-mg dose. Steady-state plasma concentrations of naproxen are achieved within 4–5 days.

Commercially available delayed-release (enteric-coated) tablets of naproxen (EC-Naprosyn®) contain the drug within a copolymer coating dispersion. Dissolution of the coating is pH-dependent, with the most rapid dissolution occurring at pH above 6; no dissolution occurs below pH 4. The coating is designed to release the drug in the higher pH environment of the small intestine, avoiding dissolution in the more acidic environment of the stomach. Naproxen is well-absorbed from the enteric-coated formulation. Peak plasma concentration usually is reached about 4–6 (range: 2–12) hours following oral administration of the first dose of the enteric-coated formulation. A crossover study of oral administration of naproxen as conventional or delayed-release tablets in a dosage of 500 mg twice daily in fasted, healthy individuals demonstrated that after one week, only time to peak plasma concentration differed between the two formulations (1.9 versus 4 hours for conventional versus delayed-release tablets, respectively); there were no differences in peak plasma concentration or extent of absorption (i.e., AUC).

Commercially available tablets of naproxen and esomeprazole magnesium (Vimovo®) contain a delayed-release (enteric-coated) naproxen core surrounded by an immediate-release layer of esomeprazole magnesium. The tablet is designed to release esomeprazole in the stomach prior to dissolution of naproxen in the small intestine. At naproxen dosages of 375 or 500 mg twice daily, the fixed-combination tablets are bioequivalent (based on AUC and peak plasma concentration) to enteric-coated preparations of naproxen. Peak steady-state plasma concentrations of naproxen are reached about 3 hours after administration of the fixed-combination tablet. Administration of the fixed-combination tablets with a high-fat meal substantially delays naproxen absorption and modestly decreases peak plasma concentrations of the drug.

Commercially available extended-release tablets of naproxen sodium (Naprelan®) contain an immediate-release component (about 30% of the total dose) and an extended-release component comprised of microparticles that slowly release the drug. The tablet matrix rapidly disintegrates in the stomach, and the microparticles are dispersed throughout the small intestine and into the proximal large intestine allowing absorption of the drug throughout the GI tract. Naproxen is well absorbed from naproxen sodium extended-release tablets, with a reported bioavailability of about 95%; peak steady-state plasma naproxen concentrations usually are reached in about 3–5 hours following oral administration. The absorption rate from extended-release naproxen sodium tablets is slower than from conventional tablets. Prolonged drug absorption from extended-release tablets allows for once-daily dosing with this formulation.

Following oral administration of fixed-combination tablets containing naproxen sodium 500 mg and sumatriptan 85 mg, peak plasma naproxen concentrations are about 36% lower and the time to peak plasma naproxen concentrations is delayed by about 4 hours compared with oral administration of naproxen sodium as conventional 550-mg tablets; the extent of exposure to naproxen (i.e., AUC) is similar for the 2 formulations. Administration of the fixed-combination tablets with food does not substantially affect the bioavailability of naproxen.

Plasma naproxen concentrations of 30–90 mcg/mL reportedly are required for anti-inflammatory or analgesic effect. In a group of patients with rheumatoid arthritis, the anti-inflammatory effect of naproxen was positively correlated with serum naproxen concentrations, although no such relationship was found for adverse effects. Onset of pain relief can begin within 1 hour in patients receiving naproxen (as conventional tablets) and within 30 minutes in patients receiving naproxen sodium (as conventional tablets), as evidenced by reduction in pain intensity scores, increase in pain relief scores, decrease in the number of patients requiring additional analgesic medication, and delay in time to remedication. In a comparative study in patients with postpartum uterine cramping, there was no difference between the drugs in onset of analgesia; both drugs provided pain relief within 1 hour. Peak analgesia occurs within 1 hour with naproxen sodium and within 2 hours with naproxen. The duration of action of both drugs is generally 7–12 hours. Because of the delayed absorption of enteric-coated naproxen tablets, onset of analgesia may be delayed.

■ **Distribution** The volume of distribution of naproxen is 0.16 L/kg. In one study, the apparent volume of distribution of naproxen averaged about 8.3 L in healthy adults and about 11.9 L in patients with severe renal failure (serum creatinine 5.4–12.5 mg/dL).

After therapeutic doses, naproxen is more than 99% bound to plasma proteins. When naproxen binding sites become saturated (at twice daily doses of 500 mg or more), plasma free drug concentrations increase and may result in increased urinary clearance rates. Therefore, plasma naproxen concentrations tend to plateau when dosage exceeds 500 mg twice daily. In a study in patients with severe renal failure, binding of naproxen to serum proteins was decreased compared to healthy adults; the decreased binding may have accounted for an increase in metabolism and apparent volume of distribution of the drug observed in these patients. In patients with chronic alcoholic liver disease, total plasma concentrations of naproxen are decreased while concentrations of the unbound drug are increased.

Naproxen crosses the placenta. Naproxen is also distributed into milk in concentrations of about 1% of simultaneous maternal plasma drug concentrations.

■ **Elimination** In healthy adults, the plasma half-life of naproxen reportedly ranges from 10–20 hours. The manufacturers state that the plasma half-life of naproxen is about 13 hours. The plasma half-life and elimination of the drug appear to be similar in children and adults. Clearance of naproxen is 0.13 mL/minute per kg.

Naproxen is extensively metabolized in the liver by cytochrome P-450 (CYP) isoenzymes 1A2 and 2C9 to 6-desmethylnaproxen. Approximately 95% of the drug is excreted in urine as unchanged naproxen (less than 1%) and 6-desmethylnaproxen (less than 1%) and their glucuronide or other conjugates (66–92%). Some data suggest that renal excretion of unchanged naproxen may be negligible or absent; previously reported concentrations of unchanged drug may reflect rapid hydrolysis of conjugates during collection, storage, and handling of urine samples. The half-life of naproxen metabolites and conjugates is shorter than 12 hours.

Naproxen metabolites may accumulate in patients with renal impairment. Elimination of naproxen is reduced in patients with severe renal impairment. A small amount (less than 5%) of the drug is excreted in feces.

Chemistry and Stability

■ **Chemistry** Naproxen, a propionic acid derivative, is a prototypical anti-inflammatory agent (NSAIA). The drug is structurally and pharmacologically related to fenoprofen and ibuprofen.

Naproxen is commercially available as the acid and as the sodium salt. Each 275 mg of naproxen sodium is approximately equivalent to 250 mg of naproxen and each 220 mg of naproxen sodium is approximately equivalent to 200 mg of naproxen. The acid occurs as a white to off-white, practically odorless, crystalline powder and is practically insoluble in water at low pH, freely soluble in water at high pH, and freely soluble in alcohol. Naproxen sodium occurs as a white to creamy white, crystalline powder and is freely soluble in water at neutral pH and sparingly soluble in alcohol. The apparent pK_a of naproxen is 4.15. Each 220-, 275-, 412.5-, or 550-mg tablet of naproxen sodium contains about 0.87, 1, 1.5, or 2 mEq of sodium, respectively, and each 5 mL of the commercially available naproxen suspension contains about 1.5 mEq each of sodium and chloride. Naproxen sodium is commercially available as conventional tablets and as extended-release tablets. Extended-release tablets of naproxen sodium (Naprelan®) contain an immediate-release component (about 30% of the total dose) and an extended-release component comprised of microparticles that slowly release the drug. Fixed-combination tablets of naproxen and esomeprazole magnesium contain a delayed-release (enteric-coated) naproxen core surrounded by an immediate-release layer of esomeprazole magnesium.

■ **Stability** Commercially available naproxen conventional and delayed-release (enteric-coated) tablets should be stored in well-closed, light-resistant containers at 15–30°C. Extended-release naproxen sodium tablets should be stored in well-closed containers at 20–25°C. Naproxen oral suspension should be stored in light-resistant containers at 15–30°C, and temperatures exceeding 40°C should be avoided. Naproxen sodium conventional tablets should be stored in well-closed containers at 15–30°C. Fixed-combination tablets containing delayed-release naproxen and immediate-release esomeprazole magnesium should be stored in well-closed containers at 25°C but may be exposed to temperatures ranging from 15–30°C. Fixed-combination tablets containing naproxen sodium and sumatriptan succinate should be stored in the original container with the desiccant packet at 25°C but may be exposed to temperatures ranging from 15–30°C; the tablets should not be repackaged.

Naproxen and naproxen sodium preparations containing the equivalent of 250 mg of naproxen or more per retail package should be stored in child-resistant containers in order to limit the potential toxicity associated with accidental ingestion in children.

Preparations

Excipients in commercially available drug preparations may have clinically important effects in some individuals; consult specific product labeling for details.

Naproxen

Oral		
Suspension	125 mg/5 mL*	**Naproxen Suspension**
Tablets	250 mg*	**Naprosyn®**, Canton **Naproxen Tablets**
	375 mg*	**Naprosyn®**, Canton **Naproxen Tablets**
	500 mg*	**Naprosyn®**, Canton **Naproxen Tablets**
Tablets, delayed-release (enteric-coated)	375 mg*	**EC-Naprosyn®**, Canton **Naproxen Delayed-release Tablets**
	500 mg*	**EC-Naprosyn®** (scored), Canton **Naproxen Delayed-release Tablets**

*available from one or more manufacturer, distributor, and/or repackager by generic (nonproprietary) name

Naproxen Combinations

Oral		
Tablets, delayed-release core (naproxen only)	375 mg with Esomeprazole Magnesium 20 mg (of esomeprazole)	**Vimovo®**, Horizon
	500 mg with Esomeprazole Magnesium 20 mg (of esomeprazole)	**Vimovo®**, Horizon

Naproxen Sodium

Oral		
Tablets	220 mg (equivalent to naproxen 200 mg)*	**Aleve® Caplets®**, Bayer **Aleve® Tablets**, Bayer **Naproxen Sodium Tablets**
Tablets, extended-release	412.5 mg (equivalent to 375 mg naproxen)	**Naprelan®**, Almatica
	550 mg (equivalent to 500 mg naproxen)	**Naprelan®**, Almatica
	825 mg (equivalent to 750 mg naproxen)	**Naprelan®**, Almatica
Tablets, film-coated	275 mg (equivalent to naproxen 250 mg)*	**Anaprox®**, Canton **Naproxen Sodium Film Coated Tablets**
	550 mg (equivalent to naproxen 500 mg)*	**Anaprox® DS** (scored), Canton **Naproxen Sodium Film Coated Tablets**

*available from one or more manufacturer, distributor, and/or repackager by generic (nonproprietary) name

Naproxen Sodium Combinations

Oral		
Tablets, extended release	220 mg (equivalent to 200 mg naproxen) with Pseudoephedrine Hydrochloride 120 mg	**Aleve® Cold and Sinus**, Roche
Tablets, film-coated	500 mg (equivalent to 455 mg naproxen) with Sumatriptan Succinate 85 mg (of sumatriptan)	**Treximet®**, GlaxoSmithKline

†Use is not currently included in the labeling approved by the US Food and Drug Administration

OPIATE AGONISTS 28:08.08

Opiate Agonists General Statement

■ Opiate agonists encompass a group of naturally occurring, semisynthetic, and synthetic drugs that stimulate opiate receptors and effectively relieve pain without producing loss of consciousness.

Uses

■ **Pain** Opiate agonists are generally used to provide temporary analgesia in the symptomatic treatment of moderate to severe pain such as that associated with acute and some chronic medical disorders including renal or biliary colic, myocardial infarction (MI), acute trauma, postoperative pain, and terminal cancer. Opiate analgesics increasingly have been used for the management of chronic noncancer pain despite uncertainty over the long-term benefits of such therapy. The drugs may also be used to provide analgesia during diagnostic and orthopedic procedures and during labor. In patients with acute pulmonary edema, opiate agonists are used for their cardiovascular effects and to relieve anxiety associated with this condition. The drugs are also used to provide preoperative sedation and as a supplement to anesthesia. Although most of the opiate agonists produce similar analgesia in equianalgesic doses, such factors as oral effectiveness, duration of action, other CNS effects such as euphoria or sedation, degree of action on smooth muscle, and individual variation in patient response should be considered in the selection of a specific opiate agonist.

Some opiates have been used in the treatment of pain in various combinations with nonsteroidal anti-inflammatory agents (NSAIAs), acetaminophen, and/or caffeine. Opiates (e.g., codeine, oxycodone, hydrocodone) given orally in combination with acetaminophen or NSAIAs may produce a greater analgesic effect than that produced by either drug used individually. There also is some evidence that acetaminophen or NSAIAs in combination with oral doses of an opiate may cause fewer adverse effects than equianalgesic doses of the individual drugs alone.

Various extended-release and long-acting opiate analgesics are used for the management of pain that is severe enough to require long-term, daily, around-the-clock use of an opiate analgesic. Because of the risks of addiction, abuse, and misuse associated with opiates, even at recommended doses, and because of the greater risks of overdose and death with extended-release and long-acting opiate formulations, these extended-release and long-acting opiate analgesics should be reserved for use in patients for whom alternative treatment options (e.g., nonopiate analgesics or immediate-release opiates) are inadequate or not tolerated. These preparations are not indicated for use on an as-needed ("prn") basis. Some extended-release or long-acting preparations or dosage strengths should be used only in opiate-tolerant patients (see the individual monographs in 28:08.08). Patients are considered opiate tolerant if they have been receiving opiate therapy consisting of at least 60 mg of morphine sulfate daily, 25 mcg of transdermal fentanyl per hour, 30 mg of oral oxycodone daily, 8 mg of oral hydromorphone hydrochloride daily, 25 mg of oxymorphone hydrochloride daily, or an equianalgesic dosage of another opiate daily for at least 1 week.

Chronic Pain **Chronic Noncancer Pain.** In patients with chronic pain (generally defined as pain lasting longer than 3 months or past the time of normal tissue healing) that is not associated with active cancer treatment, palliative care, or end-of-life care (also referred to as chronic noncancer pain), opiate analgesics generally should be used only if other appropriate pain management strategies (nonpharmacologic and nonopiate pharmacologic therapies) have been ineffective and the expected benefits of opiate analgesics for both pain relief and functional improvement are anticipated to outweigh the risks. If opiate analgesics are used, they should be part of an integrated approach that also includes appropriate nonpharmacologic modalities (e.g., cognitive-behavioral therapy, relaxation techniques, biofeedback, functional restoration, exercise therapy, certain interventional procedures) and other appropriate pharmacologic therapies (e.g., nonopiate analgesics, analgesic adjuncts such as selected anticonvulsants and antidepressants for certain neuropathic pain conditions).

Use of opiate analgesics for the management of chronic noncancer pain has increased despite uncertainty over the long-term benefits of such therapy. Clinical trials of opiate analgesics in the symptomatic treatment of chronic pain generally have been of short duration, and available evidence is insufficient to determine whether long-term opiate therapy results in sustained pain relief or improvements in function and quality of life. In addition, evidence that opiate analgesics are superior to other pharmacologic or nonpharmacologic treatments for chronic pain generally is lacking. However, use of opiate analgesics is associated with serious risks (e.g., opiate use disorder, overdose). Prior to initiation of opiate therapy for chronic noncancer pain, patients should undergo thorough evaluation, including assessment of risk factors for misuse, abuse, and addiction. Clinicians should establish treatment goals with all patients, including realistic goals for pain and function, and should consider how therapy will be discontinued if benefits do not outweigh risks. Initial opiate therapy for chronic noncancer pain should be regarded as a therapeutic trial that will be continued only if there are clinically meaningful improvements in pain and function that outweigh the risks of therapy. Prior to and periodically during therapy, clinicians should discuss with patients known risks and realistic benefits of such therapy and patient and clinician responsibilities for managing therapy.

Although specific recommendations for the management of opiate therapy for chronic noncancer pain vary across clinical practice guidelines, common elements include risk mitigation strategies, upper dosage thresholds, careful dosage titration, and consideration of risks associated with particular opiates and formulations, coexisting diseases, and concomitant drug therapy.

Some experts recommend that opiate therapy for chronic noncancer pain be initiated with conventional (immediate-release) opiate analgesics prescribed at the lowest effective dosage. Opiate selection, initial dosage, and dosage titration should be individualized according to the patient's health status, prior opiate use, attainment of therapeutic goals, and predicted or observed harms. Experts generally agree that methadone should be prescribed for the management of chronic pain only by clinicians who are knowledgeable about its risks (e.g., QT-interval prolongation) and pharmacokinetic properties, and should not be the first choice for an extended-release or long-acting opiate analgesic. Similarly, fentanyl transdermal system should be prescribed only by clinicians who are familiar with the absorption characteristics and dosing of this formulation.

Benefits and harms of opiate analgesic therapy should be evaluated within 1–4 weeks following initiation of therapy or an increase in dosage and reevaluated on an ongoing basis (e.g., at least every 3 months) throughout therapy. Monitoring should include documentation of pain intensity and level of functioning, assessment of progress toward therapeutic goals, presence of adverse effects, and adherence to prescribed therapies. Common opiate-related adverse effects (e.g., constipation, nausea and vomiting, cognitive and psychomotor impairment) should be anticipated and appropriately managed. If benefits do not outweigh harms, other therapies should be optimized and opiate therapy should be tapered to a lower dosage or tapered and discontinued.

When repeated increases in dosage are required, potential causes should be evaluated and the relative benefits and risks reassessed. Although evidence is limited, some experts state that a trial of opiate rotation may be considered in patients experiencing intolerable adverse effects or inadequate benefit despite increases in dosage. Although the dosage level that constitutes high-dose therapy varies across clinical practice guidelines, there is agreement that use of higher dosages requires particular caution, including more frequent and intensive monitoring or referral to a specialist. (See Dosage and Administration: Dosage.) Greater benefits of high-dose opiate therapy for chronic pain have not been established in controlled clinical studies, and higher dosages have been associated with increased risks of motor vehicle accidents, overdosage, and opiate use disorder.

Various strategies for managing risks associated with opiate therapy for chronic noncancer pain have been recommended, including written treatment agreements or plans (e.g., "contracts"), urine drug testing, review of state prescription drug monitoring program (PDMP) data, and risk assessment and monitoring tools. Although precise recommendations may vary, recent clinical practice guidelines generally recommend such monitoring in all patients receiving opiate therapy for chronic noncancer pain, although the frequency and intensity of monitoring may vary depending on risk assessments. Urine drug testing may be used at baseline and periodically during therapy to assess adherence to the treatment plan and to screen for use of other prescription or illicit drugs. Baseline and periodic review of the patient's history of controlled substance prescriptions using state PDMP data also may assist in reducing prescription drug abuse and in identifying opiate dosages or drug combinations (e.g., benzodiazepines) that increase the risk for overdosage. (See Drug Interactions: Benzodiazepines and Other CNS Depressants.) Opiate therapy should be tapered and discontinued in patients who engage in serious or repeated aberrant drug-related behaviors or drug abuse or diversion. Clinicians should offer or arrange treatment for patients with opiate use disorder.

Some experts state that consideration should be given to providing the opiate antagonist naloxone along with opiate analgesic therapy for patients at increased risk of opiate overdosage (e.g., those with a history of overdose or substance use disorder, those receiving opiate dosages equivalent to 50 mg or more of morphine sulfate daily, those receiving benzodiazepines concomitantly, those with medical conditions that could increase sensitivity to opiate effects).

Chronic Cancer Pain. In the management of severe, chronic pain associated with a terminal illness such as cancer, the principal goal of analgesic therapy is to make the patient relatively pain-free while maintaining as good a quality of life as possible. Analgesic therapy must be individualized and titrated according to patient response and tolerance. When nonopiate or combinations of nonopiate and opiate analgesics are ineffective, oral administration of an opiate agonist on a regular schedule generally will provide adequate relief of severe, chronic pain and the fear of its recurrence. Extended-release and long-acting preparations are used orally for the management of such pain when it is severe enough to require long-term, daily, around-the-clock use of an opiate analgesic and when alternative treatment options (e.g., nonopiate analgesics or immediate-release opiates) are inadequate or not tolerated. Although consideration of the dependence potential of opiate agonists has often limited their effective use by many clinicians in terminally ill patients with severe, chronic pain, such consideration is irrelevant in the context of terminal illness. When oral opiate agonists no longer provide adequate relief or in patients unable to swallow or tolerate oral drugs, alternative methods of administration such as subcutaneous, rectal, continuous IV infusion, patient-controlled IV infusion, epidural, intrathecal, or transdermal systems should be considered.

Acute Pain In the symptomatic treatment of acute pain, opiate analgesics generally should be reserved for pain resulting from severe injuries or medical conditions, surgical procedures, or when nonopiate alternatives for relieving pain and restoring function are expected to be ineffective or are contraindicated. Concomitant use of other appropriate therapies should be optimized. Because long-term opiate use often begins with the treatment of acute pain, conventional (immediate-release) opiates should be used in the smallest effective dosage and for the shortest possible duration when opiate analgesia is required for symptomatic treatment of acute pain. When sufficient for pain management, lower-potency opiate analgesics given in conjunction with acetaminophen or an NSAIA on an as-needed ("prn") basis have been recommended. The prescribed quantity of opiate analgesics should be limited to the amount needed for the expected duration of pain severe enough to require opiate analgesia, generally 3 days or less, and rarely more than 7 days, for acute pain not related to trauma or surgery. Clinicians should not prescribe larger quantities of opiate analgesics for use in the event that pain continues longer than expected; instead, patients should be reevaluated if severe acute pain does not remit.

When opiate analgesics are used to alleviate moderate to severe postoperative pain, opiate therapy should be provided as part of a multimodal regimen that also includes acetaminophen and/or NSAIAs and other pharmacologic (e.g., certain anticonvulsants, regional local anesthetic techniques) and nonpharmacologic therapy as appropriate. In the management of postoperative pain, scheduled administration of nonopiate analgesics is recommended to reduce use of opiate analgesics and provide more-consistent analgesia. Oral administration of conventional opiate analgesics generally is preferred over IV administration in patients who can tolerate oral therapy. Scheduled (around-the-clock) dosing of opiate analgesics frequently is required during the immediate postoperative period or following major surgery. When repeated parenteral administration is required, IV patient-controlled analgesia (PCA) generally is recommended. Routine use of continuous (basal) IV infusions of opiates in opiate-naive patients receiving PCA is not recommended. IM administration of opiate analgesics is discouraged because IM injections can cause pain and are associated with unreliable absorption, resulting in inconsistent postoperative analgesia.

Pain that will likely be of short duration, such as that associated with diagnostic procedures or orthopedic manipulation, should be controlled with a short-acting opiate agonist such as fentanyl. Severe but intermittent pain such as may occur in patients with renal colic should also be treated with an opiate agonist providing short-duration analgesia. In bronchoscopy, a drug with good antitussive activity such as morphine may be preferred. Opiate agonists have been used in the treatment of pain of biliary or pancreatic origin. Although it may seem illogical to treat pain of biliary origin with drugs that increase biliary pressure and spasm, these biliary effects do not always occur with therapeutic doses and sedation produced by opiate agonists may contribute to relief of pain.

When administered during labor, opiate agonists should effectively relieve pain without interfering with the progress of labor or normal respiration in the neonate. The closer to delivery the drug is given, the greater the possibility of respiratory depression in the neonate.

Acute Coronary Syndromes. Opiate agonists, principally morphine, are used to relieve pain and anxiety associated with acute coronary syndromes (ACS). Although morphine usually is considered the drug of choice in relieving pain associated with MI, other strong opiate agonists such as meperidine, hydromorphone, and levorphanol tartrate also have been used.

Because of its ability to alleviate the work of breathing, reduce anxiety, and favorably affect ventricular loading conditions, morphine is considered the analgesic agent of choice in patients with ST-segment-elevation MI (STEMI). In addition to its potent analgesic and anxiolytic effects, morphine also exhibits favorable hemodynamic effects by causing venodilation and modest reductions in heart rate and systolic blood pressure. These properties also may be beneficial in patients with non-ST-segment-elevation ACS (NSTE ACS; unstable angina or non-ST-segment-elevation MI [NSTEMI]); although randomized controlled studies specifically evaluating the use of morphine in patients with NSTE ACS have not been conducted, experts state that it may be reasonable to administer IV morphine in such patients who have continued pain despite treatment with maximally tolerated anti-ischemic drugs (e.g., nitrates). However, use of morphine should not preclude the use of other anti-ischemic drugs with proven benefit. Patients with acute MI typically exhibit overactivity of the sympathetic nervous system, which adversely increases myocardial oxygen demand via acceleration of heart rate, elevation in arterial blood pressure, augmentation of cardiac contractility, and heightened tendency to develop ventricular tachyarrhythmias. This increased sympathetic activity results from combined ischemic-type chest discomfort and anxiety, and the principal objective of therapy is to administer sufficient doses of an analgesic such as morphine to relieve what many patients describe as a feeling of impending doom. The dose of morphine sulfate needed to achieve adequate pain control is dependent upon several factors such as patient age (e.g., lower doses are recommended in geriatric patients), body size, blood pressure, and heart rate. In patients with STEMI, an initial morphine sulfate dose of 4–8 mg IV is recommended, with additional doses of 2–8 mg administered every 5–15 minutes as needed. In patients with NSTE ACS, experts state that a morphine sulfate dose of 1–5 mg IV may be administered during IV nitroglycerin therapy and repeated every 5–30 minutes to relieve symptoms and maintain patient comfort.

Pain in Critically Ill Patients Opiate agonists may be used in combination with sedative agents to maintain an optimal level of comfort and safety in patients in a critical care setting. Some clinicians state that pain assessment and subsequent documentation using standard assessment tools (e.g., numeric rating scale) should be performed regularly to monitor the patient's response to analgesic therapy. If patients are unable to communicate, their pain should be assessed by subjective observations of pain-related behaviors (e.g., movement, facial expression, posturing) and physiologic indicators (e.g., heart rate, blood pressure, respiratory rate). To ensure consistent analgesic therapy, a therapeutic plan and goal of analgesia should be established for each patient and communicated to all caregivers. Analgesics, including opiate agonists, should be administered on a continuous or scheduled intermittent basis, with supplemental doses given as required. If IV administration is required, some clinicians state that fentanyl, hydromorphone, or morphine are the recommended agents. In addition, fentanyl is recommended for use in acutely distressed patients because of its rapid onset of analgesia, and morphine or hydromorphone is preferred for intermittent therapy because of their longer duration of action. Fentanyl or hydromorphone also is recommended for use in critically ill patients who have hemodynamic instability or renal insufficiency. The potential for withdrawal symptoms should be considered in patients receiving high dosages of opiate agonists or longer than 7 days of continuous opiate agonist therapy and the dosage should be tapered systematically to prevent manifestations of opiate withdrawal.

Vascular Headaches Opiate agonists are not recommended for routine use in the management of acute migraine attacks because evidence of superiority over other standard therapies (e.g., serotonin type 1 [5-HT_1] receptor agonists [triptans], NSAIAs) generally is lacking and because of the risk of medication overuse headache with frequent use, risk of dependence and abuse, and potential for opiate withdrawal syndrome following drug discontinuance. Some clinicians state that infrequent use of a short-acting opiate or fixed-combination preparation (e.g., acetaminophen and tramadol, codeine-containing fixed combinations) may be considered for abortive therapy of moderate to severe acute migraine attacks when standard therapies are ineffective or not tolerated or as rescue therapy when the patient's usual therapy fails. For further information on management and classification of migraine headache, see Vascular Headaches: General Principles in Migraine Therapy, under Uses in Sumatriptan 28:32.28.

■ **Delirium** The American Psychiatric Association (APA) states that opiate agonists, including morphine, may be used in the palliative management of delirium which may have been aggravated by pain. However, some opiate agonists (e.g., fentanyl, meperidine) can exacerbate delirium, because their metabolites may exhibit anticholinergic activity. For information on the management of delirium, see Uses: Delirium, in Haloperidol 28:16.08.08.

■ **Acute Pulmonary Edema** Morphine and other strong opiate agonists including meperidine, oxymorphone, and hydromorphone have been used to relieve anxiety in patients with dyspnea associated with acute pulmonary edema and acute left ventricular failure. These drugs should *not* be used in the treatment of pulmonary edema resulting from a chemical respiratory irritant. Opiate agonists cause pooling of blood in the extremities by decreasing peripheral resistance. This effect results in decreases in venous return, cardiac work, and pulmonary venous pressure, and blood is shifted from the central to peripheral circulation.

■ **Preoperative Sedation** Routine use of opiate agonists for preoperative sedation in patients without pain is not recommended. Preoperative use of opiate agonists may cause serious complications, usually involving the respiratory or circulatory systems, during surgery and increases the incidence of adverse effects after surgery. The usefulness of mixtures of opiate agonists and antagonists in preanesthetic medication, during surgery, or postoperatively to prevent respiratory depression has not been confirmed by well-controlled clinical studies.

■ **Cough** Some opiate agonists, notably codeine and its derivative hydrocodone, are used as cough suppressants. For a discussion of opiate agonists as antitussive agents, see Codeine 48:08 and Hydrocodone 48:08. Diphenoxylate and opium preparations are used mainly as antidiarrheal agents (see 56:08).

■ **Detoxification and Maintenance of Opiate Dependence** Methadone is used in detoxification treatment as an oral substitute for heroin or other morphine-like drugs to suppress the opiate-agonist abstinence syndrome in patients who are dependent on these drugs. If more prolonged suppressive therapy is necessary, methadone or buprenorphine hydrochloride can be used as oral substitutes for maintenance treatment of opiate dependence. Levomethadyl acetate also has been used for the management of opiate dependence but is no longer commercially available in the US because of potentially severe adverse cardiac effects. (See Chronic Toxicity and also see Methadone Hydrochloride 28:08.08 and Buprenorphine Hydrochloride 28:02.12.)

■ **Neonatal Opiate Withdrawal** Opiate agonists, including morphine and methadone, have been used to manage manifestations of opiate abstinence syndrome (i.e., postnatal withdrawal) in neonates† exposed to opiates in utero. Opiates are recommended as first-line pharmacologic therapy when environmental and supportive measures (e.g., minimization of external stimuli, maximization of mother-infant contact [e.g., parental "rooming in"], breast-feeding when not contraindicated, swaddling and gentle handling) are inadequate. Other adjunctive therapy (e.g., clonidine, phenobarbital) may be added if the response to opiates is inadequate, or phenobarbital may be added if the neonate was exposed to additional substances in utero. Approximately 60–80% of neonates with opiate abstinence syndrome may require pharmacologic treatment for withdrawal symptoms. While morphine has been used more extensively than other opiates in the management of neonatal opiate abstinence syndrome, some studies suggest that use of methadone or buprenorphine (an opiate partial agonist) may be associated with shorter treatment durations and hospital stays compared with morphine use. However, additional study is needed to establish optimal dosage schedules and preferred opiate drugs and to evaluate longer-term (e.g., neurodevelopmental) outcomes.

Use of standardized protocols for identification, evaluation, and treatment of neonatal opiate abstinence syndrome is recommended since use of such protocols has been shown to improve overall response, including shorter hospital stays and durations of pharmacologic treatment. Some evidence suggests that use of a standardized protocol may be more important than use of a specific opiate agonist (e.g., methadone versus morphine) in improving outcomes. Protocols generally utilize assessment tools that were developed to quantify severity of withdrawal in term neonates to facilitate decisions regarding initiation, titration, and tapering of therapy. (See Oral Dosage for Neonatal Opiate Withdrawal under Dosage and Administration: Dosage, in Morphine Sulfate 28:08.08 and also see Neonatal Opiate Withdrawal under Dosage and Administration: Dosage, in Methadone Hydrochloride 28:08.08.)

Dosage and Administration

■ **Administration** Opiate agonists may be administered orally, rectally, IM, subcutaneously, or IV. The parenteral route is usually used for relief of severe pain, and for relief of surgical or postoperative pain and pain during labor. IV administration is used to relieve acute, unbearable pain, and as a supplement to anesthesia. The drugs should also be administered IV in patients with shock or hypothermia in whom absorption is likely to be delayed following subcutaneous or IM injection. If opiate agonists are administered IV, usual dosage should generally be reduced and the solution should be injected slowly. An opiate antagonist and facilities for administration of oxygen and control of respiration should be immediately available during and immediately following IV administration of opiate agonists. A preservative-free preparation of morphine sulfate may also be administered epidurally or intrathecally. Morphine sulfate extended-release liposomal injection is administered epidurally. Fentanyl also may be administered percutaneously (by topical application of a transdermal system or iontophoretic transdermal system) or transmucosally (intrabuccally, sublingually, intranasally).

When therapy with an extended-release or long-acting opiate formulation is initiated, all other around-the-clock opiate analgesics should be discontinued. Oral extended-release tablets or capsules should be swallowed whole, one at a time, with enough water to ensure complete swallowing of the tablet or capsule immediately after it is placed in the mouth; crushing, chewing, or dissolving the capsules or tablets will result in uncontrolled delivery of the opiate agonist and can result in overdosage and death.

■ **Dosage** Current principles of pain management indicate that opiate analgesics should be used in conjunction with appropriate nonopiate pharmacologic therapy and/or nonpharmacologic modalities in the symptomatic treatment of both acute and chronic pain. Because of the potential harms associated with opiate therapy, care is required to prevent inappropriate transition from short-term therapy for acute pain to chronic opiate therapy when other treatment modalities may be more appropriate. The lowest effective dosage and shortest duration of therapy consistent with treatment goals of the patient should be employed. Dosage of opiate agonists must be carefully adjusted according to the severity of pain and the response of the patient. Standard pain assessment tools adjusted to the patient's age and cognitive development may be employed to help the patient communicate pain intensity and to guide treatment. During long-term therapy of chronic noncancer pain, both pain intensity and functional status should be assessed regularly using validated tools, and progress toward therapeutic goals, adherence to the treatment plan, and presence of adverse effects should be monitored; when opiate therapy fails to provide clinically meaningful improvements in pain and functional status or when the risks of such therapy outweigh the benefits, other treatment approaches should be optimized and opiate analgesic therapy should be tapered and discontinued. Reduced dosage is indicated in poor-risk patients, in patients with substantial hepatic impairment, in patients with renal impairment, and in very young or very old patients. If concomitant therapy with other CNS depressants is required, the lowest effective dosages and shortest possible duration of concomitant therapy should be used. (See Drug Interactions: Benzodiazepines and Other CNS Depressants.) Following parenteral administration, adverse effects such as nausea, vomiting, dizziness, and hypotension may be alleviated by maintaining the patient in a supine position and elevating his legs. In surgical patients, dosage of opiate agonists should be based on response of the patient, premedication or concomitant medication, the anesthetics which are being used, and the nature and duration of the operation.

The following doses administered orally or IM provide analgesia comparable to that produced by 30 mg of oral morphine sulfate or 10 mg of IM morphine sulfate:

Table 1. Comparative Opiate Agonist Dosage with Oral or Parenteral Administration

	Equianalgesic Dose (in mg)[a]	
Opiate Agonist	**Oral**	**IM[b]**
Morphine	30	10
Hydrocodone	30	–
Hydromorphone	7.5	1.5
Oxycodone	20	–
Methadone	20 (acute)	10 (acute)
Levorphanol	4 (acute) 1 (chronic)	2 (acute) 1 (chronic)
Fentanyl	–	0.1
Oxymorphone	10	1
Meperidine	300	75

[a] For specific dosages for these opiate agonists, see the individual monographs in 28:08.08.

[b] These are standard IM doses for acute pain in adults and also can be used to convert doses for IV infusions and repeated small IV doses ("boluses"). For single IV doses ("boluses"), use half the IM dose.

These equivalencies were based principally on single-dose studies comparing oral and IM doses of these drugs in cancer patients and patients with postoperative pain. When such comparisons are used to convert patients already receiving opiate therapy to therapy using a different opiate agonist or a different administration route, the equianalgesic dosage estimate should be adjusted based on consideration of the clinical situation (e.g., response to the previous regimen, adverse effects) and characteristics of the specific drugs involved (e.g., elimination half-life). In patients receiving chronic opiate therapy, the calculated equianalgesic dosage of the new opiate agonist generally should be reduced by about 25–50% in order to avoid inadvertent overdosage. Equivalencies based on single-dose studies may overestimate dosage requirements for methadone during chronic therapy; such comparisons should not be used to convert patients already receiving chronic opiate therapy to therapy with methadone. For further information about transferring patients from another opiate agonist to therapy with methadone, see Dosage and Administration in Methadone Hydrochloride 28:08.08.

Orally administered oxycodone in a dose of 4.88 mg produces analgesia comparable to 30 mg of oral codeine. Orally administered oxycodone also has been described as being 7–9.5 times as potent as oral codeine. Oxycodone hydrochloride extended-release tablets are reported to be 1.5–2 times as potent as morphine sulfate extended-release tablets (MS Contin®).

When repeated increases in dosage are required, potential causes should be evaluated and the relative benefits and risks reassessed. Use of higher dosages requires particular caution, including more frequent and intensive monitoring or consultation with or referral to a pain management specialist. (See Chronic Noncancer Pain under Pain: Chronic Pain, in Uses.) The US Centers for Disease Control and Prevention (CDC) guideline for primary care clinicians who prescribe opiates for chronic noncancer pain states that clinicians should carefully reassess individual benefits and risks before prescribing dosages equivalent to 50 mg or more of morphine sulfate daily and should avoid dosages equivalent to 90 mg or more of morphine sulfate daily or carefully justify their decision to titrate dosage to such levels. Other experts have stated that a pain management specialist should be consulted before exceeding an opiate dosage equivalent to 80–120 mg of morphine sulfate daily. In contrast, guidelines developed several years earlier tended to suggest higher dosage thresholds (e.g., equivalent to 200 mg or more of morphine sulfate daily) for more frequent and intensive monitoring or consultation or referral. Clinicians should be aware that some states have established dosage thresholds for opiate prescribing (e.g., maximum daily dosages that can be prescribed, dosage thresholds at which consultation with a specialist is mandated or recommended) or have mandated certain risk-management strategies (e.g., review of state prescription drug monitoring program [PDMP] data prior to prescribing).

Extended-release and Long-acting Formulations for the Management of Chronic Pain Appropriate dosage selection and titration are essential to reduce the risk of respiratory depression associated with use of extended-release or long-acting formulations of opiate analgesics. The initial dosage must be individualized, taking into account the patient's prior analgesic use and risk factors for addiction, abuse, and misuse. Patients should be monitored closely for respiratory depression, especially during the first 24–72 hours of therapy and following any increase in dosage. Use of higher than recommended initial dosages in patients who are not opiate tolerant may result in fatal respiratory depression. Some extended-release or long-acting preparations or dosage strengths should be used only in opiate-tolerant patients. In patients who are being transferred from other oral opiates to therapy with an extended-release or long-acting opiate analgesic, all other around-the-clock opiate analgesics should be discontinued when therapy with the extended-release or long-acting formulation is initiated. Dosage must be carefully individualized since overestimation of the initial dosage in opiate-tolerant patients can result in fatal overdosage with the first dose. Because there is substantial interpatient variability in the relative potency of opiate analgesics and formulations, it is preferable to underestimate the patient's 24-hour opiate requirements and provide "rescue" therapy with an immediate-release opiate analgesic than to overestimate the requirements and manage an adverse reaction. For recommended initial dosages and titration schedules, see the individual monographs in 28:08.08.

Extended-release and long-acting formulations should be prescribed only by clinicians who are knowledgeable in the use of potent opiates for the management of chronic pain. Following transfer from other opiate analgesics to an extended-release or long-acting opiate analgesic, patients should be monitored for manifestations of opiate withdrawal and for oversedation or toxicity. Particularly close monitoring is required when patients are switched from methadone, since conversion ratios between methadone and other opiate analgesics vary widely depending on extent of prior methadone exposure and because methadone has a long half-life and tends to accumulate in plasma. Dosage of the extended-release or long-acting opiate agonist should be titrated to a level that provides adequate analgesia with minimal adverse effects. Patients should be reevaluated continually for adequacy of pain control and for adverse effects, as well as for the development of addiction, abuse, or misuse. Patients who experience breakthrough pain may require an increase in dosage of the extended-release or long-acting opiate agonist or "rescue" therapy with an appropriate dose of an immediate-release analgesic. If the pain intensity increases after dosage stabilization, an attempt should be made to identify the source of increased pain before increasing the dosage. Frequent communication is important among the prescriber, other members of the healthcare team, the patient, and the patient's caregiver or family during periods of changing analgesic requirements, including the initial dosage titration period. During long-term therapy, the continued need for opiate analgesics should be continually reevaluated.

Cautions

Respiratory depression and, to a lesser degree, circulatory depression (including orthostatic hypotension) are the chief hazards of opiate agonist therapy. Respiratory arrest, shock, and cardiac arrest have occurred. Rapid IV administration of opiate agonists increases the incidence of these serious adverse effects.

■ **Respiratory Depression** Respiratory depression is produced even with therapeutic analgesic doses of opiate agonists, but it is usually not clinically important in patients with normal respiratory capacity. It is probable that equianalgesic doses of individual opiate agonists produce similar degrees of respiratory depression; they may differ in the duration of the depressant effects they produce. Since opiate agonists may depress deep breathing and the reflex to sigh, these drugs may induce atelectasis, especially in patients with pulmonary disorders. If opiate agonists are necessary for the relief of severe pain in these patients, breathing exercises or use of forced deep inspiration with bag and mask should be encouraged. Neonates should be observed closely for signs of respiratory depression if the mother has received opiate agonists during labor.

Modified-release (e.g., extended-release) opiate agonists are associated with a greater risk of overdose and death because of the larger amount of drug contained in each dosage unit. Serious, life-threatening, or fatal respiratory depression has been reported even when these formulations were used as recommended. Although respiratory depression can occur at any time during therapy, the risk is greatest during initiation of therapy or following an increase in dosage.

■ Nervous System Effects Adverse CNS effects of opiate agonists include dizziness, visual disturbances, mental clouding or depression, sedation, coma, euphoria, dysphoria, weakness, faintness, agitation, restlessness, nervousness, seizures, and, rarely, delirium and insomnia. Opiate agonists may interfere with evaluation of CNS function, especially relative to consciousness levels, pupillary changes, and respiratory depression, thereby masking the patient's clinical course. Ambulatory patients and those patients not experiencing severe pain seem to have a higher incidence of adverse effects such as dizziness, nausea, vomiting, and hypotension than those who are in a supine position or who have severe pain. Patients with reduced blood volume, as may occur with hemorrhage or hemorrhagic shock, may be more sensitive than other patients to the hypotensive effect of opiate agonists. Although controlled studies are lacking, patients with hyperthyroidism appear to be more tolerant to the depressant effects of opiate agonists than patients with normal thyroid function.

■ GI Effects Adverse GI effects of opiate agonists include nausea, vomiting, and constipation. The use of morphine and its congeners in patients with chronic ulcerative colitis may stimulate motility in the colon; in patients with acute ulcerative colitis, toxic dilation may occur. Opiate agonist-induced increase in intraluminal pressure may endanger surgical anastomosis. Opiate agonists may obscure the diagnosis or clinical course in patients with acute abdominal conditions.

Opiate agonist-induced increase in biliary tract pressure may result in biliary spasm or colic, especially in the sphincter of Oddi. This spasm is usually accompanied by increased plasma concentrations of amylase and lipase. Because of this effect, plasma amylase and lipase determinations should not be performed within 24 hours after an opiate agonist has been given.

■ Cardiovascular Effects Several cases of QT-interval prolongation and severe cardiac arrhythmias, including torsades de pointes, have been reported during postmarketing surveillance of levomethadyl acetate hydrochloride (no longer commercially available in the US) and also have been reported in patients receiving methadone hydrochloride, especially in individuals receiving higher dosages. (For further information about cardiovascular effects in patients receiving methadone, see Cautions in Methadone Hydrochloride 28:08.08.) QT-interval prolongation also has been observed in healthy individuals receiving extended-release hydrocodone bitartrate. In addition, cardiac arrest, ST segment elevation, ventricular tachycardia, myocardial infarction, angina pectoris, and syncope have been reported during postmarketing surveillance of levomethadyl acetate hydrochloride. In a study evaluating safety, tolerability, and electrocardiographic (ECG) effects of propoxyphene (no longer commercially available in the US) in healthy individuals, QT-interval prolongation, widening of the QRS complex, and prolongation of the PR interval were observed at therapeutic dosages of the drug.

■ Genitourinary and Endocrine Effects Opiate agonists may cause urinary retention and oliguria. Patients with prostatic hypertrophy or urethral stricture may be more prone to these effects. Opiate agonists may increase the risk of water intoxication in postoperative patients because of stimulation of the release of vasopressin.

Opiate agonists inhibit release of corticotropin as reflected by a decrease in plasma and urinary concentrations of 17-hydroxysteroids and 17-ketosteroids; rarely, secondary adrenocortical hypofunction or adrenal hypertrophy associated with hyperplasia of the reticular zone may follow chronic opiate agonist therapy. Onset of adrenal insufficiency in patients receiving opiate agonists or opiate partial agonists generally has occurred after at least 1 month of opiate agonist or partial agonist use, although the time to onset has ranged from within 1 day to more than 1 year. Manifestations of adrenal insufficiency are nonspecific and may include nausea, vomiting, anorexia, fatigue, weakness, dizziness, and hypotension. In many of the reported cases, patients required hospitalization. If adrenal insufficiency is suspected, appropriate laboratory testing should be performed promptly and physiologic (replacement) dosages of corticosteroids provided; therapy with the opiate agonist or partial agonist should be tapered and discontinued to allow recovery of adrenal function. If the opiate agonist or partial agonist can be discontinued, follow-up assessment of adrenal function should be performed to determine if corticosteroid replacement therapy can be discontinued. In some patients, switching to a different opiate improved symptoms.

Hypogonadism and androgen deficiency have been reported in patients receiving long-term opiate agonist or opiate partial agonist therapy, although a causal relationship has not been established. Suppression of gonadotropic function produced by opiate agonists may cause impotence and a decline in libido, possibly accompanied by decreased plasma and urinary concentrations of 17-ketosteroids. Patients receiving long-term opiate agonist or partial agonist therapy who present with manifestations of hypogonadism (e.g., decreased libido, impotence, erectile dysfunction, amenorrhea, infertility) should undergo laboratory evaluation.

■ Cholinergic Effects Bradycardia and other cholinergic effects which may occur following administration of opiate agonists may be controlled with atropine. In contrast to cholinergic effects produced by other opiates, meperidine or its congeners may produce anticholinergic effects such as dry mouth, palpitation, and tachycardia; uncoordinated jerky movements, muscle tremors and twitches, delirium with disorientation, hallucinations, and, occasionally, tonic-clonic (grand mal) seizures may also occur.

■ Other Adverse Effects Opiate agonists can release histamine (see Pharmacology: Effects on Histamine) and may produce sweating, flushing, or warmness of the face, neck, and upper thorax; pruritus; and urticaria. True anaphylactic reactions are extremely rare. Wheals, phlebitis, and pain may occur at the site of injection and local tissue irritation and induration are common following repeated subcutaneous administration of some opiate agonists. Reversible thrombocytopenia has been reported in an opiate-dependent patient with underlying chronic hepatitis who was receiving methadone.

■ Precautions and Contraindications Concomitant use of opiate agonists and benzodiazepines or other CNS depressants (e.g., anxiolytics, sedatives, hypnotics, tranquilizers, muscle relaxants, general anesthetics, antipsychotics, other opiate agonists, alcohol) may result in profound sedation, respiratory depression, coma, and death. Concomitant use of opiate analgesics and benzodiazepines or other CNS depressants should be reserved for patients in whom alternative treatment options are inadequate; the lowest effective dosages and shortest possible duration of concomitant therapy should be used, and the patient should be monitored closely for respiratory depression and sedation. Opiate antitussives should be avoided in patients receiving CNS depressants. Patients receiving opiate agonists and/or their caregivers should be apprised of the risks associated with concomitant therapeutic or illicit use of benzodiazepines, alcohol, or other CNS depressants. Concomitant use with alcohol should be avoided. (See Drug Interactions: Benzodiazepines and Other CNS Depressants.)

Because the morbidity and mortality associated with untreated opiate addiction can outweigh the serious risks associated with concomitant use of opiates and benzodiazepines or other CNS depressants, FDA states that therapy with opiate agonists or partial agonists (e.g., methadone, buprenorphine) for opiate addiction (i.e., medication-assisted treatment [MAT]) should not be withheld from patients receiving benzodiazepines or other CNS depressants. These drugs should be tapered and discontinued, if possible, in patients receiving MAT. However, excluding or discharging patients from MAT because of benzodiazepine or CNS depressant use is not likely to prevent such concomitant use and may lead to use outside the treatment setting, which could result in more severe outcomes. Careful management can reduce the risks associated with such concomitant use. (See Cautions in Methadone Hydrochloride 28:08.08.)

Because exposure to opiate agonists may be increased in patients with renal or hepatic impairment, use of conservative initial dosages followed by slow dosage titration generally is recommended; patients should be monitored closely for respiratory and CNS depression, particularly during dosage titration.

Opiate agonists also should be used with caution in cachectic, debilitated, or geriatric patients, since pharmacokinetics of the drugs may be altered and these patients may be at increased risk for respiratory depression. These patients should be monitored closely, particularly during initiation of therapy and dosage titration and when other drugs with respiratory depressant effects are used concomitantly.

Opiate agonists are contraindicated in patients with substantial respiratory depression or with acute or severe bronchial asthma or hypercarbia in unmonitored settings or in the absence of resuscitative equipment. Opiate agonists should be used with extreme caution in patients with preexisting respiratory depression and in those with conditions accompanied by hypoxia, hypercapnia, or decreased respiratory reserve, such as asthma, chronic obstructive pulmonary disease, cor pulmonale, severe obesity, sleep apnea, myxedema, kyphoscoliosis, CNS depression, or coma. In such patients, even therapeutic doses of opiate agonists may decrease respiratory drive while simultaneously increasing airway resistance to the point of apnea. Alternative analgesics without opiate agonist activity should be considered, and opiate agonists should be used only with close monitoring and at the lowest effective dosage in such patients. The risk of respiratory depression also is increased in geriatric, cachectic, or debilitated patients; following large initial doses of opiate agonists in patients who are not opiate tolerant; and in patients receiving other agents with respiratory depressant effects.

When opiate agonists are prescribed for patients at increased risk of opiate overdosage (e.g., those with a history of overdose or substance use disorder, those receiving opiate dosages equivalent to 50 mg or more of morphine sulfate daily, those receiving benzodiazepines concomitantly, those with medical conditions that could increase sensitivity to opiate effects), some experts state that clinicians should consider offering the opiate antagonist naloxone.

Opiate agonists may cause severe hypotension in patients whose ability to maintain blood pressure has been compromised by blood volume depletion or concomitant use of certain drugs (e.g., general anesthetics, phenothiazines). Because opiate agonists may cause vasodilation that can further reduce cardiac output and blood pressure in patients with circulatory shock, the drugs should be used with caution in these patients; use of extended-release opiate agonists generally should be avoided in such patients. Opiate agonists may cause orthostatic hypotension and syncope in ambulatory patients.

The respiratory depressant effects of opiate agonists promote carbon dioxide retention, which results in elevation of intracranial pressure. The ability of opiate agonists to increase intracranial pressure may be markedly exaggerated in patients with head injury, other intracranial lesions, or preexisting elevated intracranial pressure. Opiate agonists also produce effects (e.g., pupillary changes, altered consciousness) that may obscure the clinical course and neurologic signs of further increases in intracranial pressure in patients with head injuries. Patients who may be particularly susceptible to the effects of carbon dioxide retention (e.g., those with elevated intracranial pressure, brain tumors, or impaired consciousness or coma) should be monitored closely. Use of long-acting or extended-release opiate agonists generally should be avoided in patients with impaired consciousness or coma.

Serotonin syndrome has been reported during concomitant use of opiate agonists and serotonergic drugs at recommended dosages. Manifestations of serotonin syndrome may include mental status changes (e.g., agitation, hallucinations, coma), autonomic instability (e.g., tachycardia, labile blood pressure, hyperthermia), neuromuscular aberrations (e.g., hyperreflexia, incoordination, rigidity), and/or GI symptoms (e.g., nausea, vomiting, diarrhea). Symptom onset generally occurs within several hours to a few days of concomitant use, but may occur later, particularly after dosage increases. (See Drug Interactions: Drugs Associated with Serotonin Syndrome.)

Opiate agonists are contraindicated in patients with known or suspected paralytic ileus and GI obstruction. Opiate agonists should be used with caution in patients at risk for ileus. Because opiate agonists diminish propulsive peristaltic waves in the GI tract and decrease bowel motility, postoperative patients receiving opiate analgesia should be monitored for decreased bowel motility. Chronic use of opiate agonists may result in obstructive bowel disease, especially in patients with underlying intestinal motility disorders. Opiate agonists may cause or aggravate constipation. Opiate agonists may obscure the diagnosis or clinical course of patients with acute abdominal conditions. Because opiate agonists may cause spasm of the sphincter of Oddi and diminish biliary and pancreatic secretions, patients with biliary tract disease, including those with acute pancreatitis, should be monitored for worsening symptoms.

Because of their cholinergic effects, opiate agonists should be used with caution in patients with cardiac arrhythmias.

Opiate agonists may aggravate preexisting seizures in patients with seizure disorders and may induce or aggravate seizures in some clinical settings. During long-term opiate agonist therapy, patients with seizure disorders should be monitored for worsening of seizure control.

Opiate agonists also should be used with caution in patients with hypothyroidism, adrenocortical insufficiency (e.g., Addison's disease), prostatic hyperplasia or urethral stricture, toxic psychosis, acute alcoholism, or delirium tremens.

Individuals who perform hazardous tasks requiring mental alertness or physical coordination should be warned about possible adverse CNS effects of opiate agonists.

Patients who are unable to tolerate one agent may be able to tolerate a different agent. Opiate agonists are contraindicated in patients with known hypersensitivity to the particular drug.

■ **Pediatric Precautions** Serious adverse events, including deaths, have been reported in pediatric patients receiving codeine or tramadol for management of pain; in some of these cases, ultrarapid or extensive metabolism of cytochrome P-450 (CYP) isoenzyme 2D6 substrates was confirmed or suspected. (See Pharmacogenomics under Pharmacokinetics: Elimination.) Because of the potential for serious or fatal adverse effects in pediatric patients, use of codeine or tramadol for the management of pain is *contraindicated* in children younger than 12 years of age; tramadol and codeine also are *contraindicated* in pediatric patients younger than 18 years of age for the management of postoperative pain following tonsillectomy and/or adenoidectomy. FDA also states that use of codeine or tramadol for pain management is *not* recommended in children 12–18 years of age who are obese or have conditions such as obstructive sleep apnea or compromised respiratory function, since they may be susceptible to the respiratory depressant effects of the drug. (See Codeine 28:08.08 and Tramadol Hydrochloride 28:08.08.)

Serious adverse events, including deaths, also have been reported in pediatric patients receiving opiate agonists for the management of cough and cold. For information on precautions and contraindications associated with use of codeine or hydrocodone as antitussives in pediatric patients, see Cautions: Pediatric Precautions, in Codeine 48:08 and in Hydrocodone Bitartrate 48:08.

■ **Geriatric Precautions** Geriatric patients are more likely than younger individuals to experience adverse effects, especially respiratory depressant effects, of opiate agonists and may be more sensitive to the analgesic effects of these drugs. Geriatric adults also are more likely to have prostatic hyperplasia or obstruction and renal impairment and thus may be at increased risk of opiate agonist-induced urinary retention. Clearance of opiate agonists may be decreased in geriatric patients, resulting in longer durations of action. Care should be exercised, and appropriate dosage adjustments (e.g., lower initial doses, longer dosing intervals) should be considered.

Some clinicians recommend that methadone and other opiate agonists with long elimination half-lives be used with caution in geriatric patients because of the greater frequency of decreased renal and hepatic function observed in these individuals. Meperidine should be used with caution in geriatric patients, and dosage adjustment should be considered because of the potential for adverse CNS effects (e.g., anxiety, excitation, tremors, myoclonus, seizures) secondary to accumulation of the toxic metabolite normeperidine, especially in those with decreased renal and hepatic function. Because of this risk, many experts recommend that alternative opiates be used in patients with renal impairment and in other individuals requiring large or repeated doses of opiate agonists.

■ **Pregnancy and Lactation** Analysis of data from the National Birth Defects Prevention Study, a large population-based, case-control study, suggests that therapeutic maternal use of opiate agonists during the period of organogenesis is associated with a low absolute risk of birth defects, including heart defects, spina bifida, and gastroschisis. Although there are no adequate and controlled studies to date in humans, some opiate agonists (e.g., morphine) have been shown to be teratogenic in animals. Therefore, opiate agonists should be used during pregnancy only when the potential benefits justify the possible risks to the fetus.

Prolonged maternal use of opiate agonists during pregnancy can result in neonatal opiate withdrawal syndrome with manifestations of irritability, hyperactivity and abnormal sleep pattern, high-pitched cry, tremor, vomiting, diarrhea, and failure to gain weight. In contrast to adults, the withdrawal syndrome in neonates may be life-threatening if not recognized and treated, and requires management according to protocols developed by neonatology experts. Women who require prolonged opiate agonist therapy during pregnancy should be advised of the risk of neonatal opiate withdrawal syndrome, and availability of appropriate treatment should be ensured. The onset, duration, and severity of the syndrome vary depending on the specific opiate agonist used, duration of use, timing and amount of last maternal use, and rate of drug elimination by the neonate. Use of standardized protocols for identification and management of opiate withdrawal syndrome has been shown to improve overall response, including reductions in hospital stay and duration of pharmacologic treatment. When environmental and supportive measures are inadequate, opiates are recommended as first-line pharmacologic therapy. (See Uses: Neonatal Opiate Withdrawal.)

Use of opiate agonists during late pregnancy can result in neonatal respiratory depression.

Use of long-acting or extended-release opiate agonist analgesics is not recommended immediately before or during labor, when shorter-acting analgesics or other analgesic techniques may be more appropriate. Opiate agonists may prolong labor through actions that temporarily reduce the strength, duration, and frequency of uterine contractions. However, this effect is inconsistent and may be offset by an increased rate of cervical dilatation, which tends to shorten labor.

Higher than expected concentrations of morphine (the active metabolite of codeine) may be distributed into breast milk of women taking codeine who are ultrarapid metabolizers of CYP2D6 substrates. (See Pharmacogenomics under Pharmacokinetics: Elimination.) Because of the potential for serious adverse effects in nursing infants, especially if the infant's mother is an ultrarapid metabolizer of CYP2D6 substrates, use of codeine is not recommended in nursing women. (See Codeine 48:08 and also see Codeine 28:08.08.) Because tramadol is distributed into milk and has similar risks as codeine in ultrarapid metabolizers of CYP2D6 substrates, use of tramadol also is not recommended in nursing women. (See Cautions in Tramadol Hydrochloride 28:08.08.)

Drug Interactions

■ **Benzodiazepines and Other CNS Depressants** Concomitant use of opiate agonists and benzodiazepines or other CNS depressants including other opiate agonists, anxiolytics, general anesthetics, tranquilizers, sedatives, hypnotics, muscle relaxants, antipsychotics, and alcohol can increase the risk of respiratory depression, hypotension, profound sedation, coma, and death. Opiate analgesics frequently are implicated as contributing to fatal overdoses involving other CNS depressants, and epidemiologic studies have shown that a substantial proportion of fatal opiate overdoses involve the concurrent use of benzodiazepines, alcohol, or other CNS depressants.

Whenever possible, concomitant use of opiate agonists and benzodiazepines should be avoided. Alcohol also should be avoided in patients receiving opiate agonists. Concomitant use of opiate analgesics and benzodiazepines or other CNS depressants should be reserved for patients in whom alternative treatment options are inadequate, and opiate antitussive agents should be avoided in patients receiving CNS depressant therapy. If a decision is made to prescribe opiate analgesics and CNS depressants concomitantly, the lowest effective dosages and shortest possible duration of concomitant therapy should be used, and the patient should be monitored closely for sedation, hypotension, and respiratory depressant effects. If a benzodiazepine or other CNS depressant is required for any indication other than epilepsy in a patient receiving opiate therapy for analgesia, the drug should be initiated at a lower dosage than indicated in the absence of opiate therapy and titrated based on clinical response. In patients receiving a CNS depressant, opiate analgesics, if required, should be initiated at a reduced dosage and titrated based on clinical response.

Because the morbidity and mortality associated with untreated opiate addiction can outweigh the serious risks associated with concomitant use of opiates and benzodiazepines or other CNS depressants, FDA states that therapy with opiates (e.g., methadone) for opiate addiction (i.e., medication-assisted treatment [MAT]) should not be withheld from patients receiving benzodiazepines or other CNS depressants. Clinicians should develop treatment plans that minimize the risks associated with such concomitant use. If possible, benzodiazepines or other CNS depressants should be tapered and discontinued. (See Cautions in Methadone Hydrochloride 28:08.08.)

Some experts state that consideration should be given to offering the opiate antagonist naloxone when opiates are prescribed for patients at increased risk of opiate overdosage, including those receiving benzodiazepines concomitantly.

When considering use of extended-release or long-acting opiate agonist therapy in a patient already receiving another CNS depressant, the duration of use and response to the CNS depressant, including the degree of tolerance to CNS depressant effects, as well as the patient's use of alcohol or any illicit CNS depressants, should be evaluated. Concomitant use of alcohol with some oral extended-release opiate agonist formulations can result in increased plasma concentrations of the opiate agonist and potentially fatal overdosage.

■ **Antidepressants** Opiate agonists may potentiate the effects of tricyclic antidepressants and monoamine oxidase (MAO) inhibitors, including procarbazine hydrochloride; therefore, opiate agonists should be used with great caution and in reduced dosage when used in conjunction with such drugs. Virtually all the reported incidents of opiate agonist interaction with MAO inhibitors have occurred in patients receiving meperidine. (See Meperidine Hydrochloride 28:08.08.) Because MAO inhibitors may potentiate the effects of opiate agonists and because these effects may be severe and unpredictable, use of opiate agonists during or within 14 days following treatment with an MAO inhibitor is not recommended. Meperidine is contraindicated in patients receiving MAO inhibitors. Some manufacturers state that if an opiate agonist is required in patients receiving MAO inhibitors, a sensitivity test should be performed with small increments of morphine or the opiate agonist administered over a period of several hours while the patient is kept under close medical observation.

■ **Drugs Associated with Serotonin Syndrome** Serotonin syndrome may occur in patients receiving opiate agonists in conjunction with other serotonergic drugs, including serotonin (5-hydroxytryptamine; 5-HT) type 1 receptor agonists ("triptans"), selective serotonin-reuptake inhibitors (SSRIs), selective serotonin- and norepinephrine-reuptake inhibitors (SNRIs), tricyclic antidepressants, antiemetics that are 5-HT_3 receptor antagonists, buspirone, cyclobenzaprine, dextromethorphan, lithium, St. John's wort (*Hypericum perforatum*), tryptophan, other serotonin modulators (e.g., mirtazapine, nefazodone, trazodone, vilazodone), and MAO inhibitors (both those used to treat psychiatric disorders and others, such as linezolid, methylene blue, and selegiline). Serotonin syndrome may occur within the recommended dosage ranges for these drugs. Manifestations of serotonin syndrome may include mental status changes (e.g., agitation, hallucinations, coma), autonomic instability (e.g., tachycardia, labile blood pressure, hyperthermia), neuromuscular aberrations (e.g., hyperreflexia, incoordination, rigidity), and/or GI symptoms (e.g., nausea, vomiting, diarrhea). Symptom onset generally occurs within several hours to a few days of concomitant use, but may occur later, particularly after dosage increases.

If concurrent therapy with opiate agonists and serotonergic drugs is warranted, patients should be monitored for serotonin syndrome, particularly during initiation of therapy and dosage increases. If serotonin syndrome is suspected, treatment with opiate agonists and any concurrently administered serotonergic agents should be discontinued.

For further information on serotonin syndrome, including manifestations and treatment, see Drug Interactions: Serotonergic Drugs, in Fluoxetine Hydrochloride 28:16.04.20.

■ **Opiate Antagonists and Opiate Partial Agonists** Withdrawal symptoms may occur in patients receiving opiate agonists concomitantly with opiate antagonists (e.g., naloxone, naltrexone) or opiate partial agonists (e.g., buprenorphine, butorphanol, nalbuphine, pentazocine). Partial agonists should not be administered in patients receiving opiate agonists as they may reduce the analgesic effect and/or precipitate withdrawal symptoms.

■ **Drugs Affecting Hepatic Microsomal Enzymes** Metabolism of some opiates (e.g., codeine, fentanyl, hydrocodone, methadone, oxycodone, tramadol) is mediated by the cytochrome P-450 (CYP) microsomal enzyme system. Metabolism of methadone is mediated mainly by CYP isoenzymes 2B6, 2C19, and 3A4, and, to a lesser extent, by CYP isoenzymes 2C9 and 2D6. Fentanyl, hydrocodone, and oxycodone are metabolized mainly by CYP3A4, although CYP2D6 also is involved in the metabolism of hydrocodone and oxycodone. Codeine and tramadol are metabolized by CYP2D6 and CYP3A4. Concomitant use of these opiates with drugs that induce or inhibit these isoenzymes may alter metabolism and clearance of the opiate. For further information, see Drug Interactions in the individual monographs in 28:08.08.

■ **Drugs Affecting the P-glycoprotein Transport System** Some opiate agonists (e.g., hydromorphone, morphine, tapentadol) are eliminated mainly as glucuronide conjugates. Concomitant use of morphine with P-glycoprotein inhibitors has been shown to increase systemic exposure to morphine.

■ **Drugs that Prolong QT Interval** Because of the potential for prolongation of the QT interval or serious cardiac arrhythmias, methadone should be used with extreme caution in patients receiving drugs that are known to prolong the QT interval or drugs that may result in electrolyte disturbances (e.g., hypokalemia, hypomagnesemia) that may prolong the QT interval. For further information on cardiovascular effects of methadone and associated drug interactions, see Methadone Hydrochloride 28:08.08.

■ **Anticholinergic Agents** Concomitant use of opiate agonists and drugs with anticholinergic activity may increase the risk of urinary retention or severe constipation, which can lead to paralytic ileus. Patients receiving such concomitant therapy should be monitored for signs or symptoms of urinary retention and reduced GI motility.

■ **Neuromuscular Blocking Agents** Opiate agonists may enhance the neuromuscular-blocking action of skeletal muscle relaxants.

■ **Amphetamines** Dextroamphetamine may enhance opiate agonist analgesia.

■ **Diuretics** Opiate agonists may decrease the effects of diuretics by inducing the release of vasopressin (antidiuretic hormone).

Acute Toxicity

■ **Manifestations** Opiate agonist overdosage usually produces CNS depression ranging from stupor to a profound coma; respiratory depression which may progress to Cheyne-Stokes respiration and/or cyanosis; cold, clammy skin and/or hypothermia; flaccid skeletal muscles; bradycardia; and hypotension. In patients with severe overdosage, particularly following rapid IV administration of an opiate agonist, apnea, circulatory collapse, cardiac arrest, respiratory arrest, and death may occur. Complications such as pneumonia, shock, and/or pulmonary edema may also prove fatal. Although miosis is characteristic of overdosage with morphine derivatives and methadone, mydriasis may occur in terminal narcosis or severe hypoxia. Overdosage of meperidine or its congeners may produce mydriasis rather than miosis. Toxic effects of meperidine and its derivatives may be excitatory, especially in patients who have developed tolerance to the depressant effects of the drug. These patients may exhibit dry mouth, increased muscular activity, muscle tremors and twitches, tachycardia, delirium with disorientation, hallucinations, and, occasionally, tonic-clonic seizures.

Overdosage may be caused inadvertently by delayed absorption when repeated doses of opiate agonists are administered IM or subcutaneously to a patient with hypothermia, shock, hypotension, or any other condition that might impair circulation. When circulation is restored in these patients, large amounts of the opiate agonist are absorbed into the blood stream. Therefore, such patients should receive IV rather than subcutaneous or IM injections with the consideration that IV administration may increase the already severe cardiorespiratory impairment.

Modified-release (e.g., extended-release) opiate agonists are associated with a greater risk of overdosage and death because of the larger amount of drug contained in each dosage unit. Abuse or misuse of extended-release dosage forms by crushing or chewing the extended-release capsules or tablets, snorting the contents, or injecting the dissolved contents or by intentionally compromising the transdermal system (e.g., by swallowing, snorting, or injecting drug extracted from the system) will result in uncontrolled delivery of the opiate agonist and can result in overdosage and death. Inadvertent exposure to or ingestion of these formulations, especially by a child, also can result in respiratory depression and fatal overdosage.

Neonates whose mothers have received opiate agonists during labor should be closely observed for signs of respiratory depression and treatment for opiate agonist overdosage should be instituted if necessary.

■ **Treatment** In the treatment of opiate agonist overdosage, especially in the presence of apnea, primary attention should be given to reestablishment of adequate respiratory exchange by maintaining an adequate, patent airway, using assisted or controlled respiration and oxygen as necessary. Opiate agonist-induced respiratory depression may be treated with naloxone hydrochloride (an opiate antagonist) (see 28:10); however, the duration of respiratory depression following overdosage of an opiate agonist may be longer than the duration of action of the opiate antagonist and other more immediate supportive and symptomatic treatment should also be initiated. In addition, it should be considered that use of an opiate antagonist in patients physically dependent on opiate agonists may precipitate an acute withdrawal syndrome that cannot be readily suppressed while the action of the antagonist persists. The safety and efficacy of naltrexone hydrochloride in the management of acute opiate toxicity have not been established. If respiratory depression is associated with muscular rigidity, administration of a neuromuscular blocking agent may be necessary to facilitate assisted or controlled respiration. Muscular rigidity may also respond to opiate antagonist therapy. Gastric lavage may be effective even many hours after drug ingestion since pylorospasm produced by the opiate agonist may cause much of the drug to be retained in the stomach for an extended period of time.

Chronic Toxicity

Opiate agonists have the potential to produce physical dependence and are subject to control under the Federal Controlled Substances Act of 1970. (See Preparations in the individual monographs.) Because of the drugs' opiate agonist activity at μ-receptors, tapentadol and tramadol also can produce dependence. The abuse potential of tapentadol is similar to that of hydromorphone, and tapentadol is subject to control under the Federal Controlled Substances Act of 1970. Although tramadol was *not* originally subject to control as a scheduled drug, current data suggest that the abuse potential of tramadol is less than that of morphine or oxycodone but similar to that of propoxyphene, and tramadol became subject to control under the Act effective August 18, 2014.

Tolerance, psychological dependence, and physical dependence may occur in patients receiving opiate agonists. Addiction can occur at recommended dosages or may be associated with misuse or abuse. Each patient's risk for addiction, abuse, or misuse should be assessed prior to prescribing opiate analgesics and all patients receiving the drugs should be monitored regularly for the development of these behaviors or conditions. Risks are increased in patients with a personal or family history of substance abuse (including drug or alcohol addiction or abuse) or mental illness (e.g., major depression). The potential for these risks should not prevent appropriate use of opiate agonists for the management of pain; however, use of the drugs in patients at increased risk necessitates intensive counseling about the risks and proper use, along with intensive monitoring for signs of addiction, abuse, and misuse.

Surveillance data suggest a parallel relationship between the number of opiate analgesic prescriptions dispensed in the US and the diversion and abuse of these drugs and associated adverse outcomes. Prescriptions for opiate analgesics in the US increased substantially (nearly tripling) from 1991 to 2011, and then plateaued or decreased slightly from 2011 through 2013; rates of diversion and abuse of prescription opiate analgesics followed similar patterns. Deaths associated with the use of prescription opiate analgesics increased sharply from 1999 to 2006, plateaued for several years, decreased slightly through 2013, but then increased again in 2014. From 2001 to 2014, deaths associated with the use of prescription opiate analgesics increased 3.4-fold. Fatal overdoses of heroin (diacetylmorphine, which is not available on the legitimate commercial market) have increased since 2007, with substantial increases observed each year from 2011 through 2014. Fatal heroin overdoses in 2013 were nearly quadruple the rate in the early 2000s, with most of the increase occurring after 2010. From 2001 to 2014, the number of heroin-related deaths increased sixfold. Although data suggest that only a very small proportion of individuals who abuse prescription opiate analgesics transition to heroin use, prescription opiate abuse has emerged as a growing risk factor for heroin use. In a survey of individuals entering treatment programs for heroin addiction, 80% of those who began abusing opiates in the 1960s reported that heroin was their first opiate of abuse, whereas 75% of those who began abusing opiates in the 2000s reported that their first opiate of abuse was a prescription drug. Factors that have been cited as potentially contributing to the upsurge in heroin use include the lower cost and greater accessibility of high-purity heroin, the introduction of abuse-deterrent prescription formulations, and flattening of opiate prescribing rates.

Tolerance to the analgesic, respiratory depressant, sedative, and euphoric effects of opiate agonists usually develops during prolonged therapy; however, overdosage even in patients who have developed tolerance will cause respiratory depression and death. Tolerance to all effects of opiate agonists does not develop uniformly. Meperidine-dependent patients, for example, receiving 3–4 g of the drug daily, do not develop substantial tolerance to the excitant and anticholinergic actions of meperidine and may develop stimulatory symptoms of acute meperidine toxicity.

Development of tolerance seems to depend on the degree of opiate agonist-induced CNS depression and the extent to which this depression is continued by frequent or prolonged opiate agonist administration and may occur as a result of prolonged medical use or intentional abuse. Development of tolerance in patients receiving meperidine has been reported to be more gradual than in those receiving morphine; tolerance to methadone may develop more slowly than to meperidine. Patients who have developed tolerance to one opiate agonist usually exhibit cross-tolerance to other opiate agonists. Cross-tolerance among opiate agonists may be incomplete (see Cautions in Methadone Hydrochloride 28:08.08).

Continued administration of opiate agonists may lead to physical dependence which is closely related to tolerance. Individuals who are physically dependent on opiate agonists may remain relatively asymptomatic as long as they are able to maintain their daily opiate agonist requirement. Individuals who are morphine dependent will usually continue to exhibit miosis while those who are dependent on methadone may develop some tolerance to miosis. Physical dependence results in withdrawal symptoms in patients who abruptly discontinue the drug or receive an opiate antagonist. The abstinence syndrome varies in severity according to the specific drug and the amount of drug the patient has been taking. If the abstinence syndrome is precipitated by the parenteral administration of naloxone, symptoms will be apparent within a few minutes and maximal within 30 minutes after administration; effects will usually be more severe than those following withdrawal of the opiate agonist. (Induction of methadone abstinence in this manner is especially severe.) Because of naltrexone's long duration of antagonist effect, withdrawal precipitated by the drug may be prolonged. Until the antagonist has been eliminated, large doses of opiate agonists will only partially suppress these symptoms.

In patients who have taken up to 80 mg of morphine sulfate daily for up to one month, withdrawal symptoms are usually slight and require little or no treatment. A severe abstinence syndrome occurs if the patient has received 240 mg or more of morphine sulfate for 30 days or longer. Severe opiate agonist abstinence syndrome is characterized by restlessness, lacrimation, rhinorrhea, yawning, perspiration, gooseflesh, restless sleep or "yen," and mydriasis during the first 24 hours. As the syndrome progresses, these symptoms become more severe and may be accompanied by twitching and spasms of muscles; kicking movements; severe aches in back, abdomen, and legs; abdominal and muscle cramps; hot and cold flashes; insomnia; nausea, vomiting, and diarrhea; coryza and severe sneezing; and increases in body temperature, blood pressure, respiratory rate, and heart rate. These symptoms reach peak intensity 36–72 hours following withdrawal of morphine sulfate. In addition, marked increase in urinary 17-ketosteroid concentrations and leukocytosis with leukocyte counts above 14,000/mm^3 occur frequently. Because of the excessive loss of fluids through sweating, vomiting and diarrhea, there is usually marked weight loss, dehydration, ketosis, and disturbances in acid-base balance. Cardiovascular collapse may occur especially in aged or debilitated patients. Administration of an opiate agonist will readily suppress most withdrawal symptoms except those resulting from fluid deficiency. If no treatment is given, most observable symptoms disappear in 5–14 days; however, there appears to be a phase of secondary or chronic abstinence which may last for 2–6 months after withdrawal of the drug. This phase is associated with gradually decreasing insomnia, irritability, and muscular aches. In addition, the patient may have miosis and a slight lowering of blood pressure, pulse rate, and body temperature; respiratory centers exhibit a decreased response to the stimulatory effects of carbon dioxide.

In patients who are physically dependent on meperidine, abstinence symptoms usually occur 3–4 hours after the last dose of the drug, reaching maximal intensity within 8–12 hours. Although symptoms associated with meperidine withdrawal are generally milder than those of morphine withdrawal, during the period of maximal intensity, muscle twitching, restlessness and nervousness may be worse than with morphine. Symptoms of meperidine withdrawal decline until few are apparent after 4–5 days.

Because of the cumulative effects of methadone, abstinence symptoms following its withdrawal are less intense and more prolonged than those following withdrawal of other opiate agonists and may not be manifested until 3 or 4 days after the last dose. Peak intensity of symptoms occurs on the sixth day and may include weakness, anxiety, anorexia, insomnia, abdominal discomfort, headache, sweating, and hot and cold flashes. Few symptoms are apparent after 10–14 days, although patients may exhibit lethargy and anorexia for longer periods. Other opiate agonists produce abstinence syndromes similar to those described previously. In general, the shorter the onset and duration of action of the drug, the greater the intensity and rapidity of onset of withdrawal symptoms. Those drugs which are eliminated slowly produce a mild, prolonged abstinence syndrome.

In the treatment of physical dependence, the patient may be detoxified by gradual reduction of daily opiate agonist dosage. If abstinence symptoms become severe, the patient may receive methadone (see Methadone Hydrochloride 28:08.08). Temporary administration of tranquilizers and sedatives may aid in reducing patient anxiety and opiate agonist craving. Symptoms involving GI disturbance or dehydration should be treated accordingly. Supportive social, vocational, psychiatric, and educational services should be available to the patient. For some patients, maintenance treatment with relatively stable doses of methadone or buprenorphine for relatively long periods may be necessary in the management of opiate dependence. (See Methadone Hydrochloride 28:08.08 and Buprenorphine Hydrochloride 28:08.12.) Therapy with naltrexone, an opiate antagonist, may be a useful adjunct in the maintenance of opiate cessation in some individuals formerly physically dependent on opiates who have successfully undergone detoxification. (See Naltrexone Hydrochloride 28:10.)

Alternatively, rapid detoxification has been used in the management of opiate withdrawal in opiate-dependent individuals, both in inpatient and outpatient settings. Rapid opiate detoxification involves the administration of opiate antagonists such as naloxone and naltrexone to shorten the time period of detoxification. The reported advantage of this technique is to minimize the risk of relapse and to initiate maintenance therapy with naltrexone and psychosocial interventions more quickly. Ultrarapid detoxification is similar, but involves the administration of opiate antagonists while the patient is sedated or under general anesthesia. However, the risk of adverse respiratory and cardiovascular effects associated with this procedure must be considered as well as the costs of general anesthesia and hospitalization. Safety and efficacy of these therapies have not been established and further study is needed.

Neonates born to mothers physically dependent on opiate agonists may also be opiate dependent and usually exhibit withdrawal symptoms from 1–4 days after birth. These symptoms include generalized tremors and hypertonicity with any form of tactile stimuli, hyperalertness, sleeplessness, excessive crying, vomiting, diarrhea, yawning, and, occasionally, fever. (See Pregnancy under Cautions: Pregnancy and Lactation and also see Uses: Neonatal Opiate Withdrawal.)

Pharmacology

■ **Nervous System Effects** Opiate agonists exert their principal pharmacologic effect on the CNS and on the intestines. The drugs interact as agonists at specific receptor binding sites in the CNS and other tissues. Opiate receptors are present in highest concentration in the limbic system, thalamus, striatum, hypothalamus, midbrain, and spinal cord. Several subtypes of opiate receptors have been described including the μ-receptor, which is localized in pain modulating regions of the CNS; the κ-receptor, which is localized in the deep layers of the cerebral cortex; the δ-receptor, which is localized in the limbic regions of the CNS; and the σ-receptor, which is thought to mediate the dysphoric and psychotomimetic effects of some opiate partial agonists (e.g., pentazocine). Morphine, the prototype opiate agonist, has agonist activity at the μ- and κ-receptors but has little, if any, activity at the σ-receptor; the drug is a more potent agonist at the μ- than κ-receptor. Morphine may also have some agonist activity at the δ-receptor. Agonist activity at the μ- or κ-receptor can result in analgesia, miosis, and/or decreased body temperature. Agonist activity at the μ-receptor can also result in suppression of opiate withdrawal, whereas antagonist activity can result in precipitation of withdrawal. Respiratory depression may be mediated by μ-receptors, possibly μ_2-receptors (which may be distinct from μ_1-receptors involved in analgesia); κ- and δ-receptors may also be involved in respiratory depression. Cough-suppressant opiate receptors have also been suggested.

Opiate agonists act at several sites within the CNS involving several systems of neurotransmitters to produce analgesia, but the precise mechanism of action has not been fully elucidated. Opiate agonists do not alter the threshold or responsiveness of afferent nerve endings to noxious stimuli nor the conduction of impulses along peripheral nerves; instead, the drugs alter the perception of pain at the spinal cord and higher levels in the CNS (substantia gelatinosa, spinal trigeminal nucleus, periaqueductal gray, periventricular gray, medullary raphe nuclei, hypothalamus) and the patient's emotional response to pain.

In addition to analgesia, the effects of opiate agonists on the CNS cause suppression of the cough reflex, respiratory depression, drowsiness, sedation, change in mood, euphoria, dysphoria, mental clouding, nausea, vomiting, and EEG changes. Dosages higher than usual analgesic dosages result in anesthesia;

however, prevention of awareness during and recall after opiate-agonist anesthesia may require supplementation with other agents (e.g., benzodiazepines), since awareness and recall of the surgical procedure have been reported by some patients even at high doses of an opiate agonist alone. Large doses of opiate agonists may induce excitation or seizures. Morphine and its congeners and methadone depress the cough reflex by a direct effect on the cough centers in the medulla; antitussive effects may occur with doses lower than those required for analgesia. Meperidine and its congeners generally have appreciable antitussive activity only in analgesic doses. Opiate agonists produce respiratory depression by a direct effect on the respiratory centers in the brain stem resulting in decreased sensitivity and responsiveness to increases in serum carbon dioxide tension (Pco_2). These drugs depress the pontine and medullary centers which regulate respiratory rhythm and may also alter voluntary control of respiration. Depressed respiration produces an increase in arterial Pco_2 resulting in cerebral vasodilation and a consequential rise in cerebral blood flow and CSF pressure. Increased CSF pressure is more likely to occur following IV administration of opiate agonists than following other routes of administration. Nausea is probably caused by stimulation of the chemoreceptor trigger zone (CTZ) in the medulla oblongata or by the occurrence of orthostatic hypotension. Vomiting may result from stimulation of the CTZ. In addition, the opiate agonists depress the vomiting center; therefore, subsequent doses of the drugs are unlikely to produce vomiting. Increase in vestibular sensitivity may also contribute to the high incidence of nausea and vomiting in ambulatory patients.

■ **Ocular Effects** Morphine and its congeners and, to a lesser extent, methadone cause miosis which is antagonized by atropine. Some reports state that meperidine and its congeners also produce miosis, whereas others indicate that these drugs tend to produce mydriasis or no pupillary change. Therapeutic doses of morphine and its congeners increase accommodation and sensitivity to light reflex and decrease intraocular tension in both normal and glaucomatous eyes. Opiate agonists decrease the response of the hypothalamus to afferent stimulation; slight hypothermia may also occur.

■ **GI Effects** Gastric, biliary, and pancreatic secretions are decreased by opiate agonists and the drugs delay digestion. Although the precise action of clinical doses of opiate agonists on GI smooth muscle tone is controversial, the ultimate result is constipation. Morphine congeners, meperidine and its congeners, and methadone are less constipating than morphine. Opiate agonists increase smooth muscle tone in the antral portion of the stomach, the small intestine (particularly the duodenum), the large intestine, and the sphincters. It has been generally believed that tone increases to the point of spasm. Although intensity and frequency of propulsive contractions are decreased, amplitude of nonpropulsive rhythmic contractions may be enhanced. Vigorous spasms that occur in the smooth muscle of intestinal walls and sphincters may be partially blocked by atropine. Although meperidine and its congeners have some anticholinergic properties, these drugs produce smooth muscle spasms to a similar or lesser degree than does morphine.

Tone is increased in the biliary tract, and spasms (particularly of the sphincter of Oddi) and an increase in biliary tract pressure may result. Morphine produces a greater increase in biliary pressure than does meperidine; meperidine produces a greater effect than does codeine. These biliary effects do not always occur with therapeutic doses; some patients may have no change in bile duct diameter or pressure. Biliary spasms may result in plasma amylase and lipase concentrations as much as 2–15 times the normal values.

■ **Genitourinary Effects** Opiate agonists increase smooth muscle tone in the urinary tract and induce spasms. Although the response of the ureters is quite variable, the drugs may increase tone and amplitude of contractions, especially of the lower third of the ureter. In the urinary bladder, tone of the detrusor muscle is increased, possibly resulting in urinary urgency. Opiate agonists also increase tone of the vesical sphincter which may make urination difficult. These effects, in conjunction with the central effect of the drugs on release of vasopressin, may produce oliguria; however, results of one study suggest that decreased urine output may occur without any apparent release of vasopressin and may be attributed to decreased rate of glomerular filtration and solute excretion. Some clinicians have attributed decreased urine output to decreased renal plasma flow or increased reabsorption. Large doses of opiate agonists may cause bronchoconstriction, but this effect is rarely seen with therapeutic doses.

Morphine and its congeners in therapeutic doses may prolong labor. There are conflicting reports on the effect of meperidine on the progress of labor. Generally, the effect of opiate agonists on the pregnant uterus appears to depend on the time of administration; administration of the drugs during the latent phase of the first stage of labor or before cervical dilation of 4–5 cm has occurred will probably hamper the progress of labor. In the uterus made hyperactive by oxytocics, morphine tends to restore uterine tone and contractions to a normal level. Although meperidine may have little effect on the normal contracting uterus late in pregnancy, if oxytocics have been administered, meperidine tends to increase uterine tone and contractions.

■ **Cardiovascular Effects** Most opiate agonists have little cardiovascular effect when given in therapeutic doses to supine patients. When the supine patient who has received an opiate agonist assumes a head-up position, however, orthostatic hypotension and fainting may occur as a result of peripheral vasodilation, particularly in volume-depleted patients. Dilation of peripheral blood vessels may be caused by opiate agonist-induced release of histamine or by depression of the vasomotor center in the medulla. Large doses of opiate agonists may produce hypotension, even in the supine patient. In addition, large doses and/or rapid administration of opiate agonists may produce bradycardia as a result of stimulation of medullary vagal nuclei. Meperidine may produce either bradycardia or tachycardia.

■ **Effects on Histamine** Although meperidine and its congeners may have some antihistaminic activity, these drugs also cause histamine release although it may be less than that produced by morphine. Sufentanil and fentanyl are less potent stimulators of histamine release than are meperidine or morphine. Manifestations of histamine release and/or peripheral dilation also include flushing, pruritus, red eyes, and sweating.

■ **Endocrine Effects** Opiate agonists exert endocrinologic effects, some of which may be related to CNS effects. The drugs generally stimulate release of vasopressin. Although opiate agonists have been reported to stimulate the release of corticotropin in animals, the drugs generally inhibit the stress-induced (e.g., associated with surgery) release of corticotropin and the release of gonadotropins (i.e., luteinizing hormone, follicle-stimulating hormone) from the pituitary resulting in decreased plasma and urinary 17-hydroxycorticosteroid and 17-ketosteroid concentrations; however, the functions of the adrenal gland and sex organs are not necessarily suppressed and usually exhibit a normal response to administration of exogenous corticotropin and chorionic gonadotropin. The drugs inhibit the release of thyrotropin from the adenohypophysis leading to a decrease in release of thyroid hormone. Opiate agonists may produce hyperglycemia by an action on paraventricular receptor sites near the foramen of Monro or by stimulating release of epinephrine. Basal metabolic rate may be decreased by 10–20% in patients receiving opiate agonists.

■ **Other Effects** Opiate agonists may also decrease olfactory and auditory acuity.

Pharmacokinetics

■ **Absorption and Disribution** Some opiate agonists are well absorbed following oral or rectal administration, but others must be administered parenterally. Individual opiate agonists differ in onset and duration of action. Following subcutaneous administration, rates of absorption and onset of action differ because of differences in solubility and/or rate of dissolution. Opiate agonists are rapidly removed from the blood stream and distributed in decreasing order of concentration into skeletal muscle, kidneys, liver, intestinal tract, lungs, spleen, and brain. The drugs readily penetrate the placental barrier.

■ **Elimination** Opiate agonists are metabolized mainly in the liver, the microsomes in the endoplasmic reticulum being the major site of metabolism. The drugs are also metabolized in the CNS, kidneys, lungs, and placenta. Opiate agonists undergo conjugation with glucuronic acid, hydrolysis, oxidation, and/or *N*- or *O*-dealkylation. The drugs are excreted principally in urine in the unchanged form and as metabolites; small amounts are excreted in the feces.

Some opiate agonists (e.g., codeine, fentanyl, hydrocodone, methadone, oxycodone, tramadol) undergo metabolism via the cytochrome P-450 (CYP) microsomal enzyme system. Methadone is metabolized mainly by CYP isoenzymes 2B6, 2C19, and 3A4, and, to a lesser extent, by CYP isoenzymes 2C9 and 2D6. Fentanyl, hydrocodone, and oxycodone are metabolized mainly by CYP3A4, although CYP2D6 also is involved in the metabolism of hydrocodone and oxycodone. Codeine and tramadol are metabolized by CYP2D6 and CYP3A4. Other opiate agonists (e.g., hydromorphone, morphine, tapentadol) are eliminated mainly via hepatic metabolism to glucuronide conjugates that are excreted in urine.

Pharmacogenomics Genetic polymorphism of CYP2D6 may cause variations in individual drug response and should be considered as a factor when differences in efficacy or toxicity of drugs metabolized by this pathway are observed. Serious adverse reactions have been reported in individuals who are ultrarapid metabolizers of codeine because they convert codeine to morphine (its active metabolite) at a higher rate. (See Codeine 48:08 and also see Codeine 28:08.08.)

Chemistry

Opiate agonists encompass a group of naturally occurring, semisynthetic, and synthetic drugs that stimulate opiate receptors and effectively relieve pain without producing loss of consciousness.

The term "opiate" has been used in the medical literature to describe drugs that are opium derivatives, and "opioid" has been used to describe opium derivatives as well as drugs that are not opium derivatives but are, at least to some extent, opium- or morphine-like in their effects and to describe endogenous peptides (e.g., enkephalins) that have morphine-like activity. Using these definitions, drugs with pharmacologic effects that result in part from agonist activity at opiate receptors but that are not opium derivatives nor semisynthetic derivatives of morphine or thebaine (e.g., tapentadol, tramadol) would not be considered an "opiate" but would be considered an "opioid." However, the terms "opiate" and "opioid" also have been used interchangeably to describe the receptors and associated agonist and antagonist activity of drugs (e.g., morphine) and other mediators at these receptors. In the AHFS Pharmacologic-Therapeutic Classification©, the term "opiate agonist" is applied to any drug, regardless of chemical origin, whose pharmacologic and/or toxicologic effects result to an important degree from agonist activity at opiate receptors. The emphasis in the AHFS Classification is on the actual effects of the drugs rather than on chemical derivation. While the term "opioid agonist" also has been applied to drugs that stimulate opiate receptors, the AHFS Pharmacologic-

Therapeutic Classification© employs "opiate" rather than "opioid" as the modifier for agonist (and antagonist) activity since *true* opiate receptors, not opiate-*like* (i.e., opi-*oid*) receptors, are affected. Therefore, although drugs like tapentadol and tramadol do not fit the classic definition of an opiate (i.e., if they are not opium derivatives nor semisynthetic derivatives), these drugs *are* classified as opiate agonists in *AHFS Drug Information* because they possess agonist activity at opiate receptors.

Chemically, opiate agonists may be classified as phenanthrene derivatives, phenylpiperidine derivatives, or diphenylheptane derivatives.

■ Phenanthrene Derivatives

codeine	levorphanol tartrate
concentrated opium alkaloids hydrochlorides	morphine sulfate
hydrocodone bitartrate	oxycodone
hydromorphone hydrochloride	oxymorphone hydrochloride

Morphine is the prototype of the phenanthrene-derivative opiate agonists. Etherification of the 3-hydroxyl group (e.g., codeine) decreases analgesic activity. Oxidation of the 6-hydroxyl group (e.g., hydromorphone, oxymorphone) increases analgesic activity. Although levorphanol is a morphinan derivative, it is structurally similar to the phenanthrene-derivative opiate agonists. Most phenanthrene derivatives are analgesics; however, naloxone hydrochloride and naltrexone hydrochloride are essentially pure opiate antagonists (see 28:10), which have little or no analgesic activity. Hydrocodone bitartrate is also used as an antitussive (see 48:08).

■ Phenylpiperidine Derivatives

anileridine hydrochloride	meperidine hydrochloride
fentanyl citrate	sufentanil citrate

Meperidine is the prototype of the phenylpiperidine-derivative opiate agonists. Replacement of the *N*-methyl group of meperidine with a large rigid aralkyl group (e.g., anileridine) increases analgesic activity. Replacement of the *N*-methyl group of meperidine with a diphenylcyanopropyl group produces diphenoxylate, a compound which is devoid of analgesic activity but has good antidiarrheal activity (see 56:08).

■ Diphenylheptane Derivatives

methadone hydrochloride	levomethadyl acetate hydrochloride

Methadone hydrochloride is the prototype of the diphenylheptane-derivative opiate agonists. Levomethadyl acetate hydrochloride (no longer commercially available in the US because of potentially severe adverse cardiac effects) is a synthetic congener of methadone with a delayed onset of action and prolonged duration of effect. Propoxyphene (no longer commercially available in the US), which is closely related structurally to methadone, has mild analgesic activity.

Most opiate agonists are basic in reaction and readily react with acids to form water-soluble salts. Such salts have a wide range of water solubility.

For specific dosages and additional information on chemistry and stability, pharmacology, pharmacokinetics, uses, cautions, and drug interactions of the opiate agonists, see the individual monographs in 28:08.08.

†Use is not currently included in the labeling approved by the US Food and Drug Administration

Codeine Phosphate
Codeine Sulfate

■ Codeine is a phenanthrene-derivative opiate agonist.

REMS

FDA approved a REMS for codeine to ensure that the benefits outweigh the risk. The REMS may apply to one or more preparations of codeine and consists of the following: medication guide and elements to assure safe use. See the FDA REMS page (http://www.accessdata.fda.gov/scripts/cder/rems/index.cfm).

Uses

Codeine is a mild analgesic used in the relief of mild to moderately severe pain that is not relieved by a nonopiate analgesic. Because of differing mechanisms of action, codeine and aspirin or acetaminophen in combination probably produce additive analgesic effects. Combinations containing codeine, aspirin, and caffeine are effective but produce no more analgesia than a combination of aspirin and codeine. For further information on the role of opiate analgesics in the management of acute or chronic pain, see Uses: Pain, in the Opiate Agonists General Statement 28:08.08.

For use of codeine as an antitussive agent, see 48:08.

Dosage and Administration

■ Administration Codeine sulfate and codeine phosphate are administered orally.

■ Dosage Codeine salts should be given at the lowest effective dosage and for the shortest duration of therapy consistent with the treatment goals of the patient. Reduced dosage is indicated in poor-risk patients and in very old patients. If concomitant therapy with other CNS depressants is required, the lowest effective dosages and shortest possible duration of concomitant therapy should be used.

When opiate analgesics are administered in fixed combination with nonopiate analgesics, the opiate dosage may be limited by the nonopiate component. Because commercially available preparations contain codeine and nonopiate analgesics in various fixed ratios and because these nonopiate analgesics also are available in many other prescription and OTC preparations, care should be taken to ensure that therapy is not duplicated and that dosage of the nonopiate drug does not exceed maximum recommended dosages.

The initial dosage must be individualized, taking into account the patient's prior opiate use; concurrent drug therapy; degree of opiate tolerance; medical condition; type and severity of pain; and risk factors for addiction, abuse, and misuse.

For the relief of mild to moderate pain in adults, the usual oral dosage of codeine phosphate or codeine sulfate is 30 mg every 4 hours as necessary; the usual dose range is 15–60 mg. Adult dosage should not exceed 360 mg daily.

Children may receive 3 mg/kg or 100 mg/m^2 daily in 6 divided doses. Alternatively, children may be given 0.5 mg/kg or 15 mg/m^2 every 4–6 hours. (See Cautions: Pediatric Precautions.)

For acute pain not related to trauma or surgery, the prescribed quantity should be limited to the amount needed for the expected duration of pain severe enough to require opiate analgesia (generally 3 days or less and rarely more than 7 days). When opiate analgesics are used for the management of chronic noncancer pain, the US Centers for Disease Control and Prevention (CDC) recommends that primary care clinicians carefully reassess individual benefits and risks before prescribing dosages equivalent to 50 mg or more of morphine sulfate daily (approximately 330 mg or more of codeine phosphate or codeine sulfate daily) and avoid dosages equivalent to 90 mg or more of morphine sulfate daily or carefully justify their decision to titrate the dosage to such levels. Other experts recommend consulting a pain management specialist before exceeding a dosage equivalent to 80–120 mg of morphine sulfate daily. For further information on the management of opiate analgesic therapy, see Dosage and Administration: Dosage, in the Opiate Agonists General Statement 28:08.08.

Cautions

■ Precautions and Contraindications Codeine shares the toxic potentials of the opiate agonists, and the usual precautions of opiate agonist therapy should be observed. (See Cautions in the Opiate Agonists General Statement 28:08.08.)

Codeine is contraindicated in children younger than 12 years of age for the management of pain and in pediatric patients younger than 18 years of age for the management of postoperative pain following tonsillectomy and/or adenoidectomy. In addition, FDA states that use of codeine for the management of pain is *not* recommended in pediatric patients 12–18 years of age who are obese or have conditions such as obstructive sleep apnea or compromised respiratory function. (See Cautions: Pediatric Precautions.)

Individuals who are ultrarapid metabolizers of cytochrome P-450 (CYP) 2D6 substrates are likely to have higher than expected serum concentrations of morphine, the active metabolite of codeine; therefore, FDA states that codeine should *not* be used in such patients. (See Pharmacokinetics: Pharmacogenomics.)

FDA also states that use of codeine is *not* recommended in nursing women, especially those who have evidence of ultrarapid metabolism of CYP2D6 substrates. Serious adverse events (e.g., excessive sedation, difficulty nursing, respiratory depression), including death, have been reported in nursing infants exposed to codeine. One case of opiate toxicity resulting in neonatal death has been reported in the nursing infant of a woman receiving codeine; genetic testing of the woman indicated that she was an ultrarapid metabolizer of codeine. (See Pharmacokinetics: Pharmacogenomics.) Higher than expected concentrations of morphine were found in breast milk and in the blood of the infant. Somnolence also has been reported more frequently in nursing infants whose mothers received codeine in combination with acetaminophen compared with those whose mothers received acetaminophen alone; evidence of ultrarapid metabolism of CYP2D6 substrates was identified in some of these women. Concentrations of morphine in breast milk are low and dose dependent in women who are normal metabolizers of codeine. Although not routinely used in clinical practice, FDA-approved tests (e.g., AmpliChip® CYP450 Test) are available to identify an individual's CYP2D6 genotype. However, testing alone may not adequately predict the risk of adverse reactions. Infants exposed to codeine through breast milk should be monitored closely for clinical manifestations of opiate toxicity (e.g., sedation, difficulty breast-feeding or breathing, hypotonia). If such manifestations occur, caregivers should seek immediate medical treatment for the infant.

When preparations containing codeine in fixed combination with other drugs are administered, the cautions, precautions, and contraindications applicable to each ingredient must be considered.

■ Pediatric Precautions Pediatric patients receiving codeine for the management of pain, especially those who are obese, have obstructive sleep apnea or severe lung disease, or have evidence of ultrarapid metabolism of

CYP2D6 substrates, are at increased risk of respiratory depression. Serious adverse events, including deaths, have been reported during postmarketing experience in pediatric patients receiving codeine. Between January 1969 and May 2015, the FDA Adverse Event Reporting System (AERS) received 64 reports of respiratory depression, including 24 reports of death, worldwide that were associated with codeine use in pediatric patients younger than 18 years of age; in all 10 of the reports that provided information about CYP2D6 metabolizer status, the patients were ultrarapid or extensive metabolizers of CYP2D6 substrates. (See Pharmacokinetics: Pharmacogenomics.) Most of the cases of respiratory depression, including most of the deaths, occurred in children younger than 12 years of age. Respiratory depression may occur despite serum concentrations of codeine or morphine being within the therapeutic range; one patient who had concentrations within the therapeutic range died following use of codeine for management of pain after tonsillectomy and adenoidectomy.

To minimize the risk of serious adverse events in pediatric patients, FDA states that codeine-containing preparations must *not* be used for the management of pain in children younger than 12 years of age or for the management of postoperative pain following tonsillectomy and/or adenoidectomy in pediatric patients younger than 18 years of age, and that use of codeine for the management of pain is *not* recommended in pediatric patients 12–18 years of age who are obese or have conditions such as obstructive sleep apnea or compromised respiratory function (because of potentially greater susceptibility to the respiratory depressant effects of the drug). If codeine is used for the management of pain in pediatric patients 12–18 years of age, caregivers should closely monitor the child for clinical manifestations of opiate toxicity (e.g., shallow, difficult, or noisy breathing; confusion; unusual sleepiness) and seek immediate medical treatment for the child if such manifestations occur.

Serious adverse events, including deaths, also have been reported in children receiving codeine for relief of symptoms of upper respiratory tract infection. For additional information on precautions and contraindications associated with the use of codeine as an antitussive in pediatric patients, see Cautions: Pediatric Precautions, in Codeine 48:08.

Pharmacology

Equianalgesic parenteral doses of codeine phosphate and morphine sulfate have produced similar degrees of respiratory depression. Codeine has good antitussive activity, although on a weight basis antitussive activity of codeine is less than that of morphine.

Pharmacokinetics

Codeine and its salts are well absorbed following oral administration. Following oral administration, onset of action occurs in 15–30 minutes and analgesia is maintained for 4–6 hours. Codeine is distributed into milk. Codeine is metabolized mainly in the liver where it undergoes *O*-demethylation (by cytochrome P-450 [CYP] isoenzyme 2D6), *N*-demethylation (by CYP3A4), and partial conjugation with glucuronic acid; the drug is excreted mainly in urine as norcodeine and free and conjugated morphine. Negligible amounts of codeine and its metabolites are found in feces.

Codeine is metabolized by the CYP microsomal enzyme system, principally by CYP3A4, and to a lesser extent by CYP2D6 (debrisoquine hydroxylase). Although the CYP2D6 isoenzyme accounts for only 10% of the metabolism of codeine, it plays an essential role in converting the drug to its active *O*-demethylated metabolite, morphine.

Pharmacogenomics: Metabolism of certain drugs, including codeine, is influenced by CYP2D6 polymorphism. Individuals who lack functional alleles of the CYP2D6 gene are described as poor metabolizers, those with 1 or 2 functional alleles are described as extensive metabolizers, and those who carry a duplicate or amplified gene are described as ultrarapid metabolizers. Genetically determined differences in drug metabolism can affect an individual's response to a drug or risk of having an adverse event. Individuals who are poor metabolizers experience no analgesic effects of codeine; individuals who are ultrarapid metabolizers are likely to have higher than expected serum concentrations of morphine.

Variations in CYP2D6 polymorphism occur at different frequencies among subpopulations of different ethnic or racial origin. Approximately 1–7% of Caucasians and 10–30% of Ethiopians and Saudi Arabians carry the genotype associated with ultrarapid metabolism of CYP2D6 substrates.

Chemistry and Stability

■ **Chemistry** Codeine is a phenanthrene-derivative opiate agonist. Codeine occurs as colorless or white crystals or as a white, crystalline powder; the drug is slightly soluble in water and freely soluble in alcohol. Codeine phosphate occurs as fine, white, needle-shaped crystals or as a white, crystalline powder and is freely soluble in water and slightly soluble in alcohol. Codeine sulfate occurs as white crystals, usually needle-like, or as a white, crystalline powder and is soluble in water and very slightly soluble in alcohol.

■ **Stability** Codeine sulfate tablets should be stored in well-closed, light-resistant containers at a temperature less than 40°C, preferably between 15–30°C.

For further information on chemistry, pharmacology, uses, cautions, chronic toxicity, acute toxicity, drug interactions, and dosage and administration of codeine, see the Opiate Agonists General Statement 28:08.08.

Preparations

Codeine preparations are subject to control under the Federal Controlled Substances Act of 1970.

Excipients in commercially available drug preparations may have clinically important effects in some individuals; consult specific product labeling for details.

Codeine Phosphate

Crystals

Powder

Acetaminophen and Codeine Phosphate

Oral		
Solution	120 mg/5 mL Acetaminophen and Codeine Phosphate 12 mg/5 mL*	**Acetaminophen and Codeine Phosphate Oral Solution** (C-V)
Tablets	300 mg Acetaminophen and Codeine Phosphate 15 mg*	**Acetaminophen and Codeine Phosphate Tablets** (C-III)
	300 mg Acetaminophen and Codeine Phosphate 30 mg*	**Acetaminophen and Codeine Phosphate Tablets** (C-III)
		Tylenol® with Codeine No. 3 (C-III), Janssen
	300 mg Acetaminophen and Codeine Phosphate 60 mg*	**Acetaminophen and Codeine Phosphate Tablets** (C-III)
		Tylenol® with Codeine No. 4 (C-III), Janssen

*available from one or more manufacturer, distributor, and/or repackager by generic (nonproprietary) name

Other Codeine Phosphate Combinations

Oral		
Capsules	30 mg with Acetaminophen 300 mg, Butalbital 50 mg, and Caffeine 40 mg*	**Butalbital, Acetaminophen, Caffeine, and Codeine Phosphate Capsules** (C-III)
		Fioricet® with Codeine (C-III), Actavis
	30 mg with Acetaminophen 325 mg, Butalbital 50 mg, and Caffeine 40 mg*	**Butalbital, Acetaminophen, Caffeine, and Codeine Phosphate Capsules** (C-III)
	30 mg with Aspirin 325 mg, Butalbital 50 mg, and Caffeine 40 mg*	**Ascomp® with Codeine** (C-III), Nexgen
		Butalbital, Aspirin, Caffeine, and Codeine Phosphate Capsules (C-III)
		Fiorinal® with Codeine (C-III), Allergan
Tablets	16 mg with Aspirin 325 mg and Carisoprodol 200 mg*	**Carisoprodol, Aspirin, and Codeine Phosphate Tablets** (C-III)
		Soma® Compound with Codeine (C-III), Meda

*available from one or more manufacturer, distributor, and/or repackager by generic (nonproprietary) name

Codeine Sulfate

Powder

Oral		
Tablets	15 mg*	**Codeine Sulfate Tablets** (C-II)
	30 mg*	**Codeine Sulfate Tablets** (C-II)
	60 mg*	**Codeine Sulfate Tablets** (C-II)

*available from one or more manufacturer, distributor, and/or repackager by generic (nonproprietary) name

fentaNYL
fentaNYL Citrate
fentaNYL Hydrochloride

■ Fentanyl is a synthetic phenylpiperidine-derivative opiate agonist.

REMS

FDA approved a REMS for fentanyl to ensure that the benefits outweigh the risks. The REMS may apply to one or more preparations of fentanyl and consists of some or all of the following: medication guide, elements to assure safe use, and implementation system. See the FDA REMS page (https://www.accessdata.fda.gov/scripts/cder/rems/index.cfm).

Uses

Fentanyl citrate is a strong analgesic used preoperatively, during surgery, and in the immediate postoperative period for its analgesic action. In addition, the drug may be used to prevent or relieve tachypnea and postoperative emergence delirium. Fentanyl citrate is used parenterally to provide preoperative anxiolysis and sedation and as a supplement to anesthesia. The drug may be especially useful preoperatively before surgery of short duration or minor surgery in outpatients and in diagnostic procedures or treatments that require the patient to be awake or very lightly anesthetized. Fentanyl citrate may be used as a supplement to general or regional anesthesia, including neuroleptanalgesia in which it is often used in combination with droperidol. When attenuation of the response to surgical stress is especially important, fentanyl citrate may be administered with oxygen and a skeletal muscle relaxant to provide anesthesia without the use of additional anesthetic agents.

Fentanyl citrate buccal lozenges, buccal tablets, sublingual tablets, and nasal spray, and fentanyl sublingual spray are used for the management of breakthrough pain in patients who are already being treated with, and are tolerant of, opiates used around the clock for persistent cancer pain. Patients are considered opiate tolerant if they have been receiving around-the-clock opiate therapy consisting of at least 60 mg of oral morphine sulfate daily, 25 mcg of transdermal fentanyl per hour, 30 mg of oral oxycodone daily, 8 mg of oral hydromorphone hydrochloride daily, 25 mg of oral oxymorphone hydrochloride daily, or an equianalgesic dosage of another opiate daily for at least 1 week. Patients must continue receiving around-the-clock opiate analgesic therapy while receiving these transmucosal immediate-release preparations for the relief of breakthrough pain. Because of the risk of fatal or life-threatening respiratory depression (e.g., hypoventilation), fentanyl citrate buccal lozenges, buccal tablets, sublingual tablets, and nasal spray and fentanyl sublingual spray are contraindicated in the management of acute or postoperative pain and in patients who are not opiate tolerant. The manufacturers state that these transmucosal immediate-release formulations should be administered only under the supervision of qualified clinicians who are experienced in the use of schedule II (C-II) opiates for the management of cancer pain. *Substantial pharmacokinetic differences exist among these transmucosal immediate-release formulations of fentanyl, and between these formulations and other preparations of the drug; these differences could result in clinically important differences in the rate and extent of absorption. Therefore, fentanyl citrate buccal lozenges, buccal tablets, sublingual tablets, and nasal spray and fentanyl sublingual spray must not be used interchangeably (e.g., on a mcg-per-mcg basis) with each other or with any other preparation of the drug.* Fatal overdosage may occur if these formulations are substituted on a mcg-per-mcg basis for any other fentanyl preparation. Only limited information is available for safely switching from one formulation to another. (See Dosage and Administration: Dosage.)

In clinical studies in opiate-tolerant adults with breakthrough cancer pain, transmucosal immediate-release fentanyl formulations (fentanyl citrate buccal lozenges, buccal tablets, sublingual tablets, and nasal spray; fentanyl sublingual spray) have been shown to provide substantially more pain relief than placebo. Patients enrolled in these studies received long-term maintenance dosages of opiate analgesics for persistent cancer pain; following titration of the transmucosal immediate-release formulation to an effective dose, patients received a sequence of 7 treatments with the transmucosal immediate-release fentanyl preparation and 3 treatments with placebo in a randomized double-blind manner for successive episodes of breakthrough pain. In these studies, 60–75% of patients successfully achieved an adequate dose during the titration period. The fentanyl doses evaluated in these studies ranged from 200–1600 mcg as fentanyl citrate buccal lozenges, 100–800 mcg as fentanyl citrate buccal tablets, 100–800 mcg as fentanyl citrate sublingual tablets, 100–1600 mcg as fentanyl sublingual spray, and 100–800 mcg as fentanyl citrate nasal spray.

Fentanyl also previously was available for restricted use as an intrabuccal (transmucosal) premedicant prior to anesthesia or for inducing conscious sedation prior to diagnostic or therapeutic procedures in a monitored anesthesia setting (Fentanyl Oralet®). However, this preparation no longer is commercially available for such use in the US, and the currently available buccal preparations (Actiq® lozenge, Fentora® tablet, generic oral transmucosal fentanyl citrate lozenge) are *only* labeled for use in opiate-tolerant patients with chronic cancer pain.

Fentanyl is used transdermally in opiate-tolerant patients for the management of pain that is severe enough to require long-term, daily, around-the-clock use of an opiate analgesic. Because of the risks of addiction, abuse, and misuse associated with opiates, even at recommended doses, and because of the greater risks of overdose and death with extended-release opiate formulations, therapy with fentanyl transdermal system should be reserved for use in patients for whom alternative treatment options (e.g., nonopiate analgesics, immediate-release opiates) are inadequate or not tolerated. Because of the risk of life-threatening respiratory depression, fentanyl transdermal system is contraindicated in patients who are not opiate tolerant, in those who require opiate analgesia for a short period of time, and for the management of acute, mild, intermittent, or postoperative pain. Fentanyl transdermal systems should be prescribed only by qualified clinicians who are experienced in the use of potent opiates for the management of chronic pain and are familiar with the absorption characteristics and dosing of this formulation.

In clinical studies in patients with cancer, fentanyl transdermal system was administered at dosages of 25–600 mcg/hour for variable periods of time (i.e., periods exceeding 30 days, 4 months, or 1 year in 56, 28, or 10% of patients, respectively, and extending up to 866 days in individual patients). At one month following initiation of transdermal fentanyl therapy, pain intensity generally was less than that reported with the oral morphine regimen used prior to the study.

Fentanyl hydrochloride is used transdermally as an iontophoretic transdermal system for the short-term management of acute postoperative pain in patients requiring opiate analgesia in a hospital setting. Treatment with the iontophoretic transdermal system should be initiated only after an acceptable level of analgesia has been achieved using other opiate analgesics and should be used only in patients who are sufficiently alert and have adequate cognitive ability to understand the directions for use. The iontophoretic transdermal system is intended for use in the hospital setting only and must be discontinued prior to hospital discharge. Fentanyl should be administered as an iontophoretic transdermal system only under the supervision of qualified clinicians who are experienced in the use of potent opiates for pain management and also are experienced in the detection and management of hypoventilation.

Efficacy of fentanyl hydrochloride iontophoretic transdermal system in relieving acute postoperative pain has been demonstrated in several randomized placebo-controlled studies in adults following major (mainly lower abdominal or orthopedic) surgery. In the immediate postoperative period, patients in these studies received IV opiate analgesia until they were comfortable and then were randomized to receive either the fentanyl hydrochloride iontophoretic transdermal system or a placebo system; supplemental IV fentanyl was allowed only during the initial 3-hour period following system application. From 3–24 hours following system application, 8–27% of patients receiving fentanyl as the transdermal iontophoretic system discontinued therapy because of inadequate analgesia compared with 40–57% of those receiving placebo, and those receiving active treatment reported less pain at the end of the treatment period. Among patients who completed the 24-hour treatment period, the mean number of fentanyl doses administered per patient was 29 (range: 0–93), with 56.5% of patients administering between 11 and 50 doses. Body mass index (range: less than 25 to 40 kg/m^2 or more) did not appear to affect efficacy.

For further information on the role of opiate analgesics in the management of acute or chronic pain, see Uses: Pain, in the Opiate Agonists General Statement 28:08.08.

Dosage and Administration

■ **Administration** Fentanyl citrate is administered by IM or IV injection, intrabucally as a buccal lozenge or buccal tablet, sublingually as a sublingual tablet, or by nasal inhalation as an aqueous solution. Fentanyl citrate buccal tablets also may be administered sublingually once an effective dose has been established. Fentanyl is administered percutaneously by topical application of a transdermal system or sublingually as a spray. Fentanyl hydrochloride is administered percutaneously by topical application of an iontophoretic transdermal system.

Patients receiving transmucosal immediate-release fentanyl preparations (e.g., fentanyl citrate buccal lozenges, buccal tablets, sublingual tablets, or nasal spray; fentanyl sublingual spray) or fentanyl transdermal system should be instructed carefully regarding proper use, administration, storage, and disposal of these dosage formulations. Those receiving fentanyl hydrochloride iontophoretic transdermal system should be instructed carefully regarding proper use of the system and avoidance of accidental exposure to the drug. (See Precautions Against Serious Toxicity Resulting From Fentanyl Overdosage or Accidental Exposure under Cautions: Precautions and Contraindications.)

Risk Management and Restricted Distribution Programs The US Food and Drug Administration (FDA) has approved risk evaluation and mitigation strategy (REMS) programs for most fentanyl preparations; however, the specific requirements may vary depending on the fentanyl preparation. (See REMS.)

Because of the risk of misuse, abuse, addiction, and overdosage, transmucosal immediate-release fentanyl (TIRF) preparations (e.g., fentanyl citrate buccal lozenges, buccal tablets, sublingual tablets, and nasal spray; fentanyl sublingual spray) are available only through a restricted distribution program under the TIRF Risk Evaluation and Mitigation Strategy (REMS) Access program. (See REMS.) Outpatients who receive transmucosal immediate-release preparations of the drug, clinicians who prescribe these preparations to outpatients, and pharmacies, wholesalers, and distributors that dispense or distribute these preparations must enroll in the program. Patient and prescriber enrollment is not required for inpatient administration (e.g., in hospitals, hospices, and long-term care facilities that prescribe for inpatient use). Additional information about the program can be obtained at https://www.tirfremsaccess.com or by calling 866-822-1483.

Because of the risk of respiratory depression resulting from accidental exposure, fentanyl hydrochloride iontophoretic transdermal system is available only through a restricted distribution program under the Ionsys REMS program. (See REMS.) Hospitals that dispense and administer the iontophoretic transdermal system must be certified and comply with the REMS requirements and must dispense the iontophoretic transdermal system for hospital use only. Additional information about the program can be obtained at https://www.ionsysrems.com or by calling 877-488-6835.

FDA also has approved a REMS program for opiate analgesics, including fentanyl transdermal system, used in the outpatient setting and not covered by other REMS programs. The goals of this program are to reduce the occurrence of addiction, unintentional overdosage, and death resulting from inappropriate prescribing, misuse, and abuse of opiate analgesics. The program consists of educational programs for prescribers and other health care providers, including pharmacists and nurses, who are involved in the treatment and monitoring of patients with pain; information that health care providers can use when counseling patients about opiate analgesics; and a product-specific medication guide that must be dispensed with every prescription. Additional information about the program can be obtained at https://opioidanalgesicrems.com.

Parenteral Administration An opiate antagonist and facilities for administration of oxygen and controlled respiration should be available during and immediately following IV administration of fentanyl citrate.

Preservative-free injections of fentanyl citrate also have been injected or infused epidurally†; specialized techniques are required for administration of the drug by this route, and such administration should be performed only by qualified individuals familiar with the techniques of administration, dosages, and special patient management problems associated with epidural fentanyl citrate administration.

Intrabuccal Administration Fentanyl citrate is administered intrabuccally as buccal lozenges (Actiq®, oral transmucosal fentanyl citrate lozenge) and buccal tablets (Fentora®).

Buccal Lozenges. When fentanyl citrate buccal lozenges are used, the package should be cut open with scissors just prior to administration. The lozenge should be placed in the patient's mouth (between the cheek and the lower gum) using the handle and the patient should be instructed to suck, and *not* bite or chew, the lozenge; efficacy may be reduced if the lozenge is chewed and swallowed rather than being administered as directed. (See Buccal Lozenges and Tablets under Pharmacokinetics: Absorption.) The lozenge occasionally may be moved from one side to the other using the handle. Buccal lozenges of fentanyl citrate usually should be consumed over a period of 15 minutes; longer or shorter consumption times may result in reduced efficacy compared with that reported in clinical trials.

If signs of excessive opiate effects develop before the buccal lozenge is consumed completely, the remaining portion should be removed from the patient's mouth immediately, and future doses should be decreased.

After consumption of a lozenge unit is complete and the lozenge matrix is totally dissolved, the handle should be disposed of in a trash container that is out of the reach of children; any drug matrix remaining on the handle can be removed by placing the handle under hot running tap water until the drug matrix is completely dissolved. While all units should be disposed of immediately after use, unused portions of the preparation represent a special risk, since they are no longer protected by the child-resistant blister package, and they still may contain sufficient amounts of the drug to be fatal to a child. If unused portions of the drug cannot be disposed of immediately by the patients or their caregivers, they should be stored in a temporary storage bottle (supplied by the manufacturer) according to enclosed instructions and then should be disposed of at least once a day.

Buccal Tablets. When fentanyl citrate buccal tablets are used, a single blister unit should be separated by bending and tearing along the blister card perforations. Immediately prior to administration, the single blister unit should be opened by bending the unit along the indicated line and peeling the backing to expose the buccal tablet. The buccal tablet should not be pushed through the blister, since this may damage the buccal tablet. The tablets should not be split. The fentanyl citrate buccal tablet should be placed in the patient's buccal cavity (above a rear molar, between the upper cheek and gum); alternatively, once an effective dose has been established, the tablet may be administered sublingually. The patient should be instructed *not* to crush, suck, chew, or swallow the tablet; efficacy may be reduced if the buccal tablet is crushed, sucked, chewed, or swallowed whole rather than being administered as directed. (See Buccal Lozenges and Tablets under Pharmacokinetics: Absorption.) The fentanyl citrate buccal tablet should be left between the patient's upper cheek and gum or under the tongue until it has disintegrated (generally 14–25 minutes); the disintegration time does not appear to affect early systemic exposure to the drug. If the buccal tablet has not completely disintegrated after 30 minutes, the remnants may be swallowed with a glass of water. Patients should be instructed to alternate sides of the mouth with each intrabuccal dose.

If signs of excessive opiate effects develop before the buccal tablet has disintegrated completely, the remaining portion should be removed from the patient's mouth immediately, and future doses should be decreased.

Sublingual Administration Fentanyl is administered sublingually as fentanyl citrate sublingual tablets (Abstral®) and fentanyl sublingual spray (Subsys®). The manufacturer states that fentanyl citrate buccal tablets (Fentora®) also may be administered sublingually once an effective dose of the drug has been established. (See Buccal Tablets under Administration: Intrabuccal Administration, in Dosage and Administration.)

Sublingual Tablets. When fentanyl citrate sublingual tablets are used, a single blister unit should be separated from the blister card and then the backing of the single blister should be peeled back so that the tablet can be gently removed; the sublingual tablet should not be pushed through the blister, since this may damage the tablet. Immediately after removal from the blister unit, the sublingual tablet should be placed on the floor of the mouth directly under the tongue as far back as possible. If more than one tablet is required, the tablets should be spread around the floor of the mouth under the tongue. The tablet(s) should be allowed to dissolve completely in the sublingual cavity and should not be chewed, sucked, or swallowed. Patients should not eat or drink until the sublingual tablet(s) has dissolved completely. Patients with a dry mouth may moisten the buccal mucosa with water before administering fentanyl citrate sublingual tablets.

Sublingual Spray. Immediately prior to administration of fentanyl sublingual spray, a blister package containing a single-use spray unit should be opened with scissors. The contents of the unit (100, 200, 400, 600, or 800 mcg of fentanyl) should be carefully sprayed into the mouth underneath the tongue. The drug should be held under the tongue for 30–60 seconds. The drug should not be spit out, nor should the mouth be rinsed. The spray unit will remain locked after use. Consumed units of the preparation represent a special risk, since they are no longer protected by the child-resistant blister package, and they still may contain sufficient amounts of the drug to be fatal to a child. Immediately after use, the used spray unit should be placed in a disposal bag provided by the manufacturer, and the bag should be sealed prior to disposal. The patient instructions in the medication guide should be consulted for additional information about administration and disposal of fentanyl sublingual spray.

Nasal Inhalation Fentanyl citrate is administered by nasal inhalation as an aqueous solution using a metered-dose nasal spray pump (Lazanda®).

Prior to initial use, the nasal spray pump should be primed by actuating the device 4 times into the carbon-lined disposal pouch provided by the manufacturer. If the inhaler has not been used for 5 or more days, the nasal spray pump should be primed again by actuating it one time into the disposal pouch. To administer a dose, the patient should insert the nozzle of the bottle a short distance (about ½ inch or 1 cm) into the nostril, pointing the nozzle toward the bridge of the nose and tilting the bottle slightly. The finger grips should be depressed firmly until a click is audible and the number in the counting window advances by one. The patient may not feel the mist on the nasal mucous membranes. If the prescribed dose requires more than a single spray into one nostril, the patient should be instructed to alternate nostrils with each spray. Patients should remain seated for at least 1 minute after administering the drug. Patients should be instructed carefully in the use of the nasal spray pump. As soon as the bottles are no longer required, all fully used, unused, or partially used bottles must be completely emptied of accessible fentanyl citrate by spraying the remaining contents into the disposal pouch and placing the emptied bottle and the sealed pouch in the child-resistant container provided by the manufacturer prior to disposal. The patient instructions in the medication guide should be consulted for additional information about administration and disposal of the nasal solution.

Transdermal Administration **Transdermal System.** Steps should be taken to ensure that fentanyl transdermal systems (e.g., Duragesic®) are not administered inadvertently to opiate-naive patients or for acute pain management because of the risk of potentially fatal overdosage. (See Contraindications under Cautions: Precautions and Contraindications.) If transdermal therapy is considered for the management of acute pain, the iontophoretic system (Ionsys®) should be used but only in carefully selected hospitalized patients under close medical supervision. (See Iontophoretic Transdermal System under Administration: Transdermal Administration, in Dosage and Administration.)

Patients receiving fentanyl transdermal systems (e.g., Duragesic®) should be carefully instructed in the proper use and disposal of the transdermal system.

To expose the adhesive surface of the system, the protective-liner covering should be peeled and discarded just prior to application. The transdermal system is applied to a dry, intact, nonirritated, nonirradiated flat surface on the chest, back, flank, or upper arm by firmly pressing the system with the palm of the hand for 30 seconds with the adhesive side touching the skin and ensuring that contact is complete, particularly around the edges. When the transdermal system is applied to young children or to individuals with cognitive impairment, the system should be placed on the upper back to reduce the risk that the system could be removed and placed in the mouth. The transdermal system should *not* be used if the seal of the package is broken or if the system is cut, damaged, or altered in any way.

Hair at the application site should be clipped, not shaved, prior to application of the transdermal system. If the site must be cleansed prior to application, only clear water should be used. Soaps, oils, lotions, alcohol, or any other agents that could irritate the skin or alter its characteristics should *not* be used.

Patients or caregivers who apply the transdermal system should wash their hands with soap and water immediately after application. Contact with unwashed or unclothed application sites can result in secondary exposure to the drug and should be avoided. (See Precautions Against Serious Toxicity Resulting From Fentanyl Overdosage or Accidental Exposure under Cautions: Precautions and Contraindications.) If a transdermal system accidentally adheres to the skin of another person, the system should be removed immediately, the area should be washed with water, and medical attention for the exposed person should be sought immediately.

Patients may bathe, shower, or swim while wearing a transdermal system. However, they should be advised to avoid sunbathing, taking hot baths, engaging in strenuous exercise that increases core body temperature, or exposing the application site and surrounding area to direct external heat sources (e.g., heating pads, electric blankets, heat or tanning lamps, saunas, hot tubs, heated water beds) while wearing the transdermal system, since temperature-dependent increases in percutaneous absorption of fentanyl from the system are possible under such conditions and may result in fatal overdosage. (See Precautions Against Serious Toxicity Resulting From Fentanyl Overdosage or Accidental Exposure under Cautions: Precautions and Contraindications.)

Each fentanyl transdermal system may be worn continuously for 72 hours; subsequent systems should be applied to a different site after removal of the previous system. If a system should inadvertently come off during the period of use, a new system may be applied to a different skin site and left in place for 72 hours. Patients who experience difficulty with system adhesion should be advised that they may tape the edges of the system in place with first-aid tape. If adhesion problems persist, patients may apply a transparent adhesive film dressing (e.g., Bioclusive®, Tegaderm®) over the system.

Immediately following removal, used systems should be folded so that the adhesive side adheres to itself and then should be flushed down the toilet. Used systems represent a special risk, since they may contain sufficient amounts of the drug to be fatal to children, pets, or other adults for whom the drug was not prescribed.

Iontophoretic Transdermal System. Fentanyl hydrochloride iontophoretic transdermal system (Ionsys®) should be used only in hospital settings for the management of acute postoperative pain. Patients should be carefully instructed in the proper use of the iontophoretic transdermal system; only those patients who are alert enough and have adequate cognitive ability to understand the directions for use should be allowed to use the device, and only the patient should be allowed to activate the device to administer a dose of fentanyl. Iontophoretic transdermal fentanyl therapy should be prescribed only by clinicians knowledgeable in the use of potent opiates for the management of pain and used under the supervision of medical personnel with expertise in the detection and management of respiratory depression and in the use of opiate antagonists. Before the patient leaves the hospital, the iontophoretic transdermal system must be removed and disposed of properly.

Gloves must be worn when handling fentanyl hydrochloride iontophoretic transdermal systems, since accidental contact with the hydrogels on the adhesive side of the system can result in fatal overdosage. If accidental contact with the skin occurs, the affected area should be rinsed thoroughly with water. Soap, alcohol, or other solvents should not be used to remove the gel because they may enhance percutaneous absorption of fentanyl from the hydrogel.

The unit must be assembled prior to application. The foil pouch and controller should be removed from the tray, and then the drug unit should be removed from the pouch and placed on a hard flat surface. The system should not be used if the seal of the tray or drug unit pouch is broken or damaged. The matching shapes of the drug unit and controller should be aligned and both ends of the device should be pressed to fully engage the snaps at each end. Following assembly, the digital display of the controller completes a self-test and then the system can be applied to the patient's skin. The clear plastic liner covering the adhesive and hydrogels should be removed and discarded, taking care not to pull the red tab that is used when separating the device for disposal. The iontophoretic transdermal system is then applied to healthy unbroken skin on the chest or upper outer aspect of either arm; with the adhesive side of the system touching the skin and the fingers placed along the edge of the system (taking care not to press the dosing button), the system should be pressed firmly in place for at least 15 seconds, ensuring that the system adheres to the skin. Hair at the application site should be clipped, not shaved, if necessary prior to application of the iontophoretic transdermal system. The site should be cleansed with alcohol and allowed to dry prior to application; soaps, lotions, or other agents should *not* be used.

If an iontophoretic system loosens from the skin, the system should be secured to the patient's skin by pressing the edges with fingers or securing with a nonallergenic tape to ensure that all edges make complete contact with the skin. The tape should be applied along the long edges of the system and should not be applied over the dosing button, light, or digital display. Tape should not be applied to blistered or broken skin.

The iontophoretic transdermal system provides a 40-mcg dose of fentanyl over a 10-minute period following each activation of the device. To initiate administration of a fentanyl dose, the patient must press and release the dosing button on the device twice within 3 seconds. During delivery of one dose, the system is locked and will not respond to additional attempts to activate the device. The iontophoretic transdermal system delivers a maximum of 6 doses of fentanyl per hour and 80 doses per 24 hours (40 mcg per dose). Each system is operational for 24 hours following assembly or until 80 doses have been delivered, whichever comes first. Only one system should be used at a time. If continued therapy with the iontophoretic transdermal system is desired following removal of one system, a new system should be applied at a different site. A health care professional must observe the first dose to ensure that the device is functioning properly and that the patient understands how to operate the device. Visual displays and audible beeps indicate the number of doses delivered and the functional status of the device.

Fentanyl hydrochloride iontophoretic transdermal system may be removed at any time; however, once a system has been removed, the same system must not be reapplied. Following 24 hours of use or delivery of 80 doses, the system is deactivated and should be removed. The used system should be handled by the sides and top to avoid contact with the hydrogels. If either hydrogel becomes separated from the system during removal, gloves or tweezers should be used to remove the hydrogel from the skin and the hydrogel should be properly disposed of in accordance with the institution's procedures for controlled substance disposal. The used bottom housing of the system contains sufficient fentanyl to cause fatal overdosage. Following removal of the iontophoretic transdermal system, the red tab should be pulled to separate the 2 housing units. The bottom housing unit containing fentanyl should be folded in half with the adhesive side facing inward and disposed of in accordance with the institution's procedures for disposal of controlled substances. The dosing button should be depressed until the display goes blank and the remaining part of the system containing electronics disposed of in waste designed for batteries.

The manufacturer's prescribing information should be consulted for additional information about assembly, application, and operation of the device and troubleshooting device malfunction.

Because the iontophoretic transdermal system is considered unsafe for use during magnetic resonance imaging (MRI) procedures and may be damaged by strong electromagnetic fields, the system must be removed prior to MRI or other radiographic imaging procedures, cardioversion, defibrillation, or diathermy. In addition, to prevent damage of the iontophoretic transdermal system, contact with synthetic materials (e.g., carpeted flooring) should be avoided during assembly, and the system should not be exposed to electronic security systems. The recommended separation distance between the iontophoretic transdermal system and communications equipment or radio frequency identification (RFID) transmitters is 0.12–23 meters, depending on the rated maximum output power and frequency of the transmitter. (See Precautions Related to Transdermal Iontophoretic Administration under Cautions: Precautions and Contraindications.)

■ Dosage

Dosage of fentanyl, fentanyl citrate, and fentanyl hydrochloride is expressed in terms of fentanyl. The drugs should be given at the lowest effective dosage and for the shortest duration of therapy consistent with the treatment goals of the patient. Reduced dosage is indicated initially in poor-risk patients and geriatric patients. Dosage of fentanyl should be titrated carefully in geriatric patients. If concomitant therapy with other CNS depressants is required, the lowest effective dosages and shortest possible duration of concomitant therapy should be used. (See Drug Interactions: Benzodiazepines and Other CNS Depressants.)

Parenteral Dosage For use as a preoperative medication, 50–100 mcg of fentanyl is administered IM 30–60 minutes prior to surgery.

As an adjunct to general anesthesia, fentanyl may be given in low-dose, moderate-dose, or high-dose regimens. In the low-dose regimen which is used for minor but painful surgical procedures, an IV dose of 2 mcg/kg is administered; additional doses are usually not necessary. In the moderate-dose regimen which is used in more major surgical procedures, an initial IV dose of 2–20 mcg/kg is administered; additional doses of 25–100 mcg may be given IV or IM as necessary. In the high-dose regimen which may be used during open heart surgery or certain complicated neurosurgical or orthopedic procedures where surgery is more prolonged, an initial IV dose of 20–50 mcg/kg may be given; additional doses ranging from 25 mcg to one-half the initial dose may be administered as necessary.

To provide general anesthesia without additional anesthetic agents when attenuation of the response to surgical stress is especially important, fentanyl doses of 50–100 mcg/kg may be administered IV in conjunction with oxygen and a skeletal muscle relaxant; in some cases, doses up to 150 mcg/kg may be required.

As an adjunct to regional anesthesia, 50–100 mcg of fentanyl may be administered by IM injection or by slow IV injection over 1–2 minutes when additional analgesia is required.

For the control of postoperative pain, restlessness, tachypnea, and emergence delirium, 50–100 mcg of the drug may be administered IM every 1–2 hours as needed.

During the induction and maintenance phases of general anesthesia in children 2–12 years of age, a fentanyl dose of 1.7–3.3 mcg/kg is recommended.

Intrabuccal Dosage **Buccal Lozenges.** Dosage of buccal lozenges of fentanyl citrate (Actiq®, generic oral transmucosal fentanyl citrate lozenge) should be individualized based on clinical response to provide adequate analgesia and to minimize adverse effects.

When buccal lozenges of fentanyl citrate are used for the management of breakthrough cancer pain in adults who are already receiving and are tolerant of opiates used for chronic cancer pain, the initial recommended dose is 200 mcg (of fentanyl) in *all* patients. Because of differences in pharmacokinetic properties, patients should not be switched on a mcg-per-mcg basis from any other fentanyl preparation, including fentanyl citrate buccal tablets (Fentora®), to the buccal lozenges, since the buccal lozenges are not equivalent to other fentanyl preparations and are not a generic version of the buccal tablets. The manufacturer recommends that a total of 6 lozenges be prescribed initially and that all 6 lozenges be used before the dose of fentanyl is increased. Until the appropriate dose of fentanyl citrate is attained, it may be necessary to use more than one lozenge per episode of breakthrough cancer pain; the additional lozenge may be administered 15 minutes after the previous lozenge has been consumed (i.e., 30 minutes after the first lozenge initially was placed in the mouth). The manufacturer states that, during the dosage titration phase, a maximum of 2 lozenges per breakthrough pain episode may be given, if necessary. If several consecutive breakthrough cancer pain episodes occur that require the use of more than one lozenge per episode, the dose should be increased to the next higher available strength, again prescribing only 6 lozenges.

During the titration phase, each new dose should be evaluated over several breakthrough cancer pain episodes to determine efficacy and tolerability of the drug. Patients should be instructed to record their use of buccal lozenges over several episodes of breakthrough pain and to discuss their experience with their clinician to decide whether dosage adjustment is warranted. To reduce the risk of overdosage, patients should have only one strength of the buccal lozenges available for use at any one time.

Once the patient has been titrated to an adequate fentanyl dose (average breakthrough pain episode is treated with a single lozenge), the patient should limit consumption of fentanyl citrate to a maximum of 4 lozenges daily and generally should use only one lozenge of the appropriate strength per episode of breakthrough pain. On occasion during maintenance therapy, when a breakthrough pain episode is not relieved within 15 minutes after the previous lozenge was consumed (i.e., 30 minutes after the first lozenge initially was placed in the mouth), the patient may take *only one* additional dose of the same strength during that episode of breakthrough pain.

Patients should be instructed that, after treating one episode of breakthrough pain with fentanyl citrate buccal lozenges, they must wait at least 4 hours before taking an additional dose of the buccal lozenges to treat a subsequent episode of breakthrough pain.

During maintenance therapy, dosage adjustment may be necessary to ensure that an appropriate dosage is maintained; however, dosage generally should be increased only if several consecutive episodes require administration of more than one lozenge of the current dose for pain relief. If the patient experiences more than 4 breakthrough pain episodes daily, the dosage of opiates used around the clock for persistent cancer pain should be reevaluated.

If discontinuance of opiates is required, gradual tapering of the dose is recommended to avoid signs and symptoms associated with abrupt withdrawal. The dosage level at which fentanyl citrate buccal lozenges may be discontinued without producing manifestations of opiate withdrawal is not known.

In clinical trials, geriatric (older than 65 years of age) patients were titrated to an adequate dose of fentanyl citrate buccal lozenges that generally was about 200 mcg (of fentanyl) lower than the dose required in younger patients.

Buccal Tablets. For the management of breakthrough pain in adults who are already receiving and are tolerant of opiates used for the management of chronic cancer pain, the recommended initial dose of fentanyl citrate buccal tablets (Fentora®) is 100 mcg in *all* patients except those being switched from fentanyl citrate buccal lozenges (Actiq®). In patients being switched from the buccal lozenges to the buccal tablets, the initial dose of the buccal tablets should be based on the current buccal lozenge dose (see Table 1). Because of differences in pharmacokinetic properties, patients should not be switched on a mcg-per-mcg basis from any other fentanyl preparation to the buccal tablets, since the buccal tablets are not equivalent to other fentanyl preparations. For opiate-tolerant adults who are being transferred from fentanyl citrate buccal lozenges to fentanyl citrate buccal tablets for the management of breakthrough cancer pain, the increased bioavailability of the buccal tablets must be considered. (See Buccal Lozenges and Tablets under Pharmacokinetics: Absorption.) Fatal overdosage may occur if fentanyl citrate buccal tablets are substituted on a mcg-per-mcg basis for fentanyl citrate buccal lozenges or any other fentanyl preparation.

The manufacturer's dosage conversion recommendations for patients being transferred from the buccal lozenges to the buccal tablets are shown in Table 1. The manufacturer states that these doses should be considered starting doses for the buccal tablets and are not intended to represent equianalgesic doses. If the patient previously received 600 mcg or more of fentanyl daily as the buccal lozenges, therapy with the buccal tablets should be initiated using the 200-mcg strength of buccal tablets (see Table 1), and dosage should be titrated in multiples of this tablet strength. Patients being transferred from the buccal lozenges to the buccal tablets should be instructed to discontinue use of the buccal lozenges and to dispose of any remaining lozenges.

Table 1: Initial Dosage Recommendations for Adults Being Transferred from Fentanyl Citrate Buccal Lozenges to Fentanyl Citrate Buccal Tablets for Management of Breakthrough Cancer Pain

Current Fentanyl Dose Administered as Buccal Lozenge	Initial Fentanyl Dose Administered as Buccal Tablet
200 mcg	100 mcg (as one 100-mcg tablet)
400 mcg	100 mcg (as one 100-mcg tablet)
600 mcg	200 mcg (as one 200-mcg tablet)
800 mcg	200 mcg (as one 200-mcg tablet)
1200 mcg	400 mcg (as two 200-mcg tablets)
1600 mcg	400 mcg (as two 200-mcg tablets)

If breakthrough pain is not relieved within 30 minutes following the initial dose of fentanyl citrate buccal tablets, the patient may take *only one* additional dose of the same strength during that episode of breakthrough pain. Patients should be instructed that, after treating one episode of breakthrough pain with fentanyl citrate buccal tablets, they must wait at least 4 hours before treating a subsequent episode of breakthrough pain with the buccal tablets.

Dosage should be titrated with close monitoring to a level that provides adequate analgesia with acceptable adverse effects. Patients should be instructed to record their use of buccal tablets over several episodes of breakthrough pain and to discuss their experience with their clinician to decide whether dosage adjustment is warranted. Patients receiving an initial dose of 100 mcg who require titration to a higher dosage level may be instructed to increase the dose to 200 mcg (two 100-mcg tablets, with one tablet placed on each side of the mouth in the buccal cavity) with the next episode of breakthrough pain. Patients who require a further increase in dosage may be instructed to place two 100-mcg tablets on each side of the mouth in the buccal cavity (total of four 100-mcg tablets). If doses exceeding 400 mcg (i.e., doses of 600 or 800 mcg) are required, dosage should be titrated using multiples of 200-mcg tablets. During dosage titration, one dose may include administration of 1–4 tablets of the same strength. No more than 4 tablets should be administered simultaneously. The manufacturer states that the only time that patients should take more than one tablet as a single dose (e.g., two 100-mcg tablets for a single 200-mcg dose) is during dosage titration.

During the dosage titration period, if breakthrough pain is not relieved within 30 minutes following the initial dose of fentanyl citrate buccal tablets, the patient may take *only one* additional dose of the same strength during that episode of breakthrough pain. The manufacturer states that no more than 2 doses of the buccal tablet formulation may be given during a single episode of breakthrough pain, even if the patient continues to experience pain after the second dose is administered. To reduce the risk of overdosage during titration, patients should be strongly advised to use or discard all the buccal tablets of one strength prior to obtaining tablets of a different strength. During the dosage titration phase, each new dose should be evaluated over several breakthrough cancer pain episodes to determine efficacy and tolerability of the drug.

Once the patient has been titrated to an adequate fentanyl dose, breakthrough pain episodes generally should be treated effectively with a single buccal tablet. The manufacturer states that sublingual administration of the buccal tablets is an alternative to intrabuccal administration once an effective dose has been established. On occasion during maintenance therapy, when a breakthrough pain episode is not relieved within 30 minutes after the first intrabuccal dose, the patient may take *only one* additional dose of the same strength during that episode of breakthrough pain. Some patients may require adjustment of the intrabuccal fentanyl dosage to maintain effective analgesia for breakthrough pain episodes; however, dosage generally should be increased only if several consecutive episodes require administration of more than one intrabuccal dose for pain relief. Patients should be instructed that, after treating one episode of breakthrough pain with fentanyl citrate buccal tablets, they must wait at least 4 hours before taking an additional dose of the buccal tablets to treat a subsequent episode of breakthrough cancer pain. If the patient experiences more than 4 breakthrough pain episodes daily, the dosage of opiates used around the clock for chronic cancer pain should be reevaluated.

If discontinuance of opiates is required, gradual tapering of the dose is recommended to avoid signs and symptoms associated with abrupt withdrawal. The dosage level at which fentanyl citrate buccal tablets may be discontinued without producing manifestations of opiate withdrawal is not known.

In a limited number of patients, the presence of grade 1 mucositis did not appear to substantially alter fentanyl absorption or adverse effects following intrabuccal administration of the tablets.

In clinical trials, the dosage of fentanyl citrate buccal tablets (following titration to an adequate dose) tended to be slightly lower in geriatric (older than 65 years of age) patients than in younger patients.

Sublingual Dosage **Sublingual Tablets.** For the management of breakthrough pain in adults who are already receiving and are tolerant of opiates used for the management of persistent cancer pain, the recommended initial dose of fentanyl citrate sublingual tablets (Abstral®) is 100 mcg of fentanyl in *all* patients except those being switched from fentanyl citrate buccal lozenges (Actiq®). Because of differences in pharmacokinetic properties, patients should not be switched on a mcg-per-mcg basis from any other fentanyl preparation to fentanyl citrate sublingual tablets, since the sublingual tablets are not bioequivalent to other fentanyl preparations and are not a generic version of other fentanyl preparations.

In patients being switched from the buccal lozenges to the sublingual tablets, the initial dose of the sublingual tablets should be based on the current buccal lozenge dose (see Table 2). Patients who are switching to the sublingual tablets should be instructed to discontinue use of the buccal lozenges and dispose of any remaining lozenges. If adequate analgesia is not achieved with the initial dose of sublingual tablets, dosage titration should be initiated with close monitoring using a sublingual tablet strength of 100 mcg of fentanyl in patients receiving a buccal lozenge dose of 200 mcg, a sublingual tablet strength of 200 mcg in those receiving a buccal lozenge dose of 400, 600, 800, or 1200 mcg, or a sublingual tablet strength of 400 mcg in those receiving a buccal lozenge dose of 1600 mcg; titration should then proceed in multiples of the initial sublingual tablet strength.

Table 2. Recommended Initial Dose of Fentanyl Citrate Sublingual Tablets for Patients Switching from Fentanyl Citrate Buccal Lozenges

Current Fentanyl Dose as Buccal Lozenges	Initial Fentanyl Dose as Sublingual Tablets
200 mcg	100 mcg
400 mcg	200 mcg
600 mcg	200 mcg
800 mcg	200 mcg
1200 mcg	200 mcg
1600 mcg	400 mcg

In all patients except those being switched from fentanyl citrate buccal lozenges, the recommended initial dose of fentanyl as sublingual tablets is 100 mcg. If adequate analgesia is not achieved with the first 100-mcg dose, dosage should be titrated in a stepwise manner (see Table 3) with close monitoring to a level that provides adequate analgesia and an acceptable level of adverse effects. During titration, patients can use multiples of 100- and/or 200-mcg tablets for any single dose; however, no more than 4 tablets should be administered at one time.

Table 3. Recommended Stepwise Dosage Titration of Fentanyl Citrate Sublingual Tablets

Fentanyl Dose
200 mcg (as two 100-mcg tablets or one 200-mcg tablet)
300 mcg (as three 100-mcg tablets or one 300-mcg tablet)
400 mcg (as four 100-mcg tablets, two 200-mcg tablets, or one 400-mcg tablet)
600 mcg (as three 200-mcg tablets or one 600-mcg tablet)
800 mcg (as four 200-mcg tablets or one 800-mcg tablet)

During the dosage titration period, if breakthrough pain is not relieved within 30 minutes following the initial dose of fentanyl citrate sublingual tablets, the patient may take *only one* additional dose of the same strength during that episode of breakthrough pain. No more than 2 doses of the sublingual tablets may be given during a single episode of breakthrough pain. Patients must wait at least 2 hours before treating a subsequent episode of breakthrough pain with fentanyl citrate sublingual tablets. Patients may use a rescue analgesic as directed by their clinician if the sublingual tablets do not provide adequate pain relief.

Safety and efficacy of sublingual tablet doses exceeding 800 mcg have not been established in clinical trials.

Once an appropriate dose of fentanyl citrate sublingual tablets has been achieved, patients should be instructed to use only one sublingual tablet of the appropriate strength per episode of breakthrough pain. On occasion during maintenance therapy, when a breakthrough pain episode is not relieved within 30 minutes after the first sublingual dose, the patient may take *only one* additional dose during that episode of breakthrough pain. Patients should be instructed that, after treating one episode of breakthrough pain with fentanyl citrate sublingual tablets, they must wait at least 2 hours before taking an additional dose of the sublingual tablets to treat a subsequent episode of breakthrough pain.

If the response (analgesia or adverse reactions) to the titrated sublingual tablet dosage changes markedly, dosage adjustment may be necessary to ensure that an appropriate dosage is maintained. If the patient experiences more than 4 breakthrough pain episodes daily, the dosage of opiates used around the clock for chronic cancer pain should be reevaluated. If the long-acting opiate or the dosage of the long-acting opiate is changed, the dosage of the sublingual tablets should be reevaluated and re-titrated as necessary. Use of the sublingual tablets should be limited to no more than 4 episodes of breakthrough pain daily.

In patients no longer requiring opiate analgesia, consideration should be given to discontinuing fentanyl citrate sublingual tablets along with the gradual tapering of other opiate analgesics to avoid signs and symptoms associated with abrupt withdrawal. In patients who continue to take around-the-clock opiate analgesics for persistent pain but no longer require treatment for breakthrough pain, the sublingual tablets generally can be discontinued immediately.

Sublingual Spray. Each fentanyl sublingual spray unit (Subsys®) provides 100, 200, 400, 600, or 800 mcg of the drug. Because of differences in pharmacokinetic properties, patients should not be switched on a mcg-per-mcg basis from any other fentanyl preparation to fentanyl sublingual spray, since the sublingual spray is not bioequivalent to other fentanyl preparations.

Patients with grade 1 mucositis should be monitored particularly closely, especially during treatment initiation, because of the potential for increased exposure to the drug in these patients; those with grade 2 mucositis should not receive fentanyl sublingual spray unless the benefits outweigh the potential risk of respiratory depression from increased drug exposure. (See Sublingual Tablets and Spray under Pharmacokinetics: Absorption.)

For the management of breakthrough pain in adults who are already receiving and are tolerant of opiates used for the management of persistent cancer pain, the recommended initial dose of fentanyl sublingual spray is 100 mcg in *all* patients except those being switched from fentanyl citrate buccal lozenges (Actiq®).

In patients being switched from the buccal lozenges to the sublingual spray, the initial dose of the sublingual spray should be based on the current dose of the buccal lozenge (see Table 4). Patients who are switching to the sublingual spray should be instructed to discontinue use of the buccal lozenges and dispose of any remaining lozenges. If adequate analgesia is not achieved with the initial dose of the sublingual spray, dosage titration should be initiated using a sublingual spray strength of 100 mcg in patients receiving a buccal lozenge dose of 400 mcg or less, a sublingual spray strength of 200 mcg in those receiving a buccal lozenge dose of 600 or 800 mcg, or a sublingual spray strength of 400 mcg in those receiving a buccal lozenge dose of 1200 or 1600 mcg; titration should then proceed in multiples of the initial spray unit strength.

Table 4. Recommended Initial Dose of Fentanyl Sublingual Spray for Patients Switching from Fentanyl Citrate Buccal Lozenges

Current Fentanyl Dose as Buccal Lozenges	Initial Fentanyl Dose as Sublingual Spray
200 mcg	100 mcg
400 mcg	100 mcg
600 mcg	200 mcg
800 mcg	200 mcg
1200 mcg	400 mcg
1600 mcg	400 mcg

In all patients except those being switched from fentanyl citrate buccal lozenges, the recommended initial dose of fentanyl sublingual spray is 100 mcg. If adequate analgesia is not achieved with the first 100-mcg dose of fentanyl sublingual spray, dosage should be titrated in a stepwise manner (see Table 5) with close monitoring to a level that provides adequate analgesia and an acceptable level of adverse effects with a single dose per episode of breakthrough pain. Patients should be instructed to record their use of the sublingual spray over several episodes of breakthrough pain and to discuss their experience with their clinician to decide whether dosage adjustment is warranted. To reduce the risk of overdosage during dosage titration, patients should have only one strength of fentanyl sublingual spray available at any time.

Table 5. Recommended Stepwise Dosage Titration of Fentanyl Sublingual Spray

Fentanyl Dose
100 mcg (as one 100-mcg unit)
200 mcg (as one 200-mcg unit)
400 mcg (as one 400-mcg unit)
600 mcg (as one 600-mcg unit)
800 mcg (as one 800-mcg unit)
1200 mcg (as two 600-mcg units)
1600 mcg (as two 800-mcg units)

During the dosage titration period, if breakthrough pain is not relieved within 30 minutes following the initial dose of fentanyl sublingual spray, the patient may take *only one* additional dose of the same strength during that episode of breakthrough pain. No more than 2 doses of the sublingual spray may be given during a single episode of breakthrough pain. Patients must wait at least 4 hours before treating a subsequent episode of breakthrough pain with fentanyl sublingual spray.

Once an appropriate dose of fentanyl sublingual spray has been achieved, patients generally should use only one dose of the appropriate strength per episode of breakthrough pain. On occasion during maintenance therapy, when a breakthrough pain episode is not relieved within 30 minutes after the first sublingual dose, the patient may take *only one* additional dose of the same strength during that episode of breakthrough pain. Patients should be instructed that, after treating one episode of breakthrough pain with fentanyl sublingual spray, they must wait at least 4 hours before taking an additional dose of the sublingual spray to treat a subsequent episode of breakthrough pain. Once an appropriate dose has been achieved, patients should administer no more than 4 doses of fentanyl sublingual spray daily.

Some patients may require adjustment of the sublingual fentanyl dosage to maintain effective analgesia for breakthrough pain episodes; however, dosage generally should be increased only if several consecutive episodes require administration of more than one sublingual dose for pain relief. If a single dose of the sublingual spray produces excessive opiate effects, subsequent doses should be decreased. If the patient experiences more than 4 breakthrough pain episodes daily, the dosage of opiates used around the clock for persistent cancer pain should be reevaluated. If pain worsens, the patient's condition should be reevaluated.

Intranasal Dosage After initial priming (4 sprays), each fentanyl citrate nasal inhaler (Lazanda®) delivers eight 100-μL sprays, each containing 100, 300, or 400 mcg of fentanyl per metered spray.

Dosage of fentanyl citrate nasal solution for the management of breakthrough pain in adults who are already receiving and are tolerant of opiates used for the management of persistent cancer pain should be individualized based on clinical response to provide adequate analgesia and an acceptable level of adverse effects. The dosage is not predicted from the daily maintenance dosage of opiate analgesics and must be determined by titration.

For the management of breakthrough pain in opiate-tolerant adults, the recommended initial dose of fentanyl citrate nasal solution for *all*patients, including those switching from therapy with another fentanyl preparation, is 100 mcg (1 spray) in one nostril. Because of differences in pharmacokinetic properties and individual variability, patients should not be switched on a mcg-per-mcg basis from any other fentanyl preparation to the nasal spray, since the nasal spray is not equivalent to other fentanyl preparations and is not a generic version of other fentanyl preparations. If adequate analgesia is obtained within 30 minutes of administration of the single 100-mcg dose, efficacy of the 100-mcg dose should be confirmed in the next episode of breakthrough pain and, if adequate, this dose should be used for subsequent episodes of breakthrough pain. If adequate analgesia is not achieved with the first 100-mcg dose, the dosage should be increased in a stepwise manner (see Table 6) with close monitoring over consecutive episodes of breakthrough pain until adequate analgesia with acceptable adverse effects is achieved. Safety and efficacy of doses exceeding 800 mcg have not been established in clinical trials. Different dosage strengths should not be combined to treat a single episode of breakthrough pain, since this could result in dosage errors. Once an appropriate dose has been established, that dose should be used for each subsequent episode of breakthrough pain.

Table 6. Recommended Stepwise Dosage Titration of Fentanyl Citrate Nasal Spray

Fentanyl Dose (mcg)	Recommended Mode of Administration
100	1 spray (100 mcg/spray) in 1 nostril
200	Total of 2 sprays (100 mcg/spray), as 1 spray in each nostril
300	Total of 3 sprays (100 mcg/spray), alternating between right and left nostrils
400	Total of 4 sprays (100 mcg/spray), alternating between right and left nostrils; alternatively, 1 spray (400 mcg/spray) in 1 nostril
600	Total of 2 sprays (300 mcg/spray), as 1 spray in each nostril
800	Total of 2 sprays (400 mcg/spray), as 1 spray in each nostril

Patients should be instructed that they must wait at least 2 hours after treating one episode of breakthrough pain with fentanyl citrate nasal spray before treating a subsequent episode of breakthrough pain with the nasal spray. An interval of 2 hours between consecutive doses is recommended based on pharmacokinetic data and the frequency of breakthrough pain episodes in patients with cancer. (See Nasal Spray under Pharmacokinetics: Absorption.) If breakthrough pain is not relieved within 30 minutes following a dose of fentanyl citrate nasal spray or if a separate episode of breakthrough pain occurs before the next dose of the nasal spray is permitted, the patient may use a rescue analgesic as directed by their clinician.

If the response (analgesia or adverse reactions) to the titrated nasal spray dosage changes markedly, dosage adjustment may be necessary to ensure that an appropriate dosage is maintained. If the patient experiences more than 4 breakthrough pain episodes daily, the dosage of opiates used around the clock for chronic cancer pain should be reevaluated. If the long-acting opiate or the dosage of the long-acting opiate is changed, the dosage of the nasal spray should be reevaluated and re-titrated as necessary. The nasal spray should be used to treat no more than 4 episodes of breakthrough pain daily.

In patients no longer requiring opiate analgesia, consideration should be given to discontinuing the nasal spray along with the gradual tapering of other opiate analgesics to avoid signs and symptoms associated with abrupt withdrawal. In patients who continue to take around-the-clock opiate analgesics for persistent pain but no longer require treatment for breakthrough pain, the nasal spray generally can be discontinued immediately.

Transdermal Dosage **Transdermal System.** When fentanyl transdermal system is used in opiate-tolerant patients for the management of pain that is severe enough to require long-term, daily, around-the-clock opiate analgesia, appropriate dosage selection and titration are essential to reduce the risk of respiratory depression. The initial dosage of fentanyl transdermal system must be individualized, taking into account the patient's prior analgesic use and risk factors for addiction, abuse, and misuse. Because of the risk of respiratory depression, fentanyl transdermal system should be used only in patients who are opiate tolerant. Patients are considered opiate tolerant if they have been receiving opiate therapy consisting of at least 60 mg of oral morphine sulfate daily, 30 mg of oral oxycodone daily, 8 mg of oral hydromorphone hydrochloride daily, or an equianalgesic dosage of another opiate daily for at least 1 week. Patients should be monitored closely for respiratory depression, especially during the first 24–72 hours of therapy and following any increase in dosage. All other around-the-clock opiate analgesics should be discontinued when therapy with transdermal fentanyl is initiated. Dosage must be carefully individualized since overestimation of the initial transdermal fentanyl dosage can result in fatal overdosage with the first dose. Because there is substantial interpatient variability in the relative potency of opiate analgesics and analgesic formulations, it is preferable to underestimate the patient's 24-hour opiate requirements and provide "rescue" therapy with an immediate-release opiate analgesic than to overestimate the requirements and manage an adverse reaction.

The manufacturers provide specific dosage recommendations for switching opiate-tolerant children and adults from therapy with certain oral or parenteral opiates to therapy with fentanyl transdermal system (see Tables 7 and 8).

Table 7: Dosage of Fentanyl Transdermal System Based on Current Oral Opiate Dosage

Daily Dosage of Oral Opiate (in mg/day)	Transdermal Fentanyl (in mcg/hr)
Morphine sulfate	
60–134	25
135–224	50
225–314	75
315–404	100
Oxycodone hydrochloride	
30–67	25
67.5–112	50
112.5–157	75
157.5–202	100
Codeine phosphate	
150–447	25
Hydromorphone hydrochloride	
8–17	25
17.1–28	50
28.1–39	75
39.1–51	100
Methadone hydrochloride	
20–44	25
45–74	50
75–104	75
105–134	100

Table 8: Dosage of Fentanyl Transdermal System Based on Current Parenteral Opiate Dosage

Daily Dosage of Parenteral Opiate (in mg/day)	Transdermal Fentanyl (in mcg/hr)
Morphine sulfate IV/IM	
10–22	25
23–37	50
38–52	75
53–67	100
Hydromorphone hydrochloride IV	
1.5–3.4	25
3.5–5.6	50
5.7–7.9	75
8–10	100
Meperidine hydrochloride IM	
75–165	25
166–278	50
279–390	75
391–503	100

Alternatively, to switch patients who currently are receiving other opiate therapy or dosages that are not listed in Table 7 or 8 to therapy with fentanyl transdermal system, the manufacturers state that the opiate analgesic requirements during the previous 24 hours should be calculated, an equianalgesic 24-hour dosage of oral morphine sulfate should be calculated using a reliable source, and the initial dosage of fentanyl transdermal system should be determined using Table 9. For transdermal dosages exceeding labeled delivery rates of 100 mcg/hour, multiple systems can be applied at different sites simultaneously.

Table 9: Dosage of Fentanyl Transdermal System Based on Daily Oral Morphine Equivalence

Oral 24-hr Morphine Sulfate (in mg/day)	Transdermal Fentanyl (in mcg/hr)
60–134	25
135–224	50
225–314	75
315–404	100
405–494	125
495–584	150
585–674	175
675–764	200
765–854	225
855–944	250
945–1034	275
1035–1124	300

The manufacturers consider the recommended initial dosages of transdermal fentanyl in Tables 7, 8, and 9 to be conservative estimates. *The dosage conversion guidelines in these tables should not be used to switch patients from therapy with fentanyl transdermal system to therapy with oral or parenteral opiates, since dosage of oral or parenteral opiates may be overestimated.* In clinical trials, the dosage conversion guidelines in these tables were used as a basis for switching patients to therapy with fentanyl transdermal system.

Dosage of transdermal fentanyl should be titrated to a level that provides adequate analgesia and minimizes adverse effects. Patients should be reevaluated continually for adequacy of pain control and for adverse effects, as well as for the development of addiction, abuse, or misuse. Frequent communication is important among the prescriber, other members of the healthcare team, the patient, and the patient's caregiver or family during periods of changing analgesic requirements, including the initial dosage titration period. During long-term therapy, the continued need for opiate analgesics should be continually reevaluated.

Most patients maintain adequate pain control with fentanyl transdermal systems applied at 72-hour intervals, although some patients may require application of the systems at 48-hour intervals. However, dosing intervals of less than 72 hours have not been evaluated in children and adolescents and therefore cannot be recommended for use in this population. Before shortening the dosing interval in patients not responding adequately to a given dosage, an increase in dosage should be evaluated so that patients can be maintained on a 72-hour regimen if possible. Supplemental doses of a short-acting opiate analgesic should be used as needed during the initial application period and subsequently thereafter as necessary to relieve breakthrough pain.

The initial transdermal dosage may be increased after 3 days based on the daily dose of supplemental opiate analgesics during the second or third day after initial application. Because subsequent equilibrium with an increased dose may require up to 6 days to achieve, the manufacturers recommend that further upward titration in dosage based on supplemental opiate analgesic requirements be made no more frequently than every 6 days (i.e., after two 72-hour application periods with a given dosage). The manufacturers recommend that conversion of supplemental opiate requirements to transdermal fentanyl dosage be based on a ratio of 45 mg of oral morphine sulfate (during a 24-hour period) to each 12.5-mcg/hour of transdermal fentanyl. If unacceptable adverse effects are observed, subsequent dosage should be decreased.

To switch to another opiate, the manufacturers recommend that the fentanyl transdermal system be removed and dosage of the other opiate titrated according to patient response. Substantial amounts of fentanyl continue to be absorbed from the skin for 24 hours or more after removal of the transdermal system. It generally takes 20–27 hours for serum fentanyl concentrations to decline by 50% following removal of the system. Symptoms of withdrawal (e.g., nausea, vomiting, diarrhea, anxiety, shivering) may occur in some patients after switching to another opiate agonist or following discontinuance of the fentanyl transdermal system. When transdermal fentanyl therapy is discontinued and another opiate analgesic is not initiated, fentanyl should be withdrawn gradually (e.g., by reducing the transdermal fentanyl dosage by 50% every 6 days) to avoid precipitation of withdrawal symptoms. The dosage level at which transdermal fentanyl may be discontinued without producing manifestations of opiate withdrawal is not known.

When opiate analgesics are used for the management of chronic noncancer pain, the US Centers for Disease Control and Prevention (CDC) recommends that primary care clinicians carefully reassess individual benefits and risks before prescribing dosages equivalent to 50 mg or more of morphine sulfate daily (approximately 20.8 mcg/hour or more of transdermal fentanyl) and avoid dosages equivalent to 90 mg or more of morphine sulfate daily (approximately 37.5 mcg/hour or more of transdermal fentanyl) or carefully justify their decision to titrate the dosage to such levels. Other experts recommend consulting a pain management specialist before exceeding a dosage equivalent to 80–120 mg of morphine sulfate daily. For further information on the management of opiate analgesic therapy, see Dosage and Administration: Dosage, in the Opiate Agonists General Statement 28:08.08.

Iontophoretic Transdermal System. For the short-term management of acute postoperative pain in adults who require opiate analgesia in a hospital setting, fentanyl hydrochloride may be administered via an iontophoretic transdermal system that provides a 40-mcg dose of fentanyl over a 10-minute period following each activation of the device by the patient. Therapy with the iontophoretic transdermal system should be initiated only after the patient has achieved an acceptable level of analgesia with other opiate analgesics. Only one system should be used at a time; if that system fails to provide adequate analgesia, supplemental or alternative analgesic therapy should be initiated.

The iontophoretic transdermal system delivers a maximum of 6 doses of fentanyl per hour and 80 doses per 24 hours (40 mcg per dose). During delivery of one dose, the system is locked and will not respond to additional attempts to activate the device. Each system is operational for 24 hours following assembly or until 80 doses have been delivered, whichever comes first. Therapy with fentanyl hydrochloride iontophoretic transdermal system may be continued for a maximum of 72 hours.

If continued analgesic therapy is required following discontinuance of therapy with fentanyl hydrochloride iontophoretic transdermal system, the dosage of the new analgesic should be titrated until adequate analgesia has been obtained, keeping in mind that serum fentanyl concentrations will decline slowly following removal of the iontophoretic transdermal system. During the analgesic conversion period, the patient should be monitored for respiratory and CNS depression.

■ **Dosage in Renal and Hepatic Impairment** In patients with mild to moderate renal or hepatic impairment, the initial dosage of fentanyl transdermal system should be reduced by 50%, and such patients should be monitored closely for sedation and respiratory depression, including after each increase in dosage. Because of the long half-life of fentanyl when administered as fentanyl transdermal system, the manufacturers state that this formulation should be avoided in patients with severe renal or hepatic impairment.

The manufacturers of transmucosal immediate-release fentanyl preparations (fentanyl citrate buccal lozenges, buccal tablets, sublingual tablets, and nasal spray; fentanyl sublingual spray) state that insufficient information is available to make recommendations regarding use of these preparations in patients with renal or hepatic impairment. Caution is advised if these preparations are used in patients with renal or hepatic impairment.

The manufacturer of fentanyl hydrochloride iontophoretic transdermal system also states that insufficient information is available regarding use of this preparation in patients with renal or hepatic impairment and such patients should be monitored closely for CNS and respiratory depression, especially when initiating iontophoretic transdermal therapy with the drug.

Cautions

Fentanyl shares the toxic potentials of the opiate agonists, and the usual precautions of opiate agonist therapy should be observed. (See Cautions in the Opiate Agonists General Statement 28:08.08.) The most serious adverse effect of fentanyl is respiratory depression. (See Precautions Against Serious Toxicity Resulting From Fentanyl Overdosage or Accidental Exposure under Cautions: Precautions and Contraindications.) Fentanyl citrate appears to cause a lower incidence of nausea and vomiting than do other opiate agonists. Skeletal and thoracic muscle rigidity occurs frequently, especially following rapid IV administration of fentanyl. Muscular rigidity may be associated with reduced pulmonary compliance and/or apnea, laryngospasm, and bronchoconstriction and may be managed by use of assisted or controlled respiration or, if necessary, by IV administration of a neuromuscular blocking agent. Bradycardia may occur following administration of fentanyl and may be controlled with atropine.

In addition to the usual adverse effects associated with opiate therapy, local adverse effects associated with topical application of fentanyl transdermal system include dermatitis, erythema, papules, pruritus, hypersensitivity, and edema at the site of application. Erythema at the site of application is common and may persist for 6 hours or longer following removal of the transdermal system.

Dermatologic reactions (e.g., erythema, pruritus, sweating, vesicles, papules/pustules) also may occur in patients receiving therapy with fentanyl hydrochloride iontophoretic transdermal system; such reactions generally are limited to the application site. If a severe reaction is observed, the system should be removed and further use discontinued.

Application site reactions, ranging from paresthesia to ulceration and bleeding, occurred in 10% of patients receiving fentanyl citrate buccal tablets in clinical trials. The most common application site reactions were pain, ulcer, and irritation, each occurring in 3–4% of patients receiving this preparation of fentanyl. Such reactions tended to occur early during treatment and generally were self-limited.

Dental decay, including caries, tooth loss, and gum line erosion, has occurred in patients receiving fentanyl citrate buccal lozenges, despite routine oral hygiene in some patients. (See Other Precautions under Cautions: Precautions and Contraindications.)

■ **Precautions and Contraindications** ***Precautions Against Serious Toxicity Resulting From Fentanyl Overdosage or Accidental Exposure*** The most serious adverse effect of fentanyl is respiratory depression. Fentanyl should be administered only under the supervision of qualified clinicians. (See Uses.) Patients receiving fentanyl should be advised of the importance of taking the drug exactly as prescribed.

During postmarketing experience with fentanyl transdermal system, death and life-threatening adverse effects secondary to inappropriate prescribing by clinicians (e.g., use of fentanyl transdermal system for postoperative pain, occasional or mild pain, or headaches) and incorrect use by patients (application of too many systems, application of heat to the system, replacement of systems too frequently) have been reported. These systems should be used for pain management only in opiate-tolerant patients with pain that is severe enough to require long-term, daily, around-the-clock use of an opiate analgesic and in whom alternative treatment options (e.g., nonopiate analgesics, immediate-release opiates) are inadequate or not tolerated. (See Uses.)

Death and life-threatening adverse effects also have been reported during postmarketing experience in patients receiving transmucosal immediate-release fentanyl preparations and have been attributed to improper patient selection (e.g., use of these formulations in patients who were not opiate tolerant) and/or improper dosage. Transmucosal immediate-release preparations should be used only for treatment of breakthrough pain in patients with cancer who are already receiving opiates for persistent cancer pain and are opiate tolerant. Because substantial differences exist in the pharmacokinetic profiles of transmucosal immediate-release fentanyl preparations, patients receiving one transmucosal immediate-release fentanyl preparation (e.g., fentanyl citrate buccal lozenges, buccal tablets, sublingual tablets, or nasal spray; fentanyl sublingual spray) must not be switched on a mcg-per-mcg basis to another such preparation or to any other fentanyl preparation, and one such preparation must not be dispensed as a substitute for another. (See Pharmacokinetics: Absorption.) Substitution of one transmucosal immediate-release fentanyl preparation for another may result in fatal overdosage. (See Uses.)

When fentanyl hydrochloride is administered as an iontophoretic transdermal system for the management of acute postoperative pain, the device should be used only in a hospital setting and only the patient should be allowed to activate the device.

Peak serum concentrations of fentanyl occur between 20–72 hours after application of fentanyl transdermal system; serious or life-threatening respiratory depression may occur at any time, but especially during initiation of therapy and after increases in dosage. Because serum fentanyl concentrations decline slowly following removal of the transdermal system (see Transdermal System under Pharmacokinetics: Absorption), patients who have received an overdose of transdermally administered fentanyl should be monitored for at least 72–96 hours after the overdose.

Because release of fentanyl from fentanyl transdermal systems and percutaneous permeability of the drug are temperature dependent, serum fentanyl concentrations could theoretically increase by approximately one-third in patients with a body temperature of 40°C. Patients who develop a fever while using fentanyl transdermal system should be observed closely for manifestations of opiate toxicity, and dosage of the drug should be adjusted accordingly. Patients should be cautioned to avoid strenuous exertion that leads to increased core body temperature while wearing the transdermal system. Because application of heat over the fentanyl transdermal system increases mean systemic exposure and peak plasma concentrations of the drug by 120 and 61%, respectively, and has resulted in fatal overdosage, patients wearing a fentanyl transdermal system should be advised to avoid exposing the application site or surrounding area to direct external heat sources. (See Transdermal System under Administration: Transdermal Administration, in Dosage and Administration.)

Because the presence of grade 1 mucositis can substantially increase exposure to fentanyl administered as a sublingual spray, patients with grade 1 mucositis receiving this formulation of the drug should be monitored closely for respiratory and CNS depression, particularly during initiation of therapy. Use of fentanyl sublingual spray should be avoided in patients with grade 2 or worse mucositis unless the benefits are expected to outweigh the risks of respiratory depression, since the increase in fentanyl exposure in these patients may be large and variable. (See Sublingual Tablets and Spray under Pharmacokinetics: Absorption.)

Accidental exposure to an intact fentanyl hydrochloride iontophoretic transdermal system or to the fentanyl-containing hydrogel component of the system, especially by a child, through contact with skin or mucous membranes, can result in fatal overdosage. If the system is not handled correctly using gloves, health care professionals also are at risk of accidental exposure and fatal overdosage. If accidental contact with the system or its components occurs, the affected area should be rinsed thoroughly and immediately with water.

Contact with unwashed or unclothed sites of application for fentanyl transdermal system can result in accidental exposure to the drug and should be avoided. Serious or fatal adverse effects have occurred after accidental exposure to fentanyl transdermal systems (including transfer of a transdermal system from an adult to a child while hugging, exposure of individuals sharing the same bed, inadvertently sitting on a transdermal system, exposure of the caregiver's skin to the drug during application or removal of the transdermal system, exposure to systems that were disposed of improperly). If individuals other than the patient for whom the transdermal system was prescribed are accidentally exposed to the drug or if the transdermal system accidentally adheres to the individual, the system should be removed and the area of contact should be washed with water. The accidentally exposed individual should seek medical attention immediately. Placement of fentanyl transdermal systems in the mouth, chewing or swallowing transdermal systems, or using these systems in other unintended ways may cause choking or potentially fatal overdosage of fentanyl.

Because of the risk of fatal overdosage associated with accidental exposure to fentanyl transdermal systems or ingestion of transmucosal immediate-release preparations of the drug by non-opiate-tolerant individuals or individuals for whom the drug was not prescribed, patients receiving these formulations of the drug should be advised regarding proper storage and disposal of the preparations. (See Chemistry and Stability: Stability and also see Dosage and Administration: Administration.)

For additional information on cautions associated with the use of transdermal or transmucosal fentanyl, see Uses.

Precautions Related to Transdermal Iontophoretic Administration Fentanyl hydrochloride iontophoretic transdermal system is considered to be unsafe for use with magnetic resonance imaging (MRI); the iontophoretic transdermal system contains metal components and must be removed prior to an MRI procedure to avoid patient injury and damage to the system. Whether exposure to an MRI procedure increases release of fentanyl from the iontophoretic transdermal system is unknown. Patients inadvertently exposed to MRI while wearing a fentanyl hydrochloride iontophoretic transdermal system should be monitored for CNS and respiratory depression. The iontophoretic transdermal system also can be damaged by the strong electromagnetic fields set up by cardioversion, defibrillation, radiographic imaging, computed-tomography (CT) scanning, or diathermy; because the iontophoretic transdermal system contains radiopaque components, it also may interfere with radiographic imaging or CT scanning. The iontophoretic transdermal system should be removed prior to these medical procedures. If exposure of the system to these procedures occurs and the system does not appear to function normally, the exposed system should be removed and replaced with a new system.

Contact with synthetic materials (e.g., carpeted flooring) should be avoided to reduce the possibility of electrostatic discharge and damage to the iontophoretic transdermal system; exposure to electronic security systems also should be avoided to reduce the possibility that the system may be damaged. In addition, use of the iontophoretic transdermal system near communications equipment (e.g., base stations for radio telephones and land mobile radios, amateur radio, AM and FM radio broadcast, TV broadcast, radio) and radio frequency identification (RFID) transmitters can damage the iontophoretic transdermal system; the recommended separation distance between the iontophoretic transdermal system and communications equipment or RFID transmitters ranges from 0.12–23 meters, depending on the rated maximum output power and frequency of the transmitter. If exposure to electronic security systems, electrostatic discharge, communications equipment, or RFID transmitters occurs and the iontophoretic transdermal system does not appear to function normally, the exposed system should be removed and replaced with a new system. The manufacturer's prescribing information should be consulted for additional information on electromagnetic compatibility and troubleshooting for device malfunction.

The low-level electrical current provided by the iontophoretic transdermal system does not result in electromagnetic interference with other electromechanical devices such as pacemakers or electrical monitoring equipment.

Other Precautions The high concentration of fentanyl contained in fentanyl transdermal systems may make this formulation a target for diversion and abuse. Transmucosal immediate-release preparations of the drug also may be targets for diversion and abuse. Patients should be instructed to keep these preparations in a secure place to prevent theft or misuse in the home or workplace. Patients should be informed of the risk of severe or fatal respiratory depression if these preparations of fentanyl are used in individuals for whom the drug was not prescribed.

Fentanyl should be used with caution in patients with cardiac bradyarrhythmias. Patients with bradyarrhythmias should be monitored closely for changes in heart rate, particularly during initiation of fentanyl therapy.

Because fentanyl undergoes extensive hepatic metabolism and there is some evidence that renal excretion contributes to elimination of the drug, fentanyl should be used with caution in patients with renal or hepatic impairment.

Serotonin syndrome has been reported during concomitant use of opiate agonists, including fentanyl, and serotonergic drugs at recommended dosages. Manifestations of serotonin syndrome may include mental status changes (e.g., agitation, hallucinations, coma), autonomic instability (e.g., tachycardia, labile blood pressure, hyperthermia), neuromuscular aberrations (e.g., hyperreflexia, incoordination, rigidity), and/or GI symptoms (e.g., nausea, vomiting, diarrhea). Symptom onset generally occurs within several hours to a few days of concomitant use, but may occur later, particularly after dosage increases. (See Drug Interactions: Drugs Associated with Serotonin Syndrome.)

Patients receiving fentanyl citrate buccal lozenges should be instructed to inform their dentist that they are receiving this preparation, so that appropriate dental care is provided. Each fentanyl citrate buccal lozenge contains 2 g of sugar, and frequent consumption of sugar-containing products has been associated with an increased risk of dental decay. Dental decay, including caries, tooth loss, and gum line erosion, has occurred in patients receiving fentanyl citrate buccal lozenges, despite routine oral hygiene in some patients. Dry mouth, which is frequently associated with the use of opiate agonists (e.g., fentanyl), may add to this risk.

The sugar content of fentanyl citrate buccal lozenges should be considered in patients with diabetes mellitus.

The manufacturer's patient information (e.g., medication guide) should be provided to the patient each time fentanyl transdermal system or transmucosal immediate-release fentanyl preparations (fentanyl citrate buccal tablets, buccal lozenges, sublingual tablets, and nasal spray; fentanyl sublingual spray) are dispensed. Patients should be instructed to use these preparations exactly as prescribed.

Contraindications Because of the risk of life-threatening respiratory depression, transmucosal immediate-release preparations of fentanyl (fentanyl citrate buccal lozenges, buccal tablets, sublingual tablets, and nasal spray; fentanyl sublingual spray) are contraindicated in the management of acute or postoperative pain (e.g., migraine or other headaches, dental pain, emergency department use) and in patients who are not opiate tolerant. (See Uses.)

Because of the prolonged duration of effects and risk of serious or life-threatening respiratory depression associated with fentanyl transdermal system, this dosage form is contraindicated in the management of acute, mild, intermittent, or postoperative pain (e.g., following outpatient or day surgery [e.g., tonsillectomy]); in patients who require opiate analgesia for a short period of time; and in patients who are not opiate tolerant. (See Uses.) Use of the transdermal system also is contraindicated in patients with substantial respiratory depression, especially in settings where adequate monitoring and equipment for resuscitation are not available; in patients with acute or severe bronchial asthma; and in those with known or suspected paralytic ileus.

Use of fentanyl hydrochloride iontophoretic transdermal system is contraindicated in patients with substantial respiratory depression, acute or severe bronchial asthma, or known or suspected paralytic ileus and GI obstruction.

Fentanyl preparations also are contraindicated in patients with known hypersensitivity to the drug or any component of the dosage form (e.g., cetylpyridinium chloride, an inactive ingredient in fentanyl hydrochloride iontophoretic transdermal system).

■ **Pediatric Precautions** Safety and efficacy of parenteral fentanyl citrate and fentanyl transdermal system have not been established in children younger than 2 years of age. In clinical studies evaluating the safety of fentanyl transdermal system in 289 patients 2–18 years of age with chronic pain, treatment was continued for 15 days or less in 20% of patients, 16–30 days in 46%, 31–60 days in 16%, and at least 61 days in 17% of patients. To reduce the potential for accidental ingestion, the application site in young children receiving transdermal fentanyl therapy should be carefully selected and caregivers should monitor the system for proper adhesion over the period of application. (See Transdermal System under Administration: Transdermal Administration, in Dosage and Administration.)

Safety and efficacy of fentanyl citrate buccal lozenges have not been established in children younger than 16 years of age; safety and efficacy of fentanyl sublingual spray, fentanyl hydrochloride iontophoretic transdermal system, or fentanyl citrate buccal tablets, sublingual tablets, or nasal spray have not been established in patients younger than 18 years of age.

Fentanyl transdermal systems, fentanyl hydrochloride iontophoretic transdermal systems, and transmucosal immediate-release preparations of the drug (fentanyl citrate buccal lozenges, buccal tablets, sublingual tablets, and nasal spray; fentanyl sublingual spray) contain fentanyl in amounts that can be fatal to a child. If a child accidentally ingests a transmucosal immediate-release preparation of fentanyl, the risk of respiratory depression is high. Fatal respiratory depression can occur if a transdermal system is accidentally or deliberately applied or ingested by a child or adolescent, and choking can occur if the system is ingested. Because transdermal systems can be accidentally transferred to children, patients should be instructed to take special precautions to avoid accidental contact when holding or caring for children. Patients and/or caregivers must be instructed to keep new, used, and partially used transdermal systems and transmucosal immediate-release preparations of the drug out of the reach of children and to strictly adhere to storage and disposal instructions. (See Dosage and Administration: Administration and also see Chemistry and Stability: Stability.) Clinicians should specifically question patients and/or their caregivers about the presence of children in the patient's home on a full-time or visiting basis. If a child is accidentally exposed to a fentanyl transdermal system or accidentally ingests a transmucosal immediate-release preparation of the drug, parents or caregivers should seek immediate medical treatment for the child.

■ **Geriatric Precautions** Life-threatening respiratory depression is more likely to occur in geriatric, cachectic, or debilitated patients since pharmacokinetics of fentanyl in these patients may be altered compared with that observed in younger, healthier patients. Data for IV fentanyl suggest that clearance of the drug may be decreased and the terminal half-life prolonged in geriatric patients; greater sensitivity to the effects of IV fentanyl has been observed in geriatric patients compared with younger individuals. Therefore, geriatric patients receiving fentanyl should be monitored closely for sedation and respiratory depression, particularly during initiation or titration of therapy and when other respiratory depressants are used concomitantly; dosage of fentanyl should be titrated cautiously.

Clinical studies of fentanyl transdermal system did not include sufficient numbers of patients 65 years of age or older to determine whether geriatric patients respond differently to this formulation than younger patients; however, other reported clinical experience has not identified differences in response between geriatric and younger patients. Pharmacokinetics of fentanyl transdermal system in geriatric patients did not differ substantially from that in younger adults, although peak serum concentrations tended to be lower and mean half-life was prolonged in geriatric patients.

About 23% of cancer patients included in clinical trials of fentanyl citrate buccal tablets were 65 years of age or older. Dosage of fentanyl citrate (following titration to an adequate dosage) tended to be slightly lower in geriatric patients than in younger adults. Geriatric patients receiving fentanyl citrate buccal tablets reported a slightly higher frequency of vomiting, constipation, and abdominal pain than did younger adults.

About 24% of cancer patients included in clinical trials of fentanyl citrate buccal lozenges were 65 years of age or older, and 6% of patients were 75 years of age or older. Dosage of fentanyl (following titration to an adequate dosage) generally was about 200 mcg lower in geriatric patients than in younger adults. The safety profile of fentanyl citrate buccal lozenges in geriatric patients appeared to be similar to that observed in younger adults.

About 21% of cancer patients included in phase 3 clinical trials of fentanyl citrate sublingual tablets were 65 years of age or older. The median dosage of fentanyl citrate (following titration to an adequate dosage) and the overall safety of the drug in patients 65 years of age or older did not differ from those in younger adults.

About 27% of cancer patients included in clinical trials of fentanyl sublingual spray were 60 years of age or older, while 17% were 65 years of age or older, and 3% were 75 years of age or older. No overall differences in safety were observed between patients older than 65 years of age and younger adults.

About 28% of cancer patients included in clinical trials of fentanyl citrate nasal spray were 60 years of age or older. No clinically important differences in safety were observed between these patients and younger adults.

In clinical trials of fentanyl hydrochloride iontophoretic transdermal system at the recommended dose, 499 patients were 65 years of age or older, and 174 of these patients were 75 years of age or older. Although no overall differences in safety and efficacy were observed between geriatric patients and younger adults, hypotension, confusion, hypokalemia, hypoxia, and hypoventilation occurred slightly more frequently (difference of 1–2 percentage points) in geriatric patients than in younger adults. Age did not substantially affect the extent of drug absorption following iontophoretic transdermal administration.

■ **Pregnancy and Lactation** There are no adequate and well-controlled studies of fentanyl in pregnant women. Fentanyl should be used during pregnancy only if the potential benefit justifies the potential risk to the fetus.

Transient neonatal muscular rigidity has been observed in infants whose mothers received IV fentanyl.

Analysis of data from the National Birth Defects Prevention Study, a large population-based, case-control study, suggests that therapeutic use of opiates in pregnant women during the period of organogenesis is associated with a low absolute risk of birth defects, including heart defects, spina bifida, and gastroschisis. Fentanyl was not teratogenic in rats at dosages of 10–500 mcg/kg daily when administered on days 7–21 of gestation via an implanted microosmotic minipump. In animal reproduction and developmental studies, there was an increased risk for early embryolethality, decreased pup survival, and developmental delays in surviving pups at fentanyl doses within the human dosage range. At an IV dosage of 10–30 mcg/kg daily on days 6–18 of gestation in rats, fentanyl was embryotoxic or fetotoxic and slightly increased mean delivery time in animals receiving the highest dosage, but the drug was not teratogenic. At IV doses of 30 mcg/kg or subcutaneous doses of 160 mcg/kg in rats, fentanyl increased embryonic resorptions.

Since fentanyl may cause sedation and serious respiratory depression and the drug is distributed into milk, the manufacturers of fentanyl transdermal system and transmucosal immediate-release preparations of the drug (used only in opiate-tolerant patients) state that these preparations should not be used in nursing women because of the potential for serious adverse reactions to the drug in nursing infants. However, the manufacturer of fentanyl hydrochloride iontophoretic transdermal system (used for short-term management of acute postoperative pain) states that the developmental and health benefits from breast-feeding should be considered along with the mother's need for the drug and any potential effects on the breast-fed infant from either the drug or the underlying maternal condition. Limited data suggest that breast-fed infants receive an estimated 0.38% of the maternal weight-adjusted dosage. Symptoms of withdrawal can occur in opiate-dependent infants upon cessation of breast-feeding by women receiving fentanyl.

Drug Interactions

Fentanyl shares the drug interaction potentials of the opiate agonists. (See Drug Interactions in the Opiate Agonists General Statement 28:08.08.)

■ **Drugs Affecting or Metabolized by Hepatic Microsomal Enzymes** Because fentanyl undergoes metabolism via cytochrome P-450 (CYP) isoenzyme 3A4 in the liver and the intestinal mucosa, concomitant use of inhibitors of CYP3A4 (e.g., amiodarone, aprepitant, cimetidine, clarithromycin, diltiazem, erythromycin, fluconazole, fosamprenavir, grapefruit juice, indinavir, itraconazole, ketoconazole, nefazodone, nelfinavir, ritonavir, saquinavir, telithromycin, troleandomycin, verapamil) may increase plasma concentrations of fentanyl, possibly resulting in increased or prolonged opiate effects, including potentially fatal respiratory depression. Results of a crossover study evaluating the potential interaction between ritonavir (200 mg 3 times daily on day 1, then 300 mg 3 times daily for 4 additional doses) and fentanyl citrate (single IV dose of 5 mcg/kg on day 2) in healthy individuals suggested that ritonavir might decrease clearance of fentanyl by 67% and increase exposure (area under the concentration-time curve [AUC]) to the opiate by 174% (range: 52–420%). Concomitant use of grapefruit products should be avoided. If concomitant use of fentanyl with drugs that inhibit CYP3A4 is necessary, patients should be monitored at frequent intervals and dosage adjustments should be considered until stable drug effects are achieved. Patients receiving fentanyl who initiate therapy with, or increase the dosage of, a CYP3A4 inhibitor should be monitored carefully over an extended period of time for increased opiate effects. Any increases in dosage should be conservative.

Conversely, concomitant use of drugs that induce CYP3A4 (e.g., barbiturates, carbamazepine, efavirenz, glucocorticoids, modafinil, nevirapine, oxcarbazepine, phenytoin, pioglitazone, rifabutin, rifampin, St. John's wort [*Hypericum perforatum*]) may reduce plasma concentrations of fentanyl, possibly resulting in decreased analgesic efficacy and/or development of opiate withdrawal. If concomitant use of fentanyl with CYP3A4 inducers is necessary, patients should be monitored for opiate withdrawal and dosage adjustments should be considered until stable drug effects are achieved. Discontinuance of a concomitantly used CYP3A4 inducer may result in increased plasma concentrations of fentanyl, possibly resulting in increased or prolonged therapeutic or adverse effects, including potentially fatal respiratory depression. Patients receiving fentanyl who discontinue therapy with, or decrease the dosage of, a CYP3A4 inducer should be monitored for increased opiate effects and the fentanyl dosage should be adjusted as necessary.

■ **Benzodiazepines and Other CNS Depressants** Concomitant use of opiate agonists and benzodiazepines or other CNS depressants, including other opiate agonists, anxiolytics, sedatives, hypnotics, tranquilizers, muscle relaxants, general anesthetics, antipsychotics, and alcohol, may result in hypotension, profound sedation, respiratory depression, coma, and death. (See Drug Interactions: Benzodiazepines and Other CNS Depressants, in the Opiate Agonists General Statement 28:08.08.)

Concomitant use of parenteral fentanyl and benzodiazepines or other CNS depressants also may result in decreased pulmonary arterial pressure; even relatively small dosages of diazepam may cause cardiovascular depression when used with high or anesthetic dosages of fentanyl. Clinicians should consider the potential for such concomitant therapy to decrease pulmonary arterial pressure when performing diagnostic or surgical procedures where interpretation of pulmonary arterial pressure measurements might determine patient management. If hypotension occurs, the possibility of hypovolemia should be considered and managed with appropriate fluid therapy. When operative conditions permit, repositioning of the patient to improve venous return to the heart should be considered. Because of the potential for orthostatic hypotension, care should be exercised when moving and repositioning the patient. If volume expansion and other countermeasures do not correct hypotension, administration of a pressor agent (other than epinephrine, which may cause a reduction in blood pressure in patients receiving a neuroleptic with α-adrenergic blocking activity) should be considered. If used parenterally for postoperative analgesia in conjunction with a benzodiazepine or other CNS depressant, fentanyl should be initiated at a reduced dosage and titrated based on clinical response, and the patient should be monitored closely for respiratory depression, sedation, and hypotension. Fluids or other measures to counteract hypotension should be available.

■ **Drugs Associated with Serotonin Syndrome** Serotonin syndrome has occurred in patients receiving opiate agonists, including fentanyl, in conjunction with other serotonergic drugs, including serotonin (5-hydroxytryptamine; 5-HT) type 1 receptor agonists ("triptans"), selective serotonin-reuptake inhibitors (SSRIs), selective serotonin- and norepinephrine-reuptake inhibitors (SNRIs), tricyclic antidepressants, antiemetics that are 5-HT$_3$ receptor antagonists, buspirone, cyclobenzaprine, dextromethorphan, lithium, St. John's wort, tryptophan, other serotonin modulators (e.g., mirtazapine, nefazodone, trazodone, vilazodone), and monoamine oxidase (MAO) inhibitors (both those used to treat psychiatric disorders and others, such as linezolid, methylene blue, and selegiline). Serotonin syndrome may occur within the recommended dosage ranges for these drugs. Manifestations of serotonin syndrome may include mental status changes (e.g., agitation, hallucinations, coma), autonomic instability (e.g., tachycardia, labile blood pressure, hyperthermia), neuromuscular aberrations (e.g., hyperreflexia, incoordination, rigidity), and/or GI symptoms (e.g., nausea, vomiting, diarrhea). Symptom onset generally occurs within several hours to a few days of concomitant use, but may occur later, particularly after dosage increases.

If concurrent therapy with opiate agonists and serotonergic drugs is warranted, patients should be monitored for serotonin syndrome, particularly during initiation of therapy and dosage increases. If serotonin syndrome is suspected, treatment with fentanyl, other opiate therapy, and/or any concurrently administered serotonergic agents should be discontinued.

For further information on serotonin syndrome, including manifestations and treatment, see Drug Interactions: Serotonergic Drugs, in Fluoxetine Hydrochloride 28:16.04.20.

■ **Nasal Decongestants** Concomitant administration of intranasal fentanyl citrate and a vasoactive nasal decongestant for the treatment of allergic rhinitis may alter absorption of fentanyl across the nasal mucosa. In individuals with ragweed-induced allergic (seasonal) rhinitis, concomitant intranasal administration of oxymetazoline and fentanyl citrate reduced peak plasma concentrations and AUC of fentanyl by approximately 32 and 10%, respectively, and delayed peak plasma fentanyl concentrations by approximately 30 minutes compared with pharmacokinetic parameters observed in asymptomatic (unchallenged) individuals. The presence of allergic rhinitis alone (in the absence of nasal decongestant therapy) did not substantially alter the rate or extent of fentanyl exposure. These findings suggest that intranasally administered fentanyl may be less effective in patients with allergic rhinitis who use nasal decongestants, thus potentially interfering with pain management. In addition, because titration of the intranasal fentanyl dosage in patients experiencing an acute episode of rhinitis could result in selection of an inappropriate dose for use during subsequent episodes of breakthrough pain, particularly if the patient is using a nasal decongestant, dosage titration under these circumstances must be avoided.

Pharmacology

Fentanyl citrate shares the actions of the opiate agonists. When given in equivalent analgesic doses, fentanyl is similar to morphine and meperidine in its respiratory effects except that respiration of healthy individuals returns to normal more quickly after fentanyl than after either of the other drugs. Although pharmacodynamically similar to meperidine and morphine, fentanyl exhibits little hypnotic activity, and histamine release rarely occurs.

Pharmacokinetics

The pharmacokinetics of fentanyl citrate following IV administration are best described by a 3-compartment model.

■ **Absorption** Fentanyl is well absorbed percutaneously following topical application of fentanyl transdermal system to a flat surface on the upper torso or following topical application of fentanyl hydrochloride iontophoretic transdermal system to the upper outer arm or chest. The drug also is well absorbed transmucosally following intrabuccal administration as fentanyl citrate buccal lozenge or buccal tablet, sublingual administration as fentanyl citrate sublingual tablet or fentanyl sublingual spray, or intranasal administration as fentanyl citrate nasal spray.

Following parenteral administration, the action of fentanyl is more prompt and less prolonged than that of morphine or meperidine. The onset of action following IV administration is rapid; peak analgesia occurs within several minutes and the duration of analgesia is 30–60 minutes after a single dose of up to 100 mcg. Following IM administration of fentanyl citrate, the onset of action occurs within about 7–15 minutes and the duration of action is 1–2 hours. Respiratory depressant effects may persist longer than analgesia. Residual effects of one dose of fentanyl citrate may potentiate the effects of subsequent doses. It has been suggested that redistribution is the main cause of the brief analgesic effect of fentanyl.

In opiate-naive (nontolerant) patients, minimum effective analgesic serum fentanyl concentrations range from 0.2–2 ng/mL. Adverse effects of the drug in opiate-naive patients generally increase as serum concentrations exceed 2 ng/mL, although respiratory depression (e.g., hypoventilation) can occur throughout the therapeutic range of fentanyl serum concentrations, especially in patients with underlying pulmonary conditions or those receiving concomitant therapy with respiratory depressants. CNS depression becomes prominent as serum fentanyl concentrations exceed 3 ng/mL in opiate-naive patients, and anesthesia and profound respiratory depression generally occur at concentrations of 10–20 ng/mL. With continued use, tolerance to the pharmacologic and adverse effects of the drug develop, but the rate of development of tolerance exhibits considerable interindividual variation.

Transdermal System The amount of fentanyl released from each fentanyl transdermal system is proportional to the surface area of the transdermal system. Fentanyl transdermal systems are designed to deliver fentanyl at a nearly constant rate; however, the actual amount of drug delivered to the skin during the period of application exhibits interindividual variation, and the labeled rate on each system corresponds to the average amount of drug delivered across average skin to systemic circulation per hour. Following initial application of a transdermal system of fentanyl, initial release of the drug saturates skin sites beneath the system, and a depot of drug concentrates in the upper layers of the skin. Serum fentanyl concentrations increase slowly following topical application of the system, reaching a plateau between 12–24 hours and then remaining relatively constant, but with some fluctuation, during the remainder of the application period (up to 72 hours total); peak serum concentrations of the drug generally occur 20–72 hours after initial application. Although the transdermal system was applied for 24-hour periods in most published studies, data provided by the manufacturer are for application for 72-hour periods. In healthy adults, application of heat over the transdermal system increased mean exposure and peak plasma concentrations of the drug by 120 and 61%, respectively.

Steady-state serum fentanyl concentrations achieved with sequential applications of transdermal systems exhibit considerable interindividual variation, depending on individual variation in skin permeability and body clearance of the drug. With sequential continuous use, serum fentanyl concentrations increase with the first 2 transdermal system applications. By the end of the second 72-hour application, a steady-state serum concentration is reached and is maintained during subsequent applications of systems with the same labeled rate of fentanyl delivery. Peak serum concentrations of the drug following the initial 72-hour application average 0.4, 0.9, 1.7, 2.3, or 3.4 ng/mL following topical application of transdermal systems labeled as delivering 12.5, 25, 50, 75, or 100 mcg/hour, respectively. Following use of fentanyl transdermal systems in non-opiate-tolerant children 1.5–5 years of age, plasma fentanyl concentrations were about twice the concentrations achieved in adults; however, pharmacokinetic parameters in older children were similar to those in adults. The pharmacokinetic profile of fentanyl in healthy Caucasian adults 65 years of age or older (mean age: 71 years) generally was similar to that in adults 18–45 years of age following application of a fentanyl transdermal system labeled as delivering 100 mcg/hour for 72 hours; mean peak plasma concentration was about 8% lower and area under the plasma concentration-time curve (AUC) about 7% greater in geriatric individuals compared with the younger age group, and interindividual variability in AUC was greater in geriatric individuals (58 versus 37%). Following application of a fentanyl transdermal system labeled as delivering 50 mcg/hour for 72 hours in patients with cirrhosis, peak plasma concentration and AUC of the drug were increased by 35 and 73%, respectively, compared with values in control patients. Following discontinuance of transdermal therapy, serum fentanyl concentrations decline gradually with an average half-life of about 20–27 hours; the slower decline in serum concentrations relative to that following IV administration results from the continued absorption of residual drug from the skin.

Buccal Lozenges and Tablets Following intrabuccal administration of fentanyl citrate in a lozenge matrix, the drug is absorbed transmucosally from the buccal mucosa and also from the GI tract (for any portion of the dose that is swallowed in saliva during sucking of the lozenge matrix). Thus, systemic absorption of intrabuccally administered drug is characterized by an initial rapid phase from the buccal mucosa and a more prolonged phase from the GI tract. Both the plasma concentration profile and bioavailability of the drug are variable and depend on the relative fractions of the dose that are absorbed from the buccal mucosa and the GI tract.

Generally, approximately 25% of a dose of fentanyl administered as a buccal lozenge is absorbed rapidly from the buccal mucosa and the remaining portion is swallowed with saliva and then absorbed slowly from the GI tract. Approximately one-third of the drug that is swallowed with saliva (approximately 25% of the total dose) bypasses first-pass metabolism in the liver and the intestinal mucosa and becomes systemically available. In general, the combined systemic bioavailability of fentanyl following administration of the lozenge is approximately 50%, being approximately equally divided between rapid transmucosal absorption and more prolonged GI absorption. Therefore, if a lozenge were chewed and swallowed rather than being administered as recommended, bioavailability and peak plasma concentrations of the drug might be reduced. In a limited number of adults receiving single 15-mcg/kg doses in one study, systemic bioavailability relative to IV administration averaged 50% with the lozenge. The manufacturers state that in a limited number of adults, mean peak serum concentrations and AUC of fentanyl increased in proportion to dose from the commercially available 200-, 400-, 800-, and 1600-mcg lozenges. Following intrabuccal administration of fentanyl citrate lozenges in healthy individuals (after a standardized consumption time of 15 minutes), mean peak serum concentrations of fentanyl were attained at a median of 20–40 minutes (range: 20 minutes to 8 hours) and were 0.39, 0.75, 1.55, and 2.51 ng/mL following single 200-, 400-, 800-, and 1600-mcg doses of fentanyl, respectively.

Following intrabuccal administration of fentanyl citrate buccal tablets, the drug is absorbed transmucosally from the buccal mucosa and also from the GI tract (for any portion of the dose that is swallowed). In general, the combined systemic bioavailability of fentanyl following administration of the buccal tablet is approximately 65%, being approximately equally divided between rapid transmucosal absorption and more prolonged GI absorption. Peak plasma fentanyl concentrations generally are attained within 1 hour following administration of fentanyl citrate buccal tablets. Following administration of the buccal tablets in healthy individuals, systemic exposure to fentanyl generally increased proportionally with the dose over the range of 100–800 mcg. Following administration of single 100-, 200-, 400-, and 800-mcg doses of fentanyl (as buccal tablets) in healthy individuals, peak serum concentrations of the drug were attained at a median of 35–45 minutes (range 20 minutes to 3 hours) and averaged 0.25, 0.4, 0.97, and 1.59 ng/mL, respectively. The time required for the tablet to fully disintegrate following intrabuccal administration does not appear to affect early systemic exposure to the drug. Following administration of a single 200-mcg dose of fentanyl as a buccal tablet, the absorption profile of the drug in patients with grade 1 mucositis appeared to be similar to that in patients without mucositis. Time to peak plasma concentration and AUC are similar following either sublingual or intrabuccal administration of the buccal tablet.

In a crossover study comparing the bioavailability of fentanyl citrate buccal tablets with that of fentanyl citrate buccal lozenges, the buccal tablet was more bioavailable than the lozenge (absolute bioavailability: 65 versus 47%). The tablet and lozenge formulations differed in both the rate and extent of absorption. When the dose was administered as a buccal tablet rather than a lozenge, a larger fraction of the administered dose was absorbed transmucosally (48% versus 22%). The peak plasma concentration was achieved earlier with the buccal tablet (47 minutes) than with the lozenge (91 minutes), and dose-normalized systemic exposure to the drug was approximately 30% greater when the dose was administered as a buccal tablet rather than a lozenge. In another bioavailability study, systemic exposure to fentanyl reportedly was about 50% greater with the buccal tablet compared with the lozenge.

Sublingual Tablets and Spray Following sublingual administration of fentanyl citrate sublingual tablets, the drug is absorbed mainly from the oral mucosa. Bioavailability of the sublingual tablets is estimated to be 54%. When administered at equivalent doses, multiple lower-strength tablets are bioequivalent to a single higher-strength tablet. Following administration of single 100-, 200-, 400-, and 800-mcg doses of fentanyl as fentanyl citrate sublingual tablets in healthy individuals, peak plasma concentrations of the drug were attained at a median of 30–60 minutes (range: 19 minutes to 4 hours) and averaged 0.19, 0.3, 0.77, and 1.4 ng/mL, respectively. Studies indicate that the peak plasma concentration and AUC of fentanyl increase proportionally with dose over the range of 100–1600 mcg.

Following sublingual administration of a single 400-mcg dose of fentanyl as fentanyl sublingual spray, the mean absolute bioavailability of the drug is

76%. The pharmacokinetic profile and bioavailability depend on the relative fractions of the dose that are absorbed from the sublingual mucosa and the GI tract. The peak plasma concentration and AUC of fentanyl increase in an approximately dose-proportional manner over the dose range of 100–800 mcg. Following administration of single 100-, 200-, 400-, 600-, and 800-mcg doses of fentanyl as the sublingual spray in healthy individuals, peak plasma concentrations of the drug were attained at a median of 0.7–1.3 hours (range: approximately 5 minutes to 4 hours) and averaged 0.2, 0.4, 0.8, 1.2, and 1.6 ng/mL, respectively. When fentanyl sublingual spray was administered under fasted conditions, peak plasma concentration and total exposure were not appreciably affected by pretreatment of the oral cavity with hot water or refrigerated iced water or by beverages with either low or high pH.

In a study comparing the bioavailability of fentanyl sublingual spray with that of fentanyl citrate buccal lozenges, both the rate and extent of fentanyl absorption were substantially greater with the sublingual spray; peak plasma concentration and AUC for the sublingual spray were 34 and 38% greater, respectively, than values for the buccal lozenge, and peak plasma concentrations were attained at a median of 1.5 or 2 hours following administration of the sublingual spray or buccal lozenge, respectively.

Following administration of a single 100-mcg dose of fentanyl sublingual spray in cancer patients, peak plasma concentration and AUC of the drug were 73 and 52% greater in patients with grade 1 mucositis compared with patients without mucositis. In 2 patients with grade 2 mucositis, peak plasma concentrations were fourfold and sevenfold higher and AUC values were threefold or higher than values in patients without mucositis. (See Precautions Against Serious Toxicity Resulting From Fentanyl Overdosage or Accidental Exposure under Cautions: Precautions and Contraindications.)

Nasal Spray Fentanyl is absorbed from the nasal mucosa following intranasal administration. Following administration of single 100-, 200-, 400-, and 800-mcg doses of fentanyl as fentanyl citrate nasal spray in healthy individuals, peak plasma concentrations of the drug were attained at a median of 15–21 minutes (range: approximately 5 minutes to 8 hours) and averaged 0.4, 0.8, 1.6, and 2.8 ng/mL, respectively. Peak plasma concentration and AUC increase linearly over a dose range of 100–800 mcg.

In a study evaluating the pharmacokinetics of fentanyl citrate nasal spray following administration of consecutive doses in the same nostril at intervals of 1–4 hours, the peak plasma concentration after the second dose exceeded the peak plasma concentration after the first dose by 30% when the 2 doses were administered 1 hour apart, by 25% when the 2 doses were administered 2 hours apart, and by 10% when the 2 doses were administered 4 hours apart. An interval of 2 hours between consecutive doses of fentanyl citrate nasal spray is recommended based on these data, observed times to achieve peak plasma concentrations, and the frequency of breakthrough pain episodes in patients with cancer.

The presence of allergic rhinitis does not substantially alter the rate or extent of fentanyl exposure following intranasal administration; however, use of nasal decongestants for allergic rhinitis may alter exposure to the drug. (See Drug Interactions: Nasal Decongestants.)

Bioavailability of fentanyl citrate nasal spray is approximately 20% greater than that of fentanyl citrate buccal lozenges; peak concentrations achieved after administration of a single 200-mcg dose were higher with the nasal spray than with the buccal lozenges (0.8 versus 0.3 mcg/mL) and peak plasma concentrations occurred earlier (median of 15 minutes versus 1.5 hours) after administration of the nasal spray.

Iontophoretic Transdermal System Activation of the dosing button of the fentanyl hydrochloride iontophoretic transdermal system results in activation of an electrical current for 10 minutes, which delivers a dose of fentanyl from the drug-containing reservoir through the skin and into the systemic circulation. Compared with IV administration of fentanyl citrate, blood concentrations of the drug increase slowly following activation of the device and continue to increase for approximately 5 minutes after the completion of each 10-minute dose. Systemic absorption of fentanyl increases as a function of time, independent of the frequency of dosing. Upon initiation of therapy with the iontophoretic transdermal system, the amount of fentanyl that is absorbed systemically is expected to be approximately 16 mcg; beginning about 10 hours after initiation of therapy (when the initial dose has been administered immediately after application of the system), 40 mcg of fentanyl per dose is absorbed. When patients titrated the dosage to analgesic effect, serum fentanyl concentrations over the 24-hour dosing period for the iontophoretic transdermal system ranged from 0.4–1.5 ng/mL. In patients administering the maximum number of doses in the shortest possible time period (80 doses over approximately 13 hours), the mean serum concentration of fentanyl was approximately 1.9 ng/mL (range: 1.5–2.4 ng/mL). Intersubject variability in fentanyl exposure (AUC) is similar to that observed following IV administration. Delivery of fentanyl is similar following application of the iontophoretic transdermal system to either the upper outer arm or chest (the recommended application sites), but approximately 20% lower following application to the lower inner arm; rates of drug delivery following application at other sites have not been established. Race and age do not appear to affect absorption of fentanyl from the iontophoretic transdermal system.

■ **Distribution** Fentanyl is highly lipophilic. Animal data indicate that fentanyl distributes rapidly from blood into the brain, heart, lungs, kidneys, and spleen; the drug then redistributes more slowly into skeletal muscle and fat compartments, and then redistributes slowly from these tissues into systemic circulation. Following IV administration of fentanyl citrate in healthy individuals, the estimated initial distribution half-life was about 6 minutes, the second distribution half-life was about 1 hour, and the terminal half-life was about 16 hours. Large single doses or repeated doses can result in substantial accumulation of the drug, potentially resulting in an extended duration of effect.

Fentanyl is 80–85% protein bound in plasma, binding principally to α_1-acid glycoprotein but also to albumin, lipoproteins, and erythrocytes. Binding is independent of drug concentration over the therapeutic range. However, the plasma protein-binding capacity of fentanyl decreases with increasing ionization of the drug. Alterations in blood pH may alter ionization of fentanyl and therefore its distribution between plasma and the CNS. The free fraction of fentanyl in plasma increases with acidosis. The mean volume of distribution of the drug at steady state has been reported to be 4–6 L/kg.

Fentanyl crosses the placenta and is distributed into milk in humans.

■ **Elimination** In one study, serum fentanyl concentrations decreased rapidly to about 20% of peak concentrations within 5 minutes after IV administration of the drug. Serum concentrations then decreased more slowly during the next 10–20 minutes and stabilized at low concentrations by 2 hours. Concentrations then decreased very slowly and the drug could be detected for at least 6 hours after administration. In a study comparing single 15-mcg/kg IV, oral, and buccal (transmucosal) doses in healthy adults, the elimination half-life of fentanyl averaged approximately 7.1, 7.8, and 7.7 hours, respectively. The manufacturers state that the mean half-life in adults ranges from approximately 3.2–6.4 hours following administration of fentanyl 200–1600 mcg as buccal lozenges and 5.3–12 hours following administration of fentanyl 100–800 mcg as a sublingual spray. Following administration as a nasal spray (100–800 mcg) or buccal lozenge (200 mcg), the mean elimination half-life was 15–25 or 18.6 hours, respectively. The manufacturer states that the median half-life is approximately 2.6–11.7 hours following administration of fentanyl 100–800 mcg as buccal tablets and 5–13.5 hours following administration of fentanyl 100–800 mcg as sublingual tablets. Following administration as fentanyl transdermal system, the elimination half-life of fentanyl is approximately 20–27 hours. The terminal half-life of fentanyl following administration as fentanyl hydrochloride iontophoretic transdermal system reportedly is similar to that observed following IV administration of the drug.

Studies of IV fentanyl suggest that clearance of the drug may be decreased and half-life increased in geriatric patients. Although the pharmacokinetic profile of fentanyl in healthy Caucasian adults 65 years of age or older (mean age: 71 years) generally was similar to that in adults 18–45 years of age following application of a fentanyl transdermal system labeled as delivering 100 mcg/hour for 72 hours, the mean half-life of the drug was longer in geriatric individuals compared with younger adults (34.4 versus 23.5 hours).

Fentanyl citrate is metabolized extensively in the liver and the intestinal mucosa. Animal studies indicate that the drug undergoes oxidation via the microsomal enzymes in the liver and intestinal mucosa (principally cytochrome P-450 [CYP] isoform 3A4) to form norfentanyl; the drug also undergoes hydrolysis to form 4-*N*-anilinopiperidine and propionic acid. Norfentanyl has been shown to be pharmacologically inactive in animal studies. Fentanyl is excreted in the urine as inactive metabolites and as unchanged drug. Less than 10% of a dose is excreted in urine unchanged and only about 1% is excreted in the feces as unchanged drug. In one study using ^{3}H-labeled fentanyl citrate, about 20% of the total radioactivity was excreted in the urine within 8 hours and about 70% within 4 days. Fentanyl does not appear to be metabolized in skin when administered transdermally. Data from clinical studies and from studies using a human keratinocyte cell assay indicate that about 92% of a dose delivered from the fentanyl transdermal system is accounted for as unchanged drug in systemic circulation. Total plasma clearance of fentanyl is reported to be about 500 mL/hour per kg (range: 300–700 mL/hour per kg) or 42–53 L/hour.

Chemistry and Stability

■ **Chemistry** Fentanyl is a synthetic phenylpiperidine-derivative opiate agonist. The drug is commercially available for parenteral, intrabuccal, sublingual (tablet), and intranasal use as the citrate salt; for transdermal and sublingual (spray) use as the base; and for use in an iontophoretic transdermal system as the hydrochloride salt.

Fentanyl citrate occurs as a white, crystalline powder and is sparingly soluble in water and soluble in alcohol. The commercially available injections have a pH of 4–7.5.

Fentanyl citrate buccal lozenges contain the drug in a solid drug (lozenge) matrix that is molded onto a plastic holder; the holder, which is fracture resistant under normal conditions when used as directed, allows the matrix unit to be removed from the mouth when needed.

Fentanyl citrate buccal tablets utilize the OraVescent® drug delivery system, which generates a reaction that releases carbon dioxide when the tablet comes in contact with saliva. The transient pH changes accompanying the reaction are thought to facilitate tablet dissolution and enhance drug permeation through the buccal mucosa.

Fentanyl sublingual spray is supplied in single-use spray units. Each unit-dose system consists of an actuator attached to a vial holder and delivers 100, 200, 400, 600, or 800 mcg of fentanyl.

For intranasal administration, fentanyl citrate is supplied as an aqueous solution in a multidose container attached to a metered-dose pump with a visual and audible spray counter. The nasal inhaler delivers 100 μL of solution containing 100, 300, or 400 mcg of fentanyl per metered spray.

Fentanyl transdermal systems available from various manufacturers may vary in their components and structure, size, and total fentanyl content. All are labeled as to the nominal fentanyl delivery rate per hour. The amount of fentanyl released per hour from each system in an individual manufacturer's product line is proportional to the surface area; the composition per unit area of all transdermal fentanyl systems in an individual manufacturer's product line is identical.

Each fentanyl hydrochloride iontophoretic transdermal system consists of a plastic top housing unit that contains the battery and electronics and a plastic bottom housing unit containing 2 hydrogel reservoirs and a polyisobutylene adhesive; one of the hydrogels (anode, located under the dosing button) contains fentanyl hydrochloride and inactive ingredients, while the other hydrogel (cathode) contains only pharmacologically inactive ingredients. The bottom housing unit has a red tab that is used when removing the device from the skin and during disposal. A siliconized clear plastic release liner covers the hydrogels and must be removed prior to application. The system is powered by a 3-volt lithium battery. The iontophoretic transdermal system provides a 40-mcg dose of fentanyl over 10 minutes following each activation of the device and delivers a maximum of 6 doses of fentanyl per hour and 80 doses per 24 hours. Each system is operational for 24 hours following assembly or until 80 doses have been delivered, whichever comes first.

■ **Stability** Commercially available fentanyl citrate injections should be protected from light and stored at room temperatures of 15–30°C; brief exposure to temperatures up to 40°C does not adversely affect the injection. Fentanyl citrate is hydrolyzed in acidic solutions. Specialized references should be consulted for specific compatibility information.

Fentanyl hydrochloride iontophoretic transdermal systems should be stored at 25°C, but may be exposed to temperatures ranging from 15–30°C; the system should be assembled and applied to the skin immediately after removal from the individually sealed package, and should be discarded if the seal on the tray or drug unit pouch was previously broken or damaged.

Fentanyl transdermal systems should be stored at room temperature; the system should be applied to the skin immediately after removal from the individually sealed package, and should be discarded if the seal was previously broken or if the transdermal system has been cut, damaged, or altered in any way.

Fentanyl citrate buccal lozenges, buccal tablets, and sublingual tablets and fentanyl sublingual spray should be stored at 20–25°C, but may be exposed to temperatures ranging from 15–30°C; the buccal preparations should be protected from freezing and moisture, and the sublingual tablets should be protected from moisture. The buccal lozenges, buccal tablets, sublingual tablets, and sublingual spray should be administered immediately after removal from the individually sealed blister package; these preparations should not be used if the blister package was previously opened or tampered with. Once a buccal tablet of fentanyl citrate has been removed from the blister, it should not be stored for use at a later time because the integrity of the dosage form may be compromised and because of the risk of accidental exposure to the drug. A child safety kit that includes a portable carrying case, a lock for the bag, and safety latches for securing storage spaces in the home can be requested from the manufacturer of the sublingual spray.

Fentanyl citrate nasal spray should be stored at temperatures up to 25°C and protected from light; the nasal spray should not be frozen. The nasal spray should be stored in the child-resistant container between uses, and the pouch used for disposal of priming sprays, unwanted doses, and residual fentanyl citrate nasal solution should be stored in the cardboard carton.

Buccal, transdermal, sublingual, and intranasal formulations of the drug and the multiple-use disposal pouch provided with the nasal spray should be stored in a secure place to prevent access by children and pets. Used or partially used dosage forms should be properly disposed of immediately after use. (See Dosage and Administration: Administration.) If unused portions of fentanyl citrate buccal lozenges cannot be disposed of immediately by the patients or their caregivers, they should be stored in a temporary storage bottle (supplied by the manufacturer) according to enclosed instructions and then should be disposed of at least once a day. Any drug matrix remaining on the handle can be removed by placing the handle under hot running tap water until the drug matrix is completely dissolved.

Any unused dosage forms should be properly disposed of as soon as they are no longer needed. If patients and/or their caregivers need assistance with disposal of fentanyl preparations, the respective manufacturer or, alternatively, the local office of the Drug Enforcement Administration (DEA) may be contacted.

The manufacturers state that unopened units of fentanyl citrate buccal lozenges that are no longer needed should be removed from their blister packages (using scissors) and disposed of by cutting the matrix from the handles with wire-cutting pliers over a toilet bowl and then flushing them twice down the toilet. Handles, blister packages, and cartons should *not* be flushed down the toilet, but disposed of according to instructions provided by the manufacturer.

The manufacturers state that fentanyl citrate buccal tablets or sublingual tablets that are no longer needed should be removed from their blister packages and flushed down the toilet.

Unused units of fentanyl sublingual spray that are no longer needed should be emptied by spraying the contents into a charcoal-lined disposal pouch provided by the manufacturer; the sealed pouch and the emptied spray units may then be placed in disposal bags (also provided by the manufacturer), and the bags should be sealed prior to disposal. The patient instructions in the medication guide should be consulted for additional information about disposal of fentanyl sublingual spray.

Unused, fully used, or partially used bottles of fentanyl citrate nasal spray that are no longer needed must be emptied completely of accessible drug by spraying the remaining contents into the disposal pouch and placing the emptied bottle and the sealed pouch in the child-resistant container provided by the manufacturer prior to disposal. The patient instructions in the medication guide should be consulted for additional information about disposal of the nasal solution.

The manufacturers recommend that any unused fentanyl transdermal systems that are no longer needed be removed from their packaging, folded carefully so that the adhesive side adheres to itself, and then flushed down the toilet.

For further information on chemistry, pharmacology, pharmacokinetics, uses, cautions, chronic toxicity, acute toxicity, drug interactions, and dosage and administration of fentanyl citrate, see the Opiate Agonists General Statement 28:08.08.

Preparations

Distribution of transmucosal immediate-release fentanyl and fentanyl citrate preparations and fentanyl hydrochloride iontophoretic transdermal system is restricted. (See Risk Management and Restricted Distribution Programs under Dosage and Administration: Administration.)

Fentanyl, fentanyl citrate, and fentanyl hydrochloride preparations are subject to control under the Federal Controlled Substances Act of 1970 as schedule II (C-II) drugs.

Excipients in commercially available drug preparations may have clinically important effects in some individuals; consult specific product labeling for details.

fentaNYL

Sublingual		
Solution	100 mcg	**Subsys®** (C-II; with charcoal-lined disposal pouches and disposal bags), Insys
	200 mcg	**Subsys®** (C-II; with charcoal-lined disposal pouches and disposal bags), Insys
	400 mcg	**Subsys®** (C-II; with charcoal-lined disposal pouches and disposal bags), Insys
	600 mcg	**Subsys®** (C-II; with charcoal-lined disposal pouches and disposal bags), Insys
	800 mcg	**Subsys®** (C-II; with charcoal-lined disposal pouches and disposal bags), Insys
	1200 mcg	**Subsys®** (C-II; supplied as two 600-mcg units, with charcoal-lined disposal pouches and disposal bags), Insys
	1600 mcg	**Subsys®** (C-II; supplied as two 800-mcg units, with charcoal-lined disposal pouches and disposal bags), Insys
Topical		
Transdermal System	12.5 mcg/hour (total fentanyl content and transdermal system size may vary by manufacturer)*	**Duragesic®** (C-II), Janssen **fentaNYL Transdermal System** (C-II)
	25 mcg/hour (total fentanyl content and transdermal system size may vary by manufacturer)*	**Duragesic®** (C-II), Janssen **fentaNYL Transdermal System** (C-II)
	50 mcg/hour (total fentanyl content and transdermal system size may vary by manufacturer)*	**Duragesic®** (C-II), Janssen **fentaNYL Transdermal System** (C-II)
	75 mcg/hour (total fentanyl content and transdermal system size may vary by manufacturer)*	**Duragesic®** (C-II), Janssen **fentaNYL Transdermal System** (C-II)
	100 mcg/hour (total fentanyl content and transdermal system size may vary by manufacturer)*	**Duragesic®** (C-II), Janssen **fentaNYL Transdermal System** (C-II)

*available from one or more manufacturer, distributor, and/or repackager by generic (nonproprietary) name

fentaNYL Citrate

Buccal (Transmucosal)		
Lozenge (solid drug matrix on a handle)	200 mcg (of fentanyl)*	**Actiq®** (C-II), Cephalon **Oral Transmucosal fentaNYL Citrate** (C-II)
	400 mcg (of fentanyl)*	**Actiq®** (C-II), Cephalon **Oral Transmucosal fentaNYL Citrate** (C-II)
	600 mcg (of fentanyl)*	**Actiq®** (C-II), Cephalon **Oral Transmucosal fentaNYL Citrate** (C-II)

	800 mcg (of fentanyl)*	**Actiq**® (C-II), Cephalon
		Oral Transmucosal fentaNYL Citrate (C-II)
	1200 mcg (of fentanyl)*	**Actiq**® (C-II), Cephalon
		Oral Transmucosal fentaNYL Citrate (C-II)
	1600 mcg (of fentanyl)*	**Actiq**® (C-II), Cephalon
		Oral Transmucosal fentaNYL Citrate (C-II)
Tablet	100 mcg (of fentanyl)	**Fentora**® (C-II), Teva
	200 mcg (of fentanyl)	**Fentora**® (C-II), Teva
	400 mcg (of fentanyl)	**Fentora**® (C-II), Teva
	600 mcg (of fentanyl)	**Fentora**® (C-II), Teva
	800 mcg (of fentanyl)	**Fentora**® (C-II), Teva
Nasal		
Solution	100 mcg (of fentanyl) per metered spray	**Lazanda**® (C-II; with carbon-lined disposal pouch), Depomed
	300 mcg (of fentanyl) per metered spray	**Lazanda**® (C-II; with carbon-lined disposal pouch), Depomed
	400 mcg (of fentanyl) per metered spray	**Lazanda**® (C-II; with carbon-lined disposal pouch), Depomed
Parenteral		
Injection	50 mcg (of fentanyl) per mL*	**fentaNYL Citrate Injection** (C-II)
		Sublimaze® (C-II), Taylor
Sublingual		
Tablet	100 mcg (of fentanyl)	**Abstral**® (C-II), Galena
	200 mcg (of fentanyl)	**Abstral**® (C-II), Galena
	300 mcg (of fentanyl)	**Abstral**® (C-II), Galena
	400 mcg (of fentanyl)	**Abstral**® (C-II), Galena
	600 mcg (of fentanyl)	**Abstral**® (C-II), Galena
	800 mcg (of fentanyl)	**Abstral**® (C-II), Galena

*available from one or more manufacturer, distributor, and/or repackager by generic (nonproprietary) name

fentaNYL Hydrochloride

Topical		
Transdermal System, iontophoretic	40 mcg (of fentanyl) per activation (9.7 mg/system)	**Ionsys**® (C-II; in sealed tray with 1 controller and 1 drug unit), Medicines Company

†Use is not currently included in the labeling approved by the US Food and Drug Administration

HYDROcodone Bitartrate

Dihydrocodeinone Bitartrate

■ Hydrocodone bitartrate is a phenanthrene-derivative opiate agonist that is used as an analgesic and antitussive agent.

REMS

FDA approved a REMS for hydrocodone to ensure that the benefits outweigh the risks. The REMS may apply to one or more preparations of hydrocodone and consists of the following: medication guide and elements to assure safe use. See the FDA REMS page (https://www.accessdata.fda.gov/scripts/cder/rems/index.cfm).

Uses

Extended-release hydrocodone bitartrate is used for the relief of pain that is severe enough to require long-term, daily, around-the-clock use of an opiate analgesic. Because of the risks of addiction, abuse, and misuse associated with opiates, even at recommended dosages, and because of the greater risks of overdose and death associated with extended-release opiate formulations, extended-release hydrocodone bitartrate should be reserved for use in patients for whom alternative treatment options (e.g., nonopiate analgesics or immediate-release opiates) are inadequate or not tolerated. Extended-release hydrocodone bitartrate is *not* indicated for use on an as-needed ("prn") basis.

Efficacy of hydrocodone bitartrate extended-release capsules (Zohydro® ER) was established in patients with moderate to severe chronic low back pain requiring chronic opiate therapy; the currently prescribed opiate was switched to the extended-release hydrocodone bitartrate capsules and the dosage was titrated to a stable level (up to 100 mg twice daily) during an initial open-label phase of the study; over a subsequent 12-week, randomized, placebo-controlled withdrawal phase, hydrocodone was associated with reductions in pain intensity compared with placebo.

Efficacy of extended-release tablets of hydrocodone bitartrate (Hysingla® ER) also was established in patients with moderate to severe chronic low back pain. The currently prescribed opiate and/or nonopiate analgesic(s) were switched to

extended-release hydrocodone bitartrate tablets and the dosage was titrated to a stable level (20–120 mg once daily) during an initial open-label phase of the study; over a subsequent 12-week, randomized, placebo-controlled withdrawal phase, hydrocodone provided greater analgesia compared with placebo.

Hydrocodone bitartrate in fixed combination with acetaminophen is used for the relief of moderate to moderately severe pain.

Hydrocodone bitartrate in fixed combination with ibuprofen is used short term (generally for less than 10 days) for the relief of acute pain. Efficacy was established in single-dose studies in patients with postoperative (abdominal, gynecologic, orthopedic) pain. Hydrocodone bitartrate in fixed combination with ibuprofen is not indicated for the management of pain associated with such chronic conditions as osteoarthritis or rheumatoid arthritis.

For further information on the role of opiate analgesics in the management of acute or chronic pain, see Uses: Pain, in the Opiate Agonists General Statement 28:08.08.

For use of hydrocodone as an antitussive agent, see 48:08.

Dosage and Administration

■ **Administration** Hydrocodone bitartrate is administered orally. Patients receiving hydrocodone should avoid alcohol; concomitant use may result in profound sedation, respiratory depression, coma, or death.

Hydrocodone bitartrate extended-release capsules are administered twice daily (every 12 hours). The extended-release capsules must be taken whole; crushing, breaking, cutting, chewing, or dissolving the capsules will result in uncontrolled delivery of hydrocodone and can result in overdosage and death. Patients should be advised that they must *not* consume alcoholic beverages or take prescription or nonprescription preparations containing alcohol during therapy, since concomitant ingestion of alcohol with hydrocodone bitartrate extended-release capsules may result in increased plasma concentrations of the drug and a potentially fatal overdose. (See Drug Interactions: Alcohol.)

Hydrocodone bitartrate extended-release tablets are administered once daily (every 24 hours) without regard to meals. Multiple tablets of lower-dose strengths that provide the desired total daily dosage can be taken as a once-daily dose. If a dose is missed, the next dose should be taken at the scheduled time on the following day. The extended-release tablets must be taken whole, one tablet at a time, with enough water to ensure complete swallowing of the tablet immediately after it is placed in the mouth. The tablets should not be wet (e.g., soaked, licked) before they are placed in the mouth for swallowing, since wetting the tablets results in formation of a gelatinous mass that may be difficult to swallow. (See Cautions.) Crushing, chewing, or dissolving the tablets will result in uncontrolled delivery of hydrocodone and can result in overdosage and death.

■ **Dosage** Hydrocodone bitartrate should be given at the lowest effective dosage and for the shortest duration of therapy consistent with the treatment goals of the patient. Reduced dosage is indicated in poor-risk and geriatric patients. If concomitant therapy with other CNS depressants is required, the lowest effective dosages and shortest possible duration of concomitant therapy should be used.

For acute pain not related to trauma or surgery, the prescribed quantity should be limited to the amount needed for the expected duration of pain severe enough to require opiate analgesia (generally 3 days or less and rarely more than 7 days). When opiate analgesics are used for the management of chronic noncancer pain, the US Centers for Disease Control and Prevention (CDC) recommends that primary care clinicians carefully reassess individual benefits and risks before prescribing dosages equivalent to 50 mg or more of morphine sulfate daily (approximately 50 mg or more of hydrocodone bitartrate daily) and avoid dosages equivalent to 90 mg or more of morphine sulfate daily (approximately 90 mg or more of hydrocodone bitartrate daily) or carefully justify their decision to titrate the dosage to such levels. Other experts recommend consulting a pain management specialist before exceeding a dosage equivalent to 80–120 mg of morphine sulfate daily. For further information on the management of opiate analgesic therapy, see Dosage and Administration: Dosage, in the Opiate Agonists General Statement 28:08.08.

Extended-release Capsules To reduce the risk of respiratory depression in patients receiving hydrocodone bitartrate extended-release capsules, appropriate dosage selection and titration are essential. The initial dosage must be individualized, taking into account the patient's prior analgesic use and risk factors for addiction, abuse, and misuse. Patients should be monitored closely for respiratory depression, especially during the first 24–72 hours of therapy and following any increase in dosage.

For the management of severe pain requiring long-term, around-the-clock analgesia in adults who are not opiate tolerant or not currently receiving opiate analgesics, therapy with extended-release hydrocodone bitartrate capsules (Zohydro® ER) should be initiated at a dosage of 10 mg every 12 hours. Use of higher initial dosages in patients who are not opiate tolerant may result in fatal respiratory depression. A single dose exceeding 40 mg, the 50-mg extended-release hydrocodone bitartrate capsules, or a total daily dosage exceeding 80 mg should be used only in patients in whom tolerance to an opiate of comparable potency has been established. Patients are considered opiate tolerant if they have been receiving at least 60 mg of oral morphine sulfate daily, 25 mcg of transdermal fentanyl per hour, 30 mg of oral oxycodone hydrochloride daily, 8 mg of oral hydromorphone hydrochloride daily, 25 mg of oral oxymorphone hydrochloride daily, or an equianalgesic dose of another opiate daily for at least 1 week.

In adults who are being transferred from other oral opiates to therapy with extended-release hydrocodone bitartrate capsules, all other around-the-clock opiate analgesics should be discontinued when therapy with the extended-release capsules is initiated. Dosage must be carefully individualized since overestimation of the initial dosage in opiate-tolerant patients can result in fatal overdosage. The manufacturer states that the conversion factors in Table 1 may be used as a guide for selecting an initial dosage of extended-release hydrocodone bitartrate capsules for patients being transferred from therapy with one of the oral opiates listed in the table. The manufacturer cautions that the doses in Table 1 are not equianalgesic doses and the table cannot be used to transfer patients from extended-release hydrocodone bitartrate capsules to another opiate, as this will result in overestimation of the dosage of the new opiate and possible fatal overdosage. For patients receiving a single opiate analgesic, the current total daily dosage of the opiate should be multiplied by the appropriate conversion factor in Table 1 to calculate the approximate daily dosage of extended-release hydrocodone bitartrate capsules; the calculated daily dosage should then be divided in half for administration every 12 hours. For patients receiving more than one opiate analgesic, the approximate daily dosage of extended-release hydrocodone bitartrate should be calculated for each opiate and then those totals should be summed to obtain the approximate total daily dosage of extended-release hydrocodone bitartrate capsules; the calculated total daily dosage should then be divided in half for administration every 12 hours. For patients receiving analgesics containing opiates and nonopiates in a fixed ratio, only the opiate component should be considered in the conversion. Calculated doses that do not correspond to an available capsule strength should always be rounded down to the nearest whole capsule.

Table 1. Conversion Factors for Transfer from Other Oral Opiates to Extended-release Hydrocodone Bitartrate Capsules (Zohydro® ER)

Prior Oral Opiate	Oral Dose (mg)	Approximate Oral Conversion Factor
Hydrocodone	10	1
Oxycodone	10	1
Methadone	10	1
Oxymorphone	5	2
Hydromorphone	3.75	2.67
Morphine	15	0.67
Codeine	100	0.1

Following transfer from other opiate analgesics to extended-release hydrocodone bitartrate, patients should be monitored for manifestations of opiate withdrawal and for oversedation or toxicity. Particularly close monitoring is required when patients are switched from methadone, since conversion ratios between methadone and other opiates vary widely depending on extent of prior methadone exposure and because methadone has a long half-life and tends to accumulate in plasma.

In adults who are being transferred from transdermal fentanyl to extended-release hydrocodone bitartrate capsules, therapy with the extended-release capsules can be initiated 18 hours following removal of the transdermal fentanyl system at a conservative hydrocodone bitartrate dosage of approximately 10 mg every 12 hours for each 25 mcg/hour of transdermal fentanyl. Patients should be monitored closely, as there is limited experience with this conversion.

Dosage of extended-release hydrocodone bitartrate capsules should be adjusted gradually, every 3–7 days in increments of 10 mg every 12 hours, to provide adequate analgesia and to minimize adverse effects. If discontinuance of therapy is required, gradual tapering of the dosage every 2–4 days is recommended to avoid manifestations associated with abrupt withdrawal. Patients should be monitored closely for manifestations of withdrawal, which may indicate the need for slower tapering. In a phase 3 clinical trial, dosage of extended-release hydrocodone bitartrate capsules in patients reassigned to receive placebo was tapered according to the schedule in Table 2; dosages exceeding 100 mg twice daily were not evaluated in the clinical trial.

Table 2. Dosage Taper Used in Clinical Trial of Extended-release Hydrocodone Bitartrate Capsules (Zohydro® ER)

Stable Dosage at Time of Taper Initiation	Taper Schedule
20–30 mg every 12 hours	10 mg every 12 hours for 2 days, then discontinue on day 3
40–70 mg every 12 hours	40 mg every 12 hours for 2 days, 20 mg every 12 hours for 2 days, 10 mg every 12 hours for 2 days, then discontinue on day 7
80–100 mg every 12 hours	80 mg every 12 hours for 2 days, 60 mg every 12 hours for 2 days, 40 mg every 12 hours for 2 days, 20 mg every 12 hours for 2 days, 10 mg every 12 hours for 2 days, then discontinue on day 11

Extended-release Tablets To reduce the risk of respiratory depression in patients receiving hydrocodone bitartrate extended-release tablets, appropriate dosage selection and titration are essential. The initial dosage must be individualized, taking into account the patient's prior analgesic use and risk factors for addiction, abuse, and misuse. Patients should be monitored closely for respiratory depression, especially during the first 24–72 hours of therapy and following any increase in dosage.

For the management of severe pain requiring long-term, around-the-clock analgesia in adults who are not opiate tolerant or not currently receiving opiate analgesics, therapy with extended-release hydrocodone bitartrate tablets (Hysingla® ER) should be initiated at a dosage of 20 mg every 24 hours. Use of higher initial dosages in patients who are not opiate tolerant may result in fatal respiratory depression. Dosages of 80 mg or more daily should be used only in opiate-tolerant patients. Patients are considered opiate tolerant if they have been receiving at least 60 mg of oral morphine sulfate daily, 25 mcg of transdermal fentanyl per hour, 30 mg of oral oxycodone hydrochloride daily, 8 mg of oral hydromorphone hydrochloride daily, 25 mg of oral oxymorphone hydrochloride daily, or an equianalgesic dose of another opiate daily for at least 1 week.

Patients being transferred from other oral hydrocodone-containing formulations to the extended-release tablets should receive the same total daily dosage of hydrocodone bitartrate administered once daily.

In adults who are being transferred from other oral opiates to therapy with extended-release hydrocodone bitartrate tablets, all other around-the-clock opiate analgesics should be discontinued when therapy with the extended-release tablets is initiated. Dosage must be carefully individualized since overestimation of the initial dosage in opiate-tolerant patients can result in fatal overdosage. The conversion factors in Table 3 may be used as a guide for selecting an initial dosage of extended-release hydrocodone bitartrate tablets for patients being transferred from therapy with one of the oral opiates listed in the table. The manufacturer cautions that the doses in Table 3 are not equianalgesic doses and the table cannot be used to transfer patients from extended-release hydrocodone bitartrate tablets to another opiate, as this will result in overestimation of the dosage of the new opiate and possible fatal overdosage. For patients receiving a single opiate analgesic, the current total daily dosage of the opiate should be multiplied by the appropriate conversion factor in Table 3 to calculate the approximate daily dosage of oral hydrocodone bitartrate; for patients receiving more than one opiate analgesic, the approximate daily dosage of oral hydrocodone bitartrate should be calculated for each opiate and then those totals should be summed to obtain the approximate daily dosage of oral hydrocodone bitartrate. *Initial oral hydrocodone bitartrate dosages calculated using the conversion factors in Table 3 should be reduced by 25% to account for interpatient variability in the relative potency of different opiates.* For patients receiving analgesics containing opiates and nonopiates in a fixed ratio, only the opiate component should be considered in the conversion. Calculated doses that do not correspond to an available tablet strength should always be rounded down to the nearest whole tablet. If the calculated dose is less than 20 mg, therapy should be initiated at a dosage of 20 mg once daily.

Table 3. Conversion Factors for Transfer from Other Oral Opiates to Extended-release Hydrocodone Bitartrate Tablets (Hysingla® ER)

Prior Oral Opiate	Oral Dose (mg)	Approximate Oral Conversion Factor
Codeine	133	0.15
Hydromorphone	5	4
Methadone	13.3	1.5
Morphine	40	0.5
Oxycodone	20	1
Oxymorphone	10	2
Tramadol	200	0.1

Following transfer from other opiate analgesics to extended-release hydrocodone bitartrate, patients should be monitored for manifestations of opiate withdrawal and for oversedation or toxicity. Particularly close monitoring is required when patients are switched from methadone, since conversion ratios between methadone and other opiates vary widely depending on extent of prior methadone exposure and because methadone has a long half-life and tends to accumulate in plasma.

In adults who are being transferred from transdermal fentanyl to extended-release hydrocodone bitartrate tablets, therapy with the extended-release tablets can be initiated 18 hours following removal of the transdermal fentanyl system at a conservative hydrocodone bitartrate dosage of approximately 20 mg every 24 hours for each 25 mcg/hour of transdermal fentanyl. Patients should be monitored closely, as there is limited experience with this conversion.

Adults receiving transdermal buprenorphine at a dosage of 20 mg or less per hour should be switched to extended-release hydrocodone bitartrate tablets at a dosage of 20 mg every 24 hours. Patients should be monitored closely, as there is limited experience with this conversion.

Dosage of extended-release hydrocodone bitartrate tablets should be adjusted gradually, every 3–5 days in increments of 10–20 mg every 24 hours, to provide adequate analgesia and to minimize adverse effects. If discontinuance of therapy is required, gradual tapering of the dosage every 2–4 days is recommended to avoid manifestations associated with abrupt withdrawal. As the dosage is tapered, each new dose should be at least 50% of the prior dose; once the dosage has been reduced to 20 mg daily for 2–4 days, therapy can be discontinued.

Immediate-release Fixed-combination Preparations The usual adult dosage of hydrocodone bitartrate when used in fixed combination with acetaminophen for relief of moderate to moderately severe pain is 5–10 mg every 4–6 hours as necessary. When used in fixed combination with ibuprofen for relief of acute pain, the usual adult dosage of hydrocodone bitartrate is 2.5–10 mg every 4–6 hours as needed, generally given for no longer than 10 days; the manufacturers state that the total daily dosage should not exceed 5 tablets (each providing from 2.5–10 mg of hydrocodone bitartrate and 200 mg of ibuprofen). Dosage should be adjusted according to the severity of the pain and the response and tolerance of the patient. When opiate analgesics are administered in fixed combination with nonopiate analgesics, the opiate dosage may be limited by the nonopiate component. Because commercially available preparations contain hydrocodone bitartrate and nonopiate analgesics in various fixed ratios and because these nonopiate analgesics also are available in many other prescription and OTC preparations, care should be taken to ensure that therapy is not duplicated and that dosage of the nonopiate drug does not exceed maximum recommended dosages.

■ **Dosage in Renal and Hepatic Impairment** No adjustment of initial hydrocodone bitartrate dosage is required in patients with mild or moderate hepatic impairment. Because of the potential for increased drug exposure, the manufacturer states that therapy with hydrocodone bitartrate extended-release capsules should be initiated at a dosage of 10 mg every 12 hours in patients with severe hepatic impairment. The manufacturer of hydrocodone bitartrate extended-release tablets states that dosage of this formulation should be reduced by 50% in patients with severe hepatic impairment. Patients with severe hepatic impairment should be monitored closely for adverse effects (e.g., respiratory depression, sedation).

Because of the potential for increased drug exposure, the manufacturer states that therapy with hydrocodone bitartrate extended-release capsules should be initiated at a low dose in patients with renal impairment. The manufacturer of hydrocodone bitartrate extended-release tablets states that dosage of this formulation should be reduced by 50% in patients with moderate or severe renal impairment (including end-stage renal disease); the manufacturer states that the extended-release tablets may be used without dosage adjustment in patients with mild renal impairment. Patients with renal impairment should be monitored closely for adverse effects (e.g., respiratory depression, sedation).

Cautions

Hydrocodone bitartrate shares the toxic potentials of the opiate agonists, and the usual precautions of opiate agonist therapy should be observed. (See Cautions in the Opiate Agonists General Statement 28:08.08.) For further information on cautions, precautions, and contraindications associated with the use of hydrocodone, see also Cautions in Hydrocodone Bitartrate 48:08. When hydrocodone is used as a fixed-combination preparation that includes acetaminophen or ibuprofen, the cautions, precautions, and contraindications associated with these drugs must be considered in addition to those associated with hydrocodone.

Because some patients have reported difficulty in swallowing hydrocodone bitartrate extended-release tablets, the tablets should be administered one at a time with enough water to ensure that each tablet is completely swallowed immediately after it is placed in the mouth; the extended-release tablets should not be wet (e.g., soaked, licked) before they are placed in the mouth for swallowing. Choking, dysphagia, and esophageal obstruction (in at least one case requiring medical intervention to remove the tablet) have been reported. Patients with underlying GI disorders (e.g., esophageal or colon cancer) associated with a narrow GI lumen are at greater risk of developing these complications. Use of an alternative analgesic should be considered for patients who have difficulty swallowing and in those at risk for underlying GI disorders associated with a narrow GI lumen. Because the extended-release tablets gradually form a gelatinous mass when exposed to fluids, pediatric patients may be at increased risk of esophageal obstruction, dysphagia, and choking because of their smaller GI lumen if they ingest the tablets.

Prolongation of the corrected QT (QT_c) interval was observed in healthy individuals receiving hydrocodone bitartrate 160 mg daily (as extended-release tablets). This observation should be considered when making decisions regarding patient monitoring (e.g., periodic monitoring of ECGs and electrolyte concentrations) when hydrocodone bitartrate extended-release tablets are used in patients with congestive heart failure, bradyarrhythmias, or electrolyte abnormalities or in those who are receiving drugs that are known to prolong the QT_c interval. The manufacturer states that use of the extended-release tablets should be avoided in patients with congenital long QT syndrome. If prolongation of the QT_c interval occurs, reduction of hydrocodone bitartrate dosage by 33–50% or use of an alternative analgesic should be considered.

■ **Misuse and Abuse** Because of the challenges associated with providing access to an adequate array of options for management of chronic pain while simultaneously preventing prescription opiate abuse and misuse, the decision by the US Food and Drug Administration (FDA) to approve hydrocodone bitartrate extended-release capsules (Zohydro® ER) was controversial, as the formulation lacks tamper-resistant features that might deter abuse and, like other extended-release opiates, some strengths contain substantial amounts of the drug (up to 50 mg). Hydrocodone bitartrate extended-release tablets (Hysingla® ER; containing up to 120 mg of the drug) are formulated with physical and chemical properties that are intended to make this dosage form more difficult to manipulate for IV or intranasal abuse and misuse, and some extended-release characteristics are retained if the tablets are physically compromised. In vitro studies indicate that exposing the tablets to water results in formation of a viscous hydrogel that resists passage through a needle; the tablets also are resistant to crushing, breaking, and dissolution by various tools and solvents. Results of clinical abuse potential studies suggest a reduced potential for intranasal abuse (compared with powdered hydrocodone bitartrate) or oral abuse by chewing the tablets (compared with hydrocodone bitartrate solution). However, the potential for IV, intranasal, and oral abuse still exists.

Modified-release (e.g., extended-release) opiates are associated with a greater risk of overdose and death because of the larger amount of drug contained in each dosage unit. Abuse or misuse of hydrocodone bitartrate extended-release dosage forms by cutting, breaking, crushing, chewing, or dissolving the capsules or tablets, snorting the contents, or injecting the dissolved contents will result in uncontrolled delivery of the drug and can result in overdosage and death. Inadvertent ingestion of even one dose of extended-release hydrocodone bitartrate capsules or tablets, especially by a child, also can result in a fatal overdose. Intake of alcohol with the extended-release capsules may result in increased peak plasma concentrations of hydrocodone and ingestion of a potentially toxic dose of the drug. (See Drug Interactions: Alcohol.) Extended-release preparations of hydrocodone bitartrate should be prescribed only by clinicians who are knowledgeable in the use of potent opiates for the management of chronic pain.

Hydrocodone in fixed combination with other analgesics (e.g., acetaminophen, nonsteroidal anti-inflammatory agents) is used widely in the management of pain. Hydrocodone also is used in antitussive preparations for the management of cough. Depending on the formulation, many of these fixed-combination analgesic and antitussive preparations previously were subject to control under the Federal Controlled Substances Act of 1970 as schedule III (C-III) drugs. However, because of increasing concerns about misuse, abuse, and diversion of these preparations, the US Department of Health and Human Services (HHS) recommended on December 16, 2013, that these preparations be rescheduled to schedule II (C-II) in response to an evidence-based analysis by FDA. This recommendation subsequently was accepted by the US Drug Enforcement Administration (DEA) and became effective October 6, 2014. Preparations containing hydrocodone in fixed combination with other analgesics have a clinically important and legitimate role in the management of moderate to moderately severe pain. Hydrocodone-containing combination preparations also have a clinically important and legitimate role in the symptomatic treatment of cough and upper respiratory symptoms associated with allergy and cold when they combine hydrocodone with other antitussives or antihistamines.

The conclusions of FDA and DEA considered a number of factors such as abuse potential, pharmacologic effects, history and current patterns of abuse, public health risk, dependence liability, and scope, duration, and significance of abuse. In recent years, hydrocodone-containing preparations have become the most frequently prescribed products in the US. In 2011, 131 million prescriptions totaling up to 8 billion or more tablets for fixed-combination hydrocodone analgesic preparations were prescribed and dispensed in the US to over 47 million patients, representing about 4 times the number of prescriptions written for fixed-combination oxycodone preparations and about 10 times the number of prescriptions for codeine-containing preparations. In 2011, approximately 5 million prescriptions were dispensed for hydrocodone-containing combination antitussives.

Data from 2012 showed that 37 million Americans had used analgesics nonmedically (misuse and abuse) in their lifetime, and that roughly 70% of these individuals reported lifetime nonmedical use of fixed-combination hydrocodone preparations. Further, hydrocodone is associated with substantial numbers of reports of overdose, suicide, abuse, and dependence. While the addition of non-opiate analgesic ingredients decreases the abuse potential and the rates of abuse for hydrocodone-containing combination analgesic preparations are lower than those for oxycodone-containing preparations, hydrocodone-containing combinations have a high potential for abuse that is considered similar to that of schedule II oxycodone-containing combination preparations. There also is evidence to suggest that individuals are taking sufficient amounts of hydrocodone to create a hazard to their health or the safety of others or the community, that there is considerable diversion from legitimate channels, and that individuals are taking the drug on their own initiative rather than on the basis of medical advice. Similar to the pattern for abuse are the risks of psychological and physical dependence, which can be severe. Considering this and other evidence, a decision to reschedule these hydrocodone-containing combination preparations to C-II was made. However, because of concerns about the impact of this scheduling change on public health, particularly access to effective pain management, FDA recommended that the impact of this action be assessed through close continued monitoring.

■ **Pregnancy, Fertility, and Lactation** Analysis of data from the National Birth Defects Prevention Study, a large population-based, case-control study, suggests that therapeutic use of opiates in pregnant women during the period of organogenesis is associated with a low absolute risk of birth defects, including heart defects, spina bifida, and gastroschisis. Oral hydrocodone bitartrate was not teratogenic in rats or rabbits at dosages or 25 or 50 mg/kg daily (equivalent to 2 or 10 times, respectively, a human dosage of 100 mg daily on a mg/m² basis). In studies in rats, oral administration of hydrocodone bitartrate 10 mg/kg daily (approximately equivalent to a human dosage of 100 mg daily) during gestation and lactation was associated with reduced fetal viability (increase in stillborn pups and decrease in pup survival). At a dosage of 25 mg/kg daily, reduced nursing behavior and decreased pup body weight were observed; minimal maternal toxicity was observed at this dosage. In studies in rabbits, an increase in umbilical hernias, irregularly shaped bones, and delayed fetal skeletal maturation were observed at a maternally toxic dosage of 75 mg/kg daily (equivalent to 15 times a human dosage of 100 mg daily). An oral hydrocodone bitartrate dosage of 25 mg/kg daily (equivalent to approximately

5 times a human dosage of 100 mg daily) was associated with reduced fetal weights.

No effects on fertility were observed in male rats receiving hydrocodone bitartrate at dosages equivalent to 10 times a human dosage of 100 mg daily, although decreased weight of male reproductive organs was observed at dosages equivalent to 2.4 times a human dosage of 100 mg daily. Reductions in female fertility indices observed at a dosage equivalent to twice the human dosage of 100 mg daily are not thought to be clinically relevant to humans.

Hydrocodone is distributed into breast milk. The manufacturers state that a decision should be made whether to discontinue nursing or the drug, taking into account the importance of the drug to the woman. Infants exposed to hydrocodone through breast milk should be observed for excessive sedation, respiratory depression, GI effects, and altered feeding patterns. Symptoms of withdrawal can occur in opiate-dependent infants when maternal administration of opiates is discontinued or breast-feeding is stopped.

Drug Interactions

■ **Drugs Affecting Hepatic Microsomal Enzymes** Because hydrocodone is metabolized by the cytochrome P-450 (CYP) microsomal enzyme system, principally by isoenzyme 3A4, concomitant use of hydrocodone with drugs that inhibit CYP3A4 activity may result in reduced clearance and increased plasma concentrations of the drug, possibly resulting in increased or prolonged opiate effects, including an increased risk of fatal respiratory depression. Concomitant administration of hydrocodone bitartrate (single 20-mg dose as extended-release tablets) and the potent CYP3A4 inhibitor ketoconazole (200 mg twice daily for 6 days) increased mean area under the concentration-time curve (AUC) and peak plasma concentration of hydrocodone by 135 and 78%, respectively. Conversely, concomitant use of hydrocodone with CYP3A4 inducers may result in increased clearance and decreased plasma concentrations of hydrocodone, with possible lack of efficacy or development of opiate withdrawal. If concomitant therapy with a CYP3A4 inducer is discontinued, an increase in plasma hydrocodone concentrations may occur, potentially increasing or prolonging therapeutic and adverse effects of the drug and increasing the risk of fatal overdosage. Therefore, caution should be exercised and patients who require concomitant therapy with a CYP3A4 inhibitor or inducer, or who have recently discontinued such therapy, should be monitored closely at frequent intervals, and dosage adjustments should be considered until stable drug effects are achieved.

Hydrocodone is metabolized to a lesser extent by CYP2D6; however, concomitant administration of hydrocodone bitartrate (single 20-mg dose as extended-release tablets) and the CYP2D6 inhibitor paroxetine (20 mg once daily for 12 days) did not alter systemic exposure to hydrocodone.

■ **Alcohol** Alcohol and hydrocodone may cause additive CNS depression and may result in hypotension, profound sedation, coma, respiratory depression, and death. Patients receiving hydrocodone should be instructed to avoid alcohol, including alcoholic beverages and prescription or nonprescription preparations containing alcohol.

In addition to such additive depressant effects, concomitant use of alcohol with extended-release hydrocodone bitartrate capsules can result in increased plasma concentrations of the opiate and potentially fatal overdosage. Administration of extended-release hydrocodone bitartrate capsules (Zohydro® ER) 50 mg with 40% alcohol in the fasted state increased the rate of hydrocodone absorption, increased peak plasma concentrations of the drug by an average of 2.4-fold (up to 3.9-fold in one individual), and increased the extent of absorption by an average of 1.2-fold (up to 1.7-fold in one individual).

■ **Laxatives** Concomitant use of hydrocodone bitartrate extended-release tablets with strong laxatives that rapidly increase GI motility (e.g., lactulose) may result in decreased absorption and decreased plasma concentrations of the opiate. Patients receiving such concomitant therapy should be monitored closely for adverse events and changing analgesic requirements.

For further information about drug interactions involving opiate agonists (including hydrocodone bitartrate), see Drug Interactions in the Opiate Agonists General Statement 28:08.08.

Pharmacokinetics

Overall systemic exposure or bioavailability of hydrocodone bitartrate following administration as extended-release capsules (Zohydro® ER) or tablets (Hysingla® ER) is similar to that observed following administration of immediate-release fixed-combination preparations containing the drug in the same or similar dosage; however, peak plasma concentrations of the drug are lower with the extended-release formulations. Peak plasma concentrations of hydrocodone are attained approximately 1.3–1.7 hours after administration as an immediate-release preparation, 5 hours after administration as extended-release capsules, and 6–30 hours (median: 14–16 hours) after administration as extended-release tablets.

After administration of the extended-release capsules for 7 days, area under the plasma concentration-time curve (AUC) and peak concentrations of hydrocodone are approximately twofold higher than values attained on the first day of administration. At doses of up to 50 mg, the pharmacokinetics of extended-release hydrocodone bitartrate are independent of dose. Administration of the extended-release capsules with food does not substantially affect the extent of absorption, although peak plasma hydrocodone concentrations were increased by 27% following administration of a 20-mg dose of the extended-release capsules with a high-fat meal.

After single-dose administration of hydrocodone bitartrate extended-release tablets, peak concentrations and AUC of the drug increased linearly and in a slightly more than dose-proportional manner over the dose range of 20–120 mg. With once-daily dosing, peak plasma concentrations and AUC were 1.1- and 1.3-fold higher at steady state. Higher doses (80 or 120 mg versus 30 mg) produced larger fluctuations in peak-to-trough plasma concentrations of the drug. Although administration of the 120-mg extended-release tablets with a high-fat meal increased peak plasma concentrations by 54% compared with administration in the fasted state, AUC was increased by only 20% and the manufacturer states that the extended-release tablets may be administered without regard to meals.

Hydrocodone is about 36% bound to plasma proteins.

Hydrocodone is metabolized by *N*-demethylation, *O*-demethylation, and 6-keto reduction to the corresponding 6-α- and 6-β-hydroxy metabolites. Hydrocodone is metabolized principally by cytochrome P-450 (CYP) isoenzyme 3A4 to form norhydrocodone (*N*-demethylation) and to a lesser extent by CYP2D6 to form hydromorphone (*O*-demethylation). Hydrocodone also may be metabolized to a small extent by CYP2B6 and CYP2C19. Hydromorphone accounts for less than 3% of the circulating parent drug, but may contribute to the total analgesic effect of hydrocodone. Hydrocodone and its metabolites are eliminated mainly in urine; only about 6.5% of an administered dose is excreted as unchanged drug. About 99% of an administered dose is eliminated within 72 hours. The mean plasma half-life of the drug is 3.8–4.5 hours after oral administration as an immediate-release preparation and approximately 7–9 hours after oral administration as extended-release capsules or tablets.

Following oral administration of a single 20-mg dose of hydrocodone bitartrate as extended-release capsules, peak plasma concentrations of the drug were 15, 48, or 41% higher and AUC was 15, 57, or 44% higher in patients with mild, moderate, or severe renal impairment, respectively, compared with individuals with normal renal function. Following oral administration of a single 20-mg dose of hydrocodone bitartrate as extended-release capsules, peak plasma concentrations of the drug were 8–10% higher and AUC was 10 or 26% higher in patients with mild or moderate hepatic impairment, respectively, compared with individuals with normal hepatic function; pharmacokinetics of the drug were not evaluated in patients with severe hepatic impairment. Population analyses indicated that the pharmacokinetics of the drug were not substantially affected by gender or age of 65 years or older.

Following oral administration of a single 20-mg dose of hydrocodone bitartrate as extended-release tablets, peak plasma concentrations and AUC of the drug reportedly were 6 and 14% lower, respectively, in patients with mild hepatic impairment; 5 and 13% higher, respectively, in patients with moderate hepatic impairment; and 5 and 4% higher, respectively, in patients with severe hepatic impairment compared with individuals with normal hepatic function. Hepatic impairment did not substantially alter plasma protein binding of the drug. Following oral administration of a single 60-mg dose of the drug as extended-release tablets, peak plasma concentrations reportedly were 14, 23, or 11% higher and AUC was 13, 61, or 57% higher in patients with mild, moderate, or severe renal impairment, respectively, compared with individuals with normal renal function; among patients with end-stage renal disease requiring dialysis, peak plasma concentrations of the drug reportedly were decreased by 13% and AUC was increased by 4% compared with values in individuals with normal renal function.

Age (65 years or older) and gender do not appear to substantially alter exposure to hydrocodone.

Chemistry and Stability

■ **Chemistry** Hydrocodone bitartrate is a phenanthrene-derivative opiate agonist that is used as an analgesic and antitussive agent. Hydrocodone is a hydrogenated-ketone derivative of codeine. Hydrocodone bitartrate occurs as fine, white crystals or as a crystalline powder and is soluble in water and slightly soluble in alcohol.

■ **Stability** Hydrocodone bitartrate is affected by light. Hydrocodone bitartrate preparations should be stored in tight, light-resistant containers at 15–30°C.

For further information on the chemistry, pharmacology, pharmacokinetics, uses, cautions, chronic toxicity, acute toxicity, drug interactions, and dosage and administration of hydrocodone bitartrate, see the Opiate Agonists General Statement 28:08.08 and Hydrocodone Bitartrate 48:08.

Preparations

Single-entity hydrocodone bitartrate preparations are subject to control under the Federal Controlled Substances Act of 1970 as schedule II (C-II) drugs; when available as a fixed-combination preparation in a concentration of 15 mg or less per dosage unit or 5 mL combined with a therapeutic amount of one or more non-opiate drugs or with a fourfold or greater quantity of isoquinolone opium alkaloid, hydrocodone previously was subject to control as a schedule III (C-III) drug. However, because of increasing concerns about misuse, abuse, and diversion, hydrocodone-containing preparations that previously were subject to control as schedule III drugs have been rescheduled and, effective October 6, 2014, are subject to control as schedule II (C-II) drugs. (See Cautions: Misuse and Abuse.)

Preparations containing hydrocodone in combination with more than 325 mg of acetaminophen per dosage unit have been discontinued to minimize the risk of inadvertent acetaminophen overdosage; some of these preparations may have been reformulated to limit the amount of acetaminophen to 325 mg or less per dosage unit.

Excipients in commercially available drug preparations may have clinically important effects in some individuals; consult specific product labeling for details.

HYDROcodone Bitartrate

Oral		
Capsules, extended-release	10 mg	**Zohydro® ER** (C-II), Zogenix
	15 mg	**Zohydro® ER** (C-II), Zogenix
	20 mg	**Zohydro® ER** (C-II), Zogenix
	30 mg	**Zohydro® ER** (C-II), Zogenix
	40 mg	**Zohydro® ER** (C-II), Zogenix
	50 mg	**Zohydro® ER** (C-II), Zogenix
Tablets, extended-release, film-coated	20 mg	**Hysingla® ER** (C-II), Purdue Pharma
	30 mg	**Hysingla® ER** (C-II), Purdue Pharma
	40 mg	**Hysingla® ER** (C-II), Purdue Pharma
	60 mg	**Hysingla® ER** (C-II), Purdue Pharma
	80 mg	**Hysingla® ER** (C-II), Purdue Pharma
	100 mg	**Hysingla® ER** (C-II), Purdue Pharma
	120 mg	**Hysingla® ER** (C-II), Purdue Pharma

HYDROcodone Bitartrate Combinations

Oral		
Solution	2.5 mg/5 mL with Acetaminophen 108 mg/5 mL*	**HYDROcodone Bitartrate and Acetaminophen Oral Solution** (C-II)
	3.3 mg/5 mL with Acetaminophen 100 mg/5 mL*	**HYDROcodone Bitartrate and Acetaminophen Oral Solution** (C-II)
		Lortab® Elixir (C-II), ECR
	3.3 mg/5 mL with Acetaminophen 108 mg/5 mL*	**HYDROcodone Bitartrate and Acetaminophen Oral Solution** (C-II)
Tablets	2.5 mg with Acetaminophen 325 mg*	**HYDROcodone Bitartrate and Acetaminophen Tablets** (C-II)
	5 mg with Acetaminophen 300 mg*	**HYDROcodone Bitartrate and Acetaminophen Tablets** (C-II)
		Vicodin® (C-II; scored), AbbVie
	5 mg with Acetaminophen 325 mg*	**HYDROcodone Bitartrate and Acetaminophen Tablets** (C-II)
		Lortab® (C-II; scored), UCB
		Norco® (C-II; scored), Actavis
	7.5 mg with Acetaminophen 300 mg*	**HYDROcodone Bitartrate and Acetaminophen Tablets** (C-II)
		Vicodin ES® (C-II; scored), AbbVie
	7.5 mg with Acetaminophen 325 mg*	**HYDROcodone Bitartrate and Acetaminophen Tablets** (C-II)
		Lortab® (C-II; scored), UCB
		Norco® (C-II; scored), Actavis
	10 mg with Acetaminophen 300 mg*	**HYDROcodone Bitartrate and Acetaminophen Tablets** (C-II)
		Vicodin HP® (C-II; scored), AbbVie
	10 mg with Acetaminophen 325 mg*	**HYDROcodone Bitartrate and Acetaminophen Tablets** (C-II)
		Lortab® (C-II; scored), UCB
		Norco® (C-II; scored), Actavis
Tablets, film-coated	2.5 mg with Ibuprofen 200 mg*	**HYDROcodone Bitartrate and Ibuprofen Film-coated Tablets** (C-II)
		Reprexain® (C-II), Gemini
	5 mg with Ibuprofen 200 mg*	**HYDROcodone Bitartrate and Ibuprofen Film-coated Tablets** (C-II)
		Reprexain® (C-II), Gemini
	7.5 mg with Ibuprofen 200 mg*	**HYDROcodone Bitartrate and Ibuprofen Film-coated Tablets** (C-II)
		Vicoprofen® (C-II), AbbVie
	10 mg with Ibuprofen 200 mg*	**HYDROcodone Bitartrate and Ibuprofen Film-coated Tablets** (C-II)
		Reprexain® (C-II), Gemini

*available from one or more manufacturer, distributor, and/or repackager by generic (nonproprietary) name

HYDROmorphone Hydrochloride

Dihydromorphinone

■ Hydromorphone is a semisynthetic phenanthrene-derivative opiate agonist.

REMS

FDA approved a REMS for hydromorphone to ensure that the benefits outweigh the risks. The REMS may apply to one or more preparations of hydromorphone and consists of the following: medication guide and elements to assure safe use. See the FDA REMS page (https://www.accessdata.fda.gov/scripts/cder/rems/index.cfm). .

Uses

Hydromorphone is a strong analgesic used in the relief of moderate to severe pain. Extended-release tablets of hydromorphone hydrochloride are used orally for the management of moderate to severe pain in *opiate-tolerant* patients when a continuous, around-the-clock analgesic is needed for an extended period of time; the extended-release tablets should not be used for relief of acute or postoperative pain or on an as-needed ("prn") basis. Hydromorphone hydrochloride injection containing 10 mg of the drug per mL is a highly concentrated parenteral formulation of the drug that should be used *only* in patients who are tolerant to opiate agonists and are currently receiving high dosages of an opiate agonist (e.g., patients being treated for severe chronic pain associated with cancer). Patients are considered opiate tolerant if they have been receiving at least 60 mg of oral morphine sulfate daily, 25 mcg of transdermal fentanyl per hour, 30 mg of oral oxycodone hydrochloride daily, 8 mg of oral hydromorphone hydrochloride daily, 25 mg of oral oxymorphone hydrochloride daily, or an equianalgesic dosage of another opiate daily for at least 1 week. The highly concentrated injection may be particularly useful in patients in whom IM or subcutaneous injection of large volumes of other opiate agonists is associated with discomfort or is precluded because of small muscle mass (such as in emaciated patients).

For further information on the role of opiate analgesics in the management of acute or chronic pain, see Uses: Pain, in the Opiate Agonists General Statement 28:08.08.

Dosage and Administration

■ **Reconstitution and Administration** Hydromorphone hydrochloride may be administered by subcutaneous, IM, or slow IV injection; the drug also may be administered orally as conventional (immediate-release) or extended-release tablets or as an oral solution. If rapid onset and shorter duration of analgesia are required, the drug may be given IV at a very slow rate (over at least 2–3 minutes) with special attention to the possibility of respiratory depression and hypotension. Hydromorphone hydrochloride has been administered as a continuous subcutaneous or IV infusion in selected opiate-tolerant patients with chronic pain conditions; extreme caution is advised when administering continuous infusions of opiates to patients with no prior exposure to opiate analgesics. The drug also has been administered IV via a controlled-delivery device for patient-controlled analgesia (PCA). Hydromorphone hydrochloride also has been administered epidurally†.

Parenteral Administration Parenteral preparations of hydromorphone hydrochloride are commercially available in various concentrations (1, 2, 4, and 10 mg/mL). Preparations containing lower concentrations of the drug (1, 2, or 4 mg/mL) should be used to initiate parenteral hydromorphone therapy in opiate-naive patients. **The highly concentrated (10-mg/mL) injection is intended for use only in patients who are tolerant to and already receiving high dosages of opiate agonists.** (See Uses and also Cautions.) **Confusion between the different concentrations or between mg and mL can result in accidental overdosage and/or death. To avoid such dosing errors, care should be taken to ensure that correct dosages are prescribed and dispensed. Prescriptions for hydromorphone hydrochloride injection should specify the intended total dose of the drug (in mg) along with the corresponding total volume (in mL).** The highly concentrated injection should be used only when the volume required for the intended dose can be accurately measured; this injection should not be used when low doses are required. The highly concentrated injection should be reserved for use in patients who require the reduced total volume and higher concentration of this formulation.

When the single-dose 10-mg/mL vial containing 500 mg of hydromorphone hydrochloride is used for preparation of IV infusion solutions, the manufacturer recommends that the container seal and rubber stopper of the vial be removed (not penetrated with a syringe) in a laminar flow hood or equivalent clean air compounding area. The appropriate amount should then be withdrawn for preparation of a single large-volume parenteral solution and any unused portion of the vial should be discarded. Hydromorphone hydrochloride lyophilized powder should be reconstituted immediately prior to use by adding 25 mL of sterile water for injection to a vial labeled as containing 250 mg of the drug to provide a solution containing 10 mg/mL. The drug has been diluted to a concentration of 1 mg/mL in 5% dextrose or 0.9% sodium chloride injection for continuous IV infusion in critically ill adults.

Oral Administration Commercially available conventional (immediate-release) tablets and oral solutions of hydromorphone hydrochloride are bioequivalent. Although food may decrease the rate and extent of absorption of hydromorphone hydrochloride conventional tablets (see Pharmacokinetics), the manufacturer states that these effects may not be clinically important. Patients receiving hydromorphone should avoid alcohol; concomitant use may result in profound sedation, respiratory depression, coma, and death.

When therapy with extended-release hydromorphone hydrochloride is initiated, all other extended-release opiates should be discontinued. Extended-release tablets of hydromorphone hydrochloride should not be administered more frequently than once every 24 hours. The tablets should be swallowed intact and should *not* be broken, crushed, dissolved, or chewed; ingestion of broken, crushed, chewed, or dissolved tablets may result in rapid release of the drug from the preparation and absorption of a potentially fatal dose of hydromorphone hydrochloride. Extended-release tablets of hydromorphone hydrochloride may be administered without regard to food. Intake of alcohol with the extended-release tablets may result in increased peak plasma concentrations of hydromorphone and ingestion of a potentially toxic dose of the drug.

Caution should be exercised when prescribing or dispensing oral hydromorphone hydrochloride to avoid inadvertent interchange of the 8-mg extended-release tablets and the 8-mg conventional tablets.

■ **Dosage** Hydromorphone hydrochloride should be given at the lowest effective dosage and for the shortest duration of therapy consistent with the treatment goals of the patient. Reduced dosage is indicated in geriatric or debilitated patients and in patients with hepatic or renal impairment. If concomitant therapy with other CNS depressants is required, the lowest effective dosages and shortest possible duration of concomitant therapy should be used.

Dosage of hydromorphone hydrochloride should be individualized to provide adequate analgesia and to minimize adverse effects. When selecting an initial dosage, consideration should be given to the type, severity, and frequency of the patient's pain; the age, general condition, and medical status of the patient; concurrent drug therapy; the patient's risk for abuse or addiction; prior use of opiates; and the acceptable balance between pain relief and adverse effects. In addition, in patients who are being transferred to hydromorphone from other opiate therapy, consideration should be given to the daily dosage, potency, and specific characteristics (e.g., elimination half-life) of the previously administered opiate and the reliability of the relative potency estimate used to calculate an equivalent hydromorphone hydrochloride dosage. When opiate therapy is discontinued, it should be done so gradually to avoid precipitation of withdrawal symptoms.

For acute pain not related to trauma or surgery, the prescribed quantity should be limited to the amount needed for the expected duration of pain severe enough to require opiate analgesia (generally 3 days or less and rarely more than 7 days). When opiate analgesics are used for the management of chronic noncancer pain, the US Centers for Disease Control and Prevention (CDC) recommends that primary care clinicians carefully reassess individual benefits and risks before prescribing dosages equivalent to 50 mg or more of morphine sulfate daily (approximately 12.5 mg or more of hydromorphone hydrochloride daily) and avoid dosages equivalent to 90 mg or more of morphine sulfate daily (approximately 22.5 mg or more of hydromorphone hydrochloride daily) or carefully justify their decision to titrate the dosage to such levels. Other experts recommend consulting a pain management specialist before exceeding a dosage equivalent to 80–120 mg of morphine sulfate daily. For further information on the management of opiate analgesic therapy, see Dosage and Administration: Dosage, in the Opiate Agonists General Statement 28:08.08.

Parenteral Dosage The manufacturer states that the usual initial parenteral dosage of hydromorphone hydrochloride in opiate-naive adults is 1–2 mg every 2–3 hours as needed by subcutaneous or IM injection, or 0.2–1 mg every 2–3 hours by slow (i.e., over at least 2–3 minutes) IV injection. Some patients may require lower initial dosages. The dose and/or frequency of administration should be adjusted gradually based on patient response. In critically ill adults in an intensive care unit (ICU) setting, an IV loading dose of 0.2–0.6 mg followed by a maintenance continuous IV infusion of 0.5–3 mg/hour has been used. Hydromorphone hydrochloride also has been administered in intermittent IV doses of 10–30 mcg/kg every 1–2 hours or as a continuous IV infusion of 7–15 mcg/kg per hour in critically ill adults.

To switch patients who currently are receiving other opiate therapy to therapy with parenteral hydromorphone hydrochloride, the total daily dosage of the current opiate should be converted to an equivalent daily dosage of hydromorphone hydrochloride and then administered in divided doses. An equianalgesic dosage of parenteral hydromorphone hydrochloride should be calculated using the manufacturer's suggested dosage conversions in Table 1. For opiates not in Table 1, the total daily dosage of the current opiate should first be converted to an equivalent dosage of morphine sulfate, and then the estimated daily dosage of morphine sulfate can be used to determine an equianalgesic dosage of hydromorphone hydrochloride. The manufacturer states that the estimated parenteral dosage of hydromorphone hydrochloride should be reduced by one-half because of the possibility of incomplete cross-tolerance. Dosage of parenteral hydromorphone hydrochloride should then be adjusted based on patient response.

Table 1. Equianalgesic Potency Conversion

	Equianalgesic Dose (in mg)	
Opiate Agonist or Partial Agonist	**Oral**	**Parenteral**
Morphine sulfate	40–60	10
Hydromorphone hydrochloride	6.5–7.5	1.3–2
Oxymorphone hydrochloride	6.6	1–1.1
Levorphanol tartrate	4	2–2.3
Meperidine hydrochloride	300–400	75–100
Methadone hydrochloride	10–20	10
Nalbuphine hydrochloride		10–12
Butorphanol tartrate	–	1.5–2.5

Although safety and efficacy of parenteral hydromorphone hydrochloride have not been established in pediatric patients†, some clinicians recommend an initial parenteral dosage of 0.015 mg/kg every 3–6 hours as needed in children who weigh less than 50 kg and an initial parenteral dosage of 0.2–0.6 mg IV every 2–4 hours or 0.8–1 mg by IM or subcutaneous injection every 4–6 hours as needed in children and adolescents who weigh 50 kg or more.

Oral Dosage **Conventional Preparations.** The usual initial oral dosage of hydromorphone hydrochloride conventional (immediate-release) preparations in non-opiate-tolerant adults is 2–4 mg every 4–6 hours. For adults with severe pain, initial oral doses of 4–8 mg have been used. The dose and/or frequency of administration should be adjusted gradually based on patient response. The manufacturer states that the usual oral dosage of hydromorphone hydrochloride conventional preparations in adults is 2.5–10 mg every 3–6 hours, although some patients may require higher dosages. For management of chronic pain, conventional oral preparations of the drug should be administered at regularly scheduled intervals ("around the clock"); supplemental doses equivalent to 5–15% of the total daily dosage may be administered every 2 hours as needed for breakthrough pain.

To switch patients who currently are receiving other opiate therapy to therapy with conventional oral preparations of hydromorphone hydrochloride, the total daily dosage of the current opiate should be converted to an equivalent daily dosage of hydromorphone hydrochloride and then administered in divided doses. An equianalgesic dosage of oral hydromorphone hydrochloride should be calculated using the manufacturer's suggested dosage conversions in Table 1. For opiates not in Table 1, the total daily dosage of the current opiate should first be converted to an equivalent dosage of morphine sulfate, and then the estimated daily dosage of morphine sulfate can be used to determine an equianalgesic dosage of hydromorphone hydrochloride. To account for individual variation in response to different opiate agonists, the manufacturer states that the first few doses of oral hydromorphone hydrochloride be reduced to one-half to two-thirds of the estimated equianalgesic oral dose. The dose and/or frequency of administration of oral hydromorphone hydrochloride should then be adjusted based on patient response.

Although safety and efficacy of conventional oral preparations of hydromorphone hydrochloride have not been established in pediatric patients†, some clinicians recommend an initial oral hydromorphone hydrochloride dosage of 0.03–0.08 mg/kg every 3–4 hours as needed in children who weigh less than 50 kg and a usual initial oral dosage of 1–2 mg every 3–4 hours as needed in children and adolescents who weigh 50 kg or more. For children with severe pain, initial oral doses of 0.06 mg/kg have been used.

Extended-release Tablets. When hydromorphone hydrochloride extended-release tablets are used in opiate-tolerant patients, dosage must be carefully individualized since overestimation of the initial dosage can result in fatal overdosage. The manufacturer considers the following dosage recommendations to be suggested approaches to the individual management of each patient.

Adults being transferred from conventional (immediate-release) oral hydromorphone preparations to the extended-release tablets should receive the same total daily dosage administered once every 24 hours. Dosage may be titrated every 3–4 days based on patient response. When transferring adults from other oral opiates to extended-release hydromorphone hydrochloride, clinicians should consult published dosage conversion tables (see Table 2 for estimated equianalgesic oral doses), keeping in mind that such conversion ratios are only approximate. For conversion from transdermal fentanyl, the estimated equianalgesic dosage of extended-release hydromorphone hydrochloride is 12 mg every 24 hours for each 25-mcg/hour increment in fentanyl transdermal dosage. Therapy with the extended-release tablet should be initiated no earlier than 18 hours following removal of the fentanyl transdermal system. In general, dosage of extended-release hydromorphone hydrochloride should be initiated at 50% of the calculated total daily dosage, then titrated upward (by suggested increments of 25–50% of the current daily dosage) based on patient response. Particularly close monitoring is required when patients are switched from methadone therapy, since equianalgesic conversion ratios between methadone and other opiates vary widely depending on extent of prior methadone exposure (see Dosage and Administration: Dosage, in Methadone Hydrochloride 28:08.08). Dosage of extended-release hydromorphone hydrochloride should be increased no more often than every 3–4 days to allow sufficient time for steady-state plasma concentrations of the drug to be attained at each dosage level. If more than 2 doses of supplemental (rescue) analgesic are required for breakthrough pain within a 24-hour period on 2 consecutive days, then an increase in dosage of extended-release hydromorphone hydrochloride may be needed. The extended-release tablets should be administered no more frequently than every 24 hours. Dosage of extended-release hydromorphone hydrochloride in clinical trials ranged from 8–64 mg daily.

Table 2. Approximate Equianalgesic Doses for Conversion from Oral Opiate Agonists to Extended-release Hydromorphone Hydrochloride

Opiate Agonist	Equianalgesic Oral Dose (in mg)
Hydromorphone hydrochloride	12
Codeine phosphate	200
Hydrocodone bitartrate	30
Methadone hydrochloride	20
Morphine sulfate	60
Oxycodone hydrochloride	30
Oxymorphone hydrochloride	20

Therapy with extended-release hydromorphone hydrochloride should be discontinued by reducing the dose by 25–50% every 2–3 days until a dose of 8 mg is reached.

■ **Dosage in Renal and Hepatic Impairment** Because of the potential for increased drug exposure, dosage of hydromorphone hydrochloride should be reduced in patients with renal or hepatic impairment based on the degree of impairment.

The initial oral dosage of hydromorphone hydrochloride should be reduced in patients with moderate hepatic impairment (Child-Pugh class B); because of the possibility of further increases in drug exposure, even more conservative initial dosages should be used in patients with severe hepatic impairment (Child-Pugh class C). When hydromorphone hydrochloride injection is used in patients with moderate hepatic impairment, the manufacturer recommends that the initial dosage be reduced to one-fourth to one-half the usual recommended dosage; the possibility that systemic exposure to hydromorphone may be further increased in patients with severe hepatic impairment should be taken into account when selecting an initial dosage.

The initial oral dosage of hydromorphone hydrochloride should be reduced in patients with moderate renal impairment (creatinine clearance of 40–60 mL/minute) and even further reduced in those with severe renal impairment (creatinine clearance less than 30 mL/minute). Because the extended-release preparation of the drug is intended only for once-daily administration, the manufacturer recommends that an alternative analgesic regimen with a more flexible dosing interval should be considered in patients with severe renal impairment. When hydromorphone hydrochloride injection is used in patients with renal impairment, the manufacturer states that the initial dosage be reduced to one-fourth to one-half the usual recommended dosage depending on the degree of renal impairment.

Use of the oral solution rather than conventional (immediate-release) tablets in patients with renal or hepatic impairment is recommended to facilitate dosage titration.

Patients with hepatic or renal impairment should be closely monitored during dosage titrations.

Cautions

Hydromorphone shares the toxic potentials of the opiate agonists, and the usual precautions of opiate agonist therapy should be observed. (See Cautions in the Opiate Agonists General Statement 28:08.08.) Mild to severe seizures and myoclonus have been reported in critically ill patients receiving high doses of parenterally administered hydromorphone.

Nausea, vomiting, constipation, and euphoria may be less marked with hydromorphone than with morphine.

Some commercially available preparations of hydromorphone hydrochloride contain sulfites that may cause allergic-type reactions, including anaphylaxis and life-threatening or less severe asthmatic episodes, in certain susceptible individuals. The overall prevalence of sulfite sensitivity in the general population is unknown but probably low; such sensitivity appears to occur more frequently in asthmatic than in nonasthmatic individuals.

Some packaging components of some hydromorphone hydrochloride products contain natural latex proteins in the form of dry natural rubber and/or natural rubber latex (see the manufacturers' labeling). Some individuals may be hypersensitive to natural latex proteins found in a wide range of medical devices, including such packaging components, and the level of sensitivity may vary depending on the form of natural rubber present; rarely hypersensitivity reactions to natural latex proteins have been fatal. Therefore, while the specific risk cannot necessarily be predicted, health-care professionals should take appropriate precautions when administration of such hydromorphone preparations is considered for individuals with a history of natural latex sensitivity.

Because hydromorphone hydrochloride extended-release tablets are nondeformable and do not appreciably change shape in the GI tract, they should not be administered to patients with any underlying condition that can result in narrowing of the GI tract (e.g., prior GI surgery, GI obstruction, blind loop syndrome, esophageal motility disorders, small bowel inflammatory disease, short-gut syndrome due to adhesions or decreased transit time, history of peritonitis, cystic fibrosis, chronic intestinal pseudo-obstruction, Meckel's diverticulum).

Hydromorphone hydrochloride extended-release tablets should only be used in patients who are tolerant to opiate agonists; use of this formulation in patients who are not opiate tolerant may result in fatal respiratory depression. Inadvertent ingestion of the extended-release tablets, especially by children, can result in fatal overdosage.

Patients receiving hydromorphone should avoid alcohol; intake of alcohol with the extended-release tablets may result in increased peak plasma concentrations of hydromorphone and ingestion of a potentially toxic dose of the drug.

In clinical studies, hydromorphone hydrochloride injection containing 10 mg of the drug per mL was not associated with local tissue irritation or induration at the site of subcutaneous injection but pain and/or burning occurred rarely; mild erythema occurred rarely at the site of IM injection. Because local irritation and induration have been reported with other opiate agonists, the possibility that they could occur with hydromorphone hydrochloride injection should be considered. The highly concentrated (10 mg/mL) injection should be used *only* in patients who are tolerant to opiate agonists (see Uses); use of this injection in patients who are *not* tolerant to opiate agonists may result in overdosage and/or death. Extreme caution should be taken to avoid confusing the highly concentrated injection with the less concentrated injections of the drug.

■ **Pediatric Precautions** Safety and efficacy of hydromorphone hydrochloride in children have not been established; however, conventional preparations of hydromorphone have been used in children.

■ **Geriatric Precautions** Clinical studies of hydromorphone hydrochloride did not include sufficient numbers of patients 65 years of age and older to determine whether geriatric patients respond differently than younger patients. Experience with hydromorphone hydrochloride extended-release tablets suggests that geriatric patients may be more susceptible to adverse effects of the drug. Because of the greater frequency of decreased hepatic, renal, and/or cardiac function and of concomitant disease and drug therapy in geriatric patients, the manufacturers suggest that patients in this age group receive initial dosages of the drug in the lower end of the usual range.

■ **Pregnancy and Lactation** Safe use of hydromorphone in pregnancy has not been established. Administration of hydromorphone to pregnant women during labor may result in some degree of respiratory depression in the neonate and sinusoidal fetal heart rate patterns. Neonates whose mothers received an opiate agonist such as hydromorphone during labor and delivery should be observed closely for signs of respiratory depression. The manufacturer states that hydromorphone hydrochloride injection should be used with caution during labor, and an opiate antagonist for reversal of respiratory depression should be readily available. The manufacturers of oral formulations of hydromorphone hydrochloride state that these formulations should not be used during and immediately prior to labor and delivery.

Because some opiate agonists have been detected in milk, the manufacturers state that women should not breast-feed while receiving hydromorphone hydrochloride.

Pharmacokinetics

Hydromorphone hydrochloride is well absorbed following oral, rectal, or parenteral administration. Hydromorphone has a more rapid onset and may have a shorter duration of action than does morphine. The onset of action of hydromorphone with conventional (immediate-release) preparations is usually 15–30 minutes and analgesia is maintained for 4–5 hours, depending on the route of administration. Hydromorphone is metabolized primarily in the liver where it undergoes conjugation with glucuronic acid and is excreted principally in the urine as the glucuronide conjugate. The terminal elimination half-life of hydromorphone after IV administration is about 2.3 hours.

Commercially available conventional tablets and oral solutions of hydromorphone hydrochloride are bioequivalent.

Following oral administration of hydromorphone hydrochloride as conventional tablets given 4 times daily or as extended-release tablets given once daily at the same total daily dosage, steady-state plasma concentrations of the drug are maintained within the same concentration range; however, the extended-release preparation produces less fluctuation between peak and trough concentrations. Following administration of the extended-release tablets, peak plasma concentrations of hydromorphone occur about 12–16 hours after a dose. Steady state is reached after 3–4 days of once-daily dosing of the extended-release tablets. The mean half-life of this formulation of hydromorphone is approximately 11 hours (range: 8–15 hours).

Administration of hydromorphone hydrochloride extended-release tablets with food does not alter the pharmacokinetics of the drug. Oral administration of a single 8-mg dose of hydromorphone hydrochloride (as conventional tablets) with food decreased peak plasma concentrations and increased systemic exposure of the drug by 25 and 35%, respectively, and delayed peak plasma concentrations by 0.8 hour.

Following oral administration of a single 4-mg dose of conventional hydromorphone hydrochloride tablets, systemic exposure to the drug was increased twofold in individuals with moderate renal impairment (creatinine clearance of 40–60 mL/minute), threefold to fourfold in individuals with severe renal impairment (creatinine clearance less than 30 mL/minute), and fourfold in individuals with moderate hepatic impairment (Child-Pugh class B). In addition, the elimination half-life of hydromorphone was prolonged (40 hours) in patients with severe renal impairment.

Chemistry and Stability

■ **Chemistry** Hydromorphone is a semisynthetic phenanthrene-derivative opiate agonist. The drug differs structurally from morphine in the substitution of an oxygen for the 6-hydroxyl group and hydrogenation of the 7-8 double bond of the morphine molecule. Hydromorphone is commercially available as the hydrochloride salt. Hydromorphone hydrochloride occurs as a fine, white or practically white, crystalline powder and is freely soluble in water and sparingly soluble in alcohol. Hydromorphone hydrochloride injection has a pH of 3.5–5.5.

■ **Stability** Hydromorphone hydrochloride is affected by light; although hydromorphone hydrochloride injection may develop a slight yellowish discoloration, this change apparently does not indicate loss of potency. Hydromorphone hydrochloride injection should be protected from light and stored at a controlled room temperature of 20–25°C, but may be exposed to temperatures ranging from 15–30°C. Hydromorphone hydrochloride immediate-release tablets and oral solution should be stored in tight, light-resistant containers at 25°C, but may be exposed to temperatures ranging from 15–30°C. The extended-release tablets should also be stored at 25°C, but may be exposed to temperatures ranging from 15–30°C.

Hydromorphone hydrochloride injection reportedly is physically and chemically stable for at least 24 hours in most common IV infusion solutions when protected from light at 25°C. Hydromorphone hydrochloride injection has been reported to be physically or chemically incompatible with solutions containing sodium bicarbonate and thiopental sodium (no longer commercially available in the US). Specialized references should be consulted for specific compatibility information.

For further information on chemistry, pharmacology, pharmacokinetics, uses, cautions, chronic toxicity, acute toxicity, drug interactions, and dosage and administration of hydromorphone hydrochloride, see the Opiate Agonists General Statement 28:08.08.

Preparations

Hydromorphone hydrochloride preparations are subject to control under the Federal Controlled Substances Act of 1970 as schedule II (C-II) drugs.

Excipients in commercially available drug preparations may have clinically important effects in some individuals; consult specific product labeling for details.

HYDROmorphone Hydrochloride

Powder			**HYDROmorphone Hydrochloride Powder for Prescription Compounding** (C-II)
Oral			
	Solution	5 mg/5 mL	**Dilaudid®** (C-II), Purdue Pharma
			HYDROmorphone Hydrochloride Solution (C-II)
	Tablets	2 mg*	**Dilaudid®** (C-II), Purdue Pharma
			HYDROmorphone Hydrochloride Tablets (C-II)
		4 mg*	**Dilaudid®** (C-II), Purdue Pharma
			HYDROmorphone Hydrochloride Tablets (C-II)
		8 mg*	**Dilaudid®** (C-II; scored), Purdue Pharma
			HYDROmorphone Hydrochloride Tablets (C-II)
	Tablets, extended-release	8 mg	**Exalgo®** (C-II), Mallinckrodt
		12 mg	**Exalgo®** (C-II), Mallinckrodt
		16 mg	**Exalgo®** (C-II), Mallinckrodt
Parenteral			
	For injection	250 mg	**Dilaudid-HP® Lyophilized** (C-II), Purdue Pharma
	Injection	1 mg/mL*	**Dilaudid®** (C-II), Purdue Pharma
			HYDROmorphone Hydrochloride Injection (C-II)
		2 mg/mL*	**Dilaudid®** (C-II), Purdue Pharma
			HYDROmorphone Hydrochloride Injection (C-II)
		4 mg/mL*	**Dilaudid®** (C-II), Purdue Pharma
			HYDROmorphone Hydrochloride Injection (C-II)
		10 mg/mL (10, 50, or 500 mg)*	**Dilaudid-HP®** (C-II), Purdue Pharma
			HYDROmorphone Hydrochloride Injection (C-II)

*available from one or more manufacturer, distributor, and/or repackager by generic (nonproprietary) name

†Use is not currently included in the labeling approved by the US Food and Drug Administration

Methadone Hydrochloride

■ Methadone hydrochloride is a synthetic diphenylheptane-derivative opiate agonist.

REMS

FDA approved a REMS for methadone hydrochloride to ensure that the benefits outweigh the risk. The REMS may apply to one or more preparations of methadone hydrochloride and consists of the following: medication guide and elements to assure safe use. See the FDA REMS page (https://www.accessdata.fda.gov/scripts/cder/rems/index.cfm).

Uses

Methadone is used in the relief of pain. Methadone also may be used in detoxification and maintenance treatment. Although the drug has antitussive activity, methadone is no longer approved by the US Food and Drug Administration for this indication.

■ **Pain** Methadone is a strong analgesic used parenterally for the treatment of moderate to severe pain that has not responded to non-opiate analgesics. Methadone is used orally for relief of moderate to severe pain when a continuous, around-the-clock analgesic is needed for an extended period of time. Methadone is used for relief of chronic pain in both opiate-naive patients and in individuals being switched to methadone therapy from other opiate agonists because of inadequate pain relief or adverse effects from the previous drug (opiate rotation). Most clinical studies evaluating methadone in the management of pain have involved individuals with chronic malignant pain. The manufacturers state that oral preparations of the drug are not indicated for relief of acute (including postoperative) pain, for relief of pain that is mild or is not expected to persist for an extended period of time, or for use on an as-needed ("prn") basis.

Clinical studies suggest that methadone may have efficacy similar to that of morphine and other opiates in patients with chronic malignant pain. However, experts generally agree that methadone should be prescribed for chronic pain management only by clinicians knowledgeable about its risks (e.g., QT-interval prolongation) and pharmacokinetics, and should not be the first choice for an extended-release or long-acting opiate analgesic. Benefits associated with the use of methadone for management of chronic pain include the commercial availability of multiple dosage forms of the drug, good oral bioavailability, rapid onset of action, reduced dosing frequency (because of the drug's long half-life), low cost, and lack of active metabolites. Incomplete cross-tolerance between methadone and other opiate agonists has been reported; some patients who were previously refractory to high doses of other opiate agonists have experienced pain relief with methadone therapy. This incomplete cross-tolerance may allow for successful pain relief in patients who previously were refractory to or who experienced adverse effects from increasing dosages of other opiate agonists. Disadvantages associated with the use of methadone include its increased potential for accumulation with repeated doses (which may result in toxicity), considerable interindividual variability in pharmacokinetic parameters, the potential for drug interactions, challenges associated with methadone dosage titration and with the transfer of patients from therapy with other opiate agonists to therapy with methadone, and the commercial availability and relative ease of use of extended-release preparations of other opiate agonists. (See Cautions.)

For further information on the role of opiate analgesics in the management of chronic pain, see Uses: Pain, in the Opiate Agonists General Statement 28:08.08.

■ **Detoxification and Maintenance of Opiate Dependence** Methadone is used in detoxification treatment and maintenance treatment as an oral substitute for heroin or other morphine-like drugs to suppress the opiate-agonist abstinence syndrome in patients who are dependent on these drugs. The success of such treatment programs is dependent on the selection of properly motivated patients and on the availability of social, psychologic, vocational, and educational as well as medical supportive services. In **detoxification treatment**, methadone is administered in decreasing doses over a period not exceeding either 30 days (*short-term detoxification*) or 180 days (*long-term detoxification*) in order to withdraw use of opiate agonist(s); previously (prior to enactment of Public Law 98-509 in 1984), detoxification treatment with methadone could not exceed 21 days. Patients of any age may undergo detoxification treatment. Methadone is approved by the US Food and Drug Administration (FDA) for **detoxification treatment of opiate dependence** and for **maintenance treatment of opiate dependence.** Buprenorphine hydrochloride is approved by the FDA for the management of opiate dependence. Levomethadyl acetate

(LAAM, ORLAAM®) also has been approved by the FDA for the management of opiate dependence but is no longer commercially available in the US because of potentially severe adverse cardiac effects.

Maintenance treatment consists of administration of stable doses of methadone or buprenorphine for relatively long periods (i.e., exceeding 21 days). **Maintenance treatment** with methadone is provided as *comprehensive maintenance*, which is provided in conjunction with a comprehensive range of appropriate medical and rehabilitative services, or *interim maintenance*, which is provided in conjunction with appropriate medical services while the patient is awaiting transfer to comprehensive maintenance. **Maintenance treatment** with buprenorphine is provided as office-based outpatient therapy. Office-based treatment with buprenorphine is an innovative model intended to increase access to opiate dependence treatment and may be appropriate for individuals who may not otherwise seek methadone maintenance treatment (comprehensive maintenance), do not meet enrollment criteria, do not have access to such programs, or have chosen to opt out of such programs for another reason. In the office-based treatment model, specially trained physicians prescribe buprenorphine as a take-home medication. As with detoxification treatment, the eventual goal of maintenance therapy is withdrawal of the drug.

According to federal regulations, only patients who have demonstrated current physiologic dependence on opiate drugs and at least a 1-year history of this dependence can be admitted to *comprehensive* maintenance programs. If clinically appropriate, the 1-year history of dependence can be waived for individuals released within the previous 6 months from a penal institution, pregnant women, or previously treated individuals (up to 2 years after discharge from treatment).

Detoxification or maintenance treatment with methadone is permitted to be undertaken only by opiate-dependency treatment programs certified by the Substance Abuse and Mental Health Services Administration (SAMHSA) and approved by the designated state authority; however, this does not preclude detoxification or maintenance treatment of an addict who is hospitalized or is admitted to a long-term care facility for medical conditions other than addiction and who requires detoxification or maintenance treatment during his hospitalization or stay in the long-term care facility, nor does it exclude administration of opiates for up to 72 hours (emergency treatment to relieve acute withdrawal symptoms) while care in an opiate-dependency treatment program is being sought. For information on the use of methadone for detoxification and maintenance treatment in children younger than 18 years of age and during pregnancy, see Cautions: Pediatric Precautions and also Pregnancy and Lactation.

Because of the risk of acquiring human immunodeficiency virus (HIV) infection from illicit IV drug use, the conditions for use of methadone in maintenance treatment were revised (effective January 6, 1993) to facilitate more rapid entry into treatment programs of increased numbers of opiate-dependent patients more rapidly. The revisions permit programs to provide minimum service (*interim*) maintenance treatment (which is aimed at helping to alleviate the human suffering of opiate-dependent individuals, including the risk of HIV infection, and to reduce the abuse of IV drugs) in addition to *comprehensive* maintenance treatment (which already existed). There is some evidence that the revised conditions for treatment of opiate dependence can reduce substantially the illicit use of IV drugs (and hence needles) by dependent individuals and that such reductions in IV use of these drugs will decrease the spread of HIV within this population. In addition, the revised conditions for use of methadone in detoxification and in maintenance treatment require provision of counseling for preventing HIV transmission and exposure and provision of information on the availability of, and ensuring access to, HIV testing; mandatory HIV testing is *not* a requirement of opiate-dependency treatment programs, but such testing must be made available, either on site or at another facility, to any patient requesting it.

The minimum service program serves as interim treatment until a patient can be admitted into a comprehensive program; however, such treatment cannot exceed 120 days in any 12-month period. In general, the requirements for comprehensive maintenance treatment or detoxification treatment apply to interim maintenance treatment, although the provision of a comprehensive range of services is *not* required during interim maintenance treatment. Comprehensive medical, vocational rehabilitative, employment, educational, and counseling services (e.g., formation and periodic evaluation of treatment plans, primary counselor assignments) are *not* required during interim maintenance. However, some services are required (e.g., medical treatment referrals, prenatal care referrals, HIV counseling), and sufficient counseling staff should be available to provide such services and to respond to emergencies. In addition to initial drug screening, interim programs must provide a minimum of 2 additional drug screenings to assist in assessing patient needs and priorities for transfer into comprehensive programs. Patients admitted to an interim maintenance program are required to be administered each daily methadone dose while being closely observed; take-home medication is *not* permitted. Both admission to interim treatment programs and transfer to comprehensive treatment programs are to be provided preferentially to pregnant women. Interim maintenance treatment programs can be implemented by existing maintenance programs, provided the program has filed for and received federal authorization (formerly from FDA but as of May 18, 2001, from SAMHSA) and authorization from the appropriate local (e.g., state) authority.

Federal regulations (effective May 18, 2001) concerning use of opiates in detoxification and maintenance programs transferred oversight for such programs from FDA to SAMHSA and altered the nature of the regulatory system from one that relied on inspection for compliance with process-oriented regulations to a system based on program accreditation and subsequent certification by SAMHSA. Standards for treatment programs also were modified to permit greater flexibility and professional judgment in treatment. The requirement that programs use only liquid oral formulations was modified to allow for use of either liquid or solid oral dosage forms. The requirement that treatment programs administer methadone hydrochloride dosages exceeding 100 mg daily under direct supervision at least 6 days per week regardless of length of time in the program (unless prior approval for take-home dosages exceeding 100 mg had been obtained from FDA and the state authority) was eliminated, and a more flexible schedule for unsupervised administration was allowed (see Maintenance under Dosage: Detoxification and Maintenance of Opiate Dependence, in Dosage and Administration).

Other federal initiatives were undertaken in 2000 to expand access to treatment and to involve office-based physicians in the care of opiate-dependent individuals. These initiatives were taken in response to limitations in the heavily regulated comprehensive maintenance programs and the increasing heroin use and high rates of HIV and hepatitis C virus transmission among illicit users of IV drugs. The Drug Addiction Treatment Act (DATA) of 2000 allows qualifying physicians to prescribe and dispense opiates in schedules III, IV, and V of the Federal Controlled Substances Act that have been approved by the FDA for detoxification or maintenance treatment of opiate dependence. With the approval of buprenorphine and buprenorphine in fixed combination with naloxone for the management of opiate dependence, treatment of opiate dependence can be undertaken in a system that resembles care provided for other chronic medical conditions.

■ **Neonatal Opiate Withdrawal** Methadone has been used to manage manifestations of opiate abstinence syndrome (i.e., postnatal withdrawal) in neonates† exposed to opiates in utero. Opiates are recommended as first-line pharmacologic therapy when environmental and supportive measures (e.g., minimization of external stimuli, maximization of mother-infant contact [e.g., parental "rooming in"], breast-feeding when not contraindicated, swaddling and gentle handling) are inadequate. Other adjunctive therapy (e.g., clonidine, phenobarbital) may be added if the response to opiates is inadequate, or phenobarbital be added if the neonate was exposed to additional substances in utero. Approximately 60–80% of neonates with opiate abstinence syndrome may require pharmacologic treatment for withdrawal symptoms. While morphine has been used more extensively than other opiates in the management of neonatal opiate abstinence syndrome, some studies suggest that use of methadone or buprenorphine (an opiate partial agonist) may be associated with shorter treatment durations and hospital stays compared with morphine use. However, additional study is needed to establish optimal dosage schedules and preferred opiate drugs and to evaluate longer-term (e.g., neurodevelopmental) outcomes. Conflicting findings to date may be related in part to differences in study design, nonpharmacologic care, concomitant in utero drug exposures, the stringency of institutional protocols for care, and optimization of dosage schedules.

Use of standardized protocols for identification, evaluation, and treatment of neonatal opiate withdrawal syndrome is recommended since use of such protocols has been shown to improve overall response, including shorter hospital stays and durations of pharmacologic treatment. Some evidence suggests that use of a standardized protocol may be more important than use of a specific opiate agonist (e.g., methadone versus morphine) in improving outcomes. Protocols generally utilize assessment tools that were developed to quantify severity of withdrawal in term neonates (e.g., Finnegan or modified Finnegan scoring tools) to facilitate decisions regarding initiation, titration, and tapering of therapy.

Dosage and Administration

■ **Administration** Methadone hydrochloride may be administered orally as tablets, solution, concentrated solution, or dispersible tablets or by subcutaneous, IM, or IV injection.

Methadone hydrochloride dispersible tablets are intended for dispersion in a liquid prior to oral administration. Dispersible tablets of the drug contain insoluble excipients and therefore must *not* be used to prepare solutions for injection. Each 40-mg dispersible tablet can be divided in half or in quarters; the desired dose should be dispersed in approximately 120 mL of water, orange juice, Tang®, citrus-flavored Kool-Aid®, or other acidic fruit beverage immediately prior to administration. Complete tablet dispersion occurs within 1 minute; dispersion time is slightly increased when a cold and/or acidic vehicle is used. If any residue remains in the cup after initial administration, a small amount of liquid should be added and the resulting mixture administered. Because the dispersible tablets can be administered only in increments of 10 mg, this dosage form may not be appropriate in many patients for initial dosing during detoxification and maintenance treatment or for gradual dosage reduction following short-term detoxification or a period of maintenance treatment.

When the 10-mg/mL oral concentrate solution is used for the treatment of pain, the dose must be diluted with water or other suitable liquid (e.g., Kool-Aid®, Tang®, apple juice, Crystal Light® [with aspartame]) to at least 30 mL prior to administration.

Absorption of methadone following subcutaneous or IM injection may be unpredictable and has not been fully characterized; local tissue reactions may occur.

Methadone hydrochloride also has been administered rectally† and by epidural injection†.

Restricted Distribution Manufacturers of methadone hydrochloride 40-mg dispersible tablets and the Drug Enforcement Administration (DEA) have agreed to restrict distribution of this preparation to authorized opiate-dependency treatment programs and to hospitals. This restriction is in response to reports of serious adverse effects such as cardiotoxicity and death in patients receiving methadone (see Cautions). Methadone hydrochloride 40-mg dispersible tablets are used in detoxification and maintenance treatment of opiate addiction; this preparation is *not* labeled by the US Food and Drug Administration (FDA) for the treatment of pain.

■ Dosage

Dosage of methadone hydrochloride must be carefully individualized because repeated doses may result in substantial accumulation of the drug, prolonging its duration of action and possibly resulting in adverse effects, and because there is considerable interindividual variability in absorption, metabolism, and relative analgesic potency of the drug. Patients should be carefully monitored during initiation of therapy, dosage titration, and conversion from one opiate agonist to another. Steady-state plasma concentrations and full analgesic effects of methadone generally are not achieved until completion of 3–5 days of therapy.

Pain When selecting an initial dosage of methadone hydrochloride for management of pain, consideration should be given to the type, severity, and expected duration of the patient's pain; the age, general condition, and medical status of the patient; concurrent drug therapy (see Drug Interactions); and the acceptable balance between pain relief and adverse effects. In addition, in patients who are being transferred to methadone from other opiate therapy, consideration should be given to the daily dosage, potency, and specific characteristics (e.g., elimination half-life) of the previously administered opiate; adverse effects of and response to the previous regimen; degree of opiate tolerance; and the relative potency estimate used to calculate an equianalgesic dosage of methadone hydrochloride. Appropriate dosage selection and titration are essential to prevent overdosage.

A high degree of opiate tolerance does not preclude the possibility of unintended methadone overdosage. Failure to individualize dosage has resulted in serious adverse effects, including death, in opiate-tolerant patients during conversion to methadone therapy. (See Cautions.) Overestimation of the methadone dosage when transferring patients from other opiate therapy to methadone therapy can result in fatal overdosage with the first dose.

Published equianalgesic dosage conversion ratios between methadone hydrochloride and other opiate agonists are imprecise. Dose equivalencies that are obtained from commonly used tables generally are based on single-dose studies in patients who are not opiate tolerant. When transferring patients to methadone from other opiate agonist therapy, use of single-dose equivalency tables may *overestimate* dosage requirements for methadone hydrochloride during chronic therapy, since methadone may accumulate with repeated doses secondary to the long elimination half-life of the drug (see Pharmacokinetics: Elimination). Therefore, estimates of methadone hydrochloride dosage that are based on single-dose studies should *not* be used for conversion in patients receiving chronic opiate therapy. In addition, equianalgesic dosage conversion ratios between morphine sulfate and methadone hydrochloride have been reported to vary substantially depending on the dosage of the previously administered morphine regimen; the morphine sulfate-to-methadone hydrochloride equianalgesic dosage conversion ratio has been reported to be lower in patients receiving prior opiate therapy at a lower morphine sulfate dosage and higher in those receiving prior therapy at a higher morphine sulfate dosage.

Regardless of the strategy employed to determine initial methadone dosage, methadone hydrochloride therapy is most safely initiated using small initial doses and gradual dosage adjustments. Some clinicians recommend a transition period of at least 3 days for patients being transferred from therapy with another opiate agonist to therapy with methadone; during the transition period, the dosage of the previous opiate agonist is gradually tapered while the dosage of methadone hydrochloride is slowly increased. Other clinicians state that patients receiving *low* dosages of another opiate agonist may be transferred to methadone therapy in 1 day.

As an analgesic, methadone hydrochloride should be given at the lowest effective dosage and for the shortest duration of therapy consistent with the treatment goals of the patient. Reduced dosage is indicated in poor-risk patients such as very young, very old, or debilitated patients. If concomitant therapy with other CNS depressants is required, the lowest effective dosages and shortest possible duration of concomitant therapy should be used. (See Drug Interactions: Benzodiazepines and Other CNS Depressants.)

When opiate analgesics are used for the management of chronic noncancer pain, the US Centers for Disease Control and Prevention (CDC) recommends that primary care clinicians carefully reassess individual benefits and risks before prescribing dosages equivalent to 50 mg or more of morphine sulfate daily and avoid dosages equivalent to 90 mg or more of morphine sulfate daily or carefully justify their decision to titrate the dosage to such levels. Other experts recommend consulting a pain management specialist before exceeding a dosage equivalent to 80–120 mg of morphine sulfate daily. For further information on the management of opiate analgesic therapy, see Dosage and Administration: Dosage, in the Opiate Agonists General Statement 28:08.08.

Parenteral Dosage. For the relief of moderate to severe pain, the manufacturer recommends a usual initial methadone hydrochloride dosage in opiate-naive adults of 2.5–10 mg administered IV every 8–12 hours. Dosage may be increased as necessary to provide adequate analgesia, but should be increased slowly to avoid accumulation of the drug and potential toxicity. More frequent administration may be required during initiation of therapy in order to maintain adequate analgesia, but caution is necessary to avoid overdosage.

In patients being switched from oral to parenteral methadone hydrochloride, parenteral methadone hydrochloride should be initiated at a parenteral-to-oral dosage ratio of 1:2 (e.g., 5 mg of parenteral methadone hydrochloride in patients previously receiving 10 mg of oral methadone hydrochloride).

When patients are transferred from chronic therapy with another oral or parenteral opiate to therapy with parenteral methadone hydrochloride, dosage must be selected carefully, since cross-tolerance between methadone and other opiate agonists is incomplete, dosage conversion ratios are imprecise, and substantial interindividual variability exists. The dosage conversion methods recommended by the manufacturer for converting to IV methadone hydrochloride (See Tables 1 and 2) are based on comparisons with morphine. The manufacturer states that these estimates provide a safe starting point for opiate conversion; however, the IV methadone hydrochloride dosage obtained from these comparisons must be individualized (e.g., based on prior opiate use, medical condition, concurrent drug therapy, anticipated use of analgesics for breakthrough pain). The total daily dosage should be administered in divided doses (e.g., at 8-hour intervals) based on individual patient requirements. For patients being transferred from therapy with opiate agonists other than morphine, a comparative opiate agonist dosage table (such as the table in the Opiate Agonists General Statement 28:08.08) may be consulted to determine the equivalent morphine dosage.

Table 1. Conversion of Oral Morphine Sulfate to IV Methadone Hydrochloride (for Chronic Administration)

Baseline Total Daily *Oral* Morphine Sulfate Dosage	Estimated Daily *IV* Methadone Hydrochloride Dosage (as % of Total Daily Morphine Sulfate Dosage)
<100 mg	10–15%
100–300 mg	5–10%
300–600 mg	4–6%
600–1000 mg	3–5%
>1000 mg	<3%

Table 2. Conversion of Parenteral Morphine Sulfate to IV Methadone Hydrochloride (for Chronic Administration)[a]

Baseline Total Daily *Parenteral* Morphine Sulfate Dosage	Estimated Daily *IV* Methadone Hydrochloride Dosage (as % of Total Daily Morphine Dosage)
10–30 mg	40–66%
30–50 mg	27–66%
50–100 mg	22–50%
100–200 mg	15–34%
200–500 mg	10–20%

[a] Derived from Table 1 assuming a 3:1 oral-to-parenteral morphine ratio.

Oral Dosage. When oral methadone hydrochloride is used for the relief of moderate to severe pain in opiate-naive adults who require a continuous, around-the-clock analgesic for an extended period of time, therapy should be initiated with small doses of no more than 2.5–10 mg given every 8–12 hours. Dosage must be carefully individualized according to patient response. Dosage may be titrated to provide adequate analgesia, but should be increased slowly to avoid accumulation of the drug and potential toxicity. The dosage interval during methadone therapy may range from 4–12 hours, since the duration of analgesia is relatively short during the first days of therapy but increases substantially with continued administration. Clinicians and patients must be prepared to markedly reduce the methadone hydrochloride dose and/or increase the dosing interval after the first few doses based on assessments of pain relief, sedation, and other adverse effects. Some clinicians experienced with the use of methadone may elect to initiate opiate therapy by administering methadone hydrochloride on an as-needed basis for the first 3–7 days and then establishing an around-the-clock dosage schedule based on the duration of action reported by the patient. Opiate therapy also may be initiated with a short-acting opiate agonist and then switched to methadone once adequate analgesia is established.

In patients being switched from parenteral to oral methadone hydrochloride, oral methadone hydrochloride should be initiated at an oral-to-parenteral dosage ratio of 2:1 (e.g., 10 mg of oral methadone hydrochloride in patients previously receiving 5 mg of parenteral methadone hydrochloride).

When patients are transferred to oral methadone from chronic therapy with other oral or parenteral opiates, dosage must be selected carefully because cross-tolerance between methadone hydrochloride and other opiate agonists is incomplete, dosage conversion ratios are imprecise, and considerable interindividual variability exists. The dosage conversion method shown in Table 3 is based on comparison with morphine sulfate. The oral methadone hydrochloride dosage obtained from this comparison must be individualized (e.g., based on prior opiate use, medical condition, concurrent drug therapy, anticipated use of analgesics for breakthrough pain). The total daily dosage should be administered in divided doses (e.g., at 8-hour intervals) based on individual patient requirements. For patients being transferred from therapy with opiate agonists other than morphine, a comparative opiate agonist dosage table (such as the table in the Opiate Agonists General Statement 28:08.08) may be consulted to determine the equivalent morphine dosage.

Table 3. Conversion of Oral Morphine Sulfate to Oral Methadone Hydrochloride (for Chronic Administration)

Baseline Total Daily *Oral* Morphine Sulfate Dosage	Estimated Daily *Oral* Methadone Hydrochloride Dosage (as % of Total Daily Morphine Sulfate Dosage)
<100 mg	20–30%
100–300 mg	10–20%
300–600 mg	8–12%
600–1000 mg	5–10%
>1000 mg	<5%

Dosage adjustments may be made at intervals of 1–2 days with close monitoring to achieve adequate analgesia with minimal adverse effects. Patients who experience breakthrough pain may require dosage adjustment or rescue therapy with a small dose of an immediate-release analgesic. If excessive opiate-related adverse effects are observed, the next dose of methadone hydrochloride may be reduced; if adverse effects are intolerable, either the dose or dosing interval of the drug may be adjusted. If discontinuance of opiates is required, gradual tapering of the dosage every 2–4 days is recommended to avoid manifestations of abrupt withdrawal.

Detoxification and Maintenance of Opiate Dependence In detoxification and maintenance treatment, methadone hydrochloride may be administered or dispensed only as an oral preparation (e.g., tablet, dispersible tablet, liquid) that is formulated and packaged in such a way as to reduce potential for parenteral abuse and accidental ingestion. Hospitalized patients being treated for a medical or surgical condition may receive methadone parenterally if necessary. The dosage of methadone used for detoxification or maintenance treatment should be adjusted to control abstinence symptoms without causing respiratory depression or marked sedation. Any substantial deviations from the FDA-approved labeling for methadone hydrochloride (e.g., concerning dose, frequency of administration, or conditions of use) must be documented in the patient's medical record.

If at any time during detoxification or maintenance the patient cannot tolerate oral medication because of nausea or vomiting associated with acute complicating illness, he should be hospitalized and methadone hydrochloride may be continued by the parenteral route. The patient should receive 2 injections daily by the subcutaneous or IM route; each dose should be about one-fourth of the total oral daily dosage.

Detoxification. Detoxification treatment is initiated when there are substantial opiate-agonist abstinence symptoms. The initial dose of methadone hydrochloride should be based on the opiate tolerance of the patient. A single oral dose of 20–30 mg of methadone hydrochloride will often suppress withdrawal symptoms. The initial dose should not exceed 30 mg. Initial doses should be lower for patients whose tolerance is expected to be low at treatment initiation. Loss of tolerance should be considered if more than 5 days have elapsed since the patient took opiates. Initial doses should not be based on those used during prior treatment episodes or on the patient's expenditures for illicit drugs. If there is any doubt, it is usually safer to start with a smaller dose and keep the patient under observation. Additional doses of methadone hydrochloride may be necessary if withdrawal symptoms are not suppressed or if they reappear. The manufacturer states that if same-day dosage adjustments are to be made, the patient should be reevaluated 2–4 hours after the previous dose, since peak plasma concentrations of methadone will have been attained. If an additional dose is required to suppress withdrawal symptoms, an additional 5–10 mg of methadone hydrochloride may be administered. The total dose on the first day should not exceed 40 mg unless it is documented that this total dose does not suppress withdrawal symptoms.

Dosage adjustments should be made over the first week of methadone therapy based on assessments of withdrawal-symptom suppression at times of expected peak activity (i.e., 2–4 hours after a methadone hydrochloride dose). Dosage adjustments should be cautious, in order to avoid overdosage. With continued dosing, symptoms will be suppressed for longer periods of time as the drug accumulates in body tissues. In most patients, a daily dosage of 40 mg of methadone hydrochloride in single or divided doses will usually constitute an adequate stabilizing dosage level, but higher dosage may be required. When the patient has been stabilized (i.e., substantial symptoms of withdrawal are absent) for 2 or 3 days, dosage of methadone hydrochloride can be gradually decreased daily or at 2-day intervals. Dosage must be individualized and adjusted to keep withdrawal symptoms at a tolerable level. In hospitalized patients, dosage can usually be reduced by 20% daily, but a more gradual reduction may be required in ambulatory patients.

For short-term detoxification, methadone must be administered daily while the patient is under close observation in reducing dosages over a period not exceeding 30 days. For long-term detoxification, methadone must be administered in a regimen designed to reach a drug-free state within 180 days or less. Take-home medication may be allowed during long-term detoxification if certain conditions are met (see Maintenance under Dosage: Detoxification and Maintenance of Opiate Dependence, in Dosage and Administration). Individuals with 2 or more unsuccessful detoxification episodes within a 12-month period should be evaluated for alternative forms of treatment. An opiate-dependency treatment program may not admit an individual for more than 2 detoxification treatments within one year.

Maintenance. Interim (minimum service) maintenance treatment is that which is provided in conjunction with appropriate medical services while a patient is awaiting transfer to comprehensive maintenance treatment. A maintenance program that is unable to place a patient requesting treatment into a comprehensive maintenance treatment program within 14 days of application for admission and within a reasonable geographic area may place the patient in an interim maintenance treatment program until placement in a comprehensive program is possible. A patient may *not* continue in an interim treatment program for longer than 120 days in any 12-month period, and must be transferred to a comprehensive program after 120 days in an interim program if still in need of treatment. A patient admitted to an interim maintenance program is required to be administered each daily methadone dose while being closely observed, and take-home medication is *not* allowed. Although most requirements for comprehensive maintenance treatment apply to interim maintenance treatment, some do *not* apply. (See Uses: Detoxification and Maintenance of Opiate Dependence.)

When methadone hydrochloride is used to initiate maintenance treatment, the initial dose should be based on the opiate tolerance of the patient. A single oral dose of 20–30 mg of methadone hydrochloride will often suppress withdrawal symptoms. The initial dose should not exceed 30 mg. Initial doses should be lower for patients whose tolerance is expected to be low at treatment initiation. Loss of tolerance should be considered if more than 5 days have elapsed since the patient took opiates. Initial doses should not be based on those used during prior treatment episodes or on the patient's expenditures for illicit drugs. If there is any doubt, it is usually safer to start with a smaller dose and keep the patient under observation. Additional doses of methadone hydrochloride may be necessary if withdrawal symptoms are not suppressed or if they reappear. The manufacturer states that if same-day dosage adjustments are to be made, the patient should be reevaluated 2–4 hours after the previous dose, since peak plasma concentrations of methadone will have been attained. If an additional dose is required to suppress withdrawal symptoms, an additional 5–10 mg of methadone hydrochloride may be administered. The total dose on the first day should not exceed 40 mg unless it is documented that this total dose does not suppress withdrawal symptoms.

Subsequent dosage should be adjusted according to the requirements and response of the patient. Dosage adjustments should be made over the first week of methadone treatment based on assessments of withdrawal-symptom suppression at times of expected peak activity (i.e., 2–4 hours after a methadone hydrochloride dose). Dosage adjustments should be cautious, in order to avoid overdosage. With continued dosing, symptoms will be suppressed for longer periods of time as the drug accumulates in body tissues. Dosage should be titrated to a level at which opiate symptoms are prevented for 24 hours, drug craving is reduced, the euphoric effects of self-administered opiates are blocked or attenuated, and tolerance to the sedative effect of methadone is evident. It has been suggested that trough plasma methadone concentrations exceeding 100–200 ng/mL may be necessary to optimize the success of methadone maintenance, particularly during the first 6 months of treatment. Stabilization of maintenance dosage usually occurs at 80–120 mg daily, although higher dosage is sometimes required. A single dose of methadone daily usually adequately maintains the patient and there generally is no apparent advantage to divided doses. However, rapid metabolizers of methadone may not maintain adequate plasma methadone concentrations with usual dosing regimens. Highly motivated patients may be maintained on dosage as low as 20–30 mg daily.

Because levomethadyl acetate hydrochloride is no longer commercially available in the US, patients receiving maintenance treatment with the drug should be transferred to alternative treatments. Patients maintained on levomethadyl acetate hydrochloride can be transferred to methadone. Methadone hydrochloride can be initiated at a daily dose that is 80% of the levomethadyl acetate hydrochloride dose; the initial methadone dose must be given no sooner than 48 hours after the last levomethadyl acetate hydrochloride dose. Subsequent doses of methadone hydrochloride may be increased or decreased in increments of 5–10 mg daily to control manifestations of withdrawal or excess sedation according to clinical observation.

Experience with the transfer of patients from methadone maintenance to buprenorphine is limited.

Any individual in a comprehensive maintenance treatment program, including long-term detoxification treatment, may receive one daily dose of methadone to take at home for a day that the clinic is closed. Decisions to allow additional unsupervised administration by these individuals should be based on the following factors: absence of recent abuse of drugs (including alcohol), regularity of clinic attendance, absence of serious behavioral problems at the clinic, absence of known recent criminal activity, stability of the individual's home environment and social relationships, length of time in the program, assurance that the drug can be safely stored in the individual's home, and assessment of whether the rehabilitative benefit derived from decreased clinic attendance outweighs potential risks of diversion. Individuals meeting these criteria may be permitted to receive additional supplies of the drug to take at home each week, in the following amounts: 1-day supply during the first 90 days of treatment, 2-day supply during the second 90 days, and 3-day supply during the third 90 days (each in addition to the one dose allowed for clinic closure). All other doses must be administered while the individual is closely observed. During the remainder of the first year of treatment, individuals may receive a maximum 6-day supply of methadone and must visit the clinic once weekly. After 1 year of continuous treatment, individuals may receive a maximum 2-week supply of methadone and must make twice monthly visits. After 2 years of continuous treatment, the individual may receive a maximum 1-month supply of the drug and must make monthly visits.

Maintenance dosage requirements should be reviewed regularly and reduced as indicated. In patients desiring medically supervised withdrawal from methadone maintenance treatment, there is considerable variability in the appropriate rate of methadone dosage reduction; dosage generally should be reduced at intervals of 10–14 days by an amount that is less than 10% of the established tolerance or maintenance dosage. All patients in a maintenance program should be given careful consideration for discontinuance of methadone therapy, especially after reaching a dosage of 10–20 mg daily.

Neonatal Opiate Withdrawal For the management of neonatal opiate abstinence syndrome†, use of standardized protocols that base initiation, adjustment, and tapering of methadone hydrochloride dosage on standardized patient assessments performed at regular intervals is recommended. The most commonly used tool for assessing severity of withdrawal in term neonates is the Finnegan scoring system (original or modified versions) performed every 3–4 hours. Treatment with methadone hydrochloride oral solution generally is initiated at a dose of 0.05–0.1 mg/kg based on Finnegan score (e.g., score is 8 or greater on 2 or 3 occasions, a single score or 2 consecutive scores are 12 or greater). However, protocols vary in initial dosing frequency, incremental changes and thresholds for dosage adjustment, and tapering strategies. In general, dosage may be escalated if Finnegan score remains elevated (e.g., 2 consecutive scores are 8 or greater, one score is 12 or greater), and dosage is tapered once patients are stable (e.g., no score exceeds 8 or average score is less than 8 for 24 hours).

Some protocols are based on pharmacokinetic modeling of methadone in neonates and utilize a stepwise approach to dosage escalation and tapering. Under such protocols, methadone hydrochloride may be administered at an initial dose of 0.1 mg/kg; dosing intervals are shorter during the initial steps of the protocol, but then are lengthened to and maintained at 12 hours while the dose is tapered, if tolerated, by a modest amount every 24 hours until the dosage of the drug has been reduced to 0.01 mg/kg once daily. The drug may then be discontinued. Such protocols increase early exposure to the drug, and limited experience suggests that such an approach may allow for shorter treatment durations and hospital stays. Other clinicians have recommended administration of methadone hydrochloride at an initial dosage of 0.05–0.1 mg/kg every 12 hours; dosage increases, when indicated, in increments of 0.02–0.05 mg/kg per dose or 10%; a maximum dosage of 1 mg/kg daily; and/or tapering schedules of 10–20% per week. Following discontinuance of methadone, neonates should be monitored for 48–72 hours. Specialized protocols should be consulted for further information on methadone hydrochloride dosage and monitoring of Finnegan scores in neonates with opiate abstinence syndrome. Further study is needed to define optimal dosing strategies.

Cautions

Methadone shares the toxic potentials of the opiate agonists, and the usual precautions of opiate agonist therapy should be observed. (See Cautions in the Opiate Agonists General Statement 28:08.08.)

Death and life-threatening adverse effects, including respiratory depression and cardiac arrhythmias, have occurred during initiation of methadone for the treatment of pain and in patients being transferred to methadone from other opiate therapy, possibly as a result of inadvertent overdosage, drug interactions, and adverse cardiac effects of the drug.

While serious, life-threatening, or fatal respiratory depression can occur at any time during therapy, the risk is greatest during initiation of therapy and following dosage increases. In some cases, respiratory depression has occurred when methadone was used as recommended and was not misused or abused. Deaths have been reported in patients being transferred to methadone from chronic therapy with high dosages of other opiate analgesics; deaths also have been reported during initiation of methadone maintenance treatment for opiate dependence in individuals who previously used high dosages of other opiates. An understanding of methadone's pharmacokinetic and pharmacodynamic properties is crucial for safe use of the drug. Methadone's elimination half-life (8–59 hours) is substantially longer than the duration of its analgesic action (4–8 hours); in addition, peak respiratory depressant effects of the drug typically occur later and persist longer than its peak analgesic effect, particularly during the early dosing period. The full analgesic effect usually is not attained for 3–5 days. These properties can contribute to inadvertent overdosage, particularly during treatment initiation and dosage adjustment. Methadone should be prescribed only by clinicians who are experienced in the use of potent opiates for the treatment of chronic pain. Methadone dosage should be selected carefully and titrated slowly, even in opiate-tolerant patients, and patients should be monitored carefully during treatment initiation, transfer to methadone from other opiate therapy, and dosage titration.

Prolongation of the QT interval and serious cardiac arrhythmias, including torsades de pointes, have been reported in patients receiving methadone. Most of the reported cases have occurred in patients receiving methadone at relatively high dosages (more than 200 mg daily) for the treatment of chronic pain, but cases also have been reported in patients receiving methadone maintenance therapy at lower dosages. In most cases involving patients receiving usual methadone maintenance dosages, concomitant drug therapy and/or conditions such as hypokalemia were identified as contributing factors. Methadone should be used for pain management only when the potential benefit from the drug outweighs the possible risk of QT-interval prolongation that has been reported with higher methadone dosages. Patients should be monitored closely for changes in cardiac rhythm during initiation of therapy and following increases in dosage. In addition, methadone should be used with caution and careful monitoring in patients who may be at risk for development of prolonged QT syndrome (e.g., those with cardiac hypertrophy, hypokalemia, or hypomagnesemia; those receiving methadone at relatively high dosages or receiving concomitant therapy with a drug that may cause electrolyte disturbances or prolong the QT interval [see Drug Interactions: Drugs that Prolong QT Interval]). If prolongation of the QT interval occurs in a patient receiving methadone, the patient's drug regimen should be evaluated to identify drugs that may prolong the QT interval, cause electrolyte abnormalities, or inhibit metabolism of methadone. Use of methadone in patients with known prolongation of the QT interval has not been systematically evaluated.

Profound sedation, respiratory depression, coma, and death may occur when opiate agonists are used concomitantly with benzodiazepines or other CNS depressants. Concomitant use of opiate analgesics and other CNS depressants should be reserved for patients in whom alternative treatment options are inadequate; the lowest effective dosages and shortest possible duration of concomitant therapy should be used, and the patient should be monitored closely for respiratory depression and sedation. Patients receiving methadone and/or their caregivers should be apprised of the risks associated with concomitant therapeutic or illicit use of benzodiazepines, alcohol, or other CNS depressants. Concomitant use with alcohol should be avoided. (See Drug Interactions: Alcohol and also see Drug Interactions: Benzodiazepines and Other CNS Depressants.)

Because the morbidity and mortality associated with untreated opiate addiction can outweigh the serious risks associated with concomitant use of opiates and benzodiazepines or other CNS depressants, FDA states that methadone treatment for opiate addiction (i.e., medication-assisted treatment [MAT]) should not be withheld from patients receiving benzodiazepines or other CNS depressants. These drugs should be tapered and discontinued, if possible, in patients receiving MAT. However, excluding or discharging patients from MAT because of benzodiazepine or CNS depressant use is not likely to prevent such concomitant use and may lead to use outside the treatment setting, which could result in more severe outcomes. Careful management can reduce the risks associated with concomitant use of benzodiazepines or other CNS depressants in patients receiving methadone treatment for opiate addiction. FDA states that benzodiazepines are not the treatment of choice for anxiety or insomnia in patients receiving methadone treatment for opiate addiction; other pharmacologic or nonpharmacologic therapies should be considered. FDA also states that current evidence does not support dose limitations or other arbitrary limits on methadone as a strategy for addressing concomitant benzodiazepine or other CNS depressant use in patients receiving MAT. However, in patients who are sedated at the time of a scheduled methadone dose, the cause of sedation should be evaluated and omission or reduction of the methadone dose may be appropriate.

Precautions recommended by FDA for minimizing risks associated with concomitant use of benzodiazepines or other CNS depressants in patients receiving MAT include the following:

- Patient education upon initiation of MAT regarding the risks associated with concomitant use of benzodiazepines or other CNS depressants;
- Development of strategies upon initiation of MAT for managing any prescribed or illicit use of benzodiazepines or other CNS depressants;
- Verification of the diagnosis in any patient receiving prescribed benzodiazepines or other CNS depressants for anxiety or insomnia, and consideration of other treatment options for these conditions;
- Recognition that MAT may be required indefinitely and should be continued for as long as the patient derives benefit and MAT contributes to the intended treatment goals;
- Coordination of care to minimize risks and ensure that other prescribers are aware that the patient is receiving methadone treatment; and
- Toxicology screening to monitor for prescribed or illicit drug use.

Patients should be instructed to take methadone exactly as prescribed and advised not to initiate or discontinue use of other drugs or dietary supplements without consulting their clinician; patients also should be informed of the signs and symptoms of overdosage and symptoms suggestive of a cardiac arrhythmia, and advised to seek immediate medical attention if such manifestations occur.

Serotonin syndrome has been reported during concomitant use of opiate agonists, including methadone, and serotonergic drugs at recommended dosages. Manifestations of serotonin syndrome may include mental status changes (e.g., agitation, hallucinations, coma), autonomic instability (e.g., tachycardia, labile blood pressure, hyperthermia), neuromuscular aberrations (e.g., hyperreflexia, incoordination, rigidity), and/or GI symptoms (e.g., nausea, vomiting, diarrhea). Symptom onset generally occurs within several hours to a few days of concomitant use, but may occur later, particularly after dosage increases. (See Drug Interactions: Drugs Associated with Serotonin Syndrome.)

Patients who are tolerant to other opiate agonists may have incomplete tolerance to methadone; therefore, methadone should be used with caution and at appropriately adjusted dosages in patients being transferred to methadone from other opiate therapy. Overdosage of methadone (sometimes fatal) has been reported in patients being transferred from chronic, high-dose therapy with other opiate analgesics to therapy with methadone. Pharmacokinetic parameters must be carefully considered during initiation and titration of methadone therapy in patients who previously received chronic opiate agonist therapy. (See Dosage and Administration: Dosage.)

Inadvertent ingestion of methadone, particularly by children, may result in fatal overdosage.

Deaths associated with illicit use of methadone frequently have involved concomitant abuse of benzodiazepines.

Methadone overdosage has been reported to induce pulmonary edema. During methadone maintenance treatment, most adverse effects disappear over a period of several weeks; however, constipation and excessive sweating often persist.

In patients receiving methadone maintenance treatment for opiate dependence, abrupt discontinuance of the drug can result in withdrawal symptoms and may increase the risk of relapse to illicit drug use. Anxiety in a patient receiving methadone maintenance treatment should not be confused with withdrawal syndrome and should not be treated with an increase in methadone dosage.

Patients receiving methadone maintenance treatment for opiate dependence who experience physical trauma or other acute (e.g., postoperative) pain should not be expected to derive adequate analgesia from their stable methadone regimen. Such patients should receive analgesics, including opiates, that would be appropriate for other patients experiencing similar nociceptive stimulation. Opiate doses may be somewhat higher or dosing intervals somewhat shorter than those used in non-opiate-tolerant patients.

Use of methadone has not been extensively evaluated in patients with renal or hepatic impairment. Because methadone is metabolized in the liver, patients with hepatic impairment may be at risk for accumulation of the drug with repeated administration.

■ Pediatric Precautions The manufacturers state that safety, efficacy, and pharmacokinetics of methadone in pediatric patients younger than 18 years of age have not been established.

Short- or long-term *detoxification* treatment using methadone is not subject to any age limitation. However, the effects of prolonged methadone use on the physiologic and psychologic development of children are not known; therefore, *maintenance* treatment with the drug should not be initiated indiscriminately in children younger than 18 years of age. Children younger than 18 years of age are eligible to receive maintenance treatment with methadone provided they have undergone at least 2 documented attempts at detoxification or drug-free treatment within a 12-month period and the program physician has documented that the child continues to be, or is again, physiologically dependent on opiates. In addition, signed informed consent must be obtained from a parent, legal guardian, or responsible adult designated by the appropriate local (e.g., state) authority (e.g., via emancipated minor laws).

■ Pregnancy and Lactation ***Pregnancy*** Methadone should be used during pregnancy only when the potential benefits justify the possible risks. Because of the drug's long duration of effect, use of methadone for obstetric analgesia is not recommended since there may be an increased risk of neonatal respiratory depression.

Untreated opiate addiction during pregnancy is associated with adverse obstetrical outcomes, including preeclampsia, fetal growth restriction, preterm birth, spontaneous abortion, and fetal death. In addition, untreated opiate addiction often results in continued or relapsing illicit opiate use and engagement in high-risk behaviors. The recommended treatment of opiate dependence in pregnant women is maintenance treatment with methadone or buprenorphine; this approach is superior to medically supervised withdrawal (i.e., detoxification) because withdrawal is associated with high relapse rates and poorer outcomes.

Short- or long-term *detoxification* treatment using methadone is *not* recommended during pregnancy. However, pregnant women, regardless of age, are eligible for admission into a comprehensive *maintenance* treatment program using methadone if they have a history of documented opiate dependence and are considered at risk of possibly returning to such dependence (and all its attendant risks) during pregnancy. For such women, evidence of *current* physiologic dependence is not necessary, provided the program physician certifies the pregnancy and considers such therapy medically justified using reasonable clinical judgment. All pregnant women admitted into a maintenance program with methadone must be given the opportunity for prenatal care either by the program or by referral to an appropriate health-care provider. Such women should be advised of the possible risks to them and their fetus from continued use of illicit drugs and from the use and withdrawal of methadone as part of maintenance or detoxification treatment.

Pharmacokinetic data from a limited number of pregnant women suggest that methadone clearance may be increased, trough plasma concentrations of the drug may be lower, and half-life of the drug may be decreased during the second and third trimesters of pregnancy compared with pharmacokinetic values determined for the same women postpartum or for nonpregnant opiate-dependent women. If methadone is used during pregnancy, dosage adjustment (i.e., increased dose or decreased dosing interval) may be necessary.

Studies of methadone use during pregnancy generally have compared benefits of methadone maintenance treatment with the risks of untreated dependence on illicit drugs; the relevance of these findings to use of methadone as an analgesic during pregnancy is unclear. Pregnant women in methadone maintenance programs receive better prenatal care, with fewer obstetric and fetal complications and reduced neonatal morbidity and mortality, compared with women using illicit drugs. Available data suggest that maternal use of methadone during pregnancy as part of a supervised therapeutic regimen is unlikely to pose a substantial teratogenic risk; however, data are insufficient to fully exclude such risk. Most information regarding pregnancy outcomes involves methadone exposure after the first trimester, and information on methadone dosage and duration of use during pregnancy is limited. Interpretation of available information on pregnancy outcomes also is complicated by maternal factors such as illicit drug use, nutritional status, presence of infections, and psychosocial circumstances.

In a double-blind, randomized, controlled trial (Maternal Opioid Treatment: Human Experimental Research [MOTHER]), outcomes, principally opiate withdrawal effects, were assessed in neonates born to women who received methadone or buprenorphine treatment for opiate dependence during pregnancy. Enrollment in the study occurred at an average gestational age of 18.7 weeks. Prior to the end of pregnancy, 18% of methadone-treated women and 33% of buprenorphine-treated women discontinued treatment; outcomes were evaluated for the neonates whose mothers remained in treatment until delivery. No difference was observed between methadone- and buprenorphine-exposed neonates in the proportion of neonates requiring treatment for opiate withdrawal syndrome or the peak severity of the syndrome. Buprenorphine-exposed neonates required a lower total mean morphine sulfate dosage for treatment of withdrawal (1.1 versus 10.4 mg), had shorter hospital stays (10 versus 17.5 days), and shorter duration of treatment for withdrawal (4.1 versus 9.9 days) compared with methadone-exposed neonates. The groups did not differ in other outcome measures (head circumference, weight and length at birth, preterm birth, gestational age at delivery, and 1- and 5-minute Apgar scores) or in the rates of serious maternal or neonatal adverse events. The imbalance in treatment discontinuance rates between methadone- and buprenorphine-treated women complicate interpretation of the study findings.

A retrospective review of pregnancy outcomes for women who underwent inpatient methadone detoxification did not reveal any increase in the risk of spontaneous abortion during the second trimester or premature delivery during the third trimester, although other studies have suggested an increased risk of premature delivery in opiate-dependent women who received methadone during pregnancy. Several studies have suggested that use of methadone in opiate-dependent women during pregnancy results in decreased fetal growth (with reduced birth weight, length, and/or head circumference), but this growth deficit does not appear to persist into later childhood. However, mild but persistent deficits in psychometric and behavioral test performance have been observed in children who were exposed to methadone in utero. In addition, several studies have suggested that the risk of visual developmental anomalies may be increased in children born to opiate-dependent women who received methadone during pregnancy. There are conflicting reports on whether maternal use of methadone during pregnancy is associated with a higher incidence of sudden infant death syndrome. During late pregnancy, results of fetal nonstress tests reportedly are more likely to be abnormal when the tests are performed 1–2 hours after a maintenance dose of methadone than when they are performed in control subjects.

Methadone has been detected in cord blood and amniotic fluid at concentrations proportional to maternal plasma concentrations.

Prolonged maternal use of opiate agonists during pregnancy can result in neonatal opiate withdrawal syndrome with manifestations of irritability, hyperactivity and abnormal sleep pattern, high-pitched cry, tremor, vomiting, diarrhea, and failure to gain weight. In contrast to adults, the withdrawal syndrome in neonates may be life-threatening if not recognized and treated, and requires management according to protocols developed by neonatology experts. Women who require prolonged opiate agonist therapy during pregnancy should be advised of the risk of neonatal opiate withdrawal syndrome, and availability of appropriate treatment should be ensured. The onset, duration, and severity of the syndrome vary depending on the specific opiate agonist used, duration of use, timing and amount of last maternal use, and rate of drug elimination by the neonate. Use of standardized protocols for identification and management of opiate withdrawal syndrome has been shown to improve overall response, including reductions in hospital stay and duration of pharmacologic treatment. When environmental and supportive measures are inadequate, opiates (e.g., methadone) are recommended as first-line pharmacologic therapy. (See Uses: Neonatal Opiate Withdrawal.)

Although no teratogenic effects were observed in rats or rabbits given methadone, administration of large doses of the drug in guinea pigs, hamsters, and mice resulted in teratogenic effects including exencephaly and cranioschisis. When male rodents were given methadone prior to mating, their offspring exhibited decreased weight gain after weaning, increased neonatal mortality, reduced thymus weight (male progeny), increased adrenal weight (female progeny), and physiologic and behavioral changes; increased embryolethality and preimplantation deaths also have been reported. Perinatal exposure to methadone in rats has been associated with alterations in learning ability, motor activity, thermal regulation, nociceptive responses, and sensitivity to other drugs. Animal data also indicate neurochemical changes in the brains of methadone-treated offspring, including changes to the cholinergic, dopaminergic, noradrenergic, and serotonergic systems.

Lactation Methadone is distributed into human milk. Peak concentrations in milk reportedly occur approximately 4–5 hours after an oral dose of the drug. In 2 studies in 22 nursing women who were receiving methadone maintenance treatment, methadone was present in low concentrations in milk, but no adverse effects on breast-fed infants were observed. At maternal oral dosages of 10–80 mg daily, reported concentrations of methadone in milk were

50–570 ng/mL; in most of the milk samples, methadone concentrations were lower than maternal steady-state serum concentrations of the drug. At maternal oral dosages of 20–80 mg daily, the mean infant dosage of the drug, calculated based on an assumed average milk consumption of 150 mL/kg daily, was approximately 17.4 mcg/kg daily, which was approximately 2–3.5% of the oral maternal dosage. Methadone has been detected in very low plasma concentrations in some infants whose mothers were receiving methadone. Cases of sedation and respiratory depression in infants exposed to methadone through breast milk have been reported rarely.

Experts recommend that women who are stable on methadone treatment for opiate dependence, are not using other illicit drugs, and have no contraindications to nursing be encouraged to breast-feed their infants; to lower the risk of return to substance use, women receiving methadone should be encouraged to continue treatment during the postpartum period. Breast-feeding has been associated with decreased severity of neonatal opiate withdrawal syndrome, decreased need for pharmacotherapy, and shorter hospital stays for the neonate. The manufacturers state that the benefits of breast-feeding should be considered along with the mother's clinical need for the drug and any potential adverse effects on the breast-fed infant from either the drug or the underlying maternal condition. Women who are receiving methadone and are breast-feeding or wish to breast-feed should be advised that the drug distributes into human milk, should be instructed to recognize respiratory depression and sedation in infants and to know when to seek medical care, and should be informed that nursing should be discontinued gradually (not abruptly) in order to prevent withdrawal (neonatal abstinence syndrome) in the infant.

Drug Interactions

■ Drugs Affecting Hepatic Microsomal Enzymes

Methadone is metabolized principally by the cytochrome P-450 (CYP) microsomal enzyme system, mainly by isoenzymes 3A4, 2B6, and 2C19 and to a lesser extent by isoenzymes 2C9 and 2D6. Concomitant use of methadone with drugs that induce CYP isoenzymes may result in increased metabolism and decreased plasma concentrations of methadone. Conversely, administration of methadone with drugs that inhibit CYP3A4 and/or CYP2C9 may result in decreased metabolism and increased plasma concentrations of methadone. Therefore, methadone should be used with caution in patients receiving drugs that inhibit or induce these CYP isoenzymes, and patients receiving such drugs concomitantly should be monitored carefully.

Alcohol Chronic consumption of alcohol has been reported to increase metabolism of methadone and reduce serum concentrations of the drug; however, acute consumption of alcohol has been reported to increase the area under the plasma concentration-time curve (AUC) of methadone, resulting in an increased potential for adverse effects. Concomitant use of opiate agonists and CNS depressants, including alcohol, may result in profound sedation, respiratory depression, coma, and death. (See Drug Interactions: Benzodiazepines and Other CNS Depressants.)

Anticonvulsants Administration of phenytoin, phenobarbital, or carbamazepine in patients receiving methadone may result in increased metabolism of methadone secondary to induction of CYP3A4. Concomitant use of phenytoin (250 mg twice daily for 24 hours followed by 300 mg daily for 3–4 days) in patients receiving methadone maintenance therapy reduced plasma concentrations of methadone by 50% and resulted in withdrawal symptoms. Withdrawal symptoms also may occur in patients receiving methadone concomitantly with phenobarbital or carbamazepine.

Antidepressants Concomitant use of certain selective serotonin-reuptake inhibitors (SSRIs) (e.g., sertraline, fluoxetine, fluvoxamine) may increase serum methadone concentrations and increase opiate effects secondary to inhibition of methadone metabolism.

Concomitant use of desipramine with methadone may result in increased serum desipramine concentrations. Opiate agonists (including methadone) may potentiate the effects of tricyclic antidepressants (see Drug Interactions: Antidepressants, in the Opiate Agonists General Statement 28:08.08).

Concomitant use of methadone and antidepressants also may result in serotonin syndrome. (See Drug Interactions: Drugs Associated with Serotonin Syndrome.)

Antifungals Administration of azole antifungal agents that are known to inhibit the CYP3A4 isoenzyme (e.g., fluconazole, ketoconazole, itraconazole, voriconazole) in patients receiving methadone may result in decreased clearance of methadone. Administration of fluconazole (200 mg daily) has been shown to increase the AUC and peak plasma concentrations of methadone by 35 and 27%, respectively. Administration of voriconazole increased steady-state peak plasma concentrations and AUC of the pharmacologically active *R*-isomer of methadone by 31 and 47%, respectively, in individuals receiving methadone maintenance treatment (30–100 mg daily). Because of the potential for increased or prolonged opiate agonist effects, patients receiving these agents concomitantly should be carefully monitored and methadone dosage should be adjusted as necessary.

Antimycobacterials Administration of rifampin in patients receiving methadone therapy has reduced serum methadone concentrations and resulted in withdrawal symptoms.

Antiretrovirals Approximately 25–30% of patients receiving methadone maintenance therapy are HIV-positive, and numerous drug interactions have been reported in HIV-positive patients receiving antiretroviral agents concomitantly with methadone. Clinicians should monitor patients carefully for potential adverse effects when antiretroviral agents are used concomitantly with methadone.

Abacavir. Concomitant use of methadone and abacavir increased methadone clearance by 22%. Some experts state that dosage adjustment is not necessary in patients receiving the drugs concomitantly. The manufacturer states that patients receiving concomitant therapy with abacavir and methadone should be monitored closely for opiate withdrawal, and methadone dosage should be increased as clinically indicated.

Atazanavir. Concomitant use of methadone and atazanavir does not substantially alter plasma concentrations of either drug. No dosage adjustment is necessary.

Concomitant use of methadone and *ritonavir-boosted* atazanavir decreased plasma concentrations of *R*-methadone by about 16–18%. Opiate withdrawal is unlikely but may occur. Patients should be monitored for opiate withdrawal, and methadone dosage should be increased as clinically indicated.

Darunavir. Concomitant use of methadone and *ritonavir-boosted* darunavir decreased the AUC of methadone by 16%. Opiate withdrawal is unlikely but may occur. Patients should be carefully monitored for opiate withdrawal, and methadone dosage should be increased as clinically indicated.

Delavirdine. Concomitant use of delavirdine and methadone may increase plasma concentrations of methadone. Patients receiving concomitant delavirdine and methadone therapy should be closely monitored for methadone toxicity; methadone dosage may need to be reduced.

Didanosine. Concomitant use of methadone and buffered didanosine preparations appears to decrease bioavailability of didanosine. In a limited number of individuals, concomitant use of methadone and buffered didanosine resulted in a 66% decrease in the peak serum concentration and 63% decrease in the AUC of didanosine; trough concentrations of methadone did not appear to be affected. Concomitant use of methadone and didanosine delayed-release capsules does not affect the pharmacokinetics of didanosine; dosage adjustments are not necessary with this preparation.

Efavirenz. Administration of methadone hydrochloride (35–100 mg daily) and efavirenz (600 mg daily for 14–21 days) in HIV-infected individuals with a history of drug dependence decreased the peak plasma concentration and AUC of methadone by 45 and 52%, respectively, and resulted in manifestations of opiate withdrawal. The maintenance dosage of methadone hydrochloride was increased by an average of 22% to alleviate withdrawal symptoms.

Individuals receiving concurrent methadone and efavirenz therapy should be informed of this potential interaction and closely monitored for signs of opiate withdrawal; an increase in the maintenance dosage of methadone frequently is necessary in such individuals.

Elvitegravir, Cobicistat, Tenofovir, and Emtricitabine. Concomitant use of methadone and the fixed combination of elvitegravir, cobicistat, tenofovir, and emtricitabine does not substantially affect plasma concentrations of any of the concomitantly administered drugs. No dosage adjustment is necessary.

Etravirine. Concomitant use of etravirine and methadone does not appear to affect plasma concentrations of either drug. Dosage adjustment is not needed.

Fosamprenavir. Concomitant use of methadone and amprenavir (no longer commercially available in the US) decreased trough plasma concentrations of *R*-methadone by 21% but did not substantially alter the AUC of methadone. Because fosamprenavir is metabolized to amprenavir, interactions reported with amprenavir are expected to occur in patients receiving fosamprenavir. Patients receiving methadone concomitantly with fosamprenavir should be carefully monitored and methadone dosage should be adjusted as necessary.

Concomitant use of methadone and *ritonavir-boosted* fosamprenavir decreased the AUC of *R*-methadone by 18%. Opiate withdrawal is unlikely but may occur. Patients should be monitored for opiate withdrawal, and methadone dosage should be increased as clinically indicated.

Indinavir. Concomitant use of methadone and indinavir does not appear to substantially affect exposure to either drug.

Lopinavir. Concomitant use of methadone and the fixed combination of lopinavir and ritonavir (lopinavir/ritonavir) decreased the AUC of methadone by 26–53%; opiate withdrawal symptoms may occur. Patients should be monitored closely for opiate withdrawal, and methadone dosage should be increased as clinically indicated.

Maraviroc. No data are available regarding concomitant use of maraviroc and methadone. Some experts state that maraviroc is considered safe for use in patients receiving methadone.

Nelfinavir. Concomitant use of methadone and nelfinavir may result in decreased plasma concentrations of methadone; opiate withdrawal occurs rarely. Individuals receiving concomitant methadone and nelfinavir therapy should be closely monitored for signs of opiate withdrawal; an increase in the maintenance dosage of methadone may be necessary.

Nevirapine. There have been reports of opiate withdrawal and subtherapeutic or decreased serum methadone concentrations following initiation of nevirapine therapy in individuals who were receiving long-term methadone treatment for opiate addiction. nevirapine has been reported to decrease the AUC of methadone by 37–51%.

Individuals receiving concomitant methadone and nevirapine therapy should be informed of this potential interaction, and should be closely monitored for signs of opiate withdrawal when nevirapine therapy is initiated; an increase in the maintenance dosage of methadone frequently is necessary. If methadone dosage is increased during nevirapine therapy, patients should be monitored for methadone overdosage when the antiretroviral agent is discontinued.

Raltegravir. Concomitant use of methadone and raltegravir does not substantially affect plasma concentrations of either drug. Dosage adjustment is not necessary in patients receiving the drugs concomitantly.

Rilpivirine. Rilpivirine has been reported to decrease the AUC of methadone by 16%. No dosage adjustment is necessary, but patients should be monitored for withdrawal symptoms.

Ritonavir. Administration of a single 5-mg dose of methadone hydrochloride and ritonavir (500 mg every 12 hours for 15 days) decreased the AUC of methadone by 36%. There has been at least one report of opiate withdrawal and subtherapeutic or decreased serum methadone concentrations following initiation of ritonavir therapy in an HIV-infected patient who was receiving long-term methadone treatment for opiate addiction.

Methadone should be administered with caution in patients receiving ritonavir, especially when used in combination with other drugs that may decrease plasma concentrations of methadone. Individuals receiving concomitant methadone and ritonavir therapy should be informed of this potential interaction, and should be closely monitored for manifestations of opiate withdrawal when ritonavir therapy is initiated; an increase in the maintenance dosage of methadone may be necessary. If methadone dosage is increased during ritonavir therapy, patients should be monitored for methadone overdosage when the antiretroviral agent is discontinued.

Saquinavir. Concomitant use of methadone and *ritonavir-boosted* saquinavir decreased the AUC of *R*-methadone by 19%. Opiate withdrawal is unlikely but may occur. Patients should be monitored closely for opiate withdrawal, and methadone dosage should be increased as clinically indicated.

Stavudine. Concomitant use of stavudine and methadone appears to decrease bioavailability of stavudine. In a limited number of individuals, concomitant use of stavudine and methadone resulted in a 44% decrease in peak concentrations and a 25% decrease in the AUC of stavudine; trough concentrations of methadone did not appear to be affected. Dosage adjustment is not necessary in patients receiving the drugs concomitantly.

Tenofovir. Concomitant use of tenofovir and methadone does not appear to affect plasma concentrations of either drug.

Tipranavir. Concomitant use of methadone and *ritonavir-boosted* tipranavir decreased peak plasma concentrations and AUC of *R*-methadone by 46 and 48%, respectively. Patients should be monitored closely for opiate withdrawal, and methadone dosage should be increased as clinically indicated.

Zidovudine. In one study in IV drug abusers with HIV infection who were receiving long-term methadone hydrochloride treatment for opiate addiction (30–90 mg daily), initiation of zidovudine therapy (200 mg orally every 4 hours) did not appear to have any clinically important effects on the pharmacokinetics of methadone and did not result in any evidence of opiate withdrawal. However, the AUC of zidovudine was increased about 43% in patients receiving concomitant methadone compared with those receiving zidovudine alone. In another study in HIV-infected individuals who had been receiving methadone treatment for approximately 2 months, concomitant use of oral or IV zidovudine increased the zidovudine AUC by 29 or 41%, respectively, and reduced the clearance of zidovudine by about 26%. While the mechanism of this interaction requires further study, limited data indicate that methadone inhibits zidovudine glucuronidation and also reduces renal clearance of zidovudine.

Based on the results of these studies, it appears that the maintenance dosage of methadone probably does not need to be adjusted when zidovudine therapy is initiated in patients receiving long-term methadone treatment; however, the clinical importance of the increased zidovudine AUC during concomitant therapy is unclear. Patients receiving concomitant zidovudine and methadone therapy should be monitored for dose-related zidovudine toxicity.

Macrolide Antibiotics Administration of macrolide anti-infectives that are known to inhibit CYP3A4 (e.g., clarithromycin, erythromycin, telithromycin) may result in decreased clearance of methadone. Patients receiving methadone concomitantly with macrolide anti-infectives should be carefully monitored and methadone dosage should be adjusted as necessary.

Smoking Some evidence indicates that cigarette smoking increases CYP1A2 activity and may reduce plasma methadone concentrations.

St. John's Wort Manifestations of opiate withdrawal may occur in patients receiving methadone and St. John's wort (*Hypericum perforatum*) concomitantly, since St. John's wort may increase metabolism of methadone via induction of CYP3A4. Patients receiving methadone concomitantly with St. John's wort should be carefully monitored, and methadone dosage should be adjusted as necessary.

Concomitant use of methadone and St. John's wort also may result in serotonin syndrome. (See Drug Interactions: Drugs Associated with Serotonin Syndrome.)

■ **Benzodiazepines and Other CNS Depressants.** Concomitant use of opiate agonists, including methadone, and benzodiazepines or other CNS depressants (e.g., anxiolytics, sedatives, hypnotics, tranquilizers, muscle relaxants, general anesthetics, antipsychotics, other opiate agonists, alcohol) may result in profound sedation, respiratory depression, coma, and death. (See Drug Interactions: Benzodiazepines and Other CNS Depressants, in the Opiate Agonists General Statement 28:08.08.) Concomitant use of opiate analgesics and other CNS depressants should be reserved for patients in whom alternative treatment options are inadequate; the lowest effective dosages and shortest possible duration of concomitant therapy should be used, and the patient should be monitored closely for respiratory depression and sedation. Concomitant use with alcohol should be avoided.

If a benzodiazepine or other CNS depressant is required for any indication other than epilepsy in a patient receiving methadone for analgesia, the drug should be initiated at a lower dosage than indicated in the absence of opiate therapy and titrated based on clinical response. In patients receiving a benzodiazepine or other CNS depressant, methadone, if required for analgesia, should be initiated at a reduced dosage and titrated based on clinical response.

Because the morbidity and mortality associated with untreated opiate addiction can outweigh the serious risks associated with concomitant use of opiates and benzodiazepines or other CNS depressants, FDA states that methadone treatment for opiate addiction (i.e., medication-assisted treatment [MAT]) should not be withheld from patients receiving benzodiazepines or other CNS depressants. Clinicians should develop treatment plans that minimize the risks associated with concomitant use. If possible, benzodiazepines or other CNS depressants should be tapered and discontinued. (See Cautions.)

Some experts state that consideration should be given to offering the opiate antagonist naloxone when opiates are prescribed for patients at increased risk of opiate overdosage, including those receiving benzodiazepines concomitantly.

■ **Drugs Associated with Serotonin Syndrome** Serotonin syndrome has occurred in patients receiving opiate agonists, including methadone, in conjunction with other serotonergic drugs, including serotonin (5-hydroxytryptamine; 5-HT) type 1 receptor agonists ("triptans"), selective serotonin-reuptake inhibitors (SSRIs), selective serotonin- and norepinephrine-reuptake inhibitors (SNRIs), tricyclic antidepressants, antiemetics that are 5-HT_3 receptor antagonists, buspirone, cyclobenzaprine, dextromethorphan, lithium, St. John's wort, tryptophan, other serotonin modulators (e.g., mirtazapine, nefazodone, trazodone, vilazodone), and monoamine oxidase (MAO) inhibitors (both those used to treat psychiatric disorders and others, such as linezolid, methylene blue, and selegiline). Serotonin syndrome may occur within the recommended dosage ranges for these drugs. Manifestations of serotonin syndrome may include mental status changes (e.g., agitation, hallucinations, coma), autonomic instability (e.g., tachycardia, labile blood pressure, hyperthermia), neuromuscular aberrations (e.g., hyperreflexia, incoordination, rigidity), and/or GI symptoms (e.g., nausea, vomiting, diarrhea). Symptom onset generally occurs within several hours to a few days of concomitant use, but may occur later, particularly after dosage increases.

If concurrent therapy with opiate agonists and serotonergic drugs is warranted, patients should be monitored for serotonin syndrome, particularly during initiation of therapy and dosage increases. If serotonin syndrome is suspected, treatment with methadone, other opiate therapy, and/or any concurrently administered serotonergic agents should be discontinued.

For further information on serotonin syndrome, including manifestations and treatment, see Drug Interactions: Serotonergic Drugs, in Fluoxetine Hydrochloride 28:16.04.20.

■ **Drugs that Prolong QT Interval** Drugs known to prolong the QT interval (e.g., class I or III antiarrhythmic agents, calcium-channel blocking agents, some antipsychotic agents, tricyclic antidepressants) should be used with extreme caution in patients receiving methadone because of the risk of severe and potentially life-threatening cardiac arrhythmias. Methadone also should be used with caution in patients receiving drugs (e.g., diuretics, laxatives, corticosteroid hormones with mineralocorticoid activity) that may result in electrolyte disorders (e.g., hypomagnesemia, hypokalemia) that may prolong the QT interval.

■ **Risperidone** There have been reports of opiate withdrawal following the initiation of risperidone therapy in patients receiving methadone.

For further information about drug interactions involving opiate agonists (including methadone hydrochloride), see Drug Interactions in the Opiate Agonists General Statement 28:08.08.

Laboratory Test Interferences

Chlorpromazine, clomipramine, diphenhydramine, doxylamine, quetiapine, thioridazine, and verapamil may produce false-positive results for urine screening tests for methadone.

Pharmacology

In equianalgesic doses, methadone hydrochloride may produce a similar or slightly greater degree of respiratory depression than does morphine sulfate. A single dose of methadone may produce less sedation and euphoria than does morphine; however, because of the cumulative effect of methadone, marked sedation occurs after repeated administration. Methadone causes less constipation than does morphine. Methadone has antitussive activity. Methadone inhibits cardiac potassium channels and prolongs the QT interval.

Pharmacokinetics

■ **Absorption** Methadone is well absorbed from the GI tract. Following oral administration, bioavailability is approximately 80%; however, there is considerable interindividual variability in oral bioavailability (range: 36–100%). Following IM or subcutaneous administration of a single dose of methadone, onset and duration of analgesic effect are similar to those of morphine; duration is approximately 4–8 hours. Oral administration delays the onset as compared to parenteral administration. Peak plasma concentrations of the drug occur 1–7.5 hours following oral administration. Steady-state plasma concentrations and full analgesic effects usually are not attained until completion of 3–5 days of therapy.

With repeated methadone dosing, storage in and slow release of the drug from the liver and other tissues may prolong the duration of action of methadone despite the presence of low plasma concentrations. Peak respiratory depressant effects of methadone typically occur later and persist longer than the drug's peak analgesic effects, particularly during the early dosing period. The drug has an extended duration of action in patients who are physically dependent on oral methadone. Duration of action increases with repeated administration and is approximately 22–48 hours following oral administration in patients on methadone maintenance. Depressant effects after overdosage may also continue for 36–48 hours.

■ **Distribution** Methadone is highly lipophilic and is widely distributed in body tissues. Because of its lipophilicity, methadone may persist in the liver and other tissues. Slow release of methadone from these sites may prolong the duration of action of the drug despite the presence of low plasma concentrations.

Methadone is highly bound (85–90%) to plasma proteins, mainly α_1-acid glycoprotein.

Methadone crosses the placenta and is distributed into milk.

■ **Elimination** In clinical studies, the terminal elimination half-life of methadone ranged from 8–59 hours. In clinical use, the elimination half-life of methadone has varied considerably, ranging from 9–87 hours in postoperative patients, from 8.5–75 hours in opiate-dependent patients, and up to 120 hours in outpatients receiving therapy for chronic malignant pain. In one study in 5 patients receiving 100 or 120 mg of oral methadone hydrochloride daily for maintenance treatment of opiate addiction, the drug had an apparent plasma half-life of 13–47 hours, with an average of 25 hours.

Methadone is extensively metabolized, principally by cytochrome P-450 (CYP) isoenzymes 3A4, 2B6, and 2C19 and to a lesser extent by CYP isoenzymes 2C9 and 2D6. The drug undergoes *N*-demethylation to an inactive metabolite, 2-ethylidene-1,5-dimethyl-3,3-diphenylpyrrolidene (EDDP), and other metabolites with little or no pharmacologic activity. Although methadone appears to be a substrate of the P-glycoprotein transport system, its pharmacokinetics do not appear to be substantially altered by P-glycoprotein polymorphism or inhibition.

Methadone and its metabolites are excreted to varying degrees in urine and feces. Methadone is excreted by glomerular filtration and undergoes renal reabsorption. Reabsorption of methadone decreases as urinary pH decreases. Urinary excretion of methadone and its metabolic end products is dose dependent and comprises the major route of excretion only in dosages exceeding 55 mg daily. Methadone metabolites are also excreted in the feces via the bile.

Chemistry and Stability

■ **Chemistry** Methadone hydrochloride is a synthetic diphenylheptane-derivative opiate agonist. The drug occurs as colorless crystals or a white, crystalline powder and is soluble in water and freely soluble in alcohol. Dispersible tablets of methadone hydrochloride are specially formulated with insoluble excipients to deter use of the drug by injection. Methadone hydrochloride injection has a pH of 3–6.5. Methadone hydrochloride oral concentrate has a pH of 1–6.

■ **Stability** Methadone hydrochloride preparations should be stored in tight, light-resistant containers. Methadone hydrochloride oral concentrate and oral solution should be stored at 15–30°C; the tablets and injection should be stored at a controlled room temperature of 25°C, but may be exposed to temperatures ranging from 15–30°C.

Methadone hydrochloride injection has been reported to be physically or chemically incompatible with solutions containing aminophylline, ammonium chloride, amobarbital sodium, chlorothiazide sodium, phenytoin sodium, heparin sodium, methicillin sodium (no longer commercially available in the US), nitrofurantoin sodium, pentobarbital sodium, phenobarbital sodium, sodium bicarbonate, and thiopental sodium (no longer commercially available in the US). Specialized references should be consulted for more specific compatibility information.

For further information on chemistry, pharmacology, pharmacokinetics, uses, cautions, chronic toxicity, acute toxicity, drug interactions, and dosage and administration of methadone hydrochloride, see the Opiate Agonists General Statement 28:08.08.

Preparations

Methadone hydrochloride is subject to control under the Federal Controlled Substances Act of 1970 as a schedule II (C-II) drug and, in addition, is subject to US Food and Drug Administration regulations (21 CFR 291.505) for drugs that require special studies, records, and reports when used for detoxification and maintenance of opiate dependence.

Distribution of methadone hydrochloride 40-mg dispersible tablets is restricted. (See Restricted Distribution under Dosage and Administration: Administration.)

Excipients in commercially available drug preparations may have clinically important effects in some individuals; consult specific product labeling for details.

Methadone Hydrochloride

Oral		
Solution	5 mg/5 mL*	**Methadone Hydrochloride Oral Solution** (C-II)
	10 mg/5 mL*	**Methadone Hydrochloride Oral Solution** (C-II)
Solution, concentrate	10 mg/mL*	**Methadone Hydrochloride Intensol®** (C-II), Roxane
		Methadone Hydrochloride Oral Concentrate (C-II)
		Methadose® Oral Concentrate (C-II), Mallinckrodt
Tablets	5 mg*	**Dolophine® Hydrochloride** (C-II; scored), Roxane
		Methadone Hydrochloride Tablets (C-II)
		Methadose® (C-II; scored), Mallinckrodt
	10 mg*	**Dolophine® Hydrochloride** (C-II; scored), Roxane
		Methadone Hydrochloride Tablets (C-II)
		Methadose® (C-II; scored), Mallinckrodt
Tablets, dispersible	40 mg*	**Methadone Hydrochloride Diskets®** (C-II; scored), Roxane
		Methadose® (C-II; scored), Mallinckrodt
Parenteral		
Injection	10 mg/mL*	**Methadone Hydrochloride Injection** (C-II)

*available from one or more manufacturer, distributor, and/or repackager by generic (nonproprietary) name

†Use is not currently included in the labeling approved by the US Food and Drug Administration

Morphine Sulfate

■ Morphine sulfate is a phenanthrene-derivative opiate agonist; morphine is the principal alkaloid of opium and considered to be the prototype of the opiate agonists.

REMS

FDA approved a REMS for morphine sulfate to ensure that the benefits outweigh the risk. The REMS may apply to one or more preparations of morphine sulfate and consists of the following: medication guide and elements to assure safe use. See the FDA REMS page (https://www.accessdata.fda.gov/scripts/cder/rems/index.cfm).

Uses

■ **Pain** Morphine sulfate is a strong analgesic used to relieve severe, acute pain or moderate to severe, chronic pain (e.g., in terminally ill patients). The drug is also used parenterally as a supplement to anesthesia and for analgesia during labor.

Extended-release preparations of morphine are used orally for the management of moderate to severe pain when a continuous, around-the-clock analgesic is needed for an extended period of time. Morphine sulfate extended-release oral preparations are not indicated for relief of acute pain or for use on an as-needed ("prn") basis.

Morphine sulfate is also available as a preservative-free injection (Astramorph® PF, Duramorph® PF, Infumorph®) that can be injected epidurally or intrathecally for relief of severe pain (neuraxial analgesia); administration of the drug by these routes reportedly provides pain relief for prolonged periods without attendant loss of motor, sensory, or sympathetic function. Epidural or intrathecal administration of highly concentrated injections (i.e., Infumorph®) via continuous, controlled microinfusion for the management of chronic intractable pain has been designated an orphan use by the US Food and Drug Administration (FDA). Chronic epidural or intrathecal analgesia is indicated only when adequate pain relief cannot be obtained with less invasive therapies. Morphine sulfate also is available as an extended-release liposomal injection (DepoDur®) that can be injected epidurally as a single dose for the relief of severe pain following major surgery. For epidural or intrathecal injection, the drug should only be administered by qualified individuals familiar with the techniques and patient management problems associated with these routes of morphine administration. (See Cautions: Precautions and Contraindications.)

Morphine is used to relieve pain and anxiety associated with acute coronary syndromes (ACS). Because of its ability to alleviate the work of breathing, reduce anxiety, and favorably affect ventricular loading conditions, morphine is considered the analgesic agent of choice in patients with ST-segment-elevation myocardial infarction (STEMI). In addition to its potent analgesic and anxiolytic effects, morphine also exhibits favorable hemodynamic effects by causing venodilation and modest reductions in heart rate and systolic blood pressure. These properties also may be beneficial in patients with non-ST-segment-elevation ACS (NSTE ACS; unstable angina or non-ST-segment-elevation myocardial infarction [NSTEMI]); although randomized controlled studies specifically evaluating the use of morphine in patients with NSTE ACS have not been conducted, experts state that it may be reasonable to administer IV morphine in such patients who have continued pain despite treatment with maximally tolerated anti-ischemic drugs (e.g., nitrates). However, use of morphine should not preclude the use of other anti-ischemic drugs with proven benefit. Patients with acute MI typically exhibit overactivity of the sympathetic nervous system, which adversely increases myocardial oxygen demand via acceleration of heart rate, elevation in arterial blood pressure, augmentation of cardiac contractility, and heightened tendency to develop ventricular tachyarrhythmias. This increased sympathetic activity results from combined ischemic-type chest discomfort and anxiety, and the principal objective of therapy is to administer sufficient doses of an analgesic such as morphine to relieve what many patients describe as a feeling of impending doom. The dose of morphine sulfate needed to achieve adequate pain control is dependent upon several factors such as patient age (e.g., lower doses are recommended in geriatric patients), body size, blood pressure, and heart rate. To reverse the effects of morphine (e.g., such as when respiratory depression occurs), naloxone hydrochloride may be used.

In one large study of patients undergoing open-heart surgery, IV administration of large doses (i.e., 1–3 mg/kg) of morphine sulfate alone or in combination with inhalation anesthetic agents increased cardiac index, stroke index, central venous pressure and pulmonary-artery pressure, and decreased systemic vascular resistance. This study suggested that morphine sulfate may be used in patients with minimal circulatory reserve and for production of analgesia and anesthesia in patients undergoing cardiovascular surgery. Another similar study reported that large doses of morphine produced marked antidiuresis, muscular rigidity with decreased chest compliance, and an increase in systolic blood pressure and central venous pressure. Antidiuresis was effectively relieved by IV administration of 1 L of 5% alcohol.

For further information on the role of opiate analgesics in the management of acute or chronic pain, see Uses: Pain, in the Opiate Agonists General Statement 28:08.08.

■ **Acute Pulmonary Edema** Morphine is used in patients with acute pulmonary edema for its cardiovascular effects and to allay anxiety. Morphine should not be used in the treatment of pulmonary edema resulting from a chemical respiratory irritant.

■ **Neonatal Opiate Withdrawal** Morphine has been used to manage manifestations of opiate abstinence syndrome (i.e., postnatal withdrawal) in neonates† exposed to opiates in utero. Opiates are recommended as first-line pharmacologic therapy when environmental and supportive measures (e.g., minimization of external stimuli, maximization of mother-infant contact [e.g., parental "rooming in"], breast-feeding when not contraindicated, swaddling and gentle handling) are inadequate. Other adjunctive therapy (e.g., clonidine, phenobarbital) may be added if the response to opiates is inadequate, or phenobarbital may be added if the neonate was exposed to additional substances in utero. Approximately 60–80% of neonates with opiate abstinence syndrome may require pharmacologic treatment for withdrawal symptoms. While morphine has been used more extensively than other opiates in the management of neonatal opiate abstinence syndrome, some studies suggest that use of methadone or buprenorphine (an opiate partial agonist) may be associated with shorter treatment durations and hospital stays compared with morphine use. However, additional study is needed to establish optimal dosage schedules and preferred opiate drugs and to evaluate longer-term (e.g., neurodevelopmental) outcomes. Conflicting findings to date may be related in part to differences in study design, nonpharmacologic care, concomitant in utero drug exposures, the stringency of institutional protocols for care, and optimization of dosage schedules.

Use of standardized protocols for identification, evaluation, and treatment of neonatal opiate withdrawal syndrome is recommended since use of such protocols has been shown to improve overall response, including shorter hospital stays and durations of pharmacologic treatment. Some evidence suggests that use of a standardized protocol may be more important than use of a specific opiate agonist (e.g., morphine versus methadone) in improving outcomes. Protocols generally utilize assessment tools that were developed to quantify severity of withdrawal in term neonates (e.g., Finnegan or modified Finnegan scoring tools) to facilitate decisions regarding initiation, titration, and tapering of therapy.

Dosage and Administration

■ **Administration** ***Parenteral Administration*** Morphine sulfate is administered subcutaneously, by IM or slow IV injection, or by IV infusion. The preservative-free injection (Astramorph® PF, Duramorph® PF, or Infumorph®) may also be administered epidurally or intrathecally via intermittent injection or continuous infusion. Morphine sulfate extended-release liposomal injection (DepoDur®) is administered epidurally.

Highly concentrated, conventional, preservative-free morphine sulfate injections intended for continuous epidural or intrathecal infusion via a controlled-microinfusion device (e.g., Infumorph® 10 or 25 mg/mL) are not recommended for IV, IM, or sub-Q administration of individual doses of the drug because of the large amount of morphine sulfate contained in each ampul (200 mg/20 mL, 500 mg/20 mL) and the attendant risk of substantial overdosage.

The manufacturers state that morphine sulfate for injection usually is given subcutaneously, but may be given by IM or slow IV injection. The manufacturers also state that IM administration is preferred to subcutaneous injection when repeated parenteral doses are necessary, since repeated subcutaneous injection causes local tissue irritation, pain, and induration. However, some experts state that IV injection or continuous IV or subcutaneous infusion† provides better comfort and reliability and that repeated IM injection should not be used routinely.

When morphine sulfate is administered IV, epidurally, or intrathecally, an opiate antagonist and facilities for administration of oxygen and control of respiration should be available. When the drug is administered epidurally or intrathecally as individual doses, the patient should be in a setting where adequate monitoring is possible. Because delayed respiratory depression can occur, monitoring should be continued for a specific period of time depending on patient status and the morphine sulfate preparation used. When conventional morphine sulfate injection is administered epidurally or intrathecally as individual doses, patient monitoring should be continued for at least 24 hours after each dose. When morphine sulfate extended-release liposomal injection (DepoDur®) is administered epidurally, patient monitoring should be continued for at least 48 hours after the dose. When morphine is administered via continuous, controlled microinfusion, such precautions should be continued for at least 24 hours after administration of each test dose and for several days after surgical implantation of the catheter as appropriate for additional monitoring and dosage adjustment. An opiate antagonist and resuscitative equipment also should be immediately available whenever the reservoir of the microinfusion device is refilled with morphine sulfate or is otherwise being manipulated. Facilities, drugs, and equipment necessary for the management of inadvertent intravascular injection during attempted epidural or intrathecal injection should also be readily available. Because the intrathecal dose of morphine is 1/10 the epidural dose, the risk of overdose from inadvertent intrathecal injection during attempted epidural injection should be considered and facilities, drugs, and equipment for treating morphine overdose should be readily available.

Parenteral solutions of conventional morphine sulfate injection should be inspected visually prior to administration whenever container and solution permit. Unopened solutions should be discarded if they contain a precipitate that does not disappear with shaking. In addition, solutions that are not colorless or pale yellow (outside any amber container) should be discarded.

Because of the potency of injections of morphine sulfate, such injections should be handled carefully, and accidental cutaneous exposure should be treated by removing any contaminated clothing and rinsing the affected area with water. In addition, morphine sulfate injections are subject to substantial risk of overdosage if used inappropriately and to diversion and abuse. Therefore, special control measures should be implemented within the institution, including restricted access, rigid accounting, and rigorous control of waste disposal.

IV Administration. For IV administration, morphine sulfate should be injected slowly with the patient in the recumbent position. Rapid IV injection of the drug may result in an increased frequency of opiate-induced adverse effects; severe respiratory depression, apnea, hypotension, peripheral circulatory collapse, chest wall rigidity, cardiac arrest, and anaphylactoid reactions have occurred following rapid IV injection.

For continuous IV infusion, morphine sulfate has been diluted to a concentration of 0.1–1 mg/mL in 5% dextrose and administered via a controlled-infusion device; more concentrated solutions have been used in patients whose fluid intake was restricted and/or dosage requirements were high. Morphine sulfate injections containing 25 or 50 mg/mL are intended for preparation of IV infusion solutions and should *not* be administered IV without prior dilution. Alternatively, for multiple, slow IV injections, a commercially available injection containing 1 or 5 mg/mL may be administered undiluted using a compatible patient-controlled infusion device. For continuous subcutaneous infusion†, the drug has been diluted to an appropriate concentration in 5% dextrose and administered via a portable, controlled, subcutaneous infusion device. The rate of continuous IV or subcutaneous infusion of the drug must be individualized according to the response and tolerance of the patient.

Epidural and Intrathecal Administration. Specialized techniques are required for epidural or intrathecal administration of morphine sulfate; the drug should be administered via these routes only by qualified individuals familiar with the techniques of administration and patient management problems associated with these routes of morphine administration. (See Cautions: Precautions and Contraindications.) Epidural or intrathecal administration should be limited to the lumbar region since administration in the thoracic region has been associated with a substantially increased frequency of early and late respiratory depression even at low doses. Because epidural administration of the drug has been associated with a lower potential for immediate and delayed adverse effects than intrathecal administration, the epidural rather than intrathecal route should be used whenever possible.

Parenteral morphine sulfate preparations that are appropriate for epidural or intrathecal administration must be free of preservatives (antioxidants, antimicrobial agents), alcohol, other neurotoxic ingredients, or any ingredient that could compromise the safety and performance of an infusion pump (when continuous-infusion therapy is employed); the recommended pH of solutions is 4–8. Appropriate morphine sulfate solutions (e.g., Astramorph/PF®, Duramorph®, Infumorph®) may be given epidurally or intrathecally by intermittent administration or by continuous infusion (e.g., via an implantable controlled-infusion device such as an Infusaid® or SynchroMed® pump) if necessary.

For epidural administration, the appropriate dose of the drug is injected into the epidural space after proper placement of the needle or catheter has been verified. Appropriate conventional morphine sulfate injections may be administered by continuous epidural infusion (e.g., via an implantable controlled-infusion device such as an Infusaid® or SynchroMed® pump) if necessary. For intrathecal administration, no more than 2 or 1 mL of the injection containing 0.5 or 1 mg/mL, respectively, should be injected intrathecally. The safety of injecting repeated intermittent doses of the drug intrathecally, other than for establishing initial dosage when continuous intrathecal infusion is contemplated, has not been determined and, if pain recurs and additional morphine therapy is required for patients who are not candidates for such infusion, alternative routes of administration should be considered.

For continuous epidural or intrathecal infusion of conventional morphine sulfate injection, a controlled-infusion device is used to administer the drug; familiarization with the device is essential. If the highly concentrated injections intended for such administration (e.g., Infumorph®) are used, an implantable controlled-microinfusion device is used. Dilution of the highly concentrated injections may be necessary, depending on the infusion device employed and/or individual dosage requirements; 0.9% sodium chloride injection is recommended for dilution. To minimize the risk of contamination with glass or other particles, doses of the injections should be withdrawn from the ampul through a 5-μm (or smaller pore diameter) microfilter. Filling of the drug reservoir of the device should be performed only by fully trained and qualified personnel, following the directions provided by the device's manufacturer. Care should be taken in employing the proper refill frequency so that depletion of the reservoir during use is avoided. Such depletion could result in exacerbation of severe pain and/or reflux of CSF into the reservoir of some devices. Strict aseptic filling technique is required to avoid potential microbial contamination. *Extreme caution must be employed to ensure proper placement of the syringe needle in the filling port of the device prior to refilling the reservoir; inadvertent injection outside the filling port, into the tissue surrounding the device, or, in the case of multiport devices, into a port intended for single supplementary doses could result in large, clinically important overdosage. Severe, potentially life-threatening respiratory depression could result from technical errors during refill.* Patients and/or their attendants should be instructed in proper home care of the device and the insertion site and in the recognition and practical treatment of epidural or intrathecal morphine overdosage.

Highly concentrated, preservative-free morphine sulfate injections intended for continuous epidural or intrathecal infusion via a controlled-microinfusion device (e.g., Infumorph® 10 or 25 mg/mL) should not be used for individual-dose epidural or intrathecal injection since less-concentrated, preservative-free injections can be employed more reliably for the small doses required.

Morphine sulfate extended-release liposomal injection (DepoDur®) is administered epidurally (at the lumbar level) as a single dose prior to surgery or after the umbilical cord is clamped during cesarean section. The appropriate dose of the drug is injected into the epidural space after proper placement of the needle or catheter has been verified. If a test dose (3 mL of preservative-free 1.5% lidocaine and epinephrine 1:200,000 injection) is used to verify placement of the catheter, the catheter should be flushed with 1 mL of preservative-free 0.9% sodium chloride injection; at least 15 minutes should elapse between the test dose and administration of morphine sulfate extended-release liposomal injection. Epidural administration of morphine sulfate extended-release liposomal injection at the thoracic or higher level has not been evaluated and is not recommended; the preparation is not intended for intrathecal, IV, or IM administration. Morphine sulfate extended-release liposomal injection may be administered undiluted or diluted with preservative-free 0.9% sodium chloride injection to a total volume of up to 5 mL. Morphine sulfate extended-release liposomal injection should not be administered using an inline filter; the preparation should not be admixed with other drugs, including local anesthetics. Following administration of morphine sulfate extended-release liposomal injection, no other drug should be administered into the epidural space for at least 48 hours.

Oral and Rectal Administration Morphine sulfate also is administered orally or rectally. Patients receiving morphine should avoid alcohol; concomitant use may result in profound sedation, respiratory depression, coma, or death.

The manufacturers state that certain morphine sulfate extended-release preparations (i.e., Avinza® extended-release capsules, Kadian® extended-release capsules, Oramorph® SR extended-release tablets) can be administered without regard to food; the effect of food on the GI absorption of other morphine sulfate extended-release preparations (i.e., MS-Contin® extended-release tablets) has not been fully evaluated to date. Extended-release tablets of the drug should be swallowed intact and should *not* be broken, crushed, or chewed; intake of a broken, crushed, or chewed tablet may result in too rapid a release of the drug from the preparation and absorption of a potentially toxic dose of morphine sulfate. The manufacturers of morphine sulfate extended-release capsules state that the capsules may be swallowed whole or the entire contents of the capsules may be sprinkled on a small amount of applesauce, at room temperature or cooler, immediately prior to administration; subdividing the contents of a capsule is not recommended. The patient should swallow the entire mixture. The beads or pellets should not be crushed, chewed, or dissolved; intake of crushed, chewed, or dissolved beads or pellets may result in too rapid a release of the drug from the preparation and absorption of a potentially fatal dose of morphine sulfate. Following administration, the patient should drink a glass of water to rinse the mouth and ensure that the beads or pellets are swallowed. The mixture of applesauce and beads or pellets should not be stored for future use. Patients receiving morphine sulfate extended-release capsules (Avinza®, Kadian®) must *not* consume alcoholic beverages or prescription or nonprescription preparations containing alcohol; intake of alcohol may result in rapid release of the drug from the capsules and intake of a potentially toxic dose of morphine sulfate. Additionally, one manufacturer states that the contents of the extended-release capsules (Kadian®) should not be administered through a nasogastric tube; however, the manufacturer's information may be consulted for information regarding administration through a 16 French (16F) gastrostomy tube.

Dispensing and Administration Precautions. Serious adverse events and deaths have occurred as a result of inadvertent overdosage of concentrated morphine sulfate oral solutions. In most of these cases, morphine sulfate oral solutions prescribed in mg were mistakenly interchanged for mL of the concentrated preparation, resulting in 20-fold overdoses. Clinicians should be aware that morphine sulfate oral solutions are commercially available in various concentrations, which generally are expressed in terms of mg of drug per mL (mg/mL) or per 5 mL (mg/5 mL) of solution. Oral solutions containing morphine sulfate 100 mg/5 mL should be used only in patients who are opiate tolerant (i.e., individuals who have been receiving at least 60 mg of oral morphine sulfate daily, 30 mg of oral oxycodone daily, 12 mg of hydromorphone hydrochloride daily, or an equianalgesic dosage of another opiate daily for at least one week) and have been titrated to a stable analgesic dosage using a preparation containing a lower concentration of morphine sulfate. To avoid medication errors, the prescriber should write a prescription for morphine sulfate oral solution by clearly specifying the concentration of morphine sulfate oral solution to be dispensed *and*, in the directions for use, indicating the intended dose of morphine in mg along with the corresponding volume in mL (in parentheses). It is important that the prescription be filled with the proper concentration of morphine sulfate oral solution to prevent potential medication errors; if the specified morphine sulfate oral solution is unavailable, pharmacists should contact the prescriber. Patients receiving morphine sulfate oral solution should be carefully instructed in how to measure and administer the prescribed dose; those receiving an oral solution containing morphine sulfate 100 mg/5 mL should be advised to always use the graduated oral syringe supplied by the manufacturer to ensure that the dose is measured and administered accurately. Patients receiving prescriptions for morphine sulfate oral solution should be instructed as to which concentration they have been prescribed and should be advised whenever the concentration is changed.

Dispensing errors have occurred because of similarity in spelling between Kadian® (a trade name for morphine sulfate) and Kapidex® (the former trade name for dexlansoprazole, a proton-pump inhibitor). Therefore, in April 2010, the manufacturer of Kapidex® changed the trade name for dexlansoprazole from Kapidex® to Dexilant® to avoid future dispensing errors. (See Cautions: Precautions and Contraindications.)

■ Dosage

Morphine sulfate should be given at the lowest effective dosage and for the shortest duration of therapy consistent with the treatment goals of the patient. Reduced dosage is indicated in poor-risk patients, in patients with substantial hepatic impairment, and in very young or very old patients. In addition, dosage of morphine sulfate should be reduced in patients with renal impairment, since the active metabolite morphine 6-glucuronide accumulates in such patients, which can result in enhanced and prolonged opiate activity. It has been suggested that if therapy with an opiate agonist is needed in patients with renal impairment, an alternative opiate agonist (whose excretion is independent of renal function) be used instead of morphine in such patients. If concomitant therapy with other CNS depressants is required, the lowest effective dosages and shortest possible duration of concomitant therapy should be used.

In patients with severe, chronic pain, dosage should be adjusted according to the severity of the pain and the response and tolerance of the patient.

For acute pain not related to trauma or surgery, the prescribed quantity should be limited to the amount needed for the expected duration of pain severe enough to require opiate analgesia (generally 3 days or less and rarely more than 7 days). When opiate analgesics are used for the management of chronic noncancer pain, the US Centers for Disease Control and Prevention (CDC) recommends that primary care clinicians carefully reassess individual benefits and risks before prescribing dosages equivalent to 50 mg or more of morphine sulfate daily and avoid dosages equivalent to 90 mg or more of morphine sulfate daily or carefully justify their decision to titrate the dosage to such levels. Other experts recommend consulting a pain management specialist before exceeding a dosage equivalent to 80–120 mg of morphine sulfate daily. For further information on the management of opiate analgesic therapy, see Dosage and Administration: Dosage, in the Opiate Agonists General Statement 28:08.08.

Morphine sulfate extended-release liposomal injection (DepoDur®) should *not* be substituted for conventional morphine sulfate injection.

Parenteral Dosage The usual adult parenteral dosage of morphine sulfate is 10 mg every 4 hours as necessary; dosage may range from 2.5–20 mg every 2–6 hours as necessary depending on patient requirements and response.

Adolescents 12 years of age or older may receive morphine sulfate at a dose of 3–4 mg IV, repeated in 5 minutes if needed. Infants and children may receive a parenteral morphine sulfate dosage of 0.1–0.2 mg/kg every 2–4 hours as necessary. Neonates may receive a parenteral morphine sulfate dosage of 0.05–0.2 mg/kg every 2–4 hours. Single pediatric doses should not exceed 10 mg.

To relieve pain and associated anxiety and provide potentially beneficial cardiovascular effects in adults with ST-segment-elevation myocardial infarction (STEMI), an initial morphine sulfate dose of 4–8 mg IV is recommended; additional doses of 2–8 mg may be administered every 5–15 minutes as needed. In patients with non-ST-segment-elevation acute coronary syndromes (NSTE ACS) who continue to experience pain despite maximally tolerated anti-ischemic therapy, experts state that a morphine sulfate dose of 1–5 mg IV may be administered during IV nitroglycerin therapy; additional doses may be given every 5–30 minutes to relieve symptoms and maintain patient comfort.

To provide analgesia during labor, 10 mg of morphine sulfate is usually administered subcutaneously or IM.

When morphine sulfate is administered by multiple, slow IV injections for patient-controlled analgesia (PCA), dosage is adjusted according to the severity of the pain and response of the patient; the operator's manual for the patient-controlled infusion device should be consulted for directions on administering the drug at the desired rate of infusion. Care must be exercised to avoid overdosage, which could result in respiratory depression, or abrupt cessation of therapy with the drug, which could precipitate opiate withdrawal. For adults, a standard protocol that initiates PCA with morphine sulfate interval doses of 1 mg, a time between doses of 6 minutes (lockout period), and a limit of 10 doses per hour has been used. Interval doses of 0.5–2 mg of morphine sulfate and lockout periods of 6–12 minutes generally have been used in adults. Adults may receive an initial loading dose, preferably titrated by a clinician or nurse at the bedside and generally administered in increments of 2–4 mg every 10 minutes up to a total dose of 6–16 mg, if needed to achieve more rapid control of pain. In one study that evaluated PCA postoperatively in pediatric patients 7–19 years of age undergoing orthopedic surgery, the interval dose of morphine sulfate was 25 mcg/kg, the time between doses was 10 minutes, and the 4-hour limit was 0.24 mg/kg. Interval doses of 10–20 mcg/kg of morphine sulfate and lockout periods of 6–12 minutes generally are used for developmentally mature pediatric patients 7 years of age or older. Pediatric patients may receive an initial loading dose, preferably titrated by a clinician or nurse at the bedside and generally administered in increments of 0.05 mg/kg up to a total dose of 0.05–0.2 mg/kg, if needed to achieve more rapid control of pain.

When morphine sulfate is administered by continuous IV or subcutaneous† infusion for relief of severe, chronic pain associated with cancer, the dosage of the drug must be individualized according to the response and tolerance of the patient. Continuous IV infusions of the drug have been initiated at 0.8–10 mg/hour in adults and then increased to an effective dosage as necessary; an IV loading dose of 15 mg or more can be administered for initial relief of pain prior to initiating continuous IV infusion of the drug. In adults with severe, chronic pain, maintenance dosages usually have ranged from 0.8–80 mg/hour infused IV, although higher (e.g., 150 mg/hour) maintenance dosages occasionally have been required. In addition, relatively high dosages (e.g., 275–440 mg/hour) occasionally have been infused IV for several hours or days to provide relief of exacerbations of chronic pain in adults who had been previously stabilized on lower dosages or whose dosage had been gradually titrated to relatively high levels; subsequent dosage reductions according to patient response generally were possible.

In a limited number of children with severe, chronic pain associated with cancer, maintenance morphine sulfate dosages of 0.025–2.6 mg/kg per hour (median: 0.04–0.07 mg/kg per hour) have been infused IV. Maintenance dosages of 0.03–0.15 mg/kg per hour have been infused IV in a limited number of children with severe pain associated with sickle cell crisis. Maintenance dosages of 0.025–1.79 mg/kg per hour (median: 0.06 mg/kg per hour) have been infused subcutaneously in a limited number of children with severe, chronic pain associated with cancer. For postoperative analgesia, children have received maintenance dosages by IV infusion at a rate of 0.01–0.04 mg/kg per hour. Because elimination of the drug may be slower in neonates and they may be more susceptible to CNS effects of the drug, some clinicians have suggested that the rate of IV infusion generally not exceed 0.015–0.02 mg/kg per hour in this age group. However, morphine sulfate has been administered by IV infusion for analgesia in neonates at a rate of 0.025–0.05 mg/kg per hour.

Epidural and Intrathecal Dosage. When conventional morphine sulfate injection is used for pain relief, the usual initial epidural dose for intermittent injection in adults is 5 mg. The drug should be administered epidurally in debilitated or geriatric patients with extreme caution. If adequate pain relief is not achieved within 1 hour after administration of the initial dose, additional epidural doses may be given carefully in 1- to 2-mg increments at intervals sufficient to assess efficacy, but the manufacturers state that no more than 10 mg total generally should be administered by intermittent epidural injection daily. Pain relief generally occurs within 6–30 minutes and persists for about 16–24 hours (range: 4–36 hours) after a single, effective epidural dose of morphine. For continuous epidural infusion when the device is not implanted surgically, an initial dosage of 2–4 mg per 24 hours has been recommended; epidural dosage may be increased by 1–2 mg daily if adequate relief is not achieved initially. In some patients with severe, chronic pain, epidural dosages have been titrated up to 30 mg daily via continuous epidural infusion following initiation of therapy at dosages of 0.6–0.8 mg/kg daily. If an implantable microinfusion device is to be employed for continuous epidural infusion, efficacy and adverse effects of initial dosage should be assessed for each patient using serial, intermittent epidural doses of the drug prior to implantation surgery. Once it has been determined that the patient is a suitable candidate for such chronic therapy and initial dosage has been established, implantation surgery can be performed. Most adults who are not tolerant to opiates achieve adequate relief with initial epidural dosages of 3.5–7.5 mg daily. Based on limited experience, an initial epidural dosage of 4.5–10 mg daily has been suggested for adults with some degree of opiate tolerance. Epidural dosage requirements may increase substantially during chronic therapy, frequently to 20–30 mg daily; the upper daily limit must be individualized for each patient.

When morphine sulfate extended-release liposomal injection (DepoDur®) is used for pain relief in adults undergoing major surgery, a single dose of the drug should be given. The recommended dose is 15 mg in those undergoing major orthopedic surgery of a lower extremity and 10–15 mg in those undergoing lower abdominal or pelvic surgery. While some patients may benefit from a 20-mg dose, the incidence of serious adverse respiratory effects was dose related in clinical studies. When morphine sulfate extended-release liposomal injection is used for cesarean section, the recommended dose is 10 mg.

The intrathecal dose of morphine sulfate is about 1/10 the epidural dose. A single 0.2- to 1-mg intrathecal dose (as conventional morphine sulfate injection) may provide adequate relief for up to 24 hours in adults who are not tolerant to opiates. Repeated intrathecal doses of the drug are not recommended except to establish initial intrathecal dosage when continuous intrathecal infusion is to be employed; if additional morphine therapy is necessary for patients who are not candidates for continuous intrathecal infusion, alternative routes of administration should be considered. Naloxone may be infused IV at a rate of 0.6 mg/hour for 24 hours after intrathecal morphine administration to decrease potential opiate-induced adverse effects. If an implantable microinfusion device is to be employed for continuous intrathecal infusion, efficacy and adverse effects of initial dosage should be assessed for each patient using serial, intermittent intrathecal doses of the drug prior to implantation surgery. Once it has been determined that the patient is a suitable candidate for such chronic therapy and initial dosage has been established, implantation surgery can be performed. Intrathecal dosage requirements may increase substantially during chronic therapy, but the rate of increase over time is highly variable, and the upper daily limit must be individualized for each patient. Intrathecal dosages exceeding 20 mg daily should be employed with caution since they may be associated with an increased likelihood of serious toxicity, including myoclonic spasms. Based on limited experience, continuous intrathecal dosage requirements can be expected to increase at a relatively constant rate over time to maximums averaging about 25 mg daily (95% confidence limits: maximums of 18–39 mg daily) after 40 weeks of continuous intrathecal therapy.

Morphine sulfate should be administered with extreme caution and in reduced dosage epidurally or intrathecally in geriatric or debilitated patients. Safety and efficacy of epidural or intrathecal administration in children have not been determined.

Oral and Rectal Dosage for Analgesia The usual adult dosage of morphine sulfate is 10–30 mg orally as conventional tablets, capsules, or oral solution or 10–20 mg rectally as suppositories every 4 hours as necessary or as directed by a physician. Oral or rectal dosages higher than the usual dosages may be required in some patients.

The usual oral pediatric dosage of morphine sulfate is 0.2–0.5 mg/kg (conventional tablets, oral solution) every 4–6 hours.

Most manufacturers suggest that it is preferable to initiate and stabilize oral morphine sulfate therapy with an immediate-release preparation and then transfer the patient to an extended-release preparation since titration of dosage may be more difficult with the latter preparation. The dosing regimen must be individualized based on the patient's prior analgesic therapy. The initial dosage of the morphine sulfate extended-release preparation should be based on the total daily dosage, potency, and specific characteristics of the current opiate agonist. Other considerations should include the reliability of relative potency estimates used in calculating the equivalent morphine sulfate dosage, the degree of opiate tolerance, the medical condition of the patient, concomitant drug therapy, and the nature and severity of the patient's pain. It is preferable to underestimate the initial dosage of the extended-release preparation than to inadvertently cause an overdosage of morphine sulfate. If necessary, supplemental doses of a short-acting opiate agonist can be considered if breakthrough pain occurs with dosing regimens employing extended-release preparations. When converting to another oral extended-release morphine sulfate preparation or to other oral or parenteral opiate analgesics, the manufacturer's labeling information should be consulted.

MS Contin®. Adults being transferred from an immediate-release oral morphine preparation to morphine sulfate extended-release tablets (MS Contin®) may receive the same total daily dosage given in 2 divided doses every 12 hours or in 3 divided doses every 8 hours. Dosage of morphine sulfate extended-release tablets (MS Contin®) should be individualized according to patient response and tolerance. In patients whose morphine sulfate requirement is expected to be less than 60 mg daily, use of 15-mg extended-release tablets is recommended; in patients whose morphine sulfate requirement is expected to be 60–120 mg daily, use of 30-mg extended-release tablets is recommended; and in patients whose daily morphine sulfate requirement is expected to exceed 120 mg daily, the appropriate combination of extended-release tablets should be used.

In adults who currently are receiving parenteral morphine sulfate or other oral or parenteral opiate therapy, the opiate analgesic requirements during the previous 24 hours should be calculated and converted to an equianalgesic dosage of morphine sulfate extended-release tablets (MS Contin®). Conservative dosage conversion ratios should be used to avoid toxicity. In patients whose morphine sulfate requirement is expected to be 120 mg or less daily, initial use of 30-mg extended-release tablets is recommended by the manufacturer; once a stable dosage regimen has been achieved, tablet strength may be increased as clinically appropriate.

Administration of large single doses of morphine sulfate as extended-release tablets (MS Contin®) may lead to acute overdosage, since this formulation does not release morphine sulfate at a continuous controlled rate. In order to avoid administration of large single doses, the interval between doses of morphine sulfate as extended-release tablets (MS Contin®) should not exceed 12 hours. In addition, the manufacturer states that the 100- and 200-mg strengths of this preparation should be used only in patients who are opiate tolerant and require dosages of 200 mg or greater daily. The manufacturer also recommends that the 200-mg tablets be reserved for patients who already have been titrated to a stable analgesic regimen.

Oramorph SR®. Adults being transferred from an immediate-release oral morphine preparation to morphine sulfate extended-release tablets (Oramorph SR®) may receive the same total daily dosage given in 2 divided doses every 12 hours. Dosage of morphine sulfate extended-release tablets (Oramorph SR®) should be individualized according to patient response and tolerance. In patients whose morphine sulfate requirement is expected to be 120 mg or less daily, use of 30-mg extended-release tablets is recommended.

In adults who currently are receiving parenteral morphine or other oral or parenteral opiate therapy, the opiate analgesic requirements during the previous 24 hours should be calculated and converted to an equianalgesic dosage of morphine sulfate extended-release tablets (Oramorph SR®). Conservative dosage conversion ratios should be used to avoid toxicity. In patients whose morphine sulfate requirement is expected to be 120 mg or less daily, initial use of 30-mg extended-release tablets is recommended by the manufacturer; once a stable dosage regimen has been achieved, tablet strength may be increased as clinically appropriate.

The dosing interval for morphine sulfate extended-release tablets (Oramorph SR®) should not exceed 12 hours because administration of large single doses may lead to acute overdosage. If pain is not controlled for the entire 12-hour interval, then the dosing interval may be decreased, but doses should be administered no more frequently than every 8 hours.

Kadian®. Adults being transferred from other oral morphine preparations to morphine sulfate extended-release capsules (Kadian®) may receive the same total daily dosage given in 2 divided doses every 12 hours or given as a single dose every 24 hours. Dosage of morphine sulfate extended-release capsules (Kadian®) should be individualized according to patient response and tolerance. However, the dosage should not be increased more frequently than every other day. Patients receiving once-daily dosing who experience excessive sedation with this regimen or who experience inadequate analgesia prior to the next dose should be switched to twice-daily dosing.

In adults who are currently receiving parenteral morphine sulfate or other oral or parenteral opiate therapy, the opiate analgesic requirements during the previous 24 hours should be calculated and converted to an equianalgesic dosage of morphine sulfate extended-release capsules (Kadian®). Conservative dosage conversion ratios should be used to avoid toxicity.

In adults who are not opiate tolerant, initial use of 10- or 20-mg extended-release capsules is recommended by the manufacturer; dosage generally should be increased by no more than 20 mg every other day in such patients. The 100- and 200-mg capsules should be administered only to opiate-tolerant patients.

Doses of morphine sulfate as extended-release capsules (Kadian®) should be administered no more frequently than every 12 hours. The first dose of morphine sulfate extended-release capsules (Kadian®) may be administered concurrently with the last dose of immediate-release opiate therapy because of the delayed peak plasma morphine concentrations produced by Kadian®. (See Pharmacokinetics: Absorption.)

Avinza®. Adults being transferred from other oral morphine preparations to morphine sulfate extended-release capsules (Avinza®) may receive the same total daily dosage administered once every 24 hours. Supplemental doses of a short-acting opiate analgesic may be required for up to 4 days until the patient's response to morphine sulfate extended-release capsules (Avinza®) has stabilized. Dosage of morphine sulfate extended-release capsules (Avinza®) should be individualized according to patient response and tolerance, but should not exceed 1.6 g daily. (See Cautions: Precautions and Contraindications.)

In adults who currently are receiving parenteral morphine or other oral or parenteral opiate therapy, the opiate analgesic requirements during the previous 24 hours should be calculated and converted to an equianalgesic dosage of morphine sulfate extended-release capsules (Avinza®). Conservative dosage conversion ratios should be used to avoid toxicity.

The usual initial adult dosage of morphine sulfate as extended-release capsules (Avinza®) in patients who are not opiate tolerant is 30 mg once daily; dosage should be increased by no more than 30 mg every 4 days. The 60-, 90-, and 120-mg capsules should be administered only to opiate-tolerant patients. Doses of morphine sulfate as extended-release capsules (Avinza®) should be administered no more frequently than every 24 hours.

Oral Dosage for Neonatal Opiate Withdrawal For the management of neonatal opiate abstinence syndrome†, use of standardized protocols that base initiation, adjustment, and tapering of morphine sulfate dosage on standardized patient assessments performed at regular intervals is recommended. The most commonly used tool for assessing severity of withdrawal in term neonates is the Finnegan scoring system (original or modified versions) performed every 3–4 hours. Treatment protocols vary in recommended dosages, thresholds for initiation of therapy, incremental changes and thresholds for dosage adjustment, and tapering strategies.

Under various protocols, treatment with morphine sulfate oral solution is initiated at a dosage of 0.04–0.05 mg/kg every 3–4 hours based on Finnegan score (e.g., score exceeds 8 on at least 2 or 3 occasions, the sum of 3 consecutive scores is 24 or greater, a single score or 2 consecutive scores are 12 or greater); under other protocols, initial dosage may vary depending on the severity of withdrawal manifestations, with higher initial dosages recommended for neonates with higher Finnegan scores. Some clinicians state that initial dosage usually ranges from 0.03–0.1 mg/kg every 3–4 hours. If Finnegan score remains elevated (e.g., a single score or 2 consecutive scores are 12 or greater, 2 consecutive scores are 8 or greater, the sum of 3 scores is 24 or greater), dosage may be increased, generally by 0.02–0.05 mg/kg per dose or by 10–20% depending on the protocol and/or Finnegan score, to achieve stabilization. Some clinicians have recommended a usual maximum dosage of 1.2–1.3 mg/kg daily or 0.2 mg/kg per dose. Once patients are stable (generally, no score exceeds 8) for at least 48 hours, morphine sulfate dosage typically is tapered in decrements of approximately 0.02 mg/kg per dose or approximately 10% of the highest (stabilization) dose at intervals of approximately 24–48 hours. Protocols vary in terms of the dosage at which morphine sulfate can be discontinued. However, neonates should be monitored for at least 48 hours after the drug has been discontinued. Specialized protocols should be consulted for further information on morphine sulfate dosage and monitoring of Finnegan scores in neonates with opiate abstinence syndrome. Further study is needed to define optimal dosing strategies.

Cautions

■ Precautions and Contraindications

Morphine shares the toxic potentials of the opiate agonists, and the usual precautions of opiate agonist therapy should be observed. (See Cautions in the Opiate Agonists General Statement 28:08.08.)

In patients with myocardial infarction, morphine causes a decrease in systemic vascular resistance which may result in a transient fall in systemic arterial pressure leading to severe hypotension; however, this usually is not a particular threat to supine patients. To decrease the possibility of the development of hypotension, the minimal effective dose should be given and the patient's legs should be elevated. Avoiding concomitant use of vasodilators also should be considered.

Morphine should be used with caution in patients with toxic psychoses.

Some commercially available formulations of morphine sulfate injection contain sulfites that may cause allergic-type reactions, including anaphylaxis and life-threatening or less severe asthmatic episodes, in certain susceptible individuals. The overall prevalence of sulfite sensitivity in the general population is unknown but probably low; such sensitivity appears to occur more frequently in asthmatic than in nonasthmatic individuals.

Morphine sulfate extended-release capsules (Avinza®) contain fumaric acid. Safety of dosages exceeding 1.6 g daily has not been established; such dosages contain a quantity of fumaric acid that may be associated with serious renal toxicity.

Patients receiving morphine sulfate extended-release capsules (Avinza®, Kadian®) must *not* consume alcoholic beverages or prescription or nonprescription preparations containing alcohol; intake of alcohol may result in rapid release of the drug from the capsules and intake of a potentially toxic dose of morphine sulfate.

In addition to the usual precautions associated with morphine use, for epidural or intrathecal administration, the drug should only be used by qualified individuals familiar with the techniques of administration and patient management problems associated with these routes of administration. Because chronic epidural or intrathecal therapy employing a controlled-microinfusion device is accompanied by considerable patient risk and requires a high level of skill to be accomplished successfully, such therapy should only be undertaken by experienced clinical teams who are well informed about patient selection criteria, evolving technology, and emerging standards of care. The risks of sepsis associated with urinary catheterization also should be considered when epidural or intrathecal administration of the drug is considered, especially during the perioperative period, since morphine may cause smooth-muscle hypertonicity resulting in difficulty in urination and possible urinary retention that requires catheterization. Myoclonic spasms of skeletal muscle also have been reported; treatment of opiate intoxication may be required in some cases. In some patients developing myoclonic spasms, resumption of therapy after appropriate management of the toxicity may be possible at reduced dosage and/or by replacement of epidural with intrathecal therapy.

The most serious adverse effect of morphine is respiratory depression. Bolus epidural or intrathecal administration of the drug may result in early respiratory depression because of direct venous redistribution of the drug to the respiratory centers in the CNS. Late (up to 24 hours) onset of acute respiratory depression has occurred following epidural or intrathecal administration of conventional morphine sulfate injection and is thought to result from rostral spread of the drug in the CNS. Delayed respiratory depression (48 hours or longer following injection) may occur following epidural administration of morphine sulfate extended-release liposomal injection (DepoDur®). The risk of respiratory depression may be increased in patients whose surgical procedure is cancelled after administration of morphine sulfate extended-release liposomal injection; careful patient monitoring is particularly important in these patients. Intrathecal administration of morphine has been associated with a higher incidence of respiratory depression than epidural administration. Respiratory depression may be severe, requiring maintenance of an adequate airway, use of resuscitative equipment, and administration of oxygen, an opiate antagonist, and/or other resuscitative drugs. A diminished CO_2 ventilatory response may be present for up to 22 hours following epidural or intrathecal administration of the drug, despite the absence of clinical evidence of inadequate ventilation. When chronic epidural or intrathecal therapy is employed, the patient should be monitored in an adequately equipped (e.g., resuscitative equipment, oxygen, an opiate antagonist and other resuscitative drugs) and staffed environment (hospitalization is recommended) for at least 24 hours after administration of an initial test dose and, as appropriate, for several days after catheter implantation for additional monitoring and dosage adjustment. An opiate antagonist and resuscitative equipment also should be immediately available whenever the reservoir of the microinfusion device is being refilled with morphine sulfate or is being otherwise manipulated. Orthostatic hypotension is a frequent complication of single-dose epidural or intrathecal morphine therapy, and patients with reduced circulatory volume or impaired myocardial function and those receiving sympatholytic therapy may be at particular risk.

Epidural and intrathecal administration of morphine are also frequently associated with pruritus, which is dose related but not confined to the site of administration. Urinary retention, which may persist for 10–20 hours after administration, has occurred in about 90% of males who received the drug epidurally or intrathecally and less frequently in females. Administration of low doses (i.e., 0.2 mg) of naloxone will frequently alleviate drug-induced pruritus, nausea and/or vomiting, and urinary retention; however, the risks of administering opiate antagonists should be considered in patients chronically maintained on opiate agonists. Urinary retention also has been managed with parasympathomimetic therapy and/or judicious use of urinary catheterization. Early recognition of urinary difficulty and prompt intervention in cases of retention are important, particularly in patients with prostatic enlargement. Caution should be exercised when epidural morphine therapy is undertaken in patients with reduced metabolic clearance and those with renal and/or hepatic dysfunction since accumulation (over several days) of high systemic concentrations of the drug may occur in such patients. Lumbar puncture-type headache occurs in many patients for several days after intrathecal catheter implantation but generally responds to bedrest and/or other conventional therapy. Peripheral edema, including unexplained genital swelling in males, also has occurred following infusion-device implantation surgery.

Epidural or intrathecal injection of morphine sulfate is contraindicated in patients whose concomitant drug therapy or medical condition would contraindicate administration of the drug by these routes, such as when infection is present at the injection site or the patient has uncontrolled bleeding diathesis or is receiving anticoagulants.

Morphine may cause severe hypotension in patients whose ability to maintain blood pressure has been compromised by blood volume depletion or concomitant use of certain drugs (e.g., general anesthetics, phenothiazines).

Serious adverse events and deaths have occurred as a result of inadvertent overdosage of concentrated morphine sulfate oral solutions. In most of these cases, morphine sulfate oral solutions prescribed in milligrams (mg) were mistakenly interchanged for milliliters (mL) of the concentrated preparation, resulting in 20-fold overdoses. Concentrated (100 mg/5 mL) morphine sulfate oral solutions are indicated for use only in patients who are opiate tolerant. It is important that prescriptions for morphine sulfate oral solution be written clearly and filled with the proper concentration of morphine sulfate oral solution to prevent potential medication errors. Patients receiving morphine sulfate oral solution should be carefully instructed in proper administration of the drug to avoid dosing errors, and they must be given a copy of and instructed to read the medication guide for morphine sulfate oral solution prior to initiating therapy and each time the oral solution is dispensed. (See Oral and Rectal Administration under Dosage and Administration: Administration.)

Because of similarity in spelling between Kadian® and Kapidex® (the former trade name for dexlansoprazole, a proton-pump inhibitor), dispensing errors have been reported. Therefore, in April 2010, the manufacturer of Kapidex® changed the trade name for dexlansoprazole from Kapidex® to Dexilant® to avoid future dispensing errors. The potential exists for serious adverse effects to occur if patients receive the incorrect drug. Kadian® is intended for use in managing moderate to severe pain when a continuous around-the-clock opiate analgesic is needed for an extended period of time; ingestion of the 100- or 200-mg Kadian® capsules by patients who are not opiate tolerant can cause fatal respiratory depression. Some experts recommend that pharmacists assess measures of avoiding dispensing errors and implement them as appropriate (e.g., by using computerized name alerts, matching the prescribed drug with the patient's medical history, verifying orders for these drugs) and that clinicians consider including the intended use of the drug on the prescription.

For a complete discussion of these and other precautions associated with morphine, see Cautions in the Opiate Agonists General Statement 28:08.08.

■ Pediatric Precautions Safety and efficacy of morphine in neonates have not been established. Opiate agonists generally should not be used in premature neonates since the drugs reportedly cross the immature blood-brain barrier more readily than they do the mature barrier and thereby produce disproportionate respiratory depression. Opiate agonists should be administered with caution and in carefully determined dosages to infants and small children since they may be relatively more sensitive to opiates on a body-weight basis. Safety and efficacy of epidural or intrathecal injection of morphine in children have not been established and such injections in children are not recommended. Safety and efficacy of morphine sulfate extended-release capsules in children younger than 18 years of age have not been established. In addition, the manufacturers state that commercially available strengths of morphine sulfate extended-release capsules are not appropriate for children and that the contents of the capsules should not be sprinkled onto applesauce for administration to children. Safety and efficacy of morphine sulfate extended-release tablets in children also have not been established.

■ Geriatric Precautions Clinical studies of morphine sulfate extended-release preparations did not include sufficient numbers of patients 65 years of age and older to determine whether they respond differently than younger adults. While other clinical experience generally has not revealed age-related differences in safety or response to the drug, care should be taken in dosage selection in geriatric patients. Because of the greater frequency of decreased hepatic, renal, and/or cardiac function and of concomitant disease and drug therapy in geriatric patients, some manufacturers suggest that patients in this age group receive initial dosages of morphine sulfate as extended-release preparations in the lower end of the usual range.

When the total number of patients studied in clinical trials of morphine sulfate extended-release liposomal injection (DepoDur®) is considered, 25% were 65 years of age or older, while 5% were 75 years of age or older. No overall differences in safety and efficacy were observed between geriatric patients and younger adults; geriatric patients received the same or lower doses of the drug than younger adults. Geriatric patients may have increased sensitivity to the drug; in addition, comorbid conditions may predispose geriatric patients to serious adverse events (e.g., respiratory depression, ileus, hypotension, myocardial infarction). Careful evaluation of underlying conditions, vigilant monitoring, and dosing at the low end of the recommended range are advised.

The pharmacodynamics of epidurally or intrathecally administered morphine are more variable in geriatric patients than in younger adults. Considerable interindividual variation in effective initial dosage, rate of development of tolerance, and frequency and severity of adverse effects exists for epidural or intrathecal therapy with the drug in this population. Therefore, initial dosage should be selected carefully based on clinical assessment of response to test doses and consideration of the patient's age and infirmity on their ability to clear the drug, particularly in those receiving the drug epidurally.

■ Mutagenicity and Carcinogenicity Morphine sulfate is not known to have mutagenic or carcinogenic potential at non-narcotic doses in animals; however, the mutagenic or carcinogenic potential of morphine sulfate injection has not been established.

■ Pregnancy, Fertility, and Lactation Morphine sulfate was not teratogenic in rats at dosages of 35 mg/kg daily (35 times the usual human dose), but does result in increased pup mortality and growth retardation at doses that narcotize the animal (greater than 10 mg/kg daily, 10 times the usual human dose). However, morphine has been shown to be teratogenic in mice receiving single subcutaneous doses exceeding 2000 times the recommended human therapeutic dose. Teratogenic effects resembled hypoxia-induced malformations. In addition, morphine was teratogenic in golden hamsters receiving morphine doses of 35 mg/kg (exceeding 230 times the usual therapeutic human dose). Although there are no adequate and controlled studies to date in humans, morphine should be used during pregnancy only when the potential benefits justify the possible risks to the fetus.

Although safe use of morphine has been established during labor, use of opiate agonists generally should be avoided during labor when delivery of a premature neonate is anticipated. (See Cautions: Pediatric Precautions.) Because maternally administered opiate agonists are readily distributed into fetal circulation, an opiate antagonist and resuscitative equipment for reversal of opiate-induced respiratory depression should be readily available when the drugs are used during labor and delivery. Epidurally and intrathecally administered morphine also is readily distributed into fetal circulation and may result in respiratory depression in the neonate. Controlled clinical studies have shown that epidurally administered morphine has little or no effect on labor pain. Morphine sulfate extended-release liposomal injection (DepoDur®) should not be used during labor and/or vaginal delivery. There is some evidence that intrathecally administered morphine (0.2–1 mg) provides adequate pain relief during labor in most patients, with minimal effect on the duration of the first stage of labor; the second stage of labor may be prolonged if the woman is not encouraged to bear down. If the drug is administered intrathecally during labor, naloxone may be infused IV in the woman at a rate of 0.6 mg/hour for 24 hours after intrathecal morphine administration to decrease potential opiate-induced adverse effects. Highly concentrated morphine injections intended for administration via controlled-microinfusion devices (Infumorph®) are too potent for routine obstetric use; such injections should only be used in pregnant women when no other means for controlling pain is available and facilities to manage delivery and provide perinatal care for opiate toxicity and dependence in the neonate are readily accessible.

Prolonged maternal use of opiate agonists during pregnancy can result in neonatal opiate withdrawal syndrome with manifestations of irritability, hyperactivity and abnormal sleep pattern, high-pitched cry, tremor, vomiting, diarrhea, and failure to gain weight. In contrast to adults, the withdrawal syndrome in neonates may be life-threatening if not recognized and treated, and requires management according to protocols developed by neonatology experts. Women who require prolonged opiate agonist therapy during pregnancy should be advised of the risk of neonatal opiate withdrawal syndrome, and availability of appropriate treatment should be ensured. The onset, duration, and severity of the syndrome vary depending on the specific opiate agonist used, duration of use, timing and amount of last maternal use, and rate of drug elimination by the neonate. Use of standardized protocols for identification and management of opiate withdrawal syndrome has been shown to improve overall response, including reductions in hospital stay and duration of pharmacologic treatment. When environmental and supportive measures are inadequate, opiates (e.g., morphine) are recommended as first-line pharmacologic therapy. (See Uses: Neonatal Opiate Withdrawal.)

Morphine sulfate is not known to impair fertility at non-narcotic doses in animals; however, the effects of morphine sulfate injection on fertility have not been established.

Morphine should be used with caution in nursing women, since the drug has been reported to distribute into milk. Although clinically important concentrations of the drug probably are not present in milk following usual therapeutic dosages of the drug, the possibility that clinically important concentrations may be present should be considered especially when higher than usual dosages of the drug are used and in patients who have a history of opiate agonist abuse.

Pharmacokinetics

■ **Absorption** Morphine sulfate is variably absorbed from the GI tract. Food may increase the extent of GI absorption of morphine sulfate administered as conventional preparations. Food may decrease the rate of absorption of morphine sulfate administered as extended-release capsules; however, the extent of absorption of the drug does not appear to be affected. Following administration of single 10-mg doses of morphine sulfate as an oral solution or rectal suppository in one study in a limited number of patients with pain associated with cancer, absorption of the drug from the rectal suppository was greater than that from the oral solution over a 4.5-hour period after administration. Oral bioavailability and average plasma concentrations at steady state reportedly are similar following oral administration of morphine sulfate as conventional or extended-release preparations. However, lower peak and higher trough plasma concentrations of morphine may occur with administration of some extended-release tablets and capsules compared with conventional morphine sulfate formulations. In patient-controlled analgesia studies, the minimum analgesic plasma concentration of morphine was determined to be 20–40 ng/mL.

Peak analgesia occurs within 60 minutes following oral administration of conventional preparations of the drug, and analgesia occurs within 20–60 minutes after rectal administration. Peak analgesia occurs within 50–90 minutes following subcutaneous injection, 30–60 minutes after IM injection, and 20 minutes after IV injection. Analgesia may be maintained up to 7 hours. Following IM administration of morphine sulfate, maximal respiratory depression occurs within 30 minutes. Maximal respiratory depression following IV and subcutaneous injection occurs within 7 minutes and 90 minutes, respectively. Sensitivity of the respiratory center returns to normal within 2–3 hours, but respiratory minute volume may remain below normal for 4–5 hours.

Because of the blood-brain barrier, when morphine sulfate is injected into peripheral circulation (e.g., via IV injection), systemic plasma concentrations of the drug remain higher than the corresponding CNS concentration. Morphine sulfate is absorbed slowly into systemic circulation following intrathecal administration, accounting for the prolonged duration of action by this route. Systemic absorption following epidural administration of conventional morphine sulfate injection is rapid, with plasma concentration-time profiles reportedly resembling closely those attained after IV or IM administration of the drug; however, CSF morphine concentrations exceed those in plasma within 15 minutes after epidural injection of a single 2-mg dose and are detectable for up to 20 hours after administration. Area under the plasma concentration-time curve (AUC) is similar following epidural administration of equivalent single doses of morphine sulfate as conventional injection or extended-release liposomal injection, but peak plasma concentrations achieved with the extended-release liposomal formulation are about 30% of those achieved with the conventional injection. Following epidural injection of the extended-release liposomal formulation, absorption of morphine into the intrathecal space relative to absorption into systemic circulation has not been determined.

The minimum effective CSF concentration of morphine sulfate required for postoperative analgesia averages 150 ng/mL (range: less than 1 to 380 ng/mL). During patient-controlled analgesia (PCA), the minimum analgesic plasma concentration of morphine has been reported to be 20–40 ng/mL. Following epidural administration of 3 mg of conventional morphine sulfate injection, peak plasma concentrations averaging 33–40 ng/mL (range: 5–62 ng/mL) have been reported within 10–15 minutes of injection. CSF concentrations of morphine after epidural doses of 2–6 mg (as the conventional injection) have been reported to be 50–250 times that of the corresponding plasma concentration. Maximum CSF concentration of morphine in the CSF following epidural administration of conventional morphine sulfate injection is seen within 60–90 minutes. Following intrathecal administration of 0.3 mg of morphine, mean morphine CSF concentration at 6 hours following injection was 332 ng/mL (range: 195–469 ng/mL), while the corresponding maximum plasma morphine concentration has been reported to be less than 1 to 7.8 ng/mL.

Time to peak plasma concentration following either intrathecal or epidural morphine sulfate administration is similar, approximately 5–10 minutes. Following administration of morphine sulfate extended-release liposomal injection (DepoDur®) into the epidural space, morphine sulfate is released from the multivesicular liposomes over time; following epidural administration of the extended-release liposomal preparation, time to peak plasma concentrations is about 1 hour. The time to peak plasma concentration following oral administration of morphine sulfate extended-release capsules (Kadian®) every 24 hours was 10.3 hours compared with 4.4 hours for morphine sulfate extended-release tablets (MS Contin®) administered every 12 hours.

■ **Distribution** Following IV administration, morphine has an apparent volume of distribution ranging from 1–4.7 L/kg. Protein binding is reported to be 36% and muscle tissue binding reported to be 54%. Following epidural administration as the conventional injection, the absorption half-life of morphine across the dura is approximately 22 minutes. Following intrathecal administration of morphine, there is a rapid initial distribution phase lasting approximately 15–30 minutes; the disposition period of the drug in CSF from 15 minutes to approximately 6 hours following intrathecal administration appears to represent a combination of the distribution and elimination phases. Approximately 4% of an epidurally injected dose of conventional morphine sulfate injection distributes into CSF. Distribution across the dura is slow, with peak CSF concentrations occurring 60–90 minutes after an epidural dose. The apparent volume of distribution of morphine in the intrathecal space is about 22 mL (range: 14–30 mL).

Small amounts of morphine are distributed into the milk of nursing women.

■ **Elimination** In postoperative patients, total plasma clearance of morphine is reported to range from 0.9–1.2 L/kg per hour, but is subject to considerable interindividual variation.

Following epidural injection of conventional morphine sulfate injection, plasma concentrations of morphine decline in a multiexponential fashion; the mean terminal half-life of morphine following epidural injection is 90 minutes (range: 39–349 minutes), which is similar to the half-life of the drug reported after IV or IM administration (1.5–4.5 hours). CSF concentrations of morphine decline in a biphasic manner following epidural injection of conventional morphine sulfate injection, with an early distribution half-life of 1.5 hours and a terminal half-life of about 6 hours. Following epidural administration of a 10-, 15-, or 20-mg dose of morphine sulfate extended-release liposomal injection (DepoDur®), the half-life reportedly is 16.2, 20, or 23.9 hours, respectively. Because intrathecal injection of morphine circumvents meningeal diffusion barriers, lower doses are required to achieve comparable analgesia relative to epidural injection. Following intrathecal administration of the drug, the mean reported CSF half-life is 90 minutes (range: 42–136 minutes). The analgesic contribution of morphine redistributed from systemic circulation into the CNS is thought to be minimal within 30–60 minutes after an epidural dose and virtually nonexistent after an intrathecal dose.

Morphine is metabolized principally in the liver and undergoes conjugation with glucuronic acid principally at the 3-hydroxyl group. Secondary conjugation also occurs at the 6-hydroxyl group to form the 6-glucuronide, which is pharmacologically active, and to a limited extent the 3,6-diglucuronide. Plasma concentrations of the 3-glucuronide, which is inactive, and the 6-glucuronide substantially exceed those of unchanged drug, and the latter metabolite appears to contribute substantially to the drug's pharmacologic activity. Elimination of the drug may be reduced substantially in neonates compared with older children and adults. Morphine is excreted in urine mainly as morphine-3-glucuronide. In addition to the 3,6-diglucuronide, other minor metabolites that have been described includes normorphine and the 3-ethereal sulfate. Up to 2–12% of an administered dose of morphine is eliminated unchanged in the urine. About 90% of total urinary excretion occurs within 24 hours after the last dose is given. Approximately 7–10% of a dose of morphine is excreted in feces with a large portion of this excreted via bile. In patients with renal impairment, accumulation of morphine-6-glucuronide occurs, which can result in enhanced and prolonged opiate activity.

Chemistry and Stability

■ **Chemistry** Morphine is a phenanthrene-derivative opiate agonist. Morphine is the principal alkaloid of opium and considered to be the prototype of the opiate agonists. Morphine sulfate occurs as white, feathery, silky crystals; cubical masses of crystals; or a white, crystalline powder. The drug contains five molecules of water of hydration and has solubilities of approximately 62.5 mg/mL in water and 1.75 mg/mL in alcohol at 25°C. Morphine sulfate injection has a pH of 2.5–6. Duramorph® PF injection has a pH of 3.5–7 and Infumorph® has a pH of 4.5.

Morphine sulfate extended-release liposomal injection (DepoDur®) is a sterile, nonpyrogenic, white to off-white, preservative-free suspension of multivesicular lipid-based particles containing morphine sulfate. The liposomes are suspended in 0.9% sodium chloride solution. The preparation also contains 1,2-dioleoyl-*sn*-glycero-3-phosphocholine (DOPC), cholesterol, 1,2-dipalmitoyl-*sn*-glycero-3-phospho-*rac*-(1-glycerol)(DPPG), tricaprylin, and triolein, and has a pH of 5–8.

■ **Stability** When exposed to air, morphine sulfate gradually loses its water of hydration. The drug darkens on prolonged exposure to light.

Morphine sulfate injection should be protected from light and stored at 15–30°C; the injection should not be frozen. Astramorph® PF, Duramorph® PF, and Infumorph® injections and injections for use in a compatible patient-controlled infusion device contain no preservatives and are intended for single use only; unused portions should be discarded. Morphine sulfate extended-release liposomal injection (DepoDur®) should be stored under refrigeration at 2–8°C but may be stored at 15–30°C for up to 7 days in sealed, unopened vials. Morphine sulfate extended-release liposomal injection contains no preservative; the drug must be administered within 4 hours after withdrawal of a dose from the vial; unused portions should be discarded. The extended-release liposomal injection should be protected from freezing; if freezing occurs, the injection should be discarded. The preparation should not be sterilized by heat or gas (ethylene oxide).

Morphine sulfate soluble tablets, extended-release capsules and tablets, and oral solution should be stored in tight, light-resistant containers at 15–30°C; freezing of the oral solution should be avoided.

Morphine sulfate has been reported to be physically or chemically incompatible with solutions containing aminophylline, amobarbital sodium, chlorothiazide sodium, phenytoin sodium, heparin sodium, meperidine hydrochloride, methicillin sodium (no longer commercially available in the US), nitrofurantoin sodium, pentobarbital sodium, phenobarbital sodium, sodium bicarbonate, sodium iodide, and thiopental sodium (no longer commercially available in the US). Specialized references should be consulted for specific compatibility information.

For further information on the chemistry, pharmacology, pharmacokinetics, uses, cautions, chronic toxicity, acute toxicity, drug interactions, and dosage and administration of morphine sulfate, see the Opiate Agonists General Statement 28:08.08.

Preparations

Morphine sulfate is subject to control under the Federal Controlled Substances Act of 1970 as a schedule II (C-II) drug when available as a single entity or as a schedule III (C-III) drug when available as a fixed-combination preparation in a concentration of 0.5 mg or less per mL or g combined with a therapeutic amount of one or more nonopiate drugs.

Excipients in commercially available drug preparations may have clinically important effects in some individuals; consult specific product labeling for details.

Morphine Sulfate

Oral		
Capsules, extended-release (containing beads)	30 mg (extended-release 27 mg with 3 mg immediate-release)/24 hours	**AVINza®** (C-II), Ligand (also promoted by Organon)
	60 mg (extended-release 54 mg with 6 mg immediate-release)/24 hours	**AVINza®** (C-II), Ligand (also promoted by Organon)
	90 mg (extended-release 81 mg with 9 mg immediate-release)/24 hours	**AVINza®** (C-II), Ligand (also promoted by Organon)
	120 mg (extended-release 108 mg with 12 mg immediate-release)/24 hours	**AVINza®** (C-II), Ligand (also promoted by Organon)
Capsules, extended-release (containing pellets)	10 mg/24 hours	**Kadian®** (C-II), Actavis
	20 mg/24 hours	**Kadian®** (C-II), Actavis
	30 mg/24 hours	**Kadian®** (C-II), Actavis
	50 mg/24 hours	**Kadian®** (C-II), Actavis
	60 mg/24 hours	**Kadian®** (C-II), Actavis
	80 mg/24 hours	**Kadian®** (C-II), Actavis
	100 mg/24 hours	**Kadian®** (C-II), Actavis
	200 mg/24 hours	**Kadian®** (C-II), Actavis
Solution	10 mg/5 mL	**Morphine Sulfate Oral Solution** (C-II)
	20 mg/5 mL	**Morphine Sulfate Oral Solution** (C-II)
	100 mg/5 mL	**Morphine Sulfate Oral Solution** (C-II; with graduated oral syringe)
Tablets	15 mg	**Morphine Sulfate Tablets** (C-II; scored)
	30 mg	**Morphine Sulfate Tablets** (C-II; scored)
Tablets, extended-release	15 mg/12 hours	**Oramorph® SR** (C-II), Xanodyne
	30 mg/12 hours	**Oramorph® SR** (C-II), Xanodyne
	60 mg/12 hours	**Oramorph® SR** (C-II), Xanodyne
	100 mg/12 hours	**Oramorph® SR** (C-II), Xanodyne
Tablets, extended-release, film-coated	15 mg/12 hours	**Morphine Sulfate Tablets ER** (C-II)
		MS Contin® (C-II), Purdue Pharma
	30 mg/12 hours	**Morphine Sulfate Tablets ER** (C-II)
		MS Contin® (C-II), Purdue Pharma
	60 mg/12 hours	**Morphine Sulfate Tablets ER** (C-II)
		MS Contin® (C-II), Purdue Pharma
	100 mg/12 hours	**Morphine Sulfate Tablets ER** (C-II)
		MS Contin® (C-II), Purdue Pharma
	200 mg/12 hours	**Morphine Sulfate Tablets ER** (C-II)
		MS Contin® (C-II), Purdue Pharma
Tablets, soluble	10 mg	**Morphine Sulfate Tablets** (C-II)
	15 mg	**Morphine Sulfate Tablets** (C-II)
	30 mg	**Morphine Sulfate Tablets** (C-II)
Parenteral		
Injection, for IM, IV, or subcutaneous use	0.5 mg/mL	**Morphine Sulfate Injection** (C-II)
	1 mg/mL	**Morphine Sulfate Injection** (C-II)
	2 mg/mL	**Morphine Sulfate Injection** (C-II)
	4 mg/mL	**Morphine Sulfate Injection** (C-II)
	5 mg/mL	**Morphine Sulfate Injection** (C-II)
	8 mg/mL	**Morphine Sulfate Injection** (C-II)
	10 mg/mL	**Morphine Sulfate Injection** (C-II)
	15 mg/mL	**Morphine Sulfate Injection** (C-II)
Injection, for epidural, intrathecal, or IV use	0.5 mg/mL	**Astramorph/PF®** (C-II), AstraZeneca
		Duramorph® (C-II), Baxter
		Morphine Sulfate Injection (C-II)
	1 mg/mL	**Astramorph/PF®** (C-II), AstraZeneca
		Duramorph® (C-II), Baxter
		Morphine Sulfate Injection (C-II)
Injection, for epidural or intrathecal use via continuous microinfusion device only	10 mg/mL	**Infumorph®** (C-II), Baxter
	25 mg/mL	**Infumorph®** (C-II), Baxter
		Morphine Sulfate Injection (C-II)
Injection, for IV infusion via compatible patient-controlled infusion device only	1 mg/mL	**Morphine Sulfate Injection** (C-II)

	5 mg/mL	**Morphine Sulfate Injection** (C-II)
Injection, for IV infusion	25 mg/mL	**Morphine Sulfate ADD-Vantage®** (C-II)
Injection, for preparation of IV infusion	25 mg/mL	**Morphine Sulfate Injection** (C-II)
	50 mg/mL	**Morphine Sulfate Injection** (C-II)
Rectal		
Suppositories	5 mg	**Morphine Sulfate Suppositories** (C-II)
		RMS® (C-II), Upsher-Smith
	10 mg	**Morphine Sulfate Suppositories** (C-II)
		RMS® (C-II), Upsher-Smith
	20 mg	**Morphine Sulfate Suppositories** (C-II)
		RMS® (C-II), Upsher-Smith
	30 mg	**Morphine Sulfate Suppositories** (C-II)
		RMS® (C-II), Upsher-Smith

Morphine Sulfate Liposomal

Parenteral		
Injectable suspension, extended-release, for epidural use	10 mg/mL (of morphine sulfate) (10, 15, and 20 mg)	**DepoDur®** (C-II), Endo

†Use is not currently included in the labeling approved by the US Food and Drug Administration

oxyCODONE Hydrochloride

Dihydrohydroxycodeinone, 14-Hydroxydihydrocodeinone

oxyCODONE Myristate

■ Oxycodone is a synthetic phenanthrene-derivative opiate agonist.

REMS

FDA approved a REMS for oxycodone to ensure that the benefits outweigh the risk. The REMS may apply to one or more preparations of oxycodone and consists of the following: medication guide and elements to assure safe use. See the FDA REMS page (https://www.accessdata.fda.gov/scripts/cder/rems/index.cfm).

Uses

■ **Pain** Conventional preparations of oxycodone hydrochloride are used orally for the management of moderate to severe acute or chronic pain when use of an opiate analgesic is appropriate.

Oxycodone hydrochloride extended-release tablets and oxycodone myristate extended-release capsules are used orally for the relief of pain that is severe enough to require long-term, daily, around-the-clock use of an opiate analgesic. Because of the risks of addiction, abuse, and misuse associated with opiates even at recommended dosages, and because of the greater risks of overdose and death associated with extended-release opiate formulations, these extended-release preparations of oxycodone hydrochloride or oxycodone myristate should be reserved for use in patients for whom alternative treatment options (e.g., nonopiate analgesics, immediate-release opiates) are inadequate or not tolerated. Oxycodone hydrochloride extended-release tablets may be used for the relief of such pain in pediatric patients 11 years of age or older who are opiate tolerant and already receiving and tolerating opiate agonist therapy at a dosage equivalent to 20 mg or more of oxycodone hydrochloride daily. The manufacturer states that safety and efficacy of oxycodone myristate extended-release capsules have not been established in patients younger than 18 years of age. Oxycodone hydrochloride extended-release tablets and oxycodone myristate extended-release capsules are *not* intended for use on an as-needed ("prn") basis.

Extended-release tablets containing oxycodone hydrochloride in fixed combination with acetaminophen are used for the relief of acute pain that is severe enough to require opiate therapy and for which alternative treatments (e.g., nonopiate analgesics) are inadequate or not tolerated.

For further information on the role of opiate analgesics in the management of acute or chronic pain, see Uses: Pain, in the Opiate Agonists General Statement 28:08.08.

■ **Misuse and Abuse** Oxycodone has emerged as one of the most problematic abused opiate agonists in the US; therefore, patients should be advised about the risk of theft, and clinicians should be informed about abuse and diversion issues. (See Cautions.)

Dosage and Administration

■ **Administration** Oxycodone is administered orally as the hydrochloride salt, often in combination with nonopiate analgesics (e.g., acetaminophen), or as the myristate salt.

Conventional Oxycodone Hydrochloride Formulations Some manufacturers state that their formulations of oxycodone hydrochloride conventional tablets should not be crushed and dissolved. These formulations should not be administered via gastric, nasogastric, or other feeding tube since they can obstruct the tube. Instead, these tablets should be administered intact with sufficient water to ensure that each tablet is completely swallowed immediately after it is placed in the mouth. The respective manufacturer's labeling should be consulted for specific recommendations.

Oxycodone hydrochloride is commercially available as a 5-mg/5-mL oral solution and as a 100-mg/5-mL oral concentrate solution; confusion between the different concentrations or between mg and mL can result in accidental overdosage and/or death. The oral concentrate solution should be used only in opiate-tolerant patients. Caution is required when prescribing, dispensing, and administering oral solutions of the drug to avoid dosing errors. Care should be taken to ensure that the appropriate dose is communicated and dispensed. Prescriptions should specify the intended total dose of the drug (in mg) along with the corresponding total volume (in mL). The calibrated measuring device provided with the particular formulation should always be used to ensure that the dose is measured and administered accurately.

Oxycodone Hydrochloride and Acetaminophen Fixed-combination Extended-release Tablets Extended-release tablets containing oxycodone hydrochloride in fixed combination with acetaminophen should be swallowed whole and should *not* be broken, chewed, crushed, cut, or dissolved, since such physical alteration of the tablets could result in rapid release of the drug and absorption of a potentially toxic dose. The fixed-combination extended-release tablets should be administered one at a time with enough water to ensure that each tablet is completely swallowed immediately after it is placed in the mouth; extended-release tablets should not be wet (e.g., soaked, licked) before they are placed in the mouth for swallowing. The tablets may be administered without regard to food. This formulation should not be used for administration through a nasogastric, gastric, or other feeding tube.

Oxycodone Hydrochloride Extended-release Tablets Oxycodone hydrochloride extended-release tablets should be swallowed whole and should *not* be broken, chewed, crushed, cut, split, or dissolved, since such physical alteration of the tablets could result in rapid release of the drug and absorption of a potentially toxic dose. Extended-release tablets should be administered one at a time with enough water to ensure that each tablet is completely swallowed immediately after it is placed in the mouth; extended-release tablets should not be wet (e.g., soaked, licked) before they are placed in the mouth for swallowing. Oxycodone hydrochloride extended-release tablets should not be administered rectally because of increased bioavailability and peak plasma concentrations compared with oral administration. (See Pharmacokinetics.) Food does not substantially affect the extent of oral absorption of oxycodone hydrochloride extended-release tablets.

Oxycodone Myristate Extended-release Capsules Oxycodone myristate extended-release capsules *must* be administered orally with food. Each dose should be administered with approximately the same amount of food (whether given as an intact capsule or as capsule contents sprinkled on food or directly in the mouth) in order to ensure that consistent plasma concentrations of the drug are achieved. (See Pharmacokinetics.) For patients who have difficulty swallowing, the capsules may be opened and the contents sprinkled onto a small amount of soft food (e.g., applesauce, pudding, yogurt, ice cream, jam) or into a cup and then administered directly into the mouth. The capsule contents should be swallowed immediately, and the mouth should be rinsed to ensure that the entire dose has been swallowed.

Alternatively, the capsule contents may be administered through a nasogastric or gastrostomy tube. The tube should first be flushed with water and then the capsule should be opened and the contents carefully poured directly into the tube; the capsule contents should not be premixed with the liquid that will be used to flush the tube. Following administration, the tube should be flushed with 15 mL of liquid (water, milk, or liquid nutritional supplement) and then flushed 2 more times, each time with 10 mL of liquid, to ensure that the entire dose is delivered.

■ **Dosage** Dosage of oxycodone hydrochloride is expressed in terms of the salt; dosage of oxycodone myristate is expressed in terms of oxycodone base.

Oxycodone should be given at the lowest effective dosage and for the shortest duration of therapy consistent with the treatment goals of the patient. Reduced dosage is indicated in debilitated patients and in very young or very old patients. If concomitant therapy with other CNS depressants is required, the lowest effective dosages and shortest possible duration of concomitant therapy should be used. Some manufacturers recommend that initial dosages of 33–50% of the usual dosage be employed when therapy with oxycodone hydrochloride extended-release tablets is initiated in patients receiving other CNS depressants. When therapy with extended-release tablets containing oxycodone hydrochloride in fixed combination with acetaminophen is initiated in patients receiving other CNS depressants, the manufacturer states that the initial oxycodone hydrochloride dosage should be reduced by 50% (i.e., to 7.5 mg twice daily).

For acute pain not related to trauma or surgery, the prescribed quantity should be limited to the amount needed for the expected duration of pain severe enough to require opiate analgesia (generally 3 days or less and rarely more than 7 days). When opiate analgesics are used for the management of chronic noncancer pain, the US Centers for Disease Control and Prevention (CDC) recommends that primary care clinicians carefully reassess individual benefits and risks before prescribing dosages equivalent to 50 mg or more of morphine sulfate daily (approximately 33 mg or more of oxycodone hydrochloride daily) and avoid dosages equivalent to 90 mg or more of morphine sulfate daily (approximately 60 mg or more of oxycodone hydrochloride daily) or carefully justify their decision to titrate the dosage to such levels. Other experts recommend consulting a pain management specialist before exceeding a dosage equivalent to 80–120 mg of morphine sulfate daily.

Patients receiving long-term, daily, around-the-clock opiate analgesia should be reevaluated continually for adequacy of pain control and for adverse effects, as well as for manifestations of opiate withdrawal and for the development of addiction, abuse, or misuse. To reduce the risk of respiratory depression, appropriate dosage selection and titration are essential. The initial dosage of oxycodone must be individualized, taking into account the patient's severity of pain, response, prior analgesic use, and risk factors for addiction, abuse, and misuse. Because there is substantial interpatient variability in the relative potency of opiate analgesics and analgesic formulations, it is preferable to underestimate the patient's 24-hour opiate requirements and provide "rescue" therapy with an immediate-release opiate analgesic than to overestimate the requirements and manage an adverse reaction. Patients should be monitored closely for respiratory depression, especially during the first 24–72 hours of therapy and following any increase in dosage.

In patients requiring long-term around-the-clock opiate analgesia, dosage of oxycodone should be titrated to a level that provides adequate analgesia and minimizes adverse effects. Frequent communication among the prescriber, other members of the healthcare team, the patient, and the patient's caregiver or family is important during periods of changing analgesic requirements, including the initial dosage titration period. Patients who experience breakthrough pain may require dosage adjustment or supplemental analgesia (i.e., "rescue" therapy with an immediate-release analgesic). If the level of pain increases after dosage stabilization, an attempt should be made to identify the source of increased pain before increasing the oxycodone dosage. During long-term therapy, the continued need for opiate analgesics should be continually reevaluated. If discontinuance of opiate therapy is required, the dosage should be tapered gradually to avoid manifestations of abrupt withdrawal.

For further information on the management of opiate analgesic therapy, see Dosage and Administration: Dosage, in the Opiate Agonists General Statement 28:08.08.

Conventional (Immediate-release) Preparations For the management of moderate to severe pain in patients who have not been receiving opiate analgesic therapy, the usual initial adult dosage of conventional oxycodone hydrochloride preparations is 5–15 mg every 4–6 hours as needed. Although safety and efficacy of conventional oxycodone hydrochloride preparations have not been established in children, the drug has been recommended for use in pediatric patients. For the management of moderate to severe pain in children, some experts have suggested a dosage of 0.05–0.15 mg/kg (up to 5 mg) every 4–6 hours as needed.

Dosage should be adjusted based on the response and tolerance of the patient. Patients with chronic pain may require around-the-clock rather than as-needed dosing. Because opiate analgesics given on a fixed dosage schedule have a narrow therapeutic index in certain patient populations, especially when used concomitantly with other drugs, fixed dosage schedules should be reserved for patients for whom the benefits of opiate analgesia outweigh the risks of respiratory depression, altered mental state, and orthostatic hypotension. In patients switching from other opiates or opiate formulations to therapy with conventional oxycodone hydrochloride preparations, the potency of the prior opiate relative to that of oxycodone should be considered, keeping in mind that published dosage conversion ratios are only approximations. Conservative initial dosages, patient monitoring, and dosage adjustment based on response are essential when the opiate or opiate formulation is switched.

When opiate analgesics are administered in fixed combination with nonopiate analgesics, the opiate dosage may be limited by the nonopiate component. Because commercially available preparations contain oxycodone and nonopiate analgesics in various fixed ratios and because these nonopiate analgesics also are available in many other prescription and OTC preparations, care should be taken to ensure that therapy is not duplicated and that dosage of the nonopiate drug does not exceed maximum recommended dosages.

When therapy with conventional preparations of oxycodone hydrochloride is discontinued following long-term opiate therapy, dosage generally can be reduced by 25–50% per day. If symptoms of withdrawal occur, the dosage should be increased to the prior level and tapered more slowly.

Oxycodone Hydrochloride and Acetaminophen Fixed-combination Extended-release Tablets When extended-release tablets containing oxycodone hydrochloride in fixed combination with acetaminophen are used for the management of acute pain in adults, the recommended oxycodone hydrochloride dosage is 15 mg (given in fixed combination with 650 mg of acetaminophen) every 12 hours. The second dose may be administered as soon as 8 hours after the initial dose if required for adequate analgesia, but all subsequent doses should be administered at 12-hour intervals. When therapy with this formulation is discontinued in a patient who may be opiate dependent, the dosage should be tapered gradually (i.e., reduced by 50% every 2–4 days) to avoid manifestations of abrupt withdrawal.

When opiate analgesics are administered in fixed combination with acetaminophen, the opiate dosage may be limited by the acetaminophen component. Because acetaminophen also is available in many other prescription and OTC preparations, care should be taken to ensure that therapy is not duplicated and that dosage of acetaminophen does not exceed maximum recommended dosages.

Oxycodone Hydrochloride Extended-release Tablets **Adult Dosage.** For the management of pain severe enough to require daily, around-the-clock, long-term opiate analgesia in adults who are *not* opiate tolerant, therapy with oxycodone hydrochloride extended-release tablets should be initiated at a dosage of 10 mg every 12 hours. The manufacturers state that use of higher initial dosages in patients who are not opiate tolerant may result in fatal respiratory depression. A single dose exceeding 40 mg, total daily dosages exceeding 80 mg, and 60- and 80-mg extended-release tablets should be used only in adults in whom tolerance to an opiate of comparable potency has been established. Adults are considered opiate tolerant if they have been receiving opiate therapy consisting of at least 60 mg of morphine sulfate daily, 25 mcg of transdermal fentanyl per hour, 30 mg of oral oxycodone hydrochloride daily, 8 mg of oral hydromorphone hydrochloride daily, 25 mg of oxymorphone hydrochloride daily, or an equianalgesic dosage of another opiate daily for at least 1 week.

In patients who are being switched from other opiates to oxycodone hydrochloride extended-release tablets, all other around-the-clock opiate analgesics should be discontinued when therapy with the extended-release tablets is initiated. For patients receiving conventional oxycodone preparations, the total daily dosage of the drug should be calculated and given as oxycodone hydrochloride extended-release tablets in 2 divided doses at 12-hour intervals.

For patients receiving conventional formulations of other opiates, the recommended initial dosage of oxycodone hydrochloride extended-release tablets is 10 mg every 12 hours, since dosage conversion factors have not been established in clinical trials. Particularly close monitoring is required when patients are switched from methadone, since conversion ratios between methadone and other opiates vary widely depending on extent of prior methadone exposure and because methadone has a long half-life and tends to accumulate in plasma.

Patients receiving fentanyl transdermal systems may receive oxycodone hydrochloride extended-release tablets beginning 18 hours after removal of the transdermal system. The manufacturers state that an initial oxycodone hydrochloride dosage of approximately 10 mg every 12 hours as extended-release tablets can be substituted for each 25-mcg/hour increment in fentanyl transdermal system dosage; however, patients should be monitored closely, since clinical experience with this dosage conversion ratio is limited.

Dosage adjustments in adults generally may be made in increments of 25–50% of the total daily dosage at intervals of 1–2 days, to a level that provides adequate analgesia and minimizes adverse effects. Safety and efficacy of dosing intervals shorter than 12 hours have not been established.

The manufacturer states that usual doses and dosing intervals for oxycodone hydrochloride extended-release tablets may be appropriate for geriatric patients, since no unexpected adverse effects were observed in geriatric patients receiving this preparation in clinical trials with appropriate initiation of therapy and dosage titration. However, the manufacturer recommends that initial dosages of 33–50% of the usual dosage be employed when therapy with oxycodone hydrochloride extended-release tablets is initiated in non-opiate-tolerant, debilitated geriatric patients. Dosage in geriatric patients should be titrated cautiously.

Pediatric Dosage. Extended-release oxycodone hydrochloride tablets should be used only in opiate-tolerant pediatric patients 11 years of age and older; such patients must be receiving and tolerating opiate analgesics for at least 5 consecutive days, and at a dosage of at least 20 mg of oxycodone hydrochloride (or equivalent) daily for at least 2 days immediately prior to initiation of therapy with oxycodone hydrochloride extended-release tablets. All other around-the-clock opiate analgesics should be discontinued when therapy with the extended-release tablets is initiated.

In pediatric patients who are being switched from other opiate therapy to oxycodone hydrochloride extended-release tablets, the manufacturer states that the conversion factors in Table 1 may be used as a guide for selecting an initial dosage of the extended-release tablets. The manufacturer cautions that the doses in Table 1 are not equianalgesic doses and the table cannot be used to switch patients from oxycodone hydrochloride extended-release tablets to another opiate, as this will result in overestimation of the dosage of the new opiate and possible fatal overdosage. For patients receiving a single opiate analgesic, the current total daily dosage of the opiate should be multiplied by the appropriate conversion factor in Table 1 to calculate the approximate daily dosage of oxycodone hydrochloride extended-release tablets; the calculated daily dosage should then be divided in half for administration every 12 hours. For patients receiving more than one opiate analgesic, the approximate daily dosage of extended-release oxycodone hydrochloride should be calculated for each opiate and then those totals should be summed to obtain the approximate total daily dosage of oxycodone hydrochloride extended-release tablets; the calculated total daily dosage should then be divided in half for administration every 12 hours. For patients receiving analgesics containing opiates and nonopiates in a fixed ratio, only the opiate component should be considered in the conversion. Calculated doses that do not correspond to an available tablet strength should always be rounded down to the nearest whole tablet when initiating therapy; if the calculated total daily dosage is less than 20 mg, patients should *not* be switched to the extended-release formulation.

Dosage adjustments in pediatric patients may be made in increments of 25% of the total daily dosage at intervals of 1–2 days, to a level that provides adequate analgesia and minimizes adverse effects. Safety and efficacy of dosing intervals shorter than 12 hours have not been established.

In patients receiving asymmetric dosing, the higher dose should be taken in the morning and the lower dose in the evening.

Table 1. Conversion Factors When Switching Pediatric Patients 11 Years of Age or Older to Oxycodone Hydrochloride Extended-release Tablets

	Conversion Factor	
Prior Opiate	Oral	Parenteral[a]
Oxycodone	1	
Hydrocodone	0.9	–
Hydromorphone	4	20
Morphine	0.5	3
Tramadol	0.17	0.2

[a] For patients receiving high-dose parenteral opiates, a more conservative conversion is warranted (e.g., for high-dose parenteral morphine, use 1.5 instead of 3 as a multiplication factor).

Pediatric patients receiving fentanyl transdermal systems may receive oxycodone hydrochloride extended-release tablets beginning 18 hours after removal of the transdermal system. The manufacturers state that an initial oxycodone hydrochloride dosage of approximately 10 mg every 12 hours as extended-release tablets can be substituted for each 25-mcg/hour increment in fentanyl transdermal system dosage; however, patients should be monitored closely, since clinical experience with this dosage conversion ratio is limited.

Oxycodone Myristate Extended-release Capsules **Adult Dosage.** For the management of pain that is severe enough to require long-term, daily, around-the-clock analgesia in adults who are not currently receiving opiate analgesics or are not opiate tolerant, therapy with oxycodone myristate extended-release capsules should be initiated at a dosage of 9 mg of oxycodone (equivalent to 10 mg of oxycodone hydrochloride) every 12 hours. Use of higher initial dosages in patients who are not opiate tolerant may result in fatal respiratory depression. A single dose exceeding 36 mg of oxycodone (equivalent to 40 mg of oxycodone hydrochloride) or total daily dosages exceeding 72 mg of oxycodone (equivalent to 80 mg of oxycodone hydrochloride) should be used only in patients in whom tolerance to an opiate of comparable potency has been established. Patients are considered opiate tolerant if they have been receiving at least 60 mg of oral morphine sulfate daily, 25 mcg of transdermal fentanyl per hour, 30 mg of oral oxycodone hydrochloride daily, 8 mg of oral hydromorphone hydrochloride daily, 25 mg of oral oxymorphone hydrochloride daily, 60 mg of oral hydrocodone bitartrate daily, or an equianalgesic dose of another opiate daily for at least 1 week.

In adults who are being transferred from other oral opiates to therapy with oxycodone myristate extended-release capsules, all other around-the-clock opiate analgesics should be discontinued when therapy with the extended-release capsules is initiated. Dosage must be carefully individualized since overestimation of the initial dosage in opiate-tolerant patients can result in fatal overdosage. For adults receiving other oral oxycodone preparations, the total daily dosage of the drug should be calculated and given as oxycodone myristate extended-release capsules in 2 divided doses at 12-hour intervals; because oxycodone myristate extended-release capsules are not bioequivalent to other extended-release preparations of the drug, dosage adjustment may be necessary. For patients receiving other opiate analgesics, the recommended initial dosage of oxycodone myristate extended-release capsules is 9 mg of oxycodone every 12 hours, since dosage conversion factors have not been established in clinical trials. Particularly close monitoring is required when patients are switched from methadone, since conversion ratios between methadone and other opiates vary widely depending on extent of prior methadone exposure and because methadone has a long half-life and tends to accumulate in plasma.

Adults receiving therapy with fentanyl transdermal system may receive oxycodone myristate extended-release capsules beginning 18 hours after removal of the transdermal system. The manufacturer states that a conservative initial oxycodone dosage of approximately 9 mg every 12 hours as extended-release capsules can be substituted for each 25-mcg/hour increment in transdermal fentanyl system dosage; however, patients should be monitored closely, since clinical experience with this dosage conversion ratio is limited.

Dosage adjustments generally may be made in increments of 25–50% of the total daily dosage at intervals of 1–2 days, to a level that provides adequate analgesia and minimizes adverse effects. Safety and efficacy of dosing intervals shorter than 12 hours have not been established. The maximum recommended dosage of oxycodone myristate extended-release capsules is 288 mg of oxycodone daily (eight 36-mg capsules), since safety of excipients in the formulation at dosages exceeding 288 mg daily has not been established.

The manufacturer states that usual doses and dosing intervals for oxycodone myristate extended-release capsules may be appropriate for geriatric patients, since no unexpected adverse effects were observed in geriatric patients receiving this preparation in a clinical trial with appropriate initiation of therapy and dosage titration. Nevertheless, dosage should be selected with caution because of the greater frequency of decreased hepatic, renal, and/or cardiac function and of concomitant disease and drug therapy observed in geriatric patients and titrated slowly because of the risk of respiratory depression.

■ **Dosage in Renal and Hepatic Impairment** In patients with impaired hepatic function, initial oxycodone dosages should be conservative and adjusted according to the clinical situation. The manufacturers recommend that therapy with oxycodone hydrochloride extended-release tablets or oxycodone myristate extended-release capsules be initiated at 33–50% of the usual dosage and titrated carefully. When extended-release tablets containing oxycodone hydrochloride in fixed combination with acetaminophen are used for the management of acute pain in patients with hepatic impairment, the manufacturer recommends an initial oxycodone hydrochloride dose of 7.5 mg (given in fixed combination with 325 mg of acetaminophen); dosage should be adjusted as needed with close monitoring for respiratory depression.

In patients with impaired renal function (creatinine clearance less than 60 mL/minute), initial oxycodone dosages should be conservative and adjusted according to the clinical situation. When extended-release tablets containing oxycodone hydrochloride in fixed combination with acetaminophen are used for the management of acute pain in patients with renal impairment, the manufacturer recommends an initial oxycodone hydrochloride dose of 7.5 mg (given in fixed combination with 325 mg of acetaminophen); dosage should be adjusted as needed with close monitoring for respiratory depression.

If the required dose of oxycodone myristate extended-release capsules is less than 9 mg of oxycodone, an alternative analgesic should be selected.

Cautions

Although adverse effects are milder than those of morphine, addiction liability of oxycodone is about the same as that of morphine; oxycodone shares the toxic potentials of the opiate agonists, and the usual precautions of opiate agonist therapy should be observed. (See Cautions in the Opiate Agonists General Statement 28:08.08.) When preparations containing oxycodone in combination with other drugs are administered, the cautions applicable to each ingredient must be considered.

Because oxycodone hydrochloride is commercially available as an oral solution (5 mg/5 mL) and as an oral concentrate solution (100 mg/5 mL), confusion between the different concentrations or between mg and mL can result in accidental overdosage and/or death. Caution is required to avoid confusing the formulations. (See Conventional Oxycodone Hydrochloride Formulations under Dosage and Administration: Administration.) The oral concentrate solution should be used only in opiate-tolerant patients.

Extended-release opiates are associated with a greater risk of overdose and death because of the larger amount of drug contained in each dosage unit. Oxycodone has been intentionally abused by crushing extended-release preparations and "snorting" the powder or dissolving the contents in water and injecting the solution IV. Abuse by chewing extended-release preparations also has been reported. Breaking, chewing, crushing, or dissolving of extended-release tablets containing oxycodone hydrochloride results in immediate release of the opiate and the risk of a potentially fatal overdose. Snorting or injecting the dissolved contents of oxycodone myristate extended-release capsules also can result in a potentially fatal overdose. The risk of toxicity is increased when oxycodone is used concomitantly with alcohol or other CNS depressants, including other opiates.

Oxycodone hydrochloride extended-release tablets (OxyContin®) and oxycodone myristate extended-release capsules (Xtampza® ER) are formulated with physical and chemical properties that are intended to make these dosage forms more difficult to manipulate for IV or intranasal abuse and misuse. However, abuse by these routes, as well as by the oral route, is still possible.

Because some patients have reported difficulty in swallowing oxycodone hydrochloride extended-release tablets, the tablets should be administered one at a time with enough water to ensure that each tablet is completely swallowed immediately after it is placed in the mouth; the extended-release tablets should not be wet (e.g., soaked, licked) before they are placed in the mouth for swallowing. Choking, gagging, regurgitation, tablets stuck in the throat, and, rarely, intestinal obstruction and exacerbation of diverticulitis (sometimes requiring medical intervention to remove the tablet) have been reported. Patients with underlying GI disorders (e.g., esophageal or colon cancer) associated with a narrow GI lumen are at greater risk of developing these complications. Use of an alternative analgesic should be considered for patients who have difficulty swallowing and in those at risk for underlying GI disorders associated with a narrow GI lumen. Because extended-release tablets containing oxycodone hydrochloride in fixed combination with acetaminophen swell and become sticky when wet, the same precautions apply to this formulation.

Some commercially available formulations of oxycodone hydrochloride contain sodium metabisulfite, a sulfite that may cause allergic-type reactions, including anaphylaxis and life-threatening or less severe asthmatic episodes, in certain susceptible individuals. The overall prevalence of sulfite sensitivity in the general population is unknown but probably low; such sensitivity appears to occur more frequently in asthmatic than in nonasthmatic individuals.

The presence of oxycodone is not reliably detected by all urine drug tests for opiates, especially those designed for in-office use, and laboratories may report urine drug concentrations below a specified value as negative results. If urine testing for oxycodone is used in patient management, the limitations of such testing should be considered and appropriate assay sensitivity and specificity should be ensured.

Oxycodone is distributed into milk. Because of the possibility of sedation or respiratory depression in breast-fed infants, use of oxycodone in nursing women should be avoided. Infants exposed to oxycodone through breast milk should be observed for GI effects, excessive sedation, respiratory depression, and changes in feeding patterns. Symptoms of withdrawal can occur in opiate-dependent breast-fed infants when maternal administration of opiates is discontinued or breast-feeding is stopped.

Drug Interactions

■ **Drugs Affecting Hepatic Microsomal Enzymes** Because oxycodone is metabolized by the cytochrome P-450 (CYP) microsomal enzyme system, principally by isoenzyme 3A4, concomitant use of oxycodone with drugs that inhibit CYP3A4 activity (e.g., macrolide antibiotics [e.g., erythromycin], azole antifungals [e.g., ketoconazole, voriconazole], protease inhibitors [e.g., ritonavir]) may result in reduced clearance and increased plasma concentrations of oxycodone, possibly resulting in increased or prolonged opiate effects, including an increased risk of fatal respiratory depression. These effects could be more pronounced with concomitant use of oxycodone and inhibitors of both CYP2D6 and CYP3A4 (see Pharmacokinetics), particularly when an inhibitor is added after a stable oxycodone dosage has been achieved. Concomitant administration of oxycodone hydrochloride (single 10-mg dose as extended-release tablets) and the potent CYP3A4 inhibitor ketoconazole (200 mg twice daily) increased area under the plasma concentration-time curve (AUC) and peak plasma concentration of oxycodone by 170 and 100%, respectively, while concomitant administration of voriconazole with oxycodone increased the AUC and peak plasma concentration of oxycodone by 3.6- and 1.7-fold, respectively. However, inhibition of the CYP2D6 pathway alone has not been shown to result in clinically important interactions. If concomitant therapy with a CYP3A4 inhibitor is discontinued, a decrease in plasma oxycodone concentrations may occur, potentially decreasing analgesic efficacy or resulting in withdrawal effects.

Concomitant use of oxycodone with CYP3A4 inducers (e.g., carbamazepine, phenytoin, rifampin) may result in increased clearance and decreased plasma concentrations of oxycodone, with possible lack of efficacy or development of opiate withdrawal. Concomitant administration of oxycodone and the CYP3A4 inducer rifampin decreased AUC and peak plasma concentration of oxycodone by 86 and 63%, respectively. If concomitant therapy with a CYP3A4 inducer is discontinued, an increase in plasma oxycodone concentrations may occur, potentially increasing or prolonging therapeutic and adverse effects of the drug and increasing the risk of serious respiratory depression.

Therefore, caution should be exercised and patients who require concomitant therapy with a CYP3A4 inhibitor or inducer, or who have recently discontinued such therapy, should be monitored closely at frequent intervals, and dosage adjustments should be considered until stable drug effects are achieved.

For further information about drug interactions involving opiate agonists (including oxycodone), see Drug Interactions in the Opiate Agonists General Statement 28:08.08.

Pharmacokinetics

Following oral administration of conventional preparations of oxycodone, the analgesic effect occurs within 10–15 minutes, reaches its maximum in 30–60 minutes, and persists for 3–6 hours. Following oral administration of oxycodone as an extended-release tablet, the onset of analgesia occurred within 1 hour in most patients. Oxycodone is extensively metabolized to noroxycodone, oxymorphone, and noroxymorphone and their glucuronide conjugates, with the formation of noroxycodone and oxymorphone mediated by cytochrome P-450 (CYP) isoenzymes 3A and 2D6, respectively; oxycodone and its metabolites are excreted principally in urine. Because oxymorphone is present in plasma in only low concentrations following oxycodone administration, it is not thought to contribute substantially to analgesic effects of the drug.

The oral bioavailability of oxycodone is 60–87%. The relative oral bioavailability of extended-release tablets of oxycodone hydrochloride compared with conventional oral preparations is 100%. The extended-release tablets are formulated to provide controlled delivery of oxycodone over 12 hours. Release of the drug from the extended-release tablets is pH independent. Following rectal administration of oxycodone hydrochloride extended-release tablets in healthy adults, the area under the plasma concentration-time curve (AUC) and peak plasma concentration were increased by 39 and 9%, respectively, compared with oral administration. With multiple oral dosing, steady-state plasma concentrations usually are achieved within 24–36 hours in healthy individuals receiving extended-release tablets of oxycodone hydrochloride. Administration of the extended-release tablets with food does not substantially affect the extent of absorption. The apparent elimination half-life following oral administration of the extended-release tablets or conventional preparations is 4.5 or 3.2 hours, respectively.

Oxycodone myristate extended-release capsules also are formulated to provide delivery of oxycodone over 12 hours but are not bioequivalent to oxycodone hydrochloride extended-release tablets. Under fasting conditions, both peak serum concentrations and AUC are lower for the extended-release capsules; under fed conditions, peak serum concentrations are lower, but AUC is similar to values for the extended-release tablets. Mean peak serum concentrations of oxycodone are lower (73 and 43% lower for administration under fasting and fed conditions, respectively) and the median time to peak serum concentration is approximately 3 hours longer when the drug is administered as extended-release capsules compared with administration as an oral solution in the fasting state. The relative oral bioavailability of oxycodone myristate extended-release capsules compared with an oral solution of the drug is lower in the fasting state (75%) but comparable in the fed state (114%). The time to peak plasma concentrations is approximately 4.5 hours following administration of the extended-release capsules under fed conditions. With repeated administration in healthy individuals, steady-state concentrations are achieved within 24–36 hours. The apparent elimination half-life following oral administration of the extended-release capsules under fed conditions is 5.6 hours, compared with 3.2 hours following administration of conventional preparations of the drug.

Bioavailability of oxycodone myristate extended-release capsules is increased by administration with food and is dependent on the content of the meal. When the extended-release capsules are administered following a high-fat, high-calorie meal rather than in the fasted state, peak concentrations and AUC are increased by 100–150 and 50–60%, respectively; when administered following a medium-fat, medium-calorie meal, peak concentrations and AUC are increased by 84 and 28%, respectively. When the extended-release capsules are administered following a low-fat, low-calorie meal, peak concentrations are 19% higher and AUC is comparable to values following administration under fasting conditions. The pharmacokinetic profile for the capsule contents sprinkled on food is equivalent to that for the intact capsule administered with food.

Extended-release tablets containing oxycodone hydrochloride in fixed combination with acetaminophen are available as a bilayer formulation in which a portion of the labeled oxycodone hydrochloride and acetaminophen doses is contained in an immediate-release layer and the remaining portion is contained in a layer that slowly releases the drugs. Following single or multiple doses of this formulation, the bioavailability (dose-normalized AUC and peak plasma concentration) of oxycodone is comparable to that of conventional preparations of the drug. Oxycodone is detectable in plasma within 30 minutes following administration of the fixed-combination extended-release tablets; peak concentrations are achieved in 3–4 hours. Following administration every 12 hours, steady-state concentrations are attained within 24 hours. Administration of this fixed-combination extended-release formulation with a low-fat or high-fat meal delayed peak concentrations by 1 or 2 hours, respectively; increased mean AUC by 15–16%; and increased peak concentrations by 12–25%. The apparent elimination half-life of oxycodone following oral administration of the fixed-combination extended-release tablets is 4.5 hours, compared with 3.9 hours following administration of conventional preparations of the drug.

Following oral administration of oxycodone hydrochloride extended-release tablets in patients with renal impairment (creatinine clearance less than 60 mL/minute), peak plasma concentrations of the drug and its noroxycodone metabolite were 50 and 20% higher, respectively, and AUCs of oxycodone, noroxycodone, and oxymorphone were 60, 50, and 40% higher, respectively, than values in individuals with normal renal function. The elimination half-life of oxycodone was increased by 1 hour in patients with renal impairment compared with individuals with normal renal function.

Administration of oxycodone hydrochloride extended-release tablets to patients with mild to moderate hepatic impairment resulted in increases in peak plasma concentrations and AUCs of oxycodone (50 and 95%, respectively) and noroxycodone (20 and 65%, respectively) but decreases in peak plasma concentrations and AUC of oxymorphone (30 and 40%, respectively). The elimination half-life of oxycodone was increased by 2.3 hours in patients with mild to moderate hepatic impairment compared with individuals with normal hepatic function.

Chemistry and Stability

■ **Chemistry** Oxycodone is a synthetic phenanthrene-derivative opiate agonist. The drug differs structurally from hydrocodone only in the attachment of a hydroxyl group to carbon 14 on the phenanthrene nucleus. Oxycodone occurs as long rods or as tautomeric, strongly refringent scales and is insoluble in water and soluble in alcohol. Oxycodone is commercially available as the hydrochloride or myristate salt; the hydrochloride salt is freely soluble in water and slightly soluble in alcohol. Oxycodone hydrochloride oral solution has a pH of 1.4–4.

Oxycodone myristate extended-release capsules contain extended-release microspheres in which oxycodone is present as a solid solution of a fatty acid salt (oxycodone myristate) in a hydrophobic matrix that also contains waxes. Homogeneous dispersion of the drug in the form of a solid solution in fatty acid and waxes imparts extended-release properties.

Extended-release tablets containing oxycodone hydrochloride in fixed combination with acetaminophen are available as a bilayer formulation in which a portion of the labeled oxycodone hydrochloride and acetaminophen doses is contained in an immediate-release layer and the remaining portion is contained in a layer that slowly releases the drugs. The tablets are designed to swell in gastric fluid and gradually release the extended-release components.

■ **Stability** Oxycodone preparations should be stored in tight containers and generally should be protected from light and stored at 15–30°C.

For further information on chemistry, pharmacology, pharmacokinetics, uses, cautions, chronic toxicity, acute toxicity, drug interactions, and dosage and administration of oxycodone, see the Opiate Agonists General Statement 28:08.08.

Preparations

Oxycodone preparations are subject to control under the Federal Controlled Substances Act of 1970 as schedule II (C-II) drugs.

Preparations containing oxycodone in combination with more than 325 mg of acetaminophen per dosage unit have been discontinued to minimize the risk of inadvertent acetaminophen overdosage.

Excipients in commercially available drug preparations may have clinically important effects in some individuals; consult specific product labeling for details.

oxyCODONE Hydrochloride

Oral		
Capsules	5 mg*	**oxyCODONE Hydrochloride Capsules** (C-II)
Solution	5 mg/5 mL*	**oxyCODONE Hydrochloride Oral Solution** (C-II)
	100 mg/5 mL*	**oxyCODONE Hydrochloride Oral Concentrate Solution** (C-II)
Tablets	5 mg*	**Oxaydo®** (C-II), Egalet
		Oxecta® (C-II), Pfizer
		oxyCODONE Hydrochloride Tablets (C-II)
		Roxicodone® (C-II; scored), Mallinckrodt
	7.5 mg	**Oxaydo®** (C-II), Egalet
		Oxecta® (C-II), Pfizer
	10 mg*	**oxyCODONE Hydrochloride Tablets** (C-II)
	15 mg*	**oxyCODONE Hydrochloride Tablets** (C-II)
		Roxicodone® (C-II; scored), Mallinckrodt
	20 mg*	**oxyCODONE Hydrochloride Tablets** (C-II)
	30 mg*	**oxyCODONE Hydrochloride Tablets** (C-II)
		Roxicodone® (C-II), Mallinckrodt
Tablets, extended-release	10 mg	**OxyCONTIN®** (C-II), Purdue
	15 mg	**OxyCONTIN®** (C-II), Purdue
	20 mg	**OxyCONTIN®** (C-II), Purdue
	30 mg	**OxyCONTIN®** (C-II), Purdue
	40 mg	**OxyCONTIN®** (C-II), Purdue
	60 mg	**OxyCONTIN®** (C-II), Purdue
	80 mg	**OxyCONTIN®** (C-II), Purdue

*available from one or more manufacturer, distributor, and/or repackager by generic (nonproprietary) name

oxyCODONE and Acetaminophen

Oral		
Solution	5 mg/5 mL Oxycodone Hydrochloride and Acetaminophen 325 mg/5 mL	**Roxicet®** (C-II), Roxane
Tablets	2.5 mg Oxycodone Hydrochloride and Acetaminophen 300 mg*	**oxyCODONE Hydrochloride and Acetaminophen Tablets** (C-II)
	2.5 mg Oxycodone Hydrochloride and Acetaminophen 325 mg*	**oxyCODONE Hydrochloride and Acetaminophen Tablets** (C-II)
		Percocet® (C-II), Endo
	5 mg Oxycodone Hydrochloride and Acetaminophen 300 mg*	**oxyCODONE Hydrochloride and Acetaminophen Tablets**
		Primlev® (C-II), Akrimax
	5 mg Oxycodone Hydrochloride and Acetaminophen 325 mg*	**Endocet®** (C-II; scored), Qualitest
		oxyCODONE Hydrochloride and Acetaminophen Tablets (C-II)
		Percocet® (C-II; scored), Endo
	7.5 mg Oxycodone Hydrochloride and Acetaminophen 300 mg*	**oxyCODONE Hydrochloride and Acetaminophen Tablets** (C-II)
		Primlev® (C-II), Akrimax
	7.5 mg Oxycodone Hydrochloride and Acetaminophen 325 mg*	**Endocet®** (C-II), Qualitest
		oxyCODONE Hydrochloride and Acetaminophen Tablets (C-II)
		Percocet® (C-II), Endo
	10 mg Oxycodone Hydrochloride and Acetaminophen 300 mg*	**oxyCODONE Hydrochloride and Acetaminophen Tablets** (C-II)
		Primlev® (C-II), Akrimax
	10 mg Oxycodone Hydrochloride and Acetaminophen 325 mg*	**Endocet®** (C-II), Qualitest
		oxyCODONE Hydrochloride and Acetaminophen Tablets (C-II)
		Percocet® (C-II), Endo
Tablets, extended-release, film-coated	7.5 mg Oxycodone Hydrochloride and Acetaminophen 325 mg	**Xartemis® XR** (C-II), Mallinckrodt

*available from one or more manufacturer, distributor, and/or repackager by generic (nonproprietary) name

oxyCODONE and Aspirin

Oral		
Tablets	4.835 mg Oxycodone Hydrochloride and Aspirin 325 mg*	**Endodan®** (C-II; scored), Endo
		oxyCODONE Hydrochloride and Aspirin Tablets (C-II)

*available from one or more manufacturer, distributor, and/or repackager by generic (nonproprietary) name

Other oxyCODONE Hydrochloride Combinations

Oral		
Tablets, film-coated	5 mg with Ibuprofen 400 mg*	**oxyCODONE Hydrochloride and Ibuprofen Film-coated Tablets** (C-II)

*available from one or more manufacturer, distributor, and/or repackager by generic (nonproprietary) name

oxyCODONE Myristate

Oral		
Capsules, extended-release	9 mg (of oxycodone [equivalent to 10 mg oxycodone hydrochloride])	**Xtampza® ER** (C-II), Collegium
	13.5 mg (of oxycodone [equivalent to 15 mg oxycodone hydrochloride])	**Xtampza® ER** (C-II), Collegium
	18 mg (of oxycodone [equivalent to 20 mg oxycodone hydrochloride])	**Xtampza® ER** (C-II), Collegium
	27 mg (of oxycodone [equivalent to 30 mg oxycodone hydrochloride])	**Xtampza® ER** (C-II), Collegium
	36 mg (of oxycodone [equivalent to 40 mg oxycodone hydrochloride])	**Xtampza® ER** (C-II), Collegium

oxyMORphone Hydrochloride

■ Oxymorphone hydrochloride is a semisynthetic phenanthrene-derivative opiate agonist.

REMS

FDA approved a REMS for oxymorphone hydrochloride to ensure that the benefits outweigh the risk. The REMS may apply to one or more preparations of oxymorphone hydrochloride and consists of the following: medication guide and elements to assure safe use. See the FDA REMS page (https://www.accessdata.fda.gov/scripts/cder/rems/index.cfm).

Uses

Oxymorphone hydrochloride is a strong analgesic used in the relief of moderate to severe pain. The drug is also used parenterally as a supplement to anesthesia and for analgesia during labor. Oxymorphone is used in patients with pulmonary edema for its cardiovascular effects and to allay anxiety. The drug should not be used in the treatment of pulmonary edema resulting from a chemical respiratory irritant.

Oxymorphone hydrochloride extended-release tablets are used orally for the management of moderate to severe pain when a continuous, around-the-clock analgesic is needed for an extended period of time. Oxymorphone hydrochloride extended-release tablets are not indicated for use on an as-needed ("prn") basis.

For further information on the role of opiate analgesics in the management of acute or chronic pain, see Uses: Pain, in the Opiate Agonists General Statement 28:08.08.

Dosage and Administration

■ **Administration** *Parenteral Administration* Oxymorphone hydrochloride is administered by subcutaneous, IM, or IV injection. An opiate antagonist and facilities for administration of oxygen and control of respiration should be available during and immediately following IV administration of the drug.

Oral Administration Oxymorphone hydrochloride is administered orally as conventional tablets and extended-release tablets. Because food affects oral absorption of oxymorphone administered as conventional tablets or extended-release tablets, these preparations should be taken on an empty stomach (i.e., at least 1 hour before or 2 hours after meals). Patients receiving oxymorphone should avoid alcohol; concomitant use may result in profound sedation, respiratory depression, coma, or death.

Oxymorphone hydrochloride extended-release tablets should be swallowed whole and should *not* be broken, chewed, or crushed; intake of a broken, crushed, or chewed tablet may result in too rapid a release of the drug from the preparation and absorption of a potentially toxic dose of oxymorphone hydrochloride. Patients receiving oxymorphone hydrochloride extended-release tablets must *not* consume alcoholic beverages or prescription or nonprescription preparations containing alcohol; intake of alcohol may result in rapid release of the drug from the tablet and intake of a potentially toxic dose of oxymorphone.

■ **Dosage** Oxymorphone hydrochloride should be given at the lowest effective dosage and for the shortest duration of therapy consistent with the treatment goals of the patient. Reduced dosage is indicated in poor-risk patients and in geriatric patients. If concomitant therapy with other CNS depressants is required, the lowest effective dosages and shortest possible duration of concomitant therapy should be used.

The manufacturer recommends that initial dosages of 33–50% of the usual dosage be employed when therapy with oxymorphone hydrochloride is initiated in patients receiving other CNS depressants.

For acute pain not related to trauma or surgery, the prescribed quantity should be limited to the amount needed for the expected duration of pain severe enough to require opiate analgesia (generally 3 days or less and rarely more than 7 days). When opiate analgesics are used for the management of chronic noncancer pain, the US Centers for Disease Control and Prevention (CDC) recommends that primary care clinicians carefully reassess individual benefits and risks before prescribing dosages equivalent to 50 mg or more of morphine sulfate daily (approximately 17 mg or more of oxymorphone hydrochloride daily) and avoid dosages equivalent to 90 mg or more of morphine sulfate daily (approximately 30 mg or more of oxymorphone hydrochloride daily) or carefully justify their decision to titrate the dosage to such levels. Other experts recommend consulting a pain management specialist before exceeding a dosage equivalent to 80–120 mg of morphine sulfate daily. For further information on the management of opiate analgesic therapy, see Dosage and Administration: Dosage, in the Opiate Agonists General Statement 28:08.08.

Parenteral Administration The usual initial adult subcutaneous or IM dosage of oxymorphone hydrochloride is 1–1.5 mg every 4–6 hours as necessary. The usual initial IV dose is 0.5 mg. In nondebilitated patients, the dose may be increased cautiously until satisfactory analgesia is attained. The usual dose for analgesia during labor is 0.5–1 mg by IM injection.

Conventional Tablets For opiate-naive adults, the usual initial dosage of conventional oxymorphone hydrochloride tablets is 10–20 mg every 4–6 hours. Alternatively, therapy can be initiated with 5 mg every 4–6 hours. Dosage should be adjusted according to patient tolerance and response. Therapy should *not* be initiated with an oxymorphone hydrochloride dose exceeding 20 mg.

Extended-release Tablets For opiate-naive adults, the usual initial dosage of oxymorphone hydrochloride extended-release tablets is 5 mg every 12 hours. The dosage can be titrated in increments of 5–10 mg every 12 hours every 3–7 days. Dosage should be adjusted according to patient tolerance and response.

Cautions

Oxymorphone shares the toxic potentials of the opiate agonists, and the usual precautions of opiate agonist therapy should be observed. (See Cautions in the Opiate Agonists General Statement 28:08.08.)

Oxymorphone hydrochloride is contraindicated in patients with moderate or severe hepatic impairment.

Safe use of oxymorphone hydrochloride during pregnancy, other than during labor, has not been established. Safety and efficacy of oxymorphone hydrochloride in pediatric patients younger than 18 years of age have not been established.

Pharmacology

Oxymorphone hydrochloride has little antitussive activity and may be less constipating than morphine. In equianalgesic doses, oxymorphone hydrochloride may cause more nausea, vomiting, and euphoria than does morphine sulfate.

Pharmacokinetics

Oxymorphone is well absorbed following subcutaneous, IM, or IV administration. Onset of action usually occurs within 5–10 minutes after IV administration and 10–15 minutes after subcutaneous or IM administration. Analgesia is maintained for 3–6 hours following parenteral administration.

Following oral administration of oxymorphone hydrochloride, bioavailability is approximately 10%. Following oral administration of oxymorphone hydrochloride conventional tablets with a high-fat meal, peak plasma concentrations and area under the concentration-time curve (AUC) were increased 38%. Following oral administration of oxymorphone hydrochloride extended-release tablets with food, peak plasma concentrations were increased 50%; AUC reportedly was unchanged in one study and increased 18% in another study. Bioavailability of oxymorphone was increased in patients with renal impairment, those with hepatic impairment, and in geriatric individuals following administration as extended-release tablets.

Concomitant administration of oxymorphone hydrochloride extended-release tablets with alcohol has resulted in variable effects on peak plasma concentrations of the drug. Changes in peak plasma concentrations of oxymorphone have ranged from a 50% decrease to a 270% increase. Concomitant administration of oxymorphone with alcohol *must* be avoided.

Oxymorphone hydrochloride is metabolized primarily in the liver. Like morphine, it probably undergoes conjugation with glucuronic acid and is excreted primarily in urine as oxymorphone glucuronide.

Chemistry and Stability

■ **Chemistry** Oxymorphone hydrochloride is a semisynthetic phenanthrene-derivative opiate agonist. Oxymorphone hydrochloride occurs as a white or slightly off-white powder and is freely soluble in water and sparingly soluble in alcohol. Oxymorphone hydrochloride injection has a pH of 2.7–4.5.

■ **Stability** Oxymorphone hydrochloride injection should be protected from light and stored at 15–30°C; freezing should be avoided. Oxymorphone hydrochloride conventional tablets and extended-release tablets should be stored at 15–30°C.

For further information on the chemistry, pharmacology, pharmacokinetics, uses, cautions, chronic toxicity, acute toxicity, drug interactions, and dosage and administration of oxymorphone hydrochloride, see the Opiate Agonists General Statement 28:08.08.

Preparations

Oxymorphone hydrochloride is subject to control under the Federal Controlled Substances Act of 1970 as a schedule II (C-II) drug.

In July 2017, Endo Pharmaceuticals voluntarily agreed to comply with an FDA request to remove Opana® ER extended-release tablets from the US market. FDA's request was based on postmarketing data indicating that the route of abuse of Opana® ER had shifted from nasal to injection route following reformulation in 2012; the reformulation was intended to make the extended-release tablets more resistant to physical and chemical manipulation for abuse by the nasal or injection routes. However, FDA stated that abuse by injection of the reformulated preparation had been associated with a serious outbreak of human immunodeficiency virus (HIV) infection and hepatitis C virus infection, as well as cases of thrombotic microangiopathy. FDA concluded that the benefits associated with the reformulated preparation may no longer outweigh its risks.

Excipients in commercially available drug preparations may have clinically important effects in some individuals; consult specific product labeling for details.

oxyMORphone Hydrochloride

Oral		
Tablets	5 mg*	**Opana®** (C-II), Endo
		oxyMORphone Hydrochloride Tablets (C-II)
	10 mg*	**Opana®** (C-II), Endo
		oxyMORphone Hydrochloride Tablets (C-II)
Tablet, extended-release	5 mg*	**oxyMORphone Hydrochloride Extended-release Tablets** (C-II)
	7.5 mg*	**oxyMORphone Hydrochloride Extended-release Tablets** (C-II)
	10 mg*	**oxyMORphone Hydrochloride Extended-release Tablets** (C-II)
	15 mg*	**oxyMORphone Hydrochloride Extended-release Tablets** (C-II)
	20 mg*	**oxyMORphone Hydrochloride Extended-release Tablets** (C-II)
	30 mg*	**oxyMORphone Hydrochloride Extended-release Tablets** (C-II)
	40 mg*	**oxyMORphone Hydrochloride Extended-release Tablets** (C-II)
Parenteral		
Injection	1 mg/mL	**Opana®** (C-II), Endo

*available from one or more manufacturer, distributor, and/or repackager by generic (nonproprietary) name

SUFentanil Citrate

Fentathienil Citrate, Sufentanyl Citrate, Sulfentanil Citrate

■ Sufentanil citrate is a synthetic phenylpiperidine-derivative opiate agonist.

Uses

Sufentanil citrate is a strong analgesic used as an analgesic supplement in the maintenance of balanced general anesthesia. The drug is also used to provide general anesthesia without additional anesthetic agents. When used as the primary anesthetic agent for the induction and maintenance of anesthesia, sufentanil is administered in conjunction with 100% oxygen and a skeletal muscle relaxant (e.g., pancuronium bromide, metocurine iodide [no longer commercially available in the US], succinylcholine chloride) and principally in patients undergoing major surgical procedures such as neurosurgery, occasionally performed with the patient in the sitting position, or cardiovascular surgery; the drug is particularly useful when extended postoperative ventilation is anticipated and in providing favorable myocardial and cerebral oxygen balance.

Cardiovascular parameters (i.e., heart rate, systolic and diastolic blood pressure, cardiac output, systemic vascular resistance, mean arterial pressure) are generally more stable in patients who have received sufentanil as the analgesic or anesthetic agent during surgery compared with patients who have received inhalation agents. The incidence of postoperative hypertension and requirements for administration of vasoactive agents or postoperative analgesics are generally decreased in patients who have received moderate or high doses of sufentanil as compared with patients who have received inhalation agents (e.g., enflurane, halothane, isoflurane).

Sufentanil has produced adequate analgesia and/or general anesthesia in patients undergoing various types of surgery, including cardiovascular (e.g., arteriography, coronary artery bypass, valve replacement, vascular), neurologic (e.g., craniotomy), gynecologic, abdominal, orthopedic (e.g., total hip replacement), urologic, and general surgery and thoracotomy. Sufentanil has also produced adequate analgesia and/or general anesthesia in children as young as 1 day of age undergoing cardiovascular surgery.

Sufentanil is used for epidural administration as an analgesic combined with low dose bupivacaine, usually 12.5 mg per administration, during labor and vaginal delivery. Sufentanil and bupivacaine should be mixed together before administration.

Dosage and Administration

■ **Administration** Sufentanil citrate may be administered by IV injection, intermittent or continuous IV infusion, or epidural injection. The drug has also been administered by IM injection†. Sufentanil citrate for injection and the diluted solution should be inspected visually for particulate matter and discoloration prior to administration whenever solution and container permit. Specialized techniques are required for epidural administration of the drug, and such administration should be performed only by qualified individuals familiar with the techniques of administration, dosages, and special patient management problems associated with epidural sufentanil citrate administration.

■ **Dosage** Dosage of sufentanil citrate is expressed in terms of sufentanil. Dosage must be carefully adjusted according to body weight, individual requirements and response, physical status and underlying pathologic condition, premedication or concomitant medication(s), the anesthetic(s) being used, and the nature and duration of the surgery. Additional doses of sufentanil are administered when patient movement and/or changes in vital signs indicate surgical stress or lightening of analgesia, and should be adjusted according to individual requirements, response, and the anticipated remaining duration of the surgical procedure.

The manufacturers recommend that dosage of sufentanil be based on an estimate of ideal (lean) body weight in obese patients whose body weight exceeds their ideal weight by more than 20%. Reduced dosage is indicated initially in geriatric and debilitated patients; additional doses of the drug in these patients should be adjusted according to the initial response and desired effect. Although specific recommendations for adjustment of sufentanil dosage in patients with hepatic or renal impairment have not been established, dosage should be adjusted carefully in these patients since elimination of the drug may be decreased.

The selection of preanesthetic medication(s) should be based on the individual needs of the patient. Since sufentanil may cause skeletal muscle rigidity, administration of a neuromuscular blocking agent may be necessary prior to or concomitantly with sufentanil; the neuromuscular blocking agent used should be compatible with the patient's condition, taking into account the hemodynamic effects of the drug, the cardiovascular status of the patient, existing drug therapy (e.g., preoperative use of β-adrenergic blocking agents), and the degree of skeletal muscle relaxation required. For sufentanil doses up to 8 mcg/kg, up to 25% of the full paralyzing dose of a nondepolarizing neuromuscular blocking agent should be administered just prior to sufentanil; for anesthetic doses of sufentanil greater than 8 mcg/kg that are titrated by slow IV infusion, a full paralyzing dose of a neuromuscular blocking agent should be administered following loss of consciousness (e.g., loss of eyelash reflex, loss of response to voice command). For rapidly administered anesthetic doses of sufentanil greater than 8 mcg/kg, a full paralyzing dose of a neuromuscular blocking agent should be administered simultaneously with sufentanil or immediately after loss of consciousness. However, preliminary data indicate that initial dosage requirements for neuromuscular blocking agents are generally lower in patients receiving high doses of sufentanil compared with fentanyl. (See Drug Interactions: Anesthetic Agents and Adjuncts.)

Adult Dosage In minor but painful general surgical procedures (anticipated duration of anesthesia of 1–2 hours) requiring endotracheal intubation and assisted or controlled respiration in adults, a total sufentanil dosage of 1–2 mcg/kg is administered IV in conjunction with nitrous oxide and oxygen; approximately 75% or more of the total dosage (titrated to patient response) may be administered by slow IV injection or infusion prior to intubation. Supplemental IV doses of 10–25 mcg or, alternatively, intermittent or continuous maintenance IV infusions may be given as necessary when movement and/or changes in vital signs indicate surgical stress or lightening of anesthesia. Maintenance infusion rates should be adjusted based on the induction dose so that the total sufentanil dosage does not exceed 1 mcg/kg per hour of anticipated surgical time. In the absence of evidence of lightening of anesthesia, maintenance infusion rates should be adjusted downward until there is some response to surgical stimulation.

In more complicated, major surgical procedures (anticipated duration of anesthesia of 2–8 hours) in adults, a total sufentanil dosage of 2–8 mcg/kg is administered IV in conjunction with nitrous oxide and oxygen; approximately 75% or less of the total dosage (titrated to patient response) may be administered by slow IV injection or infusion prior to intubation. Supplemental IV doses of 10–50 mcg or, alternatively, intermittent or continuous maintenance IV infusions may be given as necessary when movement and/or changes in vital signs indicate surgical stress or lightening of anesthesia. Maintenance infusion rates should be adjusted based on the induction dose so that the total sufentanil dosage does not exceed 1 mcg/kg per hour of anticipated surgical time. In the absence of evidence of lightening of anesthesia, infusion rates should be adjusted downward until there is some response to surgical stimulation.

When used as the primary anesthetic agent to provide general anesthesia in adults, a total sufentanil dosage of 8–30 mcg/kg, administered IV by slow injection, infusion, or injection followed by infusion, may be used in conjunction with oxygen and a skeletal muscle relaxant. Depending on the initial dose, maintenance IV doses of 0.5–10 mcg/kg may be given by slow IV injection in anticipation of surgical stress (e.g., incision, sternotomy, cardiopulmonary bypass); alternatively, intermittent or continuous maintenance IV infusions may be given as necessary as determined by changes in vital signs that indicate surgical stress and lightening of anesthesia. Maintenance infusion rates should be adjusted based on the induction dose so that the total sufentanil dosage for the procedure does not exceed 30 mcg/kg. In the absence of evidence of lightening of anesthesia, infusion rates should be adjusted downward until there is some response to surgical stimulation. IV doses of 8–25 mcg/kg generally attenuate catecholamine release and those of 25–30 mcg/kg generally block sympathetic responses including catecholamine release during surgery but not during cardiopulmonary bypass. High dosages are used in adults undergoing major surgical procedures such as cardiovascular surgery or neurosurgery performed with the patient in the sitting position when maintenance of favorable myocardial and cerebral oxygen consumption is preferred.

In adults undergoing surgical procedures for coronary artery bypass grafting, sufentanil has been administered by intermittent IV infusion as the primary anesthetic agent for the induction and maintenance of anesthesia in conjunction with 100% oxygen and a skeletal muscle relaxant. Following administration of preanesthetic medications, oxygen, and pancuronium bromide (0.01–0.02 mg/kg) sufentanil was infused at a rate of 300 mcg/minute until unconsciousness developed up to a total dose of 3.8–4.9 mcg/kg; following administration of a second dose of a skeletal muscle relaxant (e.g., succinylcholine) and intubation in these patients, sufentanil was infused over 30 minutes in a dose equivalent to that which previously produced unconsciousness. The surgical procedure was started and additional 50-mcg doses of sufentanil were administered by IV injection as necessary as determined by systolic blood pressure response; at the end of the surgical procedure, the total dose of sufentanil for the entire procedure ranged from 11.1–15 mcg/kg in adults.

The epidural dose for labor and delivery is 10–15 mcg of sufentanil and 10 mL of bupivacaine 0.125% with or without epinephrine. Doses may be repeated twice (for a total of 3 doses) at not less than 1-hour intervals until delivery.

Pediatric Dosage The manufacturers state that when sufentanil is used to provide induction and maintenance of anesthesia without additional anesthetic agents in children younger than 12 years of age undergoing cardiovascular surgery, an initial anesthetic dose of 10–25 mcg/kg is administered IV in conjunction with 100% oxygen and a skeletal muscle relaxant; additional IV doses of up to 25–50 mcg each (or, alternatively, 1–2 mcg/kg each) are recommended as necessary based on response to the initial dose and as determined by changes in vital signs that indicate surgical stress or lightening of anesthesia. The manufacturers state that the dosage of sufentanil should be reduced in neonates, especially in those with cardiovascular disease, because clearance of the drug is reduced in these patients. Some clinicians report use of total sufentanil doses of 5–10 mcg/kg infused at a rate of 1 mcg/kg per minute in infants with mean ages of about 8–9 months undergoing repair of complex congenital heart defects†.

Cautions

■ Adverse Effects Sufentanil shares the toxic potentials of the opiate agonists, and the usual precautions of opiate agonist therapy should be observed. (See Cautions in the Opiate Agonists General Statement 28:08.08.)

The most common adverse effects of sufentanil are respiratory depression and skeletal muscle rigidity (e.g., of the truncal muscles). Hypotension, hypertension, chest wall rigidity, and bradycardia reportedly occur in 7, 3, 3, and 3% of patients, respectively, receiving the drug. Other adverse effects, including tachycardia, arrhythmia, cardiac arrest, nausea, vomiting, apnea, postoperative respiratory depression, bronchospasm, pruritus, anaphylaxis, chills, and intraoperative muscle movement, reportedly occur in less than 1% of patients receiving the drug. Nausea, vomiting, and pruritus also have been reported with epidural† injection of the drug. Apnea occurred in 2 patients receiving epidural sufentanil doses of 200 and 350 mcg in 50-mcg increments over 20–22 hours; both patients responded to respiratory support and IV naloxone. Apnea also has been reported in several other patients after epidural injection of the drug. Other cardiovascular effects, including increases in cardiac index, changes in mean arterial pressure, and decreases in systemic vascular resistance, have been observed occasionally following administration of sufentanil; changes in cardiac index and mean arterial pressure may occur secondary to changes in systemic vascular resistance. Some cardiovascular effects may be associated with endotracheal intubation, concomitantly administered drugs, and/or surgical manipulation (e.g., incision, sternotomy) rather than with the drug itself. (See Pharmacology: Cardiovascular Effects.) Tonic-clonic movements developed in a few patients shortly after IV injection of a single dose of the drug.

■ Precautions and Contraindications Sufentanil can severely compromise respiratory function. Sufentanil should be used only by individuals who are experienced in the use of parenteral anesthetics and in the maintenance of an adequate airway and respiratory support. Facilities and personnel necessary for intubation, administration of oxygen, and assisted or controlled respiration should be immediately available whenever sufentanil is used. An opiate antagonist (e.g., naloxone) should be readily available. Vital signs should be monitored routinely during administration of sufentanil; facilities for postoperative monitoring and assisted or controlled respiration should be available following administration of anesthetic doses of the drug (i.e., 8 mcg/kg or greater). Because sufentanil is highly lipophilic, a secondary rise in plasma concentrations of the drug may occur during the recovery period as blood perfusion to peripheral tissues increases and the drug redistributes; therefore, the possibility of a recurrence of the pharmacologic effects of the drug during recovery should be considered.

For a complete discussion of these and other precautions associated with sufentanil citrate, see Cautions in the Opiate Agonists General Statement 28:08.08.

Sufentanil should be used with caution in patients with head injuries, since the drug may obscure the clinical course in these patients. The drug should be used with caution in patients with pulmonary disease, decreased respiratory reserve, or potentially compromised respiratory function, since opiate agonists may cause additional decreases in respiratory function and increases in airway resistance in these patients. These adverse respiratory effects can be managed by using assisted or controlled respiration during anesthesia. Sufentanil-induced respiratory depression can be reversed by administration of an opiate antagonist (e.g., naloxone); however, the duration of respiratory depression produced by sufentanil may be longer than the duration of the opiate antagonist and, therefore, appropriate patient monitoring should be continued following apparent initial reversal.

Sufentanil should be administered with caution in patients with hepatic or renal impairment, since the drug undergoes metabolism and excretion mainly in the liver and kidney.

Sufentanil is contraindicated in patients with known hypersensitivity to the drug.

■ Pediatric Precautions Safety and efficacy of sufentanil in children as young as 1 day of age have been documented in a limited number of patients undergoing cardiovascular surgery. Sufentanil should be administered with caution to neonates because decreased clearance may result in increased blood concentrations of the drug. (See Pharmacokinetics: Elimination.)

■ Mutagenicity and Carcinogenicity It is not known if sufentanil is mutagenic or carcinogenic in humans. Sufentanil did not exhibit mutagenic activity in the Ames microbial mutagen test with metabolic activation. In female rats receiving single IV doses up to 80 mcg/kg (about 2.5 times the maximum dose in humans), sufentanil did not produce structural chromosome mutations in the micronucleus test. Long-term animal studies to determine the carcinogenic potential of sufentanil have not been performed to date.

■ Pregnancy and Lactation Although there are no adequate and controlled studies to date in humans, reproduction studies in rats and rabbits using sufentanil doses 2.5 times the maximum human dose for a period of 10 to longer than 30 days have shown evidence of embryocidal effect; however, this effect was probably secondary to maternal toxicity (e.g., anoxia, decreased food consumption) that occurred during prolonged administration of the drug, which precludes meaningful interpretation of the findings. Sufentanil has not been shown to be teratogenic in rats or rabbits. Sufentanil should be used during pregnancy only when the potential benefits justify the possible risks to the fetus.

Since it is not known if sufentanil is distributed into milk, the drug should be administered with caution to nursing women.

Drug Interactions

■ Benzodiazepines and Other CNS Depressants Concomitant use of sufentanil and benzodiazepines or other CNS depressants may result in hypotension or decreased pulmonary arterial pressure; even relatively small dosages of diazepam may cause cardiovascular depression when used with high or anesthetic dosages of sufentanil. Clinicians should consider the potential for such concomitant therapy to decrease pulmonary arterial pressure when performing diagnostic or surgical procedures where interpretation of pulmonary arterial pressure measurements might determine patient management. If hypotension occurs, the possibility of hypovolemia should be considered and managed with appropriate fluid therapy. When operative conditions permit, repositioning of the patient to improve venous return to the heart should be considered. Because of the potential for orthostatic hypotension, care should be exercised when moving and repositioning the patient. If volume expansion and other countermeasures do not correct hypotension, administration of a pressor agent (other than epinephrine, which may cause a reduction in blood pressure in patients receiving a neuroleptic with α-adrenergic blocking activity) should be considered.

Concomitant use of opiate agonists, including sufentanil, and benzodiazepines or other CNS depressants, including other opiate agonists, anxiolytics, sedatives, hypnotics, tranquilizers, muscle relaxants, general anesthetics, antipsychotics, and alcohol, also may result in profound sedation, respiratory depression, coma, and death. If used in the immediate postoperative period for analgesia in conjunction with a benzodiazepine or other CNS depressant, sufentanil should be initiated at a reduced dosage and titrated based on clinical response, and the patient should be monitored closely for respiratory depression, sedation, and hypotension. Fluids or other measures to counteract hypotension should be available.

■ Anesthetic Agents and Adjuncts Cardiovascular depression, manifested by bradycardia and decreases in mean arterial pressure and cardiac output, may occur following administration of nitrous oxide concomitantly with high doses of sufentanil. (See Pharmacology: Cardiovascular Effects.) Bradycardia occurs infrequently during anesthesia with sufentanil and oxygen and may be corrected by administration of atropine.

The manufacturers state that preliminary data suggest that the initial dosage requirements for neuromuscular blocking agents in patients receiving high doses of sufentanil are similar to those in patients receiving enflurane but generally less than those in patients receiving fentanyl or halothane.

Because of the inhibitory effects of pancuronium on the vagus nerve, tachycardia may occur following administration of high doses of pancuronium bromide during anesthesia with sufentanil and oxygen. Hypertension and an increase in cardiac index may also occur when sufentanil and pancuronium are administered concomitantly. To maintain a stable, lower heart rate and blood pressure during anesthesia with sufentanil and oxygen, a neuromuscular blocking agent with a lesser inhibitory effect on the vagus nerve or moderate doses of pancuronium should be used.

■ β-Adrenergic Blocking Agents Patients with coronary artery disease who have received chronic preoperative therapy with β-adrenergic blocking agents appear to require lower initial and fewer supplemental doses of sufentanil during coronary artery bypass surgery in which anesthesia with sufentanil and oxygen is used than do patients who have not received preoperative therapy with β-adrenergic blocking agents. In one study in patients undergoing coronary artery bypass surgery, patients who were receiving chronic preoperative therapy with 80–240 mg of propranolol hydrochloride daily required 3.8 mcg/kg of sufentanil for induction of anesthesia and a total dose of 11.1 mcg/kg for the entire surgical procedure; those patients who were not receiving preoperative propranolol therapy required 4.9 mcg/kg of sufentanil for induction of anesthesia and a total of 15 mcg/kg for the entire surgical procedure. In addition, patients who were receiving propranolol routinely for angina or hypertension developed less hypertension with surgical manipulation (e.g., sternotomy, sternal spread) and required fewer supplemental drugs (e.g., phentolamine, sodium nitroprusside) to control hypertension than did patients not receiving propranolol preoperatively.

For further information about drug interactions involving opiate agonists (including sufentanil citrate), see Drug Interactions in the Opiate Agonists General Statement 28:08.08.

Acute Toxicity

■ Pathogenesis The IV LD_{50} of sufentanil has been reported to be 16.8–18.7, 11.8–13, 10.1–19.5, and 9.3–12.5 mg/kg in mice, guinea pigs, dogs, and rats, respectively; deaths from acute toxicity generally resulted from respiratory depression.

■ Manifestations Overdosage of sufentanil is likely to produce symptoms that are mainly extensions of the usual pharmacologic effects of opiate agonists. (See Pharmacology.)

■ Treatment In sufentanil overdosage, especially in the presence of hypoventilation or apnea, primary attention should be given to reestablishment of adequate respiratory exchange by maintaining an adequate, patent airway, using assisted or controlled respiration and oxygen as necessary. Opiate agonist-induced respiratory depression should also be treated with an opiate antagonist such as naloxone hydrochloride (see 28:10); however, the duration of respiratory depression following overdosage with sufentanil may be longer than the duration of action of the opiate agonist and other more immediate supportive and symptomatic treatment should also be initiated. In addition, it should be considered that use of an opiate antagonist in a patient who is physically dependent on opiate agonists may precipitate an acute withdrawal syndrome that cannot be readily suppressed while the action of the antagonist persists. If respiratory depression is associated with muscular rigidity, administration of a neuromuscular blocking agent may be necessary to facilitate assisted or controlled respiration. Muscular rigidity may also respond to opiate antagonist therapy. If cardiovascular support is necessary, treatment should include fluid administration and/or use of vasopressors.

Pharmacology

Sufentanil citrate shares the actions of the opiate agonists. Sufentanil has a high affinity and selectivity for the μ-opiate receptor in the CNS and reportedly is more selective and binds more tightly to this receptor than does fentanyl. Partial occupancy of the μ-receptor by naloxone (an opiate antagonist) has been shown to substantially decrease the analgesic effect of sufentanil.

■ **CNS Effects** Like other opiate agonists, sufentanil produces dose-related analgesia; at doses up to 8 mcg/kg, the drug has a potent analgesic effect. Higher doses usually produce substantial CNS depression resulting in hypnosis and anesthesia; however, hypnosis may occur at doses of 1.5 mcg/kg. The analgesic potency of sufentanil appears to be 5–12 times that of fentanyl on a weight basis. Opiate agonists do not alter the threshold or responsiveness of afferent nerve endings to noxious stimuli nor the conduction of impulses along peripheral nerves; instead, the drugs alter the perception of pain at the spinal cord and higher levels in the CNS (spinal trigeminal nucleus, periaqueductal gray, periventricular gray, medullary raphe nuclei, hypothalamus). Like fentanyl, high doses of sufentanil reportedly cause amnesia and loss of consciousness; however, prevention of awareness during and recall after opiate-agonist anesthesia may require supplementation with other agents (e.g., benzodiazepines), since awareness and recall of the surgical procedure have been reported by some patients even at high doses of an opiate agonist alone.

Like fentanyl, sufentanil, in initial doses ranging from 5–160 mcg/kg, has been shown to reduce cerebral cortical blood flow and oxygen consumption in animals. The drug also causes selective changes in regional cerebral glucose metabolism in animals following doses of 40–160 mcg/kg. The manufacturers state that in one study in patients undergoing craniotomy, sufentanil doses of 20 mcg/kg provided a more pronounced reduction in intracranial volume than equivalent doses of fentanyl, based on requirements for furosemide and supplemental anesthesia.

Sufentanil doses of 8 mcg/kg or greater result in EEG patterns indicative of a deep level of anesthesia; the drug induces a shift to the left in EEG amplitude and frequency that is consistent with central anesthetic activity. Like fentanyl and other opiate agonists, sufentanil, in initial doses ranging from 5–160 mcg/kg in animals, produces EEG patterns characterized by low frequency, high amplitude (delta) waves and burst suppression; these effects are reversed by naloxone. Brief periods of seizure activity, characterized by epileptoid patterns and spikes, occurred in animals following administration of initial doses of 40, 80, or 160 mcg/kg of the drug. Following administration of sufentanil (e.g., 15 mcg/kg) and oxygen in patients undergoing cardiovascular surgery, EEG patterns have been characterized by high voltage, slow delta waves. Surgical manipulation did not appear to alter the EEG pattern. Although the mean power in the delta band declined with time, the contribution of delta power to total power in the frequency range 0.5–40 Hz remained constant (at about 96%) until the onset of cardiopulmonary bypass (about 45 minutes after administration of sufentanil) procedure. Sharp waves of uncertain neurophysiologic importance have also been observed; however, these waves were not associated with clinical signs of seizure activity.

Sufentanil has been shown to antagonize apomorphine-induced emesis.

■ **Cardiovascular Effects** Sufentanil generally produces few cardiovascular effects. Unlike morphine, sufentanil appears to have little effect on histamine release; release of histamine contributes in part to the peripheral dilation and hypotensive effect induced by opiate agonists. Sufentanil and fentanyl are less potent stimulators of histamine release than are meperidine or morphine. When given in equianalgesic doses to supine patients, the cardiovascular effects of sufentanil are generally similar to those of fentanyl. Unlike morphine, sufentanil, in doses of 10 mcg/kg, did not affect microcirculation and peripheral perfusion or cellular function in animals. Although a hypotensive effect and/or a decrease in peripheral vascular resistance have been reported occasionally in patients receiving sufentanil, these effects do not appear to be secondary to histamine release. Like fentanyl, sufentanil may have a centrally mediated vagal effect which may occasionally result in bradycardia that can be controlled by administering atropine.

In several studies in patients undergoing cardiovascular surgery and receiving sufentanil as the primary anesthetic agent in total doses ranging from 11.4–31.7 mcg/kg concomitantly with pancuronium bromide doses of 0.02 mg/kg and succinylcholine, heart rate, cardiac output, central venous pressure, and pulmonary wedge pressure generally remained stable compared with control measurements; pulmonary artery pressure was stable or elevated and mean arterial pressure and systemic vascular resistance were stable or decreased compared with control measurements. Heart rate and cardiac output were elevated and systemic vascular resistance was decreased following administration of sufentanil as the primary anesthetic agent in doses up to 30 mcg/kg concomitantly with the neuromuscular blocking agent, pancuronium bromide, in doses of 0.1–0.12 mg/kg; initial IV doses of 1–2 mg of pancuronium bromide were administered in some patients. (See Drug Interactions: Anesthetic Agents and Adjuncts.) Anesthesia with high doses of sufentanil appears to attenuate the hemodynamic responses to endotracheal intubation and surgical manipulation (e.g., incision); although low doses of the drug may also partially or completely suppress the hemodynamic responses to surgical manipulation (e.g., sternotomy, aortic arch manipulation) in some patients, a substantial number of hypertensive episodes have occurred in other patients and have required treatment with additional doses of sufentanil, vasoactive agents (e.g., phentolamine, sodium nitroprusside), and/or other anesthetic agents (e.g., nitrous oxide). Clinically tolerable doses of sufentanil do not appear to inhibit sympathetic reflexes that may be activated during surgical manipulation. Hypertensive episodes following sternotomy or aortic arch manipulation may occur secondary to activation of sympathetic reflexes rather than secondary to inadequate analgesic doses of the drug.

■ **Hormonal and Metabolic Effects** Data on the effects of sufentanil on hormonal and metabolic responses to surgery-induced stress are conflicting.

Although opiate agonists stimulate the release of corticotropin in animals, the drugs generally inhibit the stress-induced release of corticotropin in patients undergoing surgery. Sufentanil has been reported to prevent the stress-induced increase in serum cortisol concentration that occurs during surgery; however, the drug has also been reported to lack an inhibitory effect on surgery-induced increases in serum cortisol in some patients. Plasma concentrations of vasopressin (antidiuretic hormone) and growth hormone usually increase during anesthesia and surgery. Like high doses of fentanyl, sufentanil has been reported to inhibit increases in plasma concentrations of vasopressin and growth hormone during induction of anesthesia, endotracheal intubation, sternotomy, and/or surgery; however, plasma vasopressin concentrations have been reported to be increased in some sufentanil-treated patients during cardiopulmonary bypass and after surgery. Like most other opiate agonists, sufentanil has been reported to enhance the release of prolactin. In one study, the drug inhibited surgery-induced increases in plasma insulin concentration but did not inhibit increases in plasma glucose or nonesterified fatty acid (NEFA) concentrations during cardiopulmonary bypass; plasma triglyceride concentrations decreased during cardiopulmonary bypass and returned to control concentrations after surgery. However, changes in plasma NEFA and triglyceride concentrations probably resulted from heparin administration prior to bypass, since heparin is a potent stimulator of lipoprotein lipase release. Sufentanil has been reported to lack an inhibitory effect on cardiovascular surgery-induced increases in plasma aldosterone concentration and renin activity.

The manufacturers state that sufentanil causes a dose-related decrease in catecholamine release, especially that of norepinephrine. Sufentanil-induced decreases in sympathetic responses to surgery are apparent at doses of 2–8 mcg/kg and become more prominent as the dose increases up to 25 mcg/kg; doses of 25–30 mcg/kg reportedly block surgery-induced sympathetic responses and catecholamine release. However, in several studies, the drug did not inhibit increases in plasma catecholamine (i.e., epinephrine, norepinephrine) or dopamine concentrations during cardiopulmonary bypass or after surgery, although the drug inhibited their release prior to surgery.

■ **Respiratory Effects** Sufentanil depresses respiration and increases airway resistance; the duration and degree of respiratory depression are dose-related following doses of less than 8 mcg/kg of sufentanil. Higher doses of the drug may produce pronounced hypoventilation resulting in decreased pulmonary exchange and may cause apnea. Like other opiate agonists, sufentanil suppresses the cough reflex. For further discussion of the respiratory effects of opiate agonists, see Pharmacology in the Opiate Agonists General Statement 28:08.08.

■ **Other Effects** Although specific data have not been published to date, sufentanil would be expected to produce other pharmacologic effects of opiate agonists, including constipation, urinary retention, and biliary spasm.

For complete discussion of the pharmacologic effects of opiate agonists, see the Opiate Agonists General Statement 28:08.08.

Pharmacokinetics

In all studies described in the Pharmacokinetics section, sufentanil was administered as the citrate; dosages and concentrations of the drug are expressed in terms of sufentanil.

■ **Absorption** Following IV administration, sufentanil has a more rapid onset of action than does morphine or fentanyl. The onset of action of sufentanil as determined by time to unconsciousness (i.e., loss of response to voice command) reportedly ranges from 1.2–3 minutes following total mean doses of 4.9–30 mcg/kg. Since sufentanil undergoes limited accumulation and is eliminated rapidly from tissue storage sites, recovery from anesthesia may be more rapid following administration of sufentanil than fentanyl, especially at high doses. (See Pharmacokinetics: Elimination.) The manufacturers state that although the time to recovery from anesthesia is similar following 1- to 6-mcg/kg doses of sufentanil or 7.5- to 20-mcg/kg doses of fentanyl, time to recovery from anesthesia is more rapid following 8- to 30-mcg/kg doses of sufentanil than following 50- to 100-mcg/kg doses of fentanyl. The mean duration of anesthesia is reportedly 40, 35, and 87 minutes following initial doses of 0.4 mcg/kg of sufentanil, 4 mcg/kg of fentanyl, and 400 mcg/kg of morphine, respectively; the mean duration of anesthesia of additional doses of 0.1 mcg/kg of sufentanil, 1 mcg/kg of fentanyl, and 100 mcg/kg of morphine is reportedly 41–44, 39–66, and 52–76 minutes, respectively. Patient response to verbal command and adequate ventilation have been reported to occur 0.6–1.8 and 5.6 hours, respectively, following administration of anesthetic doses (about 13–19 mcg/kg total) of sufentanil. Endotracheal extubation was performed about 5, 9, and 23 hours after administration of total mean doses of 13, 19, and 30 mcg/kg, respectively. Recovery following equipotent doses of morphine or fentanyl reportedly has been slower.

Following IM administration of single doses of 0.15, 0.3, or 0.5 mcg/kg of sufentanil in patients with pain, the approximate duration of detectable analgesia was 2.3, 3.7, and 3.8 hours, respectively.

Following IV administration of two 15-mcg/kg doses of sufentanil in patients undergoing coronary artery surgery, mean peak plasma concentrations averaged 36–43 ng/mL after injection of both doses; 17 and 22 ng/mL 2 minutes after the first and second doses, respectively; and declined to 0.33 ng/mL at 23 hours.

Following epidural administration of sufentanil 10–15 mcg and 0.125% bupivacaine with epinephrine 1:200,000 during the first stage of labor, the onset of action occurred within 10 minutes and the duration of action was 1–2 hours. After epidural administration of incremental doses totaling 5–40 mcg, maternal and neonatal plasma concentrations were approximately 0.05–0.1 mcg/mL and were slightly higher in mothers than in infants.

■ **Distribution** Distribution of sufentanil into human body tissues and fluids has not been fully characterized; however, the drug is highly lipophilic and is rapidly and extensively distributed in animals. Following administration of radiolabeled drug in rats, the drug distributes into brain, lung, liver, kidney, heart, and muscle within 2 minutes; into thymus, spleen, testis, and GI tract within 8–15 minutes; and into pancreas and adipose tissue within 30 minutes.

The volumes of distribution of sufentanil in the central compartment (V_c) and at steady-state (V_{ss}) in adults following administration of a single 5-mcg/kg dose reportedly average 0.1 and 2.48 L/kg, respectively. At plasma pH 7.4, the drug is approximately 93% bound in plasma, mainly to albumin; α-, α_1-, β-, and γ-globulins; and α_1-acid glycoprotein. At pH 7.4, approximately 8% of the drug in blood is distributed into plasma water, 22% to blood cells, and 70% is bound to plasma proteins. Because a large portion of the drug appears to be bound to α_1-acid glycoprotein, binding of the drug may be affected by disease states in which this protein is altered. Binding of sufentanil in plasma is independent of plasma drug concentration within the therapeutic range (i.e., 0.1–10 ng/mL). Binding of the drug in plasma is affected by changes in plasma pH; increases in plasma pH from 7.4 to 7.8 increase sufentanil binding by about 30% and decreases in plasma pH from 7.4 to 7.0 decrease binding by about 30%.

It is not known if sufentanil crosses the placenta; however, fentanyl has been shown to cross the placenta and peak concentrations of the drug occur in the fetus within 2 minutes following IV administration of a 1-mcg/kg dose to the mother. It also is not known if sufentanil distributes into milk.

■ **Elimination** Plasma concentrations of sufentanil decline rapidly secondary to redistribution and appear to decline in a triphasic manner. In adults with normal renal and hepatic function, the plasma half-life in the initial (distribution) phase averages 0.72–1.2 minutes, the plasma half-life in the second (redistribution) phase averages 13.7–17 minutes, and the plasma half-life in the terminal (elimination) phase averages 140–158 minutes. The elimination half-life is longer (434 minutes) in neonates but shorter in infants and children (97 minutes), compared with adults and adolescents. The clearance of sufentanil in healthy neonates is approximately one-half that reported in adults and children, and the clearance may be further reduced by up to one-third in neonates with cardiovascular disease. Like fentanyl, total plasma concentrations of sufentanil may decrease following initiation of cardiopulmonary bypass but remain relatively steady during bypass, and the terminal elimination half-life may be prolonged after bypass.

Although the metabolic fate of sufentanil in humans has not been fully characterized, the drug appears to be metabolized mainly in the liver and small intestine via *N*-dealkylation at the piperidine nitrogen and *O*-demethylation. The *O*-demethylated metabolite appears to have about 10% of the analgesic activity of the unchanged drug. The hepatic extraction ratio of the drug (E_H) has been reported to be about 0.72 following IV administration of a single 5-mcg/kg dose.

Sufentanil and its metabolites are excreted principally in urine and also in feces via biliary elimination; approximately 80% of the administered dose is excreted in urine and feces within 24 hours after administration. Only 2% of the dose is excreted unchanged in urine and feces. Following administration of 0.16 mg/kg of radiolabeled drug in rats, 86.8 and 99.4% of the dose were excreted within 24 hours and 4 days, respectively; of the 99.4% excreted, about 38 and 62% were excreted in urine and feces, respectively, but only 1.5–2.5% as unchanged drug. In dogs, however, about 60 and 40% of excreted drug appeared in urine and feces, respectively.

Plasma clearance of sufentanil is reportedly 11.8 mL/minute per kg following IV administration of a single 5-mcg/kg dose in adults.

Chemistry and Stability

■ **Chemistry** Sufentanil citrate is a synthetic phenylpiperidine-derivative opiate agonist. The drug differs structurally from fentanyl in the addition of a methoxymethyl group at the 4-position and the substitution of a thienylethyl group for a phenylethyl group at the 1-position of the piperidine ring. Sufentanil citrate occurs as a white, crystalline powder and has solubilities of 46 and 21 mg/mL in water and alcohol, respectively. The drug has a pK_a of 8.01. Commercially available sufentanil citrate injection is a sterile solution of the drug in water for injection. The injection occurs as a clear solution and has a pH of 3.5–6 with citric acid added when necessary to adjust the pH.

Potency of sufentanil citrate is expressed in terms of sufentanil.

■ **Stability** Commercially available sufentanil citrate injection should be protected from light and stored at 15–25°C. Sufentanil citrate is hydrolyzed in acidic solutions.

For further information on chemistry, pharmacology, pharmacokinetics, uses, cautions, chronic toxicity, acute toxicity, drug interactions, and dosage and administration of sufentanil citrate, see the Opiate Agonists General Statement 28:08.08.

Preparations

Sufentanil citrate is subject to control under the Federal Controlled Substances Act of 1970 as a schedule II (C-II) drug.

Excipients in commercially available drug preparations may have clinically important effects in some individuals; consult specific product labeling for details.

SUFentanil Citrate

Parenteral

Injection	50 mcg (of sufentanil) per mL*	Sufenta® (C-II), Akorn SUFentanil Citrate Injection (C-II)

*available from one or more manufacturer, distributor, and/or repackager by generic (nonproprietary) name

†Use is not currently included in the labeling approved by the US Food and Drug Administration

Tapentadol Hydrochloride

■ Tapentadol hydrochloride is a synthetic, centrally active analgesic.

REMS

FDA approved a REMS for tapentadol hydrochloride to ensure that the benefits outweigh the risk. The REMS may apply to one or more preparations of tapentadol hydrochloride and consists of the following: medication guide and elements to assure safe use. See the FDA REMS page (https://www.accessdata.fda.gov/scripts/cder/rems/index.cfm).

Uses

■ **Pain** Conventional (immediate-release) formulations of tapentadol hydrochloride are used for the relief of acute pain that is severe enough to require an opiate analgesic; because of the risks of addiction, abuse, and misuse associated with opiates even at recommended dosages, conventional preparations of tapentadol should be reserved for use in patients for whom alternative treatment options (e.g., nonopiate analgesics, opiate-containing fixed combinations) have not been, or are not expected to be, adequate or tolerated.

Tapentadol hydrochloride extended-release tablets are used for the relief of pain, including neuropathic pain associated with diabetic peripheral neuropathy, that is severe enough to require long-term, daily, around-the-clock use of an opiate analgesic. Because of the risks of addiction, abuse, and misuse associated with opiates, even at recommended dosages, and because of the greater risks of overdosage and death associated with extended-release opiate formulations, extended-release tapentadol should be reserved for use in patients for whom alternative treatment options (e.g., nonopiate analgesics, immediate-release opiates) are inadequate or not tolerated. Extended-release tapentadol is *not* intended for use on an as-needed ("prn") basis.

Acute Pain Efficacy and safety of conventional preparations of tapentadol for the relief of acute pain have been established in 2 phase 3, randomized, double-blind, placebo- and active-controlled clinical studies in adults with moderate to severe pain secondary to either bunionectomy or end-stage degenerative joint disease.

In the first study, 603 patients with moderate to severe pain (defined as a baseline pain score of at least 4 on an 11-point rating scale) following unilateral first metatarsal bunionectomy were randomized to receive conventional tablets of tapentadol (50, 75, or 100 mg), oxycodone hydrochloride (15 mg), or placebo every 4–6 hours for 72 hours. On day 1, patients were allowed a second dose of study drug as early as 1 hour after the first dose, with subsequent doses administered every 4–6 hours. At each dosage level studied, tapentadol provided a greater reduction in pain intensity, as assessed by the sum of pain intensity difference (SPID) over the first 48 hours of therapy, compared with placebo. In addition, at each dosage level studied, a greater proportion of tapentadol-treated patients experienced at least a 30 or 50% reduction in pain intensity at 48 hours compared with placebo recipients. A post-hoc noninferiority analysis found that tapentadol 100 mg was comparable to oxycodone hydrochloride 15 mg in analgesic efficacy, and tapentadol 100 mg was associated with a lower incidence of adverse GI effects (i.e., nausea, vomiting) compared with oxycodone hydrochloride 15 mg. Although analgesic efficacy of tapentadol 75 mg was inferior to that of oxycodone hydrochloride 15 mg in this study, another phase 3 study in patients undergoing bunionectomy found that tapentadol 50 and 75 mg provided analgesic efficacy comparable to that of oxycodone hydrochloride 10 mg.

In the second study, 674 patients with moderate to severe pain associated with end-stage degenerative joint disease of the hip or knee (defined as a 3-day mean pain score of at least 5 on an 11-point rating scale) were randomized to receive conventional tablets of tapentadol (50 or 75 mg), oxycodone hydrochloride (10 mg), or placebo every 4–6 hours during waking hours for 10 days. Patients who had received a stable regimen of a nonopiate analgesic for at least 28 days prior to the screening period were allowed to continue receiving that regimen throughout the study. At each dosage level studied, tapentadol provided a greater reduction in pain intensity, as assessed by the SPID over the first 5 days of therapy, compared with placebo. In addition, at each dosage level studied, a greater proportion of tapentadol-treated patients experienced at least a 30 or 50% reduction in pain intensity at day 5 of therapy compared with placebo recipients. In a prespecified noninferiority analysis, tapentadol 50 and 75 mg provided analgesic efficacy comparable to that of oxycodone hydrochloride 10 mg, and the incidence of adverse GI effects (i.e., nausea, vomiting, constipation) was lower with tapentadol compared with oxycodone.

For further information on the role of opiate analgesics in the management of acute pain, see Uses: Pain, in the Opiate Agonists General Statement 28:08.08.

Chronic Pain Efficacy of tapentadol extended-release tablets for the relief of pain requiring long-term, daily, around-the-clock use of an opiate analgesic was established in 3 randomized, double-blind studies, including one placebo- and active-controlled study in adults with chronic low back pain and 2 placebo-controlled studies in patients with diabetic peripheral neuropathy.

In the first study, 981 patients with chronic low back pain and a baseline pain score of at least 5 on an 11-point rating scale were randomized in a 1:1:1 ratio to receive tapentadol extended-release tablets (100–250 mg twice daily), extended-release oxycodone hydrochloride (20–50 mg twice daily), or placebo for 12 weeks following a 3-week dosage titration period. The mean age of patients in the study was 50 years (range: 18–89 years); the mean baseline pain score was 8, and approximately one-half of the patients had not received opiate analgesics in the past 3 months. Extended-release tapentadol was initiated at a dosage of 50 mg twice daily, increased to 100 mg twice daily after 3 days, and subsequently titrated over the 3-week titration period up to a maximum dosage of 250 mg twice daily. Approximately one-half of the patients completed the 15-week study. At week 15, patients receiving extended-release tapentadol or extended-release oxycodone had substantially greater pain reduction from baseline compared with those receiving placebo. The incidence of adverse GI effects (i.e., nausea and/or vomiting, constipation) or pruritus was lower with tapentadol compared with oxycodone.

In 2 similarly designed studies, patients with chronic pain due to diabetic peripheral neuropathy and a baseline pain score of at least 5 on an 11-point rating scale received open-label treatment with extended-release tapentadol titrated over 3 weeks to a stable dosage in the range of 100–250 mg twice daily. Patients who tolerated the drug and had at least a 1-point improvement in pain score were randomized in a 1:1 ratio to receive continued therapy with extended-release tapentadol or to receive placebo (following a taper to 100 mg twice daily for 3 days) during a 12-week double-blind withdrawal phase. In the 2 studies combined, 709 patients met criteria for entering the double-blind phase. Low-dose extended-release tapentadol (25 mg twice daily as needed for 4 days, then 25 mg once daily as needed) was available to patients in both groups throughout the double-blind phase. The mean age of patients in these studies was 59–60 years, and approximately 67% of the patients had not received opiate analgesics in the past 3 months. In both studies, reductions in pain intensity were substantially greater in patients receiving extended-release tapentadol compared with those receiving placebo during the 12-week double-blind phase.

For further information on the role of opiate analgesics in the management of chronic pain, see Uses: Pain, in the Opiate Agonists General Statement 28:08.08.

Dosage and Administration

■ **Administration** Tapentadol hydrochloride conventional tablets, extended-release tablets, and oral solution are administered orally without regard to food.

Tapentadol extended-release tablets are administered twice daily (approximately every 12 hours). The extended-release tablets should be swallowed whole, one at a time, with enough water to ensure that each tablet is completely swallowed immediately after it is placed in the mouth; crushing, chewing, or dissolving the tablets will result in uncontrolled delivery of tapentadol and can result in overdosage and death. Patients receiving tapentadol extended-release tablets should not consume alcoholic beverages or use prescription or nonprescription preparations containing alcohol; intake of alcohol with the extended-release tablets may result in increased peak plasma concentrations of tapentadol and ingestion of a potentially toxic dose of the drug. Extended-release tablets of tapentadol should be prescribed only by clinicians who are knowledgeable in the use of potent opiates for the management of chronic pain.

Caution is required when prescribing, dispensing, and administering tapentadol oral solutions to avoid dosing errors. Care should be taken to ensure that the appropriate dose is communicated and dispensed; prescriptions should specify the intended total dose of the drug (in mg) along with the corresponding total volume (in mL). The calibrated measuring device provided with the particular formulation should always be used to ensure that the dose is measured and administered accurately. Use of a household spoon as a measuring device could result in overdosage. (See Dispensing and Administration Precautions with Oral Solution under Warnings/Precautions: Warnings, in Cautions.)

■ **Dosage** Dosage of tapentadol hydrochloride is expressed in terms of tapentadol.

Opiate analgesics should be given at the lowest effective dosage and for the shortest duration of therapy consistent with the treatment goals of the patient. The dosage regimen should be individualized according to severity of pain, response, prior analgesic use, and risk factors for addiction, abuse, and misuse. If concomitant therapy with other CNS depressants is required, the lowest effective dosages and shortest possible duration of concomitant therapy should be used. (See Drug Interactions: Benzodiazepines and Other CNS Depressants.)

For acute pain not related to trauma or surgery, the prescribed quantity should be limited to the amount needed for the expected duration of pain severe enough to require opiate analgesia (generally 3 days or less and rarely more than 7 days). When opiate analgesics are used for the management of chronic noncancer pain, the US Centers for Disease Control and Prevention (CDC) recommends that primary care clinicians carefully reassess individual benefits and risks before prescribing dosages equivalent to 50 mg or more of morphine sulfate daily and avoid dosages equivalent to 90 mg or more of morphine sulfate daily or carefully justify their decision to titrate the dosage to such levels. Other experts recommend consulting a pain management specialist before exceeding a dosage equivalent to 80–120 mg of morphine sulfate daily.

Appropriate dosage selection and titration are essential to reduce the risk of respiratory depression. Patients should be monitored closely for respiratory depression, especially during the first 24–72 hours of therapy and following any increase in dosage.

Patients receiving opiate analgesia should be reevaluated continually for adequacy of pain control and for adverse effects, as well for the development of addiction, abuse, or misuse. During long-term therapy, the continued need for opiate analgesics should be periodically reevaluated. Frequent communication among the prescriber, other members of the healthcare team, the patient, and the patient's caregiver or family is important during periods of changing analgesic requirements, including the initial dosage titration period. If the level of pain increases after dosage stabilization, an attempt should be made to identify the source of increased pain before increasing the tapentadol dosage.

When tapentadol therapy is discontinued in a patient who may be physically dependent on opiates, the dosage generally should be reduced by 25–50% every 2–4 days. If manifestations of withdrawal occur, the dosage should be increased to the prior level and tapered more slowly (i.e., by increasing the interval between dosage reductions and/or reducing the amount of each incremental change in dose).

For further information on the management of opiate analgesic therapy, see Dosage and Administration: Dosage, in the Opiate Agonists General Statement 28:08.08.

Conventional (Immediate-release) Preparations For the management of acute pain that is severe enough to require use of an opiate analgesic, the recommended initial adult dosage of tapentadol as conventional (immediate-release) tablets or oral solution is 50–100 mg administered every 4–6 hours as needed. On day 1 of therapy, patients with inadequate pain relief may receive a second dose of the drug as soon as 1 hour after the first dose. Subsequent doses should be administered at intervals of 4–6 hours and should be adjusted to maintain adequate analgesia and minimize adverse effects. Dosages exceeding 700 mg daily on the first day of therapy or 600 mg daily on subsequent days have not been evaluated and are not recommended by the manufacturer.

Extended-release Tablets For the management of pain, including neuropathic pain associated with diabetic peripheral neuropathy, that is severe enough to require daily, around-the-clock, long-term opiate analgesia in adults who are opiate-naive or *not* opiate tolerant, therapy with tapentadol extended-release tablets should be initiated at a dosage of 50 mg every 12 hours. The manufacturer states that use of higher initial dosages in patients who are not opiate tolerant may result in fatal respiratory depression.

For patients receiving conventional (immediate-release) tapentadol preparations, the total daily dosage of the drug should be calculated and given as tapentadol extended-release tablets in 2 divided doses at 12-hour intervals.

In patients who are being switched from other opiate analgesics to tapentadol extended-release tablets, the recommended initial dosage of tapentadol extended-release tablets is 50 mg every 12 hours, since dosage conversion factors have not been established in clinical trials. Particularly close monitoring is required when patients are switched from methadone, since conversion ratios between methadone and other opiates vary widely depending on extent of prior methadone exposure and because methadone has a long half-life and tends to accumulate in plasma.

When therapy with tapentadol extended-release tablets is initiated, all other tapentadol- or tramadol-containing preparations should be discontinued.

Because there is substantial interpatient variability in the relative potency of opiate analgesics and analgesic formulations, it is preferable to underestimate the patient's 24-hour opiate requirements and provide "rescue" therapy with an immediate-release opiate analgesic than to overestimate the requirements and manage an adverse reaction. Patients who experience breakthrough pain may require dosage adjustment or supplemental analgesia (i.e., "rescue" therapy with an immediate-release analgesic).

Dosage adjustments may be made in increments of 50 mg no more than twice daily at intervals of every 3 days, to a level that provides adequate analgesia and minimizes adverse effects. Dosage should not exceed 500 mg daily (i.e., 250 mg twice daily). Dosage of extended-release tapentadol in clinical trials ranged from 100–250 mg twice daily.

■ **Special Populations** No dosage adjustment is needed in patients with mild or moderate renal impairment (creatinine clearance 30–90 mL/minute). Tapentadol is not recommended in patients with severe renal impairment (creatinine clearance less than 30 mL/minute) because of accumulation of a glucuronide metabolite. (See Renal Impairment under Warnings/Precautions: Specific Populations, in Cautions.)

No dosage adjustment is needed in patients with mild hepatic impairment (Child-Pugh score 5–6). In patients with moderate hepatic impairment (Child-Pugh score 7–9), conventional preparations of tapentadol should be initiated at a dosage of 50 mg given no more frequently than once every 8 hours for a maximum of 3 doses in 24 hours; if continued therapy is required, the dosage should be adjusted by lengthening or shortening the dosing interval to maintain adequate analgesia and minimize adverse effects. In patients with moderate hepatic impairment, extended-release tapentadol should be initiated at a dosage of 50 mg given no more frequently than once every 24 hours; the maximum recommended dosage of extended-release tapentadol in patients with moderate hepatic impairment is 100 mg daily. Tapentadol has not been evaluated in patients with severe hepatic impairment (Child-Pugh score 10–15) and, therefore, is not recommended for use in this population. (See Hepatic Impairment under Warnings/Precautions: Specific Populations, in Cautions.)

Geriatric patients may exhibit increased sensitivity to tapentadol. Because of the greater frequency of decreased hepatic, renal, and/or cardiac function and of concomitant disease and drug therapy in geriatric patients, dosage selection of tapentadol in such patients should be cautious, usually initiating therapy with dosages in the lower end of the usual range. Dosage of tapentadol should be titrated slowly with close monitoring for CNS and respiratory depression. (See Geriatric Use under Warnings/Precautions: Specific Populations, in Cautions.)

Cautions

■ **Contraindications** Tapentadol is contraindicated in patients with substantial respiratory depression; acute or severe bronchial asthma or hypercarbia in unmonitored settings or in the absence of resuscitative equipment; known or suspected GI obstruction, including paralytic ileus; or known hypersensitivity (e.g., anaphylaxis, angioedema) to the drug or any ingredient in the formulation. Tapentadol also is contraindicated in patients who are receiving or have recently received (i.e., within 2 weeks) therapy with a monoamine oxidase (MAO) inhibitor. (See Drug Interactions: Monoamine Oxidase Inhibitors.)

■ **Warnings/Precautions** ***Warnings*** **Addiction, Abuse, and Misuse.** Tapentadol exposes patients and other users to the risks of opiate addiction, abuse, and misuse, which can lead to overdosage and death. Tapentadol has an abuse potential similar to that of other potent opiate agonists (e.g., fentanyl, hydrocodone, hydromorphone, methadone, morphine, oxycodone, oxymorphone). (See Description.) Addiction can occur at recommended dosages or may be associated with misuse or abuse. Concurrent abuse of alcohol and other CNS depressants increases the risk of toxicity. Each patient's risk for addiction, abuse, or misuse should be assessed prior to initiating tapentadol therapy, and all patients receiving the drug should be monitored for the development of these behaviors or conditions. Personal or family history of substance abuse (including drug or alcohol addiction or abuse) or mental illness (e.g., major depression) increases risk. The potential for addiction, abuse, or misuse should not prevent opiate prescribing for appropriate pain management, but does necessitate intensive counseling about risks and proper use and intensive monitoring for signs of addiction, abuse, and misuse. Tapentadol should be prescribed in the smallest appropriate quantity and the patient should be instructed on secure storage and proper disposal to prevent theft.

Extended-release opiates are associated with a greater risk of overdosage and death because of the larger amount of drug contained in each dosage unit. Abuse or misuse of tapentadol extended-release tablets by crushing or chewing the tablets, snorting the powder, or injecting the dissolved contents results in uncontrolled release of tapentadol and can result in fatal overdosage. In addition, IV injection of excipients in extended-release tapentadol tablets can result in local tissue necrosis, infection, pulmonary granulomas, embolism, and death and increase the risk of endocarditis and valvular heart injury.

Respiratory Depression. Serious, life-threatening, or fatal respiratory depression can occur in patients receiving opiates, including tapentadol, even when the drugs are used as recommended. Carbon dioxide retention as a result of opiate-induced respiratory depression can exacerbate sedation and, in certain patients, can lead to elevated intracranial pressure. (See Increased Intracranial Pressure or Head Injury under Warnings/Precautions: Other Warnings and Precautions, in Cautions.) Although respiratory depression can occur at any time during therapy, the risk is greatest during initiation of therapy or following an increase in dosage; therefore, patients receiving tapentadol should be monitored closely for respiratory depression, especially during the first 24–72 hours of therapy and following any increase in dosage.

Appropriate dosage selection and titration are essential to reduce the risk of respiratory depression. Large initial doses in nontolerant patients, overestimation of initial tapentadol dosage when transferring patients from other opiate therapy, or accidental ingestion of even one dose of tapentadol, especially by a child, can result in respiratory depression and death. (See Dosage under Dosage and Administration.)

Geriatric, cachectic, or debilitated patients are at increased risk for life-threatening respiratory depression since pharmacokinetics of the drugs may be altered in these patients. In patients with chronic obstructive pulmonary disease or cor pulmonale, substantially decreased respiratory reserve, hypoxia, hypercapnia, or preexisting respiratory depression, even recommended doses of tapentadol may decrease respiratory drive to the point of apnea. Such patients should be monitored closely, particularly during initiation of tapentadol therapy and dosage titration and when other drugs with respiratory depressant effects are used concomitantly. Alternatively, use of nonopiate analgesics should be considered in such patients. Use of tapentadol in patients with substantial respiratory depression or in those with acute or severe bronchial asthma in unmonitored settings or in the absence of resuscitative equipment is contraindicated.

For usual guidelines for management of opiate agonist-induced respiratory depression, see Acute Toxicity: Treatment, in the Opiate Agonists General Statement 28:08.08.

When opiate agonists are prescribed for patients at increased risk of opiate overdosage (e.g., those with a history of overdose or substance use disorder, those receiving 50 mg or more of morphine sulfate [or equivalent] daily, those receiving benzodiazepines concomitantly, those with medical conditions that could increase sensitivity to opiates), some experts state that clinicians should consider offering the opiate antagonist naloxone.

Neonatal Opiate Withdrawal Syndrome. Prolonged maternal use of tapentadol during pregnancy can result in neonatal opiate withdrawal syndrome. (See Pregnancy under Warnings/Precautions: Specific Populations, in Cautions.)

Concomitant Use with Benzodiazepines or Other CNS Depressants. Profound sedation, respiratory depression, coma, and death may occur when opiate agonists are used concomitantly with benzodiazepines or other CNS depressants. Concomitant use of such drugs should be reserved for patients in whom alternative treatment options are inadequate. (See Drug Interactions: Benzodiazepines and Other CNS Depressants.)

Dispensing and Administration Precautions with Oral Solution. Caution is required when prescribing, dispensing, and administering tapentadol oral solution since dosing errors caused by confusion between milligrams (mg) and milliliters (mL) can result in overdosage and death. To avoid such medication errors, the prescriber should specify the intended total dose of the drug (in mg) along with the corresponding total volume (in mL). Patients and/or caregivers should be instructed to use extreme caution when measuring a dose of tapentadol oral solution. (See Dosage and Administration: Administration.)

Interaction of Extended-release Tablets with Alcohol. Concomitant ingestion of alcohol with tapentadol extended-release tablets may result in increased plasma concentrations of the drug and a potentially fatal overdose. Patients should not consume alcoholic beverages or use prescription or nonprescription preparations containing alcohol during therapy with tapentadol extended-release tablets.

Other Warnings and Precautions **General Opiate Agonist Precautions.** Administration of tapentadol may cause effects similar to those produced by other opiate agonist drugs, and the usual precautions of opiate agonist therapy should be observed. (See the Opiate Agonists General Statement 28:08.08.)

Serotonin Syndrome. Potentially serious, sometimes fatal serotonin syndrome may occur with serotonin- and norepinephrine-reuptake inhibitors (SNRIs), including tapentadol, particularly with concurrent use of other serotonergic drugs or drugs that impair the metabolism of serotonin (e.g., MAO inhibitors). (See Description.) Manifestations of serotonin syndrome may include mental status changes (e.g., agitation, hallucinations, coma), autonomic instability (e.g., tachycardia, labile blood pressure, hyperthermia), neuromuscular aberrations (e.g., hyperreflexia, incoordination, rigidity), and/or GI symptoms (e.g., nausea, vomiting, diarrhea). Symptom onset generally occurs within several hours to a few days of concomitant use, but may occur later, particularly after dosage increases. (See Drug Interactions: Drugs Associated with Serotonin Syndrome.)

Adrenal Insufficiency. Adrenal insufficiency has been reported in patients receiving opiate agonists or opiate partial agonists. Manifestations of adrenal insufficiency are nonspecific and may include nausea, vomiting, anorexia, fatigue, weakness, dizziness, and hypotension. In many of the reported cases, onset of adrenal insufficiency occurred after at least 1 month of opiate agonist or partial agonist use, although the time to onset has ranged from within 1 day to more than 1 year.

If adrenal insufficiency is suspected, appropriate laboratory testing should be performed promptly and physiologic (replacement) dosages of corticosteroids provided; therapy with the opiate agonist or partial agonist should be tapered and discontinued to allow recovery of adrenal function. If the opiate agonist or partial agonist can be discontinued, follow-up assessment of adrenal function should be performed to determine if corticosteroid replacement therapy can be discontinued. In some patients, switching to a different opiate improved symptoms.

Hypotension. Tapentadol may cause severe hypotension, including orthostatic hypotension and syncope, in ambulatory patients. Because the risk is increased in patients whose ability to maintain blood pressure has been compromised by blood volume depletion or concomitant use of certain CNS depressants (e.g., general anesthetics, phenothiazines), such patients should be monitored for hypotension following initiation of tapentadol therapy or an increase in dosage. Use of tapentadol should be avoided in patients with circulatory shock since the drug may cause vasodilation that can further reduce cardiac output and blood pressure.

Increased Intracranial Pressure or Head Injury. The respiratory depressant effects of tapentadol promote carbon dioxide retention, which can result in elevation of intracranial pressure. Patients who may be particularly susceptible to these effects (e.g., those with evidence of increased intracranial pressure or brain tumors) should be monitored for sedation and respiratory depression, particularly during initiation of therapy. Opiates also may obscure the clinical course in patients with head injuries. Use of tapentadol should be avoided in patients with impaired consciousness or coma.

GI Conditions. Tapentadol may increase serum amylase concentrations and cause spasm of the sphincter of Oddi. Patients with biliary tract disease, including those with acute pancreatitis, should be monitored for worsening symptoms during therapy with tapentadol.

Tapentadol is contraindicated in patients with known or suspected GI obstruction, including paralytic ileus.

Seizures. Tapentadol may increase the frequency of seizures in patients with seizure disorders and may increase the risk of seizures in some clinical settings associated with seizures. Patients with seizure disorders should be monitored for worsening of seizure control during tapentadol therapy.

Dependence and Tolerance. Both physical dependence and tolerance can develop during long-term opiate therapy. Tolerance may not develop uniformly to all opiate effects.

In patients who are physically dependent on opiates, abrupt discontinuance of tapentadol or a substantial reduction in dosage may result in manifestations of withdrawal (e.g., restlessness, lacrimation, rhinorrhea, yawning, sweating, chills, myalgia, mydriasis, irritability, anxiety, backache, joint pain, weakness, abdominal cramps, insomnia, nausea, anorexia, vomiting, diarrhea, increases in blood pressure, respiratory rate, or heart rate). Withdrawal also may be precipitated by concomitant administration of an opiate antagonist or opiate partial agonist. (See Drug Interactions: Opiate Partial Agonists.) In a study evaluating the safety of tapentadol administered for periods up to 90 days, objective manifestations of opiate withdrawal, as assessed by the Clinical Opiate Withdrawal Scale (COWS), were absent in 83% of tapentadol-treated patients who abruptly discontinued therapy and were assessed for withdrawal symptoms 2–4 days after drug discontinuance; mild to moderate withdrawal symptoms were noted in 17% of tapentadol-treated patients compared with 29% of oxycodone-treated patients. When tapentadol therapy is discontinued in a patient who may be physically dependent on opiates, the dosage should be tapered gradually.

Infants born to women who are physically dependent on opiates also will be physically dependent. (See Pregnancy under Warnings/Precautions: Specific Populations, in Cautions.)

CNS Depression. Tapentadol may impair mental alertness and/or physical coordination required to perform potentially hazardous tasks such as driving or operating machinery. (See Advice to Patients.)

Concurrent use of tapentadol and other CNS depressants may result in profound sedation, respiratory depression, coma, or death. (See Drug Interactions: Benzodiazepines and Other CNS Depressants.)

Hypogonadism. Hypogonadism or androgen deficiency has been reported in patients receiving long-term opiate agonist or opiate partial agonist therapy, although a causal relationship has not been established. Patients receiving long-term opiate agonist or partial agonist therapy who present with manifestations of hypogonadism (e.g., decreased libido, impotence, erectile dysfunction, amenorrhea, infertility) should undergo laboratory evaluation.

Specific Populations **Pregnancy.** Category C. (See Users Guide.)

Analysis of data from the National Birth Defects Prevention Study, a large population-based, case-control study, suggests that therapeutic use of opiate agonists in pregnant women during the period of organogenesis is associated with a low absolute risk of birth defects, including heart defects, spina bifida, and gastroschisis. The manufacturer states that available data regarding use of tapentadol in pregnant women are not sufficient to establish the risk of major birth defects and spontaneous abortion with the drug. In animal studies, embryofetal mortality and structural malformations were observed in rabbits and delays in skeletal maturation and increased pup mortality were observed in rats at exposure levels equivalent to or less than those associated with the maximum recommended human dosage. Based on animal data, patients should be apprised of potential risks to the fetus if tapentadol is used during pregnancy.

Use of opiates in pregnant women during labor can result in neonatal respiratory depression. Tapentadol is not recommended for use during or immediately prior to labor and delivery. Neonates exposed to opiates during labor should be monitored for respiratory depression and withdrawal symptoms; an opiate antagonist (e.g., naloxone) should be available to reverse opiate-induced respiratory depression in the neonate.

Prolonged maternal use of opiates, including tapentadol, during pregnancy can result in neonatal opiate withdrawal syndrome with manifestations of irritability, hyperactivity and abnormal sleep pattern, high-pitched cry, tremor, vomiting, diarrhea, and failure to gain weight. In contrast to adults, the withdrawal syndrome in neonates may be life-threatening if not recognized and treated, and requires management according to protocols developed by neonatology experts. Women who require prolonged opiate agonist therapy during pregnancy should be advised of the risk of neonatal opiate withdrawal syndrome, and availability of appropriate treatment should be ensured. The onset, duration, and severity of the syndrome vary depending on the specific opiate agonist used, duration of use, timing and amount of last maternal use, and rate of drug elimination by the neonate.

Lactation. Limited data suggest that tapentadol may be distributed into milk; risk to nursing infants cannot be ruled out. The benefits of breast-feeding and the importance of tapentadol therapy to the woman should be considered along with the potential adverse effects on the breast-fed infant from the drug or from the underlying maternal condition. Because of the potential for serious adverse effects (e.g., sedation, respiratory depression) in nursing infants, breast-feeding is not recommended during therapy with tapentadol extended-release tablets.

Infants exposed to tapentadol through breast milk should be monitored for excessive sedation and respiratory depression. Symptoms of withdrawal can occur in opiate-dependent infants when maternal administration of opiates is discontinued or breast-feeding is stopped.

Pediatric Use. Safety and efficacy of tapentadol in children younger than 18 years of age have not been established.

Geriatric Use. In clinical studies of tapentadol administered as conventional or extended-release tablets, 19 or 28%, respectively, of patients were 65 years of age or older and 5 or 7%, respectively, were 75 years of age or older. No overall differences in efficacy were observed between geriatric patients and younger adults; however, in patients receiving tapentadol conventional tablets, the incidence of constipation was higher in geriatric patients 65 years of age or older compared with those younger than 65 years of age (12 versus 7%). Systemic exposure to tapentadol, as measured by area under the plasma concentration-time curve (AUC), was similar in geriatric patients and young adults; the mean peak plasma tapentadol concentration was 16% lower in geriatric patients compared with young adults. (See Dosage and Administration: Special Populations.)

Hepatic Impairment. Serum concentrations and AUC of tapentadol were increased in patients with hepatic impairment compared with individuals with normal hepatic function; in addition, the rate of formation of the inactive *O*-glucuronide metabolite was reduced in patients with increased hepatic impairment. Tapentadol dosage should be reduced in patients with moderate hepatic impairment (Child-Pugh score 7–9), and the patient should be monitored closely for respiratory and CNS depression. (See Dosage and Administration: Special Populations.) Dosage adjustment is not necessary in patients with mild hepatic impairment (Child-Pugh score 5–6). The drug has not been studied in patients with severe hepatic impairment (Child-Pugh score 10–15), and use in such patients is not recommended.

Renal Impairment. Peak plasma concentrations and AUC of tapentadol were similar in individuals with normal to severely impaired renal function, but exposure to the *O*-glucuronide metabolite increased as the degree of renal impairment increased; AUC of the *O*-glucuronide metabolite was 1.5-, 2.5-, and 5.5-fold higher in patients with mild, moderate, and severe renal impairment, respectively, when compared with individuals with normal renal function. Because the clinical relevance of accumulation of the glucuronide metabolite is unknown, use of tapentadol is not recommended in patients with severe renal impairment (creatinine clearance less than 30 mL/minute). No dosage adjustment is needed in patients with mild or moderate renal impairment (creatinine clearance 30–90 mL/minute).

■ **Common Adverse Effects** Adverse effects reported in 3% or more of tapentadol-treated patients in clinical studies and more frequently with tapentadol than with placebo include nausea, dizziness, vomiting, somnolence, constipation, pruritus, dry mouth, hyperhidrosis, fatigue, headache, vomiting, diarrhea, decreased appetite, anxiety, insomnia, dyspepsia, and hot flush. In several clinical studies, adverse GI effects (nausea, vomiting, constipation) were reported more commonly with oxycodone than with tapentadol (see Uses: Pain).

Drug Interactions

■ **Drugs Affecting or Metabolized by Hepatic Microsomal Enzymes** Tapentadol is metabolized principally by glucuronidation and to a lesser extent by cytochrome P-450 (CYP) isoenzymes 2C9, 2C19, and 2D6. Tapentadol did not induce CYP isoenzymes 1A2, 2D6, or 3A4 or inhibit isoenzymes 1A2, 2A6, 2C9, 2C19, 2E1, or 3A4 in vitro; tapentadol inhibited CYP2D6 to a limited extent in vitro, but at clinically irrelevant concentrations. Clinically important interactions mediated by CYP isoenzymes are unlikely.

■ **Benzodiazepines and Other CNS Depressants** Potential pharmacologic interaction (additive CNS depressant effects and increased risk of respiratory depression, hypotension, profound sedation, coma, and death) when tapentadol is used concomitantly with benzodiazepines or other CNS depressants, including other opiate agonists, anxiolytics, sedatives, hypnotics, tranquilizers, muscle relaxants, general anesthetics, antipsychotics, and alcohol. A substantial proportion of fatal opiate overdoses involve concurrent benzodiazepine use. Whenever possible, concomitant use of opiate agonists and benzodiazepines should be avoided. Concomitant use of opiate analgesics and benzodiazepines or other CNS depressants should be reserved for patients in whom alternative treatment options are inadequate; the lowest effective dosages and shortest possible duration of concomitant therapy should be used, and the patient should be monitored closely for respiratory depression and sedation. Concomitant use with alcohol should be avoided. (See Drug Interactions: Alcohol.)

If a benzodiazepine or other CNS depressant is required for any indication other than epilepsy in a patient receiving tapentadol, the drug should be initiated at a lower dosage than indicated in the absence of opiate therapy and titrated based on clinical response. In patients receiving a CNS depressant, tapentadol, if required, should be initiated at a reduced dosage and titrated based on clinical response. Some experts state that consideration should be given to offering the opiate antagonist naloxone when opiates are prescribed for patients at increased risk of opiate overdosage, including those receiving benzodiazepines concomitantly.

■ **Monoamine Oxidase Inhibitors** Potential pharmacologic interaction (potentially serious, sometimes fatal serotonin syndrome; respiratory depression, coma, or other manifestations of opiate toxicity). Tapentadol is contraindicated in patients who are receiving or have recently (i.e., within 2 weeks) received a monoamine oxidase (MAO) inhibitor. (See Drug Interactions: Drugs Associated with Serotonin Syndrome.)

■ **Drugs Associated with Serotonin Syndrome** Potential pharmacologic interaction (potentially serious, sometimes fatal serotonin syndrome) when tapentadol is used concurrently with other serotonergic drugs, including serotonin (5-hydroxytryptamine; 5-HT) type 1 receptor agonists ("triptans"), selective serotonin-reuptake inhibitors (SSRIs), selective serotonin- and norepinephrine-reuptake inhibitors (SNRIs), tricyclic antidepressants, antiemetics that are 5-HT_3 receptor antagonists, buspirone, cyclobenzaprine, dextromethorphan, lithium, St. John's wort (*Hypericum perforatum*), tramadol, tryptophan, other serotonin modulators (e.g., mirtazapine, nefazodone, trazodone, vilazodone) and MAO inhibitors (both those used to treat psychiatric disorders and others, such as linezolid, methylene blue, and selegiline). Serotonin syndrome may occur within the recommended dosage ranges for these drugs. Manifestations of serotonin syndrome may include mental status changes (e.g., agitation, hallucinations, coma), autonomic instability (e.g., tachycardia, labile blood pressure, hyperthermia), neuromuscular aberrations (e.g., hyperreflexia, incoordination, rigidity), and/or GI symptoms (e.g., nausea, vomiting, diarrhea). Symptom onset generally occurs within several hours to a few days of concomitant use, but may occur later, particularly after dosage increases.

Tapentadol is contraindicated in patients who are receiving or have recently (i.e., within 2 weeks) received an MAO inhibitor. (See Drug Interactions: Monoamine Oxidase Inhibitors.) If concomitant use of tapentadol with other serotonergic drugs is warranted, patients should be monitored for serotonin syndrome, particularly during initiation of therapy and dosage increases. If serotonin syndrome is suspected, treatment with tapentadol, other opiate therapy, and/or any concurrently administered serotonergic agents should be discontinued.

For further information on serotonin syndrome, including manifestations and treatment, see Drug Interactions: Serotonergic Drugs, in Fluoxetine Hydrochloride 28:16.04.20.

■ **Opiate Partial Agonists** Use of opiate partial agonists (e.g., buprenorphine, butorphanol, nalbuphine, pentazocine) should be avoided in patients receiving opiate agonists, since the partial agonist may reduce the analgesic effect of the full opiate agonist and/or precipitate withdrawal symptoms.

■ **Acetaminophen** Pharmacokinetics of tapentadol were not altered when a single 80-mg dose of the drug was administered concomitantly with the fifth of 7 doses of acetaminophen (1 g every 6 hours) in healthy individuals.

■ **Aspirin** Pharmacokinetics of tapentadol were not altered when a single 80-mg dose of the drug was administered concomitantly with the second of 2 doses of aspirin (325 mg once daily) in healthy individuals.

■ **Alcohol** In addition to additive CNS depressant effects that could result in respiratory depression, hypotension, profound sedation, coma, or death (see Drug Interactions: Benzodiazepines and Other CNS Depressants), concomitant use of alcohol with extended-release tapentadol tablets can result in increased plasma tapentadol concentrations and potentially fatal overdosage. Administration of tapentadol extended-release tablets with 240 mL of 40% alcohol in the fasted state did not affect the rate of tapentadol absorption but increased mean peak plasma concentration and area under the plasma concentration-time curve (AUC) of the drug by 48 and 17%, respectively following a single 100-mg dose, and by 28 and 16%, respectively, following a single 250-mg dose.

Concomitant use of extended-release tapentadol tablets with alcohol or products containing alcohol should be avoided.

■ **Anticholinergic Agents** Concomitant use of tapentadol and drugs with anticholinergic activity may increase the risk of urinary retention and/or severe constipation, which can lead to paralytic ileus. Patients receiving such concomitant therapy should be monitored for signs or symptoms of urinary retention and reduced GI motility.

■ **Diuretics** Opiate agonists may decrease the effects of diuretics by inducing the release of vasopressin (antidiuretic hormone). Patients receiving such concomitant therapy should be monitored for decreased diuretic or hypotensive effects; dosage of the diuretic may be increased if clinically indicated.

■ **Metoclopramide** Pharmacokinetics of tapentadol were not affected by metoclopramide.

■ **Naproxen** Naproxen increased the AUC of tapentadol by 17% when a single 80-mg dose of tapentadol was administered concomitantly with the third of 4 doses of naproxen (500 mg twice daily) in healthy individuals; this change was not considered to be clinically relevant and dosage adjustments are not necessary.

■ **Neuromuscular Blocking Agents** Opiates may enhance the neuromuscular blocking action and increase the respiratory depressant effect of neuromuscular blocking agents. Patients receiving such concomitant therapy should be monitored for a greater than expected degree of respiratory depression; dosage of one or both drugs should be decreased as needed.

■ **Omeprazole** Pharmacokinetics of tapentadol were not affected by omeprazole.

■ **Probenecid** Probenecid increased the AUC of tapentadol by 57%; this change was not considered to be clinically relevant and dosage adjustments are not necessary.

■ **Protein-bound Drugs** Pharmacokinetic interactions are unlikely.

Description

Tapentadol is a synthetic, centrally active analgesic that is structurally and pharmacologically related to tramadol. Tapentadol, like tramadol, exhibits agonist activity at the μ-opiate receptor and inhibits norepinephrine and serotonin reuptake; however, animal studies indicate that the serotonergic activity of tapentadol is much lower than its noradrenergic activity. The precise mechanism of the analgesic effect of tapentadol is unknown, but is thought to be related to the drug's opiate agonist activity and inhibition of norepinephrine reuptake. Studies with selective serotonin-reuptake inhibitors (SSRIs), selective serotonin- and norepinephrine-reuptake inhibitors (SNRIs), and other mixed reuptake inhibitors have indicated that analgesia is more readily obtained by inhibiting the reuptake of norepinephrine rather than serotonin. It is thought that inhibition of norepinephrine reuptake may work synergistically with μ-receptor activation to enhance analgesic efficacy and/or attenuate adverse effects associated with traditional opiate analgesics (e.g., GI effects) by reducing the requirement for μ-receptor activation. Results of rat synaptosomal reuptake assays indicate that tapentadol is almost as potent as venlafaxine in inhibiting the reuptake of norepinephrine. In animal models, tapentadol is 2–3 times less potent than morphine in producing analgesia. Compared with morphine, tapentadol possesses a reduced emetogenic potential, and produces less physical dependence at equianalgesic doses in animal models. The drug has an abuse potential similar to that seen with other potent opiates, including fentanyl, hydrocodone, hydromorphone, methadone, morphine, oxycodone, and oxymorphone, and exhibits weak antagonist activity for muscarinic receptors. Tapentadol appears to have a greater abuse potential than tramadol; unlike tramadol (which originally was not subject to control under the Federal Controlled Substances Act of 1970, but currently is subject to control as a schedule IV drug), tapentadol is subject to control as a schedule II drug.

Tapentadol undergoes extensive first-pass metabolism with a mean absolute bioavailability following a single oral dose of approximately 32%. Peak plasma concentrations of tapentadol are attained 1.25 hours after administration as conventional (immediate-release) preparations and 3–6 hours after administration as extended-release tablets. Peak plasma tapentadol concentration and area under the plasma concentration-time curve (AUC) are dose proportional over the dosing range of 50–150 mg for conventional preparations; AUC also is dose proportional over the therapeutic dosage range for extended-release tablets. Following oral administration of extended-release tablets every 12 hours, steady-state tapentadol exposure is attained after the third dose. Administration of conventional preparations of tapentadol with a high-fat, high-calorie meal increases peak plasma concentration and AUC of the drug by 16 and 25%, respectively; when the extended-release tablets are administered with a high-fat, high-calorie meal, peak plasma concentration and AUC are increased by 17 and 6%, respectively. The manufacturer states that conventional or extended-release formulations may be administered without regard to food. The drug distributes widely throughout the body and is approximately 20% bound to plasma proteins. Tapentadol undergoes extensive metabolism, principally by glucuronidation; its major metabolite, tapentadol-*O*-glucuronide, is formed via uridine diphosphate-glucuronosyltransferase enzymes 1A9 and 2B7. The drug also is metabolized to a lesser extent by cytochrome P-450 (CYP) isoenzymes 2C9 and 2C19 to a desmethyl metabolite and by CYP2D6 to a hydroxide metabolite; both metabolites undergo secondary conjugation. None of the metabolites contribute to the analgesic activity of the drug. The average terminal half-life of tapentadol is 4 or 5 hours following oral administration of conventional preparations or extended-release tablets, respectively. Following oral administration, approximately 70% of a dose is excreted in urine as glucuronide or sulfate conjugates and only 3% is excreted unchanged. Tapentadol and its inactive metabolites are eliminated mainly by the kidneys (99%).

Advice to Patients

Importance of reading the patient information (medication guide) provided by the manufacturer before initiating therapy and each time the prescription is refilled.

Importance of taking tapentadol only as directed; importance of not adjusting the dosage of tapentadol without consulting a clinician and of not discontinuing the drug abruptly as withdrawal symptoms may occur.

Importance of instructing patients on proper administration of the drug. Importance of always using the calibrated oral syringe when administering tapentadol oral solution and of *not* using a household spoon to measure the dose.

Importance of instructing patients to swallow extended-release tablets whole with enough water to ensure complete swallowing of the tablet immediately after it is placed in the mouth. Importance of not cutting, crushing, chewing, or dissolving extended-release tablets.

Importance of informing patients that tapentadol is an opiate and carries the risk of addiction, abuse, and misuse, which can lead to overdosage and death, even when used as recommended. Importance of informing patients that this drug should never be given to anyone other than the individual for whom it was prescribed, that the drug should be protected from theft or misuse, and that any unused drug should be disposed of properly.

Risk of potentially fatal respiratory depression. Importance of informing patients that the risk is greatest following initiation of therapy and dosage increases, and may occur even at recommended dosages. Importance of advising patient to seek immediate medical attention if signs or symptoms of respiratory depression occur.

Risk of respiratory depression or death if accidentally ingested, particularly by a child. Importance of keeping tapentadol out of reach of children.

Risk of potentially fatal additive effects (e.g., profound sedation, respiratory depression, coma) if used concomitantly with benzodiazepines or other CNS depressants, including alcohol and other opiates, either therapeutically or illicitly. Importance of avoiding concomitant use unless such use is supervised by clinician. Importance of advising patients that tapentadol should not be combined with alcohol.

Risk of orthostatic hypotension and syncope.

Potential for tapentadol to impair mental alertness and/or physical coordination; driving or operating machinery should be avoided until the drug's effects on the individual are known.

Importance of informing patients that severe constipation may develop and advising patients on appropriate management.

Potential risk of serotonin syndrome with concurrent use of tapentadol and other serotonergic agents. (See Interactions.) Importance of immediately contacting clinician if manifestations of serotonin syndrome (e.g., agitation, hallucinations, tachycardia, labile BP, fever, excessive sweating, shivering, shaking, muscle stiffness, twitching, loss of coordination, nausea, vomiting, diarrhea) develop.

Potential risk of adrenal insufficiency. Importance of contacting clinician if manifestations of adrenal insufficiency (e.g., nausea, vomiting, loss of appetite, fatigue, weakness, dizziness, hypotension) develop.

Possible risk (although causality not established) of hypogonadism or androgen deficiency with long-term opiate agonist or partial agonist use. Importance of informing clinician if decreased libido, impotence, erectile dysfunction, amenorrhea, or infertility occurs.

Importance of informing clinicians of existing or contemplated concomitant therapy, including prescription and OTC drugs, as well as any concomitant illnesses. Importance of avoiding concomitant therapy with monoamine oxidase (MAO) inhibitors.

Importance of women informing clinicians if they are or plan to become pregnant or plan to breast-feed. Importance of informing women that tapentadol may cause fetal harm and that chronic use during pregnancy may result in neonatal opiate withdrawal syndrome, which can be life-threatening if not recognized and treated. Importance of immediately seeking medical attention if an infant exposed to tapentadol through breast milk exhibits symptoms of opiate overdosage (e.g., sedation, difficulty breathing, hypotonia). Importance of advising patients that breast-feeding during therapy with extended-release tapentadol is not recommended.

Importance of informing patients with a history of seizures that tapentadol may precipitate seizures and of advising them to use tapentadol with care. Importance of advising patients to discontinue tapentadol if seizures occur and to contact their clinician immediately.

Importance of informing patients of other important precautionary information. (See Cautions.)

Overview® (see Users Guide). For additional information on this drug until a more detailed monograph is developed and published, the manufacturer's labeling should be consulted. It is *essential* that the manufacturer's labeling be consulted for more detailed information on usual cautions, precautions, contraindications, potential drug interactions, laboratory test interferences, and acute toxicity.

Preparations

Tapentadol hydrochloride is subject to control under the Federal Controlled Substances Act of 1970 as a schedule II (C-II) drug.

Excipients in commercially available drug preparations may have clinically important effects in some individuals; consult specific product labeling for details.

Tapentadol Hydrochloride

Oral		
Solution	100 mg (of tapentadol) per 5 mL	**Nucynta® Oral Solution** (C-II), Depomed
Tablets, extended-release, film-coated	50 mg (of tapentadol)	**Nucynta® ER** (C-II), Depomed
	100 mg (of tapentadol)	**Nucynta® ER** (C-II), Depomed
	150 mg (of tapentadol)	**Nucynta® ER** (C-II), Depomed
	200 mg (of tapentadol)	**Nucynta® ER** (C-II), Depomed
	250 mg (of tapentadol)	**Nucynta® ER** (C-II), Depomed
Tablets, film-coated	50 mg (of tapentadol)	**Nucynta®** (C-II), Depomed
	75 mg (of tapentadol)	**Nucynta®** (C-II), Depomed
	100 mg (of tapentadol)	**Nucynta®** (C-II), Depomed

traMADol Hydrochloride

■ Tramadol hydrochloride is a synthetic opiate agonist and inhibitor of norepinephrine and serotonin uptake.

REMS

FDA approved a REMS for tramadol to ensure that the benefits outweigh the risk. The REMS may apply to one or more preparations of tramadol and consists of the following: medication guide and elements to assure safe use. See the FDA REMS page (http://www.accessdata.fda.gov/scripts/cder/rems/index.cfm).

Uses

■ **Pain** Tramadol hydrochloride conventional tablets are used orally for the relief of pain that is severe enough to require an opiate analgesic; because of the risks of addiction, abuse, and misuse associated with opiates even at recommended dosages, conventional preparations of tramadol should be reserved for use in patients for whom alternative treatment options (e.g., nonopiate analgesics) have not been, or are not expected to be, adequate or tolerated. Comparative and noncomparative clinical studies have shown that tramadol is an effective analgesic agent in the treatment of moderately severe acute or chronic pain, including postoperative, gynecologic, and obstetric pain, as well as pain of various other origins, including cancer.

Tramadol hydrochloride extended-release capsules and tablets are used for the relief of pain that is severe enough to require long-term, daily, around-the-clock use of an opiate analgesic. Because of the risks of addiction, abuse, and misuse associated with opiates even at recommended dosages, and because of the greater risks of overdose and death associated with extended-release opiate formulations, these extended-release preparations of tramadol should be reserved for use in patients for whom alternative treatment options (e.g., nonopiate analgesics, immediate-release opiates) are inadequate or not tolerated. These extended-release preparations of tramadol are *not* intended for use on an as-needed ("prn") basis.

Tramadol hydrochloride in fixed combination with acetaminophen is used for the short-term (5 days or less) management of acute pain that is severe enough to require an opiate analgesic; because of the risks of addiction, abuse, and misuse associated with opiates even at recommended dosages, preparations containing tramadol in fixed combination with acetaminophen should be reserved for use in patients for whom alternative treatment options (e.g., nonopiate analgesics) have not been, or are not expected to be, adequate or tolerated.

Single oral doses of tramadol hydrochloride ranging from 50–200 mg (as conventional tablets) have provided relief of postoperative pain in patients who have undergone various types of surgery, including orthopedic, gynecologic, and cesarean section, and in oral surgical procedures (e.g., extraction of impacted molars). In controlled clinical studies of postoperative pain, tramadol hydrochloride administered as a single oral dose of 150 mg was comparable to, or more effective than, the combination of acetaminophen 650 mg and propoxyphene napsylate 100 mg. In patients undergoing oral surgery, a single oral tramadol hydrochloride dose of 50 or 75 mg provided analgesia in some patients, and a single oral dose of 100 mg provided analgesia that was superior to that provided by 60 mg of codeine sulfate but inferior to the combination of codeine phosphate 60 mg and aspirin 650 mg. In a study of patients undergoing dental extraction, a single oral dose of tramadol hydrochloride 75 or 150 mg was more effective than codeine phosphate 60 mg, and tramadol hydrochloride 150 mg was more effective (while tramadol hydrochloride 75 mg was less effective) than acetaminophen 650 mg and propoxyphene napsylate 100 mg.

In several long-term controlled clinical studies of patients with chronic pain (e.g., low back pain, cancer pain, neuropathic pain, pain associated with orthopedic and joint disorders), tramadol hydrochloride dosages averaging 250 mg daily administered in divided doses as conventional tablets were as effective as acetaminophen 300 mg or aspirin 325 mg administered with codeine phosphate 30 mg 5 times daily or acetaminophen 500 mg administered with oxycodone hydrochloride 5 mg 2 or 3 times daily. Tramadol also may be useful in the management of cancer pain when nonopiate-agonist analgesics are no longer effective (i.e., step 2 of the WHO guidelines for cancer pain treatment).

In a study of cancer patients with severe chronic pain, tramadol hydrochloride conventional tablets provided effective analgesia but were less effective than an extended-release morphine dosage form; however, patients receiving tramadol experienced only mild adverse effects, none of which resulted in patient withdrawal from the study, while about 23% of patients receiving extended-release morphine withdrew from the study because of severe adverse effects.

Tolerance to tramadol-induced adverse effects may be increased by initiating therapy with a dosage titration regimen. In clinical studies, the rate of discontinuance of tramadol therapy (as conventional tablets) secondary to adverse effects was decreased by utilizing a 10- or 16-day dosage titration regimen for initiating therapy. Fewer patients discontinued therapy because of dizziness or vertigo when the dosage was titrated over 10 days rather than 4 days; similarly, if the dosage was titrated over 16 days rather than 10 days, fewer patients discontinued therapy because of nausea or vomiting, or any cause. When tramadol hydrochloride conventional tablets are used, the manufacturers currently recommend a dosage titration regimen in patients not requiring rapid onset of analgesic effect. (See Dosage and Administration.)

The onset and peak of analgesia occur within 1 and 2–4 hours, respectively, after oral administration of tramadol hydrochloride conventional tablets; peak plasma concentrations of racemic tramadol and its *O*-desmethyl metabolite (M1) are achieved about 2 and 3 hours, respectively, after oral administration, corresponding to the time of peak analgesic effect. The duration of analgesia produced by a single oral dose of tramadol hydrochloride conventional tablets has been reported to be about 3–6 hours. Following oral administration of the drug as extended-release tablets, peak plasma concentrations of tramadol and its M1 metabolite are achieved about 12 and 15 hours, respectively, after a dose. Following oral administration of the drug as extended-release capsules, peak plasma concentrations of tramadol and its M1 metabolite are achieved about 6 and 11 hours, respectively, after a dose.

Efficacy and safety of tramadol hydrochloride extended-release tablets have been evaluated in clinical studies in adults with chronic, moderate to moderately severe pain associated with osteoarthritis and/or low back pain. Adequate evidence of efficacy was demonstrated in 2 of 4 clinical studies. In a placebo-controlled clinical study of 12 weeks' duration in patients with moderate to moderately severe pain associated with osteoarthritis of the knee or hip, therapy with tramadol hydrochloride extended-release tablets (100 and 200 mg daily) was more effective than placebo as evaluated by changes from baseline in the Western Ontario and McMasters Universities (WOMAC) pain subscale. In a placebo-controlled, flexible-dose study of 12 weeks' duration in patients with osteoarthritis of the knee, therapy with tramadol hydrochloride extended-release tablets (average dose: 270 mg daily) was more effective than placebo as measured by change from baseline on the Arthritis Pain Intensity Visual Analog Scale. Efficacy of tramadol hydrochloride extended-release capsules (which are bioequivalent to the extended-release tablets under fasting conditions) has been evaluated in 4 randomized, placebo-controlled clinical studies of 12 weeks' duration. These studies failed to demonstrate efficacy but differed in design from the clinical studies evaluating the extended-release tablets. In 2 clinical studies, tramadol hydrochloride extended-release capsules were evaluated at dosages of 100, 200, and 300 mg daily in patients with moderate to moderately severe osteoarthritis pain of the hip and knee; the other 2 studies were similar in design, but evaluated only a fixed dosage of 300 mg daily (even in patients who responded to a lower dosage).

A variety of drugs have been used for management of pain in patients with osteoarthritis, including oral agents (e.g., acetaminophen, nonsteroidal anti-inflammatory agents [NSAIAs], tramadol), intra-articular agents (e.g., glucocorticoids, sodium hyaluronate), and topical agents (e.g., capsaicin, methylsalicylate). Factors to consider when making treatment decisions for the management of pain in patients with osteoarthritis include the presence of risk factors for serious adverse GI effects or renal toxicity (which may affect decisions regarding use of NSAIAs), existing comorbidities and concomitant therapy, and the adverse effects profiles and costs of specific therapies.

Because there is evidence that acetaminophen can be effective and because of its relative safety and low cost, the American College of Rheumatology (ACR) recommends use of the drug as the initial analgesic for many osteoarthritis patients. Acetaminophen appears to be as effective as NSAIAs for relief of mild to moderate joint pain in many patients with osteoarthritis; however, the drug is not effective in all patients and may not provide adequate relief in those with moderate to severe pain or when joint inflammation is present. An NSAIA can be considered an alternative initial drug of choice for patients with osteoarthritis, especially for those who have moderate to severe pain and signs of joint inflammation, and also can be considered in patients who fail to obtain adequate symptomatic relief with acetaminophen. Tramadol can be considered in patients in whom NSAIAs are contraindicated (e.g., those with renal impairment) or in whom acetaminophen or NSAIAs have not produced an adequate response.

In controlled single-dose studies in patients with acute pain following oral surgery, analgesia provided by tramadol hydrochloride (75 mg) in fixed combination with acetaminophen (650 mg) was comparable to that provided by ibuprofen 400 mg, and superior to that provided by monotherapy with tramadol hydrochloride 75 mg or acetaminophen 650 mg or by placebo. Onset of pain relief occurred in about 17 minutes in patients receiving the fixed combination of tramadol and acetaminophen and about 15 minutes in those receiving acetaminophen alone. Onset of pain relief occurred in about 30 minutes in patients receiving either tramadol alone or ibuprofen. Duration of pain relief was about 5 hours in patients receiving either tramadol in fixed combination with acetaminophen or ibuprofen, but was about 2 hours with administration of tramadol alone and 3 hours with acetaminophen alone.

For further information on the role of opiate analgesics in the management of acute or chronic pain, see Uses: Pain, in the Opiate Agonists General Statement 28:08.08.

Dosage and Administration

■ Administration Tramadol hydrochloride alone or in fixed combination with acetaminophen is administered orally.

Since food does not affect substantially the rate or extent of absorption of tramadol hydrochloride administered alone as conventional tablets, the manufacturers state that conventional tablets of the drug can be taken without regard to food. Food may decrease the rate and extent of absorption of tramadol when the drug is administered as extended-release tablets (delaying peak plasma concentrations by about 3 hours and decreasing the extent of absorption by about 16%); the manufacturer states that although tramadol hydrochloride extended-release tablets may be administered once daily without regard to food, the extended-release tablets should be administered in a consistent manner relative to food intake. The manufacturer also recommends that tramadol hydrochloride extended-release capsules be administered in a consistent manner relative to food intake, although the rate and extent of absorption are similar following oral administration with or without food. Food delays absorption of tramadol hydrochloride and acetaminophen administered in fixed combination, increasing times to peak plasma concentrations by about 35 and 60 minutes, respectively. However, food does not affect peak plasma concentrations achieved or the extent of absorption of the drugs, and the clinical importance of the delays in absorption is unknown. The manufacturers make no specific recommendation regarding administration of the fixed-combination preparation with food.

Tramadol hydrochloride extended-release tablets or capsules should be swallowed whole and should not be broken, crushed, chewed, split, or dissolved, since such physical alteration of the tablets or capsules could result in rapid release of the drug and absorption of a potentially fatal overdose. The extended-release preparations should not be used concomitantly with other tramadol-containing preparations.

For patients receiving tramadol hydrochloride conventional tablets alone for the relief of moderate to moderately severe pain and not requiring rapid onset of analgesic effect, the manufacturers recommend a dosage titration regimen to decrease the likelihood of discontinuance secondary to adverse effects (e.g., nausea, vomiting, dizziness, vertigo) associated with administration at higher initial dosages.

■ Dosage Opiate agonists should be given at the lowest effective dosage and for the shortest duration of therapy consistent with the treatment goals of the patient. The initial dosage of tramadol must be individualized, taking into account the patient's severity of pain, response, prior analgesic use, and risk factors for addiction, abuse, and misuse. Dosage should be titrated to a level that provides adequate analgesia and minimizes adverse effects. If concomitant therapy with other CNS depressants is required, the lowest effective dosages and shortest possible duration of concomitant therapy should be used. (See Concomitant Use with Benzodiazepines or Other CNS Depressants under Cautions: Precautions and Contraindications.)

Because of the greater frequency of decreased hepatic, renal, and/or cardiac function and of concomitant disease and/or drug therapy in geriatric patients, care should be taken in dosage selection for such patients. The manufacturers recommend that geriatric patients receive initial dosages of tramadol hydrochloride alone in the lower end of the usual range and that the dosage not exceed 300 mg daily in those older than 75 years of age. Dosage of tramadol hydrochloride should be titrated slowly in geriatric patients, with close monitoring for CNS and respiratory depression.

Appropriate dosage selection and titration are essential to reduce the risk of respiratory depression. Patients should be monitored closely for respiratory depression, especially during the first 24–72 hours of therapy and following any increase in dosage.

Patients receiving opiate analgesics should be reevaluated continually for adequacy of pain control and for adverse effects, as well as for manifestations of opiate withdrawal and for the development of addiction, abuse, or misuse. During long-term therapy, the continued need for opiate analgesics should be continually reevaluated. Frequent communication among the prescriber, other members of the healthcare team, the patient, and the patient's caregiver or family is important during periods of changing analgesic requirements, including the initial dosage titration period. Patients with chronic pain who experience episodes of breakthrough pain may require dosage adjustment or supplemental analgesia (i.e., "rescue" therapy with an immediate-release analgesic). If the level of pain increases after dosage stabilization, an attempt should be made to identify the source of increased pain before increasing the dosage.

For acute pain not related to trauma or surgery, the prescribed quantity should be limited to the amount needed for the expected duration of pain severe enough to require opiate analgesia (generally 3 days or less and rarely more than 7 days).

When opiate analgesics are used for the management of chronic noncancer pain, the US Centers for Disease Control and Prevention (CDC) recommends that primary care clinicians carefully reassess individual benefits and risks before prescribing dosages equivalent to 50 mg or more of morphine sulfate daily and avoid dosages equivalent to 90 mg or more of morphine sulfate daily or carefully justify their decision to titrate the dosage to such levels. Other experts recommend consulting a pain management specialist before exceeding a dosage equivalent to 80–120 mg of morphine sulfate daily.

If discontinuance of opiate therapy is required in a patient who may be physically dependent on opiates, the dosage should be tapered gradually to avoid manifestations of abrupt withdrawal. When tramadol therapy is discontinued in such patients, dosage generally can be reduced by 25–50% every 2–4 days. If manifestations of withdrawal occur, the dosage should be increased to the prior level and tapered more slowly (i.e., by increasing the interval between dosage reductions and/or reducing the amount of each incremental change in dose).

For further information on the management of opiate analgesic therapy, see Dosage and Administration: Dosage, in the Opiate Agonists General Statement 28:08.08.

Conventional (Immediate-release) Tablets Adults with moderate to moderately severe chronic pain not requiring rapid onset of analgesic effect may initially receive tramadol hydrochloride conventional tablets using a dosage titration regimen; the manufacturers recommend an initial dosage of 25 mg daily in the morning, increased by increments of 25 mg every 3 days as separate doses up to a dosage of 25 mg 4 times daily. Thereafter, daily dosage of conventional tablets may be increased as tolerated by 50 mg every 3 days, up to 50 mg 4 times daily. Following titration, 50–100 mg of conventional tablets may be administered every 4–6 hours as needed. Dosages exceeding 400 mg daily are not recommended by the manufacturers.

Adults requiring rapid onset of analgesia, and in whom the benefit of rapid onset of analgesia outweighs the risk of drug discontinuance secondary to adverse effects associated with higher initial dosage, may receive tramadol hydrochloride conventional tablets in a dosage of 50–100 mg every 4–6 hours. Dosages exceeding 400 mg daily are not recommended by the manufacturers.

Tramadol Hydrochloride in Fixed Combination with Acetaminophen When tramadol hydrochloride is used in fixed combination with acetaminophen for the short-term (5 days or less) management of acute pain in adults, the usual dosage is 75 mg of tramadol hydrochloride every 4–6 hours as needed, up to a maximum of 300 mg daily.

Extended-release Tablets and Capsules When tramadol hydrochloride extended-release tablets or capsules are used in the management of chronic pain in adults who are not currently receiving tramadol, the recommended initial dosage is 100 mg once daily. The daily dosage may be increased in 100-mg increments every 5 days as needed and tolerated. Dosages exceeding 300 mg daily are not recommended by the manufacturers.

Because ratios for conversion from other opiate analgesics to extended-release preparations of tramadol hydrochloride have not been established in clinical trials, the manufacturers state that patients being switched from therapy with other opiate agonists should receive an initial tramadol hydrochloride dosage of 100 mg daily as extended-release tablets or capsules. For patients receiving conventional tramadol hydrochloride preparations, the total daily dosage of the drug should be calculated and rounded down to the next lower 100-mg increment for administration as the extended-release tablets or capsules; the dosage may then be adjusted according to patient requirements. Patients being switched from immediate-release to extended-release preparations of tramadol should be monitored closely for sedation and respiratory depression since data establishing the relative bioavailability of these formulations are lacking. Because of limitations in dose selection, some patients may not be successfully switched from immediate-release to extended-release preparations of the drug. All other around-the-clock opiate analgesics should be discontinued when therapy with the extended-release preparation is initiated.

■ **Dosage in Renal and Hepatic Impairment** Dosage of tramadol hydrochloride (as conventional tablets) should be reduced in certain patients with renal or hepatic impairment by decreasing the frequency of administration. Adults with creatinine clearances less than 30 mL/minute may receive oral tramadol hydrochloride conventional tablets in a dosage of 50–100 mg every 12 hours, not to exceed 200 mg daily. Since less than 7% of a dose of tramadol hydrochloride is removed by hemodialysis, patients undergoing dialysis may receive their usual dosage on the day of dialysis. Adults with hepatic cirrhosis may receive the conventional tablets in a dosage of 50 mg every 12 hours.

Tramadol hydrochloride extended-release oral formulations should not be used in patients with severe renal impairment (creatinine clearances less than 30 mL/minute) or severe hepatic impairment (Child-Pugh class C). The available tablet or capsule strengths and once-daily dosing of these formulations do not provide sufficient dosing flexibility for safe use in these patients.

Adults with creatinine clearances of less than 30 mL/minute may receive tramadol hydrochloride in fixed combination with acetaminophen at a dosing interval of every 12 hours; in such patients, the dosage of tramadol hydrochloride administered as the fixed combination should not exceed 75 mg every 12 hours. Tramadol hydrochloride in fixed combination with acetaminophen should *not* be used in patients with impaired hepatic function.

Cautions

At recommended dosages, tramadol generally is well tolerated. Adverse effects usually have been mild and similar in incidence to active controls (i.e., acetaminophen 300 mg with codeine phosphate 30 mg and aspirin 325 mg with codeine phosphate 30 mg). The frequency of some adverse effects may be related to dose and route of administration. The most common adverse effects observed with tramadol in controlled clinical trials and open-label extension periods enrolling patients with chronic nonmalignant pain were nervous system effects (e.g., dizziness) and GI disturbances.

■ **Nervous System Effects** The most frequent adverse nervous system effect of tramadol is dizziness or vertigo, which occurred in 26, 31, and 33% of patients receiving tramadol hydrochloride conventional tablets for up to 7, 30, and 90 days, respectively, in clinical studies. In patients receiving tramadol hydrochloride as extended-release tablets in clinical studies, dizziness was reported in about 16, 20, 23, or 28% of patients receiving the drug in a dosage of 100, 200, 300, or 400 mg once daily, respectively. In patients receiving tramadol hydrochloride as extended-release capsules in clinical studies, dizziness was reported in about 10, 12, or 14% of patients receiving the drug in a dosage of 100, 200, or 300 mg once daily, respectively. The incidence of dizziness may be dose related.

Headache occurred in 18, 26, and 32% of patients, and somnolence occurred in 16, 23, and 25% of patients receiving the conventional tablets for up to 7, 30, and 90 days, respectively. Headache was reported in up to 16 or 23% of patients receiving tramadol hydrochloride as extended-release tablets or extended-release capsules, respectively, at recommended dosages (100–300 mg daily) in clinical studies. Somnolence or insomnia occurred in up to 11 or 9%, respectively, of patients receiving recommended dosages of tramadol hydrochloride extended-release tablets and in up to 16 or 5%, respectively, of patients receiving recommended dosages of tramadol hydrochloride extended-release capsules in clinical studies. Weakness has been reported in up to 4% of patients receiving the extended-release tablets in recommended dosages.

CNS stimulation (a composite of nervousness, anxiety, agitation, tremor, spasticity, euphoria, emotional lability, and hallucinations) occurred in 7, 11, and 14% of patients receiving tramadol hydrochloride conventional tablets for up to 7, 30, and 90 days, respectively. Asthenia occurred in 6, 11, and 12% of patients, and sweating occurred in 6, 7, and 9% of patients receiving the conventional tablets for up to 7, 30, and 90 days, respectively. Sweating may be more common following rapid IV injection. Asthenia or increased sweating was reported in up to 7 or 4%, respectively, of patients receiving recommended dosages of tramadol hydrochloride extended-release tablets in clinical studies. Asthenia or increased sweating was reported in up to 9% or 7%, respectively, of patients receiving recommended dosages of the extended-release capsules in clinical studies.

Anxiety, confusion, coordination disturbance, euphoria, nervousness, and sleep disorder each have been reported in 1% to less than 5% of patients receiving tramadol hydrochloride conventional tablets. Adverse nervous system effects reported in 1% to less than 5% of patients receiving tramadol hydrochloride extended-release tablets include tremor, paresthesia, hypoesthesia, nervousness, anxiety, depression, and restlessness. Paresthesia, tremor, withdrawal syndrome, agitation, anxiety, apathy, confusion, depersonalization, depression, euphoria, and nervousness each have been reported in 1% to less than 5% of patients receiving tramadol hydrochloride extended-release capsules.

Abnormal gait, amnesia, cognitive dysfunction, depression, difficulty in concentration, dysphoria, fatigue, hallucinations, motor system weakness, paresthesia, tremor, suicidal tendencies, seizures, and symptoms of serotonin syndrome (e.g., mental status change, hyperreflexia, fever, shivering, tremor, agitation, diaphoresis, seizures, coma) each were reported in less than 1% of patients receiving tramadol hydrochloride conventional tablets. (See Cautions: Precautions and Contraindications.) Migraine, syncope, disturbance in attention, vertigo, irritability, euphoric mood, sleep disorder, agitation, disorientation, and abnormal dreams each were reported in less than 1% of patients receiving the extended-release tablets in clinical studies. Emotional lability, hyperkinesia, hypertonia, abnormal thinking, twitching, and vertigo each were reported in 0.5% to less than 1% of patients receiving the extended-release capsules in clinical studies. Mania, delirium, movement disorder, and speech disorders also have been reported infrequently in patients receiving tramadol.

■ **GI Effects** Constipation is the most common adverse GI effect of tramadol, occurring in 24, 38, and 46% of patients receiving tramadol hydrochloride conventional tablets for up to 7, 30, and 90 days, respectively, in clinical studies. Nausea occurred in 24, 34, and 40% of patients, and vomiting occurred in 9, 13, and 17% of patients receiving conventional tablets of the drug for up to 7, 30, and 90 days, respectively. Nausea, constipation, vomiting, or anorexia has been reported in up to 26, 22, 9, or 5%, respectively, of patients receiving recommended dosages of tramadol hydrochloride extended-release tablets (100–300 mg daily) in clinical studies. Nausea, constipation, vomiting, or anorexia has been reported in up to 25, 21, 10, or 6%, respectively, of patients receiving recommended dosages of the extended-release capsules (100–300 mg daily) in clinical studies. Nausea and vomiting may occur more frequently with higher doses and following rapid IV injection.

Other adverse GI effects reported in patients receiving conventional tablets of the drug include dyspepsia, which occurred in 5, 9, and 13% of patients, dry mouth, which occurred in 5, 9, and 10%, and diarrhea, which occurred in 5, 6, and 10% of patients receiving tramadol for up to 7, 30, and 90 days, respectively. Dry mouth or diarrhea was reported in up to 10 or 9%, respectively, of patients receiving recommended dosages of tramadol hydrochloride extended-release tablets in clinical studies. Dry mouth also was reported in up to 13% of patients receiving recommended dosages of the extended-release capsules in clinical studies.

Abdominal pain, anorexia, and flatulence each were reported in 1% to less than 5% of patients receiving tramadol hydrochloride conventional tablets in clinical trials. Weight loss was reported in less than 1% of patients receiving conventional tablets of the drug. GI bleeding, hepatitis, liver failure, stomatitis, dysphagia, and gastritis have been reported infrequently with tramadol, although a causal relationship to the drug has not been established.

Adverse GI effects reported in 1% to less than 5% of patients receiving tramadol hydrochloride extended-release tablets include abdominal pain, dyspepsia, anorexia, and weight decrease. Flatulence and gastroenteritis each were reported in less than 1% of patients receiving extended-release tablets of the drug in clinical studies. Diarrhea and dry mouth also have been reported in patients receiving the extended-release tablets.

Adverse GI effects reported in 1% to less than 5% of patients receiving tramadol hydrochloride extended-release capsules include dyspepsia, flatulence, weight loss, and abdominal pain. Gastroenteritis was reported in 0.5% to less than 1% of patients receiving extended-release capsules of the drug in clinical studies.

■ **Sensitivity Reactions** Pruritus occurred in 8, 10, and 11% of patients receiving tramadol hydrochloride conventional tablets for up to 7, 30, and 90 days, respectively; in up to 9% of patients receiving the extended-release tablets in recommended dosages (100–300 mg daily); and in up to 7% of patients receiving the extended-release capsules in recommended dosages (100–300 mg daily). Rash or dermatitis was reported in 1% to less than 5% of patients receiving the drug in clinical trials. Serious and rarely fatal anaphylactoid reactions, often occurring after the initial dose, have been reported in patients receiving tramadol. (See Cautions: Precautions and Contraindications.) Urticaria, bronchospasm, and angioedema have occurred. Anaphylaxis, allergic reaction, Stevens-Johnson syndrome, or toxic epidermal necrolysis and vesicles each have been reported in less than 1% of patients receiving tramadol.

■ **Cardiovascular Effects** Vasodilation has been reported in 1% to less than 5% of patients receiving tramadol hydrochloride conventional tablets in clinical trials. Orthostatic hypotension, syncope, and tachycardia each were reported in less than 1% of patients receiving conventional tablets of the drug. Postural hypotension or flushing occurred in up to 4 or 10%, respectively, of patients receiving tramadol hydrochloride extended-release tablets in recommended dosages (100–300 mg daily) in clinical studies. Chest pain, hot flushes, and vasodilation each occurred in 1% to less than 5% of patients receiving extended-release tablets of the drug in clinical studies. Palpitations, myocardial infarction, hypertension, peripheral ischemia, and increased heart rate each were reported in less than 1% of patients receiving the extended-release tablets. Hypertension and vasodilation each occurred in 1% to less than 5% of patients receiving extended-release capsules of the drug in clinical trials. Abnormal ECG, hypotension, and tachycardia each were reported in 0.5% to less than 1% of patients receiving tramadol hydrochloride extended-release capsules. Abnormal ECG, hypertension, hypotension, myocardial ischemia, flushing, and palpitation also have been reported infrequently with conventional tablets of the drug, although a causal relationship to the drug has not been established.

■ **Genitourinary and Endocrine Effects** Menopausal symptoms, urinary frequency, and urinary retention each were reported in 1% to less than 5% of patients receiving tramadol hydrochloride conventional tablets in clinical trials. Dysuria and menstrual disorder each were reported in less than 1% of patients receiving conventional tablets of the drug. Micturition difficulty, urinary frequency, urinary retention, dysuria, hematuria, and decreased libido each were reported in less than 1% of patients receiving tramadol hydrochloride extended-release tablets. Urine abnormality, prostatic disorder, and urinary tract infection each were reported in 1% to less than 5% of patients receiving tramadol hydrochloride extended-release capsules in clinical trials. Cystitis, dysuria, sexual function abnormality, and urinary retention each were reported in 0.5% to less than 1% of patients receiving the extended-release capsules.

Hypoglycemia has been reported very rarely in patients receiving tramadol, mainly in patients with predisposing risk factors (e.g., diabetes mellitus, renal insufficiency) or in geriatric patients. Increased blood glucose concentrations have occurred in patients receiving tramadol hydrochloride extended-release tablets. Hyperglycemia was reported in 1% to less than 5% of patients receiving the extended-release capsules in clinical trials.

Adrenal insufficiency has been reported in patients receiving opiate agonists or opiate partial agonists. Manifestations of adrenal insufficiency are nonspecific and may include nausea, vomiting, anorexia, fatigue, weakness, dizziness, and hypotension. The onset generally has occurred after at least 1 month of opiate agonist or partial agonist use, although the time to onset has ranged from within 1 day to more than 1 year. In many of the reported cases, patients required hospitalization. If adrenal insufficiency is suspected, appropriate laboratory testing should be performed promptly and physiologic (replacement) dosages of corticosteroids provided; therapy with the opiate agonist or partial agonist should be tapered and discontinued to allow recovery of adrenal function. If the opiate agonist or partial agonist can be discontinued, follow-up assessment of adrenal function should be performed to determine if corticosteroid replacement therapy can be discontinued. In some patients, switching to a different opiate improved symptoms.

Hypogonadism and androgen deficiency have been reported in patients receiving long-term opiate agonist or opiate partial agonist therapy, although a causal relationship has not been established. Patients receiving long-term opiate agonist or partial agonist therapy who present with manifestations of hypogonadism (e.g., decreased libido, impotence, erectile dysfunction, amenorrhea, infertility) should undergo laboratory evaluation.

■ **Other Effects** Malaise, hypertonia, miosis, and visual disturbance each have been reported in 1% to less than 5% of patients receiving tramadol hydrochloride conventional tablets in clinical trials. Accidental injury, dyspnea, and dysgeusia each were reported in less than 1% of patients receiving conventional tablets of the drug. Respiratory depression has been reported rarely. Decreased serum hemoglobin concentrations, pulmonary edema, pulmonary embolism, cataracts, deafness, tinnitus, and elevated serum hepatic enzymes also have occurred in patients receiving the conventional tablets, but a causal relationship to the drug has not been established.

Blurred vision, sore throat, pain, influenza-like illness, falls, rigors, lethargy, pyrexia, certain infections (e.g., nasopharyngitis, upper respiratory tract infection, urinary tract infection), arthralgia, musculoskeletal pain, nasal symptoms, cough, dyspnea, and sneezing each have been reported in 1% to less than 5% of patients receiving tramadol hydrochloride extended-release tablets in clinical trials. Events reported in less than 1% of patients receiving extended-release tablets of the drug include tinnitus, toothache, jittery feeling, edema, joint swelling, peripheral swelling, pancreatitis, cholelithiasis, cholecystitis, certain infections (e.g., appendicitis, cellulitis, pneumonia), minor injuries (i.e., joint sprain, muscle injury), joint stiffness, myalgia, muscle cramps/spasms/twitching, osteoarthritis aggravated, malaise, yawning, contusion, clamminess, and piloerection. Increased blood creatine phosphokinase and alterations in liver function test values also have occurred in patients receiving the extended-release tablets.

Arthralgia was reported in approximately 5% of patients receiving recommended dosages (100–300 mg daily) of tramadol hydrochloride as extended-release capsules in clinical trials. Accidental injury, chills, fever, flu syndrome, neck pain, pelvic pain, peripheral edema, myalgia, bronchitis, pharyngitis, rhinitis, and sinusitis each have been reported in 1% to less than 5% of patients receiving extended-release capsules of the drug. Neck rigidity, viral infection, anemia, ecchymosis, increased BUN, increased γ-glutamyltransferase (γ-glutamyltranspeptidase, GGT, GGTP), gout, increased ALT, arthritis, arthrosis, joint disorder, leg cramps, pneumonia, hair disorder, skin disorder, eye disorder, and lacrimation disorder each have been reported in 0.5% to less than 1% of patients receiving the extended-release capsules.

Increased serum creatinine concentrations and proteinuria also have been reported infrequently with tramadol; however, a causal relationship to the drug has not been established. Mydriasis also has been reported in patients receiving tramadol.

■ **Acute Toxicity** ***Manifestations*** Tramadol taken in excessive doses, either alone or in combination with other CNS depressants, is a cause of drug-related deaths. Fatalities associated with both intentional and unintentional overdose have been reported. Estimates of ingested dose in non-US fatalities ranged from 3–5 g. A 3-g intentional overdose by a patient enrolled in a clinical trial produced emesis and no sequelae. The lowest tramadol hydrochloride dose reportedly associated with fatality was possibly between 0.5–1 g in a 40-kg woman, but details of the case are not completely known. Tramadol is intended for oral use only. Crushing, cutting, breaking, or chewing tramadol hydrochloride extended-release tablets or capsules, "snorting" the powder, or injecting dissolved contents of the tablets or capsules results in uncontrolled delivery of tramadol and poses a risk of a potentially fatal overdose. The risk of a fatal overdose is increased when tramadol is misused concurrently with other CNS depressants (e.g., alcohol, other opiates). Manifestations of overdosage are similar to those of other opiate agonists, with the most serious potential consequences being respiratory depression, lethargy, skeletal muscle flaccidity, coma, seizure, bradycardia, hypotension, pulmonary edema, partial or complete airway obstruction, cardiac arrest, cardiac collapse, and death. Death may occur within 1 hour of overdosage. Other manifestations may include miosis, vomiting, cold and clammy skin, and atypical snoring. Marked mydriasis (rather than miosis) may be observed in patients with hypoxia.

Treatment When treating tramadol overdosage, primary attention should be given to maintaining adequate ventilation along with general supportive treatment (including administration of oxygen and vasopressors as clinically indicated). Tramadol hydrochloride extended-release tablets or capsules will continue to release the drug for 24–48 hours or longer following ingestion, necessitating prolonged monitoring. An opiate antagonist should be administered if clinically important respiratory or circulatory depression is present, but should not be administered in the absence of such manifestations. Although an opiate antagonist (e.g., naloxone, nalmefene) will reverse some, but not all, manifestations of tramadol overdosage, the risk of seizures also is increased with naloxone administration. In animals, seizures following the administration of toxic tramadol doses could be suppressed with barbiturates or benzodiazepines but were increased with naloxone. Naloxone administration did not change the lethality of an overdose in mice. Hemodialysis is unlikely to be helpful in a tramadol overdosage because it removes less than 7% of the administered dose in a 4-hour dialysis period. For additional information about overdosage of opiate agonists, see Acute Toxicity in the Opiate Agonists General Statement 28:08.08.

■ **Precautions and Contraindications** ***General Opiate Agonist Precautions*** Administration of tramadol may cause effects similar to those produced by other opiate agonist drugs, and the usual precautions of opiate agonist therapy should be observed. (See Description and the manufacturers' labeling.)

Extended-release preparations of tramadol should be prescribed only by clinicians who are knowledgeable in the use of potent opiates for the management of chronic pain.

Addiction, Abuse, and Misuse Tramadol exposes patients and other users to the risks of opiate addiction, abuse, and misuse, which can lead to overdosage and death. The abuse potential of tramadol is less than that of morphine or oxycodone but similar to that of propoxyphene (see Description). Addiction can occur with appropriately prescribed or illicitly obtained opiates, and at recommended dosages or with misuse or abuse. Concurrent abuse of alcohol or other CNS depressants increases the risk of toxicity. Each patient's risk for addiction, abuse, and misuse should be assessed prior to initiating tramadol therapy, and all patients receiving the drug should be monitored for development of these behaviors or conditions. Personal or family history of substance abuse (drug or alcohol addiction or abuse) or mental illness (e.g., major depression) increases risk. The potential for addiction, abuse, and misuse should not prevent opiate prescribing for appropriate pain management, but does necessitate intensive counseling about risks and proper use and intensive monitoring for signs of addiction, abuse, and misuse. Tramadol should be prescribed in the smallest appropriate quantity and the patient should be instructed on secure storage and proper disposal to prevent theft.

Extended-release opiates are associated with a greater risk of overdosage and death because of the larger amount of drug contained in each dosage unit. Abuse or misuse of tramadol extended-release tablets or capsules by splitting, crushing, breaking, cutting, or chewing the tablets or capsules, snorting the contents, or injecting the dissolved contents will result in uncontrolled delivery of tramadol and can result in a fatal overdosage. IV injection of excipients in these formulations can result in local tissue necrosis, infection, pulmonary granulomas, embolism, and death and increase the risk of endocarditis and valvular heart injury.

Respiratory Depression Serious, life-threatening, or fatal respiratory depression can occur in patients receiving opiates, even when used as recommended. Although respiratory depression can occur at any time during therapy, the risk is greatest during initiation of therapy and following an increase in dosage; therefore, patients receiving tramadol should be monitored closely for respiratory depression, especially during the first 24–72 hours of therapy and following any increase in dosage. Appropriate dosage selection and titration are essential to reduce the risk of respiratory depression. Large initial doses in nontolerant patients, overestimation of the initial tramadol dosage when transferring patients from another opiate analgesic, or accidental ingestion of even one dose of tramadol, especially by a child, can result in respiratory depression and death. For clinically important respiratory depression resulting from tramadol overdosage, an opiate antagonist should be administered. (See Treatment under Cautions: Acute Toxicity.)

Geriatric, cachectic, or debilitated patients are at increased risk of life-threatening respiratory depression. In patients with chronic obstructive pulmonary disease or cor pulmonale, substantially decreased respiratory reserve, hypoxia, hypercapnia, or preexisting respiratory depression, even recommended doses of tramadol may decrease respiratory drive to the point of apnea. Such patients should be monitored closely, particularly following initiation of therapy, during dosage titration, and during concomitant therapy with other respiratory depressants. Alternatively, use of nonopiate analgesics should be considered in such patients. Use of tramadol in patients with substantial respiratory depression or in those with severe bronchial asthma in unmonitored settings or in the absence of resuscitative equipment is contraindicated.

When opiate agonists are prescribed for patients at increased risk of opiate overdosage (e.g., those with a history of overdose or substance use disorder, those receiving 50 mg or more of morphine sulfate [or equivalent] daily, those receiving benzodiazepines concomitantly, those with medical conditions that could increase sensitivity to opiates), some experts state that clinicians should consider offering the opiate antagonist naloxone.

Drugs Affecting Hepatic Microsomal Enzymes Because orally administered tramadol undergoes extensive hepatic metabolism, including metabolism by cytochrome P-450 (CYP) isoenzymes 2D6 and 3A4, concomitant use of drugs that inhibit or induce CYP3A4 or inhibit CYP2D6 requires careful consideration of the effects on tramadol and its active *O*-desmethyl metabolite (M1) (see Description).

Because formation of M1 is dependent on CYP2D6 activity, concomitant use of tramadol and CYP2D6 inhibitors (e.g., amiodarone, bupropion, fluoxetine, paroxetine, quinidine) may result in increased plasma concentrations of tramadol and decreased concentrations of M1, particularly when the CYP2D6 inhibitor is initiated after a stable dosage of tramadol has been achieved. The increase in tramadol concentrations can result in increased or prolonged therapeutic effects and an increased risk of serious adverse effects, including seizures and serotonin syndrome, while the decrease in M1 concentrations may result in reduced therapeutic effects and, in patients physically dependent on opiates, manifestations of opiate withdrawal. Discontinuance of the CYP2D6 inhibitor may result in a decrease in plasma concentrations of tramadol and an increase in M1 concentrations, which could increase or prolong therapeutic effects or manifestations of opiate toxicity and potentially cause fatal respiratory depression. If concomitant therapy with tramadol and a CYP2D6 inhibitor is required, patients should be monitored closely for serious tramadol-related adverse effects (including seizures and serotonin syndrome) and manifestations of opiate toxicity or opiate withdrawal. If concomitant therapy with a CYP2D6 inhibitor is discontinued, the patient should be monitored closely for adverse effects, including respiratory depression and sedation, and consideration should be given to reducing the tramadol dosage until stable drug effects are achieved.

Concomitant use of tramadol and CYP3A4 inhibitors, such as macrolide antibiotics (e.g., erythromycin), azole antifungals (e.g., ketoconazole), or HIV protease inhibitors (e.g., ritonavir), can increase plasma concentrations of tramadol, which may result in larger amounts of parent drug being metabolized by CYP2D6 and higher concentrations of M1. If concomitant therapy with tramadol and a CYP3A4 inhibitor is required, patients should be monitored closely for serious adverse effects (including seizures and serotonin syndrome) and for manifestations of opiate toxicity (including sedation and potentially fatal respiratory depression), particularly when the CYP3A4 inhibitor is initiated after a stable dosage of tramadol has been achieved, and consideration should be given to reducing the tramadol dosage until stable drug effects are achieved. If concomitant therapy with a CYP3A4 inhibitor is discontinued, the patient should be monitored for manifestations of opiate withdrawal, and consideration should be given to increasing the tramadol dosage until stable drug effects are achieved.

Concomitant use of tramadol and CYP3A4 inducers (e.g., carbamazepine, phenytoin, rifampin) can decrease plasma concentrations of tramadol, resulting in decreased efficacy and, in patients who are physically dependent on opiates, manifestations of opiate withdrawal. Discontinuance of the CYP3A4 inducer may result in increased plasma concentrations of tramadol, which could increase or prolong both the therapeutic and adverse effects of tramadol and may cause seizures, serotonin syndrome, and potentially fatal respiratory depression. If concomitant therapy with tramadol and a CYP3A4 inducer is required, patients should be monitored for manifestations of opiate withdrawal, and consideration should be given to increasing the tramadol dosage until stable drug effects are achieved. If concomitant therapy with a CYP3A4 inducer is discontinued, patients should be monitored for seizures, serotonin syndrome, sedation, and respiratory depression, and consideration should be given to decreasing the tramadol dosage until stable drug effects are achieved.

Concomitant use of tramadol with carbamazepine is not recommended because carbamazepine increases tramadol metabolism and substantially reduces tramadol's analgesic effect, and because tramadol is associated with increased risk of seizures.

Concomitant Use with Benzodiazepines or Other CNS Depressants Tramadol may potentiate the respiratory and CNS depressant effects of other CNS depressants. Concomitant use of tramadol with benzodiazepines or other CNS depressants (e.g., anxiolytics, sedatives, hypnotics, tranquilizers, muscle relaxants, general anesthetics, antipsychotics, other opiate agonists, alcohol) may result in profound sedation, respiratory depression, hypotension, coma, and death. (See Cautions: Acute Toxicity.) Concomitant use of such drugs should be reserved for patients in whom alternative treatment options are inadequate; the lowest effective dosages and shortest possible duration of concomitant therapy should be used, and the patient should be monitored closely for respiratory depression and sedation. Concomitant use with alcohol should be avoided. (See Drug Interactions: Benzodiazepines and Other CNS Depressants, in the Opiate Agonists General Statement 28:08.08.)

If a benzodiazepine or other CNS depressant is required for any indication other than epilepsy in a patient receiving tramadol, the drug should be initiated at a lower dosage than indicated in the absence of opiate therapy and titrated based on clinical response. In patients receiving a CNS depressant, tramadol, if required, should be initiated at a reduced dosage and titrated based on clinical response.

Serotonin Syndrome Potentially life-threatening serotonin syndrome may occur with tramadol, particularly with concurrent use of other serotonergic drugs, drugs that impair the metabolism of serotonin (e.g., monoamine oxidase [MAO] inhibitors), or drugs that impair the metabolism of tramadol (e.g., inhibitors of CYP2D6 and CYP3A4). Manifestations of serotonin syndrome may include mental status changes (e.g., agitation, hallucinations, coma), autonomic instability (e.g., tachycardia, labile blood pressure, hyperthermia), neuromuscular aberrations (e.g., hyperreflexia, incoordination, rigidity), and/or GI symptoms (e.g., nausea, vomiting, diarrhea). Symptom onset generally occurs within several hours to a few days of concomitant use, but may occur later, particularly after dosage increases. (See Drugs Associated with Serotonin Syndrome under Cautions: Precautions and Contraindications.)

Seizures Seizures have occurred during tramadol therapy with recommended dosages. Spontaneous postmarketing reports indicate that seizure risk is increased with tramadol doses above the recommended range. Seizures can occur following the first dose. The manufacturers warn that tramadol increases the seizure risk in patients taking selective serotonin-reuptake inhibitors (SSRIs), selective serotonin- and norepinephrine-reuptake inhibitors (SNRIs), anorectic agents, tricyclic antidepressants or other tricyclic compounds (e.g., cyclobenzaprine, promethazine), or other opiate agonists. The manufacturers also warn that the drug may enhance the risk of seizure in those receiving MAO inhibitors, antipsychotic agents, or other drugs that decrease the seizure threshold. Patients with epilepsy, those with a history of seizures, or patients with a recognized risk for seizure (e.g., head trauma, metabolic disorders, alcohol and drug withdrawal, CNS infections) may be at increased risk of seizure. Naloxone administration in patients with tramadol overdose also may increase the risk of seizure.

Suicide Tramadol should not be prescribed for individuals who are suicidal or prone to addiction. Tramadol should be used with caution in patients with a history of misuse, patients receiving concomitant therapy with CNS-active drugs including tranquilizers or antidepressants, individuals with excessive alcohol consumption, and patients with emotional disturbances or depression. The use of alternative analgesics without opiate agonist activity should be considered in suicidal or depressed patients. (See Cautions: Acute Toxicity.)

Monoamine Oxidase Inhibitors Concomitant use of opiates with MAO inhibitors (e.g., linezolid, phenelzine, tranylcypromine) may increase the risk of serotonin syndrome, seizures, and opiate toxicity (e.g., respiratory depression, coma). Use of tramadol is contraindicated in patients who are currently receiving or have recently (within 14 days) received an MAO inhibitor.

Pharmacogenomics Tramadol is metabolized by the CYP microsomal enzyme system, principally by CYP2D6 to its active M1 metabolite. Metabolism of certain drugs, including tramadol, is influenced by CYP2D6 polymorphism. Individuals who lack functional alleles of the CYP2D6 gene are described as poor metabolizers, those with one or two functional alleles are described as extensive metabolizers, and those who carry a duplicate or amplified gene are described as ultrarapid metabolizers. Population pharmacokinetic analysis of phase 1 studies of tramadol hydrochloride conventional tablets in healthy individuals indicated that concentrations of tramadol were approximately 20% higher and those of M1 were 40% lower in poor metabolizers compared with extensive metabolizers.

Genetically determined differences in drug metabolism can affect an individual's response to a drug or risk of having an adverse event. Individuals who are poor metabolizers may experience reduced analgesic effects of tramadol; individuals who are ultrarapid metabolizers are likely to have higher than expected serum concentrations of M1. To minimize the risk of adverse events in individuals who are ultrarapid metabolizers of CYP2D6, FDA states that tramadol should *not* be used in such patients. Variations in CYP2D6 polymorphism occur at different frequencies among subpopulations of different ethnic or racial origin. Approximately 1–7% of Caucasians and 10–30% of Ethiopians and Saudi Arabians carry the genotype associated with ultra-rapid metabolism of CYP2D6 substrates.

Drugs Associated with Serotonin Syndrome Serotonin syndrome may occur when tramadol is used concurrently with other serotonergic drugs, including serotonin (5-hydroxytryptamine; 5-HT) type 1 (5-HT_1) receptor agonists ("triptans"), SSRIs, SNRIs, tricyclic antidepressants, antiemetics that are 5-HT_3 receptor antagonists, buspirone, cyclobenzaprine, dextromethorphan, lithium, St. John's wort (*Hypericum perforatum*), tryptophan, other serotonin modulators (e.g., mirtazapine, nefazodone, trazodone, vilazodone), and MAO inhibitors (both those used to treat psychiatric disorders and others, such as linezolid, methylene blue, and selegiline). Serotonin syndrome may occur within the recommended dosage ranges for these drugs. Serotonin syndrome has been reported during postmarketing experience in patients receiving tramadol concomitantly with MAO inhibitors, SSRIs, SNRIs, or α_2-adrenergic blocking agents. Tramadol decreases the synaptic reuptake of the monoamine neurotransmitters norepinephrine and serotonin, and animal studies have shown increased deaths with combined administration of tramadol and MAO inhibitors. Manifestations of serotonin syndrome may include mental status changes (e.g., agitation, hallucinations, coma), autonomic instability (e.g., tachycardia, labile blood pressure, hyperthermia), neuromuscular aberrations (e.g., hyperreflexia, incoordination, rigidity), and/or GI symptoms (e.g., nausea, vomiting, diarrhea). Symptom onset generally occurs within several hours to a few days of concomitant use, but may occur later, particularly after dosage increases.

If concomitant use of other serotonergic drugs is warranted, great caution is advised and patients should be monitored for serotonin syndrome, particularly during initiation of therapy and dosage increases. If serotonin syndrome is suspected, treatment with tramadol, other opiate therapy, and/or any concurrently administered serotonergic agents should be discontinued.

For further information on serotonin syndrome, including manifestations and treatment, see Drug Interactions: Serotonergic Drugs, in Fluoxetine Hydrochloride 28:16.04.20.

Hypotension Tramadol may cause severe hypotension, including orthostatic hypotension and syncope, in ambulatory patients. Because the risk of severe hypotension is increased in patients whose ability to maintain blood pressure has been compromised by blood volume depletion or concomitant use of certain CNS depressants (e.g., phenothiazines, general anesthetics), such patients should be monitored for hypotension following initiation of tramadol therapy or an increase in tramadol dosage. Use of tramadol should be avoided in patients with circulatory shock since the drug may cause vasodilation that can further reduce cardiac output and blood pressure.

Increased Intracranial Pressure or Head Injury The respiratory depressant effects of opiate agonists promote carbon dioxide retention, which can result in elevation of intracranial pressure. Patients who may be particularly susceptible to these effects (e.g., those with evidence of elevated intracranial pressure or brain tumors) should be monitored closely for sedation and respiratory depression, particularly during initiation of therapy. Opiates also may obscure the clinical course in patients with head injuries. Use of tramadol should be avoided in patients with impaired consciousness or coma.

GI Conditions Opiates may increase serum amylase concentrations and cause spasm of the sphincter of Oddi. Patients with biliary tract disease, including those with acute pancreatitis, should be monitored for worsening symptoms. Tramadol is contraindicated in patients with known or suspected GI obstruction, including paralytic ileus.

Sensitivity Reactions Serious and rarely fatal anaphylactoid reactions have been reported in patients receiving tramadol. These reactions often occur following the first dose. Other reported hypersensitivity reactions include pruritus, urticaria, angioedema, bronchospasm, toxic epidermal necrolysis, and Stevens-Johnson syndrome. The manufacturers warn that patients with a history of anaphylactoid reactions to codeine or other opiate agonists may be at increased risk and therefore should not receive tramadol. If anaphylaxis or other hypersensitivity reaction occurs, tramadol should be discontinued immediately and permanently.

Dependence and Tolerance Both tolerance and physical dependence can develop during long-term opiate therapy. Tolerance may not develop uniformly to all opiate effects.

In patients who are physically dependent on opiates, abrupt discontinuance of tramadol or a substantial reduction in dosage may result in manifestations of withdrawal (e.g., restlessness, lacrimation, rhinorrhea, yawning, sweating, chills, myalgia, mydriasis, irritability, anxiety, backache, joint pain, weakness, abdominal cramps, insomnia, nausea, anorexia, vomiting, diarrhea, increases in blood pressure, respiratory rate, or heart rate). When tramadol therapy is discontinued in a patient who may be physically dependent on opiates, the dosage should be tapered gradually. Infants born to women who are physically dependent on opiates also will be physically dependent. (See Cautions: Pregnancy, Fertility, and Lactation.)

Concomitant use of opiate partial agonists (e.g., buprenorphine, butorphanol, nalbuphine, pentazocine) should be avoided since they may reduce the analgesic effect of tramadol and/or precipitate withdrawal symptoms.

CNS Depression Tramadol may impair mental alertness and/or physical coordination required to perform potentially hazardous activities such as driving or operating machinery; patients should be warned about possible adverse CNS effects of the drug.

Warfarin Prolongation of the international normalized ratio (INR) and prothrombin time and extensive ecchymoses have been reported in patients receiving tramadol and warfarin concomitantly. Therefore, tramadol should be used with caution in patients receiving warfarin; the INR should be closely monitored in those receiving the combination, and the warfarin dosage should be adjusted as needed.

Digoxin Digoxin toxicity has been reported rarely during postmarketing experience in patients receiving digoxin and tramadol concomitantly. Patients receiving such concomitant therapy should be monitored for digoxin toxicity, and digoxin dosage should be adjusted as needed.

Renal and Hepatic Impairment Impaired renal function results in a decreased rate and extent of excretion of tramadol and its active *O*-desmethyl metabolite (M1). Therefore, in patients with creatinine clearance less than 30 mL/minute, the manufacturers recommend dosage reduction when tramadol is used alone as conventional tablets or in fixed combination with acetaminophen. Tramadol hydrochloride extended-release tablets and capsules should *not* be used in patients with severe renal impairment (i.e., creatinine clearance less than 30 mL/minute); the available tablet and capsule strengths and once-daily dosing do not provide sufficient dosing flexibility for safe use in these patients. (See Dosage and Administration: Dosage in Renal and Hepatic Impairment.)

Tramadol and M1 metabolism are reduced in patients with advanced hepatic cirrhosis. When tramadol hydrochloride conventional tablets are used in adults with cirrhosis, dosage adjustment is recommended. Tramadol hydrochloride extended-release tablets and capsules should *not* be used in patients with severe hepatic impairment (Child-Pugh class C); the available tablet and capsule strengths and once-daily dosing do not provide sufficient dosing flexibility for safe use in these patients. The manufacturers state that pharmacokinetics and safety of tramadol in fixed combination with acetaminophen have not been studied in patients with impaired hepatic function. Therefore, because both tramadol and acetaminophen are extensively metabolized by the liver, the fixed-combination preparation should *not* be used in patients with hepatic impairment. (See Dosage and Administration: Dosage in Renal and Hepatic Impairment.)

With the prolonged half-life of tramadol in patients with renal or hepatic impairment, achievement of steady-state plasma concentrations is delayed, and it may take several days for elevated plasma concentrations to occur.

Advice to Patients Patients should be advised to read the manufacturer's patient information (e.g., medication guide) for tramadol before initiating therapy with the drug and each time the prescription is refilled. Patients should be informed that use of tramadol, even when taken as recommended, can result in addiction, abuse, and misuse, which can lead to overdosage and death. Patients also should be informed that accidental ingestion of tramadol, especially by a child, may result in respiratory depression or death. Patients should be instructed not to share the drug with others, to take steps to protect the drug from theft or misuse, to securely store the drug, to keep the drug out of reach of children, and to properly dispose of any unused drug.

Patients should be advised of the risk of life-threatening respiratory depression and instructed to seek immediate medical attention if manifestations of respiratory depression occur. Patients receiving tramadol and/or their caregivers should be advised that concomitant therapeutic or illicit use of benzodiazepines or other CNS depressants, including alcohol, can result in potentially fatal additive effects (e.g., profound sedation, respiratory depression, coma); patients should be advised to avoid concomitant use of alcohol and to avoid concomitant use of other CNS depressants unless such use is supervised by a clinician.

Patients should be informed of the risk of opiate toxicity in children, especially those who are obese, have respiratory diseases, or have evidence of ultrarapid metabolism of tramadol and advised that tramadol should *not* be given to children younger than 12 years of age for pain relief or to children younger than 18 years of age for pain relief following tonsillectomy or adenoidectomy. (See Cautions: Pediatric Precautions.)

Patients should be advised that tramadol may cause seizures and/or serotonin syndrome, particularly when used concurrently with serotonergic drugs or drugs that substantially decrease the metabolism of tramadol. (See Drugs Associated with Serotonin Syndrome and also Drugs Affecting Hepatic Microsomal Enzymes under Cautions: Precautions and Contraindications.) Patients should be advised that tramadol may impair mental or physical abilities required for the performance of potentially hazardous tasks such as driving a car or operating machinery. Patients should be advised of the importance of informing clinicians of existing or contemplated concomitant therapy, including prescription and OTC drugs, as well as any concomitant illnesses; patients should be advised that tramadol should not be used concomitantly with MAO inhibitors. Patients also should be advised that severe hypersensitivity reactions have occurred and that the drug may cause orthostatic hypotension and syncope. Because opiates can cause severe constipation, patients should be advised on appropriate management of constipation. Because of the potential risk of adrenal insufficiency, patients should be advised to immediately contact a clinician if manifestations of adrenal insufficiency (e.g., nausea, vomiting, loss of appetite, fatigue, weakness, dizziness, hypotension) develop. Although a causal relationship between hypogonadism or androgen deficiency and long-term opiate agonist use has not been established, patients should be advised of this potential risk and instructed to inform their clinician if decreased libido, impotence, erectile dysfunction, amenorrhea, or infertility occurs.

Women of childbearing potential should be instructed to inform their clinician if they are or plan to become pregnant and should be advised that use of tramadol is not recommended in nursing women. Women of childbearing potential should be advised that tramadol may cause fetal harm and that prolonged use of opiates during pregnancy may result in neonatal opiate withdrawal syndrome, which can be life-threatening if not recognized and treated. (See Cautions: Pregnancy, Fertility, and Lactation.)

Clinicians should be certain that patients understand the single-dose and 24-hour dose limit, and the recommended interval between doses of tramadol administered alone or in fixed combination with acetaminophen, since exceeding these recommendations can result in respiratory depression, seizures, acetaminophen-associated hepatic toxicity, and death. Patients receiving therapy with tramadol hydrochloride extended-release tablets or capsules should be advised that the tablets or capsules should be swallowed whole and should not be crushed, chewed, broken, split, or dissolved. Because of the risk of withdrawal syndrome, patients should be advised not to abruptly discontinue therapy with the drug without consulting their clinician.

Contraindications Tramadol is contraindicated in patients with substantial respiratory depression; acute or severe bronchial asthma in unmonitored settings or in the absence of resuscitative equipment; known or suspected GI obstruction, including paralytic ileus; or known hypersensitivity (e.g., anaphylaxis) to the drug, other opiates, or any ingredient in the formulation. Tramadol also is contraindicated during or within 14 days following treatment with an MAO inhibitor.

Tramadol is contraindicated in children younger than 12 years of age for the management of pain and in those younger than 18 years of age for the management of postoperative pain following tonsillectomy and/or adenoidectomy. (See Cautions: Pediatric Precautions.)

For a more complete discussion of the usual precautions associated with opiate agonist therapy, see the Opiate Agonists General Statement 28:08.08.

■ **Pediatric Precautions** Children receiving tramadol for the management of pain, especially those who are obese, have obstructive sleep apnea or severe lung disease, or have evidence of ultrarapid metabolism of CYP2D6 substrates, are at increased risk of respiratory depression. Between January 1969 and May 2016, the FDA Adverse Event Reporting System (AERS) received 9 reports of respiratory depression, including 3 deaths, worldwide that were associated with tramadol use in children younger than 18 years of age. Respiratory depression generally occurred within the first 24 hours of dosing and required medical intervention (e.g., naloxone). All 3 of the fatal cases occurred outside of the US in children younger than 6 years of age receiving tramadol hydrochloride oral solution for postoperative analgesia or management of fever. One 5-year-old child with obstructive sleep apnea experienced severely slowed and difficult breathing requiring emergency intervention and hospitalization after receiving a single 20-mg dose of tramadol hydrochloride oral solution (approximately 1 mg/kg) for pain relief following tonsillectomy and adenoidectomy. The child was resuscitated and later found to be a CYP2D6 ultra-rapid metabolizer and to have a high concentration of the active *O*-desmethyl metabolite (M1). In the other 8 reported cases, the CYP2D6 metabolizer status was unknown.

To minimize the risk of serious adverse events in children, FDA states that tramadol-containing preparations must *not* be used for the management of pain in children younger than 12 years of age or for the management of postoperative pain following tonsillectomy and/or adenoidectomy in children younger than 18 years of age. FDA also states that use of tramadol for the management of pain is *not* recommended in children 12–18 years of age who are obese or have conditions such as obstructive sleep apnea or compromised respiratory function (because of potentially greater susceptibility to the respiratory depressant effects of the drug). If tramadol is used for the management of pain in children 12–18 years of age, caregivers should closely monitor the child for clinical manifestations of opiate toxicity (e.g., slow, shallow, difficult, or noisy breathing; confusion; unusual sleepiness) and seek immediate medical treatment for the child if such manifestations occur.

The manufacturers state that safety and efficacy of tramadol hydrochloride conventional tablets have not been established in children younger than 16 years of age. Safety and efficacy of tramadol hydrochloride extended-release tablets and capsules and of tablets containing tramadol hydrochloride in fixed combination with acetaminophen have not been established in children younger than 18 years of age. The manufacturers state that use of tramadol in pediatric patients is not recommended.

■ **Geriatric Precautions** In general, tramadol dosage should be titrated carefully in geriatric patients, usually initiating therapy at the low end of the dosage range, considering the greater frequency of decreased hepatic, renal, and/or cardiac function and of concomitant disease and drug therapy observed in the elderly. (See Dosage and Administration: Dosage.) Because respiratory depression is the chief risk for geriatric patients receiving opiates, dosage should be titrated slowly and geriatric patients should be monitored closely for CNS and respiratory depression. Tramadol is substantially excreted by the kidneys, and the risk of adverse effects may be increased in patients with impaired renal function. Because geriatric patients may have decreased renal function, dosage should be selected carefully; it may be useful to monitor renal function in such patients.

In controlled clinical trials of tramadol hydrochloride conventional tablets, 455 patients who received the drug were 65 years of age or older, while 145 patients were 75 years of age or older. In patients older than 75 years of age receiving conventional tablets of the drug, maximum serum tramadol concentrations are elevated (208 ng/mL) and the elimination half-life is prolonged (7 hours) compared with patients 65–75 years of age (162 ng/mL and 6 hours, respectively). In clinical studies including geriatric patients receiving tramadol hydrochloride conventional tablets, treatment-limiting adverse GI effects occurred in 30% of patients older than 75 years of age compared with 17% of those younger than 65 years of age, and constipation resulted in discontinuance of treatment in 10% of those older than 75 years of age.

In clinical trials of tramadol hydrochloride extended-release tablets, 901 patients who received the drug were 65 years of age or older, while 156 patients were 75 years of age or older. In these studies, the incidence of adverse effects was higher in patients older than 65 years of age compared with younger adults; adverse effects reported more frequently in older adults include constipation, fatigue, weakness, postural hypotension, and dyspepsia. Tramadol hydrochloride extended-release tablets should be used with caution in patients older than 65 years of age and with even greater caution in those older than 75 years of age.

In clinical trials of tramadol hydrochloride extended-release capsules, 812 patients who received the drug were 65 years of age or older, while 240 patients were 75 years of age or older. In these studies, the incidence of adverse effects was higher in patients older than 65 years of age compared with younger adults; adverse effects reported more frequently in older adults include nausea, constipation, somnolence, dizziness, dry mouth, vomiting, asthenia, pruritus, anorexia, sweating, fatigue, weakness, postural hypotension, and dyspepsia. Tramadol hydrochloride extended-release capsules should be used with great caution in geriatric patients older than 75 years of age.

Limited data from a study of patients with chronic pain receiving tramadol in fixed combination with acetaminophen indicated that there were no substantial changes in pharmacokinetics of tramadol or acetaminophen in patients 65 years of age and older with normal renal and hepatic function compared with younger adults.

■ **Mutagenicity and Carcinogenicity** Tramadol did not exhibit mutagenic potential in vitro in the Ames *Salmonella* and *Escherichia coli* bacterial reverse mutation assay, mouse lymphoma assay (in the absence of metabolic activation), or chromosomal aberration assay. The drug also did not exhibit mutagenic potential in vivo in bone marrow micronucleus tests. Tramadol was mutagenic in vitro with metabolic activation in the mouse lymphoma assay.

A slight, but statistically significant, increase in pulmonary and hepatic murine tumors was observed in a mouse carcinogenicity study, particularly in aged mice who received oral tramadol hydrochloride dosages of up to 30 mg/kg daily (0.36–0.5 times the maximum daily human dosage) for approximately 2 years (the maximum tolerated dose was not studied). This finding is not believed to suggest risk in humans. No evidence of carcinogenicity was observed in p53(±)-heterozygous mice given oral tramadol hydrochloride dosages of up to 150 mg/kg daily for 26 weeks. No evidence of carcinogenicity was observed in 2 rat carcinogenicity studies; however, inadequate weight gain may have reduced the sensitivity to detect carcinogenicity of the drug.

■ **Pregnancy, Fertility, and Lactation** ***Pregnancy*** Prolonged maternal use of opiate agonists during pregnancy can result in neonatal opiate withdrawal syndrome with manifestations of irritability, hyperactivity and abnormal sleep pattern, high-pitched cry, tremor, vomiting, diarrhea, and failure to gain weight. In contrast to adults, the withdrawal syndrome in neonates may be life-threatening if not recognized and treated, and requires management according to protocols developed by neonatology experts. Women who require prolonged opiate agonist therapy during pregnancy should be advised of the risk of neonatal opiate withdrawal syndrome, and availability of appropriate treatment should be ensured. The onset, duration, and severity of the syndrome vary depending on the specific opiate agonist used, duration of use, timing and amount of last maternal use, and rate of drug elimination by the neonate. Neonatal seizures, neonatal withdrawal syndrome, fetal death, and stillbirth have been reported with tramadol during postmarketing experience. The effect of tramadol, if any, on the later growth, development, and functional maturation of the child is unknown.

Use of opiates in pregnant women during labor can result in neonatal respiratory depression. Use of tramadol is not recommended immediately before or during labor, when other analgesic techniques may be more appropriate. Opiate agonists may prolong labor through actions that temporarily reduce the strength, duration, and frequency of uterine contractions. However, this effect is inconsistent and may be offset by an increased rate of cervical dilatation, which tends to shorten labor. Neonates exposed to opiates during labor should be monitored for excessive sedation and respiratory depression. An opiate antagonist must be available for reversal of opiate-induced respiratory depression.

Tramadol has been shown to cross the placenta. The mean ratio of serum tramadol in the umbilical veins compared with maternal veins was 0.83 for women given tramadol during labor.

Analysis of data from the National Birth Defects Prevention Study, a large population-based, case-control study, suggests that therapeutic maternal use of opiate agonists during the period of organogenesis is associated with a low absolute risk of birth defects, including heart defects, spina bifida, and gastroschisis. The manufacturers state that available data regarding use of tramadol in pregnant women are insufficient to establish the risk of major birth defects and spontaneous abortion with the drug.

Based on animal data, women of childbearing potential should be advised of the potential for tramadol to cause fetal harm.

Although there are no adequate and controlled studies to date in humans, tramadol has been shown to be embryotoxic and fetotoxic in mice, rats, and rabbits at maternally toxic doses 1.4, 0.6, and 3.6 times, respectively, the maximum daily human dosage (120 mg/kg in mice, 25 mg/kg in rats, and 75 mg/kg in rabbits). Embryo and fetal toxicity consisted mainly of decreased fetal weights, decreased skeletal ossification, and increased supernumerary ribs at maternally toxic dose levels. Transient delays in developmental or behavioral parameters also were seen in pups from rat dams allowed to deliver. Embryo and fetal lethality was reported in only one rabbit study, in which rabbits received tramadol hydrochloride 300 mg/kg, a dose that would cause extreme maternal toxicity in rabbits.

Embryotoxicity and fetotoxicity have been demonstrated in rats when tramadol and acetaminophen were administered in fixed combination at maternally toxic doses of 50 and 434 mg/kg, respectively, or 1.6 times the maximum daily human dosages of these drugs. Embryonic and fetal toxicity consisted of decreased fetal weights and increased supernumerary ribs.

Tramadol was not teratogenic in mice, rats, and rabbits at maternally toxic doses 1.4, 0.6, and 3.6 times, respectively, the maximum human daily dosage (120 mg/kg in mice, 25 mg/kg in rats, and 75 mg/kg in rabbits). No drug-related teratogenic effects were observed in progeny of mice, rats, or rabbits receiving tramadol (up to 140, 80, or 300 mg/kg or 1.7, 1.9, or 14.6 times, respectively, the maximum daily human dosage) by various routes.

Tramadol and acetaminophen in fixed combination was not teratogenic in rats at a maternally toxic dose of 50 and 434 mg/kg, respectively, or 1.6 times the maximum daily human dosages of these drugs.

In perinatal and postnatal studies in rats, progeny of dams receiving oral (gavage) tramadol hydrochloride doses of 50 mg/kg or higher had decreased weights, and pup survival was decreased early in lactation at tramadol hydrochloride doses of 80 mg/kg (1.2–1.6 or 1.9–2.6 times, respectively, the maximum human dose). No toxicity was observed for progeny of dams receiving doses of 8, 10, 20, 25, or 40 mg/kg. Maternal toxicity was observed at all dose levels, but effects on progeny were evident only at higher dose levels where maternal toxicity was more severe.

Fertility Long-term use of opiates may reduce fertility in females and males of reproductive potential. It is not known whether these effects are reversible. (See Cautions: Genitourinary and Endocrine Effects.)

No effects on fertility were observed in male rats receiving oral tramadol hydrochloride doses up to 50 mg/kg or in female rats receiving oral tramadol hydrochloride doses up to 75 mg/kg or 1.2 or 1.8 times, respectively, the maximum daily human dosage based on body surface area.

Lactation Tramadol is distributed into milk. Following a single IV tramadol dose of 100 mg, the cumulative distribution into milk within 16 hours after dosing was 100 mcg of tramadol (0.1% of the maternal dose) and 27 mcg of M1.

Because the safety of tramadol in infants and neonates has not been established, the drug is not recommended for obstetrical preoperative medication or for use in nursing women, including use for post-delivery analgesia. FDA review of available medical literature did not reveal evidence of an increased frequency of adverse effects in nursing infants of women receiving tramadol; however, because the drug is distributed into milk and has similar risks as codeine in ultrarapid metabolizers of CYP2D6 substrates, FDA recommends that tramadol *not* be used in nursing women. (See Pharmacogenomics under Cautions: Precautions and Contraindications. Also see Cautions: Precautions and Contraindications, in Codeine Phosphate and Codeine Sulfate 28:08.08.) Infants exposed to tramadol through breast milk should be monitored closely for clinical manifestations of opiate toxicity (e.g., sedation, difficulty breastfeeding or breathing, hypotonia). If clinical manifestations of opiate toxicity occur, caregivers should seek immediate medical treatment for the infant.

Symptoms of withdrawal can occur in opiate-dependent infants when maternal administration of opiates is discontinued or breast-feeding is stopped.

Description

Tramadol hydrochloride is a synthetic, centrally active analgesic. The drug (and its active *O*-desmethyl metabolite [M1]) acts as an opiate agonist, apparently by selective activity at the μ-receptor. In addition to opiate agonist activity, tramadol inhibits reuptake of certain monoamines (norepinephrine, serotonin), which appears to contribute to the drug's analgesic effect. Although the relative contribution of tramadol versus its M1 metabolite to analgesia in humans is unknown, the metabolite is 6 times more potent than the parent drug in producing analgesia in animal models and 200 times more potent in μ-receptor binding. The antinociceptic effect of tramadol is antagonized only partially by naloxone in some tests in animals and healthy individuals.

Although the pharmacologic effects of tramadol result in part from agonist activity at opiate receptors, the drug is not an opium derivative nor a semisynthetic derivative of morphine or thebaine. However, because tramadol is an agonist of *true* opiate receptors, not opiate-*like* (i.e., opi-*oid*) receptors, the drug is classified as an opiate agonist in the AHFS Pharmacologic-Therapeutic Classification®. (See Chemistry in the Opiate Agonists General Statement 28:08.08.)

Because of the drug's opiate agonist activity at μ-receptors, tramadol also can produce dependence. Although tramadol and tramadol in fixed combination with acetaminophen were *not* originally subject to control under the Federal Controlled Substances Act of 1970 as scheduled drugs, these preparations became subject to such control as schedule IV (C-IV) drugs effective August 18, 2014. Current data suggest that the abuse potential of tramadol is less than that of morphine or oxycodone but similar to that of propoxyphene. Tolerance and manifestations of withdrawal also can occur, although such effects are relatively mild compared with those of other opiate agonists.

Tramadol shares many of the other pharmacologic and toxicologic effects of opiate agonists, including dizziness, somnolence, nausea, constipation, dry mouth, sweating, and pruritus. The respiratory depressant effects of the drug are less than those of morphine, and usually are not clinically important at usual oral doses. At relatively high doses (e.g., those administered parenterally), tramadol can produce respiratory depression, and even usual oral doses should be employed cautiously in patients at risk for respiratory depression. At usual oral doses, the drug exhibits minimal cardiovascular effects, although hypotension, syncope, and tachycardia can occur occasionally.

SumMon® (see Users Guide). For additional information on this drug until a more detailed monograph is developed and published, the manufacturer's labeling should be consulted. It is *essential* that the labeling be consulted for detailed information on the usual cautions, precautions, and contraindications concerning potential drug interactions and/or laboratory test interferences.

Preparations

Effective August 18, 2014, tramadol hydrochloride preparations are subject to control under the Federal Controlled Substances Act of 1970 as schedule IV (C-IV) drugs. (See Description.)

Excipients in commercially available drug preparations may have clinically important effects in some individuals; consult specific product labeling for details.

traMADol Hydrochloride

Oral

Capsules, extended-release	100 mg (with extended-release 75 mg and immediate-release 25 mg)	**Conzip®** (C-IV), Vertical
	200 mg (with extended-release 150 mg and immediate-release 50 mg)	**Conzip®** (C-IV), Vertical
	300 mg (with extended-release 250 mg and immediate-release 50 mg)	**Conzip®** (C-IV), Vertical
Tablets, extended-release	100 mg*	**traMADol Hydrochloride Extended-Release Tablets** (C-IV)
		Ultram® ER (C-IV), Janssen
	200 mg*	**traMADol Hydrochloride Extended-Release Tablets** (C-IV)
		Ultram® ER (C-IV), Janssen
	300 mg*	**traMADol Hydrochloride Extended-Release Tablets** (C-IV)
		Ultram® ER (C-IV), Janssen
Tablets, film-coated	50 mg*	**traMADol Hydrochloride Tablets** (C-IV)
		Ultram® (C-IV; scored), Janssen

*available from one or more manufacturer, distributor, and/or repackager by generic (nonproprietary) name

traMADol Hydrochloride Combinations

Oral		
Tablets, film-coated	37.5 with Acetaminophen 325 mg*	**traMADol Hydrochloride and Acetaminophen Tablets** (C-IV)
		Ultracet® (C-IV), Janssen

*available from one or more manufacturer, distributor, and/or repackager by generic (nonproprietary) name

OPIATE PARTIAL AGONISTS 28:08.12

Buprenorphine
Buprenorphine Hydrochloride

■ Buprenorphine is a synthetic opiate partial agonist analgesic.

REMS

FDA approved a REMS for buprenorphine to ensure that the benefits outweigh the risk. (See Risk Evaluation and Mitigation Strategies under Dosage and Administration: Administration.) The REMS may apply to one or more preparations of buprenorphine and may consist of the following: medication guide, elements to assure safe use, and implementation system. See the FDA REMS page (https://www.accessdata.fda.gov/scripts/cder/rems/index.cfm).

Uses

Buprenorphine hydrochloride is used parenterally for the relief of pain that is severe enough to require opiate analgesia and for which alternative treatment options are inadequate. Buprenorphine hydrochloride also is used buccally and buprenorphine is used transdermally for the management of pain that is severe enough to require daily, around-the-clock, long-term opiate analgesia and for which alternative treatment options are inadequate.

In the management of opiate dependence (opiate use disorder), buprenorphine is used parenterally as an extended-release subcutaneous injection, buprenorphine hydrochloride is used sublingually or as a subdermal implant, and buprenorphine hydrochloride in fixed combination with naloxone hydrochloride is used sublingually or buccally.

■ **Pain** ***Parenteral Therapy*** Buprenorphine hydrochloride is used parenterally as an analgesic for the relief of pain that is severe enough to require an opiate analgesic and for which alternate treatments are inadequate; because of the risks of addiction, abuse, and misuse associated with opiates even at recommended dosages, parenteral buprenorphine should be reserved for use in patients for whom alternative treatment options (e.g., nonopiate analgesics, opiate-containing fixed combinations) have not been, or are not expected to be, adequate or tolerated. The analgesic activity of 0.3 mg of parenteral buprenorphine is about equal to that of 10 mg of parenteral morphine sulfate or 75–100 mg of parenteral meperidine. In equianalgesic doses, parenteral buprenorphine generally appears to be as effective as or possibly slightly more effective than parenteral morphine, meperidine, or pentazocine in relieving moderate to severe pain. The duration of analgesia produced by a single dose of parenteral buprenorphine is generally longer than that produced by a single parenteral dose of meperidine or pentazocine and is comparable to and, in some patients, may be longer than that produced by a single parenteral dose of morphine.

Buprenorphine is used parenterally in the management of postoperative pain in patients who have undergone various types of surgery, including neurologic, cardiovascular (e.g., coronary artery bypass, valve replacement), cesarean section, gynecologic, abdominal (e.g., cholecystectomy, bowel resection), urologic, general (e.g., head and neck, breast), and orthopedic (e.g., total hip replacement, spinal fusion). Because of its limited cardiovascular effects, buprenorphine may be safer than morphine when used as an analgesic in patients with compromised cardiac function undergoing cardiovascular surgery. The drug has also been administered by epidural injection† in the management of postoperative pain in total dosages substantially less than the equivalent morphine dosages necessary to produce a comparable analgesic effect. Buprenorphine has also been used to provide preoperative sedation and analgesia† and as an adjunct to surgical anesthesia†; however, the drug should be used with caution in patients undergoing surgery of the biliary tract. (See GI Conditions under Cautions: Precautions and Contraindications.)

Buprenorphine has been used parenterally as an analgesic for the relief of moderate to severe pain associated with cancer and trigeminal neuralgia. The drug has also been used as an analgesic in critically ill patients for the relief of moderate to severe pain resulting from accidental trauma and as an analgesic for the relief of moderate to severe pain resulting from ureteral calculi. Buprenorphine has also been used as an analgesic for the relief of moderate to severe pain associated with myocardial infarction.

Transdermal Therapy Buprenorphine is used transdermally for the management of pain that is severe enough to require daily, around-the-clock, long-term opiate analgesia and for which alternative treatment options are inadequate. Because of the risks of addiction, abuse, and misuse associated with opiates, even at recommended dosages, and because of the greater risks of overdosage and death associated with extended-release opiate formulations, transdermal buprenorphine should be reserved for use in patients for whom alternative treatment options (e.g., nonopiate analgesics, immediate-release opiates) are inadequate or not tolerated. Transdermal buprenorphine is *not* intended for use on an as-needed ("prn") basis.

The safety and efficacy of transdermal buprenorphine have been evaluated in 4 double-blind, controlled trials of 12 weeks' duration. Two studies, one in patients with chronic low back pain and one in patients with osteoarthritis, failed to show efficacy for either transdermal buprenorphine or the active comparators. Efficacy and safety of transdermal buprenorphine were established in 2 studies in patients with moderate to severe chronic low back pain, including one study in adults not previously receiving opiates and one study in adults receiving chronic opiate therapy at a dosage equivalent to 30–80 mg daily of oral morphine sulfate. Chronic opiate regimens were tapered prior to initiating buprenorphine. Both studies utilized an initial open-label dose titration period of up to 3–4 weeks; buprenorphine was initiated at a dosage of 5 mcg/hour (or 10 mcg/hour in those previously receiving opiate treatment) and increased at intervals of at least 72 hours to a maximum dosage of 20 mcg/hour. Patients who achieved adequate analgesia with tolerable adverse effects (approximately 53–57% of patients) during this phase were randomized to 12 weeks of double-blind treatment. In patients who had not previously received opiates for analgesia, transdermal buprenorphine was more effective than placebo in reducing 24-hour average pain scores (measured on an 11-point numeric rating scale). Patients who previously had received opiates for analgesia also achieved greater reductions in 24-hour average pain scores with 20 mcg/hour of transdermal buprenorphine when compared with 5 mcg/hour of transdermal buprenorphine (low-dose control).

Oral Transmucosal Therapy Buprenorphine is used buccally for the management of pain that is severe enough to require daily, around-the-clock, long-term opiate analgesia and for which alternative treatment options are inadequate. Because of the risks of addiction, abuse, and misuse associated with opiates, even at recommended dosages, and because of the greater risks of overdosage and death associated with long-acting opiate formulations, intrabuccal buprenorphine should be reserved for use in patients for whom alternative treatment options (e.g., nonopiate analgesics, immediate-release opiates) are inadequate or not tolerated. Intrabuccal buprenorphine is *not* intended for use on an as-needed ("prn") basis.

The safety and efficacy of intrabuccal buprenorphine have been evaluated in 3 double-blind, controlled trials of 12 weeks' duration in patients with moderate to severe, chronic low back pain. One study failed to show efficacy. Efficacy and safety of intrabuccal buprenorphine were established in 2 studies, including one study in adults not previously receiving opiates and one study in adults receiving long-term opiate therapy at a dosage equivalent to 30–160 mg daily of oral morphine sulfate. Opiate regimens were tapered to a dosage equivalent to 30 mg daily of oral morphine sulfate prior to initiating buprenorphine. Both studies utilized an initial open-label dose-titration period with buprenorphine of up to 8 weeks' duration. Patients who achieved adequate analgesia with tolerable adverse effects (61–63% of patients) during this phase were randomized to 12 weeks of double-blind treatment with buprenorphine or placebo. In patients who had not previously received opiates for analgesia, intrabuccal buprenorphine was more effective than placebo in reducing mean pain scores (as measured on an 11-point numeric rating scale), and a greater proportion of buprenorphine-treated patients compared with placebo recipients achieved at least a 30% reduction in pain score (62 versus 47%) or at least a 50% reduction in pain score (41 versus 33%) from baseline (prior to the open-label titration period) to end of study. In patients who previously had received opiates for analgesia, intrabuccal buprenorphine also was more effective than placebo in reducing mean pain scores, and a greater proportion of buprenorphine-treated patients compared with placebo recipients achieved at least a 30% reduction in pain score (64 versus 31%) or at least a 50% reduction in pain score (39 versus 17%) from baseline (prior to the open-label titration period) to end of study.

Oral transmucosal formulations of buprenorphine or buprenorphine in fixed combination with naloxone that are intended for use in the treatment of opiate dependence should *not* be used for analgesia. Fatal overdosage has been reported following administration of 2 mg of sublingual buprenorphine for analgesia in opiate-naive individuals.

For further information on the role of opiate analgesics in the management of acute or chronic pain, see Uses: Pain, in the Opiate Agonists General Statement 28:08.08.

■ **Opiate Dependence** Buprenorphine is used parenterally as an extended-release subcutaneous injection, buprenorphine hydrochloride is used sublingually or as a subdermal implant, and buprenorphine hydrochloride in fixed combination with naloxone hydrochloride is used sublingually or buccally for the treatment of opiate dependence (opiate use disorder); buprenorphine has been designated an orphan drug by FDA for this indication. Safety and efficacy of transdermal buprenorphine for the management of opiate dependence have not been established. In the treatment of opiate dependence, buprenorphine should be used as part of a comprehensive treatment program that includes counseling and psychosocial support.

Buprenorphine and buprenorphine in fixed combination with naloxone (buprenorphine/naloxone) are available in the US for office-based outpatient medication-assisted treatment (MAT) of opiate dependence. The Drug Addiction Treatment Act of 2000 (DATA 2000) allows qualifying physicians to prescribe and dispense opiates in schedules III, IV, and V of the Federal Controlled Substances Act that have been approved by FDA for the management of opiate dependence. Prior to passage of this law, opiate dependence treatment could be provided only at specially registered clinics. The Comprehensive Addiction and Recovery Act of 2016 (CARA 2016) expands the categories of practitioners recognized under DATA 2000 to include qualifying nurse practitioners and physician assistants. Office-based treatment with buprenorphine is intended to increase access to opiate dependence treatment. Expansion of the categories of qualifying practitioners is intended to further bridge the gap between MAT providers and individuals seeking such treatment, a particular problem in rural areas. In the office-based treatment model, specially trained clinicians may prescribe buprenorphine as a take-home medication.

The choice between buprenorphine and methadone for maintenance treatment of opiate dependence should take into consideration the patient's preferences; the patient's medical, psychiatric, substance use, and treatment histories; and treatment availability and setting. Buprenorphine is preferred for many patients because it can be prescribed in an office-based setting and is considered to have a better safety profile than methadone. Methadone may be preferred for patients who would benefit from daily supervised dosing in an opiate treatment program and for those who do not have access to, or have not benefited from, buprenorphine therapy. Office-based treatment may not be suitable for patients with other concurrent substance use disorders or for those routinely using other CNS depressants.

Oral Transmucosal Therapy for Induction and Maintenance Treatment Buprenorphine and buprenorphine/naloxone are used sublingually or buccally for the treatment of opiate dependence. Although buprenorphine traditionally has been considered the preferred drug for the initial (i.e., induction) phase of treatment, additional experience indicates that either buprenorphine or buprenorphine/naloxone may be used for induction therapy in patients dependent on heroin or other short-acting opiates. Use of buprenorphine/naloxone for the induction phase of treatment in patients dependent on long-acting opiates has not been evaluated to date in adequate and well-controlled studies, and the manufacturers and some experts still recommend use of buprenorphine alone for induction in these patients. Following induction, buprenorphine/naloxone is the preferred drug for maintenance treatment when use includes unsupervised administration since the presence of naloxone (an opiate antagonist) in the formulation should discourage parenteral misuse of the oral transmucosal preparation. Administration of buprenorphine without naloxone in an unsupervised setting should be limited to pregnant women and patients who cannot tolerate naloxone. (See Dosage and Administration: Dosage in Hepatic Impairment and also see Pregnancy under Cautions: Pregnancy, Fertility, and Lactation.)

Sublingual buprenorphine and buprenorphine/naloxone have been evaluated in several placebo- and active-controlled studies in patients physically dependent on opiates. In these studies, buprenorphine therapy has been used in conjunction with psychosocial counseling as part of a comprehensive addiction treatment program. When administered sublingually, buprenorphine and buprenorphine/naloxone have similar clinical effects. Results of a dose-ranging study indicate that sublingual administration of buprenorphine dosages of 6–24 mg daily are effective in the treatment of opiate dependence. Buprenorphine and buprenorphine/naloxone were more effective than placebo in reducing illicit opiate use, as determined by urine tests for other opiates, in one placebo-controlled study that included patients randomized to receive buprenorphine 8 mg or placebo on day 1, buprenorphine 16 mg or placebo on day 2, and then buprenorphine 16 mg daily, buprenorphine 16 mg in fixed combination with naloxone 4 mg daily, or placebo daily for 4 weeks. In another study that included a 16- to 17-week maintenance phase and a 7- to 8-week detoxification phase, buprenorphine generally was more effective than low dosages of methadone hydrochloride (20 mg daily) and as effective as high dosages of methadone hydrochloride (60 mg daily) in reducing illicit opiate use and retaining patients in the program. In another comparative study, buprenorphine, levomethadyl acetate (no longer commercially available in the US because of potentially severe adverse cardiac effects), and high-dose methadone hydrochloride (60–100 mg daily) were more effective than low-dose methadone hydrochloride (20 mg daily) in reducing illicit opiate use.

Induction therapy with sublingual buprenorphine/naloxone has been evaluated in 2 blinded, randomized noninferiority studies in a total of 1068 opiate-dependent adults. In both studies, treatment retention rates at day 3 were compared following induction therapy with buprenorphine/naloxone sublingual tablets (Zubsolv®; total induction dosage of buprenorphine 5.7 mg and naloxone 1.4 mg on day 1 followed by either buprenorphine 5.7 mg and naloxone 1.4 mg or buprenorphine 11.4 mg and naloxone 2.8 mg on day 2) or generic buprenorphine sublingual tablets (total induction dosage of 8 mg on day 1 followed by 8 or 16 mg on day 2). On day 1, patients received an initial supervised dose of the assigned drug (buprenorphine 1.4 mg and naloxone 0.36 mg or buprenorphine 2 mg); at the investigator's discretion, the remainder of the day 1 dosage was administered in 1 dose or, if the first dose precipitated withdrawal manifestations, in 3 divided doses at intervals of 1–2 hours. Because of its higher bioavailability, a Zubsolv® sublingual tablet containing buprenorphine 5.7 mg and naloxone 1.4 mg provides equivalent buprenorphine exposure and 12% lower naloxone exposure as a Suboxone® sublingual tablet containing buprenorphine 8 mg and naloxone 2 mg. In the first study, the treatment retention rate at day 3 was 93% for patients receiving buprenorphine/naloxone compared with 92% for those receiving buprenorphine alone; in the second study, treatment retention rates at day 3 were 85 and 95%, respectively. The lower retention rate observed with the fixed-combination preparation compared with buprenorphine alone in the second study may have been related to infrequent use of divided dosing in this study (5%) compared with the first study (22%).

Maintenance Treatment with Buprenorphine Extended-release Subcutaneous Injection Buprenorphine extended-release subcutaneous injection is used for the treatment of moderate to severe opiate dependence in patients who have initiated treatment with an oral transmucosal buprenorphine-containing preparation followed by dosage adjustment for a minimum of 7 days.

Buprenorphine extended-release subcutaneous injection has been evaluated in an opiate challenge study and in a randomized, double-blind, placebo-controlled clinical trial.

In the opiate challenge study, efficacy of buprenorphine extended-release subcutaneous injection in blocking subjective opiate effects following hydromorphone challenge was assessed in 39 individuals with moderate to severe opiate use disorder who were not seeking treatment. Following stabilization on sublingual buprenorphine/naloxone over one week, study participants received two 300-mg subcutaneous doses of extended-release buprenorphine given 4 weeks apart. "Drug liking" scores (measured on a 100-mm visual analog scale) following challenge with placebo and hydromorphone hydrochloride (IM doses of 6 and 18 mg) were recorded weekly for 12 weeks after the first buprenorphine injection. At weeks 1–4, neither hydromorphone dose was substantially more likeable than placebo. Full blockade of the subjective effects of hydromorphone was observed at both dosage levels during each of the 12 weeks of the study, although substantial variability in isolated measurements from individual study participants was observed.

In the randomized double-blind study, 504 patients seeking treatment for moderate to severe opiate use disorder were randomized to receive buprenorphine extended-release subcutaneous injection (300 mg monthly for 6 months or 300 mg monthly for 2 months followed by 100 mg monthly for 4 months) or placebo following stabilization on buprenorphine/naloxone sublingually dissolving strips. Supplemental sublingual doses of buprenorphine/naloxone were not permitted during the study. All patients received psychosocial counseling at least weekly. Efficacy was evaluated over weeks 5–24 by means of urine drug testing and self-reports of illicit opiate use. Treatment success, defined as opiate-free status for 80% or more of the weeks during the evaluation period, was attained by 28–29% of buprenorphine-treated patients compared with 2% of placebo recipients.

Maintenance Treatment with Buprenorphine Subdermal Implants Buprenorphine hydrochloride subdermal implants are used for maintenance treatment of opiate dependence in patients who have achieved and maintained prolonged clinical stability on a low to moderate dosage of an oral transmucosal buprenorphine-containing preparation (i.e., a transmucosal dosage that provides blood buprenorphine concentrations comparable to or lower than those provided by the subdermal implants). Examples of appropriate dosages of oral transmucosal buprenorphine-containing preparations include the following: Subutex® sublingual tablets (or generic equivalent; branded formulation no longer commercially available in the US) at a dosage not exceeding buprenorphine 8 mg daily, Suboxone® sublingual tablets (or generic equivalent; branded formulation no longer commercially available in the US) at a dosage not exceeding buprenorphine 8 mg and naloxone 2 mg daily, Bunavail® buccally dissolving strips at a dosage not exceeding buprenorphine 4.2 mg and naloxone 0.7 mg daily, and Zubsolv® sublingual tablets at a dosage not exceeding buprenorphine 5.7 mg and naloxone 1.4 mg daily. Buprenorphine subdermal implants are not appropriate for individuals just initiating treatment for opiate dependence or for those who have not achieved and sustained prolonged clinical stability on a low to moderate oral transmucosal dosage of the drug. (See Implant Dosage for Maintenance Treatment under Dosage: Opiate Dependence, in Dosage and Administration.)

Efficacy of buprenorphine subdermal implants for the maintenance treatment of opiate dependence was established in a randomized, double-blind study in 177 patients who were clinically stable while receiving a sublingual buprenorphine dosage of 8 mg daily or less (as Suboxone® sublingual tablets or equivalent). Patients were randomized to receive 4 buprenorphine hydrochloride 80-mg subdermal implants (with daily placebo sublingual tablets) or daily treatment with buprenorphine/naloxone sublingual tablets administered at the prerandomization dosage (with 4 placebo subdermal implants). Supplemental doses of sublingual buprenorphine/naloxone tablets were permitted as clinically indicated. In the sublingual treatment group, supplemental dosing was considered consistent with usual treatment, whereas in the implant treatment group, supplemental dosing was interpreted as indicating that the implant dosage was inadequate. Efficacy assessments were based on urine drug testing and self-reports of illicit opiate use. During 6 months of treatment, 63% of patients with subdermal buprenorphine implants (without supplemental sublingual therapy) had no evidence of illicit opiate use, compared with 64% of patients receiving usual sublingual buprenorphine therapy. In addition, 11 patients with buprenorphine implants required supplemental sublingual dosing but had no evidence of illicit opiate use; one of these patients required supplemental dosing only at the end of the implantation period, potentially indicating the need for early implant replacement.

Two additional studies in patients who had not previously received buprenorphine therapy suggested that buprenorphine subdermal implants should not be used for patients who are new to buprenorphine treatment or who have not achieved and sustained prolonged clinical stability while receiving a low to moderate dosage of an oral transmucosal buprenorphine-containing preparation; the implant dosage appears to be too low to be effective in these populations.

■ **Other Uses** Buprenorphine has been used in a limited number of patients as an antagonist to reverse fentanyl-induced anesthesia† and provide subsequent analgesia; however, buprenorphine-induced reversal of fentanyl anesthesia may occur slowly, and usefulness of the drug in situations when rapid recovery from fentanyl anesthesia is desirable may therefore be limited.

Buprenorphine has caused substantial clinical improvement in a limited number of patients with refractory endogenous depression† when administered as a sublingual tablet for several days.

Dosage and Administration

■ **Administration** ***Risk Evaluation and Mitigation Strategies*** FDA required and approved REMS for oral transmucosal formulations of buprenorphine alone or in fixed combination with naloxone (buprenorphine/naloxone) that are used for treatment of opiate dependence (opiate use disorder), for opiate analgesics used in the outpatient setting (including buprenorphine transdermal systems and buprenorphine buccally dissolving strips), for buprenorphine subdermal implants, and for buprenorphine extended-release subcutaneous injection. (See REMS.)

The REMS programs for buprenorphine-containing oral transmucosal preparations (i.e., sublingual tablets and sublingually or buccally dissolving strips) used for the treatment of opiate dependence require that a medication guide be provided to the patient each time the formulation is dispensed and outline steps to ensure documentation of safe use conditions and proper monitoring for each patient receiving the drug. The REMS requirement does not apply when buprenorphine-containing oral transmucosal preparations are dispensed to patients admitted to an opiate treatment program. The goals are to reduce the risk of accidental overdosage, misuse, and abuse and to inform prescribers, pharmacists, and patients of the serious risks associated with these preparations. Under the REMS programs, pharmacists dispensing prescriptions for oral transmucosal buprenorphine-containing preparations for treatment of opiate dependence should verify that the prescriber is certified to prescribe the drug (see Dosage and Administration: Restricted Distribution Program for Buprenorphine Treatment of Opiate Dependence); check the state prescription drug monitoring program (PDMP), where practical, to identify behaviors that may indicate abuse; keep in mind that only a limited supply of the drug should be dispensed during treatment initiation; provide a copy of the manufacturer-provided medication guide to the patient; remind patients who are picking up induction doses of buprenorphine to return as directed to the practitioner's office to receive the dose under supervision; and to be vigilant in detecting fraudulent prescriptions or simultaneous prescriptions for the same patient from multiple prescribers. Additional information about the Suboxone® and Subutex® REMS can be obtained at http://www.suboxonerems.com, and information about the Buprenorphine-containing Transmucosal Products for Opioid Dependence (BTOD) REMS (which includes generic equivalents of Suboxone® and Subutex® sublingual tablets, buprenorphine/naloxone sublingual tablets [Zubsolv®], and buprenorphine/naloxone buccally dissolving strips [Bunavail®]) can be obtained at http://www.btodrems.com.

The Sublocade® REMS program is intended to reduce the risk of serious harm or death that could result from IV self-administration by ensuring that buprenorphine extended-release subcutaneous injection is dispensed by certified health care settings and pharmacies directly to health care providers for administration by a health care professional. The REMS includes a redistricted distribution program. Additional information about the program can be obtained at http://www.sublocaderems.com.

The goals of the Probuphine® REMS are to reduce the risks of complications of buprenorphine subdermal implant migration, protrusion, or expulsion; nerve damage associated with implant insertion and removal; and accidental overdosage, misuse, and abuse if an implant is expelled or protrudes from the skin. The program includes requirements for certification of clinicians who prescribe the implant and for those who insert the implants; monitoring and documentation of implant removal; restriction of distribution to settings with a certified prescriber; and a medication guide that must be provided with every implant prescription. Additional information about the program can be obtained at http://probuphinerems.com.

FDA also has approved a REMS program for opiate analgesics used in the outpatient setting and not covered by other REMS programs, including buprenorphine transdermal system (Butrans®) and buprenorphine buccally dissolving strips (Belbuca®). The goals of this program are to reduce the occurrence of addiction, unintentional overdosage, and death resulting from inappropriate prescribing, misuse, and abuse of opiate analgesics. The program consists of educational programs for prescribers and other health care providers, including pharmacists and nurses, who are involved in the treatment and monitoring of patients with pain; information that health care providers can use when counseling patients about opiate analgesics; and a product-specific medication guide that must be dispensed with every prescription. Additional information about the program can be obtained at http://opioidanalgesicrems.com.

In addition to the restricted distribution systems established for certain buprenorphine-containing preparations (extended-release subcutaneous injection, subdermal implants) under REMS programs, buprenorphine and buprenorphine/naloxone may be prescribed for the treatment of opiate dependence only by clinicians who meet certain requirements, have notified the Secretary of the US Department of Health and Human Services (HHS) of their intent to prescribe these preparations for this indication, and have been assigned a unique identification number that must be included on each prescription for the drug. (See Dosage and Administration: Restricted Distribution Program for Buprenorphine Treatment of Opiate Dependence.)

Parenteral Administration **Conventional Injection for Pain Management.** For the relief of pain severe enough to require opiate analgesia and for which alternative treatments are inadequate, buprenorphine hydrochloride is administered by IM or slow (over a period of at least 2 minutes) IV injection. The drug has also been administered by continuous IV infusion†, by IM or IV injection using a patient-controlled infusion device†, and by epidural injection†.

For continuous IV infusion†, buprenorphine hydrochloride injection has been diluted to a concentration of 15 mcg/mL in 0.9% sodium chloride and administered via a controlled-infusion device. For continuous IV infusion†, the drug should be administered only by qualified individuals familiar with the technique and patient management problems (i.e., respiratory depression) associated with buprenorphine administration. For epidural injection†, buprenorphine hydrochloride injection has been diluted to a concentration of 6–30 mcg/mL in 0.9% sodium chloride.

Buprenorphine hydrochloride injection and diluted solutions of the drug should be inspected visually for particulate matter and discoloration prior to administration whenever solution and container permit.

If accidental dermal exposure occurs, any contaminated clothing should be removed and the affected area rinsed with water.

Extended-release Subcutaneous Injection for Opiate Dependence. For the management of opiate dependence in patients who have initiated buprenorphine therapy with an oral transmucosal buprenorphine-containing preparation followed by dosage adjustment for at least 7 days, buprenorphine extended-release injection is administered by subcutaneous injection into the abdomen at monthly intervals (minimum of 26 days between injections); this formulation is for subcutaneous injection *only* and should *not* be administered IV or IM. (See Extended-release Subcutaneous Injection under Cautions: Precautions and Contraindications.) A clinician must prepare and administer the injection. (See Risk Evaluation and Mitigation Strategies under Dosage and Administration: Administration.)

Buprenorphine extended-release injection should be removed from the refrigerator and allowed to reach room temperature (over at least 15 minutes) prior to administration. Each injection should be administered using the manufacturer-provided syringe and safety needle. The foil pouch containing the syringe should not be opened until the patient has arrived for the injection, and the safety needle should not be attached until just prior to administration. The injection should be inspected visually for discoloration and particulate matter prior to administration; the injection should appear clear, viscous, and colorless to yellow to amber. The injection should be discarded if stored at room temperature for longer than 7 days. Injections should be made into the abdomen between the transpyloric and transtubercular planes at a site with adequate subcutaneous tissue that is free of skin conditions (e.g., nodules, lesions, excessive pigmentation). Injections should not be made into areas that are irritated, reddened, bruised, infected, or scarred. It is recommended that injections be made with the patient in the supine position. Injection sites should be rotated.

Following administration, the injection forms a solid depot from which buprenorphine is gradually released. Patients should be advised that a lump may be present at the injection site for several weeks and that it will decrease in size over time. Patient should be instructed that they should not rub or massage the injection site or allow belts or waistbands to rub the site. Injection sites should be monitored for signs of infection and for evidence of tampering or attempted depot removal. A depot can be excised surgically, if necessary, under local anesthesia within 14 days of injection.

Subdermal Implants for Opiate Dependence. For maintenance treatment of opiate dependence in patients who have achieved and maintained prolonged clinical stability on a low to moderate dosage of an oral transmucosal buprenorphine-containing preparation, buprenorphine hydrochloride implants are inserted subdermally in the inner aspect of the upper arm. Clinicians must successfully complete required training and become certified prior to prescribing buprenorphine implant therapy; those performing implant insertion or removal procedures must successfully complete training on these procedures and be certified to perform implant insertion. Patients must be monitored to ensure that buprenorphine implants are removed by a clinician with appropriate certification, and clinicians must maintain documentation of implant insertion and removal in each patient's medical record. A surgical specialist consulted to assist with a difficult implant removal does not require certification.

Each buprenorphine dose consists of 4 implants that are intended to be left in place for 6 months and then removed by the end of the sixth month. If continued implant therapy is desired at the time the initial implants are removed, new implants may be inserted subdermally in the contralateral arm. After one insertion in each arm, most patients should be transitioned back to oral transmucosal buprenorphine therapy, since experience is lacking with insertion of implants into other sites in the arm or with insertion of new implants at prior administration sites. The manufacturer's prescribing information should be consulted for proper methods of implant insertion and removal and associated precautions. The presence of each implant should always be verified by palpation or, if necessary, by ultrasound or magnetic resonance imaging (MRI) immediately after insertion and prior to attempted removal.

Proper implant placement is essential to avoid serious complications and to facilitate removal. (See Implant Complications under Cautions: Precautions and Contraindications.) The implant site should be examined one week following insertion for signs of infection, adequacy of wound healing, and evidence of implant extrusion. If an implant is expelled spontaneously, the expelled portion should be measured to ensure that it is intact; any partial implant remaining in the patient's arm should be removed, and the incision site should be examined for infection and to determine whether the remaining implants should be removed. A replacement for the expelled implant may be inserted in the same arm medially or laterally to the existing implants or, alternatively, in the contralateral arm.

Sublingual Administration **Sublingual Preparations for Opiate Dependence.** For management of opiate dependence, buprenorphine hydrochloride is administered sublingually as a single agent (as sublingual tablets) or in fixed combination with naloxone hydrochloride (as sublingual tablets and sublingually dissolving strips). Buprenorphine/naloxone sublingually dissolving strips (Suboxone®) may be administered either sublingually or buccally during maintenance treatment of opiate dependence; however, sublingual administration of this formulation is recommended during induction therapy to minimize exposure to naloxone and reduce the risk of withdrawal. (See Dosage Adjustments When Switching Between Oral Transmucosal Strengths and Preparations under Dosage: Opiate Dependence, in Dosage and Administration.)

Buprenorphine or buprenorphine/naloxone sublingual tablets are placed under the tongue and allowed to dissolve. Drinking warm fluids prior to administration may aid dissolution. For doses requiring multiple tablets, patients are advised to place all the tablets under the tongue at once. Alternatively, patients may place 2 tablets under the tongue at a time if they are unable to place more than 2 tablets comfortably under the tongue. Patients should continue to hold the tablets under the tongue until the tablets dissolve. If sequential administration is preferred, patients should adhere to the same manner of dosing with continued use to ensure consistent bioavailability. The median dissolution time for buprenorphine/naloxone (Zubsolv®) sublingual tablets is 5 minutes.

Buprenorphine/naloxone sublingually dissolving strips are placed under the tongue, on either side near the base of the tongue. The strip(s) should be kept under the tongue until completely dissolved; drinking water prior to administration may aid dissolution. Up to 2 strips may be administered at one time and should be placed under opposite sides of the tongue in a way that minimizes overlapping. When more than 2 strips are required to complete the dose, additional strips may be administered after the first 2 strips have dissolved. Strips should not be moved after placement.

To ensure consistency in bioavailability, patients should follow a consistent manner of administration. Proper administration technique should be demonstrated to the patient. The sublingual tablet or strip must be administered whole and should not be cut. Patients should not eat or drink until the tablet or strip is completely dissolved. Talking while the tablet or strip is dissolving, chewing the tablet or strip, or swallowing the tablet or strip may affect absorption and, therefore, efficacy of the drug and should be avoided. Patients should be advised to keep unused sublingual tablets or strips containing buprenorphine out of sight and reach of children. After completion of sublingual buprenorphine therapy, patients should be advised to discard any remaining tablets or strips by removing the tablets or strips from their packaging and then flushing them down the toilet.

Buccal Administration **Buccal Preparations for Pain Management.** For the relief of pain severe enough to require daily, around-the-clock, long-term opiate analgesia and for which alternative treatment options are inadequate, buprenorphine hydrochloride is administered buccally every 12 hours as buccally dissolving strips (Belbuca®). The manufacturer states that this formulation is for buccal use only.

Immediately prior to administering buprenorphine buccally dissolving strips (Belbuca®), the patient must wet the inside of the cheek with the tongue or rinse the mouth with water to wet the area for placement. The strip is then applied immediately after removal from the individually sealed package with the yellow side of the strip placed against the inside of the cheek, where it will adhere to the moist mucosa. The entire strip should be held in place with clean, dry fingers for 5 seconds and then left in place until fully dissolved (usually within 30 minutes). The strip should not be applied to areas of the mouth with open sores or lesions. The strip should not be manipulated with the tongue or fingers; eating and drinking should be avoided until the strip has dissolved. Chewing or swallowing the strip may result in lower peak plasma concentrations and reduced bioavailability of the drug. The strip should not be used if the package seal is broken or the strip is cut, damaged, or altered in any way. Proper administration technique should be demonstrated to the patient.

Patients should be advised to keep the strips out of sight and reach of children. Any strips that are no longer needed should be removed from their packaging and flushed down the toilet.

Buccal Preparations for Opiate Dependence. For the management of opiate dependence, buprenorphine/naloxone is administered buccally as buccally dissolving strips (Bunavail®). Sublingually dissolving strips containing buprenorphine/naloxone (Suboxone®) may be administered either sublingually or buccally during maintenance treatment of opiate dependence; however, sublingual administration of this formulation is recommended during induction therapy to minimize exposure to naloxone and reduce the risk of withdrawal. To ensure consistency in bioavailability, patients should follow a consistent manner of administration.

Immediately prior to administering buprenorphine/naloxone buccally dissolving strips (Bunavail®), the patient should wet the inside of the cheek with the tongue or rinse the mouth with water to moisten the area for placement. The strip is then applied immediately after removal from the individually sealed package. The strip should be held by clean, dry fingers with the text on the strip facing up and then placed against the inside of the cheek with the text side against the cheek; the strip should be pressed in place for 5 seconds. If a second strip is required to complete the dose, it should be placed on the inside of the other cheek immediately after the first strip is administered. When multiple strips are required, no more than 2 strips should be applied to the inside of one cheek at a time. The strip should not be manipulated with the tongue or fingers; eating and drinking should be avoided until the strip has dissolved. The strip must be administered whole and should not be cut or torn. Chewing or swallowing the strip may alter absorption and should be avoided.

For buccal administration of buprenorphine/naloxone sublingually dissolving strips (Suboxone®), one strip is placed on the inside of the right or left cheek. If a second strip is required to complete the dose, it is placed on the inside of the opposite cheek. If a third strip is required, it is placed on the inside of the right or left cheek after the first 2 strips have dissolved. Strips should not be moved after placement and must be left in place on the inside of the cheek until completely dissolved. Eating and drinking should be avoided until the strip has completely dissolved. The strip must be administered whole and should not be cut. Talking while the strip is dissolving, chewing the strip, or swallowing the strip may affect absorption and, therefore, efficacy of the drug and should be avoided.

Patients should be advised to keep the strips out of sight and reach of children. Any strips that are no longer needed should be removed from their packaging and flushed down the toilet.

Transdermal Administration **Transdermal System for Pain Management.** For the relief of pain severe enough to require daily, around-the-clock, long-term opiate analgesia and for which alternative treatment options are inadequate, buprenorphine is administered transdermally. Each buprenorphine transdermal system is intended to be worn continuously for 7 days; subsequent systems should be applied to a different site after removal of the previous system. The manufacturer recommends an interval of at least 21 days between applications to a particular site, since more frequent application at the same site may result in variable absorption. Rotation among 8 recommended application sites (4 on each side of the body) is advised.

Patients receiving buprenorphine transdermal systems should be carefully instructed in the proper use and disposal of the transdermal system. The transdermal system should not be used if the seal of the package is broken or if the system is cut, damaged, or altered in any way. The transdermal system should be removed from the sealed pouch and the protective-liner covering should be peeled and discarded just prior to application of the system. The transdermal system should be applied to a dry, intact, nonirritated, hairless or nearly hairless surface on the upper chest, upper back, side of chest, or upper outer arm on either side of the body by firmly pressing the system by hand for 15 seconds with the adhesive side touching the skin and ensuring that contact is complete, particularly around the edges. If 2 systems are applied for a single dose, the systems should be applied adjacently at the same site and should always be applied and removed at the same time. If needed, hair at the application site should be clipped, not shaved, prior to application of the transdermal system. If the site must be cleansed prior to application, only water should be used. Soaps, oils, lotions, alcohol, or abrasive devices could alter the absorption of buprenorphine and should not be used.

If a system should inadvertently come off during the period of use, a new system may be applied to a different skin site and left in place for 7 days. Patients who experience difficulty with system adhesion should be advised that they may tape the edges of the system in place with first-aid tape. If adhesion problems persist, patients may apply a transparent, waterproof or semipermeable adhesive film dressing that is suitable for 7 days of wear (e.g., Bioclusive®, Tegaderm®) over the system.

Although incidental exposure to water (e.g., while showering or bathing) is acceptable, the transdermal system should not be exposed to external heat sources, hot water, or prolonged direct sunlight. Patients should be advised to avoid sunbathing, taking hot baths, or exposing the application site and surrounding area to direct external heat sources (e.g., heating pads, electric blankets, heat or tanning lamps, saunas, hot tubs, heated water beds) while wearing the transdermal system, since temperature-dependent increases in percutaneous absorption of buprenorphine from the system are possible under such conditions and may result in fatal overdosage.

Patients should be advised to keep both used and unused buprenorphine transdermal systems out of the reach of children. The manufacturer states that immediately following removal, used systems should be properly discarded. In addition, following completion of a course of transdermal buprenorphine therapy, any unused systems should be removed from the package and properly discarded. Systems to be discarded should be folded carefully so that the adhesive side adheres to itself and then should be flushed down the toilet; transdermal systems may be disposed in the trash only after the system has been sealed in the manufacturer-supplied disposal unit. If the drug-containing adhesive matrix accidentally contacts the skin, the affected area should be washed with water; soap, alcohol, or other solvents should not be used to cleanse the area since they actually may enhance percutaneous absorption of bupreno rphine. Patients or caregivers should always wash their hands after applying or handling a buprenorphine transdermal system.

■ **Dosage** Dosage of buprenorphine and buprenorphine hydrochloride usually is expressed in terms of buprenorphine. Dosage of buprenorphine hydrochloride subdermal implants may be expressed as either the salt or the base.

Pain Opiate analgesics should be given at the lowest effective dosage and for the shortest duration of therapy consistent with the treatment goals of the patient. Initial dosage of buprenorphine should be individualized according to severity of pain, response, prior analgesic use, and risk factors for addiction, abuse, and misuse. Appropriate dosage selection and titration are essential to reduce the risk of respiratory depression. Overestimation of the dosage of buprenorphine when transferring patients from other opiate therapy to buprenorphine therapy can result in fatal overdosage with the first dose. Patients should be monitored closely for respiratory depression, especially during the first 24–72 hours of therapy and following any increase in dosage, and dosage should be adjusted accordingly. If concomitant therapy with other CNS depressants is required, the lowest effective dosages and shortest possible duration of concomitant therapy should be used. (See Drug Interactions: Benzodiazepines and Other CNS Depressants.)

For acute pain not related to trauma or surgery, the prescribed quantity should be limited to the amount needed for the expected duration of pain severe enough to require opiate analgesia (generally 3 days or less and rarely more than 7 days).

When opiate analgesics are used for the management of chronic noncancer pain, the US Centers for Disease Control and Prevention (CDC) recommends that primary care clinicians carefully reassess individual benefits and risks before prescribing dosages equivalent to 50 mg or more of morphine sulfate daily and avoid dosages equivalent to 90 mg or more of morphine sulfate daily or carefully justify their decision to titrate the dosage to such levels. Other experts recommend consulting a pain management specialist before exceeding a dosage equivalent to 80–120 mg of morphine sulfate daily. Some states have set prescribing limits (e.g., maximum daily dosages that can be prescribed, dosage thresholds at which consultation with a specialist is mandated or recommended).

Parenteral Dosage. For the relief of pain that is severe enough to require opiate analgesia and for which alternative treatments are inadequate, the usual IM or IV dosage of buprenorphine in patients 13 years of age and older is 0.3 mg given at intervals of up to every 6 hours as necessary. The initial dose (up to 0.3 mg) may be repeated once in 30–60 minutes, if needed. The dose should be limited to the minimum amount required in high-risk patients (e.g., geriatric or debilitated patients, those with respiratory disease) and in patients receiving other CNS depressants, including patients in the immediate postoperative period (see Respiratory and CNS Depression and also Concomitant Use of Benzodiazepines or Other CNS Depressants under Cautions: Precautions and Contraindications). Particular caution is necessary if the drug is administered IV, especially with initial doses. In some patients, it may be necessary to increase the dose up to 0.6 mg, but the manufacturer recommends that such relatively high doses *only* be administered IM and *only* to adults who are not considered high-risk patients. In some patients, a dosing interval greater than 6 hours may be adequate. For the management of postoperative pain, a recommended regimen is an initial dose of 0.3 mg IM, repeated once after 30–60 minutes and then every 4–6 hours as necessary. Alternatively, a regimen including an initial dose of 0.3 mg of buprenorphine followed by another 0.3-mg dose repeated in 3 hours has been shown to be as effective as a single 0.6-mg dose in relieving postoperative pain. There are insufficient clinical data to recommend single doses greater than 0.6 mg for long-term use.

Although children 2–12 years of age have received parenteral buprenorphine dosages of 2–6 mcg/kg every 4–6 hours, longer dosing intervals (e.g., every 6–8 hours) may be sufficient for some children, and a fixed around-the-clock dosing interval should not be used until an adequate dosing interval has been established by clinical observation of the patient. In addition, the manufacturer states that there are insufficient data in children 2–12 years of age to recommend buprenorphine doses exceeding 6 mcg/kg or administration of a repeat dose within 30–60 minutes of the initial dose.

When buprenorphine has been administered by continuous IV infusion† in the management of postoperative pain, dosages of 25–250 mcg/hour have been used in adults.

Buprenorphine has been administered epidurally† in the management of postoperative pain in single doses of 60 mcg, up to a mean total dose of 180 mcg administered over a 48-hour period. Buprenorphine has also been administered epidurally† in a dose of 0.3 mg as a supplement to surgical anesthesia with a local anesthetic. In the management of severe, chronic pain (e.g., in terminally ill patients), buprenorphine doses of 0.15–0.3 mg have been administered epidurally as frequently as every 6 hours up to a mean total daily dose of 0.86 mg (range: 0.15–7.2 mg).

The manufacturer states that data are insufficient to recommend a parenteral buprenorphine dosage for infants younger than 2 years of age. In children 9 months to 9 years of age† undergoing circumcision, some clinicians have used an initial IM buprenorphine dose of 3 mcg/kg as an adjunct to surgical anesthesia followed by additional 3-mcg/kg doses as necessary to provide analgesia postoperatively.

Transdermal Dosage. Buprenorphine transdermal system should be prescribed only by clinicians who are knowledgeable in the use of potent opiates for the management of chronic pain. Dosages of 7.5, 10, 15, and 20 mcg/hour should be reserved for patients who are opiate experienced (i.e., have been receiving oral morphine sulfate dosages of up to 80 mg or more daily [or equivalent] for one week or longer) and have developed tolerance to an opiate of comparable potency.

In opiate-naive adults with pain that is severe enough to require daily, around-the-clock, long-term opiate analgesia and for which alternative treatments are inadequate, treatment with transdermal buprenorphine should be initiated at a dosage of 5 mcg/hour.

When patients currently receiving opiate agonist therapy are switched to transdermal buprenorphine, there is a potential for buprenorphine to precipitate withdrawal. In these patients, the current opiate regimen should be tapered over a period of up to 7 days to a total 24-hour dosage equivalent to 30 mg or less of oral morphine sulfate. For patients whose prior total daily dosage of opiates was less than 30 mg of oral morphine sulfate (or equivalent), transdermal buprenorphine may be initiated at a dosage of 5 mcg/hour. For patients whose prior total daily dosage was 30–80 mg of oral morphine sulfate (or equivalent), transdermal buprenorphine may be initiated at a dosage of 10 mcg/hour. Patients may receive supplemental short-acting analgesics as needed until adequate analgesia is attained. For patients whose prior total daily dosage exceeded 80 mg of oral morphine sulfate (or equivalent), buprenorphine 20 mcg/hour may not provide adequate analgesia and an alternative analgesic should be considered. When therapy with a buprenorphine transdermal system is initiated, all other around-the-clock opiate analgesics should be discontinued. Buprenorphine may be initiated at the next dosing interval following discontinuance of the current opiate regimen. Particularly close monitoring is required when patients are switched from methadone, since conversion ratios between methadone and other opiates vary widely depending on extent of prior methadone exposure and because methadone has a long half-life and tends to accumulate in plasma.

Buprenorphine dosage may be titrated upward at minimum intervals of 72 hours to a level that provides adequate analgesia and minimizes adverse effects. The maximum recommended transdermal dosage of buprenorphine is 20 mcg/hour, since higher dosages have been shown to prolong the QT interval (see Cautions: Cardiovascular Effects). Dosage may be adjusted in increments of 5, 7.5, or 10 mcg/hour by simultaneously applying no more than two 5-, 7.5-, or 10-mcg/hour systems; the total combined dosage of the 2 transdermal systems should not exceed 20 mcg/hour.

Patients should be reevaluated continually for adequacy of pain control and for adverse effects, as well as for the development of addiction, abuse, or misuse. Patients who experience episodes of breakthrough pain may require dosage adjustment or supplemental analgesia (i.e.," rescue" therapy with an immediate-release analgesic). If the level of pain increases after dosage stabilization, an attempt should be made to identify the source of increased pain before increasing the dosage. Frequent communication is important among the prescriber, other members of the healthcare team, the patient, and the patient's caregiver or family during periods of changing analgesic requirements, including the initial dosage titration period. During long-term therapy, the continued need for opiate analgesics should be periodically reevaluated. If unacceptable adverse effects are observed, dosage reduction should be considered.

When the patient no longer requires buprenorphine therapy, the dosage should be tapered gradually every 7 days to prevent symptoms of opiate withdrawal. The use of an appropriate short-acting opiate may be considered during the tapering process. Therapy with buprenorphine transdermal system should not be discontinued abruptly.

Buccal Dosage. Buprenorphine hydrochloride buccally dissolving strips (Belbuca®) should be prescribed only by clinicians who are knowledgeable in the use of potent opiates for the management of chronic pain.

For the management of pain that is severe enough to require daily, around-the-clock, long-term opiate analgesia and for which alternative treatments are inadequate, treatment with buprenorphine bucally dissolving strips should be initiated at a dosage of 75 mcg once daily or, if tolerated, 75 mcg every 12 hours in adults who are opiate-naive or are not tolerant to opiates. After at least 4 days at this initial dosage, dosage may be increased to 150 mcg every 12 hours. Use of higher initial dosages in patients who are not opiate tolerant may cause fatal respiratory depression.

When patients currently receiving opiate agonist therapy are switched to intrabuccal buprenorphine, there is a potential for buprenorphine to precipitate withdrawal. In these patients, the current opiate regimen should be tapered to a total 24-hour dosage equivalent to 30 mg or less of oral morphine sulfate. For patients whose prior total daily dosage of opiates was less than 30 mg of oral morphine sulfate (or equivalent), intrabuccal buprenorphine may be initiated at a dosage of 75 mcg once daily or 75 mcg every 12 hours. For patients whose prior total daily dosage was 30–89 mg of oral morphine sulfate (or equivalent), intrabuccal buprenorphine may be initiated at a dosage of 150 mcg every 12 hours. For those whose prior total daily dosage was 90–160 mg of oral morphine sulfate (or equivalent), intrabuccal buprenorphine may be initiated at a dosage of 300 mcg every 12 hours. Patients may receive supplemental short-acting analgesics as needed until adequate analgesia is attained. For patients whose prior total daily dosage exceeded 160 mg of oral morphine sulfate (or equivalent), buprenorphine buccally dissolving strips may not provide adequate analgesia and an alternative analgesic should be considered. When therapy with buprenorphine buccally dissolving strips is initiated, all other around-the-clock opiate analgesics should be discontinued. Particularly close monitoring is required when patients are switched from methadone, since conversion ratios between methadone and other opiates vary widely depending on extent of prior methadone exposure and because methadone has a long half-life and tends to accumulate in plasma.

Buprenorphine dosage may be titrated upward in increments of no more than 150 mcg every 12 hours at minimum intervals of 4 days to a level that provides adequate analgesia and minimizes adverse effects. Doses of 600, 750, and 900 mcg should be used only following titration from lower intrabuccal dosages. Dosages of up to 450 mcg every 12 hours were studied in opiate-naive patients in clinical trials. The maximum recommended intrabuccal dosage is 900 mcg every 12 hours because of the risk of QT-interval prolongation (see Cautions: Cardiovascular Effects); if this dosage fails to provide adequate analgesia, an alternative analgesic should be considered.

Patients should be reevaluated continually for adequacy of pain control and for adverse effects, as well as for the development of addiction, abuse, or misuse. Patients who experience episodes of breakthrough pain may require dosage adjustment or supplemental analgesia (i.e.," rescue" therapy with an immediate-release analgesic). If the level of pain increases after dosage stabilization, an attempt should be made to identify the source of increased pain before increasing the dosage. Frequent communication is important among the prescriber, other members of the healthcare team, the patient, and the patient's caregiver or family during periods of changing analgesic requirements, including the initial dosage titration period. During long-term therapy, the continued need for opiate analgesics should be periodically reevaluated. If unacceptable adverse effects are observed, dosage should be adjusted to obtain an appropriate balance between pain control and adverse effects.

In patients with known or suspected mucositis, the usual initial dosage and each incremental dosage during titration should be reduced by one-half because of the potential for higher peak concentrations and systemic exposure to the drug. (See Oral Transmucosal Formulations Used for Analgesia under Pharmacokinetics: Absorption.)

When the patient no longer requires buprenorphine therapy, the dosage should be tapered gradually to prevent symptoms of opiate withdrawal. Intrabuccal therapy with buprenorphine should not be discontinued abruptly. If manifestations of withdrawal occur, the dosage should be increased to the prior level and tapered more slowly by increasing the interval between dosage reductions and/or reducing the amount of each incremental change in dose.

For further information on the management of opiate analgesic therapy, see Dosage and Administration: Dosage, in the Opiate Agonists General Statement 28:08.08.

Opiate Dependence Buprenorphine and buprenorphine/naloxone are prescribed and distributed in the management of opiate dependence (opiate use disorder) under a restricted distribution program. (See Dosage and Administration: Restricted Distribution Program for Buprenorphine Treatment of Opiate Dependence.)

Oral transmucosal preparations containing buprenorphine or buprenorphine/naloxone may be used during induction and/or maintenance phases of treatment, while buprenorphine extended-release subcutaneous injection and buprenorphine subdermal implants are used only during maintenance. Because all oral transmucosal formulations are *not* bioequivalent, dosage recommendations vary according to differences in bioavailability. Recommended dosage ranges (based on the buprenorphine component) are the same for generic buprenorphine sublingual tablets (i.e., generic equivalents of Subutex® sublingual tablets [branded formulation no longer commercially available in the US]), generic buprenorphine/naloxone sublingual tablets (i.e., generic equivalents of Suboxone® sublingual tablets [branded formulation no longer commercially available in the US]), and buprenorphine/naloxone sublingually dissolving strips (Suboxone®), although some strengths and dose combinations of these preparations are not bioequivalent. Dosage ranges for certain other oral transmucosal buprenorphine/naloxone preparations (i.e., Bunavail® buccally dissolving strips, Zubsolv® sublingual tablets) are lower, reflecting the greater bioavailability of these preparations. (See Dosage Adjustments When Switching Between Oral Transmucosal Strengths and Preparations under Dosage: Opiate Dependence, in Dosage and Administration.) Although generic buprenorphine/naloxone sublingual tablets are labeled in the US only for maintenance treatment, this formulation also has been used (similarly to other oral transmucosal buprenorphine/naloxone preparations) in the induction† phase of treatment.

Presence of naloxone, an opiate antagonist, in the fixed-combination preparation is intended to deter parenteral abuse of buprenorphine by individuals dependent on other opiates since a sufficient amount of the opiate antagonist is present in the formulation to precipitate opiate withdrawal if administered parenterally (but not sublingually). When administered sublingually, systemic naloxone concentrations are insufficient to elicit clinically important effects; in addition, sublingual administration of buprenorphine and buprenorphine/naloxone has been shown to elicit similar clinical, physiologic, and subjective effects.

Although buprenorphine traditionally has been considered the preferred drug for the initial (i.e., induction) phase of treatment, additional experience indicates that either buprenorphine or buprenorphine/naloxone may be used for induction in patients dependent on heroin or other short-acting opiates. Use of buprenorphine/naloxone for the induction phase of treatment in patients dependent on long-acting opiates has not been evaluated to date in adequate and well-controlled studies; the manufacturers and some experts still recommend use of buprenorphine alone for induction in these patients. Following induction, buprenorphine/naloxone is the preferred drug for maintenance treatment when use includes unsupervised administration. Administration of buprenorphine without naloxone in an unsupervised setting should be limited to pregnant women and patients who cannot tolerate naloxone. (See Dosage and Administration: Dosage in Hepatic Impairment and also see Pregnancy under Cautions: Pregnancy, Fertility, and Lactation.)

Prior to induction, the type of opiate dependence (i.e., long- or short-acting opiate), time since last opiate use, and degree of opiate dependence should be considered. Abuse of long-acting formulations by manipulation of the dosage form (e.g., crushing and snorting or injecting extended-release oral dosage forms) may cause these formulations to act as short-acting drugs. To avoid precipitating withdrawal, the first dose of buprenorphine or buprenorphine/naloxone should be given when objective and clear signs of opiate withdrawal are evident.

In individuals dependent on heroin or other short-acting opiates, the manufacturers state that the first dose of buprenorphine or buprenorphine/naloxone should be administered at least 4 or 6 hours, respectively, after the last use of the opiate. Some experts recommend waiting at least 6–12 hours after last use of short-acting opiates and recommend use of an opiate withdrawal scale (e.g., Clinical Opioid Withdrawal Scale [COWS] score of approximately 11–12 or higher) to establish that withdrawal is sufficient to allow for safe and comfortable induction. Administration of a low initial dose of buprenorphine or buprenorphine/naloxone also reduces the risk of precipitated withdrawal. Because gradual titration of buprenorphine dosage over several days has been associated with a high dropout rate during the induction phase in clinical studies, an adequate treatment dosage, titrated to clinical effectiveness, should be achieved as rapidly as possible once it has been established that the initial dose of the drug was well tolerated.

Patients dependent on methadone or other long-acting opiates may be more susceptible than those who are dependent on short-acting opiates to precipitated and prolonged withdrawal during induction. Therefore, the first dose of buprenorphine should be given when objective and clear signs of opiate withdrawal are evident, generally not less than 24 hours after the last use of the opiate. Controlled experience with the transfer of patients from methadone maintenance to buprenorphine is limited. Withdrawal symptoms appear to be more likely in those receiving higher dosages of methadone hydrochloride (greater than 30 mg daily) and when the first dose of buprenorphine is given shortly after the last methadone dose. Thus, dosage of methadone hydrochloride should be tapered to approximately 30–40 mg daily or less and maintained at this level for at least a week prior to induction. Experts state that the first dose of buprenorphine may be administered at least 24–72 hours or longer after last use of long-acting opiates such as methadone and recommend use of an opiate withdrawal scale (e.g., COWS score of approximately 11–12 or higher) to establish that withdrawal is sufficient to allow for safe and comfortable induction.

Induction in the prescribing clinician's office is recommended to reduce the risk of precipitated withdrawal; unsupervised administration may then be initiated as the patient's clinical stability allows. Although large, randomized, controlled studies are lacking, experts state that at-home induction (with early in-office follow-up) by patients dependent on short-acting opiates may be considered depending on the patient's circumstances if the patient and/or clinician is experienced with the use of buprenorphine and the patient can rate withdrawal symptoms, fully understand induction dosing instructions, and can and will contact the clinician as needed.

Patients receiving maintenance treatment should be seen at reasonable intervals (e.g., at least weekly during the first months of therapy) based on the individual's circumstances; once patients are receiving a stable buprenorphine dosage and are progressing toward treatment goals, less frequent (e.g., monthly) visits may be reasonable. Prescription quantities for unsupervised administration should take into account the patient's clinical stability, home situation, and ability to manage take-home medication. Authorization of multiple refills is not advised early in treatment or without appropriate follow-up visits. Review of state prescription drug monitoring program (PDMP) data for other prescribed drugs of concern, urine drug testing, and recall visits for "pill" counts also are recommended. If treatment goals are not being achieved, the appropriateness of the current therapy should be reevaluated. Unstable patients (e.g., those who are abusing or are dependent on various drugs or are unresponsive to psychosocial interventions) may require referral for more intensive treatment.

For the maintenance treatment of opiate dependence, oral transmucosal preparations of buprenorphine/naloxone are labeled only for once-daily administration; however, other dosage regimens (i.e., administration every other day† or 3 times weekly† at a dose higher than the individually titrated daily dose) have been used once satisfactory stabilization has been achieved.

Dosage of Lower-bioavailability Oral Transmucosal Formulations for Induction and Maintenance. When generic buprenorphine sublingual tablets (i.e., generic equivalents of Subutex® sublingual tablets), generic buprenorphine/naloxone sublingual tablets (i.e., generic equivalents of Suboxone® sublingual tablets), or buprenorphine/naloxone sublingually dissolving strips (Suboxone®) are used for induction therapy, the recommended induction dosage of buprenorphine on day 1 is up to 8 mg (alone or in fixed combination with up to 2 mg of naloxone). Induction should be initiated on day 1 with a buprenorphine dose of 2 or 4 mg (alone or in fixed combination with naloxone 0.5 or 1 mg, respectively), with additional doses of 2 or 4 mg administered at approximately 2-hour intervals if there are continued withdrawal symptoms and sedation is not observed. Use of an opiate withdrawal scale (e.g., COWS) during induction can be helpful in assessing the effects of administered doses. On day 2, a single dose of up to 16 mg of buprenorphine (alone or in fixed combination with up to 4 mg of naloxone) is given. Other induction dosages that also employ a low initial dose with rapid titration to an effective maintenance dosage have been used.

For oral transmucosal maintenance treatment, buprenorphine/naloxone is preferred over buprenorphine alone. (See initial paragraphs of Opiate Dependence under Dosage and Administration: Dosage.) From day 3 onward, buprenorphine/naloxone dosage should be adjusted in increments or decrements of 2 or 4 mg of buprenorphine in fixed combination with 0.5 or 1 mg, respectively, of naloxone daily to a dosage that suppresses opiate withdrawal symptoms and ensures that the patient continues buprenorphine treatment. The maintenance buprenorphine/naloxone dosage generally ranges from 4–24 mg of buprenorphine in fixed combination with 1–6 mg of naloxone daily. The recommended buprenorphine/naloxone target dosage during maintenance treatment is 16 mg of buprenorphine and 4 mg of naloxone as a single daily dose. Dosages exceeding 24 mg of buprenorphine in fixed combination with 6 mg of naloxone daily have not been shown to provide any additional clinical advantage.

Zubsolv® Dosage for Induction and Maintenance. When Zubsolv® sublingual tablets are used for induction and maintenance treatment, the recommended induction dosage on day 1 is up to 5.7 mg of buprenorphine in fixed combination with up to 1.4 mg of naloxone. Induction should be initiated with a buprenorphine/naloxone dose of 1.4 mg of buprenorphine in fixed combination with 0.36 mg of naloxone, with the remainder of the day 1 dosage (up to 4.2 mg of buprenorphine and up to 1.08 mg of naloxone) administered in divided doses as 1 or 2 tablets containing buprenorphine 1.4 mg and naloxone 0.36 mg at intervals of 1.5–2 hours. Some patients (e.g., those who recently received buprenorphine) may tolerate up to 3 tablets containing buprenorphine 1.4 mg and naloxone 0.36 mg as a single second dose. On day 2, a single dose of up to 11.4 mg of buprenorphine and 2.9 mg of naloxone is recommended.

From day 3 onward, buprenorphine/naloxone dosage should be adjusted in increments or decrements of no more than 2.9 mg of buprenorphine and 0.71 mg of naloxone to a level that suppresses opiate withdrawal symptoms and ensures that the patient continues buprenorphine treatment. After induction and stabilization, the maintenance buprenorphine/naloxone dosage generally ranges from 2.9–17.2 mg of buprenorphine in fixed combination with 0.71–4.2 mg of naloxone daily. The recommended buprenorphine/naloxone target dosage during maintenance treatment is 11.4 mg of buprenorphine and 2.9 mg of naloxone as a single daily dose. Dosages exceeding 17.2 mg of buprenorphine in fixed combination with 4.2 mg of naloxone daily have not been shown to provide any additional clinical advantage.

Bunavail® Dosage for Induction and Maintenance. When Bunavail® buccally dissolving strips are used for induction and maintenance treatment, the recommended induction dosage on day 1 is up to 4.2 mg of buprenorphine in fixed combination with up to 0.7 mg of naloxone. Induction should be initiated with a buprenorphine/naloxone dose of 2.1 mg of buprenorphine in fixed combination with 0.3 mg of naloxone; a second dose of the same strength is administered approximately 2 hours later based on control of acute withdrawal symptoms. On Day 2, a single dose of up to 8.4 mg of buprenorphine in fixed combination with 1.4 mg of naloxone is recommended.

From day 3 onward, buprenorphine/naloxone dosage should be adjusted in increments or decrements of 2.1 mg of buprenorphine and 0.3 mg of naloxone to a level that suppresses opiate withdrawal symptoms and ensures that the patient continues buprenorphine treatment. After induction and stabilization, the maintenance buprenorphine/naloxone dosage generally ranges from 2.1–12.6 mg of buprenorphine in fixed combination with 0.3–2.1 mg of naloxone daily. The recommended buprenorphine/naloxone target dosage during maintenance treatment is 8.4 mg of buprenorphine and 1.4 mg of naloxone as a single daily dose. Dosages exceeding 12.6 mg of buprenorphine in fixed combination with 2.1 mg of naloxone daily have not been shown to provide any additional clinical advantage.

Dosage Adjustments When Switching Between Oral Transmucosal Strengths and Preparations. Not all formulations, strengths, or dose combinations of oral transmucosal buprenorphine/naloxone preparations are bioequivalent.

Patients who currently are receiving generic buprenorphine or buprenorphine/naloxone sublingual tablets (i.e., generic equivalents of Subutex® or Suboxone® sublingual tablets) and are switching to buprenorphine/naloxone sublingually dissolving strips (Suboxone®), or vice versa, should continue to receive the same drug dosage. However, not all strengths and dose combinations of the strips and sublingual tablets are bioequivalent. Because of potentially greater bioavailability with the strips relative to the tablets, patients should be monitored for underdosage (e.g., manifestations of withdrawal) or overdosage when switching between sublingual dosage forms and the dosage should be adjusted when indicated. (See Oral Transmucosal Formulations Used for Treatment of Opiate Dependence under Pharmacokinetics: Absorption.)

The 4 strengths of Suboxone® sublingually dissolving strips differ in size and buprenorphine and naloxone concentrations (on a % [w/w] basis). Switching between various combinations of lower- and higher-strength strips to obtain the same total dose may result in changes in systemic exposure to buprenorphine and naloxone and require that the patient be monitored for underdosage or overdosage. Therefore, substitution of one or more strip strengths for another without the prescriber's approval is not recommended. Because systemic exposure to naloxone is somewhat higher after buccal compared with sublingual administration of the strips, sublingual administration is recommended during induction to minimize the risk of precipitated withdrawal. However, exposure to buprenorphine is similar following either buccal or sublingual administration, and once induction is complete, patients can switch between buccal and sublingual administration without substantial risk of underdosage or overdosage.

Bunavail® and Zubsolv® have different bioavailabilities than Suboxone® (or generic equivalent) sublingual tablets. Patients switching between these preparations should receive a different dosage strength (see Table 1 and Table 2) and should be monitored for underdosage or overdosage. Dosage adjustments may be necessary. Systemic buprenorphine exposure following administration of one Suboxone® sublingual tablet containing buprenorphine 8 mg and naloxone 2 mg is equivalent to that achieved following administration of one Bunavail® buccally dissolving strip containing buprenorphine 4.2 mg and naloxone 0.7 mg or one Zubsolv® sublingual tablet containing buprenorphine 5.7 mg and naloxone 1.4 mg. (See Oral Transmucosal Formulations Used for Treatment of Opiate Dependence under Pharmacokinetics: Absorption.)

Table 1. Corresponding Doses and Strengths of Suboxone® Sublingual Tablets and Bunavail® Buccally Dissolving Strips

Suboxone® Sublingual Dose or Tablet Strength	Corresponding Bunavail® Strip Strength
Buprenorphine 4 mg and naloxone 1 mg	Buprenorphine 2.1 mg and naloxone 0.3 mg
Buprenorphine 8 mg and naloxone 2 mg	Buprenorphine 4.2 mg and naloxone 0.7 mg
Buprenorphine 12 mg and naloxone 3 mg	Buprenorphine 6.3 mg and naloxone 1 mg

Table 2. Corresponding Dosage Strengths of Suboxone® Sublingual Tablets (or Generic Equivalent) and Zubsolv® Sublingual Tablets

Suboxone® (or Generic Equivalent) Sublingual Dose (Tablet Strength)	Corresponding Zubsolv® Sublingual Tablet Strength
Buprenorphine 2 mg and naloxone 0.5 mg (as one 2-mg/0.5-mg tablet)	One 1.4-mg/0.36-mg tablet
Buprenorphine 4 mg and naloxone 1 mg (as two 2-mg/0.5-mg tablets)	One 2.9-mg/0.71-mg tablet
Buprenorphine 8 mg and naloxone 2 mg (as one 8-mg/2-mg tablet)	One 5.7-mg/1.4-mg tablet
Buprenorphine 12 mg and naloxone 3 mg (as one 8-mg/2-mg tablet and two 2-mg/0.5-mg tablets)	One 8.6-mg/2.1-mg tablet
Buprenorphine 16 mg and naloxone 4 mg (as two 8-mg/2-mg tablets)	One 11.4-mg/2.9-mg tablet

Extended-release Subcutaneous Injection Dosage for Maintenance Treatment. Maintenance treatment with buprenorphine extended-release subcutaneous injection may be initiated in patients who have initiated buprenorphine induction therapy with an oral transmucosal buprenorphine-containing preparation followed by dosage adjustment over a least 7 days to an oral transmucosal buprenorphine dosage of 8–24 mg daily (as Subutex® or Suboxone® [or equivalent generic buprenorphine or buprenorphine/naloxone preparation]) or a dosage of another oral transmucosal preparation that provides equivalent buprenorphine exposure. One Bunavail® buccally dissolving strip containing buprenorphine 4.2 mg and naloxone 0.7 mg or one Zubsolv® sublingual tablet containing buprenorphine 5.7 mg and naloxone 1.4 mg provides equivalent buprenorphine exposure as one Suboxone® sublingual tablet containing buprenorphine 8 mg and naloxone 2 mg or one Subutex® sublingual tablet containing buprenorphine 8 mg.

The recommended dosage of buprenorphine extended-release subcutaneous injection following induction and dosage adjustment with oral transmucosal buprenorphine is 300 mg monthly for the first 2 months followed by a maintenance dosage of 100 mg monthly. The maintenance dosage may be increased to 300 mg monthly in patients who tolerate the 100-mg monthly dosage but do not achieve a satisfactory clinical response, as evidenced by self-reports or urine drug test results indicating illicit opiate use. If a dose is missed, the dose should be administered as soon as possible, with the following dose given no less than 26 days later. Occasional delays in dosing of up to 2 weeks are not expected to substantially alter the treatment effect. If a subcutaneous depot of the drug must be surgically excised, the patient should be monitored for manifestations of withdrawal and appropriate treatment (e.g., an oral transmucosal preparation of the drug) should be instituted as clinically indicated.

Implant Dosage for Maintenance Treatment. Maintenance treatment with buprenorphine subdermal implants may be initiated in patients who have achieved and maintained prolonged clinical stability on oral transmucosal buprenorphine therapy; are currently receiving an oral transmucosal buprenorphine maintenance dosage of 8 mg daily or less (as Subutex® or Suboxone® [or equivalent generic buprenorphine or buprenorphine/naloxone preparation] or a dosage of another oral transmucosal preparation that provides comparable blood buprenorphine concentrations [e.g., Bunavail® buccally dissolving strips at a dosage of buprenorphine 4.2 mg and naloxone 0.7 mg daily or less, Zubsolv® sublingual tablets at a dosage of buprenorphine 5.7 mg and naloxone 1.4 mg daily or less]); *and* have received a stable oral transmucosal buprenorphine maintenance dosage of 8 mg daily or less for at least 3 months without the need for supplemental doses of the drug or dosage adjustments. The dosage of oral transmucosal buprenorphine should not be tapered to this dosage level solely for the purpose of transitioning to implant therapy. The 8-mg oral transmucosal dosage provides blood buprenorphine concentrations that are similar to or less than those provided by the recommended implant dosage.

Each buprenorphine dose consists of 4 implants (each containing 80 mg of buprenorphine hydrochloride [equivalent to 74.2 mg of the base]) inserted subdermally in the inner aspect of the upper arm; the implants are intended to be left in place for 6 months and then removed by the end of the sixth month. If continued implant therapy is desired at the time the initial implants are removed, new implants may be inserted subdermally in the contralateral arm. If new implants are not inserted on the same day that the current ones are removed, patients should receive their previous dosage of oral transmucosal buprenorphine (i.e., the dosage they received prior to initiation of implant therapy) prior to additional implant therapy. After one insertion in each arm, most patients should be transitioned back to oral transmucosal buprenorphine therapy, since experience is lacking with insertion of implants at other sites in the arm or with insertion of new implants at prior administration sites (where potential effects of scarring and fibrosis on efficacy and safety are unknown).

Although some patients may require occasional supplemental dosing with buprenorphine, the manufacturer states that patients should not be provided with prescriptions for oral transmucosal buprenorphine-containing preparations for use on as-needed basis. Instead, patients who feel the need for supplemental dosing should be evaluated promptly by a clinician. An ongoing need for supplemental dosing indicates that the amount of buprenorphine delivered by the implants is not adequate for stable maintenance treatment; use of an alternative buprenorphine preparation for maintenance treatment should be considered. If an implant is expelled spontaneously, the patient should be carefully monitored until the implant is replaced for withdrawal manifestations or other indications that supplemental oral transmucosal dosing may be required.

Discontinuance. The decision to discontinue therapy with buprenorphine or buprenorphine/naloxone after a period of maintenance or brief stabilization should be made as part of a comprehensive treatment plan. Oral transmucosal dosage should be tapered to reduce the occurrence of withdrawal manifestations. Dosage generally is tapered over several months with close monitoring and a plan for sustaining recovery.

If therapy with buprenorphine extended-release subcutaneous injection is discontinued, the patient should be monitored for several months for manifestations of withdrawal, since the onset of any withdrawal manifestations may be delayed; if treatment of withdrawal manifestations is required, use of oral transmucosal buprenorphine should be considered. In clinical trials, withdrawal manifestations were not observed during the first month following discontinuance of treatment with buprenorphine extended-release subcutaneous injection. Plasma concentrations of buprenorphine may be detectable for 12 months or longer if therapy with this formulation is discontinued after steady state has been achieved (4–6 months of treatment); the correlation between plasma and detectable urine concentrations of buprenorphine is not known.

If therapy with buprenorphine implants is discontinued, the patient should be monitored for manifestations of withdrawal and use of a tapering dosage of oral transmucosal buprenorphine should be considered.

Other Uses To reverse fentanyl-induced anesthesia† and provide subsequent analgesia in adults, IV or IM buprenorphine doses of 0.3–0.8 mg have been administered 1–4 hours following induction of anesthesia and about 30 minutes prior to the end of surgery.

■ Restricted Distribution Program for Buprenorphine Treatment of Opiate Dependence The Drug Addiction Treatment Act of 2000 (DATA 2000) allows qualifying physicians to prescribe and dispense narcotics in schedules III, IV, and V of the Federal Controlled Substances Act that have been approved by FDA for detoxification or maintenance treatment of opiate dependence. The Comprehensive Addiction and Recovery Act of 2016 (CARA 2016) expands the categories of practitioners through October 1, 2021, to include qualifying nurse practitioners and physician assistants. Prior to passage of DATA 2000, opiate dependence treatment could be provided only at specially registered clinics. Under DATA 2000 and CARA 2016, prescription use of buprenorphine and buprenorphine/naloxone in the treatment of opiate dependence is limited to practitioners who meet certain requirements, have notified the Secretary of the US Department of Health and Human Services (HHS) of their intent to prescribe these preparations for this indication, and have been assigned a unique identification number that must be included on each prescription for the drug. (See Risk Evaluation and Mitigation Strategies under Dosage and Administration: Administration.)

Prescribers DATA 2000 limited office-based use of buprenorphine and buprenorphine/naloxone for the management of opiate dependence to physicians who meet special training criteria and can provide appropriate services. CARA 2016 expanded the categories of practitioners to include qualifying nurse practitioners and physician assistants. To qualify, physicians must meet one or more of the following training requirements: hold a subspecialty board certification in addiction psychiatry from the American Board of Medical Specialties; hold subspecialty board certification in addiction medicine from the American Osteopathic Association; hold an addiction certification from the American Society of Addiction Medicine; have completed not less than 8 hours of authorized training on the management or treatment of opiate-dependent patients; have participated as an investigator in one or more clinical trials leading to the approval of a schedule III, IV, or V opiate for maintenance or detoxification treatment; and/or have other training or experience that is deemed by HHS or the state medical licensing board to demonstrate the physician's ability to treat and manage opiate-dependent patients. To quality, nurse practitioners and physician assistants must meet all of the following requirements: be authorized under state law to prescribe schedule III, IV, or V drugs for pain management; work in collaboration with or be supervised by a qualifying physician if so required by state law; and have completed not less than 24 hours of authorized initial training. In addition, practitioners must have the capacity to provide or to refer patients for needed ancillary services (i.e., psychosocial therapy) and must agree to prescribe schedule III, IV, or V drugs for management of opiate dependence for a limited number of patients. Before prescribing buprenorphine or buprenorphine/naloxone, practitioners who meet these criteria must notify the HHS Substance Abuse and Mental Health Services Administration (SAMHSA) of their intention to prescribe these agents.

Initially, each qualifying practitioner, whether practicing individually or in a group practice, can treat no more than 30 patients at one time. Practitioners who have been certified to treat opiate dependence with buprenorphine for at least 1 year can apply to treat up to 100 patients at one time. Those who have been eligible to treat up to 100 patients at a time for at least one year without interruption can apply to increase the limit to 275 patients if they have additional credentialing or practice in a qualified setting. In addition, practitioners who currently are eligible to treat up to 100 patients but who otherwise are not eligible to increase their patient limit to 275 may request a temporary increase in certain emergency situations.

The US Drug Enforcement Administration (DEA) will issue qualifying practitioners a unique identification number; this number indicates that the practitioner is qualified under DATA 2000 or CARA 2016 to prescribe buprenorphine for the management of opiate dependence and is intended to preserve the confidentiality of the patient. The SAMHSA Center for Substance Abuse Treatment will inform the practitioner of the new DEA identification number in writing via email. The DEA requires inclusion of the new identification number along with the practitioner's usual DEA number on all prescriptions issued for the treatment of opiate dependence. Although it is anticipated that most prescribers will obtain DEA identification numbers before prescribing buprenorphine or buprenorphine/naloxone for such use, DATA 2000 allows practitioners with qualifying credentials and/or training to write prescriptions for these agents before the DEA identification number is issued if the practitioner has notified SAMHSA of their intention to begin treating a patient immediately and has verified that SAMHSA received the notification form. Immediate treatment is limited to one patient per notification form, and no more than one form may be submitted on a given day.

Practitioners should be aware that there are special federal regulations concerning confidentiality of substance abuse treatment records and the privacy of health records. Any patient-identifying information pertaining to treatment of substance abuse must be handled with a greater degree of confidentiality than patients' general medical information. Before a prescriber can disclose any information to a third party about a patient's treatment for substance abuse, that prescriber must obtain the patient's signed consent. Each disclosure made with the patient's consent must be accompanied by a statement indicating that unauthorized disclosure is prohibited.

Dispensing Pharmacies Each time a pharmacist fills a prescription for buprenorphine or buprenorphine/naloxone, the pharmacist is expected to verify that the prescription is from a prescriber who is in compliance with the provisions of DATA 2000. Practitioners who are qualified to prescribe buprenorphine and buprenorphine/naloxone and are in compliance with DATA 2000 are issued a *unique* DEA identification number; the new identification number along with the practitioner's usual DEA number is required on all prescriptions issued for the treatment of opiate dependence. If a prescription is phoned to the pharmacy, pharmacists must ensure that both numbers are on the prescription record. Pharmacists may utilize SAMHSA's online look-up tool (at https://www.samhsa.gov/bupe/lookup-form) or contact 866-287-2728 to verify whether a prescriber is in compliance with the provisions of DATA 2000.

If a pharmacist receives a prescription for buprenorphine or buprenorphine/naloxone that does not include the *unique* DEA identification number, the pharmacist should contact the prescriber for clarification and to confirm that the prescriber has notified SAMHSA of their intention to prescribe the drug. Pharmacists also may contact SAMHSA (at infobuprenorphine@samhsa.hhs.gov or 866-287-2728). It is anticipated that most prescribers will obtain DEA identification numbers before prescribing buprenorphine or buprenorphine/naloxone. However, DATA 2000 allows practitioners with qualifying credentials and/or training to write prescriptions for these agents before the DEA identification number is issued if the practitioner has notified SAMHSA of their intention to begin treating a patient immediately.

Pharmacists should be aware that there are special federal regulations concerning confidentiality of substance abuse treatment records and the privacy of health records. Any patient-identifying information pertaining to treatment of substance abuse must be handled with a greater degree of confidentiality than patients' general medical information. Before a prescriber can disclose any information to a third party about a patient's treatment for substance abuse, the prescriber must obtain the patient's signed consent. When a prescriber directly transmits a prescription for a buprenorphine-containing preparation for treatment of substance abuse to a pharmacy, the patient's signed consent must be obtained before any patient-identifying information is further disclosed by the pharmacy.

With the availability of buprenorphine for outpatient management of opiate dependence, many pharmacists have the opportunity to provide services that focus on ensuring appropriate drug administration, monitoring for adverse effects, alleviating withdrawal symptoms, treating intercurrent illnesses, minimizing diversion, and aiding in the prevention of relapse.

A potential problem with take-home outpatient opiate agonist treatment is diversion. While the addition of naloxone is intended to decrease the potential for parenteral abuse of the combination preparations, the possibility of diversion exists because the drug may be used by opiate-dependent individuals in an attempt to attenuate withdrawal symptoms when illicit substances (e.g., heroin) are not available. In addition, individuals who are not opiate dependent may acquire buprenorphine for the purpose of getting high. To address diversion, patients may be asked on a random, unannounced basis to return to the clinic or pharmacy for verification of tablet counts. Since diversion is a concern, pharmacists should be alert for signs of this activity, including presentation of simultaneous prescriptions for the same patient from multiple prescribers, requests for additional doses or refills prior to the appropriate date, calls from opiate-dependent individuals who are not patients, and accidental loss or destruction of the drug. It is important to report any suspicion of diversion to the appropriate authorities.

■ **Dosage in Hepatic Impairment** Transdermal buprenorphine has not been studied in patients with severe hepatic impairment; use of an alternative analgesic regimen that allows for greater dosage flexibility should be considered in these patients.

When buprenorphine buccally dissolving strips (Belbuca®) are used for analgesia in patients with severe hepatic impairment (i.e., Child-Pugh class C), the usual initial dosage should be reduced and each incremental change in dosage during titration should be reduced by one-half (i.e., from 150 mcg to 75 mcg). No dosage adjustment is required in patients with moderate hepatic impairment, but patients with either moderate or severe hepatic impairment should be monitored for overdosage and toxicity.

When buprenorphine or buprenorphine/naloxone is used sublingually or buccally for the management of opiate dependence in patients with mild hepatic impairment, plasma concentrations and half-lives of the drugs are not substantially altered. However, in individuals with moderate or severe hepatic impairment, plasma concentrations of both buprenorphine and naloxone are increased and half-lives of the drugs are prolonged. Naloxone is affected to a greater degree than buprenorphine, and the magnitude of the difference in effect is greater in individuals with severe hepatic impairment than in those with moderate hepatic impairment. (See Pharmacokinetics: Elimination.) This may result in an increased risk of precipitated withdrawal during induction and interference with buprenorphine's efficacy throughout treatment. Buprenorphine/naloxone should be avoided in patients with severe hepatic impairment and may not be appropriate for those with moderate hepatic impairment. In patients with moderate hepatic impairment, buprenorphine/naloxone is not recommended for induction therapy but may be used with caution and careful monitoring for maintenance treatment following induction therapy with buprenorphine alone. The manufacturer states that the initial dose and titration increments of buprenorphine administered as the single-entity sublingual tablets should be reduced by one-half in patients with severe hepatic impairment and recommends that patients with either moderate or severe hepatic impairment be monitored for buprenorphine overdosage or toxicity.

Use of buprenorphine extended-release subcutaneous injection or buprenorphine subdermal implants is not recommended in patients with preexisting moderate to severe hepatic impairment since the extended-release injection does not allow for rapid adjustment of plasma buprenorphine concentrations and the implant dosage cannot be titrated.

Cautions

Adverse effects of buprenorphine are qualitatively similar to those of morphine, meperidine, and the opiate partial agonists (e.g., pentazocine, nalbuphine); however, the frequency of specific adverse effects produced by buprenorphine may differ from that of the various opiate agonists and partial agonists. Certain adverse effects of buprenorphine, including nausea, vomiting, CNS effects, and respiratory depression, appear to be dose and plasma concentration related. In opiate-tolerant patients, this relationship may be altered by the development of tolerance to opiate-related adverse effects; however, tolerance to opiate effects does not develop uniformly.

When administered sublingually, the adverse effect profile of buprenorphine is similar to that of buprenorphine in fixed combination with naloxone (buprenorphine/naloxone). Sublingually dissolving strips and sublingual tablets containing buprenorphine/naloxone generally have similar adverse effect profiles. Following buccal administration of buprenorphine/naloxone sublingually dissolving strips, the adverse effect profile is similar to that observed following sublingual administration.

■ **Nervous System Effects** Buprenorphine may cause CNS depression, including somnolence, dizziness, alterations in judgment, and alterations in levels of consciousness, including coma.

Sedation (e.g., drowsiness) is the most common adverse effect of parenteral buprenorphine, occurring in approximately two-thirds of patients; however, patients reportedly are easily aroused to an alert state. Dizziness and vertigo have been reported in about 5–10% of patients receiving parenteral buprenorphine. Headache has been reported in about 1–5% of these patients. Confusion, euphoria, weakness, fatigue, nervousness, mental depression, slurred speech, paresthesia, dreaming, psychosis, malaise, hallucinations, depersonalization, and coma have been reported in less than 1% of patients receiving parenteral buprenorphine for pain relief. Lightheadedness, insomnia, and disorientation have also occurred. Seizures, muscle twitching, lack of muscle coordination, ataxia, dysphoria, and agitation have been reported rarely. Psychotomimetic effects occur less frequently in patients receiving buprenorphine than in patients receiving pentazocine but more frequently than in patients receiving morphine.

Buprenorphine has the potential to lower the seizure threshold and may aggravate seizure disorders and induce seizures in some clinical settings.

Frequent adverse CNS effects reported in clinical trials in patients receiving transdermal buprenorphine include headache and dizziness (each occurring in about 5–15% of patients) and somnolence (occurring in up to 15% of patients). Fatigue, asthenia, insomnia, hypoesthesia, paresthesia, tremor, migraine, anxiety, and depression have been reported in about 1–5% of patients receiving transdermal buprenorphine. Other adverse nervous system effects reported in less than 1% of patients receiving transdermal buprenorphine include affect lability, agitation, apathy, confusional state, abnormal coordination, depersonalization, depressed mood, disorientation, attention disturbance, dysarthria, euphoric mood, gait disturbance, hallucination, loss of consciousness, depressed level of consciousness, malaise, memory impairment, mental impairment, mental status changes, nervousness, nightmare, psychotic disorder, restlessness, sedation, and vertigo.

In clinical trials in patients receiving buprenorphine buccally dissolving strips for pain relief, fatigue, headache, dizziness, and somnolence were reported in at least 5% of patients receiving the buccally administered drug; anxiety, insomnia, and depression were reported in 1 to less than 5% of patients; and asthenia, hypoesthesia, lethargy, migraine, and tremor were reported in less than 1% of patients.

Adverse nervous system effects reported in clinical trials in patients receiving sublingual buprenorphine or buprenorphine/naloxone for the treatment of opiate dependence include headache, insomnia, anxiety, depression, irritability, restlessness, asthenia, dizziness, nervousness, and somnolence. Intoxication and disturbance in attention also have been reported. In clinical trials in patients receiving buprenorphine/naloxone buccally dissolving strips, headache and lethargy were reported in at least 5% of patients, and insomnia, somnolence, and fatigue were reported in more than 1 to less than 5% of patients.

In phase 3 clinical trials, headache, fatigue, somnolence, sedation, and dizziness were reported in less than 10% of patients receiving buprenorphine extended-release subcutaneous injection.

In phase 3 clinical trials, headache and depression were reported in 6–13% and dizziness, somnolence, fatigue, asthenia, migraine, sedation, and paresthesia were reported in less than 5% of patients with buprenorphine subdermal implants.

■ **GI Effects** Nausea occurs in about 5–10% of patients receiving parenteral buprenorphine for pain relief and is accompanied by vomiting in about 1–5% of patients. Vomiting alone occurs in about 1–5% of these patients. The frequency of buprenorphine-induced nausea and vomiting appears to be higher in ambulatory patients. Dry mouth, constipation, dyspepsia, abdominal cramps, and flatulence have occurred in less than 1% of patients receiving parenteral buprenorphine. Anorexia and diarrhea have been reported rarely.

In clinical trials in patients receiving transdermal buprenorphine, the most frequent adverse GI effects were nausea (10–25% of patients), constipation (5–15%), vomiting (5–10%), and dry mouth (6%). Diarrhea, dyspepsia, stomach discomfort, anorexia, and upper abdominal pain have been reported in about 1–5% of patients receiving transdermal buprenorphine. Other adverse GI effects reported in less than 1% of patients receiving transdermal buprenorphine include abdominal distension, abdominal pain, diverticulitis, dysgeusia, dysphagia, flatulence, and ileus.

In clinical trials in patients receiving buprenorphine buccally dissolving strips for pain relief, nausea, constipation, vomiting, diarrhea, and dry mouth were reported in at least 5% of patients receiving the buccally administered drug; abdominal pain, decreased appetite, and gastroenteritis were reported in 1 to less than 5% of patients; and abdominal discomfort, dyspepsia, toothache, and tooth abscess were reported in less than 1% of patients.

Nausea, abdominal pain, constipation, vomiting, diarrhea, dyspepsia, and stomach discomfort have occurred in patients receiving sublingual buprenorphine or buprenorphine/naloxone for the treatment of opiate dependence in clinical trials. Oral hypoesthesia, glossodynia, glossitis, stomatitis, blistering and ulceration of the mouth or tongue, and oral mucosal erythema also have occurred with sublingual use of the drug. Constipation and oral mucosal erythema have been reported in less than 5% of patients receiving buprenorphine/naloxone buccally dissolving strips.

In phase 3 clinical trials, constipation, nausea, and vomiting were reported in about 5–9% of patients receiving buprenorphine extended-release subcutaneous injection.

Nausea, vomiting, constipation, upper abdominal pain, flatulence, and toothache were reported in phase 3 clinical trials in 1–6% of patients with buprenorphine subdermal implants.

■ **Hepatic Effects** Cytolytic hepatitis and hepatitis with jaundice have occurred in individuals receiving buprenorphine for the treatment of opiate dependence in clinical trials and during postmarketing experience. Adverse hepatic effects that have occurred in these individuals include transient asymptomatic elevations in serum hepatic aminotransferase concentrations, hepatic failure, hepatic necrosis, hepatorenal syndrome, and hepatic encephalopathy. In some individuals, preexisting hepatic enzyme abnormalities, hepatitis B virus (HBV) or hepatitis C virus (HCV) infection, concomitant use of potentially hepatotoxic drugs, or ongoing illicit use of injectable drugs may have contributed to or caused these adverse hepatic events. Data were insufficient in some cases to determine the etiology of the adverse event. The possibility exists that buprenorphine had a causative or contributory role in some of these adverse hepatic events. (See Hepatic Impairment under Cautions: Precautions and Contraindications.)

Increased ALT concentrations have been reported in clinical trials in less than 1% of patients receiving transdermal buprenorphine.

In clinical trials in patients receiving buprenorphine buccally dissolving strips for pain relief, increased AST concentration and liver function test abnormality were reported in less than 1% of patients receiving the buccally administered drug.

In phase 3 clinical trials, increased concentrations of ALT, AST, and γ-glutamyltransferase (GGT, γ-glutamyltranspeptidase, GGTP) were reported in about 1–5% of patients receiving buprenorphine extended-release subcutaneous injection.

■ Cardiovascular Effects Buprenorphine has the potential to prolong the QT interval. In a randomized, double-blind, placebo-controlled, single-dose study in 132 healthy adults, the effect of transdermal buprenorphine on the QT interval corrected for heart rate (QT_c) was evaluated under steady-state conditions (i.e., on day 3 of treatment with buprenorphine 10 mcg/hour and day 4 of treatment with buprenorphine 40 mcg/hour). Although the 10-mcg/hour dosage had no clinically meaningful effect on the QT_c interval, the 40-mcg/hour dosage prolonged the QT_c interval by a maximum of 9.2 msec. Therefore, the maximum recommended dosage of transdermal buprenorphine is 20 mcg/hour. In controlled and open-label clinical trials, prolongation of the QT_c interval (corrected for heart rate using Fridericia's formula) to 450–480 msec occurred in 2% of patients with chronic pain receiving buprenorphine buccally dissolving strips at dosages up to 900 mcg every 12 hours, which is the maximum recommended dosage of buccally dissolving strips. (See QT-Interval Prolongation under Cautions: Precautions and Contraindications.)

Hypotension has reportedly occurred in about 1–5% of patients receiving parenteral buprenorphine for pain relief. Other adverse cardiovascular effects, including hypertension, tachycardia, bradycardia, and ECG abnormalities manifested as Wenckebach period, have occurred in less than 1% of patients receiving parenteral buprenorphine for pain relief. Shock has occurred rarely.

Peripheral edema and hypertension have been reported in clinical trials in about 1–5% of patients receiving transdermal buprenorphine. Other adverse cardiovascular effects reported in less than 1% of patients receiving transdermal buprenorphine include hypotension, orthostatic hypotension, angina pectoris, bradycardia, palpitation, syncope, tachycardia, and vasodilation. Hypotension may be severe, especially in patients with blood volume depletion and those receiving concomitant therapy with dugs that may compromise vasomotor tone (e.g., phenothiazines).

In clinical trials in patients receiving buprenorphine buccally dissolving strips for pain relief, hypertension and peripheral edema were reported in 1 to less than 5% of patients receiving the buccally administered drug, and increased blood pressure and QT-interval prolongation were reported less than 1% of patients.

Vasodilation has occurred in patients receiving sublingual buprenorphine or buprenorphine/naloxone for the treatment of opiate dependence in clinical trials. Peripheral edema and palpitations also have been reported.

■ Respiratory Effects Respiratory depression (decreased rate and depth of respiration) may occur occasionally in patients receiving parenteral buprenorphine. (See Respiratory and CNS Depression under Cautions: Precautions and Contraindications.) Respiratory depression requiring active treatment has occurred in less than 1% of patients receiving parenteral buprenorphine for pain relief. Hypoventilation has been reported in about 1–5% of these patients. Dyspnea, cyanosis, and apnea have been reported in less than 1% of these patients. Hypoxemia has occurred rarely.

Dyspnea, cough, pharyngolaryngeal pain, upper respiratory infection, nasopharyngitis, influenza, sinusitis, and bronchitis have been reported in clinical trials in about 1–5% of patients receiving transdermal buprenorphine. Other adverse respiratory effects reported in less than 1% of patients receiving transdermal buprenorphine include aggravated asthma, rhinitis, hyperventilation, hypoventilation, abnormal respiration, respiratory depression, respiratory distress, respiratory failure, and wheezing.

In clinical trials in patients receiving buprenorphine buccally dissolving strips for pain relief, upper respiratory infection was reported in at least 5% of patients receiving the buccally administered drug; nasopharyngitis, sinusitis, bronchitis, oropharyngeal pain, and sinus congestion were reported in at least 1% of patients; and acute sinusitis, cough, dyspnea, nasal congestion, and rhinorrhea were reported in less than 1% of patients.

Rhinitis, rhinorrhea, increased cough, and pharyngitis have occurred in patients receiving sublingual buprenorphine or buprenorphine/naloxone for the treatment of opiate dependence in clinical trials. In clinical trials in patients receiving buprenorphine/naloxone buccally dissolving strips, rhinorrhea was reported in more than 1 to less than 5% of patients.

Oropharyngeal pain, cough, and dyspnea were reported in phase 3 clinical trials in 1–5% of patients with buprenorphine subdermal implants.

Naloxone and doxapram have been used to reverse buprenorphine-induced respiratory depression, but these agents may be only partially effective and, rarely, completely ineffective. (See Pharmacology: Respiratory Effects.) Consequently, the principal management of respiratory depression induced by the drug should be assisted or controlled respiration and administration of oxygen as necessary.

■ Sensitivity Reactions Acute and chronic hypersensitivity reactions have been reported in patients receiving buprenorphine. Rash, urticaria, and pruritus are the most common manifestations of these hypersensitivity reactions. Bronchospasm, angioedema, and anaphylactic shock also have occurred in patients receiving the drug.

Angioedema, hypersensitivity reaction, facial edema, and urticaria have been reported in clinical trials in less than 1% of patients receiving transdermal buprenorphine.

■ Ocular Effects Miosis occurs in about 1–5% of patients receiving parenteral buprenorphine. Blurred vision, diplopia, amblyopia, mydriasis, other visual abnormalities, and conjunctivitis have been reported in less than 1% of patients receiving parenteral buprenorphine for pain relief.

Dry eye, miosis, blurred vision, and visual disturbance have been reported in clinical trials in less than 1% of patients receiving transdermal buprenorphine.

Runny eyes, increased lacrimation, and blurred vision have been reported in patients receiving sublingual buprenorphine or buprenorphine/naloxone for the treatment of opiate dependence.

■ Dermatologic Effects Adverse dermatologic effects, including pruritus, reactions at the injection site, and rash, have occurred in less than 1% of patients receiving parenteral buprenorphine for pain relief. Urticaria has been reported rarely. Stevens-Johnson syndrome occurred in at least one patient receiving concomitant radiation and drug therapy that included parenteral buprenorphine; however, a causal relationship to buprenorphine was not established.

Application site reactions, including pruritus, erythema, rash, and irritation, have been reported in about 5–15% of patients receiving transdermal buprenorphine in clinical trials. Severe application site reactions with marked inflammation, characterized by burning, discharge, or vesicles occurring days to months after initiation of therapy, also have occurred rarely. Application site dermatitis, contact dermatitis, and dry skin have been reported in less than 1% of patients receiving transdermal buprenorphine.

In clinical trials in patients receiving buprenorphine buccally dissolving strips for pain relief, pruritus and rash were reported in 1 to less than 5% of patients receiving the buccally administered drug, and cellulitis was reported in less than 1% of patients.

In phase 3 clinical trials in patients receiving buprenorphine extended-release subcutaneous injection, the most frequent injection site reactions were pain, pruritus, and erythema (each occurring in about 5–7% of patients); induration at the injection site was reported in 1.4% of patients; and bruising, swelling, discomfort, cellulitis, and infection at the injection site were reported in less than 1% of patients.

Pain, pruritus, erythema, hematoma, hemorrhage, and edema at the implant site were reported in phase 3 clinical trials in 5–13% of patients with buprenorphine subdermal implants. Rash and skin lesion were reported in 1–2% of patients with buprenorphine implants.

■ Genitourinary and Endocrine Effects Urinary retention and decreased libido have been reported in less than 1% of patients receiving parenteral buprenorphine for pain relief. Flushing, hot flush, decreased libido, sexual dysfunction, urinary hesitancy, and urinary incontinence have been reported in less than 1% of patients receiving transdermal buprenorphine.

In clinical trials in patients receiving buprenorphine buccally dissolving strips for pain relief, urinary tract infection and hot flush were reported in 1 to less than 5% of patients receiving the buccally administered drug, and decreased blood testosterone concentration was reported in less than 1% of patients.

Adrenal insufficiency has been reported in patients receiving opiate agonists or opiate partial agonists. Manifestations of adrenal insufficiency are nonspecific and may include nausea, vomiting, anorexia, fatigue, weakness, dizziness, and hypotension. The onset generally has occurred after at least 1 month of opiate agonist or partial agonist use, although the time to onset has ranged from within 1 day to more than 1 year. In many of the reported cases, patients required hospitalization. If adrenal insufficiency is suspected, appropriate laboratory testing should be performed promptly and physiologic (replacement) dosages of corticosteroids provided; therapy with the opiate agonist or partial agonist should be tapered and discontinued to allow recovery of adrenal function. If the opiate agonist or partial agonist can be discontinued, follow-up assessment of adrenal function should be performed to determine if corticosteroid replacement therapy can be discontinued. In some patients, switching to a different opiate improved symptoms.

Hypogonadism and androgen deficiency have been reported in patients receiving long-term opiate agonist or opiate partial agonist therapy, although a causal relationship has not been established. Patients receiving long-term opiate agonist or partial agonist therapy who present with manifestations of hypogonadism (e.g., decreased libido, impotence, erectile dysfunction, amenorrhea, infertility) should undergo laboratory evaluation.

■ Other Adverse Effects Diaphoresis occurs in about 1–5% of patients receiving parenteral buprenorphine for pain relief. Other adverse effects reported in less than 1% of these patients include flushing and a sensation of warmth, tremor, chills and a sensation of cold, hiccups, tinnitus, and pallor. Increased pressure in the common bile duct has occurred in some patients receiving parenteral buprenorphine for pain relief. Decreases in erythrocyte count, hemoglobin, hematocrit, sedimentation rate, and total serum protein concentration have been reported during prolonged administration of buprenorphine (1–2 months), but these effects were reversible upon discontinuance of the drug. Serum alkaline phosphatase concentrations also decreased during prolonged buprenorphine therapy and were not reversible upon discontinuance; however, values remained within the normal range.

Hyperhidrosis, falls, pain (including pain in extremity, back, neck, or chest), pyrexia, urinary tract infection, joint swelling, arthralgia, muscle spasm, musculoskeletal pain, and myalgia have been reported in clinical trials in about 1–5% of patients receiving transdermal buprenorphine. Accidental injury, chills, dehydration, hiccups, muscle weakness, tinnitus, and weight loss have been reported in less than 1% of patients receiving transdermal buprenorphine.

In clinical trials in patients receiving buprenorphine buccally dissolving strips for pain relief, anemia, contusion, falls, hyperhidrosis, muscle spasm, back pain, and pyrexia were reported in 1 to less than 5% of patients receiving the buccally administered drug, and chills, excoriation, laceration, musculoskeletal pain, and neck pain were reported in less than 1% of patients.

Pain (including back pain), sweating, cold sweat, chills, fever, infection, abscess, flu syndrome, arthralgia, piloerection, and accidental injury have been reported in patients receiving sublingual buprenorphine or buprenorphine/naloxone for the treatment of opiate dependence in clinical trials. In clinical trials in patients receiving buprenorphine/naloxone buccally dissolving strips, chills and hyperhidrosis were reported in more than 1 to less than 5% of patients.

In clinical trials, increased creatine kinase (CK, creatine phosphokinase, CPK) concentration was reported in up to about 5% of patients receiving buprenorphine extended-release subcutaneous injection.

In phase 3 clinical trials, pain (including pain in back, chest, or extremity), pyrexia, chills, feeling cold, local swelling, laceration, excoriation, and scratch were reported in 1–6% of patients with buprenorphine subdermal implants.

■ **Opiate Withdrawal** Because of buprenorphine's antagonist activity, the drug may precipitate mild to moderate signs and symptoms of withdrawal in some patients physically dependent on opiates. Signs and symptoms of mild withdrawal may also appear following discontinuance of prolonged therapy with buprenorphine alone.

■ **Precautions and Contraindications** When the fixed-combination preparation containing buprenorphine and naloxone is used, the usual cautions, precautions, and contraindications associated with naloxone should be considered in addition to those associated with buprenorphine.

Addiction, Abuse, and Misuse Buprenorphine exposes patients and other users to the risks of opiate addiction, abuse, and misuse, which can lead to overdosage and death. Addiction can occur with appropriately prescribed or illicitly obtained opiate analgesics, and at recommended dosages or with misuse or abuse. Concurrent abuse of alcohol or other CNS depressants increases the risk of toxicity. Each patient's risk for addiction, abuse, and misuse should be assessed prior to initiating buprenorphine for analgesia, and all patients receiving the drug should be monitored for development of these behaviors or conditions. Personal or family history of substance abuse (drug or alcohol addiction or abuse) or mental illness (e.g., major depression) increases risk. The potential for addiction, abuse, and misuse should not prevent opiate prescribing for appropriate pain management, but does necessitate intensive counseling about risks and proper use and intensive monitoring for signs of addiction, abuse, and misuse. Buprenorphine should be prescribed for analgesia in the smallest appropriate quantity, and the patient should be instructed on secure storage and proper disposal to prevent theft.

When used for treatment of opiate dependence, buprenorphine should be prescribed and dispensed with appropriate precautions to minimize risk of misuse, abuse, or diversion, and to ensure appropriate protection from theft, including in the patient's home. Patients should be monitored for progression of opiate use disorder and addictive behaviors. Clinical monitoring appropriate to the patient's level of stability is essential. Multiple refills should not be authorized early in treatment or without appropriate patient follow-up visits.

Extended-release opiates (e.g., buprenorphine transdermal system) are associated with a greater risk of overdosage and death because of the larger amount of drug contained in each dosage unit. Abuse or misuse of the transdermal system by placing it in the mouth, chewing it, swallowing it, or using it in other unintended ways may cause choking, overdosage, and death.

Abuse or misuse of buprenorphine buccally dissolving strips by swallowing the strips may cause choking, overdosage, and death.

Buprenorphine subdermal implants that protrude from the skin or have been expelled are subject to misuse and abuse.

Respiratory and CNS Depression Serious, life-threatening, or fatal respiratory depression may occur in patients receiving opiates, including buprenorphine, even when used as recommended. Although respiratory depression can occur at any time during therapy, the risk is greatest during initiation of therapy and following an increase in dosage; therefore, patients receiving buprenorphine should be monitored closely for respiratory depression, especially during the first 24–72 hours of therapy and following any increase in dosage. Appropriate dosage selection and titration are essential to reduce the risk of respiratory depression. Large initial doses in nontolerant patients, overestimation of the initial buprenorphine dosage when transferring patients from another opiate analgesic, or accidental exposure to buprenorphine, especially by a child, can result in respiratory depression and death. (See Accidental Exposure under Cautions: Precautions and Contraindications.)

The risk of respiratory depression is increased when opiates, including buprenorphine, are used concomitantly with other agents that cause respiratory depression. Many postmarketing reports of coma and death have involved misuse of buprenorphine by self-injection or were associated with the concomitant use of buprenorphine and benzodiazepines or other CNS depressants, including alcohol. (See Concomitant Use of Benzodiazepines or Other CNS Depressants under Cautions: Precautions and Contraindications.)

Carbon dioxide retention from opiate-induced respiratory depression can exacerbate the drug's sedative effects and, in certain patients, can lead to elevated intracranial pressure. (See Increased Intracranial Pressure or Head Injury under Cautions: Precautions and Contraindications.)

Geriatric, cachectic, or debilitated patients are at increased risk of life-threatening respiratory depression. In patients with chronic obstructive pulmonary disease or cor pulmonale, substantially decreased respiratory reserve, hypoxia, hypercapnia, or preexisting respiratory depression, even recommended doses of buprenorphine may decrease respiratory drive to the point of apnea. Such patients should be monitored closely, particularly following initiation of therapy, during dosage titration, and during concomitant therapy with other respiratory depressants. Alternatively, use of nonopiate analgesics should be considered in such patients. Use of buprenorphine formulations labeled for analgesic use is contraindicated in patients with substantial respiratory depression and in those with severe bronchial asthma in unmonitored settings or in the absence of resuscitative equipment.

If therapy with buprenorphine extended-release subcutaneous injection is discontinued because of compromised respiratory function, the patient should be monitored for continued buprenorphine effects for several months.

When opiate analgesics are prescribed for patients at increased risk of opiate overdosage (e.g., those with a history of overdose or substance use disorder, those receiving opiate dosages equivalent to 50 mg or more of morphine sulfate daily, those receiving benzodiazepines concomitantly, those with medical conditions that could increase sensitivity to opiate effects), some experts state that clinicians should consider offering naloxone. Since naloxone and doxapram may be only partially effective in reversing buprenorphine-induced respiratory depression, the use of assisted or controlled respiration may be necessary and should be considered the principal method of management.

Concomitant Use of Benzodiazepines or Other CNS Depressants Concomitant use of opiate agonists or opiate partial agonists and benzodiazepines or other CNS depressants (e.g., anxiolytics, sedatives, hypnotics, tranquilizers, muscle relaxants, general anesthetics, antipsychotics, other opiates, alcohol) may result in profound sedation, respiratory depression, coma, and death. Concomitant use of opiate analgesics and benzodiazepines or other CNS depressants should be reserved for patients in whom alternative treatment options are inadequate; the lowest effective dosages and shortest possible duration of concomitant therapy should be used, and the patient should be monitored closely for respiratory depression and sedation. Patients receiving buprenorphine and/or their caregivers should be apprised of the risks associated with concomitant therapeutic or illicit use of benzodiazepines, alcohol, or other CNS depressants. Concomitant use with alcohol should be avoided. (See Drug Interactions: Benzodiazepines and Other CNS Depressants.)

Because the morbidity and mortality associated with untreated opiate addiction can outweigh the serious risks associated with concomitant use of opiate agonists or partial agonists and benzodiazepines or other CNS depressants, buprenorphine treatment for opiate addiction (i.e., medication-assisted treatment [MAT]) should not be categorically withheld from patients receiving benzodiazepines or other CNS depressants. These drugs should be tapered and discontinued, if possible, in patients receiving MAT. However, excluding or discharging patients from MAT because of benzodiazepine or CNS depressant use is not likely to prevent such concomitant use and may lead to use outside the treatment setting, which could result in more severe outcomes. Careful management can reduce the risks associated with concomitant use of benzodiazepines or other CNS depressants in patients receiving buprenorphine treatment for opiate addiction. Benzodiazepines are not the treatment of choice for anxiety or insomnia in patients receiving buprenorphine treatment for opiate addiction; other pharmacologic or nonpharmacologic therapies should be considered. Current evidence does not support dose limitations or other arbitrary limits on buprenorphine as a strategy for addressing concomitant benzodiazepine or other CNS depressant use in patients receiving MAT. However, in patients who are sedated at the time of a scheduled buprenorphine dose, the cause of sedation should be evaluated and omission or reduction of the buprenorphine dose may be appropriate.

Precautions for minimizing risks associated with concomitant use of benzodiazepines or other CNS depressants in patients receiving MAT include the following:

- Patient education upon initiation of MAT regarding the risks associated with concomitant use of benzodiazepines or other CNS depressants;
- Development of strategies upon initiation of MAT for managing any prescribed or illicit use of benzodiazepines or other CNS depressants;
- Verification of the diagnosis in any patient receiving prescribed benzodiazepines or other CNS depressants for anxiety or insomnia, and consideration of other treatment options for these conditions;
- Possible adjustment of induction procedures and more intensive monitoring;
- Recognition that MAT may be required indefinitely and should be continued for as long as the patient derives benefit and MAT contributes to the intended treatment goals;

- Coordination of care to minimize risks and ensure that other prescribers are aware that the patient is receiving buprenorphine treatment; and
- Measures to confirm that prescribed drugs are being used as intended and are not being diverted or supplemented with illicit drugs;
- Toxicology screening to monitor for prescribed or illicit drug use.

Selection of an Appropriate Formulation Oral transmucosal preparations of buprenorphine that are intended for use in the treatment of opiate dependence should *not* be used for analgesia. Fatal overdosage has been reported following administration of 2 mg of sublingual buprenorphine for analgesia in opiate-naive individuals. Buprenorphine extended-release subcutaneous injection also should not be used in opiate-naive individuals. Safety and efficacy of transdermal buprenorphine for the management of opiate dependence have not been established.

Accidental Exposure Accidental exposure to buprenorphine can cause severe, possibly fatal, respiratory depression in children. Buprenorphine-containing preparations are involved in a disproportionate share of unsupervised prescription drug and opiate ingestions by children younger than 6 years of age. From 2004–2011, buprenorphine was involved in an estimated 24% of emergency department visits involving accidental opiate ingestion by children 1–5 years of age. Other surveillance data for 2010–2011 indicate that buprenorphine was involved in approximately 30% of emergency department visits and 60% of emergent hospitalizations involving opiate ingestion by children younger than 6 years of age. The surveillance data for 2010–2011 also indicate that approximately 96% of the reported emergency department visits involving buprenorphine ingestion in this age group involved buprenorphine/naloxone. Buprenorphine-containing preparations should be stored out of the sight and reach of children. Used transdermal systems and any drug that is no longer needed should be disposed of appropriately. Any subdermal implant that has been expelled from the skin should be kept away from others, especially from children.

QT-Interval Prolongation Prolongation of the QT interval corrected for heart rate (QT_c) has occurred in some patients receiving buprenorphine in clinical trials. In controlled and open-label clinical trials, prolongation of the QT_c interval (corrected for rate using Fridericia's formula) to 450–480 msec occurred in 2% of patients with chronic pain receiving buprenorphine buccally dissolving strips at dosages up to 900 mcg every 12 hours. In healthy adults, transdermal buprenorphine given in a dosage of 40 mcg/hour prolonged the QT interval. These findings should be taken into account when considering buprenorphine therapy in patients with hypokalemia, hypomagnesemia, or clinically unstable cardiac disease (e.g., unstable atrial fibrillation, symptomatic bradycardia, unstable congestive heart failure, active myocardial ischemia). Periodic ECG monitoring is recommended in such patients. Use of buprenorphine should be avoided in patients with a personal or family (i.e., immediate family member) history of long QT syndrome and in patients who are receiving class IA (e.g., quinidine, procainamide, disopyramide) or class III (e.g., sotalol, amiodarone, dofetilide) antiarrhythmic agents or other drugs known to prolong the QT interval. The maximum dosage of transdermal buprenorphine should not exceed 20 mcg/hour, and the maximum dosage of buprenorphine administered as buccally dissolving strips (Belbuca®) should not exceed 900 mcg every 12 hours.

Opiate Withdrawal Misuse of oral transmucosal preparations of buprenorphine/naloxone via parenteral injection by individuals who are physically dependent on opiates is likely to produce marked and intense opiate withdrawal symptoms. (See Pharmacology: Opiate Agonist and Antagonist Properties.)

Because of buprenorphine's opiate antagonist activity, it may precipitate withdrawal in patients physically dependent on opiates if administered before the agonistic effects of the full opiate agonist have subsided. To avoid precipitating withdrawal symptoms in patients currently receiving opiate analgesia, the dosage of the current opiate analgesic should be tapered to a dosage equivalent to no more than 30 mg daily of oral morphine sulfate prior to switching to buprenorphine. In patients initiating buprenorphine therapy for opiate dependence, induction therapy should be initiated when objective and clear signs of opiate withdrawal are evident. Prior to receiving therapy with buprenorphine implants or buprenorphine extended-release subcutaneous injection, patients should be stabilized on oral transmucosal therapy with the drug. (See Opiate Dependence under Dosage and Administration: Dosage.)

Because abrupt discontinuance of buprenorphine or rapid reduction in dosage may result in withdrawal symptoms in patients who are physically dependent on the drug, dosage should be tapered gradually when therapy with the drug is discontinued. (See Dosage and Administration: Dosage.)

Prolonged maternal use of opiates during pregnancy can result in neonatal opiate withdrawal syndrome. (See Clinical Experience under Pregnancy, Fertility, and Lactation: Pregnancy, in Cautions.)

Hepatic Impairment Since buprenorphine is metabolized in the liver, the activity of the drug may be increased and/or prolonged in patients with hepatic impairment. Buprenorphine injection should be used with caution in patients with severe hepatic impairment. When buprenorphine buccally dissolving strips are used for analgesia, dosage adjustment is recommended in patients with severe hepatic impairment, and patients with either moderate or severe hepatic impairment should be monitored for toxicity or overdosage. Because buprenorphine transdermal system is intended for 7-day application, use of an alternative analgesic regimen that allows for greater dosage flexibility should be considered in patients with severe hepatic impairment.

When oral transmucosal preparations of buprenorphine or buprenorphine/naloxone are used for the management of opiate dependence in patients with moderate or severe hepatic impairment, plasma concentrations of buprenorphine and naloxone are increased and half-lives of the drugs are prolonged. Naloxone is affected to a greater degree than buprenorphine, and the magnitude of the difference in effect is greater in individuals with severe hepatic impairment than in those with moderate hepatic impairment. (See Pharmacokinetics: Elimination.) This may result in an increased risk of precipitated withdrawal during the induction phase of treatment and interference with buprenorphine's efficacy throughout treatment. Buprenorphine/naloxone should be avoided in patients with severe hepatic impairment and may not be appropriate for those with moderate hepatic impairment. In patients with moderate hepatic impairment, buprenorphine/naloxone is not recommended for induction therapy but may be used with caution and careful monitoring for maintenance treatment following induction therapy with buprenorphine alone. Dosage adjustment of sublingual buprenorphine is recommended in patients with severe hepatic impairment, and patients with either moderate or severe hepatic impairment who are receiving the single-entity sublingual tablets should be monitored for toxicity or overdosage.

Use of buprenorphine extended-release subcutaneous injection or buprenorphine subdermal implants is not recommended in patients with moderate to severe hepatic impairment since the extended-release injection does not allow for rapid adjustment of plasma buprenorphine concentrations and the implant dosage cannot be titrated. (See Dosage and Administration: Dosage in Hepatic Impairment and also see Pharmacokinetics: Elimination.) If moderate or severe hepatic impairment develops during therapy with buprenorphine extended-release subcutaneous injection or buprenorphine subdermal implants, the patient should be monitored for manifestations of toxicity or overdosage. If such manifestations occur in patients with buprenorphine implants, removal of the implants may be required. Patients who have received the extended-release subcutaneous injection should be monitored for several months; if manifestations of overdosage or toxicity occur within 2 weeks following an injection, the depot containing buprenorphine may be surgically excised, if necessary.

Hepatotoxicity Serious adverse hepatic events have occurred in patients receiving buprenorphine for the treatment of opiate dependence. (See Cautions: Hepatic Effects.) While some individuals had risk factors for such adverse events (i.e., preexisting hepatic enzyme abnormalities, HBV or HCV infection, concomitant use of potentially hepatotoxic drugs, ongoing illicit use of injectable drugs), the possibility exists that buprenorphine had a causative or contributory role in some of these adverse hepatic events. In patients with opiate dependence, evaluation of liver function prior to initiation of buprenorphine therapy and periodically during treatment is recommended. The manufacturer of buprenorphine extended-release subcutaneous injection recommends monthly monitoring of liver function during treatment with this formulation, particularly in patients receiving the 300-mg dosage. Liver function also should be evaluated prior to initiation of buprenorphine therapy for analgesia and periodically during such treatment in patients at increased risk of hepatotoxicity (e.g., patients with a history of excessive alcohol intake, IV drug abuse, or liver disease). Careful biologic and etiologic evaluation is recommended in the event of an adverse hepatic event. In some patients, withdrawal of buprenorphine has resulted in amelioration of acute hepatitis; in other patients, no dosage reduction was necessary. If a decision is made to discontinue buprenorphine therapy, the drug should discontinued carefully to prevent withdrawal symptoms and, in patients being treated for opiate dependence, the return to illicit drug use; strict monitoring of the patient should be initiated.

Hypotension Buprenorphine may cause severe hypotension, including orthostatic hypotension and syncope, in ambulatory patients. Because the risk of severe hypotension is increased in patients whose ability to maintain blood pressure has been compromised by blood volume depletion or concomitant use of certain CNS depressants (e.g., phenothiazines, general anesthetics), such patients should be monitored for hypotension following initiation of buprenorphine therapy or an increase in buprenorphine dosage. Use of buprenorphine should be avoided in patients with circulatory shock since the drug may cause vasodilation that can further reduce cardiac output and blood pressure.

Increased Intracranial Pressure or Head Injury The respiratory depressant effects of opiates promote carbon dioxide retention, which can result in elevation of intracranial pressure. Patients who may be particularly susceptible to these effects (e.g., those with evidence of elevated intracranial pressure or brain tumors) should be monitored closely for sedation and respiratory depression, particularly during initiation of therapy. Opiates also may obscure the clinical course in patients with head injuries. Use of buprenorphine should be avoided in patients with impaired consciousness or coma.

Seizures Buprenorphine may increase the frequency of seizures in patients with seizure disorders and may increase the risk of seizures in some clinical settings associated with seizures. Patients with seizure disorders should be monitored for worsening of seizure control during buprenorphine therapy.

GI Conditions Opiates may increase serum amylase concentrations and cause spasm of the sphincter of Oddi. Patients with biliary tract disease, including those with acute pancreatitis, should be monitored for worsening symptoms. Buprenorphine formulations labeled for analgesic use are contraindicated in patients with known or suspected GI obstruction, including paralytic ileus.

Like other opiates, buprenorphine may obscure the diagnosis and/or clinical course of acute abdominal conditions.

Anesthesia and Analgesia in Patients Receiving Extended-release Injection or Implant Therapy for Opiate Dependence When patients with buprenorphine subdermal implants or those who have received buprenorphine extended-release subcutaneous injection within the prior 6 months require anesthesia or analgesia for acute pain, nonopiate analgesics should be used whenever possible. Those patients requiring opiate analgesia may receive a high-affinity, full opiate agonist under clinician supervision, with particular attention given to respiratory function. Because higher doses may be required for analgesia, the potential for toxicity is increased. If opiates are a required component of anesthesia, patients should be continuously monitored in an anesthesia care setting by persons not involved in the conduct of the surgical or diagnostic procedure. Opiate therapy must be provided by individuals trained in the use of anesthetic drugs and the management of respiratory effects of potent opiates, specifically the establishment and maintenance of a patent airway and assisted ventilation.

Implant Complications Improper insertion of buprenorphine subdermal implants may result in rare but serious complications including nerve damage and implant migration resulting in embolism and death. Local migration, protrusion, and expulsion of implants also may occur. Protrusion or expulsion may be caused by incomplete insertion or infection at the insertion site and may result in accidental exposure to the drug. Buprenorphine implants should be inserted in accordance with the manufacturer's instructions. It is essential for each implant to be inserted subdermally so that it is palpable following insertion and for proper placement to be confirmed by palpation immediately after insertion.

Neural or vascular injury may occur if buprenorphine implants are inserted into muscle or fascia. If an implant is inserted too deeply, cannot be palpated, or has migrated, removal may be complicated. Additional surgical procedures may be required to remove an implant that was inserted too deeply and cannot be readily localized. Injury to deeper neural or vascular structures may occur when deeply inserted implants are removed.

Excessive palpation shortly after insertion or improper removal may increase the risk of infection at the implant site.

Because of the risks associated with implant insertion and removal, buprenorphine implants are available only through a restricted distribution program (Probuphine® REMS). (See Risk Evaluation and Mitigation Strategies under Dosage and Administration: Administration.)

Extended-release Subcutaneous Injection Because buprenorphine extended-release subcutaneous injection forms a solid mass upon contact with body fluids, IV administration could result in death or serious complications (e.g., venous occlusion, local tissue damage, thromboembolic events including life-threatening pulmonary embolism). The extended-release subcutaneous injection should *not* be administered IV or by IM injection. Because of the risks associated with IV self-administration, the extended-release subcutaneous injection is available only through a restricted distribution program (Sublocade® REMS). (See Risk Evaluation and Mitigation Strategies under Dosage and Administration: Administration.)

Transdermal Therapy Patients receiving transdermal buprenorphine therapy who develop severe reactions with marked inflammation (e.g., burning, discharge, vesicles) at the application site should be advised to consult their clinician promptly about the need to remove the transdermal system.

Because the absorption of topically applied buprenorphine from the transdermal system depends in part on the temperature of the skin and increases with increased temperature, patients who develop a fever while using the transdermal system and individuals whose core body temperature increases as a result of strenuous exercise should be observed closely for manifestations of opiate toxicity, and dosage of the drug should be adjusted if respiratory or CNS depression occurs. In addition, patients wearing a transdermal system of the drug should be advised to avoid exposing the application site or surrounding area to direct external heat sources. (See Transdermal System for Pain Management under Administration: Transdermal Administration, in Dosage and Administration.)

Buccal Buprenorphine in Cancer Patients with Mucositis Cancer patients with oral mucositis may absorb buprenorphine from buccally dissolving strips (Belbuca®) more rapidly than intended and are likely to achieve higher plasma concentrations of the drug. Dosage reduction and careful monitoring for toxicity or overdosage is recommended in patients with known or suspected mucositis receiving this formulation of the drug. (See Buccal Dosage under Dosage: Pain, in Dosage and Administration and also see Oral Transmucosal Formulations Used for Analgesia under Pharmacokinetics: Absorption.)

Patient Advice Patients should be advised to read the manufacturer's patient information (e.g., medication guide and any instructions for use of the prescribed formulation) for buprenorphine before initiating therapy with the drug and each time the prescription is refilled. Patients should be informed that use of buprenorphine, even when taken as recommended, can result in addiction, abuse, and misuse, which can lead to overdosage and death. Patients also should be informed that accidental exposure to buprenorphine, especially by a child, may result in respiratory depression or death. Patients should be instructed not to share the drug with others, to take steps to protect the drug from theft or misuse, to securely store the drug, to keep the drug out of reach of children, and to properly dispose of any unused drug.

Patients should be advised of the risk of life-threatening respiratory depression and instructed to seek immediate medical attention if manifestations of respiratory depression occur. Patients receiving buprenorphine and/or their caregivers should be advised that concomitant therapeutic or illicit use of benzodiazepines or other CNS depressants, including alcohol, can result in potentially fatal additive effects (e.g., profound sedation, respiratory depression, coma); patients should be advised to avoid concomitant use of alcohol and to avoid concomitant use of other CNS depressants unless such use is supervised by a clinician. Patients should be advised that self-administration of benzodiazepines while taking buprenorphine is extremely dangerous.

Patients should be advised of the importance of informing clinicians of existing or contemplated concomitant therapy, including prescription and OTC drugs, and herbal supplements, as well as any concomitant illnesses. Patients should be advised that buprenorphine should not be used concomitantly with or within 14 days following a monoamine oxidase (MAO) inhibitor and that concomitant use of buprenorphine and serotonergic drugs may cause serotonin syndrome.

Patients should be advised that buprenorphine may impair mental or physical abilities required to perform potentially hazardous tasks such as driving a car or operating machinery and that they should avoid such activities until they know how the drug affects them. Patients also should be advised that severe hypersensitivity reactions (e.g., anaphylaxis) have occurred and that the drug may cause orthostatic hypotension and syncope. Because opiates can cause severe constipation, patients should be advised on appropriate management of constipation. Because of the potential risk of adrenal insufficiency, patients should be advised to immediately contact a clinician if manifestations of adrenal insufficiency (e.g., nausea, vomiting, anorexia, fatigue, weakness, dizziness, hypotension) develop. Although a causal relationship between hypogonadism or androgen deficiency and long-term opiate use has not been established, patients should be advised of this potential risk and instructed to inform their clinician if decreased libido, impotence, erectile dysfunction, amenorrhea, or infertility occurs.

Women of childbearing potential should be instructed to inform their clinician if they are or plan to become pregnant or plan to breast-feed. Risks and benefits of buprenorphine therapy should be discussed with pregnant and nursing women in the context of the intended use (pain management, treatment of opiate dependence). Women of childbearing potential should be advised that prolonged use of opiates during pregnancy may result in neonatal opiate withdrawal syndrome, which can be life-threatening if not recognized and treated. Nursing women should be advised to monitor their breast-fed infants for drowsiness or difficulty breathing. (See Cautions: Pregnancy, Fertility, and Lactation.)

Patients should be instructed on proper administration of the prescribed dosage form and instructed not to alter the dosage without consulting their clinician. (See Dosage and Administration: Administration.) Patients receiving oral transmucosal therapy with buprenorphine or buprenorphine/naloxone for treatment of opiate dependence should be instructed that if a dose of the drug is missed, the missed dose should be taken as soon as it is remembered; however, if it is almost time for the next dose, the missed dose should be skipped and the regular schedule resumed with the next dose.

Patients should be informed that buprenorphine can cause physical dependence and that gradual tapering of the dosage may be required to prevent withdrawal symptoms when the drug is discontinued. Patients receiving buprenorphine or buprenorphine/naloxone for maintenance treatment of opiate dependence should be advised of the potential for relapse to illicit drug use upon discontinuance of maintenance treatment.

Patients receiving buprenorphine as an analgesic should be instructed to inform their clinician of any breakthrough pain or adverse effects that occur, so that therapy may be adjusted based on individual patient requirements.

Patients receiving buprenorphine or buprenorphine/naloxone for treatment of opiate dependence should be advised to instruct their family members that, in the event of an emergency, they should inform the treating clinician or emergency department staff that the patient is physically dependent on opiates and is receiving treatment with an oral transmucosal or long-acting formulation of the drug.

Patients receiving therapy with buprenorphine extended-release subcutaneous injection should be informed that the drug may be detectable for a prolonged time after administration and that drug effects and other associated precautions and considerations (e.g., risk of drug interactions, risks associated with treatment of emergent acute pain) may persist for several months after the last injection. Patients should be informed that a lump may develop at the injection site and that it will gradually diminish in size. Patients should be instructed not to tamper with or attempt to remove the solid depot containing buprenorphine and should be advised that the extended-release subcutaneous injection is available only under a restricted distribution program because of the risk of serious harm or death if the formulation is self-administered IV.

Patients receiving buprenorphine subdermal implants should be instructed on appropriate care of the incision and should be advised of potential complications resulting from insertion or removal procedures, including neural or vascular injury, infection, and implant migration with the potential for embolism or nerve damage. Patients should be informed that complications may be more likely during removal if the implants were inserted too deeply or were manipulated by the patient or if the patient has gained substantial weight following insertion. Patients also should be informed that implant removal carries risks inherent to other minor surgical procedures, improper removal may result in infection, and premature removal may induce withdrawal symptoms. Patients should be informed that there is a risk to others of accidental overdosage, misuse, and abuse if an implant protrudes from the skin or is expelled; patients should be instructed on safety precautions that they must follow prior to seeing their clinician for such events. Patients should be advised that buprenorphine implants are available only under a restricted distribution program and must be inserted and removed in the facility of a certified prescriber.

Patients receiving buprenorphine transdermal systems should be advised to avoid exposing the application site or surrounding area to direct external heat sources, hot water, or prolonged direct sunlight since such exposure can increase absorption of the drug.

Contraindications Buprenorphine is contraindicated in patients with known hypersensitivity to the drug or any components of the formulation. In addition, buprenorphine/naloxone is contraindicated in patients with known hypersensitivity to naloxone. Buprenorphine formulations labeled for analgesic use are contraindicated in patients with known or suspected GI obstruction (including paralytic ileus), substantial respiratory depression, or acute or severe bronchial asthma in an unmonitored setting or in the absence of resuscitative equipment.

■ Pediatric Precautions Safety and efficacy of buprenorphine conventional injection in children 2–12 years of age is supported by evidence from adequate and well-controlled trials in adults, with additional data from studies including 960 children and adolescents 9 months to 18 years of age; data are available from a pharmacokinetic study, several controlled clinical trials, and several large postmarketing studies and case series. The manufacturer states that there is reasonable evidence of safety in children 2–12 years of age and efficacy similar to that observed in adults. Safety and efficacy of buprenorphine injection for pain relief in children younger than 2 years of age have not been established.

Safety and efficacy of buprenorphine buccally dissolving strips for pain relief in pediatric patients have not been established. Safety and efficacy of transdermal buprenorphine for pain relief in patients younger than 18 years of age have not been established.

Safety and efficacy of buprenorphine sublingual tablets, buprenorphine/naloxone sublingual tablets, or buprenorphine/naloxone buccally or sublingually dissolving strips for the management of opiate dependence in pediatric patients have not been established. Naloxone-containing preparations are not appropriate for management of neonatal opiate withdrawal syndrome.

Safety and efficacy of buprenorphine extended-release subcutaneous injection for the treatment of opiate dependence in pediatric patients have not been established. Safety and efficacy of buprenorphine subdermal implants for treatment of opiate dependence have not been established in pediatric patients younger than 16 years of age.

■ Geriatric Precautions When the total number of patients studied in clinical trials of transdermal buprenorphine or buprenorphine buccally dissolving strips for pain relief is considered, approximately 25 or 16%, respectively, were 65 years of age or older, while about 8 or 2%, respectively, were 75 years of age and older. The pharmacokinetic profiles of these analgesic formulations in geriatric adults appear to be similar to those in younger adults. The safety profile of transdermal buprenorphine in healthy geriatric individuals appears to be similar to that in younger adults; however, constipation and urinary retention may occur more frequently in geriatric individuals. In clinical trials of buprenorphine buccally dissolving strips in patients with chronic pain, some adverse effects also occurred more frequently in geriatric patients. Other reported clinical experience with buprenorphine has not identified differences in responses between geriatric and younger adults. While specific dosage adjustments of transdermal buprenorphine or buprenorphine buccally dissolving strips are not necessary based on age, buprenorphine should be used with caution in geriatric patients. Because geriatric patients may have increased sensitivity to the drug, the manufacturer of buprenorphine injection states that dosage in geriatric patients should be selected with caution, usually starting at the low end of the dosing range, reflecting the greater frequency of decreased hepatic, renal, and/or cardiac function and of concomitant disease or other drug therapy. Because respiratory depression is the chief risk for geriatric patients receiving opiate analgesics, buprenorphine dosage should be titrated slowly and the patient should be monitored closely for CNS and respiratory depression.

Clinical studies of buprenorphine subdermal implants for the treatment of opiate dependence did not include patients older than 65 years of age and clinical studies of buprenorphine sublingual tablets, buprenorphine/naloxone sublingual tablets, buprenorphine/naloxone buccally or sublingually dissolving strips, and buprenorphine extended-release subcutaneous injection did not include sufficient numbers of patients 65 years of age or older to determine whether geriatric patients respond differently than younger adults. However, other reported clinical experience with buprenorphine has not revealed age-related differences in response. Because of age-related decreases in hepatic, renal, and/or cardiac function and the potential for concomitant disease and drug therapy, the decision to use buprenorphine or buprenorphine/naloxone for the treatment of opiate dependence in patients 65 years of age or older should be made cautiously, and these patients should be monitored for toxicity or overdosage.

■ Mutagenicity and Carcinogenicity Studies examining the mutagenic potential of buprenorphine in in vivo and in vitro systems have shown conflicting results when high concentrations or doses of the drug were used; although the mutagenic potential of buprenorphine has not been clearly established, the manufacturer states that the possibility of mutagenicity appears remote. The combination of buprenorphine and naloxone (in a 4:1 ratio) was not mutagenic in the Ames test, nor was the combination clastogenic in an in vitro cytogenetic assay in human lymphocytes or in an IV micronucleus test in rats. Buprenorphine was not mutagenic or clastogenic in a series of tests utilizing gene, chromosome, and DNA interactions in prokaryotic and eukaryotic systems, although Ames test results were equivocal. Buprenorphine was not genotoxic in vitro in a bacterial mutagenicity test, mouse lymphoma assay, or chromosomal aberration assay in human peripheral blood lymphocytes, nor was it genotoxic in vivo in a mouse micronucleus test.

An increased incidence of benign testicular interstitial tumors was observed in rats receiving topical buprenorphine dosages of 20–200 mg/kg daily (130–350 times the human exposure [based on area under the concentration-time curve; AUC] of a transdermal dosage of 20 mcg/hour) for 100 weeks. In rats receiving dietary buprenorphine (with naloxone) in dosages of 7–123 mg/kg daily (4–44 times the human AUC after a sublingual dose of buprenorphine 16 mg and naloxone 4 mg) for 104 weeks, an increased incidence of Leydig cell carcinomas was observed at all dosages. Similar results were observed in rats receiving oral buprenorphine dosages of 0.6–56 mg/kg daily (0.4–35 times the human exposure on a mg/m^2 basis of a sublingual dosage of 16 mg daily) for 27 months.

However, in an 86-week study in mice, buprenorphine was not carcinogenic at dietary dosages up to 100 mg/kg daily (approximately 30 times the human exposure on a mg/m^2 basis of a sublingual dosage of 16 mg daily). In addition, there was no evidence of carcinogenicity in mice receiving topical buprenorphine in dosages up to 600 mg/kg daily (approximately 1000 times the human AUC after a transdermal dosage of 20 mcg/hour) for 6 months.

■ Pregnancy, Fertility, and Lactation ***Pregnancy*** **Animal Reproduction Studies.** Reproduction studies in rats and rabbits using IM or subcutaneous buprenorphine dosages up to 5 mg/kg daily (3 and 6 times, respectively, the human exposure on a mg/m^2 basis of a sublingual dosage of 16 mg daily), transdermal dosages of 20 mcg/hour in rats and 80 mcg/hour in rabbits (110 times the human exposure at a transdermal dosage of 20 mcg/hour), oral dosages of 160 mg/kg daily in rats or 25 mg/kg daily in rabbits (approximately 95 or 30 times, respectively, a human sublingual dosage of 16 mg daily), and IV dosages up to 0.8 mg/kg daily in rats and rabbits (0.5 and 1 times, respectively, the human exposure on a mg/m^2 basis of a sublingual dosage of 16 mg daily) have not revealed evidence of teratogenicity, although an increase in skeletal abnormalities (e.g., extra rib formation) occurred in rats receiving a subcutaneous dosage of 1 mg/kg daily (0.6 times the human exposure on a mg/m^2 basis of a sublingual dosage of 16 mg daily).

Studies in rats and rabbits using buprenorphine (in a 1:1 ratio with naloxone) at oral dosages up to 250 mg/kg daily in rats and 40 mg/kg daily in rabbits (approximately 150 and 50 times, respectively, the human exposure on a mg/m^2 basis of a sublingual dosage of 16 mg daily) have not revealed evidence of teratogenicity. Studies in rats and rabbits using buprenorphine (in a 3:2 ratio with naloxone) at IM dosages of up to 30 mg/kg daily (20 and 35 times, respectively, the human exposure on a mg/m^2 basis of a sublingual dosage of 16 mg daily) have not revealed definitive drug-related teratogenic effects; acephalus was observed in one rabbit fetus from the low-dose group, omphalocele was observed in 2 rabbit fetuses from the same litter in the medium-dose group, and no teratogenic effects were observed in fetuses from the high-dose group.

Buprenorphine has been shown to increase pregnancy loss in rats and rabbits. Dose-related postimplantation loss occurred in rats at oral dosages of 10 mg/kg daily (approximately 6 times the human exposure on a mg/m^2 basis of a sublingual dosage of 16 mg daily); postimplantation loss also occurred in rats at IM dosages of 30 mg/kg daily. In rabbits, increased preimplantation loss occurred at oral dosages of 1 mg/kg daily and increased postimplantation loss occurred at IV dosages of 0.2 mg/kg daily (both approximately 0.3 times the human exposure on a mg/m^2 basis of a sublingual dosage of 16 mg daily). Increased postimplantation loss also was observed in rabbits at oral dosages of 40 mg/kg daily and IM dosages of 30 mg/kg daily.

Transdermal or subcutaneous buprenorphine caused maternal toxicity in rats and increased the number of stillborns, reduced litter size, and reduced offspring growth at maternal rat exposure levels that were approximately 10 times those observed with a human transdermal dosage of 20 mcg/hour. Dystocia occurred in pregnant rats receiving IM dosages of 5 mg/kg daily (approximately 3 times the human sublingual dosage of 16 mg daily on a mg/m^2 basis). An increase in rat neonatal mortality was observed with oral, IM, or subcutaneous dosages of 0.8, 0.5, or 0.1 mg/kg daily (approximately 0.5, 0.3, or 0.06 times, respectively, the human sublingual dosage of 16 mg daily on a mg/m^2 basis). An apparent lack of milk production during reproduction studies in rats likely contributed to decreased pup survival. Oral dosages of 80 mg/kg daily (approximately 50 times the human sublingual dosage of 16 mg daily on a mg/m^2 basis) were associated with delayed occurrence of the righting reflex and startle response in rat pups.

In studies in rats using a solvent (*N*-methyl-2-pyrrolidone; NMP) contained in the Atrigel® vehicle of buprenorphine extended-release subcutaneous injection (Sublocade®), preimplantation loss, delayed ossification, reduced fetal weight, and developmental delays and impaired cognitive function in pups born to NMP-exposed animals occurred at inhaled NMP dosages approximately equivalent to the amount of NMP provided by the recommended human dose of the Sublocade® formulation; fetal malformations and resorption occurred at oral NMP dosages approximately 3 times that provided by the human dose of this buprenorphine formulation. Decreased pup survival occurred at oral maternal NMP dosages of 1.8 times that provided by the maximum recommended human dose of the Sublocade® formulation. In rabbits, postimplantation loss and increased cardiovascular and skull malformations occurred at oral NMP dosages of 3.2 times the amount of NMP provided by the maximum recommended human dose of this formulation.

In studies in rats using the Sublocade® formulation at subcutaneous buprenorphine dosages of approximately 38 times the maximum recommended human dosage, embryolethality (which appeared to be attributable principally to the vehicle), reduced fetal body weight, and increased visceral and skeletal (principally skull) malformations occurred. These effects also were observed with the Atrigel® vehicle alone, but the skeletal and visceral malformations appeared to be at least partially attributable to buprenorphine. In studies in rabbits using the Sublocade® formulation, increased skeletal malformations (which appeared to be related to buprenorphine) occurred at a subcutaneous buprenorphine dosage of 7 times the maximum recommended human dosage. Increased malformations (external malformations, visceral malformations, skeletal malformations and variations), embryolethality, and decreased fetal body weight occurred at a subcutaneous buprenorphine dosage of approximately 15 times the maximum recommended human dosage and appeared to be attributable to the vehicle.

Clinical Experience. Limited data from clinical trials, observational studies, case series, and case reports on use of buprenorphine during pregnancy do not indicate an increased risk of major malformations specifically due to the drug. However, interpretation is complicated by maternal factors such as illicit drug use, late presentation for prenatal care, poor nutritional status, presence of infections, poor compliance, and psychosocial circumstances and by the lack of comparative data for untreated opiate-dependent pregnant women. Comparisons generally have been made to women receiving a different opiate for medication-assisted treatment of opiate dependence or to women in the general population, who may differ from buprenorphine-treated women in their risk factors for poor pregnancy outcomes.

In a double-blind, randomized, controlled trial (Maternal Opioid Treatment: Human Experimental Research [MOTHER]), outcomes, principally opiate withdrawal effects, were assessed in neonates born to women who received buprenorphine or methadone treatment for opiate dependence during pregnancy. Enrollment in the study occurred at an average gestational age of 18.7 weeks. Prior to the end of pregnancy, 33% of buprenorphine-treated women and 18% of methadone-treated women discontinued treatment; outcomes were evaluated for the neonates whose mothers remained in treatment until delivery. No difference was observed between buprenorphine- and methadone-exposed neonates in the proportion of neonates requiring treatment for opiate withdrawal syndrome or the peak severity of the syndrome. Buprenorphine-exposed neonates required a lower total mean morphine sulfate dosage for treatment of withdrawal (1.1 versus 10.4 mg), had shorter hospital stays (10 versus 17.5 days), and shorter duration of treatment for withdrawal (4.1 versus 9.9 days) compared with methadone-exposed neonates. The groups did not differ in other outcome measures (head circumference, weight and length at birth, preterm birth, gestational age at delivery, and 1- and 5-minute Apgar scores) or in the rates of serious maternal or neonatal adverse events. The imbalance in treatment discontinuance rates between buprenorphine- and methadone-treated women complicate interpretation of the study findings.

Untreated opiate addiction during pregnancy is associated with adverse obstetrical outcomes, including preeclampsia, fetal growth restriction, preterm birth, spontaneous abortion, and fetal death. In addition, untreated opiate addiction often results in continued or relapsing illicit opiate use and engagement in high-risk behaviors. The recommended treatment of opiate dependence in pregnant women is maintenance treatment with buprenorphine or methadone; this approach is superior to medically supervised withdrawal because withdrawal is associated with high relapse rates and poorer outcomes.

Use of a single-entity buprenorphine preparation is recommended during pregnancy to protect the fetus from any potential exposure to naloxone, especially if the fixed-combination preparation is injected, and also to avoid precipitated withdrawal in the event of IV injection. However, expert opinion regarding use of buprenorphine versus buprenorphine/naloxone during pregnancy appears to be evolving. Recent studies suggest that neonatal outcomes are similar with buprenorphine/naloxone or buprenorphine; if additional safety data confirm these findings, buprenorphine/naloxone use during pregnancy may increase, since the single-entity preparation has a higher risk for misuse and diversion. The manufacturers of buprenorphine/naloxone preparations currently state that the extremely limited data on sublingual naloxone exposure in pregnancy are not sufficient to evaluate a drug-associated risk.

The manufacturer states that buprenorphine extended-release subcutaneous injection should be used during pregnancy only if the potential benefits justify the potential risks to the fetus. Based on animal data, pregnant women should be advised of the potential risk of this formulation to the fetus. (See Animal Reproduction Studies under Pregnancy, Fertility, and Lactation: Pregnancy, in Cautions.) There are no adequate and well-controlled studies to date with use of buprenorphine subdermal implants in pregnant women.

Dosage adjustments of buprenorphine may be required during pregnancy, even if the patient was receiving a stable dosage prior to pregnancy. Pregnant women receiving buprenorphine should be monitored closely for withdrawal manifestations and the dosage adjusted as necessary.

Opiate-dependent women receiving buprenorphine maintenance therapy may require additional analgesia during labor. When opiate analgesics are required during the intrapartum period, higher than usual dosages generally are needed to achieve adequate analgesia because of tolerance to the maintenance treatment dosage.

Opiate analgesics, including buprenorphine, cross the placenta and may produce respiratory depression in neonates. The manufacturer states that safety of buprenorphine injection when administered during labor and delivery has not been established. Opiate analgesics, including buprenorphine, may prolong labor through actions that temporarily reduce the strength, duration, and frequency of uterine contractions. However, this effect is inconsistent and may be offset by an increased rate of cervical dilatation, which tends to shorten labor. Transdermal buprenorphine and buprenorphine buccally dissolving strips should not be used for pain relief in women immediately prior to or during labor, when use of shorter-acting analgesics or other analgesic techniques is more appropriate. Neonates exposed to opiates during labor should be monitored for respiratory depression. An opiate antagonist must be available for reversal of opiate-induced respiratory depression.

Prolonged maternal use of opiates, including buprenorphine, during pregnancy can result in physical dependence in the neonate and neonatal opiate withdrawal syndrome. Manifestations may include irritability, hyperactivity and abnormal sleep pattern, high-pitched cry, tremor, vomiting, diarrhea, and failure to gain weight. In contrast to adults, the withdrawal syndrome in neonates may be life-threatening if not recognized and treated, and requires management according to protocols developed by neonatology experts. Women who require prolonged opiate agonist therapy during pregnancy should be advised of the risk of neonatal opiate withdrawal syndrome, and availability of appropriate treatment should be ensured. The onset, duration, and severity of the syndrome vary depending on the specific opiate agonist used, duration of use, timing and amount of last maternal use, and rate of drug elimination by the neonate. In neonates who have been exposed to buprenorphine, the onset of neonatal withdrawal symptoms generally occurs in the first 1–2 days after birth. Neonates born to women taking opiates chronically should be closely observed for signs of withdrawal.

Fertility Long-term use of opiates may reduce fertility in females and males of reproductive potential. It is not known whether these effects on fertility are reversible. Long-term use of opiates may influence the hypothalamic-pituitary-gonadal axis, resulting in androgen deficiency that may be manifested as low libido, impotence, erectile dysfunction, amenorrhea, or infertility. The causal role of opiates in hypogonadism is unknown because studies to date have not adequately controlled for other potential influences on gonadal hormone levels (e.g., medical or physical factors, lifestyle, psychological stressors).

Reproduction studies in rats using IM and subcutaneous buprenorphine dosages up to 5 mg/kg daily or dietary dosages up to 80 mg/kg daily (approximately 48 or 763 times, respectively, the recommended parenteral human dose of 1.2 mg on a mg/m² basis) have not revealed evidence of impaired fertility. Slight decreases in growth rate were observed in the offspring (second generation) of rats receiving buprenorphine IM; however, the offspring did not exhibit evidence of impaired fertility or reproductive performance. Reduced conception rates were observed in female rats receiving dietary buprenorphine dosages of approximately 47 mg/kg daily (approximately 28 times the human exposure on a mg/m² basis of a sublingual dosage of 16 mg daily). No evidence of impaired fertility or reproductive performance was observed in rats receiving transdermal buprenorphine in dosages resulting in AUCs up to 65 (in females) or 100 (in males) times the exposure level in humans receiving a transdermal dosage of 20 mcg/hour.

However, adverse effects on sperm (low motility, low sperm count, and higher percentage of abnormal sperm) were observed in rats at a buprenorphine dose of 600 mg/kg (as buprenorphine extended-release subcutaneous injection [Sublocade®]) and with the corresponding dose of the Atrigel® vehicle contained in the drug injection. No effects on female mating, fertility, or fecundity indices were observed at subcutaneous extended-release buprenorphine dosages up to 900 mg/kg (approximately 38 times the maximum recommended human dose based on AUC comparison). Adverse effects on testes and male fertility also have been observed in rats receiving a solvent (*N*-methyl-2-pyrrolidone; NMP) contained in the Atrigel® vehicle for 10 weeks at a daily oral dosage greater than 11.6 times the amount of solvent delivered by the maximum recommended human dosage.

Lactation Buprenorphine is distributed into milk in humans. In 2 studies that included 13 nursing women receiving maintenance treatment with sublingual buprenorphine (2.4–24 mg daily) for opiate dependence, buprenorphine and its metabolite norbuprenorphine were present in low concentrations in milk and in the breast-fed infant's urine; the infants were exposed to less than 1% of the maternal daily buprenorphine dosage. In the first study in 6 women receiving buprenorphine (median dosage of 0.29 mg/kg daily) at 5–8 days postpartum, breast milk provided a median infant dosage of 0.42 mcg/kg daily of buprenorphine and 0.33 mcg/kg daily of norbuprenorphine (0.2 and 0.12%, respectively, of the maternal weight-adjusted dosage). In the other study in 7 women receiving buprenorphine (median dosage of 7 mg daily) at an average of 1.12 months postpartum, mean milk concentrations of buprenorphine and norbuprenorphine were 3.65 and 1.94 mcg/L, respectively; based on the results of this study, an exclusively breast-fed infant consuming 150 mL/kg daily of milk would receive a mean estimated dosage of 0.55 mcg/kg daily of buprenorphine and 0.29 mcg/kg daily of norbuprenorphine (0.38 and 0.18%, respectively, of the maternal weight-adjusted dosage). Adverse reactions in nursing infants were not observed.

Experts recommend that women who are stable on buprenorphine or buprenorphine/naloxone treatment for opiate dependence, are not using other illicit drugs, and have no contraindications to nursing be encouraged to breastfeed their infants; to lower the risk of return to substance use, women receiving buprenorphine should be encouraged to continue treatment during the postpartum period. Breast-feeding has been associated with decreased severity of neonatal opiate withdrawal syndrome, decreased need for pharmacotherapy, and shorter hospital stays for the neonate. The manufacturers of buprenorphine-containing preparations used for treatment of opiate dependence state that developmental and health benefits of breast-feeding should be considered along with the mother's clinical need for buprenorphine or buprenorphine/naloxone and any potential adverse effects on the breast-fed child from the drug or from the underlying maternal condition. Because of the potential for serious adverse reactions, including excess sedation and respiratory depression in nursing infants, the manufacturers of buprenorphine preparations labeled for use as analgesics state that women should be advised not to nurse an infant while receiving the drug. Infants who are exposed to buprenorphine through breast milk should be monitored for excess sedation and respiratory depression.

Symptoms of withdrawal can occur in opiate-dependent infants when maternal administration of opiates is discontinued or breast-feeding is stopped.

Drug Interactions

Drug interactions that reportedly occur with other opiate agonists may also potentially occur during administration of buprenorphine.

■ **Benzodiazepines and Other CNS Depressants** Concomitant use of opiate agonists or opiate partial agonists, including buprenorphine, and benzodiazepines or other CNS depressants (e.g., anxiolytics, sedatives or hypnotics, tranquilizers, muscle relaxants, general anesthetics, antipsychotics, other opiates, alcohol) may result in profound sedation, respiratory depression, hypotension, coma, and death. Opiate analgesics frequently are implicated as contributing to fatal overdoses involving other CNS depressants, and epidemiologic studies have shown that a substantial proportion of fatal opiate overdoses involve the concurrent use of benzodiazepines, alcohol, or other CNS depressants. Whenever possible, concomitant use of opiates and benzodiazepines should be avoided. Alcohol also should be avoided in patients receiving opiates. Concomitant use of opiate analgesics and benzodiazepines or other CNS depressants should be reserved for patients in whom alternative treatment options are inadequate; the lowest effective dosages and shortest possible duration of concomitant therapy should be used, and the patient should be monitored closely for respiratory depression and sedation.

If a benzodiazepine or other CNS depressant is required for any indication other than epilepsy in a patient receiving buprenorphine for analgesia, the drug should be initiated at a lower dosage than indicated in the absence of opiate therapy and titrated based on clinical response. In patients receiving a CNS depressant, buprenorphine, if required for analgesia, should be initiated at a reduced dosage and titrated based on clinical response.

Because the morbidity and mortality associated with untreated opiate addiction can outweigh the serious risks associated with concomitant use of opiate agonists or partial agonists and benzodiazepines or other CNS depressants, buprenorphine treatment for opiate addiction (i.e., medication-assisted treatment [MAT]) should not be categorically withheld from patients receiving benzodiazepines or other CNS depressants. Clinicians should develop treatment plans that minimize the risks associated with concomitant use. If possible, benzodiazepines or other CNS depressants should be tapered and discontinued. (See Concomitant Use of Benzodiazepines or Other CNS Depressants under Cautions: Precautions and Contraindications.)

Some experts state that consideration should be given to offering the opiate antagonist naloxone when opiates are prescribed for patients at increased risk of opiate overdosage, including those receiving benzodiazepines concomitantly.

There have been reports of death or coma when buprenorphine was misused, often via self-injection of crushed tablets, or used concomitantly with benzodiazepines or other CNS depressants, including alcohol. In addition, results of preclinical studies indicate that the combination of benzodiazepines and buprenorphine may alter the usual ceiling on buprenorphine-induced respiratory depression, making the respiratory-depressant effects of buprenorphine, an opiate partial agonist, appear similar to those of opiate agonists. Patients receiving treatment with buprenorphine should be warned of the potential danger of self-administration of benzodiazepines or other CNS depressants, including IV self-administration.

Respiratory and cardiovascular collapse has occurred in several patients receiving usual doses of IV buprenorphine and oral diazepam concomitantly; the patients recovered following treatment that included assisted respiration and IV doxapram. Bradycardia, respiratory depression, and prolonged drowsiness occurred following IV administration of buprenorphine during surgery in a patient who had received oral lorazepam preoperatively. The patient recovered following treatment that included IV atropine and assisted respiration; however, drowsiness persisted for more than 12 hours, and lack of awareness and recall of the surgical procedure (amnesia) reportedly lasted for 48 hours.

Concomitant administration of buprenorphine and fentanyl produced satisfactory analgesia of prolonged duration, minimal respiratory depression, and allowed the patient to be aroused quickly and easily following surgery.

Concomitant administration of buprenorphine and droperidol produced satisfactory analgesia during and after surgery and also in a terminally ill patient with severe, chronic pain that was previously unresponsive to buprenorphine therapy alone. In a group of patients who received a single, high dose of buprenorphine before undergoing cholecystectomy with balanced anesthesia and experienced pain in the immediate postoperative phase, addition of naloxone reportedly resulted in adequate analgesia, possibly by counteracting dominant antagonistic effects of buprenorphine.

■ **Drugs Affecting Hepatic Microsomal Enzymes** Buprenorphine metabolism is mediated principally by cytochrome P-450 (CYP) isoenzyme 3A4. Buprenorphine and its major metabolite (norbuprenorphine) also undergo conjugation with glucuronic acid.

CYP3A4 Inhibitors Concomitant use of buprenorphine with drugs that inhibit CYP3A4 (e.g., macrolide antibiotics [e.g., erythromycin], azole antifungals [e.g., ketoconazole], protease inhibitors [e.g., ritonavir]) may increase plasma concentrations of buprenorphine, possibly resulting in increased or prolonged opiate effects, particularly when an inhibitor is added after a stable buprenorphine dosage has been achieved. If concomitant use of buprenorphine with drugs that inhibit CYP3A4 is necessary, patients should be monitored at frequent intervals for respiratory depression and sedation, and dosage adjustments should be considered until stable drug effects are achieved. Discontinuance of a concomitantly used CYP3A4 inhibitor may result in decreased plasma concentrations of buprenorphine, possibly resulting in decreased opiate effects and/or development of opiate withdrawal. Patients receiving buprenorphine who discontinue therapy with a CYP3A4 inhibitor should be monitored for opiate withdrawal, and dosage adjustments should be considered until stable drug effects are achieved.

Patients who initiate therapy with buprenorphine subdermal implants or buprenorphine extended-release subcutaneous injection after being stabilized on oral transmucosal buprenorphine administered concurrently with a CYP3A4 inhibitor should be monitored to ensure that the plasma buprenorphine concentrations provided by the implants or subcutaneous injection are adequate. Patients already receiving therapy with buprenorphine implants or buprenorphine extended-release subcutaneous injection who initiate therapy with a CYP3A4 inhibitor should be monitored for manifestations of excessive buprenorphine dosage; if there is evidence of buprenorphine toxicity or overdosage and dosage reduction or discontinuance of the concomitant CYP3A4 inhibitor is not feasible, removal of the buprenorphine implants or subcutaneous drug depot and initiation of a buprenorphine formulation that permits dosage adjustments may be necessary. Conversely, if a CYP3A4 inhibitor is discontinued following stable concomitant therapy with either the implants or extended-release subcutaneous injection, the patient should be monitored for manifestations of withdrawal; if the dosage of buprenorphine from the implants or subcutaneous depot is inadequate in the absence of the CYP3A4 inhibitor, the patient should be switched to a buprenorphine formulation that permits dosage adjustments.

The potential for interactions may depend in part on the route of buprenorphine administration. The manufacturer of transdermal buprenorphine states that the pharmacokinetics of buprenorphine administered by the transdermal route are not expected to be affected by concomitant use of CYP3A4 inhibitors.

CYP3A4 Inducers Although specific drug interaction studies have not been performed, concomitant use of drugs that induce CYP3A4 (e.g., carbamazepine, phenytoin, rifampin) may reduce plasma concentrations of buprenorphine, possibly resulting in decreased analgesic efficacy and/or development of opiate withdrawal. If concomitant use of buprenorphine with CYP3A4 inducers is necessary, patients should be monitored for opiate withdrawal, and dosage adjustments should be considered until stable drug effects are achieved. Discontinuance of a concomitantly used CYP3A4 inducer may result in increased plasma concentrations of buprenorphine, possibly resulting in increased or prolonged therapeutic or adverse effects, including serious respiratory depression. Patients receiving buprenorphine who discontinue therapy with a CYP3A4 inducer should be monitored for respiratory depression, and the buprenorphine dosage should be adjusted as necessary.

Patients who initiate therapy with buprenorphine subdermal implants or buprenorphine extended-release subcutaneous injection after being stabilized on oral transmucosal buprenorphine administered concurrently with a CYP3A4 inducer should be monitored to ensure that the plasma buprenorphine concentrations provided by the implants or subcutaneous injection are adequate but not excessive. Patients already receiving therapy with buprenorphine implants or buprenorphine extended-release subcutaneous injection who initiate therapy with a CYP3A4 inducer should be monitored for manifestations of withdrawal; if the dosage of buprenorphine from the implants or subcutaneous injection is inadequate and dosage reduction or discontinuance of the concomitant CYP3A4 inducer is not feasible, the patient should be switched to a buprenorphine formulation that permits dosage adjustments. Conversely, if a CYP3A4 inducer is discontinued following stable concomitant therapy with either the implants or extended-release subcutaneous injection, the patient should be monitored for manifestations of excessive buprenorphine dosage; if the dosage of buprenorphine from the implants or subcutaneous injection is excessive in the absence of the CYP3A4 inducer, removal of the buprenorphine implants or subcutaneous drug depot and initiation of a buprenorphine formulation that permits dosage adjustments may be necessary.

The potential for interactions may depend in part on the route of buprenorphine administration.

Antifungals Administration of ketoconazole 400 mg daily in patients receiving stable sublingual doses of buprenorphine in fixed combination with naloxone (buprenorphine/naloxone) increased peak plasma concentrations of buprenorphine by 100% and mean area under the plasma concentration-time curve (AUC) by 75–100% from baseline. However, concomitant use of ketoconazole 200 mg twice daily for 11 days and transdermal buprenorphine 10 mcg/hour for 7 days did not affect the pharmacokinetics of buprenorphine.

Antiretrovirals Some human immunodeficiency virus (HIV) protease inhibitors (PIs) with CYP3A4 inhibitory activity (i.e., lopinavir in fixed combination with ritonavir [lopinavir/ritonavir], nelfinavir, ritonavir) have been shown to have minimal pharmacokinetic and no clinically important pharmacodynamic interactions with buprenorphine. However, concomitant use of buprenorphine and other PIs with CYP3A4 inhibitory activity (i.e., *unboosted* atazanavir, *ritonavir-boosted* atazanavir) has resulted in increased plasma concentrations of buprenorphine and norbuprenorphine and excessive opiate effects. While concomitant use of *ritonavir-boosted* atazanavir and buprenorphine is not expected to affect the pharmacokinetics of atazanavir, concomitant use of *unboosted* atazanavir and buprenorphine may result in decreased plasma atazanavir concentrations. The manufacturers of buprenorphine state that patients receiving buprenorphine concomitantly with atazanavir (with or without ritonavir) should be monitored; buprenorphine dosage reduction may be warranted. The manufacturer of atazanavir states that concomitant use of *unboosted* atazanavir and buprenorphine is not recommended. If therapy with *ritonavir-boosted* or *unboosted* atazanavir must be initiated in a patient already receiving therapy with buprenorphine subdermal implants or extended-release subcutaneous injection, the patient should be monitored for manifestations of excessive buprenorphine dosage; removal of the buprenorphine implants or subcutaneous drug depot and initiation of an alternative buprenorphine formulation that permits dosage adjustments may be necessary.

Nonnucleoside reverse transcriptase inhibitors (NNRTIs) are metabolized principally by CYP3A4, and certain NNRTIs may either inhibit (e.g., delavirdine) or induce (e.g., efavirenz, etravirine, nevirapine) CYP3A enzymes. Pharmacokinetic interactions have been observed with concomitant use of buprenorphine and certain NNRTIs (i.e., efavirenz, delavirdine). However, these interactions did not result in substantial pharmacodynamic effects. Patients receiving chronic buprenorphine therapy who begin therapy with an NNRTI should have their buprenorphine dosage monitored.

Nucleoside reverse transcriptase inhibitors (NRTIs) do not appear to induce or inhibit CYP enzymes, and interactions with buprenorphine are not expected.

■ **Drugs Metabolized by Hepatic Microsomal Enzymes** In vitro studies indicate that buprenorphine inhibits activity of CYP2D6 and CYP3A4 and its major metabolite, norbuprenorphine, is a moderate inhibitor of CYP2D6. However, the relatively low plasma concentrations of buprenorphine and norbuprenorphine resulting from therapeutic doses of the drug are not expected to result in clinically important interactions.

■ **Drugs that Prolong the QT Interval** Because of the risk of QT-interval prolongation, buprenorphine should be avoided in patients receiving class IA (e.g., quinidine, procainamide, disopyramide) or class III (e.g., sotalol, amiodarone, dofetilide) antiarrhythmic agents or other drugs known to prolong the QT interval. (See Cautions: Cardiovascular Effects.)

■ **Drugs Associated with Serotonin Syndrome** Serotonin syndrome may occur in patients receiving opiate partial agonists concomitantly with other serotonergic drugs, including serotonin (5-hydroxytryptamine; 5-HT) type 1 receptor agonists ("triptans"), selective serotonin-reuptake inhibitors (SSRIs), selective serotonin- and norepinephrine-reuptake inhibitors (SNRIs), tricyclic antidepressants, antiemetics that are 5-HT_3 receptor antagonists, buspirone, cyclobenzaprine, dextromethorphan, lithium, St. John's wort (*Hypericum perforatum*), tryptophan, other serotonin modulators (e.g., mirtazapine, nefazodone, trazodone, vilazodone), and monoamine oxidase (MAO) inhibitors (both those used to treat psychiatric disorders and others, such as linezolid, methylene blue, and selegiline). Serotonin syndrome may occur within the recommended dosage ranges for these drugs. Manifestations of serotonin syndrome may include mental status changes (e.g., agitation, hallucinations, coma), autonomic instability (e.g., tachycardia, labile blood pressure, hyperthermia), neuromuscular aberrations (e.g., hyperreflexia, incoordination, rigidity), and/or GI symptoms (e.g., nausea, vomiting, diarrhea). Symptom onset generally occurs within several hours to a few days of concomitant use, but may occur later, particularly after dosage increases.

If concomitant use of other serotonergic drugs is warranted, patients should be monitored for serotonin syndrome, particularly during initiation of therapy and dosage increases. If serotonin syndrome is suspected, treatment with buprenorphine, other opiate agonist or partial agonist therapy, and/or any concurrently administered serotonergic agents should be discontinued.

For additional information on interactions with MAO inhibitors, see Drug Interactions: Monoamine Oxidase Inhibitors.

For further information on serotonin syndrome, including manifestations and treatment, see Drug Interactions: Serotonergic Drugs, in Fluoxetine Hydrochloride 28:16.04.20.

■ **Drugs Affecting Hepatic Blood Flow** When buprenorphine is administered concomitantly with a drug(s) that may reduce hepatic blood flow (e.g., halothane) and thereby reduce hepatic elimination of the partial opiate agonist, the activity of buprenorphine may be increased and/or prolonged. If such concomitant therapy is administered, buprenorphine should be used with caution and dosage of at least one of the drugs should be reduced.

■ **Anticholinergic Agents** Concomitant use of buprenorphine and drugs with anticholinergic activity may increase the risk of urinary retention and/or severe constipation, which can lead to paralytic ileus. Patients receiving such concomitant therapy should be monitored for signs or symptoms of urinary retention and reduced GI motility.

■ **Diuretics** Opiates may decrease the effects of diuretics by inducing the release of vasopressin (antidiuretic hormone). Patients receiving such concomitant therapy should be monitored for decreased diuretic or hypotensive effects; dosage of the diuretic may be increased if clinically indicated.

■ **Local Anesthetics** Buprenorphine may potentiate the effects of local anesthetics (e.g., bupivacaine hydrochloride, mepivacaine hydrochloride), and concomitant administration of the drugs may result in a more rapid onset and prolonged duration of analgesia.

■ **Monoamine Oxidase Inhibitors** Because concomitant use of opiates with MAO inhibitors (e.g., linezolid, phenelzine, tranylcypromine) may result in serotonin syndrome or manifestations of opiate toxicity (e.g., respiratory depression, coma), use of buprenorphine is not recommended in patients who are receiving or have recently (i.e., within 2 weeks) received an MAO inhibitor.

■ **Neuromuscular Blocking Agents** Buprenorphine may enhance the neuromuscular blocking action and increase the respiratory depressant effect of neuromuscular blocking agents. Patients receiving such concomitant therapy should be monitored for a greater than expected degree of respiratory depression; dosage of one or both drugs should be decreased as needed.

■ **Opiate Agonists and Partial Agonists** Opiate partial agonists (e.g., butorphanol, nalbuphine, pentazocine) may reduce the analgesic effect of buprenorphine and/or precipitate withdrawal symptoms; such concomitant use should be avoided.

Buprenorphine, which has high affinity but weaker agonistic effects at μ-opiate receptors, can displace full agonists from these receptors, with a resultant reduction in opiate agonist effects; therefore, initiation of buprenorphine therapy in individuals dependent on full opiate agonists before the agonistic effects of the opiate have subsided may precipitate withdrawal. Dosage of the full opiate agonist should be tapered before buprenorphine is initiated for analgesia. (See Dosage and Administration: Dosage.) Induction therapy with buprenorphine-containing preparations for opiate dependence should be initiated only when clear and objective signs of withdrawal are evident.

Acute Toxicity

■ **Pathogenesis** The oral LD_{50} of buprenorphine hydrochloride was 261 mg/kg (range: 233–304 mg/kg) and 600 mg/kg and higher in mice and rats, respectively, and the intraperitoneal LD_{50} was 94 mg/kg (range: 65–125 mg/kg) and 243 mg/kg (range: 145–255 mg/kg), in mice and rats, respectively. The IV LD_{50} was 26 mg/kg (range: 21–31 mg/kg) and 30 mg/kg (range: 26–51 mg/kg) in mice and rats, respectively, and the subcutaneous LD_{50} was 600 mg/kg and higher in both mice and rats. The IM LD_{50} was 100 mg/kg and higher in rats. In rodents, death from acute toxicity of buprenorphine occurs at doses at least 1000 times greater than the effective dose.

■ **Manifestations** Acute overdosage of buprenorphine may produce respiratory depression, CNS depression with somnolence progressing to stupor or coma, cardiovascular manifestations including bradycardia and hypotension, skeletal muscle flaccidity, cold and clammy skin, pinpoint pupils, partial or complete airway obstruction, pulmonary edema, atypical snoring, and death. Marked mydriasis (rather than miosis) may be observed in patients with hypoxia.

■ **Treatment** In acute buprenorphine overdosage, the patient's respiratory and cardiac status should be monitored carefully. Primary attention should be given to reestablishment of adequate respiratory exchange by maintaining an adequate, patent airway and using assisted or controlled respiration. Other supportive measures, such as oxygen and IV fluids and vasopressors, should also be used as necessary. While doxapram and naloxone may be of value in the management of buprenorphine overdosage, they also may be ineffective in, and therefore should *not* be relied on for, reversing buprenorphine-induced respiratory depression; instead, the use of assisted or controlled respiration and administration of oxygen may be necessary and should be considered the principal method of management of buprenorphine overdosage. When naloxone is used to reverse respiratory depression in patients receiving buprenorphine, larger than usual doses and repeated administration may be necessary.

An opiate antagonist (e.g., naloxone, nalmefene) should not be administered in the absence of clinically important respiratory or circulatory depression secondary to buprenorphine overdosage. In patients physically dependent on opiates, administration of the usual dose of an opiate antagonist will precipitate acute withdrawal. If a decision is made to treat serious respiratory depression in a physically dependent patient with an opiate antagonist, administration should be initiated with care and by titration using smaller than usual doses.

In cases of acute overdosage involving transdermal buprenorphine, the transdermal system should be removed immediately and the pharmacokinetic profile of transdermal administration should be considered. While patients may appear to improve with appropriate supportive measures, there is the possibility of extended buprenorphine effects as the drug continues to be absorbed from the skin. After removal of the buprenorphine transdermal system, plasma drug concentrations decrease by 50% in approximately 12 hours (range 10–24 hours) and the apparent terminal half-life is approximately 26 hours. The duration of action of transdermal buprenorphine may exceed the duration of action of the opiate antagonist used to treat the overdose. Patients may require monitoring and treatment for at least 24 hours after the buprenorphine transdermal system is removed.

In cases of overdosage potentially involving multiple agents, the potential contribution of buprenorphine versus other CNS depressants should be considered in deciding whether buprenorphine subdermal implants should be removed. In an emergency situation, the implants may be removed by a surgeon who is not REMS certified. (See Risk Evaluation and Mitigation Strategies under Dosage and Administration: Administration.) In patients who have received buprenorphine extended-release subcutaneous injection, clinical data are limited regarding possible surgical removal of the subcutaneous drug depot.

Chronic Toxicity

Patients may develop psychological dependence to the opiate agonist activity of buprenorphine; however, animal studies suggest that the reinforcing efficacy of buprenorphine may be less than that of the opiate agonists, morphine and codeine, and less than that of the other opiate partial agonists, butorphanol, nalbuphine, and pentazocine. Limited physical dependence also may occur, although infrequently, and the potential for development of tolerance to the drug's opiate agonist activity is limited. Studies in animals have suggested that cross-tolerance between buprenorphine and other opiate agonists (i.e., morphine) may develop. Studies in animals and humans have also suggested that buprenorphine may have a lesser physical dependence liability than morphine or pentazocine; however, buprenorphine has been misused by drug abusers and patients physically dependent on opiates in an attempt to substitute the drug for opiate agonists.

Administration of naloxone in a group of patients who received prolonged therapy with buprenorphine (1–2 months) and who were formerly physically dependent on opiates did not produce withdrawal. In a group of patients physically dependent on opiates who had substituted buprenorphine for the opiate agonist, discontinuance of buprenorphine slowly over several days resulted in a complete absence of signs and symptoms of withdrawal during the 30-day observation period. An initial 0.4-mg IV dose of naloxone produced no evidence of withdrawal in an individual with a history of parenteral misuse of opiate agonists who had substituted IV buprenorphine for the opiate agonist for a 6-month period and in whom a urinalysis confirmed the absence of opiate agonists in the urine; however, additional 2-mg doses of naloxone injected IV every 5 minutes up to a total dose of 10 mg precipitated signs and symptoms of opiate withdrawal which were relieved by administration of IV morphine.

Signs and symptoms of acute withdrawal following discontinuance of buprenorphine are similar to, but less intense than, those produced by morphine or methadone and may include abdominal pain, nausea, vomiting, restlessness, insomnia, diarrhea, chills, hot flushes (flashes), general aches and pains, hypertension, anorexia, malaise, tachycardia, lacrimation, rhinorrhea, diaphoresis, and piloerection. Similar signs and symptoms of withdrawal reportedly occurred following administration of naloxone in an individual with a history of buprenorphine abuse. Following abrupt discontinuance of buprenorphine after prolonged use (1–2 months), signs and symptoms of acute withdrawal were delayed and gradually appeared over 3–10 days, reached a peak after about 14 days, and continued for an additional 7–14 days.

Pharmacology

■ Opiate Agonist and Antagonist Properties Buprenorphine is an opiate partial agonist and shares many of the actions of opiate agonists. The drug exhibits analgesic and opiate antagonist activities. Buprenorphine is thought to act as a partial agonist at μ-opiate receptors in the CNS and peripheral tissues. The drug also is an antagonist at κ-opiate receptors and an agonist at δ-opiate receptors.

Buprenorphine appears to have a high affinity for both μ- and κ-receptors, and low to moderate intrinsic activity at μ- and κ-receptors; in contrast, the drug appears to have low to high affinity for and low intrinsic activity at δ-receptors. Buprenorphine binds slowly with and dissociates slowly from the μ-receptor. It is thought that the high affinity of buprenorphine for the μ-receptor and its slow binding to and dissociation from the receptor may account for the prolonged duration of analgesia and possibly in part for the limited physical dependence potential observed with the drug.

The opiate agonist and antagonist activities of buprenorphine appear to be dose related. At doses of up to 1 mg subcutaneously, buprenorphine has a potent analgesic effect; at doses greater than 1 mg subcutaneously, the opiate agonist activity of the drug decreases and the opiate antagonist activity predominates. Following IM administration, the opiate antagonist activity of buprenorphine occurs principally at doses greater than 0.8 mg. The drug may antagonize its own opiate agonist activity when administered at doses within the opiate antagonist range.

Animal studies have shown that antagonism of the opiate agonist activity of buprenorphine by other opiate antagonists may not occur once buprenorphine binds to opiate receptors in the CNS. In animals not physically dependent on opiates, administration of an opiate antagonist (e.g., naloxone) prior to or concomitantly with administration of buprenorphine results in a reduction or complete block of buprenorphine-induced opiate agonist activity. When buprenorphine is administered prior to an opiate antagonist, the agonist activity of buprenorphine is dominant. Similarly, administration of naloxone in a group of patients receiving prolonged therapy with buprenorphine (1–2 months) did not precipitate withdrawal.

On a weight basis, the opiate antagonist activity of buprenorphine is reportedly equal to or up to 3 times greater than that of naloxone when both drugs are compared as antagonists of morphine. Buprenorphine may precipitate mild to moderate withdrawal in some patients physically dependent on opiates. In patients who have received single subcutaneous morphine doses of up to 120 mg during chronic buprenorphine therapy, buprenorphine produces a block of the pharmacologic effects of morphine. Buprenorphine reportedly does not antagonize respiratory depression produced by non-opiate analgesics and other drugs.

Repeated exposure to short-acting opiates appears to result in neurobiologic changes in cellular and molecular systems; these changes include perturbations in opiate-receptor kinetics, transmembrane signaling, postreceptor signal transduction, and intracellular messengers. The physiologic dependence and addictive behavior that are characteristic of opiate dependence result from these neurobiologic changes and are the basis for use of opiate agonists for the treatment of opiate dependence. Opiate agonists stabilize brain neurochemistry by replacing short-acting euphorigenic opiates (e.g., heroin) with long-acting noneuphorigenic opiates (e.g., buprenorphine, levomethadyl acetate hydrochloride [no longer commercially available in the US], methadone). The mechanism(s) of action of these long-acting noneuphorigenic opiates include cross-tolerance at the opiate receptor, thus preventing opiate withdrawal, and competition for opiate-receptor binding sites, thus blocking the effects of exogenously administered opiates.

Like opiate agonists such as methadone or hydromorphone, sublingual administration of buprenorphine produces typical opiate agonist effects, which are limited by a ceiling effect. In individuals who were not opiate dependent, administration of a single sublingual dose of buprenorphine produced opiate agonist effects; these effects were maximal at doses of 8–16 mg. The effect of buprenorphine 16 mg was similar to that of an equivalent dose of buprenorphine given in fixed combination with naloxone.

Administration of single doses of buprenorphine produce physiologic and subjective effects that are similar to those produced by equivalent doses of buprenorphine administered in fixed combination with naloxone. When administered sublingually, the naloxone in fixed combination with buprenorphine does not have any clinically important pharmacologic effects. Buprenorphine in fixed combination with naloxone is recognized as an opiate agonist in opiate-dependent individuals when the preparation is given sublingually. However, parenteral administration of buprenorphine in conjunction with naloxone results in opiate antagonist actions similar to those of naloxone. IV administration of buprenorphine in conjunction with naloxone precipitates opiate withdrawal symptoms in opiate-dependent individuals.

■ CNS Effects Like other opiate agonists, buprenorphine produces dose-related analgesia. The exact mechanism has not been fully elucidated, but analgesia appears to result from a high affinity of buprenorphine for μ- and possibly κ-opiate receptors in the CNS. The drug may also alter the pain threshold (threshold of afferent nerve endings to noxious stimuli). On a weight basis, the analgesic potency of parenteral buprenorphine appears to be about 25–50, 200, and 600 times that of parenteral morphine, pentazocine, and meperidine, respectively. Buprenorphine may produce sex-related differences in analgesia, with females requiring substantially less drug than males to produce adequate analgesia. Following IV doses of 4 mcg/kg and higher, the drug may produce amnesia.

In patients physically dependent on opiates, buprenorphine produces many of the subjective and objective effects of opiates; however, the drug may not be a satisfactory substitute for opiate agonists for pain relief in all patients physically dependent on opiates. The potential for development of tolerance to the drug's opiate agonist activity is limited.

Buprenorphine may produce psychological dependence. Buprenorphine may also produce limited physical dependence, although infrequently. Signs and symptoms of mild withdrawal may appear following discontinuance of prolonged therapy with the drug alone. (See Chronic Toxicity.) Because buprenorphine binds slowly with and dissociates slowly from the μ-receptor, elimination of the drug from the CNS is prolonged following abrupt discontinuance; consequently, signs and symptoms of acute withdrawal are less intense than those produced by morphine and delayed in appearance. Buprenorphine is a partial opiate agonist with behavioral and psychic effects similar to morphine, and, unlike pentazocine, it rarely causes psychotomimetic effects.

Like other opiate agonists, buprenorphine may produce increases in intracranial pressure.

In rats, buprenorphine produces dose-related changes in the EEG pattern, and changes appear to be maximal at doses of 1 mg/kg. Increasing doses up to 1 mg/kg produce intense stupor and continuous high-voltage bursting activity, while doses of 0.3 and 10 mg/kg produce less intense stupor and intermittent bursting activity. In rabbits, buprenorphine produces EEG patterns characterized by increases in delta and theta wave activity. When administered in daily subcutaneous doses of 2 mg in individuals formerly receiving methadone, buprenorphine therapy was associated with EEG patterns characterized by an increase in alpha wave activity; however, the increase in activity may have resulted from a return of normal EEG patterns following discontinuance of methadone. Upon discontinuance of buprenorphine, the EEG pattern was characterized by a decrease in alpha wave activity; an increase in alpha wave activity was subsequently observed about 20 days following discontinuance of buprenorphine.

■ Cardiovascular Effects Buprenorphine generally produces few cardiovascular effects. In healthy individuals, cardiovascular effects induced by parenteral buprenorphine are similar to those following equivalent parenteral doses of morphine, including decreases in heart rate and systolic and diastolic blood pressures. Cardiovascular effects of buprenorphine appear to be of minor clinical importance in most patients, including patients with compromised cardiac function who have undergone surgery or patients who are recovering from myocardial infarction. In a limited number of patients, buprenorphine has been reported to inhibit cardiovascular effects that occur during surgery (e.g., increases in heart rate and systolic blood pressure).

Buprenorphine may decrease heart rate and systolic and/or diastolic blood pressure. In postoperative patients, decreases in heart rate reportedly may be indicative of adequate analgesia. The drug has also been shown to increase heart rate and blood pressure (principally systolic pressure) in some patients. Stroke volume and cardiac output may be slightly increased or decreased. Buprenorphine produces peripheral vasodilation, which may result in orthostatic hypotension or syncope. Cardiovascular effects of buprenorphine, including changes in heart rate, stroke volume, and systolic blood pressure, may be dose related; in several studies, buprenorphine-induced cardiovascular effects were not apparent at IV doses of 1.5 mcg/kg but appeared at IV doses of 2 mcg/kg and higher.

Prolongation of the QT interval was observed in healthy individuals receiving transdermal buprenorphine at dosages of 40 mcg/hour; dosages of 10 mcg/hour did not result in clinically relevant changes in the QT interval. Prolongation of the QT interval also was observed in patients receiving buprenorphine buccally dissolving strips at dosages of up to 900 mcg every 12 hours.(See Cautions: Cardiovascular Effects.)

■ **Respiratory Effects** Usual parenteral doses of buprenorphine potentially may depress respiration to the same degree as 10 mg of parenteral morphine sulfate. The onset of buprenorphine-induced respiratory depression is slower than that of morphine-induced respiratory depression and the duration appears to be more prolonged. Respiratory depression may be severe in individuals with compromised respiratory function or those receiving other respiratory depressant drugs concomitantly. (See Respiratory and CNS Depression and also Concomitant Use of Benzodiazepines or Other CNS Depressants under Cautions: Precautions and Contraindications.)

Buprenorphine-induced respiratory depression is dose related in single parenteral doses of up to 1.2 mg, although it appears that the dose-response curve is shallow. Unlike morphine, there appears to be a ceiling to buprenorphine-induced respiratory depression in most patients, so that higher doses of the drug do not necessarily produce a proportionate increase in respiratory depression. Respiratory depression in healthy adults generally appears to plateau or may even decrease in severity with doses greater than 1.2 mg, and changes in frequency, depth, and pattern of respiration and changes in arterial blood gas values do not appear to be clinically important in most patients. However, in animal studies, concomitant use of buprenorphine with benzodiazepines appeared to alter the usual ceiling on buprenorphine-induced respiratory depression, resulting in respiratory depressant effects similar to those of full opiate agonists.

The general absence of dose-related respiratory depression at higher than usual doses of buprenorphine may result from the drug's opiate antagonist activity at higher than usual doses. When low doses of a μ-receptor opiate agonist (e.g., fentanyl) and buprenorphine are administered concomitantly, the respiratory effects of both drugs are additive; however, when high doses of a μ-receptor opiate agonist analgesic and buprenorphine are administered concomitantly, buprenorphine may act as an opiate antagonist and antagonize the respiratory effects of the opiate agonist.

Buprenorphine-induced respiratory depression is characterized by decreases in arterial Po_2 and rate of respiration and increases in arterial Pco_2. In some patients receiving buprenorphine, decreases in rate of respiration may not be accompanied by changes in arterial blood gas values because of compensatory increases in depth of respiration. Decreases in rate of respiration in patients receiving buprenorphine may be indicative of changes in the intensity of pain and the adequacy of analgesia.

IV naloxone hydrochloride has been used to reverse signs of buprenorphine-induced respiratory depression; however, in usual doses, naloxone is substantially less effective in reversing buprenorphine-induced respiratory depression than in reversing morphine-induced respiratory depression and is occasionally only partially effective and, rarely, completely ineffective in reversing buprenorphine-induced respiratory depression. When naloxone is used to reverse signs of respiratory depression in patients receiving buprenorphine, larger than usual doses may be necessary. Doxapram has also been used with some success in reversing buprenorphine-induced respiratory depression.

The effect of buprenorphine on the cough reflex in humans has not been studied; however, in guinea pigs, the drug suppresses experimentally induced cough.

■ **Endocrine Effects** Like other opiate agonists, buprenorphine has been shown to decrease plasma concentrations of luteinizing hormone (LH) and increase plasma concentrations of prolactin. Buprenorphine has been reported to prevent the stress-induced increase in plasma cortisol concentration that occurs during surgery; however, the drug has also been reported to lack an inhibitory effect on surgery-induced increases in plasma cortisol in other patients and to increase plasma cortisol in healthy individuals. In some patients, the drug did not inhibit increases in plasma glucose concentration, but in other patients it reportedly prevented increases in plasma glucose concentration. Buprenorphine has been shown to reverse surgery-induced increases in plasma growth hormone (GH) and insulin concentrations, but the drug has produced increases in plasma GH concentration in healthy individuals.

■ **GI Effects** Buprenorphine produces minimal GI effects, including nausea, vomiting, and constipation. Like other opiate agonists, buprenorphine may produce an increase in pressure within the common bile duct, which may be followed by a rapid decrease in pressure. In healthy individuals, the drug did not alter baseline pressure of the sphincter of Oddi, and flow of biliary and pancreatic fluids was unaffected.

■ **Other Effects** Buprenorphine causes dose-related miosis, with peak miotic effects occurring at 6 hours and miosis continuing for about 72 hours after parenteral administration.

Buprenorphine produces urinary retention in some patients.

Pharmacokinetics

■ **Absorption** Plasma concentrations of buprenorphine required for analgesia are not known; some pharmacokinetic data indicate that a relationship between plasma buprenorphine concentrations and a given analgesic effect does not exist.

Buprenorphine Hydrochloride Conventional Injection Buprenorphine hydrochloride is rapidly and approximately 40–90% absorbed systemically following IM administration.

Following IV administration of a single 0.3-mg dose of buprenorphine, mean peak plasma drug concentrations of 18 ng/mL occurred within 2 minutes; plasma concentrations declined to 9 and 0.4 ng/mL after 5 minutes and 3 hours, respectively. Following IM administration of a second 0.3-mg dose 3 hours after the initial IV dose, mean peak plasma buprenorphine concentrations of 3.6 ng/mL occurred within 2–5 minutes and declined to 0.4 ng/mL after 3 hours. Approximately 10 minutes after administration, plasma concentrations of buprenorphine are similar following IV or IM injection. Plasma concentrations of buprenorphine may be increased slightly by concomitant administration of a general anesthetic (e.g., halothane) as a result of anesthesia-induced decrease in hepatic blood flow and hepatic clearance of the drug.

Following IM or IV administration of a single dose of buprenorphine, onset of analgesia is similar to that following IM or IV administration of morphine, respectively; the time of peak analgesia is similar to that of parenteral morphine, meperidine, or pentazocine. The onset of analgesia and time to peak analgesia are shorter following IV administration of buprenorphine than IM administration. The duration of analgesia produced by parenteral buprenorphine is longer than that produced by parenteral meperidine or pentazocine and is comparable to and, in some patients, may be longer than that produced by parenteral morphine. The duration of analgesia may vary according to the route of administration, with a more prolonged duration following IV or epidural administration than IM administration. The duration of analgesia may be prolonged with higher doses of buprenorphine; however, duration of analgesia did not differ substantially in a group of patients receiving 0.15- to 0.4-mg doses of the drug. The duration of analgesia induced by buprenorphine may also be affected by patient age, with the duration slightly prolonged in older patients. Following parenteral administration of single doses of 0.15–0.6 mg or 2–12 mcg/kg of buprenorphine in postoperative patients, the onset of analgesia usually occurs within 10–30 minutes, and peak analgesia usually occurs within 60 minutes; however, peak analgesia may occur within as little as 15 minutes in some patients. The mean duration of analgesia generally is 6 hours following single IM or IV doses of 0.2–0.3 mg or 2–4 mcg/kg; however, in some studies, the mean duration of analgesia reportedly ranged from 4–10 hours following single IM doses of 0.2–0.6 mg and 2–24 hours following single IV doses of 0.3 mg or 2–15 mcg/kg.

Buprenorphine Transdermal System When administered transdermally, buprenorphine has an absolute bioavailability of approximately 15%. Following application of a single transdermal system delivering buprenorphine 5, 10, or 20 mcg/hour, peak plasma concentrations of buprenorphine average 0.176, 0.191, or 0.471 ng/mL, respectively. Quantifiable buprenorphine concentrations are detectable approximately 17 hours after placement of the 10-mcg/hour transdermal system, with steady-state concentrations attained by the third day of treatment. Blood concentrations of buprenorphine increased by 26–55% when heat was applied directly to a transdermal system designed to deliver the drug at a dosage of 10 mcg/hour; concentrations returned to normal within 5 hours after the heat source was removed.

Oral Transmucosal Formulations Used for Analgesia Following administration of a single dose of buprenorphine (75–1200 mcg) as a buccally dissolving strip (Belbuca®), absolute bioavailability is 46–65% and peak plasma concentrations and area under the serum concentration-time curve (AUC) increase in a linear manner. Following single doses of 75, 300, or 1200 mcg, peak plasma concentrations of buprenorphine average 0.17, 0.47, or 1.43 ng/mL, respectively, and are achieved at a median of 2.5–3 hours. Following repeated administration at a dosage of 60–240 mcg every 12 hours, steady-state plasma concentrations are attained prior to the sixth dose, and steady-state peak plasma concentrations and AUC are proportional to dose.

Ingestion of cold, hot, or room-temperature water during buccal administration of the strips decreased systemic exposure to buprenorphine by 23–27%; concurrent ingestion of a low-pH liquid such as decaffeinated cola decreased systemic exposure to the drug by approximately 37%.

In cancer patients with grade 3 mucositis, absorption of buprenorphine from the buccally dissolving strips was more rapid and peak plasma concentrations and AUC were approximately 79 and 56% higher, respectively, compared with healthy controls.

Oral Transmucosal Formulations Used for Treatment of Opiate Dependence Not all formulations, strengths, or dose combinations of oral transmucosal preparations containing buprenorphine in fixed combination with naloxone (buprenorphine/naloxone) are bioequivalent.

Following sublingual administration of generic buprenorphine or buprenorphine/naloxone sublingual tablets (i.e., generic equivalents of Subutex® or Suboxone® sublingual tablets [branded formulations no longer commercially available in the US]), there is substantial interindividual variability in absorption of the drugs, but intraindividual variability is low. Peak plasma concentrations and AUC of buprenorphine increase with increasing dose (over the range of 4–16 mg), but the increase is not directly proportional to dose. Following sublingual administration of buprenorphine sublingual tablets at a dose of 2, 8, or 16 mg, peak plasma buprenorphine concentrations average 1.25, 2.88, or 4.7 ng/mL, respectively. Following sublingual administration of a single tablet containing buprenorphine 2 mg and naloxone 0.5 mg or containing buprenorphine 8 mg and naloxone 2 mg, peak plasma buprenorphine concentrations average 0.78 or 2.58 ng/mL, respectively. In most individuals, quantifiable amounts of naloxone are not detected in plasma beyond 2 hours after sublingual administration of buprenorphine/naloxone at naloxone doses of 1–4 mg; mean peak plasma concentrations of naloxone at these doses range from 0.11–0.28 ng/mL.

Not all strengths and combinations of buprenorphine/naloxone (Suboxone®) sublingually dissolving strips are bioequivalent to Suboxone® sublingual tablets administered at the same total dose. A dose consisting of one or two strips, each containing buprenorphine 2 mg and naloxone 0.5 mg, administered sublingually or buccally showed comparable relative bioavailability to sublingual tablets providing the same total dose. However, at a strength of buprenorphine 8 mg in fixed combination with naloxone 2 mg or a strength of buprenorphine 12 mg in fixed combination with naloxone 3 mg, a single strip administered sublingually or buccally showed higher relative bioavailability for both buprenorphine and naloxone compared with sublingual tablets providing the same total dose. A combination of one strip containing buprenorphine 8 mg and naloxone 2 mg and two strips containing buprenorphine 2 mg and naloxone 0.5 mg (total dose of buprenorphine 12 mg and naloxone 3 mg) administered sublingually showed comparable relative bioavailability as sublingual tablets providing the same total dose; however, when the strips were administered buccally, relative bioavailability was higher than that of the sublingual tablets. Pharmacokinetic parameters and systemic exposures are generally comparable following either buccal or sublingual administration of buprenorphine/naloxone strips, although systemic exposure to naloxone may be somewhat higher after buccal administration. (See Dosage Adjustments When Switching Between Oral Transmucosal Strengths and Preparations, under Dosage: Opiate Dependence, in Dosage and Administration.)

Buprenorphine/naloxone (Zubsolv®) sublingual tablets are not bioequivalent to Suboxone® sublingual tablets. One Zubsolv® sublingual tablet containing buprenorphine 5.7 mg and naloxone 1.4 mg provides 12% lower naloxone exposure and equivalent buprenorphine exposure as one Suboxone® sublingual tablet containing buprenorphine 8 mg and naloxone 2 mg. Although there is substantial interindividual variability in absorption of buprenorphine and naloxone from Zubsolv® sublingual tablets, intraindividual variability is low. Peak plasma concentrations and AUC of buprenorphine increase with increasing dose (over the range of 1.4–11.4 mg), but the increase is not directly proportional to dose.

Buprenorphine/naloxone (Bunavail®) buccally dissolving strips are not bioequivalent to Suboxone® sublingual tablets. One buccally dissolving strip containing buprenorphine 4.2 mg and naloxone 0.7 mg provides 33% lower naloxone exposure and equivalent buprenorphine exposure as one sublingual tablet containing buprenorphine 8 mg and naloxone 2 mg. Although there is substantial interindividual variability in buccal absorption of buprenorphine and naloxone from Bunavail® strips, intraindividual variability is low. Peak plasma concentrations and AUC of buprenorphine increase with increasing dose (over the range of 0.875–6.3 mg), but the increase is not directly proportional to dose. Administration of liquids with the strips reduces systemic exposure to both buprenorphine and naloxone by as much as 59 and 76%, respectively, depending on the pH of the liquid.

Concomitant administration of naloxone and buprenorphine does not affect the pharmacokinetics of buprenorphine.

Buprenorphine Extended-release Subcutaneous Injection Following subcutaneous administration of buprenorphine extended-release injection, a solid depot forms and the drug is released via diffusion from and biodegradation of the depot. Following administration of single doses of 50–200 mg and repeated doses of 50–300 mg at 28-day intervals, initial peak plasma concentrations of the drug were attained at a median of 24 hours after injection; concentrations then decreased slowly to a plateau, and steady-state concentrations were achieved at 4–6 months. Mean steady-state plasma concentrations attained following 6 doses of the extended-release subcutaneous injection (a series of two 300-mg doses followed by four 100-mg doses or a series of six 300-mg doses) administered at 28-day intervals were 3.21 or 6.54 ng/mL, respectively, compared with 2.91 ng/mL following stabilization on a buprenorphine dosage of 24 mg daily as sublingual tablets. At steady state, mean trough plasma concentrations achieved with both subcutaneous dosages and the mean peak concentration achieved with the higher-dosage subcutaneous regimen exceeded those attained with the sublingual dosage; the peak concentration attained with the lower-dosage subcutaneous regimen was approximately 59% of that attained with the sublingual dosage. Pharmacokinetic simulations suggest that therapeutic concentrations of the drug persist for 2–5 months, depending on the dosage (100 or 300 mg monthly), following the last injection of the drug.

Buprenorphine Hydrochloride Subdermal Implants Following insertion of buprenorphine hydrochloride subdermal implants, initial peak plasma concentrations of the drug were attained at a median of 12 hours after insertion; concentrations then decreased slowly, and steady-state concentrations were achieved by approximately week 4. Mean steady-state plasma concentrations of approximately 0.5–1 ng/mL were maintained for approximately 20 weeks (weeks 4–24) and were comparable to the steady-state trough buprenorphine concentrations attained with a sublingual buprenorphine dosage of 8 mg daily. In one study in patients who received sublingual buprenorphine (16 mg daily for at least 5 days) followed by insertion of 4 implants (total buprenorphine hydrochloride dose of 320 mg), overall peak plasma concentrations of buprenorphine were markedly lower after implant insertion compared with the sublingual dosing lead-in period. On day 28 of implant therapy, the steady-state AUC was 31% of the steady-state AUC achieved with the sublingual dosage, and the mean steady-state drug concentration was approximately 0.82 ng/mL (8% of the peak concentration and 52% of the trough concentration achieved at steady state with the sublingual dosage).

■ **Distribution** Distribution of buprenorphine into human body tissues and fluids has not been well characterized. Following oral or IM administration in rats, buprenorphine distributes into the liver, brain, placenta, and GI tract; highest concentrations were attained in the liver within 10 or 40 minutes following oral or IM administration, respectively. The hepatic extraction ratio of buprenorphine (E_H) is approximately 1. The drug and its metabolites are distributed into bile. Following IV administration in humans, the drug rapidly distributes into CSF (within several minutes). CSF buprenorphine concentrations appear to be approximately 15–25% of concurrent plasma concentrations.

The volume of distribution of buprenorphine following IV administration in adults is approximately 430 L.

Buprenorphine is approximately 96% bound to plasma proteins, mainly to α- and β-globulins; the drug does not appear to bind substantially to albumin.

Buprenorphine crosses the placenta, and the drug and its metabolites distribute into milk in rats in concentrations equal to or greater than those in maternal plasma. Buprenorphine distributes into milk (see Lactation under Cautions: Pregnancy, Fertility, and Lactation) and crosses the placenta in humans.

■ **Elimination** Plasma concentrations of buprenorphine generally appear to decline in a triphasic manner. Following IV administration of a single dose in postoperative patients with normal renal and hepatic function, the plasma half-life of buprenorphine reportedly averages 2 minutes in the initial (distribution) phase, 11 minutes in the second (redistribution) phase, and 2.2 hours (range: 1.2–7.2 hours) in the terminal (elimination) phase. Some pharmacokinetic data indicate that plasma concentrations of buprenorphine may decline in a biphasic manner in some patients.

Buprenorphine reportedly has a mean elimination half-life of 31–35 hours following sublingual administration as buprenorphine sublingual tablets, 24–42 hours following sublingual administration as buprenorphine/naloxone sublingual tablets or sublingual or buccal administration as buprenorphine/naloxone sublingually dissolving strips, 16–28 hours following buccal administration as buprenorphine/naloxone buccally dissolving strips, and 28 hours following buccal administration as buprenorphine buccally dissolving strips. Following transdermal administration, the terminal elimination half-life of buprenorphine is approximately 26 hours. Following administration as an extended-release subcutaneous injection, buprenorphine has an apparent elimination half-life of 43–60 days as a result of slow release from the subcutaneous depot.

Buprenorphine is almost completely metabolized in the liver, principally by *N*-dealkylation, to form norbuprenorphine (*N*-dealkylbuprenorphine). The *N*-dealkylation pathway is mediated by the cytochrome P-450 (CYP) 3A4 isoenzyme. Buprenorphine and norbuprenorphine also undergo conjugation with glucuronic acid. Buprenorphine is conjugated by uridine diphosphate-glucuronosyltransferase (UGT) isoenzymes, mainly UGT 1A1 and 2B7, to form buprenorphine 3-*O*-glucuronide; norbuprenorphine also is conjugated, mainly by UGT 1A3. Following oral administration, buprenorphine appears to undergo extensive first-pass metabolism in the GI mucosa and liver. Following transdermal administration, buprenorphine undergoes negligible metabolism in the skin.

Norbuprenorphine binds to opiate receptors in vitro, but it is not known whether norbuprenorphine contributes to the overall effects of buprenorphine. The AUC ratio of norbuprenorphine to buprenorphine is reportedly 0.2–0.4 at steady state following administration of buprenorphine extended-release subcutaneous injection and approximately 0.36–0.45 following sublingual administration of buprenorphine sublingual tablets. A norbuprenorphine half-life of 12–21 hours has been reported following sublingual administration of buprenorphine sublingual tablets.

Buprenorphine and its metabolites are excreted principally in feces (about 69%) via biliary elimination and also in urine (about 30%), almost entirely as unchanged drug, norbuprenorphine, and 2 unidentified metabolites. Most of the buprenorphine and norbuprenorphine excreted in urine is conjugated (buprenorphine: 1% unconjugated and 9.4% conjugated; norbuprenorphine: 2.7% unconjugated and 11% conjugated), whereas most of the buprenorphine and norbuprenorphine excreted in feces is unconjugated (buprenorphine: 33% unconjugated and 5% conjugated; norbuprenorphine: 21% unconjugated and 2% conjugated). Buprenorphine and its metabolites are believed to undergo enterohepatic circulation. Following IM administration of a 2-mcg/kg dose of buprenorphine, approximately 70% of the dose is excreted in feces and 27% in urine within 7 days. Following IV administration of a 0.6-mg dose, about 30% of the dose is excreted in urine within 7 days; approximately 9 and 8% of the dose are excreted in urine as buprenorphine (almost completely as conjugated drug) and norbuprenorphine (mainly as conjugated norbuprenorphine), respectively, within 4 days.

Total plasma clearance of buprenorphine reportedly is approximately 1.28 L/minute in conscious postoperative patients. Since metabolism and excretion of buprenorphine occur mainly via hepatic elimination, reductions in hepatic blood flow induced by some general anesthetics (e.g., halothane) and other drugs may result in a decreased rate of hepatic elimination of the drug. Plasma clearance of the drug is substantially reduced to 0.9 L/minute following IV administration of a single 0.3-mg dose in patients undergoing nitrous oxide and halothane anesthesia.

Limited data indicate that there is considerable interindividual variability in buprenorphine pharmacokinetics in children; however, clearance of the drug appears to be increased in children (e.g., those 5–7 years of age) compared with that in adults. Optimal dosing interval of buprenorphine may have to be decreased in pediatric patients.

No substantial relationship between estimated creatinine clearance and steady-state buprenorphine concentrations has been observed. Following IV administration, no differences in pharmacokinetics of buprenorphine have been observed between patients with renal impairment or renal failure requiring dialysis and those with normal renal function. In dialysis-dependent patients receiving transdermal buprenorphine, predialysis and postdialysis concentrations of the drug were not substantially different.

Following sublingual administration of a single buprenorphine/naloxone sublingual tablet (buprenorphine 2 mg and naloxone 0.5 mg) in patients with hepatic impairment, no clinically important changes in peak plasma concentrations, systemic exposures, and half-lives of buprenorphine or naloxone were observed in those with mild hepatic impairment. However, pharmacokinetics of the drugs were altered in patients with moderate or severe hepatic impairment; naloxone was affected to a greater degree than buprenorphine, and the magnitude of the difference in effect was greater in individuals with severe hepatic impairment than in those with moderate hepatic impairment. In those with moderate hepatic impairment, peak plasma concentrations of buprenorphine and naloxone were increased by 8 and 170%, respectively; AUC was increased by 64 and 218%, respectively; and half-life was increased by 35 and 165%, respectively, compared with individuals with normal hepatic function. In those with severe hepatic impairment, peak plasma concentrations of buprenorphine and naloxone were increased by 72 and 1030%, respectively; AUC was increased by 181 and 1302%, respectively; and half-life was increased by 57 and 122%, respectively.

The effects of hepatic impairment on the pharmacokinetics of buprenorphine administered as a 0.3-mg IV infusion have been evaluated in a limited number of patients with mild or moderate hepatic impairment (Child-Pugh class A or B). Exposure to buprenorphine and norbuprenorphine was not increased in such patients when compared with patients with normal hepatic function. Buprenorphine transdermal system and buprenorphine buccally dissolving strips have not been evaluated in patients with severe hepatic impairment (Child-Pugh class C). Data are lacking on the effects of hepatic impairment on the pharmacokinetics of buprenorphine administered as subdermal implants or as an extended-release subcutaneous injection.

In patients with hepatitis C virus (HCV) infection without evidence of hepatic impairment, no clinically important changes in peak plasma concentrations, systemic exposure, and half-lives of buprenorphine or naloxone were observed.

Chemistry and Stability

■ **Chemistry** Buprenorphine is a synthetic partial opiate agonist analgesic. Buprenorphine is derived from thebaine and is structurally related to morphine but pharmacologically similar to other currently available opiate partial agonists. Buprenorphine differs structurally from morphine in that buprenorphine contains a carbon bridge on the C ring; in addition, the methyl group on the nitrogen atom of morphine is replaced by a cyclopropylmethyl group, the C-6 position is substituted with a methoxy group rather than a hydroxyl group, the C-7 position is substituted with an alkylhydroxyl group, and there is a single rather than a double bond between C-7 and -8.

Buprenorphine hydrochloride occurs as a white, crystalline powder and has solubilities of 17 mg/mL in water (pH 4.4) at 25°C and 42 mg/mL in alcohol at room temperature. The drug has pK_as of 8.24–8.42 (amine) and 9.92–10 (phenol). Commercially available buprenorphine hydrochloride injection is a sterile solution of the drug in 5% dextrose injection. The injection occurs as a clear solution and has an osmolality of 297 mOsm/kg. The pH of the injection is adjusted to 3.5–5.5 with hydrochloric acid.

Potency of buprenorphine hydrochloride is expressed in terms of buprenorphine, calculated on the anhydrous basis. Each mL of commercially available buprenorphine hydrochloride injection contains 0.324 mg of buprenorphine hydrochloride, equivalent to 0.3 mg of buprenorphine.

The Sublocade® extended-release subcutaneous injection contains buprenorphine (18% by weight) dissolved in a biodegradable vehicle (Atrigel®) containing poly(D,L-lactide coglycolide) polymer and *N*-methyl-2-pyrrolidone (NMP) solvent in a 50:50 ratio. Following subcutaneous injection, precipitation of the polymer results in formation of a solid depot; buprenorphine is released from the depot at a controlled rate over one month via diffusion from and biodegradation of the depot.

Each Probuphine® implant is a soft, flexible rod (26 mm in length and 2.5 mm in diameter) that contains 80 mg of buprenorphine hydrochloride (equivalent to 74.2 mg of the base) and ethylene vinyl acetate. It is designed to be implanted subdermally and to provide sustained delivery of the drug for up to 6 months.

The Butrans® transdermal system consists of an outer web backing layer, an adhesive rim that does not contain buprenorphine, a separating layer over the buprenorphine-containing adhesive matrix, and a buprenorphine-containing adhesive matrix. The adhesive layer is covered by a protective strip that is removed prior to application. The amount of buprenorphine released from each system per hour is proportional to the surface area; release of the drug is designed to occur at an average rate of 5 mcg/hour per 6.25 cm². The total buprenorphine content in each 5-, 7.5-, 10-, 15-, and 20-mcg/hour system is 5, 7.5, 10, 15, and 20 mg, respectively.

■ **Stability** Buprenorphine hydrochloride injection should be protected from prolonged exposure to light and stored at a temperature of 20–25°C, but may be exposed to temperatures ranging from 15–30°C.

Buprenorphine hydrochloride is stable in solution at a pH of 3.5–5.5. The drug may undergo substantial decomposition when autoclaved. Specialized references should be consulted for specific compatibility information.

Oral transmucosal preparations of buprenorphine hydrochloride (sublingual tablets, buccally dissolving strips) or buprenorphine hydrochloride in fixed combination with naloxone hydrochloride (sublingual tablets, sublingually dissolving strips, buccally dissolving strips) should be stored at room temperature (generally 20–25°C, but may be exposed to temperatures ranging from 15–30°C). Sublingually or buccally dissolving strips should be used immediately after removal from the individually sealed package; strips that have been altered (e.g., torn, cut, damaged) should not be used. Bunavail® buccally dissolving strips should be protected from freezing and moisture.

Buprenorphine extended-release subcutaneous injection should be stored at 2–8°C. After removal from the refrigerator, the injection may be stored in its original package at 15–30°C for up to 7 days prior to administration; if not used within 7 days, the injection should be discarded.

Kits containing buprenorphine hydrochloride implants should be stored at 20–25°C, but may be exposed to temperatures ranging from 15–30°C.

Buprenorphine transdermal systems should be stored at 25°C, but may be exposed to temperatures ranging from 15–30°C. The system should be applied to the skin immediately after removal from the individually sealed package, and should be discarded if the seal was previously broken. Transdermal systems that have been cut, damaged, or altered in any way should be discarded since use of such systems may expose the patient or caregiver to the contents of the system and result in a potentially lethal overdose of the drug.

Buprenorphine preparations should be stored in a secure place to prevent access by children. (See Accidental Exposure under Cautions: Precautions and Contraindications.)

Preparations

Buprenorphine and buprenorphine hydrochloride are subject to control under the Federal Controlled Substances Act of 1970 as schedule III (C-III) drugs.

Under the Drug Addiction Treatment Act of 2000 (DATA 2000) and Comprehensive Addiction and Recovery Act of 2016 (CARA 2016), use of buprenorphine hydrochloride and buprenorphine hydrochloride in fixed combination with naloxone hydrochloride for the treatment of opiate dependence is restricted to physicians, nurse practitioners, and physician assistants who meet certain qualifying requirements; have notified the US Department of Health and Human Services (HHS) Substance Abuse and Mental Health Services Administration (SAMHSA) of their intention to prescribe these preparations for this indication; and have been assigned a unique identification number that must be included on each prescription for the drug. (See Dosage and Administration: Restricted Distribution Program for Buprenorphine Treatment of Opiate Dependence.)

Distribution of buprenorphine hydrochloride subdermal implants and buprenorphine extended-release subcutaneous injection is further restricted under risk evaluation and mitigation strategies. (See Risk Evaluation and Mitigation Strategies under Dosage and Administration: Administration.)

Excipients in commercially available drug preparations may have clinically important effects in some individuals; consult specific product labeling for details.

Buprenorphine

Parenteral

Injection, extended-release, for subcutaneous use	100 mg/0.5 mL	**Sublocade®** (C-III; available as single-use prefilled syringe), Indivior
	300 mg/1.5 mL	**Sublocade®** (C-III; available as single-use prefilled syringe), Indivior

Topical		
Transdermal System	5 mcg/hour (5 mg/6.25 cm²)	**Butrans**® (C-III), Purdue Pharma
	7.5 mcg/hour (7.5 mg/9.375 cm²)	**Butrans**® (C-III), Purdue Pharma
	10 mcg/hour (10 mg/12.5 cm²)	**Butrans**® (C-III), Purdue Pharma
	15 mcg/hour (15 mg/18.75 cm²)	**Butrans**® (C-III), Purdue Pharma
	20 mcg/hour (20 mg/25 cm²)	**Butrans**® (C-III), Purdue Pharma

Buprenorphine Hydrochloride

Buccal		
Strips, buccally dissolving	75 mcg (of buprenorphine)	**Belbuca**® (C-III), BioDelivery Sciences
	150 mcg (of buprenorphine)	**Belbuca**® (C-III), BioDelivery Sciences
	300 mcg (of buprenorphine)	**Belbuca**® (C-III), BioDelivery Sciences
	450 mcg (of buprenorphine)	**Belbuca**® (C-III), BioDelivery Sciences
	600 mcg (of buprenorphine)	**Belbuca**® (C-III), BioDelivery Sciences
	750 mcg (of buprenorphine)	**Belbuca**® (C-III), BioDelivery Sciences
	900 mcg (of buprenorphine)	**Belbuca**® (C-III), BioDelivery Sciences
Parenteral		
Implant, for subdermal use	80 mg (equivalent to buprenorphine 74.2 mg) per implant	**Probuphine**® (C-III; available as a kit containing 4 implants and 1 disposable applicator), Braeburn
Injection	0.3 mg (of buprenorphine) per mL*	**Buprenex**® (C-III), Reckitt Benckiser
		Buprenorphine Hydrochloride Injection (C-III)
Sublingual		
Tablets	2 mg (of buprenorphine)*	**Buprenorphine Hydrochloride Sublingual Tablets** (C-III)
	8 mg (of buprenorphine)*	**Buprenorphine Hydrochloride Sublingual Tablets** (C-III)

*available from one or more manufacturer, distributor, and/or repackager by generic (nonproprietary) name

Buprenorphine Hydrochloride Combinations

Buccal		
Strips, buccally dissolving	2.1 mg (of buprenorphine) with Naloxone Hydrochloride 0.3 mg (of naloxone)	**Bunavail**® (C-III), BioDelivery Sciences
	4.2 mg (of buprenorphine) with Naloxone Hydrochloride 0.7 mg (of naloxone)	**Bunavail**® (C-III), BioDelivery Sciences
	6.3 mg (of buprenorphine) with Naloxone Hydrochloride 1 mg (of naloxone)	**Bunavail**® (C-III), BioDelivery Sciences
Sublingual		
Strips, sublingually dissolving	2 mg (of buprenorphine) with Naloxone Hydrochloride 0.5 mg (of naloxone)	**Suboxone**® (C-III), Indivior
	4 mg (of buprenorphine) with Naloxone Hydrochloride 1 mg (of naloxone)	**Suboxone**® (C-III), Indivior
	8 mg (of buprenorphine) with Naloxone Hydrochloride 2 mg (of naloxone)	**Suboxone**® (C-III), Indivior
	12 mg (of buprenorphine) with Naloxone Hydrochloride 3 mg (of naloxone)	**Suboxone**® (C-III), Indivior
Tablets	0.7 mg (of buprenorphine) with Naloxone Hydrochloride 0.18 mg (of naloxone)	**Zubsolv**® (C-III), Orexo
	1.4 mg (of buprenorphine) with Naloxone Hydrochloride 0.36 mg (of naloxone)	**Zubsolv**® (C-III), Orexo
	2 mg (of buprenorphine) with Naloxone Hydrochloride 0.5 mg (of naloxone)*	**Buprenorphine Hydrochloride and Naloxone Hydrochloride Sublingual Tablets** (C-III)
	2.9 mg (of buprenorphine) with Naloxone Hydrochloride 0.71 mg (of naloxone)	**Zubsolv**® (C-III), Orexo
	5.7 mg (of buprenorphine) with Naloxone Hydrochloride 1.4 mg (of naloxone)	**Zubsolv**® (C-III), Orexo
	8 mg (of buprenorphine) with Naloxone Hydrochloride 2 mg (of naloxone)*	**Buprenorphine Hydrochloride and Naloxone Hydrochloride Sublingual Tablets** (C-III)
	8.6 mg (of buprenorphine) with Naloxone Hydrochloride 2.1 mg (of naloxone)	**Zubsolv**® (C-III), Orexo
	11.4 mg (of buprenorphine) with Naloxone Hydrochloride 2.9 mg (of naloxone)	**Zubsolv**® (C-III), Orexo

*available from one or more manufacturer, distributor, and/or repackager by generic (nonproprietary) name

†Use is not currently included in the labeling approved by the US Food and Drug Administration

Butorphanol Tartrate

Stadol

■ Butorphanol tartrate is a synthetic opiate partial agonist analgesic.

REMS

FDA approved a REMS for butorphanol tartrate to ensure that the benefits outweigh the risk. The REMS may apply to one or more preparations of butorphanol tartrate and consists of the following: medication guide and elements to assure safe use. See the FDA REMS page (http://www.accessdata.fda.gov/scripts/cder/rems/index.cfm).

Uses

Butorphanol tartrate injection is used for the relief of pain that is severe enough to require an opiate analgesic; because of the risks of addiction, abuse, and misuse associated with opiates even at recommended dosages, butorphanol should be reserved for use in patients for whom alternative treatment options (e.g., nonopiate analgesics) have not been, or are not expected to be, adequate or tolerated. Butorphanol tartrate injection also is used to provide preoperative sedation and analgesia and as a supplement to surgical anesthesia. However, butorphanol should be used with caution in patients undergoing surgery of the biliary tract. Butorphanol tartrate injection also is used for obstetric analgesia during labor.

In equianalgesic doses, parenteral butorphanol is as effective as morphine, meperidine, and pentazocine, but determination of the relative potential for abuse of butorphanol reportedly is less than that of codeine or propoxyphene.

Butorphanol tartrate nasal solution is used as an analgesic for the relief of moderate to severe postoperative (including that associated with orthopedic surgery), postpartum, and orthopedic (including musculoskeletal) pain. Butorphanol tartrate nasal solution also is used for the management of migraine headache. Some experts state that butorphanol tartrate nasal spray may be considered when other antimigraine drugs cannot be used or as rescue therapy when sedative effects will not place the patient at risk. In patients in whom butorphanol tartrate might be indicated for management of migraine headache, special attention should be given to the potential for overuse and dependence. When used to relieve postoperative pain, single intranasal butorphanol tartrate doses of 1 or 2 mg have been as effective as IM meperidine hydrochloride doses of 37.5 or 75 mg, respectively. When used to relieve migraine headache, butorphanol tartrate nasal solution administered as two 1-mg doses (given 1 hour apart) was as effective as a single 10-mg dose of IM methadone hydrochloride. (For further information on management and classification of migraine headache, see Vascular Headaches: General Principles in Migraine Therapy, under Uses in Sumatriptan 28:32.28.)

Because it does not suppress the abstinence syndrome and may induce withdrawal in opiate-dependent patients, butorphanol cannot be substituted for opiate agonists after physical dependence has been established without prior detoxification. (See Cautions: Precautions and Contraindications.) Butorphanol probably is not an effective antidote in the treatment of cardiovascular, respiratory, or behavioral depression induced by opiate agonists because of its relatively weak antagonistic effects.

For further information on the role of opiate analgesics in pain management, see Uses: Pain, in the Opiate Agonists General Statement 28:08.08.

Dosage and Administration

■ **Administration** Butorphanol tartrate is administered by IM or IV injection or by nasal inhalation using a spray pump. The nasal solution spray pump containing butorphanol tartrate should be assembled according to the manufacturer's instructions. Prior to initial use, the spray pump should be fully primed; priming of the pump should be repeated whenever the pump has not been used for 48 hours or longer. The patient instructions provided by the manufacturer should be consulted for use of the nasal solution spray pump. Since butorphanol nasal solution spray pump is an open delivery system that may increase environmental exposure of health-care personnel and visitors, the pump spray should be aimed away from such individuals.

■ **Dosage** Opiate analgesics should be given at the lowest effective dosage and for the shortest duration of therapy consistent with the treatment goals of the patient. Dosage of butorphanol tartrate should be adjusted according to the severity of pain, physical status of the patient, and other drugs that the patient is receiving. If concomitant therapy with other CNS depressants is required, the lowest effective dosages and shortest possible duration of concomitant therapy should be used. (See Cautions: Precautions and Contraindications, Chronic Toxicity, and Drug Interactions.)

The usual adult dose of butorphanol tartrate is 2 mg IM or 1 mg IV. These doses may be repeated every 3–4 hours as necessary. The usual effective dosage, depending on the severity of the pain, ranges from 1–4 mg IM or 0.5–2 mg IV, repeated every 3–4 hours. There are insufficient clinical data to recommend IM doses greater than 4 mg.

After initial priming, the nasal solution spray pump delivers about 14–15 metered doses containing 1 mg of butorphanol tartrate per spray. If repriming of the pump is necessary because of intermittent use, the spray pump will deliver about 8–10 metered doses, depending on the extent of repriming. The usual initial intranasal butorphanol tartrate dose is 1 mg (1 spray in one nostril); if adequate analgesia is not achieved, an additional 1-mg dose may be given within 60–90 minutes. This initial dose sequence may be repeated in 3–4 hours if needed. For the management of severe pain, an initial dose of 2 mg (1 spray in each nostril) may be given to patients who can remain recumbent if drowsiness or dizziness occurs; however, these patients should not receive additional 2-mg doses at intervals shorter than 3–4 hours, since the incidence of adverse effects may be increased.

In the treatment of postepisiotomy and musculoskeletal pain, 4–16 mg of butorphanol tartrate has been given orally† every 4–6 hours.

For acute pain not related to trauma or surgery, the prescribed quantity should be limited to the amount needed for the expected duration of pain severe enough to require opiate analgesia (generally 3 days or less and rarely more than 7 days).

For further information on the management of opiate analgesic therapy, see Dosage and Administration: Dosage, in the Opiate Agonists General Statement 28:08.08.

■ **Dosage in Hepatic or Renal Impairment and in Geriatric Patients** Patients with hepatic or renal impairment and geriatric patients should receive half of the recommended parenteral adult dose (i.e., 1 mg IM or 0.5 mg IV). If needed these doses may be repeated within usually not less than 6 hours. The usual initial dose of butorphanol tartrate nasal solution is 1 mg (1 spray in one nostril) in these patients; an additional 1-mg dose may be given within 90–120 minutes. This initial dose sequence may be repeated within usually not less than 6 hours.

Cautions

■ **Adverse Effects** Incidence and type of adverse effects of butorphanol tartrate (administered parenterally or intranasally) are similar to those of opiate analgesics. Sedation is the most frequent adverse reaction and occurs in about 43% of patients receiving butorphanol; sedation occurs more frequently with butorphanol than with morphine, meperidine, or pentazocine. Dizziness occurs in about 19% and nausea and/or vomiting has been reported in 13% of patients receiving butorphanol tartrate. Clamminess, sweatiness, headache, vertigo, floating feeling, asthenia, anxiety, euphoria, nervousness, paresthesia, lethargy, confusion, and lightheadedness occur in 1–10% of patients. Other adverse CNS effects, such as unusual dreams, agitation, hallucinations, seizures, hostility, transient difficulty in speaking and/or executing purposeful movements, and delusion, occur in less than 1% of patients receiving butorphanol. In equianalgesic dosage, adverse psychotomimetic effects such as hallucinations, dysphoria, unreality, depersonalization, and nervousness may occur more frequently with butorphanol than with morphine or nalbuphine. Insomnia has been reported in 11% of patients receiving butorphanol tartrate nasal solution. In addition, taste perversion, anorexia, constipation, and tinnitus occurred in 3–9% and otic pain and tremor were reported in 1% or more of patients receiving butorphanol tartrate nasal solution.

Other adverse GI effects, including vomiting, abdominal cramps, and constipation, occur in less than 1% of patients receiving butorphanol. Adverse cardiovascular effects include vasodilation and palpitation which occur in 1–9% of patients receiving the drug and chest pain, tachycardia, bradycardia and increased or decreased blood pressure which occur in less than 1% of patients. Hypotension associated with syncope (usually occurring within the first hour of administration) has been reported rarely in patients receiving butorphanol tartrate nasal solution, particularly in those who experienced similar adverse effects when receiving an opiate analgesic. Adverse dermatologic effects, such as rash or urticaria and itching, and other adverse effects, such as flushing and warmth, miosis, dry mouth, acrocyanosis, impaired urination, sensitivity to cold, tingling, diplopia, and blurred vision, also occur in less than 1% of patients receiving the drug. In addition, burning at the site of IV injection has been reported in patients receiving butorphanol tartrate injection.

Respiratory depression (decreased rate and depth of respiration) and apnea have occurred in less than 1% of patients receiving butorphanol; respiratory depression occurs mainly in patients receiving other drugs with CNS effects and in those with a history of CNS disease or respiratory impairment. In doses above the usual therapeutic range, butorphanol causes less respiratory depression than does morphine. Butorphanol-induced respiratory depression can be reversed by naloxone. The most common respiratory effects associated with the administration of butorphanol tartrate nasal solution are nasal congestion, which has been reported in 13% of patients, and dyspnea, epistaxis, nasal irritation, pharyngitis, rhinitis, sinus congestion, or upper respiratory infection, occurring in 3–9% of patients. Bronchitis, cough, and sinusitis have been reported in 1% or more of patients receiving butorphanol tartrate nasal solution.

Adrenal insufficiency has been reported in patients receiving opiate agonists or opiate partial agonists. Manifestations of adrenal insufficiency are nonspecific and may include nausea, vomiting, anorexia, fatigue, weakness, dizziness, and hypotension. The onset generally has occurred after at least 1 month of opiate agonist or partial agonist use, although the time to onset has ranged from within 1 day to more than 1 year. In many of the reported cases, patients required hospitalization. If adrenal insufficiency is suspected, appropriate laboratory testing should be performed promptly and physiologic (replacement) dosages of corticosteroids provided; therapy with the opiate agonist or partial agonist should be tapered and discontinued to allow recovery of adrenal function. If the opiate agonist or partial agonist can be discontinued, follow-up assessment of adrenal function should be performed to determine if corticosteroid replacement therapy can be discontinued. In some patients, switching to a different opiate improved symptoms.

Hypogonadism and androgen deficiency have been reported in patients receiving long-term opiate agonist or opiate partial agonist therapy, although a causal relationship has not been established. Patients receiving long-term opiate agonist or partial agonist therapy who present with manifestations of hypogonadism (e.g., decreased libido, impotence, erectile dysfunction, amenorrhea, infertility) should undergo laboratory evaluation.

■ **Precautions and Contraindications** Concomitant use of opiate agonists or opiate partial agonists and benzodiazepines or other CNS depressants (e.g., anxiolytics, sedatives, hypnotics, tranquilizers, muscle relaxants, general anesthetics, antipsychotics, other opiates, alcohol) may result in profound sedation, respiratory depression, coma, and death. Concomitant use of such drugs should be reserved for patients in whom alternative treatment options are inadequate; the lowest effective dosages and shortest possible duration of concomitant therapy should be used, and the patient should be monitored closely for respiratory depression and sedation. Patients receiving butorphanol and/or their caregivers should be apprised of the risks associated with concomitant therapeutic or illicit use of benzodiazepines, alcohol, or other CNS depressants. Concomitant use with alcohol should be avoided. (See Drug Interactions: Benzodiazepines and Other CNS Depressants.)

Because of possible adverse CNS effects such as drowsiness and dizziness, ambulatory patients receiving butorphanol should be cautioned against performing hazardous tasks requiring mental alertness or physical coordination such as driving a motor vehicle or operating machinery and warned about possible additive effects with other drugs that cause CNS depression. (See Drug Interactions: Benzodiazepines and Other CNS Depressants.) Although butorphanol appears to have a low physical dependence liability compared with codeine or propoxyphene (see Chronic Toxicity), the drug should be used cautiously in patients who are emotionally unstable or have a history of opiate abuse, and these patients should be closely supervised during long-term butorphanol therapy.

Butorphanol should be administered with caution and in low doses in patients with impaired respiration caused by other drugs, uremia, severe infection, severely limited respiratory reserve, bronchial asthma, respiratory obstruction, or cyanosis. In patients with acute myocardial infarction, ventricular dysfunction, or coronary insufficiency, butorphanol should be used only if the potential benefits justify the possible risks. Since butorphanol may slightly increase blood pressure, the drug should be used cautiously before surgery or anesthesia in hypertensive patients. If hypertension occurs, butorphanol should be discontinued and a hypotensive agent administered as necessary; butorphanol-induced hypertension reportedly has been managed with naloxone in patients who were not opiate dependent. In addition, since hypotension associated with syncope has been reported rarely in patients receiving butorphanol tartrate nasal solution, the manufacturer states that patients should be cautioned against performing activities that may pose risks if hypotension were to occur. Safe use of butorphanol in patients about to undergo biliary tract surgery has not been established, and the drug should be used with caution in these patients. Because butorphanol potentially may be associated with carbon dioxide retention and secondary elevation of CSF pressure, drug-induced miosis, and alterations in mental state (that may interfere with evaluation of CNS function), the drug should be used in patients with head injury only if the potential benefits justify the possible risks. In patients with head injury, the drug also may interfere with evaluation of CNS function.

When opiate analgesics are prescribed for patients at increased risk of opiate overdosage (e.g., those with a history of overdose or substance use disorder, those receiving opiate dosages equivalent to 50 mg or more of morphine sulfate daily, those receiving benzodiazepines concomitantly, those with medical conditions that could increase sensitivity to opiate effects), some experts state that clinicians should consider offering naloxone.

Because of the drug's partial opiate antagonistic effects, butorphanol is not recommended for use in opiate-dependent patients, and such patients should have an adequate period of withdrawal from opiates before initiating butorphanol therapy. In patients who have been taking opiate analgesics chronically, administration of butorphanol tartrate has been associated with withdrawal symptoms (e.g., anxiety, agitation, mood changes, hallucinations, dysphoria, weakness, diarrhea). In addition, because it may be difficult to assess tolerance in patients who have recently received substantial amounts of opiate agonists, butorphanol should be used with caution in these patients. The drug should be used in opiate-dependent patients only after they have been detoxified since butorphanol does not suppress the abstinence syndrome in these patients, and high doses may precipitate withdrawal symptoms as a result of opiate antagonist effect.

Butorphanol should be used with caution in patients with renal or hepatic dysfunction. The drug is contraindicated in patients with known hypersensitivity to butorphanol or to benzethonium chloride contained in the multiple-dose vials of the injection or in the nasal solution of the drug.

■ **Pediatric Precautions** Safety and efficacy of butorphanol in children younger than 18 years of age have not been established.

■ **Geriatric Precautions** Since clearance is decreased and elimination half-life of butorphanol may be increased in patients older than 65 years of age, dosage and dosage interval of butorphanol tartrate should be modified in such patients. (See Dosage in Renal or Hepatic Impairment and in Geriatric Patients, in Dosage.) In addition, geriatric patients may be more sensitive to drug-induced adverse effects than younger individuals. Results of a long-term clinical study indicate that geriatric patients may tolerate dizziness associated with intranasal butorphanol tartrate less well than younger patients.

■ **Pregnancy, Fertility, and Lactation** Safe use of butorphanol during pregnancy (except during labor) has not been established. Reproduction studies in rats, mice, and rabbits using butorphanol dosages of approximately 2.5–5 times the usual human dosage, during organogenesis, have not revealed evidence of harm to the fetus. However, subcutaneous butorphanol doses of 1 mg/kg were associated with higher incidences of stillbirths in rats. In addition, increased postimplantation losses occurred in rabbits receiving oral butorphanol doses of 30 and 60 mg/kg. There are no adequate and controlled studies to date using butorphanol tartrate in pregnant women, and the drug should be used during pregnancy only when the potential benefits justify the possible risk to the fetus. When butorphanol is administered during labor and delivery, respiratory depression may occur in the neonate; the drug should be used with caution in women delivering premature infants. In one clinical study using 1-mg IV doses of butorphanol tartrate during labor, transient (10–90 minutes) sinusoidal fetal heart rate patterns were reported; however, no adverse neonatal outcomes occurred. Butorphanol should be used with caution in the presence of abnormal fetal heart rate pattern. Because of the absence of clinical experience with butorphanol nasal solution during labor and delivery, use of the nasal preparation is not recommended in such circumstances.

Reproduction studies in rats using oral butorphanol dosages of 160 mg/kg daily revealed a decreased pregnancy rate; however, this effect was not observed in rats using subcutaneous butorphanol dosages of 2.5 mg/kg daily.

Butorphanol is distributed into human milk following parenteral administration of the drug in nursing women. The manufacturer states that the amount of the drug distributed into milk probably is clinically insignificant, estimated at 4 mcg/L of milk in a woman receiving 2 mg of butorphanol IM 4 times daily. Although there is no clinical experience with the use of butorphanol tartrate nasal solution in nursing women, it is assumed that the amount of the drug distributed into milk will be similar to that when administered parenterally.

Drug Interactions

■ **Benzodiazepines and Other CNS Depressants** Concomitant use of opiate agonists or opiate partial agonists, including butorphanol, and benzodiazepines or other CNS depressants (e.g., anxiolytics, sedatives, hypnotics, tranquilizers, muscle relaxants, general anesthetics, antipsychotics, other opiates, alcohol) may result in profound sedation, respiratory depression, hypotension, coma, and death. Opiate analgesics frequently are implicated as contributing to fatal overdoses involving other CNS depressants, and epidemiologic studies have shown that a substantial proportion of fatal opiate overdoses involve the concurrent use of benzodiazepines, alcohol, or other CNS depressants. Whenever possible, concomitant use of opiates and benzodiazepines should be avoided. Alcohol also should be avoided in patients receiving opiates. Concomitant use of opiate analgesics and benzodiazepines or other CNS depressants should be reserved for patients in whom alternative treatment options are inadequate; the lowest effective dosages and shortest possible duration of concomitant therapy should be used, and the patient should be monitored closely for respiratory depression and sedation.

If a benzodiazepine or other CNS depressant is required for any indication other than epilepsy in a patient receiving butorphanol, the drug should be initiated at a lower dosage than indicated in the absence of opiate therapy and titrated based on clinical response. In patients receiving a CNS depressant, butorphanol, if required, should be initiated at a reduced dosage and titrated based on clinical response. Some experts state that consideration should be given to offering the opiate antagonist naloxone when opiates are prescribed for patients at increased risk of opiate overdosage, including those receiving benzodiazepines concomitantly.

■ **Drugs Associated with Serotonin Syndrome** Serotonin syndrome may occur in patients receiving opiate partial agonists concomitantly with other serotonergic drugs, including serotonin (5-hydroxytryptamine; 5-HT) type 1 receptor agonists ("triptans"), selective serotonin-reuptake inhibitors (SSRIs), selective serotonin- and norepinephrine-reuptake inhibitors (SNRIs), tricyclic antidepressants, antiemetics that are 5-HT_3 receptor antagonists, buspirone, cyclobenzaprine, dextromethorphan, lithium, St. John's wort (*Hypericum perforatum*), tryptophan, other serotonin modulators (e.g., mirtazapine, nefazodone, trazodone, vilazodone), and monoamine oxidase (MAO) inhibitors (both those used to treat psychiatric disorders and others, such as linezolid, methylene blue, and selegiline). Serotonin syndrome may occur within the recommended dosage ranges for these drugs. Manifestations of serotonin syndrome may include mental status changes (e.g., agitation, hallucinations, coma), autonomic instability (e.g., tachycardia, labile blood pressure, hyperthermia), neuromuscular aberrations (e.g., hyperreflexia, incoordination, rigidity), and/or GI symptoms (e.g., nausea, vomiting, diarrhea). Symptom onset generally occurs within several hours to a few days of concomitant use, but may occur later, particularly after dosage increases.

If concomitant use of other serotonergic drugs is warranted, patients should be monitored for serotonin syndrome, particularly during initiation of therapy and dosage increases. If serotonin syndrome is suspected, treatment with butorphanol, other opiate agonist or partial agonist therapy, and/or any concurrently administered serotonergic agents should be discontinued.

For further information on serotonin syndrome, including manifestations and treatment, see Drug Interactions: Serotonergic Drugs, in Fluoxetine Hydrochloride 28:16.04.20.

■ **Other Drugs** Concomitant administration of butorphanol and pancuronium reportedly may cause an increase in conjunctival changes. In patients receiving a nasal vasoconstrictor (e.g., oxymetazoline), the rate of absorption of intranasal butorphanol may be decreased while the extent of absorption appears to be unchanged; therefore, a slower onset of analgesic action may occur in patients receiving butorphanol nasal solution immediately following or concomitantly with oxymetazoline.

Since it is not known if drugs that affect hepatic microsomal enzymes (e.g., cimetidine, erythromycin, theophylline) may interfere with the metabolism of butorphanol, the manufacturer suggests that clinicians consider decreasing doses and increasing intervals between doses of butorphanol in patients receiving such drugs.

Acute Toxicity

No instances of butorphanol overdosage have been reported, but expected symptoms would be respiratory depression, cardiovascular effects, and other CNS effects. Treatment consists of immediate IV administration of naloxone. Respiratory and cardiac status should be constantly evaluated, and appropriate supportive measures such as administration of oxygen, IV fluids and vasopressors, and assisted or controlled respiration should also be used if necessary.

Chronic Toxicity

Tolerance and psychological and physical dependence may occur in patients receiving butorphanol. Although episodes of drug abuse have been reported by all routes of administration, the potential for abuse of butorphanol tartrate is reportedly less than that of codeine or propoxyphene. In addition, butorphanol has been misused in combination with diphenhydramine by drug abusers in a manner similar to the parenteral use of pentazocine and tripelennamine (known as T's and blues), since the combination's effects are purported to be similar to those of IV heroin (diacetylmorphine).

Following abrupt discontinuance after prolonged use of butorphanol, withdrawal symptoms, which are similar to but more intense than those produced by morphine, have occurred and may include nausea, vomiting, gastric distress, decreased caloric intake, abdominal cramping, diarrhea, increased temperature, flu-like symptoms, diaphoresis, mydriasis, visual changes (including alteration of color perception), malaise, myalgia, rhinorrhea, itching, tachycardia, and "electric shocks" usually associated with a feeling of faintness. Acute withdrawal has been reported to develop within 4–24 hours after discontinuance of the drug in individuals who are dependent. Clonidine hydrochloride has been used in the management of acute butorphanol withdrawal in at least one individual.

The manufacturer states that more cases of drug abuse have been reported in patients receiving butorphanol tartrate nasal solution than in those receiving butorphanol tartrate injection. Results of a randomized, double-blind, placebo-controlled, crossover study in 7 men with a history of opiate dependence indicate that the psychopharmacologic profile of butorphanol tartrate injection is similar to that of the nasal solution. Therefore, it has been suggested that butorphanol's abuse potential may be independent of the route of administration, but might be dependent on nonpharmacologic factors (e.g., pattern of usage, alteration of the formulation).

In clinical studies, less than 1% of patients using butorphanol tartrate nasal solution had experiences suggestive of development of physical dependence or tolerance; however, patients in these studies did not receive prolonged continuous administration of the nasal solution. In 1 controlled clinical study in patients with chronic pain secondary to nonmalignant disease who were receiving butorphanol tartrate nasal solution or placebo for up to 6 months, overuse (probably associated with development of tolerance) was reported in 2.9% of patients receiving the drug, while tolerance reportedly did not occur in patients receiving placebo. In this study, following abrupt discontinuance of the nasal solution, withdrawal symptoms (e.g., anxiety, agitation, tremulousness, diarrhea, chills, diaphoresis, insomnia, confusion, incoordination, hallucinations) occurred in about 2.6% of patients, most of whom discontinued the drug after prolonged use or administration of high dosages. Such withdrawal symptoms were not reported in patients receiving placebo.

Prolonged continuous use of butorphanol tartrate injection also may result in physical dependence or tolerance and abrupt discontinuance of the injection in patients physically dependent on butorphanol may result in withdrawal symptoms.

The manufacturer states that to minimize the risk of abuse and physical dependence associated with butorphanol tartrate, careful patient selection, dosage and prescription limitations for the drug, appropriate directions for use, and frequent monitoring are important. Butorphanol tartrate should be used carefully in patients with a history of drug abuse or in those receiving the drug repeatedly for extended periods of time.

Pharmacology

Butorphanol tartrate has analgesic and opiate antagonistic effects. The exact mechanisms of actions of the drug are not known. However, the analgesic effect is believed to result from an interaction with an opiate receptor site in the CNS (probably in or associated with the limbic system); the opiate antagonistic effect may result from competitive inhibition at the opiate receptor, but other mechanisms probably also are involved. The drug exerts antagonistic or partially antagonistic effects at μ opiate receptor sites, while it is thought that butorphanol exerts its agonistic effects principally at the κ and Σ opiate receptors. On a weight basis, the analgesic activity of IM butorphanol tartrate is approximately 4–7 times that of IM morphine, 15–30 times that of IM pentazocine, and 30–50 times that of IM meperidine. Studies in animals indicate that, on a weight basis, subcutaneous butorphanol has 30 times the opiate antagonist activity of subcutaneous pentazocine and $^1/_{40}$ that of subcutaneous naloxone.

Like opiate agonists, butorphanol produces respiratory depression, sedation, miosis and, in animals, antitussive effects. In adults, a single 2-mg IV dose of butorphanol tartrate (about 0.03 mg/kg) decreases respiration to the same degree as 10 mg of morphine sulfate IV or 70 mg of meperidine hydrochloride IV. In contrast to morphine, respiratory depression in healthy adults plateaus with a 2-mg IV dose of butorphanol tartrate. However, the duration of respiratory depression produced by butorphanol is increased with increasing dosage (i.e., respiratory depression persists 1 hour after 2 mg IV and at least 90 minutes after 4 mg IV).

In one study, IV administration of butorphanol tartrate 0.025 mg/kg slightly increased pulmonary artery pressure, pulmonary wedge pressure, left ventricular end-diastolic pressure, systemic arterial pressure, pulmonary vascular resistance, and cardiac index.

In animals, butorphanol tartrate inhibits GI motility slightly, causes little increase in duodenal smooth muscle activity, and has little or no effect on bile duct flow. In dogs, butorphanol causes very little systemic histamine release as compared to equianalgesic doses of morphine. In contrast to morphine, butorphanol transiently increases urine output and decreases urine osmolality and sodium and potassium excretion in rats. These effects are caused by inhibition of release of vasopressin from the hypothalamus.

IV administration of 0.2–0.8 mg of naloxone hydrochloride reverses the respiratory depressant effects of 2–4 mg of IV butorphanol tartrate. Naloxone also reverses the analgesic, antitussive, and GI motility inhibiting effects of butorphanol; the diuretic response to butorphanol in animals is *not* reversed by naloxone.

Pharmacokinetics

■ **Absorption** Butorphanol tartrate is completely absorbed from the GI tract in healthy, fasting individuals and from IM injection sites. However, orally administered butorphanol tartrate undergoes first-pass metabolism and only 17% of a dose reaches systemic circulation unchanged. The absolute bioavailability of butorphanol following nasal inhalation may vary with age and gender; the absolute bioavailability of the nasal solution is about 50, 70, and 75% in geriatric women, young individuals, and geriatric men, respectively. Absolute bioavailability of nasally inhaled butorphanol appears to be unchanged in patients with allergic rhinitis. However, in patients receiving a nasal vasoconstrictor (e.g., oxymetazoline), rate of absorption of intranasal butorphanol may be decreased while extent of absorption appears to be unchanged. When intranasal butorphanol was administered in patients receiving oxymetazoline, peak plasma concentrations of butorphanol were reduced by about 50%.

Following oral administration of a single 8-mg dose of butorphanol tartrate to healthy, fasting individuals, peak plasma butorphanol concentrations of 0.7 ng/mL are achieved within 1–1.5 hours. Peak plasma butorphanol concentrations of approximately 2.2 ng/mL occur 30–60 minutes after IM administration of a single 2-mg dose. Peak plasma concentrations of 1.5 ng/mL occur almost immediately after a single 1-mg IV dose. Following nasal inhalation of a single 1-mg dose of butorphanol tartrate solution, mean peak blood butorphanol concentrations of 0.9–1.04 ng/mL are achieved in about 30–60 minutes. Butorphanol tartrate appears to exhibit dose-proportional, linear pharmacokinetics following inhalation of 1–4 mg of nasal solution of the drug every 6 hours for 5 days; peak plasma concentrations and the area under the plasma concentration-time curve (AUC) increased in a dose-dependent fashion, while time to achieve peak plasma concentrations remained relatively constant. Steady-state plasma concentrations of nasally inhaled butorphanol were reached within 48 hours and were about 1.8 times those reported following administration of single doses of the nasal solution; therefore, modest accumulation of the drug appears to occur. After an initial absorption/distribution phase, single-dose pharmacokinetics of butorphanol are similar following IV, IM, or intranasal administration.

After IV administration of 1 or 2 mg of butorphanol tartrate in postoperative patients, the onset of analgesic activity occurs in 1 minute, peak analgesia occurs in 4–5 minutes, and the duration of action is 2–4 hours. Following IM administration of 1 or 2 mg of butorphanol tartrate in postoperative patients, analgesic activity occurs within 10–30 minutes, peak analgesia occurs within 30–60 minutes, and duration of analgesia is 3–4 hours; after 4 mg IM, analgesic effects usually persist at least 4 hours. After nasal inhalation of 1 or 2 mg of butorphanol tartrate solution in postoperative patients, onset of analgesia occurs within 15 minutes, peak analgesia occurs in about 1–2 hours, and duration of analgesia is approximately 2.5–5 hours. In one study, oral administration of 8 or 16 mg of butorphanol tartrate produced analgesic effects within 1–2 hours and analgesia persisted 5–6 hours.

■ **Distribution** Animal studies indicate that highest concentrations of butorphanol and its metabolites are found in the liver, kidneys, and intestine; drug concentrations are higher in the lungs, spleen, heart, endocrine tissues, blood cells, and fat tissue than in plasma; brain concentrations are lower than plasma concentrations. In concentrations of 1–7 ng/mL, about 80% of butorphanol is bound to plasma proteins. Following IV administration, the mean volume of distribution of butorphanol is 487 (range: 305–901 L) and 552 L (range: 305–737 L) in young (20–40 years of age) and geriatric individuals (older than 65 years of age), respectively.

Butorphanol rapidly crosses the placenta, and neonatal serum concentrations are 0.4–1.4 times maternal concentrations. The drug is distributed into milk.

■ **Elimination** Plasma elimination half-life of butorphanol is similar following intranasal and IV administration; the plasma elimination half-life of butorphanol is about 4.6 (range: 2–8.7 hours) and 4.7 hours (range: 2.9–8.8 hours) after IV and intranasal administration, respectively. Plasma elimination half-life of butorphanol may be increased in geriatric individuals following IV and intranasal administration; elimination half-life reportedly was about 5.6 (range 3.3–8.8 hours) and 6.6 hours (range: 3.8–9.2 hours) following IV and intranasal administration, respectively. Plasma elimination half-life also may be increased in patients with renal impairment (creatinine clearance less than 30 mL/minute); elimination half-life reportedly was 10.5 hours in such patients.

Butorphanol is extensively metabolized in the liver, principally by hydroxylation to form hydroxybutorphanol, the major metabolite; *N*-dealkylation and conjugation of butorphanol and its metabolites also occur. Metabolites of butorphanol have no analgesic activity. Butorphanol and its metabolites are excreted mainly by the kidneys as unconjugated hydroxybutorphanol (60–80% of a dose), and less than 5% of a dose is excreted unchanged in urine. In 72–96 hours, 62% of a 1-mg IV dose, 72% of a 2-mg IM dose, and 75% of an 8-mg oral dose can be recovered in the urine. Glucuronides of butorphanol and/or hydroxybutorphanol are excreted in bile and undergo enterohepatic recycling. About 11–14% of a parenteral dose is excreted in feces. Following IV administration of butorphanol tartrate, mean total body clearance of butorphanol is 1650 (range: 1167–2567 mL/minute) and 1367 mL/minute (range: 867–2383 mL/minute) in young (20–40 years of age) and geriatric (older than 65 years of age) individuals, respectively. Body clearance of butorphanol also may be decreased in patients with renal impairment. Following administration of butorphanol tartrate nasal solution, total body clearance of butorphanol is about 4333 and 2500 mL/minute in healthy individuals and in patients with renal impairment (those with creatinine clearance less than 30 mL/minute), respectively.

Chemistry and Stability

■ **Chemistry** Butorphanol tartrate is a synthetic opiate partial agonist analgesic. The drug is structurally related to morphine but pharmacologically similar to pentazocine and nalbuphine. Butorphanol tartrate occurs as a white powder with a bitter taste and is sparingly soluble in water and insoluble in alcohol. The pK_a of the drug is 8.6.

Butorphanol tartrate is commercially available as an injection and as a solution for nasal inhalation. Butorphanol tartrate injection is a sterile solution of the drug in water; the injection contains sodium citrate and has a pH of 3–5.5. For intranasal use, butorphanol tartrate is available as a solution of the drug in purified water; sodium hydroxide and/or hydrochloric acid are added to adjust pH to 5. Butorphanol tartrate injection and nasal solution contain sodium chloride to adjust tonicity and citric acid; the multiple-dose vials of the injection and nasal solution also contain benzethonium chloride as a preservative. Butorphanol tartrate nasal solution is administered by a spray pump which, after initial priming, delivers metered sprays containing 1 mg of butorphanol tartrate per spray.

■ **Stability** Butorphanol tartrate injection should be protected from light and stored at temperatures below 30°C; freezing should be avoided. Butorphanol tartrate nasal solution should be stored at temperatures below 30°C.

Butorphanol tartrate reportedly is physically and chemically compatible for at least 24 hours with atropine sulfate, hydroxyzine hydrochloride, or promethazine hydrochloride. Specialized references should be consulted for specific compatibility information.

Preparations

Butorphanol tartrate (including its optical isomers) preparations are subject to control under the Federal Controlled Substances Act of 1970 as a schedule IV (C-IV) drug.

Excipients in commercially available drug preparations may have clinically important effects in some individuals; consult specific product labeling for details.

Butorphanol Tartrate

Nasal		
Solution	1 mg/metered spray (10 mg/mL)*	**Butorphanol Tartrate Nasal Spray** (C-IV)
Parenteral		
Injection	1 mg/mL*	**Butorphanol Tartrate Injection** (C-IV)
	2 mg/mL*	**Butorphanol Tartrate Injection** (C-IV)

*available from one or more manufacturer, distributor, and/or repackager by generic (nonproprietary) name

†Use is not currently included in the labeling approved by the US Food and Drug Administration

ANALGESICS AND ANTIPYRETICS, MISCELLANEOUS 28:08.92

Acetaminophen

Paracetamol

■ Acetaminophen is a synthetic nonopiate derivative of *p*-aminophenol that produces analgesia and antipyresis.

Uses

Acetaminophen is used extensively in the treatment of mild to moderate pain and fever.

■ **Pain** Acetaminophen is used to provide temporary analgesia in the treatment of mild to moderate pain. Acetaminophen also is used in fixed combination with other agents (e.g., chlorpheniramine, dextromethorphan, diphenhydramine, doxylamine, guaifenesin, phenylephrine, pseudoephedrine) for short-term relief of minor aches and pain, headache, and/or other symptoms (e.g., rhinorrhea, sneezing, lacrimation, itching eyes, oronasopharyngeal itching, nasal congestion, cough) associated with seasonal allergic rhinitis (e.g., hay fever), other upper respiratory allergies, or the common cold.

Acetaminophen is most effective in relieving low intensity pain of nonvisceral origin. Acetaminophen does *not* have antirheumatic effects. Unlike salicylates and prototypical nonsteroidal anti-inflammatory agents (NSAIAs), acetaminophen does not usually depress prothrombin levels. In addition, acetaminophen produces a lower incidence of gastric irritation, erosion, or bleeding than do salicylates or prototypical NSAIAs. Acetaminophen is a desirable alternative in patients who require a mild analgesic or antipyretic but in whom salicylates or prototypical NSAIAs are contraindicated or not tolerated. Because of its efficacy, relative safety at recommended dosages, and low cost, many experts recommend use of the drug as the initial analgesic for many patients. However, the risk of inadvertent overdosage and resultant acute liver failure must be considered, and patients should be counseled about the importance of not exceeding recommended dosages or combining acetaminophen-containing preparations.

Acetaminophen has been used in the treatment of pain in various combinations with aspirin, caffeine, opiates, and/or other agents. Acetaminophen (650-mg oral doses) in combination with oral doses of an opiate (e.g., codeine, oxycodone) produces greater analgesic effect than that produced by either acetaminophen or higher doses of the opiate alone. In patients with moderate to severe postoperative pain, single or repeated IV doses of acetaminophen (650 mg every 4 hours or 1 g every 6 hours) reduced pain intensity and rescue opiate requirements compared with placebo, but clinical benefits of the lower opiate dosages (e.g., reduction in opiate-related adverse effects) have not been established. Although some evidence suggests that the combination of acetaminophen, aspirin, and caffeine is more effective than acetaminophen alone for the treatment of tension-type headache, combinations of acetaminophen with aspirin or caffeine generally have not been shown to have greater analgesic effect than an optimal dose of acetaminophen alone. In addition, there is little evidence that such combinations cause fewer adverse effects than higher doses of the individual agents alone. In one study, the simultaneous administration of 325- or 650-mg oral doses of acetaminophen with 650-mg oral doses of aspirin resulted in increased blood concentrations of unhydrolyzed aspirin compared with 650-mg oral doses of aspirin alone; however, the clinical importance of such an effect remains to be established.

Pain Associated with Migraine Headache Acetaminophen in fixed combination with aspirin and caffeine (containing 250 mg of acetaminophen, 250 mg of aspirin, and 65 mg of caffeine) is used for the temporary relief of mild to moderate pain associated with migraine headache. Some experts state that this combination also may be used for the treatment of severe migraine headache if previous attacks have responded to similar nonopiate analgesics or nonsteroidal anti-inflammatory agents (NSAIAs). The efficacy of oral acetaminophen in fixed combination with aspirin and caffeine for the management of mild to moderate pain associated with migraine headache was established by 3 double-blind, randomized, parallel group, placebo-controlled (one of them a population-based study) studies in adult patients who had migraine with aura or migraine without aura as defined by criteria established by International Headache Society (IHS). The efficacy of therapy for management of pain associated with migraine headache in these studies was evaluated in terms of a reduction in headache severity as rated by the patient (i.e., a reduction in pain from at least moderate to mild or to absent 2 hours after dosing using a 4-point scale). Pooled analysis of data from the 3 studies indicate that about 59% of patients receiving 500 mg of acetaminophen in fixed combination with aspirin and caffeine attained relief of pain associated with migraine headache within 2 hours compared with about 33% of placebo recipients; at 6 hours, about 79 and 52%, respectively, of drug- and placebo-treated patients had mild or no headache pain. In addition, 2 hours after dosing about 21% of patients receiving the combination were pain free versus about 7% receiving placebo, and at 6 hours 51% of drug-treated patients were pain free versus 24% receiving placebo. It appears that the drug also relieves manifestations of migraine other than headache, including nausea, vomiting, photophobia, and phonophobia. Patients in whom pain associated with migraine headache is not relieved by acetaminophen in fixed combination with aspirin and caffeine should consult their clinician about possible alternatives (e.g., use of prescription drugs including ergot alkaloids or vascular serotonin type 1-like receptor agonists) based on evaluation of their medical condition. Efficacy of oral acetaminophen alone for the treatment of acute migraine headache has not been established. For further information on management and classification of migraine headache, see Vascular Headaches: General Principles in Migraine Therapy, under Uses in Sumatriptan 28:32.28.

Pain Associated with Osteoarthritis Acetaminophen is used in the symptomatic treatment of pain associated with osteoarthritis and is considered an initial drug of choice for pain management in osteoarthritis patients. Medical management of osteoarthritis of the hip and knee includes both pharmacologic therapy to reduce pain and nonpharmacologic therapy to maintain and/or improve joint mobility and limit functional impairment (e.g., patient education, weight loss when necessary, aerobic and muscle-strengthening exercise programs, physical therapy and range-of-motion exercises, assistive devices for ambulation and activities of daily living, patellar taping, appropriate footwear or bracing). Pain management is considered an adjunct to nonpharmacologic measures and is most effective when combined with nonpharmacologic strategies.

A variety of drugs have been used for management of pain in patients with osteoarthritis, including oral agents (e.g., acetaminophen, NSAIAs, tramadol), intraarticular agents (e.g., glucocorticoids, sodium hyaluronate), and topical agents (e.g., capsaicin, methylsalicylate). Factors to consider when making treatment decisions for the management of pain in patients with osteoarthritis include the presence of risk factors for serious adverse GI effects or renal toxicity (which may affect decisions regarding use of NSAIAs), existing comorbidities and concomitant therapy, and the adverse effects profiles and costs of specific therapies. Because there is evidence that acetaminophen can be effective, because of its relative safety when used at recommended dosages, and because of its low cost, the American College of Rheumatology (ACR) and other clinicians recommended use of the drug as the initial analgesic for many osteoarthritis patients.

Acetaminophen appears to be as effective as NSAIAs for relief of mild to moderate joint pain in many patients with osteoarthritis; however, the drug is not effective in all patients and may not provide adequate relief in those with moderate to severe pain or when joint inflammation is present. A NSAIA can be considered an alternative initial drug of choice for patients with osteoarthritis, especially for those who have moderate to severe pain and signs of joint inflammation, and also can be considered in patients who fail to obtain adequate symptomatic relief with acetaminophen. Because NSAIAs that selectively inhibit COX-2 (e.g., celecoxib) are associated with a lower incidence of serious adverse GI effects than prototypical NSAIAs and, unlike prototypical NSAIAs, do not affect platelet aggregation and bleeding time, one of these selective inhibitors of COX-2 may be preferred when a NSAIA is being considered for management of pain in osteoarthritis patients at risk for GI complications. (See Uses: Osteoarthritis, in Celecoxib 28:08.04.08.) In patients with osteoarthritis of the knee who have moderate to severe pain and signs of joint inflammation, some clinicians suggest that joint aspiration accompanied by intraarticular glucocorticoid injections or use of an oral NSAIA can be considered for initial therapy.

In patients with osteoarthritis of the knee who fail to respond to adequate regimens of acetaminophen or other appropriate oral analgesics given in conjunction with nonpharmacologic therapy, intraarticular sodium hyaluronate therapy may be indicated; this alternative may be especially advantageous when oral NSAIAs are contraindicated or ineffective. Intraarticular glucocorticoid injections can be used as an adjunct to oral therapy with acetaminophen or other appropriate oral analgesic or as monotherapy in selected patients with osteoarthritis of the knee; these injections also are used occasionally in patients with osteoarthritis of the hip. Intraarticular glucocorticoid injections are of value and may be particularly beneficial in patients with osteoarthritis of the knee who have signs of local inflammation with joint effusion. Use of topical analgesics can be considered as either adjunctive treatment or monotherapy in patients with osteoarthritis of the knee who have mild to moderate pain and have failed to obtain adequate symptomatic relief with acetaminophen and cannot or prefer not to receive other systemic analgesics; topical agents have not been evaluated for pain management in patients with osteoarthritis of the hip and are of questionable value in these patients because of the depth of the hip joint.

■ **Fever** Acetaminophen is used frequently to lower body temperature in febrile patients in whom fever may be deleterious or in whom considerable relief is obtained when fever is lowered. However, antipyretic therapy is generally nonspecific, does not influence the course of the underlying disease, and may obscure the patient's illness. Parents and caregivers of pediatric patients should be reassured that while some parental anxiety over fever is understandable, the principal reason for treating fever is for patient comfort and that complete normalization of body temperature is not necessary and may not be possible. To minimize the risk of acetaminophen overdosage, alternative antipyretics should be considered for children at increased risk of developing toxicity and in those with refractory fever.

Acetaminophen is used in fixed combination with other agents (e.g., chlorpheniramine, dextromethorphan, diphenhydramine, doxylamine, guaifenesin, phenylephrine, pseudoephedrine) for short-term relief of fever and/or other symptoms (e.g., rhinorrhea, sneezing, lacrimation, itching eyes, oronasopharyngeal itching, nasal congestion, cough) associated with seasonal allergic rhinitis (e.g., hay fever), other upper respiratory allergies, or the common cold.

If an antipyretic is considered necessary in children or teenagers with known or suspected varicella, influenza-like illness, or other viral illness, use of acetaminophen (not aspirin) is recommended because use of salicylates in these pediatric patients may be associated with an increased risk of developing Reye's syndrome. (See Cautions: Pediatric Precautions, in the Salicylates General Statement 28:08.04.24.) In the treatment of influenza in young children, control of fever with acetaminophen or other appropriate antipyretic may be important because the fever and other symptoms of influenza could exacerbate underlying chronic conditions.

Acetaminophen and aspirin are equally effective as antipyretics. In one study in febrile children, the combination of oral doses of acetaminophen and aspirin was at least as effective in reducing fever as either drug alone, and the duration of fever reduction was longer with the combination than with the individual drugs. However, because of the study design, it could not be concluded that the combination had additive effects. Many clinicians use regimens of alternating doses of acetaminophen and aspirin; however, combined overdosage with both drugs has occurred with such a regimen and the efficacy and safety of these regimens remain to be established.

To minimize the risk of acetaminophen overdosage, some clinicians have used pediatric regimens of alternating doses of acetaminophen and ibuprofen; however, the efficacy and safety of these regimens remain to be established. In addition, although some such clinicians have alternated acetaminophen and ibuprofen at 2-hour intervals (i.e., with each drug administered every 4 hours) in pediatric patients, there is no pharmacokinetic rationale to support such a regimen; longer alternating dosing intervals would seem more appropriate if an alternating regimen is considered, but additional study and experience are necessary.

Febrile Seizures Because febrile seizures occur only in conjunction with a fever, it has been postulated that aggressive intermittent antipyretic therapy might prevent such seizures. However, there currently is no evidence to substantiate that aggressive antipyretic therapy can prevent recurrent febrile seizures. In one study in a limited number of children, 25% of patients in whom antipyretic therapy was initiated when any rectal temperature exceeded 37.2°C (99°F) experienced seizure recurrence compared with 5% of those who received continuous phenobarbital prophylaxis. In another study comparing low-dose diazepam, acetaminophen, and placebo, there was no evidence that acetaminophen prevented recurrent febrile seizures; acetaminophen was administered in a dosage of 10 mg/kg 4 times daily. In children hospitalized after a simple febrile seizure, administration of aggressive antipyretic therapy with acetaminophen 15–20 mg/kg every 4 hours was no more effective than sporadic acetaminophen use in preventing a second febrile seizure during that admission; the 2 treatment groups also had a similar frequency, duration, and magnitude of temperature elevations.

Dosage and Administration

■ **Administration** Acetaminophen is administered orally, rectally as suppositories, and by IV infusion over 15 minutes.

Acetaminophen preparations for *self-medication* should not be used unless seals on the tamper-resistant packaging are intact.

Oral Administration Acetaminophen usually is administered orally. Extended-release acetaminophen tablets should not be crushed, chewed, or dissolved in liquid. Orally disintegrating tablets containing acetaminophen (e.g., Tylenol® Meltaways) should be allowed to dissolve in the mouth or should be chewed before swallowing.

Rectal Administration In patients who cannot tolerate oral medication, acetaminophen may be administered rectally as suppositories; however, the rectal dose required to produce the same plasma concentrations may be higher than the oral dose and rectal absorption can be erratic. Dividing suppositories in an attempt to administer lower dosages may not provide a predictable dose.

Some experts state that rectal preparations of acetaminophen should not be used for *self-medication* in children unless such use is specifically discussed with a clinician and parents or caregivers are instructed to adhere to dosage and administration recommendations; poor or variable absorption of acetaminophen following rectal administration may be associated with inadequate therapy or may result in toxicity following frequent or excessive doses.

IV Administration Acetaminophen is administered by IV infusion over 15 minutes. The commercially available acetaminophen injection may be administered without further dilution. Each vial containing 1 g/100 mL is intended for single use only; any unused portions must be discarded.

Acetaminophen doses of 1 g should be administered by inserting a vented IV set through the septum of the 100-mL vial. Doses of less than 1 g must be withdrawn from the vial and placed in a separate container for IV infusion in order to avoid inadvertent administration of the total volume of the commercially available vial. The appropriate dose of acetaminophen should be withdrawn aseptically from an intact sealed vial and transferred to an empty sterile container (e.g., glass bottle, plastic container, syringe); small-volume (up to 60 mL) pediatric doses should be drawn into a syringe and administered using a syringe pump. Once the vacuum seal of the vial has been penetrated or the vial contents have been transferred to another container, the dose of acetaminophen should be administered within 6 hours. The end of the infusion should be monitored in order to prevent the possibility of air embolism, especially when the acetaminophen solution is the primary infusion.

Acetaminophen should not be admixed with any other drugs. Acetaminophen solution should be inspected visually for particulate matter and discoloration prior to preparation and administration; if either is present, the solution should be discarded.

■ **Dosage** Acetaminophen is relatively safe when used at recommended dosages. However, acetaminophen overdosage has been the leading cause of acute liver failure in the US, United Kingdom, and most of Europe, with about 50% of US cases in recent years resulting from inadvertent overdosage (e.g., in patients not recognizing the presence of the drug in multiple over-the-counter [OTC] and/or prescription products that they may be taking). Therefore, patients should be warned about the importance of determining whether acetaminophen is present in their medications (e.g., by examining labels carefully, by consulting their clinician and pharmacist) and of not exceeding recommended dosages or combining acetaminophen-containing preparations.

Acetaminophen should not be used for *self-medication* of pain for longer than 10 days (in adults or children 12 years of age and older) or 5 days (in children 2–11 years of age), unless directed by a clinician because pain of such intensity and duration may indicate a pathologic condition requiring medical evaluation and supervised treatment.

Acetaminophen should not be used in adults or children for *self-medication* of marked fever (greater than 39.5°C), fever persisting longer than 3 days, or recurrent fever, unless directed by a clinician because such fevers may indicate serious illness requiring prompt medical evaluation.

Acetaminophen should not be used in adults or children for *self-medication* of sore throat pain (pharyngitis, laryngitis, tonsillitis) for longer than 2 days.

To minimize the risk of overdosage, recommended age-appropriate daily dosages of acetaminophen should not be exceeded. Because severe liver toxicity and death have occurred in children who received multiple excessive doses of acetaminophen as part of therapeutic administration, parents or caregivers should be instructed to use weight-based dosing for acetaminophen, to use only the calibrated measuring device provided with the particular acetaminophen formulation for measuring dosage, to ensure that the correct number of tablets required for the intended dose is removed from the package, and not to exceed the recommended daily dosage because serious adverse effects could result. In addition, patients should be warned that the risk of overdosage and severe liver damage is increased if more than one preparation containing acetaminophen are used concomitantly.

Pharmacists have an important role in preventing acetaminophen-induced hepatotoxicity by advising consumers about the risk of failing to recognize that a wide variety of OTC and prescription preparations contain acetaminophen. Failure to recognize acetaminophen as an ingredient may be particularly likely with prescription drugs because the label of the dispensed drug may not clearly state its presence. Educating consumers about the risk of exceeding recommended acetaminophen dosages also is important. The US Food and Drug Administration (FDA) recommends that pharmacists receiving prescriptions for fixed-combination preparations containing more than 325 mg of acetaminophen per dosage unit contact the prescriber to discuss use of a preparation containing no more than 325 mg of the drug per dosage unit. (See Preparations.)

Clinicians should exercise caution when prescribing, preparing, and administering IV acetaminophen to avoid dosing errors that could result in accidental overdosage and death. In particular, clinicians should ensure that the dose (in mg) and the volume (in mL) are not confused, the dose for patients weighing less than 50 kg is based on body weight, the infusion pump is programmed correctly, and the total daily dosage of acetaminophen from all sources does not exceed the maximum recommended daily dosage.

Adult Dosage **Pain and Fever.** For analgesia or antipyresis in adults or children 12 years of age or older, the usual oral dosage of acetaminophen as an immediate-release (conventional) preparation is 650 mg every 4–6 hours or 1 g every 6 hours as necessary. An oral acetaminophen dosage of 1.3 g as extended-release tablets every 8 hours can be used for the management of pain in adults. The currently recommended maximum dosage of acetaminophen is 4 g daily. Some experts recommend a maximum dosage of 3 g daily when the drug is used for long-term therapy (e.g., 2 or more weeks). The FDA is reviewing available data to determine whether it is possible to identify subgroups of patients with increased susceptibility to acetaminophen-associated hepatotoxicity and to determine whether data support establishing a lower (i.e., less than 4 g daily) maximum daily dosage for certain patients. (See Cautions: Precautions and Contraindications.) To minimize the risk of inadvertent overdosage, some manufacturers (e.g., McNeil, Tylenol®) have voluntarily revised their labeling to recommend less frequent dosing and lower total daily dosages of acetaminophen. These manufacturers now recommend that dosages in adults and children 12 years of age and older not exceed 1 g every 6 hours up to a maximum of 3 g daily.

For analgesia or antipyresis in adults or children 12 years of age or older, the usual rectal dosage of acetaminophen is 325–650 mg every 4 hours as necessary; dosage should not exceed 4 g daily.

Acetaminophen may be given IV as a single dose or as repeated doses for analgesia or antipyresis. No dosage adjustment is required when an adult or adolescent who weighs 50 kg or more is switched between oral and IV acetaminophen. The recommended IV dosage of acetaminophen for analgesia or antipyresis in adults and adolescents 13 years of age or older who weigh 50 kg or more is 1 g every 6 hours or 650 mg every 4 hours; the maximum recommended single dose is 1 g, the minimum dosing interval is 4 hours, and the maximum daily dosage is 4 g per 24-hour period, including all routes of administration and all acetaminophen-containing preparations, including fixed combinations. In adults and adolescents 13 years of age or older who weigh less than 50 kg, the recommended dosage is 15 mg/kg every 6 hours or 12.5 mg/kg every 4 hours; the maximum single dose is 15 mg/kg, the minimum dosing interval is 4 hours, and the maximum daily dosage is 75 mg/kg per 24-hour period, including all routes of administration and all acetaminophen-containing preparations, including fixed combinations.

Patients receiving acetaminophen in fixed combination with an opiate analgesic may develop tolerance to the opiate and increase the dosage of the combination not realizing the risk of inadvertent acetaminophen overdosage. Therefore, to minimize the risk of inadvertent acetaminophen overdosage, FDA has requested manufacturers to reformulate prescription combination preparations to limit the amount of acetaminophen to 325 mg or less per dosage unit. (See Preparations.) FDA also recommends that health care providers stop prescribing and dispensing prescription combination preparations containing more than 325 mg of acetaminophen per dosage unit. FDA states that doses consisting of either 1 or 2 dosage units (i.e., 325 or 650 mg of acetaminophen per dose) may be prescribed as clinically appropriate for the patient; to ensure appropriate dosages of each component of the fixed combination, the strength of each component (generally acetaminophen and an opiate analgesic) must be considered. FDA states that there are no data indicating that use of prescription combination preparations containing more than 325 mg of acetaminophen per dosage unit provides additional benefit that would outweigh the increased risk of liver injury resulting from inadvertent overdosage.

Pain Associated with Migraine Headache. For *self-medication* for the temporary relief of mild to moderate pain associated with migraine headache in adults, the recommended oral dosage is 500 mg of acetaminophen (combined with 500 mg of aspirin and 130 mg of caffeine) as a single dose of an immediate-release (conventional) preparation taken with a full glass of water; no more than 500 mg of acetaminophen (in combination with 500 mg of aspirin and 130 mg of caffeine) should be taken in any 24-hour period, unless directed by a clinician. Individuals younger than 18 years of age should consult their clinician before using this combination preparation.

Pain Associated with Osteoarthritis. For the treatment of pain associated with osteoarthritis, many clinicians recommend acetaminophen dosages in adults up to 1 g administered 4 times daily as an immediate-release (conventional) preparation. Alternatively, 1.3 g as extended-release tablets every 8 hours can be used. Some experts recommend a maximum dosage of 3 g daily when the drug is used for long-term therapy (e.g., 2 or more weeks). FDA is reviewing available data to determine whether it is possible to identify subgroups of patients with increased susceptibility to acetaminophen-associated hepatotoxicity and to determine whether data support establishing a lower (i.e., less than 4 g daily) maximum daily dosage for certain patients. (See Cautions: Precautions and Contraindications.) To minimize the risk of inadvertent overdosage, some manufacturers (e.g., McNeil, Tylenol®) have voluntarily revised their labeling to recommend less frequent dosing and lower total daily dosages of acetaminophen. These manufacturers now recommend that dosages in adults not exceed 1 g every 6 hours up to a maximum of 3 g daily.

Pediatric Dosage **Pain and Fever.** For analgesia and antipyresis in children 12 years of age or older, the usual oral dosage of acetaminophen as an immediate-release (conventional) preparation is 650 mg every 4–6 hours or 1 g every 6 hours as necessary. The currently recommended maximum dosage of acetaminophen in children 12 years of age and older is 4 g daily; however, some manufacturers recommend that dosage of acetaminophen not exceed 3 g daily in such patients. For analgesia and antipyresis, children may receive the following oral doses of acetaminophen every 4–6 hours as necessary (up to 5 times in 24 hours) as an immediate-release (conventional) preparation: children 11 years of age (33–43 kg), 480 mg; children 9–10 years of age (27–32 kg), 400 mg; children 6–8 years of age (22–27 kg), 320 mg; children 4–5 years of age (16–21 kg), 240 mg; children 2–3 years of age (11–16 kg), 160 mg; children 12–23 months of age (8–11 kg), 120 mg; children 4–11 months of age (5–8 kg), 80 mg; and children up to 3 months of age (2.7–5 kg), 40 mg. (See Cautions: Pediatric Precautions.)

For analgesia and antipyresis in children 12 years of age or older, the usual rectal dosage of acetaminophen is 325–650 mg every 4 hours as necessary; dosage should not exceed 4 g daily. For analgesia and antipyresis, children may receive the following rectal doses of acetaminophen every 4 hours as necessary (up to 5 times in 24 hours): children 11–12 years of age, 320–480 mg; children 9–11 years of age, 320–400 mg; children 6–9 years of age, 320 mg; children 4–6 years of age, 240 mg; children 2–4 years of age, 160 mg. Rectal dosages in children younger than 2 years of age must be individualized, and the possibility of erratic systemic absorption should be considered.

Acetaminophen may be given IV as a single dose or as repeated doses for analgesia or antipyresis. The recommended IV dosage of acetaminophen for analgesia or antipyresis in children 2–12 years of age is 15 mg/kg every 6 hours or 12.5 mg/kg every 4 hours; the maximum single dose is 15 mg/kg, the minimum dosing interval is 4 hours, and the maximum daily dosage is 75 mg/kg per 24-hour period, including all routes of administration and all acetaminophen-containing preparations, including fixed combinations.

■ **Dosage in Renal and Hepatic Impairment** In patients with hepatic impairment or active liver disease, reduction of the total daily dosage of acetaminophen may be warranted. In patients with severe renal impairment (creatinine clearance of 30 mL/minute or less), longer dosing intervals and a reduced total daily dosage of acetaminophen may be warranted. (See Cautions: Precautions and Contraindications.)

Cautions

Acetaminophen is relatively nontoxic in therapeutic doses when taken as directed. However, acetaminophen overdosage has been the leading cause of acute liver failure (with encephalopathy and coagulopathy) in the US, United Kingdom, and most of Europe, with about 50% of US cases in recent years resulting from inadvertent overdosage (e.g., in patients not recognizing the presence of the drug in multiple over-the-counter (OTC) and/or prescription products that they may be taking). Therefore, patients should be warned about the importance of determining whether acetaminophen is present in their medications (e.g., by examining labels carefully, by consulting their clinician and pharmacist) and of not exceeding recommended dosages or combining acetaminophen-containing preparations.

Many OTC drug products and prescription preparations contain acetaminophen. In fact, acetaminophen, alone or in combination, is one of the most commonly used drugs in the US. Simultaneous use of more than one preparation containing acetaminophen can result in adverse consequences (e.g., acetaminophen overdose). Patients should be advised not to take multiple acetaminophen-containing preparations concomitantly.

When acetaminophen is used in fixed combination with other agents (e.g., antihistamines, aspirin, caffeine, dextromethorphan, guaifenesin, nasal decongestants, opiate agonists), the usual cautions, precautions, and contraindications associated with these agents must be considered in addition to those associated with acetaminophen.

The most common adverse effects reported in clinical trials in patients receiving IV acetaminophen were nausea, vomiting, headache, and insomnia in adults and nausea, vomiting, constipation, pruritus, agitation, and atelectasis in pediatric patients.

■ **Dermatologic and Sensitivity Reactions** Serious, potentially fatal dermatologic reactions, including Stevens-Johnson syndrome, toxic epidermal necrolysis, and acute generalized exanthematous pustulosis, have been reported rarely in patients receiving acetaminophen. In several published cases, serious dermatologic reactions recurred following rechallenge with the drug; in other published cases, acetaminophen was the only drug administered prior to the reaction, or hypersensitivity to acetaminophen was demonstrated by skin testing or by other means. In addition to these published cases, the US Food and Drug Administration (FDA) identified 107 cases of Stevens-Johnson syndrome, toxic epidermal necrolysis, or acute generalized exanthematous pustulosis that had been reported to the FDA Adverse Event Reporting System (AERS) from 1969–2012 and were considered possibly or probably related to acetaminophen; 67 of the patients described in these reports were hospitalized and 12 patients died. Serious dermatologic reactions may occur at any time during acetaminophen therapy. Results of case-control studies suggest that the risk of Stevens-Johnson syndrome or toxic epidermal necrolysis associated with acetaminophen use generally is independent of the effects of other drugs. Although other analgesic and antipyretic agents (e.g., nonsteroidal anti-inflammatory agents [NSAIAs]) may cause similar reactions, cross-sensitivity with acetaminophen does not appear to occur. Acetaminophen should be discontinued immediately at the first appearance of rash or any other manifestation of hypersensitivity (e.g., urticaria, rash, pruritus, respiratory distress, swelling of the face, mouth, or throat). Patients should be advised to discontinue acetaminophen and seek immediate medical attention if rash or other manifestations of dermatologic or hypersensitivity reactions occur during therapy with the drug. Individuals with a history of such reactions should be advised *not* to take any acetaminophen-containing preparations.

Other dermatologic reactions including pruritic maculopapular rash, urticaria, rash, and periorbital edema also have been reported, and other sensitivity reactions including laryngeal edema, angioedema, and anaphylactoid reactions may occur rarely.

■ Hematologic Effects Thrombocytopenia, leukopenia, and pancytopenia have been associated with the use of *p*-aminophenol derivatives, especially with prolonged administration of large doses. Neutropenia, anemia, and thrombocytopenic purpura have been reported with acetaminophen use. Rarely, agranulocytosis has been reported in patients receiving acetaminophen.

■ Hepatic Effects Hepatotoxicity can result from ingestion of a single toxic dose or multiple excessive doses of acetaminophen, and overdosage of acetaminophen is the leading cause of acute liver failure (ALF) in adults in the US; in most cases, overdosage was inadvertent rather than intentional. (See Acute Toxicity and also see Chronic Toxicity.) While most patients who develop acetaminophen-induced acute liver failure survive without liver transplantation (60%), 9% require transplantation and 30% die.

Substantial elevations in ALT occurred in healthy individuals receiving oral acetaminophen in a dosage of 4 g daily in one randomized study. Study participants (58–59% Hispanic American, 28–31% Caucasian, 12–13% African American) were randomized to receive 4 g of acetaminophen daily (alone or in combination with an opiate) or placebo for 14 days; the study was conducted at an inpatient clinical pharmacology unit. Maximum ALT values exceeding 3 times the upper limit of normal (ULN) occurred in 38 or 31–44% of individuals receiving acetaminophen or acetaminophen in combination with an opiate, respectively; substantial elevations in ALT (i.e., values exceeding 3 times the ULN) were not observed in individuals given placebo. In clinical trials evaluating IV acetaminophen, increased AST concentrations have been reported in adults and increased hepatic enzyme concentrations have been reported in pediatric patients receiving the drug.

■ Other Adverse Effects Nausea, vomiting, headache, and insomnia were reported in clinical trials in 34, 15, 10, and 7%, respectively, of adults receiving IV acetaminophen compared with 31, 11, 9, and 5%, respectively, of placebo recipients. Other adverse effects reported in clinical trials in adults receiving IV acetaminophen include abnormal breath sounds, anxiety, dyspnea, fatigue, hypertension, hypokalemia, hypotension, infusion site pain, muscle spasms, peripheral edema, and trismus.

Adverse effects reported in clinical trials in pediatric patients receiving IV acetaminophen include cardiovascular effects (hypertension, hypotension, tachycardia), GI effects (abdominal pain, diarrhea), nervous system effects (headache, insomnia), respiratory effects (hypoxia, pleural effusion, pulmonary edema, stridor, wheezing), hypoalbuminemia, hypokalemia, hypomagnesemia, hypophosphatemia, hypervolemia, injection site pain, muscle spasm, oliguria, pain in extremity, peripheral edema, and pyrexia.

■ Precautions and Contraindications Some commercially available formulations of acetaminophen contain sulfites that may cause allergic-type reactions, including anaphylaxis and life-threatening or less severe asthmatic episodes, in certain susceptible individuals. The overall prevalence of sulfite sensitivity in the general population is unknown but probably low; such sensitivity appears to occur more frequently in asthmatic than in nonasthmatic individuals. Acetaminophen should be discontinued if hypersensitivity reactions occur.

Although psychologic dependence on acetaminophen may occur, tolerance and physical dependence do not appear to develop even with prolonged use.

The antipyretic effects of acetaminophen may mask the presence of fever.

Because concomitant administration of acetaminophen (especially when administered in high dosages or for prolonged periods) with oral anticoagulants may potentiate the effects of the oral anticoagulant, additional monitoring of prothrombin time (PT)/international normalized ratio (INR) values has been suggested for patients receiving oral anticoagulants following initiation of, or during sustained therapy with, large doses of acetaminophen. The manufacturer of acetaminophen injection states that more frequent monitoring of the INR also may be appropriate when patients receiving oral anticoagulants require short-term IV acetaminophen therapy, since the effects of such concomitant use have not been established. (See Drug Interactions: Oral Anticoagulants.)

Acetaminophen should be used with caution in patients with hepatic impairment or active liver disease and is contraindicated in those with severe hepatic impairment or severe active liver disease. Acetaminophen also should be used with caution in patients with alcoholism, chronic malnutrition, severe hypovolemia (e.g., resulting from dehydration or blood loss), or severe renal impairment (creatinine clearance of 30 mL/minute or less). Dosage reduction may be warranted in patients with hepatic impairment, active liver disease, or severe renal impairment. (See Dosage and Administration: Dosage in Renal and Hepatic Impairment.)

Because chronic, excessive consumption of alcohol may increase the risk of acetaminophen-induced hepatotoxicity, chronic alcoholics should be cautioned to avoid regular or excessive use of acetaminophen, or alternatively, to avoid chronic ingestion of alcohol. The manufacturers currently caution that patients who generally consume 3 or more alcohol-containing drinks per day should ask their clinician whether to use acetaminophen or an alternative analgesic for *self-medication*. However, FDA has proposed eliminating this statement from the labeling of OTC acetaminophen-containing preparations and adding a new warning that would highlight the potential for severe liver damage to occur in individuals who consume 3 or more alcohol-containing drinks per day while taking acetaminophen, in those who use more than one acetaminophen-containing product concomitantly, and in those who exceed the recommended daily dosage of the drug. FDA also has proposed revising the labeling of OTC acetaminophen-containing preparations to include a statement that patients should consult a clinician prior to use if they have liver disease. FDA is reviewing available data to determine whether it is possible to identify subgroups of patients with increased susceptibility to acetaminophen-associated hepatotoxicity and to determine whether data support establishing a lower (i.e., less than 4 g daily) maximum daily dosage for certain patients (e.g., those who chronically ingest alcohol).

Acetaminophen is contraindicated in patients with known hypersensitivity to the drug or any ingredient in the formulation.

■ Pediatric Precautions Because severe liver toxicity and death have occurred in children who received multiple excessive doses of acetaminophen as part of therapeutic administration (i.e., with therapeutic intent), parents or caregivers should be instructed to use weight-based dosing for acetaminophen, to use only the calibrated measuring device provided with the particular acetaminophen formulation for measuring dosage, to ensure that the correct number of tablets required for the intended dose is removed from the package, and not to exceed the recommended daily dosage because serious adverse effects could result. Parents also should be cautioned not to use other acetaminophen-containing products (e.g., some cold and cough products) concomitantly with acetaminophen in children because of the potential for overdoses.

Because acetaminophen therapy usually is begun without the direct advice of a clinician and carries the risk of potential overdosage, instruction regarding appropriate pain and fever therapy preferably should be incorporated into well-child visits. Optimally, clinicians should provide parents and/or caregivers with written, specific advice as part of well-child visits, which should be reviewed during subsequent visits. Parents and caregivers should be advised about the appropriate dose, frequency, duration of therapy, and specific strength and formulation for an individual pediatric patient. They also should be advised of the danger of substituting alternative dosage forms, particularly adult for pediatric formulations. Parents and caregivers should be warned not to exceed recommended acetaminophen dosages and cautioned that children should not be allowed to administer the drug themselves. They also should be warned to read the labeled contents of over-the-counter (OTC) preparations, particularly those recommended for cold, cough, fever, headache, and general ache and pain because simultaneous use of more than one preparation containing acetaminophen could be dangerous. In addition, they should be warned not to substitute extended-release formulations for immediate-release (conventional) ones without making appropriate changes in the dosing interval. A clinician should be contacted for advice if fever and/or other signs and symptoms amenable to acetaminophen persist.

Inadvertent acetaminophen overdosage, possibly resulting in hepatic failure and death, has been reported following confusion over different concentrations of the drug (e.g., 80 mg/0.8 mL, 80 mg/mL, 160 mg/5 mL) contained in various pediatric preparations. To minimize dosing confusion, a recommendation was made in June 2009 during a joint meeting between several FDA advisory committees to have only one concentration of liquid acetaminophen be available for *self-medication* (OTC use) in all pediatric patients. As a result, some manufacturers have decided to voluntarily change the concentration of the infants' formulation to be the same as that of the children's formulation (i.e., from 80 mg/0.8 mL or 80 mg/mL to 160 mg/5 mL). On December 22, 2011, FDA announced that a new liquid preparation marketed for infants, containing the lower concentration of acetaminophen (160 mg/5 mL), was available. This change in concentration affects the amount of liquid acetaminophen given to an infant, and should be especially noted if parents or caregivers have been accustomed to using the 80-mg/0.8-mL or 80-mg/mL concentration of liquid acetaminophen. The new preparation may be packaged with an oral syringe instead of a dropper. Because reformulation of the infants' preparation was voluntary, older, more-concentrated liquid acetaminophen preparations marketed for infants may remain available. To avoid confusion and the potential for dosing errors, clinicians should advise caregivers on product differences; clinicians also should specify both the concentration and dose of liquid acetaminophen when providing directions for use in children. Consumers, parents, and caregivers should be advised to carefully read the product labeling to identify the concentration of acetaminophen (in mg/mL), dosage, and directions for use. Parents and caregivers also should be advised to use only the measuring device provided with the particular preparation and not to mix and match measuring devices; if use of the measuring device seems confusing, or if there is any uncertainty in the proper use of the device, a clinician should be contacted. It should be noted that older, more-concentrated preparations of liquid acetaminophen (80 mg/0.8 mL or 80 mg/mL), if not expired, are safe and effective if used according to the directions specified on the product labeling that accompanies the preparation.

Overdosage and toxicity (including death) have been reported in children younger than 2 years of age receiving OTC preparations containing antihistamines, cough suppressants, expectorants, and nasal decongestants alone or in combination for relief of symptoms of upper respiratory tract infection. Such preparations also may contain analgesics and antipyretics (e.g., acetaminophen). There is limited evidence of efficacy for these preparations in this age group, and appropriate dosages (i.e., approved by FDA) have not been established. FDA recommends that parents and caregivers adhere to the dosage instructions and warnings on the product labeling that accompanies the preparation if administering to children and consult with their clinician about any concerns. Clinicians should ask caregivers about use of nonprescription cough and cold preparations to avoid overdosage. For additional information on precautions associated with the use of cough and cold preparations in pediatric patients, see Cautions: Pediatric Precautions in Pseudoephedrine 12:12.12.

Use of IV acetaminophen for analgesia or antipyresis in pediatric patients 2 years of age and older is supported by evidence from adequate and well-controlled studies of IV acetaminophen in adults and additional safety and pharmacokinetic data from 355 pediatric patients ranging in age from premature neonates (postmenstrual age of at least 32 weeks) to adolescents. Efficacy of IV acetaminophen for analgesia and antipyresis has not been established in pediatric patients younger than 2 years of age.

■ **Geriatric Precautions** When the total number of patients studied in clinical trials of IV acetaminophen is considered, 15% were 65 years of age or older, while 5% were 75 years of age and older. Although no overall differences in efficacy or safety were observed between geriatric and younger patients, and other clinical experience revealed no evidence of age-related differences, the possibility that some older patients may exhibit increased sensitivity to IV acetaminophen cannot be ruled out.

■ **Mutagenicity and Carcinogenicity** Acetaminophen was not mutagenic in the bacterial reverse mutation assay (Ames test), but positive results were observed in vitro in the mouse lymphoma assay and the chromosomal aberration assay using human lymphocytes. The drug has been reported to be clastogenic in rats at a dosage equivalent to 3.6 times the maximum recommended human daily dosage (4 g daily, based on body surface area comparison) but was not clastogenic at a dosage equivalent to 1.8 times the maximum recommended human daily dosage; these results suggest a threshold effect.

In 2-year studies in rats and mice fed a diet containing acetaminophen (up to 6000 ppm), there was no evidence of carcinogenicity in male rats or in mice given acetaminophen at dosages equivalent to 0.7 or 1.2–1.4 times, respectively, the maximum recommended human daily dosage (based on body surface area comparison). In female rats, there was equivocal evidence of carcinogenic activity based on an increased incidence of mononuclear cell leukemia at dosages equivalent to 0.8 times the maximum recommended human daily dosage.

■ **Pregnancy, Fertility, and Lactation** ***Pregnancy*** Epidemiologic data regarding oral acetaminophen use in pregnant women have shown no increased risk of major congenital malformations in infants exposed in utero to the drug. In a large population-based prospective cohort study involving more than 26,000 women with live-born singleton infants who were exposed to oral acetaminophen during the first trimester of pregnancy, no increase in the risk of congenital malformations was observed in exposed children compared with a control group of unexposed children; the rate of congenital malformations (4.3%) was similar to the rate in the general population. A population-based, case-control study from the National Birth Defects Prevention Study also found no increase in the risk of major birth defects in a group of 11,610 children who had been exposed to acetaminophen during the first trimester of pregnancy compared with a control group of 4500 children.

Animal reproduction studies in pregnant rats given oral acetaminophen during organogenesis at dosages up to 0.85 times the maximum recommended human daily dosage (4 g daily, based on body surface area comparison) showed evidence of fetotoxicity (reduced fetal weight and length) and a dose-related increase in bone variations (reduced ossification and rudimentary rib changes); the offspring showed no evidence of external, visceral, or skeletal malformations. When pregnant rats received oral acetaminophen throughout gestation at a dosage of 1.2 times the maximum recommended human daily dosage, areas of necrosis occurred in both the liver and kidney of pregnant rats and fetuses; these effects did not occur in animals given acetaminophen at dosages of 0.3 times the maximum recommended human dosage.

In a continuous breeding study in which pregnant mice were given acetaminophen at dosages approximately equivalent to 0.43, 0.87, or 1.7 times the maximum recommended human daily dosage (based on body surface area comparison), a dose-related reduction in body weight of the fourth and fifth litter offspring of the treated mating pair occurred during lactation and following weaning at all dosages studied. Animals receiving the highest dosage had a reduced number of litters per mating pair, male offspring with an increased percentage of abnormal sperm, and reduced birth weights in the next-generation pups.

Acetaminophen is commonly used during all stages of pregnancy for its analgesic and antipyretic effects. Although acetaminophen has been thought not to be associated with risk in offspring, some recent reports have questioned this assessment, especially with frequent maternal use or in cases involving genetic variability. FDA reviewed data on a possible association between acetaminophen use during pregnancy and risk of attention deficit hyperactivity disorder (ADHD) in children and announced in January 2015 that the data were inconclusive. Some experts state that as with all drug use during pregnancy, *routine* use of acetaminophen should be avoided.

The manufacturer states that there are no studies of IV acetaminophen in pregnant women and animal reproduction studies have not been conducted with this preparation. Therefore, the manufacturer states that IV acetaminophen should be used during pregnancy only when clearly needed.

Because there are no adequate and well-controlled studies of IV acetaminophen during labor and delivery, the manufacturer states that IV acetaminophen should be used in this setting only after careful assessment of potential benefits and risks.

Fertility In a continuous breeding study in mice, no effects on fertility were observed in mice given acetaminophen at dosages up to 1.7 times the maximum recommended human daily dosage (based on body surface area comparison). In mice receiving acetaminophen at a dosage of 1.7 times the maximum recommended human daily dosage, no effect on sperm motility or sperm density in the epididymis was observed, but the percentage of abnormal sperm was increased and the number of mating pairs producing a fifth litter was reduced, suggesting the potential for cumulative toxicity with chronic administration of acetaminophen near the upper limit of daily dosing.

Other studies in rodents indicate that oral administration of acetaminophen at doses equivalent to at least 1.2 times the maximum recommended human daily dosage (based on body surface area comparison) results in decreased testicular weights, reduced spermatogenesis, and reduced fertility in males and reduced implantation sites in females. These effects appeared to increase with duration of treatment. The clinical relevance of these findings is not known.

Lactation Acetaminophen is distributed into human milk in small quantities after oral administration. Data from more than 15 nursing women suggest that approximately 1–2% of the maternal daily dosage would be ingested by a nursing infant. A case of maculopapular rash in a breast-fed infant has been reported; the rash resolved when the mother discontinued acetaminophen use and recurred when she resumed acetaminophen therapy. The American Academy of Pediatrics and other experts state that acetaminophen is an acceptable choice for use in nursing women. The manufacturer states that IV acetaminophen should be used with caution in nursing women.

Drug Interactions

■ **Drugs Affecting Hepatic Microsomal Enzymes** Drugs that induce or regulate hepatic cytochrome P-450 isoenzyme 2E1 (CYP2E1) may alter the metabolism of acetaminophen and increase its hepatotoxic potential. (See Pharmacokinetics: Elimination.) The clinical importance of such effects has not been established to date.

■ **Alcohol** The effects of alcohol on acetaminophen pharmacokinetics are complex; although excessive alcohol use can induce hepatic cytochromes, alcohol also competitively inhibits the metabolism of acetaminophen. Because there is some evidence that chronic, excessive consumption of alcohol may increase the risk of acetaminophen-induced hepatotoxicity, chronic alcoholics should be cautioned to avoid regular or excessive use of acetaminophen, or alternatively, to avoid chronic ingestion of alcohol. The manufacturers currently caution that patients who generally consume 3 or more alcohol-containing drinks per day should ask their clinician whether to use acetaminophen or an alternative analgesic for *self-medication* because acetaminophen may increase the risk of hepatotoxicity. However, the US Food and Drug Administration (FDA) has proposed eliminating this statement from the labeling of OTC acetaminophen-containing preparations and adding a new warning that would highlight the potential for severe liver damage to occur under certain circumstances, including in individuals who consume 3 or more alcohol-containing drinks per day while taking acetaminophen. (See Cautions: Precautions and Contraindications.)

■ **Anticonvulsants** Anticonvulsants (including phenytoin, barbiturates, carbamazepine) that induce hepatic microsomal enzymes may increase acetaminophen-induced liver toxicity because of increased conversion of the drug to hepatotoxic metabolites. The risk of acetaminophen-induced hepatic toxicity is substantially increased in patients ingesting larger than recommended dosages of acetaminophen while receiving anticonvulsants. Usually, no dosage reduction is required in patients receiving concomitant administration of therapeutic dosages of acetaminophen and anticonvulsants; however, patients should limit self-medication with acetaminophen while receiving anticonvulsants.

■ **Aspirin** Limited data indicate that administration of acetaminophen (1 g daily) does not inhibit the antiplatelet effect of aspirin (81 mg daily).

■ **Isoniazid** Concomitant administration of isoniazid with acetaminophen may result in an increased risk of hepatotoxicity, but the exact mechanism of this interaction has not been established. The risk of hepatic toxicity is substantially increased in patients ingesting larger than recommended dosages of acetaminophen while receiving isoniazid. Therefore, patients should limit self-medication with acetaminophen while receiving isoniazid.

■ **Oral Anticoagulants** Chronic ingestion of large doses of acetaminophen has been reported to potentiate the effects of coumarin- and indandione-derivative anticoagulants, although conflicting data exist and the clinical importance of any such interaction has been questioned. The results of an observational study in patients stabilized on warfarin therapy indicate an association between ingestion of even low to moderate dosages of acetaminophen (7 or more 325-mg tablets weekly) and excessively high international normalized ratio (INR) values, and some clinicians suggest that additional monitoring of INR values may be prudent in patients receiving warfarin therapy following initiation of, and during sustained therapy with, large doses of acetaminophen.

In a case-control study, patients receiving warfarin who had an INR exceeding 6 (target INR: 2–3) were more likely to have taken acetaminophen during the week preceding the INR than patients who had actual INRs of 1.7–3.3 (i.e., controls) on warfarin therapy; this association was dose-dependent in that case patients reported ingesting greater amounts of acetaminophen in the week preceding the INR (approximately 21 acetaminophen 325-mg tablets) than did controls (approximately 9 acetaminophen 325-mg tablets). For most of these patients, the elevated INR represented a recent deterioration in control of anticoagulation. Patients who reported taking about 1.3 g of acetaminophen daily for longer than 1 week had a tenfold increase in the risk of having an INR exceeding 6 compared with those not reporting acetaminophen use. Such risk decreased with lower acetaminophen dosages (4.6 up to 9.1 g weekly) and reached baseline values at acetaminophen dosages of about 2 g weekly or less. Although the precise mechanism of the described interaction is not known, it has been suggested that acetaminophen (particularly when administered in large doses) can inhibit metabolism of warfarin probably via inhibition of the cytochrome P-450 microsomal enzyme system, resulting in increased blood concentrations of warfarin. There is controversy concerning the design of this study (e.g., presence of possibly confounding risk factors, lack of causality assessment), and some clinicians doubt the clinical importance of these findings.

Pending completion of randomized, controlled studies to assess causality and more fully determine the clinical importance of this interaction, acetaminophen generally remains preferable to nonsteroidal anti-inflammatory agents (NSAIAs) as a mild analgesic or antipyretic in patients receiving warfarin because of the potential for serious adverse effects (e.g., bleeding) associated with concomitant warfarin and NSAIA therapy. Some clinicians suggest that when long-term therapy with acetaminophen (e.g., 3–4 g daily, as may be required for pain in patients with osteoarthritis) is initiated in patients receiving warfarin, the INR or prothrombin time (PT) should be determined about 7–14 days after beginning acetaminophen therapy. As with other drugs that may interact with warfarin, when concomitant acetaminophen therapy is initiated or discontinued or acetaminophen dosage is modified, the INR or PT should be monitored more frequently and warfarin dosage adjusted if necessary until these values have stabilized.

The manufacturer of acetaminophen injection states that more frequent monitoring of the INR may also be appropriate when patients receiving oral anticoagulants require short-term IV acetaminophen therapy, since the effects of such concomitant use have not been established.

■ Phenothiazines The possibility of severe hypothermia should be considered in patients receiving concomitant phenothiazine and antipyretic (e.g., acetaminophen) therapy.

Laboratory Test Interferences

Acetaminophen may produce false-positive test results for urinary 5-hydroxyindoleacetic acid.

Acute Toxicity

■ Pathogenesis The toxicity of acetaminophen is closely linked to the drug's metabolism. With therapeutic dosing, acetaminophen is metabolized principally by sulfate and glucuronide conjugation. Small amounts (5–10%) usually are oxidized by cytochrome P-450 (CYP)-dependent pathways (mainly CYP2E1) to a toxic metabolite, *N*-acetyl-*p*-benzoquinoneimine (NAPQI). NAPQI is detoxified by glutathione and eliminated in urine and/or bile, and any remaining toxic metabolite may bind to hepatocytes and cause cellular necrosis. Because of the relatively small amount of NAPQI usually formed and the adequate supply of glutathione that usually is present in the body, acetaminophen generally has an excellent safety profile. However, with acetaminophen overdosage and occasionally with usual dosages in susceptible individuals (e.g., those with nutritional [malnutrition] or drug interactions, those consuming alcohol chronically, those with predisposing medical conditions, those with a genetic metabolic predisposition), hepatotoxic concentrations of NAPQI may accumulate.

■ Manifestations Acetaminophen toxicity may result from a single toxic dose, from repeated ingestion of large doses of acetaminophen (e.g., 7.5–10 g daily for 1–2 days), or from chronic ingestion of the drug. (See Chronic Toxicity.) Dose-dependent, hepatic necrosis is the most serious acute toxic effect associated with overdosage and is potentially fatal.

Acetaminophen toxicity usually involves 4 phases: 1) anorexia, nausea, vomiting, malaise, and diaphoresis (which inappropriately may prompt administration of additional acetaminophen); 2) resolution of phase-1 manifestations and replacement with right upper quadrant pain or tenderness, liver enlargement, elevated bilirubin and hepatic enzyme concentrations, prolongation of prothrombin time, and occasionally oliguria; 3) anorexia, nausea, vomiting, and malaise recur (usually 3–5 days after initial symptom onset) and signs of hepatic failure (e.g., jaundice, hypoglycemia, coagulopathy, encephalopathy) and possibly renal failure and cardiomyopathy develop; and 4) recovery or progression to fatal complete liver failure.

Nausea, vomiting, and abdominal pain usually occur within 2–3 hours after ingestion of toxic doses of the drug. Unlike salicylates, acetaminophen does not usually cause acid/base changes in toxic doses. In severe poisoning, CNS stimulation, excitement, and delirium may occur initially. This may be followed by CNS depression; stupor; hypothermia; marked prostration; rapid, shallow breathing; rapid, weak, irregular pulse; low blood pressure; and circulatory failure. Vascular collapse results from the relative hypoxia and from a central depressant action that occurs only with massive doses. Shock may develop if vasodilation is marked. Fatal asphyxial seizures may occur. Coma usually precedes death, which may occur suddenly or may be delayed for several days.

Fulminant, fatal hepatic failure may occur in chronic alcoholics following overdosage of acetaminophen. *p*-Aminophenol derivatives may elevate serum bilirubin concentrations, and jaundice may develop within 2–6 days after ingestion of one of the drugs. In adults, hepatic toxicity rarely has occurred with acute overdoses of less than 10 g, although hepatotoxicity has been reported in fasting patients ingesting 4–10 g of acetaminophen. (See Pharmacokinetics: Elimination.) Fatalities are rare with less than 15 g. However, the risk of severe and possibly fatal hepatic injury following acetaminophen overdosage cannot be accurately assessed based on the amount of acetaminophen ingested. Although some discordance in evidence exists, the overwhelming weight of existing evidence currently supports a relationship between chronic, excessive consumption of alcohol and an increased risk of acetaminophen-induced hepatotoxicity. When an individual has ingested a toxic dose of acetaminophen, the individual should be hospitalized for several days of observation, even if there are no apparent ill effects, because maximum liver damage usually does not become apparent until 2–4 days after ingestion of the drug. Transient azotemia and renal tubular necrosis have been reported in patients with acetaminophen poisoning; renal failure is often associated with fatality. There have been reports of acute myocardial necrosis and pericarditis in individuals with acetaminophen poisoning. Maximum cardiotoxic effects of these drugs appear to be delayed in a manner similar to hepatotoxic effects. Hypoglycemia, which can progress to coma, and metabolic acidosis have been reported in patients ingesting toxic doses of acetaminophen and cerebral edema occurred in one patient.

Young children appear to be less likely to develop hepatotoxic effects than adults, apparently because of age-related differences in acetaminophen metabolism. However, cases of severe hepatotoxicity and death have been reported in children who apparently received acetaminophen dosages exceeding those recommended (10–15 mg/kg per dose with a maximum of 5 doses per day) for children. Factors contributing to overdosage and toxicity of acetaminophen in children appear to include improper interpretation by the parent or caregiver of dosing information or failure to read such information, use of adult-strength acetaminophen preparations because of unavailability of pediatric formulations, use of excessive dosing because of the perception that desired therapeutic effects had not been achieved, and lack of knowledge about the potential toxicity of acetaminophen in excessive dosage. Current data suggest that the outcome after multiple excessive doses of acetaminophen in children under conditions of therapeutic intent may differ from the outcome observed after acute intoxications where as few as 1% of children have developed serious liver toxicity, which was successfully managed. Diagnosis and treatment may be made more difficult in cases of multiple overdoses because the parent or caregiver may not recognize acetaminophen overdose as a factor in the child's symptoms or may not accurately recall the dosage administered. The mechanism of acetaminophen toxicity in pediatric patients after multiple supratherapeutic doses remains to be elucidated. It has been suggested that certain individuals may be more susceptible to cellular injury induced by acetaminophen, and the combination of supratherapeutic doses, disease (e.g., diabetes mellitus, viral infection, febrile illness accompanied by acute malnourishment), nutritional factors (e.g., obesity, chronic undernutrition, prolonged fasting), metabolic factors (e.g., polymorphism in expression of the cytochrome P-450 enzyme system, alternate metabolic pathways under conditions of drug accumulation after multiple doses, enzyme induction), and stage of development may result in enhanced acetaminophen toxicity in these individuals. Whether hepatic injury resulting from other underlying conditions (e.g., viral infections, metabolic diseases) is exacerbated by acetaminophen has not been established.

Low prothrombin levels have been reported in patients with acetaminophen poisoning and in one patient fatal GI hemorrhage was attributed to hypoprothrombinemia. Thrombocytopenia also has been reported. Toxic doses of *p*-aminophenol derivatives may produce skin reactions of an erythematous or urticarial nature which may be accompanied by fever and oral mucosal lesions.

■ Treatment In all cases of suspected acetaminophen overdosage, a regional poison control center at 800-222-1212 may be contacted immediately for assistance in diagnosis and for directions in the use of acetylcysteine as an antidote.

Management of acetaminophen acute overdosage includes determination of the magnitude of the ingestion, classification of risk, and measures to reduce morbidity and mortality. Early recognition and treatment of overdosage are essential to prevent morbidity and mortality.

If acetaminophen has been recently ingested, activated charcoal may reduce acetaminophen absorption and should be administered as soon as possible (preferably within 1 hour of ingestion). Other methods of gastric decontamination (i.e., syrup of ipecac) are less effective and generally are not recommended. Management of acetaminophen overdose also includes general physiologic supportive measures such as control of respiration and fluid and electrolyte therapy.

Because reported or estimated quantity of acetaminophen ingestion often is inaccurate and is not a reliable guide to the therapeutic management of the overdose, the preferred method to assess the risk of toxicity after acetaminophen ingestion usually is measurement of plasma or serum acetaminophen concentrations. Plasma or serum acetaminophen concentrations should be determined as soon as possible, but no sooner than 4 hours after ingestion (to ensure that peak concentrations have occurred). If an extended-release preparation of acetaminophen was ingested, it may be appropriate to obtain an additional sample of plasma or serum 4–6 hours after the initial sample for determination of drug concentrations. Plasma or serum acetaminophen concentrations are used in conjunction with a nomogram that follows to estimate the potential for hepatotoxicity and the necessity of acetylcysteine therapy. If the initial acetaminophen concentration falls on or above the solid line in the nomogram, hepatotoxicity is probable (in the absence of acetylcysteine therapy), and if the initial concentration falls on the dashed line or between the dashed and solid lines, hepatotoxicity is possible (in the absence of acetylcysteine therapy). (To allow error on the side of safety, the dashed line is plotted 25% below the line indicating probable toxicity). If the initial plasma or serum acetaminophen concentration is below the dashed line on the nomogram, there is minimal risk of hepatotoxicity.

A full course of acetylcysteine therapy is indicated if initial plasma or serum acetaminophen concentrations fall on or above the dashed line on the nomogram. Results are optimal if acetylcysteine therapy is initiated within 8–16 hours of ingestion, but acetylcysteine is effective when given more than 24 hours after ingestion. *If plasma or serum acetaminophen concentrations cannot be obtained, it should be assumed that the overdosage is potentially toxic, and acetylcysteine therapy should be initiated.* Acetylcysteine may be withheld until acetaminophen assay results are available provided initiation of acetylcysteine is not delayed beyond 8 hours after acetaminophen ingestion. If more than 8 hours has elapsed since acetaminophen ingestion, acetylcysteine therapy should be started immediately.

When indicated (e.g., in patients in whom the initial acetaminophen concentration is toxic on the nomogram or in those in whom a toxic dose is suspected and the time of ingestion is unknown, 8 hours have elapsed since ingestion, acetaminophen concentrations cannot be obtained, or acetaminophen concentration values will not be available within 8 hours of ingestion), acetylcysteine therapy is initiated as soon as possible with an oral or IV loading dose in adults and pediatric patients. In the event that a loading dose of acetylcysteine is administered before plasma or serum acetaminophen concentration values are available, the initial plasma or serum concentration (obtained at least 4 hours after ingestion) is used in conjunction with the nomogram to determine the necessity of completing a full course of acetylcysteine therapy. In such situations, administration of a full course of acetylcysteine therapy is indicated if initial plasma or serum acetaminophen concentrations fall on or above the dashed line on the nomogram; acetylcysteine therapy is discontinued if initial acetaminophen concentrations fall below the dashed line on the nomogram.

When acetylcysteine is administered orally, a loading dose of 140 mg/kg is administered; the loading dose is followed by oral maintenance doses of 70 mg/kg every 4 hours for 17 doses (full course of therapy). Alternatively, when acetylcysteine is administered IV, a loading dose of 150 mg/kg is infused over 60 minutes; the loading dose is followed by an IV maintenance dose of 50 mg/kg infused over 4 hours and then 100 mg/kg infused over 16 hours (for a full course consisting of 300 mg/kg administered IV over 21 hours).

If a patient receiving oral acetylcysteine vomits a loading or maintenance dose within 1 hour of administration, the dose should be repeated. If the patient is persistently unable to retain orally administered acetylcysteine, the drug may be administered via a duodenal tube. Antiemetic therapy also may be used for persistent vomiting. The usual dosage of oral acetylcysteine is appropriate in patients given activated charcoal; higher dosages are not necessary in these patients.

Because acetylcysteine therapy may be useful even when instituted more than 24 hours after an overdose, a full course of acetylcysteine therapy is recommended for patients presenting 24 or more hours postingestion with measurable plasma or serum acetaminophen concentrations or biochemical evidence of hepatic injury. In a few patients with fulminant hepatic failure, IV administration of acetylcysteine has been associated with increased oxygen delivery and consumption resulting in beneficial effects on survival in such patients.

Because there is some evidence that excessive consumption of alcohol may increase the risk of acetaminophen-induced hepatotoxicity, some clinicians recommend that plasma or serum acetaminophen concentrations on the nomogram indicating the necessity for acetylcysteine therapy be lowered (by 25–70%) in chronic alcoholic patients. Some clinicians recommend that following overdosage of acetaminophen, plasma or serum acetaminophen concentrations on the nomogram indicating the necessity for acetylcysteine therapy also be lowered in patients receiving drugs that may interfere with the hepatic metabolism of acetaminophen (e.g., isoniazid; anticonvulsants including phenytoin, phenobarbital, primidone, valproic acid, carbamazepine) because the risk of acetaminophen-induced hepatotoxicity also may be increased in these patients. It has been suggested that when acetaminophen toxicity results from repeated ingestion of large doses of acetaminophen (e.g., 7.5–10 g daily for 1 or 2 days), acetylcysteine therapy should be considered irrespective of plasma or serum acetaminophen concentrations. Some experts state that early therapy with acetylcysteine should be considered when acetaminophen toxicity is a likely contributor to hepatic dysfunction. In addition, some clinicians state that if an extended-release preparation of acetaminophen has been ingested, the usefulness of the current nomogram (which is based on ingestion of immediate-release preparations) may be limited. Although area under the plasma concentration-time curve (AUC) may be increased following ingestion of an extended-release preparation, delayed absorption and decreased peak plasma acetaminophen concentrations may occur, which may lead to an underestimation of the need for antidotal therapy. Some clinicians suggest that higher than usual doses of acetylcysteine may be necessary in patients ingesting an overdosage of acetaminophen extended-release preparations. However, the manufacturer states that the standard nomogram may be used for acetaminophen extended-release tablets, but that an additional determination of plasma or serum acetaminophen concentrations from a sample obtained 4–6 hours after the initial sample also should be evaluated using the nomogram. In cases where it is unclear whether high doses of the drug were ingested as extended-release tablets or as conventional preparations of acetaminophen, the manufacturer suggests that overdosage of the drug be managed as if extended-release preparations were ingested.

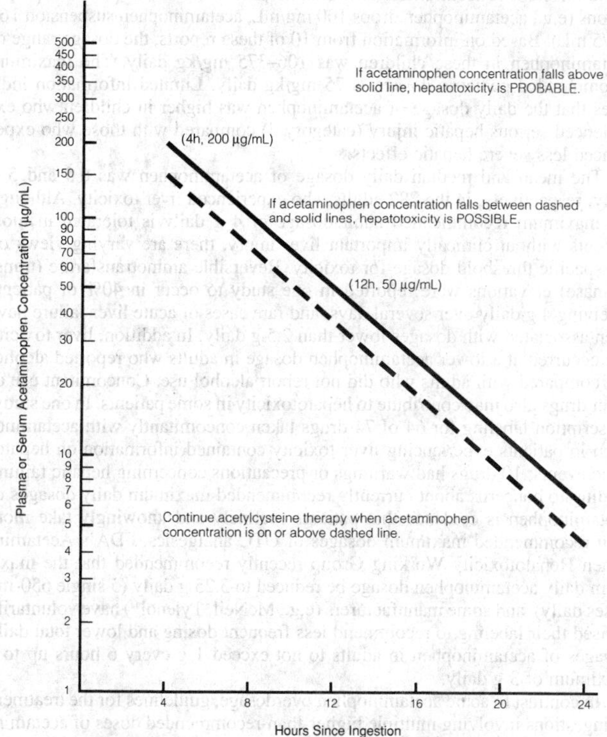

Nomogram relating plasma or serum acetaminophen concentration and probability of hepatotoxicity at varying intervals following ingestion of a single toxic dose of acetaminophen. Modified from Rumack BH, Matthew H. Acetaminophen poisoning and toxicity. Pediatrics. 1975; 55:871-6. © American Academy of Pediatrics 1975.—and from Rumack BH et al. Acetaminophen overdose. Arch Intern Med. 1981; 141:380-5. © American Medical Association.

In addition to plasma or serum acetaminophen concentrations, baseline prothrombin time, BUN, blood glucose concentration, and serum AST (SGOT), ALT (SGPT), bilirubin, creatinine, and electrolyte concentrations should be determined. Prothrombin time, blood glucose concentration, and serum AST, ALT, bilirubin, and electrolyte concentrations should be determined at 24-hour intervals for at least 96 hours after the time of ingestion; if toxicity is evident, these parameters should continue to be monitored at least daily as necessary. Fluid and electrolyte balance should be maintained; use of diuretics and forced diuresis should be avoided. Hypoglycemia should be treated as necessary. If the prothrombin time is greater than 1.5 times the control value, phytonadione should be administered; if the prothrombin time is greater than 3 times the control value, fresh frozen plasma should be given. If hepatic or renal impairment develops, appropriate laboratory parameters should be monitored until values return toward normal. A serum bilirubin concentration greater than 4 mg/dL and a prothrombin time greater than 2.2 times the control value may indicate impending hepatic encephalopathy. Hemodialysis or charcoal hemoperfusion generally are not useful in enhancing the elimination of acetaminophen from the body. Peritoneal dialysis is ineffective.

Chronic Toxicity

While some evidence from animal studies suggests that tolerance to acetaminophen may occur when the dose is increased gradually, continued increases presumably will eventually exceed a threshold resulting in toxicity that is similar in acuity and severity to single time-point overdoses. Unintentional overdosage and resultant acute liver failure often may go unrecognized for several days. Despite long-term acetaminophen ingestion histories associated with unintentional acetaminophen overdosages, such overdosage still is associated with acute hepatic injury that is indistinguishable from intentional (suicidal) ingestions. This experience suggests that there may not be a true chronic form of toxicity but instead a safety threshold that may be breached with devastating consequences.

Three hundred and seven cases of liver injury associated with acetaminophen use were reported to the US Food and Drug Administration (FDA) from January 1998 to July 2001. Sixty percent of these adverse events were categorized as severe life-threatening injury with liver failure (category 4); 40% of patients died. Review of these case reports indicates that use of higher than recommended daily dosages of acetaminophen results in adverse hepatotoxic effects more often than use of recommended dosages.

Twenty-five of these case reports involved pediatric patients 12 years of age or younger and 84% (21) of these cases involved medication errors. Administration of higher than recommended dosages of acetaminophen has occurred as a result of parents or caregivers misunderstanding the directions provided on the product label or given by a clinician. An added source of confusion is the different concentrations of acetaminophen available in pediatric preparations (e.g., acetaminophen drops 100 mg/mL, acetaminophen suspension 160 mg/5 mL). Based on information from 10 of these reports, the dosage range of acetaminophen in these children was 106–375 mg/kg daily. The maximum recommended pediatric dosage is 75 mg/kg daily. Limited information indicates that the daily dosage of acetaminophen was higher in children who experienced serious hepatic injury (category 4) compared with those who experienced less severe hepatic effects.

The mean and median daily dosage of acetaminophen was 6.5 and 5 g daily, respectively, in the 282 adults who experienced liver toxicity. Although the maximum recommended adult dosage of 4 g daily is tolerated in most patients without clinically important liver injury, there are varying views on the specific threshold dosage for toxicity. Reversible aminotransferase (transaminase) elevations were reported in one study to occur in 40% of patients receiving 4 g daily over several days, and rare cases of acute liver failure have been associated with dosages lower than 2.5 g daily. In addition, liver toxicity has occurred at a lower acetaminophen dosage in adults who reported alcohol use compared with adults who did not report alcohol use. Concomitant use of other drugs also may contribute to hepatotoxicity in some patients. In one study, prescription labeling for 64 of 74 drugs taken concomitantly with acetaminophen in patients experiencing liver toxicity contained information on hepatotoxic events; 10 drugs had warnings or precautions concerning hepatic failure. Adding to concerns about currently recommended maximum daily dosages of acetaminophen is evidence that patients routinely and knowingly take more than recommended maximum dosages of OTC analgesics. FDA's Acetaminophen Hepatotoxicity Working Group recently recommended that the maximum daily acetaminophen dosage be reduced to 3.25 g daily (5 single 650-mg doses daily), and some manufacturers (e.g., McNeil, Tylenol®) have voluntarily revised their labeling to recommend less frequent dosing and lower total daily dosages of acetaminophen in adults to not exceed 1 g every 6 hours up to a maximum of 3 g daily.

In contrast to acute acetaminophen overdosage, guidelines for the treatment of ingestions involving multiple higher-than-recommended doses of acetaminophen currently are not available. In addition, it can be difficult to recognize the onset of liver injury, with symptom onset taking several days in some patients, even in severe cases. Symptoms also may not be specific, mimicking flu symptoms, which can result in patients continuing to take acetaminophen after symptoms emerge. Some poison centers use plasma aspartate aminotransferase (AST) and/or alanine aminotransferase (ALT) concentrations and plasma or serum acetaminophen concentrations to estimate the potential for hepatotoxicity and necessity of acetylcysteine therapy. In cases of repeated supratherapeutic ingestion of acetaminophen, a regional poison center (800-222-1222) or an assistance line for acetaminophen overdosage (800-525-6115) can be contacted.

Chronic ingestion of large doses of analgesics (e.g., 1 kg or more of phenacetin [no longer commercially available in the US] and/or salicylate over any period of time) has been associated with analgesic nephropathy which is characterized by papillary necrosis and subsequent chronic interstitial nephritis, with or without pyelonephritis. Analgesic nephropathy frequently has been associated with ingestion of large amounts of combinations of aspirin, phenacetin, and caffeine (combinations containing phenacetin no longer are commercially available in the US). Because phenacetin previously was a component of many analgesic drug mixtures, this drug has been implicated as the causative agent of renal damage. Many clinicians, however, believe that nephropathy may be caused by a combination of several analgesics rather than a single drug. Cancer of the renal pelvis has been reported in patients with analgesic nephropathy and in patients following chronic ingestion of phenacetin-containing analgesic mixtures. Splenomegaly has also been associated with abuse of phenacetin-containing mixtures.

Pharmacology

Acetaminophen produces analgesia and antipyresis by a mechanism similar to that of salicylates. Unlike salicylates, however, acetaminophen does not have uricosuric activity. There is some evidence that acetaminophen has weak anti-inflammatory activity in some nonrheumatoid conditions (e.g., in patients who have had oral surgery). In equal doses, the degree of analgesia and antipyresis produced by acetaminophen is similar to that produced by aspirin.

Acetaminophen lowers body temperature in patients with fever but rarely lowers normal body temperature. The drug acts on the hypothalamus to produce antipyresis; heat dissipation is increased as a result of vasodilation and increased peripheral blood flow.

The effects of acetaminophen on cyclooxygenase activity have not been fully determined. Acetaminophen is a weak, reversible, isoform-nonspecific cyclooxygenase inhibitor at dosages of 1 g daily. The inhibitory effect of acetaminophen on cyclooxygenase-1 is limited, and the drug does not inhibit platelet function.

Therapeutic doses of acetaminophen appear to have little effect on cardiovascular and respiratory systems; however, toxic doses may cause circulatory failure and rapid, shallow breathing.

Pharmacokinetics

■ Absorption Acetaminophen is rapidly and almost completely absorbed from the GI tract following oral administration. In healthy men, steady-state oral bioavailability of 1.3-g doses of extended-release tablets of acetaminophen administered every 8 hours for a total of 7 doses was equal to 1-g doses of conventional tablets of acetaminophen given every 6 hours for a total of 7 doses. Food may delay slightly absorption of extended-release tablets of acetaminophen. Following oral administration of immediate- or extended-release acetaminophen preparations, peak plasma concentrations are attained within 10–60 or 60–120 minutes, respectively. Following oral administration of a single 500-mg conventional tablet or a single 650-mg extended-release tablet, average plasma acetaminophen concentrations of 2.1 or 1.8 μg/mL, respectively, occur at 6 or 8 hours, respectively. In addition, dissolution of the extended-release tablets may depend slightly on the gastric or intestinal pH. Dissolution appears to be slightly faster in the alkaline pH of the intestines compared with the acidic pH of the stomach; however, this is of no clinical importance. Following administration of conventional preparations of acetaminophen, only small amounts of the drug are detectable in plasma after 8 hours. The extended-release tablets of acetaminophen release the drug for up to 8 hours, but in vitro data indicate that at least 95% of the dose is released within 5 hours.

Following rectal administration of acetaminophen, there is considerable variation in peak plasma concentrations attained, and time to reach peak plasma concentrations is substantially longer than after oral administration.

Following IV administration of single 500-mg, 650-mg, and 1-g doses of acetaminophen in adults, the pharmacokinetics of the drug are proportional to the dose administered. The peak plasma concentration of acetaminophen occurs at the end of the 15-minute IV infusion and is up to 70% higher than peak concentrations observed following oral administration of the same dose; however, systemic exposure to the drug is similar following IV or oral administration. Following IV administration of a single dose of 15 mg/kg in pediatric patients or 1 g in adults, systemic exposure to acetaminophen in children and adolescents is similar to that in adults, but exposure is higher in neonates and infants. Dosing simulations using pharmacokinetic data from infants and neonates suggest that dose reductions of 33% in infants 1 month to less than 2 years of age and 50% in neonates up to 28 days of age, with a minimum dosing interval of 6 hours, would result in systemic exposures similar to those observed in children 2 years of age and older.

■ Distribution Acetaminophen is rapidly and uniformly distributed into most body tissues except fat. Acetaminophen crosses the placenta and is distributed into human milk in small quantities following oral administration. About 10–25% of acetaminophen in blood is bound to plasma proteins.

■ Elimination Acetaminophen has been reported to have a plasma half-life of 1.25–3 hours. Following IV administration of a single dose of 15 mg/kg in pediatric patients or 1 g in adults, plasma half-lives of 2.4 hours in adults, 2.9–3 hours in children and adolescents, 4.2 hours in infants, and 7 hours in neonates have been reported. Plasma half-life of acetaminophen may be prolonged following toxic doses or in patients with liver damage, although limited data indicate that following overdosage of acetaminophen the terminal plasma half-life of the drug reported with extended-release tablets is comparable to that reported with standard-release preparations.

About 80–85% of the acetaminophen in the body undergoes conjugation principally with glucuronic acid and to a lesser extent with sulfuric acid. Acetaminophen also is metabolized by microsomal enzyme systems in the liver.

In vitro and animal data indicate that small quantities of acetaminophen are metabolized by cytochrome P-450 (CYP) microsomal enzymes, mainly CYP2E1, to a reactive intermediate metabolite (*N*-acetyl-*p*-benzoquinoneimine, *N*-acetylimidoquinone, NAPQI) which is further metabolized via conjugation with glutathione and ultimately excreted in urine as a mercapturic acid. It has been suggested that this intermediate metabolite is responsible for acetaminophen-induced liver necrosis and that high doses of acetaminophen may deplete glutathione so that inactivation of this toxic metabolite is decreased. At high doses, the capacity of metabolic pathways for conjugation with glucuronic acid and sulfuric acid may be exceeded, resulting in increased metabolism of acetaminophen by alternative pathways. In addition, it also has been suggested that in fasting individuals conjugation of high doses of acetaminophen with glucuronic acid may be reduced, secondary to decreased hepatic carbohydrate reserves and microsomal oxidation may be increased, resulting in increased risk of hepatotoxicity. Drugs that potentially modify these metabolic processes are used (e.g., acetylcysteine) or are being studied (e.g., cysteine, mercaptamine) as antidotes for acetaminophen-induced hepatotoxicity.

Acetaminophen is excreted in urine principally as acetaminophen glucuronide with small amounts of acetaminophen sulfate and mercaptate and unchanged drug. Approximately 85% of a dose of acetaminophen is excreted in urine as free and conjugated acetaminophen within 24 hours after ingestion. Administration of acetaminophen to patients with moderate to severe renal impairment may result in accumulation of acetaminophen conjugates.

Chemistry and Stability

■ Chemistry Acetaminophen is a synthetic nonopiate derivative of *p*-aminophenol that produces analgesia and antipyresis. Acetaminophen is a major metabolite of phenacetin. Phenacetin, another derivative of *p*-aminophenol, has been associated with analgesic nephropathy (renal papillary necrosis with subsequent chronic interstitial nephritis) and no longer is commercially available in the US. Acetaminophen occurs as a white, crystalline powder with a slightly bitter taste. Acetaminophen is soluble in boiling water and freely soluble in alcohol.

Acetaminophen oral solution has a pH of 3.8–6.1, and the oral suspension has a pH of 4–6.9. Although an official USP acetaminophen elixir that contained 6.5–10.5% alcohol was previously available under this title, USP combined the official descriptions for the elixir and solution to just acetaminophen oral solution in 1990 to simplify compendial standards for these liquid oral dosage forms. Therefore, both preparations, regardless of whether they contain alcohol, currently are titled oral solutions; those that contain alcohol are differentiated from those that do not only by specifying the alcohol content on the labeling.

Acetaminophen 650-mg extended-release tablets (e.g., Tylenol® Arthritis Pain Extended Release, Tylenol® 8 Hour Extended-Release) are bilayer (immediate-release and extended-release layers) tablets.

Acetaminophen injection is a sterile, clear, colorless, nonpyrogenic, isotonic aqueous solution containing 10 mg of acetaminophen per mL. Hydrochloric acid and/or sodium hydroxide may be added to adjust pH to approximately 5.5. The commercially available injection also contains mannitol, cysteine hydrochloride monohydrate, and dibasic sodium phosphate and has an osmolality of approximately 290 mOsm/kg.

■ **Stability** Oral acetaminophen preparations should be stored at a controlled room temperature of 20–25°C; freezing of the oral solution or suspension should be avoided. Acetaminophen suppositories should be stored at room temperature or in a refrigerator.

Acetaminophen injection should be stored at a temperature of 20–25°C and should not be refrigerated or frozen. The injection should be used within 6 hours after the vacuum seal of the vial has been penetrated or the vial contents have been transferred to another container. Acetaminophen injection is incompatible with acyclovir sodium, diazepam, and chlorpromazine hydrochloride.

Preparations

To minimize the risk of inadvertent acetaminophen overdosage in pediatric patients, FDA has recommended that only one concentration of liquid acetaminophen be available for *self-medication* (over-the-counter [OTC] use) in all pediatric patients. As a result, some manufacturers have decided to voluntarily change the concentration of the infants' formulation to be the same as that of the children's formulation. (See Cautions: Pediatric Precautions.) However, because this change is voluntary, older, more-concentrated liquid acetaminophen preparations marketed for infants may remain available.

To minimize the risk of inadvertent acetaminophen overdosage, FDA has requested manufacturers to reformulate prescription combination preparations containing the drug to limit the acetaminophen amount to 325 mg or less per dosage unit. FDA no longer considers prescription combination preparations containing more than 325 mg of acetaminophen per dosage unit to be safe. As of March 26, 2014, all manufacturers of such preparations had discontinued marketing of the preparations, although some had not withdrawn the drug applications. FDA intends to withdraw approval of those applications if they are not voluntarily withdrawn. Therefore, availability of combination preparations with higher concentrations of acetaminophen per dose will diminish over time. Some prescription combination preparations that previously contained more than 325 mg of acetaminophen per dosage unit may have been reformulated to contain a smaller amount of acetaminophen. Pharmacists are encouraged to return any prescription combination preparations containing more than 325 mg of acetaminophen per dosage unit to the wholesaler or manufacturer. FDA has stated that the agency intends to address nonprescription acetaminophen-containing preparations in a separate regulatory action.

Excipients in commercially available drug preparations may have clinically important effects in some individuals; consult specific product labeling for details.

Acetaminophen

Oral		
Capsules, gel-coated	500 mg*	**Acetaminophen Extra Strength Gel-coated Capsules**
Solution	167 mg/5 mL*	**Tylenol® Extra-Strength Adult,** McNeil
Suspension	160 mg/5 mL*	**Tylenol® Oral Suspension Children's,** McNeil
		Tylenol® Oral Suspension Infant's, McNeil
Tablets	325 mg*	**Tylenol® Regular Strength** (scored), McNeil
Tablets, extended-release, film-coated	650 mg*	**Tylenol® Arthritis Pain Extended-Release Caplets,** McNeil
		Tylenol® 8 HR Extended-Release Caplets®, McNeil
Tablets, film-coated	500 mg*	**Tylenol® Extra Strength Caplets,** McNeil
Tablets, orally disintegrating	80 mg*	**Tylenol® Meltaways Children's,** McNeil
	160 mg*	**Tylenol® Meltaways Junior Strength,** McNeil
Parenteral		
Injection, for IV infusion	10 mg/mL (1 g)	**Ofirmev®,** Mallinckrodt
Rectal		
Suppositories	80 mg	**FeverAll® Infants',** Taro
	120 mg*	**Acephen®,** G&W
		FeverAll® Children's, Taro
	325 mg	**Acephen®,** G&W
		FeverAll® Junior Strength, Taro
	650 mg*	**Acephen®,** G&W

*available from one or more manufacturer, distributor, and/or repackager by generic (nonproprietary) name

Acetaminophen and Aspirin

Oral		
For solution	325 mg/packet Acetaminophen and Aspirin 500 mg/packet	**Goody's® Back & Body Pain Powder,** Prestige
Tablets, film-coated	250 mg Acetaminophen, Aspirin 250 mg, and buffer	**Excedrin® Back and Body Caplets,** Novartis

Acetaminophen, Aspirin, and Caffeine

Oral		
Capsules, gel-coated	250 mg Acetaminophen, Aspirin 250 mg, and Caffeine 65 mg*	**Excedrin® Menstrual Complete Gelcaps,** Novartis
For solution	260 mg/packet Acetaminophen, Aspirin 520 mg/packet, and Caffeine 32.5 mg/packet	**Goody's® Extra Strength Headache Powder,** Prestige
	325 mg/packet Acetaminophen, Aspirin 500 mg/packet, and Caffeine 65 mg/packet	**Goody's® Cool Orange Extra Strength Powder,** Prestige
Tablets, film-coated	194 mg Acetaminophen, Aspirin 227 mg, Caffeine 33 mg, and buffers	**Vanquish® Caplets,** Moberg
	250 mg Acetaminophen, Aspirin 250 mg, and Caffeine 65 mg	**Excedrin® Extra Strength Caplets,** Novartis
		Excedrin® Migraine Caplets, Novartis
		Goody's® Extra Strength Caplets, Prestige
		Pamprin® Max, Chattem

*available from one or more manufacturer, distributor, and/or repackager by generic (nonproprietary) name

Acetaminophen and Codeine Phosphate

Oral		
Solution	120 mg/5 mL Acetaminophen and Codeine Phosphate 12 mg/5 mL*	**Acetaminophen and Codeine Phosphate Oral Solution** (C-V)
Suspension	120 mg/5 mL Acetaminophen and Codeine Phosphate 12 mg/5 mL	**Capital® and Codeine** (C-V), Valeant
Tablets	300 mg Acetaminophen and Codeine Phosphate 15 mg*	**Acetaminophen and Codeine Phosphate Tablets** (C-III)
	300 mg Acetaminophen and Codeine Phosphate 30 mg*	**Tylenol® with Codeine No. 3** (C-III), Janssen
	300 mg Acetaminophen and Codeine Phosphate 60 mg*	**Tylenol® with Codeine No. 4** (C-III), Janssen

*available from one or more manufacturer, distributor, and/or repackager by generic (nonproprietary) name

Acetaminophen and Diphenhydramine Citrate

Oral		
For solution	500 mg/packet Acetaminophen and Diphenhydramine Citrate 38 mg/packet	**Goody's® PM Powder,** Prestige
Tablets, film-coated	500 mg Acetaminophen and Diphenhydramine Citrate 38 mg*	**Excedrin PM® Caplets,** Novartis
		Excedrin PM® Geltabs, Novartis
		Midol® PM Caplets, Bayer

*available from one or more manufacturer, distributor, and/or repackager by generic (nonproprietary) name

Oxycodone and Acetaminophen

Oral		
Solution	5 mg/5 mL Oxycodone Hydrochloride and Acetaminophen 325 mg/5 mL	**Roxicet®** (C-II), Roxane
Tablets	2.5 mg Oxycodone Hydrochloride and Acetaminophen 300 mg*	**Oxycodone Hydrochloride and Acetaminophen Tablets** (C-II)
	2.5 mg Oxycodone Hydrochloride and Acetaminophen 325 mg*	**Percocet®** (C-II), Endo
	5 mg Oxycodone Hydrochloride and Acetaminophen 300 mg*	**Primlev®** (C-II), Akrimax
	5 mg Oxycodone Hydrochloride and Acetaminophen 325 mg*	**Endocet®** (C-II; scored), Qualitest **Percocet®** (C-II; scored), Endo
	7.5 mg Oxycodone Hydrochloride and Acetaminophen 300 mg*	**Primlev®** (C-II), Akrimax
	7.5 mg Oxycodone Hydrochloride and Acetaminophen 325 mg*	**Endocet®** (C-II), Qualitest **Percocet®** (C-II), Endo
	10 mg Oxycodone Hydrochloride and Acetaminophen 300 mg*	**Primlev®** (C-II), Akrimax
	10 mg Oxycodone Hydrochloride and Acetaminophen 325 mg*	**Endocet®** (C-II), Qualitest **Percocet®** (C-II), Endo

*available from one or more manufacturer, distributor, and/or repackager by generic (nonproprietary) name

Other Acetaminophen Combinations

Oral		
Capsules	300 mg with Butalbital 50 mg and Caffeine 40 mg*	**Fioricet®**, Actavis
	300 mg with Butalbital 50 mg, Caffeine 40 mg, and Codeine Phosphate 30 mg*	**Fioricet® with Codeine** (C-III), Actavis
	320.5 mg with Caffeine 30 mg and Dihydrocodeine Bitartrate 16 mg	**Trezix®** (C-III), WraSer
	325 mg with Butalbital 50 mg and Caffeine 40 mg*	**Capacet®**, Magna
	325 mg with Butalbital 50 mg, Caffeine 40 mg, and Codeine Phosphate 30 mg*	**Butalbital, Acetaminophen, Caffeine, and Codeine Phosphate Capsules** (C-III)
Capsules, gel-coated	500 mg with Caffeine 60 mg and Pyrilamine Maleate 15 mg	**Midol® Complete Gelcaps**, Bayer
	500 mg with Caffeine 65 mg*	**Acetaminophen with Caffeine Gelcaps**
Solution	83 mg/5 mL with Caffeine 5.4 mg/5 mL	**Goody's® Headache Relief Shot**, Prestige
	100 mg/5 mL with Hydrocodone Bitartrate 3.3 mg/5 mL*	**Lortab® Elixir** (C-II), ECR
	108 mg/5 mL with Butalbital 16.7 mg/5 mL and Caffeine 13.3 mg/5 mL*	**Alagesic LQ®**, Poly Pharmaceuticals
	108 mg/5 mL with Hydrocodone Bitartrate 2.5 mg/5 mL*	**Hydrocodone Bitartrate and Acetaminophen Oral Solution** (C-II)
	108 mg/5 mL with Hydrocodone Bitartrate 3.3 mg/5 mL*	**Hydrocodone Bitartrate and Acetaminophen Oral Solution** (C-II)
Tablets	300 mg with Butalbital 50 mg	**Bupap®**, ECR
	300 mg with Hydrocodone Bitartrate 5 mg*	**Vicodin®** (C-II; scored), AbbVie
	300 mg with Hydrocodone Bitartrate 7.5 mg*	**Vicodin ES®** (C-II; scored), AbbVie
	300 mg with Hydrocodone Bitartrate 10 mg*	**Vicodin HP®** (C-II; scored), AbbVie
	325 mg with Butalbital 50 mg	**Butapap®**, Mikart **Phrenilin®** (scored), Valeant
	325 mg with Butalbital 50 mg and Caffeine 40 mg*	**Butalbital, Acetaminophen, and Caffeine Tablets**
	325 mg with Hydrocodone Bitartrate 2.5 mg*	**Hydrocodone and Acetaminophen Tablets** (C-II)
	325 mg with Hydrocodone Bitartrate 5 mg*	**Lortab®** (C-II; scored), UCB **Norco®** (C-II; scored), Actavis
	325 mg with Hydrocodone Bitartrate 7.5 mg*	**Lortab®** (C-II; scored), UCB **Norco®** (C-II; scored), Actavis
	325 mg with Hydrocodone Bitartrate 10 mg*	**Lortab®** (C-II; scored), UCB **Norco®** (C-II; scored), Actavis
Tablets, film-coated	325 mg with Diphenhydramine Hydrochloride 12.5 mg*	**Percogesic® Original Strength**, Prestige
	325 mg with Tramadol Hydrochloride 37.5 mg*	**Ultracet®** (C-IV), Janssen
	500 mg with Caffeine 60 mg and Pyrilamine Maleate 15 mg*	**Midol® Complete Caplets**, Bayer
	500 mg with Caffeine 65 mg*	**Excedrin® Tension Headache Caplets**, Novartis
	500 mg with Diphenhydramine Hydrochloride 12.5 mg	**Percogesic® Extra Strength Caplets®**, Prestige
	500 mg with Diphenhydramine Hydrochloride 25 mg*	**Tylenol® PM Extra Strength Caplets**, McNeil **Tylenol® PM Extra Strength Geltabs®**, McNeil
	500 mg with Pamabrom 25 mg	**Midol® Teen Caplets®**, Bayer
	500 mg with Pamabrom 25 mg and Pyrilamine Maleate 15 mg	**Pamprin® Multi-Symptom Caplets**, Chattem **Premsyn PMS® Caplets**, Chattem

Acetaminophen also is commercially available in combination with other drugs, including analgesics, antihistamines, antimuscarinics, antitussives, barbiturates, decongestants, and expectorants.

*available from one or more manufacturer, distributor, and/or repackager by generic (nonproprietary) name

Ziconotide

■ Ziconotide, a synthetic form of a conopeptide isolated from the venom of the marine snail *Conus magus*, is a potent nonopiate analgesic.

Uses

■ **Pain** Ziconotide is used intrathecally for the management of severe chronic pain in patients who are intolerant of or do not obtain adequate pain relief from other therapies (e.g., systemic analgesics, adjunctive therapies, intrathecal morphine therapy) when intrathecal therapy is warranted.

Safety and efficacy of ziconotide have been evaluated in 3 double-blind, placebo-controlled studies using 2 different dosage titration schedules. In the slow dosage titration schedule, dosage was increased 2 or 3 times per week (minimum interval between dose escalations: 24 hours) up to a maximum dosage of 19.2 mcg per 24 hours at day 21. In the fast dosage titration schedule, dosage was increased daily up to a maximum dosage of 57.6 mcg per 24 hours after 5–6 days.

Efficacy of ziconotide administered using the slow dosage titration schedule has been evaluated in one randomized, placebo-controlled, multicenter study in patients with severe chronic pain (mean baseline score of 81 on the 100-mm Visual Analog Scale of Pain Intensity [VASPI]; pain was unresponsive to other analgesic therapy in 97% of patients). Prior to randomization, all intrathecal agents were discontinued and patients received a stable regimen of analgesics (including opiates) for at least 7 days. The mean improvement in VASPI score from baseline to study completion at day 21 (the primary efficacy measure) was 12% in patients receiving ziconotide and 5% in those receiving placebo. The effect of ziconotide on pain was variable over time. Some patients experienced pain relief (i.e., improvement in VASPI score) during the first or second week, but improvement was not sustained through the end of the third week. Other patients did not show improvement in VASPI score until the third week. Sixteen or 12% of those receiving ziconotide or placebo, respectively, were classified as responders (defined as having at least a 30% improvement in VASPI score from baseline). Use of systemic opiate analgesics decreased by 24% in patients receiving ziconotide and by 17% in those receiving placebo.

Although the duration of ziconotide therapy in controlled clinical studies to date has been limited to 21 days, the drug has been used in a substantial number of patients in long-term open-label studies.

Dosage and Administration

■ **Administration** Ziconotide is administered intrathecally using a programmable implanted variable-rate microinfusion device (i.e., Medtronic SynchroMed® EL or SynchroMed® II) or an external microinfusion device and catheter (i.e., CADD-Micro® ambulatory infusion pump) by or under the supervision of a qualified clinician familiar with the drug, the techniques of intrathecal administration, and the device being used. The device manufacturer's manual should be consulted for specific instructions and precautions for performing a reservoir rinse, initial filling, refilling the reservoir or replacing the drug cartridge, and programming.

An appropriate vial strength and final concentration of the drug should be selected in accordance with the manufacturer's instructions. The commercially available preparation containing ziconotide 25 mcg/mL may be used undiluted; the preparation containing ziconotide 100 mcg/mL may be used undiluted or may be diluted with 0.9% sodium chloride injection prior to placement in the pump. Sodium chloride solutions containing preservatives are not appropriate for intrathecal administration and should not be used to dilute ziconotide. Diluted ziconotide solutions should be refrigerated; freezing should be avoided. Infusion of diluted ziconotide solutions should be initiated within 24 hours of preparation.

Ziconotide is *not* for IV administration.

■ **Dosage** Ziconotide therapy should be initiated using a slow dosage titration schedule in order to minimize the risk of adverse effects that are serious or require drug discontinuance. A faster titration schedule should be used only if an urgent need for analgesia outweighs the risk to patient safety.

The recommended initial dosage of ziconotide for management of severe chronic pain in adults is 2.4 mcg per 24 hours (0.1 mcg/hour) or less. Dosage is then titrated based on patient response. Dosage can be increased 2 or 3 times per week in increments of up to 2.4 mcg per 24 hours (0.1 mcg/hour), up to a maximum recommended dosage of 19.2 mcg per 24 hours (0.8 mcg/hour) by day 21. In a study that evaluated efficacy of ziconotide using the slow dosage titration schedule, the average dosage at day 21 was 6.9 mcg per 24 hours (0.29 mcg/hour); the maximum dosage was 19.2 mcg per 24 hours.

Ziconotide therapy can be interrupted or discontinued abruptly without withdrawal effects.

■ **Special Populations** Initiate ziconotide at the lower end of the dosage range in geriatric patients. (See Specific Populations: Geriatric Use under Cautions: Warnings/Precautions.)

Cautions

■ **Contraindications** Concomitant treatments or medical conditions (e.g., presence of infection at the microinfusion injection site, uncontrolled bleeding diathesis, spinal canal obstruction that impairs CSF circulation) that make intrathecal therapy hazardous.

History of psychosis.

Known hypersensitivity to ziconotide or any ingredient in the formulation.

■ **Warnings/Precautions** ***Warnings*** **Nervous System Effects.** Severe psychiatric symptoms and neurologic impairment may occur in patients receiving ziconotide. Patients with a history of psychosis should not receive ziconotide. (See Contraindications.) Patients should be monitored for cognitive impairment, hallucinations, and changes in mood or consciousness. If a severe adverse neurologic or psychiatric event occurs, ziconotide can be temporarily interrupted or abruptly discontinued without withdrawal effects.

Cognitive impairment (e.g., confusion, memory impairment, speech disorder, aphasia, abnormal thinking, amnesia) has been reported in patients receiving ziconotide. Cognitive impairment may appear gradually over several weeks and generally is reversible following discontinuance of the drug. If cognitive impairment develops, the dose of ziconotide should be reduced or the drug discontinued; other causes that could contribute to cognitive impairment should be considered.

Acute psychiatric disturbances (e.g., hallucinations, paranoid reactions, hostility, delirium, psychosis, manic reactions) have occurred in patients receiving ziconotide. Patients with preexisting psychiatric disorders may be at increased risk for these adverse events. Ziconotide may cause or worsen depression, resulting in the risk of suicide in certain patients. Suicide, suicide attempts, and suicidal ideation have been reported more frequently in ziconotide-treated patients than in placebo-treated patients. If psychiatric disturbances occur, ziconotide should be discontinued and the disturbances managed appropriately (e.g., psychotherapeutic agents, hospital admission). A decision to reinitiate ziconotide therapy in a patient who has experienced psychiatric symptoms should be made on an individual basis after careful evaluation.

Patients receiving ziconotide have become unresponsive or stuporous; patients sometimes appear to be conscious, and breathing is not depressed during these events. Patients receiving concomitant therapy with anticonvulsants, antipsychotics, sedatives, or diuretics may be at increased risk for this adverse effect. If reduced levels of consciousness occur, ziconotide should be discontinued until the event resolves; other etiologies (e.g., meningitis) should be considered. In addition, concomitant CNS depressants (e.g., anticonvulsants, antipsychotics, sedatives) should be discontinued as clinically appropriate if altered consciousness occurs.

Opiate Withdrawal. Ziconotide does not prevent or treat the symptoms of opiate withdrawal. For patients discontinuing intrathecal opiate therapy, the intrathecal infusion rate should be gradually tapered over a few weeks and replaced with equivalent doses of oral opiates to avoid symptoms of opiate withdrawal.

Major Toxicities **Meningitis.** Meningitis has occurred in patients receiving ziconotide, principally in individuals receiving therapy via an external microinfusion device and catheter. Meningitis may occur secondary to inadvertent contamination of the microinfusion device or as a result of CSF seeding caused by hematogenous or direct spread from an infected pump pocket or catheter tract. Patients should be monitored for signs and symptoms of meningitis (e.g., fever, headache, stiff neck, altered mental status, nausea or vomiting, seizures). Preparation of ziconotide solution and filling of the drug reservoir should be performed under aseptic conditions by trained and qualified personnel. If meningitis is suspected (especially in immunocompromised patients) or is confirmed, appropriate measures (CSF culture, anti-infective therapy, removal of the microinfusion device and catheter) should be initiated.

General Precautions **Serum Creatine Kinase.** Serum creatine kinase (CK, creatine phosphokinase, CPK) concentrations exceeding the upper limit of normal have been observed in many patients (40%) receiving ziconotide; CK concentrations 3 or more times the upper limit of normal have occurred in 11% of patients. These increases generally have been observed during the first 2 months of therapy with ziconotide and have not been associated with treatment-limiting adverse effects. Men, patients receiving concomitant therapy with antidepressants or anticonvulsants, and those who had received intrathecal morphine were more likely to have elevated serum CK values.

Symptomatic myopathy with electromyographic abnormalities has occurred in at least one patient, and acute renal failure with rhabdomyolysis and markedly elevated CK concentrations (17,000–27,000 IU/L) has been reported in at least 2 patients.

Serum CK concentrations should be monitored periodically (e.g., every other week during the first month of therapy and then monthly as appropriate). If neuromuscular symptoms (e.g., myalgias, myasthenia, muscle cramps, asthenia) develop or a reduction in physical activity occurs, the patient should be evaluated (e.g., clinical evaluation, determination of serum CK concentrations). If symptoms persist and CK concentrations remain elevated or continue to rise, dosage reduction or discontinuance of ziconotide should be considered.

Specific Populations **Pregnancy.** Category C. (See Users Guide.)

Lactation. Not known whether ziconotide is distributed into milk. Discontinue nursing or the drug, taking into account the importance of the drug to the mother.

Pediatric Use. Safety and efficacy not established in patients younger than 18 years of age.

Geriatric Use. In clinical studies, 22% of patients were 65 years of age or older and 7% were 75 years of age or older. In all studies, the incidence of confusion was higher in individuals 65 years of age or older than in younger adults. No substantial difference in efficacy in geriatric patients relative to younger adults.

Select dosage with caution, starting at the low end of the dosage range, because of age-related decreases in hepatic, renal, and/or cardiac function and potential for concomitant disease and drug therapy.

■ **Common Adverse Effects** Adverse effects reported in 25% or more of patients receiving ziconotide include dizziness, nausea, confusion, headache, somnolence, nystagmus, asthenia, and pain.

Drug Interactions

■ **Drugs Affecting or Metabolized by Hepatic Microsomal Enzymes** Pharmacokinetic interaction unlikely.

■ **Protein-bound Drugs** Pharmacokinetic interaction unlikely.

■ **CNS Agents** Used concomitantly with anticonvulsants, antidepressants, antipsychotics, anxiolytics, and sedatives in clinical studies. Potential interaction with CNS depressants (increased incidence of adverse CNS effects [e.g., dizziness, confusion, reduced levels of consciousness]). Dosage adjustment or discontinuance of ziconotide or the concomitant CNS depressant may be needed.

Potential interaction with antidepressants or anticonvulsants (elevated serum creatine kinase [CK, creatine phosphokinase, CPK]).

■ **Diuretics** Potential interaction (reduced levels of consciousness).

■ **Opiates** Used concomitantly with systemically administered opiates in clinical studies; concomitant use of ziconotide with intrathecal opiates has not been evaluated in placebo-controlled studies and is not recommended.

Potential interaction in patients who previously had received intrathecal morphine (elevated serum CK).

Description

Ziconotide, a synthetic form of a naturally occurring conopeptide found in the venom of the marine snail *Conus magus*, is a 25-amino acid polybasic peptide containing 3 disulfide bridges. Ziconotide produces potent antinociceptive effects by selectively binding to N-type voltage-sensitive calcium channels on the primary nociceptive afferent nerves in the superficial layers of the spinal cord, thus blocking neurotransmission from primary nociceptive afferents.

Ziconotide does not bind to opiate receptors, and the pharmacologic effects of the drug are not blocked by opiate antagonists. Ziconotide does not potentiate opiate-induced respiratory depression.

Intrathecal administration of ziconotide results in little systemic exposure. Following passage from the CSF into the systemic circulation, ziconotide is expected to be degraded to peptide fragments and their constituent amino acids by endopeptidases and exopeptidases present in most organs.

Advice to Patients

Risk of somnolence; avoid driving, operating machinery, or performing hazardous tasks until effects on individual are known.

Importance of informing clinician if new or worsening muscle pain, soreness, weakness, or brown urine develops.

Importance of promptly reporting any change in mental status (e.g., lethargy, confusion, disorientation, decreased alertness), mood or perception (e.g., hallucinations, unusual tactile sensations in the mouth), and symptoms of depression or suicidal ideation.

Importance of promptly informing clinician if symptoms of meningitis (i.e., nausea, vomiting, seizures, fever, headache, stiff neck) occur.

For patients receiving ziconotide via an external microinfusion device and catheter, importance of proper handling of the device and proper care of the skin at the catheter exit site.

Importance of women informing clinicians if they are or plan to become pregnant or plan to breast-feed.

Importance of informing clinicians of existing or contemplated concomitant therapy, including prescription and OTC drugs, as well as concomitant illnesses. Potential for additive CNS effects if used concomitantly with other CNS depressants.

Importance of informing patients of other important precautionary information. (See Cautions.)

Overview® (see Users Guide). For additional information on this drug until a more detailed monograph is developed and published, the manufacturer's labeling should be consulted. It is *essential* that the manufacturer's labeling be consulted for more detailed information on usual cautions, precautions, contraindications, potential drug interactions, laboratory test interferences, and acute toxicity.

Preparations

Excipients in commercially available drug preparations may have clinically important effects in some individuals; consult specific product labeling for details.

Ziconotide

Parenteral		
Injection, for intrathecal administration via compatible microinfusion device only	25 mcg/mL	Prialt®, Elan
	100 mcg/mL	Prialt®, Elan

OPIATE ANTAGONISTS 28:10

Naloxone Hydrochloride

N-Allylnoroxymorphone Hydrochloride

■ Naloxone hydrochloride is essentially a pure opiate antagonist.

Uses

■ Opiate-induced Depression and Acute Opiate Overdosage

Naloxone hydrochloride is used for the complete or partial reversal of opiate-induced depression, including respiratory depression, caused by natural and synthetic opiates (e.g., anileridine, codeine, diphenoxylate, fentanyl citrate, heroin, hydromorphone, levorphanol, meperidine, methadone, morphine, oxymorphone, concentrated opium alkaloids hydrochlorides, propoxyphene) and certain opiate partial agonists (e.g., butorphanol, nalbuphine, pentazocine, cyclazocine). However, reversal of respiratory depression resulting from overdosage of opiate partial agonists (e.g., buprenorphine, pentazocine) may be incomplete and require higher or more frequent doses of naloxone. Administration of naloxone should be accompanied by other resuscitative measures such as administration of oxygen, mechanical ventilation, or artificial respiration. Naloxone is effective for the treatment of mild or moderate as well as severe opiate-induced respiratory depression. Naloxone is also indicated for the diagnosis of suspected acute opiate overdosage.

Although naloxone historically has been administered mainly by trained medical personnel in hospitals or ambulances, naloxone increasingly is being administered by nonmedical personnel in community (nonmedical) settings for emergency treatment of known or suspected opiate overdosage, as manifested by respiratory and/or CNS depression. Commercially available naloxone hydrochloride auto-injector and nasal spray formulations facilitate administration of the drug by family members or other caregivers in such settings; such treatment is *not* a substitute for emergency medical care.

Deaths associated with the use of prescription opiate analgesics increased sharply from 1999 to 2006, plateaued for several years, decreased slightly through 2013, but then increased again in 2014. From 2001 to 2014, deaths associated with the use of prescription opiate analgesics increased 3.4-fold. Fatal overdoses of heroin have increased since 2007, with substantial increases observed each year from 2011 through 2014. Fatal heroin overdoses in 2013 were nearly quadruple the rate in the early 2000s, with most of the increase occurring after 2010. From 2001 to 2014, the number of heroin-related deaths increased sixfold. In addition, substantial increases in availability of illicitly manufactured fentanyl and highly potent fentanyl analogs (e.g., carfentanil) were reported in 2014–2016.

Distribution of naloxone through community-based programs that provide overdose education and prevention services for substance users has been shown to be associated with decreased opiate-related mortality rates, and early efforts to expand naloxone availability focused largely on this population. Experts recommend that individuals being treated for opiate use disorder and their family members also have access to naloxone. Experts also state that consideration should be given to prescribing naloxone along with opiate analgesic therapy for patients at increased risk of opiate overdosage (e.g., those with a history of overdose or substance use disorder, those receiving opiate dosages equivalent to 50 mg or more of morphine sulfate daily, those receiving benzodiazepines or other sedatives concomitantly with the opiate agonist, those with medical conditions that could increase sensitivity to opiate effects). In addition, experts recommend that additional first responders (e.g., other emergency medical service personnel, police officers, fire fighters) be trained and authorized to administer naloxone following known or suspected opiate overdosage and support greater access to naloxone by workers in settings where opiate overdoses may be witnessed (e.g., nursing homes, home visiting nurses, school nurses and college campuses, outreach programs, substance abuse treatment programs, halfway houses, homeless shelters, correctional facilities). Although barriers remain to making naloxone more widely available, many states have removed at least some legal barriers to timely administration of the drug. (See Preparations.)

There is no conclusive evidence that concomitant use of naloxone with an opiate analgesic will prevent respiratory depression while retaining the analgesic effect; in fact, analgesia and sedation may be decreased if these drugs are administered together.

Naloxone may be used in neonates for the treatment of asphyxia resulting from administration of opiates to the mother during labor and delivery. Naloxone has been given to the mother shortly before delivery†, but many clinicians believe it is preferable to administer an opiate antagonist directly to the neonate if needed after delivery.

■ Other Uses Naloxone has been used for detection of chronic opiate abuse†, but it is preferable to use chemical methods to detect the presence of opiates in the urine, since naloxone may precipitate severe withdrawal symptoms in patients who are physically dependent on opiates; however, to avoid precipitating opiate withdrawal following administration of naltrexone, administration of naloxone is recommended as a screening test (the naloxone challenge test) prior to induction of therapy with naltrexone for opiate cessation in patients formerly dependent on opiates who have completed detoxification. (See Naloxone Challenge Test in Dosage and Administration: Dosage, in Naltrexone Hydrochloride 28:10.)

When prolonged vomiting occurs after apomorphine has been used to induce vomiting in the treatment of oral poisonings (apomorphine is no longer used as an emetic), naloxone has been used to terminate the emetic effects and to help diminish respiratory depression induced by apomorphine†; however, it has been reported that the CNS and respiratory effects of apomorphine may not always be reversed by naloxone.

Naloxone has been used to reverse clonidine-induced coma and respiratory depression†.

Naloxone has been used as adjunctive therapy in a limited number of patients to increase blood pressure in the management of septic shock. Treatment with naloxone results in a rise in blood pressure that may last up to several hours; however, this pressor effect has not been demonstrated to improve patient survival. Naloxone therapy is not included in the current Surviving Sepsis Campaign International Guidelines for Management of Sepsis and Septic Shock. In some studies, use of naloxone for the management of septic shock has been associated with adverse effects, including agitation, nausea, vomiting, pulmonary edema, hypotension, cardiac arrhythmias, and seizures. If a decision is made to use naloxone for management of septic shock, the manufacturers state that the drug should be used with caution, particularly in patients who may have underlying pain or have previously received opiate therapy and may have developed opiate tolerance.

A combination of pentazocine hydrochloride and naloxone hydrochloride in a ratio of 100:1 is commercially available for oral use as an analgesic. (See Pentazocine 28:08.12.) Combinations of buprenorphine hydrochloride and naloxone hydrochloride in a ratio of 4:1 for sublingual administration or approximately 6:1 for intrabuccal administration are commercially available for use in the management of opiate dependence. (See Buprenorphine 28:08.12.) A combination of methadone hydrochloride and naloxone hydrochloride in a ratio of 20:1 has also been administered orally in the detoxification or maintenance treatment of opiate addiction in conjunction with appropriate social and medical services. The presence of naloxone in these combinations minimizes the abuse potential of pentazocine, buprenorphine, or methadone, since the antagonistic effect of naloxone will predominate if the combinations are administered parenterally and/or if usual oral doses are exceeded.

Opiate antagonists (e.g., naloxone, naltrexone) have been used for rapid or ultrarapid detoxification in the management of opiate withdrawal† in opiate-dependent individuals, both in inpatient and outpatient settings. Rapid opiate detoxification involves the administration of opiate antagonists such as naloxone and/or naltrexone to shorten the time period of detoxification. The reported advantage of this technique is to minimize the risk of relapse and to initiate maintenance therapy with naltrexone and psychosocial interventions more quickly. Ultrarapid detoxification is similar, but involves the administration of opiate antagonists (i.e., naloxone, naltrexone) while the patient is sedated or under general anesthesia. However, the risk of adverse respiratory and cardiovascular effects associated with this procedure must be considered as well as the costs of general anesthesia and hospitalization. Safety and efficacy of these therapies have not been established and further study is needed.

Dosage and Administration

■ **Administration** Naloxone hydrochloride may be administered by IV, subcutaneous, or IM injection; by IV infusion; or intranasally. The drug also has been administered via an endotracheal tube† and by intraosseous† (IO) injection.

To facilitate immediate administration of naloxone following known or suspected opiate overdosage (i.e., administration by family members or other caregivers in a community setting prior to emergency medical response), naloxone hydrochloride is commercially available as an auto-injector for IM or subcutaneous injection and as a nasal spray. When naloxone is made available for use in the community setting, patients and their family members or close contacts should be instructed carefully regarding clinical manifestations requiring naloxone administration, proper administration technique, and the importance of seeking emergency care immediately following administration of the initial dose. Although it is recommended that patients and caregivers become familiar with the training device for the auto-injector upon receiving this naloxone preparation, untrained individuals should still attempt to use the auto-injector to administer naloxone in the event of a suspected opiate overdose.

Parenteral, Endotracheal, and Intraosseous Administration IV administration of naloxone hydrochloride is recommended for emergency situations in medically supervised settings. The American Academy of Pediatrics (AAP) does not endorse subcutaneous or IM administration for emergency medical management of opiate intoxication in children or neonates since hypotension, hypoperfusion, and/or peripheral vasoconstriction may result in erratic or delayed absorption of the drug. When IV access cannot be established in emergency situations, limited evidence suggests that the drug also can be administered effectively via an endotracheal tube† in adults or pediatric patients or by IO† injection for opiate overdosage in pediatric patients. Although naloxone may be administered via an endotracheal tube, some experts state that optimal endotracheal dosages have not been established and IV or IO administration is preferred because of more predictable drug delivery and pharmacologic effect.

Naloxone hydrochloride also may be administered by continuous IV infusion. Continuous IV infusions of the drug may be most appropriate in patients who require higher doses, continue to experience recurrent respiratory or CNS depression after effective therapy with repeated doses, and/or in whom the effects of long-acting opiates are being antagonized. For continuous IV infusion, 2 mg of naloxone hydrochloride may be diluted in 500 mL of 0.9% sodium chloride or 5% dextrose injection to produce a solution containing 0.004 mg/mL (4 mcg/mL). The rate of IV infusion should be titrated in accordance with the patient's response. Diluted solutions of the drug should be used within 24 hours; unused portions should be discarded after 24 hours.

Naloxone hydrochloride also may be administered by IM or subcutaneous injection via an auto-injector. Each carton of the drug contains two 2-mg naloxone hydrochloride auto-injectors and one drug-free, needleless, reusable training device. Following known or suspected opiate overdosage, the contents of one naloxone hydrochloride auto-injector should be injected into the anterolateral aspect of the thigh and emergency care should be sought immediately; depending on the thickness of adipose tissue at the injection site, the injection may be either subcutaneous or IM. For pediatric patients younger than 1 year of age, the thigh should be pinched prior to administration of the dose to provide a thicker injection area (to minimize the risk that the needle might strike bone and break); following administration, the injection site should be observed for residual needle fragments and/or signs of infection. To administer a dose, the caregiver should remove an auto-injector from the outer case and then remove the red safety guard and firmly press the black base of the auto-injector against the anterolateral aspect of the thigh for 5 seconds until the dose is delivered. The injection may be administered through clothing if necessary. Once the red safety guard has been removed, the auto-injector must be used immediately or disposed of properly; the red safety guard should *not* be replaced once removed. Following delivery of the dose, the needle retracts into the case and the auto-injector indicates that a dose has been delivered. If the electronic voice instruction system included with the auto-injector malfunctions, the intended dose of naloxone hydrochloride will be delivered when the device is activated according to the printed instructions. If additional doses are required, a new auto-injector must be used for each dose.

Prior to administration, parenteral solutions of naloxone hydrochloride should be carefully inspected for the presence of particulate matter or discoloration.

Intranasal Administration Naloxone hydrochloride may be administered intranasally. Each carton of the commercially available drug contains 2 single-use naloxone hydrochloride nasal spray units; each unit delivers a 4-mg dose of the drug. The nasal spray units should not be removed from the carton until time of administration and should not be primed or tested prior to administration. For intranasal administration following known or suspected opiate overdosage, the patient should be placed in a supine position, and then the nasal spray unit should be removed from the carton and from the blister package. The device should be held with the thumb on the bottom of the plunger and the first and middle fingers on either side of the nozzle. The patient's head should be tilted back, with one hand supporting the patient's neck. The tip of the nasal spray unit should be gently inserted into one nostril until the fingers on either side of the nozzle are against the patient's nose, and the device plunger should be pressed firmly to administer the dose of naloxone. The nozzle should be removed from the nostril following administration of the drug, and the patient should be placed in the left lateral decubitus position and closely monitored. If additional doses are required, each dose should be administered into alternate nostrils using a new nasal spray unit.

■ **Dosage** ***Postoperative Opiate Depression*** When naloxone hydrochloride is used to partially reverse opiate depression following the use of opiates during surgery, the usual initial dosage recommended by the manufacturers is 0.1–0.2 mg IV in adults or 0.005–0.01 mg IV in children, given at 2- to 3-minute intervals until the desired response (i.e., adequate ventilation and alertness without substantial pain or discomfort) is obtained. Additional doses may be necessary at 1- to 2-hour intervals depending on the response of the patient and the dosage and duration of action of the opiate administered.

Some clinicians have recommended an adult dosage regimen of 0.005 mg/kg administered IV and repeated after 15 minutes if necessary. Alternatively, the initial IV dose may be followed in 15 minutes with an IM dose of 0.01 mg/kg. The manufacturers state that supplemental IM doses of naloxone produce a more prolonged effect than repeated IV doses of the drug. Continuous IV infusions of naloxone in a dosage of 0.0037 mg/kg per hour have also been used in adults to reverse postoperative opiate-induced respiratory depression.

Neonatal Opiate Depression When used to reverse opiate-induced asphyxia neonatorum, the usual initial dosage of naloxone hydrochloride is 0.01 mg/kg, administered into the umbilical vein of the neonate at 2- to 3-minute intervals until the desired response is obtained. Additional doses may be necessary at 1- to 2-hour intervals depending on the response of the neonate and the dosage and duration of action of the opiate administered to the mother. When the IV route cannot be used, the drug may be administered by IM or subcutaneous injection.

Known or Suspected Opiate Overdosage **Treatment in a Health Care Setting.** For the treatment of known opiate overdosage or as an aid in the diagnosis of suspected opiate overdosage, the usual initial adult dosage of naloxone hydrochloride is 0.4–2 mg IV, administered at 2- to 3-minute intervals if necessary; if no response is observed after a total of 10 mg of the drug has been administered, the depressive condition may be caused by a drug or disease process not responsive to naloxone. In patients who are physically dependent on opiates, a lower dose of naloxone hydrochloride (0.04–0.4 mg) should be used to minimize adverse cardiovascular effects and withdrawal symptoms; if the initial response is inadequate, the dose may be repeated or titrated up to 2 mg. (See Precautions and Contraindications.) Some experts state that some patients may require higher doses of naloxone following massive opiate overdosage or overdosage of certain opiates (e.g., propoxyphene [no longer commercially available in the US]). In addition, a higher dose of naloxone may be needed for the endotracheal† route as compared with other routes; however, the optimum dose of naloxone administered via an endotracheal tube† remains to be established. (See Parenteral, Endotracheal, and Intraosseous Administration under Dosage and Administration: Administration.)

Children may receive an initial IV naloxone hydrochloride dose of 0.01 mg/kg; if this dose does not produce the desired degree of response, a subsequent dose of 0.1 mg/kg may be administered. Alternatively, an initial 0.1-mg/kg IV dose, repeated as necessary, has been recommended for neonates and children younger than 5 years of age or weighing 20 kg or less. In pediatric patients 5 years of age or older or weighing more than 20 kg, a 2-mg IV dose, repeated as necessary, can be used. However, some experts state that lower doses should be used to reverse respiratory depression associated with therapeutic opiate use in pediatric patients (e.g., 0.001–0.015 mg/kg for reversal of peri-arrest respiratory depression, 0.001–0.005 mg/kg for respiratory depression during procedural sedation to maintain some opiate analgesia). Some experts suggest an endotracheal† or IO† dose of 0.1 mg/kg in pediatric patients younger than 5 years of age or weighing 20 kg or less or a dose of 2 mg in pediatric patients 5 years of age or older or weighing more than 20 kg; however, the optimum dose of naloxone administered via an endotracheal tube† remains to be established and higher (e.g., double or triple) doses may be necessary. (See Parenteral, Endotracheal, and Intraosseous Administration under Dosage and Administration: Administration.)

Since the duration of action of the opiate is often longer than that of naloxone, the depressant effects of the opiate may return as the effects of naloxone diminish, and additional doses (or a continuous IV infusion) of naloxone may be required. Continuous IV infusion dosage regimens of naloxone have not been well established, and the rate of administration must be titrated according to the patient's response. In adults, some clinicians recommend an initial IV loading dose of 0.4 mg, followed by a continuous infusion at an initial rate of 0.4 mg/hour. Alternatively, other clinicians have recommended that an IV loading dose of 0.005 mg/kg be given, followed by continuous infusion of 0.0025 mg/kg per hour. Experience with continuous IV infusions of naloxone in children is very limited, but children may require higher infusion rates on a mg/kg basis than adults. In several reports, infusion rates in children have ranged from 0.024–0.16 mg/kg per hour. Some clinicians recommend an initial pediatric infusion rate of 0.4 mg/hour.

Community-based Use. To facilitate immediate administration of naloxone following known or suspected opiate overdosage (i.e., administration by family members or other caregivers in a community setting prior to emergency medical response), naloxone hydrochloride is commercially available in a prefilled auto-injector and as a nasal spray.

The optimal dosage of naloxone hydrochloride for use in community settings has not been fully established. While large doses may increase the risk of acute opiate withdrawal, lower doses may require titration and risk further hypoxic injury to the patient. When the naloxone hydrochloride auto-injector was originally approved by FDA, each device delivered 0.4 mg of the drug; the dose delivered per auto-injector has subsequently been increased to 2 mg. Both 2- and 4-mg strengths of naloxone hydrochloride nasal spray currently are commercially available. The manufacturer states that the 2-mg strength of the nasal spray should be prescribed for opiate-dependent patients expected to be at risk for severe opiate withdrawal only when the risk for accidental or intentional opiate exposure by household contacts is low. There are limited data to indicate whether the 2-mg intranasal dose will avoid precipitation of severe opiate withdrawal in opiate-dependent patients; however, the 2-mg dose may not provide adequate and timely reversal of opiate effects in individuals exposed to an overdose involving a potent opiate or very high opiate dose.

For administration in a community (nonmedical) setting in pediatric patients (all ages) and adults, the contents of one auto-injector (naloxone hydrochloride 2 mg) should be administered by IM or subcutaneous injection. If the patient fails to respond or if the patient responds but subsequently relapses into respiratory depression, additional 2-mg doses of naloxone hydrochloride, if available, may be administered every 2–3 minutes until emergency care arrives.

For administration in a community (nonmedical) setting, the recommended initial dose of naloxone hydrochloride nasal spray in pediatric patients (all ages) and adults is one spray (2 or 4 mg) administered intranasally. If the patient fails to respond or if the patient responds but subsequently relapses into respiratory depression, additional 2- or 4-mg doses of naloxone hydrochloride, if available, should be administered every 2–3 minutes until emergency personnel arrive.

Since the duration of action of the opiate is often longer than that of naloxone, the depressant effects of the opiate may return as the effects of naloxone diminish, and additional doses of naloxone may be required. The patient should be closely observed and emergency care should be sought immediately following administration of the initial dose. If necessary, supportive and/or resuscitative measures should be performed until emergency care arrives.

Other Uses For information on the use of naloxone as a screening test (the naloxone challenge test) prior to induction of therapy with naltrexone for opiate cessation in patients formerly dependent on opiates who have completed detoxification, see Naloxone Challenge Test in Dosage and Administration: Dosage, in Naltrexone Hydrochloride 28:10.

When naloxone hydrochloride was used in the diagnosis of opiate dependence† in adults, a dose of 0.16 mg was given IM. If no withdrawal symptoms were evident after 20–30 minutes, a second dose of 0.24 mg was given IV. Negative test results were assumed if no withdrawal symptoms were apparent within 30 minutes after the second dose. Withdrawal symptoms induced by naloxone began to diminish 20–40 minutes after injection and were essentially gone within 1.5 hours.

Cautions

■ Adverse Effects

Nausea and vomiting have been reported rarely in postoperative patients who were receiving a parenteral dose of naloxone hydrochloride greater than that usually recommended; however, a causal relationship has not been established. Tremor and hyperventilation associated with an abrupt return to consciousness have occurred in some patients receiving naloxone for opiate overdosage.

Although a causal relationship to the drug has not been established, severe cardiopulmonary effects (e.g., hypotension, hypertension, ventricular tachycardia and fibrillation, dyspnea, pulmonary edema, cardiac arrest) resulting in death, coma, and encephalopathy have been reported in patients following postoperative administration of naloxone hydrochloride. Adverse cardiopulmonary effects have occurred most frequently in postoperative patients with preexisting cardiovascular disease or in those receiving other drugs that produce similar adverse cardiovascular effects. (See Cautions: Precautions and Contraindications.)

In healthy adults who participated in a pharmacokinetic study of naloxone hydrochloride nasal spray, the most common adverse effects included hypertension, musculoskeletal pain, headache, and local effects (nasal dryness, edema, congestion, and inflammation).

In healthy adults who participated in pharmacokinetic studies of naloxone hydrochloride administered by auto-injector, the most common adverse effects were dizziness and erythema at the injection site. Agitation, disorientation, confusion, and anger also have been reported with this preparation during postmarketing experience.

Seizures have occurred rarely following administration of naloxone hydrochloride; however, a causal relationship to the drug has not been established.

When high oral† doses of naloxone have been used in the treatment of opiate addiction†, some patients have experienced mental depression, apathy, inability to concentrate, sleepiness, irritability, anorexia, nausea, and vomiting. These adverse effects usually occurred in the first few days of treatment and abated rapidly with continued therapy or dosage reduction. One case of erythema multiforme cleared promptly after naloxone was discontinued.

■ Precautions and Contraindications

When naloxone hydrochloride is used in the management of acute opiate overdosage, other resuscitative measures (e.g., maintenance of an adequate airway, artificial respiration, cardiac massage, vasopressor agents) should be readily available and used when necessary. If opiate-induced cardiac arrest occurs, usual guidelines for advanced cardiovascular life support (ACLS) should be followed.

Following the use of opiates during surgery, excessive dosage of naloxone hydrochloride should be avoided, because it may result in excitement, agitation, an increase in blood pressure, and clinically important reversal of analgesia. A reversal of opiate effects achieved too rapidly may induce nausea, vomiting, sweating, tremor, tachycardia, hypotension, hypertension, seizures, ventricular tachycardia and fibrillation, pulmonary edema, and cardiac arrest, which may result in death.

Naloxone should be used with caution in patients with preexisting cardiovascular disease or in those receiving potentially cardiotoxic drugs, since serious adverse cardiopulmonary effects (e.g., ventricular tachycardia and fibrillation, pulmonary edema, cardiac arrest) resulting in death, coma, and encephalopathy have occurred in postoperative patients following administration of naloxone; such patients should be monitored for hypotension, ventricular tachycardia or fibrillation, and pulmonary edema. (See Cautions: Adverse Effects.)

Reversal of respiratory depression resulting from overdosage of opiate partial agonists (e.g., buprenorphine, pentazocine) may be incomplete and require higher or repeated doses of naloxone.

Naloxone should be given with caution to patients known or suspected to be physically dependent on opiates (including neonates born to women who are opiate dependent), particularly in patients with cardiovascular disease, because the drug may precipitate severe withdrawal symptoms. (See Cautions: Pregnancy, Fertility, and Lactation and see Pharmacology.) For additional information on opiate withdrawal, including its management, see Chronic Toxicity in the Opiate Agonists General Statement 28:08.08.

Patients who have responded to naloxone should be carefully monitored, since the duration of action of most opiates may exceed that of naloxone. Repeated doses of naloxone should be administered to these patients when necessary. Some experts state that while a brief observation period may be adequate following overdosage of certain opiates with a shorter duration of action (morphine, heroin), patients who have presented with life-threatening overdosage of a long-acting or extended-release opiate may require longer periods of observation. The manufacturers state that pediatric patients who have responded to naloxone must be carefully monitored for at least 24 hours.

Safety and efficacy of naloxone in patients with renal or hepatic impairment have not been established in well-controlled clinical trials. Naloxone should be used with caution in these patients.

Naloxone is contraindicated in patients with known hypersensitivity to the drug or any ingredient in the formulation.

■ Pediatric Precautions

Naloxone hydrochloride injection may be used to reverse the effects of opiates in infants and children. In addition, safety and efficacy of naloxone hydrochloride administered via auto-injector or nasal spray have been established in pediatric patients of all ages for the emergency treatment of known or suspected opiate overdosage manifested by respiratory and/or CNS depression. Use of naloxone for reversal of opiate effects in pediatric patients is supported by well-controlled studies in adults, additional data from controlled and uncontrolled studies in which neonates and children received parenteral naloxone hydrochloride in doses of 0.005–0.01 mg/kg, bioequivalence studies in adults, other published data, and postmarketing experience with the drug.

As in adults, naloxone may precipitate opiate withdrawal in pediatric patients who are physically dependent on opiates; however, unlike opiate withdrawal in adults, neonatal opiate withdrawal may be life-threatening and should be treated according to protocols developed by neonatology experts. To avoid abrupt precipitation of neonatal opiate withdrawal syndrome, use of a naloxone preparation that can be dosed based on weight and titrated to effect may be preferred over a preparation that delivers a fixed dose of the drug (e.g., auto-injector, nasal spray) in neonates with known or suspected exposure to maternally administered opiates (e.g., maternal illicit use, opiate therapy for chronic pain management, opiate maintenance treatment) who require naloxone for reversal of respiratory depression. In addition, in infants at risk for opiate overdosage (e.g., those receiving a tapering opiate dosage following hospital discharge), use of a naloxone formulation other than the nasal spray (e.g., naloxone auto-injector) should be considered, since there is some concern that intranasal instrumentation could induce respiratory distress in young infants.

Absorption of naloxone following intranasal administration or IM or subcutaneous injection in pediatric patients may be erratic or delayed. Pediatric patients who have responded to naloxone must be carefully monitored for at least 24 hours, since relapse may occur as the opiate antagonist is metabolized.

Safety and efficacy of naloxone in the management of hypotension associated with septic shock have not been established in pediatric patients. In a study of 2 neonates with septic shock, treatment with naloxone produced positive pressor response; however, one patient subsequently died after intractable seizures.

■ Geriatric Precautions Clinical studies of naloxone did not include sufficient numbers of patients 65 years of age and older to determine whether geriatric patients respond differently than younger patients. While other clinical experience has not revealed age-related differences in response, drug dosage generally should be titrated carefully in geriatric patients, usually initiating therapy at the low end of the dosage range. The greater frequency of decreased hepatic, renal, and/or cardiac function and of concomitant disease and drug therapy observed in the elderly also should be considered.

■ Mutagenicity and Carcinogenicity Naloxone was weakly positive in the Ames mutagenicity test and the in vitro human lymphocyte chromosome aberration test but was negative in the in vitro Chinese hamster V79 cell HGPRT mutagenicity assay and the in vivo rat bone marrow chromosome aberration study. Studies to determine the carcinogenic potential of naloxone have not been performed to date.

■ Pregnancy, Fertility, and Lactation Reproduction studies in mice and rats using naloxone hydrochloride at dosages of 4 and 8 times, respectively, a human dosage of 10 mg daily in a 50-kg individual or at dosages of 6 and 12 times, respectively, a human dosage of 8 mg daily demonstrated no embryotoxic or teratogenic effects. Furthermore, no adverse effects were reported on the offspring of rats receiving naloxone subcutaneously at dosages of 2 or 10 mg/kg (up to 12 times a human dosage of 8 mg daily) from gestation day 15 to postnatal day 21. There are limited data to date on use of the drug in pregnant women. Naloxone hydrochloride should be used during pregnancy only when clearly needed.

The risk-benefit ratio must be considered before naloxone hydrochloride is administered to a pregnant woman who is known or suspected to be dependent on opiates, since maternal dependence may often be accompanied by fetal dependence. Naloxone crosses the placenta and may precipitate withdrawal symptoms in both the fetus and the pregnant woman. Use of naloxone in opiate-dependent pregnant women should be accompanied by monitoring for fetal distress.

It is not known if naloxone affects the duration of labor and/or delivery. However, published reports indicate that administration of naloxone during labor did not adversely affect maternal or neonatal status. Patients with mild to moderate hypertension who receive naloxone during labor should be carefully monitored, as severe hypertension may occur.

Reproduction studies in mice and rats using naloxone hydrochloride at dosages of 4 and 8 times, respectively, a human dosage of 10 mg daily in a 50-kg individual (based on body surface area) revealed no evidence of impaired fertility. In addition, studies in rats using the drug at dosages of 2 or 10 mg/kg (up to 12 times a human dosage of 8 mg daily) administered for 60 days prior to mating in males or administered for 14 days prior to mating and then throughout gestation in females revealed no evidence of impaired fertility.

Since it is not known whether naloxone hydrochloride is distributed into milk or has any effect on the breast-fed infant or on milk production, the drug should be used with caution in nursing women. The drug does not affect prolactin or oxytocin concentrations in nursing women, and oral bioavailability of naloxone is minimal.

Pharmacology

Naloxone hydrochloride is essentially a pure opiate antagonist. The precise mechanism of action of the opiate antagonist effects of naloxone is not fully understood. Naloxone is thought to act as a competitive antagonist at μ, κ, and σ opiate receptors in the CNS; it is thought that the drug has the highest affinity for the μ receptor. In contrast to levallorphan or nalorphine, naloxone has little or no agonistic activity. When administered in usual doses to patients who have not recently received opiates, naloxone exerts little or no pharmacologic effect. Even extremely high doses of the drug (10 times the usual therapeutic dose) produce insignificant analgesia, only slight drowsiness, and no respiratory depression, psychotomimetic effects, circulatory changes, or miosis.

In patients who have received large doses of morphine or other analgesic drugs with morphine-like effects, naloxone antagonizes most of the effects of the opiate. There is an increase in respiratory rate and minute volume, arterial PCO_2 decreases toward normal, and blood pressure returns to normal if depressed. Unlike nalorphine or levallorphan, naloxone antagonizes mild respiratory depression caused by small doses of opiates. Because the duration of action of naloxone is generally shorter than that of the opiate, the effects of the opiate may return as the effects of naloxone dissipate. Naloxone antagonizes opiate-induced sedation or sleep. Reports are conflicting on whether or not the drug modifies opiate-induced excitement or seizures.

Naloxone does not produce tolerance or physical or psychological dependence. In patients who are dependent on opiates, parenteral administration of naloxone hydrochloride will precipitate opiate withdrawal symptoms, which may appear within minutes of naloxone administration and subside in about 2 hours. The severity and duration of the withdrawal symptoms are related to the dose of naloxone and the degree and type of opiate dependence. Oral administration of naloxone generally does not precipitate withdrawal symptoms unless the dose exceeds 10 mg. Even a 30-mg oral dose of naloxone usually induces only very mild abstinence symptoms.

Naloxone has been shown to increase blood pressure in a limited number of patients with septic shock. (See Uses: Other Uses.)

Pharmacokinetics

■ Absorption Naloxone is rapidly inactivated following oral administration. Although the drug is effective orally, doses much larger than those required for parenteral administration are required for complete antagonism. In one study, a single 3-g oral dose of naloxone hydrochloride was required to effectively antagonize the effects of 50 mg of heroin for 24 hours. Naloxone has an onset of action within 1–2 minutes following IV administration and within 2–5 minutes following subcutaneous or IM administration. The duration of action depends on the dose and route of administration and is more prolonged following IM administration than after IV administration. In one study, the duration of action was 45 minutes following IV administration of naloxone hydrochloride 0.4 mg/70 kg.

In healthy individuals, IM or subcutaneous administration of naloxone hydrochloride 0.4 mg using an auto-injector (Evzio®) or standard syringe resulted in similar overall systemic exposure to naloxone, but peak plasma concentrations of the drug were 15% higher following administration using the auto-injector. Peak plasma concentrations of naloxone were attained at a median of 15 minutes (range: 5 minutes to 1.2 hours) after administration using the auto-injector and 20 minutes (range: 5 minutes to 2.03 hours) after administration using a standard syringe. In another study, peak plasma concentrations of the drug were attained in approximately 13–15 minutes after IM or subcutaneous injection via auto-injector of naloxone hydrochloride 0.4 mg, 0.8 mg (administered as two 0.4-mg doses given 2 minutes apart), or 2 mg. Peak plasma concentrations and systemic exposure (area under the plasma concentration-time curve [AUC]) of naloxone following the 2-mg dose were approximately 5.9- and 5.2-fold higher, respectively, than values attained with the 0.4-mg dose and were approximately 3.7- and 2.7-fold higher, respectively, than values attained with the 0.8-mg dose.

Following intranasal administration of naloxone hydrochloride (Narcan®) 2 or 4 mg (single spray in one nostril) or 4 or 8 mg (one 2- or 4-mg spray, respectively, in each nostril) in healthy adults, the median time to peak plasma concentration was similar to that observed following IM injection of a 0.4-mg dose of the drug and the dose-normalized bioavailability relative to that of the IM injection ranged from 43–54%. Peak plasma concentrations and AUC of naloxone were substantially higher following intranasal administration of a 2-mg dose as a single spray in one nostril (approximately 3.3- and 2.6-fold higher, respectively), a 4-mg dose as a single spray in one nostril (approximately 5.5- and 4.4-fold higher, respectively), a 4-mg dose as one 2-mg spray in each nostril (approximately 7.2- and 5.4-fold higher, respectively), or an 8-mg dose as one 4-mg spray in each nostril (approximately 11- and 8.7-fold higher, respectively) than following IM injection of a 0.4-mg dose.

Following administration of 35 or 70 mcg of naloxone hydrochloride into the umbilical vein in neonates in one study, peak plasma naloxone concentrations occurred within 40 minutes and were 4–5.4 ng/mL and 9.2–20.2 ng/mL, respectively. After IM administration of 0.2 mg to neonates in the same study, peak plasma naloxone concentrations of 11.3–34.7 ng/mL occurred within 0.5–2 hours.

■ Distribution Following parenteral administration, naloxone is rapidly distributed into body tissues and fluids. In rats, high concentrations are observed in the brain, kidney, spleen, lung, heart, and skeletal muscle. Naloxone is weakly bound to plasma proteins (mainly albumin). In humans, the drug readily crosses the placenta. It is not known whether naloxone is distributed into milk.

■ Elimination The half-life of naloxone has been reported to be 30–81 minutes in adults and about 3 hours in neonates. The mean plasma half-life of naloxone was 1.28 hours following IM or subcutaneous injection of naloxone hydrochloride 0.4 mg using an auto-injector (Evzio®), compared with 1.36 hours following IM or subcutaneous injection using a standard syringe. In another study, the plasma half-life of naloxone was approximately 1.5 hours following IM or subcutaneous injection of naloxone hydrochloride 0.4 mg, 0.8 mg (administered as two 0.4-mg doses given 2 minutes apart), or 2 mg using an auto-injector. Following intranasal administration, naloxone exhibits a slightly longer half-life compared with the IM route (1.9–2.1 versus 1.2 hours).

Naloxone is rapidly metabolized in the liver, principally by conjugation with glucuronic acid. The major metabolite is naloxone-3-glucuronide. Naloxone also undergoes *N*-dealkylation and reduction of the 6-keto group followed by conjugation. Limited studies with radiolabeled naloxone indicate that 25–40% of an oral or IV dose of the drug is excreted as metabolites in urine in 6 hours, about 50% in 24 hours, and 60–70% in 72 hours.

Chemistry and Stability

■ Chemistry Naloxone hydrochloride is a semisynthetic opiate antagonist which is derived from thebaine. Naloxone differs structurally from oxymorphone only in that the methyl group on the nitrogen atom of oxymorphone is replaced by an allyl group.

Naloxone hydrochloride occurs as white to slightly off-white powder and is soluble in water, in dilute acids, and in strong alkali; the drug is slightly soluble in alcohol and practically insoluble in ether and chloroform. The drug has a pK_a of 7.94. The commercially available injections are adjusted to pH 3–4.5 with hydrochloric acid or sodium hydroxide; the injections also *may* contain methylparaben and propylparaben as preservatives.

Naloxone hydrochloride may be available either as the anhydrous drug or as the dihydrate; both are defined officially (USP) as simply the hydrochloride salt, and potency is expressed in terms of the salt, calculated on the dried basis. Despite this official designation, manufacturers of some preparations (e.g., Bunavail®, Suboxone®, Zubsolv®) calculate potency in terms of the base rather than the salt.

■ **Stability** Commercially available naloxone hydrochloride injection in a prefilled auto-injector should be stored in the outer case provided by the manufacturer at 15–25°C but may be exposed to temperatures ranging from 4–40°C.

Vials and ampuls containing naloxone hydrochloride injection should be stored at 20–25°C and protected from light. The injections are stable at pH 2.5–5. Following dilution in 5% dextrose or 0.9% sodium chloride injection to a concentration of 0.004 mg/mL (4 mcg/mL), naloxone hydrochloride solutions are apparently stable for 24 hours; after 24 hours, any unused solution should be discarded.

Naloxone hydrochloride injection should not be mixed with preparations containing bisulfite, metabisulfite, long-chain or high molecular weight anions, or any solution having an alkaline pH. Drugs or chemical agents should not be added to solutions of naloxone hydrochloride unless their effect on the chemical and physical stability of the solution has been established. Specialized references should be consulted for specific compatibility information.

Commercially available naloxone hydrochloride nasal spray should be stored in the original blister package and carton provided by the manufacturer at 15–20°C but may be exposed to temperatures up to 40°C. The nasal spray should not be frozen and should be protected from light.

Preparations

To facilitate timely administration of naloxone following opiate overdosages occurring in community (nonmedical) settings, many states have taken steps to make naloxone available to first responders, community-based organizations, and laypersons (e.g., through legislation permitting prescribing to third parties, prescribing by standing order, or pharmacist prescribing or dispensing in accordance with protocols or standing orders) and to limit adverse legal consequences to prescribers and to laypersons who administer the drug.

Excipients in commercially available drug preparations may have clinically important effects in some individuals; consult specific product labeling for details.

Naloxone Hydrochloride

Intranasal		
Solution	2 mg/0.1 mL	**Narcan®**, Adapt
	4 mg/0.1 mL	**Narcan®**, Adapt
Parenteral		
Injection	0.4 mg/mL*	**Naloxone Hydrochloride Injection**
	1 mg/mL*	**Naloxone Hydrochloride Injection**
	5 mg/mL (2 mg)	**Evzio®** (available as kit with 2 prefilled, single-use 0.4-mL auto-injectors and 1 drug-free, needleless, reusable training device), Kaleo

*available from one or more manufacturer, distributor, and/or repackager by generic (nonproprietary) name

Pentazocine and Naloxone Hydrochlorides

Oral		
Tablets	Pentazocine Hydrochloride 50 mg (of pentazocine) and Naloxone Hydrochloride 0.5 mg (of naloxone)*	**Pentazocine and Naloxone Hydrochlorides Tablets** (C-IV)

*available from one or more manufacturer, distributor, and/or repackager by generic (nonproprietary) name

Naloxone Hydrochloride Dihydrate Combinations

Buccal (Transmucosal)		
Strips, intrabuccally dissolving	0.3 mg (of naloxone) with Buprenorphine Hydrochloride 2.1 mg (of buprenorphine)	**Bunavail®** (C-III), BioDelivery Sciences
	0.7 mg (of naloxone) with Buprenorphine Hydrochloride 4.2 mg (of buprenorphine)	**Bunavail®** (C-III), BioDelivery Sciences
	1 mg (of naloxone) with Buprenorphine Hydrochloride 6.3 mg (of buprenorphine)	**Bunavail®** (C-III), BioDelivery Sciences
Sublingual		
Strips, sublingually dissolving	0.5 mg (of naloxone) with Buprenorphine Hydrochloride 2 mg (of buprenorphine)	**Suboxone®** (C-III), Indivior
	1 mg (of naloxone) with Buprenorphine Hydrochloride 4 mg (of buprenorphine)	**Suboxone®** (C-III), Indivior
	2 mg (of naloxone) with Buprenorphine Hydrochloride 8 mg (of buprenorphine)	**Suboxone®** (C-III), Indivior
	3 mg (of naloxone) with Buprenorphine Hydrochloride 12 mg (of buprenorphine)	**Suboxone®** (C-III), Indivior
Tablets	0.36 mg (of naloxone) with Buprenorphine Hydrochloride 1.4 mg (of buprenorphine)	**Zubsolv®** (C-III), Orexo
	0.5 mg (of naloxone) with Buprenorphine Hydrochloride 2 mg (of buprenorphine)*	**Buprenorphine Hydrochloride and Naloxone Hydrochloride Sublingual Tablets** (C-III)
	0.71 mg (of naloxone) with Buprenorphine Hydrochloride 2.9 mg (of buprenorphine)	**Zubsolv®** (C-III), Orexo
	1.4 mg (of naloxone) with Buprenorphine Hydrochloride 5.7 mg (of buprenorphine)	**Zubsolv®** (C-III), Orexo
	2 mg (of naloxone) with Buprenorphine Hydrochloride 8 mg (of buprenorphine)*	**Buprenorphine Hydrochloride and Naloxone Hydrochloride Sublingual Tablets** (C-III)
	2.1 mg (of naloxone) with Buprenorphine Hydrochloride 8.6 mg (of buprenorphine)	**Zubsolv®** (C-III), Orexo
	2.9 mg (of naloxone) with Buprenorphine Hydrochloride 11.4 mg (of buprenorphine)	**Zubsolv®** (C-III), Orexo

*available from one or more manufacturer, distributor, and/or repackager by generic (nonproprietary) name

†Use is not currently included in the labeling approved by the US Food and Drug Administration

Naltrexone
Naltrexone Hydrochloride

■ Naltrexone is essentially a pure opiate antagonist.

REMS

FDA approved a REMS for naltrexone to ensure that the benefits outweigh the risks. The REMS may apply to one or more preparations of naltrexone and consists of the following: medication guide and communication plan. See the FDA REMS page (https://www.accessdata.fda.gov/scripts/cder/rems/index.cfm).

Uses

■ **Opiate Dependence** Naltrexone hydrochloride is designated an orphan drug by the US Food and Drug Administration (FDA) and is used orally for its opiate antagonist effects as an adjunct to a medically supervised behavior modification program in the maintenance of opiate cessation (opiate-free state) in individuals formerly physically dependent on opiates and who have successfully undergone detoxification. Behavior modification is an integral component in maintaining opiate cessation when naltrexone is used, and such modification involves supervised programs of counseling, psychologic support and therapy, and education, and changes in life-style (social rehabilitation). The theoretical rationale for using naltrexone as an adjunct in opiate cessation therapy is that the drug may diminish or eliminate opiate-seeking behavior by blocking the euphoric reinforcement produced by self-administration of opiates and by preventing the conditioned abstinence syndrome (i.e., heightened sensitivity to stimuli, abnormal autonomic responses, dysphoria, and intense opiate craving) that occurs following opiate withdrawal. There are no data that unequivocally demonstrate a beneficial effect of naltrexone on the tendency to relapse (recidivism) to drug abuse in detoxified, former opiate-dependent individuals; however, by blocking opiate-induced euphoria and potentially preventing the redevelopment of opiate dependence, naltrexone therapy in conjunction with a medically supervised behavior modification program may contribute to the prevention of relapse in the postaddiction period.

In individuals formerly dependent on opiates, naltrexone reportedly decreases opiate craving within 3–5 weeks of initiation of therapy; however, decreased opiate craving has occurred during the first week of naltrexone therapy in some individuals, with further decreases occurring in subsequent weeks. The efficacy of opiate cessation therapy that includes naltrexone on long-term cessation rates appears to be low, and poor compliance appears to be the major limiting factor in opiate cessation therapy that includes naltrexone. Because noncompliance with naltrexone therapy, unlike methadone or levomethadyl acetate (LAAM; no longer commercially available in the US because of potentially severe adverse cardiac effects) maintenance therapy, is not associated with unpleasant symptoms of withdrawal, compliance with opiate cessation therapy that includes naltrexone depends more on the voluntary efforts of the individual, and successful cessation appears to be more likely in highly motivated individuals. Repeated attempts at opiate cessation therapy may increase efficacy in terms of the amount of time the individual remains opiate-free; complete cessation may not be an obtainable goal in some individuals, and cycles of relapse to opiate use and cessation may be likely.

Behavioral therapy, as a component of opiate cessation therapy, allows the patient to undergo a social and psychologic rehabilitation that will aid in maintaining opiate cessation. Naltrexone therapy in combination with behavioral therapy has been shown to be more effective than naltrexone or behavioral therapy alone in prolonging opiate cessation in patients formerly physically dependent on opiates. Individuals who are highly motivated, employed, and in a stable married or other relationship appear to be most successful with naltrexone therapy and able to maintain opiate cessation. Strong external support from family and/or employer also contributes to the success of opiate cessation therapy that includes naltrexone. Because naltrexone is used as an adjunct to the individual's own cessation efforts, individuals should be highly motivated to develop a life-style free of opiate dependence. Individuals who are psychologically healthier generally are more successful in opiate cessation than those with more baseline psychologic disturbances, including mood disorders. Potential candidates for opiate cessation therapy that involves naltrexone include former opiate-dependent individuals who are employed and socially functioning, were recently detoxified from methadone maintenance, are leaving prison or residential treatment settings, are sporadically abusing opiates but are not yet dependent, are physically dependent on opiates secondary to medical use of the drugs, and/or are ineligible for methadone maintenance; naltrexone therapy may also be useful when the waiting period for admission into a methadone maintenance program is long. Naltrexone may be particularly useful as maintenance therapy in the prevention of relapse in former opiate-dependent individuals during times of stress when relapse to drug abuse may be most likely. Adolescents who have only recently become physically dependent on opiates may benefit particularly well from opiate cessation therapy that includes naltrexone. Opiate cessation therapy that includes naltrexone may also be especially beneficial in health-care professionals physically dependent on opiates. However, individuals may differ in their specific needs for behavioral therapy (e.g., psychotherapy, counseling) or additional pharmacologic support (e.g., sedatives and hypnotics, GI drugs). Individuals from lower socioeconomic groups who have recently been detoxified from methadone maintenance appear to benefit less from naltrexone therapy than health-care professionals and white-collar workers; however, behavioral therapy in the form of strong family external support improves the beneficial results of naltrexone therapy observed in individuals from lower socioeconomic groups.

Most clinical experience with naltrexone therapy in detoxified, former opiate-dependent individuals has been reported to date in uncontrolled studies. In controlled studies, patients receiving naltrexone therapy generally appeared to decrease their consumption of opiates, participated in opiate cessation programs longer, and had greater decreases in craving for opiates than did patients receiving placebo.

Opiate antagonists (e.g., naltrexone, naloxone) have been used for rapid or ultrarapid detoxification in the management of opiate withdrawal† in opiate-dependent individuals, both in inpatient and outpatient settings. Rapid opiate detoxification involves the administration of opiate antagonists such as naltrexone and/or naloxone to shorten the time period of detoxification. When used for this purpose, naltrexone sometimes has been given in combination with clonidine, guanabenz, or lofexidine (not currently available in the US). The reported advantage of rapid detoxification is to minimize the risk of relapse and to initiate maintenance therapy with naltrexone and psychosocial interventions more quickly. Ultrarapid detoxification is similar, but involves the administration of opiate antagonists (i.e., naltrexone, naloxone) while the patient is sedated or under general anesthesia. However, the risk of adverse respiratory and cardiovascular effects associated with this procedure must be considered as well as the costs of general anesthesia and hospitalization. Safety and efficacy of these therapies have not been established and further study is needed.

Parenteral naltrexone is not approved for use for its opiate antagonist effects or for the treatment of opiate dependence.

■ **Alcohol Dependence** Naltrexone is used orally or IM in the management of alcohol dependence in conjunction with a comprehensive management program that includes psychosocial support. Naltrexone is used IM in patients with alcohol dependence who are able to abstain from alcohol in an outpatient setting prior to initiation of naltrexone therapy and are abstinent at the time such therapy is initiated.Individuals who are willing to use pharmacologic therapy as part of their treatment for alcohol dependence are candidates for naltrexone therapy. A comprehensive management program is an integral component in maintaining alcohol cessation when naltrexone is used, since the drug has not been shown to provide any therapeutic benefit except as part of an appropriate plan of addiction management. These programs involve evaluation, counseling, psychologic support and therapy, and education. Although psychosocial programs alone (i.e., without drug therapy) may be associated with moderate improvement in complete cessation rates and substantial initial rates of alcohol cessation, long-term cessation rates are low, with 50% of patients undergoing intensive inpatient and/or outpatient behavior modification usually relapsing within the first 3 months. When pharmacologic therapy (e.g., naltrexone) is used in conjunction with a comprehensive management program, benefits of such programs may be prolonged.

In general, the goals of pharmacologic therapy in alcohol dependence are to consistently reduce craving for alcohol and to reduce the motivation to drink by blunting pleasant feelings associated with alcohol consumption. In addition, pharmacologic therapy for alcohol dependence should not interact with alcohol or have addictive potential. Factors associated with positive outcomes in clinical trials in alcohol-dependent patients receiving naltrexone for alcohol dependence include type, intensity, and duration of pharmacologic therapy; use of community-based support groups; appropriate management of conditions accompanying alcoholism; and good medication compliance.

When used in conjunction with a comprehensive management program, naltrexone reportedly decreases alcohol craving, reduces alcohol consumption, decreases the number of drinking days, maintains abstinence from alcohol ingestion, and prevents, decreases, or ameliorates the severity of relapse. However, naltrexone therapy is not uniformly effective, and the expected effect is a modest improvement in the outcome of conventional therapy. The theoretical rationale for using naltrexone as an adjunct in alcohol dependence therapy is that the drug may diminish alcohol consumption by blocking the rewarding, pleasurable effects associated with alcohol ingestion. (See Pharmacology: Opiate Antagonist Effects).

In one controlled study in alcohol-dependent patients, reported abstinence rates for naltrexone hydrochloride (50 mg orally once daily for 12 weeks) compared with placebo were 51 vs 23%, while relapse (defined as consumption of 4 or 5 drinks per occasion for women or men, respectively) within 12 weeks of the study period occurred in 31 vs 60% of patients receiving the drug or placebo, respectively. In this study, psychologic behavior modification consisted either of learning coping skills to prevent relapse or of abstinence supportive therapy without coping skills training. Further analysis of these data indicates that rates of abstinence for naltrexone vs placebo were 61 vs 19% in patients receiving supportive therapy in addition to naltrexone or placebo, respectively, while in patients undergoing coping skills training, abstinence rates were 28 vs 21% in those receiving additional naltrexone or placebo therapy, respectively.

In another controlled study in alcohol-dependent patients that evaluated oral naltrexone, rates of abstinence for naltrexone vs placebo were 54 vs 43%, respectively. Although relapse (defined as drinking during 5 or more days within 1 week, having 5 or more drinks per drinking occasion, or having an alcohol blood concentration exceeding 100 mg/dL) in this study was reported in 23 or 54% of patients receiving naltrexone hydrochloride (50 mg orally once daily for 12 weeks) or placebo, respectively, reanalysis by the manufacturer found relapse rates of 21 or 41% in patients receiving the drug or placebo, respectively. In patients who reportedly had consumed at least one drink while undergoing the study, relapse occurred in 50 or 95% of patients receiving naltrexone or placebo, respectively. Results of this study also indicate that patients receiving naltrexone experienced less pleasure after alcohol ingestion and had fewer drinking days and less alcohol craving than those receiving placebo. In an uncontrolled, large multicenter study in patients with alcohol dependence, including those with psychiatric conditions, those physically dependent on other substances, and those with human immunodeficiency virus (HIV) infection, abstinence and relapse rates were similar to those in the controlled studies.

In a study in 627 US veterans (almost all men) with chronic, severe alcoholism (history of heavy drinking at least twice in a week during the previous 30 days and a DSM-IV diagnosis of alcohol dependence but who were sober for at least 5 days prior to study entry), oral naltrexone hydrochloride therapy (50 mg daily) was not effective as an adjunct to standard psychosocial therapy in the management of alcohol dependence as evidenced by no apparent benefit after 13 weeks on days to relapse (mean: 72.3 vs 62.4 days for naltrexone and placebo, respectively) nor at 52 weeks on the percentage of days on which drinking occurred or the number of drinks per drinking day. As a result, it was concluded that the use of adjunctive naltrexone therapy could not be supported in men with chronic, severe alcoholism. Whether these findings can be extrapolated to patients with less severe or less chronic alcoholism or to women or non-veterans remains to be established. Patients in this study relative to other studies typically were older, had been drinking for longer periods, and were less likely to be married or living with a partner; although employment data were not reported, about one-third were receiving disability pensions, which may have negatively affected their motivation to stop drinking. Pending further accumulation of data, some experts recommend that naltrexone continue to be prescribed for patients considered likely to benefit from such therapy such as those who have been drinking heavily for no longer than 20 years and who have stable social support and living situations.

Efficacy of oral naltrexone therapy for alcohol dependence has been established in short-term (up to 12 weeks) clinical studies involving a limited number of patients with alcohol dependence, and the long-term safety and efficacy of the drug for the management of this condition have not been established.

Efficacy of an injectable extended-release formulation of naltrexone has been evaluated in a 6-month study in individuals with alcohol dependence. Adults were randomized to receive naltrexone 380 mg, naltrexone 190 mg, or placebo administered IM monthly in conjunction with 12 sessions of psychosocial intervention. Treatment with 380 mg of naltrexone was associated with a greater reduction in days of heavy drinking (defined as 5 or more alcohol-containing drinks per day for men and 4 or more alcohol-containing drinks per day for women) than treatment with placebo. Individuals receiving 380 mg of naltrexone reported a 25% greater reduction in the rate of heavy drinking relative to placebo-treated individuals. Treatment with 190 mg of naltrexone generally was not associated with a substantial reduction in the rate of heavy drinking. Subgroup analyses suggested that treatment effects were greater in men than in women and also were greater in individuals with lead-in abstinence (about 8% of the study population) than in those who drank during the lead-in phase. Naltrexone-associated reductions in heavy drinking were observed in men and individuals with lead-in abstinence, but the same effects were not observed in women or individuals who drank during the lead-in period.

Studies sponsored by the National Institute of Alcohol Abuse and Alcoholism (NIAAA) are ongoing in an attempt to identify which alcohol-dependent patients are most likely to benefit from naltrexone therapy, to determine optimum duration and dosage of naltrexone, and to identify potential combination therapies that are most effective for use with naltrexone in these patients. *Routine* use of naltrexone in the management of alcohol dependence currently is not recommended.

■ **Obesity** For use of naltrexone hydrochloride in fixed combination with bupropion hydrochloride for weight management, see Naltrexone Hydrochloride and Bupropion Hydrochloride 28:20.08.92.

■ **Other Uses** Naltrexone has been used in dosages up to 800 mg daily for the treatment of schizophrenic disorder,† since elevated endorphin concentrations have been observed in patients with this disorder and naltrexone may inhibit the effects of endogenous endorphins. Although a few patients with schizophrenic disorder have shown some clinical improvement during naltrexone therapy, patients generally showed no improvement and psychoses worsened in some patients. Naltrexone has also been used in a patient with a psychoneurologic syndrome of unknown etiology† that included some signs and symptoms similar to those associated with mast cell disease, carcinoid disease, and dermatitis herpetiformis; the drug reversed and/or suppressed flush and organic psychosis and associated mood alterations, anxiety, and severe skin, bone, and abdominal pain in this patient.

There is preliminary evidence that opiate antagonists (i.e., naloxone, naltrexone) may cause some clinical improvement in patients with dementia of the Alzheimer's type (Alzheimer's disease), but additional study of the efficacy of these drugs in this disease is necessary. In one study in a limited number of patients, there was little evidence of cognitive or behavioral improvement following oral naltrexone dosages up to 100 mg daily.

Dosage and Administration

■ **Reconstitution and Administration** Naltrexone hydrochloride is administered orally. Adverse GI effects may be minimized by taking the drug with food or antacids or after meals.

Naltrexone extended-release injection is administered by deep IM injection into the upper outer quadrant of the gluteal muscle every 4 weeks or once a month. Subsequent injections should be made in alternate buttocks. To avoid inadvertent injection of the suspension into a blood vessel, the plunger of the syringe should be drawn back prior to IM administration to ensure that blood is not aspirated. The IM preparation should *not* be administered by IV or subcutaneous injection; the IM preparation should *not* be inadvertently administered into fatty tissue. Inadvertent subcutaneous injection may increase the likelihood of severe injection site reactions. Therefore, the patient's body habitus should be evaluated prior to each injection to ensure that the length of the needle supplied by the manufacturer (1.5 inches) is adequate for gluteal IM injection in that patient. Because the IM preparation must be administered using the manufacturer-provided needle, alternative treatment should be considered for any patient whose body habitus (i.e., thickness of gluteal adipose tissue) precludes IM injection with the provided needle. Patients should be instructed to monitor the injection site and to notify the clinician if injection site reactions (i.e., pain, swelling, tenderness, induration, bruising, pruritus, redness) worsen or if they do not improve within 2 weeks following injection. Patients should be advised to notify the clinician promptly if intense or prolonged pain, swelling, skin color changes, or signs of necrosis (e.g., hard nodule, blistering, open wound, dark scab) are present at the injection site. Patients with signs of abscess, cellulitis, necrosis, or extensive swelling at the injection site should be promptly evaluated to determine if referral to a surgeon is warranted.

Naltrexone for extended-release injectable suspension should be reconstituted prior to administration using the components of the dose pack supplied by the manufacturer. The dose pack should be allowed to reach room temperature prior to reconstitution of the injection. The preparation should be reconstituted using only the diluent supplied by the manufacturer and administered with the needle supplied by the manufacturer. The vial labeled as containing 380 mg of naltrexone extended-release microspheres should be reconstituted with 3.4 mL of diluent and shaken vigorously for 1 minute. The resulting suspension should be administered immediately. The manufacturer's prescribing information should be consulted for further details on the reconstitution and administration of this preparation.

Patients should be advised not to attempt self-administration of opiates during therapy with the drug. (See Cautions: Precautions and Contraindications.)

The US Food and Drug Administration (FDA) required and approved a Risk Evaluation and Mitigation Strategy (REMS) for parenteral naltrexone. The REMS requires that a medication guide be given to the patient each time parenteral naltrexone is dispensed. The goal of the REMS is to inform patients about serious risks associated with parenteral naltrexone (see Cautions: Precautions and Contraindications). Patients should be advised to read the medication guide prior to initiating parenteral naltrexone therapy and before each injection of the drug. Clinicians should advise patients about the risks and benefits of parenteral naltrexone therapy prior to initiating such therapy and ensure that patients understand the risks.

■ **Dosage** Prior to initiation of naltrexone therapy in patients physically dependent on opiates, detoxification should be completed. Because of the risk of precipitating opiate withdrawal (see Cautions: Opiate Withdrawal), the manufacturers recommend that a period of at least 7–10 days elapse between discontinuance of opiates and initiation of naltrexone therapy. This period varies depending on the dose and duration of the opiate used, and some clinicians recommend at least 7 days in patients using relatively short-acting opiates (e.g., heroin, hydromorphone, meperidine, morphine) and at least 10–14 days in those using longer-acting opiates (e.g., methadone). Because of the risk of relapse to drug abuse during this period, shorter periods of opiate abstinence (e.g., 2–5 days) prior to initiation of naltrexone therapy have been used in some patients. Alternatively, clonidine has been used concomitantly with naltrexone during initiation of therapy to minimize symptoms of opiate withdrawal. Some clinicians have cautiously precipitated withdrawal using repeated naloxone injections and then rapidly initiated naltrexone therapy with incremental doses of the drug; this procedure can reduce the transition period from opiate dependence to naltrexone maintenance and generally is well accepted by patients. Detoxification from opiates may be accomplished in an outpatient or supervised (e.g., hospital) setting. Detoxification in a supervised setting permits closer monitoring of patients during withdrawal, control over access to illicit drugs, and the opportunity to initiate naltrexone therapy during the period when the tendency to relapse to drug abuse may be greatest. Regardless of the setting for detoxification, it generally is preferable to detoxify the patient from all drugs on which they are dependent before initiating naltrexone therapy. In addition to patient verification of abstinence from opiates, urinalysis should be performed after the minimum 7- to 10-day waiting period, but prior to administration of naltrexone, to confirm the absence of opiates. If urinary determination is negative, a naloxone challenge test should be performed prior to administering naltrexone if the clinician believes there is a risk of precipitating a withdrawal reaction following administration of naltrexone.

Naloxone Challenge Test To avoid precipitating opiate withdrawal following administration of naltrexone, the naloxone challenge test should be performed prior to induction of naltrexone therapy in patients formerly physically dependent on opiates who have completed detoxification and in those suspected of having been dependent on opiates. *The naloxone challenge test should not be performed in patients who are exhibiting signs and/or symptoms of opiate withdrawal, those whose urine shows evidence of opiates, or those in whom there is a high degree of suspicion that opiates are still being used, since naloxone may precipitate potentially severe opiate withdrawal. If signs and/or symptoms of opiate withdrawal are evident following administration of the naloxone challenge test, naltrexone therapy should not be attempted*; the naloxone challenge test may be repeated in 24 hours in these patients.

The manufacturer of naltrexone recommends that the naloxone challenge test be performed by administering naloxone by IV or subcutaneous injection. For IV or subcutaneous administration of the test, a sterile syringe containing 0.8 mg of naloxone hydrochloride should be used. For IV administration, the manufacturer of naltrexone recommends that an initial 0. 2-mg dose of the drug be injected IV and, while the needle remains in the vein, the patient should be observed for 30 seconds for evidence of opiate withdrawal. Alternatively, some clinicians recommend that an initial 0. 2-mg dose of naloxone hydrochloride be injected IV and the patient observed for 15 minutes for evidence of withdrawal. Signs and symptoms of withdrawal include, but are not limited to, nasal stuffiness, rhinorrhea, lacrimation, yawning, sweating, tremor, abdominal cramps, vomiting, piloerection, myalgia, and skin crawling. (See Chronic Toxicity in the Opiate Agonists General Statement 28:08.08.) If no evidence of withdrawal is observed, the remaining 0. 6-mg dose of naloxone hydrochloride should be injected IV and the patient observed for an additional 20 minutes for evidence of withdrawal. Some clinicians recommend that a total IV dose of 2 mg be used in the test since withdrawal has been precipitated by the first oral dose of naltrexone despite a negative naloxone challenge test using lower doses and a false-negative test rarely occurs with the 2-mg naloxone hydrochloride dose. For subcutaneous administration, the entire 0. 8-mg dose should be injected subcutaneously and the patient observed for 20 minutes for evidence of opiate withdrawal. For further information on the chemistry and stability, pharmacology, pharmacokinetics, uses, cautions, and dosage and administration of naloxone, see Naloxone Hydrochloride 28:10.

During the appropriate period (i.e., 20 or 45 minutes) in the naloxone challenge test, the patient should be closely monitored for the appearance of signs and symptoms of opiate withdrawal and vital signs should be monitored. Although the naloxone challenge test may precipitate opiate withdrawal in a patient physically dependent on opiates, signs and symptoms will be milder and of shorter duration than those precipitated by naltrexone. If signs and/or symptoms of opiate withdrawal are evident following administration of the naloxone challenge test, a potential risk for precipitating more severe and prolonged withdrawal with naltrexone exists and naltrexone therapy should *not* be initiated; if evidence of withdrawal is absent, naltrexone therapy may be initiated. (See Induction of Therapy for Opiate Cessation in Dosage and Administration: Dosage.) Some clinicians caution that even minor and/or transient GI symptoms following naloxone challenge be considered evidence of withdrawal since patients with such symptoms will often develop severe and disturbing GI symptoms if naltrexone therapy is then initiated. If evidence of opiate withdrawal is present, naltrexone therapy should be delayed and the naloxone challenge test repeated in 24 hours with the 0. 8-mg dose and every 24 hours until results are negative.

Opiate Dependence **Induction of Therapy for Opiate Cessation.** Following completion of opiate detoxification and verification that the patient is free of opiates, oral naltrexone therapy is initiated with an induction regimen. Naltrexone therapy should be initiated carefully by slowly titrating the dose; an initial 25-mg dose of naltrexone hydrochloride is recommended by the manufacturer. Following administration of the initial dose, the patient should be observed for 1 hour for the development of opiate withdrawal. If no evidence of withdrawal is present, the usual oral dosage of 50 mg once daily can be started the next day. Alternatively, some clinicians have induced therapy by administering an initial 10- or 12. 5-mg dose of naltrexone hydrochloride, followed by incremental increases of 10 or 12.5 mg daily until the usual dosage of 50 mg daily has been achieved. Therapy has also been induced by administering an initial 5-mg dose, followed by incremental increases of 10 mg hourly until the usual total daily dose of 50 mg has been achieved.

Maintenance Therapy for Opiate Cessation. Following induction of therapy, an oral maintenance dosage of 50 mg of naltrexone hydrochloride daily produces adequate antagonist activity to block the pharmacologic effects of parenterally administered opiates (e.g., a 25-mg IV dose of heroin). Flexible naltrexone dosing schedules in which the dose and/or frequency of administration of the drug are altered in an attempt to improve compliance have been suggested. The manufacturer states that naltrexone hydrochloride may be administered in dosages of 50 mg daily Monday through Friday and 100 mg on Saturday, 100 mg every other day, or 150 mg every third day. Alternatively, the drug has been administered in a regimen of 100 mg on Monday and Wednesday and 150 mg on Friday or in a regimen of 150 mg on Monday and 200 mg on Thursday. Although the opiate antagonist activity may be somewhat reduced by the administration of larger doses of naltrexone hydrochloride at longer intervals, improved patient compliance may result from administration of the drug every 48–72 hours rather than daily. Most clinicians suggest that observed ingestion of the drug in a clinic setting or by a responsible family member generally be used to ensure compliance, in which case, regimens requiring less frequent visits may be more acceptable to the patient. Some patients, particularly those who are employed, may remain in opiate cessation programs longer if they are permitted take-home doses once they are doing well in the program. Some clinicians suggest that random testing of urine for naltrexone and 6-β-naltrexol or for the presence of opiates may be used to monitor patient compliance.

The optimum duration of naltrexone maintenance therapy has not been established, but should be based on individual requirements and response. In general, patients formerly physically dependent on opiates need a minimum of 6 months to make the behavioral changes necessary to maintain opiate cessation, and naltrexone therapy may be beneficial during this period. For patients unable to successfully deal with the temptation of opiate use, maintenance naltrexone therapy may be necessary throughout the course of a comprehensive opiate cessation program. For other patients, short-term maintenance therapy with naltrexone during the early transition from opiate use to abstinence may be all that is necessary. For other patients who are able to remain abstinent for prolonged periods after an initial period of treatment but who may revert to opiate use during a crisis or get occasional irresistible cravings for opiates, additional naltrexone therapy may only be necessary during these periods. In patients who discontinue naltrexone therapy prematurely and then desire to resume therapy following a relapse to opiate abuse, urinalysis for the presence of opiates and, if necessary, a naloxone challenge test should be performed prior to resuming naltrexone therapy; if there is evidence of opiate dependence, detoxification should be conducted prior to reinitiation of naltrexone therapy.

Management of Opiate Withdrawal. In studies of naltrexone for the management of opiate withdrawal†, various dosage regimens of the drug have been used for rapid or ultrarapid detoxification of opiate dependence. In one study evaluating naltrexone in combination with clonidine, an initial 0. 005-mg/kg dose of clonidine hydrochloride was administered on the first day of detoxification to attenuate opiate withdrawal; clonidine dosage was then titrated according to the severity of withdrawal and the adverse effects induced by clonidine. The highest mean dose of clonidine hydrochloride was 2.3 mg daily, administered on the third day of detoxification. Naltrexone therapy was initiated on the second day of detoxification and administered every 4 hours on the second and third days; the initial dose of naltrexone hydrochloride was 1 mg and was increased by 1- and 2-mg increments during the daytime on the second and third days of detoxification, respectively. Clonidine was also administered every 4 hours on the second and third days to attenuate the withdrawal induced by naltrexone; however, after the third day, clonidine was administered only as needed to reduce signs and symptoms of withdrawal. Naltrexone hydrochloride was administered at a dosage of 10 mg 3 times daily on the fourth day, and as single 50-mg daily doses thereafter.

Alcohol Dependence. Following verification that the patient is free of opiates (see Dosage: Naloxone Challenge Test, in Dosage and Administration), oral naltrexone hydrochloride therapy may be initiated for alcohol dependence. A dosage of 50 mg once daily has been recommended for patients with alcohol dependence. Since about 5–15% of patients reportedly have experienced adverse effects (mainly GI effects) with this dosage, some clinicians have recommended an initial dose of 25 mg, dividing the daily dosage, or adjusting the time of dosing in an effort to minimize such effects; however, naltrexone-associated adverse effects did not appear to be alleviated by such alterations in the recommended dosage. Safety and efficacy of naltrexone hydrochloride for alcohol dependence have been established only in short-term (up to 12 weeks) clinical studies using an oral naltrexone hydrochloride dosage of 50 mg daily, and the optimum duration of naltrexone therapy for this condition currently is not known.

When naltrexone extended-release injection is used for the treatment of alcohol dependence in patients who are free of opiates (See Dosage: Naloxone Challenge Test, in Dosage and Administration), the recommended dosage is 380 mg of naltrexone IM every 4 weeks or once a month. The IM preparation should *not* be administered by IV or subcutaneous injection; the IM preparation should not be inadvertently administered into fatty tissue (see Dosage and Administration: Reconstitution and Administration).

If the patient misses a dose, the next dose should be administered as soon as possible. Dosage adjustment is not needed in patients with mild to moderate (Child-Pugh class A or B) hepatic impairment or mild renal impairment (creatinine clearance of 50–80 mL/minute). Patients initiating therapy with naltrexone for alcohol dependence may initiate therapy with the parenteral preparation; it is not necessary to initiate therapy with oral naltrexone and then switch to the parenteral preparation. Information regarding reinitiation of naltrexone therapy in patients who discontinued such therapy is lacking; data needed to support recommendations for switching patients from oral to parenteral naltrexone therapy have not been systematically collected.

Cautions

At usual oral dosages, adverse effects of naltrexone are generally mild to moderate in severity and usually subside within a few days. Because of the potential for naltrexone to precipitate or exacerbate withdrawal in patients formerly physically dependent on opiates and who are not completely free of the drugs, adverse effects associated with naltrexone in some patients may have been secondary to opiate withdrawal. Many adverse effects reported during administration of naltrexone have occurred prior to as well as during administration of the drug and may be the result of alcohol and drug abuse and poor nutrition; in some patients, adverse effects improved or resolved during administration of the drug. Therefore, a causal relationship for many adverse reactions to naltrexone has not been clearly established.

When administered to opiate-free individuals in usual oral dosages (i.e., 50 mg daily), naltrexone generally has not caused serious adverse effects or abnormal laboratory test results (e.g., liver function). In several controlled studies, the incidence of naltrexone-associated adverse effects was similar to that reported with placebo. In addition, in uncontrolled studies, the incidence of naltrexone-induced adverse effects (e.g., lymphocytosis, increases in serum aminotransferase [transaminase] concentrations, GI effects) was similar to that expected in individuals not receiving the drug.

In controlled studies in alcohol-dependent patients receiving oral therapy with naltrexone hydrochloride 50 mg daily for 12 weeks, the drug was well tolerated. In these studies, nausea required discontinuance of therapy in about 5% of patients; however, no serious adverse effects were reported.

Adverse effects reported in patients with alcohol dependence receiving naltrexone extended-release IM injection generally have been described as mild to moderate. The most common adverse effects associated with IM therapy with the drug are injection site reactions, nausea, and headache. (See Cautions: Precautions and Contraindications.)

■ GI Effects

The most frequent adverse effects reported in individuals receiving oral naltrexone are GI effects. Abdominal pain and cramps, nausea, and vomiting reportedly occur in more than 10% of patients receiving naltrexone for opiate dependence and may occasionally be severe enough to require discontinuance of the drug. Adverse GI effects reported in 1–10% of patients receiving the drug for opiate dependence include constipation and anorexia. Other adverse GI effects reported in less than 1% of patients receiving the drug for opiate dependence include diarrhea, flatulence, upset stomach, hemorrhoids, epigastric pain or heartburn, and ulcer. Nausea and vomiting were reported in 10 and 3%, respectively, of patients receiving naltrexone for the management of alcohol dependence, and were among the most common adverse effects reported in these patients.

Nausea (most commonly following the initial dose), vomiting, or diarrhea occurred in 33, 14, or 13%, respectively, of individuals receiving naltrexone extended-release IM injection in a dosage of 380 mg every 4 weeks in clinical studies. Abdominal pain, dry mouth, or anorexia (appetite disorder) was reported in 11, 5, or 14%, respectively, of these individuals. Nausea has required discontinuance of the drug in about 2% of patients.

■ Hepatic Effects

Naltrexone reportedly can cause dose-related hepatocellular injury, manifested as increases in serum hepatic enzyme concentrations. Liver function abnormalities have been observed mainly in patients receiving high dosages (e.g., 300 mg daily) of the drug investigationally for the treatment of obesity or dementia of the Alzheimer's type (Alzheimer's disease), but increases in serum aminotransferase concentrations have also occurred following administration of dosages 2 times that recommended for blockade of pharmacologic effects of opiates. Following naltrexone hydrochloride dosages of 300 mg daily for 3–8 weeks in obese patients in one placebo-controlled study, serum ALT (SGPT) concentrations increased to up to 3–19 times the baseline values in about 20% of patients receiving the drug, but not in those receiving placebo, and decreased to or near baseline values within several weeks following discontinuance of the drug. In another placebo-controlled study in obese patients, increases in serum ALT, AST (SGOT), and/or LDH concentrations occurred in about 15% of patients receiving 50 or 100 mg of naltrexone hydrochloride daily for 8 weeks and in about 25% of those receiving placebo; in the naltrexone-treated group, hepatic enzymes decreased to at or less than baseline values over several weeks to months following discontinuance of the drug. Clinical symptoms of hepatotoxicity generally were not present in patients with liver function abnormalities. Mild liver function abnormalities are common in very obese patients, probably secondary to fatty infiltration of the liver, and were present in about 50% of obese patients at baseline in one naltrexone study. Increases in serum aminotransferase concentrations have also occurred in several patients with a history of alcohol dependence or of hepatitis.

The manufacturer states that naltrexone-induced hepatocellular injury appears to be a direct toxic rather than an idiosyncratic effect of the drug. However, some clinicians suggest that liver function abnormalities associated with naltrexone use may be caused by noroxymorphone, a minor metabolite of naltrexone that has opiate agonist activity, since opiate agonists have been shown to cause increases in serum hepatic enzyme concentrations and hepatocellular injury in animals and humans. In addition, opiate antagonists, including naltrexone, have been shown to block the increases in serum hepatic enzymes and hepatocellular injury caused by opiates. Therefore, additional study to more fully elucidate the hepatotoxic potential of naltrexone and its metabolites and any possible dose relationship is necessary.

Hepatotoxicity reportedly has not occurred at dosages recommended for blockade of pharmacologic effects of opiates, and serum concentrations of liver enzymes observed following recommended dosages of the drug have been reported to be similar to those observed in the same patients prior to administration of naltrexone. In one short-term study, the incidence of serum AST elevations in individuals receiving parenteral naltrexone was similar to the incidence in those receiving oral naltrexone (1.5% each) and higher than the incidence in those receiving placebo (0.9%). Deterioration in pretreatment liver function abnormalities in former opiate-dependent patients has not been reported to date following initiation of naltrexone therapy. However, the manufacturers state that the margin between therapeutic and hepatotoxic dosages may be less than fivefold, and the hepatotoxic potential of naltrexone must be considered prior to initiation of and during therapy with the drug. (See Cautions: Precautions and Contraindications.)

■ Nervous System Effects Adverse nervous system effects reported in more than 10% of patients receiving oral naltrexone for opiate dependence include headache, lassitude, low energy, difficulty sleeping, anxiety, and nervousness. Increased energy, mental depression, irritability, and dizziness have been reported in 1–10% of patients receiving oral naltrexone for opiate dependence. Other adverse nervous system effects reported in less than 1% of patients receiving the drug for opiate dependence include paranoia, akathisia, fatigue, restlessness, confusion, dysphoria, disorientation, hallucinations, lightheadedness, nightmares and bad dreams, talkativeness, yawning, drowsiness or somnolence, and malaise. In some patients receiving the drug for opiate dependence, severe lethargy and somnolence have developed after only one or two doses of naltrexone and persisted for 12–36 hours; several such patients were receiving a phenothiazine antipsychotic agent (thioridazine) concomitantly.

Depression, suicide, attempted suicide, and suicidal ideation (possibly associated with substance abuse) have been reported in patients receiving oral naltrexone for opiate or alcohol dependence, but the risk of suicide is known to be increased in substance abusers with or without depression, and a causal relationship to the drug has not been established. Clinicians should consider that naltrexone has not been associated with a decrease in the risk of suicide. Depression has been reported in up to 15% of patients receiving oral naltrexone for alcohol dependence. Suicidal ideation or attempted suicide has been reported in up to 1% of these individuals. Headache occurred in 7% and dizziness, nervousness, fatigue, insomnia, anxiety, and somnolence have been reported in 2–4% of patients receiving oral naltrexone for the treatment of alcohol dependence.

Headache, dizziness, and somnolence have occurred in 25, 13, and 4%, respectively, of individuals receiving naltrexone extended-release IM injection in a dosage of 380 mg every 4 weeks in clinical studies. Insomnia or sleep disorder, anxiety, and depression have been reported in 14, 12, and 8–10%, respectively, of these individuals. Headache has required discontinuance of the drug in about 1% of patients. Suicidality (i.e., suicidal ideation, suicide attempt, completed suicide) was reported more frequently in individuals receiving parenteral naltrexone than in those receiving placebo (1 versus 0%). Two completed suicides, both in naltrexone-treated individuals, occurred in controlled clinical studies.

■ Musculoskeletal Effects Joint and muscle pain reportedly occur in more than 10% of patients receiving oral or parenteral naltrexone. Other adverse musculoskeletal effects reported in less than 1% of patients receiving oral naltrexone include tremors, twitching, and painful shoulders, legs, or knees. Back pain or stiffness and muscle cramps have occurred in 6–8% of patients receiving parenteral naltrexone in the recommended dosage.

■ Dermatologic Effects Rash has been reported in 1–10% of patients receiving oral naltrexone. Oily skin, pruritus, acne, athlete's foot, cold sores, and alopecia have been reported in less than 1% of these patients.

■ Local Reactions Injection site reactions, including tenderness, induration, pain, pruritus, ecchymosis, nodules, and swelling, have been reported in 65% of patients receiving parenteral naltrexone in the recommended dosage and have required discontinuance of the drug in about 3% of patients. Cellulitis, hematoma, abscess, sterile abscess, and necrosis also have been reported during postmarketing surveillance of parenteral naltrexone. Some injection site reactions may be very severe, result in substantial scarring, or require surgical intervention, including debridement of necrotic tissue. Injection site reactions have occurred predominantly in females. Inadvertent subcutaneous injection may increase the likelihood of a severe injection reaction. (See Cautions: Precautions and Contraindications and see Dosage and Administration: Reconstitution and Administration.)

■ Respiratory and Cardiovascular Effects Respiratory symptoms, including nasal congestion, rhinorrhea, sneezing, sore throat, excessive mucus or phlegm production, sinus trouble, labored breathing, hoarseness, cough, epistaxis, and dyspnea, have been reported in less than 1% of patients receiving oral naltrexone. Adverse cardiovascular effects reported in less than 1% of these patients include phlebitis, edema, increased systolic and/or diastolic blood pressures, nonspecific ECG changes, palpitation, and tachycardia. Systolic pressures have returned to pretreatment levels after the first week of therapy in some patients.

Upper respiratory tract infection and pharyngitis have occurred in 11–13 % of patients receiving the recommended dosage of parenteral naltrexone. Eosinophilic pneumonia has been reported in at least one individual receiving parenteral naltrexone. Clinicians should consider eosinophilic pneumonia in the differential diagnosis of patients with pneumonia that has not responded to anti-infective therapy.

■ Opiate Withdrawal Naltrexone may precipitate mild to severe signs and symptoms of withdrawal in some patients physically dependent on opiates. The manufacturers recommend that a period of at least 7–10 days elapse between discontinuance of opiates and initiation of naltrexone therapy, and patients should be adequately evaluated to confirm that they are free of opiates prior to initiating therapy with the drug. (See Cautions: Precautions and Contraindications.)

Accidental ingestion of naltrexone has precipitated severe withdrawal in some patients physically dependent on opiates; signs and symptoms of withdrawal usually appeared within 5 minutes of ingestion of naltrexone and continued for up to 48 hours. Signs and symptoms of opiate withdrawal vary in severity depending on the specific opiate used, its dose and duration of use, and individual physiologic and psychologic characteristics of the patient. Signs and symptoms of opiate withdrawal reported in patients receiving naltrexone have included drug craving, confusion, drowsiness, visual hallucinations, abdominal pain, and vomiting and diarrhea which resulted in substantial fluid loss requiring IV fluid replacement therapy in some patients. Other signs and symptoms of withdrawal included fever, chills, tachypnea, perspiration, salivation, lacrimation, rhinorrhea, and mydriasis. Opiate-like withdrawal symptoms, including lacrimation, nasal symptoms, mild nausea, abdominal cramps, restlessness, bone or joint pain, and myalgia have been reported in a few healthy individuals and alcohol-dependent patients receiving naltrexone. It is not known if these symptoms were associated with occult opiate use or with naltrexone therapy. For additional information on opiate withdrawal, including its management, see Chronic Toxicity in the Opiate Agonists General Statement 28:08.08.

■ Other Adverse Effects Chills have been reported in less than 10% of patients receiving oral naltrexone. Increased thirst reportedly occurs in more than 1% of these patients.

Other adverse effects of oral naltrexone reportedly occur in less than 1% of patients. Adverse genitourinary effects include urinary frequency and dysuria. Adverse ocular effects include blurred vision, sensitivity to light, burning, swelling, and aching and strained eyes. Adverse otic effects include congestion, tinnitus, and aching ears. Other adverse effects include lymphocytosis, decreased hematocrit, increased appetite, weight loss or gain, fever, diaphoresis, dry mouth, throbbing head, inguinal pain, swollen glands, cold feet, and hot flushes (flashes).

Idiopathic thrombocytopenic purpura reportedly occurred in one patient receiving oral naltrexone; however, the patient improved without additional complications following discontinuance of the drug and initiation of corticosteroid therapy. Although the patient may have developed hypersensitivity to naltrexone during previous therapy, standard antigen-antibody studies failed to clearly establish a causal relationship to the drug.

A hypersensitivity reaction, characterized by an allergic rash, occurred in one patient receiving oral naltrexone but disappeared 5 days after discontinuance of the drug; palmar erythema, pruritus, and exfoliative dermatitis reappeared upon rechallenge with low doses of the drug.

Altered plasma proteins and increases in IgM, IgA, and IgG levels have been reported in patients receiving oral naltrexone but may have been the result of alcohol abuse or a history of hepatitis.

Asthenia has occurred in 23% of patients receiving the recommended dosage of parenteral naltrexone.

Although the manufacturers state that a dose-related causal relationship between naltrexone and abnormal liver function test results has been established (see Cautions: Hepatic Effects), other abnormal laboratory test results observed during oral naltrexone therapy have not been directly attributed to the drug. Increases in eosinophil counts (which returned to normal over several months with continued use of the drug), decreases in platelet count not associated with bleeding, and serum creatine kinase (CK, creatine phosphokinase, CPK) abnormalities have occurred in individuals receiving parenteral naltrexone. Changes in baseline concentrations of some hypothalamic, pituitary, adrenal, or gonadal hormones have occurred in patients receiving opiate antagonists; however, the clinical importance of such changes has not been established.

■ Precautions and Contraindications Naltrexone reportedly can cause dose-related hepatotoxicity. (See Cautions: Hepatic Effects.) Baseline determinations of liver function should be performed in all patients prior to initiation of naltrexone. The manufacturers state that the potential benefits of naltrexone therapy should be weighed carefully against the possible hepatotoxic risks of the drug in patients with active liver disease (e.g., liver function test values exceeding 3 times the upper limit of normal). However, some clinicians have questioned the need for considering withholding naltrexone therapy in most opiate or alcohol-dependent individuals with marginal evidence of hepatic injury or disease, since baseline serum concentrations of liver enzymes are frequently elevated in opiate- or alcohol-dependent individuals and evidence of hepatotoxic risk of naltrexone therapy at usual dosages has not been demonstrated in these individuals. Naltrexone is contraindicated in patients with acute hepatitis or liver failure. Naltrexone should be discontinued if manifestations of acute hepatitis (e.g., abdominal pain lasting more than a few days, light-colored [e.g., white] stools, dark urine, yellowing of the eyes) develop. Patients receiving naltrexone therapy should be instructed to contact a clinician if such manifestations occur and to discontinue therapy with the drug (if receiving oral therapy). Although naltrexone-associated hepatic failure has not been reported, clinicians are advised to consider the risk of naltrexone-associated hepatic failure and to use the drug with caution similar to that employed with other drugs that may cause hepatic injury. In addition, some clinicians state that the possibility that naltrexone might have synergistic toxic effects in patients with alcohol-induced hepatic disease has not been ruled out. The manufacturer of oral naltrexone recommends that liver function be monitored at regular intervals in all patients during naltrexone therapy to detect hepatic injury or disease that may develop secondary to the drug. The manufacturer states that the risk of naltrexone-induced toxicity may be increased when flexible naltrexone hydrochloride dosing schedules that involve administration of single doses greater than 50 mg (e.g., 100 mg every other day, 150 mg every third day) are used, and clinicians should balance the benefits of improved patient compliance against possible risks.

Naltrexone may precipitate mild to severe withdrawal in patients physically dependent on opiates. (See Cautions: Opiate Withdrawal.) If signs and/or symptoms of withdrawal are precipitated by naltrexone in a patient physically dependent on opiates, the patient should be closely monitored and therapy adjusted according to individual requirements and response. To minimize the risk of developing acute withdrawal, opiate-dependent individuals who are candidates for naltrexone therapy should be instructed to remain free of opiates for a minimum of 7–10 days prior to initiating therapy with the drug. A urinalysis to confirm the absence of opiates should be performed after the minimum 7- to 10-day waiting period but prior to administration of naltrexone; however, the absence of opiates in urine is frequently insufficient evidence that a patient is free of opiates, and, if opiates are absent, a naloxone challenge test should also be performed prior to administering naltrexone if the clinician believes there is a risk of precipitating a withdrawal reaction following administration of naltrexone. (See Naloxone Challenge Test in Dosage and Administration: Dosage.)

Although naltrexone is a potent opiate antagonist with a dose-dependent duration of activity that ranges from 24–72 hours following oral administration, the opiate antagonist activity produced by oral or parenteral naltrexone can be overcome by administration of opiates; overcoming the blockade of pharmacologic effects produced by naltrexone may be useful in certain patients in whom opiate analgesia is necessary. Generally, if analgesia is necessary in patients receiving naltrexone, a nonopiate analgesic, regional analgesia, conscious sedation with a benzodiazepine, or general anesthesia should be used whenever possible. In an emergency situation when adequate analgesia can only be achieved by administration of an opiate agonist in naltrexone-treated patients, cautious administration of an opiate may afford adequate analgesia, but higher than usual dosages may be required. If an opiate agonist is used in these patients, the possibility that the respiratory depression produced by the opiate may be deeper and more prolonged should be considered. If an opiate is required as a component of anesthesia or analgesia, the patient should be continuously monitored in an anesthesia care setting by individuals who are trained in the use of anesthetic agents and in the management of respiratory depressant effects of potent opiates and who are not involved in the conduct of the surgical or diagnostic procedure. In addition, patients receiving naltrexone and analgesic therapy with opiate agonists may also experience apparent non-opiate receptor-induced effects such as facial swelling, pruritus, generalized erythema, or bronchoconstriction that are probably caused by opiate-induced histamine release and/or other mechanisms. Since methods for reversing opiate overdosage in patients receiving naltrexone have not been established, use of a short-acting opiate with minimal respiratory depression is preferable and dosage of the opiate agonist should be carefully adjusted according to individual requirements and response. However, regardless of the opiate agonist used, the patient should be closely monitored in a setting equipped and staffed by health-care personnel appropriately trained in cardiopulmonary resuscitation. Prior to elective surgery in which analgesia can only be achieved by administration of an opiate, oral naltrexone should be discontinued at least 48 hours prior to the surgical procedure. Use of other opiate-agonist-containing preparations such as those used for the management of cough or diarrhea should generally be avoided, since adequate therapeutic benefit may be difficult to achieve with an opiate.

Self-administration of large doses of opiates may produce serum opiate concentrations sufficient to overcome the antagonist effects of naltrexone and may produce signs and symptoms of acute opiate overdosage, including respiratory arrest, circulatory collapse, and possibly death. For a complete discussion of opiate overdosage, see Acute Toxicity in the Opiate Agonists General Statement 28:08.08. Self-administration of smaller doses of opiate agonists than previously used may produce signs and symptoms of opiate overdosage and toxicity.

Patients undergoing naltrexone therapy should be carefully instructed that naltrexone has been prescribed as part of a comprehensive program for the treatment of their drug dependence and to carry some form of medical identification that can alert medical personnel that they are taking a long-acting opiate antagonist. Patients should be instructed to take oral naltrexone as directed; patients receiving parenteral naltrexone should be advised of the frequency of administration. Patients should be warned of the serious consequences of self-administration of opiates in an attempt to overcome the antagonist activity of naltrexone. They should be advised that self-administration of small doses of opiates (e.g., heroin) during naltrexone therapy will not result in any pharmacologic effect and that large doses may result in serious pharmacologic effects, including coma and death. Patients also should be advised that if they previously self-administered opiates, they may be more sensitive to lower doses of opiates after naltrexone therapy is discontinued.

Because naltrexone and its metabolites are eliminated principally in urine, naltrexone should be used with caution in patients with moderate to severe renal impairment.

Injection site reactions have been reported in patients receiving parenteral naltrexone. Patients should be instructed to monitor the injection site and to notify the clinician if injection site reactions (i.e., pain, swelling, tenderness, induration, bruising, pruritus, redness) worsen or if they do not improve within 2 weeks following injection. Patients should be advised to notify the clinician promptly if intense or prolonged pain, swelling, skin color changes, or signs of necrosis (e.g., hard nodule, blistering, open wound, dark scab) are present at the injection site. Patients with signs of abscess, cellulitis, necrosis, or extensive swelling at the injection site should be promptly evaluated to determine if referral to a surgeon is warranted.

As with any preparation administered IM, parenteral naltrexone should be used with caution in patients with thrombocytopenia or other coagulation disorder (e.g., hemophilia).

Because eosinophilic pneumonia has been reported rarely in patients receiving parenteral naltrexone, patients receiving this preparation should be advised to seek medical attention if symptoms of pneumonia develop.

Depression and suicidality have occurred in naltrexone-treated individuals. Patients receiving naltrexone should be closely monitored for symptoms of depression and suicidal thinking and should be advised to contact their clinician immediately if they experience new or worsening symptoms of depression or suicidal thoughts.

Because naltrexone may cause dizziness, patients should be advised to avoid driving or operating heavy machinery until they know how the drug affects them.

The US Food and Drug Administration (FDA) required and approved a Risk Evaluation and Mitigation Strategy (REMS) for parenteral naltrexone. The REMS requires that a medication guide be given to the patient each time parenteral naltrexone is dispensed. The goal of the REMS is to inform patients about serious risks associated with parenteral naltrexone. Patients should be advised to read the medication guide prior to initiating parenteral naltrexone therapy and before each injection of the drug. Clinicians should advise patients about the risks and benefits of parenteral naltrexone therapy prior to initiating such therapy and ensure that patients understand the risks.

Naltrexone is contraindicated in patients receiving opiate agonists (except for emergency situations), nondetoxified patients physically dependent on opiates (including those receiving methadone), patients experiencing acute opiate withdrawal, patients who experience opiate withdrawal following administration of the naloxone challenge test, and patients in whom urinalysis for the presence of opiates is positive. Naltrexone is also contraindicated in patients with acute hepatitis or hepatic failure and in patients with known hypersensitivity to the drug or any ingredient in the formulation. It is not known whether cross-sensitivity exists between naltrexone and naloxone or phenanthrene-derivative opiate agonists (e.g., codeine, morphine, oxymorphone).

■ **Pediatric Precautions** Safety of naltrexone in children younger than 18 years of age has not been established.

■ **Geriatric Precautions** Clinical studies of parenteral naltrexone did not include sufficient numbers of patients 65 years of age or older to determine whether geriatric patients respond differently than younger adults.

■ **Mutagenicity and Carcinogenicity** Mutagenic changes and chromosomal damage have occurred in vitro in human lymphocytes and Chinese hamster ovarian cells, in the Drosophila recessive lethal assay, and in nonspecific DNA repair tests with *Escherichia coli* and WI-38 cells. However, the importance of these findings has not been determined and naltrexone did not show evidence of mutagenic potential in many other tests using bacterial, mammalian, or tissue culture systems.

In a 2-year study of the carcinogenic potential of naltrexone, there was an increase in the frequency of mesotheliomas in male rats and tumors of vascular origin in both male and female rats. No evidence of carcinogenicity was observed in several other 2-year studies in mice or rats receiving naltrexone dosages of 30 or 100 mg/kg daily (47 or 150 times greater than the usual dosage in humans), respectively.

The possible mutagenic and carcinogenic effects of 6-β-naltrexol (an active metabolite) are unknown.

■ **Pregnancy, Fertility, and Lactation** In reproduction studies in rats and rabbits, oral naltrexone was shown to increase the incidence of early fetal loss. There are no adequate and controlled studies to date using naltrexone in pregnant women, and the drug should be used during pregnancy only when the potential benefits justify the possible risks to the fetus. It is not known whether naltrexone affects the duration of labor and delivery.

Naltrexone dosages of 100 mg/kg daily in rats (about 16 times the usual human oral dosage based on body surface area) produced an increase in pseudopregnancy and a decrease in the pregnancy rate in mated rats, but the relevance of these findings to human fertility is not known. Use of the drug has been associated with delayed ejaculation and decreased or increased sexual potency in less than 10% of patients. Increased (see Pharmacology: Other Effects) or decreased libido has been reported in less than 1% of patients.

Naltrexone and its major metabolite, 6-β-naltrexol, are distributed into human milk. Because of the potential for serious adverse effects in nursing infants, a decision should be make whether to discontinue nursing or the drug, taking into account the importance of the drug to the woman.

Drug Interactions

The manufacturer states that concomitant administration of naltrexone with drugs other than opiate agonists has not been studied; therefore, naltrexone should be used with caution in patients receiving other drugs.

■ **Opiate Agonists** Patients receiving naltrexone may not benefit therapeutically from opiate-containing preparations, including those used for the management of cough and cold, diarrhea, and pain. Use of these preparations should generally be avoided during naltrexone therapy. (See Cautions: Precautions and Contraindications.) Because naltrexone can precipitate potentially severe opiate withdrawal, naltrexone should not be used in patients receiving opiates or in nondetoxified patients physically dependent on opiates (including those receiving methadone maintenance treatment).

■ **Effects on Hepatic Clearance of Drugs** Since naltrexone is metabolized principally in the liver, other drugs that alter hepatic metabolism may increase or decrease serum naltrexone concentrations. In animals and in vitro, naltrexone and 6-β-naltrexol (an active metabolite) have been shown to inhibit hepatic metabolism of aminopyrine and aniline via hepatic microsomal mixed-function oxidase enzymes; the importance of this effect on metabolism of other drugs in humans requires further study. Naltrexone reportedly does not induce its own metabolism.

■ **Other Drugs** Naltrexone has been administered concurrently with non-opiate drugs (e.g., disulfiram, antidepressants, lithium) frequently used in the treatment of drug dependence without evidence of unusual adverse effects; however, these drug interactions have not been examined closely under a controlled clinical environment.

Because the safety and efficacy of concomitant use of naltrexone and disulfiram currently are not known but potentially hepatotoxic drugs usually are not administered concomitantly, the manufacturer recommends that the drugs be used together only if the potential benefits justify the possible risks to the patient. Augmentation of naltrexone-induced lethargy and somnolence have been reported following initial doses of naltrexone in several patients stabilized on phenothiazine therapy (thioridazine). (See Cautions: Nervous System Effects.)

In a study in healthy individuals, concomitant use of acamprosate (1 g every 12 hours) and naltrexone hydrochloride (50 mg orally once daily) resulted in an increase in the rate and extent of absorption of acamprosate but did not alter the pharmacokinetics of naltrexone or 6-β-naltrexol. Area under the plasma concentration-time curve (AUC) and peak plasma concentration of acamprosate were increased by 25 and 33%, respectively, and time to peak plasma concentration was reduced by 33% when acamprosate and naltrexone were given concomitantly. Cognitive testing indicated that, although each drug alone was associated with some adverse effects on cognitive performance, combined use of the drugs did not appear to enhance these effects.

Following abrupt discontinuance of methadone, concomitant administration of naltrexone and clonidine hydrochloride has attenuated withdrawal symptoms generally precipitated or exacerbated by naltrexone. Clonidine alone reduces the severity of opiate withdrawal symptoms by stimulation of presynaptic α_2-adrenergic receptors resulting in attenuation of rebound increases in noradrenergic activity in the CNS, which may be responsible for the behavioral symptoms of opiate withdrawal. Concomitant administration of clonidine and naltrexone may reduce the duration of opiate withdrawal by decreasing opiate-induced postsynaptic supersensitivity.

Laboratory Test Interferences

Naltrexone reportedly does not interfere with the determination of urinary morphine, methadone, or quinine using thin-layer (TLC), gas-liquid (GLC), or high-pressure liquid (HPLC) chromatography. Naltrexone may interfere with some immunoassay or enzymatic methods used for the detection of urinary opiates.

Acute Toxicity

The manufacturers state that there has been limited experience to date with overdosage of naltrexone in humans.

■ **Pathogenesis** The oral LD_{50} of naltrexone has been reported to be 1.1–1.55, 1.45, 1.49, and 3 g/kg in mice, rats, guinea pigs, and monkeys, respectively; death usually occurred within 4 hours after administration. The IV LD_{50} has been reported to be 180 mg/kg in mice, and the subcutaneous LD_{50} has been reported to be 550–590, 1930, and 200 mg/kg in mice, rats, and dogs, respectively. Acute toxicity from naltrexone in mice, rats, and dogs resulted in death secondary to tonic-clonic seizures and/or respiratory failure. Weight loss occurred in monkeys following subcutaneous administration of 100-mg/kg doses, and prostration, seizures, and death occurred following subcutaneous administration of 300-mg/kg doses. Hypoactivity, salivation, and emesis occurred in monkeys following oral administration of 1-g/kg doses, and seizures and death occurred following oral administration of 3-g/kg doses.

Patients receiving 800 mg of naltrexone hydrochloride daily for up to 1 week in one study showed no evidence of toxicity. However, lower dosages reportedly have been hepatotoxic in some patients. (See Cautions: Hepatic Effects.) No serious adverse effects were observed following administration of single naltrexone doses of up to 784 mg (as the extended-release IM injection) in several healthy individuals.

■ **Treatment** There has been limited experience to date in the treatment of naltrexone overdosage, but supportive and symptomatic treatment should be initiated as necessary. When the drug has been ingested orally, usual measures to decrease GI absorption of the drug (e.g., induction of emesis, gastric lavage) should also be employed. Clinicians should consider contacting a poison control center for the most current information on treatment of naltrexone overdosage.

Pharmacology

■ **Opiate Antagonist Effects** Naltrexone hydrochloride is essentially a pure opiate antagonist. In contrast to levallorphan or nalorphine but like naloxone, naltrexone generally has little or no agonist activity. The opiate antagonist activity of naltrexone on a weight basis is reportedly 2–9 times that of naloxone, 17 times that of nalorphine, and about one-tenth that of cyclazocine (not currently available in the US). The major metabolite of naltrexone, 6-β-naltrexol, is also an opiate antagonist and may contribute to the antagonist activity of the drug. (See Pharmacokinetics: Elimination.) When administered in usual doses to patients who have not recently received opiates, naltrexone exhibits little or no pharmacologic effect. At oral doses of 30–50 mg daily, naltrexone generally produces minimal analgesia, only slight drowsiness, and no respiratory depression. Psychotomimetic effects or circulatory changes are generally absent following administration of naltrexone. However, pharmacologic effects, including psychotomimetic effects, increased systolic and/or diastolic blood pressure, respiratory depression, and decreased oral temperature, which are suggestive of opiate agonist activity, have reportedly occurred in a few individuals. The drug has also occasionally produced a small degree of miosis in some individuals, suggesting some opiate agonist activity, but the exact mechanism of this effect is not known. It has been suggested that a metabolite of naltrexone (e.g., noroxymorphone) may be responsible for any opiate agonist activity observed with the drug. (See Pharmacokinetics: Elimination.)

In patients who have received single or repeated large doses of morphine or other opiate agonists, naltrexone attenuates or produces a complete but reversible block of the pharmacologic effects (e.g., physical dependence, analgesia, euphoria, tolerance) of the opiate. The drug antagonizes most of the subjective and objective effects of opiates, including respiratory depression, miosis, euphoria, and drug craving. Like naloxone, naltrexone probably also antagonizes the psychotomimetic effects of opiate partial agonists (e.g., pentazocine). Because the duration of action of naltrexone may be shorter than that of the opiate, the effects of the opiate may return as the effects of naltrexone dissipate. The degree of opiate antagonism produced by naltrexone depends on the dose and the time elapsed since the last dose of naltrexone and the dose of the opiate. Doses of up to 3 g daily of oral naloxone are necessary to produce the degree of antagonist activity produced by 30- to 50-mg daily doses of oral naltrexone.

Naltrexone does not produce physical or psychologic dependence, and tolerance to the drug's opiate antagonist activity reportedly does not develop. Naltrexone may precipitate mild to potentially severe withdrawal in individuals physically dependent on opiates or pentazocine.

The precise mechanism of the opiate antagonist effects of naltrexone is not known. However, naltrexone reportedly shares the actions of naloxone and is thought to act as a competitive antagonist at μ, κ, and δ receptors in the CNS; the drug appears to have the highest affinity for the μ receptor. The drug may displace opiates from opiate-occupied receptor sites by competitive binding at the receptors, and displacement of naltrexone from these receptors by opiates is also reportedly possible. In one study in dogs, naltrexone failed to antagonize the agonist effect of *N*-allylnormetazocine at the Σ receptor. Naltrexone may antagonize the pharmacologic effects of endorphins, but the effect of the drug on endorphins has not been fully elucidated. Sensitivity to the analgesic effects of morphine and the number of opiate receptors in the CNS has reportedly increased in rats following chronic subcutaneous administration of naltrexone for 8 days; sensitivity and number of receptors returned to pretreatment levels within 6 days after withdrawal of naltrexone.

The mechanism of action of naltrexone in alcohol dependence is not known. Evidence from studies in animals suggests that alcohol ingestion stimulates release of endogenous opiate agonists, which may increase some of the rewarding effects associated with alcohol ingestion through agonist activity at opiate (e.g., μ) receptors. In animals and humans, opiate antagonists (e.g., naltrexone) that competitively bind to opiate receptors may reduce alcohol consumption by blocking the effects of endogenous opiates and thus making alcohol ingestion less pleasurable. In addition, naltrexone appears to decrease substantially the subjective alcohol "high" and increase the negative or dysphoric effects associated with alcohol consumption. The drug also may decrease alcohol-associated stimulant effects and increase alcohol-associated sedative effects without altering psychomotor performance in individuals receiving an intoxicating dose of alcohol. Naltrexone does not cause disulfiram-like reactions following ingestion of alcohol.

■ **Endocrine Effects** Like naloxone, naltrexone has been shown to increase plasma concentrations of luteinizing hormone (LH), corticotropin (ACTH), and cortisol. Since corticotropin has been shown to have partial antagonist activity at opiate receptors, it has been suggested that increases in plasma concentrations of corticotropin and cortisol following administration of naltrexone may result from displacement of corticotropin and endorphins from opiate receptors by naltrexone, although other mechanisms may be responsible (e.g., naltrexone-induced release of adrenocorticotropic releasing factor). Naltrexone has been shown to have little, if any, effect on plasma concentrations of follicle-stimulating hormone (FSH) and to produce minimal increases in serum testosterone concentrations. It is believed that naltrexone may influence plasma concentrations of LH by enhancing the secretion of gonadotropin releasing hormone. When administered prior to heroin (diacetylmorphine), naltrexone prevents the decrease in plasma concentrations of LH and testosterone usually produced by heroin. However, in one study, chronic administration of naltrexone in obese individuals was shown to have little, if any, effect on plasma concentrations of LH, FSH, testosterone, estradiol, cortisol, prolactin, glucose, or insulin. Like naloxone, naltrexone generally has been shown to have little, if any, effect on plasma growth hormone (GH) or serum prolactin concentrations.

Naloxone does not affect serum concentrations of basal or stimulated glucagon. The drug does not affect serum concentrations of basal or stimulated thyrotropin (TSH) or TSH concentrations in hypothyroid patients; in animals, naltrexone has reversed the decrease in plasma TSH concentrations usually observed following exposure to acute or chronic stress. Naloxone and naltrexone indirectly block the effect of thyrotropin releasing hormone (TRH) on GI transit and fluid accumulation in rabbits and rats, presumably by blocking TRH-induced release of serotonin.

Naltrexone has increased sensory-stimulated release of acetylcholine (ACh) from the cerebral cortex in rats, but spontaneous release of ACh was unaffected by the drug. The effect of naltrexone on antidiuretic hormone (ADH, vasopressin) in humans has not been studied; in animals, naltrexone did not affect changes in plasma ADH concentrations induced by most stimuli (i.e., nicotine, osmotic stimuli, hypovolemia, hemorrhage, tail pinch, overhydration). Basal plasma concentrations of ADH have not been affected by high doses (10 mg) of naloxone. The effect of naltrexone on GI secretions has not been studied; however, naloxone has reduced basal and meal-stimulated gastric acid secretion but not postprandial gastric acid secretion or basal, meal-stimulated, or postprandial gastrin and pancreatic polypeptide secretion.

■ **Other Effects** The effect of naltrexone on catecholamines in humans has not been studied; however, in rats, naltrexone produced a decrease in the midbrain and hippocampal concentrations of norepinephrine. Increased plasma concentrations of epinephrine and norepinephrine have been reported following high (10 mg) but not low (0.4 mg) doses of naloxone.

Naltrexone has produced recurrent, spontaneous sexual arousal (i.e., penile erections) associated with dysphoric sexual ideation in several individuals. However, one study failed to confirm this finding.

In a limited number of schizophrenic patients, naltrexone hydrochloride reportedly enhanced electrical evoked potentials to somatosensory stimuli and visual evoked potentials; following administration of naltrexone (average daily dose of 500 mg at time of testing) for 8 days in schizophrenic patients, electrical evoked potentials were characterized by larger amplitude at higher stimulus intensities. These effects on evoked potentials may result from the drug's inhibition of the effects of endogenous endorphins and reversal of endorphin suppression of noradrenergic activity in the CNS.

Naltrexone, in single doses of 50 or 100 mg in healthy individuals, produced EEG patterns characterized by alpha waves of decreased frequency; in addition, 1 hour after administration of 100 mg of the drug, the EEG pattern in the fast frequency band was characterized by less power than after placebo.

Inhibition of weight gain or decreased food consumption has occurred in rats following administration of naltrexone hydrochloride in single doses ranging from 0.3–10 mg/kg or daily doses of 100 mg/kg for 1–8 weeks. Anorexia and/or weight loss have occurred in several patients following oral administration of usual dosages of naltrexone for the treatment of opiate addiction. Although the exact mechanism of the anorexic effect has not been fully determined, the drug may inhibit the effects of endogenous endorphins, and decreased concentrations of endorphins in the CNS have been associated with fasting and starvation. It has also been suggested that the anorexic effect of the drug may be characteristic of withdrawal from chronic use of opiates rather than secondary to a direct effect of naltrexone. Naltrexone, administered to mice in doses of 10 mg/kg, blocked the lack of weight gain and growth inhibition produced by 5- to 20-mg/kg doses of pentazocine administered daily for 3 weeks; in these same animals, naltrexone alone did not produce growth inhibition. In the same study, protein synthesis in brain, liver, and muscle was substantially depressed by pentazocine but was unaffected by naltrexone.

Like naloxone, naltrexone increases mean arterial pressure, cardiac output, stroke volume, and left ventricular contractility in dogs with hypovolemic shock following administration of naltrexone hydrochloride doses ranging from 2.5–10 mg/kg as a rapid IV injection or 2 mg/kg rapidly IV followed by an IV infusion of 2 mg/kg per hour for 4 hours. Pretreatment with naltrexone has blocked the potentiating effect of morphine in mice with anaphylactic shock. The effects of naltrexone in shock in humans requires further study.

Bradycardia has occurred following IV naltrexone hydrochloride doses of 5–80 mcg/kg in unanesthetized dogs; respiratory rate, blood pressure, arterial blood gases, and EEG remained unchanged throughout the dose range. Within 20 minutes of 1-mg/kg IV doses in cats, total brain oxygen consumption decreased by about 48% and blood flow to the entire brain and the pons decreased by about 40%; however, the effect of naltrexone on total oxygen consumption and blood flow in humans has not been determined.

Pharmacokinetics

■ **Absorption** Naltrexone hydrochloride is rapidly and almost completely (about 96%) absorbed from the GI tract following oral administration, but the drug undergoes extensive first-pass metabolism in the liver. (See Pharmacokinetics: Elimination.) Only 5–40% of an orally administered dose reaches systemic circulation unchanged. Considerable interindividual variation in absorption of the drug during the first 24 hours after a single dose has been reported. The bioavailability of naltrexone hydrochloride tablets is reportedly similar to that of an oral solution of the drug (not commercially available in the US).

Peak plasma concentrations of naltrexone and 6-β-naltrexol (the major metabolite of naltrexone) usually occur within 1 hour following oral administration of the tablets and 0.6 hours following oral administration of the solution. Because orally administered naltrexone undergoes substantial first-pass metabolism, plasma concentrations of 6-β-naltrexol following oral administration are substantially higher than corresponding concentrations of naltrexone. Following oral administration, the area under the serum concentration-time curve (AUC) for 6-β-naltrexol is 10–30 times greater than the AUC for naltrexone. Following single- or multiple-dose (i.e., once daily) oral administration of naltrexone hydrochloride 50 mg in healthy individuals, peak plasma concentrations of naltrexone and 6-β-naltrexol averaged 10.6–13.7 and 109–139 ng/mL, respectively.

Plasma concentrations of naltrexone and 6-β-naltrexol increase with increasing doses of the drug. The AUC and peak plasma concentrations of naltrexone and 6-β-naltrexol increase proportionally with single naltrexone hydrochloride doses of 50–200 mg. Following oral administration of single doses of a 50-mg tablet, two 50-mg tablets, or 100 mg of a solution in a study in healthy individuals, mean peak plasma naltrexone concentrations were 8.6, 19.6, or 20.7 ng/mL, and mean peak plasma concentrations of 6-β-naltrexol were 99.3, 206.8, or 206.2 ng/mL, respectively.

Little, if any, accumulation of naltrexone and/or 6-β-naltrexol appears to occur following chronic administration of the drug. Following chronic administration of naltrexone, plasma concentrations of 6-β-naltrexol are at least 40% higher than those following administration of a single dose of the drug; however, plasma concentrations of naltrexone and 6-β-naltrexol 24 hours after each dose of chronically administered drug are similar to concentrations 24 hours after a single dose of the drug in most patients.

The onset of opiate antagonism following oral administration of naltrexone has been reported to be 15–30 minutes in a limited number of patients who had been receiving morphine chronically. Administration of a single 15-mg oral dose of naltrexone hydrochloride immediately following a single 30-mg subcutaneous dose of morphine has been reported to produce opiate antagonism that is prominent within 6 hours, maximal within 12 hours, and persists for at least 24 hours. The extent and duration of antagonist activity of naltrexone appear to be directly related to plasma and tissue concentrations of the drug. Plasma naltrexone concentrations of 2 ng/mL have been reported to be associated with an 87% blockade of the pharmacologic effects of a 25-mg IV dose of heroin. In one study in former opiate-dependent individuals receiving 100 mg of naltrexone hydrochloride daily and subsequently challenged with a 25-mg IV dose of heroin, the extent of blockade of the effects of heroin was 96, 87, and 47% at 24, 48, and 72 hours after naltrexone, respectively; corresponding plasma naltrexone concentrations were 2.4, 2, and 1.7 ng/mL, respectively.

The duration of the opiate antagonist activity of naltrexone appears to be dose dependent and is longer than that of equipotent doses of naloxone. A single 50-mg oral dose of naltrexone hydrochloride effectively antagonizes the pharmacologic effects of 25 mg of IV heroin or subcutaneous morphine for up to 24 hours. Increasing the dose of naltrexone hydrochloride to 100 or 150 mg reportedly antagonizes the effects of 25 mg of IV heroin for up to 48 or 72 hours, respectively.

Bioavailability of orally administered naltrexone is altered in individuals with hepatic impairment. Following oral administration of naltrexone in patients with compensated (Child-Pugh class A or B) or decompensated liver cirrhosis (Child-Pugh class C), naltrexone AUC values are fivefold or tenfold higher, respectively, than values in individuals with normal hepatic function. Although peak plasma concentrations of 6-β-naltrexol were delayed in patients with hepatic impairment, systemic exposure to the metabolite in these patients was not altered substantially compared with that in healthy individuals.

Following IM administration of naltrexone extended-release injection, the drug is released slowly and gradually from the microspheres by diffusion and erosion as the polylactide co-glycolide polymer degrades. Following IM administration of naltrexone 380 mg, peak plasma naltrexone concentrations of

12.9 ng/mL occur in 2–3 days (there is a transient initial peak 2 hours after injection); plasma concentrations start to decline after 14 days but remain detectable for 1 month or longer. Following IM administration of naltrexone 380 mg, peak plasma concentrations of 6-β-naltrexol (the major metabolite of naltrexone) generally occur in 3 days. Exposure to 6-β-naltrexol is about twofold higher than the corresponding naltrexone exposure. Following administration of a single IM dose of naltrexone 380 mg, total naltrexone exposure is threefold to fourfold higher and 6-β-naltrexol exposure is 3.4-fold lower than exposure following oral administration of naltrexone 50 mg daily for 28 days. Steady-state plasma concentrations of naltrexone and 6-β-naltrexol are attained by the end of the dosing interval after the first injection. Minimal accumulation of naltrexone and/or 6-β-naltrexol appears to occur following repeated IM administration.

Following IM administration of naltrexone extended-release injection, plasma concentrations of naltrexone and 6-β-naltrexol achieved in individuals with mild to moderate hepatic impairment (Child-Pugh class A and B) are similar to those in healthy individuals with normal hepatic function.

■ Distribution Naltrexone hydrochloride is widely distributed throughout the body, but considerable interindividual variation in distribution parameters during the first 24 hours following a single oral dose has been reported. Following subcutaneous administration of radiolabeled drug in rats, the drug distributes into CSF within 30 minutes. In animals, CSF naltrexone concentrations are reported to be approximately 30% of concurrent peak plasma concentrations. The drug and its metabolites have been shown to distribute into saliva and erythrocytes following oral administration in humans. Following IV injection of a single 1-mg dose of the drug in healthy adults with normal renal and hepatic function, the volume of distribution of naltrexone was estimated to be 1350 L. The volume of distribution of the drug in former opiate-dependent individuals with normal renal and hepatic function reportedly averages 16.1 L/kg following oral administration of a single 100-mg dose and 14.2 L/kg following oral administration of 100 mg daily for at least 18 days.

Naltrexone is approximately 21–28% protein bound.

It is not known if naltrexone and/or its metabolites cross the placenta. Naltrexone and its major metabolite, 6-β-naltrexol, are distributed into human milk.

■ Elimination Plasma concentrations of naltrexone and 6-β-naltrexol, the major metabolite, appear to decline in a biphasic manner during the first 24 hours following a single oral dose or during chronic administration of the drug. Following oral administration of single or multiple doses of naltrexone hydrochloride, the plasma half-lives of naltrexone and 6-β-naltrexol in the initial phase ($t_{1/2\alpha}$) average 1.1–3.9 and 2.3–3.1 hours, respectively, and the plasma half-lives in the terminal phase ($t_{1/2\beta}$) average 9.7–10.3 and 11.4–16.8 hours, respectively. Plasma concentrations of naltrexone and 6-β-naltrexol have also been reported to decline in a triphasic manner following oral administration, with a terminal elimination half-life after the first 24 hours of 96 hours for naltrexone and 18 hours for 6-β-naltrexol, possibly resulting from initial distribution into body tissues and subsequent redistribution into systemic circulation.

Naltrexone is metabolized in the liver principally by reduction of the 6-keto group of naltrexone to 6-β-naltrexol (6-β-hydroxynaltrexone). Naltrexone also undergoes metabolism by catechol-*O*-methyl transferase (COMT) to form 2-hydroxy-3-methoxy-6-β-naltrexol (HMN) and 2-hydroxy-3-methoxynaltrexone. Several minor metabolites have also been identified, including noroxymorphone and 3-methoxy-6-β-naltrexol. Because oral but not IM administration of naltrexone results in substantial first-pass hepatic metabolism of the drug, 6-β-naltrexol concentrations following IM administration are substantially lower than concentrations of the metabolite obtained following oral administration. Naltrexone does not appear to inhibit or induce its own metabolism following chronic administration. Cytochrome P-450 (CYP) isoenzymes are not involved in the metabolism of naltrexone. Naltrexone and its metabolites undergo conjugation with glucuronic acid. The major fraction of total drug and metabolites in both plasma and urine consists of conjugated metabolites. The drug and its metabolites may undergo enterohepatic circulation.

Metabolites of naltrexone may contribute to the opiate antagonist activity of the drug. Like naltrexone, 6-β-naltrexol is an essentially pure opiate antagonist, with a potency of 6–8% that of naltrexone in precipitating withdrawal symptoms in dogs physically dependent on morphine and 1.25–2% that of naltrexone in mice. Because of its weak affinity for opiate receptors, HMN may not contribute appreciably to the opiate antagonist activity of naltrexone; however, the in vivo opiate antagonist activity of HMN or 2-hydroxy-3-methoxynaltrexone has not been studied. Noroxymorphone, a minor metabolite of naltrexone, is a potent opiate agonist and may be responsible for the agonist activity (e.g., miosis) that occurs infrequently in individuals receiving naltrexone.

Naltrexone and its metabolites (unconjugated and conjugated) are excreted principally in urine via glomerular filtration;6-β-naltrexol, conjugated 6-β-naltrexol, and conjugated naltrexone are also excreted via tubular secretion. Naltrexone may also undergo partial reabsorption by the renal tubules. Following single- or multiple-dose oral administration of naltrexone hydrochloride, respectively, approximately 38–60 or 70% of a dose has been recovered in urine, principally as 6-β-naltrexol (conjugated and unconjugated). Most urinary excretion of naltrexone occurs within the first 4 hours after oral administration. Less than 2% of an orally administered dose is excreted unchanged in urine within 24 hours. Approximately 5–10, 19–35, 7–16, 3.5–4.6, and 0.45% of an oral dose are excreted in urine as conjugated naltrexone, 6-β-naltrexol, conjugated 6-β-naltrexol, HMN, and 2-hydroxy-3-methoxynaltrexone, respectively, within 24 hours. Less than 5% of a dose is excreted in feces, principally as 6-β-naltrexol, within 24 hours following single- or multiple-dose oral administration of the drug. Following oral administration of 50 mg of radiolabeled naltrexone in one patient, approximately 93% of the radiolabeled dose was excreted within 133 hours; about 79 and 14% were excreted in urine and feces, respectively.

Following oral administration of a single 100-mg dose in individuals formerly dependent on opiates and in healthy individuals, renal clearance of naltrexone and 6-β-naltrexol is reported to be 67–137 and 283–318 mL/minute, respectively. Renal clearance of naltrexone and 6-β-naltrexol is reported to be 30 and 369 mL/minute, respectively, following administration of 100 mg daily for at least 18 days. Total body clearance of naltrexone following oral administration is reported to be 1.5 L/minute, while systemic clearance following IV administration reportedly is about 3.5 L/minute. Since systemic clearance exceeds hepatic blood flow, it appears that the drug also is metabolized at extrahepatic sites.

Following IM administration of naltrexone extended-release injection, the half-life of naltrexone and 6-β-naltrexol is 5–10 days.

Pharmacokinetics of parenterally administered naltrexone do not appear to be substantially altered in patients with mild renal impairment (creatinine clearance of 50–80 mL/minute).

Limited data suggest that orally administered naltrexone is not removed by hemodialysis.

Chemistry and Stability

■ Chemistry Naltrexone is a synthetic opiate antagonist that is derived from thebaine. Naltrexone differs structurally from oxymorphone only in that the methyl group on the nitrogen atom of oxymorphone is replaced by a cyclopropylmethyl group. This structural modification results in naltrexone having essentially pure opiate antagonist activity, rather than the pure opiate agonist activity of oxymorphone. Naltrexone differs structurally from naloxone, another opiate antagonist, in that the allyl group on the nitrogen atom of naloxone is replaced by a cyclopropylmethyl group. This structural modification results in increased oral activity and duration of action of naltrexone compared with naloxone.

Naltrexone hydrochloride occurs as white crystals having a bitter taste and has a solubility of 100 mg/mL in water at 25°C. The drug has a pK_a of 8.13 at 37°C.

Commercially available naltrexone for extended-release injectable suspension (Vivitrol®) contains naltrexone incorporated into microspheres composed of polylactide co-glycolide, a biodegradable polymer matrix. Following reconstitution with the diluent provided by the manufacturer, naltrexone suspension is milky white, does not contain clumps, and moves freely down the wall of the vial. The diluent provided by the manufacturer provides an appropriate vehicle for reconstitution and delivery of the drug and contains carboxymethylcellulose sodium, polysorbate 20, and sodium chloride in sterile water for injection.

■ Stability Naltrexone hydrochloride tablets should be stored in well-closed containers at 15–30°C.

The entire dose pack containing naltrexone for extended-release injectable suspension should be refrigerated at 2–8°C; the dose pack can be stored at room temperature (i.e., room temperatures not exceeding 25°C) for up to 7 days. Storage at temperatures above 25°C or freezing should be avoided.

Preparations

Excipients in commercially available drug preparations may have clinically important effects in some individuals; consult specific product labeling for details.

Naltrexone

Parenteral

For injectable suspension, extended-release, for IM use	380 mg	**Vivitrol®** (available as a dose pack containing naltrexone microspheres, diluent, needles), Alkermes

Naltrexone Hydrochloride

Oral

Tablets	50 mg*	**Naltrexone Hydrochloride**
Tablets, film-coated	50 mg*	**Naltrexone Hydrochloride**
		ReVia® (scored), Duramed

*available from one or more manufacturer, distributor, and/or repackager by generic (nonproprietary) name

†Use is not currently included in the labeling approved by the US Food and Drug Administration

ANTICONVULSANTS 28:12

Anticonvulsants General Statement

Uses

■ **Seizure Disorders** Anticonvulsant drugs are used principally in the prevention and treatment of seizures, epileptic seizures, and epilepsy syndromes. A seizure is a transient occurrence of signs and symptoms due to abnormal excessive or synchronous neuronal activity in the brain, and epilepsy is a disorder of the brain characterized by an enduring predisposition to generate epileptic seizures. While epilepsy is a common cause of seizures, not all seizures are a result of epilepsy. Because a variety of other conditions (e.g., head trauma, hypoglycemia, alcohol or drug withdrawal, high fever) and certain medications also can precipitate seizures, the cause of seizures should be sought in every case and any underlying disorder corrected when possible. It is important to recognize the factors known to lower seizure threshold (e.g., fever, hypoglycemia, hyponatremia) so that corrective measures can be taken.

Seizure Classification In 1981, the International League Against Epilepsy (ILAE) developed a working classification of seizure types that divided seizures into the following 4 major categories based on EEG and clinical findings: partial seizures (seizures beginning locally in one hemisphere); generalized seizures (seizures that are bilaterally symmetrical without local onset); unilateral seizures (seizures that are predominantly unilateral); and unclassified epileptic seizures. Partial seizures were further subdivided into those with elementary symptomatology (simple partial seizures), those with complex symptomatology (complex partial seizures), and those that were secondarily generalized. Generalized seizures included tonic-clonic (grand mal) seizures, absence (petit mal) seizures, myoclonic seizures, and akinetic seizures. Although the ILAE classification has been revised over the years, the original classification scheme remains in widespread use. The 2017 ILAE classification maintains the basic framework of the 1981 system with some modifications to recognize that some seizure types can have either a focal or generalized onset, allow classification when the onset of seizure is unknown, include new seizure subtypes, and clarify terminology.

The current 2017 ILAE seizure classification continues to categorize seizures based on the type of onset (focal, generalized, or unknown). However, the term "partial" has been replaced with "focal" to better convey a sense of location rather than a part of a seizure. For focal seizures, the next level of classification is based on the individual's level of consciousness (or awareness). If awareness of the event is impaired at any time during the seizure, the seizure is classified as a "focal impaired awareness seizure", which replaces the previous term "complex partial seizure". If awareness is not impaired, the seizure is classified as a "focal aware seizure", which replaces the previous term "simple partial seizure". Focal seizures may be further characterized by motor or nonmotor onset. Focal seizures that propagate in a bilateral pattern are classified as "focal to bilateral tonic-clonic seizures", which corresponds to the previous term "secondarily generalized tonic-clonic seizures". Generalized seizures are further subdivided into motor (e.g., tonic-clonic, clonic, tonic, myoclonic, myoclonic-tonic-clonic, myoclonic-atonic, atonic, epileptic spasms) or nonmotor (absence) subtypes, which generally have remained the same with the addition of a few new subtypes. Specialized references should be consulted for a more complete discussion of seizure classification.

Status epilepticus has been traditionally defined as more than 30 minutes of either continuous seizure activity or 2 or more seizures that occur sequentially without full recovery of consciousness between the seizures. However, seizures that persist for more than 5 minutes are not likely to stop spontaneously without intervention, and therefore treatment is commonly initiated when the seizure duration reaches 5 minutes. Status epilepticus is further characterized as convulsive or nonconvulsive based on the presence or absence, respectively, of limb stiffness and rhythmic jerking.

Principles of Anticonvulsant Drug Therapy **Initial Evaluation.** Patients presenting with a new-onset seizure should undergo a comprehensive diagnostic evaluation (with careful history, physical examination, EEG, and brain imaging) to determine whether the seizure is epileptic or nonepileptic. It is important to differentiate an epileptic seizure, which by definition is a recurring event, from an acute symptomatic seizure provoked by a transient factor (e.g., sleep deprivation, medications, alcohol, illicit drug use) because the management approach can be different. It is also important to rule out other potential causes of the patient's symptoms since other paroxysmal events (e.g., migraines, transient ischemic attacks [TIAs], syncope) can mimic seizures. The risk of seizure recurrence should be considered when determining whether to initiate anticonvulsant drug therapy. Empiric treatment with anticonvulsant drugs may not be warranted in patients with a new-onset seizure.

Choice of Anticonvulsant Therapy. Choice of anticonvulsant therapy should be individualized based primarily on the specific type of seizure and/or epilepsy. In general, broad-spectrum agents (e.g., lamotrigine, levetiracetam, topiramate, valproate, zonisamide) are effective in the management of focal (partial) seizures and most generalized seizures, but have variable efficacy for specific seizure types (e.g., absence or myoclonic seizures). Narrow-spectrum agents (e.g., carbamazepine, oxcarbazepine, phenytoin, lacosamide) are generally effective for all types of focal seizures, but some of the drugs may precipitate or aggravate absence seizures. Anticonvulsant drugs that are effective in absence seizures (e.g., ethosuximide) generally are not useful in generalized tonic-clonic or focal seizures. Although many of the currently available anticonvulsant agents have been used in children and adolescents with seizure disorders, there is generally a lack of well-designed randomized controlled studies to inform selection of anticonvulsant drugs in the pediatric population.

In addition to the seizure type, choice of anticonvulsant therapy should take into account specific patient-related (e.g., age, sex, comorbidities, renal or hepatic impairment, concomitant drugs) and drug-related (e.g., efficacy, adverse effects, cost, route of administration) factors. The older anticonvulsant agents (e.g., carbamazepine, phenobarbital, phenytoin, primidone, valproate) have complex pharmacokinetics and a high potential for drug interactions because of their potent enzyme-inducing or enzyme-inhibiting properties. In patients receiving concomitant medications, use of newer anticonvulsants with more limited drug interaction potential (e.g., gabapentin, levetiracetam, lacosamide, topiramate, zonisamide, tiagabine) may be preferred.

Treatment of epilepsy should begin with a single anticonvulsant agent. If seizures are not controlled, experts generally recommend attempting at least one and sometimes a second alternative anticonvulsant before considering adjunctive therapy. While the majority of patients are able to achieve adequate seizure control with monotherapy (if not with the initial drug, then with an alternative agent), some patients will require a combination of anticonvulsants. Many anticonvulsants, particularly the newer agents, have been evaluated as adjunctive therapy for the treatment of refractory seizures; choice of adjunctive therapy should be individualized based on efficacy, safety, and tolerability of the anticonvulsant; seizure type or epilepsy; patient age; and concomitant medications.

Status Epilepticus. Status epilepticus is a medical emergency that must be treated promptly to reduce substantial morbidity and mortality. Initial treatment should include standard critical care and supportive therapy (e.g., blood pressure and respiratory support, oxygen, IV access, identification and correction of underlying causes), followed by administration of a benzodiazepine. Benzodiazepines are considered the initial drugs of choice for the treatment of status epilepticus because of their rapid onset of action, demonstrated efficacy, safety, and tolerability. Although IV lorazepam is generally preferred because of its longer duration of action, the superiority of one benzodiazepine over another is not clear, and selection of an appropriate agent should be individualized based on local availability, route of administration, pharmacokinetics, cost, and other factors. To achieve a rapid therapeutic effect, IV administration of benzodiazepines is preferred; however, administration via other routes (e.g., IM, rectal, intranasal, buccal) may be considered when IV administration is not possible (e.g., in a prehospital setting).

If seizures continue after initial therapy with a benzodiazepine, a second-line anticonvulsant agent should be administered. There are no evidence-based recommendations to guide selection of second-line therapies; reasonable options include IV fosphenytoin (or phenytoin), IV valproate sodium, IV levetiracetam, and IV phenobarbital. Fosphenytoin is generally better tolerated than phenytoin, and some experts state that fosphenytoin is preferred when both agents are available. If refractory status epilepticus occurs, continuous IV infusion of anticonvulsants, IV barbiturates, or general anesthetics may be necessary.

Posttraumatic Seizures. The use of anticonvulsant agents for the prevention of posttraumatic seizures is controversial. Most patients suffering traumatic brain injury are not at risk of long-term sequelae; epilepsy appears to occur in 15% or less of civilians with severe head injuries (although the risk may be greater in certain subgroups [e.g., those with prolonged coma]). While some evidence suggests that the risk of developing posttraumatic epilepsy also may be related to the presence of intracranial hematoma, other evidence suggests that it is not. Other patients who have been suggested as being at increased risk include those developing early seizures and those with a depressed skull fracture or dural penetration. In most civilians who develop posttraumatic epilepsy, the disorder becomes evident during the first year after injury. Phenytoin and/or phenobarbital have been used most frequently for prophylactic anticonvulsant therapy in patients with serious head injury; carbamazepine also has been used. However, evidence of the long-term benefit of any anticonvulsant in preventing posttraumatic epilepsy currently is lacking. In one well-designed, placebo-controlled study assessing the potential benefit of phenytoin prophylaxis initiated within 24 hours of hospitalization for serious head trauma, the drug reduced the frequency of seizures during the first week of therapy but not during the second through 52nd week of therapy or after an additional year of posttreatment follow-up. Such therapy was associated with a 73% reduction in the risk of seizures during the first week compared with placebo (seizures occurred in 3.6% of treated patients versus in 14.2% of those receiving placebo). Therefore, some clinicians state that while acute therapy is indicated, routine long-term prophylaxis with phenytoin (and probably other anticonvulsants) after initial stabilization currently does not appear justified, particularly when the potential adverse effects of anticonvulsants are considered. If anticonvulsant prophylaxis is considered necessary, it generally should be limited to patients presumed to be at high risk. There currently is no consensus regarding the optimum duration of anticonvulsant prophylaxis following severe head injury, and additional study is necessary to further define the potential role of anticonvulsant agents for long-term prophylaxis in patients suffering head injuries.

Epilepsy Syndromes **Lennox-Gastaut Syndrome.** Lennox-Gastaut syndrome is a rare type of epilepsy that primarily affects young children and is usually refractory to anticonvulsant drugs. Selection of an appropriate anticonvulsant therapy should be guided by the prevalent seizure type. Anticonvulsants that have demonstrated efficacy in the management of seizures associated with Lennox-Gastaut syndrome include cannabidiol, topiramate, rufinamide, lamotrigine, clobazam, clonazepam, and felbamate. Because of serious adverse effects (e.g., aplastic anemia, liver failure), use of felbamate should be reserved for patients who do not respond adequately to other treatments and whose seizure disorder is so severe that the risks of felbamate are deemed acceptable in light of the potential benefits.

Juvenile Myoclonic Epilepsy. Juvenile myoclonic epilepsy is an inherited disorder that generally consists of 3 common seizure types (myoclonic, generalized tonic-clonic, and absence seizures); however, different combinations of these seizure types can occur because of the complex genetics of the disease. Seizures in juvenile myoclonic epilepsy usually can be controlled with the appropriate anticonvulsant drugs, but life-long treatment generally is required because of a high risk of relapse. Valproate is effective in about 90% of patients with this epilepsy syndrome. Levetiracetam also may be used in combination with other anticonvulsants for the management of myoclonic seizures in adults and adolescents with juvenile myoclonic epilepsy.

Infantile Spasms. Infantile spasms (also known as West syndrome) is a severe form of epilepsy that presents with myoclonic-tonic seizures, a characteristic EEG pattern called hypsarryhthmia, and psychomotor retardation. Vigabatrin may be used for the management of infantile spasms in patients for whom the potential benefits outweigh the risk of vision loss, a serious adverse effect of the drug.

Dravet Syndrome. Dravet syndrome (also known as severe myoclonic epilepsy of infancy) is a rare and severe type of epilepsy characterized by early onset of multiple seizure types, frequent episodes of status epilepticus, and developmental delay with cognitive and psychomotor impairment. Seizures in patients with Dravet syndrome are generally refractory to current anticonvulsant drug options, and anticonvulsants that inhibit the sodium channel (e.g., carbamazepine, oxcarbazepine, lamotrigine, phenytoin) or vigabatrin may exacerbate the condition. Because complete seizure freedom is typically not achievable, treatment is generally aimed at eliminating or significantly reducing prolonged convulsive seizures and status epilepticus. Cannabidiol is used for the management of seizures associated with Dravet syndrome; clinical studies have demonstrated that the drug can substantially reduce the frequency of convulsive seizures when used adjunctively with other anticonvulsants (e.g., clobazam, valproate, stiripentol, levetiracetam, topiramate).

Barbiturates Barbiturate-derivative anticonvulsants (e.g., phenobarbital, primidone) are used in the prophylactic management of various types of seizures. Phenobarbital is used principally in the management of tonic-clonic seizures and partial seizures. Phenobarbital also has been used in the prophylaxis of febrile seizures. (See Uses in Phenobarbital 28:12.04.) The therapeutic uses of primidone are similar to those of phenobarbital and include management of tonic-clonic seizures and various partial seizures. Primidone also may be useful in the management of partial seizures with autonomic symptoms and akinetic seizures. Because of the availability of other anticonvulsant agents, the barbiturate-derived anticonvulsants generally are not recommended as first-line drugs for the treatment of epilepsy; in addition, these drugs are associated with a higher incidence of sedation than other anticonvulsants.

Benzodiazepines Benzodiazepines are the drugs of choice for initial treatment of status epilepticus. (See Status Epilepticus under Seizure Disorders: Principles of Anticonvulsant Drug Therapy, in Uses.) Benzodiazepine anticonvulsants also have been used in the management of absence seizures, akinetic seizures, and myoclonic seizures. Oral benzodiazepines generally have been used as adjuncts to other anticonvulsants in the management of seizures refractory to other drugs. In general, benzodiazepines are less effective in the prophylactic management of seizures than in the acute treatment of status epilepticus. Tolerance often develops to the anticonvulsant effects of benzodiazepines, which can limit their usefulness in the long-term management of seizure disorders.

Clonazepam is used alone or with other anticonvulsants for the management of absence seizures, especially Lennox-Gastaut syndrome (petit mal variant epilepsy), and of akinetic or myoclonic seizures. Clonazepam also is used in the management of absence seizures that do not respond to succinimides. The drug also has been used with some success in the management of other refractory seizures†, including partial seizures with complex symptomatology and some cases of infantile spasms, as well as in the management of some patients with tonic-clonic seizures†. (See Clonazepam 28:12.08.)

Clobazam, a 1,5-benzodiazepine, is used in combination with other anticonvulsants for the management of seizures associated with Lennox-Gastaut syndrome, and also has been used as adjunctive therapy for the management of other seizure disorders, which have sometimes been refractory, including partial, generalized, and myoclonic seizures†. Compared with the 1,4-benzodiazepines (e.g., clonazepam, diazepam, lorazepam), clobazam appears to have a broader spectrum of anticonvulsant activity and an improved adverse effect profile (e.g., less sedative effects). (See Clobazam 28:12.08.)

Carboxamides Carboxamide-derivative anticonvulsants (e.g., carbamazepine, oxcarbazepine, eslicarbazepine) are used principally in the treatment of focal (partial) seizures.

Hydantoins Hydantoin-derivative anticonvulsants (e.g., ethotoin, phenytoin) are used for control of tonic-clonic seizures and focal (partial) seizures with complex symptomatology. Although efficacy of phenytoin has been well established for the management of seizure disorders, particularly for partial (focal) seizures, use of the drug may be limited because of its complicated pharmacokinetics, adverse effects, and multiple drug interactions. Phenytoin and fosphenytoin (the prodrug of phenytoin) also are used parenterally for the prevention and treatment of seizures occurring during neurosurgery and as second-line drugs of choice for the treatment of status epilepticus. The hydantoins sometimes increase the frequency of absence seizures and therefore should not be used in the treatment of such seizures.

Oxazolidinediones Oxazolidinedione-derivative anticonvulsants (e.g., trimethadione), formerly drugs of choice in the management of absence seizures, are now used only in the treatment of absence seizures refractory to other anticonvulsants (e.g., ethosuximide). Trimethadione can cause serious adverse effects including rash, blood dyscrasias, renal and ocular dysfunction, lupus and myasthenia-like syndromes, and teratogenicity. As such, the drug was discontinued from the US market in 1995 and is only available on a compassionate-use basis. Oxazolidinedione anticonvulsants are of no benefit in the management of tonic-clonic seizures and may precipitate a patient's first tonic-clonic seizure or increase the frequency of preexisting tonic-clonic seizures.

Succinimides Succinimide-derivative anticonvulsants are used mainly in the management of absence seizures. Ethosuximide is considered a drug of choice in controlling absence seizures. Some clinicians have reported good results with ethosuximide in controlling myoclonic seizures or partial seizures with complex symptomatology.

Other Anticonvulsants In addition to the barbiturates, benzodiazepines, carboxamides, hydantoins, oxazolidinediones, and succinimides, other anticonvulsants used in the management of seizures and epilepsy include brivaracetam, cannabidiol, felbamate, gabapentin/gabapentin enacarbil, lacosamide, lamotrigine, levetiracetam, perampanel, pregabalin, rufinamide, tiagabine, topiramate, valproate, vigabatrin, and zonisamide; for information on these agents, see the individual monographs in 28:12.92.

A wide variety of other drugs are occasionally used in the management of epilepsy. Parenteral magnesium sulfate is used for the prevention or control of seizures in patients with preeclampsia or eclampsia, and also may be useful in controlling seizures associated with epilepsy, glomerulonephritis, or hypothyroidism. (See Uses in Magnesium Sulfate 28:12.92.) Although generally considered obsolete, bromides have been useful in the management of tonic-clonic or myoclonic seizures in some infants and preadolescent children when other drugs were unsuitable. Acetazolamide may be useful in the management of refractory partial, myoclonic, absence, or primary generalized tonic-clonic seizures; however, tolerance develops to the anticonvulsant effect of the drug. Corticotropin and corticosteroids are sometimes used in the management of myoclonic seizures in infants.

■ **Migraine Prophylaxis** Certain anticonvulsants (e.g., topiramate, valproate) may be used for prevention of migraine headaches. The currently available evidence supports the use of topiramate and valproate for migraine prophylaxis in adults. Gabapentin, lamotrigine, and oxcarbazepine also have been evaluated for this use; however, studies with these anticonvulsants either were insufficient or showed no effect of the drug compared with placebo in reducing migraine frequency.

■ **Neuropathic Pain** Certain anticonvulsants (e.g., carbamazepine, clonazepam, gabapentin, lamotrigine, phenytoin, pregabalin, valproate) have been used for the symptomatic treatment of chronic pain arising from peripheral neuropathic syndromes such as trigeminal neuralgia†, postherpetic neuralgia (PHN)†, diabetic peripheral neuropathy (DPN)†, glossopharyngeal neuralgia†, and posttraumatic neuralgia†. Gabapentin and pregabalin are recommended by many expert guidelines for use in the treatment of neuropathic pain syndromes. The exact mechanism of action of anticonvulsants in the management of neuropathic pain has not been elucidated; however, it has been suggested that modulation of ion channels (i.e., calcium, sodium), enhanced γ-aminobutyric acid (GABA) inhibition, stabilization of neuronal cell membranes, and/or activation of *N*-methyl-D-aspartate (NMDA) receptors may be involved.

Some clinicians state that while tricyclic antidepressants traditionally have been used as initial therapy in the symptomatic treatment of neuropathic pain, certain anticonvulsant agents (e.g., carbamazepine, gabapentin, pregabalin) appear to have similar or greater safety and efficacy for this use. Results of clinical studies indicate that gabapentin is effective in the management of PHN and DPN†. (See Uses in Gabapentin and Gabapentin Enacarbil 28:12.92.) In placebo-controlled studies, pregabalin also has demonstrated efficacy in the treatment of PHN and DPN. (See Uses in Pregabalin 28:12.92.) Carbamazepine is used for the symptomatic treatment of trigeminal neuralgia. (See Uses in Carbamazepine 28:12.92.) Further comparative studies are needed to evaluate the relative efficacy of anticonvulsants in the symptomatic treatment of neuropathic pain.

■ **Psychiatric Disorders** Certain anticonvulsants have been used in the treatment of psychiatric disorders. Valproate has been used as monotherapy or as an adjunct to antipsychotic agents for the management of acute manic or mixed episodes in patients with bipolar disorder. There is some evidence suggesting greater efficacy of valproate compared with lithium in the treatment of mixed states. Other anticonvulsants, including lamotrigine, oxcarbazepine, and carbamazepine, also have demonstrated efficacy in the management of bipolar disorder, but generally are used when there is an inadequate response to first-line therapies such as lithium, valproate, and antipsychotic agents (e.g., olanzapine). For additional information on the management of bipolar disorder, see Uses: Bipolar Disorder, in Lithium Salts 28:28.

Valproate and carbamazepine also have been used as an adjunct to antipsychotic agents in the management of schizophrenia. The American Psychiatric Association (APA) states that, with the exception of patients whose illness has strong affective components, these anticonvulsants alone have not been shown to be substantially effective in the long-term treatment of schizophrenia. For additional information on the management of schizophrenia, see Uses: Psychotic Disorders, in the Phenothiazines General Statement 28:16.08.24.

■ **Restless Leg Syndrome** Certain anticonvulsants (e.g., gabapentin enacarbil, pregabalin) may be used for the symptomatic treatment of restless legs syndrome.

Dosage and Administration

■ **Administration** Anticonvulsants usually are administered orally. Some anticonvulsants also are available in an IV preparation that may be used when oral administration is temporarily not feasible.

In the treatment of status epilepticus, IV administration of a benzodiazepine is preferred to achieve rapid therapeutic drug concentrations; if IV administration is not possible, some benzodiazepines may be administered by IM, intranasal, buccal, or rectal routes.

In the prevention or control of seizures in patients with preeclampsia or eclampsia, and in the control of seizures associated with epilepsy, glomerulonephritis, or hypothyroidism, magnesium sulfate may be given parenterally (IV or IM).

Patients who are currently receiving or beginning therapy with any anticonvulsant for any indication should be closely monitored for the emergence or worsening of depression, suicidal thoughts or behavior (suicidality), and/or any unusual changes in mood or behavior. (See Suicidality under Cautions: CNS Effects and also see Cautions: Precautions and Contraindications.)

Therapeutic Drug Monitoring Measurement of serum drug concentrations may be necessary with certain anticonvulsants (e.g., carbamazepine, ethosuximide, phenytoin, valproate). Such monitoring can increase the efficacy and safety of anticonvulsant therapy, and can also be useful in assessing patient compliance or in aiding the determination of the cause of toxicity when more than one medication is used.

■ **Dosage** Dosage of anticonvulsants varies from patient to patient. On a weight basis, children require relatively large dosages of phenytoin, phenobarbital, and probably other anticonvulsants.

It is important to begin therapy with a low dosage and proceed slowly when increasing or decreasing the dosage of anticonvulsants as well as when adding, withdrawing, or replacing one anticonvulsant with another. Therapy should begin with a single anticonvulsant; other drugs should be added to the therapeutic regimen only after determining that the maximum tolerated dosage of the initial drug does not control seizures. If the patient continues to have seizures or if toxic effects appear, it is preferable to measure the plasma concentration of the drug before changing the dosage or adding another drug to the regimen. When a single drug is not effective in controlling epileptic seizures, the addition of a second or third drug may be necessary. The usual dosage of an anticonvulsant may vary depending on whether the drug is used alone or in conjunction with other drugs (including other anticonvulsants).

Some anticonvulsants require dosage adjustment for renal or hepatic impairment and other patient factors. When transitioning patients from one anticonvulsant to another, dosage adjustments may be necessary.

Anticonvulsants should be discontinued gradually following long-term administration to minimize the risk of precipitating seizures, seizure exacerbation, or status epilepticus. In long-term anticonvulsant therapy, deciding when to withdraw the drug(s) is as important as the choice of drug(s) at the beginning of therapy. Some clinicians discontinue medication for the management of absence seizures when the patient has been seizure-free for 2 years and the EEG is normal; for febrile seizures when the child is 6 years old or seizure-free for 2 years, or after 30 months in otherwise healthy children who do not experience any complex seizures or sequelae after therapy is started; and for tonic-clonic seizures when the patient is seizure-free for 4 years. Other clinicians continue anticonvulsant administration in all epileptic patients for at least 4 years after the last seizure and then for an additional 1–2 years during which time the drug(s) is gradually withdrawn.

Cautions

Adverse effects of anticonvulsants are numerous and range from those that are benign and completely reversible (e.g., drowsiness, photophobia, nystagmus) to benign but frequently irreversible (e.g., hypertrichosis) to serious reactions which can be fatal (e.g., hematologic, dermatologic, renal, or hepatic toxicity).

■ **CNS Effects** The most common adverse effects of anticonvulsants are those related to the CNS and these effects can be classified into 3 general categories: somnolence and fatigue; behavioral/psychiatric abnormalities; and impaired psychomotor and cognitive performance. Adverse CNS effects include drowsiness, somnolence, fatigue, ataxia, gait disturbances, headache, restlessness, nystagmus, tremor, dizziness, vertigo, falls, dysarthria, and paresthesia. Adverse CNS effects usually are dose related, occurring more frequently during initial therapy, and can be minimized by starting with low dosages and gradually increasing the dosage.

Other adverse CNS effects include blurred vision, diplopia, and toxic amblyopia (with phenytoin). Polyneuropathies, abducens nerve palsy, and serious periorbital edema and hyperemia have occurred with some anticonvulsants. A few cases of ophthalmoplegia from phenytoin and/or primidone have been reported. In patients receiving phenytoin, ataxia is a frequent early sign of toxicity; with prolonged usage in toxic doses, cerebellar degeneration evidenced by loss of Purkinje cells has been reported.

Adverse neuropsychiatric effects associated with some anticonvulsants include irritability, anger, agitation, anxiety, labile affect, confusional state, psychotic symptoms, hallucinations, belligerence, hostility, and aggression. Serious and potentially life-threatening hostility- and aggression-related behaviors such as homicidal ideation and/or threats and physical assaults have occurred in patients receiving perampanel. In addition, all anticonvulsant drugs have the potential to cause suicidal behavior and ideation. (See Suicidality under Cautions: CNS Effects and also see Cautions: Precautions and Contraindications.)

Phenobarbital and, to a lesser extent, primidone frequently produce paradoxical excitement and hyperactivity in children or exacerbate existing hyperactivity, often requiring replacement of the drug with another barbiturate derivative or another anticonvulsant. Geriatric patients frequently react to barbiturates with excitement, confusion, or depression.

Suicidality An analysis of suicidality reports from placebo-controlled studies using various anticonvulsants indicated that patients receiving anticonvulsants had approximately twice the risk of suicidal behavior or ideation (0.43%) compared with patients receiving placebo (0.24%). The analysis included 199 randomized, placebo-controlled studies of 11 anticonvulsants (carbamazepine, felbamate, gabapentin, lamotrigine, levetiracetam, oxcarbazepine, pregabalin, tiagabine, topiramate, valproate, and zonisamide) involving over 43,000 patients 5 years of age or older; the studies evaluated the effectiveness of the anticonvulsants in epilepsy, psychiatric disorders (e.g., bipolar disorder, depression, anxiety), and other conditions (e.g., migraine, neuropathic pain). Four of the patients who were receiving one of the anticonvulsant drugs committed suicide whereas none of the patients receiving placebo did. The increased suicidality risk was observed as early as 1 week after beginning therapy and continued through 24 weeks. Because most studies included in the analysis did not extend beyond 24 weeks, the suicidality risk beyond 24 weeks could not be reliably assessed. The results were generally consistent among the 11 drugs studied with varying mechanisms of action and across a range of indications, suggesting that the suicidality risk applies to *all* anticonvulsants used for any indication. Although patients who were treated for epilepsy, psychiatric disorders, and other conditions were all found to be at increased risk for suicidality compared with placebo, the relative risk was found to be higher in patients with epilepsy compared with those receiving anticonvulsants for other conditions. (See Cautions: Precautions and Contraindications.)

■ **GI Effects** Most anticonvulsants cause GI disturbances such as nausea and vomiting, gastric distress, dysphagia, loss of taste, constipation, diarrhea, and anorexia with or without weight loss. The severity of adverse GI reactions may be minimized by administering the drugs with water or food. The oxazolidinedione and succinimide derivatives frequently cause hiccups.

Cases of life-threatening pancreatitis have been reported in patients receiving valproate. (See Valproate Sodium, Valproic Acid, and Divalproex Sodium 28:12.92.)

■ **Dermatologic and Sensitivity Reactions** Dermatologic reactions to nearly all the anticonvulsants have occurred. Adverse dermatologic reactions range from minor erythematous maculopapular rashes to more serious dermatologic reactions (e.g., exfoliative dermatitis, Stevens-Johnson syndrome [SJS], toxic epidermal necrolysis [TEN]). Carbamazepine, eslicarbazepine acetate, ethosuximide, lamotrigine, oxcarbazepine, phenytoin, and zonisamide have been associated with serious and sometimes fatal dermatologic reactions, including SJS and TEN. (See Carbamazepine 28:12.92, Eslicarbazepine Acetate 28:12.92, Fosphenytoin Sodium 28:12.12, Lamotrigine 28:12.92, Oxcarbazepine 28:12.92, Phenytoin and Phenytoin Sodium 28:12.12, and Zonisamide 28:12.92.)

Genetic polymorphism of the human leukocyte antigen (HLA) gene has been implicated in the development of adverse cutaneous reactions to the aromatic anticonvulsants. A strong association has been found between the presence of the HLA-B*1502 allele and an increased risk of SJS or TEN in patients receiving carbamazepine. (See Carbamazepine 28:12.92.) The allelic distribution pattern for HLA-B*1502 is distinct for specific geographic areas and ethnic groups. The allele is found almost exclusively in patients with ancestry across broad areas of Asia, although marked variation exists in its prevalence among specific Asian populations. Patients with ancestry in genetically at-risk populations should be screened for HLA-B*1502 prior to initiating carbamazepine therapy; screening also should be considered prior to initiating oxcarbazepine. Patients testing positive for HLA-B*1502 should not be initiated on carbamazepine or oxcarbazepine therapy unless the benefits clearly outweigh the risks. Although evidence is more limited, HLA-B*1502 also has been associated with SJS/TEN in patients receiving other structurally similar anticonvulsants (e.g., eslicarbazepine, lamotrigine, phenytoin, fosphenytoin, phenobarbital). Avoidance of these drugs should therefore be considered in HLA-B*1502-positive patients when alternative therapies are otherwise equally acceptable.

Multi-organ hypersensitivity (also known as drug reaction with eosinophilia and systemic symptoms [DRESS]), a potentially fatal or life-threatening reaction, has been reported with several anticonvulsants (e.g., carbamazepine, eslicarbazepine, ethosuximide, gabapentin, lacosamide, oxcarbazepine, perampanel, phenytoin, rufinamide, valproate, zonisamide); the clinical presentation is variable, but typically includes eosinophilia, fever, rash, lymphadenopathy, and/or facial swelling in association with other organ system involvement such as hepatitis, nephritis, hematologic abnormalities, myocarditis, or myositis sometimes resembling an acute viral infection. Because DRESS is variable in its expression, other organ systems may be involved. In addition, early manifestations of hypersensitivity, such as fever or lymphadenopathy, may be present in some cases even when rash is not evident.

Alopecia and a chloasma-like hyperpigmentation of the face and neck (without evidence of endocrinologic abnormality) have been associated with administration of some anticonvulsants. In addition, hypersensitivity reactions, including anaphylaxis and angioedema, have occurred with some anticonvulsants (e.g., fosphenytoin, phenytoin, gabapentin, pregabalin, levetiracetam).

Phenytoin produces gingival hyperplasia, most often in children, and is occasionally so severe that it may require surgical removal. Gingival hyperplasia does not occur in edentulous areas of gums. Gingival hyperplasia has been reported only rarely with other hydantoins. Secondary inflammatory changes which result in edematous enlargement of the primary gingival lesions can be minimized by good oral hygiene and gum massage. Phenytoin also produces hypertrichosis in some patients. Hypertrichosis is usually confined to the extremities but can also occur on the trunk and face and is frequently irreversible. Because of phenytoin's androgenic effect on hair follicles, the drug also has been implicated in the production of acne.

■ **Hematologic Effects** Most anticonvulsants (e.g., carbamazepine, gabapentin, oxcarbazepine, phenytoin, primidone, valproate, phenobarbital, pregabalin, primidone, topiramate) are associated with reduced serum concentrations of folate and vitamin B_{12}. Some clinicians recommend that prophylactic supplementation with folic acid and cyanocobalamin be considered in patients receiving anticonvulsant therapy.

Hematologic abnormalities have been reported with certain anticonvulsants. Bone marrow depression which can progress to fatal aplastic anemia has occurred with nearly all the drugs. Anticonvulsants have caused anemia, leukopenia, thrombocytopenia, agranulocytosis, and pancytopenia. Aplastic anemia and agranulocytosis have been reported with the use of carbamazepine. Blood dyscrasias, sometimes fatal, have been reported with ethosuximide. Use of felbamate has been associated with a marked increase in the risk of aplastic anemia. The incidence of aplastic anemia in patients receiving felbamate may be more than 100-fold greater than that seen in the general population; although the risk of death varies with severity and etiology, the fatality rate generally ranges from 20 to 30%, but has been reported to be as high as 70%.

■ **Hepatic Effects** Acute hepatotoxicity, including cases of acute hepatic failure, have been reported with some anticonvulsants (e.g., felbamate, phenytoin, valproate). Children younger than 2 years of age, especially those receiving multiple anticonvulsants, those with congenital metabolic disorders, those with severe seizure disorders accompanied by mental retardation, and those with organic brain disease, are at particularly high risk of valproate-induced hepatotoxicity.

■ **Renal Effects** The oxazolidinedione anticonvulsants have been implicated in renal damage, which has occasionally produced fatal nephrotic syndromes. Renal involvement has been evidenced by edema, urinary frequency and burning, albuminuria, microscopic hematuria, and uremia. Succinimides also have been associated with adverse renal effects. Some patients have recovered from a severe anticonvulsant-induced nephrotic syndrome without therapy following discontinuance of the drug; others recovered following prednisone and cyclophosphamide therapy.

■ **Other Adverse Effects** There is some evidence (mostly from case-control and observational studies) indicating that anticonvulsant agents can cause clinically important reductions in bone mineral density (BMD) and increase the risk of fractures. Some epileptic patients taking anticonvulsants in high dosages over long periods have developed hypocalcemia and, very rarely, rickets or osteomalacia. These effects have been seen predominately with the older anticonvulsant agents, although studies generally are lacking with the newer agents. The enzyme-inducing anticonvulsants (e.g., carbamazepine, phenobarbital, phenytoin, primidone) can increase metabolism of 25-hydroxyvitamin D, which has been proposed as a possible mechanism of anticonvulsant-induced metabolic bone disease. However, valproate (an enzyme-inhibiting anticonvulsant) also has been associated with adverse bone effects suggesting that this may be a class effect of all anticonvulsants. Clinicians should consider monitoring vitamin D levels and other measures of bone health in patients receiving long-term anticonvulsant therapy. Some clinicians recommend that patients being treated with anticonvulsants (particularly those who may not be receiving adequate nutrition and sunlight) should receive supplemental vitamin D (e.g., 4000 units/week).

Elevations in serum total cholesterol, HDL-cholesterol, and triglycerides have occurred occasionally in patients receiving anticonvulsants.

Adverse ophthalmic effects have been reported with some anticonvulsants, including ezogabine (no longer commercially available in the US) and vigabatrin. Vigabatrin can cause progressive and permanent bilateral visual field defects with a potential risk of vision loss.

Topiramate and zonisamide inhibit carbonic anhydrase and can cause adverse effects similar to those of other carbonic anhydrase inhibitors (e.g., acetazolamide), including metabolic acidosis and kidney stone formation. Oligohidrosis and hyperthermia, characterized by decreased sweating and abnormally high body temperatures, have been reported in patients (particularly pediatric patients) receiving these anticonvulsants.

Severe cardiovascular effects, including cardiovascular collapse and death, have been reported following rapid IV administration of phenytoin or fosphenytoin; hypotension can occur if either drug is administered too rapidly by the IV route. IV phenytoin or diazepam can cause local irritation, swelling, thrombophlebitis, and, rarely, vascular impairment necessitating amputation. Purple glove syndrome (PGS), a delayed soft-tissue injury of the hand and forearm, has been reported in association with IV phenytoin and also may be possible with fosphenytoin (see Fosphenytoin Sodium 28:12.12 and Phenytoin and Phenytoin Sodium 28:12.12).

■ **Precautions and Contraindications** For additional information on adverse effects, precautions, and contraindications associated with the use of anticonvulsants, see the sections in Cautions in the individual monographs in 28:12, the Barbiturates General Statement 28:24.04, and the Benzodiazepines General Statement 28:24.08.

Patients who are currently receiving or beginning therapy with any anticonvulsant for any indication should be closely monitored for the emergence or worsening of depression, suicidal thoughts or behavior (suicidality), and/or unusual changes in mood or behavior. (See Suicidality under Cautions: CNS Effects.) Clinicians should inform patients, their families, and caregivers of the potential for an increased risk of suicidality and to pay close attention to any day-to-day changes in mood, behavior, and actions; since changes can happen very quickly, it is important to be alert to any sudden differences. In addition, patients, family members, and caregivers should be aware of common warning signs that may signal suicide risk (e.g., talking or thinking about wanting to hurt oneself or end one's life, withdrawing from friends and family, becoming depressed or experiencing worsening of existing depression, becoming preoccupied with death and dying, giving away prized possessions). If these or any new and worrisome behaviors occur, the responsible clinician should be contacted immediately. Clinicians who prescribe any anticonvulsant should balance the risk for suicidality with the risk of untreated illness. Epilepsy and many other illnesses for which anticonvulsants are prescribed are themselves associated with an increased risk of morbidity and mortality and an increased risk of suicidal thoughts and behavior. If suicidal thoughts and behavior emerge during anticonvulsant therapy, the clinician must consider whether the emergence of these symptoms in any given patient may be related to the illness being treated.

All anticonvulsants can produce drowsiness, and for this reason patients should be cautioned that these drugs may impair their ability to perform hazardous activities requiring mental alertness or physical coordination (e.g., operating machinery, driving a motor vehicle). Slower dosage escalations or adjustments in the dosage regimen (e.g., giving lower doses, but more frequently) may alleviate such adverse CNS effects of these drugs.

Clinicians should be alert to the signs, including high fever, severe headache, stomatitis, conjunctivitis, rhinitis, urethritis, or balanitis, that may precede the onset of anticonvulsant-induced cutaneous lesions and reactions. Because skin eruptions can precede potentially fatal reactions, the drugs should be discontinued immediately whenever they occur. Adverse cutaneous reactions may proceed to an irreversible stage even though the medication has been discontinued, however, because these drugs are slowly metabolized and excreted.

Some anticonvulsants (e.g., carbamazepine, felbamate) can cause serious adverse hematologic effects and blood counts should be determined prior to and during therapy with these drugs. In addition, patients should be instructed to immediately report symptoms such as sore throat, fever, easy bruising, petechiae, epistaxis, or other signs of infection or bleeding tendency, which may be indications of hematologic toxicity. The drugs should be discontinued if blood dyscrasias occur. Because of the risk of aplastic anemia, felbamate should be used only in patients whose epilepsy is so severe that the risk is deemed acceptable in light of the benefits conferred by its use. Patients generally should not be initiated on felbamate without appropriate expert hematologic consultation.

With some anticonvulsants, patients should have liver function tests before starting therapy and periodically thereafter. Patients should be instructed to report promptly any symptoms of hepatotoxicity such as jaundice, dark urine, anorexia, abdominal discomfort, or other GI symptoms. The drugs should be discontinued if evidence of liver damage occurs. Anticonvulsants generally should be administered with extreme caution in patients with evidence of liver disease or abnormal liver function test values. Felbamate should be used only in patients without active liver disease and with normal baseline serum transaminase concentrations. Patients receiving oxazolidinediones or succinimides should have periodic urinalyses, and the drugs should be discontinued if evidence of renal damage appears.

Appropriate administration procedures and precautions should be followed in patients receiving parenterally administered anticonvulsants (e.g., phenytoin) to minimize the risk of local tissue injury, including purple glove syndrome. (See Cautions: Other Adverse Effects.)

Patients receiving vigabatrin should receive appropriate ophthalmologic assessments prior to initiating therapy and periodically thereafter as recommended. (See Cautions: Other Adverse Effects.)

Specific anticonvulsants are contraindicated in patients who have exhibited hypersensitivity to any derivative of the respective anticonvulsant type. Barbiturate derivatives exacerbate acute intermittent porphyria and porphyria variegata and are contraindicated in patients with a history of porphyria.

■ **Pediatric Precautions** Anticonvulsant therapy may have adverse effects on behavior and cognition in children who have epilepsy. These effects have been shown to occur with therapeutic or supratherapeutic, but not necessarily toxic, serum anticonvulsant concentrations; large doses of virtually all anticonvulsants can affect mental function. Among the older anticonvulsant drugs, phenobarbital is the most likely to affect cognitive function in pediatric patients. Phenobarbital has been associated with hyperactivity, fussiness, lethargy, disturbed sleep, irritability, disobedience, stubbornness, depressive symptom, deficits on neuropsychologic tests, impaired short-term memory, and impaired memory concentration tasks. Cognitive effects of phenytoin have included unsteadiness, involuntary movements, tiredness, alteration of emotional state, deficits on neuropsychologic tests, impaired attention, impaired problem solving, and impaired visuomotor tasks. Carbamazepine has been associated with difficulty sleeping, agitation, irritability, emotional lability, and impaired task performance, and clonazepam has been associated with irritability, aggression, hyperactivity, disobedience, and antisocial activities. Valproate has generally been associated with a lesser effect on cognitive function than the other older anticonvulsant agents; adverse effects associated with the drug have included drowsiness (especially when used in combination with barbiturates) and minimal adverse effects on psychosocial tests. There are less data on the cognitive effects of the newer anticonvulsant agents; studies that have been conducted were performed mostly in the adult population. In general, topiramate appears to be associated with more adverse cognitive effects than most other newer anticonvulsant drugs.

Children receiving anticonvulsant therapy should be under the supervision of clinicians who are knowledgeable about seizure disorders and their management, particularly when to initiate and discontinue anticonvulsant agents. There is generally a lack of well-designed randomized controlled studies of anticonvulsant drugs in the pediatric population. When anticonvulsant therapy is necessary, clinicians should consider the specificity of a drug(s) for the type of seizure, the potential adverse effects of the drug(s), and the relative potential effect of each drug on behavioral and cognitive function. In addition to careful observation of cognitive function, mood, and behavior during follow-up examinations in children receiving anticonvulsant therapy, clinicians should consider the observations of parents and teachers; if significant behavioral or cognitive changes occur and alternative causes are not readily evident, the possibility that anticonvulsant therapy may be responsible and the need for dosage reduction or substitution of an alternative anticonvulsant(s) should be considered.

■ **Pregnancy and Lactation** Several reports suggest an association between use of anticonvulsants in pregnant, epileptic women and an increased incidence of birth defects in children born to these women. However, the risk from taking anticonvulsants during pregnancy is generally considered to be less than the risk of seizures during pregnancy. Data are most extensive with regard to trimethadione, phenobarbital, phenytoin, and valproate. Major congenital abnormalities also have been demonstrated with prenatal use of topiramate and carbamazepine. Barbiturates can cause fetal harm when administered to pregnant women. Phenytoin has been associated with a fetal hydantoin syndrome consisting of craniofacial abnormalities, nail and digital hypoplasia, prenatal growth deficiency, microcephaly, and mental deficiency. A fetal trimethadione syndrome also has been reported, which may possibly be distinguished from the fetal hydantoin syndrome by the specific anomalies of V-shaped eyebrows, low set ears with anteriorly folded helix, and lack of phalangeal hypoplasia. Other manifestations of the fetal trimethadione syndrome include developmental delay, speech difficulty, palatal anomaly, and irregular teeth. Valproate is associated with the most data to date regarding pregnancy risk. Use of valproate during pregnancy is associated with an increased risk of neural tube defects (e.g., spina bifida) and other major congenital malformations (e.g., craniofacial defects, cardiovascular malformations, malformations involving various body systems). In utero exposure to valproate also can cause decreased IQ scores in children. Exposure to topiramate in utero has been associated with an increased risk of oral clefts (cleft lip and/or palate) and for being small for gestational age.

Some retrospective studies indicate that the risk of having a malformed child is 2–3 times greater in epileptic women who received anticonvulsants in the early stages of pregnancy than in those women without a history of seizure disorders. It is not clear whether these malformations were caused by the drugs, by some manifestation of epilepsy itself, or by other factors. In addition, it is not clear whether the risk applies to all or only some of the anticonvulsant drugs. Most pregnant women receiving anticonvulsants deliver infants without birth defects. If a switch to a less teratogenic anticonvulsant agent is being considered, experts recommend that this be done well before pregnancy to ensure that the new treatment is adequate for seizure control. In most pregnant women with epilepsy, discontinuance of anticonvulsant therapy may not be a reasonable or safe option. Anticonvulsants should *not* be discontinued in pregnant women in whom the drugs are administered to prevent major seizures, because of the strong possibility of precipitating status epilepticus with attendant hypoxia and threat to life. In individual cases, when the severity and frequency of the seizure disorder are such that discontinuance of therapy does not pose a serious threat to the patient, discontinuance of the drugs may be considered prior to and during pregnancy. The clinician should carefully weigh these considerations in treating or counseling epileptic women of childbearing potential.

Valproate is contraindicated in pregnant women for the prevention of migraine headaches. The drug should not be used in pregnant women with epilepsy or bipolar disorder unless other treatments have failed to provide adequate symptom relief or are otherwise unacceptable; in these cases, the benefits of valproate may continue to outweigh its risks. Other anticonvulsants associated with the greatest risk to the fetus (e.g., trimethadione) should be used during pregnancy only when clearly shown to be essential in the management of the seizure disorder. When such anticonvulsants are used, women of childbearing age should be instructed to use an effective form of contraception during therapy and be informed of the potential hazard to the fetus should they become pregnant during therapy. If such drugs are inadvertently administered during pregnancy or if the patient becomes pregnant while receiving such drugs, the desirability of continuing the pregnancy should be considered. When anticonvulsants are administered during pregnancy, it is advisable to monitor drug concentrations closely and adjust dosage when necessary. Some experts recommend that monitoring of lamotrigine, carbamazepine, and phenytoin concentrations during pregnancy should be considered and that monitoring of levetiracetam and oxcarbazepine may be considered. Results of retrospective studies suggest that combination therapy with anticonvulsants may be associated with a higher prevalence of teratogenic effects than monotherapy with such drugs; therefore, monotherapy is recommended in pregnant women.

The barbiturates and primidone have caused postpartum hemorrhage and hemorrhagic disease of the newborn; coagulation defects have also occurred in neonates whose mothers were receiving phenytoin. The possibility that this may occur with other anticonvulsants (e.g., trimethadione) should be considered. Drug-induced hemorrhagic disease of the newborn is similar to that resulting from vitamin K deficiency and is readily reversed with vitamin K therapy. For this reason, it has been recommended that vitamin K be administered for 1 month prior to and during delivery in pregnant epileptics taking these anticonvulsants. The neonate should also receive vitamin K immediately after birth.

Women who are pregnant while receiving anticonvulsant drugs should be encouraged to enroll in the North American Antiepileptic Drug (NAAED) Pregnancy Registry by calling 888-233-2334. Information on the registry also can be found at http://www.aedpregnancyregistry.org.

Some anticonvulsants probably are distributed into milk (see Pharmacokinetics: Distribution). Because of the potential for serious adverse reactions from most anticonvulsants in nursing infants, a decision should be made whether to discontinue nursing or the drug, taking into account the importance of the drug to the woman.

Drug Interactions

Many drugs have been reported to alter the response to anticonvulsants and/or have their responses altered by the anticonvulsants. Clinically important drug interactions with anticonvulsant agents generally involve inhibition or induction of hepatic drug metabolism, but can also occur as a result of other mechanisms (e.g., GI absorption, protein binding displacement, renal elimination). The first-generation anticonvulsants (e.g., carbamazepine, phenobarbital, phenytoin, primidone, valproate) are particularly susceptible to drug interactions because of their potent enzyme-inducing and enzyme-inhibiting properties. Patients should be observed closely for loss of efficacy and clinical signs of toxicity when any drug is added to or deleted from their therapeutic regimen, giving consideration to the possible need for dosage adjustments. Therapeutic drug monitoring may be useful for confirming a suspected drug interaction and for assessing the effect of a particular interaction to determine whether dosage adjustments are needed.

■ **Drugs Affecting or Metabolized by Hepatic Microsomal Enzymes** The older anticonvulsants carbamazepine, phenobarbital, phenytoin, and primidone are potent inducers of various cytochrome P-450 (CYP) isoenzymes (e.g., CYP1A2, CYP2C9, CYP2C19, CYP3A4); these anticonvulsants can therefore decrease serum concentrations and reduce the pharmacologic effect of many drugs that are metabolized by these isoenzymes. These drugs include, but are not limited to, certain antidepressant agents (e.g., clomipramine, imipramine, nefazodone), antipsychotic agents (e.g., chlorpromazine, haloperidol, aripiprazole, clozapine, olanzapine, quetiapine, risperidone, ziprasidone), antineoplastic agents (e.g., cyclophosphamide, imatinib, lapatinib, irinotecan, methotrexate, tamoxifen), azole antifungal agents, immunosuppressive agents (e.g., cyclosporine, tacrolimus), human immunodeficiency virus (HIV) protease inhibitors, corticosteroids, HMG-CoA reductase inhibitors (statins; e.g., simvastatin, atorvastatin, fluvastatin), selective serotonin-reuptake inhibitors (SSRIs; e.g., citalopram, sertraline), calcium-channel blocking agents (e.g., verapamil, nifedipine), oral contraceptives, rifampin, vitamin D, warfarin, benzodiazepines, and other anticonvulsant agents (e.g., eslicarbazepine, ethosuximide, lamotrigine, oxcarbazepine, pregabalin, rufinamide, tiagabine, topiramate, zonisamide, valproate). Valproate is a potent inhibitor of CYP isoenzymes and can therefore increase serum concentrations of drugs (e.g., carbapenem anti-infectives, cisplatin, etoposide, amitriptyline, nortriptyline, carbamazepine, ethosuximide, lamotrigine, phenobarbital, rufinamide) metabolized by these enzymes, potentially increasing their risk of toxicity.

Among the newer anticonvulsant agents, eslicarbazepine, felbamate, rufinamide, and topiramate have CYP-inducing properties, and felbamate and topiramate have CYP-inhibiting properties; although some of these effects have been shown to be weak to moderate, there is a possibility that clinically important drug interactions may occur when these anticonvulsants are used concomitantly with drugs metabolized by CYP isoenzymes. Oxcarbazepine can inhibit CYP2C19 and induce CYP3A4/5, although enzyme induction appears to have greater clinical importance. Cannabidiol has the potential to inhibit CYP2C8, CYP2C9, and CYP2C19, and may induce or inhibit CYP1A2 and CYP2B6.

Certain antidepressant agents (e.g., sertraline) and antipsychotic agents (e.g., haloperidol, risperidone, chlorpromazine) can inhibit the metabolism of anticonvulsants (e.g., carbamazepine, valproate, phenytoin), resulting in increased serum concentrations of the anticonvulsant. Macrolide antibiotics that inhibit CYP3A4 (e.g., clarithromycin, erythromycin) can increase serum concentrations of carbamazepine and some clinicians recommend that concomitant use of these drugs be avoided. Rifampin can inhibit the metabolism of lamotrigine, and isoniazid can inhibit the metabolism of carbamazepine, ethosuximide, phenytoin, and valproic acid, resulting in increased serum concentrations of the anticonvulsant. Oral contraceptives can induce the metabolism of lamotrigine and valproic acid, and possibly also oxcarbazepine, resulting in decreased serum concentrations of the anticonvulsant.

Concurrent administration of disulfiram with barbiturates, phenytoin, or ethotoin may result in inhibition of metabolism of the anticonvulsant and an increased incidence of anticonvulsant-induced adverse effects.

■ Drugs Affected by P-glycoprotein or other Transporters Some anticonvulsant agents (e.g., carbamazepine, valproate, cannabidiol) can affect the expression of P-glycoprotein (P-gp) or other transporters such as uridine diphosphate glucuronosyltransferase (UGT), potentially altering serum concentrations of drugs affected by these transport proteins. However, additional study is needed to evaluate the role of P-gp and other transporters in anticonvulsant drug interactions.

■ Protein-bound Drugs Anticonvulsant drugs that are extensively bound to plasma proteins (e.g., phenytoin, valproate, tiagabine) can displace or be displaced by other highly protein-bound drugs (e.g., salicylates, naproxen, diazepam) when used concomitantly. The resulting interaction can lead to higher free fractions of either drug.

■ Anticonvulsants The older anticonvulsants with enzyme-inducing properties (carbamazepine, phenobarbital, phenytoin, and primidone) can increase the metabolism and reduce serum concentrations of most concomitantly administered anticonvulsant drugs, including valproate, tiagabine, ethosuximide, lamotrigine, topiramate, oxcarbazepine, zonisamide, felbamate, and many benzodiazepines. The clinical importance of these interactions is generally modest since the added anticonvulsant can usually compensate for any decrease in anticonvulsant efficacy that may occur. In some cases, however, loss of seizure control can occur and dosage adjustments may be required. Particular caution is advised when withdrawing enzyme-inducing anticonvulsants from concomitant regimens since the consequent increase in serum concentrations of the drug whose metabolism was previously induced may be significant and reach toxic levels.

Phenobarbital may induce the metabolism of phenytoin. In addition, however, phenobarbital may competitively inhibit phenytoin metabolism. Concurrent administration of these drugs may result in an increase, decrease, or no change in blood phenytoin concentrations. The effect of usual therapeutic dosages of phenobarbital on plasma phenytoin concentrations in individual patients is unpredictable and usually not of great clinical importance.

Since valproate also may interact with other anticonvulsant drugs, it is advisable to monitor plasma concentrations of concomitantly administered anticonvulsants during initial valproate therapy and adjust dosages as required. Concomitant administration of valproate and phenobarbital (or primidone which is metabolized to phenobarbital) results in increased plasma phenobarbital concentrations and excessive somnolence. A few patients have become comatose during therapy with valproate and phenobarbital. If valproate is used with a barbiturate, the patient should be closely observed for possible neurologic toxicity, plasma concentrations of the barbiturate should be monitored if possible, and the dosage of the barbiturate decreased if necessary. A reduction in phenobarbital dosage by up to 80% has been required. Valproate can inhibit the metabolism of lamotrigine, which may result in increased serum concentrations and toxicity (e.g., skin rashes, neurotoxic effects) of lamotrigine. Valproate has been associated with both decreased plasma phenytoin concentrations and increased seizure frequency and with increased plasma concentrations of free phenytoin and phenytoin toxicity. Concomitant administration of valproate and clonazepam has produced absence status; therefore, some clinicians recommend that concomitant use of these drugs be avoided.

Since succinimides (e.g., ethosuximide, methsuximide) may interact with other anticonvulsant drugs, it is advisable to monitor plasma concentrations of the drugs during concomitant therapy.

■ CNS Depressants Anticonvulsants may be additive with or may potentiate the action of other CNS depressants, including other anticonvulsants and alcohol. Concomitant use of benzodiazepine anticonvulsants with opiate agonists may result in profound sedation, respiratory depression, coma, and death.

■ Oral Contraceptives The CYP-inducing anticonvulsants carbamazepine, phenobarbital, phenytoin, and primidone can reduce serum concentrations and decrease efficacy of oral contraceptives. There have been reports of women receiving some of these anticonvulsants (e.g., phenobarbital) who became pregnant while receiving oral contraceptives. Because of the risk of contraceptive failure, some clinicians recommend that concomitant use of oral contraceptives and CYP-inducing anticonvulsants be avoided, and that alternate methods of contraception be used in patients receiving these drugs.

Oral contraceptives can induce the metabolism of lamotrigine and reduce serum concentrations of the anticonvulsant by 50%; because of the possibility that seizure control may be affected, some clinicians recommend that concomitant use of these drugs be avoided. Serum concentrations of valproate also may be reduced by oral contraceptives.

Felbamate, topiramate, oxcarbazepine, eslicarbazepine, rufinamide, clobazam, and perampanel also may decrease serum concentrations of estrogens and/or progestins to a lesser extent, which can also result in contraceptive failure. Drug interactions between oral contraceptives and gabapentin, levetiracetam, pregabalin, tiagabine, vigabatrin, and zonisamide have not been reported to date.

■ Warfarin The CYP-inducing anticonvulsants (phenobarbital, phenytoin, carbamazepine, and primidone) may reduce serum concentrations of warfarin and potentially decrease anticoagulant efficacy. Close monitoring of the international normalized ratio (INR) is recommended when warfarin is used concomitantly with these anticonvulsant drugs and dosage adjustments may be required.

Acute Toxicity

The slow rate of elimination of most anticonvulsants should be considered in the treatment of acute toxicity of any anticonvulsant.

■ Barbiturates Overdosage of barbiturate derivatives may produce profound CNS depression and shock syndrome and can result in death from respiratory depression and apnea. Treatment of overdosage is mainly supportive and includes maintenance of adequate airway and ventilation and possibly induction of emesis or gastric lavage if the patient is conscious. Oral administration of activated charcoal may be useful. If renal function is normal, forced alkaline diuresis may be of benefit (particularly in the treatment of phenobarbital intoxication) by increasing renal clearance of the drug. Peritoneal dialysis or hemodialysis may be required in severe barbiturate intoxication. For further information, see Acute Toxicity in the Barbiturates General Statement 28:24.04.

■ Hydantoins Hydantoin derivative overdosage produces ataxia, nausea, vomiting, hypotension, motor restlessness, dizziness, fatigue, hallucinations, and insomnia. Deep coma may also occur. Treatment consists of inducing emesis or gastric lavage and general supportive therapy. Peritoneal dialysis or hemodialysis may be beneficial. Forced diuresis is of little or no value in treatment of phenytoin toxicity.

■ Succinimides Acute toxicity resulting from succinimide anticonvulsants has only rarely been reported and has produced nausea, vomiting, and profound CNS depression (including coma and respiratory depression). Treatment should include induction of emesis (unless the patient is comatose, obtunded, or convulsing), gastric lavage, activated charcoal, or cathartics, and general supportive measures. Hemodialysis may be beneficial; however, forced diuresis and exchange transfusions are ineffective in removing succinimides.

■ Oxazolidinediones Symptoms of oxazolidinedione overdosage include nausea, drowsiness, dizziness, ataxia, and visual disturbances. Coma may occur following massive overdosage. Treatment should include induction of emesis or gastric lavage and general supportive measures. Alkalinization of the urine may enhance elimination of the metabolites of oxazolidinedione derivatives. Following recovery from CNS effects, a careful evaluation of hepatic and renal function should be made.

Pharmacology

The principal pharmacologic actions of the anticonvulsants are elevation of the seizure threshold of the motor cortex to electrical or chemical stimuli and/or limitation of propagation of the seizure discharge from its origin (focus) to the effector organ(s). Limitation of spread of the seizure discharge from its focus may be accomplished by depression of synaptic transmission, limiting post-tetanic potentiation (PTP) of synaptic transmission, or reducing nerve conductance. When drugs are screened in the laboratory for anticonvulsant activity, some of the simpler screening tests include ability to block pentylenetetrazol-induced and other chemically induced seizures and electrically induced seizures. These tests have been widely used and, in general, drugs that protect animals against pentylenetetrazol-induced seizures are effective in the management of absence (petit mal) seizures and drugs that protect animals against seizures produced by electrical stimulation are useful in the management of tonic-clonic (grand mal) seizures and partial seizures. Although all anticonvulsants may produce some CNS depression, the degree differs with the individual agents.

The precise mechanism(s) of action of anticonvulsants has not been confirmed at the molecular level. The basic mechanism is probably stabilization of the cell membrane secondary to modification of cation (sodium, potassium, calcium) transport either by increasing sodium efflux or inhibiting sodium influx.

The exact mechanisms of action of anticonvulsants in the management of neuropathic pain have not been elucidated; however, it has been suggested that modulation of ion channels (i.e., calcium, sodium), enhanced γ-aminobutyric acid (GABA) inhibition, stabilization of neuronal cell membranes, and/or activation of *N*-methyl-D-aspartate (NMDA) receptors may be involved.

■ Barbiturates Anticonvulsant effects of barbiturate derivatives are multiple and rather nonselective. The principal mechanism of action is believed to be reduction of monosynaptic and polysynaptic transmission resulting in decreased excitability of the entire nerve cell; depression of PTP is negligible. Barbiturates also increase the threshold for electrical stimulation of the motor cortex.

■ **Benzodiazepines** The exact mechanism by which benzodiazepines exert their anticonvulsant effects is unknown, but is thought to be related to their ability to potentiate the activity of GABA. In animals, benzodiazepines protect against seizures induced by electrical stimulation and by pentylenetetrazol; benzodiazepines appear to act, at least partly, by augmenting presynaptic inhibition. The drugs suppress the spread of seizure activity but do not abolish the abnormal discharge from a focus in experimental models of epilepsy. In usual doses, benzodiazepines appear to have very little effect on the autonomic nervous system, respiration, or the cardiovascular system.

■ **Hydantoins** Most authorities agree that the principal mechanism of action of the hydantoin anticonvulsants, particularly phenytoin, is limitation of seizure propagation by reduction of PTP, possibly by reducing the passive influx of sodium ions or by increasing the efficiency of the sodium pump so that excess accumulation of intracellular sodium does not occur during tetanic stimulation. Loss of PTP also prevents cortical seizure foci from detonating adjacent cortical areas.

■ **Oxazolidinediones and Succinimides** Oxazolidinedione and succinimide derivatives elevate seizure threshold in the cortex and basal ganglia and reduce synaptic response to low frequency repetitive stimulation. They have no appreciable effect on PTP. Oxazolidinedione and succinimide derivatives suppress the paroxysmal spike and wave pattern of the EEG, which is common in absence seizures.

Pharmacokinetics

■ **Absorption** Precise information on the rate and degree of absorption from the GI tract is lacking for most anticonvulsants. Onset and duration of action vary with each drug and frequently among patients receiving the same drug. Most anticonvulsants have a relatively long plasma half-life, and several days to several weeks of therapy may be required to achieve steady-state plasma concentrations.

■ **Distribution** Anticonvulsants are widely distributed in the body. High concentrations of barbiturates are present in brain and liver. Hydantoins, especially phenytoin, reach highest concentrations in brain, liver, and salivary glands. Succinimides are freely distributed throughout body water. Some anticonvulsants (e.g., carbamazepine, gabapentin, lamotrigine, levetiracetam, oxcarbazepine, phenobarbital, phenytoin, topiramate, valproate) may cross the placental barrier. Whether or not other anticonvulsants cross the placenta is unknown. Phenobarbital, phenytoin, carbamazepine, eslicarbazepine acetate, gabapentin, oxcarbazepine, lamotrigine, levetiracetam, primidone, topiramate, valproate, and vigabatrin are distributed into milk of nursing women. However, in some cases, the amount of drug distributed into breast milk may not be clinically important.

■ **Elimination** Most anticonvulsants are metabolized by microsomal enzyme systems in the liver. Some anticonvulsants may inhibit or induce cytochrome P-450 (CYP) isoenzymes and thus inhibit or induce metabolism of other concomitantly administered drugs metabolized by these enzymes. (See Drug Interactions.)

Anticonvulsants that are eliminated renally include gabapentin, levetiracetam, pregabalin, and vigabatrin.

Chemistry

Anticonvulsants are used to reduce the number and/or severity of seizures in patients with epilepsy; many of the principal anticonvulsants used in the management of epilepsy are derivatives of barbiturates, benzodiazepines, hydantoins, or succinimides.

■ **Barbiturates and Analogs**

mephobarbital (no longer commercially available)
metharbital (no longer commercially available)
phenobarbital
primidone

All barbiturates are useful in the management of convulsive states; however, only phenobarbital and primidone (the structure of which is closely related to that of the barbiturates) currently are used in the management of epilepsy because they are effective anticonvulsants in subhypnotic doses. Other barbiturates (e.g., secobarbital or amobarbital) are occasionally used parenterally to terminate an acute seizure episode. (See also the Barbiturates General Statement 28:24.04 and individual monographs in 28:24.04.) Primidone is a structural analog of phenobarbital in which the carbonyl group at position 2 has been replaced by a methylene group.

■ **Benzodiazepines**

clobazam
clonazepam
clorazepate
diazepam
lorazepam
midazolam

The benzodiazepines contain a benzene ring structure fused to a 7-membered diazepine ring. The classic benzodiazepines (e.g., clonazepam, diazepam, lorazepam) are referred to as 1,4-benzodiazepines because they contain nitrogen atoms at positions 1 and 4 on the diazepine ring. Clobazam, a 1,5-benzodiazepine, differs structurally from the traditional benzodiazepines in that its nitrogen atoms are at positions 1 and 5 on the diazepine ring; clobazam is the only 1,5-benzodiazepine that is currently used in clinical practice. Commercially available 1,4-benzodiazepines used as anticonvulsants, except chlordiazepoxide and midazolam, have the same characteristic structure but differ in the substitutions at the R^1, R^3, R^7, and $R^{2'}$ positions. In chlordiazepoxide, a 1,4-benzodiazepine-4-oxide, a methylamino group replaces the ketone at the 2 position and a chlorine atom is at R^7. In midazolam, an imidazobenzodiazepine, an imidazole ring fused at positions 1 and 2 of the benzodiazepine nucleus replaces the ketone at position 2 of the nucleus. For information on the chemistry of benzodiazepines, see Chemistry in the Benzodiazepines General Statement 28:24.08.

■ **Hydantoins**

ethotoin
fosphenytoin
mephenytoin (no longer commercially available)
phenacemide (no longer commercially available)
phenytoin

The hydantoins have a 5-membered ring structure containing 2 nitrogens in an ureide configuration. Phenytoin is the prototype of the hydantoin derivatives. Ethotoin differs from phenytoin in that one phenyl substituent at position 5 is replaced by hydrogen, and the hydrogen substituent at position 3 is replaced by an ethyl group. Fosphenytoin is a phosphate ester prodrug of phenytoin.

■ **Succinimides**

ethosuximide
methsuximide

Succinimide derivatives also have a 5-membered ring structure similar to the hydantoins; however, the imino nitrogen at position 3 in the hydantoin structure is replaced with a methylene group which is mono- or di-substituted with methyl, ethyl, or phenyl group(s).

■ **Oxazolidinediones**

trimethadione

Oxazolidinedione derivatives have a 5-membered ring structure like the hydantoins, but these drugs have oxygen instead of nitrogen at position 1. The only available oxazolidinedione anticonvulsant in the US is trimethadione, but only on a limited basis.

For further information on the chemistry and stability, pharmacology, pharmacokinetics, uses, cautions, drug interactions, and dosage and administration of anticonvulsants, see the individual monographs in 28:12. See also the Barbiturates General Statement 28:24.04 and the Benzodiazepines General Statement 28:24.08.

†Use is not currently included in the labeling approved by the US Food and Drug Administration

BENZODIAZEPINES 28:12.08

cloBAZam

Frisium

■ Clobazam, a 1,5-benzodiazepine, is an anticonvulsant that also demonstrates anxiolytic properties.

Uses

■ **Seizure Disorders** ***Seizures Associated with Lennox-Gastaut Syndrome*** Clobazam is used in the adjunctive treatment of seizures associated with Lennox-Gastaut syndrome in adults and pediatric patients 2 years of age or older. The drug has been designated an orphan drug by the US Food and Drug Administration (FDA) for use in this condition.

Lennox-Gastaut syndrome is a rare and severe type of epilepsy that begins in childhood and is characterized by a classic triad of manifestations that includes multiple seizure types, an EEG pattern of slow spike and wave activity, and cognitive impairment; many patients also develop comorbid behavioral and psychiatric disorders. Tonic and atypical absence seizures are the most common types of seizures in Lennox-Gastaut syndrome; at least 50% of patients experience sudden tonic or atonic falls (drop seizures; also known as "drop attacks"), which can result in substantial injury.

Management of Lennox-Gastaut syndrome can be difficult given the multiple seizure types that can occur and the refractory nature of the condition. Although several drugs (e.g., clobazam, clonazepam, felbamate, lamotrigine, levetiracetam†, rufinamide, topiramate, valproic acid, zonisamide†) have been used to treat Lennox-Gastaut syndrome, no single anticonvulsant has been shown to be completely effective in controlling seizures and a combination of anticonvulsant agents often is required. When selecting an appropriate regimen, clinicians should consider anticonvulsant combinations that maximize seizure control and improve quality of life while minimizing adverse effects and potential drug interactions; treatment should be individualized based on the expected benefits and risks of each therapy.

Efficacy and safety of clobazam for the adjunctive treatment of seizures associated with Lennox-Gastaut syndrome were established in 2 randomized, multicenter, double-blind clinical studies (one phase 3 placebo-controlled study and one phase 2 dose-finding study). Patients were included in these studies if they had a current or prior diagnosis of Lennox-Gastaut syndrome and were younger than 11 years of age at the onset of Lennox-Gastaut syndrome; valproic acid, lamotrigine, levetiracetam, and topiramate were the most commonly used anticonvulsant agents at baseline. Both studies consisted of a 4-week baseline period followed by a 3-week titration period and then a 12- or 4-week maintenance period; patients then either discontinued therapy (dosage was tapered over 2–3 weeks) or continued into an open-label extension of the studies. Efficacy of clobazam was evaluated principally by the percent reduction in the weekly frequency of drop seizures (atonic, tonic, or myoclonic) from the 4-week baseline period to the maintenance period of each study.

In the placebo-controlled study (study 1; also called the CONTAIN trial), a total of 238 pediatric and adult patients (age range: 2–54 years) with Lennox-Gastaut syndrome was enrolled. Patients were stratified by weight into 2 groups (12.5–30 kg or more than 30 kg) and then randomized to receive adjunctive therapy with placebo or one of 3 target maintenance dosages of clobazam: low dosage (5 mg daily in those weighing up to 30 kg or 10 mg daily in those weighing more than 30 kg), medium dosage (10 mg daily in those weighing up to 30 kg or 20 mg daily in those weighing more than 30 kg), or high dosage (20 mg daily in those weighing up to 30 kg or 40 mg daily in those weighing more than 30 kg). Clobazam therapy was initiated at a dosage of 5 or 10 mg daily in divided doses and increased every 7 days up to the target dosage, which was then maintained for 12 weeks; dosage reductions were permitted if intolerable adverse effects occurred. Clobazam dosages exceeding 5 mg daily were administered in 2 divided doses. A substantial reduction in the weekly drop seizure rate from baseline to the 12-week maintenance period was observed in patients receiving clobazam in all 3 dosage groups (mean reduction of approximately 41, 49, and 68% for the low-, medium-, and high-dosage groups, respectively) compared with those receiving placebo (approximately 12%); this effect appeared to be dose dependent. The average weekly rate of total (drop and nondrop) seizures, a secondary efficacy end point, also was reduced with clobazam in a dose-dependent manner. In addition, the responder rate (percentage of patients with a 50% or greater decrease from baseline to maintenance period in average weekly rate of drop seizures) was approximately 32% for the placebo group compared with approximately 43, 59, and 78% for the low-, medium-, and high-dosage clobazam groups, respectively. Patients who received clobazam also had improved symptoms (based on investigator- and caregiver-rated global evaluation scores) compared with those who received placebo.

In the double-blind comparison of high- and low-dosage clobazam (study 2), 68 patients (age range: 2–25 years) with Lennox-Gastaut syndrome were stratified by weight (12.5–30 kg or more than 30 kg) and then randomized to receive adjunctive therapy with either low target dosage clobazam (5 mg daily in those weighing up to 30 kg or 10 mg daily in those weighing more than 30 kg) or high target dosage clobazam (20 mg daily in those weighing up to 30 kg or 40 mg daily in those weighing more than 30 kg). During the 3-week titration phase, clobazam was initiated at 5 or 10 mg daily (in divided doses for dosages exceeding 5 mg daily) in both treatment groups and then increased every 7 days until the target dosage was achieved; the target dosage was then maintained during the 4-week maintenance phase. The average weekly rate of drop seizures was substantially reduced from baseline to the maintenance period in both the high- and low-dosage groups; however, the reduction was substantially greater in patients receiving the high-dosage clobazam regimen compared with those receiving the low-dosage regimen (median reductions of 93 and 29%, respectively). The rate of nondrop seizures, a secondary measure of efficacy, also was reduced with clobazam treatment in a dose-dependent manner. In addition, patients who received high-dosage clobazam had greater improvements in overall symptoms (based on investigator and parent/caregiver global evaluation scores) compared with those who received the low-dosage regimen.

Tolerance to the therapeutic effects of benzodiazepines, including clobazam, may develop over time and result in partial or complete loss of anticonvulsant activity. To evaluate the potential for tolerance with clobazam, seizure frequencies were assessed during the initial, middle, and last 4 weeks of the maintenance period in the placebo-controlled efficacy study of the drug in patients with Lennox-Gastaut syndrome. The anticonvulsant effects of clobazam generally persisted during each of the time periods suggesting that substantial tolerance to clobazam does not develop, at least for the 3-month maintenance period that was studied. In addition, clobazam was shown to maintain clinical benefit for up to 2 years in the long-term, open-label extension of the 2 principal efficacy studies of the drug. In a preliminary analysis of those results, patients who continued to receive up to 2 years of clobazam therapy had median reductions in drop seizure frequency of 71.1% at 3 months and 91.6% at 24 months; dosage requirements generally were similar across various durations of treatment.

Other Seizure Disorders Clobazam currently is FDA-labeled only for the adjunctive treatment of seizures associated with Lennox-Gastaut syndrome. However, the drug has demonstrated broad anticonvulsant activity and has been used extensively in adults and pediatric patients with a wide range of other seizure disorders, which have sometimes been refractory, including partial, generalized, and myoclonic seizures†. In several randomized controlled trials, clobazam, when used as adjunctive therapy, reduced the frequency of refractory seizures and was particularly useful in patients with partial onset seizures. However, these were short-term trials and were substantially different in terms of their study design and methodology, making it difficult to determine the practical implications of these findings. Additional studies, including large-scale randomized studies of longer duration, are needed to more clearly determine the role of clobazam in the adjunctive treatment of other refractory seizure disorders.

■ **Anxiety Disorders** Clobazam has been used in the treatment of anxiety disorders† and has been labeled for the short-term (2-4 weeks) treatment of anxiety in some countries outside the US. However, the drug currently is *not* FDA-labeled for the treatment of anxiety disorders in the US.

Dosage and Administration

■ **Administration** Clobazam is administered orally as tablets or oral suspension without regard to meals. Daily dosages greater than 5 mg should be administered in divided doses twice daily; the 5-mg daily dosage can be administered as a single daily dose.

Clobazam tablets may be swallowed whole, broken in half, or crushed and mixed in applesauce.

Clobazam oral suspension should be shaken well prior to administration. The bottle adapter and calibrated oral dosing syringe supplied by the manufacturer should be used to administer the suspension. The adapter should be inserted firmly into the neck of the bottle before first use and should remain in place as long as the bottle is in use (up to 90 days). A dose is dispensed by inserting the oral dosing syringe into the adapter, and then inverting the bottle and slowly withdrawing the appropriate dose into the syringe. The dose should then be slowly administered directly into the corner of the patient's mouth. After each use, the bottle cap (which fits over the adapter) should be replaced securely. The manufacturer's prescribing information should be consulted for more detailed instructions on administration of the oral suspension.

Clobazam therapy should be withdrawn gradually (i.e., by tapering the daily dosage by 5–10 mg every week) to minimize the risk of precipitating or exacerbating seizures, status epilepticus, or withdrawal symptoms. (See Discontinuance of Therapy under Warnings/Precautions: Other Warnings and Precautions, in Cautions.)

Patients currently receiving or beginning therapy with clobazam and/or any other anticonvulsant for any indication should be closely monitored for the emergence or worsening of depression, suicidal thoughts or behavior (suicidality), and/or any unusual changes in mood or behavior. (See Suicidality Risk under Warnings/Precautions: Other Warnings and Precautions, in Cautions.)

■ **Dosage** ***Seizures Associated with Lennox-Gastaut Syndrome*** For the adjunctive treatment of Lennox-Gastaut syndrome in adults and children 2 years of age or older, clobazam dosage should be based on patient body weight. Within each body weight group, the dosage should be individualized based on clinical response and tolerability (see Table 1). Although each dosage in Table 1 has been shown to be effective, the clinical efficacy of clobazam is dose related and increases with increasing dosage. Clobazam dosage should therefore be titrated to maximum tolerability until adequate seizure control is attained; in some patients, this may be achieved with less than the recommended total daily dosage. Dosage should not be increased more frequently than once weekly to allow sufficient time for steady-state concentrations of the drug and its active metabolite to be achieved.

Table 1. Recommended Total Daily Dosage of Clobazam in Patients 2 Years of Age or Older by Weight Group

	Body Weight ≤30 kg	Body Weight >30 kg
Initial dosage	5 mg (given as a single daily dose)	10 mg (given in 2 divided doses)
Dosage starting on day 7	10 mg (given in 2 divided doses)	20 mg (given in 2 divided doses)
Dosage starting on day 14	20 mg (given in 2 divided doses)	40 mg (given in 2 divided doses)

Anxiety Disorders For the short-term (2–4 weeks) relief of anxiety that is severe, disabling, or causes unacceptable distress†, the usual dosage of clobazam is 20–30 mg daily given either in divided doses or as a single daily dose in the evening. Dosages of up to 60 mg daily have been used in the treatment of severe anxiety in hospitalized patients.

■ **Special Populations** Because of limited pharmacokinetic data, the manufacturer recommends slow titration of clobazam dosage in patients with hepatic impairment. For patients with mild to moderate hepatic impairment (Child-Pugh class A or B), the manufacturer recommends an initial clobazam dosage of 5 mg daily regardless of body weight. Dosage should then be titrated according to weight, but to half of the recommended dosage presented in Table 1 as tolerated. If necessary and based on clinical response, an additional titration to the maximum recommended dosage of 20 mg daily (in patients weighing 30 kg or less) or 40 mg daily (in patients weighing more than 30 kg) may be initiated at 3 weeks. Data currently are insufficient to make specific dosage recommendations for patients with severe hepatic impairment (Child-Pugh class C). (See Hepatic Impairment under Warnings/Precautions: Specific Populations, in Cautions.)

Dosage adjustment is not required in patients with mild (creatinine clearance greater than 50–80 mL/minute) or moderate (creatinine clearance of 30–50 mL/minute) renal impairment. Clobazam has not been systematically evaluated in patients with severe renal impairment or end-stage renal disease. It is also not known if clobazam or its active *N*-desmethylclobazam metabolite is dialyzable; however, limited evidence suggests that clobazam concentrations are unaffected by hemodialysis.

Because clobazam plasma concentrations at any given dosage are generally higher in geriatric patients, the manufacturer recommends slow dosage titration of the drug in such patients. All geriatric patients should receive an initial dosage of 5 mg daily regardless of their body weight. Dosage should then be titrated at weekly intervals according to weight, but to half of the recommended dosage presented in Table 1. If necessary and based on clinical response, an additional titration to the maximum dosage of 20 mg daily (in patients weighing 30 kg or less) or 40 mg daily (in patients weighing more than 30 kg) may be initiated at 3 weeks. (See Geriatric Use under Warnings/Precautions: Specific Populations, in Cautions.)

Patients known to be poor metabolizers of cytochrome P-450 (CYP) 2C19 substrates should receive an initial clobazam dosage of 5 mg daily regardless of their body weight. (See Poor CYP2C19 Metabolizers under Warnings/Precautions: Specific Populations, in Cautions.) Dosage should then be titrated slowly at weekly intervals according to weight, but to half of the recommended dosage presented in Table 1 as tolerated. If necessary and based on clinical response, an additional titration to the maximum dosage of 20 mg daily (in patients weighing 30 kg or less) or 40 mg daily (in patients weighing more than 30 kg) may be initiated at 3 weeks.

Cautions

■ **Contraindications** The manufacturer states that there are no known contraindications to the use of clobazam.

■ **Warnings/Precautions** ***Warnings*** **Concomitant Use with Opiates.** Concomitant use of benzodiazepines, including clobazam, and opiate agonists or opiate partial agonists may result in profound sedation, respiratory depression, coma, and death. Concomitant use of such drugs should be reserved for patients in whom alternative treatment options are inadequate; the lowest effective dosages and shortest possible duration of concomitant therapy should be used, and the patient should be monitored closely for respiratory depression and sedation. (See Opiate Agonists and Opiate Partial Agonists under Drug Interactions: CNS Depressants.)

Other Warnings and Precautions **Concomitant Use of CNS Depressants.** Since clobazam has a CNS depressant effect, patients or their caregivers should be cautioned against concomitant use of other CNS depressant drugs or alcohol and cautioned that the effects of other CNS depressants or alcohol may be potentiated. (See Concomitant Use with Opiates under Warnings/Precautions: Warnings and also see Somnolence and Sedation under Warnings/Precautions: Other Warnings and Precautions, in Cautions.)

Somnolence and Sedation. Somnolence and sedation are among the most common adverse effects associated with clobazam therapy. These effects generally begin within the first month of treatment and may diminish with continued therapy. In a placebo-controlled study of patients with Lennox-Gastaut syndrome, somnolence or sedation was reported in 26% of patients who received clobazam compared with 15% of those who received placebo. Somnolence and sedation were observed at all effective dosages in clinical trials and were dose related. The sedative effect of clobazam is reportedly less pronounced than that of other commercially available benzodiazepines (see Description).

Patients should be monitored for somnolence and sedation during clobazam therapy, particularly if they are receiving other CNS depressants (e.g., alcohol, opiate agonists, tricyclic antidepressants, sedating antihistamines, other benzodiazepines) concomitantly. (See Advice to Patients.)

Discontinuance of Therapy. Abrupt discontinuance and rapid dosage reduction of clobazam should be avoided to minimize the risk of precipitating or exacerbating seizures, status epilepticus, and withdrawal symptoms. When therapy is discontinued, dosage of the drug should be decreased gradually (i.e., by 5–10 mg daily at weekly intervals). (See Dosage and Administration: Administration.)

Withdrawal symptoms (e.g., convulsions, psychosis, hallucinations, behavioral disorders, tremor, anxiety, irritability, dysphoria, insomnia, headache, palpitations, diarrhea) have been reported following abrupt discontinuance of benzodiazepines, including clobazam; the risk of withdrawal symptoms is greater with increasing dosage and duration of treatment. Such withdrawal reactions occur in patients who have developed physical dependence on these drugs. (See Physical and Psychological Dependence under Warnings/Precautions: Other Warnings and Precautions, in Cautions.) More severe withdrawal symptoms usually are limited to patients who abruptly discontinue therapy after receiving excessive dosages of benzodiazepines for an extended period of time. Milder withdrawal symptoms (e.g., dysphoria, anxiety, insomnia) generally have been reported following abrupt discontinuance of benzodiazepines in patients continuously receiving therapeutic dosages for several months.

Serious Dermatologic Reactions. Serious and sometimes life-threatening dermatologic reactions, including Stevens-Johnson syndrome (SJS) and toxic epidermal necrolysis (TEN), have been reported rarely in both pediatric and adult patients treated with clobazam during postmarketing experience worldwide. Although such reactions may occur at any time during clobazam therapy, the risk is greater during the first 8 weeks of therapy or when clobazam is discontinued and then reinitiated. TEN developed in skin areas exposed to sunlight in one published case. The US Food and Drug Administration (FDA) states that, as of December 2013, 21 cases of SJS or TEN associated with clobazam have been identified. Hospitalization was required in all of the patients; one case resulted in blindness and at least one death occurred. The majority of the patients were receiving concomitant therapy with other drugs associated with an increased risk of SJS and TEN (e.g., other anticonvulsant agents, beta-lactam antibiotics, sulfasalazine); however, the available evidence, including a close temporal relationship (within 2 months) between initiation of clobazam and development of the serious skin reaction in most cases, suggests that clobazam was the likely cause of the skin reactions. In addition, patients in many of the cases improved after clobazam was discontinued and, in some cases, despite continuing or reinitiating the other suspected medications.

Patients receiving clobazam therapy should be closely monitored for signs and symptoms of SJS and TEN, particularly during the initial 8 weeks of treatment or when therapy with the drug is reinitiated. Clobazam should be discontinued at the first sign of a rash unless the rash is clearly not drug related (see Discontinuance of Therapy under Warnings/Precautions: Other Warnings and Precautions, in Cautions and also see Advice to Patients). If clinical manifestations suggestive of SJS or TEN occur, clobazam therapy should not be resumed and alternative therapy should be considered. When switching from one anticonvulsant drug to another, clinicians should consider that other anticonvulsants also may be associated with a risk of serious dermatologic reactions.

Physical and Psychological Dependence. Physical and/or psychological dependence may occur in patients receiving clobazam. While the risk of dependence is greater with increasing dosage and duration of therapy, some patients can become physically or psychologically dependent even with short-term use of the drug (i.e., a few weeks) at recommended dosages. The risk of dependence also is increased in patients with a history of alcohol or substance abuse. As with all benzodiazepines, tolerance to the therapeutic effects of clobazam has been reported and may be a concern with long-term use of the drug. (See Seizures Associated with Lennox-Gastaut Syndrome under Uses: Seizure Disorders.)

Patients with a history of substance abuse should be carefully monitored while receiving clobazam or other psychotropic therapy because of their predisposition to habituation and dependence. Abrupt discontinuance of therapy or rapid dosage reduction can precipitate withdrawal symptoms in patients with physical dependence on the drug, and should therefore be avoided. (See Discontinuance of Therapy under Warnings/Precautions: Other Warnings and Precautions, in Cautions.)

Suicidality Risk. Suicidal behavior and ideation have been reported in patients receiving anticonvulsants, including clobazam. The FDA has alerted healthcare professionals about an increased risk of suicidality (suicidal behavior or ideation) observed in an analysis of studies using various anticonvulsants compared with placebo. The analysis of suicidality reports from placebo-controlled studies involving 11 anticonvulsants (i.e., carbamazepine, felbamate, gabapentin, lamotrigine, levetiracetam, oxcarbazepine, pregabalin, tiagabine, topiramate, valproate, zonisamide) in patients with epilepsy, psychiatric disorders (e.g., bipolar disorder, depression, anxiety), and other conditions (e.g., migraine, neuropathic pain) found that patients receiving anticonvulsants had approximately twice the risk of suicidal behavior or ideation (0.43%) compared with patients receiving placebo (0.24%). This increased suicidality risk was observed as early as one week after beginning therapy and continued through 24 weeks. Although patients treated with an anticonvulsant for epilepsy, psychiatric disorders, and other conditions were all found to have an increased suicidality risk compared with those receiving placebo, the relative suicidality risk was higher for patients with epilepsy compared with those receiving anticonvulsants for other conditions.

Based on the current analysis of the available data, the FDA recommends that clinicians inform patients, their families, and caregivers of the potential for an increased risk of suicidality with anticonvulsant therapy and that all patients currently receiving or beginning therapy with any anticonvulsant be closely monitored for notable changes that may indicate the emergence or worsening of suicidal thoughts or behavior or depression. Symptoms such as anxiety, agitation, hostility, insomnia, and mania may be precursors to emerging suicidality.

Clinicians who prescribe clobazam or any other anticonvulsant should balance the risk of suicidality with the clinical need for the drug and the risk associated with untreated illness. Epilepsy and many other illnesses for which anticonvulsants are prescribed are themselves associated with morbidity and mortality and an increased risk of suicidal thoughts and behavior. If suicidal thoughts or behavior emerge during anticonvulsant therapy, the clinician should consider whether these symptoms may be related to the illness being treated. (See Advice to Patients.)

Abuse Potential. Clobazam is subject to control as a schedule IV (C-IV) drug. Because of its pharmacologic similarity to other benzodiazepines, particularly its potentiating effects on γ-aminobutyric acid (GABA) through the $GABA_A$ receptor, the abuse potential of clobazam is expected to be similar to that of other benzodiazepines (e.g., diazepam). Cases of abuse, misuse, and overdosage associated with clobazam have been reported to the World Health Organization (WHO).

Specific Populations **Pregnancy.** Category C. (See Users Guide.)

North American Antiepileptic Drug (NAAED) Pregnancy Registry at 888-233-2334 (for patients or caregivers); NAAED registry information also is available on the website http://www.aedpregnancyregistry.org.

Limited animal data suggest that clobazam may produce developmental toxicity, including an increased incidence of fetal abnormalities when given orally to pregnant animals at dosages similar to those used clinically. For further information on the use of anticonvulsants and benzodiazepines during pregnancy, see Cautions: Pregnancy and Lactation in the Anticonvulsants General Statement 28:12 and also see Cautions: Pregnancy and Lactation in the Benzodiazepines General Statement 28:24.08.

Lactation. Clobazam is distributed into human milk. Since the effects of this exposure on nursing infants are unknown, the manufacturer states that a decision should be made whether to discontinue nursing or the drug.

Pediatric Use. Safety and efficacy of clobazam have not been established in pediatric patients younger than 2 years of age.

Geriatric Use. Clinical trials of clobazam did not include sufficient numbers of patients 65 years of age and older to determine whether they respond differently than younger patients. Based on a population pharmacokinetic analysis, geriatric patients appear to eliminate clobazam more slowly than younger patients (2–64 years of age). Therefore, clobazam should be initiated at a low dosage and titrated slowly in geriatric patients. (See Dosage and Administration: Special Populations.)

Hepatic Impairment. Clobazam is extensively metabolized in the liver; however, the effects of hepatic impairment on the pharmacokinetics of the drug have not been fully characterized. Results of a small single-dose study showed no substantial pharmacokinetic differences (i.e., in peak plasma concentrations and plasma clearance of clobazam and peak plasma concentrations of *N*-desmethylclobazam) between patients with hepatic impairment and healthy individuals; however, because of limitations of the data, definitive conclusions cannot be drawn from this study.

Clobazam therapy should be initiated at a dosage of 5 mg daily (regardless of patient weight) and titrated slowly in patients with mild or moderate hepatic impairment (Child-Pugh class A or B). There is insufficient information regarding the metabolism of clobazam in patients with severe hepatic impairment. (See Dosage and Administration: Special Populations.)

Renal Impairment. Results of a pharmacokinetic study showed no substantial differences in systemic exposure to clobazam or its active *N*-desmethylclobazam metabolite between patients with mild (creatinine clearance exceeding 50–80 mL/minute) or moderate (creatinine clearance of 30–50 mL/minute) renal impairment and those with normal renal function.

Dosage adjustment is not required in patients with mild or moderate renal impairment. There is no experience with clobazam in patients with severe renal impairment or end-stage renal disease. It is not known whether the drug or its active *N*-desmethylclobazam metabolite is dialyzable; however, limited evidence suggests that clobazam concentrations are unaffected by hemodialysis.

Poor CYP2C19 Metabolizers. Genetic polymorphism of the cytochrome P-450 (CYP) isoenzyme 2C19 can affect the pharmacokinetic and pharmacodynamic response to clobazam. CYP2C19 is the principal enzyme involved in the metabolism of *N*-desmethylclobazam, the pharmacologically active metabolite of clobazam. Individuals with genetic variants of this enzyme may have reduced enzymatic activity and higher than expected plasma concentrations of *N*-desmethylclobazam, predisposing them to a higher risk of adverse effects. (See Description.)

Higher concentrations of *N*-desmethylclobazam have been observed in poor CYP2C19 metabolizers compared with extensive CYP2C19 metabolizers. Dosage adjustment of clobazam is therefore recommended in patients known to be poor metabolizers of CYP2C19. (See Dosage and Administration: Special Populations.)

■ Common Adverse Effects

Adverse effects associated with clobazam generally are similar to those observed with other benzodiazepines. (See Cautions in the Benzodiazepines General Statement 28:24.08.)

Adverse effects reported in at least 5% of patients receiving clobazam and more frequently with clobazam than with placebo include somnolence or sedation, lethargy, drooling, vomiting, constipation, dysphagia, decreased or increased appetite, cough, upper respiratory tract infection, pneumonia, bronchitis, urinary tract infection, aggression, insomnia, irritability, ataxia, psychomotor hyperactivity, dysarthria, pyrexia, and fatigue.

Drug Interactions

■ Drugs Affecting Hepatic Microsomal Enzymes

Clobazam is metabolized principally by the cytochrome P-450 (CYP) isoenzyme CYP3A4, and to a lesser extent by CYP2C19 and CYP2B6. The active metabolite, *N*-desmethylclobazam, is metabolized principally by CYP2C19. Pharmacokinetic interactions with clobazam are possible with drugs that inhibit or induce CYP3A4 or CYP2C19.

Concomitant use of clobazam with potent (e.g., fluconazole, fluvoxamine, ticlopidine) or moderate (e.g., omeprazole) inhibitors of CYP2C19 may increase exposure to *N*-desmethylclobazam by up to fivefold (based on extrapolation of pharmacogenomic data) and possibly increase adverse effects. Therefore, clobazam dosage adjustment may be necessary when the drug is administered concomitantly with potent or moderate CYP2C19 inhibitors.

Concomitant use of clobazam with a potent CYP3A4 inhibitor (e.g., ketoconazole) increased exposure to clobazam, but did not substantially affect pharmacokinetics of *N*-desmethylclobazam. (See Drug Interactions: Ketoconazole.)

Population pharmacokinetic analysis of data from clinical trials showed no substantial alterations in steady-state pharmacokinetics of clobazam or its active metabolite when the drug was used concomitantly with anticonvulsants that induce CYP3A4 (carbamazepine, phenobarbital, phenytoin), induce CYP2C9 (carbamazepine, phenobarbital, phenytoin, valproic acid), or inhibit CYP2C9 (felbamate, oxcarbazepine). (See Drug Interactions: Anticonvulsants.)

■ Drugs Metabolized by Hepatic Microsomal Enzymes

In vitro studies indicate that clobazam and its active metabolite (*N*-desmethylclobazam) induce CYP3A4 in a concentration-dependent manner; in vitro studies also indicate that *N*-desmethylclobazam is a weak inhibitor of CYP2C9. Clobazam does not appear to inhibit CYP isoenzymes 1A2, 2C8, 2C9, 2C19, 2D6, and 3A4 nor substantially induce CYP1A2 and CYP2C19 in vitro.

The potential for clobazam to inhibit or induce various CYP isoenzymes in vivo was evaluated in a study using probe substrates for CYP2D6 (dextromethorphan), CYP3A4 (midazolam), CYP1A2 (caffeine), and CYP2C9 (tolbutamide). In contrast to in vitro observations, clobazam increased peak plasma concentrations and area under the concentration-time curve (AUC) of dextromethorphan by 59 and 90%, respectively, indicating inhibition of CYP2D6; therefore, dosage adjustment of drugs metabolized by CYP2D6 (e.g., dextromethorphan, fluoxetine, paroxetine) may be necessary when they are used concomitantly with clobazam. Clobazam decreased systemic exposure to midazolam by 27% and increased exposure to its 1-hydroxymidazolam metabolite by approximately fourfold; however, the manufacturer states that the extent of interaction does not warrant dosage adjustment of concomitantly used drugs that are metabolized principally by CYP3A4. Clobazam had no effect on the pharmacokinetics of caffeine or tolbutamide.

■ Drugs Metabolized by Uridine Diphosphate-glucuronosyltransferase

Clobazam does not inhibit uridine diphosphate-glucuronosyltransferase (UGT) 1A1, 1A4, 1A6, or 2B4 in vitro. Clobazam's active metabolite, *N*-desmethylclobazam, was shown to be a weak inhibitor of UGT 1A4, 1A6, and 2B4. Clobazam and *N*-desmethylclobazam also increased UGT1A1 messenger RNA (mRNA), but at concentrations much higher than therapeutic concentrations. However, a population pharmacokinetic analysis indicated that clobazam does not affect the exposure of a UGT substrate (lamotrigine).

■ CNS Depressants

Additive CNS effects can occur when clobazam is administered concomitantly with other CNS depressants (e.g., opiate agonists, tricyclic antidepressants, sedating antihistamines, alcohol, other benzodiazepines). Therefore, concomitant use of clobazam and other CNS depressants generally should be avoided. (See Somnolence and Sedation under Warnings/Precautions: Other Warnings and Precautions, in Cautions and also see Advice to Patients.)

Opiate Agonists and Opiate Partial Agonists Concomitant use of benzodiazepines, including clobazam, and opiate agonists or opiate partial agonists may result in profound sedation, respiratory depression, coma, and death. Whenever possible, such concomitant use should be avoided. Opiate antitussive agents should be avoided in patients receiving benzodiazepines, and concomitant use of opiate analgesics and benzodiazepines should be reserved for patients in whom alternative treatment options are inadequate. The lowest effective dosages and shortest possible duration of concomitant therapy should be used, and the patient should be monitored closely for respiratory depression and sedation.

If clobazam is required for any indication other than epilepsy in a patient receiving opiate therapy, the drug should be initiated at a lower dosage than indicated in the absence of opiate therapy and titrated based on clinical response. If an opiate analgesic is required in a patient receiving clobazam, the opiate analgesic should be initiated at a reduced dosage and titrated based on clinical response. For further information on potential interactions between benzodiazepines and opiates, see Opiate Agonists and Opiate Partial Agonists under Drug Interactions: CNS Agents, in the Benzodiazepines General Statement 28:24.08.

Alcohol Alcohol consumption has been reported to increase the maximum plasma exposure of clobazam by approximately 50%; clobazam does not appear to alter the pharmacokinetics of alcohol. Alcohol also can potentiate the CNS depressant effects of clobazam (e.g., sedation, somnolence). Concomitant use of clobazam and alcohol may therefore be hazardous and should be avoided.

■ Anticonvulsants

Results of a population pharmacokinetic analysis indicate that the steady-state pharmacokinetics of clobazam and its active metabolite, *N*-desmethylclobazam, are not substantially altered by concurrent use of anticonvulsants that are CYP3A4 inducers (carbamazepine, phenobarbital, phenytoin), CYP2C9 inducers (carbamazepine, phenobarbital, phenytoin, valproic acid), and CYP2C9 inhibitors (felbamate, oxcarbazepine). In addition, results from a population pharmacokinetic analysis indicate that clobazam does not substantially affect exposure of lamotrigine or valproic acid.

Some studies have shown that CYP enzyme-inducing anticonvulsants (carbamazepine, phenobarbital, phenytoin) can reduce concentrations of clobazam and increase metabolic transformation to its active metabolite, thereby increasing the risk of adverse effects (e.g., sedation). There also is some evidence suggesting that *N*-desmethylclobazam concentrations may be increased via CYP2C19 inhibition in patients receiving clobazam and felbamate concomitantly.

Some studies have shown no substantial interaction with clobazam and valproic acid, while others suggest that clobazam may inhibit the metabolism of valproic acid and increase the potential for valproic acid-related toxicities.

Concomitant administration of clobazam and carbamazepine was shown in one study to moderately increase metabolism of carbamazepine and result in higher concentrations of the carbamazepine 10,11-epoxide (CBZ-E) and *trans*-10,11-dihydro-10,11-dihydroxycarbamazepine (CBZ-T) metabolites.

■ **Cimetidine** In a pharmacokinetic study, administration of single-dose clobazam and multiple-dose cimetidine in healthy males produced small increases in the systemic exposure and elimination half-life of clobazam; plasma concentrations of *N*-desmethylclobazam were not substantially affected. These changes were not considered clinically important.

■ **Hormonal Contraceptives** Clobazam is a weak CYP3A4 inducer and may reduce the efficacy of some hormonal contraceptives that are metabolized by CYP3A4. To ensure contraceptive reliability, the manufacturer recommends that women receiving hormonal contraceptives also use nonhormonal forms of contraception during clobazam therapy and for 28 days following discontinuance of the drug. (See Advice to Patients.)

■ **Ketoconazole** Concomitant administration of clobazam and ketoconazole (a potent CYP3A4 inhibitor) in healthy individuals increased systemic exposure of clobazam by 54%, but did not substantially alter peak plasma concentrations of clobazam; pharmacokinetics of *N*-desmethylclobazam were unaffected. The observed increase in clobazam exposure is not expected to be clinically important.

■ **Omeprazole** Concomitant administration of clobazam and omeprazole (a moderate CYP2C19 inhibitor) in healthy individuals increased peak plasma concentrations and systemic exposure of *N*-desmethylclobazam by 15 and 36%, respectively, but did not substantially affect the pharmacokinetics of clobazam. Clinically important effects were not observed; however, the manufacturer states that clobazam dosage adjustment may be necessary when the drug is used concomitantly with potent or moderate CYP2C19 inhibitors such as omeprazole.

Description

Clobazam is a 1,5-benzodiazepine that has anticonvulsant as well as anxiolytic properties. The exact mechanism of clobazam's anticonvulsant and anxiolytic actions has not been fully elucidated, but is thought to involve allosteric binding of the drug to the benzodiazepine site of the γ-aminobutyric acid type A ($GABA_A$) receptor, which in turn potentiates the inhibitory effects of GABA. Although structurally similar to the 1,4-benzodiazepines (e.g., clonazepam, diazepam, lorazepam), clobazam appears to have a broader spectrum of anticonvulsant activity and an improved adverse effect profile (e.g., less sedative effects), which have been attributed to differences in binding affinity for the $GABA_A$ receptor.

Clobazam is rapidly and almost completely absorbed following oral administration; peak plasma concentrations of the drug are achieved within 0.5–4 hours after single- or multiple-dose administration of the tablets and within 0.5–2 hours following single-dose administration of the oral suspension under fasting conditions. Bioavailability of the oral suspension is similar to that of the tablets under fasting conditions. Food does not appear to substantially affect absorption of clobazam tablets; although not evaluated, bioavailability of the oral suspension also is unlikely to be altered by food. Because clobazam is highly lipophilic, it distributes rapidly throughout the body. Clobazam is extensively metabolized in the liver where it undergoes *N*-demethylation and hydroxylation; approximately 2% and 1% of an orally administered dose is present in urine and feces, respectively, as unchanged drug. At least 14 metabolites of clobazam have been identified. The main circulating metabolite, *N*-desmethylclobazam, is pharmacologically active with potency estimates ranging from one-fifth to equal potency of the parent drug; therefore, the active metabolite may contribute to the efficacy and safety of the drug. At therapeutic dosages, plasma concentrations of *N*-desmethylclobazam are approximately 3–5 times higher than those of clobazam. Biotransformation of clobazam to *N*-desmethylclobazam is mediated by the cytochrome P-450 (CYP) enzyme system, principally by CYP3A4, and to a lesser extent by CYP2C19 and CYP2B6; *N*-desmethylclobazam is further metabolized by CYP2C19 to an inactive derivative. Both clobazam and *N*-desmethylclobazam are substrates of P-glycoprotein, but do not inhibit the transport protein. Both the drug and its active metabolite also exhibit a high degree of protein binding (80–90 and 70%, respectively). Clobazam is eliminated mainly through renal excretion; following administration of a single radiolabeled dose of clobazam, approximately 82% of the dose was recovered in urine and 11% in feces. The mean elimination half-life of clobazam is approximately 36–42 hours and the mean elimination half-life of *N*-desmethylclobazam is approximately 71–82 hours.

Genetic polymorphism of the CYP2C19 isoenzyme can affect the metabolism of *N*-desmethylclobazam and result in possible increased concentrations of the active metabolite. (See Poor CYP2C19 Metabolizers under Warnings/Precautions: Specific Populations, in Cautions.) Individuals with 2 copies of the defective CYP2C19*2 allele (the *2/*2 genotype) are described as poor metabolizers, those with 1 copy (the *1/*2 genotype) are intermediate metabolizers, and those homozygous for the wild-type CYP2C19*1 allele (the *1/*1 genotype) are described as extensive metabolizers (i.e., normal enzyme activity). Systemic exposure to *N*-desmethylclobazam is approximately 3–5 and 2 times higher in poor and intermediate CYP2C19 metabolizers, respectively, than in extensive metabolizers. Systemic exposure of clobazam is similar for both poor and extensive metabolizers of CYP2C19 substrates. The prevalence of poor CYP2C19 metabolizers in the general population varies depending on ethnic and racial background and has been reported to be as high as 15–30% among Asians, with a lower prevalence in Caucasians.

Advice to Patients

Importance of providing patient or caregiver with copy of written patient information (medication guide) each time clobazam is dispensed. Importance of advising patients or caregivers to read the medication guide before the start of therapy and each time the prescription is refilled.

Importance of taking clobazam only as prescribed.

Risk of somnolence or sedation. Patients should be cautioned against driving or operating hazardous machinery until they are reasonably certain that clobazam does not adversely affect their judgment, thinking, or motor skills.

Risk of potentially fatal additive effects (e.g., profound sedation, respiratory depression, coma) if benzodiazepines, including clobazam, are used concomitantly with opiates either therapeutically or illicitly. Risk of potentiated CNS depression with concurrent use of alcohol or other CNS depressants. Importance of advising patients receiving clobazam to avoid concomitant use of opiate antitussives and to also avoid concomitant use of opiate analgesics unless such use is supervised by a clinician. Importance of advising patients or caregivers to avoid concomitant use of clobazam and alcohol and to check with their clinician before using clobazam concomitantly with other CNS depressants (e.g., other benzodiazepines, TCAs, sedating antihistamines).

Risk of rare but serious skin reactions, including Stevens-Johnson syndrome and toxic epidermal necrolysis. Importance of advising patient or caregivers to seek immediate medical attention at the first appearance of a skin rash or other signs of hypersensitivity (e.g., blistering or peeling of skin, mouth sores, hives) while receiving clobazam. Drug discontinuance may be required; however, patients should be advised not to stop the drug without first consulting with their clinician.

Importance of patients, family members, and caregivers being aware that anticonvulsants, including clobazam, may increase the risk of having suicidal thoughts or actions in a very small number of people (about 1 in 500). Advise patients, family members, and caregivers to pay close attention to any day-to-day changes in mood, behavior, and actions; these changes can happen very quickly. They should also be aware of common warning signs that may signal suicide risk (e.g., talking or thinking about wanting to hurt oneself or end one's life, withdrawing from friends and family, becoming depressed or experiencing worsening of existing depression, becoming preoccupied with death and dying, giving away prized possessions). Advise patients, family members, and caregivers to contact the responsible clinician immediately if these or any other new and worrisome behaviors occur.

Importance of advising patients or caregivers to consult their clinician before increasing or decreasing the dosage of clobazam or abruptly discontinuing the drug. Patients or caregivers should be informed that sudden discontinuance of clobazam can cause serious problems, including an increased risk of seizures and withdrawal symptoms.

Importance of women informing clinicians if they are or plan to become pregnant or plan to breast-feed. Importance of clinicians informing women about the existence of and encouraging enrollment in the pregnancy registry (see Pregnancy under Warnings/Precautions: Specific Populations, in Cautions).

Importance of informing women that clobazam may cause some hormonal contraceptives (e.g., birth control pills, patches, rings, implants, injections, intrauterine devices) to be less effective; women should be advised to use additional nonhormonal forms of contraception during clobazam therapy and for 28 days after discontinuance to ensure continued contraceptive reliability.

Importance of informing clinicians of existing or contemplated concomitant therapy, including prescription and OTC drugs and dietary or herbal supplements, as well as any concomitant illnesses (e.g., kidney or liver disease, respiratory problems, depression or other mood disorders).

Importance of informing patients of other important precautionary information. (See Cautions.)

Overview® (see Users Guide). For additional information on this drug until a more detailed monograph is developed and published, the manufacturer's labeling should be consulted. It is *essential* that the manufacturer's labeling be consulted for more detailed information on usual cautions, precautions, contraindications, potential drug interactions, laboratory test interferences, and acute toxicity.

Preparations

Clobazam is subject to control under the Federal Controlled Substances Act of 1970 as a schedule IV (C-IV) drug.

Excipients in commercially available drug preparations may have clinically important effects in some individuals; consult specific product labeling for details.

cloBAZam

Oral

Suspension	2.5 mg/mL	**Onfi®** (C-IV), Lundbeck
Tablets	10 mg	**Onfi®** (C-IV; scored), Lundbeck
	20 mg	**Onfi®** (C-IV; scored), Lundbeck

†Use is not currently included in the labeling approved by the US Food and Drug Administration

clonazePAM

■ Clonazepam is a benzodiazepine derivative that is used both as an anticonvulsant and for the treatment of panic disorder with or without agoraphobia.

Uses

■ **Seizure Disorders** Clonazepam is used in the prophylactic management of Lennox-Gastaut syndrome (petit mal variant epilepsy) and akinetic and myoclonic seizures. The drug also may be used in the management of absence (petit mal) seizures in patients who have not responded to succinimides. In some patients, use of clonazepam may permit reduction in dosage or discontinuance of other anticonvulsants; however, paradoxical increases in seizure activity also have occurred. (See Cautions: Precautions and Contraindications.) A decreased response to the drug may occur after several months or years of clonazepam therapy; however, seizures may be less severe than those before clonazepam therapy. In some patients, dosage adjustment may restore efficacy.

Most studies to date on the use of clonazepam have been uncontrolled and have involved patients with seizures refractory to other anticonvulsants. In addition, clonazepam has been used mainly as an adjunct to other drugs. For these reasons, determination of the precise role of clonazepam in the management of seizure disorders must await the results of well-controlled comparative studies.

Clonazepam has been used with some success in other refractory seizures†, including partial seizures with complex symptomatology (psychomotor seizures) and other partial (focal) seizures and some cases of infantile spasms. Clonazepam also has been useful in some patients with tonic-clonic (grand mal) seizures†; however, when used in patients with multiple types of seizure disorders, the drug may increase the frequency of or precipitate tonic-clonic seizures in some patients. If this occurs, addition of another anticonvulsant and/or increase in dosage may be required.

IV clonazepam has been used with good results in the management of status epilepticus†; however, a parenteral dosage form of the drug is not currently commercially available in the US.

■ **Panic Attacks and Disorder** Clonazepam is used in the treatment of panic disorder with or without agoraphobia. Panic disorder is characterized by the occurrence of unexpected panic attacks and associated concern about having additional attacks, worry about the implications or consequences of the attacks, and/or a clinically important change in behavior related to the attacks.

According to DSM-IV, panic disorder is characterized by recurrent unexpected panic attacks, which consist of a discrete period of intense fear or discomfort in which 4 (or more) of the following symptoms develop abruptly and reach a peak within 10 minutes: palpitations, pounding heart, or accelerated heart rate; sweating; trembling or shaking; sensations of shortness of breath or smothering; feeling of choking; chest pain or discomfort; nausea or abdominal distress; feeling dizzy, unsteady, lightheaded, or faint; derealization (feelings of unreality) or depersonalization (being detached from oneself); fear of losing control; fear of dying; paresthesias (numbness or tingling sensations); and chills or hot flushes.

The efficacy of clonazepam for the management of panic disorder has been established by 2 multicenter, double-blind, placebo-controlled studies of 6–9 weeks' duration in adult outpatients who had a primary diagnosis of panic disorder (DSM-IIIR) with or without agoraphobia. In these studies, clonazepam was found to be superior to placebo on the following measures of efficacy: change from baseline in panic attack frequency, the Clinician's Global Impression Severity of Illness Score, and the Clinician's Global Impression Improvement Score.

The first study was a fixed-dose study of 9 weeks' duration involving clonazepam dosages of 0.5, 1, 2, 3, or 4 mg daily. This study was conducted in 4 phases: a 1-week placebo run-in phase, a 3-week phase of upward titration of the dosage, a 6-week fixed-dosage maintenance phase, and a 7-week discontinuance phase. A substantial difference from placebo was observed consistently only in the group receiving 1 mg of clonazepam daily; the difference between the reduction from baseline in the number of full panic attacks was approximately 1 per week in patients receiving clonazepam 1 mg daily compared with placebo. At the study end point (the end of the fixed-dosage maintenance phase), 74% of patients receiving clonazepam 1 mg daily were free of panic attacks compared to 56% of patients receiving placebo. Daily dosages exceeding 1 mg were less effective and more commonly associated with adverse effects (e.g., somnolence and ataxia) in this study.

The second study was of 6 weeks' duration and used a flexible dosing schedule involving clonazepam dosages ranging from 0.5–4 mg daily. The study was conducted in 3 phases: a 1-week placebo run-in phase, a 6-week optimal dose-finding phase, and a 6-week discontinuance phase. The mean clonazepam dosage during the optimal dosing period was 2.3 mg daily. The difference between the reduction from baseline in the number of full panic attacks was approximately 1 per week in patients receiving clonazepam compared with placebo. At the study end point, 62% of patients receiving clonazepam were free of panic attacks compared with 37% of patients receiving placebo.

Subgroup analysis from these 2 controlled studies for possible race- or gender-related effects on treatment outcome did not suggest any difference in efficacy based on either the race or gender of the patient.

The manufacturer states that the efficacy of clonazepam for long-term use (i.e., longer than 9 weeks) has not been systematically evaluated in controlled studies. However, limited information from follow-up studies of patients with panic disorder who responded favorably to benzodiazepine therapy indicates that the benefits observed during short-term therapy are usually maintained for longer periods (e.g., up to several years) without increases in dosage. In an open study in which patients with panic disorder were treated with clonazepam over a 2-year period, clonazepam produced and maintained a therapeutic benefit without evidence of tolerance development (as manifested by dosage escalation or worsening of clinical status). The manufacturer states that there is insufficient experience concerning how long patients with panic disorder who are treated with clonazepam should remain on the drug. However, some clinicians state that panic disorder is a chronic condition; therefore, it may be reasonable to continue therapy in responding patients. If clonazepam is used for extended periods, the need for continued therapy with the drug should be reassessed periodically. (See Dosage and Administration: Dosage.)

Panic disorder can be treated with cognitive behavioral psychotherapy and/or pharmacologic therapy. Currently, there are several classes of drugs that appear to be effective in the pharmacologic management of panic disorder, including tricyclic antidepressants (e.g., imipramine, clomipramine), monoamine oxidase inhibitors (e.g., phenelzine), selective serotonin-reuptake inhibitors (e.g., citalopram, escitalopram, fluoxetine, fluvoxamine, paroxetine, sertraline), selective serotonin- and norepinephrine-reuptake inhibitors (e.g., venlafaxine), and benzodiazepines (e.g., alprazolam, clonazepam). When choosing among the available drugs in the treatment of panic disorder, clinicians should consider their acceptance and tolerability by patients; their ability to reduce or eliminate panic attacks, reduce clinically important anxiety and disability secondary to phobic avoidance, and ameliorate other common comorbid conditions (such as depression); their cost; and their ability to prevent relapse during long-term therapy.

Because of their better tolerability when compared with other agents (such as the tricyclic antidepressants, monoamine oxidase inhibitors, and benzodiazepines) and the lack of physical dependence problems commonly associated with benzodiazepines, some clinicians currently prefer selective serotonin-reuptake inhibitors as first-line therapy in the management of panic disorder. However, benzodiazepines such as clonazepam have a more rapid onset of action often with immediate reduction of panic symptoms, whereas antidepressants may require several weeks or more for therapeutic effect. Therefore, benzodiazepines can be used for early symptom control (usually in combination with another form of treatment such as cognitive behavioral therapy or antidepressant therapy) and are useful in relieving anticipatory anxiety. Benzodiazepines also can be used to treat surges of anxiety or panic, although some experts state that this as-needed use of benzodiazepines should not replace the use of adequate daily dosages when clinically necessary. In addition, some clinicians consider the anxiolytic effect of benzodiazepines advantageous in reducing anxiety between panic attacks. The most serious risk factor associated with benzodiazepines in panic disorder is physical dependence; withdrawal symptoms or a recurrence of panic symptoms may occur during drug tapering or following abrupt discontinuance of therapy. Therefore, gradual discontinuance of clonazepam therapy is advised. (See Chronic Toxicity and see also Dosage and Administration.) In addition, as with other benzodiazepines, clonazepam can produce sedation and psychomotor impairment and potentially may interact with alcohol if it is not restricted. (See Cautions: Precautions and Contraindications.)

■ **Schizophrenia** Clonazepam also has been used in patients who experience akathisia† while receiving antipsychotic drugs (e.g., for management of schizophrenia) and for the treatment of acute catatonic reactions†, whether associated with schizophrenia or other conditions. (See Uses: Schizophrenia, in the Benzodiazepines General Statement 28:24.08.)

■ **Other Uses** The efficacy of clonazepam as a hypnotic† has not been fully evaluated.

Dosage and Administration

■ **Administration** Clonazepam is administered orally.

Clonazepam conventional tablets should be administered with water and swallowed whole. The orally disintegrating tablets should be administered immediately after opening the pouch and peeling back the blister; do *not* push the tablet through the foil. The orally disintegrating tablet should be removed with a dry hand and placed on the tongue, where it disintegrates rapidly in saliva, and then subsequently can be swallowed with or without water.

In the treatment of seizure disorders, the manufacturer states that daily dosage usually is given in 3 equally divided doses. The largest dose should be given at bedtime if doses are not equally divided.

In the treatment of panic disorder, the daily dosage of clonazepam may be given in 2 equally divided doses. Alternatively, the drug may be given as one dose at bedtime to reduce the inconvenience of somnolence.

Clonazepam also has been administered IV†, but a parenteral dosage form is not currently commercially available in the US.

Patients who are currently receiving or beginning therapy with clonazepam and/or any other anticonvulsant for any indication should be closely monitored for the emergence or worsening of depression, suicidal thoughts or behavior (suicidality), and/or any unusual changes in mood or behavior. (See Cautions: CNS Effects and Cautions: Precautions and Contraindications, in the Anticonvulsants General Statement 28:12.)

■ **Dosage** Dosage of clonazepam must be carefully and slowly adjusted according to individual requirements and response. Clonazepam should be withdrawn slowly, and abrupt discontinuance of the drug should be avoided, especially during long-term, high-dose therapy to avoid precipitating seizures, status epilepticus, or withdrawal symptoms. If clonazepam is to be discontinued in patients who have received prolonged therapy with the drug, it is recommended that dosage be tapered gradually. Addiction-prone patients (e.g., alcoholic patients, individuals known to have been dependent on other drugs) should be carefully monitored while receiving clonazepam or other psychotropic therapy because of the predisposition of these patients to habituation and addiction. During clonazepam withdrawal, simultaneous substitution of another anticonvulsant may be indicated.

Seizure Disorders Various clonazepam dosage regimens have been used in published studies. The manufacturer states that the usual initial dosage for infants and children up to 10 years of age or weighing up to 30 kg is 0.01–0.03 mg/kg daily. Initial pediatric dosage should not exceed 0.05 mg/kg daily given in 2 or 3 divided doses. Dosage may be increased by no more than 0.5 mg every third day until seizure control is achieved with minimal adverse effects. Pediatric maintenance dosage should not exceed 0.2 mg/kg daily.

Initial adult dosage of clonazepam should not exceed 1.5 mg daily given in 3 equally divided doses. Dosage may be increased in increments of 0.5–1 mg every third day until seizure control is achieved with minimal adverse effects. Adult maintenance dosage should not exceed 20 mg daily.

Panic Disorder For the management of panic disorder in adults, the recommended initial dosage of clonazepam is 0.25 mg twice daily. An increase to the target dose for most patients of 1 mg daily may be made after 3 days. The manufacturer states that the recommended dosage of 1 mg daily is based on the results of a fixed-dose study in which the optimal therapeutic effect was seen at this dosage. In this study, higher dosages of 2, 3, and 4 mg daily were found to be less effective than the 1 mg daily dosage and more commonly associated with adverse effects (e.g., somnolence and ataxia). Some clinicians recommend a dosage of 1–2 mg daily in patients with panic disorder and the manufacturer states that certain individual patients may benefit from dosages up to a maximum of 4 mg daily. In such cases, the dosage of clonazepam may be increased in increments of 0.125–0.25 mg twice daily every 3 days until panic disorder is controlled or until adverse effects make further increases in dosage undesirable.

The manufacturer states that the efficacy of clonazepam for long-term use (i.e., longer than 9 weeks) has not been systematically evaluated in controlled studies. However, limited information from follow-up studies of patients with panic disorder who responded favorably to benzodiazepine therapy indicate that the benefits observed during short-term therapy usually are maintained for longer periods without increases in dosage. In an open study in which patients with panic disorder were treated with clonazepam over a 2-year period, clonazepam produced and maintained a therapeutic benefit without evidence of tolerance development (as manifested by dosage escalation or worsening of clinical status). The manufacturer states that there is insufficient experience concerning how long patients with panic disorder who are treated with clonazepam should remain on the drug. However, some clinicians state that panic disorder is a chronic condition; therefore, it may be reasonable to continue therapy in responding patients. If clonazepam is used for extended periods, the need for continued therapy with the drug should be reassessed periodically.

When clonazepam therapy is to be discontinued in patients with panic disorder, the manufacturer states that therapy should be gradually discontinued by decreasing the dosage by 0.125 mg twice daily every 3 days until the drug is completely withdrawn.

■ **Dosage in Renal and Hepatic Impairment** The effect of renal impairment on clonazepam elimination is not known.

The possibility that clonazepam dosage adjustment may be necessary in patients with hepatic impairment should be considered.

Cautions

■ **Nervous System Effects** The most frequent adverse effects of clonazepam are sedation or drowsiness, ataxia or hypotonia, and behavioral disturbances (principally in children) including aggressiveness, irritability, agitation, and hyperkinesis. In one study, some patients experienced euphoria that was followed by dysphoria. Tolerance to clonazepam varies considerably among patients and is not necessarily dose related. Behavioral disturbances are most likely to occur in patients with preexisting brain damage and/or mental retardation or a history of behavioral or psychiatric disturbances; however, the precise role of clonazepam in inducing behavioral changes in these patients is difficult to assess. It has been suggested that methylphenidate or amphetamines may be useful to control behavioral disturbances if they occur. Drowsiness, ataxia, and behavioral disturbances are most severe during initial therapy and frequently decrease or disappear during continued therapy. It has been suggested that these adverse effects may be minimized by starting with low dosages and gradually increasing dosage over a 2-week period and by administering the drug in divided doses daily. In some patients, however, these adverse effects have necessitated discontinuance of clonazepam.

Adverse neurologic effects of clonazepam include abnormal eye movements, aphonia, choreiform movements, coma, diplopia, dysarthria, dysdiadochokinesis, glassy-eyed appearance, headache, hemiparesis, nystagmus, respiratory depression, slurred speech, tremor, dizziness, and vertigo. Clonazepam also may cause confusion, mental depression, forgetfulness, hallucinations, hysteria, increased libido, insomnia, psychosis, or suicidal tendencies. (See Cautions: Precautions and Contraindications.) Muscle weakness and pains also may occur.

■ **Respiratory Effects** Increased salivation, hypersecretion in upper respiratory passages, chest congestion, rhinorrhea, and shortness of breath may occur in patients receiving clonazepam. In one study, increased salivation, mucous obstruction of the nasopharynx and bronchi, and difficulty in swallowing occurred in infants receiving the drug. The investigator reported that these effects occurred most frequently when clonazepam was used in conjunction with phenobarbital.

■ **Dermatologic Effects** Dermatologic reactions, including hair loss, hirsutism, skin rash, and ankle and facial edema, have been reported in patients receiving clonazepam. Rarely, abnormal skin pigmentation has been reported in patients receiving clonazepam and phenytoin.

■ **GI Effects** Adverse GI effects of clonazepam include constipation, diarrhea, encopresis, gastritis, increased or decreased appetite, weight gain or loss, dyspepsia, nausea, coated tongue, dry mouth, abnormal thirst, and sore gums.

■ **Genitourinary Effects** Adverse genitourinary effects of clonazepam include dysuria, enuresis, nocturia, and urinary retention.

■ **Hematologic Effects** Adverse hematologic effects of clonazepam include anemia, leukopenia, thrombocytopenia, and eosinophilia.

■ **Hepatic Effects** Hepatomegaly and transient elevations of serum aminotransferase and alkaline phosphatase concentrations may occur in patients receiving clonazepam.

■ **Other Adverse Effects** Other reported adverse effects include palpitations, dehydration, general deterioration, fever, and lymphadenopathy. Abnormal retinal vascularization without visual impairment was reported in one patient who received clonazepam and other anticonvulsants.

■ **Precautions and Contraindications** Clonazepam shares the toxic potential of other benzodiazepines, and the usual cautions, precautions, and contraindications of benzodiazepine therapy should be followed. (See Cautions in the Benzodiazepines General Statement 28:24.08.)

Concomitant use of benzodiazepines, including clonazepam, and opiate agonists or opiate partial agonists may result in profound sedation, respiratory depression, coma, and death. Patients receiving clonazepam and/or their caregivers should be apprised of the risks associated with concomitant therapeutic or illicit use of benzodiazepines and opiates. (See Opiate Agonists and Opiate Partial Agonists under Drug Interactions: CNS Depressants.)

Benzodiazepines have the potential to impair judgment, thinking, or motor skills. Therefore, patients receiving clonazepam should be cautioned that the drug may impair their ability to perform activities requiring mental alertness or physical coordination (e.g., operating machinery, driving a motor vehicle) and to avoid such activities until they experience how the drug affects them.

Patients receiving clonazepam should be advised to avoid alcohol while receiving the drug. In addition, they should be advised to notify their clinician if they are taking or plan to take nonprescription (over-the-counter) or prescription medications or alcohol-containing beverages or preparations.

Clinicians should inform patients, their families, and caregivers about the potential for an increased risk of suicidal thinking and behavior (suicidality) associated with anticonvulsant therapy. For a complete discussion, see Cautions: CNS Effects and Cautions: Precautions and Contraindications, in the Anticonvulsants General Statement 28:12.

When used in patients in whom several different types of seizure disorders coexist, clonazepam may increase the incidence or precipitate the onset of generalized tonic-clonic (grand mal) seizures. This may require the addition of appropriate anticonvulsants or an increase in their dosages. The concomitant use of valproic acid and clonazepam may produce absence status.

Because clonazepam may increase salivation, it should be used with caution in patients in whom increased secretions might be harmful. The manufacturer states that the drug also should be used with caution in patients with chronic respiratory disease or impaired renal function. Periodic blood counts and liver function tests should be performed in patients receiving long-term clonazepam therapy.

The manufacturer states that clonazepam is contraindicated in patients with clinical or biochemical evidence of significant hepatic impairment or a history of sensitivity to benzodiazepines. The manufacturer states that the drug is contraindicated in patients with acute angle-closure glaucoma, but it may be used with caution in patients with open-angle glaucoma who are receiving appropriate therapy.

■ **Pediatric Precautions** The effect of long-term administration of clonazepam on physical and mental development in children has not been established. Therefore, the drug should not be administered to pediatric patients with seizure disorders unless the potential benefits outweigh the possible risks.

The manufacturer states that the safety and efficacy of clonazepam in pediatric patients with panic disorder younger than 18 years of age have not been established. Clonazepam has been effective in a limited number of adolescents with panic disorder; however, controlled studies are needed to confirm these preliminary findings.

■ **Pregnancy and Lactation** Safe use of clonazepam during pregnancy has not been established. Adverse fetal effects have been observed in reproduction studies in rats and rabbits. Although several reports suggest an association between use of anticonvulsants in pregnant, epileptic women and an increased incidence of birth defects in children born to these women, a causal relationship to many of these drugs has not been established. The manufacturer states that the majority of women receiving anticonvulsant therapy deliver normal infants. Clonazepam should be used in pregnant women or women who might become pregnant only if the drug is considered essential in the management of their seizures. Anticonvulsants should *not* be discontinued in pregnant women in whom the drugs are administered to prevent major seizures because of the strong possibility of precipitating status epilepticus with attendant hypoxia and threat to life. In individual cases, when the severity and frequency of the seizure disorder are such that discontinuance of therapy does not pose a serious threat to the patient, discontinuance of the drugs may be considered prior to and during pregnancy; however, it cannot be said with any certainty that even minor seizures do not pose some hazard to the fetus. The clinician should carefully weigh these considerations in treating or counseling epileptic women of childbearing potential.

Safe use of clonazepam during lactation has not been established. The manufacturer states that it is inadvisable for women receiving clonazepam to nurse infants.

Drug Interactions

■ **CNS Depressants** Additive CNS depression may occur when clonazepam is administered concomitantly with other CNS depressants, including alcohol, opiate agonists, barbiturates, anxiolytics, sedatives and hypnotics, some antipsychotic agents, monoamine oxidase (MAO) inhibitors, tricyclic antidepressants, and other anticonvulsants. If clonazepam is used concomitantly with other CNS depressants, caution should be used to avoid excessive CNS depression. Patients also should be advised to avoid alcohol while receiving clonazepam therapy.

Opiate Agonists and Opiate Partial Agonists Concomitant use of benzodiazepines, including clonazepam, and opiate agonists or opiate partial agonists may result in profound sedation, respiratory depression, coma, and death. Whenever possible, such concomitant use should be avoided. Opiate antitussive agents should be avoided in patients receiving benzodiazepines, and concomitant use of opiate analgesics and benzodiazepines should be reserved for patients in whom alternative treatment options are inadequate. The lowest effective dosages and shortest possible duration of concomitant therapy should be used, and the patient should be monitored closely for respiratory depression and sedation.

If clonazepam is required for any indication other than epilepsy in a patient receiving opiate therapy, the drug should be initiated at a lower dosage than indicated in the absence of opiate therapy and titrated based on clinical response. If an opiate analgesic is required in a patient receiving clonazepam, the opiate analgesic should be initiated at a reduced dosage and titrated based on clinical response. For further information on potential interactions between benzodiazepines and opiates, see Opiate Agonists and Opiate Partial Agonists under Drug Interactions: CNS Agents, in the Benzodiazepines General Statement 28:24.08.

■ **Phenytoin** In one study, increased serum phenytoin concentrations were reported to occur when clonazepam and phenytoin were administered concomitantly. In another study, plasma clonazepam concentrations decreased when the two drugs were administered. Although the clinical importance of these reports has not been established, it may be desirable to monitor serum concentrations of both drugs during initial concomitant therapy, making dosage adjustments as necessary.

Acute Toxicity

■ **Manifestations** Overdosage of clonazepam may produce somnolence, confusion, ataxia, diminished reflexes, or coma.

■ **Treatment** Treatment of clonazepam intoxication consists of general supportive therapy. Flumazenil, a benzodiazepine antagonist, can be used in the management of benzodiazepine overdosage, but the drug is an adjunct to, not a substitute for, appropriate supportive and symptomatic therapy. (See Flumazenil 28:92.) The possibility that the antagonist could precipitate withdrawal in benzodiazepine-dependent individuals should be weighed carefully against the possible benefits. Clinicians should be aware of the risk of seizure in association with flumazenil administration, particularly in patients receiving long-term benzodiazepine therapy or following tricyclic antidepressant overdosage. The risks of flumazenil therapy should be weighed carefully when multiple-drug overdosage is possible. Flumazenil is *not* indicated in patients with epilepsy who have been treated with benzodiazepines. Antagonism of the benzodiazepine's effects in such patients may provoke seizures.

If ingestion of the benzodiazepine is recent and the patient is fully conscious, emesis should be induced. If the patient is comatose, gastric lavage may be performed if an endotracheal tube with cuff inflated is in place to prevent aspiration of gastric contents. Activated charcoal and a saline cathartic may be administered after gastric lavage and/or emesis to remove any remaining drug. The patient's heart rate, blood pressure, and respiration should be monitored and the patient closely observed. IV fluids should be administered and an adequate airway maintained. Hypotension may be controlled, if necessary, by IV administration of norepinephrine or metaraminol. Although some manufacturers of benzodiazepines recommend use of caffeine and sodium benzoate to combat CNS depression, most authorities believe caffeine and other analeptic agents should *not* be used, because these drugs have questionable benefit and transient action. Instead, administration of flumazenil, if indicated, generally would be preferred. As in overdosage with other benzodiazepines, dialysis is of no known value in clonazepam overdosage.

Chronic Toxicity

The possibility of physical or psychological dependence should be considered, particularly when clonazepam is administered to alcoholic patients or to those known to have been dependent on other drugs. Abrupt withdrawal of clonazepam following prolonged administration has resulted in severe withdrawal symptoms including seizures, psychosis, hallucinations, behavioral disturbances, tremors, abdominal and muscle cramps, vomiting, sweating, irritability, restlessness, sleeplessness, and hand tremors. In one study, patients who experienced some of these withdrawal symptoms had plasma 7-aminoclonazepam concentrations 3–4 times greater than those who did not have withdrawal symptoms. In addition, milder withdrawal symptoms such as dysphoria and insomnia have been reported following abrupt discontinuance of benzodiazepines in patients receiving therapeutic dosages for several months. Because clonazepam has a long half-life, withdrawal symptoms may not occur until several days after the drug has been discontinued.

Pharmacology

The pharmacologic actions of clonazepam are qualitatively similar to those of other benzodiazepine derivatives.

In animal studies, clonazepam has been shown to protect against seizures induced by pentylenetetrazol and, to a lesser extent, electrical stimulation. Clonazepam also appears to antagonize seizures produced by photic stimulation in animals. In humans, clonazepam can suppress the spike and wave discharge in absence seizures (petit mal) and can decrease the frequency, amplitude, duration, and spread of discharge in minor motor seizures. Clonazepam also has been shown to produce a taming effect, muscle weakness, and hypnosis in animals.

The exact mechanism(s) by which clonazepam exerts its anticonvulsant, sedative, and antipanic effects is unknown. However, it is believed to be related at least in part to the drug's ability to enhance the activity of γ-aminobutyric acid (GABA), the principal inhibitory neurotransmitter in the central nervous system.

Pharmacokinetics

■ **Absorption** Clonazepam is rapidly and well absorbed from the GI tract. The absolute bioavailability is approximately 90%. In one study, peak blood concentrations of 6.5–13.5 ng/mL were usually reached within 1–2 hours following a single 2-mg oral dose of micronized clonazepam in healthy adults. In some individuals, however, peak blood concentrations were reached at 4–8 hours. Although the plasma concentration of clonazepam required for anticonvulsant effects has not been definitely established, some studies indicate it may be 20–80 ng/mL. Plasma concentrations in this range have been reported to be maintained in adults receiving 6 mg of clonazepam daily in 3 divided doses and in children 6–13 years of age receiving 1.5–4 mg of the drug daily in 3 divided doses. The onset of anticonvulsant action usually occurs within 20–60 minutes, and the duration of action usually is 6–8 hours in infants and young children and up to 12 hours in adults.

■ **Distribution** There is little information on the distribution of clonazepam. Clonazepam is approximately 85% bound to plasma proteins. Like other benzodiazepines, the drug apparently crosses the blood-brain barrier and the placenta.

■ **Elimination** The elimination half-life of clonazepam has been reported to be 18.7–39 hours.

Clonazepam is extensively metabolized in the liver to several metabolites including 7-aminoclonazepam, 7-acetaminoclonazepam, and 3-hydroxy derivatives of these metabolites and clonazepam. Clonazepam metabolites are excreted in urine by first-order kinetics, principally as their glucuronide and/or sulfate conjugates. Only very small amounts of the drug (less than 2%) are excreted unchanged.

Chemistry and Stability

■ **Chemistry** Clonazepam is a benzodiazepine derivative that is used both as an anticonvulsant and for the treatment of panic disorder with or without agoraphobia. The drug is structurally and pharmacologically related to diazepam and other benzodiazepines. Clonazepam occurs as an off-white to light yellow, crystalline powder with a faint odor and is insoluble in water and slightly soluble in alcohol. Clonazepam has pK_as of 1.5 and 10.5.

■ **Stability** Clonazepam tablets and orally disintegrating tablets should be stored in air-tight, light-resistant containers at 25°C, but may be exposed to temperatures ranging from 15–30°C. The commercially available conventional tablets have an expiration date of 5 years following the date of manufacture.

For further information on uses, cautions, and dosage and administration of clonazepam, see the Anticonvulsants General Statement 28:12 and the Benzodiazepines General Statement 28:24.08.

Preparations

Clonazepam is subject to control under the Federal Controlled Substances Act of 1970 as a schedule IV (C-IV) drug.

Excipients in commercially available drug preparations may have clinically important effects in some individuals; consult specific product labeling for details.

clonazePAM

Oral		
Tablets	0.5 mg*	**clonazePAM Tablets** (C-IV)
		KlonoPIN® (C-IV; scored), Genentech
	1 mg*	**clonazePAM Tablets** (C-IV)
		KlonoPIN® (C-IV), Genentech
	2 mg*	**clonazePAM Tablets** (C-IV)
		KlonoPIN® (C-IV), Genentech
Tablets, orally disintegrating	0.125 mg*	**clonazePAM Orally Disintegrating Tablets** (C-IV)
	0.25 mg*	**clonazePAM Orally Disintegrating Tablets** (C-IV)
	0.5 mg*	**clonazePAM Orally Disintegrating Tablets** (C-IV)
	1 mg*	**clonazePAM Orally Disintegrating Tablets** (C-IV)
	2 mg*	**clonazePAM Orally Disintegrating Tablets** (C-IV)

*available from one or more manufacturer, distributor, and/or repackager by generic (nonproprietary) name

†Use is not currently included in the labeling approved by the US Food and Drug Administration

HYDANTOINS 28:12.12

Fosphenytoin Sodium

Phosphenytoin Sodium

■ Fosphenytoin sodium, a prodrug of phenytoin, is a hydantoin-derivative anticonvulsant.

Uses

■ **Seizure Disorders** Fosphenytoin is used for the treatment of generalized tonic-clonic status epilepticus. Benzodiazepines (e.g., diazepam, lorazepam, midazolam) are considered the drugs of choice for initial treatment of status epilepticus; IV fosphenytoin (or phenytoin) may be used as a second-line agent if seizures continue. Because the full antiepileptic effect of phenytoin (whether given as fosphenytoin or phenytoin) is not immediate, concurrent use of an IV benzodiazepine usually is necessary for rapid control of status epilepticus. If administration of fosphenytoin does not terminate seizures, the use of other anticonvulsants, IV barbiturates, general anesthesia, and/or other measures should be considered. (See Status Epilepticus under Seizure Disorders: Principles of Anticonvulsant Drug Therapy, in Uses in the Anticonvulsants General Statement 28:12.)

Fosphenytoin also can be used for the prevention and treatment of seizures occurring during neurosurgery and as a short-term parenteral replacement for oral phenytoin; because of the risks associated with parenteral administration of the drug, the manufacturer states that fosphenytoin should be used only when oral phenytoin administration is not possible.

There are insufficient data regarding the comparative efficacy of IV fosphenytoin and IV phenytoin in the management of status epilepticus. Some clinicians state that since therapeutic plasma concentrations of unbound (free) phenytoin (about 1–2 mcg/mL) are attained within about 10 minutes when IV loading doses of fosphenytoin sodium (15–20 mg PE/kg [about 1200 mg PE]) or phenytoin sodium (15–20 mg/kg [about 1200 mg]) are infused at maximally tolerated infusion rates (100–150 mg PE/minute or 50 mg/minute, respectively), the onset of action of IV fosphenytoin sodium in controlling status epilepticus is likely to be similar to that of IV phenytoin sodium. However, duration of infusion usually is longer with phenytoin than with fosphenytoin.

IV fosphenytoin appears to be better tolerated than IV phenytoin, and some experts state that fosphenytoin is preferred when both agents are available. There is some evidence indicating that IV fosphenytoin produces less adverse cardiovascular effects (e.g., cardiac arrhythmias, hypotension) than IV phenytoin. Although IV administration of fosphenytoin sodium is associated with fewer local reactions (e.g., erythema, pain, burning, swelling, pruritus, soft tissue damage, phlebitis, necrosis) at the infusion site and less frequent need for infusion rate reduction, infusion interruption, and/or changes of infusion sites than IV administration of phenytoin sodium, IV fosphenytoin is associated with a higher incidence of systemic sensory disturbances (e.g., paresthesia, burning, pruritus). The higher incidence of local reactions occurring with administration of IV phenytoin sodium is possibly due to the high alkalinity (pH of about 12) of phenytoin sodium injection and/or the presence of vehicles (propylene glycol and ethanol) necessary to solubilize the drug; the aqueous fosphenytoin sodium injection has a pH of 8.6–9 and does not contain these vehicles.

When IM administration is needed (e.g., when IV access is not possible), fosphenytoin rather than phenytoin should be used since fosphenytoin is well absorbed from IM injection sites. Following IM administration of fosphenytoin sodium, the resultant systemic phenytoin concentrations are slightly higher than those achieved with oral use of phenytoin sodium. However, IM administration of fosphenytoin sodium generally should not be used for the treatment of status epilepticus because of the delay in reaching therapeutic concentrations. Phenytoin generally should not be administered IM because of its erratic absorption and localized adverse effects.

Dosage and Administration

■ **General** The dose, concentration, and rate of infusion of fosphenytoin sodium are expressed in terms of phenytoin sodium equivalents (PE); therefore, molecular weight-based adjustments are not necessary when converting between fosphenytoin sodium and phenytoin sodium. **Fosphenytoin sodium always should be prescribed and dispensed in terms of phenytoin sodium equivalents (PE), and the amount and concentration of fosphenytoin should always be expressed in terms of mg of phenytoin sodium equivalents (mg PE).**

Inadvertent overdosage of fosphenytoin (including fatalities) has occurred when the concentration stated on the drug vial was misinterpreted as the total amount of drug in the vial. Therefore, particular care should be taken to ensure that the correct dose of the drug is administered, including careful attention to the concentration of fosphenytoin sodium (expressed in mg PE/mL) present in the vial and the volume of drug (in mL) that is withdrawn from the vial. (See Dosing Errors under Warnings/Precautions: Other Warnings and Precautions, in Cautions.)

Fosphenytoin therapy should be withdrawn gradually to minimize the possibility of increased seizure frequency, including status epilepticus. (See Discontinuance of Therapy under Warnings/Precautions: Other Warnings and Precautions, in Cautions.)

Therapeutic Drug Monitoring Therapeutic drug monitoring of serum phenytoin concentrations is recommended to guide dosing of fosphenytoin. Trough concentrations (obtained just prior to the next scheduled dose) can be used to assess therapeutic effect and patient compliance, while peak concentrations (obtained at the time of expected peak concentration) can be used to assess toxicity. The usual therapeutic range for phenytoin is 10–20 mcg/mL (or 1–2 mcg/mL based on unbound [free] phenytoin concentrations); however, some patients may achieve adequate seizure control or experience toxicity with lower or higher concentrations. To obtain an accurate measurement, serum phenytoin concentrations should not be monitored until conversion of fosphenytoin to phenytoin is essentially complete (about 2 hours after completion of an IV infusion or 4 hours after IM injection); prior to complete conversion, over-estimation of serum phenytoin concentrations may occur because of cross-reactivity between fosphenytoin and phenytoin when certain immunoanalytical assay techniques are used.

Patients with renal or hepatic impairment and those with hypoalbuminemia have an increased fraction of free phenytoin due to altered protein binding; therefore, free phenytoin concentrations rather than total serum concentrations should be monitored in these patients.

■ **Administration** Fosphenytoin sodium is administered by IV infusion or IM injection. IM administration of fosphenytoin generally is not recommended in pediatric patients, but may be used in nonemergent situations in adults (when IV administration is not possible). Fosphenytoin should not be administered IM in the treatment of status epilepticus.

IV Administration Fosphenytoin sodium is administered by IV infusion.

Prior to IV infusion, the commercially available injection must be diluted in 5% dextrose injection or 0.9% sodium chloride injection to provide a solution containing 1.5–25 mg PE/mL. The maximum recommended concentration should not exceed 25 mg PE/mL. Solutions of fosphenytoin should be inspected visually for particulate matter and discoloration prior to administration. Vials are for single dose only; any unused portions should be discarded.

The manufacturer states that continuous ECG, blood pressure, and respiratory monitoring is essential during IV administration of fosphenytoin. Patients should be observed closely during the period when peak serum phenytoin concentrations are expected (about 10–20 minutes after completion of the IV infusion).

Rate of Administration. In adults with status epilepticus, IV loading doses of fosphenytoin should be administered at a rate of 100–150 mg PE/minute. For nonemergent situations in adults, IV loading doses should be administered at a rate not exceeding 150 mg PE/minute. In pediatric patients with status epilepticus, IV loading doses of fosphenytoin should be administered at a rate of 2 mg PE/kg per minute (or 150 mg PE/minute, whichever is slower). For nonemergent situations in pediatric patients, IV loading doses should be administered at a rate not exceeding 2 mg PE/kg per minute (or 150 mg PE/minute, whichever is slower) and maintenance doses should be administered at a rate not exceeding 1–2 mg PE/kg per minute (or 100 mg PE/minute, whichever is slower).

Because of the risk of cardiovascular complications, the rate of IV administration should not exceed 150 mg PE/minute in adults and 2 mg PE/kg per minute (or 150 mg PE/minute, whichever is slower) in pediatric patients. (See Cardiovascular Toxicity under Warnings/Precautions: Warnings, in Cautions.)

IM Administration In controlled clinical trials, IM fosphenytoin was administered once daily in 1 or 2 injection sites. However, some patients may require more frequent IM dosing.

■ **Dosage** Dosage of fosphenytoin sodium is expressed in terms of phenytoin sodium equivalents (PE); 1.5 mg of fosphenytoin sodium is equivalent to 1 mg of phenytoin sodium and is referred to as 1 mg PE. (See Dosage and Administration: General.) IV and IM dosages of fosphenytoin sodium (in terms of PE) are the same, and total daily doses of parenteral fosphenytoin sodium (in terms of PE) generally are equivalent to those of oral phenytoin sodium.

Status Epilepticus For the treatment of status epilepticus in adults, the manufacturer recommends an IV fosphenytoin loading dose of 15–20 mg PE/kg infused at a rate of 100–150 mg PE/minute. Some clinicians recommend a higher initial fosphenytoin dose of 20 mg PE/kg (maximum of 1500 mg PE per dose) administered at a rate not exceeding 150 mg PE/minute; an additional dose of 5–10 mg PE/kg may be given after 10 minutes if seizures continue. The loading dose should be followed by maintenance doses of either fosphenytoin or phenytoin. Because of the risks of cardiac and local toxicity associated with IV administration of fosphenytoin, oral phenytoin should be used whenever possible for maintenance dosing. If fosphenytoin is used, the recommended initial maintenance dosage in adults is 4–6 mg PE/kg daily (administered in divided doses at an infusion rate not exceeding 150 mg PE/minute). Maintenance dosing should begin at the next identified dosing interval. Subsequent maintenance dosage should be individualized based on serum phenytoin concentrations.

For the treatment of status epilepticus in pediatric patients, the manufacturer recommends an IV fosphenytoin loading dose of 15–20 mg PE/kg infused at a rate of 2 mg PE/kg per minute (or 150 mg PE/minute, whichever is slower). The loading dose should be followed by maintenance doses of either fosphenytoin or phenytoin. Because of the risks of cardiac and local toxicity associated with IV administration of fosphenytoin, oral phenytoin should be used whenever possible for maintenance dosing. If fosphenytoin is used, the recommended initial maintenance dosage in pediatric patients is 2–4 mg PE/kg every 12 hours at an infusion rate of 1–2 mg PE/kg per minute (or 100 mg PE/minute, whichever is slower) beginning 12 hours after the loading dose. Subsequent maintenance dosage should be individualized based on serum phenytoin concentrations.

Because the onset of action of phenytoin is not immediate, concomitant therapy with an IV benzodiazepine usually is necessary for the initial control of status epilepticus. (See Uses: Seizure Disorders.)

Nonemergency Loading and Maintenance Dosages Because of the risks associated with IV fosphenytoin, oral phenytoin should be used whenever possible.

If fosphenytoin is used for a nonemergent situation (e.g., for prevention or treatment of seizures during neurosurgery), the recommended loading dose in adults is 10–20 mg PE/kg by IV infusion (at a rate not exceeding 150 mg PE/minute) or IM injection. The loading dose should be followed by an initial fosphenytoin maintenance dosage of 4–6 mg PE/kg daily, administered in divided doses at an infusion rate not exceeding 150 mg PE/minute. Maintenance dosing should begin at the next identified dosing interval. Subsequent maintenance dosage should be individualized based on serum phenytoin concentrations. (See Therapeutic Drug Monitoring under Dosage and Administration: General.)

If fosphenytoin is used for a nonemergent situation in pediatric patients, the recommended loading dose is 10–15 mg PE/kg administered by IV infusion at a rate of 1–2 mg PE/kg per minute (or 150 mg PE/minute, whichever is slower). The loading dose should be followed by an initial maintenance dosage of 2–4 mg PE/kg every 12 hours administered by IV infusion at a rate of 1–2 mg PE/kg per minute (or 100 mg PE/minute, whichever is slower) beginning 12 hours after the loading dose. Subsequent maintenance dosage should be individualized based on serum phenytoin concentrations. (See Therapeutic Drug Monitoring under Dosage and Administration: General.) IM administration of fosphenytoin generally is not recommended in pediatric patients.

Conversion from Oral Phenytoin to Parenteral Fosphenytoin Patients being transferred from oral phenytoin to IM or IV fosphenytoin sodium therapy may receive the same total daily dosage in terms of PE. When transitioning from phenytoin sodium capsules to parenteral fosphenytoin, serum phenytoin concentrations may be slightly higher because the bioavailability of the capsules is 90%.

■ **Special Populations** The manufacturer makes no specific dosage recommendations for patients with renal or hepatic impairment or those with hypoalbuminemia. (See Renal and Hepatic Impairment and Hypoalbuminemia under Warnings/Precautions: Specific Populations, in Cautions.)

Lower doses or less frequent dosing of fosphenytoin may be necessary in geriatric patients. (See Geriatric Use under Warnings/Precautions: Specific Populations, in Cautions.)

In pregnant patients, serum phenytoin concentrations should be monitored closely and dosage of fosphenytoin should be adjusted as necessary. Restoration of the original dosage will probably be necessary postpartum. (See Pregnancy under Warnings/Precautions: Specific Populations, in Cautions.)

Cautions

■ **Contraindications** History of hypersensitivity to fosphenytoin or any ingredient in the formulation, phenytoin, or other hydantoins.

Sinus bradycardia, sinoatrial block, second- or third-degree atrioventricular (AV) block, or Adams-Stokes syndrome.

History of prior acute hepatotoxicity with fosphenytoin or phenytoin.

Concomitant use with delavirdine.

■ **Warnings/Precautions** ***Warnings*** **Cardiovascular Toxicity.** Severe hypotension and cardiac arrhythmias, including bradycardia, heart block, QT-interval prolongation, ventricular tachycardia, and ventricular fibrillation, have occurred following rapid IV administration of fosphenytoin (and phenytoin), sometimes resulting in asystole, cardiac arrest, and death. Severe complications appear to be most common in critically ill patients, geriatric patients, and those with hypotension and severe myocardial insufficiency, although cardiac events also have been reported in adults and pediatric patients without underlying cardiac disease or other comorbidities and at recommended dosages and infusion rates.

To minimize the risk of cardiovascular toxicity, the rate of IV administration of fosphenytoin should not exceed 150 mg PE/minute in adults and should not exceed 2 mg PE/kg per minute (or 150 mg PE/minute, whichever is slower) in pediatric patients. While the risk of toxicity increases with infusion rates above the recommended rates, cardiac events also can occur at or below these rates. Cardiac and respiratory monitoring should be performed during and after IV administration of fosphenytoin. A reduction in the rate of administration or discontinuance of the drug may be necessary.

Fosphenytoin is contraindicated in patients with sinus bradycardia, sinoatrial block, second- and third-degree AV block, or Adams-Stokes syndrome because of the drug's effects on ventricular automaticity.

Sensitivity Reactions **Serious Dermatologic Reactions.** Serious and sometimes fatal dermatologic reactions, including acute generalized exanthematous pustulosis (AGEP), Stevens-Johnson syndrome (SJS), and toxic epidermal necrolysis (TEN), have been reported in patients receiving phenytoin, the active metabolite of fosphenytoin. The onset of these reactions is usually within the first 28 days of therapy. Fosphenytoin should be discontinued at the first sign of a rash, unless the rash is clearly not drug related. If manifestations are suggestive of SJS or TEN, fosphenytoin therapy should not be resumed and alternative therapy should be considered.

Pharmacogenomic Considerations in the Development of Cutaneous Reactions. Limited data suggest an increased risk of SJS and TEN with phenytoin (the active metabolite of fosphenytoin) in individuals of Asian ancestry who carry the human leukocyte antigen (HLA)-B*1502 allele. A strong association has been found between the presence of HLA-B*1502 and an increased risk of developing SJS and TEN in patients with Chinese ancestry receiving carbamazepine; although evidence is more limited, HLA-B*1502 also has been associated with SJS/TEN in such patients receiving structurally similar anticonvulsants such as phenytoin. These anticonvulsants generally should not be used as alternatives to carbamazepine in HLA-B*1502-positive patients. (See Cautions: Dermatologic and Sensitivity Reactions, in the Anticonvulsants General Statement 28:12.)

Multi-organ Hypersensitivity. Multi-organ hypersensitivity (also known as drug reaction with eosinophilia and systemic symptoms [DRESS]), a potentially fatal or life-threatening reaction, has been reported with several anticonvulsant drugs including fosphenytoin and phenytoin. The clinical presentation is variable, but typically includes eosinophilia, fever, rash, lymphadenopathy, and/or facial swelling associated with other organ system involvement such as hepatitis, nephritis, hematologic abnormalities, myocarditis, or myositis. However, signs and symptoms associated with other organ systems also may occur. If signs and symptoms of DRESS occur during fosphenytoin therapy, patients should be evaluated immediately; if an alternative etiology cannot be identified, the drug should be discontinued.

Hypersensitivity Reactions. Angioedema has been reported in patients receiving fosphenytoin. The drug should be discontinued immediately if manifestations of angioedema (e.g., facial, perioral, or upper airway swelling) occur.

Fosphenytoin and other hydantoins are contraindicated in patients with known hypersensitivity to phenytoin. Clinicians also should consider alternatives to structurally similar compounds such as carboxamides, barbiturates, succinimides, and oxazolidinediones in patients who have experienced phenytoin hypersensitivity. Similarly, if there is a history of hypersensitivity reactions to these structurally similar drugs in the patient or immediate family member, alternatives to fosphenytoin should be considered.

Other Warnings and Precautions **Dosing Errors.** The dose of fosphenytoin sodium should always be expressed in terms of mg of phenytoin sodium equivalents (mg PE). This eliminates the need for dose conversions when switching between phenytoin and fosphenytoin. For example, 1000 mg PE of fosphenytoin is equivalent to 1000 mg of phenytoin sodium. (See Dosage and Administration: General.)

Dosing errors, sometimes resulting in fatal overdosage, have occurred when the labeled information on the fosphenytoin vial was misinterpreted. These errors occurred when the concentration stated on the fosphenytoin vial (e.g., 50 mg PE/mL) was misinterpreted as the total amount of drug in the vial (50 mg PE). Fosphenytoin is commercially available in 2-mL vials containing a total of 100 mg PE and 10-mL vials containing a total of 500 mg PE. These errors have resulted in a two- or ten-fold overdosage since each vial actually contains a total of 100 mg PE or 500 mg PE. The total amount of drug in the vial (in mg PE) must not be confused with the concentration of the drug in the vial (in mg PE/mL).

Discontinuance of Therapy. Because of the possibility of increasing seizure frequency or status epilepticus if fosphenytoin is abruptly discontinued, the drug should be withdrawn gradually, and dosage reductions or drug substitutions should be done gradually. In the event of an allergic or hypersensitivity reaction, more rapid substitution with an alternative, non-hydantoin anticonvulsant may be considered.

Hepatotoxicity. Acute hepatotoxicity, including infrequent cases of acute hepatic failure, has been reported with phenytoin (the active metabolite of fosphenytoin). Such events may or may not occur in association with DRESS. (See Multi-organ Hypersensitivity under Warnings/Precautions: Sensitivity Reactions, in Cautions.) Other common manifestations include jaundice, hepatomegaly, elevations of serum hepatic aminotransferase concentrations, leukocytosis, and eosinophilia. The clinical course of hepatotoxicity appears to be variable and ranges from prompt recovery to fatal outcome.

If acute hepatotoxicity occurs, fosphenytoin therapy should be discontinued immediately and not resumed.

Hematologic Effects. Adverse hematologic effects (sometimes fatal), including thrombocytopenia, leukopenia, granulocytopenia, agranulocytosis, and pancytopenia (with or without bone marrow suppression), have been reported with phenytoin.

Local or generalized lymphadenopathy (e.g., benign lymph node hyperplasia, pseudolymphoma, lymphoma, Hodgkin's disease) has occurred in patients receiving phenytoin, although a causal relationship has not been established. In some cases, manifestations have resembled DRESS. (See Multi-organ Hypersensitivity under Warnings/Precautions: Sensitivity Reactions, in Cautions.) Patients who develop lymphadenopathy should be monitored and further evaluated to establish a differential diagnosis; an alternative anticonvulsant should be used if possible.

Because phenytoin may exacerbate porphyria, fosphenytoin should be used with caution in patients with this disease.

Sensory Disturbances. Severe burning, pruritus, and/or paresthesia have been reported in healthy individuals receiving IV fosphenytoin sodium (at a dosage of 1200 mg PE administered at a rate of 150 mg PE/minute). These adverse effects (mainly reported in the groin) ranged from mild to severe and persisted for up to 14 or 24 hours for severe or mild reactions, respectively. The manufacturer states that patients receiving IV fosphenytoin sodium doses of 20 mg PE/kg administered at a rate of 150 mg PE/minute are likely to experience some discomfort, although the incidence and intensity of such discomfort may be decreased by reducing or temporarily stopping the infusion. The effect of continued administration of IV fosphenytoin in the presence of these sensations is unknown, but permanent sequelae have not been reported. Although the mechanism of these sensory disturbances has not been elucidated, administration of other phosphate ester-containing drugs also has been associated with burning, pruritus, and/or tingling, predominantly in the groin area.

Local Toxicity. Purple glove syndrome (PGS), characterized by progressive pain, discoloration, and edema of the distal limb, has been reported in patients receiving peripheral IV injections of phenytoin; tissue necrosis and limb ischemia requiring fasciotomy, skin grafting, or amputation have occurred rarely. Although the risk appears to be greater with IV phenytoin, several cases also have been reported in patients receiving fosphenytoin. (See Cautions: Other Adverse Effects and also see Cautions: Precautions and Contraindications, in Phenytoin 28:12.12)

Phosphate Load. Each mg PE of fosphenytoin sodium provides 0.0037 mmol of phosphate. The amount of phosphate contained in the drug should be considered, especially in patients who require phosphate restriction (e.g., patients with severe renal impairment).

Fetal/Neonatal Morbidity and Mortality. Fosphenytoin may cause fetal harm if used during pregnancy. Major congenital malformations, including a fetal hydantoin syndrome, have been reported in children born to epileptic women who received phenytoin alone or in combination with other anticonvulsant drugs during pregnancy. In addition, phenytoin has demonstrated embryotoxic and teratogenic effects in animals. (See Cautions: Pregnancy and Lactation, in Phenytoin 28:12.12.)

Coagulation defects, which may result in life-threatening bleeding disorders, may occur in neonates exposed to phenytoin in utero; because these reactions are related to decreased concentrations of vitamin K-dependent clotting factors, administration of vitamin K to the mother prior to delivery and to the neonate after birth may prevent these complications.

Slow Metabolizers of Phenytoin. A small percentage of patients receiving phenytoin have been found to metabolize the drug slowly; this appears to be due to genetic variations in hepatic enzyme induction. Because serum concentrations of phenytoin may be higher than expected in such individuals, serum concentrations should be checked immediately if early signs of CNS toxicity occur.

Hyperglycemia. Because phenytoin inhibits insulin release, increased serum glucose concentrations may occur, resulting in hyperglycemia. Phenytoin also may increase serum glucose concentrations in patients with diabetes mellitus.

CNS Toxicity. Serum phenytoin concentrations sustained above the therapeutic range have been associated with confusional states such as delirium, psychosis, or encephalopathy; rarely, irreversible cerebellar dysfunction may develop. Since phenytoin is extensively metabolized in the liver, patients with hepatic impairment, geriatric individuals, and those who are severely ill may show early signs of such toxicity.

Serum phenytoin concentrations should be checked immediately at the first sign of toxicity. Dosage of fosphenytoin should be reduced if serum concentrations are found to be excessive; if symptoms persist, therapy should be discontinued.

Specific Populations **Pregnancy.** Use of phenytoin during pregnancy has been associated with an increased risk of congenital malformations and other adverse developmental outcomes. (See Fetal/Neonatal Morbidity and Mortality under Warnings/Precautions: Other Warnings and Precautions, in Cautions.)

Reported cases of malignancies, including neuroblastoma, have occurred in children whose mothers received phenytoin during pregnancy.

Because of altered pharmacokinetics of phenytoin during pregnancy, serum concentrations of phenytoin may decline, possibly increasing the frequency of seizures in pregnant women receiving fosphenytoin. If fosphenytoin is administered during pregnancy, serum phenytoin concentrations should be monitored and dosage of fosphenytoin should be adjusted accordingly. (See Dosage and Administration: Special Populations.) Because of altered protein binding, phenytoin concentration monitoring in pregnant women should be based on the unbound (free) phenytoin fraction.

Women who are pregnant while receiving fosphenytoin should be encouraged to enroll in the North American Antiepileptic Drug (NAAED) Pregnancy Registry at 888-233-2334; registry information also is available at http://www.aedpregnancyregistry.org.

Lactation. It is not known whether fosphenytoin is distributed into milk; however, phenytoin is distributed into milk. The known benefits of breastfeeding should be considered along with the woman's clinical need for fosphenytoin and any potential adverse effects on the breast-fed infant from the drug or underlying maternal condition.

Pediatric Use. Safety and efficacy of fosphenytoin have been established for the treatment of generalized tonic-clonic status epilepticus and for the prevention and treatment of seizures occurring during neurosurgery in pediatric patients of all age groups.

Geriatric Use. Fosphenytoin has not been evaluated systematically in geriatric patients. The pharmacokinetic profile of fosphenytoin in geriatric adults is similar to that in younger adults. However, clearance of phenytoin may be reduced in geriatric patients (20% less in patients older than 70 years of age relative to that in adults 20–30 years of age). (See Dosage and Administration: Special Populations.)

Renal and Hepatic Impairment and Hypoalbuminemia. Following IV administration of fosphenytoin sodium in patients with renal or hepatic impairment or in those with hypoalbuminemia, conversion of fosphenytoin to phenytoin may be increased without a similar increase in phenytoin clearance. The resulting increases in serum phenytoin concentrations may be associated with an increased incidence and severity of adverse effects.

Since the fraction of free phenytoin may be increased in patients with renal or hepatic impairment and in those with hypoalbuminemia, total serum phenytoin concentrations should be interpreted with caution in such patients; it is recommended that the free phenytoin fraction be monitored in such patients.

■ **Common Adverse Effects** Adverse effects occurring in 2% or more of patients receiving fosphenytoin include nystagmus, dizziness, pruritus, paresthesia, headache, somnolence, and ataxia. Sensory disturbances such as paresthesia and pruritus have been reported more frequently in patients receiving IV fosphenytoin than in those receiving IV phenytoin.

Drug Interactions

The following drug interaction information is based principally on interactions that are known or expected to occur with phenytoin. Because phenytoin is the active metabolite of fosphenytoin, the same drug interactions are expected to occur with fosphenytoin.

Phenytoin is involved in multiple drug interactions because of its extensive plasma protein binding, saturable metabolism, and potent hepatic enzyme-inducing properties.

No drugs are known to interfere with the conversion of fosphenytoin to phenytoin.

■ **Drugs Affecting or Metabolized by Hepatic Microsomal Enzymes** Phenytoin is metabolized by cytochrome P-450 (CYP) isoenzymes 2C9 and 2C19; concomitant use with drugs that inhibit or induce these CYP isoenzymes can alter serum phenytoin concentrations. Phenytoin is particularly susceptible to inhibitory interactions because of its saturable metabolism. Inhibition of phenytoin metabolism may substantially increase serum concentrations of phenytoin and increase the risk of toxicity. If a drug interaction is suspected, serum phenytoin concentrations should be monitored and dosage of fosphenytoin should be adjusted as necessary.

Drugs that can increase serum phenytoin concentrations include, but are not limited to, azole antifungals (e.g., fluconazole, itraconazole, ketoconazole, miconazole, voriconazole), certain selective serotonin-reuptake inhibitors (SSRIs; e.g., fluoxetine, fluvoxamine, sertraline), cimetidine, omeprazole, sulfonamides, amiodarone, chloramphenicol, chlordiazepoxide, disulfiram, estrogen, fluvastatin, isoniazid, methylphenidate, phenothiazines, salicylates, ticlopidine, tolbutamide, trazodone, and warfarin. Drugs that can decrease serum phenytoin concentrations include, but are not limited to, certain HIV protease inhibitors (e.g., fosamprenavir, nelfinavir, ritonavir), diazepam, diazoxide, folic acid, rifampin, St. John's wort, sucralfate, and theophylline. Certain anticonvulsants (e.g., ethosuximide, felbamate, oxcarbazepine, methsuximide, topiramate) can increase serum phenytoin concentrations, while others (e.g., carbamazepine, vigabatrin) can decrease serum concentrations of phenytoin; phenobarbital and valproate can either increase or decrease serum phenytoin concentrations. Certain antineoplastic agents (e.g., capecitabine, fluorouracil) can increase serum phenytoin concentrations, while others (e.g., bleomycin, carboplatin, cisplatin, doxorubicin, methotrexate) can decrease serum concentrations of the drug.

Phenytoin is a potent inducer of CYP isoenzymes and can therefore decrease plasma concentrations and possibly reduce efficacy of many drugs. Dosage adjustments of these drugs may be necessary when phenytoin is added to or withdrawn from concomitant therapy. Drugs whose efficacy may be impaired by phenytoin include, but are not limited to, azole antifungals (e.g, fluconazole, itraconazole, ketoconazole, posaconazole, voriconazole), certain antineoplastic agents (e.g., irinotecan, paclitaxel, teniposide), delavirdine, neuromuscular blocking agents (e.g., cisatracurium, pancuronium, rocuronium, vecuronium), warfarin, corticosteroids, doxycycline, estrogens, furosemide, oral contraceptives, paroxetine, quinidine, rifampin, sertraline, theophylline, and vitamin D. Drugs whose plasma concentrations may be decreased by phenytoin include, but are not limited to, certain anticonvulsant agents (e.g., carbamazepine, felbamate, lamotrigine, topiramate, oxcarbazepine), certain antilipemic agents (e.g., atorvastatin, fluvastatin, simvastatin), certain antiviral agents (e.g., efavirenz, lopinavir/ritonavir, indinavir, nelfinavir, ritonavir, saquinavir), calcium channel-blocking agents (e.g., nifedipine, nimodipine, nisoldipine, verapamil), albendazole, chlorpropamide, clozapine, cyclosporine, digoxin, disopyramide, folic acid, methadone, mexiletine, praziquantel, and quetiapine. The effect of phenytoin on phenobarbital and valproate concentrations is unpredictable. The effect of phenytoin on fosamprenavir varies depending on whether fosamprenavir is administered alone or in conjunction with ritonavir.

■ **Protein-bound Drugs** Fosphenytoin and phenytoin are extensively bound to plasma proteins and have the potential to displace or be displaced by other protein-bound drugs. Although the clinical importance of this interaction is not known, caution is advised.

■ **Alcohol** Chronic alcohol abuse can decrease serum phenytoin concentrations, while acute alcohol intake can increase concentrations of the drug.

■ **Delavirdine** Phenytoin can substantially reduce plasma concentrations of delavirdine and result in loss of virologic response and possible resistance to delavirdine or to the class of non-nucleoside reverse transcriptase inhibitors. Concomitant use of fosphenytoin and delavirdine is contraindicated.

■ **Neuromuscular Blocking Agents** Resistance to the nondepolarizing neuromuscular blocking agents cisatracurium, pancuronium, rocuronium, and vecuronium has occurred in patients receiving long-term phenytoin therapy. Whether the same effect occurs with other nondepolarizing neuromuscular blocking agents is not known. Patients receiving neuromuscular blocking agents should be monitored closely for more rapid than expected recovery from neuromuscular blockade; increased dosage of the neuromuscular blocking agent may be necessary.

■ **Oral Contraceptives** Phenytoin can induce the metabolism of oral contraceptives and decrease serum concentrations of estrogens and/or progestins. The resulting decrease in concentrations of the oral contraceptive may lead to contraceptive failure.

■ **Warfarin** Warfarin may inhibit phenytoin metabolism and increase serum phenytoin concentrations; in addition, phenytoin may induce hepatic metabolism of warfarin and/or displace the anticoagulant from its protein-binding sites. Depending on the response, prothrombin time (PT) and international normalized ratios (INR) may be increased or decreased. Dosage adjustments may be required when fosphenytoin is added to or withdrawn from concomitant warfarin therapy.

Description

Fosphenytoin sodium is a hydantoin-derivative anticonvulsant. Fosphenytoin sodium, a water-soluble phosphate ester of phenytoin, is a prodrug and has little, if any, anticonvulsant activity until hydrolyzed in vivo to phenytoin. The pharmacologic effects of fosphenytoin are attributed to phenytoin. The exact mechanism of action has not been established, but may be due to voltage-dependent blockade of membrane sodium channels, resulting in a reduction in sustained high-frequency neuronal discharges.

Following parenteral administration, fosphenytoin sodium is rapidly hydrolyzed (by nonspecific phosphatases) in blood and other tissues (conversion half-life of approximately 8–15 minutes after IV administration) to phenytoin, phosphate, and formaldehyde (subsequently converted to formate). While phosphate and formaldehyde (formate) have potentially important biologic effects, these effects occur at concentrations substantially higher than those attained with recommended dosages of fosphenytoin.

The dose and concentration of fosphenytoin sodium are expressed in terms of phenytoin sodium equivalents (PE) in order to avoid the need for molecular weight-based adjustments when converting from fosphenytoin sodium to phenytoin sodium or vice versa. (See Dosage and Administration: Dosage.)

IV administration of a 15- to 20-mg PE/kg (about 1200 mg PE) loading dose of fosphenytoin sodium at a rate of 100–150 mg PE/minute in adults results (within about 10–30 minutes) in therapeutic plasma concentrations of unbound phenytoin of about 1–2 mcg/mL, which are similar to those achieved with an equivalent dose (15–20 mg/kg; about 1200 mg) of phenytoin sodium administered IV at a rate of 50 mg/minute.

For further information on chemistry, pharmacology, and pharmacokinetics, see Phenytoin 28:12.12 and see the Anticonvulsants General Statement 28:12.

Advice to Patients

Risk of adverse cardiovascular reactions, including severe hypotension and cardiac arrhythmias, with rapid IV administration; advise patients to report any possible manifestations to their clinician.

Importance of not abruptly discontinuing therapy.

Importance of immediately reporting early manifestations of hematologic, dermatologic, hypersensitivity, or hepatic reactions such as fever, sore throat, infection, rash, mouth ulcers, easy bruising, lymphadenopathy, facial swelling, petechial or purpuric hemorrhage, anorexia, nausea/vomiting, or jaundice. Advise patients to report these manifestations even if they are mild in severity or occur after extended use.

Importance of seeking immediate medical care if signs or symptoms of angioedema (e.g., facial, perioral, or upper airway swelling) occur.

Importance of cautioning patients not to use other drugs or alcoholic beverages without first seeking the clinician's advice.

Importance of informing clinicians of existing or contemplated concomitant therapy, including prescription and OTC drugs and dietary or herbal supplements, as well as any concomitant illnesses.

Warn women of childbearing potential that fosphenytoin can cause teratogenic effects. Advise women of childbearing potential to use effective contraceptive methods during fosphenytoin therapy. Importance of women informing clinicians if they are or plan to become pregnant or plan to breast-feed; discuss therapeutic options with their clinician if pregnancy is planned. Importance of clinicians informing women about the existence of and encouraging enrollment in the NAAED pregnancy registry.

Importance of informing patients of other important precautionary information. (See Cautions.)

Overview® (see Users Guide). For additional information on this drug until a more detailed monograph is developed and published, the manufacturer's labeling should be consulted. It is *essential* that the manufacturer's labeling be consulted for more detailed information on usual cautions, precautions, contraindications, potential drug interactions, laboratory test interferences, and acute toxicity.

Preparations

Excipients in commercially available drug preparations may have clinically important effects in some individuals; consult specific product labeling for details.

Fosphenytoin Sodium

Parenteral		
Injection	50 mg (as phenytoin sodium equivalents [PE]) per mL*	**Cerebyx®**, Pfizer **Fosphenytoin Sodium Injection**

*available from one or more manufacturer, distributor, and/or repackager by generic (nonproprietary) name

Phenytoin — Diphenylhydantoin, DPH
Phenytoin Sodium — Diphenylhydantoin Sodium

■ Phenytoin is a hydantoin-derivative anticonvulsant.

Uses

■ **Seizure Disorders** Phenytoin is used in the management of generalized tonic-clonic (grand mal) seizures and partial seizures with complex symptomatology (psychomotor and temporal lobe seizures). Although efficacy of phenytoin has been well established for the management of seizure disorders, particularly for partial (focal) seizures, use of the drug may be limited because of its complicated pharmacokinetics, adverse effects, and multiple drug interactions. Phenytoin is not recommended for the treatment of pure absence (petit mal) seizures since the drug may increase the frequency of these seizures, but may be used in conjunction with other anticonvulsants when mixed seizure types are present.

Phenytoin sodium also is used IV for the treatment of status epilepticus; however, the usefulness of the drug in this condition is limited by the need for slow administration and its slow onset of action. Benzodiazepines (e.g., diazepam, lorazepam, midazolam) are considered the drugs of choice for initial treatment of status epilepticus; IV phenytoin or fosphenytoin (a prodrug of phenytoin) may be used as a second-line agent if seizures continue. IV fosphenytoin appears to be better tolerated than IV phenytoin, and some experts state that fosphenytoin is preferred when both drugs are available. Because the full antiepileptic effect of phenytoin is not immediate, concurrent use of an IV benzodiazepine usually is necessary for rapid control of status epilepticus. If administration of IV phenytoin does not terminate seizures, the use of other anticonvulsants, IV barbiturates, general anesthesia, and/or other measures should be considered. (See Status Epilepticus under Seizure Disorders: Principles of Anticonvulsant Drug Therapy, in the Anticonvulsants General Statement 28:12.)

Phenytoin and phenytoin sodium also may be used for the prevention and treatment of seizures occurring during or following neurosurgery.

■ **Cardiac Arrhythmias** Phenytoin is a class IB antiarrhythmic agent. Because of its potent antiarrhythmic properties, IV phenytoin sodium has been used in the treatment of cardiac arrhythmias†, particularly ventricular arrhythmias† in patients who do not respond to conventional antiarrhythmic agents or to cardioversion. However, current use of phenytoin as an antiarrhythmic agent is limited by its narrow therapeutic window, multiple drug interactions, and adverse effect profile.

IV phenytoin sodium also has been used in the treatment of arrhythmias caused by cardiac glycoside intoxication†. (See Therapeutic Measures under Acute Toxicity: Treatment, in Digoxin 24:04.08.)

■ **Other Uses** Phenytoin has been used in the treatment of some neuropathic pain conditions†. However, there is insufficient evidence from clinical studies to support this use.

Dosage and Administration

■ **Administration** Phenytoin and phenytoin sodium usually are administered orally in the management of seizure disorders. Phenytoin sodium also may be administered parenterally as a short-term replacement for oral phenytoin when oral administration is not possible. Phenytoin sodium is administered by slow IV injection or IV infusion in the treatment of status epilepticus. IM administration of phenytoin generally is not recommended because of the risk of necrosis, abscess formation, and erratic absorption. (See IM Administration under Dosage and Administration: Administration.) Because parenteral administration of phenytoin is associated with more frequent and severe complications, the oral route is preferred for maintaining therapeutic drug concentrations during nonemergency situations; patients receiving the drug parenterally should routinely be assessed for feasibility of oral therapy.

Phenytoin therapy should not be abruptly discontinued to avoid precipitating seizures or status epilepticus. (See Cautions: Precautions and Contraindications.) Dosage reduction, discontinuance of therapy, or substitution with another anticonvulsant should be done cautiously and slowly. When a patient is transferred from phenytoin to another anticonvulsant, dosage of phenytoin should be gradually reduced over a period of about 1 week while at the same time therapy is instituted with a low dosage of the replacement drug.

Patients who are currently receiving or beginning therapy with phenytoin, phenytoin sodium, and/or any other anticonvulsant should be closely monitored for notable changes in behavior that could indicate the emergence or worsening of suicidal thoughts or behavior or depression. (See Cautions: Precautions and Contraindications.)

Therapeutic Drug Monitoring Therapeutic drug monitoring of serum phenytoin concentrations usually is recommended to guide dosing of phenytoin. Trough concentrations (obtained just prior to the next scheduled dose) can be used to assess therapeutic effect and patient compliance, while peak concentrations (obtained at the time of expected peak concentration) can be used to assess toxicity. The usual therapeutic range for phenytoin is 10–20 mcg/mL (or 1–2 mcg/mL based on unbound [free] phenytoin concentrations); however, some patients may achieve adequate seizure control or experience toxicity with lower or higher concentrations.

When serum concentration determinations are necessary, they should be obtained at least 5–7 half-lives after treatment initiation, change in dosage, or addition or discontinuance of another drug to the regimen, so that steady-state drug concentrations may be achieved. Patients with renal or hepatic impairment and those with hypoalbuminemia have an increased fraction of free phenytoin due to altered protein binding; therefore, free phenytoin concentrations rather than total serum concentrations should be monitored in these patients.

Oral Administration Phenytoin is administered orally as chewable tablets, extended-release capsules, or an oral suspension; only the *extended-release* phenytoin *sodium* capsules should be used for once-daily dosing. The extended-release capsules have been specifically formulated to be given as a single daily dose, while other oral formulations (e.g., oral suspension, chewable tablets) have different dissolution characteristics and absorption rates that do not permit once-daily dosing. Careful monitoring of serum phenytoin concentrations is recommended whenever there is a change in dosage form or preparation.

Phenytoin oral suspension should be administered using a calibrated measuring device; a household teaspoon or tablespoon is not an adequate measuring device. To minimize loss of phenytoin oral suspension during oral administration via a nasogastric tube (secondary to adherence to PVC tubing), the suspension can be diluted (e.g., threefold) with a compatible diluent (e.g., sterile water, 5% dextrose, 0.9% sodium chloride) prior to administration, combined with flushing the tube with at least 20 mL of diluent after administration.

IV Administration Phenytoin sodium is administered by slow IV injection or IV infusion.

Although some clinicians have not recommended IV infusions of phenytoin, such administration is feasible provided that appropriate precautions are taken, such as using a suitable infusion fluid (e.g., 0.9% sodium chloride injection), using a sufficiently diluted solution, starting the infusion immediately after preparation and completing administration within a relatively short period, using a 0.22–0.55-μm inline filter, and carefully inspecting the admixture for any discoloration or particulate matter prior to administration. To prepare the IV infusion solution, the commercially available phenytoin sodium injection should be diluted with 0.9% sodium chloride injection to a final concentration of no less than 5 mg/mL; dextrose-containing solutions should not be used for dilution because of the possibility of precipitate formation. Specialized references should be consulted for specific compatibility information. Following dilution, the infusion should begin immediately and must be completed within 1–4 hours. (See Chemistry and Stability: Stability.)

IV administration of phenytoin sodium should be made directly into a large peripheral or central vein through a large-gauge IV catheter to minimize the risk of local toxicity. Prior to administration, the IV catheter should be flushed with sterile saline to check patency. Following administration, the IV catheter should be flushed again with saline to reduce local venous irritation caused by the alkalinity of the solution.

The manufacturer states that continuous ECG, blood pressure, and respiratory monitoring is essential during IV administration of phenytoin.

Rate of Administration. Because of the risk of cardiovascular complications, the manufacturer states that the rate of IV administration of phenytoin sodium should not exceed 50 mg/minute in adults and 1–3 mg/kg per minute (or 50 mg/minute, whichever is slower) in pediatric patients. Some clinicians recommend not exceeding a rate of 0.5 mg/kg per minute in neonates and a rate of 1 mg/kg per minute in infants, children, and adults. A slower rate of administration is recommended in nonemergent situations.

IM Administration IM administration of phenytoin sodium generally is not recommended since the drug is erratically absorbed from IM injection sites and can cause local adverse effects (e.g., pain, necrosis, abscess formation). The manufacturer states that phenytoin should not be administered IM for the treatment of status epilepticus because of the delay in reaching therapeutic concentrations. Some experts state that phenytoin should not be administered by the IM route under any circumstances. If IM administration is needed (e.g., when IV access is not possible), IM fosphenytoin rather than IM phenytoin is preferred since fosphenytoin is well absorbed from IM injection sites.

Patients transitioning from oral to an equal dosage of IM phenytoin may experience a 50–60% decrease in peak plasma phenytoin concentrations due to slower IM absorption of the drug. If IM administration of phenytoin is necessary, dosage must be increased by 50% over the previously established oral dosage to maintain therapeutic serum phenytoin concentrations. To avoid drug accumulation caused by absorption from muscle depots, dosage should be reduced once oral phenytoin therapy is resumed. (See Dosage and Administration: Dosage.) Experience with IM administration for longer than 1 week is lacking; serum phenytoin concentrations should be monitored.

■ **Dosage** Phenytoin formulations containing the free acid form of the drug (oral suspension and chewable tablets) have approximately 8% greater drug content than phenytoin sodium formulations (extended-release capsules and injection); this difference should be considered if a patient is switched from the free acid form to the sodium salt form or vice versa.

Determination of serum phenytoin concentrations may be necessary to achieve optimal dosage adjustments. (See Therapeutic Drug Monitoring under Dosage and Administration: Administration.) Concurrent administration of many drugs can increase or decrease serum concentrations of phenytoin. (See Drug Interactions.)

Seizure Disorders Dosage of phenytoin and phenytoin sodium must be carefully and slowly adjusted according to individual requirements and response. Therapy is usually initiated with a low dosage and gradually titrated over several weeks.

The recommended initial oral dosage of phenytoin for the management of seizure disorders in adults who have not previously received the drug is 100 mg 3 times daily (as chewable tablets or extended-release capsules). Subsequent dosage should be adjusted based on individual requirements up to a maximum of 200 mg 3 times daily. If the oral suspension is used, the recommended initial adult dosage is 125 mg (5 mL of the 125 mg per 5 mL suspension) 3 times daily; dosage should be adjusted based on individual requirements up to a maximum of 625 mg (25 mL) daily. For patients receiving extended-release phenytoin sodium capsules who are stabilized on a dosage of 100 mg 3 times daily, once-daily dosing with 300 mg as extended-release phenytoin sodium capsules may be considered. If necessary, daily dosage may be gradually increased in increments of 100 mg every 2–4 weeks until the desired response is obtained. A period of 7–10 days may be required to achieve steady-state concentrations of the drug, and therefore, any change in dosage should not be made sooner than this interval. Increases in dosage to greater than 300 mg daily may lead to markedly increased serum phenytoin concentrations, and therefore dosage above this level should be carefully and slowly adjusted. Some experts recommend that dosage adjustments above 300 mg daily in adults be made in 25- or 30-mg increments. The optimum daily dosage varies considerably from one patient to another but is usually in the range of 300–400 mg daily for most adults. Lower doses or less frequent dosing may be required in geriatric patients.

In pediatric patients, the recommended initial oral dosage of phenytoin is 5 mg/kg daily administered in 2 or 3 equally divided doses (as chewable tablets, extended-release capsules, or oral suspension). Subsequent dosage should be adjusted based on individual requirements up to a maximum of 300 mg daily in divided doses. Maintenance dosage for children usually ranges from 4–8 mg/kg daily (administered in 2 or 3 equally divided doses); however, usual dosages may vary depending on whether phenytoin is used alone or as adjunctive therapy. Children older than 6 years of age and adolescents may require the minimum adult dosage of 300 mg daily. Some clinicians state that the usual daily phenytoin dosage (administered in 2 or 3 divided doses) for maintenance of seizure control in pediatric patients is 8–10 mg/kg for those 6 months to 3 years of age, 7.5–9 mg/kg for those 4–6 years of age, 7–8 mg/kg for those 7–9 years of age, and 6–7 mg/kg for those 10–16 years of age.

Therapeutic serum phenytoin concentrations can be achieved more rapidly (in 2–24 hours) with an oral loading-dose regimen. Some clinicians have recommended the use of oral loading doses of phenytoin in adults to achieve rapid steady-state concentrations when IV administration is not desirable. There are few published studies evaluating oral loading-dose regimens. Various regimens have been suggested, and clinicians should consult published protocols for information on specific regimens. It is recommended that oral loading-dose regimens be reserved for patients in a clinic or hospital setting where serum phenytoin concentrations can be closely monitored. The manufacturer also recommends that patients with a history of renal or liver disease not receive an oral loading-dose regimen. In one regimen, an initial oral loading dose of 1 g in adults or 500–600 mg in children is administered in divided doses, followed by the usual maintenance dosage, beginning 24 hours after the loading dose. The 1-g oral loading dose for adults is usually administered in doses of 400, 300, and 300 mg at 2-hour intervals to minimize adverse GI effects.

When oral therapy is temporarily not feasible, phenytoin sodium may be given IV at the same total daily oral dosage (administered at a rate not exceeding 50 mg/minute in adults and 1–3 mg/kg per minute [or 50 mg/minute, whichever is slower] in pediatric patients). However, serum phenytoin concentrations may increase slightly when IV phenytoin is substituted for extended-release phenytoin sodium capsules since bioavailability of the capsules is about 90%.

Because of the risks of adverse effects associated with parenteral phenytoin, oral phenytoin should be used whenever possible. However, if IV phenytoin sodium is used in a nonemergent situation (e.g., prevention of seizures during neurosurgery), the manufacturer states that a loading dose of 10–15 mg/kg should be administered slowly in adults. An IV loading dose of 15–20 mg/kg will usually produce serum phenytoin concentrations in the generally accepted therapeutic range of 10–20 mcg/mL in pediatric patients. The rate of IV administration should not exceed 50 mg/minute in adults and 1–3 mg/kg per minute (or 50 mg/minute, whichever is slower) in pediatric patients; however, slower rates are recommended to minimize the risk of cardiovascular toxicity. Following administration of the loading dose, maintenance IV or oral doses of phenytoin should be administered every 6–8 hours.

If IM administration of phenytoin sodium is required, the IM dosage should be increased by 50% over the previously established oral dosage. To avoid drug accumulation resulting from eventual absorption from IM injection sites, it is recommended that for the first week back on oral therapy, the oral dosage be reduced to *one-half* the original oral dosage. Monitoring of serum concentrations is also recommended. Experience with IM therapy for periods longer than 1 week is lacking. (See Dosage and Administration: Administration.)

Status Epilepticus. For the treatment of status epilepticus in adults, the manufacturer recommends an IV phenytoin sodium loading dose of 10–15 mg/kg, administered slowly at a rate not exceeding 50 mg/minute. In pediatric patients, the manufacturer states that an IV phenytoin sodium loading dose of 15–20 mg/kg will usually produce serum concentrations of phenytoin within the generally accepted therapeutic range of 10–20 mcg/mL; the drug should be administered slowly at a rate not exceeding 1–3 mg/kg per minute (or 50 mg/minute, whichever is slower). Some clinicians recommend an initial IV phenytoin sodium dose of 20 mg/kg (administered at a rate not exceeding 50 mg/minute in adults or not exceeding 1 mg/kg per minute in children) in adults and children with status epilepticus; an additional dose of 5–10 mg/kg may be given after 10 minutes if seizures continue. However, individual dosage requirements may vary, and as much as 30 mg/kg may be required to achieve adequate seizure control in some patients. A maximum of 1.5 g in 24 hours has been recommended for the loading dose of phenytoin sodium in patients with status epilepticus. Following administration of the loading dose, IV or oral maintenance doses should be administered every 6–8 hours. Lower doses or less frequent dosing may be required in geriatric patients.

Because of the required slow rate of IV phenytoin administration, concurrent use of an IV benzodiazepine usually is necessary for rapid control of status epilepticus. (See Uses: Seizure Disorders.) Determination of serum phenytoin concentrations is recommended when IV phenytoin is used in the management of status epilepticus; however, treatment should not be delayed to measure serum concentrations.

Cardiac Arrhythmias For the treatment of ventricular tachycardia†, 100 mg of phenytoin sodium has been administered by direct IV injection at 5-minute intervals until the arrhythmia was abolished or undesirable effects appeared or until a total of 1 g was given. Orally, 100 mg of phenytoin or phenytoin sodium has been given 2–4 times daily in the management of cardiac arrhythmias.

For the treatment of arrhythmias associated with cardiac glycoside intoxication†, IV phenytoin sodium loading doses of 1.25 mg/kg administered every 5 minutes up to a total of 15 mg/kg have been recommended in patients of all ages; maintenance IV or oral doses of 5–10 mg/kg daily given in divided doses every 8–12 hours are recommended in pediatric patients, and a maintenance oral dosing regimen consisting of 250 mg 4 times daily for 1 day, then 250 mg every 12 hours for 2 days, then 300–400 mg (in divided or once-daily doses) is recommended in adults.

Cautions

Adverse effects produced by phenytoin are frequent, of a wide variety, and may occasionally be serious in nature, particularly when the drug is administered IV; rarely, fatalities have been reported. In some instances, adverse effects may subside as therapy is continued. Clinical signs of toxicity are more likely to occur with serum phenytoin concentrations above 20 mcg/mL (unbound [free] phenytoin concentrations of 1–2 mcg/mL); however, there is marked variability and patients may experience toxicity with lower or higher concentrations. In some patients, serum phenytoin concentrations of 25 mcg/mL are associated with nystagmus, ataxia, and diplopia. As the blood concentration exceeds 30 mcg/mL, drowsiness and lethargy, and rarely asterixis, may result; extreme lethargy and, occasionally, comatose states occur with concentrations greater than 50 mcg/mL. Some patients metabolize phenytoin slowly and thus exhibit signs of toxicity even with low to moderate dosage. This effect is believed to result from congenital enzyme deficiency.

■ Cardiovascular Effects Rapid IV administration of phenytoin has caused severe hypotension and cardiac arrhythmias, including bradycardia, heart block, ventricular tachycardia, and ventricular fibrillation, sometimes resulting in asystole, cardiac arrest, and death. (See Cautions: Precautions and Contraindications.) Severe complications appear to be most common in critically ill patients, elderly patients, and those with hypotension and severe myocardial insufficiency, although cardiac events also have been reported in patients without underlying cardiac disease or other comorbidities. Cardiovascular toxicity may be due in part to the propylene glycol (cardiac depressant) in the parenteral formulation.

■ Dermatologic and Sensitivity Reactions A scarlatiniform or morbilliform rash, sometimes accompanied by fever, has been reported in patients receiving phenytoin, usually in the first month of therapy. More serious dermatologic reactions that have occurred include bullous, exfoliative, or purpuric dermatitis; acute generalized exanthematous pustulosis (AGEP); Stevens-Johnson syndrome (SJS); and toxic epidermal necrolysis (TEN). (See Cautions: Precautions and Contraindications.)

Multi-organ hypersensitivity (also known as drug reaction with eosinophilia and systemic symptoms [DRESS]), a potentially fatal or life-threatening reaction, has been reported with several anticonvulsant drugs including phenytoin. The clinical presentation is variable, but typically includes eosinophilia, fever, rash, lymphadenopathy, and/or facial swelling associated with other organ system involvement such as hepatitis, nephritis, hematologic abnormalities, myocarditis, or myositis. However, signs and symptoms associated with other organ systems also may occur.

Phenytoin produces hypertrichosis in some patients. Hypertrichosis is usually confined to the extremities but can also occur on the trunk and face and may be irreversible. Coarsening of the facial features in one sister in each of 2 pairs of identical twins has been attributed to phenytoin.

Hypersensitivity reactions, including anaphylaxis and angioedema, also have been reported in patients receiving phenytoin.

Pharmacogenomic Considerations in the Development of Cutaneous Reactions Limited data suggest an increased risk of SJS and TEN with phenytoin in individuals of Asian ancestry who carry the human leukocyte antigen (HLA)-B*1502 allele. A strong association has been found between the presence of HLA-B*1502 and an increased risk of developing SJS and TEN in patients with Chinese ancestry receiving carbamazepine; although evidence is more limited, HLA-B*1502 also has been associated with SJS/TEN in such patients receiving structurally similar anticonvulsants such as phenytoin. These anticonvulsants (e.g., eslicarbazepine, lamotrigine, phenytoin, fosphenytoin, phenobarbital) generally should not be used as alternatives to carbamazepine in HLA-B*1502-positive patients. (See Cautions: Dermatologic and Sensitivity Reactions, in the Anticonvulsants General Statement 28:12.)

■ Hematologic Effects Adverse hematologic effects (sometimes fatal) have been associated with the use of phenytoin, including thrombocytopenia, leukopenia, granulocytopenia, agranulocytosis, and pancytopenia (with or without bone marrow suppression). Macrocytosis and megaloblastic anemia, which usually respond to folic acid therapy, also may occur.

Although a causal relationship has not been established, phenytoin administration may be associated with the development of lymphadenopathy (local or generalized), including benign lymph node hyperplasia, pseudolymphoma, lymphoma, and Hodgkin's disease. (See Cautions: Precautions and Contraindications.) Lymph node involvement may or may not occur in association with DRESS. (See Cautions: Dermatologic and Sensitivity Reactions.)

■ Hepatic Effects Acute hepatotoxicity, including infrequent cases of acute hepatic failure, has been reported with phenytoin. Such events may or may not occur in association with DRESS. (See Cautions: Dermatologic and Sensitivity Reactions.) Toxic hepatitis also has occurred.

■ Nervous System Effects Adverse CNS effects of phenytoin include mental confusion, nystagmus, ataxia, blurred vision, diplopia, toxic amblyopia, dizziness, insomnia, transient nervousness, motor twitching, and headache.

Drowsiness, ataxia, and diplopia are more likely to occur at serum phenytoin concentrations greater than 20 mcg/mL, but can also occur at lower concentrations, particularly in patients with hypoalbuminemia and in geriatric patients. Rarely, phenytoin-induced dyskinesias, including chorea, dystonia, tremor, and asterixis, have been reported. Serum phenytoin concentrations sustained above the therapeutic range may produce confusional states such as delirium, psychosis, or encephalopathy; rarely, irreversible cerebellar dysfunction may develop. A predominantly sensory peripheral polyneuropathy has been observed in patients receiving long-term phenytoin therapy.

An increased risk of suicidality (suicidal behavior or ideation) was observed in an analysis of studies using various anticonvulsants compared with placebo. (See Suicidality under Cautions: CNS Effects, in the Anticonvulsants General Statement 28:12.) This increased suicidality risk was observed as early as 1 week after beginning therapy and continued through 24 weeks. Although patients treated with an anticonvulsant for epilepsy, psychiatric disorders, and other conditions were all found to be at increased risk for suicidality compared with those receiving placebo, the relative suicidality risk was higher for patients with epilepsy compared with those receiving anticonvulsants for other conditions. (See Cautions: Precautions and Contraindications.)

■ **GI Effects** Adverse GI effects of phenytoin include nausea and vomiting, constipation, epigastric pain, dysphagia, loss of taste, anorexia, and weight loss.

■ **Other Adverse Effects** Phenytoin frequently produces gingival hyperplasia, especially in children, which is occasionally so severe that it may require surgical removal. Gingival hyperplasia does not occur in edentulous areas of gums. Secondary inflammatory changes which result in an edematous enlargement of the primary gingival lesion can be minimized by good oral hygiene and gum massage.

Phenytoin has been associated with changes in bone metabolism; decreased bone mineral density (BMD) and related bone effects (e.g., osteopenia, osteoporosis, osteomalacia, fractures) have occurred in epileptic patients receiving long-term therapy with the drug. The mechanism of this effect is thought to be due to phenytoin's interference with vitamin D metabolism.

Phenytoin, especially in large doses, may increase blood glucose concentrations resulting in hyperglycemia and glycosuria. Patients with impaired renal function may be most susceptible to this effect. Average doses do not regularly elevate blood glucose or increase insulin requirements in diabetic patients, but a few patients have experienced fatal, hyperosmolar, nonketotic coma in which phenytoin may have played at least an accessory etiologic role.

IV administration of phenytoin has been associated with local soft-tissue reactions ranging from mild irritation and inflammation to extensive tissue damage (necrosis and sloughing) at the site of injection; amputation has been required rarely. (See Cautions: Precautions and Contraindications.) Severe tissue injury can occur in the presence or absence of extravasation. Purple glove syndrome (PGS), a delayed soft-tissue injury of the hand and forearm, has been reported in patients receiving peripheral IV injections of phenytoin; in at least one case, the condition was reported following oral administration of the drug. PGS is characterized by progressive pain, discoloration, and edema of the distal limb, and may or may not be associated with extravasation. The clinical course of the syndrome typically follows 3 stages. In the initial stage, a distinctive blue or purple skin discoloration appears around the injection site 2–12 hours after phenytoin is administered. This is followed by increasing edema and progression of discoloration distally and proximally over the next 12–24 hours; local skin blistering, sloughing, and ulceration also may occur during this second stage. In the last stage, gradual healing occurs over several days to weeks. PGS generally is a mild and self-limiting condition that can be managed primarily with supportive measures (e.g., limb elevation, application of dry heat); however, in severe cases, tissue necrosis and limb ischemia have occurred requiring surgical intervention such as fasciotomy, skin grafting, or amputation. From initial marketing of the drug in 1956 until June 8, 2010, 43 cases of phenytoin-associated PGS have been reported to FDA; a few of these cases resulted in serious outcomes, including hospitalization and amputation. The specific cause of phenytoin-induced soft-tissue injury is not known, but may be related at least in part to the high alkalinity or presence of vehicles (propylene glycol and ethanol) in the parenteral formulations. Possible risk factors for PGS and other types of severe soft-tissue injury include young or advanced age, female gender, use of small-bore IV catheters, preexisting cardiovascular disease, administration of multiple or large doses, and rapid rates of infusion.

■ **Precautions and Contraindications** Phenytoin shares the toxic potentials of the hydantoin-derivative anticonvulsants, and the usual precautions of anticonvulsant therapy should be observed. (See Cautions in the Anticonvulsants General Statement 28:12.)

Clinicians should inform patients, their families, and caregivers about the potential for an increased risk of suicidal thinking and behavior (suicidality) associated with anticonvulsant therapy. For a complete discussion, see Cautions: CNS Effects and Cautions: Precautions and Contraindications, in the Anticonvulsants General Statement 28:12. If any signs of CNS toxicity (e.g., delirium, psychosis, encephalopathy, cerebellar dysfunction or atrophy) occur during therapy, serum phenytoin concentrations should be measured immediately. If the serum concentration is found to be excessive, dosage of phenytoin should be decreased; if symptoms persist, therapy should be discontinued.

Phenytoin may exacerbate porphyria, and the drug should be used with caution in patients with this disease. If lymphadenopathy occurs during phenytoin therapy, the patient should be closely observed and further evaluated to establish a differential diagnosis; alternative anticonvulsants should be used, if possible, for seizure control.

To minimize the possibility of increasing seizure frequency and status epilepticus, phenytoin should not be abruptly discontinued; therapy should be withdrawn slowly and dosage reductions or drug substitutions should be done gradually. In the event of an allergic or hypersensitivity reaction, more rapid substitution with an alternative, non-hydantoin anticonvulsant may be considered.

Because phenytoin can decrease vitamin D concentrations and cause associated bone-related effects, consideration should be given to monitoring vitamin D concentrations and other measures of bone health in patients receiving long-term therapy with the drug.

Because of altered protein binding, the fraction of unbound (free) phenytoin may be increased in patients with renal or hepatic impairment and in those with hypoalbuminemia; total serum phenytoin concentrations should be interpreted with caution, and it is recommended that the unbound (free) phenytoin concentration be monitored in these patients. A small percentage of patients receiving phenytoin has been found to metabolize the drug slowly; this appears to be due to genetic variations in hepatic enzyme induction. Because serum concentrations of phenytoin may be higher than expected in such individuals, serum concentrations should be checked immediately if early signs of CNS toxicity occur.

To minimize the risk of purple glove syndrome (PGS) and other types of soft-tissue injury, appropriate procedures and precautions for IV phenytoin sodium should be followed. (See Cautions: Other Adverse Effects.) In addition, administration of IV injections of the drug should be followed by administration of sodium chloride injection through the same IV catheter to avoid the risk of local irritation of the vein. Injection sites should be monitored frequently during and for 72 hours following administration of the drug. If PGS occurs, phenytoin should be discontinued immediately and the IV catheter removed. Appropriate supportive measures (e.g., elevation of the affected extremity, application of dry heat) should also be employed. (See Dosage and Administration: Administration.)

IV phenytoin must be administered slowly to minimize the risk of cardiovascular toxicity (see Cautions: Cardiovascular Effects and also see Rate of Administration under Administration: IV Administration, in Dosage and Administration). While the risk of toxicity increases with infusion rates above the recommended rates, cardiac events also can occur at or below these rates. Cardiac and respiratory monitoring should be performed during and after IV administration of the drug. A reduction in the rate of administration or discontinuance of the drug may be necessary. Phenytoin should be administered IV only with extreme caution to patients with respiratory depression, myocardial infarction, frank or impending congestive heart failure, or otherwise damaged myocardium, and in patients in whom a sudden change in blood pressure may lead to serious complications. IV use of the drug is contraindicated in patients with sinus bradycardia, sinoatrial block, second- or third-degree atrioventricular block, or Adams-Stokes syndrome because of the drug's effects on ventricular automaticity.

If a rash appears during phenytoin therapy, the drug should be discontinued unless the rash is clearly not drug related. If manifestations suggestive of SJS or TEN occur, phenytoin therapy should not be resumed and alternative therapy should be considered. Because of the risk of developing SJS and TEN, consideration should be given to avoiding the use of phenytoin as an alternative to carbamazepine in HLA-B*1502-positive patients. (See Pharmacogenomic Considerations in the Development of Cutaneous Reactions under Cautions: Dermatologic and Sensitivity Reactions.) If signs and symptoms of DRESS occur during phenytoin therapy, patients should be evaluated immediately; if an alternative etiology cannot be identified, the drug should be discontinued. (See Cautions: Dermatologic and Sensitivity Reactions.)

Phenytoin is contraindicated in patients with a history of hypersensitivity to the drug, any of its ingredients, or other hydantoins. Clinicians should consider alternatives to structurally similar compounds such as carboxamides, barbiturates, succinimides, and oxazolidinediones in patients who have experienced phenytoin hypersensitivity. Similarly, if there is a history of hypersensitivity to these structurally similar drugs in the patient or immediate family member, alternatives to phenytoin should be considered. If manifestations of angioedema (e.g., facial, perioral, or upper airway swelling) occur during phenytoin therapy, the drug should be discontinued immediately.

Concomitant use of phenytoin and delavirdine is contraindicated because of possible loss of virologic response and resistance to delavirdine or to the class of non-nucleoside reverse transcriptase inhibitors. (See Drug Interactions: Delavirdine.) Phenytoin also is contraindicated in patients who have experienced previous acute hepatotoxicity with the drug.

■ **Pregnancy and Lactation** Phenytoin may cause fetal harm (e.g., congenital malformations, adverse developmental outcomes) if used during pregnancy. However, the risk-to-benefit ratio generally favors continued use in pregnant women whose seizure control depends on the drug. (See Cautions: Pregnancy and Lactation, in the Anticonvulsants General Statement 28:12.) Phenytoin has been associated with a fetal hydantoin syndrome consisting of craniofacial abnormalities, nail and digital hypoplasia, prenatal growth deficiency, microcephaly, and cognitive deficiency; such effects have been observed in children born to epileptic women who received phenytoin alone or in combination with other anticonvulsant drugs during pregnancy. In addition to reports of a fetal hydantoin syndrome, there have been rare reports of malignancies, including neuroblastoma, in children whose mothers received phenytoin during pregnancy. Fetal malformations (e.g., craniofacial, cardiovascular, neural, limb, and digit abnormalities) and other evidence of developmental toxicity (e.g., embryofetal death, growth impairment, behavioral abnormalities) have been observed in animal reproductive studies.

Coagulation defects which have resulted in life-threatening bleeding disorders have been reported in neonates born to women receiving phenytoin during pregnancy; because these reactions are related to decreased concentrations of vitamin K-dependent clotting factors, administration of vitamin K to the mother prior to delivery and to the neonate after birth may prevent these complications.

Women who are pregnant while receiving phenytoin should be encouraged to enroll in the North American Antiepileptic Drug (NAAED) Pregnancy Registry by calling 888-233-2334; registry information also is available at http://www.aedpregnancyregistry.org.

Because of altered pharmacokinetics of phenytoin during pregnancy, serum concentrations of phenytoin may decline, possibly increasing the frequency of seizures in pregnant women receiving the drug. If phenytoin is administered during pregnancy, serum phenytoin concentrations should be monitored and dosage of phenytoin should be adjusted accordingly; however, restoration of the patient's usual dosage will probably be necessary postpartum. Because of potential changes in protein binding of phenytoin during pregnancy, it is recommended that unbound (free) phenytoin concentrations be monitored in pregnant women.

Phenytoin is distributed into milk; however, use of phenytoin is generally considered compatible with breast-feeding. The known benefits of breast-feeding should be considered along with the woman's clinical need for phenytoin and any potential adverse effects on the breast-fed infant from the drug or underlying maternal condition.

Drug Interactions

Phenytoin is involved in multiple drug interactions because of its extensive plasma protein binding, saturable metabolism, and potent hepatic enzyme-inducing properties.

■ **Drugs Affecting or Metabolized by Hepatic Microsomal Enzymes** Phenytoin is metabolized by cytochrome P-450 (CYP) isoenzymes 2C9 and 2C19; concomitant use of drugs that inhibit or induce these CYP isoenzymes can alter serum phenytoin concentrations. Phenytoin is particularly susceptible to inhibitory interactions because of its saturable metabolism. Inhibition of phenytoin metabolism may substantially increase serum concentrations of phenytoin and increase the risk of toxicity. If a drug interaction is suspected, serum phenytoin concentrations should be monitored and dosage of phenytoin should be adjusted as necessary.

Drugs that can increase serum phenytoin concentrations include, but are not limited to, azole antifungals (e.g., fluconazole, itraconazole, ketoconazole, miconazole, voriconazole), certain selective serotonin-reuptake inhibitors (SSRIs; fluoxetine, fluvoxamine, sertraline), cimetidine, omeprazole, sulfonamides, amiodarone, chloramphenicol, chlordiazepoxide, disulfiram, estrogen, fluvastatin, isoniazid, methylphenidate, phenothiazines, salicylates, ticlopidine, tolbutamide, trazodone, and warfarin. Drugs that can decrease serum phenytoin concentrations include, but are not limited to, certain HIV protease inhibitors (e.g., fosamprenavir, nelfinavir, ritonavir), diazepam, diazoxide, folic acid, rifampin, St. John's wort, sucralfate, and theophylline. Certain anticonvulsants (e.g., ethosuximide, felbamate, oxcarbazepine, methsuximide, topiramate) can increase serum phenytoin concentrations, while others (e.g., carbamazepine, vigabatrin) can decrease serum concentrations of phenytoin; phenobarbital and valproate can either increase or decrease serum phenytoin concentrations. Certain antineoplastic agents (e.g., capecitabine, fluorouracil) can increase serum phenytoin concentrations, while others (e.g., bleomycin, carboplatin, cisplatin, doxorubicin, methotrexate) can decrease serum concentrations of the drug.

Phenytoin is a potent inducer of CYP isoenzymes and can therefore decrease plasma concentrations and possibly reduce efficacy of many drugs. Dosage adjustments of these drugs may be necessary when phenytoin is added to or withdrawn from concomitant therapy. Drugs whose efficacy may be impaired by phenytoin include, but are not limited to, azole antifungals (e.g., fluconazole, itraconazole, ketoconazole, posaconazole, voriconazole), certain antineoplastic agents (e.g., irinotecan, paclitaxel, teniposide), delavirdine, neuromuscular blocking agents (e.g., cisatracurium, pancuronium, rocuronium, vecuronium), warfarin, corticosteroids, doxycycline, estrogens, furosemide, oral contraceptives, paroxetine, quinidine, rifampin, sertraline, theophylline, and vitamin D. Drugs whose plasma concentrations may be decreased by phenytoin include, but are not limited to, certain anticonvulsant agents (e.g., carbamazepine, felbamate, lamotrigine, topiramate, oxcarbazepine), certain antilipemic agents (e.g., atorvastatin, fluvastatin, simvastatin), certain antiviral agents (e.g., efavirenz, lopinavir/ritonavir, indinavir, nelfinavir, ritonavir, saquinavir), calcium channel-blocking agents (e.g., nifedipine, nimodipine, nisoldipine, verapamil), albendazole, chlorpropamide, clozapine, cyclosporine, digoxin, disopyramide, folic acid, methadone, mexiletine, praziquantel, and quetiapine. The effect of phenytoin on phenobarbital and valproate concentrations is unpredictable. The effect of phenytoin on fosamprenavir varies depending on whether fosamprenavir is administered alone or in conjunction with ritonavir.

■ **Protein-bound Drugs** Phenytoin is extensively bound to plasma proteins and has the potential to displace or be displaced by other protein-bound drugs.

■ **Alcohol** Chronic alcohol abuse can decrease serum phenytoin concentrations, while acute alcohol intake can increase concentrations of the drug.

■ **Amiodarone** Concomitant administration of phenytoin and amiodarone has resulted in a twofold to threefold increase in steady-state serum concentrations of phenytoin and subsequent signs of phenytoin toxicity (e.g., nystagmus, ataxia, lethargy) in a limited number of patients. The increase in serum phenytoin concentrations occurred within 3–4 weeks of initiating amiodarone therapy. Patients receiving phenytoin should be monitored closely for signs of phenytoin toxicity when amiodarone is administered concomitantly; serum phenytoin concentrations should be monitored and dosage of phenytoin reduced as necessary.

■ **Antacids** Antacids (e.g., calcium carbonate, aluminum hydroxide, magnesium hydroxide) may interfere with absorption and decrease serum concentrations of phenytoin. Antacids should not be taken at the same time of day as phenytoin.

■ **Delavirdine** Phenytoin can substantially reduce plasma concentrations of delavirdine and result in loss of virologic response and possible resistance to delavirdine or to the class of non-nucleoside reverse transcriptase inhibitors. Concomitant use of phenytoin and delavirdine is contraindicated.

■ **Folic Acid** In folate-deficient patients, folic acid therapy may increase phenytoin metabolism resulting in decreased serum phenytoin concentrations. Although this interaction is not usually clinically important, an increase in seizure frequency may occur in some patients.

■ **Isoniazid** Isoniazid appears to inhibit metabolism of phenytoin, thereby increasing serum phenytoin concentrations, decreasing urinary excretion of 5-(*p*-hydroxyphenyl)-5-phenylhydantoin, and resulting in phenytoin toxicity in about 25% of patients receiving concomitant therapy. Phenytoin toxicity occurs mainly in slow isoniazid inactivators and in patients receiving both isoniazid and aminosalicylic acid or cycloserine.

Patients receiving isoniazid and phenytoin should be closely observed for signs of phenytoin intoxication. If clinical evidence of intoxication occurs, reduction of phenytoin dosage to 100 or 200 mg daily may decrease toxicity while maintaining adequate serum phenytoin concentrations. Serum phenytoin concentrations may be less stable in patients receiving isoniazid and aminosalicylic acid, and periodic dosage adjustment may be required.

■ **Neuromuscular Blocking Agents** Resistance to the nondepolarizing neuromuscular blocking agents cisatracurium, pancuronium, rocuronium, and vecuronium has occurred in patients receiving long-term phenytoin therapy. Whether the same effect occurs with other nondepolarizing neuromuscular blocking agents is not known. Patients receiving neuromuscular blocking agents should be monitored closely for more rapid than expected recovery from neuromuscular blockade; increased dosage of the neuromuscular blocking agent may be necessary.

■ **Oral Contraceptives** Phenytoin can induce the metabolism of oral contraceptives and decrease serum concentrations of estrogens and/or progestins. The resulting decrease in concentrations of the oral contraceptive may lead to contraceptive failure.

■ **Warfarin** Several interactions are possible in patients receiving phenytoin and warfarin, and the net effects are difficult to predict. Warfarin may inhibit phenytoin metabolism and increase serum phenytoin concentrations; in addition, phenytoin may induce hepatic metabolism of warfarin and/or displace the anticoagulant from its protein-binding sites. Depending on the response, prothrombin time (PT) and international normalized ratios (INR) may be increased or decreased.

If warfarin and phenytoin are used concomitantly, the patient should be closely monitored. Dosage adjustments may be required when phenytoin is added to or withdrawn from concomitant warfarin therapy.

Laboratory Test Interferences

Patients receiving phenytoin have shown reduced protein-bound iodine (PBI) test values without lowered triiodothyronine (T_3) values and without clinical symptoms of hypothyroidism; free thyroxine concentrations may also be decreased. The 24-hour I 131 thyroidal uptake is apparently not affected. Phenytoin may produce increased resin or red cell T_3 uptake values. Lowered PBI values do not occur unless phenytoin is administered for 1 week or longer, and altered values persist for 7–10 days after phenytoin is discontinued.

Phenytoin administration may cause slight decreases in urinary 17-hydroxycorticosteroids and 17-ketosteroids while urinary 6-β-hydroxycortisol excretion is increased. The drug may produce lower than normal values for dexamethasone or metyrapone tests.

Phenytoin may produce increased serum alkaline phosphatase or γ-glutamyl transferase (γ-glutamyltranspeptidase, GGT, GGTP) concentrations.

Pharmacology

The principal pharmacologic effects of phenytoin are similar to those of other hydantoin-derivative anticonvulsants. The exact mechanism of action of phenytoin has not been established, but may be due to voltage-dependent blockade of membrane sodium channels resulting in a reduction in sustained high-frequency neuronal discharges. In addition, phenytoin exhibits antiarrhythmic properties similar to those of quinidine or procainamide. Although the drug has little effect on the electrical excitability of cardiac muscle, it decreases the force of contraction, depresses pacemaker action, and improves atrioventricular conduction, particularly when it has been depressed by digitalis glycosides. Phenytoin, like quinidine, prolongs the effective refractory period relative to the action potential duration. The drug may produce hypotension following IV administration. Phenytoin has little hypnotic activity.

Pharmacokinetics

■ **Absorption** Studies using Dilantin® have shown that phenytoin and its sodium salt are usually completely absorbed from the GI tract. Bioavailability may vary enough among oral phenytoin sodium preparations of different manufacturers to result in toxic serum concentrations or a loss of seizure control (subtherapeutic serum concentrations), and this should be considered before dispensing a brand or dosage form which differs from that currently taken by a patient. The current edition of FDA's *Approved Drug Products with Therapeutic Equivalence Evaluations* (Orange Book; http://www.accessdata.fda.gov/scripts/cder/ob/default.cfm) should be consulted to determine which specific manufacturers' phenytoin sodium preparations the FDA has evaluated and deemed as being therapeutically equivalent (i.e., as bioequivalent and expected to have the same clinical effect and safety profile when administered appropriately). Extended phenytoin sodium capsules are more slowly absorbed and generally produce peak serum concentrations in 4–12 hours. When phenytoin sodium is administered IM, absorption may be erratic; this may result from crystallization of the drug at the injection site because of the change in pH.

Therapeutic serum concentrations of phenytoin are usually 10–20 mcg/mL, but can be variable depending on the patient. In some patients, seizure control is not achieved when serum concentrations are maintained in this range, and therefore clinical response of the patient is more meaningful than serum concentrations. When serum concentration determinations are necessary, they should be obtained at least 5–7 half-lives after treatment initiation, change in dosage, or addition or elimination of another drug to the regimen, so that steady-state drug levels may be achieved. Trough phenytoin concentrations provide information on clinically effective serum concentration range and confirm patient compliance; trough concentrations should be obtained just before the patient's next scheduled dose. Peak concentrations indicate an individual's threshold for emergence of dose-related adverse effects and are obtained at the time of expected peak concentration. In general, therapeutic serum phenytoin concentrations are achieved after about 1 week of therapy with an oral dosage of 300 mg daily in adults. Alternatively, therapeutic plasma concentrations can be obtained more rapidly (in 2–24 hours) and maintained by administering an initial oral loading dose of 1 g in adults or 500–600 mg in children, followed by 300–500 mg daily in adults or 200 mg daily in children. Following IV administration of 1–1.5 g of phenytoin sodium at a rate not exceeding 50 mg/minute, therapeutic plasma concentrations can be attained within 1–2 hours.

■ **Distribution** In patients with normal renal function, phenytoin is approximately 95% protein bound. In vitro studies of plasma from patients with renal and/or hepatic disease show substantially less protein binding of phenytoin. Since customary plasma assay procedures measure total phenytoin concentration, these measurements may be misleading in patients whose protein binding characteristics differ from normal (e.g., patients with renal and/or hepatic disease), and phenytoin intoxication may occur at lower total phenytoin concentrations than usual.

Phenytoin appears to be distributed into milk in small amounts.

■ **Elimination** Following oral administration, the plasma half-life of phenytoin averages about 22 hours, although the half-life has ranged from 7–42 hours in individual patients. The plasma half-life of phenytoin in humans following IV administration ranges from 10–15 hours.

Phenytoin is metabolized by hepatic cytochrome P-450 (CYP) isoenzymes. The drug is principally oxidized to the inactive metabolite 5-(*p*-hydroxyphenyl)-5-phenylhydantoin (HPPH). Because this metabolism is a saturable process, small increases in dosage may produce substantial increases in plasma phenytoin concentrations; the steady-state plasma concentration may double or triple from a 10% or more increase in dosage, possibly resulting in toxicity. HPPH undergoes enterohepatic circulation and is excreted in urine via glomerular filtration and tubular secretion, mainly as the glucuronide. Approximately 60–75% of the daily dose of the drug is excreted in this form. Other minor metabolites also appear in urine. In therapeutic doses, approximately 1% is excreted unchanged in urine; in toxic doses, up to 10% of the ingested drug may be excreted unchanged by the kidneys.

Following equal doses of phenytoin, total plasma phenytoin concentrations are lower in chronic uremic patients than in non-uremic patients which suggests an altered metabolic disposition of the drug in patients with uremia.

Chemistry and Stability

■ **Chemistry** Phenytoin is a hydantoin-derivative anticonvulsant. Phenytoin occurs as a white powder and is practically insoluble in water, soluble in hot alcohol, and slightly soluble in cold alcohol. The drug has an apparent pK_a of 8.06–8.33. Phenytoin sodium occurs as a white, hygroscopic powder and is freely soluble in water, soluble in alcohol, and freely soluble in warm propylene glycol.

Aqueous solutions of phenytoin sodium gradually absorb carbon dioxide, and the drug undergoes partial hydrolysis to phenytoin, resulting in turbid solutions. The drug is more stable in propylene glycol. Commercially available phenytoin sodium injection is a sterile solution of the drug containing 40% propylene glycol and 10% alcohol in water for injection. Sodium hydroxide is added during manufacture of the injection to adjust the pH to 12. Each 100-mg phenytoin sodium capsule contains approximately 0.35 mEq of sodium, and phenytoin sodium injection contains about 0.2 mEq of sodium per mL.

■ **Stability** Commercially available phenytoin oral suspension and tablets, and the extended-release phenytoin sodium capsules should be stored at room temperature (20–25°C); the tablets should be protected from moisture, the extended-release capsules should be protected from light and moisture, and the oral suspension should be protected from freezing and light. Phenytoin sodium injection should be stored at 20–25°C, but may be exposed to temperatures ranging from 15–30°C. Diluted solutions of phenytoin sodium injection should not be refrigerated. A precipitate may form if the injection is refrigerated or frozen; however, this will dissolve after warming to room temperature and the injection may still be used. Slight yellowish discoloration of the injection will not affect potency, but the injection should not be used if the solution is not clear or if a precipitate is present. Precipitation of free phenytoin will occur at a pH of 11.5 or less.

Phenytoin sodium injection is physically and/or chemically incompatible with some drugs, but the compatibility depends on several factors (e.g., concentrations of the drugs, specific diluents used, resulting pH, temperature). Specialized references should be consulted for specific compatibility information.

For further information on chemistry and stability, pharmacology, pharmacokinetics, uses, cautions, acute toxicity, drug interactions, and dosage and administration of phenytoin, see the Anticonvulsants General Statement 28:12.

Preparations

Excipients in commercially available drug preparations may have clinically important effects in some individuals; consult specific product labeling for details.

Phenytoin

Oral		
Suspension	125 mg/5 mL*	**Dilantin-125®**, Pfizer **Phenytoin Oral Suspension**
Tablets, chewable	50 mg*	**Dilantin® Infatabs®**, Pfizer **Phenytoin Chewable Tablets**

*available from one or more manufacturer, distributor, and/or repackager by generic (nonproprietary) name

Phenytoin Sodium

Oral		
Capsules, extended-release	30 mg	**Dilantin®**, Pfizer
	100 mg*	**Dilantin®**, Pfizer **Phenytoin Sodium Extended-release Capsules**
	200 mg*	**Phenytek®**, Mylan
	300 mg*	**Phenytek®**, Mylan
Parenteral		
Injection	50 mg/mL*	**Phenytoin Sodium Injection**

*available from one or more manufacturer, distributor, and/or repackager by generic (nonproprietary) name

†Use is not currently included in the labeling approved by the US Food and Drug Administration

ANTICONVULSANTS, MISCELLANEOUS 28:12.92

Cannabidiol CBD

■ Cannabidiol, a naturally occurring cannabinoid derived from the *Cannabis sativa L.* plant, is an anticonvulsant.

Uses

■ **Seizure Disorders** ***Seizures Associated with Lennox-Gastaut Syndrome*** Cannabidiol oral solution is used for the treatment of seizures associated with Lennox-Gastaut syndrome in adults and pediatric patients 2 years of age or older. The drug is designated an orphan drug by FDA for use in this condition.

Lennox-Gastaut syndrome is a rare and severe form of epilepsy characterized by early childhood onset (usually between 3–5 years of age), multiple seizure types including drop seizures, an EEG pattern of slow spike and wave activity, and cognitive impairment. Management of Lennox-Gastaut syndrome can be difficult given the multiple seizure types that can occur and the refractory nature of the condition.

Efficacy of cannabidiol for the treatment of seizures associated with Lennox-Gastaut syndrome was established in 2 randomized, multicenter, double-blind, placebo-controlled studies (GWPCARE3 and GWPCARE4). The studies included patients 2–55 years of age with Lennox-Gastaut syndrome whose seizures were inadequately controlled with stable dosages of at least one anticonvulsant, with or without vagal nerve stimulation and/or a ketogenic diet. Patients who had experienced at least 2 drop seizures (atonic, tonic, or tonic-clonic seizures that resulted or could have resulted in a fall or injury) per week during a 4-week baseline period were randomized to receive add-on therapy with cannabidiol (10 or 20 mg/kg daily) or placebo for 14 weeks in addition to their existing pharmacologic and nonpharmacologic therapy. In both studies, 94% of patients were taking at least 2 concomitant anticonvulsants (most frequently clobazam, valproate, lamotrigine, levetiracetam, and rufinamide). The primary measure of efficacy was the percent change from baseline in monthly (i.e., over 28 days) frequency of drop seizures during the 14-week treatment period.

In both studies, drop seizure frequency was substantially reduced in patients receiving cannabidiol compared with those receiving placebo. The median reduction in seizure frequency was 42–44% with cannabidiol 20 mg/kg daily, 37% with cannabidiol 10 mg/kg daily, and 17–22% with placebo. The treatment effect was observed within 4 weeks of initiating cannabidiol therapy and generally remained consistent over the 14-week treatment period. Total seizure frequency (including drop seizures and other seizure types) also was substantially reduced with cannabidiol (median decrease of 36–41%) compared with placebo (median decrease of 14–18%) in both studies. In addition, cannabidiol was more effective than placebo in improving scores on a patient- or caregiver-rated global impression of change scale in both studies.

Seizures Associated with Dravet Syndrome Cannabidiol oral solution is used for the treatment of seizures associated with Dravet syndrome in adults and pediatric patients 2 years of age or older. The drug is designated an orphan drug by FDA for use in this condition.

Dravet syndrome (also known as severe myoclonic epilepsy of infancy) is a rare and severe type of epilepsy characterized by early onset of multiple refractory seizure types, frequent episodes of status epilepticus, and developmental delay with cognitive and psychomotor impairment. Up to 85% of patients with Dravet syndrome have mutations in the *SCN1A* gene encoding the voltage-gated sodium channel. Patients typically present within the first year of life with recurrent generalized tonic-clonic or hemiconvulsive seizures, which are often prolonged and triggered by fever (i.e., febrile seizures). Early mortality is high; the leading causes of death are sudden unexplained death in epilepsy (SUDEP) and status epilepticus. Seizures in patients with Dravet syndrome are generally refractory to current anticonvulsant drug options, and anticonvulsants that inhibit the sodium channel (e.g., carbamazepine, oxcarbazepine, lamotrigine, phenytoin) or vigabatrin may exacerbate the condition. Because complete seizure freedom is typically not achievable, treatment is generally aimed at eliminating or significantly reducing prolonged convulsive seizures and status epilepticus.

Efficacy of cannabidiol for the treatment of seizures associated with Dravet syndrome was established in a randomized, double-blind, placebo-controlled study (GWPCARE1) in 120 patients 2–18 years of age with Dravet syndrome who had inadequately controlled seizures despite receiving stable dosages of at least one anticonvulsant, with or without vagal nerve stimulation and/or a ketogenic diet. Patients who had experienced at least 4 convulsive seizures during the 4-week baseline period were randomized to receive add-on therapy with cannabidiol (20 mg/kg daily) or placebo for 14 weeks in addition to their existing pharmacologic and nonpharmacologic regimen. The majority (93%) of patients were taking at least 2 concomitant anticonvulsants (most frequently clobazam, valproate, stiripentol, levetiracetam, and topiramate). The primary measure of efficacy was the percent change from baseline in monthly (e.g., over 28 days) frequency of convulsive seizures (i.e., all countable atonic, tonic, and tonic-clonic seizures) during the 14-week treatment period.

Patients receiving cannabidiol experienced a substantially greater reduction in convulsive seizure frequency compared with those receiving placebo (median reduction of 39 versus 13%, respectively). Seizure freedom was achieved in 4 patients in the cannabidiol group and no patients in the placebo group. The treatment effect was observed within 4 weeks of initiating cannabidiol therapy and generally remained consistent over the 14-week treatment period. In addition, patients receiving cannabidiol were more likely than those receiving placebo to be judged by their caregivers as experiencing an overall improvement in their condition as assessed by a global impression of change scale.

Interim results of an ongoing open-label extension study indicate that the reductions in convulsive seizure frequency observed in the GWPCARE1 study were maintained with continued cannabidiol therapy and that long-term cannabidiol therapy had an acceptable safety profile.

Dosage and Administration

■ General Because cannabidiol may cause hepatocellular injury, serum aminotransferase (ALT and AST) and total bilirubin concentrations should be assessed prior to initiating therapy. (See Hepatic Effects under Cautions: Warnings/Precautions.)

As with all anticonvulsant agents, cannabidiol should be withdrawn gradually to minimize the potential for increased seizure frequency and status epilepticus. (See Discontinuance of Therapy under Cautions: Warnings/Precautions.)

Patients receiving therapy with an anticonvulsant, including cannabidiol, for any indication should be closely monitored for the emergence or worsening of depression, suicidal thoughts or behavior (suicidality), or any unusual changes in mood or behavior. (See Suicidality Risk under Cautions: Warnings/Precautions.)

Restricted Distribution Cannabidiol can only be obtained through designated specialty pharmacies. Clinicians may contact the manufacturer at 833-426-4243 or consult the Epidiolex® website (https://www.epidiolex.com) for additional information.

■ Administration Cannabidiol is administered orally twice daily as an oral solution. Because food may increase exposure to cannabidiol, some clinicians suggest that the drug be administered consistently in either the fed or fasting state. (See Description.)

A calibrated measuring device (i.e., oral dosing syringe) should be used to measure and administer the prescribed dose of cannabidiol oral solution; a household teaspoon or tablespoon is not an adequate measuring device. If the prescribed dose is less than 1 mL, the manufacturer states that a 1-mL oral syringe should be obtained (e.g., from the pharmacy). If the prescribed dose is greater than 5 mL, the total dose should be administered in portions using the 5-mL oral syringe supplied by the manufacturer. The dose should be administered directly into the patient's mouth against the inside of the cheek.

Any unused portions of cannabidiol oral solution should be discarded 12 weeks after the container is first opened.

■ Dosage ***Lennox-Gastaut Syndrome*** For the treatment of seizures associated with Lennox-Gastaut syndrome in adults and pediatric patients 2 years of age or older, the recommended initial dosage of cannabidiol is 5 mg/kg daily (given as 2.5 mg/kg twice daily). After 1 week, the dosage may be increased to the recommended maintenance dosage of 10 mg/kg daily (given as 5 mg/kg twice daily). Patients who require further reduction of seizures and are tolerating a dosage of 10 mg/kg daily may benefit from an additional increase to the maximum recommended dosage of 20 mg/kg daily (given as 10 mg/kg twice daily). Dosage should be titrated in weekly increments of 5 mg/kg daily (2.5 mg/kg twice daily) as tolerated. However, if a more rapid titration is necessary, dosage may be increased in increments of 5 mg/kg daily no more frequently than every other day.

In clinical studies, a cannabidiol dosage of 20 mg/kg daily demonstrated slightly greater efficacy than the recommended maintenance dosage of 10 mg/kg daily, but was associated with an increased incidence of adverse effects.

Dravet Syndrome For the treatment of seizures associated with Dravet syndrome in adults and pediatric patients 2 years of age or older, the recommended initial dosage of cannabidiol is 5 mg/kg daily (given as 2.5 mg/kg twice daily). After 1 week, the dosage may be increased to the recommended maintenance dosage of 10 mg/kg daily (given as 5 mg/kg twice daily). Patients who require further reduction of seizures and are tolerating a dosage of 10 mg/kg daily may benefit from an additional increase to the maximum recommended dosage of 20 mg/kg daily (given as 10 mg/kg twice daily). Dosage should be titrated in weekly increments of 5 mg/kg daily (2.5 mg/kg twice daily) as tolerated. However, if a more rapid titration is necessary, dosage may be increased in increments of 5 mg/kg daily no more frequently than every other day.

In clinical studies, a cannabidiol dosage of 20 mg/kg daily demonstrated slightly greater efficacy than the recommended maintenance dosage of 10 mg/kg daily, but was associated with an increased incidence of adverse effects.

■ Special Populations Dosage reductions of cannabidiol are recommended in patients with moderate (Child-Pugh class B) or severe (Child-Pugh class C) hepatic impairment, and slower dosage titration may be necessary in these patients. In patients with moderate hepatic impairment, the manufacturer recommends an initial cannabidiol dosage of 2.5 mg/kg daily (given as 1.25 mg/kg twice daily), a maintenance dosage of 5 mg/kg daily (given as 2.5 mg/kg twice daily), and a maximum dosage of 10 mg/kg daily (given as 5 mg/kg twice daily). In patients with severe hepatic impairment, the manufacturer recommends an initial cannabidiol dosage of 1 mg/kg daily (given as 0.5 mg/kg twice daily), a maintenance dosage of 2 mg/kg daily (given as 1 mg/kg twice daily), and a maximum dosage of 4 mg/kg daily (given as 2 mg/kg twice daily). Dosage adjustment is not necessary in patients with mild hepatic impairment (Child-Pugh class A). (See Hepatic Impairment under Warnings/Precautions: Specific Populations, in Cautions.)

Dosage adjustment is not necessary in patients with renal impairment. (See Renal Impairment under Warnings/Precautions: Specific Populations, in Cautions.)

In geriatric patients, dosage should be selected cautiously, usually starting at the lower end of the dosage range.

Cautions

■ Contraindications Known hypersensitivity to cannabidiol or any excipient in the formulation, including sesame seed oil. (See Sensitivity Reactions under Cautions: Warnings/Precautions.)

■ Warnings/Precautions ***Hepatic Effects*** Dose-related elevations in serum aminotransferase concentrations (mainly ALT) have been reported in patients receiving cannabidiol, in some cases requiring hospitalization.

In controlled studies in patients with Lennox-Gastaut syndrome or Dravet syndrome, ALT concentrations exceeding 3 times the upper limit of normal

(ULN) occurred in 13% of cannabidiol-treated patients compared with 1% of those who received placebo. Elevations of ALT or AST concentrations to more than 20 times the ULN occurred in less than 1% of cannabidiol-treated patients. Such liver enzyme elevations typically occurred in the first 2 months of therapy; however, some cases were reported up to 18 months after initiation of treatment, particularly in patients receiving valproate concomitantly. Increases in liver enzymes were not associated with any clinical manifestations of liver injury and were generally reversible following discontinuance or dosage reduction of cannabidiol and/or concomitant valproate. Although small increases in bilirubin concentrations were observed in these studies, these levels generally remained within normal limits.

Risk factors for the development of treatment-emergent hepatic enzyme elevations include use of higher dosages of cannabidiol, concomitant use of valproate or clobazam, and baseline aminotransferase concentrations above the ULN. The majority of ALT elevations occurred in patients who were also receiving valproate; concomitant use of clobazam also increased the incidence of hepatic enzyme elevations, but to a lesser extent. In clinical studies, ALT elevations greater than 3 times the ULN occurred in 30% of cannabidiol-treated patients receiving both valproate and clobazam concomitantly, 21% of patients receiving concomitant valproate (without clobazam), 4% of patients receiving concomitant clobazam (without valproate), and 3% of patients not receiving either of these anticonvulsants concomitantly. (See Clobazam and also see Valproate under Drug Interactions: Anticonvulsants.) In patients receiving cannabidiol 20 mg/kg daily in controlled studies, ALT concentrations exceeding 3 times the ULN occurred in 30% of patients who had baseline ALT concentrations above the ULN compared with 12% of those who had baseline ALT concentrations within the normal range. In patients receiving cannabidiol 10 mg/kg daily, ALT concentrations exceeding 3 times the ULN occurred in none of the patients who had baseline ALT concentrations above the ULN and in 2% of patients who had baseline ALT concentrations within the normal range.

Serum aminotransferase (ALT and AST) and total bilirubin concentrations should be assessed prior to initiating cannabidiol therapy; such monitoring should be repeated at 1, 3, and 6 months after initiation of therapy, and then periodically thereafter or as clinically indicated. Serum aminotransferase and bilirubin concentrations also should be assessed within 1 month following any change in cannabidiol dosage or any addition or change to concomitant therapy with other potentially hepatotoxic drugs. More frequent monitoring should be considered in patients receiving concomitant therapy with valproate or who have elevated liver enzymes at baseline.

Patients with baseline ALT or AST concentrations exceeding 3 times the ULN with concurrent bilirubin concentrations exceeding 2 times the ULN should be evaluated prior to initiating cannabidiol. Cannabidiol therapy should be discontinued in patients with ALT or AST concentrations exceeding 3 times the ULN and bilirubin concentrations exceeding 2 times the ULN, and also in patients with sustained aminotransferase elevations exceeding 5 times the ULN. If signs or symptoms suggestive of liver injury occur (e.g., unexplained nausea, vomiting, right upper quadrant pain, fatigue, anorexia, jaundice, and/or dark urine), serum aminotransferase and total bilirubin concentrations should be assessed promptly and cannabidiol therapy should be interrupted or discontinued as appropriate. Patients with prolonged elevations of ALT or AST should be evaluated for other possible causes.

If cannabidiol is used concomitantly with other potentially hepatotoxic drugs (e.g., valproate, clobazam), dosage adjustment of the coadministered drug should be considered. (See Drug Interactions.)

Somnolence and Sedation Cannabidiol can cause dose-related somnolence and sedation. These effects generally occur early in treatment and may diminish with continued therapy. In controlled studies of patients with Lennox-Gastaut syndrome or Dravet syndrome, somnolence or sedation (including lethargy) was reported in 27 or 34% of patients receiving cannabidiol 10 or 20 mg/kg daily, respectively, compared with 11% of those receiving placebo. The incidence of somnolence and sedation was higher in patients who were also receiving clobazam compared with those not receiving clobazam (46 versus 16%, respectively). (See Clobazam under Drug Interactions: Anticonvulsants.)

Patients should be monitored for somnolence and sedation during cannabidiol therapy, particularly if they are receiving other CNS depressants (including alcohol) concomitantly. (See Advice to Patients.)

Suicidality Risk The risk of suicidality (suicidal behavior or ideation) is increased in patients receiving anticonvulsants, including cannabidiol, for any indication. An analysis of suicidality reports from 199 placebo-controlled studies involving 11 different anticonvulsants in patients with epilepsy, psychiatric disorders, and other conditions found that patients receiving anticonvulsants had approximately twice the risk of suicidal behavior or ideation (0.43%) compared with patients receiving placebo (0.24%). This increased suicidality risk was consistent among anticonvulsants with varying mechanisms of actions and across a range of indications, and was observed as early as 1 week after beginning therapy. Because most of these studies did not extend beyond 24 weeks, the risk of suicidal thoughts or behavior with anticonvulsant treatment beyond 24 weeks is not known. Although patients treated with an anticonvulsant for epilepsy, psychiatric disorders, and other conditions were all found to have an increased suicidality risk compared with those receiving placebo, the relative risk was higher for patients with epilepsy compared with those receiving anticonvulsants for other conditions.

Clinicians who prescribe cannabidiol or any other anticonvulsant should balance the risk of suicidality with the risk of untreated illness. Epilepsy and many other illnesses for which anticonvulsants are prescribed are themselves associated with morbidity and mortality and an increased risk of suicidal thoughts and behavior. All patients treated with an anticonvulsant for any indication should be closely monitored for the emergence or worsening of suicidal thoughts and behavior. If any such symptoms emerge during anticonvulsant therapy, the clinician should consider whether they may be related to the illness being treated. (See Advice to Patients.)

Sensitivity Reactions **Hypersensitivity.** Hypersensitivity reactions may occur with cannabidiol. In the principal efficacy studies, one patient developed a hypersensitivity reaction with symptoms of pruritus, erythema, and angioedema that responded to antihistamine treatment. If a hypersensitivity reaction occurs, cannabidiol oral solution should be discontinued and appropriate therapy initiated; the oral solution should not resumed in patients who have previously experienced a hypersensitivity reaction. (See Cautions: Contraindications.)

Discontinuance of Therapy As with all anticonvulsant agents, cannabidiol therapy should be withdrawn gradually to reduce the risk of increased seizure frequency and status epilepticus. Abrupt discontinuance of the drug should be avoided when possible unless safety concerns require rapid withdrawal. In clinical studies, dosage of cannabidiol was tapered over a period of 10 days at the end of the treatment period.

Abuse Potential and Dependence Cannabidiol is subject to control under the Federal Controlled Substances Act of 1970 as a schedule V (C-V) drug.

Abuse-related adverse events were not observed in phase 1 clinical studies of cannabidiol. However, since cannabidiol is derived from the *Cannabis sativa* plant, a thorough evaluation of the drug's abuse potential has been conducted. Receptor binding studies have not identified any affinity of cannabidiol for cannabinoid (CB_1 or CB_2) receptors or other receptors associated with abuse potential. In a drug discrimination study in animals, cannabidiol did not produce cannabinoid-like behavioral responses, including generalization to tetrahydrocannabinol (THC; the psychoactive component of *Cannabis sativa*); self-administration of cannabidiol also was not observed, suggesting that the drug does not possess rewarding properties. In an abuse potential study that compared cannabidiol to dronabinol (synthetic THC), alprazolam, and placebo in recreational drug users, administration of therapeutic and supratherapeutic doses of cannabidiol (equivalent to 10–60 mg/kg in an adult weighing 75 kg) produced positive subjective responses (e.g., "drug liking," "take drug again") that were comparable to placebo. In contrast, dronabinol (10 and 30 mg) and alprazolam (2 mg) produced substantially greater positive subjective responses than cannabidiol.

Cannabidiol is not likely to produce physical dependence. In a physical dependence study in humans, no withdrawal symptoms were observed following discontinuance of cannabidiol after 28 days of administration.

Laboratory Test Interferences. Treatment with cannabidiol may result in positive drug tests for cannabis.

Specific Populations **Pregnancy.** There are no adequate data on the developmental risks associated with the use of cannabidiol in pregnant women. Cannabidiol produced developmental toxicity (e.g., embryofetal mortality, decreased fetal body weight, decreased growth, delayed sexual maturation, long-term neurobehavioral changes) when administered orally to pregnant animals at exposure levels similar to or higher than those associated with the recommended human dosage.

Women who are pregnant while receiving cannabidiol should be encouraged to enroll in the North American Antiepileptic Drug (NAAED) Pregnancy Registry at 888-233-2334 or http://www.aedpregnancyregistry.org/.

Lactation. It is not known whether cannabidiol or its metabolites are distributed into milk, affects milk production, or affects the breast-fed infant. The benefits of breast-feeding should be considered along with the importance of cannabidiol to the woman and any potential adverse effects on the breast-fed infant from the drug or underlying maternal condition.

Pediatric Use. Safety and efficacy of cannabidiol for the treatment of seizures associated with Lennox-Gastaut syndrome or Dravet syndrome have been established in pediatric patients 2 years of age or older.

Safety and efficacy of cannabidiol have not been established in pediatric patients younger than 2 years of age.

Geriatric Use. There is no experience with cannabidiol in patients 55 years of age and older to determine whether these patients respond differently than younger adults. (See Dosage and Administration: Special Populations.)

Hepatic Impairment. Systemic exposure to cannabidiol is increased by approximately 2.5- to 5.2-fold in patients with moderate (Child-Pugh class B) or severe (Child-Pugh class C) hepatic impairment compared with individuals with normal hepatic function; dosage adjustments are recommended in such patients. (See Dosage and Administration: Special Populations.)

Mild hepatic impairment (Child-Pugh class A) does not have a clinically important effect on systemic exposure to cannabidiol or its metabolites; therefore, dosage adjustment is not necessary in such patients.

Renal Impairment. Renal impairment (mild, moderate, or severe) does not have a clinically important effect on systemic exposure to cannabidiol; therefore, dosage adjustment is not necessary in patients with renal impairment.

■ **Common Adverse Effects** Adverse effects reported in at least 5% of patients with Lennox-Gastaut syndrome or Dravet syndrome receiving cannabidiol in controlled clinical trials and more frequently than with placebo include somnolence, decreased appetite, diarrhea, elevated aminotransferase concentrations, fatigue/malaise/asthenia, rash, insomnia/sleep disorder/poor quality sleep, infection, irritability/agitation, lethargy, sedation, decreased weight, aggression/anger, vomiting, upper respiratory tract infection, status epilepticus, convulsion, pyrexia, and anemia.

The incidences of adverse effects were similar among patients with Lennox-Gastaut syndrome and Dravet syndrome, and also in pediatric and adult patients.

Drug Interactions

Cannabidiol is metabolized by cytochrome P-450 (CYP) isoenzymes 3A4 and 2C19, and also by uridine 5'-diphospho-glucuronosyltransferase (UGT) isoenzymes 1A7, 1A9, and 2B7.

Cannabidiol has the potential to inhibit CYP isoenzymes 2C8, 2C9, and 2C19, and may induce or inhibit CYP1A2 and CYP2B6 at clinically relevant concentrations.

Cannabidiol also inhibits UGT1A9 and UGT2B7, but does not inhibit UGT 1A1, 1A3, 1A4, 1A6, or 2B17.

Cannabidiol and its active metabolite (7-OH-CBD) are not expected to affect breast cancer resistance protein (BCRP) and bile salt export pump (BSEP), P-glycoprotein (P-pg), organic anion transporters (OAT) 1 and OAT3, organic cation transporters (OCT) 1 and OCT2, multidrug and toxin extrusion transporters (MATE) 1 and MATE2K, or organic anion transport proteins (OATP) 1B1 or OATP1B3. The inactive metabolite, 7-COOH-CBD, inhibits BCRP and BSEP transport at clinically relevant concentrations.

■ **Drugs Affecting Hepatic Microsomal Enzymes** ***Moderate or Potent Inhibitors of CYP3A4 or CYP2C19*** Concomitant use of cannabidiol with moderate or potent inhibitors of CYP3A4 or CYP2C19 may increase plasma concentrations and adverse effects of cannabidiol. Dosage reduction of cannabidiol should be considered if the drug is used concomitantly with a moderate or potent inhibitor of CYP3A4 or CYP2C19.

Potent Inducers of CYP3A4 or CYP2C19 Concomitant use of cannabidiol with potent inducers of CYP3A4 or CYP2C19 may decrease plasma cannabidiol concentrations and reduce efficacy of the drug. Dosage increase of cannabidiol should be considered (based on clinical response and tolerability) if the drug is used concomitantly with a potent inducer of CYP3A4 or CYP2C19.

■ **Drugs Metabolized by Hepatic Microsomal Enzymes** ***CYP1A2 and CYP2B6 Substrates*** Drug interactions are expected when cannabidiol is administered concomitantly with drugs metabolized by CYP1A2 (e.g., theophylline, caffeine) or CYP2B6 (e.g., bupropion, efavirenz) because cannabidiol can inhibit or induce these CYP isoenzymes. Dosage adjustment of the CYP substrate should be considered as clinically appropriate during concomitant use.

CYP2C8 and CYP2C9 Substrates Clinically important interactions are expected when cannabidiol is administered concomitantly with drugs metabolized by CYP2C8 and CYP2C9 (e.g., phenytoin) because of the potential for cannabidiol to inhibit these CYP isoenzymes. A reduction in dosage of the CYP substrate should be considered as clinically appropriate if adverse effects occur during concomitant use.

CYP2C19 Substrates Cannabidiol has been shown to increase plasma concentrations of sensitive CYP2C19 substrates (e.g., diazepam, clobazam) and may increase the risk of adverse effects with these substrates. Dosage reduction of the CYP2C19 substrate should be considered as clinically appropriate during concomitant use. (See Clobazam under Drug Interactions: Anticonvulsants.)

CYP3A4 Substrates Coadministration of cannabidiol with midazolam (a sensitive CYP3A4 substrate) did not alter plasma midazolam concentrations.

■ **Drugs Metabolized by Uridine Diphosphate-glucuronosyltransferase Enzymes** Drug interactions are expected when cannabidiol is administered concomitantly with UGT1A9 substrates (e.g., diflunisal, propofol, fenofibrate) or UGT2B7 substrates (e.g., gemfibrozil, lamotrigine, morphine, lorazepam) because cannabidiol can inhibit these UGT enzymes. Potential increased concentrations of the UGT substrate may occur; therefore, a reduction in dosage of the substrate drug should be considered as clinically appropriate if adverse effects occur during concomitant use.

■ **Anticonvulsants** ***Clobazam*** Concomitant use of cannabidiol and clobazam can increase the risk of hepatic enzyme elevations.

In addition, a clinically important pharmacokinetic interaction has been observed between cannabidiol and clobazam. Cannabidiol has been shown to increase peak plasma concentrations and area under the plasma concentration-time curve (AUC) of the active metabolite of clobazam, *N*-desmethylclobazam, by approximately threefold; such increased concentrations of *N*-desmethylclobazam can increase the risk of clobazam-related adverse effects. In clinical studies, the incidence of somnolence was higher in cannabidiol-treated patients who were also receiving clobazam compared with those patients who were not receiving clobazam. (See Somnolence and Sedation under Cautions: Warnings/Precautions.) Clobazam also had an effect on the pharmacokinetics of cannabidiol, increasing peak plasma concentrations and AUC of the active cannabidiol metabolite by 73 and 47%, respectively.

The manufacturer states that dosage reduction of clobazam should be considered if clobazam-related adverse effects occur during concomitant use with cannabidiol. If hepatic enzyme elevations occur in a patient receiving cannabidiol and clobazam concomitantly, dosage reduction or discontinuance of clobazam therapy should be considered. (See Hepatic Effects under Cautions: Warnings/Precautions.)

Stiripentol Concomitant use of cannabidiol and stiripentol in healthy individuals increased peak plasma concentrations and AUC of stiripentol by 1.28- and 1.55-fold, respectively.

Valproate Concomitant use of cannabidiol and valproate may increase the risk of hepatic enzyme elevations. Dosage reduction or discontinuance of cannabidiol and/or valproate should be considered if hepatic enzyme elevations occur. (See Hepatic Effects under Cautions: Warnings/Precautions.)

In healthy individuals, cannabidiol did not have any effect on systemic exposure of valproate.

Other Anticonvulsants In an open-label study evaluating potential pharmacokinetic interactions between cannabidiol and some commonly used anticonvulsant agents in patients with treatment-resistant epilepsy, cannabidiol did not appear to have a clinically important effect on serum concentrations of carbamazepine, clonazepam, ethosuximide, ezogabine, lacosamide, lamotrigine, levetiracetam, oxcarbazepine, perampanel, phenobarbital, phenytoin, pregabalin, or vigabatrin. However, a substantial increase in serum concentrations of topiramate, rufinamide, *N*-desmethylclobazam (active metabolite of clobazam), zonisamide, and eslicarbazepine was observed when these drugs were administered concomitantly with cannabidiol.

■ **CNS Depressants** Concomitant use of cannabidiol with other CNS depressants, including alcohol, may increase the risk of sedation and somnolence. Patients receiving cannabidiol and other CNS depressants concomitantly should be monitored for sedation and somnolence.

■ **Hepatotoxic Drugs** Concomitant use of cannabidiol and valproate may increase the risk of hepatic enzyme elevations. (See Hepatic Effects under Cautions: Warnings/Precautions.) Dosage reduction or discontinuance of cannabidiol and/or valproate should be considered if hepatic enzyme elevations occur. There are insufficient data to determine the risk of concomitant administration of other hepatotoxic drugs and cannabidiol.

Description

Cannabidiol is a highly purified cannabinoid extracted from the naturally occurring *Cannabis sativa L.* plant. Cannabidiol is structurally distinct from other currently available anticonvulsant drugs. The exact mechanism of action by which cannabidiol exerts its anticonvulsant activity in humans has not been fully elucidated, but does not appear to be related to a direct effect on cannabinoid receptors. Cannabidiol and tetrahydrocannabinol (THC) are the 2 major pharmacologically active cannabinoids. Unlike THC, cannabidiol has little to no affinity for cannabinoid receptors CB_1 or CB_2 and does not possess psychoactive properties resulting in a lower potential for abuse. (See Abuse Potential and Dependence under Cautions: Warnings/Precautions.) Cannabidiol has exhibited anticonvulsant activity in several animal seizure models, including maximal electroshock, audiogenic seizures, and chemically induced seizures (e.g., pentylenetetrazole, 3-mercaptopropionic acid). Cannabidiol also has been shown to modulate various receptors and ion channels; however, further study is needed to determine whether these effects are responsible for the anticonvulsant properties of the drug.

Systemic exposure to cannabidiol increases in a less than proportional manner over a dosage range of 5–20 mg/kg daily. At steady state, peak plasma cannabidiol concentrations occur 2.5–5 hours following administration of the oral solution. Oral bioavailability of cannabidiol is low due to first-pass metabolism. Administration of cannabidiol with a high-fat, high-calorie meal increased area under the plasma concentration-time curve (AUC) and peak plasma concentrations of the drug by fourfold and fivefold, respectively, and decreased total variability, compared with administration in the fasted state. (See Dosage and Administration: Administration.) Plasma protein binding of cannabidiol and its metabolites exceeds 94%. The drug is highly lipophilic and rapidly distributes into the CNS and adipose tissue. Cannabidiol is extensively metabolized in the liver and gut, principally by the cytochrome P-450 (CYP) enzyme system (CYP2C19 and CYP3A4) and uridine diphosphate-glucuronosyltransferase (UGT) enzymes (1A7, 1A9, and 2B7). The active metabolite, 7-hydroxy-cannabidiol (7-OH-CBD), is equipotent to cannabidiol in seizure models and has a systemic exposure that is approximately 38% lower than the parent drug. Systemic exposure to the inactive metabolite 7-carboxy-cannabidiol (7-COOH-CBD) is approximately 40-fold higher than that of the parent drug. Cannabidiol is excreted primarily in feces, with minor renal clearance. Following administration of a radiolabeled dose of cannabidiol, approximately 84% of the radioactivity was recovered in feces and 8% in urine. The mean elimination half-life of cannabidiol following repeated dosing is 56–61 hours.

Advice to Patients

Importance of advising patients and/or caregivers to read the patient information (medication guide) and the instructions for use.

Importance of instructing patients and/or caregivers regarding administration of cannabidiol oral solution. Importance of advising patients to discard any unused oral solution 12 weeks after the container is first opened. (See Dosage and Administration: Administration.)

Risk of hepatic injury; importance of informing patients and/or caregivers of the need for specific monitoring during therapy. Importance of advising patients to inform their clinician promptly if any signs or symptoms of liver injury (e.g., unexplained nausea, vomiting, abdominal pain, fatigue, anorexia, jaundice, dark urine) occur.

Risk of somnolence and sedation, and impairment of judgment, thinking, or motor skills. Importance of advising patients not to drive or operate machinery until the effects of the drug are known.

Anticonvulsants, including cannabidiol, may increase the risk of suicidal thoughts or behavior. Importance of patients, caregivers, and family members being alert to and immediately reporting emergence or worsening of depression, any unusual changes in mood or behavior, or emergence of suicidal thoughts, behavior, or thoughts of self harm.

Importance of advising patients not to discontinue cannabidiol therapy without consulting with their clinician. The drug should be gradually withdrawn to minimize the risk of increased seizure frequency and status epilepticus.

Importance of informing patients that cannabidiol may cause positive cannabis drug screens.

Importance of informing clinicians of existing or contemplated concomitant therapy, including prescription (e.g., clobazam, valproate) and OTC drugs, vitamins, herbal supplements, or any other cannabis-based products, as well as any concomitant illnesses (e.g., liver disease).

Importance of women informing clinicians if they are or plan to become pregnant or plan to breast-feed. Importance of clinicians informing women about the existence of and encouraging enrollment in the North American Antiepileptic Drug Pregnancy Registry. (See Pregnancy under Warnings/Precautions: Specific Populations, in Cautions.)

Importance of informing patients of other important precautionary information. (See Cautions.)

Overview® (see Users Guide). For additional information on this drug until a more detailed monograph is developed and published, the manufacturer's labeling should be consulted. It is *essential* that the manufacturer's labeling be consulted for more detailed information on usual cautions, precautions, contraindications, potential drug interactions, laboratory test interferences, and acute toxicity.

Preparations

Cannabidiol oral solution is subject to control under the Federal Controlled Substances Act of 1970 as a schedule V (C-V) drug.

Cannabidiol can only be obtained through designated specialty pharmacies. (See Restricted Distribution under Dosage and Administration: General.)

Excipients in commercially available drug preparations may have clinically important effects in some individuals; consult specific product labeling for details.

Cannabidiol

Oral

Solution	100 mg/mL	**Epidiolex®** (C-V), Greenwich Biosciences

Selected Revisions October 2019,

carBAMazepine

■ Carbamazepine is an iminostilbene derivative that is used as an anticonvulsant, as a specific analgesic for the relief of pain associated with trigeminal neuralgia (tic douloureux), as well as for various psychiatric disorders.

Uses

■ **Seizure Disorders** Carbamazepine is used in adults and children in the management of partial seizures with complex symptomatology (psychomotor or temporal lobe seizures), generalized tonic-clonic (grand mal) seizures, and mixed seizure patterns that include partial seizures with complex symptomatology, generalized tonic-clonic seizures, or other partial or generalized seizures. Patients with partial seizures with complex symptomatology appear to show greater improvement during carbamazepine therapy than patients with other types of seizures. Although the drug is useful in the management of mixed seizures, the response in patients with mixed seizures may be variable. Carbamazepine is ineffective in the management of absence (petit mal) seizures or myoclonic and akinetic seizures.

Carbamazepine may be used as monotherapy or adjunctive therapy (i.e., in combination with other anticonvulsants) for the management of seizure disorders. Carbamazepine has been used concomitantly with various other anticonvulsants such as phenytoin, phenobarbital, and primidone. When carbamazepine is used in combination with other anticonvulsants, the potential for drug interactions should be considered. (See Drug Interactions: Anticonvulsants.)

■ **Neuropathic Pain** Carbamazepine is used in the symptomatic treatment of pain associated with true trigeminal neuralgia. *Carbamazepine is not a simple analgesic and should not be administered casually for relief of trivial facial pain.* Although some patients with glossopharyngeal neuralgia may respond to carbamazepine, the drug usually does not provide relief in facial pain from causes other than trigeminal neuralgia. Some patients with trigeminal neuralgia who did not respond to carbamazepine have been successfully treated with combined carbamazepine-phenytoin therapy.

Like certain other anticonvulsants, carbamazepine also has been used for the symptomatic treatment of chronic pain arising from other peripheral neuropathic syndromes†, including pain of diabetic neuropathy†. (See Uses: Neuropathic Pain, in the Anticonvulsants General Statement 28:12.)

■ **Bipolar Disorder** Carbamazepine is used in the treatment of acute manic or mixed episodes in patients with bipolar I disorder. The American Psychiatric Association (APA) considers carbamazepine an alternative treatment option for patients who do not respond adequately to first-line drugs (e.g., lithium, valproate, antipsychotic agents [e.g., olanzapine]). For additional information on the management of bipolar disorder, see Uses: Bipolar Disorder, in Lithium Salts 28:28.

Efficacy of carbamazepine in the management of bipolar disorder has been established in 2 short-term (3-week) multicenter, double-blind, randomized placebo-controlled studies in over 400 adults who met the DSM-IV criteria for bipolar I disorder with manic or mixed episodes. In both studies, patients received carbamazepine (200–800 mg twice daily as extended-release capsules) or placebo. Carbamazepine was substantially more effective than placebo in reducing manic symptoms as assessed by the Young Mania Rating Scale (YMRS); the onset of effect was observed as early as 1–2 weeks. Improvements in scores on the Clinical Global Impression-Severity (CGI-S) scale and Hamilton Rating Scale for Depression (HAM-D) also were noted with carbamazepine therapy.

■ **Schizophrenia** Carbamazepine has been used in the symptomatic management of the acute phase of schizophrenia† as an adjunct to therapy with an antipsychotic agent in patients who fail to respond to an adequate trial of the antipsychotic agent alone. For adjunctive therapy with an antipsychotic agent, carbamazepine generally is administered at the same range in dosage and therapeutic plasma concentrations as in the management of seizure disorders and bipolar disorder. APA states that, with the exception of schizophrenic patients whose illness has strong affective components, carbamazepine therapy *alone* (i.e., monotherapy rather than adjunctive therapy) has not been shown to be substantially effective in the long-term treatment of schizophrenia. For additional information on the management of schizophrenia, see Uses: Psychotic Disorders, in the Phenothiazines General Statement 28:16.08.24.

■ **Other Uses** Carbamazepine has been used for the management of aggression (e.g., uncontrolled rage outbursts) and/or loss of control (dyscontrol) in patients with or without an underlying seizure disorder (e.g., as features of intermittent explosive disorder, conduct disorder, antisocial personality disorder, borderline personality disorder, dementia)†, alcohol withdrawal syndrome†, relief of neurogenic pain and/or control of seizures in a variety of conditions including "lightning" pains of tabes dorsalis†, pain and control of paroxysmal symptoms of multiple sclerosis†, paroxysmal kinesigenic choreoathetosis†, Klüver-Bucy syndrome†, post-hypoxic action myoclonus†, acute idiopathic polyneuritis (Landry-Guillain-Barré syndrome)†, pain of posttraumatic paresthesia†, and, in children, hemifacial spasm† and dystonia†. The drug also has been used for its antidiuretic effects in the management of neurohypophyseal diabetes insipidus†; however, other less toxic agents are available, and patients with primary polydipsia and polyuria have shown signs of water intoxication during carbamazepine therapy.

Dosage and Administration

■ **Administration** Carbamazepine is usually administered orally; however, an IV preparation is available for temporary (i.e., no longer than 7 days) use in the management of seizure disorders in adults when oral administration is not feasible.

Patients who are currently receiving or beginning therapy with carbamazepine and/or any other anticonvulsant for any indication should be closely monitored for the emergence or worsening of depression, suicidal thoughts or behavior (suicidality), and/or any unusual changes in mood or behavior. (See Cautions: Nervous System Effects and see Cautions: Precautions and Contraindications.)

Pharmacogenetic Testing Because of a strong association between the presence of the variant HLA-B*1502 allele and risk of developing carbamazepine-induced Stevens-Johnson syndrome (SJS) and toxic epidermal necrolysis (TEN), pharmacogenetic testing for HLA-B*1502 is recommended. (See Pharmacogenomics of Carbamazepine-induced Cutaneous Reactions under Cautions: Dermatologic and Sensitivity Reactions.) Prior to initiating carbamazepine therapy, patients with ancestry in high-risk populations (e.g., Han Chinese and other Asian populations) should be screened for the presence of HLA-B*1502. High-resolution HLA-B*1502 typing is recommended; the test is considered positive if 1 or 2 copies of HLA-B*1502 are detected and negative if no copies of the variant allele are detected. Patients who test positive for HLA-B*1502 should not be initiated on carbamazepine therapy unless the benefits clearly outweigh the risks. Genetic testing for the presence of HLA-A*3101, another variant allele associated with a wider range of carbamazepine hypersensitivity reactions, also may be considered.

Application of HLA genotyping as a screening tool has important limitations and must never substitute for appropriate clinical vigilance and patient management. Many HLA-B*1502- and HLA-A*3101-positive patients who are treated with carbamazepine will never develop SJS, TEN, or other hypersensitivity reactions, and such reactions may develop infrequently in HLA-B*1502- and HLA-A*3101-negative patients of any ethnicity. For additional information and guidance on how to interpret and apply the results of HLA-

B*1502 and HLA-A*3101 testing, the Clinical Pharmacogenetics Implementation Consortium (CPIC) guideline for HLA genotype and use of carbamazepine and oxcarbazepine should be consulted.

Dispensing and Administration Precautions Because of similarity in spelling between Tegretol® or Tegretol®-XR (trade names for carbamazepine) and Toprol-XL® (a trade name for metoprolol succinate, a β-adrenergic blocking agent), the potential exists for dispensing errors involving these drugs. According to medication error reports, the overlapping tablet strengths (100 and 200 mg) between Tegretol® or Tegretol®-XR and Toprol-XL® and the fact that these drugs were stored closely together in pharmacies also may have been contributing factors in causing these errors. Therefore, extra care should be exercised to ensure the accuracy of both oral and written prescriptions for these drugs. The manufacturer of Toprol-XL® also recommends that pharmacists assess various measures of avoiding dispensing errors and implement them as appropriate (e.g., by verifying all orders for these drugs by citing both the trade and generic names to prescribers, attaching reminders to pharmacy shelves, separating the drugs on pharmacy shelves, counseling patients). (See Cautions: Precautions and Contraindications.)

Oral Administration Carbamazepine is administered orally as conventional tablets, chewable tablets, extended-release tablets, extended-release capsules, or oral suspension.

Conventional or chewable tablets of carbamazepine are administered 2–4 times daily with meals.

Carbamazepine extended-release tablets are administered (usually twice daily) with meals. When administered at the same total daily dosage, steady-state plasma concentrations of carbamazepine from the extended-release tablet administered twice daily are comparable to concentrations from the conventional tablets given 4 times daily. Bioavailability of the extended-release tablet is 89% of that of the oral suspension. Carbamazepine extended-release tablets must be swallowed whole and not crushed, chewed, or broken. Prior to administration, the tablets should be inspected for chips or cracks; damaged tablets or tablets without a release portal should not be used. Because the coating of the extended-release tablet is not absorbed, it may be noticeable in the stool.

Carbamazepine extended-release capsules are administered (usually twice daily) without regard to meals. The extended-release capsules should be swallowed whole or administered by opening the capsule and sprinkling the contents over food (e.g., teaspoonful of applesauce). Carbamazepine extended-release capsules and their contents should not be chewed or crushed.

Carbamazepine oral suspension is administered 3 or 4 times daily with meals. The suspension should be shaken well before administration. Because coadministration of carbamazepine suspension with certain liquid preparations (e.g., chlorpromazine, thioridazine) has resulted in formation of a precipitate, the manufacturer states that the oral suspension should not be administered simultaneously with other liquid medications or diluents.

IV Administration Carbamazepine is administered by IV infusion over 30 minutes. When patients are switched from oral to IV therapy, the corresponding total daily IV dosage (equivalent to 70% of the total daily oral dosage) should be administered in 4 equally divided 30-minute infusions every 6 hours. Bioequivalence has been demonstrated between oral carbamazepine and 30-minute IV infusions of the drug. IV carbamazepine is intended for temporary use only; patients should be switched back to oral therapy at the previously administered oral dose and frequency as soon as clinically appropriate. Use of IV carbamazepine for periods longer than 7 days has not been studied and is not recommended.

Prior to administration, carbamazepine concentrate for injection must be diluted in a compatible diluent. The appropriate volume of the concentrate for injection (based on the prescribed dose) should be withdrawn from the vial(s) and diluted in 100 mL of 0.9% sodium chloride injection, lactated Ringer's injection, or 5% dextrose injection. Following dilution, the infusion solution may be stored for up to 4 hours at room temperature (20–25°C) or up to 24 hours in the refrigerator (2–8°C) if not used immediately.

IV solutions of carbamazepine should be inspected visually for particulate matter, cloudiness, and discoloration prior to administration whenever solution and container permit; the drug should not be used if the solution is discolored, cloudy, or contains any particulate matter. Vials are for single dose only; unused portions should be discarded.

■ Dosage

Dosage of carbamazepine must be carefully and slowly adjusted according to individual requirements and response. Therapy should be initiated with a low dosage and increased gradually. Once a therapeutic effect has been achieved, efforts should be made to reduce the dosage to the minimum effective dosage.

When transferring patients from conventional, immediate-release formulations to extended-release capsules or tablets, the same total daily dosage should be administered in 2 divided doses. Following the transition, patients should be closely monitored and dosage adjusted as necessary. Because a given dose of carbamazepine administered as the oral suspension will produce higher peak concentrations of the drug than when administered as tablets, therapy with the oral suspension should be initiated with low, frequent doses (e.g., 50 mg 4 times daily for children 6–12 years of age) and increased slowly to reduce the risk of adverse effects (e.g., sedation). When transferring patients from therapy with oral tablets to the oral suspension, the total daily dose administered as tablets should be divided into smaller, more frequent doses of the suspension (e.g., transfer from twice-daily divided dosing of tablets to thrice [3 times]-daily divided dosing of the suspension).

Seizure Disorders When carbamazepine is added to an existing anticonvulsant regimen, the drug should be introduced gradually while dosage of the other anticonvulsant(s) is maintained or gradually decreased, except for certain enzyme-inducing anticonvulsants (e.g., phenytoin) that may require an increase in dosage. (See Drug Interactions.) Carbamazepine should be withdrawn slowly to avoid precipitating seizures or status epilepticus.

Monitoring of plasma concentrations has increased efficacy and safety of anticonvulsants and may be particularly useful for optimizing dosage selection, minimizing adverse effects and risk of drug toxicity, and for verification of drug compliance, particularly in patients who are more likely to experience alterations in plasma concentrations (e.g., those with hepatic impairment, those receiving concomitant enzyme-inducing or -inhibiting drugs).

Adult Dosage. The recommended initial oral dosage of carbamazepine for the management of seizure disorders in adults is 200 mg twice daily (as chewable, conventional, or extended-release tablets, or extended-release capsules) or 100 mg 4 times daily (as the oral suspension). Dosage should be increased by increments of up to 200 mg daily at weekly intervals using a twice-daily divided dosing regimen (if using extended-release dosage forms) or a 3- or 4-times-daily divided dosing regimen (if using conventional or chewable tablets or oral suspension) until the optimum response is obtained. Dosage generally should not exceed 1.2 g daily in adults; however, some patients have required dosages up to 1.6 g daily. Once adequate seizure control is achieved, dosage of carbamazepine should be adjusted to the minimum effective level, which is usually 800 mg to 1.2 g daily in adults.

When oral therapy is temporarily not feasible in adults, carbamazepine may be administered by IV infusion in a total daily dosage equivalent to 70% of the total daily oral dosage; the total daily IV dosage should be administered in 4 equally divided 30-minute infusions at 6-hour intervals (e.g., a patient receiving an oral dosage of 400 mg daily would be switched to a corresponding IV dosage of 280 mg daily, administered as 70 mg every 6 hours). Because of a reduction in first-pass metabolism, elevated plasma concentrations of carbamazepine may occur when switching from oral to IV therapy in patients with hepatic impairment; plasma carbamazepine concentrations should be monitored in such patients.

Pediatric Dosage. The recommended initial oral dosage of carbamazepine for the management of seizure disorders in children older than 12 years of age is 200 mg twice daily (as chewable, conventional, or extended-release tablets, or extended-release capsules) or 100 mg 4 times daily (as the oral suspension). Dosage should be increased by increments of up to 200 mg daily at weekly intervals using a twice-daily divided dosing regimen (if using extended-release dosage forms) or a 3- or 4-times-daily dosing regimen (if using conventional or chewable tablets or oral suspension) until the optimum response is obtained. Dosage generally should not exceed 1 g daily in children 12–15 years of age or 1.2 g daily in children older than 15 years of age. Once adequate seizure control is achieved, dosage of carbamazepine should be adjusted to the minimum effective level, which is usually 800 mg to 1.2 g daily in children older than 12 years of age.

Dosage recommendations for the management of seizure disorders in children younger than 12 years of age differ based on the specific preparation of carbamazepine used. When using tablets or the oral suspension, the recommended initial dosage of carbamazepine in children 6–12 years of age is 100 mg twice daily (as conventional, chewable, or extended-release tablets) or 50 mg 4 times daily (as the oral suspension). Dosage should be increased by increments of up to 100 mg daily at weekly intervals using a twice-daily divided dosing regimen (if using extended-release tablets) or a 3- or 4-times-daily divided dosing regimen (if using conventional or chewable tablets or oral suspension) until the optimum response is obtained. Dosage generally should not exceed 1 g daily in children 6–12 years of age; once adequate seizure control is achieved, dosage should be adjusted to the minimum effective level, which is usually 400–800 mg daily in this age group. In children younger than 6 years of age, the recommended initial oral dosage of carbamazepine is 10–20 mg/kg daily in 2 or 3 divided doses (as conventional or chewable tablets) or 4 divided doses (as the oral suspension). Dosage should be increased weekly (administered 3 or 4 times daily) until the optimum response is obtained. The manufacturers state that optimal clinical response in children younger than 6 years of age generally is achieved at daily maintenance dosages less than 35 mg/kg. If satisfactory clinical response has not been achieved, plasma carbamazepine concentrations should be obtained to determine whether they are in the therapeutic range; safety of carbamazepine dosages exceeding 35 mg/kg in 24 hours in children younger than 6 years of age has not been established.

When using extended-release carbamazepine capsules for the management of seizure disorders in children younger than 12 years of age, the manufacturers state that optimal clinical response generally is achieved at daily dosages of less than 35 mg/kg. If satisfactory response has not been achieved, plasma carbamazepine concentrations should be measured to determine whether they are in the therapeutic range; safety of carbamazepine dosages exceeding 35 mg/kg in 24 hours using the extended-release capsule formulation in children younger than 12 years of age has not been established.

Therapeutic carbamazepine concentrations have been achieved more rapidly (in about 2 hours) in pediatric patients with a loading-dose regimen using the oral suspension. In this regimen, an initial oral loading dose (as the oral suspension) of 8 mg/kg in children 12 years of age and older or 10 mg/kg in children younger than 12 years of age has been administered. Loading doses should preferably be administered in a clinic or hospital setting where plasma concentrations and the patient can be monitored closely.

Neuropathic Pain For the symptomatic treatment of pain associated with trigeminal neuralgia in adults, the recommended initial oral dosage of carbamazepine on the first day of therapy is 100 mg twice daily as tablets (conventional, chewable, or extended-release), 200 mg once daily as extended-release capsules, or 50 mg 4 times daily as the oral suspension. Dosage may be increased gradually by up to 200 mg daily using 100-mg increments every 12 hours (if using tablets or capsules) or 50-mg increments 4 times daily (if using the oral suspension) until pain is relieved. Maintenance dosages of 400–800 mg daily usually are adequate; however, some patients may require as little as 200 mg daily while others may require as much as 1.2 g daily. The manufacturers state that a carbamazepine dosage of 1.2 g daily should not be exceeded for the treatment of pain associated with trigeminal neuralgia. At least once every 3 months, an attempt should be made to decrease dosage to the minimum effective level or to discontinue the drug.

Bipolar Disorder For the management of acute manic and mixed episodes associated with bipolar I disorder, the recommended initial oral dosage of carbamazepine in adults is 200 mg twice daily (as extended-release capsules). Although the manufacturer states that efficacy and safety of carbamazepine for such use in pediatric patients have not been established, initial dosages of 200–600 mg daily, given in 3 or 4 divided doses, have been used in children older than 12 years of age†. Dosage should be increased as tolerated by increments of 200 mg daily until optimal clinical response is achieved. In hospitalized patients with acute mania, some experts state that dosage may be increased as tolerated in 200-mg daily increments up to 800 mg to 1 g daily, with slower increases thereafter as indicated. In less acutely ill outpatients, dosage should be adjusted at a slower rate because rapid increases may cause patients to develop adverse GI (e.g., nausea, vomiting) or CNS (e.g., drowsiness, dizziness, ataxia, clumsiness, diplopia) effects. If such adverse effects occur, temporary dosage reduction should be considered. Dosage may be increased again more slowly once these adverse effects resolve. Maintenance dosages of carbamazepine in patients with bipolar disorder average about 1 g daily, but may range from 200 mg to 1.6 g daily in routine clinical practice.

Cautions

■ **Hematologic Effects** Although transient or persistent, minor hematologic changes (e.g., decreased leukocyte counts) are not uncommon, the risk of serious carbamazepine-induced hematologic toxicity appears to be low. Deaths from aplastic anemia have occurred rarely following carbamazepine therapy. Other hematopoietic complications associated with the drug include leukopenia, agranulocytosis, eosinophilia, leukocytosis, thrombocytopenia, pancytopenia, bone marrow depression, and purpura. Although data from a population-based, case-control study indicate that the risk of developing aplastic anemia or agranulocytosis in patients receiving carbamazepine is 5–8 times greater than that in the general population, the overall risk of these reactions in the untreated general population is low (about 6 cases per million population per year for agranulocytosis and about 2 cases per million population per year for aplastic anemia). Transient or persistent decreases in platelet or leukocyte counts are not uncommonly associated with carbamazepine use, but currently available data do not permit accurate estimates of the incidence or outcome of these effects; however, the vast majority of cases of leukopenia reportedly have not progressed to aplastic anemia or agranulocytosis. In addition, because the apparent frequency of minor hematologic changes progressing to agranulocytosis and aplastic anemia is very low, the vast majority of such changes observed during routine, periodic hematologic monitoring of carbamazepine-treated patients are unlikely to be signaling the impending development of either abnormality. Nonetheless, determination of baseline hematologic function should be performed prior to initiation of carbamazepine therapy, and patients exhibiting abnormalities during therapy with the drug should be monitored closely. (See Cautions: Precautions and Contraindications.)

■ **Dermatologic and Sensitivity Reactions** Serious and sometimes fatal dermatologic reactions, including toxic epidermal necrolysis (TEN) and Stevens-Johnson syndrome (SJS), have been reported in patients receiving carbamazepine. These reactions are estimated to occur in 1–6 per 10,000 new users of the drug in countries with mainly Caucasian populations; however, the risk in some Asian countries is estimated to be approximately 10 times higher. (See Pharmacogenomics of Carbamazepine-induced Cutaneous Reactions under Cautions: Dermatologic and Sensitivity Reactions.)

Other adverse dermatologic effects of carbamazepine include pruritic, erythematous, and maculopapular rashes (e.g., maculopapular eruption); urticaria; photosensitivity reactions; alterations in skin pigmentation; and exfoliative dermatitis. In addition, erythema multiforme and nodosum and development of a lupus erythematosus-like syndrome or aggravation of systemic lupus erythematosus have been reported. Alopecia also may occur. Although a causal relationship has not been established, hirsutism has been reported rarely in patients receiving carbamazepine.

Multi-organ hypersensitivity (also known as drug reaction with eosinophilia and systemic symptoms [DRESS]), a potentially fatal or life-threatening reaction, has been reported with carbamazepine. The clinical presentation is variable, but typically includes eosinophilia, fever, rash, lymphadenopathy, and/or facial swelling associated with other organ system involvement such as hepatitis, nephritis, hematologic abnormalities, myocarditis, or myositis. However, signs and symptoms associated with other organ systems also may occur.

Anaphylaxis and angioedema involving the larynx, glottis, lips, and eyelids have been reported rarely following administration of the first or subsequent doses of carbamazepine; such reactions may be fatal. Other hypersensitivity reactions, including fever, rash, peripheral eosinophilia, and reversible aseptic meningitis (manifested by confusion, myoclonus, and CSF pleocytosis), also have been reported rarely.

Pharmacogenomics of Carbamazepine-induced Cutaneous Reactions Retrospective, case-control studies in patients of Chinese ancestry have demonstrated a strong association between the risk of developing carbamazepine-induced SJS and TEN and the presence of human leukocyte antigen (HLA)-B*1502, an inherited allelic variant of the HLA-B gene. The allelic distribution pattern for HLA-B*1502 is distinct for specific geographic areas and ethnic groups. The allele is found almost exclusively in patients with ancestry across broad areas of Asia, although marked variation exists in its prevalence among specific Asian populations. Greater than 15% of the population is reportedly HLA-B*1502-positive in Hong Kong, Thailand, Malaysia, and parts of the Philippines compared with about 10% in Taiwan and 4% in North China. South Asians, including Indians, appear to have an intermediate prevalence of HLA-B*1502, which averages about 2–4% but may be higher in some groups. HLA-B*1502 is present in less than 1% of the population in Japan and Korea and is largely absent in individuals not of Asian origin (e.g., Caucasians, African-Americans, Hispanics, Native Americans). While these distribution frequencies may be helpful in predicting broad population risk, they should not be used in place of individual genotyping.

The manufacturers, FDA, and other experts recommend that patients with ancestry in genetically at-risk populations be screened for the presence of the HLA-B*1502 allele prior to initiating carbamazepine therapy. (See Pharmacogenetic Testing under Dosage and Administration: Administration.) In deciding which patients to screen, the rates provided above for the prevalence of the HLA-B*1502 allele may provide a rough guide; however, clinicians should keep in mind the limitations of these figures because of the wide variability in rates even within ethnic groups, the difficulty in ascertaining ethnic ancestry, and the likelihood of mixed ancestry. Patients testing positive for HLA-B*1502 should not receive carbamazepine therapy unless the benefits clearly outweigh the risks. Patients who are found to be negative for the allele are thought to have a low risk of developing SJS and TEN. In addition, over 90% of carbamazepine-induced SJS and TEN cases will develop within the first few months of therapy and, thus, the risk of these serious dermatologic events in patients who have been taking carbamazepine for longer than 3 months without experiencing a cutaneous reaction is extremely low; this information may be considered in determining the need for screening genetically at-risk patients currently receiving the drug.

The HLA-B*1502 allele has not been found to predict risk of less severe adverse dermatologic reactions associated with carbamazepine (e.g., multi-organ hypersensitivity, non-serious rash such as maculopapular eruption). However, limited evidence suggests that HLA-B*1502 may be a risk factor for the development of SJS and TEN in patients of Chinese ancestry who are receiving other anticonvulsants associated with these reactions (e.g., lamotrigine, fosphenytoin, phenytoin). Avoidance of such drugs should therefore be considered in HLA-B*1502-positive patients when alternative therapies are otherwise equally acceptable.

The HLA-A*3101 allele is a variant of the HLA-A gene that has been implicated in the development of a wider range of carbamazepine-induced hypersensitivity reactions. Retrospective, case-control studies in patients of European, Korean, and Japanese ancestry have demonstrated a moderate association between the risk of carbamazepine-induced hypersensitivity reactions (including multi-organ hypersensitivity, maculopapular exanthema, SJS, and TEN) and the presence of HLA-A*3101. Similar to HLA-B*1502, the allelic distribution of HLA-A*3101 varies considerably based on region and ethnic populations, with frequency ranging from more than 15% in patients with Japanese, Native American, South Indian, and some Arabic ancestry to no more than 5–10% of patients with Chinese, Korean, European, Latin American, African American, Thai, Taiwanese, and other Indian ancestry. In populations with low rates of the HLA-B*1502 allele (e.g., European, African, Japanese), the presence of HLA-A*3101 appears to be the primary determinant of carbamazepine-induced SJS and TEN and other hypersensitivity reactions. The risks versus benefits of carbamazepine therapy should be considered in patients who test positive for HLA-A*3101. Experts recommend that carbamazepine should not be used in treatment-naive, HLA-A*3101-positive patients if alternative therapies are available; however, cautious use of the drug may be considered in HLA-A*3101-positive patients who have previously received carbamazepine for longer than 3 months without experiencing a cutaneous reaction.

Application of HLA genotyping as a screening tool has important limitations and must never substitute for appropriate clinical vigilance and patient management. The role of other possible factors, such as anticonvulsant dosage, compliance, concomitant medications and illnesses, in the development of, and morbidity from, these reactions and the level of dermatologic monitoring have not been adequately studied to date.

■ **Cardiovascular Effects** Adverse cardiovascular effects (some of which may be fatal), including congestive heart failure, aggravation of hypertension, hypotension, syncope and collapse, edema, thrombophlebitis, thromboembolism, aggravation of coronary artery disease, arrhythmias, and AV block, have been reported with carbamazepine therapy. Such effects generally occurred in patients with underlying risk factors. Myocardial infarction has been associated with tricyclic compounds.

■ **Hepatic Effects** Hepatic complications associated with carbamazepine include abnormalities in liver function test results, cholestatic and hepatocellular jaundice, hepatitis, and very rare cases of hepatic failure. Such hepatic effects have sometimes progressed despite discontinuance of the drug. Vanishing bile duct, a cholestatic condition with a variable clinical course, has been reported rarely and in some cases had overlapping manifestations with immune-mediated hypersensitivity reactions (e.g., multi-organ hypersensitivity). (See Cautions: Precautions and Contraindications.)

■ **Genitourinary Effects** Genitourinary complications associated with carbamazepine include urinary frequency, acute urinary retention, oliguria with elevated blood pressure, azotemia, renal failure, and impotence. Albuminuria, glycosuria, elevated BUN concentrations, and microscopic deposits in the urine also have been reported.

■ **Nervous System Effects** Adverse neurologic and sensory effects of carbamazepine include dizziness, vertigo, drowsiness, fatigue, ataxia, disturbances of coordination, confusion, headache, nystagmus, blurred vision, transient diplopia, visual hallucinations, hyperacusis, oculomotor disturbances, speech disturbances, and abnormal involuntary movements. Rarely, peripheral neuritis and paresthesia, depression with agitation, talkativeness, and tinnitus may occur. Reports of associated paralysis and other symptoms of cerebral arterial insufficiency have been described, but the exact relationship of these reactions to the administration of carbamazepine has not been established.

An increased risk of suicidality (suicidal behavior or ideation) was observed in an analysis of studies using various anticonvulsants, including carbamazepine, compared with placebo. The analysis of suicidality reports from 199 placebo-controlled studies involving 11 anticonvulsants (i.e., carbamazepine, felbamate, gabapentin, lamotrigine, levetiracetam, oxcarbazepine, pregabalin, tiagabine, topiramate, valproate, and zonisamide) in patients with epilepsy, psychiatric disorders (e.g., bipolar disorder, depression, anxiety), and other conditions (e.g., migraine, neuropathic pain) found that patients receiving anticonvulsants had approximately twice the risk of suicidal behavior or ideation (0.43%) compared with patients receiving placebo (0.24%). This increased suicidality risk was observed as early as one week after beginning therapy and continued through 24 weeks. The results were generally consistent among the 11 drugs studied. Although patients treated with an anticonvulsant for epilepsy, psychiatric disorders, and other conditions were all found to be at increased risk for suicidality when compared with those receiving placebo, the relative suicidality risk was higher for patients with epilepsy compared with those receiving anticonvulsants for other conditions. (See Cautions: Precautions and Contraindications.)

Initiation of carbamazepine for the management of complex partial seizures has been associated with exacerbation of seizures, principally atypical absence and/or generalized convulsive seizures, in some children with mixed seizure disorders. In one group of children, video-EEG monitoring revealed a generalized paroxysmal spike-and-wave discharge in all of the children in whom exacerbation of seizures occurred during carbamazepine therapy. Children who developed frequent generalized convulsive seizures had a pattern of spikes and slow waves with a frequency of 1–2 cycles/second, and those who developed more frequent and severe atypical absence seizures had a generalized spike-and-wave discharge of 2.5–3 cycles/second. Although the mechanism is not known, it was suggested that exacerbation of seizures in these children may result from carbamazepine-induced activation of epileptiform discharges. It has been suggested that carbamazepine be used with caution for the management of complex partial seizures in children with mixed seizure disorders, particularly those who have a generalized absence or atypical absence component, and that the drug be avoided when there is generalized, synchronous, spike-and-wave discharges of 2.5–3 cycles/second in association with clinical seizures regardless of their clinical manifestation. The possibility that a worsening of atypical absence and/or generalized convulsive seizures following initiation of carbamazepine therapy may be drug induced rather than the natural history of the child's epilepsy should be considered.

■ **GI Effects** Adverse GI effects of carbamazepine include nausea, vomiting, gastric distress, abdominal pain, diarrhea, constipation, anorexia, dryness of the mouth and pharynx, glossitis, and stomatitis.

■ **Other Adverse Effects** Other adverse effects reported during carbamazepine therapy include diaphoresis, fever and chills, adenopathy or lymphadenopathy, acute intermittent porphyria, aching joints and muscles, leg cramps, and conjunctivitis. Decreased plasma calcium concentrations and hyponatremia have been reported. Syndrome of inappropriate antidiuretic hormone secretion (SIADH) and cases of frank water intoxication, with hyponatremia and confusion, have also been reported. Geriatric patients and patients receiving diuretics appear to be at greater risk of hyponatremia. Pulmonary hypersensitivity, characterized by fever, dyspnea, pneumonitis, or pneumonia, also has occurred. Isolated cases of neuroleptic malignant syndrome have been reported with concomitant use of carbamazepine and psychotropic drugs.

Although scattered, punctate lens opacities have occurred only rarely in patients receiving carbamazepine, other drugs such as the phenothiazines have caused various ocular changes.

■ **Precautions and Contraindications** Carbamazepine may produce serious adverse effects, principally consisting of hematopoietic, dermatologic, cardiovascular, hepatic, and renal disturbances. The drug also shares the toxic potentials of the hydantoin-derivative anticonvulsants, and the usual precautions of anticonvulsant administration should be observed. When serious adverse effects occur requiring discontinuance of the drug, it is important to remember that abrupt withdrawal of any anticonvulsant drug in epileptic patients may precipitate seizures or status epilepticus. Carbamazepine therapy should be withdrawn gradually to minimize the potential for increased seizure frequency. Patients must be carefully examined prior to initiation of carbamazepine therapy and should remain under close medical supervision throughout therapy with the drug. Carbamazepine should be prescribed only after careful benefit-to-risk evaluation in patients with a history of cardiac conduction disturbances; cardiac, hepatic, or renal damage; or adverse hematologic or hypersensitivity reaction to other drugs (e.g., other anticonvulsants) or who have had interrupted therapy with carbamazepine.

Close attention by the patient and clinician to signs and symptoms of the possible development of adverse hematologic, dermatologic, or hypersensitivity reactions is important in patients receiving carbamazepine. Patients should be informed of the early signs and symptoms of these potential problems, such as fever, sore throat, infection, rash, mouth ulcers, easy bruising, lymphadenopathy, and petechial or purpuric hemorrhage, and should be instructed to report to their clinician immediately if any such sign or symptom occurs. In addition, patients should be advised that these manifestations should be reported even if they are mild in severity or if they occur after extended use.

Pharmacogenetic testing is recommended in patients who may have a genetic predisposition to carbamazepine-induced cutaneous reactions. (See Pharmacogenetic Testing under Dosage and Administration: Administration.) If manifestations of multi-organ hypersensitivity occur during carbamazepine therapy, patients should be evaluated immediately; if an alternative cause cannot be identified, the drug should be discontinued. Because anaphylactic reactions and angioedema have occurred during carbamazepine therapy, patients should be advised to stop taking the drug and immediately report any signs or symptoms of hypersensitivity to their clinician. If anaphylaxis or angioedema develops during carbamazepine therapy, the drug should be discontinued and alternative therapy initiated; patients who experience severe hypersensitivity reactions should not be rechallenged with the drug. Because cross-hypersensitivity between carbamazepine and other anticonvulsants (e.g., phenytoin, phenobarbital, primidone) has been reported, a detailed drug history should be obtained from patients and their immediate family members. The benefits versus risks of carbamazepine therapy should be carefully considered in patients with a history of previous hypersensitivity to other anticonvulsants. Approximately one-third of patients with a history of carbamazepine hypersensitivity will develop hypersensitivity to oxcarbazepine.

Complete blood counts, including platelet and possibly reticulocyte counts and serum iron determinations, should be performed prior to initiating carbamazepine therapy; subsequent monitoring should be individualized by the clinician. Guidelines for periodic monitoring of hematologic function have been suggested by some clinicians, and clinicians experienced in the use of carbamazepine and knowledgeable about the drug's potential toxicity can be consulted for more specific information. Patients exhibiting baseline abnormalities and those receiving other potentially myelotoxic drugs or with a history of adverse hematologic reactions to any drug should be considered at special risk, and carbamazepine therapy should be monitored closely or avoided in these patients. Patients with a history of bone marrow depression should *not* receive the drug. Patients who exhibit low or decreased leukocyte or platelet counts during the course of carbamazepine therapy should be monitored closely. Discontinuance of carbamazepine therapy should be considered if any evidence of significant bone marrow depression develops. In addition, if such evidence develops, particularly if it occurs as a result of overdosage, it has been suggested that complete blood counts, platelet counts, and reticulocyte counts be performed daily and bone marrow aspiration and trephine biopsy be done immediately and repeated as often as necessary to monitor recovery. Other special periodic hematologic studies may also be helpful in patients with evidence of significant bone marrow depression. Fully developed aplastic anemia requires appropriate, intensive monitoring and therapy for which specialized consultation should be sought. Some clinicians also advise hematologic consultation if neutropenia and depressed platelet and reticulocyte counts occur during therapy with the drug.

Adverse hepatic effects, ranging from slight elevations in hepatic enzymes to rare cases of hepatic failure, have been reported. (See Cautions: Hepatic Effects.) Liver function tests must be performed prior to carbamazepine therapy and periodically thereafter, particularly in patients with a history of liver disease. Discontinuance of the drug should be considered based on clinical judgment in patients with evidence of liver disease; some manufacturers recommend immediate discontinuance if worsening liver dysfunction or active liver disease is observed. In addition, patients should be advised of the early manifestations of adverse hepatic effects (e.g., anorexia, nausea/vomiting, jaundice) and instructed to report such symptoms to their clinician immediately, even if the symptoms are mild or occur after extended use.

Because acute attacks of porphyria have been reported, carbamazepine should not be used in patients with a history of hepatic porphyria.

Because impairment of renal function has been observed in patients receiving carbamazepine, renal function (e.g., complete urinalysis and BUN determinations) should be performed prior to and periodically during therapy. Because of potential accumulation of the cyclodextrin excipient present in the IV formulation of carbamazepine, the manufacturer states that the drug generally should not be used in patients with moderate or several renal impairment. Such patients may be at greater risk of adverse renal effects and should be closely monitored if IV carbamazepine therapy is necessary.

Patients who are currently receiving or beginning therapy with any anticonvulsant for any indication should be closely monitored for the emergence or worsening of depression, suicidal thoughts or behavior (suicidality), and/or unusual changes in mood or behavior. (See Cautions: Nervous System Effects.) Clinicians should inform patients, their families, and caregivers of the potential for an increased risk of suicidality with anticonvulsant therapy and advise them to pay close attention to any day-to-day changes in mood, behavior, and actions; since changes can happen very quickly, it is important to be alert to any sudden differences. In addition, patients, family members, and caregivers should be aware of common warning signs that may signal suicide risk (e.g., talking or thinking about wanting to hurt oneself or end one's life, withdrawing from friends and family, becoming depressed or experiencing worsening of existing depression, becoming preoccupied with death and dying, giving away prized possessions). If these or any new and worrisome behaviors occur, the responsible clinician should be contacted immediately. Clinicians who prescribe carbamazepine or any other anticonvulsant should balance the risk of suicidality with the risk of untreated illness. Epilepsy and many other illnesses for which anticonvulsants are prescribed are themselves associated with an increased risk of morbidity and mortality and an increased risk of suicidal thoughts and behavior. If suicidal thoughts and behavior emerge during anticonvulsant therapy, the clinician should consider whether these symptoms may be related to the illness being treated.

Carbamazepine may exacerbate seizures in some children with mixed seizure disorders. Some clinicians recommend that prolonged video-EEG monitoring be performed prior to initiating carbamazepine therapy in children with mixed seizure disorders in an attempt to identify those children who may be at risk for carbamazepine-induced exacerbation of seizures. (See Cautions: Nervous System Effects.)

Persons who perform hazardous tasks requiring mental alertness or physical coordination should be warned about the possible adverse neurologic and sensory effects of carbamazepine. Patients receiving carbamazepine also should be advised that there is a potential for additive CNS effects if alcohol is used concomitantly with carbamazepine. Because of the relationship of carbamazepine to other tricyclic compounds, the possibility of activation of a latent psychosis or, in geriatric patients, confusion or agitation should be kept in mind.

Baseline and periodic eye examinations including slit-lamp, funduscopy, and tonometry are recommended in patients receiving carbamazepine. Carbamazepine has shown mild anticholinergic activity; therefore, patients with a history of increased intraocular pressure should be assessed for such condition prior to and periodically during carbamazepine therapy.

Because of similarity in spelling between Tegretol® or Tegretol®-XR (trade names for carbamazepine) and Toprol-XL® (metoprolol succinate, a β-adrenergic blocking agent), the potential exists for dispensing errors involving these drugs. These medication errors have been associated with serious adverse events sometimes requiring hospitalization as a result of either lack of the intended medication (e.g., seizure recurrence, return of hallucinations, suicide attempt, hypertension recurrence) or exposure to the wrong drug (e.g., bradycardia in a patient erroneously receiving metoprolol). Therefore, extra care should be exercised to ensure the accuracy of both oral and written prescriptions for these drugs. (See Dispensing and Administration Precautions under Dosage and Administration: Administration.) Dispensing errors involving Tegretol® or Tegretol®-XR (carbamazepine) and Toprol-XL® (metoprolol succinate) should be reported to the manufacturers, the USP/ISMP (Institute for Safe Medication Practices) Medication Errors Reporting Program by phone (800-233-7767), or directly to the FDA MedWatch program by phone (800-FDA-1088), fax (800-FDA-0178), or internet (http://www.fda.gov/Safety/MedWatch).

Carbamazepine is contraindicated in patients with a history of bone marrow depression or hypersensitivity to the drug or any of the tricyclic antidepressants (e.g., amitriptyline, desipramine, imipramine, nortriptyline, protriptyline). The drug also is contraindicated in patients currently receiving, or having recently received (i.e., within 2 weeks), monoamine oxidase (MAO) inhibitor therapy. (See Drug Interactions: Monoamine Oxidase Inhibitors.) Concomitant use of carbamazepine and nefazodone is contraindicated. (See Drug Interactions: Nefazodone.) In addition, the manufacturer of voriconazole states that concomitant use of carbamazepine and voriconazole is contraindicated. (See Drug Interactions: Azole Antifungal Agents.)

■ **Pediatric Precautions** Efficacy of carbamazepine for management of seizures in children is based on extrapolation of the demonstrated efficacy of carbamazepine in adults and also on in vitro studies that confirmed that the pathogenetic mechanisms associated with seizure propagation in adults are essentially the same as those in children; in addition, mechanism of action of carbamazepine in the treatment of seizures is the same in adults and children. The therapeutic range for plasma carbamazepine concentrations (i.e., 4–12 mcg/mL) is the same in children and adults. Safety of carbamazepine in children is based on clinical studies in which the drug was administered for up to 6 months. Data from long-term clinical studies in children are not available.

■ **Mutagenicity and Carcinogenicity** Bacterial and mammalian mutagenicity studies using carbamazepine have shown no evidence of mutagenicity. Carbamazepine has produced dose-related increases in the incidence of hepatocellular tumors in female rats and benign interstitial cell adenomas in male rats. The clinical importance of these findings is not known.

■ **Pregnancy and Lactation** Safe use of carbamazepine during pregnancy has not been established. Adverse fetal effects have been observed in reproduction studies in rats. Although several reports suggest an association between use of anticonvulsants in pregnant, epileptic women and an increased incidence of birth defects in children born to these women, a causal relationship to many of these drugs has not been established. However, epidemiologic data suggest that an association between carbamazepine use during pregnancy and certain congenital abnormalities such as spina bifida may exist. Other congenital anomalies and developmental disorders (e.g., craniofacial defects, cardiovascular malformations, anomalies involving various body systems) also have been reported in association with carbamazepine use.

Anticonvulsants should *not* be discontinued in pregnant women in whom the drugs are administered to prevent major seizures because of the strong possibility of precipitating status epilepticus with attendant hypoxia and threat to life. In individual cases, when the severity and frequency of the seizure disorder are such that discontinuance of therapy does not pose a serious threat to the patient, discontinuance of the drugs may be considered prior to and during pregnancy; however, it cannot be said with any certainty that even minor seizures do not pose some hazard to the fetus. Clinicians should carefully weigh these considerations in treating or counseling epileptic women of childbearing potential. Because carbamazepine can cause fetal harm when administered to pregnant women, the benefits of therapy must be weighed against the risks in women of childbearing potential. If carbamazepine is used during pregnancy, or if the patient becomes pregnant while receiving the drug, the patient should be apprised of the potential hazard to the fetus. Tests to detect fetal abnormalities using currently accepted procedures should be considered part of routine prenatal care in women of childbearing potential receiving carbamazepine.

There have been a few cases of seizures and/or respiratory depression in neonates born to women receiving carbamazepine concomitantly with other anticonvulsant agents. A few cases of vomiting, diarrhea, and/or decreased feeding also have been reported in neonates born to women receiving carbamazepine; these symptoms may represent a neonatal withdrawal syndrome.

Women who are pregnant while receiving carbamazepine should be encouraged to enroll in the North American Antiepileptic Drug (NAAED) Pregnancy Registry by calling 888-233-2334. Information on the registry also can be found on the website http://www.aedpregnancyregistry.org.

Carbamazepine and its epoxide metabolite (carbamazepine 10,11-epoxide [CBZ-E]) are distributed into milk. Safe use of carbamazepine during lactation has not been established. Because of the potential for serious adverse reactions from carbamazepine in nursing infants, a decision should be made whether to discontinue nursing or the drug, taking into account the importance of the drug to the woman. Following daily oral administration of carbamazepine in nursing women, the milk-to-maternal plasma ratio of carbamazepine is about 0.4 and that of CBZ-E is about 0.5; it is estimated that neonates may receive about 2–5 and 1–2 mg of carbamazepine and CBZ-E, respectively, daily.

Drug Interactions

■ **Drugs Affecting or Metabolized by Hepatic Microsomal Enzymes** Carbamazepine is a substrate for and potent inducer of cytochrome P-450 (CYP) isoenzyme 3A4. The drug also induces CYP1A2, 2B6, and 2C9/19.

Concomitant use of carbamazepine with drugs that inhibit CYP3A4 may increase plasma concentrations of carbamazepine, resulting in possible increased risk of adverse effects. CYP3A4 inhibitors that have been shown, or would be expected, to increase plasma carbamazepine concentrations to a clinically important extent include (but are not limited to) acetazolamide, aprepitant, azole antifungals, cimetidine, ciprofloxacin, danazol, dantrolene, delavirdine, diltiazem, fluoxetine, fluvoxamine, grapefruit juice, ibuprofen, isoniazid, loratadine, macrolide antibiotics, nefazodone, niacinamide, olanzapine, omeprazole, oxybutynin, propoxyphene, protease inhibitors, quinine, quinupristin/dalfopristin, ticlopidine, trazodone, valproate, verapamil, and zileuton. When carbamazepine is used concomitantly with CYP3A4 inhibitors, close monitoring of plasma carbamazepine concentrations is recommended; dosage adjustment may be necessary.

Concomitant use of carbamazepine with drugs that induce CYP3A4 may decrease plasma concentrations of carbamazepine, resulting in possible reduced efficacy of the drug. CYP3A4 inducers that have been shown, or would be expected, to decrease plasma carbamazepine concentrations to a clinically important extent include (but are not limited to) cisplatin, doxorubicin, felbamate, fosphenytoin, methsuximide, phenobarbital, phenytoin, primidone, rifampin, and theophylline. When carbamazepine is used concomitantly with CYP3A4 inducers, close monitoring of plasma carbamazepine concentrations is recommended; dosage adjustment may be necessary.

Carbamazepine may reduce plasma concentrations of drugs metabolized by CYP3A4, 1A2, 2B6, or 2C9/19 through its enzyme-inducing effects. These drugs include (but are not limited to) acetaminophen, albendazole, alprazolam, aprepitant, aripiprazole, buprenorphine, bupropion, citalopram, clonazepam, clozapine, corticosteroids (e.g., dexamethasone, prednisolone), cyclosporine, dihydropyridine calcium-channel blocking agents, doxycycline, eslicarbazepine, ethosuximide, everolimus, haloperidol, hormonal contraceptives, imatinib, itraconazole, lamotrigine, lapatinib, levothyroxine, methadone, methsuximide, midazolam, mirtazapine, nefazodone, olanzapine, oxcarbazepine, paliperidone, phenytoin, praziquantel, protease inhibitors, risperidone, sertraline, simvastatin, sirolimus, tacrolimus, tadalafil, temsirolimus, theophylline, tiagabine, topiramate, tramadol, trazodone, tricyclic antidepressants, valproate, warfarin, ziprasidone, and zonisamide. When carbamazepine is used concomitantly with these drugs, monitoring of plasma concentrations or dosage adjustment of the concomitantly administered drug may be necessary.

■ **Drugs Affected by P-glycoprotein Transport** Carbamazepine is an inducer of P-glycoprotein (P-gp) and can reduce plasma concentrations of drugs affected by this transport protein.

■ **Drugs Metabolized by Uridine Diphosphate Glucuronosyltransferase** Carbamazepine is a potent inducer of uridine diphosphate glucuronosyltransferase (UGT) 1A1 and can reduce plasma concentrations of drugs metabolized by this enzyme.

■ **Drugs Associated with Stevens-Johnson Syndrome and Toxic Epidermal Necrolysis** Avoidance of other drugs associated with Stevens-Johnson syndrome and toxic epidermal necrolysis should be considered in HLA-B*1502-positive patients when alternative therapies are available. (See Cautions: Dermatologic and Sensitivity Reactions and see Cautions: Precautions and Contraindications.)

■ **Drugs that Inhibit Epoxide Hydrolase** The active metabolite of carbamazepine (carbamazepine 10,11-epoxide [CBZ-E]) is metabolized by epoxide hydrolase. Drugs that inhibit this enzyme (e.g., clarithromycin, erythromycin, loxapine, quetiapine, valproic acid) can increase plasma concentrations of CBZ-E; if carbamazepine is used concomitantly with drugs that inhibit epoxide hydrolase, plasma concentrations of carbamazepine should be monitored and dosage of the drug adjusted as necessary.

■ **Alcohol** Because of the risk of additive sedative effects, caution should be exercised if carbamazepine is used concomitantly with alcohol.

■ **Alprazolam** In healthy individuals, concomitant administration of alprazolam and carbamazepine substantially increased oral clearance and decreased elimination half-life of alprazolam, but did not substantially alter peak plasma concentrations of the drug.

■ **Anticoagulants** ***Warfarin*** Carbamazepine may decrease plasma concentrations of warfarin through hepatic enzyme induction. The effects of warfarin should be monitored and dosage of the drug adjusted as necessary.

Direct Oral Anticoagulants Carbamazepine may decrease plasma concentrations of apixaban, dabigatran, edoxaban, and rivaroxaban and reduce efficacy of these anticoagulants. Some manufacturers recommend that concomitant use of carbamazepine and these drugs generally should be avoided.

■ **Anticonvulsants** Carbamazepine can induce the metabolism of and decrease plasma concentrations of certain anticonvulsants (e.g., clonazepam, eslicarbazepine, ethosuximide, lamotrigine, methsuximide, oxcarbazepine, phenytoin, tiagabine, topiramate, valproate, zonisamide). Plasma concentration monitoring or dosage adjustment of the concomitantly administered anticonvulsant may be necessary.

Concomitant use of carbamazepine with other anticonvulsants that induce CYP3A4 (e.g., felbamate, fosphenytoin, methsuximide, phenobarbital, phenytoin, primidone) may decrease plasma carbamazepine concentrations. Close monitoring of plasma carbamazepine concentrations is recommended and dosage should be adjusted as necessary.

Felbamate and valproic acid apparently can affect plasma concentrations of both carbamazepine and CBZ-E, but the interactions appear to be complex and resultant changes may be unpredictable. The effect of valproic acid on carbamazepine concentrations may depend principally on increases in plasma CBZ-E concentrations relative to parent drug (possibly secondary to inhibition of epoxide hydrolase activity), but other mechanisms (e.g., displacement of carbamazepine from protein binding sites) also have been suggested and may contribute to the overall effect. The importance of determining CBZ-E concentrations in patients exhibiting toxicity during concomitant carbamazepine and valproic acid therapy should be considered.

Carbamazepine can inhibit the metabolism of and increase plasma concentrations of primidone. Patients receiving stable dosages of primidone may require a dosage reduction when initiating concomitant therapy with carbamazepine.

Because the effect of carbamazepine on phenytoin pharmacokinetics is complex and can result in either increased or decreased concentrations of phenytoin, close monitoring of plasma phenytoin concentrations is recommended during concomitant therapy.

Results of a pharmacokinetic study in children with epilepsy showed no effect of levetiracetam on plasma carbamazepine concentrations.

No substantial pharmacokinetic interaction was observed in healthy individuals who received lacosamide and carbamazepine concomitantly.

In healthy individuals, concomitant administration of brivaracetam and carbamazepine decreased peak plasma concentrations and systemic exposure of brivaracetam by a modest degree (13 and 29%, respectively); systemic exposure to carbamazepine was not substantially altered, but exposure to CBZ-E was markedly increased by 2.6-fold.

Alterations of thyroid function have been reported with concomitant use of carbamazepine and other anticonvulsants.

■ **Antimalarial Agents** Quinine (a CYP3A4 inhibitor) can increase plasma concentrations of carbamazepine; dosage adjustment of carbamazepine may be required.

The antimalarial agents chloroquine and mefloquine may antagonize the activity of carbamazepine.

■ **Antimycobacterial Agents** ***Isoniazid*** Isoniazid (a CYP3A4 inhibitor) can increase plasma concentrations of carbamazepine. Close monitoring of plasma carbamazepine concentrations is recommended during concomitant therapy; dosage adjustment of carbamazepine may be required.

Carbamazepine has been reported to increase isoniazid-induced hepatotoxicity.

Rifampin Rifampin (a CYP3A4 inducer) can decrease plasma concentrations of carbamazepine. Close monitoring of plasma carbamazepine concentrations is recommended during concomitant therapy; dosage adjustment of carbamazepine may be required.

■ **Antipsychotic Agents** Loxapine and quetiapine can inhibit epoxide hydrolase activity and increase plasma concentrations of CBZ-E. If carbamazepine is used concomitantly with loxapine or quetiapine, plasma concentrations of carbamazepine should be monitored closely; dosage adjustment of carbamazepine may be required.

Carbamazepine may induce the metabolism of and decrease plasma concentrations of certain antipsychotic agents (e.g., aripiprazole, clozapine, haloperidol, paliperidone, quetiapine, risperidone, ziprasidone). Reductions in antipsychotic efficacy with reemergence of symptoms has occurred in some, but not all, cases. Plasma concentration monitoring of the antipsychotic agent may be necessary during concomitant therapy and dosage should be adjusted accordingly.

Aripiprazole In a study in patients with schizophrenia, concomitant administration of aripiprazole and carbamazepine substantially reduced plasma concentrations of aripiprazole and its metabolite by 64 and 68%, respectively. If carbamazepine therapy is initiated in a patient receiving aripiprazole, dosage of aripiprazole should be doubled and additional increases made based on clinical evaluation; if carbamazepine is withdrawn from therapy, dosage of aripiprazole should be reduced accordingly.

Clozapine Concomitant use of carbamazepine and clozapine has been shown to decrease clozapine concentrations by about 40–50%. Both carbamazepine and clozapine also have the potential to cause adverse hematologic effects, including agranulocytosis. In addition, neuroleptic malignant syndrome (NMS) has been reported rarely during concomitant therapy with these drugs. Therefore, the American Psychiatric Association (APA) states that concomitant use of carbamazepine and clozapine generally is not recommended. However, if carbamazepine and clozapine are used concomitantly, it should be considered that discontinuance of carbamazepine may result in increased plasma concentrations of clozapine.

Haloperidol Concomitant use of carbamazepine and haloperidol has resulted in substantially decreased plasma concentrations of haloperidol and reduced efficacy of the drug. Patients receiving carbamazepine and haloperidol concomitantly should be monitored carefully for loss of antipsychotic efficacy and, if an interaction is suspected, haloperidol dosage should be adjusted accordingly; the possibility that haloperidol toxicity may occur following discontinuance of carbamazepine also should be considered.

Olanzapine Olanzapine (a CYP3A4 inhibitor) may increase plasma concentrations of carbamazepine. Close monitoring of plasma carbamazepine concentrations is recommended during concomitant therapy; dosage adjustment of carbamazepine may be required. In addition, carbamazepine may decrease plasma concentrations of olanzapine through hepatic enzyme induction.

Quetiapine In a pharmacokinetic study in patients receiving quetiapine and carbamazepine concomitantly, peak plasma concentrations and systemic exposure of quetiapine were substantially decreased by 80 and 87%, respectively.

Risperidone In a study in patients with schizophrenia, concomitant administration of risperidone and carbamazepine substantially reduced plasma concentrations of risperidone and its active 9-hydroxyrisperidone metabolite.

Ziprasidone In healthy individuals, concomitant use of ziprasidone and carbamazepine resulted in modest reductions in peak plasma concentrations and systemic exposure of ziprasidone (by 27 and 36%, respectively); these changes were not considered to be clinically important.

■ **Antiretroviral Agents** ***Dolutegravir*** In healthy individuals, concomitant use of dolutegravir (a UGT1A1 and CYP3A4 substrate) and carbamazepine reduced peak plasma concentrations and systemic exposure of dolutegravir by 33 and 49%, respectively. An increase in dolutegravir dosage is recommended when the drug is administered concomitantly with carbamazepine.

HIV Nonnucleoside Reverse Transcriptase Inhibitors Carbamazepine can induce the metabolism of and decrease plasma concentrations of concomitantly administered HIV nonnucleoside reverse transcriptase inhibitors (NNRTIs) that are metabolized by CYP3A4 (e.g., delavirdine, efavirenz); possible loss of virologic response and resistance to the NNRTI may occur. Carbamazepine has been shown to decrease delavirdine concentrations by 90%. Some manufacturers state that concomitant use of carbamazepine and delavirdine or other NNRTIs metabolized by CYP3A4 is contraindicated.

Delavirdine (a CYP3A4 inhibitor) may increase plasma concentrations of carbamazepine. Efavirenz may decrease plasma concentrations of carbamazepine, but exposure to its active metabolite does not appear to be substantially altered.

HIV Protease Inhibitors Concomitant use of carbamazepine with HIV protease inhibitors (PIs) that inhibit CYP3A4 may result in increased plasma concentrations of carbamazepine. If used concomitantly, plasma concentrations of carbamazepine should be monitored closely and dosage of the drug adjusted as necessary.

Carbamazepine can induce the metabolism of and decrease plasma concentrations of PIs. Monitoring of plasma concentrations or dosage adjustment of the PI may be necessary.

■ **Aprepitant** Aprepitant (a CYP3A4 inhibitor) may increase plasma concentrations of carbamazepine. Close monitoring of plasma carbamazepine concentrations is recommended during concomitant therapy; dosage adjustment of carbamazepine may be required.

Carbamazepine may induce metabolism of and decrease plasma concentrations of aprepitant; plasma concentration monitoring or dosage adjustment of aprepitant may be necessary.

■ **Azole Antifungal Agents** Azole antifungal agents that inhibit CYP3A4 (e.g., fluconazole, itraconazole, ketoconazole, voriconazole) may increase plasma concentrations of carbamazepine. Close monitoring of plasma carbamazepine concentrations is recommended during concomitant therapy; dosage adjustment of carbamazepine may be required.

Carbamazepine can induce the metabolism of and decrease plasma concentrations of itraconazole and voriconazole, resulting in possible loss of antifungal efficacy. Increased dosage of itraconazole may be necessary when used concomitantly with carbamazepine. The manufacturer of voriconazole states that concomitant use of carbamazepine and voriconazole is contraindicated.

■ **Bupropion** Carbamazepine can induce the metabolism of bupropion and has been shown to decrease peak plasma concentrations and systemic exposure of the drug by 87 and 90%, respectively. Monitoring of plasma concentrations or dosage adjustment of bupropion may be necessary.

■ **Calcium-channel Blocking Agents** Concomitant use of carbamazepine and calcium-channel blocking agents that inhibit CYP3A4 may increase plasma concentrations and subsequent toxicity of carbamazepine. In several patients receiving carbamazepine (1–2 g daily), initiation of verapamil hydrochloride (360 mg daily) resulted in development of neurologic manifestations (e.g., dizziness, ataxia, nystagmus) of carbamazepine toxicity within 36–96 hours. Plasma total and unbound carbamazepine concentrations increased by a mean of 46 and 33%, respectively, but returned to baseline values within 1 week after discontinuance of verapamil; manifestations of toxicity also resolved during this period. The ratio of plasma CBZ-E to unchanged drug decreased during verapamil therapy but returned toward pretreatment levels following discontinuance of verapamil. Limited experience suggests that a similar interaction also may occur when diltiazem, but not nifedipine, is administered concomitantly with carbamazepine. It appears that verapamil and diltiazem inhibit hepatic metabolism of carbamazepine via the CYP3A4 isoenzyme.

Patients should be monitored closely for manifestations of carbamazepine toxicity and for alterations in the pharmacokinetics of carbamazepine during concomitant therapy, and carbamazepine dosage should be adjusted accordingly. If verapamil is initiated in patients receiving carbamazepine, a 40–50% reduction in carbamazepine dosage may be necessary. If verapamil is discontinued, dosage of carbamazepine should be increased to avoid loss of seizure control.

Carbamazepine can induce the metabolism of and decrease plasma concentrations of dihydropyridine calcium-channel blocking agents (e.g., felodipine). Monitoring of plasma concentrations or dosage adjustment of the calcium-channel blocking agent may be necessary.

■ **Cyclophosphamide** Carbamazepine may increase the rate of metabolism of cyclophosphamide prodrug to its active metabolite, resulting in possible increased toxicity.

■ **Diuretics** Concomitant use of diuretics (e.g., hydrochlorothiazide, furosemide) may increase the risk of carbamazepine-induced symptomatic hyponatremia.

■ **Fexofenadine** In healthy individuals, concomitant administration of fexofenadine and carbamazepine substantially decreased peak plasma concentrations and systemic exposure of fexofenadine.

■ **Grapefruit Juice** Grapefruit juice (a CYP3A4 inhibitor) has been shown to substantially increase peak plasma concentrations, trough concentrations, and systemic exposure of carbamazepine. Plasma concentrations of carbamazepine should be monitored and dosage adjusted as necessary.

■ **Hormonal Contraceptives** Carbamazepine can induce the metabolism of and reduce plasma concentrations of hormonal contraceptives. Breakthrough bleeding and unintended pregnancies have been reported in patients receiving carbamazepine and hormonal contraceptives concomitantly. In a study in healthy women, concomitant use of carbamazepine and an oral contraceptive containing ethinyl estradiol and levonorgestrel decreased systemic exposure of both components of the contraceptive and increased the incidence of breakthrough bleeding.

Because the reliability of hormonal contraceptive therapy may be adversely affected by carbamazepine, alternative or additional methods of contraception should be considered in patients receiving carbamazepine.

■ **Immunosuppressive Agents** Carbamazepine may induce the metabolism of and decrease plasma concentrations of cyclosporine, sirolimus, and tacrolimus. Plasma concentration monitoring or dosage adjustment of the immunosuppressive agent may be necessary.

■ **Lapatinib** Carbamazepine may induce the metabolism of and decrease plasma concentrations of lapatinib. In healthy individuals, carbamazepine decreased peak plasma concentrations and systemic exposure of lapatinib by 59 and 72%, respectively.

The manufacturer of carbamazepine recommends that concomitant use of carbamazepine and lapatinib generally should be avoided. If carbamazepine is initiated in a patient receiving lapatinib, dosage of lapatinib should be gradually increased; if carbamazepine is withdrawn from therapy, dosage of lapatinib should be decreased.

■ **Lithium** Concomitant use of carbamazepine with lithium may increase the risk of adverse neurologic effects.

■ **Macrolides** Concomitant use of carbamazepine with certain macrolide antibiotics that inhibit CYP3A4 (e.g., clarithromycin, erythromycin) may increase plasma carbamazepine concentrations. Clarithromycin and erythromycin also may increase concentrations of CBZ-E secondary to inhibition of epoxide hydrolase activity. Increased plasma concentrations of carbamazepine and subsequent signs of carbamazepine toxicity (e.g., ataxia, dizziness, drowsiness, vomiting) have occurred in adults or children following concomitant use of carbamazepine and erythromycin. Studies in adults indicate that erythromycin can substantially decrease serum clearance of carbamazepine, presumably by inhibiting hepatic metabolism of the drug.

Close monitoring of plasma carbamazepine concentrations is recommended when carbamazepine is used concomitantly with macrolide antibiotics that inhibit CYP3A4; dosage adjustment of carbamazepine may be required. In addition, patients receiving carbamazepine and erythromycin concomitantly should be monitored for evidence of carbamazepine toxicity. Some clinicians suggest that use of an alternative anti-infective agent, instead of erythromycin, may be necessary in patients receiving carbamazepine.

■ **Monoamine Oxidase Inhibitors** Concomitant use of carbamazepine and monoamine oxidase (MAO) inhibitors is contraindicated based on a theoretical concern of serotonin syndrome. At least 14 days should elapse between discontinuance of an MAO inhibitor and initiation of carbamazepine.

■ **Nefazodone** Concomitant use of carbamazepine and nefazodone is contraindicated; plasma concentrations of nefazodone and its active metabolite may decrease substantially, reducing the drug's therapeutic effect.

■ **Neuromuscular Blocking Agents** Resistance to the nondepolarizing neuromuscular blocking agents cisatracurium, pancuronium, rocuronium, and vecuronium has been reported in patients receiving long-term carbamazepine therapy. It is not known whether the same effect occurs with other neuromuscular blocking agents. Carbamazepine-treated patients who are receiving these nondepolarizing neuromuscular blocking agents should be monitored closely for more rapid than normal recovery from neuromuscular blockade; higher dosages of the neuromuscular blocking agent may be required.

■ **Omeprazole** In healthy individuals, concomitant use of omeprazole and carbamazepine resulted in increased peak plasma concentrations and systemic exposure of carbamazepine. Close monitoring of plasma carbamazepine concentrations is recommended during concomitant therapy; dosage adjustment of carbamazepine may be required.

■ **Selective Serotonin-reuptake Inhibitors** Fluoxetine can increase plasma carbamazepine and CBZ-E concentrations, and carbamazepine toxicity (e.g., ocular changes, vertigo, tremor) has been reported in some patients maintained on carbamazepine following initiation of fluoxetine. It has been suggested that fluoxetine-induced inhibition of hepatic metabolism (e.g., inhibition of epoxide hydrolase) of carbamazepine and/or CBZ-E may be principally responsible for such increases; alteration in protein binding does not appear to be principally responsible for this interaction. The patient and plasma concentrations of carbamazepine and its metabolite should be monitored closely whenever fluoxetine therapy is initiated or discontinued; carbamazepine dosage should be adjusted accordingly.

Concomitant use of carbamazepine with fluvoxamine (a CYP3A4 inhibitor) may result in increased plasma carbamazepine concentrations. Close monitoring of plasma carbamazepine concentrations is recommended during concomitant therapy; dosage adjustment of carbamazepine may be required.

Carbamazepine may induce the metabolism of and decrease plasma concentrations of citalopram and sertraline; plasma concentration monitoring or dosage adjustment of the selective serotonin-reuptake inhibitor (SSRI) may be necessary. Citalopram does not appear to alter plasma concentrations of carbamazepine.

■ **Simvastatin** In healthy individuals, systemic exposure of simvastatin and simvastatin acid were reduced by 75 and 82%, respectively, with carbamazepine; peak plasma concentrations of both simvastatin and its metabolite were reduced by 68%. Some experts recommend that concomitant use of carbamazepine and simvastatin be avoided; if concomitant use is necessary, dosage of simvastatin should be increased.

■ **Temsirolimus** Carbamazepine can induce the metabolism of and decrease plasma concentrations of temsirolimus. Such concomitant therapy generally should be avoided. If carbamazepine and temsirolimus must be used concomitantly, dosage adjustment of temsirolimus should be considered.

■ **Theophylline** Concomitant use of carbamazepine and theophylline may induce each other's metabolism, with resultant changes in elimination half-life and plasma concentrations. If carbamazepine and theophylline are used concomitantly, plasma concentrations of the drugs should be monitored and dosages adjusted accordingly.

■ **Trazodone** Carbamazepine can induce the metabolism of and decrease plasma concentrations of trazodone. Concomitant use of carbamazepine (400 mg daily) with trazodone (100–300 mg daily) decreased plasma concentrations of trazodone and an active metabolite, *m*-chlorophenylpiperazine, by 76 and 60%, respectively. Patients receiving carbamazepine and trazodone concomitantly should be closely monitored and dosage of trazodone increased if necessary.

Trazodone also is a CYP3A4 inhibitor and can increase plasma concentrations of carbamazepine. Close monitoring of plasma carbamazepine concentrations is recommended during concomitant therapy; dosage adjustment of carbamazepine may be required.

■ **Tricyclic Antidepressants** Carbamazepine may induce the metabolism of and decrease plasma concentrations of certain tricyclic antidepressants (e.g., amitriptyline, imipramine, nortriptyline). Monitoring of plasma concentrations or dosage adjustment of the tricyclic antidepressant may be necessary.

Carbamazepine can inhibit the metabolism of and increase plasma concentrations of clomipramine. In patients receiving stable dosages of clomipramine, dosage reduction may be required when initiating carbamazepine therapy.

■ **Zolpidem** In healthy individuals, concomitant administration of zolpidem and carbamazepine reduced bioavailability of zolpidem by 57%; the clinical importance of this interaction is not known.

Laboratory Test Interferences

■ **Pregnancy Tests** Carbamazepine interferes with some pregnancy tests.

Acute Toxicity

■ **Pathogenesis** The lowest known lethal dose of carbamazepine is 3.2 and 1.6 g in adults and children, respectively.

■ **Manifestations** Carbamazepine overdosage produces dizziness, ataxia, drowsiness, stupor, nausea, vomiting, opisthotonos, restlessness, agitation, disorientation, tremor, involuntary movements, adiadochokinesis, abnormal reflexes (hypoactive or hyperactive), mydriasis, nystagmus, flushing, cyanosis, and urinary retention. Hypotension or hypertension may develop. Coma may follow. Laboratory findings in some cases of overdosage have included leukocytosis, reduced leukocyte count, glycosuria, and acetonuria. EEG may show dysrhythmias.

A 24-year-old woman who ingested 3.2 g of carbamazepine died of cardiac arrest, and a 24-year-old man died of pneumonia and hypoxic encephalopathy ingesting the same dose. A 14-year-old girl who ingested 4 g of carbamazepine died of cardiac arrest, and a 3-year-old girl who ingested 1.6 g of carbamazepine died of aspiration pneumonia.

■ **Treatment** Treatment of carbamazepine overdosage generally consists of supportive and symptomatic therapy. Because of the relationship of carbamazepine to the tricyclic antidepressants, the ECG should be monitored, especially in children, to detect cardiac dysfunction.

Pharmacology

The pharmacologic actions of carbamazepine appear to be similar to those of the hydantoin-derivative anticonvulsants. The anticonvulsant activity of carbamazepine, like phenytoin, principally involves limitation of seizure propagation by reduction of posttetanic potentiation (PTP) of synaptic transmission. Carbamazepine appears to provide relief of pain in trigeminal neuralgia by reducing synaptic transmission within the trigeminal nucleus. The exact mechanism of carbamazepine in bipolar disorder is not known, although various pharmacologic effects have been described (e.g., modulation of sodium and calcium channels, receptor-mediated neurotransmission [e.g., GABAergic, glutamatergic, monoaminergic], and intracellular signaling pathways in experimental preparations). Carbamazepine also has demonstrated sedative, anticholinergic, antidepressant, muscle relaxant, antiarrhythmic, antidiuretic, and neuromuscular transmission-inhibitory actions. Carbamazepine has only slight analgesic properties.

Pharmacokinetics

The pharmacokinetic parameters of carbamazepine disposition are similar in children and in adults; however, there is a poor correlation between dosage and plasma concentrations of carbamazepine in children. The effects of race and gender on carbamazepine pharmacokinetics have not been systematically evaluated. However, retrospective, case-control studies in patients of Chinese ancestry have demonstrated a strong pharmacogenomic association between the risk of developing Stevens-Johnson syndrome and toxic epidermal necrolysis and the presence of HLA-B*1502, an inherited allelic variant of the HLA-B gene. (See Cautions: Dermatologic and Sensitivity Reactions.)

■ **Absorption** Carbamazepine is slowly absorbed from the GI tract. Following chronic oral administration of carbamazepine tablets, suspension, extended-release tablets, or extended-release capsules, peak plasma concentrations are reached in 4–5, 1.5, 3–12, or 4.1–7.7 hours, respectively. The oral bioavailabilities of carbamazepine conventional (immediate-release) tablets and suspension reportedly are equivalent, although the rate of absorption is faster for the suspension. The bioavailability of the extended-release tablets is reportedly 89% of that of the suspension, and the absorption of the extended-release tablets is slightly slower than that of the conventional tablets. Peak plasma concentrations of the drug are higher and trough concentrations are lower for the suspension compared with tablets when the drug is administered once or twice daily, but steady-state concentrations reportedly are comparable when the suspension is administered in 3 divided doses daily and the tablets are administered in 2 divided doses daily. Following oral administration of carbamazepine extended-release capsules or tablets every 12 hours, steady-state plasma carbamazepine concentrations were comparable to those achieved with corresponding dosages of the conventional tablets every 6 hours. Although one manufacturer states that peak plasma concentrations may be higher with chewable tablets than with conventional tablets, a crossover study employing this manufacturer's tablets in adults with seizure disorders showed no such difference. In this study, the oral pharmacokinetics, including bioavailability, and peak and trough plasma concentrations, were comparable for conventional and chewable tablets of the drug, although individual patients may have achieved somewhat higher concentrations for one or the other tablet formulation.

Following IV administration of carbamazepine at a dosage adjusted by the 70% oral-to-IV conversion factor, systemic exposure was comparable to that observed following oral administration. The pharmacokinetics of the principal metabolite of carbamazepine (carbamazepine-10,11-epoxide [CBZ-E]) were similar following oral and IV dosing.

Following oral administration, a period of 2–4 days of therapy may be required to achieve steady-state plasma concentrations. Although optimal therapeutic plasma concentrations suitable for all patients have not yet been determined, therapeutic plasma concentrations of carbamazepine (for both anticonvulsant effects and relief of pain of trigeminal neuralgia) are usually 3–14 mcg/mL. Some investigators have noted that nystagmus frequently occurs when plasma concentrations are greater than 4 mcg/mL and that ataxia, dizziness, and anorexia often occur when plasma concentrations are 10 mcg/mL or greater. There appears to be wide variation in steady-state plasma concentrations produced by specific daily dosages of carbamazepine (e.g., daily dosages of 800 mg, 1.2 g, or 1.6 g may produce plasma concentrations of 2–10 mcg/mL).

In one study, when carbamazepine extended-release capsules were administered as a single 400-mg dose with a high-fat meal, the rate, but not the extent, of carbamazepine absorption was increased when compared with administration of the capsules in the fasting state. Results of a multiple-dose study of the extended-release capsules indicate that when these capsules are administered in the fed state, peak steady-state plasma concentrations are within the therapeutic range. When the extended-release capsules of carbamazepine are broken and the beads sprinkled over applesauce prior to administration, the pharmacokinetic profile of the drug is similar to that following oral administration of the intact capsule to fasting individuals. The manufacturer of carbamazepine extended-release capsules states that the elimination half-life of the drug does not differ substantially between fasted and nonfasted conditions of administration.

■ **Distribution** Carbamazepine is widely distributed in the body; the drug has been detected in CSF (approximately 15–22% of serum concentrations), the brain (at autopsy), duodenal fluids, bile, and saliva. CBZ-E has also been detected in CSF. Carbamazepine rapidly crosses the placenta (i.e., 30–60 minutes) and accumulates in fetal tissues, with higher concentrations in the liver and kidney than in brain and lungs. Carbamazepine and its epoxide metabolite are distributed into breast milk. The ratio of the concentration in breast milk to that in plasma is approximately 0.4 for the drug and 0.5 for the epoxide metabolite.

In vitro studies indicate that at plasma concentrations of 1–50 mcg/mL, 75–90% of the drug is bound to plasma proteins.

■ **Elimination** Carbamazepine has a relatively long plasma half-life, variously reported to be 8–72 hours. The variability results in part because carbamazepine can induce its own metabolism; autoinduction of metabolism usually is completed after 3–5 weeks of a fixed dosing regimen. The plasma half-life generally ranges from 25–65 hours initially and from 12–17 hours with multiple dosing.

The metabolic fate of carbamazepine has not been completely elucidated. A major metabolic pathway appears to be oxidation by microsomal enzymes in the liver (principally cytochrome P-450 isoform 3A4) to form CBZ-E, which is almost completely metabolized to *trans*-10,11-dihydroxy-10,11-dihydrocarbamazepine (*trans*-CBZ-diol) and excreted in urine mainly unconjugated. CBZ-E has anticonvulsant activity in animals and potent analgesic activity in patients with trigeminal neuralgia. CBZ-E also has been implicated as contributing to adverse neurologic effects of the drug. Carbamazepine is more rapidly metabolized to CBZ-E in children than in adults. In children younger than 15 years of age, there is an inverse relationship between the CBZ-E/CBZ ratio and increasing age; this ratio was reported to be 0.44 in children younger than 1 year old and 0.18 in children 10–15 years of age. Carbamazepine also undergoes aromatic hydroxylation to form 2-hydroxycarbamazepine and 3-hydroxycarbamazepine. The pathway is not clearly determined, but the drug also undergoes metabolism to form 9-hydroxymethyl-10-carbamoyl-acridan. Carbamazepine and its metabolites are excreted in urine. Only about 1–3% of the drug is excreted in urine unchanged. Carbamazepine induces liver microsomal enzymes and thus may accelerate its own metabolism and that of other concomitantly administered drugs that are metabolized by these enzymes. (See Drug Interactions.)

Clearance of carbamazepine is unchanged in patients with mild renal impairment (creatinine clearance 60–89 mL/minute); the effects of moderate or severe renal impairment (creatinine clearance 15–59 mL/minute) on the pharmacokinetics of carbamazepine are not known. The effects of hepatic impairment on carbamazepine pharmacokinetics are not known; however, patients with hepatic impairment may exhibit increased plasma concentrations of the drug when switching from oral to IV therapy because of a reduction in first-pass metabolism.

Chemistry and Stability

■ **Chemistry** Carbamazepine is an iminostilbene derivative that is used as both an anticonvulsant and for the relief of pain associated with trigeminal neuralgia (tic douloureux). Carbamazepine is structurally related to the tricyclic antidepressants such as amitriptyline and imipramine. Carbamazepine occurs as a white to off-white powder and is practically insoluble in water and soluble in alcohol and in acetone.

The multi-compartment, extended-release capsule formulation of carbamazepine (e.g., Carbatrol®, Equetro®) contains 3 different types of beads: immediate-, extended-, and enteric-release beads. The 3 bead types are combined in a specific ratio to allow for twice-daily dosing.

■ **Stability** Carbamazepine conventional tablets and chewable tablets should be stored in tight containers at temperatures not exceeding 30°C and protected from moisture. The chewable tablets should additionally be protected from light (e.g., with storage in a light-resistant container). Carbamazepine extended-release tablets should be stored in tight containers at 25°C (but may be exposed to temperatures ranging from 15–30°C) and protected from moisture. Carbamazepine extended-release capsules should be stored at 25°C (but may be exposed to temperatures ranging from 15–30°C) and protected from moisture and light.

Because dissolution characteristics and associated oral bioavailability of carbamazepine tablets may be affected substantially by moisture, patients should be cautioned to keep containers of the tablets tightly closed and in a dry location, away from areas with excessive moisture (e.g., showers, bathrooms, humidifiers). Carbamazepine tablets may lose one-third or more of their oral bioavailability when exposed to excessive moisture. Tablets continuously exposed to 97% relative humidity at room temperature for 2 weeks become hardened and dissolve poorly.

Carbamazepine oral suspension should be stored in tight, light-resistant containers at temperatures not exceeding 30°C; freezing of the oral suspension should be avoided.

Carbamazepine concentrate for injection should be stored at 20–25°C (but may be exposed to temperatures ranging from 15–30°C).

Testing has shown that mixing carbamazepine oral suspension with chlorpromazine oral solution or liquid thioridazine preparations results in a rubbery, orange precipitate. Because the extent to which this interaction occurs with other liquid preparations is not known, the manufacturer recommends that carbamazepine oral suspension not be administered simultaneously with other liquid preparations.

For further information on pharmacology, cautions, and dosage and administration of carbamazepine, see the Anticonvulsants General Statement 28:12.

Preparations

Excipients in commercially available drug preparations may have clinically important effects in some individuals; consult specific product labeling for details.

carBAMazepine

Oral		
Capsules, extended-release	100 mg*	**carBAMazepine Extended-release Capsules**
		Carbatrol®, Shire
		Equetro®, Validus
	200 mg*	**carBAMazepine Extended-release Capsules**
		Carbatrol®, Shire
		Equetro®, Validus
	300 mg*	**carBAMazepine Extended-release Capsules**
		Carbatrol®, Shire
		Equetro®, Validus
Suspension	100 mg/5 mL*	**carBAMazepine Suspension**
		TEGretol®, Novartis
Tablets	200 mg*	**carBAMazepine Tablets**
		Epitol® (scored), Teva
		TEGretol® (scored), Novartis
Tablets, chewable	100 mg*	**carBAMazepine Chewable Tablets**
		TEGretol® (scored), Novartis
	200 mg*	**carBAMazepine Chewable Tablets**
Tablets, extended-release	100 mg*	**carBAMazepine Extended-release Tablets**
		TEGretol®-XR, Novartis
	200 mg*	**carBAMazepine Extended-release Tablets**
		TEGretol®-XR, Novartis
	400 mg*	**carBAMazepine Extended-release Tablets**
		TEGretol®-XR, Novartis
Parenteral		
Concentrate, for injection, for IV infusion	10 mg/mL	**Carnexiv®**, Lundbeck

*available from one or more manufacturer, distributor, and/or repackager by generic (nonproprietary) name

†Use is not currently included in the labeling approved by the US Food and Drug Administration

Gabapentin
Gabapentin Enacarbil

■ Gabapentin is an anticonvulsant structurally related to the inhibitory CNS neurotransmitter γ-aminobutyric acid (GABA); the drug also possesses analgesic activity. Gabapentin enacarbil is a prodrug of gabapentin.

Uses

Conventional (immediate-release) preparations of gabapentin are used in the management of seizure disorders. Conventional preparations also are used in the treatment of postherpetic neuralgia (PHN). Gabapentin also is commercially available as a gastroretentive tablet formulation (Gralise®) for once-daily administration in the treatment of PHN. Because of differences in pharmacokinetic properties, gabapentin gastroretentive tablets are *not* interchangeable with other gabapentin preparations.

Gabapentin enacarbil, a prodrug of gabapentin, is commercially available as an extended-release tablet formulation (Horizant®) for once-daily administration in the treatment of PHN and primary restless legs syndrome. Because of differences in pharmacokinetic properties, gabapentin enacarbil extended-release tablets are *not* interchangeable with other gabapentin preparations.

■ **Seizure Disorders** Gabapentin (as conventional preparations) is used in combination with other anticonvulsant agents in the management of partial seizures with or without secondary generalization. The anticonvulsant potential of gabapentin has been established in studies in which gabapentin or placebo was administered as adjunctive therapy in adults and children 3 years of age or older with refractory partial seizures; comparative efficacy of therapeutically effective dosages of gabapentin versus other anticonvulsants remains to be established.

In several placebo-controlled clinical studies, gabapentin (as conventional preparations) was effective in reducing seizure frequency, including that of secondarily generalized tonic-clonic seizures, in 17–26% of patients with partial seizures refractory to therapy with conventional anticonvulsant drugs (e.g., phenytoin, carbamazepine, phenobarbital, valproic acid). Patients in these studies had a history of at least 4 partial seizures (with or without secondary tonic-clonic generalization) per month despite optimum therapy with one or more anticonvulsants and were eligible for study entry if they continued to have at least 2–4 seizures per month during a 12-week baseline period while receiving their established anticonvulsant regimen. Efficacy of gabapentin in these studies was evaluated principally in terms of the percentage of patients with a reduction in seizure frequency of 50% or greater compared with baseline values (i.e., responder rate) and the change in seizure frequency associated with the addition of gabapentin or placebo to existing anticonvulsant treatment (i.e., response ratio, calculated as treatment seizure frequency minus baseline seizure frequency divided by the sum of the treatment and baseline seizure frequencies). Combined analysis of these response parameters in patients receiving various dosages of gabapentin (600, 900, 1200, or 1800 mg in 3 divided doses daily as conventional preparations) or placebo indicated a dose-related reduction in the frequency of partial seizures with gabapentin, although a dose-response relationship was not consistently found in the individual studies. The efficacy of adjunctive therapy with gabapentin for the management of partial seizures does not appear to be affected by patient gender or age, although the influence of these characteristics on efficacy has not been studied systematically.

Efficacy of gabapentin (as conventional preparations) in children 3–12 years of age with partial seizures was established in a multicenter randomized controlled trial. Response ratios were substantially better in patients receiving gabapentin 25–35 mg/kg daily (as conventional preparations) compared with those receiving placebo; for the same population, the responder rate for the drug (21%) was not substantially different from placebo (18%). Another study in children 1 month to 3 years of age reported no substantial difference in either the response ratio or responder rate for those receiving gabapentin compared with those receiving placebo.

Safety and efficacy of gabapentin gastroretentive tablets (Gralise®) and gabapentin enacarbil (Horizant®) have not been established in patients with seizure disorders.

■ Neuropathic Pain ***Postherpetic Neuralgia*** Gabapentin (as conventional preparations or gastroretentive tablets) and gabapentin enacarbil are used in the management of postherpetic neuralgia (PHN) in adults. Gabapentin is considered one of several first-line therapies for the management of neuropathic pain associated with PHN; other options include tricyclic antidepressants, pregabalin, opiate analgesics, and topical lidocaine patches. When selecting an appropriate regimen, clinicians should consider the relative efficacy and safety of the specific drugs as well as individual patient-related factors (e.g., age, preference, tolerance, contraindications, comorbid conditions, concomitant medications).

Efficacy of conventional (immediate-release) preparations of gabapentin for the management of PHN was established in 2 placebo-controlled studies of 7–8 weeks' duration in patients who were continuing to experience pain for longer than 3 months after healing of their herpes zoster rash. In these studies, gabapentin was titrated over several weeks up to a target dosage of 1.8, 2.4, or 3.6 g daily (administered in 3 divided doses as conventional preparations). Gabapentin substantially reduced weekly mean pain scores from baseline compared with placebo (assessed by an 11-point numeric rating scale); improvement was noted at 1 week and maintained throughout the duration of these studies. In addition, a greater proportion of patients receiving gabapentin compared with placebo achieved at least a 50% reduction in pain from baseline, and this was observed at all dosages evaluated.

Efficacy of gabapentin gastroretentive tablets (Gralise®) for the management of PHN was established in an 11-week double-blind, placebo-controlled study in patients who were experiencing persistent pain for at least 6 months after healing of their herpes zoster rash. Gabapentin (at a dosage of 1.8 g once daily as gastroretentive tablets) was substantially more effective than placebo in improving average pain scores from baseline; the extent of improvement was similar to that achieved with the conventional (immediate-release) formulation of the drug. In this study, the proportion of patients who experienced at least a 50% reduction in pain with gabapentin (29.5%) was not substantially different from placebo (22.6%).

Efficacy of gabapentin enacarbil for the management of PHN was established in a 12-week randomized, double-blind, placebo-controlled multicenter study that evaluated 3 different dosages of the drug (600 mg, 1.2 g, or 1.8 g twice daily as extended-release tablets) in patients who were experiencing persistent pain for at least 3 months after healing of their herpes zoster rash. Compared with placebo, treatment with gabapentin enacarbil substantially reduced mean pain scores and increased the proportion of patients with at least a 50% reduction in pain intensity from baseline; improvements were noted as early as 1 week following initiation of therapy and were maintained throughout the duration of the study. Although benefits of gabapentin enacarbil were observed at all dosages evaluated, the 1.2-g daily dosage (administered as 600 mg twice daily) appeared to provide the greatest benefit-to-risk ratio.

Other Types of Neuropathic Pain Gabapentin is used for the treatment of pain associated with diabetic neuropathy†. In an 8-week controlled clinical study in patients with diabetic neuropathy, gabapentin was more effective than placebo in improving pain (based on an 11-point numeric rating scale), sleep, and mood during weeks 2–8 of the study. Most patients in this study (67%) received gabapentin in dosages of 3.6 g daily. In addition, 2 comparative studies reported that gabapentin was at least as effective as amitriptyline in relieving pain associated with diabetic neuropathy. Analysis of data from randomized studies in patients with pain associated with diabetic neuropathy indicates that 40% of patients who received gabapentin for neuropathic pain obtained good pain relief.

Gabapentin also has been used with some evidence of benefit for the relief of chronic neurogenic pain† in a variety of conditions including trigeminal neuralgia†, pain and control of paroxysmal symptoms of multiple sclerosis†, complex regional pain syndromes† (CRPS), HIV-related peripheral neuropathy†, and neuropathic pain associated with cancer†. Additional study and experience are needed to further elucidate the precise role of gabapentin in the management of these conditions. Limited evidence indicates that gabapentin is not effective for the management of acute pain.

■ Restless Legs Syndrome Gabapentin enacarbil is used for the symptomatic treatment of moderate-to-severe primary restless legs syndrome in adults. The drug is not recommended in patients who are required to sleep during the daytime and remain awake at night.

Restless legs syndrome (also known as Ekbom syndrome) is a sensorimotor disorder characterized by a distressing urge to move the legs accompanied by sensations deep in the limbs that have been variously described as tingling, pulling, itching, aching, or jittering. These symptoms are present at rest, especially in the evening and at night, and are relieved by movement. Dopamine receptor agonists (e.g., pramipexole, ropinirole) traditionally have been considered the drugs of choice for patients with restless legs syndrome, particularly those with symptoms that occur nightly. Current evidence from randomized placebo-controlled studies also supports the use of gabapentin enacarbil for this condition. Although direct comparison studies have not been conducted to date, efficacy of gabapentin enacarbil appears to be comparable to that of the dopamine receptor agonists.

Efficacy of gabapentin enacarbil for the management of restless legs syndrome was established in 2 randomized, placebo-controlled studies of 12 weeks' duration in adults with moderate-to-severe restless legs syndrome (defined as a score of at least 15 on the International Restless Legs Syndrome [IRLS] scale, and a history of symptoms for at least 15 days in the month prior to screening). The primary measure of efficacy in these studies was a composite of the change from baseline in IRLS total score and the proportion of patients considered to be responders (i.e., those with a "much improved" or "very much improved" rating on the Clinical Global Impression-Global Improvement [CGI-I] scale) at 12 weeks. Gabapentin enacarbil (600 mg or 1.2 g once daily as extended-release tablets) substantially improved both measures of efficacy compared with placebo; improvements were noted as early as 1 week and were maintained throughout the duration of the studies. At 12 weeks, the mean change in IRLS score was a reduction of 13–13.8 with gabapentin enacarbil (versus a reduction of 8.8–9.8 with placebo), and 73–77% of patients receiving gabapentin enacarbil compared with 39–45% of those receiving placebo were described as responders. The 1.2-g daily dosage of gabapentin enacarbil appeared to provide no additional benefit over the 600-mg daily dosage, and was associated with an increased incidence of adverse effects.

Gabapentin also has been used in the treatment of restless legs syndrome†; however, the drug currently is not labeled by the FDA for this use. Although evidence supporting the use of gabapentin for restless legs syndrome alone generally is insufficient, some experts state that the analgesic effects of the drug may provide some benefit in patients with both restless legs syndrome and pain.

■ Vasomotor Symptoms Gabapentin has been used for the management of vasomotor symptoms† in women with breast cancer and in postmenopausal women. Therapy with the drug has improved both the frequency and severity of vasomotor symptoms (e.g., hot flushes or flashes) in these women.

Most women receiving systemic antineoplastic therapy for breast cancer experience vasomotor symptoms, particularly those receiving tamoxifen therapy. In a randomized, double-blind, placebo-controlled study in 420 women with breast cancer (68–75% were receiving tamoxifen) who were experiencing 2 or more episodes of hot flushes daily, the percentage reductions in hot flush severity score at 4 and 8 weeks of treatment were 21 and 15%, respectively, for placebo; 33 and 31%, respectively, for gabapentin 300 mg daily (100 mg 3 times daily), and 49 and 46%, respectively, for gabapentin 900 mg daily (300 mg 3 times daily). Comparisons among treatment groups showed that only the 900-mg daily dosage was associated with a statistically significant reduction in hot flush frequency and severity. Whether higher dosages will provide further reductions in vasomotor symptoms remains to be determined. The role of gabapentin in managing vasomotor symptoms in women with breast cancer relative to other nonhormonal therapies (e.g., selective serotonin-reuptake inhibitors [SSRIs], selective serotonin- and norepinephrine-reuptake inhibitors [SNRIs]) remains to be determined. Well-designed, comparative studies are needed to establish optimum nonhormonal therapy, both in terms of efficacy and patient tolerance of adverse effects, in these women.

Because of the risks associated with hormone replacement therapy (HRT) for vasomotor symptoms in perimenopausal and postmenopausal women, alternative nonhormonal therapies are being investigated. In a randomized, double-blind, placebo-controlled study in 59 postmenopausal women who were experiencing 7 or more hot flushes daily, intent-to-treat analysis revealed that 12 weeks of gabapentin 900 mg daily (300 mg 3 times daily) was associated with a 45% reduction in hot flush frequency and a 54% reduction in composite hot flush score (frequency and severity). In a continuation open-label phase in which patients were permitted upward titration of dosage as needed to a maximum of 2.7 g daily (25% received 900 mg or less daily, 61% received 900 mg–1.8 g daily, 14% received 1.8–2.7 g daily), the associated reductions in hot flush frequency and composite score were 54 and 67%, respectively. The role of gabapentin therapy relative to other nonhormonal therapies (e.g., SSRIs, SNRIs) for postmenopausal vasomotor symptoms, both in terms of efficacy and safety, as well as the optimum dosage remain to be established.

Current evidence indicates that gabapentin is effective and well tolerated in the short-term treatment of vasomotor symptoms associated with breast cancer treatment and with menopause. The principal adverse effects associated with gabapentin therapy in women with vasomotor symptoms have been somnolence, fatigue, dizziness, and rash (with or without peripheral edema). Additional study and experience are needed to further elucidate the role of gabapentin relative to other nonhormonal therapies, and to establish longer-term (i.e., beyond 17 weeks) efficacy and safety.

The possible role of gabapentin in the management of vasomotor symptoms† associated with antiandrogenic therapy in men with prostate cancer remains to be established. Current evidence of efficacy is limited; well-designed, controlled studies are under way in this population.

Dosage and Administration

■ Administration Gabapentin and gabapentin enacarbil are administered orally.

If discontinuance of gabapentin or gabapentin enacarbil therapy is required, gradual tapering of the dosage generally is recommended to avoid manifestations of abrupt withdrawal. (See Dosage and Administration: Dosage, and also see Cautions: Precautions and Contraindications.)

Patients who are currently receiving or beginning therapy with gabapentin, gabapentin enacarbil, and/or any other anticonvulsant for any indication should be closely monitored for the emergence or worsening of depression, suicidal thoughts or behavior (suicidality), and/or any unusual changes in mood or behavior. (See Suicidality under Cautions: Nervous System Effects and see Cautions: Precautions and Contraindications.)

Gabapentin Gabapentin is commercially available as conventional (immediate-release) capsules, tablets, or oral solution (e.g., Neurontin®). The drug also is available as a gastroretentive tablet (Gralise®) for once-daily administration in the treatment of postherpetic neuralgia (PHN). Although the gastroretentive tablet is not considered by the FDA to be an extended-release formulation, it is sometimes referred to in this manner because of similar pharmacokinetic properties to an extended-release dosage form (see Description). Because of differences in pharmacokinetics that affect frequency of administration, gabapentin gastroretentive tablets are not interchangeable with other gabapentin preparations.

Conventional (immediate-release) preparations of gabapentin should be administered orally in divided doses (3 times daily) without regard to meals; food does not substantially affect the bioavailability of gabapentin when administered as an immediate-release formulation. Gabapentin capsules should be swallowed whole with water. If film-coated scored tablets containing 600 or 800 mg of gabapentin are divided to allow administration of a 300- or 400-mg dose, the remaining half tablet should be used for the next dose; half tablets that are not used within 28 days should be discarded.

Gabapentin gastroretentive tablets should be administered orally once daily with the evening meal; food increases the rate and extent of absorption of gabapentin when administered as the gastroretentive formulation. The gastroretentive tablets should be swallowed intact and not chewed, crushed, or split.

If use of an antacid containing aluminum hydroxide and magnesium hydroxide is necessary in a patient receiving gabapentin, it is recommended that gabapentin be administered at least 2 hours after the antacid.

Gabapentin Enacarbil Gabapentin enacarbil is commercially available as extended-release tablets (Horizant®) for administration once or twice daily depending on the indication. When used for the treatment of restless legs syndrome, the drug should be administered once daily at about 5 p.m.; if a dose is missed, the next dose should be taken the following day as scheduled. When used for the management of PHN, gabapentin enacarbil extended-release tablets should be administered twice daily; if a dose is missed, the dose should be skipped and the next dose taken at the regularly scheduled time. Gabapentin enacarbil extended-release tablets should be swallowed intact and not crushed, chewed, or cut.

Because of differences in pharmacokinetics that affect frequency of administration, gabapentin enacarbil extended-release tablets are not interchangeable with other gabapentin preparations.

■ **Dosage** ***Seizure Disorders*** For adjunctive therapy in the management of partial seizures with or without secondary generalization in adults and children 12 years of age or older, the manufacturer recommends an initial gabapentin dosage of 300 mg 3 times daily and a maintenance dosage of 300–600 mg 3 times daily (as conventional capsules, tablets, or oral solution). Dosages up to 2.4 g daily have been well tolerated in long-term clinical studies, and a small number of patients have tolerated dosages of 3.6 g daily for short periods. When administered 3 times daily, the interval between doses should not exceed 12 hours.

In pediatric patients 3–11 years of age, the recommended initial dosage of gabapentin (as conventional capsules, tablets, or oral solution) for the management of partial seizures is 10–15 mg/kg daily in 3 divided doses. Dosage should be titrated upward over a period of approximately 3 days until an effective maintenance dosage is achieved. The recommended maintenance dosage of gabapentin in pediatric patients 5–11 years of age is 25–35 mg/kg daily administered in 3 divided doses; for children 3–4 years of age, the recommended maintenance dosage is 40 mg/kg daily administered in 3 divided doses. Dosages up to 50 mg/kg daily have been well tolerated by pediatric patients 3–12 years of age in a long-term clinical study. When administered 3 times daily, the interval between doses should not exceed 12 hours.

Gabapentin may be used concomitantly with other anticonvulsant agents without concern for alterations in plasma drug concentrations; additional monitoring of plasma concentrations of anticonvulsant agents is not necessary during such concomitant therapy.

If gabapentin dosage reduction or discontinuance or substitution of an alternative anticonvulsant is necessary, such changes in therapy should be made gradually over a period of at least 1 week.

Postherpetic Neuralgia For the management of postherpetic neuralgia (PHN) in adults, the initial dosage regimen of gabapentin as conventional (immediate-release) preparations is 300 mg once daily on the first day, 300 mg twice daily on the second day, and 300 mg 3 times daily on the third day. Subsequently, the dosage may be increased as needed for relief of pain up to a total dosage of 1.8 g daily administered in 3 divided doses. The recommended dosage of gabapentin as gastroretentive tablets in adults with PHN is 1.8 g once daily; dosage should be titrated gradually over 2 weeks up to the recommended maintenance dosage as follows: 300 mg once daily on the first day, 600 mg once daily on the second day, 900 mg once daily on days 3–6, 1.2 g once daily on days 7–10, 1.5 g once daily on days 11–14, and 1.8 g once daily on day 15. In clinical studies evaluating gabapentin for the treatment of PHN, dosages of the drug ranging from 1.8–3.6 g daily were effective, but there was no evidence that dosages exceeding 1.8 g daily provided any additional benefit. If gabapentin dosage reduction or discontinuance or substitution of an alternative drug is necessary, such changes in therapy should be made gradually over a period of at least 1 week.

If gabapentin enacarbil is used for the management of PHN in adults, the recommended dosage is 600 mg twice daily (as extended-release tablets); dosage should be initiated at 600 mg once daily in the morning for 3 days, then increased to 600 mg twice daily on day 4. In the principal efficacy study of gabapentin enacarbil in patients with PHN, dosages exceeding 1.2 g daily provided no additional benefit and were associated with an increased incidence of adverse effects. When discontinuing gabapentin enacarbil therapy, patients receiving a dosage of 600 mg twice daily should reduce their dosage to 600 mg once daily for 1 week prior to withdrawing therapy. (See Cautions: Precautions and Contraindications.)

Restless Legs Syndrome For the treatment of restless legs syndrome, the recommended adult dosage of gabapentin enacarbil (as extended-release tablets) is 600 mg once daily, administered at approximately 5 p.m. In clinical studies, a higher dosage of 1.2 g daily provided no additional benefit and was associated with an increased incidence of adverse effects.

When discontinuing gabapentin enacarbil therapy in patients with restless legs syndrome, gradual tapering of the dosage is not necessary in patients receiving a dosage of 600 mg or less once daily; however, in patients receiving higher than recommended dosages, dosage should be reduced to 600 mg once daily for 1 week prior to withdrawing therapy. (See Cautions: Precautions and Contraindications.)

Diabetic Neuropathy For the symptomatic treatment of diabetic neuropathy† in adults, gabapentin dosages of 900 mg to 3.6 g daily have been used; however, pain relief generally has been observed in patients receiving dosages exceeding 1.8 g daily.

Vasomotor Symptoms Although the optimum dosage remains to be established, a gabapentin dosage of 300 mg 3 times daily (as conventional [immediate-release] preparations) has been effective in reducing both the severity and frequency of vasomotor symptoms† in women with breast cancer and in postmenopausal women. Some clinicians recommend that therapy be initiated with a dosage of 300 mg once daily at bedtime. If needed, the dosage can be increased to 300 mg twice daily, and then to 300 mg 3 times daily, at 3- to 4-day intervals. A dosage of 100 mg 3 times daily appears to be no more effective than placebo, whereas dosages exceeding 900 mg daily (e.g., up to 2.7 g daily administered as 900 mg 3 times daily) may provide additional benefit in some women.

■ **Dosage in Renal Impairment** ***Gabapentin*** In adults and children 12 years of age or older with impaired renal function or undergoing hemodialysis, dosage of gabapentin (as conventional preparations) should be reduced from the effective dosages for each indication based on the patient's creatinine clearance (see Table 1). In patients with a creatinine clearance of less than 15 mL/minute, dosage should be reduced in proportion to creatinine clearance (e.g., a patient with a creatinine clearance of 7.5 mL/minute should receive one-half the dosage that a patient with a creatinine clearance of 15 mL/minute should receive). Patients undergoing hemodialysis should receive a supplemental dose of gabapentin 125–350 mg immediately following each 4-hour hemodialysis session in addition to their renally adjusted daily dosage of the drug. The use of gabapentin conventional preparations in children younger than 12 years of age with impaired renal function has not been evaluated.

Table 1. Dosage Adjustments for Renal Impairment in Adults and Children 12 Years of Age or Older Receiving Conventional (Immediate-release) Gabapentin

Creatinine Clearance (mL/minute)	Adjusted Dosage Regimen
>30 to 59	200–700 mg twice daily (i.e., up to a total dosage of 1.4 g daily)
>15 to 29	200–700 mg once daily
15	100–300 mg once daily

If gabapentin gastroretentive tablets are used in adults with a creatinine clearance of 30–60 mL/minute, dosage of the drug should be reduced to a target daily dosage between 600 mg and 1.8 g once daily; dosage must be initiated at 300 mg once daily in these patients and may be titrated according to the same schedule recommended for those with normal renal function based on individual patient response and tolerability. Gabapentin gastroretentive tablets should not be used in patients with a creatinine clearance of less than 30 mL/minute or in those undergoing hemodialysis.

Gabapentin Enacarbil In patients with renal impairment, dosage of gabapentin enacarbil should be modified based on the degree of impairment as assessed by creatinine clearance (see Tables 2 or 3 depending on indication).

Table 2. Dosage Adjustments for Renal Impairment in Adults Receiving Gabapentin Enacarbil for Postherpetic Neuralgia

Creatinine Clearance (mL/minute)	Titration Schedule	Maintenance Dosage	Tapering Schedule
30–59	300 mg once daily in the morning for 3 days	300 mg twice daily; increase to 600 mg twice daily as necessary based on patient response and tolerability	Reduce maintenance dosage to once daily in the morning for 1 week
15–29	300 mg once daily in the morning on days 1 and 3	300 mg once daily in the morning; increase to 300 mg twice daily if necessary based on patient response and tolerability	In patients currently receiving a maintenance dosage of 300 mg twice daily, reduce to 300 mg once daily in the morning for 1 week; in patients currently receiving a maintenance dosage of 300 mg once daily, no taper needed
<15 not on hemodialysis	None	300 mg every other day in the morning; increase to 300 mg once daily if necessary based on patient response and tolerability	None
<15 on hemodialysis	None	300 mg following each hemodialysis session; increase to 600 mg following each hemodialysis session if necessary based on patient response and tolerability	None

Table 3. Dosage Adjustments for Renal Impairment in Adults Receiving Gabapentin Enacarbil for Restless Legs Syndrome

Creatinine Clearance (mL/minute)	Target Dosage
30–59	Initiate at 300 mg once daily, then increase to 600 mg once daily as needed
15–29	300 mg once daily
<15 not on hemodialysis	300 mg every other day
<15 on hemodialysis	Use not recommended

Cautions

Gabapentin generally is well tolerated, and adverse effects of the drug usually are mild to moderate in severity and may be self-limiting. Nervous system effects are the most frequently reported adverse affects of gabapentin and those most frequently requiring discontinuance of the drug. The most frequent adverse effects of conventional (immediate-release) gabapentin as adjunctive therapy in the treatment of partial seizures in adults and children older than 12 years of age are somnolence, dizziness, ataxia, fatigue, and nystagmus. Discontinuance of gabapentin because of adverse effects was required in 7% of adults and children older than 12 years of age receiving the drug as adjunctive therapy in the treatment of partial seizures in premarketing uncontrolled and controlled clinical trials; the adverse effects most frequently associated with discontinuance of gabapentin were somnolence (1.2% of patients), ataxia (0.8% of patients), fatigue (0.6% of patients), nausea and/or vomiting (0.6% of patients), and dizziness (0.6% of patients). The most frequent adverse effects of conventional (immediate-release) gabapentin as adjunctive therapy in the treatment of partial seizures in patients 3–12 years of age were viral infection, fever, nausea and/or vomiting, somnolence, and hostility. Discontinuance of gabapentin because of adverse effects was required in approximately 7% of patients 3–12 years of age in clinical trials; the adverse effects most frequently associated with discontinuance of gabapentin were emotional lability (1.6%), hostility (1.3%), and hyperkinesia (1.1%).

Because clinical trials of gabapentin therapy in the treatment of partial seizures involved specific patient populations and use of the drug as adjunctive therapy, it is difficult to determine whether a causal relationship exists for many reported adverse effects, to compare adverse effect frequencies with other clinical reports, and/or to extrapolate the adverse effect experience from controlled clinical trials to usual clinical practice.

In placebo-controlled studies of gabapentin for the management of postherpetic neuralgia (PHN), adverse effects most frequently reported in adults receiving conventional (immediate-release) preparations of the drug were dizziness, somnolence, and peripheral edema. Discontinuance of gabapentin because of adverse effects was required in 16% of patients receiving the drug for the management of PHN in 2 clinical trials; adverse effects most frequently associated with discontinuance of therapy were dizziness, somnolence, and nausea. In placebo-controlled studies using the gastroretentive tablet formulation of gabapentin, dizziness was reported as the most frequent adverse effect (10.9% of patients); in these trials, 9.7% of patients required premature discontinuance of therapy because of adverse effects, the most common of which was dizziness.

Similar to gabapentin, the most frequently reported adverse effects of gabapentin enacarbil are nervous system effects. In the principal efficacy study of gabapentin enacarbil for the management of PHN, the most common adverse effects reported were dizziness, somnolence, and headache. Adverse effects resulted in discontinuance of gabapentin enacarbil therapy in 6% of patients with PHN, which was lower than the rate of discontinuance with placebo. The most common adverse effects observed in patients receiving gabapentin enacarbil for the treatment of restless legs syndrome in placebo-controlled trials were somnolence/sedation and dizziness; in these trials, 7% of patients required premature discontinuance of therapy because of adverse effects.

■ **Nervous System Effects** Nervous system effects were among the most frequent adverse effects reported in patients with epilepsy receiving conventional (immediate-release) gabapentin as adjunctive therapy in controlled clinical trials in adults and children older than 12 years of age. Somnolence was the most frequent adverse nervous system effect, occurring in about 19% of those receiving the drug; the incidence and severity of somnolence appear to be dose related. Dizziness or ataxia was reported in about 17 or 12.5%, respectively, of patients receiving conventional (immediate-release) gabapentin as adjunctive therapy for seizures in controlled trials; the incidence and severity of ataxia also appear to be dose related. Fatigue reportedly occurred in about 11% of patients receiving conventional (immediate-release) gabapentin as adjunctive therapy for seizures in placebo-controlled trials. Nystagmus was reported in 8%, tremor in 7%, dysarthria in 2%, amnesia in 2%, depression in 2%, abnormal thinking in 2%, and abnormal coordination in 1% of patients receiving the drug.

Somnolence, hostility (including aggressive behavior), and emotional lability were reported in 8, 8, and 4%, respectively, of children 3–12 years of age receiving conventional (immediate-release) gabapentin as adjunctive therapy for seizures in controlled clinical trials. Fatigue, hyperkinesia, and dizziness each were reported in 3% of these patients receiving the drug. Headache and convulsions were reported in more than 2% and equally or more frequently than among those receiving placebo in children 3–12 years of age receiving the drug. Thought disorders (e.g., concentration difficulty, change in school performance) have been reported in 1.7% of children 3–12 years of age receiving the drug.

Dizziness was reported in 28%, somnolence in 21%, asthenia in 6%, ataxia in 3%, and abnormal thinking in 3% of adults receiving conventional (immediate-release) gabapentin for the management of PHN in controlled clinical trials. Abnormal gait and incoordination occurred in 2% of patients receiving the drug. Pain, tremor, and neuralgia were reported in greater than 1% of patients receiving gabapentin in clinical studies for the management of PHN but occurred with equal or greater frequency in patients receiving placebo. Dizziness, somnolence, headache, and lethargy were reported in 10.9, 4.5, 4.2, and 1.1% of adults receiving gabapentin gastroretentive tablets for PHN in controlled clinical studies; vertigo occurred in 1.4% of patients receiving the drug.

In the placebo-controlled study of gabapentin enacarbil for the management of PHN, dizziness was reported in 17–30%, somnolence was reported in 10–14%, and headache was reported in 7–10% of patients receiving the drug. Fatigue or asthenia occurred in 4–10% and insomnia occurred in 3–7% of these patients. Somnolence/sedation (20–27%) and dizziness (13–22%) were the most common adverse effects reported in patients receiving gabapentin enacarbil for the treatment of restless legs syndrome in placebo-controlled studies. Headache occurred in 12–15%, fatigue in 6–7%, and irritability in 4% of patients receiving the drug; 1–3% of these patients reported feeling intoxicated. Depression and decreased libido were reported in up to 3% and up to 2% of these patients, respectively.

The effect of gabapentin enacarbil on driving performance was evaluated in several driving simulation studies. In one study in healthy individuals, gabapentin enacarbil (600 mg once daily for 5 days) did not appear to affect driving performance (as assessed by lane position variability) when tested at various time points after dosing. However, results of another driving simulation study in patients with moderate-to-severe primary restless legs syndrome showed evidence of substantial driving impairment with gabapentin enacarbil administration (1.2 or 1.8 g daily); patients receiving gabapentin enacarbil had greater lane position variability and a higher incidence of simulated crashes compared with those receiving placebo or an active comparator (diphenhydramine). There is some evidence, however, that patients with restless legs syndrome may have impaired driving ability in the absence of medication.

Suicidality The US Food and Drug Administration (FDA) has analyzed suicidality reports from placebo-controlled studies involving 11 anticonvulsants, including gabapentin, and found that patients receiving anticonvulsants had approximately twice the risk of suicidal behavior or ideation (0.43%) compared with patients receiving placebo (0.24%).

FDA's analysis included 199 randomized, placebo-controlled studies of 11 anticonvulsants (carbamazepine, felbamate, gabapentin, lamotrigine, levetiracetam, oxcarbazepine, pregabalin, tiagabine, topiramate, valproate, and zonisamide) involving over 43,000 patients 5 years of age or older; the studies evaluated the effectiveness of the anticonvulsants in epilepsy, psychiatric disorders (e.g., bipolar disorder, depression, anxiety), and other conditions (e.g., migraine, neuropathic pain). The increased suicidality risk was observed as early as one week after beginning therapy and continued through 24 weeks. The results were generally consistent among the 11 drugs studied. In addition, patients who were treated for epilepsy, psychiatric disorders, and other conditions were all found to be at increased risk for suicidality when compared with placebo; there did not appear to be a specific demographic subgroup of patients to which the increased risk could be attributed. However, the relative risk for suicidality was found to be higher in patients with epilepsy compared with patients who were given one of the drugs for psychiatric or other conditions. (See Cautions: Precautions and Contraindications.)

■ **GI Effects** Dyspepsia, dry mouth or throat, constipation, and dental abnormalities each occurred in 2% of adults and children older than 12 years of age receiving conventional (immediate-release) gabapentin as adjunctive therapy for seizures in controlled clinical trials.

Nausea and/or vomiting was reported in 8% of children 3–12 years of age receiving conventional (immediate-release) gabapentin as adjunctive therapy for seizures in controlled clinical trials. Diarrhea and anorexia were reported in more than 2% of children 3–12 years of age receiving the drug in these trials.

Diarrhea was reported in 6%, dry mouth in 5%, constipation in 4%, nausea in 4%, and vomiting in 3% of adults receiving conventional (immediate-release) gabapentin for the management of PHN in controlled clinical trials. Dyspepsia was reported in greater than 1% of patients receiving conventional (immediate-release) gabapentin for the management of PHN in clinical studies, but occurred with equal or greater frequency in patients receiving placebo. In controlled clinical trials evaluating gabapentin gastroretentive tablets for the management of PHN, diarrhea was reported in 3.3%, dry mouth in 2.8%, constipation in 1.4%, and dyspepsia in 1.4% of adults receiving the drug.

In the principal efficacy study of gabapentin enacarbil in the management of PHN, nausea occurred in 4–9% of adults receiving the drug. Nausea, dry mouth, and flatulence were reported in 6–7%, 3–4%, and 2–3%, respectively, of patients receiving gabapentin enacarbil in placebo-controlled studies of the drug for restless legs syndrome.

■ **Cardiovascular Effects** Peripheral edema was reported in 2% and vasodilation in 1% of adults and children older than 12 years of age receiving conventional (immediate-release) gabapentin as adjunctive therapy for seizures in controlled clinical trials.

Peripheral edema was reported in 8% of adults receiving conventional (immediate-release) gabapentin and in 3.9% of adults receiving gabapentin gastroretentive tablets for the management of PHN in controlled clinical trials.

In controlled clinical studies, peripheral edema was reported in 6–7% of adults receiving gabapentin enacarbil for the management of PHN and in up to 3% of adults receiving the drug for restless legs syndrome.

■ **Respiratory Effects** Pharyngitis occurred in 3% and coughing in 2% of adults and children older than 12 years of age receiving conventional (immediate-release) gabapentin as adjunctive therapy for seizures in controlled clinical trials.

Bronchitis and respiratory infection each were reported in 3% of children 3–12 years of age receiving conventional (immediate-release) gabapentin as adjunctive therapy for seizures in controlled clinical trials. Pharyngitis, upper respiratory infection, rhinitis, and coughing were reported in more than 2% of these children in these studies.

Pharyngitis was reported in 1% of adults receiving conventional (immediate-release) gabapentin for the management of PHN in controlled clinical trials; dyspnea was reported in greater than 1% of patients receiving the drug, but occurred with equal or greater frequency in patients receiving placebo. Nasopharyngitis was reported in 2.5% of adults receiving gabapentin gastroretentive tablets for PHN in controlled clinical trials.

■ **Ocular and Otic Effects** Diplopia was reported in 6% and amblyopia in 4% of adults and children older than 12 years of age receiving conventional (immediate-release) gabapentin as adjunctive therapy for seizures in controlled clinical trials.

Otitis media was reported in more than 2% of children 3–12 years of age receiving conventional (immediate-release) gabapentin as adjunctive therapy for seizures in clinical studies.

Amblyopia occurred in 3%, and conjunctivitis, diplopia, and otitis media each occurred in 1% of adults receiving conventional (immediate-release) gabapentin for the management of PHN in controlled clinical trials. In the placebo-controlled study of gabapentin enacarbil for the management of PHN, blurred vision occurred in 2–5% of adults receiving the drug.

■ **Musculoskeletal Effects** Back pain was reported in 2% of adults and children older than 12 years of age receiving conventional (immediate-release) gabapentin as adjunctive therapy for seizures in controlled clinical trials.

Elevated creatine kinase, rhabdomyolysis, and movement disorders have been reported during postmarketing experience with conventional (immediate-release) gabapentin; however, the manufacturers state that data are insufficient to provide an estimate of the incidence of such effects or to establish a causal relationship to the drug.

Back pain was reported in greater than 1% of adults receiving conventional (immediate-release) gabapentin in clinical studies for the management of PHN but occurred with equal or greater frequency in patients receiving placebo. Back pain and extremity pain were reported in 1.7 and 1.9%, respectively, of adults receiving gabapentin gastroretentive tablets for PHN in controlled clinical trials.

■ **Genitourinary Effects** Impotence was reported in 2% of patients receiving conventional (immediate-release) gabapentin as adjunctive therapy for seizures in controlled clinical trials.

■ **Dermatologic and Sensitivity Reactions** Abrasion occurred in 1% of adults and children older than 12 years of age receiving conventional (immediate-release) gabapentin as adjunctive therapy for seizures in controlled clinical trials.

Angioedema, erythema multiforme, and Stevens-Johnson syndrome have been reported during postmarketing experience with conventional (immediate-release) gabapentin; however, the manufacturers state that data are insufficient to provide an estimate of the incidence of such effects or to establish a causal relationship to gabapentin.

Multiorgan hypersensitivity reactions (also known as drug reaction with eosinophilia and systemic symptoms or DRESS) have been reported in patients receiving anticonvulsants, including gabapentin. The clinical presentation is variable, but typically includes fever, rash, eosinophilia, and/or lymphadenopathy in association with other organ system involvement (e.g., hepatitis, nephritis, hematologic abnormalities, myositis, myocarditis). In some cases, these reactions have been life-threatening or fatal. Early manifestations of hypersensitivity (e.g., fever, lymphadenopathy) may be present even if a rash is not evident.

■ **Hepatic Effects** Elevated liver function test results and jaundice have been reported during postmarketing experience with conventional (immediate-release) gabapentin; however, the manufacturers state that data are insufficient to provide an estimate of the incidence of such effects or to establish a causal relationship to gabapentin.

■ **Electrolyte and Metabolic Effects** Weight gain has been reported in 3% of patients receiving conventional (immediate-release) gabapentin as adjunctive therapy for seizures in clinical trials.

Weight gain and hyperglycemia were reported in 2 and 1%, respectively, of adults receiving conventional (immediate-release) gabapentin for the management of PHN in controlled clinical trials. In studies evaluating gabapentin gastroretentive tablets for the management of PHN, weight gain was reported in 1.9% of adults receiving the drug.

Fluctuation in blood glucose concentrations and hyponatremia have been reported during postmarketing experience with conventional (immediate-release) gabapentin; however, the manufacturers state that data are insufficient to provide an estimate of the incidence of such effects or to establish a causal relationship to the drug.

Weight increase was reported in 3% of children 3–12 years of age receiving conventional (immediate-release) gabapentin in controlled clinical trials.

In placebo-controlled studies of gabapentin enacarbil for the treatment of restless legs syndrome, weight gain occurred in 2–3% and increased appetite occurred in 2% of patients receiving the drug; weight gain was reported in 3–5% of patients receiving gabapentin enacarbil for the management of PHN in the principal efficacy study.

■ **Other Adverse Effects** Breast enlargement has been reported during postmarketing experience with conventional (immediate-release) gabapentin; however, the manufacturers state that data are insufficient to provide an estimate of the incidence of such an effect or to establish a causal relationship to the drug.

Viral infection and fever were reported in 11 and 10%, respectively, of children 3–12 years of age receiving conventional (immediate-release) gabapentin as adjunctive therapy for seizures in controlled clinical trials.

Infection and accidental injury were reported in 5 and 3%, respectively, of adults receiving conventional (immediate-release) gabapentin for the management of PHN in controlled clinical trials. Flu syndrome was reported in greater than 1% of patients receiving conventional (immediate-release) gabapentin for the management of PHN, but occurred with equal or greater frequency in patients receiving placebo. In controlled clinical trials evaluating gabapentin gastroretentive tablets for the management of PHN, urinary tract infection was reported in 1.7% of adults receiving the drug.

In placebo-controlled studies of gabapentin enacarbil for the treatment of restless legs syndrome, up to 3% of patients reported feeling abnormal.

■ **Precautions and Contraindications** The FDA has informed healthcare professionals about an increased risk of suicidality (suicidal behavior or ideation) observed in an analysis of studies using various anticonvulsants, including gabapentin, compared with placebo. (See Suicidality under Cautions: Nervous System Effects.) Because gabapentin enacarbil is a prodrug of gabapentin, a similar risk with gabapentin enacarbil cannot be ruled out. Based on the current analysis of the available data, FDA recommends that all patients who are currently receiving or beginning therapy with any anticonvulsant for any indication be closely monitored for the emergence or worsening of depression, suicidal thoughts or behavior (suicidality), and/or any unusual changes in mood or behavior. Symptoms such as anxiety, agitation, hostility, mania, and hypomania may be precursors to emerging suicidality. Clinicians should inform patients, their families, and caregivers of the potential for an increased risk of suicidality so that they are aware and able to notify their clinician of any unusual behavioral changes. Patients, family members, and caregivers also should be advised not to make any changes to the drug regimen without first consulting with the responsible clinician. They should pay close attention to any day-to-day changes in mood, behavior, and actions; since changes can happen very quickly, it is important to be alert to any sudden differences. In addition, patients, family members, and caregivers should be aware of common warning signs that may signal suicide risk (e.g., talking or thinking about wanting to hurt oneself or end one's life, withdrawing from friends and family, becoming depressed or experiencing worsening of existing depression, becoming preoccupied with death and dying, giving away prized possessions). If these or any new and worrisome behaviors occur, the responsible clinician should be contacted immediately.

FDA recommends that clinicians who prescribe gabapentin or any other anticonvulsant balance the risk for suicidality with the risk of untreated illness. Epilepsy and many other illnesses for which anticonvulsants are prescribed are themselves associated with an increased risk of morbidity and mortality and an increased risk of suicidal thoughts and behavior. If suicidal thoughts and behavior emerge during anticonvulsant therapy, the clinician must consider whether the emergence of these symptoms in any given patient may be related to the illness being treated.

Because of the possibility of increased seizure frequency and other withdrawal symptoms (e.g., anxiety, insomnia, nausea), anticonvulsant drugs, including gabapentin and gabapentin enacarbil, should not be discontinued suddenly. In controlled studies of gabapentin as conventional (immediate-release) formulations, the incidence of status epilepticus was 0.6% in adults and children older than 12 years of age receiving gabapentin and 0.5% in those receiving placebo. In all (uncontrolled and controlled) clinical studies of gabapentin as adjunctive therapy in adults and children older than 12 years of age, the incidence of status epilepticus was 1.5%. Because adequate historical data are unavailable for comparison, it has not been established whether the incidence of status epilepticus in patients with epilepsy treated with gabapentin is higher or lower than would be expected in a similar population of patients not treated with the drug. Discontinuance of gabapentin and gabapentin enacarbil should be done gradually. (See Dosage and Administration: Dosage.)

During the premarketing development of conventional (immediate-release) gabapentin, 8 sudden and unexplained deaths were reported among a cohort of 2203 patients with epilepsy (2103 patient-years of exposure). Although the rate of these deaths exceeds that expected to occur in a healthy (nonepileptic) population matched for age and gender, this rate was similar to that occurring in a similar population of epileptic patients not receiving gabapentin. This evidence suggests, but does not prove that the incidence of sudden, unexplained death observed with adjunctive gabapentin therapy may be reflective of the population itself rather than the effects of gabapentin.

Gabapentin and gabapentin enacarbil can produce drowsiness and dizziness, and patients should be cautioned that the drug may impair their ability to perform hazardous activities requiring mental alertness or physical coordination (e.g., operating machinery, driving a motor vehicle) or cause accidental injury (e.g., falls). Gabapentin enacarbil has been shown to cause substantial impairment in driving performance, which may be related to somnolence or other CNS effects of the drug; the duration of such impairment following administration of the drug is not known. The manufacturers state that patients should not drive a car (or operate other complex machinery) until they have gained sufficient experience with gabapentin or gabapentin enacarbil; clinicians should consider that a patient's ability to assess their performance on these tasks or their degree of somnolence may not be reliable.

Patients should be evaluated immediately if manifestations of a multiorgan hypersensitivity reaction (or DRESS) occur during gabapentin or gabapentin enacarbil therapy; the drug should be discontinued if an alternative etiology cannot be identified.

Concomitant use of alcohol or other drugs that can cause sedation or dizziness can potentiate the CNS effects of gabapentin and generally should be avoided. In addition, alcohol can increase the rate of drug release from gabapentin enacarbil extended-release tablets and should be avoided in patients receiving this formulation. Concomitant use of opiate analgesics in patients receiving gabapentin may result in increased plasma concentrations of gabapentin and increase the risk of adverse CNS effects and respiratory depression; dosage adjustments may be required with such concomitant use.

Gabapentin is contraindicated in patients with known hypersensitivity to the drug or any ingredient in the formulation. The manufacturer of gabapentin enacarbil states that there are no known contraindications to the use of this preparation.

■ **Pediatric Precautions** Safety and efficacy of conventional (immediate-release) gabapentin as adjunctive therapy in the management of partial seizures in children younger than 3 years of age have not been established. Safety and efficacy of conventional (immediate-release) gabapentin in the management of PHN have not been established in pediatric patients. Safety and efficacy of gabapentin gastroretentive tablets and gabapentin enacarbil have not been established in pediatric patients.

■ **Geriatric Precautions** Safety and efficacy of conventional (immediate-release) gabapentin in the management of partial seizures in geriatric patients have not been evaluated systematically, and clinical trials did not include sufficient numbers of patients 65 years of age and older to determine whether they respond differently than do younger patients. However, in clinical studies of the drug in patients ranging from 20–80 years of age, gabapentin plasma clearance, renal clearance, and renal clearance adjusted for body surface area declined with age. Although safety and efficacy of conventional (immediate-release) gabapentin in geriatric patients with PHN have not been established specifically, 30% of the patients receiving the drug in clinical studies were 65–74 years of age and 50% were 75 years of age and older. In these studies, gabapentin appeared to be more effective for the management of PHN in patients older than 75 years of age than in younger patients. The manufacturers state that the apparent greater efficacy in geriatric patients may be related to decreased renal function in this age group. Although adverse effects reported in older patients receiving conventional (immediate-release) gabapentin generally were similar to those reported in younger adults, the incidence of peripheral edema and ataxia appeared to increase with age. Among patients receiving the gastroretentive formulation of gabapentin in clinical studies, 63% were 65 years of age or older. Adverse effects reported in these studies generally were similar across all age groups except for the incidence of peripheral edema, which tended to increase with age.

Clinical trials of gabapentin enacarbil for the treatment of restless legs syndrome did not include sufficient numbers of patients 65 years of age or older to determine whether they respond differently than younger patients. In the principal efficacy study of gabapentin enacarbil for the treatment of PHN, 37% of the patients were 65–74 years of age and 13% were 75 years of age and older. No overall differences in safety and efficacy were observed between these geriatric patients and younger patients.

If gabapentin or gabapentin enacarbil is used in geriatric patients, dosage reduction may be required because of age-related compromised renal function; caution should be exercised since renal, hepatic, and cardiovascular dysfunction and concomitant disease or other drug therapy are more common in this age group than in younger patients. (See Dosage and Administration: Dosage in Renal Impairment.)

■ **Mutagenicity and Carcinogenicity** Gabapentin has not been shown to be mutagenic or genotoxic in various in vitro and in vivo tests.

An increased incidence of pancreatic acinar cell tumors was observed with gabapentin and gabapentin enacarbil in rat carcinogenicity studies; the clinical importance of these findings to humans is not known. In clinical studies of gabapentin in patients older than 12 years of age with seizure disorders, new tumors or worsening of preexisting tumors was reported in 21 patients (based on 2085 patient-years of exposure); however, a causal relationship to the drug has not been established.

■ **Pregnancy, Fertility, and Lactation** ***Pregnancy*** Although there are no adequate and controlled studies to date in pregnant women, gabapentin and gabapentin enacarbil have been shown to cause developmental toxicity when administered to pregnant animals during the period of organogenesis at doses similar to or lower than those used clinically. Such effects include skeletal abnormalities, hydroureter and hydronephrosis, and increased embryofetal mortality. In addition, abnormal or decreased synaptic formation was observed in neonatal mice exposed to intraperitoneal injections of gabapentin during the first postnatal week (corresponding to the last trimester of pregnancy in humans); the clinical importance of these findings is not known.

Gabapentin and gabapentin enacarbil should be used during pregnancy only when the potential benefits justify the possible risks to the fetus. Women who become pregnant while receiving gabapentin should be encouraged to enroll in the North American Antiepileptic Drug (NAAED) Pregnancy Registry by calling 888-233-2334; registry information also is available on the website at http://www.aedpregnancyregistry.org.

Fertility Animal reproduction studies revealed no adverse effects on fertility or reproduction with gabapentin exposure levels 8 times that achieved in humans at the maximum recommended dosages.

Lactation Gabapentin is distributed into milk following oral administration. Because of the potential for serious adverse reactions to gabapentin in nursing infants, the drug should be administered to nursing women only if the potential benefits justify the risk to the infant. The manufacturer of gabapentin enacarbil states that a decision should be made whether to discontinue nursing or the drug, taking into account the importance of the drug to the woman.

Description

Gabapentin is an anticonvulsant agent structurally related to the inhibitory CNS neurotransmitter γ-aminobutyric acid (GABA). Gabapentin enacarbil is a prodrug of gabapentin that is rapidly converted to gabapentin following oral administration; the therapeutic effects of gabapentin enacarbil are attributed to gabapentin. Although gabapentin was developed as a structural analog of GABA that would penetrate the blood-brain barrier (unlike GABA) and mimic the action of GABA at inhibitory neuronal synapses, the drug has no direct GABA-mimetic action and its precise mechanism of action has not been elucidated.

Results of some studies in animals indicate that gabapentin protects against seizure and/or tonic extensions induced by the GABA antagonists picrotoxin and bicuculline or by GABA synthesis inhibitors (e.g., 3-mercaptopropionic acid, isonicotinic acid, semicarbazide). However, gabapentin does not appear to bind to GABA receptors nor affect GABA reuptake or metabolism and does not act as a precursor of GABA or of other substances active at GABA receptors. Gabapentin also has no affinity for binding sites on common neuroreceptors (e.g., benzodiazepine; glutamate; quisqualate; kainate; strychnine-insensitive or -sensitive glycine; α_1-, α_2-, or β-adrenergic; adenosine A_1 or A_2; cholinergic [muscarinic or nicotinic]; dopamine D_1 or D_2; histamine H_1; type 1 or 2 serotonergic [5-HT_1 or 5-HT_2]; opiate μ, δ, or κ) or ion channels (e.g., voltage-sensitive calcium channel sites labeled with nitrendipine or diltiazem, voltage-sensitive sodium channel sites labeled with batrachotoxinin A 20α-benzoate). Conflicting results have been reported in studies of gabapentin affinity for and activity at *N*-methyl-D-aspartic acid (NMDA) receptors.

In animal test systems, gabapentin exhibits anticonvulsant activity similar to that of other commonly used anticonvulsant drugs. The drug protects against seizures induced in animals by electrical stimulation or pentylenetetrazole, suggesting that it may be effective in the management of tonic-clonic (grand mal) and partial seizures or absence (petit mal) seizures, respectively. However, available data in animals and humans are conflicting regarding the effect of gabapentin on EEG spike and wave activity associated with absence (petit mal) seizures. Gabapentin also prevents seizures in some animals with congenital epilepsy and protects against audiogenic tonic extensions and clonic seizures in mice.

Although the exact mechanism by which gabapentin exerts its analgesic effects is not known, the drug has been shown to prevent allodynia (pain-related behavior in response to normally innocuous stimuli) and hyperalgesia (exaggerated response to painful stimuli) in several models of neuropathic pain. Gabapentin also has been shown to decrease pain-related responses after peripheral inflammation in animals; however, the drug has not altered immediate pain-related behaviors. The clinical relevance of these findings is not known. In vitro studies demonstrate that gabapentin binds to the $\alpha_2\delta$ subunit of voltage-activated calcium channels; however, the clinical importance of this effect is not known.

The pharmacokinetic properties of gabapentin vary based on the specific formulation of the drug. (See Dosage and Administration: Administration.) Following oral administration, gabapentin is absorbed principally in the proximal small intestine via a saturable L-amino acid transport system; as a result, the bioavailability of the drug decreases with increasing doses. Gabapentin gastroretentive tablets are specifically formulated to swell upon contact with gastric fluid to a size that promotes gastric retention for approximately 8–10 hours when taken with a meal; this allows for gradual and slow release of the drug to the proximal small intestine, its principal site of absorption. Following administration of gabapentin gastroretentive tablets in healthy individuals, time to peak plasma concentrations of the drug was increased (about 4–6 hours longer), peak plasma concentrations were increased, and systemic exposure was decreased relative to conventional (immediate-release) gabapentin. Gabapentin enacarbil, a prodrug of gabapentin, is rapidly and efficiently converted to gabapentin by first-pass hydrolysis following oral administration. Unlike gabapentin, gabapentin enacarbil is absorbed via high-capacity transporters throughout the GI tract and is not affected by saturable absorption; this improves bioavailability of the drug and allows for dose-proportional exposure. Food has only a minimal effect on the pharmacokinetics of conventional (immediate-release) formulations of gabapentin, but increases the bioavailability of gabapentin gastroretentive tablets. Administration of gabapentin enacarbil extended-release tablets with food also increases systemic exposure of the drug compared with exposure under fasted conditions. Gabapentin does not bind to plasma proteins, is not appreciably metabolized, does not induce hepatic enzyme activity, and does not appear to alter the pharmacokinetics of commonly used anticonvulsant drugs (e.g., carbamazepine, phenytoin, valproate, phenobarbital, diazepam) or oral contraceptives. In addition, the pharmacokinetics of gabapentin are not altered substantially by concomitant administration of other anticonvulsant drugs.

SumMon® (see Users Guide). For additional information on this drug until a more detailed monograph is developed and published, the manufacturer's labeling should be consulted. It is *essential* that the labeling be consulted for detailed information on the usual cautions, precautions, and contraindications concerning potential drug interactions and/or laboratory test interferences and for information on acute toxicity.

Preparations

Excipients in commercially available drug preparations may have clinically important effects in some individuals; consult specific product labeling for details.

Gabapentin

Oral		
Capsules	100 mg*	**Gabapentin Capsules**
		Neurontin®, Pfizer
	300 mg*	**Gabapentin Capsules**
		Neurontin®, Pfizer
	400 mg*	**Gabapentin Capsules**
		Neurontin®, Pfizer
Solution	250 mg/5 mL*	**Neurontin®**, Pfizer
Tablets	100 mg*	**Gabapentin Tablets**
	300 mg*	**Gabapentin Tablets**
		Gralise®, Depomed
	400 mg*	**Gabapentin Tablets**
	600 mg*	**Gabapentin Tablets**
		Gralise®, Depomed
	800 mg*	**Gabapentin Tablets**
Tablets, film-coated	600 mg*	**Gabapentin Tablets**
		Neurontin®, Pfizer
	800 mg*	**Gabapentin Tablets**
		Neurontin®, Pfizer

*available from one or more manufacturer, distributor, and/or repackager by generic (nonproprietary) name

Gabapentin Enacarbil

Oral		
Tablets, extended-release	300 mg	**Horizant®**, XenoPort
	600 mg	**Horizant®**, XenoPort

†Use is not currently included in the labeling approved by the US Food and Drug Administration

Selected Revisions November 2015, © Copyright, June 1993, American Society of Health-System Pharmacists, Inc.

Lacosamide

Erlosamide, Harkoseride, Lacosamida, Lacosamidum

■ Lacosamide, a functionalized amino acid, is an anticonvulsant.

Uses

■ **Seizure Disorders** *Partial Seizures* Lacosamide is used orally as monotherapy or adjunctive therapy (i.e., in combination with other anticonvulsants) in the management of partial-onset seizures in adults and pediatric patients 4 years of age or older. IV lacosamide is used in adults with partial-onset seizures when oral administration is temporarily not feasible; use of the IV formulation has not been evaluated in pediatric patients.

Efficacy of lacosamide monotherapy in the treatment of partial-onset seizures has been established in a historically controlled, conversion-to-monotherapy study. Patients 16–70 years of age who were receiving stable dosages of 1 or 2 anticonvulsant drugs and experienced at least 2 partial-onset seizures every 28 days during an initial 8-week baseline period were transferred to lacosamide monotherapy and compared with a historical control group derived from the low-dose active control groups of 8 similarly designed conversion-to-monotherapy studies. The study design required the inclusion of 2 effective dosage groups; however, the primary analysis was based on an oral lacosamide dosage of 400 mg daily. Following randomization, lacosamide was added to the baseline anticonvulsant regimen over a 3-week titration period and then continued for an additional 16 weeks while background anticonvulsant drugs were withdrawn. The primary efficacy end point was the proportion of lacosamide-treated patients who met a predefined "exit" criteria (defined as doubling of the mean monthly seizure count; doubling of the highest consecutive 2-day seizure frequency; occurrence of a single generalized tonic-clinic seizure; clinically important prolongation or worsening of overall seizure duration, frequency, type, or pattern requiring discontinuance from the study; or status epilepticus or new onset of serial or cluster seizures) during the maintenance period compared with historical controls. Among patients receiving lacosamide 400 mg daily, the estimated percentage of patients meeting at least one exit criterion (30%) was lower than the expected rate in historical controls (65%), which met the statistical criteria for efficacy.

Efficacy of lacosamide as adjunctive therapy of partial-onset seizures has been established in three 12-week, randomized, double-blind, placebo-controlled clinical studies in adults. Patients enrolled in these trials had refractory partial-onset seizures with or without secondary generalization while receiving a regimen of 1–3 concomitant anticonvulsants and had experienced at least 4 partial-onset seizures every 28 days (with no seizure-free period exceeding 21 days) during an 8-week baseline period. In these 3 studies, which included a total of 1294 evaluable patients, patients had epilepsy for an average of 24 years and a median baseline seizure frequency ranging from 10 to 17 seizures over a 28-day period; 84% of the patients were concurrently receiving 2 or 3 anticonvulsants with or without concurrent vagal nerve stimulation. The studies compared oral lacosamide dosages of 200, 400, or 600 mg daily with placebo. Following an initial 4- to 6-week titration phase, patients were maintained on stable dosages of lacosamide for 12 weeks.

In these studies, patients receiving lacosamide 400 or 600 mg daily experienced substantially greater percent reduction in 28-day seizure frequency from baseline compared with those receiving placebo. A statistically significant effect was observed with lacosamide 200 mg daily in only one of the studies that evaluated this dosage. Across all 3 studies, lacosamide demonstrated consistently higher 50% responder rates (defined as the proportion of patients experiencing a reduction in seizure frequency of 50% or greater) relative to placebo. Subset evaluations did not demonstrate important differences in response based on gender or race in these studies; however, data on race were limited (about 10% of patients were non-Caucasian). In long-term, open-label extensions of the placebo-controlled studies, lacosamide (100–800 mg daily based on individual tolerability and response) was generally well tolerated and effective in maintaining seizure reduction in patients receiving the drug for periods of up to 8 years.

The safety and tolerability of IV lacosamide (200–600 mg daily for 2 days) as a temporary replacement for oral lacosamide have been demonstrated in a randomized, double-blind, multicenter study in patients with partial-onset seizures. In addition, the safety and tolerability of IV lacosamide (200–800 mg daily for 2–5 days) as a short-term replacement for oral lacosamide in hospitalized patients with partial-onset seizures have been demonstrated in a larger, open, multicenter study.

■ **Neuropathic Pain** Lacosamide has been used orally in the management of pain associated with diabetic peripheral neuropathy (DPN)† and has been evaluated for this use in adults in several short-term and long-term (up to approximately 2.5 years) clinical trials; however, additional controlled trials are needed to confirm the drug's efficacy and safety in this condition.

Dosage and Administration

■ **Administration** Lacosamide is administered orally (as tablets or oral solution). The drug may be administered by IV infusion in adults when oral administration is temporarily not feasible (e.g., after surgery or in patients with dysphagia or acute GI disorders); safety of the IV formulation has not been established in pediatric patients.

Bioequivalence has been demonstrated between the oral tablets and the 30- and 60-minute IV infusions (but not the 15-minute IV infusion) of lacosamide. The commercially available oral solution containing 50 mg/5 mL of lacosamide is bioequivalent to the tablets.

Lacosamide therapy should be withdrawn gradually (e.g., by discontinuing therapy over at least one week) to minimize the potential for increased seizure frequency in patients with seizure disorders.

Patients currently receiving or beginning therapy with lacosamide and/or any other anticonvulsant for any indication should be closely monitored for the emergence or worsening of depression, suicidal thoughts or behavior (suicidality), and/or any unusual changes in mood or behavior. (See Suicidality Risk under Cautions: Warnings/Precautions.)

Oral Administration Lacosamide tablets and oral solution are administered orally (usually twice daily) without regard to food.

A calibrated dosing device should be used to measure and administer the oral solution; a household teaspoon or tablespoon is not an adequate measuring device. Any unused portions of the oral solution should be discarded after 7 weeks of first opening the bottle. Lacosamide oral solution may be administered through a nasogastric or gastrostomy tube.

IV Administration Lacosamide injection may be administered IV without further dilution or may be mixed with a compatible diluent (5% dextrose injection, lactated Ringer's injection, or 0.9% sodium chloride injection). Following dilution, the infusion solution may be stored for up to 4 hours at room temperature.

Lacosamide injection should be inspected visually for particulate matter and discoloration prior to administration whenever solution and container permit; the drug should not be used if discoloration or particulate matter is observed. Vials are for single use only; unused portions should be discarded.

Cardiac conduction abnormalities have been observed in patients receiving lacosamide by IV infusion; the manufacturer recommends ECG monitoring prior to initiating therapy and after reaching steady-state maintenance dosage in patients who may be at risk. (See PR-Interval Prolongation under Cautions: Warnings/Precautions.)

Rate of Administration. IV infusions of lacosamide are usually administered over 30–60 minutes. Because shorter infusion times have been used safely in clinical trials, the manufacturer states that the drug may be administered as rapidly as over 15 minutes if necessary. The risk of adverse CNS effects may be increased with shorter durations of infusion.

■ **Dosage** ***Partial Seizures*** Patients being transferred from monotherapy with another anticonvulsant to lacosamide should receive both anticonvulsant agents concomitantly until the therapeutic dosage of lacosamide is reached and has been administered for at least 3 days. Withdrawal of the concomitant anticonvulsant should then be done gradually over at least 6 weeks.

Adult Dosage. In adults 17 years of age or older, the recommended initial oral dosage of lacosamide for the management of partial-onset seizures is 200 mg daily (administered as 100 mg twice daily) as *monotherapy* or 100 mg daily (administered as 50 mg twice daily) as *adjunctive therapy*. Dosage should be increased by 100 mg daily (50 mg twice daily) based on individual patient response and tolerability, no more frequently than once a week, up to the recommended maintenance dosage of 300–400 mg daily (150–200 mg twice daily) as *monotherapy* or 200–400 mg daily (100–200 mg twice daily) as *adjunctive therapy*.

Alternatively, lacosamide therapy may be initiated with a single oral loading dose of 200 mg in adults, followed 12 hours later by a dosage of 100 mg twice daily for 1 week; subsequent dosage may be increased by 100 mg daily (50 mg twice daily) based on individual patient response and tolerability, no more frequently than once a week, up to the recommended maintenance dosage of 300–400 mg daily (150–200 mg twice daily) as *monotherapy* or 200–400 mg daily (100–200 mg twice daily) as *adjunctive therapy*. Steady-state concentrations produced by a single lacosamide loading dose of 200 mg are comparable to those produced by an oral dosage of 100 mg twice daily. The loading dose should be administered under medical supervision because of an increased risk of adverse CNS effects.

When oral therapy is temporarily not feasible, lacosamide may be administered by IV infusion in adults at the same dosages recommended for oral administration, including the alternative loading dosage. The manufacturer states that clinical experience with IV dosing of lacosamide is limited to 5 consecutive days.

The maximum recommended dosage of lacosamide for the management of partial-onset seizures is 400 mg daily (200 mg twice daily). In clinical studies evaluating adjunctive therapy, lacosamide dosages exceeding 400 mg daily were not more effective than lower dosages and were associated with a substantially higher incidence of adverse effects.

Pediatric Dosage. Dosage of lacosamide in pediatric patients is based on weight.

In pediatric patients 4 years of age or older weighing at least 50 kg, the recommended initial oral dosage of lacosamide for *monotherapy* or *adjunctive therapy* of partial-onset seizures is 100 mg daily (administered as 50 mg twice daily). Dosage should be increased by 100 mg daily (50 mg twice daily) based on individual patient response and tolerability, no more frequently than once a week, up to the recommended maintenance dosage of 300–400 mg daily (150–200 mg twice daily) as *monotherapy* or 200–400 mg daily (100–200 mg twice daily) as *adjunctive therapy*.

In pediatric patients 4 years of age or older weighing 30 kg to less than 50 kg, the recommended initial oral dosage of lacosamide for monotherapy or adjunctive therapy of partial-onset seizures is 2 mg/kg daily (administered as 1 mg/kg twice daily). Dosage should be increased by 2 mg/kg daily (1 mg/kg twice daily) based on individual patient response and tolerability, no more frequently than once a week, up to the recommended maintenance dosage of 4–8 mg/kg daily (2–4 mg/kg twice daily) as monotherapy or adjunctive therapy.

In pediatric patients 4 years of age or older weighing 11 kg to less than 30 kg, the recommended initial oral dosage of lacosamide for monotherapy or adjunctive therapy of partial-onset seizures is 2 mg/kg daily (administered as 1 mg/kg twice daily). Dosage should be increased by 2 mg/kg daily (1 mg/kg twice daily) based on individual patient response and tolerability, no more frequently than once a week, up to the recommended maintenance dosage of 6–12 mg/kg daily (3–6 mg/kg twice daily) as monotherapy or adjunctive therapy.

The maximum recommended dosage of lacosamide for the management of partial-onset seizures is 400 mg daily (200 mg twice daily). In clinical studies evaluating adjunctive therapy, lacosamide dosages exceeding 400 mg daily were not more effective than lower dosages and were associated with a substantially higher incidence of adverse effects.

Neuropathic Pain For the management of pain associated with diabetic peripheral neuropathy† in adults, lacosamide usually has been given in an initial oral dosage of 100 mg daily (given as 50 mg twice daily) in clinical trials, with subsequent weekly increases to reach maintenance dosages of 400–600 mg daily (given as 200–300 mg twice daily) based on individual patient response and tolerability.

■ **Special Populations** Dosage adjustment of lacosamide is not necessary in patients with mild to moderate renal impairment. In patients with severe renal impairment (creatinine clearance of 30 mL/minute or less) or end-stage renal disease, the maximum dosage of lacosamide should be reduced by 25%. Dosage titration should be undertaken with caution in patients with any degree of renal impairment. In patients undergoing hemodialysis, dosage supplementation of up to 50% following hemodialysis should be considered.

In patients with mild or moderate hepatic impairment, the maximum dosage of lacosamide should be reduced by 25% and dosage titration should be undertaken with caution. Use of lacosamide is *not* recommended in patients with severe hepatic impairment.

Patients with renal or hepatic impairment who are taking potent inhibitors of cytochrome P-450 (CYP) 3A4 and/or CYP2C9 may require dosage reduction of lacosamide. (See Drug Interactions: Drugs Affecting or Metabolized by Hepatic Microsomal Enzymes.)

Dosage adjustment based solely on age is not considered necessary in geriatric patients; however, the manufacturer recommends cautious dosage titration in such patients, usually starting at the low end of the dosing range because of the greater frequency of decreased hepatic and renal function in this age group.

Cautions

■ **Contraindications** The manufacturer states that there are no known contraindications to the use of lacosamide.

■ **Warnings/Precautions** ***Suicidality Risk*** An increased risk of suicidality (suicidal behavior or ideation) was observed in an analysis of 199 studies using various anticonvulsants compared with placebo. The analysis of suicidality reports from placebo-controlled studies involving 11 anticonvulsants (carbamazepine, felbamate, gabapentin, lamotrigine, levetiracetam, oxcarbazepine, pregabalin, tiagabine, topiramate, valproate, and zonisamide) in patients with epilepsy, psychiatric disorders (e.g., bipolar disorder, depression, anxiety), and other conditions (e.g., migraine, neuropathic pain) found that patients receiving anticonvulsants had approximately twice the risk of suicidal behavior or ideation (0.43%) compared with patients receiving placebo (0.24%). This increased suicidality risk was observed as early as one week after beginning therapy and continued through 24 weeks. Although patients treated with an anticonvulsant for epilepsy, psychiatric disorders, and other conditions were all found to have an increased suicidality risk compared with those receiving placebo, the relative suicidality risk was higher for patients with epilepsy compared with those receiving anticonvulsants for other conditions.

Clinicians should inform patients, their families, and caregivers of the potential for an increased risk of suicidality with anticonvulsant therapy; all patients currently receiving or beginning therapy with any anticonvulsant should be closely monitored for the emergence or worsening of suicidal thoughts or behavior or depression.

Clinicians who prescribe lacosamide or any other anticonvulsant should balance the risk of suicidality with the risk of untreated illness. Epilepsy and many other illnesses for which anticonvulsants are prescribed are themselves associated with morbidity and mortality and an increased risk of suicidal thoughts and behavior. If suicidal thoughts or behavior emerge during anticonvulsant therapy, the clinician should consider whether these symptoms may be related to the illness being treated. (See Advice to Patients.)

Dizziness and Ataxia Dizziness and ataxia were reported in 25 and 6%, respectively, of patients with partial-onset seizures receiving lacosamide dosages of 200–400 mg daily and 1–3 concomitant anticonvulsants in clinical studies compared with 8 and 2% of placebo recipients, respectively; dizziness was the adverse effect most frequently leading to drug discontinuance (3%). The onset of dizziness and ataxia was most commonly observed during dosage titration. A substantial increase in these adverse effects was reported with lacosamide dosages exceeding 400 mg daily. (See Advice to Patients.)

PR-Interval Prolongation Like some other anticonvulsants (e.g., carbamazepine, lamotrigine, pregabalin), lacosamide can cause PR-interval prolongation. Dose-dependent increases in the PR interval have been observed in patients and in healthy individuals receiving lacosamide in clinical studies. At steady state, the timing of the maximum observed mean PR interval coincided with the peak plasma lacosamide concentrations. In clinical trials, asymptomatic, first-degree AV block was observed in 0.4% of patients with partial-onset epilepsy and in 0.5% of patients with diabetic neuropathy; none of the patients receiving placebo experienced asymptomatic, first-degree AV block. When lacosamide is given concomitantly with other drugs that prolong the PR interval, further PR prolongation is possible. (See Drugs that Prolong PR Interval under Drug Interactions.)

Profound bradycardia has been reported in a patient who received lacosamide 150 mg by IV infusion over 15 minutes. In addition, third-degree AV block has been reported during postmarketing experience in 2 patients with preexisting cardiac conditions who were receiving IV infusions of lacosamide at higher than recommended doses and also receiving metoprolol and amlodipine.

Lacosamide should be used with caution in patients with known cardiac conduction abnormalities (e.g., marked first-degree AV block, second- or third-degree AV block, sick sinus syndrome without a pacemaker), sodium channelopathies (e.g., Brugada syndrome), or severe cardiovascular disease (e.g., myocardial ischemia, heart failure) and in patients receiving concomitant drugs that prolong the PR interval. The manufacturer recommends obtaining an ECG before initiating lacosamide therapy and after the drug is titrated to steady state in such patients. In addition, patients who are receiving lacosamide by the IV route should be closely monitored.

Atrial Fibrillation and Atrial Flutter In short-term trials of lacosamide in patients with partial-onset seizures, there were no cases of atrial fibrillation or flutter. In patients with diabetic neuropathy, 0.5% of lacosamide-treated patients experienced atrial fibrillation or flutter compared with none of the placebo recipients. Lacosamide may predispose patients to develop atrial arrhythmias (i.e., atrial fibrillation or flutter), particularly in patients with diabetic neuropathy and/or cardiovascular disease. Patients should therefore be made aware of the symptoms of atrial fibrillation and flutter (e.g., palpitations, rapid pulse, shortness of breath). (See Advice to Patients.)

Syncope In short-term controlled trials in patients with partial-onset seizures without significant systemic illness, there was no increase in syncope with lacosamide compared with placebo; however, cases of syncope have been reported in open-label partial-onset seizure studies in adults and pediatric patients with preexisting cardiac risk factors. In short-term controlled trials of lacosamide in patients with diabetic neuropathy, syncope or loss of consciousness was reported in 1.2% of patients receiving the drug compared with none of the placebo recipients. Most of the syncope cases were observed in patients receiving lacosamide dosages exceeding 400 mg daily. Although the cause of syncope was not determined in most cases, several cases were associated with orthostatic changes in blood pressure, atrial fibrillation/flutter (and associated tachycardia), or bradycardia. (See Advice to Patients.)

Discontinuance of Anticonvulsants To minimize the risk of increased seizure frequency in patients with seizure disorders, anticonvulsant drugs, including lacosamide, should not be abruptly discontinued. The manufacturer recommends that oral lacosamide therapy be withdrawn gradually (e.g., over at least 1 week). (See Dosage and Administration: Administration.)

Phenylketonuria Individuals with phenylketonuria (i.e., homozygous genetic deficiency of phenylalanine hydroxylase) and other individuals who must restrict their intake of phenylalanine should be warned that lacosamide oral solution contains aspartame, which is metabolized in the GI tract following oral administration to provide 0.32 mg of phenylalanine per 20 mL of solution. The combined daily amount of phenylalanine from all sources, including from lacosamide oral solution, should be considered in patients with phenylketonuria.

Sensitivity Reactions **Multi-organ Hypersensitivity.** Multi-organ hypersensitivity (also known as drug reaction with eosinophilia and systemic symptoms [DRESS]), a potentially fatal or life-threatening reaction, has been reported with some anticonvulsant drugs. The clinical presentation is variable, but typically includes eosinophilia, fever, rash, lymphadenopathy, and/or facial swelling associated with other organ system involvement such as hepatitis, nephritis, hematologic abnormalities, myocarditis, or myositis. However, signs and symptoms associated with other organ systems also may occur.

One case of symptomatic hepatitis and nephritis, which was consistent with a delayed multi-organ hypersensitivity reaction, was reported in a healthy individual 10 days after discontinuing lacosamide. Full recovery occurred within 1 month without specific treatment; potential known viral etiologies for hepatitis were ruled out and the individual was not receiving any concomitant therapy. Additional cases of possible multi-organ hypersensitivity with lacosamide include 2 patients with rash and elevated hepatic enzyme concentrations and one patient with myocarditis and hepatitis of uncertain etiology.

If manifestations of a multi-organ hypersensitivity reaction occur, patients should be evaluated immediately; if an alternative cause cannot be identified, lacosamide should be discontinued.

Specific Populations **Pregnancy.** There are no adequate data in humans to determine if there is any risk associated with the use of lacosamide during pregnancy. In animal studies, lacosamide produced developmental toxicity (i.e., increased embryofetal and perinatal mortality, growth deficit) when given orally to pregnant rats. Developmental neurotoxicity was observed in animals given lacosamide during a period of postnatal development corresponding to the third trimester of human pregnancy. These effects were observed at dosages associated with clinically relevant plasma exposures.

Women who are pregnant while receiving lacosamide should be encouraged to enroll in the North American Antiepileptic Drug (NAAED) Pregnancy Registry; patients can enroll by calling 888-233-2334. Information on the registry also can be found on the website http://www.aedpregnancyregistry.org.

Lactation. Lacosamide and/or its metabolites are distributed into milk of lactating rats. It is not known if lacosamide is distributed into human milk. The effects of lacosamide on the nursing infant or on milk production also are not known. The known benefits of breast-feeding should be considered along with the mother's clinical need for lacosamide and any potential adverse effects on the infant from the drug or underlying maternal condition.

Pediatric Use. Safety and efficacy of lacosamide in pediatric patients younger than 4 years of age have not been established. Use of lacosamide tablets and oral solution in pediatric patients 4 years of age and older is supported by data from partial-onset seizure studies in adults, pharmacokinetic studies in adults and pediatric patients, and safety data in pediatric patients. Safety of lacosamide injection has not been established in pediatric patients.

Lacosamide has been shown in vitro to interfere with the activity of collapsin response mediator protein-2 (CRMP-2), a protein involved in neuronal differentiation and control of axonal outgrowth; potential adverse effects on CNS development cannot be ruled out. (See Description.) Administration of lacosamide to rats during the neonatal and juvenile periods of postnatal development resulted in decreased brain weights and long-term neurobehavioral changes (e.g., altered open field performance, deficits in learning and memory). The no-effect dosage for developmental neurotoxicity in rats was associated with an area under the plasma concentration-time curve (AUC) less than that in humans at the maximum recommended dosage of 400 mg daily.

Geriatric Use. Clinical studies of lacosamide did not include sufficient numbers of geriatric patients to determine whether they respond differently than younger patients. Systemic exposure and peak plasma concentrations of lacosamide (normalized for dosage and body weight) were approximately 20% higher in geriatric individuals compared with younger individuals, which may be related to differences in body weight and renal clearance. (See Dosage and Administration: Special Populations.)

Renal Impairment. Lacosamide and its principal metabolite are eliminated from the systemic circulation mainly by renal excretion. Systemic exposure of lacosamide was increased by approximately 25% in individuals with mild or moderate renal impairment and by 60% in individuals with severe renal impairment compared with individuals with normal renal function; however, peak plasma concentrations of the drug were unaffected. Dosage adjustments may be required in some patients with renal impairment. (See Dosage and Administration: Special Populations.)

Lacosamide is removed by hemodialysis. Following a 4-hour hemodialysis session, systemic exposure of lacosamide is reduced by approximately 50%. (See Dosage and Administration: Special Populations.)

Hepatic Impairment. Lacosamide undergoes hepatic metabolism. Individuals with moderate hepatic impairment (Child-Pugh class B) had approximately 50–60% higher systemic exposure of lacosamide compared with healthy individuals. The pharmacokinetics of lacosamide have not been specifically studied in individuals with severe hepatic impairment, and use of the drug in patients with severe hepatic impairment is *not* recommended.

Dosage adjustments may be required in some patients with hepatic impairment. (See Dosage and Administration: Special Populations.)

■ **Common Adverse Effects** Adverse reactions occurring in 5% or more of patients receiving oral lacosamide as adjunctive therapy in controlled clinical trials for partial-onset seizures and reported more frequently than with placebo include dizziness, headache, diplopia, nausea, vomiting, fatigue, blurred vision, ataxia, somnolence, tremor, nystagmus, memory impairment, balance disorder, vertigo, and diarrhea.

Adverse effects reported in the study evaluating lacosamide monotherapy generally were similar to those reported in the adjunctive placebo-controlled studies with the exception of insomnia (occurring in 2% or more of patients receiving lacosamide monotherapy).

Systemic adverse effects associated with short-term IV lacosamide therapy in patients with partial-onset seizures generally appear to be consistent with those associated with oral administration of the drug; local adverse effects include injection site pain or discomfort, irritation, and erythema.

Drug Interactions

Lacosamide generally appears to have a low potential for pharmacokinetic drug interactions with other anticonvulsants or other drugs.

■ **Drugs Affecting or Metabolized by Hepatic Microsomal Enzymes** Lacosamide is metabolized by cytochrome P-450 (CYP) isoenzymes 3A4, 2C9, and 2C19. Increased exposure to lacosamide is possible in patients with renal or hepatic impairment receiving potent inhibitors of CYP3A4 and/or CYP2C9.

Lacosamide does not substantially induce CYP 1A2, 2B6, 2C9, 2C19, or 3A4 in vitro; pharmacokinetic interaction is unlikely.

Lacosamide does not substantially inhibit CYP isoenzymes 1A1, 1A2, 2A6, 2B6, 2C8, 2C9, 2D6, 2E1, 3A4, or 3A5 at plasma concentrations observed in clinical studies; pharmacokinetic interaction is unlikely.

In vitro data suggest that lacosamide may inhibit CYP 2C19 at therapeutic concentrations; however, an in vivo study with omeprazole suggested minimal or no inhibitory effect (see Drug Interactions: Omeprazole).

■ **Drugs Affecting or Affected by P-glycoprotein Transport** Lacosamide is not an inhibitor or substrate of the P-glycoprotein transport system; pharmacokinetic interactions are unlikely.

■ **Drugs that Prolong PR Interval** The risk of AV block or bradycardia may be increased when lacosamide is administered concomitantly with other drugs that prolong the PR interval (e.g., certain β-adrenergic blocking agents, calcium-channel blocking agents, digoxin, pregabalin). These drugs should be used concomitantly with caution. (See PR-Interval Prolongation under Cautions: Warnings/Precautions.) The manufacturer recommends ECG monitoring prior to initiating lacosamide therapy and after the drug is titrated to steady state in patients receiving concomitant drugs that prolong the PR interval. In addition, such patients who are receiving lacosamide by the IV route should be closely monitored.

■ **Alcohol** No data are currently available concerning an interaction between lacosamide and alcohol.

■ **Anticonvulsants** ***Carbamazepine*** Concomitant administration of lacosamide (400 mg daily) and carbamazepine (400 mg daily) did not alter the pharmacokinetics of either drug in healthy individuals. In placebo-controlled studies in patients with partial-onset seizures, steady-state plasma concentrations of carbamazepine and its epoxide metabolite were not affected by concurrent lacosamide administered at any dosage. Population pharmacokinetic studies in patients with partial-onset seizures demonstrated small reductions (15–20% lower) in plasma lacosamide concentrations during concurrent administration of the enzyme-inducing anticonvulsants carbamazepine, phenobarbital, or phenytoin. (See Drug Interactions: Drugs that Prolong PR Interval.)

Phenobarbital In placebo-controlled studies in patients with partial-onset seizures, steady-state plasma concentrations of phenobarbital were not affected by concurrent lacosamide administered at any dosage. Population pharmacokinetic studies in patients with partial-onset seizures demonstrated small reductions (15–20% lower) in plasma lacosamide concentrations during concurrent administration of the enzyme-inducing anticonvulsants carbamazepine, phenobarbital, or phenytoin.

Phenytoin In placebo-controlled studies in patients with partial-onset seizures, steady-state plasma concentrations of phenytoin were not affected by concurrent lacosamide administered at any dosage. Population pharmacokinetic studies in patients with partial-onset seizures demonstrated small reductions (15–20% lower) in plasma lacosamide concentrations during concurrent administration of the enzyme-inducing anticonvulsants carbamazepine, phenobarbital, or phenytoin.

Valproic Acid Concomitant administration of lacosamide (400 mg daily) and valproic acid (600 mg daily) did not alter the pharmacokinetics of either drug in healthy individuals. In placebo-controlled studies in patients with partial-onset seizures, steady-state plasma concentrations of valproic acid were not affected by concurrent lacosamide at any dosage.

Other Anticonvulsants Steady-state plasma concentrations of clonazepam, gabapentin, lamotrigine, levetiracetam, oxcarbazepine's active monohydroxy metabolite (MHD), topiramate, and zonisamide were not altered by concomitant lacosamide administration at any dosage.

■ **Digoxin** Lacosamide (400 mg daily) did not alter the pharmacokinetics of digoxin (0.5 mg once daily) in a study in healthy individuals. A small increase in the PR interval was observed when the drugs were administered concomitantly compared with digoxin alone.

Because of possible additive effects on PR-interval prolongation, lacosamide and digoxin should be administered concomitantly with caution. The manufacturer recommends ECG monitoring prior to initiating lacosamide therapy and after the drug is titrated to steady state in patients receiving lacosamide with drugs that prolong the PR interval. In addition, such patients who are receiving lacosamide by the IV route should be closely monitored. (See Drug Interactions: Drugs that Prolong PR Interval.)

■ **Metformin** Clinically important changes in metformin concentrations were not observed during concurrent administration of lacosamide 400 mg daily. Metformin hydrochloride (500 mg given 3 times daily) did not alter the pharmacokinetics of lacosamide (400 mg daily).

■ **Midazolam** When lacosamide (single dose of 200 mg or repeated doses of 400 mg daily) was co-administered with the CYP3A4 substrate midazolam (single dose of 7.5 mg), no changes in the pharmacokinetics of midazolam were observed.

■ **Omeprazole** Lacosamide (600 mg daily) did not alter the pharmacokinetics of a single 40-mg dose of omeprazole (a CYP2C19 substrate and inhibitor) in healthy individuals, suggesting that lacosamide has little in vivo inhibitory or inducing effect on CYP2C19. Omeprazole (40 mg once daily) did not alter the pharmacokinetics of a single 300-mg dose of lacosamide; however, peak plasma concentrations of lacosamide's inactive *O*-desmethyl metabolite were reduced by about 60%.

■ **Oral Contraceptives** Lacosamide (400 mg daily) did not substantially affect the pharmacodynamics and pharmacokinetics of an oral contraceptive containing 0.03 mg of ethinyl estradiol and 0.15 mg of levonorgestrel in healthy individuals, except that a 20% increase in peak plasma ethinyl estradiol concentrations was observed.

■ **Protein-bound Drugs** Since less than 15% of lacosamide is bound to plasma proteins, a clinically relevant interaction with other drugs through competition for protein binding sites is considered unlikely.

■ **Warfarin** In healthy individuals, concomitant administration of lacosamide (400 mg daily) and warfarin sodium (single dose of 25 mg) did not result in any clinically relevant changes in the pharmacokinetics or pharmacodynamics of warfarin. These results suggest that dosage adjustments are not necessary when lacosamide and warfarin are used concomitantly.

Description

Lacosamide, a functionalized amino acid structurally related to serine, is an anticonvulsant. Although the precise mechanism(s) of its anticonvulsant action remains to be fully elucidated, available data suggest that lacosamide may have a dual mechanism of action, including modulation of the slow inactivation of sodium channels and modulation of collapsin response mediator protein-2 (CRMP-2)-mediated enurotropic signals. In vitro electrophysiologic studies have shown that lacosamide selectively enhances the slow inactivation of voltage-gated sodium channels without affecting fast inactivation. This selective slow inactivation of sodium channels may result in stabilization of hyperexcitable neuronal membranes and inhibition of repetitive neuronal firing. In addition, in preclinical testing, lacosamide was found to bind to CRMP-2, a phosphoprotein expressed mainly in the nervous system that is involved in neuronal differentiation, polarization, gene expression, and control of axonal outgrowth. However, in subsequent testing, such binding was not confirmed.

Lacosamide has demonstrated analgesic, antinociceptive, and anxiolytic activity in preclinical studies. The drug does not exhibit binding affinity for γ-aminobutyric acid (GABA), *N*-methyl-D-aspartate (NMDA), adenosine, muscarinic, serotonin, histamine, dopamine, or other receptors. In addition, lacosamide does not affect the reuptake or metabolism of norepinephrine, dopamine, serotonin, or GABA. The drug does not affect voltage-activated calcium channels (L-, N-, P/Q-, or T-type) or voltage-activated potassium channels and does not modulate delayed-rectifier or A-type potassium currents.

Lacosamide is rapidly and completely absorbed following oral administration. The oral bioavailability of lacosamide tablets is approximately 100%; food does not affect the rate and extent of absorption. Peak plasma concentrations of lacosamide occur approximately 0.5–4 hours following oral dosing and steady-state plasma concentrations are achieved after 3 days of twice-daily oral administration. Following IV administration, peak plasma lacosamide concentrations are reached at the end of the infusion. When infused IV over 30 or 60 minutes, the IV formulation is bioequivalent to the oral tablets. The pharmacokinetics of both oral and IV lacosamide are dose-proportional over a dosage range of 100–800 mg and exhibit low intra- and intersubject variability. Lacosamide is less than 15% bound to plasma proteins and has an elimination half-life of approximately 12–13 hours.

Lacosamide is primarily eliminated by renal excretion and biotransformation. Following oral and IV administration of a 100-mg radiolabeled dose of lacosamide, approximately 95% of the dose was recovered in the urine and less than 0.5% in the feces; the principal compounds excreted were unchanged lacosamide (approximately 40%), *O*-desmethyl-lacosamide (approximately 30%; inactive metabolite), and a structurally unknown polar fraction (approximately 20%; possibly serine derivatives). Lacosamide is a substrate of the cytochrome P-450 (CYP) isoenzyme 2C19; the relative contribution of other CYP isoenzymes or non-CYP enzymes in the metabolism of the drug is unclear. No clinically relevant differences in the pharmacokinetics of lacosamide were observed between poor and extensive metabolizers of CYP2C19 substrates; however, plasma concentrations and the amount excreted in the urine of the *O*-desmethyl metabolite were reduced by about 70% in poor metabolizers compared with extensive metabolizers.

Advice to Patients

Importance of advising patients or their caregivers to read the patient information (medication guide).

Importance of patients, family members, and caregivers being aware that anticonvulsants, including lacosamide, may increase the risk of having suicidal thoughts or actions in a very small number of people (about 1 in 500). Advise patients, family members, and caregivers to pay close attention to any day-to-day changes in mood, behavior, and actions; these changes can happen very quickly. They should also be aware of common warning signs that may signal suicide risk (e.g., talking or thinking about wanting to hurt oneself or end one's life, withdrawing from friends and family, becoming depressed or experiencing worsening of existing depression, becoming preoccupied with death and dying, giving away prized possessions). Advise patients, family members, and caregivers to contact the responsible clinician immediately if these or any other new and worrisome behaviors occur.

Importance of taking lacosamide only as prescribed.

Importance of informing patients that lacosamide may cause dizziness, drowsiness, blurred vision, or problems with coordination and balance. Importance of advising patients not to drive, operate complex machinery, or engage in other hazardous activities until they have become accustomed to any such effects.

Importance of informing patients that lacosamide may be associated with dizziness, lightheadedness, fainting, or irregular heart beat, particularly in patients with underlying cardiovascular disease, those with cardiac conduction abnormalities, and those who are taking drugs that affect the heart. These symptoms are more likely to occur when rising too quickly from a recumbent position. Importance of advising patients to lie down with their legs raised until they feel better if such symptoms develop and to contact their clinician promptly. Importance of patients also being aware of the possible symptoms of cardiac rhythm and conduction abnormalities (e.g., atrial fibrillation and flutter), including palpitations, rapid heart beat, and shortness of breath, and importance of contacting their clinician should any of these symptoms occur.

Serious hypersensitivity reactions affecting multiple organs (e.g., liver, kidney) may occur; lacosamide should be discontinued if serious hypersensitivity reactions are suspected. Importance of informing patients to contact their clinician promptly if symptoms suggestive of liver damage occur (e.g., fatigue, jaundice, dark urine).

Importance of women informing clinicians if they are or plan to become pregnant or plan to breast-feed. Importance of clinicians informing women about the existence of and encouraging enrollment in pregnancy registries (see Pregnancy under Warnings/Precautions: Specific Populations, in Cautions).

Importance of informing patients not to stop taking lacosamide without first talking to their clinician since stopping the drug suddenly can cause serious problems, including seizures.

Importance of informing clinicians of existing or contemplated concomitant therapy, including prescription and OTC drugs and dietary or herbal supplements, as well as any concomitant illness (e.g., heart disease, kidney disease, liver disease, depression, bipolar disorder) or family history of suicidality or bipolar disorder.

Importance of informing patients of other important precautionary information. (See Cautions.)

Overview® (see Users Guide). For additional information on this drug until a more detailed monograph is developed and published, the manufacturer's labeling should be consulted. It is *essential* that the manufacturer's labeling be consulted for more detailed information on usual cautions, precautions, contraindications, potential drug interactions, laboratory test interferences, and acute toxicity.

Preparations

Lacosamide is subject to control under the Federal Controlled Substances Act of 1970 as a schedule V (C-V) drug.

Excipients in commercially available drug preparations may have clinically important effects in some individuals; consult specific product labeling for details.

Lacosamide

Oral		
Solution	50 mg/5 mL	**Vimpat®** (C-V), UCB
Tablets, film-coated	50 mg	**Vimpat®** (C-V), UCB
	100 mg	**Vimpat®** (C-V), UCB
	150 mg	**Vimpat®** (C-V), UCB
	200 mg	**Vimpat®** (C-V), UCB
Parenteral		
Injection, for IV infusion	10 mg/mL	**Vimpat®** (C-V; available in single-use glass vials), UCB

†Use is not currently included in the labeling approved by the US Food and Drug Administration

lamoTRIgine

■ Lamotrigine is a phenyltriazine anticonvulsant.

Uses

■ **Seizure Disorders** ***Partial Seizures*** Lamotrigine (given as immediate-release formulations) is used in combination with other anticonvulsant agents in the management of partial seizures, with or without secondary generalization, in adults and children 2 years of age or older. Lamotrigine (given as immediate-release formulations) also is used as monotherapy in patients converting from monotherapy with a hepatic enzyme-inducing anticonvulsant agent (e.g., phenytoin, carbamazepine, phenobarbital, primidone) or valproic acid in the management of partial seizures in patients 16 years of age or older. Extended-release lamotrigine is used in combination with other anticonvulsant agents in the management of partial seizures, with or without secondary generalization, in adults and children 13 years of age or older.

In 3 multicenter, double-blind, placebo-controlled clinical studies, adjunctive therapy with immediate-release lamotrigine was effective in reducing seizure frequency in adults with simple and/or complex partial seizures refractory to therapy with one or more conventional anticonvulsant drugs (e.g., phenytoin, carbamazepine, phenobarbital, valproic acid); the median reduction in seizure frequency was 20–36%. In a multicenter, double-blind, placebo-controlled clinical study in children 2–16 years of age with partial seizures, the median reduction in frequency of all partial seizures was 36 or 7% in patients receiving immediate-release lamotrigine or placebo, respectively, in addition to their current therapy (up to 2 conventional anticonvulsant drugs). In a multicenter, double-blind, placebo-controlled clinical study in adults and children 13 years of age or older with partial seizures and receiving 1 or 2 anticonvulsants, adjunctive treatment with extended-release lamotrigine substantially reduced the median weekly seizure frequency compared with placebo (by 47 versus 25%, respectively).

The effectiveness of lamotrigine monotherapy (given as immediate-release formulations) in adults with partial seizures who are converting from monotherapy with a hepatic enzyme-inducing anticonvulsant drug (e.g., phenytoin, carbamazepine, phenobarbital, primidone) was established in a controlled clinical study of patients who experienced at least 4 simple or complex partial seizures, with or without secondary generalization, during each of 2 consecutive 4-week baseline periods; during the baseline periods, patients were receiving either phenytoin or carbamazepine monotherapy. Patients were randomized either to lamotrigine (target dosage: 500 mg daily) or valproic acid (1000 mg daily) therapy, which was added to their baseline regimen over a 4-week period. Patients were then converted to either lamotrigine or valproic acid monotherapy over another 4-week period and monotherapy continued for another 12-week period. Study end points were either successful completion of the 12-week monotherapy period or meeting a study "escape" criterion, relative to baseline. Escape criteria were defined as doubling of the mean monthly seizure count; doubling of the highest consecutive 2-day seizure frequency; emergence of a new seizure type (defined as a seizure that did not occur during the 8-week baseline period) that was more severe than the other seizure types occurring during the study period; or clinically important prolongation of generalized tonic-clonic seizures. The proportion of lamotrigine- or valproic acid-treated patients meeting escape criteria was 42 or 69%, respectively; no differences in efficacy were detected based on age, race, or gender. It was noted that the patients in the valproic acid control arm were treated intentionally with a relatively low valproic acid dosage because the intent of the study was to establish the effectiveness of lamotrigine monotherapy, and that the study results cannot be interpreted to imply the superiority of lamotrigine therapy to adequate valproic acid therapy. In addition, the manufacturers state that the use of lamotrigine therapy for the management of partial seizures has not been established as initial monotherapy; for conversion from monotherapy from anticonvulsant drugs other than hepatic enzyme-inducing anticonvulsant drugs or valproate; or for simultaneous conversion to monotherapy from 2 or more concomitant anticonvulsant drugs.

Primary Generalized Tonic-Clonic Seizures Lamotrigine (given as immediate-release formulations) is used in combination with other anticonvulsant agents in the management of primary generalized tonic-clonic seizures in adults and children 2 years of age and older. Efficacy of the drug as adjunctive therapy was established in a placebo-controlled trial in adult and pediatric patients at least 2 years of age who had experienced at least 3 primary generalized tonic-clonic seizures during an 8-week baseline phase. Patients were randomized to receive either placebo or immediate-release lamotrigine in a fixed-dose regimen (target dosages of 200–400 mg daily in adults and 3–12 mg/kg daily in children) for 19–24 weeks, which was added to their current anticonvulsant regimen of up to 2 anticonvulsant drugs. Patients receiving lamotrigine experienced a substantially greater median reduction in seizure frequency compared with baseline than did patients receiving placebo (66 and 34%, respectively).

Extended-release lamotrigine is used in combination with other anticonvulsants in the management of primary generalized tonic-clonic seizures in adults and adolescents 13 years of age and older. Efficacy of the extended-release formulation of the drug as adjunctive therapy was established in a multicenter, double-blind, placebo-controlled trial in adult and pediatric patients at least 13 years of age who had experienced at least 3 primary generalized tonic-clonic seizures during an 8-week baseline phase. Patients were randomized to receive either placebo or extended-release lamotrigine in a fixed-dose regimen (target dosages of 200–500 mg daily based on concomitant anticonvulsant therapy) for 19 weeks, which was added to their current anticonvulsant regimen of up to 2 anticonvulsant drugs. Patients receiving extended-release lamotrigine experienced a substantially greater median reduction in seizure frequency compared with baseline than did patients receiving placebo (75 and 32%, respectively).

Seizures Associated with Lennox-Gastaut Syndrome Lamotrigine (given as immediate-release formulations) is used in combination with other anticonvulsant agents in the management of generalized seizures associated with Lennox-Gastaut syndrome in pediatric patients and adults. In a controlled clinical trial in patients with Lennox-Gastaut syndrome, adjunctive therapy with immediate-release lamotrigine resulted in a 32, 34, and 36% decrease in major motor seizures, drop attacks, and tonic-clonic seizures, respectively.

■ **Bipolar Disorder** Lamotrigine (given as immediate-release formulations) is used in the maintenance therapy of bipolar 1 disorder to prevent or attenuate recurrences of bipolar episodes in adult patients who remain at high risk of relapse following treatment of an acute depressive or manic episode. The American Psychiatric Association (APA) currently recommends use of lamotrigine as an alternative to first-line maintenance therapies (e.g., lithium, valproic acid, or divalproex). The APA also states that both lamotrigine and lithium are effective in the maintenance treatment of bipolar 1 disorder; however, the results of two randomized, double-blind, placebo-controlled studies of 18 months' duration indicate that lamotrigine may be more effective in preventing depressive episodes while lithium may be more effective in preventing manic episodes.

Although efficacy of the drug in the acute treatment of mood episodes has yet to be fully established, lamotrigine is considered a first-line agent by the APA for the management of acute depressive episodes in patients with bipolar disorder†. The APA also recommends the use of lamotrigine as an alternative to lithium, valproic acid, or divalproex in the management of patients with rapid cycling bipolar disorder†, particularly in those with the bipolar 2 form of rapid cycling.

For further information on the management of bipolar disorder, see Uses: Bipolar Disorder, in Lithium Salts 28:28.

Dosage and Administration

■ **Administration** Lamotrigine is administered orally as conventional tablets, chewable/dispersible tablets, extended-release tablets, or orally disintegrating tablets. Immediate-release formulations of the drug (e.g., conventional tablets, chewable/dispersible tablets, orally disintegrating tablets) are administered once or twice daily; the extended-release tablets (Lamictal® XR) are administered once daily. Lamotrigine may be administered without regard to meals.

Lamotrigine conventional tablets should be swallowed whole.

Lamotrigine chewable/dispersible tablets may be swallowed whole, chewed (and consumed with a small amount of water or diluted fruit juice to aid swallowing), or dispersed in water or diluted fruit juice. To disperse the tablets, they should be added to a small volume (i.e., 5 mL or enough to cover the tablet) of liquid and allowed to disperse completely (over approximately 1 minute); the solution then should be swirled and consumed immediately. Administration of partial quantities of the dispersed tablets should *not* be attempted; calculated doses that do not correspond to available strengths of whole tablets should be rounded down to the nearest whole tablet.

Lamotrigine extended-release tablets should be swallowed whole and should *not* be chewed, crushed, or divided.

Lamotrigine orally disintegrating tablets should be placed on the tongue and moved around in the mouth, where the tablet disintegrates rapidly in saliva, and then subsequently can be swallowed with or without water.

Patients who are currently receiving or beginning therapy with lamotrigine and/or any other anticonvulsant for any indication should be closely monitored for the emergence or worsening of depression, suicidal thoughts or behavior (suicidality), and/or any unusual changes in mood or behavior. (See Suicidality Risk under Cautions: Precautions and Contraindications.)

Conversion from Immediate-release Lamotrigine to Extended-release Lamotrigine Patients may be converted directly from immediate-release formulations to extended-release lamotrigine tablets (Lamictal® XR). The initial dosage of extended-release lamotrigine should be the same as the total daily dosage of immediate-release lamotrigine. However, some patients receiving concomitant therapy with enzyme-inducing drugs may have lower plasma concentrations of lamotrigine on conversion and should be monitored. Following conversion to extended-release lamotrigine, all patients (particularly those receiving drugs that induce lamotrigine glucuronidation) should be closely monitored for seizure control. Depending on the therapeutic response following conversion, the total daily dosage of extended-release lamotrigine may require adjustment within the recommended dosing guidelines.

Dispensing and Administration Precautions Dispensing errors have occurred because of the similarity in spelling between Lamictal® (the trade name for lamotrigine) and Lamisil® (terbinafine hydrochloride), lamivudine, labetalol hydrochloride, Lomotil® (the fixed combination of atropine sulfate and diphenoxylate hydrochloride), and Ludiomil® (the former trade name for maprotiline hydrochloride; no longer commercially available under this trade name in the US). Medication errors also may occur between the different formulations of lamotrigine (Lamictal®, Lamictal® XR, generic lamotrigine tablets). Therefore, extra care should be exercised in ensuring the accuracy of both oral and written prescriptions for lamotrigine and these other drugs. The manufacturers recommend that clinicians consider including the intended use of the particular drug on the prescription, in addition to alerting patients to carefully check that they are receiving the correct drug as well as the correct formulation of the drug each time they fill their prescription and to promptly bring any question or concern to the attention of the dispensing pharmacist. The manufacturer of Lamictal® also recommends that pharmacists assess various measures of avoiding dispensing errors and implement them as appropriate (e.g., by computerized filling and handling of prescriptions, patient counseling). (See Possible Prescribing and Dispensing Errors under Cautions: Precautions and Contraindications.)

■ **Dosage** Because of the possibility of increasing seizure frequency, anticonvulsant drugs, including lamotrigine, should *not* be discontinued abruptly, particularly in patients with preexisting seizure disorders. Discontinuance of lamotrigine therapy should be done gradually over at least 2 weeks, in a stepwise fashion (e.g., achieving a 50% reduction in the daily dosage of lamotrigine each week). However, concerns for patient safety with continued use of lamotrigine may require more rapid withdrawal of the drug.

The dosage regimen of lamotrigine used in combination with other anticonvulsant drugs depends on whether valproic acid, hepatic enzyme-inducing anticonvulsant drugs, other anticonvulsants, or a combination of these is administered concomitantly. Addition to lamotrigine therapy of an anticonvulsant drug that induces hepatic microsomal enzymes (e.g., carbamazepine, phenobarbital, phenytoin, primidone) may be expected to increase the clearance (i.e., reduce plasma concentrations) of lamotrigine; conversely, discontinuance of such a concomitantly administered anticonvulsant drug may result in decreased clearance (i.e., increased plasma concentrations) of lamotrigine. Addition of valproate sodium to lamotrigine therapy also decreases the clearance (i.e., increases plasma concentrations) of lamotrigine. Therefore, clinicians should be aware that addition of hepatic enzyme-inducing anticonvulsant drugs or valproic acid to, or their discontinuance from, an anticonvulsant regimen including lamotrigine may require modification of the dosage of lamotrigine and/or the other anticonvulsant agent(s). Exceeding the recommended initial dosage and subsequent dosage escalations of lamotrigine may increase the risk of developing a rash and is *not* recommended.

Estrogen-containing oral contraceptives have been shown to increase the clearance of lamotrigine. The manufacturers state that no dosage adjustment to the recommended dosage escalation guidelines for lamotrigine should be necessary based solely on concomitant use of estrogen-containing oral contraceptives. Dosage escalation should follow the recommended guidelines for initiating adjunctive lamotrigine therapy based on the concomitant anticonvulsant(s) or other concomitant medications. *In women currently receiving estrogen-containing oral contraceptives* and not receiving carbamazepine, phenobarbital, phenytoin, primidone, or other drugs that induce lamotrigine glucuronidation (e.g., rifampin), the maintenance dosage of lamotrigine will in most cases need to be increased as much as twofold over the recommended target maintenance dosage in order to maintain a consistent plasma lamotrigine concentration. *In women starting estrogen-containing oral contraceptives*, receiving a stable lamotrigine dosage, and not receiving carbamazepine, phenobarbital, phenytoin, primidone, or other drugs that induce lamotrigine glucuronidation (e.g., rifampin), the maintenance dosage of lamotrigine will in most cases need to be increased as much as twofold in order to maintain a consistent plasma lamotrigine level. The dosage increases should begin at the same time that the oral contraceptive is added and continue, based on clinical response, no more rapidly than by 50–100 mg daily every week. Dosage increases should not exceed the recommended rate unless plasma lamotrigine concentrations or clinical response supports larger increases. Gradual transient increases in plasma lamotrigine concentrations may occur during the week of inactive hormonal preparation (i.e., the "pill-free" week); these increases will be greater if dosage increases are made during the days before or during the week of the inactive hormonal preparation. Such increased lamotrigine levels could potentially result in additional adverse effects (such as dizziness, ataxia, and diplopia). If such adverse effects consistently occur during the "pill-free" week, dosage adjustments to the overall maintenance dosage may be necessary; however, dosage adjustments limited to the "pill-free" week are not recommended. In women starting estrogen-containing oral contraceptives and receiving lamotrigine in addition to carbamazepine, phenobarbital, phenytoin, primidone, or other drugs that induce lamotrigine glucuronidation (e.g., rifampin), no adjustment to the lamotrigine dosage should be necessary.

When discontinuing estrogen-containing oral contraceptives in women not concurrently receiving carbamazepine, phenobarbital, phenytoin, primidone, or other drugs that induce lamotrigine glucuronidation (e.g., rifampin), the maintenance dosage of lamotrigine will in most cases need to be decreased by as much as 50% in order to maintain a consistent plasma lamotrigine concentration. The decrease in lamotrigine dosage should not exceed 25% of the total daily dosage per week over a 2-week period unless clinical response or plasma lamotrigine concentrations indicate otherwise. In women receiving lamotrigine in addition to carbamazepine, phenobarbital, phenytoin, primidone, or other drugs that induce lamotrigine glucuronidation (e.g., rifampin), adjustment of the maintenance dosage of lamotrigine should not be necessary upon discontinuance of estrogen-containing oral contraceptives. The effects of other hormonal contraceptive preparations or hormone replacement therapy on the pharmacokinetics of lamotrigine have not been systematically evaluated. Ethinyl estradiol, but not progestins, reportedly increased lamotrigine clearance up to twofold, and progestin-only formulations did not affect lamotrigine plasma concentrations. Therefore, adjustment of lamotrigine dosage in patients receiving progestins alone is unlikely to be necessary.

Seizure Disorders **Adjunctive Therapy.** For adjunctive therapy in the management of partial seizures, primary generalized tonic-clonic seizures, or Lennox-Gastaut syndrome in adults and children older than 12 years of age who are receiving hepatic enzyme-inducing anticonvulsant drugs *without* concomitant valproic acid therapy, the usual initial dosage of lamotrigine given as immediate-release formulations (e.g., conventional tablets, chewable/dispersible tablets, orally disintegrating tablets) is 50 mg daily for 2 weeks, then 100 mg daily in 2 divided doses for 2 weeks. The daily dosage may then be increased by 100 mg every 1–2 weeks until an effective maintenance dosage of 300–500 mg daily given in 2 divided doses is reached.

If extended-release tablets of lamotrigine (Lamictal® XR) are used for the management of partial seizures or primary generalized tonic-clonic seizures in adults and children 13 years of age or older who are receiving hepatic enzyme-inducing anticonvulsant drugs *without* concomitant valproic acid therapy, the usual initial dosage of lamotrigine is 50 mg once daily for 2 weeks, then 100 mg once daily for 2 weeks. The daily dosage may then be increased by 100 mg every week for the next 3 weeks (weeks 5 through 7), with subsequent increases made as necessary until an effective maintenance dosage of 400–600 mg once daily is reached. Dosage increases from week 8 and onward should not exceed 100 mg daily at weekly intervals.

For adjunctive therapy in the management of partial seizures, primary generalized tonic-clonic seizures, or Lennox-Gastaut syndrome in adults and children older than 12 years of age who are receiving an anticonvulsant regimen containing valproic acid, the usual initial dosage of lamotrigine given as immediate-release formulations (e.g., conventional tablets, chewable/dispersible tablets, orally disintegrating tablets) is 25 mg every *other* day for 2 weeks, followed by 25 mg once daily for 2 weeks. The initial dosage of lamotrigine in patients also receiving valproic acid should not exceed 25 mg every other day because of an increased incidence of rash with concomitant lamotrigine and valproic acid therapy. After the initial 4 weeks of therapy, the daily dosage of lamotrigine may be increased by 25–50 mg every 1–2 weeks until an effective maintenance dosage of 100–400 mg daily given in 1 or 2 divided doses is reached. The usual maintenance dosage of lamotrigine when added to valproic acid alone in adults and children older than 12 years of age is 100–200 mg daily given in 1 or 2 divided doses. The usual maintenance dosage of lamotrigine when added to valproic acid and other drugs that induce glucuronidation in adults and children older than 12 years of age is 100–400 mg daily given in 1 or 2 divided doses.

If extended-release tablets of lamotrigine (Lamictal® XR) are used for adjunctive therapy in the management of partial seizures or primary generalized tonic-clonic seizures in adults and children 13 years of age or older who are receiving an anticonvulsant regimen containing valproic acid, the usual initial dosage of lamotrigine is 25 mg every *other* day for 2 weeks, followed by 25 mg once daily for 2 weeks. The daily dosage may then be increased to 50 mg once daily at week 5, 100 mg once daily at week 6, and 150 mg once daily at week 7. The usual maintenance dosage of lamotrigine when added to valproic acid alone in adults and children 13 years of age or older is 200–250 mg once daily. Dosage increases from week 8 and onward should not exceed 100 mg daily at weekly intervals.

For adjunctive therapy in the management of partial seizures, primary generalized tonic-clonic seizures, or Lennox-Gastaut syndrome in adults and children older than 12 years of age who are receiving an anticonvulsant regimen that does not include carbamazepine, phenytoin, phenobarbital, primidone, or valproic acid, the usual initial dosage of lamotrigine given as immediate-release formulations (e.g., conventional tablets, chewable/dispersible tablets, orally disintegrating tablets) is 25 mg once daily for 2 weeks, followed by 50 mg daily for 2 weeks. After the initial 4 weeks of therapy, the daily dosage of lamotrigine may be increased by 50 mg every 1–2 weeks until an effective maintenance dosage of 225–375 mg daily given in 2 divided doses is reached.

If extended-release tablets of lamotrigine (Lamictal® XR) are used for adjunctive therapy in the management of partial seizures or primary generalized tonic-clonic seizures in adults and children 13 years of age or older who are receiving an anticonvulsant regimen that does not include carbamazepine, phenytoin, phenobarbital, primidone, or valproic acid, the usual initial dosage of lamotrigine is 25 mg once daily for 2 weeks, then 50 mg once daily for 2 weeks. The daily dosage may then be increased by 50 mg every week for the next 3 weeks (weeks 5 through 7), with subsequent increases made as necessary until an effective maintenance dosage of 300–400 mg once daily is reached. Dosage increases from week 8 and onward should not exceed 100 mg daily at weekly intervals.

Although maintenance dosages of immediate-release lamotrigine as high as 700 mg daily have been used in anticonvulsant drug regimens that included hepatic enzyme-inducing anticonvulsants but *not* valproic acid or as high as 200 mg daily in drug regimens that included valproic acid alone, dosages exceeding 300–500 mg daily (in regimens *not* containing valproic acid) or exceeding 200 mg daily (in regimens containing valproic acid alone) have not been evaluated in controlled studies.

For adjunctive therapy in the management of partial seizures, primary generalized tonic-clonic seizures, or Lennox-Gastaut syndrome in patients 2–12 years of age who are receiving hepatic enzyme-inducing anticonvulsant drugs *without* concomitant valproic acid therapy, the usual initial dosage of lamotrigine given as immediate-release formulations (e.g., conventional tablets, chewable/dispersible tablets, orally disintegrating tablets) is 0.6 mg/kg daily (rounded down to the nearest whole tablet) in 2 divided doses for 2 weeks. During the subsequent 2 weeks of therapy, the usual dosage is 1.2 mg/kg daily (rounded down to the nearest whole tablet) in 2 divided doses. Subsequent daily dosages should be increased every 1–2 weeks by 1.2 mg/kg (rounded down to the nearest whole tablet) until an effective daily maintenance dosage of 5–15 mg/kg (maximum of 400 mg/day in 2 divided doses) is reached. In patients weighing less than 30 kg, increases in maintenance dosages of up to 50% may be required based on the response and tolerance of the patient.

For adjunctive therapy in the management of partial seizures, primary generalized tonic-clonic seizures, or Lennox-Gastaut syndrome in patients 2–12 years of age who are receiving an anticonvulsant regimen containing valproic acid, the usual initial dosage of lamotrigine given as immediate-release formulations (e.g., conventional tablets, chewable/dispersible tablets, orally disintegrating tablets) is 0.15 mg/kg daily (rounded down to the nearest whole tablet) in 1 or 2 divided doses for 2 weeks. During the subsequent 2 weeks of therapy, the usual dosage is 0.3 mg/kg daily (rounded down to the nearest whole tablet) in 1 or 2 divided doses. Subsequent daily dosages should be increased every 1–2 weeks by 0.3 mg/kg (rounded down to the nearest whole tablet) until an effective daily maintenance dosage of 1–5 mg/kg (maximum of 200 mg/day in 1 or 2 divided doses) is reached. Usual maintenance dosages range from 1–3 mg/kg daily in patients receiving lamotrigine and valproic acid alone. In patients weighing less than 30 kg, increases in maintenance dosages of up to 50% may be required based on the response and tolerance of the patient.

For adjunctive therapy in the management of partial seizures, primary generalized tonic-clonic seizures, or Lennox-Gastaut syndrome in patients 2–12 years of age who are receiving an anticonvulsant regimen that does not include carbamazepine, phenytoin, phenobarbital, primidone, or valproic acid, the usual initial dosage of lamotrigine given as immediate-release formulations (e.g., conventional tablets, chewable/dispersible tablets, orally disintegrating tablets) is 0.3 mg/kg daily (rounded down to the nearest whole tablet) in 1 or 2 divided doses for 2 weeks. During the subsequent 2 weeks of therapy, the usual dosage is 0.6 mg/kg daily (rounded down to the nearest whole tablet) in 2 divided doses. Subsequent daily dosages should be increased every 1–2 weeks by 0.6 mg/kg (rounded down to the nearest whole tablet) until an effective daily maintenance dosage of 4.5–7.5 mg/kg (maximum of 300 mg/day in 2 divided doses) is reached. In patients weighing less than 30 kg, increases in maintenance dosages of up to 50% may be required based on the response and tolerance of the patient.

Monotherapy for Partial Seizures. For subsequent monotherapy in the management of partial seizures in patients converted from monotherapy with a hepatic enzyme-inducing anticonvulsant drug, the recommended maintenance dosage of lamotrigine given as immediate-release formulations (e.g., conventional tablets, chewable/dispersible tablets, orally disintegrating tablets) in adults and children 16 years of age or older is 500 mg daily given in 2 divided doses. The transition regimen for converting patients from monotherapy with a hepatic enzyme-inducing anticonvulsant drug to lamotrigine monotherapy is a 2-step process; the goal of the transition regimen is to ensure adequate seizure control while minimizing the possibility of developing a serious rash associated with the rapid titration of lamotrigine.

In the first step of the process, immediate-release lamotrigine therapy is added to the current drug regimen (which should be maintained at a fixed dosage) at a dosage of 50 mg once daily for 2 weeks, followed by 100 mg daily in 2 divided doses for 2 weeks; the daily dosage is then increased by 100 mg every 1–2 weeks until the maintenance dosage of 500 mg daily (in 2 divided doses) is reached. Once the maintenance lamotrigine dosage is reached, the concomitant hepatic enzyme-inducing anticonvulsant drug can then be withdrawn gradually over a period of 4 weeks; based on experience from the controlled clinical trial, the concomitant drug was withdrawn by 20% decrements each week over a 4-week period.

Bipolar Disorder For monotherapy in the maintenance treatment of bipolar disorder, the recommended initial adult dosage of lamotrigine given as immediate-release formulations (e.g., conventional tablets, chewable/dispersible tablets, orally disintegrating tablets) is 25 mg once daily for 2 weeks, followed by 50 mg once daily for 2 weeks. After the initial 4 weeks of therapy, the daily dosage of lamotrigine may be doubled at weekly intervals until an effective maintenance dosage of 200 mg daily is reached. Because 400-mg daily dosages were shown to be no more effective than 200-mg daily dosages in clinical studies of immediate-release lamotrigine monotherapy, the manufacturers recommend that daily dosages not exceed 200 mg daily.

For adjunctive therapy in the maintenance treatment of bipolar disorder in patients who are receiving carbamazepine or other hepatic enzyme-inducing drugs *without* concomitant valproic acid therapy, the usual initial adult dosage of immediate-release lamotrigine is 50 mg once daily for 2 weeks, followed by 100 mg daily in 2 divided doses for 2 weeks; the daily dosage is then increased in 100-mg increments at weekly intervals until the maintenance dosage of 400 mg daily (in 2 divided doses) is reached.

For adjunctive therapy in the maintenance treatment of bipolar disorder in adults who are receiving valproic acid, the usual initial dosage of immediate-release lamotrigine is 25 mg every other day for 2 weeks, followed by 25 mg once daily for 2 weeks. After the initial 4 weeks of therapy, the daily dosage of lamotrigine may be doubled at weekly intervals until an effective maintenance dosage of 100 mg daily is reached. To minimize the risk of potentially serious rash in patients receiving lamotrigine in conjunction with valproic acid, the recommended initial dosages and subsequent dose escalations of lamotrigine should not be exceeded.

Addition of hepatic enzyme-inducing drugs (e.g., carbamazepine) or hepatic enzyme-inhibiting drugs (e.g., valproic acid) to a regimen including immediate-release lamotrigine may require modification of the dosage of lamotrigine and/or the hepatic enzyme-inducing or -inhibiting drug. In pivotal clinical studies, dosages of lamotrigine were halved immediately following the addition of valproic acid to treat an acute mood episode and maintained at that dosage as long as valproic acid was administered concomitantly with lamotrigine. Following addition of carbamazepine or other hepatic enzyme-inducing drugs to treat an acute mood episode, dosages of lamotrigine were gradually doubled (e.g., over a period of at least 3 weeks) and maintained at that dosage as long as these drugs were administered concomitantly with lamotrigine. Following the addition of other psychotropic agents with no known clinical pharmacokinetic interactions with lamotrigine, patients were maintained at current maintenance dosages of lamotrigine.

Discontinuance of hepatic enzyme-inducing drugs (e.g., carbamazepine) or hepatic enzyme-inhibiting drugs (e.g., valproic acid) from a regimen including immediate-release lamotrigine may require modification of the dosage of lamotrigine. For patients discontinuing carbamazepine or other enzyme-inducing agents following resolution of the acute mood episode and achievement of a maintenance lamotrigine dosage, lamotrigine dosage should remain constant for the first week and then should be decreased in 100-mg daily increments at weekly intervals until an effective maintenance dosage of 200 mg daily is reached. For patients discontinuing valproic acid following resolution of the acute mood episode and achievement of a maintenance lamotrigine dosage, lamotrigine dosage should be increased in 50-mg daily increments at weekly intervals until an effective maintenance dosage of 200 mg daily is reached.

The optimum duration of lamotrigine therapy for the management of bipolar disorder has not been established, and the usefulness of the drug during prolonged therapy (i.e., longer than 18 months) should be reevaluated periodically.

■ **Dosage in Renal and Hepatic Impairment** Because clinical experience with lamotrigine is limited in patients with concomitant illness, the drug should be used with caution in patients with conditions (e.g., renal, hepatic, cardiac impairment) that may affect metabolism and elimination of the drug.

The manufacturers state that lamotrigine should be used with caution in patients with severe renal impairment because there is insufficient information from controlled clinical studies to establish the safety and efficacy of therapy with the drug in such patients. The initial dosage of lamotrigine in patients with renal impairment should be based on the patient's existing anticonvulsant drug regimen (see Dosage and Administration: Dosage). The manufacturers state that a reduced maintenance dosage of lamotrigine may be effective in patients with substantial renal impairment; however, the manufacturers currently make no specific recommendations for dosage adjustment in such patients.

The manufacturers state that experience with lamotrigine therapy in patients with hepatic impairment is limited. Based on a clinical pharmacology study of the drug in a small number of patients with moderate to severe hepatic dysfunction, the manufacturers make the general recommendation that initial, escalation, and maintenance dosages of lamotrigine therapy should be decreased by approximately 25% in patients with moderate (e.g., Child-Pugh class B) or severe (e.g., Child-Pugh class C) hepatic impairment without ascites and by 50% in patients with severe hepatic impairment with ascites. Escalation and maintenance dosages should be adjusted according to clinical response. Dosage adjustment is not necessary in patients with mild (e.g., Child-Pugh class A) hepatic impairment.

Cautions

Lamotrigine generally is well tolerated. However, there have been rare reports of serious dermatologic reactions (including some fatalities) in adults and children receiving lamotrigine. Nervous system and dermatologic effects are among the most frequently reported adverse effects of lamotrigine and among those most frequently requiring discontinuance of the drug. The most frequently occurring adverse effects associated with lamotrigine as adjunctive therapy in adults in controlled clinical trials include dizziness, ataxia, somnolence, headache, diplopia, blurred vision, nausea, vomiting, and rash. Discontinuance of lamotrigine because of adverse effects was required in about 11% of adult patients receiving immediate-release lamotrigine as adjunctive therapy in uncontrolled and controlled clinical trials; the adverse effects most frequently associated with discontinuance of lamotrigine in these trials were rash (3% of patients), dizziness (2.8% of patients), and headache (2.5% of patients). In children receiving immediate-release lamotrigine as adjunctive therapy in controlled clinical trials, the most commonly reported adverse effects were infection, vomiting, rash, fever, somnolence, accidental injury, dizziness, diarrhea, abdominal pain, nausea, ataxia, tremor, asthenia, bronchitis, flu syndrome, and diplopia. Approximately 11.5% of pediatric patients receiving immediate-release lamotrigine as adjunctive therapy in clinical trials discontinued the drug because of an adverse effect; the adverse effects most frequently associated with discontinuance of lamotrigine therapy in these patients were rash (4.4% of patients), reaction aggravated (1.7% of patients), and ataxia (0.6% of patients).

The most common adverse effects associated with extended-release lamotrigine given as adjunctive anticonvulsant therapy in adults and adolescents 13 years of age or older in 2 controlled clinical trials included dizziness, tremor/intention tremor, nausea, vomiting, diarrhea, diplopia, asthenia and fatigue, and somnolence. Discontinuance of lamotrigine because of adverse effects was required in 5% of patients receiving extended-release lamotrigine as adjunctive therapy in these trials; the adverse effects most frequently associated with discontinuance of therapy were dizziness (3% of patients), rash (1% of patients), headache (1% of patients), nausea (1% of patients), and nystagmus (1% of patients).

The most common adverse effects associated with immediate-release lamotrigine as monotherapy in adults in the controlled clinical trial were vomiting, coordination abnormality, dyspepsia, nausea, dizziness, rhinitis, anxiety, insomnia, infection, pain, weight decrease, chest pain, and dysmenorrhea; during the conversion period (i.e., when lamotrigine was initially added on to an existing monotherapy regimen consisting of a hepatic enzyme-inducing anticonvulsant drug), the most commonly reported adverse effects were dizziness, headache, nausea, asthenia, coordination abnormality, vomiting, rash, somnolence, diplopia, ataxia, accidental injury, tremor, blurred vision, insomnia, nystagmus, diarrhea, lymphadenopathy, pruritus, and sinusitis. The adverse effects most commonly associated with discontinuance of the drug in this trial were rash (4.5% of patients), headache (3.1% of patients), and asthenia (2.4% of patients).

The adverse effect profiles in males and females in clinical trials of immediate-release lamotrigine were similar and were independent of age; the rates of discontinuance of lamotrigine for individual adverse effects also were similar for males and females. In general, females receiving adjunctive therapy with immediate-release lamotrigine or placebo in controlled trials were more likely to report adverse effects than were males; however, dizziness was the only adverse effect reported with at least 10% greater frequency (i.e., 16.5% greater frequency) in females than in males (without a corresponding difference by gender with placebo) in controlled trials.

Because clinical trials of lamotrigine therapy involved specific patient populations and use of the drug as adjunctive therapy or monotherapy following conversion from therapy with another single hepatic enzyme-inducing anticonvulsant drug, it is difficult to determine whether a causal relationship exists for many reported adverse effects, to compare adverse effect frequencies with those in other clinical reports, and/or to extrapolate the adverse effects experience from controlled clinical trials to usual clinical practice.

■ **Nervous System Effects** Nervous system effects were among the most frequent adverse effects reported in patients receiving lamotrigine as adjunctive therapy in controlled clinical trials. Dizziness, headache, and ataxia were the most frequent adverse nervous system effects, occurring in 38, 29, and 22% of adults, respectively, in controlled trials of immediate-release lamotrigine adjunctive therapy. The frequency of dizziness and ataxia and the rate of discontinuance of lamotrigine because of these adverse effects were dose related in clinical trials; in a dose-response study, dizziness occurred in 54, 31, or 27% of patients receiving lamotrigine 500 mg/day, lamotrigine 300 mg/day, or placebo, respectively, while ataxia occurred in 28, 10, or 10% of those receiving these respective regimens. Limited data also suggest an increased incidence of adverse nervous system effects in patients receiving carbamazepine concomitantly with lamotrigine. (See Drug Interactions under Cautions: Precautions and Contraindications.)

Somnolence or insomnia occurred in 14 or 6%, respectively, of adults receiving immediate-release lamotrigine as adjunctive therapy in controlled clinical trials. Incoordination or tremor was reported in 6 or 4%, respectively, of lamotrigine-treated adults; limited evidence suggests that incoordination and tremor may be dose related, and tremor may occur more frequently with concomitant administration of valproic acid and lamotrigine. Depression occurred in 4%, anxiety in 4%, irritability in 3%, speech disorder in 3%, and concentration disturbance in 2% of adults receiving lamotrigine as adjunctive therapy in controlled clinical trials. Seizure or seizure exacerbation has been reported in 3 or 2% of adults, respectively, receiving lamotrigine as adjunctive therapy in controlled trials; an increase in seizure frequency also has been reported with lamotrigine therapy. Treatment-emergent seizures diagnosed unequivocally as status epilepticus were reported in 7 of 2343 adults receiving adjunctive therapy with immediate-release lamotrigine in clinical trials; however, the manufacturers state that valid estimates of the incidence of treatment-emergent status epilepticus are difficult to obtain because of variations in the definitions used by different investigators to identify such cases.

Coordination abnormality, dizziness, anxiety, and insomnia occurred in 7, 7, 5, and 5%, respectively, of adults receiving immediate-release lamotrigine as monotherapy in a controlled trial; amnesia, ataxia, asthenia, depression, hypesthesia, libido increase, decreased or increased reflexes, nystagmus, and irritability each occurred in 2% of such patients. Paresthesia or asthenia occurred in more than 1% of adults receiving lamotrigine as adjunctive therapy in controlled clinical trials but with equal or greater frequency in those receiving placebo.

Somnolence occurred in 17%, dizziness in 14%, ataxia in 11%, tremor in 10%, and asthenia in 8% of children receiving immediate-release lamotrigine as adjunctive therapy in controlled clinical trials. Emotional lability, gait abnormality, thinking abnormality, seizures, nervousness, and vertigo each occurred in 2–4% of children receiving lamotrigine as adjunctive therapy in controlled clinical trials.

Amnesia, confusion, hostility, decreased memory, nervousness, nystagmus, thinking abnormality, or vertigo was reported in at least 1% of patients receiving immediate-release lamotrigine in uncontrolled and controlled clinical trials. Abnormal dreams, abnormal gait, agitation, akathisia, apathy, aphasia, CNS depression, depersonalization, dysarthria, dyskinesia, dysphoria, emotional lability, euphoria, faintness, grand mal seizures, hallucinations, hyperkinesia, hypertonia, hypesthesia, increased libido, mind racing, myoclonus, panic attack, paranoid reaction, personality disorder, psychosis, migraine, sleep disorder, or stupor occurred in at least 0.1% but in less than 1% of such patients. Cerebellar syndrome, choreoathetosis, CNS stimulation, delirium, delusions, dystonia, hypoesthesia, hypotonia, hemiplegia, hyperalgesia, hyperesthesia, hypokinesia, hypomania, decreased libido, manic-depressive reaction, movement disorder, neuralgia, neurosis, or paralysis occurred in less than 0.1% of patients.

Suicidal ideation has been reported in 2–5% of adult patients receiving immediate-release lamotrigine monotherapy for partial seizures in a controlled clinical trial and in less than 1% of pediatric and adult patients receiving the drug in uncontrolled and controlled clinical trials; suicide and/or suicide attempt has been reported rarely. In an analysis of suicidality reports from placebo-controlled studies involving 11 anticonvulsants, including lamotrigine, patients receiving anticonvulsants had approximately twice the risk of suicidal behavior or ideation (0.43%) compared with patients receiving placebo (0.24%). (See Suicidality Risk under Cautions: Precautions and Contraindications.)

Lamotrigine therapy increases the risk of developing aseptic meningitis. FDA states that a total of 40 cases of aseptic meningitis have been identified in pediatric and adult lamotrigine-treated patients from December 1994 through November 2009. Symptoms in these cases included headache, fever, nausea, vomiting, nuchal rigidity, skin rash, photophobia, chills, altered consciousness, and/or somnolence and occurred 1–42 days (mean of 16 days) after beginning therapy with the drug. There was one death reported; however, the death was not thought to be caused by aseptic meningitis. Hospitalization was required in 35 of the patients. In most of the cases, symptoms resolved following discontinuance of lamotrigine. In 15 cases, however, symptoms rapidly returned (within 0.5–24 hours; mean: 5 hours) following reinitiation of lamotrigine. In these rechallenge cases, symptoms were frequently more severe following reexposure to the drug. Data on CSF findings were available in 25 cases; CSF analyses were characterized by mild to moderate pleocytosis, normal glucose concentrations, and mild to moderate increases in protein. CSF white blood cell differentials showed a predominance of neutrophils in the majority of cases; however, a predominance of lymphocytes was reported in approximately one-third of the cases. Some of the lamotrigine-treated patients who developed aseptic meningitis had underlying diagnoses of systemic lupus erythematosus or other autoimmune diseases. In addition, some of the patients had new onset of signs and symptoms of involvement of other organs (predominantly hepatic and renal involvement), which may suggest that some of the reported cases of lamotrigine-associated meningitis were part of a hypersensitivity or generalized drug reaction. (See Aseptic Meningitis under Cautions: Precautions and Contraindications.)

Exacerbation of parkinsonian manifestations in patients with preexisting parkinsonian syndrome and the occurrence of tics have been reported during postmarketing experience with lamotrigine and/or in worldwide uncontrolled clinical trials; however, the data are insufficient to provide an estimate of the incidence of such effects or to establish a causal relationship to lamotrigine.

■ **Immune System Effects** Hemophagocytic lymphohistiocytosis (HLH), a rare but potentially life-threatening condition involving pathologic activation of the immune system, has been reported in adults and children receiving lamotrigine. If not recognized and treated promptly, HLH is associated with high mortality. HLH can occur within days to weeks after starting lamotrigine therapy and is characterized by clinical signs and symptoms of uncontrolled systemic inflammation; manifestations include, but are not limited to, persistent fever (usually greater than 101°F), rash, hepatosplenomegaly, lymphadenopathy, neurologic effects (e.g., seizures, visual disturbances, difficulty ambulating), cytopenias, hepatic dysfunction, high serum ferritin concentrations, and coagulation abnormalities. Diagnosis may be difficult because early signs and symptoms (particularly fever and rash) are nonspecific and may be confused with other immune-related adverse reactions such as drug reaction with eosinophilia and systemic symptoms (DRESS). Since 1994, at least 8 cases of confirmed or suspected HLH have been reported among patients receiving lamotrigine worldwide; serious outcomes included hospitalization in all cases and death in one patient. In the reported cases, a temporal relationship was observed between administration of lamotrigine and development of HLH, with symptoms presenting 8–24 days following initiation of the drug. (See Hemophagocytic Lymphohistiocytosis under Cautions: Precautions and Contraindications.)

■ **GI Effects** GI effects were among the most frequent adverse effects reported in adults receiving immediate-release lamotrigine as adjunctive therapy in controlled clinical trials. Nausea was the most frequent adverse GI effect, occurring in 19% of adults in controlled clinical trials; vomiting was reported in 9% of patients in these trials. The frequency of nausea and vomiting appears to be dose related; in a dose-response study, nausea occurred in 25, 18, or 11% of patients receiving lamotrigine 500 mg daily, lamotrigine 300 mg daily, or placebo, respectively, while vomiting occurred in 18, 11, or 4% of those receiving these respective regimens. Diarrhea occurred in 6%, dyspepsia in 5%, abdominal pain in 5%, constipation in 4%, tooth disorder in 3%, and anorexia in 2% of adults receiving lamotrigine as adjunctive therapy in controlled clinical trials. Flatulence was reported in more than 1% of adults receiving lamotrigine as adjunctive therapy in controlled clinical trials but occurred with equal or greater frequency in patients receiving placebo. Vomiting, dyspepsia, and nausea occurred in 9, 7, and 7%, respectively, of adults receiving lamotrigine as monotherapy in a controlled trial; anorexia, dry mouth, rectal hemorrhage, and peptic ulcer each occurred in 2% of such patients.

Vomiting occurred in 20%, diarrhea in 11%, abdominal pain in 10%, and nausea in 10% of children receiving immediate-release lamotrigine as adjunctive therapy in controlled clinical trials. Constipation, dyspepsia, and tooth disorder each occurred in 2–4% of children receiving lamotrigine as adjunctive therapy in controlled clinical trials.

Halitosis, dry mouth, dysphagia, gingivitis, glossitis, gum hyperplasia, increased appetite, increased salivation, mouth ulceration, stomatitis, taste perversion, thirst, or tooth disorder occurred in at least 0.1% but in less than 1% of patients receiving immediate-release lamotrigine in uncontrolled and controlled clinical trials. Eructation, gastritis, GI hemorrhage, gum hemorrhage, hematemesis, hemorrhagic colitis, melena, gastric ulcer, taste loss, or tongue edema was reported in less than 0.1% of patients.

Esophagitis and pancreatitis have been reported during postmarketing experience with lamotrigine and/or in worldwide uncontrolled clinical trials; however, data are insufficient to provide an estimate of the incidence of such effects or to establish a causal relationship to lamotrigine.

■ **Dermatologic and Sensitivity Reactions** Serious dermatologic reactions (including some fatalities) have been reported in adults and children receiving lamotrigine therapy. Rash occurred in 10% of adults and 14% of children receiving immediate-release lamotrigine as adjunctive therapy in controlled clinical trials. The incidence of severe rash associated with lamotrigine also appears to be higher in pediatric patients than in adults; severe rash, including Stevens-Johnson syndrome, has been reported in approximately 0.8% of children younger than 16 years of age and in 0.3% of adults receiving immediate-release lamotrigine as adjunctive therapy in epilepsy clinical trials. In clinical trials of bipolar disorder and other mood disorders, the incidence of serious rash was 0.08% in adults receiving immediate-release lamotrigine as initial monotherapy and 0.13% in adults receiving the drug as adjunctive therapy. The risk of serious rashes associated with extended-release lamotrigine therapy is not expected to differ from that with the immediate-release formulations of the drug; however, the relatively limited treatment experience makes it difficult to characterize the incidence and risk of such rashes with the extended-release formulation.

There is evidence that most cases of rash associated with lamotrigine therapy are associated with transiently high plasma concentrations of the drug occurring during the initial weeks of therapy or with high plasma concentrations occurring during concomitant valproic acid therapy. Cases of life-threatening rashes associated with lamotrigine almost always have occurred within 2–8 weeks of treatment initiation; however, severe rashes rarely have presented following prolonged treatment (e.g., 6 months). Lamotrigine-associated rashes do not appear to have distinguishing features. Because it is not possible to distinguish benign rashes from those that may become severe and/or life-threatening, lamotrigine generally should be discontinued at the first sign of rash (unless the rash is known not to be drug related). However, a rash may become life-threatening or permanently disabling or disfiguring despite discontinuance of the drug. Discontinuance of immediate-release lamotrigine because of rash was required in 3% of adults receiving the drug as adjunctive therapy and 4.5% of adults receiving the drug as monotherapy in controlled clinical trials; 4.4% of pediatric patients receiving immediate-release lamotrigine in controlled clinical trials discontinued the drug because of the development of rash. The potential for development of a rash at the beginning of lamotrigine therapy may be decreased by employing low initial dosages and by gradual escalation of dosage to avoid initially high plasma concentrations of the drug.

Rash, including serious and potentially life-threatening rash, appears to be more likely to occur in patients receiving concomitant valproic acid. Valproic acid can decrease clearance and increase plasma concentrations of lamotrigine more than twofold; exceeding the recommended reduced initial dosage of lamotrigine or the subsequent recommended schedule for escalation of lamotrigine dosage (see Dosage and Administration: Dosage and see Drug Interactions under Cautions: Precautions and Contraindications), particularly in patients receiving valproic acid, may increase the incidence of rash, including serious rash, in lamotrigine-treated patients. In clinical trials, 1% of adults and 1.2% of children receiving a drug regimen including immediate-release lamotrigine concomitantly with valproic acid experienced a rash requiring hospitalization, while 0.16% of adults and 0.6% of children receiving a drug regimen of lamotrigine without valproic acid were hospitalized because of rash.

Rashes severe enough to cause hospitalization, including Stevens-Johnson syndrome, toxic epidermal necrolysis, erythema multiforme, angioedema, and a hypersensitivity syndrome (usually consisting of fever, rash, facial swelling, and hematologic, hepatic, and/or lymphatic involvement), occurred in 0.3% of adults receiving immediate-release lamotrigine in premarketing controlled and uncontrolled clinical trials and in about 0.8% of pediatric patients receiving the drug in clinical trials; death associated with rash has been reported rarely in postmarketing use of lamotrigine. Erythema multiforme has been reported in patients receiving lamotrigine in premarketing controlled and uncontrolled clinical trials in the US, while lupus-like syndrome and vasculitis have been reported during postmarketing experience with the drug and/or in worldwide uncontrolled clinical trials.

Pruritus occurred in 3% of adults receiving immediate-release lamotrigine as adjunctive therapy in controlled clinical trials. Contact dermatitis, dry skin, peripheral edema, and sweating each occurred in 2% of adults receiving lamotrigine as monotherapy in a controlled trial. Eczema, facial edema, photosensitivity, and pruritus each were reported in 2% of children receiving immediate-release lamotrigine as adjunctive therapy in controlled clinical trials. Acne, alopecia, facial edema, dry skin, erythema, hirsutism, maculopapular rash, peripheral edema, skin discoloration, Stevens-Johnson syndrome, sweating, urticaria, or vesiculobullous rash occurred in at least 0.1% but in less than 1% of patients receiving lamotrigine in uncontrolled and controlled clinical trials. Angioedema, erythema multiforme, fungal dermatitis, herpes zoster, leukoderma, petechial rash, pustular rash, seborrhea, or photosensitivity occurred in less than 0.1% of patients.

Hypersensitivity reactions, which can be fatal or life-threatening, have been reported in patients treated with lamotrigine. In some cases, manifestations of these reactions have included multiorgan dysfunction (including hepatic abnormalities and disseminated intravascular coagulation) (see Cautions: Hepatic Effects). Early signs of a possible hypersensitivity reaction, such as fever and lymphadenopathy, should prompt immediate evaluation of the patient; a rash may or may not be present. Unless another cause for the signs or symptoms is found, lamotrigine should be discontinued.

■ Cardiovascular Effects Hemorrhage was reported in 2% of pediatric patients receiving immediate-release lamotrigine as adjunctive therapy in controlled clinical trials. Chest pain occurred in more than 1% of adults receiving lamotrigine as adjunctive therapy in controlled clinical trials but occurred with equal or greater frequency in patients receiving placebo. Chest pain also occurred in 5% of adults receiving lamotrigine as monotherapy in a controlled clinical trial. Flushing, hot flushes, palpitations, postural hypotension, syncope, tachycardia, or vasodilation occurred in at least 0.1% but in less than 1% of patients receiving lamotrigine in uncontrolled and controlled clinical trials. Cerebrovascular accident, cerebral sinus thrombosis, deep thrombophlebitis, myocardial infarction, atrial fibrillation, angina pectoris, hemorrhage, or hypertension occurred in less than 0.1% of patients receiving lamotrigine in uncontrolled and controlled clinical trials.

■ Respiratory Effects Rhinitis occurred in 14%, pharyngitis in 10%, increased cough in 8%, and flu-like syndrome in 7% of adults receiving immediate-release lamotrigine as adjunctive therapy in controlled clinical trials. Respiratory disorder was reported in more than 1% of adults receiving lamotrigine as adjunctive therapy in controlled clinical trials but occurred with equal or greater frequency in patients receiving placebo. Rhinitis occurred in 7% of adults receiving lamotrigine as monotherapy in a controlled trial; epistaxis, bronchitis, and dyspnea each occurred in 2% of such patients. Pharyngitis, bronchitis, and increased cough occurred in 14, 7, and 7%, respectively, of children receiving immediate-release lamotrigine as adjunctive therapy in controlled clinical trials. Sinusitis and bronchospasm each were reported in 2% of children in these trials. Dyspnea, epistaxis, or hyperventilation occurred in at least 0.1% but in less than 1% of patients in uncontrolled and controlled clinical trials, and bronchospasm, hiccups, or sinusitis occurred in less than 0.1% of patients. Apnea has been reported during postmarketing experience with lamotrigine and/or in worldwide uncontrolled clinical trials; however, data are insufficient to provide an estimate of the incidence of this adverse effect or to establish a causal relationship to lamotrigine.

■ Ocular and Otic Effects Ocular effects were among the most frequent adverse effects reported in patients receiving lamotrigine as adjunctive therapy in controlled clinical trials. Diplopia was the most frequent adverse ocular effect reported in adults receiving immediate-release lamotrigine as adjunctive therapy in controlled trials, occurring in 28% of such patients, and blurred vision occurred in 16% of patients. The frequency of diplopia and blurred vision appears to be dose related; in a dose-response study, diplopia occurred in 49, 24, or 8% of patients receiving lamotrigine 500 mg daily, lamotrigine 300 mg daily, or placebo, respectively, while blurred vision occurred in 25, 11, or 10% of patients receiving these respective regimens. Limited data also indicate an increased incidence of some adverse effects, including diplopia and blurred vision, in patients receiving carbamazepine concomitantly with lamotrigine. (See Drug Interactions under Cautions: Precautions and Contraindications.)

Vision abnormality occurred in 3% of adults receiving immediate-release lamotrigine as adjunctive therapy in controlled clinical trials and in 2% of adults receiving immediate-release lamotrigine as monotherapy in a controlled trial. Diplopia, blurred vision, or vision abnormality occurred in 5, 4, or 2%, respectively, of children receiving lamotrigine as adjunctive therapy in controlled clinical trials. Abnormality of accommodation, conjunctivitis, oscillopsia, or photophobia occurred in at least 0.1% but in less than 1% of patients in uncontrolled and controlled clinical trials, and dry eyes, lacrimation disorder, strabismus, ptosis, or uveitis occurred in less than 0.1% of patients.

Ear disorder was reported in 2% of children receiving immediate-release lamotrigine as adjunctive therapy in controlled clinical trials. Otic pain or tinnitus occurred in at least 0.1% but in less than 1% of patients in uncontrolled and controlled clinical trials. Deafness was reported in less than 0.1% of patients in uncontrolled and controlled clinical trials.

■ Musculoskeletal Effects Neck pain and arthralgia each occurred in 2% of adults receiving immediate-release lamotrigine as adjunctive therapy in controlled clinical trials. Back pain or myalgia occurred in more than 1% of patients receiving lamotrigine as adjunctive therapy in controlled trials but with equal or greater frequency in patients receiving placebo. Joint disorder, myasthenia, muscle spasm, or twitching occurred in at least 0.1% but in less than 1% of patients in uncontrolled and controlled trials, and arthritis, bursitis, leg cramps, tendinous contracture, or pathological fracture occurred in less than 0.1% of patients. Rhabdomyolysis has been observed in patients experiencing hypersensitivity reactions during postmarketing experience with lamotrigine and/or in worldwide uncontrolled trials; however, data are insufficient to provide an estimate of the incidence of this adverse effect or to establish a causal relationship to lamotrigine.

■ Genitourinary Effects Dysmenorrhea occurred in 7%, vaginitis in 4%, and amenorrhea in 2% of women receiving immediate-release lamotrigine as adjunctive therapy in controlled clinical trials. Dysmenorrhea occurred in 5% of women receiving lamotrigine as monotherapy in a controlled trial. Menstrual disorder or urinary tract infection occurred in more than 1% of adults receiving adjunctive lamotrigine therapy in controlled trials but with equal or greater frequency in patients receiving placebo. Urinary tract infection occurred in 3% of children receiving lamotrigine as adjunctive therapy in controlled clinical trials; penis disorder was reported in 2% of male pediatric patients receiving lamotrigine in these trials.

Lactation (in females), vaginal candidiasis, hematuria, polyuria, urinary frequency, urinary incontinence, or urinary retention occurred in at least 0.1% but in less than 1% of patients receiving immediate-release lamotrigine therapy in uncontrolled and controlled clinical trials. Abnormal ejaculation, impotence, epididymitis, cystitis, urine abnormality, dysuria, kidney pain, kidney failure, acute kidney failure, or menorrhagia occurred in less than 0.1% of patients in uncontrolled and controlled clinical trials.

■ Endocrine and Metabolic Effects Goiter or hyperthyroidism occurred in less than 0.1% of patients receiving immediate-release lamotrigine in uncontrolled and controlled clinical trials. Weight decrease occurred in 5% of adults receiving lamotrigine as monotherapy in a controlled trial. Weight loss or weight gain occurred in at least 0.1% but in less than 1% of patients in uncontrolled and controlled clinical trials. Edema occurred in 2% of children receiving lamotrigine as adjunctive therapy in controlled clinical trials. Edema or hyperglycemia occurred in less than 0.1% of patients in uncontrolled and controlled clinical trials.

■ Hepatic Effects Fatalities associated with multiorgan failure and various degrees of hepatic failure have been reported rarely during premarketing trials of immediate-release lamotrigine as adjunctive therapy. A young woman receiving concomitant valproic acid and carbamazepine developed a possible hypersensitivity syndrome consisting of headache, fever, and a maculopapular rash 3 weeks following addition of lamotrigine to therapy; fulminant hepatic failure and hepatic coma developed within 3 days, and despite subsequent clinical improvement, the patient died of a massive pulmonary embolus 2 months later. Multiorgan (including renal and/or hepatic) failure and disseminated intravascular coagulation associated with frequent generalized seizures or status epilepticus have been reported in several patients receiving immediate-release lamotrigine; it has been suggested that this syndrome may have resulted from rhabdomyolysis caused by uncontrolled generalized seizures. The majority of these cases of hepatic and/or multiorgan failure occurred in association with other serious medical events (e.g., status epilepticus, overwhelming sepsis), making it difficult to identify the initiating cause. However, disseminated intravascular coagulation, rhabdomyolysis, renal failure, maculopapular rash, ataxia, and increased liver enzymes (e.g., AST [SGOT]) in the absence of generalized seizures also have been reported rarely with lamotrigine as adjunctive therapy. Abnormal liver function test results occurred in at least 0.1% but in less than 1% of patients receiving immediate-release lamotrigine in uncontrolled and controlled clinical trials, and hepatitis, increased alkaline phosphatase, or bilirubinemia occurred in less than 0.1% of patients.

■ Hematologic Effects Blood dyscrasias that may or may not be associated with hypersensitivity reactions, including neutropenia, leukopenia, anemia, thrombocytopenia, pancytopenia, and rarely, aplastic anemia and pure red cell aplasia (PRCA), have been reported with lamotrigine. Lymphadenopathy occurred in 2% of children receiving immediate-release lamotrigine as adjunctive therapy in controlled clinical trials. Anemia, ecchymosis, petechiae, leukocytosis, leukopenia, or lymphadenopathy occurred in at least 0.1% but in less than 1% of patients receiving immediate-release lamotrigine in uncontrolled and controlled clinical trials. Eosinophilia, fibrin decrease, fibrinogen decrease, iron deficiency anemia, lymphocytosis, macrocytic anemia, or thrombocytopenia occurred in less than 0.1% of patients receiving immediate-release lamotrigine in uncontrolled and controlled clinical trials.

Disseminated intravascular coagulation has been reported rarely in conjunction with multiorgan (e.g., renal and/or hepatic) failure in patients receiving lamotrigine as adjunctive therapy. (See Cautions: Hepatic Effects.) Agranulocytosis, aplastic anemia, hemolytic anemia, neutropenia, pancytopenia, red cell aplasia, and progressive immunosuppression have been reported during postmarketing experience with lamotrigine and/or in worldwide uncontrolled clinical trials; however, data are insufficient to provide an estimate of the incidence of such effects or to establish a causal relationship to lamotrigine.

■ Other Adverse Effects Flu syndrome or fever occurred in 7 or 6%, respectively, of adults receiving immediate-release lamotrigine as adjunctive therapy in controlled clinical trials. Pain and infection each occurred in 5% and fever in 2% of adults receiving lamotrigine as monotherapy in a controlled trial. Infection occurred in 20%, fever in 15%, accidental injury in 14%, flu syndrome in 7%, and pain in 5% of children receiving immediate-release lamotrigine as adjunctive therapy in controlled clinical trials. Pain occurred in at least 1% of patients receiving immediate-release lamotrigine in uncontrolled and controlled clinical trials. Accidental injury, infection, chills, and malaise occurred in at least 0.1% but in less than 1% of patients receiving immediate-release lamotrigine in uncontrolled and controlled clinical trials. Breast pain, breast abscess, breast neoplasm, enlarged abdomen, increase in serum creatinine concentration, parosmia, or alcohol intolerance occurred in less than 0.1% of patients.

■ Precautions and Contraindications

Risk Evaluation and Mitigation Strategy A Risk Evaluation and Mitigation Strategy (REMS) has been required and approved by the US Food and Drug Administration (FDA) for lamotrigine. The goal of this REMS program is to inform patients about the serious risks associated with use of the drug, including an increased risk of suicidal thoughts and behavior. (See Cautions.) The REMS program consists of a medication guide to be dispensed with every lamotrigine prescription.

Withdrawal Seizures Because of the possibility of increased seizure frequency, anticonvulsant drugs, including lamotrigine, should not be discontinued suddenly, particularly in patients with preexisting seizure disorders. Unless safety concerns dictate a more rapid withdrawal of the drug, discontinuance of lamotrigine should be done gradually over a period of at least 2 weeks. (See Dosage and Administration: Dosage.) Seizure exacerbation and/or status epilepticus have been reported in patients receiving lamotrigine as adjunctive therapy in the management of seizure disorders, although the incidence of these adverse effects has been difficult to determine conclusively. (See Cautions: Nervous System Effects.) The use and dosage of all anticonvulsant drugs in a regimen including lamotrigine should be reevaluated if there is a change in seizure control or appearance or worsening of adverse effects, and patients should be instructed to report immediately any worsening of seizure control.

Suicidality Risk An increased risk of suicidality (suicidal behavior or ideation) was observed in an analysis of 199 randomized, placebo-controlled studies evaluating 11 anticonvulsants (carbamazepine, felbamate, gabapentin, lamotrigine, levetiracetam, oxcarbazepine, pregabalin, tiagabine, topiramate, valproate, and zonisamide) in patients with epilepsy, psychiatric disorders (e.g., bipolar disorder, depression, anxiety), and other conditions (e.g., migraine, neuropathic pain). The analysis revealed that patients receiving these anticonvulsants had approximately twice the risk of suicidal behavior or ideation (0.43%) compared with patients receiving placebo (0.24%); this increased suicidality risk was observed as early as one week after beginning therapy and continued through 24 weeks. The results were generally consistent among the 11 drugs studied. In addition, patients who were treated for epilepsy, psychiatric disorders, and other conditions were all found to be at increased risk for suicidality when compared with placebo; there did not appear to be a specific demographic subgroup of patients to which the increased risk could be attributed. However, the relative risk for suicidality was found to be higher in patients with epilepsy compared with patients who were given one of the drugs for psychiatric or other conditions.

All patients who are currently receiving or beginning therapy with any anticonvulsant for any indication should be closely monitored for the emergence or worsening of depression, suicidal thoughts or behavior (suicidality), and/or unusual changes in mood or behavior. Clinicians should inform patients, their families, and caregivers of the potential for an increased risk of suicidality so that they are aware and able to notify their clinician of any unusual behavioral changes. Patients, family members, and caregivers also should be advised not to make any changes to the anticonvulsant regimen without first consulting with the responsible clinician. They should pay close attention to any day-to-day changes in mood, behavior, and actions; since changes can happen very quickly, it is important to be alert to any sudden differences. In addition, patients, family members, and caregivers should be aware of common warning signs that may signal suicide risk (e.g., talking or thinking about wanting to hurt oneself or end one's life, withdrawing from friends and family, becoming depressed or experiencing worsening of existing depression, becoming preoccupied with death and dying, giving away prized possessions). If these or any new and worrisome behaviors occur, the responsible clinician should be contacted immediately. Clinicians who prescribe lamotrigine or any other anticonvulsant should balance the risk for suicidality with the risk of untreated illness. Epilepsy and many other illnesses for which anticonvulsants are prescribed are themselves associated with an increased risk of morbidity and mortality and an increased risk of suicidal thoughts and behavior. If suicidal thoughts and behavior emerge during anticonvulsant therapy, the clinician must consider whether the emergence of these symptoms in any given patient may be related to the illness being treated.

Sudden Death in Epilepsy During the premarketing development of lamotrigine, 20 sudden and unexplained deaths were reported among a cohort of 4700 patients with epilepsy receiving adjunctive therapy with immediate-release lamotrigine (5747 patient-years of exposure). Although the rate of these deaths exceeds that expected to occur in a healthy (nonepileptic) population matched for age and gender, this rate was similar to that occurring in a similar population of epileptic patients receiving a chemically unrelated anticonvulsant agent. This evidence suggests, but does not prove, that the incidence of sudden, unexplained death observed with lamotrigine adjunctive therapy may be reflective of the population itself rather than the effects of lamotrigine.

Hemophagocytic Lymphohistiocytosis Hemophagocytic lymphohistiocytosis (HLH), a potentially fatal immune system reaction, has been reported rarely with lamotrigine. (See Cautions: Immune System Effects.) Patients receiving lamotrigine should be advised to seek immediate medical attention if they develop any manifestations suggestive of HLH (e.g., fever, usually exceeding 101°F; rash; enlarged liver and lymph nodes; unusual bleeding; yellowing of the skin or eyes; neurologic effects including seizures, difficulty walking, and visual disturbances). An evaluation for possible HLH should be performed based on published international diagnostic criteria. Unless an alternative etiology for the observed signs or symptoms can be established, lamotrigine should be discontinued.

Serious Skin Rash Some evidence suggests that use of lamotrigine concomitantly with valproic acid increases the risk of serious rash. The incidence of rash also appears to increase with the magnitude of the initial dosage of lamotrigine and the subsequent rate of dosage escalation; exceeding the recommended dosage of lamotrigine at initiation of therapy appears to increase the risk of rash requiring withdrawal of therapy. (See Dosage and Administration: Dosage.) A benign initial appearance of a rash in a patient receiving lamotrigine therapy cannot predict an entirely benign outcome. Patients receiving lamotrigine, especially in conjunction with valproic acid, should be cautioned that rash, in some cases potentially life-threatening, may occur, and that any occurrence of rash should immediately be reported by the patient to their clinician.

Drug Interactions The concomitant use of valproic acid and/or hepatic enzyme-inducing anticonvulsant drugs (e.g., phenobarbital, primidone, carbamazepine, phenytoin) can increase or decrease the metabolism and elimination of lamotrigine, requiring dosage adjustments to maintain efficacy and/or avoid toxicity. (See Dosage and Administration: Dosage.) Addition of valproic acid to lamotrigine therapy reduces lamotrigine clearance and increases steady-state plasma lamotrigine concentrations by slightly more than 50% whether or not hepatic enzyme-inducing anticonvulsant drugs are given concomitantly. Conversely, steady-state plasma concentrations of lamotrigine are decreased by about 40% when phenobarbital, primidone, or carbamazepine is added to lamotrigine therapy and by about 45–54% when phenytoin is added to lamotrigine therapy; the magnitude of the effect with phenytoin is dependent on the total daily dosage of phenytoin (from 100–400 mg daily). Discontinuance of an enzyme-inducing anticonvulsant drug can be expected to increase, and discontinuance of valproic acid can be expected to decrease, the elimination half-life and plasma concentrations of lamotrigine. Although the manufacturers state that a therapeutic plasma concentration range has not been established for lamotrigine and that dosage should be based on therapeutic response, the change in plasma lamotrigine concentrations resulting from addition or discontinuance of enzyme-inducing anticonvulsant drugs or valproic acid should be considered when these drugs are added to or withdrawn from an existing anticonvulsant drug regimen that includes lamotrigine.

Addition of lamotrigine to existing therapy with phenytoin or carbamazepine generally does *not* appreciably alter the steady-state plasma concentrations of these concomitantly administered drugs. Addition of lamotrigine to carbamazepine therapy reportedly has resulted in increased plasma concentrations of a pharmacologically active metabolite of carbamazepine (carbamazepine-10,11-epoxide) and an increased incidence of some adverse effects (e.g., dizziness, headache, diplopia, blurred vision, ataxia, nausea, nystagmus). However, elevations in carbamazepine-10,11-epoxide plasma concentrations and/or increased toxicity have not been consistently observed with concomitant administration of lamotrigine and carbamazepine, and the mechanism of the interaction between these drugs remains unclear.

Addition of lamotrigine to valproic acid therapy in healthy individuals resulted in a 25% reduction in trough steady-state plasma concentrations of valproic acid over a 3-week period, followed by stabilization of these concentrations.

The effects of adding lamotrigine to an existing regimen including valproic acid, phenytoin, and/or carbamazepine may be expected to be similar to those associated with addition of each drug independently (i.e., valproic acid concentrations decrease, phenytoin and carbamazepine concentrations do not change).

Some estrogen-containing oral contraceptives have been shown to decrease plasma concentrations of lamotrigine. Therefore, dosage adjustment of lamotrigine will be necessary in most patients who begin or stop estrogen-containing oral contraceptives while receiving lamotrigine therapy. During the week of inactive hormonal preparation (i.e., "pill-free" week) of oral contraceptive therapy, plasma lamotrigine concentrations are expected to increase by as much as twofold by the end of the week. Adverse effects associated with elevated plasma lamotrigine concentrations (such as dizziness, ataxia, and diplopia) may occur. (See Dosage and Administration: Dosage.)

Lamotrigine is a weak inhibitor of dihydrofolate reductase. Although clinically important alterations in blood folate concentrations or hematologic parameters have not been documented in clinical studies of lamotrigine therapy of at least 5 years duration, the manufacturers state that clinicians should be aware of this effect when prescribing other drugs that inhibit folate metabolism.

Acute Multiorgan Failure Multiorgan failure and various degrees of hepatic failure, in some cases fatal or irreversible, have been reported rarely with immediate-release lamotrigine therapy. (See Cautions: Hepatic Effects.) The possibility of such potentially fatal adverse effects should be considered in patients who exhibit signs and symptoms associated with multiorgan and/or hepatic impairment following initiation of lamotrigine as adjunctive therapy.

Aseptic Meningitis Lamotrigine may cause aseptic meningitis. (See Cautions: Nervous System Effects.) Patients receiving the drug should be instructed to immediately contact their clinician if they experience headache, fever, chills, nausea, vomiting, stiff neck, rash, abnormal sensitivity to light, myalgia, drowsiness, and/or confusion. If meningitis is suspected, patients should be evaluated and treated, as indicated, for other possible causes of meningitis. Discontinuance of lamotrigine should be considered if no other clear cause of meningitis is identified.

Somnolence and Dizziness Lamotrigine can produce drowsiness and dizziness, and patients should be cautioned that the drug may impair their ability to perform hazardous activities requiring mental alertness or physical coordination (e.g., operating machinery, driving a motor vehicle).

Renal Impairment Limited information indicates that the elimination half-life of immediate-release lamotrigine is prolonged in patients with severe chronic renal failure (mean creatinine clearance of 13 mL/minute) not receiving other anticonvulsant drugs. In a study of a limited number of patients and healthy individuals receiving a single 100-mg dose of immediate-release lamotrigine, the mean plasma half-life of the drug was 42.9 hours in patients with chronic renal failure, 57.4 hours between treatments in dialysis patients, and 26.2 hours in healthy individuals. The mean plasma half-life of lamotrigine was decreased to 13 hours during hemodialysis; an average of 20% (range: 5.6–35.1%) of the total body load of lamotrigine was eliminated during a 4-hour hemodialysis treatment. The manufacturers state that a reduced maintenance dosage of lamotrigine may be effective in patients with substantial renal impairment; however, the manufacturers currently make no specific recommendations for dosage adjustment in such patients. (See Dosage and Administration: Dosage in Renal and Hepatic Impairment.)

Hepatic Impairment The manufacturers state that experience with use of lamotrigine in patients with impaired liver function is limited. Following a single 100-mg dose of immediate-release lamotrigine, the mean half-life of the drug in patients with hepatic impairment that was mild (Child-Pugh class A), moderate (Child-Pugh class B), severe (Child-Pugh class C) without ascites, or severe with ascites was 46, 72, 67, or 100 hours, respectively, compared with 33 hours in healthy individuals. The manufacturers recommend reduction of initial, escalation, and maintenance dosages of lamotrigine in patients with moderate or severe hepatic impairment. (See Dosage and Administration: Dosage in Renal and Hepatic Impairment.)

Concomitant Diseases Because lamotrigine is transformed in the liver principally to glucuronide metabolites that are eliminated renally, the drug should be used with caution in patients with diseases or conditions (e.g., renal, hepatic, or cardiac impairment) that could affect metabolism and/or elimination of the drug. In dogs, lamotrigine is extensively metabolized to its 2-*N*-methyl metabolite, which has caused dose-dependent prolongations of the PR interval, widening of the QRS complex, and at high dosages, complete AV block. There have been no consistent effects of lamotrigine metabolites on cardiac conduction in humans. Trace amounts of the 2-*N*-methyl metabolite of lamotrigine have been found in urine, but not in plasma, with chronic dosing of lamotrigine in humans. However, the manufacturers state that it is possible that increased plasma concentrations of the 2-*N*-methyl metabolite could occur in patients with hepatic disease who have decreased ability to glucuronidate lamotrigine.

Binding to Melanin-Rich Tissues Lamotrigine binds to melanin-containing ocular tissue in pigmented rats and cynomolgus monkeys, but evidence of this manifestation has not been reported in humans. Although ophthalmologic testing was conducted in one controlled clinical trial of lamotrigine therapy, the manufacturers state that it was inadequate to detect subtle effects or injury resulting from long-term administration of lamotrigine and that the ability of available tests to detect potentially adverse effects associated with the binding of lamotrigine to melanin is unknown. The manufacturers further state that while no specific recommendations for periodic ophthalmologic monitoring of patients receiving long-term lamotrigine therapy can be provided, prolonged administration of the drug could potentially result in its accumulation and possible toxic effects in melanin-rich tissues, including those of the eye, and that clinicians should be aware of possible adverse ophthalmologic effects occurring as a result of binding of the drug to melanin.

Possible Prescribing and Dispensing Errors Because of similarity in spelling between Lamictal® (the trade name for lamotrigine) and labetalol, Lamisil® (terbinafine hydrochloride), lamivudine, Lomotil® (the fixed combination of atropine sulfate and diphenoxylate hydrochloride), and Ludiomil® (no longer commercially available under this trade name in the US; maprotiline hydrochloride), dispensing errors have been reported to the manufacturer of Lamictal® (GlaxoSmithKline). These medication errors may be associated with serious adverse events either due to lack of appropriate therapy for seizures (e.g., in patients not receiving the prescribed anticonvulsant, lamotrigine, which may lead to status epilepticus) or, alternatively, to the risk of developing adverse effects (e.g., serious rash) associated with the use of lamotrigine in patients for whom the drug was not prescribed and consequently was not properly titrated. Therefore, extra care should be exercised in ensuring the accuracy of both oral and written prescriptions for Lamictal® and these other drugs. When appropriate, clinicians might consider including the intended use of the particular drug on the prescription in addition to alerting patients to carefully check the drug they receive and promptly bring any question or concern to the attention of the dispensing pharmacist. The manufacturer of Lamictal® also recommends that pharmacists assess various measures of avoiding dispensing errors and implement them as appropriate (e.g., by computerized filling and handling of prescriptions, patient counseling). Medication errors also may occur between the different formulations of lamotrigine. Depictions of Lamictal® conventional tablets, chewable/dispersible tablets, and orally disintegrating tablets, Lamictal® XR extended-release tablets, and generic lamotrigine tablets may be found in the medication guide; patients are strongly advised to visually inspect their tablets to verify that they are lamotrigine as well as the correct formulation of the drug each time they fill their prescription.

Contraindications Lamotrigine is contraindicated in patients with known hypersensitivity to the drug or any ingredient in the formulation.

■ **Pediatric Precautions** Safety and efficacy of immediate-release formulations of lamotrigine have not been established in pediatric patients younger than 2 years of age. Safety and efficacy of immediate-release lamotrigine in children 2–16 years of age have not been established for uses other than adjunctive therapy of partial seizures, primary generalized tonic-clonic seizures, or seizures associated with Lennox-Gastaut syndrome.

Safety and efficacy of extended-release lamotrigine tablets for adjunctive therapy of partial seizures and primary generalized tonic-clonic seizures have not been established in pediatric patients younger than 13 years of age.

Safety and efficacy of immediate-release lamotrigine for the management of bipolar disorder in patients younger than 18 years of age have not been established.

The incidence of severe rashes requiring hospitalization and discontinuance of immediate-release lamotrigine appears to be higher in pediatric patients compared with adults (about 0.8% versus 0.3%, respectively). (See Cautions: Dermatologic and Sensitivity Reactions.)

Analyses of population pharmacokinetic data for children 2–18 years of age demonstrated that lamotrigine clearance is influenced mainly by total body weight and concomitant anticonvulsant therapy. Oral clearance of lamotrigine is higher in children than adults when calculated on the basis of body weight; patients weighing less than 30 kg have a higher clearance on a weight-adjusted basis than patients weighing more than 30 kg and may require increases in maintenance dosage. (See Dosage and Administration: Dosage.)

■ **Geriatric Precautions** The manufacturers state that clinical trials of lamotrigine in epilepsy and in bipolar disorder did not include sufficient numbers of patients older than 65 years of age to determine whether they respond differently than younger patients or exhibit a different safety profile than that of younger patients. Because of the greater frequency of decreased hepatic, renal, and/or cardiac function and of concomitant diseases and drug therapy in geriatric patients, the manufacturers recommend cautious dosage selection in patients in this age group, usually beginning at the lower end of the usual range.

■ **Mutagenicity and Carcinogenicity** No evidence of mutagenicity was demonstrated by lamotrigine in vitro in the Ames *Salmonella* microbial mutagen test or the mammalian mouse lymphoma assay. Lamotrigine also did not increase the incidence of structural or numerical chromosomal abnormalities in the in vitro human lymphocyte assay and the in vivo rat bone marrow assay.

No evidence of carcinogenicity was demonstrated by lamotrigine in studies in mice receiving 30 mg/kg daily and in rats receiving 10–15 mg/kg daily for up to 2 years. Steady-state plasma lamotrigine concentrations produced by these dosages ranged from 1–4 mcg/mL in mice and from 1–10 mcg/mL in rats. In humans receiving the recommended lamotrigine dosage of 300–500 mg daily, plasma lamotrigine concentrations generally are in the range of 2–5 mcg/mL, although plasma concentrations up to 19 mcg/mL have been reported.

■ **Pregnancy, Fertility, and Lactation** The safety of lamotrigine when used during pregnancy in humans is unknown, and the drug should be used during pregnancy only when the potential benefits justify the possible risks to the fetus. Patients should be advised to notify their clinician if they become pregnant or intend to become pregnant. The manufacturer of Lamictal®, in collaboration with the US Centers for Disease Control and Prevention (CDC), maintains a lamotrigine pregnancy registry to monitor fetal outcomes of pregnant women exposed to lamotrigine. Clinicians aware of patients who have received lamotrigine at any time during their pregnancy and who wish to register these cases before fetal outcome is known (e.g., through ultrasound, amniocentesis, birth) may obtain information by calling the Lamotrigine Pregnancy Registry at 800-336-2176. Patients can enroll themselves in the North American Antiepileptic Drug (NAAED) Pregnancy Registry by calling 888-233-2334; registry information also is available on the website at http://www.aedpregnancyregistry.org/.

Preliminary information from the NAAED Pregnancy Registry suggests a possible association between exposure to lamotrigine monotherapy during the first trimester of pregnancy and an increased incidence of cleft lip or cleft palate in infants. Of 564 pregnant women listed in the NAAED Pregnancy Registry who received lamotrigine monotherapy during the first trimester, 5 cases of oral clefts (2 cases of isolated cleft lips, 3 cases of isolated cleft palate) occurred, yielding a total prevalence of 8.9 cases per 1000 exposures compared with a prevalence of 0.5–2.16 reported among infants of nonepileptic women who were not receiving lamotrigine. However, other pregnancy registries of similar size have not replicated this observation, and the validity of this association cannot be established until additional data are collected in the NAAED Pregnancy Registry, in other pregnancy registries, or by additional research. The US Food and Drug Administration (FDA) states that the clinical importance of this preliminary report remains uncertain pending further data collection and more research is needed. FDA recommends that women who are pregnant should not begin or discontinue lamotrigine therapy without first talking to their clinician.

Although there are no adequate and controlled studies to date in humans, lamotrigine has been shown to produce maternal toxicity and secondary fetal toxicity (e.g., reduced fetal weight and/or delayed ossification) in mice and rats receiving oral dosages up to 1.2 or 0.5 times (on a mg/m^2 basis), respectively, the maximum usual human maintenance dosage of 500 mg daily during the period of organogenesis. However, no evidence of teratogenicity was found in mice, rats, or rabbits receiving the drug orally in dosages up to 1.2, 0.5, or 1.1 times (on a mg/m^2 basis), respectively, the maximum usual human daily maintenance dosage. Maternal toxicity and fetal death occurred in rats receiving lamotrigine orally during late gestation (days 15–20) in dosages of 0.1, 0.14, or 0.3 times (on a mg/m^2 basis) the maximum usual human daily maintenance dosage; food consumption and weight gain were reduced in dams, and the gestation period was slightly prolonged. Stillborn pups were found in all three groups of rats receiving lamotrigine, with the greatest number of stillborn pups in the group receiving the highest dosage. Postnatal death of pups occurred between days 1 and 20 only in the group of rats receiving 0.14 or 0.3 times (on a mg/m^2 basis) the maximum usual human daily maintenance dosage. Some of these deaths appeared to be drug related and not secondary to maternal toxicity. No evidence of teratogenicity was demonstrated in rats receiving lamotrigine in dosages 0.4 times (on a mg/m^2 basis) the maximum usual human daily maintenance dosage prior to and during mating and throughout gestation and lactation. However, the incidence of intrauterine death without signs of teratogenicity was increased in rat dams receiving lamotrigine isethionate by rapid IV injection in a dosage 0.6 times (on a mg/m^2 basis) the maximum usual human daily maintenance dosage. In a study designed to determine the effects of lamotrigine on postnatal development, pregnant rats received lamotrigine orally in dosages 0.1 and 0.5 times (on a mg/m^2 basis) the recommended human daily dosage during the period of organogenesis. At day 21 postpartum, pups born to dams receiving the lower dosage (5 mg/kg daily) exhibited a longer latent period for open field exploration and a lower frequency of rearing. Pups born to dams receiving the higher dosage (25 mg/kg daily) demonstrated an increased time to completion of a swimming maze test performed 39–44 days postpartum. No evidence of adverse effects on development of pups was demonstrated by lamotrigine in a group of rats receiving the drug in dosages 0.4 times (on a mg/m^2 basis) the maximum usual human daily maintenance dosage prior to and during mating, and throughout gestation and lactation.

Because lamotrigine is a dihydrofolate reductase inhibitor, it decreases fetal folate concentrations in rats, an effect known to be associated with teratogenesis in animals and humans. However, there are no adequate and well-controlled studies in pregnant women, and animal reproduction studies are not always predictive of human response. Decreased plasma folate concentrations in rats were partially returned to normal by administration of leucovorin. Clinicians should be aware of lamotrigine's dihydrofolate reductase inhibiting activity, especially when prescribing other drugs that inhibit folate metabolism.

The effect of lamotrigine on labor and delivery in humans is unknown.

Physiologic changes during pregnancy may affect plasma lamotrigine concentrations and/or therapeutic effect. Decreased lamotrigine concentrations during pregnancy and restoration of prepartum concentrations after delivery have been reported. Dosage adjustment of lamotrigine may be necessary to maintain clinical response.

Reproduction studies revealed no adverse effects on fertility in rats receiving lamotrigine in oral dosages 0.4 times (on a mg/m^2 basis) the maximum usual human daily maintenance dosage prior to and during mating, and throughout gestation and lactation. The effect of lamotrigine on human fertility is unknown.

Lamotrigine is distributed into milk. Because of the potential for serious adverse reactions to lamotrigine in nursing infants, a decision should be made whether to discontinue nursing or the drug, taking into account the importance of the drug to the woman.

Description

Lamotrigine is a phenyltriazine anticonvulsant agent. The drug differs structurally from other currently available anticonvulsant agents. Although the precise mechanism of anticonvulsant action of lamotrigine is unknown, studies in animals indicate that the drug may stabilize neuronal membranes by blocking voltage-sensitive sodium channels, which inhibits the release of excitatory amino acid neurotransmitters (e.g., glutamate, aspartate) that play a role in the generation and spread of epileptic seizures. In animal test systems, lamotrigine exhibits anticonvulsant activity similar to that of phenytoin, phenobarbital, and carbamazepine. The drug protects against seizures induced by electrical stimulation or pentylenetetrazole, suggesting that it may be effective in the management of tonic-clonic (grand mal) and partial seizures or absence (petit mal) seizures, respectively. Lamotrigine also is active in electrically evoked afterdischarge tests, indicating activity against simple and complex partial seizures, and in rat cortical kindling tests, which may indicate activity against complex partial seizures. The mechanism(s) of action of lamotrigine in bipolar disorder has not been established.

In vitro studies indicate that lamotrigine has weak inhibitory effects on type 3 serotonergic (5-HT$_3$) receptors, and does not exhibit high affinity for type 2 serotonergic (5-HT$_2$), adenosine A_1 or A_2, α_1- or α_2-adrenergic, β-adrenergic, dopamine D_1 or D_2, γ-aminobutyric acid (GABA) A or B, histamine H_1, opiate κ, or cholinergic muscarinic receptors. The drug has weak agonist effects at opiate σ receptors. Lamotrigine apparently has no effect on dihydropyridine-sensitive calcium channels or *N*-methyl-d-aspartate (NMDA) receptors and does not inhibit the uptake of norepinephrine, dopamine, serotonin, or aspartic acid.

SumMon® (see Users Guide). For additional information on this drug until a more detailed monograph is developed and published, the manufacturer's labeling should be consulted. It is *essential* that the labeling be consulted for detailed information on the usual cautions, precautions, and contraindications concerning potential drug interactions and/or laboratory test interferences and for information on acute toxicity.

Preparations

Excipients in commercially available drug preparations may have clinically important effects in some individuals; consult specific product labeling for details.

lamoTRIgine

Oral		
Tablets	25 mg*	**LaMICtal®** (scored), GlaxoSmithKline
		Lamotrigine Tablets
	100 mg*	**LaMICtal®** (scored), GlaxoSmithKline
		Lamotrigine Tablets
	150 mg*	**LaMICtal®** (scored), GlaxoSmithKline
		Lamotrigine Tablets
	200 mg*	**LaMICtal®** (scored), GlaxoSmithKline
		Lamotrigine Tablets
Tablets, chewable/ dispersible	2 mg	**LaMICtal®**, GlaxoSmithKline
	5 mg	**LaMICtal®**, GlaxoSmithKline
	25 mg	**LaMICtal®**, GlaxoSmithKline
Tablets, extended-release, film-coated	25 mg	**LaMICtal® XR**, GlaxoSmithKline
	50 mg	**LaMICtal® XR**, GlaxoSmithKline
	100 mg	**LaMICtal® XR**, GlaxoSmithKline
	200 mg	**LaMICtal® XR**, GlaxoSmithKline
Tablets, orally disintegrating	25 mg	**LaMICtal® ODT**, GlaxoSmithKline
	50 mg	**LaMICtal® ODT**, GlaxoSmithKline
	100 mg	**LaMICtal® ODT**, GlaxoSmithKline
	200 mg	**LaMICtal® ODT**, GlaxoSmithKline

*available from one or more manufacturer, distributor, and/or repackager by generic (nonproprietary) name

†Use is not currently included in the labeling approved by the US Food and Drug Administration

levETIRAcetam

■ Levetiracetam, a pyrrolidine derivative, is an anticonvulsant.

Uses

■ **Seizure Disorders** Levetiracetam is used orally in combination with other anticonvulsants in the management of partial onset, myoclonic, and primary generalized tonic-clonic seizures. The drug also is commercially available as an IV formulation for the management of such seizure disorders when oral therapy is temporarily not feasible. Efficacy of IV levetiracetam is supported by studies using oral formulations of the drug since the oral and parenteral formulations are bioequivalent.

Partial Seizures Levetiracetam conventional (immediate-release) tablets, oral solution, and injection are used in combination with other anticonvulsants in the management of partial onset seizures in adults and pediatric patients 1 month of age and older with epilepsy.

Efficacy of levetiracetam for this use was established in 3 double-blind, placebo-controlled trials in patients who had refractory partial onset seizures with or without secondary generalization while receiving a stable regimen of 1 or 2 anticonvulsants and had experienced at least 2 partial seizures during each 4-week interval of the baseline period (8–12 weeks). Patients received levetiracetam (1, 2, or 3 g daily as a conventional oral preparation) or placebo for 12 weeks after a 4- to 6-week titration period. The weekly frequency of partial seizures was reduced in patients receiving levetiracetam relative to placebo. More patients receiving levetiracetam experienced a reduction in seizure frequency of 50% or greater from baseline (i.e., responder rate) compared with placebo-treated patients. Clinical benefit was evident within 2 weeks in one study.

Data from open-label extension periods of phase 1, 2, and 3 studies with oral levetiracetam (as conventional preparations) in 1422 adult patients with epilepsy indicate that 39% of patients experienced a 50% or greater decrease in seizure frequency, while 13 and 8% of patients were seizure-free for at least 6 and 12 months, respectively, during therapy with the drug. Continuation rates for levetiracetam therapy in these patients were estimated to be 60, 37, and 32% after 1, 3, and 5 years, respectively.

Efficacy of levetiracetam as adjunctive therapy in pediatric patients with partial onset seizures was established in 2 randomized, double-blind, placebo-controlled studies. The first study was conducted in children 4–16 years of age who had refractory partial onset seizures with or without secondary generalization while receiving a stable regimen of 1 or 2 anticonvulsants and had experienced at least 4 partial seizures during the 4 weeks prior to screening as well as at least 4 partial seizures during each of the two 4-week baseline periods. Patients received levetiracetam (20–60 mg/kg daily as a conventional oral preparation) or placebo for 10 weeks after a 4-week titration period. Pediatric patients receiving levetiracetam experienced a reduction of 26.8% in mean weekly partial seizure frequency relative to placebo. The second study was conducted in infants and children 1 month to less than 4 years of age with refractory partial onset seizures (with or without secondary generalization). Seizures were assessed in this study using video electroencephalography (EEG). Patients who had experienced at least 2 partial seizures during a 48-hour baseline period while receiving a stable regimen of 1 or 2 anticonvulsants were randomized to receive levetiracetam oral solution (20–50 mg/kg daily based on age) or placebo; after an initial 1-day dose titration period, treatment was continued for an additional 4 days. The responder rate (i.e., proportion of patients experiencing a reduction in seizure frequency of 50% or greater from baseline) was substantially higher in pediatric patients receiving levetiracetam (43.1%) compared with those receiving placebo (19.6%), and these results were consistent across age groups in this study.

Levetiracetam also is commercially available as extended-release tablets for once-daily administration in the management of partial onset seizures in adults and pediatric patients 12 years of age and older. Efficacy of levetiracetam (as extended-release tablets) was established in a double-blind, placebo-controlled study in patients 12–70 years of age who had refractory partial onset seizures with or without secondary generalization. Patients who had experienced at least 8 partial seizures during an 8-week baseline period and at least 2 seizures during each 4-week interval of the baseline period while receiving a stable regimen of 1–3 anticonvulsants were randomized to receive levetiracetam 1 g daily (as extended-release tablets) or placebo for 12 weeks. The median percent reduction in weekly seizure frequency from baseline was 46.1% in patients receiving levetiracetam compared with 33.4% in those receiving placebo.

Myoclonic Seizures Levetiracetam conventional (immediate-release) tablets, oral solution, and injection are used in combination with other anticonvulsants in the management of myoclonic seizures in adults and adolescents 12 years of age and older with juvenile myoclonic epilepsy.

Efficacy of levetiracetam for this use was established in a randomized, double-blind, placebo-controlled study in patients who had myoclonic seizures while receiving a stable regimen of 1 anticonvulsant and had experienced at least one myoclonic seizure daily for at least 8 days during the 8-week baseline period. Patients received levetiracetam 3 g daily (as a conventional oral preparation) or placebo for 12 weeks after a 4-week titration period. More patients receiving levetiracetam (60.4%) experienced a reduction in seizure frequency of 50% or greater from baseline (i.e., responder rate) compared with placebo-treated patients (23.7%).

Primary Generalized Tonic-Clonic Seizures Levetiracetam conventional (immediate-release) tablets, oral solution, and injection are used in combination with other anticonvulsants in the management of primary generalized tonic-clonic seizures in adults and children 6 years of age and older with idiopathic generalized epilepsy.

Efficacy of levetiracetam for this use was established in a randomized, double-blind, placebo-controlled study in patients who had primary generalized tonic-clonic seizures while receiving a stable regimen of 1 or 2 anticonvulsants and had experienced at least 3 primary generalized tonic-clonic seizures during the 8-week combined baseline period (4-week pre-prospective baseline period and 4-week prospective baseline period). Patients received levetiracetam 3 g daily (adult dosage) or 60 mg/kg daily (pediatric dosage) as a conventional oral preparation or placebo for 20 weeks after a 4-week titration period. The median percent reduction in weekly seizure frequency from baseline was 77.6% in patients receiving levetiracetam compared with 44.6% in those receiving placebo. In addition, more patients receiving levetiracetam (72.2%) experienced a reduction in seizure frequency of 50% or greater from baseline (i.e., responder rate) compared with placebo-treated patients (45.2%).

Dosage and Administration

■ Administration

Levetiracetam is administered orally (as immediate-release tablets, extended-release tablets, or oral solution). The drug also may be administered by IV infusion in patients in whom oral therapy is temporarily not feasible.

Commercially available levetiracetam conventional (immediate-release) tablets, extended-release tablets, oral solution, and IV formulations have been shown to be bioequivalent.

Patients currently receiving or beginning therapy with levetiracetam and/or any other anticonvulsant for any indication should be closely monitored for the emergence or worsening of depression, suicidal thoughts or behavior (suicidality), and/or any unusual changes in mood or behavior. (See Suicidality Risk under Warnings/Precautions: Warnings, in Cautions.)

Oral Administration Levetiracetam immediate-release tablets and oral solution are administered orally twice daily without regard to meals. The immediate-release tablets should be swallowed whole and not chewed or crushed. A calibrated dosing device (e.g., medicine dropper, medicine cup) should be used to measure and administer doses of the oral solution; a household teaspoon or tablespoon is not an adequate measuring device.

Levetiracetam extended-release tablets are administered once daily; the tablets must be swallowed intact and not chewed, broken, or crushed.

IV Administration For IV administration, levetiracetam is commercially available as an injection concentrate that must be diluted prior to use and as a premixed solution in sodium chloride injection that is administered without further dilution; the premixed injection is indicated for use only in adults 16 years of age or older.

When using the injection concentrate, the appropriate dose should be diluted in 100 mL of a compatible IV solution (e.g., 0.9% sodium chloride injection, lactated Ringer's, 5% dextrose injection) and administered by IV infusion over 15 minutes. A smaller volume of diluent may be used (e.g., in pediatric patients or patients who may be susceptible to fluid volume overload), but the final concentration of the diluted solution should not exceed 15 mg/mL. Following dilution, the infusion solution may be stored in polyvinyl chloride (PVC) bags for up to 4 hours at controlled room temperature (15–30°C). Unused contents of the levetiracetam injection vial should be discarded after use.

When using the premixed solution, a single 100-mL bag containing 500 mg, 1 g, or 1.5 g of levetiracetam in sodium chloride 0.82, 0.75, or 0.54%, respectively, should be administered by IV infusion over 15 minutes without further dilution. Doses that are not commercially available as a premixed solution (e.g., 250 or 750 mg) should be prepared by transferring the appropriate volume of solution from an intact commercial infusion bag into a separate sterile, empty infusion bag; any unused contents of the original infusion bag should be discarded and should not be reused or stored. Levetiracetam in sodium chloride injection should not be used in series connections.

Levetiracetam injection and diluted solutions of the drug should be inspected visually for particulate matter and discoloration prior to administration whenever solution and container permit. Levetiracetam injection solutions may be mixed with diazepam, lorazepam, or valproate sodium.

Dispensing and Administration Precautions Because of similarity in spelling between Keppra® (a trade name for levetiracetam) and Kaletra® (the trade name for the fixed combination of lopinavir and ritonavir, both antiretroviral agents), the potential exists for dispensing errors involving these drugs. Therefore, extra care should be exercised in ensuring the accuracy of both oral and written prescriptions for Keppra® and Kaletra®. The manufacturer of Keppra® recommends that clinicians consider including the intended use of the particular drug on the prescription, in addition to alerting patients to carefully check the drug they receive and promptly bring any question or concern to the attention of the dispensing pharmacist. Some experts also recommend that pharmacists assess various measures of avoiding dispensing errors and implement them as appropriate (e.g., by verifying all orders for these drugs by spelling both the trade and generic names to prescribers, using computerized name alerts, attaching reminders to drug containers and pharmacy shelves, separating the drugs on pharmacy shelves, employing independent checks in the dispensing process, counseling patients). (See Dispensing and Administration Precautions under Warnings/Precautions: General Precautions, in Cautions.)

■ Dosage

Levetiracetam therapy should not be discontinued abruptly. The manufacturer recommends that oral levetiracetam be withdrawn gradually (e.g., by reducing the dosage by 1 g daily at 2-week intervals).

When switching from oral to IV levetiracetam therapy, the initial total daily dosage of IV levetiracetam should be equivalent to the daily dose and frequency of oral levetiracetam. At the completion of the IV treatment period, the patient may be switched back to oral levetiracetam at the equivalent daily dose and frequency that was administered IV.

Partial Seizures **Adult Dosage.** In adults 16 years of age and older, the recommended initial oral dosage of levetiracetam for adjunctive therapy of partial seizures is 1 g daily (administered as 500 mg twice daily as conventional tablets or oral solution, or 1 g once daily as extended-release tablets). Dosage may be increased in increments of 1 g daily at 2-week intervals up to the maximum recommended dosage of 3 g daily. However, some clinicians reportedly have initiated therapy with oral dosages of 2–4 g daily. Dosages exceeding 3 g daily have been used in open-label studies for periods of 6 months or longer; however, the manufacturers state that there is no evidence that these higher dosages provide additional therapeutic benefit.

When oral therapy is temporarily not feasible, levetiracetam may be administered by IV infusion at the same dosages recommended for conventional oral preparations.

Pediatric Dosage. When conventional oral preparations of levetiracetam are used in pediatric patients, the manufacturer recommends that children weighing 20 kg or less receive the oral solution; children weighing more than 20 kg may receive either the immediate-release tablets or oral solution. Extended-release levetiracetam tablets are indicated for use only in pediatric patients 12 years of age and older.

In pediatric patients 1 to younger than 6 months of age, the recommended initial oral dosage of levetiracetam for adjunctive therapy of partial seizures is 14 mg/kg daily, administered as 7 mg/kg twice daily (as immediate-release preparations). Dosage should be increased in increments of 14 mg/kg daily at 2-week intervals up to the recommended dosage of 42 mg/kg daily, given as 21 mg/kg twice daily. In the clinical trial, the mean daily dosage was 35 mg/kg in this age group; efficacy of lower dosages has not been established.

In pediatric patients 6 months to younger than 4 years of age, the recommended initial oral dosage of levetiracetam is 20 mg/kg daily, administered as 10 mg/kg twice daily (as immediate-release preparations). Dosage should be increased in increments of 20 mg/kg daily at 2-week intervals up to the recommended dosage of 50 mg/kg daily, given as 25 mg/kg twice daily. Dosage may be reduced if the patient is unable to tolerate a dosage of 50 mg/kg daily. In the clinical trial, the mean daily dosage was 47 mg/kg in this age group.

In pediatric patients 4 years to younger than 16 years of age, the recommended initial oral dosage of levetiracetam is 20 mg/kg daily, administered as 10 mg/kg twice daily (as immediate-release preparations). Dosage should be increased in increments of 20 mg/kg daily at 2-week intervals up to the recommended dosage of 60 mg/kg daily, given as 30 mg/kg twice daily. Dosage may be reduced if the patient is unable to tolerate a dosage of 60 mg/kg daily. In the clinical trial, the mean daily dosage was 44 mg/kg and the maximum daily dosage was 3 g daily. If levetiracetam immediate-release tablets are used in pediatric patients weighing 20–40 kg, the recommended initial dosage is 500 mg daily, given as 250 mg twice daily; dosage may be increased in increments of 500 mg daily every 2 weeks up to a maximum of 1.5 g daily, given as 750 mg twice daily. If levetiracetam immediate-release tablets are used in pediatric patients weighing more than 40 kg, the recommended initial dosage is 1 g daily, given as 500 mg twice daily; dosage may be increased in increments of 1 g daily every 2 weeks up to a maximum of 3 g daily, given as 1.5 g twice daily.

In pediatric patients 12 years of age and older, the recommended initial dosage of levetiracetam (as extended-release tablets) is 1 g once daily. Dosage may be increased in increments of 1 g daily at 2-week intervals up to the maximum recommended dosage of 3 g daily.

When oral therapy is temporarily not feasible, levetiracetam may be administered by IV infusion at the same dosages recommended for conventional oral preparations.

Myoclonic Seizures The recommended initial dosage of oral levetiracetam as adjunctive therapy for myoclonic seizures in patients 12 years of age and older is 1 g daily, given as 500 mg twice daily (as immediate-release preparations). Dosage should be increased in increments of 1 g daily at 2-week intervals up to the recommended dosage of 3 g daily, given as 1.5 g twice daily. Efficacy of dosages lower than 3 g daily has not been established.

When oral therapy is temporarily not feasible, levetiracetam may be administered by IV infusion at the same dosages recommended above.

Primary Generalized Tonic-Clonic Seizures **Adult Dosage.** The recommended initial dosage of oral levetiracetam as adjunctive therapy for primary generalized tonic-clonic seizures in adults 16 years of age and older is 1 g daily, given as 500 mg twice daily (as immediate-release preparations). Dosage should be increased in increments of 1 g daily at 2-week intervals up to the recommended dosage of 3 g daily, given as 1.5 g twice daily. Efficacy of dosages lower than 3 g daily has not been established.

When oral therapy is temporarily not feasible, levetiracetam may be administered by IV infusion at the same dosages recommended above.

Pediatric Dosage. The recommended initial dosage of oral levetiracetam as adjunctive therapy for primary generalized tonic-clonic seizures in pediatric patients 6 to younger than 16 years of age is 20 mg/kg daily, given as 10 mg/kg twice daily (as immediate-release preparations). Children weighing 20 kg or less should receive the oral solution; children weighing more than 20 kg may receive either the tablets (administered whole) or the oral solution. Dosage should be increased in increments of 20 mg/kg daily at 2-week intervals up to the recommended dosage of 60 mg/kg daily, given as 30 mg/kg twice daily. Efficacy of dosages lower than 60 mg/kg daily has not been established.

When oral therapy is temporarily not feasible, levetiracetam may be administered by IV infusion at the same dosages recommended above.

■ **Special Populations** In adults with impaired renal function, dosage of levetiracetam must be modified according to the degree of impairment. Dosage should be based on the patient's creatinine clearance adjusted for body surface area. (See Tables 1 and 2.)

Table 1. Immediate-release Levetiracetam Dosage Adjustment in Adults with Impaired Renal Function

Renal Function	Creatinine Clearance (mL/minute per 1.73 m²)	Dosage (mg)	Interval (hours)
Normal	>80	500–1500	12
Mild	50–80	500–1000	12
Moderate	30–50	250–750	12
Severe	<30	250–500	12
Patients with end-stage renal disease undergoing dialysis	–	500–1000	24[a]

[a] Following dialysis, a 250–500 mg supplemental dose is recommended.

Table 2. Extended-release Levetiracetam Dosage Adjustment in Adults with Impaired Renal Function

Renal Function	Creatinine Clearance (mL/minute per 1.73 m²)	Dosage (mg)	Interval (hours)
Normal	>80	1000–3000	24
Mild	50–80	1000–2000	24
Moderate	30–50	500–1500	24
Severe	<30	500–1000	24

Dosage should be selected carefully and renal function monitoring should be considered in geriatric patients 65 years of age and older because of the greater frequency of decreased renal function observed in this age group. Total body clearance was reduced by 38% and half-life was increased by 2.5 hours in geriatric patients with creatinine clearances of 30–74 mL/minute.

No dosage adjustment is necessary in patients with hepatic impairment. Levetiracetam pharmacokinetics were unchanged in patients with mild (Child-Pugh class A) to moderate (Child-Pugh class B) hepatic impairment. Total body clearance was reduced by 50% in patients with severe hepatic impairment (Child-Pugh class C), principally because of decreased renal clearance.

Cautions

■ **Contraindications** Levetiracetam is contraindicated in patients with known hypersensitivity to the drug.

■ **Warnings/Precautions** ***Warnings*** **Nervous System Effects.** Adverse neuropsychiatric effects reported during levetiracetam therapy are classified into 3 categories: somnolence and fatigue, coordination difficulties, and behavioral/psychiatric abnormalities. Patients should be monitored for these adverse effects during therapy. In addition, patients should be advised not to drive or operate machinery until the effects of levetiracetam are known.

In controlled studies in adults, approximately 15% of patients with partial onset seizures who received levetiracetam (as an oral conventional preparation) experienced somnolence compared with 8% of placebo-treated patients, and about 3% of levetiracetam-treated patients discontinued treatment because of somnolence. Pediatric patients and adults with other seizure types who receive levetiracetam appear to experience similar rates of somnolence and fatigue. In controlled studies in adults, asthenia was reported in about 15% of patients who received levetiracetam (as conventional preparations) compared with 9% of placebo-treated patients, and 0.8% of levetiracetam-treated patients discontinued treatment because of asthenia. Coordination difficulties (e.g., ataxia, abnormal gait, incoordination) were experienced by 3.4% of patients receiving levetiracetam (as conventional preparations) compared with 1.6% of placebo-treated patients. Somnolence, asthenia, and coordination difficulties occurred most frequently within the first 4 weeks of treatment. In studies with extended-release levetiracetam, somnolence was reported in 8% of patients receiving the drug compared with 3% of patients receiving placebo; however, the number of patients exposed to the extended-release preparation is considerably less than that of the immediate-release preparation.

In clinical studies, psychotic symptoms were reported in 1% of adults, 2% of children 4–16 years of age, and 17% of children younger than 4 years of age receiving conventional levetiracetam preparations compared with 0.2, 2, and 5% of the corresponding age groups receiving placebo, respectively. At least 2 adults who received levetiracetam in these studies were hospitalized as a result of psychosis. Nonpsychotic behavioral symptoms (e.g., aggression, agitation, anger, anxiety, apathy, depersonalization, depression, emotional lability, hostility, hyperkinesias, irritability, nervousness, neurosis, personality disorder) were reported in 13% of adults and 38% of children 4–16 years of age receiving conventional levetiracetam preparations in clinical studies compared with 6 and 19% of placebo-treated patients, respectively. Exploratory analysis of a placebo-controlled study that evaluated neurocognitive and behavioral effects of conventional levetiracetam in children 4–16 years of age indicated possible worsening of aggression in pediatric patients receiving the drug. Increased irritability was reported in clinical studies of younger children (1 month to younger than 4 years of age). In studies with extended-release levetiracetam, behavioral abnormalities (irritability and aggression) were reported in 7% of patients receiving the drug compared with none of the patients receiving placebo; however, the number of patients exposed to the extended-release preparation is considerably less than that of the immediate-release preparation. (See Suicidality Risk under Warnings/Precautions: Warnings, in Cautions.)

Suicidality Risk. The FDA has alerted healthcare professionals about an increased risk of suicidality (suicidal behavior or ideation) observed in an analysis of studies using various anticonvulsants, including levetiracetam, compared with placebo. The analysis of suicidality reports from placebo-controlled studies involving 11 anticonvulsants (i.e., carbamazepine, felbamate, gabapentin, lamotrigine, levetiracetam, oxcarbazepine, pregabalin, tiagabine, topiramate, valproate, zonisamide) in patients with epilepsy, psychiatric disorders (e.g., bipolar disorder, depression, anxiety), and other conditions (e.g., migraine, neuropathic pain) found that patients receiving anticonvulsants had approximately twice the risk of suicidal behavior or ideation (0.43%) compared with patients receiving placebo (0.24%). This increased suicidality risk was observed as early as one week after beginning therapy and continued through 24 weeks. Although patients treated with an anticonvulsant for epilepsy, psychiatric disorders, and other conditions were all found to have an increased suicidality risk compared with those receiving placebo, the relative suicidality risk was higher for patients with epilepsy compared with those receiving anticonvulsants for other conditions.

Based on the current analysis of the available data, FDA recommends that clinicians inform patients, their families, and caregivers about the potential for an increase in the risk of suicidality with anticonvulsant therapy and that all patients currently receiving or beginning therapy with any anticonvulsant for any indication be closely monitored for the emergence or worsening of depression, suicidal thoughts or behavior (suicidality), and/or unusual changes in mood or behavior. Symptoms such as anxiety, agitation, hostility, hypomania, and mania may be precursors to emerging suicidality.

Clinicians who prescribe levetiracetam or any other anticonvulsant should balance the risk of suicidality with the risk of untreated illness. Epilepsy and many other illnesses for which anticonvulsants are prescribed are themselves associated with an increased risk of morbidity and mortality and an increased risk of suicidal thoughts and behavior. If suicidal thoughts and behavior emerge during anticonvulsant therapy, the clinician should consider whether these symptoms may be related to the illness being treated. (See Nervous System Effects under Warnings/Precautions: Warnings, in Cautions, and also see Advice to Patients.)

Dermatologic Reactions. Serious dermatologic reactions, including Stevens-Johnson syndrome and toxic epidermal necrolysis, have been reported in both adults and pediatric patients receiving levetiracetam. The median time of onset is reported to be between 14 and 17 days, although cases have occurred at least 4 months after initiation of therapy.

Levetiracetam should be discontinued at the first sign of a rash, unless the rash is clearly not drug-related. If manifestations suggestive of Stevens-Johnson syndrome or toxic epidermal necrolysis occur, levetiracetam therapy should be permanently discontinued and alternative therapy considered.

Discontinuance of Therapy. Because of the possibility of increased seizure frequency, anticonvulsant drugs, including levetiracetam, should not be discontinued suddenly. The manufacturer recommends that oral levetiracetam be withdrawn gradually by reducing the dosage by 1 g daily at 2-week intervals.

Hematologic Effects. Hematologic abnormalities (e.g., decreased red blood cell, white blood cell, and neutrophil counts) were reported in patients receiving levetiracetam in clinical studies. Agranulocytosis, leukopenia, neutropenia, pancytopenia, and thrombocytopenia also have occurred during postmarketing experience.

A complete blood count (CBC) is recommended in patients who experience any signs or symptoms of hematologic abnormalities (e.g., severe weakness, pyrexia, recurrent infections, coagulation disorders) during levetiracetam therapy.

Increased Blood Pressure. In a study of pediatric patients 1 month to younger than 4 years of age, increased diastolic blood pressure was observed in levetiracetam-treated patients (17%) compared with those receiving placebo (2%). However, there was no overall difference in mean diastolic blood pressure between the treatment groups. These findings were not observed in older children or adults receiving the drug.

Pediatric patients younger than 4 years of age should be monitored for increased diastolic blood pressure during levetiracetam therapy.

Seizure Control During Pregnancy. Physiologic changes that occur during pregnancy may gradually decrease plasma levels of levetiracetam in pregnant women. This effect is most notable during the third trimester.

Patients should be closely monitored during pregnancy and throughout the postpartum period, especially if levetiracetam dosage is adjusted during pregnancy.

Sensitivity Reactions **Anaphylaxis and Angioedema.** Anaphylaxis and angioedema, in some cases life-threatening and/or requiring emergency treatment, have been reported during postmarketing experience in patients receiving levetiracetam. (See Cautions: Contraindications.) Manifestations have included hypotension, hives, rash, respiratory distress, facial swelling, and swelling of the tongue, throat, and feet. Such reactions can occur at any time during therapy.

If any signs or symptoms of anaphylaxis or angioedema occur, patients should discontinue levetiracetam immediately and seek medical attention. Levetiracetam therapy should be permanently discontinued if an alternative etiology cannot be identified.

General Precautions **Dispensing and Administration Precautions.** Because of similarity in spelling between Keppra® (a trade name for levetiracetam) and Kaletra® (the trade name for the fixed combination of lopinavir and ritonavir, both antiretroviral agents), the potential exists for dispensing errors involving these drugs. These medication errors may be associated with serious adverse events (e.g., status epilepticus) due to lack of appropriate therapy for seizures or with the risk of developing adverse effects associated with the use of levetiracetam or lopinavir and ritonavir in patients for whom the drug was not prescribed. Therefore, extra care should be exercised in ensuring the accuracy of both oral and written prescriptions for these drugs. The manufacturer of Keppra® recommends that clinicians consider including the intended use of the particular drug on the prescription in addition to alerting patients to carefully check the drug they receive and promptly bring any question or concern to the attention of the dispensing pharmacist. Some experts also recommend that pharmacists assess various measures of avoiding dispensing errors and implement them as appropriate (e.g., by verifying all orders for these drugs by spelling both the trade and generic names to prescribers, using computerized name alerts, attaching reminders to drug containers and pharmacy shelves, separating the drugs on pharmacy shelves, employing independent checks in the dispensing process, counseling patients).

Dispensing errors involving Keppra® and Kaletra® should be reported to the manufacturers, the USP Medication Errors Reporting Program by phone (800-233-7767), or directly to the FDA MedWatch program by phone (800-FDA-1088), fax (800-FDA-0178), internet (http://www.fda.gov/Safety/MedWatch/default.htm), or mail.

Specific Populations **Pregnancy.** Category C. (See Users Guide.) Seizure control during pregnancy should be carefully monitored. (See Seizure Control During Pregnancy under Warnings/Precautions: Warnings, in Cautions.)

North American Antiepileptic Drug (NAAED) Pregnancy Registry at 888-233-2334 (for patients); NAAED registry information also available at http://www.aedpregnancyregistry.org.

The effect of levetiracetam on labor and delivery is unknown.

Lactation. Levetiracetam is distributed into milk. Because of the potential for serious adverse reactions to levetiracetam in nursing infants, a decision should be made whether to discontinue nursing or the drug, taking into account the importance of the drug to the woman.

Pediatric Use. Safety and efficacy of levetiracetam immediate-release tablets, oral solution, and injection for the management of partial onset seizures have not been established in pediatric patients younger than 1 month of age. Behavioral abnormalities (e.g., paranoia, confusional state, increased aggression) have been observed in pediatric patients 4–16 years of age with partial onset seizures receiving the drug. (See Nervous System Effects under Warnings/Precautions: Warnings, in Cautions.)

Safety and efficacy of levetiracetam immediate-release tablets, oral solution, and injection for the management of myoclonic seizures have not been established in pediatric patients younger than 12 years of age.

Safety and efficacy of levetiracetam immediate-release tablets, oral solution, and injection for the management of primary generalized tonic-clonic seizures have not been established in pediatric patients younger than 6 years of age.

Safety and efficacy of extended-release levetiracetam tablets have not been established in pediatric patients younger than 12 years of age. Use of the extended-release tablets in children 12 years of age and older is supported by a placebo-controlled study using the immediate-release preparation in patients 4–16 years of age.

Safety and efficacy of levetiracetam in sodium chloride injection have not been established in pediatric patients younger than 16 years of age.

Geriatric Use. Controlled clinical studies evaluating levetiracetam have not included sufficient numbers of patients 65 years of age and older to determine whether geriatric patients respond differently than younger adults. No substantial differences in safety have been observed in geriatric patients relative to younger adults. (See Dosage and Administration: Special Populations.)

Renal Impairment. Dosage adjustment is recommended for patients with decreased creatinine clearance. (See Dosage and Administration: Special Populations.)

Hepatic Impairment. Safety and efficacy of levetiracetam have been demonstrated in a limited number of epileptic patients with chronic liver disease. No dosage adjustment is necessary in patients with hepatic impairment. (See Dosage and Administration: Special Populations.)

■ **Common Adverse Effects** Adverse effects occurring in 1% or more of adults receiving oral levetiracetam (as conventional preparations) for adjunctive management of partial seizures include somnolence, asthenia, headache, infection, dizziness, pain, pharyngitis, depression, nervousness, rhinitis, anorexia, ataxia, vertigo, amnesia, anxiety, emotional lability, hostility, paresthesia, increased cough, sinusitis, and diplopia.

Adverse effects occurring in 2% or more of pediatric patients older than 4 years of age receiving oral levetiracetam (as conventional preparations) for adjunctive management of partial seizures include headache, vomiting, nasopharyngitis, somnolence, fatigue, aggression, upper abdominal pain, cough, nasal congestion, decreased appetite, dizziness, pharyngolaryngeal pain, abnormal behavior, dizziness, irritability, diarrhea, lethargy, insomnia, head injury, anorexia, agitation, constipation, influenza, contusion, fall, depression, altered mood, ear pain, conjunctivitis, gastroenteritis, rhinitis, joint sprain, arthralgia, neck pain, sedation, labile affect, anxiety, confusional state, and mood swing. The most common adverse effects in patients younger than 4 years of age were somnolence and irritability.

The adverse effect profile of levetiracetam (as conventional preparations) in patients with myoclonic seizures or primary generalized tonic-clonic seizures is generally similar to that of patients with partial seizures.

Adverse effects occurring in 5% or more of patients receiving extended-release levetiracetam tablets for adjunctive management of partial seizures include influenza, somnolence, irritability, nasopharyngitis, dizziness, and nausea.

Adverse effects associated with IV levetiracetam generally appear to be consistent with those associated with oral administration of the drug.

Drug Interactions

■ **Drugs Affecting or Metabolized by Hepatic Microsomal Enzymes** Because levetiracetam is neither a substrate nor inhibitor of cytochrome P-450 (CYP), pharmacokinetic interactions are unlikely with drugs affecting or metabolized by CYP isoenzymes.

■ **Anticonvulsants** Clinically important pharmacokinetic interactions are unlikely when levetiracetam is administered concomitantly with other anticonvulsants (e.g., carbamazepine, gabapentin, lamotrigine, phenobarbital, phenytoin, primidone, valproic acid).

In pediatric patients, an approximate 22% increase in levetiracetam clearance was observed when the drug was administered concurrently with hepatic enzyme-inducing anticonvulsants (e.g., carbamazepine); however, dosage adjustment is not recommended by the manufacturer. Levetiracetam did not alter plasma concentrations of carbamazepine, lamotrigine, topiramate, or valproic acid in pediatric patients with epilepsy.

■ **Digoxin** Levetiracetam does not appear to affect the pharmacokinetics or pharmacodynamics (e.g., cardiac rhythm effects) of digoxin; digoxin also does not affect the pharmacokinetics of levetiracetam.

■ **Oral Contraceptives** Pharmacokinetic interactions are unlikely when levetiracetam is coadministered with oral contraceptives.

■ **Probenecid** When levetiracetam was administered concomitantly with probenecid, no effect on levetiracetam pharmacokinetics was observed, but steady-state plasma concentrations of the principal inactive metabolite were approximately doubled due to a 60% reduction in renal clearance. The manufacturer states, however, that this effect is not clinically important.

■ **Protein-bound Drugs** Pharmacokinetic interactions are unlikely with protein-bound drugs.

■ **Warfarin** Levetiracetam does not appear to affect the pharmacokinetics or pharmacodynamics (e.g., prothrombin time) of warfarin; warfarin also does not affect the pharmacokinetics of levetiracetam.

Description

Levetiracetam, a pyrrolidine derivative, is an anticonvulsant agent that is structurally unrelated to other currently available anticonvulsants. The mechanism of anticonvulsant action of levetiracetam is unknown. In animal models, levetiracetam conferred no protection against single seizures induced by electrical current or different chemoconvulsants and offered only limited protection in submaximal stimulation and threshold tests. Protection was observed against secondarily generalized activity from focal seizures induced by 2 chemoconvulsants known to induce seizures that mimic some features of human complex partial seizures with secondary generalization. Levetiracetam also showed inhibitory properties in the kindling model in rats, another model of human complex partial seizures.

Levetiracetam does not exhibit binding affinity for benzodiazepine, γ-aminobutyric acid (GABA), glycine, or *N*-methyl-D-aspartate (NMDA) receptors, reuptake sites, or second messenger systems. Levetiracetam does not appear to directly facilitate GABA-mediated neurotransmission or have an effect on neuronal voltage-gated sodium or T-type calcium currents. However, the drug has been shown to oppose the activity of negative modulators of GABA- and glycine-gated currents in neuronal cell culture.

Levetiracetam is not extensively metabolized in humans, with 66% of an administered dose excreted unchanged in urine. About 24% of an administered dose is metabolized to an inactive metabolite by enzymatic hydrolysis of the acetamide group, which does not depend on hepatic cytochrome P-450 (CYP) isoenzymes. Levetiracetam is not a high-affinity substrate for or inhibitor of CYP isoenzymes.

Advice to Patients

Importance of providing copy of written patient information (medication guide) each time levetiracetam is dispensed.

Risk of adverse neuropsychiatric effects (e.g., somnolence, fatigue, dizziness, coordination difficulties, behavioral changes), especially during the initial weeks of therapy. Avoid driving, operating machinery, or performing hazardous tasks while taking levetiracetam until the drug's effects on the individual are known.

Importance of patients, family members, and caregivers being aware that anticonvulsants, including levetiracetam, may increase the risk of having suicidal thoughts or actions in a very small number of people (about 1 in 500). Advise patients, family members, and caregivers to pay close attention to any day-to-day changes in mood, behavior, and actions; these changes can happen very quickly. They should also be aware of common warning signs that may signal suicide risk (e.g., talking or thinking about wanting to hurt oneself or end one's life, withdrawing from friends and family, becoming depressed or experiencing worsening of existing depression, becoming preoccupied with death and dying, giving away prized possessions). Advise patients, family members, and caregivers to contact the responsible clinician immediately if these or any new and worrisome behaviors occur.

Risk of serious dermatologic reactions. Importance of patients immediately notifying their clinician if a rash develops.

Risk of anaphylaxis and angioedema. Importance of patients discontinuing therapy and seeking medical care if any signs and symptoms of these reactions occur.

Importance of adhering to prescribed directions for use. Importance of not discontinuing levetiracetam abruptly. Levetiracetam is used in combination with other anticonvulsants, not as monotherapy.

Importance of informing patients who are taking levetiracetam oral solution not to use a household teaspoon or tablespoon to measure the dose; a calibrated measuring device (such as a medicine dropper, spoon, cup, or syringe) should be obtained and used when administering the oral solution.

Importance of women informing clinicians if they are or plan to become pregnant or plan to breast-feed. Importance of clinicians informing women about the existence of and encouraging enrollment in pregnancy registries (see Pregnancy under Warnings/Precautions: Specific Populations, in Cautions).

Importance of informing clinicians of existing or contemplated concomitant therapy, including prescription and OTC drugs, dietary supplements, and/or herbal products, as well as any concomitant illness (e.g., renal disease).

Importance of informing patients of other important precautionary information. (See Cautions.)

Overview (see Users Guide). For additional information until a more detailed monograph is developed and published, the manufacturer's labeling should be consulted. It is *essential* that the manufacturer's labeling be consulted for more detailed information on usual cautions, precautions, contraindications, potential drug interactions, laboratory test interferences, and acute toxicity.

Preparations

Excipients in commercially available drug preparations may have clinically important effects in some individuals; consult specific product labeling for details.

levETIRAcetam

Oral		
Solution	100 mg/mL*	**Keppra® Oral Solution**, UCB **Levetiracetam Oral Solution**
Tablets, film-coated	250 mg*	**Keppra®** (scored), UCB **Levetiracetam Tablets**
	500 mg*	**Keppra®** (scored), UCB **Levetiracetam Tablets**
	750 mg*	**Keppra®** (scored), UCB **Levetiracetam Tablets**
	1 g*	**Keppra®** (scored), UCB **Levetiracetam Tablets**
Tablets, extended-release, film-coated	500 mg*	**Keppra XR®**, UCB **Levetiracetam Extended-release Tablets**
	750 mg*	**Keppra XR®**, UCB **Levetiracetam Extended-release Tablets**
Parenteral		
Concentrate, for injection, for IV infusion	100 mg/mL*	**Keppra®**, UCB **Levetiracetam Injection**

*available from one or more manufacturer, distributor, and/or repackager by generic (nonproprietary) name

levETIRAcetam in Sodium Chloride

Parenteral		
Injection, for IV infusion	5 mg/mL (500 mg in 0.82% sodium chloride injection)*	**Levetiracetam in Sodium Chloride Injection**
	10 mg/mL (1 g in 0.75% sodium chloride injection)*	**Levetiracetam in Sodium Chloride Injection**
	15 mg/mL (1.5 g in 0.54% sodium chloride injection)*	**Levetiracetam in Sodium Chloride Injection**

*available from one or more manufacturer, distributor, and/or repackager by generic (nonproprietary) name

Magnesium Sulfate

Epsom Salt

■ Parenteral magnesium sulfate exhibits anticonvulsant properties.

Uses

■ **Prevention and Control of Seizures** Magnesium sulfate is used parenterally as an anticonvulsant for the prevention and control of seizures in severe toxemias (preeclampsia or eclampsia) of pregnancy and in various other conditions.

Preeclampsia and Eclampsia Magnesium sulfate generally is considered the drug of choice for the prevention and control of seizures in *severe* preeclampsia or in eclampsia. The American College of Obstetricians and Gynecologists (ACOG) strongly recommends the administration of intrapartum/postpartum magnesium sulfate in women with severe preeclampsia to prevent eclampsia. In a systematic review of 6 randomized clinical studies that compared magnesium sulfate with placebo or no anticonvulsant therapy in more than 11,000 women with preeclampsia, prophylactic use of magnesium sulfate was associated with an approximate 50% reduction in the rate of eclampsia. While routine use of magnesium sulfate is not recommended in women with preeclampsia who do not have severe features (e.g., systolic blood pressure of 160 mm Hg or higher, diastolic blood pressure of 110 mm Hg or higher, thrombocytopenia, impaired liver or renal function, pulmonary edema, new-onset cerebral or visual disturbances), the decision to initiate therapy in these patients should be individualized based on the presence of certain warning signs and symptoms of imminent seizures (e.g., headache, altered mental state, blurred vision, scotomata, clonus, right upper quadrant pain). Because the clinical course of preeclampsia can change rapidly and unexpectedly during labor, patients with mild disease at presentation should be monitored closely and magnesium sulfate therapy should be initiated if progression to severe disease occurs.

ACOG strongly recommends the administration of parenteral magnesium sulfate in women with eclampsia; treatment should be continued for at least 24 hours after the last seizure. Clinical studies have demonstrated that magnesium sulfate is superior to phenytoin for the prevention of eclampsia, and superior to phenytoin and diazepam for the treatment and further prevention of eclamptic seizures.

Other Seizure Etiologies Parenterally administered magnesium sulfate may be useful in controlling seizures associated with epilepsy, glomerulonephritis, or hypothyroidism.

Magnesium sulfate also has been used for the immediate control of life-threatening seizures associated with acute nephritis in children.

■ Prevention and Treatment of Hypomagnesemia Magnesium sulfate is used parenterally to correct or prevent hypomagnesemia in patients receiving total parenteral nutrition. In such patients, magnesium sulfate usually is added to the nutrient admixture to correct or prevent hypomagnesemia, which can arise during the course of therapy.

Magnesium sulfate also is used in the treatment of acute hypomagnesemia accompanied by signs of tetany similar to those observed in hypocalcemia. In such cases, serum magnesium concentrations usually are below the lower limits of normal (1.5–2.5 mEq/L) and the serum calcium concentrations are either normal (4.3–5.3 mEq/L) or elevated.

■ Preterm Labor and Fetal Neuroprotection Magnesium sulfate has been used in pregnant women to inhibit uterine contractions in preterm labor (tocolysis)† and thus prolong gestation when such prolongation of intrauterine life would be expected to benefit pregnancy outcome; however, efficacy and safety of magnesium sulfate for this use have not been established and the drug is not labeled by the FDA for this use. ACOG and the Society for Maternal-Fetal Medicine support the short-term (up to 48 hours) obstetric use of magnesium sulfate for appropriate conditions and durations of therapy. This includes the use of magnesium sulfate for short-term (i.e., up to 48 hours) prolongation of pregnancy to allow for the administration of antenatal corticosteroids in women who are at risk of preterm delivery within 7 days; corticosteroid administration prior to anticipated preterm birth is strongly associated with decreased neonatal morbidity and mortality. However, there currently is no evidence that tocolytic therapy has a direct favorable effect on neonatal outcomes or that any prolongation of pregnancy provided by tocolytic agents translates into substantial neonatal benefit. (See Antenatal Use in Preterm Labor under Uses: Complications of Prematurity, in the Corticosteroids General Statement 68:04.)

While short-term use of magnesium sulfate injection may effectively delay delivery, prolonged administration of the drug (i.e., beyond 5–7 days) has been associated with hypocalcemia and bone abnormalities (e.g., skeletal demineralization, osteopenia, fractures) in the developing fetus and is never indicated according to ACOG obstetric use guidelines. (See Cautions: Pregnancy and Lactation.) Certain maternal or fetal conditions may contraindicate tocolytic therapy (e.g., nonreassuring fetal status, chorioamnionitis, fetal demise, lethal congenital or chromosomal abnormalities, maternal bleeding with hemodynamic instability, severe preeclampsia or eclampsia, preterm premature rupture of membranes [may consider use in the absence of maternal infection for maternal transport and/or corticosteroid administration]) in general and magnesium sulfate specifically (e.g., myasthenia gravis).

Few placebo-controlled studies have evaluated the tocolytic efficacy of magnesium sulfate. Instead, most studies have compared the efficacy and toxicity profile of magnesium sulfate with those of other tocolytic agents. Clinical studies indicate that IV magnesium sulfate (4–6 g infused IV over 20 minutes as a loading dose, followed by maintenance infusions of 2–4 g per hour for 12–24 hours after contractions cease) generally appears to be as effective as IV ritodrine, sublingual and/or oral nifedipine, or rectal or oral indomethacin for the short-term management of preterm labor. Magnesium sulfate-induced prolongation of pregnancy is less successful when preterm labor is complicated by premature rupture of membranes. Some clinicians have suggested that the lack of efficacy observed in some studies with magnesium sulfate tocolysis may be the result of subtherapeutic dosing regimens. Substitution of another tocolytic agent in patients experiencing failure with a given drug may result in effective tocolysis.

ACOG guidelines for the management of preterm labor state that maintenance treatment with tocolytic drugs is not effective for preventing preterm birth and improving neonatal outcomes and is not recommended. Limited data indicate that combination therapy with magnesium sulfate and another tocolytic agent may be more effective in arresting preterm labor than a single tocolytic agent; however, combination therapy also may be associated with an increased risk of adverse maternal effects. β-Adrenergic agonists and calcium-channel blocking agents should be used with caution in combination with magnesium sulfate because of the risk of potentially serious maternal complications; concurrent use of magnesium sulfate and nifedipine may be particularly risky. (See Drug Interactions.) Additional study and experience are needed to confirm the safety and efficacy of combined tocolytic therapy and to establish the role, if any, of such therapy.

In addition to magnesium sulfate's efficacy in delaying delivery, data from several population-based observational studies and large clinical trials have indicated an association between the predelivery use of magnesium sulfate and a reduction in the incidence and severity of cerebral palsy among surviving infants if the drug is administered when birth is anticipated before 32 weeks of gestation. Based on these findings, ACOG recommends the use of magnesium sulfate for fetal neuroprotection† before anticipated preterm birth (less than 32 weeks of gestation). A possible mechanism for the neuroprotective effect of magnesium sulfate may be that the drug reduces the incidence of neonatal intraventricular hemorrhage, which is a risk factor for the development of these neurodevelopmental defects. If magnesium sulfate is being used in the preterm labor setting for fetal neuroprotection and the patient is still experiencing preterm labor, ACOG recommends that a different tocolytic agent be considered for short-term use. ACOG also recommends that hospitals that use magnesium sulfate for fetal neuroprotection† develop uniform and specific guidelines for such use, including inclusion criteria, treatment regimens, concomitant use of tocolytic agents, and patient monitoring, in accordance with one of the larger clinical trials.

■ Arrhythmias IV magnesium sulfate has been used successfully for the treatment of life-threatening arrhythmias such as atypical ventricular tachycardia† (torsades de pointes). IV magnesium sulfate is considered one of several preferred drugs in the treatment of polymorphic ventricular tachycardia suspected of being torsades de pointes† in patients in whom initial attempts at correcting or managing potential precipitating factors (e.g., ischemic cardiac events, electrolyte imbalance, drugs known to prolong the QT interval) have not been successful. Because polymorphic ventricular tachycardias other than torsades de pointes generally are unresponsive to magnesium therapy, use of β-adrenergic blocking agents or IV amiodarone generally is preferred in patients in whom polymorphic ventricular tachycardia (not suspected of being torsades de pointes) may be precipitated by myocardial ischemia.

Antiarrhythmic drugs are used during cardiac arrest to facilitate the restoration and maintenance of a spontaneous perfusing rhythm in patients with refractory (i.e., persisting or recurring after at least one shock) ventricular fibrillation or pulseless ventricular tachycardia; however, there is no evidence that these drugs increase survival to hospital discharge when given routinely during cardiac arrest. High-quality cardiopulmonary resuscitation (CPR) and defibrillation are integral components of advanced cardiovascular life support (ACLS) and the only proven interventions to increase survival to hospital discharge. Other resuscitative efforts, including drug therapy, are considered secondary and should be performed without compromising the quality and timely delivery of chest compressions and defibrillation. The principal goal of pharmacologic therapy during cardiac arrest is to facilitate return of spontaneous circulation (ROSC), and epinephrine is the drug of choice for this use. (See Uses: Advanced Cardiovascular Life Support and Cardiac Arrhythmias, in Epinephrine 12:12.12.) If an antiarrhythmic agent is needed for the treatment of ventricular fibrillation or pulseless ventricular tachycardia during cardiac resuscitation, experts generally recommend the use of amiodarone (or lidocaine). In several randomized controlled studies, administration of magnesium sulfate during cardiac arrest did not improve rates of ROSC, survival to hospital discharge, or neurologic outcome for any presenting rhythm. The American Heart Association (AHA) therefore states that IV magnesium sulfate should not be used routinely during cardiac arrest; however, the drug may be considered when the arrest rhythm is associated with torsades de pointes.

IV magnesium sulfate also has been used in the management of paroxysmal atrial tachycardia when other measures have failed and when there is no evidence of myocardial damage.

■ Acute Myocardial Infarction Magnesium sulfate has been administered IV as adjunctive therapy to reduce cardiovascular morbidity and mortality (e.g., through reduction in ventricular arrhythmias and/or limitation of infarct size and reperfusion injury) associated with acute myocardial infarction (MI)†; however, contradictory evidence of such beneficial effects has been reported.

Pooled analyses of several small, controlled studies and results of a few other randomized, controlled studies have indicated a reduction in ventricular arrhythmias and/or mortality with early IV magnesium administration in patients with acute MI; in some studies, mortality rates in magnesium-treated patients have been similar to those reported with thrombolytic therapy. In a randomized, placebo-controlled study (the Second Leicester Intravenous Magnesium Intervention Trial; LIMIT-2) in more than 2000 patients with suspected acute MI and baseline serum magnesium concentrations in the normal range, adjunctive therapy with magnesium sulfate administered as a single IV injection (2 g) within 24 hours of onset of symptoms, followed by continuous IV infusion of the drug (16 g) over the next 24 hours, was associated with a reduction in all-cause mortality of 24% at 4 weeks (7.8% mortality) compared with that in placebo recipients (10.3% mortality). Approximately one-third of patients in the LIMIT-2 study also received a thrombolytic agent, and two-thirds received concomitant aspirin. Patients receiving IV magnesium had a 25% lower rate of congestive heart failure during hospitalization and a 21% reduction in ischemic heart disease-related mortality during long-term follow-up of at least 4.5 years. The benefit of IV magnesium therapy in this study was consistent with data from several previous, smaller, controlled studies in patients with acute MI in whom thrombolytic agents, aspirin, or β-blockers were not administered routinely; subsequent analysis of pooled data from these studies and the LIMIT-2 study indicated an overall reduction in early mortality of approximately 35% in patients who received IV magnesium treatment generally within 12 hours following infarction.

In contrast to these findings, in the Fourth International Study of Infarct Survival (ISIS-4), a randomized, multicenter study in more than 58,000 patients, administration of IV magnesium sulfate in a regimen similar to that used in the LIMIT-2 study (single 2-g IV dose followed by 18 g infused over 24 hours) was not associated with a reduction in mortality or other appreciable benefit on cardiac function at 5 weeks in patients with acute MI. While the reasons for these discrepant results remain to be elucidated, some clinicians suggest that differences in the timing of IV magnesium administration in relation to onset of symptoms of MI and different patient characteristics may have accounted for the opposing outcomes of these studies. In the LIMIT-2 study, magnesium was administered *concomitantly* with thrombolytic therapy and randomization to treatment occurred within a median of 3 hours from the onset of chest pain; in ISIS-4, thrombolytic therapy was initiated *before* IV magnesium and the corresponding time to treatment randomization was a median of 8 hours. Since data in animals with experimentally induced MI indicate that elevated magnesium concentrations must be present prior to or shortly (e.g., within 1 hour) after the onset of coronary artery reperfusion in order for substantial myocardial salvage to occur, the lack of benefit on mortality reduction in the ISIS-4 study has been attributed to the late initiation of magnesium treatment in these patients relative to that in the LIMIT-2 study. In addition, it has been suggested that the low (7.2%) mortality rate in the control group in ISIS-4 may have been indicative of a relatively low-risk patient population in whom any additional mortality-reducing effects of IV magnesium (i.e., beyond those associated with the concurrently administered fibrinolytic and antiplatelet therapy) would have been difficult to detect.

In a more recent randomized controlled study (the Magnesium in Coronaries [MAGIC] trial) that was designed to evaluate the effects of early administration of IV magnesium sulfate in high-risk patients with acute ST-elevation MI (STEMI), there was no difference in 30-day mortality (the primary end point) between patients who received magnesium sulfate and those who received placebo. Based on the currently available evidence, routine prophylactic administration of magnesium sulfate in patients with acute MI is not recommended; since there is no apparent harm associated with its use, however, magnesium may still be used in patients with documented magnesium deficiency or torsades de pointes-type ventricular tachycardia.

■ **Acute Asthma** Magnesium sulfate has been used parenterally in the management of acute asthma† in both pediatric patients and adults. There is some evidence indicating that the drug may modestly improve bronchodilation and pulmonary function when given in conjunction with standard bronchodilating agents (e.g., nebulized β-adrenergic agents) and corticosteroids; patients with the most severe exacerbations of asthma appear to derive the most benefits. In one randomized, placebo-controlled, double-blind study in children with severe persistent asthma (peak expiratory flow rate less than 60% of predicted) who failed to respond to an adequate trial of conventional therapy (3 doses of albuterol administered via nebulization), use of IV magnesium sulfate (25 mg/kg up to 2 g) substantially improved pulmonary function in such children as compared with those who received placebo. Children who received IV magnesium sulfate also were less likely to be hospitalized for treatment than those who received placebo. The benefit of IV magnesium sulfate therapy in this study was consistent with data from similarly designed controlled studies in adults and children in whom IV infusion of magnesium sulfate (2 g over 20 minutes) produced a beneficial effect only in the most severely ill patients. A systematic review of 7 randomized controlled studies in adults and pediatric patients with acute asthma found that magnesium sulfate improved pulmonary function (peak expiratory flow rate and forced expiratory volume in 1 second) and reduced hospitalizations in patients with the most severe exacerbations. In another systematic review of 14 randomized controlled studies in adults presenting to the emergency department with acute asthma, treatment with a single IV infusion of magnesium sulfate (1.2 or 2 g) reduced hospital admissions and improved lung function in patients who were unresponsive to conventional therapy. Although the currently available evidence does not support routine use of IV magnesium sulfate in all patients with acute asthma, the drug may be beneficial, and thus may be considered, in some patients with severe exacerbations.

■ **Other Uses** Magnesium sulfate has been administered IV to counteract the intense muscle stimulating effects of barium poisoning.

Parenteral magnesium sulfate also has been used in the management of other clinical situations including cerebral edema (as an osmotic agent) and tetanus. The efficacy of parenteral magnesium sulfate therapy in these situations has not been conclusively demonstrated.

Although some evidence suggests an association between lower dietary intake of magnesium and higher blood pressure, there currently are no convincing data to justify increased magnesium intake as a means of lowering blood pressure.

For use of magnesium sulfate as a cathartic, see Saline Laxatives 56:12.

Dosage and Administration

■ **Administration** Magnesium sulfate is usually administered IV or IM.

For IV administration, the concentration of magnesium sulfate should not be greater than 200 mg/mL (20%) and the rate of injection generally should not exceed 150 mg/minute (e.g., 1.5 mL/minute of a 10% concentration or equivalent) except in patients with seizures associated with severe eclampsia.

For IM administration in adults, magnesium sulfate solution in concentrations of 250 mg/mL (25%) or 500 mg/mL (50%) is generally used. For IM use in infants and children, the drug concentration usually should not exceed 200 mg/mL (20%); however, higher concentrations (e.g., 50%) have been used.

Magnesium sulfate also has been administered by intraosseous (IO) infusion† in the setting of advanced cardiovascular life support (ACLS), generally when IV access is not readily available; onset of action and systemic concentrations of the drug are comparable to those achieved with venous administration.

Magnesium sulfate 50% injection must be diluted prior to IV administration; alternatively, a commercially available prediluted solution of magnesium sulfate in 5% dextrose injection or sterile water for injection may be used.

When used in pregnant women for conditions other than those labeled by the FDA, such as for the prevention of preterm labor†, magnesium sulfate injection should be administered only by trained obstetric personnel in a hospital setting with appropriate obstetrical care facilities.

■ **Dosage** Dosage of magnesium sulfate must be carefully adjusted according to individual requirements and response, and administration of the drug should be discontinued as soon as the desired effect is obtained.

Clinicians should use caution when switching between different formulations of magnesium sulfate injection to ensure that patients receive the correct dose.

Prevention and Control of Seizures **Preeclampsia and Eclampsia.** Various dosing regimens for magnesium sulfate have been recommended for the management of preeclampsia or eclampsia. IV infusions of dilute solutions of magnesium sulfate (1–8%) are often given in combination with IM injections of 50% magnesium sulfate. In severe preeclampsia or eclampsia, the manufacturer states that the total initial dose of magnesium sulfate is 10–14 g. An initial IV dose of 4–5 g of magnesium sulfate in 250 mL of 5% dextrose injection or 0.9% sodium chloride injection may be given simultaneously with IM doses of up to 10 g (5 g or 10 mL of the undiluted 50% solution of magnesium sulfate administered into each buttock). Alternatively, the initial IV dose of 4 g may be given by diluting the 50% magnesium sulfate injection to a concentration of 10 or 20% and the diluted solution (40 mL of a 10% solution or 20 mL of a 20% solution) injected IV over a period of 3–4 minutes; subsequent doses of 4–5 g (8–10 mL of the undiluted 50% magnesium sulfate injection) may then be administered IM into alternate buttocks every 4 hours as needed, depending on the continuing presence of the patellar reflex and adequate respiratory function. After the initial IV dose, some clinicians administer a maintenance IV infusion of 1–2 g/hour. For the prevention or treatment of eclamptic seizures, the American College of Obstetricians and Gynecologists (ACOG) recommends an IV loading dose of 4–6 g of magnesium sulfate, followed by a maintenance IV infusion of 1–2 g/hour for at least 24 hours.

Therapy should continue until paroxysms cease. A serum magnesium concentration of 6 mg per 100 mL is considered optimal for control of seizures. The manufacturer states that total dosage of magnesium sulfate should not exceed 30–40 g daily. In the presence of severe renal insufficiency, frequent serum magnesium concentrations must be obtained and the maximum dosage of magnesium sulfate is 20 g per 48 hours.

Other Seizure Etiologies. For controlling seizures associated with epilepsy, glomerulonephritis, or hypothyroidism, the usual adult dose is 1 g administered IM or IV.

Hypomagnesemia **Prevention.** Maintenance requirements for magnesium in total parenteral nutrition are not precisely known. As a part of total parenteral nutrition, adults are usually given 8–24 mEq of magnesium daily and infants are usually given 2–10 mEq of magnesium sulfate daily. (See Chemistry and Stability: Chemistry.)

Treatment. For the treatment of mild magnesium deficiency, the usual adult dosage of magnesium sulfate is 1 g (8.12 mEq or 2 mL of the 50% solution of magnesium sulfate) administered IM every 6 hours for 4 doses. For deficiency that is not severe in adults and older children, some manufacturers have recommended a magnesium sulfate dosage of 1 g (2 mL of the 50% solution) once or twice daily by IM injection using serum magnesium values to guide continued dosing. In patients with severe hypomagnesemia, as much as 250 mg (2 mEq or 0.5 mL of the 50% solution) of magnesium sulfate per kg of body weight may be administered IM within a 4-hour period if necessary. For severe hypomagnesemia, some manufacturers have recommended a daily magnesium sulfate dose of 1–5 g (2–10 mL of the 50% solution) given in divided doses by IM injection. Alternatively, 5 g of magnesium sulfate (approximately 40 mEq) may be added to 1 L of 5% dextrose injection or 0.9% sodium chloride injection and administered by slow IV infusion over a 3-hour period. In the treatment of deficiency states, caution must be observed to prevent exceeding the renal excretory capacity.

For the treatment of hypomagnesemia in pediatric patients, some experts recommend a magnesium sulfate dosage of 25–50 mg/kg (maximum single dose of 2 g) every 4–6 hours for 3–4 doses by IV or IM injection; doses may be repeated as needed.

Preterm Labor and Fetal Neuroprotection For use as a tocolytic agent in the management of preterm labor†, the rate and duration of magnesium sulfate infusion should be carefully adjusted according to the patient's response, as indicated by uterine response, and the maternal and fetal tolerance. Monitoring serum magnesium concentrations may be useful in minimizing the risk of magnesium toxicity (e.g., respiratory depression, cardiotoxicity, maternal tetany, muscular paralysis, hypotension) and in determining the maximum safe infusion rate. For acute tocolytic therapy, IV magnesium sulfate dosages of 4–6 g infused over 20 minutes as a loading dose, followed by maintenance infusions of 2–4 g per hour for 12–24 hours as tolerated after contractions cease, have been used. However, prolonged administration of the drug (i.e., more than 5–7 days) for tocolysis has been associated with hypocalcemia and bone abnormalities in the developing fetus. (See Cautions: Pregnancy and Lactation.) Monitoring the amount of administered IV fluids and the rate of administration is necessary to avoid circulatory fluid overload. Patients should be observed for signs and symptoms of pulmonary edema. (See Cautions: Adverse Effects.)

Hospitals that use magnesium sulfate for fetal neuroprotection† should develop uniform and specific guidelines for such use, including inclusion criteria, treatment regimens, concomitant use of tocolytic agents, and patient monitoring in accordance with one of the larger clinical trials.

Arrhythmias **Ventricular Tachycardia.** In adults with polymorphic ventricular tachycardia associated with QT interval prolongation (torsades de pointes†), some experts recommend an IV magnesium sulfate dose of 1–2 g administered over 15 minutes. A dose of 1–6 g of magnesium sulfate (8.1–48.6 mEq) administered over several minutes also has been used, followed in some cases by IV infusion of the drug at a rate of approximately 3–20 mg/minute for 5–48 hours depending on patient response and serum magnesium concentrations. For cardiac arrest associated with torsades de pointes†, some experts recommend an adult IV or IO† bolus dose of 1–2 g of magnesium sulfate, diluted in 10 mL of 5% dextrose injection.

When used in pediatric advanced life support (PALS) for the treatment of torsades de pointes or suspected hypomagnesemia, some experts recommend an IV or IO† magnesium sulfate dose of 25–50 mg/kg (maximum single dose of 2 g) over 10–20 minutes (or faster in torsades de pointes).

Paroxysmal Atrial Tachycardia. When magnesium sulfate was used in the management of paroxysmal atrial tachycardia, the usual dose was 3–4 g (e.g., 30–40 mL of a 10% solution) administered IV over 30 seconds *with extreme caution*.

Acute Asthma For the management of severe refractory asthma† in adults, some experts state that the standard magnesium sulfate dose of 2 g may be given by IV infusion over 20 minutes.

In children with moderate to severe exacerbation of reactive airway disease, a single magnesium sulfate dose of 25–75 mg/kg (maximum 2 g) over 20 minutes by IV infusion has been recommended.

Barium Poisoning In counteracting the muscle-stimulating effects of barium poisoning, the usual dose of magnesium sulfate is 1–2 g given IV.

■ Dosage in Geriatric Patients

Geriatric patients often require a reduced dosage of magnesium sulfate because of renal impairment. In geriatric patients with severe renal impairment, dosage of the drug should not exceed 20 g in a 48-hour period; serum magnesium concentrations should be monitored in such patients.

Cautions

■ Adverse Effects

Adverse effects associated with parenteral magnesium sulfate therapy are caused by magnesium intoxication. Signs of hypermagnesemia, which may begin at serum magnesium concentrations of 4 mEq/L, include neurologic symptoms (e.g., muscular weakness, flaccid paralysis, ataxia, drowsiness, confusion, depression of reflexes), flushing, sweating, vasodilation, hypotension, hypothermia, depression of cardiac function, bradycardia, cardiac arrhythmias, circulatory collapse, hypoventilation, and CNS depression. These symptoms can proceed to fatal respiratory paralysis. Hypocalcemia with signs of tetany secondary to magnesium sulfate therapy for eclampsia has been reported.

To minimize the risk of magnesium toxicity (e.g., respiratory depression, cardiotoxicity, maternal tetany, muscular paralysis, hypotension) during tocolytic therapy, serum magnesium concentrations should be monitored. In addition to the usual cautions and precautions of magnesium sulfate therapy, tocolytic therapy with the drug is associated with some risk of maternal pulmonary edema. The etiology of pulmonary edema associated with tocolytic therapy remains to be more fully elucidated. Maternal risk factors for its development include excessive hydration, multiple gestation, occult sepsis, and underlying cardiac disease. Although adjunctive corticosteroid therapy also has been suggested as contributing to the risk of developing pulmonary edema, most evidence suggests that this is not an important risk factor. The risk of maternal pulmonary edema associated with tocolytic therapy may be reduced by limiting fluid intake to 2.5–3 L daily, limiting sodium intake, and maintaining maternal pulse below 130 beats/minute. Development of pulmonary edema during the initial 24 hours of tocolytic therapy is uncommon.

■ Precautions and Contraindications

Patients receiving parenteral magnesium sulfate should be observed carefully, and serum magnesium concentration should be monitored to avoid overdosage. Disappearance of the patellar reflex is a useful clinical sign to detect the onset of magnesium intoxication. When repeated doses of the drug are given parenterally, knee jerk reflexes should be tested before each dose and if they are absent, no additional magnesium should be given until they return. In addition, the respiration rate should be at least 16 per minute prior to parenteral administration of each dose of magnesium sulfate, and therapy should not be continued unless urine output is 100 mL or more during the 4 hours preceding each dose. In the event of overdosage, artificial ventilation must be provided until a calcium salt can be given IV. Clinically important hypocalcemia including hypocalcemic tetany has occurred following parenteral magnesium sulfate therapy for eclampsia. Changes in calcium and phosphorus balance should be anticipated in each case of parenteral magnesium administration.

In adults, IV administration of 5–10 mEq of calcium (e.g., 10–20 mL of 10% calcium gluconate) will usually reverse respiratory depression or heart block caused by magnesium intoxication.

Magnesium sulfate should be administered with caution to patients with impaired renal function because of the danger of magnesium intoxication.

Some preparations of magnesium sulfate contain aluminum; aluminum accumulation and associated toxicity (e.g., CNS and bone toxicities) can occur with prolonged parenteral administration of the drug in patients with impaired renal function. Premature neonates are at particularly high risk of aluminum toxicity.

Parenteral administration of magnesium sulfate is contraindicated in patients with heart block or myocardial damage.

For precautions and contraindications associated with tocolytic use of magnesium sulfate, see Uses: Preterm Labor and Fetal Neuroprotection and also see Cautions: Adverse Effects.

■ Geriatric Precautions

Geriatric patients often require a reduced dosage of magnesium sulfate because of renal impairment. (See Dosage and Administration: Dosage in Geriatric Patients.)

■ Pregnancy and Lactation

The neonate is usually not compromised by excess magnesium when IM magnesium sulfate is administered to the toxemic mother; however, when magnesium sulfate therapy is administered by continuous IV infusion (especially if for more than 24 hours preceding delivery), the possibility that the neonate may show signs of magnesium toxicity, including neuromuscular or respiratory depression, is increased. In addition, prolonged use of parenteral magnesium sulfate during pregnancy has been associated with fetal hypocalcemia and skeletal abnormalities. IV magnesium should not be given during the 2 hours preceding delivery. Management of the neonate with hypermagnesemia may require resuscitation and assisted ventilation via endotracheal intubation and/or intermittent positive-pressure ventilation, as well as IV calcium. For additional information on the risks of tocolysis with magnesium sulfate, see Cautions: Adverse Effects.

Epidemiologic studies and case reports indicate that prolonged use (i.e., longer than 5–7 days) of magnesium sulfate injection during pregnancy may cause hypocalcemia and related skeletal abnormalities (e.g., osteopenia, bone demineralization, fractures) in the developing fetus. Such bone abnormalities have been described in case reports of neonates exposed in utero to magnesium sulfate; as of May 30, 2013, 18 cases were identified in the FDA's Adverse Event Reporting System (AERS). All of these cases were previously described in the medical literature. In these case reports, magnesium sulfate was parenterally administered for prolonged periods for the prevention of preterm labor (tocolysis)†, which is not an FDA-labeled indication for the drug. According to an FDA analysis of data obtained from AERS, the average duration of in utero exposure to magnesium sulfate was 9.6 weeks (range: 8–12 weeks). Complete or near complete resolution of the bone abnormalities occurred in cases where outcomes were reported. Results of several epidemiologic studies, most of which were retrospective chart reviews, also have indicated an increased incidence of skeletal abnormalities in infants born to mothers who had received IV magnesium sulfate for prolonged tocolysis (more than 5–7 days). Some of these studies also reported changes in serum biochemistry related to bone metabolism (e.g., hypermagnesemia, hyperphosphatemia, hypocalcemia, increased alkaline phosphatase concentrations) and radiographic changes consistent with the bone abnormalities observed; however, the long-term consequences of such findings are not known. Although a causal relationship has not been conclusively established, FDA states that the available evidence to date supports an association between prolonged (i.e., longer than 5–7 days) maternal administration of IV magnesium sulfate therapy and neonatal hypocalcemia and skeletal abnormalities.

Magnesium sulfate injection should be used during pregnancy only if clearly needed. If magnesium sulfate is administered to a pregnant woman for the prevention of preterm labor, the patient should be informed that efficacy and safety of such use have not been established and that use of the drug for more than 5–7 days in this setting may cause fetal harm; the shortest duration of use that can result in fetal harm is not known.

Since magnesium is distributed into milk during parenteral magnesium sulfate administration, the drug should be used with caution in nursing women. However, magnesium sulfate generally is considered to be compatible with breastfeeding. Milk concentrations of magnesium are increased for only about 24 hours after discontinuance of parenteral magnesium sulfate therapy; the amount of magnesium ingested by a nursing infant during this period is probably too small to be of clinical importance.

Drug Interactions

■ β-Adrenergic Agonists

Although limited data indicate that combination therapy with magnesium sulfate and another tocolytic agent may be more effective in arresting preterm labor† than a single tocolytic agent alone, American College of Obstetricians and Gynecologists (ACOG) guidelines currently state that β-adrenergic agonists should be used with caution in combination with magnesium sulfate because of the risk of potentially serious maternal complications.

■ **Calcium-channel Blocking Agents** Although limited data indicate that combination therapy with magnesium sulfate and another tocolytic agent may be more effective in arresting preterm labor† than a single tocolytic agent alone, concurrent use of magnesium sulfate and calcium-channel blocking agents (e.g., nifedipine) may be particularly risky and is potentially harmful (e.g., reduced heart rate, contractility, and left ventricular systolic pressure; neuromuscular blockade). ACOG guidelines currently state that calcium-channel blocking agents should be used with caution in combination with magnesium sulfate because of the risk of potentially serious maternal complications.

■ **CNS Depressants** When barbiturates, opiates, general anesthetics, or other CNS depressants are administered concomitantly with magnesium sulfate, dosage of these agents must be carefully adjusted because of the additive central depressant effects.

■ **Neuromuscular Blocking Agents** Excessive neuromuscular blockade has occurred in patients receiving parenteral magnesium sulfate and a neuromuscular blocking agent; these drugs should be administered concomitantly only with caution.

■ **Cardiac Glycosides** Magnesium salts should be administered with extreme caution in digitalized patients, because serious changes in cardiac conduction which can result in heart block may occur if administration of calcium is required to treat magnesium toxicity.

Pharmacology

Magnesium is the fourth most abundant cation in the body and is essential for the function of important enzymes, including those related to the transfer of phosphate groups, all reactions involving ATP, and every step related to the replication and transcription of DNA and the translation of mRNA. Magnesium also is required for cellular energy metabolism and is involved in membrane stabilization, nerve conduction, iron transport, and calcium-channel activity.

When administered parenterally in doses sufficient to produce hypermagnesemia (serum magnesium concentrations greater than 2.5 mEq/L), the drug may depress the CNS and block peripheral neuromuscular transmission, producing anticonvulsant effects. The exact mechanism of this depressant activity is not fully known; however, excess magnesium appears to decrease the amount of acetylcholine liberated by the motor nerve impulse. When serum concentrations of magnesium exceed 4 mEq/L, deep-tendon reflexes may be depressed. At serum concentrations of 10 mEq/L, deep-tendon reflexes may disappear and respiratory paralysis may occur. Serum magnesium concentrations in excess of 12 mEq/L may be fatal. Complete heart block can also occur at high serum concentrations of magnesium (approximately 10 mEq/L). Animal studies suggest that the effect of magnesium ions on cardiac muscle is to slow the rate of the sinoatrial node impulse formation and prolong conduction time. Limited data in patients with no evidence of heart disease indicate that IV infusion of magnesium prolongs PR interval, H (atria-His bundle) interval, antegrade AV nodal effective refractory period, and sinoatrial conduction time. Available data also suggest that magnesium produces systemic and coronary vasodilatation, possesses antiplatelet activity, suppresses automaticity in partially depolarized cells, and protects myocytes against calcium overload under conditions of ischemia by inhibiting calcium influx especially at the time of reperfusion. However, the clinical benefit of administering magnesium in patients with acute myocardial infarction has not been fully determined. (See Uses: Acute Myocardial Infarction.) Magnesium also acts peripherally, producing vasodilation. Moderate doses produce flushing and sweating, and higher doses lower blood pressure. Both the CNS depression and the peripheral neuromuscular transmission blockade produced by hypermagnesemia can be antagonized by administration of excess calcium.

Pharmacokinetics

When magnesium sulfate is administered IV, the onset of action is immediate and the duration of action is about 30 minutes. Following IM administration of the drug, the onset of action occurs in about 1 hour and the duration of action is 3–4 hours. As an anticonvulsant, effective serum concentrations of magnesium have been reported to range from 2.5–7.5 mEq/L.

Magnesium readily crosses the placenta and is distributed into milk following parenteral administration of magnesium sulfate. Milk concentrations of magnesium are increased for only about 24 hours after discontinuance of parenteral magnesium sulfate therapy; the amount of magnesium ingested by a nursing infant during this period is probably too small to be of clinical importance.

Magnesium sulfate is excreted by the kidneys at a rate that varies from one patient to another but that is directly proportional to the serum concentration and glomerular filtration.

Chemistry and Stability

■ **Chemistry** Parenteral magnesium sulfate exhibits anticonvulsant properties. Magnesium sulfate occurs as small, colorless crystals, usually needle-like, with a cooling, saline, bitter taste and is freely soluble in water and sparingly soluble in alcohol. The drug effloresces in warm, dry air. Each gram of magnesium sulfate heptahydrate contains 8.1 mEq of magnesium. The pHs of commercially available magnesium sulfate injection and magnesium sulfate in 5% dextrose injection are adjusted with sodium hydroxide and/or sulfuric acid; the injections have pHs of 3.5–7.

■ **Stability** Magnesium sulfate injection and magnesium sulfate in 5% dextrose injection should be stored at 20–25°C; freezing should be avoided.

Magnesium sulfate is converted to the monohydrate when heated to 150–160°C. Magnesium sulfate is incompatible with alkali hydroxides (forming insoluble magnesium hydroxide), with alkali carbonates (forming basic carbonates), and with salicylates (forming basic salicylates). The drug reacts with arsenates, phosphates, and tartrates, precipitating the corresponding magnesium salts. Lead, barium, strontium, and calcium react with magnesium sulfate resulting in precipitation of the respective sulfates. Specialized references should be consulted for specific compatibility information. Following withdrawal of a dose from one of the solutions which do not contain preservatives, any unused portion should be discarded.

Preparations

Excipients in commercially available drug preparations may have clinically important effects in some individuals; consult specific product labeling for details.

Magnesium Sulfate

Crystals

Parenteral

Injection	50%*	Magnesium Sulfate Injection
Injection, for IV use only	4% (2, 4, 20, and 40 g)*	Magnesium Sulfate Injection
	8% (4 g)*	Magnesium Sulfate Injection

*available from one or more manufacturer, distributor, and/or repackager by generic (nonproprietary) name

Magnesium Sulfate in Dextrose

Parenteral

Injection, for IV use only	1% (1 g) in 5% Dextrose*	Magnesium Sulfate in 5% Dextrose Injection
	2% (10 and 20 g) in 5% Dextrose*	Magnesium Sulfate in 5% Dextrose Injection

*available from one or more manufacturer, distributor, and/or repackager by generic (nonproprietary) name

†Use is not currently included in the labeling approved by the US Food and Drug Administration

OXcarbazepine

■ Oxcarbazepine is an anticonvulsant agent.

Uses

■ **Seizure Disorders** ***Partial Seizures*** Oxcarbazepine is used as monotherapy or adjunctive therapy (i.e., in combination with other anticonvulsants) in the management of partial seizures.

Monotherapy. Oxcarbazepine conventional (immediate-release) tablets and oral suspension are used as monotherapy of partial seizures in adults and pediatric patients 4 years of age or older.

Efficacy of oxcarbazepine monotherapy in patients with partial seizures has been established in several multicenter, randomized controlled studies using immediate-release preparations of the drug. In one placebo-controlled study in patients 11–62 years of age with refractory partial seizures (undergoing evaluation for epilepsy surgery) who had been withdrawn from anticonvulsants prior to randomization, oxcarbazepine at dosages up to 2.4 g daily for 10 days was more effective than placebo. Results of another placebo-controlled study in previously untreated patients 8–69 years of age with newly diagnosed or recent-onset partial seizures indicated that oxcarbazepine dosages up to 1.2 g daily for 84 days were more effective than placebo. In 2 conversion-to-monotherapy studies, therapy with oxcarbazepine 2.4 g daily for up to 126 days was substantially more effective than oxcarbazepine 300 mg daily in patients 11–66 years of age with partial seizures who had been withdrawn from previous therapy with 1 or 2 anticonvulsants because of inadequate control. An additional evaluator-blinded monotherapy trial was conducted in pediatric patients 1 month to 16 years of age with inadequately controlled or new-onset partial seizures. In this study, oxcarbazepine 40–60 mg/kg daily was not more effective than oxcarbazepine 10 mg/kg daily; however, due to several limitations in the study design, the results were considered uninterpretable. Efficacy of oxcarbazepine monotherapy in pediatric patients 4 years of age or older is based on pharmacokinetic and pharmacodynamic data.

Results of several multicenter, randomized, double-blind monotherapy trials in patients with newly diagnosed or previously untreated partial or generalized seizures indicate that oxcarbazepine exhibits anticonvulsant activity similar to carbamazepine, phenytoin, or valproic acid.

Adjunctive Therapy. Oxcarbazepine conventional (immediate-release) tablets and oral suspension are used as adjunctive therapy (i.e., in combination with other anticonvulsants) of partial seizures in adults and pediatric patients 2 years of age or older. Efficacy of oxcarbazepine for this use was established in 2 multicenter, randomized, double-blind, placebo-controlled studies (one in adults and one in children 3–17 years of age) and an additional evaluator-blinded study that compared 2 dosages of oxcarbazepine in infants and children 1 month to less than 4 years of age. In the placebo-controlled studies, patients initially were stabilized on optimum dosages of 1–3 anticonvulsants during an 8-week baseline period; those experiencing at least 8 (minimum 1–4 per month) partial seizures during this phase were randomized to receive oxcarbazepine (as an immediate-release preparation) or placebo during a dosage titration period of 2 weeks followed by a 14- or 24-week maintenance period in children or adults, respectively. Efficacy of oxcarbazepine in these studies was evaluated in terms of the change in seizure frequency (i.e., the median decrease [or increase] in average monthly [28-day] seizure rate). Adults receiving oxcarbazepine 600 mg, 1.2 g, or 2.4 g daily or placebo experienced a median decrease in seizure frequency of about 26, 40, 50, or 8%, respectively, while pediatric patients receiving oxcarbazepine dosages ranging from 30–46 mg/kg daily (depending on baseline body weight) or placebo experienced a median decrease in seizure frequency of about 35 or 9%, respectively. In the dose comparison study, infants and children who were receiving stable dosages of up to 2 anticonvulsants prior to study entry and who had experienced at least 2 partial seizures during a 72-hour baseline period were randomized to receive adjunctive therapy with low-dose oxcarbazepine (10 mg/kg daily with no titration period) or high-dose oxcarbazepine (60 mg/kg daily after a 26-day titration period) as an oral suspension. Patients in both groups received their target dosage for 9 days and seizures were assessed during the last 72 hours of the maintenance period with video electroencephalography (EEG). Oxcarbazepine 60 mg/kg daily was substantially more effective than oxcarbazepine 10 mg/kg daily in reducing seizure frequency. Efficacy of oxcarbazepine was not demonstrated in children younger than 2 years of age in this study.

Oxcarbazepine also is commercially available as extended-release tablets for once-daily administration in the adjunctive management of partial seizures in adults and pediatric patients 6 years of age and older. Efficacy of the extended-release tablets in adults was evaluated in a randomized, double-blind, placebo-controlled study in patients 18–65 years of age with refractory partial epilepsy. Patients who experienced at least 3 partial seizures every 28 days during an 8-week baseline period despite receiving stable dosages of 1–3 anticonvulsants were randomized to receive adjunctive therapy with oxcarbazepine (1.2 or 2.4 g daily as extended-release tablets) or placebo. Patients receiving oxcarbazepine 1.2 g daily, oxcarbazepine 2.4 g daily, or placebo experienced a median decrease in seizure frequency of about 38, 43, or 29%, respectively. Although the comparison between the 1.2-g daily dosage and placebo did not reach statistical significance in this study, the effectiveness of this dosage is supported by exposure-response analyses. Efficacy of oxcarbazepine extended-release tablets in pediatric patients is based on a pharmacokinetic study in children 4–16 years of age and studies with the immediate-release preparation in pediatric patients in addition to clinical studies performed in the adult population with both immediate-release and extended-release preparations of the drug. (See Pediatric Use under Warnings/Precautions: Specific Populations, in Cautions.)

■ **Bipolar Disorder** Oxcarbazepine has been used alone or in combination with other drugs (e.g., antipsychotic agents) for the treatment and prevention of acute manic or mixed episodes in patients with bipolar disorder†. Limited data suggest that oxcarbazepine may have equivalent efficacy and better tolerability than carbamazepine for this indication. The American Psychiatric Association (APA) considers oxcarbazepine an alternative treatment option for patients who do not respond adequately to first-line therapies such as lithium, valproic acid, and antipsychotic agents (e.g., olanzapine). For additional information on the management of bipolar disorder, see Uses: Bipolar Disorder, in Lithium Salts 28:28.

Dosage and Administration

■ **Administration** Oxcarbazepine is administered orally as conventional (immediate-release) tablets, oral suspension, or extended-release tablets.

Oxcarbazepine conventional tablets and oral suspension are administered twice daily without regard to meals. Oxcarbazepine extended-release tablets are administered once daily on an empty stomach (i.e., at least 1 hour before or 2 hours after a meal). (See Description.) The extended-release tablet should be swallowed whole with water or other liquid, and should not be cut, chewed, or crushed; because of these limitations, the extended-release tablet formulation is not recommended for use in children younger than 6 years of age.

Oxcarbazepine oral suspension should be shaken well immediately prior to administration. The appropriate dose should be administered using the oral dosing syringe supplied by the manufacturer. The oral suspension may be added to a small glass of water or swallowed directly from the syringe. After each use, the oral syringe should be rinsed with warm water and allowed to dry thoroughly.

The oral bioavailability of oxcarbazepine immediate-release tablets appears to be similar to that of the oral suspension and, therefore, these preparations can be used interchangeably on a mg-for-mg basis. At steady state, the extended-release tablets administered once daily are not bioequivalent to the immediate-release tablets administered twice daily; when converting from immediate-release preparations of oxcarbazepine to the extended-release tablets, a higher daily dosage may be required.

Patients currently receiving or beginning therapy with oxcarbazepine and/or any other anticonvulsant for any indication should be closely monitored for the emergence or worsening of depression, suicidal thoughts or behavior (suicidality), and/or any unusual changes in mood or behavior. (See Suicidality Risk under Cautions: Warnings/Precautions.)

Oxcarbazepine therapy should be withdrawn gradually to minimize the potential for increased seizure frequency and status epilepticus.

Pharmacogenetic Testing Because of a strong association between the presence of the variant HLA-B*1502 allele and risk of developing oxcarbazepine-induced Stevens-Johnson syndrome (SJS) and toxic epidermal necrolysis (TEN), pharmacogenetic testing for HLA-B*1502 should be considered prior to initiating oxcarbazepine therapy. (See Pharmacogenomics of Oxcarbazepine-induced Cutaneous Reactions under Warnings/Precautions: Serious Dermatologic Reactions, in Cautions.) The test is considered positive if 1 or 2 copies of HLA-B*1502 are detected and negative if no copies of the variant allele are detected. Patients who test positive for HLA-B*1502 should not be initiated on oxcarbazepine therapy unless the benefits clearly outweigh the risks. Application of HLA-B*1502 genotyping as a screening tool has important limitations and must never substitute for appropriate clinical vigilance and patient management. For additional information and guidance on how to interpret and apply the results of HLA-B*1502 testing, the Clinical Pharmacogenetics Implementation Consortium (CPIC) guideline for HLA genotype and use of carbamazepine and oxcarbazepine should be consulted.

■ **Dosage** ***Partial Seizures*** **Monotherapy.** In adults with partial seizures who are being transferred from other anticonvulsant drug therapy to monotherapy with oxcarbazepine, the recommended initial dosage of oxcarbazepine as conventional preparations is 600 mg daily (administered as 300 mg twice daily). Dosage may be increased in increments of up to 600 mg daily at approximately weekly intervals to the maximum recommended dosage of 2.4 g daily (administered as 1.2 g twice daily), usually within 2–4 weeks. As oxcarbazepine is being initiated, dosage of the other anticonvulsant(s) should be simultaneously reduced and discontinued over 3–6 weeks. Patients should be closely observed during this transition phase.

In adults with partial seizures who are not currently receiving any anticonvulsant drug therapy, the recommended initial dosage of oxcarbazepine as conventional preparations is 600 mg daily (administered as 300 mg twice daily). Dosage should be increased in increments of 300 mg daily every third day to a dosage of 1.2 g daily (administered as 600 mg twice daily).

In children 4–16 years of age with partial seizures who are being transferred from other anticonvulsant drug therapy to monotherapy with oxcarbazepine, the recommended initial dosage of oxcarbazepine as conventional preparations is approximately 8–10 mg/kg daily (administered as 4–5 mg/kg twice daily). Dosage may be increased in increments of up to 10 mg/kg daily at approximately weekly intervals to achieve the recommended maintenance dosage based on weight (see Table 1). As oxcarbazepine is being initiated, dosage of the other anticonvulsant(s) should be simultaneously reduced and discontinued over 3–6 weeks. Patients should be closely observed during this transition phase.

Children 4–16 years of age with partial seizures who are not currently receiving any anticonvulsant drug therapy may initiate oxcarbazepine therapy as conventional preparations at a dosage of 8–10 mg/kg daily (administered as 4–5 mg/kg twice daily). Dosage should be increased in increments of 5 mg/kg daily every third day until the recommended maintenance dosage based on weight is achieved (see Table 1).

Table 1. Recommended Maintenance Dosages in Pediatric Patients Receiving Oxcarbazepine Monotherapy (as Conventional Preparations)

Weight (kg)	Dosage Range
20	600–900 mg daily
25	900 mg to 1.2 g daily
30	900 mg to 1.2 g daily
35	900 mg to 1.5 g daily
40	900 mg to 1.5 g daily
45	1.2–1.5 g daily
50	1.2–1.8 g daily
55	1.2–1.8 g daily
60	1.2–2.1 g daily
65	1.2–2.1 g daily
70	1.5–2.1 g daily

Adjunctive Therapy. For adjunctive therapy of partial seizures in adults, the initial dosage of oxcarbazepine as conventional preparations is 600 mg daily (administered as 300 mg twice daily). Subsequent dosage may be increased in increments of up to 600 mg daily at approximately weekly intervals; the maximum recommended dosage is 1.2 g daily (administered as 600 mg twice daily). Although efficacy was somewhat greater in patients receiving dosages exceeding 1.2 g daily in clinical studies, most patients were not able to tolerate a dosage of 2.4 g daily, mainly because of adverse CNS effects.

If oxcarbazepine extended-release tablets are used for adjunctive therapy of partial seizures in adults, the manufacturer recommends an initial dosage of 600 mg once daily for 1 week. In patients receiving concomitant enzyme-inducing anticonvulsants (e.g., carbamazepine, phenobarbital, phenytoin), a higher initial dosage of 900 mg once daily may be considered. Subsequent dosage may be increased in increments of 600 mg daily at weekly intervals up to the recommended dosage of 1.2–2.4 g once daily. Although efficacy was somewhat greater with a daily dosage of 2.4 g compared with 1.2 g in clinical studies, the higher dosage was associated with an increased incidence of adverse effects.

Dosage requirements for adjunctive oxcarbazepine therapy in pediatric patients may be increased compared with adults because of increased clearance of the drug. (See Pediatric Use under Warnings/Precautions: Specific Populations, in Cautions.) For adjunctive therapy of partial seizures in children 2 to less than 4 years of age, the recommended initial dosage of oxcarbazepine as conventional preparations is 8–10 mg/kg (generally not exceeding 600 mg) daily (administered as 4–5 mg/kg twice daily). For children weighing less than 20 kg, an initial dosage of 16–20 mg/kg daily (administered as 8–10 mg/kg twice daily) may be considered. Dosage should be increased over 2–4 weeks to achieve the maximum maintenance dosage. In clinical trials in children 2–4 years of age, the target dosage was 60 mg/kg daily; however, only 50% of patients reached a final dosage of at least 55 mg/kg daily.

For adjunctive therapy of partial seizures in children 4–16 years of age, the recommended initial dosage of oxcarbazepine as conventional preparations is 8–10 mg/kg (generally not exceeding 600 mg) daily (administered as 4–5 mg/kg twice daily). Dosage should be increased over 2 weeks to the recommended target maintenance dosage based on weight (900 mg daily in children weighing 20–29 kg, 1.2 g daily in children weighing 29.1–39 kg, and 1.8 g daily in children weighing more than 39 kg).

If oxcarbazepine extended-release tablets are used for adjunctive therapy of partial seizures in children 6 years of age or older, the recommended initial dosage is 8–10 mg/kg once daily (not to exceed 600 mg once daily in the first week). Dosage may be increased over 2–3 weeks in increments of 8–10 mg/kg daily at weekly intervals up to the recommended target dosage based on weight (900 mg daily in children weighing 20–29 kg, 1.2 g daily in children weighing 29.1–39 kg, and 1.8 g daily in children weighing more than 39 kg).

Dosage adjustments may be required in patients receiving concomitant therapy with enzyme-inducing drugs. (See Drug Interactions.)

■ **Special Populations** The manufacturers make no specific dosage recommendations for patients with hepatic impairment. Use of oxcarbazepine is not recommended for patients with severe hepatic impairment. (See Hepatic Impairment under Warnings/Precautions: Specific Populations, in Cautions.)

In patients with severe renal impairment (creatinine clearance less than 30 mL/minute), the initial dosage of oxcarbazepine should be reduced to 300 mg daily (given in divided doses twice daily as conventional preparations or once daily as extended-release tablets); dosage should be increased slowly to achieve the desired clinical response. (See Renal Impairment under Warnings/Precautions: Specific Populations, in Cautions.) The manufacturer of oxcarbazepine extended-release tablets recommends that dosage be increased in increments of 300–450 mg daily at weekly intervals in patients with severe renal impairment. Use of conventional oxcarbazepine preparations (instead of the extended-release tablets) is recommended in patients with end-stage renal disease on dialysis.

The manufacturer of conventional oxcarbazepine preparations makes no specific dosage recommendations for geriatric patients. The manufacturer of oxcarbazepine extended-release tablets recommends that a lower initial dosage of 300 or 450 mg daily be considered in geriatric patients, with subsequent dosage increases made in increments of 300–450 mg daily at weekly intervals to achieve the desired response.

Cautions

■ **Contraindications** Known hypersensitivity to oxcarbazepine or any ingredient in the formulation, or to eslicarbazepine acetate.

■ **Warnings/Precautions** ***Hyponatremia*** Clinically important hyponatremia (serum sodium concentrations less than 125 mEq/L) has been reported in 2.5% of patients receiving oxcarbazepine (as conventional preparations) in clinical studies, compared with 0% in patients receiving placebo or active controls (i.e., carbamazepine, phenobarbital, phenytoin, valproic acid). Generally, hyponatremia occurred during the first 3 months of oxcarbazepine therapy, although this adverse effect was reported in some patients more than 1 year after initiation of such therapy. In clinical studies, most patients with hyponatremia were asymptomatic. However, it should be considered that these patients were monitored frequently, and in some patients dosage of oxcarbazepine was reduced or discontinued or the fluid intake restricted. It is not known whether these measures prevented development of hyponatremia. Symptomatic hyponatremia and syndrome of inappropriate antidiuretic hormone secretion (SIADH) were reported in some patients during postmarketing experience with oxcarbazepine. In clinical trials in which patients developed hyponatremia, serum sodium concentrations returned to baseline values a few days after discontinuance of the drug.

The manufacturers state that monitoring serum sodium concentrations should be considered during maintenance therapy with oxcarbazepine, particularly in patients concurrently receiving other drugs known to decrease serum sodium concentrations (e.g., drugs associated with SIADH) or in those with symptoms of hyponatremia (e.g., nausea, malaise, headache, lethargy, confusion, obtundation, increase in seizure frequency or severity).

Serious Dermatologic Reactions Serious and sometimes fatal dermatologic reactions, including Stevens-Johnson syndrome (SJS) and toxic epidermal necrolysis (TEN), have been reported in adults and children receiving oxcarbazepine. The incidence of SJS and TEN in patients receiving oxcarbazepine exceeds the rate in the general population by threefold to tenfold. The median time to onset of these reactions was 19 days after initiation of the drug.

If a skin reaction develops during oxcarbazepine therapy, consideration should be given to discontinuing the drug and initiating an alternative anticonvulsant agent.

Pharmacogenomics of Oxcarbazepine-induced Cutaneous Reactions. Studies have found that the risk of developing SJS and TEN with carbamazepine (a drug that is closely related to oxcarbazepine) is strongly associated with the presence of human leukocyte antigen (HLA)-B*1502, an inherited allelic variant of the HLA-B gene. The HLA-B*1502 allele is found almost exclusively in patients with ancestry across broad areas of Asia, although marked variation exists in its prevalence among specific Asian populations. (See Cautions: Dermatologic and Sensitivity Reactions, in Carbamazepine 28:12.92.) The frequency of this allele ranges from 2–12% in the Han Chinese population to more than 15% in the Philippines and some Malaysian populations; lower frequencies of about 1–6% have been reported in the Korean, Indian, and Japanese populations. HLA-B*1502 is largely absent in individuals not of Asian origin (e.g., Caucasians, African-Americans, Hispanics, Native Americans). Although data are more limited, the available evidence also suggests that the HLA-B*1502 allele is a risk factor for the development of SJS and TEN in patients receiving oxcarbazepine.

The manufacturers recommend that testing for the presence of HLA-B*1502 be considered in patients with ancestry in genetically at-risk populations prior to initiating oxcarbazepine therapy. (See Pharmacogenetic Testing under Dosage and Administration: Administration.) Screening generally is not recommended in populations with low prevalence of HLA-B*1502 or in patients who are currently receiving oxcarbazepine therapy since the risk of SJS and TEN usually develops within the first 4–28 days of therapy, regardless of HLA-B*1502 status. Patients testing positive for HLA-B*1502 should not receive oxcarbazepine therapy unless the benefits clearly outweigh the risks.

Application of HLA genotyping as a screening tool has important limitations and must never substitute for appropriate clinical vigilance and patient management. The role of other possible factors, such as anticonvulsant drug dosage, compliance, concomitant medications and illnesses, in the development of, and morbidity from, these reactions and the level of dermatologic monitoring have not been adequately studied to date.

Suicidality Risk An increased risk of suicidality (suicidal behavior or ideation) was observed in an analysis of studies using various anticonvulsants, including oxcarbazepine, compared with placebo. The analysis of suicidality reports from 199 placebo-controlled studies involving 11 anticonvulsants (i.e., carbamazepine, felbamate, gabapentin, lamotrigine, levetiracetam, oxcarbazepine, pregabalin, tiagabine, topiramate, valproate, and zonisamide) in patients with epilepsy, psychiatric disorders (e.g., bipolar disorder, depression, anxiety), and other conditions (e.g., migraine, neuropathic pain) found that patients receiving anticonvulsants had approximately twice the risk of suicidal behavior or ideation (0.43%) compared with patients receiving placebo (0.24%). This increased suicidality risk was observed as early as one week after beginning therapy and continued through 24 weeks. Although patients treated with an anticonvulsant for epilepsy, psychiatric disorders, and other conditions were all found to have an increased suicidality risk compared with those receiving placebo, the relative suicidality risk was higher for patients with epilepsy compared with those receiving anticonvulsants for other conditions.

Clinicians should inform patients, their families, and caregivers about the potential for an increase in the risk of suicidality with anticonvulsant therapy; all patients currently receiving or beginning therapy with any anticonvulsant for any indication be closely monitored for the emergence or worsening of depression, suicidal thoughts or behavior (suicidality), and/or unusual changes in mood or behavior. Clinicians who prescribe oxcarbazepine or any other anticonvulsant should balance the risk of suicidality with the risk of untreated illness. Epilepsy and many other illnesses for which anticonvulsants are prescribed are themselves associated with an increased risk of morbidity and mortality and an increased risk of suicidal thoughts and behavior. If suicidal thoughts and behavior emerge during anticonvulsant therapy, the clinician should consider whether these symptoms may be related to the illness being treated. (See Advice to Patients.)

Discontinuance of Therapy Because of the possibility of increased seizure frequency and status epilepticus, anticonvulsant drugs, including oxcarbazepine, should be withdrawn gradually. The manufacturer of oxcarbazepine conventional preparations states that if withdrawal is necessary because of a serious adverse event, rapid discontinuance can be considered.

Cognitive and Neuropsychiatric Effects Neuropsychiatric effects reported during oxcarbazepine treatment are classified into 3 categories: impaired cognitive or psychomotor performance including difficulties in concentrating, language, and speech; somnolence or fatigue; and coordination difficulties (e.g., ataxia, gait disturbances).Patients should be monitored for such effects during oxcarbazepine therapy. (See Advice to Patients.)

Hematologic Effects Pancytopenia, agranulocytosis, and leukopenia have been reported rarely during postmarketing experience with oxcarbazepine. Discontinuance of therapy should be considered if such hematologic abnormalities develop.

Seizure Control During Pregnancy Plasma concentrations of the active metabolite of oxcarbazepine may decrease during pregnancy. Patients should be monitored for possible loss of seizure control during pregnancy and throughout the postpartum period. (See Pregnancy under Warnings/Precautions: Specific Populations, in Cautions.)

Risk of Seizure Exacerbation Seizure exacerbation or new-onset primary generalized seizures have been reported during oxcarbazepine therapy; this has been observed particularly in children. If seizure aggravation occurs, oxcarbazepine should be discontinued.

Sensitivity Reactions **Hypersensitivity.** Anaphylaxis and angioedema involving the larynx, glottis, lips, and eyelids, sometimes fatal, have been reported rarely following administration of the first or subsequent doses of oxcarbazepine (as conventional preparations). If anaphylaxis or angioedema occurs during oxcarbazepine therapy, the drug should be discontinued and alternative therapy initiated. Patients who experience these hypersensitivity reactions should not be rechallenged with the drug.

Approximately 25–30% of patients with a history of carbamazepine hypersensitivity will develop hypersensitivity to oxcarbazepine. Oxcarbazepine should only be used in patients with previous hypersensitivity to carbamazepine if the potential benefits outweigh the risks. If a hypersensitivity reaction develops, oxcarbazepine should be discontinued immediately.

Multi-organ Hypersensitivity. Multi-organ hypersensitivity (also known as drug reaction with eosinophilia and systemic symptoms [DRESS]), a potentially fatal or life-threatening reaction, has been reported with oxcarbazepine. The clinical presentation is variable, but typically includes eosinophilia, fever, rash, lymphadenopathy, and/or facial swelling associated with other organ system involvement such as hepatitis, nephritis, hematologic abnormalities, myocarditis, or myositis. However, signs and symptoms associated with other organ systems also may occur.

If manifestations of multi-organ hypersensitivity occur during oxcarbazepine therapy, patients should be evaluated immediately; if an alternative cause cannot be identified, the drug should be discontinued.

Specific Populations **Pregnancy.** Category C. (See Users Guide.)

There are no adequate and well-controlled studies of oxcarbazepine in pregnant women; however, the drug is closely related to carbamazepine, which has been associated with teratogenic effects in humans. Limited data from pregnancy registries suggest that use of oxcarbazepine during pregnancy may be associated with congenital malformations. The drug should be used during pregnancy only if the potential benefit justifies the potential risk to the fetus.

Because of physiologic changes that occur during pregnancy, plasma concentrations of the active metabolite of oxcarbazepine (MHD) may gradually decrease during pregnancy; patients should be monitored during pregnancy and throughout the postpartum period.

Women who are pregnant while receiving oxcarbazepine should be encouraged to enroll in the North American Antiepileptic Drug (NAAED) Pregnancy Registry at 888-233-2334 (for patients); registry information also can be found on the website http://www.aedpregnancyregistry.org.

Lactation. Both oxcarbazepine and its active MHD metabolite are distributed into milk in humans. Because of the potential for serious adverse reactions to oxcarbazepine in nursing infants, a decision should be made whether to discontinue nursing or the drug, taking into account the importance of the drug to the woman.

Pediatric Use. Safety and efficacy of oxcarbazepine conventional preparations as monotherapy of partial seizures have not been established in children younger than 4 years of age.

Safety and efficacy of oxcarbazepine conventional preparations as adjunctive therapy of partial seizures have not been established in children younger than 2 years of age.

Oxcarbazepine extended-release tablets are not recommended for use in children younger than 6 years of age because of administration difficulties and lack of studies in children younger than 4 years of age. (See Dosage and Administration: Administration.)

Clearance of the active MHD metabolite of oxcarbazepine decreases as age and weight increase. In children 2 to younger than 4 years of age, mean weight-adjusted clearance is approximately 80% higher than that of adults. In children 4–12 years of age, mean weight-adjusted clearance is approximately 40% higher than that of adults. In children 13 years of age or older, weight-adjusted MHD clearance is expected to be similar to that of adults.

Oxcarbazepine has been studied as adjunctive therapy and monotherapy for partial seizures in children 1 month to 17 years of age in controlled clinical trials.

As in adults, severe dermatologic and other sensitivity reactions have been reported in pediatric patients.

Geriatric Use. Peak plasma concentrations of MHD and the area under the plasma concentration-time curve (AUC) may be 30–60% higher in geriatric patients 60 years of age or older than in younger adults (possibly related to decreases in renal function with age).

Close monitoring of serum sodium concentrations is recommended in geriatric patients at risk for hyponatremia.

Hepatic Impairment. In patients with mild to moderate hepatic impairment, the pharmacokinetics of oxcarbazepine and its active MHD metabolite were unaffected based on studies with immediate-release oxcarbazepine.

Renal Impairment. In patients with renal impairment (creatinine clearance less than 30 mL/min), half-life of the active MHD metabolite of oxcarbazepine is increased to 19 hours and systemic exposure is increased twofold based on studies with immediate-release formulations of the drug. Dosage modification is necessary in patients with renal impairment. (See Dosage and Administration: Special Populations.)

■ **Common Adverse Effects** Adverse effects occurring in 10% or more of patients receiving conventional oxcarbazepine include dizziness, somnolence, diplopia, fatigue, nausea, vomiting, ataxia, abnormal vision, abdominal pain, nystagmus, tremor, dyspepsia, and abnormal gait.

Adverse effects occurring in 5% or more of patients receiving oxcarbazepine extended-release tablets include dizziness, somnolence, headache, balance disorder, tremor, vomiting, diplopia, asthenia, and fatigue.

Drug Interactions

■ **Drugs Affecting or Metabolized by Hepatic Microsomal Enzymes** In vitro studies indicate that oxcarbazepine and its active MHD metabolite can inhibit cytochrome P-450 (CYP) isoenzyme 2C19 and can therefore potentially increase plasma concentrations of drugs metabolized by this isoenzyme. Oxcarbazepine and MHD do not appear to inhibit other CYP isoenzymes, including CYP3A4/5, 1A2, 2A6, 2C9, 2D6, 2E1, 4A9, and 4A11, at clinically relevant concentrations.

In vitro studies indicate that oxcarbazepine can induce CYP3A4/5 and can therefore potentially reduce plasma concentrations of drugs metabolized by this isoenzyme (e.g., dihydropyridine calcium-channel blocking agents, oral contraceptives, cyclosporine).

Potent inducers of CYP3A4 (e.g., carbamazepine, phenytoin, phenobarbital, rifampin) may decrease plasma concentrations of MHD. If oxcarbazepine is used concomitantly with a potent CYP3A4 inducer, the manufacturer recommends that plasma MHD concentrations be monitored during titration of oxcarbazepine therapy; dosage adjustment of oxcarbazepine may be required when initiating, discontinuing, or modifying dosage of potent CYP3A4 inducers.

■ **Drugs Affecting or Metabolized by Uridine Diphosphate Glucuronosyltransferase** In vitro studies indicate that MHD exhibits only weak induction of uridine diphosphate glucuronosyltransferase (UGT) and is therefore not likely to interact with drugs that are metabolized by UGT (e.g., valproic acid, lamotrigine).

Potent inducers of UGT may decrease plasma concentrations of MHD. If oxcarbazepine is used concomitantly with a potent UGT inducer, the manufacturer recommends that plasma MHD concentrations be monitored during titration of oxcarbazepine therapy; dosage adjustment of oxcarbazepine may be required when initiating, discontinuing, or modifying dosage of potent UGT inducers.

■ **Drugs Associated with Stevens-Johnson Syndrome and Toxic Epidermal Necrolysis** Because of the risk of Stevens-Johnson syndrome and toxic epidermal necrolysis in HLA-B*1502-positive patients receiving oxcarbazepine, avoidance of other drugs associated with these serious dermatologic reactions should be considered in such patients when alternative therapies are available.

■ **Alcohol** Additive sedative effects may occur with concomitant use of alcohol and oxcarbazepine. Caution is advised.

■ **Anticonvulsants** CYP-inducing anticonvulsants (e.g., carbamazepine, phenytoin, phenobarbital) may decrease plasma concentrations of MHD. In clinical studies, MHD concentrations were decreased by approximately 40, 25, or 30% with concomitant administration of carbamazepine, phenobarbital, or phenytoin, respectively. Dosage adjustments may be necessary. Oxcarbazepine dosages exceeding 1.2 g daily have been shown to increase plasma phenytoin concentrations by up to 40%; dosage reduction of phenytoin may be necessary.

With regard to other anticonvulsants evaluated, lamotrigine did not affect plasma MHD concentrations and valproic acid reduced plasma MHD concentrations by only 18%.

■ **Calcium-channel Blocking Agents** Concomitant administration of oxcarbazepine and felodipine resulted in a 28% decrease in systemic exposure of felodipine.

Concomitant administration of oxcarbazepine and verapamil resulted in a 20% decrease in plasma concentrations of MHD.

■ **Cimetidine** When cimetidine and oxcarbazepine were administered concomitantly, no effect on the pharmacokinetics of MHD was observed.

■ **Erythromycin** When erythromycin and oxcarbazepine were administered concomitantly, no effect on the pharmacokinetics of MHD was observed.

■ **Oral Contraceptives** Oxcarbazepine may reduce the efficacy of hormonal contraceptives. When oxcarbazepine was administered concomitantly with an oral contraceptive, systemic exposures of the estrogen and progestin components were decreased by 48–52 and 32–52%, respectively. Women of childbearing potential should use additional nonhormonal methods of contraception during oxcarbazepine therapy.

■ **Protein-bound Drugs** Clinically important interactions are not likely to occur when oxcarbazepine is administered concomitantly with protein-bound drugs.

■ **Warfarin** An interaction between oxcarbazepine and warfarin is not likely.

Description

Oxcarbazepine is an anticonvulsant agent that is structurally and chemically related to carbamazepine. Although the exact mechanism of action of oxcarbazepine is unknown, in vitro electrophysiologic studies indicate that the drug may stabilize excitatory neuronal membranes, inhibit repetitive neuronal firing, and decrease propagation of synaptic impulses by blocking voltage-sensitive sodium channels, actions that may prevent spread of epileptic seizures. Increased potassium conductance and modulation of high-voltage activated calcium channels also may contribute to the anticonvulsant activity of oxcarbazepine. No substantial interactions between the drug and neurotransmitter receptors in the brain have been observed to date.

Oxcarbazepine and its active 10-monohydroxy metabolite (MHD [10,11-dihydro-10-hydroxy-5*H*-dibenz[*b*, *f*]azepine-5-carboxamide]) exhibit anticonvulsant activity in several animal seizure models. Oxcarbazepine protects against electrically induced tonic extension seizures and, to a lesser degree, chemically induced clonic seizures and may abolish or reduce frequency of chronically recurring focal seizures.

Following oral administration, oxcarbazepine is completely absorbed and extensively metabolized in the liver by cytosolic enzymes to MHD, which is believed to be responsible for the pharmacologic activity of oxcarbazepine. Food does not affect the rate or extent of absorption of the immediate-release tablets; although not specifically studied, food is also not expected to alter bioavailability of the oral suspension. Administration of oxcarbazepine extended-release tablets with a high-fat meal increased peak plasma concentrations of MHD by about 60%.

The oral bioavailabilities of oxcarbazepine immediate-release tablets and oral suspension appear to be similar; however, the extended-release tablets (administered once daily) are not bioequivalent to the same total daily dose of the immediate-release formulation (administered twice daily). More than 95% of an oral dose of oxcarbazepine is excreted in urine, mainly as metabolites with less than 1% as unchanged drug; less than 4% is excreted in feces.

Advice to Patients

Importance of advising patients to read the patient information (medication guide).

Risk of hypersensitivity reaction; patients who have had previous hypersensitivity reaction to carbamazepine at increased risk. Importance of immediately reporting any manifestations of hypersensitivity reactions (swelling of the face, eyes, lips, or tongue, or difficulty swallowing or breathing), skin reactions, or fever accompanied by signs and/or symptoms of other organ system involvement (e.g., rash, lymphadenopathy).

Risk of dizziness and somnolence; avoid driving or operating machinery while taking oxcarbazepine until effects of the drug on the individual are known.

Risk of hematologic effects; importance of advising patients to immediately report any manifestations suggestive of a blood disorder.

Risk of hyponatremia; manifestations may include nausea, extreme drowsiness and/or fatigue, lack of energy, headache, confusion, or increase in seizure frequency or severity.

Importance of patients, family members, and caregivers being aware that anticonvulsants, including oxcarbazepine, may increase the risk of having suicidal thoughts or actions in a very small number of people (about 1 in 500). Advise patients, family members, and caregivers to pay close attention to any day-to-day changes in mood, behavior, and actions; these changes can happen very quickly. They should also be aware of common warning signs that may signal suicide risk (e.g., talking or thinking about wanting to hurt oneself or end one's life, withdrawing from friends and family, becoming depressed or experiencing worsening of existing depression, becoming preoccupied with death and dying, giving away prized possessions). Advise patients, family members, and caregivers to contact the responsible clinician immediately if these or any new and worrisome behaviors occur.

Caution if alcohol is used concomitantly because additive sedative effects may occur.

Importance of taking oxcarbazepine as prescribed and not abruptly discontinuing therapy.

Importance of women informing clinicians if they are or plan to become pregnant or plan to breast-feed. Importance of informing women of childbearing age that concomitant use of oxcarbazepine with oral contraceptives may result in decreased efficacy of the contraceptives.

Importance of informing clinicians of existing or contemplated concomitant therapy, including prescription and OTC drugs, as well as concomitant illnesses.

Importance of advising patients of other important precautionary information. (See Cautions.)

Overview® (see Users Guide). For additional information on this drug until a more detailed monograph is developed and published, the manufacturer's labeling should be consulted. It is *essential* that the manufacturer's labeling be consulted for more detailed information on usual cautions, precautions, contraindications, potential drug interactions, laboratory test interferences, and acute toxicity.

Preparations

Excipients in commercially available drug preparations may have clinically important effects in some individuals; consult specific product labeling for details.

OXcarbazepine

Oral		
Suspension	300 mg/5 mL*	**OXcarbazepine Oral Suspension**
		Trileptal®, Novartis
Tablets, extended-release	150 mg	**Oxtellar XR®**, Supernus
	300 mg	**Oxtellar XR®**, Supernus
	600 mg	**Oxtellar XR®**, Supernus
Tablets, film-coated	150 mg*	**OXcarbazepine Tablets**
		Trileptal® (scored), Novartis
	300 mg*	**OXcarbazepine Tablets**
		Trileptal® (scored), Novartis
	600 mg*	**OXcarbazepine Tablets**
		Trileptal® (scored), Novartis

*available from one or more manufacturer, distributor, and/or repackager by generic (nonproprietary) name

†Use is not currently included in the labeling approved by the US Food and Drug Administration

Pregabalin

■ Pregabalin is an anticonvulsant structurally related to the inhibitory CNS neurotransmitter γ-aminobutyric acid (GABA); the drug also possesses analgesic activity.

Uses

■ **Seizure Disorders** Pregabalin is used in combination with other anticonvulsant agents in the management of partial seizures in adults.

Efficacy of pregabalin as adjunctive therapy was established in three 12-week, multicenter, randomized, double-blind, placebo-controlled studies in adults who had refractory partial onset seizures with or without secondary generalization while receiving a regimen of 1–3 anticonvulsants, and had experienced at least 6 partial seizures (with no seizure-free period exceeding 4 weeks) during an 8-week baseline period. In these studies, patients receiving pregabalin 150, 300, or 600 mg daily (administered in 2 or 3 divided doses) experienced a median decrease in seizure frequency of 17–35, 37, or 36–51%, respectively, while those receiving placebo experienced no appreciable change in seizure frequency. In one study, 15, 31, 40, or 51% of patients receiving pregabalin 50, 150, 300, or 600 mg daily, respectively, and 14% of those receiving placebo experienced at least a 50% reduction in seizure frequency; in another study, 43 or 49% of those receiving pregabalin 600 mg daily in 2 or 3 divided doses, respectively, and 9% of those receiving placebo experienced at least a 50% reduction in seizure frequency.

■ **Neuropathic Pain** ***Postherpetic Neuralgia*** Pregabalin is used for the management of postherpetic neuralgia (PHN) in adults.

Efficacy of pregabalin in postherpetic neuralgia has been established in 3 multicenter, double-blind, placebo-controlled studies in adults with neuralgia persisting for at least 3 months following healing of herpes zoster rash. In these studies, mean pain scores (assessed on an 11-point numerical rating scale) at the end of 8 or 13 weeks of treatment were improved in patients receiving pregabalin compared with those receiving placebo; in addition, a greater proportion of patients receiving pregabalin, compared with those receiving placebo, achieved at least a 50% reduction (improvement) in pain score from baseline. In these studies, pregabalin was administered at dosages of 150 or 300 mg daily in patients with renal impairment (i.e., creatinine clearance of 30–60 mL/minute) and at dosages of 150, 300, or 600 mg daily in patients with normal renal function (i.e., creatinine clearance greater than 60 mL/minute).

Diabetic Neuropathy Pregabalin is used for the management of pain associated with diabetic peripheral neuropathy (DPN) in adults.

Efficacy of pregabalin for the management of diabetic peripheral neuropathy has been established in 3 multicenter, double-blind, placebo-controlled studies in adults with type 1 or 2 diabetes mellitus and painful distal symmetrical sensorimotor polyneuropathy of 1–5 years' duration. In 2 studies that excluded patients with renal impairment (i.e., creatinine clearance of 60 mL/minute or less), treatment with pregabalin 300 mg daily (given in 3 divided doses) for 5 or 8 weeks improved the mean pain score (assessed on an 11-point numeric rating scale) compared with placebo; in addition, a greater proportion of patients receiving pregabalin 300 mg daily, compared with those receiving placebo, achieved at least a 50% reduction (improvement) in pain score from baseline. One of these studies also evaluated pregabalin at dosages of 75 and 600 mg daily. The 600-mg daily dosage did not provide additional benefit, but was associated with an increased risk of dose-dependent adverse effects when compared with the 300-mg daily dosage. The 75-mg daily dosage was not effective.

■ **Fibromyalgia** Pregabalin is used for the management of fibromyalgia in adults.

Efficacy of pregabalin for the management of fibromyalgia has been established in one 14-week multicenter, randomized, double-blind, placebo-controlled study and in one 6-month, randomized, withdrawal study in adults with a diagnosis of fibromyalgia based on the American College of Rheumatology (ACR) classification criteria (i.e., history of widespread pain for 3 months and pain present at 11 or more of the 18 specific tender point sites). In the 14-week study, treatment with pregabalin 300, 450, or 600 mg daily (administered in 2 divided doses) improved the mean end-of-treatment pain score (assessed on an 11-point numeric rating scale) compared with placebo; in addition, a greater proportion of patients receiving pregabalin at all 3 dosages, compared with those receiving placebo, achieved at least a 30 and 50% reduction (improvement) in pain score from baseline. However, the 600-mg daily dosage did not appear to provide additional improvement in pain scores when compared with the 450-mg daily dosage, but dose-dependent adverse effects were observed.

In the 6-month withdrawal study, patients who responded to treatment with pregabalin 300, 450, or 600 mg daily (i.e., at least 50% reduction in open-label baseline visual analog scale [VAS] pain score and a self-rating of overall improvement on the Patient Global Impression of Change [PGIC] scale of "much improved" or "very much improved") following a 6-week, open-label, dose optimization period were randomized to the 26-week, double-blind treatment period to remain on their optimal pregabalin dosage or receive placebo. In the double-blind treatment period, patients receiving pregabalin had a longer time to loss of therapeutic response (i.e., less than 30% reduction in pain score from open-label baseline at 2 consecutive visits during the double-blind period or worsening of fibromyalgia symptoms requiring alternate treatment) than did those receiving placebo.

Dosage and Administration

■ **Administration** Pregabalin capsules and oral solution are administered orally without regard to meals. If pregabalin is discontinued, dosage should be tapered gradually over at least 1 week.

Pregabalin oral solution should be used within 45 days of first opening the bottle.

Patients currently receiving or beginning therapy with pregabalin and/or any other anticonvulsant for any indication should be closely monitored for the emergence or worsening of depression, suicidal thoughts or behavior (suicidality), and/or any unusual changes in mood or behavior. (See Suicidality Risk under Cautions: Warnings/Precautions.)

■ **Dosage** Pregabalin oral solution contains 20 mg of pregabalin per milliliter and prescriptions should be written in milligrams (mg). The pharmacist should calculate the applicable dose in mL for dispensing (e.g., 150 mg equals 7.5 mL of oral solution).

Seizure Disorders For adjunctive therapy in the management of partial seizures in adults, the effective dosage of pregabalin is 150–600 mg daily administered in 2 or 3 divided doses. Pregabalin therapy generally is initiated at a dosage of 75 mg twice daily or 50 mg 3 times daily (initial dosage not to exceed 150 mg daily); based on individual patient response and tolerability, dosage may be increased to a maximum dosage of 600 mg daily.

Both the efficacy and adverse effects of pregabalin are dose related, but the effect of dosage escalation rate on the tolerability of the drug has not been specifically studied.

Dosage recommendations for use of pregabalin in conjunction with gabapentin are not available, because such regimens have not been evaluated in controlled clinical studies.

Neuropathic Pain **Postherpetic Neuralgia.** For the management of postherpetic neuralgia (PHN) in adults, the recommended dosage of pregabalin is 150–300 mg daily administered in 2 or 3 divided doses. Pregabalin therapy generally is initiated at a dosage of 150 mg daily (75 mg twice daily or 50 mg 3 times daily); dosage may be increased to 300 mg daily within 1 week based on efficacy and tolerability.

Patients who tolerate the drug but do not experience adequate pain relief following 2–4 weeks of treatment with pregabalin 300 mg daily may receive dosages of up to 600 mg daily administered in 2 or 3 divided doses. Dosages exceeding 300 mg daily should be reserved for patients who have continuing pain and are tolerating the 300-mg daily dosage because of the potential for dose-dependent adverse effects and higher rates of treatment discontinuance secondary to adverse effects.

Diabetic Neuropathy. For the management of pain associated with diabetic peripheral neuropathy (DPN) in adults, the initial dosage of pregabalin is 150 mg daily administered in 3 divided doses; dosage may be increased within 1 week based on efficacy and tolerability to the maximum recommended dosage of 300 mg daily administered in 3 divided doses. Clinical studies in patients with DPN indicate that higher pregabalin dosages (i.e., 600 mg daily) provide no additional benefit but may increase the risk of adverse effects.

Fibromyalgia For the management of fibromyalgia in adults, the recommended dosage of pregabalin is 300–450 mg daily. Pregabalin therapy generally is initiated at a dosage of 150 mg daily (75 mg twice daily); dosage may be increased to 300 mg daily (150 mg twice daily) within 1 week based on efficacy and tolerability. Patients who do not experience adequate benefit with pregabalin 300 mg daily may have dosage further increased to the maximum recommended dosage of 450 mg daily (225 mg twice daily). Clinical studies in patients with fibromyalgia indicate that higher pregabalin dosages (i.e., 600 mg daily) provide no additional benefit but may increase the risk of adverse effects.

■ **Special Populations** In patients with renal impairment (creatinine clearance of less than 60 mL/minute), dosage of pregabalin should be modified based on creatinine clearance (see Table 1).

Table 1. Pregabalin Dosage Adjustment in Patients with Renal Impairment

Usual Dosage Regimen (for Patients with Creatinine Clearances of ≥60 mL/min)	Creatinine Clearance (mL/min)	Adjusted Dosage Regimen
150 mg daily given in 2 or 3 divided doses	30–60	75 mg daily given in 2 or 3 divided doses
	15–30	25–50 mg daily given as a single dose or in 2 divided doses
	<15	25 mg once daily
300 mg daily given in 2 or 3 divided doses	30–60	150 mg daily given in 2 or 3 divided doses
	15–30	75 mg daily given as a single dose or in 2 divided doses
	<15	25–50 mg once daily
450 mg daily given in 2 or 3 divided doses	30–60	225 mg daily given in 2 or 3 divided doses
	15–30	100–150 mg daily given as a single dose or in 2 divided doses
	<15	50–75 mg once daily
600 mg daily given in 2 or 3 divided doses	30–60	300 mg daily given in 2 or 3 divided doses
	15–30	150 mg daily given as a single dose or in 2 divided doses
	<15	75 mg once daily

Because pregabalin is removed by hemodialysis, the manufacturer recommends that, in addition to the adjusted daily dosage, patients undergoing hemodialysis receive a supplemental dose of the drug immediately following each 4-hour dialysis session. Individuals receiving the 25-mg once daily dosage regimen should receive a supplemental dose of 25 or 50 mg, those receiving the 25- to 50-mg once daily dosage regimen should receive a supplemental dose of 50 or 75 mg, those receiving the 50- to 75-mg once daily dosage regimen should receive a supplemental dose of 75 or 100 mg, and those receiving the 75-mg once daily dosage regimen should receive a supplemental dose of 100 or 150 mg.

Cautions

■ **Contraindications** Known hypersensitivity to pregabalin or any ingredient in the formulation.

■ **Warnings/Precautions** ***Angioedema*** Angioedema, including life-threatening angioedema with respiratory compromise requiring emergency treatment, has been reported during postmarketing surveillance in patients receiving initial and chronic pregabalin therapy. Specific symptoms included swelling of the face, mouth (e.g., tongue, lips, gums), and neck (e.g., throat, larynx). Pregabalin should be immediately discontinued in patients with these symptoms.

Caution should be exercised when using pregabalin in patients who have had a previous episode of angioedema. In addition, patients who are using other drugs associated with angioedema (e.g., angiotensin-converting enzyme [ACE] inhibitors) may be at increased risk of developing angioedema.

Hypersensitivity Reactions Hypersensitivity reactions (i.e., skin redness, blisters, hives, rash, dyspnea, wheezing) have been reported during postmarketing surveillance in patients shortly after initiation of pregabalin therapy. Pregabalin should be immediately discontinued in patients with these symptoms.

Discontinuance, Abuse Potential, and Dependence Because of the possibility of increased seizure frequency, anticonvulsant drugs, including pregabalin, should be withdrawn gradually and dosage reduced slowly over at least 1 week. In clinical studies, abrupt or rapid discontinuance of pregabalin has been associated with insomnia, nausea, headache, or diarrhea, suggestive of physical dependence.

In controlled clinical studies, 4 or 1% of patients receiving pregabalin or placebo, respectively, reported euphoria as an adverse event, although in some patient populations studied, this rate of euphoria was higher and ranged from 1–12%.

Pregabalin is not known to be active at receptor sites associated with drugs of abuse. However, the Drug Enforcement Administration (DEA) has placed pregabalin into schedule V of the Federal Controlled Substances Act (CSA) of 1970 subsequent to a recommendation for control from the Department of Health and Human Services (DHHS).

As with any CNS active drug, clinicians should carefully evaluate patients for history of drug abuse and observe them for signs of pregabalin misuse or abuse (e.g., development of tolerance, dose escalation, drug-seeking behavior).

Suicidality Risk The US Food and Drug Administration (FDA) has alerted healthcare professionals about an increased risk of suicidality (suicidal behavior or ideation) observed in an analysis of studies using various anticonvulsants, including pregabalin, compared with placebo. The analysis of suicidality reports from placebo-controlled studies involving 11 anticonvulsants (i.e., carbamazepine, felbamate, gabapentin, lamotrigine, levetiracetam, oxcarbazepine, pregabalin, tiagabine, topiramate, valproate, zonisamide) in patients with epilepsy, psychiatric disorders (e.g., bipolar disorder, depression, anxiety), and other conditions (e.g., migraine, neuropathic pain) found that patients receiving anticonvulsants had approximately twice the risk of suicidal behavior or ideation (0.43%) compared with patients receiving placebo (0.24%). This increased suicidality risk was observed as early as one week after beginning therapy and continued through 24 weeks. Although patients treated with an anticonvulsant for epilepsy, psychiatric disorders, and other conditions were all found to have an increased suicidality risk compared with those receiving placebo, the relative suicidality risk was higher for patients with epilepsy compared to those receiving anticonvulsants for other conditions.

Based on the current analysis of the available data, FDA recommends that clinicians inform patients, their families, and caregivers of the potential for an increased risk of suicidality with anticonvulsant therapy and that all patients currently receiving or beginning therapy with any anticonvulsant be closely monitored for notable changes that may indicate the emergence or worsening of suicidal thoughts or behavior or depression. Symptoms such as anxiety, agitation, aggression, hostility, mania, and insomnia may be precursors to emerging suicidality.

Clinicians who prescribe pregabalin or any other anticonvulsant should balance the risk of suicidality with the risk of untreated illness. Epilepsy and many other illnesses for which anticonvulsants are prescribed are themselves associated with morbidity and mortality and an increased risk of suicidal thoughts and behavior. If suicidal thoughts or behavior emerge during anticonvulsant therapy, the clinician should consider whether these symptoms may be related to the illness being treated. (See Advice to Patients.)

Peripheral Edema Pregabalin may cause peripheral edema. In short-term clinical trials of patients without clinically important cardiac or peripheral vascular disease, there was no apparent association between peripheral edema and cardiovascular complications (e.g., hypertension, congestive heart failure). Peripheral edema was not associated with deterioration of renal or hepatic function.

Concomitant use of pregabalin with a thiazolidinedione antidiabetic agent has been associated with a greater risk of developing weight gain and peripheral edema than either drug alone.

Because there are limited data regarding use of pregabalin in patients with New York Heart Association (NYHA) class III or IV congestive heart failure, the drug should be used with caution in these patients.

Dizziness and Somnolence Pregabalin may cause dizziness and somnolence. In controlled studies, 31 or 22% of patients who received pregabalin experienced dizziness or somnolence, respectively, compared with 9 or 7% of those receiving placebo, respectively. In controlled studies, dizziness and somnolence were the most frequent adverse effects requiring discontinuance of the drug (each in 4% of patients).

Weight Gain Pregabalin may cause weight gain. Pregabalin-associated weight gain appeared to be related to dosage and duration of exposure; however, weight gain did not appear to be associated with baseline body mass index (BMI), gender, or age and was not limited to patients with edema.

Although weight gain was not associated with clinically important changes in blood pressure in short-term controlled studies, the long-term cardiovascular effects of such weight gain have not been elucidated. In addition, while the effects of pregabalin-associated weight gain on glycemic control have not been systematically assessed in controlled and longer-term open label clinical trials in diabetic patients, pregabalin therapy did not appear to be associated with loss of glycemic control.

Carcinogenicity Carcinogenicity (e.g., hemangiosarcoma) has been demonstrated in animals.

In clinical studies across various patient populations, comprising 6396 patient-years of exposure in those 12 years of age or older, new or worsening-preexisting tumors were reported in 57 patients; however, a causal relationship to the drug has not been established.

Ocular Effects In controlled studies, blurred vision, which was reported in 7 or 2% of patients receiving pregabalin or placebo, respectively, resolved in the majority of cases with continued dosing; less than 1% of patients required discontinuance of the drug. In addition, decreased visual acuity was reported in 7 or 5% of patients receiving pregabalin or placebo, respectively, while visual field changes were detected in 13 or 12% of patients receiving the drug or placebo, respectively, and funduscopic changes were observed in 2% of patients receiving pregabalin or placebo. The clinical importance of these ophthalmologic findings has not been elucidated.

If visual disturbance persists, further ocular assessment should be considered, while more frequent assessment is recommended in patients who already are monitored for ocular conditions.

Creatine Kinase Elevations In clinical trials, increases in serum creatinine kinase (CK, creatine phosphokinase, CPK) concentrations at least 3 times the upper limit of normal have been reported in 1.5 or 0.7% of patients receiving pregabalin or placebo, respectively.

Rhabdomyolysis has been reported rarely in premarketing clinical trials. However, a definite causal relationship between these musculoskeletal effects and the drug has not been fully elucidated because the cases had documented factors that may have caused or contributed to these events.

Pregabalin treatment should be discontinued if myopathy is diagnosed or suspected or if markedly elevated CK (CPK) concentrations occur.

Thrombocytopenia In controlled clinical trials, potentially clinically important decreases in platelet count (thrombocytopenia; defined as 20% below baseline value and less than 150,000/mm^3) have been reported in 3 or 2% of patients receiving pregabalin or placebo, respectively. Pregabalin-treated patients experienced a mean maximal decrease in platelet count of 20,000/mm^3 compared with 11,000/mm^3 in placebo-treated patients. Severe thrombocytopenia with a platelet count less than 20,000/mm^3 has been reported in at least one patient who received pregabalin. In randomized controlled trials, pregabalin was not associated with an increase in bleeding-related adverse effects.

PR Interval Prolongation Prolongation of the PR interval (mean increase: 3–6 msec) has been reported in patients receiving pregabalin dosages of at least 300 mg daily. Subgroup analyses in a limited number of patients suggest that those with preexisting PR prolongation at baseline or those receiving drugs that prolong the PR interval do not appear to have an increased risk for developing prolongation of the PR interval.

Specific Populations **Pregnancy.** Category C. (See Users Guide.)

North American Antiepileptic Drug (NAAED) Pregnancy Registry at 888-233-2334 (for patients); registry information also available on the website http://www.aedpregnancyregistry.org/.

The effect of pregabalin on labor and delivery is not known.

Lactation. It is not known whether pregabalin is distributed into human milk. Pregabalin is distributed into milk in rats. Because many drugs are distributed into human milk, and because of the potential for tumorigenicity shown for pregabalin in animal studies, a decision should be made whether to discontinue nursing or the drug, taking into account the importance of the drug to the woman.

Pediatric Use. Safety and efficacy not established in children younger than 18 years of age.

Geriatric Use. No substantial differences in safety and efficacy relative to younger adults. However, in controlled clinical studies of patients with fibromyalgia, neurological adverse reactions including dizziness, blurred vision, balance disorder, tremor, confusional state, abnormal coordination, and lethargy occurred more frequently in patients 65 years of age and older than in younger adults.

It should be considered that pregabalin is substantially excreted by the kidneys, and the risk of severe adverse reactions to the drug may be increased in patients with impaired renal function. The dosage should be adjusted for geriatric patients with renal impairment. (See Dosage and Administration: Special Populations.)

Renal Impairment. In patients with renal impairment (e.g., those with creatinine clearances of less than 60 mL/minute), dosage of pregabalin should be modified according to the degree of renal impairment. Pregabalin is removed from plasma by hemodialysis. Plasma pregabalin concentrations are reduced by approximately 50% following a 4-hour hemodialysis treatment. (See Dosage and Administration: Special Populations.)

■ **Common Adverse Effects** Adverse effects reported in 2% or more of patients receiving pregabalin in combination with other anticonvulsant agents in the management of partial seizures include dizziness, somnolence, ataxia, abnormal thinking, tremor, confusion, twitching, myoclonus, amnesia, speech disorder, incoordination, abnormal gait, dry mouth, constipation, increased appetite, weight gain, peripheral edema, blurred vision, diplopia, abnormal vision, accidental injury, and pain.

Adverse effects reported in 2% or more of patients receiving pregabalin for the management of postherpetic neuralgia (PHN) include dizziness, somnolence, headache, confusion, abnormal thinking, ataxia, incoordination, amnesia, abnormal gait, dry mouth, constipation, flatulence, vomiting, weight gain, peripheral edema, edema, facial edema, blurry vision, diplopia, abnormal vision, infection, flu syndrome, accidental injury, and pain.

Adverse effects reported in 2% or more of patients receiving pregabalin for the management of pain associated with diabetic peripheral neuropathy (DPN) include dizziness, somnolence, asthenia, neuropathy, ataxia, vertigo, abnormal thinking, confusion, euphoria, incoordination, dry mouth, constipation, flatulence, weight gain, peripheral edema, edema, hypoglycemia, accidental injury, back pain, chest pain, blurry vision, and dyspnea.

Adverse effects reported in 2% or more of patients receiving pregabalin for the management of fibromyalgia include dizziness, somnolence, headache, euphoric mood, attention disturbance, balance disorder, memory impairment, confusional state, abnormal coordination, hypoaesthesia, lethargy, tremor, anxiety, disorientation, depression, dry mouth, constipation, vomiting, flatulence, abdominal distention, weight gain, fatigue, peripheral edema, chest pain, abnormal feeling, edema, fluid retention, drunk feeling, increased appetite, blurred vision, sinusitis, vertigo, pharyngolaryngeal pain, arthralgia, muscle spasms, back pain.

Drug Interactions

■ **Drugs Affecting Hepatic Microsomal Enzymes** Based on results of in vitro studies, pregabalin does not appear to inhibit cytochrome P-450 (CYP) isoenzymes 1A2, 2A6, 2C9, 2C19, 2D6, 2E1, and 3A4 or induce CYP1A2 or CYP3A4. The manufacturer states that an increase in metabolism of concomitantly administered CYP1A2 substrates (e.g., caffeine, theophylline) or CYP3A4 substrates (e.g., midazolam, testosterone) is not anticipated.

Since pregabalin undergoes negligible metabolism in humans, pharmacokinetics of the drug are unlikely to be affected by other agents through metabolic interactions.

■ **Protein-bound Drugs** Because pregabalin does not bind to plasma proteins, a pharmacokinetic interaction with drugs that are highly protein bound is unlikely.

■ **Alcohol** Pharmacokinetic interaction unlikely. Potential pharmacologic interaction (e.g., additive effects on cognitive and gross motor functioning); no clinically important effects on respiration.

■ **Angiotensin-converting Enzyme Inhibitors** Potential pharmacologic interaction with angiotensin-converting enzyme (ACE) inhibitors (e.g., increased risk of developing angioedema).

■ **Anticonvulsants** Pharmacokinetic interaction unlikely with anticonvulsants (e.g., phenytoin, carbamazepine, valproate, lamotrigine, phenobarbital, topiramate).

Concomitant administration of gabapentin with pregabalin did not alter pharmacokinetics of gabapentin although the rate, but not the extent, of absorption of pregabalin was decreased slightly.

Tiagabine does not appear to affect the pharmacokinetics of pregabalin.

■ **Antidiabetic Agents** Glyburide, insulin, and metformin do not appear to affect the pharmacokinetics of pregabalin.

Potential pharmacologic interaction with thiazolidinediones (e.g., increased risk of weight gain and peripheral edema).

■ **CNS Depressants** Potential pharmacologic interaction (e.g., additive CNS depressant effects) with concurrent administration of CNS depressants, including opiates and benzodiazepines.

■ **Furosemide** Furosemide does not appear to affect the pharmacokinetics of pregabalin.

■ **Lorazepam** Pharmacokinetic interaction unlikely. Potential pharmacologic interaction (e.g., additive effects on cognitive and gross motor functioning); no clinically important effects on respiration.

■ **Oral Contraceptives** Pharmacokinetic interaction unlikely.

■ **Oxycodone** Pharmacokinetic interaction unlikely. Potential pharmacologic interaction (e.g., additive effects on cognitive and gross motor functioning); no clinically important effects on respiration.

Description

Pregabalin is an anticonvulsant that is structurally related to the inhibitory CNS neurotransmitter γ-aminobutyric acid (GABA). Pregabalin also has demonstrated analgesic activity. Although pregabalin was developed as a structural analog of GABA, the drug does not bind directly to $GABA_A$, $GABA_B$, or benzodiazepine receptors; does not augment $GABA_A$ responses in cultured neurons; and does not alter brain concentrations of GABA in rats or affect GABA uptake or degradation. However, in cultured neurons, prolonged application of pregabalin increases the density of GABA transporter protein and increases the rate of functional GABA transport.

Pregabalin binds with high affinity to the α_2-δ site (an auxiliary subunit of voltage-gated calcium channels) in CNS tissues. Although the exact mechanism of action of pregabalin has not been elucidated, binding to the α_2-δ subunit may be involved in pregabalin's analgesic and anticonvulsant effects. In vitro, pregabalin reduces the calcium-dependent release of several neurotransmitters, including glutamate, norepinephrine, calcitonin gene-related peptide, and substance P, possibly by modulation of calcium channel function.

Pregabalin is not appreciably metabolized. Following administration of a single radiolabeled dose of pregabalin, approximately 90% of the administered dose was recovered in urine as unchanged drug.

Advice to Patients

Importance of adhering to prescribed directions for use and not altering the anticonvulsant regimen without first consulting with the clinician. Importance of providing copy of written patient information (medication guide) each time pregabalin is dispensed, and importance of reading this information prior to taking pregabalin.

Importance of patients, family members, and caregivers being aware that anticonvulsants, including pregabalin, may increase the risk of having suicidal thoughts or actions in a very small number of people (about 1 in 500). Advise patients, family members, and caregivers to pay close attention to any day-to-day changes in mood, behavior, and actions; these changes can happen very quickly. They also should be aware of common warning signs that may signal suicide risk (e.g., talking or thinking about wanting to hurt oneself or end one's life, withdrawing from friends and family, becoming depressed or experiencing worsening of existing depression, becoming preoccupied with death and dying, giving away prized possessions). Advise patients, family members, and caregivers to contact the responsible clinician immediately if these or any other new and worrisome behaviors occur.

Risk of angioedema (e.g., swelling of the face, mouth [e.g., tongue, lips, gums], and neck [e.g., throat, larynx] with or without life-threatening respiratory compromise) and other hypersensitivity reactions (e.g., wheezing, dyspnea, rash, hives, blisters); importance of discontinuing the drug and reporting suggestive manifestations (e.g., edema of face, eyes, lips, or tongue; swallowing or breathing with difficulty) to a clinician. Concomitant administration with an angiotensin-converting enzyme (ACE) inhibitor may increase such risk.

Risk of dizziness, somnolence, blurred vision, and other neuropsychiatric effects. Avoid driving or operating machinery while taking pregabalin until experience is gained with the drug's effects.

Avoid alcohol-containing beverages or products; pregabalin may potentiate impairment of motor skills and sedation associated with ingestion of alcohol.

Risk of visual disturbances. Importance of informing clinician if changes in vision occur.

Importance of not discontinuing pregabalin abruptly, since insomnia, nausea, headache, or diarrhea may occur.

Risk of edema and weight gain; concomitant administration with a thiazolidinedione antidiabetic agent may increase such risk. In patients with preexisting cardiac conditions, risk of heart failure may be increased.

Importance of patients promptly informing clinicians of any unexplained muscle pain, tenderness, or weakness, particularly if accompanied by malaise or fever.

Advise diabetic patients to watch for skin damage while receiving pregabalin therapy, since increased risk of skin ulcerations associated with pregabalin therapy has been observed in animal studies.

Importance of women informing clinicians if they are or plan to become pregnant or plan to breast-feed. Importance of clinicians informing women about the existence of and encouraging enrollment in pregnancy registries (see Pregnancy under Warnings/Precautions: Specific Populations, in Cautions).

Advise patients of male-mediated teratogenicity. Importance of men informing clinicians if they plan to father a child.

Importance of informing clinicians of existing or contemplated concomitant therapy, including prescription and OTC drugs, as well as any concomitant illnesses. Potential for additive CNS effects if used concomitantly with other CNS depressants (e.g., opiates, benzodiazepines).

Importance of informing patients of other important precautionary information. (See Cautions.)

Overview® (see Users Guide). For additional information on this drug until a more detailed monograph is developed and published, the manufacturer's labeling should be consulted. It is *essential* that the manufacturer's labeling be consulted for more detailed information on usual cautions, precautions, contraindications, potential drug interactions, laboratory test interferences, and acute toxicity.

Preparations

Pregabalin is subject to control under the Federal Controlled Substances Act of 1970 as a schedule V (C-V) drug. (See Discontinuance, Abuse Potential, and Dependence under Cautions: Warnings/Precautions.)

Excipients in commercially available drug preparations may have clinically important effects in some individuals; consult specific product labeling for details.

Pregabalin

Oral		
Capsules	25 mg	Lyrica® (C-V), Pfizer
	50 mg	Lyrica® (C-V), Pfizer
	75 mg	Lyrica® (C-V), Pfizer
	100 mg	Lyrica® (C-V), Pfizer
	150 mg	Lyrica® (C-V), Pfizer
	200 mg	Lyrica® (C-V), Pfizer
	225 mg	Lyrica® (C-V), Pfizer
	300 mg	Lyrica® (C-V), Pfizer
Solution	20 mg/mL	Lyrica® (C-V), Pfizer

Topiramate

■ Topiramate, a sulfamate-substituted derivative of D-fructose, is an anticonvulsant and antimigraine agent.

Uses

■ **Seizure Disorders** Topiramate is used as *initial* monotherapy or as adjunctive therapy (i.e., in combination with other anticonvulsants) in the management of seizure disorders. Efficacy of the drug in the management of seizure disorders was evaluated principally using topiramate immediate-release tablets. Efficacy of extended-release preparations of topiramate has been established based on experience with the immediate-release formulation and demonstration of pharmacokinetic equivalence between the formulations.

Initial Monotherapy **Partial Seizures or Primary Generalized Tonic-Clonic Seizures.** Topiramate is used as *initial* monotherapy in the management of partial-onset seizures or primary generalized tonic-clonic seizures in adults and pediatric patients 2 years of age or older.

Safety and efficacy of topiramate as initial monotherapy in adults and pediatric patients 10 years of age or older have been established in a randomized, double-blind study in 487 patients (age range: 6–83 years) with epilepsy who had 1 or 2 well-documented seizures within 3 months prior to enrollment and were not receiving anticonvulsant therapy at the time of randomization. Of those enrolled, 49% had no prior treatment with anticonvulsant drugs. During the initial open-label phase, any anticonvulsant being used for temporary or emergency purposes was withdrawn before the patients were randomized. During this phase, all patients received an initial topiramate dosage of 25 mg daily for 7 days (as an immediate-release preparation). This was followed by a double-blind phase, in which 470 patients were randomized to receive topiramate titrated to a target maintenance dosage of 50 or 400 mg daily for a median of 9 months; if the target dosage could not be achieved, patients were maintained on the maximum tolerated dosage. Patients randomized to the target dosage of 400 mg daily received a mean of 275 mg daily; 58% of patients achieved the maximum dosage of 400 mg daily for at least 2 weeks. In this study, the 400-mg daily dosage was superior to the 50-mg daily dosage in delaying time to first seizure. Substantial differences in efficacy between the 2 treatment groups were observed at day 14, when patients randomized to receive target dosages of 400 or 50 mg daily were actually receiving 100 or 25 mg daily, respectively. At 6 months following initiation of treatment, 83% of patients randomized to the 400-mg daily dosage target were seizure free, compared with 71% of those randomized to the 50-mg daily dosage target. At 12 months, 76 or 59% of patients randomized to the 400- or 50-mg daily dosage targets, respectively, were seizure free. Treatment effects were consistent across various patient subgroups defined by age, gender, geographic region, baseline body weight, baseline seizure type, time since diagnosis, and baseline anticonvulsant use.

Topiramate's efficacy as initial monotherapy in pediatric patients 2–9 years of age with partial seizures or primary generalized tonic-clonic seizures was concluded based on a pharmacometric bridging approach using data from controlled epilepsy studies conducted with an immediate-release formulation of the drug. This approach consisted of first demonstrating that the exposure-response relationships in pediatric patients (as young as 2 years of age) and adults were similar when immediate-release topiramate was given as adjunctive therapy; similarity of the exposure-response was then demonstrated in pediatric patients (6 to younger than 16 years of age) and adults when topiramate was used as initial monotherapy. Specific dosage recommendations in children 2–9 years of age were derived from simulations using plasma exposure ranges observed in pediatric and adult patients receiving topiramate as initial monotherapy. (See Dosage and Administration: Dosage.)

Adjunctive Therapy **Partial Seizures.** Topiramate is used as adjunctive therapy (i.e., in combination with other anticonvulsants) in the management of partial-onset seizures in adults and pediatric patients 2 years of age or older.

Efficacy of topiramate as adjunctive therapy in adults with partial (including simple and complex partial) seizures with or without secondarily generalized tonic-clonic seizures has been established in 6 controlled clinical studies. In these studies, patients initially were stabilized with optimum dosages of 1 or 2 conventional anticonvulsant drugs (e.g., carbamazepine, clonazepam, phenobarbital, phenytoin, primidone, valproic acid) during a 4- to 12-week baseline period; those experiencing a prespecified minimum number of partial seizures (with or without secondary generalization) during this baseline period (12 seizures for a 12-week baseline, 8 for an 8-week baseline, or 3 for a 4-week baseline) were randomized to receive topiramate (as an immediate-release preparation) or placebo during a dosage titration period of 3–6 weeks followed by a 4-, 8-, or 12-week stabilization period during which the maximally achieved dosage of topiramate or placebo was maintained. Efficacy of topiramate in these studies principally was evaluated in terms of the change in seizure frequency and the responder rate. The change in seizure frequency with the addition of topiramate or placebo to the existing anticonvulsant regimen was the median percentage decrease (or increase) in average monthly (28 day) seizure rate. The responder rate was the percentage of patients with a reduction in seizure frequency of 50% or greater compared with baseline values.

Patients receiving topiramate 200 mg daily or placebo in 2 of the studies experienced a decrease in seizure frequency of 27–44 or 12–20%, respectively, and the responder rate was 24–45 or 18–24%, respectively. In 2 of the studies, patients receiving topiramate 400 mg daily or placebo experienced a decrease in seizure frequency of 41–48 or 1–13%, respectively, and the responder rate was 35–47 or 8–18%, respectively. Patients receiving 600 mg of topiramate daily in 3 of the studies experienced a decrease in seizure frequency of 41–46%, and patients receiving placebo experienced a decrease in seizure frequency of 1–13% in 2 of the studies, and an *increase* in seizure frequency of 12% in the third study. In the 3 studies in which patients received topiramate 600 mg daily or placebo, 40–47 or 9–18%, respectively, were considered responders. Patients receiving topiramate 800 mg daily in 2 studies experienced a decrease in seizure frequency of 24–41%, and patients receiving placebo experienced a decrease in monthly seizure rate of 1–2% in one study or an 18–21% *increase* in seizure frequency in the other study. In the studies of patients receiving topiramate 800 mg daily or placebo, 40–43 or 0–9%, respectively, were considered responders. Patients receiving 1 g of topiramate or placebo daily in one study experienced a decrease in seizure frequency of 36–38 or 1–2%, respectively, and 36–38 or 8–9% of patients, respectively, were reported to be responders. Overall, topiramate dosages exceeding 600 mg daily did not result in substantially improved efficacy, although individual patients may have benefited from such relatively high dosages.

Efficacy of topiramate as adjunctive therapy in pediatric patients (2–16 years of age) with partial seizures with or without secondarily generalized seizures has been established in a multicenter, randomized controlled trial. In this study, patients initially were stabilized with optimum dosages of 1 or 2 conventional anticonvulsant drugs; patients who experienced 6 or more partial seizures with or without secondarily generalized seizures during an 8-week baseline period were randomized either to topiramate or to placebo. Patients received topiramate initially at a dosage of 25 or 50 mg daily (as an immediate-release preparation), after which the daily dosage was increased in increments of 25–150 mg every other week until the assigned dosage of 125, 175, 225, or 400 mg daily (approximately 6 mg/kg of topiramate daily, based on the patient's body weight) was reached, or until the development of adverse effects precluded increases in dosage. The 8-week dosage titration period was then followed by an 8-week maintenance period. Patients receiving topiramate 6 mg/kg daily or placebo experienced a decrease in seizure frequency of 33.1 or 10.5%, respectively, and the responder rate was 39 or 20%, respectively.

Efficacy of topiramate extended-release capsules (Qudexy® XR) was evaluated in a double-blind placebo-controlled study in adults with partial-onset seizures with or without secondary generalization who were experiencing at least 8 partial seizures during an 8-week baseline period while receiving stable dosages of 1–3 anticonvulsant agents. Topiramate was administered at an initial dosage of 50 mg once daily (as extended-release capsules) and increased at weekly intervals during a 3-week titration period up to a dosage of 200 mg daily; the maintenance dosage was continued for an additional 8 weeks. Patients receiving topiramate experienced a substantial reduction in seizure frequency from baseline compared with those receiving placebo (mean percent reduction of 39.5 versus 21.7%).

Primary Generalized Tonic-Clonic Seizures. Topiramate is used as adjunctive therapy (i.e., in combination with other anticonvulsants) in the management of primary generalized tonic-clonic seizures in adults and pediatric patients 2 years of age or older.

Efficacy of topiramate as adjunctive therapy in patients with primary generalized tonic-clonic seizures has been established in a multicenter, randomized controlled trial. In this study, patients (age range: 3–59 years) initially were stabilized with optimum dosages of 1 or 2 conventional anticonvulsant drugs; patients who experienced 3 or more primary generalized tonic-clonic seizures during an 8-week baseline period were randomized either to topiramate or to placebo. Therapy was targeted to a dosage of 6 mg/kg daily during an 8-week dosage titration period; patients received topiramate initially at a dosage of 50 mg daily (as an immediate-release preparation) for 4 weeks, after which the daily dosage was increased in increments of 50–150 mg every other week until the assigned dosage of 175, 225, or 400 mg daily (approximately 6 mg/kg of topiramate daily, based on the patient's body weight) was reached, or until the development of adverse effects precluded increases in dosage. The dosage titration period was then followed by a 12-week maintenance period. Efficacy of topiramate was evaluated in terms of the change in seizure frequency (i.e., median percent reduction in primary generalized tonic-clonic seizures) and by the responder rate (i.e., percentage of patients with a reduction in primary generalized tonic-clonic seizure frequency of 50% or greater compared with baseline values). Patients receiving topiramate 6 mg/kg daily or placebo experienced a decrease in seizure frequency of 56.7 or 9%, respectively, and the responder rate was 56 or 20%, respectively. Preliminary data from the open-label extension period of a double-blind, placebo-controlled study in a limited number of patients with resistant primary generalized seizures indicate that 92% of patients experienced a 50% or greater decrease in seizures, while 58% of patients were seizure-free during this extension period.

Seizures Associated with Lennox-Gastaut Syndrome. Topiramate is used as adjunctive therapy (i.e., in combination with other anticonvulsants) in the management of seizures associated with Lennox-Gastaut syndrome in adults and pediatric patients 2 years of age or older. Efficacy of topiramate as adjunctive therapy in patients with Lennox-Gastaut syndrome has been established in a multicenter, randomized, controlled trial. In this study, patients (age range: 2–42 years) who experienced 60 or more seizures per month prior to study entry were stabilized with optimum dosages of 1 or 2 conventional anticonvulsant drugs for 4 weeks. Following the 4-week baseline period, patients were randomized either to topiramate or to placebo. Patients received topiramate (as an immediate-release preparation) initially at a dosage of 1 mg/kg daily for 1 week, after which the dosage was increased to 3 mg/kg daily for 1 week, and then to the target dosage of 6 mg/kg daily. The dosage titration period was then followed by an 8-week maintenance period. Efficacy of topiramate was evaluated in terms of the change in seizure frequency (i.e., median percent reduction in drop attacks), the responder rate (i.e., percentage of patients with a reduction in seizure frequency of 50% or greater compared with baseline values), and the overall improvement in seizure severity (i.e., percentage of patients who were improved from baseline). Patients receiving topiramate 6 mg/kg daily experienced a decrease in seizure frequency of 14.8%, while those receiving placebo experienced an *increase* of 5.1%. Overall improvement in seizure severity was reported in more patients receiving topiramate (52%) than in those receiving placebo (28%). Responder rates were not significantly different between patients receiving topiramate (28%) and those receiving placebo (14%).

■ **Migraine Prophylaxis** Topiramate is used in the *prophylaxis* of migraine headache in adults and adolescents 12 years of age or older.

Efficacy of topiramate for migraine prophylaxis in adults has been established in 2 randomized, double-blind, placebo-controlled trials in over 900 patients with at least a 6-month history of migraine, with or without associated aura. Patients also had to experience 3–12 migraines over 4 weeks in the baseline phase; patients were excluded if they had cluster headaches or basilar, ophthalmoplegic, hemiplegic, or transformed migraine headaches. In both studies, after a 4-week baseline placebo period, patients were randomized to receive either topiramate (as an immediate-release preparation) or placebo during a 26-week treatment period consisting of an 8-week titration period and an 18-week maintenance period. Patients randomized to receive topiramate were given an initial dosage of 25 mg daily for 1 week, after which the dosage was increased by 25-mg increments every week until the target dosage of 50, 100, or 200 mg daily was achieved or the maximum tolerated dosage was reached (administered twice daily). Efficacy of prophylaxis was assessed by the reduction in migraine headache frequency, as measured by the change in the 4-week migraine headache rate from the baseline phase to the 26-week treatment period in each topiramate treatment group compared with placebo. The mean migraine headache frequency at baseline in all treatment groups in both studies was approximately 5.5 migraines per 28 days. In the first study, the reduction in the mean 4-week migraine headache frequency from baseline was 1.3, 2.1, or 2.2 for topiramate dosages of 50, 100, or 200 mg daily, respectively, and 0.8 for placebo. In the second study, the reduction in the mean 4-week migraine headache frequency from baseline was 1.4, 2.1, or 2.4 for topiramate dosages of 50, 100, or 200 mg daily, respectively, and 1.1 for placebo. In both studies, there were no apparent differences in treatment effect with respect to age or gender. Because most patients were Caucasian, there were insufficient numbers of patients from different races to make a meaningful comparison of the effectiveness of topiramate with respect to race.

Efficacy of topiramate for the prophylaxis of migraine headache in adolescents has been established in a randomized double-blind study in patients 12–17 years of age with episodic migraine headaches with or without aura. Patients who experienced 3–12 migraines with no more than 14 headache days (including nonmigraine headaches) over a 4-week baseline period were randomized to receive topiramate (50 or 100 mg daily as an immediate-release preparation) or placebo for 16 weeks (4-week titration period followed by a 12-week maintenance period). Topiramate was initiated at a dosage of 25 mg daily for one week and then increased by 25-mg increments every week until the target dosage or maximum tolerated dosage was reached (administered twice daily). Patients receiving topiramate 100 mg daily experienced a substantially greater percent reduction in monthly migraine attacks from baseline compared with those receiving placebo (72 versus 44%); no substantial difference was observed between topiramate 50 mg daily and placebo.

■ **Alcohol Dependence** Topiramate has been used successfully in adults for the management of alcohol dependence†. Efficacy of the drug in this condition has been evaluated in 2 randomized, double-blind, placebo-controlled studies in adults who met DSM-IV criteria for alcohol dependence; the initial trial was of 12 weeks' duration and was conducted at a single site, while the subsequent trial was of 14 weeks' duration and was conducted at multiple sites. Patients in both studies received escalating dosages of topiramate (initially, 25 mg daily and gradually increased up to 300 mg daily) or placebo in conjunction with a weekly medication compliance intervention. Topiramate was found to be more effective than placebo in improving self-reported drinking outcomes (e.g., number of drinks per day, number of drinks per drinking day, percentage of heavy drinking days, percentage of days abstinent) as well as the objective laboratory measure of alcohol consumption (reduced plasma γ-glutamyltransferase) in both of these studies. In addition, topiramate was shown to reduce self-reported alcohol craving to a greater extent than placebo in the 12-week study. Additional analyses of these 2 studies found topiramate to be more effective than placebo at improving physical and psychosocial well-being and some aspects of quality of life in these alcoholic individuals. In an open-label, longer-term study comparing topiramate with naltrexone in alcohol-dependent patients, topiramate was found to be at least as effective at reducing drinking behaviors as naltrexone during 6 months of therapy and appeared superior to naltrexone at reducing alcohol-related cravings.

Topiramate is one of several drugs currently recommended by the National Institute of Alcohol Abuse and Alcoholism (NIAAA) for treating alcohol dependence; however, unlike the other recommended drugs (naltrexone, acamprosate, disulfiram), topiramate has not been approved by the FDA for this indication. Topiramate also differs from the other recommended drug therapies because it has been administered to patients who were still drinking alcohol, and a period of abstinence from alcohol does not appear to be necessary before starting therapy with the drug. Additional studies, including longer-term trials, are needed to more clearly determine topiramate's efficacy, safety, and potential role in treating alcohol dependence, including its use in different populations and alcoholic subtypes, its potential use in combination with other drugs, and the optimal dosage and duration of therapy. For further information on the use of topiramate and other medications in the management of alcohol dependence, the NIAAA's web site at http://www.niaaa.nih.gov/Publications/EducationTrainingMaterials/guide.htm should be consulted.

Topiramate has been effective in the management of alcohol withdrawal† in a limited number of patients in uncontrolled studies; however, larger, well-controlled studies are needed to confirm these initial findings.

Dosage and Administration

■ **Administration** Topiramate is administered orally as immediate-release tablets, sprinkle capsules, or extended-release capsules. The immediate-release tablets and sprinkle capsules are administered in 2 divided doses; the extended-release capsules are administered once daily.

The manufacturer states that the sprinkle capsule formulation of topiramate is bioequivalent to the immediate-release tablet and may be substituted as a therapeutic equivalent. At steady state, the extended-release capsules administered once daily are bioequivalent to the immediate-release tablets administered twice daily. Because the bioavailability of topiramate is not affected by food, the drug may be administered without regard to meals.

Because of the bitter taste, immediate-release tablets of topiramate should be swallowed intact and *not* broken or chewed. If the tablets are broken, they should be used immediately since stability of exposed drug beyond a brief period cannot be ensured; any unused portion should be discarded. For patients experiencing difficulty in swallowing the tablets, contents of the capsule/sprinkle formulation may be sprinkled on a small amount of food as described below.

The sprinkle capsule formulation of topiramate may be taken whole, or may be administered by opening the capsule and sprinkling the entire contents on a small amount (e.g., a teaspoonful) of soft food (e.g., applesauce, custard, ice cream, oatmeal, pudding, yogurt). The patient should swallow the entire spoonful of the sprinkle/food mixture immediately; chewing should be avoided. It may be helpful to have the patient drink fluids immediately after administration in order to make sure that all of the mixture is swallowed. The sprinkle/food mixture must not be stored for use at a later time.

Qudexy® XR extended-release capsules may be swallowed whole or may be administered by opening the capsule and sprinkling the contents on a small amount of soft food; the sprinkle/food mixture should be swallowed immediately and not chewed, crushed, or stored for later use.

Trokendi XR® extended-release capsules must be swallowed whole and may not be sprinkled on food, crushed, or chewed; because of these limitations, Trokendi XR® is not recommended for use in children younger than 6 years of age. The manufacturer of Trokendi XR® states that patients should completely avoid consumption of alcohol at least 6 hours prior to and 6 hours after administration of the drug.

Patients who are currently receiving or beginning therapy with topiramate and/or any other anticonvulsant for any indication should be closely monitored for the emergence or worsening of depression, suicidal thoughts or behavior (suicidality), and/or any unusual changes in mood or behavior. (See Cautions: Precautions and Contraindications.)

Dispensing and Administration Precautions Because of similarity in spelling between Topamax® (the trade name for topiramate) and Toprol-XL® (a trade name for metoprolol succinate, a β-adrenergic blocking agent), the potential exists for dispensing or prescribing errors involving these drugs. According to medication error reports, the overlapping tablet strengths (25, 50, 100, and 200 mg) between Topamax® and Toprol-XL® and the fact that these drugs were stored closely together in pharmacies also may have been contributing factors in causing these errors. Another contributing factor to dispensing errors may be the use of mnemonic abbreviations in computerized listings incorporating the first 3 letters and dose of Topamax® and Toprol-XL® (e.g., "TOP25"). Extra care should be exercised to ensure the accuracy of both oral and written prescriptions for these drugs. The manufacturers of Topamax® and Toprol-XL® also recommend that pharmacists assess various measures of avoiding dispensing errors and implement them as appropriate (e.g., by verifying all orders for these drugs by citing both the trade and generic names to prescribers, attaching reminders to pharmacy shelves, separating the drugs on pharmacy shelves, counseling patients). (See Cautions: Precautions and Contraindications.)

■ **Dosage** Dosage of topiramate must be adjusted carefully and individualized according to patient response and tolerance and the condition being treated. The manufacturer states that titration of topiramate dosages too rapidly (e.g., over 3–6 weeks) to achieve target dosages and/or excessive target dosages may have contributed to an unnecessarily high incidence of adverse effects in clinical studies.

In patients with or without a history of seizures or epilepsy, anticonvulsant drugs, including topiramate, should be withdrawn gradually to minimize the risk of seizures or increased seizure frequency. In clinical studies for seizure disorders, daily dosages of topiramate were decreased in weekly intervals by 50–100 mg in adults and over a 2–8 week period in pediatric patients; transition to a new anticonvulsant regimen was permitted when clinically indicated. In clinical studies for migraine prophylaxis, daily dosages were decreased in weekly intervals by 25–50 mg. However, in situations where more rapid withdrawal of topiramate is clinically necessary, the manufacturers recommend appropriate monitoring.

Seizure Disorders The manufacturers state that it is not necessary to monitor plasma topiramate concentrations to achieve optimal clinical effect with the drug.

Addition or withdrawal of phenytoin and/or carbamazepine during adjunctive therapy may require adjustment of topiramate dosage. Addition of topiramate to an anticonvulsant regimen containing phenytoin may require adjustment of the dosage of phenytoin. (See Drug Interactions: Anticonvulsants.)

Initial Monotherapy. The recommended dosage of topiramate as initial monotherapy for management of partial-onset seizures or primary generalized tonic-clonic seizures in adults and pediatric patients 10 years of age or older is 400 mg daily (administered in 2 divided doses as immediate-release tablets or sprinkle capsules, or once daily as extended-release capsules). The dosage of topiramate should be titrated using the schedule in Table 1 or 2.

Table 1. Topiramate (Immediate-release Tablets and Sprinkle Capsules) Dosage Titration Schedule for Monotherapy of Partial Seizures or Primary Generalized Tonic-Clonic Seizures in Adults and Pediatric Patients 10 Years of Age or Older

Week	Morning Dose	Evening Dose
1	25 mg	25 mg
2	50 mg	50 mg
3	75 mg	75 mg
4	100 mg	100 mg
5	150 mg	150 mg
6	200 mg	200 mg

Table 2. Topiramate (Extended-release Capsules) Dosage Titration Schedule for Monotherapy of Partial Seizures or Primary Generalized Tonic-Clonic Seizures in Adults and Pediatric Patients 10 Years of Age or Older

Week	Dosage
1	50 mg once daily
2	100 mg once daily
3	150 mg once daily
4	200 mg once daily
5	300 mg once daily
6	400 mg once daily

In a controlled study evaluating safety and efficacy of topiramate (titrated up to 50 or 400 mg daily as an immediate-release preparation) as initial monotherapy, approximately 58% of patients randomized to receive the 400-mg daily dosage achieved this maximum dosage. Because a therapeutic effect emerges during titration, the investigators of this study recommend that topiramate dosages should be titrated in a stepwise fashion with intermediate stopping points (e.g., 100 mg daily) to evaluate patient response and achieve the optimal maintenance dosage, and to avoid possibly exceeding an appropriate dosage for an individual patient.

Dosage of topiramate as initial monotherapy for the management of partial-onset seizures or primary generalized tonic-clonic seizures in pediatric patients 2–9 years of age (or 6–9 years of age if using Trokendi XR®) is based on body weight. (See Dosage and Administration: Administration.) During the titration period, the recommended initial dosage of topiramate is 25 mg daily (administered in the evening) for the first week. Based on tolerability, dosage can be increased to 50 mg daily (administered in 2 divided doses as immediate-release tablets or sprinkle capsules, or once daily as extended-release capsules) during the second week. The total daily dosage can then be increased by 25–50 mg daily each subsequent week as tolerated. Titration to the minimum recommended dosage (see Table 3) should be attempted over 5–7 weeks of the total titration period. Based upon tolerability and seizure control, additional titration to a higher dosage (up to the maximum recommended maintenance dosage) can be attempted in weekly increments of 25–50 mg daily. The total daily dosage of topiramate should not exceed the maximum recommended maintenance dosage for each range of body weight (see Table 3).

Table 3. Target Maintenance Topiramate Dosage for Monotherapy of Partial Seizures or Primary Generalized Tonic-Clonic Seizures in Pediatric Patients 2–9 Years of Age

Weight (kg)	Minimum Total Daily Dosage (mg/day)*	Maximum Total Daily Dosage (mg/day)*
Up to 11	150	250
12–22	200	300
23–31	200	350
32–38	250	350
>38	250	400

* Administered in 2 equally divided doses if using the immediate-release tablets or sprinkle capsule formulation of the drug.

Adjunctive Therapy. In adults 17 years of age or older, the recommended dosage of topiramate as adjunctive therapy for management of partial-onset seizures or Lennox-Gastaut Syndrome is 200–400 mg daily (administered in 2 divided doses as immediate-release tablets or sprinkle capsules, or once daily as extended-release capsules). The recommended adult dosage for adjunctive management of primary generalized tonic-clonic seizures is 400 mg daily (administered in 2 divided doses as immediate-release tablets or sprinkle capsules, or once daily as extended-release capsules). Topiramate therapy should be initiated at 25–50 mg daily, titrating the daily dosage upward in increments of 25–50 mg at weekly intervals to an optimal level, but generally not exceeding 400 mg daily. Limited data indicate that upward titration in increments of 25 mg per week may delay the time to reach an effective dosage; however, such a titration schedule appears to be associated with a lower incidence of neurocognitive and/or psychiatric adverse effects and a lower discontinuance rate. Maintenance dosages less than 400 mg daily may be optimally effective in some patients and therefore should be individualized; however, results from clinical studies in adults with partial-onset seizures indicate that a daily dosage of 200 mg may produce inconsistent effects and appears to be less effective than a daily dosage of 400 mg. Dosages exceeding 400 mg daily have not improved response to topiramate substantially, although seizure control may be improved in some patients from such relatively high dosages if tolerated. Dosages exceeding 1.6 g daily have not been studied.

In pediatric patients 2–16 years of age (or 6–16 years of age if using Trokendi XR®), the recommended dosage of topiramate as adjunctive therapy for the management of partial-onset seizures, primary generalized tonic-clonic seizures, or seizures associated with Lennox-Gastaut syndrome is approximately 5–9 mg/kg daily (administered in 2 divided doses as immediate-release tablets or sprinkle capsules, or once daily as extended-release capsules). (See Dosage and Administration: Administration.) An initial dose of 25 mg (or less, based on a range of 1–3 mg/kg daily) should be given nightly for the first week. The dosage should then be increased at 1- or 2-week intervals in increments of 1–3 mg/kg daily (administered in 2 divided doses as immediate-release tablets or sprinkle capsules, or once daily as extended-release capsules) to achieve optimal clinical response. Dosage titration should be guided by clinical outcome; some manufacturers recommend that the total daily dose should not exceed 400 mg. Alternatively, some clinicians recommend that the initial topiramate dosage should range from 0.5–1 mg/kg daily and that the drug should be titrated slowly (e.g., followed by incremental increases of 1–3 mg/kg every other week or incremental increases of 0.5–1 mg/kg per week) to obtain optimal efficacy with minimal adverse effects.

Migraine Prophylaxis The recommended dosage of topiramate for prophylaxis of migraine headache in adults and adolescents 12 years of age or older is 100 mg daily (administered in 2 divided doses as immediate-release tablets or sprinkle capsules, or once daily as extended-release capsules). The dosage of topiramate should be titrated using the schedule in Table 4 or 5.

Table 4. Topiramate (Immediate-release Tablets and Sprinkle Capsules) Dosage Titration Schedule for Migraine Prophylaxis in Adults and Adolescents

Week	Morning Dose	Evening Dose
1	None	25 mg
2	25 mg	25 mg
3	25 mg	50 mg
4	50 mg	50 mg

Table 5. Topiramate (Extended-release Capsules) Dosage Titration Schedule for Migraine Prophylaxis in Adults and Adolescents

Week	Dosage
1	25 mg once daily
2	50 mg once daily
3	75 mg once daily
4	100 mg once daily

Titration of topiramate dosage should be guided by clinical outcome. If required, longer intervals between dosage adjustments can be used.

Alcohol Dependence The optimal dosage regimen of topiramate for the management of alcohol dependence† remains to be established; however, initial dosages of 25 mg given once daily in the afternoon or evening (e.g., at bedtime) followed by gradual dosage titration (e.g., increasing dosage in increments of 25–50 mg daily each week, given in 2 divided doses) to target maintenance dosages of 200–300 mg daily were found to be effective in short-term, controlled clinical trials in adults and have been recommended by some authorities. Patients who are unable to tolerate the target dosage may respond to lower dosages.

Results from clinical studies in alcohol dependence suggest that a more gradual titration (e.g., over 8 weeks) to achieve target dosages of 200–300 mg daily may be better tolerated than more rapid titration (e.g., over 6 weeks). A period of abstinence from alcohol prior to initiating topiramate therapy for alcohol dependence does not appear to be necessary.

Although the optimal duration of topiramate therapy for the management of alcohol dependence remains to be established, some authorities recommend an initial period of at least 3 months to prevent relapse in alcohol-dependent patients. These authorities also recommend continuing drug therapy for 12 months or longer if the patient responds to the medication during this initial period when the risk of relapse is highest.

■ **Dosage in Renal and Hepatic Impairment** Dosage of topiramate should be adjusted according to the degree of renal impairment. In patients with a creatinine clearance less than 70 mL/minute per 1.73 m^2, the daily dosage of topiramate should be decreased by 50%. Dosage adjustment also may be required in patients undergoing hemodialysis since clearance of topiramate is 4–6 times more rapid in such patients. Therefore, to avoid rapid decreases of plasma topiramate concentrations in patients undergoing hemodialysis, a supplemental dose of the drug may be required; selection of the supplemental dose should take into account the duration of dialysis, clearance rate of the dialysis system being used, and the patient's effective renal clearance of topiramate.

Although topiramate clearance may decrease in patients with hepatic impairment, the manufacturers make no specific recommendations for dosage adjustment in such patients.

Cautions

CNS effects including somnolence, fatigue, dizziness, paresthesia, cognitive-related dysfunction, and neuropsychiatric abnormalities are among the most commonly reported adverse effects in adults and pediatric patients receiving topiramate for seizure disorders. (See Cautions: CNS Effects.) Other common adverse effects of topiramate reported in this population include anorexia, weight loss, abnormal vision, and fever.

The most common adverse effects reported in adults and pediatric patients receiving topiramate for migraine prophylaxis and occurring more frequently with the drug than with placebo include paresthesia, anorexia, weight loss, difficulty with memory, taste perversion, diarrhea, hypoesthesia, nausea, abdominal pain, and upper respiratory tract infection.

In controlled clinical trials evaluating topiramate for alcohol dependence†, paresthesia, taste perversion, fatigue, anorexia, insomnia, concentration and attention difficulties, memory impairment, nervousness, somnolence, diarrhea, dizziness, and pruritus were reported more frequently in patients receiving topiramate than in patients receiving placebo.

■ **CNS Effects** Adverse CNS effects are frequently reported with topiramate and generally can be classified into 3 categories: cognitive-related dysfunction (e.g., confusion, psychomotor slowing, difficulty with concentration or attention, difficulty with memory, speech or language problems, particularly word-finding difficulties); psychiatric or behavioral disturbances (e.g., depression, mood problems); and somnolence or fatigue.

The risk of adverse cognitive effects is increased with rapid titration and higher initial dosages of topiramate.

Somnolence and fatigue were the most commonly reported adverse effects in patients receiving topiramate for adjunctive therapy of seizure disorders. In patients receiving topiramate as initial monotherapy for seizure disorders, the incidence of somnolence appeared to be dose related. In patients receiving topiramate as adjunctive therapy for seizure disorders, the incidence of fatigue appeared to be dose related. In patients receiving topiramate for migraine prophylaxis, both somnolence and fatigue appeared to be dose related and occurred more frequently during the titration phase.

Psychiatric or behavioral disturbances reported with topiramate in the adjunctive epilepsy and migraine populations were dose related. Suicide attempts also have been reported in patients receiving the drug. (See Cautions: Precautions and Contraindications.)

Other common adverse psychiatric effects reported with topiramate include nervousness, anxiety, aggression, insomnia, decreased libido, personality disorder, and anorexia; other frequently reported CNS effects include dizziness, ataxia, paresthesia, hypoesthesia, nystagmus, tremor, and abnormal gait or coordination.

■ **Hematologic Effects** Bleeding (e.g., epistaxis, ecchymosis, increased menstrual bleeding, life-threatening hemorrhage) was reported in about 4.5% of adults and pediatric patients receiving topiramate in controlled studies; serious bleeding events occurred in about 0.3–0.4% of patients receiving the drug. Patients who experienced a serious bleeding event generally had underlying conditions that increase the risk of bleeding or were receiving concomitant drugs that affect platelet function or coagulation.

■ **Ocular Effects** A syndrome consisting of acute myopia associated with secondary angle-closure glaucoma has been reported in some adults and pediatric patients receiving topiramate. This syndrome may be associated with supraciliary effusion, resulting in anterior displacement of the lens and iris and, subsequently, secondary angle-closure glaucoma. Symptoms include acute onset of decreased visual acuity and/or ocular pain and typically occur within one month of initiating topiramate therapy. Ophthalmologic findings include myopia, anterior chamber shallowing, ocular hyperemia, and increased intraocular pressure; mydriasis may or may not be present. (See Cautions: Precautions and Contraindications.)

Visual field defects not associated with elevated intraocular pressure also have been reported in patients receiving topiramate in clinical trials and during postmarketing experience.

■ **Precautions and Contraindications** Hyperchloremic, non-anion gap, metabolic acidosis (i.e., decreased serum bicarbonate concentrations to below the normal reference range in the absence of chronic respiratory alkalosis) has been reported in adults and pediatric patients receiving topiramate. Such electrolyte imbalance can occur at any time during therapy. Metabolic acidosis is caused by renal bicarbonate loss due to the inhibitory effect of topiramate on carbonic anhydrase. Decreases in serum bicarbonate concentrations usually are mild to moderate (average decrease of 4 mEq/L at daily topiramate dosages of 400 mg in adults and at approximately 6 mg/kg daily in pediatric patients); marked decreases in serum bicarbonate concentrations (to below 10 mEq/L) may rarely occur. Manifestations of acute or chronic metabolic acidosis may include hyperventilation, nonspecific symptoms such as fatigue and anorexia, or more severe sequelae including cardiac arrhythmias or stupor. Because chronic, untreated metabolic acidosis may have potentially serious sequelae (e.g., increased risk of nephrolithiasis or nephrocalcinosis, development of osteomalacia and/or osteoporosis with an increased risk for fractures), the manufacturers state that serum bicarbonate concentrations should be measured at baseline and periodically during topiramate therapy. If metabolic acidosis develops and persists, consideration should be given to reducing the dosage or discontinuing topiramate therapy (by gradually tapering the dosage). If a decision is made to continue topiramate therapy in the presence of persistent acidosis, alkali treatment should be considered.

Because of the risk of acute myopia associated with secondary angle-closure glaucoma and other visual defects, patients receiving topiramate should be advised to seek immediate medical attention if they experience blurred vision, visual disturbances, or periorbital pain during therapy with the drug. Such manifestations generally resolve after the drug is discontinued. If any adverse ocular effects or visual problems occur during topiramate therapy, discontinuance of the drug should be considered.

Oligohidrosis, which rarely may require hospitalization, has been reported in patients receiving topiramate; most cases have occurred in pediatric patients. Manifestations include decreased sweating and an elevation in body temperature above normal (hyperthermia). Some cases occurred following exposure to elevated environmental temperatures. The manufacturers state that patients, particularly pediatric patients, receiving topiramate should be monitored closely for evidence of decreased sweating and increased body temperature, especially in hot weather. Caution is advised if topiramate is used concomitantly with other drugs that predispose patients to heat-related disorders (e.g., carbonic anhydrase inhibitors, drugs with anticholinergic activity).

In patients with or without a history of seizures or epilepsy, anticonvulsant drugs, including topiramate, should be gradually withdrawn to minimize the potential for seizures or increased seizure frequency. (See Dosage and Administration: Dosage.) The manufacturers recommend appropriate monitoring in situations where more rapid withdrawal of topiramate is required.

Patients should be informed that topiramate may cause adverse CNS or ocular effects (e.g., somnolence, dizziness, confusion, difficulty concentrating, visual disturbances) and that they should not drive a motor vehicle or operate other complex machinery until they have gained sufficient experience with the drug to determine whether it has adverse effects on their mental performance, motor performance, and/or vision. Cognitive-related adverse effects are more likely to occur during the dose titration phase, but may persist into maintenance therapy.

Patients with seizure disorders who are receiving anticonvulsant agents, including topiramate, may continue to experience unpredictable seizures. Therefore, the manufacturers recommend that all patients receiving topiramate for seizure disorders be advised to exercise caution when engaging in any activities where loss of consciousness could result in serious danger to themselves or those around them (including swimming, driving a motor vehicle, and climbing in high places). Some patients with refractory seizure disorders may need to avoid such activities altogether.

An increased risk of suicidality (suicidal behavior or ideation) was observed in an analysis of studies using various anticonvulsants compared with placebo. The analysis of suicidality reports from 199 placebo-controlled studies involving 11 anticonvulsants (carbamazepine, felbamate, gabapentin, lamotrigine, levetiracetam, oxcarbazepine, pregabalin, tiagabine, topiramate, valproate, and zonisamide) in patients with epilepsy, psychiatric disorders (e.g., bipolar disorder, depression, anxiety), and other conditions (e.g., migraine, neuropathic pain) found that patients receiving anticonvulsants had approximately twice the risk of suicidal behavior or ideation (0.43%) compared with patients receiving placebo (0.24%); this increased suicidality risk was observed as early as one week after beginning therapy and continued through 24 weeks. Although patients treated with an anticonvulsant for epilepsy, psychiatric disorders, and other conditions were all found to be at increased risk for suicidality compared with those receiving placebo, the relative risk for suicidality was found to be higher in patients with epilepsy compared with those receiving anticonvulsants for other conditions.

All patients who are currently receiving or beginning therapy with any anticonvulsant for any indication should be closely monitored for the emergence or worsening of depression, suicidal thoughts or behavior (suicidality), and/or unusual changes in mood or behavior. Clinicians should inform patients, their families, and caregivers of the potential for an increased risk of suicidality with anticonvulsant therapy and advise them to pay close attention to any day-to-day changes in mood, behavior, and actions; since changes can happen very quickly, it is important to be alert to any sudden differences. In addition, patients, family members, and caregivers should be aware of common warning signs that may signal suicide risk (e.g., talking or thinking about wanting to hurt oneself or end one's life, withdrawing from friends and family, becoming depressed or experiencing worsening of existing depression, becoming preoccupied with death and dying, giving away prized possessions). If these or any new and worrisome behaviors occur, the responsible clinician should be contacted immediately. Clinicians who prescribe topiramate or any other anticonvulsant should balance the risk for suicidality with the risk of untreated illness. Epilepsy and many other illnesses for which anticonvulsants are prescribed are themselves associated with an increased risk of morbidity and mortality and an increased risk of suicidal thoughts and behavior. If suicidal thoughts and behavior emerge during anticonvulsant therapy, the clinician should consider whether these symptoms may be related to the illness being treated.

Dose-related hyperammonemia with or without encephalopathy has been reported in patients receiving topiramate in clinical studies and during postmarketing experience. In adolescents 12–17 years of age who received topiramate monotherapy in the migraine prophylaxis studies, hyperammonemia was reported in 26, 14, or 9% of those receiving topiramate 100 mg daily, topiramate 50 mg daily, or placebo, respectively. In some cases, ammonia concentrations were markedly increased in patients receiving the highest dosage of 100 mg daily. Concomitant administration of topiramate and valproic acid also has been associated with hyperammonemia with or without encephalopathy in patients who have previously tolerated either drug alone. Although topiramate is not labeled for use in pediatric patients 1–24 months of age, dose-related hyperammonemia was observed in such patients who were receiving topiramate and valproic acid concomitantly in partial-onset seizure studies. Although patients may be asymptomatic, manifestations of hyperammonemic encephalopathy include acute alterations in the level of consciousness and/or cognitive function with lethargy or vomiting; in most cases, manifestations abated after discontinuance of therapy. Patients with inborn errors of metabolism or reduced hepatic mitochondrial activity may be at an increased risk for hyperammonemia with or without encephalopathy. Although it has not been studied, it is possible that an interaction between topiramate and valproic acid may exacerbate existing defects or unmask deficiencies in susceptible individuals. If unexplained lethargy, vomiting, or changes in mental status occur, hyperammonemic encephalopathy should be considered, and an ammonia concentration should be measured.

Formation of kidney stones has been reported in approximately 1.5% of adults receiving topiramate in clinical trials. As in the general population, the incidence of kidney stone formation among topiramate-treated patients appears to be higher in men than in women; kidney stones also have been reported in pediatric patients receiving topiramate. Although the mechanism of this adverse effect has not been fully elucidated, it has been suggested that topiramate exhibits weak inhibition of carbonic anhydrase and, similar to other carbonic anhydrase inhibitors (e.g., acetazolamide), may promote stone formation by reducing urinary citrate excretion and increasing urinary pH. The manufacturers state that use of topiramate in patients on a ketogenic diet or concomitant use of the drug with other carbonic anhydrase inhibitors may increase the risk of kidney stone formation and, therefore, should be avoided. Because increased fluid intake may increase urinary output and reduce the concentration of substances involved in stone formation, patients receiving topiramate, particularly those with predisposing factors, should be instructed to maintain adequate fluid intake to prevent kidney stone formation.

Hypothermia (defined as an unintentional drop in body core temperature to less than 35°C), both in conjunction with and in the absence of hyperammonemia, has been reported in patients receiving concurrent topiramate and valproic acid therapy. Hypothermia may be manifested by a variety of clinical abnormalities including lethargy, confusion, coma, and substantial alterations in other major organ systems such as the cardiovascular and respiratory systems. Hypothermia may occur after initiating topiramate therapy or following a dosage increase. Discontinuance of topiramate or valproic acid therapy should be considered in patients who develop hypothermia. Since hypothermia also may be a manifestation of hyperammonemia, clinical management and assessment of hypothermia should include determination of plasma ammonia concentrations.

Serum electrolyte abnormalities have been reported in controlled clinical trials of adults with partial onset seizures receiving topiramate. Hypokalemia and hypophosphatemia were reported in 0.4 and 6% of topiramate-treated patients, respectively, compared with 0.1 and 2% of placebo-treated patients in double-blind clinical trials. Markedly increased serum alkaline phosphatase concentrations were reported in 3% of patients receiving topiramate compared with 1% of placebo recipients in these studies. The clinical importance of these abnormalities has not been clearly established.

Because of similarity in spelling between Topamax® (the trade name for topiramate) and Toprol-XL® (a trade name for metoprolol succinate, a β-adrenergic blocking agent), the potential exists for dispensing or prescribing errors involving these drugs. These medication errors have been associated with serious adverse events sometimes requiring hospitalization as a result of either lack of the intended medication (e.g., seizure or hypertension recurrence) or exposure to the wrong drug (e.g., bradycardia in a patient erroneously receiving metoprolol). Therefore, extra care should be exercised to ensure the accuracy of both oral and written prescriptions for these drugs. Patients should be advised to carefully check their medications and to bring any questions or concerns to the attention of the dispensing pharmacist. Dispensing errors involving Topamax® (topiramate) and Toprol-XL® (metoprolol succinate) should be reported to the manufacturers, the USP/ISMP (Institute for Safe Medication Practices) Medication Errors Reporting Program by phone (800-233-7767), or directly to the FDA MedWatch program by phone (800-FDA-1088), fax (800-FDA-0178), or internet (http://www.fda.gov/Safety/MedWatch/default.htm).

The manufacturer of immediate-release topiramate states there are no known contraindications to the use of the drug. Trokendi XR® extended-release topiramate capsules are contraindicated in patients with recent alcohol use, and Qudexy® XR extended-release topiramate capsules are contraindicated in patients with metabolic acidosis receiving topiramate and metformin concomitantly. (See Drug Interactions: Antidiabetic Agents.)

■ **Pediatric Precautions** Safety and efficacy of topiramate for the management of seizure disorders have not been established in children younger than 2 years of age. In a randomized, double-blind, placebo-controlled study in infants 1–24 months of age, topiramate in fixed dosages of 5, 15, and 25 mg/kg daily was not shown to be more effective than placebo in controlling seizures after 20 days of treatment. Results of this study in addition to a long-term open-label study in infants and toddlers suggest that very young children may experience adverse effects not previously observed in older pediatric patients and adults or that occur with greater frequency or severity than in these older age groups. Such adverse effects included growth/length retardation, changes in certain laboratory parameters (e.g., increased serum creatinine concentrations, increased BUN, increased protein concentrations, decreased potassium concentrations, increased eosinophil count, increased alkaline phosphatase concentrations), and impairment of adaptive behavior. Although other preparations of topiramate may be used in children as young as 2 years of age for the management of seizure disorders, use of Trokendi XR® extended-release capsules is recommended only in children 6 years of age or older because this capsule formulation must be swallowed whole and cannot be sprinkled on food, crushed, or chewed.

Safety and efficacy of topiramate for migraine prophylaxis have not been established in pediatric patients younger than 12 years of age. In a controlled study in pediatric patients 6–16 years of age, topiramate 2–3 mg/kg daily was not more effective than placebo for preventing migraine headaches.

As in adults, cognitive/neuropsychiatric effects are commonly reported in pediatric patients receiving topiramate, although the incidence appears to be lower than that observed in adults. Such effects include psychomotor slowing, difficulty with concentration or attention, speech disorders, and language problems. The most common adverse CNS effects reported in pediatric patients receiving topiramate as initial monotherapy for seizure disorders include dizziness, headache, anorexia, and somnolence. The most common adverse CNS effects reported in pediatric patients receiving the drug as adjunctive therapy for seizure disorders include somnolence and fatigue. In migraine prophylaxis studies in pediatric patients 12–17 years of age, difficulty with concentration/attention was the most commonly reported adverse CNS effect. Adverse cognitive effects observed in pediatric migraine studies were dose dependent and occurred with greater frequency in younger (6–11 years of age) compared with older (12–17 years of age) children. Topiramate may cause psychomotor slowing and decreased verbal fluency based on results of a standard neuropsychological test that was administered to adolescents 12–17 years of age.

Hyperchloremic, non-anion gap, metabolic acidosis (i.e. decreased serum bicarbonate concentrations to below the normal reference range in the absence of chronic respiratory alkalosis) has been reported in pediatric patients receiving topiramate. (See Cautions: Precautions and Contraindications.) In pediatric studies evaluating topiramate as adjunctive therapy for refractory partial-onset seizures or Lennox-Gastaut syndrome, the incidence of decreased serum bicarbonate concentrations was as high as 67 or 10% for patients receiving topiramate (approximately 6 mg/kg daily) or placebo, respectively. *Markedly* abnormally low serum bicarbonate concentrations (defined as concentrations of less than 17 mEq/L and a decrease from pretreatment values exceeding 5 mEq/L) were observed in up to 11% of patients receiving topiramate in these studies compared with no more than 2% of those receiving placebo. Chronic, untreated metabolic acidosis may have potentially serious sequelae, including development of osteomalacia (rickets), reduction of growth rates, and a decrease in maximal height achieved in pediatric patients. Although the effects of topiramate on growth and bone-related sequelae have not been systematically evaluated in long-term, placebo-controlled trials, results of an open-label study demonstrated that pediatric patients 1–24 months old who received topiramate for up to 1 year had reduced length, weight, and head circumference compared with age- and sex-matched normative data; reductions in length and weight were correlated with the degree of acidosis. Because of the potential risk of metabolic acidosis, the manufacturers state that serum bicarbonate concentrations should be measured at baseline and periodically during topiramate therapy. (See Cautions: Precautions and Contraindications.)

Oligohidrosis (decreased sweating) and hyperthermia have been reported in clinical trials and during postmarketing surveillance of topiramate. Because oligohidrosis and hyperthermia typically occurred in children and may have potentially serious sequelae, the manufacturers state that patients, particularly pediatric patients, receiving topiramate should be monitored closely for evidence of decreased sweating and increased body temperature, especially in hot weather. (See Cautions: Precautions and Contraindications.)

Clearance of topiramate is higher in pediatric patients than in adults, and also higher in younger versus older pediatric patients, presumably because of age-related changes in the rate of drug metabolism. Pediatric patients (2 to younger than 16 years of age) receiving adjunctive therapy with topiramate exhibited higher oral topiramate clearance than those receiving topiramate monotherapy; the observed difference was presumably due to concomitant use of enzyme-inducing anticonvulsant agents.

■ **Geriatric Precautions** While clinical studies evaluating topiramate did not include sufficient numbers of adults 65 years of age or older to determine whether geriatric patients respond differently than younger adults, approximately 3% of patients receiving the drug in clinical trials were older than 60 years of age. Although no age-related differences in efficacy or safety were evident in these patients, pharmacokinetic data from one controlled clinical study revealed a decreased clearance of topiramate in geriatric patients with reduced renal function (i.e., creatinine clearance reduced by 20% compared with that in younger adults). Following administration of a single 100-mg dose of topiramate in these patients, plasma clearance and renal clearance of topiramate were reduced by 21 and 19%, respectively; half-life was prolonged by 13%; and peak plasma concentrations and area under the plasma concentration-time curve (AUC) were increased by 23 or 25%, respectively, compared with younger adults. Therefore, the manufacturers state that it may be useful to monitor renal function in geriatric patients; dosage adjustment may be necessary in geriatric patients with impaired renal function (i.e., creatinine clearance less than 70 mL/minute per 1.73 m^2).

■ **Pregnancy and Lactation** Topiramate can cause fetal harm when administered to pregnant women. Exposure to the drug in utero has been associated with an increased risk of oral clefts (cleft lip and/or palate) and for neonates being small for gestational age (i.e., birth weight less than 10th percentile). Data from pregnancy registries, including the North American Antiepileptic Drug (NAAED) pregnancy registry, indicate that infants exposed to topiramate in utero have a higher prevalence of oral cleft birth defects than those with no such exposure. The prevalence of oral clefts among infants in the NAAED registry who were exposed to topiramate in utero was 1.1% compared with a prevalence of 0.36% in infants exposed to a reference anticonvulsant and a prevalence of 0.12% in infants born to women without epilepsy and without exposure to anticonvulsant agents. For comparison, the estimated background rate of oral clefts in the US as estimated by the US Centers for Disease Control and Prevention (CDC) is 0.17%. Based on NAAED data, the relative risk of developing an oral cleft defect in topiramate-exposed pregnancies was 9.6 compared with the risk in a background population of untreated women. The United Kingdom Epilepsy and Pregnancy Registry reported a similarly increased prevalence of oral clefts of 3.2% among infants exposed in utero to topiramate monotherapy; the reported rate was 16 times higher than the background rate in the United Kingdom, which is approximately 0.2%.

Data from the NAAED registry indicate that 19.7% of infants who were exposed to topiramate in utero were small for gestational age compared with 7.9% of infants exposed to a reference anticonvulsant and 5.4% of infants born to women without epilepsy and without exposure to anticonvulsant agents. In another population-based birth registry, 25% of topiramate-exposed infants were small for gestational age compared with 9% of infants who were not exposed to anticonvulsants. The long-term consequences of these findings are not known.

Topiramate has demonstrated selective developmental toxicity, including teratogenicity and embryotoxicity, in multiple species of animals (rats, rabbits, mice). Structural malformations, including craniofacial defects, and reduced fetal weights have occurred in offspring of pregnant animals that received topiramate at clinically relevant dosages. There also was some evidence of maternal toxicity (e.g., decreased maternal body weight gain, increased mortality).

Topiramate therapy can cause metabolic acidosis (see Cautions: Precautions and Contraindications). The effect of topiramate-induced metabolic acidosis has not been specifically studied during pregnancy; however, metabolic acidosis from other causes during pregnancy can result in decreased fetal growth, decreased fetal oxygenation, and fetal death, and also may affect the ability of the fetus to tolerate labor. Therefore, pregnant women receiving topiramate should be monitored and treated for metabolic acidosis in the same manner as nonpregnant patients. In addition, neonates born to women treated with topiramate should be monitored for metabolic acidosis because of possible drug transfer to the fetus and possible occurrence of transient metabolic acidosis following birth.

The benefits and risks of topiramate therapy should be carefully considered when use of the drug in women of childbearing potential is contemplated, particularly for conditions not usually associated with permanent injury or death. Alternative drugs that have a lower risk of oral clefts and other adverse birth outcomes should be considered in such patients. If a decision is made to use topiramate in a woman of childbearing potential, clinicians should recommend use of effective contraception for those who are not planning a pregnancy. The potential for decreased efficacy of estrogen-containing oral contraceptives should be considered. (See Drug Interactions: Oral Contraceptives.) Topiramate should be used during pregnancy only when the potential benefits outweigh the possible risks. If topiramate is used during pregnancy or if the patient becomes pregnant while receiving the drug, the patient should be apprised of the potential hazard to the fetus.

Women who become pregnant while receiving topiramate should be encouraged to enroll in the NAAED pregnancy registry; patients can enroll by calling 888-233-2334. Information on the registry also can be found on the website http://www.aedpregnancyregistry.org.

Limited data indicate that topiramate distributes into human milk at concentrations equal to approximately 10–20% of maternal plasma concentrations. Because the effects of this exposure on infants are unknown, caution should be exercised when topiramate is used in nursing women.

Drug Interactions

■ **Drugs Metabolized by Hepatic Microsomal Enzymes** In vitro studies indicate that topiramate is a mild inhibitor of cytochrome P-450 (CYP) isoenzyme 2C19 and a mild inducer of CYP3A4. Pharmacokinetic interactions with drugs metabolized by these isoenzymes, including some anticonvulsants, CNS depressants, and oral contraceptives, are therefore possible. Topiramate does not inhibit CYP1A2, 2A6, 2B6, 2C9, 2D6, 2E1, or 3A4/5.

■ **Amitriptyline** In healthy individuals, concomitant administration of topiramate (200 mg daily) and amitriptyline (25 mg daily) increased both peak plasma concentrations and area under the plasma concentration-time curve (AUC) of amitriptyline by 12%. Because some patients may experience a large increase in amitriptyline concentrations in the presence of topiramate, any adjustments in amitriptyline dosage should be made according to the patient's clinical response and not on the basis of plasma concentrations.

■ **Anticonvulsants** Clinically important decreases in plasma concentrations of topiramate have been observed in patients receiving concomitant therapy with phenytoin or carbamazepine. Plasma concentrations of topiramate were reduced by 48% with concomitant administration of phenytoin and topiramate compared with topiramate given alone. Plasma concentrations of phenytoin increased by 25% in some patients (generally in those receiving a twice-daily dosage regimen of phenytoin) and did not change substantially in others who received these drugs in combination. Concomitant administration of carbamazepine and topiramate decreased plasma concentrations of topiramate by 40% compared with topiramate given alone, but did not substantially alter plasma concentrations of carbamazepine or its active metabolite, carbamazepine-10,11-epoxide. Neither phenytoin nor carbamazepine alters the protein binding of topiramate.

Concomitant administration of valproic acid and topiramate decreased topiramate plasma concentrations by 14% and valproic acid plasma concentrations by 11%. In addition, concomitant use of topiramate and valproic acid has been associated with hyperammonemia with or without encephalopathy in patients who have previously tolerated either drug alone. (See Cautions: Precautions and Contraindications.) Although not studied, the interaction between valproic acid and topiramate may exacerbate existing defects or unmask deficiencies in susceptible patients. Concomitant use of topiramate with valproic acid also has been associated with hypothermia (with and without hyperammonemia) (see Cautions: Precautions and Contraindications). Discontinuance of topiramate or valproic acid therapy should be considered in patients who develop hypothermia. Valproic acid (at concentrations 5–10 times higher than therapeutic concentrations) decreases protein binding of topiramate from 23 to 13%; topiramate does not affect protein binding of valproic acid.

Concomitant administration of topiramate and phenobarbital or primidone altered plasma concentrations of the concomitantly administered anticonvulsant by less than 10%; the effects of phenobarbital or primidone on the pharmacokinetics of topiramate were not evaluated.

Lamotrigine pharmacokinetics are unlikely to be substantially affected by concurrent topiramate administration at dosages of up to 400 mg daily; however, plasma topiramate concentrations decreased by 13% during concurrent lamotrigine administration.

■ **Antidiabetic Agents** Concomitant administration of topiramate and glyburide (5 mg daily) in patients with type 2 diabetes mellitus decreased steady-state peak plasma concentrations and AUC of glyburide by 22 and 25%, respectively, compared with administration of glyburide alone. Systemic exposure of the active metabolites, 4-*trans*-hydroxyglyburide and 3-*cis*-hydroxyglyburide, also were reduced by 18 and 25%, respectively. Steady-state pharmacokinetics of topiramate were not affected by concomitant glyburide administration.

Concurrent administration of topiramate and pioglitazone in healthy individuals resulted in a nonsignificant decrease in steady-state pioglitazone AUC with no change in peak plasma concentrations. Decreases in systemic exposure to the active hydroxy- and keto-metabolites of pioglitazone also were observed; however, the clinical importance of these findings is not known. When topiramate therapy is initiated in patients receiving pioglitazone or vice versa, careful attention should be given to the routine monitoring of patients for adequate glycemic control.

In a drug interaction study in healthy individuals, mean peak plasma concentrations and AUC of metformin were increased by 18 and 25%, respectively, following concomitant administration of topiramate; however, time to reach peak plasma concentrations of metformin was not affected. Oral clearance of topiramate appears to be reduced when administered in conjunction with metformin. The clinical importance of these pharmacokinetic interactions is not known. However, topiramate can cause metabolic acidosis, a condition for which the use of metformin is contraindicated. The manufacturer of Qudexy® XR extended-release topiramate capsules states that the drug is contraindicated in patients with metabolic acidosis who are receiving metformin concomitantly.

■ **Drugs Predisposing to Heat-related Disorders** Increased risk of hyperthermia is possible with concomitant use of topiramate and drugs that predispose patients to heat-related disorders (e.g., carbonic anhydrase inhibitors, drugs with anticholinergic activity); caution is advised when topiramate is used in combination with such drugs.

■ **Carbonic Anhydrase Inhibitors** Concomitant use of topiramate with other carbonic anhydrase inhibitors (e.g., acetazolamide, dichlorphenamide, zonisamide) may increase the risk or severity of metabolic acidosis and may also increase the risk of kidney stone formation. If topiramate is used concomitantly with another carbonic anhydrase inhibitor, the patient should be monitored for the onset or worsening of metabolic acidosis.

■ **CNS Depressants** Concomitant administration of topiramate and CNS depressants (including alcohol) has not been evaluated in clinical studies. Because of the potential for topiramate to cause CNS depression as well as other cognitive and/or neuropsychiatric adverse effects, the drug should be used with extreme caution if administered concurrently with alcohol or other CNS depressants.

In vitro data indicate that in the presence of alcohol, plasma concentrations of Trokendi XR® extended-release topiramate capsules may be markedly increased soon after dosing and become subtherapeutic later in the day. Use of Trokendi XR® is contraindicated in patients with recent alcohol use (i.e., within 6 hours prior to or 6 hours after topiramate use).

■ **Digoxin** Serum digoxin AUC was decreased by 12% with concomitant use of topiramate in a single-dose study; however, the clinical importance of this interaction is unknown.

■ **Dihydroergotamine** Concomitant administration of topiramate (200 mg daily) and a single dose of dihydroegotamine (1 mg subcutaneously) in healthy individuals did not affect the pharmacokinetics of either drug.

■ **Diltiazem** Concomitant administration of topiramate (150 mg daily) and diltiazem (240 mg as extended-release capsules [Cardizem® CD]) decreased peak plasma concentrations and AUC of diltiazem by 10 and 25%, respectively. Systemic exposure to deacetyldiltiazem also was decreased, but there was no effect on *N*-monodesmethyldiltiazem. Diltiazem increased peak plasma concentrations and AUC of topiramate by 16 and 19%, respectively.

■ **Haloperidol** Pharmacokinetics of haloperidol (administered as a single 5-mg dose) were not affected by multiple doses of topiramate (100 mg every 12 hours) in healthy individuals.

■ **Hydrochlorothiazide** In a drug interaction study in healthy individuals, peak plasma concentrations and AUC of topiramate increased by 27 and 29%, respectively, following the addition of hydrochlorothiazide (25 mg daily). Steady-state pharmacokinetics of hydrochlorothiazide were not substantially altered by concomitant administration of topiramate. Although the clinical importance of this interaction is not known, a reduction in topiramate dosage may be necessary when hydrochlorothiazide is initiated.

In addition, both topiramate and hydrochlorothiazide have been shown to decrease serum potassium concentrations, and the decrease is greater when hydrochlorothiazide and topiramate are given in combination.

■ **Lithium** Although the pharmacokinetics of lithium were not affected during concurrent topiramate therapy at a dosage of 200 mg daily, an increase in lithium exposure (peak concentrations and AUC increased by 27 and 26%, respectively) has been reported in patients concurrently receiving topiramate dosages of up to 600 mg daily. Serum lithium concentrations should therefore be monitored in patients receiving concurrent lithium and high-dose topiramate therapy.

■ **Oral Contraceptives** In a pharmacokinetic study in healthy individuals, mean exposure to either component of an oral contraceptive containing 35 mcg of ethinyl estradiol and 1 mg of norethindrone was not substantially altered by concomitant administration of topiramate (given in the absence of other drugs). However, substantially decreased exposure to ethinyl estradiol was observed in patients receiving an oral contraceptive containing ethinyl estradiol and norethindrone in conjunction with topiramate and valproic acid therapy; exposure to norethindrone was not substantially affected.

The possibility of contraceptive failure and increased breakthrough bleeding should be considered in patients receiving combination oral contraceptives with topiramate. Such patients should be advised to report any changes in bleeding patterns to a clinician; contraceptive efficacy can be decreased even in the absence of breakthrough bleeding. (See Cautions: Pregnancy and Lactation.)

■ **Propranolol** Concomitant administration of topiramate (200 mg daily) and propranolol (160 mg daily) in healthy individuals did not affect the pharmacokinetics of either drug.

■ **Risperidone** Risperidone systemic exposure was decreased by 16 and 33% during concomitant topiramate therapy at dosages of 250 and 400 mg daily, respectively; no alterations of 9-hydroxyrisperidone (the active metabolite of risperidone; paliperidone) concentrations were observed. Concurrent administration of topiramate and risperidone increased peak plasma concentrations and AUC of topiramate by 14 and 12%, respectively. There were no clinically important changes in the systemic exposure of risperidone plus 9-hydroxyrisperidone or of topiramate; therefore, this interaction is unlikely to be clinically important.

■ **Sumatriptan** In healthy individuals, topiramate (100 mg every 12 hours) did not affect the pharmacokinetics of single-dose sumatriptan (100 mg orally or 6 mg subcutaneously).

■ **Venlafaxine** Concomitant multiple-dose administration of topiramate (150 mg daily) and venlafaxine (150 mg as extended-release capsules) in healthy individuals did not affect pharmacokinetics of venlafaxine, its active metabolite (O-desmethylvenlafaxine), or topiramate.

Pharmacokinetics

■ **Absorption** Topiramate is rapidly absorbed; peak plasma concentrations occur about 2 hours following an oral dose of 400 mg (as an immediate-release formulation) or approximately 20–24 hours following a single oral dose of 200 mg (as an extended-release formulation). The sprinkle capsule formulation of the drug is bioequivalent to the immediate-release tablet and, therefore, may be substituted as a therapeutic equivalent. The relative bioavailability of topiramate from the tablet formulation is about 80% compared with a solution. At steady state, the extended-release capsules administered once daily are bioequivalent to the immediate-release tablets administered twice daily. Topiramate exhibits linear, dose-proportional increases in plasma concentration over the dosage ranges evaluated (50 mg to 1.4 g daily depending on the formulation). Food may affect time to peak concentrations of the drug (depending on the formulation), but does not appear to affect systemic exposure.

■ **Distribution** Topiramate crosses the placenta and is distributed into breast milk. Approximately 15–41% of topiramate is bound to plasma proteins, with the fraction of protein binding decreasing as blood concentration increases.

■ **Elimination** The mean elimination half-life of topiramate is 21 hours following single or multiple doses of the drug as immediate-release formulations; the mean elimination half-life of Trokendi XR® extended-release capsules is approximately 31 hours following multiple doses, and the mean effective half-life of Qudexy® XR extended-release capsules is 56 hours. Approximately 70% of an administered dose is eliminated principally in urine as unchanged drug. Topiramate is not extensively metabolized; six minor metabolites have been identified, none of which constitutes more than 5% of an administered dose.

In patients with moderate (creatinine clearance 30–69 mL/minute per 1.73 m^2) or severe (creatinine clearance less than 30 mL/minute per 1.73 m^2) renal impairment, clearance of topiramate was reduced by 42 or 54%, respectively. However, since topiramate also undergoes substantial tubular reabsorption, the manufacturers state that creatinine clearance may not always predict clearance of topiramate. Geriatric patients with age-related renal impairment also may exhibit reduced clearance of the drug. (See Cautions: Geriatric Precautions.) In patients undergoing hemodialysis, clearance of topiramate is 4–6 times more rapid than in healthy individuals. (See Dosage and Administration: Dosage in Renal and Hepatic Impairment.)

Although the mechanism is not well understood, patients with hepatic impairment may have decreased clearance of topiramate.

Changes in topiramate clearance also have been observed in pediatric patients. (See Cautions: Pediatric Precautions.)

Description

Topiramate, a sulfamate-substituted derivative of the monosaccharide D-fructose, is an anticonvulsant agent that also is used for prophylaxis of migraine headache and management of alcohol dependence. The drug differs structurally from other currently available anticonvulsant agents. The spectrum of topiramate's anticonvulsant activity resembles that of carbamazepine and phenytoin, although differences in certain animal models have been observed and additive effects appear to occur when the drug is combined with these anticonvulsants.

Although the precise mechanism of action of topiramate is unknown, data from electrophysiologic and biochemical studies have revealed 4 properties that may contribute to the drug's efficacy for seizure disorders and migraine prophylaxis. At pharmacologically relevant concentrations, topiramate blocks voltage-dependent sodium channels; augments the activity of γ-aminobutyric acid (GABA) at some subtypes of the GABA-A receptor; antagonizes the AMPA/kainate subtype of the glutamate receptor; and inhibits carbonic anhydrase (particularly the CA-II and CA-IV isoenzymes). In general, anticonvulsant drugs are thought to act by one or more of the following mechanisms: modulating voltage-dependent ion (e.g., sodium) channels involved in action potential propagation or burst generation, enhancement of GABA inhibitory activity, and/or inhibition of excitatory amino acid neurotransmitter (e.g., glutamate, aspartate) activity.

Topiramate exhibits effects on cultured neurons similar to those observed with phenytoin and carbamazepine, and such effects are suggestive of an inactive state-dependent block of voltage-dependent sodium channels. Topiramate reduces the duration of epileptiform bursts of neuronal firing and decreases the number of action potentials in studies of cultured rat hippocampal neurons with spontaneous epileptiform burst activity. Topiramate also decreases the frequency of action potentials elicited by depolarizing electric current in cultured rat hippocampal neurons. Depolarization and firing of an action potential results from the rapid inflow of sodium ions through voltage-dependent sodium channels in the neuronal cell membrane. After firing, a neuron enters a period of inactivation during which it is unable to fire again even if the sodium channel is open. A slow action potential firing rate allows the neuron sufficient time to recover from inactivation, and the normal period of inactivation has a minimal effect on low-frequency firing. During a partial seizure, neurons characteristically undergo high-frequency depolarization and firing of action potentials which is uncommon during normal physiologic neuronal activity. Some anticonvulsant drugs (e.g., phenytoin, carbamazepine) preferentially bind to voltage-dependent sodium channels during their inactivated state, slow the rate of recovery of sodium channels from their period of inactivation, and limit the ability of the neuron to depolarize and fire at high frequencies.

Topiramate enhances the activity of the inhibitory neurotransmitter GABA at a nonbenzodiazepine site on $GABA_A$ receptors. Activation of the postsynaptic $GABA_A$ receptor by GABA causes inhibition by increasing the inward flow of chloride ions, resulting in hyperpolarization of the postsynaptic cell; in chloride ion-depleted murine cerebellar granule cells, therapeutic concentrations of topiramate (in combination with GABA) enhance GABA-evoked inward flux of chloride ions in a concentration-dependent manner. Benzodiazepines act at $GABA_A$ receptors to enhance GABA-evoked inward flow of chloride ions, but the benzodiazepine antagonist flumazenil does not appear to inhibit topiramate enhancement of GABA-evoked currents in $GABA_A$ cortical neuronal receptors. Topiramate also does not appear to increase duration of chloride ion channel opening. Therefore, topiramate may potentiate $GABA_A$-evoked chloride ion flux by a mechanism other than $GABA_A$-receptor modulation.

Topiramate antagonizes a non-*N*-methyl-d-aspartate (NMDA) glutamate receptor and the kainate/α-amino-3-hydroxy-5-methylisoxazole-4-propionic acid (AMPA) receptor subtype. Although topiramate had no apparent effect on glutamate receptors of the NMDA subtype in cultured rat hippocampal neurons, topiramate antagonized the ability of kainate to activate the kainate/AMPA glutamate receptor subtype, and these effects were shown to be concentration dependent. Glutamate, the principal excitatory neurotransmitter amino acid in the brain, interacts with specific neuronal membrane receptors, including ion channel coupled (ionotropic) (e.g., NMDA, kainate/AMPA, kainate) receptor subtypes and with G-protein coupled (metabotropic) receptors that modulate intracellular second-messengers. Glutamate is responsible for a variety of neurologic functions, including cognition, memory, movement, and sensation, and excessive activation of glutamate receptors may mediate injury or destruction of neurons in some acute neurologic disorders and chronic neurodegenerative diseases. The pathogenesis of seizures is thought to be mediated at least in part through excessive stimulation of glutamate receptors. In spontaneously epileptic rats, topiramate has reduced extracellular hippocampal concentrations of both glutamate and aspartate, and a correlation existed between reduction in glutamate concentrations and suppression of tonic seizures.

In animals, topiramate exhibits anticonvulsant activity in the maximal electroshock seizure (MES) test, suggesting that, like phenytoin, it may be effective in the management of partial and tonic-clonic (grand mal) seizures in humans. Topiramate also exhibited dose-dependent inhibition of absence-like seizures, which was antagonized by pretreatment with haloperidol. In animals, topiramate was ineffective or weakly effective in blocking clonic seizures induced by pentylenetetrazole, indicating that the drug may not enhance GABA inhibitory activity substantially.

Although the precise mechanism(s) of action of topiramate in the management of alcohol dependence is unclear, topiramate enhances GABA-mediated inhibitory neurotransmission and inhibits glutamatergic stimulatory neurotransmission; such changes appear to decrease dopaminergic activity in the mesocorticolimbic areas of the brain, which have been associated with alcohol dependence.

Topiramate inhibits carbonic anhydrase CA-II and CA-IV isoenzymes and, like other carbonic anhydrase inhibitors (e.g., acetazolamide, dichlorphenamide, zonisamide), the drug may promote the formation of renal calculi by increasing urinary pH and decreasing the excretion of urinary citrates. In premarketing studies, renal calculi were reported to occur in 1.5% of patients receiving topiramate, an incidence 2–4 times that expected in a similar untreated population, but most patients who developed calculi elected to continue therapy with the drug. Use of topiramate with other carbonic anhydrase inhibitors may increase the risk of renal calculi (see Drug Interactions: Carbonic Anhydrase Inhibitors).

Preparations

Excipients in commercially available drug preparations may have clinically important effects in some individuals; consult specific product labeling for details.

Topiramate

Oral		
Capsules (containing coated particles)	15 mg*	Topamax® Sprinkle Capsules, Janssen
		Topiramate Sprinkle Capsules
	25 mg*	Topamax® Sprinkle Capsules, Janssen
		Topiramate Sprinkle Capsules
Capsules, extended-release	25 mg*	Qudexy® XR, Upsher-Smith
		Topiramate Extended-release Capsules
		Trokendi XR®, Supernus
	50 mg*	Qudexy® XR, Upsher-Smith
		Topiramate Extended-release Capsules
		Trokendi XR®, Supernus
	100 mg*	Qudexy® XR, Upsher-Smith
		Topiramate Extended-release Capsules
		Trokendi XR®, Supernus
	150 mg*	Qudexy® XR, Upsher-Smith
		Topiramate Extended-release Capsules
	200 mg*	Qudexy® XR, Upsher-Smith
		Topiramate Extended-release Capsules
		Trokendi XR®, Supernus
Tablets, film-coated	25 mg*	Topamax®, Janssen
		Topiramate Tablets
	50 mg*	Topamax®, Janssen
		Topiramate Tablets
	100 mg*	Topamax®, Janssen
		Topiramate Tablets
	200 mg*	Topamax®, Janssen
		Topiramate Tablets

*available from one or more manufacturer, distributor, and/or repackager by generic (nonproprietary) name

†Use is not currently included in the labeling approved by the US Food and Drug Administration

Valproate Sodium
Sodium Dipropylacetate, Sodium α-Propylvalerate, DPA Sodium

Valproic Acid
Dipropylacetic Acid, 2-Propylvaleric Acid, DPA

Divalproex Sodium
Valproate Semisodium

■ Valproic acid, valproate sodium, and divalproex sodium are carboxylic acid-derivative anticonvulsants that also are used to treat acute manic episodes or for prophylaxis of migraine headache as well as certain other psychiatric disorders.

Uses

■ **Seizure Disorders** Valproic acid, valproate sodium, and divalproex sodium are used for the management of various seizure disorders, including complex partial seizures, absence seizures, and other seizure types. Because there are only minor differences in the pharmacokinetics of the formulations and because all forms of the drug circulate in plasma as valproic acid, the term "valproic acid" will mainly be used in the following discussion.

Valproic acid is used alone or with other anticonvulsants (e.g., ethosuximide) in the prophylactic management of simple and complex absence (petit mal) seizures. The drug also may be used in conjunction with other anticonvulsants in the management of multiple seizure types that include absence seizures. Valproic acid is considered a drug of choice for absence or atypical absence seizures.

Valproic acid is used alone or with other anticonvulsants (e.g., carbamazepine, phenytoin) in the prophylactic management of complex partial seizures that occur either by themselves or in association with other seizure types. Some clinicians state that valproic acid may be considered a drug of choice for the management of complex partial seizures. Two randomized, placebo-controlled trials, one of valproic acid as monotherapy and one of valproic acid as adjunctive therapy, demonstrated that the drug decreased the frequency of seizures in patients inadequately controlled by other therapies (e.g., carbamazepine, phenytoin, phenobarbital).

Valproic acid has been used and is considered by some clinicians as a drug of choice for management of other generalized seizures, including primary generalized tonic-clonic seizures†, myoclonic seizures†, or atonic seizures†, especially for those patients with more than one type of generalized seizure. In addition, some clinicians state that valproic acid may be used as a drug of choice for the management of simple partial seizures†. Valproic acid also has been administered rectally† or by intragastric drip† with some success in the management of status epilepticus refractory to IV diazepam†. A parenteral formulation of valproic acid has been studied and has been effective when administered IV† in the management of status epilepticus.

Valproic acid has been used with some success in the treatment of Lennox-Gastaut syndrome and infantile spasms.

Valproate sodium has been used for the prevention of posttraumatic seizures in patients with acute head injuries†. In a randomized, double-blind study comparing the efficacy of IV valproate sodium (administered for 1 week followed by oral valproic acid for 1 or 6 months) with that of IV phenytoin (administered for 1 week followed by placebo) for this use, the mortality rate was found to be higher in patients treated with valproate sodium followed by valproic acid compared with those receiving phenytoin (13 versus 8.5%, respectively). Many of these patients were critically ill with multiple and/or severe injuries and a causal relationship to valproic acid has not been established. However, pending further study, the manufacturer and some clinicians state that it is prudent to not use IV valproate sodium in patients with acute head trauma for posttraumatic seizure prophylaxis.

■ **Bipolar Disorder** Divalproex sodium and valproic acid are used in the treatment of acute manic or mixed episodes associated with bipolar disorder; valproate sodium† also has been used. Because there are only minor differences in the pharmacokinetics of the formulations and because all forms of the drug circulate in plasma as valproic acid, the term "valproic acid" will mainly be used in the following discussion.

Valproic acid has been used as monotherapy or as part of combination therapy (e.g., with lithium, antipsychotic agents [e.g., olanzapine], antidepressants, carbamazepine) in the treatment of acute manic episodes. The American Psychiatric Association (APA) currently recommends combined therapy with valproic acid plus an antipsychotic agent or with lithium plus an antipsychotic agent as first-line drug therapy for the acute treatment of more severe manic or mixed episodes and monotherapy with one of these drugs for less severe episodes. For mixed episodes, valproic acid may be preferred over lithium. Valproic acid or lithium also is recommended for the initial acute treatment of rapid cycling.

A manic episode is a distinct period of abnormally and persistently elevated, expansive, or irritable mood. Typical symptoms include pressure of speech, motor hyperactivity, reduced need for sleep, flight of ideas, grandiosity, poor judgment, aggressiveness, and possible hostility.

Efficacy of divalproex sodium (given as Depakote® or Depakote® ER tablets) in the treatment of manic episodes has been established in several short-term, placebo-controlled, parallel-group trials in patients who were hospitalized for acute mania; response to therapy was assessed using objective rating scales such as the Young Mania Rating Scale (YMRS), an augmented Brief Psychiatric Rating Scale (BPRS-A), the Mania Rating Scale (MRS), and the Global Assessment Scale (GAS). In these studies, valproic acid was found to be substantially superior to placebo in all of the outcome measures assessed. One study specifically enrolled patients who were intolerant of or unresponsive to previous lithium therapy. Up to 40% of patients fail to respond to or are intolerant of lithium therapy for manic episodes; such patients may demonstrate a response to valproic acid, although response to valproic acid appears to be independent of prior response to lithium therapy. Valproic acid therapy appears to be about as effective as lithium for the treatment of manic episodes. In one placebo-controlled trial, 48% of patients receiving valproic acid demonstrated a response to the drug as measured by changes in the Manic Syndrome subscale of the MRS; 49% of patients receiving lithium responded to therapy, while 25% of patients receiving placebo responded. Antimanic response to valproic acid typically occurs within 1–2 weeks of initiating therapy. Valproic acid therapy also appears to be effective in specific types of mania, including rapid-cycling mania and dysphoric mania, which have been reported to be poorly responsive to lithium.

Although the manufacturers state that safety and efficacy of long-term (i.e., longer than 3 weeks) valproic acid therapy have not been established in the treatment of manic episodes, valproic acid also has been used, alone or in combination therapy, for long-term or maintenance antimanic therapy†, and APA currently considers the best empiric evidence to support the use of valproic acid or lithium for maintenance therapy. Antimanic efficacy has been maintained from several months to more than 10 years, and such long-term therapy appears to decrease the frequency and severity of bipolar episodes over extended periods of time; however, further study is required to establish the efficacy of valproic acid as maintenance therapy of manic episodes. Valproic acid does not appear to be as effective for the management of the depressive component of bipolar disorder†; although some evidence suggests that long-term valproic acid therapy may be moderately effective in the prophylaxis of depressive episodes, its acute effects on depression appear to be limited. Some clinicians recommend that valproic acid therapy be used in patients with bipolar disorder or schizoaffective disorder, bipolar type, who have responded inadequately to or have been unable to tolerate treatment with lithium salts or other therapy (e.g., carbamazepine), particularly if the patient displays residual manic symptoms, or in the presence of rapid cycling, dysphoric mania or hypomania, associated neurologic abnormalities, or organic brain disorder.

■ **Migraine** ***Prophylaxis of Chronic Attacks*** Divalproex sodium and valproic acid are used in the prophylaxis of migraine headache; sodium valproate† also has been used. Because there are only minor differences in the pharmacokinetics of the formulations, and because all forms of the drug circulate in plasma as valproic acid, the term "valproic acid" will mainly be used in the following discussion.

Valproic acid should *not* be used in pregnant women for the prevention of migraine headaches; in such patients, the risks of the drug (e.g., major congenital malformations and cognitive impairment in prenatally exposed children) outweigh any possible benefits (see Pregnancy under Cautions: Pregnancy, Fertility, and Lactation). Valproic acid also should not be used in women of childbearing potential unless the drug is clearly shown to be essential in the management of their medical condition; this is especially important when the drug is being contemplated or used for the management of a condition not ordinarily associated with permanent injury or risk of death such as migraine headaches.

The US Headache Consortium states that there is good evidence from multiple well-designed clinical trials that valproic acid and divalproex sodium have medium to high efficacy for the prophylaxis of migraine headache. Divalproex sodium (given as Depakote® tablets) was demonstrated to be effective in the prophylaxis of migraine headache in 2 randomized, double-blind, placebo-controlled trials in patients with at least a 6-month history of migraine, with or without associated aura. Patients also had to experience at least 2 migraines per month in the 3 months prior to enrollment in the studies; patients were excluded if they had cluster headaches. Although women of childbearing potential were excluded from one study because of the teratogenic properties of valproic acid, they were included in the other, provided that they were practicing an effective form of contraception. In both studies, after a 4-week single-blind placebo baseline period, patients were randomized to receive either valproic acid or placebo during a 12-week treatment period consisting of a 4-week titration period and an 8-week maintenance period. Assessment of treatment outcome was based on 4-week migraine headache rates during the 12-week treatment period. In the first study, dosage titration was guided by the use of actual or sham trough total serum valproate concentrations for patients receiving valproic acid or placebo, respectively. The mean dosage of valproic acid was 1087 mg daily (range: 500–2500 mg daily), with dosages of more than 500 mg being given in 3 divided doses daily. Patients receiving valproic acid experienced a substantial decrease in the mean 4-week migraine headache rate compared with those receiving placebo (3.5 versus 5.7, respectively). In the second study, patients were randomized to receive (after titration from an initial dosage of 250 mg daily) 500, 1000, or 1500 mg of valproic acid daily or placebo, administered as 2 daily doses. Efficacy of valproic acid in the second study was to be determined by comparing the 4-week migraine headache rate in the combined groups of patients receiving 1000 and 1500 mg of valproic acid to that of patients receiving placebo. However, the manufacturer reports that the mean 4-week migraine headache rates in patients receiving valproic acid 500, 1000, or 1500 mg daily were 3.3, 3, or 3.3, respectively, compared to a rate of 4.5 in patients receiving placebo, and that the rate in the combined groups of patients receiving 1000 or 1500 mg daily was substantially lower than that of the placebo group.

In addition, divalproex sodium (given once daily as Depakote® ER extended-release tablets) was demonstrated to be effective in the prophylaxis of migraine headache in a 12-week, multicenter, double-blind, placebo-controlled clinical trial in patients with a history of migraine headaches with or without associated aura. In this study, patients receiving extended-release divalproex sodium tablets (initiated at 500 mg once daily for 1 week, then increased to 1 g once daily if tolerated) experienced a substantial mean reduction in 4-week migraine headache rate compared with those receiving placebo (reduction of 1.2 from a baseline mean of 4.4 versus a reduction of 0.6 from a baseline mean of 4.2, respectively).

Other studies also have shown valproic acid to be effective in the prophylaxis of migraine. In one comparative, single-blind, placebo-controlled, crossover study, valproic acid was shown to be as effective in migraine prophylaxis as propranolol.

Acute Attacks IV† valproate sodium has been used for the acute† management of migraine headache; however, the role of the drug relative to other acute therapies (selective serotonin type 1-like receptor agonists ["triptans"], ergot alkaloids, antiemetics, nonsteroidal anti-inflammatory agents [NSAIAs], butalbital-containing analgesics, opiate analgesics) requires further elucidation. Results of several studies, including open-label, comparative, randomized, prospective, retrospective, and/or double-blind, studies and at least one placebo-controlled study, as well as case reports, indicate that IV valproate sodium may alleviate acute migraine attacks in patients with or without aura and generally appears to be well tolerated. Efficacy generally was evaluated in terms of a reduction in headache severity as rated by the patient (i.e., a reduction in pain from severe or moderately severe to mild or absent usually using a 3- or 4-point scale) or by a visual analog pain score (VAS). Limited data indicate that 300-mg to 1-g IV valproate sodium doses (some of which were repeated at the same initial dose or less) were associated with relief of migraine headache, usually within 1 to several hours.

IV valproate sodium also has been used in the management of chronic daily headache† in a limited number of patients some of whom have had an inadequate response to dihydroergotamine or when dihydroergotamine was contraindicated.

Further study and experience are needed to more clearly define the role of IV valproate sodium in the management of acute migraine attacks and other headaches.

There is no evidence that orally administered valproic acid or divalproex sodium is useful in the acute† treatment of migraine headaches.

For further information on management and classification of migraine headache, see Vascular Headaches: General Principles in Migraine Therapy, under Uses, in Sumatriptan 28:32.28.

■ **Schizophrenia** Valproic acid or divalproex sodium has been used as an adjunct to antipsychotic agents in the symptomatic management of schizophrenia† in patients who fail to respond sufficiently to an adequate trial of an antipsychotic agent alone. The American Psychiatric Association (APA) and some clinicians state that anticonvulsant agents such as valproic acid or divalproex sodium may be useful adjuncts in schizophrenic patients with prominent mood lability or with agitated, aggressive, hostile, or violent behavior. In general, for such adjunctive therapy, valproic acid or divalproex sodium is administered in the same dosage and with the same resulting therapeutic plasma concentrations as that in the management of seizure disorders. The APA states that, with the exception of patients with schizophrenia whose illness has strong affective components, valproic acid or divalproex sodium alone has not been shown to be substantially effective in the long-term treatment of schizophrenia. For additional information on the management of schizophrenia, see Uses: Psychotic Disorders, in the Phenothiazines General Statement 28:16.08.24.

While some evidence suggested potential benefit of valproic acid in relieving tardive dyskinesia in patients receiving long-term antipsychotic drug therapy†, recent systematic review of randomized controlled trials with nonbenzodiazepine γ-aminobutyric acid (GABA) agonists such as valproic acid found the evidence for such benefit unconvincing, and indicated that any possible benefit may be outweighed by adverse effects.

■ **Other Uses** Some experts recommend use of valproic acid for the treatment of aggressive outbursts in children with ADHD. For a more detailed discussion on the management of ADHD, see Uses: Attention Deficit Hyperactivity Disorder, in Methylphenidate 28:20.04.

Valproic acid used alone or in conjunction with GABA was ineffective in the treatment of chorea† (including Huntington's chorea). Valproic acid has been effective in a limited number of patients with organic brain syndrome†.

Dosage and Administration

■ **Administration** Valproate sodium can be administered orally or by IV infusion and valproic acid and divalproex sodium are administered orally. Valproic acid also has been administered rectally† by enema or in wax-based suppositories.

Patients who are currently receiving or beginning therapy with valproic acid, valproate sodium, or divalproex sodium and/or any other anticonvulsant for any indication should be closely monitored for the emergence or worsening of depression, suicidal thoughts or behavior (suicidality), and/or any unusual changes in mood or behavior. (See Cautions: Nervous System Effects and Cautions: Precautions and Contraindications.)

A medication guide explaining the risks and benefits of valproic acid therapy should be distributed to patients receiving valproic acid, valproate sodium, or divalproex sodium.

Oral Administration Valproic acid, valproate sodium, and divalproex sodium are administered orally. Valproic acid capsules should be swallowed whole, not chewed, in order to prevent local irritation to the mouth and throat. If GI irritation occurs, the drug may be administered with food or the dosage may be gradually increased from an initially low dosage. Patients who are unable to tolerate the GI effects of valproic acid or valproate sodium may tolerate divalproex sodium.

Delayed-release capsules of valproic acid (Stavzor®) should be swallowed whole, and not crushed, chewed, or broken.

Delayed-release tablets of divalproex sodium (e.g., Depakote®) should be swallowed intact, and not crushed or chewed.

When switching to divalproex sodium delayed-release tablets (e.g., Depakote®) or valproic acid delayed-release capsules (Stavzor®) in patients receiving conventional valproic acid (e.g., Depakene®), the same daily dosage and schedule should be used. After stabilization with the delayed-release formulation, the daily dosage may be divided and administered 2 or 3 times daily in selected patients.

Extended-release tablets of divalproex sodium (e.g., Depakote® ER) are administered once daily; patients should be advised that the extended-release tablets must be swallowed intact and not chewed or crushed.

If a patient misses a dose of valproic acid or divalproex sodium, the dose should be taken as soon as possible, unless it is almost time for the next dose. However, if the patient skips a dose, a double dose should *not* be taken to make up for the missed dose.

Valproate sodium oral solution should not be administered in carbonated drinks because valproic acid will be liberated and may cause local irritation to the mouth and throat as well as an unpleasant taste.

The commercially available capsules containing coated particles of divalproex sodium (e.g., Depakote® Sprinkle Capsules) may be swallowed intact or the entire contents of the capsule(s) may be sprinkled on a small amount (about 5 mL) of soft food (e.g., applesauce, pudding) and swallowed (not chewed) immediately. The mixture of coated particles and food should not be stored for future use. Patients receiving divalproex sodium capsules containing coated particles may notice coated particles in their stool because these particles do not completely dissolve and may be passed in the stool. (See Cautions: Precautions and Contraindications.)

Although the extent of GI absorption of valproic acid from capsules containing coated particles or delayed-release tablets of divalproex sodium is equivalent, peak and trough plasma concentrations achieved with these dosage forms may vary (e.g., higher peak valproic acid concentrations generally are achieved with the delayed-release tablets). These differences are unlikely to be clinically important; however, increased monitoring of plasma valproic acid concentrations is recommended if one dosage form is substituted for the other.

IV Administration Valproate sodium injection is intended for IV use only.

For IV use, the manufacturer states that the appropriate dose of valproate sodium injection should be diluted with at least 50 mL of a compatible IV solution (e.g., 5% dextrose injection, 0.9% sodium chloride injection, lactated Ringer's injection). Diluted IV solutions of the drug should be infused IV over 60 minutes; the manufacturer recommends that the rate not exceed 20 mg/minute.

Rapid IV infusion of valproate sodium has been associated with an increased risk of adverse effects and is not currently included in the manufacturer's labeling. However, rates exceeding 20 mg/minute or infusion periods less than 60 minutes have been studied in a limited number of patients with seizure disorders and in patients with acute migraine headaches, and such administration generally appeared to be well tolerated. In a study of the safety of initial 5- to 10-minute IV infusions of valproate sodium (1.5–3 mg/kg per minute of valproic acid), patients generally tolerated such rapid infusions of the drug; the study was not designed to assess the efficacy of the regimen. The drug also appeared to be well tolerated in studies evaluating efficacy in the management of acute migraine attacks† when valproate sodium doses of 300 mg to 1 g were infused IV at rates ranging from 17–250 mg/minute or occasionally by direct rapid ("bolus") IV injection (100-mg doses).

Use of rapid infusions in patients receiving the IV preparation as a parenteral replacement for oral valproic acid has not been established.

Valproate sodium injection and diluted solutions of the drug should be inspected visually for particulate matter and discoloration prior to administration whenever solution and container permit.

■ Dosage

Dosage of valproate sodium and divalproex sodium is expressed in terms of valproic acid. Dosage must be carefully and slowly adjusted according to individual requirements and response.

Seizure Disorders **IV Dosage.** IV valproate sodium therapy may be employed in patients in whom oral therapy is temporarily not feasible, but therapy should be switched to oral administration as soon as clinically possible. IV administration of the drug can be used for monotherapy or as adjunctive therapy in the management of seizure disorders. The manufacturer states that the usual total daily dosages of valproic acid are equivalent for IV or oral administration, and the doses and frequency of administration employed with oral therapy in seizures disorders are expected to be the same with IV therapy, although plasma concentration monitoring and dosage adjustment may be necessary. The use of IV therapy for longer than 14 days has not been studied to date. The manufacturer also states that the use of IV valproate sodium for initial monotherapy has not been systematically studied; however, usual dosages and titration employed with oral therapy can be employed with parenteral therapy. Patients receiving dosages near the maximum recommended dosage of 60 mg/kg daily should be monitored closely, particularly when enzyme-inducing drugs are not used concomitantly.

Oral Dosage. Various valproic acid dosage regimens have been used in published studies. A correlation between plasma valproic acid concentration and therapeutic effect has not been established; however, an anticonvulsant therapeutic range of 50–100 mcg/mL of total (bound and unbound) valproic acid has been suggested.

For the management of complex partial seizures, the manufacturers state that the usual initial dosage of valproic acid as monotherapy or as adjunctive therapy, when being added to a current therapeutic regimen, for adults and children 10 years of age and older is 10–15 mg/kg daily. For the management of simple or complex absence seizures, the manufacturers state that the usual initial dosage of valproic acid is 15 mg/kg daily. Dosage may be increased by 5–10 mg/kg daily at weekly intervals until seizures are controlled or adverse effects prevent further increases in dosage. The manufacturers state that the maximum recommended dosage is 60 mg/kg daily. These dosage recommendations also apply when anticonvulsant therapy is being initiated with divalproex sodium as delayed- or extended-release formulations. If the total daily dose exceeds 250 mg, the drug (with the exception of the extended-release tablet formulation [e.g., Depakote® ER]) should be administered in divided doses.

When converting a patient from a current anticonvulsant to valproic acid therapy for the treatment of complex partial seizures, valproic acid therapy should be initiated at usual starting dosages. The dosage of the current anticonvulsant may be decreased by 25% every 2 weeks, either starting concomitantly with the initiation of valproic acid therapy or delayed by 1–2 weeks if there is a concern that seizures are likely to occur with a reduction. The speed and duration of withdrawal of the current anticonvulsant can be highly variable, and patients should be monitored closely during this period for increased seizure frequency. When divalproex sodium delayed-release tablets are administered, a twice-daily dosing regimen is suggested whenever feasible and appears to adequately maintain plasma valproic acid concentrations in most patients receiving the drug. The frequency of adverse effects (particularly hepatic effects) may be dose related. The benefit of improved seizure control which may accompany higher dosages should therefore be weighed carefully against the risk of adverse effects.

When converting a patient whose seizure disorder is controlled with delayed-release divalproex sodium tablets (e.g., Depakote®) to the extended-release tablets (e.g., Depakote® ER), the drug should be administered once daily using a total daily dosage that is 8–20% higher than the corresponding delayed-release dosage that the patient was receiving. For patients whose delayed-release daily dosage cannot be directly converted to a corresponding commercially available extended-release dosage, clinicians may consider increasing the delayed-release total daily dosage to the next higher dosage before converting to the appropriate extended-release dosage.

For the management of status epilepticus refractory to IV diazepam†, 400–600 mg of valproic acid has been administered rectally† by enema or in wax base suppositories at 6-hour intervals.

Bipolar Disorder The recommended initial dosage of valproic acid or divalproex sodium in the acute treatment of manic or mixed episodes is 750 mg daily in divided doses, which may be given as delayed-release tablets (e.g., Depakote®) or delayed-release capsules (Stavzor®), or 25 mg/kg once daily when given as extended-release tablets (e.g., Depakote® ER). The dosage of valproic acid or divalproex sodium should be increased as quickly as possible to achieve the lowest therapeutic dosage producing the desired clinical effect or desired serum concentration; however, the manufacturers recommend that the dosage not exceed 60 mg/kg daily. In placebo-controlled studies of patients receiving divalproex sodium as the delayed-release tablet for the treatment of acute mania, the trough serum valproic acid concentration that produced the desired clinical effect ranged from 50–125 mcg/mL; maximum serum concentrations generally were achieved within 14 days after initiating therapy. In a placebo-controlled study of patients receiving divalproex sodium as the extended-release tablet for the treatment of manic or mixed-type episodes, dosage was adjusted to achieve trough serum valproic acid concentrations of 85–125 mcg/mL.

The manufacturers state that although it is agreed that pharmacologic treatment beyond an initial response in patients with manic episodes is desirable, both for the maintenance of initial response and for prevention of new manic episodes, the safety and efficacy of long-term (i.e., longer than 3 weeks) valproic acid and divalproex sodium therapy for manic episodes have not been established in controlled clinical trials. Clinicians who elect to use such therapy for extended periods (i.e., longer than 3 weeks) should continually reevaluate the usefulness of valproic acid therapy in the individual patient. The manufacturers state that the safety of valproic acid for longer-term therapy is supported by data from record reviews involving approximately 360 patients treated with valproic acid for longer than 3 months.

Dosing guidelines for maintenance therapy† with valproic acid are less evidence-based than those for acute therapy, and dosages lower than those employed for acute therapy occasionally have been used. A 1-year study with divalproex sodium found an association between higher serum concentrations and increased appetite and decreased platelet and leukocyte counts.

Migraine **Prophylaxis of Chronic Attacks.** In the prophylaxis of migraine headache, the recommended initial dosage of divalproex sodium or valproic acid is 250 mg twice daily given as delayed-release tablets (e.g., Depakote®) or delayed-release capsules (Stavzor®), respectively, or 500 mg once daily given as extended-release divalproex sodium tablets (e.g., Depakote® ER). Some patients may benefit from dosages of up to 1 g daily; in clinical trials, there was no evidence of additional benefit with higher dosages . After 1 week at the initial dosage of 500 mg daily in patients receiving the extended-release tablets (e.g., Depakote® ER), dosage may be increased to 1 g once daily. Although maintenance dosages other than 1 g once daily have not been evaluated in patients with migraine headache, the effective dosage range for these patients is 500 mg to 1 g daily. It should be considered that divalproex sodium extended-release tablets and divalproex sodium delayed-release tablets are *not* bioequivalent. If a patient requires smaller dosage adjustment than that available using the extended-release tablets, the delayed-release tablets should be used instead.

Acute Attacks. For the acute management of migraine headache† in adults and adolescents, the optimum IV dosage, frequency, and rate of administration have not been established. In most reports, IV valproate sodium was given in doses of 300 mg to 1 g diluted in a compatible IV infusion (e.g., 5% dextrose injection, 0.9% sodium chloride injection) solution (usually about 100–250 mL) and infused IV at rates ranging from 17–100 mg/minute. In some patients, the dose was administered more rapidly (e.g., 500 mg over 2 minutes, 100 mg by direct ["bolus"] IV injection). A repeat dose (equal to the initial dose or less) was given to some patients within a few hours, if reduction of pain was not sufficient. In one study, 500-mg doses of valproate sodium were administered every 8 hours for 2 days. Some patients have received direct IV injections of 100-mg doses repeated at 5-minute intervals or infusions of a single 500-mg dose (diluted in 5 mL of 0.9% sodium chloride injection) into a free-flowing IV line of 0.9% sodium chloride injection.

When IV valproate sodium has been used in the management of chronic daily headache, an initial dose of 15 mg/kg was administered over 30 minutes followed by a dose of 5 mg/kg (infused over 15 minutes) given every 8 hours.

Dosage in Geriatric Patients Because of a decrease in clearance of free (unbound) valproic acid and the possibility of increased sensitivity to adverse effects (e.g., somnolence) in geriatric patients, the initial dosage should be reduced. Subsequent dosage should be increased more slowly in geriatric patients. In addition, the manufacturer recommends regular monitoring of fluid and nutritional intake, dehydration, somnolence, and other adverse effects in these individuals. Dosage reduction or discontinuance of valproic acid should be considered in geriatric patients with decreased food or fluid intake and in those with excessive somnolence. The ultimate therapeutic dosage in these patients should be determined on the basis of tolerability and clinical response.

Cautions

The adverse effect profile of parenteral valproate sodium can be expected to include all of the effects associated with oral administration of the drug. In addition, IV infusion of valproate sodium may cause local effects at the injection site and effects associated with the rate of infusion. (See Cautions: Local and Infusion-related Effects.)

■ **GI Effects** Nausea, vomiting, abdominal pain, anorexia, diarrhea, and dyspepsia may occur in patients receiving valproic acid. The most frequent adverse effects of valproic acid following initiation of therapy with the drug are nausea, vomiting, and indigestion. These adverse effects usually are transient, rarely require discontinuance of therapy, and can be minimized by administering the drug with meals or by beginning therapy with low dosages and increasing the dosage very gradually. While divalproex sodium shares the toxic GI potential of valproic acid, the frequency of adverse GI effects appears to be lower and the effects possibly less severe with divalproex sodium than with valproic acid; patients who are unable to tolerate the GI effects of valproic acid or valproate sodium may tolerate divalproex sodium, but GI intolerance to divalproex sodium can also occur. Both anorexia with some weight loss and increased appetite with weight gain have been reported in patients receiving valproic acid. Eructation, fecal incontinence, gastroenteritis, glossitis, flatulence, hematemesis, periodontal abscess, tooth disorder, dry mouth, stomatitis, and constipation were reported in 1–5% of patients receiving valproic acid in clinical trials. Dysphagia, gum hemorrhage, and mouth ulceration also have occurred in greater than 1% of patients receiving the drug.

Medication residue in the stool has been reported rarely with divalproex sodium (e.g., Depakote®, Depakote® ER) formulations; in some reports, the residue occurred in the presence of diarrhea. Some of the patients in the reported cases had anatomic (e.g., ileostomy, colostomy) or functional GI disorders that decrease GI transit times. (See Cautions: Precautions and Contraindications.)

■ **Pancreatitis** Cases of life-threatening pancreatitis have been reported in children and adults shortly after initial use or after several years of therapy with valproic acid. Pancreatitis may be hemorrhagic with a rapid progression from initial symptoms to death. Development of manifestations suggestive of pancreatitis (e.g., abdominal pain, nausea, vomiting, and/or anorexia) requires prompt medical evaluation. (See Cautions: Precautions and Contraindications.) It should be considered that patients receiving valproic acid are at greater risk of developing pancreatitis than that expected in the general population; in addition, pancreatitis recurred on rechallenge with the drug in several patients. In clinical trials involving 2416 patients, 2 cases of pancreatitis without alternative etiology were reported, representing 1044 patient-years experience.

■ **Nervous System Effects** Sedation and drowsiness may occur with valproic acid therapy, especially in patients receiving other anticonvulsants. (See Drug Interactions: CNS Depressants, Antidepressants, and Anticonvulsants.) Somnolence, asthenia, dizziness, and tremor generally are the most frequently reported adverse nervous system effects in patients receiving valproic acid in clinical trials. Ataxia, emotional lability, abnormal thinking, amnesia, and depression have been reported in up to 5–8% of patients receiving the drug. Some patients have reported increased alertness, insomnia, and nervousness during valproic acid therapy. Coma has been reported rarely in patients receiving valproic acid as monotherapy or in combination with phenobarbital.

Between 1–5% of patients receiving valproic acid in clinical trials experienced anxiety, confusion, headache, myasthenia, abnormal gait, paresthesia, hypertonia, incoordination, abnormal dreams, personality disorder, hallucinations, euphoria, agitation, catatonia, dysarthria, speech disorder, hypokinesia, increased reflexes, tardive dyskinesia, or vertigo. Asterixis, hypesthesia, parkinsonism, hostility, emotional upset, and psychosis/acute psychosis also have occurred rarely. Hyperactivity, aggressiveness, and other behavioral disturbances have been reported in a few children receiving valproic acid.

Patients have rarely developed encephalopathy with or without fever, without evidence of hepatic dysfunction or abnormal valproic acid plasma concentrations, shortly after the introduction of valproic acid therapy. Although this condition can be reversible upon discontinuance of the drug, there have been fatalities in patients with hyperammonemic encephalopathy, often in patients with underlying urea cycle disorder. (See Cautions: Endocrine and Metabolic Effects and see also Cautions: Precautions and Contraindications.)

Reversible and irreversible cerebral or cerebellar atrophy (or pseudoatrophy), temporally associated with the use of valproic acid and often accompanied by cognitive decline, has been reported during postmarketing experience. In some cases, patients recovered with permanent sequelae. (See Cautions: Precautions and Contraindications.)

The US Food and Drug Administration (FDA) has analyzed suicidality reports from placebo-controlled studies involving 11 anticonvulsants, including valproic acid, and found that patients receiving anticonvulsants had approximately twice the risk of suicidal behavior or ideation (0.43%) compared with patients receiving placebo (0.24%). FDA's analysis included 199 randomized, placebo-controlled studies of 11 anticonvulsants (carbamazepine, felbamate, gabapentin, lamotrigine, levetiracetam, oxcarbazepine, pregabalin, tiagabine, topiramate, valproate, and zonisamide) involving over 43,000 patients 5 years of age or older; the studies evaluated the effectiveness of the anticonvulsants in epilepsy, psychiatric disorders (e.g., bipolar disorder, depression, anxiety), and other conditions (e.g., migraine, neuropathic pain). This increased suicidality risk was observed as early as one week after beginning therapy and continued through 24 weeks. The results were generally consistent among the 11 drugs studied. In addition, patients who were treated for epilepsy, psychiatric disorders, and other conditions were all found to be at increased risk for suicidality when compared with placebo; there did not appear to be a specific demographic subgroup of patients to which the increased risk could be attributed. However, the relative risk for suicidality was found to be higher in patients with epilepsy compared with patients who were given one of the drugs for psychiatric or other conditions. (See Cautions: Precautions and Contraindications.)

■ **Hepatic Effects** Minor elevations in serum concentrations of aminotransferases (transaminases) and lactate dehydrogenase occur frequently in patients receiving valproic acid and appear to be dose related. In clinical trials, increased ALT (SGPT) and increased AST (SGOT) concentrations occurred in 1–5% of patients receiving valproic acid. Occasionally, increases in serum bilirubin concentration and abnormal changes in other hepatic function test results occur; these results may reflect potentially serious hepatotoxicity. (See Cautions: Precautions and Contraindications.)

Hepatic failure resulting in death has occurred in patients receiving valproic acid, usually during the first 6 months of therapy. Patients receiving multiple anticonvulsants, children, those with congenital metabolic disorders, those with severe seizure disorders accompanied by mental retardation, and those with organic brain disease may be at particularly high risk of valproic acid-induced hepatotoxicity. Clinical experience indicates that children younger than 2 years of age, especially those with the previously mentioned conditions, have a considerably increased risk of developing fatal hepatotoxicity. (See Cautions: Precautions and Contraindications.) In patients older than 2 years of age, clinical experience in epilepsy indicates that the frequency of fatal hepatotoxicity decreases considerably in progressively older patient groups.

An increased risk of valproic acid-induced acute liver failure and resultant deaths have been observed in patients with hereditary neurometabolic syndromes caused by mutations in the mitochondrial DNA polymerase gamma (*POLG*) gene (e.g., Alpers-Huttenlocher syndrome) compared with those without these conditions. Most of the cases were reported in children and adolescents. (See Cautions: Precautions and Contraindications.)

Severe or fatal hepatotoxicity induced by valproic acid may be preceded by nonspecific symptoms such as malaise, weakness, lethargy, facial edema, anorexia, and vomiting. In epileptic patients, loss of seizure control also may precede the development of hepatotoxicity. (See Cautions: Precautions and Contraindications.)

■ **Endocrine and Metabolic Effects** Hyperammonemic encephalopathy, including some fatalities, has been reported in patients with urea cycle disorders (UCD), particularly ornithine transcarbamylase deficiency, following initiation of valproic acid therapy. Hyperammonemia may occur in patients receiving valproic acid and may occur in the absence of abnormal hepatic function test results. Development of symptoms of unexplained hyperammonemic encephalopathy (e.g., lethargy, vomiting, changes in mental status) requires prompt medical evaluation. (See Cautions: Precautions and Contraindications.)

Plasma ammonia concentrations have not been systematically evaluated following IV administration of valproate sodium; however, hyperammonemia with encephalopathy has been reported in at least 2 patients who received IV infusions of the drug.

Concomitant administration of valproic acid and topiramate has been associated with hyperammonemia with or without encephalopathy in patients who have previously tolerated either drug alone. (See Drug Interactions: CNS Depressants, Antidepressants, and Anticonvulsants.) Patients with inborn errors of metabolism or reduced hepatic mitochondrial activity may be at increased risk of hyperammonemia with or without encephalopathy.

Hypothermia (defined as an unintentional drop in body core temperature to less than 35°C) has been reported in association with valproic acid therapy, both in conjunction with and in the absence of hyperammonemia. Hypothermia may be manifested by a variety of clinical abnormalities including lethargy, confusion, coma, and substantial alterations in other major organ systems such as the cardiovascular and respiratory systems. Hypothermia also may occur in patients receiving concurrent topiramate and valproic acid therapy after initiating topiramate therapy or following an increase in the daily dosage of topiramate.

Hyponatremia and inappropriate antidiuretic hormone (ADH) secretion also have been reported. Hyperglycinemia has been reported in patients receiving valproic acid and was associated with a fatal outcome in one patient with preexisting nonketotic hyperglycinemia. Between 1–5% of patients receiving valproic acid in clinical trials experienced dysmenorrhea, amenorrhea, vaginitis, metrorrhagia, or vaginal hemorrhage. Breast enlargement, galactorrhea, irregular menses, polycystic ovaries, hyperandrogenism, weight gain, Fanconi's syndrome (principally reported in children), and parotid gland swelling have occurred in some patients receiving valproic acid. Abnormal thyroid function test results and decreased carnitine concentrations also have been reported; however, the clinical importance of these abnormalities has not been elucidated.

■ **Hematologic Effects** Valproic acid inhibits the secondary phase of platelet aggregation and may prolong bleeding time. In one study of valproic acid monotherapy for seizures, 27% of patients receiving approximately 50 mg/kg per day had at least one platelet count of 75,000/mm^3 or less. Approximately half of the patients discontinued therapy, with their platelet counts returning to normal; the remaining patients experienced normalization of their platelet counts with continued valproic acid therapy. In this study, the probability of thrombocytopenia appeared to increase significantly at total trough valproate plasma concentrations of 110 mcg/mL or greater (females) or 135 mcg/mL or greater (males). (See Cautions: Precautions and Contraindications.)

Ecchymosis, petechiae, bruising, hematoma formation, epistaxis, frank hemorrhage, lymphocytosis, leukopenia, eosinophilia, macrocytosis, acute intermittent porphyria, decreased fibrinogen concentrations, anemia (including macrocytic anemia, with or without folate deficiency), bone marrow suppression, pancytopenia, and aplastic anemia have been reported in patients receiving valproic acid therapy.

■ **Dermatologic and Sensitivity Reactions** Between 1–5% of patients receiving valproic acid in clinical trials experienced seborrhea, dry skin, pruritus, furunculosis, rash (including maculopapular), or discoid lupus erythematosus. Transient alopecia, cutaneous vasculitis, generalized pruritus, anaphylaxis, photosensitivity, Stevens-Johnson syndrome, erythema nodosum, and erythema multiforme have been reported in patients receiving valproic acid therapy. Rare cases of toxic epidermal necrolysis have been reported, including a fatal case in a 6-month-old infant receiving valproic acid therapy; however, the infant was receiving other drugs concomitantly. An additional case of fatal toxic epidermal necrosis was reported in a 35-year-old patient with acquired immunodeficiency syndrome (AIDS) who was taking several concomitant drugs and who had a history of multiple cutaneous drug reactions.

Multi-organ hypersensitivity reactions have been reported rarely in close temporal association (median time to detection: 21 days; range: 1–40 days) to initiation of valproic acid therapy in adult and pediatric patients. Many of these cases resulted in hospitalization and at least one death has been reported.

Although signs and symptoms are diverse, patients with multi-organ hypersensitivity typically, although not exclusively, present with fever and rash associated with other organ system involvement. Other associated manifestations may include lymphadenopathy, hepatitis, liver function test abnormalities, hematologic abnormalities (e.g., eosinophilia, thrombocytopenia, neutropenia), pruritus, nephritis, oliguria, hepatorenal syndrome, arthralgia, and asthenia. Because multi-organ hypersensitivity reactions are variable in their expression, signs and symptoms associated with other organ systems also may occur. Although the existence of cross sensitivity with other drugs that produce this syndrome is unclear, experience with drugs associated with multi-organ hypersensitivity indicates that this may be a possibility. (See Cautions: Precautions and Contraindications.)

■ **Local and Infusion-related Effects** In addition to the usual adverse effects associated with oral therapy, IV infusion of valproate sodium can produce local effects at the site of injection as well as adverse effects associated with the rate of IV infusion. In clinical trials involving healthy adults as well as patients with seizure disorders at total IV dosages of 120–6000 mg daily, adverse local effects at the site of infusion were reported in up to 2.6% of patients and included pain (2.6%), injection site reaction (2.4%), and inflammation (0.6%). In these trials, about 2% of patients discontinued parenteral therapy with the drug because of adverse effects, principally because of nausea and vomiting and elevated amylase. Other reasons for discontinuing parenteral valproate sodium therapy included hallucinations, pneumonia, headache, injection site reaction, and abnormal gait.

Dizziness and injection site pain were reported more frequently when valproate sodium was infused IV at a rate of 100 mg/minute relative to slower rates that ranged up to 33 mg/minute. At an IV infusion rate of 200 mg/minute, dizziness and taste perversion occurred more frequently than at an IV infusion rate of 100 mg/minute. In clinical trials, the maximum IV infusion rate studied was 200 mg/minute.

■ **Ocular and Otic Effects** Diplopia, amblyopia, nystagmus, and tinnitus have been reported in up to 7–16% of patients receiving valproic acid in clinical trials. Other adverse ocular and otic effects reported in patients receiving valproic acid include abnormal vision, otitis media, conjunctivitis, dry eyes, ocular pain, ocular disorder, photophobia, otic pain, and otic disorder. Reversible and irreversible hearing loss (including deafness) has been reported; however, a casual relationship has not been established.

■ **Other Adverse Effects** Infection has been reported in up to 20% of patients receiving valproic acid in clinical trials. Back pain, fever, flu syndrome, bronchitis, rhinitis, pharyngitis, dyspnea, and peripheral edema have been reported in up to 5–12% of patients receiving the drug in clinical trials. Increased cough, chest pain, tachycardia, hypertension, palpitation, arrhythmia, bradycardia, hypotension, postural hypotension, taste perversion, hiccups, facial edema, pneumonia, sinusitis, dysuria, urinary incontinence, cystitis, urinary frequency, arthralgia, myalgia, arthrosis, leg cramps, twitching, malaise, chills, fever with chills, sweating, vasodilation, cyst, neck pain, neck rigidity, and accidental injury also may occur. Adverse effects reported rarely in patients receiving valproic acid include muscular weakness, interstitial nephritis, enuresis, urinary tract infection, bone pain, lupus erythematosus, and fatigue. A case of reversible skeletal muscle weakness and ventilatory failure also has been reported in a geriatric patient receiving valproic acid therapy.

■ **Precautions and Contraindications** Since divalproex sodium is a prodrug of valproate, it shares the toxic potentials of valproic acid, and the usual cautions, precautions, and contraindications of valproic acid therapy should be observed with divalproex sodium therapy.

Patients should be warned that valproic acid may impair ability to perform hazardous activities requiring mental alertness or physical coordination (e.g., operating machinery or driving a motor vehicle).

FDA has informed healthcare professionals about an increased risk of suicidality (suicidal behavior or ideation) observed in an analysis of studies using various anticonvulsants compared with placebo. (See Cautions: Nervous System Effects.) FDA recommends that all patients who are currently receiving or beginning therapy with any anticonvulsant for any indication be closely monitored for the emergence or worsening of depression, suicidal thoughts or behavior (suicidality), and/or unusual changes in mood or behavior. Symptoms such as anxiety, agitation, hostility, mania, and hypomania may be precursors to emerging suicidality. Clinicians should inform patients, their families, and caregivers of the potential for an increased risk of suicidality so that they are aware and able to notify their clinician of any unusual behavioral changes. Patients, family members, and caregivers also should be advised not to make any changes to the anticonvulsant regimen without first consulting with the responsible clinician. They should pay close attention to any day-to-day changes in mood, behavior, and actions; since changes can happen very quickly, it is important to be alert to any sudden differences. In addition, patients, family members, and caregivers should be aware of common warning signs that may signal suicide risk (e.g., talking or thinking about wanting to hurt oneself or end one's life, withdrawing from friends and family, becoming depressed or experiencing worsening of existing depression, becoming preoccupied with death and dying, giving away prized possessions). If these or any new and worrisome behaviors occur, the responsible clinician should be contacted immediately. FDA also recommends that clinicians who prescribe valproic acid or any other anticonvulsant balance the risk for suicidality with the risk of untreated illness. Epilepsy and many other illnesses for which anticonvulsants are prescribed are themselves associated with an increased risk of morbidity and mortality and an increased risk of suicidal thoughts and behavior. If suicidal thoughts and behavior emerge during anticonvulsant therapy, the clinician must consider whether the emergence of these symptoms in any given patient may be related to the illness being treated.

Results of in vitro studies indicate that valproate appears to stimulate replication of human immunodeficiency virus (HIV) and cytomegalovirus (CMV) under certain experimental conditions. The clinical importance of these in vitro findings, including any relevance to patients receiving maximally suppressive antiretroviral therapy, is not known. (See Pharmacology: Antiviral Effects.) It has been suggested that these in vitro effects should be considered when interpreting test results concerning the clinical condition of HIV-infected patients (e.g., plasma HIV RNA levels) or patients with CMV infection receiving valproic acid.

Since valproic acid may cause serious and potentially fatal hepatotoxicity, patients receiving the drug should be closely monitored for possible nonspecific symptoms of hepatic dysfunction (e.g., malaise, weakness, lethargy, facial edema, anorexia, vomiting, loss of seizure control). In addition, hepatic function tests should be performed before and at frequent intervals during therapy, especially during the first 6 months. (See Cautions: Hepatic Effects.) Since results of hepatic function tests may not be abnormal in all instances, clinicians must also consider the results of careful interim medical history and physical examination of the patient. Valproic acid therapy should be discontinued immediately in the presence of suspected or apparent substantial hepatic dysfunction. In some patients, hepatic dysfunction has progressed despite discontinuance of the drug. Since elevations in hepatic enzyme concentrations may be dose related, the benefit of improved seizure control which may accompany higher doses of the drug must be weighed against the potential risks. Valproic acid should be used with caution in patients with a history of hepatic disease. Children and patients receiving multiple anticonvulsants or those with congenital metabolic disorders, severe seizure disorders accompanied by mental retardation, or organic brain disease may be at particular risk of hepatotoxicity. Because children younger than 2 years of age, especially those with the previously listed conditions, have a considerably increased risk of developing fatal hepatotoxicity compared with older patient groups, valproic acid should be used in these patients only with extreme caution and as a single agent; the benefits of therapy must be weighed against the potential risks. In patients older than 2 years of age, experience in epilepsy indicates that the frequency of fatal hepatotoxicity decreases considerably in progressively older patient groups. Valproic acid should *not* be used in patients with hepatic disease or substantial hepatic dysfunction.

Valproic acid is contraindicated in patients known to have a mitochondrial disorder caused by mutations in the *POLG* gene (e.g., Alpers-Huttenlocher syndrome) and in children younger than 2 years of age in whom there is a clinical suspicion of such a disorder. In patients older than 2 years of age with suspected hereditary mitochondrial disease, valproic acid should be used only if other anticonvulsant therapies have failed; such patients should be closely monitored during valproic acid therapy for the development of acute liver injury with regular clinical assessments and liver function test monitoring. *POLG*-related disorders should be suspected in any patient with a family history and/or symptoms suggestive of such a disorder (e.g., unexplained encephalopathy, refractory epilepsy [focal, myoclonic], status epilepticus at presentation, developmental delays, psychomotor regression, axonal sensorimotor neuropathy, myopathy, cerebellar ataxia, ophthalmoplegia, complicated migraine with occipital aura). *POLG* screening should be performed, if necessary, in accordance with current clinical practice. The A467T and W748S mutations are present in approximately two-thirds of patients with autosomal recessive *POLG*-related disorders. Valproic acid therapy should be discontinued immediately in the presence of suspected or apparent substantial hepatic dysfunction. In some patients, hepatic dysfunction has progressed despite discontinuance of the drug. (See Cautions: Hepatic Effects.)

Because the use of valproic acid has been associated with life-threatening pancreatitis in children and adults (see Cautions: Pancreatitis), patients and guardians should be instructed that if symptoms of pancreatitis (e.g., abdominal pain, nausea, vomiting, anorexia) develop, prompt medical evaluation is needed. If pancreatitis is diagnosed, valproic acid usually should be discontinued and alternative therapy for the underlying medical condition should be initiated as clinically indicated.

Because the use of valproic acid has been associated with hyperammonemic encephalopathy, patients should be advised that if symptoms of this disorder (e.g., lethargy, vomiting, changes in mental status) develop, they should notify their clinician promptly. (See Cautions: Endocrine and Metabolic Effects.) If such symptoms are present, plasma ammonia concentrations should be determined, and, if these concentrations are increased, valproic acid therapy should be discontinued. Appropriate treatment of hyperammonemia should be initiated and the patient should be evaluated for urea cycle disorders. Asymptomatic elevation of ammonia concentrations is more common than symptomatic hyperammonemia. In patients with asymptomatic elevations, plasma ammonia concentrations should be closely monitored and, if elevations persist, discontinuance of valproic acid therapy should be considered. Prior to the initiation of valproic acid therapy, an evaluation for urea cycle disorders should be considered in patients with a history of unexplained encephalopathy or coma, encephalopathy associated with a protein load, pregnancy-related or postpartum encephalopathy, unexplained mental retardation, or history of elevated plasma ammonia or glutamine concentrations; patients with cyclical vomiting and lethargy, episodic extreme irritability, ataxia, low BUN concentration, or protein avoidance; patients with a family history of urea cycle disorders or unexplained infant deaths (particularly males); and patients with other signs or symptoms of urea cycle disorders.

Discontinuance of valproic acid therapy should be considered in patients who develop hypothermia, which can be manifested by a variety of clinical abnormalities including lethargy, confusion, coma, and substantial alterations in other major organ systems such as the cardiovascular and respiratory systems. Since hypothermia also may be a symptom of hyperammonemia, clinical management and assessment of the condition should include determination of blood ammonia concentrations.

In a randomized, double-blind study comparing the efficacy of IV valproate sodium (administered for one week followed by oral valproic acid for 1 or 6 months) with that of IV phenytoin (administered for 1 week followed by placebo) for the prevention of posttraumatic seizures in patients with acute head injuries†, the mortality rate was found to be higher in patients treated with valproate sodium followed by valproic acid compared with those receiving phenytoin (13 versus 8.5%, respectively). Many of these patients were critically ill with multiple and/or severe injuries and a causal relationship to the drug has not been established. However, pending further information, the manufacturer and some clinicians state that it is prudent to not use IV valproate sodium in patients with acute head trauma for posttraumatic seizure prophylaxis.

Anticonvulsant drugs (including valproic acid) should not be discontinued abruptly in patients, including in pregnant women, receiving the drugs to prevent major seizures because of the strong possibility of precipitating status epilepticus with attendant hypoxia and threat to life. (See Pregnancy under Cautions: Pregnancy, Fertility, and Lactation.)

Since valproic acid may cause thrombocytopenia and inhibit platelet aggregation, platelet counts and coagulation studies should be determined before and periodically during therapy with the drug and before planned (i.e., elective) surgery is performed in patients receiving the drug. Some clinicians have recommended thromboelastography as a more reliable method to assess the effects of valproic acid on coagulation. If clinical evidence of hemorrhage, bruising, or a disorder of hemostasis/coagulation occurs during valproic acid therapy, dosage should be reduced or the drug withdrawn pending further evaluation.

Because the use of valproic acid has been associated with multi-organ hypersensitivity reactions (see Cautions: Dermatologic and Sensitivity Reactions), patients should be advised that a fever associated with other organ system involvement (e.g., rash, lymphadenopathy) may be drug-related and should be reported immediately to the clinician. If a multi-organ hypersensitivity reaction is suspected, valproic acid should be discontinued and alternative treatment initiated.

Since valproic acid may interact with concurrently administered drugs that are capable of hepatic enzyme induction, periodic determinations of plasma concentrations of valproic acid and concomitant drugs are recommended during the early course of therapy. (See Drug Interactions.)

Because of the possibility of cerebral and cerebellar atrophy associated with the use of valproic acid, patients should be routinely monitored for motor and cognitive impairments during therapy; if any manifestations of brain atrophy develop or are suspected, continued use of the drug should be evaluated. (See Cautions: Nervous System Effects.)

Patients receiving divalproex sodium formulations (e.g., Depakote®, Depakote® ER, Depakote® Sprinkle Capsules) should be instructed to notify their clinician if they notice any medication residue in their stool. It is recommended that plasma valproic acid concentrations and clinical status be monitored in such patients; if clinically indicated, alternative therapy may be considered.

Valproic acid is contraindicated in patients with hepatic disease or substantial hepatic dysfunction. Valproic acid also is contraindicated in patients with known mitochondrial disorders caused by *POLG* mutations and in children younger than 2 years of age suspected of having a *POLG*-related disorder. (See Cautions: Hepatic Effects.)

Valproic acid is contraindicated in patients with known hypersensitivity to the drug. Valproic acid also is contraindicated in patients with known urea cycle disorders. (See Cautions: Endocrine and Metabolic Effects.) In addition, use of valproic acid is contraindicated for prophylaxis of migraine headaches in pregnant women. (See Cautions: Pregnancy, Fertility, and Lactation.)

■ Pediatric Precautions Experience with oral valproic acid therapy in the management of seizures indicates that children younger than 2 years of age are at an increased risk of developing fatal hepatotoxicity. The drug should be used with extreme caution and as single-agent therapy in such children, and the benefits of valproic acid therapy weighed against the risks. Experience in epilepsy indicates that the incidence of fatal hepatotoxicity decreases considerably in progressively older patient groups (i.e., older than 2 years of age). (See Cautions: Hepatic Effects and see also Cautions: Precautions and Contraindications.)

Younger children, especially those receiving enzyme-inducing drugs, will require larger maintenance dosages to attain targeted total and unbound valproic acid concentrations for the management of seizures. The variability in free fraction limits the clinical usefulness of monitoring total serum valproic acid concentrations alone. Interpretation of valproic acid concentration in children should include consideration of factors that affect hepatic metabolism and protein binding.

The safety and efficacy of valproic acid in the treatment of complex partial seizures have not been established in pediatric patients younger than 10 years of age. Available data from placebo-controlled clinical trials failed to demonstrate efficacy of extended-release divalproex sodium tablets for the treatment of mania in pediatric patients 10–17 years of age and for the prevention of migraine headaches in adolescent patients 12–17 years of age. Safety and tolerability of divalproex sodium in pediatric patients appear to be similar to those observed in adults.

The safety of valproate sodium injection has not been studied in pediatric patients younger than 2 years of age. If a decision is made to use the injection in this age group, the manufacturer states that it should be used with extreme caution and only as monotherapy, and the potential benefits should be weighed against the possible risks. No unusual adverse effects were observed in clinical trials employing IV valproate sodium for the management of seizure disorders in 35 pediatric patients 2–17 years of age.

■ Geriatric Precautions No geriatric patients older than 65 years of age were enrolled in controlled trials of oral valproic acid for the treatment of manic episodes associated with bipolar disorder. In a case review of almost 600 patients treated with valproic acid for manic episodes, approximately 12% of patients were older than 65 years of age. A higher percentage of these patients reported accidental injury, infection, pain, somnolence, or tremor during valproic acid therapy compared with younger patients. Discontinuance of valproic acid therapy occasionally was associated with somnolence or tremor. The manufacturer states that it is unclear whether these events indicate additional risks of drug therapy or whether they result from preexisting medical conditions or concomitant medication use in these geriatric patients.

Results of a double-blind, multicenter study of geriatric patients (mean age: 83 years) with dementia who were receiving valproic acid (dosages increased by 125 mg daily up to a target daily dosage of 20 mg/kg) indicate that the incidence of somnolence was higher in patients receiving valproic acid than in those receiving placebo and discontinuance of therapy because of somnolence was higher in those receiving valproic acid than in those receiving placebo. In about 50% of patients with somnolence, a reduced nutritional intake and weight loss also were observed. The incidence of dehydration also appeared to be higher in geriatric patients receiving valproic acid than in those receiving placebo. In the patients who experienced the mentioned adverse effects, a trend for lower baseline albumin concentration, lower valproic acid clearance, and higher BUN was observed. Therefore, it is recommended that initial dosage of valproic acid be reduced and subsequent dosages be increased more slowly in geriatric patients. In addition, the manufacturers recommend regular monitoring of fluid and nutritional intake, dehydration, somnolence, and other adverse effects in these individuals. Dosage reduction or discontinuance of valproic acid should be considered in geriatric patients with decreased food or fluid intake and in those with excessive somnolence.

The safety and efficacy of valproic acid for the prevention of migraine headaches in geriatric patients older than 65 years of age have not been established.

No unique safety concerns were identified in geriatric patients older than 65 years of age receiving IV valproate sodium in clinical trials.

■ Mutagenicity and Carcinogenicity Studies of valproic acid that used bacterial and mammalian test systems have shown no evidence to date of a mutagenic potential for the drug.

In rats and mice receiving valproic acid dosages of 80 and 170 mg/kg daily for 2 years, an increased incidence of subcutaneous fibrosarcomas occurred in male rats at the higher dosage level and a dose-related trend for an increased incidence of benign pulmonary adenomas was observed in male mice. The importance of these findings to humans is not known.

■ Pregnancy, Fertility, and Lactation Use of valproic acid during pregnancy is associated with an increased risk of neural tube defects (NTDs; e.g., spina bifida) and other major congenital malformations (e.g., craniofacial defects, cardiovascular malformations, malformations involving various body systems). In utero exposure to valproic acid also can cause decreased intelligence quotient (IQ) scores and other adverse cognitive effects in children.

Adverse fetal effects similar to those observed in humans have been observed in developmental toxicity studies in animals. Administration of valproic acid to mice, rats, rabbits, and monkeys during the period of organogenesis resulted in an increased incidence of fetal structural malformations (e.g., skeletal, cardiac, urogenital), intrauterine growth retardation, and embryofetal death. Such effects were observed at clinically relevant dosages of valproic acid. In addition, fetal NTDs were observed in mice following valproic acid administration during critical periods of organogenesis; this teratogenic response correlated with maximum maternal drug concentrations. Behavioral abnormalities (e.g., cognitive, locomotor, and social interaction deficits) and brain histopathologic changes also have been observed in mice and rats following prenatal exposure to clinically relevant dosages of valproic acid.

Valproic acid can cause major congenital malformations in humans, particularly NTDs, and this risk appears to be greatest during the first trimester of pregnancy. Recent data indicate that the risk of major congenital malformations is substantially greater with use of valproic acid than with use of other anticonvulsant agents during pregnancy. To monitor maternal-fetal outcomes of pregnant women exposed to anticonvulsant agents, including valproic acid, the North American Antiepileptic Drug (NAAED) pregnancy registry has been established. Data obtained from the NAAED registry indicate that the rate of major malformations in infants exposed in utero to valproic acid as monotherapy is about fourfold higher than the rate of major malformations in infants exposed to monotherapy with another anticonvulsant agent. Among 149 women in the registry who received valproic acid (average daily dosage of 1 g) for epilepsy during the first trimester of pregnancy, 16 infants were born with a birth defect, including NTDs (3 cases), craniofacial defects, cardiovascular defects, and other malformations involving various body systems. The rate of major malformations in infants exposed to valproic acid was 10.7% compared with a rate of 2.9% among infants born to a control group of women in the registry who received another anticonvulsant drug during the first trimester of pregnancy. The strongest association between maternal use of valproic acid and congenital anomalies is with the development of NTDs (e.g., spina bifida). Use of valproic acid during pregnancy is associated with an approximate 1–2% fetal risk of congenital spinal bifida (based on data from the US Centers for Disease Control and Prevention [CDC]); according to data from the CDC's National Birth Defects Prevention Network, the estimated risk of spina bifida in the general population is about 0.06–0.07%. Evidence suggests that prophylactic use of folic acid prior to conception and during pregnancy decreases the incidence of congenital NTDs in the general population, and folic acid supplementation prior to conception and during pregnancy should be routinely recommended in women receiving valproic acid. It is not known whether folic acid supplementation specifically reduces the risk of NTDs or decreased IQ in the offspring of women receiving valproic acid therapy.

In utero exposure to valproic acid also appears to be associated with an increased risk of adverse cognitive effects in children. Several epidemiologic studies have shown that children born to women who received valproic acid during pregnancy score lower on IQ tests and other cognitive function tests measuring a variety of mental and developmental abilities than those exposed in utero to other anticonvulsant agents or to no anticonvulsant therapy. In one large, prospective, observational cohort study (the Neurodevelopmental Effects of Antiepileptic Drugs [NEAD] study), children who had been exposed to valproic acid in utero had significantly lower IQ scores at 6 years of age than those exposed in utero to lamotrigine, phenytoin, or carbamazepine monotherapy. After adjustment for potentially confounding factors, IQ scores were on average 8–11 points lower in valproic acid-exposed children compared with those exposed to the other anticonvulsant drugs. These findings of reduced IQ were consistent with those reported in 2 interim analyses that were conducted when the children were 2–3 and 4.5 years of age, although overall IQ scores tended to improve with age. Fetal exposure to valproic acid also was associated with impairments in a range of other cognitive domains (e.g., memory, verbal and nonverbal abilities, executive functions, cognitive fluency and originality); in general, the effects of the drug were dose dependent, with higher dosages associated with worse cognitive outcomes. Other observational studies also have demonstrated poorer cognitive outcomes, including delayed mental development, increased special education needs, and reduced verbal IQ, in cohorts of children exposed in utero to valproic acid compared with other anticonvulsant agents. Despite the methodologic limitations of these studies (e.g., lack of randomization, small sample size), the weight of available evidence currently supports a correlation between prenatal valproic acid exposure and an increased risk of cognitive deficits, including decreased IQ, in children. The long-term effects of prenatal valproic acid exposure on cognitive development have not been established. It is also not known whether these effects occur when fetal exposure is limited with respect to duration or timing (e.g., to the first trimester) during pregnancy. Therefore, the risk for development of adverse cognitive effects in valproic acid-exposed children should be considered at any time during pregnancy. In the NEAD study, a positive association was found between periconceptional use of folic acid and IQ scores; however, this finding should be interpreted with caution because the study was not specifically designed to evaluate this outcome. Folic acid supplementation prior to conception and during pregnancy should be routinely recommended in all women of childbearing age receiving valproic acid to decrease the risk of birth defects.

There also is a possible association between in utero valproic acid exposure and developmental delay, autism, or autism spectrum disorders. Results of a population-based cohort study using national register data from Denmark found that maternal use of valproic acid during pregnancy was associated with an increased risk of autism spectrum disorders and childhood autism in the offspring. The study identified a cohort of children (total of 655,615) born during a 10-year period and followed these children from birth until death, emigration, diagnosis of autism spectrum disorder or childhood autism, or study end. Among 508 children who were identified as having been exposed to valproic acid in utero, the absolute risk of autism spectrum disorder was 4.42% (adjusted hazard ratio of 2.9) and the absolute risk of childhood autism was 2.5% (adjusted hazard ratio of 5.2); the estimated absolute risk of these disorders in the entire population of children studied was 1.53 and 0.48%, respectively, after 14 years of follow-up.

Valproic acid is contraindicated in pregnant women for the prevention of migraine headaches. The drug should not be used in pregnant women with epilepsy or bipolar disorder unless other treatments have failed to provide adequate symptom relief or are otherwise unacceptable; in these cases, the benefits of valproic acid may continue to outweigh its risks. It should be kept in mind that untreated or inadequately treated epilepsy or bipolar disorder during pregnancy increases the risk of complications in both the pregnant woman and her developing fetus.

Because of the risk of major congenital malformations and other adverse pregnancy outcomes (e.g., decreased IQ in offspring) which may occur very early in pregnancy, use of valproic acid should be avoided whenever possible in women of childbearing potential. Alternative therapies to valproic acid should be considered, especially if the drug is being used for the treatment of migraines or other conditions not usually considered life-threatening, in women of childbearing potential. If valproic acid is necessary in a woman of childbearing potential, some experts suggest that the lowest possible dosage be employed. Effective contraception should be used in such women during valproic acid therapy. If pregnancy occurs during therapy, the clinician should be notified immediately; valproic acid should not be discontinued abruptly in a pregnant woman with epilepsy because of the risk of precipitating seizures. In individual cases when the severity and frequency of the seizure disorder are such that discontinuance of therapy does not pose a serious threat to the patient, discontinuance of the drug may be considered prior to and during pregnancy; however, even minor seizures can pose some hazard to the developing embryo or fetus.

In women who are contemplating pregnancy, alternative therapies to valproic acid should be considered; clinicians should review and revise the treatment plan with the patient well before conception. Women who become pregnant while receiving valproic acid should be encouraged to enroll in the NAAED pregnancy registry by calling 888-233-2334; information on the NAAED registry also is available on the website http://www.aedpregnancyregistry.org. Tests to detect neural tube and other malformations using current accepted procedures should be considered a part of routine prenatal care and be offered to all women who become pregnant while receiving valproic acid.

Patients receiving valproic acid may develop clotting abnormalities. A pregnant patient taking multiple anticonvulsant agents, including valproic acid, developed hypofibrinogenemia; the patient then gave birth to an infant with afibrinogenemia, who subsequently died of hemorrhage. If valproic acid is to be used during pregnancy, clotting parameters should be monitored closely.

Cerebral atrophy has been reported in children following prenatal exposure to valproic acid. In addition, fatal cases of hepatic failure in infants exposed to valproic acid in utero have been reported. (See Cautions: Hepatic Effects and see also Cautions: Precautions and Contraindications.)

The effect of valproic acid on the development of the testes and on sperm production and fertility in humans is not known. Chronic toxicity studies in rats and dogs demonstrated reduced spermatogenesis and testicular atrophy. Further animal studies are ongoing.

Valproic acid is distributed into milk; caution is advised when administering the drug to nursing women.

Drug Interactions

■ **Drugs Affecting Hepatic Microsomal Enzymes** Drugs that affect the level of expression of hepatic enzymes, particularly those that elevate the levels of glucuronyltransferases, may increase valproic acid clearance. Carbamazepine, phenobarbital (or primidone), or phenytoin can double the clearance of valproic acid. Therefore, patients receiving valproic acid monotherapy generally will have longer elimination half-lives and higher plasma concentrations than patients who are concurrently receiving more than one anticonvulsant. (See Drug Interactions: CNS Depressants, Antidepressants, and Anticonvulsants.)

Drugs that inhibit cytochrome P450 (CYP450) isoenzymes, including some antidepressants, are unlikely to substantially affect valproic acid clearance because CYP450-mediated oxidation is a relatively minor secondary metabolic pathway compared with glucuronidation and β-oxidation. (See Drug Interactions: CNS Depressants, Antidepressants, and Anticonvulsants.)

Because of possible alterations in clearance of valproate, increased monitoring of plasma valproic acid concentrations and concomitant drug concentrations is recommended whenever enzyme-inducing drugs are introduced or withdrawn in valproic acid-treated patients.

■ **CNS Depressants, Antidepressants, and Anticonvulsants** Additive CNS depression may occur when valproic acid is administered concomitantly with other CNS depressants including other anticonvulsants (particularly phenobarbital and primidone) and alcohol. If valproic acid is used in conjunction with other CNS depressant drugs including alcohol, caution should be used to avoid overdosage.

Valproic acid displaces diazepam from its albumin binding sites and also inhibits its metabolism. In a study in a limited number of healthy individuals, coadministration of valproic acid (1.5 g daily) increased the free fraction of diazepam (10 mg) by 90%; plasma clearance and volume of distribution of free diazepam were decreased by 25% and 20%, respectively. The elimination half-life of diazepam was unaffected by concomitant valproic acid administration.

Concomitant use of amitriptyline (a single 50-mg oral dose) and valproic acid (500 mg twice daily) resulted in a 21% decrease in the plasma clearance of amitriptyline and a 34% decrease in the net clearance of nortriptyline (the pharmacologically active metabolite of amitriptyline). In addition, increased amitriptyline concentrations have been reported rarely in patients receiving amitriptyline concomitantly with valproic acid; concomitant use has rarely been associated with toxicity. The manufacturers state that monitoring of amitriptyline concentrations should be considered for patients receiving valproic acid concomitantly with amitriptyline/nortriptyline.

Because valproic acid may potentiate the effects of monoamine oxidase inhibitors and other antidepressants, dosage reduction of these drugs may be necessary if valproic acid is administered to patients receiving antidepressants.

Valproic acid inhibits the metabolism of ethosuximide. Administration of a single 500-mg dose of ethosuximide to a limited number of healthy individuals receiving valproic acid (800–1600 mg daily) resulted in a 25% increase in ethosuximide elimination half-life and a 15% decrease in total ethosuximide clearance when compared with ethosuximide administration alone. Patients receiving concomitant valproic acid and ethosuximide therapy, especially if receiving other concomitant anticonvulsant therapy, should have their serum drug concentrations monitored carefully.

Concomitant administration of valproic acid with felbamate (1.2 g daily) in a limited number of patients with epilepsy resulted in a 35% increase in mean peak serum valproic acid concentration, from 86 to 115 mcg/mL when compared with administration of valproic acid alone. Increasing the felbamate dose to 2.4 g daily resulted in another 16% increase in mean peak valproic acid concentration to 133 mcg/mL. A decrease in valproic acid dosage may be required when initiating concomitant felbamate therapy.

Valproic acid inhibits lamotrigine metabolism. In a steady-state study in healthy individuals, the elimination half-life of lamotrigine increased from 26 to 70 hours when concomitant valproic acid was administered. Serious skin reactions (e.g., Stevens-Johnson syndrome, toxic epidermal necrolysis) also have been reported following concomitant use of lamotrigine and valproic acid. Lamotrigine dosage should be decreased when valproic acid therapy is initiated. For detailed information on dosing lamotrigine during concurrent valproic acid therapy, see Dosage and Administration: Dosage, in Lamotrigine 28:12.92.

Concomitant administration of valproic acid and phenobarbital (or primidone which is metabolized to phenobarbital) can result in increased phenobarbital plasma concentrations and excessive somnolence. This combination can produce CNS depression (possibly severe) even without substantial increases in serum concentrations of either drug. A few patients have become comatose during therapy with valproic acid and phenobarbital. In a study of concomitant valproic acid (250 mg twice daily for 14 days) and single-dose phenobarbital (60 mg) administration in a limited number of healthy individuals, a 50% increase in phenobarbital half-life, a 30% decrease in phenobarbital clearance, and a 50% increase in unchanged phenobarbital excreted in the urine were observed. If valproic acid is used with a barbiturate, the patient should be closely observed for possible neurologic toxicity, plasma concentrations of the barbiturate should be monitored if possible, and the dosage of the barbiturate decreased if necessary.

Serum concentrations of carbamazepine have been reported to decrease by 17% and concentrations of the metabolite carbamazepine-10,11-epoxide have been reported to increase by 45% during concomitant therapy with valproic acid; such interaction may result in carbamazepine CNS toxicity (e.g., acute psychotic reaction). In addition, carbamazepine has been reported to decrease plasma valproic acid concentrations by altering its clearance during concomitant therapy, which may be clinically important. Discontinuance of carbamazepine following concomitant carbamazepine/valproic acid therapy has been reported to result in increased valproic acid concentrations. If concomitant therapy is being undertaken, or if a patient currently is receiving concomitant carbamazepine/valproic acid therapy and one agent is to be discontinued, careful therapeutic drug monitoring should be considered.

Concomitant administration of valproic acid and clonazepam has produced absence status; therefore, some clinicians recommend that concomitant use of these drugs be avoided.

Concomitant administration of valproic acid and lorazepam in healthy males decreased plasma lorazepam clearance by 17%; however, this pharmacokinetic interaction is unlikely to be clinically important.

Concomitant administration of valproic acid and topiramate has been associated with hyperammonemia with or without encephalopathy in patients who have previously tolerated either drug alone. In most cases, manifestations resolved with discontinuance of either drug. It is not known if topiramate monotherapy is associated with hyperammonemia. Although not studied, the interaction between valproic acid and topiramate may exacerbate existing defects or unmask deficiencies in susceptible patients. (See Cautions: Endocrine and Metabolic Effects and see also Cautions: Precautions and Contraindications.)

Valproic acid has been associated both with decreased plasma phenytoin concentrations and increased seizure frequency and with increased plasma concentrations of free phenytoin and phenytoin intoxication. Therefore, it is important to monitor plasma phenytoin concentrations whenever valproic acid is added to or withdrawn from the patient's therapy and adjust the dosage of phenytoin as required. Since valproic acid also may interact with other anticonvulsants, it is advisable to monitor plasma concentrations of concomitantly administered anticonvulsants during initial valproic acid therapy.

■ **Anti-infective Agents** ***Acyclovir*** In a child receiving both phenytoin and valproic acid, short-term oral therapy with acyclovir apparently reduced the plasma concentrations of both anticonvulsant agents to subtherapeutic levels; an increase in seizure frequency and a worsening in the EEG were observed. Although further study is needed to confirm the effects of acyclovir on the pharmacokinetics of anticonvulsant agents, such concomitant therapy should be undertaken with caution.

Antiretroviral Agents Concomitant use of valproic acid (250 or 500 mg every 8 hours) and oral zidovudine (100 mg every 8 hours) for 4 days in a limited number of adults with human immunodeficiency virus (HIV) infection resulted in an 80% increase in the area under the concentration-time curve (AUC) of zidovudine. The effect of concomitant zidovudine on the pharmacokinetics of valproic acid was not evaluated. Although the clinical importance of this interaction between zidovudine and valproic acid is not known, patients receiving both drugs should be monitored more closely for zidovudine-related adverse effects. Severe anemia has been reported following initiation of valproic acid therapy (500 mg twice daily) in an HIV-infected adult who was receiving an antiretroviral regimen that contained zidovudine, lamivudine, and abacavir; the patient had stable hematologic status at the time valproic acid was started. The manufacturer of zidovudine states that a reduction in zidovudine dosage may be considered if a patient experiences substantial anemia or other severe adverse effect while receiving zidovudine concomitantly with valproic acid.

Hepatotoxicity was reported in an HIV-infected adult receiving valproic acid concomitantly with an antiretroviral regimen containing ritonavir, saquinavir, stavudine, and nevirapine. It has been suggested that this may have occurred as the result of a pharmacokinetic interaction between valproic acid and ritonavir and/or nevirapine.

Concomitant use of efavirenz and valproic acid in HIV-infected adults does not appear to affect the pharmacokinetics of either drug.

Concomitant use of the fixed combination of lopinavir and ritonavir with valproic acid may result in slightly increased lopinavir concentrations, but does not affect valproic acid concentrations. It has been suggested that this pharmacokinetic interaction is not clinically important.

Carbapenem Antibiotics Carbapenem antibiotics (e.g., ertapenem, imipenem, meropenem) may reduce plasma valproic acid concentrations to subtherapeutic levels, resulting in loss of seizure control. The mechanism of this interaction is not fully understood, but may involve a combination of factors affecting the absorption, distribution, and metabolism of valproic acid.

Concomitant use of valproic acid with a carbapenem antibiotic should generally be avoided, if possible. If concomitant therapy is necessary, plasma valproic acid concentrations should be monitored frequently after the carbapenem antibiotic is initiated or discontinued; more frequent monitoring during concurrent therapy also is recommended by some clinicians. Alternative anti-infective or anticonvulsant therapy should be considered if plasma valproic acid concentrations decrease substantially or seizure control deteriorates.

Rifampin A study of administration of a single dose of valproic acid (7 mg/kg) given 36 hours after short-term rifampin administration (600 mg daily for 5 days) revealed a 40% increase in the clearance of valproic acid. Valproic acid dosage adjustment may be required when rifampin therapy is initiated.

■ **Other Drugs** Since valproic acid may affect bleeding time (see Cautions: Hematologic Effects), it should be administered with caution in patients receiving drugs which affect coagulation such as aspirin or warfarin. In addition, valproic acid potentially may displace warfarin from its plasma albumin binding sites. Although the clinical relevance of this interaction is unknown, coagulation tests should be monitored if concomitant valproic acid and anticoagulant therapy is undertaken.

In a study of a limited number of pediatric patients receiving valproic acid and antipyretic aspirin therapy (11–16 mg/kg), a decrease in valproic acid protein binding and metabolism was observed. Free valproic acid concentration increased fourfold, compared with valproic acid therapy alone. The oxidative metabolic pathway of valproic acid was inhibited, resulting in a decrease in excretion of valproic acid metabolites, from 25% to 8.3% of total metabolites excreted. Concomitant aspirin and valproic acid therapy should be instituted with caution.

In vitro studies demonstrated that addition of tolbutamide to plasma samples of patients receiving valproic acid therapy resulted in an increase in the unbound tolbutamide fraction from 20% to 50%. The clinical importance of this displacement is unknown.

Limited pharmacokinetic studies reveal either no interaction or a clinically unimportant interaction following concomitant administration of valproic acid with the following drugs: antacids, chlorpromazine, haloperidol, H_2-receptor antagonists (i.e., ranitidine, cimetidine), acetaminophen, clozapine, lithium, or oral contraceptives.

Laboratory Test Interferences

■ **Tests for Urinary Ketones** A ketone metabolite in the urine of patients receiving valproic acid may produce false-positive results for urine ketones.

■ **Tests for Thyroid Function** Valproic acid reportedly alters thyroid function test results, but the clinical importance of this effect is not known.

Acute Toxicity

■ **Manifestations** Overdosage of valproic acid may produce somnolence, heart block, or deep coma. One adult who ingested 36 g of valproic acid (as valproate sodium) in addition to 1 g of phenobarbital and 300 mg of phenytoin experienced deep coma 4 hours after ingestion of the drugs. The patient recovered following supportive therapy. Fatalities have been reported following valproic acid overdosage; however, patients have recovered from serum valproic acid concentrations as high as 2.12 mg/mL.

■ **Treatment** Treatment of valproic acid intoxication consists of general supportive therapy, particularly maintenance of adequate urinary output. Because the drug is rapidly absorbed, gastric lavage may be of limited value; since absorption of divalproex sodium delayed-release tablets is delayed, the value of gastric lavage or emesis will vary with time since ingestion if this form of the drug has been ingested. In overdose situations, the free or unbound serum valproic acid concentration is high. Hemodialysis or tandem hemodialysis with hemoperfusion may result in significant removal of drug. Naloxone has been reported to reverse the CNS depressant effects of valproic acid overdosage; however, naloxone should be used with caution since it could also theoretically reverse the anticonvulsant effects of valproic acid.

Pharmacology

■ **Anticonvulsant Effects** The mechanism of the anticonvulsant effects of valproic acid is not known. Effects of the drug may be related, at least in part, to increased brain concentrations of the inhibitory neurotransmitter, γ-aminobutyric acid (GABA). Animal studies have shown that valproic acid inhibits GABA transferase and succinic aldehyde dehydrogenase, enzymes which are important for GABA catabolism. Results of one study indicate the drug inhibits neuronal activity by increasing potassium conductance. In animals, valproic acid protects against seizures induced by electrical stimulation as well as those induced by pentylenetetrazol.

■ **Antiviral Effects** Valproic acid inhibits histone deacetylase 1 (HDAC1) (an enzyme that maintains latency of human immunodeficiency virus [HIV] in resting $CD4^+$ T-cells) and induces HIV expression from resting $CD4^+$ T-cells ex vivo. It has been suggested that this effect may be useful in depleting latent infection in resting $CD4^+$ T-cells in HIV-infected patients. Although highly active antiretroviral therapy (HAART) suppresses plasma HIV-1 RNA levels and restores immune function, the presence of replication-competent provirus in resting $CD4^+$ T-cells and persistent HIV replication prevents HAART from eradicating HIV infection. Efficacy of valproic acid in depleting HIV from resting $CD4^+$ T-cells has been evaluated in a small proof-of-concept pilot study in 4 HIV-infected adults (plasma HIV-1 RNA levels less than 50 copies/mL for at least 2 years) receiving HAART. Enfuvirtide was added to the HAART regimens (to prevent the spread of virus in the presence of valproic acid) and, after 4–6 weeks of this intensified regimen, valproic acid (500–750 mg twice daily) was added. After 16–18 weeks of combined valproic acid and enfuvirtide-intensified HAART, there was a substantial decline in the frequency of replication-competent HIV in circulating resting $CD4^+$ T-cells. These preliminary findings suggest that use of valproic acid with HAART and enfuvirtide may represent a new therapeutic approach that possibly represents a step toward the elimination of HIV infection in resting $CD4^+$ T-cells and eventual cure of HIV infection. However, it is unclear whether latently infected $CD4^+$ T-cells are the only reservoir for HIV, and larger, controlled studies are needed to investigate the possible benefits of valproic acid in HIV-infected patients.

Pharmacokinetics

■ **Absorption** ***Oral Administration*** Following oral administration, valproate sodium is rapidly converted to valproic acid in the stomach. Valproic acid is rapidly and almost completely absorbed from the GI tract. Absorption of the drug is delayed but not decreased by administration with meals; administration of the drug with milk products does not affect the rate or degree of absorption. Following oral administration of divalproex sodium extended-release tablets, divalproex sodium dissociates into valproic acid in the GI tract. Following oral administration of divalproex sodium delayed-release tablets and passage of the tablets into the upper small intestine, divalproex sodium dissociates into valproic acid, which is then absorbed; because of the enteric coating, absorption is delayed compared with that following oral administration of valproic acid capsules or valproate sodium solution.

The bioavailability of valproate from divalproex sodium delayed-release tablets and capsules containing coated particles has been shown to be equivalent to that of valproic acid capsules. The absolute bioavailability of divalproex sodium extended-release tablets following oral administration of a single dose after a meal is about 90%. The manufacturer states that divalproex sodium extended-release tablets and delayed-release tablets are not bioequivalent. Results of 5 multiple-dose studies in healthy individuals and in patients with epilepsy indicate that divalproex sodium extended-release tablets (administered either in the fasting or nonfasting state) have an average bioavailability of 89% relative to an equal, total daily dose of divalproex sodium delayed-release tablets given 2–4 times daily. Administration of divalproex sodium with food would be expected to slow absorption but not affect the extent of absorption. In a single-dose study, divalproex sodium delayed-release tablets and valproic acid delayed-release capsules demonstrated similar plasma concentration-time profiles under fasting conditions.

Peak plasma concentrations of valproic acid are usually attained 1–4 hours following a single oral dose of the acid or the sodium salt, 3–5 hours following a single oral dose of divalproex sodium, and 7–14 hours following oral administration of multiple doses of divalproex sodium extended-release tablets. There is wide interindividual variation in plasma concentrations of the drug with a specific dose. Results of a multiple-dose study indicate that following oral administration of divalproex sodium extended-release tablets once daily average plasma concentrations of the drug are 10–20% lower than those achieved with twice-daily administration of divalproex sodium delayed-release tablets. Plasma concentrations of valproic acid required for therapeutic or toxic effects have not been definitely established. Some reports indicate that therapeutic plasma concentrations may be 50–100 mcg/mL of total (bound and unbound) valproic acid and that concentrations in this range are maintained in most adults receiving 1.2–1.5 g of valproic acid daily. However, the possibility that some patients may be controlled with lower or higher plasma concentrations and that the free fraction of valproic acid increases with increasing dosage should be considered. (See Pharmacokinetics: Distribution.) The onset of therapeutic effects is several days to more than one week following initiation of valproic acid therapy.

The relationship between dose and total valproic acid concentration is nonlinear; concentration does not increase proportionally with dose, because of saturable protein binding. The pharmacokinetics of unbound drug are linear.

Parenteral Administration Equivalent valproic acid dosages as the IV injection (available as valproate sodium), administered over 1 hour, or various conventional or delayed-release oral formulations (available as valproate sodium or divalproex sodium) are expected to result in equivalent peak and trough plasma concentrations and total systemic exposure to the valproic acid. Although the rate of valproic acid absorption may vary with the specific formulation, any such differences should be of minor clinical importance under steady-state conditions achieved with chronic therapy for seizure disorders.

When oral divalproex sodium delayed-release tablets or IV valproate sodium (as a 1-hour infusion) was administered at a dosage of 250 mg of valproic acid every 6 hours for 4 days in healthy males, the resulting area under the plasma concentration-time curves (AUCs) and peak and trough plasma concentrations of the drug were equivalent at steady state as well as after the initial dose. However, the time to reach peak plasma concentrations was delayed with the tablets, occurring at approximately 4 hours after an oral dose versus at the end of the 1-hour infusion with the IV dose. Because the pharmacokinetics of unbound valproic acid are linear, bioequivalence between IV valproate sodium and oral delayed-release divalproex sodium can be expected up to maximum dosages of 60 mg/kg daily. The AUCs and peak plasma concentrations also were equivalent in healthy males receiving single 500-mg doses as the IV injection (infused over 1 hour) or valproate sodium oral solution. In addition, patients maintained on valproic acid dosages of 750–4250 mg daily (given in divided doses every 6 hours) as oral delayed-release divalproex sodium tablets alone or while stabilized on another anticonvulsant (e.g., carbamazepine, phenytoin, or phenobarbital) exhibited comparable plasma concentrations when switched from oral divalproex sodium to IV valproate sodium (as 1-hour infusions).

When valproate sodium (at a dosage of 1 g of valproic acid) was administered IV over 5, 10, 30, and 60 minutes in healthy individuals, peak plasma concentrations of the drug averaged 145 mcg/mL after the 5-minute infusion compared with 115 mcg/mL after the 60-minute infusion. However, plasma concentrations measured at 90–120 minutes after initiation of the valproate sodium infusions were similar for the 4 rates of infusion.

■ **Distribution** Valproic acid is rapidly distributed; distribution appears to be restricted to plasma and rapidly exchangeable extracellular water. Volume of distribution of total or free valproic acid is 11 or 92 L/1.73 m^2, respectively. Valproic acid has been detected in CSF (approximately 10% of serum concentrations), saliva (about 1% of plasma concentrations), and milk (about 1–10% of plasma concentrations). The drug crosses the placenta.

Plasma protein binding of valproic acid is concentration dependent; the free fraction of drug increases from 10% at a concentration of 40 mcg/mL to 18.5% at a concentration of 130 mcg/mL. Protein binding of valproic acid is decreased in geriatric patients, in patients with renal impairment or hepatic disease, or in the presence of other protein-bound drugs. Conversely, valproic acid may displace other drugs from protein binding sites. Because of decreased protein binding of the drug in special patient populations (i.e., patients with renal or hepatic disease), monitoring of total drug concentrations may be misleading, owing to the increased free fraction of valproic acid.

■ **Elimination** Valproic acid is eliminated by first-order kinetics and reportedly has an elimination half-life of 5–20 hours (average 10.6 hours). Elimination half-lives in the lower portion of the range are usually observed in patients receiving other anticonvulsants concomitantly. Half-lives of up to 30 hours have been reported following overdosage of valproate sodium.

Mean plasma clearance of total or free valproic acid is 0.56 or 4.6 L/hour per 1.73 m^2, respectively. Drug clearance may be decreased in special patient populations (e.g., patients with renal failure, geriatric patients). Because hemodialysis typically reduces plasma valproic acid concentration by about 20%, generally there is no dosage adjustment required in patients with renal failure (i.e., creatinine clearance less than 10 mL/min). Geriatric patients should receive lower initial dosages of the drug. (See Dosage and Administration: Dosage.)

Pediatric patients (i.e., age range 3 months to 10 years) have 50% higher clearance of the drug expressed by weight (i.e., mL/minute per kg); over the age of 10 years, pharmacokinetic parameters of valproic acid approximate those in adults. Neonates (i.e., younger than 2 months) have a markedly decreased clearance of valproic acid compared with older children and adults, possibly because of delayed development of metabolic enzyme systems and an increased volume of distribution. In one study, the elimination half-life in children younger than 10 days old ranged from 10–67 hours, compared with 7–13 hours in children older than 2 months.

Valproic acid is metabolized principally in the liver by *beta* (over 40%) and *omega* oxidation (up to 15–20%). Valproic acid metabolites are excreted in urine; 30–50% of an administered dose is excreted as glucuronide conjugates. Less than 3% of an administered dose is excreted in urine unchanged. The major metabolite in urine is 2-propyl-3-ketopentanoic acid; minor urinary metabolites are 2-propylglutaric acid, 2-propyl-5-hydroxypentanoic acid, 2-propyl-3-hydroxypentanoic acid, and 2-propyl-4-hydroxypentanoic acid. Small amounts of the drug are also excreted in feces and in expired air. Results of studies in rats suggest the drug may undergo enterohepatic circulation.

Liver disease impairs the ability to eliminate valproic acid. In one study, the clearance of free valproic acid was decreased by 50% in a limited number of patients with cirrhosis and by 16% in a limited number of patients with acute hepatitis, compared with healthy individuals. Half-life of valproic acid was increased from 12 to 18 hours.

Chemistry and Stability

■ **Chemistry** Valproic acid, valproate sodium, and divalproex sodium are carboxylic acid-derivative anticonvulsants. Valproic acid is structurally unrelated to other commercially available anticonvulsants; it lacks nitrogen and/or an aromatic moiety found in most anticonvulsants. Divalproex sodium is a stable coordination compound consisting of valproic acid and valproate sodium in a 1:1 molar ratio and is formed during partial neutralization of valproic acid with sodium hydroxide. Divalproex sodium is a prodrug of valproate, dissociating into valproate in the GI tract.

Valproic Acid Valproic acid occurs as a colorless to pale yellow, slightly viscous, clear liquid with a characteristic odor and is slightly soluble in water and freely soluble in alcohol. Valproic acid has a pK_a of 4.8.

Valproate Sodium Valproate sodium occurs as a white, crystalline, very hygroscopic powder with a saline taste and is very soluble in water and in alcohol.

Valproate sodium injection is a sterile solution of the drug in water for injection. The injection occurs as a clear, colorless solution; sodium hydroxide and/or hydrochloric acid may be added to adjust the pH to 7.6.

Divalproex Sodium Divalproex sodium occurs as a white powder with a characteristic odor and is insoluble in water and very soluble in alcohol.

■ **Stability** ***Valproic Acid*** USP recommends that valproic acid capsules be stored in tight containers at 15–30°C; however, the manufacturer of Depakene® recommends that the capsules be stored in tight containers at 15–25°C.

The manufacturer of valproic acid delayed-release capsules (Stavzor®) states that the capsules should be stored at 25°C, but may be exposed to temperatures ranging from 15–30°C.

Valproate Sodium Valproate sodium oral solution has a pH of 7–8. Valproate sodium oral solution should be stored in tight containers at a temperature less than 30°C; freezing should be avoided.

Valproate sodium injection should be stored at a controlled room temperature of 15–30°C. Because the injection does not contain a preservative, unused portions of the solution should be discarded. When stored in glass or PVC containers at 15–30°C, valproate sodium injection that has been further diluted with at least 50 mL of 5% dextrose injection, 0.9% sodium chloride injection, or lactated Ringer's injection is stable for at least 24 hours.

Divalproex Sodium Divalproex sodium delayed-release tablets should be stored at a temperature less than 30°C; divalproex sodium capsules containing coated particles should be stored at a temperature less than 25°C. Divalproex sodium extended-release tablets should be stored at 25°C, but may be exposed to temperatures ranging from 15–30°C.

For further information on uses and dosage and administration of valproic acid, see the Anticonvulsants General Statement 28:12.

Preparations

Excipients in commercially available drug preparations may have clinically important effects in some individuals; consult specific product labeling for details.

Valproate Sodium

Oral		
Solution	250 mg (of valproic acid) per 5 mL*	**Depakene®**, AbbVie **Valproate Sodium Oral Solution**
Parenteral		
Injection, for IV use	100 mg (of valproic acid) per mL*	**Depacon®**, AbbVie **Valproate Sodium Injection**

*available from one or more manufacturer, distributor, and/or repackager by generic (nonproprietary) name

Valproic Acid

Oral		
Capsules, delayed-release	125 mg	**Stavzor®**, Noven Therapeutics
	250 mg	**Stavzor®**, Noven Therapeutics
	500 mg	**Stavzor®**, Noven Therapeutics
Capsules, liquid-filled	250 mg*	**Depakene®**, AbbVie **Valproic Acid Capsules**

*available from one or more manufacturer, distributor, and/or repackager by generic (nonproprietary) name

Divalproex Sodium

Oral		
Capsules (containing coated particles)	equivalent to valproic acid 125 mg*	**Depakote® Sprinkle**, AbbVie **Divalproex Sodium Capsules (Sprinkle)**
Tablets, delayed-release	equivalent to valproic acid 125 mg*	**Depakote®**, AbbVie **Divalproex Sodium Delayed-Release Tablets**
	equivalent to valproic acid 250 mg*	**Depakote®**, AbbVie **Divalproex Sodium Delayed-Release Tablets**
	equivalent to valproic acid 500 mg*	**Depakote®**, AbbVie **Divalproex Sodium Delayed-Release Tablets**
Tablets, extended-release	equivalent to valproic acid 250 mg*	**Depakote® ER**, AbbVie **Divalproex Sodium Extended-Release Tablets**
	equivalent to valproic acid 500 mg*	**Depakote® ER**, AbbVie **Divalproex Sodium Extended-Release Tablets**

*available from one or more manufacturer, distributor, and/or repackager by generic (nonproprietary) name

†Use is not currently included in the labeling approved by the US Food and Drug Administration

PSYCHOTHERAPEUTIC AGENTS 28:16
ANTIDEPRESSANTS 28:16.04
MONOAMINE OXIDASE INHIBITORS 28:16.04.12

Monoamine Oxidase Inhibitors General Statement

■ Nonselective monoamine oxidase inhibitors block oxidative deamination of naturally occurring monoamines and are used as antidepressants.

Uses

■ **Major Depressive Disorder** Monoamine oxidase (MAO) inhibitors with antidepressant action (phenelzine, tranylcypromine) are used in the treatment of major depressive disorder. A major depressive episode implies a prominent and relatively persistent depressed or dysphoric mood that usually interferes with daily functioning (nearly every day for at least 2 weeks). According to DSM-IV criteria, a major depressive episode includes at least 5 of the following 9 symptoms (with at least one of the symptoms being depressed mood or loss of interest or pleasure): depressed mood most of the day as indicated by subjective report (e.g., feels sad or empty) or observation made by others; markedly diminished interest or pleasure in all, or almost all, activities most of the day; significant weight loss (when not dieting) or weight gain (e.g., a change of more than 5% of body weight in a month) or decrease or increase in appetite; insomnia or hypersomnia; psychomotor agitation or retardation (observable by others, not merely subjective feelings of restlessness or being slowed down); fatigue or loss of energy; feelings of worthlessness or excessive or inappropriate guilt (not merely self-reproach or guilt about being sick); diminished ability to think or concentrate or indecisiveness (either by subjective account or as observed by others); and recurrent thoughts of death, recurrent suicidal ideation without a specific plan, or a suicide attempt or specific plan for committing suicide.

Treatment of major depressive disorder generally consists of an acute phase (to induce remission), a continuation phase (to preserve remission), and a maintenance phase (to prevent recurrence). Various interventions (e.g., psychotherapy, antidepressant drug therapy, electroconvulsive therapy [ECT]) are used alone or in combination to treat major depressive episodes. Treatment should be individualized and the most appropriate strategy for a particular patient is determined by clinical factors such as severity of depression (e.g., mild, moderate, severe), presence or absence of certain psychiatric features (e.g., suicide risk, catatonia, psychotic or atypical features, alcohol or substance abuse or dependence, panic or other anxiety disorder, cognitive dysfunction, dysthymia, personality disorder, seasonal affective disorder), and concurrent illness (e.g., asthma, cardiac disease, dementia, seizure disorder, glaucoma, hypertension). Demographic and psychosocial factors as well as patient preference also are used to determine the most effective treatment strategy.

While use of psychotherapy alone may be considered as an initial treatment strategy for patients with mild to moderate major depressive disorder (based on patient preference and presence of clinical features such as psychosocial stressors), combined use of antidepressant drug therapy and psychotherapy may be useful for initial treatment of patients with moderate to severe major depressive disorder with psychosocial issues, interpersonal problems, or a comorbid axis II disorder. In addition, combined use of antidepressant drug therapy and psychotherapy may be beneficial in patients who have a history of poor compliance or only partial response to adequate trials of either antidepressant drug therapy or psychotherapy alone.

Antidepressant drug therapy can be used alone for initial treatment of patients with mild major depressive disorder (if preferred by the patient) and usually is indicated alone or in combination with psychotherapy for initial treatment of patients with moderate to severe major depressive disorder (unless ECT is planned). ECT is not generally used for initial treatment of uncomplicated major depression, but is recommended as first-line treatment for severe major depressive disorder when it is coupled with psychotic features, catatonic stupor, severe suicidality, food refusal leading to nutritional compromise, or other situations when a rapid antidepressant response is required. ECT also is recommended for patients who have previously shown a positive response or a preference for this treatment modality and can be considered for patients with moderate or severe depression who have not responded to or cannot receive antidepressant drug therapy. In certain situations involving severely depressed patients unresponsive to adequate trials of individual antidepressant agents, adjunctive therapy with another agent (e.g., buspirone, lithium) or concomitant use of a second antidepressant agent (e.g., bupropion) has been used; however, such combination therapy is associated with an increased risk of adverse reactions, may require dosage adjustments, and (if not contraindicated) should be undertaken only after careful consideration of the relative risks and benefits. (See Drug Interactions: Drugs Associated with Serotonin Syndrome and see Drug Interactions: Tricyclic Antidepressants.)

A variety of antidepressant drugs are available for the treatment of major depressive disorder, including selective serotonin-reuptake inhibitors (SSRIs) (e.g., citalopram, escitalopram, fluoxetine, paroxetine, sertraline), tricyclic antidepressants (e.g., amitriptyline, amoxapine, desipramine, doxepin, imipramine, nortriptyline, protriptyline, trimipramine), MAO inhibitors (e.g., phenelzine, tranylcypromine), and other antidepressants (e.g., bupropion, duloxetine, maprotiline, nefazodone, trazodone, venlafaxine). Most clinical studies have shown that the antidepressant effect of usual dosages of various antidepressant agents in patients with major depression are similar. Therefore, the choice of antidepressant agent for a given patient depends principally on other factors such as potential adverse effects, safety or tolerability of these adverse effects in the individual patient, psychiatric and medical history, patient or family history of response to specific therapies, patient preference, quantity and quality of available clinical data, cost, and relative acute overdose safety. No single antidepressant can be recommended as optimal for all patients because of substantial heterogeneity in individual responses and in the nature, likelihood, and severity of adverse effects. In addition, patients vary in the degree to which certain adverse effects and other inconveniences of drug therapy (e.g., cost, dietary restrictions) affect their preferences.

Because of the potential for serious adverse effects, MAO inhibitors generally are not used as initial therapy in the management of depression, but are reserved for patients who do not respond adequately to other antidepressant agents (e.g., SSRIs, tricyclic antidepressants) or in whom other therapies are contraindicated. It has been suggested that patients most likely to respond to MAO inhibitors are those who have depression with atypical features, including those who exhibit reactivity of mood and weight gain or increased appetite, sleep, and libido; those with a history of agoraphobia with secondary depression or agoraphobia with panic attacks; those with primary depression in whom pain or other somatic discomfort is the major complaint; and those with psychogenic pain or hypochondriasis and secondary depression. Phenelzine has been found to be effective in depressed patients clinically characterized as atypical, nonendogenous, or neurotic (these patients often have mixed anxiety and depression and phobic or hypochondriacal features), but there is less conclusive evidence that phenelzine is useful in severely depressed patients with endogenous features. Tranylcypromine is indicated for the treatment of major depressive episodes without melancholia, and effectiveness of the drug in patients who have major depressive episodes with melancholia (endogenous features) has not been established. MAO inhibitors appear to be particularly effective in reducing psychomotor retardation and morbid preoccupation. Somatic signs and symptoms associated with depression, including sleep and eating disturbances, also are reduced during MAO inhibitor therapy.

For further information on treatment of major depressive disorder and considerations in choosing the most appropriate antidepressant agent for a particular patient, including considerations related to patient tolerance, patient age, and cardiovascular, sedative, and suicidal risks, see Considerations in Choosing Antidepressants under Uses: Major Depressive Disorder, in the Tricyclic Antidepressants General Statement 28:16.04.28.

■ **Parkinsonian Syndrome** Certain MAO inhibitors that have increased selectivity for MAO-B (i.e., rasagiline, safinamide, selegiline) are used for the symptomatic treatment of parkinsonian syndrome (e.g., parkinsonism, Parkinson disease [paralysis agitans]); these drugs generally are *not* used for the management of major depressive disorder. For additional information on the use of MAO-B inhibitors in the management of parkinsonian syndrome, see the individual monographs for Rasagiline Mesylate, Safinamide Mesylate, and Selegiline Hydrochloride in 28:36.32.

■ **Eating Disorders** MAO inhibitors (e.g., phenelzine) have been used with some success in the management of bulimia nervosa†. However, MAO inhibitors potentially are dangerous in patients with chaotic binge eating and purging behaviors and the American Psychiatric Association (APA) states that MAO inhibitors should be used with caution in the management of bulimia nervosa. For information on the diagnosis and treatment of bulimia nervosa and other eating disorders, see Uses: Eating Disorders, in Fluoxetine Hydrochloride 28:16.04.20.

Dosage and Administration

■ **Administration** Monoamine oxidase (MAO) inhibitors are administered orally.

■ **Dosage** There is a wide range of individual requirements for MAO inhibitor dosage, and dosage must be carefully adjusted according to individual requirements and response, using the lowest possible effective dosage. The initial dosage may be increased gradually according to the patient's tolerance and therapeutic response; however, because therapeutic response to the drugs may be delayed for several days to up to 4 weeks or more, sufficient time should be allowed between increases in dosage. Some manufacturers recommend that at least 1–2 weeks elapse between dosage adjustments. Dosage should be increased more gradually in debilitated, emaciated, or geriatric patients.

Patients receiving MAO inhibitors should be monitored for possible worsening of depression, suicidality, or unusual changes in behavior, especially at the beginning of therapy or during periods of dosage adjustment. (See Worsening of Depression and Suicidality Risk under Cautions: Precautions and Contraindications.)

Cautions

The potential adverse effects of monoamine oxidase (MAO) inhibitors are more varied and potentially more serious than those reported for most other classes of antidepressant agents. Because monoamine oxidase is widely distributed throughout the body, MAO inhibitor therapy can be expected to cause diverse pharmacologic effects. Many adverse effects of MAO inhibitors are mild to moderate in severity and often subside as therapy is continued. However, serious reactions requiring discontinuance of therapy can occur and usually involve the cardiovascular, CNS, and hepatic systems. Some of the most serious adverse effects reported with MAO inhibitors (e.g., hypertensive crisis, serotonin syndrome) have occurred when MAO inhibitors were administered concomitantly with certain foods or prescription or nonprescription (OTC) drugs.

The adverse effect profiles of phenelzine and tranylcypromine are similar; reports of differences among the individual MAO inhibitors have been poorly substantiated.

■ **Cardiovascular Effects** ***Orthostatic Hypotension*** Orthostatic hypotension is a common adverse effect of MAO inhibitors. Although it has been reported most frequently in patients with preexisting hypertension, it also has occurred in normotensive and hypotensive patients. Hypertensive patients may occasionally experience a transient moderate rise in blood pressure while receiving MAO inhibitors, but these patients more commonly exhibit symptoms of orthostatic hypotension. Unlike hypotension reported with tricyclic antidepressants, hypotension related to MAO inhibitors affects both supine and postural blood pressure changes.

Orthostatic hypotension reported with MAO inhibitors is dose related, and may result in syncope at high doses. In patients who show some hypotensive response during initiation of MAO inhibitor therapy, dosage should be increased gradually. Postural hypotension may be relieved by having the patient lie down until blood pressure returns to normal. If orthostatic hypotension persists or is severe, dosage should be reduced or therapy with the drugs discontinued.

Hypertensive Crisis One of the most serious adverse effects associated with MAO inhibitor therapy is hypertensive crisis, which has been fatal in some patients. Several cases of spontaneous hypertension or significant increases in supine blood pressure without similar changes in standing blood pressure have been reported in patients receiving phenelzine or tranylcypromine, and it has been suggested that a family history of hypertension may be a risk factor for MAO inhibitor-induced hypertensive events. However, most reported cases of hypertensive crisis in patients receiving MAO inhibitor therapy usually have occurred when the drugs were used concomitantly with certain food or prescription or nonprescription drugs. (See Drug Interactions: Food and Drugs Associated with Hypertensive Crisis.)

Hypertensive crisis is characterized by severe headache (occipital headache which may radiate frontally); palpitation; neck stiffness or soreness; nausea or vomiting; sweating (sometimes with fever and sometimes with cold, clammy skin); and mydriasis and/or visual disturbances such as photophobia. Tachycardia or bradycardia may be present, and associated constricting chest pain and dilated pupils may occur. Intracranial hemorrhage, which may be fatal, has also been reported to occur in some patients with hypertensive crisis.

If a hypertensive crisis or prodromal signs of a hypertensive crisis occur, MAO inhibitor therapy should be discontinued and appropriate therapy to lower blood pressure should be instituted immediately. Phentolamine has been considered the hypotensive drug of choice for the management of MAO inhibitor-induced hypertensive crisis. Phentolamine should be given by IV injection; the drug should be administered slowly to avoid producing an excessive hypotensive effect. The usual adult dose of phentolamine for the treatment of hypertensive crisis is 5 mg. In general, headache tends to subside as blood pressure is lowered. Fever should be managed by external cooling. Other symptomatic and supportive measures may be necessary in some patients; however, administration of parenteral reserpine should be avoided. (See Sympathomimetic Agents and Catecholamine-releasing Agents under Drug Interactions: Food and Drugs Associated with Hypertensive Crisis.)

■ **Nervous System Effects** The most common adverse CNS effects of MAO inhibitors include dizziness, headache (without increases in blood pressure), drowsiness, sleep disturbances (e.g., insomnia, hypersomnia), fatigue, weakness, tremors, twitching, myoclonic movements, and hyperreflexia. In addition, confusion, disorientation, memory loss, palilalia, euphoria, nystagmus, akinesia, and paresthesias have been reported.

Hyperexcitability, increased anxiety, agitation, restlessness, manic symptoms, and precipitation of schizophrenia, have occurred in some patients receiving high dosages of MAO inhibitors. If these symptoms occur, dosage should be reduced or a phenothiazine agent should be administered concomitantly.

Worsening of depression and/or emergence of suicidal ideation and behavior (suicidality) or unusual changes in behavior may occur with antidepressants. (See Worsening of Depression and Suicidality Risk under Cautions: Precautions and Contraindications.)

Rarely, ataxia, shock-like coma, toxic delirium, manic reactions, seizures, and acute anxiety reaction have occurred in patients receiving MAO inhibitors.

Serotonin syndrome has occurred rarely in patients receiving MAO inhibitors when other drugs that increase serotonin availability were used concomitantly. Although serotonin syndrome occurs only rarely, it has the potential to cause fatalities. (See Drug Interactions: Drugs Associated with Serotonin Syndrome.)

■ **GI Effects** Adverse GI effects reported with MAO inhibitors include constipation, dry mouth, and GI disturbances. Anorexia, nausea, vomiting, arthralgia, increased appetite, and weight gain also have been reported.

■ **Hepatic Effects** Although the potential for hepatotoxicity with commercially available MAO inhibitors is lower than with prototypical MAO inhibitors (iproniazid), such toxicities, when they do occur, can be serious because the hydrazine derivatives cause cellular damage to the hepatic parenchyma. A carefully controlled study has shown that patients with impaired liver function may be especially sensitive to tranylcypromine. The manufacturers of commercially available MAO inhibitors report that the most common adverse hepatic effect is elevated plasma transaminase concentrations (without accompanying signs or symptoms of hepatotoxicity). Reversible jaundice and fatal progressive necrotizing hepatocellular damage have been reported rarely.

■ **Genitourinary Effects** Impotence, ejaculatory disturbances, and anorgasmia have been reported in patients receiving phenelzine or tranylcypromine. Urinary frequency, urinary retention, and urinary incontinence also have been reported in patients receiving MAO inhibitors.

■ **Dermatologic Effects** Although a causal relationship to MAO inhibitors has not been established, localized scleroderma, flare-up of cystic acne, rash, pruritus, urticaria, purpura, increased sweating, and photosensitivity have been reported in patients receiving MAO inhibitors.

■ **Metabolic Effects** A hypermetabolic syndrome, which may include, but is not limited to, hyperpyrexia, tachycardia, tachypnea, muscular rigidity, elevated creatine kinase (CK, creatine phosphokinase, CPK) concentrations, metabolic acidosis, hypoxia, and coma and may resemble an overdose, has been described in patients receiving MAO inhibitors.

■ **Ocular Effects** Rarely, therapy with MAO inhibitors has been associated with adverse ocular effects (e.g., amblyopia, visual disturbances, blurred vision). Aggravation of glaucoma has also occurred. Retinal degradation, retinal scarring, cataracts, and loss of photoreceptor cells have been observed in animal toxicity studies with safinamide.

■ **Hematologic Effects** A normocytic, normochromic anemia has reportedly developed in some patients receiving MAO inhibitors. Leukopenia, agranulocytosis, and thrombocytopenia also have been reported.

■ **Other Effects** Other adverse effects of MAO inhibitors include arthralgia, lupus-like syndrome, edema of the glottis, fissuring in the corner of the mouth, and impaired water excretion resembling syndrome of inappropriate secretion of antidiuretic hormone (SIADH).

■ **Precautions and Contraindications** MAO inhibitors can cause potentially serious adverse effects, and should only be used in carefully selected patients who can be closely supervised and only by clinicians who are completely familiar with the proper use, potential adverse effects, and associated precautions and contraindications of the drugs. MAO inhibitors generally are not used as initial therapy in the management of depression, but are reserved for patients who do not respond adequately to other antidepressant agents (e.g., selective serotonin-reuptake inhibitors [SSRIs], tricyclic antidepressants) or in whom other therapies are contraindicated.

Hypertensive Crisis Potentially fatal hypertensive crisis has been reported in patients receiving MAO inhibitors, and blood pressure should be monitored closely in all patients to detect any evidence of a pressor response; however, full reliance should not be placed on blood pressure determinations alone. The patient's clinical status should be observed frequently, particularly for signs and symptoms of hypertension. In addition, all patients receiving MAO inhibitors should be warned to contact their clinician promptly if headache or other unusual symptoms occur (e.g., palpitation and/or tachycardia, a sense of constriction of the throat or chest, sweating, dizziness, neck stiffness, nausea or vomiting). If palpitation or frequent or severe headaches occur during MAO inhibitor therapy, the drug should be discontinued immediately, since these may be prodromal symptoms of a hypertensive reaction. (See Cautions: Cardiovascular Effects.)

Because hypertensive crisis may occur if MAO inhibitors are used concomitantly with certain foods that contain large amounts of tyramine or tryptophan, patients receiving MAO inhibitors should be warned against eating food that has a high tyramine or tryptophan content and also should be advised not to consume alcohol (since tyramine is present in certain alcoholic beverages) or excessive amounts of caffeine in any form. (See Drug Interactions: Food and Drugs Associated with Hypertensive Crisis.)

Because of the potential for hypertensive crisis, concomitant use of MAO inhibitors and some sympathomimetic agents (e.g., amphetamines, dopamine, epinephrine, norepinephrine, methylphenidate) or related substances (e.g., methyldopa, levodopa, L-tryptophan, L-tyrosine, phenylalanine) is contraindicated. In addition, patients receiving MAO inhibitors should be cautioned not to take prescription or nonprescription (OTC) cold, hay fever, or weight-reducing preparations unless under the direction of a clinician, since many of these preparations contain pressor agents. (See Drug Interactions: Food and Drugs Associated with Hypertensive Crisis.) To help avoid possible drug interactions, patients receiving MAO inhibitors should be instructed to inform their other clinicians and their dentist that they are receiving an MAO inhibitor.

MAO inhibitors are contraindicated in patients with pheochromocytoma. The drugs also are contraindicated in patients with confirmed or suspected cerebrovascular or cardiovascular disease, including hypertension and congestive heart failure. Since headache may be the first symptom of a hypertensive reaction during MAO inhibitor therapy, the drugs should not be used in patients with a history of severe or frequent headaches.

Worsening of Depression and Suicidality Risk Worsening of depression and/or the emergence of suicidal ideation and behavior (suicidality) or unusual changes in behavior may occur in both adult and pediatric (see Cautions: Pediatric Precautions) patients with major depressive disorder or other psychiatric disorders, whether or not they are taking antidepressants. This risk may persist until clinically important remission occurs. Suicide is a known risk of depression and certain other psychiatric disorders, and these disorders themselves are the strongest predictors of suicide. However, there has been a long-standing concern that antidepressants may have a role in inducing worsening of depression and the emergence of suicidality in certain patients during the early phases of treatment. Pooled analyses of short-term, placebo-controlled studies of antidepressants (i.e., selective serotonin-reuptake inhibitors and other antidepressants) have shown an increased risk of suicidality in children, adolescents, and young adults (18–24 years of age) with major depressive disorder and other psychiatric disorders. An increased suicidality risk was not demonstrated with antidepressants compared with placebo in adults older than 24 years of age, and a reduced risk was observed in adults 65 years of age or older. It is currently unknown whether the suicidality risk extends to longer-term use (i.e., beyond several months); however, there is substantial evidence from placebo-controlled maintenance trials in adults with major depressive disorder that antidepressants can delay the recurrence of depression.

The US Food and Drug Administration (FDA) recommends that all patients being treated with antidepressants for any indication be appropriately monitored and closely observed for clinical worsening, suicidality, and unusual changes in behavior, particularly during initiation of therapy (i.e., the first few months) and during periods of dosage adjustments. Families and caregivers of patients being treated with antidepressants for major depressive disorder or other indications, both psychiatric and nonpsychiatric, also should be advised to monitor patients on a daily basis for the emergence of agitation, irritability, or unusual changes in behavior, as well as the emergence of suicidality, and to report such symptoms immediately to a health-care provider.

Although a causal relationship between the emergence of symptoms such as anxiety, agitation, panic attacks, insomnia, irritability, hostility, aggressiveness, impulsivity, akathisia, hypomania, and/or mania and either the worsening of depression and/or the emergence of suicidal impulses has not been established, there is concern that such symptoms may represent precursors to emerging suicidality. Consequently, consideration should be given to changing the therapeutic regimen or discontinuing therapy in patients whose depression is persistently worse or in patients experiencing emergent suicidality or symptoms that might be precursors to worsening depression or suicidality, particularly if such manifestations are severe, abrupt in onset, or were not part of the patient's presenting symptoms. FDA also recommends that the drugs be prescribed in the smallest quantity consistent with good patient management, in order to reduce the risk of overdosage.

Bipolar Disorder It is generally believed (though not established in controlled trials) that treating a major depressive episode with an antidepressant alone may increase the likelihood of precipitating a mixed or manic episode in patients at risk for bipolar disorder. Therefore, patients should be adequately screened for bipolar disorder prior to initiating treatment with an antidepressant; such screening should include a detailed psychiatric history (e.g., family history of suicide, bipolar disorder, and depression). MAO inhibitors are *not* approved for use in treating bipolar depression in adults.

When MAO inhibitors are used in patients with bipolar disorder, there may be a mood swing to mania. If such a mood swing occurs, MAO inhibitor therapy should be temporarily withheld and subsequently resumed at a reduced dosage.

Other Precautions and Contraindications Since MAO inhibitors may suppress anginal pain that would otherwise serve as a warning sign of myocardial ischemia, patients with angina pectoris or coronary artery disease should be warned against overexertion.

MAO inhibitors should be used with caution in patients with impaired renal function, since the drugs may accumulate in plasma in these patients.

Since MAO inhibitors have a variable effect on the seizure threshold, the drugs should be used with caution in patients with a history of seizures.

Nonselective MAO inhibitors should be used with caution in patients with parkinsonian syndrome, since the drugs may increase the frequency and severity of signs and symptoms associated with this disorder. Selective MAO-B inhibitors (e.g., rasagiline, safinamide, selegiline), on the other hand, have been used principally for the management of parkinsonian syndrome.

Since hepatic damage (e.g., progressive necrotizing hepatocellular damage) has occurred in some patients receiving MAO inhibitors (e.g., isocarboxazid [no longer commercially available in the US], phenelzine), periodic evaluation of liver function (i.e., bilirubin, serum alkaline phosphatase, serum aminotransferases [transaminases]) is recommended in patients receiving high dosages and in those receiving prolonged therapy with the drugs. MAO inhibitors are contraindicated in patients with a history of liver disease or abnormal liver function tests.

There is conflicting evidence regarding whether MAO inhibitors affect glucose metabolism or potentiate antidiabetic agents. Use of MAO inhibitors in patients receiving insulin or oral antidiabetic agents has been associated with hypoglycemic episodes. MAO inhibitors should be used with caution in diabetic patients who are receiving insulin or oral antidiabetic agents.

MAO inhibitors should be used with caution in patients with hyperthyroidism, since these patients have an increased sensitivity to pressor amines.

Since inhibition of monoamine oxidase may persist for several days following discontinuance of therapy, it is suggested that MAO inhibitors be discontinued for at least 10 days prior to elective surgery to allow time for recovery of enzymatic activity before general anesthetics are used. (See Drug Interactions: Anesthetics.)

MAO inhibitors are contraindicated in patients currently receiving, or having recently received, SSRIs or tricyclic antidepressants. (See Drug Interactions: Drugs Associated with Serotonin Syndrome and see Drug Interactions: Tricyclic Antidepressants.)

MAO inhibitors are contraindicated in patients who are hypersensitive to the drugs or any ingredients in the formulations.

■ **Pediatric Precautions** Safety and efficacy of phenelzine in children younger than 16 years of age have not been established. Safety and efficacy of tranylcypromine in pediatric patients have not been established.

FDA warns that antidepressants increase the risk of suicidal thinking and behavior (suicidality) in children and adolescents with major depressive disorder and other psychiatric disorders. The risk of suicidality for these drugs was identified in a pooled analysis of data from a total of 24 short-term (4–16 weeks), placebo-controlled studies of 9 antidepressants (i.e., bupropion, citalopram, fluoxetine, fluvoxamine, mirtazapine, nefazodone, paroxetine, sertraline, venlafaxine) in over 4400 children and adolescents with major depressive disorder, obsessive-compulsive disorder (OCD), or other psychiatric disorders. The analysis revealed a greater risk of adverse events representing suicidal behavior or thinking (suicidality) during the first few months of treatment in pediatric patients receiving antidepressants than in those receiving placebo. The average risk of such events was 4% among children and adolescents receiving these drugs, twice the risk (2%) that was observed among those receiving placebo. However, a more recent meta-analysis of 27 placebo-controlled trials of 9 antidepressants (SSRIs and others) in patients younger than 19 years of age with major depressive disorder, OCD, or non-OCD anxiety disorders suggests that the benefits of antidepressant therapy in treating these conditions may outweigh the risks of suicidal behavior or suicidal ideation. No suicides occurred in these pediatric trials.

The risk of suicidality in FDA's pooled analysis differed across the various psychiatric indications, with the highest incidence observed in the major depressive disorder studies. In addition, although there was considerable variation in risk among the antidepressants, a tendency toward an increase in suicidality risk in younger patients was found for almost all drugs studied. It is currently unknown whether the suicidality risk in pediatric patients extends to longer-term use (i.e., beyond several months).

As a result of this analysis and public discussion of the issue, FDA has directed manufacturers of all antidepressants to add a boxed warning to the labeling of their products to alert clinicians of this suicidality risk in children and adolescents and to recommend appropriate monitoring and close observation of patients receiving these agents. (See Worsening of Depression and Suicidality Risk under Cautions: Precautions and Contraindications.) The drugs that are the focus of the revised labeling are all drugs included in the general class of antidepressants, including those that have not been studied in controlled clinical trials in pediatric patients, since the available data are not adequate to exclude any single antidepressant from an increased risk. In addition to the boxed warning and other information in professional labeling on antidepressants, FDA currently recommends that a patient medication guide explaining the risks associated with the drugs be provided to the patient each time the drugs are dispensed.

Anyone considering the use of antidepressants in a child or adolescent for any clinical use must balance the potential risk of therapy with the clinical need.

■ **Geriatric Precautions** Clinical experience to date with MAO inhibitors in geriatric patients has not identified any differences in responses between geriatric and younger adults. However, geriatric patients appear to be more susceptible to adverse effects of MAO inhibitors (e.g., episodes of hypertension, malignant hyperthermia) than younger patients, and these adverse effects are associated with increased morbidity in geriatric patients since they have less compensatory reserve to cope with any serious adverse reactions. Therefore, MAO inhibitor therapy should be initiated cautiously in geriatric patients using a low initial dosage and patients observed closely since renal, hepatic, and cardiovascular dysfunction and concomitant disease or other drug therapy are more common in this age group than in younger patients.

In pooled data analyses, a *reduced* risk of suicidality was observed in adults 65 years of age or older with antidepressant therapy compared with placebo. (See Precautions and Contraindications: Worsening of Depression and Suicidality Risk, in Cautions.)

■ **Pregnancy, Fertility, and Lactation** Safety of MAO inhibitors during pregnancy has not been established. Administration of phenelzine to pregnant mice resulted in a decrease in the number of viable offspring, and the growth of young dogs and rats has been retarded by phenelzine dosages exceeding the maximum human dosage. Tranylcypromine has been shown to cross the placenta in rats. It is not known whether MAO inhibitors can cause fetal harm when administered to pregnant women, and the drugs should be used during pregnancy only when the potential benefits justify the possible risks to the fetus.

The effect of MAO inhibitors on fertility in humans is not known. Sexual disturbances including impotence and delayed ejaculation have occurred in some individuals during MAO inhibitor therapy.

It is not known if MAO inhibitors are distributed into human milk; however, tranylcypromine is distributed into the milk of lactating dogs. MAO inhibitors should be used with caution in nursing women.

Drug Interactions

■ Food and Drugs Associated with Hypertensive Crisis Concomitant use of MAO inhibitors and certain food or prescription or nonprescription (over-the-counter, OTC) drugs can result in interactions that have the potential to cause hypertensive crisis due to the release and potentiation of catecholamines similar to that experienced in pheochromocytoma. The severity and consequences of such interactions vary among individuals. If only minor increases in blood pressure occur, patients may be unaware of the interactions. However, if substantial and rapid increases in blood pressure (an increase of 30 mm Hg or more in systolic blood pressure within 20 minutes) occur, patients may experience symptoms associated with subarachnoid hemorrhage or cardiac failure (sudden severe occipital headache, palpitations) if the cerebral vasculature or cardiac musculature are already weakened. (See Hypertensive Crisis under Cautions: Cardiovascular Effects.)

Food Hypertensive crises have occurred following ingestion of foods containing large amounts of tyramine or tryptophan in some patients receiving MAO inhibitors. In general, patients should avoid protein foods that have undergone protein breakdown by aging, fermentation, pickling, smoking, or bacterial contamination; protein extracts and liquid or powdered dietary supplements also should be avoided. Patients should be specifically instructed not to eat foods such as cheese, particularly strong or aged varieties (e.g., cheddar, Camembert, Stilton) and processed cheese; sour cream; wine, especially chianti, champagne, and alcohol-free or reduced-alcohol wine products; beer, including alcohol-free and reduced-alcohol beers; pickled herring; anchovies; caviar; shrimp paste; liver, especially chicken liver; dry sausage (e.g., Genoa salami, hard salami, pepperoni, Lebanon bologna); figs, particularly if overripe, or canned figs; raisins; bananas or avocados, particularly if overripe; chocolate; soy sauce; bean curd; yeast extracts (including brewer's yeast in large quantities); yogurt; papaya products, including certain meat tenderizers; and pods of broad beans (e.g., fava beans). Excessive amounts of caffeine may also reportedly precipitate hypertensive crisis. Specialized references on food constituents or a dietician should be consulted for more specific information on the tyramine content of foods and beverages.

Sympathomimetic Agents and Catecholamine-releasing Agents Because some patients appear to be particularly sensitive to the hypertensive effects of sympathomimetic agents during MAO inhibitor therapy, centrally acting sympathomimetic agents (e.g., amphetamines) or peripherally acting sympathomimetic agents, including prescription or nonprescription cold, hay fever, or weight-reducing preparations that contain pressor agents (e.g., ephedrine) generally should not be administered concomitantly with an MAO inhibitor. The manufacturer of rasagiline states that concomitant use of the drug with sympathomimetic agents should be employed with caution. The manufacturer of safinamide states that concomitant use of the drug with methylphenidate or amphetamines is contraindicated and that patients receiving safinamide in conjunction with other prescription or nonprescription sympathomimetics should be monitored for hypertension.

Parenteral or oral administration of reserpine or guanethidine in patients receiving MAO inhibitors may cause a severe pressor response as a result of a sudden release of accumulated catecholamines. Therefore, the manufacturers of MAO inhibitors do not recommend concomitant use of guanethidine in patients receiving an MAO inhibitor and also recommend that reserpine be administered cautiously in patients receiving MAO inhibitors.

Levodopa and other Catecholamines Hypertension, headache, hyperexcitability, and related symptoms reportedly have occurred in patients receiving MAO inhibitors concurrently with methyldopa, dopamine, or levodopa. It has been suggested that use of a decarboxylase inhibitor (e.g., carbidopa) with levodopa may prevent hypertensive reactions during concomitant therapy with an MAO inhibitor.

■ Drugs Associated with Serotonin Syndrome Serotonin syndrome may occur in patients receiving MAO inhibitors in combination with other serotonergic drugs. Although the syndrome appears to be relatively uncommon and usually mild in severity, serious complications, including seizures, disseminated intravascular coagulation, respiratory failure, severe hyperthermia, and death occasionally have been reported. The precise mechanism of the syndrome is not fully understood; however, it appears to result from excessive serotonergic activity in the CNS, probably mediated by activation of serotonin 5-HT_{1A} receptors. The possible involvement of dopamine and 5-HT_2 receptors also has been suggested, although their roles remain unclear.

The syndrome most commonly occurs when 2 or more serotonergic agents with different mechanisms of action are administered either concurrently or in close succession. Serotonergic agents include those that increase serotonin synthesis (e.g., the serotonin precursor tryptophan), stimulate synaptic serotonin release (e.g., some amphetamines, dexfenfluramine [no longer commercially available in the US], fenfluramine [no longer commercially available in the US]), inhibit the reuptake of serotonin after release (e.g., selective serotonin-reuptake inhibitors [SSRIs], tricyclic antidepressants, trazodone, dextromethorphan, meperidine, tramadol), decrease the metabolism of serotonin (e.g., MAO inhibitors), have direct serotonin postsynaptic receptor activity (e.g., buspirone), or nonspecifically induce increases in serotonergic neuronal activity (e.g., lithium salts).

The combination of MAO inhibitors and SSRI antidepressants (e.g., fluoxetine) appears to be responsible for most of the recent case reports of serotonin syndrome. The syndrome also has been reported when MAO inhibitors have been combined with tricyclic antidepressants, tryptophan, meperidine, or dextromethorphan. In rare cases, serotonin syndrome reportedly has occurred with the recommended dosage of a single serotonergic agent (e.g., clomipramine) or during accidental overdosage (e.g., sertraline intoxication in a child). Some other drugs that have been implicated in certain circumstances include buspirone, bromocriptine, dextropropoxyphene, methylenedioxymethamphetamine (MDMA; "ecstasy"), and selegiline (a selective MAO-B inhibitor). Other drugs that have been associated with the syndrome but for which less convincing data are available include carbamazepine, fentanyl, and pentazocine.

Clinicians should be aware of the potential for serious, possibly fatal reactions associated with serotonin syndrome in patients receiving 2 or more drugs that increase the availability of serotonin in the CNS, even if no such interactions with the specific drugs have been reported to date in the medical literature. Pending further data, all drugs with serotonergic activity should be used cautiously in combination and such combinations avoided whenever clinically possible. Some clinicians state that patients who have experienced serotonin syndrome may be at higher risk for recurrence of the syndrome upon reinitiation of serotonergic drugs. Pending further experience in such cases, some clinicians recommend that therapy with serotonergic agents be limited following recovery. In cases in which the potential benefit of the drug is thought to outweigh the risk of serotonin syndrome, lower potency agents and reduced dosages should be used, combination serotonergic therapy should be avoided, and patients should be monitored carefully for symptoms of serotonin syndrome. For further information on serotonin syndrome, including manifestations and treatment, see Serotonin Syndrome under Drug Interactions: Drugs Associated with Serotonin Syndrome, in Fluoxetine Hydrochloride 28:16.04.20.

Selective Serotonin-reuptake Inhibitors Concurrent use of SSRIs and MAO inhibitors potentially is hazardous and may result in serotonin syndrome. Probably because of its extensive clinical use and the prolonged elimination half-life of both fluoxetine and norfluoxetine, fluoxetine has been the SSRI most commonly implicated in serotonin syndrome when combined with MAO inhibitor therapy. In at least 2 cases, serotonin syndrome has developed when MAO inhibitor therapy has been initiated after the discontinuance of fluoxetine therapy. Shivering, diplopia, nausea, confusion, and anxiety reportedly occurred in one patient 6 days after discontinuance of fluoxetine therapy and 4 days after initiation of tranylcypromine therapy; signs and symptoms resolved without apparent sequelae within 24 hours following discontinuance of the MAO inhibitor in this patient. In another case, the initiation of tranylcypromine therapy more than 5 weeks after discontinuance of fluoxetine reportedly resulted in serotonin syndrome. The manufacturer of fluoxetine, the manufacturers of MAO inhibitors, and some clinicians state that concurrent use of fluoxetine with MAO inhibitors is contraindicated or generally should be avoided. Because both fluoxetine and its principal metabolite have relatively long half-lives, the manufacturer of fluoxetine, the manufacturers of MAO inhibitors, and some clinicians recommend that at least 5 weeks elapse between discontinuance of fluoxetine therapy and initiation of MAO inhibitor therapy, since administration of an MAO inhibitor prior to elapse of this time may increase the risk of serious adverse effects. Although the manufacturers of some MAO inhibitors (i.e., phenelzine) recommend that at least 10 days elapse following discontinuance of MAO inhibitor therapy prior to initiation of fluoxetine therapy, based on clinical experience with concurrent administration of tricyclic antidepressants and MAO inhibitors, the manufacturers of fluoxetine and the manufacturers of some MAO inhibitors (e.g., selegiline, tranylcypromine) recommend that at least 2 weeks elapse following discontinuance of an MAO inhibitor prior to initiation of fluoxetine therapy.

Other SSRI antidepressants, including sertraline and citalopram, also have been associated with serotonin syndrome when given in combination with MAO inhibitors. Because of the potential risk of serotonin syndrome when SSRIs are combined with MAO inhibitor therapy, the manufacturers of fluvoxamine, paroxetine, and sertraline currently recommend that a drug-free interval of at least 2 weeks elapse when switching from an MAO inhibitor to these agents or when switching from these agents to an MAO inhibitor. The manufacturer of the selective MAO-B inhibitor safinamide states that if safinamide is used concomitantly with an SSRI, the lowest effective dosage of the SSRI should be used.

Moclobemide, a selective and reversible MAO-A inhibitor (not commercially available in the US), also has been associated with serotonin syndrome and such reactions have been fatal in several cases in which the drug was given in combination with citalopram or with clomipramine. Pending further experience with such combinations, some clinicians recommend that concurrent therapy with moclobemide and SSRIs be used only with extreme caution and that the SSRI should have been discontinued for some time (depending on the elimination half-lives of the drug and its active metabolites) before initiating moclobemide therapy.

Tryptophan Although tryptophan sometimes has been used to enhance the antidepressant activity of MAO inhibitors, serotonin syndrome, which was fatal in at least one case, has been reported in a limited number of patients receiving these drugs in combination either with or without concurrent lithium therapy. While the mechanism for this interaction has not been fully elucidated, it has been suggested that these adverse effects resemble serotonin syndrome and therefore may result from a marked increase in serotonin availability in the CNS when these agents are administered concurrently. Behavioral and neurologic syndromes, including disorientation, confusion, amnesia, delirium, agitation, hypomanic signs, ataxia, myoclonus, hyperreflexia, shivering, ocular oscillations, and Babinski signs, also have been reported in patients receiving MAO inhibitors and tryptophan concomitantly. Pending further evaluation of this potential interaction, clinicians should be aware that toxic reactions may occur when MAO inhibitors and tryptophan are administered concomitantly.

Buspirone Elevations in blood pressure have been observed in several patients receiving an MAO inhibitor and buspirone concomitantly; no adverse sequelae were associated with these elevations. Buspirone may have been partially responsible for a case of serotonin syndrome that resulted in the death of a patient receiving buspirone, an MAO inhibitor (tranylcypromine), and fluoxetine concomitantly. Pending accumulation of additional data, it is recommended that MAO inhibitors not be used concomitantly with buspirone. Some manufacturers recommend that at least 10 days elapse between discontinuance of MAO inhibitor therapy and administration of buspirone.

■ **Tricyclic Antidepressants** Concomitant use of MAO inhibitors with tricyclic antidepressants is contraindicated or generally should be avoided, and it generally is recommended that at least 2 weeks should elapse between discontinuance of tricyclic antidepressant therapy or MAO inhibitor therapy and initiation of therapy with the other class of drugs. Serious, sometimes fatal, reactions including hyperpyrexia, confusion, diaphoresis, myoclonus, rigidity, seizures, cardiovascular disturbances, and coma have occurred in patients who received an MAO inhibitor and a tricyclic antidepressant concomitantly. Patients receiving therapeutic dosages of an oral MAO inhibitor and an oral tricyclic antidepressant concomitantly generally have experienced nonfatal hyperpyrexia, hypertension, tachycardia, confusion, and seizures; most reported cases of hyperpyretic crises, severe seizures, or death occurred following overdosage or parenteral administration of one or both drugs. Although the mechanism has not been clearly established, these reactions resemble serotonin syndrome and may be caused by excessive serotonergic activity in CNS. (See Drug Interactions: Drugs Associated with Serotonin Syndrome.)

■ **CNS Depressants** Several manufacturers caution that MAO inhibitors may be additive with, or may potentiate the action of, CNS depressants such as opiates or other analgesics, barbiturates or other sedatives, anesthetics, or alcohol. CNS depressants should be administered cautiously to patients receiving MAO inhibitors in order to avoid excessive sedation and acute hypotension; a reduction in dosage of the CNS depressant agent(s) may be necessary. One manufacturer recommends that, if emergency surgery is necessary in a patient receiving an MAO inhibitor, the dose of opiate, sedative, analgesic, and other premedication be reduced to one-fourth to one-fifth the usual dose.

Meperidine Meperidine should *not* be used in patients receiving MAO inhibitors since severe, generally immediate reactions, including excitation, sweating, rigidity, and hypertension, suggestive of serotonin syndrome, have occurred. Circulatory collapse and death have also occurred following administration of a single dose of meperidine in some patients receiving an MAO inhibitor.

Dextromethorphan Concomitant use of MAO inhibitors and dextromethorphan (ingested as a lozenge) has been reported to cause brief episodes of psychosis or bizarre behavior. Cases of apparent serotonin syndrome, including at least 2 fatalities, have been reported in patients receiving concurrent MAO inhibitor and dextromethorphan therapy. Dextromethorphan preparations should *not* be used in patients receiving an MAO inhibitor.

■ **Bupropion** Studies in animals using phenelzine have shown that the acute toxicity of bupropion is enhanced by the MAO inhibitor. Concomitant use of an MAO inhibitor and bupropion is contraindicated, and it is suggested that at least 14 days elapse between discontinuance of MAO inhibitor therapy and initiation of bupropion therapy.

■ **Anesthetics** The hypotensive and CNS depressant effects of general anesthetics may be exaggerated in patients receiving MAO inhibitors. Since inhibition of monoamine oxidase may persist for several days following discontinuance of therapy, some manufacturers suggest that MAO inhibitors be discontinued for at least 7–14 days prior to elective surgery to allow time for recovery of enzymatic activity before general anesthetics are used. If emergency surgery is necessary in a patient receiving an MAO inhibitor, the dose of the general anesthetic should be carefully adjusted.

Patients receiving MAO inhibitors should not be given cocaine or local anesthetics that contain sympathomimetic vasoconstrictors, since hypertension may result.

Because MAO inhibitors may potentiate the hypotensive effect of local anesthetics used in spinal anesthesia, these agents should be used with caution in patients receiving MAO inhibitors.

■ **Disulfiram** MAO inhibitors should probably be used with caution in patients receiving disulfiram. In one study in animals receiving large intraperitoneal doses of disulfiram and the *d*- or *l*-isomer of tranylcypromine, severe toxicity, including seizures and death, occurred. However, in other studies in animals receiving large oral doses of disulfiram and racemic tranylcypromine, no adverse interaction was reported.

■ **Diuretics and Hypotensive Agents** In general, MAO inhibitor antidepressants should not be administered concomitantly with diuretics or hypotensive agents since a marked hypotensive effect may occur.

■ **Drugs with Anticholinergic Activity** Some manufacturers state that anticholinergic antiparkinsonian drugs should be used with caution in patients receiving MAO inhibitors, since severe reactions have reportedly occurred when these drugs were used concurrently; however, additional information is needed to determine the clinical importance of this potential interaction. It also should be considered that MAO inhibitors may prolong and intensify some anticholinergic effects (e.g., dryness) of antihistamines.

Acute Toxicity

■ **Manifestations** In general, overdosage of monoamine oxidase (MAO) inhibitors may be expected to produce effects that are extensions of common adverse reactions. Patients with early or mild intoxication may experience drowsiness, dizziness (sometimes severe), ataxia, headache (sometimes severe), insomnia, restlessness, anxiety, and irritability. Other reported effects associated with severe overdosage include mental confusion, incoherence, tachycardia, rapid and irregular pulse, hypotension, coma, seizures, respiratory depression, hyporeflexia or hyperreflexia, fever, diaphoresis (sometimes perfuse and associated with cool, clammy skin), precordial pain, and shock. A few patients have developed hypertension, which rarely may be associated with twitching or myoclonic fibrillation of skeletal muscles and with hyperpyrexia, sometimes progressing to generalized rigidity and coma. In addition, trismus and opisthotonus have been reported to occur in some patients. Hyperactivity with marked agitation may occur. Signs and symptoms following acute overdosage may be delayed for 12–24 hours. Although signs and symptoms usually resolve within 3–4 days, they may persist for up to 2 weeks in some patients. Careful observation of patients for at least 1 week after overdosage is generally recommended.

■ **Treatment** Treatment of MAO inhibitor overdosage generally involves symptomatic and supportive care; there is no specific antidote for intoxication. In acute overdosage, the stomach should be emptied immediately by inducing emesis or by gastric lavage with instillation of charcoal slurry. If the patient is comatose, having seizures, or lacks the gag reflex, gastric lavage may be performed if an endotracheal tube with cuff inflated is in place to prevent aspiration of gastric contents. Hemodialysis, peritoneal dialysis, and charcoal hemoperfusion may be of value in cases of massive overdosage, but data are insufficient to recommend the routine use of these procedures in MAO inhibitor overdosage.

Because of the potential for interactions with other drugs, extreme caution should be used in the management of patients following MAO inhibitor overdosage. Conservative measures to maintain normal body temperature (e.g., external cooling), respiration, and blood pressure and to correct fluid and electrolyte abnormalities have generally been successful. Appropriate therapy (e.g., volume expansion) should be instituted if hypotension occurs; however, administration of pressor amines (e.g., norepinephrine) may be of limited value and should be used with caution, since the hypertensive effects of these agents may be potentiated by MAO inhibitors (see Sympathomimetic Agents and Catecholamine-releasing Agents under Drug Interactions: Food and Drugs Associated with Hypertensive Crisis). Appropriate therapy should be instituted if severe hypertension (i.e., hypertensive crisis) occurs. For the management of hypertensive crisis, see Hypertensive Crisis under Cautions: Cardiovascular Effects. Signs and symptoms of CNS stimulation, including seizures, should be treated with diazepam. Appropriate therapy should be instituted if excessive sedation occurs. Phenothiazines and CNS stimulants should be avoided (see Sympathomimetic Agents and Catecholamine-releasing Agents under Drug Interactions: Food and Drugs Associated with Hypertensive Crisis). Evaluation of liver function is recommended at the time of overdosage and for 4–6 weeks following recovery.

Chronic Toxicity

Although MAO inhibitors are not usually associated with dependence and addiction, drug dependence has occurred in some patients receiving tranylcypromine doses substantially in excess of the usual therapeutic range. Some of these patients had a history of previous substance abuse. Following discontinuance of the drug, symptoms of withdrawal, including restlessness, anxiety, depression, confusion, hallucinations, headache, weakness, and diarrhea have occurred. A withdrawal syndrome also has been reported to occur infrequently after abrupt discontinuance of phenelzine. In reported cases, signs and symptoms of withdrawal ranging from vivid nightmares with agitation to frank psychosis and seizures have been evident within 24–72 hours after phenelzine was discontinued; the syndrome generally responds to reinitiation of MAO inhibitor therapy followed by cautious downward titration and discontinuance.

Pharmacology

The discovery of monoamine oxidase (MAO) inhibitors resulted from a search for derivatives of isoniazid (isonicotinic acid hydrazide) with antitubercular activity. During clinical trials with these hydrazine derivatives, a rather consistent beneficial effect of mood elevation was noted in depressed patients with tuberculosis receiving the drugs. Iproniazid, the first derivative synthesized, was found to be too toxic (principally hepatotoxicity) at the dosage level required for antitubercular activity. Although its antidepressant effect was still pronounced at lower dosage, toxicity was also eventually observed at the lower dosage level and use of iproniazid was finally discontinued. However, the antidepressant activity of iproniazid prompted a search for other MAO inhibitors and resulted in the synthesis of several agents, both hydrazine and nonhydrazine compounds, that were relatively less toxic than iproniazid.

Monoamine oxidase, an enzyme found mainly in nerve tissue and in the liver and lungs, catalyzes the oxidative deamination of various amines, including epinephrine, norepinephrine, dopamine, and serotonin (5-HT). There appear to be at least 2 isoforms of monoamine oxidase, monoamine oxidase-A (MAO-A) and monoamine oxidase-B (MAO-B), with differences in substrate preference, inhibitor specificity, tissue distribution, immunologic properties, and amino acid sequence. MAO-A substrates include serotonin; MAO-B substrates include phenylethylamine. Tyramine, epinephrine, norepinephrine, and dopamine are substrates for both MAO-A and MAO-B. Inhibition of monoamine oxidase results in increased concentrations of these amines. Currently available MAO inhibitor antidepressants (phenelzine, tranylcypromine) are considered nonselective inhibitors of MAO. Phenelzine binds irreversibly to monoamine oxidase; tranylcypromine binds reversibly to the enzyme. Selective inhibitors of monoamine oxidase-A (e.g., clorgiline) are being investigated. Rasagiline, safinamide, and selegiline are considered selective MAO-B inhibitors and are used for the symptomatic treatment of parkinsonian syndrome. (See Rasagiline Mesylate 28:36.32, see Safinamide Mesylate 28:36.32, and see Selegiline Hydrochloride 28:36.32.)

Although the precise mechanism of antidepressant action of MAO inhibitors is unclear, it has been suggested that the increase in free serotonin and norepinephrine and/or alterations in other amine concentrations within the CNS are mainly responsible for the antidepressant effect of the drugs. Although this concept offers a useful working hypothesis, it should be remembered that definite proof of the mode of action of MAO inhibitors is lacking. Attempts have been made to correlate inhibition of platelet monoamine oxidase (a possible index of a drug's effect on brain monoamine oxidase) with therapeutic effect; preliminary evidence suggests that a dose-related effect of phenelzine on platelet monoamine oxidase correlates with a beneficial effect on mood in depressed patients.

MAO inhibitors may cause hypotension or hypertension, probably by the same mechanism of action. The reduction in blood pressure induced by MAO inhibitors is mainly an orthostatic (postural) effect; reduction in supine blood pressure is minimal in most patients. Although the precise mechanism of hypotensive action of MAO inhibitors is not fully understood, it has been postulated that this paradoxical effect may result from gradual accumulation of false neurotransmitters (phenylethylamines) in peripheral adrenergic neurons. Phenylethylamines (e.g., tyramine) are usually oxidatively deaminated in the GI tract and liver; however, inhibition of monoamine oxidase in the GI tract and liver may result in substantial systemic absorption of these indirect-acting amines. Gradual accumulation of octopamine in the adrenergic neurons may result from MAO inhibition in the neurons with subsequent alternate hydroxylation of tyramine to octopamine. It has been suggested that octopamine gradually displaces norepinephrine from storage granules. Stimulation of norepinephrine release may result in release of some norepinephrine and some octopamine, the latter amine having minimal activity at α- or β-adrenergic receptors. Thus, gradual MAO inhibitor-induced displacement of norepinephrine from adrenergic neurons may result in a functional block of sympathetic neurotransmission. Similarly, MAO inhibitors may cause severe hypertension when foods containing large amounts of tyramine are ingested. (See Drug Interactions: Food and Drugs Associated with Hypertensive Crisis.) Following systemic absorption of large amounts of tyramine, there may be a rapid, massive displacement and release of norepinephrine from adrenergic neurons resulting in severe hypertension. It has been suggested that selective inhibitors of monoamine oxidase-B (e.g., rasagiline, selegiline) may be less likely than nonselective MAO inhibitors to cause hypertension; however, hypertensive reactions have been reported rarely with selegiline at recommended doses as a result of dietary influences.

MAO inhibitors interfere with the hepatic metabolism of many drugs and may potentiate the actions of such agents as general anesthetics, barbiturates, morphine, alcohol, corticosteroids, and atropine. (See Drug Interactions.)

The pharmacologic effects of MAO inhibitors are cumulative; a latent period of a few days to several months may occur before the onset of antidepressant or hypotensive activity, and effects may persist for up to 3 weeks following discontinuance of therapy.

Chemistry

Monoamine oxidase (MAO) inhibitors are a chemically heterogeneous group of drugs that can block oxidative deamination of naturally occurring monoamines. Various MAO inhibitors have been found to have antidepressant action (e.g., isocarboxazid, iproniazid, phenelzine, tranylcypromine); however, the only MAO inhibitors currently commercially available in the US for use as antidepressant agents are phenelzine and tranylcypromine.

Based on their structure, MAO inhibitors can be classified as hydrazines (e.g., phenelzine) and nonhydrazines (e.g., tranylcypromine). Although no longer used clinically, the prototype hydrazine MAO inhibitor is iproniazid. (See Pharmacology.) MAO inhibitors also can be classified according to their ability to selectively or nonselectively inhibit monoamine oxidase. (See Pharmacology.)

For further information on chemistry and stability, pharmacology, pharmacokinetics, uses, cautions, and dosage and administration of MAO inhibitors, see the individual monographs on Phenelzine Sulfate and Tranylcypromine Sulfate in 28:16.04.12 and see Rasagiline Mesylate, Safinamide Mesylate, and Selegiline Hydrochloride in 28:36.32.

†Use is not currently included in the labeling approved by the US Food and Drug Administration

SELECTIVE SEROTONIN- AND NOREPINEPHRINE-REUPTAKE INHIBITORS 28:16.04.16

Desvenlafaxine Succinate

DVS, *O*-desmethylvenlafaxine

■ Desvenlafaxine succinate, the succinate salt of the principal active metabolite of venlafaxine, is a selective serotonin- and norepinephrine-reuptake inhibitor (SNRI) and an antidepressant.

Uses

■ **Major Depressive Disorder** Desvenlafaxine succinate is used in the treatment of major depressive disorder in adults. The antidepressant efficacy of desvenlafaxine has been established in 4 randomized, double-blind, placebo-controlled, fixed-dose studies of 8 weeks' duration in adult outpatients who met DSM-IV criteria for major depressive disorder. In all of these studies, patients receiving desvenlafaxine (50–400 mg daily as extended-release tablets) demonstrated greater improvement in the 17-item Hamilton Rating Scale for Depression (HAMD-17) total score than did patients receiving placebo. Patients receiving desvenlafaxine also demonstrated greater overall improvement as measured by the Clinical Global Impressions Scale-Improvement (CGI-I) compared with placebo recipients in 3 out of 4 of these studies. In the 2 studies that directly compared 50 mg and 100 mg of desvenlafaxine given once daily, there was no evidence of a greater therapeutic effect at the higher 100-mg dosage. In addition, adverse effects and drug discontinuances were reported more frequently at higher dosages of the drug in these studies. No age- or gender-related differences in efficacy were noted in these studies; data were insufficient to determine whether there were race-related differences in efficacy.

The manufacturer states that the efficacy of desvenlafaxine for long-term use (i.e., exceeding 8 weeks) has not been established by controlled studies. If desvenlafaxine is used for extended periods, the need for continued therapy should be reassessed periodically.

For further information on treatment of major depressive disorder and considerations in choosing the most appropriate antidepressant for a particular patient, including considerations related to patient tolerance, patient age, and cardiovascular, sedative, and suicidal risks, see Considerations in Choosing Antidepressants under Uses: Major Depressive Disorder, in Fluoxetine Hydrochloride 28:16.04.20.

■ **Vasomotor Symptoms** Like some other SNRIs and SSRIs, desvenlafaxine succinate has been studied for the management of vasomotor symptoms† in postmenopausal women.

For further information on treatment of vasomotor symptoms in postmenopausal women and women with breast cancer, see Vasomotor Symptoms under Uses in Venlafaxine Hydrochloride 28:16.04.16.

Dosage and Administration

■ **Administration** Desvenlafaxine succinate is administered orally once daily with or without food at approximately the same time each day. Extended-release tablets of the drug should be swallowed whole with fluid and should *not* be divided, crushed, chewed, or dissolved.

Patients receiving desvenlafaxine should be monitored for possible worsening of depression, suicidality, or unusual changes in behavior, especially at the beginning of therapy or during periods of dosage adjustment. (See Worsening of Depression and Suicidality Risk under Warnings/Precautions: Warnings, in Cautions.)

Discontinuance symptoms have been reported when switching patients from other antidepressants, including venlafaxine, to desvenlafaxine. When switching from another antidepressant to desvenlafaxine, it may be necessary to taper the dosage of the previous antidepressant to minimize discontinuance symptoms. (See Withdrawal of Therapy under Warnings/Precautions: Other Warnings and Precautions, in Cautions.)

The manufacturer recommends that at least 2 weeks elapse between discontinuance of a monoamine oxidase (MAO) inhibitor and initiation of desvenlafaxine and that at least 7 days elapse between discontinuance of desvenlafaxine and initiation of MAO inhibitor therapy. (See Serotonin Syndrome or Neuroleptic Malignant Syndrome [NMS]-like Reactions under Warnings/Precautions: Other Warnings and Precautions, in Cautions and see also Drug Interactions: Monoamine Oxidase Inhibitors.)

■ **Dosage** Dosage of desvenlafaxine succinate is expressed in terms of desvenlafaxine.

Because withdrawal effects may occur, abrupt discontinuance of desvenlafaxine should be avoided whenever possible. When desvenlafaxine therapy is discontinued, dosage should be tapered gradually and the patient monitored to reduce the risk of withdrawal symptoms. If intolerable symptoms occur following dosage reduction or upon discontinuance of treatment, consider reinstituting desvenlafaxine therapy at the previously prescribed dosage until symptoms abate. Clinicians may resume dosage reductions at that time but at a more gradual rate. (See Withdrawal of Therapy under Warnings/Precautions: Other Warnings and Precautions, in Cautions.)

Major Depressive Disorder For the management of major depressive disorder, the recommended dosage of desvenlafaxine in adults is 50 mg once daily. Although efficacy has been established at dosages of 50–400 mg once daily in clinical studies, no additional benefit was observed with dosages greater than 50 mg once daily, and adverse effects and discontinuances were more frequent at higher dosages.

While the optimum duration of desvenlafaxine succinate therapy has not been established, many experts state that acute depressive episodes require several months or longer of sustained antidepressant therapy. However, the manufacturer states that long-term efficacy (i.e., exceeding 8 weeks) of desvenlafaxine at a dosage of 50 mg once daily has not been studied. If desvenlafaxine therapy is prolonged, the need for continued therapy should be reassessed periodically.

■ **Special Populations** Although there are no specific dosage recommendations for desvenlafaxine in geriatric patients, the possibility of reduced renal clearance of the drug should be considered when determining dosage. If desvenlafaxine is poorly tolerated in such patients, administering the drug every other day can be considered.

In patients with hepatic impairment, the recommended desvenlafaxine dosage is 50 mg given once daily. Dosages exceeding 100 mg daily are *not* recommended.

In patients with mild renal impairment, desvenlafaxine dosage adjustment is not necessary. In patients with moderate renal impairment (creatinine clearance of 30–50 mL/minute), the recommended desvenlafaxine dosage is 50 mg given once daily. The recommended dosage in patients with severe renal impairment (creatinine clearance less than 30 mL/minute) or end-stage renal disease is 50 mg given every other day. Desvenlafaxine dosage should *not* be increased in patients with moderate or severe renal impairment or end-stage renal disease. Supplemental doses should not be administered to patients after dialysis.

Treatment of Pregnant Women during the Third Trimester Because some neonates exposed to venlafaxine and other SNRIs or SSRIs late in the third trimester of pregnancy have developed severe complications, consideration may be given to cautiously tapering desvenlafaxine therapy in the third trimester prior to delivery if the drug is administered during pregnancy. (See Pregnancy under Warnings/Precautions: Specific Populations, in Cautions.)

Cautions

■ **Contraindications** Known hypersensitivity to desvenlafaxine succinate, venlafaxine hydrochloride, or any ingredient in the desvenlafaxine succinate formulation.

Concurrent or recent (i.e., within 2 weeks) therapy with a monoamine oxidase (MAO) inhibitor. At least 7 days should elapse between discontinuance of desvenlafaxine and initiation of MAO inhibitor therapy. (See Serotonin Syndrome or Neuroleptic Malignant Syndrome [NMS]-like Reactions under Warnings/Precautions: Other Warnings and Precautions, in Cautions.)

■ **Warnings/Precautions** ***Warnings*** **Worsening of Depression and Suicidality Risk.** Worsening of depression and/or the emergence of suicidal ideation and behavior (suicidality) or unusual changes in behavior may occur in both adult and pediatric (see Pediatric Use under Cautions: Specific Populations) patients with major depressive disorder or other psychiatric disorders, whether or not they are taking antidepressants. This risk may persist until clinically important remission occurs. Suicide is a known risk of depression and certain other psychiatric disorders, and these disorders themselves are the strongest predictors of suicide. However, there has been a long-standing concern that antidepressants may have a role in inducing worsening of depression and the emergence of suicidality in certain patients during the early phases of treatment. Pooled analyses of short-term, placebo-controlled studies of antidepressants (i.e., selective serotonin-reuptake inhibitors and other antidepressants) have shown an increased risk of suicidality in children, adolescents, and young adults (18–24 years of age) with major depressive disorder and other psychiatric disorders. An increased suicidality risk was not demonstrated with antidepressants compared with placebo in adults older than 24 years of age, and a reduced risk was observed in adults 65 years of age or older.

The US Food and Drug Administration (FDA) recommends that all patients being treated with antidepressants for any indication be appropriately monitored and closely observed for clinical worsening, suicidality, and unusual changes in behavior, particularly during initiation of therapy (i.e., the first few months) and during periods of dosage adjustments. Families and caregivers of patients being treated with antidepressants for major depressive disorder or other indications, both psychiatric and nonpsychiatric, also should be advised to monitor patients on a daily basis for the emergence of agitation, irritability, or unusual changes in behavior as well as the emergence of suicidality, and to report such symptoms immediately to a health-care provider.

Although a causal relationship between the emergence of symptoms such as anxiety, agitation, panic attacks, insomnia, irritability, hostility, aggressiveness, impulsivity, akathisia, hypomania, and/or mania and either the worsening of depression and/or the emergence of suicidal impulses has not been established, there is concern that such symptoms may represent precursors to emerging suicidality. Consequently, consideration should be given to changing the therapeutic regimen or discontinuing therapy in patients whose depression is persistently worse or in patients experiencing emergent suicidality or symptoms that might be precursors to worsening depression or suicidality, particularly if such manifestations are severe, abrupt in onset, or were not part of the patient's presenting symptoms. FDA also recommends that the drugs be prescribed in the smallest quantity consistent with good patient management, in order to reduce the risk of overdosage.

Other Warnings and Precautions **Serotonin Syndrome or Neuroleptic Malignant Syndrome (NMS)-like Reactions.** Potentially life-threatening serotonin syndrome or neuroleptic malignant syndrome (NMS)-like reactions have been reported with selective serotonin-reuptake inhibitors (SSRIs) and SNRIs alone, including desvenlafaxine, but particularly with concurrent use of other serotonergic drugs (including serotonin [5-hydroxytryptamine; 5-HT] type 1 receptor agonists ["triptans"]), drugs that impair the metabolism of serotonin (e.g., MAO inhibitors), or antipsychotics or other dopamine antagonists. Symptoms of serotonin syndrome may include mental status changes (e.g., agitation, hallucinations, coma), autonomic instability (e.g., tachycardia, labile blood pressure, hyperthermia), neuromuscular aberrations (e.g., hyperreflexia, incoordination), and/or GI symptoms (e.g., nausea, vomiting, diarrhea). In its most severe form, serotonin syndrome may resemble neuroleptic malignant syndrome (NMS), which is characterized by hyperthermia, muscle rigidity, autonomic instability with possible rapid fluctuation of vital signs, and mental status changes. Patients receiving desvenlafaxine should be monitored for the development of serotonin syndrome or NMS-like signs and symptoms. (See Contraindications and see also Drug Interactions.)

Concurrent or recent (i.e., within 2 weeks) therapy with MAO inhibitors used for treatment of depression is contraindicated. (See Contraindications and see also Drug Interactions: Monoamine Oxidase Inhibitors.)

If concurrent therapy with desvenlafaxine and a 5-HT_1 receptor agonist (triptan) is clinically warranted, the patient should be observed carefully, particularly during initiation of therapy, when dosage is increased, or when another serotonergic agent is initiated.

Concomitant use of desvenlafaxine and serotonin precursors (e.g., tryptophan) is not recommended.

If serotonin syndrome or NMS signs and symptoms occur, treatment with desvenlafaxine and any concurrently administered serotonergic or antidopaminergic agents, including antipsychotic agents, should immediately be discontinued, and supportive and symptomatic treatment initiated.

Risk of Sustained Hypertension. Sustained increases in blood pressure have been reported. In controlled studies, sustained hypertension occurred in 0.7–2.3% of patients receiving desvenlafaxine dosages from 50–400 mg daily, with a suggestion of a higher incidence (2.3%) in those receiving 400 mg of the drug daily. In addition, some cases of elevated blood pressure requiring immediate treatment have been reported with desvenlafaxine.

Sustained blood pressure increases could have adverse consequences in patients receiving the drug. Therefore, the manufacturer recommends that preexisting hypertension be controlled before initiating desvenlafaxine therapy and that regular blood pressure monitoring be performed in patients receiving the drug. Desvenlafaxine should be used cautiously in patients with preexisting hypertension or other underlying conditions that may be compromised by increases in blood pressure. Dosage reduction or drug discontinuance should be considered in patients who experience a sustained increase in blood pressure during therapy.

Abnormal Bleeding. SSRIs and SNRIs, including desvenlafaxine, may increase the risk of bleeding events. Concurrent administration of aspirin, nonsteroidal anti-inflammatory agents, warfarin, and other anticoagulants may add to this risk. Case reports and epidemiologic studies have demonstrated an association between the use of drugs that interfere with serotonin reuptake and the occurrence of GI bleeding. Bleeding events related to SSRI and SNRI use have ranged from ecchymoses, hematomas, epistaxis, and petechiae to life-threatening hemorrhages. The manufacturer recommends that patients be advised of the risk of bleeding associated with the concomitant use of desvenlafaxine and aspirin or other nonsteroidal anti-inflammatory agents, warfarin, or other drugs that affect coagulation or bleeding. (See Drug Interactions: Drugs Affecting Hemostasis.)

Mydriasis. Mydriasis has been reported in association with desvenlafaxine therapy. Therefore, patients with elevated intraocular pressure or those at risk of angle-closure glaucoma should be monitored during treatment with the drug.

Activation of Mania/Hypomania. Activation of mania and hypomania reported in approximately 0.1% of desvenlafaxine-treated patients during clinical studies for major depressive disorder and vasomotor symptoms†. Use with caution in patients with a personal or family history of mania or hypomania.

Patients with Cardiovascular/Cerebrovascular Disease. Increases in blood pressure and small increases in heart rate were reported in clinical studies. Desvenlafaxine has not been systematically evaluated in patients with a recent history of myocardial infarction, unstable cardiovascular disease, uncontrolled hypertension, or cerebrovascular disease; patients with these diagnoses, except for cerebrovascular disease, were excluded from clinical studies. Therefore, the manufacturer advises using desvenlafaxine with caution in patients with cardiovascular, cerebrovascular, or lipid metabolism disorders.

Effects on Lipoproteins. Dose-dependent, possibly clinically significant increases in fasting serum total cholesterol, low-density lipoprotein (LDL) cholesterol, and triglycerides reported in controlled studies. Consider measuring serum lipid concentrations during desvenlafaxine therapy.

Withdrawal of Therapy. In clinical studies, abrupt discontinuance or dosage reduction of desvenlafaxine has been associated with the appearance of withdrawal effects, including dizziness, nausea, headache, irritability, insomnia, diarrhea, anxiety, fatigue, abnormal dreams, and hyperhidrosis, in patients with major depressive disorder. These symptoms generally occurred more frequently with longer duration of therapy. Withdrawal effects have also been reported upon discontinuance of other SNRIs and SSRIs, particularly when abrupt; these effects have included dysphoric mood, irritability, agitation, dizziness, sensory disturbances (e.g., paresthesia, such as electric shock sensations), anxiety, confusion, headache, lethargy, emotional lability, insomnia, hypomania, tinnitus, and seizures. While these events are generally self-limiting, there have been serious cases. Therefore, patients should be monitored for possible withdrawal symptoms when discontinuing desvenlafaxine therapy. A gradual reduction in dosage rather than abrupt cessation is recommended whenever possible. (See Dosage and Administration: Dosage.)

Seizures. Seizures have been reported in premarketing clinical studies of desvenlafaxine. Desvenlafaxine has not been systematically evaluated in patients with seizure disorders; such patients were excluded from premarketing clinical studies. The manufacturer states that the drug should be used with caution in patients with a seizure disorder.

Hyponatremia/Syndrome of Inappropriate Antidiuretic Hormone Secretion. Treatment with SSRIs and SNRIs, including desvenlafaxine, may result in hyponatremia. In many cases, hyponatremia appears to be due to the syndrome of inappropriate antidiuretic hormone secretion (SIADH). Cases with serum sodium concentrations lower than 110 mmol/L have been reported. Geriatric individuals and patients receiving diuretics or who are otherwise volume depleted may be at greater risk of developing hyponatremia. Signs and symptoms of hyponatremia include headache, difficulty concentrating, memory impairment, confusion, weakness, and unsteadiness, which may lead to falls; more severe and/or acute cases have been associated with hallucinations, syncope, seizures, coma, respiratory arrest, and death. Initiate appropriate medical intervention and consider drug discontinuance in patients with symptomatic hyponatremia.

Concomitant Administration of Drugs Containing Desvenlafaxine and Venlafaxine. Desvenlafaxine is the major active metabolite of venlafaxine. The manufacturer states that products containing desvenlafaxine and products containing venlafaxine should not be used concomitantly with desvenlafaxine extended-release tablets (Pristiq®). (See Serotonin Syndrome or Neuroleptic Malignant Syndrome [NMS]-like Reactions under Warnings/Precautions: Other Warnings and Precautions, in Cautions.)

Interstitial Lung Disease and Eosinophilic Pneumonia. Interstitial lung disease and eosinophilic pneumonia associated with venlafaxine (the parent drug of desvenlafaxine) have been reported rarely. The possibility of such adverse effects should be considered in patients treated with desvenlafaxine who present with progressive dyspnea, cough, or chest discomfort. Such patients should be evaluated promptly and discontinuance of desvenlafaxine should be considered.

Specific Populations **Pregnancy.** Category C. (See Users Guide.)

Some neonates exposed to SNRIs or SSRIs late in the third trimester of pregnancy have developed complications that have sometimes been severe and required prolonged hospitalization, respiratory support, enteral nutrition, and other forms of supportive care in special-care nurseries. Such complications may arise immediately upon delivery and usually last several days or up to 2–4 weeks. Clinical findings reported to date in the neonates have included respiratory distress, cyanosis, apnea, seizures, temperature instability or fever, feeding difficulty, dehydration, excessive weight loss, vomiting, hypoglycemia, hypotonia, hypertonia, hyperreflexia, tremor, jitteriness, irritability, lethargy, reduced or lack of reaction to pain stimuli, and constant crying. These clinical features appear to be consistent with either a direct toxic effect of the SNRI or SSRI or, possibly, a drug withdrawal syndrome. It should be noted that, in some cases, the clinical picture was consistent with serotonin syndrome. (For additional information, see Cautions: Pregnancy, Fertility, and Lactation, in Fluoxetine Hydrochloride 28:16.04.20.) When treating a pregnant woman with desvenlafaxine during the third trimester of pregnancy, the clinician should carefully consider the potential risks and benefits of such therapy. Consideration may be given to cautiously tapering desvenlafaxine therapy in the third trimester prior to delivery if the drug is administered during pregnancy. (See Treatment of Pregnant Women during the Third Trimester under Dosage and Administration: Special Populations.)

Lactation. Desvenlafaxine is excreted into human milk. Because of the potential for serious advere effects in nursing infants from desvenlafaxine, discontinue nursing or the drug, taking into account the importance of the drug to the woman. The manufacturer states that desvenlafaxine should only be administered to nursing women if the expected benefits outweigh any possible risk.

Pediatric Use. Safety and effectiveness of desvenlafaxine in pediatric patients younger than 18 years of age have not been established.

FDA warns that a greater risk of suicidal thinking or behavior (suicidality) occurred during the first few months of antidepressant treatment compared with placebo in children and adolescents with major depressive disorder, obsessive-compulsive disorder (OCD), or other psychiatric disorders based on pooled analyses of 24 short-term, placebo-controlled trials of 9 antidepressant drugs (SSRIs and other antidepressants). However, a more recent meta-analysis of 27 placebo-controlled trials of 9 antidepressants (SSRIs and others) in patients younger than 19 years of age with major depressive disorder, OCD, or non-OCD anxiety disorders suggests that the benefits of antidepressant therapy in treating these conditions may outweigh the risks of suicidal behavior or suicidal ideation. No suicides occurred in these pediatric trials.

These findings should be carefully considered when assessing potential benefits and risks of desvenlafaxine in a child or adolescent for any clinical use. (See Worsening of Depression and Suicidality Risk under Warnings/Precautions: Warnings, in Cautions.)

Geriatric Use. In clinical studies of desvenlafaxine, 5% of patients studied were 65 years of age or older. Although no overall differences in safety or efficacy were observed between geriatric and younger patients in these studies, a higher incidence of systolic orthostatic hypotension was reported in patients 65 years of age or older compared with younger patients in the short-term, placebo-controlled studies. Consider possible reduced renal clearance of the drug in geriatric patients. (See Dosage and Administration: Special Populations.) The possibility that some older patients may exhibit increased sensitivity to the drug cannot be ruled out.

SSRIs and SNRIs, including desvenlafaxine, have been associated with clinically important hyponatremia in geriatric patients, who may be at greater risk for this adverse effect. (See Hyponatremia/Syndrome of Inappropriate Antidiuretic Hormone Secretion under Warnings/Precautions: Other Warnings and Precautions, in Cautions.)

In pooled data analyses, a *reduced* risk of suicidality was observed in adults 65 years of age or older with antidepressant therapy compared with placebo. (See Worsening of Depression and Suicidality Risk under Warnings/Precautions: Warnings, in Cautions.)

Hepatic Impairment. Mean elimination half-life of desvenlafaxine is increased in patients with moderate or severe hepatic impairment compared with healthy individuals and patients with mild hepatic impairment. The recommended desvenlafaxine dosage in patients with hepatic impairment is 50 mg daily; dosages exceeding 100 mg daily are not recommended in such patients. (See Dosage and Administration: Special Populations.)

Renal Impairment. In patients with moderate or severe renal impairment or end-stage renal disease, clearance of desvenlafaxine was decreased, resulting in potentially clinically significant increases in drug exposure. Dosage adjustment is necessary in such patients. (See Dosage and Administration: Special Populations.)

■ **Common Adverse Effects** Adverse effects reported in at least 5% of patients with major depressive disorder receiving desvenlafaxine (50 or 100 mg daily) and at an incidence of at least twice that reported with placebo in short-term clinical studies include nausea, dizziness, insomnia, hyperhidrosis, constipation, somnolence, decreased appetite, anxiety, and sexual function disorders in males (e.g., anorgasmia, decreased libido, abnormal orgasm, delayed ejaculation, erectile dysfunction, ejaculation disorder, ejaculation failure, and sexual dysfunction).

Drug Interactions

■ **Drugs Metabolized by Hepatic Microsomal Enzymes** Desvenlafaxine minimally inhibits the cytochrome P-450 (CYP) 2D6 isoenzyme. In a study in healthy adults, concurrent administration of desvenlafaxine (100 mg daily) and desipramine (single 50-mg dose), a CYP2D6 substrate, increased peak plasma concentrations and AUCs of desipramine by approximately 25 and 17%, respectively. The manufacturer states that concomitant use of desvenlafaxine with a drug metabolized by CYP2D6 can result in higher plasma concentrations of that drug.

Desvenlafaxine does not inhibit or induce the CYP3A4 isoenzyme in vitro. Concurrent administration of desvenlafaxine (400 mg daily; 8 times the recommended dosage) and midazolam (single 4-mg dose), a CYP3A4 substrate, decreased the AUC and peak plasma concentrations of midazolam by approximately 31 and 16%, respectively. The manufacturer states that concurrent use of desvenlafaxine with a drug metabolized by CYP3A4 can result in lower exposures to that drug.

Desvenlafaxine does not inhibit CYP isoenzymes 1A2, 2A6, 2C8, 2C9, and 2C19 in vitro and is unlikely to affect the pharmacokinetics of drugs that are metabolized by these CYP isoenzymes.

■ **Drugs Affecting Hepatic Microsomal Enzymes** CYP3A4 is a minor pathway for the metabolism of desvenlafaxine. Concomitant administration of ketoconazole (200 mg twice daily), a CYP3A4 inhibitor, and a single 400-mg dose of desvenlafaxine resulted in a 43% increase in AUC and an 8% increase in peak plasma concentrations of desvenlafaxine. The manufacturer states that concurrent use of desvenlafaxine with other potent CYP3A4 inhibitors may result in higher plasma concentrations of desvenlafaxine.

Inhibitors of CYP isoenzymes 1A1, 1A2, 2A6, 2D6, 2C8, 2C9, 2C19, and 2E1: clinically important pharmacokinetic interaction is unlikely.

■ **CNS-active Drugs** The risk of concurrent administration of desvenlafaxine and other CNS-active drugs has not been systematically evaluated to date; use with caution.

■ **Monoamine Oxidase Inhibitors** Potential pharmacologic interaction (potentially serious, sometimes fatal serotonin syndrome or NMS-like reactions). Concomitant use of monoamine oxidase (MAO) inhibitors with desvenlafaxine is contraindicated. In addition, at least 2 weeks should elapse between discontinuance of an MAO inhibitor and initiation of desvenlafaxine and at least 7 days should elapse between discontinuance of desvenlafaxine and initiation of MAO inhibitor therapy. (See Serotonin Syndrome or Neuroleptic Malignant Syndrome [NMS]-like Reactions under Warnings/Precautions: Other Warnings and Precautions, in Cautions.)

■ **Serotonergic Drugs** Potential pharmacologic interaction (potentially serious, sometimes fatal serotonin syndrome or NMS-like reactions) with drugs affecting serotonergic neurotransmission, including linezolid (an anti-infective agent that is an MAO inhibitor), lithium, tramadol, and St. John's wort (*Hypericum perforatum*); use concomitantly with caution. If serotonin syndrome or NMS signs and symptoms occur, immediately discontinue treatment with desvenlafaxine and any concurrently administered serotonergic or antidopaminergic agents and initiate supportive and symptomatic treatment. Concurrent administration of desvenlafaxine and serotonin precursors (such as tryptophan) is not recommended. (See Serotonin Syndrome or Neuroleptic Malignant Syndrome [NMS]-like Reactions under Warnings/Precautions: Other Warnings and Precautions, in Cautions.)

■ **Selective Serotonin-reuptake Inhibitors and Selective Serotonin- and Norepinephrine-reuptake Inhibitors** Potential pharmacologic interaction (potentially serious, sometimes fatal serotonin syndrome or NMS-like reactions). (See Serotonin Syndrome or Neuroleptic Malignant Syndrome [NMS]-like Reactions under Warnings/Precautions: Other Warnings and Precautions, in Cautions.)

Desvenlafaxine is the major active metabolite of venlafaxine. The manufacturer states that products containing desvenlafaxine and products containing venlafaxine should not be used concomitantly with commercially available desvenlafaxine succinate extended-release tablets (Pristiq®).

■ **5-HT$_1$ Receptor Agonists ("Triptans")** Potential pharmacologic interaction (potentially serious, sometimes fatal serotonin syndrome or NMS-like reactions) if used concurrently with 5-HT$_1$ receptor agonists (e.g., almotriptan, eletriptan, frovatriptan, naratriptan, rizatriptan, sumatriptan, zolmitriptan). If concomitant therapy is clinically warranted, the patient should be observed carefully, particularly during treatment initiation, when dosage is increased, or when another serotonergic agent is initiated. (See Serotonin Syndrome or Neuroleptic Malignant Syndrome [NMS]-like Reactions under Warnings/Precautions: Other Warnings and Precautions, in Cautions.)

■ **Drugs Affecting Hemostasis** Potential pharmacologic interaction (increased risk of bleeding) if used concurrently with aspirin or other nonsteroidal anti-inflammatory agents, warfarin, or other drugs that affect coagulation or bleeding; use with caution.

Altered anticoagulant effects, including increased bleeding, have been reported when SSRIs or SNRIs were concurrently administered with warfarin or other anticoagulants. The manufacturer recommends carefully monitoring patients receiving warfarin during initiation and discontinuance of desvenlafaxine therapy.

■ **Antipsychotic Agents and Other Dopamine Antagonists** Potential pharmacologic interaction (potentially serious, sometimes fatal serotonin syndrome or NMS-like reactions) if used concurrently with antipsychotic agents or other dopamine antagonists. If serotonin syndrome or NMS signs and symptoms occur, immediately discontinue treatment with desvenlafaxine and any concurrently administered antidopaminergic or serotonergic agents and initiate supportive and symptomatic treatment. (See Serotonin Syndrome or Neuroleptic Malignant Syndrome [NMS]-like Reactions under Warnings/Precautions: Other Warnings and Precautions, in Cautions.)

■ **Drugs that are Substrates of or Inhibitors of P-glycoprotein Transport System** Desvenlafaxine is not a substrate or an inhibitor for the P-glycoprotein transporter in vitro. The pharmacokinetics of desvenlafaxine are unlikely to be affected by drugs that inhibit the P-glycoprotein transporter, and desvenlafaxine is not likely to affect the pharmacokinetics of drugs that are substrates of the P-glycoprotein transporter.

■ **Alcohol** In a clinical study, desvenlafaxine did not increase impairment of mental and motor skills caused by alcohol. However, the manufacturer recommends avoiding concomitant alcohol consumption during desvenlafaxine therapy.

■ **Electroconvulsive Therapy** The risks and/or benefits of combined use of electroconvulsive therapy and desvenlafaxine have not been evaluated.

Description

Desvenlafaxine succinate, a selective serotonin- and norepinephrine-reuptake inhibitor (SNRI), is an antidepressant. The drug is the principal active metabolite of venlafaxine and is pharmacologically related to duloxetine, another SNRI.

The exact mechanism of antidepressant action of desvenlafaxine has not been fully elucidated but appears to be associated with the drug's potentiation of serotonergic and noradrenergic activity in the CNS. Like venlafaxine and duloxetine, desvenlafaxine is a potent inhibitor of neuronal serotonin and norepinephrine reuptake; however, inhibition of dopamine reuptake at concentrations that inhibit serotonin and norepinephrine reuptake appears unlikely in most patients. The drug does not inhibit monoamine oxidase (MAO) and has not demonstrated significant affinity for muscarinic cholinergic, H$_1$-histaminergic, α_1-adrenergic, dopaminergic, γ-aminobutyric acid (GABA), glutamate, and opiate receptors in vitro.

Desvenlafaxine is principally metabolized via conjugation by uridine disphosphoglucuronosyltransferase (UGT) isoenzymes and, to a lesser extent, through oxidation (by the cytochrome P-450 [CYP] 3A4 isoenzyme). The drug minimally inhibits the CYP2D6 isoenzyme and does not inhibit the CYP 1A2, 2A6, 2C8, 2C9, or 2C19 isoenzymes. Desvenlafaxine is not an inhibitor of CYP3A4, nor is it an inducer of CYP3A4. The drug exhibits a low degree of protein binding (30%) and has a mean elimination half-life of approximately 11 hours. Approximately 45% of a single oral dose of desvenlafaxine is eliminated unchanged in the urine at 72 hours, approximately 19% of the dose is excreted as the glucuronide metabolite, and less than 5% is excreted as the oxidative metabolite (N,O-didesmethylvenlafaxine).

Advice to Patients

Risk of suicidality; importance of patients, family, and caregivers being alert to and immediately reporting emergence of suicidality, worsening depression, or unusual changes in behavior, especially during the first few months of therapy or during periods of dosage adjustment. (See Worsening of Depression and Suicidality Risk under Warnings/Precautions: Warnings, in Cautions.) FDA recommends providing written patient information (medication guide) explaining risks of suicidality each time the drug is dispensed. Importance of advising patients about importance of reading the patient information before taking desvenlafaxine and each time the prescription is refilled.

Importance of informing patients of potential risk of serotonin syndrome and neuroleptic malignant syndrome (NMS)-like reactions, particularly with concurrent use of desvenlafaxine and 5-HT$_1$ receptor agonists (also called triptans), tramadol, tryptophan, other serotonergic agents, or antipsychotic agents. Importance of immediately contacting clinician if signs and symptoms of these syndromes develop (e.g., restlessness, hallucinations, loss of coordination, fast heart beat, increased body temperature, muscle stiffness, increased blood pressure, diarrhea, coma, nausea, vomiting, confusion).

Importance of advising patients not to concurrently take other products containing desvenlafaxine or venlafaxine.

Importance of instructing patients not to take desvenlafaxine with a monoamine oxidase (MAO) inhibitor or within 14 days of stopping the drug, and to allow at least 7 days after stopping desvenlafaxine before starting therapy with an MAO inhibitor.

Risk of discontinuance symptoms when switching from other antidepressants, including venlafaxine, to desvenlafaxine. Importance of advising patients that tapering of the previous antidepressant may be necessary to minimize the risk of such symptoms.

Importance of advising patients that they should have regular monitoring of blood pressure while taking desvenlafaxine.

Importance of advising patients with raised intraocular pressure or those at risk of acute narrow-angle glaucoma (angle-closure glaucoma) that mydriasis has been reported with desvenlafaxine and that they should be monitored.

Importance of advising patients, their families, and caregivers to observe desvenlafaxine-treated patients for signs of activation or mania/hypomania.

Importance of advising patients that elevations in total cholesterol, LDL, and triglycerides may occur and that measurement of lipid levels may be considered during therapy.

Importance of advising patients to notify their clinician if they develop any allergic signs or symptoms during therapy (e.g., rash, hives, swelling, difficulty breathing).

Risk of cognitive and motor impairment; importance of exercising caution while operating hazardous machinery, including automobile driving, until patients are reasonably certain that desvenlafaxine therapy does not adversely affect their ability to engage in such activities.

Importance of avoiding alcohol during desvenlafaxine therapy.

Importance of informing clinicians of existing or contemplated concomitant therapy, including prescription and OTC drugs or herbal supplements, as well as any concomitant illnesses (e.g., cardiovascular, cerebrovascular, or lipid metabolism disorders; glaucoma) or personal or family history of suicidality or bipolar disorder. Importance of advising patients about the risk of bleeding associated with concomitant use of desvenlafaxine with aspirin or other nonsteroidal anti-inflammatory agents, warfarin, or other drugs that affect coagulation.

Importance of women informing clinicians if they are or plan to become pregnant or plan to breast-feed.

Importance of advising patients with depression that it usually takes several weeks of antidepressant therapy before they will start to feel better. Advise patients not to stop taking the drug if they do not feel the results right away.

Importance of advising patients not to stop taking taking desvenlafaxine without first talking with their clinician. Importance of patients being aware that discontinuance effects may occur when stopping the drug.

Importance of informing patients to swallow desvenlafaxine tablets whole with fluid, and not to crush, cut, chew, or dissolve the tablets because the tablets are timed-released.

Importance of informing patients that they may notice an inert matrix tablet passing in the stool or via colostomy, and that the active medication has already been absorbed by the time the patient sees the inert matrix tablet.

Importance of informing patients of other important precautionary information. (See Cautions.)

Overview® (see Users Guide). For additional information on this drug until a more detailed monograph is developed and published, the manufacturer's labeling should be consulted. It is *essential* that the manufacturer's labeling be consulted for more detailed information on usual cautions, precautions, contraindications, potential drug interactions, laboratory test interferences, and acute toxicity.

Preparations

Excipients in commercially available drug preparations may have clinically important effects in some individuals; consult specific product labeling for details.

Desvenlafaxine Succinate

Oral		
Tablet, extended-release, film-coated	50 mg (of desvenlafaxine)	Pristiq®, Wyeth
	100 mg (of desvenlafaxine)	Pristiq®, Wyeth

†Use is not currently included in the labeling approved by the US Food and Drug Administration

DULoxetine Hydrochloride

■ Duloxetine hydrochloride, a selective serotonin- and norepinephrine-reuptake inhibitor (SNRI), is an antidepressant and anxiolytic agent.

Uses

■ **Major Depressive Disorder** Duloxetine hydrochloride is used for the acute and maintenance treatment of major depressive disorder in adults.

Efficacy of duloxetine for the acute treatment of major depression has principally been established by 4 double-blind, placebo-controlled studies of 8–9 weeks' duration in outpatient settings in adults. In these studies, patients receiving duloxetine (40–120 mg daily) had greater improvements in the 17-item Hamilton depression rating scale (HAMD-17) total score than did patients receiving placebo. No age-, race-, or gender-related differences in efficacy were noted in these studies.

Efficacy of duloxetine for the maintenance treatment of major depressive disorder has been established in a randomized, placebo-controlled relapse prevention study in which 533 adult outpatients who met DSM-IV criteria for major depressive disorder initially received duloxetine 60 mg once daily in a 12-week, open-label acute phase. Patients who responded to treatment during the acute phase were then randomized to continue receiving duloxetine at the same dosage or to receive placebo for 26 weeks in the continuation phase. The duloxetine-treated patients experienced a longer time to relapse of depression compared with the placebo recipients. In addition, more placebo recipients relapsed compared with patients receiving duloxetine (approximately 29% and 17%, respectively).

The manufacturer states that if duloxetine is used for extended periods, the need for continued therapy should be reassessed periodically.

Antidepressant efficacy of duloxetine in hospital settings has not been adequately studied to date.

For further information on treatment of major depressive disorder and considerations in choosing the most appropriate antidepressant for a particular patient, including considerations related to patient tolerance, patient age, and cardiovascular, sedative, and suicidal risk, see Considerations in Choosing Antidepressants under Uses: Major Depressive Disorder, in Fluoxetine Hydrochloride 28:16.04.20.

■ **Generalized Anxiety Disorder** Duloxetine hydrochloride is used for the acute management of generalized anxiety disorder in adults. Efficacy of duloxetine for this indication has been established by 3 placebo-controlled trials of 9–10 weeks' duration in outpatient settings in adults who met DSM-IV criteria for generalized anxiety disorder. In these studies, patients receiving duloxetine (60–120 mg daily) had greater improvements in the Hamilton anxiety scale (HAM-A) total score and the Sheehan Disability Scale (SDS) global functional impairment score than did patients receiving placebo. No age- or gender-related differences in efficacy were noted in these studies.

The manufacturer states that the anxiolytic efficacy of duloxetine for long-term use (i.e., exceeding 10 weeks) has not been established by controlled studies to date. If duloxetine is used for extended periods, the need for continued therapy should be reassessed periodically.

■ **Neuropathic Pain** Duloxetine hydrochloride is used for the management of neuropathic pain associated with diabetic peripheral neuropathy in adults. Efficacy of duloxetine for this indication has been established by 2 controlled studies of 12 weeks' duration in adults with type 1 or 2 diabetes mellitus and a diagnosis of painful distal symmetrical sensorimotor polyneuropathy for at least 6 months. Patients were excluded from the studies if they met DSM-IV-TR criteria for major depressive disorder and dysthymia. In these studies, 51% of patients receiving duloxetine (60–120 mg daily) and up to 4 g of acetaminophen daily (as needed) reported at least a 30% sustained reduction in pain compared with 31% of those receiving placebo plus acetaminophen (as needed). Some patients in the study experienced a decrease in pain as early as week 1, which persisted throughout the study.

■ **Fibromyalgia** Duloxetine hydrochloride is used for the management of fibromyalgia in adults. Efficacy of duloxetine for this indication has been established by 2 randomized, double-blind, placebo-controlled, fixed-dose studies in adults with a diagnosis of fibromyalgia based on the American College of Rheumatology (ACR) criteria (i.e., history of widespread pain for 3 months and pain present in 11 or more of the 18 specific tender point sites). The first study was of 3 months' duration and enrolled female patients only while the second study was of 6 months' duration and enrolled both male and female patients. Approximately 25% of the patients had concurrent major depressive disorder. Both of these studies compared duloxetine 60 mg once daily or 120 mg daily (given in divided doses in study 1 and as a single daily dose in study 2) with placebo. In addition, Study 2 compared duloxetine 20 mg daily with placebo during the initial 3 months of the 6-month study; after 3 months, the duloxetine dosage was titrated up to 60 mg once daily for the remainder of the study. In these studies, duloxetine therapy in dosages of 60 or 120 mg daily significantly improved the endpoint mean pain scores from baseline and increased the number of patients who had at least a 50% reduction in pain score compared with baseline. Although pain reduction was observed in patients both with and without major depressive disorder, the degree of pain reduction may be greater in patients with major depressive disorder. Some patients experienced a reduction in pain as early as week 1, which persisted throughout the study. Improvement also was noted on measures of function as well as on the Patient Global Impression of Improvement (PGI) scale. Neither study demonstrated an additional therapeutic benefit of 120 mg daily compared with 60 mg daily, and the higher dosage was associated with more frequent adverse effects and early discontinuance of therapy.

The manufacturer states that the efficacy of duloxetine for long-term use (i.e., exceeding 3 months) has not been established by controlled studies to date. However, longer-term efficacy of the drug has been demonstrated for up to 6 months in extension phases of 2 controlled studies to date. The manufacturer recommends that the decision to continue therapy with the drug be based on individual patient response.

■ **Stress Urinary Incontinence** Duloxetine has been used for the management of moderate to severe stress urinary incontinence (SUI)† in women. In a number of placebo-controlled clinical trials involving women with predominantly SUI receiving duloxetine or placebo for up to 12 weeks, duloxetine was significantly better than placebo in reducing the frequency of incontinence episodes (which were reduced by approximately 50% in patients receiving duloxetine) and improving patients' quality of life (as assessed by Incontinence Quality of Life questionnaire scores). Therapy with the drug generally was well tolerated in these studies, with nausea being the most commonly reported adverse effect.

Data from one subsequent analysis suggest that the beneficial effects of duloxetine in women with SUI are maintained for up to 30 months. In addition, some data suggest that combining duloxetine and pelvic floor muscle training exercises may be more effective than either treatment alone. The potential role of duloxetine therapy relative to other forms of treatment (including pelvic floor muscle training, management of fluid intake and voiding, weight loss, devices, and surgery) remains to be established and requires additional study.

Dosage and Administration

■ **Administration** Duloxetine hydrochloride is administered orally without regard to meals. Duloxetine hydrochloride delayed-release capsules should be swallowed whole and should *not* be chewed or crushed, nor should the contents be sprinkled on food or mixed with liquids.

■ **Dosage** Dosage of duloxetine hydrochloride is expressed in terms of duloxetine.

Patients receiving duloxetine should be monitored for possible worsening of depression, suicidality, or unusual changes in behavior, especially at the beginning of therapy or during periods of dosage adjustment. (See Worsening of Depression and Suicidality Risk under Warnings/Precautions: Warnings, in Cautions.)

The manufacturer recommends that an interval of at least 2 weeks elapse when switching a patient from a monoamine oxidase (MAO) inhibitor to duloxetine. In addition, an interval of at least 5 days should elapse when switching from duloxetine to an MAO inhibitor.

Because withdrawal effects may occur (see Withdrawal Effects under Warnings/Precautions: Other Warnings and Precautions in Cautions), abrupt discontinuance of duloxetine should be avoided. When duloxetine therapy is discontinued, dosage should be tapered gradually and the patient carefully monitored to reduce the risk of withdrawal symptoms. If intolerable symptoms occur following dosage reduction or upon discontinuance of treatment, duloxetine therapy may be reinstituted at the previously prescribed dosage until such symptoms abate. Clinicians may resume dosage reductions at that time but at a more gradual rate.

Major Depressive Disorder For the management of major depressive disorder, the recommended initial dosage of duloxetine in adults is 40 mg daily (given as 20 mg twice daily) to 60 mg daily (given either as 60 mg once daily or 30 mg twice daily). In some patients, it may be desirable to initiate therapy with a dosage of 30 mg once daily given for 1 week, followed by an increase to 60 mg once daily. Although duloxetine dosages of 120 mg daily have been effective, there is no evidence that dosages exceeding 60 mg daily provide additional therapeutic benefit. Safety of dosages exceeding 120 mg daily has not been adequately evaluated.

While the optimum duration of duloxetine therapy has not been established, it generally is agreed that acute depressive episodes require several months or longer of sustained antidepressant therapy. Systematic evaluation of duloxetine has shown that its antidepressant efficacy is maintained for periods of up to 26 weeks in patients receiving 60 mg daily. The manufacturer recommends a maintenance dosage of 60 mg once daily in adults. The manufacturer also recommends that the usefulness of duloxetine be reevaluated periodically in patients receiving long-term therapy.

Generalized Anxiety Disorder For the management of generalized anxiety disorder, the recommended initial adult dosage of duloxetine is 60 mg once daily. In some patients, it may be desirable to initiate therapy with a dosage of 30 mg once daily given for 1 week, followed by an increase to 60 mg once daily. Dosage may be increased in increments of 30 mg once daily (up to a maximum dosage of 120 mg once daily). However, no additional benefit has been demonstrated from duloxetine dosages exceeding 60 mg once daily.

While the optimum duration of duloxetine therapy has not been established, it generally is agreed that generalized anxiety disorder is a chronic condition. The manufacturer states that the efficacy of duloxetine for long-term use (i.e., exceeding 10 weeks) has not been established by controlled studies and that the usefulness of the drug in patients receiving prolonged therapy should be reevaluated periodically.

Neuropathic Pain For the management of neuropathic pain associated with diabetic peripheral neuropathy, the recommended adult dosage of duloxetine is 60 mg once daily. Duloxetine dosages exceeding 60 mg daily do not appear to provide substantially greater therapeutic benefit and clearly are less well tolerated. For patients for whom tolerability is a concern, a lower initial dosage may be considered. Because progression of diabetic peripheral neuropathy is highly variable and management of pain is empirical, efficacy of the drug must be assessed individually. The manufacturer states that the efficacy of duloxetine for long-term use (i.e., exceeding 12 weeks) has not been established by controlled studies.

Fibromyalgia For the management of fibromyalgia, the recommended adult dosage of duloxetine is 60 mg once daily. The manufacturer states that treatment should be initiated at 30 mg once daily for one week to allow patients to adjust to the drug before increasing the dosage to 60 mg once daily. Some patients may respond to the initial dosage of 30 mg once daily. Duloxetine dosages exceeding 60 mg daily do not appear to provide greater therapeutic benefit, even in patients not responding to a dosage of 60 mg daily, and are associated with a higher incidence of adverse effects.

Fibromyalgia is recognized as a chronic condition. The manufacturer states that efficacy of duloxetine in the management of fibromyalgia has been demonstrated in placebo-controlled studies lasting up to 3 months, and that the efficacy of the drug for longer-term use (i.e., exceeding 3 months) has not been established in controlled studies. However, efficacy of the drug has been demonstrated for up to 6 months in extension phases of 2 controlled studies. The manufacturer recommends that the decision to continue therapy with the drug be based on individual patient response.

Stress Urinary Incontinence Although the optimum dosage and duration of duloxetine therapy for the treatment of stress urinary incontinence† in women remain to be established, the most commonly used dosage in controlled trials has been 80 mg daily, usually given as 40 mg twice daily (dosage range: 20–120 mg daily). Some patients may benefit (i.e., reduced risk of nausea and dizziness) from initiating therapy with a duloxetine dosage of 20 mg twice daily for 2 weeks before increasing to the usual dosage of 40 mg twice daily. If adverse effects are bothersome during the first few weeks of therapy at the usual dosage, the dosage may be reduced to 20 mg twice daily. The safety of higher dosages (i.e., 120 mg daily), which have been used in a limited number of women with more severe cases of stress urinary incontinence, requires additional study.

■ **Special Populations** Although there are no specific dosage recommendations for geriatric patients, extra caution is recommended when the duloxetine dosage is increased in elderly patients.

Although the manufacturer makes no specific dosage recommendation for smoking patients, some clinicians recommend a slightly increased duloxetine dosage (by about 15%) in patients who smoke. (See Drug Interactions: Smoking.)

In patients with mild to moderate renal impairment (creatinine clearance 30–80 mL/minute), a lower initial dosage and gradual increase in dosage may be considered. The manufacturer recommends that duloxetine *not* be administered to patients with end-stage renal disease (requiring dialysis), severe renal impairment (creatinine clearance less than 30 mL/minute), or any hepatic insufficiency. (See Specific Populations under Cautions: Warnings/Precautions.)

Treatment of Pregnant Women during the Third Trimester Because some neonates exposed to duloxetine and other selective serotonin- and norepinephrine-reuptake inhibitors (SNRIs) or selective serotonin-reuptake inhibitors late in the third trimester of pregnancy have developed severe complications, consideration may be given to cautiously tapering duloxetine therapy in the third trimester prior to delivery if the drug is administered during pregnancy. (See Pregnancy under Warnings/Precautions: Specific Populations, in Cautions.)

Cautions

■ **Contraindications** Concurrent or recent (i.e., within 2 weeks) therapy with a monoamine oxidase (MAO) inhibitor. (See Drug Interactions: Monoamine Oxidase Inhibitors.)

Uncontrolled angle-closure glaucoma.

Known hypersensitivity to duloxetine or any ingredient in the formulation.

■ **Warnings/Precautions** ***Warnings*** **Worsening of Depression and Suicidality Risk.** Worsening of depression and/or the emergence of suicidal ideation and behavior (suicidality) or unusual changes in behavior may occur in both adult and pediatric (see Pediatric Use under Cautions: Specific Populations) patients with major depressive disorder or other psychiatric disorders, whether or not they are taking antidepressants. This risk may persist until clinically important remission occurs. Suicide is a known risk of depression and certain other psychiatric disorders, and these disorders themselves are the strongest predictors of suicide. However, there has been a long-standing concern that antidepressants may have a role in inducing worsening of depression and the emergence of suicidality in certain patients during the early phases of treatment. Pooled analyses of short-term, placebo-controlled studies of antidepressants (i.e., selective serotonin-reuptake inhibitors and other antidepressants) have shown an increased risk of suicidality in children, adolescents, and young adults (18–24 years of age) with major depressive disorder and other psychiatric disorders. An increased suicidality risk was not demonstrated with antidepressants compared with placebo in adults older than 24 years of age and a reduced risk was observed in adults 65 years of age or older.

The US Food and Drug Administration (FDA) recommends that all patients being treated with antidepressants for any indication be appropriately monitored and closely observed for clinical worsening, suicidality, and unusual changes in behavior, particularly during initiation of therapy (i.e., the first few months) and during periods of dosage adjustments. Families and caregivers of patients being treated with antidepressants for major depressive disorder or other indications, both psychiatric and nonpsychiatric, also should be advised to monitor patients on a daily basis for the emergence of agitation, irritability, or unusual changes in behavior as well as the emergence of suicidality, and to report such symptoms immediately to a health-care provider.

Although a causal relationship between the emergence of symptoms such as anxiety, agitation, panic attacks, insomnia, irritability, hostility, aggressiveness, impulsivity, akathisia, hypomania, and/or mania and either the worsening of depression and/or the emergence of suicidal impulses has not been established, there is concern that such symptoms may represent precursors to emerging suicidality. Consequently, consideration should be given to changing the therapeutic regimen or discontinuing therapy in patients whose depression is persistently worse or in patients experiencing emergent suicidality or symptoms that might be precursors to worsening depression or suicidality, particularly if such manifestations are severe, abrupt in onset, or were not part of the patient's presenting symptoms. FDA also recommends that the drugs be prescribed in the smallest quantity consistent with good patient management, in order to reduce the risk of overdosage.

Other Warnings and Precautions **Hepatic Effects.** Hepatic failure, sometimes fatal, has been reported in duloxetine-treated patients. The cases presented as hepatitis accompanied by abdominal pain, hepatomegaly, and markedly elevated serum transaminase concentrations (more than 20 times the upper limit of normal) with or without jaundice, reflecting a mixed or hepatocellular pattern of hepatic injury. Duloxetine should be discontinued in any patient who develops jaundice or other evidence of clinically important hepatic dysfunction; therapy should not be resumed unless another cause for the hepatic dysfunction can be established.

Cases of cholestatic jaundice with minimal elevation of serum transaminase concentrations also have been reported. Postmarketing reports indicate that elevated serum transaminase, bilirubin, and alkaline phosphatase concentrations have occurred in duloxetine-treated patients with chronic hepatic disease or cirrhosis.

Duloxetine has been shown to increase the risk of serum transaminase elevations in clinical trials; such elevations resulted in discontinuance of the drug in 0.3% of patients. The median time to detection of the transaminase elevation was about 2 months. In placebo-controlled trials, elevations in serum ALT concentrations to more than 3 times the upper limit of normal occurred in 1.1% of the duloxetine-treated patients compared with 0.2% of those receiving placebo. There was evidence of a dose-response relationship for ALT (SGPT) and AST (SGOT) elevations of more than 3 times the upper limit of normal and more than 5 times the upper limit of normal, respectively.

Because of the possibility that duloxetine and alcohol may interact to cause hepatic injury or that duloxetine may aggravate preexisting hepatic disease, duloxetine should not ordinarily be prescribed to patients with a history of excessive alcohol consumption or evidence of chronic hepatic disease. Patients and clinicians should be aware of the signs and symptoms of hepatic injury (e.g., pruritus, dark urine, jaundice, right upper quadrant tenderness, unexplained flu-like symptoms), and clinicians should promptly investigate such manifestations in patients receiving the drug.

Orthostatic Hypotension and Syncope. Orthostatic hypotension and syncope reported with therapeutic dosages; although these effects tend to occur within the first week of therapy, they may occur at any time during therapy, particularly following increases in dosage. Risk of decreased blood pressure may be greater in patients concomitantly receiving other drugs that produce orthostatic hypotension (such as antihypertensive agents); in patients receiving potent inhibitors of the cytochrome P-450 (CYP) 1A2 isoenzyme (see Drug Interactions: Drugs Affecting Hepatic Microsomal Enzymes); or in those receiving duloxetine dosages exceeding 60 mg daily. Discontinuance of the drug should be considered in patients experiencing symptomatic orthostatic hypotension and/or syncope during duloxetine therapy.

Serotonin Syndrome. Potentially life-threatening serotonin syndrome reported with selective serotonin- and norepinephrine-reuptake inhibitors (SNRIs), including duloxetine, or selective serotonin-reuptake inhibitors (SSRIs), particularly with concurrent administration of other serotonergic drugs (e.g., serotonin [5-hydroxytryptamine; 5-HT] type 1 receptor agonists ["triptans"]) or drugs that impair serotonin metabolism (e.g., monoamine oxidase [MAO] inhibitors). Symptoms of serotonin syndrome may include mental status changes (e.g., agitation, hallucinations, coma), autonomic instability (e.g., tachycardia, labile blood pressure, hyperthermia), neuromuscular aberrations (e.g., hyperreflexia, incoordination), and/or GI symptoms (e.g., nausea, vomiting, diarrhea).

Concurrent therapy with MAO inhibitors used for treatment of depression is contraindicated. (See Drug Interactions: Monoamine Oxidase Inhibitors.)

If concurrent therapy with duloxetine and a 5-HT_1 receptor agonist is clinically warranted, the patient should be observed carefully, particularly during initiation of therapy, when dosage is increased, or when another serotonergic agent is initiated.

Concomitant use of duloxetine and serotonin precursors (e.g., tryptophan) is not recommended.

Abnormal Bleeding. SSRIs and SNRIs, including duloxetine, may increase the risk of bleeding events. Concurrent administration of aspirin, nonsteroidal anti-inflammatory agents, warfarin, and other anticoagulants may add to this risk. Case reports and epidemiologic studies have demonstrated an association between the use of drugs that interfere with serotonin reuptake and the occurrence of GI bleeding. Bleeding events related to SSRI and SNRI use have ranged from ecchymoses, hematomas, epistaxis, and petechiae to life-threatening hemorrhages. The manufacturer recommends that patients be advised of the risk of bleeding associated with the concomitant use of duloxetine and aspirin or other nonsteroidal anti-inflammatory agents, warfarin, or other drugs that affect coagulation. (See Drug Interactions: Drugs Affecting Hemostasis.)

Withdrawal Effects. Because withdrawal effects (e.g., dysphoric mood, irritability, agitation, nausea/vomiting, dizziness, sensory disturbances, anxiety, confusion, headache, lethargy, emotional lability, insomnia, nightmares, hypomania, tinnitus, seizures) may occur, abrupt discontinuance of duloxetine should be avoided. (See Dosage and Administration: Dosage.)

If intolerable symptoms occur following dosage reduction or discontinuance, reinstitute previously prescribed dosage until symptoms abate, then resume more gradual dosage reductions.

Activation of Mania/Hypomania. Activation of mania and hypomania has occurred in patients with major depressive disorder receiving duloxetine. Use with caution in patients with a history of mania.

Seizures. The risk of seizures associated with duloxetine use has not been systematically evaluated, but seizures have been reported in patients receiving the drug; therefore, use with caution in patients with a history of seizures.

Blood Pressure. May increase blood pressure. Monitor blood pressure prior to and periodically during duloxetine therapy.

Clinically Important Drug Interactions. Because both CYP1A2 and CYP2D6 are responsible for duloxetine metabolism, the potential exists for clinically important drug interactions when duloxetine is concurrently administered with CYP1A2 inhibitors, CYP2D6 inhibitors, and CYP2D6 substrates.

Concurrent therapy with MAO inhibitors used for treatment of depression is contraindicated. (See Serotonin Syndrome under Warnings/Precautions: Other Warnings and Precautions, in Cautions and also see Drug Interactions: Monoamine Oxidase Inhibitors.)

Because of the possibility that duloxetine and alcohol may interact to cause hepatic injury, duloxetine should not ordinarily be prescribed to patients with a history of excessive alcohol consumption or evidence of chronic hepatic disease. (See Hepatic Effects under Warnings/Precautions: Other Warnings and Precautions, in Cautions and also see Drug Interactions: Alcohol.)

Potential pharmacologic interaction when duloxetine is given with or substituted for other centrally acting drugs, including those with a similar mechanism of action; CNS-active drugs should be used with caution in patients receiving duloxetine.

Hyponatremia/Syndrome of Inappropriate Antidiuretic Hormone Secretion. Treatment with SSRIs and SNRIs, including duloxetine, may result in hyponatremia. In many cases, hyponatremia appears to be due to the syndrome of inappropriate antidiuretic hormone secretion (SIADH). Cases with serum sodium concentrations lower than 110 mmol/L have been reported and hyponatremia appeared reversible when duloxetine was discontinued. Geriatric individuals and patients receiving diuretics or who are otherwise volume depleted may be at greater risk of developing hyponatremia. Signs and symptoms of hyponatremia include headache, difficulty concentrating, memory impairment, confusion, weakness, and unsteadiness, which may lead to falls; more severe and/or acute cases have been associated with hallucinations, syncope, seizures, coma, respiratory arrest, and death. Initiate appropriate medical intervention and consider drug discontinuance in patients with symptomatic hyponatremia.

Concomitant Illnesses. Experience with duloxetine in patients with concomitant diseases is limited. (See Hepatic Impairment and see Renal Impairment under Warnings/Precautions: Specific Populations, in Cautions.)

Because alterations in gastric motility may affect the stability of the enteric coating of the pellets contained in duloxetine capsules, the drug should be used with caution in patients with conditions that may slow gastric emptying (e.g., in some patients with diabetes mellitus).

Duloxetine has not been systematically evaluated in patients with a recent history of myocardial infarction or unstable coronary artery disease; such patients were generally excluded from clinical studies. The manufacturer states that duloxetine use was not associated with the development of clinically important ECG abnormalities in controlled clinical studies of up to 13 weeks' duration.

Duloxetine worsens glycemic control in some patients with diabetes. In the 12-week acute treatment phase of 3 clinical studies in patients with diabetic peripheral neuropathy, small increases in fasting blood glucose were observed in the duloxetine-treated patients compared with those receiving placebo. In the extension phase of these studies, which lasted up to 52 weeks, fasting blood glucose increased by 12 mg/dL in the duloxetine-treated patients and decreased by 11.5 mg/dL in the routine care group; increases in glycosylated hemoglobin (hemoglobin A_{1c}) were observed in both groups of patients although the average increase was 0.3% greater in the duloxetine-treated patients compared with those receiving routine care.

Controlled Narrow-Angle Glaucoma. Possible increased risk of mydriasis; use with caution in patients with *controlled* narrow-angle glaucoma. Contraindicated in patients with such glaucoma that is not controlled.

Urinary Hesitation and Retention. Duloxetine belongs to a class of drugs known to affect urethral resistance. If symptoms of urinary hesitation develop during therapy, consider possibility that they may be drug-related. (See Uses: Stress Urinary Incontinence.)

Cases of urinary retention have been reported during postmarketing experience; in some of these cases, hospitalization and/or catheterization has been necessary.

Specific Populations **Pregnancy.** Category C. (See Users Guide.)

Some neonates exposed to selective serotonin- and norepinephrine-reuptake inhibitors (SNRIs) or selective serotonin-reuptake inhibitors late in the third trimester of pregnancy have developed complications that have sometimes been severe and required prolonged hospitalization, respiratory support, enteral nutrition, and other forms of supportive care in special-care nurseries. Such complications can arise immediately upon delivery and usually last several days or up to 2–4 weeks. Clinical findings reported to date in the neonates have included respiratory distress, cyanosis, apnea, seizures, temperature instability or fever, feeding difficulty, dehydration, excessive weight loss, vomiting, hypoglycemia, hypotonia, hyperreflexia, tremor, jitteriness, irritability, lethargy, reduced or lack of reaction to pain stimuli, and constant crying. These clinical features appear to be consistent with either a direct toxic effect of the SNRI or selective serotonin-reuptake inhibitor or, possibly, a drug withdrawal syndrome. It should be noted that, in some cases, the clinical picture was consistent with serotonin syndrome (see Drug Interactions: Drugs Associated with Serotonin Syndrome, in Fluoxetine Hydrochloride 28:16.04.20). When treating a pregnant woman with duloxetine during the third trimester of pregnancy, the clinician should carefully consider the potential risks and benefits of such therapy. Consideration may be given to cautiously tapering duloxetine therapy in the third trimester prior to delivery if the drug is administered during pregnancy. (See Treatment of Pregnant Women during the Third Trimester under Dosage and Administration: Special Populations.)

Lactation. Duloxetine is distributed into human milk. At steady state, concentrations in breast milk are approximately one-fourth the maternal plasma concentrations. Because the safety of duloxetine in infants is not known, use in nursing women is not recommended. However, if the clinician determines that the potential benefits of duloxetine therapy for the mother outweigh the potential risks to the infant, dosage adjustment is not required since lactation does not affect pharmacokinetics.

Pediatric Use. Safety and efficacy of duloxetine in children younger than 18 years of age have not been established.

FDA warns that a greater risk of suicidal thinking or behavior (suicidality) occurred during first few months of antidepressant treatment (4%) compared with placebo (2%) in children and adolescents with major depressive disorder, obsessive-compulsive disorder (OCD), or other psychiatric disorders based on pooled analyses of 24 short-term, placebo-controlled trials of 9 antidepressant drugs (selective serotonin-reuptake inhibitors [SSRIs] and other antidepressants). However, a more recent meta-analysis of 27 placebo-controlled trials of 9 antidepressants (SSRIs and others) in patients younger than 19 years of age with major depressive disorder, OCD, or non-OCD anxiety disorders suggests that the benefits of antidepressant therapy in treating these conditions may outweigh the risks of suicidal behavior or suicidal ideation. No suicides occurred in these pediatric trials.

Carefully consider these findings when assessing potential benefits and risks of duloxetine in a child or adolescent for any clinical use. (See Worsening of Depression and Suicidality Risk under Warnings/Precautions: Warnings, in Cautions.)

Geriatric Use. Approximately 5.9, 33, and 7.9% of patients studied in clinical trials of duloxetine for major depressive disorder, diabetic peripheral neuropathy, and fibromyalgia, respectively, were 65 years of age or older. The generalized anxiety disorder clinical trials did not include sufficient numbers of patients 65 years of age or older to determine whether they respond differently than younger adults. Although no overall differences in efficacy or safety were observed between geriatric and younger patients in the major depressive disorder, diabetic peripheral neuropathic pain, and fibromyalgia clinical trials and other clinical experience has not revealed any evidence of age-related differences, the possibility that some older patients may exhibit increased sensitivity to the drug cannot be ruled out.

Clinically important hyponatremia has been reported in geriatric patients, who may be at greater risk for this adverse effect. (See Hyponatremia/Syndrome of Inappropriate Antidiuretic Hormone Secretion under Warnings/Precautions: Other Warnings and Precautions, in Cautions.)

In pooled data analyses, a *reduced* risk of suicidality was observed in adults 65 years of age or older with antidepressant therapy compared with placebo. (See Worsening of Depression and Suicidality Risk under Warnings/Precautions: Other Warnings and Precautions, in Cautions.)

Hepatic Impairment. Substantially increased exposure to duloxetine; use is not recommended in patients with hepatic insufficiency or with substantial alcohol use. (See Hepatic Effects under Warnings/Precautions: Other Warnings and Precautions, in Cautions.)

Renal Impairment. Increased plasma concentrations of duloxetine and its metabolites; use is not recommended in patients with end-stage renal disease (requiring dialysis) or severe renal impairment (creatinine clearance less than 30 mL/minute).

Population pharmacokinetic analyses suggest that mild to moderate renal impairment has no clinically important effect on duloxetine apparent clearance.

■ **Common Adverse Effects** Adverse effects reported in 5% or more of patients with major depressive disorder receiving duloxetine and at an incidence at least twice that reported with placebo include nausea, dry mouth, constipation, decreased appetite, fatigue, somnolence, and increased sweating.

Adverse effects reported in 5% or more of patients with generalized anxiety disorder receiving duloxetine and at an incidence at least twice that reported with placebo include nausea, fatigue, dry mouth, somnolence, constipation, insomnia, decreased appetite, vomiting, hyperhidrosis, decreased libido, delayed ejaculation, and erectile dysfunction.

Adverse effects reported in 5% or more of patients with diabetic peripheral neuropathy receiving duloxetine and at an incidence at least twice that reported with placebo include nausea, somnolence, dizziness, dry mouth, constipation, hyperhidrosis, decreased appetite, and asthenia.

Adverse effects reported in 5% or more of patients with fibromyalgia receiving duloxetine and at an incidence at least twice that reported with placebo include nausea, dry mouth, constipation, decreased appetite, somnolence, agitation, and hyperhidrosis.

Drug Interactions

■ **Drugs Metabolized by Hepatic Microsomal Enzymes** Substrates of cytochrome P-450 (CYP) 2D6 isoenzyme (e.g., tricyclic antidepressants [TCAs; amitriptyline, desipramine, imipramine, nortriptyline], phenothiazines, class IC antiarrhythmics [flecainide, propafenone]): potential pharmacokinetic (increased AUC of the substrate) interactions. Use with caution. Consider monitoring plasma TCA concentrations and reducing the TCA dosage if a TCA is administered concurrently with duloxetine.

Substrates of CYP1A2, CYP3A, CYP2C9, or CYP2C19 isoenzymes: clinically important pharmacokinetic interaction generally is considered unlikely.

■ **Drugs Affecting Hepatic Microsomal Enzymes** Potent inhibitors of CYP1A2 (e.g., fluvoxamine, some quinolone anti-infective agents [e.g., ciprofloxacin, enoxacin]): potential pharmacokinetic (increased plasma duloxetine concentrations) interaction. Avoid concomitant use.

Potent inhibitors of CYP2D6 (e.g., fluoxetine, paroxetine, quinidine) isoenzymes: potential pharmacokinetic interaction (increased plasma duloxetine concentrations).

Concomitant administration of duloxetine and fluvoxamine, a potent CYP1A2 inhibitor, in poor CYP2D6 metabolizers resulted in a sixfold increase in duloxetine area under the plasma concentration-time curve (AUC) and peak plasma concentrations.

■ **Drugs Affecting Hemostasis** Altered anticoagulant effects, including increased bleeding, have been reported when selective serotonin-reuptake inhibitors (SSRIs) or selective serotonin- and norepinephrine-reuptake inhibitors (SNRIs), including duloxetine, were concurrently administered with warfarin or other anticoagulants. The manufacturer recommends carefully monitoring patients receiving warfarin during initiation and discontinuance of duloxetine therapy.

Potential pharmacologic (increased risk of bleeding) interaction with aspirin or other nonsteroidal anti-inflammatory agents; use with caution.

■ **Drugs that Affect Gastric Acidity** Theoretical risk of altered duloxetine bioavailability if administered with drugs that increase gastric pH. However, no clinically important effect was demonstrated when duloxetine was administered with aluminum- and magnesium-containing antacids or famotidine.

Whether the concomitant administration of proton-pump inhibitors affects duloxetine absorption is currently unknown.

■ **Alcohol** Potential pharmacologic (increased risk of hepatotoxicity) interaction; avoid concomitant use in patients with substantial alcohol use. (See Hepatic Effects under Warnings/Precautions: Other Warnings and Precautions, in Cautions.)

Duloxetine has not been shown to potentiate the impairment of mental and motor skills caused by alcohol.

■ **Antihypertensive Agents** Potential pharmacologic (increased risk of hypotension and syncope) interaction.

■ **Benzodiazepines** Lorazepam does not appear to affect the pharmacokinetics of duloxetine.

Temazepam does not appear to affect the pharmacokinetics of duloxetine.

■ **CNS-active Drugs** Potential pharmacologic interaction when given with or substituted for other centrally acting drugs, including those with a similar mechanism of action; use with caution.

■ **5-HT$_1$ Receptor Agonists ("Triptans")** Pharmacologic interaction (potentially life-threatening serotonin syndrome) if used concurrently with 5-HT$_1$ receptor agonists (e.g., almotriptan, eletriptan, frovatriptan, naratriptan, rizatriptan, sumatriptan, zolmitriptan). If concomitant use is clinically warranted, the patient should be observed carefully, particularly during treatment initiation, when dosage is increased, or when another serotonergic agent is initiated. (See Serotonin Syndrome under Warnings/Precautions:Other Warnings and Precautions, in Cautions.)

■ **Monoamine Oxidase (MAO) Inhibitors** Pharmacologic interaction (potentially fatal serotonin syndrome); concomitant use is contraindicated. The manufacturer recommends that at least 2 weeks should elapse between discontinuance of an MAO inhibitor and initiation of duloxetine and that at least 5 days elapse between discontinuance of duloxetine therapy and initiation of MAO inhibitor therapy. (See Serotonin Syndrome under Warnings/Precautions:Other Warnings and Precautions, in Cautions.)

■ **Selective Serotonin-reuptake Inhibitors and Selective Serotonin- and Norepinephrine-reuptake Inhibitors** Potential pharmacologic interaction (potentially life-threatening serotonin syndrome); concurrent administration not recommended. (See Serotonin Syndrome under Warnings/Precautions:Other Warnings and Precautions, in Cautions.)

Concomitant administration of duloxetine and fluvoxamine, a potent CYP1A2 inhibitor, in poor CYP2D6 metabolizers resulted in a six-fold increase in duloxetine AUCs and peak plasma concentrations.

■ **Serotonergic Drugs** Potential pharmacologic interaction (potentially life-threatening serotonin syndrome) with drugs affecting serotonergic neurotransmission, including linezolid (an anti-infective agent that is a nonselective, reversible MAO inhibitor), lithium, tramadol, and St. John's wort *(Hypericum perforatum)*; use with caution. Concurrent administration of serotonin precursors (such as tryptophan) is not recommended. (See Serotonin Syndrome under Warnings/Precautions: Other Warnings and Precautions, in Cautions.)

■ **Smoking** Potential pharmacokinetic interaction (reduced duloxetine bioavailability and plasma concentrations). The manufacturer states that routine dosage adjustment is not necessary. However, some clinicians recommend a small increase in duloxetine dosage (about 15%) in patients who smoke.

■ **Theophylline** Although small increases (averaging from 7–20%) in theophylline AUCs have been reported during concurrent administration of theophylline and duloxetine, combined use of these drugs reportedly has been well tolerated and routine theophylline dosage adjustment does not appear to be necessary during concomitant administration.

■ **Thioridazine** Potential pharmacokinetic (increased plasma thioridazine concentrations) interaction with resulting increased risk of serious ventricular arrhythmias and sudden death; concomitant use is not recommended by manufacturer of duloxetine.

Description

Duloxetine hydrochloride, a selective serotonin- and norepinephrine-reuptake inhibitor (SNRI), is an antidepressant and anxiolytic agent. The drug also has demonstrated analgesic activity in animal models of chronic and persistent pain and in clinical trials evaluating the drug's activity in conditions associated with chronic pain (e.g., neuropathic pain, fibromyalgia). Duloxetine hydrochloride is pharmacologically related to venlafaxine hydrochloride and desvenlafaxine succinate.

The exact mechanisms of the antidepressant, anxiolytic, and central pain inhibitory actions of duloxetine have not been fully elucidated, but appear to be associated with the drug's potentiation of serotonergic and noradrenergic activity in the CNS. Like venlafaxine and desvenlafaxine, duloxetine is a potent inhibitor of neuronal serotonin and norepinephrine reuptake and a less potent inhibitor of dopamine reuptake. Duloxetine does not inhibit monoamine oxidase (MAO) and has not demonstrated significant affinity for dopaminergic, adrenergic, cholinergic, γ-aminobutyric acid (GABA), glutamate, histaminergic, and opiate receptors in vitro.

Although the precise mechanism of action of duloxetine in stress urinary incontinence is unknown, it is thought to be related to potentiation of serotonin and norepinephrine activity in the sacral spinal cord, which increases urethral closure forces and thereby reduces involuntary urine loss.

Duloxetine is extensively metabolized in the liver, principally via oxidation by the cytochrome P-450 (CYP) 2D6 and 1A2 isoenzymes. Duloxetine is a moderate inhibitor of CYP2D6 and a somewhat weak inhibitor of CYP1A2. The drug is not an inhibitor of CYP2C9, CYP2C19, or CYP3A, nor is it an inducer of CYP1A2 or CYP3A.

Advice to Patients

Risk of suicidality; importance of patients, family, and caregivers being alert to and immediately reporting emergence of suicidality, worsening depression, or unusual changes in behavior, especially during the first few months of therapy or during periods of dosage adjustment. FDA recommends providing written patient information (medication guide) explaining risks of suicidality each time the drug is dispensed.

Importance of promptly reporting any manifestations of liver dysfunction (e.g., pruritus, dark urine, jaundice, right upper quadrant tenderness, unexplained flu-like symptoms) to clinician.

Importance of informing patient of risk of severe liver injury associated with concomitant use of duloxetine and heavy alcohol intake. (See Hepatic Effects under Warnings/Precautions: Other Warnings and Precautions and also see Drug Interactions: Alcohol.)

Risk of psychomotor impairment; importance of exercising caution while operating hazardous machinery, including automobile driving, until patient gains experience with the drug's effects.

Importance of advising patients of risk of orthostatic hypotension and syncope, particularly during initial therapy and subsequent dosage escalation and during concomitant therapy with drugs that may potentiate the orthostatic effect of duloxetine.

Importance of informing patients of risk of serotonin syndrome with concurrent use of duloxetine and 5-HT_1 receptor agonists (also called triptans), tramadol, or other serotonergic agents. Importance of seeking immediate medical attention if symptoms of serotonin syndrome develop.

Importance of taking medication exactly as prescribed by the clinician. Importance of informing patients that the delayed-release capsules should be swallowed whole and should not be chewed or crushed, nor should the capsule contents be sprinkled on food or mixed with liquids.

Importance of continuing duloxetine therapy even if a response is not evident within 1–4 weeks, unless directed otherwise.

Importance of women informing clinicians if they are or plan to become pregnant or plan to breast-feed.

Importance of informing clinicians of existing or contemplated concomitant therapy, including prescription and OTC drugs, as well as any concomitant illnesses (e.g., bipolar disorder, liver disease) or family history of suicidality or bipolar disorder. Risk of bleeding associated with concomitant use of duloxetine with aspirin or other nonsteroidal anti-inflammatory agents, warfarin, or other drugs that affect coagulation.

Importance of informing patients of other important precautionary information. (See Cautions.)

Overview® (see Users Guide). For additional information on this drug until a more detailed monograph is developed and published, the manufacturer's labeling should be consulted. It is *essential* that the manufacturer's labeling be consulted for more detailed information on usual cautions, precautions, contraindications, potential drug interactions, laboratory test interferences, and acute toxicity.

Preparations

Excipients in commercially available drug preparations may have clinically important effects in some individuals; consult specific product labeling for details.

DULoxetine Hydrochloride

Oral		
Capsules, delayed-release (containing enteric-coated pellets)	20 mg (of duloxetine)	**Cymbalta®**, Lilly
	30 mg (of duloxetine)	**Cymbalta®**, Lilly
	60 mg (of duloxetine)	**Cymbalta®**, Lilly

†Use is not currently included in the labeling approved by the US Food and Drug Administration

Levomilnacipran Hydrochloride

1*S*,2*R*-Milnacipran

■ Levomilnacipran hydrochloride, the 1*S*,2*R*-enantiomer of racemic milnacipran hydrochloride, is a selective serotonin- and norepinephrine-reuptake inhibitor (SNRI) and an antidepressant.

Uses

■ **Major Depressive Disorder** Levomilnacipran hydrochloride is used for the treatment of major depressive disorder in adults. The short-term antidepressant efficacy of levomilnacipran was mainly established in 3 multicenter, randomized, double-blind, placebo-controlled studies of 8 weeks' duration in 1709 adult outpatients who met DSM-IV-TR criteria for major depressive disorder. Two of the studies compared multiple fixed doses of levomilnacipran and the third was flexible dose in design. In all 3 of these studies, levomilnacipran (40–120 mg once daily given as extended-release capsules) was found to be more effective than placebo in improving depressive symptoms as measured by the mean change from baseline to week 8 on the Montgomery-Asberg Depression Rating Scale (MADRS) total score (the primary efficacy end point). Levomilnacipran was also found to be more effective than placebo in improving the Sheehan Disability Scale (SDS) functional impairment total score (the secondary efficacy end point) in these studies. In the flexible-dose study, 21, 34, and 44% of the levomilnacipran-treated patients were receiving 40, 80, or 120 mg once daily of the drug, respectively, at the end of the treatment; the mean daily dosage was approximately 73 mg. No age-, race-, or gender-related differences in efficacy were noted in these studies.

In a long-term (24-week), double-blind relapse prevention study comparing fixed-dose extended-release levomilnacipran (40, 80, or 120 mg daily) with placebo in 345 adults with major depressive disorder, the relapse rate for levomilnacipran (14%) was lower than that for placebo (21%), but the difference did not achieve statistical significance (possibly because of lower than predicted relapse rates). In a longer-term (48-week), multicenter, open-label, flexible-dose study, extended-release levomilnacipran (40–120 mg daily) was found to be generally well tolerated in adults with major depressive disorder. Most of the adverse effects were mild or moderate in severity and similar to those reported in the short-term studies; in addition, levomilnacipran did not appear to be associated with weight gain during long-term use.

The manufacturer states that the efficacy of levomilnacipran for long-term use (i.e., exceeding 8 weeks) has not been established. If the drug is used for extended periods, the need for continued therapy and the appropriate dosage should be reassessed periodically.

The American Psychiatric Association (APA) states that the effectiveness of antidepressants in the treatment of major depressive disorder is generally comparable between and within classes of these medications, including selective serotonin-reuptake inhibitors (SSRIs), serotonin- and norepinephrine-reuptake inhibitors (SNRIs), tricyclic antidepressants, monoamine oxidase (MAO) inhibitors, and other antidepressants (e.g., bupropion, mirtazapine, trazodone). Therefore, the initial selection of an antidepressant can be based mainly on the following factors: patient preference; nature of prior response to medication; safety, tolerability, and anticipated adverse effects; concurrent psychiatric and medical conditions; specific properties of the medication (e.g., half-life, actions on cytochrome P-450 [CYP] isoenzymes, other drug interactions); and cost. For most patients, an SSRI, SNRI, mirtazapine, or bupropion is considered optimal based on these considerations. Clinicians may consult APA's Practice Guidelines for the Treatment of Patients with Major Depressive Disorder (at http://www.psychiatryonline.com/pracGuide/pracGuideTopic_7.aspx) for additional information.

■ **Fibromyalgia** Levomilnacipran is the more active 1*S*,2*R*-enantiomer of racemic milnacipran (Savella®), which is labeled by the US Food and Drug Administration (FDA) for the management of fibromyalgia. (See Description.) However, the manufacturer states that levomilnacipran (Fetzima®) is not approved for the management of fibromyalgia†, and that the efficacy and safety of the drug for the management of this condition have not been established.

Dosage and Administration

■ **Administration** Levomilnacipran hydrochloride is commercially available as extended-release capsules, which are administered orally once daily, with or without food, at approximately the same time each day. Extended-release capsules of the drug should be swallowed whole and should *not* be opened, chewed, cut, or crushed.

Patients receiving levomilnacipran should be monitored for possible worsening of depression, suicidality, or unusual changes in behavior, especially at the beginning of therapy or during periods of dosage adjustment. (See Worsening of Depression and Suicidality Risk under Warnings/Precautions: Warnings, in Cautions.)

The manufacturer states that at least 2 weeks must elapse between discontinuance of a monoamine oxidase (MAO) inhibitor intended to treat psychiatric disorders and initiation of levomilnacipran therapy and that at least 7 days should elapse between discontinuance of levomilnacipran and initiation of MAO inhibitor therapy. (See Contraindications, Serotonin Syndrome under Warnings/Precautions: Other Warnings and Precautions, in Cautions, and Drug Interactions: Monoamine Oxidase Inhibitors.)

■ **Dosage** Dosage of levomilnacipran hydrochloride is expressed in terms of levomilnacipran.

Major Depressive Disorder For the management of major depressive disorder in adults, the recommended initial dosage of levomilnacipran is 20 mg once daily for 2 days, followed by an increase to 40 mg once daily. Depending on efficacy and tolerability, the daily dosage of levomilnacipran may be increased in increments of 40 mg at intervals of 2 or more days. The maximum recommended dosage of the drug is 120 mg once daily. In a short-term, flexible-dose clinical study of levomilnacipran in major depressive disorder, 21, 34, and 44% of the patients were receiving 40, 80, or 120 mg of the drug once daily, respectively, at the end of the treatment; the mean daily dosage was approximately 73 mg. A titration pack of levomilnacipran hydrochloride (Fetzima®) capsules is commercially available for the initial 1-month dosage titration period.

The dosage of levomilnacipran should not exceed 80 mg once daily when used concurrently with potent CYP3A4 inhibitors (e.g., clarithromycin, ketoconazole, ritonavir). (See Drug Interactions: Drugs Affecting Hepatic Microsomal Enzymes.)

While the optimum duration of levomilnacipran therapy has not been established, it generally is agreed that acute depressive episodes require several months or longer of sustained antidepressant therapy. In addition, some clinicians recommend that long-term antidepressant therapy be considered in certain patients at risk for recurrence of depressive episodes (such as those with chronic and recurrent major depressive disorder). The manufacturer states that the efficacy of levomilnacipran for long-term use (i.e., exceeding 8 weeks) has not been established. If levomilnacipran is used for extended periods, the need for continued maintenance therapy and the appropriate dosage of the drug should be reassessed periodically.

Discontinuance of Therapy Because withdrawal effects may occur with discontinuance of serotonergic drugs such as levomilnacipran, abrupt discontinuance should be avoided whenever possible. When levomilnacipran therapy is discontinued, the dosage should be reduced gradually and the patient monitored for possible withdrawal symptoms. If intolerable symptoms occur following dosage reduction or upon discontinuance of therapy, reinstitution of levomilnacipran therapy at the previously prescribed dosage may be considered until symptoms abate. The clinician may resume dosage reduction at that time, but at a more gradual rate. (See Withdrawal of Therapy under Warnings/Precautions: Other Warnings and Precautions, in Cautions.)

■ **Special Populations** Dosage adjustment is not necessary in patients with mild renal impairment (creatinine clearance of 60–89 mL/minute). In patients with moderate renal impairment (creatinine clearance of 30–59 mL/minute), the maintenance dosage of levomilnacipran should not exceed 80 mg once daily. In patients with severe renal impairment (creatinine clearance of 15–29 mL/minute), the maintenance dosage should not exceed 40 mg once daily. Levomilnacipran is *not* recommended for use in patients with end-stage renal disease.

Dosage adjustment is not necessary in patients with mild (Child-Pugh score of 1–6), moderate (Child-Pugh score of 7–9), or severe (Child-Pugh score of 10–13) hepatic impairment.

Routine dosage adjustment is not necessary in geriatric patients; however, the renal clearance of levomilnacipran should be considered when determining the dosage in such patients. (See Geriatric Use under Warnings/Precautions: Specific Populations, in Cautions.)

Dosage adjustment based on gender is not recommended.

Cautions

■ **Contraindications** Known hypersensitivity to levomilnacipran hydrochloride, milnacipran hydrochloride, or any ingredient in the formulation.

Concurrent or recent (i.e., within 2 weeks) therapy with a monoamine oxidase (MAO) inhibitor intended to treat psychiatric disorders. Use of an MAO inhibitor intended to treat psychiatric disorders within 7 days of levomilnacipran discontinuance. (See Serotonin Syndrome under Warnings/Precautions: Other Warnings and Precautions, in Cautionsand also see Drug Interactions: Monoamine Oxidase Inhibitors.)

Initiation of levomilnacipran therapy in patients receiving MAO inhibitors such as linezolid or IV methylene blue. (See Drug Interactions: Linezolid and also see Drug Interactions: Methylene Blue.)

■ **Warnings/Precautions** ***Warnings*** **Worsening of Depression and Suicidality Risk.** Worsening of depression and/or the emergence of suicidal ideation and behavior (suicidality) or unusual changes in behavior may occur in both adult and pediatric (see Pediatric Use under Warnings/Precautions: Specific Populations, in Cautions) patients with major depressive disorder or other psychiatric disorders, whether or not they are taking antidepressants. This risk may persist until clinically important remission occurs. Suicide is a known risk of depression and certain other psychiatric disorders, and these disorders themselves are the strongest predictors of suicide. However, there has been a long-standing concern that antidepressants may have a role in inducing worsening of depression and the emergence of suicidality in certain patients during the early phases of treatment. Pooled analyses of short-term, placebo-controlled studies of antidepressants (i.e., selective serotonin-reuptake inhibitors [SSRIs] and other antidepressants) have shown an increased risk of suicidality in children, adolescents, and young adults (18–24 years of age) with major depressive disorder and other psychiatric disorders. An increased suicidality risk was not demonstrated with antidepressants compared with placebo in adults older than 24 years of age, and a reduced risk was observed in adults 65 years of age or older.

The US Food and Drug Administration (FDA) recommends that all patients being treated with antidepressants for any indication be appropriately monitored and closely observed for clinical worsening, suicidality, and unusual changes in behavior, particularly during initiation of therapy (i.e., the first few months) and during periods of dosage adjustments. Families and caregivers of patients being treated with antidepressants for major depressive disorder or other indications, both psychiatric and nonpsychiatric, also should be advised to monitor patients on a daily basis for the emergence of agitation, irritability, or unusual changes in behavior as well as the emergence of suicidality, and to report such symptoms immediately to a health-care provider.

Although a causal relationship between the emergence of symptoms such as anxiety, agitation, panic attacks, insomnia, irritability, hostility, aggressiveness, impulsivity, akathisia, hypomania, and/or mania and either the worsening of depression and/or the emergence of suicidal impulses has not been established, there is concern that such symptoms may represent precursors to emerging suicidality. Consequently, consideration should be given to changing the therapeutic regimen or discontinuing therapy in patients whose depression is persistently worse or in patients experiencing emergent suicidality or symptoms that might be precursors to worsening depression or suicidality, particularly if such manifestations are severe, abrupt in onset, or were not part of the patient's presenting symptoms. If a decision is made to discontinue therapy, levomilnacipran dosage should be tapered as rapidly as is feasible but consideration should be given to the risks of abrupt discontinuance. FDA also recommends that the drugs be prescribed in the smallest quantity consistent with good patient management, in order to reduce the risk of overdosage.

Other Warnings and Precautions **Serotonin Syndrome.** Potentially life-threatening serotonin syndrome has been reported with SSRIs and SNRIs alone, but particularly with concurrent use of other serotonergic drugs (including serotonin [5-hydroxytryptamine; 5-HT] type 1 receptor agonists ["triptans"], tricyclic antidepressants, buspirone, fentanyl, lithium, tramadol, tryptophan, and St. John's wort [*Hypericum perforatum*]) and with drugs that impair the metabolism of serotonin (particularly MAO inhibitors, both those used to treat psychiatric disorders and others, such as linezolid and methylene blue). Manifestations of serotonin syndrome may include mental status changes (e.g., agitation, hallucinations, delirium, coma), autonomic instability (e.g., tachycardia, labile blood pressure, dizziness, diaphoresis, flushing, hyperthermia), neuromuscular symptoms (e.g., tremor, rigidity, myoclonus, hyperreflexia, incoordination), seizures, and/or GI symptoms (e.g., nausea, vomiting, diarrhea). Patients receiving levomilnacipran should be monitored for the development of serotonin syndrome.

Concurrent or recent (i.e., within 2 weeks) therapy with MAO inhibitors intended to treat psychiatric disorders is contraindicated. (See Contraindications and also see Drug Interactions: Monoamine Oxidase Inhibitors.) Levomilnacipran also should not be initiated in patients who are being treated with other MAO inhibitors such as linezolid or IV methylene blue. (See Drug Interactions: Linezolid and also see Drug Interactions: Methylene Blue.)

If concurrent therapy with levomilnacipran and other serotonergic drugs is clinically warranted, the patient should be made aware of the potential increased risk for serotonin syndrome, particularly during initiation of therapy or when dosage is increased. (See Drug Interactions.)

If manifestations of serotonin syndrome occur, treatment with levomilnacipran and any concurrently administered serotonergic agents should be immediately discontinued and supportive and symptomatic treatment initiated.

For further information on serotonin syndrome, including manifestations and treatment, see Drug Interactions: Serotonergic Drugs, in Fluoxetine Hydrochloride 28:16.04.20.

Elevated Blood Pressure. SNRIs, including levomilnacipran, have been associated with increases in blood pressure. In short-term controlled studies, mean increases in systolic and diastolic blood pressure from initiation of treatment to end of treatment were 3 and 3.2 mm Hg, respectively, in levomilnacipran-treated patients compared with no change in the placebo group. In patients receiving long-term (1 year), open-label treatment with levomilnacipran (40–120 mg once daily), the mean increase from initiation of treatment in systolic blood pressure was 3.9 mm Hg and diastolic blood pressure was 3.1 mm Hg.

In short-term, placebo-controlled studies, 11.6% of patients receiving levomilnacipran met orthostatic hypotension criteria (systolic or diastolic blood pressure) compared with 9.7% of patients receiving placebo. Orthostatic reductions in diastolic blood pressure of 10 mm Hg or greater occurred in 5.8, 6.1, and 9.8% of patients receiving 40, 80, and 120 mg daily of levomilnacipran, respectively, compared with 6.2% of those receiving placebo.

Concurrent use of levomilnacipran with other drugs that increase blood pressure and heart rate has not been evaluated, and the manufacturer recommends that such combinations be used with caution. (See Drug Interactions: Drugs that Increase Blood Pressure and Heart Rate.)

Effects of levomilnacipran on blood pressure in patients with clinically important hypertension or cardiovascular disease have not been systematically evaluated; the drug should be used with caution in such patients.

The manufacturer states that preexisting hypertension should be controlled before initiating levomilnacipran therapy. In addition, blood pressure should be measured prior to initiating levomilnacipran and then monitored periodically throughout treatment. Caution should be used in treating patients with preexisting hypertension, cardiovascular conditions, or cerebrovascular conditions that might be compromised by increases in blood pressure.

Drug discontinuance or other appropriate medical intervention should be considered in patients who experience a sustained increase in blood pressure during levomilnacipran therapy.

Elevated Heart Rate. SNRIs, including levomilnacipran, have been associated with increases in heart rate. In short-term clinical trials, levomilnacipran was associated with a mean increase in heart rate of 7.4 beats per minute compared with a mean decrease of 0.3 beats per minute with placebo. The heart rate increase was 7.2, 7.2, and 9.1 beats per minute in patients receiving 40, 80, and 120 mg of levomilnacipran daily, respectively.

Concurrent use of levomilnacipran with other drugs that increase blood pressure and heart rate has not been evaluated, and the manufacturer recommends that such combinations be used with caution. (See Drug Interactions: Drugs that Increase Blood Pressure and Heart Rate.)

Levomilnacipran has not been systematically evaluated in patients with cardiac rhythm disorders.

The manufacturer states that preexisting tachyarrhythmias and other cardiovascular disease should be treated before initiating levomilnacipran therapy. In addition, heart rate should be measured prior to initiating levomilnacipran and periodically during therapy with the drug.

Drug discontinuance or other appropriate medical intervention should be considered in patients who experience a sustained increase in heart rate during levomilnacipran therapy.

Abnormal Bleeding. SNRIs and SSRIs, including levomilnacipran, may increase the risk of bleeding events. Concurrent use of aspirin, nonsteroidal anti-inflammatory agents (NSAIAs), warfarin, and other anticoagulants may add to this risk. Case reports and epidemiologic studies have demonstrated an association between the use of drugs that interfere with serotonin reuptake and the occurrence of GI bleeding. Bleeding events related to SNRI and SSRI use have ranged from ecchymoses, hematomas, epistaxis, and petechiae to life-threatening hemorrhages. The manufacturer recommends that patients be advised of the risk of bleeding associated with the concomitant use of levomilnacipran and aspirin or other NSAIAs, warfarin, or other drugs that affect coagulation. (See Drug Interactions: Drugs Affecting Hemostasis.)

Angle-closure Glaucoma. The pupillary dilation (mydriasis) that occurs following the use of many antidepressant agents, including levomilnacipran, may trigger an acute attack of angle-closure glaucoma (narrow-angle glaucoma) in patients with anatomically narrow angles who do not have a patent iridectomy. (See Advice to Patients.)

Urinary Hesitation and Retention. Because of their noradrenergic effect, SNRIs, including levomilnacipran, may affect urethral resistance. In controlled short-term trials, urinary hesitation occurred in 4, 5, and 6% of patients receiving levomilnacipran daily dosages of 40, 80, and 120 mg, respectively, compared with none of those receiving placebo.

The manufacturer recommends exercising caution if levomilnacipran is used in patients prone to obstructive urinary disorders. If a patient develops symptoms of urinary hesitation, urinary retention, or dysuria during levomilnacipran therapy, the possibility that such effects might be drug-related should be considered; in such cases, discontinuance of the drug or other appropriate medical intervention should be considered.

Activation of Mania/Hypomania. Symptoms of mania or hypomania were reported in 0.2% of patients receiving levomilnacipran and in 0.2% of patients receiving placebo in clinical studies. Activation of mania and hypomania also have been reported in a small proportion of patients with mood disorders who were treated with other antidepressants. Levomilnacipran should therefore be used with caution in patients with a personal or family history of bipolar disorder, mania, or hypomania.

Seizures. Levomilnacipran has not been systematically evaluated in patients with seizure disorders; patients with a history of seizures were excluded from clinical trials. One case of seizure has been reported during premarketing clinical trials with the drug. Levomilnacipran therapy should be used with caution in patients with a history of a seizure disorder.

Withdrawal of Therapy. Adverse effects have been reported following discontinuance of serotonergic antidepressants, particularly when discontinuance was abrupt. These withdrawal effects include dysphoric mood, irritability, agitation, dizziness, sensory disturbances (e.g., paresthesias, such as electric shock sensations), anxiety, confusion, headache, lethargy, emotional lability, insomnia, hypomania, tinnitus, and seizures. While these events generally are self-limiting, there have been serious discontinuance symptoms.

Patients should be monitored for possible withdrawal symptoms when discontinuing levomilnacipran therapy. A gradual reduction in dosage rather than abrupt cessation is recommended whenever possible. If intolerable symptoms occur following dosage reduction or discontinuance of levomilnacipran, the previously prescribed dosage should be reinstituted until symptoms abate; dosage reductions may then be resumed at a more gradual rate. (See Dosage and Administration: Dosage.)

Hyponatremia/Syndrome of Inappropriate Antidiuretic Hormone Secretion. Although no cases of hyponatremia were reported in levomilnacipran-treated patients in the main clinical trials, treatment with SSRIs and SNRIs may result in hyponatremia. In many cases, hyponatremia appears to be due to the syndrome of inappropriate antidiuretic hormone secretion (SIADH). Cases with serum sodium concentrations lower than 110 mmol/L have been reported. Geriatric individuals and patients receiving diuretics or who are otherwise volume depleted may be at greater risk of developing hyponatremia. Signs and symptoms of hyponatremia include headache, difficulty concentrating, memory impairment, confusion, weakness, and unsteadiness, which may lead to falls; more severe and/or acute cases have been associated with hallucinations, syncope, seizures, coma, respiratory arrest, and death. Levomilnacipran should be discontinued and appropriate medical intervention should be instituted in patients with symptomatic hyponatremia.

Specific Populations **Pregnancy.** Category C. (See Users Guide.)

Some neonates exposed to SNRIs or SSRIs late in the third trimester of pregnancy have developed complications, which have sometimes been severe and required prolonged hospitalization, respiratory support, enteral nutrition, and other forms of supportive care in special-care nurseries. Such complications may arise immediately upon delivery and usually last several days or up to 2–4 weeks. Clinical findings reported to date in the neonates have included respiratory distress, cyanosis, apnea, seizures, temperature instability or fever, feeding difficulty, dehydration, excessive weight loss, vomiting, hypoglycemia, hypotonia, hypertonia, hyperreflexia, tremor, jitteriness, irritability, lethargy, reduced or lack of reaction to pain stimuli, and constant crying. These clinical features appear to be consistent with either a direct toxic effect of these classes of drugs or, possibly, a drug withdrawal syndrome. In some cases, the clinical picture was consistent with serotonin syndrome (see Serotonin Syndrome under Warnings/Precautions: Other Warnings and Precautions, in Cautions).

For additional information on the management of depression in women prior to conception and during pregnancy, including treatment algorithms, clinicians may consult the joint American Psychiatric Association and American College of Obstetricians and Gynecologists guidelines (at https://www.ncbi.nlm.nih.gov/pmc/articles/PMC3103063/pdf/nihms293836.pdf).

Lactation. It is not known whether levomilnacipran is distributed into human milk. Levomilnacipran is distributed into milk in rats. Because of the potential for serious adverse reactions to levomilnacipran in nursing infants, a decision should be made whether to discontinue the drug, taking into account the importance of the drug to the woman.

Pediatric Use. Clinical studies of levomilnacipran in pediatric patients have not been conducted; therefore, the safety and effectiveness of the drug in pediatric patients have not been established.

FDA warns that a greater risk of suicidal thinking or behavior (suicidality) occurred during the first few months of antidepressant treatment compared with placebo in children and adolescents with major depressive disorder, obsessive-compulsive disorder (OCD), or other psychiatric disorders based on pooled analyses of 24 short-term, placebo-controlled trials of 9 antidepressant drugs (SSRIs and other antidepressants). However, a later meta-analysis of 27 placebo-controlled trials of 9 antidepressants (SSRIs and others) in patients younger than 19 years of age with major depressive disorder, OCD, or non-OCD anxiety disorders suggests that the benefits of antidepressant therapy in treating these conditions may outweigh the risks of suicidal behavior or ideation. No suicides occurred in these pediatric trials. These findings should be carefully considered when assessing potential benefits and risks of levomilnacipran in a child or adolescent for any clinical use. (See Worsening of Depression and Suicidality Risk under Warnings/Precautions: Warnings, in Cautions.)

The manufacturer states that levomilnacipran is not approved for use in pediatric patients.

Geriatric Use. In clinical trials with levomilnacipran, 2.8% of patients were 65 years of age or older.

In a multiple-dose clinical pharmacokinetic study, individuals older than 65 years of age had slightly higher exposure to levomilnacipran (peak plasma concentration increased by 24% and area under the concentration-time curve [AUC] increased by 26%) than younger individuals (18–45 years of age).

Because levomilnacipran is primarily eliminated by renal excretion, renal clearance of levomilnacipran should be considered when determining the dosage in geriatric patients.

SSRIs and SNRIs, including levomilnacipran, have been associated with clinically important hyponatremia in geriatric patients, who may be at greater risk for this adverse effect. (See Hyponatremia/Syndrome of Inappropriate Antidiuretic Hormone Secretion under Warnings/Precautions: Other Warnings and Precautions, in Cautions.)

In pooled data analyses, a *reduced* risk of suicidality was observed in adults 65 years of age or older with antidepressant therapy compared with placebo. (See Worsening of Depression and Suicidality Risk under Warnings/Precautions: Warnings, in Cautions.)

Hepatic Impairment. Hepatic elimination of levomilnacipran is low, and the pharmacokinetics of the drug are not substantially affected by hepatic impairment. Therefore, dosage adjustment of levomilnacipran is not necessary in patients with mild (Child-Pugh score of 1–6), moderate (Child-Pugh score of 7–9), or severe (Child-Pugh score of 10–13) hepatic impairment.

Renal Impairment. Levomilnacipran is primarily eliminated by renal excretion.

Dosage adjustment is not necessary in patients with mild renal impairment (creatinine clearance of 60–89 mL/minute). However, dosage adjustment is recommended in patients with moderate (creatinine clearance of 30–59 mL/minute) or severe renal impairment (creatinine clearance of 15–29 mL/minute). Levomilnacipran use is *not* recommended in patients with end-stage renal disease. (See Dosage and Administration: Special Populations.)

Because of levomilnacipran's large volume of distribution, hemodialysis is not expected to reduce plasma concentrations of the drug.

■ **Common Adverse Effects** Adverse effects reported in at least 5% of patients with major depressive disorder receiving levomilnacipran and at an incidence of at least twice that reported with placebo in controlled studies include nausea, constipation, hyperhidrosis, increased heart rate, erectile dysfunction, tachycardia (including sinus tachycardia and postural orthostatic tachycardia syndrome), vomiting, and palpitations. The incidence of erectile dysfunction was dose related in a pooled analysis of these studies.

Drug Interactions

Levomilnacipran is metabolized primarily by cytochrome P-450 (CYP) isoenzyme 3A4 with minor contributions by CYP isoenzymes 2C8, 2C19, 2D6, and 2J2. In vitro studies demonstrate that levomilnacipran does not inhibit CYP isoenzymes 1A2, 2A6, 2C8, 2C9, 2C19, 2D6, or 2E1. Other than CYP3A4-mediated drug interactions, levomilnacipran has a low potential to be involved in clinically important pharmacokinetic drug interactions.

Levomilnacipran is not a substrate or inhibitor of breast cancer resistance protein (BCRP), organic anion-transporting polypeptides (OATP) 1B1 and 1B3, organic cation transporter (OCT) 2, and organic anion transporters (OAT) 1 and 3. No dosage adjustment is necessary when levomilnacipran is used concomitantly with a substrate or inhibitor of BCRP, OATP1B1, OATP1B3, OAT1, OAT3, or OCT2.

■ **Drugs Affecting Hepatic Microsomal Enzymes** ***Ketoconazole and Other Potent CYP3A4 Inhibitors*** Concomitant administration of levomilnacipran and ketoconazole substantially increased levomilnacipran exposure in an in vivo study.

The manufacturer states that the dosage of levomilnacipran should not exceed 80 mg once daily if administered concomitantly with potent CYP3A4 inhibitors (e.g., clarithromycin, ketoconazole, ritonavir).

Inhibitors of Other CYP Isoenzymes In vitro studies suggest that CYP isoenzymes 2C8, 2C19, 2D6, and 2J2 have minimal contributions to the metabolism of levomilnacipran; therefore, no dosage adjustment of levomilnacipran is necessary when the drug is used concomitantly with inhibitors of these isoenzymes.

Carbamazepine and Other CYP3A4 Inducers No clinically important changes in levomilnacipran exposure occurred when the drug was administered concomitantly with carbamazepine (a CYP3A4 inducer) in vivo. The manufacturer of levomilnacipran states that dosage adjustment of the drug is not necessary when used concomitantly with a CYP3A4 inducer.

■ **Drugs Metabolized by Hepatic Microsomal Enzymes** ***Alprazolam and Other CYP3A4 Substrates*** No clinically important changes in levomilnacipran exposure occurred when the drug was administered concomitantly with alprazolam (a CYP3A4 substrate) in vivo; alprazolam exposure also was not substantially changed by levomilnacipran (also a CYP3A4 substrate). The manufacturer states that no dosage adjustment of levomilnacipran is necessary when the drug is used concomitantly with a CYP3A4 substrate.

Substrates of Other CYP Isoenzymes In vitro studies have shown that levomilnacipran does not inhibit CYP isoenzymes 1A2, 2A6, 2C8, 2C9, 2C19, 2D6, or 2E1. No dosage adjustment of concomitantly administered substrates of these isoenzymes is recommended in patients receiving levomilnacipran.

■ **Drugs Affecting P-glycoprotein Transport** Levomilnacipran is a weak substrate of P-glycoprotein (P-gp), but did not inhibit P-gp in in vitro studies. No dosage adjustment of concomitantly administered P-gp substrates is recommended in patients receiving levomilnacipran.

■ **Drugs Affecting Hemostasis** Altered anticoagulant effects, including increased bleeding, have been reported when SSRIs or SNRIs were administered concurrently with warfarin or other anticoagulants. The manufacturer of levomilnacipran recommends carefully monitoring patients receiving warfarin during initiation and discontinuance of levomilnacipran therapy.

The risk of bleeding may be increased if levomilnacipran is used concurrently with aspirin or other nonsteroidal anti-inflammatory agents (NSAIAs); levomilnacipran and drugs that affect hemostasis should be used concomitantly with caution.

■ **Monoamine Oxidase Inhibitors** Concomitant use of SSRIs and SNRIs (e.g., levomilnacipran) and monoamine oxidase (MAO) inhibitors is associated with a risk of serious, sometimes fatal, serotonin syndrome. Concomitant use of MAO inhibitors intended to treat psychiatric disorders with levomilnacipran is contraindicated. In addition, at least 2 weeks should elapse between discontinuance of an MAO inhibitor and initiation of levomilnacipran and at least 7 days should elapse between discontinuance of levomilnacipran and initiation of MAO inhibitor therapy. (See Contraindications and also see Serotonin Syndrome under Warnings/Precautions: Other Warnings and Precautions, in Cautions.)

■ **Linezolid** Linezolid, an anti-infective agent that is also a reversible MAO inhibitor, has been associated with drug interactions resulting in serotonin syndrome, including some associated with SSRIs and SNRIs. Because of this potential risk, linezolid generally should not be used in patients receiving levomilnacipran. However, the manufacturer and the US Food and Drug Administration (FDA) state that certain life-threatening or urgent situations may necessitate immediate linezolid treatment in a patient receiving a serotonergic drug such as levomilnacipran. In such emergency situations, the availability of alternative anti-infectives should be considered and the benefits of linezolid should be weighed against the risk of serotonin syndrome. If linezolid is indicated in such emergency situations, levomilnacipran must be immediately discontinued and the patient monitored for symptoms of CNS toxicity for 2 weeks or until 24 hours after the last linezolid dose, whichever comes first. Treatment with levomilnacipran may be resumed 24 hours after the last linezolid dose.

If nonemergency use of linezolid is being planned for a patient receiving levomilnacipran, levomilnacipran should be withheld for at least 2 weeks prior to initiating linezolid.

Treatment with levomilnacipran should not be initiated in a patient receiving linezolid. In patients who require more urgent treatment of a psychiatric condition, other interventions, including hospitalization, should be considered. Levomilnacipran may be started 24 hours after the last linezolid dose. (See Contraindications and also see Serotonin Syndrome under Warnings/Precautions: Other Warnings and Precautions, in Cautions.)

■ **Methylene Blue** Methylene blue, a potent and reversible inhibitor of MAO-A, has been associated with drug interactions resulting in serotonin syndrome, including some associated with SSRIs and SNRIs. Most of these cases occurred when methylene blue was used as a diagnostic (visualizing) dye† (1–8 mg/kg IV) during parathyroid surgery; it is unclear whether there is a risk of serotonin syndrome when methylene blue is administered by other routes or in lower IV doses in patients receiving serotonergic drugs. Because of this potential risk, methylene blue generally should not be used in patients receiving levomilnacipran. However, the manufacturer and the FDA state that certain life-threatening or urgent situations may necessitate immediate IV methylene blue treatment in a patient receiving a serotonergic drug such as levomilnacipran. In such emergency situations, the availability of alternative interventions should be considered and the benefits of methylene blue should be weighed against the risk of serotonin syndrome. If methylene blue is indicated in such emergency situations, levomilnacipran must be immediately discontinued and the patient monitored for symptoms of CNS toxicity for 2 weeks or until 24 hours after the last methylene blue dose, whichever comes first. Treatment with levomilnacipran may be resumed 24 hours after the last methylene blue dose.

If nonemergency use of methylene blue is being planned for a patient receiving levomilnacipran, levomilnacipran should be withheld for at least 2 weeks prior to initiating methylene blue treatment.

Treatment with levomilnacipran should not be initiated in a patient receiving IV methylene blue. In patients who require more urgent treatment of a psychiatric condition, other interventions, including hospitalization, should be considered. Levomilnacipran may be started 24 hours after the last IV methylene blue dose. (See Contraindications and also see Serotonin Syndrome under Warnings/Precautions: Other Warnings and Precautions, in Cautions.)

The manufacturer of levomilnacipran states that the risk of administering methylene blue by non-IV routes (e.g., oral tablets, local injection) or in IV doses much lower than 1 mg/kg in patients receiving levomilnacipran is unclear. Clinicians should be aware of the possibility of the emergent symptoms of serotonin syndrome with concomitant use.

■ **Selective Serotonin-reuptake Inhibitors and Selective Serotonin- and Norepinephrine-reuptake Inhibitors** Concomitant use of levomilnacipran and a selective serotonin-reuptake inhibitor (SSRI) or another selective serotonin- and norepinephrine-reuptake inhibitor (SNRI) is associated with a risk of serious, sometimes fatal, serotonin syndrome. If concomitant use of levomilnacipran and an SSRI or another SNRI is clinically warranted, patients should be advised of the increased risk for serotonin syndrome, particularly during treatment initiation and dosage increases (see Advice to Patients). If serotonin syndrome manifestations occur, treatment with levomilnacipran and the concurrently administered SSRI or SNRI should be discontinued immediately and supportive and symptomatic treatment should be initiated. (See Serotonin Syndrome under Warnings/Precautions: Other Warnings and Precautions, in Cautions.)

■ **Tricyclic Antidepressants** Concomitant use of levomilnacipran and a tricyclic antidepressant is associated with a risk of serious, sometimes fatal, serotonin syndrome. If concomitant use of levomilnacipran and tricyclic antidepressants is clinically warranted, patients should be advised of the increased risk for serotonin syndrome, particularly during treatment initiation and dosage increases (see Advice to Patients). If serotonin syndrome manifestations occur, treatment with levomilnacipran, the tricyclic antidepressant, and any other concurrently administered serotonergic agents should be discontinued immediately and supportive and symptomatic treatment should be initiated. (See Serotonin Syndrome under Warnings/Precautions: Other Warnings and Precautions, in Cautions.)

■ **5-HT$_1$ Receptor Agonists ("Triptans")** Concomitant use of levomilnacipran and a triptan is associated with a risk of serious, sometimes fatal, serotonin syndrome. If concomitant use of levomilnacipran and triptans is clinically warranted, patients should be advised of the increased risk for serotonin syndrome, particularly during treatment initiation and dosage increases (see Advice to Patients). If serotonin syndrome manifestations occur, treatment with levomilnacipran, the triptan, and any other concurrently administered serotonergic agents should be discontinued immediately and supportive and symptomatic treatment should be initiated. (See Serotonin Syndrome under Warnings/Precautions: Other Warnings and Precautions, in Cautions.)

■ **Tryptophan** Concomitant use of levomilnacipran and tryptophan is associated with a risk of serious, sometimes fatal, serotonin syndrome. If concomitant use of levomilnacipran and tryptophan is clinically warranted, patients should be advised of the increased risk for serotonin syndrome, particularly during treatment initiation and dosage increases (see Advice to Patients). If serotonin syndrome manifestations occur, treatment with levomilnacipran, tryptophan, and any other concurrently administered serotonergic agents should be discontinued immediately and supportive and symptomatic treatment should be initiated. (See Serotonin Syndrome under Warnings/Precautions: Other Warnings and Precautions, in Cautions.)

■ **Serotonergic Drugs** Concomitant use of levomilnacipran and other serotonergic drugs is associated with a risk of serious, sometimes fatal, serotonin syndrome. If concomitant use of levomilnacipran and other serotonergic drugs is clinically warranted, patients should be advised of the increased risk for serotonin syndrome, particularly during treatment initiation and dosage increases (see Advice to Patients). If serotonin syndrome manifestations occur, treatment with levomilnacipran and any concurrently administered serotonergic agents should be discontinued immediately and supportive and symptomatic treatment should be initiated. (See Serotonin Syndrome under Warnings/Precautions: Other Warnings and Precautions, in Cautions.)

■ **CNS-active Drugs** The risk of concurrent use of levomilnacipran and other CNS-active drugs has not been systematically evaluated. The manufacturer of levomilnacipran recommends using caution when the drug is used in combination with other centrally-acting drugs, including those with a similar mechanism of action. (See Drug Interactions: Alcohol.)

■ **Alcohol** In an in vitro study, alcohol interacted with the extended-release properties of levomilnacipran. If levomilnacipran is taken with alcohol, a pronounced accelerated release of the drug may occur. The manufacturer therefore recommends that levomilnacipran extended-release capsules not be taken with alcohol. (See Drug Interactions: CNS-active Drugs and also see Advice to Patients.)

■ **Buspirone** Concomitant use of levomilnacipran and buspirone is associated with a risk of serious, sometimes fatal, serotonin syndrome. If concomitant use of levomilnacipran and buspirone is clinically warranted, patients should be advised of the increased risk for serotonin syndrome, particularly during treatment initiation and dosage increases (see Advice to Patients). If serotonin syndrome manifestations occur, treatment with levomilnacipran, buspirone, and any other concurrently administered serotonergic agents should be discontinued immediately and supportive and symptomatic treatment should be initiated. (See Serotonin Syndrome under Warnings/Precautions: Other Warnings and Precautions, in Cautions.)

■ **Diuretics** Concomitant use of levomilnacipran and diuretics may increase the risk of hyponatremia. (See Hyponatremia/Syndrome of Inappropriate Antidiuretic Hormone Secretion under Warnings/Precautions: Other Warnings and Precautions, in Cautions.)

■ **Fentanyl** Concomitant use of levomilnacipran and fentanyl is associated with a risk of serious, sometimes fatal, serotonin syndrome. If concomitant use of levomilnacipran and fentanyl is clinically warranted, patients should be advised of the increased risk for serotonin syndrome, particularly during treatment initiation and dosage increases (see Advice to Patients). If serotonin syndrome manifestations occur, treatment with levomilnacipran, fentanyl, and any other concurrently administered serotonergic agents should be discontinued immediately and supportive and symptomatic treatment should be initiated. (See Serotonin Syndrome under Warnings/Precautions: Other Warnings and Precautions, in Cautions.)

■ **Lithium** Concomitant use of levomilnacipran and lithium is associated with a risk of serious, sometimes fatal, serotonin syndrome. If concomitant use of levomilnacipran and lithium is clinically warranted, patients should be advised of the increased risk for serotonin syndrome, particularly during treatment initiation and dosage increases (see Advice to Patients). If serotonin syndrome manifestations occur, treatment with levomilnacipran, lithium, and any other concurrently administered serotonergic agents should be discontinued immediately and supportive and symptomatic treatment should be initiated. (See Serotonin Syndrome under Warnings/Precautions: Other Warnings and Precautions, in Cautions.)

■ **Drugs that Increase Blood Pressure and Heart Rate** Concurrent use of levomilnacipran with other drugs that increase blood pressure and heart rate has not been evaluated; such combinations should be used with caution.

■ **Tramadol** Concomitant use of levomilnacipran and tramadol is associated with a risk of serious, sometimes fatal, serotonin syndrome. If concomitant use of levomilnacipran and tramadol is clinically warranted, caution should be exercised and patients should be advised of the increased risk for serotonin syndrome, particularly during treatment initiation and dosage increases (see Advice to Patients). If serotonin syndrome manifestations occur, treatment with levomilnacipran, tramadol, and any other concurrently administered serotonergic agents should be discontinued immediately and supportive and symptomatic treatment should be initiated. (See Serotonin Syndrome under Warnings/Precautions: Other Warnings and Precautions, in Cautions.)

■ **St. John's Wort** Concomitant use of levomilnacipran and St. John's wort (*Hypericum perforatum*) is associated with a risk of serious, sometimes fatal, serotonin syndrome. If concomitant use of levomilnacipran and St. John's wort is clinically warranted, patients should be advised of the increased risk for serotonin syndrome, particularly during treatment initiation and dosage increases (see Advice to Patients). If serotonin syndrome manifestations occur, treatment with levomilnacipran, St. John's wort, and any other concurrently administered serotonergic agents should be discontinued immediately and supportive and symptomatic treatment should be initiated. (See Serotonin Syndrome under Warnings/Precautions: Other Warnings and Precautions, in Cautions.)

Description

Levomilnacipran hydrochloride is a selective serotonin- and norepinephrine-reuptake inhibitor (SNRI). Levomilnacipran is the more active 1*S*,2*R* enantiomer of the SNRI milnacipran, which is a racemic mixture of the 1*S*,2*R* and 1*R*,2*S* enantiomers that is used in the management of fibromyalgia. The precise mechanism of the antidepressant effect of levomilnacipran is not fully understood, but is thought to be related to potentiation of serotonin and norepinephrine activity in the CNS through selective inhibition of serotonin and norepinephrine reuptake.

Levomilnacipran potently and selectively inhibits the reuptake of serotonin and norepinephrine, with preferential activity at the norepinephrine transporters. Levomilnacipran demonstrated a twofold preference for norepinephrine- over serotonin-reuptake inhibition in vitro. In in vitro studies, the drug lacked substantial affinity for other receptors, ion channels, or transporters tested, including serotonergic (5-HT_{1-7}), α- and β-adrenergic, muscarinic, and histaminergic receptors, and calcium, sodium, potassium, and chloride channels. Levomilnacipran does not inhibit monoamine oxidase (MAO).

Relative oral bioavailability of levomilnacipran hydrochloride extended-release capsules is 92% compared with the oral solution. Administration of the drug with food did not substantially affect levomilnacipran concentrations. The median time to achieve peak plasma concentrations of levomilnacipran is 6–8 hours following oral administration of the drug. Interconversion between levomilnacipran and its stereoisomer does not appear to occur in humans. Levomilnacipran is widely distributed and 22% protein bound. The elimination half-life of the drug is approximately 12 hours. Levomilnacipran undergoes desethylation, which is catalyzed primarily by cytochrome P-450 (CYP) isoenzyme 3A4 with minor contributions by CYP isoenzymes 2C8, 2C19, 2D6, and 2J2, to form desethyl levomilnacipran; the drug also undergoes hydroxylation to form *p*-hydroxy-levomilnacipran. Both of these oxidative metabolites further undergo glucuronide conjugation. Following oral administration of a single dose of radiolabeled levomilnacipran solution, approximately 58% of the dose is excreted in urine as unchanged drug. The principal metabolite excreted in urine is *N*-desethyl levomilnacipran, which accounted for approximately 18% of the dose; other metabolites excreted in urine include levomilnacipran glucuronide (4%), desethyl levomilnacipran glucuronide (3%), *p*-hydroxy levomilnacipran glucuronide (1%), and *p*-hydroxy levomilnacipran (1%). All of these metabolites are inactive.

Advice to Patients

Importance of providing a copy of written patient information (medication guide) each time levomilnacipran hydrochloride is dispensed. Importance of advising patients to read the patient information before taking levomilnacipran and each time the prescription is refilled.

Risk of suicidality; importance of patients, family, and caregivers being alert to and immediately reporting emergence of suicidality, worsening depression, or unusual changes in behavior, especially during the first few months of therapy or during periods of dosage adjustment. (See Worsening of Depression and Suicidality Risk under Warnings/Precautions: Warnings, in Cautions.)

Importance of informing patients of potential risk of serotonin syndrome, particularly with concurrent use of levomilnacipran and 5-HT_1 receptor agonists (also called triptans), tramadol, tryptophan, other serotonergic agents, or antipsychotic agents. Importance of immediately contacting clinician if signs and symptoms of this syndrome develop (e.g., restlessness, hallucinations, delirium, loss of coordination, tachycardia, increased body temperature, sweating, muscle stiffness, labile blood pressure, diarrhea, coma, nausea, vomiting, confusion).

Importance of instructing patients not to take levomilnacipran with or within 14 days of discontinuing a monoamine oxidase (MAO) inhibitor and to allow 7 days after discontinuing levomilnacipran before initiating an MAO inhibitor.

Importance of advising patients that levomilnacipran can be taken with or without food. Importance of advising patients to swallow levomilnacipran extended-release capsules whole and not to chew, cut, crush, or open the capsules. Importance of also informing patients that the dosage of levomilnacipran should be titrated when initiating therapy.

If a dose of levomilnacipran is missed, it should be taken as soon as it is remembered. However, if a dose is missed and it is almost time for the next scheduled dose, the missed dose should be skipped and the next dose should be taken at the regularly scheduled time. Importance of advising patients not to take 2 doses of the drug at the same time.

Risk of seizures; importance of cautioning patients about use of levomilnacipran if they have a history of a seizure disorder.

Importance of advising patients not to stop taking levomilnacipran without first talking with their clinician. Importance of patients being aware that withdrawal symptoms may occur when stopping levomilnacipran, especially with abrupt discontinuance of the drug.

Importance of informing patients that if they receive diuretics, are otherwise volume depleted, or are elderly, that they may be at greater risk of developing hyponatremia during levomilnacipran therapy.

Risk of cognitive and motor impairment; importance of patients exercising caution while operating hazardous machinery, including driving a motor vehicle, until they are reasonably certain that levomilnacipran therapy does not adversely affect their ability to engage in such activities.

Importance of advising patients to avoid alcohol consumption during levomilnacipran therapy.

Risk of increased blood pressure and heart rate; importance of advising patients that their blood pressure and heart rate should be measured prior to initiating levomilnacipran and periodically during therapy.

Importance of advising patients that levomilnacipran can cause mild pupillary dilation, which can lead to an episode of angle-closure glaucoma in susceptible individuals. Possible symptoms include eye pain, vision changes, and swelling or redness in or around the eye. Preexisting glaucoma is almost always open-angle glaucoma since angle-closure glaucoma can be treated definitively with iridectomy when diagnosed; open-angle glaucoma is not a risk factor for angle-closure glaucoma. Patients may wish to be examined to determine whether they are susceptible to angle-closure glaucoma and have a prophylactic procedure (e.g., iridectomy) if they are susceptible.

Importance of cautioning patients about the risk of urinary hesitation or retention while taking levomilnacipran, particularly in patients prone to obstructive urinary disorders.

Importance of advising patients to notify their clinician if any signs or symptoms of an allergic reaction develop during levomilnacipran therapy (e.g., rash, hives, swelling, difficulty breathing).

Importance of advising patients and their caregivers to watch for signs of activation of mania/hypomania.

Importance of informing clinicians of existing or contemplated concomitant therapy, including prescription and OTC drugs or herbal supplements, as well as any concomitant illnesses (e.g., hypertension, cardiovascular or cerebrovascular disease, seizure disorder, glaucoma) or personal or family history of suicidality or bipolar disorder. Importance of advising patients about the risk of bleeding associated with concomitant use of levomilnacipran with aspirin or other nonsteroidal anti-inflammatory agents, warfarin, or other drugs that affect coagulation.

Importance of women informing clinicians if they are or plan to become pregnant or plan to breast-feed.

Importance of informing patients of other important precautionary information. (See Cautions.)

Overview® (see Users Guide). For additional information on this drug until a more detailed monograph is developed and published, the manufacturer's labeling should be consulted. It is *essential* that the manufacturer's labeling be consulted for more detailed information on usual cautions, precautions, contraindications, potential drug interactions, laboratory test interferences, and acute toxicity.

Preparations

Excipients in commercially available drug preparations may have clinically important effects in some individuals; consult specific product labeling for details.

Levomilnacipran Hydrochloride

Oral		
Capsules, extended-release	20 mg (of levomilnacipran)	**Fetzima®**, Forest
	40 mg (of levomilnacipran)	**Fetzima®**, Forest
	80 mg (of levomilnacipran)	**Fetzima®**, Forest
	120 mg (of levomilnacipran)	**Fetzima®**, Forest
Titration Pack	2 Capsules, extended-release, Levomilnacipran Hydrochloride 20 mg (of levomilnacipran; Fetzima®) 26 Capsules, extended-release, Levomilnacipran Hydrochloride 40 mg (of levomilnacipran; Fetzima®)	**Fetzima® Titration Pack (available as blister package for first month of therapy)**, Forest

†Use is not currently included in the labeling approved by the US Food and Drug Administration

Venlafaxine Hydrochloride

■ Venlafaxine hydrochloride, a selective serotonin- and norepinephrine-reuptake inhibitor (SNRI), is a phenylethylamine-derivative antidepressant and anxiolytic agent.

Uses

■ **Major Depressive Disorder** Venlafaxine hydrochloride is used in the treatment of major depressive disorder. Efficacy of venlafaxine conventional tablets for the management of major depression has been established in several placebo-controlled studies in outpatient settings in patients who had major depression and in 1 placebo-controlled study in a hospital setting in patients who had major depression with melancholia. Efficacy of venlafaxine extended-release capsules for the treatment of major depression also has been established by controlled studies of 8–12 weeks' duration in outpatient settings; however, the safety and efficacy of venlafaxine extended-release capsules in hospitalized patients with major depression have not been adequately evaluated.

In 4 studies of 6 weeks' duration in adult outpatients with major depression, venlafaxine in dosages of 75–225 mg daily administered in 2 or 3 divided doses as conventional tablets was found to be superior to placebo on at least 2 of the following 3 clinical measures of depression: Hamilton Depression Rating Scale (HAM-D) total score, HAM-D depressed mood item, and the Clinical Global Impression (CGI) Severity of Illness Scale. In these studies, higher dosages (i.e., dosages exceeding 225 mg daily) were not associated with greater response. In 2 short-term (8 or 12 weeks), placebo-controlled, flexible-dose (75–225 mg daily) studies with venlafaxine extended-release capsules in adult outpatients, venlafaxine was found to be superior to placebo on the same clinical measures of depression that were used in the studies of venlafaxine conventional tablets, as well as on the Montgomery-Asberg Depression Rating Scale (MADRS) total score and certain factors of the HAM-D, including the anxiety/somatization factor, the cognitive disturbance factor, the retardation factor, and the psychic anxiety score.

Venlafaxine also has been shown to be superior to placebo in the management of major depression with melancholia in a hospital setting. In a study of 4 weeks' duration, 65% of hospitalized patients with major depressive disorder and melancholia who received venlafaxine 150–375 mg daily (mean dosage of 350 mg daily) administered in 3 divided doses as conventional tablets had at least a 50% reduction in MADRS total score compared with 28% of those who received placebo. Patients who participated in this study had a mean baseline MADRS total score of 35 (range: 26–48); those with a baseline score of 4 or greater on the suicidal thought item of the MADRS were excluded from the study.

Results of long-term, relapse prevention studies in outpatients with major depression indicate that venlafaxine's antidepressant effects are maintained for up to 1 year. In these studies, patients who responded to an initial 8-week course of venlafaxine 75–225 mg once daily (as extended-release capsules) or an initial 26-week course of venlafaxine 100–200 mg daily in 2 divided doses (as conventional tablets) were randomized to receive either venlafaxine (same dosage range) or placebo. Patients receiving venlafaxine experienced substantially lower relapse rates than those receiving placebo. Relapse was defined in clinical studies with venlafaxine conventional tablets as a score of 4 or greater on the CGI Severity of Illness Scale and in clinical studies with venlafaxine extended-release capsules as a reappearance of major depressive disorder as defined by DSM-IV criteria and a CGI Severity of Illness score of 4 or greater (i.e., moderately severe depression), 2 consecutive scores of 4 or greater on the CGI Severity of Illness Scale, or a final CGI Severity of Illness score of 4 or greater for any patient who withdrew from the study for any reason.

For further information on treatment of major depressive disorder and considerations in choosing the most appropriate antidepressant for a particular patient, including considerations related to patient tolerance, patient age, and cardiovascular, sedative, and suicidal risk, see Considerations in Choosing Antidepressants under Uses: Major Depressive Disorder, in Fluoxetine Hydrochloride 28:16.04.20.

■ **Generalized Anxiety Disorder** Venlafaxine hydrochloride is used in the treatment of generalized anxiety disorder. Efficacy of venlafaxine extended-release capsules for the management of generalized anxiety disorder has been established in 4 randomized, multicenter, placebo-controlled studies of 2 or 6 months' duration in adult outpatients who met DSM-IV criteria for generalized anxiety disorder. Three studies employed fixed venlafaxine dosages, and the other employed a flexible dosing schedule. In the flexible-dose study, approximately 69% of patients receiving venlafaxine (75–225 mg daily as extended-release capsules) were categorized as responders (defined as a 40% or greater reduction from baseline in the Hamilton Rating Scale for Anxiety [HAM-A] total score or a score of 1 ["very much improved"] or 2 ["much improved"] on the Clinical Global Impressions [CGI] Global Improvement Scale) during weeks 6–28 of therapy compared with 42–46% of those receiving placebo. In separate clinical studies of 2 or 6 months' duration employing fixed dosages of venlafaxine (37.5, 75, 150, or 225 mg daily as extended-release capsules), venlafaxine was shown to be substantially more effective than placebo on HAM-A total score, both the HAM-A anxiety and tension items, and the CGI Scale. While a relationship between dosage (over the dosage range of 75–225 mg daily) and efficacy in generalized anxiety disorder has not been definitively established, dosages of 37.5 mg daily were not as consistently effective in one study as dosages of 75 or 150 mg daily.

■ **Social Phobia** Venlafaxine hydrochloride is used in the treatment of social phobia (social anxiety disorder). Efficacy of venlafaxine extended-release capsules in the treatment of social phobia has been established in 2 multicenter, placebo-controlled studies of 12 weeks' duration in adult outpatients who met DSM-IV criteria for social phobia. In these studies, venlafaxine (75–225 mg daily administered as extended-release capsules) was substantially more effective than placebo, as determined by change from baseline in the Liebowitz Social Anxiety Scale (LSAS) total score.

Subgroup analysis of these controlled studies in adult outpatients with social anxiety disorder did not reveal any evidence of gender-related differences in treatment outcome; there was insufficient information to determine the effect of age or race on outcome in these studies.

■ **Panic Disorder** Venlafaxine hydrochloride is used in the treatment of panic disorder with or without agoraphobia. Efficacy of venlafaxine extended-release capsules in the treatment of panic disorder has mainly been established in 2 multicenter, double-blind, placebo-controlled studies of 12 weeks' duration in adult outpatients who met DSM-IV criteria for panic disorder with or without agoraphobia. Venlafaxine was given in a fixed dosage of 75 or 150 mg once daily as extended-release capsules in one study and in a fixed dosage of 75 or 225 mg once daily as extended-release capsules in the other study. Venlafaxine was found to be substantially more effective than placebo, as determined by percentage of patients free of full-symptom attacks on the Panic and Anticipatory Anxiety Scale (PAAS), mean change from baseline on the Panic Disorder Severity Scale (PDSS) total score, and the percentage of patients rated as responders on the Clinical Global Impressions (CGI) Improvement Scale. While a relationship between dosage (over the dosage range of 75–225 mg daily) and efficacy in panic disorder has not been definitively established, efficacy was established for each dosage studied in these 2 trials.

Subgroup analysis of these controlled studies in adult outpatients with panic disorder did not reveal any evidence of gender-related differences in treatment outcome; there was insufficient information to determine the effect of age or race on outcome in these studies.

In a longer-term study, patients meeting DSM-IV criteria for panic disorder who had responded during the 12-week open phase of a clinical trial with venlafaxine (75, 150, or 225 mg once daily as extended-release capsules) were randomly assigned to either continue receiving venlafaxine in the same dosage range or be switched to placebo and observed for relapse. Relapse was defined as having 2 or more full-symptom panic attacks per week for 2 consecutive weeks or having discontinued therapy due to loss of effectiveness as determined by the study investigators. Patients who continued receiving venlafaxine therapy experienced a significantly longer time to relapse than those receiving placebo in this study.

■ **Vasomotor Symptoms** Venlafaxine has been used for the management of vasomotor symptoms† in women with breast cancer and in postmenopausal women. Therapy with the drug has improved both the frequency and severity of vasomotor symptoms (hot flushes [flashes]) in these women.

Most women receiving systemic antineoplastic therapy for breast cancer experience vasomotor symptoms, particularly those receiving tamoxifen therapy. In a randomized, double-blind, placebo-controlled study in 191 women with breast cancer (69% were receiving tamoxifen) who were experiencing 2 or more episodes of hot flushes daily, the percentage reductions in hot flush severity score at 4 weeks of treatment were 27% for placebo, 37% for venlafaxine 37.5 mg daily, 61% for venlafaxine 75 mg daily, and 61% for venlafaxine 150 mg daily. Comparisons among treatment groups showed that all 3 venlafaxine dosages were associated with a statistically significant reduction in hot flush frequency and severity; in addition, the 75-mg dosage was more effective than the 37. 5-mg dosage, but the 150-mg dosage provided no additional benefit. The role of venlafaxine in managing vasomotor symptoms in women with breast cancer relative to other nonhormonal therapies (e.g., selective serotonin-reuptake inhibitors [SSRIs], gabapentin) remains to be determined. Well-designed, comparative studies are needed to establish optimum nonhormonal therapy, both in terms of efficacy and patient tolerance of adverse effects in these women.

Because of the risks associated with hormone replacement therapy (HRT) for vasomotor symptoms in perimenopausal and postmenopausal women, alternative nonhormonal therapies are being investigated. In a randomized, double-blind, placebo-controlled study in 80 postmenopausal women who were experiencing more than 14 hot flushes weekly, 12 weeks of venlafaxine 75 mg daily was associated with a 51% reduction in hot flush score (patient's perception of hot flush interference with daily living). Although there also was a reduction in hot flush severity, the difference did not reach statistical significance. The role of venlafaxine therapy relative to other nonhormonal therapies (e.g., SSRIs, gabapentin) for postmenopausal vasomotor symptoms, both in terms of efficacy and safety, remains to be established.

Current evidence indicates that venlafaxine is well tolerated in the short-term treatment of vasomotor symptoms associated with breast cancer treatment and with menopause. The principal adverse effects associated with venlafaxine therapy in women with vasomotor symptoms have been dry mouth, decreased appetite, nausea, constipation, and difficulty sleeping. Additional study and experience are needed to further elucidate the role of venlafaxine relative to other nonhormonal therapies and to establish longer-term (i.e., beyond 4–12 weeks) efficacy and safety.

The possible role of venlafaxine in the management of vasomotor symptoms† associated with antiandrogenic therapy in men with prostate cancer remains to be determined.

■ **Obesity** Although substantial changes in appetite and weight have been reported in clinical studies of venlafaxine for the management of major depression, generalized anxiety disorder, social phobia, and panic disorder, the manufacturer states that the drug, alone or in combination with weight loss agents such as phentermine, is *not* indicated for the management of exogenous obesity†. Concomitant use of venlafaxine and weight loss agents also is not recommended by the manufacturer because the safety and efficacy of these agents when used concomitantly have not been established.

Dosage and Administration

■ **Administration** Venlafaxine hydrochloride is administered orally. To minimize GI intolerance (e.g., nausea), the manufacturer recommends that conventional venlafaxine tablets be taken with food. Food does not appear to affect GI absorption of the drug. Venlafaxine extended-release capsules should be administered as a single daily dose with food at approximately the same time each day (in the morning or evening). The extended-release capsules should be swallowed whole with fluid or the entire contents of a capsule(s) may be sprinkled on a small amount of applesauce immediately prior to administration. The extended-release capsules of venlafaxine and their contents should not be divided, crushed, chewed, or placed in water. If the capsule contents are administered by sprinkling on applesauce, the patient should drink some water after swallowing the entire mixture without chewing to ensure that the pellets are completely swallowed.

Risk of Sustained Hypertension Venlafaxine therapy has been associated with sustained increases in blood pressure in some patients. An analysis of patients with sustained hypertension and patients whose hypertension resulted in discontinuance of the drug revealed that most blood pressure elevations were modest in severity (i.e., 10–15 or 8–28 mm Hg increases in supine diastolic blood pressure among patients receiving conventional or extended-release venlafaxine, respectively). However, sustained blood pressure increases of this magnitude could have adverse consequences in patients receiving the drug. In addition, some cases of elevated blood pressure requiring immediate treatment have been reported during postmarketing surveillance of the drug. Therefore, the manufacturer recommends that preexisting hypertension be controlled before initiating venlafaxine therapy and that regular blood pressure monitoring be performed in patients receiving the drug. In patients who experience a sustained increase in blood pressure during venlafaxine therapy, dosage reduction or discontinuance of the drug should be considered.

Risk of Serotonin Syndrome or Neuroleptic Malignant Syndrome (NMS)-like Reactions Potentially life-threatening serotonin syndrome or neuroleptic malignant syndrome (NMS)-like reactions have been reported with selective serotonin- and norepinephrine-reuptake inhibitors (SNRIs), including venlafaxine, and selective serotonin-reuptake inhibitors (SSRIs) alone, but particularly with concurrent use of other serotonergic drugs (including serotonin [5-hydroxytryptamine; 5-HT] type 1 receptor agonists ["triptans"], drugs that impair the metabolism of serotonin [e.g., monoamine oxidase inhibitors], or antipsychotics or other dopamine antagonists). Manifestations of serotonin syndrome may include mental status changes (e.g., agitation, hallucinations, coma), autonomic instability (e.g., tachycardia, labile blood pressure, hyperthermia), neuromuscular aberrations (e.g., hyperreflexia, incoordination), and/or GI symptoms (e.g., nausea, vomiting, diarrhea). In its most severe form, serotonin syndrome may resemble NMS, which is characterized by hyperthermia, muscle rigidity, autonomic instability with possible rapid fluctuation in vital signs, and mental status changes. Patients receiving venlafaxine should be monitored for the development of serotonin syndrome or NMS-like signs and symptoms.

Serious (sometimes fatal) adverse reactions, possibly related to serotonin syndrome or NMS, have been reported in patients who received a monoamine oxidase (MAO) inhibitor shortly before or after venlafaxine therapy. Therefore, concomitant use of venlafaxine and MAO inhibitors is *contraindicated.* It is recommended that at least 2 weeks elapse between discontinuance of an MAO inhibitor and initiation of venlafaxine and that an interval of at least 1 week elapse between discontinuance of venlafaxine and initiation of an MAO inhibitor.

If concurrent therapy with venlafaxine and a 5-HT_1 receptor agonist (triptan) is clinically warranted, the patient should be observed carefully, particularly during initiation of therapy, when dosage is increased, or when another serotonergic agent is initiated. Concurrent use of venlafaxine and serotonin precursors (e.g., tryptophan) is not recommended.

If signs and symptoms of serotonin syndrome or NMS develop during venlafaxine therapy, treatment with venlafaxine and any concurrently administered serotonergic or antidopaminergic agents, including antipsychotic agents, should be discontinued immediately and supportive and symptomatic treatment should be initiated.

For additional information on serotonin syndrome, see Drug Interactions: Serotonergic Drugs, in Fluoxetine Hydrochloride 28:16.04.20.

Risk of Suicidality and Overdosage Worsening of depression and/or the emergence of suicidal ideation and behavior (suicidality) or unusual changes in behavior may occur in both adult and pediatric (see Administration: Pediatric Precautions, in Dosage and Administration) patients with major depressive disorder or other psychiatric disorders, whether or not they are taking antidepressants. This risk may persist until clinically important remission occurs. Suicide is a known risk of depression and certain other psychiatric disorders, and these disorders themselves are the strongest predictors of suicide. However, there has been a long-standing concern that antidepressants may have a role in inducing worsening of depression and the emergence of suicidality in certain patients during the early phases of treatment. Pooled analyses of short-term, placebo-controlled studies of antidepressants (i.e., selective serotonin-reuptake inhibitors and other antidepressants) have shown an increased risk of suicidality in children, adolescents, and young adults (18–24 years of age) with major depressive disorder and other psychiatric disorders. An increased suicidality risk was not demonstrated with antidepressants compared with placebo in adults older than 24 years of age and a reduced risk was observed in adults 65 years of age or older. It is currently unknown whether the suicidality risk extends to longer-term use (i.e., beyond several months); however, there is substantial evidence from placebo-controlled maintenance trials in adults with major depressive disorder that antidepressants can delay the recurrence of depression.

The US Food and Drug Administration (FDA) recommends that all patients being treated with antidepressants for any indication be appropriately monitored and closely observed for clinical worsening, suicidality, and unusual changes in behavior, particularly during initiation of therapy (i.e., the first few months) and during periods of dosage adjustments. Families and caregivers of patients being treated with antidepressants for major depressive disorder or other indications, both psychiatric and nonpsychiatric, should be advised to monitor patients on a daily basis for the emergence of agitation, irritability, or unusual changes in behavior, as well as the emergence of suicidality, and to report such symptoms immediately to a health-care provider.

Although a causal relationship between the emergence of symptoms such as anxiety, agitation, panic attacks, insomnia, irritability, hostility, aggressiveness, impulsivity, akathisia, hypomania, and/or mania and either the worsening of depression and/or the emergence of suicidal impulses has not been established, there is concern that such symptoms may represent precursors to emerging suicidality. Consequently, consideration should be given to changing the therapeutic regimen or discontinuing therapy in patients whose depression is persistently worse or in patients experiencing emergent suicidality or symptoms that might be precursors to worsening depression or suicidality, particularly if such manifestations are severe, abrupt in onset, or were not part of the patient's presenting symptoms. If a decision is made to discontinue therapy, venlafaxine dosage should be tapered as rapidly as is feasible but with recognition of the risks of abrupt discontinuance. (See Discontinuance of Therapy under Dosage and Administration: Dosage.)

The results of retrospective studies indicate that venlafaxine overdosage may be associated with an increased risk of fatal outcome compared with that observed with SSRIs but lower than that associated with tricyclic antidepressants. Epidemiologic studies have shown that venlafaxine-treated patients have a higher preexisting burden of suicide risk factors than patients treated with SSRIs. The extent to which the finding of an increased risk of fatal outcomes can be attributed to the toxicity of venlafaxine in an overdosage as opposed to other characteristics of these venlafaxine-treated patients is not clear. As with other antidepressants, FDA and the manufacturer of venlafaxine recommend that the drug be prescribed in the smallest quantity consistent with good patient management, in order to reduce the risk of overdosage.

Risk of Bipolar Disorder It is generally believed (though not established in controlled trials) that treating a major depressive episode with an antidepressant alone may increase the likelihood of precipitating a mixed or manic episode in patients at risk for bipolar disorder. Therefore, patients should be adequately screened for bipolar disorder prior to initiating treatment with an antidepressant; such screening should include a detailed psychiatric history (e.g., family history of suicide, bipolar disorder, and depression). Venlafaxine is *not* approved for use in treating bipolar depression.

Risk of Mydriasis Mydriasis has been reported in association with venlafaxine therapy. Therefore, patients with elevated intraocular pressure or those at risk of angle-closure glaucoma should be monitored during treatment with the drug.

Pediatric Precautions Safety and efficacy of venlafaxine in children younger than 18 years of age have not been established.

Although clinical studies designed to primarily assess the effect of venlafaxine on the growth, development, and maturation of children and adolescents have not been conducted to date, the results from available studies suggest that the drug may adversely affect weight, height, and appetite. Should the decision be made to prescribe venlafaxine for unlabeled (off-label) uses in pediatric patients, the manufacturer recommends regular monitoring of height and weight during therapy, particularly during long-term administration of the drug. In addition, the manufacturer states that the long-term safety of therapy with venlafaxine extended-release capsules (beyond 6 months) has not been systematically evaluated to date. Because the results of clinical studies indicate that the occurrence of blood pressure elevations considered to be clinically important in children and adolescents was similar to that observed in adults receiving venlafaxine, the manufacturer advises that the precautions for adults also should apply to pediatric patients receiving the drug. (See Risk of Sustained Hypertension under Dosage and Administration: Administration.)

In placebo-controlled clinical studies in children and adolescents† 6–17 years of age, efficacy of venlafaxine (administered as extended-release capsules) was *not* established for major depressive disorder or generalized anxiety disorder, and there were increased reports of hostility and suicide-related adverse events such as suicidal ideation and self-harm. Hostility and suicidal ideation were the most common adverse effects leading to discontinuance of the drug in clinical studies in pediatric patients with major depressive disorder, each occurring in 2% of children and adolescents receiving venlafaxine extended-release capsules compared with less than 1 or 0% of those receiving placebo, respectively. In addition, abnormal/changed behavior was the most common adverse effect leading to discontinuance of the drug in clinical studies in pediatric patients with generalized anxiety disorder, occurring in 1% of children and adolescents receiving venlafaxine extended-release capsules compared with none of those receiving placebo. There were no suicides reported in any of these clinical studies.

FDA has determined that antidepressants increase the risk of suicidal thinking and behavior (suicidality) in children and adolescents with major depressive disorder and other psychiatric disorders. However, the FDA also states that depression and certain other psychiatric disorders are themselves associated with an increased risk of suicide. (See Cautions: Pediatric Precautions, in Fluoxetine Hydrochloride 28:16.04.20.) Anyone considering the use of venlafaxine in a child or adolescent for any clinical use must therefore balance the potential risks with the clinical need. (See Risk of Suicidality and Overdosage under Dosage and Administration: Administration.)

■ Dosage

Dosage of venlafaxine hydrochloride is expressed in terms of venlafaxine.

Although no overall differences in efficacy or safety were observed between geriatric and younger adults receiving venlafaxine, the possibility that some older patients may exhibit increased sensitivity to the drug cannot be ruled out. No age-related differences in the pharmacokinetics of venlafaxine have been identified and dosage adjustments are not necessary for geriatric patients on the basis of age alone; however, as with any drug used for the treatment of depression, generalized anxiety disorder, social phobia, or panic disorder, caution should be used when treating geriatric patients and dosage should be increased cautiously. In addition, the greater frequency of decreased hepatic and renal function observed in the elderly should be considered. (See Dosage and Administration: Dosage in Renal and Hepatic Impairment.)

Venlafaxine also should be used with caution in patients whose underlying medical condition might be compromised by increases in heart rate (e.g., patients with hyperthyroidism, heart failure, or recent myocardial infarction), particularly when the venlafaxine dosage exceeds 200 mg daily.

Patients should be monitored for possible worsening of depression, suicidality, or unusual changes in behavior, especially at the beginning of therapy or during periods of dosage adjustment. (See Risk of Suicidality and Overdosage under Dosage and Administration: Administration.)

Major Depressive Disorder For the treatment of major depressive disorder in adults, the recommended initial dosage of venlafaxine is 75 mg daily administered in 2 or 3 divided doses as conventional tablets or as a single daily dose when using the extended-release capsules. According to the manufacturer, an initial dosage of 37.5 mg daily (as extended-release capsules) for the first 4–7 days (followed by an increase to 75 mg daily) may be considered for some patients. If no clinical improvement is apparent, the dosage may be increased by increments of up to 75 mg daily at intervals of not less than 4 days. If clinically necessary, dosage can be increased up to 225 mg daily in divided doses as conventional tablets or in a single daily dose when using the extended-release capsules. Although studies with venlafaxine conventional tablets in outpatient settings did not demonstrate additional benefit from dosages exceeding 225 mg daily in moderately depressed patients, patients with more severe depression responded to a mean dosage of 350 mg daily. Whether higher dosages of venlafaxine extended-release capsules are needed for more severely depressed patients is unknown; however, the manufacturer states that experience with dosages of venlafaxine extended-release capsules exceeding 225 mg daily is very limited. The manufacturer states that venlafaxine dosage should not exceed 375 mg daily (usually administered in 3 divided doses) as conventional tablets or 225 mg daily as extended-release capsules.

If desired, patients with depression who are undergoing treatment with a therapeutic dose of conventional tablets may be switched to the extended-release capsules at the nearest equivalent daily venlafaxine dose (e.g., change 37.5 mg twice daily administered as conventional tablets to a 75-mg extended-release capsule administered once daily).

Although the optimum duration of venlafaxine therapy has not been established, the manufacturer states that acute depressive episodes require several months or longer of sustained antidepressant therapy. Results of 2 relapse prevention trials indicate that the antidepressant efficacy of venlafaxine is maintained for up to 6 months in patients receiving 75–225 mg once daily as extended-release capsules and for up to 12 months in those receiving 100–200 mg daily in 2 divided doses as conventional tablets. In these studies, the same dosage of venlafaxine was used for both acute-phase and maintenance treatment. Based on these limited data, it is not known whether the dosage required to induce remission of depression would be comparable to that required to maintain euthymia. The usefulness of the drug in patients receiving prolonged therapy should be reevaluated periodically.

Generalized Anxiety Disorder For the management of generalized anxiety disorder in adults, the initial dosage of venlafaxine as extended-release capsules recommended for most patients is 75 mg once daily. In some patients, it may be desirable to initiate therapy with a dosage of 37.5 mg daily given for the first 4–7 days, followed by an increase to 75 mg daily. Although a dose-response relationship for effectiveness in generalized anxiety disorder was not clearly established in clinical studies, certain patients not responding to a venlafaxine dosage of 75 mg daily may benefit from a higher dosage. Dosage in these patients may be increased in increments of up to 75 mg daily at intervals of not less than 4 days up to a maximum dosage of 225 mg daily.

The optimum duration of venlafaxine therapy for the management of generalized anxiety disorder has not been established. Although the drug has been used for up to 6 months in controlled clinical studies, the usefulness of the drug in patients receiving prolonged therapy should be reevaluated periodically.

Social Phobia For the management of social phobia in adults, the recommended initial dosage of venlafaxine for most patients is 75 mg once daily as extended-release capsules. In some patients, it may be desirable to initiate therapy with a dosage of 37.5 mg daily given for the first 4–7 days, followed by an increase to 75 mg daily. Although a dose-response relationship for effectiveness in social phobia was not clearly established in clinical studies, certain patients not responding to a venlafaxine dosage of 75 mg daily may benefit from a higher dosage. Dosage in these patients may be increased in increments of up to 75 mg daily at intervals of not less than 4 days up to a maximum dosage of 225 mg daily.

The optimum duration of venlafaxine therapy for the management of social phobia has not been established. The efficacy of venlafaxine for long-term therapy (i.e., longer than 12 weeks) has not been demonstrated in controlled clinical studies to date. The usefulness of the drug in patients receiving prolonged therapy should be reevaluated periodically.

Panic Disorder For the management of panic disorder in adults, the recommended initial dosage of venlafaxine is 37.5 mg once daily as extended-release capsules for 7 days, followed by 75 mg once daily as extended-release capsules for another 7 days. In clinical trials, 37.5 mg once daily was given initially for 7 days, then 75 mg once daily for 7 days; thereafter, dosage was increased in increments of 75 mg once daily every 7 days if necessary up to a maximum dosage of 225 mg daily. Although a dose-response relationship for effectiveness in panic disorder was not clearly established in fixed-dose clinical studies, certain patients not responding to a venlafaxine dosage of 75 mg daily may benefit from a higher dosage. Dosage in these patients may be increased in increments of up to 75 mg daily at intervals of not less than 7 days up to a maximum dosage of approximately 225 mg daily.

The optimum duration of venlafaxine therapy for the management of panic disorder has not been established. The efficacy of venlafaxine for long-term therapy (i.e., longer than 12 weeks) in prolonging time to relapse in responding patients has been demonstrated in a controlled clinical trial. However, the usefulness of the drug in patients receiving prolonged therapy should be reevaluated periodically.

Vasomotor Symptoms Although the optimum dosage for the treatment of vasomotor symptoms† in women with breast cancer and in postmenopausal women remains to be established, some clinicians suggest that venlafaxine be initiated at a dosage of 37.5 mg once daily as extended-release capsules, increasing as necessary to 75 mg once daily. In one clinical study, 75 mg once daily as extended-release capsules appeared to be optimal. Further increases in dosage do not appear to provide substantially increased benefit but are potentially more toxic.

Discontinuance of Therapy Because withdrawal effects may occur, abrupt discontinuance of venlafaxine should be avoided. When venlafaxine therapy is discontinued, dosage should be tapered gradually and the patient carefully monitored to reduce the risk of withdrawal symptoms. If intolerable symptoms occur following dosage reduction or upon discontinuance of treatment, venlafaxine therapy may be reinstituted at the previously prescribed dosage until such symptoms abate. Clinicians may resume dosage reductions at that time but at a more gradual rate.

Withdrawal symptoms reported in clinical studies in adults receiving venlafaxine for major depression or generalized anxiety disorder include agitation, anorexia, anxiety, confusion, impaired coordination, diarrhea, dizziness, dry mouth, dysphoric mood, fasciculation, fatigue, headaches, hypomania, insomnia, nausea, nervousness, nightmares, sensory disturbances (including shock-like electrical sensations), somnolence, sweating, tremor, vertigo, and vomiting. Abrupt discontinuance or dosage reduction of venlafaxine has been associated with the appearance of new symptoms, the frequency of which increased with increased dosage and longer duration of treatment.

In clinical studies, venlafaxine hydrochloride extended-release capsules were discontinued by reducing the daily dosage by 75 mg at intervals of 1 week; however, individualized tapering may be necessary.

■ **Dosage in Renal and Hepatic Impairment** Since clearance of venlafaxine is decreased and elimination half-life is increased in patients with renal impairment, the manufacturer states that dosage of the drug should be reduced by 25–50% in patients with mild-to-moderate renal impairment and by 50% in those undergoing hemodialysis and administration of the dose withheld until the dialysis period is complete (4 hours). Venlafaxine dosage also should be reduced by 50% in patients with moderate hepatic impairment. The manufacturer's labeling should be consulted for more detailed information on the dosage modifications in these patient populations.

■ **Treatment of Pregnant Women during the Third Trimester** Some neonates exposed to venlafaxine, other selective serotonin- and norepinephrine-reuptake inhibitors (SNRIs), or selective serotonin-reuptake inhibitors late in the third trimester of pregnancy have developed complications, which have sometimes been severe and required prolonged hospitalization, respiratory support, enteral nutrition, and other forms of supportive care in special care nurseries. (For additional information, see Cautions: Pregnancy, Fertility, and Lactation, in Fluoxetine Hydrochloride 28:16.04.20.) Therefore, the clinician should carefully consider the potential risks and benefits of treating a pregnant woman with venlafaxine during the third trimester of pregnancy. In addition, consideration should be given to cautiously tapering venlafaxine therapy in the third trimester prior to delivery if the drug is administered during pregnancy.

Description

Venlafaxine hydrochloride, a selective serotonin- and norepinephrine-reuptake inhibitor (SNRI), is a phenylethylamine-derivative antidepressant and anxiolytic agent. Venlafaxine differs structurally and pharmacologically from other commercially available antidepressants, including tricyclic and tetracyclic antidepressants, and also differs from other commercially available agents used to treat generalized anxiety disorder.

The exact mechanisms of antidepressant and anxiolytic actions of venlafaxine have not been fully elucidated but appear to be associated with the drug's potentiation of neurotransmitter activity in the CNS. Venlafaxine and its active metabolite, O-desmethylvenlafaxine (ODV), are potent inhibitors of neuronal serotonin and norepinephrine reuptake and weak inhibitors of dopamine reuptake. In vitro studies have demonstrated that venlafaxine and ODV do not possess any significant affinity for muscarinic cholinergic, H_1-histaminergic, or α_1-adrenergic receptors.

SumMon® (see Users Guide). For additional information on this drug until a more detailed monograph is developed and published, the manufacturer's labeling should be consulted. It is *essential* that the labeling be consulted for detailed information on the usual cautions, precautions, and contraindications.

Preparations

Excipients in commercially available drug preparations may have clinically important effects in some individuals; consult specific product labeling for details.

Venlafaxine Hydrochloride

Oral		
Tablets	25 mg (of venlafaxine)*	**Effexor®** (scored), Wyeth
		Venlafaxine Hydrochloride Tablets
	37.5 mg (of venlafaxine)*	**Effexor®** (scored), Wyeth
		Venlafaxine Hydrochloride Tablets
	50 mg (of venlafaxine)*	**Effexor®** (scored), Wyeth
		Venlafaxine Hydrochloride Tablets
	75 mg (of venlafaxine)*	**Effexor®** (scored), Wyeth
		Venlafaxine Hydrochloride Tablets
	100 mg (of venlafaxine)*	**Effexor®** (scored), Wyeth
		Venlafaxine Hydrochloride Tablets
Capsules, extended-release	37.5 mg (of venlafaxine)	**Effexor® XR,** Wyeth
	75 mg (of venlafaxine)	**Effexor® XR,** Wyeth
	150 mg (of venlafaxine)	**Effexor® XR,** Wyeth

*available from one or more manufacturer, distributor, and/or repackager by generic (nonproprietary) name

†Use is not currently included in the labeling approved by the US Food and Drug Administration

Selective Serotonin-reuptake Inhibitors 28:16.04.20

Citalopram Hydrobromide

■ Citalopram hydrobromide, a selective serotonin-reuptake inhibitor (SSRI), is an antidepressant.

Uses

Citalopram hydrobromide is used in the treatment of major depressive disorder. In addition, citalopram has been used for the treatment of obsessive-compulsive disorder†, panic disorder†, social phobia† (social anxiety disorder), alcohol dependence†, premenstrual dysphoric disorder†, premature ejaculation†, eating disorders†, diabetic neuropathy†, and posttraumatic stress disorder†.

■ **Major Depressive Disorder** Citalopram hydrobromide is used in the treatment of major depressive disorder. A major depressive episode implies a prominent and relatively persistent depressed or dysphoric mood that usually interferes with daily functioning (nearly every day for at least 2 weeks). According to DSM-IV criteria, a major depressive episode includes at least 5 of the following 9 symptoms (with at least one of the symptoms being either depressed mood or loss of interest or pleasure): depressed mood most of the day as indicated by subjective report (e.g., feels sad or empty) or observation made by others; markedly diminished interest or pleasure in all, or almost all, activities most of the day; significant weight loss (when not dieting) or weight gain (e.g., a change of more than 5% of body weight in a month), or decrease or increase in appetite; insomnia or hypersomnia; psychomotor agitation or retardation (observable by others, not merely subjective feelings of restlessness or being slowed down); fatigue or loss of energy; feelings of worthlessness or excessive or inappropriate guilt (not merely self-reproach or guilt about being sick); diminished ability to think or concentrate or indecisiveness (either by subjective account or as observed by others); and recurrent thoughts of death, recurrent suicidal ideation without a specific plan, or a suicide attempt or specific plan for committing suicide.

Treatment of major depressive disorder generally consists of an acute phase (to induce remission), a continuation phase (to preserve remission), and a maintenance phase (to prevent recurrence). Various interventions (e.g., psychotherapy, antidepressant drug therapy, electroconvulsive therapy [ECT]) are used alone or in combination to treat major depressive episodes. Treatment should be individualized, and the most appropriate strategy for a particular patient is determined by clinical factors such as severity of depression (e.g., mild, moderate, severe), presence or absence of certain psychiatric features (e.g., suicide risk, catatonia, psychotic or atypical features, alcohol or substance abuse or dependence, panic or other anxiety disorder, cognitive dysfunction, dysthymia, personality disorder, seasonal affective disorder), and concurrent illness (e.g., asthma, cardiac disease, dementia, seizure disorder, glaucoma, hypertension). Demographic and psychosocial factors as well as patient preference also are used to determine the most effective treatment strategy.

While use of psychotherapy alone may be considered as an initial treatment strategy for patients with mild to moderate major depressive disorder (based on patient preference and presence of clinical features such as psychosocial stressors), combined use of antidepressant drug therapy and psychotherapy may be useful for initial treatment of patients with moderate to severe major depressive disorder with psychosocial issues, interpersonal problems, or a comorbid axis II disorder. In addition, combined use of antidepressant drug therapy and psychotherapy may be beneficial in patients who have a history of poor compliance or only partial response to adequate trials of either antidepressant drug therapy or psychotherapy alone.

Antidepressant drug therapy can be used alone for initial treatment of patients with mild major depressive disorder (if preferred by the patient) and usually is indicated alone or in combination with psychotherapy for initial treatment of patients with moderate to severe major depressive disorder (unless ECT is planned). ECT is not generally used for initial treatment of uncomplicated major depression, but is recommended as first-line treatment for severe major depressive disorder when it is coupled with psychotic features, catatonic stupor, severe suicidality, food refusal leading to nutritional compromise, or other situations when a rapid antidepressant response is required. ECT also is recommended for patients who have previously shown a positive response to or a preference for this treatment modality and can be considered for patients with moderate or severe depression who have not responded to or cannot receive antidepressant drug therapy. In certain situations involving depressed patients unresponsive to adequate trials of several individual antidepressant agents, adjunctive therapy with another agent (e.g., buspirone, lithium) or concomitant use of a second antidepressant agent (e.g., bupropion) has been used; however, such combination therapy is associated with an increased risk of adverse reactions, may require dosage adjustments, and (if not contraindicated) should be undertaken only after careful consideration of the relative risks and benefits. (See Drug Interactions: Serotonergic Drugs, Tricyclic and Other Antidepressants under Drug Interactions: Drugs Undergoing Hepatic Metabolism or Affecting Hepatic Microsomal Enzymes, and Drug Interactions: Lithium.)

The efficacy of citalopram for the management of major depression has been established in short-term (4–6 weeks' duration), placebo-controlled studies in outpatients 18–66 years of age who met DSM-III or -III-R criteria for major depressive disorder. In a 6-week study in which patients received fixed citalopram dosages of 10, 20, 40, or 60 mg daily, the drug was effective at dosages of 40 and 60 mg daily as measured by the Hamilton Depression Rating Scale (HAM-D) Total Score, the HAM-D Depressed Mood Item (Item 1), the Montgomery Asberg Depression Rating Scale, and the Clinical Global Impression (CGI) Severity Scale. This study showed no clear antidepressant effect of the 10 or 20 mg daily dosages, and the 60 mg daily dosage was not more effective than the 40 mg daily dosage.

In a 4-week, placebo-controlled study in depressed adult patients, of whom 85% met criteria for melancholia, those who were treated with citalopram (at an initial dosage of 20 mg daily, titrated to the maximum tolerated dosage or to a maximum daily dosage of 80 mg) showed greater improvement than patients receiving placebo on the HAM-D Total Score, HAM-D Item 1, and the CGI Severity score. In 3 additional placebo-controlled depression trials, the difference in response to treatment between patients receiving citalopram and patients receiving placebo was not statistically significant, possibly due at least in part to a high spontaneous response rate, a high placebo response rate, small sample size, or, in the case of one study, too low a dosage.

In 2 placebo-controlled studies, depressed adult patients who had responded to an initial 6- to 8-week course of citalopram (fixed dosage of 20 or 40 mg daily in one study and flexible dosages ranging from 20–60 mg daily in the second study) were randomized to continue receiving citalopram or placebo for up to 6 months. In both of these studies, patients receiving citalopram experienced substantially lower relapse rates over the subsequent 6 months compared with those receiving placebo. In the fixed-dose study, the decreased rate of depression relapse was similar in patients receiving 20 or 40 mg daily of citalopram. An analysis of these data for possible age-, gender-, and race-related effects on treatment outcome did not suggest any difference in antidepressant efficacy based on the age, gender, and race of the patient. In a placebo-controlled trial, citalopram also was shown to help prevent recurrences of depression in patients with recurrent major depression receiving the drug for up to 6–18 months.

While the optimum duration of citalopram therapy has not been established, many experts state that acute depressive episodes require several months or longer of sustained antidepressant therapy. In addition, some clinicians recommend that long-term antidepressant therapy be considered in certain patients at risk for recurrence of depressive episodes (such as those with highly recurrent unipolar depression). In placebo-controlled studies, citalopram has been shown to be effective for the long-term (e.g., up to 18 months) management of depression. In addition, the drug has been used in some patients for longer periods (e.g., up to 28 months) without apparent loss of clinical effect or increased toxicity. However, when citalopram is used for extended periods, the need for continued therapy should be reassessed periodically. (See Dosage and Administration: Dosage.)

The manufacturer states that efficacy of citalopram as an antidepressant in hospital settings has not been studied adequately to date; however, the drug has been shown to be effective in hospitalized patients with depression, including severe depression, in several studies.

As with other antidepressants, the possibility that citalopram may precipitate hypomanic or manic attacks in patients with bipolar or other major affective disorder should be considered. Citalopram is *not* approved for use in treating bipolar depression.

Considerations in Choosing an Antidepressant A variety of antidepressant drugs are available for the treatment of major depressive disorder, including selective serotonin-reuptake inhibitors (SSRIs; e.g., citalopram, fluoxetine, paroxetine, sertraline), selective serotonin- and norepinephrine-reuptake inhibitors (SNRIs; e.g., desvenlafaxine, duloxetine, venlafaxine), tricyclic antidepressants (e.g., amitriptyline, amoxapine, desipramine, doxepin, imipramine, nortriptyline, protriptyline, trimipramine), monoamine oxidase (MAO) inhibitors (e.g., phenelzine, tranylcypromine), and other antidepressants (e.g., bupropion, maprotiline, nefazodone, trazodone, vilazodone). Most clinical studies have shown that the antidepressant effect of usual dosages of citalopram in patients with depression is greater than that of placebo and comparable to that of usual dosages of tricyclic antidepressants (e.g., amitriptyline, imipramine, clomipramine), other SSRIs (e.g., fluoxetine, fluvoxamine, paroxetine, sertraline), and other antidepressants (e.g., mirtazapine, venlafaxine). Escitalopram, the active *S*-enantiomer of citalopram, also is commercially available for the treatment of depression. Although there is some evidence that escitalopram may offer some clinical advantages compared with citalopram or other SSRIs (e.g., increased efficacy, more rapid onset of therapeutic effect, fewer adverse effects), additional studies are needed to confirm these initial findings. The onset of antidepressant action of citalopram appears to be comparable to that of tricyclic antidepressants and other SSRIs, although there is some evidence that the onset of action may occur slightly earlier with citalopram than with some other antidepressants, including sertraline. However, additional study is needed to confirm these findings.

In general, response rates in patients with major depression are similar for currently available antidepressants, and the choice of antidepressant agent for a given patient depends principally on other factors such as potential adverse effects, safety or tolerability of these adverse effects in the individual patient, psychiatric and medical history, patient or family history of response to specific therapies, patient preference, quantity and quality of available clinical data, cost, and relative acute overdose safety. No single antidepressant can be recommended as optimal for all patients because of substantial heterogeneity in individual responses and in the nature, likelihood, and severity of adverse effects. In addition, patients vary in the degree to which certain adverse effects and other inconveniences of drug therapy (e.g., cost, dietary restrictions) affect their preferences.

In the large-scale Sequenced Treatment Alternatives to Relieve Depression (STAR*D) effectiveness trial, patients with major depressive disorder who did not respond to or could not tolerate citalopram therapy were randomized to switch to extended-release ("sustained-release") bupropion, sertraline, or extended-release venlafaxine as a second step of treatment (level 2). Remission rates as assessed by the 17-item Hamilton Rating Scale for Depression (HRSD-17) and the Quick Inventory of Depressive Symptomatology—Self Report (QIDS-SR-16) were approximately 21 and 26% for extended-release bupropion, 18 and 27% for sertraline, and 25 and 25% for extended-release venlafaxine therapy, respectively; response rates as assessed by the QIDS-SR-16 were 26, 27, and 28% for extended-release bupropion, sertraline, and extended-release venlafaxine therapy, respectively. These results suggest that after unsuccessful initial treatment of depressed patients with an SSRI, approximately 25% of patients will achieve remission after therapy is switched to another antidepressant, and either another SSRI (e.g., sertraline) or an agent from another class (e.g., bupropion, venlafaxine) may be reasonable alternative antidepressants in patients not responding to initial SSRI therapy.

Patient Tolerance Considerations. Because of differences in the adverse effect profile between selective serotonin-reuptake inhibitors and tricyclic antidepressants, particularly less frequent anticholinergic effects, cardiovascular effects, and/or weight gain with selective serotonin-reuptake inhibitors, these drugs may be preferred in patients in whom such effects are not tolerated or are of potential concern. The decreased incidence of anticholinergic effects associated with citalopram and other selective serotonin-reuptake inhibitors compared with tricyclic antidepressants is a potential advantage, since such effects may result in discontinuance of the drug early during therapy in unusually sensitive patients. In addition, some anticholinergic effects may become troublesome during long-term tricyclic antidepressant therapy (e.g., persistent dry mouth may result in tooth decay). Although selective serotonin-reuptake inhibitors share the same overall tolerability profile, certain patients may tolerate one drug in this class better than another. Antidepressants other than selective serotonin-reuptake inhibitors may be preferred in patients in whom certain adverse GI effects (e.g., nausea, anorexia), nervous system effects (e.g., anxiety, nervousness, insomnia), and/or weight loss are not tolerated or are of concern, since such effects appear to occur more frequently with citalopram and other drugs in this class.

Pediatric Considerations. The clinical presentation of depression in children and adolescents† can differ from that in adults and generally varies with the age and developmental stages of the child. Younger children may exhibit behavioral problems such as social withdrawal, aggressive behavior, apathy, sleep disruption, and weight loss; adolescents may present with somatic complaints, self-esteem problems, rebelliousness, poor performance in school, or a pattern of engaging in risky or aggressive behavior.

Only limited data are available to date from controlled clinical studies evaluating various antidepressant agents in children and adolescents, and many of these studies have methodologic limitations (e.g., nonrandomized or uncontrolled, small sample size, short duration, nonspecific inclusion criteria). However, there is some evidence that the response to antidepressants in pediatric patients may differ from that seen in adults, and caution should be used in extrapolating data from adult studies when making treatment decisions for pediatric patients.

Results of several studies evaluating tricyclic antidepressants (e.g., amitriptyline, desipramine, imipramine, nortriptyline) in preadolescent and adolescent patients with major depression indicate a lack of overall efficacy in this age group. Based on the lack of efficacy data regarding use of tricyclic antidepressants and MAO inhibitors in pediatric patients and because of the potential for life-threatening adverse effects associated with the use of these drugs, many experts consider selective serotonin-reuptake inhibitors, including citalopram, the drugs of choice when antidepressant therapy is indicated for the treatment of major depressive disorder in children and adolescents. However, the US Food and Drug Administration (FDA) states that, while efficacy of fluoxetine has been established in pediatric patients, efficacy of other newer antidepressants (i.e., citalopram, desvenlafaxine, duloxetine, escitalopram, fluvoxamine, mirtazapine, nefazodone, paroxetine, sertraline, venlafaxine) was not conclusively established in clinical trials in pediatric patients with major depressive disorder. In addition, FDA now warns that antidepressants increase the risk of suicidal thinking and behavior (suicidality) in children and adolescents with major depressive disorder and other psychiatric disorders. (See Cautions: Pediatric Precautions.) FDA currently states that anyone considering using an antidepressant in a child or adolescent for any clinical use must balance the potential risk of therapy with the clinical need. (See Cautions: Precautions and Contraindications.)

Geriatric Considerations. The response to antidepressants in depressed geriatric patients without dementia is similar to that reported in younger adults, but depression in geriatric patients often is not recognized and is not treated. In geriatric patients with major depressive disorder, SSRIs appear to be as effective as tricyclic antidepressants but may cause fewer overall adverse effects than these other agents. Geriatric patients appear to be especially sensitive to anticholinergic (e.g., dry mouth, constipation, vision disturbance), cardiovascular, orthostatic hypotensive, and sedative effects of tricyclic antidepressants. The low incidence of anticholinergic effects associated with citalopram and other SSRIs compared with tricyclic antidepressants is a potential advantage in geriatric patients, since such effects (e.g., constipation, dry mouth, confusion, memory impairment) may be particularly troublesome in these patients. However, SSRI therapy may be associated with other troublesome adverse effects (e.g., nausea and vomiting, agitation and akathisia, parkinsonian adverse effects, sexual dysfunction, weight loss, and hyponatremia). Some clinicians state that SSRIs including citalopram may be preferred for treating depression in geriatric patients in whom the orthostatic hypotension associated with many antidepressants (e.g., tricyclics) potentially may result ininjuries (such as severe falls). However, despite the fewer cardiovascular and anticholinergic effects associated with SSRIs, these drugs did not show any advantage over tricyclic antidepressants with regard to hip fracture in a case-control study. In addition, there was little difference in the rates of falls between nursing home residents receiving SSRIs and those receiving tricyclic antidepressants in a retrospective study. Therefore, all geriatric patients receiving either type of antidepressant should be considered at increased risk of falls and appropriate measures should be taken. In addition, clinicians prescribing SSRIs in geriatric patients should be aware of the many possible drug interactions associated with these drugs, including those involving metabolism of the drugs through the cytochrome P-450 system. (See Drug Interactions.)

Patients with dementia of the Alzheimer's type (Alzheimer's disease, presenile or senile dementia) often present with depressive symptoms, such as depressed mood, appetite loss, insomnia, fatigue, irritability, and agitation. Most experts recommend that patients with dementia of the Alzheimer's type who present with clinically significant and persistent depressive symptoms be considered as candidates for pharmacotherapy even if they fail to meet the criteria for a major depressive syndrome. The goals of such therapy are to improve mood, functional status (e.g., cognition), and quality of life. Treatment of depression also may reduce other neuropsychiatric symptoms associated with depression in patients with dementia, including aggression, anxiety, apathy, and psychosis. Although patients may present with depressed mood alone, the possibility of more extensive depressive symptomatology should be considered. Therefore, patients should be evaluated and monitored carefully for indices of major depression, suicidal ideation, and neurovegetative signs since safety measures (e.g., hospitalization for suicidal ideations) and more vigorous and aggressive therapy (e.g., relatively high dosages, multiple drug trials) may be needed in some patients.

Although placebo-controlled trials of antidepressants in depressed patients with concurrent dementia have shown mixed results, the available evidence and experience with the use of antidepressants in patients with dementia of the Alzheimer's type and associated depressive manifestations indicate that depressive symptoms (including depressed mood alone and with neurovegetative changes) in such patients are responsive to antidepressant therapy. In some patients, cognitive deficits may partially or fully resolve during antidepressant therapy, but the extent of response will be limited to the degree of cognitive impairment that is directly related to depression. SSRIs such as citalopram, escitalopram, fluoxetine, paroxetine, or sertraline generally are considered first-line agents in the treatment of depressed patients with dementia since they usually are better tolerated than some other antidepressants (e.g., tricyclic antidepressants, monoamine oxidase inhibitors). Some possible alternative agents to SSRIs include bupropion, mirtazapine, and venlafaxine. Some geriatric patients with dementia and depression may be unable to tolerate the antidepressant dosages needed to achieve full remission. When a rapid antidepressant response is not critical, some experts therefore recommend a very gradual dosage titration to increase the likelihood that a therapeutic dosage of the SSRI or other antidepressant will be reached and tolerated. In a controlled study comparing citalopram and placebo in elderly patients with dementia, citalopram was found to improve depression as well as cognitive and emotional functioning more than placebo. In an open study in a limited number of patients with dementia and behavioral disturbances, citalopram was found to improve the behavioral complications associated with dementia†.

Cardiovascular Considerations. Clinical studies of citalopram for the management of depression generally did not include individuals with cardiovascular disease (e.g., those with a recent history of myocardial infarction or unstable cardiovascular disease).

Citalopram causes dose-dependent QT_c-interval prolongation, and torsades de pointes, ventricular tachycardia, and sudden death have been reported in postmarketing experience in patients receiving the drug. Patients with congenital long QT syndrome, uncompensated heart failure, bradyarrhythmias, recent acute myocardial infarction, or hypokalemia or hypomagnesemia or who are receiving other drugs that prolong the QT interval are at higher risk of developing torsades de pointes. (See Cautions: Cardiovascular Effects, Cautions: Precautions and Contraindications, and Drug Interactions: Drugs that Prolong the QT Interval.)

Sedative Considerations. Because citalopram and other selective serotonin-reuptake inhibitors generally are less sedating than some other antidepressants (e.g., tricyclics), some clinicians state that these drugs may be preferable in patients who do not require the sedative effects associated with many antidepressant agents or in patients who are prone to accidents; however, an antidepressant with more prominent sedative effects (e.g., trazodone) may be preferable in certain patients (e.g., those with insomnia).

Suicidal Risk Considerations. Suicide is a known risk of depression and certain other psychiatric disorders, and these disorders themselves are the strongest predictors of suicide. However, there has been a long-standing concern that antidepressants may have a role in inducing worsening of depression and the emergence of suicidal thinking and behavior (suicidality) in certain patients during the early phases of treatment. FDA states that antidepressants increased the risk of suicidality in short-term studies in children, adolescents, and young adults (18–24 years of age) with major depressive disorder and other psychiatric disorders. (See Cautions: Pediatric Precautions.) An increased suicidality risk was not demonstrated with antidepressants compared with placebo in adults older than 24 years of age and a reduced risk was observed in adults 65 years of age or older. It currently is unknown whether the suicidality risk extends to longer-term antidepressant use (i.e., beyond several months); however, there is substantial evidence from placebo-controlled maintenance trials in adults with major depressive disorder that antidepressants can delay the recurrence of depression. Because the risk of suicidality in depressed patients may persist until substantial remission of depression occurs, appropriate monitoring and close observation of patients of all ages who are receiving antidepressant therapy are recommended. (See Cautions: Precautions and Contraindications.)

Other Considerations. Citalopram has been effective in patients with moderate to severe depression, endogenous depression, post-stroke depression and pathologic crying, and depression associated with chronic hepatitis C virus infection.

In an open study in a limited number of patients with bipolar depression† (mainly bipolar I disorder), citalopram was effective and well tolerated when added to monotherapy or combined therapy with lithium, divalproex sodium, and/or carbamazepine. Controlled studies are needed to confirm these preliminary findings. The manufacturer states that citalopram is *not* approved for use in treating bipolar depression, and that the possibility that the drug may precipitate hypomanic or manic attacks in patients with bipolar or other major affective disorder should be considered. For detailed information on bipolar disorder, including its management, see Uses: Bipolar Disorder, in Lithium Salts 28:28.

In patients with refractory depression, citalopram was more effective when given in combination with buspirone in one placebo-controlled study. However, combined citalopram and buspirone therapy was not found to be more effective than citalopram monotherapy in another placebo-controlled study. In the Sequenced Treatment Alternatives to Relieve Depression (STAR*D) level 2 trial, patients with major depressive disorder who did not respond to or could not tolerate citalopram therapy were randomized to receive either extended-release ("sustained-release") bupropion or buspirone therapy in addition to citalopram. Although both extended-release bupropion and buspirone were found to produce similar remission rates, extended-release bupropion produced a greater reduction in the number and severity of symptoms and a lower rate of drug discontinuance than buspirone in this large-scale effectiveness trial. These results suggest that augmentation of SSRI therapy with extended-release bupropion may be useful in some patients with refractory depression. The addition of lithium to citalopram in depressed patients not responding to citalopram alone also has been found to be effective and well tolerated in a double-blind, placebo-controlled trial. (See Drug Interactions: Lithium.)

In a limited number of depressed patients not responding to citalopram alone, the addition of carbamazepine was effective and well tolerated in an open study. However, the possibility of serotonin syndrome and drug interactions should be considered pending further clinical experience with this combination. (See Drug Interactions: Serotonergic Drugs and Carbamazepine under Drug Interactions: Drugs Undergoing Hepatic Metabolism or Affecting Hepatic Microsomal Enzymes.)

Citalopram was found to improve personality disturbances† (decrease in anxiety and aggression-related symptoms and increase in social desirability and socialization) in depressed patients in one study.

■ **Obsessive-Compulsive Disorder** Citalopram has been used in the treatment of obsessive-compulsive disorder†. In a large, double-blind, placebo-controlled trial evaluating citalopram (20, 40, or 60 mg daily for 12 weeks) in adults with obsessive-compulsive disorder, the drug was more effective than placebo as measured by Yale-Brown Obsessive-Compulsive Scale score changes at all 3 dosages. The highest response rate (65%) was observed in those who received 60 mg daily; this compared with 52 or 57% in those receiving 40 or 20 mg daily, respectively. An analysis of predictors of response to citalopram therapy from this trial suggested that patients with a longer duration of obsessive-compulsive disorder, more severe symptoms, or a history of previous selective serotonin-reuptake inhibitor therapy were less likely to respond to therapy with citalopram. In an open trial, 76% of patients with obsessive-compulsive disorder receiving citalopram therapy (usually 40 or 60 mg daily) for 24 weeks demonstrated improved symptoms associated with this condition. In another open study, citalopram (40 mg daily) was effective in a limited number of patients with refractory obsessive-compulsive disorder who had failed to respond to therapy with other selective serotonin-reuptake inhibitors. Clinical experience to date indicates that citalopram is well tolerated in patients with obsessive-compulsive disorder. Additional study is needed to determine the long-term efficacy of citalopram in the treatment of this condition.

For additional information on the use of selective serotonin-reuptake inhibitors in the treatment of obsessive-compulsive disorder, see Uses: Obsessive-Compulsive Disorder, in Sertraline Hydrochloride 28:16.04.20.

■ **Panic Disorder** Citalopram has been used in the treatment of panic disorder with or without agoraphobia†. In a randomized, single-blind study comparing citalopram and paroxetine in adults with panic disorder, both drugs were found to be effective and well tolerated, with 86% of the citalopram-treated patients and 84% of the paroxetine-treated patients responding well to 2 months of therapy. In a limited number of adults with panic disorder, citalopram therapy (20–60 mg daily) produced a full remission in 66% of the patients and improved symptomatology.

In a large, double-blind, placebo-controlled trial evaluating the efficacy and tolerability of long-term therapy (up to 1 year) with citalopram at 3 dosages (10–15 mg daily, 20–30 mg daily, 40–60 mg daily) or clomipramine in adult outpatients with panic disorder with or without agoraphobia, both drugs were more effective than placebo. Citalopram was more effective than placebo at all dosages studied, with a dosage of 20–30 mg daily being the most effective maintenance dosage in most patients.

For additional information on the use of selective serotonin-reuptake inhibitors in the treatment of panic disorder, see Uses: Panic Disorder, in Sertraline Hydrochloride 28:16.04.20.

■ **Social Phobia** Like some other selective serotonin-reuptake inhibitors, citalopram has been used in the treatment of social phobia† (social anxiety disorder). However, additional evidence from well-designed studies is needed to more fully elucidate the role of the drug in this disorder.

In an open study in a limited number of patients with social phobia, 86% of patients responded to citalopram 40 mg daily after 12 weeks as rated by the Clinical Global Impressions (CGI) score and the Liebowitz Social Anxiety Scale (LSAS).

In an open, flexible-dose study in patients with social anxiety disorder with comorbid major depression, response rates after 12 weeks of citalopram therapy (mean dosage: 38 mg daily) were approximately 67 and 76% for social anxiety disorder and depression, respectively. However, the depression symptoms responded more rapidly and completely than the social anxiety symptoms after 12 weeks of citalopram therapy, suggesting that a longer duration of therapy may be necessary to fully assess the clinical efficacy of the drug in such patients.

In a randomized, open trial comparing citalopram and moclobemide (not commercially available in the US) in patients with social phobia, similar improvements in the CGI-improvement score and LSAS were noted with these drugs. Clinical experience to date suggests that citalopram generally is well tolerated in patients with social phobia. However, well controlled studies are needed to confirm the efficacy and safety and to determine the optimal dosage of citalopram in patients with this condition.

■ **Alcohol Dependence** Like some other selective serotonin-reuptake inhibitors (fluoxetine, zimelidine [not commercially available in the US]), citalopram has been used in the management of alcohol dependence†. In clinical studies, citalopram has been shown to reduce alcohol consumption in alcohol-dependent, nondepressed drinkers receiving short-term therapy with 40 mg of the drug daily. In clinical studies conducted to date with selective serotonin-reuptake inhibitors in alcoholic patients, considerable interindividual variability in response has been observed, with reduction in alcohol consumption ranging from 10 to more than 70%. Several factors, including gender, alcoholic subtype, presence or absence of depression, and extent of drinking, appear to affect the clinical efficacy of selective serotonin-reuptake inhibitors in the management of alcohol dependence. Additional study is required to fully determine the safety and efficacy of citalopram in the management of alcohol dependence. (See Pharmacology: Effects on Alcohol Intake and also see Drug Interactions: Alcohol.)

■ **Premenstrual Dysphoric Disorder** Like some other selective serotonin-reuptake inhibitors (e.g., fluoxetine, paroxetine, sertraline), citalopram has been used in a limited number of women with premenstrual dysphoric disorder† (previously late luteal phase dysphoric disorder). Clinical experience to date suggests that the onset of action of serotonin-reuptake inhibitors in women with premenstrual dysphoric disorder is more rapid than when used for other psychiatric conditions; therefore, administration only during the luteal phase of the menstrual cycle may potentially be effective in this condition.

In a placebo-controlled trial, intermittent administration of citalopram (10–30 mg daily during the luteal phase) for 3 menstrual cycles appeared to be more effective than continuous (10–30 mg daily throughout the menstrual cycle) or semi-intermittent administration (5 mg daily during the follicular phase and 10–30 mg daily during the luteal phase) of the drug and substantially more effective than placebo. Citalopram was well tolerated in all 3 regimens, and adverse effects generally were mild and transient. Additional controlled studies are needed to determine whether the efficacy of the drug is sustained during longer-term, maintenance therapy in women with this condition.

■ **Premature Ejaculation** Like some other selective serotonin-reuptake inhibitors, citalopram has been used for the treatment of premature ejaculation†. However, studies with citalopram to date have only involved a limited number of patients and there is some evidence that the drug may be less effective than certain other selective serotonin-reuptake inhibitors (e.g., paroxetine). In a double-blind study in men with premature ejaculation, citalopram 20 mg daily delayed ejaculation to a slight degree (1. 8-fold increase in intravaginal ejaculation latency time) compared with a marked increase (8. 9-fold increase) with paroxetine 20 mg daily following 6 weeks of therapy. These preliminary findings suggest that paroxetine may be more effective than citalopram in the treatment of premature ejaculation.

■ **Eating Disorders** Citalopram has been used in a limited number of patients for the treatment of bulimia nervosa† or anorexia nervosa†. Although citalopram reportedly has been effective in some patients with these eating disorders, underweight patients with anorexia nervosa who received citalopram in conjunction with psychotherapy did worse (i.e., experienced greater weight loss) than those receiving psychotherapy alone in one open-label study. Because of limited evidence and experience to date, the role if any of citalopram in the management of eating disorders remains to be elucidated. For information on the use of selective serotonin-reuptake inhibitors in the treatment of eating disorders, see Uses: Eating Disorders, in Fluoxetine Hydrochloride 28:16.04.20.

■ **Diabetic Neuropathy** Tricyclic antidepressants generally have been considered a mainstay of therapy for the treatment of diabetic neuropathy. However, because of potentially improved patient tolerability, therapy with selective serotonin-reuptake inhibitors or selective serotonin- and norepinephrine-reuptake inhibitors (e.g., duloxetine, venlafaxine) has been attempted as an alternative. In a double-blind, placebo-controlled trial, citalopram (40 mg daily) substantially reduced the symptoms associated with diabetic neuropathy† (pain, paresthesia, and dysesthesia) in a limited number of patients and generally was well tolerated. When compared with earlier results obtained with imipramine in the management of this condition, selective serotonin-reuptake inhibitors such as citalopram, fluoxetine, paroxetine, and sertraline appear to be less effective but better tolerated overall. Additional study and experience are needed to elucidate the relative roles of selective serotonin-reuptake inhibitors versus tricyclic antidepressants, selective serotonin- and norepinephrine-reuptake inhibitors, anticonvulsants (e.g., pregabalin, gabapentin), and other forms of treatment in the management of this condition.

■ **Posttraumatic Stress Disorder** Citalopram has been used in a limited number of adults with civilian- or combat-related posttraumatic stress disorder† (PTSD). In an open study, patients treated with citalopram for 8 weeks showed marked improvement in PTSD manifestations (reexperiencing, hyperarousal, and avoidance) as well as in depression and anxiety. Well-designed, controlled studies are needed to confirm these preliminary findings.

For additional information on the use of selective serotonin-reuptake inhibitors in the treatment of PTSD, see Uses: Posttraumatic Stress Disorder, in Prazosin Hydrochloride 24:20, Paroxetine 28:16.04.20, and Sertraline Hydrochloride 28:16.04.20.

Dosage and Administration

■ **Administration** Citalopram hydrobromide is administered orally. Citalopram also has been administered by IV infusion†, but a parenteral dosage form is not commercially available in the US.

Citalopram usually is administered once daily in the morning or evening. Since food does not substantially affect the absorption of citalopram, the drug may be administered without regard to meals.

Hypokalemia and hypomagnesemia, if present, should be corrected prior to initiation of citalopram therapy and electrolytes should be monitored periodically during therapy as needed. (See Cautions: Cardiovascular Effects and also see Cautions: Precautions and Contraindications.)

Dispensing and Administration Precautions Because of similarity in spelling of Celexa® (citalopram hydrobromide), Celebrex® (celecoxib), and Cerebyx® (fosphenytoin sodium), extra care should be exercised in ensuring the accuracy of prescriptions for these drugs.

■ **Dosage** Dosage of citalopram hydrobromide is expressed in terms of citalopram.

Patients receiving citalopram should be monitored for possible worsening of depression, suicidality, or unusual changes in behavior, especially at the beginning of therapy or during periods of dosage adjustment. (See Cautions: Precautions and Contraindications.)

The manufacturers state that at least 2 weeks must elapse between discontinuance of a monoamine oxidase (MAO) inhibitor intended to treat psychiatric disorders and initiation of citalopram therapy and that at least 2 weeks must elapse between discontinuance of citalopram and initiation of MAO inhibitor therapy intended to treat psychiatric disorders. For additional information on potentially serious drug interactions that may occur between citalopram and MAO inhibitors or other serotonergic agents, see Cautions: Precautions and Contraindications and also see Drug Interactions: Serotonergic Drugs.

Because withdrawal effects may occur with discontinuance of citalopram, other selective serotonin-reuptake inhibitors (SSRIs), and selective serotonin- and norepinephrine-reuptake inhibitors (SNRIs), abrupt discontinuance of these drugs should be avoided whenever possible. When citalopram therapy is discontinued, the dosage should be reduced gradually (e.g., over a period of several weeks) and the patient monitored for possible withdrawal symptoms. If intolerable symptoms occur following a dosage reduction or upon discontinuance of therapy, the drug may be reinstituted at the previously prescribed dosage. Subsequently, the clinician may continue decreasing the dosage, but at a more gradual rate. (See Cautions: Nervous System Effects and see Chronic Toxicity.)

Major Depressive Disorder For the management of major depressive disorder in adults, the recommended initial dosage of citalopram is 20 mg once daily, with an increase to a maximum dosage of 40 mg once daily at an interval of not less than 1 week. Previously, the prescribing information for citalopram stated that certain patients may require a dosage of 60 mg daily. However, *citalopram dosages above 40 mg once daily no longer are recommended because of the risk of QT-interval prolongation* (see Cautions: Cardiovascular Effects and see also Cautions: Precautions and Contraindications) and because they provide no additional therapeutic benefit. A dose-response study did not show the 60-mg daily dosage to be more effective than the 40-mg daily dosage overall. Although antidepressant effects may be evident within 1 week in some patients, the full antidepressant effect of citalopram may not be observed for several weeks.

While the optimum duration of citalopram therapy has not been established, many experts state that acute depressive episodes require several months or longer of sustained antidepressant therapy. In addition, some clinicians recommend that long-term antidepressant therapy be considered in certain patients at risk for recurrence of depressive episodes (such as those with highly recurrent unipolar depression). Whether the dosage of citalopram required to induce remission is identical to the dosage needed to maintain and/or sustain euthymia is unknown. In placebo-controlled studies, the antidepressant efficacy of citalopram was maintained for up to 8 months in patients receiving 20–60 mg daily. In addition, the drug has been used in some patients for longer periods (e.g., up to 28 months) without apparent loss of clinical effect or increased toxicity.

If troublesome adverse effects occur during maintenance therapy, the manufacturer states that a decrease in dosage to 20 mg daily can be considered. If citalopram is used for extended periods, the need for continued therapy should be reassessed periodically.

Obsessive-Compulsive Disorder For the management of obsessive-compulsive disorder† in adults, citalopram usually has been given orally in an initial dosage of 20 mg daily and the dosage was then gradually increased according to clinical response. The usual maintenance dosage in adults has been 40 or 60 mg daily; however, citalopram dosages exceeding 40 mg daily no longer are recommended due to the risk of QT prolongation.

Panic Disorder For the management of panic disorder† in adults, the usual initial dosage of citalopram is 10 mg daily. After an interval of at least 1 week, the dosage may be gradually increased in increments of 10–20 mg up to a dosage of 20–40 mg daily, depending on individual patient response and tolerability. The usual maintenance dosage in adults has been 20–30 mg daily. Citalopram dosages exceeding 40 mg daily no longer are recommended due to the risk of QT prolongation.

■ **Dosage in Geriatric Patients** ***Major Depressive Disorder*** For the management of depression in geriatric patients over 60 years of age, the maximum recommended citalopram dosage is 20 mg once daily due to the risk of QT-interval prolongation. (See Cautions: Cardiovascular Effects.)

For the management of depressive symptoms associated with dementia of the Alzheimer's type in geriatric patients, some experts recommend a lower initial citalopram dosage of 5–10 mg once daily. The dosage may then be gradually increased at intervals of at least several weeks up to the maximum recommended dosage of 20 mg once daily.

■ **Dosage in Hepatic and Renal Impairment** In depressed patients with hepatic impairment, the maximum recommended citalopram dosage is 20 mg once daily due to the risk of QT-interval prolongation. (See Cautions: Cardiovascular Effects and also see Pharmacokinetics: Elimination.)

Dosage adjustment is not necessary in depressed patients with mild to moderate renal impairment. Severe renal failure did not substantially affect the pharmacokinetics of citalopram in one study, suggesting that dosage adjustment also may be unnecessary in patients with severe renal impairment. However, the manufacturer recommends that the drug be used with caution in patients with severe renal impairment. (See Pharmacokinetics: Elimination.)

■ **Dosage in Poor CYP2C19 Metabolizers or Patients Receiving CYP2C19 Inhibitors** For the management of major depressive disorder in patients who are poor metabolizers of the cytochrome P-450 (CYP) isoenzyme 2C19 and in patients receiving cimetidine or another CYP2C19 inhibitor, the maximum recommended dosage of citalopram is 20 mg once daily due to the risk of QT-interval prolongation. (See CYP2C19 Inhibitors under Drug Interactions: Drugs Undergoing Hepatic Metabolism or Affecting Hepatic Microsomal Enzymes and see also Pharmacokinetics: Elimination.)

■ **Treatment of Pregnant Women during the Third Trimester** Some neonates exposed to citalopram and other SSRIs or SNRIs late in the third trimester of pregnancy have developed severe complications. When treating pregnant women with citalopram during the third trimester, the clinician should carefully consider the potential risks and benefits of therapy. (See Pregnancy under Cautions: Pregnancy, Fertility, and Lactation.)

Cautions

The adverse effect profile of citalopram is similar to that of other selective serotonin-reuptake inhibitors (SSRIs) (e.g., escitalopram, fluoxetine, fluvoxamine, paroxetine, sertraline). Because citalopram is a highly selective serotonin-reuptake inhibitor with little or no effect on other neurotransmitters, the incidence of some adverse effects commonly associated with tricyclic antidepressants, such as anticholinergic effects (e.g., dry mouth, constipation), certain cardiovascular effects (e.g., orthostatic hypotension), drowsiness, and weight gain, is lower in patients receiving citalopram. However, certain adverse GI (e.g., nausea, anorexia), nervous system (e.g., somnolence, anxiety, nervousness, insomnia), and sexual function effects appear to occur more frequently with citalopram and other SSRIs than with tricyclic antidepressants.

In controlled studies, the most common adverse effects occurring more frequently in patients receiving citalopram than in those receiving placebo included nervous system effects such as somnolence, insomnia, anxiety, agitation, fatigue, tremor, and yawning; GI effects such as nausea, dry mouth, diarrhea, dyspepsia, anorexia, vomiting, and abdominal pain; sweating; ejaculation dysfunction (principally ejaculation delay) and impotence in male patients, decreased libido, and dysmenorrhea; fever, arthralgia, and myalgia; and upper respiratory tract infection, rhinitis, and sinusitis.

The results of a fixed-dose clinical study in depressed patients suggest that somnolence, insomnia, increased sweating, fatigue, impotence, and yawning are dose-related adverse effects of citalopram.

In short-term, placebo-controlled trials (6 weeks or less), discontinuance of citalopram therapy was required in approximately 16% of depressed patients, principally because of adverse psychiatric (e.g., insomnia, somnolence, agitation), other nervous system (e.g., dizziness, asthenia), or GI (e.g., nausea, vomiting, dry mouth) effects.

■ **Nervous System Effects** Somnolence and insomnia, which appear to be dose related, are the most common adverse nervous system effects of citalopram, occurring in approximately 18 and 15% of depressed patients, respectively, receiving the drug and in approximately 10 and 14% of those receiving placebo, respectively, in short-term controlled clinical trials. Insomnia or somnolence required discontinuance of therapy in about 3 or 2% of patients, respectively. However, because insomnia is a symptom also associated with depression, relief of insomnia and improvement in sleep patterns may occur when clinical improvement in depression becomes apparent during antidepressant therapy. Sleep disorders have been reported in at least 2% of citalopram-treated patients in clinical trials, although a causal relationship to the drug has not been established.

Fatigue, which appeared to be dose related, occurred in approximately 5% of patients receiving citalopram in short-term clinical studies. Asthenia has been reported in at least 2% of citalopram-treated patients in clinical trials and required discontinuance of therapy in about 1% of patients.

Tremor occurred in about 8%, anxiety in about 4%, and agitation in about 3% of patients receiving citalopram in short-term clinical studies; agitation resulted in discontinuance of therapy in about 1% of patients receiving the drug. Nervousness, headache, yawning, and dizziness have been reported in at least 2% of citalopram-treated patients in clinical trials. Yawning appeared to be dose related. Dizziness required discontinuance of therapy in 2% of patients.

Impaired concentration, amnesia, apathy, depression and aggravated depression, confusion, paresthesia, and migraine each have been reported in at least 1% of patients receiving citalopram; however, these adverse effects have not been definitely attributed to the drug.

Adverse nervous system effects reported in at least 0.1% of patients receiving citalopram include aggressive reaction, paroniria (disagreeable or terrifying dreams), depersonalization, hallucinations, euphoria, psychotic depression, delusion, paranoid reaction, emotional lability, panic reaction, psychosis, vertigo, neuralgia, abnormal gait, hyperkinesia, hypertonia, hypoesthesia, and ataxia; a causal relationship to the drug has not been clearly established.

Seizures occurred in 0.3% of patients receiving citalopram and in 0.5% of patients receiving placebo in clinical studies. A causal relationship to citalopram remains to be established in these cases. (See Cautions: Precautions and Contraindications.) Nonconvulsive status epilepticus also has been reported in a geriatric patient receiving citalopram for poststroke depression. In addition, involuntary muscle contractions have been reported in less than 1% of patients receiving the drug.

Activation of mania and hypomania have occurred in 0.2% of depressed patients receiving citalopram in placebo-controlled trials; some of these trials included patients with bipolar disorder. In an analysis of postmarketing clinical trials, manic episodes were reported in 0.62% of unipolar depressed patients. (See Cautions: Precautions and Contraindications.) Such reactions have been reported in patients receiving other antidepressant agents and may be caused by antidepressant-induced functional increases in catecholamine activity within the CNS, resulting in a "switch" from depressive to manic behavior. There is some evidence that patients with bipolar disorder may be more likely to experience antidepressant-induced hypomanic or manic reactions than patients without evidence of this disorder. In addition, limited evidence suggests that such reactions may occur more frequently in bipolar depressed patients receiving tricyclics and tetracyclics (e.g., maprotiline, mianserin [not commercially available in the US]) than in those receiving selective serotonin-reuptake inhibitors (e.g., citalopram, escitalopram, fluoxetine, fluvoxamine, paroxetine, sertraline). However, further studies are needed to confirm these findings.

Extrapyramidal reactions associated with citalopram, which are uncommon, appear to be a class effect of selective serotonin-reuptake inhibitors and dose related. Reactions occurring early during therapy with the drug may be secondary to preexisting parkinsonian syndrome and/or concomitant therapy. Although a causal relationship to citalopram has not been established, extrapyramidal symptoms reported in at least 0.1% of patients receiving the drug include tremor, hypokinesia, and dystonia. Choreoathetosis also has been reported rarely. Pending further clinical experience, some clinicians recommend that extrapyramidal reactions developing in patients receiving selective serotonin-reuptake inhibitors be managed by reducing the dosage or discontinuing the drug; if necessary, the symptoms appear to respond to the same treatment as antipsychotic-induced extrapyramidal reactions.

Adverse nervous system effects reported in less than 0.1% of patients receiving citalopram include abnormal coordination, hyperesthesia, melancholia, catatonic reaction, and stupor. Although a causal relationship to the drug has not been established, serotonin syndrome also has been reported in patients receiving citalopram, other selective serotonin-reuptake inhibitors (SSRIs), and selective serotonin- and norepinephrine-reuptake inhibitors (SNRIs). (See Cautions: Precautions and Contraindications, Drug Interactions: Serotonergic Drugs, and see also Acute Toxicity.)

Withdrawal Reactions Withdrawal symptoms, including dysphoric mood, irritability, agitation, dizziness, sensory disturbances (e.g., paresthesias such as electric shock sensations), anxiety, confusion, headache, lethargy, emotional lability, insomnia, hypomania, tinnitus, and seizures, have been reported upon discontinuance of citalopram, other SSRIs, and SNRIs, particularly when discontinuance of these drugs is abrupt. While these reactions are generally self-limiting, there have been reports of serious discontinuance symptoms. Therefore, patients should be monitored for such symptoms when discontinuing citalopram therapy. A gradual reduction in the dosage rather than abrupt cessation is recommended whenever possible. (See Dosage and Administration: Dosage.)

Withdrawal reactions have been reported rarely in citalopram-treated patients following discontinuance of the drug. Data from a controlled study evaluating citalopram in preventing depression relapse suggest that the symptoms associated with abrupt discontinuance of therapy generally are mild and transient. Overall clinical experience to date suggests that the risk of withdrawal effects may be somewhat lower with citalopram, fluoxetine, and sertraline compared with paroxetine. These differences may be due at least in part to the prolonged elimination half-lives of the parent drugs and/or their active metabolites. In addition, drug dependence has been reported in at least 0.1% of patients receiving citalopram, although a causal relationship to the drug remains to be established. (See Chronic Toxicity.)

Suicidality Suicide and suicide attempts have been reported in less than 1% of depressed adults receiving citalopram. The US Food and Drug Administration (FDA) has determined that antidepressants increase the risk of suicidal thinking and behavior (suicidality) in children, adolescents, and young adults (18–24 years of age) with major depressive disorder and other psychiatric disorders. Patients, therefore, should be appropriately monitored and closely observed for clinical worsening, suicidality, and unusual changes in behavior, particularly during initiation of citalopram therapy (i.e., the first few months) and during periods of dosage adjustments. (See Cautions: Precautions and Contraindications, see Cautions: Pediatric Precautions, and see also Acute Toxicity.)

■ **GI Effects** Like other selective serotonin-reuptake inhibitors (e.g., escitalopram, fluoxetine, fluvoxamine, paroxetine, sertraline), citalopram therapy is associated with a relatively high incidence of GI disturbances, principally nausea, dry mouth, diarrhea, dyspepsia, anorexia, vomiting, and abdominal pain. The most frequent adverse GI effect associated with citalopram therapy is nausea, which occurred in about 21% of patients receiving the drug in controlled clinical trials. Nausea generally is mild to moderate in severity. In clinical trials, nausea required discontinuance of citalopram in about 4% of patients and was the most frequent adverse effect requiring discontinuance of the drug. While the mechanism(s) of citalopram-induced GI effects has not been fully elucidated, such effects appear to arise at least in part because of increased serotonergic activity in the GI tract (which may result in stimulation of small intestine motility and inhibition of gastric and large intestine motility) and possibly because of the drug's effect on central serotonergic type 3 ($5-HT_3$) receptors.

Dry mouth occurred in about 20%, diarrhea in about 8%, and dyspepsia in about 5% of patients receiving citalopram in short-term controlled clinical trials. Other adverse GI effects associated with citalopram therapy include vomiting and anorexia, which both occurred in 4% of patients, and abdominal pain, which occurred in about 3% of patients receiving the drug in short-term controlled clinical trials. Vomiting and dry mouth each resulted in discontinuance of citalopram in about 1% of patients. Constipation was reported in at least 2% of citalopram-treated patients in clinical trials.

As with some other selective serotonin-reuptake inhibitors, bruxism (involuntary clenching or grinding of the teeth) has been reported in at least 0.1% of patients receiving citalopram. The cases of bruxism reported to date with citalopram and other serotonin-reuptake inhibitors suggest that bruxism may be dose dependent and that buspirone therapy may be helpful in relieving this symptom.

Although a causal relationship to citalopram has not been established, increased salivation and flatulence have been reported in at least 1% of patients receiving the drug. Gastritis, gastroenteritis, stomatitis, eructation, hemorrhoids, dysphagia, gingivitis, and esophagitis have been reported in at least 0.1% of patients receiving citalopram. However, a causal relationship to the drug has not been established for these effects.

Epidemiologic case-control and cohort design studies have suggested that selective serotonin-reuptake inhibitors may increase the risk of upper GI bleeding. Although the precise mechanism for this increased risk remains to be clearly established, serotonin release by platelets is known to play an important role in hemostasis, and selective serotonin-reuptake inhibitors decrease serotonin uptake from the blood by platelets thereby decreasing the amount of serotonin in platelets. In addition, concurrent use of aspirin or other nonsteroidal anti-inflammatory agents was found to substantially increase the risk of GI bleeding in patients receiving selective serotonin-reuptake inhibitors in 2 of these studies. Although these studies focused on upper GI bleeding, there is some evidence suggesting that bleeding at other sites may be similarly potentiated. Further clinical studies are needed to determine the clinical importance of these findings. (See Cautions: Hematologic Effects and see also Drug Interactions: Drugs Affecting Hemostasis.)

Colitis, gastric ulcer, duodenal ulcer, cholecystitis, cholelithiasis, gastroesophageal reflux, glossitis, diverticulitis, and rectal hemorrhage have been reported in less than 0.1% of patients receiving citalopram. However, these adverse effects have not been definitely attributed to the drug.

■ **Dermatologic and Sensitivity Reactions** Increased sweating, which appears to be dose related, occurred in approximately 11% of patients receiving citalopram in short-term clinical studies. Rash and pruritus have been reported in at least 1% of patients receiving citalopram; however, these adverse effects have not been definitely attributed to the drug.

Photosensitivity reaction, urticaria, acne, skin discoloration, eczema, alopecia, dermatitis, dry skin, and psoriasis have been reported in less than 1% of patients receiving citalopram; however, these adverse effects have not been definitely attributed to the drug.

Hypertrichosis, decreased sweating, melanosis, keratitis, cellulitis, pruritus ani, hay fever, and facial edema have occurred in less than 0.1% of citalopram-treated patients, although a causal relationship to the drug has not been established. Allergic reactions, anaphylaxis, and angioedema also have been reported in patients receiving citalopram, although a causal relationship to the drug has not been established.

Severe adverse dermatologic effects such as erythema multiforme and epidermal necrolysis have occurred rarely in patients receiving citalopram. In addition, a case of extensive papular and purpuric erythema with keratinocytes, necrosis, and dermal leukocytoclastic vasculitis has been reported in a patient receiving citalopram; improvement occurred slowly following discontinuance of the drug.

■ **Metabolic and Endocrine Effects** Weight loss and weight gain each occurred in at least 1% of patients receiving citalopram in controlled clinical trials; obesity has occurred rarely. Increased appetite also has been reported in at least 1% of patients receiving the drug, although a causal relationship has not been established. While clinically important weight loss may occur in some patients receiving citalopram, only minimal weight loss (averaging 0.5 kg) generally occurred in patients receiving the drug in controlled clinical trials. In addition, while decreased appetite was reported in about 4% of patients receiving citalopram in short-term clinical trials, the drug, unlike fluoxetine, does not appear to exhibit clinically important anorectic effects nor to produce clinically important long-term weight changes. In addition, short-term citalopram therapy did not produce substantial weight loss in severely obese individuals in one study.

Taste perversion has occurred in more than 1% of patients, and thirst and abnormal glucose tolerance have been reported in less than 1% of citalopram-treated patients, although a causal relationship to the drug has not been established. Taste loss has been reported rarely. Adverse metabolic and endocrine effects reported in less than 0.1% of patients receiving the drug include hypoglycemia, hypothyroidism, and goiter.

■ **Ocular and Otic Effects** Vision abnormalities occurred in about 2% and abnormality of accommodation in at least 1% of patients receiving citalopram in short-term controlled clinical trials. Ocular dryness, conjunctivitis, and ocular pain have been reported in less than 1% of citalopram-treated patients, although a causal relationship to the drug has not been established. Mydriasis, photophobia, diplopia, ptosis, abnormal lacrimation, and cataract have been reported in less than 0.1% of patients receiving the drug; these adverse effects have not been definitely attributed to the drug. Angle-closure glaucoma (narrow-angle glaucoma) also has been reported in citalopram-treated patients. (See Cautions: Precautions and Contraindications.)

Tinnitus occurred in less than 1% of patients receiving citalopram; this adverse effect has not been definitely attributed to the drug.

■ **Cardiovascular Effects** Citalopram does not exhibit clinically important anticholinergic activity, and current evidence suggests that the drug generally is less cardiotoxic than many older antidepressants (e.g., tricyclic antidepressants, monoamine oxidase inhibitors) at the usual recommended dosages.

No clinically important changes in vital signs (systolic and diastolic blood pressure and heart rate) were observed in patients receiving citalopram in controlled trials.

Citalopram causes dose-dependent prolongation of the corrected QT (QT_c) interval, an ECG abnormality that has been associated with torsades de pointes, ventricular tachycardia, and sudden death, all of which have been reported in postmarketing experience in patients receiving the drug. In a study of the effects of citalopram on the QT interval, use of the drug was associated with a dose-dependent increase in the corrected QT_c interval. In this placebo-controlled study, a change from baseline in QT_cF (Fridericia's formula) greater than 60 msec occurred in 1.9% of patients receiving citalopram compared with 1.2% of patients receiving placebo. None of the patients receiving placebo had a post-dose QT_cF greater than 500 msec compared with 0.5% of patients receiving citalopram. The incidence of tachycardic and bradycardic outliers was 0.5 and 0.9% in the citalopram group, respectively, and 0.4% in the placebo group. Individually corrected QT_c (QT_cNi) interval was evaluated in a randomized, double-blind, placebo- and active-controlled, crossover study in healthy individuals. In this study, the maximum mean differences from placebo were 8.5 and 18.5 msec for daily dosages of 20 and 60 mg of citalopram, respectively. Based on these results, the predicted QT_cNi for citalopram 40 mg daily is 12.6 msec. ECG changes, including QT-interval prolongation, also have been reported in individuals receiving overdosages of the drug (more than 400–600 mg). (See Dosage and Administration: Dosage, Cautions: Precautions and Contraindications, and see also Acute Toxicity.)

Palpitation was reported in at least 2% of citalopram-treated patients in clinical trials, although a causal relationship to the drug remains to be established. A comparison of supine and standing vital signs in depressed patients receiving citalopram indicated that the drug generally does not produce orthostatic changes such as hypotension. Although postural hypotension and hypotension occurred in at least 1% of patients receiving citalopram in short-term controlled clinical trials, a causal relationship to the drug has not been established.

Tachycardia, hypertension, bradycardia, peripheral edema, syncope, angina pectoris, extrasystoles, cardiac failure, flushing and hot flushes, myocardial infarction, cerebrovascular accident, myocardial ischemia, transient ischemic attack, phlebitis, atrial fibrillation, ventricular arrhythmia, cardiac arrest, and bundle branch block have been reported in premarketing studies of citalopram or during postmarketing surveillance; these adverse effects have not been definitely attributed to the drug.

■ **Musculoskeletal Effects** Arthralgia and myalgia each occurred in about 2% of patients receiving citalopram in short-term controlled clinical trials. In addition, back pain was reported in at least 2% of citalopram-treated patients in clinical trials, although a causal relationship to the drug remains to be established.

Arthritis, muscle weakness, leg cramps, and skeletal pain have been reported in at least 0.1% of citalopram-treated patients; these adverse effects have not been definitely attributed to the drug. Bursitis and osteoporosis have been reported in less than 0.1% of patients receiving citalopram, although a causal relationship has not been established.

■ **Hematologic Effects** Purpura, anemia, leukocytosis, and leukopenia have been reported in at least 0.1% of patients receiving citalopram, although a causal relationship to the drug has not been established.

Adverse hematologic effects reported in less than 0.1% of patients receiving citalopram include pulmonary embolism, granulocytopenia, lymphocytosis, lymphopenia, hypochromic anemia, coagulation disorders, and gingival bleeding; however, a causal relationship to the drug has not been established. In addition, thrombocytopenia has been reported.

Bleeding complications (e.g., ecchymosis, purpura, menorrhagia, rectal bleeding) have been reported infrequently in patients receiving citalopram and other selective serotonin-reuptake inhibitors. Although the precise mechanism for these reactions has not been established, it has been suggested that impaired platelet aggregation and prolonged bleeding time may be due at least in part to inhibition of serotonin reuptake into platelets and/or that increased capillary fragility and vascular tone may contribute to these cases. (See Cautions: GI Effects and see also Drug Interactions: Drugs Affecting Hemostasis.)

■ **Respiratory Effects** Respiratory disorders have been reported in patients receiving citalopram in short-term controlled clinical trials. Upper respiratory tract infections and rhinitis both have been reported in about 5% of citalopram-treated patients and sinusitis has occurred in about 3% of patients receiving the drug. Yawning and pharyngitis each occurred in about 2% of patients receiving citalopram. In addition, coughing has been reported in at least 1% of citalopram-treated patients.

Adverse respiratory effects reported in at least 0.1% of patients receiving citalopram in controlled trials include bronchitis, dyspnea, epistaxis, and pneumonia; however, a causal relationship to the drug remains to be established. Other adverse effects reported in less than 0.1% of citalopram-treated patients include asthma, laryngitis, bronchospasm, pneumonitis, and increased sputum; these adverse effects have not been definitely attributed to the drug.

■ **Renal, Electrolyte, and Genitourinary Effects** ***Sexual Dysfunction*** Like other selective serotonin-reuptake inhibitors, adverse effects on sexual function have been reported in both men and women receiving citalopram. Although changes in sexual desire, sexual performance, and sexual satisfaction often occur as manifestations of a psychiatric disorder, they also may occur as the result of pharmacologic therapy. It is difficult to determine the true incidence and severity of adverse effects on sexual function during citalopram therapy, in part because patients and clinicians may be reluctant to discuss these effects. Therefore, incidence data reported in product labeling and earlier studies are most likely underestimates of the true incidence of adverse sexual effects. Recent reports indicate that up to 50% of patients receiving selective serotonin-reuptake inhibitors describe some form of sexual dysfunction during treatment and the actual incidence may be even higher.

Ejaculatory disturbances (principally ejaculatory delay) are the most common adverse urogenital effects associated with citalopram in males, occurring in about 6% of male patients receiving the drug compared with 1% of depressed patients receiving placebo in controlled clinical studies. However, the adverse effect of ejaculatory delay associated with serotonin-reuptake inhibitors has been used for therapeutic benefit in the treatment of premature ejaculation. (See Uses: Premature Ejaculation.) Results of some (but not all) studies in men and women suggest that paroxetine may be associated with a higher incidence of sexual dysfunction than some other currently available selective serotonin-reuptake inhibitors, including citalopram and sertraline. Since it is difficult to know the precise risk of sexual dysfunction associated with citalopram and other serotonin-reuptake inhibitors, clinicians should routinely inquire about such possible adverse effects in patients receiving these drugs.

Decreased libido was reported in about 4% of depressed male patients receiving citalopram in short-term placebo-controlled studies compared with less than 1% of patients receiving placebo. In these studies, impotence, which appears to be dose related, was reported in about 3% of male patients receiving citalopram compared with less than 1% of males receiving placebo. In female patients receiving citalopram in controlled clinical studies for the treatment of depression, decreased libido and anorgasmia were reported in about 1% of those receiving citalopram. Increased libido has been reported in up to 1% of patients receiving citalopram. Priapism also has been reported during postmarketing surveillance in male patients, and clitoral priapism has been reported in at least 3 female patients receiving the drug.

The long-term effects of selective serotonin-reuptake inhibitors on sexual function have not been fully determined to date. In a double-blind study evaluating 6 months of citalopram or sertraline therapy in depressed patients, sexual desire and overall sexual functioning (as measured on the UKU Side Effect Scale) substantially improved in women and sexual desire improved in men. In men, no change in orgasmic dysfunction, erectile dysfunction, or overall sexual functioning was reported after 6 months of therapy with citalopram or sertraline, although there was a trend toward worsening of ejaculatory dysfunction. However, in the subgroups of women and men reporting no sexual problems at baseline, approximately 12% of women reported decreased sexual desire and 14% reported orgasmic dysfunction after 6 months of citalopram therapy; the corresponding figures in the same subgroup of men were approximately 17 and 19%, respectively, and as many as 25% experienced ejaculatory dysfunction after 6 months. No substantial differences between citalopram and sertraline were reported in this study.

Management of sexual dysfunction caused by selective serotonin-reuptake inhibitor therapy includes waiting for tolerance to develop; using a lower dosage of the drug; using drug holidays; delaying administration of the drug until after coitus; or changing to another antidepressant. Although further study is needed, there is some evidence that adverse sexual effects of the selective serotonin-reuptake inhibitors may be reversed by concomitant use of certain drugs, including buspirone, 5-hydroxytryptamine-2 ($5-HT_2$) receptor antagonists (e.g., nefazodone), $5-HT_3$ receptor inhibitors (e.g., granisetron), or α_2-adrenergic receptor antagonists (e.g., yohimbine), selective phosphodiesterase (PDE) inhibitors (e.g., sildenafil), or dopamine receptor agonists (e.g., amantadine, dextroamphetamine, pemoline [no longer commercially available in the US], methylphenidate). In most patients, sexual dysfunction is fully reversed 1–3 days after discontinuance of the antidepressant.

Other Renal, Electrolyte, and Genitourinary Effects Treatment with SSRIs, including citalopram, or selective serotonin- and norepinephrine-reuptake inhibitors (SNRIs) may result in hyponatremia. In many cases, this hyponatremia appeared to be due to the syndrome of inappropriate antidiuretic hormone secretion (SIADH) and was reversible when citalopram was discontinued. Cases with serum sodium concentrations lower than 110 mmol/L have been reported. Prolonged coma caused by hyponatremia has been reported in a patient with multiple sclerosis receiving citalopram therapy. Severe postoperative hyponatremia has been reported in an elderly female patient receiving the drug. Hyponatremia and SIADH usually develop an average of 2 weeks after initiating therapy (range: 3–120 days). Geriatric individuals and patients receiving diuretics or who are otherwise volume depleted may be at greater risk of developing hyponatremia during therapy with SSRIs or SNRIs. Discontinuance of citalopram should be considered in patients with symptomatic hyponatremia and appropriate medical intervention should be instituted. Because geriatric patients may be at increased risk for hyponatremia associated with these drugs, clinicians prescribing citalopram in such patients should be aware of the possibility that such reactions may occur. In addition, periodic monitoring of serum sodium concentrations (particularly during the first several months) in geriatric patients receiving selective serotonin-reuptake inhibitors has been recommended by some clinicians.

Hypokalemia and dehydration have occurred in less than 0.1% of patients receiving citalopram; these adverse effects have not been definitely attributed to the drug.

Urinary disorders (e.g., micturition disorders) have been reported in at least 2% of patients receiving citalopram in short-term controlled trials. In addition, polyuria has been reported in at least 1% of patients receiving the drug. Although a definite causal relationship to citalopram has not been established, urinary frequency, urinary incontinence, urinary retention, and dysuria have been reported in at least 0.1% of patients receiving the drug. Other adverse urologic effects reported in less than 0.1% of citalopram-treated patients include hematuria, oliguria, pyelonephritis, renal calculus, and renal pain; these adverse effects have not been definitely attributed to the drug.

Dysmenorrhea has been reported in at least 3% of female patients receiving citalopram in short-term controlled trials. In addition, amenorrhea has been reported in at least 1% of patients receiving the drug. Galactorrhea, breast pain, breast enlargement, and vaginal hemorrhage have been reported in less than 1% of patients receiving citalopram, and spontaneous abortion has been reported rarely; however, these adverse effects have not been definitely attributed to the drug. Breast enlargement also has been reported in some women receiving chronic therapy with other selective serotonin-reuptake inhibitors. In one study, approximately 40% of patients receiving selective serotonin-reuptake inhibitors (e.g., fluoxetine, paroxetine, sertraline) or venlafaxine reported some degree of breast enlargement; most patients with breast enlargement also experienced weight gain. In addition, serum prolactin concentrations were increased in the women receiving other selective serotonin-reuptake inhibitors in this study. Gynecomastia has been reported rarely.

■ **Hepatic Effects** Abnormal liver function test results, including elevations in serum hepatic enzyme concentrations, and increased serum alkaline phosphatase concentrations have been reported in at least 0.1% of patients receiving citalopram. Hepatitis, jaundice, and hyperbilirubinemia have been reported in less than 0.1% of patients receiving citalopram; however, these adverse effects have not been definitely attributed to the drug. Hepatic necrosis has also been reported during postmarketing surveillance in citalopram-treated patients.

■ **Other Adverse Effects** Fever occurred in about 2% of patients receiving citalopram in short-term controlled clinical trials. Rigors, alcohol intolerance, lymphadenopathy, and influenza-like symptoms have been reported in less than 1% of patients receiving citalopram; however, these adverse effects have not been definitely attributed to the drug. Pancreatitis also has occurred in association with citalopram, although a causal relationship to the drug has not been clearly established.

■ **Precautions and Contraindications** Worsening of depression and/or the emergence of suicidal ideation and behavior (suicidality) or unusual changes in behavior may occur in both adult and pediatric (see Cautions: Pediatric Precautions) patients with major depressive disorder or other psychiatric disorders, whether or not they are taking antidepressants. This risk may persist until clinically important remission occurs. Suicide is a known risk of depression and certain other psychiatric disorders, and these disorders themselves are the strongest predictors of suicide. However, there has been a long-standing concern that antidepressants may have a role in inducing worsening of depression and the emergence of suicidality in certain patients during the early phases of treatment. Pooled analyses of short-term, placebo-controlled studies of antidepressants (i.e., selective serotonin-reuptake inhibitors and other antidepressants) have shown an increased risk of suicidality in children, adolescents, and young adults (18–24 years of age) with major depressive disorder and other psychiatric disorders. An increased suicidality risk was not demonstrated with antidepressants compared with placebo in adults older than 24 years of age and a reduced risk was observed in adults 65 years of age or older. It currently is unknown whether the suicidality risk extends to longer-term use (i.e., beyond several months); however, there is substantial evidence from placebo-controlled maintenance trials in adults with major depressive disorder that antidepressants can delay the recurrence of depression.

The US Food and Drug Administration (FDA) recommends that all patients being treated with antidepressants for any indication be appropriately monitored and closely observed for clinical worsening, suicidality, and unusual changes in behavior, particularly during initiation of therapy (i.e., the first few months) and during periods of dosage adjustments. Families and caregivers of patients being treated with antidepressants for major depressive disorder or other indications, both psychiatric and nonpsychiatric, also should be advised to monitor patients on a daily basis for the emergence of agitation, irritability, or unusual changes in behavior as well as the emergence of suicidality, and to report such symptoms immediately to a health-care provider. (See Suicidality under Cautions: Nervous System Effects, in Paroxetine 28:16.04.20.)

Although a causal relationship between the emergence of symptoms such as anxiety, agitation, panic attacks, insomnia, irritability, hostility, aggressiveness, impulsivity, akathisia, hypomania, and/or mania and either the worsening of depression and/or the emergence of suicidal impulses has not been established, there is concern that such symptoms may represent precursors to emerging suicidality. Consequently, consideration should be given to changing the therapeutic regimen or discontinuing therapy in patients whose depression is persistently worse or in patients experiencing emergent suicidality or symptoms that might be precursors to worsening depression or suicidality, particularly if such manifestations are severe, abrupt in onset, or were not part of the patient's presenting symptoms. If a decision is made to discontinue therapy, citalopram dosage should be tapered as rapidly as is feasible but with recognition of the risks of abrupt discontinuance. (See Dosage and Administration: Dosage.) FDA also recommends that the drugs be prescribed in the smallest quantity consistent with good patient management, in order to reduce the risk of overdosage.

Citalopram causes dose-dependent QT_c-interval prolongation, an ECG abnormality that has been associated with torsades de pointes, ventricular tachycardia, and sudden death, all of which have been reported in postmarketing experience in patients receiving the drug. On August 24, 2011, the US Food and Drug Administration (FDA) notified healthcare professionals that *citalopram should no longer be used at dosages exceeding 40 mg daily due to the risk of QT-interval prolongation and torsades de pointes*; previously, the prescribing information for the drug stated that certain patients may require a dosage of 60 mg daily. On March 28, 2012, the FDA provided the following revised recommendations for citalopram use related to the potential risk of abnormal heart rhythms associated with higher dosages of the drug. The FDA advised that citalopram therapy is not recommended in patients with congenital long QT syndrome, bradycardia, hypokalemia or hypomagnesemia, recent acute myocardial infarction, or uncompensated heart failure. The FDA also stated that citalopram should not be used in patients receiving other drugs known to prolong the QT_c interval. Such drugs include class IA (e.g., quinidine, procainamide) or class III (e.g., amiodarone, sotalol) antiarrhythmic agents, certain antipsychotic agents (e.g., chlorpromazine, thioridazine), some anti-infective agents (e.g., gatifloxacin, moxifloxacin), and other drugs (e.g., pentamidine, levomethadyl acetate, methadone). In addition, the *maximum* dosage of citalopram should be limited to 20 mg once daily in patients who are poor metabolizers of the cytochrome P-450 (CYP) isoenzyme 2C19; patients receiving cimetidine or another CYP2C19 inhibitor; patients with hepatic impairment; and in patients older than 60 years of age; higher citalopram exposures in such patients increase the risk of QT-interval prolongation and torsades de pointes. Furthermore, electrolyte and/or ECG monitoring is recommended in certain situations. Patients being considered for citalopram therapy who are at risk for clinically important electrolyte disturbances should have baseline measurements of serum potassium and magnesium concentrations with subsequent periodic monitoring. Because hypokalemia and/or hypomagnesemia may increase the risk of QT_c-interval prolongation and arrhythmias, hypokalemia and hypomagnesemia should be corrected prior to citalopram administration and serum concentrations of these electrolytes should be periodically monitored. In addition, ECG monitoring is recommended in patients for whom citalopram use is not recommended but nevertheless considered essential, including those with the above-mentioned cardiovascular conditions (e.g., congenital long QT syndrome, bradycardia, recent acute myocardial infarction, uncompensated heart failure) and those concurrently receiving other drugs that may prolong the QT_c interval. Citalopram should be discontinued in any patient who has persistent QT_c measurements exceeding 500 msec. Patients receiving citalopram should be informed of the possible symptoms of QT-interval prolongation and torsades de pointes (e.g., chest pain, irregular heartbeat, shortness of breath, dizziness or fainting) and advised to seek immediate medical attention should such symptoms occur. If a citalopram-treated patient experiences such symptoms, further evaluation should be initiated, including cardiac monitoring.

It is generally believed (though not established in controlled trials) that treating a major depressive episode with an antidepressant alone may increase the likelihood of precipitating a mixed or manic episode in patients at risk for bipolar disorder. Therefore, patients should be adequately screened for bipolar disorder prior to initiating treatment with an antidepressant; such screening should include a detailed psychiatric history (e.g., family history of suicide, bipolar disorder, and depression).

Potentially life-threatening serotonin syndrome has been reported with SSRIs, including citalopram, and selective serotonin- and norepinephrine-reuptake inhibitors (SNRIs) when used alone, but particularly with concurrent use of other serotonergic drugs (including serotonin [5-hydroxytryptamine; 5-HT] type 1 receptor agonists ["triptans"], tricyclic antidepressants, buspirone, fentanyl, lithium, tramadol, tryptophan, and St. John's wort [*Hypericum perforatum*]) and with drugs that impair the metabolism of serotonin (particularly monoamine oxidase [MAO] inhibitors, both those used to treat psychiatric disorders and others, such as linezolid and methylene blue). Manifestations of serotonin syndrome may include mental status changes (e.g., agitation, hallucinations, delirium, coma), autonomic instability (e.g., tachycardia, labile blood pressure, dizziness, diaphoresis, flushing, hyperthermia), neuromuscular symptoms (e.g., tremor, rigidity, myoclonus, hyperreflexia, incoordination), seizures, and/or GI symptoms (e.g., nausea, vomiting, diarrhea). Patients receiving citalopram should be monitored for the development of serotonin syndrome.

Concomitant use of citalopram and MAO inhibitors intended to treat psychiatric disorders is contraindicated. Citalopram also should not be initiated in patients who are being treated with other MAO inhibitors such as linezolid or IV methylene blue. In patients who require more urgent treatment of a psychiatric condition, other interventions, including hospitalization, should be considered. Citalopram may be started 24 hours after the last dose of linezolid or IV methylene blue.

If concurrent therapy with citalopram and other serotonergic drugs is clinically warranted, the patient should be made aware of the potential increased risk for serotonin syndrome, particularly during initiation of therapy or when dosage is increased. If manifestations of serotonin syndrome occur, treatment with citalopram and any concurrently administered serotonergic agents should be discontinued immediately and supportive and symptomatic treatment should be initiated. (See Drug Interactions: Serotonergic Drugs.) For further information on serotonin syndrome, including manifestations and treatment, see Drug Interactions: Serotonergic Drugs, in Fluoxetine Hydrochloride 28:16.04.20.

The pupillary dilation (mydriasis) that occurs following the use of many antidepressant agents, including citalopram, may trigger an acute attack of angle-closure glaucoma (narrow-angle glaucoma) in patients with anatomically narrow angles who do not have a patent iridectomy. Possible symptoms of angle-closure glaucoma include eye pain, vision changes, and swelling or redness in or around the eye. Preexisting glaucoma is almost always open-angle glaucoma since angle-closure glaucoma can be treated definitively with iridectomy when diagnosed; open-angle glaucoma is not a risk factor for angle-closure glaucoma. Patients should be advised that citalopram can cause mild pupillary dilation, which can lead to an episode of angle-closure glaucoma in susceptible individuals. In addition, patients may wish to be examined to determine whether they are susceptible to angle-closure glaucoma and have a prophylactic procedure (e.g., iridectomy) if they are susceptible.

Citalopram should be used with caution and a lower maximum dosage (20 mg once daily) is recommended in patients with hepatic impairment, since decreased clearance and increased plasma concentrations of the drug may occur in such patients. (See Dosage and Administration: Dosage in Hepatic and Renal Impairment and see also Pharmacokinetics: Elimination.)

Because citalopram is extensively metabolized, excretion of unchanged drug in urine is a minor route of elimination. Severe renal failure did not markedly affect the pharmacokinetics of citalopram in one study, suggesting that dosage adjustment may not be necessary in patients with severe renal impairment. However, until long-term citalopram therapy has been more fully evaluated in such patients, citalopram should be used with caution in patients with severe renal impairment. (See Dosage and Administration: Dosage in Hepatic and Renal Impairment and see also Pharmacokinetics: Elimination.)

Because of the potential for adverse drug interactions, patients receiving citalopram should be advised to notify their clinician if they are taking or plan to take nonprescription (over-the-counter) or prescription medications. Although citalopram has not been shown to potentiate the impairment of mental and motor skills caused by alcohol, patients should be advised to avoid alcohol while receiving the drug.

Citalopram generally is less sedating than many other currently available antidepressants and does not appear to produce substantial impairment of cognitive or psychomotor function nor to potentiate psychomotor impairment induced by other CNS depressants (e.g., alcohol). However, patients should be cautioned that citalopram may impair their ability to perform activities requiring mental alertness or physical coordination (e.g., operating machinery, driving a motor vehicle) and to avoid such activities until they gain experience with the drug's effects.

Patients receiving citalopram should be advised that while they may notice improvement within 1–4 weeks after starting therapy, they should continue therapy with the drug as directed by their clinician.

Although anticonvulsant effects have been observed in animal studies with citalopram, the drug has not been systematically evaluated in patients with a seizure disorder. In addition, patients with seizure disorders were excluded from premarketing clinical trials with the drug. In clinical studies of citalopram, seizures occurred in 0.3% of patients receiving citalopram and in 0.5% of patients receiving placebo; a causal relationship to the drug remains to be established. However, as with other antidepressants, citalopram should be initiated and used with caution in patients with a history of seizures.

Activation of mania and hypomania have occurred in patients receiving therapeutic dosages of citalopram. The drug should be used with caution in patients with a history of mania. (See Cautions: Nervous System Effects.)

Treatment with SSRIs, including citalopram, or SNRIs may result in hyponatremia. In many cases, this hyponatremia appears to be due to the syndrome of inappropriate antidiuretic hormone secretion (SIADH) and was reversible when the SSRI or SNRI was discontinued. Geriatric individuals and patients receiving diuretics or who are otherwise volume depleted may be at greater risk of developing hyponatremia during therapy with SSRIs or SNRIs. Signs and symptoms of hyponatremia include headache, difficulty concentrating, memory impairment, confusion, weakness, and unsteadiness, which may lead to falls; more severe and/or acute cases have been associated with hallucinations, syncope, seizures, coma, respiratory arrest, and death. Discontinuance of citalopram should be considered in patients with symptomatic hyponatremia and appropriate medical intervention should be instituted. (See Cautions: Renal, Electrolyte, and Genitourinary Effects and see also see Cautions: Geriatric Precautions.)

Because of similarity in spelling of Celexa® (citalopram hydrobromide), Celebrex® (celecoxib), and Cerebyx® (fosphenytoin sodium), extra care should be exercised in ensuring the accuracy of prescriptions for these drugs.

Use of citalopram is contraindicated in patients who are currently receiving or have recently (i.e., within 2 weeks) received therapy with an MAO inhibitor intended to treat psychiatric disorders because of an increased risk of serotonin syndrome. Conversely, use of an MAO inhibitor intended to treat psychiatric disorders is contraindicated within 2 weeks of citalopram discontinuance. (See Drug Interactions: Serotonergic Drugs.)

Initiation of citalopram therapy in patients receiving MAO inhibitors such as linezolid or IV methylene blue also is contraindicated because of an increased risk of serotonin syndrome. (See Drug Interactions: Serotonergic Drugs.)

Concurrent use of citalopram in patients receiving pimozide is contraindicated. (See Drug Interactions: Pimozide.)

Citalopram is contraindicated in patients who are hypersensitive to the drug, escitalopram, or any ingredient in the formulation.

■ **Pediatric Precautions** Safety and efficacy of citalopram in pediatric patients have not been established. Two placebo-controlled trials involving 407 children and adolescents with major depressive disorder have been conducted with citalopram; the results of these trials were not sufficient to support a claim of efficacy for use of the drug in pediatric patients with this condition. (See Pediatric Considerations under Uses: Major Depressive Disorder.)

Decreased appetite and weight loss have been observed in patients receiving SSRIs. Therefore, regular monitoring of weight and growth should be performed in children and adolescents receiving citalopram therapy.

FDA warns that antidepressants increase the risk of suicidal thinking and behavior (suicidality) in children and adolescents with major depressive disorder and other psychiatric disorders. The risk of suicidality for these drugs was identified in a pooled analysis of data from a total of 24 short-term (4–16 weeks), placebo-controlled studies of 9 antidepressants (i.e., citalopram, bupropion, fluoxetine, fluvoxamine, mirtazapine, nefazodone, paroxetine, sertraline, venlafaxine) in over 4400 children and adolescents with major depressive disorder, obsessive-compulsive disorder (OCD), or other psychiatric disorders. The analysis revealed a greater risk of adverse events representing suicidal behavior or thinking (suicidality) during the first few months of treatment in pediatric patients receiving antidepressants than in those receiving placebo. However, a more recent meta-analysis of 27 placebo-controlled trials of 9 antidepressants (SSRIs and others) in patients younger than 19 years of age with major depressive disorder, OCD, or non-OCD anxiety disorders suggests that the benefits of antidepressant therapy in treating these conditions may outweigh the risks of suicidal behavior or suicidal ideation. No suicides occurred in these pediatric trials.

The risk of suicidality in the FDA's pooled analysis differed across the different psychiatric indications, with the highest incidence observed in the major depressive disorder studies. In addition, although there was considerable variation in risk among the antidepressants, a tendency toward an increase in suicidality risk in younger patients was found for almost all drugs studied. It currently is unknown whether the suicidality risk in pediatric patients extends to longer-term use (i.e., beyond several months). (See Suicidality under Cautions: Nervous System Effects, in Paroxetine 28:16.04.20.)

As a result of this analysis and public discussion of the issue, FDA has directed manufacturers of all antidepressants to add a boxed warning to the labeling of their products to alert clinicians of this suicidality risk in children and adolescents and to recommend appropriate monitoring and close observation of patients receiving these agents. (See Cautions: Precautions and Contraindications.) The drugs that are the focus of the revised labeling are all drugs included in the general class of antidepressants, including those that have not been studied in controlled clinical trials in pediatric patients, since the available data are not adequate to exclude any single antidepressant from an increased risk. In addition to the boxed warning and other information in professional labeling on antidepressants, FDA currently recommends that a patient medication guide explaining the risks associated with the drugs be provided to the patient each time the drugs are dispensed. Caregivers of pediatric patients whose depression is persistently worse or who are experiencing emergent suicidality or symptoms that might be precursors to worsening depression or suicidality during antidepressant therapy should consult their clinician regarding the best course of action (e.g., whether the therapeutic regimen should be changed or the drug discontinued). *Patients should not discontinue use of selective serotonin-reuptake inhibitors without first consulting their clinician; it is very important that the drugs not be abruptly discontinued, as withdrawal effects may occur.* (See Dosage and Administration: Dosage.)

Anyone considering the use of citalopram in a child or adolescent for any clinical use must balance the potential risk of therapy with the clinical need.

■ **Geriatric Precautions** While safety and efficacy of citalopram in geriatric patients have not been established specifically, approximately 31% of patients receiving the drug for depression in clinical trials were 60 years of age or older, approximately 23% were 65 years of age or older, and approximately 10% were 75 years of age or older.

Although no overall differences in the efficacy or adverse effect profile of citalopram were observed between geriatric and younger patients and other clinical experience revealed no evidence of age-related differences in response, pharmacokinetic studies in healthy geriatric individuals and depressed patients 60 years of age or older have revealed higher areas under the plasma concentration-time curve (AUC) values and longer elimination half-lives compared with those in younger individuals. (See Pharmacokinetics: Absorption and Elimination.) Therefore, the manufacturer and some clinicians recommend a maximum citalopram dosage of 20 mg once daily for geriatric patients older than 60 years of age with major depressive disorder. (See Dosage and Administration: Dosage in Geriatric Patients.)

In pooled data analyses, a *reduced* risk of suicidality was observed in adults 65 years of age or older with antidepressant therapy compared with placebo. (See Cautions: Precautions and Contraindications.)

Limited evidence suggests that geriatric patients also may be more likely than younger patients to develop citalopram-induced hyponatremia and transient syndrome of inappropriate secretion of antidiuretic hormone (SIADH). Therefore, clinicians prescribing citalopram in geriatric patients should be aware of the possibility that such reactions may occur. In addition, periodic monitoring (especially during the first several months) of serum sodium concentrations in geriatric patients receiving selective serotonin-reuptake inhibitors has been recommended by some clinicians.

In a double-blind, multicenter trial, citalopram (20 or 40 mg daily) was found to be as effective as and better tolerated than amitriptyline in depressed geriatric patients. In a small study comparing citalopram and nortriptyline in depressed geriatric patients, citalopram was found to be somewhat less effective but better tolerated than nortriptyline.

In a controlled study comparing citalopram and placebo in elderly patients with dementia†, citalopram (20–30 mg daily) was found to improve depression as well as cognitive and emotional functioning more than placebo. In an open study in a limited number of patients with dementia and behavioral disturbances†, citalopram was found to improve the behavioral complications associated with dementia†.

As with other psychotropic drugs, geriatric patients receiving antidepressants appear to have an increased risk of hip fracture. Despite the decreased incidence of cardiovascular and anticholinergic effects associated with selective serotonin-reuptake inhibitors, these drugs did not show any advantage over tricyclic antidepressants with regard to hip fracture in a case-control study. In addition, there was little difference in the rates of falls between nursing home residents receiving selective serotonin-reuptake inhibitors and those receiving tricyclic antidepressants in a retrospective study. Therefore, all geriatric individuals receiving either type of antidepressant should be considered at increased risk of falls, and appropriate measures should be taken.

■ **Mutagenicity and Carcinogenicity** Citalopram was mutagenic in the in vitro bacterial reverse mutation assay (Ames test) in 2 out of 5 bacterial strains (Salmonella TA98 and TA1537) in the absence of metabolic activation. In the in vitro Chinese hamster lung cell assay for chromosomal aberrations, citalopram was clastogenic in the presence and absence of metabolic activation. The drug was not mutagenic in the in vitro mammalian forward gene mutation assay (HPRT) in mouse lymphoma cells or in a coupled in vitro/in vivo unscheduled DNA synthesis (UDS) assay in rat liver. Citalopram was not found to be clastogenic in the in vitro chromosomal aberration assay in human lymphocytes or in 2 in vivo mouse micronucleus assays.

Studies to determine the carcinogenic potential of citalopram were performed in mice receiving oral dosages of up to 240 mg/kg daily for 18 months and in rats receiving 8 or 24 mg/kg daily for 24 months. These dosages were approximately 20 times the maximum recommended human daily dosage of 60 mg on a surface area (mg/m^2) basis in mice and approximately 1.3 and 4 times the maximum recommended human daily dosage on a mg/m^2 basis in rats, respectively. No evidence of carcinogenicity was found in the mice. In rats receiving 8 or 24 mg/kg daily of citalopram, an increased incidence of small intestine carcinoma was reported. The manufacturer states that a no-effect dosage for this finding was not established; the relevance of this finding to humans is not known.

■ **Pregnancy, Fertility, and Lactation** ***Pregnancy*** Some neonates exposed to citalopram and other selective serotonin-reuptake inhibitors (SSRIs) or selective serotonin- and norepinephrine-reuptake inhibitors (SNRIs) late in the third trimester of pregnancy have developed complications that have sometimes been severe and required prolonged hospitalization, respiratory support, enteral nutrition, and other forms of supportive care in special-care nurseries. Such complications can arise immediately upon delivery and usually last several days or up to 2–4 weeks. Clinical findings reported to date in the neonates have included respiratory distress, cyanosis, apnea, seizures, temperature instability or fever, feeding difficulty, dehydration, excessive weight loss, vomiting, hypoglycemia, hypotonia, hypertonia, hyperreflexia, tremor, jitteriness, irritability, lethargy, reduced or lack of reaction to pain stimuli, and constant crying. These clinical features appear to be consistent with either a direct toxic effect of the SSRI or SNRI or, possibly, a drug withdrawal syndrome. It should be noted that, in some cases, the clinical picture was consistent with serotonin syndrome (see Drug Interactions: Serotonergic Drugs).

Infants exposed to SSRIs in late pregnancy may have an increased risk of persistent pulmonary hypertension of the newborn (PPHN). PPHN is a rare heart and lung condition occurring in an estimated 1–2 infants per 1000 live births in the general population; it occurs when a neonate does not adapt to breathing outside the womb. Some experts have suggested that respiratory distress in neonates exposed to SSRIs may occur along a spectrum of seriousness in association with maternal use of SSRIs, with PPHN among the most serious consequences. Neonates with PPHN may require intensive care support, including mechanical ventilation; in severe cases, multiple organ damage, including brain damage, and even death may occur. Although several epidemiologic studies have suggested an increased risk of PPHN with SSRI use during pregnancy, other studies did not demonstrate a statistically significant association. Thus, the FDA states that it is currently unclear whether use of SSRIs, including citalopram, during pregnancy can cause PPHN and recommends that clinicians not alter their current clinical practice of treating depression during pregnancy.

Clinicians should consider that in a prospective longitudinal study of 201 women with a history of recurrent major depression who were euthymic in the context of antidepressant therapy at the beginning of pregnancy, women who discontinued their antidepressant medication (SSRIs, tricyclic antidepressants, or others) during pregnancy were found to be substantially more likely to have a relapse of depression than were women who continued to receive their antidepressant therapy while pregnant. When treating a pregnant woman with citalopram, the clinician should carefully consider the potential risks of taking an SSRI along with the established benefits of treating depression with an antidepressant; this decision can only be made on a case-by-case basis. (See Dosage and Administration: Treatment of Pregnant Women during the Third Trimester.)

For additional information on the management of depression in women prior to conception and during pregnancy, including treatment algorithms, the FDA advises clinicians to consult the joint American Psychiatric Association and American College of Obstetricians and Gynecologists guidelines (at https://www.ncbi.nlm.nih.gov/pmc/articles/PMC3103063/pdf/nihms293836.pdf).

Most epidemiologic studies of pregnancy outcome following first-trimester exposure to SSRIs, including citalopram, conducted to date have not revealed evidence of an increased risk of major congenital malformations. Analysis of data collected in 531 Swedish women who received SSRIs during early pregnancy (citalopram accounted for 375 of these exposures) found that no increase in congenital abnormalities was observed during the neonatal period compared with the general population. In a prospective, controlled, multicenter study, maternal use of several SSRIs (fluvoxamine, paroxetine, sertraline) did not appear to increase the risk of congenital malformation, miscarriage, stillbirth, or premature delivery when used during pregnancy at recommended dosages. Birth weight and gestational age in neonates exposed to the drugs were similar to those in the control group. In another small study based on medical records review, the incidence of congenital anomalies reported in infants born to women who were treated with several other SSRIs (fluoxetine, paroxetine, sertraline) during pregnancy was comparable to that observed in the general population.

Citalopram and its metabolites have been shown to cross the placenta in humans. In 11 women who received 20–40 mg of citalopram daily during pregnancy, trough plasma citalopram, demethylcitalopram, and didemethylcitalopram concentrations in the infants at the time of delivery were found to be 64, 66, and 68%, respectively, of maternal concentrations. No significant difference in pregnancy outcome was observed between the group of women who received citalopram during pregnancy and a similar control group of pregnant women who did not receive the drug. In addition, the body weight and neurologic status of the infants in both groups were all assessed as normal after 12 months. However, the results of epidemiologic studies indicate that exposure to paroxetine during the first trimester of pregnancy may increase the risk for congenital malformations, particularly cardiovascular malformations. (See Pregnancy, under Cautions: Pregnancy, Fertility, and Lactation, in Paroxetine 28:16.04.20.) Additional epidemiologic studies are needed to more thoroughly evaluate the relative safety of citalopram and other SSRIs during pregnancy, including their potential teratogenic risks and possible effects on neurobehavioral development.

There are no adequate and well-controlled studies to date using citalopram in pregnant women and the drug should be used during pregnancy only when the potential benefits justify the potential risks to the fetus. Women should be advised to notify their clinician if they become pregnant or plan to become pregnant during therapy with the drug. FDA states that women who are pregnant or thinking about becoming pregnant should not discontinue any antidepressant, including citalopram, without first consulting their clinician. The decision whether or not to continue antidepressant therapy should be made only after careful consideration of the potential benefits and risks of antidepressant therapy for each individual pregnant patient. If a decision is made to discontinue treatment with citalopram or other SSRIs before or during pregnancy, discontinuance of therapy should be done in consultation with the clinician in accordance with the prescribing information for the antidepressant, and the patient should be closely monitored for possible relapse of depression.

The effect of citalopram on labor and delivery is not known.

In animal reproduction studies, citalopram has been shown to have adverse effects on embryo/fetal and postnatal development, including teratogenic effects, when administered at dosages that exceeded the recommended human dosage. Teratogenic effects were observed in rats receiving dosages of citalopram that were toxic to the dams but were not observed in rabbits. In 2 rat embryo/fetal development studies, oral administration of citalopram dosages of 32, 56, or 112 mg/kg daily to pregnant animals during the period of organogenesis resulted in decreased embryo/fetal growth and survival and an increased incidence of fetal abnormalities, including cardiovascular and skeletal defects, at the highest dosage (equivalent to approximately 18 times the maximum recommended human daily dosage on a mg/m^2 basis). This dosage also was associated with maternal toxicity. The developmental no-effect dosage was 56 mg/kg daily, which is approximately 9 times the maximum recommended human daily dosage on a mg/m² basis. No adverse effects on embryo/fetal development were observed in rabbits receiving citalopram dosages of up to 16 mg/kg daily (equivalent to approximately 5 times the maximum recommended human dosage on a mg/m² basis).

In female rats receiving citalopram dosages of 4.8, 12.8, or 32 mg/kg daily from late gestation through weaning, increased offspring mortality during the first 4 days following birth and persistent offspring growth retardation were observed at the highest dosage, which is equivalent to approximately 5 times the maximum recommended human dosage on a mg/m² basis. The no-effect dosage of 12.8 mg/kg daily is approximately 2 times the maximum recommended human dosage on a mg/m² basis. Similar effects on offspring mortality and growth were seen when dams were treated with the drug throughout gestation and early lactation at daily dosages of 24 mg/kg or more (approximately 4 or more times the maximum recommended human dosage on a mg/m² basis). A no-effect dosage was not determined in this study.

Fertility In reproduction studies in male and female rats receiving oral citalopram dosages of 16/24 (males/females), 32, 48, and 72 mg/kg daily, decreased mating was observed at all dosages. Fertility was decreased at daily dosages of 32 mg/kg or more (approximately 5 times the maximum recommended human dosage on a mg/m² basis). Gestation duration was increased in rats receiving 48 mg/kg daily of the drug, which is equivalent to approximately 8 times the maximum recommended human dosage.

Lactation Like other SSRIs, citalopram and its principal metabolite, demethylcitalopram, are distributed into milk. (See Pharmacokinetics: Distribution.) Limited data indicate that milk-to-plasma ratios of citalopram and demethylcitalopram range from 1.7–3. Available data indicate that citalopram and fluoxetine are the serotonin-reuptake inhibitors with the highest relative exposure for breast-fed infants. Excessive somnolence, decreased feeding, and weight loss were reported in 2 nursing infants whose mothers received citalopram. In one of these cases, the infant reportedly recovered completely upon discontinuance of citalopram by its mother, and in the second case, no follow-up information is available. Disturbed sleep has been reported in another breast-feeding infant whose mother was receiving citalopram 40 mg daily. The infant's sleep normalized once the citalopram dosage was reduced and 2 breast-feedings were replaced with artificial nutrition.

Women should be advised to notify their clinician if they plan to breast-feed. Because of the potential for adverse reactions to citalopram in nursing infants, a decision should be made whether to discontinue nursing or the drug, taking into account the importance of the drug to the woman. If a decision is made to continue citalopram therapy in a nursing woman, some clinicians recommend that the lowest effective dosage of citalopram be used and that breast-feeding during the period of drug absorption be avoided.

Drug Interactions

■ Drugs that Prolong the QT Interval

Citalopram use is not recommended in patients concurrently receiving other drugs known to prolong the QT_c interval, including class IA (e.g., quinidine, procainamide) or class III (e.g., amiodarone, sotalol) antiarrhythmic agents, certain antipsychotic agents (e.g., chlorpromazine, thioridazine), some anti-infective agents (e.g., gatifloxacin, moxifloxacin), and other drugs (e.g., pentamidine, levomethadyl acetate, methadone). However, if citalopram therapy is considered essential in such patients, ECG monitoring is recommended. (See Cautions: Cardiovascular Effects and see Drug Interactions: Pimozide.)

■ Serotonergic Drugs

Use of selective serotonin-reuptake inhibitors (SSRIs) such as citalopram concurrently or in close succession with other drugs that affect serotonergic neurotransmission may result in potentially life-threatening serotonin syndrome. Manifestations of serotonin syndrome may include mental status changes (e.g., agitation, hallucinations, delirium, coma), autonomic instability (e.g., tachycardia, labile blood pressure, dizziness, diaphoresis, flushing, hyperthermia), neuromuscular symptoms (e.g., tremor, rigidity, myoclonus, hyperreflexia, incoordination), seizures, and/or GI symptoms (e.g., nausea, vomiting, diarrhea). The precise mechanism of serotonin syndrome is not fully understood; however, it appears to result from excessive serotonergic activity in the CNS, probably mediated by activation of serotonin 5-HT_{1A} receptors. The possible involvement of dopamine and 5-HT_2 receptors also has been suggested, although their roles remain unclear.

Serotonin syndrome most commonly occurs when 2 or more drugs that affect serotonergic neurotransmission are administered either concurrently or in close succession. Serotonergic agents include those that increase serotonin synthesis (e.g., the serotonin precursor tryptophan), stimulate synaptic serotonin release (e.g., some amphetamines, dexfenfluramine [no longer commercially available in the US], fenfluramine [no longer commercially available in the US]), inhibit the reuptake of serotonin after release (e.g., SSRIs, selective serotonin- and norepinephrine-reuptake inhibitors [SNRIs], tricyclic antidepressants, trazodone, dextromethorphan, meperidine, tramadol), decrease the metabolism of serotonin (e.g., monoamine oxidase [MAO] inhibitors), have direct serotonin postsynaptic receptor activity (e.g., buspirone), or nonspecifically induce increases in serotonergic neuronal activity (e.g., lithium salts). Selective agonists of serotonin (5-hydroxytryptamine; 5-HT) type 1 (5-HT_1) receptors ("triptans") and dihydroergotamine, agents with serotonergic activity used in the management of migraine headache, and St. John's wort (*Hypericum perforatum*) also have been implicated in cases of serotonin syndrome.

The combination of SSRIs and MAO inhibitors may result in serotonin syndrome. Such reactions also have been reported in patients receiving SSRIs concomitantly with tryptophan, lithium, dextromethorphan, sumatriptan, or dihydroergotamine. In rare cases, serotonin syndrome reportedly has occurred in patients receiving the recommended dosage of a single serotonergic agent (e.g., clomipramine) or during accidental overdosage (e.g., sertraline intoxication in a child). Some other drugs that have been implicated in precipitating symptoms suggestive of serotonin syndrome include buspirone, bromocriptine, dextropropoxyphene, linezolid, methylene blue, methylenedioxymethamphetamine (MDMA; "ecstasy"), selegiline (a selective MAO-B inhibitor), and sibutramine (an SNRI used for the management of obesity [no longer commercially available in the US]). Other drugs that have been associated with the syndrome but for which less convincing data are available include carbamazepine, fentanyl, and pentazocine.

Clinicians should be aware of the potential for serious, possibly fatal reactions associated with serotonin syndrome in patients receiving 2 or more drugs that affect serotonergic neurotransmission, even if no such interactions with the specific drugs have been reported to date in the medical literature. Such patients should be monitored for the emergence of serotonin syndrome. Serotonin syndrome may be more likely to occur when initiating therapy, increasing the dosage, or following the addition of another serotonergic drug. Some clinicians state that patients who have experienced serotonin syndrome may be at higher risk for recurrence of the syndrome upon reinitiation of serotonergic drugs. Pending further experience in such cases, some clinicians recommend that therapy with serotonergic agents be limited following recovery. If concomitant use of citalopram and other serotonergic drugs is clinically warranted, patients should be advised of the increased risk for serotonin syndrome, particularly during treatment initiation and dosage increases. If manifestations of serotonin syndrome occur, treatment with citalopram and any concurrently administered serotonergic agents should be discontinued immediately and supportive and symptomatic treatment should be initiated.

For further information on serotonin syndrome, including manifestations and treatment, see Drug Interactions: Serotonergic Drugs, in Fluoxetine Hydrochloride 28:16.04.20.

Monoamine Oxidase Inhibitors Concomitant use of citalopram and MAO inhibitors, both those used to treat psychiatric disorders and others such as linezolid and methylene blue, is associated with a risk of potentially life-threatening serotonin syndrome. Such reactions also have been reported in patients who recently have discontinued an SSRI and have initiated therapy with an MAO inhibitor.

Because of the potential risk of serotonin syndrome, concomitant use of citalopram and MAO inhibitors intended to treat psychiatric disorders is contraindicated. At least 2 weeks should elapse between discontinuance of MAO inhibitors intended to treat psychiatric disorders and initiation of citalopram therapy and vice versa.

Linezolid. Linezolid, an anti-infective agent that is a nonselective and reversible MAO inhibitor, has been associated with drug interactions resulting in serotonin syndrome, including some associated with SSRIs. Because of this potential risk, linezolid generally should *not* be used in patients receiving citalopram. However, certain life-threatening or urgent situations may necessitate immediate linezolid treatment in a patient receiving a serotonergic drug, including citalopram. In such emergency situations, the availability of acceptable alternative anti-infectives should be considered and the benefits of linezolid should be weighed against the risk of serotonin syndrome. If linezolid is indicated in such emergency situations, citalopram must be immediately discontinued and the patient monitored for symptoms of serotonin syndrome for 2 weeks or until 24 hours after the last linezolid dose, whichever comes first. Treatment with citalopram may be resumed 24 hours after the last linezolid dose.

If nonemergency use of linezolid is being planned for a patient receiving citalopram, citalopram should be withheld for at least 2 weeks prior to initiating linezolid.

Initiation of citalopram in a patient receiving linezolid is contraindicated; when necessary, citalopram may be started 24 hours after the last linezolid dose. (See Drug Interactions: Serotonergic Drugs, in Linezolid 8:12.28.24.)

Methylene Blue. Methylene blue, a potent and reversible inhibitor of MAO-A, has been associated with drug interactions resulting in serotonin syndrome, including some associated with SSRIs. All of the reports of serotonin syndrome with methylene blue that provided information on the route of administration involved IV administration of doses of 1–8 mg/kg (e.g., when used as a diagnostic [visualizing] dye† during parathyroid surgery); none of the reports to date involved administration of methylene blue by other routes (such as oral tablets or by local tissue injection) or at lower doses. Because of this potential risk, methylene blue generally should *not* be used in patients receiving citalopram. However, certain life-threatening or urgent situations may necessitate immediate IV methylene blue administration in a patient receiving a serotonergic drug, including citalopram. In such emergency situations, the availability of acceptable alternatives to methylene blue should be considered and the benefits of IV methylene blue should be weighed against the risk of serotonin syndrome. If methylene blue is indicated in such emergency situations, citalopram must be immediately discontinued and the patient monitored for symptoms of serotonin syndrome for 2 weeks or until 24 hours after the last methylene blue dose, whichever comes first. Treatment with citalopram may be resumed 24 hours after the last methylene blue dose.

If nonemergency use of methylene blue is being planned for a patient receiving citalopram, citalopram should be withheld for at least 2 weeks prior to initiating methylene blue treatment.

Initiation of citalopram in a patient receiving IV methylene blue is contraindicated; when necessary, citalopram may be started 24 hours after the last IV methylene blue dose.

Moclobemide. Moclobemide (not commercially available in the US), a selective and reversible MAO-A inhibitor, has been associated with serotonin syndrome, and such reactions have been fatal in several cases in which the drug was given in combination with citalopram or with clomipramine. Pending further experience with such combinations, some clinicians recommend that concurrent therapy with moclobemide and a selective serotonin-reuptake inhibitor be used only with extreme caution and serotonin-reuptake inhibitors should have been discontinued for some time (depending on the elimination half-lives of the drug and its active metabolites) before initiating moclobemide therapy.

Selegiline. Selegiline, a selective MAO-B inhibitor used in the management of parkinsonian syndrome, has been reported to cause serotonin syndrome when given concurrently with selective serotonin-reuptake inhibitors (e.g., fluoxetine, paroxetine, sertraline). Although selegiline is a selective MAO-B inhibitor at therapeutic dosages, the drug appears to lose its selectivity for the MAO-B enzyme at higher dosages (e.g., those exceeding 10 mg/kg), thereby increasing the risk of serotonin syndrome in patients receiving higher dosages of the drug either alone or in combination with other serotonergic agents.

In a double-blind, placebo-controlled study in healthy individuals receiving citalopram and selegiline concurrently, no clinically important differences in vital signs or in the frequency of adverse events between the study groups were reported. In addition, no evidence of a clinically relevant pharmacokinetic interaction between the 2 drugs was found. Pending further accumulation of data, the manufacturer of selegiline recommends avoiding concurrent selegiline and selective serotonin-reuptake inhibitor therapy. In addition, the manufacturer of selegiline recommends that at least 2 weeks elapse between discontinuance of selegiline and initiation of selective serotonin-reuptake inhibitor therapy.

Isoniazid. Isoniazid, an antituberculosis agent, appears to have some MAO-inhibiting activity. In addition, iproniazid (not commercially available in the US), another antituberculosis agent structurally related to isoniazid that also possesses MAO-inhibiting activity, reportedly has resulted in serotonin syndrome in at least 2 patients when given in combination with meperidine. Pending further experience, clinicians should be aware of the potential for serotonin syndrome when isoniazid is given in conjunction with selective serotonin-reuptake inhibitor therapy (such as citalopram) or other serotonergic agents.

Tryptophan An interaction between paroxetine (another SSRI) and tryptophan (a serotonin precursor) has been reported during concurrent use. Adverse reactions reported to date during combined therapy with these drugs resemble serotonin syndrome and have consisted principally of headache, nausea, sweating, and dizziness. If concomitant use of citalopram and tryptophan is clinically warranted, patients should be advised of the increased risk for serotonin syndrome, particularly during treatment initiation and dosage increases. If serotonin syndrome manifestations occur, treatment with citalopram, tryptophan, and any other concurrently administered serotonergic agents should be discontinued immediately and supportive and symptomatic treatment should be initiated. (See Cautions: Precautions and Contraindications.)

5-HT$_1$ Receptor Agonists ("Triptans") Weakness, hyperreflexia, and incoordination have been reported rarely during postmarketing surveillance in patients receiving sumatriptan concomitantly with an SSRI (e.g., citalopram, escitalopram, fluoxetine, fluvoxamine, paroxetine, sertraline); these reactions resembled serotonin syndrome. Oral or subcutaneous sumatriptan and SSRIs were used concomitantly in some clinical studies without unusual adverse effects. However, an increase in the frequency of migraine attacks and a decrease in the effectiveness of sumatriptan in relieving migraine headache have been reported in a patient receiving subcutaneous injections of sumatriptan intermittently while undergoing fluoxetine therapy.

Clinicians prescribing triptans, SSRIs, and SNRIs should consider that triptans often are used intermittently and that either the triptan, SSRI, or SNRI may be prescribed by a different clinician. Clinicians also should weigh the potential risk of serotonin syndrome with the expected benefit of using a triptan concurrently with SSRI or SNRI therapy. If concomitant treatment with a triptan and citalopram is clinically warranted, patients should be advised of the increased risk of serotonin syndrome, particularly during treatment initiation and dosage increases. If serotonin syndrome manifestations occur, treatment with citalopram, the triptan, and any other concurrently administered serotonergic agents should be discontinued immediately and supportive and symptomatic treatment should be initiated. (See Cautions: Precautions and Contraindications.)

Other Selective Serotonin-reuptake Inhibitors and Selective Serotonin- and Norepinephrine-reuptake Inhibitors Concomitant use of citalopram and other SSRIs or SNRIs potentially may result in serotonin syndrome. If concomitant use of citalopram and other SSRIs or SNRIs is clinically warranted, patients should be advised of the increased risk for serotonin syndrome, particularly during treatment initiation and dosage increases. If serotonin syndrome manifestations occur, treatment with citalopram, the other SSRI or SNRI, and any other concurrently administered serotonergic agents should be discontinued immediately and supportive and symptomatic treatment should be initiated. (See Cautions: Precautions and Contraindications.)

Clinical experience regarding the optimal timing of switching from other SSRIs to citalopram therapy is limited. Therefore, care and prudent medical judgment should be exercised when switching from other SSRIs to citalopram, particularly from long-acting agents (e.g., fluoxetine). Because some adverse reactions resembling serotonin syndrome have developed when fluoxetine therapy has been abruptly discontinued and therapy with another SSRI (sertraline) was initiated immediately afterward, a washout period may be advisable when transferring a patient from fluoxetine to another SSRI. However, the appropriate duration of the washout period when switching from other SSRIs to citalopram has not been clearly established. Pending further experience in patients being transferred from therapy with another SSRI to citalopram and as the clinical situation permits, it generally is recommended that the previous antidepressant be discontinued according to the recommended guidelines for the specific SSRI prior to initiation of citalopram therapy.

■ **Drugs Undergoing Hepatic Metabolism or Affecting Hepatic Microsomal Enzymes** In vitro enzyme inhibition data did not reveal an inhibitory effect of citalopram on cytochrome P-450 (CYP) isoenzyme 3A4, 2C9, or 2E1 but did suggest that it is a weak inhibitor of 1A2, 2D6, and 2C19. Citalopram would be expected to have little inhibitory effect on in vivo metabolism mediated by these isoenzymes. However, in vivo data to address this question are very limited.

In vitro studies have indicated that CYP3A4 and CYP2C19 are the principal isoenzymes involved in the metabolism of citalopram. Therefore, it is expected that potent inhibitors of CYP3A4 (e.g., ketoconazole, itraconazole, macrolide antibiotics) and potent inhibitors of CYP2C19 (e.g., omeprazole) might decrease the clearance of citalopram. However, concurrent administration of citalopram and ketoconazole, a potent inhibitor of CYP3A4, did not substantially affect the pharmacokinetics of citalopram. (See Ketoconazole under Drug Interactions: Drugs Undergoing Hepatic Metabolism or Affecting Hepatic Microsomal Enzymes.)

Steady-state plasma citalopram concentrations were not substantially different in healthy individuals with poor or extensive CYP2D6 metabolizer phenotypes following multiple-dose administration of citalopram, suggesting that coadministration of citalopram with a drug that inhibits CYP2D6 is unlikely to have clinically important effects on citalopram metabolism.

Carbamazepine Concurrent administration of citalopram (40 mg daily for 14 days) and carbamazepine (titrated up to 400 mg daily for a total of 35 days) in healthy individuals did not significantly affect the pharmacokinetics of carbamazepine, a CYP3A4 substrate. Trough plasma citalopram concentrations were unaffected in this study, which suggests that the initiation of citalopram therapy in patients stabilized on carbamazepine should not produce clinically important changes in plasma carbamazepine concentrations. However, in an open study in depressed patients, the addition of carbamazepine to citalopram therapy resulted in a decrease in the plasma concentrations of escitalopram, the active enantiomer with the 1-(*S*) absolute configuration. In addition, 2 cases of increased plasma citalopram concentrations and altered antidepressant response have been reported when carbamazepine was discontinued. Because of the enzyme-inducing properties of carbamazepine, the possibility that carbamazepine might increase the clearance of citalopram should be considered if the 2 drugs are administered concomitantly or if carbamazepine therapy is initiated or discontinued in a patient receiving citalopram.

CYP2C19 Inhibitors Cimetidine is known to inhibit many CYP oxidative enzymes, including CYP2C19, and can affect the pharmacokinetics of citalopram. In a study in which oral citalopram (40 mg daily) was given for 3 weeks, the area under the plasma concentration-time curve (AUC) and peak plasma concentrations of citalopram were increased by approximately 43 and 39%, respectively, during concomitant use of oral cimetidine (400 mg daily) for the final 8 days. The possible effects of citalopram on the pharmacokinetics of cimetidine have not been studied.

Because of the potential risk of QT-interval prolongation and torsades de pointes, the maximum recommended dosage of citalopram is 20 mg once daily in patients concomitantly receiving citalopram and cimetidine or other CYP2C19 inhibitors.

Ketoconazole In a randomized, double-blind study, concurrent administration of single doses of citalopram (40 mg) and ketoconazole (200 mg), a potent inhibitor of CYP3A4, in healthy individuals decreased the peak plasma ketoconazole concentrations and AUC by 21 and 10%, respectively. The pharmacokinetics of citalopram and demethylcitalopram were not substantially affected during concomitant administration of these two drugs in this study. Therefore, citalopram dosage adjustment is unlikely to be necessary in patients receiving ketoconazole concurrently.

Triazolam Concurrent administration of citalopram (titrated to 40 mg daily for 28 days) and a single dose of triazolam (0.25 mg), a CYP3A4 substrate, in healthy individuals did not substantially affect the pharmacokinetics of either drug. However, triazolam appeared to be absorbed slightly more quickly during citalopram coadministration.

Tricyclic and Other Antidepressants The extent to which selective serotonin-reuptake inhibitor interactions with tricyclic antidepressants may pose clinical problems depends on the degree of inhibition and the pharmacokinetics of the serotonin-reuptake inhibitor involved. In vitro studies suggest that citalopram is a relatively weak inhibitor of CYP2D6 and CYP2C19. In one study in healthy adults receiving citalopram (40 mg once daily for 10 days), concurrent administration of a single 100-mg dose of imipramine hydrochloride, a CYP2D6 and CYP2C19 substrate, did not substantially affect the plasma concentrations of either citalopram or imipramine. However, the plasma concentration of the principal imipramine metabolite, desipramine, increased by approximately 50%; the clinical importance of this change is not known. The manufacturer of citalopram recommends that caution be exercised during concurrent use of tricyclic antidepressants with citalopram.

In addition, concomitant use of citalopram and tricyclic antidepressants potentially may result in serotonin syndrome. If concomitant use of citalopram and a tricyclic antidepressant is clinically warranted, patients should be advised of the increased risk for serotonin syndrome, particularly during treatment initiation and dosage increases. If serotonin syndrome manifestations occur, treatment with citalopram, the tricyclic antidepressant, and any concurrently administered serotonergic agents should be discontinued immediately and supportive and symptomatic treatment should be initiated. (See Cautions: Precautions and Contraindications and also see Drug Interactions: Serotonergic Drugs.)

Clinical experience regarding the optimal timing of switching from other antidepressants to citalopram therapy is limited. Therefore, care and prudent medical judgment should be exercised when switching from other antidepressants to citalopram. Pending further experience in patients being transferred from therapy with another antidepressant to citalopram and as the clinical situation permits, it generally is recommended that the previous antidepressant be discontinued according to the recommended guidelines for the specific antidepressant prior to initiation of citalopram therapy.

■ **Alcohol** Citalopram has not been shown to potentiate the impairment of mental and motor skills caused by alcohol. However, the drug's ability to reduce alcohol consumption in animals and humans suggests that there may be a serotonergically mediated, pharmacodynamic interaction between citalopram and alcohol within the CNS. (See Pharmacology: Effects on Alcohol Intake, and also see Uses: Alcohol Dependence.) The manufacturer recommends that patients be advised to avoid alcohol while receiving citalopram.

■ **Lithium** The manufacturer states that coadministration of lithium and citalopram did not substantially affect the pharmacokinetics of either drug in healthy individuals. In a placebo-controlled trial in depressed patients refractory to citalopram therapy alone, there also was no evidence of a pharmacokinetic interaction when lithium therapy (800 mg daily) was added; the combination was found to be well tolerated. However, pending further accumulation of data, the manufacturer of citalopram recommends that plasma lithium concentrations be monitored in patients receiving citalopram concurrently and that the lithium dosage be adjusted accordingly. Lithium also may enhance the serotonergic effects of citalopram, potentially resulting in serotonin syndrome. Caution should be exercised in patients receiving these two drugs concomitantly. (See Drug Interactions: Serotonergic Drugs.)

■ **Drugs Affecting Hemostasis** ***Warfarin*** The administration of a single, 25-mg dose of warfarin, a CYP3A4 substrate, in healthy individuals receiving citalopram 40 mg daily for 15 days did not affect the pharmacokinetics of warfarin. However, the prothrombin time increased by an average of 5% compared with baseline. The clinical importance, if any, of these findings is not known.

Other Drugs that Interfere with Hemostasis Epidemiologic case-control and cohort design studies that have demonstrated an association between selective serotonin-reuptake inhibitor therapy and an increased risk of upper GI bleeding also have shown that concurrent use of aspirin or other nonsteroidal anti-inflammatory agents substantially increases the risk of GI bleeding. Although these studies focused on upper GI bleeding, there is some evidence suggesting that bleeding at other sites may be similarly potentiated. The precise mechanism for this increased risk remains to be clearly established; however, serotonin release by platelets is known to play an important role in hemostasis, and selective serotonin-reuptake inhibitors decrease serotonin uptake from the blood by platelets, thereby decreasing the amount of serotonin in platelets. Patients receiving citalopram should be cautioned about the concomitant use of drugs that interfere with hemostasis, including aspirin and other nonsteroidal anti-inflammatory agents.

■ **Pimozide** In a controlled study, concurrent administration of a single 2-mg dose of pimozide in individuals receiving citalopram (40 mg once daily for 11 days) was associated with mean increases in the QT_c interval of approximately 10 msec compared with pimozide given alone. Citalopram did not substantially affect the mean AUC or peak plasma concentrations of pimozide. The mechanism for this potential pharmacodynamic interaction is not known. In addition, concomitant use of citalopram and pimozide rarely may result in potentially serious, sometimes fatal serotonin syndrome.

The manufacturers of citalopram hydrobromide state that concurrent administration of citalopram and pimozide is contraindicated.

■ **Other CNS-active Agents** The manufacturers state that, given the primary CNS effects of citalopram, caution should be used when it is given concurrently with other centrally acting drugs.

■ **Digoxin** In healthy adults who received citalopram (40 mg daily for 3 weeks), the concurrent administration of a single, 1-mg dose of digoxin did not significantly affect the pharmacokinetics of citalopram or digoxin. Concurrent administration of the 2 drugs was well tolerated, with no serious adverse events and no clinically important ECG changes reported. These data suggest that concomitantly administered citalopram is unlikely to substantially affect serum digoxin concentrations in patients who are receiving chronic digoxin therapy.

■ **Diuretics** Concomitant use of citalopram and diuretics may increase the risk of hyponatremia. (See Other Renal, Electrolyte, and Genitourinary Effects under Cautions: Renal, Electrolyte, and Genitourinary Effects.)

■ **Electroconvulsive Therapy** The manufacturer states that there are no clinical studies on the concurrent use of citalopram and electroconvulsive therapy (ECT). In a limited number of depressed women given either citalopram 20 mg or placebo before their third and fourth ECT sessions, no adverse effects were reported after citalopram administration and the length of the electrically induced seizures and neurohormonal responses did not substantially differ between the 2 groups. However, additional studies are needed to confirm the safety and efficacy of ECT in patients receiving citalopram.

■ **Metoprolol** Administration of citalopram 40 mg daily for 22 days resulted in a twofold increase in the plasma concentrations of metoprolol in one study. Increased plasma concentrations of metoprolol have been associated with decreased cardioselectivity. Concurrent administration of citalopram and metoprolol had no clinically important effects on blood pressure or heart rate.

■ **Theophylline** In an open, multiple-dose study, concurrent administration of citalopram (40 mg daily) for 21 days and theophylline (single, 300-mg dose), a CYP1A2 substrate, in healthy individuals did not substantially affect the pharmacokinetics of theophylline. Therefore, some clinicians state that dosage adjustment of theophylline may not be necessary in patients receiving citalopram concurrently. The effect of theophylline on the pharmacokinetics of citalopram was not evaluated.

■ **Cyclosporine** Limited evidence suggests that citalopram does not substantially affect the pharmacokinetics of cyclosporine; further study is needed to confirm these preliminary findings.

Acute Toxicity

Limited information is available on the acute toxicity of citalopram.

■ **Pathogenesis** The acute lethal dose of citalopram in humans is not known. The manufacturer states that no fatalities were reported among patients taking overdosages of up to 2 g during clinical trials. However, postmarketing reports of citalopram overdosage have included ingestions of up to 6 g; as with other selective serotonin-reuptake inhibitors, fatalities have been reported rarely following citalopram overdosage.

■ **Manifestations** In general, overdosage of citalopram may be expected to produce effects that are extensions of the drug's pharmacologic and adverse effects. Case reports in humans indicate that the possible effects of citalopram overdosage (either alone or in combination with other drugs and/or alcohol) include dizziness, sweating, nausea, vomiting, tremor, somnolence, and sinus tachycardia. In rare cases, observed symptoms have included amnesia, confusion, coma, seizures, hyperventilation, cyanosis, and rhabdomyolysis.

ECG changes, including QT_c prolongation, sinus bradycardia, nodal rhythm, ventricular arrhythmias, left bundle branch block, and torsades de pointes, have been reported rarely in citalopram overdosage. In a young, healthy female who ingested 400 mg of citalopram, QT_c prolongation was reported. In most cases of pure citalopram overdosage at doses exceeding 600 mg, ECG changes, including QT prolongation and sinus bradycardia, gradually resolved 12–24 hours following the intoxication. However, severe sinus bradycardia developed within about 4 hours following ingestion of 800 mg of citalopram alone in one female patient and lasted up to 6 days during intensive care unit (ICU) treatment; hypotension and syncope also occurred but no QT-interval prolongation was observed. A temporary pacemaker was necessary for treatment of this patient. In another case, a woman developed life-threatening cardiac toxicity, including torsades de pointes with cardiac arrest, approximately 32 hours following ingestion of 1 g of citalopram; her corrected QT interval remained abnormal for 24 hours after presentation.

Manifestations resembling serotonin syndrome also have been reported following citalopram overdosage either alone or in combination with other serotonergic drugs (e.g., moclobemide [not commercially available in the US]). (See Cautions: Precautions and Contraindications and also see Drug Interactions: Serotonergic Drugs.)

In one fatal case involving a 47-year-old man who ingested an unknown amount of citalopram in combination with other drugs, postmortem citalopram concentrations were 0.88 mg/L in femoral blood, 1.16 mg/L in heart blood, and 0.9 mg/L in urine. In another fatal case involving a 53-year-old woman who ingested an unknown amount of citalopram and trimipramine, postmortem analysis revealed a citalopram concentration of 4.81 mg/L and a trimipramine concentration of 2.33 mg/L in femoral blood. The citalopram to demethylcitalopram ratios were 1.96 and 2.02 in femoral blood and hepatic tissue, respectively.

■ **Treatment** Because fatalities and severe toxicity have been reported following overdosage of citalopram and other selective serotonin-reuptake inhibitors, particularly in large overdosage and when taken with other drugs or alcohol, some clinicians recommend that any overdosage involving these drugs be managed aggressively. Because suicidal ingestion often involves more than one drug, clinicians treating citalopram overdosage should be alert to possible manifestations caused by drugs other than citalopram.

Clinicians also should consider the possibility of serotonin syndrome in patients presenting with similar clinical features and a recent history of citalopram ingestion and/or ingestion of other serotonergic agents. (See Cautions: Precautions and Contraindications and also see Drug Interactions: Serotonergic Drugs.)

Management of citalopram overdosage generally requires symptomatic and supportive care. A patent airway should be established and maintained, and adequate oxygenation and ventilation should be ensured. An ECG should be obtained and monitoring of cardiac function instituted. Frequent vital sign monitoring and close observation of the patient is necessary. Clinicians should consider that development of cardiac toxicity following citalopram overdosage may be delayed. There is no specific antidote for citalopram intoxication.

Following recent (i.e., within 4 hours) ingestion of a potentially toxic amount of citalopram and in the absence of signs and symptoms of cardiac toxicity, the stomach should be emptied immediately by inducing emesis or by gastric lavage. However, some clinicians recommend avoidance of emesis in patients who have ingested overdoses of selective serotonin-reuptake inhibitors because of the potential for unexpected changes in mental status. If the patient is comatose, having seizures, or lacks the gag reflex, gastric lavage may be performed if an endotracheal tube with cuff inflated is in place to prevent aspiration of gastric contents. However, some clinicians note that gastric lavage generally is not necessary because of the low incidence of fatalities associated with selective serotonin-reuptake inhibitor overdoses. In one study, activated charcoal alone or gastric lavage followed by activated charcoal demonstrated similar efficacy in preventing the absorption of citalopram. In another study, single-dose activated charcoal administration given an average of 2.1 hours after citalopram ingestion was found to be effective in reducing the risk of QT-interval prolongation associated with overdosage of the drug. Since administration of activated charcoal (which may be used in conjunction with sorbitol) may be as or more effective than induction of emesis or gastric lavage, its use has been recommended either in the initial management of selective serotonin-reuptake inhibitor overdosage or following induction of emesis or gastric lavage in patients who have ingested a potentially toxic quantity of these drugs.

Because of the large volume of distribution of citalopram, hemodialysis, peritoneal dialysis, forced diuresis, hemoperfusion, and/or exchange transfusion are unlikely to be effective in removing substantial amounts of citalopram from the body.

Clinicians should consult a poison control center for additional information on the management of citalopram overdosage.

Chronic Toxicity

The results of animal studies suggest that the abuse potential for citalopram is low. Citalopram has not been studied systematically in humans to determine whether therapy with the drug is associated with abuse, tolerance, or physical dependence.

The premarketing clinical experience with citalopram did not reveal any drug-seeking behavior. However, these observations were not systematic, and it is not possible to accurately predict from the limited data currently available the extent to which a CNS-active drug like citalopram will be misused, diverted, and/or abused.

Experience with citalopram, other selective serotonin-reuptake inhibitors (SSRIs), and selective serotonin- and norepinephrine-reuptake inhibitors (SNRIs) suggests that a withdrawal syndrome may occur within several days following discontinuance of these drugs, particularly when abrupt. The most commonly observed manifestations are those that resemble influenza, such as fatigue, lethargy, GI complaints (e.g., nausea), dizziness or lightheadedness, impaired sleep, tremor, anxiety, insomnia, chills, sweating, and incoordination. Other reported manifestations include dysphoric mood, irritability, emotional lability, hypomania, memory impairment, sensory disturbances (such as paresthesias, including electric shock-like sensations), confusion, headache, palpitations, agitation, and aggression. Although the mechanism(s) for such withdrawal reactions is not fully understood, it has been suggested that they may be caused by a sudden decrease in serotonin availability at the synapse or cholinergic rebound; other neurotransmitters (e.g., dopamine, norepinephrine, GABA) also may be involved. These manifestations may in some cases be mistaken for physical illness or relapse into depression. While these reactions generally appear to be self-limiting and improve over one to several weeks, there have been reports of serious discontinuance symptoms. Manifestations of withdrawal also may be improved by restarting therapy with citalopram or another antidepressant with a similar pharmacologic profile.

Withdrawal reactions have been reported rarely in citalopram-treated patients. Data from a controlled study evaluating citalopram in preventing depression relapse indicate that the symptoms associated with abrupt discontinuance of therapy generally are mild and transient. Overall clinical experience to date suggests that the risk of withdrawal effects may be somewhat lower with citalopram, fluoxetine, and sertraline compared with paroxetine. These differences may be due at least in part to the prolonged elimination half-lives of the parent drugs and/or their active metabolites. The manufacturer and some clinicians recommend that citalopram, like other SSRIs, be discontinued gradually (e.g., over a period of several weeks) rather than abruptly whenever possible to prevent the possible development of withdrawal reactions.

As with other CNS-active drugs, clinicians should carefully evaluate patients for a history of substance abuse prior to initiating citalopram therapy. If citalopram therapy is initiated in patients with a history of substance abuse, such patients should be monitored closely for signs of misuse or abuse of the drug (e.g., development of tolerance, use of increasing doses, drug-seeking behavior).

Pharmacology

The pharmacology of citalopram is complex and in many ways resembles that of other antidepressant agents, particularly those agents (e.g., escitalopram, fluoxetine, fluvoxamine, paroxetine, sertraline, clomipramine, trazodone) that predominantly potentiate the pharmacologic effects of serotonin (5-hydroxytryptamine [5-HT]). Like other selective serotonin-reuptake inhibitors (SSRIs), citalopram is a potent and highly selective inhibitor of serotonin reuptake and has little or no effect on other neurotransmitters.

■ **Nervous System Effects** The precise mechanism of antidepressant action of citalopram is unclear, but the drug has been shown to selectively inhibit the reuptake of serotonin at the presynaptic neuronal membrane. Citalopram-induced inhibition of serotonin reuptake causes increased synaptic concentrations of serotonin in the CNS, resulting in numerous functional changes associated with enhanced serotonergic neurotransmission. Like other selective serotonin-reuptake inhibitors (e.g., fluoxetine, fluvoxamine, paroxetine, sertraline), citalopram appears to have only very weak effects on the reuptake of norepinephrine or dopamine and does not exhibit clinically important anticholinergic, antihistaminic, or adrenergic (α_1, α_2, β) blocking activity at usual therapeutic dosages.

Although the mechanism of antidepressant action of antidepressant agents may involve inhibition of the reuptake of various neurotransmitters (e.g., serotonin, norepinephrine) at the presynaptic neuronal membrane, it has been suggested that postsynaptic receptor modification is mainly responsible for the antidepressant action observed during long-term administration of antidepressant agents. During long-term therapy with most antidepressants (e.g., tricyclic antidepressants, monoamine oxidase [MAO] inhibitors), these adaptive changes mainly consist of subsensitivity of the noradrenergic adenylate cyclase system in association with a decrease in the number of β-adrenergic receptors; such effects on noradrenergic receptor function are commonly referred to as "down regulation." However, selective serotonin-reuptake inhibitors have not consistently demonstrated the ability to downregulate β-adrenergic receptors despite being effective antidepressant agents clinically. Thus, downregulation of β-adrenergic receptors does not appear to be an absolute prerequisite for antidepressant action. Long-term administration of desipramine but not citalopram substantially decreased β-adrenergically mediated cyclic adenosine monophosphate accumulation. In addition, some antidepressants (e.g., amitriptyline) reportedly decreased the number of serotonergic binding sites following chronic administration.

The exact mechanism of action of citalopram in panic disorder has not been fully elucidated but appears to involve at least in part changes in serotonergic neurotransmission.

The precise mechanism of action that is responsible for the efficacy of citalopram in the treatment of obsessive-compulsive disorder is unclear. However, because of the potency of clomipramine and other selective serotonin-reuptake inhibitors (e.g., fluoxetine, fluvoxamine, paroxetine, sertraline) in inhibiting serotonin reuptake and their efficacy in the treatment of obsessive-compulsive disorder, a serotonin hypothesis has been developed to explain the pathogenesis of the condition. The hypothesis postulates that a dysregulation of serotonin is responsible for obsessive-compulsive disorder and that citalopram and these other agents are effective because they correct this imbalance. Although considerable evidence supports the serotonergic hypothesis of obsessive-compulsive disorder, additional studies are necessary to confirm this hypothesis. Regardless of the precise pathogenesis of obsessive-compulsive disorder, the clinical efficacy of long-term therapy with selective serotonin-reuptake inhibitors such as citalopram appears to be due at least in part to alterations in serotonergic neurotransmission.

Serotonergic mechanisms also appear to be involved at least in part in a number of other pharmacologic effects associated with selective serotonin-reuptake inhibitors, including citalopram, such as decreased alcohol intake and regulation of food intake.

Serotonergic Effects Citalopram is a highly selective inhibitor of serotonin reuptake at the presynaptic neuronal membrane. Citalopram-induced inhibition of serotonin reuptake causes increased synaptic concentrations of the neurotransmitter, resulting in numerous functional changes associated with enhanced serotonergic neurotransmission.

Based on in vitro studies, the relative potency of citalopram as an inhibitor of serotonin reuptake compared with norepinephrine and dopamine reuptake inhibition is 3400 and 22,000, respectively, making the drug the most selective serotonin-reuptake inhibitor currently available. These findings have been confirmed by the results of in vivo and ex vivo studies demonstrating that citalopram inhibits the uptake of serotonin without appreciably inhibiting the uptake of norepinephrine or dopamine. In an initial study in rats, tolerance to the serotonin-reuptake inhibiting effect was not induced following long-term (14 days) citalopram administration.

Citalopram occurs as a racemic mixture and data from in vitro and in vivo studies indicate that the serotonin-reuptake blocking activity of citalopram is principally due to escitalopram, the (+)-enantiomer with the 1-(*S*) absolute configuration. Escitalopram is at least 100-fold more potent as an inhibitor of the reuptake of serotonin at the presynaptic membranes and the 5-HT neuronal firing rate than the *R*-enantiomer and is twice as potent as the racemic mixture. However, further studies are needed to determine whether these differences result in any clinical superiority of escitalopram. For additional information on escitalopram, see Escitalopram Oxalate 28:16.04.20.

Unlike some other serotonin-reuptake inhibitors, the demethylated metabolites of citalopram, demethylcitalopram and didemethylcitalopram, are substantially less active than the parent compound as inhibitors of serotonin reuptake and have negligible affinity for various neurotransmitter receptor-binding sites. In vitro studies have shown that citalopram is at least 8 times more potent than its metabolites in inhibiting serotonin reuptake; therefore, the drug's metabolites are unlikely to contribute to the clinical activity of the drug.

At therapeutic dosages in humans, citalopram has been shown to inhibit the reuptake of serotonin into platelets.

Like other selective serotonin-reuptake inhibitors, in vitro data have demonstrated that citalopram has no or very low affinity for serotonergic receptor subtypes (5-HT_{1A} and 5-HT_{2A} receptors).

Effects on Other Neurotransmitters The results of in vitro and in vivo studies indicate that citalopram has little effect on the neuronal reuptake of norepinephrine and dopamine. In addition, in vivo and in vitro data suggest that citalopram does not substantially inhibit MAO. However, citalopram has demonstrated some inhibitory activity towards MAO-A and MAO-B, with clear selectivity for MAO-B, in one in vivo study.

Unlike tricyclic and some other antidepressants, citalopram does not exhibit clinically important anticholinergic, α- or β-adrenergic blocking, or antihistaminic activity at usual therapeutic dosages. As a result, the incidence of adverse effects commonly associated with blockade of muscarinic cholinergic receptors (e.g., dry mouth, blurred vision, urinary retention, constipation, confusion), α-adrenergic receptors (e.g., orthostatic hypotension), and histamine H_1- and H_2-receptors (e.g., sedation) is lower in citalopram-treated patients. In vitro studies have demonstrated that citalopram possesses no or very low affinity for α_1- or α_2-adrenergic, β-adrenergic, histaminergic (H_1), GABA, muscarinic, benzodiazepine, dopamine D_1 and D_2, or opiate receptors.

Effects on Sleep Like tricyclic and most other antidepressants, citalopram suppresses rapid eye movement (REM) sleep. In animals, citalopram has been shown to suppress REM sleep and increase deep slow wave sleep. In one study in humans, single doses of the drug suppressed REM sleep in a dose-dependent manner while chronic therapy produced more sustained REM sleep inhibition. Single doses of citalopram resulted in only minor changes in non-REM sleep as well as in non-REM EEG power spectral density in this study. However, chronic administration of the drug resulted in a major shift from slow-wave sleep stage 2 to slow-wave sleep stage 1. In another study, citalopram prolonged REM latency and increased non-REM stage 2 sleep.

Although not clearly established, there is some evidence that the REM-suppressing effects of antidepressant agents may contribute to the antidepressant activity of these drugs. Although the precise mechanism has not been fully elucidated, available data suggest that citalopram's effects on REM sleep may be serotonergically mediated.

Effects on EEG Limited data currently are available regarding the effects of citalopram on the EEG. In animals, EEG studies have revealed an activating effect associated with behavioral arousal. In healthy individuals receiving single 20- and 40-mg doses, citalopram decreased slow-wave EEG activity in one study. However, the overall EEG changes were considered minimal in this study, particularly following repeated doses of the drug. EEG changes in healthy individuals receiving single, 10- to 50-mg oral doses of citalopram were dose-related and similar to those produced by desipramine, protriptyline, and fluvoxamine in another study.

Effects on Psychomotor Function Citalopram generally does not appear to cause clinically important sedation and generally does not adversely affect psychomotor performance. In studies in healthy individuals, citalopram did not produce impairment of psychomotor function or intellectual function when given in doses of 40 mg daily. In one controlled study, improved psychomotor responses to sensory stimuli and sustained attention, with substantial decreases in movement times of the choice reaction time test and an increase in critical flicker fusion threshold, were reported in healthy individuals receiving single doses of the drug.

■ **Cardiovascular Effects** No clinically important changes in vital signs (systolic and diastolic blood pressure and heart rate) were observed in patients receiving citalopram in controlled trials. In addition, a comparison of supine and standing vital signs in depressed patients receiving citalopram indicated that the drug generally does not produce orthostatic changes. Adverse cardiovascular effects, including QT-interval prolongation and torsades de pointes, have occasionally been reported in healthy individuals and in depressed patients receiving citalopram. (See Cautions: Cardiovascular Effects and see also Cautions: Precautions and Contraindications.)

In a thorough QT study, citalopram was associated with a dose-dependent increase in the corrected QT (QT_c) interval. In a placebo-controlled study, a change from baseline in QT_cF (Fridericia's formula) greater than 60 msec occurred in 1.9% of patients receiving citalopram compared with 1.2% of patients receiving placebo. None of the patients receiving placebo had a post-dose QT_cF greater than 500 msec compared with 0.5% of patients receiving citalopram. The incidence of tachycardic and bradycardic outliers was 0.5 and 0.9% in the citalopram group, respectively, and 0.4% in the placebo group. ECG changes also have been reported in individuals receiving overdosages of the drug. (See Acute Toxicity.)

Citalopram did not induce any substantial change in cardiovascular autonomic function tests (such as heart rate variability) in a limited number of healthy individuals receiving the drug.

■ **Effects on Appetite and Body Weight** Citalopram appears to possess some anorexigenic activity, although to a lesser degree than certain other serotonergic agents (e.g., fenfluramine [no longer commercially available in the US], fluoxetine, sertraline, zimelidine [not commercially available in the US]). Although the precise mechanism has not been clearly established, results from animal studies indicate that the appetite-inhibiting action of these drugs may result at least in part from serotonin-reuptake blockade and enhancement of serotonin release thereby increasing serotonin availability at the neuronal synapse.

Only minimal weight loss (averaging 0.5 kg) generally occurred in patients receiving citalopram in controlled clinical trials. In addition, while decreased appetite was reported in about 4% of patients receiving citalopram in short-term clinical trials, the drug, unlike fluoxetine, does not appear to exhibit clinically important anorectic effects nor to produce clinically important long-term weight changes. Short-term citalopram therapy did not produce substantial weight loss in severely obese individuals in one study. Paradoxical weight gain and obesity also have been reported in some patients receiving the drug.

■ **Effects on Alcohol Intake** Like some other serotonergic agents, citalopram produces a substantial decrease in voluntary alcohol intake in animals; however, development of tolerance to this effect has been reported. Like some other serotonin-reuptake inhibitors (fluoxetine, zimelidine), citalopram also has been shown to reduce alcohol consumption in alcohol-dependent, nondepressed drinkers receiving short-term therapy with 40 mg of the drug daily. Because serotonin appears to be involved in the regulation of alcohol intake, it has been suggested that selective serotonin-reuptake inhibitors may attenuate alcohol consumption via enhanced serotonergic neurotransmission. (See Uses: Alcohol Dependence and see Drug Interactions: Alcohol.)

■ **Neuroendocrine Effects** Limited data currently are available regarding the effects of citalopram on the neuroendocrine system. In a controlled study in healthy individuals, plasma prolactin concentrations reportedly were increased by 40% following 10 days of treatment with citalopram 20 mg daily. In addition, in healthy individuals receiving low-dose IV citalopram (parenteral dosage form not commercially available in the US), plasma prolactin and cortisol concentrations increased in a dose-dependent manner.

■ **Other Effects** Like some other antidepressants that are amphiphilic cationic compounds, citalopram has been found to cause a generalized lipidosis in animal studies. Lipidosis-like changes in lymph nodes, adrenal cortex and medulla, kidney, lung, and sympathetic ganglia have been noted in animals receiving 140 mg/kg daily of the drug for 7 weeks; however, the clinical importance of these findings remains to be established.

Limited data in animals suggest that citalopram may possess anticonvulsant activity during chronic administration.

Pharmacokinetics

In all human studies described in the Pharmacokinetics section, citalopram was administered as the hydrobromide salt; dosages and concentrations are expressed in terms of citalopram.

A concentration of 1 nmol/L of citalopram is approximately equivalent to 0.32 ng/mL.

■ **Absorption** Like other selective serotonin-reuptake inhibitors, citalopram is a highly lipophilic compound that appears to be rapidly and well absorbed from the GI tract following oral administration. Following a single 40-mg oral dose of citalopram as a tablet, the manufacturer states that peak plasma concentrations averaging approximately 44 ng/mL occur at about 4 hours.

The absolute bioavailability of citalopram is approximately 80% relative to an IV dose. The oral tablets and solution of citalopram reportedly are bioequivalent. Food does not substantially affect the absorption of citalopram.

The single- and multiple-dose pharmacokinetics of citalopram are linear and dose-proportional in a dosage range of 10–60 mg daily. With once-daily dosing, steady-state plasma concentrations are achieved within approximately 1 week. In one study, the steady-state plasma concentrations ranged from about 30–230 ng/mL in depressed patients receiving dosages of 30–60 mg daily and agreed well with predicted values. The mean plasma concentration was approximately 80 ng/mL at the usual dosage of 40 mg daily. At steady state, the extent of accumulation of citalopram in plasma, based on the half-life, is expected to be about 2.5 times higher than the plasma concentrations observed after a single dose of the drug.

In depressed patients receiving 20–60 mg daily of citalopram, steady-state plasma concentrations of racemic citalopram and demethylcitalopram, a principal metabolite, ranged from 9–200 ng/mL and 10–105 ng/mL, respectively. When using a stereoselective analysis method, plasma concentrations ranged from 9–106 ng/mL for escitalopram (*S*-citalopram), 20–186 ng/mL for *R*-citalopram, 4–38 ng/mL for *S*-demethylcitalopram, and 3–75 ng/mL for *R*-demethylcitalopram in depressed patients receiving citalopram therapy (20–80 mg daily). The mean ratio between *R*-citalopram and escitalopram was 0.56 (range: 0.32–0.97).

The effect of age on the pharmacokinetics of citalopram has not been fully elucidated. Studies in healthy individuals and depressed patients 60 years of age or older have found higher areas under the plasma concentration-time curves (AUC) and longer elimination half-lives compared with those in younger individuals. (See Pharmacokinetics: Elimination.) In healthy individuals 60 years of age or older, the AUC of citalopram was increased by an average of approximately 30% in a single-dose study and by an average of approximately 23% in a multiple-dose study. Steady-state plasma citalopram concentrations were up to 4 times higher in geriatric patients receiving 20 mg of the drug once daily in one multiple-dose study than expected based on data in younger patients and healthy individuals. (See Dosage and Administration: Dosage in Geriatric Patients and see Cautions: Geriatric Precautions.)

The effect of gender on the pharmacokinetics of citalopram has not been fully elucidated to date. The manufacturer states that in 3 pharmacokinetic studies, the AUC of citalopram in women was 1.5–2 times higher than that found in men; however, this difference was not observed in 5 other pharmacokinetic studies performed with the drug. In clinical studies, no differences in steady-state plasma citalopram concentrations were observed between men and women. In addition, there were no gender differences in the pharmacokinetics of the principal metabolites of citalopram, demethylcitalopram and didemethylcitalopram. Therefore, the manufacturer states that no adjustment of citalopram dosage on the basis of gender is necessary.

The onset of antidepressant activity following oral administration of citalopram hydrobromide usually occurs within 1–4 weeks.

As with other selective serotonin-reuptake inhibitors, the relationship between plasma citalopram concentrations and the therapeutic and/or toxic effects of the drug has not been clearly established. Since citalopram is administered as a racemic mixture with the pharmacologic effect of the drug associated mainly with escitalopram, the *S*-enantiomer, it may be important to take the stereoselective metabolism of the drug into account when evaluating the relationship between the clinical effect of the drug and plasma concentrations of citalopram.

■ Distribution Distribution of citalopram and its metabolites into human body tissues and fluids has not been fully characterized. However, limited pharmacokinetic data suggest that the drug, which is highly lipophilic, is widely distributed in body tissues.

The volume of distribution of citalopram is approximately 12 L/kg. The drug crosses the blood-brain barrier in humans and animals.

The binding of citalopram, demethylcitalopram, and didemethylcitalopram to human plasma proteins in vitro is about 80%.

Citalopram and demethylcitalopram are distributed into milk and also cross the placenta. In a study involving 7 lactating women who received median oral citalopram doses of 0.36 mg/kg daily for the treatment of depression, mean milk-to-plasma AUC values of 1.8 were calculated for both citalopram and demethylcitalopram. Depending on the method of calculation, mean infant exposure was estimated to be 3.2 or 3.7% for citalopram and 1.2 or 1.4% for demethylcitalopram in this study. In 9 lactating women receiving 20–40 mg daily of citalopram in another study, maternal milk-to-plasma ratios of the drug ranged from approximately 2–3; however, plasma citalopram concentrations in the neonates were found to be very low or below the limit of detection. In a lactating woman receiving 40 mg daily of citalopram, concentrations of the drug in milk and serum were about 205 ng/mL and 99 ng/mL, respectively, and the drug concentration in the infant's serum was about 13 ng/mL. In another lactating woman receiving 20 mg daily of citalopram, peak milk concentrations of the drug occurred 3–9 hours following maternal drug intake; the milk-to-serum concentration ratio was approximately 3 for both citalopram and demethylcitalopram. Accordingly, the infant received approximately 5% of the mother's dose when adjusted for weight. (See Cautions: Pregnancy, Fertility, and Lactation.)

■ Elimination The elimination half-life of citalopram averages approximately 35 hours in adults with normal renal and hepatic function.

The exact metabolic fate of citalopram has not been fully elucidated; however, metabolism of citalopram is mainly hepatic and involves *N*-demethylation. Citalopram is metabolized to demethylcitalopram, didemethylcitalopram, citalopram-*N*-oxide, and a deaminated propionic acid derivative. In vitro studies have indicated that cytochrome P-450 (CYP) 3A4 and 2C19 isoenzymes are the principal enzymes involved in the *N*-demethylation of citalopram to demethylcitalopram and that demethylcitalopram is further *N*-demethylated to didemethylcitalopram by CYP2D6. Because citalopram is metabolized by multiple enzyme systems, inhibition of a single enzyme is unlikely to appreciably decrease the clearance of citalopram. Unlike some other selective serotonin-reuptake inhibitors, the demethylated metabolites of citalopram, demethylcitalopram and didemethylcitalopram, are substantially less active than the parent compound as inhibitors of serotonin reuptake. Thus, citalopram's metabolites are unlikely to contribute to the antidepressant and other clinical actions of the drug.

In humans, unchanged citalopram is the predominant compound in plasma. At steady state, the concentrations of demethylcitalopram and didemethylcitalopram in plasma are approximately one-half and one-tenth, respectively, that of the parent drug. Following IV (parenteral dosage form not commercially available in the US) administration of citalopram, the fraction of drug recovered in urine as citalopram and demethylcitalopram was about 10 and 5%, respectively.

Following oral administration of a single, radiolabeled dose of citalopram in healthy individuals, approximately 75% of the dose was excreted in urine and approximately 10% was eliminated in feces within 17 days. An analysis of the urinary composition showed that besides the known metabolites of citalopram, 3 glucuronides were present. The relative amounts of citalopram, demethylcitalopram, didemethylcitalopram, and the *N*-oxide metabolite present in urine collected for 7 days were 26, 19, 9, and 7%, respectively, with glucuronidated metabolites accounting for the remainder.

Following IV administration, the mean systemic clearance of citalopram is approximately 330 mL/minute, with approximately 20% of that due to renal clearance.

The effect of age on the elimination of citalopram has not been fully elucidated. Studies in healthy geriatric individuals and depressed geriatric patients have found higher AUC values and longer elimination half-lives compared with younger individuals. (See Pharmacokinetics: Absorption.) In healthy individuals 60 years of age or older, the elimination half-life of citalopram was increased by 50% in a single-dose study and by 30% in a multiple-dose study. It has been suggested that these differences in pharmacokinetic parameters may reflect declining liver and kidney function. In addition, the stereoselective metabolism of the enantiomers for citalopram and demethylcitalopram in older individuals appears to differ from that reported in younger patients, suggesting possible age-associated changes in CYP2C19 activities. (See Dosage and Administration: Dosage in Geriatric Patients and see Cautions: Geriatric Precautions.)

Because citalopram is extensively metabolized in the liver, hepatic impairment can affect the elimination of the drug. Following oral administration, the clearance of citalopram in patients with impaired hepatic function was reduced by 37% and the elimination half-life was increased twofold compared with that in healthy individuals. Therefore, the manufacturer recommends that in depressed patients with hepatic impairment, the maximum recommended dosage of citalopram is 20 mg once daily due to the risk of QT-interval prolongation. (See Dosage and Administration: Dosage in Hepatic and Renal Impairment and see Cautions: Precautions and Contraindications.)

In poor metabolizers of CYP2C19, steady-state peak concentrations and AUC values of citalopram increased by 68 and 107%, respectively. Therefore, the manufacturer recommends that in poor metabolizers of CYP2C19, the maximum recommended dosage of citalopram is 20 mg once daily due to the risk of QT-interval prolongation. (See Dosage and Administration: Dosage in Poor CYP2C19 Metabolizers or Patients Receiving CYP2C19 Inhibitors and see Cautions: Precautions and Contraindications.) Steady-state plasma citalopram concentrations were not substantially different in healthy individuals with poor or extensive CYP2D6 metabolizer phenotypes following multiple-dose administration of the drug.

The effect of renal impairment on the pharmacokinetics of citalopram has not been fully evaluated to date. In patients with moderate renal impairment, the renal clearance of citalopram and its 2 principal metabolites was reduced and the elimination half-life of citalopram was slightly prolonged to an average of about 50 hours. In a study comparing the pharmacokinetics of citalopram in a limited number of patients with severe renal failure undergoing hemodialysis and in healthy individuals, no substantial differences were found between the 2 groups in any of the pharmacokinetic parameters, with the exception of the renal clearance of citalopram, which was significantly lower in the renal failure group than in the control group (1.7 mL/minute versus 66 mL/minute). Therefore, moderate to severe renal failure does not appear to markedly affect the pharmacokinetics of citalopram suggesting that dosage adjustment in such patients may not be necessary. Additional studies evaluating long-term citalopram therapy in patients with severe renal impairment are necessary to confirm these findings. (See Dosage and Administration: Dosage in Hepatic and Renal Impairment.)

Limited data indicate that citalopram and demethylcitalopram are not appreciably removed by hemodialysis. In a limited number of patients, hemodialysis cleared only about 1% of an oral dose of citalopram as the parent drug and 1% as demethylcitalopram. Because of the large volume of distribution of citalopram, hemodialysis, peritoneal dialysis, forced diuresis, hemoperfusion, and/or exchange transfusion also are unlikely to be effective in removing substantial amounts of citalopram from the body.

Chemistry and Stability

■ Chemistry Citalopram hydrobromide, a selective serotonin-reuptake inhibitor (SSRI), is a bicyclic phthalane-derivative antidepressant. The drug differs structurally from most other selective serotonin-reuptake inhibitors (e.g., fluoxetine, fluvoxamine, paroxetine, sertraline) and also differs structurally and pharmacologically from tricyclic and tetracyclic antidepressants. The commercially available drug is a 50:50 racemic mixture of the *R*- and *S*-enantiomers. The inhibition of serotonin reuptake by citalopram is principally due to the *S*-enantiomer, escitalopram (see Escitalopram Oxalate 28:16.04.20).

Citalopram hydrobromide occurs as a fine white to off-white powder that is sparingly soluble in water and soluble in ethanol. The drug has a pK_a of 9.5.

Citalopram hydrobromide is commercially available for oral administration as tablets and as an oral solution. Commercially available citalopram hydrobromide oral solution is a clear, colorless solution with a peppermint flavor and contains 10 mg of citalopram per 5 mL. Citalopram hydrobromide oral solution contains methylparabens and propylparabens as preservatives. Citalopram also is commercially available in some countries as an IV injection†; however, this dosage form currently is not available in the US.

■ Stability Citalopram hydrobromide tablets should be stored at a temperature of 25°C but may be exposed to temperatures ranging from 15–30°C. When stored as directed, the tablets have an expiration date of 2 years following the date of manufacture.

Citalopram hydrobromide oral solution should be stored at 20–25°C but may be exposed to temperatures ranging from 15–30°C.

Preparations

Because of similarity in spelling of Celexa® (citalopram hydrobromide), Celebrex® (celecoxib), and Cerebyx® (fosphenytoin sodium), extra care should be exercised in ensuring the accuracy of prescriptions for these drugs.

Excipients in commercially available drug preparations may have clinically important effects in some individuals; consult specific product labeling for details.

Citalopram Hydrobromide

Oral		
Tablets, film-coated	10 mg (of citalopram)*	**CeleXA®**, Forest
		Citalopram Hydrobromide Tablets
	20 mg (of citalopram)*	**CeleXA®** (scored), Forest
		Citalopram Hydrobromide Tablets
	40 mg (of citalopram)*	**CeleXA®** (scored), Forest
		Citalopram Hydrobromide Tablets
Solution	10 mg (of citalopram) per 5 mL*	**Citalopram Hydrobromide Oral Solution**

*available from one or more manufacturer, distributor, and/or repackager by generic (nonproprietary) name

†Use is not currently included in the labeling approved by the US Food and Drug Administration

Escitalopram Oxalate

■ Escitalopram, the *S*-enantiomer of citalopram, is a selective serotonin-reuptake inhibitor (SSRI) and an antidepressant.

Uses

■ Major Depressive Disorder Escitalopram oxalate is used for the acute and maintenance treatment of major depressive disorder in adults and adolescents 12–17 years of age.

Efficacy of escitalopram for the acute management of major depression in adults was established in 3 placebo-controlled studies of 8 weeks' duration in adult outpatients who met DSM-IV criteria for major depressive disorder. In these studies, 10- and 20-mg daily dosages of escitalopram were more effective than placebo in improving scores on the Montgomery Asberg Depression Rating Scale (MADRS), the Hamilton Rating Scale for Depression (HAM-D), and the Clinical Global Impression Improvement and Severity of Illness Scale. Escitalopram also was more effective than placebo in improving other aspects of depressive disorder, including anxiety, social functioning, and overall quality of life. Substantial improvement in MADRS and HAM-D scores was noted in patients receiving either dosage of escitalopram compared with those receiving placebo after 1–2 weeks of therapy. In addition, escitalopram dosages of 10–20 mg daily appeared to be at least as effective as racemic citalopram dosages of 20–40 mg daily. No age-, race-, or gender-related differences in efficacy were noted in these studies.

Efficacy of escitalopram for the acute management of major depressive disorder in adolescents 12–17 years of age was established in an 8-week, flexible-dose, placebo-controlled study in outpatients who met DSM-IV criteria for major depressive disorder. Escitalopram-treated patients in this study demonstrated substantially greater improvement on the Children's Depression Rating Scale–Revised (CDRS-R) compared with those receiving placebo. Efficacy of escitalopram in the acute treatment of major depressive disorder in adolescents was also established on the basis of extrapolation from an 8-week, flexible-dose, placebo-controlled study with racemic citalopram 20–40 mg daily. In this outpatient study conducted in children and adolescents 7–17 years of age who met DSM-IV criteria for major depressive disorder, citalopram-treated patients demonstrated substantially greater improvement on the CDRS-R compared with those receiving placebo; the positive results in this trial came largely from the adolescent subgroup. Two additional flexible-dose, placebo-controlled depression studies (one for escitalopram in patients 7–17 years of age and one for citalopram in adolescents) did not demonstrate efficacy.

In a longer-term study, 274 adults with major depressive disorder who had responded to escitalopram 10 or 20 mg daily during an initial 8-week, open-label, flexible dosage treatment phase were randomized to continue escitalopram at the same dosage or receive placebo for up to 36 weeks of observation for relapse in the double-blind phase. Relapse during the double-blind phase was defined as an increase in the MADRS total score to 22 or greater or discontinuance due to insufficient clinical response. Escitalopram-treated patients experienced a substantially longer time to relapse of depression compared with those receiving placebo. In addition, more placebo recipients relapsed compared with patients receiving escitalopram (cumulative relapse rates were approximately 40 and 26%, respectively).

Although efficacy of escitalopram as maintenance therapy in adolescent patients has not been systematically evaluated, such efficacy can be extrapolated from adult data along with comparisons of escitalopram pharmacokinetic parameters in adults and adolescent patients.

The manufacturers state that if escitalopram is used for extended periods, the need for continued therapy should be reassessed periodically.

There is some evidence that escitalopram may offer some clinical advantages compared with citalopram or other selective serotonin-reuptake inhibitors (e.g., increased efficacy, more rapid onset of therapeutic effect, fewer adverse effects); however, additional studies are needed to confirm these initial findings.

For further information on use of SSRIs in the treatment of major depressive disorder and considerations in choosing the most appropriate antidepressant agent for a particular patient, see Uses: Major Depressive Disorder, in Citalopram Hydrobromide 28:16.04.20.

■ Generalized Anxiety Disorder Escitalopram is used in the management of generalized anxiety disorder in adults. Efficacy for the management of generalized anxiety disorder was established in 3 multicenter, flexible-dose, placebo-controlled studies of 8-weeks' duration in adult outpatients who met DSM-IV criteria for generalized anxiety disorder. In these studies, patients receiving 10–20 mg daily of escitalopram had substantially greater mean improvements in scores on the Hamilton Anxiety Scale (HAM-A) than those receiving placebo.

For further information on the treatment of generalized anxiety disorder, see Uses: Anxiety Disorders, in Paroxetine 28:16.04.20.

Dosage and Administration

■ Administration Escitalopram oxalate is administered orally once daily, in the morning or evening, without regard to meals. Commercially available escitalopram oxalate tablets and oral solution are bioequivalent.

Patients receiving escitalopram should be monitored for possible worsening of depression, suicidality, or unusual changes in behavior, especially at the beginning of therapy or during periods of dosage adjustment. (See Worsening of Depression and Suicidality Risk under Warnings/Precautions: Warnings, in Cautions.)

The manufacturers recommend that at least 2 weeks elapse between discontinuance of a monoamine oxidase (MAO) inhibitor and initiation of escitalopram and vice versa. (See Serotonin Syndrome or Neuroleptic Malignant Syndrome-like Reactions under Warnings/Precautions: Other Warnings and Precautions, in Cautions and also see Drug Interactions: Monoamine Oxidase Inhibitors.)

■ Dosage Dosage of escitalopram oxalate is expressed in terms of escitalopram.

Major Depressive Disorder For the acute management of major depressive disorder in adults, the recommended initial dosage of escitalopram is 10 mg once daily. Although efficacy has been established at dosages of 10 or 20 mg once daily, no additional benefit was observed with the 20-mg dosage in a fixed-dose study. If a dosage exceeding 10 mg daily is considered necessary, dosage may be increased to 20 mg daily after a minimum of 1 week.

For the acute management of major depressive disorder in adolescents 12–17 years of age, the recommended initial dosage of escitalopram is 10 mg once daily. Efficacy has been established at dosages of 10–20 mg daily in a flexible-dose study. If dosage is increased to 20 mg daily, this should occur after a minimum of 3 weeks.

While the optimum duration of escitalopram oxalate therapy has not been established, many experts state that acute depressive episodes require several months or longer of sustained antidepressant therapy. In addition, some clinicians recommend that long-term antidepressant therapy be considered in certain patients at risk for recurrence of depressive episodes (such as those with highly recurrent unipolar depression). Whether the dosage of escitalopram oxalate required to induce remission is identical to the dosage needed to maintain and/or sustain euthymia is unknown. Systematic evaluation of escitalopram oxalate has shown that its antidepressant efficacy is maintained for periods of up to 36 weeks in adults receiving 10–20 mg daily. Nevertheless, the manufacturers recommend that the usefulness of escitalopram be reevaluated periodically in patients receiving long-term therapy.

Generalized Anxiety Disorder For the management of generalized anxiety disorder in adults, the recommended initial dosage of escitalopram is 10 mg once daily. If no clinical improvement is apparent, dosage may be increased to 20 mg daily after a minimum of 1 week.

Although the manufacturers state that the efficacy of escitalopram for long-term therapy (i.e., longer than 8 weeks) has not been demonstrated in controlled studies to date, generalized anxiety disorder is a chronic condition. If escitalopram is used for extended periods, the need for continued therapy with the drug should be reassessed periodically.

Discontinuance of Therapy Because withdrawal effects may occur with discontinuance of escitalopram and other SSRIs and selective serotonin- and norepinephrine-reuptake inhibitors (SNRIs), abrupt discontinuance should be avoided whenever possible. When escitalopram therapy is discontinued, the dosage should be reduced gradually and the patient monitored for possible withdrawal symptoms. If intolerable symptoms occur following dosage reduction or upon discontinuance of therapy, the drug may be reinstituted at the previously prescribed dosage. Subsequently, the clinician may continue decreasing the dosage, but at a more gradual rate. (See Withdrawal of Therapy under Warnings/Precautions: Other Warnings and Precautions, in Cautions.)

■ Special Populations The recommended dosage of escitalopram in most geriatric patients and those with hepatic impairment is 10 mg once daily.

Dosage adjustment in patients with mild to moderate renal impairment is not necessary, but the drug should be used with caution in those with severe renal impairment.

Cautions

■ **Contraindications** Concurrent or recent (i.e., within 2 weeks) therapy with a monoamine oxidase (MAO) inhibitor. At least 14 days should elapse between discontinuance of escitalopram and initiation of MAO inhibitor therapy and vice versa. (See Serotonin Syndrome or Neuroleptic Malignant Syndrome-like Reactions under Warnings/Precautions: Other Warnings and Precautions, in Cautions and also see Drug Interactions: Monoamine Oxidase Inhibitors.)

Concomitant use with pimozide. (See Drug Interactions: Antipsychotic Agents and Other Dopamine Antagonists.)

Known hypersensitivity to escitalopram, citalopram, or any ingredient in the formulation.

■ **Warnings/Precautions** ***Warnings*** **Worsening of Depression and Suicidality Risk.** Worsening of depression and/or the emergence of suicidal ideation and behavior (suicidality) or unusual changes in behavior may occur in both adult and pediatric (see Pediatric Use under Warnings/Precautions: Specific Populations, in Cautions) patients with major depressive disorder or other psychiatric disorders, whether or not they are taking antidepressants. This risk may persist until clinically important remission occurs. Suicide is a known risk of depression and certain other psychiatric disorders, and these disorders themselves are the strongest predictors of suicide. However, there has been a long-standing concern that antidepressants may have a role in inducing worsening of depression and the emergence of suicidality in certain patients during the early phases of treatment. Pooled analyses of short-term, placebo-controlled studies of antidepressants (i.e., selective serotonin-reuptake inhibitors [SSRIs] and other antidepressants) have shown an increased risk of suicidality in children, adolescents, and young adults (18–24 years of age) with major depressive disorder and other psychiatric disorders. An increased suicidality risk was not demonstrated with antidepressants compared with placebo in adults older than 24 years of age and a reduced risk was observed in adults 65 years of age or older.

The US Food and Drug Administration (FDA) recommends that all patients being treated with antidepressants for any indication be appropriately monitored and closely observed for clinical worsening, suicidality, and unusual changes in behavior, particularly during initiation of therapy (i.e., the first few months) and during periods of dosage adjustments. Families and caregivers of patients being treated with antidepressants for major depressive disorder or other indications, both psychiatric and nonpsychiatric, also should be advised to monitor patients on a daily basis for the emergence of agitation, irritability, or unusual changes in behavior as well as the emergence of suicidality, and to report such symptoms immediately to a health-care provider.

Although a causal relationship between the emergence of symptoms such as anxiety, agitation, panic attacks, insomnia, irritability, hostility, aggressiveness, impulsivity, akathisia, hypomania, and/or mania and either the worsening of depression and/or the emergence of suicidal impulses has not been established, there is concern that such symptoms may represent precursors to emerging suicidality. Consequently, consideration should be given to changing the therapeutic regimen or discontinuing therapy in patients whose depression is persistently worse or in patients experiencing emergent suicidality or symptoms that might be precursors to worsening depression or suicidality, particularly if such manifestations are severe, abrupt in onset, or were not part of the patient's presenting symptoms. If a decision is made to discontinue therapy, taper escitalopram dosage as rapidly as is feasible but consider the risks of abrupt discontinuance. (See Discontinuance of Therapy, under Dosage and Administration: Dosage.) FDA also recommends that the drugs be prescribed in the smallest quantity consistent with good patient management, in order to reduce the risk of overdosage.

Other Warnings and Precautions **Serotonin Syndrome or Neuroleptic Malignant Syndrome-like Reactions.** Potentially life-threatening serotonin syndrome or neuroleptic malignant syndrome (NMS)-like reactions have been reported with SSRIs, including escitalopram, and selective serotonin- and norepinephrine-reuptake inhibitors (SNRIs) alone, but particularly with concurrent use of other serotonergic drugs (including serotonin [5-hydroxytryptamine; 5-HT] type 1 receptor agonists ["triptans"]), drugs that impair the metabolism of serotonin (e.g., MAO inhibitors), or antipsychotics or other dopamine antagonists. Manifestations of serotonin syndrome may include mental status changes (e.g., agitation, hallucinations, coma), autonomic instability (e.g., tachycardia, labile blood pressure, hyperthermia), neuromuscular aberrations (e.g., hyperreflexia, incoordination), and/or GI symptoms (e.g., nausea, vomiting, diarrhea). In its most severe form, serotonin syndrome may resemble NMS, which is characterized by hyperthermia, muscle rigidity, autonomic instability with possible rapid fluctuation in vital signs, and mental status changes. Patients receiving escitalopram should be monitored for the development of serotonin syndrome or NMS-like signs and symptoms. (See Contraindications and also see Drug Interactions.)

Concurrent or recent (i.e., within 2 weeks) therapy with MAO inhibitors intended to treat depression is contraindicated. (See Contraindications and also see Drug Interactions: Monoamine Oxidase Inhibitors.)

If concurrent therapy with escitalopram and a 5-HT_1 receptor agonist (triptan) is clinically warranted, the patient should be observed carefully, particularly during initiation of therapy, when dosage is increased, or when another serotonergic agent is initiated.

Concomitant use of escitalopram and serotonin precursors (e.g., tryptophan) is not recommended.

If signs and symptoms of serotonin syndrome or NMS occur, treatment with escitalopram and any concurrently administered serotonergic or antidopaminergic agents, including antipsychotic agents, should be immediately discontinued and supportive and symptomatic treatment initiated.

Withdrawal of Therapy. Withdrawal symptoms, including dysphoric mood, irritability, agitation, dizziness, sensory disturbances (e.g., paresthesias such as electric shock sensations), anxiety, confusion, headache, lethargy, emotional lability, insomnia, hypomania, tinnitus, and seizures, have been reported upon discontinuance of escitalopram and other SSRIs and SNRIs, particularly when discontinuance of these drugs is abrupt. While these reactions are generally self-limiting, there have been reports of serious discontinuance symptoms. Therefore, patients should be monitored for such symptoms when discontinuing escitalopram therapy. A gradual reduction in dosage rather than abrupt cessation is recommended whenever possible. (See Discontinuance of Therapy under Dosage and Administration: Dosage.)

If intolerable symptoms occur following dosage reduction or discontinuance of escitalopram, the previously prescribed dosage should be reinstituted until symptoms abate; dosage reductions may then be resumed at a more gradual rate.

Seizures. Although anticonvulsant effects of racemic citalopram have been observed in animal studies, escitalopram has not been systematically evaluated in patients with seizure disorders. Seizures have been reported in patients receiving escitalopram in clinical trials; therefore, as with other antidepressants, escitalopram therapy should be initiated with caution in patients with a history of seizure disorder.

Activation of Mania/Hypomania. Activation of mania and hypomania has occurred in patients receiving escitalopram or citalopram. Escitalopram should be used with caution in patients with a history of mania.

Hyponatremia/Syndrome of Inappropriate Antidiuretic Hormone Secretion. Treatment with SNRIs and SSRIs, including escitalopram, may result in hyponatremia. In many cases, hyponatremia appears to be due to the syndrome of inappropriate antidiuretic hormone secretion (SIADH). Cases with serum sodium concentrations lower than 110 mEq/L have been reported. Geriatric individuals and patients receiving diuretics or who are otherwise volume depleted may be at greater risk of developing hyponatremia. Signs and symptoms of hyponatremia include headache, difficulty concentrating, memory impairment, confusion, weakness, and unsteadiness, which may lead to falls; more severe and/or acute cases have been associated with hallucinations, syncope, seizures, coma, respiratory arrest, and death. Discontinuance of escitalopram should be considered and appropriate medical intervention should be initiated in patients with symptomatic hyponatremia.

Abnormal Bleeding. SNRIs and SSRIs, including escitalopram, may increase the risk of bleeding events. Concurrent use of aspirin, nonsteroidal anti-inflammatory agents (NSAIAs), warfarin, and other anticoagulants may add to this risk. Case reports and epidemiologic studies have demonstrated an association between the use of drugs that interfere with serotonin reuptake and the occurrence of GI bleeding. Bleeding events related to SNRI and SSRI use have ranged from ecchymoses, hematomas, epistaxis, and petechiae to life-threatening hemorrhages. The manufacturers recommend that patients be advised of the risk of bleeding associated with the concomitant use of escitalopram and aspirin or other NSAIAs, warfarin, or other drugs that affect coagulation. (See Drug Interactions: Drugs Affecting Hemostasis.)

Interference with Cognitive and Motor Performance. In a study in healthy volunteers, escitalopram 10 mg daily did not impair intellectual function or psychomotor performance. However, because any psychoactive drug may impair judgment, thinking, or motor skills, caution patients about operating hazardous machinery, including driving a motor vehicle, until they are reasonably certain that the drug does not affect their ability to engage in such activities.

Concomitant Illnesses. Experience with escitalopram in patients with certain concomitant diseases is limited. (See Renal Impairment and see Hepatic Impairment under Warnings/Precautions: Specific Populations, in Cautions.)

Escitalopram has not been systematically evaluated in patients with a recent history of myocardial infarction or unstable cardiovascular disease; such patients were generally excluded from clinical studies. The drug should be used with caution in patients with diseases or conditions that produce altered metabolism or hemodynamic responses.

Concomitant use of SSRIs and MAO inhibitors has been associated with serious, sometimes fatal, reactions, including hyperthermia, rigidity, myoclonus, autonomic instability, and mental status changes; these reactions have resembled serotonin syndrome or NMS. (See Contraindications and Serotonin Syndrome or Neuroleptic Malignant Syndrome-like Reactions under Warnings/Precautions: Other Warnings and Precautions, in Cautions and see also Drug Interactions: Monoamine Oxidase Inhibitors.)

Specific Populations **Pregnancy.** Category C. (See Users Guide.)

Some neonates exposed to serotonergic antidepressants (e.g., SSRIs, SNRIs) late in the third trimester of pregnancy have developed complications that have sometimes been severe and required prolonged hospitalization, respiratory support, enteral nutrition, and other forms of supportive care in special-care nurseries. Such complications may arise immediately upon delivery and usually last several days or up to 2–4 weeks. Clinical findings reported in the neonates have included respiratory distress, cyanosis, apnea, seizures, temperature instability or fever, feeding difficulty, dehydration, excessive weight loss, vomiting, hypoglycemia, hypotonia, hypertonia, hyperreflexia, tremor, jitteriness, irritability, and constant crying. These features appear to be consistent with either a direct toxic effect of serotonergic antidepressants or, possibly, a drug withdrawal syndrome. In some cases, the clinical picture was consistent with serotonin syndrome.

Infants exposed to SSRIs in late pregnancy may have an increased risk of persistent pulmonary hypertension of the newborn (PPHN), a rare heart and lung condition associated with substantial neonatal morbidity and mortality. Although several epidemiologic studies have suggested an increased risk of PPHN with SSRI use during pregnancy, other studies did not demonstrate a statistically significant association. The US Food and Drug Administration (FDA) states that it is currently unclear whether the use of SSRIs, including escitalopram, during pregnancy can cause PPHN and recommends that clinicians not alter their current clinical practice of treating depression during pregnancy.

For additional information on the management of depression in women prior to conception and during pregnancy, including treatment algorithms, clinicians may consult the joint American Psychiatric Association and American College of Obstetricians and Gynecologists guidelines (at https://www.ncbi.nlm.nih.gov/pmc/articles/PMC3103063/pdf/nihms293836.pdf).

Lactation. Escitalopram is distributed into human milk. Because of the potential for serious adverse effects (e.g., excessive somnolence, decreased feeding, weight loss) in nursing infants, caution should be exercised and nursing infants should be observed for adverse reactions when escitalopram is administered to a nursing woman.

Pediatric Use. Safety and efficacy of escitalopram have not been established in pediatric patients younger than 12 years of age with major depressive disorder. Safety and effectiveness have been established in adolescents 12–17 years of age for the acute treatment of major depressive disorder. Although efficacy of escitalopram as maintenance therapy in adolescent patients with major depressive disorder has not been systematically evaluated, such efficacy can be extrapolated from adult data along with comparisons of pharmacokinetic parameters in adults and adolescent patients. (See Uses: Major Depressive Disorder.)

Safety and efficacy of escitalopram have not been established in pediatric patients younger than 18 years of age with generalized anxiety disorder.

Decreased appetite and weight loss have been observed in association with the use of SSRIs. Therefore, regular monitoring of weight and growth should be performed in children and adolescents treated with an SSRI such as escitalopram.

FDA warns that a greater risk of suicidal thinking or behavior (suicidality) occurred during first few months of antidepressant treatment compared with placebo in children and adolescents with major depressive disorder, obsessive-compulsive disorder (OCD), or other psychiatric disorders based on pooled analyses of 24 short-term, placebo-controlled trials of 9 antidepressant drugs (SSRIs and other antidepressants). However, a more recent meta-analysis of 27 placebo-controlled trials of 9 antidepressants (SSRIs and others) in patients younger than 19 years of age with major depressive disorder, OCD, or non-OCD anxiety disorders suggests that the benefits of antidepressant therapy in treating these conditions may outweigh the risks of suicidal behavior or suicidal ideation. No suicides occurred in these pediatric trials. These findings should be carefully considered when assessing potential benefits and risks of escitalopram in a child or adolescent for any clinical use. (See Worsening of Depression and Suicidality Risk under Warnings/Precautions: Warnings, in Cautions.)

Geriatric Use. Approximately 6% of patients studied in clinical trials of escitalopram for major depressive disorder and generalized anxiety disorder were 60 years of age or older; geriatric patients in these trials received daily dosages of 10–20 mg daily. Experience in geriatric patients in these trials was insufficient to determine whether they respond differently from younger adults; however, increased sensitivity cannot be ruled out.

In 2 pharmacokinetic studies, the mean area under the plasma concentration-time curve (AUC) and elimination half-life of escitalopram were increased by approximately 50% in geriatric individuals compared with younger individuals and peak escitalopram concentrations were unchanged. Therefore, the manufacturers state that the recommended dosage of escitalopram in geriatric patients is 10 mg once daily.

SNRIs and SSRIs, including escitalopram, have been associated with clinically important hyponatremia in geriatric patients, who may be at greater risk for this adverse effect. (See Hyponatremia/Syndrome of Inappropriate Antidiuretic Hormone Secretion under Warnings/Precautions: Other Warnings and Precautions, in Cautions.)

In pooled data analyses, a *reduced* risk of suicidality was observed in adults 65 years of age or older with antidepressant therapy compared with placebo. (See Worsening of Depression and Suicidality Risk under Warnings/Precautions: Warnings, in Cautions.)

Renal Impairment. Escitalopram should be used with caution in patients with severe renal impairment (i.e., creatinine clearance less than 20 mL/minute). (See Dosage and Administration: Special Populations.)

Hepatic Impairment. In clinical studies, clearance of racemic citalopram was decreased by 37% and elimination half-life was doubled relative to that in patients with normal hepatic function. Dosage reduction is recommended for patients with hepatic impairment. (See Dosage and Administration: Special Populations.)

■ **Common Adverse Effects** Adverse effects reported in approximately 5% or more of patients with generalized anxiety or major depressive disorder receiving escitalopram and with an incidence of at least twice that of placebo include insomnia, nausea, increased sweating, sexual dysfunction (ejaculation disorder [primarily ejaculatory delay], decreased libido, anorgasmia), fatigue, and somnolence.

Drug Interactions

■ **Drugs Affecting or Metabolized by Hepatic Microsomal Enzymes** Inhibitors or inducers of cytochrome P-450 (CYP) 3A4 (e.g., carbamazepine, ketoconazole, ritonavir, triazolam) and 2C19 isoenzymes: clinically important pharmacokinetic interaction unlikely since escitalopram is metabolized by multiple enzyme systems. However, possibility that carbamazepine may increase clearance of escitalopram should be considered.

Substrates of CYP2D6 isoenzyme (e.g., desipramine, metoprolol): potential pharmacokinetic (increased peak plasma concentrations and AUC of the substrate) interactions. Use with caution. Increased plasma concentrations of metoprolol have been associated with decreased cardioselectivity.

■ **Drugs Affecting Hemostasis** Pharmacokinetics of warfarin were not affected by racemic citalopram; however, prothrombin time increased by 5%. The effects of escitalopram have not been evaluated, and the clinical importance of this interaction is unknown.

Altered anticoagulant effects, including increased bleeding, have been reported when SSRIs or selective serotonin- and norepinephrine-reuptake inhibitors (SNRIs) were concurrently administered with warfarin or other anticoagulants. The manufacturers of escitalopram recommend carefully monitoring patients receiving warfarin during initiation and discontinuance of escitalopram therapy.

Potential pharmacologic (increased risk of bleeding) interaction with aspirin or other nonsteroidal anti-inflammatory agents (NSAIAs); escitalopram and drugs that affect hemostasis should be used concomitantly with caution.

■ **Antipsychotic Agents and Other Dopamine Antagonists** Potential pharmacologic interaction (potentially serious, sometimes fatal serotonin syndrome or NMS-like reactions) if used concurrently with antipsychotic agents or other dopamine antagonists. If signs and symptoms of serotonin syndrome or NMS occur, immediately discontinue treatment with escitalopram and any concurrently administered antidopaminergic or serotonergic agents and initiate supportive and symptomatic treatment. (See Serotonin Syndrome or Neuroleptic Malignant Syndrome-like Reactions under Warnings/Precautions: Other Warnings and Precautions, in Cautions.)

Pimozide In a controlled study, concurrent administration of a single, 2-mg dose of pimozide in individuals receiving citalopram (40 mg once daily for 11 days) was associated with mean increases in the corrected QT (QT_c) interval of approximately 10 msec compared with pimozide given alone. Citalopram did not substantially affect the mean area under the plasma concentration-time curve (AUC) or peak plasma concentrations of pimozide. The mechanism for this potential pharmacodynamic interaction is not known. In addition, concomitant use of citalopram and pimozide rarely may result in potentially serious, sometimes fatal serotonin syndrome or NMS-like reactions. The manufacturers of escitalopram state that concurrent use of escitalopram and pimozide is contraindicated.

■ **5-HT$_1$ Receptor Agonists ("Triptans")** Potential pharmacologic interaction (potentially serious, sometimes fatal serotonin syndrome or NMS-like reactions) if used concurrently with 5-HT$_1$ receptor agonists (e.g., almotriptan, eletriptan, frovatriptan, naratriptan, rizatriptan, sumatriptan, zolmitriptan). If concomitant use is clinically warranted, the patient should be observed carefully, particularly during treatment initiation, when dosage is increased, or when another serotonergic agent is initiated. (See Serotonin Syndrome or Neuroleptic Malignant Syndrome-like Reactions under Warnings/Precautions: Other Warnings and Precautions, in Cautions.)

■ **Monoamine Oxidase Inhibitors** Potential pharmacologic interaction (potentially serious, sometimes fatal serotonin syndrome or NMS-like reactions). Concomitant use of monoamine oxidase (MAO) inhibitors with escitalopram is contraindicated. In addition, at least 2 weeks should elapse between discontinuance of an MAO inhibitor and initiation of escitalopram and vice versa. (See Serotonin Syndrome or Neuroleptic Malignant Syndrome-like Reactions under Warnings/Precautions: Other Warnings and Precautions, in Cautions.)

Isoniazid Potential pharmacologic interaction (potentially serious serotonin syndrome) when isoniazid, an antituberculosis agent that appears to have some MAO-inhibiting activity, is used concomitantly with escitalopram.

■ **Linezolid** Linezolid, an anti-infective agent that is also a reversible MAO inhibitor, has been associated with drug interactions resulting in serotonin syndrome, including some associated with SSRIs. Because of this potential risk, linezolid generally should not be used in patients receiving escitalopram. However, the FDA states that certain life-threatening or urgent situations may necessitate immediate linezolid treatment in a patient receiving a serotonergic drug. In such emergency situations, the availability of alternative anti-infectives should be considered and the benefits of linezolid should be weighed against the risk of serotonin syndrome. If linezolid is indicated in such emergency situations, escitalopram must be immediately discontinued and the patient monitored for symptoms of CNS toxicity for 2 weeks or until 24 hours after the last linezolid dose, whichever comes first. Treatment with escitalopram may be resumed 24 hours after the last linezolid dose. If nonemergency use of linezolid is being planned for a patient receiving escitalopram, escitalopram should be withheld for at least 2 weeks prior to initiating linezolid. Treatment with escitalopram should not be initiated in a patient receiving linezolid; when necessary, escitalopram may be started 24 hours after the last linezolid dose. (See Drug Interactions: Serotonergic Drugs, in Linezolid 8:12.28.24.)

■ **Selective Serotonin-reuptake Inhibitors and Selective Serotonin- and Norepinephrine-reuptake Inhibitors** Potential pharmacologic interaction (potentially serious, sometimes fatal serotonin syndrome or NMS-like reactions); concurrent administration not recommended. (See Serotonin Syndrome or Neuroleptic Malignant Syndrome-like Reactions under Warnings/Precautions: Other Warnings and Precautions, in Cautions.)

■ **Other Serotonergic Drugs** Potential pharmacologic interaction (potentially serious, sometimes fatal serotonin syndrome or NMS-like reactions) with drugs affecting serotonergic neurotransmission, including tramadol and St. John's wort (*Hypericum perforatum*); use concomitantly with caution. If signs and symptoms of serotonin syndrome or NMS occur, immediately discontinue treatment with escitalopram and any concurrently administered serotonergic or antidopaminergic agents and initiate supportive and symptomatic treatment. Concurrent administration of escitalopram and serotonin precursors (such as tryptophan) is not recommended. (See Serotonin Syndrome or Neuroleptic Malignant Syndrome-like Reactions under Warnings/Precautions: Other Warnings and Precautions, in Cautions.)

■ **Alcohol** Concomitant use not recommended.

■ **Cimetidine** Potential pharmacokinetic interaction (increased AUC and peak plasma concentrations of citalopram have been observed); effects on escitalopram have not been evaluated. Clinical importance of this interaction is unknown.

■ **Citalopram** Potential pharmacologic interaction (potentially serious, sometimes fatal serotonin syndrome or NMS-like reactions).

Because escitalopram is the more active isomer of racemic citalopram, the 2 agents should not be used concomitantly.

■ **CNS-active Drugs** Potential pharmacologic interaction when given with other centrally acting drugs; use concomitantly with caution.

■ **Digoxin** Pharmacokinetic interaction unlikely based on studies with racemic citalopram.

■ **Lithium** Concurrent administration of racemic citalopram and lithium did not substantially affect the pharmacokinetics of either drug. However, pending further accumulation of data, the manufacturers of escitalopram recommend that plasma lithium concentrations be monitored in patients concurrently receiving escitalopram and that lithium dosage be adjusted accordingly.

Potential pharmacologic interaction (enhanced serotonergic effects of escitalopram and potentially serious, sometimes fatal serotonin syndrome or NMS-like reactions); use concomitantly with caution.

■ **Ritonavir** Combined administration of a single 600-mg dose of ritonavir, a CYP3A4 substrate and potent inhibitor of CYP3A4, and escitalopram 20 mg did not substantially affect the pharmacokinetics of either drug.

■ **Sibutramine** Potential pharmacologic interaction (potentially serious, sometimes fatal serotonin syndrome or NMS-like reactions). Use concomitantly with caution.

■ **Theophylline** Pharmacokinetics of theophylline were not affected by racemic citalopram. The effect of theophylline on the pharmacokinetics of racemic citalopram, however, has not been evaluated.

■ **Electroconvulsive Therapy** The combined use of electroconvulsive therapy and escitalopram has not been evaluated.

Description

Escitalopram, a selective serotonin-reuptake inhibitor (SSRI), is a bicyclic phthalane-derivative antidepressant. Escitalopram is the *S*-enantiomer of citalopram, an SSRI that occurs as a 50:50 racemic mixture of the *R*- and *S*-enantiomers. Escitalopram and citalopram differ structurally from other SSRIs (e.g., fluoxetine, fluvoxamine, paroxetine, sertraline) and other currently available antidepressants (e.g., monoamine oxidase inhibitors, tricyclic and tetracyclic antidepressants). Escitalopram is at least 100-fold more potent as an inhibitor of the reuptake of serotonin (5-hydroxytryptamine [5-HT]) at the presynaptic membranes and the 5-HT neuronal firing rate than the *R*-enantiomer and is twice as potent as the racemic mixture. However, further studies are needed to determine whether these differences result in any clinical superiority of escitalopram compared with citalopram.

Like other SSRIs, escitalopram's antidepressant effect is believed to involve potentiation of serotonin activity in the CNS. Escitalopram appears to have little or no effect on reuptake of other neurotransmitters such as norepinephrine and dopamine. In vitro studies also have demonstrated that escitalopram possesses little or no affinity for α- or β-adrenergic, dopamine D_{1-5}, histamine H_{1-3}, GABA-benzodiazepine, muscarinic M_{1-5}, or 5-HT_{1-7} receptors or various ion channels (e.g., calcium, chloride, potassium, sodium channels).

Escitalopram is extensively metabolized, principally by the hepatic cytochrome P-450 (CYP) 2C19 and 3A4 isoenzymes. The principal metabolites are less potent inhibitors of serotonin reuptake, suggesting that the metabolites do not substantially contribute to the antidepressant activity of escitalopram.

Advice to Patients

Importance of providing a copy of written patient information (medication guide) each time escitalopram is dispensed. Importance of advising patients to read the patient information before taking escitalopram and each time the prescription is refilled.

Risk of suicidality; importance of patients, family, and caregivers being alert to and immediately reporting emergence of suicidality, worsening depression, or unusual changes in behavior, especially during the first few months of therapy or during periods of dosage adjustment. (See Worsening of Depression and Suicidality Risk under Warnings/Precautions: Warnings, in Cautions.)

Importance of informing patients of potential risk of serotonin syndrome and neuroleptic malignant syndrome (NMS)-like reactions, particularly with concurrent use of escitalopram and 5-HT_1 receptor agonists (also called triptans), tramadol, tryptophan, other serotonergic agents, or antipsychotic agents. Importance of immediately contacting clinician if signs and symptoms of these syndromes develop (e.g., restlessness, hallucinations, loss of coordination, fast heart beat, increased body temperature, muscle stiffness, labile blood pressure, diarrhea, coma, nausea, vomiting, confusion).

Risk of psychomotor impairment; importance of exercising caution while operating hazardous machinery, including driving a motor vehicle, until the drug's effects on the individual are known.

Importance of patients being aware that withdrawal effects may occur when stopping escitalopram, especially with abrupt discontinuance of the drug.

Risks associated with concomitant use of escitalopram with alcohol or racemic citalopram.

Importance of informing clinicians of existing or contemplated concomitant therapy, including prescription and OTC drugs or herbal supplements, as well as any concomitant illnesses (e.g., bipolar disorder) or personal or family history of suicidality or bipolar disorder. Importance of advising patients about the risk of bleeding associated with concomitant use of escitalopram with aspirin or other nonsteroidal anti-inflammatory agents, warfarin, or other drugs that affect coagulation.

Importance of women informing clinicians if they are or plan to become pregnant or plan to breast-feed.

Importance of advising patients that, although they may notice improvement with escitalopram therapy within 1–4 weeks, they should continue therapy as directed.

Importance of informing patients of other important precautionary information. (See Cautions.)

Overview® (see Users Guide). For additional information on this drug until a more detailed monograph is developed and published, the manufacturer's labeling should be consulted. It is *essential* that the manufacturer's labeling be consulted for more detailed information on usual cautions, precautions, contraindications, potential drug interactions, laboratory test interferences, and acute toxicity.

Preparations

Excipients in commercially available drug preparations may have clinically important effects in some individuals; consult specific product labeling for details.

Escitalopram Oxalate

Oral		
Solution	5 mg (of escitalopram) per 5 mL	**Lexapro®**, Forest
Tablets, film-coated	5 mg (of escitalopram)*	**Escitalopram Oxalate Tablets**
		Lexapro®, Forest
	10 mg (of escitalopram)*	**Escitalopram Oxalate Tablets**
		Lexapro® (scored), Forest
	20 mg (of escitalopram)*	**Escitalopram Oxalate Tablets**
		Lexapro® (scored), Forest

*available from one or more manufacturer, distributor, and/or repackager by generic (nonproprietary) name

FLUoxetine Hydrochloride

■ Fluoxetine, a selective serotonin-reuptake inhibitor (SSRI), is an antidepressant.

Uses

Fluoxetine is used in the treatment of major depressive disorder, obsessive-compulsive disorder, premenstrual dysphoric disorder, bulimia nervosa, and panic disorder with or without agoraphobia. In addition, fluoxetine has been used for the treatment of depression associated with bipolar disorder†; obesity†; anorexia nervosa†; myoclonus†; cataplexy†; alcohol dependence†; and premature ejaculation†.

■ **Major Depressive Disorder** Fluoxetine is used in the acute and maintenance treatment of major depressive disorder in adults and pediatric patients 8 years of age and older. If fluoxetine is used for extended periods, the need for continued therapy should be reassessed periodically.

A major depressive episode implies a prominent and relatively persistent depressed or dysphoric mood that usually interferes with daily functioning (nearly every day for at least 2 weeks). According to DSM-IV criteria, a major depressive episode includes at least 5 of the following 9 symptoms (with at least one of the symptoms being either depressed mood or loss of interest or pleasure): depressed mood most of the day as indicated by subjective report (e.g., feels sad or empty) or observation made by others; markedly diminished interest or pleasure in all, or almost all, activities most of the day; significant weight loss (when not dieting) or weight gain (e.g., a change of more than 5% of body weight in a month), or decrease or increase in appetite; insomnia or hypersomnia; psychomotor agitation or retardation (observable by others, not merely subjective feelings of restlessness or being slowed down); fatigue or loss of energy; feelings of worthlessness or excessive or inappropriate guilt (not merely self-reproach or guilt about being sick); diminished ability to think or concentrate or indecisiveness (either by subjective account or as observed by others); and recurrent thoughts of death, recurrent suicidal ideation without a specific plan, or a suicide attempt or specific plan for committing suicide.

Treatment of major depressive disorder generally consists of an acute phase (to induce remission), a continuation phase (to preserve remission), and a maintenance phase (to prevent recurrence). Various interventions (e.g., psychotherapy, antidepressant drug therapy, electroconvulsive therapy [ECT]) are used alone or in combination to treat major depressive episodes. Treatment should be individualized and the most appropriate strategy for a particular patient is determined by clinical factors such as severity of depression (e.g., mild, moderate, severe), presence or absence of certain psychiatric features (e.g., suicide risk, catatonia, psychotic or atypical features, alcohol or substance abuse or dependence, panic or other anxiety disorder, cognitive dysfunction, dysthymia, personality disorder, seasonal affective disorder), and concurrent illness (e.g., asthma, cardiac disease, dementia, seizure disorder, glaucoma, hypertension). Demographic and psychosocial factors as well as patient preference also are used to determine the most effective treatment strategy.

While use of psychotherapy alone may be considered as an initial treatment strategy for patients with mild to moderate major depressive disorder (based on patient preference and presence of clinical features such as psychosocial stressors), combined use of antidepressant drug therapy and psychotherapy may be useful for initial treatment of patients with moderate to severe major depressive disorder with psychosocial issues, interpersonal problems, or a comorbid axis II disorder. In addition, combined use of antidepressant drug therapy and psychotherapy may be beneficial in patients who have a history of poor compliance or only partial response to adequate trials of either antidepressant drug therapy or psychotherapy alone.

Antidepressant drug therapy can be used alone for initial treatment of patients with mild major depressive disorder (if preferred by the patient) and usually is indicated alone or in combination with psychotherapy for initial treatment of patients with moderate to severe major depressive disorder (unless ECT is planned). ECT is not generally used for initial treatment of uncomplicated major depression, but is recommended as first-line treatment for severe major depressive disorder when it is coupled with psychotic features, catatonic stupor, severe suicidality, food refusal leading to nutritional compromise, or other situations when a rapid antidepressant response is required. ECT also is recommended for patients who have previously shown a positive response or a preference for this treatment modality and can be considered for patients with moderate or severe depression who have not responded to or cannot receive antidepressant drug therapy. In certain situations involving depressed patients unresponsive to adequate trials of several individual antidepressant agents, adjunctive therapy with another agent (e.g., buspirone, lithium) or concomitant use of a second antidepressant agent (e.g., bupropion) has been used; however, such combination therapy is associated with an increased risk of adverse reactions, may require dosage adjustments, and (if not contraindicated) should be undertaken only after careful consideration of the relative risks and benefits. (See Drug Interactions: Serotonergic Drugs, see Drug Interactions: Tricyclic and Other Antidepressants, and see Drug Interactions: Lithium.)

Efficacy of fluoxetine for the management of major depression has been established principally in outpatient settings. Most patients evaluated in clinical studies with fluoxetine had major depressive episodes of at least moderate severity, had no evidence of bipolar disorder, and had experienced either single or recurrent episodes of depressive illness. Limited evidence suggests that mildly depressed patients may respond less well to fluoxetine than moderately depressed patients. There also is some evidence that patients with atypical depression (which usually is characterized by atypical signs and symptoms such as hypersomnia and hyperphagia), a history of poor response to prior antidepressant therapy, chronic depressive symptomatology with or without episodic worsening of depressive symptoms, a longer duration of depression in the current episode, and/or a younger age of onset of depression may be more likely to respond to fluoxetine than to tricyclic antidepressant therapy.

As with other antidepressants, the possibility that fluoxetine may precipitate hypomanic or manic attacks in patients with bipolar or other major affective disorder should be considered. Fluoxetine monotherapy is *not* approved for use in treating depressive episodes associated with bipolar disorder. However, fluoxetine is used in combination with olanzapine for the treatment of acute depressive episodes in patients with bipolar disorder. (See Uses: Bipolar Disorder.)

Considerations in Choosing Antidepressants A variety of antidepressant drugs are available for the treatment of major depressive disorder, including selective serotonin-reuptake inhibitors (SSRIs; e.g., citalopram, escitalopram, fluoxetine, paroxetine, sertraline), selective serotonin- and norepinephrine-reuptake inhibitors (SNRIs; e.g., desvenlafaxine, duloxetine, venlafaxine), tricyclic antidepressants (e.g., amitriptyline, amoxapine, desipramine, doxepin, imipramine, nortriptyline, protriptyline, trimipramine), monoamine oxidase (MAO) inhibitors (e.g., phenelzine, tranylcypromine), and other antidepressants (e.g., bupropion, maprotiline, nefazodone, trazodone, vilazodone). Most clinical studies have shown that the antidepressant effect of usual dosages of fluoxetine in patients with moderate to severe depression is greater than that of placebo and comparable to that of usual dosages of tricyclic antidepressants, maprotiline, other selective serotonin-reuptake inhibitors (e.g., paroxetine, sertraline), and other antidepressants (e.g., trazodone). Fluoxetine appears to be as effective as tricyclic antidepressants in reducing most of the signs and symptoms associated with major depressive disorder, including depression, anxiety, cognitive disturbances, and somatic symptoms. However, in some studies, the drug did not appear to be as effective as tricyclic antidepressants or trazodone in reducing sleep disturbances associated with depression. In geriatric patients with major depressive disorder, fluoxetine appears to be as effective as and to cause fewer overall adverse effects than doxepin. The onset of action of fluoxetine appears to be comparable to that of tricyclic antidepressants, although the onset of action has been variably reported to be somewhat faster or slower than that of tricyclic antidepressants in some studies.

Because response rates in patients with major depression are similar for most currently available antidepressants, the choice of antidepressant agent for a given patient depends principally on other factors such as potential adverse effects, safety or tolerability of these adverse effects in the individual patient, psychiatric and medical history, patient or family history of response to specific therapies, patient preference, quantity and quality of available clinical data, cost, and relative acute overdose safety. No single antidepressant can be recommended as optimal for all patients because of substantial heterogeneity in individual responses and in the nature, likelihood, and severity of adverse effects. In addition, patients vary in the degree to which certain adverse effects and other inconveniences of drug therapy (e.g., cost, dietary restrictions) affect their preferences.

In the large-scale Sequenced Treatment Alternatives to Relieve Depression (STAR*D) effectiveness trial, patients with major depressive disorder who did not respond to or could not tolerate therapy with one SSRI (citalopram) were randomized to switch to extended-release ("sustained-release") bupropion, sertraline, or extended-release venlafaxine as a second step of treatment (level 2). Remission rates as assessed by the 17-item Hamilton Rating Scale for Depression (HRSD-17) and the Quick Inventory of Depressive Symptomatology—Self Report (QIDS-SR-16) were approximately 21 and 26% for extended-release bupropion, 18 and 27% for sertraline, and 25 and 25% for extended-release venlafaxine therapy, respectively; response rates as assessed by the QIDS-SR-16 were 26, 27, and 28% for extended-release bupropion, sertraline, and extended-release venlafaxine therapy, respectively. These results suggest that after unsuccessful initial treatment of depressed patients with an SSRI, approximately 25% of patients will achieve remission after therapy is switched to another antidepressant, and either another SSRI (e.g., sertraline) or an agent from another class (e.g., bupropion, venlafaxine) may be reasonable alternative antidepressants in patients not responding to initial SSRI therapy.

Patient Tolerance Considerations. Because of differences in the adverse effect profile between selective serotonin-reuptake inhibitors and tricyclic antidepressants, particularly less frequent anticholinergic effects, cardiovascular effects, and weight gain with selective serotonin-reuptake inhibitors, these drugs may be preferred in patients in whom such effects are not tolerated or are of potential concern. The decreased incidence of anticholinergic effects associated with fluoxetine and other selective serotonin-reuptake inhibitors compared with tricyclic antidepressants is a potential advantage, since such effects may result in discontinuance of the drug early during therapy in unusually sensitive patients. In addition, some anticholinergic effects may become troublesome during long-term tricyclic antidepressant therapy (e.g., persistent dry mouth may result in tooth decay). Although selective serotonin-reuptake inhibitors share the same overall tolerability profile, certain patients may tolerate one drug in this class better than another. In an open study, most patients who had discontinued fluoxetine therapy because of adverse effects subsequently tolerated sertraline therapy. Antidepressants other than selective serotonin-reuptake inhibitors may be preferred in patients in whom certain adverse GI effects (e.g., nausea, anorexia) or nervous system effects (e.g., anxiety, nervousness, insomnia, weight loss) are not tolerated or are of concern, since such effects appear to occur more frequently with fluoxetine and other drugs in this class.

Pediatric Considerations. The clinical presentation of depression in children and adolescents can differ from that in adults and generally varies with the age and developmental stages of the child. Younger children may exhibit behavioral problems such as social withdrawal, aggressive behavior, apathy, sleep disruption, and weight loss; adolescents may present with somatic complaints, self esteem problems, rebelliousness, poor performance in school, or a pattern of engaging in risky or aggressive behavior.

Data from controlled clinical studies evaluating various antidepressant agents in children and adolescents are less extensive than with adults, and many of these studies have methodologic limitations (e.g., nonrandomized or uncontrolled, small sample size, short duration, nonspecific inclusion criteria). However, there is some evidence that the response to antidepressants in pediatric patients may differ from that seen in adults, and caution should be used in extrapolating data from adult studies when making treatment decisions for pediatric patients. Results of several studies evaluating tricyclic antidepressants (e.g., amitriptyline, desipramine, imipramine, nortriptyline) in preadolescent and adolescent patients with major depression indicate a lack of overall efficacy in this age group.

Based on the lack of efficacy data regarding use of tricyclic antidepressants and MAO inhibitors in pediatric patients and because of the potential for life-threatening adverse effects associated with the use of these drugs, many experts consider selective serotonin-reuptake inhibitors, including fluoxetine, the drugs of choice when antidepressant therapy is indicated for the treatment of major depressive disorder in children and adolescents. However, the US Food and Drug Administration (FDA) states that, while efficacy of fluoxetine has been established in pediatric patients, efficacy of other newer antidepressants (i.e., citalopram, desvenlafaxine, duloxetine, escitalopram, fluvoxamine, mirtazapine, nefazodone, paroxetine, sertraline, venlafaxine) was not conclusively established in clinical trials in pediatric patients with major depressive disorder. In addition, FDA now warns that antidepressants increase the risk of suicidal thinking and behavior (suicidality) in children and adolescents with major depressive disorder and other psychiatric disorders. (See Cautions: Pediatric Precautions.) FDA currently states that anyone considering using an antidepressant in a child or adolescent for any clinical use must balance the potential risk of therapy with the clinical need. (See Cautions: Precautions and Contraindications.)

Geriatric Considerations. The response to antidepressants in depressed geriatric patients without dementia is similar to that reported in younger adults, but depression in geriatric patients often is not recognized and is not treated. In geriatric patients with major depressive disorder, SSRIs appear to be as effective as tricyclic antidepressants (e.g., amitriptyline) but may cause fewer overall adverse effects than these other agents. Geriatric patients appear to be especially sensitive to anticholinergic (e.g., dry mouth, constipation, vision disturbance), cardiovascular, orthostatic hypotensive, and sedative effects of tricyclic antidepressants. The low incidence of anticholinergic effects associated with fluoxetine and other SSRIs compared with tricyclic antidepressants is a potential advantage in geriatric patients, since such effects (e.g., constipation, dry mouth, confusion, memory impairment) may be particularly troublesome in these patients. However, SSRI therapy may be associated with other troublesome adverse effects (e.g., nausea and vomiting, agitation and akathisia, parkinsonian adverse effects, sexual dysfunction, weight loss, hyponatremia). Some clinicians state that SSRIs including fluoxetine may be preferred for treating depression in geriatric patients in whom the orthostatic hypotension associated with many antidepressants (e.g., tricyclics) potentially may result in injuries (such as severe falls). However, despite the fewer cardiovascular and anticholinergic effects associated with SSRIs, these drugs did not show any advantage over tricyclic antidepressants with regard to hip fracture in a case-control study. In addition, there was little difference in the rates of falls between nursing home residents receiving SSRIs and those receiving tricyclic antidepressants in a retrospective study. Therefore, all geriatric individuals receiving either type of antidepressant should be considered at increased risk of falls and appropriate measures should be taken. In addition, clinicians prescribing SSRIs in geriatric patients should be aware of the many possible drug interactions associated with these drugs, including those involving metabolism of the drugs through the cytochrome P-450 system. (See Drug Interactions.)

Patients with dementia of the Alzheimer's type (Alzheimer's disease, presenile or senile dementia) often present with depressive symptoms, such as depressed mood, appetite loss, insomnia, fatigue, irritability, and agitation. Most experts recommend that patients with dementia of the Alzheimer's type who present with clinically important and persistent depressive symptoms be considered as candidates for pharmacotherapy even if they fail to meet the criteria for a major depressive syndrome. The goals of such therapy are to improve mood, functional status (e.g., cognition), and quality of life. Treatment of depression also may reduce other neuropsychiatric symptoms associated with depression in patients with dementia, including aggression, anxiety, apathy, and psychosis. Although patients may present with depressed mood alone, the possibility of more extensive depressive symptomatology should be considered. Therefore, patients should be evaluated and monitored carefully for indices of major depression, suicidal ideation, and neurovegetative signs since safety measures (e.g., hospitalization for suicidality) and more vigorous and aggressive therapy (e.g., relatively high dosages, multiple drug trials) may be needed in some patients.

Although placebo-controlled trials of antidepressants in depressed patients with concurrent dementia have shown mixed results, the available evidence and experience with the use of antidepressants in patients with dementia of the Alzheimer's type and associated depressive manifestations indicate that depressive symptoms (including depressed mood alone and with neurovegetative changes) in such patients are responsive to antidepressant therapy. In some patients, cognitive deficits may partially or fully resolve during antidepressant therapy, but the extent of response will be limited to the degree of cognitive impairment that is directly related to depression. SSRIs such as fluoxetine, citalopram, escitalopram, paroxetine, or sertraline are generally considered as first-line agents in the treatment of depressed patients with dementia since they are usually better tolerated than some other antidepressants (e.g., tricyclic antidepressants, monoamine oxidase inhibitors). Some possible alternative agents to SSRIs include bupropion, mirtazapine, and venlafaxine. Some geriatric patients with dementia and depression may be unable to tolerate the antidepressant dosages needed to achieve full remission. When a rapid antidepressant response is not critical, some experts therefore recommend a very gradual dosage increase to increase the likelihood that a therapeutic dosage of the SSRI or other antidepressant will be reached and tolerated. In a randomized, double-blind study comparing fluoxetine and amitriptyline in a limited number of patients with major depression complicating Alzheimer's disease, fluoxetine and amitriptyline were found to be equally effective; however, fluoxetine was better tolerated.

Cardiovascular Considerations. The relatively low incidence of adverse cardiovascular effects, including orthostatic hypotension and conduction disturbances, associated with fluoxetine and most other selective serotonin-reuptake inhibitors may be advantageous in patients in whom cardiovascular effects associated with tricyclic antidepressants may be hazardous. However, most clinical studies of fluoxetine for the management of depression did not include individuals with cardiovascular disease (e.g., those with a recent history of myocardial infarction or unstable heart disease), and further experience in such patients is necessary to confirm the reported relative lack of cardiotoxicity with the drug. (See Cautions: Precautions and Contraindications.)

Sedative Considerations. Because fluoxetine and other SSRIs generally are less sedating than some other antidepressants (e.g., tricyclics), some clinicians state that these drugs may be preferable in patients who do not require the sedative effects associated with many antidepressant agents; however, an antidepressant with more prominent sedative effects (e.g., trazodone) may be preferable in some patients (e.g., those with insomnia).

Suicidal Risk Considerations. Suicide is a known risk of depression and certain other psychiatric disorders, and these disorders themselves are the strongest predictors of suicide. However, there has been a long-standing concern that antidepressants may have a role in inducing worsening of depression and the emergence of suicidal thinking and behavior (suicidality) in certain patients during the early phases of treatment. FDA states that antidepressants increased the risk of suicidality in short-term studies in children, adolescents, and young adults (18–24 years of age) with major depressive disorder and other psychiatric disorders. (See Cautions: Pediatric Precautions.) An increased suicidality risk was not demonstrated with antidepressants compared with placebo in adults older than 24 years of age and a reduced risk was observed in adults 65 years of age or older. It currently is unknown whether the suicidality risk extends to longer-term antidepressant use (i.e., beyond several months); however, there is substantial evidence from placebo-controlled maintenance trials in adults with major depressive disorder that antidepressants can delay the recurrence of depression. Because the risk of suicidality in depressed patients may persist until substantial remission of depression occurs, appropriate monitoring and close observation of patients of all ages who are receiving antidepressant therapy are recommended. (See Cautions: Precautions and Contraindications.)

Dosing Interval Considerations. Fluoxetine can be administered once weekly as delayed-release capsules for continuing management of major depressive disorder. Whether the weekly regimen is equivalent to daily therapy with conventional preparations for preventing relapse has not been established. In a double-blind study in adults who responded to daily fluoxetine therapy for major depressive disorder, the relapse rate for continuing therapy with fluoxetine 20-mg conventional capsules administered daily, fluoxetine 90-mg delayed-release capsules administered once weekly, or placebo was 26, 37, or 50%, respectively.

Other Considerations. Fluoxetine has been effective for the treatment of depression in adults with human immunodeficiency virus (HIV) infection. In one randomized, placebo-controlled study, analysis of patients who completed the study showed a statistically significant benefit in patients receiving fluoxetine compared with those receiving placebo. However, results of intent-to-treat analysis did not show a statistically significant benefit in those receiving the antidepressant, possibly because of a high attrition rate and substantial placebo response. There was no evidence that the degree of immunosuppression affected the response to antidepressant therapy.

Fluoxetine has been effective when used in combination with lithium in a limited number of patients with refractory depression who had not responded to prior therapy (including tricyclic antidepressants and MAO inhibitors administered alone or in combination with lithium), suggesting that lithium may potentiate the antidepressant activity of fluoxetine. (See Drug Interactions: Lithium.) In the Sequenced Treatment Alternatives to Relieve Depression (STAR*D) level 2 trial, patients with major depressive disorder who did not respond to or could not tolerate therapy with citalopram (another SSRI) were randomized to receive either extended-release ("sustained-release") bupropion or buspirone therapy in addition to citalopram. Although both extended-release bupropion and buspirone were found to produce similar remission rates, extended-release bupropion produced a greater reduction in the number and severity of symptoms and a lower rate of drug discontinuance than buspirone in this large-scale, effectiveness trial. These results suggest that augmentation of SSRI therapy with extended-release bupropion may be useful in some patients with refractory depression.

Fluoxetine has been used safely for the management of depression in at least one patient with established susceptibility to malignant hyperthermia, suggesting that the drug may be useful in depressed patients susceptible to malignant hyperthermia and in whom tricyclics and MAO inhibitors are potentially hazardous; however, additional experience is necessary to confirm this preliminary finding.

Because fluoxetine possesses anorectic and weight-reducing properties, some clinicians state that the drug may be preferred in obese patients and/or patients in whom the increase in appetite, carbohydrate craving, and weight gain associated with tricyclic antidepressant therapy may be undesirable (e.g., potentially hazardous to the patient's health; result in possible discontinuance of or noncompliance with therapy). However, the possibility that some patients with concurrent eating disorders or those who may desire to lose weight may misuse fluoxetine for its anorectic and weight-reducing effects should be considered. (See Uses: Eating Disorders and also see Chronic Toxicity.)

■ **Obsessive-Compulsive Disorder** Fluoxetine is used in the acute and maintenance treatment of obsessive-compulsive disorder in adults and pediatric patients 7 years of age and older when the obsessions or compulsions cause marked distress, are time consuming, or interfere substantially with social or occupational functioning. Obsessions are recurrent and persistent ideas, thoughts, impulses, or images that, at some time during the disturbance, are experienced as intrusive and inappropriate (i.e., "ego dystonic") and that cause marked anxiety or distress but that are not simply excessive worries about real-life problems. Compulsions are repetitive, intentional behaviors (e.g., hand washing, ordering, checking) or mental acts (e.g., praying, counting, repeating words silently) performed in response to an obsession or according to rules that must be applied rigidly (e.g., in a stereotyped fashion). Although the behaviors or acts are aimed at preventing or reducing distress or preventing some dreaded event or situation, they either are not connected in a realistic manner with what they are designed to neutralize or prevent or are clearly excessive. At some time during the course of the disturbance, the patient, if an adult, recognizes that the obsessions or compulsions are excessive or unreasonable; children may not make such a recognition.

The efficacy of fluoxetine for the management of obsessive-compulsive disorder has been established in several multicenter, placebo-controlled studies, including 2 studies of 13 weeks' duration in adults and one study of 13 weeks' duration in children and adolescents 7–17 years of age. Patients in these studies had moderate to severe obsessive-compulsive disorder with average baseline total scores on the Yale-Brown Obsessive-Compulsive Scale (YBOCS) of 22–26 in adults and 25–26 in children and adolescents (measured on the Children's Yale-Brown Obsessive-Compulsive Scale [CY-BOCS]).

In 2 fixed-dose studies of 13 weeks' duration, adults receiving fluoxetine dosages of 20, 40 and 60 mg daily experienced substantially greater reductions in the YBOCS total score than those receiving placebo. Mean reductions in total scores on the YBOCS in fluoxetine-treated patients were approximately 4–6 units in one study and 4–9 units in the other study compared with a 1-unit reduction in patients receiving placebo. In these 2 studies, a positive clinical response (much or very much improved on the Clinical Global Impressions improvement scale) occurred in 36–47 or 11% of patients receiving fluoxetine or placebo, respectively. While there was no indication of a dose-response relationship for effectiveness in one study, a dose-response relationship was observed in the other study, with numerically better responses in patients receiving 40 or 60 mg of fluoxetine daily compared with those receiving 20 mg of the drug daily. No age- or gender-related differences in outcome were noted in either of these studies.

In another randomized, placebo-controlled study of 13 weeks' duration, children and adolescents 7–17 years of age with obsessive-compulsive disorder who received mean fluoxetine dosages of approximately 25 mg daily (range: 10–60 mg daily) demonstrated substantially greater reductions in the CY-BOCS total score than those receiving placebo. In this study, a positive clinical response (much or very much improved on the Clinical Global Impressions improvement scale) occurred in approximately 55–58 or 9–19% of patients receiving fluoxetine or placebo, respectively. In addition, 49% of patients who received fluoxetine were classified as responders (i.e., patients with a 40% or greater reduction in their CY-BOCS total score from baseline) compared with 25% of those who received placebo. Subgroup analyses on outcome did not suggest any differential responsiveness on the basis of age or gender.

Results from comparative studies to date suggest fluoxetine and other selective serotonin-reuptake inhibitors (SSRIs; e.g., fluvoxamine, paroxetine, sertraline) are as effective or somewhat less effective than clomipramine in the management of obsessive-compulsive disorder. In a pooled analysis of separate short-term (10–13 weeks) studies comparing clomipramine, fluoxetine, fluvoxamine, or sertraline with placebo, clomipramine was calculated as being more effective (as determined by measures on the YBOC scale) than SSRIs, although all drugs were superior to placebo.

Many clinicians consider an SSRI (e.g., fluoxetine, fluvoxamine, paroxetine, sertraline) or clomipramine to be the drugs of choice for the pharmacologic treatment of obsessive-compulsive disorder. The decision whether to initiate therapy with an SSRI or clomipramine often is made based on the adverse effect profile of these drugs. For example, some clinicians prefer clomipramine in patients who may not tolerate the adverse effect profile of SSRIs (e.g., nausea, headache, overstimulation, sleep disturbances) while SSRIs may be useful alternatives in patients unable to tolerate the adverse effects associated with clomipramine therapy (e.g., anticholinergic effects, cardiovascular effects, sedation). Consideration of individual patient characteristics (age, concurrent medical conditions), pharmacokinetics of the drug, potential drug interactions, and cost of therapy may also influence decisions regarding use of SSRIs or clomipramine as first-line therapy in patients with obsessive-compulsive disorder. Although not clearly established, it has been suggested that the mechanism of action of fluoxetine and other drugs (e.g., clomipramine) used in the management of obsessive-compulsive disorder may be related to their serotonergic activity.

Other Disorders with an Obsessive-Compulsive Component Experience in a limited number of patients suggests that fluoxetine also reduces obsessive-compulsive symptoms associated with Tourette's disorder† (Gilles de la Tourette's syndrome); however, the drug did not appear to be effective in suppressing motor and vocal tics associated with the condition.

Trichotillomania† (an urge to pull out one's hair) has some features in common with those of obsessive-compulsive disorder and some studies have suggested that antiobsessional agents such as SSRIs and clomipramine may be useful in treating this condition. Successful treatment with fluoxetine has been reported in some patients with trichotillomania, including in 2 short-term, open studies in which dosages of up to 80 mg daily were given. However, fluoxetine's efficacy in the management of this disorder was not demonstrated in 2 double-blind, placebo-controlled, crossover studies. In addition, behavioral therapy was found to be more effective than fluoxetine in treating trichotillomania in a short-term, controlled study. Further studies are needed to more clearly determine the role of fluoxetine and other serotonin-reuptake blockers in the management of this condition.

■ **Premenstrual Dysphoric Disorder** Fluoxetine is used in the treatment of premenstrual dysphoric disorder (previously late luteal phase dysphoric disorder). DSM-IV criteria for premenstrual dysphoric disorder (PMDD) require that in most menstrual cycles of the previous year at least 5 of the following 11 symptoms must have been present for most of the time during the last week of the luteal phase (with at least one of the symptoms being the first 4 listed): marked depressed mood, feelings of hopelessness, or self-deprecating thoughts; marked anxiety, tension, feelings of being "keyed up" or on "edge"; marked affective lability (e.g., feeling suddenly sad or tearful or increased sensitivity to rejection); persistent and marked anger or irritability or increased interpersonal conflicts; decreased interest in usual activities (e.g., work, school, friends, hobbies); a subjective sense of difficulty in concentrating; lethargy, easy fatigability, or marked lack of energy; marked change in appetite, overeating, or specific food cravings; hypersomnia or insomnia; a subjective sense of being overwhelmed or out of control; and other physical symptoms, such as breast tenderness or swelling, headaches, joint or muscle pain, or a sensation of "bloating" or weight gain. Such symptoms should begin to remit within a few days of the onset of menses (follicular phase) and are always absent in the week following menses. The presence of this cyclical pattern of symptoms must be confirmed by at least 2 consecutive months of prospective daily symptom ratings. PMDD should be distinguished from the more common premenstrual syndrome (PMS) by prospective daily ratings and the strict criteria listed above.

There is some evidence that serotonergic agents (e.g., fluoxetine, paroxetine) have greater efficacy compared with non-serotonergic agents (e.g., bupropion, maprotiline) in relieving the physical and/or emotional symptoms of PMDD. In published studies, the response rates to fluoxetine therapy in women with PMDD appear to be similar to those described in patients with depression, panic disorder, and obsessive-compulsive disorder. However, unlike the onset of action of fluoxetine in other psychiatric conditions (6–8 weeks), some clinicians have observed a rapid onset of response to fluoxetine (approximately 2–4 weeks) in women with PMDD, suggesting that the mechanism of action of these agents in PMDD is not mediated by the drug's antidepressant or antiobsessive effects. In addition, use of fluoxetine in the treatment of PMDD does not appear to produce the sustained remission typically seen in the treatment of major depressive disorder. PMDD symptoms recur soon after discontinuance of fluoxetine therapy (e.g., within 2 menstrual cycles), even in women who have received the drug for more than 1 year. It has been suggested that a past history of major depression may be associated with a partial or absent response to lower dosages of fluoxetine therapy. Because patients on oral contraceptives were excluded from most clinical studies to date, efficacy of fluoxetine used in conjunction with oral contraceptives for the treatment of PMDD has not been determined.

The efficacy of fluoxetine for the management of PMDD has been established in 3 randomized, placebo-controlled (1 intermittent- and 2 continuous-dosing) studies of 3 or 6 months' duration in adult women who met DSM-III-R or DSM-IV criteria for PMDD. One study involved over 300 women (20–40 years of age) who were randomized to receive either fluoxetine (at fixed dosages of 20 or 60 mg daily) or placebo continuously throughout the full menstrual cycle, beginning on the first day of their cycle. In this study, fixed doses of fluoxetine were shown to be substantially more effective than placebo in decreasing the mean total of 3 visual analog scale scores (tension, irritability, dysphoria); total scores decreased by 36–39% on 20 or 60 mg of fluoxetine and 7% on placebo. However, marked (greater than 50% reduction from baseline) improvement in total luteal phase visual analog scale scores occurred only in 18% of patients receiving 60 mg of fluoxetine and in 6 or 4% of those receiving 20 mg of fluoxetine or placebo, respectively. Fluoxetine therapy appeared to be well tolerated in patients receiving dosages of 20 mg daily, but approximately 33% of women receiving 60 mg daily discontinued the drug because of adverse reactions and 86% of those receiving this dosage who remained in the study reported one or more adverse effects attributable to the drug.

In a second double-blind, placebo-controlled, crossover study, women with PMDD who received flexible doses of fluoxetine (20–60 mg daily; mean dosage of 27 mg daily) throughout the menstrual cycle for a total of 3 cycles had an average visual analog scale total score (follicular to luteal phase increase) that was 3.8 times lower than that of patients receiving placebo. However, results of another double-blind, parallel study indicated that the response rate in women receiving fluoxetine 20 mg daily or bupropion 300 mg daily continuously for 2 cycles was not substantially superior to placebo on the Clinical Global Impressions scale.

The efficacy of intermittent dosing (defined as initiation of daily dosage 14 days prior to the anticipated onset of menstruation and continuing through the first full day of menses) was established in a double-blind, parallel group study of 3 months' duration. In this study, women receiving intermittent dosing of 20 mg daily dosages of fluoxetine had substantially greater improvements on the Daily Record of Severity of Problems, a patient-rated instrument that mirrors the diagnostic criteria for PMDD as identified in the DSM-IV, than those receiving placebo. Further studies are needed to evaluate the comparative efficacy of continuous and intermittent dosing regimens.

■ **Eating Disorders** Fluoxetine is used in the acute and maintenance treatment of bulimia nervosa in adults; the drug also has been used in a limited number of patients with other eating disorders (e.g., anorexia nervosa).

Although DSM-IV criteria provide guidelines for establishing a diagnosis of a specific eating disorder, the symptoms frequently occur along a continuum between those of anorexia nervosa and bulimia nervosa. The primary features in both anorexia nervosa and bulimia nervosa are weight preoccupation and excessive self-evaluation (i.e., disturbed perception) of body weight and shape, and many patients exhibit a mixture of both anorexic and bulimic behaviors.

The American Psychiatric Association (APA) states that psychiatric management forms the foundation of treatment for patients with eating disorders and should be instituted for all patients in combination with other specific treatment modalities (e.g., nutritional rehabilitation and pharmacotherapy). Because patients with eating disorders often exhibit comorbid conditions and/or associated psychiatric features that may compromise clinical outcome, treatment programs should identify and address all comorbid conditions before initiating therapy. Clinicians should recognize that patients with concurrent diabetes mellitus often underdose their insulin in order to lose weight, and that pregnant patients with disturbed eating behaviors (e.g., inadequate nutritional intake, binge eating, purging, abuse of teratogenic medications) may be at high risk for fetal or maternal complications. Results from several studies indicate that patients with associated psychiatric features such as substance abuse/dependence or personality disorder may require longer-term therapy than those without these comorbid conditions. Although the presence of depression at initial presentation has no predictive value for treatment outcome, many clinicians suggest that severe depression can impair the patient's involvement in and/or response to psychotherapy, and such patients should receive initial pharmacologic therapy to improve mood symptoms.

Bulimia Nervosa Fluoxetine is used in the acute and maintenance treatment of binge-eating and self-induced vomiting behaviors in patients with moderate to severe bulimia nervosa (e.g., at least 3 bulimic episodes per week for 6 months).

According to DSM-IV, bulimia nervosa is characterized by recurrent episodes of binge eating and recurrent inappropriate compensatory behaviors to prevent weight gain (e.g., self-induced vomiting; misuse of laxatives, diuretics, enemas, or other medications; fasting; excessive exercise) and binge eating and compensatory behaviors both occur at least twice a week for 3 months.

Treatment strategies for bulimia nervosa include psychosocial interventions, nutritional counseling and rehabilitation, and pharmacotherapy. The primary goals in treating bulimia nervosa are to reduce binge eating and purging. Although antidepressants initially were used only in bulimic patients who were clinically depressed, evidence from recent studies indicates that nondepressed patients also respond to these agents, and that the presence of depression is not predictive of therapeutic response. Therefore, antidepressants are included as one component of initial treatment regimens for patients with bulimia nervosa. Because selective serotonin-reuptake inhibitors have a more favorable adverse effects profile, these drugs usually are preferred and may be especially useful for patients with symptoms of depression, anxiety, obsessions, or certain impulse disorder symptoms or for those who previously failed to achieve optimal response to psychosocial therapy. Other antidepressants also may be used to reduce the symptoms of binge eating and purging and help prevent relapse. However, the APA cautions against the use of tricyclic antidepressants in patients who are suicidal and cautions against use of MAO inhibitors in those with chaotic binge eating and purging.

The APA states that in patients who fail to respond to initial antidepressant therapy, it may be necessary to assess whether the patient has taken the drug shortly before vomiting or to determine whether effective drug concentrations have been achieved. Although only limited data are available regarding use of antidepressants for maintenance therapy, there appears to be a high rate of relapse during the treatment phase and an even higher rate following discontinuance of therapy. However, limited data indicate that the rate of relapse appears to correlate with the time at which drug therapy is initiated. In one small, open-label study, patients who received drug treatment within 13 weeks of diagnosis were more likely to exhibit sustained recovery during the first year than those who did not receive pharmacotherapy. Furthermore, continuing cognitive behavior therapy following discontinuance of drug therapy appears to prevent relapse in patients with bulimia nervosa. Additional study is needed to determine the effects of sequential use of psychotherapy and pharmacotherapy in the treatment of bulimia nervosa.

The efficacy of fluoxetine for the management of bulimia nervosa has been established in several multicenter, placebo-controlled studies, including 2 studies of 8 weeks' duration (using fluoxetine dosages of 20 or 60 mg daily) and one study of 16 weeks' duration (using fluoxetine dosages of 60 mg once daily) in patients with moderate to severe bulimia nervosa with median binge eating and self-induced vomiting of 7–10 and 5–9 times a week, respectively. In these studies, fluoxetine given in dosages of 60 mg daily (but not in dosages of 20 mg daily) was substantially more effective than placebo in reducing the number of binge-eating and self-induced vomiting episodes weekly. The superiority of fluoxetine compared with placebo was evident as early as within 1 week of therapy and persisted throughout each study period. The drug-related reduction in bulimic episodes appeared to be independent of baseline depression as assessed by the Hamilton Depression Rating Scale. The beneficial effect of fluoxetine therapy (compared with placebo), as measured by median reductions in the frequency of bulimic behaviors at the end of therapy compared with baseline, ranged from 1–2 and 2–4 episodes per week for binge eating and self-induced vomiting, respectively. The magnitude of clinical effect was related to baseline frequency of bulimic behaviors since greater reductions in such behaviors were observed in patients with higher baseline frequencies. Although binge eating and purging resolved completely in some patients who received fluoxetine therapy, the majority of fluoxetine-treated patients only experienced a partial reduction in the frequency of bulimic behaviors.

In an uncontrolled study in patients with bulimia nervosa, fluoxetine substantially reduced the frequency of binge eating and self-induced vomiting but did not affect bodily dissatisfaction in patients receiving 60–80 mg of the drug for 4 weeks; in several patients, therapeutic effects of the drug appeared to be maintained during chronic therapy. In another uncontrolled study, fluoxetine reduced the frequency of binge eating and self-induced vomiting in several patients with bulimia nervosa who were unresponsive to previous therapy with imipramine. The drug also reportedly improved bulimic symptoms, expanded food preferences, and resulted in weight gain in one underweight patient with anorexia nervosa and bulimia who was unresponsive to or unable to tolerate previous therapy for her eating disorder (including tricyclic antidepressants, monoamine oxidase inhibitors, bupropion, nomifensine, or lithium). In addition, fluoxetine used in combination with lithium was effective in improving bulimic symptoms in a patient with major depression and bulimia who was unresponsive to prior therapy.

The efficacy of fluoxetine for long-term use in the treatment of bulimia nervosa has been established in a placebo-controlled study of up to 52 weeks' duration in patients who responded to an initial single-blind, 8-week acute treatment phase with fluoxetine 60 mg daily for bulimia nervosa. In this study, fluoxetine decreased the likelihood of relapse and improved the clinical outcome. However, symptoms of bulimia gradually worsened over time in patients in both the fluoxetine and placebo groups in this study, suggesting that fluoxetine alone may not be an adequate maintenance treatment after acute response in some patients with bulimia nervosa. Additional management strategies, such as psychotherapy, may be required to augment or to sustain initial improvement in this condition.

Pending further accumulation of data, most clinicians recommend that antidepressant therapy, including fluoxetine, be continued for at least 6–12 months in patients with bulimia nervosa before attempting to discontinue therapy. If fluoxetine is used for extended periods, the need for continued therapy with the drug should be reassessed periodically.

Anorexia Nervosa Fluoxetine has been used in a limited number of patients with anorexia nervosa†. According to DSM-IV, anorexia nervosa is characterized by refusal to maintain body weight at or above a minimally normal weight for age and height (e.g., weight loss leading to maintenance of body weight less than 85% of that expected or failure to make expected weight gain during periods of growth, leading to body weight less than 85% of that expected); intense fear of gaining weight or becoming fat (even though underweight); disturbance in the perception of body weight and shape, undue influence of body weight or shape on self-evaluation, or denial of the seriousness of the current low body weight; and amenorrhea in postmenarchal females (i.e., absence of at least 3 consecutive menstrual cycles). Patients with anorexia nervosa often exhibit depressive (e.g., depressed mood, social withdrawal, irritability, insomnia, and diminished interest in sex) and obsessive-compulsive symptoms that may be associated with or exacerbated by undernutrition.

The APA recommends that a program of nutritional rehabilitation, including vitamin (e.g., potassium and phosphorus) supplementation, be established for all patients who are significantly underweight. The APA states that pharmacologic measures (e.g., antidepressants) may be considered in patients with anorexia nervosa to maintain weight and normal eating behaviors; to treat psychiatric symptoms associated with the disorder (e.g., depression, anxiety, or obsessive-compulsive symptoms); and to prevent relapse. However, such therapy should not be used as the sole or primary treatment for anorexia nervosa. Because associated psychiatric symptoms of anorexia nervosa (e.g., depression) often improve with weight gain, the APA states that the decision to initiate antidepressant therapy should be deferred until weight gain has been restored, and that the choice of an antidepressant agent depends on the remaining symptoms. According to the APA, selective serotonin-reuptake inhibitors commonly are considered in patients with anorexia nervosa whose depressive, obsessive, or compulsive symptoms persist in spite of or in the absence of weight gain.

Although there are few well-controlled, clinical studies of antidepressants for the treatment of anorexia nervosa, data from one study indicate that weight-restored patients with anorexia nervosa who received fluoxetine (40 mg daily) after hospital discharge had less weight loss, depression, and fewer rehospitalizations for anorexia nervosa during the subsequent year than those who received placebo. However, it should be noted that fluoxetine has been misused for its anorectic and weight-reducing effects in a patient with a history of chronic depression, anorexia nervosa, and laxative abuse who was receiving the drug for the treatment of depression; therefore, the misuse potential of fluoxetine in depressed patients with concurrent eating disorders or in other patients who may desire to lose weight should be considered. (See Chronic Toxicity.)

■ **Panic Disorder** Fluoxetine is used in the acute treatment of panic disorder with or without agoraphobia in adults. Panic disorder is characterized by the occurrence of unexpected panic attacks and associated concern about having additional attacks, worry about the implications or consequences of the attacks, and/or a clinically important change in behavior related to the attacks.

According to DSM-IV, panic disorder is characterized by recurrent unexpected panic attacks, which consist of a discrete period of intense fear or discomfort in which 4 (or more) of the following symptoms develop abruptly and reach a peak within 10 minutes: palpitations, pounding heart, or accelerated heart rate; sweating; trembling or shaking; sensations of shortness of breath or smothering; feeling of choking; chest pain or discomfort; nausea or abdominal distress; feeling dizzy, unsteady, lightheaded, or faint; derealization (feelings of unreality) or depersonalization (being detached from oneself); fear of losing control; fear of dying; paresthesias (numbness or tingling sensations); and chills or hot flushes.

The efficacy of fluoxetine for the management of panic disorder with or without agoraphobia has been established by 2 randomized, double-blind, placebo-controlled studies in adult outpatients who met DSM-IV criteria for panic disorder with or without agoraphobia. These studies were of 12 weeks' duration and used a flexible dosing schedule. Fluoxetine therapy in both studies was initiated in a dosage of 10 mg daily for the first week and then the dosage was escalated to 20–60 mg daily depending on clinical response and tolerability. In these studies, 42–62% of patients receiving fluoxetine were free from panic attacks at week 12 compared with 28–44% of those receiving placebo. The mean fluoxetine dosage in one of these studies was approximately 30 mg daily.

The optimum duration of fluoxetine therapy required to prevent recurrence of panic disorder has not been established to date. The manufacturer states that the efficacy of fluoxetine for long-term use (i.e., longer than 12 weeks) has not been demonstrated in controlled studies. However, in a 10-week, placebo-controlled, fixed-dose study, patients responding to fluoxetine 10 or 20 mg daily were randomized to receive continued therapy with their previous fluoxetine dosage or placebo during a 6-month continuation phase. The patients who received an additional 6 months of fluoxetine therapy in this study demonstrated continued clinical improvement.. The manufacturer and some clinicians state that panic disorder is a chronic condition and requires several months or longer of sustained therapy. Therefore, it is reasonable to continue therapy in responding patients. The manufacturer recommends, however, that patients be reassessed periodically to determine the need for continued therapy.

Panic disorder can be treated with cognitive and behavioral psychotherapy and/or pharmacologic therapy. There are several classes of drugs that appear to be effective in the pharmacologic management of panic disorder, including tricyclic antidepressants (e.g., imipramine, clomipramine), monoamine oxidase (MAO) inhibitors (e.g., phenelzine), selective serotonin-reuptake inhibitors (SSRIs), and benzodiazepines (e.g., alprazolam, clonazepam). When choosing among the available drugs, clinicians should consider their acceptance and tolerability by patients; their ability to reduce or eliminate panic attacks, reduce clinically important anxiety and disability secondary to phobic avoidance, and ameliorate other common comorbid conditions (such as depression); and their ability to prevent relapse during long-term therapy. Because of their better tolerability when compared with other agents (such as the tricyclic antidepressants and benzodiazepines), the lack of physical dependence problems commonly associated with benzodiazepines, and efficacy in panic disorder with comorbid conditions (e.g., depression, other anxiety disorders such as obsessive-compulsive disorder, alcoholism), many clinicians prefer SSRIs as first-line therapy in the management of panic disorder. If SSRI therapy is ineffective or is not tolerated, use of a tricyclic antidepressant or a benzodiazepine is recommended.

■ **Bipolar Disorder** Fluoxetine monotherapy has been used for the short-term treatment of acute depressive episodes† in a limited number of patients with bipolar depression† (bipolar disorder, depressed). In one poorly controlled study, fluoxetine was more effective than imipramine, and each drug was more effective than placebo in the management of depression in patients with bipolar disorder; fluoxetine appeared to be particularly effective in reducing anxiety and somatic symptoms in these patients. However, because the drug has been reported to cause manic reactions in some patients, the possibility that hypomanic or manic attacks may be precipitated in patients with bipolar disorder must be considered. In addition, some experts have reported an association between use of antidepressants and the development of rapid cycling and mixed affective states in patients with bipolar disorder, suggesting that such use may worsen the overall course of bipolar disorder in these patients. Consequently, the American Psychiatric Association (APA) does not recommend use of antidepressant monotherapy in patients with bipolar disorder. Initiation or optimization of dosages of maintenance agents (i.e., lithium, lamotrigine) are considered first-line therapies for the management of acute episodes of depression in patients with bipolar disorder. While the addition of either lamotrigine, bupropion, or paroxetine currently is recommended as the next step for patients who fail to respond to optimum dosages of maintenance agents, the APA states that other SSRIs (e.g., fluoxetine) can be used as an alternative to these agents. For further information on the management of bipolar disorder, see Uses: Bipolar Disorder, in Lithium Salts 28:28.

Fluoxetine also is used in combination with olanzapine for the treatment of acute depressive episodes in patients with bipolar I disorder. In 2 randomized, double-blind studies of 8 weeks' duration comparing a fixed combination of fluoxetine and olanzapine with olanzapine monotherapy and placebo, the fixed combination (flexible daily dosages of 6 mg olanzapine and 25 or 50 mg of fluoxetine or of 12 mg of olanzapine and 50 mg of fluoxetine) was more effective than olanzapine monotherapy (5–20 mg daily) or placebo in improvement in depressive symptoms as assessed by the Montgomery-Asberg Depression Rating Scale (MADRS). Although the manufacturer states that efficacy beyond 8 weeks' duration remains to be established, patients have received the fixed combination for up to 24 weeks in clinical trials. Clinicians who elect to extend therapy beyond 8 weeks should reevaluate the risks and benefits of continued therapy periodically.

■ **Obesity** Fluoxetine has been used in a limited number of patients for the short-term management of exogenous obesity†. In a controlled study, obese (i.e., more than 20% overweight), nondepressed individuals receiving fluoxetine (average dosage: 64.9 mg daily), benzphetamine hydrochloride (average dosage: 97 mg daily), or placebo concurrently with reduced food intake and increased exercise for 8 weeks lost an average of about 4.8, 4, and 1.7 kg, respectively. Fluoxetine-treated patients who usually experienced carbohydrate cravings reportedly lost more weight during this study than those who did not experience such cravings. (See Pharmacology: Effects on Appetite and Body Weight.)

In a study evaluating the safety of fluoxetine therapy in the management of exogenous obesity, the drug was generally well tolerated. The adverse effect profile of the drug in nondepressed obese patients appeared to differ somewhat from that in depressed patients receiving similar dosages of the drug; obese patients reportedly had a higher incidence of fatigue and a lower incidence of nausea, anxiety, and tremor. Unlike amphetamines, the potential for addiction to or abuse of fluoxetine appears to be minimal (see Chronic Toxicity), and tolerance to the drug's anorectic and weight-reducing effects has not been reported to date following short-term administration. However, long-term studies are necessary to fully determine whether tolerance develops during chronic fluoxetine therapy and to fully establish the relative efficacy and safety of fluoxetine in the management of exogenous obesity.

■ **Cataplexy** Fluoxetine has been used for the symptomatic management of cataplexy† in a limited number of patients with cataplexy and associated narcolepsy. In one study, the drug appeared to be as effective as clomipramine in reducing the number of cataplexy attacks in patients concurrently receiving CNS stimulants (e.g., dextroamphetamine) for the symptomatic management of associated narcolepsy.

■ **Alcohol Dependence** Like some other selective serotonin-reuptake inhibitors (SSRIs; e.g., citalopram, zimeldine [not commercially available in the US]), fluoxetine has been used in the management of alcohol dependence†. However, studies of SSRIs have generally shown modest effects on alcohol consumption. In a limited number of early-stage problem drinkers (who drank an average of about 8 drinks daily prior to therapy), alcohol consumption was reduced by an average of 17% in patients receiving 60 mg of fluoxetine daily; however, response showed considerable interindividual variability, and alcohol consumption was not altered substantially in problem drinkers receiving 40 mg of the drug daily. It has been suggested that the clinical effects of SSRIs in the management of alcohol dependence may only be transient. In patients with mild to moderate alcohol dependence, alcohol consumption is substantially decreased for only the first 1–4 weeks of fluoxetine therapy or first 12 weeks of citalopram therapy. Additional study is required to fully determine the safety and efficacy of fluoxetine in the management of alcohol dependence. (See Pharmacology: Effects on Alcohol Intake and also see Drug Interactions: Alcohol.)

■ **Myoclonus** Fluoxetine has been used for the management of intention myoclonus†, including postanoxic action myoclonus† and progressive action myoclonus†, in a limited number of patients. Although fluoxetine alone was not effective in improving myoclonus, speech abnormalities, gait abnormalities, or overall performance on neurological examination in such patients, the drug did appear to potentiate the therapeutic effects of combined oxitriptan (l-5-hydroxytryptophan, l-5HTP) and carbidopa therapy in some patients. In addition, fluoxetine reportedly reduced the dosage requirement of oxitriptan and the incidence of adverse GI effects (e.g., diarrhea, abdominal cramps) associated with such therapy. Fluoxetine used in combination with oxitriptan also has exhibited antimyoclonic activity in animals. (See Pharmacology: Other Effects.) However, because toxic effects have been reported in some patients concurrently receiving fluoxetine and tryptophan, a serotonergic agent that is structurally similar to oxitriptan (see Tryptophan and Other Serotonin Precursors under Drug Interactions: Serotonergic Drugs), further study and experience are needed to fully determine the safety and efficacy of combined therapy with fluoxetine and oxitriptan-carbidopa in the management of intention myoclonus.

■ **Premature Ejaculation** Like some other SSRIs, fluoxetine has been used with some success in the treatment of premature ejaculation†. In a placebo-controlled study, fluoxetine produced substantial improvements compared with placebo in time to ejaculation and was well tolerated in most patients. However, in a comparative study, patients receiving either clomipramine or sertraline reported a greater increase in mean intravaginal ejaculation latency time and a greater patient sexual satisfaction rating than those receiving either fluoxetine or placebo. Although the mechanism of action of SSRIs in delaying ejaculation is unclear, it has been suggested that these drugs may be particularly useful in patients who fail or refuse behavioral or psychotherapeutic treatment or when partners are unwilling to cooperate with such therapy.

Dosage and Administration

■ **Administration** Fluoxetine hydrochloride is administered orally without regard to meals.

Fluoxetine hydrochloride conventional capsules, tablets, and solution are administered once or twice daily; the delayed-release capsules are administered once weekly. For the initial management of depression, obsessive-compulsive disorder, premenstrual dysphoric disorder, or bulimia nervosa, the drug generally is administered once daily in the morning. If the dosage exceeds 20 mg daily, the manufacturer and some clinicians state that fluoxetine should be administered in 2 divided doses daily (preferably in the morning and at noon). However, limited evidence suggests that no clinically important differences in either the efficacy or incidence of adverse effects exist with once-daily (in the morning) versus twice-daily (in the morning and at noon) administration of the drug. If sedation occurs during fluoxetine therapy, administering the second dose at bedtime rather than at noon may be useful. Because fluoxetine and its principal active metabolite have relatively long half-lives, the drug has been administered less frequently than once daily (e.g., every 2–7 days), particularly during maintenance therapy. Fluoxetine delayed-release capsules are administered once weekly as maintenance therapy in the management of major depressive disorder in patients who have responded to daily administration of the drug. Some clinicians have suggested that conventional fluoxetine preparations administered less frequently than once daily (i.e., three 20-mg capsules once weekly) may also be effective as maintenance therapy in the management of major depressive disorder, but such dosing regimens should be considered investigational at this time and require additional study to confirm their safety and efficacy.

Because of the prolonged elimination of fluoxetine and its active metabolite from the body, missing a dose of the drug once steady-state concentrations have been achieved is unlikely to result in substantial alterations in plasma fluoxetine or norfluoxetine concentrations.

■ Dosage

Dosage of fluoxetine hydrochloride is expressed in terms of fluoxetine.

In titrating dosage of or discontinuing fluoxetine therapy, the prolonged elimination half-life of fluoxetine and norfluoxetine should be considered. Several weeks will be required before the full effect of such alterations is realized.

The manufacturers and some clinicians recommend that an interval of at least 5 weeks elapse between discontinuance of fluoxetine therapy and initiation of monoamine oxidase (MAO) inhibitor therapy, and that at least 2 weeks elapse following discontinuance of an MAO inhibitor prior to initiation of fluoxetine therapy. For additional information on potentially serious drug interactions that may occur between fluoxetine and MAO inhibitors or other serotonergic agents, see Cautions: Precautions and Contraindications and also see Drug Interactions: Serotonergic Drugs.

Because withdrawal effects may occur with discontinuance of fluoxetine, other selective serotonin-reuptake inhibitors (SSRIs), and selective serotonin- and norepinephrine-reuptake inhibitors (SNRIs), abrupt discontinuance of these drugs should be avoided whenever possible. When fluoxetine therapy is discontinued, the dosage should be reduced gradually (e.g., over a period of several weeks) and the patient monitored for possible withdrawal symptoms. If intolerable symptoms occur following a dosage reduction or upon discontinuance of therapy, the drug may be reinstituted at the previously prescribed dosage. Subsequently, the clinician may continue decreasing the dosage, but at a more gradual rate. Plasma concentrations of fluoxetine and norfluoxetine (the principal metabolite) decline gradually after cessation of therapy, which may minimize the risk of withdrawal symptoms. (See Withdrawal Reactions under Cautions: Nervous System Effects and also see Chronic Toxicity.)

Patients receiving fluoxetine should be monitored for possible worsening of depression, suicidality, or unusual changes in behavior, especially at the beginning of therapy or during periods of dosage adjustment. (See Cautions: Precautions and Contraindications.)

Major Depressive Disorder

Adult Dosage. For the management of major depression, the recommended initial dosage of fluoxetine in adults is 20 mg daily administered in the morning. However, some clinicians suggest that fluoxetine therapy be initiated with lower dosages (e.g., 5 mg daily or 20 mg every 2 or 3 days). Although symptomatic relief may be apparent within the first 1–3 weeks of fluoxetine therapy, optimum antidepressant effect usually requires at least 4 weeks or more of therapy with the drug. If insufficient clinical improvement is apparent after several weeks of fluoxetine therapy at 20 mg daily, an increase in dosage may be considered. Efficacy of fluoxetine for major depression was demonstrated in clinical trials employing 10–80 mg daily. Studies comparing fluoxetine 20, 40, and 60 mg daily to placebo indicate that a dosage of 20 mg daily is sufficient to obtain a satisfactory response in most adults with major depression. Fluoxetine dosages up to 80 mg daily have been administered in some patients, and dosages as low as 5 mg daily may be effective in some patients with depression. In addition, in a study in moderately depressed patients, increasing the dosage of fluoxetine from 20 mg to 40 or 60 mg daily did not result in substantial improvement in depression but was associated with an increase in certain adverse effects (e.g., nausea, anxiety, diarrhea, dry mouth, weight loss). The manufacturer states that the maximum dosage of fluoxetine in adults with major depression should not exceed 80 mg daily; however, somewhat higher dosages (e.g., 100–120 mg daily) occasionally have been used in patients who did not respond adequately to lower dosages.

When fluoxetine hydrochloride delayed-release capsules are used for the continuing management of major depressive disorder, the recommended dosage of fluoxetine is 90 mg once weekly beginning 7 days after the last dose of fluoxetine 20 mg daily. If a satisfactory response is not maintained with once weekly administration, consideration may be given to reestablishing a daily dosage schedule.

As with the use of fluoxetine for other indications, lower dosages or less frequent dosing regimens should be considered for geriatric patients, patients with concurrent disease, and patients receiving multiple concomitant drug therapies.

Pediatric Dosage. For the management of major depressive disorder in children and adolescents 8–18 years of age, the recommended initial dosage of fluoxetine is 10 or 20 mg daily. If therapy is initiated at 10 mg daily, it should be increased after 1 week to 20 mg daily. Because higher plasma fluoxetine concentrations occur in lower weight children, the manufacturer states that both the initial and target dosage in lower weight children may be 10 mg daily. An increase in dosage to 20 mg daily may be considered after several weeks in lower weight children if insufficient clinical improvement is observed. Because a rare but serious drug interaction may occur in depressed children and adolescents with comorbid attention-deficit hyperactivity disorder (ADHD) who receive stimulants and selective serotonin-reuptake inhibitors concomitantly, some experts recommend a maximum fluoxetine dosage of 20 mg daily in such patients. (See Tramadol and Other Serotonergic Drugs under Drug Interactions: Serotonergic Drugs.)

Duration of Therapy. The optimum duration of fluoxetine therapy required to prevent recurrence of depressive symptoms has not been established to date. However, many experts state that acute depressive episodes require several months or longer of sustained antidepressant therapy. Systematic evaluation of fluoxetine has shown that its antidepressant efficacy is maintained for periods of up to approximately 9 months following 3 months of open-label acute treatment (12 months total) in adults receiving 20 mg daily as conventional fluoxetine capsules or for periods of up to approximately 6 months with once-weekly dosing of the 90 mg delayed-release fluoxetine capsules following 3 months of open-label treatment with 20 mg once daily as conventional fluoxetine capsules. However, the therapeutic equivalence of once-weekly administration of the 90-mg delayed-release capsules with that of once-daily administration of the 20-mg conventional preparations for delaying time to relapse has not been established. In addition, it has not been determined to date whether the dosage of the antidepressant necessary to treat acute symptoms of depression is the same as the dosage necessary to prevent recurrence of such symptoms. If therapy with the drug is prolonged, the need for continued therapy should be reassessed periodically.

Switching To or From Other Antidepressants. Because concurrent use of fluoxetine and a tricyclic antidepressant may result in greater than two- to 10-fold elevations in plasma tricyclic antidepressant concentrations, dosage of the tricyclic antidepressant may need to be reduced and plasma tricyclic concentrations may need to be monitored temporarily when fluoxetine is administered concurrently or has been recently discontinued. (See Drug Interactions: Tricyclic and Other Antidepressants.)

Because of the potential risk of serotonin syndrome, the manufacturer recommends that an interval of at least 2 weeks elapse when switching a patient from a monoamine oxidase (MAO) inhibitor to fluoxetine. Because both fluoxetine and its principal metabolite have relatively long half-lives, the manufacturers and some clinicians recommend that at least 5 weeks elapse between discontinuance of fluoxetine therapy and initiation of MAO inhibitor therapy. (See Drug Interactions: Serotonergic Drugs.)

Obsessive-Compulsive Disorder

Adult Dosage. For the management of obsessive-compulsive disorder, the recommended initial dosage of fluoxetine in adults is 20 mg daily administered in the morning. Because a possible dose-response relationship for effectiveness was suggested in one clinical study, an increase in dosage may be considered following several weeks of therapy if insufficient clinical improvement is observed. The manufacturer recommends fluoxetine dosages of 20–60 mg daily for the treatment of obsessive-compulsive disorder; dosages up to 80 mg daily have been well tolerated in clinical studies evaluating the drug in adults with obsessive-compulsive disorder. The manufacturer states that fluoxetine dosage should not exceed 80 mg daily. Like fluoxetine's antidepressant effect, the full therapeutic effect of the drug in patients with obsessive-compulsive disorder may be delayed until 5 weeks of fluoxetine therapy or longer.

Pediatric Dosage. For the management of obsessive-compulsive disorder, the recommended initial dosage of fluoxetine in children and adolescents 7–17 years of age is 10 mg once daily. In adolescents and higher weight children, the dosage should be increased to 20 mg daily after 2 weeks; additional dosage increases may be considered after several more weeks if insufficient clinical improvement is observed. In lower weight children, dosage increases may be considered after several weeks if insufficient clinical improvement is observed. The manufacturer recommends fluoxetine dosages of 20–60 mg daily for adolescents and higher weight children and fluoxetine dosages of 20–30 mg daily for lower weight children for the treatment of obsessive-compulsive disorder. In lower weight children, the manufacturer states that clinical experience with fluoxetine dosages exceeding 20 mg daily is minimal and that there is no experience with dosages exceeding 60 mg daily in such patients.

Duration of Therapy. Although the efficacy of fluoxetine for long-term use (i.e., longer than 13 weeks) has not been demonstrated in controlled studies, patients have been continued on the drug under double-blind conditions for up to an additional 6 months without loss of benefit. The manufacturer and many experts state that obsessive-compulsive disorder is chronic and requires several months or longer of sustained therapy. Therefore, it is reasonable to continue therapy in responding patients. If fluoxetine is used for extended periods, dosage should be adjusted so that the patient is maintained on the lowest effective dosage, and the need for continued therapy with the drug should be reassessed periodically.

Premenstrual Dysphoric Disorder

For the management of premenstrual dysphoric disorder (previously late luteal phase dysphoric disorder), the recommended dosage of fluoxetine is 20 mg once daily given continuously throughout the menstrual cycle or intermittently (i.e., only during the luteal phase, starting 14 days prior to the anticipated onset of menstruation and continuing through the first full day of menses). The intermittent dosing regimen is then repeated with each new menstrual cycle. Decisions regarding which dosing regimen to use should be individualized. In a clinical study evaluating continuous dosing of fluoxetine dosages of 20 or 60 mg once daily for the treatment of premenstrual dysphoric disorder (PMDD), both dosages were effective but there was no evidence that the higher dosage provided any additional benefit. The manufacturer states that dosages exceeding 60 mg daily have not been systematically studied in patients with PMDD and that 80 mg daily is the maximum dosage of fluoxetine for the management of PMDD.

Clinical studies using fluoxetine dosages of 20 mg daily given intermittently or continuously have shown that the efficacy of the drug in the treatment of PMDD is maintained for up to 3 or 6 months, respectively. Patients should be periodically reassessed to determine the need for continued treatment. Discontinuance of the drug (even after more than 1 year of therapy) has resulted in relapse of PMDD within approximately 2 menstrual cycles.

Eating Disorders **Bulimia Nervosa.** For the management of bulimia nervosa in adults, the recommended dosage of fluoxetine is 60 mg daily, administered as a single dose in the morning. The manufacturer states that in some patients, oral dosage of the drug may be carefully titrated up to the recommended initial dosage over a period of several days. However, since 60-mg doses of fluoxetine were found to be well tolerated, the APA states that many clinicians initiate treatment for bulimia nervosa at the higher dosage, titrating downward as necessary to minimize adverse effects. Fluoxetine dosages exceeding 60 mg daily have not been evaluated in patients with bulimia.

Systematic evaluation of fluoxetine has demonstrated that its efficacy in the treatment of bulimia nervosa is maintained for periods of up to 12 months following 2 months of acute treatment in patients receiving 60 mg daily as conventional fluoxetine capsules. Pending further accumulation of data, most clinicians recommend that antidepressant therapy, including fluoxetine, be continued for at least 6–12 months in patients with bulimia nervosa before attempting to discontinue therapy. If fluoxetine is used for extended periods, the manufacturer states that the need for continued therapy should be reassessed periodically.

Anorexia Nervosa. Although safety and efficacy of fluoxetine for the management of anorexia nervosa† and optimal dosage of the drug for this disorder have not been established, fluoxetine has been given in a dosage of 40 mg daily in weight-restored patients with anorexia nervosa.

Panic Disorder For the management of panic disorder, the recommended initial dosage of fluoxetine in adults is 10 mg daily. After 1 week, the dosage should be increased to 20 mg once daily. If no clinical improvement is apparent after several weeks of fluoxetine therapy at 20 mg daily, an increase in dosage may be considered. Efficacy of the drug was demonstrated in clinical trials employing 10–60 mg daily. However, the most frequently administered dosage in flexible-dose clinical studies was 20 mg daily. As with the use of fluoxetine for other indications, lower dosages or less frequent dosing regimens should be considered for geriatric patients and patients with concurrent disease or those receiving multiple concomitant drug therapies. The manufacturer states that fluoxetine dosages exceeding 60 mg daily have not been systematically evaluated in patients with panic disorder.

The optimum duration of fluoxetine therapy required to prevent recurrence of panic disorder has not been established to date. The manufacturer states that the efficacy of fluoxetine beyond 12 weeks of therapy has not been demonstrated in controlled studies. However, the manufacturer and some clinicians state that panic disorder is chronic and requires several months or longer of sustained therapy. Therefore, it is reasonable to continue therapy in responding patients. The manufacturer recommends, however, that patients be reassessed periodically to determine the need for continued therapy.

Bipolar Disorder **Monotherapy.** For the short-term treatment of acute depressive episodes in patients with bipolar disorder†, fluoxetine has been given in a dosage of 20–60 mg daily. Because of the risk of developing manic episodes associated with antidepressant therapy in patients with bipolar disorder, many clinicians recommend using the lowest effective dosage of fluoxetine for the shortest time necessary using the antidepressant in conjunction with a mood-stabilizing agent (e.g., lithium).

Combination Therapy. When used in fixed combination with olanzapine for acute depressive episodes associated with bipolar I disorder, fluoxetine is administered once daily in the evening, usually initiating therapy with a dosage of 6 mg of olanzapine and 25 mg of fluoxetine. A dosage of 3 mg of olanzapine and 25 mg of fluoxetine or 6 mg of olanzapine and 25 mg of fluoxetine should be used as initial therapy in patients with a predisposition to hypotensive reactions, patients with hepatic impairment, those with a combination of factors that may slow metabolism of the drugs(s) (e.g., female gender, geriatric age, nonsmoking status), or those patients who may be pharmacodynamically sensitive to olanzapine; when indicated, dosage should be escalated with caution. In other patients, dosage can be increased according to patient response and tolerance as indicated. In clinical trials, antidepressive efficacy was demonstrated at olanzapine dosages ranging from 6–12 mg daily and fluoxetine dosages ranging from 25–50 mg daily. Dosages exceeding 18 mg of olanzapine and 75 mg of fluoxetine have not been evaluated in clinical studies.

Alternatively, when using fluoxetine and olanzapine in combination as the single-ingredient components for acute depressive episodes associated with bipolar I disorder, the drugs should be given once daily in the evening, generally initiating therapy with 5 mg of olanzapine and 20 mg of fluoxetine. When indicated, dosage adjustments may be made within the dosage ranges of 20–50 mg for fluoxetine and 5–12.5 mg for olanzapine. An initial dosage of 2.5–5 mg of olanzapine with fluoxetine 20 mg should be used in patients with a predisposition to hypotensive reactions, patients with hepatic impairment, those with a combination of factors that may slow metabolism of the drugs(s) (e.g., female gender, geriatric age, nonsmoking status), or those patients who may be pharmacodynamically sensitive to olanzapine; when indicated, dosage increases should be escalated with caution.

Cataplexy For the management of cataplexy†, fluoxetine has been given in a dosage of 20 mg once or twice daily in conjunction with CNS stimulant therapy (e.g., methylphenidate, dextroamphetamine).

Alcohol Dependence For the management of alcohol dependence†, fluoxetine has been given in a dosage of 60 mg daily. Studies have shown that reductions in alcohol intake occur only with dosages of selective serotonin-reuptake inhibitors that are higher than the average therapeutic dosages used in depression. Alcohol intake in patients receiving lower dosages of fluoxetine (40 mg daily) was comparable to that of patients receiving placebo.

■ **Dosage in Renal and Hepatic Impairment** In depressed patients on hemodialysis, chronic fluoxetine administration produced steady-state plasma fluoxetine and norfluoxetine concentrations that were comparable with those observed in patients with normal renal function. The manufacturer therefore states that a reduction in dosage and/or frequency of administration of fluoxetine is not routinely required in patients with renal impairment. Supplemental doses of fluoxetine during hemodialysis also do not appear to be necessary since the drug and its active metabolite norfluoxetine are not removed substantially by hemodialysis. (See Pharmacokinetics: Elimination.)

Since fluoxetine is extensively metabolized in the liver, elimination may be prolonged in patients with hepatic impairment. Therefore, the manufacturer and some clinicians recommend a reduction in dosage and/or frequency of administration of fluoxetine in patients with hepatic impairment. Some clinicians recommend a 50% reduction in initial fluoxetine dosage for patients with well-compensated cirrhosis; however, patients with more substantial hepatic impairment, particularly those with severe disease, will require careful individualization of dosage. Subsequent dosage adjustment based on the tolerance and therapeutic response of the patient has been recommended in patients with hepatic impairment.

■ **Treatment of Pregnant Women during the Third Trimester** Because some neonates exposed to fluoxetine and other SSRIs or selective serotonin- and norepinephrine-reuptake inhibitors (SNRIs) late in the third trimester of pregnancy have developed severe complications, consideration may be given to cautiously tapering fluoxetine therapy in the third trimester prior to delivery if the drug is administered during pregnancy. (See Pregnancy under Cautions: Pregnancy, Fertility, and Lactation.)

Cautions

The adverse effect profile of fluoxetine is similar to that of other selective serotonin-reuptake inhibitors (SSRIs; e.g., citalopram, escitalopram, fluvoxamine, paroxetine, sertraline). Because fluoxetine is a highly selective serotonin-reuptake inhibitor with little or no effect on other neurotransmitters, the incidence of some adverse effects commonly associated with tricyclic antidepressants, such as anticholinergic effects (dry mouth, dizziness, constipation), adverse cardiovascular effects, drowsiness, and weight gain, is lower in patients receiving fluoxetine. However, certain adverse GI (e.g., nausea) and nervous system (e.g., anxiety, nervousness, insomnia) effects appear to occur more frequently during fluoxetine therapy than during therapy with tricyclic antidepressants.

In controlled studies, the most common adverse reactions occurring more frequently in adults receiving fluoxetine than in those receiving placebo included nervous system effects such as anxiety, nervousness, insomnia, somnolence, asthenia, tremor, and abnormal dreams; GI effects such as anorexia, nausea, diarrhea, and dyspepsia; abnormal ejaculation, decreased libido, and impotence; dry mouth; flu syndrome; pharyngitis; rash; sinusitis; sweating; vasodilation; and yawn. Discontinuance of fluoxetine therapy was required principally because of adverse psychiatric (e.g., nervousness, anxiety, insomnia) and dermatologic (e.g., rash) effects. Because of the relatively long elimination half-lives of fluoxetine and its principal metabolite norfluoxetine, the possibility that some adverse effects may resolve slowly following discontinuance of the drug should be considered.

In controlled clinical trials, adverse effects reported in adults with weekly administration of fluoxetine delayed-release capsules were similar to those reported with daily administration of conventional capsules. Diarrhea and cognitive problems occurred more frequently with the delayed-release formulation compared with the conventional capsules.

Common adverse effects associated with fluoxetine therapy for major depressive disorder or obsessive-compulsive disorder in children and adolescents 7 years of age and older are generally similar to those observed in adults and include nausea, tiredness, nervousness, dizziness, and difficulty concentrating. However, manic reactions, including mania and hypomania, were the most common adverse events associated with discontinuance of the drug in 3 pivotal, pediatric, placebo-controlled studies. These reactions occurred in 2.6% of pediatric patients receiving fluoxetine compared with 0% of those receiving placebo and resulted in the discontinuance of fluoxetine in 1.8% of the patients during the acute phases of the studies combined. Consequently, regular monitoring for the occurrence of mania and hypomania in pediatric patients is recommended by the manufacturer.

The usual cautions and precautions of olanzapine should be observed when fluoxetine is used in fixed combination with the antipsychotic.

■ **Nervous System Effects** Headache has occurred in approximately 21% of patients receiving fluoxetine. Nervousness and anxiety have occurred in about 13 and 12% of patients, respectively, and insomnia has occurred in about 19% of patients receiving the drug; such effects appear to be dose-related and have required discontinuance of therapy in approximately 1–2% of fluoxetine-treated patients. The manufacturer and some clinicians state that a sedative (e.g., a short-acting benzodiazepine) may be administered to patients who experience insomnia or nervousness early in therapy; however, the possibility that fluoxetine may interact with some benzodiazepines (e.g., diazepam) should be considered. (See Drug Interactions: Benzodiazepines.)

Drowsiness or somnolence and asthenia reportedly occur in about 12 and 11%, respectively, of patients receiving fluoxetine therapy. Tremor and dizziness have both occurred in about 9% of patients; the incidence of dizziness may be dose-related. Abnormal thinking and abnormal dreams have been reported in about 2 and 1–5% of patients receiving fluoxetine therapy, respectively, and emotional lability has been reported in at least 1% of patients treated with the drug.

Hypomania, mania, and manic reaction have been reported in 1% or less of patients receiving fluoxetine, including those with depression or obsessive-compulsive disorder. In addition, mania reportedly occurred following administration of a higher than recommended dosage (140 mg daily) in a patient with major depression refractory to conventional antidepressant therapy; this patient subsequently responded to a fluoxetine dosage of 60 mg daily without apparent adverse effects. Such reactions have occurred in patients receiving other antidepressant agents and may be caused by antidepressant-induced functional increases in catecholamine activity within the CNS, resulting in a "switch" from depressive to manic behavior. There is some evidence that patients with bipolar disorder may be more likely to experience antidepressant-induced hypomanic or manic reactions than patients without evidence of this disorder. In addition, limited evidence suggests that such reactions may occur more frequently in bipolar depressed patients receiving tricyclics and tetracyclics (e.g., maprotiline, mianserin [not commercially available in the US]) than in those receiving SSRIs (e.g., citalopram, escitalopram, fluoxetine, fluvoxamine, paroxetine, sertraline). However, further studies are needed to confirm these findings.

Extrapyramidal reactions, including acute dystonic reactions, torticollis, dyskinesia (including buccolingual and buccoglossal syndrome), hypertonia, and akathisia, have occurred in 1% or less of patients receiving fluoxetine. An extrapyramidal reaction consisting of torticollis, jaw rigidity, cogwheel rigidity, and loss of fluid motion in gait reportedly occurred in one patient several days after initiation of fluoxetine therapy, but responded rapidly to an anticholinergic antiparkinsonian agent (i.e., trihexyphenidyl) and did not recur despite continued fluoxetine therapy. Serum prolactin concentrations were increased and CSF 3-methoxy-4-hydroxyphenylacetic acid (homovanillic acid, HVA) concentrations were decreased in this patient, suggesting that a decrease in dopaminergic activity (possibly as a result of enhanced serotonergic neurotransmission) may have contributed to the reaction.

Although a causal relationship to the drug has not been established, serotonin syndrome and neuroleptic malignant syndrome (NMS)-like reactions also have been reported rarely in patients receiving fluoxetine, other SSRIs, and selective serotonin- and norepinephrine-reuptake inhibitors (SNRIs). (See Cautions: Precautions and Contraindications and also see Drug Interactions: Serotonergic Drugs.)

The incidence of seizures during fluoxetine therapy appears to be similar to that observed during therapy with most other currently available antidepressants. Seizures or events that were described as possible seizures have been reported in approximately 0.2% of patients receiving fluoxetine therapy to date. (See Cautions: Precautions and Contraindications.) In addition, seizures have occurred following acute overdosage of the drug (see Acute Toxicity) and in at least one patient undergoing electroconvulsive therapy (ECT) concomitantly.

Adverse nervous system effects occurring in less than 1% of fluoxetine-treated patients include ataxia, balance disorder, and bruxism; however, a causal relationship to the drug has not been established. Depersonalization, euphoria, myoclonus, and paranoid reaction also have been reported in less than 1% of patients receiving the drug and delusions have been reported rarely, although these adverse effects have not been definitely attributed to fluoxetine. Rarely reported adverse nervous system effects for which a causal relationship has not been established include violent behavior, precipitation or worsening of depression, hypertonia, myoclonus, dyskinesia, and exacerbation of multiple sclerosis. Interference with facial nerve conduction, manifesting as ocular tics and impaired hearing, and memory impairment also have been reported. In some patients developing movement disorders with fluoxetine, there were underlying risk factors such as predisposing drug therapy and/or the disorder was an exacerbation of a preexisting disorder.

Withdrawal Reactions Withdrawal symptoms, including dysphoric mood, irritability, agitation, dizziness, sensory disturbances (e.g., paresthesias such as electric shock sensations), anxiety, confusion, headache, lethargy, emotional lability, insomnia, and hypomania, have been reported upon discontinuance of fluoxetine, other SSRIs, and SNRIs, particularly when discontinuance of these drugs is abrupt. While these reactions are generally self-limiting, there have been reports of serious discontinuance symptoms. Therefore, patients should be monitored for such symptoms when discontinuing fluoxetine therapy. A gradual reduction in the dosage rather than abrupt cessation is recommended whenever possible. Plasma concentrations of fluoxetine and norfluoxetine (the principal metabolite) decline gradually after cessation of therapy, which may minimize the risk of withdrawal symptoms. (See Dosage and Administration: Dosage and also see Chronic Toxicity.)

Suicidality Suicide attempts have been reported in less than 1% of fluoxetine-treated patients in clinical trials. The US Food and Drug Administration (FDA) has determined that antidepressants increase the risk of suicidal thinking and behavior (suicidality) in children, adolescents, and young adults (18–24 years of age) with major depressive disorder and other psychiatric disorders. Suicidal ideation, which can manifest as persistent, obsessive, and violent suicidal thoughts, has emerged occasionally in adults receiving fluoxetine. In a report of several fluoxetine-associated cases, severe suicidal ideation developed within 2–7 weeks after initiation of fluoxetine therapy and resolved within several days to months after discontinuance of the drug; however, the patients were unresponsive to fluoxetine and had received monoamine oxidase inhibitor therapy previously, and most had a history of suicidal ideation, were receiving relatively high dosages (60–80 mg daily) of fluoxetine, and were receiving other psychotropic therapy concomitantly. Suicidal ideation also has been reported in patients who reportedly had no history of such ideation, but the drug also has been used without recurrence of suicidal ideation in a few patients in whom such ideation emerged during tricyclic antidepressant therapy. Because of the possibility of suicidality, patients should be appropriately monitored and closely observed for clinical worsening, suicidality, and unusual changes in behavior, particularly during initiation of fluoxetine therapy (i.e., the first few months) and during periods of dosage adjustments. (See Cautions: Precautions and Contraindications and see Cautions: Pediatric Precautions and see Acute Toxicity.)

■ **GI Effects** The most frequent adverse effect associated with fluoxetine therapy is nausea, which occurs in about 22% of patients. Nausea generally is mild, occurs early in therapy, and usually subsides after a few weeks of continued therapy with the drug. Limited evidence suggests that the incidence of nausea may be dose-related, but additional experience with the drug is necessary to confirm this finding. Although the incidence of vomiting appears to be similar in patients receiving fluoxetine or tricyclic antidepressants (e.g., imipramine), the incidence of nausea appears to be higher with fluoxetine. While the mechanism(s) of fluoxetine-induced GI effects has not been fully elucidated, serotonin has been shown to have complex effects on the GI tract (e.g., stimulation of small intestine motility, inhibition of gastric and large intestine motility).

Diarrhea occurs in about 11%, anorexia in about 10%, and dyspepsia in about 8% of patients receiving fluoxetine; limited evidence suggests that the incidence of anorexia may be dose-related. Other adverse GI effects associated with fluoxetine therapy include vomiting and flatulence, which both reportedly occur in about 3% of patients receiving the drug. Change in taste perception has been reported in at least 1% of fluoxetine-treated patients.

Other adverse GI effects, including dysphagia, gastritis, gastroenteritis, melena, and stomach ulcer, have been reported in less than 1% of fluoxetine-treated patients; however, a causal relationship to the drug has not been established. Bloody diarrhea, duodenal or esophageal ulcer, GI hemorrhage, hematemesis, hepatitis, peptic ulcer, and stomach ulcer hemorrhage have occurred rarely, but have not been definitely attributed to fluoxetine.

Epidemiologic case-control and cohort design studies have suggested that selective serotonin-reuptake inhibitors may increase the risk of upper GI bleeding. Although the precise mechanism for this increased risk remains to be clearly established, serotonin release by platelets is known to play an important role in hemostasis, and selective serotonin-reuptake inhibitors decrease serotonin uptake from the blood by platelets thereby decreasing the amount of serotonin in platelets. In addition, concurrent use of aspirin or other nonsteroidal anti-inflammatory agents was found to substantially increase the risk of GI bleeding in patients receiving selective serotonin-reuptake inhibitors in 2 of these studies. Although these studies focused on upper GI bleeding, there is some evidence suggesting that bleeding at other sites may be similarly potentiated. Further clinical studies are needed to determine the clinical importance of these findings. (See Cautions: Hematologic Effects and also see Drug Interactions: Drugs Affecting Hemostasis.)

■ **Dermatologic and Sensitivity Reactions** Rash (including purpuric rash and erythema multiforme) and/or urticaria occurs in about 7% and pruritus occurs in about 3% of patients receiving fluoxetine. Adverse dermatologic effects, principally rash and pruritus, generally occur during the first few weeks of therapy and have required discontinuance of the drug in approximately 1% of patients.

Fluoxetine-induced rash and/or urticaria have been associated with systemic signs or symptoms such as fever, leukocytosis, arthralgia, edema, carpal tunnel syndrome, respiratory distress, lymphadenopathy, proteinuria, and mild elevation in serum aminotransferase (transaminase) concentrations in some patients. Serious systemic illnesses have developed rarely in patients with fluoxetine-induced dermatologic reactions to date. Although the diagnosis was equivocal in at least 2 of these patients, one patient was diagnosed as having a leukocytoclastic vasculitis and the other patient exhibited a severe desquamating syndrome that was variably diagnosed as either vasculitis or erythema multiforme. In addition, serum sickness reactions have developed in several other patients who experienced adverse dermatologic effects in association with fluoxetine therapy. Additional cases of systemic reactions possibly related to vasculitis have been reported in patients with rash. Although systemic reactions appear to occur rarely in patients receiving fluoxetine, such reactions may be serious and potentially may involve the lung, kidney, or liver; death reportedly has occurred in association with such reactions.

Anaphylactoid reactions (including bronchospasm, angioedema, and/or urticaria) have been reported in fluoxetine-treated patients; adverse pulmonary effects (including inflammatory processes of varying histopathology and/or fibrosis), which have occurred with dyspnea as the only preceding symptom, have been reported rarely. It has not been established whether the systemic reactions and associated skin rash in fluoxetine-treated patients share a common underlying cause or are due to different etiologies or pathogenic processes; in addition, a specific, underlying immunologic basis for these effects has not been identified. However, such systemic reactions are of potential concern since zimeldine (another selective serotonin-reuptake inhibitor that previously was commercially available outside the US) reportedly was associated with the development of Guillain-Barré syndrome following flu-like, hypersensitivity reactions to the drug; because of such reactions, zimeldine no longer is commercially available. Most patients with fluoxetine-induced rash and/or urticaria improve soon after discontinuance of therapy and/or administration of an antihistamine or corticosteroid, and most patients with such reactions to date have recovered completely without serious adverse sequelae. In addition, several patients who developed hypersensitivity reactions while receiving zimeldine subsequently received fluoxetine with no recurrence of a similar reaction. However, because of associated severe adverse systemic effects with fluoxetine and pharmacologically similar antidepressants (e.g., zimeldine), it is recommended that fluoxetine be discontinued if rash and/or other possible manifestations of hypersensitivity (e.g., fever, flu-like symptoms), for which alternative etiologies cannot be identified, occur during therapy with the drug.

Sweating occurs in about 7% of patients receiving fluoxetine. Adverse dermatologic and hypersensitivity reactions occurring in less than 1% of patients receiving fluoxetine include dry skin, alopecia, and photosensitivity reaction; however, these effects have not been definitely attributed to the drug. Although a causal relationship has not been established, erythema nodosum, epidermal necrolysis, exfoliative dermatitis, and Stevens-Johnson syndrome have also been reported.

■ Metabolic Effects Weight loss occurs in approximately 2% of patients receiving fluoxetine therapy. Normal-weight and overweight (i.e., body mass index exceeding 25 kg/m^2) depressed patients lost an average of 0.9–1.8 kg and 1.8 kg, respectively, following 6 weeks of therapy with the drug. Weight loss associated with fluoxetine therapy appears to be reversible, with a gradual increase in body weight occurring following discontinuance of the drug. Such weight loss appears to result from decreased food consumption rather than adverse GI effects associated with the drug; there is some evidence that fluoxetine-induced weight loss may be dose-related. (See Pharmacology: Effects on Appetite and Body Weight.) In addition, weight loss appears to occur independent of the antidepressant effect of the drug. Although weight loss is commonly associated with fluoxetine therapy, less than 1% of patients discontinue the drug because of this effect. In some cases, however, substantial weight loss may be an undesirable effect of therapy with the drug, particularly in underweight depressed or bulimic patients.

Fluoxetine potentially may alter blood glucose concentrations. Hypoglycemia has occurred during fluoxetine therapy. In addition, hyperglycemia has developed following discontinuance of the drug. Therefore, the possibility that insulin and/or oral antidiabetic agent dosage adjustments may be necessary when fluoxetine therapy is initiated or discontinued in patients with diabetes mellitus should be considered.

■ Ocular Effects Vision abnormalities, including blurred vision, occur in approximately 2% of patients receiving fluoxetine. In addition, cataract and optic neuritis have been reported in patients treated with fluoxetine, although a causal relationship to the drug remains to be established.

Mydriasis has been reported in less than 1% of patients receiving fluoxetine. (See Cautions: Precautions and Contraindications.)

■ Cardiovascular Effects Current evidence suggests that fluoxetine is less cardiotoxic than most antidepressant agents (e.g., tricyclic antidepressants, monoamine oxidase inhibitors). Unlike tricyclic antidepressants, which may cause characteristic ECG changes such as prolongation of PR, QRS, and QT intervals and ST-segment and T-wave abnormalities, clinically important ECG changes (such as conduction abnormalities) have not been commonly reported during controlled studies in fluoxetine-treated patients without preexisting cardiac disease. In addition, while tricyclic antidepressants commonly cause an increase in heart rate, heart rate reportedly is reduced by an average of approximately 3 beats/minute in patients receiving fluoxetine. (See Pharmacology: Cardiovascular Effects.)

Vasodilation has been reported in approximately 2% and palpitations have been reported in at least 1% of patients receiving fluoxetine. Unlike tricyclic antidepressants, fluoxetine has been associated with hypotension relatively infrequently. Cardiac arrhythmia also has occurred infrequently in fluoxetine-treated patients. Atrial fibrillation, ventricular tachycardia (including torsades de pointes-type arrhythmias), QT-interval prolongation, cardiac arrest, pulmonary hypertension, and cerebrovascular accident have occurred rarely, but these adverse effects have not been definitely attributed to the drug.

■ Hematologic Effects Ecchymosis has been reported in less than 1% of patients receiving fluoxetine. Lymphadenopathy and anemia also have been reported in patients receiving fluoxetine. Blood dyscrasia, leukopenia, pancytopenia, aplastic anemia, immune-related hemolytic anemia, petechiae, and purpura have occurred rarely, although a causal relationship to the drug has not been established. Thrombocytopenia and thrombocytopenic purpura also have been reported.

SNRIs and SSRIs, including fluoxetine, may increase the risk of bleeding events. Concomitant use of aspirin, nonsteroidal anti-inflammatory agents, warfarin, and other anticoagulants may add to this risk. Bleeding complications (e.g., ecchymosis, purpura, menorrhagia, rectal bleeding) have been reported infrequently in patients receiving SSRIs. Although the precise mechanism for these reactions has not been established, it has been suggested that impaired platelet aggregation and prolonged bleeding time may be due at least in part to inhibition of serotonin reuptake into platelets and/or that increased capillary fragility and vascular tone may contribute to these cases. (See Cautions: GI Effects and also see Drug Interactions: Drugs Affecting Hemostasis.)

■ Respiratory Effects Flu-like syndrome (see Cautions: Dermatologic and Sensitivity Reactions), pharyngitis, and sinusitis have occurred in approximately 1–11% of patients receiving fluoxetine in controlled clinical trials. Adverse respiratory effects reportedly occurring in at least 1% of patients but not directly attributable to the drug include rhinitis and yawning. Laryngeal edema has occurred rarely in patients receiving fluoxetine. Pulmonary fibrosis, pulmonary embolism, and eosinophilic pneumonia also have been reported in fluoxetine-treated patients; however, these adverse effects have not been definitely attributed to the drug.

■ Renal, Electrolyte, and Genitourinary Effects ***Sexual Dysfunction*** Like other SSRIs, adverse effects on sexual function have been reported in both men and women receiving fluoxetine. Although changes in sexual desire, sexual performance, and sexual satisfaction often occur as manifestations of a psychiatric disorder, they also may occur as the result of pharmacologic therapy. It is difficult to determine the true incidence and severity of adverse effects on sexual function during fluoxetine therapy, in part because patients and clinicians may be reluctant to discuss these effects. Therefore, incidence data reported in product labeling and earlier studies are most likely underestimates of the true incidence of adverse sexual effects. Recent reports indicate that up to 50% of patients receiving SSRIs describe some form of sexual dysfunction during treatment and the actual incidence may be even higher.

Ejaculatory disturbances (principally ejaculatory delay) are the most common adverse urogenital effects associated with fluoxetine in men, occurring in up to 7% of men receiving the drug compared with less than 1% of those receiving placebo in controlled clinical studies for the treatment of obsessive-compulsive disorder or bulimia. In some cases, the adverse effect of ejaculatory delay has been used for therapeutic benefit in the treatment of premature ejaculation. (See Uses: Premature Ejaculation.) Other genital disorders reported in patients receiving the drug include impotence, increased libido, penile (of the glans) anesthesia, and anorgasmy (in both males and females). Decreased libido also reportedly occurs in up to 11% of patients. In addition, clitoral engorgement, sexual arousal, and orgasm reportedly occurred in at least one female patient receiving fluoxetine.

Management of sexual dysfunction caused by selective SSRI therapy includes waiting for tolerance to develop; using a lower dosage of the drug; using drug holidays; delaying administration of the drug until after coitus; or changing to another antidepressant. Although further study is needed, there is some evidence that adverse sexual effects of the SSRIs may be reversed by concomitant use of certain drugs, including buspirone, 5-hydroxytryptamine-2 (5-HT$_2$) receptor antagonists (e.g., nefazodone), 5-HT$_3$ receptor inhibitors (e.g., granisetron), or α_2-adrenergic receptor antagonists (e.g., yohimbine), selective phosphodiesterase (PDE) inhibitors (e.g., sildenafil), or dopamine receptor agonists (e.g., amantadine, dextroamphetamine, pemoline [no longer commercially available in the US], methylphenidate). In most patients, sexual dysfunction is fully reversed 1–3 days after discontinuance of the antidepressant. Ejaculatory dysfunction associated with fluoxetine therapy also has responded to concomitant cyproheptadine therapy in a few patients.

Other Renal, Electrolyte, and Genitourinary Effects Treatment with SSRIs, including fluoxetine, and SNRIs may result in hyponatremia. In many cases, this hyponatremia appears to be due to the syndrome of inappropriate antidiuretic hormone secretion (SIADH) and was reversible when fluoxetine was discontinued. Cases with serum sodium concentrations lower than 110 mEq/L have been reported. Geriatric individuals and patients receiving diuretics or who are otherwise volume depleted may be at greater risk of developing hyponatremia during therapy with SSRIs or SNRIs. Signs and symptoms of hyponatremia include headache, difficulty concentrating, memory impairment, confusion, weakness, and unsteadiness, which may lead to falls; more severe and/or acute cases have been associated with hallucinations, syncope, seizures, coma, respiratory arrest, and death. Discontinuance of fluoxetine should be considered in patients with symptomatic hyponatremia and appropriate medical intervention should be instituted. Because geriatric patients may be at increased risk for hyponatremia associated with these drugs, clinicians prescribing fluoxetine in such patients should be aware of the possibility that such reactions may occur. In addition, periodic monitoring of serum sodium concentrations (particularly during the first several months) in geriatric patients receiving SSRIs has been recommended by some clinicians.

Micturition disorder has occurred in at least 1% of patients receiving fluoxetine. Gynecological bleeding and dysuria have been reported in less than 1% of fluoxetine-treated patients, although these adverse effects have not been definitely attributed to the drug. Menorrhagia, gynecomastia, uterine hemorrhage, vaginal hemorrhage, and vaginal bleeding also have occurred, although a causal relationship to the drug has not been established.

■ Anticholinergic Effects Although bothersome anticholinergic effects occur commonly in patients receiving tricyclic antidepressant agents, such effects occur less frequently with fluoxetine. Dry mouth, dizziness, and constipation have been reported in about 9, 9, and 5% of patients receiving the drug, respectively. Blurred vision also has been reported.

■ Other Adverse Effects Chills have occurred in more than 1% of patients receiving fluoxetine. (See Cautions: Dermatologic and Sensitivity Reactions.)

Abnormal liver function test results, lymphadenopathy, and epistaxis have been reported in less than 1% of fluoxetine-treated patients, although such effects have not been definitely attributed to the drug. Adverse effects occurring rarely in patients receiving fluoxetine include hepatitis, jaundice (including cholestatic jaundice), acute abdominal syndrome, serum sickness, and lupus erythematosus syndrome. Pancreatitis and hyperprolactinemia also have occurred in patients receiving the drug. Although a causal relationship to fluoxetine has not been established for these effects, serotonin has been implicated as a possible physiologic factor in the release of prolactin. (See Pharmacology: Neuroendocrine Effects.)

■ Precautions and Contraindications Worsening of depression and/or the emergence of suicidal ideation and behavior (suicidality) or unusual changes in behavior may occur in both adult and pediatric (see Cautions: Pediatric Precautions) patients with major depressive disorder or other psychiatric disorders, whether or not they are taking antidepressants. This risk may persist until clinically important remission occurs. Suicide is a known risk of depression and certain other psychiatric disorders, and these disorders themselves are the strongest predictors of suicide. However, there has been a long-standing concern that antidepressants may have a role in inducing worsening of depression and the emergence of suicidality in certain patients during the early phases of treatment. Pooled analyses of short-term, placebo-controlled studies of antidepressants (i.e., selective serotonin-reuptake inhibitors [SSRIs] and other antidepressants) have shown an increased risk of suicidality in children, adolescents, and young adults (18–24 years of age) with major depressive disorder and other psychiatric disorders. An increased suicidality risk was not demonstrated with antidepressants compared with placebo in adults older than 24 years of age, and a reduced risk was observed in adults 65 years of age or older. It currently is unknown whether the suicidality risk extends to longer-term use (i.e., beyond several months); however, there is substantial evidence from placebo-controlled maintenance trials in adults with major depressive disorder that antidepressants can delay the recurrence of depression.

The US Food and Drug Administration (FDA) recommends that all patients being treated with antidepressants for any indication be appropriately monitored and closely observed for clinical worsening, suicidality, and unusual changes in behavior, particularly during initiation of therapy (i.e., the first few months) and during periods of dosage adjustments. Families and caregivers of patients being treated with antidepressants for major depressive disorder or other indications, both psychiatric and nonpsychiatric, also should be advised to monitor patients on a daily basis for the emergence of agitation, irritability, or unusual changes in behavior, as well as the emergence of suicidality, and to report such symptoms immediately to a health care provider.

Although a causal relationship between the emergence of symptoms such as anxiety, agitation, panic attacks, insomnia, irritability, hostility, aggressiveness, impulsivity, akathisia, hypomania, and/or mania and either the worsening of depression and/or the emergence of suicidal impulses has not been established, there is concern that such symptoms may represent precursors to emerging suicidality. Consequently, consideration should be given to changing the therapeutic regimen or discontinuing therapy in patients whose depression is persistently worse or in patients experiencing emergent suicidality or symptoms that might be precursors to worsening depression or suicidality, particularly if such manifestations are severe, abrupt in onset, or were not part of the patient's presenting symptoms. FDA also recommends that the drugs be prescribed in the smallest quantity consistent with good patient management, in order to reduce the risk of overdosage.

It is generally believed (though not established in controlled trials) that treating a major depressive episode with an antidepressant alone may increase the likelihood of precipitating a mixed or manic episode in patients at risk for bipolar disorder. Therefore, patients should be adequately screened for bipolar disorder prior to initiating treatment with an antidepressant; such screening should include a detailed psychiatric history (e.g., family history of suicide, bipolar disorder, and depression).

Potentially life-threatening serotonin syndrome or neuroleptic malignant syndrome (NMS)-like reactions have been reported with SSRIs, including fluoxetine, and selective serotonin- and norepinephrine-reuptake inhibitors (SNRIs) alone, but particularly with concurrent administration of other serotonergic drugs (including serotonin [5-hydroxytryptamine; 5-HT] type 1 receptor agonists [triptans]), drugs that impair the metabolism of serotonin (e.g., monoamine oxidase [MAO] inhibitors), or antipsychotic agents or other dopamine antagonists. Symptoms of serotonin syndrome may include mental status changes (e.g., agitation, hallucinations, coma), autonomic instability (e.g., tachycardia, labile blood pressure, hyperthermia), neuromuscular aberrations (e.g., hyperreflexia, incoordination), and/or GI symptoms (e.g., nausea, vomiting, diarrhea). In its most severe form, serotonin syndrome may resemble NMS, which is characterized by hyperthermia, muscle rigidity, autonomic instability with possible rapid fluctuation in vital signs, and mental status changes. Patients receiving fluoxetine should be monitored for the development of serotonin syndrome or NMS-like signs and symptoms.

Fluoxetine is contraindicated in patients who currently are receiving or recently (i.e., within 2 weeks) have received therapy with MAO inhibitors used for treatment of depression. If concurrent therapy with fluoxetine and a 5-HT_1 receptor agonist (triptan) is clinically warranted, the patient should be observed carefully, particularly during initiation of therapy, when dosage is increased, or when another serotonergic agent is initiated. Concomitant use of fluoxetine and serotonin precursors (e.g., tryptophan) is not recommended. If signs and symptoms of serotonin syndrome or NMS develop during therapy, treatment with fluoxetine and any concurrently administered serotonergic or antidopaminergic agents, including antipsychotic agents, should be discontinued immediately and supportive and symptomatic treatment should be initiated. (See Drug Interactions: Serotonergic Drugs.)

Because clinical experience with fluoxetine in patients with concurrent systemic disease, including cardiovascular disease, hepatic impairment, and renal impairment, is limited, caution should be exercised when fluoxetine is administered to patients with any systemic disease or condition that may alter metabolism of the drug or adversely affect hemodynamic function. (See Dosage and Administration: Dosage.) Fluoxetine should be used with caution in patients with hepatic impairment, since prolonged elimination of the drug and its principal metabolite has been reported to occur in patients with liver cirrhosis. Because the safety of long-term fluoxetine therapy in patients with severe renal impairment has not been adequately evaluated to date, fluoxetine also should be used with caution in patients with severe renal impairment. (See Dosage and Administration: Dosage in Renal and Hepatic Impairment.) Although current evidence suggests that fluoxetine is less cardiotoxic than most older antidepressant agents (see Cautions: Cardiovascular Effects), the safety of fluoxetine in patients with a recent history of myocardial infarction or unstable cardiovascular disease has not been adequately evaluated to date.

Patients receiving fluoxetine should be advised to notify their clinician if they are taking or plan to take nonprescription (over-the-counter), including herbal supplements, or prescription medications or alcohol-containing beverages or products. (See Drug Interactions.)

Patients receiving fluoxetine should be cautioned about the concurrent use of nonsteroidal anti-inflammatory agents (including aspirin), warfarin, or other drugs that affect coagulation since combined use of SSRIs and these drugs has been associated with an increased risk of bleeding. Patients should be advised to contact their physician if they experience any increased or unusual bruising or bleeding while taking fluoxetine. (See Cautions: GI Effects and also see Drug Interactions: Drugs Affecting Hemostasis.)

Fluoxetine generally is less sedating than many other currently available antidepressants and does not appear to produce substantial impairment of cognitive or psychomotor function. However, patients should be cautioned that fluoxetine may impair their ability to perform activities requiring mental alertness or physical coordination (e.g., operating machinery, driving a motor vehicle) and to avoid such activities until they experience how the drug affects them.

Patients receiving fluoxetine should be advised to notify their clinician if they develop a rash or other possible signs of an allergic reaction during therapy with the drug. Pending further accumulation of data, monitoring for such effects is particularly important since these effects have been associated with the development of potentially serious systemic reactions in patients receiving fluoxetine or pharmacologically similar antidepressants (e.g., zimeldine). (See Cautions: Dermatologic and Sensitivity Reactions.)

Seizures have been reported in patients receiving therapeutic dosages and following acute overdosage of fluoxetine. Because of limited experience with fluoxetine in patients with a history of seizures, therapy with the drug should be initiated with caution in such patients.

Because fluoxetine may alter blood glucose concentrations in patients with diabetes mellitus (see Cautions: Metabolic Effects), the possibility that insulin and/or oral antidiabetic agent dosage adjustments may be necessary when fluoxetine therapy is initiated or discontinued should be considered.

Because fluoxetine therapy has been commonly associated with anorexia and weight loss, the drug should be used with caution in patients who may be adversely affected by these effects (e.g., underweight or bulimic patients).

Because mydriasis has been reported in association with fluoxetine therapy (see Cautions: Ocular Effects), the drug should be used with caution in patients elevated intraocular pressure or those at risk of acute narrow-angle glaucoma.

Treatment with SSRIs, including fluoxetine, or SNRIs may result in hyponatremia. In many cases, this hyponatremia appears to be due to the syndrome of inappropriate antidiuretic hormone secretion (SIADH) and was reversible when the SSRI or SNRI was discontinued. Cases with serum sodium concentrations lower than 110 mEq/L have been reported. Geriatric individuals and patients receiving diuretics or who are otherwise volume depleted may be at greater risk of developing hyponatremia during therapy with SSRIs or SNRIs. Signs and symptoms of hyponatremia include headache, difficulty concentrating, memory impairment, confusion, weakness, and unsteadiness, which may lead to falls; more severe and/or acute cases have been associated with hallucinations, syncope, seizures, coma, respiratory arrest, and death. Discontinuance of fluoxetine should be considered in patients with symptomatic hyponatremia and appropriate medical intervention should be instituted. (See Cautions: Renal, Electrolyte, and Genitourinary Effects and also see Cautions: Geriatric Precautions.)

Fluoxetine therapy is contraindicated in patients concurrently receiving thioridazine therapy. The manufacturer recommends that an interval of at least 5 weeks elapse between discontinuance of fluoxetine therapy and initiation of thioridazine. In addition, concurrent use of fluoxetine in patients receiving pimozide is contraindicated. (See Thioridazine and also see Pimozide under Drug Interactions: Antipsychotic Agents.)

■ **Pediatric Precautions** Safety and efficacy of fluoxetine in pediatric patients have not been established in children younger than 8 years of age for the management of major depressive disorder (see Pediatric Considerations under Uses: Major Depressive Disorder) or in children younger than 7 years of age for the management of obsessive-compulsive disorder.

FDA warns that antidepressants increase the risk of suicidal thinking and behavior (suicidality) in children and adolescents with major depressive disorder and other psychiatric disorders. The risk of suicidality for these drugs was identified in a pooled analysis of data from a total of 24 short-term (4–16 weeks), placebo-controlled studies of 9 antidepressants (i.e., fluoxetine, bupropion, citalopram, fluvoxamine, mirtazapine, nefazodone, paroxetine, sertraline, venlafaxine) in over 4400 children and adolescents with major depressive disorder, obsessive-compulsive disorder (OCD), or other psychiatric disorders. The analysis revealed a greater risk of adverse events representing suicidal behavior or thinking (suicidality) during the first few months of treatment in pediatric patients receiving antidepressants than in those receiving placebo. However, a more recent meta-analysis of 27 placebo-controlled trials of 9 antidepressants (SSRIs and others) in patients younger than 19 years of age with major depressive disorder, OCD, or non-OCD anxiety disorders suggests that the benefits of antidepressant therapy in treating these conditions may outweigh the risks of suicidal behavior or suicidal ideation. No suicides occurred in these pediatric trials.

The risk of suicidality in FDA's pooled analysis differed across the different psychiatric indications, with the highest incidence observed in the major depressive disorder studies. In addition, although there was considerable variation in risk among the antidepressants, a tendency toward an increase in suicidality risk in younger patients was found for almost all drugs studied. It is currently unknown whether the suicidality risk in pediatric patients extends to longer-term use (i.e., beyond several months).

As a result of this analysis and public discussion of the issue, FDA has directed manufacturers of all antidepressants to add a boxed warning to the labeling of their products to alert clinicians of this suicidality risk in children and adolescents and to recommend appropriate monitoring and close observation of patients receiving these agents. (See Cautions: Precautions and Contraindications.) The drugs that are the focus of the revised labeling are all drugs included in the general class of antidepressants, including those that have not been studied in controlled clinical trials in pediatric patients, since the available data are not adequate to exclude any single antidepressant from an increased risk. In addition to the boxed warning and other information in professional labeling on antidepressants, FDA currently recommends that a patient medication guide explaining the risks associated with the drugs be provided to the patient each time the drugs are dispensed. Caregivers of pediatric patients whose depression is persistently worse or who are experiencing emergent suicidality or symptoms that might be precursors to worsening depression or suicidality during antidepressant therapy should consult their clinician regarding the best course of action (e.g., whether the therapeutic regimen should be changed or the drug discontinued). *Patients should not discontinue use of selective serotonin-reuptake inhibitors without first consulting their clinician; it is very important that the drugs not be abruptly discontinued, as withdrawal effects may occur.* (See Dosage and Administration: Dosage.)

Anyone considering the use of fluoxetine in a child or adolescent for any clinical use must balance the potential risks of therapy with the clinical need.

Important toxicity, including myotoxicity, long-term neurobehavioral and reproductive toxicity, and impaired bone development, has been observed following exposure of juvenile animals to fluoxetine; some of these effects occurred at clinically relevant exposures to the drug. In a study in which fluoxetine (3, 10, or 30 mg/kg) was orally administered to young rats from weaning (postnatal day 21) through adulthood (day 90), male and female sexual development was delayed at all dosages, and growth (body weight gain, femur length) was decreased during the dosing period in animals receiving the highest dosage. At the end of the treatment period, serum levels of creatine kinase (a marker of muscle damage) were increased in animals receiving the intermediate and highest dosage, and abnormal muscle and reproductive organ histopathology (skeletal muscle degeneration and necrosis, testicular degeneration and necrosis, epididymal vacuolation and hypospermia) was observed at the highest dosage. When animals were evaluated after a recovery period (up to 11 weeks after drug cessation), neurobehavioral abnormalities (decreased reactivity at all dosages and learning deficit at the highest dosage) and reproductive functional impairment (decreased mating at all dosages and impaired fertility at the highest dosage) were noted; testicular and epididymal microscopic lesions and decreased sperm concentrations were observed in the high-dosage group indicating that the reproductive organ effects seen at the end of treatment were irreversible. Reversibility of fluoxetine-induced muscle damage was not assessed in this study. Adverse effects similar to those observed in rats treated with fluoxetine during the juvenile period have not been reported after administration of fluoxetine to adult animals. Plasma exposures (AUC) to fluoxetine in juvenile rats receiving the low, intermediate, and high dosages in this study were approximately 0.1–0.2, 1–2, and 5–10 times, respectively, the average exposure in pediatric patients receiving the maximum recommended dosage of 20 mg daily. Exposures to norfluoxetine, the principal active metabolite of fluoxetine, in rats were approximately 0.3–0.8, 1–8, and 3–20 times the pediatric exposure at the maximum recommended dosage, respectively.

A specific effect of fluoxetine on bone development has been reported in mice treated with fluoxetine during the juvenile period. In mice treated with fluoxetine (5 or 20 mg/kg given intraperitoneally) for 4 weeks beginning at 4 weeks of age, bone formation was reduced resulting in decreased bone mineral content and density. These dosages did not affect overall growth (e.g., body weight gain or femoral length). The dosages given to juvenile mice in this study were approximately 0.5 and 2 times the maximum recommended dose for pediatric patients on a mg/m^2 basis.

In a study conducted in mice, fluoxetine administration (10 mg/kg intraperitoneally) during early postnatal development (postnatal days 4 to 21) produced abnormal emotional behaviors (decreased exploratory behavior in elevated plus-maze, increased shock avoidance latency) in adulthood (12 weeks of age). The dosage used in this study was approximately equal to the pediatric maximum recommended dosage on a mg/m^2 basis. Because of the early dosing period in this study, the clinical importance of these findings for the labeled pediatric use in humans is unknown.

As with other SSRIs, decreased weight gain has been observed in association with the use of fluoxetine in children and adolescents. In one clinical trial in pediatric patients 8–17 years of age, height gain averaged about 1.1 cm less and weight gain averaged about 1 kg less after 19 weeks of fluoxetine therapy relative to placebo-treated patients. In addition, fluoxetine therapy was associated with a decrease in plasma alkaline phosphatase concentrations. Because the safety of fluoxetine in pediatric patients has not been systematically assessed for chronic therapy longer than several months in duration and studies that directly evaluate the long-term effects of fluoxetine on the growth, development, and maturation of children and adolescents are lacking, height and weight should be monitored periodically in pediatric patients receiving fluoxetine. The clinical importance of these findings on long-term growth currently is not known, but the manufacturer will conduct a phase IV study to evaluate any potential impact of fluoxetine therapy on long-term pediatric growth. For further information on adverse effects associated with the use of fluoxetine in pediatric patients, see the opening discussion in Cautions.

■ **Geriatric Precautions** The efficacy of fluoxetine has been established in clinical studies in geriatric patients. Although no overall differences in efficacy or safety were observed between geriatric and younger patients, the possibility that some older patients particularly those with systemic disease or those who are receiving other drugs concomitantly (see Pharmacokinetics: Elimination and also see Uses: Major Depressive Disorder) may exhibit increased sensitivity to the drug cannot be ruled out.

In pooled data analyses, a *reduced* risk of suicidality was observed in adults 65 years of age or older with antidepressant therapy compared with placebo. (See Cautions: Precautions and Contraindications.)

Limited evidence suggests that geriatric patients may be more likely than younger patients to develop fluoxetine-induced hyponatremia and transient syndrome of inappropriate secretion of antidiuretic hormone (SIADH). Therefore, clinicians prescribing fluoxetine in geriatric patients should be aware of the possibility that such reactions may occur. In addition, periodic monitoring (especially during the first several months) of serum sodium concentrations in geriatric patients receiving the drug has been recommended by some clinicians.

As with other psychotropic drugs, geriatric patients receiving antidepressants appear to have an increased risk of hip fracture. Despite the fewer cardiovascular and anticholinergic effects associated with SSRIs, these drugs did not show any advantage over tricyclic antidepressants with regard to hip fracture in a case-control study. In addition, there was little difference in the rates of falls between nursing home residents receiving SSRIs and those receiving tricyclic antidepressants in a retrospective study. Therefore, all geriatric individuals receiving either type of antidepressant should be considered at increased risk of falls, and appropriate measures should be taken.

■ **Mutagenicity and Carcinogenicity** Fluoxetine and norfluoxetine did not exhibit mutagenic activity in vitro in mammalian cell (e.g., mouse lymphoma, rat hepatocyte DNA repair) or microbial (the *Salmonella* microbial mutagen [Ames]) test systems, or with the in vivo sister chromatid-exchange assay in Chinese hamster bone marrow cells. No evidence of carcinogenesis was seen in rats or mice receiving oral fluoxetine dosages of about 7.5 or 9 times the maximum recommended human dosage of the drug, respectively, for 24 months.

■ **Pregnancy, Fertility, and Lactation** ***Pregnancy*** Some neonates exposed to fluoxetine and other selective serotonin-reuptake inhibitors (SSRIs) or selective serotonin- and norepinephrine-reuptake inhibitors (SNRIs) late in the third trimester of pregnancy have developed complications that have sometimes been severe and required prolonged hospitalization, respiratory support, enteral nutrition, and other forms of supportive care in special care nurseries. Such complications can arise immediately upon delivery and usually last several days or up to 2–4 weeks. Clinical findings reported to date in the neonates have included respiratory distress, cyanosis, apnea, seizures, temperature instability or fever, feeding difficulty, dehydration, excessive weight loss, vomiting, hypoglycemia, hypotonia, hypertonia, hyperreflexia, tremor, jitteriness, irritability, lethargy, reduced or lack of reaction to pain stimuli, and constant crying. These clinical features appear to be consistent with either a direct toxic effect of the SSRI or SNRI or, possibly, a drug withdrawal syndrome. It should be noted that, in some cases, the clinical picture was consistent with serotonin syndrome (see Drug Interactions: Serotonergic Drugs).

Infants exposed to SSRIs in late pregnancy may have an increased risk of persistent pulmonary hypertension of the newborn (PPHN). PPHN is a rare heart and lung condition occurring in an estimated 1–2 infants per 1000 births in the general population; it occurs when a neonate does not adapt to breathing outside the womb. Some experts have suggested that respiratory distress in neonates exposed to SSRIs may occur along a spectrum of seriousness in association with maternal use of SSRIs, with PPHN among the most serious consequences. Neonates with PPHN may require intensive care support, including mechanical ventilation; in severe cases, multiple organ damage, including brain damage, and even death may occur. Although several epidemiologic studies have suggested an increased risk of PPHN with SSRI use during pregnancy, other studies did not demonstrate a statistically significant association. Thus, the FDA states that it is currently unclear whether the use of SSRIs, including fluoxetine, during pregnancy can cause PPHN and recommends that clinicians not alter their current clinical practice of treating depression during pregnancy.

When treating a pregnant woman with fluoxetine, the clinician should carefully consider the potential risks and benefits of such therapy. Clinicians should consider that in a prospective longitudinal study of 201 women with a history of recurrent major depression who were euthymic in the context of antidepressant therapy at the beginning of pregnancy, women who discontinued their antidepressant medication (SSRIs, tricyclic antidepressants, or others) during pregnancy were found to be substantially more likely to have a relapse of depression than were women who continued to receive their antidepressant therapy while pregnant. Consideration may be given to cautiously tapering fluoxetine therapy in the third trimester prior to delivery if the drug is administered during pregnancy. (See Dosage and Administration: Treatment of Pregnant Women during the Third Trimester.)

Fluoxetine and its principal metabolite norfluoxetine have been shown to cross the placenta in animals. There are no adequate and controlled studies to date using fluoxetine in pregnant women, and the drug should be used during pregnancy only if the potential benefit justifies the potential risk to the fetus. Women should be advised to notify their clinician if they are or plan to become pregnant. FDA states that women who are pregnant or thinking about becoming pregnant should not discontinue any antidepressant, including fluoxetine, without first consulting their clinician. The decision whether or not to continue antidepressant therapy should be made only after careful consideration of the potential benefits and risks of antidepressant therapy for each individual pregnant patient. If a decision is made to discontinue treatment with fluoxetine or other SSRIs before or during pregnancy, discontinuance of therapy should be done in consultation with the clinician in accordance with the prescribing information for the antidepressant, and the patient should be closely monitored for possible relapse of depression. In addition, the prolonged elimination of the drug and its active metabolite from the body after discontinuance of therapy should be considered when a woman of childbearing potential receiving fluoxetine plans to become pregnant.

For additional information on the management of depression in women prior to conception and during pregnancy, including treatment algorithms, the FDA advises clinicians to consult the joint American Psychiatric Association and American College of Obstetricians and Gynecologists guidelines (at https://www.ncbi.nlm.nih.gov/pmc/articles/PMC3103063/pdf/nihms293836.pdf).

Results of a number of epidemiologic studies assessing the risk of fluoxetine exposure during the first trimester of pregnancy have demonstrated inconsistent results. Although more than 10 cohort studies and case-control studies failed to demonstrate an increased risk of congenital malformations with fluoxetine overall, one prospective cohort study conducted by the European Network of Teratology Information Services reported an increased risk of cardiovascular malformations in infants born to women exposed to fluoxetine during the first trimester of pregnancy compared with those born to women who were not exposed to the drug. There was no specific pattern of cardiovascular malformations observed in this trial. Overall, a causal relationship between fluoxetine exposure during early pregnancy and congenital malformations has not been established. However, the results of epidemiologic studies indicate that exposure to paroxetine during the first trimester of pregnancy may increase the risk for congenital malformations, particularly cardiovascular malformations. (See Pregnancy, under Cautions: Pregnancy, Fertility, and Lactation, in Paroxetine 28:16.04.20.) Additional epidemiologic studies are needed to more thoroughly evaluate the relative safety of fluoxetine and other SSRIs during pregnancy, including their potential teratogenic risks and possible effects on neurobehavioral development.

The effect of fluoxetine on labor and delivery is not known.

Fertility Reproduction studies in rats using fluoxetine dosages 5–9 times the maximum recommended human daily dosage have not revealed evidence of impaired fertility. However, a slight decrease in neonatal survival that probably was related to reduced maternal food consumption and suppressed weight gain was reported in the offspring. Like some other SSRIs, pretreatment with fluoxetine inhibits methoxydimethyltryptamine-induced ejaculation in rats; this effect is blocked by metergoline, a serotonin antagonist. Alterations in sexual function also have been reported in patients receiving the drug. (See Sexual Dysfunction under Cautions: Renal, Electrolyte, and Genitourinary Effects and also see Cautions: Pediatric Precautions.)

Lactation Fluoxetine and its metabolites distribute into human milk. Limited data indicate that fluoxetine and norfluoxetine concentrations are 20–30% of concurrent maternal plasma drug concentrations. Crying, sleep disturbance, vomiting, and watery stools developed in an infant who nursed from a woman receiving fluoxetine; plasma fluoxetine and norfluoxetine concentrations in the infant on the second day of feeding were 340 and 208 ng/mL, respectively. Therefore, fluoxetine should not be used in nursing women, and women should be advised to notify their physician if they plan to breast-feed. In addition, the slow elimination of fluoxetine and norfluoxetine from the body after discontinuance of the drug should be considered.

Drug Interactions

As with other drugs, the possibility that fluoxetine may interact with any concomitantly administered drug by a variety of mechanisms, including pharmacodynamic and pharmacokinetic interactions, should be considered. The potential for interactions exists not only with concomitantly administered drugs but also with drugs administered for several weeks after discontinuance of fluoxetine therapy due to the prolonged elimination of fluoxetine and its principal metabolite, norfluoxetine. (See Pharmacokinetics: Elimination.)

■ **Serotonergic Drugs** Use of selective serotonin-reuptake inhibitors (SSRIs) such as fluoxetine concurrently or in close succession with other drugs that affect serotonergic neurotransmission may result in serotonin syndrome or neuroleptic malignant syndrome (NMS)-like reactions. Symptoms of serotonin syndrome may include mental status changes (e.g., agitation, hallucinations, coma), autonomic instability (e.g., tachycardia, labile blood pressure, hyperthermia), neuromuscular aberrations (e.g., hyperreflexia, incoordination), and/or GI symptoms (e.g., nausea, vomiting, diarrhea). Although the syndrome appears to be relatively uncommon and usually mild in severity, serious and potentially life-threatening complications, including seizures, disseminated intravascular coagulation, respiratory failure, and severe hyperthermia, as well as death occasionally have been reported. In its most severe form, serotonin syndrome may resemble NMS, which is characterized by hyperthermia, muscle rigidity, autonomic instability with possible rapid fluctuation in vital signs, and mental status changes. The precise mechanism of these reactions is not fully understood; however, they appear to result from excessive serotonergic activity in the CNS, probably mediated by activation of serotonin 5-HT_{1A} receptors. The possible involvement of dopamine and 5-HT_2 receptors also has been suggested, although their roles remain unclear.

Serotonin syndrome most commonly occurs when 2 or more drugs that affect serotonergic neurotransmission are administered either concurrently or in close succession. Serotonergic agents include those that increase serotonin synthesis (e.g., the serotonin precursor tryptophan), stimulate synaptic serotonin release (e.g., some amphetamines, dexfenfluramine [no longer commercially available in the US], fenfluramine [no longer commercially available in the US]), inhibit the reuptake of serotonin after release (e.g., SSRIs, selective serotonin- and norepinephrine-reuptake inhibitors [SNRIs], tricyclic antidepressants, trazodone, dextromethorphan, meperidine, tramadol), decrease the metabolism of serotonin (e.g., monoamine oxidase [MAO] inhibitors), have direct serotonin postsynaptic receptor activity (e.g., buspirone), or nonspecifically induce increases in serotonergic neuronal activity (e.g., lithium salts). Selective agonists of serotonin (5-hydroxytryptamine; 5-HT) type 1 receptors ("triptans") and dihydroergotamine, agents with serotonergic activity used in the management of migraine headache, and St. John's wort (*Hypericum perforatum*) also have been implicated in serotonin syndrome.

The combination of SSRIs and MAO inhibitors may result in serotonin syndrome or NMS-like reactions. Such reactions have also been reported when SSRIs have been used concurrently with tryptophan, lithium, dextromethorphan, sumatriptan, dihydroergotamine, or antipsychotics or other dopamine antagonists. In rare cases, the serotonin syndrome reportedly has occurred in patients receiving the recommended dosage of a single serotonergic agent (e.g., clomipramine) or during accidental overdosage (e.g., sertraline intoxication in a child). Some other drugs that have been implicated in precipitating symptoms suggestive of serotonin syndrome or NMS-like reactions include buspirone, bromocriptine, dextropropoxyphene, linezolid, methylene blue, methylenedioxymethamphetamine (MDMA; "ecstasy"), selegiline (a selective MAO-B inhibitor), and sibutramine (an SNRI used for the management of obesity [no longer commercially available in the US]). Other drugs that have been associated with the syndrome but for which less convincing data are available include carbamazepine, fentanyl, and pentazocine.

Clinicians should be aware of the potential for serious, possibly fatal reactions associated with serotonin syndrome or NMS-like reactions in patients receiving 2 or more drugs that affect serotonergic neurotransmission, even if no such interactions with the specific drugs have been reported to date in the medical literature. Pending further accumulation of data, serotonergic drugs should be used cautiously in combination and such combinations avoided whenever clinically possible. Serotonin syndrome may be more likely to occur when initiating therapy with a serotonergic agent, increasing the dosage, or following the addition of another serotonergic drug. Some clinicians state that patients who have experienced serotonin syndrome may be at higher risk for recurrence of the syndrome upon reinitiation of serotonergic drugs. Pending further experience in such cases, some clinicians recommend that therapy with serotonergic agents be limited following recovery. In cases in which the potential benefit of the drug is thought to outweigh the risk of serotonin syndrome, lower potency agents and reduced dosages should be used, combination serotonergic therapy should be avoided, and patients should be monitored carefully for manifestations of serotonin syndrome. If signs and symptoms of serotonin syndrome or NMS develop during therapy, treatment with fluoxetine and any concurrently administered serotonergic or antidopaminergic agents, including antipsychotic agents, should be discontinued immediately and supportive and symptomatic treatment should be initiated.

Serotonin Syndrome **Manifestations.** Serotonin syndrome is characterized by mental status and behavioral changes, altered muscle tone or neuromuscular activity, autonomic instability with rapid fluctuations of vital signs, hyperthermia, and diarrhea. Some clinicians have stated that the diagnosis of serotonin syndrome can be made based on the presence of at least 3 of the following manifestations: mental status changes (e.g., confusion, hypomania), agitation, myoclonus, hyperreflexia, fever, shivering, tremor, diaphoresis, ataxia, and diarrhea in the setting of a recent addition or an increase in dosage of a serotonergic agent; the absence of other obvious causes of mental status changes and fever (e.g., infection, metabolic disorders, substance abuse or withdrawal); and no recent initiation or increase in dosage of an antipsychotic agent prior to the onset of the signs and symptoms (in order to rule out NMS). In some cases, features of the serotonin syndrome have resembled those associated with NMS, which may occur in patients receiving phenothiazines or other antipsychotic agents. (See Extrapyramidal Reactions in Cautions: Nervous System Effects, in the Phenothiazines General Statement 28:16.08.24.)

Other signs and symptoms associated with serotonin syndrome have included restlessness, irritability, insomnia, aggressive behavior, headache, drowsiness, dizziness, disorientation, loss of coordination, anxiety, euphoria, hallucinations, dilated pupils, nystagmus, paresthesias, rigidity, clonus, seizures, and coma. Nausea, vomiting, abdominal cramping, flushing, hypertension, hypotension, tachycardia, tachypnea, and hyperventilation also have occurred.

The onset of the serotonin syndrome can range from minutes after initiating therapy with a second serotonergic agent to several weeks after receiving a stable dosage. Preliminary evidence to date suggests that neither the occurrence nor the severity of serotonin syndrome is related to the dose or duration of serotonergic drug therapy.

The incidence of serotonin syndrome is unknown, but it is likely that the syndrome is underreported because it is not recognized or appears in various degrees of severity (mild, moderate, or severe). In addition, serotonin syndrome may be confused with or resemble NMS in some cases.

Treatment. Mild cases of serotonin syndrome generally respond within 12–24 hours to the immediate discontinuance of serotonergic agents and general supportive therapy. Symptoms rarely last more than 72–96 hours in the absence of complications. Supportive therapy in such cases may include hospitalization, adequate hydration, control of myoclonus and hyperreflexia with benzodiazepines such as clonazepam (and possibly propranolol), and control of fever with acetaminophen and external cooling, if necessary. Other possible causes of altered mental status and fever also should be considered and treated accordingly.

Patients with severe hyperthermia (i.e., a temperature of more than 40.5°C) are considered to have more severe cases of serotonin syndrome which are associated with more serious complications and mortality. Muscular rigidity often accompanies hyperthermia and may respond to benzodiazepine therapy. Such patients should be managed with aggressive cooling measures, including external cooling, the institution of muscular paralysis (to decrease body temperature, help prevent rhabdomyolysis and disseminated intravascular coagulation from muscular rigidity refractory to benzodiazepines, and facilitate intubation), and maintenance of a patent airway with endotracheal intubation. Seizures may be treated with benzodiazepines and, if necessary, other anticonvulsants (e.g., barbiturates). Patients who develop hypertension, cardiac arrhythmias, and other serious complications such as disseminated intravascular coagulation or rhabdomyolysis associated with serotonin syndrome should receive appropriate therapy for these conditions.

Although there is no specific therapy for serotonin syndrome, nonspecific serotonin (5-HT_1 and 5-HT_2) receptor antagonists such as cyproheptadine and methysergide and drugs with 5-HT_{1A} receptor affinity such as propranolol have been used with some success in a limited number of patients whose symptoms persisted or were unusually severe. Dantrolene, bromocriptine, and chlorpromazine (for sedation, to help reduce fever, and because of its 5-HT-receptor blocking activity) also have been used in a limited number of patients with serotonin syndrome but with inconsistent results; the possibility that chlorpromazine may lower the seizure threshold in this setting should be considered.

Monoamine Oxidase Inhibitors Potentially serious, sometimes fatal serotonin syndrome or NMS-like reactions have been reported in patients receiving serotonin-reuptake inhibitors in combination with an MAO inhibitor. Such reactions also have been reported in patients who recently have discontinued a selective serotonin-reuptake inhibitor and have been started on an MAO inhibitor.

Probably because of its extensive clinical use and the prolonged elimination half-life of both fluoxetine and norfluoxetine, fluoxetine has been the selective serotonin-reuptake inhibitor most commonly implicated in serotonin syndrome. In at least 2 cases, serotonin syndrome developed when MAO inhibitor therapy was initiated after the discontinuance of fluoxetine therapy. Shivering, diplopia, nausea, confusion, and anxiety reportedly occurred in one patient 6 days after discontinuance of fluoxetine therapy and 4 days after initiation of tranylcypromine therapy; signs and symptoms resolved without apparent sequelae within 24 hours following discontinuance of the MAO inhibitor in this patient. In another case, the initiation of tranylcypromine therapy more than 5 weeks after discontinuance of fluoxetine reportedly resulted in serotonin syndrome.

Concurrent administration of fluoxetine and MAO inhibitors is contraindicated. Because both fluoxetine and its principal metabolite have relatively long half-lives, at least 5 weeks should elapse between discontinuance of fluoxetine therapy and initiation of MAO inhibitor therapy, since administration of an MAO inhibitor prior to elapse of this time may increase the risk of serious adverse effects. Based on clinical experience with concurrent administration of tricyclic antidepressants and MAO inhibitors, at least 2 weeks should elapse following discontinuance of an MAO inhibitor prior to initiation of fluoxetine therapy.

Linezolid. Linezolid, an anti-infective agent that is a nonselective and reversible MAO inhibitor, has been associated with drug interactions resulting in serotonin syndrome, including some associated with SSRIs, and potentially may also cause NMS-like reactions. Because of the risk of serotonin syndrome, linezolid generally should *not* be used in patients receiving fluoxetine. The US Food and Drug Administration (FDA) states that certain life-threatening or urgent situations may necessitate immediate linezolid treatment in a patient receiving a serotonergic drug, including SSRIs. In such emergency situations, the availability of alternative anti-infectives should be considered and the benefits of linezolid should be weighed against the risk of serotonin syndrome. If linezolid is indicated in such emergency situations, fluoxetine must be immediately discontinued and the patient monitored for symptoms of CNS toxicity (e.g., mental changes, muscle twitching, excessive sweating, shivering/shaking, diarrhea, loss of coordination, fever) for 5 weeks or until 24 hours after the last linezolid dose, whichever comes first. Treatment with fluoxetine may be resumed 24 hours after the last linezolid dose. If nonemergency use of linezolid is being planned for a patient receiving fluoxetine, fluoxetine should be withheld for at least 5 weeks prior to initiating linezolid. Treatment with fluoxetine should not be initiated in a patient receiving linezolid; when necessary, fluoxetine may be started 24 hours after the last linezolid dose. (See Drug Interactions: Serotonergic Drugs, in Linezolid 8:12.28.24.)

Methylene Blue. There have been case reports of serotonin syndrome in patients who received methylene blue, which is a potent and selective inhibitor of MAO-A, while receiving serotonergic drugs, including SSRIs (e.g., citalopram, escitalopram, fluoxetine, fluvoxamine, paroxetine, sertraline). Therefore, methylene blue generally should *not* be used in patients receiving fluoxetine. However, the FDA states that certain emergency situations (e.g., methemoglobinemia, ifosfamide-induced encephalopathy†) may necessitate immediate use of methylene blue in a patient receiving fluoxetine.

Moclobemide. Moclobemide, a selective and reversible MAO-A inhibitor (not commercially available in the US), also has been associated with serotonin syndrome and such reactions have been fatal in several cases in which the drug was given in combination with the selective serotonin-reuptake inhibitor citalopram or with clomipramine. Pending further experience with such combinations, some clinicians recommend that concurrent therapy with moclobemide and selective serotonin-reuptake inhibitors be used only with extreme caution and serotonin-reuptake inhibitors should have been discontinued for some time (depending on the elimination half-lives of the drug and its active metabolites) before initiating moclobemide therapy.

Selegiline. Selegiline, a selective MAO-B inhibitor used in the management of parkinsonian syndrome, also has been reported to cause serotonin syndrome when given concurrently with selective serotonin-reuptake inhibitors (fluoxetine, paroxetine, sertraline). Although selegiline is a selective MAO-B inhibitor at therapeutic dosages, the drug appears to lose its selectivity for the MAO-B enzyme at higher dosages (e.g., those exceeding 10 mg/kg), thereby increasing the risk of serotonin syndrome in patients receiving higher dosages of the drug either alone or in combination with other serotonergic agents. The manufacturer of selegiline recommends avoiding concurrent selegiline and selective serotonin-reuptake inhibitor therapy. In addition, the manufacturer of selegiline recommends that a drug-free interval of at least 2 weeks elapse between discontinuance of selegiline and initiation of selective serotonin-reuptake inhibitor therapy. Because of the long half-lives of fluoxetine and its principal metabolite, at least 5 weeks should elapse or even longer (particularly if fluoxetine has been prescribed chronically and/or at higher dosages) between discontinuance of fluoxetine and initiation of selegiline therapy.

Isoniazid. Isoniazid, an antituberculosis agent, appears to have some MAO-inhibiting activity. In addition, iproniazid (not commercially available in the US), another antituberculosis agent structurally related to isoniazid that also possesses MAO-inhibiting activity, reportedly has resulted in serotonin syndrome in at least 2 patients when given in combination with meperidine. Pending further experience, clinicians should be aware of the potential for serotonin syndrome when isoniazid is given in combination with selective serotonin-reuptake inhibitor therapy or other serotonergic agents.

Tryptophan and Other Serotonin Precursors Adverse nervous system effects (e.g., agitation, restlessness, aggressive behavior, insomnia, poor concentration, headache, paresthesia, incoordination, worsening of symptoms of obsessive-compulsive disorder), adverse GI effects (e.g., nausea, abdominal cramps, diarrhea), palpitation, and/or chills reportedly have occurred in a limited number of patients receiving fluoxetine concurrently with tryptophan, a serotonin precursor. Such symptoms generally resolved within several weeks following discontinuance of tryptophan despite continued fluoxetine therapy. Although the mechanism for this interaction has not been fully elucidated, it has been suggested that these adverse effects resemble the serotonin syndrome observed in animals and therefore may result from a marked increase in serotonin availability when tryptophan and potent serotonin-reuptake inhibitors such as fluoxetine are administered concurrently. Because of the potential risk of serotonin syndrome or NMS-like reactions, concurrent use of tryptophan or other serotonin precursors should be avoided in patients receiving fluoxetine.

Sibutramine Because of the possibility of developing potentially serious, sometimes fatal serotonin syndrome or NMS-like reactions, sibutramine (no longer commercially available in the US) should be used with caution in patients receiving fluoxetine.

5-HT₁ Receptor Agonists ("Triptans") Weakness, hyperreflexia, and incoordination have been reported rarely during postmarketing surveillance in patients receiving sumatriptan concomitantly with an SSRI (e.g., fluoxetine, citalopram, escitalopram, fluvoxamine, paroxetine, sertraline). Oral or subcutaneous sumatriptan and SSRIs were used concomitantly in some clinical studies without unusual adverse effects. However, an increase in the frequency of migraine attacks and a decrease in the effectiveness of sumatriptan in relieving migraine headache have been reported in a patient receiving subcutaneous injections of sumatriptan intermittently while undergoing fluoxetine therapy.

Clinicians prescribing 5-HT_1 receptor agonists, SSRIs, and SNRIs should consider that triptans often are used intermittently and that either the 5-HT_1 receptor agonist, SSRI, or SNRI may be prescribed by a different clinician. Clinicians also should weigh the potential risk of serotonin syndrome or NMS-like reactions with the expected benefit of using a triptan concurrently with SSRI or SNRI therapy. If concomitant treatment with fluoxetine and a triptan is clinically warranted, the patient should be observed carefully, particularly during treatment initiation, dosage increases, and following the addition of other serotonergic agents. Patients receiving concomitant triptan and fluoxetine therapy should be informed of the possibility of serotonin syndrome or NMS-like reactions and advised to immediately seek medical attention if they experience symptoms of these syndromes.

Other Selective Serotonin-reuptake Inhibitors and Selective Serotonin- and Norepinephrine-reuptake Inhibitors Concomitant administration of fluoxetine with other SSRIs or SNRIs potentially may result in serotonin syndrome or NMS-like reactions and is therefore not recommended.

Antipsychotic Agents and Other Dopamine Antagonists Concomitant use of antipsychotic agents and other dopamine antagonists with fluoxetine potentially may result in serotonin syndrome or NMS-like reactions. If signs and symptoms of serotonin syndrome or NMS occur, treatment with fluoxetine and any concurrently administered antidopaminergic or serotonergic agents should be immediately discontinued and supportive and symptomatic treatment initiated. (See Drug Interactions: Antipsychotic Agents.)

Tramadol and Other Serotonergic Drugs Because of the potential risk of serotonin syndrome or NMS-like reactions, caution is advised whenever SSRIs, including fluoxetine, and SNRIs are concurrently administered with other drugs that may affect serotonergic neurotransmitter systems, including tramadol and St. John's wort (*Hypericum perforatum*).

Pentazocine, an opiate partial agonist analgesic, has been reported to cause transient symptoms of diaphoresis, ataxia, flushing, and tremor suggestive of the serotonin syndrome when used concurrently with fluoxetine.

Serotonin syndrome rarely may occur following concomitant use of fluoxetine and stimulants because stimulants can release serotonin, and amphetamine is metabolized by the cytochrome P-450 (CYP) 2D6 isoenzyme, which is inhibited by some SSRIs (e.g., fluoxetine, paroxetine).

■ **Drugs Undergoing Metabolism by Hepatic Microsomal Enzymes** ***Drugs Metabolized by Cytochrome P-450 (CYP) 2D6*** Fluoxetine, like many other antidepressants (e.g., other selective serotonin-reuptake inhibitors, many tricyclic antidepressants), is metabolized by the drug-metabolizing cytochrome P-450 (CYP) 2D6 isoenzyme (debrisoquine hydroxylase). In addition, like many other drugs metabolized by CYP2D6, fluoxetine inhibits the activity of CYP2D6 and potentially may increase plasma concentrations of concomitantly administered drugs that also are metabolized by this enzyme. Fluoxetine may make normal CYP2D6 metabolizers resemble "poor metabolizers". Although similar interactions are possible with other selective serotonin-reuptake inhibitors, there is considerable variability among the drugs in the extent to which they inhibit CYP2D6; fluoxetine and paroxetine appear to be more potent in this regard than sertraline.

Concomitant use of fluoxetine with other drugs metabolized by CYP2D6 has not been systematically studied. The extent to which this potential interaction may become clinically important depends on the extent of inhibition of CYP2D6 by the antidepressant and the therapeutic index of the concomitantly administered drug. The drugs for which this potential interaction is of greatest concern are those that are metabolized principally by CYP2D6 and have a narrow therapeutic index, such as tricyclic antidepressants, class IC antiarrhythmics (e.g., propafenone, flecainide, encainide), vinblastine, and some phenothiazines (e.g., thioridazine).

Caution should be exercised whenever concurrent therapy with fluoxetine and other drugs metabolized by CYP2D6 is considered. If fluoxetine therapy is initiated in a patient already receiving a drug metabolized by CYP2D6, the need for decreased dosage of that drug should be considered. In addition, a low initial dosage should be used whenever a drug that is predominantly metabolized by CYP2D6 and has a relatively narrow therapeutic margin (e.g., tricyclic antidepressants, class IC antiarrhythmics) is initiated in a patient who is receiving or has received fluoxetine during the previous 5 weeks. Because of the risk of serious ventricular arrhythmias and sudden death potentially associated with increased plasma concentrations of thioridazine, thioridazine is contraindicated in any patient who is receiving or has received fluoxetine during the previous 5 weeks. (See Thioridazine under Drug Interactions: Antipsychotic Agents.)

Drugs Metabolized by Cytochrome P-450 (CYP) 3A4 Although fluoxetine can inhibit the cytochrome P-450 (CYP) 3A4 isoenzyme, results of in vitro and in vivo studies indicate that the drug is a much less potent inhibitor of this enzyme than many other drugs. In one in vivo drug interaction study, concomitant administration of single doses of the CYP3A4 substrate terfenadine (no longer commercially available in the US) and fluoxetine did not increase plasma concentrations of terfenadine. In addition, in vitro studies have shown that ketoconazole, a potent inhibitor of CYP3A4 activity, is at least 100 times more potent than fluoxetine or norfluoxetine as an inhibitor of several substrates of this enzyme (e.g., astemizole [no longer commercially available in the US], cisapride, midazolam). Some clinicians state that concomitant use of fluoxetine with astemizole or terfenadine is not recommended since substantially increased plasma concentrations of unchanged astemizole or terfenadine could occur, resulting in an increased risk of serious adverse cardiac effects. However, the manufacturer of fluoxetine states that the extent of fluoxetine's inhibition of CYP3A4 activity is unlikely to be of clinical importance.

■ **Tricyclic and Other Antidepressants** Concurrent administration of fluoxetine and a tricyclic antidepressant (e.g., nortriptyline, desipramine, imipramine) reportedly has resulted in adverse effects associated with tricyclic toxicity (including sedation, decreased energy, lightheadedness, psychomotor retardation, dry mouth, constipation, memory impairment). In patients receiving imipramine or desipramine, initiation of fluoxetine therapy reportedly resulted in plasma concentrations of these tricyclic antidepressants that were at least 2–10 times higher; this effect persisted for 3 weeks or longer after fluoxetine was discontinued. Elevated plasma trazodone concentrations and adverse effects possibly associated with trazodone toxicity (e.g., sedation, unstable gait) also have been reported during concomitant fluoxetine and trazodone therapy. Although the mechanism for this possible interaction has not been established, it has been suggested that fluoxetine may inhibit the hepatic metabolism of tricyclic antidepressants. (See Drugs Metabolized by Cytochrome P-450 [CYP] 2D6 under Drug Interactions: Drugs Undergoing Metabolism by Hepatic Microsomal Enzymes.) Further study of this potential interaction is needed, but current evidence suggests that patients receiving fluoxetine and a tricyclic antidepressant or trazodone concomitantly should be closely observed for adverse effects; monitoring of plasma tricyclic or trazodone concentrations also should be considered and their dosage reduced as necessary. Because fluoxetine may increase plasma concentrations and prolong the elimination half-life of tricyclic antidepressants, the need for more prolonged monitoring following combined tricyclic and fluoxetine overdose should be considered. In addition, because of the prolonged elimination of fluoxetine and norfluoxetine, the possibility that the drug may interact with tricyclic antidepressants after recent discontinuance of fluoxetine also should be considered.

■ **Antipsychotic Agents** Concomitant use of antipsychotic agents with fluoxetine potentially may result in serotonin syndrome or NMS-like reactions. If signs and symptoms of serotonin syndrome or NMS occur, treatment with fluoxetine and any concurrently administered antipsychotic agent should be immediately discontinued and supportive and symptomatic treatment initiated. (See Drug Interactions: Serotonergic Drugs.)

Some clinical data suggest a possible pharmacodynamic and/or pharmacokinetic interaction between SSRIs, including fluoxetine, and some antipsychotic agents.

Clozapine Concomitant use of fluoxetine and clozapine can increase plasma concentrations of clozapine and enhance clozapine's pharmacologic effects secondary to suspected inhibition of clozapine metabolism by fluoxetine. Increased plasma clozapine concentrations also have been reported in patients receiving other SSRIs (e.g., fluvoxamine, paroxetine). There has been at least one fatality related to clozapine toxicity following ingestion of clozapine, fluoxetine, and alcohol. The manufacturer of clozapine states that caution should be used and patients closely monitored if clozapine is used in patients receiving SSRIs, and a reduction in clozapine dosage should be considered.

Haloperidol Elevated plasma concentrations of haloperidol have been observed in patients receiving concomitant fluoxetine therapy. Severe extrapyramidal symptoms (e.g., tongue stiffness, parkinsonian symptoms, akathisia), which required hospitalization and were refractory to conventional therapy (including anticholinergic antiparkinsonian agents, diphenhydramine, and diazepam), reportedly occurred in a patient receiving fluoxetine and haloperidol concurrently; this patient previously had experienced only mild adverse extrapyramidal effects with haloperidol therapy alone. The extrapyramidal symptoms gradually abated following discontinuance of both drugs, and the patient subsequently tolerated haloperidol therapy with evidence of only a slight parkinsonian gait. The clinical importance of this possible interaction has not been established, and additional study is required to determine the safety of combined fluoxetine and antipsychotic therapy.

Olanzapine Concomitant administration of fluoxetine (60 mg as a single dose or 60 mg daily for 8 days) with a single 5-mg dose of oral olanzapine caused a small increase in peak plasma olanzapine concentrations (averaging 16%) and a small decrease (averaging 16%) in olanzapine clearance; the elimination half-life was not substantially affected. Fluoxetine is an inhibitor of CYP2D6, and thereby may affect a minor metabolic pathway for olanzapine. Although the changes in pharmacokinetics are statistically significant when olanzapine and fluoxetine are given concurrently, the changes are unlikely to be clinically important in comparison to the overall variability observed between individuals; therefore, routine dosage adjustment is not recommended.

When fluoxetine is used in fixed combination with olanzapine, the drug interactions associated with olanzapine also should be considered. (See Drug Interactions in Olanzapine 28:16.08.04.)

Pimozide Clinical studies evaluating pimozide in combination with other antidepressants have demonstrated an increase in adverse drug interactions or QT_c prolongation during combined therapy. In addition, rare case reports have suggested possible additive cardiovascular effects of fluoxetine and pimozide, resulting in bradycardia. Marked changes in mental status (e.g., stupor, inability to think clearly) and hypersalivation also were reported in one woman who received both drugs concurrently. Although a specific study evaluating concurrent fluoxetine and pimozide therapy has not been performed to date, concurrent use of these drugs is contraindicated because of the potential for adverse drug interactions or QT_c prolongation.

Risperidone Extrapyramidal symptoms followed by persistent tardive dyskinesia (dyskinetic tongue movements) have occurred in one 18-year-old who received risperidone concomitantly with fluoxetine; however, a causal relationship has not been established. The AUC of risperidone increased during concomitant fluoxetine therapy in one study in psychotic patients, and the AUC of active drug (risperidone plus 9-hydroxyrisperidone) increased in poor and extensive metabolizers (determined by CYP2D6 genotyping); there was no evidence of increased severity or incidence of extrapyramidal symptoms in this 30-day study.

Thioridazine Although specific drug interaction studies evaluating concomitant use of fluoxetine and thioridazine are not available, concomitant use of other SSRIs (e.g., fluvoxamine) has resulted in increased plasma concentrations of the antipsychotic agent. Because of the risk of serious ventricular arrhythmia and sudden death associated with elevated plasma concentrations of thioridazine, thioridazine is contraindicated in any patient who is receiving or has received fluoxetine during the previous 5 weeks. (See Drugs Metabolized by Cytochrome P-450 [CYP] 2D6 under Drug Interactions: Drugs Undergoing Metabolism by Hepatic Microsomal Enzymes.)

■ **Benzodiazepines** Fluoxetine appears to inhibit the metabolism of diazepam, as evidenced by increases in the elimination half-life and plasma concentration of diazepam and decreases in diazepam clearance and the rate of formation of desmethyldiazepam (an active metabolite of diazepam) during concomitant use of the drugs. Although clinically important increase in psychomotor impairment has not been noted when fluoxetine and diazepam were administered concomitantly as compared with administration of diazepam alone, concomitant administration of alprazolam and fluoxetine has resulted in increased plasma concentrations of alprazolam and further psychomotor performance impairments. Pending further accumulation of data, the possibility that a clinically important interaction could occur in geriatric or other susceptible patients should be considered.

■ **Buspirone** Buspirone has serotonergic activity and may have been partially responsible for a case of serotonin syndrome that resulted in the death of a patient receiving fluoxetine, buspirone, and an MAO inhibitor (tranylcypromine) concomitantly. (See Drug Interactions: Serotonergic Drugs.)

In a patient with depression, generalized anxiety disorder, and panic attacks who was receiving concomitant buspirone and trazodone therapy, an increase in anxiety symptoms to a level comparable to that observed prior to buspirone therapy occurred when fluoxetine was added to the regimen. Although the mechanism of this possible interaction has not been established, it was suggested that fluoxetine may have either directly antagonized the therapeutic activity of buspirone or may have precipitated the anxiety symptoms through a separate mechanism. However, combined use of the drugs also has been reported to potentiate therapeutic efficacy in patients with obsessive-compulsive disorder.

■ **Lithium** Fluoxetine and lithium have been used concurrently in a limited number of patients without apparent adverse effects. However, both increased and decreased serum lithium concentrations and adverse neuromuscular effects possibly associated with lithium toxicity and/or serotonin syndrome (e.g., ataxia, dizziness, dysarthria, stiffness of the extremities) have been reported during combined therapy with the drugs. Lithium appears to have some serotonergic activity, and serotonin syndrome has been reported following the initiation of lithium therapy in at least one patient receiving fluoxetine. (See Drug Interactions: Serotonergic Drugs.) The clinical importance of this potential interaction remains to be determined and further substantiation is required; however, caution should be exercised when fluoxetine and lithium are administered concurrently. It is recommended that serum lithium concentrations be monitored closely during concomitant fluoxetine therapy.

■ **Anticonvulsants** ***Carbamazepine*** Fluoxetine can increase plasma carbamazepine and carbamazepine 10,11-epoxide (CBZ-E, an active metabolite) concentrations, and carbamazepine toxicity (e.g., ocular changes, vertigo, tremor) has been reported in some patients maintained on carbamazepine following initiation of fluoxetine. It has been suggested that fluoxetine-induced inhibition of hepatic metabolism (e.g., inhibition of epoxide hydrolase) of carbamazepine and/or CBZ-E may be principally responsible for such increases; alteration in protein binding does not appear to be principally responsible for this interaction. The patient and plasma concentrations of carbamazepine and its metabolite should be monitored closely whenever fluoxetine therapy is initiated or discontinued; carbamazepine dosage should be adjusted accordingly.

Phenytoin Initiation of fluoxetine in patients stabilized on phenytoin has resulted in increased plasma phenytoin concentrations and clinical manifestations of phenytoin toxicity.

■ **β-Adrenergic Blocking Agents** Concomitant use of fluoxetine and a β-adrenergic blocking agent has resulted in increased plasma concentrations that have enhanced the β-adrenergic blocking effects of the drug, possibly resulting in cardiac toxicity. Metoprolol is metabolized by the CYP2D6 isoenzyme and fluoxetine is known to potently inhibit this enzyme. Although specific data are lacking, β-adrenergic blocking agents that are renally eliminated (e.g., atenolol) may be a safer choice. Patients who were previously stabilized on propranolol or metoprolol should be monitored for toxicity (e.g., bradycardia, conduction defects, hypotension, heart failure, central nervous system disturbances) following initiation of fluoxetine therapy.

■ **Protein-bound Drugs** Because fluoxetine is highly protein bound, the drug theoretically could be displaced from binding sites by, or it could displace from binding sites, other protein-bound drugs such as oral anticoagulants and digitoxin (no longer commercially available in the US). Pending further accumulation of data, patients receiving fluoxetine with any highly protein-bound drug should be observed for potential adverse effects associated with such therapy. (See Drug Interactions: Drugs Affecting Hemostasis.)

■ **Drugs Affecting Hemostasis** ***Warfarin*** Concomitant use of fluoxetine and warfarin has resulted in altered anticoagulant effects, including increased bleeding. Therefore, patients receiving warfarin should be carefully monitored whenever fluoxetine is initiated or discontinued.

Other Drugs that Interfere with Hemostasis Epidemiologic case-control and cohort design studies that have demonstrated an association between selective serotonin-reuptake inhibitor therapy and an increased risk of upper GI bleeding also have shown that concurrent use of aspirin or other nonsteroidal anti-inflammatory agents substantially increases the risk of GI bleeding. Although these studies focused on upper GI bleeding, there is some evidence suggesting that bleeding at other sites may be similarly potentiated. The precise mechanism for this increased risk remains to be clearly established; however, serotonin release by platelets is known to play an important role in hemostasis, and selective serotonin-reuptake inhibitors decrease serotonin uptake from the blood by platelets, thereby decreasing the amount of serotonin in platelets. Patients receiving fluoxetine should be cautioned about the concomitant use of drugs that interfere with hemostasis, including aspirin and other nonsteroidal anti-inflammatory agents.

■ **Alcohol** Concurrent administration of single or multiple doses of fluoxetine and alcohol does not appear to alter blood or Breathalyzer® alcohol, plasma fluoxetine, or plasma norfluoxetine concentrations in healthy individuals, suggesting that there is no pharmacokinetic interaction between fluoxetine and alcohol. In addition, fluoxetine does not appear to potentiate the psychomotor and cognitive impairment or cardiovascular effects induced by alcohol. However, the drug's ability to reduce alcohol consumption in animals and humans suggests that there may be a serotonergically mediated, pharmacodynamic interaction between fluoxetine and alcohol within the CNS. (See Pharmacology: Effects on Alcohol Intake, and also see Uses: Alcohol Dependence.)

■ **Electroconvulsive Therapy** The effects of fluoxetine in conjunction with electroconvulsive therapy (ECT) for the management of depression have not been evaluated to date in clinical studies. Prolonged seizures reportedly have occurred rarely during concurrent use of fluoxetine and ETC.

■ **Antidiabetic Agents** Fluoxetine potentially may alter blood glucose concentrations in patients with diabetes mellitus. (See Cautions: Metabolic Effects.) Therefore, dosage adjustments of insulin and/or oral antidiabetic agents may be necessary when fluoxetine therapy is initiated or discontinued in such patients.

Acute Toxicity

Limited information is available on the acute toxicity of fluoxetine.

■ **Pathogenesis** The acute lethal dose of fluoxetine in humans is not known. The median oral LD_{50} of fluoxetine has been reported to be approximately 452 and 248 mg/kg in rats and mice, respectively. In animals, oral administration of single large doses of the drug has resulted in hyperirritability and seizures. Tonic-clonic seizures occurred in 5 of 6 dogs given a toxic dose of fluoxetine orally; the seizures ceased immediately after IV administration of diazepam. In these dogs, the lowest plasma fluoxetine concentration at which seizures occurred reportedly was only twice the maximum plasma concentration reported in humans receiving 80 mg of the antidepressant daily during long-term therapy. Single large oral doses of fluoxetine reportedly do not cause QT- or PR-interval prolongation or widening of the QRS complex in dogs, although tachycardia and an increase in blood pressure have occurred.

The risk of fluoxetine overdosage may be increased in patients with a genetic deficiency in the cytochrome P-450 (CYP) isoenzyme 2D6.

■ **Manifestations** In general, overdosage of fluoxetine may be expected to produce effects that are extensions of the drug's pharmacologic and adverse effects. Animal studies and case reports in humans indicate that possible effects of overdosage include agitation, restlessness, hypomania, vertigo, insomnia, tremor, and other signs of CNS excitation; nausea and vomiting; and tachycardia and/or increased blood pressure. Seizures have been reported in at least one patient after overdosage of fluoxetine. Acute overdosage of fluoxetine alone reportedly has resulted in nystagmus, drowsiness, coma, urticaria, spontaneous emesis, and ST-segment depression. Nausea and vomiting appear to occur commonly following acute ingestion of relatively large single doses of the drug.

Several fatalities following fluoxetine overdosage have been reported to date. One of the deaths occurred in a patient who reportedly ingested 1.8 g of fluoxetine and an unknown quantity of maprotiline; plasma fluoxetine and maprotiline concentrations in this patient were approximately 4570 and 4180 ng/mL, respectively. Another patient died after concomitantly ingesting fluoxetine, codeine, and temazepam; plasma fluoxetine, norfluoxetine, codeine, and temazepam concentrations in this patient reportedly were 1930, 1110, 1800, and 3800 ng/mL, respectively. A fatal overdose also has been reported in a patient ingesting fluoxetine and alcohol concomitantly. There also are a few reported cases of overdose in which fatality was attributed to fluoxetine alone. In one such case, death was associated with extracted blood fluoxetine and norfluoxetine concentrations of 6000 and 5000 ng/mL, respectively, and biliary concentrations of 13,000 ng/mL each for the drug and metabolite. A patient enrolled in a clinical study of fluoxetine reportedly died following intentional ingestion of an unknown quantity of amitriptyline, clobazam, and pentazocine; however, it is not known whether this patient also ingested fluoxetine with the other drugs.

A patient with a history of seizures who reportedly ingested 3 g of fluoxetine and an unknown quantity of aspirin experienced 2 tonic-clonic seizures, tachycardia, dizziness, blurred vision, unsustained clonus, and ECG changes. The seizures occurred about 9 hours post-ingestion, lasted approximately 2–3 minutes, and remitted spontaneously without anticonvulsant therapy. Although the actual amount of fluoxetine absorbed by this patient may have been less than expected because of vomiting and gastric lavage, the plasma fluoxetine concentration reportedly was 2461 ng/mL when seizures occurred; the patient recovered with no apparent sequelae. Another patient reported that he experienced sleepiness and nausea that lasted for several days following the intentional ingestion of 840 mg of fluoxetine with alcohol; this patient did not seek medical treatment. Drowsiness, lethargy, and nausea occurred in a patient who reportedly ingested 1.4 g of fluoxetine and 15 mg of clonazepam. No ECG abnormalities were reported in 2 patients who intentionally ingested 200 mg and 1 g of fluoxetine.

A child with a genetic deficiency in the CYP2D6 isoenzyme died following prolonged therapy with fluoxetine, methylphenidate, and clonidine. Autopsy findings revealed blood, brain, and other tissue concentrations of fluoxetine and norfluoxetine that were several-fold higher than expected. Poor metabolism of fluoxetine via CYP2D6 was the likely cause of fluoxetine intoxication in this child.

■ **Treatment** Because fatalities and severe toxicity have been reported following overdosage of selective serotonin-reuptake inhibitors, particularly in large overdosage and when taken with other drugs or alcohol, some clinicians recommend that any overdosage involving these drugs be managed aggressively. Because suicidal ingestion often involves more than one drug, clinicians treating fluoxetine overdosage should be alert to possible toxic manifestations caused by drugs other than fluoxetine.

Clinicians also should consider the possibility of serotonin syndrome or NMS-like reactions in patients presenting with similar clinical features and a recent history of fluoxetine ingestion and/or ingestion of other serotonergic and/or antipsychotic agents or other dopamine antagonists. (See Cautions: Precautions and Contraindications and also see Drug Interactions: Serotonergic Drugs.)

Management of fluoxetine overdosage generally involves symptomatic and supportive care. A patent airway should be established and maintained, and adequate oxygenation and ventilation should be assured. ECG and vital sign monitoring is recommended following acute overdosage with the drug, although the value of ECG monitoring in predicting the severity of fluoxetine-induced cardiotoxicity is not known. (See Acute Toxicity: Manifestations, in the Tricyclic Antidepressants General Statement.) There is no specific antidote for fluoxetine intoxication.

Following recent (i.e., within 4 hours) ingestion of a potentially toxic amount of fluoxetine and in the absence of signs and symptoms of cardiac toxicity, the stomach should be emptied immediately by inducing emesis or by gastric lavage. If the patient is comatose, having seizures, or lacks the gag reflex, gastric lavage may be performed if an endotracheal tube with cuff inflated is in place to prevent aspiration of gastric contents. Since administration of activated charcoal (which may be used in conjunction with sorbitol or a saline cathartic) may be as effective or more effective than induction of emesis or gastric lavage, its use has been recommended either in the initial management of fluoxetine overdosage or following induction of emesis or gastric lavage in patients who have ingested a potentially toxic quantity of the drug.

Based on data from animal studies, IV diazepam should be considered for the management of fluoxetine-induced seizures that do not remit spontaneously. If seizures are not controlled or recur following administration of diazepam, administration of phenytoin or phenobarbital has been recommended by some clinicians.

Fluoxetine and norfluoxetine are not substantially removed by hemodialysis. Because of the large volume of distribution and extensive protein binding of the drug and its principal metabolite, peritoneal dialysis, forced diuresis, hemoperfusion, and/or exchange transfusion probably are also ineffective in removing substantial amounts of fluoxetine and norfluoxetine from the body. Clinicians should consider consulting a poison control center for additional information on the management of fluoxetine overdosage.

Chronic Toxicity

Fluoxetine has not been studied systematically in animals or humans to determine whether therapy with the drug is associated with tolerance or psychologic and/or physical dependence. One patient receiving the drug for the management of obesity reportedly experienced nervousness 2 days following discontinuance of fluoxetine therapy. However, it is unclear whether this adverse effect represented a withdrawal reaction since both the parent drug and its principal metabolite have relatively long half-lives, and withdrawal reactions following discontinuance of fluoxetine therapy may therefore be more delayed. Although clinical experience to date has not revealed substantial evidence of drug-seeking behavior or a withdrawal syndrome associated with discontinuance of fluoxetine therapy, it is difficult to predict from the limited data currently available the extent to which a CNS-active drug like fluoxetine may be misused, diverted, and/or abused.

Despite the lack of substantial evidence for abuse potential or dependence liability, clinicians should carefully evaluate patients for a history of substance abuse prior to initiating fluoxetine therapy. If fluoxetine therapy is initiated in patients with a history of substance abuse, such patients should be monitored closely for signs of misuse or abuse of the drug (e.g., development of tolerance, use of increasing doses, drug-seeking behavior).

The potential for misuse of fluoxetine by depressed patients with concurrent eating disorders and/or those who may seek the drug for its appetite-suppressant effects also should be considered. One patient with an undisclosed history of anorexia nervosa and laxative abuse who was given fluoxetine for depression ingested larger-than-prescribed doses (e.g., 90–120 mg/day) and lost 9.1 kg within 2 months; this patient falsely claimed mood improvement in order to continue receiving the drug for its anorectic and weight-reducing effects.

Fluoxetine has produced phospholipidosis following long-term administration in animals; however, no evidence of phospholipidosis has been reported in humans receiving the drug to date. Additional study is needed to determine the clinical importance of these findings in patients receiving long-term fluoxetine therapy. (See Pharmacology: Effects on Phospholipids.)

Pharmacology

The pharmacology of fluoxetine is complex and in many ways resembles that of other antidepressant agents, particularly those agents (e.g., citalopram, clomipramine, escitalopram, fluvoxamine, paroxetine, sertraline, trazodone) that predominantly potentiate the pharmacologic effects of serotonin (5-HT). Like other selective serotonin-reuptake inhibitors (SSRIs), fluoxetine is a potent and highly selective reuptake inhibitor of serotonin and has little or no effect on other neurotransmitters.

■ **Nervous System Effects** The precise mechanism of antidepressant action of fluoxetine is unclear, but the drug has been shown to selectively inhibit the reuptake of serotonin at the presynaptic neuronal membrane. Fluoxetine-induced inhibition of serotonin reuptake causes increased synaptic concentrations of serotonin in the CNS, resulting in numerous functional changes associated with enhanced serotonergic neurotransmission. Like other selective serotonin-reuptake inhibitors (fluvoxamine, paroxetine, sertraline), fluoxetine appears to have minimal or no effect on the reuptake of norepinephrine or dopamine and does not exhibit clinically important anticholinergic, antihistaminic, or α_1-adrenergic blocking activity at usual therapeutic dosages.

Although the mechanism of antidepressant action of antidepressant agents may involve inhibition of the reuptake of various neurotransmitters (i.e., norepinephrine, serotonin) at the presynaptic neuronal membrane, it has been suggested that postsynaptic receptor modification is mainly responsible for the antidepressant action observed during long-term administration of antidepressant agents. During long-term therapy with most antidepressants (e.g., tricyclic antidepressants, monoamine oxidase [MAO] inhibitors), these adaptive changes generally consist of subsensitivity of the noradrenergic adenylate cyclase system in association with a decrease in the number of β-adrenergic receptors; such effects on noradrenergic receptor function commonly are referred to as "down-regulation." In addition, some antidepressants reportedly decrease the number of 5-HT binding sites following chronic administration. Fluoxetine may exert its antidepressant activity by somewhat different mechanisms than those usually associated with tricyclic and some other antidepressants. Although some evidence indicates that long-term administration of fluoxetine does not substantially decrease the number of β-adrenergic binding sites or reduce the sensitivity of β-adrenergic receptors, a decrease in the number of β-adrenergic binding sites in the brain has been reported in at least one study in animals. Data regarding the effects of fluoxetine on the number of serotonin (5-HT_1 and/or 5-HT_2) binding sites have been conflicting, with either no change or a reduction in the number of binding sites being reported during chronic administration of the drug. Increased postsynaptic receptor binding of GABA B also has been reported following prolonged administration of many antidepressants, including fluoxetine. The clinical importance of these findings for fluoxetine has not been fully elucidated to date, and further study is needed to determine the role, if any, of binding site alteration in the antidepressant action of fluoxetine and other antidepressants.

The precise mechanism of action responsible for the efficacy of fluoxetine in the treatment of obsessive-compulsive disorder is unclear. However, based on the efficacy of other selective serotonin-reuptake inhibitors (e.g., fluvoxamine, paroxetine, sertraline) and clomipramine in the treatment of obsessive-compulsive disorder and the potency of these drugs in inhibiting serotonin reuptake, a serotonergic hypothesis has been developed to explain the pathogenesis of the condition. The hypothesis postulates that a dysregulation of serotonin is responsible for obsessive-compulsive disorder and that fluoxetine and these other agents are effective because they correct this imbalance. Although the available evidence supports the serotonergic hypothesis of obsessive-compulsive disorder, additional studies are necessary to confirm this hypothesis.

Serotonergic Effects Fluoxetine is a highly selective inhibitor of serotonin reuptake at the presynaptic neuronal membrane. In addition, the potency and selectivity of serotonin-reuptake inhibition exhibited by fluoxetine's principal metabolite, norfluoxetine, appear to be similar to those of the parent drug. Fluoxetine- and norfluoxetine-induced inhibition of serotonin reuptake causes increased synaptic concentrations of serotonin, resulting in numerous functional changes associated with enhanced serotonergic neurotransmission.

Data from in vitro studies suggest that fluoxetine is approximately equivalent to or less potent than clomipramine as a serotonin-reuptake inhibitor; however, in vivo studies indicate that the serotonin-reuptake inhibiting effect of fluoxetine may be more potent than that of clomipramine on a weight as well as an equimolar basis. This apparent discrepancy may be explained at least in part by the relatively long elimination half-lives of fluoxetine and norfluoxetine. In addition, metabolism via *N*-demethylation decreases the potency and specificity of serotonin-reuptake inhibition of clomipramine but not fluoxetine. Data from both in vivo and in vitro studies indicate that fluoxetine also is a more potent serotonin-reuptake inhibitor than other currently available antidepressant agents, including imipramine and trazodone. Fluoxetine appears to have practically no affinity for serotonin (e.g., 5-HT_1 and 5-HT_2) receptors in vitro, although limited in vivo data suggest that the drug may bind to low-affinity sites on 5-HT receptors.

Fluoxetine appears to decrease the turnover of serotonin in the CNS, probably as a result of a decrease in the rate of serotonin synthesis. The drug reportedly decreases brain concentrations of 5-hydroxyindoleacetic acid (5-HIAA), the principal metabolite of serotonin; reduces the uptake of radiolabeled tryptophan by synaptosomes; and reduces the rate of conversion of tryptophan to serotonin. Fluoxetine also inhibits spontaneous firing of serotonergic neurons in the dorsal raphe nucleus.

Like other serotonin-reuptake inhibitors, administration of fluoxetine alone does not produce the serotonin behavioral syndrome (a characteristic behavioral pattern caused by central stimulation of serotonin activity) in animals. However, the drug potentiates the serotonin behavioral syndrome induced by oxitriptan (l-5-hydroxytryptophan, l-5HTP), MAO inhibitors, and MAO inhibitors combined with tryptophan.

Effects on Other Neurotransmitters Like other selective serotonin-reuptake inhibitors, fluoxetine appears to have little or no effect on the reuptake of other neurotransmitters such as norepinephrine or dopamine. In addition, the drug appears to have a substantially higher selectivity ratio of serotonin-to-norepinephrine reuptake inhibiting activity than tricyclic antidepressant agents, including clomipramine.

Unlike tricyclic and some other antidepressants, fluoxetine does not exhibit clinically important anticholinergic, α_1-adrenergic blocking, or antihistaminic activity at usual therapeutic dosages. As a result, the incidence of adverse effects commonly associated with blockade of muscarinic cholinergic receptors (e.g., dry mouth, blurred vision, urinary retention, constipation, confusion), α_1-adrenergic receptors (e.g., orthostatic hypotension), and histamine H_1- and H_2-receptors (e.g., sedation) is lower in fluoxetine-treated patients. In vitro studies have demonstrated that the drug possesses only weak affinity for α_1- and α_2-adrenergic, β-adrenergic, H_1 and H_2, muscarinic, opiate, GABA-benzodiazepine, and dopamine receptors.

Effects on Sleep Like tricyclic and most other antidepressants, fluoxetine suppresses rapid eye movement (REM) sleep. Although not clearly established, there is some evidence that the REM-suppressing effects of antidepressant agents may contribute to the antidepressant activity of these drugs. In animal studies, fluoxetine produces a dose-related suppression of REM sleep; the drug generally appears to reduce the amount of REM sleep by increasing REM latency (the time to onset of REM sleep) and by decreasing the number rather than the duration of REM episodes. Limited data in animals suggest that REM rebound does not occur following discontinuance of fluoxetine. The precise mechanism has not been fully elucidated, but results of animal studies indicate that fluoxetine's effects on REM sleep are serotonergically mediated. Like other specific serotonin-reuptake inhibitors (e.g., zimeldine [previously zimelidine]), the effects of fluoxetine on non-REM sleep reported to date have been variable and do not appear to be as clearly defined as those of tricyclic antidepressants, which usually increase slow-wave sleep.

Effects on EEG Limited data currently are available regarding the effects of fluoxetine on the EEG. Substantial EEG changes did not occur following oral administration of single 30-mg doses of the drug in healthy individuals. An increase in alpha activity and a decrease in fast beta activity and slow activity were noted following single oral 60-mg doses in this study; such changes are characteristic of desipramine-type antidepressants and appear to indicate increased vigilance. Single 75-mg doses of fluoxetine produced an increase in slow and fast activity and a decrease in alpha activity; such EEG changes are similar to those observed with amitriptyline and imipramine and suggest possible sedative activity.

Effects on Psychomotor Function Fluoxetine does not appear to cause clinically important sedation and does not interfere with psychomotor performance. Controlled studies in healthy young adults 21–45 of years and in adults with major depression did not demonstrate any adverse effects on psychomotor performance in those receiving the drug. No adverse effects on psychomotor performance or cognitive function were observed in men with depression older than 60 years of age who received 20-mg doses of fluoxetine in a controlled study. Results of this study showed that overall cognition, as assessed by the critical flicker fusion thresholds test, generally was better in patients receiving fluoxetine than in those receiving amitriptyline (a tricyclic antidepressant); however, less sedating tricyclic antidepressants (e.g., desipramine) were not included in the study and it is possible that fluoxetine may not have such an advantage over these other agents. In a controlled study evaluating the effects of fluoxetine (20 mg daily for 22 days) on psychomotor performance and car driving in healthy adults, the drug did not affect the highway driving or the car following tests but slightly impaired performance in correctly detecting changes in visual signals was evident in the sustained attention test.

Analgesic Effects Like other serotonin-reuptake inhibitors (e.g., zimeldine), fluoxetine exhibits analgesic activity in some analgesic test systems when administered alone in animals, but the lack of such effects observed in other test systems suggests that demonstration of analgesic activity may be test-dependent. Fluoxetine has potentiated opiate agonist-induced analgesia in most but not all studies, possibly as a result of the drug's ability to enhance serotonergic neurotransmission. The clinical importance of these effects in the management of acute and chronic pain remains to be determined.

Effects on Respiration Usual therapeutic dosages of fluoxetine do not appear to affect respiration substantially in humans; however, the effect of higher dosages of the drug on respiratory function remains to be established. In animals, administration of single 20-mg/kg doses of fluoxetine reportedly increased blood Po_2 concentrations but did not alter blood Pco_2 concentrations. The drug also has been shown to attenuate morphine-induced respiratory depression, although the precise mechanism for this effect has not been established.

Effects on Thermoregulation Data are conflicting regarding the effect of fluoxetine on thermoregulation. In animals, fluoxetine has produced dose-dependent hypothermia in some studies, suggesting that serotonin may play a role in thermoregulation, but the drug has produced only slight or minimal hypothermia in other studies.

The drug has been used safely in at least one patient with established susceptibility to malignant hyperthermia; however, additional experience with the drug is needed to confirm the safety of fluoxetine in patients known to be susceptible to this condition.

■ **Cardiovascular Effects** The cardiovascular effects of fluoxetine have been studied in animals and to a limited extent in humans. Unlike some other antidepressant agents (e.g., tricyclic antidepressants, MAO inhibitors), fluoxetine has been associated with only minimal cardiovascular effects. The absence of substantial anticholinergic activity, α_1-adrenergic blocking activity, catecholamine-potentiating effects, and quinidine-like cardiotoxic effects appears to be the principal reason for the general lack of cardiovascular effects associated with fluoxetine.

Fluoxetine does not exhibit clinically important α_1-adrenergic blocking activity and does not inhibit catecholamine reuptake. Unlike tricyclic antidepressants, fluoxetine does not block the neuronal reuptake of norepinephrine and therefore does not potentiate the pressor response associated with administration of norepinephrine. In addition, the drug does not inhibit the reuptake of and has no effect on the pressor response to tyramine.

Fluoxetine does not appear to have substantial arrhythmogenic activity; however, safety of the drug in patients with a recent history of myocardial infarction or unstable cardiovascular disease has not been adequately evaluated to date. Fluoxetine generally does not appear to affect cardiac conduction, and clinically important ECG changes have not been reported in patients without preexisting heart disease receiving therapeutic dosages of the drug. Unlike tricyclic antidepressants, which commonly cause an increase in heart rate, fluoxetine reportedly reduces heart rate by an average of about 3 beats/minute in patients receiving usual therapeutic dosages of the antidepressant. (See Cautions: Cardiovascular Effects.) Unlike tricyclics, the drug does not appear to exhibit direct quinidine-like cardiotoxic activity, although the cardiovascular effects associated with fluoxetine overdosage have not been fully established to date. (See Acute Toxicity.)

■ **Effects on Appetite and Body Weight** Like some other serotonergic agents (e.g., fenfluramine [no longer commercially available in the US], zimeldine), fluoxetine possesses anorectic activity. Although the precise mechanism has not been clearly established, results of animal studies indicate that the drug's appetite-inhibiting action may result from serotonin-reuptake blockade and the resultant increase in serotonin availability at the neuronal synapse. Following administration of single and multiple doses of fluoxetine in both meal-fed and free-feeding animals, a reduction in food intake usually occurs, particularly at relatively high doses of the drug (i.e., 10 mg/kg). The anorectic effect of fluoxetine appears to be potentiated by oxitriptan. Tolerance to the anorectic effect of fluoxetine has not developed following short-term administration in humans and animals; however, long-term studies in humans are necessary to fully determine whether tolerance develops during chronic therapy with the drug.

In animal studies, fluoxetine has been shown to suppress palatability-induced food consumption (as determined by the volume of sweetened versus plain water ingested). Like fenfluramine, fluoxetine also appears to selectively suppress carbohydrate and overall food intake while maintaining protein intake. Such carbohydrate intake-suppressing and protein-sparing effects may be of potential clinical importance in the management of obesity; however, additional study is necessary. (See Uses: Obesity.) Fluoxetine therapy also has resulted in decreases in body weight in normal-weight and obese animals as well as in depressed, nondepressed, and obese individuals receiving the drug. (See Uses: Obesity and also see Cautions: Metabolic Effects.)

■ **Effects on Alcohol Intake** Like some other serotonergic agents, fluoxetine produces a dose-dependent decrease in voluntary alcohol intake in normal and alcohol-preferring animals. Like some other serotonin-reuptake inhibitors (e.g., citalopram, zimeldine), fluoxetine has been shown to reduce alcohol consumption in a limited number of heavy drinkers receiving 60 mg of the drug daily. Because serotonin appears to be involved in the regulation of alcohol intake, it has been suggested that fluoxetine may attenuate alcohol consumption via enhanced serotonergic neurotransmission. In addition, there is some evidence that such effects may be at least partially mediated by the renin-angiotensin-aldosterone system. (See Uses: Alcohol Dependence and see Drug Interactions: Alcohol.)

■ **Neuroendocrine Effects** Fluoxetine affects the endocrine system. Like other selective inhibitors of serotonin reuptake, the drug has produced a dose-related increase in serum corticosterone concentrations in animals. Fluoxetine also reportedly potentiates oxitriptan-induced elevation in serum corticosterone concentrations. Such effects appear to be serotonergically mediated. Following parenteral administration of fluoxetine in animals, the elevation in serum corticosterone concentration generally lasts only a few hours, although fluoxetine-induced inhibition of serotonin reuptake is known to persist for longer than 24 hours. Therefore, it has been suggested that other compensatory mechanisms, possibly including decreased firing of serotonergic neurons, may contribute to the restoration of normal hypothalamic-pituitary-adrenal (HPA) axis function despite prolonged blockade of serotonin reuptake by the drug. Fluoxetine also has increased corticotropin (ACTH) and vasopressin (antidiuretic hormone, ADH) concentrations in peripheral plasma and has increased corticotropin and corticotropin-releasing factor (CRF, corticoliberin) concentrations in hypophysial portal blood. These effects may represent the initial step in fluoxetine-induced elevation of plasma corticosterone concentrations.

The effects of fluoxetine on serum prolactin concentrations have not been clearly established. In some animal studies, fluoxetine potentiated tryptophan-induced increases in serum prolactin concentrations, although administration of the drug alone in animals and humans usually does not substantially alter prolactin concentrations. However, administration of fluoxetine alone reportedly increased serum prolactin concentrations in young but not old male rats in one study. Fluoxetine-induced effects on prolactin secretion appear to be serotonergically mediated.

■ **Effects on Phospholipids** Like many other cationic, amphiphilic drugs (e.g., amiodarone, fenfluramine, imipramine, ranitidine), fluoxetine reportedly increases tissue phospholipid concentrations following chronic administration in animal studies; however, such effects have not been demonstrated in humans receiving fluoxetine to date. Histologic examination following long-term (i.e., 1–12 months) fluoxetine administration in animals has revealed the presence of characteristic concentric, lamellar inclusion bodies associated with phospholipidosis in alveolar macrophages of the lung, Kupffer cells of the liver, and adrenal cortical cells; an increase in phospholipid content of the lung also has been reported. Fluoxetine-induced phospholipid accumulation in these animals was reversible within 1–2 months following discontinuance of the drug.

Studies in humans receiving fluoxetine have not revealed biochemical or clinical evidence of drug-induced phospholipidosis to date. There was no evidence of increased phospholipid content or changes in lamellar inclusion bodies in peripheral blood lymphocytes of either healthy individuals receiving 1 month of fluoxetine therapy or depressed patients receiving long-term (0.9–2.6 years) therapy with the drug. In addition, ophthalmologic examination and chest radiographs in patients receiving fluoxetine during clinical studies have not revealed evidence of phospholipidosis induced by the drug. Although data from clinical studies suggest that fluoxetine-induced phospholipidosis is unlikely to occur in humans receiving long-term therapy with the drug, further study is needed to fully determine whether the phospholipidosis observed in animal studies is clinically important in humans receiving therapeutic dosages of the drug.

■ **Other Effects** Fluoxetine has demonstrated some antimyoclonic activity in animals and humans when used in combination with oxitriptan. Although the mechanism of fluoxetine's antimyoclonic activity has not been fully elucidated, some forms of myoclonus appear to be related to impaired serotonergic neurotransmission. Therefore, it has been suggested that fluoxetine-induced enhancement of serotonergic neurotransmission via serotonin-reuptake blockade potentially may contribute to oxitriptan-induced increases in CNS serotonin concentrations in the management of this condition. (See Uses: Myoclonus.)

Fluoxetine also has reduced cataplexy in both humans and animals. (See Uses: Cataplexy.)

Fluoxetine reportedly has produced a dose-related elevation in plasma β-endorphin and β-lipotropin concentrations in healthy individuals receiving single oral doses of the drug.

Pharmacokinetics

In all human studies described in the Pharmacokinetics section, fluoxetine was administered as the hydrochloride salt.

■ **Absorption** Fluoxetine hydrochloride appears to be well absorbed from the GI tract following oral administration. The oral bioavailability of fluoxetine in humans has not been fully elucidated to date, but at least 60–80% of an oral dose appears to be absorbed. However, the relative proportion of an oral dose reaching systemic circulation unchanged currently is not known. The conventional and delayed-release capsules, tablets, and solution of fluoxetine hydrochloride reportedly are bioequivalent. However, onset of absorption of fluoxetine hydrochloride delayed-release capsules (Prozac® Weekly®) is delayed 1–2 hours relative to the onset of absorption when the drug is administered as a conventional preparation. Limited data from animals suggest that the drug may undergo first-pass metabolism and extraction in the liver and/or lung following oral administration. In these animals (beagles), approximately 72% of an oral dose reached systemic circulation unchanged. Food appears to cause a slight decrease in the rate, but not the extent, of absorption of fluoxetine in humans.

Peak plasma fluoxetine concentrations usually occur within 4–8 hours (range: 1.5–12 hours) after oral administration of conventional preparations. Following oral administration of a single 40-mg dose of the drug in healthy fasting adults, peak plasma concentrations of approximately 15–55 ng/mL are attained. Peak plasma fluoxetine concentrations following administration of single oral doses of 20–80 mg are approximately proportional and are linearly related to dose, although there appears to be considerable interindividual variation in plasma concentrations attained with a given dose. The manufacturer states that the peak plasma concentrations achieved following weekly administration of fluoxetine 90-mg delayed-release capsules are in the range of the average concentrations achieved following daily administration of 20-mg conventional preparations; however, average trough concentrations are reported to be lower following weekly administration of the delayed-release preparation. Peak-to-trough fluctuations in plasma concentrations of fluoxetine and norfluoxetine (the principal metabolite) reportedly are greater following weekly administration of the delayed-release capsules (164 and 43%, respectively) compared with daily administration of conventional preparations (24 and 17%, respectively).

Preliminary data suggest that fluoxetine may exhibit nonlinear accumulation following multiple dosing. (See Pharmacokinetics: Elimination.) The relatively slow elimination of fluoxetine and its active metabolite, norfluoxetine, leads to clinically important accumulation of these active species in chronic use and delayed attainment of steady state, even when a fixed dose is used. In healthy adults receiving 40 mg of fluoxetine daily for 30 days, plasma concentrations of 91–302 and 72–258 ng/mL of fluoxetine and norfluoxetine, respectively, were attained. These plasma concentrations of fluoxetine were higher than those predicted by single-dose studies because fluoxetine's metabolism is not proportional to dose. In addition, prolonged administration of the drug and/or patient's disease states did not appear to affect steady-state concentrations. In one study, steady-state plasma fluoxetine and norfluoxetine concentrations did not differ substantially among healthy individuals receiving 4 weeks of fluoxetine therapy, depressed patients receiving 5 weeks of fluoxetine therapy, or depressed patients receiving more than a year of fluoxetine therapy.

Average steady-state fluoxetine and norfluoxetine concentrations, however, were affected by patient age. In pediatric patients with major depressive disorder or obsessive-compulsive disorder (OCD) who received fluoxetine 20 mg daily for up to 62 days, average steady-state concentrations of fluoxetine and norfluoxetine in children 6–12 years of age were 2- and 1.5-fold higher, respectively, than in adolescents 13–17 years of age who received the same fluoxetine regimen. These results are consistent with those observed in another study in 94 pediatric patients 8–17 years of age diagnosed with major depressive disorder, and can be almost entirely explained by differences in children's weight. Higher average steady-state fluoxetine and norfluoxetine concentrations also were observed in children relative to adults; however, these concentrations were within the range of concentrations observed in the adult population. As in adults, fluoxetine and norfluoxetine accumulated extensively following multiple oral dosing. Following daily oral administration of the drug, steady-state plasma fluoxetine and norfluoxetine concentrations generally are achieved within about 2–4 weeks.

The manufacturer states that average steady-state plasma fluoxetine concentrations are approximately 50% lower with weekly administration of the 90-mg delayed-release capsules compared with daily administration of a 20-mg conventional preparation. In patients being switched from daily therapy with fluoxetine 20-mg conventional preparations to weekly therapy with fluoxetine 90-mg delayed-release capsules, peak plasma fluoxetine concentrations reportedly were 1.7 times higher with the weekly regimen than with the established daily regimen when there was no transition period (i.e., therapy with delayed-release fluoxetine was initiated the day after the last daily dose of fluoxetine 20 mg). When weekly therapy was initiated one week after the last daily dose of fluoxetine 20 mg, peak plasma fluoxetine concentrations for the 2 regimens were similar. (See Dosage and Administration: Dosage.)

The onset of antidepressant activity following oral administration of fluoxetine hydrochloride usually occurs within the first 1–3 weeks of therapy, but optimum therapeutic effect usually requires 4 weeks or more of therapy with the drug. Maximal EEG changes and behavioral changes on psychometric tests reportedly occur about 8–10 hours after single oral doses of the drug; the delay in maximal CNS effects compared with achievement of peak plasma fluoxetine concentrations may relate to formation of an active metabolite or to delayed distribution of the parent drug and its principal metabolite into the CNS.

The relationship between plasma fluoxetine and norfluoxetine concentrations and the therapeutic and/or toxic effects of the drug has not been clearly established. In a group of patients receiving fluoxetine for the management of major depressive disorder, there was no correlation between plasma fluoxetine, norfluoxetine, or total fluoxetine plus norfluoxetine concentrations and either the antidepressant response or the weight-reducing effect of the drug.

■ **Distribution** Distribution of fluoxetine and its metabolites into human body tissues and fluids has not been fully characterized. Limited pharmacokinetic data obtained during long-term administration of fluoxetine to animals suggest that the drug and some of its metabolites, including norfluoxetine, are widely distributed in body tissues, with highest concentrations occurring in the lungs and liver. The drug crosses the blood-brain barrier in humans and animals. In animals, fluoxetine:norfluoxetine ratios reportedly were similar in the cerebral cortex, corpus striatum, hippocampus, hypothalamus, brain stem, and cerebellum 1 hour after administration of a single dose of the drug.

The apparent volumes of distribution of fluoxetine and norfluoxetine in healthy adults each reportedly average 20–45 L/kg. Limited data suggest that the volume of distribution of fluoxetine is not altered substantially following multiple dosing. The apparent volume of distribution of norfluoxetine reportedly is higher in patients with cirrhosis than in healthy individuals, although this difference may reflect decreases in the rates of formation and elimination of the metabolite rather than changes in volume of distribution. The volumes of distribution of fluoxetine and norfluoxetine do not appear to be altered substantially in patients with renal impairment.

At in vitro plasma concentrations of 200–1000 ng/mL, fluoxetine is approximately 94.5% bound to plasma proteins, including albumin and α_1-acid glycoprotein (α_1-AGP); the extent of protein binding appears to be independent of plasma concentration. The extent of fluoxetine protein binding does not appear to be altered substantially in patients with hepatic cirrhosis or renal impairment, including those undergoing hemodialysis.

It is not known whether fluoxetine or its metabolites cross the placenta in humans, but fluoxetine and norfluoxetine reportedly cross the placenta in rats following oral administration. Fluoxetine and norfluoxetine are distributed into milk. Limited data indicate that concentrations of the drug and this metabolite in milk are about 20–30% of concurrent plasma concentrations.

■ **Elimination** Fluoxetine and norfluoxetine, the principal metabolite, are eliminated slowly. Following a single oral dose of fluoxetine in healthy adults, the elimination half-life of fluoxetine reportedly averages approximately 2–3 days (range: 1–9 days) and that of norfluoxetine averages about 7–9 days (range: 3–15 days). The plasma half-life of fluoxetine exhibits considerable interindividual variation, which may be related to genetic differences in the rate of *N*-demethylation of the drug in the liver. The absence of either a bimodal or trimodal distribution of clearance values suggests that the rate of such metabolism may be under polygenic control. The half-life of fluoxetine reportedly is prolonged (to approximately 4–5 days) after administration of multiple versus single doses, suggesting a nonlinear pattern of drug accumulation during long-term administration. Norfluoxetine appears to exhibit dose-proportional pharmacokinetics following multiple dosing, although limited data indicate that the rate of formation of the metabolite is decreased slightly once steady-state plasma concentrations have been achieved.

Following oral administration of single doses of fluoxetine in healthy individuals, total apparent plasma clearances of fluoxetine and norfluoxetine average approximately 346 mL/minute (range: 94–703 mL/minute) and 145 mL/minute (range: 61–284 mL/minute), respectively. Limited data suggest that plasma clearance of fluoxetine decreases by approximately 75% following multiple oral doses of the drug once steady-state plasma fluoxetine concentrations have been achieved. Plasma clearances of fluoxetine and norfluoxetine also reportedly are decreased in patients with chronic liver disease (e.g., cirrhosis). Evidence from single-dose studies indicates that clearances of the drug and its principal metabolite are not altered substantially in patients with renal impairment.

The exact metabolic fate of fluoxetine has not been fully elucidated. The drug appears to be metabolized extensively, probably in the liver, to norfluoxetine and several other metabolites. Norfluoxetine (desmethylfluoxetine), the principal metabolite, is formed by *N*-demethylation of fluoxetine, which may be under polygenic control. The potency and selectivity of norfluoxetine's serotonin-reuptake inhibiting activity appear to be similar to those of the parent drug. Both fluoxetine and norfluoxetine undergo conjugation with glucuronic acid in the liver, and limited evidence from animals suggests that both the parent drug and its principal metabolite also undergo *O*-dealkylation to form *p*-trifluoromethylphenol, which subsequently appears to be metabolized to hippuric acid.

Following oral administration, fluoxetine and its metabolites are excreted principally in urine. In healthy individuals, approximately 60% of an orally administered, radiolabeled dose of fluoxetine is excreted in urine within 35 days, with approximately 72.8% of excreted drug as unidentified metabolites, 10% as norfluoxetine, 9.5% as norfluoxetine glucuronide, 5.2% as fluoxetine glucuronide, and 2.5% as unchanged drug. Approximately 12% of the dose was eliminated in feces within 28 days following oral administration, but the relative proportion of unabsorbed versus absorbed drug that is excreted in feces (e.g., via biliary elimination) is not known.

The effect of age on the elimination of fluoxetine has not been fully elucidated. Single-dose studies suggest that the pharmacokinetics of fluoxetine in healthy geriatric individuals do not differ substantially from those in younger adults. However, because the drug has a relatively long half-life and nonlinear disposition following multiple-dose administration, single-dose studies are not sufficient to exclude the possibility of altered pharmacokinetics in geriatric individuals, particularly those with systemic disease and/or in those receiving multiple medications concomitantly. The elimination half-lives of fluoxetine and norfluoxetine may be prolonged in patients with hepatic impairment. Following a single oral dose of the drug in patients with hepatic cirrhosis, the elimination half-lives of fluoxetine and norfluoxetine reportedly average approximately 7 and 12 days, respectively.

The elimination half-lives of fluoxetine and norfluoxetine do not appear to be altered substantially in patients with renal impairment following oral administration of single doses of fluoxetine. In addition, chronic fluoxetine administration in depressed patients on hemodialysis produced steady-state plasma fluoxetine and norfluoxetine concentrations that were comparable with those observed in patients with normal renal function.

Fluoxetine and norfluoxetine are not removed substantially by hemodialysis. Because of the large volume of distribution and extensive protein binding of the drug and its principal metabolite, peritoneal dialysis, forced diuresis, hemoperfusion, and/or exchange transfusion also are likely to be ineffective in removing substantial amounts of fluoxetine and norfluoxetine from the body.

Chemistry and Stability

■ **Chemistry** Fluoxetine, a selective serotonin-reuptake inhibitor (SSRI) antidepressant, is a phenylpropylamine-derivative. The drug differs structurally from other selective serotonin-reuptake inhibitor antidepressants (e.g., citalopram, paroxetine, sertraline) and also differs structurally and pharmacologically from other currently available antidepressant agents (e.g., tricyclic antidepressants, monoamine oxidase inhibitors).

Fluoxetine contains a *p*-trifluoromethyl substituent that appears to contribute to the drug's high selectivity and potency for inhibiting serotonin reuptake, possibly as a result of its electron-withdrawing effect and lipophilicity. The commercially available drug is a racemic mixture of 2 optical isomers. Limited in vivo and in vitro data suggest that the pharmacologic activities of the optical isomers do not differ substantially, although the dextrorotatory isomer appears to have slightly greater serotonin-reuptake inhibiting activity and a longer duration of action than the levorotatory isomer.

Fluoxetine is commercially available as the hydrochloride salt, which occurs as a white to off-white crystalline solid and has a solubility of 14 mg/mL in water.

■ **Stability** Fluoxetine hydrochloride conventional and delayed-release capsules should be stored at 15–30°C and protected from light. Fluoxetine hydrochloride tablets and oral solution should be stored at 20–25°C and protected from light.

Preparations

Excipients in commercially available drug preparations may have clinically important effects in some individuals; consult specific product labeling for details.

FLUoxetine Hydrochloride

Oral		
Capsules	10 mg (of fluoxetine)*	**FLUoxetine Hydrochloride Capsules**
		PROzac® Pulvules®, Dista
		Sarafem® Pulvules®, Lilly
	20 mg (of fluoxetine)*	**FLUoxetine Hydrochloride Capsules**
		PROzac® Pulvules®, Dista
		Sarafem® Pulvules®, Lilly
	40 mg (of fluoxetine)*	**FLUoxetine Hydrochloride Capsules**
		PROzac® Pulvules®, Dista
Capsules, delayed-release (containing enteric-coated pellets)	90 mg (of fluoxetine)	**PROzac® Weekly**, Dista
Solution	20 mg (of fluoxetine) per 5 mL*	**FLUoxetine Hydrochloride Oral Solution**

Tablets	10 mg (of fluoxetine)*	**FLUoxetine Hydrochloride Tablets**
		Sarafem®, Warner Chilcott
	15 mg (of fluoxetine)*	**Sarafem®**, Warner Chilcott
	20 mg (of fluoxetine)*	**FLUoxetine Hydrochloride Tablets**
		Sarafem®, Warner Chilcott
	60 mg (of fluoxetine)*	**FLUoxetine Hydrochloride Tablets**

*available from one or more manufacturer, distributor, and/or repackager by generic (nonproprietary) name

FLUoxetine Hydrochloride Combinations

Oral		
Capsules	25 mg (of fluoxetine) with Olanzapine 3 mg*	**Symbyax®**, Lilly
	25 mg (of fluoxetine) with Olanzapine 6 mg*	**Symbyax®**, Lilly
	25 mg (of fluoxetine) with Olanzapine 12 mg*	**Symbyax®**, Lilly
	50 mg (of fluoxetine) with Olanzapine 6 mg*	**Symbyax®**, Lilly
	50 mg (of fluoxetine) with Olanzapine 12 mg*	**Symbyax®**, Lilly

*available from one or more manufacturer, distributor, and/or repackager by generic (nonproprietary) name

†Use is not currently included in the labeling approved by the US Food and Drug Administration

PARoxetine

■ Paroxetine hydrochloride and paroxetine mesylate, selective serotonin-reuptake inhibitors (SSRIs), are antidepressant agents.

Uses

Paroxetine is commercially available in the US as paroxetine hydrochloride (e.g., Paxil®, Paxil CR®) and as paroxetine mesylate (i.e., Pexeva®). The US Food and Drug Administration (FDA) considers paroxetine mesylate (Pexeva®) conventional tablets to be a pharmaceutical *alternative* (as described in section 505[b][2] of the Federal Food, Drug, and Cosmetic Act) and not a pharmaceutical (generic) equivalent to paroxetine hydrochloride conventional tablets (e.g., Paxil®), since both contain the same active moiety (paroxetine) but have different salts. The clinical studies that established efficacy of paroxetine in various conditions have been conducted with paroxetine hydrochloride. Because paroxetine hydrochloride and paroxetine mesylate contain the same active moiety (paroxetine), clinical efficacy is expected to be similar between the 2 different salts.

Paroxetine hydrochloride conventional tablets and oral suspension are used in the treatment of major depressive disorder, obsessive-compulsive disorder, panic disorder with or without agoraphobia, social phobia (social anxiety disorder), generalized anxiety disorder, and posttraumatic stress disorder. Paroxetine hydrochloride extended-release tablets are used in the treatment of major depressive disorder, panic disorder with or without agoraphobia, social phobia, and premenstrual dysphoric disorder (PMDD). Paroxetine mesylate conventional tablets are used in the treatment of major depressive disorder, obsessive-compulsive disorder, and panic disorder with or without agoraphobia. In addition, paroxetine has been used in the treatment of premature ejaculation†, diabetic neuropathy†, chronic headache†, and depression associated with bipolar disorder†.

■ **Major Depressive Disorder** Paroxetine is used in the treatment of major depressive disorder. A major depressive episode implies a prominent and relatively persistent depressed or dysphoric mood that usually interferes with daily functioning (nearly every day for at least 2 weeks). According to DSM-IV criteria, a major depressive episode includes at least 5 of the following 9 symptoms (with at least one of the symptoms being either depressed mood or loss of interest or pleasure): depressed mood most of the day as indicated by subjective report (e.g., feels sad or empty) or observation made by others; markedly diminished interest or pleasure in all, or almost all, activities most of the day; significant weight loss (when not dieting) or weight gain (e.g., a change of more than 5% of body weight in a month), or decrease or increase in appetite; insomnia or hypersomnia; psychomotor agitation or retardation (observable by others, not merely subjective feelings of restlessness or being slowed down); fatigue or loss of energy; feelings of worthlessness or excessive or inappropriate guilt (not merely self-reproach or guilt about being sick); diminished ability to think or concentrate or indecisiveness (either by subjective account or as observed by others); and recurrent thoughts of death, recurrent suicidal ideation without a specific plan, or a suicide attempt or specific plan for committing suicide.

Treatment of major depressive disorder generally consists of an acute phase (to induce remission), a continuation phase (to preserve remission), and a maintenance phase (to prevent recurrence). Various interventions (e.g., psychotherapy, antidepressant drug therapy, electroconvulsive therapy [ECT]) are used alone or in combination to treat major depressive episodes. Treatment should be individualized and the most appropriate strategy for a particular patient is determined by clinical factors such as severity of depression (e.g., mild, moderate, severe), presence or absence of certain psychiatric features (e.g., suicide risk, catatonia, psychotic or atypical features, alcohol or substance abuse or dependence, panic or other anxiety disorder, cognitive dysfunction, dysthymia, personality disorder, seasonal affective disorder), and concurrent illness (e.g., asthma, cardiac disease, dementia, seizure disorder, glaucoma, hypertension). Demographic and psychosocial factors as well as patient preference also are used to determine the most effective treatment strategy.

While use of psychotherapy alone may be considered as an initial treatment strategy for patients with mild to moderate major depressive disorder (based on patient preference and presence of clinical features such as psychosocial stressors), combined use of antidepressant drug therapy and psychotherapy may be useful for initial treatment of patients with moderate to severe major depressive disorder with psychosocial issues, interpersonal problems, or a comorbid axis II disorder. In addition, combined use of antidepressant drug therapy and psychotherapy may be beneficial in patients who have a history of poor compliance or only partial response to adequate trials of either antidepressant drug therapy or psychotherapy alone.

Antidepressant drug therapy can be used alone for initial treatment of patients with mild major depressive disorder (if preferred by the patient) and usually is indicated alone or in combination with psychotherapy for initial treatment of patients with moderate to severe major depressive disorder (unless ECT is planned). ECT is not generally used for initial treatment of uncomplicated major depression, but is recommended as first-line treatment for severe major depressive disorder when it is coupled with psychotic features, catatonic stupor, severe suicidality, food refusal leading to nutritional compromise, or other situations when a rapid antidepressant response is required. ECT also is recommended for patients who have previously shown a positive response or a preference for this treatment modality and can be considered for patients with moderate or severe depression who have not responded to or cannot receive antidepressant drug therapy. In certain situations involving depressed patients unresponsive to adequate trials of several individual antidepressant agents, adjunctive therapy with another agent (e.g., buspirone, lithium) or concomitant use of a second antidepressant agent (e.g., bupropion) has been used; however, such combination therapy is associated with an increased risk of adverse reactions, may require dosage adjustments, and (if not contraindicated) should be undertaken only after careful consideration of the relative risks and benefits. (See Drug Interactions: Serotonergic Drugs, see Drug Interactions: Tricyclic and Other Antidepressants, and see Drug Interactions: Lithium.)

The efficacy of paroxetine for the management of major depression has been established by placebo-controlled studies of 6 weeks' duration in adult outpatients from 18–73 years of age who met DSM-III criteria for major depressive disorder. In these studies, paroxetine hydrochloride was found to be more effective than placebo in improving scores by at least 2 on the Hamilton Depression Rating Scale (HDRS) and the Clinical Global Impression and Severity of Illness Scale. Paroxetine hydrochloride also was more effective than placebo in improving HDRS subfactor scores, including the depressed mood item, sleep disturbance factor, and the anxiety factor.

The efficacy of paroxetine hydrochloride extended-release tablets for the management of depression has been established in 2 flexible-dosage, controlled studies of 12-weeks' duration in adults 18–88 years of age who met DSM-IV criteria for major depressive disorder. In these studies, paroxetine was more effective than placebo in improving scores on the HDRS, the Hamilton depressed mood item, and the Clinical Global Impression-Severity of Illness Scale.

In a study of depressed outpatients who had responded by the end of an initial 8-week open treatment phase to paroxetine (mean dosage: approximately 30 mg daily; HDRS total score of less than 8) and were randomized to continue paroxetine or receive placebo for 1 year, the relapse rate in the paroxetine-treated patients (15%) was substantially lower than that in those who received placebo (39%). An analysis of these data for possible gender-related effects on treatment outcome did not suggest any difference in efficacy based on the gender of the patient. In controlled studies of depressed patients who had responded to a 6-week course of paroxetine or imipramine and were randomized to receive either the same antidepressant or placebo for up to 1 year, both paroxetine and imipramine were more effective than placebo in maintaining euthymia; however, paroxetine was better tolerated than imipramine during long-term therapy. While the optimum duration of paroxetine therapy has not been established, many experts state that acute depressive episodes require several months or longer of sustained antidepressant therapy. In addition, some clinicians recommend that long-term antidepressant therapy be considered in certain patients at risk for recurrence of depressive episodes (such as those with highly recurrent unipolar depression). In placebo-controlled studies, paroxetine has been shown to be effective for the long-term (e.g., up to 1 year) management of depression. In addition, the drug has been used in some patients for longer periods (e.g., up to 4 years) without apparent loss of clinical effect or increased toxicity. However, when paroxetine is used for extended periods, the need for continued therapy should be reassessed periodically. (See Dosage and Administration: Dosage.)

The efficacy of paroxetine as an antidepressant in hospital settings has not been studied adequately to date; however, the drug has been shown to be effective in hospitalized patients with severe depression in at least one controlled study.

As with other antidepressants, the possibility that paroxetine may precipitate hypomanic or manic attacks in patients with bipolar or other major affective disorder should be considered. Paroxetine is *not* approved for use in treating bipolar depression.

Considerations in Choosing Antidepressants A variety of antidepressant drugs are available for the treatment of major depressive disorder, including selective serotonin-reuptake inhibitors (SSRIs; e.g., citalopram, escitalopram, fluoxetine, paroxetine, sertraline), selective serotonin- and norepinephrine-reuptake inhibitors (SNRIs; e.g., desvenlafaxine, duloxetine, venlafaxine), tricyclic antidepressants (e.g., amitriptyline, amoxapine, desipramine, doxepin, imipramine, nortriptyline, protriptyline, trimipramine), monoamine oxidase (MAO) inhibitors (e.g., phenelzine, tranylcypromine), and other antidepressants (e.g., bupropion, maprotiline, nefazodone, trazodone, vilazodone). Most clinical studies have shown that the antidepressant effect of usual dosages of paroxetine in patients with depression is greater than that of placebo and comparable to that of usual dosages of tricyclic antidepressants (e.g., amitriptyline, imipramine, doxepin), other SSRIs (e.g., fluoxetine, fluvoxamine, sertraline), and other antidepressants (e.g., nefazodone). The onset of antidepressant action of paroxetine appears to be comparable to that of tricyclic antidepressants and other SSRIs, although there is some evidence that the onset of action may occur slightly earlier with paroxetine than with imipramine and fluoxetine.

In general, response rates in patients with major depression are similar for currently available antidepressants, and the choice of antidepressant agent for a given patient depends principally on other factors such as potential adverse effects, safety or tolerability of these adverse effects in the individual patient, psychiatric and medical history, patient or family history of response to specific therapies, patient preference, quantity and quality of available clinical data, cost, and relative acute overdose safety. No single antidepressant can be recommended as optimal for all patients because of substantial heterogeneity in individual responses and in the nature, likelihood, and severity of adverse effects. In addition, patients vary in the degree to which certain adverse effects and other inconveniences of drug therapy (e.g., cost, dietary restrictions) affect their preferences.

In the large-scale Sequenced Treatment Alternatives to Relieve Depression (STAR*D) effectiveness trial, patients with major depressive disorder who did not respond to or could not tolerate therapy with one SSRI (citalopram) were randomized to switch to extended-release ("sustained-release") bupropion, sertraline, or extended-release venlafaxine as a second step of treatment (level 2). Remission rates as assessed by the 17-item Hamilton Rating Scale for Depression (HRSD-17) and the Quick Inventory of Depressive Symptomatology—Self Report (QIDS-SR-16) were approximately 21 and 26% for extended-release bupropion, 18 and 27% for sertraline, and 25 and 25% for extended-release venlafaxine therapy, respectively; response rates as assessed by the QIDS-SR-16 were 26, 27, and 28% for extended-release bupropion, sertraline, and extended-release venlafaxine therapy, respectively. These results suggest that after unsuccessful initial treatment of depressed patients with an SSRI, approximately 25% of patients will achieve remission after therapy is switched to another antidepressant and that either another SSRI (e.g., sertraline) or an agent from another class (e.g., bupropion, venlafaxine) may be reasonable alternative antidepressants in patients not responding to initial SSRI therapy.

Patient Tolerance Considerations. Because of differences in the adverse effect profile between SSRIs and tricyclic antidepressants, particularly less frequent anticholinergic effects, cardiovascular effects, and/or weight gain with SSRIs, these drugs may be preferred in patients in whom such effects are not tolerated or are of potential concern. The decreased incidence of anticholinergic effects associated with paroxetine and other SSRIs compared with tricyclic antidepressants is a potential advantage, since such effects may result in discontinuance of the drug early during therapy in unusually sensitive patients. In addition, some anticholinergic effects may become troublesome during long-term tricyclic antidepressant therapy (e.g., persistent dry mouth may result in tooth decay). Although SSRIs share the same overall tolerability profile, certain patients may tolerate one drug in this class better than another. Antidepressants other than SSRIs may be preferred in patients in whom certain adverse GI effects (e.g., nausea, anorexia), nervous system effects (e.g., anxiety, nervousness, insomnia), and/or weight loss are not tolerated or are of concern, since such effects appear to occur more frequently with paroxetine and other drugs in this class.

Pediatric Considerations. The clinical presentation of depression in children and adolescents can differ from that in adults and generally varies with the age and developmental stages of the child. Younger children may exhibit behavioral problems such as social withdrawal, aggressive behavior, apathy, sleep disruption, and weight loss; adolescents may present with somatic complaints, self esteem problems, rebelliousness, poor performance in school, or a pattern of engaging in risky or aggressive behavior.

Data from controlled clinical studies evaluating various antidepressant agents in children and adolescents are less extensive than with adults, and many of these studies have methodologic limitations (e.g., nonrandomized or uncontrolled, small sample size, short duration, nonspecific inclusion criteria). However, there is some evidence that the response to antidepressants in pediatric patients may differ from that seen in adults, and caution should be used in extrapolating data from adult studies when making treatment decisions for pediatric patients. Results of several studies evaluating tricyclic antidepressants (e.g., amitriptyline, desipramine, imipramine, nortriptyline) in preadolescent and adolescent patients with major depression indicate a lack of overall efficacy in this age group. Based on the lack of efficacy data regarding use of tricyclic antidepressants and MAO inhibitors in pediatric patients and because of the potential for life-threatening adverse effects associated with the use of these drugs, many experts consider selective serotonin-reuptake inhibitors the drugs of choice when antidepressant therapy is indicated for the treatment of major depressive disorder in children and adolescents. However, the US Food and Drug Administration (FDA) states that, while efficacy of fluoxetine has been established in pediatric patients, efficacy of other newer antidepressants (i.e., paroxetine, citalopram, desvenlafaxine, duloxetine, escitalopram, fluvoxamine, mirtazapine, nefazodone, sertraline, venlafaxine) was not conclusively established in clinical trials in pediatric patients with major depressive disorder. In addition, FDA warns that antidepressants increase the risk of suicidal thinking and behavior (suicidality) in children and adolescents with major depressive disorder and other psychiatric disorders. (See Cautions: Pediatric Precautions.) FDA currently states that anyone considering using an antidepressant in a child or adolescent for any clinical use must balance the potential risk of therapy with the clinical need. (See Cautions: Precautions and Contraindications.)

Geriatric Considerations. The response to antidepressants in depressed geriatric patients without dementia is similar to that reported in younger adults, but depression in geriatric patients often is not recognized and is not treated. In geriatric patients with major depressive disorder, SSRIs appear to be as effective as tricyclic antidepressants but may cause fewer overall adverse effects than these other agents. Geriatric patients appear to be especially sensitive to anticholinergic (e.g., dry mouth, constipation, vision disturbance), cardiovascular, orthostatic hypotensive, and sedative effects of tricyclic antidepressants. The low incidence of anticholinergic effects associated with paroxetine and other SSRIs compared with tricyclic antidepressants is a potential advantage in geriatric patients, since such effects (e.g., constipation, dry mouth, confusion, memory impairment) may be particularly troublesome in these patients. However, SSRI therapy may be associated with other troublesome adverse effects (e.g., nausea and vomiting, agitation and akathisia, parkinsonian adverse effects, sexual dysfunction, weight loss, and hyponatremia). Some clinicians state that SSRIs including paroxetine may be preferred for treating depression in geriatric patients in whom the orthostatic hypotension associated with many antidepressants (e.g., tricyclics) potentially may result in injuries (such as severe falls). However, despite the fewer cardiovascular and anticholinergic effects associated with SSRIs, these drugs did not show any advantage over tricyclic antidepressants with regard to hip fracture in a case-control study. In addition, there was little difference in the rates of falls between nursing home residents receiving SSRIs and those receiving tricyclic antidepressants in a retrospective study. Therefore, all geriatric individuals receiving either type of antidepressant should be considered at increased risk of falls and appropriate measures should be taken. In addition, clinicians prescribing SSRIs in geriatric patients should be aware of the many possible drug interactions associated with these drugs, including those involving metabolism of the drugs through the cytochrome P-450 system. (See Drug Interactions.)

Patients with dementia of the Alzheimer's type (Alzheimer's disease, presenile or senile dementia) often present with depressive symptoms, such as depressed mood, appetite loss, insomnia, fatigue, irritability, and agitation. Most experts recommend that patients with dementia of the Alzheimer's type who present with clinically important and persistent depressive symptoms be considered as candidates for pharmacotherapy even if they fail to meet the criteria for a major depressive syndrome. The goals of such therapy are to improve mood, functional status (e.g., cognition), and quality of life. Treatment of depression also may reduce other neuropsychiatric symptoms associated with depression in patients with dementia, including aggression, anxiety, apathy, and psychosis. Although patients may present with depressed mood alone, the possibility of more extensive depressive symptomatology should be considered. Therefore, patients should be evaluated and monitored carefully for indices of major depression, suicidal ideation, and neurovegetative signs since safety measures (e.g., hospitalization for suicidal ideation) and more vigorous and aggressive therapy (e.g., relatively high dosages, multiple drug trials) may be needed in some patients.

Although placebo-controlled trials of antidepressants in depressed patients with concurrent dementia have shown mixed results, the available evidence and experience with the use of antidepressants in patients with dementia of the Alzheimer's type and associated depressive manifestations indicate that depressive symptoms (including depressed mood alone and with neurovegetative changes) in such patients are responsive to antidepressant therapy. In some patients, cognitive deficits may partially or fully resolve during antidepressant therapy, but the extent of response will be limited to the degree of cognitive impairment that is directly related to depression. SSRIs such as citalopram, escitalopram, fluoxetine, paroxetine, or sertraline are generally considered as first-line agents in the treatment of depressed patients with dementia since they usually are better tolerated than some other antidepressants (e.g., tricyclic antidepressants, monoamine oxidase inhibitors). Some possible alternative agents to SSRIs include bupropion, mirtazapine, and venlafaxine. Some geriatric patients with dementia and depression may be unable to tolerate the antidepressant dosages needed to achieve full remission. When a rapid antidepressant response is not critical, some experts therefore recommend a very gradual dosage increase to increase the likelihood that a therapeutic dosage of the SSRI or other antidepressant will be reached and tolerated. In a controlled study comparing paroxetine and imipramine in patients with coexisting depression and dementia, both drugs were found to be effective; however, paroxetine was better tolerated (fewer anticholinergic and serious adverse effects).

Cardiovascular Considerations. The relatively low incidence of adverse cardiovascular effects, including orthostatic hypotension and conduction disturbances, associated with paroxetine and most other SSRIs may be advantageous in patients in whom the cardiovascular effects associated with tricyclic antidepressants may be hazardous. In a controlled trial comparing paroxetine and nortriptyline in patients with stable ischemic disease, both antidepressants were found to be effective in treating depression and neither drug substantially affected blood pressure or conduction intervals; however, paroxetine did not produce sustained effects on heart rate or rhythm or heart rate variability whereas nortriptyline increased heart rate and reduced heart rate variability. Most clinical studies of paroxetine for the management of depression did not include individuals with cardiovascular disease (e.g., those with a recent history of myocardial infarction or unstable cardiovascular disease), and further experience in such patients is necessary to confirm the relative lack of cardiotoxicity reported with the drug to date. (See Cautions: Cardiovascular Effects and see Cautions: Precautions and Contraindications.)

Sedative Considerations. Because paroxetine and other SSRIs generally are less sedating than some other antidepressants (e.g., tricyclics), some clinicians state that these drugs may be preferable in patients who do not require the sedative effects associated with many antidepressant agents or in patients who are prone to accidents; however, an antidepressant with more prominent sedative effects (e.g., trazodone) may be preferable in certain patients (e.g., those with insomnia).

Suicidal Risk Considerations. Suicide is a known risk of depression and certain other psychiatric disorders, and these disorders themselves are the strongest predictors of suicide. However, there has been a long-standing concern that antidepressants may have a role in inducing worsening of depression and the emergence of suicidal thinking and behavior (suicidality) in certain patients during the early phases of treatment. FDA states that antidepressants increased the risk of suicidality in short-term studies in children, adolescents, and young adults (18–24 years of age) with major depressive disorder and other psychiatric disorders. (See Cautions: Pediatric Precautions.) An increased suicidality risk was not demonstrated with antidepressants compared with placebo in adults older than 24 years of age and a reduced risk was observed in adults 65 years of age or older. It is currently unknown whether the suicidality risk extends to longer-term antidepressant use (i.e., beyond several months); however, there is substantial evidence from placebo-controlled maintenance trials in adults with major depressive disorder that antidepressants can delay the recurrence of depression. Because the risk of suicidality in depressed patients may persist until substantial remission of depression occurs, appropriate monitoring and close observation of patients of all ages who are receiving antidepressant therapy are recommended. (See Suicidality under Cautions: Nervous System Effects, and see Cautions: Precautions and Contraindications.)

Other Considerations. Paroxetine has been effective in patients with moderate to severe depression, endogenous depression, reactive depression (including traumatic grief), depression associated with human immunodeficiency virus (HIV) infection, and depression associated with anxiety and/or agitation.

■ Obsessive-Compulsive Disorder

Paroxetine is used in the treatment of obsessive-compulsive disorder when obsessions or compulsions cause marked distress, are time-consuming (take longer than 1 hour daily), or interfere substantially with the patient's normal routine, occupational or academic functioning, or usual social activities or relationships. Obsessions are recurrent and persistent thoughts, impulses, or images that, at some time during the disturbance, are experienced as intrusive and inappropriate (i.e., "ego dystonic") and that cause marked anxiety or distress but that are not simply excessive worries about real-life problems. Compulsions are repetitive behaviors (e.g., hand washing, ordering, checking) or mental acts (e.g., praying, counting, repeating words silently) performed in response to an obsession or according to rules that must be applied rigidly (e.g., in a stereotyped fashion). Although the behaviors or acts are aimed at preventing or reducing distress or preventing some dreaded event or situation, they either are not connected in a realistic manner with what they are designed to neutralize or prevent or are clearly excessive. At some time during the course of the disturbance, the patient, if an adult, recognizes that the obsessions or compulsions are excessive or unreasonable; children may not make such recognition.

The efficacy of paroxetine hydrochloride for the management of obsessive-compulsive disorder in adults has been established by 2 multicenter, placebo-controlled studies of 12 weeks' duration. In these clinical studies, paroxetine was more effective than placebo in reducing the severity of obsessive-compulsive manifestations in adult outpatients with moderate to severe obsessive-compulsive disorder (Yale-Brown Obsessive-Compulsive Scale [YBOCS] baseline values of 23–26). In a fixed-dose study of 12 weeks' duration involving paroxetine dosages of 20, 40, or 60 mg daily, patients receiving 40 or 60 mg of the drug daily experienced substantially greater reductions in the YBOCS total score (approximately 6 and 7 points, respectively) than those receiving paroxetine 20 mg daily (approximately 4 points) or placebo (approximately 3 points). The effective dosage of paroxetine was 40 or 60 mg daily. In a 12-week study with flexible dosing of paroxetine (20–60 mg daily) or clomipramine (25–250 mg daily) compared with placebo, paroxetine-treated patients exhibited a mean reduction of approximately 7 points on the YBOCS total score, which was substantially greater than the mean reduction of approximately 4 points in patients receiving placebo. No age- or gender-related differences in outcome were noted in either of these studies.

The efficacy of paroxetine for long-term use (i.e., longer than 12 weeks) has been demonstrated in a 6-month relapse prevention trial, which was an extension of the fixed-dose study of 12 weeks' duration in patients who had responded to paroxetine. Patients who received paroxetine relapsed substantially less frequently than those receiving placebo in a double-blind placebo-controlled study. The manufacturers and many experts state that obsessive-compulsive disorder is chronic and requires several months or longer of sustained therapy. Therefore, it is reasonable to continue therapy in responding patients. If paroxetine is used for extended periods, dosage should be adjusted so that patients are maintained on the lowest effective dosage, and the need for continued therapy with the drug should be reassessed periodically.

Results from comparative studies to date suggest that paroxetine and other SSRIs (e.g., fluoxetine, fluvoxamine, sertraline) are as effective as or somewhat less effective than clomipramine in the management of obsessive-compulsive disorder. In a pooled analysis of separate short-term (10–13 weeks) studies comparing clomipramine, fluoxetine, fluvoxamine, or sertraline with placebo, clomipramine was calculated as being more effective (as determined by measures on the YBOC scale) than SSRIs, although all drugs were superior to placebo. Like clomipramine, SSRIs reduce but do not completely eliminate obsessions and compulsions.

Many clinicians consider an SSRI (e.g., paroxetine, fluoxetine, fluvoxamine, sertraline) or clomipramine to be the drugs of choice for the pharmacologic treatment of obsessive-compulsive disorder. The decision whether to initiate therapy with an SSRI or clomipramine often is made based on the adverse effect profile of these drugs. For example, some clinicians prefer clomipramine in patients who may not tolerate the adverse effect profile of SSRIs (nausea, headache, overstimulation, sleep disturbances) while SSRIs may be useful alternatives in patients unable to tolerate the adverse effects (anticholinergic effects, cardiovascular effects, sedation) associated with clomipramine therapy. Consideration of individual patient characteristics (age, concurrent medical conditions), pharmacokinetics of the drug, potential drug interactions, and cost of therapy may also influence clinicians when selecting between SSRIs and clomipramine as first-line therapy in patients with obsessive-compulsive disorder.

Pediatric Considerations In children† with obsessive-compulsive disorder, cognitive behavioral therapy and/or serotonin-reuptake inhibitors (such as clomipramine and SSRIs) may be beneficial. Controlled studies evaluating paroxetine in this setting currently are lacking and it remains to be established whether one serotonin-reuptake inhibitor is more effective than another. Pending further data, some experts state that the choice of an agent may depend on their adverse effect profile, potential for adverse drug interactions, and the presence of comorbid conditions. Although clomipramine has been more extensively studied to date than SSRIs, it has the most prominent anticholinergic effects, requires electrocardiographic (ECG) monitoring, and is the most toxic following acute overdosage. SSRIs do not require ECG monitoring; however, they are associated with headache, nausea, insomnia, and agitation. If a decision is made to initiate SSRI therapy in a child with obsessive-compulsive disorder, some experts recommend starting with a low initial dosage and then gradually increasing the dosage as tolerated. If there is no clinical response after 10–12 weeks, consideration should be given to switching to another SSRI or clomipramine. (See Cautions: Pediatric Precautions.)

Although combined clomipramine and SSRI therapy has been effective in a limited number of children and adolescents with obsessive-compulsive disorder, very close monitoring of the ECG, blood clomipramine concentrations, and vital signs is necessary because of the risks of potentially dangerous drug interactions (including serotonin syndrome) and adverse effects with such combinations. (See Drug Interactions: Serotonergic Drugs.) As in adults, the optimal duration of pharmacologic therapy in children with obsessive-compulsive disorder remains unclear. Although periodic trials of gradual withdrawal from drug therapy are advisable, some children appear to require long-term maintenance therapy to prevent relapse.

■ Panic Disorder

Paroxetine is used in the treatment of panic disorder with or without agoraphobia. Panic disorder is characterized by the occurrence of unexpected panic attacks and associated concern about having additional attacks, worry about the implications or consequences of the attacks, and/or a clinically important change in behavior related to the attacks.

According to DSM-IV, panic disorder is characterized by recurrent unexpected panic attacks, which consist of a discrete period of intense fear or discomfort in which 4 (or more) of the following symptoms develop abruptly and reach a peak within 10 minutes: palpitations, pounding heart, or accelerated heart rate; sweating; trembling or shaking; sensations of shortness of breath or smothering; feeling of choking; chest pain or discomfort; nausea or abdominal distress; feeling dizzy, unsteady, lightheaded, or faint; derealization (feelings of unreality) or depersonalization (being detached from oneself); fear of losing control; fear of dying; paresthesias (numbness or tingling sensations); and chills or hot flushes.

The efficacy of paroxetine hydrochloride for the management of panic disorder with or without agoraphobia has been established by multicenter, double-blind, placebo-controlled studies in adult outpatients who met DSM-IIIR criteria for panic disorder with or without agoraphobia. In a fixed-dose study of 10 weeks' duration in which paroxetine was given in dosages of 10, 20, and 40 mg daily, a substantially greater reduction in panic attack frequency from placebo was noted only in the patients receiving paroxetine 40 mg daily; at the end of the study, 76% of patients receiving paroxetine 40 mg daily were free of panic attacks compared with 44% of those receiving placebo. In 2 studies of 12 weeks' duration employing a flexible dosing schedule, greater improvement was reported in patients receiving paroxetine 10–60 mg daily than in those receiving placebo. In one study, 51% of the paroxetine recipients compared with 32% of the placebo recipients were free of panic attacks at the end of the study, and in the other study which was conducted in patients receiving standardized cognitive behavioral therapy, 33% of patients receiving paroxetine 10–60 mg daily had a reduction in panic attack frequency to 0 or 1 panic attacks during the study period compared with 14% of those receiving placebo. The mean paroxetine dosage for those completing these 2 flexible-dose studies was approximately 40 mg daily.

In these studies, paroxetine was found to be substantially more effective than placebo in the treatment of panic disorder in at least 2 out of 3 measures of panic attack frequency and on the Clinical Global Impression Severity of Illness Scale. The results of the studies conducted to date demonstrate that paroxetine reduces global anxiety, depressive symptoms, phobic avoidance, and improves overall impairment associated with panic disorder.

The efficacy of paroxetine hydrochloride extended-release tablets for the management of panic disorder with or without agoraphobia has been established in multicenter, placebo-controlled, flexible-dosage studies in patients with panic disorder with or without agoraphobia. In 2 studies, paroxetine extended-release tablets were more effective than placebo, but a third study failed to show any benefit compared with placebo.

The efficacy of paroxetine for long-term use (i.e., longer than 12 weeks) has been demonstrated in controlled studies. In a 3-month relapse prevention trial which was an extension of the 10-week, fixed-dose study, patients who were responders to paroxetine were randomized to receive either paroxetine (10, 20, or 40 mg daily) or placebo. The patients receiving long-term therapy with paroxetine relapsed substantially less frequently than those receiving placebo. In another controlled study, patients receiving paroxetine therapy for 1 year demonstrated not only long-term efficacy but also continued improvement. The manufacturers and some clinicians state that panic disorder is a chronic condition; therefore, it is reasonable to continue therapy in responding patients. Dosage adjustment may be necessary to maintain the patient on the lowest effective dosage, and patients should be reassessed periodically to determine the need for continued therapy.

Subgroup analysis in controlled studies for possible age- or gender-related effects on treatment outcome did not suggest any difference in efficacy based on either the age or sex of the patient.

The results of controlled studies suggest that paroxetine is as effective as and better tolerated than clomipramine in the treatment of panic disorder. In addition, paroxetine was found to have a more rapid onset of action than clomipramine in reducing the number of panic attacks in one study.

Unlike imipramine which reduces heart rate variability in patients with panic disorder (a condition associated with decreased heart rate variability and consequently an increased risk of serious cardiovascular problems including sudden cardiac death), paroxetine has been shown to normalize heart rate variability in a limited number of patients with panic disorder. The clinical importance of these findings with regard to potentially decreasing cardiovascular mortality in patients with panic disorder remains to be determined.

Panic disorder can be treated with cognitive and behavioral psychotherapy and/or pharmacologic therapy. There are several classes of drugs that appear to be effective in the pharmacologic management of panic disorder, including tricyclic antidepressants (e.g., imipramine, clomipramine), monoamine oxidase (MAO) inhibitors (e.g., phenelzine), selective serotonin-reuptake inhibitors (SSRIs; e.g., citalopram, fluoxetine, sertraline, paroxetine), and benzodiazepines (e.g., alprazolam, clonazepam). When choosing among the available drugs, clinicians should consider their acceptance and tolerability by patients; their ability to reduce or eliminate panic attacks, reduce clinically important anxiety and disability secondary to phobic avoidance, and ameliorate other common comorbid conditions (such as depression); and their ability to prevent relapse during long-term therapy. Because of their better tolerability when compared with other agents (such as the tricyclic antidepressants and benzodiazepines), the lack of physical dependence problems commonly associated with benzodiazepines, and efficacy in panic disorder with comorbid conditions (e.g., depression, other anxiety disorders such as obsessive-compulsive disorder, alcoholism), many clinicians prefer SSRIs as first-line therapy in the management of panic disorder. If SSRI therapy is ineffective or is not tolerated, use of a tricyclic antidepressant or a benzodiazepine is recommended.

■ **Social Phobia** Paroxetine hydrochloride is used in the treatment of social phobia (social anxiety disorder). According to DSM-IV, social phobia is characterized by a marked and persistent fear of one or more social or performance situations in which the person is exposed to unfamiliar people or to possible scrutiny by others. Exposure to the feared situation almost invariably provokes anxiety, which may approach the intensity of a panic attack. The feared situations are avoided or endured with intense anxiety or distress. The avoidance, fear, or anxious anticipation of encountering the social or performance situation interferes significantly with the person's daily routine, occupational or academic functioning, or social activities or relationships, or there is marked distress about having the phobias. Lesser degrees of performance anxiety or shyness generally do not require psychotherapy or pharmacologic treatment.

The efficacy of paroxetine hydrochloride in the treatment of social phobia has been established in 3 multicenter, placebo-controlled studies in adult outpatients who met DSM-IV criteria for social phobia. In 2 studies of 12 weeks' duration in which paroxetine was given in dosages ranging from 20–50 mg daily, significant improvement in the Clinical Global Impressions (CGI) Improvement score and Liebowitz Social Anxiety Scale (LSAS) were noted. In these studies, 69 or 77% of paroxetine-treated patients were CGI Improvement responders compared with 29 or 42% of placebo-treated patients. In the third study, paroxetine was given in fixed dosages of 20, 40, or 60 mg daily for 12 weeks. There was significant improvement in the CGI Improvement responder criterion and LSAS Total Score in patients receiving 20 mg daily compared with placebo. Although there were trends in superiority noted in those receiving 40 or 60 mg daily compared with placebo, the results did not reach statistical significance and there was no indication that dosages exceeding 20 mg daily provide any additional benefit.

Subgroup analysis of these controlled studies in adult outpatients with social anxiety disorder did not reveal any evidence of age- or gender-related differences in treatment outcome. Safety and efficacy of paroxetine for the treatment of social phobia in children or adolescents have not been established to date.

■ **Anxiety Disorders** Paroxetine hydrochloride is used in the management of generalized anxiety disorder. According to DSM-IV-TR, generalized anxiety disorder is characterized by excessive anxiety and worry (apprehensive expectation), occurring more days than not for at least 6 months, about a number of events or activities (e.g., work or school performance). Patients with generalized anxiety disorder find it difficult to control the worry. The anxiety and worry are accompanied by at least 3 of the following somatic symptoms in adults and at least 1 of these symptoms in children: restlessness or feeling keyed up or on edge, being easily fatigued, difficulty concentrating or mind going blank, irritability, muscle tension, and sleep disturbance (e.g., difficulty falling or staying asleep, restless unsatisfying sleep). These symptoms cause clinically important distress or impairment in social, occupational, or other important areas of functioning and are not caused by direct physiologic effects of substances (e.g., medications, drugs of abuse, toxin exposure) or by a general medical condition (e.g., hyperthyroidism). Although patients with generalized anxiety disorder may have another underlying mental disorder (axis I disorder), the focus of the anxiety and worry is unrelated to the latter disorder and does not occur only during the course of a mood, psychotic, or pervasive developmental disorder.

Selective serotonin-reuptake inhibitors (SSRIs) are among several classes of antidepressants recommended by some clinicians as first-line treatment for generalized anxiety disorder because of their safety, tolerability (e.g., lack of physical dependence problems commonly associated with benzodiazepines), and proven efficacy in the treatment of depression and other anxiety disorders (e.g., obsessive-compulsive disorder, panic disorder) that frequently present as comorbid conditions in patients with generalized anxiety disorder. Because an estimated 80% of patients with generalized anxiety disorder will have a comorbid mood disorder (e.g., depression) during their lifetime, an SSRI or a drug that predominantly inhibits serotonin and norepinephrine reuptake (e.g., venlafaxine) is preferred by some clinicians for treatment of patients with long-standing generalized anxiety disorder and in those with several comorbid mood or anxiety disorders. However, the efficacy of antidepressants, including paroxetine, in the management of generalized anxiety disorder in patients with comorbid conditions such as depression has yet to be established, since such patients have been excluded from study entry, and therefore further research is needed.

Efficacy of paroxetine hydrochloride for the management of generalized anxiety disorder has been established in 2 randomized, multicenter, placebo-controlled studies of 8 weeks' duration in adult outpatients who met DSM-IV criteria for generalized anxiety disorder. One study employed fixed paroxetine dosages, and the other employed a flexible dosing schedule. In the flexible-dose study, approximately 62% of patients receiving paroxetine (20–50 mg daily; mean dosage of 26.8 mg daily) had a score of 1 ("very much improved") or 2 ("much improved") on the Clinical Global Impressions (CGI) Global Improvement scale, and approximately 36% of these patients had complete or nearly complete resolution of anxiety (defined as a Hamilton Rating Scale for Anxiety [HAM-A] total score of 7 or less), compared with approximately 47 and 23%, respectively, of patients receiving placebo. These results were similar to those seen in the fixed-dose study, in which a score of 1 or 2 on the CGI Global Improvement scale was attained by 62, 68, or 46%, respectively, and a HAM-A total score of 10 or less was attained by 49, 52, or 33%, respectively, of patients receiving paroxetine 20 or 40 mg daily or placebo. However, in a third study, reductions in HAM-A total score attained by patients receiving flexible dosages of paroxetine (20–50 mg daily; mean dosage of 23.8 mg daily) were not substantially different than those attained by patients receiving placebo. Subgroup analysis of these controlled studies in adult outpatients with generalized anxiety disorder did not reveal any evidence of gender- or race-related differences in treatment outcome.

Systematic evaluation of continuing paroxetine for periods of up to 6 months in patients with generalized anxiety disorder who had responded while taking paroxetine during an 8-week acute treatment phase has demonstrated a benefit of such maintenance therapy. In a double-blind, 24-week relapse prevention trial that was an extension of a single-blind, 8-week acute treatment study, patients who had responded to paroxetine 20–50 mg daily were randomized to receive either paroxetine at the same dosage or placebo. Relapse during the double-blind phase was defined as an increase of 2 or more points on the

CGI-Severity of Illness scale to a score of 4 or higher or drug discontinuance due to lack of efficacy. The paroxetine-treated patients experienced a significantly lower relapse rate over the 24-week period compared with those receiving placebo. In addition, 73% of patients receiving a total of 32 weeks of paroxetine therapy achieved remission (defined as a HAM-A total score of 7 or less) compared with about 34% of those who received 8 weeks of therapy and then received 24 weeks of placebo. Because generalized anxiety disorder is a chronic condition, it is reasonable to continue therapy in responding patients. Dosage adjustment may be necessary to maintain patients receiving long-term paroxetine therapy on the lowest effective dosage, and patients should be reassessed periodically to determine the need for continued therapy.

Results of a comparative study indicate that the anxiolytic effects of paroxetine are comparable to those of imipramine, a tricyclic antidepressant, and slightly superior to those of 2′-chlordesmethyldiazepam, a benzodiazepine (not commercially available in the US). In this study, during the first 2 weeks of therapy, 2′-chlordesmethyldiazepam displayed greater anxiolytic efficacy, as measured by HAM-A score, than paroxetine or imipramine; however, following 8 weeks of therapy, a 50% or greater decrease in HAM-A score was attained by 68, 72, or 55% of patients receiving paroxetine, imipramine, or 2′-chlordesmethyldiazepam, respectively. Antidepressants such as paroxetine appear to affect predominantly psychic symptoms, whereas benzodiazepines such as 2′-chlordesmethyldiazepam appear to affect predominately somatic symptoms associated with generalized anxiety disorder.

■ **Posttraumatic Stress Disorder** Paroxetine hydrochloride is used in the treatment of posttraumatic stress disorder (PTSD). PTSD is an anxiety disorder that involves the development of certain characteristic symptoms following personal exposure to an extreme traumatic stressor. According to DSM-IV, PTSD requires exposure to a traumatic event(s) that involved actual or threatened death or serious injury, or threat to the physical integrity of self or others, and the response to the event must involve intense fear, helplessness, or horror (in children the response may be expressed by disorganized or agitated behavior). PTSD is characterized by persistent symptoms of *reexperiencing* the trauma (e.g., intrusive, distressing recollections of the event; recurrent distressing dreams of the event; acting or feeling as if the event were recurring including illusions, hallucinations, or flashbacks; intense distress at exposure to internal or external cues that symbolize or resemble an aspect of the event; physiologic reactivity on exposure to internal or external cues that symbolize or resemble an aspect of the event), persistent *avoidance* of stimuli associated with the trauma and numbing of general responsiveness (e.g., efforts to avoid thoughts, feelings, or conversations related to the event; efforts to avoid activities, places, or people that arouse recollections of the event; inability to recall an important aspect of the event; markedly diminished interest or participation in significant activities; feeling of detachment or estrangement from others; restricted emotions and/or range of affect not present before the event; sense of a foreshortened future); and persistent symptoms of *increased arousal* (e.g., difficulty sleeping; irritability/outbursts of anger; difficulty concentrating; hypervigilance; exaggerated startle response). According to DSM-IV, a PTSD diagnosis requires the presence of 1 or more symptoms of *reexperiencing*, 3 or more symptoms of *avoidance*, and 2 or more symptoms of *increased arousal*, all of which must be present for at least 1 month and cause clinically important distress or impairment in social, occupational, or other important areas of functioning. PTSD, like other anxiety disorders, rarely occurs alone, and patients with PTSD often present with comorbid disorders (e.g., major depressive disorder, substance abuse disorders, panic disorder, generalized anxiety disorders, obsessive-compulsive disorder, social phobia); it is unknown whether these comorbid disorders precede or follow the onset of PTSD.

Psychotherapy alone or in combination with pharmacotherapy generally is considered the treatment of choice for PTSD. Pharmacologic therapy may be indicated in addition to psychotherapy for initial treatment of PTSD in patients who have comorbid disorders (e.g., major depressive disorder, bipolar disorder, other anxiety disorders) and also may be indicated in those who do not respond to initial treatment with psychotherapy alone. If pharmacotherapy is indicated in patients with PTSD, selective serotonin-reuptake inhibitors (SSRIs; e.g., fluoxetine, paroxetine, sertraline) usually are considered the drugs of choice (except in patients with bipolar disorder who require treatment with mood-stabilizing agents).

Efficacy of paroxetine hydrochloride in the treatment of PTSD has been established in 2 multicenter, placebo-controlled studies of 12 weeks' duration in adult outpatients (66–68% women) with a primary diagnosis (DSM-IV) of PTSD following physical or sexual assault (48–54%), witnessing injury or death (17–19%), serious accident or injury (6–13%), or exposure to combat (5–8%). The mean duration of PTSD for these patients was approximately 13 years and 41 or 40% of patients had secondary depressive disorders or non-PTSD anxiety disorders, respectively. In these studies, patients receiving fixed (20 or 40 mg daily) or flexible (20–50 mg daily; mean: 27.6 mg daily) dosages of paroxetine had substantially greater changes from baseline on the Clinician-Administered PTSD Scale Part 2 (CAPS-2) score, a multi-item instrument that measures 3 aspects of PTSD with the following symptom clusters: reexperiencing/intrusion, avoidance/numbing, and hyperarousal, and were more likely to have a score of 1 (very much improved) or 2 (much improved) on the Clinical Global Impression-Global Improvement Scale (CGI-I) compared with those receiving placebo. Treatment response in the fixed-dose study appeared to be unaffected by patient's gender, type of trauma, duration of PTSD, or severity of baseline PTSD or comorbid conditions. A third study, also a flexible-dose study comparing paroxetine (20–50 mg daily) with placebo, demonstrated paroxetine to be substantially superior to placebo as assessed by improvement from baseline for CAPS-2 total score, but not by proportion of responders on the CGI-I.

Use of paroxetine in the treatment of chronic PTSD did not appear to produce a complete remission in a substantial proportion of patients receiving the drug in clinical studies. Therefore, some clinicians suggest combined use of psychotherapy with pharmacotherapy in order to optimize treatment outcome; however, further studies are needed.

■ **Premenstrual Dysphoric Disorder** Like some other selective serotonin-reuptake inhibitors (SSRIs; e.g., fluoxetine, sertraline), paroxetine is used in the treatment of premenstrual dysphoric disorder (previously late luteal phase dysphoric disorder). In women suffering from severe premenstrual dysphoric disorder treated daily for 3 menstrual cycles with paroxetine, maprotiline, or placebo, paroxetine was found to be superior to maprotiline or placebo in improving symptoms associated with this disorder. In women with severe premenstrual dysphoric disorder receiving paroxetine 5–30 mg daily for 10 consecutive menstrual cycles, paroxetine also markedly reduced symptoms (premenstrual irritability, depressed mood, increase in appetite, anxiety/tension). The improvement in symptoms continued throughout the entire treatment period; sedation, dry mouth, and nausea occurred commonly but declined during therapy whereas adverse sexual effects (reduced libido, anorgasmia) persisted. Additional controlled studies are needed to determine whether the efficacy of the drug is sustained during longer-term, maintenance therapy in women with this condition. For further information on use of SSRIs in the treatment of premenstrual dysphoric disorder, see Uses: Premenstrual Dysphoric Disorder, in Fluoxetine Hydrochloride 28:16.04.20.

■ **Premature Ejaculation** Like some other SSRIs, paroxetine has been used with some success in the treatment of premature ejaculation†. In a placebo-controlled study in men with premature ejaculation, paroxetine (20 mg daily for the first week followed by 40 mg daily for 5 additional weeks) produced substantially greater clinical improvement (increased intravaginal ejaculation latency time, increased number of thrusts before ejaculation) than placebo. Nearly all the patients in this study reported some improvement in ejaculatory latency during the first week of paroxetine therapy. In an open study, paroxetine 20 mg daily improved premature ejaculation within about 14 days with all patients studied reporting a longer interval before ejaculation. When dosages of 20 or 40 mg daily were compared in patients with primary premature ejaculation, 20 mg daily was found to be sufficient; further study is needed to determine whether higher dosages may further increase ejaculation latency. In a study comparing paroxetine 20 mg daily for 6 months with paroxetine 20 mg daily for 14 days followed by 10 mg daily for a total of 6 months, both regimens were found to be similarly effective in improving premature ejaculation and were well tolerated. There is some evidence that paroxetine may be more effective than other SSRIs in terms of increasing intravaginal ejaculation latency time.

Additional studies have investigated the use of paroxetine on an "as needed" basis for the treatment of premature ejaculation. In one study, men with premature ejaculation (mean age: 39.5 years; mean pretreatment ejaculatory latency time: 0.3 minutes) were randomized to receive 20 mg of paroxetine or placebo 3–4 hours before planned intercourse; at 4 weeks, the mean ejaculatory latency time was 3.2–3.5 minutes in those receiving the drug compared with 0.45–0.6 minutes in those receiving placebo. However, mean ejaculatory latency time was even longer in another group of men (mean age: 40.5 years; mean pretreatment ejaculatory latency time: 0.5 minutes) who received an initial regimen of paroxetine 10 mg daily for 3 weeks and then received paroxetine 20 mg on an as needed basis for 4 weeks.

Further controlled studies are necessary to confirm these findings, to determine the optimal dosage regimen, and to evaluate the long-term efficacy of paroxetine in patients with this condition. Some clinicians advise that a trial with drug therapy may be particularly useful in patients with premature ejaculation who fail or refuse behavioral or psychotherapeutic treatment or when partners are unwilling to cooperate with such therapy.

■ **Diabetic Neuropathy** Tricyclic antidepressants generally have been considered a mainstay of therapy for the treatment of diabetic neuropathy. However, because of potentially improved patient tolerability, therapy with selective serotonin-reuptake inhibitors (SSRIs) or selective serotonin- and norepinephrine-reuptake inhibitors (SNRIs; e.g., duloxetine, venlafaxine) has been attempted as an alternative. In a controlled study, paroxetine (40 mg daily) was effective in a limited number of patients in substantially reducing the symptoms associated with diabetic neuropathy† and was somewhat less effective but better tolerated than imipramine. Because patients who did not respond as well to paroxetine as to imipramine had lower plasma paroxetine concentrations, it was suggested that dosage adjustment based on plasma concentration monitoring potentially may be useful in the management of this condition. When compared with earlier results obtained with imipramine in the management of diabetic neuropathy, SSRIs such as citalopram, fluoxetine, paroxetine, and sertraline generally appear to be less effective but better tolerated overall. Additional study and experience are needed to elucidate the relative roles of SSRIs versus tricyclic antidepressants, SNRIs, anticonvulsants (e.g., pregabalin, gabapentin), and other forms of treatment in the management of this condition.

■ **Chronic Headache** Paroxetine has been used in a limited number of patients with chronic headache† with some success. In an open study, patients with chronic daily headache unresponsive to previous therapy were treated with paroxetine 10–50 mg daily for 3–9 months; most of the patients showed reductions in the number of headache days per month. Fatigue, insomnia, and urogenital disturbances were the most common adverse effects reported in this study. In a double-blind, crossover study in nondepressed patients with chronic tension-type headache comparing paroxetine (20–30 mg daily) and sulpiride (a dopamine antagonist; not commercially available in the US), both drugs improved headache although sulpiride appeared to provide greater relief. Additional controlled studies are needed to confirm these preliminary findings.

■ **Bipolar Disorder** Paroxetine has been used for the short-term management of acute depressive episodes in patients with bipolar disorder†. While antidepressants such as selective serotonin-reuptake inhibitors (SSRIs) have shown good efficacy in the treatment of unipolar depression, the drugs generally have been studied as adjuncts to mood stabilizing agents such as lithium or valproate in the management of bipolar disorder; antidepressant monotherapy is *not* recommended, given the risk of precipitating a switch into mania. The American Psychiatric Association (APA) currently recommends that paroxetine be reserved for patients who had an inadequate therapeutic response to optimal therapy with first-line agents (i.e., lithium, lamotrigine) or who do not tolerate these drugs. If paroxetine was effective for the management of an acute depressive episode, including during the continuation phase, then maintenance therapy with the drug should be considered to prevent recurrence of major depressive episodes. For further information on the management of bipolar disorder, see Uses: Bipolar Disorder, in Lithium Salts 28:28.

Dosage and Administration

■ **Administration** Paroxetine hydrochloride and paroxetine mesylate are administered orally.

Paroxetine hydrochloride conventional tablets, extended-release tablets, and suspension usually are administered once daily in the morning. Since food does not appear to substantially affect GI absorption of paroxetine hydrochloride, the drug generally can be administered without regard to meals; however, administration with food may minimize adverse GI effects. The manufacturer of paroxetine hydrochloride makes no specific recommendations about administration of paroxetine with regard to food.

Paroxetine mesylate conventional tablets are administered once daily, usually in the morning, without regard to meals.

Paroxetine hydrochloride oral suspension should be shaken well just prior to administration of each dose.

Extended-release tablets of paroxetine hydrochloride should be swallowed whole and should *not* be chewed or crushed.

■ **Dosage** Paroxetine is commercially available in the US as paroxetine hydrochloride (e.g., Paxil®, Paxil CR®) and as paroxetine mesylate (i.e., Pexeva®). Conventional tablets of Paxil® and Pexeva® are *not* bioequivalent. The US Food and Drug Administration (FDA) considers paroxetine mesylate (Pexeva®) conventional tablets to be a pharmaceutical *alternative* (as described in section 505[b][2] of the Federal Food, Drug, and Cosmetic Act) and *not* a pharmaceutical (generic) equivalent to paroxetine hydrochloride conventional tablets (e.g., Paxil®), since both contain the same active moiety (paroxetine) but have different salts.

Dosages of paroxetine hydrochloride and paroxetine mesylate are expressed in terms of paroxetine.

Patients receiving paroxetine should be monitored for possible worsening of depression, suicidality, or unusual changes in behavior, especially at the beginning of therapy or during periods of dosage adjustment. (See Cautions: Precautions and Contraindications.)

The manufacturers recommend that an interval of at least 2 weeks elapse when switching a patient from a monoamine oxidase (MAO) inhibitor intended to treat psychiatric disorders to paroxetine or when switching from paroxetine to an MAO inhibitor intended to treat psychiatric disorders. For additional information on potentially serious drug interactions that may occur between paroxetine and MAO inhibitors or other serotonergic agents, see Cautions: Precautions and Contraindications and see also Drug Interactions: Serotonergic Drugs.

Clinical experience regarding the optimal timing of switching from other antidepressants to paroxetine therapy is limited. Therefore, care and prudent medical judgment should be exercised when switching from other antidepressants, particularly from long-acting agents (e.g., fluoxetine), to paroxetine. Because some adverse reactions resembling serotonin syndrome have developed when fluoxetine therapy has been abruptly discontinued and therapy with another serotonin-reuptake inhibitor (sertraline) initiated immediately afterward, a washout period may be advisable when transferring a patient from fluoxetine to another SSRI. However, the appropriate duration of the washout period when switching from other serotonin-reuptake inhibitors to paroxetine has not been clearly established. Pending further experience in patients being transferred from therapy with another antidepressant to paroxetine and as the clinical situation permits, it generally is recommended that the previous antidepressant be discontinued according to the recommended guidelines for the specific antidepressant prior to initiation of paroxetine therapy.

Because withdrawal effects may occur with discontinuance of paroxetine, other SSRIs, and selective serotonin- and norepinephrine-reuptake inhibitors (SNRIs), abrupt discontinuance of these drugs should be avoided whenever possible. When paroxetine therapy is discontinued, the dosage should be reduced gradually (e.g., over a period of several weeks) and the patient monitored for possible withdrawal symptoms. If intolerable symptoms occur following dosage reduction or upon discontinuance of therapy, the drug may be reinstituted at the previously prescribed dosage. Subsequently, the clinician may continue decreasing the dosage, but at a more gradual rate. (See Withdrawal Reactions under Cautions: Nervous System Effects and see Chronic Toxicity.)

Major Depressive Disorder For the management of major depressive disorder in adults, the recommended initial dosage of paroxetine is 20 mg daily as conventional tablets or suspension or 25 mg daily as extended-release tablets. If no clinical improvement is apparent, dosage may be increased in increments of 10 mg daily for conventional tablets or suspension or 12.5 mg daily for extended-release tablets at intervals of not less than 1 week up to a maximum of 50 mg daily for conventional tablets or suspension or 62.5 mg daily for extended-release tablets. While a relationship between dosage and antidepressant effect has not been established, efficacy of the drug was demonstrated in clinical trials employing 20–50 mg daily dosages as conventional tablets or suspension and 25–62.5 daily dosages as extended-release tablets. Like with other antidepressants, the full antidepressant effects may be delayed.

While the optimum duration of paroxetine therapy has not been established, many experts state that acute depressive episodes require several months or longer of sustained antidepressant therapy. In addition, some clinicians recommend that long-term antidepressant therapy be considered in certain patients at risk for recurrence of depressive episodes (such as those with highly recurrent unipolar depression). Whether the dosage of paroxetine required to induce remission is identical to the dosage needed to maintain and/or sustain euthymia is unknown. In a controlled study, a paroxetine dosage of 40 mg daily was more effective in preventing recurrences of depression than 20 mg daily in patients with recurrent, unipolar depression. Systematic evaluation of paroxetine hydrochloride has shown that its antidepressant efficacy is maintained for periods of up to 1 year in patients receiving a mean dosage of 30 mg daily as conventional tablets or suspension, which corresponds to a 37.5 mg dosage of paroxetine extended-release tablets. In addition, the drug has been used in some patients for longer periods (e.g., up to 4 years) without apparent loss of clinical effect or increased toxicity. If paroxetine is used for extended periods, dosage should be adjusted so that the patient is maintained on the lowest effective dosage, and the need for continued therapy should be reassessed periodically.

Obsessive-Compulsive Disorder For the management of obsessive-compulsive disorder in adults, the recommended initial dosage of paroxetine is 20 mg daily as conventional tablets or suspension. If no clinical improvement is apparent, dosage may be increased in 10-mg increments at intervals of not less than 1 week. The manufacturers recommend a paroxetine dosage of 40 mg daily in the treatment of obsessive-compulsive disorder. Efficacy of the drug was demonstrated in clinical trials employing paroxetine dosages of 20–60 mg daily. The manufacturers state that paroxetine dosage should not exceed 60 mg daily.

Although the optimum duration of paroxetine therapy required to prevent recurrence of obsessive-compulsive symptoms has not been established to date, the efficacy of paroxetine for long-term use (i.e., longer than 12 weeks) has been demonstrated in a 6-month relapse prevention trial. Patients who received paroxetine relapsed substantially less frequently than those receiving placebo. The manufacturers and many clinicians state that obsessive-compulsive disorder is chronic and requires several months or longer of sustained therapy. Therefore, it is reasonable to continue therapy in responding patients. If paroxetine is used for extended periods, dosage should be adjusted so that the patient is maintained on the lowest effective dosage, and the need for continued therapy with the drug should be reassessed periodically.

Panic Disorder For the management of panic disorder in adults, the recommended initial dosage of paroxetine is 10 mg daily as conventional tablets or suspension or 12.5 mg daily as extended-release tablets. Dosage should be increased in 10-mg increments for those receiving conventional tablets or suspension or in 12.5-mg increments for those receiving extended-release tablets at intervals of not less than 1 week. The manufacturers recommend dosages of 40 mg daily for paroxetine conventional tablets or suspension in the treatment of panic disorder. Efficacy of the drug was demonstrated in clinical trials employing 10–60 mg daily as conventional tablets or suspension or 12.5–75 mg daily as extended-release tablets. The manufacturers state that paroxetine dosages should not exceed 60 mg daily for conventional tablets or suspension and 75 mg daily for extended-release tablets.

Although the optimum duration of paroxetine therapy required to prevent recurrence of panic disorder has not been established to date, the efficacy of paroxetine for long-term use (i.e., longer than 12 weeks) has been demonstrated in a 3-month relapse prevention trial. Patients who were treated with paroxetine hydrochloride conventional tablets or suspension (10–40 mg daily) relapsed substantially less frequently than those receiving placebo. The manufacturers and some clinicians state that panic disorder is a chronic condition; therefore, it is reasonable to continue therapy in responding patients. Dosage adjustment may be necessary to maintain the patient on the lowest effective dosage, and patients receiving the drug for extended periods should be reassessed periodically to determine the need for continued therapy.

Social Phobia For the management of generalized social phobia (social anxiety disorder) in adults, the recommended dosage of paroxetine (administered as paroxetine hydrochloride) is 20 mg daily as conventional tablets or suspension or 12.5 mg daily as extended-release tablets. Dosage of the extended-release tablets may be increased in increments of 12.5 mg daily at intervals of not less than 1 week. Efficacy of the drug was demonstrated in clinical trials employing dosages of 20–60 mg daily as conventional tablets or suspension or 12.5–37.5 mg daily as extended-release tablets. The manufacturer of paroxetine hydrochloride states that no additional clinical benefit was observed at dosages exceeding 20 mg daily for conventional tablets or suspension and that the maximum dosage for extended-release tablets should not exceed 37.5 mg daily.

Although the efficacy of paroxetine for long-term therapy (i.e., longer than 12 weeks) has not been demonstrated in controlled studies to date, the manufacturer of paroxetine hydrochloride states that it is reasonable to consider continuation of therapy for a patient who responds to the drug. If paroxetine is used for extended periods, dosage should be adjusted so that the patient is maintained on the lowest effective dosage, and the need for continued therapy should be reassessed periodically.

Anxiety Disorder For the management of generalized anxiety disorder in adults, the recommended initial dosage of paroxetine (administered as paroxetine hydrochloride) is 20 mg daily as conventional tablets or suspension. Although dosages of 20–50 mg daily were effective in clinical studies, there is insufficient evidence to indicate that dosages exceeding 20 mg daily provide additional clinical benefit. Dosage of paroxetine should be increased in 10-mg increments at intervals of not less than 1 week.

The optimum duration of paroxetine therapy for the management of generalized anxiety disorder has not been established to date. Because this disorder is chronic, it is reasonable to continue therapy in responding patients. In general, patients with generalized anxiety disorder usually require at least 8 weeks of treatment to achieve a Hamilton Rating Scale for Anxiety (HAM-A) score of 10 or less, which has been shown to be the score at which specific treatment effects can begin to be distinguished from nonspecific placebo effects. However, available data suggest that some patients may require an extended duration of treatment in order to achieve a HAM-A score of 7–10 or less. In a 32-week, multicenter, relapse-prevention study in outpatients with generalized anxiety disorder and a mean baseline HAM-A score of 26.5, about 34% of patients achieved remission (defined as a HAM-A total score of 7 or less) following 8 weeks of paroxetine therapy compared with 73% of patients following 32 weeks of paroxetine therapy. In addition, patients receiving long-term therapy with the drug relapsed substantially less frequently than those receiving placebo.

Because of the prolonged nature of depressive episodes in patients with generalized anxiety disorder and comorbid depression, some clinicians currently recommend that such patients be treated for at least 12 months to ensure remission of both anxiety and depression. If paroxetine is used for extended periods, dosage should be adjusted so that patients are maintained on the lowest effective dosage, and the need for continued therapy with the drug should be reassessed periodically.

Posttraumatic Stress Disorder For the management of posttraumatic stress disorder (PTSD) in adults, the recommended dosage of paroxetine (administered as paroxetine hydrochloride) is 20 mg daily as conventional tablets or suspension. Although efficacy has been established for dosages ranging from 20–50 mg daily, there is insufficient evidence to suggest a greater benefit with 40 mg daily compared with 20 mg daily. If a dosage increase above 20 mg daily is considered necessary, it should be in increments of 10 mg daily at intervals of at least 1 week.

Some clinicians suggest that an adequate trial period for determining the effectiveness of paroxetine in patients with PTSD is 8 weeks; patients who have not achieved at least a 25% reduction in PTSD symptoms at week 8 generally are unlikely to respond to continued paroxetine therapy and use of alternative agents is recommended in such patients. In addition, although the optimum duration of paroxetine therapy required to prevent recurrence of PTSD has not been established to date, some clinicians recommend up to 24 months of drug therapy in patients who achieve good response (i.e., greater than 75% reduction in PTSD symptoms and response maintained for at least 3 months). Although the efficacy of paroxetine for long-term therapy (i.e., longer than 12 weeks) has not been demonstrated in controlled studies to date, PTSD is a chronic condition for which it is reasonable to continue paroxetine therapy as long as a response is maintained. If paroxetine is used for extended periods, dosage should be adjusted so that the patient is maintained on the lowest possible effective dosage, and the need for continued therapy with the drug should be reassessed periodically.

Premenstrual Dysphoric Disorder For the treatment of premenstrual dysphoric disorder (previously late luteal phase dysphoric disorder), the recommended initial dosage of paroxetine (administered as paroxetine hydrochloride) is 12.5 mg daily as extended-release tablets. Dosage should be increased at intervals of not less than 1 week. In clinical trials, both the 12.5-mg and 25-mg daily dosages were shown to be effective.

Efficacy of paroxetine for long-term therapy (i.e., longer than 3 menstrual cycles) has not been demonstrated in controlled studies to date. However, women commonly report that symptoms worsen with age until relieved by the onset of menopause. Therefore, the manufacturer of paroxetine hydrochloride states that it is reasonable to consider continuation of therapy for a patient who responds to the drug. Patients should be periodically reassessed to determine the need for continued treatment.

Premature Ejaculation For the treatment of premature ejaculation†, paroxetine has been given in a dosage of 10–40 mg daily to increase ejaculatory latency time. Alternatively, patients have taken paroxetine on an "as needed" basis for the treatment of premature ejaculation using 20-mg doses of the drug 3–4 hours before planned intercourse. However, one study noted more prolonged ejaculatory latency time if patients received paroxetine in a dosage of 10 mg daily for 3 weeks prior to using 20-mg doses of the drug on an as needed basis.

Diabetic Neuropathy In patients with diabetic neuropathy†, paroxetine has been given in a dosage of 40 mg daily to reduce the symptoms associated with the disease.

Chronic Headache In the management of chronic headache†, paroxetine has been given in a dosage of 10–50 mg daily for 3–9 months to reduce the number of headaches per month.

■ **Dosage in Geriatric and Debilitated Patients** In geriatric or debilitated patients, an initial paroxetine dosage of 10 mg daily as conventional tablets or suspension or 12.5 mg daily as extended-release tablets is recommended; if no clinical improvement is apparent, dosage may be titrated up to a maximum of 40 mg daily (for conventional tablets or suspension) or 50 mg (for extended-release tablets).

■ **Dosage in Renal and Hepatic Impairment** In patients with severe renal or hepatic impairment, an initial paroxetine dosage of 10 mg daily as conventional tablets or suspension or 12.5 mg daily as extended-release tablets is recommended. If no clinical improvement is apparent, dosage may be titrated with caution up to a maximum of 40 mg daily (for conventional tablets or suspension) or 50 mg (for extended-release tablets). (See Pharmacokinetics: Elimination and see Cautions: Precautions and Contraindications.)

Cautions

The adverse effect profile of paroxetine is similar to that of other selective serotonin-reuptake inhibitors (SSRIs; e.g., citalopram, escitalopram, fluoxetine, fluvoxamine, sertraline). Paroxetine is commercially available in the US as paroxetine hydrochloride (e.g., Paxil®, Paxil CR®) and as paroxetine mesylate (i.e., Pexeva®). The main clinical studies with paroxetine have been conducted with paroxetine hydrochloride, and the incidences of adverse effects reported in this section are from clinical trials using the hydrochloride salt. Because paroxetine hydrochloride and paroxetine mesylate contain the same active moiety (paroxetine), tolerability is expected to be similar between the 2 different salts. However, direct comparison studies have not been conducted to date, and the possibility that differences in tolerability between paroxetine hydrochloride and paroxetine mesylate may exist should be taken into consideration.

Because paroxetine is a highly selective serotonin-reuptake inhibitor with little or no effect on other neurotransmitters, the incidence of some adverse effects commonly associated with tricyclic antidepressants, such as anticholinergic effects (dry mouth, constipation), cardiovascular effects, drowsiness, and weight gain, is lower in patients receiving paroxetine. However, certain adverse GI (e.g., nausea, anorexia) and nervous system (e.g., somnolence, anxiety, nervousness, insomnia) effects appear to occur more frequently with paroxetine and other SSRIs than with tricyclic antidepressants.

Overall, the adverse effect profile of paroxetine in patients with depression, obsessive-compulsive disorder, panic disorder, social phobia, generalized anxiety disorder, or posttraumatic stress disorder (PTSD) appears to be similar. In controlled studies, the most common adverse effects occurring more frequently in patients receiving paroxetine than in those receiving placebo included nervous system effects such as asthenia, somnolence, dizziness, insomnia, tremor, and nervousness; GI effects such as nausea, decreased appetite, constipation, diarrhea, and dry mouth; impotence, ejaculatory dysfunction (principally ejaculatory delay), and other male genital disorders; female genital disorders (principally anorgasmia or difficulty reaching climax/orgasm); and sweating. The incidence of many of these adverse effects appears to be dose related in patients with depression; however, there was no clear evidence of dose-related adverse events in patients with obsessive-compulsive disorder or social phobia. In addition, there was no clear relationship between the incidence of adverse events and dose except for asthenia, dry mouth, anxiety, decreased libido, tremor, and abnormal ejaculation in the treatment of panic disorder and asthenia, constipation, and abnormal ejaculation in the treatment of generalized anxiety disorder.

Patients receiving paroxetine may develop tolerance to some adverse effects (e.g., nausea, dizziness) with continued therapy (e.g., after 4–6 weeks); however, tolerance is less likely to develop to other adverse effects such as dry mouth, somnolence, and asthenia. During short-term (6 weeks or less) studies, nausea was the most common adverse effect, whereas during long-term studies, headache, sweating, weight gain, and constipation were among the most common. Discontinuance of paroxetine therapy was required in 20% of patients with depression, about 16% of patients with social phobia, about 12% of patients with obsessive-compulsive disorder or PTSD, about 11% of patients with generalized anxiety disorder, and about 9% of patients with panic disorder in clinical trials, principally because of adverse psychiatric (e.g., somnolence, insomnia, agitation, tremor), other nervous system (e.g., dizziness, asthenia), GI (e.g., nausea, vomiting, diarrhea, constipation, dry mouth), or male urogenital (e.g., abnormal ejaculation, impotence) effects or because of sweating.

■ **Nervous System Effects** Somnolence, which appears to be dose related, is among the most common adverse effects of paroxetine, occurring in approximately 23% of depressed patients receiving the drug in short-term controlled clinical trials. Somnolence required discontinuance of therapy in about 2% of patients. Headache occurred in about 18 or 15% of patients receiving paroxetine in short- or long-term controlled clinical trials, respectively. In addition, migraine or vascular headache has been reported in up to 1% or less than 0.1% of paroxetine-treated patients, respectively. Asthenia, which also appears to be dose related, occurred in 15% of depressed patients receiving the drug in short-term controlled clinical trials and required discontinuance of therapy in about 2% of patients.

Dizziness, which appears to be dose related, occurred in about 13% of patients receiving paroxetine in short-term controlled clinical trials. Insomnia occurred in about 13 or 8% of patients receiving the drug in short- or long-term controlled clinical trials, respectively. However, because insomnia is a symptom also associated with depression, relief of insomnia and improvement in sleep patterns may occur when clinical improvement in depression becomes apparent during antidepressant therapy. In clinical trials, less than 2% of patients discontinued paroxetine because of insomnia.

Tremor occurred in about 8%, nervousness or anxiety each in about 5%, paresthesia in about 4%, and agitation in about 2% of patients receiving paroxetine in short-term controlled clinical trials. The incidence of tremor and paresthesia may be dose related. Agitation and tremor each resulted in discontinuance of the drug in about 1% of patients receiving the drug in clinical trials. Drugged feeling or confusion occurred in about 2 or 1% of patients, respectively.

The incidence of seizures during paroxetine therapy appears to be similar to that observed during therapy with most other currently available antidepressants. Seizures, including tonic-clonic (grand mal) seizures, occurred in less than 0.1% of patients receiving paroxetine in clinical trials. (See Cautions: Precautions and Contraindications.) In addition, myoclonus has been reported in about 1% of patients receiving the drug.

Hypomania, mania, manic reaction, and manic-depressive reaction have been reported in approximately 1% of patients receiving paroxetine in short- or long-term controlled clinical trials, which is similar to the incidence reported in patients receiving active control agents (i.e., other antidepressants). The incidence of these adverse effects was 0.3% in unipolar patients receiving placebo. In a subset of patients classified as having bipolar disorder, the incidence of manic episodes was 2.2% in patients receiving paroxetine and 11.6% in patients receiving other antidepressants. (See Cautions: Precautions and Contraindications.) Such reactions have occurred in patients receiving other antidepressant agents and may be caused by antidepressant-induced functional increases in catecholamine activity within the CNS, resulting in a "switch" from depressive to manic behavior. There is some evidence that patients with bipolar disorder may be more likely to experience antidepressant-induced hypomanic or manic reactions than patients without evidence of this disorder. In addition, limited evidence suggests that such reactions may occur more frequently in bipolar depressed patients receiving tricyclics and tetracyclics (e.g., maprotiline, mianserin [not commercially available in the US]) than in those receiving SSRIs (e.g., citalopram, escitalopram, fluoxetine, fluvoxamine, paroxetine, sertraline). However, further studies are needed to confirm these initial findings.

Amnesia, CNS stimulation, impaired concentration, precipitation or worsening of depression, emotional lability, and vertigo each have been reported in at least 1% of patients receiving paroxetine; however, a causal relationship to the drug has not been established. Abnormal thinking, lack of emotion, neurosis, paralysis, paranoid reaction, alcohol abuse, depersonalization, delirium, euphoria, hallucinations, hostility, ataxia, dyskinesia, hyperkinesia, hypesthesia, hypokinesia, and incoordination have been reported in up to 1% of patients receiving the drug, although these adverse effects have not been definitely attributed to paroxetine.

Extrapyramidal reactions associated with paroxetine, which are uncommon, appear to be a class effect of SSRIs and dose related. Reactions occurring *early* during therapy with the drug may be secondary to preexisting parkinsonian syndrome and/or concomitant therapy. Paroxetine and other SSRIs have been associated with the development of akathisia, which is characterized by an inner sense of restlessness and psychomotor agitation such as an inability to sit or stand still usually associated with subjective distress. Akathisia is most likely to occur within the first few weeks of therapy with these drugs. Other extrapyramidal symptoms reported in patients receiving paroxetine include dystonia, bradykinesia, cogwheel rigidity, hypertonia, oculogyric crisis (associated with concomitant use of pimozide), tremor, and trismus; however, a causal relationship to the drug has not been established.

Adverse nervous system effects reported in less than 0.1% of patients receiving paroxetine include akinesia, antisocial reaction, aphasia, choreoathetosis, circumoral paresthesias, delusions, drug dependence, dysarthria, fasciculations, gait abnormalities, hyperalgesia, hyperreflexia, decreased reflexes, hysteria, meningitis, myelitis, neuralgia, neuropathy, nystagmus, psychotic depression, stupor, and torticollis; these effects have not been definitely attributed to the drug. Fatigue also has been reported. Although a causal relationship to the drug has not been established, serotonin syndrome and neuroleptic malignant syndrome (NMS)-like reactions also have been reported rarely in patients receiving paroxetine, other SSRIs, and selective serotonin- and norepinephrine-reuptake inhibitors. (See Cautions: Precautions and Contraindications, Drug Interactions: Serotonergic Drugs, and Acute Toxicity.)

Status epilepticus has been reported during postmarketing surveillance in patients receiving paroxetine, although a causal relationship to the drug has not been established. Guillain-Barré syndrome has been reported rarely in association with paroxetine; however, a causal relationship to the drug has not been clearly established.

Withdrawal Reactions Withdrawal symptoms, including dysphoric mood, irritability, agitation, dizziness, sensory disturbances (e.g., paresthesias such as electric shock sensations), anxiety, confusion, headache, lethargy, emotional lability, insomnia, and hypomania, have been reported upon discontinuance of paroxetine, other SSRIs, and SNRIs, particularly when discontinuance of these drugs is abrupt. While these reactions are generally self-limiting, there have been reports of serious discontinuance symptoms. Therefore, patients should be monitored for such symptoms when discontinuing paroxetine therapy. A gradual reduction in the dosage rather than abrupt cessation is recommended whenever possible. (See Dosage and Administration: Dosage.)

Withdrawal syndrome, manifested as dizziness, blurred vision, sweating, nausea, insomnia, tremor, confusion, lethargy, insomnia, sensory disturbances, anxiety or nervousness, headache, paresthesias, hypomanic-like symptoms (including hyperactivity, decreased need for sleep, irritability, agitation, aggressiveness, volatility, explosive vocal and temper outbursts), and ego-dystonic impulsive behavior (including shoplifting, homicidal impulses, suicidal impulses and gestures) following discontinuance of the drug, has been reported in less than 0.1% of patients receiving paroxetine in early clinical trials. Later clinical trials employed a taper-phase regimen rather than abrupt discontinuance of paroxetine, which involved an incremental decrease in the daily dosage by 10 mg daily at weekly intervals. When a daily dosage of 20 mg daily was reached, patients continued to receive this dosage for one week before stopping the drug. Using this taper regimen, abnormal dreams, paresthesia, and dizziness were reported in 2% or more of patients treated with paroxetine. In the majority of these cases, the withdrawal reactions were mild to moderate in severity and were self-limiting and did not require medical intervention.

Some evidence suggests that the risk of withdrawal effects may be somewhat greater with paroxetine than sertraline; fluoxetine appears to be associated with the fewest withdrawal effects, possibly because of its prolonged elimination half-life. Additional clinical experience is necessary to confirm these findings. (See Chronic Toxicity.)

Suicidality The US Food and Drug Administration (FDA) has determined that antidepressants increase the risk of suicidal thinking and behavior (suicidality) in children, adolescents, and young adults (18–24 years of age) with major depressive disorder and other psychiatric disorders. Patients, therefore, should be appropriately monitored and closely observed for clinical worsening, suicidality, and unusual changes in behavior, particularly during initiation of paroxetine therapy (i.e., the first few months) and during periods of dosage adjustments. (See Cautions: Precautions and Contraindications, Cautions: Pediatric Precautions, and Acute Toxicity.)

■ **GI Effects** Like other SSRIs (e.g., citalopram, escitalopram, fluoxetine, fluvoxamine, sertraline), paroxetine therapy is associated with a relatively high incidence of GI disturbances, principally nausea, dry mouth, and bowel abnormalities. The most frequent adverse effect associated with paroxetine therapy is nausea, which occurred in about 26% of patients receiving the drug in controlled clinical trials. Nausea generally is mild to moderate in severity and usually subsides after a few weeks of continued therapy with the drug. The incidence of nausea appears to be dose related. In clinical trials, nausea required discontinuance of paroxetine in about 3% of patients and was the most frequent adverse effect requiring discontinuance of the drug. Overall, adverse GI effects, principally nausea, required discontinuance of paroxetine therapy in about 6% of patients receiving the drug in clinical trials. While the mechanism(s) of paroxetine-induced GI effects has not been fully elucidated, they appear to arise at least in part because of increased serotonergic activity in the GI tract (which may result in stimulation of small intestine motility and inhibition of gastric and large intestine motility) and possibly because of the drug's effect on central serotonergic type 3 (5-HT_3) receptors.

Dry mouth occurred in about 18%, constipation in about 14%, diarrhea in about 12%, and decreased appetite in about 6% of patients receiving paroxetine in short-term controlled clinical trials. Other adverse GI effects associated with paroxetine therapy include flatulence, which occurred in 4%, and vomiting, which occurred in about 2% of patients receiving the drug in short-term controlled clinical trials. Vomiting generally is mild to moderate in severity and required discontinuance of the drug in about 1% of patients receiving the drug in controlled trials. Oropharyngeal disorders (principally lump or tightness in the throat), taste perversion, and dyspepsia were reported in about 2% and abdominal pain and increased appetite were reported in at least 1% of patients receiving paroxetine. The incidence of constipation, anorexia, decreased appetite, and dry mouth appear to be dose related.

Although a causal relationship to paroxetine has not been established, bruxism, colitis, dysphagia, eructation, gastroenteritis, gingivitis, glossitis, increased salivation, rectal hemorrhage, and ulcerative stomatitis have been reported in up to 1% of patients receiving the drug. Aphthous stomatitis, stomatitis, esophagitis, duodenitis, enteritis, peptic or gastric ulcer, ileus, peritonitis, hematemesis, bloody diarrhea, intestinal obstruction, fecal impaction or incontinence, melena, bulimia, cholelithiasis, tongue discoloration, tongue edema, mouth ulceration, loss of taste, gingival hemorrhage, salivary gland enlargement, and dental caries have been reported in less than 0.1% of patients receiving paroxetine. In addition, laryngismus has been reported during postmarketing surveillance. However, these adverse effects have not been definitely attributed to the drug.

Epidemiologic case-control and cohort design studies have suggested that SSRIs may increase the risk of upper GI bleeding. Although the precise mechanism for this increased risk remains to be clearly established, serotonin release by platelets is known to play an important role in hemostasis, and SSRIs decrease serotonin uptake from the blood by platelets thereby decreasing the amount of serotonin in platelets. In addition, concurrent use of aspirin or other nonsteroidal anti-inflammatory drugs was found to substantially increase the risk of GI bleeding in patients receiving SSRIs in 2 of these studies. Although these studies focused on upper GI bleeding, there is evidence suggesting that bleeding at other sites may be similarly potentiated. Further clinical studies are needed to determine the clinical importance of these findings. (See Cautions: Hematologic Effects and see also Drug Interactions: Drugs Affecting Hemostasis.)

■ **Dermatologic and Sensitivity Reactions** Rash, which may be maculopapular or vesiculobullous, has been reported in about 2% of patients receiving paroxetine in short-term controlled clinical trials. Pruritus has been reported in at least 1% of patients receiving the drug. In addition, allergic reactions have been reported in up to 1% of patients in clinical trials, and allergic alveolitis and anaphylaxis have been reported during postmarketing surveillance. However, these adverse effects have not been definitely attributed to paroxetine.

Adverse dermatologic effects reported in up to 1% of patients receiving paroxetine include acne, alopecia, contact dermatitis, dry skin, eczema, herpes simplex, photosensitivity, and urticaria; however, these adverse effects have not been definitely attributed to the drug. Angioedema, erythema nodosum, erythema multiforme, exfoliative dermatitis, fungal dermatitis, furunculosis, herpes zoster, hirsutism, maculopapular rash, seborrhea, skin discoloration, skin hypertrophy, decreased sweating, and skin ulcer have been reported in less than 0.1% of patients receiving the drug. In addition, Stevens-Johnson syndrome and toxic epidermal necrolysis have been reported in paroxetine-treated patients.

Sweating occurred in about 11–12% of patients receiving paroxetine in short- or long-term controlled clinical trials and required discontinuance of therapy in approximately 1% of patients. The incidence of sweating appears to be dose related.

■ **Metabolic and Endocrine Effects** Weight gain occurred in at least 1% of patients receiving paroxetine in controlled clinical trials. While clinically important weight loss may occur in some patients, only minimal weight loss (averaging 0.45 kg) generally occurred in up to 17% of patients receiving paroxetine in controlled clinical trials. In addition, while decreased appetite was reported in about 6% of patients receiving paroxetine in short-term clinical trials, the drug, unlike fluoxetine, does not appear to exhibit clinically important anorectic effects.

Ketosis and increased LDH concentrations have also been reported in less than 1% of paroxetine-treated patients, although a causal relationship to the drug has not been established. Thirst has been reported in up to 1% of patients receiving paroxetine, although a causal relationship to the drug has not been established. Adverse effects reported in less than 0.1% of patients receiving the drug include gout, hypercholesterolemia, hyperglycemia, hypoglycemia, and increased creatine kinase (CK, creatine phosphokinase, CPK), gamma globulin and nonprotein nitrogen concentrations; however, these adverse effects also have not been definitely attributed to paroxetine.

Diabetes mellitus, goiter, hyperthyroidism, hypothyroidism, thyroiditis, and symptoms suggestive of prolactinemia and galactorrhea have been reported in less than 0.1% of patients receiving paroxetine; however, these adverse effects have not been definitely attributed to the drug.

■ **Ocular and Otic Effects** Blurred vision, which appears to be dose related, occurred in about 4% of patients receiving paroxetine in controlled clinical trials. Adverse ocular effects reported in up to 1% of patients receiving paroxetine include abnormality of accommodation, conjunctivitis, ocular pain, mydriasis, and keratoconjunctivitis. Although a causal relationship to paroxetine has not been established, amblyopia, blepharitis, diplopia, cataract, conjunctival edema, corneal ulcer, exophthalmos, ocular hemorrhage, glaucoma, photophobia, night blindness, ptosis, retinal hemorrhage, and visual field defect, have been reported in less than 0.1% of patients receiving the drug. Anisocoria and optic neuritis also have been reported in at least one paroxetine-treated patient; these adverse effects have not been definitely attributed to the drug.

Tinnitus occurred in at least 1% of patients receiving paroxetine in controlled clinical trials. Otic pain or otitis media has been reported in up to 1% of patients receiving paroxetine. Deafness, hyperacusis, otitis externa, and parosmia have been reported in less than 0.1% of patients.

■ **Cardiovascular Effects** Paroxetine does not exhibit clinically important anticholinergic activity, and current evidence suggests that paroxetine is less cardiotoxic than most older antidepressant agents (e.g., tricyclic antidepressants, monoamine oxidase inhibitors).

No clinically important changes in vital signs (systolic and diastolic blood pressure, heart rate) were observed in patients receiving paroxetine in controlled trials. Unlike tricyclic antidepressants, which may cause characteristic ECG changes such as prolongation of PR, QRS, and QT intervals and ST-segment and T-wave abnormalities, clinically important ECG changes have not been reported during controlled clinical trials in paroxetine-treated patients. However, small but statistically significant QRS widening was reported with paroxetine relative to placebo in one study, and ECG changes occasionally have been reported in healthy individuals and patients receiving the drug. In addition, the relative safety of paroxetine in patients with underlying cardiac disease remains to be more fully elucidated.

Palpitation and vasodilation each have been reported in about 3% of patients receiving paroxetine in short-term controlled clinical trials. Unlike tricyclic antidepressants, paroxetine has been associated with hypotension (e.g., orthostatic) infrequently; in short-term controlled clinical trials, orthostatic hypotension occurred in at least 1% of patients receiving the drug. Chest pain also occurred in about 1–2% of patients in such trials. Hypertension, syncope, and tachycardia also have been reported in at least 1% of patients receiving paroxetine. Bradycardia and generalized peripheral and facial edema have been reported in up to 1% of patients receiving the drug, although a definite causal relationship to paroxetine has not been established. Angina pectoris, myocardial ischemia, myocardial infarction, cerebral ischemia, cerebrovascular accident, pallor, congestive heart failure, low cardiac output, arrhythmia nodal, supraventricular or ventricular extrasystoles, atrial fibrillation, heart block, bundle-branch block, pulmonary embolus, thrombosis, phlebitis, and varicose veins have been reported in less than 0.1% of patients receiving paroxetine; these adverse effects have not been definitely attributed to the drug.

In addition, ventricular fibrillation, ventricular tachycardia (including torsades de pointes), and pulmonary hypertension have been reported during postmarketing surveillance; however, these adverse effects have not been definitely attributed to paroxetine.

■ **Musculoskeletal Effects** Myopathy or myalgia occurred in about 2% of patients receiving paroxetine in short-term controlled clinical trials. In addition, arthralgia has been reported in at least 1% of patients receiving the drug. Myasthenia or back pain was reported in about 1% of patients receiving the drug in such trials. Arthritis or neck pain has been reported in up to 1% of patients receiving paroxetine, although a causal relationship to the drug has not been established. Arthrosis, bursitis, myositis, neck rigidity, osteoporosis, generalized spasm, tenosynovitis, and tetany have been reported in less than 0.1% of patients receiving paroxetine; these adverse effects have not been definitely attributed to the drug.

■ **Hematologic Effects** Anemia, eosinophilia, leukocytosis, leukopenia, ecchymosis, and purpura have been reported in up to 1% of patients receiving paroxetine, although a causal relationship to the drug has not been established. Altered platelet function and abnormal bleeding also have been reported. The manufacturers state that there have been several cases of abnormal bleeding (mostly ecchymosis and purpura) and a case of impaired platelet aggregation in patients receiving paroxetine to date. In one woman, widespread bruising developed on the arms, legs, and hips 15 days after paroxetine therapy was begun; the bruising subsided following discontinuance of the drug. In another female patient, spontaneous bruising of the arms and legs and excessive menstrual blood loss developed 2 weeks after starting paroxetine therapy; addition of ascorbic acid 500 mg daily improved the bleeding after 3 weeks but subsequent discontinuance of ascorbic acid led to a gradual recurrence of these symptoms. Similar reactions have been reported in several patients receiving other SSRIs (e.g., fluoxetine, fluvoxamine, sertraline). Although the precise mechanism for these reactions has not been established, it has been suggested that impaired platelet aggregation caused by platelet serotonin depletion and/or increased capillary fragility may contribute to these cases. (See Cautions: GI Effects and see also Drug Interactions: Drugs Affecting Hemostasis.)

Although a causal relationship to the drug has not been established, hemolytic anemia, impaired hematopoiesis (including aplastic anemia, pancytopenia, bone marrow aplasia, and agranulocytosis), porphyria, and thrombocytopenia have been reported during postmarketing surveillance in patients receiving paroxetine. Abnormal erythrocytes or lymphocytes; prolonged bleeding time; hypochromic anemia, iron-deficiency anemia, microcytic anemia, or normocytic anemia; eosinophilia, leukocytosis, lymphocytosis, and monocytosis each have been reported in less than 0.1% of patients receiving paroxetine; these adverse effects have not been definitely attributed to the drug.

■ **Respiratory Effects** Respiratory disorders (principally cold symptoms and upper respiratory infections), pharyngitis and other oropharyngeal disorders (sensation of having a lump or tightness in the throat), increased cough, rhinitis, and sinusitis have been reported in at least 1% of patients receiving paroxetine in short-term controlled clinical trials. Yawning occurred in about 4% of patients receiving the drug.

Adverse effects reported in up to 1% of patients receiving paroxetine include asthma, dyspnea, epistaxis, hyperventilation, bronchitis, pneumonia, and respiratory influenza; however, a causal relationship to the drug has not been established. Other adverse respiratory effects reported in less than 0.1% of patients receiving paroxetine include emphysema, hemoptysis, hiccups, lung fibrosis, pulmonary edema, increased sputum production, stridor, and voice alteration; these adverse effects have not been definitely attributed to the drug. Pulmonary alveolitis has been reported rarely.

■ **Renal, Electrolyte, and Genitourinary Effects** ***Sexual Dysfunction*** Like other SSRIs, adverse effects on sexual function have been reported in both men and women receiving paroxetine. Although changes in sexual desire, sexual performance, and sexual satisfaction often occur as manifestations of a psychiatric disorder, they also may occur as the result of pharmacologic therapy. It is difficult to determine the true incidence and severity of adverse effects on sexual function during paroxetine therapy, in part because patients and clinicians may be reluctant to discuss these effects. Therefore, incidence data reported in product labeling and earlier studies are most likely underestimates of the true incidence of adverse sexual effects. Recent reports indicate that up to 50% of patients receiving SSRIs describe some form of sexual dysfunction during treatment and the actual incidence may be even higher. Results of some (but not all) studies in men and women suggest that paroxetine may be associated with a higher incidence of sexual dysfunction than some other currently available SSRIs.

Ejaculatory disturbances (principally ejaculatory delay), which appear to be dose related, are the most common adverse urogenital effects associated with paroxetine in males, reported by the manufacturer as occurring in about 13–28% of male patients receiving the drug compared with 0–2% of patients receiving placebo in controlled clinical studies for the treatment of depression, obsessive-compulsive disorder, panic disorder, social phobia, generalized anxiety disorder, or posttraumatic stress disorder. Abnormal ejaculation was a reason for drug discontinuance in up to about 5% of patients in these controlled clinical studies. However, the adverse effect of ejaculatory delay has been used for therapeutic benefit in the treatment of premature ejaculation. (See Uses: Premature Ejaculation.)

Decreased libido was reported in 6–15% of male patients receiving paroxetine in controlled clinical studies for the treatment of depression, obsessive-compulsive disorder, panic disorder, social phobia, generalized anxiety disorder, or PTSD compared with 0–5% of males receiving placebo. In these studies, impotence was reported in 2–9% of male patients receiving paroxetine compared with 0–3% of males receiving placebo.

In female patients receiving paroxetine in controlled clinical studies for the treatment of depression, obsessive-compulsive disorder, panic disorder, social phobia, generalized anxiety disorder, or PTSD, decreased libido was reported in 0–9% of those receiving paroxetine compared with 0–2% of women receiving placebo. In these studies, orgasmic disturbances were reported in 2–9% of female patients receiving the drug compared with 0–1% of female patients receiving placebo.

Increased libido has been reported in up to 1% of patients receiving paroxetine. Other reported adverse sexual effects include anorgasmia, erectile difficulties, and delayed orgasm. Priapism also has been reported in male patients receiving the drug.

Results of some (but not all) studies in men and women suggest that paroxetine may be associated with a higher incidence of sexual dysfunction than some other currently available SSRIs, including citalopram and sertraline. Since it is difficult to know the precise risk of sexual dysfunction associated with serotonin-reuptake inhibitors, clinicians should routinely inquire about such possible adverse effects in patients receiving these drugs.

Management of sexual dysfunction caused by SSRI therapy includes waiting for tolerance to develop; using a lower dosage of the drug; using drug holidays; delaying administration of the drug until after coitus; or changing to another antidepressant. Although further study is needed, there is some evidence that adverse sexual effects of SSRIs may be reversed by concomitant use of certain drugs, including buspirone, 5-hydroxytryptamine-2 (5-HT_2) receptor antagonists (e.g., nefazodone), 5-HT_3 receptor inhibitors (e.g., granisetron), or α_2-adrenergic receptor antagonists (e.g., yohimbine), selective phosphodiesterase (PDE) inhibitors (e.g., sildenafil), or dopamine receptor agonists (e.g., amantadine, dextroamphetamine, pemoline [no longer commercially available in the US], methylphenidate). In most patients, sexual dysfunction is fully reversed 1–3 days after discontinuance of the antidepressant.

Other Renal, Electrolyte, and Genitourinary Effects Treatment with SSRIs, including paroxetine, and selective serotonin- and norepinephrine-reuptake inhibitors (SNRIs) may result in hyponatremia. In many cases, this hyponatremia appears to be due to the syndrome of inappropriate antidiuretic hormone secretion (SIADH) and was reversible when the SSRI or SNRI was discontinued. Cases with serum sodium concentrations lower than 110 mEq/L have been reported. Hyponatremia has been reported following paroxetine overdosage in a geriatric patient. Hyponatremia and SIADH in patients receiving SSRIs usually develop an average of 2 weeks after initiating therapy (range: 3–120 days). Geriatric individuals and patients receiving diuretics or who are otherwise volume depleted may be at greater risk of developing hyponatremia during therapy with SSRIs or SNRIs. Discontinuance of paroxetine should be considered in patients with symptomatic hyponatremia and appropriate medical intervention should be instituted. Because geriatric patients may be at increased risk for hyponatremia associated with these drugs, clinicians prescribing paroxetine in such patients should be aware of the possibility that such reactions may occur. In addition, periodic monitoring of serum sodium concentrations (particularly during the first several months) in geriatric patients receiving SSRIs has been recommended by some clinicians.

Hyperkalemia, hypercalcemia, hyperphosphatemia, dehydration, increased BUN, hypocalcemia, and hypokalemia have been reported in less than 0.1% of patients receiving the drug; however, these adverse effects have not been definitely attributed to paroxetine.

Urinary frequency and urinary disorders (principally difficulty with micturition or urinary hesitancy) have been reported in about 3% of patients receiving paroxetine in short-term controlled clinical trials. Although a definite causal relationship to paroxetine has not been established, amenorrhea, breast pain, menorrhagia, cystitis, urinary tract infection, dysuria, hematuria, nocturia, polyuria, pyuria, urinary incontinence, urinary retention, urinary urgency, and vaginitis have been reported in up to 1% of patients receiving the drug. In addition, spontaneous abortion, breast atrophy, vaginal hemorrhage, metrorrhagia, uterine spasm, oliguria, urethritis, salpingitis, urinary casts, renal calculus, renal pain, nephritis, vaginal candidiasis, female lactation, fibrocystic breast, mastitis, and epididymitis have been reported in less than 0.1% of patients receiving paroxetine; however, these adverse effects have not been definitely attributed to paroxetine. Breast enlargement also has been reported in some women receiving chronic therapy with paroxetine or other selective serotonin-reuptake inhibitors. In one study, approximately 40% of patients receiving either selective serotonin-reuptake inhibitors or venlafaxine reported some degree of breast enlargement; most patients with breast enlargement also experienced weight gain, and serum prolactin concentrations were increased in the paroxetine-treated women in this study.

In addition, acute renal failure and eclampsia also have been reported during postmarketing surveillance in patients receiving paroxetine; however, these adverse effects have not been definitely attributed to the drug.

■ **Hepatic Effects** Abnormal liver function test results, including elevations in serum ALT (SGOT) and AST (SGPT) concentrations, have been reported in up to 1% of patients receiving paroxetine, and rarely have been a reason for drug discontinuance. Elevated serum alkaline phosphatase concentrations, bilirubinemia, hepatitis, ascites, and jaundice have been reported in less than 0.1% of patients receiving the drug. In addition, death resulting from liver necrosis and substantially elevated serum aminotransferase (transaminase) concentrations associated with severe liver dysfunction have been reported rarely.

■ **Other Adverse Effects** Fever, influenza-like symptoms, infections, and trauma occurred in at least 2% of patients receiving paroxetine. In addition, chills, influenza, lymphadenopathy, and malaise have been reported in up to 1% of patients receiving the drug. Adrenergic syndrome, cellulitis, lymphedema, moniliasis, pelvic pain, and sepsis have been reported in less than 0.1% of patients receiving the drug, but a definite causal relationship to paroxetine has not been established. Pancreatitis and restless legs syndrome also have been reported during postmarketing surveillance in paroxetine-treated patients; however, a causal relationship to the drug has not been clearly established.

■ **Precautions and Contraindications** Worsening of depression and/or the emergence of suicidal ideation and behavior (suicidality) or unusual changes in behavior may occur in both adult and pediatric (see Cautions: Pediatric Precautions) patients with major depressive disorder or other psychiatric disorders, whether or not they are taking antidepressants. This risk may persist until clinically important remission occurs. Suicide is a known risk of depression and certain other psychiatric disorders, and these disorders themselves are the strongest predictors of suicide. However, there has been a long-standing concern that antidepressants may have a role in inducing worsening of depression and the emergence of suicidality in certain patients during the early phases of treatment. Pooled analyses of short-term, placebo-controlled studies of antidepressants (i.e., selective serotonin-reuptake inhibitors and other antidepressants) have shown an increased risk of suicidality in children, adolescents, and young adults (18–24 years of age) with major depressive disorder and other psychiatric disorders. An increased suicidality risk was not demonstrated with antidepressants compared with placebo in adults older than 24 years of age and a reduced risk was observed in adults 65 years of age or older. It is currently unknown whether the suicidality risk extends to longer-term use (i.e., beyond several months); however, there is substantial evidence from placebo-controlled maintenance trials in adults with major depressive disorder that antidepressants can delay the recurrence of depression.

The US Food and Drug Administration (FDA) recommends that all patients being treated with antidepressants for any indication be appropriately monitored and closely observed for clinical worsening, suicidality, and unusual changes in behavior, particularly during initiation of therapy (i.e., the first few months) and during periods of dosage adjustments. Families and caregivers of patients being treated with antidepressants for major depressive disorder or other indications, both psychiatric and nonpsychiatric, also should be advised to monitor patients on a daily basis for the emergence of agitation, irritability, or unusual changes in behavior, as well as the emergence of suicidality, and to report such symptoms immediately to a health-care provider.

Although a causal relationship between the emergence of symptoms such as anxiety, agitation, panic attacks, insomnia, irritability, hostility, aggressiveness, impulsivity, akathisia, hypomania, and/or mania and either the worsening of depression and/or the emergence of suicidal impulses has not been established, there is concern that such symptoms may represent precursors to emerging suicidality. Consequently, consideration should be given to changing the therapeutic regimen or discontinuing therapy in patients whose depression is persistently worse or in patients experiencing emergent suicidality or symptoms that might be precursors to worsening depression or suicidality, particularly if such manifestations are severe, abrupt in onset, or were not part of the patient's presenting symptoms. If a decision is made to discontinue therapy, paroxetine dosage should be tapered as rapidly as is feasible but with recognition of the risks of abrupt discontinuance. (See Dosage and Administration: Dosage.) FDA also recommends that the drugs be prescribed in the smallest quantity consistent with good patient management, in order to reduce the risk of overdosage.

It is generally believed (though not established in controlled trials) that treating a major depressive episode with an antidepressant alone may increase the likelihood of precipitating a mixed or manic episode in patients at risk for bipolar disorder. Therefore, patients should be adequately screened for bipolar disorder prior to initiating treatment with an antidepressant; such screening should include a detailed psychiatric history (e.g., family history of suicide, bipolar disorder, and depression).

Potentially life-threatening serotonin syndrome or neuroleptic malignant syndrome (NMS)-like reactions have been reported with SSRIs, including paroxetine, and selective serotonin- and norepinephrine-reuptake inhibitors (SNRIs) alone, but particularly with concurrent administration of other serotonergic drugs (including serotonin [5-hydroxytryptamine; 5-HT] type 1 receptor agonists ["triptans"]), drugs that impair the metabolism of serotonin (e.g., monoamine oxidase [MAO] inhibitors), or antipsychotic agents or other dopamine antagonists. Manifestations of serotonin syndrome may include mental status changes (e.g., agitation, hallucinations, coma), autonomic instability (e.g., tachycardia, labile blood pressure, hyperthermia), neuromuscular aberrations (e.g., hyperreflexia, incoordination), and/or GI symptoms (e.g., nausea, vomiting, diarrhea). In its most severe form, serotonin syndrome may resemble NMS, which is characterized by hyperthermia, muscle rigidity, autonomic instability with possible rapid fluctuation in vital signs, and mental status changes. Patients receiving paroxetine should be monitored for the development of serotonin syndrome or NMS-like signs and symptoms.

Concurrent or recent (i.e., within 2 weeks) therapy with MAO inhibitors used for treatment of depression is contraindicated in patients receiving paroxetine. If concurrent therapy with paroxetine and a 5-HT_1 receptor agonist (triptan) is clinically warranted, the patient should be observed carefully, particularly during initiation of therapy, when dosage is increased, or when another serotonergic agent is initiated. Concomitant use of paroxetine and serotonin precursors (e.g., tryptophan) is not recommended. If signs and symptoms of serotonin syndrome or NMS develop during therapy, treatment with paroxetine and any concurrently administered serotonergic or antidopaminergic agents, including antipsychotic agents, should be discontinued immediately and supportive and symptomatic treatment should be initiated. (See Drug Interactions: Serotonergic Drugs.)

Because clinical experience with paroxetine in patients with concurrent systemic disease, including cardiovascular disease, hepatic impairment, or renal impairment, is limited, caution should be exercised when paroxetine is administered to patients with any systemic disease or condition that may alter metabolism of the drug or adversely affect hemodynamic function. (See Dosage and Administration: Dosage.)

Because paroxetine may cause mydriasis, the drug should be used with caution in patients with angle-closure glaucoma.

Paroxetine should be used with caution in patients with severe renal or hepatic impairment, since increased plasma concentrations of the drug may occur in such patients. (See Pharmacokinetics: Elimination and see Dosage and Administration: Dosage in Renal and Hepatic Impairment.)

Although current evidence suggests that paroxetine is less cardiotoxic than most older antidepressant agents (see Cautions: Cardiovascular Effects), the safety of paroxetine in patients with a recent history of myocardial infarction or unstable cardiovascular disease has not been adequately evaluated to date.

Because of the potential for adverse drug interactions, the manufacturers recommend that patients receiving paroxetine be advised to notify their clinician if they are taking or plan to take nonprescription (over-the-counter) or prescription medications or alcohol-containing beverages or preparations. Although paroxetine has not been shown to potentiate the impairment of mental and motor skills caused by alcohol, the manufacturers recommend that patients be advised to avoid alcohol while receiving the drug.

Paroxetine generally is less sedating than most other currently available antidepressants and does not appear to produce substantial impairment of cognitive or psychomotor function nor to potentiate psychomotor impairment induced by other CNS depressants. However, patients should be cautioned that paroxetine may impair their ability to perform activities requiring mental alertness or physical coordination (e.g., operating machinery, driving a motor vehicle), particularly at dosages of 40 mg or more daily, and to avoid such activities until they experience how the drug affects them. In addition, the possibility that paroxetine may potentiate other (i.e., nonpsychomotor) adverse nervous system effects of CNS depressants should be considered.

The manufacturers recommend that patients receiving paroxetine be advised that while they may notice improvement within 1–4 weeks after starting therapy, they should continue therapy with the drug as directed by their physician.

Seizures have been reported in patients receiving therapeutic dosages of paroxetine. Because of limited experience with paroxetine in patients with a history of seizures, the drug should be used with caution in such patients and should be discontinued if seizures occur.

Activation of mania and hypomania has occurred in patients receiving therapeutic dosages of paroxetine. The drug should be used with caution in patients with a history of mania. (See Cautions: Nervous System Effects.)

Concomitant administration of paroxetine with tamoxifen, a prodrug requiring metabolic activation by CYP2D6, may result in reduced plasma concentrations of an active metabolite of tamoxifen (endoxifen) and thereby reduce the clinical efficacy of tamoxifen. (See Cautions: Precautions and Contraindications.) When tamoxifen is used for the treatment or prevention of breast cancer, clinicians should consider using an alternative antidepressant with little or no CYP2D6 inhibition potential.

Paroxetine and other SSRIs have been associated with the development of akathisia, which is characterized by an inner sense of restlessness and psychomotor agitation such as an inability to sit or stand still usually associated with subjective distress. Akathisia is most likely to occur within the first few weeks of therapy with these drugs.

Treatment with SSRIs, including paroxetine, and selective serotonin- and norepinephrine-reuptake inhibitors (SNRIs) may result in hyponatremia. In many cases, this hyponatremia appears to be due to the syndrome of inappropriate antidiuretic hormone secretion (SIADH) and was reversible when paroxetine was discontinued. Cases with serum sodium concentrations lower than 110 mEq/L have been reported. Geriatric individuals and patients receiving diuretics or who are otherwise volume depleted may be at greater risk of developing hyponatremia during therapy with SSRIs or SNRIs. Signs and symptoms of hyponatremia include headache, difficulty concentrating, memory impairment, confusion, weakness, and unsteadiness, which may lead to falls; more severe and/or acute cases have been associated with hallucinations, syncope, seizures, coma, respiratory arrest, and death. Discontinuance of paroxetine should be considered in patients with symptomatic hyponatremia and appropriate medical intervention should be instituted. (See Cautions: Renal, Electrolyte, and Genitourinary Effects and see also Cautions: Geriatric Precautions.)

The manufacturers state that there have been several cases of abnormal bleeding (mostly ecchymosis and purpura) and a case of impaired platelet aggregation in patients receiving paroxetine. (See Cautions: Hematologic Effects.)

Epidemiologic studies of bone fracture risk following exposure to various antidepressants, including SSRIs, have revealed an association between antidepressant treatment and fractures. There are a number of possible causes for this observation and it is currently unknown to what extent fracture risk is directly attributable to SSRI therapy. Pending further accumulation of data, the possibility of a pathological fracture (i.e., a fracture produced by minimal trauma in a patient with decreased bone mineral density) should be considered in paroxetine-treated patients who present with unexplained bone pain, point tenderness, swelling, or bruising.

Because paroxetine is the active moiety in both paroxetine mesylate conventional tablets (Pexeva®) and commercially available paroxetine hydrochloride preparations (e.g., Paxil®, nonproprietary [generic] preparations), concurrent administration of paroxetine hydrochloride and paroxetine mesylate should be avoided.

Paroxetine is contraindicated in patients concurrently receiving pimozide. (See Drug Interactions: Pimozide.)

Paroxetine is contraindicated in patients concomitantly receiving thioridazine. (See Drugs Metabolized by Cytochrome P-450 [CYP] 2D6 under Drug Interactions: Drugs Undergoing Hepatic Metabolism or Affecting Hepatic Microsomal Enzymes.)

Paroxetine should not be initiated in patients concurrently receiving linezolid or methylene blue. (See Monoamine Oxidase Inhibitors under Drug Interactions: Serotonergic Drugs.)

Paroxetine also is contraindicated in patients hypersensitive to the drug or any ingredient in the formulation.

■ **Pediatric Precautions** Safety and efficacy of paroxetine in children younger than 18 years of age have not been established.

Paroxetine has not demonstrated efficacy in several placebo-controlled trials in 752 children and adolescents with major depressive disorder. Adverse effects reported in at least 2% of the paroxetine-treated pediatric patients in these trials and that occurred at least twice as frequently as in pediatric patients receiving placebo included emotional lability (including self-harm, suicidal thoughts, attempted suicide, crying, and mood fluctuations), hostility, decreased appetite, tremor, sweating, hyperkinesia, and agitation. Upon discontinuance of paroxetine in these pediatric trials following a taper phase regimen, adverse events that occurred in at least 2% of the paroxetine-treated pediatric patients and occurred at least twice as frequently as in pediatric patients receiving placebo included emotional lability (including suicidal ideation, suicide attempt, mood changes, and tearfulness), nervousness, dizziness, nausea, and abdominal pain.

In June 2003, the United Kingdom (UK) regulatory agency warned clinicians to avoid the off-label use of paroxetine for the treatment of depression in children younger than 18 years of age. This action was taken in response to concern about a possible association between selective serotonin-reuptake inhibitors and suicidal behavior, which includes a broad range of symptoms ranging from episodes of self-harm to attempted suicide. Proprietary data examined by the UK regulatory agency showed a slight increase in suicidal behavior among patients who were randomly assigned to selective serotonin-reuptake inhibitor treatment, as compared with subjects who received placebo.

The US Food and Drug Administration (FDA) determined that the available data at that time were not sufficient either to establish or to rule out an association between the use of these drugs and increased suicidal thoughts or actions by pediatric patients. However, following the results of independent classification and analysis of the suicidal events and behaviors observed in controlled studies, FDA now warns that antidepressants increase the risk of suicidal thinking and behavior (suicidality) in children and adolescents with major depressive disorder and other psychiatric disorders. The risk of suicidality for these drugs was identified in a pooled analysis of data from a total of 24 short-term (4–16 weeks), placebo-controlled studies of 9 antidepressants (i.e., paroxetine, bupropion, citalopram, fluoxetine, fluvoxamine, mirtazapine, nefazodone, sertraline, venlafaxine) in over 4400 children and adolescents with major depressive disorder, obsessive-compulsive disorder (OCD), or other psychiatric disorders. The analysis revealed a greater risk of adverse events representing suicidal behavior or thinking (suicidality) during the first few months of treatment in pediatric patients receiving antidepressants than in those receiving placebo. However, a more recent meta-analysis of 27 placebo-controlled trials of 9 antidepressants (SSRIs and others) in patients younger than 19 years of age with major depressive disorder, OCD, or non-OCD anxiety disorders suggests that the benefits of antidepressant therapy in treating these conditions may outweigh the risks of suicidal behavior or suicidal ideation. No suicides occurred in these pediatric trials.

The risk of suicidality in the FDA's pooled analysis differed across the different psychiatric indications, with the highest incidence observed in the major depressive disorder studies. In addition, although there was considerable variation in risk among the antidepressants, a tendency toward an increase in suicidality risk in younger patients was found for almost all drugs studied. It is currently unknown whether the suicidality risk in pediatric patients extends to longer-term use (i.e., beyond several months).

As a result of this analysis and public discussion of the issue, FDA has directed manufacturers of all antidepressants to add a boxed warning to the labeling of their products to alert clinicians of this suicidality risk in children and adolescents and to recommend appropriate monitoring and close observation of patients receiving these agents. (See Cautions: Precautions and Contraindications.) The drugs that are the focus of the revised labeling are all drugs included in the general class of antidepressants, including those that have not been studied in controlled clinical trials in pediatric patients, since the available data are not adequate to exclude any single antidepressant from an increased risk. In addition to the boxed warning and other information in professional labeling on antidepressants, FDA currently recommends that a patient medication guide explaining the risks associated with the drugs be provided to the patient each time the drugs are dispensed. Caregivers of pediatric patients whose depression is persistently worse or who are experiencing emergent suicidality or symptoms that might be precursors to worsening depression or suicidality during antidepressant therapy should consult their clinician regarding the best course of action (e.g., whether the therapeutic regimen should be changed or paroxetine discontinued). *Patients should not discontinue use of paroxetine without first consulting their clinician; it is very important that paroxetine not be abruptly discontinued (see Dosage and Administration: Dosage), as withdrawal effects may occur.*

Decreased appetite and weight loss have been observed in association with SSRI therapy. Therefore, regular monitoring of weight and growth should be performed in children and adolescents receiving an SSRI, including paroxetine.

Anyone considering the use of paroxetine in a child or adolescent for any clinical use must balance the potential risk of therapy with the clinical need.

■ **Geriatric Precautions** While safety and efficacy of paroxetine in geriatric patients have not been established specifically, 17% of patients (approximately 700) receiving the drug for depression in clinical trials were 65 years of age or older. Although no overall differences in efficacy or the adverse effect profile of paroxetine were observed between geriatric and younger patients and other clinical experience revealed no evidence of age-related differences, pharmacokinetic studies have revealed a decreased clearance of paroxetine in geriatric patients. (See Pharmacokinetics: Elimination.) For this reason, the manufacturers and some clinicians recommend initiating paroxetine therapy in patients 65 years of age or older at a lower dosage than in younger patients. (See Dosage and Administration: Dosage in Geriatric or Debilitated Patients.)

Geriatric patients appear to be more likely than younger patients to develop paroxetine-induced hyponatremia and transient syndrome of inappropriate secretion of antidiuretic hormone (SIADH). Therefore, clinicians prescribing paroxetine in geriatric patients should be aware of the possibility that such reactions may occur. Periodic monitoring (especially during the first several months) of serum sodium concentrations in geriatric patients receiving the drug has been recommended by some clinicians.

In studies comparing paroxetine and various tricyclic antidepressants, including amitriptyline, clomipramine, and doxepin, in geriatric patients, paroxetine was at least as effective and as well tolerated as or better tolerated than tricyclic antidepressants. In addition, serum anticholinergicity of paroxetine was found to be substantially lower than that of nortriptyline in geriatric depressed patients; complaints of dry mouth and tachycardia also occurred more frequently in nortriptyline-treated patients than in those receiving paroxetine. These findings indicate that, at therapeutic plasma concentrations, paroxetine has approximately 20% the anticholinergic potential of nortriptyline in older patients. Overall, paroxetine was less frequently associated with dry mouth, somnolence, constipation, tachycardia, or confusion than tricyclic antidepressants, although certain adverse effects (e.g., nausea, diarrhea, headache) were more common with paroxetine. In geriatric patients with depression, paroxetine appears to be at least as effective as fluoxetine.

In pooled data analyses, a *reduced* risk of suicidality was observed in adults 65 years of age or older with antidepressant therapy compared with placebo. (See Cautions: Precautions and Contraindications.)

As with other psychotropic drugs, geriatric patients receiving antidepressants appear to have an increased risk of hip fracture. Despite the fewer cardiovascular and anticholinergic effects associated with selective serotonin-reuptake inhibitors (SSRIs), these drugs did not show any advantage over tricyclic antidepressants with regard to hip fracture in a case-control study. In addition, there was little difference in the rates of falls between nursing home residents receiving SSRIs and those receiving tricyclic antidepressants in a retrospective study. Therefore, all geriatric individuals receiving either type of antidepressant should be considered to be at increased risk of falls and appropriate measures should be taken.

■ **Mutagenicity and Carcinogenicity** Paroxetine was not mutagenic in several in vitro tests including the bacterial mutation assay, mouse lymphoma mutation assay, and unscheduled DNA synthesis assay. The drug also was not mutagenic in tests for cytogenetic aberrations in vivo in mouse bone marrow, in vitro in human lymphocytes, and in a dominant lethal test in rats.

Studies to determine the carcinogenic potential of paroxetine were performed in mice receiving oral dosages of 1, 5, and 25 mg/kg daily and in rats receiving dosages of 1, 5, and 20 mg/kg daily for 2 years. In mice, the maximum dosage was up to approximately 2.4 times the maximum human dose for depression, social anxiety disorder, generalized anxiety disorder, and PTSD on a mg/m^2 basis. In rats, the maximum dosage was up to approximately 3.9 times the maximum human dose for depression on a mg/m^2 basis. Because the maximum recommended human dosage for depression, social anxiety disorder, generalized anxiety disorder, and PTSD is slightly lower than that for obsessive-compulsive disorder (50 versus 60 mg daily, respectively), the dosages used in these carcinogenicity studies were only about 2 and 3.2 times the maximum recommended human dosage for obsessive-compulsive disorder in mice and rats, respectively. A substantially greater number of male rats in the high-dose group had reticulum cell sarcomas (1/100, 0/50, 0/50, and 4/50 for control, low-, middle-, and high-dose groups, respectively), and a substantially increased linear trend across dose groups was evident for the occurrence of lymphoreticular tumors in male rats. Female rats were not affected. Although there was a dose-related increase in the number of tumors in mice, there was no drug-related increase in the number of mice with tumors. The relationship of these findings to human exposure to paroxetine is not known.

■ **Pregnancy, Fertility, and Lactation** ***Pregnancy*** Some neonates exposed to paroxetine and other selective serotonin-reuptake inhibitors (SSRIs) or selective serotonin- and norepinephrine-reuptake inhibitors (SNRIs) late in the third trimester of pregnancy have developed complications that occasionally have been severe and required prolonged hospitalization, respiratory support, enteral nutrition, and other forms of supportive care in special care nurseries. Such complications can arise immediately upon delivery and usually last for several days or up to 2–4 weeks. Clinical findings reported to date in the neonates have included respiratory distress, cyanosis, apnea, seizures, temperature instability or fever, feeding difficulty, dehydration, excessive weight loss, vomiting, hypoglycemia, hypotonia, hypertonia, hyperreflexia, tremor, jitteriness, irritability, lethargy, reduced or lack of reaction to pain stimuli, and constant crying. These clinical features appear to be consistent with either a direct toxic effect of the SSRI or SNRI or, possibly, a drug withdrawal syndrome. It should be noted that, in some cases, the clinical picture was consistent with serotonin syndrome (see Drug Interactions: Serotonergic Drugs).

Infants exposed to SSRIs in late pregnancy may have an increased risk of persistent pulmonary hypertension of the newborn (PPHN). PPHN is a rare heart and lung condition occurring in an estimated 1–2 infants per 1,000 births in the general population; it occurs when a neonate does not adapt to breathing outside the womb. Some experts have suggested that respiratory distress in neonates exposed to SSRIs may occur along a spectrum of seriousness in association with maternal use of SSRIs, with PPHN among the most serious consequences. Neonates with PPHN may require intensive care support, including mechanical ventilation; in severe cases, multiple organ damage, including brain damage, and even death may occur. Although several epidemiologic studies have suggested an increased risk of PPHN with SSRI use during pregnancy, other studies did not demonstrate a statistically significant association. Thus, the FDA states that it is currently unclear whether use of SSRIs, including paroxetine, during pregnancy can cause PPHN and recommends that clinicians not alter their current clinical practice of treating depression during pregnancy.

When treating a pregnant woman with paroxetine during the third trimester of pregnancy, the clinician should carefully consider the potential risks and benefits of such therapy. Clinicians should consider that in a prospective longitudinal study of 201 women with a history of recurrent major depression who were euthymic in the context of antidepressant therapy at the beginning of pregnancy, women who discontinued their antidepressant medication (SSRIs, tricyclic antidepressants, or others) during pregnancy were found to be substantially more likely to have a relapse of depression than were women who continued to receive their antidepressant therapy while pregnant.

For additional information on the management of depression in women prior to conception and during pregnancy, including treatment algorithms, the FDA advises clinicians to consult the joint American Psychiatric Association and American College of Obstetricians and Gynecologists guidelines (at https://www.ncbi.nlm.nih.gov/pmc/articles/PMC3103063/pdf/nihms293836.pdf).

Reproduction studies in rats receiving oral paroxetine dosages of 50 mg/kg daily and in rabbits receiving 6 mg/kg daily during organogenesis have been conducted. These dosages correspond to approximately 9.7 and 2.2 times the maximum recommended human dose for depression, social anxiety disorder, generalized anxiety disorder, and PTSD and approximately 8.1 and 1.9 times the maximum recommended human dose for obsessive-compulsive disorder on a mg/m^2 basis in rats and rabbits, respectively. Although these studies have not revealed evidence of teratogenicity, an increase in pup deaths was observed in rats during the first 4 days of lactation when dosing occurred during the last trimester of gestation and continued throughout lactation. This effect occurred at a dose of 1 mg/kg daily, which corresponds to 0.19 times the maximum recommended human dose for depression, social anxiety disorder, generalized anxiety disorder, and PTSD and 0.16 times the maximum recommended human dose for obsessive-compulsive disorder on a mg/m^2 basis. The no-effect dose for rat pup mortality has not been determined and the cause of these deaths is not known.

Preliminary analyses from 2 epidemiologic studies have shown that infants born to women exposed to paroxetine during the first trimester of pregnancy had an increased risk of cardiovascular malformations, principally ventricular and atrial septal defects. In one of these studies using Swedish national registry data, infants born to 6896 women exposed to antidepressants during the first trimester of pregnancy were evaluated; 5175 of the infants born to 5123 of these women were exposed to SSRIs, including 822 infants born to 815 women reporting first trimester use of paroxetine. An analysis of these data indicated that infants exposed to paroxetine during early pregnancy had an increased risk of cardiovascular malformations (principally ventricular and atrial septal defects) compared to the entire registry population. The rate of cardiovascular malformations following early pregnancy exposure to paroxetine was approximately 2% compared with 1% in the entire registry population. An analysis of the data from the same paroxetine-exposed infants revealed no increase in the overall risk of congenital malformations.

A separate retrospective cohort epidemiologic study using U.S. United Healthcare data evaluated 5956 infants born to women dispensed paroxetine (822 infants born to 815 women) or other antidepressants during the first trimester of pregnancy showed a trend toward an increased risk for cardiovascular malformations for paroxetine compared with other antidepressants. The prevalence of cardiovascular malformations following first trimester dispensing was 1.5% for paroxetine compared with 1% for other antidepressants; most of the observed cardiovascular malformations (in 9 out of 12 paroxetine-exposed infants) were ventricular septal defects. This study also demonstrated an increased risk of overall major congenital malformations (inclusive of cardiovascular malformations) for paroxetine compared with other antidepressants; the prevalence of all congenital malformations following first trimester exposure was 4% for paroxetine compared with 2% for other antidepressants.

In addition, a smaller study examining pregnancy outcomes in pregnant women exposed to paroxetine or fluoxetine who contacted two teratogen information services in Israel and Italy reported a higher overall rate of congenital malformations in infants exposed to paroxetine in the first trimester compared with infants in the control group with exposures to drugs not known to be teratogenic (5.1% and 2.6%, respectively). A higher rate of cardiovascular anomalies was also observed in the paroxetine group (1.9%) compared with the control group (0.6%) in this study. Similar trends were reported in the fluoxetine group but these did not achieve statistical significance.

Previous epidemiologic studies of pregnancy outcome following first trimester exposure to SSRIs, including paroxetine, had not revealed evidence of an increased risk of major congenital malformations. In a prospective, controlled, multicenter study, maternal use of SSRIs (paroxetine, fluvoxamine, sertraline) in a limited number of pregnant women did not appear to increase the risk of congenital malformation, miscarriage, stillbirth, or premature delivery when used during pregnancy at recommended dosages. Birth weight and gestational age in neonates exposed to the drugs were similar to those in the control group. In addition, an increased risk of major congenital malformations was not observed in infants in 2 small, case-control studies based on prospectively gathered epidemiologic data collected in women exposed to paroxetine during the first trimester of pregnancy. In another small study based on medical records review, the incidence of congenital anomalies reported in infants born to women who were treated with paroxetine and other SSRIs during pregnancy was comparable to that observed in the general population.

Based on the conflicting preliminary findings reported to date from the available studies, the manufacturer of paroxetine hydrochloride states that it is unclear whether a causal relationship exists between these congenital malformations and maternal paroxetine exposure. However, the available data indicate that the individual risk of a mother having an infant with a cardiovascular malformation following first trimester paroxetine exposure is approximately 1/50, compared with an expected rate for such defects of approximately 1/100 infants in the general population. In general, septal defects range from those that are symptomatic and require surgical intervention to those that are asymptomatic and may resolve spontaneously. The final results of recent studies and additional data relating to the use of paroxetine during pregnancy will be analyzed further once they become available to better characterize the risk for congenital malformations with paroxetine.

The manufacturers of paroxetine state that if a woman becomes pregnant while receiving paroxetine, she should be informed of the potential hazard to the fetus. Unless the potential benefits to the mother justify continuing treatment, consideration should be given to either discontinuing paroxetine therapy or switching to another antidepressant. For women who intend to become pregnant or are in their first trimester of pregnancy, the manufacturer of paroxetine hydrochloride states that paroxetine should only be initiated after consideration of the other available treatment options.

The effect of paroxetine on labor and delivery is not known. However, there have been postmarketing reports of premature births in pregnant women who have received paroxetine or other selective serotonin-reuptake inhibitors.

Fertility Reproduction studies in rats receiving paroxetine dosages of 15 mg/kg daily, which corresponds to 2.9 times the highest recommended human daily dose for depression, social anxiety disorder, generalized anxiety disorder, and PTSD and 2.4 times the highest recommended human daily dose for obsessive-compulsive disorder on a mg/m^2 basis, revealed evidence of a reduced pregnancy rate. In toxicity studies performed for 2–52 weeks in male rats receiving paroxetine, irreversible lesions in the reproductive tract were reported. These lesions consisted of vacuolation of epididymal tubular epithelium in male rats receiving paroxetine dosages of 50 mg/kg daily (9.8 times the highest recommended human daily dose in major depressive disorder, social anxiety disorder, and generalized anxiety disorder and 8.2 times the highest recommended human daily dose in obsessive-compulsive disorder and panic disorder on a mg/m^2 basis). In male rats receiving paroxetine dosages of 25 mg/kg daily (4.9 times the highest recommended human daily dose in major depressive disorder, social anxiety disorder, and generalized anxiety disorder and 4.1 times the highest recommended human daily dose in obsessive-compulsive disorder and panic disorder on a mg/m^2 basis), atrophic changes in the seminiferous tubules of the testes with arrested spermatogenesis were observed.

Some clinical studies have shown that SSRIs, including paroxetine, may affect sperm quality during therapy, which may affect fertility in some men.

Lactation Paroxetine is distributed into human milk. (See Pharmacokinetics: Distribution.) Paroxetine should be used with caution in nursing women, and women should be advised to notify their clinician if they plan to breast-feed.

Drug Interactions

■ **Serotonergic Drugs** Use of selective serotonin-reuptake inhibitors (SSRIs) such as paroxetine concurrently or in close succession with other drugs that affect serotonergic neurotransmission may result in serotonin syndrome or neuroleptic malignant syndrome (NMS)-like reactions. Manifestations of serotonin syndrome may include mental status changes (e.g., agitation, hallucinations, coma), autonomic instability (e.g., tachycardia, labile blood pressure, hyperthermia), neuromuscular aberrations (e.g., hyperreflexia, incoordination), and/or GI symptoms (e.g., nausea, vomiting, diarrhea). Although the syndrome appears to be relatively uncommon and usually mild in severity, serious and potentially life-threatening complications, including seizures, disseminated intravascular coagulation, respiratory failure, and severe hyperthermia, as well as death occasionally have been reported. In its most severe form, serotonin syndrome may resemble NMS, which is characterized by hyperthermia, muscle rigidity, autonomic instability with possible rapid fluctuation in vital signs, and mental status changes. The precise mechanism of these reactions is not fully understood; however, they appear to result from excessive serotonergic activity in the CNS, probably mediated by activation of serotonin 5-HT$_{1A}$ receptors. The possible involvement of dopamine and 5-HT$_2$ receptors also has been suggested, although their roles remain unclear.

Serotonin syndrome most commonly occurs when 2 or more drugs that affect serotonergic neurotransmission are administered either concurrently or in close succession. Serotonin syndrome also has been reported when paroxetine was given together with another drug that impairs the hepatic metabolism of paroxetine. Serotonergic agents include those that increase serotonin synthesis (e.g., the serotonin precursor tryptophan), stimulate synaptic serotonin release (e.g., some amphetamines, dexfenfluramine [no longer commercially available in the US], fenfluramine [no longer commercially available in the US]), inhibit the reuptake of serotonin after release (e.g., SSRIs, selective serotonin- and norepinephrine-reuptake inhibitors [SNRIs], tricyclic antidepressants, trazodone, dextromethorphan, meperidine, tramadol), decrease the metabolism of serotonin (e.g., monoamine oxidase [MAO] inhibitors), have direct serotonin postsynaptic receptor activity (e.g., buspirone), or nonspecifically induce increases in serotonergic neuronal activity (e.g., lithium salts). Selective agonists of serotonin (5-hydroxytryptamine; 5-HT) type 1 receptors ("triptans") and dihydroergotamine, agents with serotonergic activity used in the management of migraine headache, and St. John's wort (*Hypericum perforatum*) also have been implicated in several cases of serotonin syndrome.

The combination of SSRIs and MAO inhibitors may result in serotonin syndrome or NMS-like reactions. Such reactions also have been reported in patients receiving SSRIs concomitantly with tryptophan, lithium, dextromethorphan, sumatriptan, dihydroergotamine, or antipsychotics or other dopamine antagonists. In rare cases, serotonin syndrome reportedly has occurred in patients receiving the recommended dosage of a single serotonergic agent (e.g., clomipramine) or during accidental overdosage (e.g., sertraline intoxication in a child). Some other drugs that have been implicated in precipitating symptoms suggestive of serotonin syndrome or NMS-like reactions include buspirone, bromocriptine, dextropropoxyphene, fentanyl, linezolid, methylene blue, methylenedioxymethamphetamine (MDMA; "ecstasy"), selegiline (a selective MAO-B inhibitor), and sibutramine (an SNRI used for the management of obesity [no longer commercially available in the US]). Other drugs that have been associated with the syndrome but for which less convincing data are available include carbamazepine and pentazocine.

Clinicians should be aware of the potential for serious, possibly fatal reactions associated with serotonin syndrome or NMS-like reactions in patients receiving 2 or more drugs that affect serotonergic neurotransmission, even if no such interactions with the specific drugs have been reported to date in the medical literature. Pending further accumulation of data, drugs that affect serotonergic neurotransmission should be used cautiously in combination and such combinations should be avoided whenever clinically possible. Serotonin syndrome may be more likely to occur when initiating therapy with a serotonergic agent, increasing the dosage, or following the addition of another serotonergic agent. Some clinicians state that patients who have experienced serotonin syndrome may be at higher risk for recurrence of the syndrome upon reinitiation of serotonergic drugs. Pending further experience in such cases, some clinicians recommend that therapy with serotonergic agents be limited following recovery. In cases in which the potential benefit of the drug is thought to outweigh the risk of serotonin syndrome, lower potency agents and reduced dosages should be used, combination serotonergic therapy should be avoided, and patients should be monitored carefully for manifestations of serotonin syndrome. If signs and symptoms of serotonin syndrome or NMS develop during therapy, treatment with paroxetine and any concurrently administered serotonergic or antidopaminergic agents, including antipsychotic agents, should be discontinued immediately and supportive and symptomatic treatment should be initiated.

For further information on serotonin syndrome, including manifestations and treatment, see Serotonin Syndrome under Drug Interactions: Serotonergic Drugs, in Fluoxetine Hydrochloride 28:16.04.20.

Monoamine Oxidase Inhibitors Potentially serious, sometimes fatal serotonin syndrome or NMS-like reactions have been reported in patients receiving SSRIs in combination with an MAO inhibitor. Such reactions also have been reported in patients who recently have discontinued an SSRI and have been started on an MAO inhibitor. While there are no human data to date demonstrating such interactions with paroxetine, limited data from animal studies evaluating the effects of concomitant use of paroxetine and an MAO inhibitor suggest that these drugs may act synergistically to elevate blood pressure and produce behavioral excitation.

Because of the potential risk of serotonin syndrome or NMS-like reactions, concomitant use of paroxetine and MAO inhibitors is contraindicated. At least 2 weeks should elapse between discontinuance of MAO inhibitor therapy and initiation of paroxetine therapy and vice versa.

Linezolid. Linezolid, an anti-infective agent that is a nonselective and reversible MAO inhibitor, has been associated with drug interactions resulting in serotonin syndrome, including some associated with SSRIs, and potentially may also cause NMS-like reactions. Because of the risk of serotonin syndrome, linezolid generally should *not* be used in patients receiving paroxetine. The US Food and Drug Administration (FDA) states that certain life-threatening or urgent situations may necessitate immediate linezolid treatment in a patient receiving a serotonergic drug, including SSRIs. In such emergency situations, the availability of alternative anti-infectives should be considered and the benefits of linezolid should be weighed against the risk of serotonin syndrome. If linezolid is indicated in such emergency situations, paroxetine must be immediately discontinued and the patient monitored for symptoms of CNS toxicity (e.g., mental changes, muscle twitching, excessive sweating, shivering/shaking, diarrhea, loss of coordination, fever) for 2 weeks or until 24 hours after the last linezolid dose, whichever comes first. Treatment with paroxetine may be resumed 24 hours after the last linezolid dose.

If nonemergency use of linezolid is being planned for a patient receiving paroxetine, paroxetine should be withheld for at least 2 weeks prior to initiating linezolid.

Treatment with paroxetine should not be initiated in a patient receiving linezolid; when necessary, paroxetine may be started 24 hours after the last linezolid dose. (See Drug Interactions: Serotonergic Drugs, in Linezolid 8:12.28.24.)

Methylene Blue. There have been case reports of serotonin syndrome in patients who received methylene blue, which is a potent and selective inhibitor of MAO-A, while receiving serotonergic drugs, including SSRIs (e.g., citalopram, escitalopram, fluoxetine, fluvoxamine, paroxetine, sertraline). Therefore, methylene blue generally should *not* be used in patients receiving paroxetine. The FDA states that certain emergency situations (e.g., methemoglobinemia, ifosfamide-induced encephalopathy†) may necessitate immediate use of methylene blue in a patient receiving paroxetine. In such emergency situations, the availability of alternative interventions should be considered and the benefits of methylene blue should be weighed against the risk of serotonin syndrome. If methylene blue is indicated in such emergency situations, paroxetine must be immediately discontinued and the patient monitored for symptoms of CNS toxicity (e.g., mental changes, muscle twitching, excessive sweating, shivering/shaking, diarrhea, loss of coordination, fever) for 2 weeks or until 24 hours after the last methylene blue dose, whichever come first. Treatment with paroxetine may be resumed 24 hours after the last methylene blue dose.

If nonemergency use of methylene blue is being planned for a patient receiving paroxetine, paroxetine should be withheld for at least 2 weeks prior to initiating methylene blue.

Treatment with paroxetine should not be initiated in a patient receiving methylene blue; when necessary, paroxetine may be started 24 hours after the last methylene blue dose.

Moclobemide. Moclobemide (not commercially available in the US), a selective and reversible MAO-A inhibitor, has been associated with serotonin syndrome, and such reactions have been fatal in several cases in which the drug was given in combination with the SSRI citalopram or with clomipramine. Pending further experience with such combinations, some clinicians recommend that concurrent therapy with moclobemide and SSRIs be used only with extreme caution and that these drugs should have been discontinued for some time (depending on the elimination half-lives of the drug and its active metabolites) before initiating moclobemide therapy.

Selegiline. Selegiline, a selective MAO-B inhibitor used in the management of parkinsonian syndrome, has been reported to cause serotonin syndrome when used concomitantly with SSRIs (e.g., fluoxetine, paroxetine, sertraline). Although selegiline is a selective MAO-B inhibitor at therapeutic dosages, the drug appears to lose its selectivity for the MAO-B enzyme at higher dosages (e.g., those exceeding 10 mg/kg), thereby increasing the risk of serotonin syndrome in patients receiving higher dosages of the drug either alone or in combination with other serotonergic agents. The manufacturer of selegiline recommends avoiding concurrent selegiline and SSRI therapy. In addition, the manufacturer of selegiline recommends that at least 2 weeks elapse between discontinuance of selegiline and initiation of SSRI therapy.

Isoniazid. Isoniazid, an antituberculosis agent, appears to have some MAO-inhibiting activity. In addition, iproniazid (not commercially available in the US), another antituberculosis agent structurally related to isoniazid that also possesses MAO-inhibiting activity, reportedly has resulted in serotonin syndrome in at least 2 patients when given in combination with meperidine. Pending further experience, clinicians should be aware of the potential for serotonin syndrome when isoniazid is given in conjunction with SSRI therapy (such as paroxetine) or other serotonergic agents.

Other Selective Serotonin-reuptake Inhibitors and Selective Serotonin- and Norepinephrine-reuptake Inhibitors Concomitant administration of paroxetine with other SSRIs or SNRIs potentially may result in serotonin syndrome or NMS-like reactions and is therefore not recommended.

Antipsychotic Agents and Other Dopamine Antagonists Concomitant use of antipsychotic agents and other dopamine antagonists with paroxetine rarely may result in potentially serious, sometimes fatal serotonin syndrome or NMS-like reactions. If signs and symptoms of serotonin syndrome or NMS occur, treatment with paroxetine and any concurrently administered antidopaminergic or serotonergic agents should be immediately discontinued and supportive and symptomatic treatment initiated. (See Drugs Metabolized by Cytochrome P-450 [CYP] 2D6 under Drug Interactions: Drugs Undergoing Hepatic Metabolism or Affecting Hepatic Microsomal Enzymes and see Drug Interactions: Clozapine and see Drug Interactions: Pimozide.)

Tryptophan and Other Serotonin Precursors As with other serotonin-reuptake inhibitors, an interaction between paroxetine and tryptophan, a serotonin precursor, may occur during concurrent use. Adverse reactions reported to date during concomitant therapy resembled serotonin syndrome and have consisted principally of headache, nausea, sweating, and dizziness. Because of the potential risk of serotonin syndrome or NMS-like reactions, concurrent use of tryptophan or other serotonin precursors should be avoided in patients receiving paroxetine.

Sibutramine Because of the possibility of developing potentially serious, sometimes fatal serotonin syndrome or NMS-like reactions, sibutramine (no longer commercially available in the US) should be used with caution in patients receiving paroxetine.

5-HT$_1$ Receptor Agonists ("Triptans") Weakness, hyperreflexia, and incoordination have been reported rarely during postmarketing surveillance in patients receiving sumatriptan concomitantly with an SSRI (e.g., citalopram, escitalopram, fluoxetine, fluvoxamine, paroxetine, sertraline). Oral or subcutaneous sumatriptan and SSRIs were used concomitantly in some clinical studies without unusual adverse effects. However, an increase in the frequency of migraine attacks and a decrease in the effectiveness of sumatriptan in relieving migraine headache have been reported in a patient receiving subcutaneous injections of sumatriptan intermittently while undergoing fluoxetine therapy.

Clinicians prescribing 5-HT$_1$ receptor agonists, SSRIs, and SNRIs should consider that triptans often are used intermittently and that either the 5-HT$_1$ receptor agonist, SSRI, or SNRI may be prescribed by a different clinician. Clinicians also should weigh the potential risk of serotonin syndrome or NMS-like reactions with the expected benefit of using a triptan concurrently with SSRI or SNRI therapy. If concomitant treatment with paroxetine and a triptan is clinically warranted, the patient should be observed carefully, particularly during treatment initiation, dosage increases, and following the addition of other serotonergic agents. Patients receiving concomitant triptan and SSRI or SNRI therapy should be informed of the possibility of serotonin syndrome or NMS-like reactions and advised to immediately seek medical attention if they experience signs or symptoms of these syndromes.

Fentanyl Because cases of serotonin syndrome have been reported in patients concurrently receiving fentanyl and SSRIs, including paroxetine, clinicians should be aware of this potential interaction and monitor patients receiving these drugs in combination for possible signs and symptoms of serotonin syndrome.

Tramadol and Other Serotonergic Drugs Because of the potential risk of serotonin syndrome or NMS-like reactions, caution is advised whenever SSRIs, including paroxetine, and SNRIs are concurrently administered with other drugs that may affect serotonergic neurotransmitter systems, including tramadol and St. John's wort (*Hypericum perforatum*).

■ **Drugs Undergoing Hepatic Metabolism or Affecting Hepatic Microsomal Enzymes** The metabolism and pharmacokinetics of paroxetine may be affected by a number of drugs that induce (e.g., phenobarbital) or inhibit (e.g., cimetidine, tricyclic antidepressants) drug-metabolizing enzymes.

Drugs Metabolized by Cytochrome P-450 (CYP) 2D6 Paroxetine, like many other antidepressants (e.g., other SSRIs, many tricyclic antidepressants), is metabolized by the drug-metabolizing cytochrome P-450 (CYP) 2D6 isoenzyme (debrisoquine hydroxylase). In addition, like many other drugs metabolized by CYP2D6, paroxetine inhibits the activity of CYP2D6 and potentially may increase plasma concentrations of concomitantly administered drugs that also are metabolized by this isoenzyme. Although similar interactions are possible with other SSRIs, there is considerable variability among the drugs in the extent to which they inhibit CYP2D6; fluoxetine and paroxetine appear to be more potent in this regard than sertraline. In most patients (greater than 90%), the CYP2D6 isoenzyme is saturated early during paroxetine therapy. At steady state when the CYP2D6 pathway is essentially saturated, paroxetine is cleared by alternative cytochrome P-450 isoenzymes which, unlike CYP2D6, show no evidence of saturation.

Concomitant administration of paroxetine with risperidone, a CYP2D6 substrate, was evaluated in one study. In 10 patients with schizophrenia or schizoaffective disorder stabilized on risperidone therapy (4–8 mg daily) who also received paroxetine (20 mg daily) for 4 weeks, mean plasma concentrations of risperidone increased approximately fourfold, mean plasma concentrations of 9-hydroxyrisperidone (the active metabolite of risperidone) decreased by approximately 10%, and concentrations of the active moiety (the sum of the plasma concentrations of risperidone and 9-hydroxyrisperidone) increased by approximately 1.4 fold. These drugs were generally well tolerated when administered concurrently, with the exception of one patient who developed parkinsonian symptoms. Although the precise mechanism for this interaction remains to be fully established, it appears that paroxetine may impair the elimination of risperidone, principally by inhibiting CYP2D6-mediated 9-hydroxylation and, to a lesser extent, by simultaneously affecting the further metabolism of 9-hydroxyrisperidone or other pathways of risperidone biotransformation. Pending further accumulation of data, some clinicians recommend careful clinical observation and possible monitoring of plasma risperidone concentrations when paroxetine and risperidone are given concurrently. Consideration also should be given to using a lower initial dosage of paroxetine (10–20 mg daily) since the inhibitory effect of paroxetine on CYP2D6 is concentration dependent.

The steady-state pharmacokinetics of atomoxetine were altered when the drug was administered at a dosage of 20 mg twice daily concurrently with paroxetine 20 mg daily in healthy adults who were extensive CYP2D6 metabolizers. Concurrent administration with paroxetine increased maximum plasma atomoxetine concentrations threefold to fourfold and steady-state area under the plasma concentration curve was increased sixfold to eightfold compared with administration of atomoxetine alone. The pharmacokinetics of paroxetine were not altered. The manufacturers of paroxetine and atomoxetine recommend that atomoxetine be administered at a reduced dosage when the drugs are administered concurrently.

Concomitant use of paroxetine with other drugs metabolized by CYP2D6 has not been systematically studied. The extent to which this potential interaction may become clinically important depends on the extent of inhibition of CYP2D6 by the antidepressant and the therapeutic index of the concomitantly administered drug. The drugs for which this potential interaction is of greatest concern are those that are metabolized principally by CYP2D6 and have a narrow therapeutic index, such as tricyclic antidepressants, class IC antiarrhythmics (e.g., propafenone, flecainide, encainide), risperidone, and some phenothiazines (e.g., perphenazine, thioridazine).

In one study, chronic dosing of paroxetine (20 mg once daily) under steady-state conditions increased single-dose desipramine (100 mg) peak plasma concentrations, AUC, and elimination half-life by an average of approximately two-, five-, and threefold, respectively. (See Drug Interactions: Tricyclic and Other Antidepressants.)

Administration of perphenazine in patients receiving paroxetine 20 mg daily for 10 days increased plasma concentrations and the adverse CNS effects of perphenazine. This interaction appears to result principally from paroxetine-induced inhibition of the CYP2D6 isoenzyme. Pending further experience with combined therapy, a reduction in perphenazine dosage may be necessary to prevent adverse CNS effects in patients receiving paroxetine.

For information on a potential interaction between paroxetine and metoprolol, see Drug Interactions: β-Adrenergic Blocking Agents.

Concurrent use of paroxetine with other drugs metabolized by CYP2D6, including certain antidepressants (e.g., nortriptyline, amitriptyline, imipramine, desipramine, fluoxetine), phenothiazines (e.g., perphenazine), and class IC antiarrhythmics, or drugs that inhibit CYP2D6 should be approached with caution. Because concomitant use of paroxetine and thioridazine may result in increased plasma concentrations of the phenothiazine and increase the risk of serious, potentially fatal, adverse cardiac effects (e.g., ventricular arrhythmias, sudden death), thioridazine should not be used concomitantly with paroxetine (see Cautions: Precautions and Contraindications). The manufacturer of paroxetine states that concurrent use of a drug metabolized by CYP2D6 may necessitate the administration of dosages of the other drugs that are lower than those usually prescribed. Furthermore, whenever paroxetine therapy is discontinued (and plasma concentrations of the drug are decreased) during concurrent therapy with another drug metabolized by CYP2D6, an increased dosage of the concurrently administered drug may be necessary.

Some studies have shown that the clinical efficacy of tamoxifen (as measured by the risk of breast cancer relapse/mortality) may be reduced when administered concurrently with paroxetine as a result of paroxetine's irreversible inhibition of cytochrome P-450 (CYP) isoenzyme 2D6; however, other studies have failed to demonstrate such a risk. Therefore, it remains uncertain whether concurrent administration of paroxetine has a significant adverse effect on the clinical efficacy of tamoxifen. One study suggests that the risk may increase with longer duration of concurrent administration of the drugs. (See Drug Interactions: Drugs Undergoing Hepatic Metabolism or Affecting Hepatic Microsomal Enzymes.)

Drugs Metabolized by Cytochrome P-450 (CYP) 3A4 Although paroxetine can inhibit the cytochrome P-450 (CYP) 3A4 isoenzyme, results of in vitro and in vivo studies indicate that the drug is a much less potent inhibitor of this enzyme than many other drugs. In an in vivo drug interaction study, concomitant administration of paroxetine and the cytochrome P-450 3A4 substrate, terfenadine (no longer commercially available in the US), had no effect on the pharmacokinetics of terfenadine. In another in vivo interaction study, ketoconazole, which is a potent inhibitor of CYP3A4 activity, was found to be at least 100 times more potent than paroxetine as an inhibitor of the metabolism of several substrates for this enzyme, including terfenadine, astemizole (no longer commercially available in the US), cisapride, triazolam, and cyclosporine. Based on the assumption that the relationship between paroxetine's inhibitory activity in vitro and its lack of effect on terfenadine's clearance in vivo predicts its effect on other CYP3A4 substrates, the manufacturer states that these data suggest that the extent of paroxetine's inhibition of CYP3A4 activity is unlikely to be of clinical importance.

Drugs Metabolized by Other Cytochrome P-450 Isoenzymes Unlike fluvoxamine, in vitro data indicate that paroxetine does not substantially inhibit the CYP1A2 isoenzyme, which is responsible for the metabolism of caffeine and numerous other substances.

Cimetidine Cimetidine is known to inhibit many cytochrome P-450 oxidative enzymes and can affect the pharmacokinetics of paroxetine. In a study in which oral paroxetine (30 mg once daily) was given for 4 weeks, steady-state plasma paroxetine concentrations were increased by approximately 50% during concomitant use of oral cimetidine (300 mg 3 times daily) for the final week. The possible effects of paroxetine on the pharmacokinetics of cimetidine have not been studied. If paroxetine and cimetidine are used concurrently, dosage adjustment of paroxetine after the initial 20-mg dose should be guided by clinical effect.

Phenobarbital Phenobarbital is known to induce many cytochrome P-450 oxidative enzymes and can affect the pharmacokinetics of paroxetine. Following administration of a single 30-mg oral dose of paroxetine in individuals who had achieved steady-state serum phenobarbital concentrations (100 mg of phenobarbital daily for 14 days), the AUC and elimination half-life of paroxetine were reduced by an average of 25 and 38%, respectively, compared with administration of paroxetine alone. The influence of paroxetine on the pharmacokinetics of phenobarbital has not been studied to date. Since paroxetine exhibits nonlinear pharmacokinetics, the results of this study may not apply in situations in which both drugs are administered chronically. The manufacturer of paroxetine states that initial dosage adjustment of paroxetine is not considered necessary in patients receiving phenobarbital, and any subsequent dosage adjustment should be guided by clinical effect.

■ **Tricyclic and Other Antidepressants** The extent to which SSRI interactions with tricyclic antidepressants may pose clinical problems depends on the degree of inhibition and the pharmacokinetics of the serotonin-reuptake inhibitor involved. In one study, daily dosing of paroxetine (20 mg once daily) under steady-state conditions increased single-dose desipramine (100 mg) peak plasma concentrations, AUC, and elimination half-life by an average of approximately 2-, 5-, and 3-fold, respectively. This interaction appears to result from paroxetine-induced inhibition of CYP2D6. Thus, the manufacturers recommend that caution be exercised during concomitant use of tricyclics with paroxetine since paroxetine may inhibit the metabolism of the tricyclic antidepressant. In addition, plasma tricyclic concentrations may need to be monitored and the dosage of the tricyclic reduced during concomitant use. (See Drugs Metabolized by Cytochrome P-450 [CYP] 2D6 under Drug Interactions: Drugs Undergoing Hepatic Metabolism or Affecting Hepatic Microsomal Enzymes.)

Clinical experience regarding the optimal timing of switching from other antidepressants to paroxetine therapy is limited. Therefore, care and prudent medical judgment should be exercised when switching from other antidepressants to paroxetine. (See Dosage and Administration: Dosage and see also Drug Interactions: Serotonergic Drugs.)

■ **Lithium** In a multiple-dose study, there was no evidence of a pharmacokinetic interaction between lithium and paroxetine. However, because there is little clinical experience with combined therapy and because lithium may enhance the serotonergic effects of paroxetine, potentially resulting in serotonin syndrome or NMS-like reactions, concurrent use of lithium and paroxetine should be undertaken with caution. (See Drug Interactions: Serotonergic Drugs.)

■ **Protein-bound Drugs** Because paroxetine is highly protein bound, the drug theoretically could be displaced from binding sites by, or it could displace from binding sites, other protein-bound drugs such as oral anticoagulants or digitoxin (no longer commercially available in the US). In vitro studies to date have shown that paroxetine has no effect on the protein binding of 2 highly protein-bound drugs, phenytoin and warfarin; however, preliminary data suggest that there may be a pharmacodynamic interaction between paroxetine and warfarin. Pending further accumulation of data, patients receiving paroxetine concomitantly with any highly protein-bound drug should be observed for potential adverse effects associated with combined therapy. (See Warfarin under Drug Interactions: Drugs Affecting Hemostasis.)

■ **Drugs Affecting Hemostasis** ***Warfarin*** In vitro data have shown that paroxetine has no effect on the protein binding of warfarin. However, preliminary data suggest that there may be a pharmacodynamic interaction between these drugs that causes an increased bleeding diathesis while the prothrombin time remains unchanged. An increase in mild but clinically important bleeding was observed in healthy individuals receiving paroxetine and warfarin for several days. Because of limited clinical experience to date, the concurrent use of paroxetine and warfarin should be undertaken with caution. (See Drug Interactions: Protein-bound Drugs.)

Other Drugs that Interfere with Hemostasis Epidemiologic case-control and cohort design studies that have demonstrated an association between selective serotonin-reuptake inhibitor therapy and an increased risk of upper GI bleeding also have shown that concurrent use of aspirin or other nonsteroidal anti-inflammatory drugs substantially increases the risk of GI bleeding. Although these studies focused on upper GI bleeding, there is some evidence suggesting that bleeding at other sites may be similarly potentiated. The precise mechanism for this increased risk remains to be clearly established; however, serotonin release by platelets is known to play an important role in hemostasis, and selective serotonin-reuptake inhibitors decrease serotonin uptake from the blood by platelets, thereby decreasing the amount of serotonin in platelets. Patients receiving paroxetine should be cautioned about the concomitant use of drugs that interfere with hemostasis, including aspirin and other nonsteroidal anti-inflammatory agents.

■ **Digoxin** The steady-state pharmacokinetics of paroxetine were not altered when administered concurrently with digoxin at steady state. The mean AUC of digoxin at steady state decreased by 15% in the presence of paroxetine. Because there is limited clinical experience to date, the manufacturers state that combined therapy with paroxetine and digoxin should be undertaken with caution.

■ **Alcohol** Paroxetine has not been shown to potentiate the impairment of mental and motor skills caused by alcohol. However, the drug's ability to reduce alcohol consumption in animals and humans suggests that there may be a serotonergically mediated, pharmacodynamic interaction between paroxetine and alcohol within the CNS. The manufacturers recommend that patients be advised to avoid alcohol while receiving paroxetine.

■ **Benzodiazepines** Under steady-state conditions, diazepam does not appear to affect the pharmacokinetics of paroxetine. The effect of paroxetine on diazepam pharmacokinetics has not been evaluated to date. Paroxetine does not appear to potentiate the CNS depressant effects of diazepam, lorazepam, or oxazepam.

■ **Clozapine** Concomitant use of SSRIs such as paroxetine in patients receiving clozapine can increase plasma concentrations of the antipsychotic agent. In a study in schizophrenic patients receiving clozapine under steady-state conditions, initiation of paroxetine therapy resulted in only minor changes in plasma concentrations of clozapine and its metabolites; however, initiation of fluvoxamine therapy resulted in increases that were threefold compared with baseline. In other published reports, concomitant use of clozapine and SSRIs (fluvoxamine, paroxetine, sertraline) resulted in modest increases (less than twofold) in clozapine and metabolite concentrations. The manufacturer of clozapine states that caution should be exercised and patients closely monitored if clozapine is used in patients receiving SSRIs, and a reduction in clozapine dosage should be considered. (See Antipsychotic Agents and Other Dopamine Antagonists under Drug Interactions: Serotonergic Drugs.)

■ **Pimozide** In a controlled study, concurrent administration of a single 2-mg dose of pimozide in healthy individuals receiving paroxetine (dosage titrated up to 60 mg daily) was associated with mean increases in the AUC and peak plasma concentrations of pimozide of 151 and 62%, respectively, compared with pimozide given alone. Because of the narrow therapeutic index of pimozide and its known ability to prolong the QT interval, concurrent administration of paroxetine and pimozide is contraindicated. (See Antipsychotic Agents and Other Dopamine Antagonists under Drug Interactions: Serotonergic Drugs.)

■ **Electroconvulsive Therapy** The effects of paroxetine in conjunction with electroconvulsive therapy (ECT) have not been systematically evaluated to date in clinical studies.

■ **β-Adrenergic Blocking Agents** In a study in which propranolol (80 mg twice daily) was given orally for 18 days, the steady-state plasma concentrations of propranolol were not affected when paroxetine (30 mg once daily) was used concurrently during the last 10 days. The manufacturers state that the effect(s) of propranolol on paroxetine have not been systematically evaluated.

Severe hypotension has been reported following the initiation of paroxetine therapy in a patient who had been receiving chronic metoprolol therapy. Metoprolol is metabolized by the CYP2D6 isoenzyme and paroxetine is known to potently inhibit this enzyme. Pending further experience with this combination, caution should be exercised when paroxetine and metoprolol are used concomitantly.

■ **Phenytoin** In vitro studies to date have shown that paroxetine has no effect on the protein binding of phenytoin. When a single 30-mg oral dose of paroxetine was administered in individuals in whom steady-state plasma phenytoin concentrations (300 mg once daily for 14 days) had been achieved, the AUC and elimination half-life of paroxetine were reduced by an average of 50 and 35%, respectively, compared with paroxetine administered alone. In another study, when a single 300-mg oral dose of phenytoin was administered to individuals in whom steady-state plasma paroxetine concentrations (30 mg once daily for 14 days) had been achieved, the AUC of phenytoin was slightly reduced (by an average of 12%) compared with phenytoin administered alone. However, because both paroxetine and phenytoin exhibit nonlinear pharmacokinetics, these studies may not address the case in which both drugs are given chronically. Elevated plasma phenytoin concentration has been reported in one patient 4 weeks after concurrent therapy with paroxetine and phenytoin. Pending further experience, the manufacturers state that initial dosage adjustments are not considered necessary during concurrent use and that any subsequent adjustments in dosage should be guided by clinical effects.

■ **Theophylline** Elevated serum theophylline concentrations associated with paroxetine therapy have been reported. Although this interaction has not been systematically studied to date, the manufacturers recommend that serum concentrations of theophylline be monitored during concomitant paroxetine therapy.

■ **Procyclidine** Multiple oral doses of paroxetine (30 mg once daily) have increased the steady-state AUC, peak concentrations, and trough concentrations of procyclidine (5 mg once daily) by 35, 37, and 67%, respectively, compared with procyclidine alone at steady state. If anticholinergic effects are observed in patients receiving concurrent therapy with these drugs, the manufacturers recommend that the procyclidine dosage be reduced.

■ **Antacids** Limited data indicate that antacids do not substantially interfere with the absorption of paroxetine following oral administration.

■ **Fosamprenavir and Ritonavir** Concurrent administration of fosamprenavir and ritonavir with paroxetine substantially decreased plasma paroxetine concentrations. The manufacturers recommend that dosage adjustments in patients receiving these drugs concurrently be guided by clinical effect (tolerability and efficacy).

Acute Toxicity

Limited information is available on the acute toxicity of paroxetine.

■ **Pathogenesis** The acute lethal dose of paroxetine in humans is not known.

■ **Manifestations** In general, overdosage of paroxetine may be expected to produce effects that are extensions of the drug's pharmacologic and adverse effects. Overdosages of paroxetine may result in somnolence, coma, nausea, tremor, tachycardia, confusion, vomiting, and dizziness. Other signs and symptoms observed in patients who received overdosages of paroxetine alone or in combination with other substances include mydriasis, convulsions (including status epilepticus), ventricular arrhythmias (including torsades de pointes), hypertension, aggressive reactions, syncope, hypotension, stupor, bradycardia, dystonia, rhabdomyolysis, symptoms of hepatic dysfunction (including hepatic failure, hepatic necrosis, jaundice, hepatitis, and hepatic steatosis), serotonin syndrome, manic reactions, myoclonus, acute renal failure, and urinary retention.

The manufacturers state that, since introduction of paroxetine in the US, 48 fatalities involving overdosages of paroxetine alone or in combination with other substances have been reported worldwide. In 145 nonfatal overdosages, most patients recovered without sequelae. One patient recovered after ingesting 2 g of paroxetine (33 times the maximum recommended daily dosage).

In a geriatric woman who ingested 360 mg of paroxetine, the initial sign of overdosage was excessive vomiting; hyponatremia developed 5 days later and was associated with somnolence, confusion, muscle spasms, dehydration, and slow reflexes. Ecchymoses and myxedema also were observed in this patient.

In 28 children aged 10.5 months to 17 years of age who ingested an overdosage of paroxetine alone, less sedation and fewer adverse cardiovascular effects were observed when compared with tricyclic antidepressant overdosage. In children 5 years of age and younger, ingestions of 120 mg or less of paroxetine were treated with GI evacuation and minimal supportive care with favorable outcomes. In children 12 years of age and younger who ingested 100–800 mg of the drug alone, most of the patients remained asymptomatic.

■ **Treatment** Because fatalities and severe toxicity have been reported following paroxetine overdosage, particularly in large overdosage and when taken with other drugs or alcohol, some clinicians recommend that any overdosage involving the drug be managed aggressively. Because suicidal ingestion often involves more than one drug, clinicians treating paroxetine overdosage should be alert to possible manifestations caused by drugs other than paroxetine. The manufacturers specifically caution about patients who are currently receiving or recently have taken paroxetine who might ingest either accidentally or intentionally excessive quantities of a tricyclic antidepressant. In such cases, accumulation of both the tricyclic and its active metabolite may increase the possibility of clinically important sequelae and lengthen the time needed for close medical supervision. (See Drug Interactions: Tricyclic and Other Antidepressants.)

Clinicians also should consider the possibility of serotonin syndrome or NMS-like reactions in patients presenting with similar clinical features and a recent history of paroxetine ingestion and/or ingestion of other serotonergic and/or antipsychotic agents or other dopamine antagonists. (See Cautions: Precautions and Contraindications and see also Drug Interactions: Serotonergic Drugs.)

Management of paroxetine overdosage generally involves symptomatic and supportive care. A patent airway should be established and maintained, and adequate oxygenation and ventilation should be ensured. An ECG should be taken and monitoring of cardiac function should be instituted if there is any evidence of abnormality. Frequent vital sign monitoring and close observation of the patient is necessary. There is no specific antidote for paroxetine intoxication.

Following recent (i.e., within 4 hours) ingestion of a potentially toxic amount of paroxetine and in the absence of signs and symptoms of cardiac toxicity, the stomach should be emptied immediately by inducing emesis or by gastric lavage. If the patient is comatose, having seizures, or lacks the gag reflex, gastric lavage may be performed if an endotracheal tube with cuff inflated is in place to prevent aspiration of gastric contents. Since administration of activated charcoal (which may be used in conjunction with sorbitol) may be as or more effective than induction of emesis or gastric lavage, its use has been recommended either in the initial management of paroxetine overdosage or following induction of emesis or gastric lavage in patients who have ingested a potentially toxic quantity of the drug. In the past, the manufacturer of paroxetine hydrochloride suggested that 20–30 g of activated charcoal be administered following gastric evacuation every 4–6 hours during the first 24–48 hours following ingestion.

Because of the large volume of distribution of paroxetine and its principal metabolite, peritoneal dialysis, forced diuresis, hemoperfusion, and/or exchange transfusion are unlikely to be effective in removing substantial amounts of paroxetine from the body.

Clinicians should consult a poison control center for additional information on the management of paroxetine overdosage.

Chronic Toxicity

Paroxetine has not been studied systematically in animals or humans to determine whether therapy with the drug is associated with abuse, tolerance, or physical dependence.

The clinical trials conducted with paroxetine did not reveal any tendency for drug-seeking behavior. However, withdrawal syndrome, manifested as dizziness, sensory disturbances, blurred vision, sweating, nausea, insomnia, tremor, confusion, lethargy, insomnia, nervousness or anxiety, headache, paresthesias, hypermanic-like symptoms (including hyperactivity, decreased need for sleep, irritability, agitation, aggressiveness, volatility, explosive vocal and temper outbursts), and egodystonic impulsive behavior (including shoplifting, homicidal impulses, suicidal impulses and gestures), has been reported following discontinuance of paroxetine therapy.

Some evidence suggests that the risk of withdrawal effects may be somewhat greater with paroxetine than with sertraline; fluoxetine appears to associated with the fewest withdrawal effects, possibly due at least in part to its prolonged elimination half-life. Additional clinical experience is necessary to confirm these findings.

Experience with paroxetine, other serotonin-reuptake inhibitors (SSRIs), and selective serotonin- and norepinephrine-reuptake inhibitors (SNRIs) suggests that a withdrawal syndrome may occur within several days following discontinuance of these drugs, particularly when abrupt. The most commonly observed manifestations are those that resemble influenza, such as fatigue, GI complaints (e.g., nausea), dizziness or lightheadedness, tremor, anxiety, insomnia, chills, sweating, and incoordination. Other reported manifestations include dysphoric mood, irritability, emotional lability, hypomania, memory impairment, sensory disturbances (such as paresthesias, including electric shock-like sensations), confusion, headache, palpitations, agitation, and aggression. Although the mechanism(s) for such withdrawal reactions is not fully understood, it has been suggested that they may be caused by a sudden decrease in serotonin availability at the synapse or cholinergic rebound; other neurotransmitters (e.g., dopamine, norepinephrine, GABA) also may be involved. These manifestations may in some cases be mistaken for physical illness or relapse into depression. While these reactions generally appear to be self-limiting and improve over one to several weeks, there have been reports of serious discontinuance symptoms. Manifestations of withdrawal also may be improved by restarting therapy with paroxetine or another antidepressant with a similar pharmacologic profile. Paroxetine therapy should be discontinued gradually (e.g., over a period of several weeks) to prevent the possible development of withdrawal reactions. (See Dosage and Administration: Dosage.)

As with other CNS-active drugs, clinicians should carefully evaluate patients for a history of substance abuse prior to initiating paroxetine therapy. If paroxetine therapy is initiated in patients with a history of substance abuse, such patients should be monitored closely for signs of misuse or abuse of the drug (e.g., development of tolerance, use of increasing doses, drug-seeking behavior).

Pharmacology

The pharmacology of paroxetine is complex and in many ways resembles that of other antidepressant agents, particularly those agents (e.g., citalopram, escitalopram, fluoxetine, fluvoxamine, sertraline, clomipramine, trazodone) that predominantly potentiate the pharmacologic effects of serotonin (5-HT). Like other selective serotonin-reuptake inhibitors (SSRIs), paroxetine is a potent and highly selective reuptake inhibitor of serotonin and has little or no effect on other neurotransmitters.

■ **Nervous System Effects** The precise mechanism of antidepressant action of paroxetine is unclear, but the drug has been shown to selectively inhibit the reuptake of serotonin at the presynaptic neuronal membrane. Paroxetine-induced inhibition of serotonin reuptake causes increased synaptic concentrations of serotonin in the CNS, resulting in numerous functional changes associated with enhanced serotonergic neurotransmission. Like other SSRIs (e.g., citalopram, fluoxetine, fluvoxamine, sertraline), paroxetine appears to have only very weak effects on the reuptake of norepinephrine or dopamine and does not exhibit clinically important anticholinergic, antihistaminic, or adrenergic (α_1, α_2, β) blocking activity at usual therapeutic dosages.

Although the mechanism of antidepressant action of antidepressant agents may involve inhibition of the reuptake of various neurotransmitters (i.e., serotonin, norepinephrine) at the presynaptic neuronal membrane, it has been suggested that postsynaptic receptor modification is mainly responsible for the antidepressant action observed during long-term administration of antidepressant agents. During long-term therapy with most antidepressants (e.g., tricyclic antidepressants, monoamine oxidase [MAO] inhibitors), these adaptive changes mainly consist of subsensitivity of the noradrenergic adenylate cyclase system in association with a decrease in the number of β-adrenergic receptors; such effects on noradrenergic receptor function are commonly referred to as "down regulation". However, in an animal study, long-term administration of paroxetine was not shown to downregulate noradrenergic receptors in the CNS as has been observed with many other clinically effective antidepressants. In addition, some antidepressants (e.g., amitriptyline) reportedly decrease the number of serotonergic (5-HT) binding sites following chronic administration.

The precise mechanism of action that is responsible for the efficacy of paroxetine in the treatment of obsessive-compulsive disorder is unclear. However, because of the potency of clomipramine and SSRIs (e.g., citalopram, fluoxetine, fluvoxamine, sertraline) in inhibiting serotonin reuptake and their efficacy in the treatment of obsessive-compulsive disorder, a serotonin hypothesis has been developed to explain the pathogenesis of the condition. The hypothesis postulates that a dysregulation of serotonin is responsible for obsessive-compulsive disorder and that paroxetine and these other agents are effective because they correct this imbalance. Although the available evidence supports the serotonergic hypothesis of obsessive-compulsive disorder, additional studies are necessary to confirm this hypothesis.

The exact mechanism of action of paroxetine in panic disorder, social phobia, or generalized anxiety disorder has not been fully elucidated but appears to involve inhibition of reuptake of serotonin at the presynaptic membrane.

Animal data indicate that serotonergic mechanisms also appear to be involved at least in part in a number of other pharmacologic effects associated with SSRIs, such as decreased food intake and altered food selection as well as decreased alcohol intake.

Serotonergic Effects Paroxetine is a highly selective inhibitor of serotonin reuptake at the presynaptic neuronal membrane. Paroxetine-induced inhibition of serotonin reuptake causes increased synaptic concentrations of the neurotransmitter, resulting in numerous functional changes associated with enhanced serotonergic neurotransmission.

Data from in vitro studies suggest that paroxetine is more potent than citalopram, clomipramine, fluoxetine, fluvoxamine, and sertraline as a serotonin-reuptake inhibitor. Unlike some other serotonin-reuptake inhibitors, the metabolites of paroxetine have been shown to possess no more than 2% of the potency of the parent compound as inhibitors of serotonin reuptake; therefore, they are unlikely to contribute to the clinical activity of the drug.

At therapeutic dosages in humans, paroxetine has been shown to inhibit the reuptake of serotonin into platelets.

Effects on Other Neurotransmitters Like other serotonin-reuptake inhibitors, paroxetine has been shown to have little or no activity in inhibiting the reuptake of norepinephrine. Paroxetine appears to have only very weak activity on neuronal reuptake of dopamine. In addition, paroxetine does not inhibit monoamine oxidase (MAO).

Unlike tricyclic and some other antidepressants, paroxetine does not exhibit clinically important anticholinergic, α- or β-adrenergic blocking, or antihistaminic activity at usual therapeutic dosages. As a result, the incidence of adverse effects commonly associated with blockade of muscarinic cholinergic receptors (e.g., dry mouth, blurred vision, urinary retention, constipation, confusion), α-adrenergic receptors (e.g., orthostatic hypotension), and histamine H_1- and H_2-receptors (e.g., sedation) is lower in paroxetine-treated patients than tricyclic-treated patients. In vitro studies have demonstrated that paroxetine does not possess clinically important affinity for α_1- or α_2-adrenergic, β- adrenergic, histaminergic (H_1-, GABA, benzodiazepine, or dopamine D_2-receptors.

Although paroxetine has demonstrated weak affinity for muscarinic cholinergic receptors in vitro and has caused mydriasis in vivo, these effects generally occurred only at dosages greatly exceeding those required for increasing serotonergic activity in the CNS. Limited data indicate that mydriasis may also be serotonergically mediated. In addition, serum anticholinergicity of paroxetine was found to be substantially lower than that of nortriptyline in depressed geriatric patients in one study; complaints of dry mouth and tachycardia also occurred more frequently in the nortriptyline-treated patients than in those treated with paroxetine. These findings indicate that, at therapeutic plasma concentrations, paroxetine has approximately 20% the anticholinergic potential of nortriptyline in older patients. Therefore, it appears unlikely that paroxetine will produce adverse anticholinergic events when given in the usual recommended dosage.

Effects on Sleep Like tricyclic and most other antidepressants, paroxetine suppresses rapid eye movement (REM) sleep. Some evidence suggests that the drug may suppress REM sleep in a dose-dependent manner. Although not clearly established, there is some evidence that the REM-suppressing effects of antidepressant agents may contribute to the antidepressant activity of these drugs. While the precise mechanism has not been fully elucidated, results of animal studies indicate that paroxetine's effects on REM sleep may be serotonergically mediated.

In some studies, paroxetine prolonged REM latency, increased awakenings, increased stage 1 sleep, and/or reduced actual sleep time and sleep efficiency. In one study, administration of single, 40-mg doses of paroxetine in the morning increased sleep latency; however, the drug did not affect sleep latency when given at bedtime. In addition, sleep maintenance parameters (such as nocturnal wake time, total sleep time, and sleep efficiency) deteriorated in a dose-dependent manner both when a single dose of the drug was given in the morning and when given as a single 30-mg dose at bedtime. Overall, the changes in sleep observed with paroxetine are relatively small and are unlikely to be of clinical importance during prolonged administration. In addition, the changes noted with paroxetine are similar to those reported with other SSRIs and suggest an alerting effect on sleep that has not been shown to adversely affect sleep quality.

Effects on EEG Limited data currently are available regarding the effects of paroxetine on the EEG. In animals, EEG studies have revealed an activating effect associated with slight behavioral arousal and weak locomotor stimulation at dosages higher than those required to inhibit serotonin reuptake in the CNS. EEG changes in healthy individuals receiving single, 70-mg oral doses of paroxetine revealed a decrease in delta and theta activity and an increase in beta activity; these changes were still evident after 72 hours. Overall, available data in humans suggest that paroxetine generally does not produce clinically relevant changes on the EEG.

Effects on Psychomotor Function Paroxetine generally does not appear to cause clinically important sedation and generally does not interfere with psychomotor performance. Controlled studies in healthy young individuals and in patients with major depression did not demonstrate any adverse effects on psychomotor performance in those receiving 20-mg doses of the drug. No adverse effects on psychomotor performance or cognitive function were observed in healthy men older than 60 years of age who received single and repeated doses of paroxetine 20 mg in a controlled study; in some tests (e.g., critical flicker fusion thresholds), paroxetine improved information processing ability. In a controlled study evaluating the effects of paroxetine (20 or 40 mg administered daily for 8 days) on psychomotor performance and car driving in healthy males, the 20-mg dosage was found to have no effect while the 40-mg dosage was not found to affect road tracking but slightly impaired performance in some psychomotor tests in a persistent manner. Further study is needed to clarify whether paroxetine may adversely affect psychomotor performance at dosages of 40 mg daily or more.

■ **Cardiovascular Effects** No clinically important changes in vital signs (systolic and diastolic blood pressure, heart rate, temperature) were observed in patients receiving paroxetine in controlled trials. Paroxetine also appears to have little effect on the ECG. In controlled studies, paroxetine did not produce clinically important changes in heart rate, cardiac conduction, or other ECG parameters in patients receiving the drug. In depressed patients with stable ischemic heart disease, paroxetine did not substantially affect blood pressure or conduction intervals and did not produce sustained effects on heart rate, heart rhythm, or indexes of heart rate variability. However, a small but statistically significant QRS widening relative to placebo was reported in one study, and ECG changes occasionally have been reported in healthy individuals and patients receiving the drug. In addition, the relative safety of paroxetine in patients with underlying cardiac disease, particularly those with severe cardiovascular disease and immediately following a myocardial infarction, remains to be more fully elucidated.

Paroxetine did not demonstrate any substantial change in cardiovascular autonomic function tests (such as heart rate variability) in a limited number of depressed patients receiving the drug for 14 days. On the other hand, paroxetine has been shown to increase heart rate variability in a limited number of patients with panic disorder, a condition associated with decreased heart rate variability and consequently an increased risk of serious cardiovascular problems including sudden cardiac death.

■ **Effects on Appetite and Body Weight** Paroxetine appears to possess some anorexigenic activity, although to a lesser degree than certain other serotonergic agents (e.g., fenfluramine [no longer commercially available in the US], fluoxetine, sertraline, zimelidine). Limited data from animal studies suggest that fenfluramine is the most effective inhibitor of food intake followed by fluoxetine, then sertraline, and then paroxetine. Although the precise mechanism has not been clearly established, results from animal studies indicate that the appetite-inhibiting action of these antidepressants may result at least in part from serotonin-reuptake blockade and enhancement of serotonin release thereby increasing serotonin availability at the neuronal synapse.

While clinically important weight loss may occur in some patients receiving paroxetine, only minimal weight loss (averaging 0.45 kg) generally occurred in patients receiving the drug in controlled clinical trials. In addition, while decreased appetite was reported in about 6% of patients receiving paroxetine in short-term clinical trials, the drug, unlike fluoxetine, does not appear to exhibit clinically important anorectic effects. (See Cautions: Metabolic and Endocrine Effects.)

■ **Neuroendocrine Effects** Limited data currently are available regarding the effects of paroxetine on the endocrine system. Elevated serum prolactin concentrations have been reported in some women receiving chronic paroxetine therapy.

Pharmacokinetics

Paroxetine is commercially available in the US as paroxetine hydrochloride (e.g., Paxil®, Paxil CR®) and as paroxetine mesylate (i.e., Pexeva®). Conventional tablets of Paxil® and Pexeva® are *not* bioequivalent. The U.S. Food and Drug Administration (FDA) considers paroxetine mesylate (Pexeva®) conventional tablets to be a pharmaceutical *alternative* (as described in section 505[b][2] of the Federal Food, Drug, and Cosmetic Act) and not a pharmaceutical (generic) equivalent to paroxetine hydrochloride conventional tablets (e.g., Paxil®), since both contain the same active moiety (paroxetine) but have different salts.

In all human studies described in the Pharmacokinetics section, paroxetine was administered as either the hydrochloride or the mesylate salt; dosages and concentrations are expressed in terms of paroxetine.

■ **Absorption** Paroxetine hydrochloride appears to be slowly but well absorbed from the GI tract following oral administration. Although the oral bioavailability of paroxetine hydrochloride in humans has not been fully elucidated to date, the manufacturer states that paroxetine is completely absorbed after oral dosing of a solution of the hydrochloride salt. However, the relative proportion of an oral dose that reaches systemic circulation unchanged appears to be relatively small because paroxetine undergoes extensive first-pass metabolism. The oral tablets and suspension of paroxetine hydrochloride reportedly are bioequivalent.

Paroxetine mesylate is completely absorbed following oral administration of the tablets.

Food does not substantially affect the absorption of paroxetine. In one study, no substantial differences in pharmacokinetic parameters were noted when paroxetine hydrochloride was administered under fasting and nonfasting conditions or with a low- or high-fat diet, milk, water, or antacids. In another study, administration of a single dose of paroxetine hydrochloride with food resulted in a 6% increase in the area under the concentration-time curve (AUC), a 29% increase in peak plasma concentrations of the drug, and a decrease in the time to peak plasma concentrations from 6.4 to 4.9 hours.

In healthy males receiving one 30-mg tablet of paroxetine (administered as paroxetine hydrochloride) once daily for 30 days, steady-state plasma paroxetine concentrations were achieved after approximately 10 days in most patients, although achievement of steady-state concentrations may take substantially longer in some patients. At steady-state, mean peak plasma paroxetine concentrations of 61.7 ng/mL occurred after an average of 5.2 hours following oral administration; corresponding mean trough concentrations of 30.7 ng/mL were reported. However, wide interindividual variation in peak plasma concentrations of paroxetine has been observed in both single- and multiple-dose studies. In geriatric individuals receiving multiple daily doses of 20–40 mg daily of paroxetine (administered as paroxetine hydrochloride), trough plasma concentrations were 70–80% higher than trough concentrations in nongeriatric individuals. In another multiple-dose study, mean steady-state trough concentrations were approximately 3 times higher in geriatric individuals than in younger adults receiving paroxetine (administered as paroxetine hydrochloride) 20 mg daily, although there was considerable overlap between the 2 groups. Therefore, the manufacturers and some clinicians recommend that paroxetine be administered in a reduced dosage (i.e., 10 mg daily) initially in geriatric patients. (See Cautions: Geriatric Precautions and see Dosage and Administration: Dosage in Geriatric and Debilitated Patients.)

In healthy males receiving one 30-mg tablet of paroxetine (administered as paroxetine mesylate) once daily for 24 days, steady-state plasma paroxetine concentrations were achieved after approximately 13 days in most patients, although achievement of steady-state concentrations may take substantially longer in some patients. At steady-state, mean peak plasma paroxetine concentrations of 81.3 ng/mL occurred after an average of 8.1 hours following oral administration of paroxetine mesylate tablets; corresponding mean trough concentrations of 43.2 ng/mL were reported.

When compared with administration of a single dose of paroxetine hydrochloride, steady-state peak and trough paroxetine concentrations following multiple dosing were approximately 6 and 14 times higher than would be expected from single-dose values. In addition, steady-state drug exposure based on AUC (0–24 hour) was about 8 times greater than would have been predicted based on the single-dose data in these individuals. When compared with administration of a single dose of paroxetine mesylate, steady-state peak and trough paroxetine concentrations following multiple dosing were approximately 7 and 10 times higher than would be expected from single-dose values. In addition, steady-state drug exposure based on AUC (0–24 hour) was about 8 and 10 times greater than would have been predicted based on the single-dose data in these individuals receiving the hydrochloride and mesylate salts of paroxetine, respectively. The manufacturers attributed this excess accumulation to the fact that one of the enzymes that metabolizes paroxetine, the cytochrome P-450 isoenzyme CYP2D6, is saturable.

In steady-state, dose-proportionality studies involving geriatric and nongeriatric patients receiving 20–40 and 20–50 mg daily of paroxetine (administered as paroxetine hydrochloride), respectively, some nonlinearity was observed in both groups, which also suggests a saturable metabolic pathway. When compared with trough paroxetine concentrations after 20 mg of the drug daily, trough concentrations after 40 mg daily were approximately 2–3 times higher than doubled.

In a meta-analysis of paroxetine pharmacokinetics from 4 studies performed in healthy individuals following multiple dosing of 20–40 mg daily, males did not exhibit a substantially lower peak plasma concentration or AUC of paroxetine than females.

As with other serotonin-reuptake inhibitors, the relationship between plasma paroxetine concentrations and the therapeutic and/or toxic effects of the drug has not been clearly established.

■ **Distribution** Distribution of paroxetine and its metabolites into human body tissues and fluids has not been fully characterized. However, limited pharmacokinetic data suggest that the parent drug, which is highly lipophilic, and some of its metabolites are widely distributed throughout body tissues, including the CNS. Only 1% of paroxetine remains in plasma.

Although the apparent volume of distribution of paroxetine has not been determined in humans, values ranging from 3.1–28 L/kg have been reported in animal studies. The drug crosses the blood-brain barrier in humans and animals.

In vitro, approximately 95 and 93% of paroxetine is bound to plasma proteins at plasma concentrations of 100 and 400 ng/mL, respectively. Under usual clinical conditions, plasma paroxetine concentrations would be less than 400 ng/mL. In vitro, paroxetine does not alter the plasma protein binding of 2 other highly protein-bound drugs, phenytoin and warfarin.

Paroxetine is distributed into human milk. In one lactating woman receiving paroxetine (administered as paroxetine hydrochloride) 20 mg daily for 1 week, the concentration of paroxetine in breast milk was 7.6 ng/mL 4 hours after the daily dose; no adverse effects were observed in the infant during lactation. Based on an estimated weight-adjusted dose to the infant of 0.34% of the maternal dose, the exposure of infants during breastfeeding appears to be lower for paroxetine and fluvoxamine than for fluoxetine; however, further study is needed to clarify the clinical importance of these findings.

■ **Elimination** The elimination half-life of paroxetine when administered as paroxetine hydrochloride averages approximately 21–24 hours, although there is wide interpatient variation with half-lives (ranging from 7–65 hours in one study). In healthy males receiving one 30-mg tablet of paroxetine (administered as paroxetine mesylate) once daily for 24 days, the mean paroxetine half-life was 33.2 hours. In geriatric individuals, elimination half-life of paroxetine (administered as paroxetine hydrochloride) may be increased (e.g., to about 36 hours).

The exact metabolic fate of paroxetine has not been fully elucidated; however, paroxetine is extensively metabolized, probably in the liver. The principal metabolites are polar and conjugated products of oxidation and methylation, which are readily cleared by the body. Conjugates with glucuronic acid and sulfate predominate, and the principal metabolites have been isolated and identified. The metabolites of paroxetine have been shown to possess no more than 2% of the potency of the parent compound as inhibitors of serotonin reuptake; therefore, they are essentially inactive.

Like some other serotonin-reuptake inhibitors, paroxetine is partially metabolized by the drug metabolizing isoenzyme CYP2D6 (a cytochrome P-450 isoenzyme implicated in sparteine/debrisoquine polymorphism). Saturation of this enzyme at dosages used clinically appears to account for the nonlinearity of paroxetine kinetics observed with increasing dosage and duration of treatment. The role of the CYP2D6 enzyme in paroxetine metabolism also suggests potential drug-drug interactions. (See Drug Interactions: Drugs Undergoing Hepatic Metabolism or Affecting Hepatic Microsomal Enzymes.)

Following oral administration, paroxetine and its metabolites are excreted in both urine and feces. Following oral administration of a single, 30-mg dose of paroxetine (administered as paroxetine hydrochloride) as an oral solution (not commercially available), approximately 64% of the dose was excreted in the urine within 10 days; unchanged paroxetine accounted for 2% of the dose and metabolites accounted for the remaining 62% of the dose. During the same period, approximately 36% of the dose was eliminated in feces (probably via the bile), mostly as metabolites and less than 1% as the parent drug.

The effect of age on the elimination of paroxetine has not been fully elucidated. In healthy geriatric adults, hepatic clearance of paroxetine was mildly impaired leading to slower elimination and increased plasma concentrations of the drug. (See Pharmacokinetics: Absorption.) Studies in depressed, geriatric patients confirm these findings with higher steady-state concentrations and longer elimination half-lives reported compared with younger individuals. These results suggest that older patients may be more susceptible to saturation of hepatic metabolic activity resulting in nonlinear kinetics and higher plasma concentrations occurring at lower dosages of paroxetine. Therefore, the manufacturers and some clinicians recommend that paroxetine initially be administered in a reduced dosage in geriatric patients. (See Cautions: Geriatric Precautions and see Dosage and Administration: Dosage in Geriatric and Debilitated Patients.)

Because paroxetine is extensively metabolized by the liver, hepatic impairment can affect the elimination of the drug. In cirrhotic patients with moderate hepatic impairment who received a single 20-mg dose of paroxetine (administered as paroxetine hydrochloride), no significant difference in plasma paroxetine concentrations and pharmacokinetic parameters was observed when compared with corresponding data in healthy individuals. However, accumulation potentially may occur in patients receiving multiple daily doses of paroxetine. The manufacturers state that patients with impaired hepatic function have approximately twofold higher peak plasma concentrations and AUC values. Therefore, the manufacturers recommend that paroxetine be administered in a reduced dosage initially in patients with severe hepatic impairment; caution also should be exercised when increasing the dosage of paroxetine in such patients. (See Cautions: Precautions and Contraindications and see Dosage and Administration: Dosage in Renal and Hepatic Impairment.)

The effect of renal impairment on the pharmacokinetics of paroxetine has not been fully evaluated to date. Following oral administration of multiple daily doses of paroxetine as paroxetine hydrochloride in patients with creatinine clearances less than 30 mL/minute, mean plasma concentrations of paroxetine were approximately 4 times greater than those seen in healthy individuals. In patients with creatinine clearances of 30–60 mL/minute, peak plasma concentrations and AUC values were approximately twofold higher when compared with healthy individuals. The influence of renal impairment in patients receiving multiple daily doses of paroxetine has not been evaluated to date. Pending further accumulation of data, the manufacturers and some clinicians recommend that paroxetine be administered in a reduced dosage initially in patients with severe renal impairment. (See Cautions: Precautions and Contraindications and see Dosage and Administration: Dosage in Renal and Hepatic Impairment.)

Because of the large volume of distribution of paroxetine and its principal metabolite, peritoneal dialysis, forced diuresis, hemoperfusion, and/or exchange transfusion are unlikely to be effective in removing substantial amounts of paroxetine from the body.

Chemistry and Stability

■ **Chemistry** Paroxetine, a selective serotonin-reuptake inhibitor (SSRI) antidepressant agent, is a phenylpiperidine-derivative. Paroxetine differs structurally from other SSRIs (e.g., citalopram, fluoxetine, sertraline) and also differs structurally and pharmacologically from other currently available antidepressants (e.g., tricyclic antidepressants, monoamine oxidase inhibitors).

Paroxetine is commercially available in the US as the hydrochloride and mesylate salts. Paroxetine hydrochloride occurs as an odorless, off-white powder and has a solubility of 5.4 mg/mL in water. The drug has a pK_a of approximately 9.9. Paroxetine mesylate also occurs as an odorless, off-white powder but has a solubility of more than 1 g/mL in water.

The commercially available extended-release tablets of paroxetine hydrochloride contain the drug in a biodegradable polymeric delivery system, consisting of a hydrophilic core surrounded by a biodegradable barrier layer. This delivery system is designed to release the drug gradually over a period of 4–5 hours after ingestion; in addition, an enteric coating delays the release of drug until after the extended-release tablet has left the stomach.

■ **Stability** Paroxetine hydrochloride conventional tablets should be stored at 15–30°C. The oral suspension and extended-release tablets of paroxetine hydrochloride should be stored at or below 25°C. When stored as directed, paroxetine hydrochloride conventional tablets and oral suspension have an expiration date of 3 and 2 years following the date of manufacture, respectively.

Paroxetine mesylate conventional tablets should be stored at a temperature of 25°C but may be exposed to temperatures ranging from 15–30°C; the tablets should be protected from humidity.

Preparations

Excipients in commercially available drug preparations may have clinically important effects in some individuals; consult specific product labeling for details.

PARoxetine Hydrochloride

Oral		
Suspension	10 mg (of paroxetine) per 5 mL	**Paxil**®, GlaxoSmithKline
Tablets, extended-release, film-coated	12.5 mg (of paroxetine)	**Paxil CR**®, GlaxoSmithKline
	25 mg (of paroxetine)	**Paxil CR**®, GlaxoSmithKline
	37.5 mg (of paroxetine)	**Paxil CR**®, GlaxoSmithKline
Tablets, film-coated	10 mg (of paroxetine)*	**Paroxetine Hydrochloride Film-coated Tablets**
		Paxil® (scored), GlaxoSmithKline
	20 mg (of paroxetine)*	**Paroxetine Hydrochloride Film-coated Tablets**
		Paxil® (scored), GlaxoSmithKline
	30 mg (of paroxetine)*	**Paroxetine Hydrochloride Film-coated Tablets**
		Paxil®, GlaxoSmithKline
	40 mg (of paroxetine)*	**Paroxetine Hydrochloride Film-coated Tablets**
		Paxil®, GlaxoSmithKline

*available from one or more manufacturer, distributor, and/or repackager by generic (nonproprietary) name

PARoxetine Mesylate

Oral		
Tablets, film-coated	10 mg (of paroxetine)	**Pexeva**®, Noven Therapeutics
	20 mg (of paroxetine)	**Pexeva**® (scored), Noven Therapeutics
	30 mg (of paroxetine)	**Pexeva**®, Noven Therapeutics
	40 mg (of paroxetine)	**Pexeva**®, Noven Therapeutics

†Use is not currently included in the labeling approved by the US Food and Drug Administration

Sertraline Hydrochloride

■ Sertraline, a selective serotonin-reuptake inhibitor (SSRI), is an antidepressant agent.

Uses

■ **Major Depressive Disorder** Sertraline is used in the treatment of major depressive disorder. A major depressive episode implies a prominent and relatively persistent depressed or dysphoric mood that usually interferes with daily functioning (nearly every day for at least 2 weeks). According to DSM-IV criteria, a major depressive episode includes at least 5 of the following 9 symptoms (with at least one of the symptoms being either depressed mood or loss of interest or pleasure): depressed mood most of the day as indicated by subjective report (e.g., feels sad or empty) or observation made by others; markedly diminished interest or pleasure in all, or almost all, activities most of the day; significant weight loss (when not dieting) or weight gain (e.g., a change of more than 5% of body weight in a month), or decrease or increase in appetite; insomnia or hypersomnia; psychomotor agitation or retardation (observable by others, not merely subjective feelings of restlessness or being slowed down); fatigue or loss of energy; feelings of worthlessness or excessive or inappropriate guilt (not merely self-reproach or guilt about being sick); diminished ability to think or concentrate or indecisiveness (either by subjective account or as observed by others); and recurrent thoughts of death, recurrent suicidal ideation without a specific plan, or a suicide attempt or specific plan for committing suicide.

Treatment of major depressive disorder generally consists of an acute phase (to induce remission), a continuation phase (to preserve remission), and a maintenance phase (to prevent recurrence). Various interventions (e.g., psychotherapy, antidepressant drug therapy, electroconvulsive therapy [ECT]) are used alone or in combination to treat major depressive episodes. Treatment should be individualized and the most appropriate strategy for a particular patient is determined by clinical factors such as severity of depression (e.g., mild, moderate, severe), presence or absence of certain psychiatric features (e.g., suicide risk, catatonia, psychotic or atypical features, alcohol or substance abuse or dependence, panic or other anxiety disorder, cognitive dysfunction, dysthymia, personality disorder, seasonal affective disorder), and concurrent illness (e.g., asthma, cardiac disease, dementia, seizure disorder, glaucoma, hypertension). Demographic and psychosocial factors as well as patient preference also are used to determine the most effective treatment strategy.

While use of psychotherapy alone may be considered as an initial treatment strategy for patients with mild to moderate major depressive disorder (based on patient preference and presence of clinical features such as psychosocial stressors), combined use of antidepressant drug therapy and psychotherapy may be useful for initial treatment of patients with moderate to severe major depressive disorder with psychosocial issues, interpersonal problems, or a comorbid axis II disorder. In addition, combined use of antidepressant drug therapy and psychotherapy may be beneficial in patients who have a history of poor compliance or only partial response to adequate trials of either antidepressant drug therapy or psychotherapy alone.

Antidepressant drug therapy can be used alone for initial treatment of patients with mild major depressive disorder (if preferred by the patient) and usually is indicated alone or in combination with psychotherapy for initial treatment of patients with moderate to severe major depressive disorder (unless ECT is planned). ECT is not generally used for initial treatment of uncomplicated major depression, but is recommended as first-line treatment for severe major depressive disorder when it is coupled with psychotic features, catatonic stupor, severe suicidality, food refusal leading to nutritional compromise, or other situations when a rapid antidepressant response is required. ECT also is recommended for patients who have previously shown a positive response or a preference for this treatment modality and can be considered for patients with moderate or severe depression who have not responded to or cannot receive antidepressant drug therapy. In certain situations involving depressed patients unresponsive to adequate trials of several individual antidepressant agents, adjunctive therapy with another agent (e.g., buspirone, lithium) or concomitant use of a second antidepressant agent (e.g., bupropion) has been used; however, such combination therapy is associated with an increased risk of adverse reactions, may require dosage adjustments, and (if not contraindicated) should be undertaken only after careful consideration of the relative risks and benefits. (See Drug Interactions: Serotonergic Drugs, Drug Interactions: Tricyclic and Other Antidepressants, and Drug Interactions: Lithium.)

The efficacy of sertraline for the acute treatment of major depression has been established by 2 placebo-controlled studies in adult outpatients who met DSM-III criteria for major depression. In the first study of 8 weeks' duration, sertraline was administered with flexible dosing in a range of 50–200 mg daily; the mean daily dosage for patients completing the study was 145 mg daily. In the second study of 6 weeks' duration, sertraline was administered in fixed doses of 50, 100, and 200 mg daily. Overall, these 2 studies demonstrated that sertraline was superior to placebo in improving scores on the Hamilton Depression Rating Scale and the Clinical Global Impression Severity and Improvement Scales. However, the second study was not readily interpretable regarding whether there was a dose-response relationship for the drug's efficacy.

In a third study, depressed outpatients who had responded by the end of an initial 8-week open treatment phase to sertraline 50–200 mg daily were randomized to continue sertraline in the same dosage range or placebo for 44 weeks in a double-blind manner. The mean daily dosage of sertraline in those who completed this long-term study was 70 mg daily, and the relapse rate in the sertraline-treated patients was substantially lower than in those who received placebo.

An analysis of these 3 controlled studies for possible gender-related effects on treatment outcome did not suggest any difference in efficacy based on the gender of the patient.

While the optimum duration of sertraline therapy has not been established, many experts state that acute depressive episodes require several months or longer of sustained antidepressant therapy. In addition, some clinicians recommend that long-term antidepressant therapy be considered in certain patients at risk for recurrence of depressive episodes (such as those with highly recurrent unipolar depression). The efficacy of sertraline in maintaining an antidepressant response for up to 1 year without increased toxicity has been demonstrated in a controlled setting. The manufacturers state that the usefulness of the drug in patients receiving prolonged therapy should be reevaluated periodically. (See Dosage and Administration: Dosage.)

The manufacturers state that the drug's antidepressant efficacy in hospital settings has not been adequately studied to date.

As with certain other antidepressants, the possibility that sertraline may precipitate hypomanic or manic attacks in patients with bipolar or other major affective disorder should be considered. Sertraline is *not* approved for use in treating bipolar depression in adults.

Considerations in Choosing an Antidepressant A variety of antidepressant drugs is available for the treatment of major depressive disorder, including selective serotonin-reuptake inhibitors (SSRIs; e.g., citalopram, escitalopram, fluoxetine, paroxetine, sertraline), selective serotonin- and norepinephrine-reuptake inhibitors (SNRIs; e.g., desvenlafaxine, duloxetine, venlafaxine), tricyclic antidepressants (e.g., amitriptyline, amoxapine, desipramine, doxepin, imipramine, nortriptyline, protriptyline, trimipramine), monoamine oxidase (MAO) inhibitors (e.g., phenelzine, tranylcypromine), and other antidepressants (e.g., bupropion, maprotiline, nefazodone, trazodone, vilazodone). Most clinical studies have shown that the antidepressant effect of usual dosages of sertraline in patients with depression is greater than that of placebo and comparable to that of usual dosages of tricyclic antidepressants (e.g., amitriptyline), other SSRIs (e.g., fluoxetine), and other antidepressants (e.g., nefazodone). In geriatric patients with major depression, sertraline appears to be as effective as amitriptyline. The onset of action of sertraline appears to be comparable to that of tricyclic antidepressants.

In general, response rates in patients with major depression are similar for currently available antidepressants, and the choice of antidepressant agent for a given patient depends principally on other factors such as potential adverse effects, safety or tolerability of these adverse effects in the individual patient, psychiatric and medical history, patient or family history of response to specific therapies, patient preference, quantity and quality of available clinical data, cost, and relative acute overdose safety. No single antidepressant can be recommended as optimal for all patients because of substantial heterogeneity in individual responses and in the nature, likelihood, and severity of adverse effects. In addition, patients vary in the degree to which certain adverse effects and other inconveniences of drug therapy (e.g., cost, dietary restrictions) affect their preferences.

In the large-scale Sequenced Treatment Alternatives to Relieve Depression (STAR*D) effectiveness trial, patients with major depressive disorder who did not respond to or could not tolerate therapy with one SSRI (citalopram) were randomized to switch to extended-release ("sustained-release") bupropion, sertraline, or extended-release venlafaxine as a second step of treatment (level 2). Remission rates as assessed by the 17-item Hamilton Rating Scale for Depression (HRSD-17) and the Quick Inventory of Depressive Symptomatology—Self Report (QIDS-SR-16) were approximately 21 and 26% for extended-release bupropion, 18 and 27% for sertraline, and 25 and 25% for extended-release venlafaxine therapy, respectively; response rates as assessed by the QIDS-SR-16 were 26, 27, and 28% for extended-release bupropion, sertraline, and extended-release venlafaxine therapy, respectively. These results suggest that after unsuccessful initial treatment of depressed patients with an SSRI, approximately 25% of patients will achieve remission after therapy is switched to another antidepressant and that either another SSRI (e.g., sertraline) or an agent from another class (e.g., bupropion, venlafaxine) may be reasonable alternative antidepressants in patients not responding to initial SSRI therapy.

Patient Tolerance Considerations. Because of differences in the adverse effect profile between SSRIs and tricyclic antidepressants, particularly less frequent anticholinergic effects, cardiovascular effects, and weight gain with SSRIs, these drugs may be preferred in patients in whom such effects are not tolerated or are of potential concern. The decreased incidence of anticholinergic effects associated with sertraline and other SSRIs compared with tricyclic antidepressants is a potential advantage, since such effects may result in discontinuance of the drug early during therapy in unusually sensitive patients. In addition, some anticholinergic effects may become troublesome during long-term tricyclic antidepressant therapy (e.g., persistent dry mouth may result in tooth decay). Although SSRIs share the same overall tolerability profile, certain patients may tolerate one drug in this class better than another. In an open study, most patients who had discontinued fluoxetine therapy because of adverse effects subsequently tolerated sertraline therapy. Antidepressants other than SSRIs may be preferred in patients in whom certain adverse GI effects (e.g., nausea, anorexia), nervous system effects (e.g., anxiety, nervousness, insomnia), and/or weight loss are not tolerated or are of concern, since such effects appear to occur more frequently with this class of drugs.

Pediatric Considerations. The clinical presentation of depression in children and adolescents can differ from that in adults and generally varies with the age and developmental stages of the child. Younger children may exhibit behavioral problems such as social withdrawal, aggressive behavior, apathy, sleep disruption, and weight loss; adolescents may present with somatic complaints, self esteem problems, rebelliousness, poor performance in school, or a pattern of engaging in risky or aggressive behavior.

Only limited data are available to date from controlled clinical studies evaluating various antidepressant agents in children and adolescents, and many of these studies have methodologic limitations (e.g., nonrandomized or uncontrolled, small sample size, short duration, nonspecific inclusion criteria). However, there is some evidence that the response to antidepressants in pediatric patients may differ from that seen in adults, and caution should be used in extrapolating data from adult studies when making treatment decisions for pediatric patients. Results of several studies evaluating tricyclic antidepressants (e.g., amitriptyline, desipramine, imipramine, nortriptyline) in preadolescent and adolescent patients with major depression indicate a lack of overall efficacy in this age group. Based on the lack of efficacy data regarding use of tricyclic antidepressants and MAO inhibitors in pediatric patients and because of the potential for life-threatening adverse effects associated with the use of these drugs, many experts consider selective serotonin-reuptake inhibitors, including sertraline, the drugs of choice when antidepressant therapy is indicated for the treatment of major depressive disorder in children and adolescents. However, the US Food and Drug Administration (FDA) states that, while efficacy of fluoxetine has been established in pediatric patients, efficacy of other newer antidepressants (i.e., sertraline, citalopram, desvenlafaxine, duloxetine, escitalopram, fluvoxamine, mirtazapine, nefazodone, paroxetine, venlafaxine) was not conclusively established in clinical trials in pediatric patients with major depressive disorder. In addition, FDA now warns that antidepressants increase the risk of suicidal thinking and behavior (suicidality) in children and adolescents with major depressive disorder and other psychiatric disorders. (See Cautions: Pediatric Precautions.) FDA currently states that anyone considering using an antidepressant in a child or adolescent for any clinical use must balance the potential risk of therapy with the clinical need. (See Cautions: Precautions and Contraindications.)

Geriatric Considerations. The response to antidepressants in depressed geriatric patients without dementia is similar to that reported in younger adults, but depression in geriatric patients often is not recognized and is not treated. In geriatric patients with major depressive disorder, selective serotonin-reuptake inhibitors (SSRIs) appear to be as effective as tricyclic antidepressants (e.g., amitriptyline) but generally are associated with fewer overall adverse effects than these other agents. Geriatric patients appear to be especially sensitive to anticholinergic (e.g., dry mouth, constipation, vision disturbance), cardiovascular, orthostatic hypotensive, and sedative effects of tricyclic antidepressants. The low incidence of anticholinergic effects associated with sertraline and other SSRIs compared with tricyclic antidepressants also is a potential advantage in geriatric patients, since such effects (e.g., constipation, dry mouth, confusion, memory impairment) may be particularly troublesome in these patients. However, SSRI therapy may be associated with other troublesome adverse effects (e.g., nausea and vomiting, agitation and akathisia, parkinsonian adverse effects, sexual dysfunction, weight loss, hyponatremia). Some clinicians state that SSRIs such as sertraline may be preferred for treating depression in geriatric patients in whom the orthostatic hypotension associated with many antidepressants (e.g., tricyclics) potentially may result in injuries (such as severe falls). However, despite the fewer cardiovascular and anticholinergic effects associated with SSRIs, these drugs did not show any advantage over tricyclic antidepressants with regard to hip fracture in a case-control study. In addition, there was little difference in the rates of falls between nursing home residents receiving SSRIs and those receiving tricyclic antidepressants in a retrospective study. Therefore, all geriatric individuals receiving either type of antidepressant should be considered at increased risk of falls and appropriate measures should be taken. In addition, clinicians prescribing SSRIs in geriatric patients should be aware of the many possible drug interactions associated with these drugs, including those involving metabolism of the drugs through the cytochrome P-450 system. (See Drug Interactions.)

Patients with dementia of the Alzheimer's type (Alzheimer's disease, presenile or senile dementia) often present with depressive symptoms, such as depressed mood, appetite loss, insomnia, fatigue, irritability, and agitation. Most experts recommend that patients with dementia of the Alzheimer's type who present with clinically important and persistent depressive symptoms be considered as candidates for pharmacotherapy even if they fail to meet the criteria for a major depressive syndrome. The goals of such therapy are to improve mood, functional status (e.g., cognition), and quality of life. Treatment of depression also may reduce other neuropsychiatric symptoms associated with depression in patients with dementia, including aggression, anxiety, apathy, and psychosis. Although patients may present with depressed mood alone, the possibility of more extensive depressive symptomatology should be considered. Therefore, patients should be evaluated and monitored carefully for indices of major depression, suicidal ideation, and neurovegetative signs since safety measures (e.g., hospitalization for suicidality) and more vigorous and aggressive therapy (e.g., relatively high dosages, multiple drug trials) may be needed in some patients.

Although placebo-controlled trials of antidepressants in depressed patients with concurrent dementia have shown mixed results, the available evidence and experience with the use of antidepressants in patients with dementia of the Alzheimer's type and associated depressive manifestations indicate that depressive symptoms (including depressed mood alone and with neurovegetative changes) in such patients are responsive to antidepressant therapy. In some patients, cognitive deficits may partially or fully resolve during antidepressant therapy, but the extent of response will be limited to the degree of cognitive impairment that is directly related to depression. SSRIs such as sertraline, citalopram, escitalopram, fluoxetine, or paroxetine are generally considered as first-line agents in the treatment of depressed patients with dementia since they are better tolerated than some other antidepressants (e.g., tricyclic antidepressants, monoamine oxidase inhibitors). Some possible alternative agents to SSRIs include bupropion, mirtazapine, and venlafaxine. Some geriatric patients with dementia and depression may be unable to tolerate the antidepressant dosages needed to achieve full remission. When a rapid antidepressant response is not critical, some experts therefore recommend a very gradual dosage increase to increase the likelihood that a therapeutic dosage of the SSRI or other antidepressant will be reached and tolerated. In a randomized, placebo-controlled study in a limited number of patients with major depression and Alzheimer's disease, sertraline was found to be superior to placebo; depression reduction in this study was accompanied by lessened behavior disturbance and improved activities of daily living but not improved cognition.

Cardiovascular Considerations. The relatively low incidence of adverse cardiovascular effects, including orthostatic hypotension and conduction disturbances, associated with sertraline and most other SSRIs may be advantageous in patients in whom the cardiovascular effects associated with tricyclic antidepressants may be hazardous. Patients with a recent history of myocardial infarction or unstable cardiovascular disease were excluded from premarketing clinical studies with sertraline. However, the cardiovascular safety of sertraline (50–200 mg daily for 24 weeks; mean dosage of 89 mg daily) was evaluated in a postmarketing, double-blind, placebo-controlled study in adult outpatients with major depressive disorder and a recent history of myocardial infarction or unstable angina pectoris requiring hospitalization but who were otherwise free of life-threatening medical conditions. When therapy was initiated during the acute phase of recovery (within 30 days after a myocardial infarction or hospitalization for unstable angina), sertraline therapy did not differ from placebo on the following cardiovascular end points at week 16: left ventricular ejection fraction and total cardiovascular events (angina, chest pain, edema, palpitations, syncope, postural dizziness, chronic heart failure, myocardial infarction, tachycardia, bradycardia, blood pressure changes). Although not statistically significant, approximately 20% fewer major cardiovascular events involving death or requiring hospitalization (e.g., for myocardial infarction, chronic heart failure, stroke, angina) occurred in the sertraline-treated patients compared with those receiving placebo. (See Cautions: Cardiovascular Effects and also see Cautions: Precautions and Contraindications.)

Sedative Considerations. Because sertraline and other SSRIs are generally less sedating than some other antidepressants (e.g., tricyclics), some clinicians state that these drugs may be preferable in patients who do not require the sedative effects associated with many antidepressant agents; however, an antidepressant with more prominent sedative effects (e.g., trazodone) may be preferable in certain patients (e.g., those with insomnia).

Suicidal Risk Considerations. Suicide is a known risk of depression and certain other psychiatric disorders, and these disorders themselves are the strongest predictors of suicide. However, there has been a long-standing concern that antidepressants may have a role in inducing worsening of depression and the emergence of suicidal thinking and behavior (suicidality) in certain patients during the early phases of treatment. FDA states that antidepressants increased the risk of suicidality in short-term studies in children, adolescents, and young adults (18–24 years of age) with major depressive disorder and other psychiatric disorders. (See Cautions: Pediatric Precautions.) An increased suicidality risk was not demonstrated with antidepressants compared with placebo in adults older than 24 years of age and a reduced risk was observed in adults 65 years of age or older. It currently is unknown whether the suicidality risk extends to longer-term antidepressant use (i.e., beyond several months); however, there is substantial evidence from placebo-controlled maintenance trials in adults with major depressive disorder that antidepressants can delay the recurrence of depression. Because the risk of suicidality in depressed patients may persist until substantial remission of depression occurs, appropriate monitoring and close observation of all patients who are receiving antidepressant therapy is recommended. (See Cautions: Precautions and Contraindications.)

Other Considerations. Sertraline has been effective in patients with moderate to severe depression.

In the Sequenced Treatment Alternatives to Relieve Depression (STAR*D) level 2 trial, patients with major depressive disorder who did not respond to or could not tolerate therapy with citalopram (another SSRI) were randomized to receive either extended-release ("sustained-release") bupropion or buspirone therapy in addition to citalopram. Although both extended-release bupropion and buspirone were found to produce similar remission rates, extended-release bupropion produced a greater reduction in the number and severity of symptoms and a lower rate of drug discontinuance than buspirone in this large-scale, effectiveness trial. These results suggest that augmentation of SSRI therapy with extended-release bupropion may be useful in some patients with refractory depression.

Sertraline has been effective in patients with depression and concurrent human immunodeficiency virus (HIV) infection and depression with anxiety.

In a double-blind, placebo-controlled study, both sertraline and imipramine were found to be more effective than placebo in reducing the depressive symptoms and improving psychosocial functioning in patients with dysthymia† without concurrent major depression; moreover, fewer patients treated with sertraline than those treated with imipramine or placebo discontinued therapy because of adverse effects. The results of several other studies, both controlled and uncontrolled, also suggest that sertraline may be effective in patients with dysthymia. Because dysthymia is a chronic condition and requires prolonged antidepressant therapy, the good tolerability demonstrated in clinical studies to date may be advantageous. Sertraline also has been used in the treatment of anger attacks associated with atypical depression and dysthymia† in a limited number of patients.

■ **Obsessive-Compulsive Disorder** Sertraline is used in the treatment of obsessive-compulsive disorder when the obsessions or compulsions cause marked distress, are time consuming (take longer than 1 hour daily), or interfere substantially with the patient's normal routine, occupational or academic functioning, or usual social activities or relationships. Obsessions are recurrent and persistent ideas, thoughts, impulses, or images that, at some time during the disturbance, are experienced as intrusive and inappropriate (i.e., "ego dystonic") and that cause marked anxiety or distress but that are not simply excessive worries about real-life problems. Compulsions are repetitive, intentional behaviors (e.g., hand washing, ordering, checking) or mental acts (e.g., praying, counting, repeating words silently) performed in response to an obsession or according to rules that must be applied rigidly (e.g., in a stereotyped fashion). Although the behaviors or acts are aimed at preventing or reducing distress or preventing some dreaded event or situation, they either are not connected in a realistic manner with what they are designed to neutralize or prevent or are clearly excessive. At some time during the course of the disturbance, the patient, if an adult, recognizes that the obsessions or compulsions are excessive or unreasonable; children may not make such a recognition.

The efficacy of sertraline for the management of obsessive-compulsive disorder has been established in several multicenter, placebo-controlled studies, including one study of 8 weeks' duration and 2 studies of 12 weeks' duration in adults and one study of 12 weeks' duration in children and adolescents 6–17 years of age. Patients in these studies had moderate to severe obsessive-compulsive disorder with mean baseline total scores on the Yale-Brown Obsessive-Compulsive Scale (YBOCS) of 23–25 in adults and 22 in children and adolescents (measured in the Children's Yale-Brown Obsessive-Compulsive Scale [CY-BOCS]). In the 8-week study with flexible dosing, adult patients received sertraline in dosages ranging from 50–200 mg daily; the mean dosage for those completing the study was 186 mg daily. Total scores on the YBOCS decreased by an average of approximately 4 points in sertraline-treated patients and 2 points in patients receiving placebo; this difference was statistically significant.

In a fixed-dose study of 12 weeks' duration involving sertraline dosages of 50, 100, and 200 mg daily, adult patients receiving 50 and 200 mg of the drug daily experienced substantially greater reductions in the YBOCS total score than those receiving placebo (approximately 6 to approximately 3 points, respectively). In a 12-week study with flexible dosing in the range of 50–200 mg daily, the mean sertraline dosage in adult patients completing the study was 185 mg daily. YBOCS total scores in the sertraline-treated patients were reduced by a mean of approximately 7 points, which was better than the mean reduction of approximately 4 points reported in the placebo-treated patients.

In a 12-week study with flexible dosing, sertraline therapy was initiated at dosages of 25 or 50 mg daily in children 6–12 years of age or adolescents 13–17 years of age, respectively. Subsequent dosage was titrated according to individual tolerance over the first 4 weeks to a maximum dosage of 200 mg daily; the mean dosage for those completing the study was 178 mg daily. The drug produced substantially greater reductions in scores in the Children's Yale-Brown Obsessive-Compulsive Scale (CY-BOCS), the National Institute of Mental Health Global Obsessive-Compulsive Scale (NIMH-OC), and the Clinical Global Impressions (CGI) Improvement Scale; total scores on the CY-BOCS decreased by an average of approximately 7 units in sertraline-treated patients and 3 units in patients receiving placebo. An analysis of these controlled studies for possible age- and gender-related effects on treatment outcome did not suggest any difference in efficacy based on either the age or gender of the patient.

In addition, in an uncontrolled 6-week study with flexible dosing (50–200 mg daily) in children or adolescents 6–17 years of age with obsessive-compulsive disorder or major depression†, those with a diagnosis of obsessive-compulsive disorder had mean baseline total scores on the CY-BOCS, NIMH-OC, and CGI of about 24.9, 10.2, and 5.2, respectively. Sertraline produced substantial reductions in all 3 of the scales; total scores on CY-BOCS, NIMH-OC, and CGI decreased to 12.9, 6.7, and 3.4, respectively. In another uncontrolled, 6-week study employing a sertraline dosage that was escalated from 25 to 200 mg daily over 3 weeks, the drug combined with behavioral therapy was effective in a limited number of adolescents 13–17 years of age with obsessive-compulsive disorder refractory to other therapies; total scores on the CY-BOCS at the end of the study decreased by 11 points (from 25.4 to 14.4).

Results from comparative studies to date suggest sertraline and other selective serotonin-reuptake inhibitors (SSRIs; e.g., fluoxetine, fluvoxamine, paroxetine) are as effective or somewhat less effective than clomipramine and more effective than tricyclic antidepressants (e.g., amitriptyline, desipramine, imipramine, nortriptyline) in the management of obsessive-compulsive disorder. In a pooled analysis of separate short-term (10–13 weeks) studies comparing clomipramine, fluoxetine, fluvoxamine, or sertraline with placebo, clomipramine was calculated as being more effective (as determined by measures on the YBOC scale) than SSRIs, although all drugs were superior to placebo. Like clomipramine, SSRIs reduce but do not completely eliminate obsessions and compulsions.

Many clinicians consider an SSRI (e.g., sertraline, fluoxetine, fluvoxamine, paroxetine) or clomipramine to be the drugs of choice for the pharmacologic treatment of obsessive-compulsive disorder. The decision whether to initiate therapy with an SSRI or clomipramine often is made based on the adverse effect profile of these drugs. For example, some clinicians prefer clomipramine in patients who may not tolerate the adverse effect profile of SSRIs (nausea, headache, overstimulation, sleep disturbances) while SSRIs may be useful alternatives in patients unable to tolerate the adverse effects (anticholinergic effects, cardiovascular effects, sedation) associated with clomipramine therapy. Consideration of individual patient characteristics (age, concurrent medical conditions), pharmacokinetics of the drug, potential drug interactions, and cost of therapy may also influence clinicians when selecting between SSRIs and clomipramine as first-line therapy in patients with obsessive-compulsive disorder. Although not clearly established, it has been suggested that the mechanism of action of sertraline and other potent serotonin-reuptake inhibitors (e.g., clomipramine, fluoxetine, fluvoxamine, paroxetine) used in the management of obsessive-compulsive disorder may be related to their serotonergic activity.

■ **Panic Disorder** Sertraline is used in the treatment of panic disorder with or without agoraphobia. Panic disorder is characterized by the occurrence of unexpected panic attacks and associated concern about having additional attacks, worry about the implications or consequences of the attacks, and/or a clinically important change in behavior related to the attacks.

According to DSM-IV, panic disorder is characterized by recurrent unexpected panic attacks, which consist of a discrete period of intense fear or discomfort in which 4 (or more) of the following symptoms develop abruptly and reach a peak within 10 minutes: palpitations, pounding heart, or accelerated heart rate; sweating; trembling or shaking; sensations of shortness of breath or smothering; feeling of choking; chest pain or discomfort; nausea or abdominal distress; feeling dizzy, unsteady, lightheaded, or faint; derealization (feelings of unreality) or depersonalization (being detached from oneself); fear of losing control; fear of dying; paresthesias (numbness or tingling sensations); and chills or hot flushes.

The efficacy of sertraline for the management of panic disorder has been established by 3 double-blind, placebo-controlled studies in adult outpatients who met DSM-III-R criteria for panic disorder with or without agoraphobia. The first 2 studies were of 10 weeks' duration and used a flexible dosing schedule. Sertraline therapy was initiated in a dosage of 25 mg daily for the first week and then dosage was escalated to 50–200 mg daily depending on clinical response and tolerability. The mean sertraline dosages for completers were 131 and 144 mg daily for the first 2 studies. Overall, these 2 studies demonstrated that sertraline was superior to placebo in decreasing the frequency of panic attacks and in improving scores on the Clinical Global Impression Severity of Illness and Global Improvement Scales. The difference between sertraline and placebo in reduction in the number of full panic attacks per week compared with baseline was approximately 2 in both studies.

The third study was a fixed-dose study of 12 weeks' duration. Sertraline was given in dosages of 50, 100, and 200 mg daily. The patients receiving sertraline demonstrated a substantially greater reduction in panic attack frequency than patients receiving placebo. However, the results of this study were not readily interpretable regarding a dose-response relationship for efficacy in this condition.

An analysis of these 3 controlled studies for possible age-, race-, or gender-related effects on treatment outcome did not suggest any difference in efficacy based on these patient characteristics.

Panic disorder can be treated with cognitive and behavioral psychotherapy and/or pharmacologic therapy. There are several classes of drugs that appear to be effective in the pharmacologic management of panic disorder, including tricyclic antidepressants, MAO inhibitors (e.g., phenelzine), selective serotonin-reuptake inhibitors (SSRIs; e.g., citalopram, fluoxetine, paroxetine, sertraline), and benzodiazepines (e.g., alprazolam, clonazepam). When choosing among the available drugs, clinicians should consider their acceptance and tolerability by patients; their ability to reduce or eliminate panic attacks, reduce clinically important anxiety and disability secondary to phobic avoidance, and ameliorate other common comorbid conditions (such as depression); and their ability to prevent relapse during long-term therapy. Because of their better tolerability when compared with other agents (such as the tricyclic antidepressants and benzodiazepines), the lack of physical dependence problems commonly associated with benzodiazepines, and efficacy in panic disorder with comorbid conditions (e.g., depression, other anxiety disorders such as obsessive-compulsive disorder, alcoholism), many clinicians prefer SSRIs as first-line therapy in the management of panic disorder. If SSRI therapy is ineffective or not tolerated, use of a tricyclic antidepressant or a benzodiazepine is recommended.

Sertraline has improved chronic idiopathic urticaria† associated with panic disorder in at least one patient, but further study is needed to determine whether serotonin is involved in the pathogenesis of urticaria and whether SSRIs are effective in this condition.

■ **Posttraumatic Stress Disorder** Sertraline is used in the treatment of posttraumatic stress disorder (PTSD). PTSD is an anxiety disorder that involves the development of certain characteristic symptoms following personal exposure to an extreme traumatic stressor. According to DSM-IV, PTSD requires exposure to a traumatic event(s) that involved actual or threatened death or serious injury, or threat to the physical integrity of self or others, and the response to the event must involve intense fear, helplessness, or horror (in children the response may be expressed by disorganized or agitated behavior). PTSD is characterized by persistent symptoms of *reexperiencing* the trauma (e.g., intrusive distressing recollections of the event; recurrent distressing dreams of the event; acting or feeling as if the event were recurring including illusions, hallucinations, or flashbacks; intense distress at exposure to internal or external cues that symbolize or resemble an aspect of the event; physiologic reactivity on exposure to internal or external cues that symbolize or resemble an aspect of the event), persistent *avoidance* of stimuli associated with the trauma and numbing of general responsiveness (e.g., efforts to avoid thoughts, feelings, or conversations related to the event; efforts to avoid activities, places, or people that arouse recollections of the event; inability to recall an important aspect of the event; markedly diminished interest or participation in significant activities; feeling of detachment or estrangement from others; restricted emotions and/or range of affect not present before the event; sense of a foreshortened future), and persistent symptoms of *increased arousal* (e.g., difficulty sleeping; irritability/outbursts of anger; difficulty concentrating; hypervigilance; exaggerated startle response). According to DSM-IV, a PTSD diagnosis requires the presence of 1 or more symptoms of *reexperiencing*, 3 or more symptoms of *avoidance*, and 2 or more symptoms of *increased arousal*, all of which must be present for at least one month and cause clinically important distress or impairment in social, occupational, or other important areas of functioning. PTSD, like other anxiety disorders, rarely occurs alone, and patients with PTSD often present with comorbid disorders (e.g., major depressive disorder, substance abuse disorders, panic disorder, generalized anxiety disorders, obsessive-compulsive disorder, social phobia); it is unknown whether these comorbid disorders precede or follow the onset of PTSD.

Psychotherapy alone or in combination with pharmacotherapy generally is considered the treatment of choice for PTSD. Pharmacologic therapy may be indicated in addition to psychotherapy for initial treatment of PTSD in patients who have comorbid disorders (e.g., major depressive disorder, bipolar disorder, other anxiety disorders) and also may be indicated in those who do not respond to initial treatment with psychotherapy alone. If pharmacotherapy is indicated in patients with PTSD, selective serotonin-reuptake inhibitors (SSRIs; e.g., sertraline, fluoxetine, paroxetine) usually are considered the drugs of choice (except in patients with bipolar disorder who require treatment with mood stabilizing agents).

The efficacy of sertraline for the management of PTSD has been established in 2 placebo-controlled studies of 12 weeks' duration in adult outpatients (76% women) who met DSM-III-R criteria for chronic PTSD (duration of symptoms 3 months or longer). The mean duration of PTSD for these patients was approximately 12 years and 44% of patients had secondary depressive disorders. Sertraline therapy was initiated at a dosage of 25 mg daily for the first week and then dosage was escalated (using a flexible dosage schedule) to 50–200 mg daily based on clinical response and tolerability. The mean sertraline dosage for patients who completed studies 1 and 2 was 146 mg and 151 mg daily, respectively. Overall, these 2 studies showed that sertraline was superior to placebo in improving scores on the Clinician-Administered PTSD Scale Part 2 total severity scale (a measure of the intensity and frequency of all 3 PTSD diagnostic symptom clusters [reexperiencing/intrusion, avoidance/numbing, and hyperarousal]), Impact of Event Scale (a patient rated measurement of the intrusion and avoidance symptoms), and the Clinical Global Impressions Severity of Illness and Global Improvement Scales.

However, in 2 additional placebo-controlled studies of similar design and duration, the difference in response to treatment on key assessment scales between patients receiving sertraline and those receiving placebo was not statistically significant. In one study of mostly female patients who met the DSM-III-R criteria for PTSD related to sexual/physical trauma, those receiving placebo experienced substantially greater improvement on the Impact of Event Scale than those receiving sertraline therapy. Although this study enrolled a higher proportion of patients with comorbid anxiety disorders and a higher proportion of patients receiving placebo with a successful response to previous psychotropic therapies than the studies demonstrating efficacy of the drug, it is unknown whether these factors alone account for the high placebo response in the study.

Efficacy of sertraline for the management of PTSD related to war or combat was evaluated in a study involving primarily white men in a VA medical center outpatient setting (mean duration of PTSD approximately 18 years). At the end of this study, patients receiving sertraline did not differ from those receiving placebo on any of the key efficacy assessment scales (e.g., Clinician-Administered PTSD scale, Davidson Self-Rating Trauma scale, Impact of Event Scale). In addition, the mean change from baseline for both treatment groups in this study was of a lesser magnitude than those of patients receiving placebo in the other reported studies. The lack of response to sertraline treatment in these combat veterans is consistent with controlled studies evaluating other selective serotonin-reuptake inhibitors (e.g., fluoxetine, brofaromine [not commercially available in the US]) in Vietnam veterans with PTSD. Some experts suggest that patients with combat- or war-related PTSD may be less responsive to treatment than patients with PTSD related to other traumatic events (e.g., sexual assault, accidents, natural disasters) because of some factor inherent in combat- or war-related trauma. However, other experts suggest that the poor treatment response in studies evaluating use in veterans may be the result of sampling error since veterans receiving treatment at VA hospitals may constitute a self-selected group of patients with chronic PTSD who have multiple impairments (comorbid disorders, substance abuse) that make them less responsive to treatment.

Since PTSD is a more common disorder in women than men, the majority (76%) of patients in reported studies were women. A retrospective analysis of pooled data has shown a substantial difference between sertraline and placebo on key efficacy assessment scales (e.g., Clinician-Administered PTSD scale, Impact of Event Scale, Clinical Global Impressions Severity of Illness Scale) in women (regardless of a baseline diagnosis of comorbid depression), but essentially no effect in the limited number of men studied. The clinical importance of this apparent gender effect is unknown; however, only limited data are available to date regarding use of SSRIs in men who have PTSD related to noncombat-related trauma (e.g., sexual assault, accidents, natural disasters). There are insufficient data to date to determine whether race or age has any effect on the efficacy of sertraline in the management of PTSD.

For additional information on the use of SSRIs in the treatment of PTSD, see Uses: Posttraumatic Stress Disorder, in Prazosin Hydrochloride 24:20 and Paroxetine 28:16.04.20.

■ **Premenstrual Dysphoric Disorder** Sertraline is used in the treatment of premenstrual dysphoric disorder (previously late luteal phase dysphoric disorder). DSM-IV criteria for premenstrual dysphoric disorder (PMDD) require that in most menstrual cycles of the previous year at least 5 of the following 11 symptoms must have been present for most of the time during the last week of the luteal phase (with at least one of the symptoms being one of the first 4 listed): marked depressed mood, feelings of hopelessness, or self-deprecating thoughts; marked anxiety, tension, feelings of being "keyed up" or on "edge"; marked affective lability (e.g., feeling suddenly sad or tearful or increased sensitivity to rejection); persistent and marked anger or irritability or increased interpersonal conflicts; decreased interest in usual activities (e.g., work, school, friends, hobbies); a subjective sense of difficulty in concentrating; lethargy, easy fatigability, or marked lack of energy; marked change in appetite, overeating, or specific food cravings; hypersomnia or insomnia; a subjective sense of being overwhelmed or out of control; and other physical symptoms, such as breast tenderness or swelling, headaches, joint or muscle pain, or a sensation of "bloating" or weight gain. Such symptoms should begin to remit within a few days of the onset of menses (follicular phase) and are always absent in the week following menses. The presence of this cyclical pattern of symptoms must be confirmed by at least 2 consecutive months of prospective daily symptom ratings. PMDD should be distinguished from the more common premenstrual syndrome (PMS) by prospective daily ratings and the strict criteria listed above.

The efficacy of sertraline for the management of PMDD has been established in 2 randomized, placebo-controlled studies over 3 menstrual cycles in adult women who met DSM-III-R or DSM-IV criteria for PMDD. In these studies, flexible dosages (range: 50–150 mg daily) of sertraline administered continuously throughout the menstrual cycle or during the luteal phase only (i.e., for 2 weeks prior to the onset of menses) were shown to be substantially more effective than placebo in improving scores from baseline on the Daily Record of Severity of Problems (DRSP), the Clinical Global Impression of Severity of Illness (CGI-S) and Improvement (CGI-I), and/or the Hamilton Depression Rating Scales (HAMD-17). The mean dosage of sertraline in patients completing these trials was 102 or 74 mg daily for those receiving continuous or luteal-phase dosing of the drug, respectively.

When given in a flexible dosage of 50–150 mg daily in a separate double-blind, placebo-controlled study, sertraline was substantially better than placebo in improving symptoms (depressive symptoms, physical symptoms, anger/irritability) and functional impairment associated with this disorder. The beneficial effect of the drug was apparent by the first treatment cycle. In an open study comparing sertraline and desipramine in the treatment of premenstrual dysphoric disorder, sertraline and possibly desipramine were found to be effective; however, sertraline was better tolerated than desipramine. Additional controlled studies are needed to determine whether the efficacy of the drug is sustained during longer-term, maintenance therapy in women with this condition. In addition, efficacy of sertraline used in conjunction with oral contraceptives for the treatment of PMDD has not been determined since patients receiving oral contraceptives were excluded from most clinical studies to date.

■ **Social Phobia** Sertraline is used in the treatment of social phobia (social anxiety disorder). According to DSM-IV, social phobia is characterized by a marked and persistent fear of one or more social or performance situations in which the person is exposed to unfamiliar people or to possible scrutiny by others. Exposure to the feared situation almost invariably provokes anxiety, which may approach the intensity of a panic attack. The feared situations are avoided or endured with intense anxiety or distress. The avoidance, fear, or anxious anticipation of encountering the social or performance situation interferes significantly with the person's daily routine, occupational or academic functioning, or social activities or relationships, or there is marked distress about having the phobias. Lesser degrees of performance anxiety or shyness generally do not require psychotherapy or pharmacologic treatment.

The efficacy of sertraline in the treatment of social phobia has been established in 2 multicenter, placebo-controlled studies in adult outpatients who met DSM-IV criteria for social phobia. In one study of 12 weeks' duration, 47% of patients receiving flexible dosages of sertraline (50–200 mg daily; mean dosage of 144 mg daily) were characterized as responders (defined as a score of 1 or 2 on the Clinical Global Impressions [CGI] Global Improvement Scale) compared with 26% of those receiving placebo (intent-to-treat analysis). Sertraline also was found to be superior to placebo on the Liebowitz Social Anxiety Scale (LSAS), a 24-item clinician administered measure of fear, anxiety, and avoidance of social and performance situation, and on most secondary efficacy measures, including the Duke Brief Social Phobia Scale (BSPS) total score, fear and avoidance subscales of BSPS, and fear/anxiety and avoidance subscales of LSAS. These results were similar to those seen in a flexible-dose study of 20 weeks' duration, in which a score of 1 ("very much improved") or 2 ("much improved") on the CGI Global Improvement Scale was attained by the end of the treatment period by 53 or 29% of patients receiving sertraline (50–200 mg daily; mean dosage of 147 mg daily) or placebo, respectively (intent-to-treat analysis). Sixty-five patients in this study subsequently were enrolled in a separate controlled study, including 50 patients who had responded to sertraline in the initial study and then were randomized to receive either continued treatment with sertraline or placebo in the subsequent study and 15 patients who had responded to placebo in the initial study and continued to receive placebo in the subsequent study. Based on an intent-to-treat analysis, 4% of patients who continued treatment with sertraline, 36% of patients randomized to receive placebo, and 27% of those who continued treatment with placebo relapsed (defined as an increase of 2 or more points from baseline in the CGI Severity of Illness score or discontinuance of the study drug because of lack of efficacy) at the end of the 24-week treatment period. Similar to results of pivotal, short-term clinical studies, sertraline also was shown to be substantially more effective than placebo on the CGI Severity of Illness Scale, Marks Fear Questionnaire (MFQ) Social Phobia subscale, and BSPS total score.

Subgroup analysis of short-term, controlled studies in adult outpatients with social anxiety disorder did not reveal any evidence of gender-related differences in treatment outcome. There was insufficient information to determine the effect of race or age on treatment outcome. Safety and efficacy of sertraline for the treatment of social phobia in children or adolescents have not been established to date.

■ **Premature Ejaculation** Like some other serotonin-reuptake inhibitors, sertraline has been used with some success in the treatment of premature ejaculation†. In a placebo-controlled study, sertraline produced substantial improvements compared with placebo in time to ejaculation, number of successful attempts at intercourse, and incidence of ejaculation during foreplay, as well as overall clinical judgment of improvement. In addition, the drug was well tolerated in most patients. A trial with drug therapy may be particularly useful in patients who fail or refuse behavioral or psychotherapeutic treatment or when partners are unwilling to cooperate with such therapy.

■ **Other Uses** Sertraline has been used in a limited number of patients with various types of headache† with variable results; however, its use in this condition may be limited by frequent adverse effects.

Dosage and Administration

■ **Administration** Sertraline is administered orally. The drug usually is administered once daily in the morning or evening. The extent of GI absorption of sertraline reportedly may be increased slightly, the peak concentration increased by about 25%, and the time to peak concentration after a dose decreased from about 8 to 5.5 hours when the drug is administered with food, but such changes do not appear to be clinically important.

When sertraline hydrochloride concentrate for oral solution (Zoloft®) is used, doses of the drug should be measured carefully using the calibrated dropper provided by the manufacturer. The appropriate dose of the oral solution should be diluted in 120 mL of water, ginger ale, lemon/lime soda, lemonade, or orange juice before administration. The diluted solution containing sertraline hydrochloride should be mixed and administered immediately and should not be allowed to stand before administration. A slight haze may occasionally appear in the diluted oral solution, but the manufacturer states that this is normal.

■ **Dosage** Dosage of sertraline hydrochloride is expressed in terms of sertraline.

Patients receiving sertraline should be monitored for possible worsening of depression, suicidality, or unusual changes in behavior, especially at the beginning of therapy or during periods of dosage adjustment. (See Cautions: Precautions and Contraindications.)

Because withdrawal effects may occur with discontinuance of sertraline, other selective serotonin-reuptake inhibitors (SSRIs), and selective serotonin- and norepinephrine-reuptake inhibitors (SNRIs), abrupt discontinuance of these drugs should be avoided whenever possible. In addition, patients may experience a worsening of psychiatric status when the drug is discontinued abruptly. When sertraline therapy is discontinued, the dosage should be reduced gradually (e.g., over a period of several weeks) and the patient monitored for possible withdrawal symptoms. If intolerable symptoms occur following a dosage reduction or upon discontinuance of therapy, the drug may be reinstituted at the previously prescribed dosage. Subsequently, the clinician may continue decreasing the dosage, but at a more gradual rate. (See Cautions: Nervous System Effects and see Chronic Toxicity.)

The manufacturers recommend that an interval of at least 2 weeks elapse when switching a patient from a monoamine oxidase (MAO) inhibitor to sertraline or when switching from sertraline to an MAO inhibitor. For additional information on potentially serious drug interactions that may occur between sertraline and MAO inhibitors or other serotonergic agents, see Cautions: Precautions and Contraindications and also see Drug Interactions: Serotonergic Drugs.

Clinical experience regarding the optimal timing of switching from other drugs used in the treatment of major depressive disorder, obsessive-compulsive disorder, panic disorder, posttraumatic stress disorder, premenstrual dysphoric disorder, and social anxiety disorder to sertraline therapy is limited. Therefore, the manufacturers recommend that care and prudent medical judgment be exercised when switching from other drugs to sertraline, particularly from long-acting agents (such as fluoxetine). Because some adverse reactions resembling serotonin syndrome have developed when fluoxetine therapy was discontinued abruptly and sertraline therapy was initiated immediately afterward, a washout period appears to be advisable when transferring a patient from fluoxetine to sertraline therapy. However, the appropriate duration of the washout period when switching from one selective serotonin-reuptake inhibitor to another has not been clearly established. Pending further experience in patients being transferred from therapy with another antidepressant to sertraline, it generally is recommended that the previous antidepressant be discontinued according to the recommended guidelines for the specific antidepressant prior to initiation of sertraline therapy. (See Drug Interactions: Serotonergic Drugs and see Drug Interactions: Tricyclic and Other Antidepressants.)

Major Depressive Disorder For the management of major depressive disorder in adults, the recommended initial dosage of sertraline is 50–100 mg once daily. If no clinical improvement is apparent, dosage may be increased at intervals of not less than 1 week up to a maximum of 200 mg daily. Clinical experience with the drug to date suggests that many patients will respond to 50–100 mg of the drug once daily. While a relationship between dose and antidepressant effect has not been established, efficacy of the drug was demonstrated in clinical trials employing 50–200 mg daily.

While the optimum duration of sertraline therapy has not been established, many experts state that acute depressive episodes require several months or longer of sustained antidepressant therapy. In addition, some clinicians recommend that long-term antidepressant therapy be considered in certain patients at risk for recurrence of depressive episodes (such as those with highly recurrent unipolar depression). Whether the dose of sertraline required to induce remission is identical to the dose needed to maintain and/or sustain euthymia is unknown. Systematic evaluation of sertraline has shown that its antidepressant efficacy is maintained for periods of up to 1 year in patients receiving 50–200 mg daily (mean dose of 70 mg daily). The usefulness of the drug in patients receiving prolonged therapy should be reevaluated periodically.

Obsessive-Compulsive Disorder For the management of obsessive-compulsive disorder in adults and adolescents 13–17 years of age, the recommended initial dosage of sertraline is 50 mg once daily. In children 6–12 years of age, the recommended initial dosage of sertraline is 25 mg once daily. If no clinical improvement is apparent, dosage may be increased at intervals of not less than 1 week up to a maximum of 200 mg daily. However, it should be considered that children usually have a lower body weight than adults and particular care should be taken to avoid excessive dosage in children. While a relationship between dose and efficacy in obsessive-compulsive disorder has not been established, efficacy of the drug was demonstrated in clinical trials employing 50–200 mg daily in adults and 25–200 mg daily in children and adolescents.

While the optimum duration of sertraline therapy required to prevent recurrence of obsessive-compulsive symptoms has not been established to date, the manufacturer and many experts state that this disorder is chronic and requires several months or longer of sustained therapy. Whether the dose of sertraline required to induce remission is identical to the dose needed to maintain and/or sustain remission in patients with this disorder is unknown. Systematic evaluation of sertraline has shown that its efficacy in the management of obsessive-compulsive disorder is maintained for periods of up to 28 weeks in patients receiving 50–200 mg daily. The usefulness of the drug in patients receiving prolonged therapy should be reevaluated periodically.

Panic Disorder For the management of panic disorder in adults, the recommended initial dosage of sertraline is 25 mg once daily. After 1 week, the dosage should be increased to 50 mg once daily. If no clinical improvement is apparent, dosage may then be increased at intervals of not less than 1 week up to a maximum of 200 mg daily.

While the optimum duration of sertraline therapy required to prevent recurrence of panic disorder has not been established to date, the manufacturer and many experts state that this disorder is chronic and requires several months or longer of sustained therapy. Whether the dose of sertraline required to induce remission is identical to the dose needed to maintain and/or sustain remission in patients with this disorder is unknown. Systematic evaluation of sertraline has shown that its efficacy in the management of panic disorder is maintained for periods of up to 28 weeks in patients receiving 50–200 mg daily. The usefulness of the drug in patients receiving prolonged therapy should be reevaluated periodically.

Posttraumatic Stress Disorder For the management of posttraumatic stress disorder (PTSD) in adults, the recommended initial dosage of sertraline is 25 mg once daily. After 1 week, dosage should be increased to 50 mg once daily. If no clinical improvement is apparent, dosage may then be increased at intervals of not less than 1 week up to a maximum of 200 mg daily.

While the optimum duration of sertraline therapy required to prevent recurrence of PTSD has not been established to date, this disorder is chronic and it is reasonable to continue therapy in responding patients. Whether the dose of sertraline required to induce remission is identical to the dose needed to maintain and/or sustain remission in patients with this disorder is unknown. Systematic evaluation of sertraline has shown that its efficacy in the management of posttraumatic stress disorder is maintained for periods of up to 28 weeks in patients receiving 50–200 mg daily. The usefulness of the drug in patients receiving prolonged therapy should be reevaluated periodically.

Premenstrual Dysphoric Disorder For the treatment of premenstrual dysphoric disorder (previously late luteal phase dysphoric disorder), the recommended initial dosage of sertraline is 50 mg daily given continuously throughout the menstrual cycle or given during the luteal phase only (i.e., starting 2 weeks prior to the anticipated onset of menstruation and continuing through the first full day of menses). If no clinical improvement is apparent, dosage may be increased in 50-mg increments at the onset of each new menstrual cycle up to a maximum of 150 mg daily when administered continuously or 100 mg daily when administered during the luteal phase only. If a dosage of 100 mg daily has been established with luteal phase dosing, dosages should be increased gradually over the first 3 days of each luteal phase dosing period. While a relationship between dose and effect in premenstrual dysphoric disorder (PMDD) has not been established, efficacy of the drug was demonstrated in clinical trials employing 50–150 mg daily.

The optimum duration of sertraline therapy required to treat PMDD has not been established to date. The manufacturer states that the efficacy of sertraline therapy beyond 3 menstrual cycles has not been demonstrated in controlled studies. However, because women commonly report that symptoms of PMDD worsen with age until relieved by the onset of menopause, the manufacturer recommends that long-term sertraline therapy be considered in responding women. Dosage adjustments, which may include transfers between dosing regimens (e.g., continuous versus luteal phase dosing), may be needed to maintain the patient on the lowest effective dosage, and patients should be periodically reassessed to determine the need for continued treatment.

Social Phobia For the management of social phobia in adults, the recommended initial dosage of sertraline is 25 mg once daily. After 1 week, the dosage should be increased to 50 mg once daily. If no clinical improvement is apparent, dosage may then be increased at intervals of not less than 1 week up to a maximum of 200 mg daily.

While the optimum duration of sertraline therapy required to prevent recurrence of social phobia symptoms has not been established to date, the manufacturer states that this disorder is chronic and requires several months or longer of sustained therapy. Whether the dose of sertraline required to induce remission is identical to the dose needed to maintain and/or sustain remission in patients with this disorder is unknown. Systematic evaluation of sertraline has shown that its efficacy in the management of social phobia is maintained for periods of up to 24 weeks following 20 weeks of therapy at dosages of 50–200 mg daily. Dosages should be adjusted so that the patient is maintained on the lowest effective dosage, and patients should be reassessed periodically to determine the need for continued therapy.

Premature Ejaculation For the management of premature ejaculation†, sertraline has been given in a dosage of 25–50 mg daily. Alternatively, patients have taken sertraline on an "as needed" basis using doses of 25–50 mg daily.

■ Dosage in Geriatric Patients

Major Depressive Disorder For the management of depressive symptoms associated with dementia of the Alzheimer's type in geriatric patients, some experts recommend an initial sertraline dosage of 12.5–25 mg once daily. The dosage may then be gradually increased at intervals of 1–2 weeks up to a maximum dosage of 150–200 mg once daily.

■ Dosage in Renal and Hepatic Impairment

The manufacturers state that, based on the pharmacokinetics of sertraline, there is no need for dosage adjustment in patients with renal impairment. Because sertraline does not appear to be removed substantially by dialysis, supplemental doses of the drug probably are unnecessary after dialysis.

Because sertraline is metabolized extensively by the liver, hepatic impairment can affect the elimination of the drug. (See Pharmacokinetics: Elimination.) Therefore, the manufacturers recommend that sertraline be administered with caution and in a reduced dosage or less frequently in patients with hepatic impairment.

■ Treatment of Pregnant Women during the Third Trimester

Because some neonates exposed to sertraline and other SSRIs or SNRIs late in the third trimester of pregnancy have developed severe complications, consideration may be given to cautiously tapering sertraline therapy in the third trimester prior to delivery if the drug is administered during pregnancy. (See Pregnancy, under Cautions: Pregnancy, Fertility, and Lactation.)

Cautions

The adverse effect profile of sertraline is similar to that of other selective serotonin-reuptake inhibitors (SSRIs) (e.g., citalopram, escitalopram, fluoxetine, fluvoxamine, paroxetine). Because sertraline is a highly selective serotonin-reuptake inhibitor with little or no effect on other neurotransmitters, the incidence of some adverse effects commonly associated with tricyclic antidepressants, such as anticholinergic effects (dry mouth, constipation), certain cardiovascular effects (e.g., orthostatic hypotension), drowsiness, and weight gain, is lower in patients receiving sertraline. However, certain adverse GI (e.g., nausea, diarrhea, anorexia) and nervous system (e.g., tremor, insomnia) effects appear to occur more frequently with sertraline and other SSRIs than with tricyclic antidepressants.

Overall, the adverse effect profile of sertraline in adults with depression, obsessive-compulsive disorder, or panic disorder appears to be similar. In controlled studies, the most common adverse effects occurring more frequently in adults receiving sertraline than in those receiving placebo included GI effects such as nausea, diarrhea or loose stools, dyspepsia, and dry mouth; nervous system effects such as somnolence, dizziness, insomnia, and tremor; sexual dysfunction in males (principally ejaculatory delay); and sweating. Discontinuance of sertraline therapy was required in about 15% of adults in clinical trials, principally because of adverse psychiatric (e.g., somnolence, insomnia, agitation, tremor), other nervous system (e.g., dizziness, headache), GI (e.g., nausea, diarrhea or loose stools, anorexia), or male sexual dysfunction (e.g., ejaculatory delay) effects or because of fatigue.

■ Nervous System Effects

Headache is the most common adverse nervous system effect of sertraline, occurring in approximately 26% of patients receiving the drug in controlled clinical trials; headache occurred in 23% of those receiving placebo in these trials. Somnolence or drowsiness occurred in about 14% of patients receiving sertraline in controlled clinical trials. Headache or somnolence each required discontinuance of therapy in about 2% of patients. Fatigue has been reported in approximately 12% of patients receiving the drug in clinical trials and required discontinuance of therapy in about 1% of patients; this effect was reported in 8% of those receiving placebo in these trials.

Dizziness occurred in about 13% of patients receiving sertraline in controlled clinical trials and required discontinuance of therapy in less than 1% of patients. Insomnia occurred in about 22% of patients receiving the drug in controlled clinical trials. However, because insomnia is a symptom also associated with depression, relief of insomnia and improvement in sleep patterns may occur when clinical improvement in depression becomes apparent during antidepressant therapy. In clinical trials, about 2% of patients discontinued sertraline because of insomnia.

Tremor occurred in about 9%, nervousness in about 6%, anxiety (which occasionally may be severe [e.g., panic]) in about 4%, paresthesia in about 3%, and agitation in about 6% of patients receiving sertraline in controlled clinical trials. Tremor, agitation, and nervousness resulted in discontinuance of sertraline in about 1% of patients while anxiety resulted in discontinuance in less than 1% of patients in clinical trials. Agitation and anxiety may subside with continued therapy. Hypoesthesia, hypertonia, or malaise occurred in at least 1% of patients receiving sertraline in clinical trials. Impaired concentration, dystonia, or twitching occurred in approximately 0.1–1% of patients receiving sertraline, although these adverse effects have not been definitely attributed to the drug.

The incidence of seizures during sertraline therapy appears to be similar to or less than that observed during therapy with most other currently available antidepressants. Seizures occurred in less than 0.1% of patients receiving sertraline in clinical trials. (See Cautions: Precautions and Contraindications.)

Hypomania and mania have been reported in approximately 0.4% of patients receiving sertraline in controlled clinical trials, which is similar to the incidence reported in patients receiving active control agents (i.e., other antidepressants). In at least 2 patients, hypomanic symptoms occurred after they were receiving sertraline 200 mg daily for approximately 9 weeks. In both patients, the adverse reaction was obviated by a reduction in sertraline dosage. (See Cautions: Precautions and Contraindications.) Such reactions have occurred in patients receiving other antidepressant agents and may be caused by antidepressant-induced functional increases in catecholamine activity within the CNS, resulting in a "switch" from depressive to manic behavior. There is some evidence that patients with bipolar disorder may be more likely to experience antidepressant-induced hypomanic or manic reactions than patients without evidence of this disorder. In addition, limited evidence suggests that such reactions may occur more frequently in bipolar depressed patients receiving tricyclics and tetracyclics (e.g., maprotiline, mianserin [not commercially available in the US]) than in those receiving SSRIs (e.g., citalopram, escitalopram, fluoxetine, paroxetine, sertraline). However, further studies are needed to confirm these findings.

Asthenia has been reported in at least 1% of patients receiving sertraline; however, a causal relationship to the drug has not been established. Confusion, migraine, abnormal coordination, abnormal gait, hyperesthesia, ataxia, depersonalization, hallucinations, hyperkinesia, hypokinesia, nystagmus, vertigo, abnormal dreams, aggressive reaction, amnesia, apathy, paroniria, delusion, depression or aggravated depression, emotional lability, euphoria, abnormal thinking, or paranoid reaction have been reported in 0.1–1% of patients receiving the drug, although these adverse effects have not been definitely attributed to sertraline.

Adverse nervous system effects reported in less than 0.1% of patients receiving sertraline include dysphoria, choreoathetosis, dyskinesia, coma, dysphonia, hyporeflexia, hypotonia, ptosis, somnambulism, and illusion; these effects have not been definitely attributed to the drug. Although a causal relationship has not been established, psychosis, extrapyramidal symptoms, and oculogyric crisis have been reported during postmarketing surveillance. Forgetfulness, panic attacks, and unspecified pain also have been reported rarely, although a causal relationship to sertraline has not been established. Sertraline also has been reported to precipitate or exacerbate "flashbacks" in patients who previously had used lysergic acid diethylamide (LSD).

Serotonin syndrome and neuroleptic malignant syndrome (NMS)-like reactions have been reported in patients receiving sertraline, other SSRIs, and selective serotonin- and norepinephrine-reuptake inhibitors (SNRIs). (See Cautions: Precautions and Contraindications, Drug Interactions: Serotonergic Drugs, and Acute Toxicity.)

Extrapyramidal reactions, including akathisia, stuttering (which may be a speech manifestation of akathisia), bilateral jaw stiffness, and torticollis, have been reported rarely with sertraline use, and such reactions appear to be a class effect of SSRIs and dose related. Reactions occurring *early* during therapy with these drugs may be secondary to preexisting parkinsonian syndrome and/or concomitant therapy.

Withdrawal Reactions Withdrawal symptoms, including dysphoric mood, irritability, agitation, dizziness, sensory disturbances (e.g., paresthesias such as electric shock sensations), anxiety, confusion, headache, lethargy, emotional lability, insomnia, and hypomania, have been reported upon discontinuance of sertraline, other SSRIs, and SNRIs, particularly when discontinuance of these drugs is abrupt. While these reactions are generally self-limiting, there have been reports of serious discontinuance symptoms. Therefore, patients should be monitored for such symptoms when discontinuing sertraline therapy. A gradual reduction in the dosage rather than abrupt cessation is recommended whenever possible. (See Dosage and Administration: Dosage.)

A withdrawal syndrome has been reported in less than 0.1% of sertraline-treated patients. Fatigue, severe abdominal cramping, memory impairment, and influenza-like symptoms were reported 2 days following abrupt discontinuance of sertraline in one patient; when sertraline was restarted, the symptoms remitted. Electric shock-like sensations occurred in another patient 1 day after the last administered dose of sertraline; these sensations became less intense and eventually disappeared 13 weeks after sertraline therapy was discontinued. (See Chronic Toxicity.)

Suicidality Suicidal ideation has been reported in less than 0.1% of adults receiving sertraline. The US Food and Drug Administration (FDA) has determined that antidepressants increase the risk of suicidal thinking and behavior (suicidality) in children, adolescents, and young adults (18–24 years of age) with major depressive disorder and other psychiatric disorders. (See Suicidality, under Cautions: Nervous System Effects, in Paroxetine 28:16.04.20.) Patients, therefore, should be appropriately monitored and closely observed for clinical worsening, suicidality, and unusual changes in behavior, particularly during initiation of sertraline therapy (i.e., the first few months) and during periods of dosage adjustments. (See Cautions: Precautions and Contraindications and see Cautions: Pediatric Precautions.)

■ **GI Effects** Like other selective serotonin-reuptake inhibitors (e.g., citalopram, escitalopram, fluoxetine, fluvoxamine, paroxetine), sertraline therapy is associated with a relatively high incidence of GI disturbances, principally nausea, dry mouth, and diarrhea/loose stools. The most frequent adverse effect associated with sertraline therapy is nausea, which occurred in about 28% of patients receiving the drug in controlled clinical trials. In clinical trials, nausea required discontinuance of sertraline in about 4% of patients. In general, the incidence of nausea associated with selective serotonin-reuptake inhibitors appears to be higher when therapy is initiated with high doses but decreases as therapy with these drugs is continued. While the mechanism(s) of sertraline-induced GI effects has not been fully elucidated, they appear to arise at least in part because of increased serotonergic activity in the GI tract (which may result in stimulation of small intestine motility and inhibition of gastric and large intestine motility) and possibly because of the drug's effect on central serotonergic type 3 (5-HT_3) receptors.

Diarrhea or loose stools occurred in about 20%, dry mouth in about 15%, constipation in about 7%, dyspepsia in about 8%, or anorexia in about 6% of patients receiving sertraline in controlled clinical trials. Other adverse GI effects associated with sertraline therapy include vomiting which occurred in about 4% and flatulence which occurred in about 3% of patients receiving the drug in controlled clinical trials. Abdominal pain was reported in approximately 2% and taste perversion in about 1% of patients receiving sertraline. In clinical trials, diarrhea or loose stools required discontinuance of sertraline in about 3% of patients and dry mouth required discontinuance of therapy in about 1% of patients.

Epidemiologic case-control and cohort design studies have suggested that selective serotonin-reuptake inhibitors may increase the risk of upper GI bleeding. Although the precise mechanism for this increased risk remains to be clearly established, serotonin release by platelets is known to play an important role in hemostasis, and selective serotonin-reuptake inhibitors decrease serotonin uptake from the blood by platelets thereby decreasing the amount of serotonin in platelets. In addition, concurrent use of aspirin or other nonsteroidal anti-inflammatory drugs was found to substantially increase the risk of GI bleeding in patients receiving selective serotonin-reuptake inhibitors in 2 of these studies. Although these studies focused on upper GI bleeding, there is some evidence suggesting that bleeding at other sites may be similarly potentiated. Further clinical studies are needed to determine the clinical importance of these findings. (See Cautions: Hematologic Effects and also see Drug Interactions: Drugs Affecting Hemostasis.)

Although a causal relationship to sertraline has not been established, dysphagia, esophagitis, aggravation of dental caries, gastroenteritis, eructation, and increased salivation have been reported in 0.1–1% of patients receiving the drug. Aphthous stomatitis, ulcerative stomatitis, stomatitis, tongue ulceration or edema, glossitis, diverticulitis, gastritis, hemorrhagic peptic ulcer, rectal hemorrhage, colitis, proctitis, fecal incontinence, melena, or tenesmus has been reported in less than 0.1% of patients receiving sertraline; however, these adverse effects have not been definitely attributed to the drug. Pancreatitis also has been reported rarely in association with sertraline; however, a causal relationship to the drug has not been clearly established.

Although a causal relationship has not been established, nocturnal bruxism (clenching and/or grinding of the teeth during sleep) has developed within 2–4 weeks following initiation of sertraline or fluoxetine therapy in several patients. The bruxism remitted upon reduction in dosage of the serotonin-reuptake inhibitor and/or the addition of buspirone therapy.

Speech blockage also has been reported in at least one sertraline-treated patient.

■ **Dermatologic and Sensitivity Reactions** Sweating occurred in about 7% of patients receiving sertraline in controlled clinical trials.

Rash, which may be erythematous, follicular, maculopapular, or pustular, has been reported in about 3% of patients receiving sertraline in controlled clinical trials. Adverse dermatologic effects reported in 0.1–1% of patients receiving sertraline in controlled clinical trials include acne, alopecia, dry skin, urticaria, pruritus, and photosensitivity reaction (which may be severe); however, these adverse effects have not been definitely attributed to sertraline. Bullous eruption, eczema, contact dermatitis, skin discoloration, and hypertrichosis have been reported in less than 0.1% of patients receiving the drug, although a causal relationship to sertraline has not been established. Allergy, allergic reaction, and angioedema also have been reported rarely.

Other dermatologic and sensitivity events, which can be severe and potentially may be fatal, reported during the postmarketing surveillance of sertraline have included anaphylactoid reaction, angioedema, Stevens-Johnson syndrome, erythema multiforme, and vasculitis.

■ **Metabolic Effects** Thirst has been reported in 0.1–1% of patients receiving sertraline in controlled clinical trials.

Weight loss occurred in 0.1–1% of patients receiving sertraline. In controlled clinical trials, patients lost an average of about 0.45–0.9 kg while receiving sertraline. Rarely, weight loss has required discontinuance of therapy. Like fluoxetine, sertraline exhibits anorexigenic activity and can cause anorexia, which may be more pronounced in overweight patients and those with carbohydrate craving. Anorexia occurred in about 3% of patients receiving sertraline in controlled clinical trials and required discontinuance in at least 1% of patients. Increased appetite and weight gain have been reported in at least 1% of patients receiving sertraline in controlled clinical trials, although a causal relationship to the drug has not been established. (See Cautions: Pediatric Precautions.)

Sertraline use has been associated with small mean decreases (approximately 7%) in serum uric acid concentration as a result of a weak uricosuric effect; the clinical importance is not known and there have been no cases of acute renal failure associated with the drug. Small mean increases in serum total cholesterol (about 3%) and triglyceride (about 5%) concentrations also have been reported in patients receiving sertraline. Hypercholesterolemia has been reported in less than 0.1% of patients. Other adverse effects reported in less than 0.1% of patients receiving the drug include dehydration and hypoglycemia. These adverse effects have not been definitely attributed to sertraline.

■ **Ocular and Otic Effects** Abnormal vision (including blurred vision) occurred in about 4% of patients receiving sertraline in controlled clinical trials. Adverse ocular effects reported in 0.1–1% of patients receiving sertraline include abnormality of accommodation, conjunctivitis, and ocular pain. Although a causal relationship to sertraline has not been established, anisocoria, abnormal lacrimation, xerophthalmia, diplopia, scotoma, visual field defect, exophthalmos, hemorrhage of the anterior chamber of the eye, or photophobia has been reported in less than 0.1% of patients receiving the drug. Other adverse ocular effects reported during postmarketing surveillance of sertraline have included blindness, optic neuritis, and cataract; however, a causal relationship to the drug has not been established.

SSRIs, including sertraline, may have an effect on pupil size resulting in mydriasis. This mydriatic effect potentially can narrow the eye angle resulting in increased intraocular pressure and angle-closure glaucoma, particularly in predisposed patients. Mydriasis has been reported in 0.1–1% of patients receiving sertraline and glaucoma has been reported in less than 0.1% of patients receiving the drug. (See Cautions: Precautions and Contraindications.)

Tinnitus occurred in at least 1% of patients receiving sertraline in controlled clinical trials. Earache has been reported in 0.1–1% of patients, and hyperacusis and labyrinthine disorder have been reported in less than 0.1% of patients.

■ **Cardiovascular Effects** Sertraline does not exhibit clinically important anticholinergic activity, and current evidence suggests that sertraline is less cardiotoxic than many antidepressant agents (e.g., tricyclic antidepressants, monoamine oxidase inhibitors). (See Cardiovascular Considerations in Uses: Major Depressive Disorder and also see Pharmacology: Cardiovascular Effects.) However, bradycardia, AV block, atrial arrhythmias, QT-interval prolongation, and ventricular tachycardia (including torsades de pointes-type arrhythmias) have been reported during postmarketing surveillance evaluations of the drug.

Hot flushes occurred in about 2% of patients receiving sertraline in controlled clinical trials. Palpitation and chest pain have been reported in at least 1% of patients receiving sertraline in controlled clinical trials. In one patient with underlying coronary artery disease, chest pain developed suddenly and was relieved with sublingual nitroglycerin but was not associated with ECG changes; the mechanism of this effect, particularly regarding any potential cardiovascular effect, is unclear and alternative mechanisms (e.g., GI) for the chest pain have been proposed.

Unlike tricyclic antidepressants, sertraline has been associated with hypotension (e.g., orthostatic) infrequently; in controlled clinical trials, postural effects (e.g., dizziness, hypotension [which can also be nonpostural]) occurred in 0.1–1% of patients receiving sertraline. Syncope also occurred in at least 0.1% of patients.

Hypertension, peripheral ischemia, and tachycardia have been reported in 0.1–1% of patients receiving the drug, although a definite causal relationship to sertraline has not been established. Precordial or substernal chest pain, aggravated hypertension, myocardial infarction, pallor, vasodilation, and cerebrovascular disorder have been reported in less than 0.1% of patients receiving sertraline; these adverse effects have not been definitely attributed to the drug. Cerebrovascular spasm (including reversible cerebral vasoconstriction syndrome and Call-Fleming Syndrome) also has been reported during postmarketing experience with sertraline.

Generalized, dependent, periorbital, or peripheral edema has been reported in at least 0.1% of patients receiving sertraline, and facial edema has been reported rarely. However, a causal relationship to the drug has not been established.

■ **Musculoskeletal Effects** Myalgia or back pain occurred in at least 1% of patients receiving sertraline in controlled clinical trials. Arthralgia, arthrosis, leg or other muscle cramps, or muscle weakness has been reported in 0.1–1% of patients receiving sertraline; these adverse effects have not been definitely attributed to the drug.

■ **Hematologic Effects** Purpura, aplastic anemia, pancytopenia, leukopenia, thrombocytopenia, and abnormal bleeding have been reported occasionally in patients receiving sertraline; however, these adverse effects have not been definitely attributed to the drug.

Altered platelet function and/or abnormal platelet laboratory results have been reported rarely, but a causal relationship to sertraline remains to be established. In addition, in at least one patient with idiopathic thrombocytopenic purpura, sertraline therapy was associated with an increase in platelet counts. Anemia has been reported in less than 0.1% of patients receiving sertraline, although a causal relationship to the drug has not been established. Neutropenia also has been reported rarely with sertraline use and has been a reason for drug discontinuance. Agranulocytosis and septic shock developed in a geriatric woman who had been receiving sertraline for about 1 month in addition to atenolol, bendroflumethiazide, and thioridazine; the patient responded to anti-infective and granulocyte colony-stimulating factor therapy and made a full recovery within 10 days.

Bleeding complications (e.g., ecchymosis, purpura, menorrhagia, rectal bleeding) have been reported infrequently in patients receiving selective serotonin-reuptake inhibitors. Although the precise mechanism for these reactions has not been established, it has been suggested that impaired platelet aggregation and prolonged bleeding time may be due at least in part to inhibition of serotonin reuptake into platelets and/or that increased capillary fragility and vascular tone may contribute to these cases. (See Cautions: GI Effects and also see Drug Interactions: Drugs Affecting Hemostasis.)

■ **Respiratory Effects** Rhinitis or yawning has been reported in at least 1% of patients receiving sertraline in controlled clinical trials. Adverse respiratory effects reported in 0.1–1% of patients receiving the drug include bronchospasm, dyspnea, epistaxis, upper respiratory tract infection, sinusitis, and coughing; however, a definite causal relationship to sertraline has not been established. Adverse respiratory effects reported in less than 0.1% of patients receiving sertraline include bradypnea, hypoventilation, hyperventilation, apnea, stridor, hiccups, hemoptysis, bronchitis, laryngismus, and laryngitis. Pulmonary hypertension also has been reported during postmarketing surveillance evaluations of the drug. However, these adverse effects have not been definitely attributed to the drug.

■ **Renal, Electrolyte, and Genitourinary Effects** ***Sexual Dysfunction*** Like other selective serotonin-reuptake inhibitors, adverse effects on sexual function have been reported in both men and women receiving sertraline. Although changes in sexual desire, sexual performance, and sexual satisfaction often occur as manifestations of a psychiatric disorder, they also may occur as the result of pharmacologic therapy. It is difficult to determine the true incidence and severity of adverse effects on sexual function during sertraline therapy, in part because patients and clinicians may be reluctant to discuss these effects. Therefore, incidence data reported in product labeling and earlier studies are most likely underestimates of the true incidence of adverse sexual effects. Recent reports indicate that up to 50% of patients receiving selective serotonin-reuptake inhibitors describe some form of sexual dysfunction during treatment and the actual incidence may be even higher.

Sexual dysfunction (principally ejaculatory delay) is the most common adverse urogenital effect of sertraline in males, occurring in about 14% of male patients receiving the drug in controlled clinical trials. In some cases, this effect has been used for therapeutic benefit in the treatment of premature ejaculation. (See Uses: Premature Ejaculation.) Impotence has occurred in at least 1% of male patients receiving sertraline in controlled trials, and priapism has been reported rarely. Female sexual dysfunction (e.g., anorgasmia) has been reported in at least 1% of female patients receiving the drug in controlled clinical trials. Decreased libido has been reported in males and females, occurring in 6% of patients in controlled clinical studies. Sexual dysfunction (principally ejaculatory delay) required discontinuance of therapy in at least 1% of patients in controlled clinical trials. Increased libido has been reported in less than 1% of patients receiving the drug.

Results of some (but not all) studies in men and women suggest that paroxetine may be associated with a higher incidence of sexual dysfunction than some other currently available selective serotonin-reuptake inhibitors, including sertraline and citalopram. Since it is difficult to know the precise risk of sexual dysfunction associated with serotonin-reuptake inhibitors, clinicians should routinely inquire about such possible adverse effects in patients receiving these drugs.

The long-term effects of selective serotonin-reuptake inhibitors on sexual function have not been fully determined to date. In a double-blind study evaluating 6 months of sertraline or citalopram therapy in depressed patients, sexual desire and overall sexual functioning (as measured on the UKU Side Effect Scale) substantially improved in women and sexual desire improved in men. In men, no change in orgasmic dysfunction, erectile dysfunction, or overall sexual functioning was reported after 6 months of therapy with sertraline or citalopram, although there was a trend toward worsening of ejaculatory dysfunction. However, in the subgroups of women and men reporting no sexual problems at baseline, approximately 12% of women reported decreased sexual desire and 14% reported orgasmic dysfunction after 6 months of citalopram therapy; the corresponding figures in the same subgroup of men were approximately 17 and 19%, respectively, and as many as 25% experienced ejaculatory dysfunction after 6 months. No substantial differences between sertraline and citalopram were reported in this study.

Management of sexual dysfunction caused by selective serotonin-reuptake inhibitor therapy includes waiting for tolerance to develop; using a lower dosage of the drug; using drug holidays; delaying administration of the drug until after coitus; or changing to another antidepressant. Although further study is needed, there is some evidence that adverse sexual effects of the selective serotonin-reuptake inhibitors may be reversed by concomitant use of certain drugs, including buspirone, 5-hydroxytryptamine-2 (5-HT_2) receptor antagonists (e.g., nefazodone), 5-HT_3 receptor inhibitors (e.g., granisetron), or α_2-adrenergic receptor antagonists (e.g., yohimbine), selective phosphodiesterase (PDE) inhibitors (e.g., sildenafil), or dopamine receptor agonists (e.g., amantadine, dextroamphetamine, pemoline [no longer commercially available in the US], methylphenidate). In most patients, sexual dysfunction is fully reversed 1–3 days after discontinuance of the antidepressant.

Other Renal, Electrolyte, and Genitourinary Effects Although a definite causal relationship to sertraline has not been established, menstrual disorders, dysmenorrhea, intermenstrual bleeding, amenorrhea, vaginal hemorrhage, and leukorrhea have been reported in 0.1–1% of patients receiving sertraline. In addition, menorrhagia, breast enlargement, female breast pain or tenderness, acute mastitis in females, gynecomastia, and atrophic vaginitis have been reported in less than 0.1% of patients receiving sertraline; however, a causal relationship to the drug has not been clearly established.

Treatment with SSRIs, including sertraline, and selective serotonin- and norepinephrine-reuptake inhibitors (SNRIs) may result in hyponatremia. In many cases, this hyponatremia appears to be due to the syndrome of inappropriate antidiuretic hormone secretion (SIADH) and was reversible when the SSRI or SNRI was discontinued. Cases with serum sodium concentrations lower than 110 mEq/L have been reported. Hyponatremia and SIADH in patients receiving SSRIs usually develop an average of 2 weeks after initiating therapy (range: 3–120 days). Geriatric individuals and patients receiving diuretics or who are otherwise volume depleted may be at greater risk of developing hyponatremia during therapy with SSRIs or SNRIs. Discontinuance of sertraline should be considered in patients with symptomatic hyponatremia and appropriate medical intervention should be instituted. Because geriatric patients may be at increased risk for hyponatremia associated with these drugs, clinicians prescribing sertraline in such patients should be aware of the possibility that such reactions may occur. In addition, periodic monitoring of serum sodium concentrations (particularly during the first several months) in geriatric patients receiving SSRIs has been recommended by some clinicians.

A variety of urinary disorders, including urinary frequency, polyuria, urinary hesitancy and/or retention, dysuria, nocturia, and urinary incontinence, has been reported in 0.1–1% of patients receiving sertraline; however, these effects have not been definitely attributed to the drug. In addition, cystitis, oliguria, pyelonephritis, hematuria, renal pain, strangury, and balanoposthitis have been reported in less than 0.1% of patients receiving sertraline, although a causal relationship to the drug has not been clearly established.

■ **Hepatic Effects** Impaired hepatic function has been reported in less than 1% of patients receiving sertraline in controlled clinical trials; in most cases, such reactions appeared to be reversible upon discontinuance of sertraline therapy. Asymptomatic elevations in serum AST (SGOT) and ALT (SGPT) concentrations have been reported in approximately 0.8% of patients receiving the drug and occasionally have been a reason for drug discontinuance. Elevations in aminotransferase concentrations usually occurred within the first 1–9 weeks of sertraline therapy and were rapidly reversible following discontinuance of the drug. In addition, in at least 2 patients, elevated liver enzymes returned to normal levels with continued therapy.

Increased serum alkaline phosphatase and bilirubin concentrations occurred rarely in patients receiving sertraline in clinical trials and required discontinuance of therapy in some cases. Other clinical features associated with adverse hepatic reactions that have been reported in at least one patient include hepatitis, hepatomegaly, jaundice, abdominal pain, vomiting, hepatic failure, and death. However, these effects have not been definitely attributed to the drug.

■ **Endocrine Effects** Low levels of total thyroxine developed in a depressed adolescent who had been receiving sertraline therapy; however, it appears that sertraline only displaced the bound fraction of total thyroxine but was not associated with true hypothyroidism. In a limited number of hypothyroid patients receiving thyroxine therapy, elevated serum thyrotropin and reduced serum thyroxine concentrations have been observed following the initiation of sertraline therapy. Hypothyroidism also has been reported. (See Cautions: Precautions and Contraindications.)

Diabetes mellitus, hyperglycemia, hyperprolactinemia, and galactorrhea have been reported rarely in sertraline-treated patients; however, a causal relationship to the drug has not been established.

■ **Other Adverse Effects** Cold clammy skin, flushing, fever, or rigors has been reported in 0.1–1% of patients receiving the drug, although a causal relationship to sertraline has not been established. In addition, lupus-like syndrome and serum sickness have been reported during postmarketing surveillance evaluations of the drug; however, a causal relationship has not been definitively established.

■ **Precautions and Contraindications** Worsening of depression and/or the emergence of suicidal ideation and behavior (suicidality) or unusual changes in behavior may occur in both adult and pediatric (see Cautions: Pediatric Precautions) patients with major depressive disorder or other psychiatric disorders, whether or not they are taking antidepressants. This risk may persist until clinically important remission occurs. Suicide is a known risk of depression and certain other psychiatric disorders, and these disorders themselves are the strongest predictors of suicide. However, there has been a long-standing concern that antidepressants may have a role in inducing worsening of depression and the emergence of suicidality in certain patients during the early phases of treatment. Pooled analyses of short-term, placebo-controlled studies of antidepressants (i.e., selective serotonin-reuptake inhibitors [SSRIs] and other antidepressants) have shown an increased risk of suicidality in children, adolescents, and young adults (18–24 years of age) with major depressive disorder and other psychiatric disorders. An increased suicidality risk was not demonstrated with antidepressants compared to placebo in adults older than 24 years of age and a reduced risk was observed in adults 65 years of age or older. It currently is unknown whether the suicidality risk extends to longer-term use (i.e., beyond several months); however, there is substantial evidence from placebo-controlled maintenance trials in adults with major depressive disorder that antidepressants can delay the recurrence of depression.

The US Food and Drug Administration (FDA) recommends that all patients being treated with antidepressants for any indication be appropriately monitored and closely observed for clinical worsening, suicidality, and unusual changes in behavior, particularly during initiation of therapy (i.e., the first few months) and during periods of dosage adjustments. Families and caregivers of patients being treated with antidepressants for major depressive disorder or other indications, both psychiatric and nonpsychiatric, also should be advised to monitor patients on a daily basis for the emergence of agitation, irritability, or unusual changes in behavior as well as the emergence of suicidality, and to report such symptoms immediately to a health-care provider. (See Suicidality under Cautions: Nervous System Effects, in Paroxetine 28:16.04.20.)

Although a causal relationship between the emergence of symptoms such as anxiety, agitation, panic attacks, insomnia, irritability, hostility, aggressiveness, impulsivity, akathisia, hypomania, and/or mania and either the worsening of depression and/or the emergence of suicidal impulses has not been established, there is concern that such symptoms may represent precursors to emerging suicidality. Consequently, consideration should be given to changing the therapeutic regimen or discontinuing therapy in patients whose depression is persistently worse or in patients experiencing emergent suicidality or symptoms that might be precursors to worsening depression or suicidality, particularly if such manifestations are severe, abrupt in onset, or were not part of the patient's presenting symptoms. If a decision is made to discontinue therapy, sertraline dosage should be tapered as rapidly as is feasible but with recognition of the risks of abrupt discontinuance. (See Dosage and Administration: Dosage.) FDA also recommends that the drugs be prescribed in the smallest quantity consistent with good patient management, in order to reduce the risk of overdosage.

It is generally believed (though not established in controlled trials) that treating a major depressive episode with an antidepressant alone may increase the likelihood of precipitating a mixed or manic episode in patients at risk for bipolar disorder. Therefore, patients should be adequately screened for bipolar disorder prior to initiating treatment with an antidepressant; such screening should include a detailed psychiatric history (e.g., family history of suicide, bipolar disorder, and depression).

Potentially life-threatening serotonin syndrome or neuroleptic malignant syndrome (NMS)-like reactions have been reported with SSRIs, including sertraline, and selective serotonin- and norepinephrine-reuptake inhibitors (SNRIs) alone, but particularly with concurrent administration of other serotonergic drugs (including serotonin [5-hydroxytryptamine; 5-HT] type 1 receptor agonists ["triptans"]), drugs that impair the metabolism of serotonin (e.g., monoamine oxidase [MAO] inhibitors), or antipsychotic agents or other dopamine antagonists. Symptoms of serotonin syndrome may include mental status changes (e.g., agitation, hallucinations, coma), autonomic instability (e.g., tachycardia, labile blood pressure, hyperthermia), neuromuscular aberrations (e.g., hyperreflexia, incoordination), and/or GI symptoms (e.g., nausea, vomiting, diarrhea). In its most severe form, serotonin syndrome may resemble NMS, which is characterized by hyperthermia, muscle rigidity, autonomic instability with possible rapid fluctuation in vital signs, and mental status changes. Patients receiving sertraline should be monitored for the development of serotonin syndrome or NMS-like signs and symptoms.

Concurrent or recent (i.e., within 2 weeks) therapy with MAO inhibitors used for treatment of depression is contraindicated in patients receiving sertraline and vice versa. If concurrent therapy with sertraline and a 5-HT_1 receptor agonist (triptan) is clinically warranted, the patient should be observed carefully, particularly during initiation of therapy, when dosage is increased, or when another serotonergic agent is initiated. Concomitant use of sertraline and serotonin precursors (e.g., tryptophan) is not recommended. If signs and symptoms of serotonin syndrome or NMS develop during sertraline therapy, treatment with sertraline and any concurrently administered serotonergic or antidopaminergic agents, including antipsychotic agents, should be discontinued immediately and supportive and symptomatic treatment should be initiated. (See Drug Interactions: Serotonergic Drugs.)

The dropper dispenser provided with Zoloft® oral solution contains natural latex proteins in the form of dry natural rubber which may cause sensitivity reactions in susceptible individuals.

Because clinical experience with sertraline in patients with certain concurrent systemic disease, including cardiovascular disease and renal impairment, is limited, caution should be exercised when sertraline is administered to patients with any systemic disease or condition that may alter metabolism of the drug or adversely affect hemodynamic function. (See Dosage and Administration: Dosage.)

Sertraline should be used with caution in patients with hepatic impairment, since prolonged elimination of the drug has been reported to occur in patients with liver cirrhosis. (See Pharmacokinetics: Elimination and see Dosage and Administration: Dosage in Renal and Hepatic Impairment.)

The manufacturers recommend that patients receiving sertraline be advised to notify their clinician if they are taking or plan to take nonprescription (over-the-counter) or prescription medications or alcohol-containing beverages or preparations. Although no interactions with nonprescription medications have been reported to date, the potential for such adverse drug interactions exists. Therefore, the use of any nonprescription medication should be initiated cautiously according to the directions of use provided on the nonprescription medication. Although sertraline has not been shown to potentiate the impairment of mental and motor skills caused by alcohol, the manufacturers recommend that patients be advised to avoid alcohol while receiving the drug.

Sertraline generally is less sedating than most other currently available antidepressants and does not appear to produce substantial impairment of cognitive or psychomotor function. However, patients should be cautioned that sertraline may impair their ability to perform activities requiring mental alertness or physical coordination (e.g., operating machinery, driving a motor vehicle) and to avoid such activities until they experience how the drug affects them. Because the risk of using sertraline concomitantly with other CNS active drugs has not been evaluated systematically to date, the manufacturers recommend that such therapy be employed cautiously.

Seizures have been reported in patients receiving therapeutic dosages of sertraline. Because of limited experience with sertraline in patients with a history of seizures, the drug should be used with caution in such patients.

Activation of mania and hypomania has occurred in patients receiving therapeutic dosages of sertraline. The drug should be used with caution in patients with a history of mania or hypomania.

Treatment with SSRIs, including sertraline, and selective serotonin- and norepinephrine-reuptake inhibitors (SNRIs) may result in hyponatremia. In many cases, this hyponatremia appears to be due to the syndrome of inappropriate antidiuretic hormone secretion (SIADH) and was reversible when sertraline was discontinued. Cases with serum sodium concentrations lower than 110 mEq/L have been reported. Geriatric individuals and patients receiving diuretics or who are otherwise volume depleted may be at greater risk of developing hyponatremia during therapy with SSRIs or SNRIs. Signs and symptoms of hyponatremia include headache, difficulty concentrating, memory impairment, confusion, weakness, and unsteadiness, which may lead to falls; more severe and/or acute cases have been associated with hallucinations, syncope, seizures, coma, respiratory arrest, and death. Discontinuance of sertraline should be considered in patients with symptomatic hyponatremia and appropriate medical intervention should be instituted. (See Cautions: Renal, Electrolyte, and Genitourinary Effects and also see Cautions: Geriatric Precautions.)

Altered platelet function has been reported rarely in patients receiving sertraline. In addition, use of the drug has been associated with several reports of abnormal bleeding or purpura. While a causal relationship to sertraline remains to be established, pending such establishment, the drug should be used with caution in patients with an underlying coagulation defect since the possible effects on hemostasis may be exaggerated in such patients. (See Cautions: Hematologic Effects.)

SSRIs, including sertraline, may have an effect on pupil size resulting in mydriasis. This mydriatic effect potentially can narrow the eye angle resulting in increased intraocular pressure and angle-closure glaucoma, particularly in predisposed patients. Sertraline should therefore by used with caution in patients with angle-closure glaucoma or a history of glaucoma.

Sertraline has a weak uricosuric effect. (See Cautions: Metabolic Effects.)

Pending further elucidation of the clinical importance, if any, of this effect, the drug should be used with caution in patients who may be adversely affected (e.g., those at risk for acute renal failure).

Because sertraline therapy has been associated with anorexia and weight loss (see Cautions: Metabolic Effects), the drug should be used with caution in patients who may be adversely affected by these effects (e.g., underweight patients).

Like many other antidepressant drugs, sertraline has been associated with hypothyroidism, elevated serum thyrotropin, and/or reduced serum thyroxine concentrations in a limited number of patients. Because of reports with other antidepressant agents and the complex interrelationship between the hypothalamic-pituitary-thyroid axis and affective (mood) disorders, at least one manufacturer recommends that thyroid function be reassessed periodically in patients with thyroid disease who are receiving sertraline.

Commercially available sertraline hydrochloride oral solution (Zoloft®) contains alcohol. Therefore, concomitant use of sertraline hydrochloride oral solution and disulfiram is contraindicated.

Sertraline is contraindicated in patients concurrently receiving pimozide. (See Drug Interactions: Pimozide.)

Sertraline also is contraindicated in patients who are hypersensitive to the drug or any ingredient in the formulation.

■ Pediatric Precautions Safety and efficacy of sertraline in children with obsessive-compulsive disorder (OCD) younger than 6 years of age have not been established. Safety and efficacy of sertraline in pediatric patients with other disorders (e.g., major depressive disorder, panic disorder, posttraumatic stress disorder, premenstrual dysphoric disorder, social phobia) have not been established. The overall adverse effect profile of sertraline in over 600 pediatric patients who received sertraline in controlled and uncontrolled clinical trials was generally similar to that seen in the adult clinical studies. As with other SSRIs, decreased appetite and weight loss have been observed in association with sertraline therapy.

Efficacy of sertraline in pediatric patients with major depressive disorder was evaluated in 2 randomized, 10-week, double-blind, placebo-controlled, flexible-dose (50–200 mg daily) trials in 373 children and adolescents with major depressive disorder, but data from these studies were not sufficient to establish efficacy in pediatric patients. In a safety analysis of the pooled data from these 2 studies, a difference in weight change between the sertraline and placebo groups was noted of approximately 1 kg for both pediatric patients (6–11 years of age) and adolescents (12–17 years of age) representing a slight weight loss for those receiving sertraline and a slight weight gain for those receiving placebo. In addition, a larger difference was noted in children than in adolescents between the sertraline and placebo groups in the proportion of outliers for clinically important weight loss; about 7% of the children and about 2% of the adolescents receiving sertraline in these studies experienced a weight loss of more than 7% of their body weight compared with none of those receiving placebo.

A subset of patients who completed these controlled trials was continued into a 24-week, flexible-dose, open-label, extension study. A mean weight loss of approximately 0.5 kg was observed during the initial 8 weeks of treatment for those pediatric patients first exposed to sertraline during the extension study, which was similar to the weight loss observed among sertraline-treated patients during the first 8 weeks of the randomized controlled trials. The patients continuing in the extension study began gaining weight relative to their baseline weight by week 12 of sertraline therapy, and patients who completed the entire 34 weeks of therapy with the drug had a weight gain that was similar to that expected using data from age-adjusted peers. The manufacturers state that periodic monitoring of weight and growth is recommended in pediatric patients receiving long-term therapy with sertraline or other selective serotonin-reuptake inhibitors (SSRIs).

FDA warns that antidepressants increase the risk of suicidal thinking and behavior (suicidality) in children and adolescents with major depressive disorder and other psychiatric disorders. The risk of suicidality for these drugs was identified in a pooled analysis of data from a total of 24 short-term (4–16 weeks), placebo-controlled studies of 9 antidepressants (i.e., sertraline, bupropion, citalopram, fluoxetine, fluvoxamine, mirtazapine, nefazodone, paroxetine, venlafaxine) in over 4400 children and adolescents with major depressive disorder, OCD, or other psychiatric disorders. The analysis revealed a greater risk of adverse events representing suicidal behavior or thinking (suicidality) during the first few months of treatment in pediatric patients receiving antidepressants than in those receiving placebo. However, a more recent meta-analysis of 27 placebo-controlled trials of 9 antidepressants (SSRIs and others) in patients younger than 19 years of age with major depressive disorder, OCD, or non-OCD anxiety disorders suggests that the benefits of antidepressant therapy in treating these conditions may outweigh the risks of suicidal behavior or suicidal ideation. No suicides occurred in these pediatric trials.

The risk of suicidality in FDA's pooled analysis differed across the different psychiatric indications, with the highest incidence observed in the major depressive disorder studies. In addition, although there was considerable variation in risk among the antidepressants, a tendency toward an increase in suicidality risk in younger patients was found for almost all drugs studied. It is currently unknown whether the suicidality risk in pediatric patients extends to longer-term use (i.e., beyond several months). (See Suicidality, under Cautions: Nervous System Effects, in Paroxetine 28:16.04.20.)

As a result of this analysis and public discussion of the issue, FDA has directed manufacturers of all antidepressants to add a boxed warning to the labeling of their products to alert clinicians of this suicidality risk in children and adolescents and to recommend appropriate monitoring and close observation of patients receiving these agents. (See Cautions: Precautions and Contraindications.) The drugs that are the focus of the revised labeling are all drugs included in the general class of antidepressants, including those that have not been studied in controlled clinical trials in pediatric patients, since the available data are not adequate to exclude any single antidepressant from an increased risk. In addition to the boxed warning and other information in professional labeling on antidepressants, FDA currently recommends that a patient medication guide explaining the risks associated with the drugs be provided to the patient each time the drugs are dispensed. Caregivers of pediatric patients whose depression is persistently worse or who are experiencing emergent suicidality or symptoms that might be precursors to worsening depression or suicidality during antidepressant therapy should consult their clinician regarding the best course of action (e.g., whether the therapeutic regimen should be changed or the drugs discontinued). *Patients should not discontinue use of selective serotonin-reuptake inhibitors without first consulting their clinician; it is very important that the drugs not be abruptly discontinued (see Dosage and Administration: Dosage), as withdrawal effects may occur.*

Anyone considering the use of sertraline in a child or adolescent for any clinical use must balance the potential risk of therapy with the clinical need.

■ Geriatric Precautions In clinical studies in geriatric patients, 660 patients receiving sertraline for the treatment of depression were 65 years of age or older, and 180 were 75 years of age or older. No overall differences in efficacy or adverse effects were observed for geriatric patients in these studies relative to younger patients, and other clinical experience has revealed no evidence of age-related differences in safety. In addition, no adverse effects on psychomotor performance were observed in geriatric individuals who received the drug in one controlled study. However, the possibility that older patients may exhibit increased sensitivity to the drug cannot be excluded. (See Dosage in Geriatric Patients under Dosage and Administration.)

Limited evidence suggests that geriatric patients may be more likely than younger patients to develop sertraline-induced hyponatremia and transient syndrome of inappropriate secretion of antidiuretic hormone (SIADH). Therefore, clinicians prescribing sertraline in geriatric patients should be aware of the possibility that such reactions may occur. Periodic monitoring (especially during the first several months) of serum sodium concentrations in geriatric patients receiving the drug has been recommended by some clinicians. (See Cautions: Precautions and Contraindications.)

As with other psychotropic drugs, geriatric patients receiving antidepressants appear to have an increased risk of hip fracture. Despite the fewer cardiovascular and anticholinergic effects associated with selective serotonin-reuptake inhibitors (SSRIs), these drugs did not show any advantage over tricyclic antidepressants with regard to hip fracture in a case-control study. In addition, there was little difference in the rates of falls between nursing home residents receiving SSRIs and those receiving tricyclic antidepressants in a retrospective study. Therefore, all geriatric individuals receiving either type of antidepressant should be considered to be at increased risk of falls and appropriate measures should be taken.

In pooled data analyses, a *reduced* risk of suicidality was observed in adults 65 years of age or older with antidepressant therapy compared with placebo. (See Cautions: Precautions and Contraindications.)

Plasma clearance of sertraline may be decreased in geriatric patients; plasma clearance of the less active metabolite, *N*-desmethylsertraline, also may be decreased in older males.

■ Mutagenicity and Carcinogenicity Sertraline was not mutagenic, with or without metabolic activation, in several in vitro tests including the bacterial mutation assay and the mouse lymphoma mutation assay. Sertraline also was not mutagenic in tests for cytogenetic aberrations in vivo in mouse bone marrow and in vitro in human lymphocytes.

Lifetime studies to determine the carcinogenic potential of sertraline were performed in CD-1 mice and Long-Evans rats receiving dosages up to 40 mg/kg daily. This dosage corresponded to 1 and 2 times the maximum recommended human dose on a mg/m² basis in mice and rats, respectively. There was a dose-related increase in the incidence of hepatic adenomas in male mice receiving sertraline dosages of 10–40 mg/kg (0.25–1 times the maximum recommended human dose on a mg/m² basis). No increase was seen in female mice or in rats of either gender receiving the same dosages, nor was there an increase in hepatocellular carcinomas. Hepatic adenomas have a variable rate of spontaneous occurrence in this strain of mice, and the relevance of this finding to humans is not known. There was an increase in follicular adenomas of the thyroid, not accompanied by thyroid hyperplasia, in female rats receiving a sertraline dosage of 40 mg/kg (2 times the maximum recommended human dose on a mg/m² basis). There also was an increase in uterine adenocarcinomas in rats receiving sertraline dosages of 10–40 mg/kg (0.5–2 times the maximum recommended human dose on a mg/m² basis); however, this effect could not be directly attributed to the drug.

■ Pregnancy, Fertility, and Lactation ***Pregnancy*** Some neonates exposed to sertraline and other SSRIs or SNRIs late in the third trimester of pregnancy have developed complications that have sometimes been severe and required prolonged hospitalization, respiratory support, enteral nutrition, and other forms of supportive care in special-care nurseries. Such complications can arise immediately upon delivery and usually last several days or up to 2–4 weeks. Clinical findings reported in the neonates have included respiratory distress, cyanosis, apnea, seizures, temperature instability or fever, feeding difficulty, dehydration, excessive weight loss, vomiting, hypoglycemia, hypotonia, hypertonia, hyperreflexia, tremor, jitteriness, irritability, lethargy, reduced or lack of reaction to pain stimuli, and constant crying. These clinical features appear to be consistent with either a direct toxic effect of the SSRI or SNRI or, possibly, a drug withdrawal syndrome. It should be noted that in some cases the clinical picture was consistent with serotonin syndrome (see Drug Interactions: Serotonergic Drugs).

Infants exposed to SSRIs in late pregnancy may have an increased risk of persistent pulmonary hypertension of the newborn (PPHN). PPHN is a rare heart and lung condition occurring in an estimated 1–2 infants per 1000 live births in the general population; it occurs when a neonate does not adapt to breathing outside the womb. Some experts have suggested that respiratory distress in neonates exposed to SSRIs may occur along a spectrum of seriousness in association with maternal use of SSRIs, with PPHN among the most serious consequences. Neonates with PPHN may require intensive care support, including mechanical ventilation; in severe cases, multiple organ damage, including brain damage, and even death may occur. Although several epidemiologic studies have suggested an increased risk of PPHN with SSRI use during pregnancy, other studies did not demonstrate a statistically significant association. Thus, the FDA states that it is currently unclear whether use of SSRIs, including sertraline, during pregnancy can cause PPHN and recommends that clinicians not alter their current clinical practice of treating depression during pregnancy.

When treating a pregnant woman with sertraline during the third trimester of pregnancy, the clinician should carefully consider the potential risks and benefits of such therapy. Clinicians should consider that in a prospective longitudinal study of 201 women with a history of recurrent major depression who were euthymic in the context of antidepressant therapy at the beginning of pregnancy, women who discontinued their antidepressant medication (SSRIs, tricyclic antidepressants, or others) during pregnancy were found to be substantially more likely to have a relapse of depression than were women who continued to receive their antidepressant therapy while pregnant. Consideration may be given to cautiously tapering sertraline therapy in the third trimester prior to delivery if the drug is administered during pregnancy. (See Treatment of Pregnant Women during the Third Trimester under Dosage and Administration: Dosage.)

For additional information on the management of depression in women prior to conception and during pregnancy, including treatment algorithms, the FDA advises clinicians to consult the joint American Psychiatric Association and American College of Obstetricians and Gynecologists guidelines (at https://www.ncbi.nlm.nih.gov/pmc/articles/PMC3103063/pdf/nihms293836.pdf).

Most epidemiologic studies of pregnancy outcome following first-trimester exposure to SSRIs, including sertraline, conducted to date have not revealed evidence of an increased risk of major congenital malformations. In a prospective, controlled, multicenter study, maternal use of several SSRIs (sertraline, fluvoxamine, paroxetine) in a limited number of pregnant women did not appear to increase the risk of congenital malformation, miscarriage, stillbirth, or premature delivery when used during pregnancy at recommended dosages. Birth weight and gestational age in neonates exposed to the drugs were similar to those in the control group. In another small study based on medical records review, the incidence of congenital anomalies reported in infants born to women who were treated with sertraline and other SSRIs during pregnancy was comparable to that observed in the general population. However, the results of epidemiologic studies indicate that exposure to paroxetine during the first trimester of pregnancy may increase the risk for congenital malformations, particularly cardiovascular malformations. (See Cautions: Pregnancy, Fertility, and Lactation, in Paroxetine 28:16.04.20.) Additional epidemiologic studies are needed to more thoroughly evaluate the relative safety of sertraline and other SSRIs during pregnancy, including their potential teratogenic risks and possible effects on neurobehavioral development.

The manufacturers state that there are no adequate and controlled studies to date using sertraline in pregnant women, and the drug should be used during pregnancy only when the potential benefits justify the potential risks to the fetus. Women should be advised to notify their clinician if they become pregnant or plan to become pregnant during therapy with the drug. FDA states that women who are pregnant or thinking about becoming pregnant should not discontinue any antidepressant, including sertraline, without first consulting their clinician. The decision whether or not to continue antidepressant therapy should be made only after careful consideration of the potential benefits and risks of antidepressant therapy for each individual pregnant patient. If a decision is made to discontinue treatment with sertraline or other SSRIs before or during pregnancy, discontinuance of therapy should be done in consultation with the clinician in accordance with the prescribing information for the antidepressant and the patient should be closely monitored for possible relapse of depression.

Reproduction studies in rats using sertraline dosages up to 80 mg/kg daily and in rabbits using dosages up to 40 mg/kg daily have not revealed evidence of teratogenicity; these dosages correspond to approximately 4 times the maximum recommended human dosage on a mg/m² basis. No evidence of teratogenicity was observed at any dosage studied. When pregnant rats and rabbits were given sertraline during the period of organogenesis, delayed ossification was observed in fetuses at doses of 10 mg/kg (0.5 times the maximum recommended human dose on a mg/m² basis) in rats and 40 mg/kg (4 times the maximum recommended human dose on a mg/m² basis) in rabbits. When female rats received sertraline during the last third of gestation and throughout lactation, there was an increase in the number of stillborn pups and in the number of pups dying during the first 4 days after birth. The body weights of the pups also were decreased during the first 4 days after birth. These effects occurred at a dose of 20 mg/kg (approximately the same as the maximum recommended human dose on a mg/m² basis). At 10 mg/kg (0.5 times the maximum recommended human dose on a mg/m² basis), no effect on rat pup mortality was observed. The decrease in pup survival was shown to result from in utero exposure to the drug. The clinical importance of these effects is not known.

The effect of sertraline on labor and delivery is not known.

Fertility A decrease in fertility was observed in 1 of 2 reproduction studies in rats using sertraline dosages of 80 mg/kg (4 times the maximum recommended human dose on a mg/m² basis).

Lactation Sertraline and its principal metabolite, *N*-desmethylsertraline, are distributed into milk. Sertraline should be used with caution in nursing women, and women should be advised to notify their physician if they plan to breast-feed.

Drug Interactions

■ Serotonergic Drugs Use of selective serotonin-reuptake-inhibitors (SSRIs) such as sertraline concurrently or in close succession with other drugs that affect serotonergic neurotransmission may result in serotonin syndrome or neuroleptic malignant syndrome (NMS)-like reactions. Symptoms of serotonin syndrome may include mental status changes (e.g., agitation, hallucinations, coma), autonomic instability (e.g., tachycardia, labile blood pressure, hyperthermia), neuromuscular aberrations (e.g., hyperreflexia, incoordination), and/or GI symptoms (e.g., nausea, vomiting, diarrhea). Although the syndrome appears to be relatively uncommon and usually mild in severity, serious and potentially life-threatening complications, including seizures, disseminated intravascular coagulation, respiratory failure, and severe hyperthermia as well as death occasionally have been reported. In its most severe form, serotonin syndrome may resemble NMS, which is characterized by hyperthermia, muscle rigidity, autonomic instability with possible rapid fluctuation in vital signs, and mental status changes. The precise mechanism of these reactions is not fully understood; however, they appear to result from excessive serotonergic activity in the CNS, probably mediated by activation of serotonin 5-HT_{1A} receptors. The possible involvement of dopamine and 5-HT_2 receptors also has been suggested, although their roles remain unclear.

Serotonin syndrome most commonly occurs when 2 or more drugs that affect serotonergic neurotransmission are administered either concurrently or in close succession. Serotonergic agents include those that increase serotonin synthesis (e.g., the serotonin precursor tryptophan), stimulate synaptic serotonin release (e.g., some amphetamines, dexfenfluramine [no longer commercially available in the US], fenfluramine [no longer commercially available in the US]), inhibit the reuptake of serotonin after release (e.g., SSRIs, selective serotonin- and norepinephrine-reuptake inhibitors [SNRIs], tricyclic antidepressants, trazodone, dextromethorphan, meperidine, tramadol), decrease the metabolism of serotonin (e.g., MAO inhibitors), have direct serotonin postsynaptic receptor activity (e.g., buspirone), or nonspecifically induce increases in serotonergic neuronal activity (e.g., lithium salts). Selective agonists of serotonin (5-hydroxytryptamine; 5-HT) type 1 receptors ("triptans") and dihydroergotamine, agents with serotonergic activity used in the management of migraine headache, and St. John's wort (*Hypericum perforatum*) also have been implicated in serotonin syndrome.

The combination of SSRIs and MAO inhibitors may result in serotonin syndrome or NMS-like reactions. Such reactions have also been reported in patients receiving SSRIs concomitantly with tryptophan, lithium, dextromethorphan, sumatriptan, dihydroergotamine, or antipsychotics or other dopamine antagonists. In rare cases, serotonin syndrome reportedly has occurred in patients receiving the recommended dosage of a single serotonergic agent (e.g., clomipramine) or during accidental overdosage (e.g., sertraline intoxication in a child). Some other drugs that have been implicated in precipitating symptoms suggestive of serotonin syndrome or NMS-like reactions include buspirone, bromocriptine, dextropropoxyphene, linezolid, methylene blue, methylenedioxymethamphetamine (MDMA; "ecstasy"), selegiline (a selective MAO-B inhibitor), and sibutramine (an SNRI used for the management of obesity [no longer commercially available in the US]). Other drugs that have been associated with the syndrome but for which less convincing data are available include carbamazepine, fentanyl, and pentazocine.

Clinicians should be aware of the potential for serious, possibly fatal reactions associated with serotonin syndrome or NMS-like reactions in patients receiving 2 or more drugs that affect serotonergic neurotransmission, even if no such interactions with the specific drugs have been reported to date in the medical literature. Pending further accumulation of data, serotonergic drugs should be used cautiously in combination and such combinations avoided whenever clinically possible. Serotonin syndrome may be more likely to occur when initiating therapy, increasing the dosage, or following the addition of another serotonergic drug. Some clinicians state that patients who have experienced serotonin syndrome may be at higher risk for recurrence of the syndrome upon reinitiation of serotonergic drugs. Pending further experience in such cases, some clinicians recommend that therapy with serotonergic agents be limited following recovery. In cases in which the potential benefit of the drug is thought to outweigh the risk of serotonin syndrome, lower potency agents and reduced dosages should be used, combination serotonergic therapy should be avoided, and patients should be monitored carefully for manifestations of serotonin syndrome. If signs and symptoms of serotonin syndrome or NMS develop during therapy, treatment with sertraline and any concurrently administered serotonergic or antidopaminergic agents, including antipsychotic agents, should be discontinued immediately and supportive and symptomatic treatment should be initiated.

For further information on serotonin syndrome, including manifestations and treatment, see Drug Interactions: Serotonergic Drugs, in Fluoxetine Hydrochloride 28:16.04.20.

Monoamine Oxidase Inhibitors Potentially serious, sometimes fatal serotonin syndrome or NMS-like reactions have been reported in patients receiving SSRIs, including sertraline, in combination with an MAO inhibitor. Severe serotonin syndrome reaction developed several hours after initiating sertraline in a woman already receiving phenelzine, lithium, thioridazine, and doxepin. Such reactions also have been reported in patients who recently have discontinued an SSRI and have been started on an MAO inhibitor.

Because of the potential risk of serotonin syndrome or NMS-like reactions, concomitant use of sertraline and MAO inhibitors is contraindicated. At least 2 weeks should elapse between discontinuance of MAO inhibitor therapy and initiation of sertraline therapy and vice versa.

Linezolid. Linezolid, an anti-infective agent that is a nonselective and reversible MAO inhibitor, has been associated with drug interactions resulting in serotonin syndrome, including some associated with SSRIs, and potentially may also cause NMS-like reactions. Because of the risk of serotonin syndrome, linezolid generally should *not* be used in patients receiving sertraline. The US Food and Drug Administration (FDA) states that certain life-threatening or urgent situations may necessitate immediate linezolid treatment in a patient receiving a serotonergic drug, including SSRIs. In such emergency situations, the availability of alternative anti-infectives should be considered and the benefits of linezolid should be weighed against the risk of serotonin syndrome. If linezolid is indicated in such emergency situations, sertraline must be immediately discontinued and the patient monitored for symptoms of CNS toxicity (e.g., mental changes, muscle twitching, excessive sweating, shivering/shaking, diarrhea, loss of coordination, fever) for 2 weeks or until 24 hours after the last linezolid dose, whichever comes first. Treatment with sertraline may be resumed 24 hours after the last linezolid dose.

If nonemergency use of linezolid is being planned for a patient receiving sertraline, sertraline should be withheld for at least 2 weeks prior to initiating linezolid.

Treatment with sertraline should not be initiated in a patient receiving linezolid; when necessary, sertraline may be started 24 hours after the last linezolid dose. (See Drug Interactions: Serotonergic Drugs, in Linezolid 8:12.28.24.)

Methylene Blue. There have been case reports of serotonin syndrome in patients who received methylene blue, which is a potent and selective inhibitor of MAO-A, while receiving serotonergic drugs, including SSRIs (e.g., citalopram, escitalopram, fluoxetine, fluvoxamine, paroxetine, sertraline). Therefore, methylene blue generally should *not* be used in patients receiving sertraline. The FDA states that certain emergency situations (e.g., methemoglobinemia, ifosfamide-induced encephalopathy†) may necessitate immediate use of methylene blue in a patient receiving sertraline. In such emergency situations, the availability of alternative interventions should be considered and the benefits of methylene blue should be weighed against the risk of serotonin syndrome. If methylene blue is indicated in such emergency situations, sertraline must be immediately discontinued and the patient monitored for symptoms of CNS toxicity (e.g., mental changes, muscle twitching, excessive sweating, shivering/shaking, diarrhea, loss of coordination, fever) for 2 weeks or until 24 hours after the last methylene blue dose, whichever come first. Treatment with sertraline may be resumed 24 hours after the last methylene blue dose.

If nonemergency use of methylene blue is being planned for a patient receiving sertraline, sertraline should be withheld for at least 2 weeks prior to initiating methylene blue.

Treatment with sertraline should not be initiated in a patient receiving methylene blue; when necessary, sertraline may be started 24 hours after the last methylene blue dose.

Moclobemide. Moclobemide (not commercially available in the US), a selective and reversible MAO-A inhibitor, has been associated with serotonin syndrome, and such reactions have been fatal in several cases in which the drug was given in combination with the SSRI citalopram or with clomipramine. Pending further experience with such combinations, some clinicians recommend that concurrent therapy with moclobemide and SSRIs be used only with extreme caution and that SSRIs should have been discontinued for some time (depending on the elimination half-lives of the drug and its active metabolites) before initiating moclobemide therapy.

Selegiline. Selegiline, a selective MAO-B inhibitor used in the management of parkinsonian syndrome, has been reported to cause serotonin syndrome when given concurrently with SSRIs (e.g., fluoxetine, paroxetine, sertraline). Although selegiline is a selective MAO-B inhibitor at therapeutic dosages, the drug appears to lose its selectivity for the MAO-B enzyme at higher dosages (e.g., those exceeding 10 mg/kg), thereby increasing the risk of serotonin syndrome in patients receiving higher dosages of the drug either alone or in combination with other serotonergic agents. The manufacturer of selegiline recommends avoiding concurrent selegiline and SSRI therapy. In addition, the manufacturer of selegiline recommends that at least 2 weeks elapse between discontinuance of selegiline and initiation of SSRI therapy.

Isoniazid. Isoniazid, an antituberculosis agent, appears to have some MAO-inhibiting activity. In addition, iproniazid (not commercially available in the US), another antituberculosis agent structurally related to isoniazid that also possesses MAO-inhibiting activity, reportedly has resulted in serotonin syndrome in at least 2 patients when given in combination with meperidine. Pending further experience, clinicians should be aware of the potential for serotonin syndrome when isoniazid is given in combination with SSRI therapy (such as sertraline) or other serotonergic agents.

Tryptophan and Other Serotonin Precursors Because of the potential risk of serotonin syndrome or NMS-like reactions, concurrent use of tryptophan or other serotonin precursors should be avoided in patients receiving sertraline.

5-HT$_1$ Receptor Agonists ("Triptans") Weakness, hyperreflexia, and incoordination have been reported rarely during postmarketing surveillance in patients receiving sumatriptan concomitantly with an SSRI (e.g., citalopram, escitalopram, fluoxetine, fluvoxamine, paroxetine, sertraline); these reactions resembled serotonin syndrome. Oral or subcutaneous sumatriptan and SSRIs were used concomitantly in some clinical studies without unusual adverse effects. However, an increase in the frequency of migraine attacks and a decrease in the effectiveness of sumatriptan in relieving migraine headache have been reported in a patient receiving subcutaneous injections of sumatriptan intermittently while undergoing fluoxetine therapy.

Clinicians prescribing 5-HT$_1$ receptor agonists, SSRIs, and SNRIs should consider that 5-HT$_1$ receptor agonists often are used intermittently and that either the 5-HT$_1$ receptor agonist, SSRI, or SNRI may be prescribed by a different clinician. Clinicians also should weigh the potential risk of serotonin syndrome or NMS-like reactions with the expected benefit of using a 5-HT$_1$ receptor agonist concurrently with SSRI or SNRI therapy. If concomitant treatment with sumatriptan or another 5-HT$_1$ receptor agonist and sertraline is clinically warranted, the patient should be observed carefully, particularly during treatment initiation, dosage increases, and following the addition of other serotonergic agents. Patients receiving concomitant 5-HT$_1$ receptor agonist and SSRI or SNRI therapy should be informed of the possibility of serotonin syndrome or NMS-like reactions and advised to immediately seek medical attention if they experience signs or symptoms of these syndromes.

Sibutramine Because of the possibility of developing potentially serious, sometimes fatal serotonin syndrome or NMS-like reactions, sibutramine (no longer commercially available in the US) should be used with caution in patients receiving sertraline.

Other Selective Serotonin-reuptake Inhibitors and Selective Serotonin- and Norepinephrine-reuptake Inhibitors Concomitant administration of sertraline with other SSRIs or SNRIs potentially may result in serotonin syndrome or NMS-like reactions and is therefore not recommended. (See Dosage and Administration: Dosage.)

Antipsychotic Agents and Other Dopamine Antagonists Concomitant use of antipsychotic agents and other dopamine antagonists with sertraline rarely may result in potentially serious, sometimes fatal serotonin syndrome or NMS-like reactions. If signs and symptoms of serotonin syndrome or NMS occur, treatment with sertraline and any concurrently administered antidopaminergic or serotonergic agents should be immediately discontinued and supportive and symptomatic treatment initiated. (See Drug Interactions: Clozapine and also see Drug Interactions: Pimozide.)

Tramadol and Other Serotonergic Drugs Because of the potential risk of serotonin syndrome or NMS-like reactions, caution is advised whenever SSRIs, including sertraline, and SNRIs are concurrently administered with other drugs that may affect serotonergic neurotransmitter systems, including tramadol and St. John's wort (*Hypericum perforatum*).

■ **Drugs Undergoing Hepatic Metabolism or Affecting Hepatic Microsomal Enzymes** Animal studies have demonstrated that sertraline induces hepatic microsomal enzymes. In humans, microsomal enzyme induction by sertraline was minimal as determined by a small (5%) but statistically significant decrease in antipyrine half-life following sertraline administration (200 mg daily) for 21 days. The manufacturers state that this small change in antipyrine half-life reflects a clinically unimportant change in hepatic metabolism. Nonetheless, caution should be exercised when sertraline is given to patients receiving drugs that are hepatically metabolized and that have a low therapeutic ratio, such as warfarin. (See Drug Interactions: Protein-bound Drugs and also see Anticoagulants under Drug Interactions: Drugs Affecting Hemostasis.)

Drugs Metabolized by Cytochrome P-450 (CYP) 2D6 Sertraline, like many other antidepressants (e.g., other SSRIs, many tricyclic antidepressants) is metabolized by the drug-metabolizing cytochrome P-450 (CYP) 2D6 isoenzyme (debrisoquine hydroxylase). In addition, like many other drugs metabolized by CYP2D6, sertraline inhibits the activity of CYP2D6 and potentially may increase plasma concentrations of concomitantly administered drugs that also are metabolized by this isoenzyme. Although similar interactions are possible with other SSRIs, there is considerable variability among the drugs in the extent to which they inhibit CYP2D6. At lower doses, sertraline has demonstrated a less prominent inhibitory effect on CYP2D6 than some other SSRIs. Nevertheless, even sertraline has the potential for clinically important CYP2D6 inhibition.

Concomitant use of sertraline with other drugs metabolized by CYP2D6 has not been systematically studied. The extent to which this potential interaction may become clinically important depends on the extent of inhibition of CYP2D6 by the antidepressant and the therapeutic index of the concomitantly administered drug. The drugs for which this potential interaction is of greatest concern are those that are metabolized principally by CYP2D6 and have a narrow therapeutic index, such as tricyclic antidepressants, class IC antiarrhythmics (e.g., propafenone, flecainide, encainide), and some phenothiazines (e.g., thioridazine).

Caution should be used whenever concurrent therapy with sertraline and other drugs metabolized by CYP2D6 is considered. Because concomitant use of sertraline and thioridazine may result in increased plasma concentrations of the phenothiazine and increase the risk of serious, potentially fatal, adverse cardiac effects (e.g., cardiac arrhythmias), the manufacturer of thioridazine states that the drug should not be used concomitantly with any drug that inhibits the CYP2D6 isoenzyme. The manufacturers of sertraline state that concurrent use of a drug metabolized by CYP2D6 may necessitate the administration of dosages of the other drug that are lower than those usually prescribed. Furthermore, whenever sertraline therapy is discontinued (and plasma concentrations of sertraline are decreased) during concurrent therapy with another drug metabolized by CYP2D6, an increased dosage of the concurrently administered drug may be necessary.

Drugs Metabolized by Cytochrome P-450 (CYP) 3A4 Although sertraline can inhibit the cytochrome P-450 (CYP) 3A4 isoenzyme, results of in vitro and in vivo studies indicate that the drug is a much less potent inhibitor of this enzyme than many other drugs. In an in vivo drug interaction study, concomitant use of sertraline and the CYP3A4 substrate, carbamazepine, under steady-state conditions had no effect on plasma concentrations of carbamazepine. The manufacturers of sertraline state that these data suggest that the extent of sertraline's inhibition of CYP3A4 activity is unlikely to be of clinical importance. However, a marked increase in plasma concentrations (ranging from 80–250%) and bone marrow suppression developed within 1–2 months of initiating sertraline in a patient previously stabilized on carbamazepine and flecainide therapy. Although the precise mechanism for this possible interaction and the role of the cytochrome P-450 enzyme system are unclear, some clinicians recommend that carbamazepine concentrations be monitored during concomitant sertraline therapy.

Results of an in vivo drug interaction study with cisapride indicate that concomitant use of sertraline (200 mg daily) induces the metabolism of cisapride; peak plasma concentrations and area under the plasma concentration-time curve (AUC) of cisapride were decreased by about 35% in the study. However, the manufacturers of sertraline state that the extent of sertraline's inhibition of CYP3A4 activity is unlikely to be of clinical importance.

Results of another drug interaction study in which sertraline was used concomitantly with terfenadine (no longer commercially available in the US), a drug metabolized principally by the cytochrome P-450 microsomal enzyme system (mainly by the CYP3A4 isoenzyme), indicate that concurrent use of sertraline did not increase plasma concentrations of terfenadine and, therefore, the manufacturers state that these data suggest that the extent of sertraline's inhibition of CYP3A4 activity is unlikely to be of clinical importance. However, the manufacturer of astemizole (no longer commercially available in the US) and some clinicians state that until the clinical importance of these findings is established, concomitant use of sertraline with astemizole or terfenadine is not recommended since substantially increased plasma concentrations of unchanged astemizole or terfenadine could occur resulting in an increased risk of serious adverse cardiac effects.

■ Tricyclic and Other Antidepressants The extent to which SSRI interactions with tricyclic antidepressants may pose clinical problems depends on the degree of inhibition and the pharmacokinetics of the serotonin-reuptake inhibitor involved. In healthy individuals, sertraline has been shown to substantially reduce the clearance of two tricyclic antidepressants, desipramine and imipramine. This interaction appears to result from sertraline-induced inhibition of CYP2D6. Thus, the manufacturers and some clinicians recommend that caution be exercised during concurrent use of tricyclics with sertraline since sertraline may inhibit the metabolism of the tricyclic antidepressant. In addition, plasma tricyclic concentrations may need to be monitored and the dosage of the tricyclic reduced during concomitant administration. (See Dosage and Administration: Dosage and also see Drugs Metabolized by Cytochrome P-450 [CYP] 2D6 under Drug Interactions: Drugs Undergoing Hepatic Metabolism or Affecting Hepatic Microsomal Enzymes.)

Clinical experience regarding the optimal timing of switching from other antidepressants to sertraline therapy is limited. Therefore, the manufacturers recommend that care and prudent medical judgment be exercised when switching from other antidepressants to sertraline, particularly from long-acting agents (e.g., fluoxetine). Pending further experience in patients being transferred from therapy with another antidepressant to sertraline and as the clinical situation permits, it generally is recommended that the previous antidepressant be discontinued according to the recommended guidelines for the specific antidepressant prior to initiation of sertraline therapy. (See Drug Interactions: Serotonergic Drugs.)

■ Protein-bound Drugs Because sertraline is highly protein bound, the drug theoretically could be displaced from binding sites by, or it could displace from binding sites, other protein-bound drugs such as oral anticoagulants or digitoxin. In vitro studies to date have shown that sertraline has no effect on the protein binding of 2 other highly protein-bound drugs, propranolol or warfarin; these findings also have been confirmed in clinical studies. However, pending further accumulation of data, patients receiving sertraline concomitantly with any highly protein-bound drug should be observed for potential adverse effects associated with combined therapy. (See Anticoagulants under Drug Interactions: Drugs Affecting Hemostasis.)

■ Drugs Affecting Hemostasis ***Anticoagulants*** In a study comparing prothrombin time AUC (0–120 hour) following a dose of warfarin (0.75 mg/kg) or placebo prior to and after 21 days of either sertraline (50–200 mg daily) or placebo, prothrombin time increased by an average of 8% compared with baseline in the sertraline group and decreased by an average of 1% in those receiving placebo. In addition, the normalization of prothrombin time was slightly delayed in those receiving sertraline when compared with those receiving placebo. Because the clinical importance of these findings is not known, prothrombin time should be monitored carefully whenever sertraline therapy is initiated or discontinued in patients receiving anticoagulants. (See Drug Interactions: Protein-bound Drugs.)

Other Drugs That Interfere with Hemostasis Epidemiologic case-control and cohort design studies that have demonstrated an association between selective serotonin-reuptake inhibitor therapy and an increased risk of upper GI bleeding also have shown that concurrent use of aspirin or other nonsteroidal anti-inflammatory agents substantially increases the risk of GI bleeding. Although these studies focused on upper GI bleeding, there is some evidence suggesting that bleeding at other sites may be similarly potentiated. The precise mechanism for this increased risk remains to be clearly established; however, serotonin release by platelets is known to play an important role in hemostasis, and selective serotonin-reuptake inhibitors decrease serotonin uptake from the blood by platelets, thereby decreasing the amount of serotonin in platelets. Patients receiving sertraline should be cautioned about the concomitant use of drugs that interfere with hemostasis, including aspirin and other nonsteroidal anti-inflammatory agents.

■ Alcohol Sertraline administration did not potentiate the cognitive and psychomotor effects induced by alcohol in healthy individuals. In addition, no apparent additive CNS depressant effects were observed in geriatric patients receiving sertraline together with moderate amounts of alcohol. Nonetheless, the manufacturers state that concurrent use of sertraline and alcohol is not recommended.

■ Electroconvulsive Therapy The effects of sertraline in conjunction with electroconvulsive therapy (ECT) have not been evaluated to date in clinical studies.

■ Cimetidine In a study evaluating the effect of the addition of a single dose of sertraline (100 mg) on the second of 8 days of cimetidine administration (800 mg daily), the mean AUC, peak concentration, and elimination half-life of sertraline increased substantially (by 50, 24, and 26%, respectively) compared with the placebo group. The clinical importance of these changes is unknown.

■ Benzodiazepines In a study comparing the disposition of diazepam administered IV before and after 21 days of sertraline therapy (dosage titrated from 50–200 mg daily) or placebo, there was a 32% decrease in diazepam clearance in the sertraline recipients and a 19% decrease in those receiving placebo when compared with baseline. There was a 23% increase in the time to maximal plasma concentration for desmethyldiazepam in the sertraline group compared with a 20% decrease in the placebo group. The clinical importance of these findings is unknown; however, they suggest that sertraline and *N*-desmethylsertraline are not likely to substantially inhibit the CYP2C19 and CYP3A3/4 hepatic isoenzymes involved in the metabolism of diazepam.

■ Clozapine Concomitant use of SSRIs such as sertraline in patients receiving clozapine can increase plasma concentrations of the antipsychotic agent. In a study in schizophrenic patients receiving clozapine under steady-state conditions, initiation of paroxetine therapy resulted in only minor changes in plasma concentrations of clozapine and its metabolites; however, initiation of fluvoxamine therapy resulted in increases that were threefold compared with baseline. In other published reports, concomitant use of clozapine and SSRIs (fluvoxamine, paroxetine, sertraline) resulted in modest increases (less than twofold) in clozapine and metabolite concentrations. The manufacturer of clozapine states that caution should be exercised and patients closely monitored if clozapine is used in patients receiving SSRIs, and a reduction in clozapine dosage should be considered. (See Antipsychotic Agents and Other Dopamine Antagonists under Drug Interactions: Serotonergic Drugs.)

■ Lithium In a placebo-controlled trial, the administration of 2 doses of sertraline did not substantially alter steady-state plasma lithium concentrations or the renal clearance of lithium. Pending further accumulation of data, however, the manufacturers recommend that plasma lithium concentrations be monitored following initiation of sertraline in patients receiving lithium and that lithium dosage be adjusted accordingly. In addition, because of the potential risk of serotonin syndrome or NMS-like reactions, caution is advised during concurrent sertraline and lithium use. (See Drug Interactions: Serotonergic Drugs.)

■ Hypoglycemic Drugs In a placebo-controlled study in healthy male volunteers, sertraline administration for 22 days (including 200 mg daily for the final 13 days) caused a small but statistically significant decrease (16%) in the clearance of a 1-g IV dose of tolbutamide compared with baseline values and an increase in the terminal elimination half-life (from 6.9 to 8.6 hours). The decrease in clearance was not accompanied by any substantial changes in the plasma protein binding or the apparent volume of distribution of tolbutamide, which suggests that the change in tolbutamide clearance may be caused by a slight inhibition of the cytochrome P-450 isoenzyme CYP2C9/10 when sertraline is given in the maximum recommended dosage. The clinical importance of these findings remains to be determined.

■ **Digoxin** In a placebo-controlled trial in healthy volunteers, sertraline administration for 17 days (including 200 mg daily for the final 10 days) did not alter serum digoxin concentrations or renal clearance of digoxin. The results of this study suggest that dosage adjustment of digoxin may not be necessary in patients receiving concomitant sertraline.

■ **Atenolol** In a double-blind, placebo-controlled, randomized, crossover study, a single, 100-mg dose of sertraline had no effect on the β-adrenergic blocking activity of atenolol when administered to a limited number of healthy males.

■ **Amiodarone** A decrease in the plasma concentrations of amiodarone and its active metabolite, desmethylamiodarone, to 82 and 85% of the baseline values, respectively, occurred in one patient following the discontinuance of sertraline and carbamazepine therapy, suggesting that sertraline may have been inhibiting the metabolism of amiodarone by CYP3A4.

■ **Phenytoin** In a randomized, double-blind, placebo-controlled trial, chronic administration of high dosages of sertraline (200 mg daily) did not substantially affect the pharmacokinetics or pharmacodynamics of phenytoin when the 2 drugs were given concurrently in healthy volunteers. However, substantial reductions in plasma sertraline concentrations have been observed in sertraline-treated patients concurrently receiving phenytoin; it was suggested that induction of the cytochrome P-450 isoenzymes may be responsible. In addition, concurrent administration of sertraline and phenytoin reportedly resulted in elevated phenytoin concentrations in 2 geriatric patients. Pending further accumulation of data, the manufacturers and some clinicians recommend that plasma phenytoin concentrations be monitored following initiation of sertraline therapy and that phenytoin dosage should be adjusted as necessary, particularly in patients with multiple underlying medical conditions and/or those receiving multiple concomitant drugs.

■ **Pimozide** Concomitant use of sertraline and pimozide has resulted in substantial increases in peak plasma concentrations and area under the plasma concentration-time curve (AUC) of pimozide. In one controlled study, administration of a single 2-mg dose of pimozide in individuals receiving sertraline 200 mg daily resulted in a mean increase in pimozide AUC and peak plasma concentrations of about 40%, but was not associated with changes in ECG parameters. The effects on QT interval and pharmacokinetic parameters of pimozide administered in higher doses (i.e., doses exceeding 2 mg) in combination with sertraline are as yet unknown. Concomitant use of sertraline and pimozide is contraindicated because of the low therapeutic index of pimozide and because the reported interaction between the 2 drugs occurred at a low dose of pimozide. The mechanism of this interaction is as yet unknown. (See Antipsychotic Agents and Other Dopamine Antagonists under Drug Interactions: Serotonergic Drugs.)

■ **Valproic Acid** The effect of sertraline on plasma valproic acid concentrations remains to be evaluated in clinical studies. In the absence of such data, the manufacturers recommend monitoring plasma valproic acid concentrations following initiation of sertraline therapy and adjusting the dosage of valproic acid as necessary.

Acute Toxicity

■ **Pathogenesis** The acute lethal dose of sertraline in humans is not known. One patient who ingested 13.5 g of sertraline alone subsequently recovered. However, death occurred in another patient who ingested 2.5 g of the drug alone.

In general, overdosage of sertraline may be expected to produce effects that are extensions of the drug's pharmacologic and adverse effects. The most common signs and symptoms associated with nonfatal sertraline overdosage include somnolence, nausea, vomiting, tachycardia, dizziness, agitation, and tremor. Other adverse events observed in patients who received overdosages of sertraline (alone or in combination with other drugs) include bradycardia, bundle branch block, coma, seizures, delirium, hallucinations, hypertension, hypotension, manic reaction, pancreatitis, QT-interval prolongation, serotonin syndrome, stupor, and syncope. Prolonged tachycardia, hypertension, hallucinations, hyperthermia, tremors of the extremities, and skin flushing have occurred in a child after accidental sertraline ingestion; the reaction resembled serotonin syndrome. Flushing, anger, emotional lability, and distractability developed 1 hour after an adult female ingested 2 g of sertraline; recovery was uneventful apart from watery bowel movements.

■ **Treatment** Because fatalities and severe toxicity have been reported when sertraline was ingested alone or in combination with other drugs and/or alcohol, the manufacturers and some clinicians recommend that any overdosage involving sertraline be managed aggressively. Clinicians also should consider the possibility of serotonin syndrome or NMS-like reactions in patients presenting with similar clinical features and a recent history of sertraline and/or ingestion of other serotonergic agents and/or antipsychotic agents or other dopamine antagonists. (See Cautions: Precautions and Contraindications and also see Drug Interactions: Serotonergic Drugs.)

Management of sertraline overdosage generally involves symptomatic and supportive care. A patent airway should be established and maintained, and adequate oxygenation and ventilation should be ensured. ECG and vital sign monitoring is recommended following acute overdosage with the drug, although the value of ECG monitoring in predicting the severity of sertraline-induced cardiotoxicity is not known. (See Acute Toxicity: Manifestations, in the Tricyclic Antidepressants General Statement 28:16.04.28.) There is no specific antidote for sertraline intoxication. Because suicidal ingestion often involves more than one drug, clinicians treating sertraline overdosage should be alert to possible manifestations caused by drugs other than sertraline.

If the patient is comatose, having seizures, or lacks the gag reflex, gastric lavage may be performed if an endotracheal tube with cuff inflated is in place to prevent aspiration of gastric contents. Since administration of activated charcoal (which may be used in conjunction with sorbitol) may be as effective as or more effective than induction of emesis or gastric lavage, its use has been recommended either in the initial management of sertraline overdosage or following induction of emesis or gastric lavage in patients who have ingested a potentially toxic quantity of the drug.

Limited data indicate that sertraline is not appreciably removed by hemodialysis. Because of the large volume of distribution of sertraline and its principal metabolite, peritoneal dialysis, forced diuresis, hemoperfusion, and/or exchange transfusion also are likely to be ineffective in removing substantial amounts of sertraline and *N*-desmethylsertraline from the body.

Clinicians should consult a poison control center for additional information on the management of sertraline overdosage.

Chronic Toxicity

Sertraline has not been studied systematically in animals or humans to determine whether therapy with the drug is associated with abuse, tolerance, or physical dependence.

The premarketing clinical experience with sertraline did not reveal any tendency for a withdrawal syndrome or any drug-seeking behavior. However, fatigue, severe abdominal cramping, memory impairment, and influenza-like symptoms were reported 2 days following abrupt discontinuance of sertraline in one patient; when sertraline was restarted, the symptoms remitted. Electric shock-like sensations occurred in another patient 1 day after the last administered dose of sertraline; these sensations became less intense and eventually disappeared 13 weeks after sertraline therapy was discontinued. When evaluating these cases and those reported with other serotonin-reuptake inhibitors, it appears that a withdrawal syndrome may occur within several days following abrupt discontinuance of these drugs. The most commonly observed symptoms are those that resemble influenza, such as fatigue, stomach complaints (e.g., nausea), dizziness or lightheadedness, tremor, anxiety, chills, sweating, and incoordination. Other reported symptoms include memory impairment, insomnia, paresthesia, shock-like sensations, headache, palpitations, agitation, or aggression. Such reactions appear to be self-limiting and improve over 1 to several weeks. Pending further experience, sertraline therapy should be discontinued gradually to prevent the possible development of withdrawal reactions.

As with other CNS-active drugs, clinicians should carefully evaluate patients for a history of substance abuse prior to initiating sertraline therapy. If sertraline therapy is initiated in patients with a history of substance abuse, such patients should be monitored closely for signs of misuse or abuse of the drug (e.g., development of tolerance, use of increasing doses, drug-seeking behavior).

The potential for misuse of sertraline in patients with concurrent eating disorders and/or those who may seek the drug for its appetite-suppressant effects also may be considered.

Pharmacology

The pharmacology of sertraline is complex and in many ways resembles that of other antidepressant agents, particularly those agents (e.g., fluoxetine, fluvoxamine, paroxetine, clomipramine, trazodone) that predominantly potentiate the pharmacologic effects of serotonin (5-HT). Like other selective serotonin-reuptake inhibitors (SSRIs), sertraline is a potent and highly selective reuptake inhibitor of serotonin and has little or no effect on other neurotransmitters.

■ **Nervous System Effects** The precise mechanism of antidepressant action of sertraline is unclear, but the drug has been shown to selectively inhibit the reuptake of serotonin at the presynaptic neuronal membrane. Sertraline-induced inhibition of serotonin reuptake causes increased synaptic concentrations of serotonin in the CNS, resulting in numerous functional changes associated with enhanced serotonergic neurotransmission. Like other SSRIs (e.g., fluoxetine, fluvoxamine, paroxetine), sertraline appears to have only very weak effects on the reuptake of norepinephrine or dopamine and does not exhibit clinically important anticholinergic, antihistaminic, or adrenergic (α_1, α_2, β) blocking activity at usual therapeutic dosages.

Although the mechanism of antidepressant action of antidepressant agents may involve inhibition of the reuptake of various neurotransmitters (i.e., serotonin, norepinephrine) at the presynaptic neuronal membrane, it has been suggested that postsynaptic receptor modification is mainly responsible for the antidepressant action observed during long-term administration of antidepressant agents. During long-term therapy with most antidepressants (e.g., tricyclic antidepressants, monoamine oxidase [MAO] inhibitors), these adaptive changes mainly consist of subsensitivity of the noradrenergic adenylate cyclase system in association with a decrease in the number of β-adrenergic receptors; such effects on noradrenergic receptor function are commonly referred to as "down regulation." In animal studies, long-term administration of sertraline has been shown to downregulate noradrenergic receptors in the CNS as has been observed with many other clinically effective antidepressants. In addition, some antidepressants (e.g., amitriptyline) reportedly decrease the number of serotonergic (5-HT) binding sites following chronic administration. Although changes in the density of type 2 serotonergic (5-HT_2) binding sites were not observed during chronic administration of sertraline in animals in one study, the drug caused desensitization of the 5-HT_2 receptor transmembrane signaling system; the clinical importance of these findings requires further study.

The precise mechanism of action that is responsible for the efficacy of sertraline in the treatment of obsessive-compulsive disorder is unclear. However, because of the potency of clomipramine and other selective serotonin-reuptake inhibitors (e.g., fluoxetine, fluvoxamine, paroxetine) in inhibiting serotonin reuptake and their efficacy in the treatment of obsessive-compulsive disorder, a serotonin hypothesis has been developed to explain the pathogenesis of the condition. The hypothesis postulates that a dysregulation of serotonin is responsible for obsessive-compulsive disorder and that sertraline and these other agents are effective because they correct this imbalance. Although the available evidence supports the serotonergic hypothesis of obsessive-compulsive disorder, additional studies are necessary to confirm this hypothesis.

Serotonergic mechanisms also appear to be involved at least in part in a number of other pharmacologic effects associated with selective serotonin-reuptake inhibitors, including sertraline, such as decreased food intake and altered food selection as well as decreased alcohol intake.

Serotonergic Effects Sertraline is a highly selective inhibitor of serotonin reuptake at the presynaptic neuronal membrane. Sertraline-induced inhibition of serotonin reuptake causes increased synaptic concentrations of the neurotransmitter, resulting in numerous functional changes associated with enhanced serotonergic neurotransmission.

Data from in vitro studies suggest that sertraline is more potent than fluvoxamine, fluoxetine, or clomipramine as a serotonin-reuptake inhibitor. Like some other serotonin-reuptake inhibitors, sertraline undergoes metabolism via *N*-demethylation to form *N*-desmethylsertraline, the principal metabolite. Data from in vivo and in vitro studies have shown that *N*-desmethylsertraline is approximately 5–10 times less potent as an inhibitor of serotonin reuptake than sertraline; however, the metabolite retains selectivity for serotonin reuptake compared with either norepinephrine or dopamine reuptake.

At therapeutic dosages (50–200 mg daily) in healthy individuals, sertraline has been shown to inhibit the reuptake of serotonin into platelets in a dose-dependent manner. Like other serotonin-reuptake inhibitors, sertraline inhibits the spontaneous firing of serotonergic neurons in the dorsal raphe nucleus. In vitro data have demonstrated that sertraline has substantial affinity for serotonergic (5-HT_{1A}, 5-HT_{1B}, 5-HT_2) receptors.

Effects on Other Neurotransmitters Like other serotonin-reuptake inhibitors, sertraline has been shown to have little or no activity in inhibiting the reuptake of norepinephrine. In addition, the drug has demonstrated a substantially higher selectivity ratio of serotonin-to-norepinephrine reuptake inhibiting activity than fluoxetine or tricyclic antidepressant agents, including clomipramine.

Although sertraline has only weak activity in inhibiting the reuptake of dopamine, the relative selectivity of sertraline for inhibiting serotonin reuptake relative to dopamine reuptake appears to be somewhat less than that of fluoxetine, fluvoxamine, zimelidine, or clomipramine. In addition, sertraline does not inhibit monoamine oxidase.

Unlike tricyclic and some other antidepressants, sertraline does not exhibit clinically important anticholinergic, α- or β-adrenergic blocking, or antihistaminic activity at usual therapeutic dosages. As a result, the incidence of adverse effects commonly associated with blockade of muscarinic cholinergic receptors (e.g., dry mouth, blurred vision, urinary retention, constipation, confusion), α-adrenergic receptors (e.g., orthostatic hypotension), and histamine H_1- and H_2-receptors (e.g., sedation) is lower in sertraline-treated patients. In vitro studies have demonstrated that sertraline does not possess clinically important affinity for α_1- or α_2-adrenergic, β-adrenergic, histaminergic, muscarinic, GABA, benzodiazepine, or dopamine receptors.

Effects on Sleep Like tricyclic and most other antidepressants, sertraline suppresses rapid eye movement (REM) sleep. Although not clearly established, there is some evidence that the REM-suppressing effects of antidepressant agents may contribute to the antidepressant activity of these drugs. In animal studies, sertraline suppressed REM sleep; the drug appears to reduce the amount of REM sleep by decreasing the number as well as the duration of REM episodes. Although the precise mechanism has not been fully elucidated, results of animal studies indicate that sertraline's effects on REM sleep are serotonergically mediated.

Effects on EEG Limited data currently are available regarding the effects of sertraline on the EEG. EEG changes in healthy individuals receiving single, 100-mg doses of sertraline resembled the EEG profiles of patients receiving desipramine-type antidepressants (increased alpha and decreased but accelerated delta activity) and suggest improved vigilance and psychometric performance. In individuals receiving higher single doses (200 and 400 mg) of the drug, sertraline produced EEG changes similar to imipramine-type antidepressants (reduced alpha and low beta activity and increased theta and fast beta activity), which reflect vigilance changes of the dissociative type and therefore possible sedative activity.

Effects on Psychomotor Function Sertraline does not appear to cause clinically important sedation and does not interfere with psychomotor performance. The drug did not appear to have any adverse effects on psychomotor performance when given to healthy women in single doses up to 100 mg. In healthy individuals over 50 years of age, single, 100-mg doses of sertraline increased the critical flicker fusion frequency slightly and the subjective perception of sedation; however, the drug had no depressant effect on objective tests of psychomotor performance. In addition, no adverse effects on psychomotor performance were observed in geriatric individuals who received the drug in a controlled study.

■ **Cardiovascular Effects** Sertraline appears to have little effect on the ECG. Data from controlled studies indicate sertraline does not produce clinically important changes in heart rate, cardiac conduction, or other ECG parameters in depressed patients.

■ **Effects on Appetite and Body Weight** Like some other serotonergic agents (e.g., fenfluramine [no longer commercially available in the US], fluoxetine, zimelidine), sertraline possesses anorexigenic activity. Limited data from animal studies suggest that fenfluramine has been the most effective inhibitor of food intake followed by fluoxetine and then sertraline. Although the precise mechanism has not been clearly established, results from animal studies indicate that sertraline's appetite-inhibiting action may result at least in part from serotonin-reuptake blockade and the resultant increase in serotonin availability at the neuronal synapse. Because sertraline's anorexigenic activity was not antagonized by prior administration of serotonergic antagonists, other mechanisms also may be involved but require further study. Following administration of single doses of sertraline in meal-fed animals, food intake was reduced in a dose-dependent manner. At a dose of 3 mg/kg, the reduction in food intake was substantially reduced and higher doses of 10 or 30 mg/kg reduced food intake by 45 or 74%, respectively.

Sertraline therapy has resulted in dose-dependent decreases in body weight in animals receiving the drug for 3 days; the weight loss was not accompanied by any overt signs of behavioral abnormality. Sertraline therapy also has resulted in decreases in body weight in individuals receiving the drug. However, weight loss is usually minimal and averaged about 0.45–0.9 kg in individuals treated with the drug in controlled clinical trials. (See Cautions: Metabolic Effects and see also Cautions: Pediatric Precautions.) Rarely, weight loss has required discontinuance of therapy.

■ **Effects on Alcohol Intake** Like some other serotonergic agents, sertraline produces a substantial decrease in voluntary alcohol intake in animals. Because serotonin appears to be involved in the regulation of alcohol intake, it has been suggested that selective serotonin-reuptake inhibitors may attenuate alcohol consumption via enhanced serotonergic neurotransmission. (See Cautions.)

■ **Neuroendocrine Effects** Limited data currently are available regarding the effects of sertraline on the endocrine system. In one animal study, sertraline did not demonstrate substantial neuroendocrine effects at a dose that substantially reduced gross activity.

Although a causal relationship has not been established, hypothyroidism, decreased serum thyroxine concentrations, and/or increased serum thyrotropin (thyroid-stimulating hormone, TSH) concentrations have been reported in a limited number of sertraline patients, some of whom were receiving thyroxine concurrently. (See Cautions: Other Adverse Effects and also see Precautions and Contraindications.)

■ **Other Effects** Sertraline appears to have a weak uricosuric effect; mean decreases in serum uric acid of approximately 7% have been reported in patients receiving the drug. The clinical importance of these findings is unknown, and there have been no reports of acute renal failure associated with the drug. (See Cautions: Precautions and Contraindications.)

Pharmacokinetics

In all human studies described in the Pharmacokinetics section, sertraline was administered as the hydrochloride salt; dosages and concentrations are expressed in terms of sertraline.

■ **Absorption** Sertraline appears to be slowly but well absorbed from the GI tract following oral administration. The oral bioavailability of sertraline in humans has not been fully elucidated to date because a preparation for IV administration is not available. However, the relative proportion of an oral dose that reaches systemic circulation unchanged appears to be relatively small because sertraline undergoes extensive first-pass metabolism. In animals, the oral bioavailability of sertraline ranges from 22–36%. The manufacturers state that the bioavailability of a single dose of sertraline hydrochloride tablets is approximately equal to that of an equivalent dose of sertraline hydrochloride oral solution. In a study in healthy adults who received a single 100-mg dose of sertraline as a tablet or oral solution, the solution to tablet ratios of the mean geometric AUC and peak plasma concentration were 114.8 and 120.6%, respectively.

The effect of food on the absorption of sertraline hydrochloride given as tablets or the oral solution has been studied in single-dose studies. Administration of a sertraline hydrochloride tablet with food slightly increased the area under the concentration-time curve (AUC) of sertraline, increased peak plasma concentrations by approximately 25%, and decreased the time to achieve peak plasma concentrations from about 8 to 5.5 hours. Administration of sertraline hydrochloride oral solution with food increased the time to achieve peak plasma concentrations from 5.9 to 7.0 hours.

Peak plasma sertraline concentrations usually occur within 4.5–8.4 hours following oral administration of 50–200 mg once daily for 14 days. Peak plasma sertraline concentrations following administration of single oral doses of 50–200 mg are proportional and linearly related to dose. Peak plasma concentrations and bioavailability are increased in geriatric individuals.

Following multiple dosing, steady-state plasma sertraline concentrations should be achieved after approximately 1 week of once-daily dosing. When compared with a single dose, there is an approximate twofold accumulation of sertraline after multiple daily dosing in dosages ranging from 50–200 mg daily. *N*-Desmethylsertraline, sertraline's principal metabolite, exhibits time-related, dose-dependent increases in AUC (0–24 hour), peak plasma concentrations, and trough plasma concentrations with about a 5- to 9-fold increase in these parameters between day 1 and 14.

As with other serotonin-reuptake inhibitors, the relationship between plasma sertraline and *N*-desmethylsertraline concentrations and the therapeutic and/or toxic effects of the drug has not been clearly established.

■ **Distribution** Distribution of sertraline and its metabolites into human body tissues and fluids has not been fully characterized. However, limited pharmacokinetic data suggest that the drug and some of its metabolites are widely distributed in body tissues. Although the apparent volume of distribution of sertraline has not been determined in humans, values exceeding 20 L/kg have been reported in rats and dogs. The drug crosses the blood-brain barrier in humans and animals.

At in vitro plasma concentrations ranging from 20–500 ng/mL, sertraline is approximately 98% bound to plasma proteins, principally to albumin and α_1-acid glycoprotein. Protein binding is independent of plasma concentrations from 20–2000 mcg/mL. However, sertraline and *N*-desmethylsertraline did not alter the plasma protein binding of 2 other highly protein bound drugs, warfarin or propranolol, at concentrations of 300 and 200 ng/mL, respectively.

Sertraline and *N*-desmethylsertraline are distributed into milk. In a study involving 12 lactating women who received oral dosages of sertraline ranging from 25–200 mg daily, both sertraline and *N*-desmethylsertraline were present in all breast milk samples, with the highest concentrations observed in hind milk 7–10 hours after the maternal dose. Detectable concentrations of sertraline were found in 3 and *N*-desmethylsertraline in 6, respectively, out of 11 nursing infants.

■ **Elimination** The elimination half-life of sertraline averages approximately 25–26 hours and that of desmethylsertraline averages about 62–104 hours. In geriatric adults elimination half-life may be increased (e.g., to about 36 hours); however, such prolongation does not appear clinically important and does not warrant dosing alterations.

The exact metabolic fate of sertraline has not been fully elucidated. Sertraline appears to be extensively metabolized, probably in the liver, to *N*-desmethylsertraline and several other metabolites. Like some other serotonin-reuptake inhibitors, sertraline undergoes metabolism via *N*-demethylation to form *N*-desmethylsertraline, the principal metabolite. Unlike some other serotonin-reuptake inhibitors, the drug metabolizing isoenzyme CYP2D6 (a cytochrome P-450 isoenzyme implicated in the sparteine/debrisoquine polymorphism) does not appear to have a major role in the conversion of sertraline to *N*-desmethylsertraline. Nonetheless, sertraline has the potential for clinically important inhibition of this enzyme. (See Drug Interactions: Drugs Undergoing Hepatic Metabolism or Affecting Hepatic Microsomal Enzymes.) In vitro, the conversion of sertraline to *N*-desmethylsertraline correlates more with CYP3A3/4 activity than with CYP2D6 activity. Data from in vivo and in vitro studies have shown that *N*-desmethylsertraline is approximately 5–10 times less potent as an inhibitor of serotonin reuptake than sertraline; however, the metabolite retains selectivity for serotonin reuptake compared with either norepinephrine or dopamine reuptake. Both sertraline and desmethylsertraline undergo oxidative deamination and subsequent reduction, hydroxylation, and glucuronide conjugation. Desmethylsertraline has an elimination half-life approximately 2.5 times that of sertraline.

Following oral administration, sertraline and its metabolites are excreted in both urine and feces. Following oral administration of a single, radiolabeled dose in 2 healthy males, unchanged sertraline accounted for less than 5% of plasma radioactivity. Approximately 40–45% of the radiolabeled dose was excreted in urine within 9 days. Unchanged sertraline was not detectable in urine. During the same period, approximately 40–45% of the radiolabeled drug was eliminated in feces, including 12–14% of unchanged sertraline.

The effect of age on the elimination of sertraline has not been fully elucidated. Plasma clearance of sertraline was approximately 40% lower in a group of 16 geriatric patients (8 males and 8 females) who received 100 mg of the drug for 14 days than that reported in a similar study involving younger individuals (from 25–32 years of age). Based on these results, the manufacturers state that steady-state should be achieved in about 2–3 weeks in older individuals. In addition, decreased clearance of *N*-desmethylsertraline was noted in older males but not in older females. (See Dosage and Administration: Dosage in Geriatric Patients.)

Because sertraline is extensively metabolized by the liver, hepatic impairment can affect the elimination of the drug. In one study in patients with chronic mild hepatic impairment (Child-Pugh scores of 5–8) who received 50 mg of sertraline daily for 21 days, sertraline clearance was reduced resulting in a 2–3 times greater exposure to the drug and its metabolite (desmethylsertraline) than that reported for age-matched individuals without hepatic impairment. In a single-dose study in patients with mild, stable cirrhosis, the elimination half-life of sertraline was prolonged to a mean of 52 hours compared with 22 hours in individuals without hepatic disease. In addition, peak plasma concentrations and AUC values for sertraline were 1.7- and 4.4-fold higher, respectively, in patients with hepatic impairment when compared with healthy individuals without liver disease, reflecting decreased clearance of the drug. The pharmacokinetics of sertraline have not been studied to date in patients with moderate and severe hepatic impairment; therefore, the manufacturers recommend that sertraline be administered with caution and in reduced dosage or less frequently in patients with hepatic impairment. (See Cautions: Precautions and Contraindications and see Dosage and Administration: Dosage in Renal and Hepatic Impairment.)

Because sertraline is extensively metabolized in the liver and renal clearance of the drug is negligible, the manufacturers state that clinically important decreases in sertraline clearance are not anticipated if the drug is used in patients with renal impairment. Results of a multiple-dose study indicate that the pharmacokinetics of sertraline are not affected by renal impairment. In this study, individuals with mild to moderate renal impairment (creatinine clearance: 30–60 mL/minute), moderate to severe renal impairment (creatinine clearance: 10–29 mL/minute), or severe renal impairment (undergoing hemodialysis) received 200 mg of sertraline daily for 21 days; the pharmacokinetics and protein binding of the drug in these patients were similar to those reported for age-matched individuals without renal impairment. (See Cautions: Precautions and Contraindications and see Dosage and Administration: Dosage in Renal and Hepatic Impairment.)

Limited data indicate that sertraline is not appreciably removed by hemodialysis. Because of the large volume of distribution of sertraline and its principal metabolite, peritoneal dialysis, forced diuresis, hemoperfusion, and/or exchange transfusion also are likely to be ineffective in removing substantial amounts of sertraline and *N*-desmethylsertraline from the body.

Chemistry and Stability

■ **Chemistry** Sertraline, a selective serotonin-reuptake inhibitor antidepressant agent, is a naphthalenamine (naphthylamine)-derivative. Sertraline differs structurally from other selective serotonin-reuptake inhibitor antidepressants (e.g., citalopram, fluoxetine, paroxetine) and also differs structurally and pharmacologically from other currently available antidepressants (e.g., tricyclic antidepressants, monoamine oxidase inhibitors). Like most other serotonin-reuptake inhibitors, sertraline contains an asymmetric carbon; therefore, there are 2 existing optical isomers of the drug. However, only one of the optical isomers is present in the commercially available form of the drug.

Sertraline is commercially available as the hydrochloride salt, which occurs as a white, crystalline powder that is slightly soluble in water and isopropyl alcohol and sparingly soluble in ethanol. Commercially available sertraline hydrochloride oral solution is a clear, colorless solution with a menthol scent containing 20 mg of sertraline per mL and 12% alcohol.

■ **Stability** Commercially available sertraline hydrochloride tablets and oral solution should be stored at 25°C, but may be exposed to temperatures ranging from 15–30°C. Sertraline hydrochloride oral solution should be diluted only in the liquids specified by the manufacturer, and should be used immediately after dilution.

Preparations

Excipients in commercially available drug preparations may have clinically important effects in some individuals; consult specific product labeling for details.

Sertraline Hydrochloride

Oral		
For solution, concentrate	20 mg (of sertraline) per mL*	**Sertraline Hydrochloride Oral Solution**
		Zoloft® (with calibrated dropper dispenser containing latex rubber), Pfizer
Tablets, film-coated	25 mg (of sertraline)*	**Sertraline Hydrochloride Tablets**
		Zoloft® (scored), Pfizer
	50 mg (of sertraline)*	**Sertraline Hydrochloride Tablets**
		Zoloft® (scored), Pfizer
	100 mg (of sertraline)*	**Sertraline Hydrochloride Tablets**
		Zoloft® (scored), Pfizer
	150 mg (of sertraline)*	**Sertraline Hydrochloride Tablets,** Ranbaxy
	200 mg (of sertraline)*	**Sertraline Hydrochloride Tablets,** Ranbaxy

*available from one or more manufacturer, distributor, and/or repackager by generic (nonproprietary) name

†Use is not currently included in the labeling approved by the US Food and Drug Administration

SEROTONIN MODULATORS 28:16.04.24

traZODone Hydrochloride

■ Trazodone hydrochloride is a triazolopyridine-derivative antidepressant that is chemically and structurally unrelated to tricyclic or tetracyclic antidepressants or to selective serotonin-reuptake inhibitors.

Uses

■ **Major Depressive Disorder** Trazodone is used in the treatment of major depressive disorder. The drug is used in patients who exhibit a prominent and relatively persistent (nearly every day for at least 2 weeks) depressed or dysphoric mood that usually interferes with daily functioning and is manifested as a change in appetite, psychomotor agitation or retardation, a loss of interest in usual activities, a decrease in sexual drive, increased fatigability, a change in sleep, feelings of guilt or worthlessness, slowed thinking or impaired concentration, and/or suicidal ideation or attempts. Trazodone has been used effectively in the treatment of patients who have major depression with or without prominent anxiety. In addition, trazodone has been used effectively in patients with major depression in hospital, institutional, and outpatient settings. Unlike tricyclic antidepressants, trazodone generally has not been reported to precipitate hypomanic or manic attacks in patients with bipolar disorder; however, further study is needed to determine the safety and efficacy of trazodone when used alone as an antidepressant in these patients.

Trazodone is particularly effective in reducing affective and ideational manifestations of depression, especially anxiety, apathy, irritability, and suicidal thoughts. Somatic signs and symptoms associated with depression, including sleep disturbances and fatigue, are also reduced during trazodone therapy. Most clinical studies have shown that the antidepressant effect of usual dosages of trazodone in patients with moderate to severe depression is about equal to that of usual dosages of amitriptyline, imipramine, or doxepin. However, trazodone has reportedly caused fewer adverse effects (e.g., anticholinergic effects) than these tricyclic antidepressants. (See Cautions: Anticholinergic Effects.) Although trazodone has been reported to have a slightly more rapid onset of action than amitriptyline, desipramine, or imipramine, this has not been established.

Trazodone has been used in patients with major depression who have associated anxiety. Based on limited data, the antidepressant effect of usual dosages of trazodone appears to be greater than that of amitriptyline or imipramine in these patients. Trazodone is particularly effective in reducing anxiety, tension, somatic symptoms, insomnia, and psychomotor retardation in these patients.

For further information on treatment of major depressive disorder and considerations in choosing the most appropriate antidepressant for a particular patient, including considerations related to patient tolerance, patient age, and cardiovascular, sedative, and suicidal risk, see Considerations in Choosing Antidepressants under Uses: Major Depressive Disorder, in Fluoxetine Hydrochloride 28:16.04.20.

■ **Schizophrenic Disorder** Although trazodone has been used in the treatment of schizophrenic disorder†, the drug is less effective than chlorpromazine. Depressive symptomatology may improve during trazodone therapy, but the drug does not appear to relieve psychotic symptoms in most schizophrenic patients. Based on limited data, trazodone has little value when used alone in patients with chronic schizophrenic disorder without depression; however, it may be a useful adjunct to antipsychotic agents (e.g., phenothiazines) in patients with chronic schizophrenic disorder and associated depression. Unlike tricyclic antidepressants, trazodone does *not* appear to worsen psychotic symptoms in these patients.

■ **Alcohol Dependence** Trazodone has been used in the adjunctive treatment of alcohol dependence†. In a limited number of patients with alcohol dependence, oral (50–75 mg daily) or IV (50 mg twice daily) trazodone has reduced tremor, depression, and anxiety. In one study, trazodone was more effective in patients who had pronounced affective symptomatology during periods of intoxication and abstention than in those who only had affective symptomatology during intoxication. Further study is needed to determine the efficacy of trazodone in the treatment of alcohol dependence.

■ **Erectile Dysfunction** Trazodone has been used in a limited number of patients for the treatment of erectile dysfunction† (ED, impotence); however, the American Urological Association (AUA) states that such therapy currently is not recommended. Although some studies indicated that trazodone was more effective than placebo for the treatment of erectile dysfunction, other comparative studies did not. In addition, pooled analysis of these studies failed to show a statistically beneficial effect of the drug on sexual function, although subgroup analysis suggested possible benefit in those with psychogenic erectile dysfunction.

■ **Other Uses** Trazodone may be useful in the treatment of some patients with anxiety states† (anxiety neuroses). In one study, the drug reduced anxiety, tension, somatic symptoms, and insomnia in most of these patients. Based on limited data, trazodone appears to have a greater anxiolytic effect than some other antidepressant agents (e.g., tricyclic antidepressants); however, further study is needed to confirm this finding.

Trazodone has been used in the symptomatic treatment of a limited number of patients with drug-induced dyskinesias†. In one placebo-controlled study in patients with levodopa-induced dyskinesias, oral trazodone (60–120 mg daily) reduced signs and symptoms of dyskinesia by up to 50%. In this study, most patients showed some improvement, with greatest improvement in facial, orobuccal-facial, and neck dyskinesias. In another study, IV trazodone (50 mg twice daily) eliminated chronic chlorpromazine- and haloperidol-induced tardive dyskinesias in some patients. The decrease in tremor was accompanied by a reduction in anxiety, which may be partly responsible for the favorable effect of trazodone on tremor in these patients. Additional studies are required to determine the efficacy of trazodone in the treatment of drug-induced dyskinesias.

Dosage and Administration

■ **Administration** Trazodone hydrochloride is administered orally. The drug should be taken shortly after a meal or light snack. If drowsiness occurs, a major portion of the daily dose may be given at bedtime or dosage may be reduced.

■ **Dosage** There is a wide range of individual trazodone hydrochloride dosage requirements, and dosage must be carefully adjusted according to individual tolerance and response, using the lowest possible effective dosage.

Patients receiving trazodone should be monitored for possible worsening of depression, suicidality, or unusual changes in behavior, especially at the beginning of therapy or during periods of dosage adjustment. (See Cautions: Precautions and Contraindications.)

Major Depressive Disorder For the treatment of major depressive disorder, the usual initial adult dosage of trazodone hydrochloride is 150 mg daily given in divided doses. Dosage may be increased by 50 mg/day every 3 or 4 days, depending on the patient's therapeutic response and tolerance. The maximum dosage for outpatients usually should not exceed 400 mg daily. Dosages up to 600 mg daily may be required in hospitalized, institutionalized, or severely depressed patients. Dosages up to 800 mg daily have been used in the treatment of some patients with severe depression; however, the manufacturers do not recommend exceeding a dosage of 600 mg daily.

Although symptomatic relief may be seen in some patients during the first week of therapy, optimum antidepressant effect usually occurs within 2 weeks. About 25% of patients who respond to trazodone require up to 4 weeks of therapy to reach optimum response.

To avoid recurrence of depressive symptoms, trazodone therapy may be required for several months following optimum therapeutic response. Dosage during prolonged maintenance therapy should be kept at the lowest effective level; once an adequate response has been achieved, dosage should be gradually reduced and subsequently adjusted according to the patient's therapeutic response and tolerance.

Cautions

Trazodone hydrochloride apparently causes fewer adverse anticholinergic effects than currently available tricyclic antidepressant agents. Other adverse effects, including cardiovascular effects, also appear to occur less frequently with trazodone than with currently available tricyclic antidepressants.

The incidence and severity of adverse reactions to trazodone in relation to dosage and duration of therapy have not been fully characterized; however, adverse effects appear to occur more frequently at dosages greater than 300 mg/day. Total trazodone hydrochloride dosages up to 800 mg daily have been well tolerated by some patients. Adverse effects appear to be mild to moderate in severity and may decrease after the first few weeks of trazodone therapy. Adverse effects may be obviated by a reduction in dosage or alteration in dosage schedule. Serious reactions requiring discontinuance of therapy are relatively rare.

■ **Nervous System Effects** Adverse nervous system effects occur frequently during the first few weeks of therapy with trazodone. The most frequent adverse effect associated with trazodone therapy is drowsiness, which occurs in 20–50% of patients receiving the drug. Other less frequent adverse nervous system effects of trazodone include dizziness and lightheadedness, nervousness, fatigue, malaise, weakness, heaviness or fullness of the head, headache, and insomnia. Confusion, incoordination, anger or hostility, agitation, decreased concentrating ability, impaired memory, impaired speech, disorientation, hallucinations or delusions, and excitement have also occurred. Hypomania, nightmares or vivid dreams, tonic-clonic seizures, tremors, and paresthesias and akathisia occur rarely.

■ **Anticholinergic Effects** Although bothersome anticholinergic effects commonly occur with tricyclic antidepressants, these effects appear to occur less frequently with trazodone. Dry mouth has been reported in about 15–30% of patients during trazodone therapy; it has been suggested that this effect may result from an α-adrenergic blocking effect rather than an anticholinergic effect of trazodone. In several placebo-controlled studies, the incidence of dry mouth was similar in trazodone- and placebo-treated patients. Other anticholinergic effects such as blurred vision, constipation, and urinary retention have been reported less frequently.

■ **Genitourinary Effects** Trazodone therapy has been associated with priapism, with surgical intervention required in approximately one-third of reported cases; in some cases, permanent impairment of erectile function or impotence has resulted. Male patients receiving trazodone who experience prolonged or inappropriate penile erections should immediately discontinue the drug and consult their physician. Decreased or increased libido, retrograde ejaculation, impotence, inhibited female orgasm (anorgasmia), increased urinary frequency, delayed urine flow, and hematuria have also been associated with trazodone therapy.

■ **GI Effects** Adverse GI effects of trazodone include nausea and vomiting, dysgeusia, and abdominal and gastric disorders. Flatulence and diarrhea have also been reported.

■ **Cardiovascular Effects** Trazodone is thought to be less cardiotoxic than currently available tricyclic antidepressant agents. (See Pharmacology: Cardiovascular Effects.) Hypotension (including orthostatic hypotension) is the most frequent adverse cardiovascular effect of trazodone, occurring in about 5% of patients receiving the drug. In most patients, hypotension is mild and not dose related. Syncope, shortness of breath, chest pain, tachycardia, palpitations, and hypertension have also occurred. Bradycardia has occurred in a few patients during long-term therapy.

Various ECG changes have occurred in patients receiving trazodone. In patients with preexisting cardiac disease, trazodone may be arrhythmogenic. PVCs, ventricular couplets, and short episodes (3 or 4 beats) of ventricular tachycardia have occurred in these patients. Arrhythmias have also been reported in patients without preexisting cardiac disease. Cardiac arrest has also been reported. Myocardial infarction has been reported, but this effect has not been attributed directly to trazodone.

■ **Hematologic Effects** Occasional decreases in leukocyte and neutrophil counts have occurred in some patients receiving trazodone. These changes were not considered clinically important and did not require discontinuance of the drug. Anemia has also been associated with trazodone therapy in a few patients.

■ **Other Adverse Effects** Musculoskeletal aches and pains have occurred in about 5% of patients receiving trazodone. A few patients have developed muscle twitches. Pruritus, rash, urticaria, acne, photosensitivity, edema, nasal or sinus congestion, eye irritation, sweating or clamminess, early or absent menses, and tinnitus have been reported in some patients receiving trazodone. Allergic reactions and hypersalivation have rarely occurred. Minimal increases in serum concentrations of alkaline phosphatase, AST (SGOT), and ALT (SGPT) have occurred in some patients receiving trazodone.

■ **Precautions and Contraindications** Worsening of depression and/or the emergence of suicidal ideation and behavior (suicidality) or unusual changes in behavior may occur in both adult and pediatric (see Cautions: Pediatric Precautions) patients with major depressive disorder or other psychiatric disorders, whether or not they are taking antidepressants. This risk may persist until clinically important remission occurs. Suicide is a known risk of depression and certain other psychiatric disorders, and these disorders themselves are the strongest predictors of suicide. However, there has been a long-standing concern that antidepressants may have a role in inducing worsening of depression and the emergence of suicidality in certain patients during the early phases of treatment. Pooled analyses of short-term, placebo-controlled studies of antidepressants (i.e., selective serotonin-reuptake inhibitors and other antidepressants) have shown an increased risk of suicidality in children, adolescents, and young adults (18–24 years of age) with major depressive disorder and other psychiatric disorders. An increased suicidality risk was not demonstrated with antidepressants compared with placebo in adults older than 24 years of age, and a reduced risk was observed in adults 65 years of age or older. It currently is unknown whether the suicidality risk extends to longer-term use (i.e., beyond several months); however, there is substantial evidence from placebo-controlled maintenance trials in adults with major depressive disorder that antidepressants can delay the recurrence of depression.

The US Food and Drug Administration (FDA) recommends that all patients being treated with antidepressants for any indication be appropriately monitored and closely observed for clinical worsening, suicidality, and unusual changes in behavior, particularly during initiation of therapy (i.e., the first few months) and during periods of dosage adjustments. Families and caregivers of patients being treated with antidepressants for major depressive disorder or other indications, both psychiatric and nonpsychiatric, also should be advised to monitor patients on a daily basis for the emergence of agitation, irritability, or unusual changes in behavior as well as the emergence of suicidality, and to report such symptoms immediately to a health-care provider.

Although a causal relationship between the emergence of symptoms such as anxiety, agitation, panic attacks, insomnia, irritability, hostility, aggressiveness, impulsivity, akathisia, hypomania, and/or mania and either the worsening of depression and/or the emergence of suicidal impulses has not been established, there is concern that such symptoms may represent precursors to emerging suicidality. Consequently, consideration should be given to changing the therapeutic regimen or discontinuing therapy in patients whose depression is persistently worse or in patients experiencing emergent suicidality or symptoms that might be precursors to worsening depression or suicidality, particularly if such manifestations are severe, abrupt in onset, or were not part of the patient's presenting symptoms. FDA also recommends that the drugs be prescribed in the smallest quantity consistent with good patient management, in order to reduce the risk of overdosage. Because of the possibility of comorbidity between major depressive disorder and other psychiatric and nonpsychiatric disorders, the same precautions observed when treating patients with major depressive disorder should be observed when treating patients with other psychiatric and nonpsychiatric disorders.

It is generally believed (though not established in controlled trials) that treating a major depressive episode with an antidepressant alone may increase the likelihood of precipitating a mixed or manic episode in patients at risk for bipolar disorder. Therefore, patients should be adequately screened for bipolar disorder prior to initiating treatment with an antidepressant; such screening should include a detailed psychiatric history (e.g., family history of suicide, bipolar disorder, and depression).

Patients should be warned that trazodone may impair their ability to perform activities requiring mental alertness or physical coordination (e.g., operating machinery, driving a motor vehicle). Patients also should be warned that trazodone may enhance their response to alcohol, barbiturates, or other CNS depressants. Since the risk of dizziness or lightheadedness may be increased during fasting conditions, patients should be advised to take trazodone shortly after a meal or light snack. In addition, total drug absorption may be up to 20% greater when the drug is taken with food rather than on an empty stomach. Because priapism has been associated with trazodone therapy, patients should be instructed to discontinue the drug and consult a physician if prolonged or inappropriate penile erection occurs.

Until additional clinical experience on the safety of trazodone in patients with cardiovascular disease is obtained, it is recommended that these patients be closely monitored, particularly for arrhythmias, while receiving the drug. (See Cautions: Cardiovascular Effects.) It is also recommended that trazodone *not* be used during the initial recovery phase of myocardial infarction.

Leukocyte and differential counts should be performed in patients who develop fever and sore throat or other signs of infection while receiving trazodone. The drug should be discontinued in patients whose leukocyte or absolute neutrophil count decreases to less than normal levels. (See Cautions: Hematologic Effects.)

Trazodone is contraindicated in patients who are hypersensitive to the drug.

■ **Pediatric Precautions** Safety and efficacy of trazodone in children younger than 18 years of age have not been established.

FDA warns that antidepressants increase the risk of suicidal thinking and behavior (suicidality) in children and adolescents with major depressive disorder and other psychiatric disorders. The risk of suicidality for these drugs was identified in a pooled analysis of data from a total of 24 short-term (4–16 weeks), placebo-controlled studies of 9 antidepressants (i.e., bupropion, citalopram, fluoxetine, fluvoxamine, mirtazapine, nefazodone, paroxetine, sertraline, venlafaxine) in over 4400 children and adolescents with major depressive disorder, obsessive-compulsive disorder (OCD), or other psychiatric disorders. The analysis revealed a greater risk of adverse events representing suicidal behavior or thinking (suicidality) during the first few months of treatment in pediatric patients receiving antidepressants than in those receiving placebo. The average risk of such events was 4% among children and adolescents receiving these drugs, twice the risk (2%) that was observed among those receiving placebo. However, a more recent meta-analysis of 27 placebo-controlled trials of 9 antidepressants (SSRIs and others) in patients younger than 19 years of age with major depressive disorder, OCD, or non-OCD anxiety disorders suggests that the benefits of antidepressant therapy in treating these conditions may outweigh the risks of suicidal behavior or suicidal ideation. No suicides occurred in these pediatric trials.

The risk of suicidality in FDA's pooled analysis differed across the different psychiatric indications, with the highest incidence observed in the major depressive disorder studies. In addition, although there was considerable variation in risk among the antidepressants, a tendency toward an increase in suicidality risk in younger patients was found for almost all drugs studied. It is currently unknown whether the suicidality risk in pediatric patients extends to longer-term use (i.e., beyond several months).

As a result of this analysis and public discussion of the issue, FDA has directed manufacturers of all antidepressants to add a boxed warning to the labeling of their products to alert clinicians of this suicidality risk in children and adolescents and to recommend appropriate monitoring and close observation of patients receiving these agents. (See Cautions: Precautions and Contraindications.) The drugs that are the focus of the revised labeling are all drugs included in the general class of antidepressants, including those that have not been studied in controlled clinical trials in pediatric patients, since the available data are not adequate to exclude any single antidepressant from an increased risk of suicidality. In addition to the boxed warning and other information in professional labeling on antidepressants, FDA currently recommends that a patient medication guide explaining the risks associated with the drugs be provided to the patient each time the drugs are dispensed.

Anyone considering the use of trazodone in a child or adolescent for any clinical use must balance the potential risk of therapy with the clinical need.

■ **Mutagenicity and Carcinogenicity** In vitro tests have *not* shown trazodone to be mutagenic. No evidence of carcinogenesis was seen in animals receiving oral trazodone dosages up to 300 mg/kg daily for 18 months.

■ **Pregnancy, Fertility, and Lactation** Trazodone has been shown to be teratogenic in rats and rabbits when given at dosages 15–50 times the maximum human dosage. The drug also caused increased fetal resorption and other adverse fetal effects in rats when given at dosages approximately 30–50 times the suggested maximum human dosage. There are no adequate and controlled studies to date using trazodone in pregnant women, and the drug should be used during pregnancy only when the potential benefits justify the possible risks to the fetus.

The effect of trazodone on fertility in humans is not known. Impotence, retrograde ejaculation, and decreased or increased libido have occurred in some individuals during trazodone therapy. Reproduction studies in male and female rats using trazodone dosages up to 150 times the usual human dosage have not revealed evidence of impaired fertility.

Because trazodone is distributed into milk, the drug should be used with caution in nursing women.

Drug Interactions

■ **Drugs Affecting Hepatic Microsomal Enzymes** Results of in vitro studies indicate that metabolism of trazodone is mediated by the cytochrome P-450 (CYP) 3A4 isoenzyme, and the possibility exists that drugs that inhibit or induce this isoenzyme may affect the pharmacokinetics of trazodone. Other metabolic pathways that may be involved in the metabolism of trazodone have not been well characterized.

Concomitant use of trazodone with inhibitors of CYP3A4 can result in substantially increased plasma concentrations of trazodone and increase the potential for adverse effects. In one study, concomitant use of ritonavir (200 mg twice daily for 2 days) and trazodone (a single 50-mg dose) in healthy individuals increased maximum plasma concentrations and decreased clearance of trazodone by 34 and 52%, respectively, and increased area under the plasma concentration-time curve (AUC) and half-life of trazodone by greater than twofold. Adverse effects (e.g., nausea, hypotension, syncope) also were observed with concomitant use of trazodone and ritonavir. The manufacturers of trazodone state that a reduction in trazodone dosage should be considered in patients receiving a potent inhibitor of the CYP3A4 isoenzyme (e.g., indinavir, itraconazole, ketoconazole, nefazodone, ritonavir) concomitantly with trazodone.

Concomitant use of trazodone (100–300 mg daily) with carbamazepine (400 mg daily), an inducer of CYP3A4, decreased plasma concentrations of trazodone and an active metabolite, *m*-chlorophenylpiperazine, by 76 and 60%, respectively. Patients receiving trazodone and carbamazepine concomitantly should be closely monitored and dosage of trazodone increased if necessary.

■ **Serotonergic Agents** ***Fluoxetine*** Elevated plasma trazodone concentrations and adverse effects possibly associated with trazodone toxicity have been reported occasionally during concomitant trazodone and fluoxetine therapy. Although the exact mechanism has not been established, it has been suggested that fluoxetine may inhibit the hepatic metabolism of many antidepressant agents, including trazodone. In addition, both trazodone and fluoxetine possess serotonergic activity; therefore, the possibility of serotonin syndrome also should be considered in patients receiving trazodone and fluoxetine or other selective serotonin-reuptake inhibitor therapy concurrently. For detailed information on serotonin syndrome, see Drug Interactions: Drugs Associated with Serotonin Syndrome in Fluoxetine Hydrochloride 28:16.04.20 and the Monoamine Oxidase Inhibitors General Statement 28:16.04.12. Further study is needed, but current evidence suggests that patients receiving trazodone and fluoxetine concomitantly should be observed closely for adverse effects; monitoring of plasma trazodone concentrations also should be considered and trazodone dosage reduced as necessary.

Monoamine Oxidase Inhibitors It is not known whether interactions between trazodone and monoamine oxidase (MAO) inhibitors can occur. Unlike tricyclic antidepressants, trazodone does not interfere with catecholamine uptake by the adrenergic neuron or the pressor response to tyramine. Therefore, an interaction between trazodone and MAO inhibitors is unlikely. However, both trazodone and MAO inhibitors possess serotonergic activity; therefore, the possibility that serotonin syndrome may occur during concurrent therapy should be considered. For detailed information on serotonin syndrome, see Drug Interactions: Drugs Associated with Serotonin Syndrome in Fluoxetine Hydrochloride 28:16.04.20 and the Monoamine Oxidase Inhibitors General Statement 28:16.04.12. Because of the absence of clinical experience, if MAO inhibitors are discontinued shortly before or are to be given concomitantly with trazodone, it is recommended that trazodone therapy be initiated cautiously and dosage increased gradually until optimum response is achieved.

Other Serotonergic Agents Trazodone possesses serotonergic activity and rarely has been associated with serotonin syndrome when combined with other serotonergic agents, including buspirone, phenelzine, and dextropropoxyphene. Because severe complications and even fatalities have accompanied the serotonin syndrome, trazodone probably should be used with caution in patients receiving or who recently have received other serotonergic agents. For additional information on potentially serious drug interactions that may occur between trazodone and other serotonergic agents, see Drug Interactions: Drugs Associated with Serotonin Syndrome, in Fluoxetine Hydrochloride 28:16.04.20 and the Monoamine Oxidase Inhibitors General Statement 28:16.04.12.

■ **General Anesthetics** Since little is known about the interaction between trazodone and general anesthetics, it is recommended that trazodone be discontinued for as long as clinically feasible prior to elective surgery.

■ **Electroconvulsive Therapy** Pending further accumulation of clinical data on the concurrent use of trazodone and electroconvulsive therapy (ECT), concurrent use of these therapies should be avoided.

■ **CNS Depressants** Trazodone may be additive with, or may potentiate the action of, other CNS depressants such as opiates or other analgesics, barbiturates or other sedatives, anesthetics, or alcohol. When trazodone is used concomitantly with other CNS depressants, caution should be used to avoid excessive sedation.

■ **Hypotensive Agents** Because trazodone can cause hypotension, including orthostatic hypotension and syncope, concomitant administration of antihypertensive therapy may require a reduction in dosage of the antihypertensive agent(s). Trazodone has been shown to inhibit the hypotensive effect of various antihypertensive agents (e.g., clonidine, methyldopa) in animals; however, this inhibition has not always been reproducible. It is not known whether trazodone can inhibit the hypotensive effect of these agents in humans, and the clinical importance of this potential interaction has not been determined.

■ **Other Drugs** Increased serum digoxin or phenytoin concentrations have reportedly occurred in patients receiving trazodone concurrently with either drug.

■ **Food** The rate and extent of absorption of trazodone are affected by the presence of food. When trazodone is taken shortly after the ingestion of food, there may be a slight increase in the amount of drug absorbed, a decrease in peak plasma concentration of the drug, and a lengthening of the time to reach the peak plasma concentration. Total drug absorption may be up to 20% greater when the drug is taken with food rather than on an empty stomach. In animals, the rate of absorption has been delayed when trazodone was administered concomitantly with food because of a decrease in the rate of transfer of the drug from the stomach to the small intestine.

The effect of food on absorption of trazodone during long-term administration of the drug is not considered clinically important. Concomitant administration of trazodone with food is generally recommended since it appears to decrease the incidence of dizziness or lightheadedness.

Acute Toxicity

Limited information is available on the acute toxicity of trazodone.

■ **Pathogenesis** The acute lethal dose of trazodone in humans is not known. In addition, there is no clearly defined relationship between plasma trazodone concentration and severity of intoxication. The oral LD_{50} of trazodone is 610 mg/kg in mice, 486 mg/kg in rats, 560 mg/kg in rabbits, and 500 mg/kg in dogs. In animals, lethal doses produced dyspnea, salivation, prostration, and clonic seizures.

■ **Manifestations** One patient who intentionally ingested 7.5 g of trazodone experienced only drowsiness and weakness; the patient was aroused at the time of hospitalization and emesis was induced. Another patient had an uneventful recovery after ingesting 9.2 g of trazodone. There have been several reports of accidental ingestion in children; however, the exact amounts ingested are unknown. Each of these children exhibited only lethargy and drowsiness, and recoveries were uneventful. Fatalities have occurred in adults who intentionally ingested trazodone and other drugs (e.g., alcohol, chloral hydrate, amobarbital, chlordiazepoxide, meprobamate) concurrently.

In general, overdosage of trazodone may be expected to produce effects that are extensions of common adverse reactions; vomiting, drowsiness, and lethargy have been the principal effects reported. Other reported effects associated with acute trazodone overdosage have included orthostatic hypotension, tachycardia, coma, headache, tinnitus, dizziness, dyspnea, shivering, aching muscles, incontinence, and dry mouth. Unlike tricyclic antidepressant overdosage, seizures and arrhythmias do not appear to be associated with trazodone overdosage.

■ **Treatment** Treatment of trazodone overdosage generally involves symptomatic and supportive care; there is no specific antidote for trazodone intoxication. In acute overdosage, the stomach should be emptied immediately by inducing emesis or by gastric lavage. If the patient is comatose, having seizures, or lacks the gag reflex, gastric lavage may be performed if an endotracheal tube with cuff inflated is in place to prevent aspiration of vomitus. Although administration of activated charcoal after gastric lavage and/or emesis has been useful in the treatment of acute overdosage with tricyclic antidepressants, the effect of activated charcoal on the absorption of trazodone is not currently known. Appropriate therapy should be instituted if hypotension or excessive sedation occurs. Forced diuresis may be useful in facilitating elimination of the drug. It is not known if trazodone is dialyzable; however, because of extensive protein binding of the drug, hemodialysis is probably *not* effective in enhancing elimination of trazodone.

Pharmacology

The pharmacology of trazodone is complex and in some ways resembles that of tricyclic antidepressants, benzodiazepines, and phenothiazines; however, the overall pharmacologic profile of trazodone differs from each of these classes of drugs.

■ **Nervous System Effects** The precise mechanism of antidepressant action of trazodone is unclear, but the drug has been shown to selectively block the reuptake of serotonin (5-HT) at the presynaptic neuronal membrane. The effects of serotonin may thus be potentiated. Unlike other antidepressant agents (e.g., tricyclic antidepressants), trazodone may have a dual effect on the central serotonergic system. Animal studies indicate that trazodone acts as a serotonin agonist at high doses (6–8 mg/kg), while at low doses (0.05–1 mg/kg), it antagonizes the actions of serotonin. Trazodone does not appear to influence the reuptake of dopamine or norepinephrine within the CNS; however, animal studies indicate that trazodone may enhance release of norepinephrine from neuronal tissue. Trazodone does not cause serotonin release in vitro.

Although the mechanism of action of antidepressant agents may involve inhibition of the reuptake of various neurotransmitters at the presynaptic neuronal membrane, long-term therapy with antidepressant agents also affects postsynaptic neuronal receptor binding sites, resulting in some adaptive changes in neurotransmission. Long-term administration of trazodone reportedly decreases the number of postsynaptic serotonergic (i.e., serotonin$_2$) and β-adrenergic binding sites in the brain of animals. Although the clinical importance of these effects is not known, the decrease in binding sites is associated with a functional increase in serotonergic activity and a reduction in the sensitivity of adenylate cyclase to stimulation by β-adrenergic agonists. It has been suggested that postsynaptic receptor modification is mainly responsible for the antidepressant action observed during long-term administration of trazodone. Further study is needed to determine the role of binding site alteration in the antidepressant action of trazodone and other antidepressants.

In animals, trazodone's effect on various avoidance behaviors is similar to that of phenothiazines. Unlike phenothiazines, however, trazodone potentiates the effects of serotonin. Trazodone does not potentiate the actions of levodopa or alter neuronal concentrations of acetylcholine. Trazodone does not inhibit monoamine oxidase, and unlike amphetamine-like drugs, does not stimulate the CNS.

Unlike many currently available antidepressants, trazodone exhibits little, if any, anticholinergic activity in vitro. Clinical studies show a lower incidence of anticholinergic effects (e.g., dry mouth, blurred vision, urinary retention, constipation) associated with trazodone use than with tricyclic antidepressant use. (See Cautions: Anticholinergic Effects.)

Trazodone produces varying degrees of sedation in normal and mentally depressed patients. The sedative effect is thought to result principally from central α_1-adrenergic blocking activity and possibly from a histamine blocking action of the drug. Trazodone may cause EEG changes, including increased slow-wave and alpha-wave activity. Some increase in fast-wave activity also occurs. Trazodone increases total sleep time, decreases the number and duration of awakenings in depressed patients, and decreases rapid eye movement (REM) sleep. Unlike tricyclic antidepressants, trazodone does not increase stage 4 sleep.

Although the exact mechanism of action has not been determined, trazodone has an anxiolytic effect. This finding is supported by animal studies in which trazodone is active in certain antianxiety test systems. In addition, the drug has demonstrated anxiolytic activity in patients with major depression who also have associated anxiety. (See Uses: Major Depressive Disorder.)

Therapeutic dosages of trazodone do not appear to affect respiration; however, the effect of higher dosages of trazodone in patients with ventilatory insufficiency is not known.

Like many other centrally acting agents, trazodone exhibits analgesic activity in a variety of analgesic test systems. Trazodone also has weak skeletal muscle relaxant activity but lacks anticonvulsant effects.

Trazodone possesses potent peripheral α-adrenergic blocking activity in animals following IV administration of 3–10 mg/kg. In addition, in animals, the drug blocks the peripheral effects of serotonin, epinephrine, norepinephrine, and histamine. The peripheral antihistaminic effects of trazodone are weaker than those of tricyclic antidepressants.

■ Cardiovascular Effects The cardiovascular effects of trazodone have been studied in animals and to a limited extent in humans. Unlike other antidepressant agents (e.g., tricyclic antidepressants, monoamine oxidase inhibitors), trazodone has been associated with only minimal cardiovascular effects. (See Cautions: Cardiovascular Effects.) The absence of substantial anticholinergic activity and catecholamine-potentiating effects appears to be the principal reason for the general lack of cardiovascular effects of trazodone.

Trazodone exhibits α-adrenergic blocking activity and does not inhibit catecholamine reuptake. Unlike tricyclic antidepressants, trazodone blocks the pressor response to norepinephrine and lowers arterial blood pressure. However, in one study in normotensive patients with endogenous depression, the effect of trazodone on systemic blood pressure was equivocal. Trazodone does not block the neuronal uptake of tyramine; thus, unlike tricyclic antidepressants, the drug has no effect on the pressor response to this sympathomimetic amine.

Although trazodone does *not* appear to have substantial arrhythmogenic activity, arrhythmias have occurred in some patients with preexisting cardiac disease during trazodone therapy. (See Cautions: Cardiovascular Effects.) In animals, trazodone does *not* affect intra-atrial, ventricular septal, ventricular free-wall, His-Purkinje, or AV nodal conduction. At doses up to 30 mg/kg in animals, trazodone produces only minimal ECG changes, including prolongation of the QT interval and a decrease in heart rate. Unlike tricyclic antidepressants, trazodone does not exert direct quinidine-like cardiotoxic properties. In addition, trazodone does *not* exert a negative inotropic effect at therapeutic dosages; the drug may decrease aortic blood flow as a result of a decrease in heart rate.

To date, there have been no published studies comparing the cardiovascular effects of therapeutic dosages of trazodone with those of antidepressants such as mianserin, nomifensine, or zimelidine. Although available data suggest that trazodone is less cardiotoxic than tricyclic antidepressant agents at therapeutic dosages, the cardiovascular effects of trazodone overdosage have not been well described.

■ Other Effects Trazodone may affect the endocrine system. Following oral administration of a single 50-mg dose in one study in healthy adults, trazodone caused a decrease in mean serum prolactin concentration. However, in another study in depressed patients, trazodone did not alter mean serum prolactin concentration following oral administration of 200 mg daily for 2 weeks.

Trazodone-induced antagonism of α_2-adrenergic receptors may relax the tissues and enhance arterial inflow in penile vascular and corporal smooth muscle resulting in an erection.

Pharmacokinetics

In all studies described in the Pharmacokinetics section, trazodone was administered as the hydrochloride salt.

■ Absorption Trazodone is rapidly and almost completely absorbed from the GI tract following oral administration. The rate and extent of absorption are affected by the presence of food. When trazodone is taken shortly after the ingestion of food, there may be a slight increase (up to 20%) in the amount of drug absorbed, a decrease in peak plasma concentration of the drug, and a lengthening of the time to reach the peak plasma concentration.

Peak plasma concentrations of trazodone occur approximately 1 hour after oral administration when the drug is taken on an empty stomach or 2 hours after oral administration when taken with food. Following oral administration of multiple doses of trazodone (25 mg 2 or 3 times daily), steady-state plasma concentrations of the drug are usually attained within 4 days and exhibit wide interpatient variation. Following oral administration of a single 25-mg dose of radiolabeled trazodone to healthy adults in one study, mean peak plasma drug concentrations of 650 and 480 ng/mL occurred at 1.5 and 2.5 hours after ingestion, in the fasted and nonfasted state, respectively. Following oral administration of single doses of 25, 50, or 100 mg of trazodone to healthy, fasted adults in another study, mean peak plasma trazodone concentrations were 490, 860, and 1620 ng/mL, respectively. The areas under the plasma concentration-time curves (AUCs) were 3.44, 5.95, and 11.19 mcg-h/mL, for the 25-, 50-, and 100-mg doses, respectively. Limited crossover data are available comparing AUCs in fasted and nonfasted patients; however, it appears that the presence of food slightly increases the AUC for trazodone.

The therapeutic range for plasma trazodone concentrations and the relationship of plasma concentrations to clinical response and toxicity have not been established.

■ Distribution Distribution of trazodone into human body tissues and fluids has not been determined. Following oral administration of trazodone in animals, the drug and its metabolites are distributed mainly into the liver, kidneys, small intestine, lungs, adrenal glands, and pancreas, with lower concentrations being distributed into adipose tissue, heart, and skeletal muscle. Trazodone crosses the blood-brain barrier in animals, and concentrations of the drug in the brain are higher than those in plasma during the first 8 hours after oral ingestion.

In vitro, trazodone is 89–95% bound to plasma proteins at plasma trazodone concentrations of 100–1500 ng/mL.

Although it is not known if trazodone crosses the placenta in humans, the drug crosses the placenta in animals. Following a single oral dose of 50 mg, trazodone is distributed into milk in concentrations approximately 10% of maternal plasma concentrations, with a milk-to-plasma ratio (based on areas under the plasma and milk concentration-time curves) of about 0.1–0.2. Based on these data, it is estimated that a nursing infant would ingest less than 0.1% of the dose. It is not known whether trazodone metabolites are distributed into milk.

■ Elimination Plasma concentrations of trazodone decline in a biphasic manner. The half-life of trazodone in the initial phase ($t_{1/2\alpha}$) is about 3–6 hours and the half-life in the terminal phase ($t_{1/2\beta}$) is about 5–9 hours. The clearance of trazodone from the body shows wide interindividual variation. The manufacturers state that the drug may accumulate in plasma in some individuals.

Trazodone is extensively metabolized in the liver via hydroxylation, oxidation, *N*-oxidation, and splitting of the pyridine ring. A hydroxylated metabolite and oxotriazolopyridinpropionic acid (an inactive metabolite excreted in urine) are conjugated with glucuronic acid. Results of in vitro studies indicate that metabolism of trazodone to an active metabolite, *m*-chlorophenylpiperazine, is mediated by the cytochrome P-450 (CYP) 3A4 isoenzyme. The manufacturers state that other metabolic pathways involved in metabolism of trazodone have not been well characterized. Results from animal studies indicate that trazodone does not induce its own metabolism.

Approximately 70–75% of an oral dose of trazodone is excreted in urine within 72 hours of administration, principally as metabolites. About 20% of an oral dose of trazodone is excreted in urine as oxotriazolopyridinpropionic acid and its conjugates, and about 10% as a dihydrodiol metabolite; less than 1% of a dose is excreted unchanged. The remainder of an oral dose of the drug is excreted in feces via biliary elimination, principally as metabolites.

Chemistry and Stability

■ Chemistry Trazodone hydrochloride is a triazolopyridine-derivative antidepressant. The drug is chemically and structurally unrelated to tricyclic or tetracyclic antidepressants or to selective serotonin-reuptake inhibitors. Trazodone hydrochloride occurs as a white, odorless, crystalline powder with a bitter taste and is freely soluble in water and sparingly soluble in alcohol. The drug has a pK_a of 6.7.

■ Stability Commercially available trazodone hydrochloride tablets should be stored at room temperature in tight, light-resistant containers and protected from temperatures greater than 40°C.

Preparations

Excipients in commercially available drug preparations may have clinically important effects in some individuals; consult specific product labeling for details.

traZODone Hydrochloride

Oral		
Tablets	50 mg*	**traZODone Hydrochloride Tablets**
	100 mg*	**traZODone Hydrochloride Tablets**
	150 mg*	**traZODone Hydrochloride Dividose®** (scored), Sandoz
		traZODone Hydrochloride Tablets
	300 mg*	**traZODone Hydrochloride Tablets**

*available from one or more manufacturer, distributor, and/or repackager by generic (nonproprietary) name

†Use is not currently included in the labeling approved by the US Food and Drug Administration

Selected Revisions October 2014,

Vortioxetine Hydrobromide

■ Vortioxetine hydrobromide is a serotonin-reuptake inhibitor with several other activities, including serotonin type 3 (5-hydroxytryptamine [5-HT_3]) receptor antagonism and serotonin type 1A (5-HT_{1A}) receptor agonism; the drug is an antidepressant agent.

Uses

■ **Major Depressive Disorder** Vortioxetine hydrobromide is used for the treatment of major depressive disorder in adults.

The American Psychiatric Association (APA) states that the effectiveness of antidepressants in the treatment of major depressive disorder is generally comparable between and within classes of these medications, including selective serotonin-reuptake inhibitors (SSRIs), serotonin- and norepinephrine-reuptake inhibitors (SNRIs), tricyclic antidepressants, monoamine oxidase (MAO) inhibitors, and other antidepressants (e.g., bupropion, mirtazapine, trazodone). Therefore, the initial selection of an antidepressant can be based mainly on the following factors: patient preference; nature of prior response to medication; safety, tolerability, and anticipated adverse effects; concurrent psychiatric and medical conditions; specific properties of the medication (e.g., half-life, actions on cytochrome P-450 [CYP] isoenzymes, other drug interactions); and cost. For most patients, an SSRI, SNRI, mirtazapine, or bupropion is considered optimal based on these considerations. Clinicians may consult APA's Practice Guidelines for the Treatment of Patients with Major Depressive Disorder (at http://www.psychiatryonline.com/pracGuide/pracGuideTopic_7.aspx) for additional information.

The short-term antidepressant efficacy of vortioxetine was established in 6 randomized, double-blind, placebo-controlled, fixed-dose studies of 6–8 weeks' duration in adult inpatients and outpatients who met DSM-IV-TR criteria for major depressive disorder, including one study in geriatric patients. In 5 of these studies, adult patients 18–75 years of age were randomized to receive either vortioxetine 5, 10, 15, or 20 mg or placebo given once daily. The primary efficacy measure was the Hamilton Depression Scale (HAMD-24) total score in one study (study 2) and the Montgomery-Asberg Depression Rating Scale (MADRS) total score in the other studies. In each of these studies, at least one dosage group of vortioxetine was found to be more effective than placebo in improving depressive symptoms as measured by the mean change from baseline to end point visit on the HAMD-24 or MADRS total score. The remaining study (study 6) demonstrated the antidepressant efficacy of vortioxetine (5 mg once daily) in geriatric patients 64–88 years of age with recurrent major depressive disorder (with at least one previous episode before the age of 60 years) and without concomitant cognitive impairment. (See Geriatric Use under Warnings/Precautions: Specific Populations, in Cautions.) An antidepressant effect was generally observed in vortioxetine-treated patients beginning at week 2 and increased during subsequent weeks; the full antidepressant effect generally was not seen until week 4 or later. No age-, gender-, or race-related differences in response to vortioxetine were noted in the adult studies.

Two randomized, double-blind, placebo-controlled studies of vortioxetine 5 mg once daily conducted in the US failed to demonstrate effectiveness of this dosage in the treatment of major depressive disorder in adults.

In a long-term, multicenter, non-US maintenance study, 639 adult inpatients or outpatients who met DSM-IV-TR criteria for major depressive disorder initially received open-label vortioxetine therapy (given in a flexible dosage of 5 or 10 mg once daily during the first 8 weeks of the initial 12-week treatment phase; dosage was fixed between weeks 8–12). Patients in remission at weeks 10 and 12 were then randomized either to continue fixed-dosage vortioxetine therapy at the final dosage they had responded to (approximately 75% were receiving 10 mg daily) or to receive placebo for 24–64 weeks. Patients receiving vortioxetine experienced a longer time to recurrence of depressive episodes compared with patients receiving placebo. In addition, fewer patients receiving vortioxetine (13%) experienced a relapse compared with those receiving placebo (26%). In 2 additional long-term (52-week), multicenter, open-label, extension studies, vortioxetine (2.5–10 mg once daily) was found to be effective and well tolerated in adults with major depressive disorder. Laboratory, vital sign, and ECG findings in these 2 studies did not reveal any clinically important safety issues with long-term vortioxetine therapy.

Dosage and Administration

■ **Administration** Vortioxetine hydrobromide is commercially available as immediate-release tablets, which are administered orally once daily without regard to meals, at approximately the same time each day.

Patients receiving vortioxetine should be monitored for possible worsening of depression, suicidality, or unusual changes in behavior, especially at the beginning of therapy or during periods of dosage adjustments. (See Worsening of Depression and Suicidality Risk under Warnings/Precautions: Warnings, in Cautions.)

The manufacturer states that at least 2 weeks must elapse between discontinuance of a monoamine oxidase (MAO) inhibitor intended to treat psychiatric disorders and initiation of vortioxetine therapy and at least 3 weeks must elapse between discontinuance of vortioxetine and initiation of MAO inhibitor therapy intended to treat psychiatric disorders. (See Contraindications, Serotonin Syndrome under Warnings/Precautions: Other Warnings and Precautions, in Cautions, and Drug Interactions: Monoamine Oxidase Inhibitors.)

Prescribing and Dispensing Precautions Prescribing and dispensing errors have been reported because of similarities in the spelling and pronunciation of Brintellix® (the former trade name for vortioxetine hydrobromide) and Brilinta® (the trade name for ticagrelor, a platelet-aggregation inhibitor). To avoid such errors, the manufacturer of Brintellix® changed the trade name for vortioxetine hydrobromide from Brintellix® to Trintellix®, which became commercially available in June 2016. (See Prescribing and Dispensing Precautions under Warnings/Precautions: Other Warnings and Precautions, in Cautions.)

■ **Dosage** Dosage of vortioxetine hydrobromide is expressed in terms of vortioxetine.

Major Depressive Disorder For the management of major depressive disorder in adults, the recommended initial dosage of vortioxetine is 10 mg orally once daily, which should then be increased to 20 mg once daily, as tolerated, because higher dosages demonstrated better efficacy in clinical trials conducted in the US. In the main clinical trials, dosage increases were made after the first week. The manufacturer states that the efficacy and safety of dosages greater than 20 mg daily have not been evaluated in controlled clinical trials. A dosage decrease to 5 mg daily should be considered in patients who do not tolerate higher dosages of the drug.

In known poor metabolizers of the cytochrome P-450 (CYP) isoenzyme 2D6, the maximum recommended dosage of vortioxetine is 10 mg once daily.

The dosage of vortioxetine should be reduced by 50% when used concurrently with potent CYP2D6 inhibitors (e.g., bupropion, fluoxetine, paroxetine, quinidine). The dosage should then be increased back to the original dosage when the CYP2D6 inhibitor is discontinued. (See Drug Interactions.)

During concomitant use with potent CYP inducers (e.g., carbamazepine, phenytoin, rifampin) for longer than 14 days, an increase in the vortioxetine dosage should be considered. However, the manufacturer recommends that the maximum dosage not exceed 3 times the original dosage. The dosage should then be reduced back to the original dosage when the CYP inducer is discontinued. (See Drug Interactions.)

It is generally agreed that acute depressive episodes require several months or longer of sustained antidepressant therapy in responding patients. In addition, some clinicians recommend that long-term antidepressant therapy be considered in certain patients at risk for recurrence of depressive episodes (such as those with chronic and recurrent major depressive disorder).

Discontinuance of Therapy Although vortioxetine can be abruptly discontinued, patients in placebo-controlled trials experienced transient adverse reactions (including headache, muscle tension, mood swings, sudden outbursts of anger, dizziness, runny nose) in the first week following abrupt discontinuance of vortioxetine 15 or 20 mg daily. To avoid such possible adverse reactions, the manufacturer recommends that the dosage be decreased to 10 mg daily for one week before full discontinuance of vortioxetine if given at a dosage of 15 or 20 mg daily, if possible.

■ **Special Populations** Dosage adjustment is not necessary in patients with renal impairment (ranging from mild renal impairment to end-stage renal disease). (See Renal Impairment under Warnings/Precautions: Specific Populations, in Cautions.)

In patients with mild or moderate hepatic impairment, dosage adjustment is not necessary. Because vortioxetine has not been studied in patients with severe hepatic impairment, the manufacturer states that use in such patients is not recommended.

No dosage adjustment is necessary in geriatric patients. In addition, dosage adjustment is not recommended based on gender, race, or ethnicity.

Cautions

■ **Contraindications** Known hypersensitivity to vortioxetine or any ingredients in the formulation. Angioedema has been reported in vortioxetine-treated patients.

Concurrent or recent (i.e., within 2 weeks) therapy with a monoamine oxidase (MAO) inhibitor intended to treat psychiatric disorders. Use of an MAO inhibitor intended to treat psychiatric disorders within 3 weeks of vortioxetine discontinuance. (See Serotonin Syndrome under Warnings/Precautions: Other Warnings and Precautions, in Cautions and also see Drug Interactions: Monoamine Oxidase Inhibitors.)

Initiation of vortioxetine therapy in patients receiving MAO inhibitors such as linezolid or IV methylene blue. (See Drug Interactions: Linezolid and also see Drug Interactions: Methylene Blue.)

■ **Warnings/Precautions** ***Warnings*** **Worsening of Depression and Suicidality Risk.** Worsening of depression and/or the emergence of suicidal ideation and behavior (suicidality) or unusual changes in behavior may occur in both adult and pediatric (see Pediatric Use under Warnings/Precautions: Specific Populations, in Cautions) patients with major depressive disorder or other psychiatric disorders, whether or not they are taking antidepressants. This risk may persist until clinically important remission occurs. Suicide is a known risk of depression and certain other psychiatric disorders, and these disorders themselves are the strongest predictors of suicide. However, there has been a long-standing concern that antidepressants may have a role in inducing worsening of depression and the emergence of suicidality in certain patients during the early phases of treatment. Pooled analyses of short-term, placebo-controlled studies of antidepressants (i.e., selective serotonin-reuptake inhibitors [SSRIs] and other antidepressants) have shown an increased risk of suicidality in children, adolescents, and young adults (18–24 years of age) with major depressive disorder and other psychiatric disorders. An increased suicidality risk was not demonstrated with antidepressants compared with placebo in adults older than 24 years of age, and a reduced risk was observed in adults 65 years of age or older.

The US Food and Drug Administration (FDA) recommends that all patients being treated with antidepressants for any indication be appropriately monitored and closely observed for clinical worsening, suicidality, and unusual changes in behavior, particularly during initiation of therapy (i.e., the first few months) and during periods of dosage adjustments. Families and caregivers of patients being treated with antidepressants for major depressive disorder or other indications, both psychiatric and nonpsychiatric, also should be advised to monitor patients on a daily basis for the emergence of agitation, irritability, or unusual changes in behavior as well as the emergence of suicidality, and to report such symptoms immediately to a health-care provider.

Although a causal relationship between the emergence of symptoms such as anxiety, agitation, panic attacks, insomnia, irritability, hostility, aggressiveness, impulsivity, akathisia, hypomania, and/or mania and either the worsening of depression and/or the emergence of suicidal impulses has not been established, there is concern that such symptoms may represent precursors to emerging suicidality. Consequently, consideration should be given to changing the therapeutic regimen or discontinuing therapy in patients whose depression is persistently worse or in patients experiencing emergent suicidality or symptoms that might be precursors to worsening depression or suicidality, particularly if such manifestations are severe, abrupt in onset, or were not part of the patient's presenting symptoms.

Other Warnings and Precautions **Serotonin Syndrome.** Potentially life-threatening serotonin syndrome has been reported with serotonergic antidepressants, including vortioxetine, when used alone, but particularly with concurrent use of other serotonergic drugs (including serotonin [5-hydroxytryptamine; 5-HT] type 1 receptor agonists ["triptans"], tricyclic antidepressants, buspirone, fentanyl, lithium, tramadol, tryptophan, and St. John's wort [*Hypericum perforatum*]) and with drugs that impair the metabolism of serotonin (particularly MAO inhibitors, both those used to treat psychiatric disorders and others, such as linezolid and methylene blue). Manifestations of serotonin syndrome may include mental status changes (e.g., agitation, hallucinations, delirium, coma), autonomic instability (e.g., tachycardia, labile blood pressure, dizziness, diaphoresis, flushing, hyperthermia), neuromuscular symptoms (e.g., tremor, rigidity, myoclonus, hyperreflexia, incoordination), seizures, and/or GI symptoms (e.g., nausea, vomiting, diarrhea). Patients receiving vortioxetine should be monitored for the development of serotonin syndrome.

Concurrent or recent (i.e., within 2 weeks) therapy with MAO inhibitors intended to treat psychiatric disorders is contraindicated. Use of an MAO inhibitor intended to treat psychiatric disorders within 3 weeks of vortioxetine discontinuance also is contraindicated. (See Contraindications and also see Drug Interactions: Monoamine Oxidase Inhibitors.) Vortioxetine also should not be initiated in patients who are being treated with other MAO inhibitors such as linezolid or IV methylene blue. (See Drug Interactions: Linezolid and also see Drug Interactions: Methylene Blue.)

If concurrent therapy with vortioxetine and other serotonergic drugs is clinically warranted, the patient should be made aware of the potential increased risk for serotonin syndrome, particularly during initiation of therapy or when dosage is increased. (See Drug Interactions.)

If manifestations of serotonin syndrome occur, treatment with vortioxetine and any concurrently administered serotonergic agents should be immediately discontinued and supportive and symptomatic treatment initiated.

For further information on serotonin syndrome, including manifestations and treatment, see Drug Interactions: Serotonergic Drugs, in Fluoxetine Hydrochloride 28:16.04.20.

Abnormal Bleeding. Serotonergic antidepressants, including vortioxetine, may increase the risk of bleeding events. Concomitant use of aspirin, nonsteroidal anti-inflammatory agents (NSAIAs), warfarin, and other anticoagulants may add to this risk. Case reports and epidemiologic studies have demonstrated an association between use of drugs that interfere with serotonin reuptake and the occurrence of GI bleeding. Bleeding events related to drugs that inhibit serotonin reuptake have ranged from ecchymoses, hematomas, epistaxis, and petechiae to life-threatening hemorrhages. The manufacturer recommends that patients be advised of the increased risk of bleeding associated with concomitant use of vortioxetine and aspirin or other NSAIAs, warfarin, or other drugs that affect coagulation or bleeding. (See Drug Interactions: Drugs Affecting Hemostasis.)

Activation of Mania/Hypomania. Symptoms of mania and hypomania have been reported in less than 0.1% of patients receiving vortioxetine in clinical studies. Activation of mania and hypomania also have been reported in a small proportion of patients with major affective disorder who were treated with other antidepressants. Vortioxetine should therefore be used with caution in patients with a personal or family history of bipolar disorder, mania, or hypomania.

Angle-closure Glaucoma. The pupillary dilation (mydriasis) that occurs following the use of many antidepressant agents, including vortioxetine, may trigger an acute attack of angle-closure glaucoma (narrow-angle glaucoma) in patients with anatomically narrow angles who do not have a patent iridectomy. (See Advice to Patients.)

Hyponatremia/Syndrome of Inappropriate Antidiuretic Hormone Secretion. Treatment with serotonergic drugs, including vortioxetine, may result in hyponatremia. In many cases, hyponatremia appears to be due to the syndrome of inappropriate antidiuretic hormone secretion (SIADH). One case of hyponatremia with a serum sodium concentration lower than 110 mmol/L has been reported with vortioxetine in a premarketing study. Geriatric individuals and patients receiving diuretics or who are otherwise volume depleted may be at greater risk of developing hyponatremia with serotonergic antidepressants. Signs and symptoms of hyponatremia include headache, difficulty concentrating, memory impairment, confusion, weakness, and unsteadiness, which may lead to falls; more severe and/or acute cases have been associated with hallucinations, syncope, seizures, coma, respiratory arrest, and death. Vortioxetine should be discontinued and appropriate medical intervention should be instituted in patients with symptomatic hyponatremia.

Prescribing and Dispensing Precautions. Because of similarities in the spelling and pronunciation of Brintellix® (the former trade name for vortioxetine hydrobromide) and Brilinta® (the trade name for ticagrelor, a platelet-aggregation inhibitor), prescribing and dispensing errors have been reported to FDA for these drugs. As of June 2015, the FDA had received 50 medication error reports describing trade name confusion with Brintellix® and Brilinta®. In most cases, Brintellix® was mistaken for Brilinta®. The wrong drug was actually dispensed in 12 of the reported cases of name confusion; however, none of the reports indicated that a patient ingested the wrong drug. To avoid future prescribing and dispensing errors, FDA approved a change in the trade name for vortioxetine in May 2016; the manufacturer of Brintellix® changed the trade name for vortioxetine hydrobromide to Trintellix®; the drug became commercially available under this trade name in June 2016. To reduce the risk of medication errors (e.g., during the transition period to the new name), FDA recommends that clinicians include both the trade (brand) and generic (nonproprietary) names of the drug and the indication for use, as well as the correct dosage, and directions for use in each prescription. In addition, patients should be advised to check their prescriptions to ensure that the correct drug was dispensed and to carefully read the medication guide provided with their prescriptions.

Specific Populations **Pregnancy.** Category C. (See Users Guide.)

Some neonates exposed to SSRIs or SNRIs late in the third trimester of pregnancy have developed complications, which have sometimes been severe and required prolonged hospitalization, respiratory support, enteral nutrition, and other forms of supportive care in special-care nurseries. Such complications may arise immediately upon delivery and usually last several days or up to 2–4 weeks. Clinical findings reported to date in the neonates have included respiratory distress, cyanosis, apnea, seizures, temperature instability or fever, feeding difficulty, dehydration, excessive weight loss, vomiting, hypoglycemia, hypotonia, hypertonia, hyperreflexia, tremor, jitteriness, irritability, and constant crying. These features appear to be consistent with either a direct toxic effect of these classes of drugs or, possibly, a drug withdrawal syndrome. In some cases, the clinical picture was consistent with serotonin syndrome (see Serotonin Syndrome under Warnings/Precautions: Other Warnings and Precautions, in Cautions).

For additional information on the management of depression in women prior to conception and during pregnancy, including treatment algorithms, clinicians may consult the joint American Psychiatric Association and American College of Obstetricians and Gynecologists guidelines (at https://www.ncbi.nlm.nih.gov/pmc/articles/PMC3103063/pdf/nihms293836.pdf).

Lactation. Vortioxetine is distributed into milk in rats. It is not known whether the drug is distributed into human milk. Because many drugs are present in human milk and because of the potential for serious adverse reactions, a decision should be made whether to discontinue nursing or to discontinue the drug, taking into account the importance of the drug to the mother.

Pediatric Use. Clinical studies of vortioxetine in pediatric patients have not been conducted; therefore, the safety and effectiveness of the drug in pediatric patients have not been established.

FDA warns that a greater risk of suicidal thinking or behavior (suicidality) occurred during the first few months of antidepressant treatment compared with placebo in children and adolescents with major depressive disorder, obsessive-compulsive disorder (OCD), or other psychiatric disorders based on pooled analyses of 24 short-term, placebo-controlled trials of 9 antidepressant drugs (SSRIs and other antidepressants). However, a later meta-analysis of 27 placebo-controlled trials of 9 antidepressants (SSRIs and others) in patients younger than 19 years of age with major depressive disorder, OCD, or non-OCD anxiety disorders suggests that the benefits of antidepressant therapy in treating these conditions may outweigh the risks of suicidal behavior or ideation. No suicides occurred in these pediatric trials. These findings should be carefully considered when assessing potential benefits and risks of vortioxetine in a child or adolescent for any clinical use. (See Worsening of Depression and Suicidality Risk under Warnings/Precautions: Warnings, in Cautions.)

Geriatric Use. In clinical trials with vortioxetine, 11% of the patients were 65 years of age or older, including in a placebo-controlled study conducted specifically in geriatric patients. No overall differences in safety or effectiveness were observed between geriatric and younger adults in these studies; other reported clinical experience has not identified any differences in response to the drug between geriatric and younger adults.

No dosage adjustment is necessary in geriatric patients. In a single-dose pharmacokinetic study, the pharmacokinetics of vortioxetine generally were similar between geriatric individuals older than 65 years of age and younger individuals (24–45 years of age).

Serotonergic antidepressants, including vortioxetine, have been associated with clinically important hyponatremia in geriatric patients, who may be at greater risk for this adverse effect. (See Hyponatremia/Syndrome of Inappropriate Antidiuretic Hormone Secretion under Warnings/Precautions: Other Warnings and Precautions, in Cautions.)

In pooled data analyses, a *reduced* risk of suicidality was observed in adults 65 years of age or older with antidepressant therapy compared with placebo. (See Worsening of Depression and Suicidality Risk under Warnings/Precautions: Warnings, in Cautions.)

Hepatic Impairment. Dosage adjustment of vortioxetine is not necessary in patients with mild or moderate hepatic impairment. However, vortioxetine has not been studied in patients with severe hepatic impairment and use in such patients is not recommended.

Renal Impairment. The presence of mild, moderate, or severe renal impairment or end-stage renal disease does not affect the apparent clearance or the plasma protein binding of vortioxetine. Dosage adjustment of vortioxetine is not necessary in patients with renal impairment (ranging from mild renal impairment to end-stage renal disease).

Only a small fraction of a single, 10-mg dose of vortioxetine was removed by dialysis; area under the concentration-time curve and peak plasma concentrations were 13 and 27% lower postdialysis, respectively.

■ **Common Adverse Effects** Adverse effects reported in at least 5% of patients with major depressive disorder receiving vortioxetine and at an incidence of at least twice that reported with placebo in controlled clinical studies include nausea, constipation, and vomiting. Nausea was the most common adverse effect in these studies and it occurred most often during the first week of treatment; the incidence of nausea was dose related and higher in females than in males.

Drug Interactions

Vortioxetine is metabolized principally by cytochrome P-450 (CYP) isoenzyme 2D6 with lesser contributions from CYP3A4/5, 2C19, 2C9, 2A6, 2C8, and 2B6. In vitro and in vivo studies have demonstrated that vortioxetine and its metabolites are unlikely to inhibit CYP1A2, 2A6, 2B6, 2C8, 2C9, 2C19, 2D6, 2E1, or 3A4/5. In an in vitro study, vortioxetine did not induce CYP1A2, 2A6, 2B6, 2C8, 2C9, 2C19, or 3A4/5.

■ **Drugs Affecting Hepatic Microsomal Enzymes** ***Potent CYP2D6 Inhibitors*** The dosage of vortioxetine should be reduced by 50% when used concurrently with potent CYP2D6 inhibitors (e.g., bupropion, fluoxetine, paroxetine, quinidine). The dosage should be increased back to the original dosage when the CYP2D6 inhibitor is discontinued.

Potent CYP Inducers When administered with a potent CYP inducer (e.g., carbamazepine, phenytoin, rifampin) for longer than 14 days, increasing the dosage of vortioxetine should be considered. The manufacturer recommends that the maximum dosage of vortioxetine not exceed 3 times the original dosage. Following discontinuance of the potent CYP inducer, the original vortioxetine dosage should be resumed within 14 days.

■ **Drugs Metabolized by Hepatic Microsomal Enzymes** The manufacturer states that clinically important pharmacokinetic interactions are unlikely and that dosage adjustment of the concurrently administered drug is not necessary when vortioxetine is used concurrently with substrates of CYP1A2 (e.g., duloxetine), CYP2A6, CYP2B6 (e.g., bupropion), CYP2C8 (e.g., repaglinide), CYP2C9 (e.g., *S*-warfarin), CYP2C19 (e.g., diazepam), CYP2D6 (e.g., venlafaxine), or CYP3A4/5 (e.g., budesonide). Clinically important pharmacokinetic drug interactions also are unlikely during concurrent administration of substrates of CYP2E1.

In an in vivo study, no clinically important pharmacokinetic interaction was observed during concomitant administration of vortioxetine and caffeine (a CYP1A2 substrate), tolbutamide (a CYP2C9 substrate), or midazolam (a CYP3A4 substrate).

No clinically important pharmacokinetic interaction has been observed during concomitant administration of vortioxetine and warfarin (a CYP2C9 substrate) or diazepam (a CYP2C19 substrate).

Chronic administration of vortioxetine is unlikely to induce the metabolism of drugs metabolized by CYP isoenzymes 1A2, 2A6, 2B6, 2C8, 2C9, 2C19, or 3A4/5.

■ **Drugs Affecting or Affected by P-glycoprotein Transport** Vortioxetine is a poor P-glycoprotein (P-gp) substrate and inhibitor. The manufacturer states that no dosage adjustment is necessary when a P-gp substrate is concurrently administered with vortioxetine.

■ **Monoamine Oxidase Inhibitors** Potentially serious, sometimes fatal adverse reactions may occur in patients who are receiving or have recently received a monoamine oxidase (MAO) inhibitor and then initiate therapy with serotonergic antidepressants or in those who received SSRI or SNRI therapy shortly before initiation of an MAO inhibitor. Concomitant use of MAO inhibitors intended to treat psychiatric disorders with vortioxetine is contraindicated. In addition, at least 2 weeks should elapse between discontinuance of an MAO inhibitor intended to treat psychiatric disorders and initiation of vortioxetine and at least 3 weeks should elapse between discontinuance of vortioxetine and initiation of an MAO inhibitor intended to treat psychiatric disorders. (See Contraindications and also see Serotonin Syndrome under Warnings/Precautions: Other Warnings and Precautions, in Cautions.)

Linezolid Linezolid, an anti-infective agent that is also a reversible MAO inhibitor, has been associated with drug interactions resulting in serotonin syndrome, including some associated with SSRIs and SNRIs. Because of this potential risk, linezolid generally should not be used in patients receiving vortioxetine. However, the manufacturer and the US Food and Drug Administration (FDA) state that certain life-threatening or urgent situations necessitate immediate linezolid treatment in a patient receiving a serotonergic drug such as vortioxetine. In such emergency situations, the availability of alternative anti-infectives should be considered and the benefits of linezolid should be weighed against the risk of serotonin syndrome. If linezolid is indicated in such emergency situations, vortioxetine must be immediately discontinued and the patient monitored for symptoms of CNS toxicity for 3 weeks or until 24 hours after the last linezolid dose, whichever comes first. Treatment with vortioxetine may be resumed 24 hours after the last linezolid dose.

If nonemergency use of linezolid is being planned for a patient receiving vortioxetine, vortioxetine should be withheld for at least 2 weeks prior to initiating linezolid.

Treatment with vortioxetine should not be initiated in a patient receiving linezolid. In patients who require more urgent treatment of a psychiatric condition, other interventions, including hospitalization, should be considered. Vortioxetine may be started 24 hours after the last linezolid dose. (See Contraindications and also see Serotonin Syndrome under Warnings/Precautions: Other Warnings and Precautions, in Cautions.)

Methylene Blue Methylene blue, a potent and reversible inhibitor of MAO-A, has been associated with drug interactions resulting in serotonin syndrome, including some associated with SSRIs and SNRIs. Most of these cases occurred when methylene blue was used as a diagnostic (visualizing) dye† (1–8 mg/kg IV) during parathyroid surgery; it is unclear whether there is a risk of serotonin syndrome when methylene blue is administered by other routes or in lower IV doses in patients receiving serotonergic drugs. Because of this potential risk, methylene blue generally should not be used in patients receiving vortioxetine. However, the manufacturer and the FDA state that certain life-threatening or urgent situations may necessitate immediate IV methylene blue treatment in a patient receiving a serotonergic drug such as vortioxetine. In such emergency situations, the availability of alternative interventions should be considered and the benefits of methylene blue should be weighed against the risk of serotonin syndrome. If methylene blue is indicated in such emergency situations, vortioxetine must be immediately discontinued and the patient monitored for symptoms of CNS toxicity for 3 weeks or until 24 hours after the last methylene blue dose, whichever comes first. Treatment with vortioxetine may be resumed 24 hours after the last methylene blue dose.

If nonemergency use of methylene blue is being planned for a patient receiving vortioxetine, vortioxetine should be withheld for at least 2 weeks prior to initiating methylene blue treatment.

Treatment with vortioxetine should not be initiated in a patient receiving IV methylene blue. In patients who require more urgent treatment of a psychiatric condition, other interventions, including hospitalization, should be considered. Vortioxetine may be started 24 hours after the last IV methylene blue dose. (See Contraindications and also see Serotonin Syndrome under Warnings/Precautions: Other Warnings and Precautions, in Cautions.)

The manufacturer of vortioxetine states that the risk of administering methylene blue by non-IV routes (e.g., oral tablets, local injection) or in IV doses much lower than 1 mg/kg in patients receiving vortioxetine is unclear. Clinicians should be aware of the possibility of the emergent symptoms of serotonin syndrome with concomitant use.

■ **Serotonergic Drugs** Concomitant use of vortioxetine and other serotonergic drugs is associated with a risk of serious, sometimes fatal, serotonin syndrome. If concomitant use of vortioxetine and other serotonergic drugs is clinically warranted, patients should be advised of the increased risk for serotonin syndrome, particularly during treatment initiation and dosage increases (see Advice to Patients). If serotonin syndrome manifestations occur, treatment with vortioxetine and any concurrently administered serotonergic agents should be discontinued immediately and supportive and symptomatic treatment should be initiated. (See Serotonin Syndrome under Warnings/Precautions: Other Warnings and Precautions, in Cautions.)

■ **Selective Serotonin-reuptake Inhibitors and Selective Serotonin- and Norepinephrine-reuptake Inhibitors** Concomitant use of vortioxetine and a selective serotonin-reuptake inhibitor (SSRI) or selective serotonin- and norepinephrine-reuptake inhibitor (SNRI) is associated with a risk of serious, sometimes fatal, serotonin syndrome. If concomitant use of vortioxetine and an SSRI or SNRI is clinically warranted, patients should be advised of the increased risk for serotonin syndrome, particularly during treatment initiation and dosage increases (see Advice to Patients). If serotonin syndrome manifestations occur, treatment with vortioxetine and the concurrently administered SSRI or SNRI should be discontinued immediately and supportive and symptomatic treatment should be initiated. (See Serotonin Syndrome under Warnings/Precautions: Other Warnings and Precautions, in Cautions.)

Duloxetine The manufacturer states that dosage adjustment of duloxetine (a CYP1A2 substrate) is not necessary when used concomitantly with vortioxetine.

Fluoxetine and Paroxetine The dosage of vortioxetine should be reduced by 50% when used concurrently with fluoxetine or paroxetine, which are both potent CYP2D6 inhibitors. The dosage should be increased back to the original dosage when fluoxetine or paroxetine is discontinued. (See Potent CYP2D6 Inhibitors under Drug Interactions: Drugs Affecting Hepatic Microsomal Enzymes.)

Venlafaxine The manufacturer states that dosage adjustment of venlafaxine (a CYP2D6 substrate) is not necessary when used concomitantly with vortioxetine.

■ **Tricyclic Antidepressants** Concomitant use of vortioxetine and a tricyclic antidepressant is associated with a risk of serious, sometimes fatal, serotonin syndrome. If concomitant use of vortioxetine and a tricyclic antidepressant is clinically warranted, patients should be advised of the increased risk for serotonin syndrome, particularly during treatment initiation and dosage increases (see Advice to Patients). If serotonin syndrome manifestations occur, treatment with vortioxetine, the tricyclic antidepressant, and any other concurrently administered serotonergic agents should be discontinued immediately and supportive and symptomatic treatment should be initiated. (See Serotonin Syndrome under Warnings/Precautions: Other Warnings and Precautions, in Cautions.)

■ **5-HT$_1$ Receptor Agonists ("Triptans")** Concomitant use of vortioxetine and a triptan is associated with a risk of serious, sometimes fatal, serotonin syndrome. If concomitant use of vortioxetine and triptans is clinically warranted, patients should be advised of the increased risk for serotonin syndrome, particularly during treatment initiation and dosage increases (see Advice to Patients). If serotonin syndrome manifestations occur, treatment with vortioxetine, the triptan, and any other concurrently administered serotonergic agents should be discontinued immediately and supportive and symptomatic treatment should be initiated. (See Serotonin Syndrome under Warnings/Precautions: Other Warnings and Precautions, in Cautions.)

■ **Tryptophan** Concomitant use of vortioxetine and tryptophan is associated with a risk of serious, sometimes fatal, serotonin syndrome. If concomitant use of vortioxetine and tryptophan is clinically warranted, patients should be advised of the increased risk for serotonin syndrome, particularly during treatment initiation and dosage increases (see Advice to Patients). If serotonin syndrome manifestations occur, treatment with vortioxetine, tryptophan, and any other concurrently administered serotonergic agents should be discontinued immediately and supportive and symptomatic treatment should be initiated. (See Serotonin Syndrome under Warnings/Precautions: Other Warnings and Precautions, in Cautions.)

■ **Buspirone** Concomitant use of vortioxetine and buspirone is associated with a risk of serious, sometimes fatal, serotonin syndrome. If concomitant use of vortioxetine and buspirone is clinically warranted, patients should be advised of the increased risk for serotonin syndrome, particularly during treatment initiation and dosage increases (see Advice to Patients). If serotonin syndrome manifestations occur, treatment with vortioxetine, buspirone, and any other concurrently administered serotonergic agents should be discontinued immediately and supportive and symptomatic treatment should be initiated. (See Serotonin Syndrome under Warnings/Precautions: Other Warnings and Precautions, in Cautions.)

■ **Fentanyl** Concomitant use of vortioxetine and fentanyl is associated with a risk of serious, sometimes fatal, serotonin syndrome. If concomitant use of vortioxetine and fentanyl is clinically warranted, patients should be advised of the increased risk for serotonin syndrome, particularly during treatment initiation and dosage increases (see Advice to Patients). If serotonin syndrome manifestations occur, treatment with vortioxetine, fentanyl, and any other concurrently administered serotonergic agents should be discontinued immediately and supportive and symptomatic treatment should be initiated. (See Serotonin Syndrome under Warnings/Precautions: Other Warnings and Precautions, in Cautions.)

■ **St. John's Wort** Concomitant use of vortioxetine and St. John's wort (*Hypericum perforatum*) is associated with a risk of serious, sometimes fatal, serotonin syndrome. If concomitant use of vortioxetine and St. John's wort is clinically warranted, patients should be advised of the increased risk for serotonin syndrome, particularly during treatment initiation and dosage increases (see Advice to Patients). If serotonin syndrome manifestations occur, treatment with vortioxetine, St. John's wort, and any other concurrently administered serotonergic agents should be discontinued immediately and supportive and symptomatic treatment should be initiated. (See Serotonin Syndrome under Warnings/Precautions: Other Warnings and Precautions, in Cautions.)

■ **Tramadol** Concomitant use of vortioxetine and tramadol is associated with a risk of serious, sometimes fatal, serotonin syndrome. If concomitant use of vortioxetine and tramadol is clinically warranted, patients should be advised of the increased risk for serotonin syndrome, particularly during treatment initiation and dosage increases (see Advice to Patients). If serotonin syndrome manifestations occur, treatment with vortioxetine, tramadol, and any other concurrently administered serotonergic agents should be discontinued immediately and supportive and symptomatic treatment should be initiated. (See Serotonin Syndrome under Warnings/Precautions: Other Warnings and Precautions, in Cautions.)

■ **Drugs Affecting Hemostasis** Altered anticoagulant effects, including increased bleeding, have been reported when SSRIs or SNRIs were administered concurrently with warfarin.

Following concurrent administration of stable doses of warfarin (1–10 mg daily) with multiple daily doses of vortioxetine (10 mg daily), no clinically important effects were observed on international normalized ratio (INR), prothrombin values, or warfarin pharmacokinetics (protein-bound and free drug) for both *R*- and *S*-warfarin. The manufacturer of vortioxetine states that dosage adjustment of warfarin is not necessary when these drugs are given in combination.

The risk of bleeding may be increased if vortioxetine is used concurrently with aspirin or other nonsteroidal anti-inflammatory agents (NSAIAs).

Concurrent administration of aspirin (150 mg daily) with multiple daily doses of vortioxetine did not have a clinically important inhibitory effect on platelet aggregation or the pharmacokinetics of aspirin and salicylic acid. The manufacturer states that dosage adjustment of aspirin is not necessary when these drugs are given in combination.

Patients receiving other drugs that interfere with hemostasis should be carefully monitored when vortioxetine is initiated or discontinued.

■ **Drugs Highly Bound to Plasma Protein** Vortioxetine is highly bound to plasma proteins and concurrent administration of vortioxetine in patients receiving another drug that is highly protein bound potentially may result in increased free concentrations of the other drug. (See Drug Interactions: Drugs Affecting Hemostasis.)

■ **Alcohol** In a clinical study, vortioxetine (single 20- or 40-mg dose) did not increase impairment of mental and motor skills caused by alcohol. However, the manufacturer recommends avoiding concomitant alcohol consumption during vortioxetine therapy.

■ **Budesonide** The manufacturer of vortioxetine states that dosage adjustment of budesonide (a CYP3A4/5 substrate) is not necessary during concurrent administration of vortioxetine.

■ **Bupropion** Concurrent administration of vortioxetine (10 mg once daily) and bupropion (75 or 150 mg twice daily), a potent CYP2D6 inhibitor and CYP2B6 substrate, in healthy individuals increased peak plasma concentrations of bupropion by 18%, and increased vortioxetine peak plasma concentrations and area under the concentration-time curve (AUC) by 114 and 128%, respectively. Increased adverse effects also were observed when vortioxetine and bupropion were given in combination, probably as a result, at least in part, of increased vortioxetine exposure.

Dosage adjustment of bupropion is not necessary when concomitantly administered with vortioxetine. However, the dosage of vortioxetine should be reduced by 50% when used concurrently with bupropion. The dosage of vortioxetine should be increased back to the original dosage when bupropion is discontinued. (See Potent CYP2D6 Inhibitors under Drug Interactions: Drugs Affecting Hepatic Microsomal Enzymes.)

■ **Caffeine** Multiple doses of vortioxetine did not have a clinically important effect on the pharmacokinetics of caffeine (a CYP1A2 substrate) in healthy individuals.

■ **Carbamazepine** When vortioxetine is administered concurrently with carbamazepine (a potent CYP inducer) for longer than 14 days, increasing the dosage of vortioxetine should be considered. The manufacturer recommends that the maximum dosage of vortioxetine not exceed 3 times the original dosage. Following discontinuance of carbamazepine, the original vortioxetine dosage should be resumed within 14 days.

■ **Diazepam** Multiple daily doses of vortioxetine did not affect the pharmacokinetics or pharmacodynamics (i.e., composite cognitive score) of diazepam (a CYP2C19 substrate). The manufacturer of vortioxetine states that dosage adjustment of diazepam is not necessary during concurrent administration of vortioxetine.

■ **Diuretics** Concomitant use of vortioxetine and diuretics may increase the risk of hyponatremia. (See Hyponatremia/Syndrome of Inappropriate Antidiuretic Hormone Secretion under Warnings/Precautions: Other Warnings and Precautions, in Cautions.)

■ **Fluconazole** Administration of a single dose of vortioxetine (10 mg) to healthy individuals receiving fluconazole (200 mg once daily) increased peak plasma concentrations and AUC of vortioxetine by 15 and 46%, respectively; these increases were not considered clinically important. Dosage adjustment of fluconazole therefore is not necessary when administered concomitantly with vortioxetine.

■ **Ketoconazole** Administration of a single dose of vortioxetine (10 mg) to healthy individuals receiving ketoconazole (400 mg once daily) increased peak plasma concentration and AUC of vortioxetine by 26 and 30%, respectively; these increases were not considered clinically important. Dosage adjustment of ketoconazole therefore is not necessary when administered concomitantly with vortioxetine.

■ Lithium Administration of multiple daily doses of vortioxetine with lithium (at steady state) did not have a clinically important effect on lithium exposure. The manufacturer of vortioxetine states that dosage adjustment of lithium is not necessary when these drugs are given in combination.

Concomitant use of vortioxetine and lithium is associated with a risk of serious, sometimes fatal, serotonin syndrome. If concomitant use of vortioxetine and lithium is clinically warranted, patients should be advised of the increased risk for serotonin syndrome, particularly during treatment initiation and dosage increases (see Advice to Patients). If serotonin syndrome manifestations occur, treatment with vortioxetine, lithium, and any other concurrently administered serotonergic agents should be discontinued immediately and supportive and symptomatic treatment should be initiated. (See Serotonin Syndrome under Warnings/Precautions: Other Warnings and Precautions, in Cautions.)

■ Midazolam Multiple doses of vortioxetine did not have a clinically important effect on the pharmacokinetics of midazolam (a CYP3A4 substrate) in healthy individuals.

■ Omeprazole Administration of a single 40-mg dose of omeprazole (a CYP2C19 inhibitor and substrate) to healthy individuals receiving vortioxetine (10 mg once daily) did not have a clinically important effect on the pharmacokinetics of either drug.

■ Oral Contraceptives Vortioxetine (10 mg once daily) did not have a clinically important effect on the pharmacokinetics of concurrently administered ethinyl estradiol (0.03 mg) and levonorgestrel (0.15 mg).

■ Phenytoin When vortioxetine is administered concurrently with phenytoin (a potent CYP inducer) for longer than 14 days, increasing the dosage of vortioxetine should be considered. The manufacturer of vortioxetine recommends that the maximum dosage of vortioxetine not exceed 3 times the original dosage. Following discontinuance of phenytoin, the original vortioxetine dosage should be resumed within 14 days.

■ Quinidine The dosage of vortioxetine should be reduced by 50% when used concurrently with quinidine, a potent CYP2D6 inhibitor. The dosage should be increased back to the original dosage when quinidine is discontinued. (See Potent CYP2D6 Inhibitors under Drug Interactions: Drugs Affecting Hepatic Microsomal Enzymes.)

■ Repaglinide The manufacturer of vortioxetine states that dosage adjustment of repaglinide (a CYP2C8 substrate) is not necessary during concurrent administration of vortioxetine.

■ Rifampin Administration of a single dose of vortioxetine (20 mg) to healthy individuals receiving rifampin (a potent CYP inducer; 600 mg once daily for 10 days) decreased peak plasma concentrations and AUC of vortioxetine by 51 and 72–77%, respectively. When vortioxetine is administered concurrently with rifampin for longer than 14 days, increasing the dosage of vortioxetine should be considered. The manufacturer of vortioxetine recommends that the maximum dosage of vortioxetine not exceed 3 times the original dosage. Following discontinuance of rifampin, the original vortioxetine dosage should be resumed within 14 days.

■ Tolbutamide Multiple doses of vortioxetine did not have a clinically important effect on the pharmacokinetics of tolbutamide (a CYP2C9 substrate) in healthy individuals.

Description

Vortioxetine hydrobromide is a serotonergic antidepressant. Although the precise mechanism of the drug's antidepressant effect is not fully understood, it is thought to be related to enhancement of serotonergic activity in the CNS through inhibition of serotonin reuptake. Vortioxetine also possesses several other activities, including serotonin type 3A (5-hydroxytryptamine [5-HT_{3A}]) receptor antagonism and 5-HT_{1A} receptor agonism; however, the contribution of these activities to the drug's antidepressant effect has not been established.

Vortioxetine binds with high affinity to the human serotonin transporter, but not to norepinephrine or dopamine transporters. The drug potently and selectively inhibits the reuptake of serotonin. Vortioxetine binds to 5-HT_3, 5-HT_{1A}, 5-HT_7, 5-HT_{1D}, and 5-HT_{1B} receptors and is a 5-HT_3, 5-HT_{1D}, and 5-HT_7 receptor antagonist; a 5-HT_{1B} receptor partial agonist; and a 5-HT_{1A} receptor agonist.

Vortioxetine is slowly but well absorbed following oral administration. Peak plasma vortioxetine concentrations are reached within 7–11 hours, and the drug has an absolute bioavailability of 75%. Administration with food does not affect the pharmacokinetics of vortioxetine. The drug is widely distributed and 98% protein bound. Vortioxetine is extensively metabolized through oxidation by cytochrome P-450 (CYP) isoenzymes, principally by CYP2D6 with lesser contributions from CYP3A4/5, 2C19, 2C9, 2A6, 2C8, and 2B6, and subsequent glucuronic acid conjugation. CYP2D6 is the main enzyme catalyzing the metabolism of vortioxetine to its principal carboxylic acid metabolite, which is pharmacologically inactive. The plasma concentration of vortioxetine was approximately 2 times higher in poor metabolizers of CYP2D6 than in extensive metabolizers. (See Dosage and Administration: Dosage.) Following administration of a single dose of radiolabeled vortioxetine, approximately 59 and 26% of administered radioactivity was recovered in the urine and feces, respectively, as metabolites. Negligible amounts of unchanged vortioxetine were excreted in the urine. The mean terminal half-life of vortioxetine is approximately 66 hours, and steady-state concentrations of the drug usually are achieved within 2 weeks.

Advice to Patients

Importance of providing a copy of written patient information (medication guide) each time vortioxetine hydrobromide is dispensed. Importance of advising patients and their caregivers to read the patient information before taking vortioxetine and each time the prescription is refilled.

Importance of advising patients to check their prescription carefully to ensure that they have received the correct drug; prescribing and dispensing errors have been reported due to similarities in the spelling and pronunciation of Brintellix® (the former trade name for vortioxetine hydrobromide, which was changed to Trintellix® in May 2016) and Brilinta® (the trade name for ticagrelor, a platelet aggregation inhibitor). (See Prescribing and Dispensing Precautions under Warnings/Precautions: Other Warnings and Precautions, in Cautions.)

Risk of suicidality; importance of patients, family, and caregivers being alert to and immediately reporting emergence of suicidality, worsening depression, or unusual changes in behavior, especially during the first few months of therapy or during periods of dosage adjustment. (See Worsening of Depression and Suicidality Risk under Warnings/Precautions: Warnings, in Cautions.)

Importance of informing patients who are receiving vortioxetine 15 or 20 mg daily that they may experience possible withdrawal reactions (e.g., headache, muscle tension, mood swings, sudden outbursts of anger, dizziness, runny nose) if they abruptly stop the drug. Patients should be advised not to stop taking vortioxetine without first talking with their clinician.

Importance of instructing patients not to take vortioxetine with or within 2 weeks of discontinuing a monoamine oxidase (MAO) inhibitor and to allow 3 weeks after stopping vortioxetine before initiating an MAO inhibitor.

Importance of informing patients of potential risk of serotonin syndrome, particularly with concurrent use of vortioxetine and other serotonergic agents or antipsychotic agents. (See Drug Interactions.) Importance of immediately contacting clinician if signs and symptoms of this syndrome develop (e.g., restlessness, hallucinations, delirium, loss of coordination, fast heart beat, increased body temperature, sweating, muscle stiffness, labile blood pressure, diarrhea, coma, nausea, vomiting, confusion).

Importance of advising patients that vortioxetine can be taken with or without food, and should be taken at about the same time every day.

Importance of informing patients that if they receive diuretics, are otherwise volume depleted, or are elderly, that they may be at greater risk of developing hyponatremia during vortioxetine therapy.

Importance of informing patients that nausea is the most common adverse effect associated with vortioxetine, and that it is dose related. Nausea commonly occurs within the first week of treatment then decreases in frequency, but can persist in some patients.

Risk of cognitive and motor impairment; although not observed in a trial in healthy individuals, importance of patients exercising caution while operating hazardous machinery, including driving a motor vehicle, until they are reasonably certain that vortioxetine therapy does not adversely affect their ability to engage in such activities.

Importance of advising patients to avoid alcohol consumption during vortioxetine therapy.

Importance of advising patients to notify their clinician if any signs or symptoms of an allergic reaction develop during vortioxetine therapy (e.g., rash, hives, swelling, difficulty breathing).

Importance of advising patients and their caregivers to watch for signs of activation of mania/hypomania.

Importance of advising patients that vortioxetine can cause mild pupillary dilation, which can lead to an episode of angle-closure glaucoma in susceptible individuals. Possible symptoms include eye pain, vision changes, and swelling or redness in or around the eye. Preexisting glaucoma is almost always open-angle glaucoma since angle-closure glaucoma can be treated definitively with iridectomy when diagnosed; open-angle glaucoma is not a risk factor for angle-closure glaucoma. Patients may wish to be examined to determine whether they are susceptible to angle-closure glaucoma and have a prophylactic procedure (e.g., iridectomy) if they are susceptible.

Importance of informing clinicians of existing or contemplated concomitant therapy, including prescription and OTC drugs or herbal supplements, as well as any concomitant illnesses (e.g., liver disease, glaucoma) or personal or family history of suicidality or bipolar disorder. Importance of advising patients about the risk of bleeding associated with concomitant use of vortioxetine with aspirin or other nonsteroidal anti-inflammatory agents, warfarin, or other drugs that affect coagulation.

Importance of women informing clinicians if they are or plan to become pregnant or plan to breast-feed.

Importance of informing patients of other important precautionary information. (See Cautions.)

Overview® (see Users Guide). For additional information on this drug until a more detailed monograph is developed and published, the manufacturer's labeling should be consulted. It is *essential* that the manufacturer's labeling be consulted for more detailed information on usual cautions, precautions, contraindications, potential drug interactions, laboratory test interferences, and acute toxicity.

Preparations

Excipients in commercially available drug preparations may have clinically important effects in some individuals; consult specific product labeling for details.

Vortioxetine Hydrobromide

Oral		
Tablets, film-coated	5 mg (of vortioxetine)	**Trintellix®**, Takeda
	10 mg (of vortioxetine)	**Trintellix®**, Takeda
	15 mg (of vortioxetine)	**Trintellix®**, Takeda
	20 mg (of vortioxetine)	**Trintellix®**, Takeda

†Use is not currently included in the labeling approved by the US Food and Drug Administration

TRICYCLICS AND OTHER NOREPINEPHRINE-REUPTAKE INHIBITORS 28:16.04.28

Tricyclic Antidepressants General Statement

■ Tricyclic antidepressants contain a 3-ring structure and differ structurally and pharmacologically from other currently available antidepressants (e.g., selective serotonin-reuptake inhibitors, monoamine oxidase inhibitors).

Uses

■ **Major Depressive Disorder** Tricyclic antidepressants are used in the treatment of major depressive disorder. A major depressive episode implies a prominent and relatively persistent depressed or dysphoric mood that usually interferes with daily functioning (nearly every day for at least 2 weeks). According to DSM-IV criteria, a major depressive episode includes at least 5 of the following 9 symptoms (with at least one of the symptoms being depressed mood or loss of interest or pleasure): depressed mood most of the day as indicated by subjective report (e.g., feels sad or empty) or observation made by others; markedly diminished interest or pleasure in all, or almost all, activities most of the day; significant weight loss (when not dieting) or weight gain (e.g., a change of more than 5% of body weight in a month), or decrease or increase in appetite; insomnia or hypersomnia; psychomotor agitation or retardation (observable by others, not merely subjective feelings of restlessness or being slowed down); fatigue or loss of energy; feelings of worthlessness or excessive or inappropriate guilt (not merely self-reproach or guilt about being sick); diminished ability to think or concentrate or indecisiveness (either by subjective account or as observed by others); and recurrent thoughts of death or a suicide attempt or suicidal ideation.

Treatment of major depressive disorder generally consists of an acute phase (to induce remission), a continuation phase (to preserve remission), and a maintenance phase (to prevent recurrence). Various interventions (e.g., psychotherapy, antidepressant drug therapy, electroconvulsive therapy [ECT]) are used alone or in combination to treat major depressive episodes. Treatment should be individualized and the most appropriate strategy for a particular patient is determined by clinical factors such as severity of depression (e.g., mild, moderate, severe), presence or absence of certain psychiatric features (e.g., suicide risk, catatonia, psychotic or atypical features, alcohol or substance abuse or dependence, panic or other anxiety disorder, cognitive dysfunction, dysthymia, personality disorder, seasonal affective disorder), and concurrent illness (e.g., asthma, cardiac disease, dementia, seizure disorder, glaucoma, hypertension). Demographic and psychosocial factors as well as patient preference also are used to determine the most effective treatment strategy.

While use of psychotherapy alone may be considered as an initial treatment strategy for patients with mild to moderate major depressive disorder (based on patient preference and presence of clinical features such as psychosocial stressors), combined use of antidepressant drug therapy and psychotherapy may be useful for initial treatment of patients with moderate to severe major depressive disorder with psychosocial issues, interpersonal problems, or a comorbid axis II disorder. In addition, combined use of antidepressant drug therapy and psychotherapy may be beneficial in patients who have a history of poor compliance or only partial response to adequate trials of either antidepressant drug therapy or psychotherapy alone.

Antidepressant drug therapy can be used alone for initial treatment of patients with mild major depressive disorder (if preferred by the patient) and usually is indicated alone or in combination with psychotherapy for initial treatment of patients with moderate to severe major depressive disorder (unless ECT is planned). ECT is not generally used for initial treatment of uncomplicated major depression, but is recommended as first-line treatment for severe major depressive disorder when it is coupled with psychotic features, catatonic stupor, severe suicidality, food refusal leading to nutritional compromise, or other situations when a rapid antidepressant response is required. ECT also is recommended for patients who have previously shown a positive response or a preference for this treatment modality and can be considered for patients with moderate or severe depression who have not responded to or cannot receive antidepressant drug therapy. In certain situations involving severely depressed patients unresponsive to adequate trials of several individual antidepressant agents, adjunctive therapy with another agent (e.g., buspirone, lithium) or concomitant use of a second antidepressant agent (e.g., bupropion) has been used; however, such combination therapy is associated with an increased risk of adverse reactions, may require dosage adjustments, and (if not contraindicated) should be undertaken only after careful consideration of the relative risks and benefits. (See Drug Interactions: Monoamine Oxidase Inhibitors and see Selective Serotonin-Reuptake Inhibitors under Drug Interactions: Drugs Affecting Hepatic Microsomal Enzymes.)

Considerations in Choosing Antidepressants A variety of antidepressant drugs are available for the treatment of major depressive disorder, including tricyclic antidepressants, selective serotonin-reuptake inhibitors (SSRIs) (e.g., citalopram, escitalopram, fluoxetine, paroxetine, sertraline), monoamine oxidase (MAO) inhibitors (e.g., phenelzine, tranylcypromine), and other antidepressants (e.g., bupropion, desvenlafaxine, duloxetine, maprotiline, nefazodone, trazodone, venlafaxine). Most clinical studies have shown that the antidepressant effect of usual dosages of tricyclic antidepressants in patients with major depression is comparable to that of usual dosages of SSRIs (e.g., fluoxetine, paroxetine, sertraline) or other antidepressants (e.g., nefazodone, trazodone). Studies that have compared various tricyclic antidepressants have not conclusively demonstrated superiority of one agent over another. The onset of action of tricyclic antidepressants appears to be comparable to that of SSRIs, although the onset of action of these drugs has been variably reported to be somewhat faster or slower than that of tricyclic antidepressants in some studies.

Because response rates in patients with major depression are similar for most currently available antidepressants, the choice of antidepressant agent for a given patient depends principally on other factors such as potential adverse effects, safety or tolerability of these adverse effects in the individual patient, psychiatric and medical history, patient or family history of response to specific therapies, patient preference, quantity and quality of available clinical data, cost, and relative acute overdose safety. No single antidepressant can be recommended as optimal for all patients because of substantial heterogeneity in individual responses and in the nature, likelihood, and severity of adverse effects. In addition, patients vary in the degree to which certain adverse effects and other inconveniences of drug therapy (e.g., cost, dietary restrictions) affect their preferences.

Patient Tolerance Considerations. Because of differences in the adverse effect profile between tricyclic antidepressants and SSRIs, particularly more frequent anticholinergic effects, cardiovascular effects, and weight gain with tricyclic antidepressants, SSRIs such as citalopram, escitalopram, fluoxetine, paroxetine, or sertraline may be preferred in patients in whom such effects are not tolerated or are of potential concern. The decreased incidence of anticholinergic effects associated with SSRIs compared with tricyclic antidepressants is a potential advantage, since tricyclic antidepressants may be discontinued early in unusually sensitive patients. In addition, some anticholinergic effects may become troublesome during long-term tricyclic antidepressant therapy (e.g., persistent dry mouth may result in tooth decay). Although MAO inhibitors are not anticholinergic, many of their adverse effects resemble anticholinergic symptoms. Certain adverse GI effects (e.g., nausea, anorexia) or nervous system effects (e.g., anxiety, nervousness, insomnia, weight loss) appear to occur more frequently with SSRIs than with other antidepressant agents and alternatives may be preferred in patients who cannot tolerate these effects or when these effects are a concern.

Pediatric Considerations. The clinical presentation of depression in children and adolescents can differ from that in adults and generally varies with the age and developmental stages of the child. Younger children may exhibit behavioral problems such as social withdrawal, aggressive behavior, apathy, sleep disruption, and weight loss; adolescents may present with somatic complaints, self esteem problems, rebelliousness, poor performance in school, or a pattern of engaging in risky or aggressive behavior.

Only limited data are available to date from controlled clinical studies evaluating various antidepressant agents in children and adolescents, and many of these studies have methodologic limitations (e.g., nonrandomized or uncontrolled, small sample size, short duration, nonspecific inclusion criteria). However, there is some evidence that the response to antidepressants in pediatric patients may differ from that seen in adults, and caution should be used in extrapolating data from adult studies when making treatment decisions for pediatric patients. Results of several studies evaluating tricyclic antidepressants (e.g., amitriptyline, desipramine, imipramine, nortriptyline) in preadolescent and adolescent patients with major depression indicate a lack of overall efficacy in this age group. Based on the lack of efficacy data regarding use of tricyclic antidepressants and MAO inhibitors in pediatric patients and because of the potential for life-threatening adverse effects associated with the use of these drugs, many experts consider SSRIs the drugs of choice when antidepressant therapy is indicated for the treatment of major depressive disorder in children and adolescents. However, the US Food and Drug Administration (FDA) states that, while efficacy of fluoxetine in major depressive disorder has been established in pediatric patients, efficacy of other newer antidepressants (i.e., citalopram, duloxetine, escitalopram, fluvoxamine, mirtazapine, nefazodone, paroxetine, sertraline, venlafaxine) was not conclusively established in clinical trials in pediatric patients with major depressive disorder. In addition, FDA now warns that antidepressants increase the risk of suicidal thinking and behavior (suicidality) in children and adolescents with major depressive disorder and other psychiatric disorders. (See Cautions: Pediatric Precautions.) FDA currently states that anyone considering using an antidepressant in a child or adolescent for any clinical use must balance the potential risk of therapy with the clinical need. (See Cautions: Precautions and Contraindications.)

Geriatric Considerations. The response to antidepressants in geriatric patients is similar to that reported in younger adults, but depression in geriatric patients often is not recognized and is not treated. In geriatric patients with major depressive disorder, tricyclic antidepressants (e.g., amitriptyline) appear to be as effective as SSRIs (e.g., citalopram, escitalopram, fluoxetine, paroxetine, sertraline) but may cause more overall adverse effects than these other agents. Geriatric patients appear to be more susceptible to adverse effects of MAO inhibitors (e.g., episodes of hypertension, malignant hyperthermia) than younger patients, and these adverse effects are associated with increased morbidity in geriatric patients since they have less compensatory reserve to cope with any serious adverse reactions. Geriatric patients appear to be especially sensitive to anticholinergic (e.g., dry mouth, constipation, vision disturbance), cardiovascular, orthostatic hypotension, and sedative effects of tricyclic antidepressants. The low incidence of anticholinergic effects associated with SSRIs compared with tricyclic antidepressants is a potential advantage in geriatric patients, since some of these effects (e.g., constipation, dry mouth, confusion, memory impairment) may be particularly troublesome in these patients. Some clinicians state that SSRIs may be preferred for treating depression in geriatric patients in whom the orthostatic hypotension associated with tricyclic antidepressants potentially may result in injuries (such as severe falls). However, despite the fewer cardiovascular and anticholinergic effects associated with SSRIs, these drugs did not show any advantage over tricyclic antidepressants with regard to hip fracture in a case-control study. In addition, there was little difference in the rates of falls between nursing home residents receiving tricyclic antidepressants and SSRIs in a retrospective study. Therefore, all geriatric individuals receiving either type of antidepressant should be considered at increased risk of falls and appropriate measures should be taken.

Patients with dementia of the Alzheimer's type (Alzheimer's disease, presenile or senile dementia) often present with depressive symptoms, such as depressed mood, appetite loss, insomnia, fatigue, irritability, and agitation. Most experts recommend that patients with dementia of the Alzheimer's type and depressive symptoms be considered as candidates for pharmacotherapy even if they fail to meet the criteria for a major depressive syndrome. The goals of such therapy are to improve mood, functional status (e.g., cognition), and quality of life. Although patients may present with depressed mood alone, the possibility of more extensive depressive symptomatology should be considered. Therefore, patients should be monitored carefully for indices of major depression, suicidal ideation, and neurovegetative signs since safety measures (e.g., hospitalization for suicidal ideation) and more vigorous and aggressive therapy (e.g., relatively high dosages, multiple drug trials) may be needed in some patients.

If pharmacotherapy is initiated for depressive symptoms in Alzheimer's patients, most experts recommend SSRIs such as citalopram, escitalopram, fluoxetine, paroxetine, or sertraline as first-line therapy because of their favorable adverse effect profile in this population compared with other currently available antidepressants (e.g., tricyclic antidepressants, MAO inhibitors). Although evidence of efficacy from controlled studies currently is limited, the available evidence and experience with the use of antidepressants in patients with dementia of the Alzheimer's type and associated depressive manifestations indicate that depressive symptoms (including depressive mood alone and with neurovegetative changes) in such patients are responsive to antidepressant therapy. In some patients, cognitive deficits may partially or fully resolve during antidepressant therapy, but the extent of response will be limited to the degree of cognitive impairment that is directly related to depression. In a controlled study comparing paroxetine and imipramine in patients with coexisting depression and dementia, both drugs were found to be effective; however, paroxetine was better tolerated (fewer anticholinergic and serious adverse effects).

Cardiovascular Considerations. Tricyclic antidepressants, MAO inhibitors, duloxetine, and trazodone are associated with orthostatic hypotension and tricyclic antidepressants also are associated with certain other cardiovascular effects (see Cautions: Cardiovascular Effects). The relatively low incidence of orthostatic hypotension and conduction disturbances reported to date with SSRIs may be advantageous in patients in whom cardiovascular effects may be hazardous. However, most clinical studies evaluating citalopram, escitalopram, fluoxetine, paroxetine, or sertraline for the management of depression did not include individuals with cardiovascular disease (e.g., those with a recent history of myocardial infarction or unstable heart disease) and further experience in such patients is necessary to confirm the reported relative lack of cardiotoxicity with SSRIs.

Sedative Considerations. Because most tricyclic antidepressants frequently cause drowsiness and SSRIs are less sedating, some clinicians state that SSRIs may be preferable in patients who do not require sedative effects; however, a tricyclic antidepressant or some other agent with more prominent sedative effects may be preferable in some patients (e.g., those with insomnia).

Suicidal Risk Considerations. Suicide is a known risk of depression and certain other psychiatric disorders, and these disorders themselves are the strongest predictors of suicide. However, there has been a long-standing concern that antidepressants may have a role in inducing worsening of depression and the emergence of suicidal thinking and behavior (suicidality) in certain patients during the early phases of treatment. FDA states that antidepressants increased the risk of suicidality in short-term studies in children, adolescents, and young adults (18–24 years of age) with major depressive disorder and other psychiatric disorders. (See Cautions: Pediatric Precautions.) An increased suicidality risk was not demonstrated with antidepressants compared with placebo in adults older than 24 years of age, and a reduced risk was observed in adults 65 years of age or older. It is currently unknown whether the suicidality risk extends to longer-term antidepressant use (i.e., beyond several months); however, there is substantial evidence from placebo-controlled maintenance trials in adults with major depressive disorder that antidepressants can delay the recurrence of depression. Because the risk of suicidality in depressed patients may persist until substantial remission of depression occurs, appropriate monitoring and close observation of patients of all ages who are receiving antidepressant therapy are recommended. (See Cautions: Precautions and Contraindications.) Tricyclic antidepressants may produce potentially life-threatening cardiotoxicity following overdosage. Desipramine overdosage, in particular, has resulted in a higher death rate compared with overdosages of other tricyclic antidepressants. (See Acute Toxicity.)

Other Considerations. Tricyclic antidepressants and MAO inhibitors have the capacity to induce weight gain. In obese patients and/or patients in whom the increase in appetite, carbohydrate craving, and weight gain associated with tricyclic antidepressant therapy may be undesirable (e.g., potentially hazardous to the patient's health, result in possible discontinuance of or noncompliance with therapy), some clinicians state that other drugs (e.g., SSRIs) may be preferred since they possess anorectic and weight-reducing properties. However, the possibility that some patients with concurrent eating disorders or those who may desire to lose weight may misuse such drugs for their anorectic and weight-reducing effects should be considered.

■ **Panic Disorder** Tricyclic antidepressants (e.g., clomipramine, desipramine, imipramine) have been used effectively for the treatment of panic disorder with or without agoraphobia†. Although not clearly established, the antiphobic and antipanic effects of the drugs appear to be independent of their antidepressive action.

Panic disorder can be treated with cognitive and behavioral psychotherapy and/or pharmacologic therapy. There are several classes of drugs that appear to be effective in the pharmacologic management of panic disorder, including tricyclic antidepressants, MAO inhibitors (e.g., phenelzine), SSRIs (e.g., citalopram, fluoxetine, paroxetine, sertraline), and benzodiazepines (e.g., alprazolam, clonazepam). When choosing among the available drugs, clinicians should consider their acceptance and tolerability by patients; their ability to reduce or eliminate panic attacks, reduce clinically important anxiety and disability secondary to phobic avoidance, and ameliorate other common comorbid conditions (such as depression); and their ability to prevent relapse during long-term therapy. Because of their better tolerability when compared with other agents (such as the tricyclic antidepressants and benzodiazepines), the lack of physical dependence problems commonly associated with benzodiazepines, and efficacy in panic disorder with comorbid conditions (e.g., depression, other anxiety disorders such as obsessive-compulsive disorder, alcoholism), many clinicians prefer SSRIs as first-line therapy in the management of panic disorder. If SSRI therapy is ineffective or not tolerated, use of a tricyclic antidepressant or a benzodiazepine is recommended.

In many patients receiving clomipramine, complete or nearly complete relief from panic attacks has been reported during therapy. For further information on use of clomipramine for the treatment of panic disorder, see Uses: Panic Disorder, in Clomipramine Hydrochloride 28:16.04.24.

■ **Obsessive-Compulsive Disorder** Clomipramine is used in the treatment of obsessive-compulsive disorder. For information on use of clomipramine for the treatment of obsessive-compulsive disorder, see Uses: Obsessive-compulsive Disorder, in Clomipramine Hydrochloride 28:16.04.24.

■ **Attention Deficit Hyperactivity Disorder** Tricyclic antidepressants have been used for the treatment of attention deficit hyperactivity disorder† (ADHD). Several studies that carefully evaluated the effect of tricyclic antidepressants (desipramine, imipramine) demonstrated positive effects on ADHD manifestations. Although tricyclic antidepressants generally have been shown to be effective in the management of ADHD, further evaluation of their safety and efficacy is needed and the drugs should be used cautiously in appropriately selected patients.

Stimulants (e.g., methylphenidate, amphetamines) remain the drugs of choice for the management of ADHD. For patients who are intolerant of or unresponsive to stimulants, various other drugs (e.g., tricyclic antidepressants, bupropion, clonidine, guanfacine) have proven useful in clinical practice. These alternatives also may be useful in patients with comorbid conditions. However, experience with such alternative drug therapy is far less extensive than with stimulants, and conclusions regarding relative efficacy currently cannot be made.

Tricyclic antidepressants generally have been shown to be effective in the management of ADHD in children and adolescents, but are associated with a narrower margin of safety than some other drugs. In addition, although a causal relationship has not been established, several cases of sudden death have been reported in children who received desipramine for ADHD† and have raised concerns about the use of this tricyclic in pediatric patients. (See Cautions: Pediatric Precautions.) Several clinical studies comparing tricyclic antidepressants with methylphenidate indicated either no difference in response or slightly better results with stimulants. Tricyclic antidepressants appear to be less effective than stimulants in improving attentional and cognitive symptoms, but may be useful for impulsive or hyperactive behavior. Tricyclic antidepressant therapy may be indicated as second-line therapy in patients who do not respond to stimulants or who develop clinically important depression or otherwise do not tolerate stimulants, but antidepressant therapy should be under the direction of a clinician familiar with use of the drugs. These antidepressants also may be useful for patients with tics or Tourette's disorder or in whom these conditions are exacerbated or not adequately controlled during stimulant therapy. Regardless of which tricyclic antidepressant is considered for use in the management of ADHD, the drugs should be used only if clearly indicated and with careful monitoring, including baseline and subsequent determinations of ECG and other parameters. For a more detailed discussion on the management of ADHD, see Uses: Attention Deficit Hyperactivity Disorder, in Methylphenidate 28:20.92.

■ **Migraine** Tricyclic antidepressants also have been used for the prophylaxis of migraine headache†. The US Headache Consortium states that there is good evidence from multiple well-designed clinical trials that amitriptyline has medium to high efficacy for the prophylaxis of migraine headache and considers the drug to have mild to moderate adverse effects when used for this indication. Consistent evidence of efficacy is lacking for other antidepressants. For further information on management and classification of migraine headache, see Vascular Headaches: General Principles in Migraine Therapy, under Uses in Sumatriptan 28:32.28.

■ **Enuresis** Imipramine hydrochloride is used as temporary adjunctive therapy in the treatment of functional enuresis in children 6 years of age or older. Other tricyclic antidepressants also have been used effectively for the treatment of enuresis†. Organic causes of enuresis should be ruled out before treatment with tricyclic antidepressants is begun, as the effects of the drugs may mask underlying genitourinary disease. When patients exhibit symptoms such as daytime urgency and frequency, appropriate examinations such as voiding cystourethrography and cystoscopy should be conducted. Relapses may occur following discontinuance of tricyclic antidepressants or even during therapy. Safety of imipramine or other tricyclic antidepressants for long-term, chronic use as adjunctive therapy for nocturnal enuresis has not been established; therefore, after a satisfactory response has been maintained, the drugs should be withdrawn gradually.

■ **Eating Disorders** Tricyclic antidepressants (e.g., amitriptyline, desipramine, imipramine) have been used effectively in the management of eating disorders†, principally bulimia nervosa†. In patients with bulimia nervosa, therapy with the drugs has reduced substantially the frequency of binge eating, vomiting, and purging (laxative abuse) and the preoccupation with food. Although tricyclic antidepressant therapy also has improved associated depressed mood in many patients with this condition, reduction of bulimic manifestations by the drugs does not appear to depend on improvement in mood or the presence of concomitant depression.

Experience with tricyclic antidepressants in the management of anorexia nervosa† is limited, and the possible role of the drugs in the management of this condition remains to be more fully elucidated. However, some clinicians state that tricyclic antidepressants may be useful for associated depression.

Because malnourished depressed patients may be particularly susceptible to the adverse cardiovascular effects or other severe toxicities (including death) of tricyclic antidepressants, the American Psychiatric Association (APA) states that these agents should be avoided in underweight individuals and in those exhibiting suicidal ideation. For further information on use of antidepressants in the treatment of eating disorders, see Uses: Eating Disorders, in Fluoxetine Hydrochloride 28:16.04.20.

■ **Smoking Cessation** Tricyclic (e.g., nortriptyline) and other (e.g., extended-release bupropion) antidepressants have been used for the management of nicotine (tobacco) dependence†. Although bupropion currently is considered first-line therapy for the management of nicotine dependence, the US Public Health Service (USPHS) currently recommends tricyclic antidepressant therapy with nortriptyline as second-line therapy for use under the supervision of a clinician. This recommendation is based on evidence from pooled analysis of 2 clinical studies on smoking cessation showing that nortriptyline therapy increased abstinence rates relative to placebo. Second-line pharmacotherapy (e.g., clonidine, nortriptyline, combined therapy with 2 forms of nicotine replacement) is of a more limited role than first-line pharmacotherapy (i.e., bupropion [as extended-release tablets], nicotine polacrilex gum, transdermal nicotine, nicotine nasal spray, nicotine nasal inhaler) in part because of more concerns about potential adverse effects with second-line drugs than with first-line drugs. The use of second-line pharmacotherapy should be considered after first-line pharmacotherapy was attempted or considered and should be individualized based on patient considerations. Use of second-line pharmacotherapy for smoking cessation should be considered for patients who received first-line drugs but were not able to quit smoking or in whom these drugs are contraindicated. (See Guidelines under Uses: Smoking Cessation, in Nicotine 12:92.)

Nicotine dependence therapy with an antidepressant may be particularly useful when a depressive disorder is included in the current or past history of patients attempting to quit smoking.

Although it is not necessary to assess for possible comorbid psychiatric disorders prior to initiating therapy for nicotine dependence, such comorbidity is important in the assessment and treatment of nicotine-dependent patients since psychiatric disorders are common in this population, smoking cessation or nicotine withdrawal may exacerbate the comorbid condition, and patients with psychiatric comorbidities have an increased risk for relapse to smoking after a cessation attempt. However, even though some smokers may experience exacerbation of a comorbid condition with smoking cessation, most evidence suggests that abstinence entails little adverse impact. In addition, while psychiatric comorbidity places smokers at increased relapse risk, smoking cessation therapy still can be beneficial. Treatment of nicotine dependence can be provided concurrently with treatment of other chemical dependencies (alcohol and other drugs), and there currently is little evidence that patients with such dependencies relapse to other drug use when they stop smoking.

■ **Bipolar Disorder** Tricyclic antidepressants have been used to treat the depressive phase of bipolar disorder†, but do not prevent and may precipitate hypomanic or manic attacks in patients with this disorder. Tricyclic antidepressants appear to be associated with response rates equivalent to or poorer than other antidepressants (e.g., selective serotonin-reuptake inhibitors [SSRIs], bupropion) (although superior to placebo) and also may carry a greater risk of precipitating hypomania or manic episodes in patients with bipolar disorder than other classes of antidepressants.

■ **Depression Associated with Schizophrenia** Tricyclic antidepressants may be beneficial in the treatment of depressive stages of schizophrenia† or in the treatment of depression with psychotic features, although when given alone, they may precipitate psychotic or hostile behavior in individuals with these disorders. If the drugs are used for these patients, they should be administered with antipsychotic drugs such as phenothiazines.

■ **Anxiety Disorders** Tricyclic antidepressants have been used to alleviate anxiety† in patients with psychoneurotic anxiety, anxiety associated with organic disease or alcoholism, and mixed symptoms of anxiety and depression. Occasionally, concurrent administration of tricyclic antidepressants with anxiolytics, sedatives, or antipsychotic drugs may be used in the treatment of depression with symptoms of anxiety, but treatment with an anxiolytic alone may also be successful. Detoxified alcoholics with mixed anxiety and depression and anxious depressed patients with a history of alcohol abuse appear more closely analogous to endogenous depressives than to reactive depressives and may respond better to tricyclic antidepressants than to conventional anxiolytics.

■ **Postherpetic Neuralgia** Tricyclic antidepressants are considered by some clinicians to be among the drugs of choice for the symptomatic treatment of postherpetic neuralgia†. The analgesic effects of these drugs appear to be independent of their antidepressant action. Although most studies of antidepressant use in the symptomatic treatment of postherpetic neuralgia have involved amitriptyline, nortriptyline has been shown to have equivalent analgesic effects and generally is better tolerated than amitriptyline. Alternatively, desipramine may be used in patients who experience unacceptable sedation while receiving nortriptyline.

■ **Insomnia** Doxepin is used for the treatment of insomnia characterized by difficulties with sleep maintenance. Although other tricyclic antidepressants have occasionally been used as hypnotics in nondepressed patients†, conventional hypnotics generally are more effective and cause fewer serious adverse reactions.

Dosage and Administration

■ **Administration** Tricyclic antidepressants are administered orally. Amitriptyline hydrochloride and imipramine hydrochloride also have been given IM, but parenteral dosage forms of these drugs no longer are commercially available in the US. Clomipramine hydrochloride has been administered IM† or IV†, but a parenteral dosage form is not commercially available in the US.

Although tricyclic antidepressants have been administered in up to 4 divided doses throughout the day, the drugs are long-acting and the entire oral daily dose may be administered at one time. Administration of single daily doses may improve patient compliance. Administration of the entire daily dose at bedtime may promote sleep, reduce daytime sedation, and possibly reduce the awareness of other adverse effects. Patients who experience insomnia and stimulation from the drugs may receive the entire daily dose in the morning.

■ **Dosage** There is a wide range of tricyclic antidepressant dosage requirements among patients, and dosage must be carefully individualized. Monitoring of plasma drug concentrations may be useful depending on the specific drug administered and clinical situation. Initially, tricyclic antidepressants are usually given in small dosages which are gradually increased according to the response and tolerance of the patient. Hospitalized patients under close supervision may generally be given higher dosages than outpatients; geriatric and adolescent patients should usually be given lower than average dosages. Maximum antidepressant effects may not occur for 2 or more weeks after therapy is begun.

After symptoms are controlled, dosage should be gradually reduced to the lowest level which will maintain relief of symptoms. The duration of tricyclic antidepressant therapy depends on the condition being treated, but maintenance therapy is usually continued for several months after a remission is achieved. To avoid the possibility of precipitating withdrawal symptoms, tricyclic antidepressants should not be terminated abruptly in patients who have received a high dosage for a prolonged period.

Patients receiving tricyclic antidepressants should be monitored for possible worsening of depression, suicidality, or unusual changes in behavior, especially at the beginning of therapy or during periods of dosage adjustment. (See Cautions: Precautions and Contraindications.)

Cautions

Minor adverse effects associated with tricyclic antidepressants generally reflect the drugs' anticholinergic and CNS activities. Serious reactions requiring discontinuance of therapy are relatively rare. Tolerance usually develops to sedative and anticholinergic effects and to postural hypotension; therefore, these adverse effects can be minimized by starting therapy with a low dosage and gradually increasing the dosage. Although all of the following adverse effects have not been reported for each tricyclic antidepressant, the possibility that each reaction may occur with any of the drugs should be kept in mind.

■ **Anticholinergic Effects** The most common adverse effects of tricyclic antidepressants are those which result from anticholinergic activity. These include dry mucous membranes (occasionally associated with sublingual adenitis), blurred vision resulting from mydriasis and cycloplegia, increased intraocular pressure, hyperthermia, constipation, adynamic ileus, urinary retention, delayed micturition, and dilation of the urinary tract. The drugs have been reported to reduce the tone of the esophagogastric sphincter and to induce hiatal hernia in susceptible individuals or to exacerbate the condition in patients with preexisting hiatal hernias. Tricyclic antidepressants should be withdrawn if symptoms of esophageal reflux develop; if antidepressant therapy is essential, a cautious trial of a cholinergic agent such as bethanechol used concomitantly with the antidepressant may be warranted. Anticholinergic effects appear to occur most frequently in geriatric patients, but constipation is frequent in children receiving tricyclic antidepressants for functional enuresis.

■ **Nervous System Effects** Adverse CNS and neuromuscular effects occur frequently. Drowsiness is the most frequent adverse reaction to tricyclic antidepressants; weakness, lethargy, and fatigue are also common. Conversely, agitation, excitement, nightmares, restlessness, and insomnia have occurred. Headache also has been reported. Confusion, disturbed concentration, disorientation, delusions, and hallucinations may occur, most commonly in geriatric patients. Children receiving tricyclic antidepressants for functional enuresis may experience drowsiness, anxiety, emotional instability, nervousness, and sleep disorders. Although effects differ among individual patients, sedative effects are usually greatest with amitriptyline or doxepin and least with protriptyline.

Worsening of depression and/or emergence of suicidal ideation and behavior (suicidality) or unusual changes in behavior may occur with antidepressants. (See Cautions: Precautions and Contraindications.)

Exacerbation of hypomania, panic, troublesome hostility, anxiety, or euphoria may occur in patients receiving tricyclic antidepressants. Exacerbation of psychosis has occurred in patients with schizophrenia or paranoid symptoms treated with the drugs; patients with bipolar depression may shift to the manic phase. Such psychotic manifestations should be treated by decreasing the dosage of tricyclic antidepressant or by administering an antipsychotic agent with the antidepressant. Alteration in EEG patterns and occasionally seizures have occurred. Seizures are more common in children than in adults. Coma also has occurred.

Extrapyramidal symptoms, including abnormal involuntary movements and tardive dyskinesia, may occur in patients receiving tricyclic antidepressants. A persistent fine tremor may occur in young as well as older patients, while the parkinsonian syndrome, when it occurs, is most common in geriatric patients receiving high dosages. Other extrapyramidal effects include rigidity, akathisia, dystonia, oculogyric crisis, opisthotonos, dysarthria, and dysphagia. Like antipsychotic agents, amoxapine and amitriptyline (with or without concomitant drugs known to cause neuroleptic malignant syndrome [NMS]) have been associated with NMS, a potentially fatal syndrome requiring immediate discontinuance of the drug and intensive symptomatic treatment. For additional information on NMS, see Extrapyramidal Reactions under Cautions: Nervous System Effects, in the Phenothiazines General Statement 28:16.08.24.

Peripheral neuropathy, dizziness, tinnitus, dysarthria, numbness, tingling and paresthesia, incoordination, ataxia or unsteadiness, and falling also have been reported in patients receiving tricyclic antidepressants.

■ **Cardiovascular Effects** Postural hypotension may occur during tricyclic antidepressant therapy. Other cardiovascular effects of the drugs include T-wave abnormalities (primarily flattening of the T-wave) and other alterations in ECG patterns; conduction disturbances such as bundle branch blocks and atrioventricular blocks; various arrhythmias such as palpitation, tachycardia (including ventricular tachycardia and torsades de pointes), bradycardia, ventricular fibrillation, ventricular premature complexes, and ventricular extrasystoles; syncope; collapse; sudden death; hypotension; hypertension; thrombosis and thrombophlebitis; stroke; and congestive heart failure. In at least one patient (an 8-year-old boy) receiving desipramine for 2 years for hyperactivity†, collapse and sudden death occurred; sudden death also has been reported in other children receiving desipramine. (See Cautions: Precautions and Contraindications and see also Pediatric Precautions.)

Patients with preexisting cardiovascular disease may be especially sensitive to the cardiotoxicity of tricyclic antidepressants. In addition, those with disturbed eating behaviors (e.g., purging) that result in inadequate hydration and/or compromised cardiac status also may be at greater risk of severe adverse cardiovascular effects (e.g., hypotension, increased cardiac conduction time, arrhythmia).

Hypertensive episodes have occurred during surgery in patients receiving tricyclic antidepressants, and the drugs should be discontinued several days prior to elective surgery. In patients with cardiovascular disease receiving therapeutic dosages of tricyclic antidepressants, the drugs have been reported to increase the incidence of sudden death. Although myocardial infarction has been attributed to therapy with tricyclic antidepressants, a causal relationship has not been established.

■ **Hematologic Effects** Rarely, agranulocytosis, thrombocytopenia, eosinophilia, leukopenia, and purpura have been reported and may be hypersensitivity reactions. Death related to eosinophilia has been reported in at least one adolescent (14 years of age) receiving desipramine therapy. Leukocyte and differential counts should be performed in all patients who develop symptoms of blood dyscrasias, such as sore throat and fever, and tricyclic antidepressants should be discontinued if evidence of pathologic neutrophil depression is found.

■ **Hepatic Effects** Asymptomatic increases in serum aminotransferase (transaminase) concentrations, changes in serum alkaline phosphatase concentrations, obstructive-type jaundice, and hepatitis which appear to be allergic in nature have also occurred during therapy with tricyclic antidepressants. Elevated values on liver function tests indicate the need for repeat tests; if progressive elevations occur, the drugs should be discontinued. Jaundice and hepatitis are reversible following discontinuance of the drugs; however, deaths resulting from hepatitis have occurred when tricyclic antidepressants were continued. Hepatic failure has been reported in patients receiving amitriptyline; however, a causal relationship to the drug could not be established.

■ **Sensitivity Reactions** Allergic manifestations have included rash and erythema, petechiae, urticaria, pruritus, eosinophilia, edema (general or of face and tongue), drug fever, and photosensitivity. Patients who demonstrate photosensitivity should avoid exposure to sunlight. A lupus-like syndrome (migratory arthritis, positive ANA and rheumatoid factor) has been reported in patients receiving amitriptyline; however, a causal relationship to the drug could not be established.

■ **GI Effects** Adverse GI effects such as anorexia, nausea and vomiting, diarrhea, abdominal cramps, increases in pancreatic enzymes, epigastric distress, stomatitis, peculiar taste, and black tongue have been reported in patients receiving tricyclic antidepressants. Ageusia has been reported in patients receiving amitriptyline; however, a causal relationship to the drug could not be established.

■ **Endocrine and Genitourinary Effects** Endocrine and genitourinary effects that have occurred in patients receiving tricyclic antidepressants include increased or decreased libido, impotence, testicular swelling, painful ejaculation, anorgasmia, breast engorgement and galactorrhea in females, gynecomastia in males, and elevation or lowering of blood glucose concentrations. The syndrome of inappropriate secretion of antidiuretic hormone (SIADH) also has been reported.

Paradoxically, urinary frequency and nocturia have been reported.

■ **Other Adverse Effects** In addition, some patients have developed headache, alopecia, flushing, chills, diaphoresis, interstitial pneumonitis, parotid swelling, nasal congestion, increased appetite, and weight gain or loss.

■ **Precautions and Contraindications** Worsening of depression and/or the emergence of suicidal ideation and behavior (suicidality) or unusual changes in behavior may occur in both adult and pediatric (see Cautions: Pediatric Precautions) patients with major depressive disorder or other psychiatric disorders, whether or not they are taking antidepressants. This risk may persist until clinically important remission occurs. Suicide is a known risk of depression and certain other psychiatric disorders, and these disorders themselves are the strongest predictors of suicide. However, there has been a long-standing concern that antidepressants may have a role in inducing worsening of depression and the emergence of suicidality in certain patients during the early phases of treatment. Pooled analyses of short-term, placebo-controlled studies of antidepressants (i.e., selective serotonin-reuptake inhibitors and other antidepressants) have shown an increased risk of suicidality in children, adolescents, and young adults (18–24 years of age) with major depressive disorder and other psychiatric disorders. An increased suicidality risk was not demonstrated with antidepressants compared with placebo in adults older than 24 years of age, and a reduced risk was observed in adults 65 years of age or older. It currently is unknown whether the suicidality risk extends to longer-term use (i.e., beyond several months); however, there is substantial evidence from placebo-controlled maintenance trials in adults with major depressive disorder that antidepressants can delay the recurrence of depression.

The US Food and Drug Administration (FDA) recommends that all patients being treated with antidepressants for any indication be appropriately monitored and closely observed for clinical worsening, suicidality, and unusual changes in behavior, particularly during initiation of therapy (i.e., the first few months) and during periods of dosage adjustments. Families and caregivers of patients being treated with antidepressants for major depressive disorder or other indications, both psychiatric and nonpsychiatric, also should be advised to monitor patients on a daily basis for the emergence of agitation, irritability, or unusual changes in behavior as well as the emergence of suicidality, and to report such symptoms immediately to a health-care provider.

Although a causal relationship between the emergence of symptoms such as anxiety, agitation, panic attacks, insomnia, irritability, hostility, aggressiveness, impulsivity, akathisia, hypomania, and/or mania and either the worsening of depression and/or the emergence of suicidal impulses has not been established, there is concern that such symptoms may represent precursors to emerging suicidality. Consequently, consideration should be given to changing the therapeutic regimen or discontinuing therapy in patients whose depression is persistently worse or in patients experiencing emergent suicidality or symptoms that might be precursors to worsening depression or suicidality, particularly if such manifestations are severe, abrupt in onset, or were not part of the patient's presenting symptoms. If a decision is made to discontinue therapy, tricyclic antidepressant dosage should be tapered as rapidly as is feasible but with recognition of the risks of abrupt discontinuance. (See Dosage and Administration: Dosage.) FDA also recommends that the drugs be prescribed in the smallest quantity consistent with good patient management, in order to reduce the risk of overdosage.

It is generally believed (though not established in controlled trials) that treating a major depressive episode with an antidepressant alone may increase the likelihood of precipitating a mixed or manic episode in patients at risk for bipolar disorder. Therefore, patients should be adequately screened for bipolar disorder prior to initiating treatment with an antidepressant; such screening should include a detailed psychiatric history (e.g., family history of suicide, bipolar disorder, and depression). Tricyclic antidepressants are *not* approved for use in treating bipolar depression. (See Uses: Bipolar Disorder.)

Tricyclic antidepressants should be used with caution in patients for whom excess anticholinergic activity could be harmful, such as those with benign prostatic hypertrophy, a history of urinary retention, increased intraocular pressure, or angle-closure glaucoma. Patients who exhibit symptoms of angle-closure glaucoma should not receive the drugs until the cause of the symptoms is determined, and glaucoma should be corrected before treatment with tricyclic antidepressants is initiated. Patients whose glaucoma is adequately controlled by drugs should be closely monitored during therapy with tricyclic antidepressants, because tricyclic antidepressants may precipitate an attack of angle-closure glaucoma. The risk of hyperthermia should be considered when tricyclic antidepressants are used concomitantly with other drugs possessing anticholinergic activity and/or that affect thermoregulation (e.g., antimuscarinics, phenothiazines), particularly during hot weather. The toxic potential of tricyclic antidepressants (e.g., cardiotoxic effects with overdosage) relative to available alternative therapies should be considered in clinical decisions.

Patients should be warned that tricyclic antidepressants may impair their ability to perform hazardous activities requiring mental alertness or physical coordination such as operating machinery or driving a motor vehicle.

Tricyclic antidepressants should be administered with caution to patients with thyroid disease or patients receiving thyroid agents. (See Drug Interactions: Thyroid Agents.)

Respiratory failure resulting from CNS depression has occurred in a patient with chronic bronchitis receiving a tricyclic antidepressant, and the drugs should be used cautiously in individuals with respiratory difficulties.

Tricyclic antidepressants may lower the seizure threshold and should be used with caution in patients with a history of seizure disorders, organic brain disease, or who may be predisposed to seizures (e.g., in the acute withdrawal phase of alcoholism). The manufacturers of desipramine state that seizures may precede cardiac arrhythmias and death in some patients.

Tricyclic antidepressants are contraindicated in the acute recovery phase following myocardial infarction. The drugs should be used with extreme caution in patients with preexisting cardiovascular disease because tricyclic antidepressants may cause adverse cardiovascular effects. The manufacturers of desipramine also state that the drug should be used with extreme caution in patients who have a family history of sudden death, cardiac arrhythmias, or cardiac conduction disturbances. (See Cautions: Cardiovascular Effects.) If use of tricyclic antidepressants in patients with preexisting cardiovascular disease is deemed essential, patients should be closely monitored and ECG tracings performed periodically. In addition, all patients receiving higher than usual dosages should have periodic ECG tracings, regardless of the presence or absence of cardiac abnormalities prior to treatment.

Individual tricyclic antidepressants are contraindicated in patients who have demonstrated hypersensitivity to them. Cross-sensitivity among the drugs has been reported, and should be considered when switching patients from one tricyclic antidepressant to another because of a hypersensitivity reaction.

The manufacturers of amitriptyline hydrochloride and protriptyline hydrochloride state that these drugs are contraindicated in patients taking cisapride because of the possibility of adverse cardiac effects, including cardiac arrhythmias and conduction disturbances (e.g., prolongation of the QT interval).

■ **Pediatric Precautions** Safety and efficacy of amitriptyline, amoxapine, clomipramine, desipramine, nortriptyline, protriptyline, or trimipramine in pediatric patients have not been established. The manufacturers state that amoxapine should not be used in children younger than 16 years of age, amitriptyline should not be used in children younger than 12 years of age, and clomipramine should not be used in children younger than 10 years of age. Use of doxepin in children younger than 12 years of age for depressive and/or anxiety disorders is not recommended because safety has not been established; safety and efficacy of doxepin for insomnia in pediatric patients have not been established.

Imipramine is used for the treatment of enuresis in children 6 years of age or older, but safety and efficacy of the drug for the treatment of enuresis in younger children or for the treatment of any other condition in pediatric patients have not been established.

Collapse and sudden death occurred in at least one child (an 8-year-old boy) receiving desipramine for 2 years for attention deficit hyperactivity disorder† and sudden death also has been reported in other children receiving the drug. Although a causal relationship between the use of desipramine and the risk of sudden death has not been established, many clinicians recommend that desipramine *not* be used for the treatment of attention deficit hyperactivity disorder in children when tricyclic antidepressant therapy is contemplated.

In addition, FDA warns that antidepressants increase the risk of suicidal thinking and behavior (suicidality) in children and adolescents with major depressive disorder and other psychiatric disorders. The risk of suicidality for these drugs was identified in a pooled analysis of data from a total of 24 short-term (4–16 weeks), placebo-controlled studies of 9 antidepressants (i.e., bupropion, citalopram, fluoxetine, fluvoxamine, mirtazapine, nefazodone, paroxetine, sertraline, venlafaxine) in over 4400 children and adolescents with major depressive disorder, obsessive-compulsive disorder (OCD), or other psychiatric disorders. The analysis revealed a greater risk of adverse events representing suicidal behavior or thinking (suicidality) during the first few months of treatment in pediatric patients receiving antidepressants than in those receiving placebo. The average risk of such events was 4% among children and adolescents receiving these drugs, twice the risk (2%) that was observed among those receiving placebo. However, a more recent meta-analysis of 27 placebo-controlled trials of 9 antidepressants (SSRIs and others) in patients younger than 19 years of age with major depressive disorder, OCD, or non-OCD anxiety disorders suggests that the benefits of antidepressant therapy in treating these conditions may outweigh the risks of suicidal behavior or suicidal ideation. No suicides occurred in these pediatric trials.

The risk of suicidality in the FDA's pooled analysis differed across the various psychiatric indications, with the highest incidence observed in the major depressive disorder studies. In addition, although there was considerable variation in risk among the antidepressants, a tendency toward an increase in suicidality risk in younger patients was found for almost all drugs studied. It is currently unknown whether the suicidality risk in pediatric patients extends to longer-term use (i.e., beyond several months).

As a result of this analysis and public discussion of the issue, FDA has directed manufacturers of all antidepressants to add a boxed warning to the labeling of their products to alert clinicians of this suicidality risk in children and adolescents and to recommend appropriate monitoring and close observation of patients receiving these agents. (See Cautions: Precautions and Contraindications.) The drugs that are the focus of the revised labeling are all drugs included in the general class of antidepressants, including those that have not been studied in controlled clinical trials in pediatric patients, since the available data are not adequate to exclude any single antidepressant from an increased risk. In addition to the boxed warning and other information in professional labeling on antidepressants, FDA currently recommends that a patient medication guide explaining the risks associated with the drugs be provided to the patient each time the drugs are dispensed.

Anyone considering the use of an antidepressant in a child or adolescent for any clinical use must balance the potential risk of therapy with the clinical need.

■ **Geriatric Precautions** Clinical experience to date with the various tricyclic antidepressants in geriatric patients has not identified any differences in responses between geriatric and younger adults. However, safety and efficacy of tricyclic antidepressants have not been systematically studied in geriatric patients.

In pooled data analyses, a *reduced* risk of suicidality was observed in adults 65 years of age or older with antidepressant therapy compared with placebo. (See Cautions: Precautions and Contraindications.)

Most manufacturers recommend that therapy in geriatric patients be initiated cautiously using a low initial dosage and that patients be observed closely since renal, hepatic, and cardiovascular dysfunction and concomitant disease or other drug therapy are more common in this age group than in younger patients. Cardiovascular function, particularly arrhythmias and fluctuations in blood pressure, should be monitored. Geriatric patients appear to be especially sensitive to anticholinergic (e.g., dry mouth, constipation, vision disturbance), cardiovascular, orthostatic hypotension, and sedative effects of tricyclic antidepressants. Adverse hepatic events (principally characterized by jaundice and elevated liver enzymes) have been observed very rarely in geriatric patients and deaths associated with cholestatic liver damage have been reported in isolated instances.

Renal damage manifested by confusion, disorientation, and increased BUN and serum creatinine concentration was reported in a geriatric patient receiving 300 mg of imipramine hydrochloride daily.

Plasma concentrations of the active nortriptyline metabolite, 10-hydroxynortriptyline, have been reported to be higher in geriatric patients than in younger patients.

Geriatric patients may be at risk of drug-induced toxicity when treated with desipramine, a tricyclic antidepressant that is known to be eliminated mainly by the kidneys. In this patient population, the ratio of the principal metabolite, 2-hydroxydesipramine, to desipramine appears to be increased, most likely because of decreased renal elimination that occurs with aging. Therefore, particular attention should be paid to desipramine dosage and it may be useful to monitor renal function in these patients. Desipramine use in geriatric patients also has been associated with an increased risk of falling and mental confusion.

■ **Pregnancy and Lactation** Safe use of tricyclic antidepressants in pregnancy has not been established. Teratogenic effects occurred in reproduction studies evaluating amitriptyline in mice, rats, and rabbits, and embryotoxicity, fetotoxic effects (intrauterine death, stillbirth, decreased birth weight), or decreased postnatal survival have been reported in reproduction studies in animals evaluating amoxapine, clomipramine, or trimipramine. Although a causal relationship was not established, fetal malformations (including limb deformities) and developmental delay have been reported in neonates whose mothers received a tricyclic antidepressant (e.g., amitriptyline, imipramine) during pregnancy. In addition, urinary retention, CNS effects (including lethargy), and withdrawal symptoms (including jitteriness, tremor, seizures) have occurred in neonates whose mothers received a tricyclic antidepressant during pregnancy. Tricyclic antidepressants should not be used in pregnant women or women who may become pregnant unless the possible benefits outweigh the potential risks to the fetus.

Smoking cessation programs consisting of behavioral and educational rather than pharmacologic interventions should be tried in pregnant women before drug therapy is considered. Smoking cessation† therapy with a tricyclic antidepressant (e.g., nortriptyline), which is a second-line agent, should be used during pregnancy only if the increased likelihood of smoking cessation, with its potential benefits, justifies the potential risk to the fetus and patient of tricyclic therapy and possible continued smoking, and first-line pharmacotherapy (e.g., bupropion, nicotine replacement) has failed. Although smoking cessation prior to conception or early in pregnancy is most beneficial, health benefits result from cessation at anytime; therefore, effective smoking cessation interventions should be offered at the first prenatal visit and persist throughout the course of pregnancy for women who continue smoking after conception.

Amitriptyline, amoxapine, clomipramine, desipramine, doxepin, imipramine, and nortriptyline are distributed into milk, and it is likely that other tricyclic antidepressants also are distributed into milk. There has been at least one report of apnea and drowsiness in a nursing infant whose mother was receiving doxepin. Because of the potential for serious adverse reactions to tricyclic antidepressants in nursing infants, a decision should be made whether to discontinue nursing or the drug, taking into account the importance of the drug to the woman.

Drug Interactions

■ **Monoamine Oxidase Inhibitors** Concomitant administration of tricyclic antidepressants and monoamine oxidase (MAO) inhibitors is contraindicated, and it generally is recommended that at least 2 weeks should elapse between discontinuance of tricyclic antidepressant therapy or MAO inhibitor therapy and initiation of therapy with the other class of drugs. Serious, sometimes fatal, reactions including hyperpyrexia, confusion, diaphoresis, myoclonus, rigidity, seizures, cardiovascular disturbances, and coma have occurred in patients who received a tricyclic antidepressant and an MAO inhibitor concomitantly. Patients receiving therapeutic dosages of an oral tricyclic antidepressant and an oral MAO inhibitor concomitantly generally have experienced nonfatal hyperpyrexia, hypertension, tachycardia, confusion, and seizures; most reported cases of hyperpyretic crises, severe seizures, or death occurred following overdosage or parenteral administration of 1 or both drugs. Although the mechanism has not been clearly established, these reactions resemble serotonin syndrome and may be caused by excessive serotonergic activity in the CNS. The possibility of these reactions should also be considered in patients receiving tricyclic antidepressants and other drugs with MAO inhibitor activity (e.g., procarbazine).

For further information on serotonin syndrome, including manifestations and treatment, see Serotonin Syndrome under Drug Interactions: Drugs Associated with Serotonin Syndrome, in Fluoxetine Hydrochloride 28:16.04.20.

■ **Hypotensive Agents** With the exception of doxepin in dosages less than 150 mg daily, tricyclic antidepressants block the uptake of guanethidine and similarly acting compounds into adrenergic neurons, and thus prevent their hypotensive activity.

Tricyclic antidepressants (i.e., imipramine, desipramine) have reportedly inhibited the hypotensive effect of clonidine. The increase in blood pressure usually occurs during the second week of tricyclic antidepressant therapy, but occasionally may occur during the first several days of concomitant therapy. The possibility of this interaction should be considered in patients receiving tricyclic antidepressants and clonidine concomitantly; blood pressure should be closely monitored during the first several weeks of concurrent therapy, and dosage of clonidine should be increased to adequately control hypertension if necessary. Alternatively, other hypotensive agents that do not interact with tricyclic antidepressants may be substituted, but clonidine therapy should *not* be discontinued abruptly. If tricyclic antidepressant therapy is discontinued in patients receiving clonidine, the hypotensive effect of clonidine may increase; blood pressure should be monitored and dosage of clonidine reduced if necessary. The possibility that this interaction may also occur in patients receiving guanabenz and tricyclic antidepressants concomitantly should also be considered. In rats, concurrent administration of clonidine and amitriptyline has produced corneal lesions within 5 days.

Tricyclic antidepressants may decrease the antihypertensive effect of rauwolfia alkaloids (no longer commercially available in the US). A stimulating effect has been reported in some depressed patients receiving tricyclic therapy after administration of reserpine.

■ **CNS Depressants** Tricyclic antidepressants may be additive with or may potentiate the action of CNS depressants such as alcohol, sedatives, or hypnotics. Barbiturates may potentiate the adverse effects, including respiratory depression, produced by toxic doses of tricyclic antidepressants. With therapeutic doses of tricyclic antidepressants, barbiturates appear to stimulate metabolism and decrease blood concentrations of tricyclic antidepressants. The clinical importance of this effect has not been established, but the possibility of reduced therapeutic efficacy must be considered.

Concomitant administration of ethchlorvynol and amitriptyline has been reported to produce transient delirium. Pending further documentation of this interaction, ethchlorvynol should be used with caution in patients receiving tricyclic antidepressants.

Although some studies showed no substantial alteration of plasma tricyclic antidepressant concentrations during simultaneous administration of benzodiazepines, one study indicated that the half-life and steady-state plasma concentrations of amitriptyline may be increased in patients receiving diazepam. The clinical importance of this possible interaction has not been determined. There have been reports of impaired motor function when tricyclic antidepressants were used with benzodiazepines, but these have not been confirmed and the drugs have often been administered concomitantly with no adverse effects.

The manufacturer of protriptyline states that tricyclic antidepressants may increase the seizure risk in patients taking tramadol hydrochloride.

■ **Antipsychotic Agents** Various phenothiazines and haloperidol have been shown to inhibit metabolism and increase blood concentrations of tricyclic antidepressants. Although the clinical importance has not been established, dosages of both drugs should be carefully adjusted whenever antipsychotics are given with tricyclic antidepressants.

■ **Sympathomimetic and Anticholinergic Agents** Concomitant administration of tricyclic antidepressants with sympathomimetic drugs such as isoproterenol, phenylephrine, norepinephrine, epinephrine, or amphetamines may increase sympathetic activity to the extent that pressor and cardiac effects of the sympathomimetics could be fatal. If tricyclic antidepressants are used with adrenergic agents, dosage must be monitored closely.

Additive anticholinergic effects of tricyclic antidepressants and other agents with parasympatholytic activity require careful dosage adjustment if the drugs are given concomitantly. Concomitant administration of tricyclic antidepressants and anticholinergic agents has been reported to produce hyperthermia, particularly during hot weather, and paralytic ileus.

■ **Drugs Affecting Hepatic Microsomal Enzymes** Tricyclic antidepressants are metabolized by various isoenzymes of the cytochrome P-450 (CYP) microsomal enzyme system, including CYP1A2, CYP2D6, CYP3A4, and CYP2C isoenzymes. (See Pharmacokinetics: Elimination.) Drugs that inhibit the activity of the cytochrome P-450 2D6 (CYP2D6) isoenzyme may increase plasma concentrations of tricyclic antidepressants to such an extent that extensive metabolizers of tricyclics may resemble poor metabolizers of the drugs. Drugs that inhibit cytochrome CYP2D6 include some drugs that are not metabolized by the enzyme (e.g., quinidine, cimetidine) and many that are substrates for CYP2D6 (e.g., flecainide, phenothiazines, propafenone, selective serotonin-reuptake inhibitors [SSRIs], other antidepressants). A patient who is stable on a given dose of a tricyclic antidepressant may abruptly experience symptoms of toxicity when given concomitant therapy with a drug that inhibits CYP2D6. Concomitant use of tricyclic antidepressants with drugs that inhibit CYP2D6 may necessitate lower dosages than usually prescribed for either the tricyclic or the other drug. In addition, whenever such drugs are discontinued, an increased dosage of the tricyclic antidepressant may be necessary. The manufacturers recommend that plasma concentrations of tricyclics be monitored whenever a tricyclic is coadministered with another drug known to be an inhibitor of CYP2D6.

Quinidine Concomitant administration of quinidine and nortriptyline may result in a substantially longer plasma half-life, increased area under the plasma concentration-time curve, and decreased clearance of nortriptyline. In addition, quinidine reportedly decreased the clearance of desipramine and imipramine.

Selective Serotonin-Reuptake Inhibitors While all the selective serotonin-reuptake inhibitors (SSRIs) (e.g., citalopram, fluoxetine, paroxetine, sertraline) inhibit CYP2D6, there appears to be considerable variability among the SSRIs in the extent to which they inhibit this isoenzyme. Paroxetine and fluoxetine appear to be more potent in this regard than sertraline, fluvoxamine, venlafaxine, or citalopram (only weakly inhibitory).

Fluvoxamine is a potent inhibitor of CYP1A2, and increased plasma concentrations (increases ranging from 1- to 8-fold) and clinical signs of tricyclic toxicity have occurred when the drug was administered in patients receiving amitriptyline, clomipramine, desipramine, or imipramine.

The extent to which the interaction between SSRIs and tricyclic antidepressants may become clinically important depends on the extent of inhibition of the cytochrome isoenzymes and the pharmacokinetics of the concomitantly administered SSRI. Nevertheless, tricyclics and SSRIs should be used concomitantly with caution, and the dosage of the tricyclic should be reduced. In addition, the manufacturers of several tricyclics recommend a drug-free interval when switching from therapy with an SSRI to a tricyclic antidepressant. In particular, at least 5 weeks should elapse before initiating tricyclic antidepressant therapy in a patient being withdrawn from fluoxetine, given the long half-life of fluoxetine and its active metabolite.

Concurrent use of a tricyclic antidepressant (e.g., nortriptyline, desipramine, imipramine) and fluoxetine reportedly has resulted in adverse effects associated with tricyclic toxicity (including sedation, decreased energy, lightheadedness, psychomotor retardation, dry mouth, constipation, memory impairment) and/or greater than twofold elevations in plasma tricyclic antidepressant concentrations. There have been very rare cases of serotonin syndrome reported in patients receiving amitriptyline in conjunction with other serotonergic drugs.

Cimetidine Cimetidine, apparently through inhibition of hepatic microsomal enzyme systems, reduces the hepatic metabolism of some tricyclic antidepressants (i.e., amitriptyline, desipramine, imipramine). Concomitant administration of cimetidine and these tricyclic antidepressants may result in decreased tricyclic antidepressant clearance and increased bioavailabilities, elimination half-lives, or peak plasma and/or steady-state concentrations. Frequency and severity of antidepressant-induced adverse effects, especially anticholinergic effects, have increased during concomitant administration of cimetidine and tricyclic antidepressants. A reduction in tricyclic antidepressant dosage may be necessary if cimetidine is initiated in a patient receiving one of these antidepressants; conversely, an increase in dosage of the antidepressant may be necessary if cimetidine is discontinued. Ranitidine appears to be less likely to interact with tricyclic antidepressants than cimetidine.

■ **Levodopa** Tricyclic antidepressants may delay gastric emptying as a result of their anticholinergic activity. Absorption of drugs such as levodopa, which is absorbed from the intestine, may be delayed sufficiently to permit inactivation in the stomach. Careful dosage monitoring is essential when such drugs are administered with tricyclic antidepressants.

■ **Anticoagulants** Nortriptyline and amitriptyline have been reported to increase plasma concentrations of dicumarol, and amitriptyline has also increased the prothrombin time in patients stabilized on warfarin. The mechanism is as yet unknown but may involve inhibition of anticoagulant metabolism or decrease in intestinal motility, thereby increasing the time available for absorption of the anticoagulant.

■ **Cisapride** The manufacturers of amitriptyline hydrochloride and protriptyline hydrochloride state that these drugs are contraindicated in patients taking cisapride because of the possibility of adverse cardiac effects, including cardiac arrhythmias and conduction disturbances (e.g., prolongation of the QT interval).

■ **Thyroid Agents** Levothyroxine and liothyronine have been reported to accelerate the onset of therapeutic effects of tricyclic antidepressants; however, concomitant use may also produce cardiovascular toxicity, including arrhythmias. Tricyclic antidepressants should be administered with extreme caution to patients who have thyroid disease or who are receiving thyroid agents.

■ **Methylphenidate** Methylphenidate has been reported to inhibit the metabolism of tricyclic antidepressants and to increase their effectiveness; presumably, the toxicity of tricyclic antidepressants could also be increased.

■ **Antidiabetic Agents** Substantial hypoglycemia occurred in one patient with type 2 diabetes mellitus receiving chlorpropamide 250 mg daily after nortriptyline 125 mg daily was initiated.

Acute Toxicity

■ **Pathogenesis** The toxic dose of tricyclic antidepressants varies considerably. Generally, tricyclic antidepressant doses of approximately 10–20 mg/kg are associated with moderate to severe toxicity, and doses of 30–40 mg/kg are often fatal in adults. The lowest known fatal adult dose of amitriptyline is 500 mg, but 1 patient survived after ingesting 10 g of the drug. Although the average acute lethal dose of imipramine for adults has been estimated to be 30 mg/kg, fatalities have occurred in adults who received 500 mg of the drug. Some patients have survived reported nortriptyline ingestions of up to 525 mg. Severe symptoms or death occur in children who receive more than 20 mg/kg of imipramine. Death was reported in a 5-year-old child who inadvertently received a single 500-mg dose of imipramine for the treatment of enuresis. Desipramine overdosage has resulted in a higher death rate compared with overdosages of other tricyclic antidepressants. Patients with preexisting cardiac disease, patients with disturbed eating behaviors (e.g., purging) that result in inadequate hydration and/or compromised cardiac status, and children appear to be somewhat more susceptible to tricyclic antidepressant-induced cardiotoxicity than healthy adults.

The manufacturers state that ingestion of multiple drugs, including alcohol, is common in patients who deliberately ingest overdoses of tricyclic antidepressants.

■ **Manifestations** Overdosage of tricyclic antidepressants produces symptoms that are primarily extensions of common adverse reactions.

Following a latent period that may last approximately 1–12 hours, CNS stimulation, which may result in part from excess anticholinergic activity, usually occurs initially. Peripheral anticholinergic symptoms which occur in overdose include urinary retention, dry mucous membranes, mydriasis, constipation, and occasionally adynamic ileus.

Severe CNS depression usually follows the initial stimulation. The patient may exhibit extreme drowsiness, areflexia, hypothermia, respiratory depression, cyanosis, severe hypotension, depressed level of consciousness, and coma.

The most important cardiovascular effects of tricyclic antidepressants in overdosage are their quinidine-like effects on cardiac conduction, particularly decreased intraventricular conduction as manifested by QRS interval prolongation. Data suggest that ECG changes, particularly in the QRS axis or width (i.e., prolongation of the QRS interval to 100 msec or greater), may be clinically important indicators of the severity of tricyclic antidepressant overdosage (although possibly not in the case of amoxapine). The manufacturers of desipramine state that early changes in the QRS complex include a widening of the terminal 40 msec with a rightward axis in the frontal plane, which is recognized by the presence of a terminal S wave in lead 1 and AVL and an R wave in AVR. The manufacturers of desipramine further state that prolongation of the maximal limb-lead QRS interval to greater than 100 msec is a clinically significant indicator of desipramine toxicity, particularly for the risk of seizures and, eventually, cardiac dysrhythmias. Although QRS prolongation usually is associated with total plasma tricyclic concentrations greater than 1000 ng/mL, it is possible to have high plasma tricyclic concentrations without evidence of substantial ECG abnormalities. A fatal arrhythmia, which occurred as late as 56 hours after an amitriptyline overdose, has been reported.

Acid-base disturbances may occur in acute tricyclic intoxication. Acidosis, which appears to be the most frequent acid-base disturbance, may be metabolic and/or respiratory in origin and usually results from hypotension, hypoventilation, and/or seizures. Occasional manifestations of tricyclic antidepressant overdosage have included ataxia, dysarthria, bullous cutaneous lesions, vermiculation, polyradiculoneuropathy, renal failure, vomiting, and pulmonary consolidation.

■ **Treatment** Treatment of tricyclic overdosage generally involves aggressive symptomatic and supportive care and serum alkalinization. Because signs and symptoms of toxicity may develop rapidly following tricyclic overdosage, hospital monitoring usually is required as soon as possible after ingestion. An ECG should be obtained and cardiac monitoring initiated immediately. Patients should be closely observed for a minimum of 6 hours for signs of CNS or respiratory depression, hypotension, seizures, and cardiac dysthythmias and/or conduction block. If signs of toxicity develop at any time during this period, extended monitoring is necessary. Late-onset, fatal dysrhythmias have been reported after an overdose; these patients had clinical evidence of substantial poisoning prior to death and most had received inadequate GI decontamination. Plasma concentrations of tricyclic antidepressants should not guide management of the patient. Support of cardiovascular and respiratory functions is critical. An adequate airway should be maintained; respiratory assistance may be necessary. The patient's temperature should be maintained; initial hyperthermia may be treated with ice packs, while patients with hypothermia should be kept warm. Fluid, acid-base, and electrolyte balance should be monitored frequently and corrected if necessary. In addition, renal function and plasma creatinine phosphokinase (CPK) concentrations should be monitored if clinically needed. External stimulation should be minimized to reduce the tendency to seizures.

Physical removal of tricyclic antidepressants from the GI tract generally should be attempted and activated charcoal administered to decrease absorption even several hours after ingestion, because the anticholinergic effects of the tricyclic antidepressants may delay gastric emptying and the drugs also may be secreted into the stomach. Gastric lavage, preferably followed by the instillation of activated charcoal, is sometimes recommended (since CNS depression can develop rapidly) if an endotracheal tube with cuff inflated is in place to prevent aspiration of gastric contents. Emesis generally is contraindicated in tricyclic intoxication. Tricyclic antidepressants are highly protein bound, so peritoneal dialysis and hemodialysis are not effective in removing the drugs. Forced diuresis also eliminates very little drug and may be dangerous if cardiac function is impaired.

IV benzodiazepines (e.g., diazepam) generally are considered to be the drugs of choice for treatment of seizures; however, they should be used with caution since respiratory and CNS depression may result. If benzodiazepines are ineffective or if seizures recur, other drugs with anticonvulsant activity (e.g., phenobarbital, propofol) may be used. Barbiturates generally should *not* be used as they may enhance respiratory depression, but the drugs may be useful in seizures refractory to diazepam.

In patients with substantial cardiovascular toxicity (e.g., QRS widening greater than 100 msec on the ECG, cardiac conduction disturbances and arrhythmias, hypotension), serum alkalinization with IV sodium bicarbonate (i.e., to achieve a systemic pH of 7.4–7.55) is recommended. Hyperventilation may be used to increase the pH if the response to sodium bicarbonate alone is inadequate. Some experts and manufacturers state that class IA (e.g., disopyramide, procainamide, quinidine), IC (e.g., flecainide, propafenone), and III (e.g., amiodarone, sotalol) antiarrhythmics and other antiarrhythmic agents that block the fast sodium channel generally are contraindicated in cases of poisoning with tricyclic antidepressants or other fast sodium channel blockers and in the management of conduction abnormalities and cardiac arrhythmias, because of the risk of synergistic toxicity (e.g., further depressed myocardial conduction and contractility). Administration of more than one antiarrhythmic agent may be required. Insertion of a temporary transvenous cardiac pacemaker may be necessary in patients with advanced AV block, severe bradycardia, and/or life-threatening ventricular arrhythmias unresponsive to drug therapy.

Tricyclic overdosage may result in central (e.g., delirium, agitation, myoclonus, coma) and peripheral (e.g., urinary retention, constipation) anticholinergic manifestations, but these signs and symptoms are generally not life-threatening. Although physostigmine has been used successfully in the treatment of tricyclic-induced anticholinergic toxicity, the drug currently is rarely used because of its potential to cause serious adverse effects, including seizures, bronchospasm, and bradyarrhythmias (including asystole). The precise role of physostigmine in the management of tricyclic overdosage remains controversial; most clinicians advise against the routine use of physostigmine in such cases, and some clinicians recommend that the drug be reserved only for treatment of life-threatening anticholinergic symptoms refractory to other forms of treatment.

Because the management of tricyclic antidepressant overdosage is complex and changing, clinicians should consult a poison control center for the most current information on treatment.

Patients whose overdosage was deliberate should be monitored especially carefully during recovery to prevent additional suicide attempts, and mental health counseling is usually necessary prior to and following medical discharge.

Chronic Toxicity

Abrupt withdrawal of tricyclic antidepressants following prolonged therapy and/or treatment with high doses may precipitate a syndrome consisting of akathisia, anxiety, chills, coryza, malaise, myalgia, headache, dizziness, nausea, and/or vomiting. In addition, irritability, restlessness, and dream and sleep disturbances reportedly may occur within 2 weeks when tricyclic antidepressant dosage is gradually reduced. Mania and hypomania have occurred rarely within 2–7 days following discontinuance of chronic tricyclic antidepressant therapy. Whether or not these symptoms are indicative of physical dependence is unclear.

Pharmacology

■ **Nervous System Effects** ***Antidepressant Effect*** The precise mechanism of antidepressant action of the tricyclic antidepressants is unclear, but the drugs have been shown to block, in varying degrees, the reuptake of various neurotransmitters at the neuronal membrane. The effects of norepinephrine and serotonin may thus be potentiated. In addition, tricyclic antidepressants exhibit strong anticholinergic activity. The antidepressant activity of these drugs may be related to any or all of these effects, although effects on norepinephrine and serotonin are generally regarded as the most important.

Effects on Animal Behavior In animals, tricyclic antidepressants are similar to phenothiazines in their effects on various avoidance behavior. Unlike the phenothiazines, however, tricyclic antidepressants potentiate the effects of norepinephrine, serotonin, amphetamines, and certain other CNS stimulants. Tricyclic antidepressants do not inhibit monoamine oxidase (MAO).

Effects on Sleep Tricyclic antidepressants produce varying degrees of sedation in patients with or without a history of depression. Tricyclic antidepressants decrease the number of awakenings, increase stage-4 sleep, and substantially increase the latency and decrease the total time spent in rapid eye movement (REM) sleep, which is typically more prominent and occurs earlier in the sleep of patients with depression. Tricyclic antidepressants appear to have greater sedative effects than secondary-amine antidepressants (bupropion) or selective serotonin-reuptake inhibitors (e.g., fluoxetine).

Effects on EEG Tricyclic antidepressants may produce abnormal EEG patterns in which the *alpha* activity decreases while *theta* activity increases. Some increase in *delta, beta*, and burst activity also occurs. The drugs also may lower the seizure threshold.

■ **Enuresis** The mechanism of action of the tricyclic antidepressants in the treatment of enuresis is not known but may involve inhibition of urination due to anticholinergic activity, CNS stimulant activity resulting in easier arousal by the stimulus of a full bladder, and/or other mechanisms which are presently unknown.

■ **Cardiovascular Effects** Tricyclic antidepressants have direct quinidine-like cardiotoxic properties which, in conjunction with indirect cardiac effects resulting from anticholinergic activity and potentiation of norepinephrine, may produce a variety of cardiovascular disturbances, such as ECG changes, tachycardia, and postural hypotension. (See Cautions: Cardiovascular Effects and see also Acute Toxicity.)

■ **Other Effects** Therapeutic doses of tricyclic antidepressants do not affect respiration, but respiratory depression may occur following toxic doses. Tricyclic antidepressants may also affect the endocrine system, producing changes in the concentrations of sex hormones and blood glucose. In toxic doses, the drugs may alter temperature regulation; hyperpyrexia or hypothermia may result.

Pharmacokinetics

■ **Absorption** Tricyclic antidepressants are well absorbed from the GI tract. Plasma concentrations exhibit considerable interpatient variation apparently because of genetic differences in rate of metabolism and differences in the amount of drug bound to proteins. Plasma concentrations of tricyclics may be elevated in patients with the poor-metabolizer phenotype. (See Pharmacokinetics: Elimination.) Such elevations may be slight or quite large (e.g., an eightfold increase in area under the plasma concentration-time curve) depending on the fraction of the drug that is metabolized by the cytochrome P-450 (CYP) 2D6 (CPY2D6) isoenzyme. Poor metabolizers may have an increased risk of adverse effects (e.g., cardiac toxicity) when receiving tricyclics that are metabolized principally by CYP2D.

The relationship of plasma concentrations to clinical response and acute toxicity has not been fully established. A Task Force of the American Psychiatric Association concluded on the basis of available evidence that monitoring plasma concentrations of imipramine and nortriptyline (and probably desipramine) is definitely useful in patients who do not respond to usual dosages, in those at particular risk of toxicity because of age or existing illness, and in those whose treatment is considered urgent (e.g., potentially suicidal patients or those whose illness may jeopardize their work or ability to care for their family) and may be helpful in other situations (e.g., assessing compliance). The Task Force also concluded that for other currently available tricyclic antidepressants there were generally insufficient data to date to assess the value of and/or formulate recommendations for monitoring plasma concentrations. Adverse effects appear within a few hours after administration of the drugs, but full antidepressant effects may not occur for several weeks.

■ **Distribution** Tricyclic antidepressants are distributed to the lungs, heart, brain, and liver. Tricyclic antidepressants and their active metabolites are highly bound to plasma and tissue proteins. Clomipramine, nortriptyline, and probably other tricyclic antidepressants, readily cross the placenta. Amitriptyline, amoxapine, clomipramine, desipramine, doxepin, imipramine, and nortriptyline are distributed into milk. It is likely that other tricyclic antidepressants are also distributed into milk.

■ **Elimination** Steady-state half-lives of tricyclic antidepressants exhibit wide interpatient variation.

Clomipramine, imipramine, and nortriptyline undergo first-pass metabolism in the liver when administered orally. Metabolism of tricyclic antidepressants by *N*-demethylation, *N*-oxidation, aromatic and aliphatic hydroxylation, dealkylation, and conjugation occurs in the liver.

Tricyclic antidepressants are metabolized by various isoenzymes of the cytochrome P-450 (CYP) microsomal enzyme system, including CYP1A2, CYP2D6, CYP3A4, and CYP2C isoenzymes, which are under genetic control. Genetic absence or inhibition of one isoenzyme may lead to compensation through a secondary isoenzyme pathway. However, genetic absence or inhibition of an isoenzyme may lead to increased drug toxicity. The ability to metabolize tricyclics via CYP2D6 is associated with the ability to oxidatively metabolize debrisoquin or dextromethorphan. Approximately 90–93% of Caucasians exhibit the extensive-oxidizer phenotype and about 7–10% the poor-oxidizer phenotype. The percentage of extensive- and poor-metabolizer phenotypes among Asian, African, and other populations has not been precisely determined, although it has been estimated that 1–3% of Asians and African-Americans are poor metabolizers of dextromethorphan. Individuals who extensively metabolize tricyclics via the CYP2D6 pathway exhibit the extensive-metabolizer phenotype, while those who have an impaired ability to metabolize the drugs by this pathway exhibit the poor-metabolizer phenotype.

Metabolites which are lipophilic, such as *N*-monodemethylated derivatives, can cross the blood-brain barrier and are pharmacologically active; metabolites formed by oxidation or hydroxylation and their glucuronide conjugates, however, are more polar and are probably pharmacologically less active. Enterohepatic circulation and secretion of the drugs and their metabolites into gastric juice may occur. Only small amounts of unchanged drugs and active metabolites are excreted; lipophilic metabolites are largely reabsorbed and further metabolized, while more polar derivatives are excreted. The primary route of elimination of the tricyclic antidepressants and their metabolites is urinary excretion, but they may also be excreted in feces via the bile. The rate of elimination varies among the drugs.

Chemistry

Amitriptyline, amoxapine, clomipramine, desipramine, doxepin, imipramine, nortriptyline, protriptyline, and trimipramine are classified as tricyclic antidepressants since they contain a 3-ring structure and possess antidepressant action. Maprotiline is a tetracyclic antidepressant that shares many of the pharmacologic actions and toxic potentials of the tricyclic antidepressants. Tricyclic antidepressants differ structurally and pharmacologically from other currently available antidepressants (e.g., selective serotonin-reuptake inhibitors, monoamine oxidase inhibitors).

Amitriptyline, desipramine, doxepin, imipramine, nortriptyline, and protriptyline contain 2 aromatic rings connected by a 7-membered ring to which is joined a propylamino side chain. Amoxapine, clomipramine, and trimipramine also contain 2 aromatic rings connected by a 7-membered ring, but these drugs have other side groups joined to the 7-membered ring. Maprotiline differs structurally from tricyclic antidepressants by the presence of an ethylene bridge in its center ring, resulting in a rigid flexure of its molecular structure.

Based on structure, the tricyclic antidepressants can be subdivided into dibenzazepine (iminodibenzyl), dibenzocycloheptene, or dibenzoxepin derivatives.

■ **Dibenzazepine Derivatives** Imipramine, desipramine, clomipramine, and trimipramine are dibenzazepine-derivative tricyclic antidepressants. Desipramine is the *N*-monodemethylated metabolite of imipramine; clomipramine is the 3-chloro analog of imipramine. The dibenzazepine-derivative tricyclic antidepressants differ structurally from the antipsychotic phenothiazines in that an ethylene bridge replaces the sulfur atom in the phenothiazine nucleus.

■ **Dibenzocycloheptene Derivatives** Amitriptyline, nortriptyline, and protriptyline are dibenzocycloheptene-derivative tricyclic antidepressants. Nortriptyline is the *N*-monodemethylated metabolite of amitriptyline. The dibenzocycloheptene-derivative tricyclic antidepressants differ structurally from the antipsychotic thioxanthenes in that an ethylene bridge replaces the sulfur atom in the thioxanthene nucleus. In protriptyline, the ethylene bridge in the center ring is unsaturated while the carbon atoms joining the propylamino group to the ring nucleus are saturated.

■ **Dibenzoxepin Derivatives** Amoxapine and doxepin are dibenzoxepin-derivative tricyclic antidepressants. Amoxapine differs structurally from other currently available tricyclic antidepressants in that it has both a nitrogen and an oxygen atom in its 7-membered ring and a piperazinyl ring attached to the center ring. Doxepin differs structurally from amitriptyline in that an oxygen atom is substituted for a carbon atom in the center ring.

For further information on the chemistry and stability, pharmacokinetics, uses, and dosage and administration of tricyclic antidepressants, see the individual monographs in 28:16.04.24.

†Use is not currently included in the labeling approved by the US Food and Drug Administration

Amitriptyline Hydrochloride

■ Amitriptyline hydrochloride is a dibenzocycloheptene-derivative tricyclic antidepressant.

Dosage and Administration

■ **Administration** Amitriptyline hydrochloride is given orally. Although amitriptyline has been administered in up to 4 divided doses throughout the day, it is long-acting and the entire oral daily dose may be administered at one time. Administration of the entire daily dose at bedtime may reduce daytime sedation.

In patients who were unwilling or unable to take amitriptyline orally, the drug also has been given IM. However, a parenteral dosage form is no longer commercially available in the US. Oral therapy should replace IM administration as soon as possible.

■ **Dosage** There is a wide range of oral amitriptyline hydrochloride dosage requirements, and dosage must be carefully individualized.

Patients should be monitored for possible worsening of depression, suicidality, or unusual changes in behavior, especially at the beginning of therapy or during periods of dosage adjustment. (See Cautions: Precautions and Contraindications, in the Tricyclic Antidepressants General Statement 28:16.04.28.)

Initial dosages should be low and generally range from 75–100 mg daily, depending on the severity of the condition being treated. Dosage may be gradually adjusted (preferably the late-afternoon and/or bedtime doses) to the level that produces maximal therapeutic effect with minimal toxicity and may range from 150–300 mg daily. Alternatively, the manufacturers recommend an initial amitriptyline hydrochloride dosage of 50–100 mg daily at bedtime. Dosage then can be increased by 25 or 50 mg as necessary to a suggested maximum of 150 mg daily. Hospitalized patients under close supervision may generally be given higher dosages than outpatients. Hospitalized patients generally may receive an initial amitriptyline dosage of 100 mg daily; dosage may be increased gradually to 200 mg daily as needed. Some patients may require dosages as high as 300 mg daily. Geriatric and adolescent patients should usually be given lower than average dosages. Manufacturers state that these patients may obtain satisfactory improvement with 10 mg of amitriptyline hydrochloride 3 times daily plus 20 mg at bedtime. Maximum antidepressant effects may not occur for 30 days after therapy is begun.

After symptoms are controlled, dosage should be gradually reduced to the lowest level that will maintain relief of symptoms. If maintenance therapy is necessary, the manufacturers recommend 50–100 mg of amitriptyline hydrochloride daily; however, 25–40 mg daily may be sufficient for some patients. During maintenance therapy, the total daily dosage may be administered as a single daily dose, preferably at bedtime. The manufacturers recommend that maintenance therapy be continued for at least 3 months to prevent relapse. To avoid the possibility of precipitating withdrawal symptoms, amitriptyline should not be terminated abruptly in patients who have received a high dosage for prolonged periods.

When amitriptyline is used in conjunction with a phenothiazine, commercially available fixed-ratio combination preparations should not be used initially. Dosage should first be adjusted by administering each drug separately. If it is determined that the optimum maintenance dosage corresponds to the ratio in a commercial combination, such a preparation may be used. However, whenever dosage adjustment is necessary, the drugs should be administered separately.

Cautions

Amitriptyline shares the pharmacologic actions, uses, and toxic potentials of the tricyclic antidepressants, and the usual precautions of tricyclic antidepressant administration should be observed. Patients should be fully advised about the risks, especially suicidal thinking and behavior (suicidality), associated with tricyclic antidepressant therapy. For a complete discussion, see Cautions: Precautions and Contraindications and Cautions: Pediatric Precautions, in the Tricyclic Antidepressants General Statement 28:16.04.28.

■ **Pediatric Precautions** Safety and efficacy of amitriptyline in children younger than 12 years of age have not been established. Therefore, the manufacturers state that the drug should not be used in this age group.

The US Food and Drug Administration (FDA) has determined that antidepressants increase the risk of suicidal thinking and behavior (suicidality) in children and adolescents with major depressive disorder and other psychiatric disorders, However, the FDA also states that depression and certain other psychiatric disorders are themselves associated with an increased risk of suicide. Anyone considering the use of amitriptyline in a child or adolescent for any clinical use must therefore balance the potential risk of therapy with the clinical need. (See Cautions: Precautions and Contraindications and Cautions: Pediatric Precautions, in the Tricyclic Antidepressants General Statement 28:16.04.28.)

Pharmacokinetics

■ **Absorption** Amitriptyline hydrochloride is rapidly absorbed from the GI tract and from parenteral sites. Peak plasma concentrations occur within 2–12 hours after oral or IM (a parenteral dosage form no longer is commercially available in the US) administration.

■ **Distribution** Amitriptyline and its active metabolite, nortriptyline, are distributed into milk. Amitriptyline and nortriptyline concentrations in milk appear to be similar to or slightly greater than those present in maternal serum. It is estimated that a nursing infant would ingest less than 1% of the daily maternal dose of amitriptyline, and the drug was not detected in the serum of several nursing infants whose mothers were receiving 75–100 mg daily.

■ **Elimination** The plasma half-life of amitriptyline ranges from 10–50 hours. Amitriptyline is metabolized via the same pathways as are other tricyclic antidepressants; nortriptyline, its *N*-monodemethylated metabolite, is pharmacologically active. Approximately 25–50% of a dose of amitriptyline is excreted in urine as inactive metabolites within 24 hours; small amounts are excreted in feces via biliary elimination.

Chemistry and Stability

■ **Chemistry** Amitriptyline hydrochloride is a dibenzocycloheptene-derivative tricyclic antidepressant. Amitriptyline hydrochloride occurs as a white or practically white, odorless or practically odorless, crystalline powder or small crystals with a bitter, burning taste and is freely soluble in water and in alcohol. The drug has a pK_a of 9.4.

■ **Stability** Amitriptyline hydrochloride tablets should be stored in well-closed containers at a temperature preferably between 15–30°C; exposure to temperatures exceeding 30°C should be avoided. Perphenazine and amitriptyline hydrochloride tablets should be stored at 2–25°C; in addition, unit-dose packages of these tablets should be protected from excessive moisture. Following the date of manufacture, amitriptyline hydrochloride preparations have expiration dates of 3–5 years depending on the manufacturer and dosage form.

For further information on chemistry, pharmacology, pharmacokinetics, uses, cautions, acute toxicity, drug interactions, and dosage and administration of amitriptyline, see the Tricyclic Antidepressants General Statement 28:16.04.28.

Preparations

Excipients in commercially available drug preparations may have clinically important effects in some individuals; consult specific product labeling for details.

Amitriptyline Hydrochloride

Oral

Tablets, film-coated	10 mg*	**Amitriptyline Hydrochloride Film-coated Tablets**
	25 mg*	**Amitriptyline Hydrochloride Film-coated Tablets**
	50 mg*	**Amitriptyline Hydrochloride Film-coated Tablets**
	75 mg*	**Amitriptyline Hydrochloride Film-coated Tablets**
	100 mg*	**Amitriptyline Hydrochloride Film-coated Tablets**
	150 mg*	**Amitriptyline Hydrochloride Film-coated Tablets**

*available from one or more manufacturer, distributor, and/or repackager by generic (nonproprietary) name

Chlordiazepoxide and Amitriptyline Hydrochloride

Oral

Tablets, film-coated	5 mg Chlordiazepoxide and Amitriptyline Hydrochloride 12.5 mg (of amitriptyline)*	**Chlordiazepoxide and Amitriptyline Hydrochloride Tablets** (C-IV)
		Limbitrol® (C-IV), Valeant
	10 mg Chlordiazepoxide and Amitriptyline Hydrochloride 25 mg (of amitriptyline)*	**Chlordiazepoxide and Amitriptyline Hydrochloride Tablets** (C-IV)
		Limbitrol® DS (C-IV), Valeant

*available from one or more manufacturer, distributor, and/or repackager by generic (nonproprietary) name

Perphenazine and Amitriptyline Hydrochloride

Oral		
Tablets, film-coated	2 mg Perphenazine and Amitriptyline Hydrochloride 10 mg*	**Perphenazine and Amitriptyline Hydrochloride Tablets**
	2 mg Perphenazine and Amitriptyline Hydrochloride 25 mg*	**Perphenazine and Amitriptyline Hydrochloride Tablets**
	4 mg Perphenazine and Amitriptyline Hydrochloride 10 mg*	**Perphenazine and Amitriptyline Hydrochloride Tablets**
	4 mg Perphenazine and Amitriptyline Hydrochloride 25 mg*	**Perphenazine and Amitriptyline Hydrochloride Tablets**
	4 mg Perphenazine and Amitriptyline Hydrochloride 50 mg*	**Perphenazine and Amitriptyline Hydrochloride Tablets**

*available from one or more manufacturer, distributor, and/or repackager by generic (nonproprietary) name

clomiPRAMINE Hydrochloride

Chlorimipramine Hydrochloride, Chloroimipramine Hydrochloride, CMI

■ Clomipramine, a dibenzazepine-derivative tricyclic antidepressant, is the 3-chloro analog of imipramine.

Uses

■ **Obsessive-Compulsive Disorder** Clomipramine is used in the treatment of obsessive-compulsive disorder when obsessions or compulsions cause marked distress, are time-consuming (take longer than 1 hour daily), or interfere substantially with the patient's normal routine, occupational or academic functioning, or usual social activities or relationships. Obsessions are recurrent and persistent thoughts, impulses, or images that, at some time during the disturbance, are experienced as intrusive and inappropriate (i.e., "ego dystonic") and that cause marked anxiety or distress but that are not simply excessive worries about real-life problems. Compulsions are repetitive behaviors (e.g., hand washing, ordering, checking) or mental acts (e.g., praying, counting, repeating words silently) performed in response to an obsession or according to rules that must be applied rigidly (e.g., in a stereotyped fashion). Although the behaviors or acts are aimed at preventing or reducing distress or preventing some dreaded event or situation, they either are not connected in a realistic manner with what they are designed to neutralize or prevent or are clearly excessive. At some time during the course of the disturbance, the patient, if an adult, recognizes that the obsessions or compulsions are excessive or unreasonable; children may not make such recognition.

The efficacy of clomipramine for the management of obsessive-compulsive disorder has been established in several multicenter, placebo-controlled, parallel-group studies, including 2 studies of 10 weeks' duration in adults and one study of 8 weeks' duration in children and adolescents 10–17 years of age. In these clinical studies, clomipramine was more effective than placebo in reducing the severity of obsessive-compulsive manifestations in patients with moderate to severe obsessive-compulsive disorder. The drug produced substantial improvement in scores on both the Yale-Brown Obsessive-Compulsive Scale (YBOCS) and the National Institute of Mental Health (NIMH) Clinical Global Obsessive-Compulsive Scale (NIMH-OC), while the response with placebo was clinically insignificant. Scores on the YBOCS decreased by an average of approximately 10 from baseline values of 26–28, representing an average improvement of 35–42% in adults and 37% in children and adolescents treated with clomipramine. Scores on the NIMH-OC were reduced by an average of 3.5 units from a mean baseline of 10 in adults, children, and adolescents treated with clomipramine, which represents an improvement in obsessive-compulsive disorder from severe at baseline to subclinical after treatment with the drug. The maximum dosage of clomipramine hydrochloride was 250 mg daily for most adults and 3 mg/kg (up to 200 mg) daily for children and adolescents.

Although obsessive-compulsive manifestations often persist to some extent in patients who respond to clomipramine, responders generally find it easier to resist the manifestations and spend less time engaged in the associated behavior. Data from a retrospective analysis suggest that clomipramine may be more effective in patients who developed obsessive-compulsive disorder during middle age (35–62 years of age) than in those in whom onset occurred during early adulthood (16–23 years old), independent of the length of illness.

Therapeutic response to clomipramine in patients with obsessive-compulsive disorder generally is evident within 2–6 weeks but may not be maximal until 3–4 months after beginning therapy with the drug. Thus, it is essential that patients receive an adequate trial of clomipramine at a therapeutic dosage in order to determine efficacy.

Many clinicians consider clomipramine or a serotonin-reuptake inhibitor (e.g., fluoxetine, fluvoxamine) to be the drugs of choice in obsessive-compulsive disorder. In addition, behavior therapy often is recommended in patients with obsessive-compulsive disorder even when pharmacologic therapy alone has been partially effective.

Results from comparative studies to date suggest that clomipramine is more effective than other tricyclic antidepressants (e.g., amitriptyline, desipramine, imipramine, nortriptyline) and as or more effective than selective serotonin-reuptake inhibitors (e.g., fluoxetine, fluvoxamine) in the management of obsessive-compulsive disorder. In a pooled analysis of separate short-term (10–13 weeks) studies comparing clomipramine, fluoxetine, fluvoxamine, or sertraline with placebo, clomipramine was calculated as being more effective (as determined by measures on the YBOC scale) than selective serotonin-reuptake inhibitors, although all drugs were superior to placebo. Like clomipramine, selective serotonin-reuptake inhibitors reduce but do not completely eliminate obsessions and compulsions. The decision whether to initiate therapy with clomipramine or a selective serotonin-reuptake inhibitor often is made based on the adverse effect profile of these drugs. For example, some clinicians prefer clomipramine in patients who may not tolerate the adverse effect profile of selective serotonin-reuptake inhibitors (nausea, headache, overstimulation, sleep disturbances) while selective serotonin-reuptake inhibitors may be useful alternatives in patients unable to tolerate the adverse effects (anticholinergic effects, cardiovascular effects, sedation) associated with clomipramine therapy. Consideration of individual patient characteristics (age, concurrent medical conditions), the pharmacokinetics of the drug, potential drug interactions, and cost of therapy may also influence clinicians when selecting between clomipramine and selective serotonin-reuptake inhibitors as first-line therapy in patients with obsessive-compulsive disorder. Although not clearly established, it has been suggested that the mechanism of action of clomipramine and other drugs (fluoxetine, fluvoxamine) used in the management of obsessive-compulsive disorder may be related to their serotonergic activity. Clomipramine also has been effective when used in combination with clonidine in several patients with obsessive-compulsive disorder; however, additional experience is needed to confirm the safety and efficacy of this combination.

The manufacturers state that the efficacy of clomipramine for long-term use (i.e., longer than 10 weeks) in the treatment of obsessive-compulsive disorder has not been established in placebo-controlled studies. After 36 weeks of treatment with clomipramine, improvement compared with placebo was observed on measures of rituals, mood, and social adjustment, although such effects were more substantial after 18 weeks of treatment. At follow-up 22 weeks after treatment ended, clomipramine differed from placebo on one measure of rituals. Clomipramine was not distinguishable from placebo in efficacy at follow-up 6 years after the conclusion of treatment. The combination of clomipramine or placebo with the same behavioral therapy resulted in greater improvement with clomipramine on measures of rituals, mood, and social adjustment at 8 weeks of treatment, but thereafter through the last 15 weeks of treatment and at follow-up through 52 weeks, clomipramine was indistinguishable from placebo. However, clomipramine has been used in some patients for prolonged periods (e.g., up to 1 year) without apparent loss of clinical effect. If clomipramine is used for extended periods, dosage should be adjusted so that patients are maintained on the lowest effective dosage, and the need for continued therapy with the drug should be reassessed periodically.

Discontinuance of clomipramine frequently results in a progressive recurrence of symptoms in patients with obsessive-compulsive disorder, and therefore long-term continued therapy with the drug may be advisable on an individual basis. In a study conducted under double-blind conditions, most patients with obsessive-compulsive disorder who had improved clinically following 5–27 months of clomipramine therapy experienced profound worsening of manifestations after discontinuance of the drug. This worsening started at 4 weeks and continued for the rest of the 7-week placebo period and appeared to be unrelated to the duration of clomipramine therapy or to the type of obsessive-compulsive manifestations originally present. However, readministration of clomipramine resulted in clinical improvement similar to that obtained prior to discontinuance of the drug.

Disorders with an Obsessive-Compulsive Component Depressive episodes may be associated with obsessive-compulsive disorder. Clomipramine and selective serotonin-reuptake inhibitors are effective antidepressants when obsessive manifestations accompany an episode of major depression. However, the antiobsessional effectiveness of clomipramine does not appear to depend on the presence of depression.

Clomipramine also may reduce obsessive-compulsive manifestations in some patients with schizophrenia and such accompanying manifestations. However, exacerbation of psychosis has been reported in some patients treated with clomipramine. Therefore, the possibility of exacerbating psychosis should be considered in patients with obsessive-compulsive manifestations and schizophrenia, and such patients receiving clomipramine should be observed closely for early signs of worsening psychosis.

There is a high incidence of obsessive-compulsive disorder in patients with Tourette's disorder (Gilles de la Tourette's syndrome), and clomipramine can reduce obsessive-compulsive manifestations associated with Tourette's and suppress associated motor and vocal tics. However, in at least one controlled study, clomipramine did not differ from placebo in the number of tics observed during 4 weeks of treatment.

Obsessive thoughts were decreased with the combination of clomipramine and lithium carbonate in a limited number of patients who had obsessive manifestations that previously failed to respond to clomipramine therapy alone. However, in a study of patients with obsessive-compulsive disorder treated with clomipramine for at least 6 months and who were partial responders to the drug, the addition of lithium carbonate for 4 weeks did not result in improvement in scores on the YBOCS.

■ **Panic Disorder** Clomipramine has been used effectively for the treatment of panic disorder† with or without agoraphobia†. In an uncontrolled study, clomipramine reduced both the weekly frequency and severity of panic attacks when given in an average dosage of 45 mg daily (range: 6.25–75 mg daily). In many patients, complete or nearly complete relief from panic attacks was reported during therapy. The number of days that panic attacks occurred was less with clomipramine (mean dosage of 83 mg daily) than with placebo after 8 weeks of treatment in one study. Therapeutic response generally is seen within about 1–3 weeks but may take up to 6 weeks. Although clomipramine therapy generally is well tolerated, a transient increase in the number and intensity of panic attacks may occur during initial therapy with the drug. (See Dosage and Administration: Dosage.) Clomipramine (mean dosage of 109 mg daily; range: 25–200 mg daily) was at least as effective as imipramine (mean dosage of 109 mg daily; range: 25–200 mg daily) in patients with panic disorder and had a faster onset of action in reducing panic attacks and improving phobic avoidance and associated anxiety.

Clomipramine generally is equally effective in patients with panic disorder with or without agoraphobia. In a limited number of patients whose panic disorder with agoraphobia did not respond to exposure-based behavioral treatment, measures of fear (i.e., fear of bodily incapacitation, fear of losing control), state and trait anxiety, depression, severity of condition, and avoidance of separation situations indicated improvement compared with placebo after receiving clomipramine for about 5 weeks (3 weeks at the maximum dosage of 150 mg daily). Despite such improvement, the efficacy of clomipramine in the treatment of such patients was uncertain. A clinical response, as indicated by improvement by at least 50% on assessment of avoidance of separation situations with the Phobic Avoidance Rating Scale, was produced by clomipramine in 29% of the patients, while such response was observed with behavioral treatment in 47% of the patients.

Preliminary results from an uncontrolled study suggest that clomipramine is effective in patients with panic disorder or agoraphobia with panic attacks who have concurrent mitral valve prolapse.

Although it has been suggested that the mechanism of action of clomipramine in patients with panic disorder may be related to the drug's serotonergic activity, the absence of clear superiority compared with less selective antidepressants (e.g., desipramine) suggests that this may not be the case.

For further information on treatment of panic disorder, see Uses: Panic Disorder, in the Tricyclic Antidepressants General Statement 28:16.04.28.

■ **Major Depressive Disorder** Clomipramine has been used effectively in the treatment of major depressive disorder†. Clinical studies have shown that the antidepressant effect of clomipramine exceeds that of placebo and is comparable to that of usual dosages of other tricyclic antidepressants (e.g., amitriptyline, doxepin, imipramine) or selective serotonin-reuptake inhibitors (e.g., fluoxetine, paroxetine). Several (e.g., 4–6) weeks may be required for optimal antidepressant effect at a given clomipramine dosage. Despite comparable efficacy, the adverse effect profile (e.g., anticholinergic effects) of clomipramine may limit its usefulness relative to other antidepressants, and antidepressant therapy should be individualized based on patient response and tolerance. Clomipramine appears to offer no substantial advantage over other tricyclic antidepressants for the management of typical depression in the absence of obsessive-compulsive manifestations and may be more poorly tolerated, particularly compared with tricyclics exhibiting only mild to moderate anticholinergic effects. Although some clinicians have preferred clomipramine to other tricyclic antidepressants for atypical depression (e.g., because of clomipramine's dopaminergic activity), other agents (e.g., selective serotonin-reuptake inhibitors such as fluoxetine) generally have replaced this preference for clomipramine in such depression.

For further information on treatment of major depressive disorder and considerations in choosing the most appropriate antidepressant for a particular patient, including considerations related to patient tolerance, patient age, and cardiovascular, sedative, and suicidal risks, see Considerations in Choosing Antidepressants under Uses: Major Depressive Disorder, in the Tricyclic Antidepressants General Statement 28:16.04.28.

■ **Chronic Pain** Like other tricyclic antidepressants, clomipramine has been used for the treatment of chronic pain†, including central pain, idiopathic pain disorder, tension headache, diabetic peripheral neuropathy, and pain of other neuropathic origin (e.g., cancer pain). Antidepressants have been used alone or as adjuncts to conventional analgesics in the management of such pain. In patients with central pain (e.g., phantom or stump pain, post-herpetic neuralgia, deafferentation pain secondary to posttraumatic nerve lesions), reduction in pain intensity, as indicated by scores on a visual analog scale for pain, was greater during treatment with clomipramine for 3 weeks than with placebo. Treatment of idiopathic pain disorder with clomipramine (mean dosage of 97 mg daily) for 6 weeks resulted in improvement, as indicated by the physicians' global assessment, in 63% of patients. The patients' scores on visual analog scales that included assessment of pain also were improved. In patients with tension headache, a greater decrease in headache pain, as indicated by scores on a visual analog scale, occurred with clomipramine administered for 6 weeks than with placebo. Treatment of diabetic peripheral neuropathy with clomipramine for 2 weeks resulted in a greater decrease compared with placebo in the severity of symptoms overall, as evaluated by a physician through use of a scale that quantified pain, paresthesia, dyesthesia, numbness, nightly deterioration, and sleep disturbances.

■ **Cataplexy and Associated Narcolepsy** Clomipramine has been used for the symptomatic management of cataplexy† in a limited number of patients with cataplexy and associated narcolepsy. Cataplexy attacks and sleep paralysis resolved or were reduced in frequency during clomipramine therapy (25–200 mg daily); however, the drug did not consistently improve sleep attacks. Although the precise mechanism of clomipramine's anticataplectic action is not known, it has been suggested that its serotonergic and REM-suppressing activity may be involved.

■ **Autistic Disorder** Clomipramine has been effective in a limited number of patients with autistic disorder†. In a double-blind study, clomipramine therapy (mean dosage: 152 mg daily) was superior to both desipramine and placebo in improving standardized ratings of autistic manifestations, including repetitive and obsessive-compulsive behaviors and hyperactivity in a limited number of pediatric outpatients aged 6–18 years with autistic disorder. However, in an open study involving younger inpatients aged 3–9 years with autistic disorder but with relatively low intellectual functioning and without prominent obsessive-compulsive manifestations, clomipramine was not found to be effective and was commonly associated with adverse effects, including acute urinary retention.

■ **Trichotillomania** Clomipramine has been used in a limited number of patients with trichotillomania† (an urge to pull out one's hair). In one double-blind, crossover study, clomipramine (mean dosage of 181 mg daily; range: 100–250 mg daily) was shown to be more effective than desipramine (mean dosage of 173 mg daily; range: 150–200 mg daily) in the short-term management of trichotillomania. However, relapse has been reported in some patients receiving long-term treatment with clomipramine.

■ **Onychophagia** Clomipramine has been used in a limited number of patients with severe onychophagia† (nail biting) and no history of obsessive-compulsive disorder. In one study, the severity of nail biting decreased in patients treated with clomipramine hydrochloride 25–200 mg daily for 5 weeks. However, the relatively high dropout rate secondary to adverse effects and drug intolerance suggests that clomipramine should not be considered as first-line therapy in most patients with onychophagia.

■ **Stuttering** Clomipramine has been used in a limited number of patients with stuttering†. Following 5 weeks of therapy (mean dosage: 147 mg daily), clomipramine improved the severity of stuttering, preoccupation with thoughts about stuttering, amount of energy spent resisting stuttering, and expectancy of stuttering. Additional study of the efficacy of clomipramine in the management of stuttering is necessary.

■ **Eating Disorders** Clomipramine has been used in a limited number of patients with anorexia nervosa†. In a placebo-controlled study, clomipramine therapy was associated with increased appetite, hunger, and calorie consumption during initial therapy; however, the drug was not associated with improved eating behavior after 8 weeks of therapy or greater weight gain. In addition, body weight did not differ between the clomipramine and placebo groups at 1-year follow-up and a measure of outcome based on nutritional status, sexual adjustment, socioeconomic adjustment, and mental state did not differ between the 2 groups at 4-year follow-up. Few controlled studies on the pharmacotherapy for anorexia nervosa have been published, and results with most drugs have been unimpressive. Because malnourished depressed patients may be particularly susceptible to the adverse cardiovascular effects or other severe toxicities (including death) of tricyclic antidepressants, the American Psychiatric Association (APA) states that tricyclic antidepressants should be avoided in underweight individuals and in those exhibiting suicidal ideation. For further information on use of antidepressants in the treatment of eating disorders see Uses: Eating Disorders, in Fluoxetine Hydrochloride 28:16.04.20.

■ **Premature Ejaculation** Clomipramine has been used with some success in the treatment of premature ejaculation†. In a controlled study, mean ejaculatory latency was prolonged in patients receiving 25 or 50 mg of the drug daily. Sexual and relationship satisfaction also was improved. A trial with drug therapy may be particularly useful in patients who fail or refuse behavioral or psychotherapeutic treatment or when partners are unwilling to cooperate with such therapy.

■ **Premenstrual Syndrome** Clomipramine has been used in the management of premenstrual syndrome†. In a limited number of women with severe premenstrual irritability and/or depressed mood, clomipramine given either continuously or intermittently (i.e., premenstrual administration) during 3 menstrual cycles at a dosage of 25–75 mg daily was more effective than placebo in reducing premenstrual irritability and depressed mood. However, preliminary data suggest that patients with premenstrual syndrome may be particularly sensitive to the adverse effects associated with the drug.

Dosage and Administration

■ **Administration** Clomipramine hydrochloride is administered orally. The drug also has been administered IM† or IV†, but a parenteral dosage form is not commercially available in the US.

During initial therapy when the dosage is being titrated, the manufacturers recommend that clomipramine be given in divided doses with meals to lessen adverse GI effects. After dosage titration, the total daily dose may be given once daily at bedtime to minimize adverse effects such as sedation during waking hours and enhance patient compliance.

■ **Dosage** Dosage of clomipramine hydrochloride is expressed in terms of the hydrochloride.

Because there is wide interindividual variation in dosage and dosage may differ in various disease states, the dosage of clomipramine hydrochloride must be individualized carefully.

Patients receiving clomipramine should be monitored for possible worsening of depression, suicidality, or unusual changes in behavior, especially at the beginning of therapy or during periods of dosage adjustment. (See Cautions: Precautions and Contraindications.)

Obsessive-Compulsive Disorder For the management of obsessive-compulsive disorder in adults, children, or adolescents, the recommended initial dosage of clomipramine hydrochloride is 25 mg daily. During the first 2 weeks of therapy, dosage should be increased gradually as tolerated to approximately 100 mg daily in adults. In children and adolescents, dosage should be increased gradually, as tolerated, during the first 2 weeks of therapy up to a maximum of 3 mg/kg or 100 mg daily, whichever is lower. This initial period of titration is intended to minimize adverse effects by permitting tolerance to develop or allowing the patient time to adapt if tolerance does not develop.

During the next several weeks, the dosage of clomipramine hydrochloride may be increased gradually up to a maximum of 250 mg daily in adults and 3 mg/kg or 200 mg daily (whichever is lower) in children and adolescents. Daily clomipramine hydrochloride dosages exceeding 250 mg in adults or 3 mg/kg (up to 200 mg) in children and adolescents should be avoided because of the increased risk of seizures (see Cautions: Nervous System Effects).

Because of the long elimination half-lives of both clomipramine and its active metabolite, desmethylclomipramine, clinicians should take into consideration that steady-state plasma concentrations may not be achieved for 2–3 weeks or even longer. Therefore, the manufacturers state that it may be appropriate to wait 2–3 weeks between any further dosage adjustments after the initial dosage titration period.

Although the optimum duration of clomipramine therapy has not been established, obsessive-compulsive disorder is a chronic condition and it seems reasonable to consider continuation of therapy in responding patients. Although the manufacturers state that the efficacy of clomipramine when given for periods exceeding 10 weeks has not been established systematically in controlled studies, the drug has been given under double-blind conditions for up to 1 year without loss of clinical efficacy. Pending further accumulation of data, some clinicians recommend that clomipramine therapy be continued for at least 18 months in patients with obsessive-compulsive disorder before attempting to discontinue therapy. However, the dosage should be adjusted during maintenance therapy so that patients are maintained on the minimum effective dosage and patients should be reassessed periodically to determine the need for continued therapy.

Clomipramine should not be used concomitantly with MAO inhibitors and it is recommended that at least 2 weeks elapse between discontinuance of therapy with a MAO inhibitor and initiation of clomipramine therapy and vice versa. A similar interval is recommended between discontinuance of therapy with a selective serotonin-reuptake inhibitor (e.g., citalopram, escitalopram, fluvoxamine, paroxetine, sertraline) and initiation of therapy with a tricyclic antidepressant agent such as clomipramine and vice versa. However, because fluoxetine and its active metabolite have a long half-life, at least 5 weeks should elapse between discontinuance of fluoxetine therapy and initiation of clomipramine therapy.

Abrupt discontinuance of clomipramine therapy should be avoided since a variety of withdrawal symptoms have been reported. (See Cautions: Nervous System Effects and also see Chronic Toxicity.) In addition, patients may experience a worsening of psychiatric status when the drug is discontinued abruptly. Therefore, it is recommended that dosage be tapered gradually (e.g., over a period of approximately 2 weeks) and the patient monitored carefully when clomipramine therapy is discontinued.

Panic Disorder For the management of panic disorder† with or without agoraphobia†, clomipramine hydrochloride usually has been effective in dosages ranging from 12.5–150 mg (maximum: 200 mg) daily. Most patients with panic attacks respond to a clomipramine hydrochloride dosage of less than 50 mg daily; however, patients with agoraphobia may require a higher dosage. Because clomipramine may worsen anxiety symptoms during initial therapy, some clinicians recommend that patients be started on a low dosage initially, and then the dosage can be increased gradually until therapeutic response or bothersome adverse effects occur.

Other Uses For the management of major depressive disorder† or chronic pain†, clomipramine hydrochloride is generally given in dosages ranging from 100–250 mg daily.

For the management of cataplexy and associated narcolepsy†, clomipramine hydrochloride has been given in dosages ranging from 25–200 mg daily.

■ **Dosage in Geriatric Patients** The manufacturers and some clinicians recommend selecting an initial clomipramine dosage at the lower end of the recommended range since decreased hepatic, renal, or cardiac function and concomitant illness and medications are more frequent in geriatric patients.

Cautions

Clomipramine shares the toxic potentials of the tricyclic antidepressants, and the usual precautions of tricyclic antidepressant administration should be observed. (See Cautions in the Tricyclic Antidepressants General Statement 28:16.04.28.)

Common adverse effects of clomipramine are extensions of its pharmacologic activity, principally anticholinergic effects; adverse effects secondary to antihistaminic and α-adrenergic activity also may occur. Like other tricyclics, adverse effects of clomipramine could affect compliance and result in dosage reduction; however, the possibility that such reductions could affect response should be considered.

In controlled studies, the most common adverse effects occurring more frequently in patients receiving clomipramine than in those receiving placebo included GI effects such as dry mouth, constipation, nausea, dyspepsia, anorexia, and increased appetite; nervous system effects such as somnolence, tremor, dizziness, nervousness, fatigue, and myoclonus; genitourinary effects such as changed libido, ejaculatory failure, impotence, and micturition disorder; sweating; weight gain; and visual changes. Approximately 20% of the 3616 patients who participated in US premarketing clinical trials for obsessive-compulsive or other disorders discontinued clomipramine therapy because of an adverse effect. About one-half of those who discontinued therapy (9% of the total) experienced multiple adverse effects, none of which could be classified as the principal reason. However, in the cases in which a principal reason for discontinuing therapy could be identified, most of the patients did so because of nervous system effects (5.4%), mainly somnolence, and GI effects (1.3%), mainly nausea and vomiting.

The incidences of adverse effects reported by the manufacturers to have occurred in at least 1% of clomipramine-treated patients were obtained from pooled data from placebo-controlled clinical trials involving 322 adults and 46 children or adolescents who received clomipramine for the treatment of obsessive-compulsive disorder. However, clinicians prescribing clomipramine should be aware that these figures cannot be used to predict the incidence of adverse effects during usual medical practice, in which patient characteristics and other factors differ from those that prevailed during these trials. Similarly, the cited incidences cannot be compared with the incidences obtained from other trials involving different treatments, uses, and investigators. However, the incidences from these trials provide the clinician with a basis for estimating the relative contribution of both drug and nondrug factors to the incidence of adverse effects in the populations studied. Various other adverse effects have been reported in 3525 out of approximately 3600 individuals who received multiple doses of clomipramine for obsessive-compulsive or other disorders during premarketing trials in the US; however, these adverse effects have not been definitely attributed to the drug.

Some evidence suggests that patients with depression may tolerate clomipramine relative to placebo more poorly than those with obsessive-compulsive disorder.

■ **Nervous System Effects** ***Seizures*** Seizure is the most clinically important risk associated with clomipramine therapy. However, seizure remains a relatively uncommon adverse effect of clomipramine therapy. The cumulative incidence of seizures in patients treated with clomipramine hydrochloride dosages of up to 300 mg daily was 0.64, 1.12, and 1.45% at 90, 180, and 365 days, respectively. The cumulative rates correct the crude incidence of 0.7% (25 of 3519 patients) for the variable duration of exposure to clomipramine in clinical trials. Seizures also have been associated with abrupt withdrawal of the drug.

Dose appears to be a predictor of the development of seizures. However, the influence of dose is confounded by the duration of exposure to the drug, making independent assessment of the effect of either factor alone difficult. Seizures occurred in about 0.5 or 2% of patients who received a maximum daily dose of 250 mg or higher than 250 mg, respectively, of the drug. The ability to predict seizures with daily doses exceeding 250 mg is limited because plasma concentrations achieved during clomipramine therapy may be dose dependent and vary considerably among individuals administered the same dosage.

Rare reports of fatalities in association with clomipramine-associated seizures have been reported in foreign postmarketing surveillance, but not in US clinical trials. In some of these cases, clomipramine had been administered with other epileptogenic agents, while in other cases the patients had possible predisposing medical conditions. Thus, a causal relationship between clomipramine therapy and these fatalities has not been established. (See Cautions: Precautions and Contraindications.)

Withdrawal Effects Withdrawal syndrome has been reported rarely in patients receiving clomipramine. In a limited number of patients, abrupt discontinuance of clomipramine resulted in a variety of withdrawal manifestations, including dizziness, nausea, vomiting, headache, malaise, sleep disturbance, hyperthermia, sweating, and irritability. Abrupt discontinuance of the drug also reportedly has resulted in seizures. In addition, some patients have experienced a worsening of psychiatric status when the drug was discontinued abruptly. Therefore, abrupt discontinuance of clomipramine therapy should be avoided. (See Cautions: Precautions and Contraindications.)

Serotonin Syndrome The manifestation of a group of adverse effects (e.g., tremor, myoclonus, diaphoresis, shivering, restlessness, fever, mental status changes, diarrhea) that resembles the serotonin syndrome observed in animals has been reported with clomipramine monotherapy. In an open study in which patients received clomipramine 150 mg daily for about 4 weeks for the treatment of depression, tremor of the tongue and myoclonus occurred most commonly (42 and 36% of patients, respectively). Tremor of the tongue or fingers and myoclonus were accompanied by diaphoresis and shivering in over a quarter of the patients. In most cases, these manifestations were transient and resolved despite continued therapy. More severe and sometimes fatal reactions resembling the serotonin syndrome have been reported when clomipramine has been given concurrently with other serotonergic agents such as MAO inhibitors, fluoxetine, lithium, or alprazolam. (See Drug Interactions.)

Other Nervous System Effects In controlled trials, somnolence, dizziness, or tremor was each reported in about 54% of adults and in about 46, 41, or 33%, respectively, of children and adolescents receiving clomipramine. Headache occurred in about 52% of adults and 28% of children and adolescents receiving clomipramine. Fatigue occurred in about 39% of adults and 35% of children and adolescents receiving the drug. Insomnia occurred in about 25% of adults and 11% of children and adolescents and nervousness occurred in about 18% of adults and 4% of children and adolescents treated with clomipramine.

Myoclonus occurred in about 13% of adults and 2% of children and adolescents receiving clomipramine. Motor hyperactivity that included jerking of the arms and legs during nocturnal sleep also has been reported. Memory impairment occurred in about 9 or 7% of adults or children and adolescents, respectively, receiving clomipramine. Paresthesia and anxiety each occurred in about 9 or 2% of adults or children and adolescents, respectively, receiving the drug. Twitching occurred in about 7 or 4% of adults or children and adolescents, respectively, receiving clomipramine. Impaired concentration and depression each occurred in about 5% of adults receiving clomipramine. Sleep disorder occurred in about 4 or 9% of adults or children and adolescents, respectively, treated with the drug. Disturbance of sleep by fright that was accompanied by myoclonus also has been reported in association with clomipramine therapy. Hypertonia occurred in about 4 or 2% of adults or children and adolescents, respectively, receiving the drug.

Confusion occurred in about 3 or 2% of adults or children and adolescents, respectively, receiving clomipramine. Psychosomatic disorder, speech disorder, dream abnormalities, agitation, or migraine occurred in about 3% of adults treated with the drug. Depersonalization or irritability occurred in about 2% of both adults and children or adolescents receiving clomipramine. Emotional lability occurred in about 2% of adults and aggressive reaction occurred in about 2% of children and adolescents treated with the drug. Paresis and asthenia each occurred in about 2% of children and adolescents and panic reaction occurred in about 1 or 2% of adults or children and adolescents, respectively, receiving clomipramine.

During premarketing clinical trials in patients with affective disorder, hypomania or mania was precipitated infrequently in patients receiving clomipramine therapy. Activation of mania or hypomania also has been reported in patients treated with other tricyclic antidepressants.

More than 30 cases of hyperthermia with clomipramine have been reported by foreign postmarketing surveillance systems. Most of these cases occurred in patients receiving clomipramine in combination with other drugs (e.g., antipsychotic agents). When clomipramine and an antipsychotic agent were used concomitantly, the cases sometimes were considered to be examples of neuroleptic malignant syndrome (NMS).

Abnormal thinking and vertigo each occurred in 1% or more of patients receiving clomipramine; however, a causal relationship to the drug has not been established.

Dyskinesia occurred in less than 1% of patients receiving clomipramine, although a causal relationship to the drug has not been established. Persistent tardive dyskinesia has been reported after initiation of clomipramine in a patient who was already receiving dextroamphetamine. A severe tardive dyskinesia-like syndrome consisting of orobuccal movements, choreoathetosis of the arms and other abnormal movements of the extremities, motor restlessness, and incoordination has been reported in another patient who was receiving clomipramine concurrently with thiothixene, buspirone, and trihexyphenidyl.

Other adverse nervous system effects occurring in less than 1% of clomipramine-treated patients include apathy, ataxia, coma, abnormal coordination, delirium, delusions, dysphonia, EEG abnormalities, encephalopathy, euphoria, extrapyramidal disorder, abnormal gait, hallucinations, hostility, hyperkinesia, hypnagogic hallucinations, hypokinesia, neuralgia, paranoia, phobic disorder, psychosis, sensory disturbance, somnambulism, stimulation, and teeth grinding; however, a causal relationship to the drug has not been established.

Rarely reported adverse nervous system effects for which a causal relationship to clomipramine has not been established include anticholinergic syndrome, aphasia, apraxia, catalepsy, cholinergic syndrome, choreoathetosis, hemiparesis, hyperesthesia, hyperreflexia, hypoesthesia, illusion, impaired impulse control, indecisiveness, mutism, neuropathy, nystagmus, oculogyric crisis, oculomotor nerve paralysis, schizophrenic reaction, generalized spasm, stupor, and torticollis. Dystonia has been reported rarely in clomipramine-treated patients, although a causal relationship to the drug has not been established. Acute dystonia that included oculogyric crisis, torticollis, and lead-pipe rigidity has occurred in a patient receiving clomipramine. Exacerbation of motor tics and development of vocal tics also have been reported in a patient receiving the drug.

Suicidal ideation and suicide attempt have been reported in less than 1% of patients receiving clomipramine and suicide has been reported rarely. (See Cautions: Precautions and Contraindications.)

■ **Cardiovascular Effects** During clinical trials, modest orthostatic decreases in blood pressure and modest tachycardia each occurred in about 20% of patients receiving clomipramine, although patients frequently were asymptomatic. Postural hypotension occurred in about 6 or 4% of adults or children and adolescents, respectively, and tachycardia occurred in about 4 or 2% of adults or children and adolescents, respectively, receiving clomipramine in controlled clinical trials. Flushing occurred in about 8 or 7% of adults or children and adolescents, respectively, treated with the drug in controlled clinical trials.

Palpitations occurred in about 4% of both adults and children or adolescents receiving clomipramine in controlled clinical trials. Chest pain occurred in about 4 or 7% of adults or children and adolescents, respectively, and syncope occurred in about 2% of children and adolescents receiving clomipramine in controlled clinical trials.

Among approximately 1400 patients who received clomipramine during the premarketing evaluation, ECG abnormalities were observed in about 1.5% of the patients compared with 3.1% of those who received an active control and 0.7% of those receiving placebo. The most commonly observed ECG changes were ventricular premature contractions, ST-T wave changes, and intraventricular conduction abnormalities. These changes rarely were associated with clinically important symptoms; nevertheless, caution is necessary when treating patients with known cardiovascular disease with clomipramine, and gradual dosage titration is recommended in such patients.

Arrhythmia, bradycardia, cardiac arrest, extrasystoles, and pallor occurred in less than 1% of patients receiving clomipramine, although a causal relationship to the drug has not been established. Aneurysm, atrial flutter, bundle-branch block, cardiac failure, cerebral hemorrhage, heart block, myocardial infarction, myocardial ischemia, peripheral ischemia, thrombophlebitis, vasospasm, and ventricular tachycardia have occurred rarely, but these adverse effects also have not been attributed definitely to the drug. Hypertension also has been reported.

General edema, greater susceptibility to infection, malaise, and parosmia have been reported in less than 1% of clomipramine-treated patients and dependent edema has been reported rarely, although these adverse effects have not been attributed definitely to the drug.

There have been reports of fatigue and dizziness during physical exertion in children and adolescents receiving clomipramine. Because the cardiovascular effects of the drug have not been studied during such stress in this age group, some clinicians state that clomipramine should be used with caution in children and adolescents who participate in active sports.

■ **GI Effects** Adverse GI effects are encountered commonly during initial clomipramine therapy and in some cases can lead to early withdrawal of the drug. Dry mouth occurs in about 84 or 63% of adults or children and adolescents, respectively, and constipation occurs in about 47 or 22% of adults or children and adolescents, respectively, receiving clomipramine.

Nausea has been reported in about 33 or 9% of adults or children and adolescents, respectively, receiving clomipramine. Dyspepsia occurred in about 22 or 13% of adults or children and adolescents, respectively, and diarrhea occurred in about 13 or 7% of adults or children and adolescents, respectively, receiving the drug. Anorexia occurred in about 12 or 22% of adults or children and adolescents, respectively, receiving the drug. Abdominal pain occurred in about 11 or 13% of adults or children and adolescents, respectively, receiving clomipramine. Increase in appetite occurred in 11% of adults treated with the drug. Taste perversion occurred in about 8 or 4% of adults or children and adolescents, respectively, receiving clomipramine. Vomiting occurred in about 7% of clomipramine-treated adults, children, and adolescents. Flatulence has been reported in about 6% of adults receiving the drug. GI disorder or dysphagia occurred in about 2% of clomipramine-treated adults, and eructation, ulcerative stomatitis, or halitosis occurred in about 2% of children and adolescents receiving the drug. Esophagitis occurred in about 1% of adults receiving clomipramine.

Blood in stool, colitis, duodenitis, gastric ulcer, gastritis, gastroesophageal reflux, gingivitis, glossitis, hemorrhoids, increased salivation, irritable bowel syndrome, peptic ulcer, rectal hemorrhage, taste loss, and tongue ulceration were reported in less than 1% of patients receiving clomipramine, but a causal relationship to the drug has not been established. Cheilitis, chronic enteritis, discolored feces, gastric dilatation, gingival bleeding, intestinal obstruction, oral/pharyngeal edema, paralytic ileus, and salivary gland enlargement have occurred rarely but have not been attributed definitely to clomipramine.

■ **Dermatologic and Sensitivity Reactions** In controlled trials, increased sweating occurred in about 29 or 9% of adults or children and adolescents, respectively, receiving clomipramine. Rash occurred in about 8% of adults and 4% of children and adolescents treated with the drug. Pruritus occurred in about 6% of adults and 2% of children and adolescents receiving clomipramine. Dermatitis, acne, or dry skin occurred in about 2% of clomipramine-treated adults. Abnormal skin odor occurred in about 2% of children and adolescents receiving clomipramine therapy. Urticaria occurred in about 1% of adults and allergy occurred in about 3% of adults and 7% of children and adolescents treated with the drug.

Alopecia, cellulitis, cyst, eczema, genital pruritus, psoriasis, and rash that was erythematous, maculopapular, or pustular have been reported in less than 1% of patients receiving clomipramine, but these effects have not been attributed definitely to the drug. Lupus erythematosus rash has occurred rarely. Photosensitivity reaction or skin discoloration has occurred in less than 1% of patients receiving clomipramine, although a causal relationship to the drug has not been established. Pseudocyanotic (e.g., slate-gray, blue-black, purplish) pigmentation that affected areas of the body exposed to sunlight and therefore may have been a photosensitivity reaction also has occurred with clomipramine. Chloasma has been reported rarely. Folliculitis, hypertrichosis, piloerection, polyarteritis nodosa, seborrhea, skin hypertrophy, or skin ulceration has been reported rarely in patients receiving clomipramine, although a causal relationship has not been established.

■ **Metabolic and Electrolyte Effects** In controlled studies, weight gain occurred in about 18% of adults who received clomipramine therapy for the treatment of obsessive-compulsive disorder compared with 1% of those receiving placebo. In these studies, a weight gain of at least 7% of initial body weight occurred in about 28% of clomipramine-treated patients compared with 4% of those receiving placebo. In several patients, weight gain exceeded 25% of the initial body weight. Conversely, weight losses of at least 7% of initial body weight occurred in about 5% of clomipramine-treated patients compared with 1% of those who received placebo. In controlled studies, weight gain or weight loss occurred in about 2 or 7% of children and adolescents, respectively, receiving clomipramine.

Thirst occurred in about 2% of adults receiving clomipramine. Dehydration, gout, hypercholesterolemia, hyperglycemia, hyperuricemia, and hypokalemia have been reported in less than 1% of patients receiving clomipramine, although a causal relationship to the drug has not been established. Fat intolerance and glycosuria have been reported rarely in patients receiving clomipramine, although these adverse effects have not been attributed definitely to the drug.

■ **Ocular and Otic Effects** Abnormal vision occurred in about 18 or 7% of adults or children and adolescents, respectively, receiving clomipramine. Abnormal lacrimation, mydriasis, and conjunctivitis occurred in about 3, 2, and 1% of adults, respectively, receiving the drug. Anisocoria, blepharospasm, and ocular allergy occurred in about 2% of children and adolescents receiving clomipramine. Adverse ocular effects reported in less than 1% of clomipramine-treated patients include abnormal accommodation, diplopia, ocular pain, foreign body sensation, photophobia, and scleritis; however, a causal relationship to the drug has not been established.

Glaucoma has been reported rarely in patients receiving clomipramine, although a causal relationship to the drug has not been established. Angle-closure glaucoma that presented clinically as amaurosis fugax (transient monocular blindness) attacks that were precipitated by rising from a sitting or supine position has been reported in at least one female patient treated with the drug. Although the precise mechanism is unclear, it was suggested that an abnormally large fall in blood pressure upon standing up combined with an increase in intraocular pressure may have been responsible. Blepharitis, chromatopsia, conjunctival hemorrhage, exophthalmos, keratitis, night blindness, retinal disorder, strabismus, and visual field defect occurred rarely in patients receiving clomipramine, but have not been attributed definitely to the drug.

Tinnitus occurred in about 6 or 4% of adults or children and adolescents, respectively, receiving clomipramine. Otitis media or vestibular disorder occurred in about 4 or 2% of children and adolescents, respectively, receiving clomipramine. Adverse otic effects reported in less than 1% of clomipramine-treated patients include hyperacusis, deafness, earache, and labyrinth disorder; however, these effects have not been attributed definitely to the drug.

■ **Musculoskeletal Effects** Myalgia occurred in about 13% of adults receiving clomipramine. Back pain and arthralgia occurred in about 6 and 3% of adults, respectively, receiving clomipramine. Muscle weakness occurred in about 1 or 2% of adults or children and adolescents, respectively, receiving clomipramine. Arthrosis and leg cramps have been reported in less than 1% of patients receiving clomipramine, although a causal relationship to the drug has not been established. Exostosis, bruising, myopathy, and myositis have been reported rarely in clomipramine-treated patients, although these effects have not been attributed definitely to the drug.

■ **Hematologic Effects** Purpura has been reported in about 3% of adults receiving clomipramine. Although no cases of severe hematologic toxicity were reported during the premarketing evaluation of clomipramine, there subsequently have been rare reports of bone marrow depression in patients receiving the drug, including leukopenia, agranulocytosis, thrombocytopenia, anemia, and pancytopenia. In controlled trials, anemia occurred in about 2% of children and adolescents receiving the drug.

■ **Respiratory Effects** Pharyngitis occurred in about 14% of adults receiving clomipramine. Rhinitis occurred in about 12 or 7% of adults or children and adolescents, respectively, receiving clomipramine. Cough occurred in about 6 or 4% of adults or children and adolescents, respectively, receiving clomipramine. Sinusitis occurred in about 6 or 2% of adults or children and adolescents, respectively, treated with the drug. Yawning occurred in about 3% of adults receiving clomipramine. Bronchospasm occurred in about 2 or 7% of adults or children and adolescents, respectively, receiving clomipramine.

Epistaxis occurred in about 2% of adults receiving clomipramine. Dyspnea or laryngitis occurred in about 2% of clomipramine-treated children and adolescents. The development of adverse respiratory effects (e.g., dry sore throat, cough) severe enough to result in aphonia also has been reported.

Although a causal relationship has not been established, bronchitis, hyperventilation, increased sputum, and pneumonia have been reported in less than 1% of patients receiving clomipramine, and cyanosis, hemoptysis, hiccup, hypoventilation, and laryngismus have been reported rarely.

■ **Genitourinary Effects** ***Sexual Dysfunction*** One characteristic of clomipramine therapy that may be troublesome to some patients is its relatively high incidence of sexual dysfunction. The incidence of sexual dysfunction in male patients receiving clomipramine therapy for obsessive-compulsive disorder during premarketing clinical trials was substantially higher than in those receiving placebo. Normal sexual functioning usually returns within a few days after discontinuing clomipramine therapy.

Libido change occurred in about 21% of adults receiving clomipramine. Ejaculatory failure occurred in about 42% of adult males treated with clomipramine compared with 2% of those receiving placebo, and impotence occurred in 20% of clomipramine-treated adult males compared with about 3% of those receiving placebo. Approximately 85% of adult males who experienced sexual dysfunction during clomipramine therapy chose to continue therapy with the drug. About 6% of adolescent males experienced ejaculation failure while receiving clomipramine. Premature ejaculation has been reported rarely but has not been attributed definitely to the drug. On the other hand, clomipramine has been used in the treatment of premature ejaculation† in a limited number of patients. Painful ejaculation or orgasm has been reported in a limited number of male patients receiving the drug.

Anorgasmy has been reported in both male and female patients receiving clomipramine. In a controlled trial, difficulty or inability to reach orgasm was the most common adverse sexual effect in clomipramine-treated patients; sexual function generally returned to normal within 3 days after discontinuance of the drug. Anorgasmy associated with clomipramine has responded to anticipatory administration of yohimbine in several patients. Orgasm during yawning also has been reported in a limited number of patients receiving clomipramine.

Other Genitourinary Effects Micturition disorder occurred in about 14 or 4% of adults or children and adolescents, respectively, receiving clomipramine. Urinary tract infection and frequent micturition occurred in about 6 and 5%, respectively, of adults receiving the drug. Urinary retention occurred in about 2 or 7% of adults or children and adolescents, respectively, receiving clomipramine while dysuria, including painful urination in men, and cystitis have been reported in about 2% of adults receiving clomipramine.

Dysmenorrhea has been reported in about 12 and 10% of adult and adolescent females, respectively, receiving clomipramine, and menstrual disorder (including irregular menstruation) has been reported in about 4% of adult females receiving the drug. Vaginitis and leukorrhea each occurred in about 2% of adult females receiving clomipramine therapy. Amenorrhea occurred in about 1% of adult females receiving clomipramine.

Although not attributed definitely to the drug, endometriosis, epididymitis, hematuria, nocturia, oliguria, ovarian cyst, perineal pain, polyuria, prostatic disorder, urethral disorder, urinary incontinence, uterine hemorrhage, or vaginal hemorrhage has been reported in less than 1% of clomipramine-treated patients. Albuminuria, cervical dysplasia, endometrial hyperplasia, pyuria, uterine inflammation, and vulvar disorder have occurred rarely; however, a causal relationship to the drug has not been established.

■ **Hepatic Effects** During premarketing evaluation, potentially clinically important elevations in serum ALT (SGOT) and AST (SGPT) concentrations exceeding 3 times the upper limit of normal were reported in approximately 1 and 3%, respectively, of patients receiving clomipramine. In most cases, these elevations in hepatic enzyme concentrations were not associated with other clinical findings suggestive of hepatic injury, and jaundice was not observed. Severe hepatic injury that was fatal in some cases has been reported rarely in foreign postmarketing experience. (See Cautions: Precautions and Contraindications.) Abnormal hepatic function and hepatitis have been reported in less than 1% of patients receiving clomipramine, although a causal relationship to the drug has not been established. Cross hepatotoxicity (e.g., elevated values on hepatic function tests, abdominal pain) involving different tricyclic antidepressants including clomipramine also has been reported.

■ **Other Adverse Effects** Hot flushes occurred in about 5% of adults and 2% of children and adolescents receiving clomipramine. Fever occurred in about 4% of adults and 2% of children and adolescents treated with the drug. Pain has been reported in about 3% of adults and 4% of children and adolescents receiving clomipramine therapy. Chills and local edema each occurred in about 2% of adults receiving the drug.

Tooth disorder occurred in about 5% of clomipramine-treated adults, and dental caries has been reported in less than 1% of patients receiving the drug. Although the exact mechanism for these effects is unclear, it has been suggested that long-term therapy with clomipramine or other antidepressants with prominent anticholinergic activity can lead to dental caries through inhibition of saliva secretion.

Elevations in serum prolactin concentrations have been reported following single and multiple doses of clomipramine. Nonpuerperal lactation has been reported in about 4% of adult females receiving clomipramine therapy. Breast enlargement and breast pain have been reported in about 2 and 1% of adult females, respectively, receiving the drug. Breast engorgement, breast fibroadenosis, and gynecomastia have been reported rarely in patients receiving clomipramine; however; these effects have not been attributed definitely to the drug.

Lymphadenopathy has been reported in less than 1% of clomipramine-treated patients, and leukemoid reaction and lymphoma-like disorder have been reported rarely, although a causal relationship to the drug has not been established.

Diabetes mellitus and hypothyroidism each have been reported in less than 1% of patients receiving clomipramine, and goiter and hyperthyroidism have been reported rarely; however, these effects have not been attributed definitely to the drug.

Oliguria, renal calculus, and renal pain have been reported in less than 1% of patients receiving clomipramine, and pyelonephritis and renal cyst have been reported rarely; however, a causal relationship to the drug has not been established. Hyponatremia also has occurred with clomipramine.

■ Precautions and Contraindications

Worsening of depression and/or the emergence of suicidal ideation and behavior (suicidality) or unusual changes in behavior may occur in both adult and pediatric (see Cautions: Pediatric Precautions) patients with major depressive disorder or other psychiatric disorders, whether or not they are taking antidepressants. This risk may persist until clinically important remission occurs. Suicide is a known risk of depression and certain other psychiatric disorders, and these disorders themselves are the strongest predictors of suicide. However, there has been a long-standing concern that antidepressants may have a role in inducing worsening of depression and the emergence of suicidality in certain patients during the early phases of treatment. Pooled analyses of short-term, placebo-controlled studies of antidepressants (i.e., selective serotonin-reuptake inhibitors and other antidepressants) have shown an increased risk of suicidality in children, adolescents, and young adults (18–24 years of age) with major depressive disorder and other psychiatric disorders. An increased suicidality risk was not demonstrated with antidepressants compared with placebo in adults older than 24 years of age, and a reduced risk was observed in adults 65 years of age or older. It currently is unknown whether the suicidality risk extends to longer-term use (i.e., beyond several months); however, there is substantial evidence from placebo-controlled maintenance trials in adults with major depressive disorder that antidepressants can delay the recurrence of depression.

The US Food and Drug Administration (FDA) recommends that all patients being treated with antidepressants for any indication be appropriately monitored and closely observed for clinical worsening, suicidality, and unusual changes in behavior, particularly during initiation of therapy (i.e., the first few months) and during periods of dosage adjustments. Families and caregivers of patients being treated with antidepressants for major depressive disorder or other indications, both psychiatric and nonpsychiatric, also should be advised to monitor patients on a daily basis for the emergence of agitation, irritability, or unusual changes in behavior as well as the emergence of suicidality, and to report such symptoms immediately to a health-care provider.

Although a causal relationship between the emergence of symptoms such as anxiety, agitation, panic attacks, insomnia, irritability, hostility, aggressiveness, impulsivity, akathisia, hypomania, and/or mania and either the worsening of depression and/or the emergence of suicidal impulses has not been established, there is concern that such symptoms may represent precursors to emerging suicidality. Consequently, consideration should be given to changing the therapeutic regimen or discontinuing therapy in patients whose depression is persistently worse or in patients experiencing emergent suicidality or symptoms that might be precursors to worsening depression or suicidality, particularly if such manifestations are severe, abrupt in onset, or were not part of the patient's presenting symptoms. If a decision is made to discontinue therapy, clomipramine dosage should be tapered as rapidly as is feasible but with recognition of the risks of abrupt discontinuance. (See Dosage and Administration.) FDA also recommends that the drugs be prescribed in the smallest quantity consistent with good patient management, in order to reduce the risk of overdosage.

It is generally believed (though not established in controlled trials) that treating a major depressive episode with an antidepressant alone may increase the likelihood of precipitating a mixed or manic episode in patients at risk for bipolar disorder. Therefore, patients should be adequately screened for bipolar disorder prior to initiating treatment with an antidepressant; such screening should include a detailed psychiatric history (e.g., family history of suicide, bipolar disorder, and depression). Clomipramine is *not* approved for use in treating bipolar depression.

As with closely related tricyclic antidepressants, clomipramine should be used with caution in patients with concurrent cardiovascular disease; hyperthyroidism; increased intraocular pressure, a history of angle-closure glaucoma, or urinary retention; tumors of the adrenal medulla; clinically important renal impairment; or hepatic disease.

In patients with cardiovascular disease, gradual dosage titration of clomipramine is recommended. In hyperthyroid patients or patients receiving thyroid agents, the possibility of cardiac toxicity also should be considered. The manufacturers state that clomipramine should be used with caution in patients with increased intraocular pressure, a history of angle-closure glaucoma, or urinary retention, since its anticholinergic effects may exacerbate these conditions. Caution also should be exercised in patients with tumors of the adrenal medulla (e.g., pheochromocytoma, neuroblastoma), since hypertensive crises may be provoked by clomipramine.

Clomipramine should be used with caution in patients with known hepatic disease, and the manufacturers recommend periodic monitoring of hepatic enzyme concentrations in such patients.

A variety of neuropsychiatric manifestations, including delusions, hallucinations, psychotic episodes, confusion, and paranoia, have been reported in patients receiving clomipramine. (See Cautions: Nervous System Effects.) However, because of the uncontrolled design of many of these studies, it is not possible to provide a precise estimate of the extent of the risk of such effects in clomipramine-treated patients. In patients whose schizophrenia has been unrecognized, an acute psychotic episode may be precipitated by clomipramine or other antidepressants. Another possibility is that clomipramine, like other antidepressants, may precipitate mania or hypomania in patients with affective disorder.

As with other tricyclic antidepressants, the development of fever and sore throat in any patient receiving clomipramine therapy should prompt the clinician to obtain leukocyte and differential blood cell counts. (See Cautions: Hematologic Effects.)

Male patients for whom clomipramine therapy is considered should be informed about the relatively high incidence of sexual dysfunction associated with the drug. Sexual dysfunction occurred in more males with obsessive-compulsive disorder treated with clomipramine than with placebo in premarketing experience. (See Cautions: Genitourinary Effects.)

As with closely related tricyclic antidepressants, the risks associated with electroconvulsive therapy (ECT) may be increased during concurrent clomipramine therapy. Because of the limited clinical experience to date, the manufacturers recommend that the combination of clomipramine and ECT be limited to those patients for whom it is essential.

Prior to elective surgery with general anesthetics, the manufacturers state that clomipramine therapy should be discontinued for as long as is clinically feasible, and the anesthetist should be so advised.

The withdrawal effects of clomipramine have not been systematically evaluated in controlled studies, although such effects have been reported following abrupt withdrawal of closely related tricyclic antidepressants. (See Cautions: Nervous System Effects and also see Chronic Toxicity in the Tricyclic Antidepressants General Statement 28:16.04.28.) Therefore, gradual tapering of clomipramine dosage and careful monitoring of the patient is recommended during discontinuance of clomipramine therapy.

Clomipramine can produce somnolence and impaired concentration, and patients should be cautioned that the drug may impair the mental and/or physical abilities required for the performance of these complex tasks. Patients also should be cautioned about the use of alcohol, barbiturates, or other CNS depressants because the effects of these agents may be exaggerated during concurrent clomipramine therapy.

The possibility of seizure is the most clinically important risk associated with clomipramine therapy (see Cautions: Nervous System Effects), and the drug should be used with caution in patients with a history of seizures or other predisposing factors (e.g., brain damage of various etiology, alcoholism, concurrent use of other drugs that lower the seizure threshold). The ability to predict the occurrence of seizures with daily doses exceeding 250 mg is limited because plasma concentrations may be dose dependent and may vary considerably among individuals administered the same dosage. Nevertheless, the manufacturers recommend limiting the daily dose of clomipramine to a maximum of 250 mg in adults or 3 mg/kg (up to 200 mg) in children and adolescents. Patients receiving clomipramine should be informed about the risk of seizures associated with the drug. In addition, physicians should discuss with patients the risk and the possibility of serious injury to themselves or other people resulting from sudden loss of consciousness while engaged in certain complex and hazardous activities (e.g., operation of complex machinery, driving a motor vehicle, swimming, climbing).

Clomipramine is contraindicated in patients with known hypersensitivity to the drug or other tricyclic antidepressants. The drug also is contraindicated in patients currently receiving, or having recently received (i.e., within 2 weeks), monoamine oxidase (MAO) inhibitor therapy. (See Drugs Associated with Serotonin Syndrome: Monoamine Oxidase Inhibitors, under Drug Interactions.) Clomipramine also is contraindicated during the acute recovery phase following myocardial infarction.

■ Pediatric Precautions

Safety and efficacy of clomipramine in children younger than 10 years of age have not been established. Therefore, the manufacturers state that no specific recommendations can be made for the use of the drug in this age group.

Safe use of clomipramine in pediatric patients 10 years of age or older for the treatment of obsessive-compulsive disorder (OCD) is based on relatively short-term studies in this patient population and from extrapolation of experience gained with adult patients. The potential risks associated with long-term clomipramine therapy have not been systematically evaluated in children and adolescents. Although there is no evidence that the drug adversely affects growth, development, or maturation in these patients, the absence of such findings does not rule out a potential for such effects with long-term use.

In a controlled study, clomipramine has been administered for up to 8 weeks to 46 children and adolescents 10–17 years of age. In addition, 150 adolescent patients have received clomipramine therapy for periods ranging from several months to several years in uncontrolled studies. Out of a total of 196 children and adolescents studied, 50 patients were 13 years of age or younger and 146 patients were 14–17 years of age. The adverse effect profile in this age group is similar to that observed in adults.

FDA warns that antidepressants increase the risk of suicidal thinking and behavior (suicidality) in children and adolescents with major depressive disorder and other psychiatric disorders. The risk of suicidality for these drugs was identified in a pooled analysis of data from a total of 24 short-term (4–16 weeks), placebo-controlled studies of 9 antidepressants (i.e., bupropion, citalopram, fluoxetine, fluvoxamine, mirtazapine, nefazodone, paroxetine, sertraline, venlafaxine) in over 4400 children and adolescents with major depressive disorder, OCD, or other psychiatric disorders. The analysis revealed a greater risk of adverse events representing suicidal behavior or thinking (suicidality) during the first few months of treatment in pediatric patients receiving antidepressants than in those receiving placebo. The average risk of such events was 4% among children and adolescents receiving these drugs, twice the risk (2%) that was observed among those receiving placebo. However, a more recent meta-analysis of 27 placebo-controlled trials of 9 antidepressants (SSRIs and others) in patients younger than 19 years of age with major depressive disorder, OCD, or non-OCD anxiety disorders suggests that the benefits of antidepressant therapy in treating these conditions may outweigh the risks of suicidal behavior or suicidal ideation. No suicides occurred in these pediatric trials.

The risk of suicidality in FDA's pooled analysis differed across the different psychiatric indications, with the highest incidence observed in the major depressive disorder studies. In addition, although there was considerable variation in risk among the antidepressants, a tendency toward an increase in suicidality risk in younger patients was found for almost all drugs studied. It is currently unknown whether the suicidality risk in pediatric patients extends to longer-term use (i.e., beyond several months).

As a result of this analysis and public discussion of the issue, FDA has directed manufacturers of all antidepressants to add a boxed warning to the labeling of their products to alert clinicians of this suicidality risk in children and adolescents and to recommend appropriate monitoring and close observation of patients receiving these agents. (See Cautions: Precautions and Contraindications.) The drugs that are the focus of the revised labeling are all drugs included in the general class of antidepressants, including those that have not been studied in controlled clinical trials in pediatric patients, since the available data are not adequate to exclude any single antidepressant from an increased risk. In addition to the boxed warning and other information in professional labeling on antidepressants, FDA currently recommends that a patient medication guide explaining the risks associated with the drugs be provided to the patient each time the drugs are dispensed.

Anyone considering the use of clomipramine in a child or adolescent for any clinical use must balance the potential risk of therapy with the clinical need.

■ **Geriatric Precautions** The manufacturers state that clinical studies with clomipramine did not include sufficient numbers of patients 65 years of age or older to determine whether they respond differently than younger patients. No unusual age-related adverse effects were identified in 152 patients at least 60 years of age participating in US clinical studies who received the drug for periods of several months to several years. In addition, other clinical experience revealed no evidence of age-related differences in response to clomipramine.

In pooled data analyses, a *reduced* risk of suicidality was observed in adults 65 years of age or older with antidepressant therapy compared with placebo. (See Cautions: Precautions and Contraindications.)

Clomipramine is eliminated more slowly in geriatric patients. In addition, older patients may not tolerate the drug's adverse effects as well as younger patients. The manufacturers and some clinicians recommend cautiously selecting a clomipramine dosage regimen in geriatric patients, usually starting at the lower end of the recommended dosage range, since decreased hepatic, renal, or cardiac function and concomitant illnesses and medications are more frequent in this population.

■ **Mutagenicity and Carcinogenicity** No clear evidence of carcinogenicity was seen in rats receiving oral clomipramine hydrochloride dosages of 20 times the maximum recommended human daily dosage in a 2-year bioassay. Hemangioendothelioma was observed in 3 out of 235 rats administered clomipramine; the relationship between this rare tumor and the drug is not known.

■ **Pregnancy, Fertility, and Lactation** Teratogenic effects were not observed in rats and mice receiving clomipramine hydrochloride dosages up to 20 times the maximum human daily dosage. Slight, nonspecific fetotoxic effects were observed in the offspring of pregnant mice receiving 10 times the maximum human daily dosage. Slight, nonspecific embryotoxicity occurred in rats receiving 5–10 times the maximum human daily dosage.

There are no adequate and controlled studies using clomipramine in pregnant women, and the drug should be used during pregnancy only if the possible benefits justify the potential risk to the fetus. Women should be advised to notify their physician if they are or plan to become pregnant during clomipramine therapy. Neonates whose mothers had received clomipramine throughout pregnancy in dosages of 75–250 mg daily have exhibited withdrawal manifestations or adverse effects, including jitteriness, tremor, seizures, twitching, hypertonia, hypotonia, tachypnea, respiratory acidosis, cyanosis, feeding difficulties, hypothermia, lethargy, and diaphoresis. Phenobarbital has been recommended by some clinicians for the management of neurologic withdrawal symptoms. Abrupt discontinuance of clomipramine at 32 weeks of pregnancy resulted in premature birth of a neonate who developed seizures soon after delivery. Because of the risk of neonatal withdrawal, some clinicians state that clomipramine therapy particularly should be avoided during late pregnancy.

Reproduction studies in rats using clomipramine hydrochloride dosages approximately 5 times the maximum human daily dosage have not revealed evidence of impaired fertility.

Clomipramine is distributed into milk. (See Pharmacokinetics: Distribution.) Adverse effects were absent in an infant who was breast-feeding from a woman who continued treatment with clomipramine at a dosage of 150 mg daily. However, because of the potential for adverse reactions, including concern about the potential for tricyclic antidepressants to affect development of the CNS of infants, a decision should be made whether to discontinue nursing or clomipramine, taking into account the importance of the drug to the woman. Women should be advised to notify their physician if they are breast-feeding.

Drug Interactions

Because of the similarity of clomipramine to other tricyclic antidepressants, all drug interactions that may occur with this class of drugs should be considered when clomipramine is used. (See Drug Interactions in the Tricyclic Antidepressants General Statement 28:16.04.28.) In addition, the possibility that clomipramine may interact with any concomitantly administered drug has not been evaluated systematically but should be considered.

■ **Drugs Associated with Serotonin Syndrome** ***Serotonin Syndrome*** Use of clomipramine concurrently or in close succession with other serotonergic drugs may result in serotonin syndrome. Although the syndrome appears to be relatively uncommon and usually mild in severity, serious complications, including seizures, disseminated intravascular coagulation, respiratory failure, severe hyperthermia, and death occasionally have been reported.

The syndrome most commonly occurs when 2 or more serotonergic agents with different mechanisms of action are administered either concurrently or in close succession. Serotonergic agents include those that increase serotonin synthesis (e.g., the serotonin precursor tryptophan), stimulate synaptic serotonin release (e.g., some amphetamines, dexfenfluramine, fenfluramine), inhibit the reuptake of serotonin after release (e.g., selective serotonin-reuptake inhibitors, tricyclic antidepressants, trazodone, dextromethorphan, meperidine, tramadol), decrease the metabolism of serotonin (e.g., monoamine oxidase [MAO] inhibitors), have direct serotonin postsynaptic receptor activity (e.g., buspirone), or nonspecifically induce increases in serotonergic neuronal activity (e.g., lithium salts).

The combination of selective serotonin-reuptake inhibitors and MAO inhibitors appears to be responsible for most of the recent case reports of serotonin syndrome. The syndrome also has been reported when MAO inhibitors have been combined with tricyclic antidepressants such as clomipramine, tryptophan, meperidine, or dextromethorphan. In rare cases, the serotonin syndrome reportedly has occurred with the recommended dosage of a single serotonergic agent (e.g., clomipramine) or during accidental overdosage (e.g., sertraline intoxication in a child). Some other drugs that have been implicated in certain circumstances include buspirone, bromocriptine, dextropropoxyphene, methylenedioxymethamphetamine (MDMA; ecstasy), selegiline (a selective MAO-B inhibitor), and sumatriptan. Other drugs that have been associated with the syndrome but for which less convincing data are available include carbamazepine, fentanyl, and pentazocine.

Clinicians should be aware of the potential for serious, possibly fatal reactions associated with the serotonin syndrome in patients receiving 2 or more drugs that increase the availability of serotonin in the CNS, even if no such interactions with the specific drugs have been reported to date in the medical literature. Pending further accumulation of data, all drugs with serotonergic activity should be used cautiously in combination and such combinations avoided whenever clinically possible. Some clinicians state that patients who have experienced serotonin syndrome may be at higher risk for recurrence of the syndrome upon reinitiation of serotonergic drugs. Pending further experience in such cases, some clinicians recommend that therapy with serotonergic agents be limited following recovery. In cases in which the potential benefit of the drug is thought to outweigh the risk of serotonin syndrome, lower potency agents and reduced dosages should be used, combination serotonergic therapy should be avoided, and patients should be monitored carefully for symptoms of serotonin syndrome.

For further information on serotonin syndrome, including manifestations and treatment, see Serotonin Syndrome under Drug Interactions: Drugs associated with Serotonin Syndrome, in Fluoxetine Hydrochloride 28:16.04.20.

Monoamine Oxidase Inhibitors Concomitant administration of clomipramine and MAO inhibitors is contraindicated, and at least 2 weeks elapse between discontinuance of clomipramine therapy and initiation of MAO inhibitor therapy and vice versa. Concomitant administration of clomipramine and an MAO inhibitor is potentially hazardous and may result in severe adverse effects associated with serotonin syndrome such as hyperpyrexia, seizures, and coma. Other adverse effects that have occurred with this combination of drugs include confusion, agitation, myoclonus, tremor, diaphoresis, shivering, rigors, rigidity, hypotension, tachycardia, cardiac arrhythmia, and disseminated intravascular coagulation. Some reactions occurring in patients receiving clomipramine and an MAO inhibitor have been fatal.

Clonus, hyperreflexia, tremor, rigidity, and diaphoresis were observed in some patients after administration of clomipramine about 1 month after discontinuance of a selective inhibitor of monoamine oxidase-A. Status epilepticus developed in a patient after treatment with clomipramine was started approximately 24 hours after discontinuance of phenelzine sulfate. Although the mechanism has not been clearly established, the reactions resemble serotonin syndrome and may be caused by excessive serotonergic activity in the CNS.

Other Serotonergic Agents Concurrent administration of clomipramine and other serotonergic drugs (e.g., lithium, alprazolam) has resulted in the development of adverse effects similar to those reported with the combination of clomipramine and an MAO inhibitor and which resemble the serotonin syndrome.

Concurrent administration of clomipramine and fluoxetine has resulted in seizures. Concurrent administration of clomipramine and fluvoxamine has resulted in a severalfold elevation of the plasma clomipramine concentration.

■ **CNS Depressants** Like other tricyclic antidepressants, clomipramine may be additive with or may potentiate the action of other CNS depressants such as alcohol and barbiturates. In addition, concomitant administration of clomipramine with phenobarbital reportedly resulted in an increase in the plasma concentration of phenobarbital.

■ **Drugs Affecting the Seizure Threshold** Caution should be observed with concurrent administration of clomipramine and drugs (e.g., other antidepressants, antipsychotic agents) that lower the seizure threshold. (See Cautions: Nervous System Effects.)

■ **Haloperidol** Concomitant administration of clomipramine with haloperidol reportedly resulted in increases in the plasma concentrations of clomipramine, presumably because of haloperidol-induced inhibition of clomipramine metabolism.

■ **Valproic Acid** The initiation of clomipramine therapy in a patient with a seizure disorder that was well controlled by valproic acid resulted in status epilepticus. The serum clomipramine concentration at the time of the seizures was elevated despite the relatively small dosage of clomipramine received (75 mg daily for 12 days). Although the mechanism has not been established clearly, it was suggested that valproic acid may have inhibited the metabolism and/or elimination of clomipramine. Pending further experience, it should be kept in mind that elevated serum concentrations of clomipramine and possibly its metabolites may occur when clomipramine and valproic acid are used concomitantly and that these changes may precipitate seizures in predisposed individuals.

■ **Other CNS Agents** The risks associated with concurrent administration of clomipramine and other CNS-active agents have not been fully evaluated to date; therefore, caution should be exercised when such agents are administered concomitantly.

■ **Oral Contraceptives** Limited data suggest that oral contraceptives do not interfere with the therapeutic effects of clomipramine. No difference in adverse effects or depression was observed in patients receiving clomipramine and oral contraceptives compared with those receiving clomipramine alone in one study. However, the clomipramine dosage given (25 mg daily) was lower than those commonly used in the treatment of obsessive-compulsive disorder or depression. Further study to confirm the safety and efficacy of combined clomipramine and oral contraceptive therapy is necessary.

■ **Smoking** Substantially lower plasma clomipramine concentrations have been reported in cigarette smokers receiving clomipramine when compared with nonsmokers. The presumed mechanism appears to be induction of clomipramine metabolism by nicotine or other substances present in cigarette smoke.

■ **Protein-bound Drugs** Clomipramine and its active metabolite, desmethylclomipramine, are highly protein bound; therefore, they theoretically could be displaced from binding sites by or could displace from binding sites other protein-bound drugs such as oral anticoagulants (e.g., warfarin) and digoxin. Pending further accumulation of data, patients receiving clomipramine with any highly protein-bound drug should be observed for potential adverse effects associated with combined therapy.

■ **Other Drugs** Concomitant use of clomipramine with anticholinergic or sympathomimetic drugs requires close supervision and careful adjustment of the dosage of clomipramine because of potential additive effects.

Consideration of the structural similarity of clomipramine with other tricyclic antidepressants would suggest that blockade of the pharmacologic effects (such as hypotension) and possibly the adverse effects of guanethidine, clonidine, or other similar hypotensive agents, as has been reported with several other tricyclic antidepressants, may be anticipated with clomipramine.

The plasma concentrations of several tricyclic antidepressants closely related to clomipramine reportedly were increased with concomitant administration of methylphenidate or drugs that inhibit hepatic microsomal enzyme systems (e.g., cimetidine, fluoxetine) and were decreased with concomitant administration of drugs that induce hepatic microsomal enzymes (e.g., barbiturates, phenytoin). Such effects also may be anticipated with clomipramine.

Acute Toxicity

Limited information is available on the acute toxicity of clomipramine.

■ **Pathogenesis** Postmarketing reports from the UK suggest that clomipramine overdosage results in lethality similar to that reported for other closely related tricyclic antidepressants.

In 10 out of 12 patients who overdosed on clomipramine taken alone or with other drugs during US clinical studies, complete recovery occurred with overdosages of up to 5 g that produced plasma concentrations of up to 1010 ng/mL. In the 2 remaining patients, who were suspected of ingesting overdosages of 7 g and 5.75 g, death occurred. Other fatalities have been reported after overdosages of clomipramine were ingested. The lowest dosage of clomipramine associated with fatality outside of the US is 750 mg.

■ **Manifestations** Overdosage with clomipramine produces signs and symptoms similar to that with other tricyclic antidepressants. (See Acute Toxicity: Manifestations, in the Tricyclic Antidepressants General Statement 28:16.04.28.) Acute pancreatitis accompanied by prolonged ileus has occurred following an overdose of clomipramine in one patient.

The signs and symptoms of clomipramine overdosage vary in severity depending on a number of factors, including the amount of drug absorbed, the patient's age, and the amount of time elapsed since ingestion. Plasma concentrations of clomipramine should not guide management of the patient. However, they may be of qualitative value when the diagnosis is not clear. In addition, evidence from one patient who experienced biphasic absorption (delayed) and elimination of clomipramine in which, after an initial decline, the serum concentration of clomipramine and desmethylclomipramine increased to a peak and declined subsequently, suggests that monitoring such concentrations until the patient is stable may be of diagnostic benefit, since manifestations of severe toxicity and the need for aggressive management also were biphasic, recurring 3–4 days after the initial toxic episode. Although clomipramine and desmethylclomipramine have low cross-reactivity (e.g., 40–50% to antibody for clomipramine at concentrations of 189–472 ng/mL) with a fluorescent polarization immunoassay (FPIA) for tricyclic antidepressants, clomipramine concentrations of 100 ng/mL are detectable by the assay, and therefore this nonspecific assay may still be useful in diagnosing overdosage with the drug.

■ **Treatment** For information on the management of tricyclic antidepressant overdosage, see Acute Toxicity: Treatment, in the Tricyclic Antidepressants General Statement 28:16.04.28. In addition, clinicians should consult a poison control center for current information about therapy for overdoses of tricyclic antidepressants because such treatment is complex and changeable.

Chronic Toxicity

Clomipramine has not been evaluated systematically in animals or humans to determine its potential for abuse, tolerance, or physical dependence. Although discontinuance of therapy has been associated with a variety of withdrawal manifestations (see Cautions: Nervous System Effects), there is no evidence of drug-seeking behavior, except for one patient with a history of dependence on codeine, benzodiazepines, and multiple psychoactive drugs. This patient received clomipramine for depression and panic attacks and appeared to become dependent on the drug after hospital discharge.

Although foreign clinical experience has not revealed substantial evidence for abuse potential with clomipramine, it is impossible to predict the extent to which the drug may be misused or abused. Because of such uncertainty, clinicians should carefully evaluate patients for a history of substance abuse and such patients who receive clomipramine should be monitored closely.

Pharmacology

The pharmacology of clomipramine is complex and in many ways resembles that of other antidepressants, particularly those agents (e.g., selective serotonin-reuptake inhibitors, trazodone) that predominantly potentiate the pharmacologic effects of serotonin (5-HT). Although clomipramine's principal pharmacologic effect in vitro is the selective inhibition of serotonin reuptake, in vivo the drug's pharmacologic activity is not so selective because of the action of its demethylated metabolite, desmethylclomipramine, as an inhibitor of norepinephrine reuptake. As a result of this and other effects, clomipramine also shares the pharmacologic profile of other tricyclic antidepressants.

■ **Nervous System Effects** The precise mechanism of action that is responsible for the efficacy of clomipramine in the treatment of obsessive-compulsive disorder is unclear. However, because of its pronounced potency in blocking serotonin reuptake at the presynaptic neuronal membrane and its efficacy in the treatment of obsessive-compulsive disorder, a serotonin hypothesis has been developed to explain the pathogenesis of the condition. The hypothesis postulates that a dysregulation of serotonin is responsible for obsessive-compulsive disorder and that clomipramine is effective because it corrects this imbalance. The potency of clomipramine relative to other tricyclic antidepressants as a serotonin-reuptake inhibitor and its superiority in obsessive-compulsive disorder provide additional support to this hypothesis. Although the available evidence supports the serotonergic hypothesis of obsessive-compulsive disorder (see Pharmacology: Serotonergic Effects), additional studies are necessary to confirm this hypothesis.

Like other tricyclic antidepressants, the exact mechanism of clomipramine's antidepressant action is unclear. Clomipramine and its principal metabolite, desmethylclomipramine, have been shown to block the reuptake of serotonin and norepinephrine, respectively, at the presynaptic neuronal membrane. The effects of serotonin and norepinephrine may thus be potentiated. However, it has been suggested that postsynaptic receptor modification is mainly responsible for the antidepressant action observed during long-term administration of antidepressant agents. During long-term therapy with most antidepressants (e.g., tricyclic antidepressants, monoamine oxidase [MAO] inhibitors), these adaptive changes generally consist of subsensitivity of the noradrenergic adenylate cyclase system in association with a decrease in the number of β-adrenergic receptors; such effects on noradrenergic receptor function commonly are referred to as "down-regulation." In addition, some antidepressants reportedly decrease the number of 5-HT binding sites following chronic administration.

Like other tricyclic antidepressants, clomipramine may produce sedation. The drug also may lower the seizure threshold, particularly at relatively high dosages. (See Cautions: Nervous System Effects.)

Serotonergic Effects Clomipramine is a potent and somewhat selective inhibitor of serotonin reuptake at the presynaptic neuronal membrane. Clomipramine-induced inhibition of serotonin reuptake causes increased synaptic concentrations of the neurotransmitter, resulting in numerous functional changes associated with enhanced serotonergic neurotransmission.

Clomipramine is the most potent inhibitor of serotonin reuptake among currently available tricyclic antidepressants. Data from in vitro studies suggest that clomipramine is approximately equivalent to or more potent than fluoxetine as a serotonin-reuptake inhibitor; however, in vivo studies indicate that the serotonin-reuptake inhibiting effect of fluoxetine may be more potent than that of clomipramine on a weight as well as an equimolar basis. This apparent discrepancy may be explained at least in part by the relatively long elimination half-lives of fluoxetine and its principal metabolite, norfluoxetine. In addition, metabolism by *N*-demethylation decreases the potency and specificity of serotonin-reuptake inhibition by clomipramine but not fluoxetine.

Clomipramine appears to decrease the turnover of serotonin in the CNS, probably as a result of a decrease in the release and/or synthesis of serotonin. Several studies have investigated the effects of clomipramine on serotonin concentrations in patients with obsessive-compulsive disorder. The concentration of serotonin in platelets has been shown to be substantially lower in patients with obsessive-compulsive disorder treated with the drug, and this decrease has been shown to correlate with clinical improvement in obsessive-compulsive manifestations in these patients.

Clomipramine reportedly decreases the concentration of 5-hydroxyindoleacetic acid (5-HIAA), the principal metabolite of serotonin, in the CSF of patients with obsessive-compulsive disorder or depression. Limited data suggest a possible relationship between improvement of obsessive-compulsive manifestations and decreased concentrations of 5-HIAA in the CSF.

Manifestations of obsessive-compulsive disorder worsened after administration of a serotonin agonist, metachlorophenylpiperazine (mCPP), compared with placebo. Manifestations of obsessive-compulsive disorder also appeared to worsen after administration of a nonselective serotonin antagonist, metergoline, compared with placebo in patients receiving clomipramine. In contrast, such exacerbation was not observed with administration of mCPP in patients treated with clomipramine for several weeks or longer. If obsessive-compulsive disorder is related to increased serotonergic responsiveness, then these data suggest that clomipramine's efficacy following long-term administration may be related to induction of subsensitivity in the serotonergic system; such an effect has been referred to as "down-regulation" of serotonin receptors.

Effects on Other Neurotransmitters Clomipramine's principal metabolite, desmethylclomipramine, is an inhibitor of norepinephrine reuptake. Clomipramine decreases the concentration of 3-methoxy-4-hydroxyphenylglycol (MHPG), a metabolite of norepinephrine, in CSF in patients with obsessive-compulsive disorder. Patients with depressive affective (mood) disorders (e.g., major depressive episode) also exhibit decreases in concentrations of 5-HIAA and MHPG in CSF during treatment with clomipramine. The decrease in the concentration of 5-HIAA in CSF was correlated with inhibition of the in vitro uptake of ^{3}H-serotonin in plasma. The change in concentration of MHPG in CSF during clomipramine therapy was correlated with amelioration of depression.

Preliminary evidence suggests that clomipramine may inhibit dopaminergic activity. Unlike many other antidepressants, clomipramine exhibited extensive binding to postsynaptic receptors of dopamine antagonists (^{3}H-spiroperidol) in vitro. In animals, dopamine antagonism has been demonstrated by clomipramine's ability to reduce apomorphine-induced behavioral stereotypy. The drug also increases the CSF concentration of the dopamine metabolite homovanillic acid secondary to increased dopamine turnover. Because obsessive-compulsive disorder is common in patients with certain disorders of dopamine regulation (e.g., Sydenham's chorea, Tourette's disorder [Gilles de la Tourette's syndrome]), additional studies are needed to determine whether these initial findings are clinically important. (See Uses: Obsessive-Compulsive Disorder.)

Like other tricyclic antidepressants, clomipramine binds to cholinergic receptors and exhibits marked anticholinergic activity. As a result, clomipramine therapy may cause adverse effects commonly associated with blockade of muscarinic cholinergic receptors (e.g., dry mouth, blurred vision, urinary retention, constipation, confusion). In addition, clomipramine binds to α_1-adrenergic and histaminergic receptors and consequently exhibits α_1-adrenergic blocking and antihistaminic activity at usual therapeutic dosages. The drug also has been shown to bind to α_2-adrenoceptors and opiate receptors.

CNS Metabolic Effects Brain imaging studies using positron emission tomography (PET) have demonstrated metabolic abnormalities (usually hypermetabolism) in certain regions of the brain (including the orbitofrontal cortex, caudate nucleus, and prefrontal gyri) in patients with obsessive-compulsive disorder. Clomipramine appears to produce a return of metabolism to a more normal level in the regions of the brain that may be involved in the pathology of obsessive-compulsive disorder (orbitofrontal cortex and the caudate nucleus). For example, the metabolic rate of glucose was decreased in regions of the orbitofrontal cortex and the left caudate nucleus and was increased in other areas of the basal ganglia, including the right anterior putamen, in patients with obsessive-compulsive disorder treated with clomipramine compared with pretreatment measurements.

Other limited data suggest a relationship between decreases in the metabolic rate of glucose in the orbitofrontal cortex and the efficacy of clomipramine in obsessive-compulsive disorder. The decrease from baseline in the metabolic rate of glucose in the left orbitofrontal region was greater in patients whose obsessive-compulsive symptoms improved during clomipramine or fluoxetine therapy than in nonresponders to such therapy. In these patients, the decrease from baseline in the metabolic rate of glucose in the right orbitofrontal region was correlated with improvement in the manifestations of obsessive-compulsive disorder.

Effects on Sleep Like tricyclic and most other antidepressants, clomipramine suppresses rapid eye movement (REM) sleep. The drug appears to be the most potent suppressor of REM sleep in the tricyclic antidepressant class. The REM-suppressing effect may be sustained following discontinuance of clomipramine therapy, and chronic therapy leads to substantial REM rebound upon withdrawal of the drug.

■ **Cardiovascular Effects** Clomipramine shares the cardiovascular effects of other tricyclic antidepressants (see Pharmacology in the Tricyclic Antidepressants General Statement 28:16.04.24) and may produce ECG changes (e.g., increases from baseline in QRS duration, QT interval corrected for rate [QT_c], and QRS axis; inversion or flattening of the T waves), cardiac arrhythmias, tachycardia, and postural hypotension.

■ **Neuroendocrine Effects** Clomipramine affects the endocrine system. IV administration of clomipramine produced a dose-related increase in plasma prolactin and corticotropin (ACTH) concentrations in healthy individuals; an increase in the plasma cortisol concentration also was observed. Patients with depressive affective (mood) disorders (e.g., major depressive episode) also exhibited increases in plasma prolactin, ACTH, and cortisol concentrations following IV administration of clomipramine; however, the increase in plasma prolactin noted in patients with a major depressive episode was less than in nondepressed individuals. Clomipramine-induced increases in prolactin secretion appear to be serotonergically mediated.

Clomipramine appears to affect the CSF concentration of neuropeptides that are elevated in patients with obsessive-compulsive disorder. The concentrations of such neuropeptides (e.g., corticotropin-releasing hormone, vasopressin) are decreased during long-term (e.g., 20 months) therapy with the drug. In addition, an increase in the CSF concentration, corrected for age, of oxytocin has been observed.

For further information on the pharmacology of clomipramine, see Pharmacology in the Tricyclic Antidepressants General Statement 28:16.04.24.

Pharmacokinetics

In all human studies described in the Pharmacokinetics section, clomipramine was administered as the hydrochloride salt.

■ **Absorption** Clomipramine hydrochloride appears to be well absorbed from the GI tract following oral administration. However, extensive first-pass metabolism decreases its oral bioavailability to about 50%. The oral capsules and solution of clomipramine hydrochloride reportedly are bioequivalent. Food does not appear to substantially affect the bioavailability of clomipramine from the capsules.

Peak plasma clomipramine concentrations of approximately 56–154 ng/mL (mean: 92 ng/mL) usually occur within 2–6 hours (mean: 4.7 hours) following oral administration of a single 50-mg dose of clomipramine hydrochloride. Like other tricyclic antidepressants, clomipramine exhibits considerable interindividual variation in plasma concentrations achieved with a given dose due, at least in part, to genetic differences in the metabolism of the drug. (See Pharmacokinetics: Elimination.)

Following multiple-dose oral administration of clomipramine, steady-state plasma concentrations of the drug generally are achieved within about 1–2 weeks. Steady-state plasma desmethylclomipramine (the principal metabolite) concentrations may be achieved at about the same time as steady-state plasma clomipramine concentrations or later. In some cases, plasma desmethylclomipramine concentrations have been observed to continue to increase during 4–6 weeks of administration of a constant dosage of clomipramine hydrochloride. Plasma concentrations of desmethylclomipramine generally exceed those of the parent drug following multiple daily dosing of clomipramine hydrochloride.

The manufacturers state that, after multiple daily dosing of clomipramine hydrochloride 150 mg, the accumulation factors for clomipramine and desmethylclomipramine are approximately 2.5 and 4.6, respectively. However, it may take 2 weeks or more to achieve this extent of accumulation at a constant dosage because of the relatively long elimination half-lives of clomipramine and desmethylclomipramine. At steady state, peak plasma concentrations of 94–339 (mean: 218) and 134–532 (mean: 274) ng/mL of clomipramine and desmethylclomipramine, respectively, were attained following multiple daily doses of 150 mg of clomipramine hydrochloride. Pharmacokinetic data in patients receiving clomipramine hydrochloride dosages ranging from 150–250 mg daily are lacking.

In a dose-proportionality study involving multiple dosing, steady-state plasma concentrations and the areas under the plasma concentration-time curve (AUCs) of clomipramine and desmethylclomipramine were not proportional to dose at dosages ranging from 25–150 mg daily. However, at dosages ranging from 100–150 mg daily there was an approximately linear relationship between these variables and dose. The manufacturers state that the relationship between dose and plasma clomipramine or desmethylclomipramine concentrations has not been systematically evaluated at higher dosages. However, if there is a substantial dose dependency at dosages exceeding 150 mg daily, the potential exists for dramatically higher steady-state plasma concentrations and AUCs of clomipramine and desmethylclomipramine even in patients receiving dosages within the recommended range. Such an effect may pose a potential risk in some patients. (See Cautions: Precautions and Contraindications.)

The effect of age on plasma concentrations of clomipramine and desmethylclomipramine is not fully known. However, substantially lower plasma concentrations of clomipramine and desmethylclomipramine have been reported in younger adults (18–40 years of age) compared with those obtained in individuals older than 65 years of age. Children younger than 15 years of age also had substantially lower plasma concentration-dose ratios of clomipramine when compared with adults. In addition, clomipramine appears to be better tolerated in younger than in older patients.

Substantially lower steady-state plasma clomipramine concentrations have been reported in smokers when compared with nonsmokers. However, smoking appears to have less effect on plasma concentrations of desmethylclomipramine.

The relationship between plasma clomipramine and desmethylclomipramine concentrations and the therapeutic and/or toxic effects of the drug has not been clearly established. The results of studies involving plasma concentration monitoring in patients with obsessive-compulsive disorder and/or depression have been equivocal. In some studies, the sum of plasma clomipramine and desmethylclomipramine concentrations has been used as the drug concentration. In depressed patients, preliminary evidence suggests that lower plasma concentrations of clomipramine plus desmethylclomipramine (less than 150 ng/mL) are associated with nonresponse while higher concentrations (exceeding 450 ng/mL) may be associated with an increased risk of adverse effects and perhaps nonresponse. In patients with obsessive-compulsive disorder, the results of 2 studies in which a relationship between plasma concentration and therapeutic response was found suggested that optimal therapeutic response may be obtained in patients with plasma clomipramine concentrations ranging from 100–250 ng/mL and plasma desmethylclomipramine concentrations ranging from 230–550 ng/mL.

■ **Distribution** Distribution of clomipramine and its metabolites into human body tissues and fluids has not been fully characterized. However, both clomipramine and desmethylclomipramine are highly lipophilic and are widely distributed in body tissues, with moderate to high concentrations occurring in organs such as the lungs, adrenals, kidneys, heart, and brain. The apparent volume of distribution of clomipramine in healthy adults averages 17 L/kg (range: 9–25 L/kg).

Both clomipramine and desmethylclomipramine cross the blood-brain barrier; the manufacturers state that desmethylclomipramine is distributed into CSF at a concentration about 2.6 times higher than in plasma. However, in one study of patients with depression or obsessive-compulsive disorder, the concentration of desmethylclomipramine in CSF was 2.6% that of the plasma concentration, corresponding to the fraction of desmethylclomipramine not bound to plasma proteins.

Clomipramine is approximately 97–98% bound to plasma proteins, principally to albumin and possibly to α_1-acid glycoprotein (α_1-AGP). The extent of protein binding of clomipramine appears to be independent of plasma concentration. Desmethylclomipramine is approximately 97–99% bound to plasma proteins. Because protein binding of both clomipramine and desmethylclomipramine is extensive, the manufacturers state that, while the possibility that clomipramine interacts with other highly protein-bound drugs has not been fully evaluated, such interactions may be important. (See Drug Interactions: Protein-bound Drugs.)

Clomipramine crosses the placenta and also is distributed into human milk. In one case report, plasma clomipramine concentrations were measured in an infant whose mother was receiving clomipramine hydrochloride 125 mg daily during pregnancy. The plasma clomipramine concentration in the infant was 267 ng/mL at birth; subsequently, the plasma concentration in the infant decreased although nursing began 7 days after delivery and continued. After the first week postpartum, the mother's dosage of clomipramine hydrochloride was increased to 150 mg daily and the concentration of clomipramine in milk was 80–160% of the concurrent plasma clomipramine concentration at steady state. The infant's plasma concentration of clomipramine was at the limit of detection (9.8 ng/mL) 35 days postpartum. Serum concentrations of clomipramine and its metabolites (i.e., desmethylclomipramine, 8-hydroxyclomipramine, 8-hydroxydesmethylclomipramine) were not observed or were below the limit of detection in a limited number of healthy, full-term neonates and infants who were breast-fed by mothers whose only medication was clomipramine administered at a constant dosage for at least 3 weeks.

■ **Elimination** Evidence that the steady-state plasma concentrations and AUCs of clomipramine and desmethylclomipramine may increase disproportionately with increasing oral doses of the drug suggests that the metabolism of clomipramine and desmethylclomipramine may be capacity-limited (saturable). The manufacturers caution that this fact should be considered when evaluating the available data concerning the pharmacokinetic parameters of clomipramine as these data often were obtained in individuals receiving 150-mg daily doses. If clomipramine and desmethylclomipramine exhibit nonlinear pharmacokinetics at dosages exceeding 150 mg daily, their elimination half-lives may be considerably prolonged at dosages near the upper limit of the recommended dosage range (i.e., 200–250 mg daily). At such dosages, clomipramine and desmethylclomipramine may accumulate, which may increase the incidence of any dose- or plasma concentration-dependent adverse effects, particularly seizures.

The elimination half-life of clomipramine averages approximately 32 hours (range: 19–37 hours) and that of desmethylclomipramine averages about 69 hours (range: 54–77 hours) following a single, 150-mg oral dose of the drug.

The exact metabolic fate of clomipramine has not been fully elucidated. Clomipramine appears to be extensively metabolized to desmethylclomipramine and other metabolites and their glucuronide conjugates. Desmethylclomipramine, the principal metabolite, is formed by *N*-demethylation of clomipramine. Other metabolites of clomipramine include 8-hydroxyclomipramine, 2-hydroxyclomipramine, and clomipramine *N*-oxide, which appear to be formed via 8-hydroxylation, 2-hydroxylation, and *N*-oxidation, respectively. The metabolites of desmethylclomipramine include 8-hydroxydesmethylclomipramine and didesmethylclomipramine, which apparently are formed via 8-hydroxylation and *N*-demethylation, respectively. Although desmethylclomipramine is pharmacologically active, its efficacy in obsessive-compulsive disorder is not known. 8-Hydroxyclomipramine and 8-hydroxydesmethylclomipramine also are pharmacologically active but the clinical importance of their presence remains unknown.

The hydroxylation of clomipramine and desmethylclomipramine appears to be under genetic control (similar to that of debrisoquine and sparteine). In healthy adults who were phenotyped for debrisoquine hydroxylation, extensive metabolizers were distinguishable from poor metabolizers with regard to the extent of hydroxylation of desmethylclomipramine. Blood concentrations of desmethylclomipramine were higher than expected in a limited number of patients who subsequently were found to be poor metabolizers. Limited data suggest that CYP2D6, a cytochrome P-450 isoenzyme implicated in the sparteine/debrisoquine oxidation polymorphism, is involved in the 8-hydroxylation of clomipramine and desmethylclomipramine and in the 2-hydroxylation of clomipramine. In addition, demethylation of clomipramine may involve CYP2C, which is implicated in the *S*-mephenytoin oxidation polymorphism, and CYP1A2.

Possible differences in the metabolism of clomipramine among ethnic populations were suggested by a study in a limited number of healthy individuals that showed plasma clomipramine concentrations after a single oral dose of the drug to be higher in Asians (e.g., Indian, Pakistani) than in whites (e.g., British). In Japanese patients treated with clomipramine, substantial interindividual variation in demethylation and hydroxylation was observed; however, the prevalence of possibly poor demethylators and poor hydroxylators of clomipramine was estimated to be 0 and 1%, respectively. Further study is needed to clarify whether the pharmacokinetics of clomipramine truly differ in individuals of various ethnic backgrounds.

Following oral administration, clomipramine and its metabolites are excreted in urine and in feces (via biliary elimination). In 2 healthy individuals, approximately 51–60 and 24–32% of an orally administered, radiolabeled, 25-mg dose of clomipramine hydrochloride were excreted in urine and feces, respectively, after 14 days. Unchanged clomipramine and desmethylclomipramine were excreted in urine in quantities that together comprised approximately 0.8–1.3% of the dose. In a limited number of healthy individuals who received a single oral dose of clomipramine, 8-hydroxyclomipramine glucuronide was the principal metabolite found in urine. Although the urinary recovery of 8-hydroxyclomipramine glucuronide in these individuals who were phenotyped for metabolism of sparteine and mephenytoin was lower in poor metabolizers of sparteine compared with extensive metabolism of sparteine, estimates of clearance via glucuronidation did not differ between phenotypes, suggesting that the capacity for glucuronidation is not contingent on the capacity for 8-hydroxylation of clomipramine.

The effects of renal and hepatic impairment on the disposition of clomipramine have not been fully elucidated.

Limited data suggest that demethylation of clomipramine may be reduced with chronic alcohol consumption. In one study, the clearance of clomipramine via demethylation was decreased substantially and the ratio of blood clomipramine to desmethylclomipramine concentrations at steady state was higher in recently detoxified alcoholic patients (abstinence periods ranged from 4–20 weeks) compared with a control group of patients with no history of alcoholism.

Induction of drug-metabolizing enzymes (as measured by antipyrine half-life) does not appear to occur with clomipramine.

Hemodialysis, peritoneal dialysis, forced diuresis, and/or exchange transfusion are unlikely to remove clomipramine and desmethylclomipramine substantially because of the drug s rapid distribution into body tissues.

Chemistry and Stability

■ **Chemistry** Clomipramine, a dibenzazepine-derivative tricyclic antidepressant, is the 3-chloro analog of imipramine. Clomipramine is commercially available as the hydrochloride salt, which occurs as a white to off-white crystalline powder. The drug is freely soluble in water, methanol, and methylene chloride, and insoluble in ethyl ether and hexane. The drug has a pK_a of 9.5.

■ **Stability** Clomipramine hydrochloride capsules should be stored in tight containers at a temperature of 20–25°C and protected from moisture. When stored as directed, the capsules have an expiration date of 3 years following the date of manufacture.

For further information on chemistry, pharmacology, pharmacokinetics, uses, cautions, acute toxicity, drug interactions, and dosage and administration of clomipramine, see the Tricyclic Antidepressants General Statement 28:16.04.28.

Preparations

Excipients in commercially available drug preparations may have clinically important effects in some individuals; consult specific product labeling for details.

clomiPRAMINE Hydrochloride

Oral		
Capsules	25 mg*	Anafranil®, Mallinckrodt
		clomiPRAMINE Hydrochloride Capsules
	50 mg*	Anafranil®, Mallinckrodt
		clomiPRAMINE Hydrochloride Capsules
	75 mg*	Anafranil®, Mallinckrodt
		clomiPRAMINE Hydrochloride Capsules

*available from one or more manufacturer, distributor, and/or repackager by generic (nonproprietary) name

†Use is not currently included in the labeling approved by the US Food and Drug Administration

Doxepin Hydrochloride

■ Doxepin hydrochloride is a dibenzoxepin-derivative tricyclic antidepressant.

Uses

■ **Depressive and Anxiety Disorders** Doxepin shares the pharmacologic actions of the other tricyclic antidepressants and is used principally in the treatment of depression and/or anxiety in psychoneurotic patients, depression and/or anxiety associated with alcoholism or organic disease, and psychotic depressive disorders with associated anxiety, including involutional depression and manic-depressive disorders. Symptoms of psychoneurosis that respond well to doxepin include anxiety, tension, depression, somatic symptoms and concerns, sleep disturbances, guilt, lack of energy, fear, apprehension, and worry.

For further information on treatment of major depression and considerations in choosing the most appropriate antidepressant for a particular patient, including considerations related to patient tolerance, patient age, and cardiovascular, sedative, and suicidality risks, see Considerations in Choosing Antidepressants under Uses: Major Depressive Disorder, in the Tricyclic Antidepressants General Statement 28:16.04.28.

■ **Chronic Idiopathic Urticaria** Doxepin also has been effective in the management of chronic idiopathic urticaria† and may be used as an alternative to antihistamines, which generally are considered as first-line therapy in patients with this condition.

Dosage and Administration

■ **Administration** Doxepin hydrochloride is administered orally. Although doxepin has been administered in up to 3 divided doses throughout the day, it is long-acting and the entire daily dose may be administered at one time. Administration of the entire daily dose at bedtime may reduce daytime sedation.

Each dose of the oral concentrate should be diluted with approximately 120 mL of water, whole or skimmed milk, or orange, grapefruit, tomato, prune, or pineapple juice just prior to administration; the solution is physically incompatible with many carbonated beverages. For patients requiring doxepin therapy while on methadone maintenance, doxepin solution and methadone syrup can be mixed together with Gatorade®, lemonade, orange juice, sugar water, Tang®, or water, but not with grape juice. Bulk dilution and storage are not recommended by the manufacturers.

Doxepin is applied topically to the skin as an antipruritic. (See Doxepin Hydrochloride 84:08.)

■ **Dosage** Dosage of doxepin hydrochloride is expressed in terms of doxepin. There is a wide range of dosage requirements, and dosage must be carefully individualized. Initial dosages should be low and generally range from 30–150 mg daily, depending on the severity of the condition being treated. Dosage may be gradually adjusted to the level which produces maximal therapeutic effect with minimal toxicity and may range up to 300 mg daily. The manufacturers state that dosages exceeding 300 mg daily rarely produce additional therapeutic benefits. Hospitalized patients under close supervision may generally be given higher dosages than outpatients. Patients with very mild symptomatology or organic brain syndrome should usually be given lower than average dosages and may obtain satisfactory improvement with 25–50 mg of doxepin daily. The manufacturers state that appropriate dosage in geriatric patients should be selected with caution, usually initiating therapy at the low end of the dosage range since decreased hepatic, renal, or cardiac function occurs more frequently in these patients.

When doxepin is administered as a single daily dose, the maximum daily dose recommended by the manufacturers is 150 mg. Commercially available 150-mg capsules of doxepin are intended for maintenance therapy only and are not recommended for initial therapy. Maximum antidepressant effects may not occur for 2 or more weeks after therapy is begun, although anxiolytic effects may develop more rapidly.

After symptoms are controlled, dosage should be gradually reduced to the lowest level which will maintain relief of symptoms. To avoid the possibility of precipitating withdrawal symptoms, doxepin should not be terminated abruptly in patients who have received high dosages for prolonged periods.

Patients should be monitored for possible worsening of depression, suicidality, or unusual changes in behavior, especially at the beginning of therapy or during periods of dosage adjustment. (See Cautions: Precautions and Contraindications, in the Tricyclic Antidepressants General Statement 28:16.04.28.)

Cautions

Doxepin shares the pharmacologic actions and toxic potentials of the tricyclic antidepressants, and the usual precautions of tricyclic antidepressant administration should be observed. Patients should be fully advised about the risks, especially suicidal thinking and behavior (suicidality), associated with tricyclic antidepressant therapy. For a complete discussion, see Cautions: Precautions and Contraindications and Cautions: Pediatric Precautions, in the Tricyclic Antidepressants General Statement 28:16.04.28.

■ **Pediatric Precautions** Safety of doxepin in children younger than 12 years of age has not been established.

The US Food and Drug Administration (FDA) has determined that antidepressants increase the risk of suicidal thinking and behavior (suicidality) in children and adolescents with major depressive disorder and other psychiatric disorders. However, FDA also states that depression and certain other psychiatric disorders are themselves associated with an increased risk of suicide. Anyone considering the use of doxepin in a child or adolescent for any clinical use must therefore balance the potential risk of therapy with the clinical need. (See Cautions: Precautions and Contraindications and Cautions: Pediatric Precautions, in the Tricyclic Antidepressants General Statement 28:16.04.28.)

■ **Lactation** Limited data indicate that doxepin and its active *N*-demethylated metabolite are distributed into milk. Sedation and serious respiratory depression were reported in a nursing infant whose mother was receiving 75 mg of doxepin daily; substantial concentrations of the active metabolite of the drug were detected in the infant's serum and urine. In addition, poor sucking and swallowing while nursing, drowsiness, muscle hypotonia, and vomiting were reported in a nursing infant whose mother was receiving 35 mg of doxepin daily. Because of the potential for serious adverse reactions to doxepin and/or its active metabolite in nursing infants, a decision should be made whether to discontinue nursing or the drug, taking into account the importance of the drug to the woman.

Pharmacokinetics

■ **Absorption** The pharmacokinetics of doxepin have not been extensively studied, but the drug is well absorbed from the GI tract in animals. Peak plasma concentrations usually occur within 2 hours after oral administration of the drug.

■ **Distribution** Doxepin is highly bound to plasma proteins.

Limited data indicate that doxepin and its active *N*-demethylated metabolite are distributed into milk in concentrations reportedly ranging from about 30–140% and 10–115%, respectively, of those in maternal serum and that substantial concentrations of the active metabolite have been detected in the serum and urine of nursing infants whose mothers were receiving 75–150 mg of doxepin daily.

■ **Elimination** The plasma half-life of doxepin is 6–24.5 hours. The drug appears to be metabolized via the same pathways as are other tricyclic antidepressants; its *N*-demethylated metabolite is pharmacologically active.

Chemistry and Stability

■ **Chemistry** Doxepin hydrochloride is a dibenzoxepin-derivative tricyclic antidepressant. The drug occurs as a white powder, is freely soluble in water and in alcohol, and has a pK_a of 8. Doxepin hydrochloride oral concentrate has a pH of 4–7.

■ **Stability** Doxepin hydrochloride capsules should be stored in tight, light-resistant containers at a temperature between 15–30°C and the oral concentrate should be stored at a temperature between 20–25°C. Commercially available doxepin hydrochloride capsules have an expiration date of 36 months and the oral concentrate has an expiration date of 24 months following the date of manufacture.

Doxepin hydrochloride oral concentrate is physically incompatible with many carbonated beverages, but is compatible with some other beverages. (See Dosage and Administration: Administration.) Bulk preparation and storage of dilutions of the commercially available oral concentrate are not recommended by the manufacturers.

For further information on chemistry, pharmacology, pharmacokinetics, uses, cautions, acute toxicity, drug interactions, and dosage and administration of doxepin, see the Tricyclic Antidepressants General Statement 28:16.04.28.

Preparations

Excipients in commercially available drug preparations may have clinically important effects in some individuals; consult specific product labeling for details.

Doxepin Hydrochloride

Oral		
Capsules	10 mg (of doxepin)*	**Doxepin Hydrochloride Capsules**
		SINEquan®, Pfizer
	25 mg (of doxepin)*	**Doxepin Hydrochloride Capsules**
		SINEquan®, Pfizer
	50 mg (of doxepin)*	**Doxepin Hydrochloride Capsules**
		SINEquan®, Pfizer
	75 mg (of doxepin)*	**Doxepin Hydrochloride Capsules**
		SINEquan®, Pfizer
	100 mg (of doxepin)*	**Doxepin Hydrochloride Capsules**
		SINEquan®, Pfizer
	150 mg (of doxepin)*	**Doxepin Hydrochloride Capsules**
		SINEquan®, Pfizer
Solution, concentrate	10 mg (of doxepin) per mL*	**Doxepin Hydrochloride Oral Solution (Concentrate)**
		SINEquan® Oral Concentrate, Pfizer

*available from one or more manufacturer, distributor, and/or repackager by generic (nonproprietary) name

ANTIDEPRESSANTS, MISCELLANEOUS 28:16.04.92

buPROPion Hydrochloride

Amfebutamone Hydrochloride

■ Bupropion hydrochloride is an aminoketone-derivative antidepressant agent that is chemically unrelated to tricyclic, tetracyclic, or other currently available antidepressants (e.g., selective serotonin-reuptake inhibitors) and also is chemically unrelated to nicotine or other agents currently used in the treatment of nicotine dependence.

Uses

■ **Major Depressive Disorder** Bupropion hydrochloride is used in the treatment of major depressive disorder. Efficacy of conventional bupropion tablets for long-term use (i.e., exceeding 6 weeks) as an antidepressant has not been established by controlled studies; if conventional or extended-release tablets of the drug are used for extended periods, the need for continued therapy should be reassessed periodically. Systematic evaluation of bupropion hydrochloride extended-release tablets has shown that antidepressant efficacy is maintained for periods of up to 44 weeks in patients receiving 150 mg twice daily.

Efficacy of bupropion for the management of major depression has been established by a controlled study of approximately 6 weeks' duration in an outpatient setting and by 2 controlled studies of approximately 4 weeks' duration in inpatient settings. Bupropion hydrochloride was administered as conventional tablets in these studies, and the dosage received by 78% of the patients in one of the studies of 4 week's duration was 450 mg or less daily, although the dosage was titratable to 600 mg daily. Efficacy of bupropion in these studies was demonstrated by improvement in total score on the Hamilton rating scale for depression (HAM-D), in item 1 of the HAM-D that measures depressed mood, and in the Clinical Global Impressions of Severity of Illness (CGI-S) scale. Patients received 300 or 450 mg daily of bupropion hydrochloride in the second study of 4 weeks' duration, which demonstrated efficacy only of the higher dosage, as indicated by improvement in total score on the HAM-D and in the CGI-S scale. However, in the study of 6 weeks' duration that evaluated the efficacy of 300 mg daily of bupropion hydrochloride, the drug was superior to placebo in improvement of total score on the HAM-D, which was the primary measure of efficacy. In addition, depressed mood, as measured by item 1 on the HAM-D, was improved in patients treated with bupropion. The drug also was superior to placebo in improvement of scores on the Montgomery-Asberg Depression Rating Scale, the CGI-S scale, and the Clinical Global Impressions of Improvement (CGI-I) scale. Although clinical studies specifically establishing the efficacy of extended-release tablets of bupropion in the management of major depression have not been performed to date, the extended-release, film-coated tablet (e.g., Wellbutrin® SR) formulation of the drug has been shown to be bioequivalent at steady state to conventional tablets of bupropion, and antidepressant efficacy was maintained for up to 44 weeks in a placebo-controlled study. In addition, the extended-release tablet (Wellbutrin® XL) has been shown to be bioequivalent to the conventional and the extended-release, film-coated tablets. (See Pharmacokinetics: Absorption.)

A major depressive episode is characterized principally by a relatively persistent depressed mood and/or loss of interest or pleasure in all or almost all activities; such symptoms differ from previous functioning and occur for most of the day nearly every day for at least 2 weeks. In addition, the episode may be manifested as a change in appetite, substantial weight loss or gain, a change in sleep, psychomotor agitation or retardation, fatigue or loss of energy, feelings of guilt or worthlessness, difficulty in thinking or concentrating, and/or suicidal ideation or attempts.

Clinical studies have shown that the antidepressant effect of usual dosages of bupropion in patients with moderate to severe depression is greater than that of placebo and comparable to that of usual dosages of tricyclic antidepressants, fluoxetine, or trazodone. Bupropion generally was not distinguishable from these antidepressant agents in measures of efficacy that included the HAM-D scale, the CGI-S scale, the CGI-I scale, and the Hamilton rating scale for anxiety (HAM-A). However, other antidepressants were associated with greater improvement on the HAM-D rating scale during some weeks of the evaluations principally because of the greater improvement in the sleep factor of this scale observed with tricyclic antidepressants or trazodone in comparison to bupropion.

Because of differences in the adverse effect profile between bupropion and tricyclic antidepressants, particularly less frequent anticholinergic effects, cardiovascular effects, antihistaminic effects, and weight gain with bupropion therapy, bupropion may be preferred for patients in whom such effects are not tolerated or are of potential concern. In a study that compared bupropion with doxepin, discontinuance of therapy because of adverse effects resulted mainly from anticholinergic effects, particularly drowsiness, in patients treated with doxepin but from a variety of adverse effects in patients treated with bupropion. After 13 weeks of therapy, patients who received doxepin had gained 2.73 kg while those who received bupropion had lost 1.36 kg. Orthostatic hypotension that required discontinuance of the antidepressant agent occurred with some frequency with imipramine but not with bupropion. In addition, in a large open study, 54% of patients who responded poorly to previous antidepressant therapy responded to bupropion therapy, and 63% of patients who poorly tolerated previous antidepressant therapy tolerated bupropion; 81% of patients who completed an initial 8-week treatment phase in this study elected to receive maintenance therapy with bupropion. Although the possibility of bupropion-induced seizures should be considered in weighing the benefits versus risks compared with alternative therapies, the risk of seizures appears to be within clinically acceptable parameters in patients without preexisting risk. (See Cautions: Nervous System Effects.)

Bupropion also may be preferable because of its minimal adverse effects and possibly beneficial effects on sexual functioning. Most men with depression who experienced sexual dysfunction (e.g., decreased libido, partial erectile failure) during therapy with another antidepressant (e.g., tricyclic antidepressant, maprotiline, trazodone, tranylcypromine) did not have such impairment with bupropion. In a study comparing the adverse sexual effects of bupropion with those of selective serotonin-reuptake inhibitors (i.e., fluoxetine, paroxetine, and sertraline), statistically significant increases in libido, sexual arousal, intensity of orgasm, and/or duration of orgasm were reported in most bupropion-treated patients compared with those reported before the onset of illness, while selective serotonin-reuptake inhibitor therapy significantly reduced these aspects of sexual functioning in most of the patients studied. In another study, dysfunctional orgasm resolved when antidepressant therapy was changed from fluoxetine to bupropion in most men and women who developed orgasm failure and/or delay with fluoxetine. Libido and satisfaction with overall sexual functioning also were improved with bupropion. Limited experience suggests that bupropion also may be useful in the management of sexual dysfunction associated with fluoxetine. Sexual dysfunction (e.g., decreased libido, erectile and orgasmic impairment) associated with fluoxetine was reported to respond to concomitant administration of 75 mg daily of bupropion hydrochloride.

Bupropion administered alone or concurrently with other antidepressant agents may be useful in patients with refractory depression. In the large-scale Sequenced Treatment Alternatives to Relieve Depression (STAR*D) effectiveness trial, patients with major depressive disorder who did not respond to or could not tolerate citalopram, a selective serotonin-reuptake inhibitor (SSRI), were randomized to switch to extended-release ("sustained-release") bupropion, sertraline (another SSRI), or extended-release venlafaxine (a selective serotonin- and norepinephrine-reuptake inhibitor) as a second step of treatment (level 2). Remission rates as assessed by the 17-item Hamilton Rating Scale for Depression (HRSD-17) and the Quick Inventory of Depressive Symptomatology—Self Report (QIDS-SR-16) were approximately 21 and 26% for extended-release bupropion, 18 and 27% for sertraline, and 25 and 25% for extended-release venlafaxine therapy, respectively; response rates as assessed by the QIDS-SR-16 were 26%, 27%, and 28% for extended-release bupropion, sertraline, and extended-release venlafaxine therapy, respectively. These results suggest that after unsuccessful initial treatment of depressed patients with an SSRI, approximately 25% of patients will achieve remission after therapy is switched to another antidepressant, and either another SSRI (e.g., sertraline) or an agent from another class (e.g., bupropion, venlafaxine) may be reasonable alternative antidepressants in patients not responding to initial SSRI therapy.

In a second STAR*D level 2 trial, patients with major depressive disorder who did not respond to or could not tolerate SSRI therapy (citalopram) were randomized to receive either extended-release ("sustained-release") bupropion or buspirone therapy in addition to citalopram. Although both extended-release bupropion and buspirone were found to produce similar remission rates, extended-release bupropion produced a greater reduction in the number and severity of symptoms and a lower rate of drug discontinuance than buspirone in this large-scale, effectiveness trial. These results suggest that augmentation of SSRI therapy with extended-release bupropion may be useful in some patients with refractory depression.

For further information on treatment of major depressive disorder and considerations in choosing the most appropriate antidepressant for a particular patient, including considerations related to patient tolerance, patient age, and cardiovascular, sedative, and suicidal risks, see Considerations in Choosing Antidepressants under Uses: Major Depressive Disorder, in the Tricyclic Antidepressants General Statement 28:16.04.28.

■ Seasonal Affective Disorder Bupropion, as extended-release tablets (Wellbutrin® XL), is used in the prevention of seasonal major depressive episodes in patients with a diagnosis of seasonal affective disorder (SAD; also referred to as winter depression). Seasonal affective disorder is characterized by recurrent major depressive episodes, most commonly occurring during the autumn and/or winter months. Episodes may last up to 6 months and typically begin in the autumn and remit in the springtime. Although patients with seasonal affective disorder may have depressive episodes during other times of the year, the number of seasonal episodes should substantially outnumber the number of nonseasonal episodes during the individual's lifetime for a diagnosis of seasonal affective disorder to be considered.

Efficacy of bupropion, as extended-release tablets, for the prevention of seasonal major depressive episodes associated with seasonal affective disorder has been established in 3 double-blind, placebo-controlled trials in adult outpatients with a history of major depressive disorder with an autumn-winter seasonal pattern (as defined by DSM-IV criteria). Bupropion therapy was initiated prior to symptom onset during the autumn (September to November), continued through the winter months, and discontinued following a 2-week tapering period beginning the first week of spring (the fourth week of March), which resulted in a treatment duration of approximately 4 to 6 months for the majority of patients. Patients were randomized to receive either placebo or 150 mg of bupropion as extended-release tablets (Wellbutrin® XL) once daily for 1 week, then the dosage was titrated upward to 300 mg once daily. Patients judged by the investigator to be unlikely or unable to tolerate the 300-mg daily dosage were allowed to continue to receive 150 mg daily or to have their dosage reduced to 150 mg once daily; mean dosages in the 3 studies ranged from 257–280 mg once daily. In these 3 trials, a substantially higher percentage of patients receiving bupropion extended-release tablets were depression-free at the end of treatment compared with those receiving placebo (81.4 vs 69.7%, 87.2 vs 78.7%, and 84 vs 69%, respectively, for studies 1, 2, and 3, respectively); the depression-free rate for the 3 studies combined was 84.3% for extended-release bupropion tablets and 72% for placebo.

■ Smoking Cessation Bupropion, as extended-release tablets, is used as an adjunct in the cessation of smoking. Such therapy may be combined with nicotine replacement therapy if necessary. However, the manufacturer states that before patients receive this combination of therapies, the labeling for both bupropion and nicotine should be consulted and recommends that patients who receive bupropion and nicotine concurrently be monitored for the development of hypertension related to such therapy. (See Cautions: Cardiovascular Effects.)

The US Public Health Service (USPHS) guideline for the treatment of tobacco use and dependence recommends bupropion (as extended-release tablets) as one of several first-line drugs that may reliably increase long-term smoking abstinence rates. Nicotine (tobacco) dependence is a chronic relapsing disorder that requires ongoing assessment and often repeated intervention. Because effective nicotine dependence therapies are available, every patient should be offered effective treatment, and those who are unwilling to attempt cessation should be provided at least brief interventions designed to increase their motivation to stop tobacco use. Delineated in the current USPHS guideline for the treatment of tobacco use and dependence are 5 brief strategies of intervention that can be provided by any clinician; these strategies consist of asking patients if they use tobacco, advising those who use tobacco to quit, assessing their willingness to quit, assisting those who attempt to quit, and arranging follow-up to prevent relapse. Also included in the USPHS guideline are recommendations for the use of pharmacotherapy in general, first-line drugs (i.e., extended-release bupropion, buccal [gum or lozenge] nicotine polacrilex, transdermal nicotine, nicotine nasal spray, nicotine oral inhaler, varenicline) that should be considered initially as part of treatment for tobacco dependence, unless contraindicated, and second-line drugs (i.e., clonidine, nortriptyline). Clinicians should encourage all patients attempting to quit smoking to use effective pharmacotherapy, except when contraindicated or in specific populations for which there is insufficient evidence of efficacy (e.g., pregnant women, smokeless tobacco users, light smokers [e.g., less than 10 cigarettes daily], adolescents). For additional information on smoking cessation, see Guidelines under Uses: Smoking Cessation, in Nicotine 12:92, and also consult the most current USPHS Clinical Practice Guideline on Treating Tobacco Use and Dependence available at http://www.ahrq.gov/professionals/clinicians-providers/guidelines-recommendations/index.html.

Bupropion (extended-release) may be particularly useful in patients greatly concerned about gaining weight after cessation of smoking since therapy with the drug has been shown to result in delay in such gain in weight. Nicotine dependence therapy with an antidepressant such as bupropion also may be particularly useful when a depressive disorder is included in the current or past history of patients attempting to quit smoking. Although it is not necessary to assess for possible comorbid psychiatric disorders prior to initiating therapy for nicotine dependence, awareness of such comorbidity is important in the assessment and treatment of nicotine-dependent patients since psychiatric disorders are common in this population, smoking cessation or nicotine withdrawal may exacerbate the comorbid condition, bupropion and varenicline therapy have been associated with worsening of preexisting psychiatric disorders in some cases, and patients with psychiatric comorbidities have an increased risk for relapse to smoking after a cessation attempt.

It should be considered that serious neuropsychiatric adverse effects (including but not limited to depression, suicidal ideation, suicide attempt, and completed suicide) have been reported during postmarketing experience in patients being treated with bupropion or varenicline (another smoking cessation drug). (See Neuropsychiatric Symptoms and Suicidality in Smoking Cessation Treatment under Cautions: Nervous System Effects and Cautions: Precautions and Contraindications.) The possible risk of serious adverse effects during bupropion therapy should always be weighed against the significant health benefits of its use for smoking cessation, including a reduction in the risk of developing pulmonary disease, cardiovascular disease, and cancer.

Patients should begin receiving bupropion while they are still smoking since steady-state plasma concentrations of the drug are not achieved until after about 1 week. A date on which patients quit smoking (cessation date) should be scheduled within the first 2 weeks of therapy with bupropion and generally should be set for the second week (e.g., day 8). Counseling and support are important interventions for patients to receive throughout therapy with bupropion and for a period after its discontinuance. Achievement of cessation of smoking and maintenance of abstinence are more likely with frequent follow-ups and the provision of support by the clinician and other health-care professionals. The importance of participation in behavioral therapies, counseling, and/or support services to which bupropion is adjunctive therapy should be discussed with the patient. The overall program of interventions to enable cessation of smoking should be reviewed by clinicians. The choice of adjunctive therapy (e.g., nicotine replacement, bupropion) should consider factors such as ease of administration, compliance, and potential adverse effects and risks.

Clinical Studies The efficacy of bupropion, as extended-release tablets, as an adjunct in the cessation of smoking has been established in controlled studies of smokers of at least 15 cigarettes daily, who did not have an underlying depressive disorder. Patients were treated with bupropion in conjunction with individual counseling. Cessation of smoking was defined as total abstinence, as determined with patients' daily diaries and verified by measurement of expiratory carbon monoxide, during the fourth through seventh week of treatment. Treatment over 7 weeks with bupropion or placebo resulted in 1-year cessation of smoking in a greater proportion of patients treated with the drug at a dosage of 150 or 300 mg daily but not in those receiving 100 mg daily. Cessation of smoking was achieved at the end of 7 weeks of treatment in 36–44, 27–39, or 17–19% of patients who received 300 mg daily of bupropion hydrochloride, 150 mg daily of the drug, or placebo, respectively. Maintenance of abstinence was observed with bupropion hydrochloride at a dosage of 300 mg daily. At follow-up during the twelfth week, abstinence continued in 25–30 or 14% of patients who had received bupropion hydrochloride at 300 mg daily or placebo, respectively, and at follow-up during the twenty-sixth week, abstinence continued in 19–27 or 11–16% of patients who had received bupropion hydrochloride at 300 mg daily or placebo, respectively.

Treatment over 9 weeks with bupropion at a dosage of 300 mg daily, transdermal nicotine at a dosage of 21 mg/24 hours, the combination of 300 mg daily of bupropion and transdermal nicotine at 21 mg/24 hours, or placebo resulted in cessation of smoking in a greater proportion of patients treated with bupropion, transdermal nicotine, or the combination of bupropion and transdermal nicotine than in those receiving placebo. Cessation of smoking was achieved during weeks 4–7 in 49, 36, 58, or 23% of patients who received bupropion, transdermal nicotine, the combination of bupropion and transdermal nicotine, or placebo, respectively. At follow-up during the tenth week, abstinence was observed in 46, 32, 51, or 20% of patients who had received bupropion, transdermal nicotine, the combination of bupropion and transdermal nicotine, or placebo, respectively. Additionally, when these patients were assessed at 26 weeks, cessation of smoking continued to be observed in 30, 33, and 13% of patients who received bupropion, the combination of bupropion and transdermal nicotine, or placebo, respectively. A final assessment was performed at 52 weeks and abstinence continued to be observed in 23, 28, and 8% of patients who received bupropion, the combination of bupropion and nicotine, or placebo, respectively. The manufacturer states that because the comparisons between bupropion extended-release tablets, transdermal nicotine, or the combination of these products have not been replicated, these data should not be interpreted as demonstrating superiority of any individual treatment protocol.

Another clinical study also reviewed long-term maintenance treatment with bupropion. Patients received bupropion hydrochloride extended-release tablets at a dosage of 300 mg daily for 7 weeks; therapy was continued in the patients who achieved cessation of smoking at 7 weeks with either bupropion hydrochloride extended-release tablets or placebo. At 6-month follow-up, abstinence continued in 55% of patients receiving bupropion compared with 44% of patients who received placebo therapy.

The safety and efficacy of bupropion extended-release tablets as an adjunct in the cessation of smoking in patients with chronic obstructive pulmonary disease (COPD) was established in a clinical trial in adults with mild to moderate COPD (FEV_1 at least 35%, FEV_1/FVC 70% or less, and a diagnosis of chronic bronchitis, emphysema, and/or small airways disease). Treatment over a 12 week period with bupropion or placebo resulted in cessation of smoking during the final four weeks of the study in 22 or 12% of patients, respectively.

Since efficacy in clinical studies is influenced by the population selected, a lower rate of cessation of smoking is possible with use of bupropion in an unselected population. The reported cessation rates in patients receiving bupropion were similar in patients who had and had not previously received nicotine replacement therapy for the cessation of smoking. Withdrawal symptoms, especially irritability, frustration, anger, anxiety, difficulty concentrating, restlessness, and depressed mood or negative affect, were reduced with bupropion compared with placebo. Craving for cigarettes or urge to smoke appeared to be reduced with bupropion in comparison with placebo.

■ **Obesity** For use of bupropion hydrochloride in fixed combination with naltrexone hydrochloride for weight management, see Naltrexone Hydrochloride and Bupropion Hydrochloride 28:20.08.92.

■ **Bipolar Disorder** Bupropion has been used for the treatment of bipolar depression† (bipolar disorder, depressive episode). Lithium preferably or lamotrigine alternatively are considered first-line agents by the American Psychiatric Association (APA) for the treatment of acute depressive episode of bipolar disorder, and lamotrigine (if not used initially), bupropion, or paroxetine are considered second-line agents when first-line agents are ineffective or not tolerated. If bupropion was effective for the management of an acute depressive episode, including during the continuation phase, then maintenance therapy with the drug should be considered to prevent recurrences of major depressive episodes. In a comparative study, bupropion (mean dosage of 358 mg daily) was as effective as desipramine (mean dosage of 140 mg daily) in the management of depression in patients with bipolar disorder. Hypomania or mania occurred less frequently with bupropion than with desipramine in patients treated for up to 1 year with either drug and concomitant lithium, carbamazepine, or valproate sodium.

Because bupropion may be less likely than some other antidepressants to cause a switch to mania or rapid cycling in patients with bipolar disorder, many experts consider bupropion a preferred antidepressant for use in combination with a mood-stabilizing agent in patients with severe (nonpsychotic) depression that is unresponsive to therapy with mood-stabilizing agents alone. However, the possibility that manic attacks may be precipitated in patients with bipolar disorder who receive bupropion still must be considered. To reduce the risk of developing mania, antidepressants should not be used alone in patients with depression associated with bipolar disorder and the lowest effective dosage of the antidepressant should be used for the shortest time necessary.

For further information on the management of bipolar disorder, see Uses: Bipolar Disorder, in Lithium Salts 28:28.

■ **Attention Deficit Hyperactivity Disorder** Bupropion has been used in a limited number of children with attention deficit hyperactivity disorder† (ADHD). Although stimulants (e.g., methylphenidate, dextroamphetamine) usually are considered the drugs of first choice when pharmacotherapy is indicated as an adjunct to psychological, educational, social, and other remedial measures in the treatment of ADHD in children, some clinicians recommend use of bupropion or tricyclic antidepressants as second-line therapy when there has been no response to at least 2 stimulants or when the patient is intolerant of stimulants. In controlled studies, bupropion was more effective than placebo and comparably effective to methylphenidate. In addition, in a comparative study, bupropion hydrochloride (mean dosage of 3.3 mg/kg daily; range: 1.4–5.7 mg/kg daily) was comparably effective to methylphenidate hydrochloride (mean dosage of 31 mg daily; range: 20–60 mg daily) in overall improvement of symptoms, as evaluated with the Iowa-Conners Abbreviated Parent and Teacher Questionnaire, although a trend favoring methylphenidate was noted in almost all rating scales.

Bupropion also has been used in a limited number of adults with ADHD. In an uncontrolled study in adults, bupropion (mean dosage of 359 mg daily; range: 150–450 mg daily) administered for 6–8 weeks reduced the severity of signs and symptoms of attention deficit hyperactivity disorder, as evaluated with the Targeted Attention Deficit Disorder Symptoms Scale. Additional study and experience are needed to establish the role of antidepressants versus CNS stimulants in the treatment of this disorder.

For further information on management of ADHD, see Uses: Attention Deficit Hyperactivity Disorder, in Methylphenidate 28:20.92.

■ **Other Uses** Bupropion does not appear to be effective in the treatment of panic disorder and concomitant phobic disorder†. However, the drug generally improves symptoms of panic and depression in patients with major depression who have superimposed panic symptoms.

Although bupropion has been used effectively in some patients with bulimia nervosa†, the American Psychiatric Association (APA) states that the drug has been associated with seizures in purging bulimic patients and cautions against its use in the management of this disorder. For information on the use of antidepressants in the treatment of bulimia nervosa and other eating disorders, see Uses: Eating Disorders, in Fluoxetine Hydrochloride 28:16.04.20.

Dosage and Administration

■ **Administration** Bupropion hydrochloride is administered orally. As conventional tablets, the drug usually is administered 3 times daily, preferably with 6 or more hours separating doses, or in the morning, at midday, and in the evening.

Bupropion hydrochloride extended-release tablets should be swallowed whole so that the slow drug-release characteristics are maintained. Patients should be instructed not to chew, divide, or crush the extended-release tablets. As extended-release, film-coated tablets (e.g., Wellbutrin® SR, Zyban®), bupropion hydrochloride usually is administered twice daily with an interval of at least 8 hours between doses. Extended-release tablets commercially available as Wellbutrin® XL are administered once daily in the morning with an interval of at least 24 hours between doses. For patients who develop insomnia while receiving extended-release bupropion twice daily, taking the evening dose earlier (e.g., in the afternoon, but at least 8 hours after the morning dose) rather than at bedtime may provide some relief.

Bupropion therapy with conventional tablets usually is initiated with administration twice daily, in the morning and in the evening. As extended-release tablets, bupropion hydrochloride therapy usually is initiated with administration of a single daily dose in the morning.

A retrospective analysis of clinical experience suggests that the risk of seizures during bupropion therapy may be minimized by increasing dosages gradually, by not exceeding the recommended maximum daily dosage (400 mg as extended-release, film-coated tablets [e.g., Wellbutrin® SR]) or 450 mg as conventional tablets or as extended-release tablets of Wellbutrin® XL), and by administering the daily dosage in 2 divided doses with a maximum single dose of 200 mg (as extended-release tablets) or in 3 divided doses with a maximum single dose of 150 mg (as conventional tablets). Increasing the dosage gradually also lessens the occurrence of agitation, motor restlessness, and insomnia commonly experienced when bupropion therapy is initiated. If any of these adverse effects occur and are troublesome, temporarily reducing dosage or delaying any dosage increases may be useful.

Avoiding bedtime administration of the evening dose of bupropion may lessen the occurrence of insomnia (commonly experienced during initiation of bupropion therapy). Short-term administration of an intermediate- to long-acting sedative hypnotic also may be useful during the first week of therapy but thereafter generally is not needed.

Dosages exceeding 300 mg daily as conventional tablets are administered as divided doses that should not exceed 150 mg. Conventional tablets of 75 or 100 mg can be used to create the divided doses. If the components of a larger dosage include 4 whole conventional tablets of 100 mg, the divided doses are administered 4 times daily separated by 4 or more hours so that none of the doses exceed 150 mg. Dosages exceeding 150 mg daily as extended-release, film-coated tablets (e.g., Wellbutrin® SR) should be administered as divided doses twice daily, preferably with 8 or more hours separating the doses.

■ **Dosage** Dosage of bupropion hydrochloride is expressed in terms of the salt.

All patients receiving bupropion for any indication should be monitored appropriately and observed closely for clinical worsening, suicidality, or unusual changes in behavior, particularly during initial therapy or following any change (increase or decrease) in dosage. (See Clinical Worsening and Suicide Risk in Treating Psychiatric Disorders under Cautions: Nervous System Effects, and see also Cautions: Precautions and Contraindications.)

All patients receiving bupropion for smoking cessation should be monitored for serious neuropsychiatric symptoms or worsening of preexisting psychiatric illness. (See Neuropsychiatric Symptoms and Suicidality in Smoking Cessation Treatment under Cautions: Nervous System Effects, and see also Cautions: Precautions and Contraindications.)

Major Depressive Disorder For the management of depressive disorder in adults, the recommended initial dosage of bupropion hydrochloride as conventional tablets is 100 mg twice daily. Alternatively, dosage also has been initiated at 75 mg 3 times daily. If no clinical improvement is apparent, dosage may be increased to 100 mg 3 times daily as conventional tablets after at least 3 days of therapy with the initial dosage. Bupropion hydrochloride dosages exceeding 300 mg daily should not be considered until several weeks of therapy at this dosage level have been completed since maximum effects of a given dosage of antidepressant, in general, may not be fully apparent until after 4 or more weeks of therapy. Beyond this time, if no clinical improvement is apparent, dosage of the conventional preparation may be increased to a maximum of 450 mg daily as divided doses not exceeding 150 mg each.

Bupropion hydrochloride dosage as conventional tablets should not be increased by more than 100 mg daily every 3 days. Such cautious adjustment of dosage is particularly important in lessening the risk of bupropion-induced seizures. If clinical improvement is not apparent after an appropriate trial of 450 mg daily as conventional tablets, the drug should be discontinued since further increases may be associated with an unacceptable risk of toxicity.

If extended-release, film-coated tablets of bupropion hydrochloride (e.g., Wellbutrin® SR) are used for the management of depression in adults, the recommended initial dosage is 150 mg once daily given as a single dose. If the initial dosage is tolerated adequately, it may be increased to the target dosage of 150 mg twice daily (with at least 8 hours between doses) as early as the fourth day of therapy. However, the full therapeutic effect of a given dosage may not be apparent for 4 weeks or longer, and caution is recommended when increasing dosages to minimize the risk of bupropion-induced seizures. For patients not exhibiting clinical improvement with 300 mg daily, dosage of the extended-release, film-coated tablets may be increased to 400 mg daily, given as divided doses of 200 mg twice daily (with at least 8 hours between doses). Dosages exceeding 400 mg daily as extended-release, film-coated tablets are not recommended.

Alternatively, for management of depression in adults, extended-release tablets of bupropion hydrochloride (Wellbutrin® XL) may be used. The recommended initial adult dosage of Wellbutrin® XL extended-release tablets is 150 mg given as a single dose once daily in the morning. If the initial dosage is tolerated adequately, the dosage may be increased to the target dosage of 300 mg once daily given as a single dose as early as the fourth day of therapy. However, the full therapeutic effect of a given dosage may not be apparent for 4 weeks or longer, and caution is recommended when increasing dosages to minimize the risk of bupropion-induced seizures. At least 24 hours should elapse between successive doses. For patients not exhibiting clinical improvement with a dosage of 300 mg daily, the dosage may be increased to 450 mg once daily as a single dose. Dosages exceeding 450 mg daily as Wellbutrin® XL extended-release tablets are not recommended.

If therapy is to be switched from conventional bupropion (e.g., Wellbutrin®) or from the extended-release, film-coated tablets (e.g., Wellbutrin® SR) to the once-daily Wellbutrin® XL extended-release tablets, the same total daily dosage should be given when possible, but as a single daily dose.

Although the optimum duration of bupropion hydrochloride therapy has not been established, acute depressive episodes are thought to require several months or longer of sustained antidepressant therapy. In addition, some clinicians recommend that long-term antidepressant therapy be considered in certain patients at risk for recurrence of depressive episodes (such as those with highly recurrent unipolar depression). Whether the dosage of bupropion required to induce remission is identical to the dosage needed to maintain and/or sustain euthymia is unknown. Systematic evaluation of bupropion hydrochloride extended-release, film-coated tablets (Wellbutrin® SR) has shown that antidepressant efficacy is maintained for periods of up to 44 weeks in patients receiving 150 mg twice daily. Efficacy of bupropion hydrochloride conventional tablets beyond 6 weeks has not been established systematically in controlled studies. The usefulness of the drug in patients receiving prolonged therapy with conventional or extended-release tablets should be reevaluated periodically.

Seasonal Affective Disorder For the prevention of seasonal major depressive episodes associated with seasonal affective disorder in adults, therapy with extended-release tablets of bupropion hydrochloride (Wellbutrin® XL) generally is initiated in the autumn prior to the onset of depressive symptoms; treatment should continue through the winter season and should be tapered and discontinued in the early spring. The timing of initiation and duration of treatment should be individualized based on the patient's historical pattern of seasonal major depressive episodes. Patients whose seasonal depressive episodes are infrequent or not associated with clinically important impairment generally should not be treated prophylactically.

The recommended initial adult dosage of bupropion hydrochloride, as extended-release tablets (Wellbutrin® XL), is 150 mg once daily in the morning. If the 150-mg once-daily dosage is adequately tolerated, the dosage may be increased to 300 mg once daily after 1 week. If the 300-mg once daily dosage is not adequately tolerated, the dosage may be reduced to 150 mg once daily. The usual target dosage is 300 mg given once daily in the morning. For patients receiving 300 mg of bupropion hydrochloride as extended-release tablets during the autumn-winter season, the dosage should be tapered to 150 mg once daily for 2 weeks prior to discontinuance. Dosages exceeding 300 mg daily as extended-release tablets have not been studied for prevention of episodes of seasonal major depression.

Smoking Cessation For use in adults as an adjunct in smoking cessation, the initial dosage of bupropion hydrochloride, as extended-release tablets, is 150 mg daily for the first 3 days of therapy. The dosage subsequently is increased in most patients to the usual recommended dosage of 150 mg twice daily, which also is the maximum recommended dosage. Dosages exceeding 300 mg daily should not be used for smoking cessation because of the risk of seizures. Because steady-state plasma concentrations of the drug are not achieved for about 1 week, bupropion therapy for smoking cessation should be initiated 1–2 weeks prior to discontinuance of cigarette smoking. Patients should continue to receive bupropion hydrochloride for 7–12 weeks; the need for more prolonged therapy should be individualized depending on benefits and risks to the patient. Discontinuance of therapy does not require that the dosage be tapered.

For some patients, it may be appropriate to continue pharmacotherapy with bupropion for smoking cessation for periods longer than usually recommended since nicotine dependence is a chronic condition. Use of bupropion hydrochloride as an adjunct in smoking cessation has been studied systematically as maintenance therapy at 150 mg twice daily for up to 6 months. The decision to continue therapy beyond 12 weeks for smoking cessation must be individualized. Although weaning should be encouraged for all smoking cessation pharmacotherapies, continued use of such therapy is clearly preferable to a return to smoking with respect to health consequences.

Patients have received the combination of bupropion, as extended-release tablets, and transdermal nicotine. Patients treated with this combination have been started on bupropion hydrochloride at a dosage of 150 mg daily, while they were still smoking. After 3 days, the dosage of bupropion hydrochloride was increased to 150 mg twice daily. Patients received concomitant transdermal nicotine therapy at a dosage of 21 mg/24 hours after about 1 week of therapy with bupropion, when the date scheduled for patients to stop smoking was reached. The dosage of transdermal nicotine was tapered to 14 and 7 mg/24 hours during the eighth and ninth weeks of therapy, respectively.

Complete smoking abstinence is the goal of therapy with bupropion hydrochloride. Cessation of smoking is unlikely in patients who do not show substantial progress toward abstinence after receiving bupropion hydrochloride for 7 weeks, so such therapy probably should be discontinued at that time in these patients. Unsuccessful patients may benefit from interventions to enhance the possibility for success on the next attempt. Such patients should be evaluated to determine why failure occurred, and another attempt to quit smoking should be encouraged by a more favorable context that includes elimination or reduction of the factors responsible for failure.

Depression Associated With Bipolar Disorder While comparative efficacy of various dosages in the usual range have not been established in the management of depression associated with bipolar disorder†, some experts recommend that dosages of antidepressants, including bupropion, be titrated to levels comparable to those used in the treatment of unipolar depression. In clinical studies in patients with depression associated with bipolar disorder, bupropion hydrochloride has been given in a dosage of 75–400 mg daily in conjunction with a mood-stabilizing agent (e.g., carbamazepine, lithium, valproate). Antidepressants should be used in these patients for the shortest time necessary.

Attention Deficit Hyperactivity Disorder For the treatment of attention deficit hyperactivity disorder† (ADHD) in adults, bupropion hydrochloride therapy has been initiated with a dosage of 150 mg daily as conventional tablets. Dosage was then titrated to a maximum daily dosage of 450 mg as conventional tablets.

Although safety and efficacy of bupropion hydrochloride in pediatric patients younger than 18 years of age have not been established, if bupropion is used for the treatment of ADHD in children†, some experts recommend that those weighing 20 kg or more receive an initial dosage of 1 mg/kg daily in 2–3 divided doses. This initial dosage should be given for the first 3 days of therapy, then dosage should be titrated up to 3 mg/kg daily in 2–3 divided doses by day 7 and up to 6 mg/kg daily in 2–3 divided doses or 300 mg (whichever is smaller) by the third week of therapy. Alternatively, some experts suggest that pediatric patients with ADHD receive bupropion hydrochloride beginning with an initial dosage of 37.5 mg or 50 mg twice daily with dosage titration over 2 weeks up to a maximum dosage of 250 mg daily (300–400 mg daily in adolescents). Up to 4 weeks of bupropion therapy may be necessary to attain maximum effects of the drug. Pediatric dosage for ADHD generally has ranged from 50–100 mg 3 times daily. If extended-release tablets are used for ADHD, the pediatric dosage generally has ranged from 100–150 mg twice daily.

■ **Dosage in Renal and Hepatic Impairment** Bupropion should be used with caution in patients with renal impairment, and a reduction in dosage and/or frequency of administration should be considered. Although bupropion is extensively metabolized in the liver to active metabolites, its active metabolites are renally excreted and may accumulate to a greater extent in patients with renal impairment than in those with normal renal function. (See Pharmacokinetics.) Therefore, patients with renal impairment should be closely monitored for possible adverse effects (e.g., seizures) that could indicate higher than recommended drug or metabolite concentration and necessitate a reduction in dose and/or frequency of administration of bupropion. Based on limited pharmacokinetic data obtained in a single-dose study, some clinicians suggest that patients undergoing hemodialysis should receive 150 mg of bupropion hydrochloride as extended-release tablets every 3 days instead of daily for smoking cessation; a multiple-dose study is needed to confirm these findings. (See Pharmacokinetics: Elimination.)

Because substantial increases in peak plasma bupropion concentrations and accumulation of the drug may occur in patients with severe hepatic cirrhosis, bupropion should be used with extreme caution in these patients. Dosage of the drug in these patients should not exceed 75 mg once daily as conventional tablets, 100 mg once daily or 150 mg every other day as extended-release, film-coated tablets (e.g., Wellbutrin® SR), or 150 mg every other day as Wellbutrin® XL extended-release tablets or Zyban® extended-release, film-coated tablets. The drug should also be used with caution in patients with hepatic impairment (including mild to moderate hepatic cirrhosis) and a reduction in dose and/or frequency of administration of bupropion should be considered in these patients.

Cautions

Bupropion generally is well tolerated. Common adverse effects of the drug include agitation, dry mouth, insomnia, headache/migraine, nausea/vomiting, constipation, and tremor. Discontinuance of bupropion therapy was required in about 10% of patients and healthy individuals who participated in clinical trials with conventional tablets during the drug's initial development, principally secondary to adverse neuropsychiatric (mainly agitation and abnormal mental status), GI (mainly nausea and vomiting), neurologic (mainly seizures, headaches, and sleep disturbances), and dermatologic (mainly rashes) effects in 3, 2.1, 1.7, and 1.4% of patients, respectively. However, these adverse effects often occurred at dosages exceeding the daily dosages currently recommended for major depression.

The incidences of most adverse effects in controlled trials were reported for bupropion hydrochloride dosages ranging from 300–600 mg daily for 3–4 weeks as conventional tablets, and often such effects were reported regardless of whether any attempt was made to attribute them to therapy. While the manufacturer's labeling includes comparative incidences for patients receiving placebo, reporting apparently similar incidences between bupropion and placebo groups for many of the effects, no information is provided on whether significant differences in the incidences of adverse effects exist between the groups. Because of the nature and conditions of reporting these effects in clinical trials, the incidences may not predict precisely the likelihood of encountering adverse reactions under usual medical practice where patient characteristics and other factors differ from those prevailing in the trials. In one report of several placebo-controlled trials, only dry mouth was found to occur with an incidence significantly greater than that reported for placebo, occurring in 13.1% more of patients receiving bupropion than placebo, and other adverse effects occurring at incidences that exceeded those for placebo by at least 3% included syncope/dizziness, constipation, tremor, nausea/vomiting, blurred vision, excitement/agitation, and increased motor activity.

In patients receiving 300 mg daily of bupropion hydrochloride extended-release, film-coated tablets (as Wellbutrin® SR), anorexia, dry mouth, rash, sweating, tinnitus, and tremor were reported in 5% or more of patients and at least twice as often as in patients receiving placebo in clinical trials. Abdominal pain, agitation, anxiety, dizziness, dry mouth, insomnia, myalgia, nausea, palpitation, pharyngitis, sweating, tinnitus, and urinary frequency were reported in 5% or more of patients receiving 400 mg daily (as Wellbutrin® SR) and at least twice as often as in patients receiving placebo in clinical trials.

Bupropion therapy was discontinued by 9% of patients with seasonal affective disorder receiving bupropion hydrochloride extended-release tablets (as Wellbutrin® XL) in clinical studies, compared with 5% of patients receiving placebo. Adverse effects leading to discontinuance of bupropion in at least 1% of patients and at a rate that was numerically greater than that reported with placebo included insomnia and headache, which resulted in discontinuance in 2 and 1%, respectively, of those receiving bupropion, compared with less than 1% of those receiving placebo. Constipation and flatulence were reported in 5% or more of patients and at least twice as often as in patients receiving placebo in controlled clinical trials.

In patients receiving bupropion as an adjunct in the cessation of smoking, the most commonly observed adverse effects consistently associated with the drug were dry mouth and insomnia. These adverse effects may be related in incidence to dosage so reduction of the dosage may minimize their occurrence; however, dosages less than 150 mg daily may not be effective. (See Uses: Smoking Cessation.) Although headache was a commonly reported effect, the incidences between placebo and various bupropion dosages were comparable. Therapy was discontinued in 8% of patients commonly because of neurologic (mainly tremors) or dermatologic (mainly rashes) effects, which resulted in discontinuance in 3.4 or 2.4% of patients, respectively. Other common reasons for discontinuing therapy included headache and urticaria. In 2 studies of patients receiving bupropion therapy as an adjunct for cessation of smoking, one in patients with mild to moderate chronic obstructive pulmonary disease (COPD) for 12 weeks and another that evaluated long-term administration of bupropion therapy (up to 1 year), the incidence and nature of the adverse effects reported were similar to those reported in previous studies.

■ **Nervous System Effects** ***Seizures*** One of the potentially most serious adverse effects of bupropion is reduction in the seizure threshold. However, despite the potential seriousness of this effect, seizures remain a relatively uncommon adverse effect of bupropion therapy, particularly when currently recommended dosages for depression are not exceeded and underlying predisposing factors are not present.

Seizures reportedly occurred in about 1% or more of patients overall receiving bupropion as conventional tablets, many of whom had predisposing factors; however, the risk appears to be strongly associated with predisposing factors and with dosage, with seizures occurring in only approximately 0.4% of patients receiving dosages not exceeding 450 mg daily of bupropion as conventional tablets. Seizures reportedly occurred in about 0.1% of patients treated with the extended-release, film-coated tablets of bupropion hydrochloride (as Wellbutrin® SR) at dosages of 100–300 mg daily. Whether this lower incidence of seizures is related to administration of the extended-release preparation or to lower dosages is not known, although since most observed seizures reportedly occurred during steady state, a pertinent consideration in the estimation of incidence is that the extended-release and conventional tablets are bioequivalent in terms of both the rate and extent of absorption of drug at steady state. The maximum dosages recommended for the extended-release, film-coated tablets (e.g., Wellbutrin® SR), extended-release tablets (Wellbutrin® XL), and conventional tablets are close at 400, 450, and 450 mg daily, respectively, and result in the same incidence of seizures, about 0.4%.

Of approximately 2400 patients who participated in early clinical trials with bupropion as conventional tablets, 25 patients developed seizures. The incidence of seizures was 2.8%, 2.3%, or 0.3%, respectively, in patients treated with dosages of 600–900, 600, or 450 mg and lower daily as conventional tablets. In a prospective study of the incidence of seizures in approximately 3200 patients treated with dosages up to 450 mg daily of bupropion, the total incidence of seizures was 0.1 or 0.4% for patients treated for 8 weeks or longer with dosages up to 300 mg daily as extended-release tablets (as Wellbutrin® SR) or 300–450 mg daily as conventional tablets, respectively, but most patients experiencing seizures had a predisposing factor (e.g., seizure or head trauma history, current seizure disorder, concomitant use of drugs that lower the seizure threshold). The manufacturer warns that this risk of 0.4% may be up to 4 times that of other currently available antidepressants, including bupropion as extended-release tablets administered at dosages not exceeding 300 mg daily (at a dosage of 400 mg daily, the risk is the same); however, the relative risk of seizures with antidepressant agents is not clearly defined and can be affected by a number of factors, including dosage and dosing schedule, concomitantly administered drugs, age, and underlying predisposing factors (e.g., seizure history). In addition, most patients in this prospective study received the maximum dosage of 450 mg daily. Seizures often occurred during the early phase of bupropion therapy and sometimes occurred several weeks after establishment of dosage. Although one study reported that age did not influence the risk of seizures, this study did not adequately control for potentially confounding risk factors, and it has been suggested that the risk of seizures may decrease with advancing age.

Other Nervous System Effects Many other adverse nervous system effects of bupropion occur more commonly than seizures. Agitation, insomnia, and anxiety occurred in about 32, 19, and 6% of patients, respectively, receiving bupropion. These adverse effects and restlessness occur, to some extent, in a substantial number of patients, particularly at the beginning of bupropion therapy. Such adverse effects required treatment with sedative/hypnotic drugs in some patients in clinical trials in major depressive disorder, while discontinuance of bupropion was required in about 2% of patients treated with conventional tablets of bupropion and in about 1 or 3% of patients treated with extended-release, film-coated tablets (as Wellbutrin® SR) of the drug at 300 or 400 mg daily, respectively, in these studies. A limited number of patients with insomnia derived improvement in sleep with concomitant administration of a low dosage of trazodone hydrochloride (e.g., 100 mg daily). Impairment in sleep quality and asthenia each occurred in about 4% of patients receiving bupropion, and fatigue occurred in about 5% of patients. In patients receiving extended-release, film-coated tablets of bupropion hydrochloride (as Wellbutrin® SR), agitation occurred in 3 or 9%, insomnia occurred in 11 or 16%, and anxiety occurred in 5 or 6% with 300 or 400 mg daily, respectively. In patients receiving extended-release tablets of bupropion hydrochloride (as Wellbutrin® XL) for seasonal affective disorder, agitation occurred in 2%, anxiety occurred in 7%, and insomnia occurred in 20% at a dosage of 150–300 mg daily. In patients receiving bupropion hydrochloride as an adjunct in smoking cessation, insomnia occurred in 29 or 35% of patients receiving 150 or 300 mg daily, respectively, and discontinuance of therapy was required in 0.6% of patients. Insomnia occurred in 40 or 45% of patients receiving 300 mg daily of bupropion hydrochloride alone or in combination with transdermal nicotine in a dosage of 21 mg/24 hours, respectively, and discontinuance of therapy was required in 0.8% of patients who received bupropion alone. Avoidance of administering bupropion at bedtime or reducing the dosage, if necessary, may minimize insomnia. Anxiety occurred in about 11 or 5–8% of patients receiving placebo or bupropion, respectively, as an adjunct in smoking cessation.

A variety of neuropsychiatric manifestations reportedly have emerged in patients receiving bupropion. However, because of the uncontrolled nature of many studies with the drug, it is not possible to provide a precise estimate of the risk of such effects imposed by bupropion therapy. Confusion and delusions occurred in about 8 and 1% of patients, respectively, receiving bupropion. In several cases, these and other adverse neuropsychiatric effects, such as hallucinations, psychosis, disturbance in concentration, and paranoid ideation, reportedly abated when bupropion dosage was reduced, although discontinuance of the drug may be necessary. In clinical trials, administration of bupropion as an adjunct in smoking cessation or placebo resulted in a generally comparable incidence of adverse neuropsychiatric effects in smokers without a depressive disorder. However, in postmarketing experience, patients receiving bupropion for smoking cessation have reported similar types of neuropsychiatric symptoms as those reported by patients in clinical trials of bupropion for depression. (See Neuropsychiatric Symptoms and Suicidality in Smoking Cessation Treatment and see also Clinical Worsening and Suicide Risk in Treating Psychiatric Disorders under Cautions: Nervous System Effects, and see Cautions: Precautions and Contraindications.)

Headache/migraine occurred in up to about 26% of patients receiving bupropion, and dizziness (which may be secondary to cardiovascular effects), tremor, and sedation occurred in 22, 21, and 20% of patients, respectively. Akinesia/bradykinesia occurred in about 8% of patients receiving the drug. Hostility, nervousness, and sensory disturbance occurred in about 6, 5, and 4% of patients, respectively. Disturbed concentration, somnolence, irritability, and a decrease in memory occurred in about 3% of patients. Adverse nervous system effects reportedly occurring in about 1–2% of patients include akathisia, pseudoparkinsonism, euphoria, paresthesia, and CNS stimulation. Therapy with bupropion as an adjunct in smoking cessation resulted in dizziness, disturbed concentration, dream abnormalities, or nervousness in up to about 10, 9, 5, or 4% of patients, respectively. Tremor and somnolence each occurred in up to about 2% of patients receiving bupropion as an adjunct in smoking cessation, and abnormality in thinking occurred in about 1% of patients.

Mania/hypomania reportedly occurred in up to 1% or more of patients receiving bupropion, but a causal relationship to the drug has not been established. Limited data suggest that in comparison to tricyclic antidepressants or fluoxetine, mania associated with bupropion is less severe, as indicated by the Clinical Global Impression severity rating. Therapy with bupropion as an adjunct in smoking cessation has not resulted in precipitation of mania in smokers without a depressive disorder.

Psychosis reportedly occurred in less than 1% of patients receiving bupropion, but a causal relationship to the drug has not been established. Exacerbation of psychotic behavior in patients with schizoaffective disorder, depressed type also has been reported, and catatonia, manifested as mutism, waxy flexibility, staring, rigidity, withdrawal, refusal to eat, and negativism, also has been reported in patients receiving the drug. Therapy with bupropion as an adjunct in smoking cessation has not resulted in activation of psychosis in smokers without a depressive disorder.

In at least one patient who was receiving bupropion for smoking cessation (300 mg daily), extreme irritability, restlessness, anger, anxiety, and cravings occurred soon after cigarettes were withdrawn. Within 2 days after discontinuing bupropion and initiating transdermal nicotine replacement therapy, these manifestations resolved.

Ataxia/incoordination, myoclonus, dyskinesia, dystonia, and depression occurred in 1% or more of patients receiving bupropion; however, a causal relationship to the drug has not been established. Adverse nervous system effects occurring in less than 1% of bupropion-treated patients include vertigo, dysarthria, hyperkinesia, hypesthesia, hypertonia, memory impairment, depersonalization, dysphoria, mood instability, labile emotions, paranoia, and formal thought disorder; however, a causal relationship to the drug has not been established. Rarely reported adverse nervous system effects for which a causal relationship has not been established include EEG abnormalities, abnormal neurologic exam, neuropathy, impaired attention, amnesia, neuralgia, sciatica, derealization, aggression, and aphasia. Coma, delirium, dream abnormalities, akinesia, hypokinesia, extrapyramidal syndrome, and unmasking of tardive dyskinesia also have been reported, although a causal relationship to bupropion has not been established. Exacerbation of tics in patients with attention-deficit hyperactivity disorder and coexistent Tourette's syndrome has been reported, but such exacerbation also has been observed with stimulants (e.g., amphetamine, methylphenidate) in such patients.

Clinical Worsening and Suicide Risk in Treating Psychiatric Disorders Suicidal ideation has emerged rarely in patients receiving bupropion. Suicide also is a known risk of depression and certain other psychiatric disorders, and these disorders themselves are the strongest predictors of suicide. However, there has been a long-standing concern that antidepressants may have a role in inducing worsening of depression and the emergence of suicidality in certain patients during the early phases of treatment. Pooled analyses of short-term, placebo-controlled studies of antidepressants (i.e., selective serotonin-reuptake inhibitors and other antidepressants) have shown an increased risk of suicidality in children, adolescents, and young adults (18–24 years of age) with major depressive disorder and other psychiatric disorders. An increased suicidality risk was not demonstrated with antidepressants compared with placebo in adults older than 24 years of age, and a reduced risk was observed in adults 65 years of age or older. It is currently unknown whether the suicidality risk extends to longer-term use (i.e., beyond several months); however, there is substantial evidence from placebo-controlled maintenance trials in adults with major depressive disorder that antidepressants can delay the recurrence of depression. The US Food and Drug Administration (FDA) recommends that all patients being treated with antidepressants for any indication be appropriately monitored and closely observed for clinical worsening, suicidality, and unusual changes in behavior, particularly during initiation of therapy (i.e., the first few months) and during periods of dosage adjustments. (See Cautions: Precautions and Contraindications and see Cautions: Pediatric Precautions.)

Neuropsychiatric Symptoms and Suicidality in Smoking Cessation Treatment Serious neuropsychiatric symptoms, including changes in mood (including depression and mania), psychosis, hallucinations, paranoia, delusions, homicidal ideation, hostility, agitation, aggression, anxiety, and panic as well as suicidal ideation, suicide attempt, and completed suicide, have been reported during postmarketing experience in patients receiving bupropion or varenicline for smoking cessation. Such events have occurred in patients with or without preexisting psychiatric disease, and some patients experienced worsening of their psychiatric illness. While some of the cases may have been confounded by symptoms of nicotine withdrawal typically seen in individuals who have stopped smoking, these effects also were observed in patients who continued to smoke. As a postmarketing requirement to further assess the neuropsychiatric safety of bupropion and varenicline, the manufacturers conducted a large, randomized, double-blind, placebo- and active-controlled study (EAGLES) in more than 8000 smokers with or without a history of psychiatric disorders. Patients were stratified into a nonpsychiatric or psychiatric cohort and randomized to receive varenicline (1 mg twice daily), extended-release bupropion (150 mg twice daily), transdermal nicotine (21 mg/day with taper), or placebo; treatment was continued for a total of 12 weeks and patients were followed for an additional 12 weeks posttreatment. In this study, use of varenicline or bupropion was not associated with an increased risk of clinically important psychiatric events (as assessed by a composite safety end point of anxiety, depression, feeling abnormal, hostility, agitation, aggression, delusions, hallucinations, homicidal ideation, mania, panic, paranoia, psychosis, suicidal ideation, and suicidal behavior or completed suicide) compared with nicotine replacement therapy or placebo. However, patients with a psychiatric disorder were more likely than those without such a disorder to experience a clinically important neuropsychiatric event. In the psychiatric cohort, clinically important neuropsychiatric events occurred in 12.2, 11.8, or 9.8% of patients receiving varenicline, bupropion, or nicotine, respectively, and these event rates were greater for each of the active treatments compared with placebo (9.5%). In the nonpsychiatric cohort, such events occurred in approximately 3% of patients across treatment groups. Serious neuropsychiatric events, including those requiring hospitalization, were reported in less than 1% of patients with or without a psychiatric history in all treatment groups; one completed suicide occurred in a placebo-treated patient in the nonpsychiatric cohort. (See Cautions: Precautions and Contraindications.)

■ **Metabolic Effects** Weight loss exceeding 2.27 kg occurred in about 28% of patients receiving bupropion as conventional tablets. Such weight loss occurred in about 23% of patients who were heavier than normal body weight at baseline compared with about 10% of those who were lighter than normal body weight at baseline. Patients with weight loss symptomatic of a major depressive episode were not affected differently from patients without weight loss at baseline. In patients receiving extended-release, film-coated tablets of bupropion hydrochloride (as Wellbutrin® SR) for major depressive disorder, weight loss exceeding 2.27 kg occurred in about 14 or 19% with dosages of 300 or 400 mg daily, respectively. In patients receiving extended-release tablets of bupropion hydrochloride (as Wellbutrin® XL) for seasonal affective disorder, weight loss exceeding 2.27 kg occurred in about 23% with dosages of 150–300 mg daily.

Weight gain occurred in about 14% of patients receiving bupropion as conventional tablets. A gain of at least 2.27 kg occurred in 6 or 9% of patients who were overweight or underweight, respectively, at baseline. In patients receiving extended-release, film-coated tablets of bupropion hydrochloride (as Wellbutrin® SR) for major depressive disorder, weight gain exceeding 2.27 kg occurred in about 3 or 2% with dosages of 300 or 400 mg daily, respectively. In patients receiving extended-release tablets of bupropion hydrochloride (as Wellbutrin® XL) for seasonal affective disorder, weight gain exceeding 2.27 kg occurred in about 11% with dosages of 150–300 mg daily.

Although most smokers who quit smoking gain weight, bupropion appears to be effective in delaying postcessation weight gain and therefore may be particularly useful in patients greatly concerned about gaining weight after cessation of smoking. However, once bupropion therapy is discontinued, the quitting smoker on average will gain an amount of weight that is about the same as if they had not used the drug. In patients receiving bupropion for smoking cessation, weight gain from baseline was inversely related to dose at the end of treatment in patients who abstained from smoking, with gains averaging 2.3 kg in those receiving 100 or 150 mg of the drug daily and 1.5 kg in those receiving 300 mg daily; weight gain was 2.9 kg in those receiving placebo. However, in those who remained abstinent from smoking 25 weeks after discontinuance of bupropion, weight gain was not dose related, averaging 6.6, 4.4, or 4.5 kg at dosages of 100, 150, or 300 mg daily and 5.5 kg for placebo.

■ **Cardiovascular Effects** Tachycardia occurred in up to 11% of patients receiving bupropion, and cardiac arrhythmias occurred in 5% of patients. Palpitations occurred in up to about 6% of patients receiving bupropion. Hypertension, chest pain, and flushing each occurred in about 4% of patients receiving the drug. Hypotension and syncope occurred in 3 and 1% of patients, respectively. Orthostatic hypotension also has been reported. Dizziness, possibly secondary to cardiovascular effects, has been reported commonly in patients receiving bupropion. (See Cautions: Nervous System Effects.) Bupropion generally was well tolerated in a limited number of inpatients with depression and stable congestive heart failure, although an increase in supine blood pressure was associated with the drug that resulted in discontinuance of therapy in some patients because of exacerbation of hypertension present at baseline.

In patients receiving the drugs as adjunctive therapy in smoking cessation, 300 mg daily of bupropion hydrochloride alone or combined with transdermal nicotine in a dosage of 21 mg/24 hours, hypertension emergent to either treatment was observed in 2.5 or 6.1% of patients, respectively, most of whom had evidence of preexisting hypertension. Therapy was discontinued because of hypertension in 1.2% of patients who received the combination of bupropion and transdermal nicotine. Palpitations, hypertension, or chest pain occurred in about 2, 1, or less than 1% of patients, respectively, receiving bupropion as an adjunct in smoking cessation. In some cases, the hypertension reported was severe. (See Cautions: Precautions and Contraindications.)

ECG abnormalities (e.g., premature beats, nonspecific ST-T wave changes) occurred in less than 1% of patients receiving bupropion, although a causal relationship to the drug has not been established. Pallor, phlebitis, and myocardial infarction occurred rarely, but these adverse effects also have not been definitely attributed to the drug. Third-degree heart block also has been reported.

Edema occurred in 1% or more of patients receiving bupropion but has not been definitely attributed to the drug. Peripheral edema occurred in less than 1% of patients receiving bupropion, and facial edema occurred rarely. Therapy with bupropion as an adjunct in smoking cessation resulted in facial edema in less than 1% of patients. In a patient with preexisting cardiomyopathy and hypertension who had received bupropion hydrochloride (300 mg daily) for smoking cessation, cardiac and pulmonary arrest occurred 4 days after completing therapy, and the patient died 9 days later. The safety of bupropion for smoking cessation in patients with underlying coronary heart disease remains to be established.

■ **GI Effects** Dry mouth and constipation occurred in up to about 28 and 26% of patients, respectively, receiving bupropion, and the possibility exists that such effects may result from adverse nervous system effects; however, the anticholinergic activity of the drug reportedly is substantially less than that of tricyclic antidepressants. Nausea/vomiting occurred in up to about 23% of patients. Although anorexia occurred in up to about 18% of patients receiving the drug, an increase in appetite was reported in up to about 4% of patients. Abdominal pain occurred in up to about 9% of patients receiving bupropion. Diarrhea occurred in up to about 7% of patients and dyspepsia, increased salivation, and gustatory disturbance each occurred in up to about 3% of patients receiving bupropion. Dysphagia occurred in up to about 2% of patients receiving bupropion. Mouth ulcer occurred in 2% of patients receiving bupropion as an adjunct in smoking cessation.

Stomatitis has been reported in 1% or more of patients receiving bupropion, but has not been definitely attributed to the drug. Thirst disturbance, gum irritation, and oral edema were reported in less than 1% of patients receiving the drug, but a causal relationship also has not been established. Rectal complaints, colitis, GI bleeding, intestinal perforation, stomach ulcer, gingivitis, lingual edema, glossitis, and esophagitis have occurred rarely but have not been definitely attributed to bupropion.

■ **Dermatologic and Sensitivity Reactions** Excessive sweating occurred in up to about 22% of patients receiving bupropion. Rash, pruritus, and urticaria occurred in up to about 8, 4, and 2% of patients, respectively. Cutaneous temperature disturbance occurred in about 2% of patients receiving the drug. Nonspecific rashes occurred in 1% or more of patients receiving bupropion, and alopecia, photosensitivity, and dry skin have occurred in less than 1% of patients receiving the drug, but these effects have not been definitely attributed to bupropion. Although a causal relationship has not been established, a change in hair color, hirsutism, maculopapular rash, and acne have been reported rarely, and Stevens-Johnson syndrome, angioedema, exfoliative dermatitis, and ecchymosis also have been reported. Symptoms resembling serum sickness, including arthralgia, myalgia, and fever with rash and other symptoms suggestive of delayed hypersensitivity, have been reported in association with bupropion. Anaphylactoid reactions (e.g., pruritus, urticaria, angioedema, dyspnea) that required medical management occurred rarely in patients receiving bupropion; other concomitantly administered drugs may have confounded attributing these effects to bupropion. Application site reaction occurred in 15% of patients receiving bupropion combined with transdermal nicotine as adjunctive therapy in the cessation of smoking. Dry skin or allergic reaction occurred in about 2 or 1% of patients receiving bupropion as an adjunct in smoking cessation.

■ **Ocular and Otic Effects** Blurred vision occurred in about 15% of patients receiving bupropion. Amblyopia occurred in up to about 3% of patients receiving bupropion. Adverse ocular effects reported in less than 1% of bupropion-treated patients include visual disturbance, accommodation abnormality, dry eye, increased intraocular pressure, and mydriasis; however, a causal relationship to the drug has not been established. Diplopia also has occurred but has not been definitely attributed to bupropion.

Tinnitus occurred in up to about 6% of patients receiving bupropion. Auditory disturbance occurred in 5% of patients receiving the drug. Deafness has occurred but has not definitely been attributed to bupropion.

■ **Musculoskeletal Effects** Myalgia and arthralgia occurred in up to about 6 and 5%, respectively, of patients receiving bupropion. Arthritis and muscle spasm or twitch occurred in up to about 3 and 2% of patients, respectively, receiving the drug. Musculoskeletal chest pain has been reported rarely in less than 1% of patients receiving bupropion. Leg cramps, muscle weakness, and muscle rigidity/fever/rhabdomyolysis also have been reported, although a causal relationship also has not been established. Neck pain occurred in 2% of patients receiving bupropion as an adjunct in smoking cessation.

■ **Respiratory Effects** Pharyngitis occurred in up to about 11% of patients receiving bupropion. Upper respiratory complaints occurred in about 5% of patients receiving bupropion. Sinusitis and an increase in coughing each occurred in up to about 3% of patients receiving bupropion. Although a causal relationship has not been established, bronchitis and shortness of breath/dyspnea each have occurred in less than 1% of patients receiving bupropion, and respiratory rate or rhythm disorder, bronchospasm, pneumonia, and pulmonary embolism have occurred rarely. Therapy with bupropion as an adjunct in smoking cessation resulted in rhinitis, bronchitis, or dyspnea in 12, 2, or 1% of patients, respectively.

■ **Genitourinary Effects** Menstrual complaints occurred in about 5% of patients receiving bupropion, and impotence and decreased libido each occurred in about 3% of patients. Urinary frequency, urgency, and retention occurred in up to about 5, 2, and 2% of patients, respectively, receiving the drug. Vaginal hemorrhage occurred in up to about 2% of female patients receiving bupropion. Urinary tract infection occurred in up to about 1% of patients receiving bupropion. Nocturia, increased libido, and a decrease in sexual function have occurred in 1% or more of patients receiving bupropion, although a causal relationship to the drug has not been established. Although not definitely attributed to the drug, vaginal irritation, vaginitis, testicular swelling, polyuria, painful erection, retarded ejaculation, and frigidity have been reported in less than 1% of bupropion-treated patients, and dysuria, enuresis, urinary incontinence, glycosuria, menopause, ovarian disorder, salpingitis, pelvic infection, cystitis, dyspareunia, and painful or abnormal ejaculation have occurred rarely. Clitoral priapism and sexual arousal prolonged to about 24 hours reportedly occurred in at least one female receiving bupropion; she previously had experienced anorgasmia while receiving sertraline. Substantial increases in libido, level of sexual arousal, and intensity and duration of orgasm also have been reported in some bupropion-treated patients.

■ **Other Adverse Effects** Infection occurred in up to about 9% of patients receiving bupropion. Hot flashes and pain each occurred in up to about 3% of patients receiving the drug. Fever/chills occurred in up to about 2% of patients receiving bupropion. Accidental injury or epistaxis each occurred in about 2% of patients receiving bupropion as an adjunct in smoking cessation.

Flu-like symptoms occurred in 1% or more of patients receiving bupropion but have not been definitely attributed to the drug. Although a causal relationship also has not been established, gynecomastia, abnormal liver function test results, liver damage/jaundice, toothache, and bruxism have been reported in less than 1% of bupropion-treated patients, and hormone concentration change, lymphadenopathy, anemia, pancytopenia, epistaxis, body odor, surgically related pain, drug reaction, malaise, and overdose have occurred rarely in patients receiving the drug. Syndrome of inappropriate antidiuretic hormone secretion (SIADH), hyperglycemia, hypoglycemia, hepatitis, thrombocytopenia, leukocytosis, and leukopenia also have been reported, although these adverse effects have not been definitely attributed to bupropion. Eosinophilia has also been reported. In addition, altered prothrombin time and/or international normalized ratio (INR), which have been infrequently associated with hemorrhagic or thrombotic complications, has been reported when bupropion and warfarin were administered concomitantly.

■ **Precautions and Contraindications** Worsening of depression and/or the emergence of suicidal ideation and behavior (suicidality) or unusual changes in behavior may occur in both adult and pediatric (see Cautions: Pediatric Precautions) patients with major depressive disorder or other psychiatric disorders, whether or not they are taking antidepressants. This risk may persist until clinically important remission occurs. Suicide is a known risk of depression and certain other psychiatric disorders, and these disorders themselves are the strongest predictors of suicide. However, there has been a long-standing concern that antidepressants may have a role in inducing worsening of depression and the emergence of suicidality in certain patients during the early phases of treatment. Pooled analyses of short-term, placebo-controlled studies of antidepressants (i.e., selective serotonin-reuptake inhibitors and other antidepressants) have shown an increased risk of suicidality in children, adolescents, and young adults (18–24 years of age) with major depressive disorder and other psychiatric disorders. An increased suicidality risk was not demonstrated with antidepressants compared with placebo in adults older than 24 years of age, and a reduced risk was observed in adults 65 years of age or older. It is currently unknown whether the suicidality risk extends to longer-term use (i.e., beyond several months); however, there is substantial evidence from placebo-controlled maintenance trials in adults with major depressive disorder that antidepressants can delay the recurrence of depression.

FDA recommends that all patients being treated with antidepressants for any indication be appropriately monitored and closely observed for clinical worsening, suicidality, and unusual changes in behavior, particularly during initiation of therapy (i.e., the first few months) and during periods of dosage adjustments. Families and caregivers of patients being treated with antidepressants for major depressive disorder or other indications, both psychiatric and nonpsychiatric, also should be advised to monitor patients on a daily basis for the emergence of agitation, irritability, or unusual changes in behavior, as well as the emergence of suicidality, and to report such symptoms immediately to a health-care provider.

Although a causal relationship between the emergence of symptoms such as anxiety, agitation, panic attacks, insomnia, irritability, hostility, aggressiveness, impulsivity, akathisia, hypomania, and/or mania and either the worsening of depression and/or the emergence of suicidal impulses has not been established, there is concern that such symptoms may represent precursors to emerging suicidality. Consequently, consideration should be given to changing the therapeutic regimen or discontinuing therapy in patients whose depression is persistently worse or in patients experiencing emergent suicidality or symptoms that might be precursors to worsening depression or suicidality, particularly if such manifestations are severe, abrupt in onset, or were not part of the patient's presenting symptoms. FDA also recommends that the drugs be prescribed in the smallest quantity consistent with good patient management, in order to reduce the risk of overdosage.

It is generally believed (though not established in controlled trials) that treating a major depressive episode with an antidepressant alone may increase the likelihood of precipitating a mixed or manic episode in patients at risk for bipolar disorder. Therefore, patients should be adequately screened for bipolar disorder prior to initiating treatment with an antidepressant; such screening should include a detailed psychiatric history (e.g., family history of suicide, bipolar disorder, and depression). Bupropion is *not* approved for use in treating bipolar depression.

Serious neuropsychiatric symptoms, including changes in mood (including depression and mania), psychosis, hallucinations, paranoia, delusions, homicidal ideation, hostility, agitation, aggression, anxiety, and panic as well as suicidal ideation, suicide attempt, and completed suicide, have been reported in patients receiving bupropion or varenicline for smoking cessation. (See Neuropsychiatric Symptoms and Suicidality in Smoking Cessation Treatment under Cautions: Nervous System Effects.) Patients receiving bupropion for smoking cessation should be informed that it is not unusual to experience symptoms such as irritability, anxiety, depressed mood, and difficulty sleeping while withdrawing from nicotine. Patients with serious psychiatric illness (e.g., schizophrenia, bipolar disorder, major depressive disorder) should also be advised that they may experience an exacerbation of their illness when withdrawing from nicotine, regardless of whether they are receiving bupropion therapy.

Before initiating therapy with bupropion for smoking cessation, patients should inform their clinicians about any previous psychiatric history and about any symptoms they experienced during previous attempts at smoking cessation, with or without bupropion.

Based on findings from a large randomized controlled postmarketing study indicating that the risk of serious neuropsychiatric effects with bupropion and varenicline is lower than previously thought, FDA has removed the associated boxed warning that was included in the approved labeling for these drugs. Results of the study also confirmed the benefits of these smoking cessation therapies, which were observed regardless of whether patients had a history of psychiatric illness. Although the risk remains, particularly in individuals with current or past psychiatric illnesses (e.g., depression, anxiety disorder, schizophrenia), patients generally do not experience serious consequences such as hospitalization and, therefore, the benefits of smoking cessation (e.g., reduction in the risk of developing pulmonary disease, cardiovascular disease, or certain types of cancer) continue to outweigh the risks of these drugs. The health benefits of smoking cessation are immediate and substantial.

Patients receiving bupropion for smoking cessation should be monitored for neuropsychiatric symptoms or for worsening of preexisting psychiatric conditions. Patients who experience agitation, hostility, depressed mood, or changes in behavior or thinking that are not typical for the patient or who develop suicidal ideation or suicidal behavior should discontinue bupropion therapy and immediately contact a clinician. Although resolution of symptoms after bupropion discontinuance was reported in many postmarketing reports, manifestations persisted in some cases. Therefore, ongoing patient monitoring and supportive care should be provided until symptoms resolve.

Hypertension (sometimes severe) has been reported in patients with or without evidence of preexisting hypertension who were receiving bupropion alone or in combination with nicotine replacement therapy. Bupropion should be used cautiously in patients with cardiovascular disease as the safety of bupropion in patients with a recent history of myocardial infarction or unstable heart disease has not been established because of a lack of clinical experience. However, patients who developed orthostatic hypotension with tricyclic antidepressants have tolerated bupropion well. Since hypertension occurred with the combination of bupropion and transdermal nicotine as adjunctive therapy in smoking cessation, monitoring for hypertension as an adverse effect is recommended in recipients of such concurrent therapy. (See Cautions: Cardiovascular Effects.)

Bupropion should be used with extreme caution in patients with severe hepatic impairment and the dosing interval should be increased and/or the dosage reduced. Bupropion also should be used with caution in patients with mild to moderate hepatic impairment and consideration should be given to increasing the dosing interval. (See Dosage and Administration: Dosage.) Bupropion is extensively metabolized in the liver, and pharmacokinetics of the drug and its metabolites may be altered in patients with hepatic impairment. Patients with hepatic impairment who receive bupropion should be closely monitored for adverse effects that could indicate higher than recommended drug or metabolite concentrations.

Limited information is available on the pharmacokinetics of bupropion in patients with renal impairment. An interstudy comparison between healthy individuals and patients with end-stage renal failure demonstrated that the peak concentrations and AUC values for the parent drug were comparable in the 2 groups of patients; however, the AUC values of the hydroxybupropion and threohydrobupropion metabolites were increased 2.3- and 2.8-fold, respectively, in patients with end-stage renal failure. Bupropion should be used with caution in patients with renal impairment because of potential increased accumulation of the drug and its active metabolites, which principally are excreted in urine. A reduction in dosage and/or frequency of administration of bupropion should be considered in patients with renal impairment, and the patients should be closely monitored for adverse effects (e.g., seizures) that could indicate higher than recommended drug or metabolite concentrations.

Patients should be informed that since alcohol may alter the seizure threshold, minimal drinking is advisable while abstinence is optimal during bupropion therapy. Additionally, patients should be informed that if they discontinue alcohol or sedatives (e.g., benzodiazepines) abruptly during bupropion therapy, there is an increased risk of seizures. Patients also should be cautioned that bupropion may impair their ability to perform activities requiring mental alertness or physical coordination (operating machinery, driving a motor vehicle) and to avoid such activities until they experience how the drug affects them. Counseling about bupropion as an adjunct in smoking cessation should include review of information provided by the manufacturer for patients. Ensuring that patients read the instructions provided and answering their questions are important. Patients should be warned that preparations of bupropion for use as an adjunct in smoking cessation (e.g., Zyban®) contain the same drug as preparations of bupropion for use in the treatment of psychiatric disorders (e.g., various Wellbutrin® formulations) and that they should not receive such preparations concurrently.

Patients should be advised to discontinue taking bupropion and to consult a clinician if they experience allergic, anaphylactoid or anaphylactic symptoms (e.g., skin rash, pruritus, hives, chest pain, edema, shortness of breath) during treatment with the drug. Anaphylactic or anaphylactoid reactions with symptoms including pruritus, urticaria, angioedema, and dyspnea have occurred in clinical trials of bupropion. Also, rare reports of erythema multiforme, Stevens-Johnson syndrome, and anaphylactic shock associated with use of bupropion have occurred.

Patients receiving bupropion should be advised to notify their clinician if they are taking or plan to take nonprescription (over-the-counter) or prescription drugs. The metabolism of bupropion and other drugs might be affected by such concomitant use.

Because bupropion therapy has been associated with weight loss exceeding 2.27 kg at twice the incidence with tricyclic antidepressants or placebo in comparable patients and because fewer patients gained weight with bupropion than with tricyclic antidepressants (9 versus 35%), such effects should be considered in patients whose depression includes weight loss as a major manifestation.

As with other antidepressants, the possibility should be considered that bupropion may precipitate manic attacks in patients with bipolar disorder. Another consideration is that in other susceptible patients the drug may activate latent psychosis.

The hepatotoxic potential, if any, of bupropion in humans is unclear. Hepatic hyperplastic nodules and hepatocellular hypertrophy were increased in incidence in rats chronically administered large doses of bupropion, and various histologic changes in the liver and mild hepatocellular injury suggested by laboratory tests occurred in dogs chronically administered large doses of the drug. However, despite scattered abnormalities in liver function test results observed during clinical trials with bupropion, there currently is no clinical evidence that the drug is a hepatotoxin in humans.

The manufacturer states that the incidence of seizures during therapy with bupropion administered as conventional tablets has been estimated to exceed, by as much as fourfold (e.g., 0.4 versus 0.1%), that observed during therapy with other currently available antidepressants, including bupropion hydrochloride as extended-release, film-coated tablets (e.g., Wellbutrin® SR) administered at dosages not exceeding 300 mg daily. However, the relative risk of seizures with various antidepressants, including bupropion, has not been clearly defined. In addition, the incidence of seizures at dosages of 400 mg daily as extended-release, film-coated tablets (e.g., Wellbutrin® SR) reportedly increases to 0.4%. (See Seizures under Cautions: Nervous System Effects.) The risk of seizures may be higher with sudden and large increases in dosage. Estimations of the incidence of seizures increase almost tenfold with dosages between 450–600 mg daily. Because of this disproportionate increase in the incidence of seizures and in consideration of interindividual variability in the metabolism and elimination of drugs, bupropion dosage should be titrated cautiously. While many seizures occurred early in the course of therapy, some seizures have occurred after several weeks of fixed dosage bupropion therapy. The manufacturer states that bupropion should be discontinued and not restarted in patients who experience a seizure during bupropion therapy.

Besides dose, factors that are predispositions to the development of seizures (e.g., history of head trauma or prior seizure, CNS tumor, the presence of severe hepatic cirrhosis, concomitant drugs that lower seizure threshold) appear to be strongly associated with the risk of seizures with bupropion. Presence of such predisposing factors characterized approximately one-half of the patients affected with a seizure. In addition, the patient's clinical situation may be characterized by circumstances that are associated with an increase in the risk of seizures (e.g., diabetes mellitus treated with oral antidiabetic agents or insulin, excessive use of alcohol or sedatives [e.g., benzodiazepines], abrupt withdrawal from alcohol or other sedatives, use of over-the-counter stimulants and anorexigenic agents, addiction to opiate agonists, cocaine, or stimulants). Bupropion should be used with extreme caution in patients with a history of seizure, cranial trauma, or other relevant factors or who are receiving other drugs (e.g., antipsychotics, other antidepressants, theophylline, systemic corticosteroids) or therapeutic regimens (e.g., abrupt discontinuance of a benzodiazepine) that lower the seizure threshold.

For patients being treated with bupropion for psychiatric disorders other than nicotine dependence, minimization of the risk of seizures may be possible with measures that were retrospectively identified, including gradual dosage escalation and restriction of the total dosage to 400 mg daily as extended-release, film-coated tablets (e.g., Wellbutrin® SR) or 450 mg daily as extended-release tablets (Wellbutrin® XL) or as conventional tablets. In addition, administration of the daily dose in 3 divided doses each not exceeding 150 mg is recommended when the conventional tablets are used or in 2 divided doses each not exceeding 200 mg when extended-release, film-coated tablets (e.g., Wellbutrin® SR) are used to avoid high peak concentrations of bupropion and/or its metabolites. For patients receiving bupropion for smoking cessation, such measures for minimizing the risk of seizures include restriction of the total dosage to 300 mg daily, administration of the daily dose recommended for most patients (i.e., 300 mg daily) in divided doses (i.e., 150 mg twice daily), and restriction of each dose to 150 mg so that high peak concentrations of bupropion and/or its metabolites are avoided. The decision to use bupropion as an adjunct in smoking cessation must involve consideration of whether the patient is at risk for seizures through the presence of factors that are predispositions to the development of seizures, drugs already being taken, or clinical situation of the patient. The dosage of bupropion as an adjunct in smoking cessation should not exceed 300 mg daily because the risk of seizures associated with the drug depends on dose. If patients experience a seizure while receiving bupropion for smoking cessation, the drug should be discontinued and should not be restarted.

Bupropion is contraindicated in patients with a seizure disorder. Concurrent use of any bupropion-containing medication also is contraindicated in patients already receiving any other bupropion-containing formulation (e.g., Wellbutrin®, Wellbutrin® SR, Wellbutrin® XL, Zyban®) because the incidence of seizures is dose dependent. Current or past diagnosis of bulimia or anorexia nervosa also contraindicates bupropion therapy because of the increased incidence of seizures observed in patients with bulimia treated with conventional bupropion tablets. Bupropion is contraindicated in patients undergoing abrupt discontinuance of alcohol or sedatives (including benzodiazepines). Bupropion therapy also is contraindicated in patients currently receiving, or having recently received (i.e., within 2 weeks), monoamine oxidase (MAO) inhibitor therapy and in patients with known hypersensitivity to the drug or to any other component in the formulation.

■ **Pediatric Precautions** Safety and efficacy of bupropion in children younger than 18 years of age have not been established. However, the drug has been used in a limited number of children 7–16 years of age with attention deficit hyperactivity disorder† (ADHD) without unusual adverse effect, and use of the antidepressant currently is included in recommendations of the American Academy of Pediatrics (AAP) as possible second-line therapy for the treatment of this condition as directed by clinicians familiar with its use.

The US Public Health Service (USPHS) Guideline for the treatment of tobacco use and dependence states that there is insufficient evidence to support the effectiveness of extended-release bupropion in promoting long-term smoking abstinence rates in adolescents.

FDA warns that antidepressants increase the risk of suicidal thinking and behavior (suicidality) in children and adolescents with major depressive disorder and other psychiatric disorders. The risk of suicidality for these drugs was identified in a pooled analysis of data from a total of 24 short-term (4–16 weeks), placebo-controlled studies of 9 antidepressants (i.e., bupropion, citalopram, fluoxetine, fluvoxamine, mirtazapine, nefazodone, paroxetine, sertraline, venlafaxine) in over 4400 children and adolescents with major depressive disorder, obsessive-compulsive disorder (OCD), or other psychiatric disorders. The analysis revealed a greater risk of adverse events representing suicidal behavior or thinking (suicidality) during the first few months of treatment in pediatric patients receiving antidepressants than in those receiving placebo. However, a more recent meta-analysis of 27 placebo-controlled trials of 9 antidepressants (SSRIs and others) in patients younger than 19 years of age with major depressive disorder, OCD, or non-OCD anxiety disorders suggests that the benefits of antidepressant therapy in treating these conditions may outweigh the risks of suicidal behavior or suicidal ideation. No suicides occurred in these pediatric trials.

The risk of suicidality in FDA's pooled analysis differed across the different psychiatric indications, with the highest incidence observed in the major depressive disorder studies. In addition, although there was considerable variation in risk among the antidepressants, a tendency toward an increase in suicidality risk in younger patients was found for almost all drugs studied. It is currently unknown whether the suicidality risk in pediatric patients extends to longer-term use (i.e., beyond several months).

As a result of this analysis and public discussion of the issue, FDA has directed manufacturers of all antidepressants to add a boxed warning to the labeling of their products to alert clinicians of this suicidality risk in children, adolescents, and young adults and to recommend appropriate monitoring and close observation of patients receiving these agents. (See Cautions: Precautions and Contraindications.) The drugs that are the focus of the revised labeling are all drugs included in the general class of antidepressants, including those that have not been studied in controlled clinical trials in pediatric patients, since the available data are not adequate to exclude any single antidepressant from an increased risk. In addition to the boxed warning and other information in professional labeling on antidepressants, FDA currently recommends that a patient medication guide explaining the risks associated with the drugs be provided to the patient each time the drugs are dispensed.

Anyone considering the use of bupropion in a child or adolescent for any clinical use must balance the potential risk of therapy with the clinical need.

For information on serious neuropsychiatric effects in patients receiving bupropion for smoking cessation, see Neuropsychiatric Symptoms and Suicidality in Smoking Cessation Treatment under Cautions: Nervous System Effects, and see also Cautions: Precautions and Contraindications.

■ **Geriatric Precautions** Bupropion has not been evaluated systematically in geriatric patients. The adverse effect profile in several hundred patients at least 60 years old who participated in clinical trials did not differ from that in younger patients. However, geriatric patients generally metabolize drugs slower and are more sensitive to the anticholinergic, sedative, and cardiovascular adverse effects of antidepressants. In addition, the effects of age on the pharmacokinetics of bupropion and it metabolites have not been fully elucidated. Although a single-dose pharmacokinetic study demonstrated that the disposition of bupropion and its metabolites was similar in geriatric and younger individuals, another pharmacokinetic study has suggested that geriatric patients are at increased risk for accumulation of bupropion and its metabolites following administration of single and multiple doses of the drug. (See Pharmacokinetics.)

Of the approximately 6000 patients studied in clinical trials of extended-release bupropion for smoking cessation or depression, 275 were 65 years of age or older, while 47 were 75 years of age and older. In addition, several hundred patients 65 years of age and older participated in clinical studies using conventional tablets of the drug for depression. Although no overall differences in efficacy or safety were observed between geriatric and younger patients, and other clinical experience revealed no evidence of age-related differences, the possibility that some older patients may exhibit increased sensitivity to the drug cannot be ruled out. In general, smoking cessation interventions that have been shown to be effective in the general population also have been shown to be effective in adults 50 years of age and older.

In pooled data analyses, a *reduced* risk of suicidality was observed in adults 65 years of age or older with antidepressant therapy compared with placebo. (See Cautions: Precautions and Contraindications.)

■ **Mutagenicity and Carcinogenicity** Bupropion exhibited mutagenic activity in the *Salmonella* microbial mutagen (Ames) test system; the mutation rate was 2–3 times control in 2 of 5 strains. An increase in chromosomal aberrations was observed in one of 3 in vivo cytogenetic studies conducted with the bone marrow of rats.

In lifetime carcinogenicity studies of rats or mice receiving bupropion hydrochloride dosages of 100–300 (about 2–7 times the maximum dosage in mg/m^2 recommended in humans) or 150 mg/kg daily (about 2 times the maximum dosage in mg/m^2 recommended in humans), respectively, an increase in nodular proliferative lesions of the liver was observed in rats but not in mice. The relationship of these lesions to the development of neoplasms of the liver is unclear. An increase in malignant tumors of the liver and other organs was not observed in either rats or mice.

■ **Pregnancy, Fertility, and Lactation** ***Pregnancy*** In studies performed in rats and rabbits, bupropion was administered orally in dosages up to 450 and 150 mg/kg daily, respectively (equivalent to 11 and 7 times the maximum recommended human dosage [MRHD] as an antidepressant on a mg/m^2 basis, respectively, or 14 and 10 times the MRHD for smoking cessation on a mg/m^2 basis, respectively) during the period of organogenesis. Although no clear evidence of teratogenic activity was found in either species, slightly increased incidences of fetal malformations and skeletal variations were observed in rabbits receiving the lowest dosage tested (25 mg/kg daily, which is approximately equivalent to the antidepressant MRHD and twice the MRHD for smoking cessation on a mg/m^2 basis) and higher dosages. Decreased fetal weights were observed at dosages of 50 mg/kg daily and at higher dosages.

In rats receiving oral dosages of bupropion of up to 300 mg/kg daily (approximately 7 or 10 times the MRHD on a mg/m^2 basis as an antidepressant or for smoking cessation, respectively) prior to mating and throughout pregnancy and lactation, there were no apparent adverse effects on offspring development.

One study evaluating the teratogenic potential of bupropion in humans has been conducted. This retrospective, managed-care database study assessed the risk of congenital malformations overall and cardiovascular malformations specifically following bupropion exposure in the first trimester compared with the risk of such malformations following exposure to other antidepressants in the first trimester and bupropion outside of the first trimester. This study included 7,005 infants exposed to antidepressants in utero; 1,213 of these infants were exposed to bupropion during the first trimester. The study demonstrated no increased risk for congenital malformations overall or cardiovascular malformations specifically following first-trimester bupropion exposure compared with exposure to all other antidepressants in the first trimester or bupropion outside of the first trimester. The results of this study have not been corroborated.

The effect of bupropion on labor and delivery is not known.

Bupropion should be used during pregnancy only when the potential benefits justify the potential risks to the fetus. Women should be advised to notify their physician if they are or plan to become pregnant.

To monitor fetal outcomes of pregnant women exposed to bupropion in the US, the manufacturer maintains a Bupropion Pregnancy Registry. Clinicians are encouraged to register patients by calling 800-336-2176.

Fertility A fertility study in rats using oral bupropion hydrochloride dosages of up to 300 mg/kg daily did not reveal evidence of impaired fertility.

Lactation Bupropion, hydroxybupropion, and the threo-amino alcohol metabolite are distributed into milk. Limited data indicate that milk concentrations of the drug exceed concurrent plasma concentrations by as much as severalfold. Concentrations in milk of hydroxybupropion are about 10% of, and concentrations of the threo-amino alcohol metabolite are moderately higher than, the respective concurrent plasma concentrations. Bupropion, hydroxybupropion, the threo-amino alcohol, and the erythro-amino alcohol were not detected in the plasma of an infant 3.7 hours after breast-feeding that was done 9.5 hours after the mother received her last dose of the drug for the day. Because data are limited and because of the potential for adverse effects in nursing infants, a decision should be made as to whether to discontinue nursing or bupropion, taking into account the importance of the drug to the woman and the potential for serious adverse reactions to the drug in nursing infants.

Drug Interactions

■ **Smoking Cessation** Smoking, via enzyme induction, can increase the metabolism of some drugs. Cessation of smoking, with or without adjunctive use of bupropion, may alter the pharmacokinetics of and response to various drugs that the patient also may be taking, thereby possibly necessitating adjustment of dosage. (For further information on drug interactions associated with smoking cessation, see Drug Interactions: Smoking Cessation, in Nicotine 12:92.)

■ **Hepatic Microsomal Enzyme Induction** Data from animal studies suggest that bupropion may be an inducer of hepatic microsomal enzymes, which may have potential pharmacokinetic and clinical consequences in patients receiving bupropion concomitantly with drugs that depend on the microsomal enzyme system for metabolism. The possibility of an interaction between other drugs and bupropion (which is extensively metabolized) that might affect its metabolism and clinical effects also should be considered. Particular caution should be observed when bupropion is administered concomitantly with drugs that may induce its metabolism (e.g., carbamazepine, phenobarbital, phenytoin) or that may inhibit its metabolism (e.g., cimetidine).

Drugs that are substrates of or that inhibit the cytochrome P-450 (CYP) 2B6 isoenzyme (e.g., cyclophosphamide, orphenadrine, thiotepa) have the potential to interact with bupropion since in vitro studies indicate that metabolism of bupropion to hydroxybupropion (morpholinol) is principally via this isoenzyme. In addition, in vitro studies suggest that fluvoxamine, norfluoxetine (the principal metabolite of fluoxetine), paroxetine, and sertraline as well as efavirenz, nelfinavir, and ritonavir may inhibit the hydroxylation of bupropion. The threohydrobupropion metabolite of bupropion does not appear to be produced by the CYP isoenzymes.

Concomitant administration of bupropion and cimetidine resulted in 16% increases in the 24-hour area under the combined plasma concentration-time curve (AUC) and 32% increases in combined peak plasma concentration of the erythro- and threo-amino metabolites of bupropion. However, the pharmacokinetics of bupropion and hydroxybupropion were not affected.

Concomitant administration of bupropion and carbamazepine resulted in decreases in the peak plasma concentration of bupropion and in the 24-hour area under the plasma concentration-time curve (AUC) by 87 and 90%, respectively; the peak plasma concentration and 24-hour AUC of the metabolite, hydroxybupropion, were increased by 71 and 50%, respectively. In contrast, concomitant administration of bupropion and valproate sodium resulted only in an increase by 94% in 24-hour AUC of hydroxybupropion.

Steady-state bupropion did not substantially affect the pharmacokinetics of a single dose of lamotrigine in healthy individuals.

Limited data indicate that bupropion decreases the clearance of imipramine and its metabolite, desipramine, when the drugs are used concomitantly. Plasma concentrations of imipramine and desipramine were about fourfold higher with concomitant use of bupropion and imipramine than with imipramine alone. The mechanism of this interaction currently is not known, but it was suggested that studies be performed to determine whether specific cytochrome P-450 isoenzymes (e.g., CYP2D6) are involved. Pending further accumulation of data, caution should be exercised if bupropion and drugs that are metabolized by the CYP2D6 isoenzyme, including certain antidepressants (e.g., nortriptyline, imipramine, desipramine, paroxetine, fluoxetine, sertraline), antipsychotic agents (e.g., haloperidol, risperidone, thioridazine), β-adrenergic blocking agents (e.g., metoprolol), and class IC antiarrhythmic agents (e.g., propafenone, flecainide), are used concomitantly. When drugs that are metabolized by CYP2D6 are added to existing bupropion therapy or if bupropion is added to the treatment regimen of a patient already receiving one of these drugs, a reduction in dosages of the drugs that are metabolized by CYP2D6 should be considered, particularly for those with a narrow therapeutic index.

■ **Monoamine Oxidase Inhibitors** Evidence from animal studies suggests that concomitant administration of bupropion and monoamine oxidase (MAO) inhibitors is potentially hazardous. In animals, phenelzine enhanced the acute toxicity of bupropion, as indicated by an increase in mortality and a decrease in time to death. The manufacturer states that concurrent administration of bupropion and MAO inhibitors is contraindicated and that at least 2 weeks elapse following discontinuance of an MAO inhibitor prior to initiation of bupropion therapy.

■ **Levodopa and Amantadine** A limited number of patients with parkinsonian syndrome treated with either amantadine or levodopa appeared to have a high incidence of adverse effects (e.g., nausea and vomiting, excitement and restlessness, postural tremor) when bupropion was used concurrently. Caution should be exercised if bupropion therapy is initiated in a patient receiving levodopa or amantadine, including use of low initial dosage and increasing the dosage gradually in small increments.

■ **Alcohol** Adverse neuropsychiatric events or reduced alcohol tolerance have been reported rarely in patients who ingested alcohol during bupropion therapy. Because of concerns that excessive use of alcohol or abrupt withdrawal from alcohol may be associated with an increased risk of seizures during bupropion therapy, patients receiving the drug should be advised to minimize or, if possible, avoid alcohol consumption.

Concurrent administration of single doses of bupropion and alcohol did not result in alteration of blood alcohol concentrations, plasma bupropion concentrations, or other pharmacokinetic variables in healthy individuals, indicating that there is no pharmacokinetic interaction between bupropion and alcohol.

■ **Drugs Affecting the Seizure Threshold** Extreme caution should be observed with concurrent administration of bupropion and drugs (e.g., other antidepressants, antipsychotic agents, theophylline, systemic corticosteroids) or treatment regimens (e.g., abrupt discontinuance of benzodiazepines) that lower the seizure threshold. Therapy should be initiated with low doses and dosage should be increased gradually.

■ **Benzodiazepines** Concurrent administration of single doses of bupropion and diazepam to healthy individuals did not result in potentiation of the mental impairment induced by diazepam. The impairment of performance on the auditory vigilance test observed with diazepam alone was absent with the combination of diazepam and bupropion. Individuals did not feel more drowsy with the combination of diazepam and bupropion than with placebo or bupropion alone but subjective assessment indicated an increase in drowsiness with diazepam alone.

■ **Electroconvulsive Therapy** Administration of bupropion in conjunction with electroconvulsive therapy (ECT) was reported to result in an increase in the duration of motor and EEG seizures associated with ECT in at least one patient. However, such an effect was absent in 2 other patients who received the drug at the same dosage concomitantly with ECT, and some clinicians suggest that ECT can be performed safely 48 hours after discontinuance of bupropion.

■ **Nicotine** The manufacturer states that patients can receive bupropion concomitantly with transdermal nicotine therapy if indicated for smoking cessation. In a clinical study, concurrent use of bupropion extended-release tablets and nicotine transdermal systems resulted in similar plasma concentrations of bupropion and its active metabolites compared with patients receiving only bupropion extended-release tablets. However, the manufacturer reported a possible increased risk of hypertension during combined use (see Cautions: Cardiovascular Effects), and the possibility of treatment-emergent hypertension should be considered when bupropion is used concomitantly with nicotine replacement therapy.

■ **Warfarin** Concomitant use of bupropion with warfarin has resulted in altered prothrombin time/international normalized ratio (INR) that has been rarely associated with hemorrhagic or thrombotic complications.

Acute Toxicity

■ **Manifestations** The oral LD_{50} of bupropion in male and female rats has been reported to be 607 and 482 mg/kg, respectively, and in male and female mice it has been reported to be 544 and 636 mg/kg, respectively. Manifestations of acute toxicity included labored breathing, salivation, arched back, ptosis, ataxia, and seizures.

Patients reportedly have overdosed with 30 g or more of bupropion hydrochloride. Serious effects of overdosage have included seizures in about one-third of such patients, hallucinations, loss of consciousness, sinus tachycardia, and ECG changes such as conduction disturbances (e.g., widened QRS interval, prolonged QT_c interval) or arrhythmias. Lethargy, grogginess, tremors, jitteriness, confusion, lightheadedness, paresthesias, visual hallucinations, blurred vision, nausea, and vomiting also have occurred. Overdosage of bupropion (mainly as part of multiple drug overdoses) reportedly has resulted in fever, muscle rigidity, rhabdomyolysis, hypotension, stupor, coma, and respiratory failure. Recovery without sequelae has been reported in most individuals following an overdose of bupropion alone. However, massive overdosage of bupropion alone has been reported rarely to result in death preceded by multiple uncontrolled seizures, bradycardia, cardiac failure, and cardiac arrest.

■ **Treatment** Because of the dose-related risk of seizures, the manufacturer states that hospitalization for patients suspected of bupropion overdosage should be considered. Adequate respiratory exchange should be established by maintaining an adequate, patent airway, using assisted or controlled respiration and oxygen as necessary. Treatment should include supportive and symptomatic measures; in addition, cardiac rhythm and vital signs should be monitored. EEG monitoring is recommended for the first 48 hours after ingestion. Activated charcoal should be administered, but induction of emesis is *not* recommended. Gastric lavage with a large-bore orogastric tube (and appropriate airway protection, if needed) may be indicated if performed soon after ingestion, or in symptomatic patients.

Data based on animal and few human studies indicate that administration of an IV benzodiazepine (e.g., diazepam) and other appropriate supportive measures are recommended for the management of bupropion-induced seizures. Phenytoin has been effective for treatment of seizures unresponsive to an IV benzodiazepine.

Experience is lacking regarding the effect of diuresis, dialysis, hemoperfusion, or exchange transfusion in the management of bupropion overdosage. Clinicians should consider the possibility of multiple drug ingestion, and consider consulting a poison control center for additional information on the management of bupropion overdosage. No specific antidote for bupropion is known.

Chronic Toxicity

The potential for abuse or misuse of bupropion is unclear, but most evidence to date suggests that the potential is low. On several scales measuring feelings of euphoria and drug desirability, there was limited evidence of abuse potential. There also was some evidence of stimulant effects in clinical studies. However, findings from clinical studies are not known to reliably predict the abuse potential of drugs. Although the potential for abuse of bupropion is likely to be low, possible development of dependence on the drug should be considered in deciding whether to use it as an adjunct in smoking cessation in individual patients.

Some increase in motor activity and agitation or excitement occurred in clinical studies in healthy individuals, patients with depression, and individuals with a history of multiple-drug abuse. Based on single-dose studies, bupropion when dosed and administered as recommended is unlikely to be especially reinforcing to abusers of amphetamines or other stimulants, although such individuals may find higher than recommended doses, which were not studied because of seizure risk, to be modestly attractive. No evidence of psychostimulation was observed with single bupropion hydrochloride doses of up to 200 mg as determined by auditory vigilance and visual analog testing.

In multiple-drug abusers who received a single dose of bupropion, dextroamphetamine, or placebo, 400 mg of bupropion hydrochloride produced mild amphetamine-like activity (e.g., feelings of activation, general feelings of well-being) as indicated by a measure of general euphoria in the morphine-benzedrine group subscale of the Addiction Research Center Inventory (ARCI). In addition, these individuals rated 400 mg of bupropion hydrochloride with a score intermediate between those of placebo and the amphetamine on a measure of the drug desirability on the Liking Scale of the ARCI.

Bupropion has been shown to exhibit dose-related CNS-stimulant effects. In animals, some pharmacologic effects common to cerebral stimulants were manifested with the drug, including increases in locomotor activity and the production of a mild stereotyped behavior as well as increases in the rates of responding in several schedule-controlled behavior paradigms. In addition, drug discrimination studies in rats showed stimulus generalization between abusable psychostimulants (e.g., amphetamine, cocaine) and bupropion at high doses. Rhesus monkeys were shown to self-administer IV bupropion.

Pharmacology

■ **Nervous System Effects** The precise mechanism of antidepressant action of bupropion is unclear, although noradrenergic and/or dopaminergic pathways appear to be principally involved. Bupropion doses that were active in animal models of depression selectively inhibit firing of noradrenergic neurons in the locus ceruleus in animals; hydroxybupropion, an active metabolite, produces similar inhibition. In patients with depression receiving bupropion, whole-body turnover of norepinephrine is reduced, which also has been observed with various other therapies for depression. However, the reduction in whole-body turnover of this neurotransmitter observed with bupropion may not be related principally to inhibition of norepinephrine uptake, and the drug is substantially less potent than tricyclic antidepressants (e.g., amitriptyline, imipramine) in inhibiting such uptake. In addition, unlike tricyclic antidepressants, bupropion appears to have little effect on the reuptake of norepinephrine and does not inhibit the reuptake of serotonin at the presynaptic neuronal membrane. Although reuptake of dopamine is inhibited to some extent and more extensively than by these tricyclic antidepressants, such inhibition with bupropion occurs at dosages higher than those required for antidepressant activity.

Circulating concentrations of prolactin or growth hormone are not altered by bupropion or its metabolites, and neither type A nor B monoamine oxidase (MAO-A, MAO-B) is inhibited by the drug. In addition, bupropion does not exhibit clinically important anticholinergic, antihistaminic, or α-adrenergic blocking activity. Unlike most other antidepressants, bupropion also does not appear to suppress rapid eye movement (REM) sleep.

The precise mechanism of action responsible for the efficacy of bupropion as an adjunct in the cessation of smoking is unclear, although noradrenergic and/or dopaminergic effects presumably are involved. It has been suggested that CNS effects of dopamine might be involved in the reinforcement properties of addictive drugs and that nicotine withdrawal manifestations may involve the absence of CNS effects of norepinephrine that are mediated by nicotine. Efficacy of bupropion in smoking cessation does not appear to depend on the presence of underlying depression.

Dose-related CNS stimulation occurs with bupropion in animals, which exhibit increases in locomotor activity and in the rates of responding in various schedule-controlled operant behavior tasks, and, at high doses, induction of mild stereotyped behavior. Seizures occur in animals at doses approximately tenfold greater than the usual antidepressant dose in humans.

■ **Cardiovascular Effects** The cardiovascular effects of bupropion have been studied in animals and to a limited extent in humans. Unlike most other antidepressant agents (e.g., tricyclic antidepressants), bupropion has been associated with only minimal cardiovascular effects. In animals, bupropion was substantially weaker than imipramine in potentiating the pressor response associated with administration of norepinephrine. In healthy humans, bupropion did not affect the pressor response to tyramine whereas imipramine decreased the sensitivity of systolic blood pressure to this amine. The depressant effect of bupropion on canine Purkinje fibers and ventricular muscle in vitro occurred with concentrations of the drug that were substantially higher than those that would be expected after administration of usual dosages of the drug in humans.

Bupropion did not affect heart rate in short- and long-term studies of patients with depression, whereas amitriptyline commonly caused modest increases in heart rate. Likewise, nortriptyline produced greater increases in heart rate, including tachycardia, than did bupropion.

Little or no effect on supine or standing blood pressure was observed with bupropion. Bupropion does not appear to affect cardiac conduction, and clinically important ECG changes generally have not been reported during therapy with the drug. QT interval corrected for rate (QT_c) also was not affected by bupropion but appeared to be increased by nortriptyline.

Limited evaluation of the cardiovascular effects of bupropion (mean dosage of 442 mg daily) administered for 3 weeks in patients with congestive heart failure, conduction disturbances, and/or ventricular arrhythmias showed that, relative to baseline, supine systolic and diastolic blood pressures and orthostatic differences were increased, although the changes were not clinically important. Left ventricular ejection fraction was not changed and no ECG abnormalities were observed after treatment with the drug.

■ **Effects on Appetite and Body Weight** Bupropion does not appear to have a substantial effect on appetite and does not affect caloric intake. However, the drug reportedly has reduced the craving for chocolate, and bupropion therapy has been associated with decreases in body weight in depressed patients. (See Cautions: Metabolic Effects.)

Pharmacokinetics

■ **Absorption** Bupropion hydrochloride appears to be well absorbed from the GI tract following oral administration. The oral bioavailability of bupropion in humans has not been elucidated because a preparation for IV administration is not available. However, the relative proportion of an oral dose reaching systemic circulation unchanged appears likely to be small. In animals, the oral bioavailability of bupropion varies from 5–20%. Food does not appear to affect substantially the peak plasma concentration or area under the plasma concentration-time curve of bupropion achieved with extended-release tablets of the drug; these measures reportedly were increased with food by 11 or 17%, respectively.

Peak plasma bupropion concentrations usually occur within 2 or 3 hours after oral administration of the conventional or extended-release, film-coated tablets (Wellbutrin® SR, Zyban®), respectively, to healthy individuals. Plasma bupropion concentrations following administration of single oral doses of 100–250 mg and with chronic administration of up to 450 mg daily are proportional to dose. Steady-state plasma concentrations of bupropion are achieved within 8 days. During chronic administration of bupropion hydrochloride as conventional or extended-release, film-coated tablets at a dosage of 100 mg 3 times daily or 150 mg twice daily, respectively, peak plasma concentrations of the drug at steady state with extended-release tablets were about 85% of measurements for the conventional tablets. Equivalence in area under the plasma concentration-time curve (AUC) of bupropion was shown for the formulations, which demonstrated that at steady state the conventional and extended-release tablets are essentially bioequivalent. The drug exhibits linear pharmacokinetics during chronic administration of bupropion hydrochloride dosages of 300–450 mg daily.

The relationship between plasma concentrations of bupropion and its metabolites and the therapeutic and/or toxic effects of the drug has not been clearly established. Limited data suggest a curvilinear relationship between plasma concentrations of bupropion or its metabolites and antidepressant response.

■ **Distribution** Bupropion is at least 80% bound to human albumin at in vitro plasma concentrations of up to 200 mcg/mL.

Bupropion, hydroxybupropion, and the threo-amino alcohol metabolite are distributed into milk. Limited data indicate that milk concentrations of the drug exceed concurrent plasma concentrations by as much as severalfold. Concentrations in milk of hydroxybupropion are about 10% of, and concentrations of the threo-amino alcohol metabolite are moderately higher than, the respective concurrent plasma concentrations. However, bupropion, hydroxybupropion, the threo-amino alcohol, and the erythro-amino alcohol were not detected in the plasma of a nursing infant 3.7 hours after breast-feeding, which was done 9.5 hours after the mother received her last dose of the drug for the day.

■ **Elimination** Plasma concentrations of bupropion decline in a biphasic manner. A decline to approximately 30% of the peak plasma bupropion concentration is observed 6 hours after administration of a single oral dose of the drug. The half-life of bupropion in the terminal phase ($t_{1/2\beta}$) averages about 14 hours (range: 8–24 hours) following single doses; with multiple dosing, $t_{1/2\beta}$ reportedly averages 21 hours (range: 8–39 hours). In a limited number of geriatric patients with a major depressive episode, the $t_{1/2\beta}$ of bupropion averaged about 34 hours after a single oral dose of the drug.

Bupropion appears to be metabolized extensively, probably in the liver. The 3 active metabolites that have been identified are formed through reduction of the carbonyl group and/or hydroxylation. The basic metabolites identified include the erythro- and threo-amino alcohols of bupropion, and a morpholinol metabolite. The amino-alcohol isomers threohydrobupropion and erythrohydrobupropion are formed by reduction of the carbonyl group of bupropion, and the morpholinol metabolite, hydroxybupropion, is formed by hydroxylation of the *tert*-butyl group of bupropion. The metabolites of bupropion exhibit linear pharmacokinetics during chronic administration of the drug at dosages of 300–450 mg daily.

Following a single oral dose of bupropion as conventional tablets, hydroxybupropion and bupropion are detectable in systemic circulation with nearly similar rapidity, although the metabolite's peak plasma concentration and area under the plasma concentration-time curve (AUC) from 0–60 hours are higher by 3 and 15 times, respectively. The half-life of hydroxybupropion is about 24 hours. In a limited number of geriatric patients with a major depressive episode, the apparent half-life of hydroxybupropion averaged about 34 hours after a single oral dose of the drug. Hydroxybupropion and the threo-amino alcohol have similar plasma concentration-time profiles, whereas the erythro-amino alcohol and the erythro-amino diol generally cannot be detected in systemic circulation following a single oral dose of bupropion. Animal screening tests for antidepressant agents showed that hydroxybupropion is half as potent as bupropion, while threohydrobupropion and erythrohydrobupropion are fivefold less potent than bupropion. Hydroxybupropion was approximately equipotent to bupropion in other tests in animals.

Following a single oral dose of bupropion hydrochloride as extended-release, film-coated tablets (e.g., Wellbutrin® SR, Zyban®), peak plasma concentrations of hydroxybupropion occur in about 6 hours. The metabolite's peak plasma concentration achieved with extended-release tablets is about 10 times higher than the peak plasma concentration of bupropion achieved with this dosage form. At steady state, the AUC is 17 times greater for hydroxybupropion than for bupropion with extended-release tablets. The half-life of hydroxybupropion is about 20 hours. With extended-release tablets, peak plasma concentrations of the erythro- and threo-amino alcohols occur at about the same time as for hydroxybupropion, although these metabolites have longer half-lives of 33 and 37 hours, respectively. At steady state, the AUCs are 1.5 and 7 times greater for the erythro- and threo-amino alcohols, respectively, than for bupropion.

During chronic administration of bupropion hydrochloride as the conventional or extended-release, film-coated tablets (e.g., Wellbutrin® SR, Zyban®), equivalence between these formulations was shown for the peak plasma concentration and AUC of hydroxybupropion, the erythro-amino alcohol, and the threo-amino alcohol, which demonstrated that at steady state the conventional and extended-release tablets are essentially bioequivalent for these metabolites.

Although several of the identified metabolites are pharmacologically active, the contribution of these metabolites to the therapeutic and/or toxic effects of bupropion is not fully known. The longer half-lives of at least two known metabolites is a potential clinical consideration because of the expectation of very much higher plasma concentrations of the metabolites than of bupropion, especially with chronic administration. Factors or conditions (e.g., liver disease, congestive heart failure, age, concomitant drugs) that affect metabolism or elimination would be expected to alter the degree and extent of accumulation of these metabolites. The extent to which the clinical effects of bupropion are related to the parent drug or to the metabolites also could be altered with chronic administration if bupropion induces its own metabolism in humans. In animals, bupropion induced its own metabolism following subchronic administration, although such an effect was not evident in healthy individuals receiving up to 450 mg daily of the drug over 14 days.

Approximately 87 and 10% of an orally administered, radiolabeled dose of bupropion are excreted in urine and feces, respectively. Unchanged drug comprised 0.5% of the dose excreted.

The effect of age on the plasma concentrations of bupropion and its metabolites has not been fully elucidated; however, data from studies of efficacy suggest that plasma concentrations of bupropion are not affected substantially by age. Evaluation of plasma concentrations of bupropion at steady state that were obtained from these studies in which patients who were 18–83 years in age received 300–750 mg of the drug in 3 divided doses daily did not identify a relationship between age and plasma concentration of bupropion. However, in a limited number of patients 63–76 years of age with a major depressive episode, the ratio of the AUC for combined metabolites (i.e., hydroxybupropion, the erythro- and threo-amino alcohols of bupropion) to that for bupropion after about 10 days of therapy was greater than twice that after a single dose of the drug. Differences in the pharmacokinetics of bupropion related to gender were not identified in a study of healthy males and females who received a single dose of the drug. Limited data suggest that accumulation of the metabolites of bupropion occurs with multiple doses of the drug.

Because bupropion is extensively metabolized by the liver, hepatic impairment can affect elimination of the drug. In a single-dose study in patients with alcoholic liver disease, the half-life of hydroxybupropion was substantially increased to a mean of 32 hours compared with 21 hours in healthy individuals. In addition, the AUC values and other pharmacokinetic parameters were reported to be more variable for bupropion and its active metabolites in the patients with mild to moderate hepatic impairment, although the differences were not found to be significant. The pharmacokinetics of bupropion also have been studied in patients with severe hepatic impairment. The peak plasma concentration and elimination half-life of bupropion were substantially increased by 70 and 40%, respectively, and AUC increased threefold in these patients compared with healthy individuals. Additionally, the AUC and elimination half-life of the metabolites of bupropion also were increased, but the peak plasma concentration was decreased in patients with severe hepatic impairment compared with healthy individuals. Therefore, the manufacturer recommends that bupropion be administered with caution and less frequently in patients with hepatic impairment. (See Cautions: Precautions and Contraindications and see Dosage and Administration: Dosage in Renal and Hepatic Impairment.)

Limited data are available on the pharmacokinetics of bupropion in patients with renal impairment. Elimination of the principal active metabolites of bupropion may be reduced by impaired renal function. An interstudy comparison between healthy individuals and patients with end-stage renal failure who received a single oral dose of 150 mg of bupropion hydrochloride administered as an extended-release ("sustained-action"), film-coated tablet (Zyban®) demonstrated that the peak concentrations and AUC values for the parent drug were comparable in the 2 groups of patients; however, the AUC values of the hydroxybupropion and threohydrobupropion metabolites were increased 2.3- and 2.8-fold, respectively, in patients with end-stage renal failure. (See Cautions: Precautions and Contraindications and see Dosage and Administration: Dosage in Renal and Hepatic Impairment.)

In patients with left ventricular dysfunction (e.g., history of congestive heart failure, radiographic evidence of enlarged heart) who received chronic dosing of bupropion, substantial interindividual variability (e.g., twofold to fivefold) characterized trough steady-state plasma concentrations of bupropion, hydroxybupropion, and the threo-amino alcohol, although such variability was observed to a similar extent (e.g., threefold to eightfold) in healthy individuals. Steady-state plasma concentrations of the metabolites were 10–100 times greater than those for bupropion.

Whether other diseases affect metabolism and/or elimination of bupropion is unclear.

Chemistry and Stability

■ **Chemistry** Bupropion hydrochloride is an aminoketone-derivative antidepressant agent. The drug is chemically unrelated to tricyclic, tetracyclic, or other currently available antidepressants (e.g., selective serotonin-reuptake inhibitors) and also is chemically unrelated to nicotine or other agents currently used in the treatment of nicotine dependence. Bupropion and diethylpropion hydrochloride have closely similar structures and bupropion is related to the phenylethylamines (e.g., chloromethamphetamine, chlorphentermine).

The absence of complex heterocyclic fused rings in bupropion as well as other structural differences result in reduced propensity for, or absence of, certain adverse effects typically associated with polycyclic antidepressants. The presence of a carbonyl functional group in the side chain distinguishes bupropion from common stimulants, and the α-aminoketone group contributes substantially to the metabolic fate of the drug; this latter group prevents reduction to a chloromonoarylalkylamine metabolite, which possibly would possess CNS stimulant activity. Likewise, the presence of the tertiary butyl group in bupropion prevents *N*-dealkylation to metabolites that could possess sympathomimetic and/or anorexigenic properties. Therefore, despite structural similarities with certain CNS stimulants, several structural differences result in pharmacologic and therapeutic effects of bupropion that are distinct from those of stimulants.

Bupropion hydrochloride is commercially available as conventional or extended-release tablets. Bupropion hydrochloride occurs as a white, crystalline powder and is highly soluble in water. The powder has a bitter taste and produces the sensation of local anesthesia on the oral mucosa.

■ **Stability** Conventional tablets of bupropion hydrochloride should be stored at a temperature of 15–25°C and protected from light and moisture. Extended-release, film-coated tablets of bupropion hydrochloride (e.g., Wellbutrin® SR, Zyban®) should be stored in tight, light-resistant containers at a temperature of 20–25°C. Wellbutrin® XL extended-release tablets should be stored at a temperature of 25°C, but may be exposed to temperatures ranging from 15–30°C.

Preparations

Excipients in commercially available drug preparations may have clinically important effects in some individuals; consult specific product labeling for details.

buPROPion Hydrochloride

Oral		
Tablets, extended-release	150 mg*	**Wellbutrin® XL,** GlaxoSmithKline
	300 mg*	**Wellbutrin® XL,** GlaxoSmithKline
Tablets, extended-release, film-coated	100 mg*	**buPROPion Hydrochloride SR**
		Wellbutrin® SR, GlaxoSmithKline
	150 mg*	**buPROPion Hydrochloride SR**
		Wellbutrin® SR, GlaxoSmithKline
		Zyban® (available as 60-tablet Advantage Pack® or refill), GlaxoSmithKline
	200 mg*	**buPROPion Hydrochloride SR**
		Wellbutrin® SR, GlaxoSmithKline
Tablets, film-coated	75 mg*	**buPROPion Hydrochloride**
		Wellbutrin®, GlaxoSmithKline
	100 mg*	**buPROPion Hydrochloride**
		Wellbutrin®, GlaxoSmithKline

*available from one or more manufacturer, distributor, and/or repackager by generic (nonproprietary) name

†Use is not currently included in the labeling approved by the US Food and Drug Administration

Esketamine Hydrochloride

■ Esketamine hydrochloride, the *S*-enantiomer of racemic ketamine, is an *N*-methyl-D-aspartate (NMDA) receptor antagonist and an antidepressant.

REMS

FDA approved a REMS for esketamine to ensure that the benefits outweigh the risks. The REMS may apply to one or more preparations of esketamine and consists of the following: elements to assure safe use and implementation system. See the FDA REMS page (https://www.accessdata.fda.gov/scripts/cder/rems/index.cfm).

Uses

■ **Treatment-resistant Depression** Esketamine hydrochloride is used intranasally in conjunction with an oral antidepressant for the treatment of treatment-resistant depression. Although there are various definitions of treatment-resistant depression, the condition often has been defined as the failure of at least 2 trials of first-line antidepressants given in an adequate dosage for an adequate duration of therapy.

Efficacy of intranasal esketamine in conjunction with an oral antidepressant was established in 2 randomized controlled trials (one short-term trial of 4 weeks' duration and one maintenance trial) in adults younger than 65 years of age with treatment-resistant depression. Short-term efficacy of the drug was established in a double-blind, placebo-controlled, multicenter trial of 4 weeks' duration (TRANSFORM-2) in 223 patients who met DSM-5 criteria for major depressive disorder (without psychotic features) and who did not adequately respond to 2 separate trials of different antidepressants of adequate dosage and duration in their current episode. Patients with suicidal ideation with intent to act or suicidal behavior within the past year were excluded from the study. The median age of patients in this study was 47 years; 62% were female and 93% were Caucasian. After discontinuing all prior antidepressants, patients were randomized to receive either flexible-dose esketamine (initially 56 mg twice weekly and increased to 84 mg twice weekly based on tolerability and efficacy) or placebo intranasally in conjunction with open-label treatment with a newly initiated oral antidepressant (duloxetine, escitalopram, sertraline, or extended-release venlafaxine) chosen by the investigator based on the patient's treatment history. The primary efficacy end point was the change from baseline in the Montgomery-Asberg Depression Rating Scale (MADRS) total score, a 10-item clinician-rated scale used to assess the degree of depressive symptomatology, at the end of the 4-week induction phase. Scores on the MADRS range from 0 to 60; higher scores indicate more severe depression. After 4 weeks of treatment, the mean MADRS total score was substantially lower in patients who received esketamine compared with placebo. Most of the treatment effect was evident by 24 hours after the first dose. Between 24 hours and day 28, patients in both groups continued to improve; the difference between the groups remained generally the same but did not appear to increase during the 4-week treatment period. Of the patients randomized to receive esketamine, about 46% were receiving the 84-mg dosage by day 4 and about 67% were receiving the 84-mg dosage by the end of the treatment period.

In the longer-term maintenance study (SUSTAIN-1), continued treatment with intranasal esketamine was found to be effective in delaying the time to relapse compared with placebo in adult patients who had responded to at least 16 weeks of intranasal esketamine therapy. In this study, patients (newly enrolled or recruited from short-term controlled trials) initially received at least 16 weeks of treatment with intranasal esketamine 56 or 84 mg (flexibly dosed) twice weekly for 4 weeks, followed by a fixed dose once weekly for 4 weeks, then weekly or every other week (based on depressive symptoms) in conjunction with a new oral antidepressant. Patients who achieved stable remission (i.e., MADRS total score or 12 or less for at least 3 of the last 4 weeks) or stable response (i.e., at least 50% reduction in MADRS total score but MADRS score above 12 for at least 3 of the last 4 weeks and not in remission) were randomized to continue receiving intranasal esketamine (56 or 84 mg once weekly or every other week based on depressive symptoms) or to be switched to placebo for the maintenance phase and monitored for relapse (defined as MADRS total score of 22 or higher for 2 consecutive weeks or hospitalization for worsening depression or any other clinically relevant event indicative of relapse). All patients continued to receive an oral antidepressant throughout the study. Overall, 39 or 61% of patients who continued esketamine therapy received the 56- or 86-mg dose, respectively. Time to relapse of depressive symptoms in patients who had achieved stable remission (the primary end point) was substantially longer in those receiving continued intranasal esketamine therapy plus an oral antidepressant compared with those who were switched to placebo plus an oral antidepressant. Of these patients (i.e., those who had achieved stable remission) who received continued esketamine therapy, 69% received every-other-week dosing and 23% received weekly dosing the majority of time during the maintenance phase. In addition, time to relapse also was substantially longer in patients who had achieved stable response and continued intranasal esketamine therapy compared with those who were switched to placebo. Of these patients (i.e., those who had achieved stable response) who received continued esketamine therapy, 34% received every-other-week dosing and 55% received weekly dosing the majority of time during the maintenance phase.

In a randomized, placebo-controlled, double-blind, multicenter study in 68 patients considered to be at imminent risk of suicide, patients receiving intranasal esketamine 84 mg twice weekly for 4 weeks in addition to comprehensive standard-of-care treatment had a substantially greater reduction in MADRS scores than those receiving placebo and comprehensive standard-of-care treatment at 4 hours and approximately 24 hours, but not at 25 days. The esketamine-treated patients in this study also demonstrated substantially greater improvement in suicidal thinking (as assessed by their score on the MADRS suicidal thoughts item) compared with those receiving placebo at 4 hours, but not at 24 hours or 25 days. These preliminary results suggest that, like ketamine, intranasal esketamine may potentially be effective in rapidly reducing symptoms of depression, including suicidal ideation, in depressed patients at imminent risk of suicide. However, larger controlled studies are needed to more thoroughly evaluate the efficacy and safety of esketamine in such patients. (See Uses: Treatment-resistant Depression and Suicidality, in Ketamine Hydrochloride 28:04.)

■ **Other Uses** Esketamine is the *S*-enantiomer of racemic ketamine, which is used as an anesthetic agent. (See Description.) However, esketamine nasal solution is *not* labeled for use as an anesthetic agent and the manufacturer states that the safety and efficacy of the drug for this use have not been established.

Dosage and Administration

■ **General** Because esketamine nasal spray can cause increases in systolic and/or diastolic blood pressure, blood pressure should be monitored prior to intranasal administration, approximately 40 minutes after administration (which corresponds to peak plasma concentrations of the drug), and as clinically indicated thereafter until blood pressure values decline. If baseline blood pressure is elevated (i.e., systolic or diastolic blood pressure exceeding 140 or 90 mm Hg, respectively), the risks of short-term increases in blood pressure and the benefit of esketamine treatment in patients with treatment-resistant depression should be considered. Esketamine should *not* be administered in patients in whom an increase in blood pressure or intracranial pressure would constitute a serious risk. If blood pressure is decreasing and the patient appears clinically stable for at least 2 hours, the patient may be discharged at the end of the post-dose monitoring period; if not, patient monitoring should continue. (See Cautions: Contraindications and see also Increases in Blood Pressure under Warnings/Precautions: Other Warnings and Precautions, in Cautions.)

Because some patients may experience nausea and vomiting after administration of esketamine nasal spray, patients should be advised to avoid eating food for at least 2 hours before administration and avoid drinking liquids for at least 30 minutes prior to administration.

Prior to administration, patients should be instructed not to engage in potentially hazardous activities (e.g., driving a motor vehicle, operating machinery) until the next day after a restful sleep. (See Impaired Ability to Drive or Operate Machinery under Warnings/Precautions: Other Warnings and Precautions, in Cautions and see also Advice to Patients.)

If use of an intranasal corticosteroid or intranasal decongestant is required on the same day as treatment with esketamine nasal solution, they should be administered at least 1 hour prior to esketamine. (See Drug Interactions: Intranasally administered Corticosteroids and Decongestants.)

Patients receiving esketamine therapy should be monitored for possible worsening of depression or emergence of suicidality, especially at the beginning of therapy or during periods of dosage adjustments. (See Suicidality under Warnings/Precautions: Warnings, in Cautions.)

Restricted Distribution Program Because of the risks of serious adverse outcomes from sedation, dissociation, abuse, and misuse (see Cautions), esketamine nasal spray is available only through a restricted distribution program (Spravato® REMS). Healthcare settings and pharmacies must be certified with the program before they can dispense and supervise patient self-administration of esketamine nasal solution; patients must be enrolled in the program to receive treatment. Esketamine nasal solution must be administered under the direct observation of a healthcare provider in a certified healthcare setting. (See Dosage and Administration: Administration.) Further information about the Spravato® REMS program, including a list of certified pharmacies, is available at https://www.SPRAVATOrems.com or at 855-382-6022.

■ **Administration** Esketamine hydrochloride is administered intranasally using a nasal spray device. The drug is intended for patient self-administration *under the direct supervision of a healthcare provider*. A treatment session consists of intranasal administration of esketamine and post-administration observation under supervision. Patients should be instructed on use of the nasal spray device and advised to read the patient instructions for use provided by the manufacturer. Following administration of each dose, patients must be monitored at the healthcare facility by a healthcare provider for at least 2 hours and then assessed for clinical stability and readiness to be discharged from the healthcare facility. (See Postadministration Observation under Dosage and Administration: Administration.) Patients should not drive after the treatment session. (See Impaired Ability to Drive or Operate Machinery under Warnings/Precautions: Other Warnings and Precautions, in Cautions and see also Advice to Patients.)

Esketamine nasal solution is commercially available in kits containing either 2 (56-mg dose kit) or 3 (84-mg dose kit) stoppered glass vials within a nasal spray device. Each nasal spray device delivers a total of 28 mg of esketamine and delivers 2 sprays containing 14 mg of esketamine per spray. Two devices should be used for a 56-mg dose and 3 devices should be used for an 84-mg dose. An indicator on the device displays one green dot for each spray remaining in the device. Prior to administration of esketamine nasal spray, a healthcare provider should confirm the number of nasal spray devices required for the dose and check that each device indicator displays 2 green dots prior to use. To prevent loss of the drug, esketamine nasal spray devices should *not* be primed before use.

Patients should be instructed to blow the nose to clear the nasal passages before the initial spray from the first device at each treatment session. During administration, patients should recline their head to about 45 degrees to help keep the solution inside the nose.

The patient should insert the tip of the device straight into one nostril; the nose rest should touch the skin between the nostrils. While holding the other nostril closed, the patient should concurrently inspire through the nose while pushing on the plunger to activate the spray. The patient should then sniff gently to keep the solution in the nose. This procedure should be repeated for the other nostril.

The procedure should then be repeated for each device until the full dose of esketamine nasal spray has been administered. Following administration of esketamine in each device (i.e., 2 sprays), the patient should rest in a comfortable position (preferably semi-reclined) for 5 minutes to allow the drug to be absorbed. Following use, each device should be checked by the healthcare provider to ensure that both sprays have been delivered; if a green dot appears in the device indicator, the patient should spray again into the second nostril. If liquid drips out of the nostril, the nose should be dabbed with a tissue.

Used nasal spray devices should be properly disposed of in accordance with the facility's procedures and federal, state, and local regulations for controlled substance disposal. (See Abuse and Misuse under Warnings/Precautions: Warnings, in Cautions.)

Post-administration Observation During and following administration of esketamine nasal spray at each treatment session, patients must be observed (i.e., for sedation, dissociation, and increased blood pressure). Patient observation should continue for at least 2 hours until the patient can safely leave the healthcare setting. (See Cautions.)

■ **Dosage** Dosage of esketamine hydrochloride is expressed in terms of esketamine.

Treatment-resistant Depression For the treatment of treatment-resistant depression in combination with an oral antidepressant in adults, the recommended intranasal dosage of esketamine during the *induction phase (weeks 1–4)* is 56 mg initially on day 1, followed by 56- or 84-mg doses administered twice weekly. Dosage adjustments should be made based on efficacy and tolerability.

The recommended dosage during the *maintenance phase (weeks 5–8)* is 56 or 84 mg administered once weekly followed by 56 or 84 mg administered every 2 weeks or once weekly during week 9 and the following weeks. Dosing frequency during week 9 and thereafter should be individualized to the least frequent dosing interval that maintains remission or response. In the short- and long-term efficacy trials of esketamine nasal spray, approximately one-third of patients received 56-mg doses of esketamine and two-thirds received 84-mg doses of the drug.

The clinical benefit of esketamine should be assessed at the end of the induction phase (i.e., week 4) to determine the need for continued therapy.

If a treatment session is missed and worsening of depression occurs, the dosing frequency may be increased back to the patient's previous dosing schedule (i.e., every 2 weeks to once weekly, once weekly to twice weekly) based on clinical judgment.

■ **Special Populations** The manufacturer makes no specific dosage recommendations for esketamine in patients with mild hepatic impairment. Although no specific dosage adjustments are recommended for patients with moderate hepatic impairment, such patients may require prolonged monitoring for adverse effects. The drug is not recommended for use in patients with severe hepatic impairment. (See Hepatic Impairment under Warnings/Precautions: Specific Populations, in Cautions.)

The manufacturer makes no specific dosage recommendations for geriatric patients or patients with renal impairment. (See Specific Populations under Cautions: Warnings/Precautions.)

Cautions

■ **Contraindications** Esketamine in contraindicated in patients in whom an increase in blood pressure or intracranial pressure poses a serious risk such as in patients with aneurysmal vascular disease (including that affecting the thoracic and abdominal aorta and intracranial and peripheral arterial vessels) or arteriovenous malformation and those with a history of intracerebral hemorrhage. (See Increases in Blood Pressure under Warnings/Precautions: Other Warnings and Precautions, in Cautions.)

Esketamine is also contraindicated in patients who are hypersensitive to esketamine, ketamine, or any excipient in the formulation.

■ **Warnings/Precautions** ***Warnings*** **Sedation.** Esketamine can cause dose-related sedation and, rarely, loss of consciousness. Sedation (defined as any decrease from baseline in the Modified Observer's Alertness/Sedation scale [MOAA/s]) was reported in 49–61% of patients and loss of consciousness (MOAA/s score of 0) was reported in 0.3% of patients receiving esketamine nasal spray in conjunction with an oral antidepressant in clinical trials.

Because of the possibility of delayed or prolonged sedation, patients receiving esketamine must be monitored by a healthcare provider for at least 2 hours at each treatment session, followed by an assessment to determine if the patient is considered clinically stable and ready to leave the healthcare setting. (See Post-administration Observation under Dosage and Administration: Administration.)

Patients concomitantly receiving esketamine and CNS depressants should be closely monitored. (See Drug Interactions: CNS Depressants.)

Dissociation. Intranasal esketamine may cause dissociative effects (e.g., derealization, depersonalization) and perceptual changes (e.g., distortion of time and space and illusions); these adverse effects appear to be dose related. Dissociative (dissociation was defined as a Clinician-administered Dissociative States Scale [CADSS] total score of 4 or greater) or perceptual changes were reported in 61–75% of patients receiving esketamine nasal spray in clinical trials. In these trials, dissociation was transient and occurred on the day of intranasal esketamine administration.

Because of the risk of dissociative effects, patients with psychosis should be carefully assessed prior to treatment with esketamine; therapy should be initiated in such patients only if the benefit outweighs the risks.

In addition, patients receiving esketamine must be monitored by a healthcare provider for at least 2 hours at each treatment session, followed by an assessment to determine if the patient is considered clinically stable and ready to leave the healthcare setting. (See Post-administration Observation under Dosage and Administration: Administration.)

Abuse and Misuse. Esketamine is a schedule III (C-III) drug and has the potential to be abused or misused. Esketamine is the *S*-enantiomer of racemic ketamine, which is also a C-III drug with known abuse potential. For further information on abuse and misuse of ketamine, see Uses: Misuse and Abuse, in Ketamine Hydrochloride 28:04.

Intranasal esketamine may produce a variety of symptoms, including anxiety, dysphoria, disorientation, insomnia, flashbacks, hallucinations, and feelings of floating, detachment, and being "spaced out". In a double-blind, crossover abuse potential study in recreational polydrug users who had experience with perception-altering drugs, including ketamine, administration of single 84- and 112-mg intranasal doses of esketamine (the maximum recommended dose and 1.3 times the maximum recommended dose, respectively) produced scores for "drug liking at the moment" and "take drug again" that were similar to scores in patients receiving an IV infusion of ketamine (0.5 mg/kg). These scores were higher for both esketamine and ketamine compared with placebo.

Physical dependence has been reported with prolonged use of ketamine, and withdrawal symptoms have been reported following the discontinuance of frequently used large doses of the drug when given for prolonged periods of time. The manufacturer of esketamine states that although withdrawal symptoms have not been observed after cessation of esketamine treatment, such withdrawal symptoms are likely to occur if esketamine is similarly abused. Tolerance has been reported with prolonged use of ketamine, and similar tolerance would be expected with prolonged use of esketamine.

Each patient's risk for abuse or misuse should be assessed prior to prescribing esketamine, and all patients receiving the drug should be monitored for the development of these behaviors or conditions, including drug-seeking behavior, during therapy. Individuals with a history of drug abuse or dependence are at greater risk for abuse and misuse of esketamine. Therefore, the manufacturer states that careful consideration is advised prior to esketamine use in individuals with a history of substance use disorder, including alcohol. Patients receiving esketamine therapy should also be monitored for signs and symptoms of physical dependence following discontinuance of therapy.

Following use, esketamine nasal spray devices must be handled with adequate security and accountability, and disposal must be in accordance with the facility's procedures and federal, state, and local regulations for C-III drug products.

Suicidality. Pooled analyses of short-term, placebo-controlled studies of antidepressants (i.e., selective serotonin-reuptake inhibitors [SSRIs] and other antidepressants) have shown an increased risk of suicidal thoughts and behaviors (suicidality) in pediatric patients and young adults up to 24 years of age receiving antidepressants for major depressive disorder and other indications. An increased suicidality risk was not demonstrated with antidepressants compared with placebo in adults older than 24 years of age, and a reduced risk was observed in adults 65 years of age or older. It is not known whether the risk of suicidality in children, adolescents, and young adults extends to longer-term use (i.e., longer than 4 months) of antidepressants; however, substantial evidence from placebo-controlled maintenance studies in adults with major depressive disorder indicates that antidepressants delay the recurrence of depression and that depression itself is a risk factor for suicidality.

All patients being treated with antidepressants should be monitored for clinical worsening and emergence of suicidality, particularly during initiation of therapy (i.e., the first few months) and during periods of dosage adjustments. Families and caregivers of patients being treated with antidepressants also should be advised to monitor patients for changes in behavior and to report such changes immediately to a health-care provider. Consideration should be given to changing the therapeutic regimen, including possible discontinuance of esketamine and/or the concomitant oral antidepressant, in patients whose depression is persistently worse or in patients experiencing emergent suicidality.

Esketamine is not labeled for use in pediatric patients. (See Pediatric Use under Warnings/Precautions: Specific Populations, in Cautions.)

Other Warnings and Precautions **Increases in Blood Pressure.** Increases in systolic and/or diastolic blood pressure can occur following intranasal administration of esketamine at all recommended dosages. A substantial increase in blood pressure could occur after any intranasal dose of esketamine even if smaller blood pressure effects were observed with previous administration of the drug. Blood pressure increases peak approximately 40 minutes after intranasal administration of esketamine and last for approximately 4 hours. In short-term clinical trials, mean placebo-adjusted increases in systolic and diastolic blood pressure were approximately 7–9 and 4–6 mm Hg, respectively, at 40 minutes and 2–5 and 1–3 mm Hg, respectively, at 1.5 hours following intranasal administration of esketamine. Increases of more than 40 mm Hg in systolic blood pressure and/or 25 mm Hg in diastolic blood pressure in the first 1.5 hours after administration occurred at least once during the first 4 weeks of treatment in approximately 8–17% of patients receiving esketamine compared with 1–3% of placebo recipients.

Blood pressure should be assessed prior to each esketamine treatment session, approximately 40 minutes after administration of each dose, and as clinically warranted until values decline for at least 2 hours following administration. If blood pressure is elevated prior to esketamine administration (i.e., systolic or diastolic blood pressure exceeding 140 or 90 mm Hg, respectively), a decision to delay therapy should be individualized and take into consideration the potential benefit and risk of esketamine in the patient.

If blood pressure is decreasing following esketamine administration and the patient appears clinically stable for at least 2 hours, the patient may be discharged from the healthcare setting; otherwise, monitoring should be continued. If blood pressure remains elevated, clinicians experienced in blood pressure management should be consulted promptly. Patients experiencing symptoms of hypertensive crisis (e.g., chest pain, shortness of breath) or hypertensive encephalopathy (e.g., sudden severe headache, visual disturbances, seizures, diminished consciousness, focal neurologic deficits) should be immediately referred for emergency care.

Patients with a history of hypertensive encephalopathy are at increased risk for developing encephalopathy with even small increases in blood pressure and should be monitored more intensively, including more frequent blood pressure monitoring and symptom assessment.

Esketamine is contraindicated in patients in whom an increase in blood pressure or intracranial pressure would constitute a serious risk (e.g., aneurysmal vascular disease, arteriovenous malformation, history of intracerebral hemorrhage). Patients with other cardiovascular or cerebrovascular conditions should be carefully assessed to determine whether the potential benefits of esketamine treatment outweigh the risks.

Blood pressure should be closely monitored if esketamine is used concomitantly with psychostimulants or monoamine oxidase (MAO) inhibitors. (See Drug Interactions.)

Cognitive Impairment. Esketamine may cause short-term impairment in attention, judgment, thinking, reaction speed, and motor skills. In a double-blind, placebo-controlled, crossover study in 24 healthy individuals, esketamine (given as a single 84-mg intranasal dose) was associated with a greater decline in cognitive function and greater mental effort was required to complete cognitive tests compared with placebo at 40 minutes post-dose. Cognitive performance and mental effort were comparable between the esketamine and placebo groups at 2 hours post-dose. Esketamine also was associated with increased sleepiness at 40 minutes and 2 hours post-dose, but was comparable to placebo by 4 hours post-dose. (See Sedation under Warnings/Precautions: Warnings, in Cautions.)

Long-term cognitive and memory impairment have been reported with repeated ketamine misuse or abuse (see Chronic Toxicity in Ketamine Hydrochloride 28:04). Although no adverse cognitive effects of esketamine nasal spray were observed in a 1-year, open-label safety study, the long-term cognitive effects of the drug have not been evaluated beyond 1 year.

Impaired Ability to Drive or Operate Machinery. Esketamine may impair the ability to drive a motor vehicle or operate machinery. The effect of esketamine on driving performance was evaluated in 2 driving simulation studies; one study was conducted in adults with major depressive disorder and the other was conducted in healthy individuals. In a single-blind, placebo-controlled study in adults with major depressive disorder, next-day driving performance following a single 84-mg intranasal dose of esketamine was similar to that observed with placebo at 18 hours post-dose. Following twice-weekly dosing of intranasal esketamine in the same study, driving performance was evaluated once weekly on days 11, 18, and 25 and was found to be similar to that observed with placebo at 6 hours post-dose.

In a double-blind, placebo-controlled, crossover study in healthy adults, driving performance after administration of esketamine (single 84-mg intranasal dose) or placebo did not differ substantially when evaluated at 8 hours post-dose; however, 2 individuals in the study discontinued their driving tests prematurely after receiving intranasal esketamine because of a perceived inability to drive after experiencing post-dose adverse reactions.

Following treatment with esketamine, patients should not engage in potentially hazardous activities requiring full mental alertness and motor coordination, such as driving or operating machinery, until the next day after a restful sleep. Patients should also arrange their transportation home following each esketamine treatment session. (See Advice to Patients.)

Ulcerative or Interstitial Cystitis. Cases of ulcerative or interstitial cystitis have been reported with long-term, off-label use or misuse/abuse of ketamine. In clinical studies with esketamine nasal spray, a higher incidence of lower urinary tract symptoms, including pollakiuria, dysuria, urgency, nocturia, and cystitis, was observed in esketamine-treated patients compared with those receiving placebo. However, no cases of esketamine-associated interstitial cystitis were observed in any of these studies, which included treatment of up to 1 year's duration.

Patients receiving esketamine should be monitored for urinary tract and bladder symptoms (e.g., dysuria, urinary frequency or urgency, nocturia) during treatment. If urinary symptoms occur, patients should be evaluated by an appropriate healthcare provider as clinically warranted.

For further information on the urinary effects of ketamine, see Cautions: Genitourinary Effects and also see Chronic Toxicity in Ketamine Hydrochloride 28:04.

Embryofetal Toxicity. Based on published findings in pregnant animals exposed to ketamine, esketamine may cause fetal harm if administered to pregnant women. The clinical relevance of these findings to humans treated with esketamine nasal spray at the recommended dosage is not known.

Skeletal malformations were observed with intranasal administration of ketamine to pregnant rabbits; the no observed adverse effect level (NOAEL) for these malformations was associated with a plasma esketamine exposure that was 0.3 times the exposure at the maximum recommended human dosage (MRHD) of 84 mg daily. Intranasal administration of esketamine to pregnant rats produced delays in sensorimotor development and decreased motor activity at dosages that are associated with exposures that are less than the MRHD.

Studies in primates have demonstrated that use of anesthetic and sedation drugs that block *N*-methyl-D-aspartate (NMDA) receptors during the period of peak brain growth or synaptogenesis results in widespread neuronal and oligodendrocyte cell loss in the developing brain and alterations in synaptic morphology and neurogenesis in the developing brain of offspring. This period of brain development in animals is thought to correlate with the third trimester of pregnancy through the first several months of life in humans, but may extend to approximately 3 years of age. The clinical relevance of these findings to humans is not known; however, studies in juvenile animals suggest that neuroapoptosis results in long-term cognitive deficits. There are no data on pregnancy exposures in primates corresponding to periods prior to the third trimester in humans.

For further information on the effects of ketamine during pregnancy, see Neurodevelopmental and Cognitive Effects under Cautions: Pediatric Precautions, in Ketamine Hydrochloride 28:04.

Esketamine is not recommended for use during pregnancy. The manufacturer states that women of reproductive potential should consider pregnancy planning and contraception during esketamine therapy. If a woman becomes pregnant while receiving esketamine therapy, the drug should be discontinued and the patient apprised of the potential risk to the fetus.

Specific Populations

Pregnancy. Data on esketamine use in pregnant women are insufficient to inform a drug-associated risk. However, based on published findings from pregnant animals exposed to ketamine, esketamine may cause fetal harm. Esketamine is not recommended for use during pregnancy. (See Embryofetal Toxicity under Warnings/Precautions: Other Warnings and Precautions, in Cautions.)

A pregnancy registry has been established to monitor fetal outcomes of pregnant women exposed to antidepressants, including esketamine. For more information, patients or their clinicians may contact the National Pregnancy Registry for Antidepressants at 844-405-6185 or visit https://womensmentalhealth.org/research/pregnancyregistry/antidepressants/.

For additional information on the management of depression in women prior to conception and during pregnancy, including treatment algorithms, clinicians may consult the joint American Psychiatric Association and American College of Obstetricians and Gynecologists guidelines (at https://www.ncbi.nlm.nih.gov/pmc/articles/PMC3103063/pdf/nihms293836.pdf).

Lactation. Esketamine is distributed into milk in humans. It is not known if the drug has any effect on the nursing infant or on milk production.

Because of the potential for neurotoxicity in nursing infants (see Embryofetal Toxicity under Warnings/Precautions: Other Warnings and Precautions, in Cautions), the manufacturer states that breast-feeding during esketamine therapy is not recommended.

Pediatric Use. Safety and efficacy of esketamine nasal spray have not been established in pediatric patients.

Increased risk of suicidality has been observed in children and adolescents receiving antidepressants for major depressive disorder and other indications in short-term studies. (See Suicidality under Warnings/Precautions: Warnings, in Cautions.)

Results of animal studies indicate that repeated or prolonged use of drugs that block NMDA receptors, including ketamine and esketamine, in children younger than approximately 3 years of age potentially may adversely affect brain development. The clinical relevance of these findings to humans treated with esketamine nasal solution at the recommended clinical dosage is not known. (See Embryofetal Toxicity under Warnings/Precautions: Other Warnings and Precautions, in Cautions.)

For further information about the neurodevelopmental effects of ketamine in children, see Neurodevelopmental and Cognitive Effects under Cautions: Pediatric Precautions, in Ketamine Hydrochloride 28:04.

Geriatric Use. In phase 3 trials in the clinical development program for esketamine nasal spray in treatment-resistant depression, 12% of patients were 65 years of age or older and 2% were 75 years of age or older. No overall differences in the safety profile of esketamine were observed between geriatric patients and younger adults.

Higher peak plasma concentrations and systemic exposure of esketamine have been observed in geriatric patients compared with younger adults.

In a double-blind, placebo-controlled trial of 4 weeks' duration in patients 65 years of age or older with treatment-resistant depression, a reduction in the Montgomery-Asberg Depression Rating Scale (MADRS) total score was observed with esketamine treatment (initial dosage of 28 mg intranasally twice weekly then titrated to 56 or 84 mg twice weekly) in conjunction with a newly initiated oral antidepressant at the end of 4 weeks. However, the difference in the reduction in the MADRS total score between the esketamine and placebo groups did not achieve statistical significance in this study.

Hepatic Impairment. In a pharmacokinetic study of esketamine nasal spray, systemic exposure to esketamine was higher and the elimination half-life of the drug was longer in individuals with moderate hepatic impairment (Child-Pugh class B) compared with individuals with normal hepatic function. Although the manufacturer provides no specific dosage recommendations for patients with moderate hepatic impairment, the manufacturer states that such patients may require prolonged monitoring for possible adverse effects.

Peak plasma concentrations and exposure to esketamine were slightly increased in patients with mild hepatic impairment (Child-Pugh class A); these changes were not considered clinically important.

Esketamine has not been studied in patients with severe hepatic impairment (Child-Pugh class C) and is not recommended for use in such patients.

Renal Impairment. In a single-dose pharmacokinetic study, systemic exposure to esketamine was slightly higher in individuals with mild to severe renal impairment (creatinine clearance of 5–77 mL/minute; not requiring dialysis) compared with individuals with normal renal function; this difference was not considered clinically important.

Esketamine has not been studied in patients requiring dialysis to date.

■ **Common Adverse Effects** Adverse effects reported in at least 2% of patients with treatment-resistant depression receiving intranasal esketamine and an oral antidepressant and at a higher incidence than reported with placebo and an oral antidepressant in controlled trials include dissociation (including derealization and depersonalization) and perceptual changes (including distortion of time and space and illusions), dizziness, nausea, sedation, vertigo, headache, dysgeusia, hypoesthesia, anxiety, lethargy, increased blood pressure, vomiting, insomnia, diarrhea, nasal discomfort, throat irritation, dry mouth, feeling drunk, dysarthria, euphoric mood, hyperhidrosis, constipation, abnormal feeling, mental impairment, tremor, pollakiuria, oropharyngeal pain, and tachycardia.

Drug Interactions

Esketamine is metabolized principally by cytochrome P-450 (CYP) isoenzymes 2B6 and 3A4 and, to a lesser extent, by CYP2C9 and CYP2C19. The drug's major active metabolite, noresketamine, also is metabolized via CYP-mediated pathways.

In vitro, esketamine is a modest inducer of CYP2B6 and CYP3A4 and noresketamine weakly and reversibly inhibits CYP3A4. Esketamine and its major metabolites are unlikely to substantially inhibit other CYP isoenzymes or uridine diphosphate-glucuronosyltransferases (UGTs). Esketamine and its major metabolites do not induce CYP1A2 in vitro.

Esketamine is not a substrate for P-glycoprotein (P-gp), breast cancer resistance protein (BCRP), organic anion transport protein (OATP) 1B1, or OATP1B3 in vitro. The drug and its principal metabolites do not inhibit P-gp, BCRP, OATP1B1, OATP1B3, multidrug and toxin extrusion transporter (MATE) 1, MATE2K, organic cation transporter (OCT) 2, organic anion transporter (OAT) 1, or OAT3.

■ **Drugs Affecting or Metabolized by Hepatic Microsomal Enzymes** ***Inhibitors or Inducers of CYP2B6 or CYP3A*** No clinically important pharmacokinetic interactions occurred when intranasal esketamine was administered concomitantly with rifampin (a potent CYP inducer), ticlopidine (a CYP2B6 inhibitor), or clarithromycin (a potent CYP3A inhibitor).

The manufacturer states that dosage adjustment of esketamine is not necessary in patients concurrently receiving inhibitors or inducers of CYP2B6 or CYP3A4.

Clarithromycin. Concomitant administration of the potent CYP3A4 inhibitor clarithromycin (500 mg orally twice daily) with esketamine (84 mg intranasally) increased peak plasma concentrations and systemic exposure to esketamine by 11 and 4%, respectively; this pharmacokinetic interaction was not considered clinically important.

Rifampin. Concomitant administration of the potent CYP inducer rifampin (600 mg daily orally) with esketamine (56 mg intranasally) decreased peak plasma concentrations and systemic exposure to esketamine by 17 and 28%, respectively; this pharmacokinetic interaction was not considered clinically important.

Ticlopidine. Concomitant administration of the CYP2B6 inhibitor ticlopidine (250 mg orally twice daily) with esketamine (56 mg intranasally) increased peak plasma concentrations and systemic exposure to esketamine by 2 and 29%, respectively; this pharmacokinetic interaction was not considered clinically important.

Substrates of CYP2B6 or CYP3A Esketamine did not have any clinically important effect on the pharmacokinetics of oral bupropion (a CYP2B6 substrate) and its metabolite hydroxybupropion or oral midazolam (a CYP3A substrate).

■ **CNS Depressants** Concomitant use of esketamine with other CNS depressants (e.g., alcohol, benzodiazepines, opiates) may increase the risk of CNS depression. Patients should be closely monitored for sedation if esketamine is used concurrently with other CNS depressants.

■ **Hormonal Contraceptives** Based on physiologically based pharmacokinetic modeling, multiple dosing of esketamine is not expected to affect systemic exposure to ethinyl estradiol in combination oral contraceptives.

■ **Intranasally administered Corticosteroids and Decongestants** The pharmacokinetics of esketamine were not substantially altered when an intranasal corticosteroid (mometasone furoate administered daily) or intranasal decongestant (oxymetazoline hydrochloride) was administered intranasally 1 hour prior to intranasal administration of esketamine.

The manufacturer states that esketamine dosage adjustment is not necessary in patients concurrently receiving intranasal corticosteroids or decongestants. However, patients who require a nasal corticosteroid or nasal decongestant on an esketamine dosing day should administer these drugs at least 1 hour prior to intranasal esketamine.

■ **Psychostimulants** Concomitant use of esketamine with psychostimulants (e.g., amphetamines, methylphenidate, modafinil, armodafinil) may result in increased blood pressure. Blood pressure should therefore be closely monitored if esketamine is used concurrently with psychostimulants. (See Increases in Blood Pressure under Warnings/Precautions: Other Warnings and Precautions, in Cautions.)

■ **Monoamine Oxidase Inhibitors** Concomitant use of esketamine with monoamine oxidase (MAO) inhibitors may result in increased blood pressure. Blood pressure should therefore be closely monitored if esketamine is used concurrently with MAO inhibitors. (See Increases in Blood Pressure under Warnings/Precautions: Other Warnings and Precautions, in Cautions.)

Description

Esketamine is the *S*-enantiomer of racemic ketamine, which is a derivative of phencyclidine (PCP). The drug is a nonselective, noncompetitive antagonist of the *N*-methyl-D-aspartate (NMDA) receptor, which is an inotropic glutamate receptor. Esketamine has a higher affinity for the NMDA receptor than the *R*-enantiomer of racemic ketamine. The precise mechanism of action of esketamine in major depressive disorder has not been fully elucidated; however, the drug is thought to preferentially block NMDA receptors on inhibitory γ-aminobutyric acid (GABA)-ergic interneurons and transiently enhance the activity of glutamatergic neurons, leading to improved synaptic connectivity. The mechanism of antidepressant activity of esketamine is thought to be similar to that of ketamine and is not thought to directly involve serotonin, norepinephrine, or dopamine reuptake, nor is it believed to directly involve μ opiate receptor stimulation.

For detailed information on the pharmacologic effects of ketamine, see Pharmacology in Ketamine Hydrochloride 28:04.

Esketamine is rapidly absorbed following intranasal administration. The mean absolute bioavailability of the drug is approximately 48% and peak plasma concentrations occur in 20–40 minutes following the last nasal spray of a treatment session. The pharmacokinetics of esketamine increase in a less than dose-proportional manner over an intranasal dosage range of 28–84 mg; however, between 56–84 mg the pharmacokinetics are approximately dose proportional. *Interpatient* variation in peak plasma concentration and area under the concentration-time curve (AUC) ranges from 27–66 and 18–45%, respectively. The *intrapatient* variation in peak plasma concentration and AUC is 15 and 10%, respectively. Esketamine is approximately 43–45% bound to plasma proteins. The drug distributes into the brain; the brain-to-plasma ratio of noresketamine (the principal active metabolite of esketamine) is 4–6 times lower than that of esketamine. Esketamine is metabolized principally by CYP2B6 and CYP3A4 and, to a lesser extent, by CYP2C9 and CYP2C19 to its principal active metabolite noresketamine. Noresketamine has demonstrated activity at the same NMDA receptor as its parent drug but with less affinity. Noresketamine also is metabolized via CYP-mediated pathways. Plasma esketamine and noresketamine concentrations decline in a biphasic manner, with a rapid initial phase (2–4 or 4 hours for esketamine or noresketamine, respectively) and a longer elimination phase (mean terminal half-life of 7–12 or 8 hours for esketamine or noresketamine, respectively). Following IV or oral administration of radiolabeled esketamine, metabolites were mainly recovered in the urine (over 78% of the dose) and, to a lesser extent, in feces (less than 2%). Less than 1% of the dose is excreted unchanged in urine.

Advice to Patients

Importance of advising patients to read the manufacturer's medication guide and instructions for use.

Esketamine nasal spray is only available through the Spravato® REMS program. Importance of informing patients that they must be enrolled in the REMS program prior to drug administration. Importance of also informing patients that esketamine treatment must be administered under the direct supervision of a healthcare provider and that patients must be monitored by a healthcare provider for at least 2 hours following intranasal administration of the drug.

Risk of sedation, dissociative symptoms, disturbances in perception, dizziness, vertigo, and/or anxiety. Importance of advising patients to notify a healthcare provider immediately if they feel like they cannot stay awake or feel like they may lose consciousness. Importance of informing patients that they will be monitored by a healthcare provider until these potential adverse effects resolve.

Importance of advising patients that esketamine is a federally controlled substance because of its potential for abuse, misuse, and dependence.

Risk of suicidal thoughts and behaviors (suicidality); importance of patients and caregivers being alert to emergence of suicidality, especially early during therapy or during periods of dosage adjustments. (See Suicidality under Warnings/Precautions: Warnings, in Cautions.)

Risk of blood pressure increases. Importance of informing patients that they may require observation by a healthcare provider until the blood pressure elevation resolves. Importance of advising patients to notify a healthcare provider immediately if they experience chest pain, shortness of breath, sudden severe headache, changes in vision, or seizures after intranasal administration of esketamine.

Nausea and vomiting may occur in some patients. Importance of advising patients not to eat for at least 2 hours before administering esketamine nasal spray and to avoid drinking liquids for at least 30 minutes before administering the drug.

Importance of informing patients that esketamine may impair their ability to drive or operate machinery. Following a treatment session, importance of advising patients not to drive, operate machinery, or engage in potentially hazardous activities requiring full mental alertness and motor coordination until the next day after a restful sleep. Patients should be advised that they will need someone to drive them home after each treatment session.

Importance of women informing clinicians if they are or plan to become pregnant or plan to breast-feed; importance of advising women to avoid breast-feeding during esketamine therapy. Importance of informing patients about the potential fetal risk and informing women who become pregnant while taking esketamine about the existence of the national pregnancy registry for antidepressants. (See Pregnancy under Warnings/Precautions: Specific Populations, in Cautions.)

Importance of informing clinicians of existing or contemplated concomitant therapy, including prescription, OTC, and recreational drugs and dietary or herbal supplements (see Drug Interactions), as well as any concomitant or past illnesses (e.g., cardiovascular or cerebrovascular disease, hepatic disease, psychosis, substance abuse or dependence).

Importance of informing patients of other important precautionary information. (See Cautions.)

Overview® (see Users Guide). For additional information on this drug until a more detailed monograph is developed and published, the manufacturer's labeling should be consulted. It is *essential* that the manufacturer's labeling be consulted for more detailed information on usual cautions, precautions, contraindications, potential drug interactions, laboratory test interferences, and acute toxicity.

Preparations

Esketamine is subject to control under the Federal Controlled Substances Act of 1970 as a schedule III (C-III) drug.

Distribution of esketamine is restricted. (See Restricted Distribution Program under Dosage and Administration: General.)

Excipients in commercially available drug preparations may have clinically important effects in some individuals; consult specific product labeling for details.

Esketamine Hydrochloride

Nasal		
Solution	14 mg (of esketamine) per metered spray (14 mg/0.1 mL)	**Spravato® 56 mg Dose Kit** (C-III; contains two 28-mg nasal spray devices), Janssen
		Spravato® 84 mg Dose Kit (C-III; contains three 28-mg nasal spray devices), Janssen

Mirtazapine

■ Mirtazapine is a piperazinoazepine-derivative tetracyclic antidepressant agent.

Uses

■ **Major Depressive Disorder** Mirtazapine is used in the treatment of major depressive disorder. Efficacy of mirtazapine for the management of major depression has been established by controlled studies of 6 weeks' duration in outpatient settings. Results of these studies indicate that the antidepressant effect of mirtazapine (5–35 mg daily) is greater than placebo and comparable to that of tricyclic antidepressants (e.g., amitriptyline [40–280 mg daily]). In these studies, no age- or gender-related differences in efficacy were noted. The manufacturer states that the efficacy of mirtazapine for long-term use (i.e., exceeding 6 weeks) has not been established by controlled studies and that the drug's antidepressant efficacy in hospital settings has not been adequately studied to date. However, acute depressive episodes generally require several months or longer of sustained antidepressant therapy. (See Dosage and Administration: Dosage.) If mirtazapine is used for extended periods, the need for continued therapy should be reassessed periodically. For further information on treatment of major depressive disorder and considerations in choosing the most appropriate antidepressant for a particular patient, including considerations related to patient tolerance, patient age, and cardiovascular, sedative, and suicidal risks, see Considerations in Choosing Antidepressants under Uses: Major Depressive Disorder, in Fluoxetine Hydrochloride 28:16.04.20.

Since hypomanic or manic attacks have been reported rarely in patients receiving mirtazapine, the drug should be used with caution in patients with a history of hypomanic or manic attacks.

Individuals with phenylketonuria (i.e., homozygous genetic deficiency of phenylalanine hydroxylase) and other individuals who must restrict their intake of phenylalanine should be warned that mirtazapine orally disintegrating tablets (Remeron® SolTab®) contain aspartame (NutraSweet®), which is metabolized in the GI tract to provide about 2.6, 5.2, or 7.8 mg of phenylalanine following oral administration of a 15-, 30-, or 45-mg tablet, respectively, of mirtazapine.

Dosage and Administration

■ **Administration** Mirtazapine is administered orally as conventional or orally disintegrating tablets. The drug is administered once daily, usually at bedtime. Since food does not appear to substantially affect GI absorption of mirtazapine, the drug generally can be administered without regard to meals.

Patients receiving mirtazapine orally disintegrating tablets should be instructed not to remove a tablet from the blister until just prior to dosing; once removed, it cannot be stored. With dry hands, the blister backing should be peeled completely off the blister. The tablet should then be gently removed and immediately placed on the tongue to dissolve and be swallowed with the saliva; administration with liquid is not necessary. In addition, patients should be advised not to break the tablet.

■ **Dosage** For the management of major depressive disorder in adults, the recommended initial dosage of mirtazapine is 15 mg daily. If no clinical improvement is apparent, dosage may be increased up to a maximum of 45 mg daily at intervals of not less than 1–2 weeks since elimination half-life of the drug is about 20–40 hours. Although clearance of mirtazapine may decrease in geriatric patients, the manufacturer does not make specific recommendations for dosage adjustment in such patients. However, the manufacturer states that since plasma mirtazapine concentrations may be increased in geriatric patients, the drug should be used with caution in such patients. While a relationship between dosage and antidepressant effect has not been established, the effective dosage of mirtazapine in controlled clinical studies generally ranged from 15–45 mg daily. Patients should be advised that although some improvement in their condition may occur within 1–4 weeks, therapy should be continued as directed.

Although the optimum duration of mirtazapine therapy has not been established, acute depressive episodes may require 6 months or longer of sustained antidepressant medication. Whether the dosage of mirtazapine required to induce remission of depression would be comparable to that required to maintain euthymia currently is not known.

Patients should be monitored for possible worsening of depression, suicidality, or unusual changes in behavior, especially at the beginning of therapy or during periods of dosage adjustment. (See Suicidality Precautions under Dosage and Administration: Dosage.)

The manufacturer recommends that a drug-free interval of at least 2 weeks elapse when switching a patient from a monoamine oxidase (MAO) inhibitor to mirtazapine or when switching from mirtazapine to an MAO inhibitor. For additional information on potentially serious drug interactions that may occur between mirtazapine and MAO inhibitors or other serotonergic agents, see Drug Interactions: Drugs Associated with Serotonin Syndrome in Fluoxetine Hydrochloride 28:16.04.20 and the Monoamine Oxidase Inhibitors General Statement 28:16.04.12.

Suicidality Precautions Worsening of depression and/or the emergence of suicidal ideation and behavior (suicidality) or unusual changes in behavior may occur in both adult and pediatric (see Dosage and Administration: Pediatric Precautions) patients with major depressive disorder or other psychiatric disorders, whether or not they are taking antidepressants. This risk may persist until clinically important remission occurs. Suicide is a known risk of depression and certain other psychiatric disorders, and these disorders themselves are the strongest predictors of suicide. However, there has been a long-standing concern that antidepressants may have a role in inducing worsening of depression and the emergence of suicidality in certain patients during the early phases of treatment. Pooled analyses of short-term, placebo-controlled studies of antidepressants (i.e., selective serotonin-reuptake inhibitors and other antidepressants) have shown an increased risk of suicidality in children, adolescents, and young adults (18–24 years of age) with major depressive disorder and other psychiatric disorders. An increased suicidality risk was not demonstrated with antidepressants compared with placebo in adults older than 24 years of age, and a reduced risk was observed in adults 65 years of age or older. It is currently unknown whether the suicidality risk extends to longer-term use (i.e., beyond several months); however, there is substantial evidence from placebo-controlled maintenance trials in adults with major depressive disorder that antidepressants can delay the recurrence of depression.

The US Food and Drug Administration (FDA) recommends that all patients being treated with antidepressants for any indication be appropriately monitored and closely observed for clinical worsening, suicidality, and unusual changes in behavior, particularly during initiation of therapy (i.e., the first few months) and during periods of dosage adjustments. Families and caregivers of patients being treated with antidepressants for major depressive disorder or other indications, both psychiatric and nonpsychiatric, should be advised to monitor patients on a daily basis for the emergence of agitation, irritability, or unusual changes in behavior as well as the emergence of suicidality, and to report such symptoms immediately to a health-care provider.

Although a causal relationship between the emergence of symptoms such as anxiety, agitation, panic attacks, insomnia, irritability, hostility, aggressiveness, impulsivity, akathisia, hypomania, and/or mania and either the worsening of depression and/or the emergence of suicidal impulses has not been established, there is concern that such symptoms may represent precursors to emerging suicidality. Consequently, consideration should be given to changing the therapeutic regimen or discontinuing therapy in patients whose depression is persistently worse or in patients experiencing emergent suicidality or symptoms that might be precursors to worsening depression or suicidality, particularly if such manifestations are severe, abrupt in onset, or were not part of the patient's presenting symptoms. FDA also recommends that the drugs be prescribed in the smallest quantity consistent with good patient management, in order to reduce the risk of overdosage.

Bipolar Disorder Precautions It is generally believed (though not established in controlled trials) that treating a major depressive episode with an antidepressant alone may increase the likelihood of precipitating a mixed or manic episode in patients at risk for bipolar disorder. Therefore, patients should be adequately screened for bipolar disorder prior to initiating treatment with an antidepressant; such screening should include a detailed psychiatric history (e.g., family history of suicide, bipolar disorder, and depression).

■ **Pediatric Precautions** Safety and efficacy of mirtazapine in children have not been established.

FDA has determined that antidepressants increase the risk of suicidal thinking and behavior (suicidality) in children and adolescents with major depressive disorder and other psychiatric disorders. However, FDA also states that depression and certain other psychiatric disorders are themselves associated with an increased risk of suicide. (See Cautions: Pediatric Precautions, in Fluoxetine Hydrochloride 28:16.04.20) Anyone considering the use of mirtazapine in a child or adolescent for any clinical use must therefore balance the potential risks with the clinical need. (See Suicidality Precautions under Dosage and Administration: Dosage.)

■ **Dosage in Renal and Hepatic Impairment** Although clearance of mirtazapine may decrease in patients with hepatic or moderate to severe renal impairment, the manufacturer does not make specific recommendations for dosage adjustment in such patients. However, the manufacturer states that since plasma concentrations of mirtazapine may be increased in patients with hepatic or moderate to severe renal impairment, the drug should be used with caution in such patients.

Description

Mirtazapine is a piperazinoazepine-derivative antidepressant agent. As a tetracyclic antidepressant agent, the drug differs structurally from selective serotonin-reuptake inhibitors (e.g., fluoxetine, sertraline), monoamine oxidase inhibitors, and tricyclic antidepressant agents.

The exact mechanism of antidepressant action of mirtazapine has not been fully elucidated, but the drug appears to act as an antagonist at central presynaptic α_2-adrenergic autoreceptors and heteroreceptors resulting in enhanced central noradrenergic and serotonergic activity. Mirtazapine is a potent antagonist of serotonin type 2 (5-HT_2) and type 3 (5-HT_3) receptors, but the drug does not exhibit high affinity for serotonin type 1A (5-HT_{1A}) or type 1B (5-HT_{1B}) receptors. Mirtazapine is a potent antagonist of histamine H_1 receptors, which may account for the prominent sedative effects of the drug. In addition, the drug exhibits moderate peripheral α_1-adrenergic blocking activity that may explain the occasional orthostatic hypotension that reportedly has been associated with mirtazapine. The drug is a moderate antagonist at muscarinic receptors, which may account for the relatively low incidence of anticholinergic effects associated with mirtazapine.

SumMon® (see Users Guide). For additional information on this drug until a more detailed monograph is developed and published, the manufacturer's labeling should be consulted. It is *essential* that the labeling be consulted for detailed information on the usual cautions, precautions, and contraindications.

Preparations

Excipients in commercially available drug preparations may have clinically important effects in some individuals; consult specific product labeling for details.

Mirtazapine

Oral		
Tablets, film-coated	15 mg*	**Mirtazapine Film-coated Tablets**
		Remeron® (scored), Organon
	30 mg*	**Mirtazapine Film-coated Tablets**
		Remeron® (scored), Organon
	45 mg*	**Mirtazapine Film-coated Tablets**
		Remeron®, Organon
Tablets, orally disintegrating	15 mg*	**Mirtazapine Orally Disintegrating Tablets**
		Remeron® SolTab, Organon
	30 mg*	**Mirtazapine Orally Disintegrating Tablets**
		Remeron® SolTab, Organon
	45 mg*	**Mirtazapine Orally Disintegrating Tablets**
		Remeron® SolTab, Organon

*available from one or more manufacturer, distributor, and/or repackager by generic (nonproprietary) name

ANTIPSYCHOTICS 28:16.08

ATYPICAL ANTIPSYCHOTICS 28:16.08.04

ARIPiprazole

■ Aripiprazole is considered an atypical or second-generation antipsychotic agent.

Uses

Aripiprazole is used orally for the symptomatic management of psychotic disorders (e.g., schizophrenia). Aripiprazole also is used orally for the treatment of bipolar I disorder, as an adjunct to antidepressants for the acute treatment of major depressive disorder, for the acute treatment of irritability associated with autistic disorder, and for the treatment of Tourette's syndrome (Gilles de la Tourette's syndrome). Short-acting (immediate-release) aripiprazole injection (Abilify®; no longer commercially available in the US) has been used IM for the management of acute agitation in patients with bipolar disorder or schizophrenia. Extended-release aripiprazole injection (Abilify Maintena®) is used IM for the treatment of schizophrenia and maintenance treatment of bipolar I disorder. Extended-release aripiprazole lauroxil injection (Aristada®; available as prefilled syringes in 441-mg, 662-mg, 882-mg, and 1064-mg strengths) is used IM for the treatment of schizophrenia; the 675-mg strength of extended-release aripiprazole lauroxil injection (Aristada Initio®) is used IM in combination with oral aripiprazole for the initiation of extended-release aripiprazole lauroxil therapy for the treatment of schizophrenia.

Aripiprazole tablets with sensor (Abilify MyCite®) is part of a digital ingestion tracking system intended to provide objective data on drug ingestion. (See Tablets with Sensor under Administration: Oral Administration, in Dosage and Administration and also see Description: Aripiprazole Tablets with Sensor.) The ability of the system to improve patient compliance or help guide aripiprazole dosage adjustments has not been established. The manufacturer states that the use of Abilify MyCite® to track drug ingestion in "real time" or during an emergency is not recommended because detection of tablet ingestion may be delayed or may not occur. Abilify MyCite® is used orally for the treatment of schizophrenia, for the treatment of bipolar I disorder, and as an adjunct to antidepressants for the treatment of major depressive disorder.

■ **Psychotic Disorders** Aripiprazole is used orally and parenterally for the symptomatic management of psychotic disorders (e.g., schizophrenia). Drug therapy is integral to the management of acute psychotic episodes in patients with schizophrenia and generally is required for long-term stabilization to sustain symptom remission or control and to minimize the risk of relapse. Antipsychotic agents are the principal class of drugs used for the management of all phases of schizophrenia. Patient response and tolerance to antipsychotic agents are variable, and patients who do not respond to or tolerate one drug may be successfully treated with an agent from a different class or with a different adverse effect profile.

Schizophrenia Aripiprazole is used orally for the acute and maintenance treatment of schizophrenia. In addition, extended-release formulations of aripiprazole (Abilify Maintena®) and aripiprazole lauroxil (Aristada®, Aristada Initio®) are used IM for the treatment of schizophrenia. Schizophrenia is a major psychotic disorder that frequently has devastating effects on various aspects of the patient's life and carries a high risk of suicide and other life-threatening behaviors. Manifestations of schizophrenia involve multiple psychologic processes, including perception (e.g., hallucinations), ideation, reality testing (e.g., delusions), emotion (e.g., flatness, inappropriate affect), thought processes (e.g., loose associations), behavior (e.g., catatonia, disorganization), attention, concentration, motivation (e.g., avolition, impaired intention and planning), and judgment. The principal manifestations of this disorder usually are described in terms of positive and negative (deficit) symptoms and, more recently, disorganized symptoms. Positive symptoms include hallucinations, delusions, bizarre behavior, hostility, uncooperativeness, and paranoid ideation, while negative symptoms include restricted range and intensity of emotional expression (affective flattening), reduced thought and speech productivity (alogia), anhedonia, apathy, and decreased initiation of goal-directed behavior (avolition). Disorganized symptoms include disorganized speech (thought disorder) and behavior and poor attention.

Short-term efficacy of oral aripiprazole monotherapy in the acute treatment of schizophrenia in adults was evaluated in 5 placebo-controlled studies of 4 and 6 weeks' duration principally in acutely relapsed, hospitalized patients who predominantly met DSM-III/IV criteria for schizophrenia. Four of the 5 studies were able to distinguish aripiprazole from placebo, but the smallest study did not. In the 4 positive studies, assessment of improvement in manifestations of schizophrenia was based on results of psychiatric rating scales, including the Positive and Negative Syndrome Scale (PANSS), the PANSS positive subscale, the PANSS negative subscale, and the Clinical Global Impressions (CGI) scale. Aripiprazole generally was found to be superior to placebo in improving both positive and negative manifestations in acute exacerbations of schizophrenia in these 4 studies. Efficacy of 10-, 15-, 20-, and 30-mg daily dosages of aripiprazole was established in 2 studies for each dosage; however, there was no evidence that higher dosages offered any therapeutic advantage over lower dosages in these studies. Active controls (haloperidol or risperidone) were used in addition to placebo controls in 3 of these studies, but study design did not allow for comparison between aripiprazole and the active controls. An examination of population subgroups did not reveal any clear evidence of differential responsiveness to the drug based on age, gender, or race.

In a longer-term study, adult inpatients or outpatients who met DSM-IV criteria for schizophrenia and who were, by history, symptomatically stable on other antipsychotic agents for at least 3 months were discontinued from those other agents and randomized to receive either oral aripiprazole 15 mg daily or placebo for up to 26 weeks of observation for relapse in the double-blind phase. Relapse was based on results of the CGI-Improvement and PANSS psychiatric rating scales. Patients receiving aripiprazole experienced a significantly longer time to relapse over the subsequent 26 weeks compared with those receiving placebo. In addition, pooled data from 2 double-blind, multicenter studies in acutely ill patients with schizophrenia in whom therapy with aripiprazole or haloperidol was continued for 52 weeks demonstrated a substantially higher rate of symptomatic remission across 52 weeks in the aripiprazole-treated patients compared with the haloperidol-treated patients; improved tolerability with aripiprazole may have contributed to the higher overall remission rates observed in this pooled analysis.

Short-term efficacy of oral aripiprazole in the acute treatment of schizophrenia in adolescents 13–17 years of age was evaluated in a double-blind, placebo-controlled trial of 6 weeks' duration in 302 outpatients who met DSM-IV criteria for schizophrenia and had a PANSS total score of 70 or more at baseline. Patients were randomized to receive a fixed dosage of aripiprazole 10 mg daily or 30 mg daily or to receive placebo. Both dosages of aripiprazole were found to be superior to placebo in reducing the PANSS total score, which was the primary efficacy measure; the 10-mg daily dosage also demonstrated superiority over placebo on the PANSS negative subscale score at the study end point. However, the 30-mg daily dosage failed to demonstrate superiority over the 10-mg daily dosage. The drug was generally well tolerated.

Short-term efficacy of the extended-release IM formulation of aripiprazole (Abilify Maintena®) in the treatment of schizophrenia in adults was established in a multicenter, double-blind, placebo-controlled study of 12 weeks' duration in acutely relapsed inpatients who met DSM-IV-TR criteria for schizophrenia and who were experiencing an acute psychotic episode. Patients in this study were randomized to receive IM injections of extended-release aripiprazole (400 mg) or placebo every 4 weeks. Patients receiving extended-release IM aripiprazole were also given oral aripiprazole (10–20 mg daily) for 14 days beginning on the day of the first injection to provide therapeutic plasma concentrations, which may take longer to achieve in some patients; patients who received placebo injections were given placebo tablets for the first 14 days. The IM dosage of extended-release aripiprazole could be adjusted down to 300 mg and increased back to 400 mg on a one-time basis. The primary efficacy measure in this study was the change in PANSS total score from baseline to end point (week 10). Patients treated with extended-release IM aripiprazole injection demonstrated substantially greater improvement in mean PANSS total scores compared with those receiving placebo.

In a longer-term maintenance study, adults who met DSM-IV-TR criteria for schizophrenia and who were receiving at least one antipsychotic agent were treated with open-label oral aripiprazole for 4–6 weeks followed by extended-release aripiprazole (Abilify Maintena®) 400 mg IM once every 4 weeks with oral aripiprazole continued for the first 2 weeks after the initial injection. The IM extended-release aripiprazole dosage could be adjusted down to 300 mg based on tolerability and increased back to 400 mg on a one-time basis. Patients who remained stable on the extended-release IM injection for at least 12 weeks were then randomized either to continue receiving extended-release IM aripiprazole at the same dosage or to receive placebo injection IM every 4 weeks for up to 52 weeks and observed for relapse in the double-blind withdrawal phase. The primary efficacy measure was the time from randomization to relapse, and patients who received extended-release IM aripiprazole had a substantially longer time to relapse than those who received placebo.

Efficacy of extended-release aripiprazole lauroxil IM injection (Aristada®) in the treatment of schizophrenia was established, in part, based on extrapolation of efficacy data from clinical trials with oral aripiprazole. In addition, efficacy was established in a multicenter, double-blind, placebo-controlled, fixed-dose study of 12 weeks' duration in adults who met DSM-IV-TR criteria for schizophrenia and were experiencing an acute exacerbation or relapse. Patients were randomized to receive extended-release aripiprazole lauroxil 441 mg, aripiprazole lauroxil 882 mg, or placebo by IM injection every 4 weeks. After establishing tolerability to oral aripiprazole, patients concomitantly received oral aripiprazole 15 mg daily (if randomized to aripiprazole) or placebo for the first 3 weeks. The primary efficacy measure in this study was the change in PANSS total score from baseline to end point (week 12). At the study end point, both dosages of extended-release aripiprazole lauroxil injection resulted in substantially greater improvement in the PANSS total score compared with placebo. Substantial improvements in the PANSS total score were evident as early as day 8 with extended-release aripiprazole lauroxil therapy and continued through the end of the treatment period. The secondary efficacy end point was the Clinical Global Impression-Improvement (CGI-I) score on day 85. Both groups of patients receiving extended-release aripiprazole lauroxil therapy demonstrated substantially better CGI-I scores compared with the placebo group. An examination of population subgroups did not reveal any clear evidence of differential responsiveness to the drug based on age, gender, race, or body weight.

Aripiprazole tablets with sensor (Abilify MyCite®) is part of a digital ingestion tracking system intended to provide objective data on drug ingestion. (See Tablets with Sensor under Administration: Oral Administration, in Dosage and Administration and also see Description: Aripiprazole Tablets with Sensor.) The usability (i.e., ease of use, helpfulness) of this digital ingestion tracking system was evaluated in a multicenter, open-label study in 67 adults with a primary diagnosis of schizophrenia. Patients who had been stabilized on oral aripiprazole therapy were switched to the same dosage of aripiprazole tablets with sensor (Abilify MyCite®) for 8 weeks. Patients received training at baseline and weekly as needed for the first 3 weeks then were instructed to change the wearable sensor and pair it with their mobile device independently or with the assistance of a caregiver weekly for the next 5 weeks. The majority of patients in this study were male (74.6%) and black or African-American (76.1%), and 70.1% had mild disease (i.e., Clinical Global Impression-Severity [CGI-S] score of 3) and a higher range of function (indicated by relatively high mean scores on the Instrumental Activities of Daily Living and Personal and Social Performance scales). Forty-nine patients (73.1%) completed the 8-week study; by the end of the study period or at the time of withdrawal from the study, 55.2% of patients were able to apply and pair a wearable sensor with their mobile device independently and 82.1% completed the tasks independently or with minimal assistance (as rated by a clinician using a standardized scale). Of the 60 patients who rated the ease of use and helpfulness of the digital ingestion tracking system at the end of study or at the time of withdrawal from the study, 78% reported that they were somewhat satisfied to extremely satisfied with the digital ingestion tracking system, 70% rated the system as at least somewhat helpful in management of their condition, 77% rated the system as at least somewhat helpful in improving discussions with their healthcare provider, and 65% rated the system as somewhat easy to extremely easy to use.

Although the efficacy of oral aripiprazole as maintenance therapy in pediatric patients with schizophrenia has not been systematically evaluated, the manufacturer states that such efficacy can be extrapolated from adult data in addition to comparisons of aripiprazole pharmacokinetic parameters in adult and pediatric patients.

If aripiprazole is used for extended periods as maintenance therapy for schizophrenia, the need for continued therapy should be reassessed periodically. (See Dosage and Administration: Dosage and see also Pediatric Use under Warnings/Precautions: Specific Populations, in Cautions.)

The American Psychiatric Association (APA) considers most atypical antipsychotic agents first-line drugs for the management of the acute phase of schizophrenia (including first psychotic episodes), principally because of the decreased risk of adverse extrapyramidal effects and tardive dyskinesia, with the understanding that the relative advantages, disadvantages, and cost-effectiveness of conventional and atypical antipsychotic agents remain controversial. The APA states that, with the possible exception of clozapine for the management of treatment-resistant symptoms, there currently is no definitive evidence that one atypical antipsychotic agent will have superior efficacy compared with another agent in the class, although meaningful differences in response may be observed in individual patients. Conventional antipsychotic agents may be considered first-line therapy in patients who have been treated successfully in the past with or who prefer conventional agents. The choice of an antipsychotic agent should be individualized, considering past response to therapy, adverse effect profile (including the patient's experience of subjective effects such as dysphoria), and the patient's preference for a specific drug, including route of administration.

For additional information on the symptomatic management of schizophrenia, including treatment recommendations, see Schizophrenia and Other Psychotic Disorders under Uses: Psychotic Disorders, in the Phenothiazines General Statement 28:16.08.24.

■ Bipolar Disorder Aripiprazole is used orally as monotherapy or as an adjunct to either lithium or valproate for the acute treatment of manic or mixed episodes associated with bipolar I disorder with or without psychotic features. The drug also is used orally as monotherapy or as adjunctive therapy with lithium or valproate for the maintenance treatment of bipolar I disorder. Extended-release aripiprazole injection (Abilify Maintena®) is used IM as monotherapy for the maintenance treatment of bipolar I disorder. According to DSM-IV criteria, manic episodes are distinct periods lasting 1 week or longer (or less than 1 week if hospitalization is required) of abnormally and persistently elevated, expansive, or irritable mood accompanied by at least 3 (or 4 if the mood is only irritability) of the following 7 symptoms: grandiosity, reduced need for sleep, pressure of speech, flight of ideas, distractability, increased goal-directed activity (either socially, at work or school, or sexually) or psychomotor agitation, and engaging in high-risk behavior (e.g., unrestrained buying sprees, sexual indiscretions, foolish business investments).

Efficacy of oral aripiprazole monotherapy in the treatment of acute manic and mixed episodes has been demonstrated in 4 short-term (i.e., 3 weeks' duration), placebo-controlled trials in hospitalized adults who met DSM-IV criteria for bipolar I disorder with manic or mixed episodes. These studies included patients with or without psychotic features and 2 of the studies also included patients with or without a rapid cycling course. The principal rating instrument used for assessing manic symptoms in these trials was the Young Mania Rating Scale (Y-MRS), an 11-item clinician-rated scale traditionally used to assess the degree of manic symptomatology in a range from 0 (no manic features) to 60 (maximum score). The main secondary rating instrument used in these trials was the Clinical Global Impression-Bipolar (CGI-BP) scale. In these trials, aripiprazole 15–30 mg once daily (with an initial dosage of 15 mg daily in 2 studies and an initial dosage of 30 mg daily in the other 2 studies) was found to be superior to placebo in the reduction of the Y-MRS total score and the CGI-BP Severity of Illness score (mania). In the 2 studies with an initial aripiprazole dosage of 15 mg daily, 48 and 44% of patients were receiving 15 mg daily at the study end point; in the 2 studies with an initial dosage of 30 mg daily, 86 and 85% of patients were receiving 30 mg daily at end point.

Aripiprazole is used orally as monotherapy for the acute treatment of manic and mixed episodes associated with bipolar I disorder with or without psychotic features in pediatric patients 10–17 years of age. Efficacy of aripiprazole in the acute treatment of manic and mixed episodes has been demonstrated in a double-blind, placebo-controlled study of 4 weeks' duration in pediatric outpatients who met DSM-IV criteria for bipolar I disorder manic or mixed episodes (with or without psychotic features) and who had Y-MRS scores of 20 or greater at baseline. Patients in this study received aripiprazole 10 mg daily, aripiprazole 30 mg daily, or placebo. Aripiprazole was initiated at a dosage of 2 mg daily, then titrated to 5 mg daily after 2 days, and to the target dosage of 10 mg daily in 5 days or 30 mg daily in 13 days. Both dosages of aripiprazole were found to be superior to placebo in the reduction of the Y-MRS total score from baseline to week 4.

Efficacy of oral aripiprazole as an adjunct to lithium or valproate in the treatment of acute manic and mixed episodes has been demonstrated in a placebo-controlled study of 6 weeks' duration in adult outpatients who met DSM-IV criteria for bipolar I disorder manic or mixed type (with or without psychotic features). Patients initially received open-label lithium (dosage producing a serum lithium concentration of 0.6–1 mEq/L) or valproate (dosage producing a serum valproic acid concentration of 50–125 mcg/mL) monotherapy for 2 weeks during the lead-in phase. At the end of 2 weeks, patients demonstrating an inadequate response to lithium or valproate were randomized to receive either aripiprazole (15 mg daily or increased to 30 mg daily as early as day 7) or placebo as adjunctive therapy with open-label lithium or valproate during the 6-week, placebo-controlled phase. Patients who received adjunctive aripiprazole with lithium or valproate demonstrated greater reductions in the Y-MRS total score and the CGI-BP Severity of Illness score (mania) compared with patients who received adjunctive placebo with lithium or valproate.

The use of oral aripiprazole as an adjunct to lithium or valproate in the acute treatment of manic or mixed episodes associated with bipolar I disorder has not been evaluated in the pediatric population. However, the manufacturer states that such efficacy can be extrapolated from adult data in addition to comparisons of aripiprazole pharmacokinetic parameters in adult and pediatric patients.

For the initial management of less severe manic or mixed episodes in patients with bipolar disorder, current APA recommendations state that monotherapy with lithium, valproate (e.g., valproate sodium, valproic acid, divalproex), or an antipsychotic such as olanzapine may be adequate. For more severe manic or mixed episodes, combination therapy with an antipsychotic and lithium or valproate is recommended as first-line therapy. For further information on the management of bipolar disorder, see Uses: Bipolar Disorder, in Lithium Salts 28:28.

Efficacy of oral aripiprazole as monotherapy for the maintenance treatment of bipolar I disorder was evaluated in a 26-week, double-blind, placebo-controlled trial in patients with a recent manic or mixed episode who had been stabilized on open-label aripiprazole monotherapy (15–30 mg daily); patients who maintained clinical response with the drug for at least 6 weeks were randomized to either continue aripiprazole at the same dosage or be switched to placebo and monitored for manic or depressive relapse. In this study, time to relapse to any mood episode, particularly manic episode, was substantially longer and there were fewer manic relapses among patients receiving aripiprazole than in those receiving placebo. There were no differences between aripiprazole and placebo in time to relapse to depressive or mixed episodes or in the number of depressive episodes. A 74-week extension of the study also found that time to relapse to any mood episode, particularly manic episode, was substantially longer with aripiprazole than placebo at 100 weeks of treatment; however, the design and interpretation of these study findings suggesting aripiprazole's efficacy in the maintenance therapy of bipolar disorder have been criticized (i.e., insufficient duration to demonstrate prophylactic efficacy, use of an "enriched" patient sample consisting of aripiprazole responders, abrupt discontinuance of aripiprazole in patients randomized to placebo, and low study completion rate). Time to relapse to depressive episode was not substantially different between treatment groups during the 74-week extension phase.

Oral aripiprazole as adjunctive maintenance therapy in adults with bipolar I disorder was evaluated in a double-blind, placebo-controlled trial in patients with a recent manic or mixed episode. Patients in this study had received lithium or valproate therapy for at least 2 weeks, and those with an inadequate response to the mood stabilizer also received adjunctive aripiprazole therapy (10–30 mg daily) and were maintained on the combined regimen for at least 12 weeks. Patients who maintained clinical response with aripiprazole and a mood stabilizer during this period were randomized to either continue aripiprazole or be switched to placebo (combined with lithium or valproate therapy) and monitored for manic, mixed, or depressive relapse for a maximum of 52 weeks. Patients receiving adjunctive aripiprazole therapy with lithium or valproate experienced a significant delay in time to relapse to any mood episode compared with those receiving placebo plus lithium or valproate, particularly for relapse to manic episode; no difference between the treatment groups was observed for time to relapse to depressive episode.

Efficacy of extended-release IM aripiprazole injection (Abilify Maintena®) as monotherapy for the maintenance treatment of bipolar I disorder has been established in a randomized, double-blind, placebo-controlled withdrawal study of 52 weeks' duration in adults with bipolar I disorder. This study included patients currently experiencing a manic episode and who had experienced at least 1 prior manic or mixed episode with manic symptoms necessitating treatment (e.g., hospitalization, mood stabilizer, antipsychotic agent) who were converted to oral aripiprazole monotherapy over 4–6 weeks. Patients successfully converted to oral aripiprazole monotherapy or patients already receiving oral aripiprazole monotherapy continued receiving the drug orally for a stabilization phase of 2–8 weeks at a target dosage of 15–30 mg daily, and those who remained stable were subsequently converted to extended-release aripiprazole 400 mg IM once every 4 weeks for 12–28 weeks. Oral aripiprazole was continued for the first 2 weeks after the initial injection during the stabilization phase. Patients who remained stable on the extended-release IM injection for at least 8 consecutive weeks were then randomized either to continue receiving extended-release IM aripiprazole at the same dosage or placebo for up to 52 weeks during the double-blind withdrawal phase. The monthly IM aripiprazole dosage could be adjusted down to 300 mg based on tolerability and increased back to 400 mg on a one-time basis. The primary efficacy measure was the time from randomization to recurrence of any mood episode, which was defined as hospitalization for any mood episode; Y-MRS total score 15 or higher; Montgomery-Asberg Depression Rating Scale (MADRS) total score 15 or higher; CGI-BP scale overall score over 4; worsening of bipolar I disorder; withdrawal from the study because of lack of efficacy, adverse event, or worsening disease; clinical worsening with the need for addition of a mood stabilizer, antidepressant, or antipsychotic agent, and/or increase in benzodiazepine dosage above the highest permitted dosage (i.e., exceeding 2 mg of lorazepam or equivalent per day); or active suicidality. Patients who received extended-release IM aripiprazole had a substantially longer time to recurrence of any mood episode than those who received placebo. Time to recurrence of manic or mixed episodes was substantially longer in patients receiving extended-release IM aripiprazole compared with those receiving placebo; no difference between the treatment groups was observed for time to relapse to depressive episodes.

■ **Major Depressive Disorder** Aripiprazole is used orally as an adjunct to antidepressants for the treatment of major depressive disorder. The adjunctive efficacy of aripiprazole has been demonstrated in 2 short-term, double-blind, placebo-controlled trials of 6 weeks' duration in adults who met DSM-IV criteria for major depressive disorder and who had an inadequate response to previous antidepressant therapy (1–3 courses) in the current episode and who had also demonstrated an inadequate response during a prospective treatment period to 8 weeks of antidepressant therapy with extended-release paroxetine, extended-release venlafaxine, fluoxetine, escitalopram, or sertraline. The primary instrument used for assessing depressive symptoms was the MADRS, a 10-item clinician-rated scale used to assess the degree of depressive symptomatology. The principal secondary instrument was the Sheehan Disability Scale (SDS), a 3-item self-rated instrument used to assess the impact of depression on three domains of functioning (work/school, social life, and family life), with each item scored from 0 (not at all) to 10 (extreme). In both of these trials, aripiprazole was found to be superior to placebo in reducing mean MADRS total scores; aripiprazole was also superior to placebo in reducing the mean SDS score in one study. Patients in both trials initially received an aripiprazole dosage of 5 mg daily; subsequent dosage adjustments, based on efficacy and tolerability, could be made in 5-mg increments 1 week apart. Allowable aripiprazole dosages were 2, 5, 10, and 15 mg daily; patients who were not receiving the potent cytochrome P-450 (CYP) isoenzyme 2D6 inhibitors fluoxetine and paroxetine could also receive 20 mg daily.

An analysis of population subgroups did not reveal evidence of differential response based on age, choice of prospective antidepressant, or race. With regard to gender, a smaller mean reduction in the MADRS total score was observed in males than in females.

■ **Irritability Associated with Autistic Disorder** Aripiprazole is used orally for the acute treatment of irritability associated with autistic disorder. Efficacy of aripiprazole was established in 2 double-blind, placebo-controlled trials of 8 weeks' duration in pediatric patients 6–17 years of age who met DSM-IV criteria for autistic disorder and demonstrated behaviors such as aggression towards others, self-injurious behavior, quickly changing moods, or a combination of these behaviors. Over 75% of the enrolled patients were under 13 years of age. The primary instruments used for assessing clinical efficacy were the Aberrant Behavior Checklist (ABC) and the Clinical Global Impression-Improvement (CGI-I) scale. The primary outcome measure in both trials was the change from baseline to end point in the irritability subscale of the ABC (ABC-I). In one of the trials, 98 children and adolescents with autistic disorder received flexible daily dosages of aripiprazole ranging from 2–15 mg daily, starting at 2 mg daily with increases allowed up to 15 mg daily based on clinical response, or placebo. In this trial, aripiprazole improved scores on both the ABC-I subscale and on the CGI-I scale compared with placebo. The mean daily dosage of aripiprazole at the end of the 8-week treatment period was approximately 9 mg daily.

In the other trial, 218 children and adolescents with autistic disorder received one of 3 fixed dosages of aripiprazole (5, 10, or 15 mg daily) or placebo. Aripiprazole therapy was started at 2 mg daily and was increased to 5 mg daily after 1 week. After the second week, the dosage was increased to 10 mg daily for patients in the 10- and 15-mg daily dosage arms; after the third week, the dosage was increased to 15 mg daily in the 15-mg daily treatment arm. Patients receiving all 3 aripiprazole dosages in this study demonstrated improved ABC-I subscale and CGI-I scores compared with placebo.

■ **Tourette's Syndrome** Aripiprazole is used orally for the treatment of Tourette's syndrome (Gilles de la Tourette's syndrome). Efficacy of aripiprazole was established in 2 controlled trials (one 8-week and one 10-week) in pediatric patients who met DSM-IV criteria for Tourette's disorder and who had a total tic score (TTS) of at least 20–22 on the Yale Global Tic Severity Scale (YGTSS). The YGTSS is a fully validated scale that measures current tic severity. The primary outcome measure in both trials was the change from baseline to end point in the TTS on the YGTSS (YGTSS TTS). Over 65% of the enrolled patients were under 13 years of age.

In the 8-week, placebo-controlled, fixed-dose trial, 133 patients 7–17 years of age were randomized to receive high-dose aripiprazole (target daily dosage of 10 mg for patients weighing less than 50 kg and 20 mg for those weighing 50 kg or more), low-dose aripiprazole (target daily dosage of 5 mg for those weighing less than 50 kg and 10 mg for those weighing 50 kg or more), or placebo. Aripiprazole was initiated at 2 mg daily and increased to 5 mg after 2 days with subsequent increases of 5 mg on day 7 and weekly thereafter when the target dosage was 10 mg daily or higher. Patients receiving aripiprazole in both the high-dose and low-dose groups demonstrated substantially improved scores on the YGTSS TTS compared with patients receiving placebo.

In the 10-week, placebo-controlled, flexible-dose study, which was conducted in Korea, 61 patients 6–18 years of age with Tourette's syndrome were randomized to receive flexible daily dosages of aripiprazole, starting at 2 mg daily with increases allowed up to 20 mg daily based on clinical response, or placebo. The aripiprazole-treated patients in this study demonstrated substantially improved scores on the YGTSS TTS compared with patients receiving placebo. The mean daily dosage of aripiprazole at the end of the 10-week treatment period was approximately 6.5 mg daily.

For further information on Tourette's syndrome, including clinical manifestations, diagnosis, and management of the disorder, see Uses: Tourette's Syndrome, in Pimozide 28:16.08.92.

■ **Agitation Associated with Schizophrenia or Bipolar Mania** Aripiprazole has been used IM for the acute management of agitation associated with schizophrenia or bipolar disorder, manic or mixed, in patients for whom treatment with aripiprazole is appropriate and who require an IM antipsychotic agent for rapid control of behaviors that interfere with diagnosis and care (e.g., threatening behaviors, escalating or urgently distressing behavior, self-exhausting behavior). However, immediate-release aripiprazole IM injection (Abilify®) has been discontinued by the manufacturer and is no longer commercially available in the US.

Dosage and Administration

■ **Administration** Aripiprazole is administered orally or by IM injection. Aripiprazole lauroxil is administered *only* by IM injection.

Patients receiving aripiprazole should be monitored for possible worsening of depression, suicidality, or unusual changes in behavior, especially at the beginning of therapy or during periods of dosage adjustment. (See Worsening of Depression and Suicidality Risk under Warnings/Precautions: Warnings, in Cautions.)

Oral Administration Aripiprazole conventional tablets, tablets with sensor (Abilify MyCite®), orally disintegrating tablets, and oral solution are administered orally once daily without regard to meals.

Orally Disintegrating Tablets. Patients receiving aripiprazole orally disintegrating tablets should be instructed not to remove a tablet from the blister package until just prior to dosing. The tablet should not be pushed through the foil, since this may damage the tablet. With dry hands, the blister package should be peeled open to expose a tablet. The tablet should then be removed and placed on the tongue, where it rapidly disintegrates in saliva. The manufacturer recommends that the orally disintegrating tablets be taken without liquid; however, they may be taken with liquid, if necessary. Aripiprazole orally disintegrating tablets should *not* be split.

Tablets with Sensor. Aripiprazole is available as part of a digital ingestion tracking system comprised of the following components: aripiprazole tablets embedded with an ingestible event marker sensor (IEM; Abilify MyCite®); a wearable sensor (MyCite® patch), which detects the signal from the IEM sensor after ingestion and transmits data to a compatible mobile device (i.e., a smart phone); a software application (app) for compatible mobile devices (e.g., smart phones; MyCite® App), which displays information for the patient; and a web-based portal for healthcare professionals and caregivers.

Prior to initial patient use of the Abilify MyCite® system, use of the combination product and its components (patch, app, portal) should be facilitated. Clinicians should ensure that patients are capable and willing to use a mobile device (e.g., smart phone) and the software application (app). Before using any component of the system, clinicians should instruct patients to download the mobile software application and follow all the instructions for use and to ensure that the software is compatible with their specific mobile device.

Aripiprazole tablets with sensor are administered orally once daily without regard to meals; tablets with sensor should be swallowed whole and *not* divided, crushed, or chewed.

Prior to use of the software application, the patient's mobile device should be powered on and Bluetooth® enabled. The accompanying wearable sensor should be applied when prompted by the mobile software application; the application will instruct patients to apply and remove the sensor correctly. Patients should confirm that their mobile device is paired with the wearable sensor prior to use; the mobile software application will display a status icon on the mobile device to indicate that the wearable sensor is properly adhered and functioning. For further information, clinicians and patients may refer to the information provided in the product packaging as well as the instructions for use within the mobile software application.

Most ingestions of aripiprazole tablets with sensor will be detected within 30 minutes following ingestion; however, it may take up to 2 hours for the smart phone application and web portal to detect the ingestion of the tablet with sensor. In some cases, ingestion of the tablet with sensor may not be detected. If the tablet with sensor is not detected following ingestion, the dose should *not* be repeated.

The wearable sensor should be applied topically to the left side of the body just above the lower edge of the rib cage. Application to areas where the skin is scraped, cracked, inflamed, or irritated or areas overlapping the area of the most recently removed wearable sensor should be avoided. The wearable sensor should be changed weekly or sooner as needed; the mobile software application will remind patients when to change the sensor. Patients should be instructed keep the sensor in place while showering, swimming, or exercising. However, the sensor should be removed before undergoing magnetic resonance imaging (MRI) and replaced with a new sensor as soon as possible following the procedure. If skin irritation occurs, the wearable sensor should be removed. (See Skin Irritation associated with Abilify MyCite® Wearable Sensor under Warnings/Precautions: Other Warnings and Precautions, in Cautions.)

IM Administration *Clinicians should be aware that there are several different IM formulations of aripiprazole with different indications, dosages, and dosing frequencies. A short-acting, immediate-release IM formulation of aripiprazole (Abilify®) has been used for agitation associated with schizophrenia and bipolar mania, but is no longer commercially available in the US. The extended-release IM formulation of aripiprazole (Abilify Maintena®) is available in 300- and 400-mg vials and prefilled syringes and is used for the treatment of schizophrenia and maintenance monotherapy of bipolar I disorder. The extended-release IM formulation of aripiprazole lauroxil (Aristada®) is available in 441-, 662-, 882-, and 1064-mg prefilled syringes and is used for the treatment of schizophrenia.*

Extended-release aripiprazole lauroxil injection also is available in 675-mg prefilled syringes (Aristada Initio®), which are used IM as a single dose to initiate treatment of schizophrenia or to re-initiate therapy following a missed dose; this formulation is not intended for repeated dosing.

Aristada Initio® is not interchangeable with Aristada® because of their different pharmacokinetic profiles.

Extended-release aripiprazole injection and extended-release aripiprazole lauroxil injection are administered *only* by IM injection by a healthcare professional. Extended-release aripiprazole injection (Abilify Maintena®) is administered monthly. The 441- and 662-mg doses of extended-release aripiprazole lauroxil injection (Aristada®) are administered monthly, the 882-mg dose may be administered every month or every 6 weeks, and the 1064-mg dose is administered every 2 months. Extended-release aripiprazole lauroxil injection available in 675-mg prefilled syringes (Aristada Initio®) is used as a single dose only and is not intended for repeated dosing.

The manufacturers state that tolerability with oral aripiprazole therapy should be established prior to initiating IM therapy with extended-release formulations of the drug.

Extended-release Aripiprazole Injection. Extended-release aripiprazole injection (Abilify Maintena®) is administered by deep IM injection monthly into the deltoid or gluteal muscle. The manufacturer states that at least 26 days should elapse between doses. Each injection should be administered only by IM injection by a healthcare professional.

Aripiprazole extended-release IM injection must be reconstituted with sterile water for injection prior to administration. The drug is commercially available in 2 types of kits that contain aripiprazole lyophilized powder in either single-use vials or prefilled dual-chamber syringes with all the components required for reconstitution and administration (e.g., sterile water for injection diluent, needles, syringes). Because the entire contents of the prefilled syringe should be administered following reconstitution, only vials of the drug should be used for dosages smaller than 300 mg (e.g., for the 160- and 200-mg dosage adjustments recommended in patients concurrently receiving certain cytochrome P-450 [CYP] isoenzyme inhibitors or inducers; see Dosage and Administration: Special Populations). Kits containing prefilled dual-chamber syringes should be stored below 30°C and not frozen; the syringe should be protected from light by storing in the original package until the time of use. Kits containing single-use vials should be stored at 25°C, but may be exposed to temperatures ranging from 15–30°C. The manufacturer's instructions for use should be consulted for specific information on the preparation, reconstitution, and administration of aripiprazole extended-release injection using these single-use kits.

Following reconstitution, the prefilled syringe or vial should be shaken vigorously for 20 or 30 seconds, respectively, to ensure a uniform suspension. The reconstituted suspension should be inspected visually for particulate matter and discoloration prior to administration; the suspension should appear to be a uniform, homogeneous suspension that is opaque and milky-white in color. If using vials, the appropriate dose of aripiprazole should be drawn from the vial into the syringe supplied by the manufacturer and injected immediately. If a vial of reconstituted suspension is not administered immediately, the vial should be shaken vigorously for at least 60 seconds to resuspend the drug; reconstituted suspension should not be stored in a syringe. If using prefilled syringes, the entire contents of the prefilled syringe should be injected immediately following reconstitution; the manufacturer states that the contents of the prefilled syringe should be administered within 30 minutes of reconstitution.

Extended-release aripiprazole should be administered slowly by deep IM injection into the deltoid or gluteal muscle using the appropriate length needle (based on body type and injection site) supplied by the manufacturer. Injection sites should be rotated between the 2 deltoid or gluteal muscles. Following IM administration, the injection site should *not* be massaged.

Extended-release Aripiprazole Lauroxil Injection. Both formulations of extended-release aripiprazole lauroxil injectable suspension (Aristada® and Aristada Initio®) are administered by IM injection into the deltoid (441- and 675-mg doses only) or gluteal muscle (441-, 662-, 675-, 882-, or 1064-mg doses). The 441-, 662-, and 882-mg doses are administered monthly; the 882-mg dose also may be administered every 6 weeks; and the 1064-mg dose is administered every 2 months. The manufacturer states that if a dose of Aristada® is given earlier than the scheduled time, at least 14 days should elapse between doses. Each injection should be administered only by IM injection by a healthcare professional.

Extended-release aripiprazole lauroxil injection in 675-mg prefilled syringes (Aristada Initio®) is used *only* as a single dose to initiate treatment of schizophrenia or to re-initiate therapy following a missed dose; this formulation is *not* intended for repeated dosing. *Aristada Initio® is not interchangeable with Aristada® because of their different pharmacokinetic profiles.*

Aripiprazole lauroxil injectable suspension (Aristada® and Aristada Initio®) is commercially available in a kit containing the drug in a prefilled syringe and safety needles for IM injection. The kit should be stored at room temperature. Prior to use, the prefilled syringe should be tapped at least 10 times to dislodge any material that may have settled. The syringe should then be shaken vigorously for at least 30 seconds to ensure a uniform suspension. If the drug is not administered within 15 minutes, the syringe should be shaken again for 30 seconds.

The entire contents of the syringe should be administered rapidly and continuously by IM injection into either the deltoid (for 441- and 675-mg doses only) or gluteal muscle (for 441-, 662-, 675-, 882-, and 1064-mg doses) using the appropriate length needle supplied by the manufacturer. The manufacturer states that the longer needles provided should be used in patients with a larger amount of subcutaneous tissue over the injection site muscle. Concurrent administration of the 2 different aripiprazole lauroxil injection formulations (Aristada Initio® and Aristada®) in the same muscle should be avoided.

For patients receiving aripiprazole lauroxil injection 441 mg monthly, supplementation with oral aripiprazole is *not* required if the time elapsed since the last injection does not exceed 6 weeks; however, if the time elapsed since the last injection exceeds 6 weeks, but not 7 weeks, oral aripiprazole should be given for 7 days, and if the time elapsed since the last injection exceeds 7 weeks, oral aripiprazole should be given for 21 days. In patients receiving aripiprazole lauroxil injection 662 mg monthly, 882 mg monthly, or 882 mg every 6 weeks, supplementation with oral aripiprazole is *not* required if the time elapsed since the last injection does not exceed 8 weeks; however, if the time elapsed since the last injection exceeds 8 weeks, but not 12 weeks, oral aripiprazole should be given for 7 days, and if the time elapsed since the last injection exceeds 12 weeks, oral aripiprazole should be given for 21 days. In patients receiving aripiprazole lauroxil injection 1064 mg every 2 months, supplementation with oral aripiprazole is *not* required if the time elapsed since the last injection does not exceed 10 weeks; however, if the time elapsed since the last injection exceeds 10 weeks, but not 12 weeks, oral aripiprazole should be given for 7 days, and if the time elapsed since the last injection exceeds 12 weeks, oral aripiprazole should be given for 21 days. The dosage of oral aripiprazole supplementation should be the same as when the patient started receiving aripiprazole lauroxil injection. (See IM Dosage of Aripiprazole Lauroxil under Dosage: Schizophrenia, in Dosage and Administration.)

■ Dosage

Aripiprazole oral solution may be given at the same dose on a mg-per-mg basis as the tablet strengths of the drug up to a dose of 25 mg. However, if the oral solution is used in patients who were receiving aripiprazole 30 mg as tablets, a dose of 25 mg of the oral solution should be used.

Conventional tablets and orally disintegrating tablets of aripiprazole are bioequivalent; therefore, dosing for the orally disintegrating tablets is the same as for the conventional tablets.

Dosage of aripiprazole lauroxil is expressed in terms of aripiprazole lauroxil.

Extended-release aripiprazole lauroxil (Aristada®) doses of 441, 662, 882, and 1064 mg correspond to aripiprazole doses of 300, 450, 600, and 724 mg, respectively.

Schizophrenia **Oral Dosage.** For the management of schizophrenia in adults, the recommended initial and target dosage of aripiprazole is 10 or 15 mg orally once daily. Although dosages ranging from 10–30 mg daily administered as conventional tablets were effective in clinical trials, the manufacturer states that dosages exceeding 10–15 mg daily did not result in greater efficacy. The maximum recommended dosage is 30 mg daily. Because steady-state plasma concentrations of aripiprazole and dehydro-aripiprazole, its active metabolite, may not be attained for 2 weeks, dosage adjustments generally should be made at intervals of not less than 2 weeks.

For the management of schizophrenia in adolescents 13–17 years of age, the recommended target dosage of aripiprazole is 10 mg orally once daily. Therapy was initiated in a dosage of 2 mg once daily in these patients, with subsequent titration to 5 mg once daily after 2 days and to the target dosage of 10 mg once daily after 2 additional days. The manufacturer recommends that any subsequent dosage increases be made in 5-mg, once-daily increments. Although aripiprazole dosages of 10 and 30 mg once daily administered as conventional tablets have been studied in adolescents, the 30-mg daily dosage was not found to be more effective than the 10-mg daily dosage.

The optimum duration of oral aripiprazole therapy in patients with schizophrenia currently is not known, but maintenance therapy with aripiprazole 15 mg once daily as conventional tablets has been shown to be effective in preventing relapse for up to 26 weeks in adults. In addition, a combined analysis of data from 2 double-blind, multicenter studies indicates that maintenance therapy with the drug may be effective for up to 52 weeks in adults.

Although the efficacy of oral aripiprazole as maintenance therapy in pediatric patients with schizophrenia has not been systematically evaluated, the manufacturer states that such efficacy can be extrapolated from adult data in addition to comparisons of aripiprazole pharmacokinetic parameters in adult and pediatric patients.

The American Psychiatric Association (APA) states that prudent long-term treatment options in patients with schizophrenia with remitted first episodes or multiple episodes include either indefinite maintenance therapy or gradual discontinuance of the antipsychotic agent with close follow-up and a plan to reinstitute treatment upon symptom recurrence. Discontinuance of antipsychotic therapy should be considered only after a period of at least 1 year of symptom remission or optimal response while receiving the antipsychotic agent. In patients who have had multiple previous psychotic episodes or 2 psychotic episodes within 5 years, indefinite maintenance antipsychotic treatment is recommended.

The manufacturer states that the need for continued therapy with the drug should be reassessed periodically.

There are no systematically collected data to specifically address switching patients with schizophrenia from other antipsychotic agents to aripiprazole or concerning concomitant administration with other antipsychotic agents. Immediate discontinuance of the previous antipsychotic agent may be acceptable in some patients with schizophrenia, and more gradual discontinuance may be most appropriate for other patients. In all patients, the period of overlapping antipsychotic administration should be minimized.

IM Dosage of Aripiprazole (Abilify Maintena®). In patients who have never received aripiprazole, the manufacturer recommends that tolerability with oral aripiprazole be established prior to initiating IM therapy with extended-release aripiprazole injection (Abilify Maintena®). Because of the half-life of oral aripiprazole, it may take up to 2 weeks to fully assess tolerability.

For the treatment of schizophrenia in adults, the recommended dosage of extended-release aripiprazole injection (Abilify Maintena®) is 400 mg administered by IM injection every month (no sooner than 26 days following the previous injection). In patients experiencing adverse effects, a reduction in dosage to 300 mg every month may be considered.

To maintain therapeutic antipsychotic concentrations during initiation of therapy with extended-release aripiprazole injection, oral aripiprazole at a dosage of 10–20 mg daily or another oral antipsychotic agent (for patients already stable on another oral antipsychotic agent and known to tolerate aripiprazole) should be given after the first IM injection of extended-release aripiprazole and continued for 14 days.

If a dose of extended-release aripiprazole injection is missed, the next dose should be administered as soon as possible. Supplementation with oral aripiprazole may be required depending on the time elapsed. If the second or third doses are missed, supplementation with oral aripiprazole is *not* required if the time elapsed since the last injection does not exceed 5 weeks; however, if the time elapsed since the last injection exceeds 5 weeks, supplementation with oral aripiprazole should be given for 14 days with the next administered injection. If the fourth or subsequent doses are missed, supplementation with oral aripiprazole is *not* required if the time elapsed since the last injection does not exceed 6 weeks; however, if the time elapsed since the last injection exceeds 6 weeks, supplementation with oral aripiprazole should be given for 14 days with the next administered injection.

IM Dosage of Aripiprazole Lauroxil (Aristada®). In patients who have never received aripiprazole, the manufacturer recommends that tolerability with oral aripiprazole therapy be established prior to initiating IM therapy with extended-release aripiprazole lauroxil (Aristada®). Because of the half-life of oral aripiprazole, it may take up to 2 weeks to fully assess tolerability.

For the treatment of schizophrenia in adults, extended-release aripiprazole lauroxil injection (Aristada®) may be initiated at a dosage of 441, 662, or 882 mg every month; 882 mg every 6 weeks; or 1064 mg every 2 months by IM injection. Oral aripiprazole should be administered with the first IM injection of aripiprazole lauroxil and continued for 21 days.

For *patients established on oral aripiprazole 10 mg daily*, the recommended IM dosage of extended-release aripiprazole lauroxil is 441 mg every month.

For *patients established on oral aripiprazole 15 mg daily*, the recommended IM dosage of extended-release aripiprazole lauroxil is 662 mg every month, 882 mg every 6 weeks, or 1064 mg every 2 months.

For *patients established on oral aripiprazole 20 mg or higher daily*, the recommended IM dosage of extended-release aripiprazole lauroxil is 882 mg every month.

Subsequent dosage adjustments may be made if needed. If dosage adjustments are required, the manufacturer states that the pharmacokinetics and prolonged-release characteristics of extended-release aripiprazole lauroxil injection should be considered when making dosage and dosing interval adjustments.

If a dose of aripiprazole lauroxil injection is missed, the next dose should be administered as soon as possible. Supplementation with oral aripiprazole and/or a 675-mg IM dose of extended-release aripiprazole lauroxil (Aristada Initio®) may be required depending on the dosage and the time elapsed (see Tables 1 and 2).

Table 1. Recommended Oral Aripiprazole Supplementation Following Missed Doses of Extended-release Aripiprazole Lauroxil Injection (Aristada®)[a].

Dosage of Patient's Last Injection	No Oral Supplementation Required	Supplement with Oral Aripiprazole for 7 Days	Supplement with Oral Aripiprazole for 21 Days
441 mg monthly	≤6 weeks since last injection	>6 and ≤7 weeks since last injection	>7 weeks since last injection
662 mg monthly	≤8 weeks since last injection	>8 and ≤12 weeks since last injection	>12 weeks since last injection
882 mg monthly	≤8 weeks since last injection	>8 and ≤12 weeks since last injection	>12 weeks since last injection
882 mg every 6 weeks	≤8 weeks since last injection	>8 and ≤12 weeks since last injection	>12 weeks since last injection
1064 mg every 2 months	≤10 weeks since last injection	>10 and ≤12 weeks since last injection	>12 weeks since last injection

[a] Dosage of oral aripiprazole supplementation should be same as when patient began extended-release aripiprazole lauroxil therapy.

Table 2. Recommended IM Aripiprazole Lauroxil Supplementation with Aristada Initio® Following Missed Doses of Extended-release Aripiprazole Lauroxil Injection (Aristada®).

Dose of Patient's Last Injection	No IM Supplementation Required	Supplement with a Single 675-mg IM Dose of Aripiprazole Lauroxil	Reinitiate with a Single 675-mg IM Dose of Aripiprazole Lauroxil and a Single 30-mg Dose of Oral Aripiprazole
441 mg	≤6 weeks since last injection	>6 and ≤7 weeks since last injection	>7 weeks since last injection
662 mg	≤8 weeks since last injection	>8 and ≤12 weeks since last injection	>12 weeks since last injection
882 mg	≤8 weeks since last injection	>8 and ≤12 weeks since last injection	>12 weeks since last injection
1064 mg	≤10 weeks since last injection	>10 and ≤12 weeks since last injection	>12 weeks since last injection

IM Dosage of Aripiprazole Lauroxil (Aristada Initio®). In patients who have never received aripiprazole, the manufacturer recommends that tolerability with oral aripiprazole therapy be established prior to initiating IM therapy with extended-release aripiprazole lauroxil (Aristada Initio®). Because of the half-life of oral aripiprazole, it may take up to 2 weeks to fully assess tolerability.

The 675-mg strength of extended-release aripiprazole lauroxil injection (Aristada Initio®) is *only* used as a single dose to initiate aripiprazole lauroxil therapy or as a single dose to reinitiate therapy following a missed dose of extended-release aripiprazole lauroxil injection (Aristada®). The 675-mg strength of extended-release aripiprazole lauroxil injection (Aristada Initio®) is *not* used for repeated dosing of the drug.

For the initiation of aripiprazole lauroxil therapy for the treatment of schizophrenia in adults and after establishing tolerability with oral aripiprazole, the first IM injection of aripiprazole lauroxil (Aristada®; 441 mg, 662 mg, 882 mg, or 1064 mg) may be administered in conjunction with *both* one 675-mg IM injection of aripiprazole lauroxil (Aristada Initio®) into the deltoid or gluteal muscle (this dosage is equivalent to 459 mg of aripiprazole) and one 30-mg dose of oral aripiprazole.

The first dosage of aripiprazole lauroxil (Aristada®) may be administered on the same day as Aristada Initio® or up to 10 days thereafter. Clinicians should avoid injecting both IM formulations of aripiprazole lauroxil concurrently into the same deltoid or gluteal muscle.

For re-initiation of aripiprazole lauroxil (Aristada®) therapy following a missed dose, the next injection of aripiprazole lauroxil (Aristada®) should be administered as soon as possible. Depending on the time elapsed since the last Aristada® injection, the next Aristada® injection may be supplemented as recommended in Table 2.

Bipolar Disorder **Oral Dosage.** For the acute management of manic and mixed episodes associated with bipolar I disorder in adults, the recommended initial aripiprazole dosage is 15 mg given orally once daily as monotherapy or 10–15 mg given orally once daily as adjunctive therapy with lithium or valproate. The recommended target dosage of aripiprazole is 15 mg daily whether the drug is given as monotherapy or as adjunctive therapy with lithium or valproate. Based on clinical response, the dosage can be increased to the maximum recommended dosage of 30 mg daily. Safety of aripiprazole dosages exceeding 30 mg daily has not been established in clinical trials.

For the acute management of manic and mixed episodes associated with bipolar I disorder in pediatric patients 10–17 years of age, the recommended initial aripiprazole dosage when given as monotherapy is 2 mg orally once daily, with subsequent titration to 5 mg once daily after 2 days and to the target dosage of 10 mg once daily after 2 additional days. The recommended dosage when aripiprazole is given as adjunctive therapy with lithium or valproate is the same as that for monotherapy. Subsequent increases in the daily dosage of aripiprazole, if necessary, should be made in 5-mg increments. In pediatric clinical studies, oral aripiprazole dosages of 10 and 30 mg daily were effective.

IM Dosage of Aripiprazole. In patients who have never received aripiprazole, the manufacturer recommends that tolerability with oral aripiprazole be established prior to initiating IM therapy with extended-release aripiprazole injection (Abilify Maintena®). Because of the half-life of oral aripiprazole, it may take up to 2 weeks to fully assess tolerability.

For the maintenance treatment of bipolar I disorder in adults, the recommended dosage of extended-release aripiprazole injection (Abilify Maintena®) is 400 mg administered by IM injection every month (no sooner than 26 days following the previous injection). In patients experiencing adverse effects, a reduction in dosage to 300 mg every month may be considered.

To maintain therapeutic antipsychotic concentrations during initiation of therapy with extended-release aripiprazole injection, oral aripiprazole at a dosage of 10–20 mg daily or another oral antipsychotic agent (for patients already stable on another oral antipsychotic agent and known to tolerate aripiprazole) should be given after the first IM injection of extended-release aripiprazole and continued for 14 days.

If a dose of extended-release aripiprazole injection is missed, the next dose should be administered as soon as possible. Supplementation with oral aripiprazole may be required depending on the time elapsed. If the second or third doses are missed, supplementation with oral aripiprazole is *not* required if the time elapsed since the last injection does not exceed 5 weeks; however, if the time elapsed since the last injection exceeds 5 weeks, supplementation with oral aripiprazole should be given for 14 days with the next administered injection. If the fourth or subsequent doses are missed, supplementation with oral aripiprazole is *not* required if the time elapsed since the last injection does not exceed 6 weeks; however, if the time elapsed since the last injection exceeds 6 weeks, supplementation with oral aripiprazole should be given for 14 days with the next administered injection.

Major Depressive Disorder For adjunctive management of major depressive disorder in adults already receiving an antidepressant, the manufacturer recommends an initial aripiprazole dosage of 2–5 mg orally once daily for acute treatment. Subsequent dosage adjustments of up to 5 mg daily should occur gradually at intervals of at least 1 week; the recommended dosage range is 2–15 mg once daily. The maximum recommended dosage is 15 mg daily. Efficacy of the drug was established within a dosage range of 2–15 mg daily in clinical studies; mean maintenance dosage in these studies was approximately 11 mg daily.

The manufacturer states that if aripiprazole is used for maintenance therapy, the need for continued therapy with the drug should be reassessed periodically.

Irritability Associated with Autistic Disorder For the treatment of irritability associated with autistic disorder in pediatric patients 6–17 years of age, efficacy of oral aripiprazole was established within a dosage range of 5–15 mg daily in clinical studies. Dosing should be initiated at 2 mg daily, then increased to 5 mg daily, with subsequent increases to 10 mg daily or 15 mg daily, if necessary. Dosage increases should be gradual, at intervals of at least 1 week.

The manufacturer states that the need for continued therapy with the drug should be reassessed periodically.

Tourette's Syndrome For the treatment of Tourette's syndrome in pediatric patients 6–18 years of age, the recommended dosage range of oral aripiprazole is 5–20 mg once daily.

In pediatric patients weighing less than 50 kg, therapy should be initiated at 2 mg once daily, then increased to the recommended target dosage of 5 mg once daily after 2 days. In patients who do not achieve optimal control of tics, the dosage may be increased to 10 mg once daily. Dosage adjustments should be made gradually at intervals of at least 1 week.

In pediatric patients weighing 50 kg or more, therapy should be initiated at 2 mg once daily for 2 days and then increased to 5 mg once daily for 5 days, with a recommended target dosage of 10 mg once daily on day 8. In patients who do not achieve optimal control of tics, the dosage may be increased up to 20 mg once daily. Dosage adjustments should be made gradually in increments of 5 mg daily at intervals of at least 1 week.

The manufacturer states that the need for continued maintenance therapy with aripiprazole should be reassessed periodically.

■ **Special Populations** No dosage adjustment is necessary in patients with renal or hepatic impairment or in geriatric patients. In addition, no dosage adjustment is recommended based on gender, race, or smoking status.

Pharmacogenomics and Poor CYP2D6 Metabolizer Phenotype Patients who are known poor metabolizers of cytochrome P-450 isoenzyme 2D6 (CYP2D6) should receive one-half (50%) of the usual oral aripiprazole dosage. Such patients who are also taking a potent CYP3A4 inhibitor should receive 25% of the usual oral aripiprazole dosage. (See Drug Interactions: Drugs Affecting Hepatic Microsomal Enzymes.) Dosage adjustment is *not* necessary when oral aripiprazole is used as adjunctive treatment of major depressive disorder.

The manufacturer of aripiprazole extended-release injection (Abilify Maintena®) recommends a dosage of 300 mg every month in patients who are poor CYP2D6 metabolizers. In such patients who are also receiving a potent CYP3A4 inhibitor for longer than 14 days, a dosage of 200 mg every month is recommended.

Dosage of extended-release aripiprazole lauroxil injection (Aristada®) in patients who are poor CYP2D6 metabolizers should be based on the patient's established oral aripiprazole dosage. In such patients receiving a concomitant potent CYP3A4 inhibitor for longer than 2 weeks, dosage should be reduced to 441 mg every month; in patients already receiving 441 mg every month, no dosage adjustment is necessary, if tolerated. If the potent CYP3A4 inhibitor is used for less than 2 weeks, this dosage adjustment is not necessary. No further dosage adjustment is necessary in patients who are poor CYP2D6 metabolizers receiving a concomitant potent CYP2D6 inhibitor.

Extended-release aripiprazole lauroxil injection (Aristada Initio®) is only available in a single strength (675 mg) in a single-dose prefilled syringe; therefore, dosage adjustments in patients who are poor CYP2D6 metabolizers are not possible. Use of this extended-release formulation should therefore be avoided in patients who are poor CYP2D6 metabolizers.

Drugs Affecting Hepatic Microsomal Enzymes In patients receiving concomitant therapy with potent CYP3A4 inhibitors (e.g., clarithromycin, itraconazole, ketoconazole) *or* potent CYP2D6 inhibitors (e.g., quinidine, fluoxetine, paroxetine), dosage of oral aripiprazole should be reduced to 50% of the usual dosage, except when oral aripiprazole is used in the adjunctive treatment of major depressive disorder. Dosage adjustment is *not* necessary when oral aripiprazole is used as adjunctive treatment of major depressive disorder.

In patients receiving concomitant therapy with potent CYP3A4 *or* CYP2D6 inhibitors for longer than 14 days, dosage of extended-release aripiprazole injection (Abilify Maintena®) should be reduced from 400 mg to 300 mg every month, or from 300 mg to 200 mg every month. In such patients, dosage of extended-release aripiprazole lauroxil injection (Aristada®) should be reduced to the next available lower strength; in patients tolerating the 441-mg dosage, dosage reduction is not necessary. A dosage of 882 mg every 6 weeks or 1064 mg every 2 months should be reduced to 441 mg every 4 weeks. If the potent CYP3A4 or 2D6 inhibitor is used for less than 14 days, dosage adjustment of extended-release aripiprazole or aripiprazole lauroxil injection is *not* necessary.

In patients receiving concomitant therapy with potent CYP3A4 inhibitors *and* potent CYP2D6 inhibitors, oral aripiprazole dosage should be reduced to 25% of the usual dosage, except when aripiprazole is used in the adjunctive treatment of major depressive disorder. Dosage adjustment is *not* necessary when oral aripiprazole is used as adjunctive treatment of major depressive disorder.

In patients receiving concomitant therapy with potent CYP3A4 inhibitors *and* potent CYP2D6 inhibitors for longer than 14 days, dosage of extended-release aripiprazole injection (Abilify Maintena®) should be reduced from 400 mg to 200 mg every month, or from 300 mg to 160 mg every month. In such patients tolerating the 441-mg dosage of extended-release aripiprazole lauroxil injection (Aristada®), dosage adjustment is not necessary; however, the manufacturer states that concomitant therapy with potent CYP2D6 inhibitors *and* potent CYP3A4 inhibitors for longer than 2 weeks should be avoided in patients receiving 662-, 882-, or 1064-mg dosages of extended-release aripiprazole lauroxil injection. If such therapy is used for less than 14 days, dosage adjustment of extended-release aripiprazole or aripiprazole lauroxil injection is *not* necessary.

Dosage of oral aripiprazole should be reduced to 25% of the usual dosage in patients receiving aripiprazole concurrently with a combination of potent, moderate, or weak inhibitors of CYP3A4 and CYP2D6 (e.g., a potent CYP3A4 inhibitor and a moderate CYP2D6 inhibitor or a moderate CYP3A4 inhibitor and a moderate CYP2D6 inhibitor). The oral aripiprazole dosage may then be adjusted based on clinical response. (See Drug Interactions: Drugs Affecting Hepatic Microsomal Enzymes.)

Aripiprazole dosages should be increased back to the original dosage when the CYP2D6 and/or CYP3A4 inhibitor is discontinued.

In patients receiving potent CYP3A4 inducers (e.g., carbamazepine, rifampin), dosage of oral aripiprazole should be doubled over 1–2 weeks of concomitant therapy. When the CYP3A4 inducer is discontinued, the dosage should be reduced back to the original dosage over 1–2 weeks. (See Drug Interactions: Drugs Affecting Hepatic Microsomal Enzymes.)

The manufacturer recommends avoiding use of potent CYP3A4 inducers for longer than 14 days in patients receiving extended-release aripiprazole injection (Abilify Maintena®).

In patients receiving extended-release aripiprazole lauroxil injection (Aristada®), if a potent CYP3A4 inducer is used for longer than 2 weeks, dosage of aripiprazole lauroxil should be increased from 441 mg to 662 mg every month; dosage adjustment is *not* necessary in patients receiving 662-, 882-, or 1064-mg dosages. If a potent CYP3A4 inducer is used for less than 2 weeks, dosage adjustment is *not* necessary.

Extended-release aripiprazole lauroxil injection (Aristada Initio®) is only available in a single strength (675 mg); therefore, dosage adjustments in patients receiving potent CYP3A4 inhibitors, potent CYP2D6 inhibitors, or potent CYP3A4 inducers are not possible. Use of this extended-release formulation of the drug should be avoided in such patients. (See Drug Interactions: Drugs Affecting Hepatic Microsomal Enzymes.)

Cautions

■ **Contraindications** Known hypersensitivity to aripiprazole; hypersensitivity reactions have ranged from pruritus/urticaria to anaphylaxis. (See Sensitivity Reactions under Cautions: Warnings/Precautions.)

■ **Warnings/Precautions** ***Warnings*** **Increased Mortality in Geriatric Patients with Dementia-related Psychosis.** Geriatric patients with dementia-related psychosis treated with antipsychotic drugs are at an increased risk of death. Analyses of 17 placebo-controlled trials (modal duration of 10 weeks) revealed a 1.6- to 1.7-fold increase in mortality among geriatric patients receiving atypical antipsychotic drugs (i.e., aripiprazole, olanzapine, quetiapine, risperidone) compared with that observed in patients receiving placebo. Over the course of a typical 10-week controlled trial, the rate of death in drug-treated patients was about 4.5% compared with a rate of about 2.6% in the placebo group. Although the causes of death were varied, most of the deaths appeared to be either cardiovascular (e.g., heart failure, sudden death) or infectious (e.g., pneumonia) in nature. Observational studies suggest that, similar to atypical antipsychotics, treatment with conventional (first-generation) antipsychotics may increase mortality; the extent to which the findings of increased mortality in observational studies may be attributed to the antipsychotic drug as opposed to some characteristic(s) of the patients remains unclear.

The manufacturers state that aripiprazole is *not* approved for the treatment of patients with dementia-related psychosis. If the clinician elects to treat such patients with aripiprazole, patients should be assessed for the emergence of difficulty swallowing or excessive somnolence, which could predispose to accidental injury or aspiration. (See Adverse Cerebrovascular Events, including Stroke, in Geriatric Patients with Dementia-related Psychosis and see Dysphagia under Warnings/Precautions: Other Warnings and Precautions, in Cautions, and also see Geriatric Use under Warnings/Precautions: Specific Populations, in Cautions.)

Worsening of Depression and Suicidality Risk. Worsening of depression and/or the emergence of suicidal ideation and behavior (suicidality) or unusual changes in behavior may occur in both adult and pediatric (see Pediatric Use under Warnings/Precautions: Specific Populations, in Cautions) patients with major depressive disorder or other psychiatric disorders, whether or not they are taking antidepressants. This risk may persist until clinically important remission occurs. Suicide is a known risk of depression and certain other psychiatric disorders, and these disorders themselves are the strongest predictors of suicide. However, there has been a long-standing concern that antidepressants may have a role in inducing worsening of depression and the emergence of suicidality in certain patients during the early phases of treatment. Pooled analyses of short-term, placebo-controlled studies of antidepressants (i.e., selective serotonin-reuptake inhibitors [SSRIs] and other antidepressants) have shown an increased risk of suicidality in children, adolescents, and young adults (18–24 years of age) with major depressive disorder and other psychiatric disorders. An increased suicidality risk was not demonstrated with antidepressants compared with placebo in adults older than 24 years of age and a reduced risk was observed in adults 65 years of age or older.

The US Food and Drug Administration (FDA) recommends that all patients being treated with antidepressants for any indication be appropriately monitored and closely observed for clinical worsening, suicidality, and unusual changes in behavior, particularly during initiation of therapy (i.e., the first few months) and during periods of dosage adjustments. Families and caregivers of patients being treated with antidepressants for major depressive disorder or other indications, both psychiatric and nonpsychiatric, also should be advised to monitor patients on a daily basis for the emergence of agitation, irritability, or unusual changes in behavior as well as the emergence of suicidality, and to report such symptoms immediately to a health-care provider.

Although a causal relationship between the emergence of symptoms such as anxiety, agitation, panic attacks, insomnia, irritability, hostility, aggressiveness, impulsivity, akathisia, hypomania, and/or mania and either the worsening of depression and/or the emergence of suicidal impulses has not been established, there is concern that such symptoms may represent precursors to emerging suicidality. Consequently, consideration should be given to changing the therapeutic regimen or discontinuing therapy in patients whose depression is persistently worse or in patients experiencing emergent suicidality or symptoms that might be precursors to worsening depression or suicidality, particularly if such manifestations are severe, abrupt in onset, or were not part of the patient's presenting symptoms. FDA also recommends that the drugs be prescribed in the smallest quantity consistent with good patient management, in order to reduce the risk of overdosage.

It is generally believed (though not established in controlled trials) that treating a major depressive episode with an antidepressant alone may increase the likelihood of precipitating a mixed or manic episode in patients at risk for bipolar disorder. Therefore, patients with depressive symptoms should be adequately screened for bipolar disorder prior to initiating treatment with an antidepressant; such screening should include a detailed psychiatric history (e.g., family history of suicide, bipolar disorder, and depression).

Aripiprazole is not approved for use in treating depression in the pediatric population. (See Pediatric Use under Warnings/Precautions: Specific Populations, in Cautions.)

Sensitivity Reactions Allergic and sensitivity reactions (e.g., anaphylactic reaction, angioedema, laryngospasm, pruritus/urticaria, photosensitivity, rash, oropharyngeal spasm) have been reported in patients receiving aripiprazole. (See Cautions: Contraindications.)

Other Warnings and Precautions

Adverse Cerebrovascular Events, including Stroke, in Geriatric Patients with Dementia-related Psychosis. An increased incidence of adverse cerebrovascular events (cerebrovascular accidents and transient ischemic attacks), including fatalities, has been observed in geriatric patients with dementia-related psychosis treated with oral aripiprazole in several placebo-controlled studies (2 flexible-dose studies and one fixed-dose study). A statistically significant dose-response relationship for adverse cerebrovascular events was observed in patients receiving oral aripiprazole in the fixed-dose study. The manufacturers state that aripiprazole is *not* approved for the treatment of patients with dementia-related psychosis. (See Increased Mortality in Geriatric Patients with Dementia-related Psychosis under Warnings/Precautions: Warnings, and also see Geriatric Use under Warnings/Precautions: Specific Populations, in Cautions.)

Potential for Dosing and Medication Errors. Medication errors, including substitution and dispensing errors, may occur between the 2 different extended-release IM formulations of aripiprazole lauroxil (e.g., Aristada Initio® and Aristada®).

Aristada Initio® is for single-dose administration only. Aristada Initio® should not be substituted for Aristada® because of their different pharmacokinetic profiles.

Neuroleptic Malignant Syndrome. Neuroleptic malignant syndrome (NMS), a potentially fatal syndrome requiring immediate discontinuance of the drug and intensive symptomatic treatment, has been reported in patients receiving antipsychotic agents, including rare cases associated with aripiprazole therapy. (See Advice to Patients.) For additional information on NMS, see Neuroleptic Malignant Syndrome under Cautions: Nervous System Effects, in the Phenothiazines General Statement 28:16.08.24.

Tardive Dyskinesia. Because use of antipsychotic agents, including aripiprazole, may be associated with tardive dyskinesia (a syndrome of potentially irreversible, involuntary, dyskinetic movements), aripiprazole should be prescribed in a manner that is most likely to minimize the occurrence of this syndrome. Chronic antipsychotic treatment generally should be reserved for patients who suffer from a chronic illness that is known to respond to antipsychotic agents, and for whom alternative, equally effective, but potentially less harmful treatments are not available or appropriate. In patients who do require chronic treatment, the lowest dosage and the shortest duration of treatment producing a satisfactory clinical response should be sought, and the need for continued treatment should be reassessed periodically.

The American Psychiatric Association (APA) currently recommends that patients receiving atypical antipsychotic agents be assessed clinically for abnormal involuntary movements every 12 months and that patients considered to be at increased risk for tardive dyskinesia be assessed every 6 months. If signs and symptoms of tardive dyskinesia appear in an aripiprazole-treated patient, aripiprazole discontinuance should be considered; however, some patients may require continued treatment with the drug despite the presence of the syndrome. For additional information on tardive dyskinesia, see Tardive Dyskinesia under Cautions: Nervous System Effects, in the Phenothiazines General Statement 28:16.08.24.

Metabolic Changes. Atypical antipsychotic agents have been associated with metabolic changes, including hyperglycemia and diabetes mellitus, dyslipidemia, and body weight gain. While all of these drugs produce some metabolic changes, each drug has its own specific risk profile. (See Hyperglycemia and Diabetes Mellitus, see Dyslipidemia, and also see Weight Gain under Warnings/Precautions: Other Warnings and Precautions, in Cautions.)

Hyperglycemia and Diabetes Mellitus. Hyperglycemia, sometimes severe and associated with ketoacidosis, hyperosmolar coma, or death, has been reported in patients receiving atypical antipsychotic agents. Hyperglycemia has been reported in patients treated with aripiprazole. In short- and longer-term clinical trials in adult and pediatric patients, clinically important differences between oral aripiprazole and placebo in mean change from baseline to end point in fasting glucose concentrations were not observed. While confounding factors such as an increased background risk of diabetes mellitus in patients with schizophrenia and the increasing incidence of diabetes mellitus in the general population make it difficult to establish with certainty the relationship between use of agents in this drug class and glucose abnormalities, epidemiologic studies suggest an increased risk of treatment-emergent hyperglycemia-related adverse events in patients treated with atypical antipsychotic agents.

Patients with preexisting diabetes mellitus in whom therapy with an atypical antipsychotic is initiated should be periodically monitored for worsening of glucose control; those with risk factors for diabetes (e.g., obesity, family history of diabetes) should undergo fasting blood glucose testing upon therapy initiation and periodically throughout treatment. Any patient who develops manifestations of hyperglycemia (including polydipsia, polyuria, polyphagia, and weakness) during treatment with an atypical antipsychotic should undergo fasting blood glucose testing. (See Advice to Patients.) In some cases, patients who developed hyperglycemia while receiving an atypical antipsychotic have required continuance of antidiabetic treatment despite discontinuance of the atypical antipsychotic; in other cases, hyperglycemia resolved with discontinuance of the antipsychotic.

For further information on managing the risk of hyperglycemia and diabetes mellitus associated with atypical antipsychotic agents, see Hyperglycemia and Diabetes Mellitus under Cautions: Precautions and Contraindications, in Clozapine 28:16.08.04.

Dyslipidemia. Undesirable changes in lipid parameters have been observed in patients treated with some atypical antipsychotic agents; however, aripiprazole generally does not appear to adversely affect the lipid profile in patients receiving the drug. Pooled data from short- and longer-term clinical studies in adult and pediatric patients indicate no clinically important differences from baseline to end point in the proportion of patients with changes in fasting/nonfasting total cholesterol, fasting triglycerides, fasting low-density lipoprotein (LDL)-cholesterol, and fasting/nonfasting high-density lipoprotein (HDL)-cholesterol between aripiprazole-treated patients and those receiving placebo.

Weight Gain. Weight gain has been observed with atypical antipsychotic therapy. Clinical monitoring of weight is recommended in patients receiving aripiprazole.

In an analysis of 13 placebo-controlled monotherapy studies in adults primarily with schizophrenia or bipolar disorder, mean weight gain in aripiprazole-treated patients was 0.3 kg compared with a loss of 0.1 kg in those receiving placebo (with a median exposure of 21–25 days); at 24 weeks, patients receiving aripiprazole or placebo lost an average of 1.5 or 0.2 kg, respectively. In 2 placebo-controlled trials in pediatric patients with schizophrenia or bipolar disorder, mean weight gain was 1.6 kg in patients receiving oral aripiprazole and 0.3 kg in those receiving placebo (with a median exposure of 42–43 days); at 24 weeks, mean weight gain was 5.8 and 1.4 kg in aripiprazole- and placebo-treated patients, respectively.

For additional information on metabolic effects associated with atypical antipsychotic agents, see Hyperglycemia and Diabetes Mellitus under Warnings/Precautions: Other Warnings and Precautions, in Cautions.

Pathological Gambling and Other Compulsive Behaviors. Serious impulse-control and compulsive behaviors, particularly pathological gambling, have been reported rarely in adult and pediatric patients treated with aripiprazole. In May 2016, FDA reported that a total of 184 cases of impulse-control problems associated with aripiprazole use have been identified since November 2002; most of these cases (89%) involved pathological gambling. Other impulse-control and compulsive behaviors reported less frequently than gambling include compulsive or binge eating, compulsive spending or shopping, and compulsive sexual behaviors. The majority of patients in these cases had no history of compulsive behaviors and experienced the uncontrollable urges only after beginning treatment with aripiprazole. Impulse-control symptoms may also be associated with the underlying disorder. The results of a large pharmacoepidemiologic study suggest that patients with bipolar disorder who are receiving aripiprazole have a higher risk of gambling compared with patients with bipolar disorder who are not receiving aripiprazole. In some, but not all, cases, these uncontrollable urges reportedly stopped within days to weeks when the aripiprazole dosage was reduced or the drug was discontinued; recurrence of compulsive behaviors following rechallenge with the drug has been reported.

Aripiprazole-associated compulsive behaviors may result in harm to the patient or others if not recognized. Because patients may not recognize such behaviors as abnormal, clinicians should specifically ask patients or caregivers whether any new or intense gambling urges, compulsive sexual urges, compulsive shopping, binge or compulsive eating, or other urges have developed during treatment with the drug. If a patient develops new or increased impulsive or compulsive behaviors while receiving aripiprazole, consideration should be given to reducing the dosage or discontinuing the drug. (See Advice to Patients.)

Orthostatic Hypotension. Orthostatic hypotension and associated adverse effects (e.g., postural dizziness, syncope, tachycardia) have been reported in patients receiving oral or IM aripiprazole and IM aripiprazole lauroxil, perhaps because of the drug's α_1-adrenergic blocking activity. The risk of orthostatic hypotension generally appears to be greatest during initiation of therapy and dosage titration. The drug should be used with caution in patients with known cardiovascular disease (e.g., heart failure, history of myocardial infarction or ischemia, conduction abnormalities), cerebrovascular disease, and/or conditions that would predispose patients to hypotension (e.g., dehydration, hypovolemia, concomitant antihypertensive therapy), as well as in patients who are antipsychotic naive. In such patients, the manufacturer of extended-release IM aripiprazole lauroxil states that use of a lower initial dosage of the drug and monitoring of vital signs should be considered.

Falls. Aripiprazole therapy may cause somnolence, postural hypotension, and motor and sensory instability, which may lead to falls; as a consequence, fractures or other injuries may occur. For patients with diseases or conditions or receiving other drugs that could exacerbate these effects, fall risk assessments should be completed when initiating antipsychotic treatment and periodically during long-term therapy.

Leukopenia, Neutropenia, and Agranulocytosis. In clinical trial and/or postmarketing experience, leukopenia and neutropenia have been temporally related to antipsychotic agents, including aripiprazole. Agranulocytosis also has been reported.

Possible risk factors for leukopenia and neutropenia include preexisting low leukocyte count and a history of drug-induced leukopenia and neutropenia. Patients with a preexisting low leukocyte count or a history of drug-induced leukopenia or neutropenia should have their complete blood count monitored frequently during the first few months of therapy. Aripiprazole should be discontinued at the first sign of a decline in leukocyte count in the absence of other causative factors.

Patients with clinically significant neutropenia should be carefully monitored for fever or other signs or symptoms of infection and promptly treated if such signs and symptoms occur. In patients with severe neutropenia (absolute neutrophil count [ANC] less than 1000/mm^3), aripiprazole should be discontinued and the leukocyte count monitored until recovery occurs. Lithium has reportedly been used successfully in the treatment of several cases of leukopenia associated with aripiprazole, clozapine, and some other drugs; however, further clinical experience is needed to confirm these anecdotal findings.

Seizures. As with other antipsychotic agents, aripiprazole may cause seizures. Seizures have occurred in 0.1% of adult and pediatric patients (6–18 years of age) treated with oral aripiprazole. Aripiprazole should be used with caution in patients with a history of seizures or other conditions that may lower the seizure threshold; conditions that lower the seizure threshold may be more prevalent in geriatric patients 65 years of age or older.

Cognitive and Motor Impairment. Like other antipsychotic agents, aripiprazole potentially may impair judgment, thinking, or motor skills. In short-term clinical trials, somnolence (including sedation) was reported in 11% of adults treated with oral aripiprazole compared with 6% of those receiving placebo. In pediatric patients 6–17 years of age, somnolence (including sedation) was reported in 24% of aripiprazole-treated patients compared with 6% of those receiving placebo. (See Advice to Patients.)

Body Temperature Regulation. Disruption of the body's ability to reduce core body temperature has been attributed to antipsychotic agents. The manufacturers recommend appropriate caution when aripiprazole is used in patients who will be experiencing conditions that may contribute to an elevation in core body temperature (e.g., strenuous exercise, extreme heat, concomitant use of agents with anticholinergic activity, dehydration).

Suicide. Attendant risk with psychotic illnesses, bipolar disorder, and major depressive disorder; high-risk patients should be closely supervised. Aripiprazole should be prescribed in the smallest quantity consistent with good patient management to reduce the risk of overdosage. (See Worsening of Depression and Suicidality Risk under Warnings/Precautions: Warnings, in Cautions.)

Dysphagia. Esophageal dysmotility and aspiration have been associated with the use of antipsychotic agents, including aripiprazole. Aspiration pneumonia is a common cause of morbidity and mortality in geriatric patients, particularly in those with advanced Alzheimer's dementia. Aripiprazole should be used with caution in patients at risk for aspiration pneumonia. (See Increased Mortality in Geriatric Patients with Dementia-related Psychosis under Warnings/Precautions: Warnings, in Cautions.)

Phenylketonuria. Individuals with phenylketonuria (i.e., homozygous genetic deficiency of phenylalanine hydroxylase) and other individuals who must restrict their intake of phenylalanine should be warned that each aripiprazole 10- or 15-mg orally disintegrating tablet contains aspartame, which is metabolized in the GI tract to provide about 1.12 or 1.68 mg of phenylalanine, respectively, following oral administration. Aripiprazole conventional tablets and oral solution do not contain aspartame.

Skin Irritation associated with Abilify MyCite® Wearable Sensor. Symptoms of skin irritation (e.g., rash, pruritus, skin discoloration) may occur at the application site of the wearable sensor (MyCite® patch). In clinical studies, 12.4% of the patients receiving aripiprazole tablets with sensor experienced rashes at the site of wearable sensor placement. If skin irritation occurs, the manufacturer states that the wearable sensor should be removed.

Specific Populations

Pregnancy. Neonates exposed to antipsychotic agents during the third trimester of pregnancy are at risk for extrapyramidal and/or withdrawal symptoms following delivery. Symptoms reported to date have included agitation, hypertonia, hypotonia, tardive dyskinetic-like symptoms, tremor, somnolence, respiratory distress, and feeding disorder. Neonates exhibiting such symptoms should be monitored. The complications have varied in severity; some neonates recovered within hours to days without specific treatment, while others have required intensive care unit support and prolonged hospitalization. For further information on extrapyramidal and withdrawal symptoms in neonates, see Cautions: Pregnancy, Fertility, and Lactation, in the Phenothiazines General Statement 28:16.08.24.

National Pregnancy Registry for Atypical Antipsychotics: 866-961-2388 and http://womensmentalhealth.org/clinical-and-research-programs/pregnancyregistry/atypicalantipsychotic/.

Lactation. Aripiprazole is distributed into milk in humans. However, data are insufficient to determine the amount present in human milk, the effects of the drug on breast-fed infants, or the effects on milk production. Because of the potential for serious adverse reactions to aripiprazole in nursing infants, the manufacturer of aripiprazole tablets states that a decision should be made whether to discontinue nursing or the drug, taking into consideration the importance of the drug to the woman. The manufacturers of extended-release IM formulations of aripiprazole and aripiprazole lauroxil state that the benefit of aripiprazole therapy to the woman as well as the benefits of breast-feeding to the infant should be weighed against the potential risk to the infant resulting from exposure to the drug or from the underlying maternal condition.

Pediatric Use. Safety and efficacy of aripiprazole tablets with sensor have not been established in pediatric patients.

Safety and efficacy of oral aripiprazole have not been established in pediatric patients with major depressive disorder.

Safety and efficacy of extended-release IM formulations of aripiprazole and aripiprazole lauroxil have not been evaluated in pediatric patients younger than 18 years of age.

Safety and efficacy of oral aripiprazole for the acute management of schizophrenia in pediatric patients 13–17 years of age have been established in a placebo-controlled study of 6 weeks' duration. Although the efficacy of oral aripiprazole for maintenance treatment of schizophrenia in pediatric patients has not been systematically evaluated, the manufacturer states that such efficacy can be extrapolated from adult data in addition to comparisons of aripiprazole pharmacokinetic parameters in adult and pediatric patients. (See Schizophrenia under Uses: Psychotic Disorders.)

Safety and efficacy of oral aripiprazole monotherapy for the acute management of bipolar mania in pediatric patients 10–17 years of age have been established in a placebo-controlled study of 4 weeks' duration.

The efficacy of oral aripiprazole as an adjunct to lithium or valproate for the acute treatment of manic or mixed episodes associated with bipolar disorder in pediatric patients has not been systematically evaluated. However, efficacy can be extrapolated from adult data in addition to pharmacokinetic comparisons of aripiprazole between adult and pediatric populations.

Safety and efficacy of oral aripiprazole for the treatment of irritability associated with autistic disorder have been established in 2 placebo-controlled clinical trials of 8 weeks' duration in pediatric patients 6–17 years of age. Efficacy of the drug as maintenance therapy for irritability associated with autistic disorder was not established in a longer-term, placebo-controlled relapse prevention trial in pediatric patients 6–17 years of age.

Safety and efficacy of oral aripiprazole for the treatment of Tourette's syndrome have been established in one 8-week, placebo-controlled trial in pediatric patients 7–17 years of age and one 10-week, placebo-controlled trial in pediatric patients 6–18 years of age. Efficacy of the drug as maintenance therapy in pediatric patients with Tourette's syndrome has not been systematically evaluated. (See Uses: Tourette's Syndrome.)

The pharmacokinetics of aripiprazole and dehydro-aripiprazole in pediatric patients 10–17 years of age are similar to those in adults after correcting for differences in body weight.

Mean weight gain of 1.6 kg was reported in pediatric patients with schizophrenia or bipolar disorder receiving oral aripiprazole compared with a gain of 0.3 kg in those receiving placebo in 2 short-term studies. After 24 weeks of therapy, the mean change from baseline in body weight in the aripiprazole-treated patients was 5.8 kg compared with 1.4 kg in placebo recipients. Similar gains in weight were observed in short-term studies in pediatric patients with irritability associated with autistic disorder and Tourette's syndrome.

FDA warns that a greater risk of suicidal thinking or behavior (suicidality) occurred during the first few months of antidepressant treatment compared with placebo in children and adolescents with major depressive disorder, obsessive-compulsive disorder (OCD), or other psychiatric disorders based on pooled analyses of 24 short-term, placebo-controlled trials of 9 antidepressant drugs (SSRIs and other antidepressants). However, a more recent meta-analysis of 27 placebo-controlled trials of 9 antidepressants (SSRIs and others) in patients younger than 19 years of age with major depressive disorder, OCD, or non-OCD anxiety disorders suggests that the benefits of antidepressant therapy in treating these conditions may outweigh the risks of suicidal behavior or suicidal ideation. No suicides occurred in these pediatric trials. These findings should be carefully considered when assessing potential benefits and risks of aripiprazole in a child or adolescent for any clinical use. (See Worsening of Depression and Suicidality Risk under Warnings/Precautions: Warnings, in Cautions.)

Geriatric Use. In clinical studies, approximately 8% of over 13,000 patients treated with oral aripiprazole were 65 years of age or older and approximately 6% were 75 years of age or older. Experience from placebo-controlled trials with oral aripiprazole in patients with schizophrenia, bipolar mania, or major depressive disorder who are 65 years of age and older is insufficient to determine whether they respond differently than younger adults.

The manufacturer of oral and extended-release IM formulations of aripiprazole states that dosage adjustment is not necessary in geriatric patients on the basis of age alone. The manufacturer of extended-release IM aripiprazole lauroxil states that the safety and efficacy of the drug have not been evaluated in patients older than 65 years of age and makes no specific dosage recommendations for geriatric patients.

Geriatric patients with dementia-related psychosis treated with antipsychotic agents are at an increased risk of death. In addition, an increased incidence of adverse cerebrovascular events (cerebrovascular accidents and transient ischemic attacks), including fatalities, has been observed in geriatric patients with dementia-related psychosis treated with aripiprazole in placebo-controlled studies. Aripiprazole is *not* approved for the treatment of dementia-related psychosis. (See Increased Mortality in Geriatric Patients with Dementia-related Psychosis under Warnings/Precautions: Warnings, in Cautions and see also Adverse Cerebrovascular Events, including Stroke, in Geriatric Patients with Dementia-related Psychosis and see Dysphagia under Warnings/Precautions: Other Warnings and Precautions, in Cautions.) For additional information on the use of antipsychotic agents in the management of dementia-related psychosis, see Geriatric Considerations under Uses: Psychotic Disorders, in the Phenothiazines General Statement 28:16.08.24.

In pooled data analyses, a *reduced* risk of suicidality was observed in adults 65 years of age or older with antidepressant therapy compared with placebo. (See Worsening of Depression and Suicidality Risk under Warnings/Precautions: Warnings, in Cautions.)

Pharmacogenomics and Poor CYP2D6 Metabolizers. Because higher concentrations of aripiprazole have been observed in poor metabolizers of cytochrome P-450 (CYP) isoenzyme 2D6 than in normal CYP2D6 metabolizers, dosage adjustment of the drug is recommended in patients known to be poor metabolizers of CYP2D6. Approximately 8% of Caucasians and 3–8% of Blacks/African Americans cannot metabolize CYP2D6 substrates and are classified as poor CYP2D6 metabolizers. (See Pharmacogenomics and Poor CYP2D6 Metabolizer Phenotype under Dosage and Administration: Special Populations.)

■ **Common Adverse Effects** Adverse effects occurring in 10% or more of adults receiving oral aripiprazole in clinical trials include nausea, vomiting, constipation, headache, dizziness, akathisia, anxiety, insomnia, and restlessness.

Adverse effects occurring in 10% or more of pediatric patients receiving oral aripiprazole in clinical trials include somnolence, headache, vomiting, extrapyramidal disorder, fatigue, increased appetite, insomnia, nausea, nasopharyngitis, and increased weight.

In clinical trials with aripiprazole tablets with sensor and other components of the digital ingestion tracking system (Abilify MyCite®), skin rash localized at the application site of the wearable sensor (patch) was reported in 12.4% of patients. Other symptoms of skin irritation (e.g., pruritus, skin discoloration) have also been reported.

Adverse effects occurring in 5% or more of adults receiving extended-release IM aripiprazole injection (Abilify Maintena®) for schizophrenia in clinical trials and at an incidence at least twice that for placebo include increased weight, akathisia, injection site pain, and sedation.

In patients receiving extended-release IM aripiprazole lauroxil injection (Aristada®) in clinical trials, akathisia was the only adverse effect that occurred in 5% of more of patients and at an incidence at least twice that for placebo. Other extrapyramidal adverse effects (e.g., parkinsonism, dystonia) and injection site reactions (e.g., pain) were reported in 5–7% and 4–5% of patients in the clinical trials, respectively.

Drug Interactions

■ **Drugs Affecting Hepatic Microsomal Enzymes** Cytochrome P-450 (CYP) isoenzyme 3A4 (CYP3A4) inducers (e.g., carbamazepine, rifampin), CYP3A4 inhibitors (e.g., clarithromycin, itraconazole, ketoconazole), or CYP2D6 inhibitors (e.g., fluoxetine, paroxetine, quinidine): Potential pharmacokinetic interaction (altered aripiprazole metabolism); dosage adjustment generally is recommended. (See Drugs Affecting Hepatic Microsomal Enzymes under Dosage and Administration: Special Populations.)

Inhibitors or inducers of CYP isoenzymes 1A1, 1A2, 2A6, 2B6, 2C8, 2C9, 2C19, or 2E1: Pharmacokinetic interaction is unlikely.

Ketoconazole and Other CYP3A4 Inhibitors Concurrent oral administration of aripiprazole and ketoconazole, a potent CYP3A4 inhibitor, substantially increased peak serum concentrations and area under the plasma concentration-time curve (AUC) values of aripiprazole and its active metabolite, dehydro-aripiprazole. Concomitant use of aripiprazole with other potent CYP3A4 inhibitors (e.g., clarithromycin, itraconazole) would also be expected to result in substantially increased systemic exposure to aripiprazole.

Except when used in the adjunctive treatment of major depressive disorder, dosage of oral aripiprazole should be reduced by 50% when used concurrently with potent CYP3A4 inhibitors. IM dosages of extended-release aripiprazole (Abilify Maintena®) and aripiprazole lauroxil (Aristada®) should be reduced when used concurrently with potent CYP3A4 inhibitors for longer than 14 days. When the potent CYP3A4 inhibitor is withdrawn from combined therapy, the aripiprazole dosage should be increased. Use of the 675-mg strength of extended-release aripiprazole lauroxil injection (Aristada Initio®) should be avoided in patients receiving potent CYP3A4 inhibitors. (See Dosage and Administration: Special Populations.)

Quinidine and Other CYP2D6 Inhibitors Concurrent oral administration of aripiprazole and quinidine, a potent CYP2D6 inhibitor, substantially increased the AUC of aripiprazole but decreased the AUC of its active metabolite, dehydro-aripiprazole. Concomitant use of aripiprazole with other potent CYP2D6 inhibitors (e.g., fluoxetine, paroxetine) would also be expected to result in substantially increased systemic exposure to aripiprazole.

Except when used in the adjunctive treatment of major depressive disorder, dosage of oral aripiprazole should be reduced by 50% when used concurrently with potent CYP2D6 inhibitors. IM dosages of extended-release aripiprazole (Abilify Maintena®) and aripiprazole lauroxil (Aristada®) should be reduced when used concurrently with potent CYP2D6 inhibitors for longer than 14 days. When the potent CYP2D6 inhibitor is withdrawn from combined therapy, the aripiprazole dosage should be increased. Use of the 675-mg strength of extended-release aripiprazole lauroxil injection (Aristada Initio®) should be avoided in patients receiving potent CYP2D6 inhibitors. (See Dosage and Administration: Special Populations.)

Carbamazepine and Other CYP3A4 Inducers Concurrent administration of aripiprazole and carbamazepine, a potent CYP3A4 inducer, substantially decreased peak plasma concentrations and AUC of aripiprazole and its active metabolite, dehydro-aripiprazole. Concomitant use of aripiprazole with other potent CYP3A4 inducers (e.g., rifampin) may result in substantially decreased systemic exposure to aripiprazole.

Oral aripiprazole dosage should be doubled over 1–2 weeks of concurrent use with potent CYP3A4 inducers. Concurrent use of CYP3A4 inducers and extended-release aripiprazole injection (Abilify Maintena®) should be avoided since aripiprazole concentrations may fall below therapeutic concentrations. The 441-mg dose of extended-release aripiprazole lauroxil (Aristada®) should be increased to 662 mg when used concurrently with potent CYP3A4 inducers for longer than 2 weeks; dosage adjustment is not required in patients receiving 662-, 882-, or 1064-mg doses of the drug. When the potent CYP3A4 inducer is withdrawn from combined therapy, the aripiprazole dosage should be reduced to the original dosage over 1–2 weeks. Use of the 675-mg strength of extended-release aripiprazole lauroxil injection (Aristada Initio®) should be avoided in patients receiving potent CYP3A4 inducers. (See Dosage and Administration: Special Populations.)

■ **Drugs Metabolized by Hepatic Microsomal Enzymes** Substrates of CYP isoenzymes 2C9, 2C19, 2D6, and 3A4: Clinically important pharmacokinetic interaction is unlikely; dosage adjustment is not necessary.

■ **Anticholinergic Agents** Potential pharmacologic interaction (possible disruption of body temperature regulation); aripiprazole should be used with caution in patients concurrently receiving drugs with anticholinergic activity. (See Body Temperature Regulation under Warnings/Precautions: Other Warnings and Precautions, in Cautions.)

■ **Hypotensive Agents** Potential pharmacologic interaction (additive hypotensive effects due to α-adrenergic antagonism); aripiprazole should be used with caution in patients receiving hypotensive agents. During concomitant use, blood pressure should be monitored and antihypertensive dosage(s) adjusted accordingly.

■ **Lorazepam and Other Benzodiazepines** Clinically important pharmacokinetic changes have not been reported during concurrent administration of lorazepam and aripiprazole. The manufacturers state that routine dosage adjustment of aripiprazole or lorazepam is not necessary when the drugs are concurrently administered. However, increased sedative and orthostatic hypotensive effects have been reported in patients receiving these drugs in combination. If aripiprazole therapy in conjunction with a benzodiazepine is considered necessary, the patient should be carefully monitored for excessive sedation and orthostatic hypotension and dosage of the drug(s) adjusted, if necessary. (See Orthostatic Hypotension and see also Cognitive and Motor Impairment under Warnings/Precautions: Other Warnings and Precautions, in Cautions.)

■ **Alcohol** Concomitant administration of ethanol and oral aripiprazole in healthy individuals did not have clinically important effects on gross motor skills or stimulus response compared with administration of ethanol with placebo. The manufacturer of the extended-release IM formulation of aripiprazole (Abilify Maintena®) states that alcohol should be avoided during therapy. The manufacturers of other commercially available formulations of aripiprazole and aripiprazole lauroxil do not provide specific recommendations concerning alcohol use in the prescribing information for the drugs.

■ **Dextromethorphan** Clinically important pharmacokinetic interaction is unlikely. Dosage adjustment of dextromethorphan (a CYP2D6 and CYP3A4 substrate) is not necessary when administered concomitantly with aripiprazole.

■ **Escitalopram** Concurrent administration of aripiprazole 10 mg orally daily for 14 days in healthy individuals did not substantially alter the steady-state pharmacokinetics of 10 mg daily of escitalopram, a CYP2C19 and CYP3A4 substrate. Dosage adjustment of escitalopram is not necessary when administered concurrently with aripiprazole.

■ **Famotidine** Concomitant use of aripiprazole and famotidine may result in decreased peak plasma concentrations and systemic exposure of aripiprazole and its active metabolite, dehydro-aripiprazole; however, a clinically important pharmacokinetic interaction between the drugs appears unlikely. No dosage adjustment of aripiprazole is necessary when administered concurrently with famotidine.

■ **Fluoxetine, Paroxetine, and Sertraline** A population pharmacokinetic analysis in patients with major depressive disorder did not demonstrate substantial changes in the pharmacokinetics of fluoxetine, paroxetine, or sertraline (dosed to steady state) following the addition of aripiprazole therapy. Therefore, dosage adjustment of fluoxetine, paroxetine, and sertraline is not necessary in patients concomitantly receiving aripiprazole therapy.

However, fluoxetine and paroxetine are potent inhibitors of CYP2D6 and the manufacturer recommends that oral aripiprazole dosage be reduced to one-half the usual dosage in patients receiving concomitant therapy with potent inhibitors of CYP2D6, including fluoxetine and paroxetine. When fluoxetine or paroxetine is withdrawn from combined therapy with aripiprazole, the aripiprazole dosage should be increased back to the original dosage. When adjunctive aripiprazole is concurrently administered to patients with major depressive disorder receiving fluoxetine or paroxetine, aripiprazole should be given without dosage adjustment. (See Dosage and Administration: Special Populations.)

■ **Lamotrigine** Combined aripiprazole and lamotrigine therapy appears to be well tolerated in patients with bipolar disorder. Pharmacokinetic interaction is unlikely; no dosage adjustment of lamotrigine is necessary when aripiprazole is administered concurrently.

■ **Lithium** Clinically important pharmacokinetic interaction is unlikely; no dosage adjustment of aripiprazole or lithium is necessary during concurrent administration.

■ **Omeprazole** Clinically important pharmacokinetic interaction is unlikely; dosage adjustment of omeprazole is not necessary when administered concurrently with aripiprazole.

■ **Valproate** Clinically important pharmacokinetic interaction is unlikely; no dosage adjustment of aripiprazole or valproate is necessary during concurrent administration.

■ **Venlafaxine** Concurrent administration of oral aripiprazole (10–20 mg daily for 14 days) in healthy individuals did not substantially alter the steady-state pharmacokinetics of venlafaxine and O-desmethylvenlafaxine following 75 mg daily of extended-release venlafaxine, a CYP2D6 substrate. Dosage adjustment of venlafaxine is not necessary during concurrent use of aripiprazole.

■ **Warfarin** Concurrent administration of aripiprazole did not substantially affect warfarin pharmacokinetics, suggesting a lack of a clinically important effect of aripiprazole on CYP2C9 and CYP2C19 metabolism. Warfarin dosage adjustment is not necessary when administered concurrently with aripiprazole.

Description

Aripiprazole is a quinolinone derivative antipsychotic agent that differs chemically from other currently available antipsychotic agents (e.g., butyrophenones, phenothiazines) and has been referred to as an atypical or second-generation antipsychotic agent. The exact mechanism of action of aripiprazole in schizophrenia, bipolar disorder, major depressive disorder, irritability associated with autistic disorder, Tourette's syndrome, and agitation associated with schizophrenia or bipolar mania has not been fully elucidated but, like that of other drugs with efficacy in these conditions (e.g., olanzapine, risperidone, ziprasidone), may involve the drug's activity at dopamine D_2 and serotonin type 1 (5-HT_{1A}) and type 2 (5-HT_{2A}) receptors. However, aripiprazole appears to differ from other atypical antipsychotic agents because the drug demonstrates partial agonist activity at D_2 and 5-HT_{1A} receptors and antagonist activity at 5-HT_{2A} receptors. Antagonism at other receptors (e.g., α_1-adrenergic receptors, histamine H_1 receptors) may contribute to other therapeutic and adverse effects (e.g., orthostatic hypotension, somnolence) observed with aripiprazole.

Aripiprazole is well absorbed following oral administration; peak plasma concentrations following oral administration of conventional tablets occur within 3–5 hours. Administration with a high-fat meal does not affect peak plasma concentration or systemic exposure of aripiprazole or dehydro-aripiprazole. Absolute oral bioavailability of conventional tablets is 87%. Following administration of the oral solution, plasma aripiprazole concentrations are higher than those after administration of equivalent dosages of the conventional tablets. Steady-state plasma concentrations of both aripiprazole and dehydro-aripiprazole are achieved within 14 days with oral administration. Aripiprazole is extensively metabolized in the liver principally via dehydrogenation, hydroxylation, and *N*-dealkylation by the cytochrome P-450 (CYP) 2D6 and 3A4 isoenzymes. The major active metabolite of aripiprazole, dehydro-aripiprazole, exhibits affinity for D_2 receptors similar to that of the parent compound and represents approximately 40% of aripiprazole area under the concentration-time curve (AUC) in plasma. Poor CYP2D6 metabolizers have substantially increased aripiprazole and dehydro-aripiprazole exposures compared with extensive metabolizers (see Dosage and Administration: Special Populations). Approximately 18% of an orally administered dose of aripiprazole is excreted unchanged in feces and less than 1% is excreted unchanged in urine.

Following IM administration of immediate-release aripiprazole injection (no longer commercially available in the US), peak plasma concentrations were achieved within 1–3 hours and were an average of 19% higher than those achieved following oral administration of conventional tablets. Systemic exposure is similar following IM and oral administration of aripiprazole; however, in the first 2 hours after administration, AUC was 90% higher following IM administration of the injection compared with oral administration of the conventional tablets.

Following IM administration of extended-release aripiprazole (Abilify Maintena®), the low solubility of aripiprazole particles results in prolonged aripiprazole absorption. Following multiple IM doses, peak plasma aripiprazole concentrations occur after a median of 4 or 5–7 days when administered into the deltoid or gluteal muscle, respectively. Single IM injections into the deltoid result in 31% higher peak plasma concentrations compared with the gluteal site; however, aripiprazole systemic exposures and peak plasma concentrations at steady state were similar for both injection sites. Dose-proportional increases in aripiprazole and dehydro-aripiprazole systemic exposures were observed following extended-release aripiprazole IM doses of 300 or 400 mg given every 4 weeks. Steady-state plasma concentrations of aripiprazole are achieved by the fourth dose of extended-release aripiprazole for both sites of administration. Following gluteal administration of multiple 300- or 400-mg doses of extended-release aripiprazole every 4 weeks, the mean terminal half-life of aripiprazole is 29.9 or 46.5 days, respectively.

Aripiprazole lauroxil is a prodrug of aripiprazole. Following IM injection, aripiprazole lauroxil is probably converted by enzyme-mediated hydrolysis to *N*-hydroxymethyl aripiprazole, which is then hydrolyzed to aripiprazole. Following IM administration of extended-release aripiprazole lauroxil (Aristada®), aripiprazole begins to appear in the systemic circulation in 5–6 days and is continually released for an additional 36 days. Plasma concentrations of aripiprazole increase with consecutive doses and reach steady-state concentrations following the fourth monthly injection. When administered with oral aripiprazole for 21 days following the first injection, therapeutic plasma concentrations of aripiprazole are achieved within 4 days. IM injection of extended-release aripiprazole lauroxil (441 mg) into the deltoid and gluteal areas results in similar systemic exposure; therefore, these injection sites are considered interchangeable. In addition, IM administration of aripiprazole lauroxil 882 mg every 6 weeks or 1064 mg every 2 months results in plasma aripiprazole concentrations that are within the established therapeutic range for dosages of 441 and 882 mg once monthly. The mean terminal half-life of aripiprazole ranges from about 54–57 days following monthly, every 6 week, or every 2 month injections of extended-release aripiprazole lauroxil.

■ **Aripiprazole Tablets with Sensor** Aripiprazole is available as part of a digital ingestion tracking system comprised of the following components: aripiprazole tablets embedded with an ingestible event marker sensor (IEM; Abilify MyCite®); a wearable sensor (MyCite® patch), which detects the signal from the IEM sensor after ingestion and transmits data to a compatible mobile device (i.e., a smart phone); a software application (app) for compatible mobile devices (e.g., smart phones; MyCite® App), which displays information for the patient; and a web-based portal for healthcare professionals and caregivers.

Following oral administration of aripiprazole tablets with sensor, magnesium and cuprous chloride within the sensor react with gastric fluid to activate and power the sensor. Once activated, the ingestible sensor communicates with the wearable sensor within a 9-foot proximity using Bluetooth® technology. The wearable sensor records the date and time of ingestions and transmits the data to the mobile software application. The mobile software application records and displays ingestion data for patients to review; subjective data such as activity level, mood, and quality of rest also may be reported to the software application. Healthcare professionals, caregivers, and/or family members may access ingestion data shared by the patient through a web-based portal or dashboard. The manufacturer states that this access is granted by the patient and may be withdrawn by the patient at any time.

Most ingestions of aripiprazole tablets with sensor are detected within 30 minutes of oral administration; however, it may take up to 2 hours for the mobile device and web portal to detect ingestion of the sensor and, in some cases, the ingestion may not be detected at all. In a study to assess accuracy and latency of post-ingestion detection of the ingestible sensor in 29 healthy individuals, a wearable sensor was placed and paired with a mobile device provided and monitored by investigators. Placebo tablets with embedded ingestible sensors were then administered under observation every 2 hours for 4 doses without regard to food. The overall ingestion detection rate was 96.6%; approximately 90% of ingestions were detected by the mobile software application within 30 minutes of ingestion. Mean time from ingestion to detection by the wearable sensor was 1.1–1.3 minutes and from detection by the wearable sensor to detection on the cloud-based server was 6.2–10.3 minutes.

Advice to Patients

Importance of providing copy of written patient information (medication guide) each time aripiprazole is dispensed. Importance of advising patients to read the patient information before taking aripiprazole and each time the prescription is refilled.

Importance of advising patients and caregivers that geriatric patients with dementia-related psychosis treated with antipsychotic agents are at an increased risk of death. Patients and caregivers also should be informed that aripiprazole is *not* approved for treating geriatric patients with dementia-related psychosis.

Risk of suicidality; importance of patients, family, and caregivers being alert to and immediately reporting emergence of suicidality, worsening depression, manic or hypomanic symptoms, irritability, agitation, or unusual changes in behavior, especially during the first few months of therapy or during periods of dosage adjustment. (See Worsening of Depression and Suicidality Risk under Warnings/Precautions: Warnings, in Cautions.)

Because somnolence and impairment of judgment, thinking, or motor skills may be associated with aripiprazole, avoid driving, operating machinery, or performing hazardous tasks while taking aripiprazole until the drug's effects on the individual are known.

Importance of avoiding alcohol during extended-release IM aripiprazole (Abilify Maintena®) therapy.

Importance of informing patients and caregivers about the risk of neuroleptic malignant syndrome (NMS); importance of immediately contacting clinician or seeking emergency medical attention if signs and symptoms of this rare but potentially life-threatening syndrome develop (e.g., high fever, muscle stiffness, sweating, fast or irregular heart beat, change in blood pressure, confusion, kidney damage).

Importance of clinicians informing patients in whom chronic aripiprazole use is contemplated of risk of tardive dyskinesia. Importance of informing patients to report any muscle movements that cannot be stopped to a healthcare professional.

Risk of leukopenia, neutropenia, and agranulocytosis. Importance of advising patients with a preexisting low leukocyte count or a history of drug-induced leukopenia/neutropenia that they should have their complete blood cell (CBC) count monitored during aripiprazole therapy.

Importance of informing patients about the risk of metabolic changes (e.g., hyperglycemia and diabetes mellitus, dyslipidemia, weight gain), how to recognize symptoms of hyperglycemia and diabetes mellitus, and the need for specific monitoring, including blood glucose, lipids, and weight, for such changes during therapy.

Risk of pathological gambling and other compulsive behaviors. Importance of advising patients and caregivers of the possibility that they may experience compulsive urges to shop, intense urges to gamble, compulsive sexual urges, binge eating, and/or other compulsive urges and the inability to control these urges during aripiprazole therapy. In some cases, but not all, the urges reportedly stopped when the dosage was reduced or the drug was discontinued. Importance of advising patients or their caregivers to contact a clinician promptly if they experience any such urges that seem out of the ordinary; importance of also advising patients not to abruptly stop taking aripiprazole without first consulting their clinician.

Importance of informing patients about the risk of orthostatic hypotension and syncope, especially when initiating or reinitiating treatment or increasing the dosage.

Importance of informing clinicians of existing or contemplated concomitant therapy, including prescription and OTC drugs and dietary or herbal supplements, as well as any concomitant illnesses (e.g., cardiovascular or cerebrovascular disease, diabetes mellitus, seizures).

Importance of women informing clinicians if they are or plan to become pregnant or plan to breast-feed. Importance of clinicians informing patients about the benefits and risks of taking antipsychotics during pregnancy, including that third trimester use of aripiprazole may cause extrapyramidal and/or withdrawal symptoms in a neonate, and about the pregnancy exposure registry (see Pregnancy under Warnings/Precautions: Specific Populations, in Cautions). Importance of advising patients not to stop taking aripiprazole if they become pregnant without consulting their clinician; abruptly discontinuing antipsychotic agents may cause complications. Importance of advising patients that aripiprazole can pass into breast milk and to consult with their clinician about the best way to feed their infant during aripiprazole therapy.

Importance of avoiding overheating or dehydration.

For patients taking aripiprazole orally disintegrating tablets, importance of not removing a tablet from the blister package until just before administering a dose; importance of peeling blister open with dry hands and placing tablet on tongue to dissolve and be swallowed with saliva.

Importance of informing patients with phenylketonuria that aripiprazole orally disintegrating 10- and 15-mg tablets (Abilify Discmelt®) contain 1.12 and 1.68 mg of phenylalanine, respectively.

Importance of informing patients of other important precautionary information. (See Cautions.)

Aripiprazole Tablets with Sensor. Importance of instructing patients to download the MyCite® App prior to initial use of aripiprazole tablets with sensor and ensure that the software is compatible with their mobile device (i.e., smart phone). Patients should refer to the information provided by the manufacturer and within the MyCite® App for instructions regarding applying and changing the wearable sensor (i.e., MyCite® patch) and pairing the wearable sensor to their mobile device. Importance of advising patients that initial use of the MyCite® system should be facilitated by a healthcare professional.

Importance of advising patients that most ingestions of the tablets with sensor will be detected within 30 minutes; however, it may sometimes take over 2 hours for the mobile device and web portal to detect the ingestion of the tablet with sensor, and, in some cases, ingestion may not be detected at all. Importance of advising patients not to repeat a dose if the tablet with sensor is not detected after ingestion.

Importance of advising patients that if their mobile device is lost, impaired, or otherwise rendered unusable, patients should change the wearable sensor immediately and connect to a new mobile device using their current account information. Inform patients that some data collected by the system may be lost; however, data that have been previously synchronized to the patient's account will be available.

Importance of informing patients that in order for the wearable sensor to communicate with the mobile device, the device must be powered on and Bluetooth®-enabled. Importance of advising patients that the wearable sensor will communicate with a paired device when it is within a 9-foot proximity. Advise patients to keep the wearable sensor in place while showering, swimming, or exercising since it is intended to tolerate exposure to water and perspiration. However, the wearable sensor should be removed before magnetic resonance imaging (MRI) and replaced with a new wearable sensor as soon as possible following the MRI. Importance of advising patients to remove the wearable sensor if skin irritation occurs. (See Tablets with Sensor under Administration: Oral Administration, in Dosage and Administration.)

Importance of instructing patients to swallow aripiprazole tablets with sensor whole. Do not divide, crush, or chew the tablets.

Overview® (see Users Guide). For additional information on this drug until a more detailed monograph is developed and published, the manufacturer's labeling should be consulted. It is *essential* that the manufacturer's labeling be consulted for more detailed information on usual cautions, precautions, contraindications, potential drug interactions, laboratory test interferences, and acute toxicity.

Preparations

Excipients in commercially available drug preparations may have clinically important effects in some individuals; consult specific product labeling for details.

ARIPiprazole

Oral		
Solution*	5 mg/5 mL	**Aripiprazole Oral Solution**
Tablets	2 mg*	**Abilify®**, Otsuka
	5 mg*	**Abilify®**, Otsuka
	10 mg*	**Abilify®**, Otsuka
	15 mg*	**Abilify®**, Otsuka
	20 mg*	**Abilify®**, Otsuka
	30 mg*	**Abilify®**, Otsuka
Tablets, orally disintegrating	10 mg*	**Abilify Discmelt®**, Otsuka
	15 mg*	**Abilify Discmelt®**, Otsuka
Tablets with sensor	2 mg	**Abilify MyCite®** (available as kit containing 30 tablets embedded with sensor and 7 wearable sensor patches), Otsuka
	5 mg	**Abilify MyCite®** (available as kit containing 30 tablets embedded with sensor and 7 wearable sensor patches), Otsuka
	10 mg	**Abilify MyCite®** (available as kit containing 30 tablets embedded with sensor and 7 wearable sensor patches), Otsuka
	15 mg	**Abilify MyCite®** (available as kit containing 30 tablets embedded with sensor and 7 wearable sensor patches), Otsuka
	20 mg	**Abilify MyCite®** (available as kit containing 30 tablets embedded with sensor and 7 wearable sensor patches), Otsuka
	30 mg	**Abilify MyCite®** (available as kit containing 30 tablets embedded with sensor and 7 wearable sensor patches), Otsuka
Parenteral		
For injectable suspension, extended-release, for IM use	300 mg	**Abilify Maintena®** (available as kit containing either a single-dose vial, sterile water for injection, needles, and syringe or a prefilled dual-chamber syringe, sterile water for injection, and needles), Otsuka (also promoted by Lundbeck)
	400 mg	**Abilify Maintena®** (available as kit containing either a single-dose vial, sterile water for injection, needles, and syringe or a prefilled dual-chamber syringe, sterile water for injection, and needles), Otsuka (also promoted by Lundbeck)

*available from one or more manufacturer, distributor, and/or repackager by generic (nonproprietary) name

ARIPiprazole Lauroxil

Parenteral		
Injectable suspension, extended-release, for IM use	441 mg/1.6 mL	**Aristada®** (available as kit containing prefilled syringe and needles), Alkermes
	662 mg/2.4 mL	**Aristada®** (available as kit containing prefilled syringe and needles), Alkermes
	675 mg/2.4 mL	**Aristada Initio®** (available as kit containing prefilled syringe and needles), Alkermes
	882 mg/3.2 mL	**Aristada®** (available as kit containing prefilled syringe and needles), Alkermes
	1064 mg/3.9 mL	**Aristada®** (available as kit containing prefilled syringe and needles), Alkermes

Asenapine Maleate

■ Asenapine maleate is considered an atypical or second-generation antipsychotic agent.

Uses

■ **Psychotic Disorders** Drug therapy is integral to the management of acute psychotic episodes in patients with schizophrenia and generally is required for long-term stabilization to sustain symptom remission or control and to minimize the risk of relapse. Antipsychotic agents are the principal class of drugs used for the management of all phases of schizophrenia. Patient response and tolerance to antipsychotic agents are variable, and patients who do not respond to or tolerate one drug may be successfully treated with an agent from a different class or with a different adverse effect profile.

Schizophrenia Asenapine maleate is an antipsychotic agent that is administered sublingually in the acute and maintenance treatment of schizophrenia. Schizophrenia is a major psychotic disorder that frequently has devastating effects on various aspects of the patient's life and carries a high risk of suicide and other life-threatening behaviors. Manifestations of schizophrenia involve multiple psychologic processes, including perception (e.g., hallucinations), ideation, reality testing (e.g., delusions), emotion (e.g., flatness, inappropriate affect), thought processes (e.g., loose associations), behavior (e.g., catatonia, disorganization), attention, concentration, motivation (e.g., avolition, impaired intention and planning), and judgment. The principal manifestations of this disorder usually are described in terms of positive and negative (deficit) symptoms and, more recently, disorganized symptoms. Positive symptoms include hallucinations, delusions, bizarre behavior, hostility, uncooperativeness, and paranoid ideation, while negative symptoms include restricted range and intensity of emotional expression (affective flattening), reduced thought and speech productivity (alogia), anhedonia, apathy, and decreased initiation of goal-directed behavior (avolition). Disorganized symptoms include disorganized speech (thought disorder) and behavior and poor attention.

The short-term efficacy of sublingual asenapine in the acute management of schizophrenia was evaluated in 4 placebo-controlled and active comparator (haloperidol, olanzapine, or risperidone)-controlled, fixed- or flexible-dose clinical trials of 6 weeks' duration in adults who met DSM-IV criteria for schizophrenia and were experiencing an acute exacerbation of their schizophrenic illness. In 2 of the 4 studies, asenapine was found to be more effective than placebo. In the third study, asenapine could not be distinguished from placebo; however, the active control (olanzapine) in the trial was found to be superior to placebo. In the fourth study, which was flexible dosage in design, neither asenapine nor the active comparator olanzapine demonstrated superior efficacy when compared with placebo.

In the 2 positive studies for asenapine, the main efficacy rating scale was the Positive and Negative Syndrome Scale (PANSS), which assesses schizophrenia symptoms and general psychopathology, and the primary endpoint was change from baseline to the end of treatment on the PANSS total score. In the first trial, which compared asenapine (5 mg sublingually twice daily) with placebo, asenapine was found to be superior to placebo in improving the PANSS total score. In the second trial, which compared fixed dosages of asenapine (5 mg or 10 mg sublingually twice daily) with placebo, asenapine was also found to be superior to placebo in improving the PANSS total score; however, the 10-mg twice-daily dosage did not demonstrate an additional therapeutic benefit compared with the 5-mg twice-daily dosage and did not differ substantially from placebo. An examination of population subgroups did not reveal any clear evidence of differential responsiveness to the drug based on age, gender, or race.

In a longer-term (52-week), double-blind study in adult patients with schizophrenia or schizoaffective disorder who were randomized to receive either sublingual asenapine (5 or 10 mg twice daily) or olanzapine (10–20 mg once daily), asenapine was found to be effective and well tolerated and caused less frequent weight gain but more frequent extrapyramidal symptoms (primarily akathisia) than olanzapine. The long-term efficacy of asenapine (5 or 10 mg twice daily based on tolerability) in prevention of relapse in schizophrenia patients was demonstrated in a 26-week, randomized, placebo-controlled trial that followed 26 weeks of open-label treatment; asenapine was found to be more effective than placebo in prevention of relapse or impending relapse in these patients and was well tolerated over the course of this 52-week trial.

The American Psychiatric Association (APA) considers most atypical antipsychotic agents first-line drugs for the management of the acute phase of schizophrenia (including first psychotic episodes), principally because of the decreased risk of adverse extrapyramidal effects and tardive dyskinesia, with the understanding that the relative advantages, disadvantages, and cost-effectiveness of conventional and atypical antipsychotic agents remain controversial. The APA states that, with the possible exception of clozapine for the management of treatment-resistant symptoms, there currently is no definitive evidence that one atypical antipsychotic agent will have superior efficacy compared with another agent in the class, although meaningful differences in response may be observed in individual patients. Conventional antipsychotic agents also may be an appropriate first-line option for some patients, including those who have been treated successfully in the past with or who prefer conventional agents. The choice of an antipsychotic agent should be individualized, considering past response to therapy, current symptomatology, concurrent medical conditions, other medications and treatments, adverse effect profile, and the patient's preference for a specific drug, including route of administration.

For additional information on the symptomatic management of schizophrenia, including treatment recommendations and results of the Clinical Antipsychotic Trials of Intervention Effectiveness (CATIE) research program, see Schizophrenia and Other Psychotic Disorders under Uses: Psychotic Disorders, in the Phenothiazines General Statement 28:16.08.24.

■ **Bipolar Disorder** Asenapine maleate sublingual tablets are used as monotherapy or adjunctive therapy with lithium or valproate for the acute treatment of manic or mixed episodes associated with bipolar I disorder (with or without psychotic features). The drug also is used for the maintenance monotherapy of bipolar I disorder. According to DSM-IV criteria, manic episodes are distinct periods lasting 1 week or longer (or less than 1 week if hospitalization is required) of abnormally and persistently elevated, expansive, or irritable mood accompanied by at least 3 (or 4 if the mood is only irritability) of the following 7 symptoms: grandiosity, reduced need for sleep, pressure of speech, flight of ideas, distractability, increased goal-directed activity (either socially, at work or school, or sexually) or psychomotor agitation, and engaging in high-risk behavior (e.g., unrestrained buying sprees, sexual indiscretions, foolish business investments).

Efficacy of sublingual asenapine monotherapy in the treatment of acute mania has been demonstrated in 2 similarly designed, short-term (i.e., 3 weeks' duration), placebo-controlled and active comparator-controlled trials in adults who met the DSM-IV criteria for bipolar I disorder with manic or mixed episodes with or without psychotic features. The principal rating instrument used for assessing manic symptoms in these trials was the Young Mania Rating Scale (Y-MRS), an 11-item clinician-rated scale traditionally used to assess the degree of manic symptomatology in a range from 0 (no manic features) to 60 (maximum score). A secondary rating instrument used in these trials was the Clinical Global Impression-Bipolar (CGI-BP) scale. In both trials, asenapine was initially administered in a sublingual dosage of 10 mg twice daily and the dosage could then be adjusted to 5 or 10 mg twice daily from day 2 onward based on efficacy and tolerability; 90% of patients remained on the 10-mg twice-daily dosage. Asenapine was found to be superior to placebo in the reduction of the Y-MRS total score and the CGI-BP Severity of Illness score (mania) in both studies; improvements in the Y-MRS total score were observed as early as day 2 in these studies. An active control arm (olanzapine) was used in addition to placebo controls in both of these studies; however, study design did not allow for direct comparison between asenapine and olanzapine. In another short-term (3 weeks' duration), placebo-controlled study that compared 2 fixed dosages of asenapine monotherapy (5 or 10 mg twice daily) with placebo in adults with manic or mixed episodes associated with bipolar I disorder, both dosages of asenapine were found to be substantially superior to placebo in improving the Y-MRS total score and the CGI-BP Severity of Illness overall score. An examination of population subgroups did not reveal any clear evidence of differential responsiveness to the drug based on age, gender, or race.

Following completion of either of the similarly designed, short-term monotherapy efficacy studies, patients with bipolar I disorder experiencing acute manic or mixed episodes were eligible for a 9-week, double-blind extension study evaluating the efficacy and safety of asenapine versus olanzapine. In this study, no significant difference in efficacy between asenapine and olanzapine was found and asenapine was well tolerated during the extended treatment. Patients completing either of the two 3-week acute efficacy trials and the subsequent 9-week, double-blind extension trial could then enter a longer-term (40-week) extension that was designed to evaluate asenapine therapy over one year of treatment; long-term asenapine therapy (5 or 10 mg twice daily sublingually) was found to be generally well tolerated in this study.

Efficacy and safety of sublingual asenapine monotherapy in the treatment of acute mania in pediatric patients were established in a short-term (i.e., 3 weeks' duration), placebo-controlled, fixed-dosage trial in 403 pediatric patients 10–17 years of age with bipolar I disorder who were currently experiencing manic or mixed episodes. Asenapine (2.5, 5, or 10 mg twice daily) was initiated at a dosage of 2.5 mg twice daily in all the patients and titrated up to a target fixed dosage of 5 and then 10 mg twice daily at intervals of 3 days in the patients receiving these higher dosages. All dosages of asenapine evaluated in this study were found to be superior to placebo in improving the Y-MRS total score and the CGI-BP Severity of Illness overall score from baseline to week 3.

Efficacy of sublingual asenapine as adjunctive therapy in acute mania has been established in a 12-week, placebo-controlled trial with a 3-week primary efficacy endpoint in adults with bipolar I disorder with a manic or mixed episode with or without psychotic features who were partially responsive to lithium or valproate monotherapy after at least 2 weeks of treatment. Asenapine was found to be more effective than placebo in the reduction of manic symptoms (as measured by the Y-MRS total score) when given as an adjunctive therapy to either lithium or valproate at week 3 in this study.

The manufacturer states that if asenapine is used for extended periods in bipolar disorder, the long-term risks and benefits of the drug should be reassessed periodically on an individualized basis. (See Dosage and Administration: Dosage.)

For the initial management of less severe manic or mixed episodes in patients with bipolar disorder, current APA recommendations state that monotherapy with lithium, valproate (e.g., valproate sodium, valproic acid, divalproex), or an antipsychotic agent such as olanzapine may be adequate. For more severe manic or mixed episodes, combination therapy with an antipsychotic agent and lithium or valproate is recommended as first-line therapy. For further information on the management of bipolar disorder, see Uses: Bipolar Disorder, in Lithium Salts 28:28.

Dosage and Administration

■ Administration Asenapine maleate is commercially available as rapidly dissolving sublingual tablets, since the oral bioavailability of the drug after sublingual administration is much higher than following oral administration (see Description). The tablets are administered sublingually twice daily.

Patients should be instructed not to remove a sublingual tablet from the blister pack until just prior to administration. With dry hands, the blister pack should be pulled out of the case and the colored tab should be peeled back to expose the sublingual tablet; the tablet should not be pushed through the blister pack. The tablet should then be gently removed and placed *under* the tongue and allowed to dissolve completely (this usually takes about 10 seconds). The blister pack should then be slid back into the case until it clicks. *Because ingestion of food or water following asenapine administration decreases the drug's exposure, patients should be instructed not to eat or drink for 10 minutes following administration of the sublingual tablets.* The sublingual tablets should *not* be split, crushed, chewed, or swallowed.

■ Dosage Available as asenapine maleate; dosage expressed in terms of asenapine.

Schizophrenia For the acute management of schizophrenia in adults, the recommended initial and target dosage of asenapine is 5 mg given sublingually twice daily. If tolerated, the dosage may be increased to 10 mg twice daily after 1 week. In short-term controlled studies, there was no indication of additional clinical benefit with a higher dosage (10 mg sublingually twice daily) of the drug, but the higher dosage clearly was associated with an increase in certain adverse effects. The manufacturer states that the safety of asenapine dosages exceeding 10 mg twice daily has not been evaluated.

For the maintenance management of schizophrenia in adults, the recommended target dosage range of asenapine is 5–10 mg given sublingually twice daily. Asenapine 5 or 10 mg given twice daily has been shown to be effective and well tolerated for up to 52 weeks in patients with schizophrenia or schizoaffective disorder.

The American Psychiatric Association (APA) states that prudent long-term treatment options in patients with schizophrenia with remitted first or multiple episodes include either indefinite maintenance therapy or gradual discontinuance of the antipsychotic agent with close follow-up and a plan to reinstitute treatment upon symptom recurrence. Discontinuance of antipsychotic therapy should be considered only after a period of at least 1 year of symptom remission or optimal response while receiving the antipsychotic agent. In patients who have had multiple previous psychotic episodes or 2 psychotic episodes within 5 years, indefinite maintenance antipsychotic treatment is recommended.

Bipolar Disorder As monotherapy for the acute management of manic or mixed episodes associated with bipolar I disorder in adults, the recommended initial and target asenapine dosage is 5–10 mg given sublingually twice daily. The manufacturer states that the safety of asenapine dosages exceeding 10 mg twice daily has not been evaluated in clinical trials.

As monotherapy for the maintenance treatment of manic or mixed episodes associated with bipolar I disorder in adults, the same dosage used during stabilization (5–10 mg twice daily) should be continued. Based on clinical response and tolerability in the individual patient, a dosage of 10 mg twice daily can be decreased to 5 mg twice daily. The manufacturer states that the safety of asenapine dosages exceeding 10 mg twice daily has not evaluated in clinical trials.

In short-term monotherapy clinical trials in adults, the initial dosage of asenapine was 10 mg given sublingually twice daily. On the second and subsequent days of the studies, the dosage could be lowered to 5 mg twice daily based on tolerability; however, less than 10% of patients had their dosage reduced during these trials. In a 1-year extension study, the mean total daily dosage in the asenapine-treated patients was approximately 16 mg and the total daily modal dosage was 20 mg.

For the acute management of manic or mixed episodes associated with bipolar I disorder in pediatric patients 10–17 years of age, the initial dosage of asenapine is 2.5 mg given sublingually twice daily and the recommended target dosage is 2.5–10 mg given sublingually twice daily. Dosage may be adjusted based on individual response and tolerability. After 3 days, the dosage may be increased to 5 mg twice daily; after 3 additional days, the dosage may be increased to 10 mg twice daily. Because pediatric patients appear to be more sensitive to dystonia with initial dosing, asenapine should be titrated according to the manufacturer's recommended titration schedule. (See Pediatric Use under Warnings/Precautions: Specific Populations, in Cautions.) The manufacturer states that the safety of asenapine dosages exceeding 10 mg twice daily has not been evaluated in pediatric patients.

When administered as adjunctive therapy with lithium or valproate for the acute management of manic or mixed episodes associated with bipolar I disorder in adults, the recommended initial asenapine dosage is 5 mg given sublingually twice daily. The dosage may then be increased to 10 mg sublingually twice daily based on clinical response and tolerability. The manufacturer states that the safety of asenapine dosages exceeding 10 mg twice daily has not been evaluated.

For patients receiving asenapine as either monotherapy or as adjunctive therapy with lithium or valproate, it is generally recommended that patients responding to therapy continue to receive the drug beyond the acute response. Asenapine 5 or 10 mg given sublingually twice daily has been shown to be well tolerated for up to 52 weeks in adults with bipolar disorder.

■ Special Populations Dosage adjustment is not routinely required in patients with renal impairment or in geriatric patients. (See Renal Impairment under Warnings/Precautions: Specific Populations, in Cautions and also see Geriatric Use under Warnings/Precautions: Specific Populations, in Cautions.)

Dosage adjustment is not necessary in patients with mild or moderate hepatic impairment. Asenapine is contraindicated in patients with severe hepatic impairment. (See Hepatic Impairment under Warnings/Precautions: Specific Populations, in Cautions.)

Dosage adjustment is not routinely required based on gender, race, or smoking status.

Cautions

■ Contraindications Asenapine maleate is contraindicated in patients with severe hepatic impairment (Child-Pugh class C).

Asenapine also is contraindicated in patients with known hypersensitivity to the drug or any components in the formulation. Anaphylaxis, angioedema, hypotension, tachycardia, swollen tongue, dyspnea, wheezing, and rash have been reported in patients receiving asenapine. (See Hypersensitivity Reactions under Warnings/Precautions: Sensitivity Reactions, in Cautions.)

■ Warnings/Precautions ***Warnings*** **Increased Mortality in Geriatric Patients with Dementia-related Psychosis.** Geriatric patients with dementia-related psychosis treated with antipsychotic drugs are at an increased risk of death. Analyses of 17 placebo-controlled trials (modal duration of 10 weeks) revealed a 1.6- to 1.7-fold increase in mortality among geriatric patients who were mainly receiving atypical antipsychotic drugs (i.e., aripiprazole, olanzapine, quetiapine, risperidone) compared with that observed in patients receiving placebo. Over the course of a typical 10-week controlled trial, the rate of death in drug-treated patients was about 4.5% compared with a rate of about 2.6% in the placebo group. Although the causes of death were varied, most of the deaths appeared to be either cardiovascular (e.g., heart failure, sudden death) or infectious (e.g., pneumonia) in nature. The manufacturer states that asenapine is *not* approved for the treatment of patients with dementia-related psychosis. (See Adverse Cerebrovascular Events, including Stroke, in Geriatric Patients with Dementia-related Psychosis and see Dysphagia under Warnings/Precautions: Other Warnings and Precautions, in Cautions and also see Geriatric Use under Warnings/Precautions: Specific Populations, in Cautions.)

Sensitivity Reactions **Hypersensitivity Reactions.** Hypersensitivity reactions have been reported in patients treated with asenapine. From August 2009 to September 2010, the US Food and Drug Administration's (FDA) Adverse Event Reporting System (AERS) received 52 reports of type I hypersensitivity reactions associated with asenapine. Clinical manifestations reported included anaphylaxis, angioedema, hypotension, tachycardia, swollen tongue, dyspnea, wheezing, and rash. Some of the cases reported occurrence of more than one hypersensitivity reaction following asenapine administration. Several cases reported hypersensitivity reactions (possible angioedema, respiratory distress, and possible anaphylaxis) occurring after the first dose. In some patients, symptoms resolved after asenapine discontinuance while others required hospitalization or emergency room visits and therapeutic interventions. (See Cautions: Contraindications and also see Advice to Patients.)

Other Warnings and Precautions **Adverse Cerebrovascular Events, including Stroke, in Geriatric Patients with Dementia-related Psychosis.** An increased incidence of adverse cerebrovascular events (cerebrovascular accidents and transient ischemic attacks), including fatalities, has been observed in geriatric patients with dementia-related psychosis treated with certain atypical antipsychotic agents (aripiprazole, olanzapine, risperidone) in placebo-controlled studies. The manufacturer states that asenapine is *not* approved for the treatment of patients with dementia-related psychosis. (See Increased Mortality in Geriatric Patients with Dementia-related Psychosis under Warnings/Precautions: Warnings and also see Geriatric Use under Warnings/Precautions: Specific Populations, in Cautions.)

Neuroleptic Malignant Syndrome. Neuroleptic malignant syndrome (NMS), a potentially fatal symptom complex characterized by hyperpyrexia, muscle rigidity, delirium, and autonomic instability, has been reported with antipsychotic agents, including asenapine. If NMS is suspected, antipsychotic therapy should be immediately discontinued and intensive symptomatic treatment and monitoring should be provided. (See Advice to Patients.) For additional information on NMS, see Neuroleptic Malignant Syndrome under Cautions: Nervous System Effects, in the Phenothiazines General Statement 28:16.08.24.

Tardive Dyskinesia. Because use of antipsychotic agents, including asenapine, may be associated with tardive dyskinesia (a syndrome consisting of potentially irreversible, involuntary, dyskinetic movements), asenapine should be prescribed in a manner that is most likely to reduce the risk of this syndrome. Chronic antipsychotic treatment generally should be reserved for patients who suffer from a chronic illness that is known to respond to antipsychotic agents, and for whom alternative, effective, but potentially less harmful treatments are not available or appropriate. In patients who do require chronic treatment, the lowest dosage and the shortest duration of treatment needed to achieve a satisfactory clinical response should be used, and the need for continued treatment should be reassessed periodically.

The American Psychiatric Association (APA) currently recommends that patients receiving atypical antipsychotic agents be assessed clinically for abnormal involuntary movements every 12 months and that patients considered to be at increased risk for tardive dyskinesia be assessed every 6 months. If signs and symptoms of tardive dyskinesia appear in an asenapine-treated patient, asenapine discontinuance should be considered; however, some patients may require continued treatment with the drug despite the presence of the syndrome. For additional information on tardive dyskinesia, see Tardive Dyskinesia under Cautions: Nervous System Effects, in the Phenothiazines General Statement 28:16.08.24.

Metabolic Changes. Atypical antipsychotic agents, including asenapine, have caused metabolic changes including hyperglycemia and diabetes mellitus, dyslipidemia, and body weight gain. While all of these drugs produce some metabolic changes, each drug has its own specific risk profile. (See Hyperglycemia and Diabetes Mellitus, see Dyslipidemia, and also see Weight Gain under Warnings/Precautions: Other Warnings and Precautions, in Cautions.)

Hyperglycemia and Diabetes Mellitus. Hyperglycemia, sometimes severe and associated with ketoacidosis, hyperosmolar coma, or death, has been reported in patients receiving atypical antipsychotic agents. Hyperglycemia has been reported in patients treated with asenapine. In short-term controlled trials in patients with schizophrenia or bipolar mania, approximately 0–5 and 6–16% of asenapine-treated patients experienced shifts from normal to high and from borderline to high fasting glucose concentrations, respectively. In a longer-term (one-year), comparator-controlled, double-blind study, the mean increase in fasting glucose concentrations from baseline was 2.4 mg/dL in the asenapine-treated patients.

Fasting blood glucose testing should be performed before or soon after initiation of antipsychotic therapy and then periodically during long-term therapy. (See Advice to Patients.)

For further information on managing the risk of hyperglycemia and diabetes mellitus associated with atypical antipsychotic agents, see Hyperglycemia and Diabetes Mellitus under Cautions: Precautions and Contraindications, in Clozapine 28:16.08.04.

Dyslipidemia. Undesirable changes in lipid parameters have been observed in patients treated with some atypical antipsychotic agents. Asenapine appears to minimally affect the lipid profile in patients receiving short-term therapy with the drug. In short-term, placebo-controlled studies of asenapine in adults with schizophrenia, the proportion of patients with total cholesterol elevations of 240 mg/dL or more at study end point was approximately 8% for asenapine-treated patients compared with 7% for placebo recipients and the proportion of patients with elevations in triglycerides of 200 mg/dL or more at study end point was 13.2% for asenapine-treated patients compared with 10.5% for placebo recipients. In short-term, placebo-controlled bipolar mania trials in adults, the proportion of patients with total cholesterol elevations of 240 mg/dL or more at study end point was 7.8% for asenapine-treated patients compared with 7.9% for placebo recipients and the proportion of patients with elevations in triglycerides of 200 mg/dL or more at end point was 13.1% for asenapine-treated patients compared with 8.6% for placebo recipients.

The manufacturer recommends baseline (i.e., before or soon after initiation of therapy) and periodic follow-up fasting lipid evaluations in patients receiving asenapine therapy.

Weight Gain. Weight gain has been observed with atypical antipsychotic therapy, including asenapine. In short-term schizophrenia studies in adults, mean weight gain of 1.1 kg was reported in patients receiving asenapine compared with no change in weight in those receiving placebo; 4.9% of asenapine-treated patients gained 7% or more of their baseline body weight compared with 1.6% of those receiving placebo. In short-term bipolar mania studies in adults, mean weight gain of 1.3 kg was reported in patients receiving asenapine compared with a gain of 0.2 kg in those receiving placebo; 5.5% of patients receiving asenapine gained 7% or more of their baseline body weight compared with 0.4% of those receiving placebo.

During long-term asenapine therapy (52 weeks) in adults primarily with schizophrenia, mean weight gain in asenapine-treated patients was 0.9 kg. 22% of patients receiving asenapine with a baseline body mass index (BMI) less than 23 gained 7% or more of their baseline body weight compared with 13% of patients with a baseline BMI of 23–27 and 9% of patients with a BMI exceeding 27 at baseline.

In a short-term bipolar mania trial in pediatric patients, mean weight gain of 1.4–1.7 kg was reported in patients receiving asenapine compared with a gain of 0.5 kg in those receiving placebo; 8–12% of asenapine-treated patients gained 7% or more of their baseline body weight compared with 1.1% of those receiving placebo.

The manufacturer recommends baseline and frequent monitoring of weight in all patients receiving asenapine. In pediatric patients, weight gain should be monitored and assessed against that expected for normal growth.

Orthostatic Hypotension, Syncope, and Other Hemodynamic Effects. Atypical antipsychotic agents can cause orthostatic hypotension and syncope. The risk is usually the greatest during initial dosage titration and when dosage is increased. In premarketing clinical trials in adults, including long-term trials without comparison with placebo, syncope was reported in 0.6% of patients treated with asenapine. In short-term bipolar mania trials in pediatric patients, syncope was reported in 1% of patients receiving asenapine 2.5 or 5 mg twice daily and in no patients receiving asenapine 10 mg twice daily or placebo.

Orthostatic vital signs should be monitored in patients receiving asenapine who are susceptible to hypotension (e.g., geriatric patients, patients with dehydration or hypovolemia, patients concomitantly receiving antihypertensive therapy), patients with cardiovascular disease (e.g., history of myocardial infarction, ischemic heart disease, heart failure, or conduction abnormalities), and patients with cerebrovascular disease. Asenapine should be used with caution in patients receiving other drugs that can cause hypotension, bradycardia, respiratory depression, or CNS depression (see Drug Interactions). In all such patients, consideration should be given to monitoring orthostatic vital signs, and dosage reduction should be considered if hypotension develops.

Falls. Asenapine therapy may cause somnolence, postural hypotension, and motor and sensory instability, which may lead to falls; as a consequence, fractures or other injuries may occur. For patients with diseases or conditions or receiving other drugs that could exacerbate these effects, fall risk assessments should be completed when initiating antipsychotic treatment and periodically during long-term therapy.

Leukopenia, Neutropenia, and Agranulocytosis. In clinical trial and/or postmarketing experience, leukopenia and neutropenia have been temporally related to antipsychotic agents, including asenapine. Agranulocytosis (including fatal cases) also has been reported with other antipsychotic agents.

Possible risk factors for leukopenia and neutropenia include preexisting low leukocyte count or absolute neutrophil count (ANC) or a history of drug-induced leukopenia and neutropenia. Patients with a preexisting low leukocyte count or ANC or a history of drug-induced leukopenia or neutropenia should have their complete blood count monitored during the first few months of therapy. Discontinuance of asenapine should be considered at the first sign of a clinically important decline in leukocyte count in the absence of other causative factors.

Patients with clinically important neutropenia should be monitored for fever or other signs or symptoms of infection and promptly treated if such signs and symptoms occur. In patients with severe neutropenia (ANC less than 1000/mm^3), asenapine should be discontinued and the leukocyte count monitored until recovery occurs. Lithium reportedly has been used successfully in the treatment of several cases of leukopenia associated with aripiprazole, clozapine, and some other drugs; however, further clinical experience is needed to confirm these anecdotal findings.

Prolongation of QT Interval. In adult patients with schizophrenia, asenapine (in sublingual dosages of 5, 10, 15, or 20 mg twice daily) was associated with relatively small increases in the corrected QT (QT_c) interval of 2–5 msec compared with placebo in a controlled and dedicated QT study; these increases were slightly lower than those observed in patients receiving quetiapine. None of the asenapine-treated patients in this study experienced a QT_c-interval prolongation of 60 msec or greater compared with baseline, nor did any patient experience a QT_c interval of 500 msec or greater. During short-term clinical trials in patients receiving 5 or 10 mg of asenapine sublingually twice daily, post-baseline QT-interval prolongation exceeding 500 msec was reported at similar rates for asenapine and placebo. There were no reports of torsades de pointes or any adverse effects associated with delayed ventricular repolarization during these studies.

The manufacturer states that asenapine should be avoided in patients concurrently receiving other drugs known to prolong the QT_c interval (see Drug Interactions: Drugs that Prolong QT Interval). The manufacturer also states that asenapine should be avoided in patients with a history of cardiac arrhythmias and in other circumstances that may increase the risk of torsades de pointes and/or sudden death in association with the use of drugs that prolong the QT_c interval, including bradycardia, hypokalemia or hypomagnesemia, and presence of congenital prolongation of the QT interval.

Hyperprolactinemia. Similar to other antipsychotic agents and drugs with dopamine D_2 antagonistic activity, asenapine can cause elevated serum prolactin concentrations, which may persist during chronic use of the drug. In premarketing clinical trials in adults, adverse effects related to abnormal prolactin concentrations occurred in 0.4% of asenapine-treated patients compared with none of those receiving placebo. In a 3-week clinical trial in pediatric patients with bipolar mania, such adverse effects were reported in 0, 2, or 1% of patients receiving asenapine 2.5, 5, or 10 mg sublingually twice daily compared with 1% of patients receiving placebo. Clinical disturbances such as galactorrhea, amenorrhea, gynecomastia, and impotence have been associated with prolactin-elevating drugs. In addition, chronic hyperprolactinemia associated with hypogonadism may lead to decreased bone density in both female and male patients.

If asenapine therapy is considered in a patient with previously detected breast cancer, clinicians should consider that approximately one-third of human breast cancers are prolactin-dependent in vitro.

Seizures. Seizures occurred in 0 and 0.3% of adult patients with schizophrenia and bipolar mania receiving asenapine sublingual dosages of 5 and 10 mg twice daily, respectively, in premarketing short-term clinical trials. In adult premarketing clinical trials, including long-term trials without comparison to placebo, seizures were reported in 0.3% of patients treated with asenapine. There were no reports of seizures in asenapine-treated pediatric patients in a 3-week bipolar mania trial.

As with other antipsychotic agents, asenapine should be used with caution in patients with a history of seizures or with conditions that may lower the seizure threshold; such conditions may be more prevalent in patients 65 years of age or older.

Cognitive and Motor Impairment. Somnolence, usually transient with the highest incidence reported during the first week of therapy, has been reported in patients receiving asenapine. In short-term, placebo-controlled schizophrenia trials in adults, somnolence was reported in 15 and 13% of patients receiving asenapine sublingual dosages of 5 mg and 10 mg twice daily, respectively, compared with 7% of placebo recipients. In short-term, placebo-controlled bipolar mania trials in adults, somnolence was reported in 23% of asenapine-treated patients (5–10 mg sublingually twice daily) compared with 5% of placebo recipients. In the 3-week, fixed-dose study, somnolence occurred in fewer patients receiving 5 mg of asenapine sublingually twice daily (20%) compared with those receiving 10 mg of the drug sublingually twice daily (26%). Somnolence was reported in 18% of asenapine-treated adults during premarketing clinical trials, including long-term trials without placebo comparison. Somnolence led to discontinuance of the drug in 0.6% of patients in short-term, placebo-controlled trials. In a 3-week, placebo-controlled bipolar trial in pediatric patients, somnolence (including sedation and hypersomnia) occurred in 46–53% of patients receiving 2.5–10 mg sublingually twice daily. (See Drug Interactions: Other CNS Agents and see also Advice to Patients.)

Body Temperature Regulation. Disruption of the body's ability to reduce core body temperature has been attributed to atypical antipsychotic agents. In premarketing, short-term, placebo-controlled trials for schizophrenia and acute bipolar I disorder, the incidence of adverse reactions suggestive of body temperature increases was low (1% or less) and comparable to placebo. During premarketing clinical trials with asenapine, including long-term trials without comparison to placebo, up to 1% of asenapine-treated patients experienced adverse effects suggestive of body temperature increases (e.g., pyrexia, feeling hot).

The manufacturer recommends caution when asenapine is used in patients who will be experiencing conditions that may contribute to an elevation in core body temperature (e.g., strenuous exercise, extreme heat, concomitant use of agents with anticholinergic activity, dehydration).

Dysphagia. Esophageal dysmotility and aspiration have been associated with the use of antipsychotic agents. Dysphagia has been reported in patients receiving asenapine. Asenapine and other antipsychotic agents should be used with caution in patients at risk for aspiration.

Specific Populations

Pregnancy. *Pregnancy registry:* There is a pregnancy exposure registry that monitors pregnancy outcomes in women exposed to asenapine during pregnancy. For more information, clinicians may contact the National Pregnancy Registry for Atypical Antipsychotics at 866-961-2388 or visit http://womensmentalhealth.org/clinical-and-research-programs/pregnancyregistry/atypicalantipsychotic/.

Risk summary: Studies have not been conducted with asenapine in pregnant women. There are no available human data informing the drug-associated risk. Asenapine was not teratogenic in animal reproduction studies with IV administration to rats and rabbits during organogenesis at dosages 0.7 and 0.4 times, respectively, the maximum recommended human dosage (MRHD) of 10 mg sublingually twice daily. In a pre- and postnatal study in rats, IV administration of asenapine at dosages up to 0.7 times the MRHD produced increases in post-implantation loss and early pup deaths and decreases in subsequent pup survival and weight gain. The background risk of major birth defects and miscarriage for the indicated populations is unknown. In the U.S. general population, the estimated background risk of major birth defects and miscarriage in clinically recognized pregnancies is 2–4 and 15–20%, respectively. Pregnant women should be advised of the potential risk to the fetus with asenapine exposure.

Fetal/neonatal adverse reactions: Neonates exposed to antipsychotic agents during the third trimester of pregnancy are at risk for extrapyramidal and/or withdrawal symptoms following delivery. Symptoms reported to date have included agitation, hypertonia, hypotonia, tremor, somnolence, respiratory distress, and feeding disorder. The symptoms have varied in severity; some neonates recovered within hours to days without specific treatment, while others have required prolonged hospitalization. Neonates should be monitored for extrapyramidal and/or withdrawal symptoms and managed appropriately if symptoms occur.

Lactation. It is not known whether asenapine is distributed into milk in humans. The drug is distributed into milk in rats. The effects of asenapine on breast-fed infants and on milk production also are not known. The benefit of asenapine therapy to the woman as well as the benefits of breast-feeding to the infant should be weighed against the potential risk to the infant from exposure to the drug or from the underlying maternal condition.

Pediatric Use. Safety and efficacy of asenapine in pediatric patients younger than 10 years of age have not been established.

Safety and efficacy of asenapine *monotherapy* for the management of bipolar I disorder in pediatric patients 10–17 years of age have been established in a double-blind, placebo-controlled trial of 3 weeks' duration. (See Bipolar Disorder under Uses.) In a phase I study, pediatric patients 10–17 years of age appeared to be more sensitive to dystonia when the initial dosage titration schedule was not followed. Similar safety findings were reported in a long-term, open-label, uncontrolled safety trial in pediatric patients with bipolar I disorder treated with asenapine monotherapy. To reduce the risk of dystonia in pediatric patients, asenapine should be titrated according to the manufacturer's recommended schedule. (See Bipolar Disorder under Dosage and Administration: Dosage.) Safety and efficacy of asenapine as *adjunctive* therapy for the treatment of bipolar disorder have not been established in pediatric patients to date.

Efficacy of asenapine for the treatment of schizophrenia has not been established in pediatric patients younger than 18 years of age. In a short-term (i.e., 8 weeks' duration), double-blind, placebo-controlled trial in adolescents 12–17 years of age with schizophrenia, asenapine did not substantially improve the PANSS total score compared with placebo. Tolerability of asenapine in this trial generally was similar to that observed in pediatric bipolar and adult bipolar and schizophrenia trials. In addition, no important safety findings were reported in a 26-week, open-label, uncontrolled safety trial in pediatric patients with schizophrenia treated with asenapine monotherapy.

Pharmacokinetics of asenapine in pediatric patients 10–17 years of age are similar to those observed in adults.

Geriatric Use. Clinical trial experience with asenapine in patients with schizophrenia or bipolar mania who are 65 years of age and older is insufficient to determine whether they respond differently from younger adults. In premarketing clinical studies, 1.1% of approximately 2250 asenapine-treated patients were 65 years of age and older.

Asenapine exposure is 30–40% higher in geriatric patients compared with younger adult patients. Routine dosage adjustment of asenapine is not necessary based on age alone. However, multiple factors that may increase the pharmacodynamic response to asenapine, resulting in poorer tolerance and orthostasis, could be present in geriatric patients, and such patients should be monitored carefully during therapy.

Geriatric patients with dementia-related psychosis treated with asenapine are at an increased risk of death compared with those treated with placebo. In addition, an increased incidence of adverse cerebrovascular events (cerebrovascular accidents and transient ischemic attacks), including fatalities, has been observed in geriatric patients with dementia-related psychosis treated with certain atypical antipsychotic agents (aripiprazole, olanzapine, risperidone) in placebo-controlled studies. The manufacturer of asenapine states that the drug is *not* approved for the treatment of patients with dementia-related psychosis (see Increased Mortality in Geriatric Patients with Dementia-related Psychosis under Warnings/Precautions: Warnings, in Cautions and see also Dysphagia under Warnings/Precautions: Other Warnings and Precautions, in Cautions). For additional information on the use of antipsychotic agents in the management of dementia-related psychosis, see Geriatric Considerations under Uses: Psychotic Disorders, in the Phenothiazines General Statement 28:16.08.24.

Hepatic Impairment. In individuals with severe hepatic impairment (Child-Pugh class C), asenapine exposures were an average of 7 times higher than the exposures in individuals with normal hepatic function. Asenapine is therefore contraindicated in patients with severe hepatic impairment.

Following a single 5-mg sublingual dose of asenapine in individuals with mild (Child-Pugh class A) or moderate (Child-Pugh class B) hepatic impairment, asenapine exposure was not substantially altered compared with that in individuals with normal hepatic function; therefore, dosage adjustment is not required in patients with mild or moderate hepatic impairment.

Renal Impairment. The exposure of asenapine following a single 5-mg dose was similar in individuals with varying degrees of renal impairment and individuals with normal renal function; therefore, dosage adjustment is not required in renally impaired patients. The effect of renal impairment on the elimination of the drug's metabolites and the effect of dialysis on the pharmacokinetics of asenapine have not been evaluated.

■ Common Adverse Effects

Adverse effects occurring in 5% or more of adult patients receiving sublingual asenapine therapy for acute treatment of schizophrenia and at a frequency at least twice that reported with placebo in short-term clinical trials include akathisia (including hyperkinesia), oral hypoesthesia, and somnolence (including sedation and hypersomnia). Akathisia was found to be dose related in these studies. The tolerability profile of asenapine in the maintenance treatment of schizophrenia in adults was similar to that seen with acute treatment.

Adverse effects occurring in 5% or more of adult patients receiving sublingual asenapine therapy for acute monotherapy of manic or mixed episodes associated with bipolar I disorder and at a frequency at least twice that reported with placebo in short-term clinical trials include somnolence (including sedation and hypersomnia), oral hypoesthesia, dizziness, extrapyramidal symptoms other than akathisia (e.g., dystonia, blepharospasm, torticollis, dyskinesia, tardive dyskinesia, muscle rigidity, parkinsonism, gait disturbance, masked facies, tremor), and akathisia. The most common adverse effects reported during the adjunctive therapy trial in adults with bipolar 1 disorder were somnolence and oral hypoesthesia. The incidence of the most common adverse effects was lower at the 5-mg twice-daily dosage than at the 10-mg twice-daily dosage. The tolerability profile of asenapine in the maintenance treatment of manic or mixed episodes associated with bipolar 1 disorder in adults was similar to that seen with acute treatment.

Adverse effects occurring in 5% or more of pediatric patients receiving sublingual asenapine therapy for acute monotherapy of manic or mixed episodes associated with bipolar I disorder and at a frequency at least twice that reported with placebo in short-term clinical trials include somnolence (including sedation and hypersomnia), dizziness, dysgeusia, oral hypoesthesia, nausea, increased appetite, fatigue, and weight gain. Frequency of fatigue was found to be dose related in the pediatric study.

Drug Interactions

Asenapine is cleared mainly through direct glucuronidation by uridine diphosphate-glucuronosyltransferase (UGT) enzyme 1A4 and oxidative metabolism by cytochrome P-450 (CYP) isoenzymes, principally by CYP1A2 and, to a lesser extent, by CYP3A4 and CYP2D6.

Asenapine is a weak inhibitor of CYP2D6; the drug does not induce CYP1A2 or CYP3A4.

■ **Drugs Affecting or Metabolized by Hepatic Microsomal Enzymes** Clinically important pharmacokinetic interactions are possible when asenapine is used concomitantly with drugs that are both substrates and inhibitors of CYP2D6 (e.g., paroxetine) or that are inhibitors of CYP1A2 (e.g., ciprofloxacin, fluvoxamine). Because of possible increased asenapine exposure with potent CYP1A2 inhibitors, asenapine dosage reduction based on clinical response may be necessary. (See Drug Interactions: Ciprofloxacin, Drug Interactions: Fluvoxamine, and Drug Interactions: Paroxetine.)

■ **Anticholinergic Agents** Potential pharmacologic interaction (possible disruption of body temperature regulation); asenapine should be used with caution in patients concurrently receiving drugs with anticholinergic activity. (See Body Temperature Regulation under Warnings/Precautions: Other Warnings and Precautions, in Cautions.)

■ **Drugs that Prolong QT Interval** Potential pharmacologic interaction (additive effect on QT-interval prolongation); concomitant use of asenapine and other drugs known to prolong the corrected QT (QT_c) interval, including class Ia antiarrhythmics (e.g., quinidine, procainamide), class III antiarrhythmics (e.g., amiodarone, sotalol), some antipsychotic agents (e.g., chlorpromazine, thioridazine, haloperidol, olanzapine, paliperidone, pimozide, quetiapine, ziprasidone), some antibiotics (e.g., gatifloxacin, moxifloxacin), and tetrabenazine should be avoided. (See Prolongation of QT Interval under Warnings/Precautions: Other Warnings and Precautions, in Cautions.)

■ **Hypotensive Agents and Drugs causing Bradycardia** Because of its α_1-adrenergic blocking activity and potential to cause hypotension, the manufacturer cautions that asenapine may enhance the hypotensive effects of certain antihypertensive agents and other drugs that can cause hypotension. Asenapine also has been associated with bradycardia. The manufacturer recommends that asenapine be used with caution in patients receiving other drugs that can cause hypotension or bradycardia, and that monitoring of orthostatic vital signs be considered in such patients.

Monitoring of blood pressure is recommended during concurrent use of hypotensive agents and asenapine. If hypotension develops, dosage adjustment of hypotensive agents may be necessary. (See Orthostatic Hypotension, Syncope, and Other Hemodynamic Effects under Warnings/Precautions: Other Warnings and Precautions, in Cautions and also see Advice to Patients.)

■ **Other CNS Agents** Potential pharmacologic interaction (additive CNS depressant effects; increased fall risk). Asenapine should be used with caution in patients receiving other drugs that can produce CNS or respiratory depression.

■ **Carbamazepine** Concomitant administration of carbamazepine, a CYP3A4 inducer, and asenapine slightly decreased both peak plasma concentrations and the area under the plasma concentration-time curve (AUC) of asenapine in healthy individuals. Asenapine dosage adjustment is not required in patients receiving these drugs concurrently.

■ **Cimetidine** Concomitant administration of cimetidine, an inhibitor of CYP3A4, CYP2D6, and CYP1A2, and asenapine slightly decreased peak plasma asenapine concentrations and very slightly increased the drug's AUC. Asenapine dosage adjustment is not necessary in patients concurrently receiving cimetidine.

■ **Ciprofloxacin** An acute dystonic reaction was reported in an asenapine-treated patient after ciprofloxacin, a CYP1A2 inhibitor, was initiated. Because of the risk of increased asenapine exposure, a reduced dosage of asenapine based on clinical response may be necessary during concurrent use.

■ **Fluvoxamine** Concomitant administration of fluvoxamine, a potent CYP1A2 inhibitor, at a dosage of 25 mg twice daily and asenapine slightly increased peak plasma asenapine concentrations and AUCs. The manufacturer states that the full therapeutic dosage of fluvoxamine would be expected to cause a greater increase in plasma concentrations of asenapine, and that a dosage reduction of asenapine may be necessary based on clinical response during concurrent use.

■ **Imipramine** Concomitant administration of imipramine, an inhibitor of CYP1A2, CYP2C19, and CYP3A4, and asenapine slightly increased peak plasma asenapine concentrations and AUCs. Asenapine did not affect plasma concentrations of imipramine's metabolite, desipramine, which is a CYP2D6 substrate. Asenapine dosage adjustment is not required in patients concurrently receiving imipramine.

■ **Lithium** In a population pharmacokinetic analysis, concurrent administration of lithium did not affect the pharmacokinetics of asenapine. In addition, pre-dose serum concentrations of lithium collected during an adjunctive therapy study were comparable between patients receiving asenapine and those receiving placebo, indicating that asenapine does not affect serum concentrations of lithium. Asenapine dosage adjustment is not required in patients concurrently receiving lithium.

■ **Paroxetine** Concomitant administration of paroxetine, which is both a CYP2D6 substrate and inhibitor, and asenapine resulted in a twofold increase in peak plasma concentrations and exposure of paroxetine. Concomitant administration of paroxetine and asenapine slightly decreased peak plasma asenapine concentrations and AUCs. The manufacturer states that asenapine may increase the inhibitory effects of paroxetine on its own metabolism by CYP2D6. Paroxetine dosage should be reduced by one-half during concurrent administration of asenapine; asenapine dosage adjustment is not required.

■ **Valproate** Pre-dose serum concentrations of valproate collected during an adjunctive therapy study were comparable between patients receiving asenapine and those receiving placebo, indicating that asenapine does not affect plasma concentrations of valproate. Concomitant administration of valproate and asenapine slightly increased peak plasma asenapine concentrations and slightly decreased the drug's AUC; asenapine dosage adjustment is not required in patients receiving valproate concurrently.

■ **Smoking** In a population pharmacokinetic analysis, smoking had no effect on asenapine exposure in smokers. Dosage adjustment of asenapine is therefore not necessary based on smoking status.

Description

Asenapine is a dibenzo-oxepino pyrrole-derivative antipsychotic agent and has been referred to as an atypical or second-generation antipsychotic agent. Although the exact mechanism of action of asenapine in schizophrenia and bipolar disorder is unknown, it has been suggested that the efficacy of asenapine in schizophrenia may be mediated through a combination of antagonist activity at central dopamine type 2 (D_2) and serotonin type 2 (5-hydroxytryptamine [5-HT_{2A}]) receptors.

Asenapine exhibits high affinity for serotonin 5-HT_{1A}, 5-HT_{1B}, 5-HT_{2A}, 5-HT_{2B}, 5-HT_{2C}, 5-HT_{5A}, 5-HT_6, and 5-HT_7 receptors; dopamine D_1, D_{2A}, D_{2B}, D_3, and D_4 receptors; α_{1A}-, α_{2A}-, α_{2B}-, and α_{2C}-adrenergic receptors; and histamine H_1 receptors (moderate affinity for H_2 receptors). Asenapine acts as an antagonist at these receptors in vitro. Asenapine possesses no appreciable affinity for muscarinic cholinergic receptors; the drug also does not exhibit affinity for β-adrenergic receptors.

Asenapine is administered sublingually because of the low bioavailability (less than 2%) and extensive first-pass metabolism observed following oral administration. Sublingual tablets of the drug are rapidly absorbed in the sublingual, supralingual, and buccal mucosa following sublingual administration, with peak plasma concentrations occurring within 0.5–1.5 hours. The absolute bioavailability of sublingual asenapine (5 mg) is 35%. Steady-state plasma concentrations are reached within 3 days with twice-daily sublingual administration. Asenapine appears to undergo extensive extravascular distribution and is 95% bound to plasma proteins (including albumin and α_1-acid glycoprotein). The drug is cleared mainly through direct glucuronidation by uridine diphosphate-glucuronosyltransferase (UGT) enzyme 1A4 and oxidative metabolism by cytochrome P-450 (CYP) isoenzymes, principally by CYP1A2 and, to a lesser extent, by CYP3A4 and CYP2D6 in vitro. The mean terminal half-life of the drug is approximately 24 hours. Following administration of a single radiolabeled dose of asenapine, approximately 50 and 40% of the dose was excreted in urine and feces, respectively.

Advice to Patients

Importance of advising patients and caregivers that elderly patients with dementia-related psychosis treated with antipsychotic agents are at an increased risk of death. Patients and caregivers also should be informed that asenapine is *not* approved for treating elderly patients with dementia-related psychosis.

Risk of serious allergic reactions. Importance of informing patients of the signs and symptoms of such reactions (e.g., difficulty breathing; swelling of the face, tongue, or throat; lightheadedness; itching) and to immediately seek emergency medical attention if they develop any of these signs and symptoms.

Importance of informing patients that application site reactions, primarily in the sublingual area, have been reported with asenapine, including oral ulcers, blisters, peeling/sloughing, and inflammation. Patients should be instructed to monitor for such reactions during therapy.

Because somnolence (i.e., sleepiness, drowsiness) may be associated with asenapine, patients should be cautioned about performing activities requiring mental alertness, such as driving or operating hazardous machinery, while taking asenapine until they gain experience with the drug's effects.

Importance of informing patients and caregivers about the risk of a rare but life-threatening nervous system problem called neuroleptic malignant syndrome (NMS), which can cause high fever, stiff muscles, sweating, fast or irregular heart beat, change in blood pressure, confusion, and kidney damage.

Importance of informing patients about the risk of metabolic changes (e.g., hyperglycemia and diabetes mellitus, dyslipidemia, weight gain), how to recognize symptoms of hyperglycemia and diabetes mellitus, and the need for specific monitoring for such changes, including blood glucose, lipids, and weight, during therapy.

Risk of orthostatic hypotension and syncope (fainting), especially when initiating or reinitiating treatment or increasing the dosage. Importance of informing patients about interventions that may help to reduce the occurrence of orthostatic hypotension (e.g., sitting on the edge of the bed for several minutes before attempting to stand in the morning, slowly rising from a seated position).

Risk of leukopenia/neutropenia. Importance of advising patients with a preexisting low leukocyte count or a history of drug-induced leukopenia/neutropenia that they should have their complete blood cell (CBC) count monitored during asenapine therapy.

Importance of clinicians informing patients in whom chronic asenapine use is contemplated about the risk of a movement problem called tardive dyskinesia. Importance of informing patients to report any muscle movements that cannot be stopped to a healthcare professional.

Importance of informing patients that oral hypoesthesia, oral paresthesia, and/or dysgeusia (abnormal or altered taste) may occur with asenapine therapy and that these effects are not serious and are typically transient (i.e., resolving within 1 hour) following sublingual administration of the drug.

Importance of informing clinicians of existing or contemplated concomitant therapy, including prescription (see Drug Interactions) and OTC drugs, as well as any concomitant illnesses (e.g., cardiovascular disease, diabetes mellitus, seizures).

Importance of women informing clinicians if they are or plan to become pregnant or plan to breast-feed. Importance of clinicians informing patients about the benefits and risks of taking antipsychotics during pregnancy, including that third trimester use of asenapine may cause extrapyramidal and/or withdrawal symptoms in a neonate, and about the pregnancy exposure registry (see Pregnancy under Warnings/Precautions: Specific Populations, in Cautions). Importance of advising patients not to stop taking asenapine if they become pregnant without consulting their clinician; abruptly discontinuing antipsychotic agents may cause complications.

Importance of avoiding overheating or dehydration.

Importance of not removing a sublingual tablet from the blister pack until just before administering a dose; importance of pulling blister pack out of the case with dry hands and then peeling back the colored tab on the pack and gently removing the sublingual tablet. The sublingual tablet should then be placed *under* the tongue and allowed to dissolve completely. Importance of not eating or drinking for 10 minutes following administration. Importance of sliding the blister pack back into the case until it clicks after use. (See Dosage and Administration: Administration.)

Importance of informing patients of other important precautionary information. (See Cautions.)

Overview® (see Users Guide). For additional information on this drug until a more detailed monograph is developed and published, the manufacturer's labeling should be consulted. It is *essential* that the manufacturer's labeling be consulted for more detailed information on usual cautions, precautions, contraindications, potential drug interactions, laboratory test interferences, and acute toxicity.

Preparations

Excipients in commercially available drug preparations may have clinically important effects in some individuals; consult specific product labeling for details.

Asenapine Maleate

Sublingual		
Tablets	2.5 mg (of asenapine)	**Saphris® Black Cherry Flavor,** Allergan
	5 mg (of asenapine)	**Saphris® Black Cherry Flavor,** Allergan
	10 mg (of asenapine)	**Saphris® Black Cherry Flavor,** Allergan

Brexpiprazole

■ Brexpiprazole is considered an atypical or second-generation antipsychotic agent.

Uses

■ Adjunctive Therapy of Major Depressive Disorder Brexpiprazole is used orally as an adjunct to antidepressants for the treatment of major depressive disorder.

The adjunctive antidepressant efficacy of brexpiprazole was established in 2 short-term, double-blind, placebo-controlled, fixed-dose studies of 6 weeks' duration (studies 1 and 2) in adults who met DSM-IV-TR criteria for major depressive disorder with or without symptoms of anxiety and who had an inadequate response to previous antidepressant therapy (1–3 courses) in the current episode and had also demonstrated an inadequate response during an 8-week prospective treatment period of antidepressant therapy with delayed-release duloxetine, escitalopram, fluoxetine, extended-release paroxetine, sertraline, or extended-release venlafaxine. The primary efficacy end point in these studies was change from baseline to week 6 on the Montgomery-Asberg Depression Rating Scale (MADRS) total score. In study 1, patients were randomized to receive either brexpiprazole 2 mg once daily or placebo in addition to their antidepressant therapy; in study 2, patients were randomized to receive brexpiprazole 1 or 3 mg once daily or placebo as adjunctive therapy. Brexpiprazole therapy was initiated at a dosage of 0.5 mg once daily in all patients, then the dosage was increased to 1 mg once daily at week 2 in all treatments groups; the dosage was then either maintained at 1 mg once daily or increased to 2 or 3 mg once daily, based on treatment assignment, from week 3 onward. In studies 1 and 2, brexpiprazole at a dosage of 2 or 3 mg daily was superior to placebo in reducing mean MADRS total scores at week 6 and was generally well tolerated. An analysis of population subgroups did not reveal evidence of differential response to adjunctive brexpiprazole therapy based on age, gender, race, or choice of prospective antidepressant.

The manufacturer states that the need for continued therapy and appropriate dosage of brexpiprazole should be reassessed periodically in patients with major depressive disorder. (See Dosage and Administration: Dosage.)

■ Psychotic Disorders Drug therapy is integral to the management of acute psychotic episodes in patients with schizophrenia and generally is required for long-term stabilization to sustain symptom remission or control and to minimize the risk of relapse. Antipsychotic agents are the principal class of drugs used for the management of all phases of schizophrenia. Patient response and tolerance to antipsychotic agents are variable, and patients who do not respond to or tolerate one drug may be successfully treated with an agent from a different class or with a different adverse effect profile.

Schizophrenia Brexpiprazole is an atypical antipsychotic that is administered orally in the treatment of schizophrenia. Schizophrenia is a major psychotic disorder that frequently has devastating effects on various aspects of the patient's life and carries a high risk of suicide and other life-threatening behaviors. Manifestations of schizophrenia involve multiple psychologic processes, including perception (e.g., hallucinations), ideation, reality testing (e.g., delusions), emotion (e.g., flatness, inappropriate affect), thought processes (e.g., loose associations), behavior (e.g., catatonia, disorganization), attention, concentration, motivation (e.g., avolition, impaired intention and planning), and judgment. The principal manifestations of this disorder usually are described in terms of positive and negative (deficit) symptoms and, more recently, disorganized symptoms. Positive symptoms include hallucinations, delusions, bizarre behavior, hostility, uncooperativeness, and paranoid ideation, while negative symptoms include restricted range and intensity of emotional expression (affective flattening), reduced thought and speech productivity (alogia), anhedonia, apathy, and decreased initiation of goal-directed behavior (avolition). Disorganized symptoms include disorganized speech (thought disorder) and behavior and poor attention.

Short-term efficacy of oral brexpiprazole monotherapy in the acute treatment of schizophrenia has been established in 2 randomized, multicenter, double-blind, placebo-controlled, fixed-dose studies of 6 weeks' duration (studies 3 and 4) in adults who met DSM-IV-TR criteria for schizophrenia and were experiencing an acute exacerbation of psychotic symptoms. Both studies evaluated fixed brexpiprazole dosages of 2 or 4 mg once daily. Brexpiprazole therapy was initiated at a dosage of 1 mg once daily, given on days 1 through 4, then the dosage was increased to 2 mg once daily on days 5 to 7; the dosage was then either maintained at 2 mg once daily or increased to 4 mg once daily, based on treatment assignment, for 5 weeks. The primary efficacy end point in these studies was the change from baseline to week 6 on the Positive and Negative Syndrome Scale (PANSS) total score. In both studies, brexpiprazole 4 mg once daily was found to be more effective than placebo in improving the PANSS total score at week 6; the 2-mg daily dosage of brexpiprazole was more effective than placebo only in study 3. An examination of population subgroups did not reveal any clear evidence of differential responsiveness to the drug based on age, gender, or race.

Efficacy and safety of brexpiprazole in the maintenance treatment of schizophrenia have been established in a randomized, multicenter withdrawal study (study 5). Adults with schizophrenia were stabilized for at least 12 weeks on 1–4 mg daily of brexpiprazole and were then randomized in the double-blind treatment phase to either continue brexpiprazole at their achieved stable dosage or to switch to placebo for up to 52 weeks. The primary efficacy end point in this study was time from randomization to impending relapse during the double-blind phase. A prespecified interim analysis demonstrated a substantially longer time to relapse in patients randomized to brexpiprazole therapy compared with the placebo recipients. The study was therefore terminated early because maintenance of efficacy had been demonstrated. Long-term brexpiprazole therapy also was found to be well tolerated in this study.

The American Psychiatric Association (APA) considers most atypical antipsychotic agents first-line drugs for the management of the acute phase of schizophrenia (including first psychotic episodes), principally because of the decreased risk of adverse extrapyramidal effects and tardive dyskinesia, with the understanding that the relative advantages, disadvantages, and cost-effectiveness of conventional and atypical antipsychotic agents remain controversial. The APA states that, with the possible exception of clozapine for the management of treatment-resistant symptoms, there currently is no definitive evidence that one atypical antipsychotic agent will have superior efficacy compared with another agent in the class, although meaningful differences in response may be observed in individual patients. Conventional antipsychotic agents also may be an appropriate first-line option for some patients, including those who have been treated successfully in the past with or who prefer conventional agents. The choice of an antipsychotic agent should be individualized, considering past response to therapy, current symptomatology, concurrent medical conditions, other medications and treatments, adverse effect profile, and the patient's preference for a specific drug, including route of administration.

For additional information on the symptomatic management of schizophrenia, including treatment recommendations, see Schizophrenia and Other Psychotic Disorders under Uses: Psychotic Disorders, in the Phenothiazines General Statement 28:16.08.24.

Dosage and Administration

■ **Administration** Brexpiprazole is commercially available as tablets, which are administered orally once daily without regard to meals. (See Description.)

Patients receiving brexpiprazole should be monitored for possible worsening of depression, suicidality, or unusual changes in behavior, especially at the beginning of therapy or during periods of dosage adjustments. (See Worsening of Depression and Suicidality Risk under Warnings/Precautions: Warnings, in Cautions.)

■ **Dosage** ***Adjunctive Therapy of Major Depressive Disorder*** For adjunctive treatment of major depressive disorder in adults already receiving an antidepressant, the recommended initial dosage of brexpiprazole is 0.5 or 1 mg orally once daily. The dosage should be titrated to 1 mg once daily and then up to the target dosage of 2 mg once daily; dosage adjustments should be made at weekly intervals based on individual patient response and tolerability. The maximum recommended dosage of brexpiprazole for the adjunctive treatment of major depressive disorder is 3 mg daily.

The manufacturer states that the need for continued therapy with brexpiprazole and the appropriate dosage of the drug should be reassessed periodically.

Schizophrenia For the management of schizophrenia in adults, the recommended initial dosage of brexpiprazole is 1 mg orally once daily on days 1–4, followed by an increase in dosage to 2 mg once daily on days 5–7. Based on individual patient response and tolerability, the dosage may be increased to 4 mg once daily on day 8. The recommended target dosage of brexpiprazole for the treatment of schizophrenia is 2–4 mg once daily. The maximum recommended dosage of the drug for the treatment of schizophrenia is 4 mg daily.

The American Psychiatric Association (APA) states that prudent long-term treatment options in patients with schizophrenia with remitted first or multiple episodes include either indefinite maintenance therapy or gradual discontinuance of the antipsychotic agent with close follow-up and a plan to reinstitute treatment upon symptom recurrence. Discontinuance of antipsychotic therapy should be considered only after a period of at least 1 year of symptom remission or optimal response while receiving the antipsychotic agent. In patients who have had multiple previous psychotic episodes or 2 psychotic episodes within 5 years, indefinite maintenance antipsychotic treatment is recommended.

■ **Special Populations** In patients with moderate, severe, or end-stage renal impairment (creatinine clearance less than 60 mL/minute), the maximum recommended dosage of brexpiprazole is 2 mg once daily for adjunctive treatment of major depressive disorder and 3 mg once daily for the treatment of schizophrenia. (See Renal Impairment under Warnings/Precautions: Specific Populations, in Cautions.)

The manufacturer does not provide any specific dosage recommendations for brexpiprazole in patients with mild hepatic impairment. In patients with moderate to severe hepatic impairment (Child-Pugh score of 7 or higher), the maximum recommended dosage of brexpiprazole is 2 mg once daily for adjunctive treatment of major depressive disorder and 3 mg once daily for the treatment of schizophrenia. (See Hepatic Impairment under Warnings/Precautions: Specific Populations, in Cautions.)

In geriatric patients, the manufacturer states that dosage selection of brexpiprazole should be cautious, usually starting at the lower end of the recommended dosage range, reflecting the greater frequency of decreased hepatic, renal, and cardiac function and concomitant illness and other drug therapy in this population. (See Geriatric Use under Warnings/Precautions: Specific Populations, in Cautions.)

Dosage adjustment is not required based on gender, race, or smoking status.

Hepatic Microsomal Enzyme Considerations Dosage adjustments of brexpiprazole are recommended in patients who are known poor metabolizers of the cytochrome P-450 (CYP) isoenzyme 2D6 and in patients concomitantly receiving CYP3A4 and/or CYP2D6 inhibitors or potent CYP3A4 inducers. (See Drug Interactions: Drugs Affecting Hepatic Microsomal Enzymes.)

Patients who are known poor metabolizers of CYP2D6 should receive 50% of the usual brexpiprazole dosage, since poor CYP2D6 metabolizers have higher concentrations of brexpiprazole than extensive metabolizers (see Description). Such patients who are also taking moderate or potent CYP3A4 inhibitors should receive 25% of the usual brexpiprazole dosage.

For the treatment of schizophrenia, brexpiprazole dosage should be reduced to 50% of the usual dosage when used concurrently with potent CYP2D6 inhibitors (e.g., fluoxetine, paroxetine, quinidine). When the potent CYP2D6 inhibitor is withdrawn from combined therapy, the original brexpiprazole dosage may be resumed. For adjunctive therapy of major depressive disorder, brexpiprazole dosage adjustment is *not* necessary when used concomitantly with potent CYP2D6 inhibitors because CYP-related considerations have already been taken into account for the general dosage recommendations. (See Adjunctive Therapy of Major Depressive Disorder under Dosage and Administration: Dosage and also see Drug Interactions: Drugs Affecting Hepatic Microsomal Enzymes.)

Brexpiprazole dosage should be reduced to 50% of the usual dosage when used concurrently with potent CYP3A4 inhibitors (e.g., clarithromycin, itraconazole, ketoconazole). When the potent CYP3A4 inhibitor is withdrawn from combined therapy, the original brexpiprazole dosage may be resumed.

When used concurrently with a combination of moderate or potent CYP2D6 inhibitors and moderate or potent CYP3A4 inhibitors, brexpiprazole dosage should be reduced to 25% of the usual dosage. When the moderate or potent CYP2D6 inhibitor(s) and moderate or potent CYP3A4 inhibitor(s) are withdrawn from combined therapy, the original brexpiprazole dosage may be resumed.

If brexpiprazole is used concurrently with potent CYP3A4 inducers (e.g., rifampin, St. John's wort [*Hypericum perforatum*]), the usual brexpiprazole dosage should be doubled over 1–2 weeks, with further dosage adjustments based on clinical response. When the potent CYP3A4 inducer is withdrawn from combined therapy, the original brexpiprazole dosage may be resumed over 1–2 weeks.

Cautions

■ **Contraindications** Known hypersensitivity to brexpiprazole or any components in the formulation. Rash, facial swelling, urticaria, and anaphylaxis have been reported in patients receiving brexpiprazole.

■ **Warnings/Precautions** ***Warnings*** **Increased Mortality in Geriatric Patients with Dementia-related Psychosis.** Geriatric patients with dementia-related psychosis treated with antipsychotic drugs are at an increased risk of death. Analyses of 17 placebo-controlled trials (modal duration of 10 weeks) revealed a 1.6- to 1.7-fold increase in mortality among geriatric patients who were mainly receiving atypical antipsychotic drugs (i.e., aripiprazole, olanzapine, quetiapine, risperidone) compared with that observed in patients receiving placebo. Over the course of a typical 10-week controlled trial, the rate of death in drug-treated patients was about 4.5% compared with a rate of about 2.6% in the placebo group. Although the causes of death were varied, most of the deaths appeared to be either cardiovascular (e.g., heart failure, sudden death) or infectious (e.g., pneumonia) in nature. The manufacturer states that brexpiprazole is *not* approved for the treatment of patients with dementia-related psychosis. (See Adverse Cerebrovascular Events, including Stroke, in Geriatric Patients with Dementia-related Psychosis and see Dysphagia under Warnings/Precautions: Other Warnings and Precautions, in Cautions, and also see Geriatric Use under Warnings/Precautions: Specific Populations, in Cautions.)

Worsening of Depression and Suicidality Risk. Worsening of depression and/or the emergence of suicidal ideation and behavior (suicidality) or unusual changes in behavior may occur in both adult and pediatric (see Pediatric Use under Warnings/Precautions: Specific Populations, in Cautions) patients with major depressive disorder or other psychiatric disorders, whether or not they are taking antidepressants. This risk may persist until clinically important remission occurs. Suicide is a known risk of depression and certain other psychiatric disorders, and these disorders themselves are the strongest predictors of suicide. However, there has been a long-standing concern that antidepressants may have a role in inducing worsening of depression and the emergence of suicidality in certain patients during the early phases of treatment. Pooled analyses of short-term, placebo-controlled studies of antidepressants (i.e., selective serotonin-reuptake inhibitors [SSRIs] and other antidepressants) have shown an increased risk of suicidality in children, adolescents, and young adults (18–24 years of age) with major depressive disorder and other psychiatric disorders. An increased suicidality risk was not demonstrated with antidepressants compared with placebo in adults older than 24 years of age, and a reduced risk was observed in adults 65 years of age or older.

All patients being treated with antidepressants for any indication should be appropriately monitored for clinical worsening, suicidality, and unusual changes in behavior, particularly during initiation of therapy (i.e., the first few months) and during periods of dosage adjustments. Families and caregivers of patients being treated with antidepressants for major depressive disorder or other indications, both psychiatric and nonpsychiatric, also should be advised to monitor patients on a daily basis for the emergence of agitation, irritability, or unusual changes in behavior as well as the emergence of suicidality, and to report such symptoms immediately to a health-care provider.

Although a causal relationship between the emergence of symptoms such as anxiety, agitation, panic attacks, insomnia, irritability, hostility, aggressiveness, impulsivity, akathisia, hypomania, and/or mania and either the worsening of depression and/or the emergence of suicidal impulses has not been established, there is concern that such symptoms may represent precursors to emerging suicidality. Consequently, consideration should be given to changing the therapeutic regimen or discontinuing therapy in patients whose depression is persistently worse or in patients experiencing emergent suicidality. FDA also recommends that the drugs be prescribed in the smallest quantity consistent with good patient management, in order to reduce the risk of overdosage.

Other Warnings and Precautions **Adverse Cerebrovascular Events, including Stroke, in Geriatric Patients with Dementia-related Psychosis.** In placebo-controlled studies in geriatric patients with dementia, patients randomized to risperidone, aripiprazole, and olanzapine had a higher incidence of adverse cerebrovascular events (cerebrovascular accidents and transient ischemic attacks), including fatalities. The manufacturer states that brexpiprazole is *not* approved for the treatment of patients with dementia-related psychosis. (See Increased Mortality in Geriatric Patients with Dementia-related Psychosis under Warnings/Precautions: Warnings and also see Geriatric Use under Warnings/Precautions: Specific Populations, in Cautions.)

Neuroleptic Malignant Syndrome. Neuroleptic malignant syndrome (NMS), a potentially fatal syndrome characterized by hyperpyrexia, muscle rigidity, altered mental status, and autonomic instability, has been reported with antipsychotic agents. If NMS is suspected, antipsychotic therapy should be immediately discontinued and intensive symptomatic treatment and monitoring should be provided. (See Advice to Patients.) For additional information on NMS, see Neuroleptic Malignant Syndrome under Cautions: Nervous System Effects, in the Phenothiazines General Statement 28:16.08.24.

Tardive Dyskinesia. Because use of antipsychotic agents, including brexpiprazole, may be associated with tardive dyskinesia (a syndrome consisting of potentially irreversible, involuntary, dyskinetic movements), brexpiprazole should be prescribed in a manner that is most likely to reduce the risk of this syndrome. Chronic antipsychotic treatment generally should be reserved for patients who suffer from a chronic illness that is known to respond to antipsychotic agents, and for whom alternative, effective, but potentially less harmful treatments are not available or appropriate. In patients who do require chronic treatment, the lowest dosage and the shortest duration of treatment needed to achieve a satisfactory clinical response should be used, and the need for continued treatment should be reassessed periodically.

The American Psychiatric Association (APA) currently recommends that patients receiving atypical antipsychotic agents be assessed clinically for abnormal involuntary movements every 12 months and that patients considered to be at increased risk for tardive dyskinesia be assessed every 6 months. If signs and symptoms of tardive dyskinesia appear in a brexpiprazole-treated patient, brexpiprazole discontinuance should be considered; however, some patients may require continued treatment with the drug despite the presence of the syndrome. For additional information on tardive dyskinesia, see Tardive Dyskinesia under Cautions: Nervous System Effects, in the Phenothiazines General Statement 28:16.08.24.

Metabolic Changes. Atypical antipsychotic agents, including brexpiprazole, have caused metabolic changes, including hyperglycemia and diabetes mellitus, dyslipidemia, and body weight gain. While all of these drugs produce some metabolic changes, each drug has its own specific risk profile. (See Hyperglycemia and Diabetes Mellitus, see Dyslipidemia, and also see Weight Gain under Warnings/Precautions: Other Warnings and Precautions, in Cautions.)

Hyperglycemia and Diabetes Mellitus. Hyperglycemia, sometimes severe and associated with ketoacidosis, hyperosmolar coma, or death, has been reported in patients receiving atypical antipsychotic agents. Hyperglycemia has been reported in patients treated with brexpiprazole. While confounding factors such as an increased background risk of diabetes mellitus in patients with schizophrenia and the increasing incidence of diabetes mellitus in the general population make it difficult to establish with certainty the relationship between use of agents in this drug class and glucose abnormalities, epidemiologic studies suggest an increased risk of treatment-emergent hyperglycemia-related adverse events in patients treated with atypical antipsychotic agents. In short-term clinical studies, clinically important differences between brexpiprazole and placebo in the proportion of patients experiencing an increase in fasting glucose concentrations were not observed. In longer-term studies, 9–10% of brexpiprazole-treated patients with normal or borderline fasting glucose concentrations experienced shifts to high fasting glucose concentrations.

Patients with preexisting diabetes mellitus in whom therapy with an atypical antipsychotic is initiated should be periodically monitored for worsening of glucose control; those with risk factors for diabetes (e.g., obesity, family history of diabetes) should undergo fasting blood glucose testing upon therapy initiation and periodically throughout treatment. Any patient who develops manifestations of hyperglycemia (including polydipsia, polyuria, polyphagia, and weakness) during treatment with an atypical antipsychotic should undergo fasting blood glucose testing. (See Advice to Patients.) In some cases, patients who developed hyperglycemia while receiving an atypical antipsychotic have required continuance of antidiabetic treatment despite discontinuance of the atypical antipsychotic; in other cases, hyperglycemia resolved with discontinuance of the antipsychotic.

For further information on managing the risk of hyperglycemia and diabetes mellitus associated with atypical antipsychotic agents, see Hyperglycemia and Diabetes Mellitus under Cautions: Precautions and Contraindications, in Clozapine 28:16.08.04.

Dyslipidemia. Atypical antipsychotics cause adverse alterations in lipid parameters. In short-term clinical studies. a higher incidence of hypertriglyceridemia was reported with brexpiprazole than with placebo while changes in fasting total cholesterol, low-density lipoprotein (LDL)-cholesterol, and high-density lipoprotein (HDL)-cholesterol were similar between brexpiprazole-treated patients and those receiving placebo. In uncontrolled, longer-term depression studies, 14% of brexpiprazole-treated patients experienced a shift from normal baseline HDL-cholesterol concentrations to low HDL-cholesterol concentrations and 17% of brexpiprazole-treated patients with normal baseline triglyceride concentrations experienced shifts to high and 0.2% experienced shifts to very high triglyceride concentrations. In uncontrolled, longer-term schizophrenia studies, 13% of brexpiprazole-treated patients with normal baseline triglyceride concentrations experienced shifts to high and 0.4% experienced shifts to very high triglyceride concentrations.

Weight Gain. Weight gain has been observed with atypical antipsychotic therapy. Monitoring of weight at baseline and frequently thereafter is recommended in patients receiving brexpiprazole.

Brexpiprazole generally appears to be associated with moderate weight gain. Mean weight gain during short-term studies in patients receiving brexpiprazole for depression or schizophrenia was 1–1.6 kg compared with 0.2–0.3 kg in those receiving placebo. In longer-term, open-label studies, 20–30% of brexpiprazole-treated patients gained 7% or more of their baseline body weight while 4–10% of patients receiving the drug lost 7% or more.

For additional information on metabolic effects associated with atypical antipsychotic agents, see Hyperglycemia and Diabetes Mellitus under Warnings/Precautions: Other Warnings and Precautions, in Cautions.

Leukopenia, Neutropenia, and Agranulocytosis. Leukopenia and neutropenia have been reported during therapy with antipsychotic agents. Agranulocytosis (including fatal cases) has been reported with other antipsychotic agents.

Possible risk factors for leukopenia and neutropenia include preexisting low leukocyte count or absolute neutrophil count (ANC) or a history of drug-induced leukopenia or neutropenia. Patients with a preexisting low leukocyte count or ANC or a history of drug-induced leukopenia or neutropenia should have their complete blood count monitored frequently during the first few months of therapy. Brexpiprazole should be discontinued at the first sign of a clinically important decline in leukocyte count in the absence of other causative factors.

Patients with neutropenia should be carefully monitored for fever or other signs or symptoms of infection and promptly treated if such signs and symptoms occur. In patients with severe neutropenia (ANC less than 1000/mm^3), brexpiprazole should be discontinued and the leukocyte count monitored until recovery occurs. Lithium reportedly has been used successfully in the treatment of several cases of leukopenia associated with aripiprazole, clozapine, and some other drugs; however, further clinical experience is needed to confirm these anecdotal findings.

Orthostatic Hypotension and Syncope. Atypical antipsychotic agents cause orthostatic hypotension and syncope, perhaps because of their α_1-adrenergic blocking activity. The risk of these adverse effects generally is greatest during initial dosage titration and when the dosage is increased.

In short-term depression studies, dizziness and orthostatic hypotension were reported as adverse events in 2 and 0.1%, respectively, of patients receiving brexpiprazole with an antidepressant compared with 2% and none, respectively, of patients receiving placebo with an antidepressant. In short-term schizophrenia studies, dizziness, orthostatic hypotension, and syncope were reported in 2 and 2%, 0.4 and 0.2%, and 0.1% and none of the patients receiving brexpiprazole or placebo, respectively.

The manufacturer recommends monitoring orthostatic vital signs in patients who are susceptible to hypotension (e.g., geriatric patients, patients with dehydration or hypovolemia, patients receiving concomitant antihypertensive therapy), patients with known cardiovascular disease (e.g., history of myocardial infarction, ischemic heart disease, heart failure, or conduction abnormalities), and patients with cerebrovascular disease. The manufacturer states that brexpiprazole has not been evaluated in patients with a recent history of myocardial infarction or unstable cardiovascular disease. Such patients were excluded from premarketing clinical trials.

Falls. Brexpiprazole therapy may cause somnolence, postural hypotension, and motor and sensory instability, which may lead to falls; as a consequence, fractures or other injuries may occur. For patients with diseases or conditions or receiving other drugs that could exacerbate these effects, fall risk assessments should be completed when initiating antipsychotic treatment and periodically during long-term therapy.

Seizures. As with other antipsychotic agents, brexpiprazole may cause seizures. The risk of seizures is greatest in patients with a history of seizures or with conditions that lower the seizure threshold; such conditions may be more prevalent in older patients.

Body Temperature Dysregulation. Atypical antipsychotics may disrupt the body's ability to reduce core body temperature. The manufacturer recommends using brexpiprazole with caution in patients who may experience conditions that contribute to an elevation in core body temperature (e.g., strenuous exercise, extreme heat, dehydration, concomitant use of agents with anticholinergic activity). (See Advice to Patients.)

Dysphagia. Esophageal dysmotility and aspiration have been associated with the use of antipsychotic agents. Brexpiprazole should be used with caution in patients at risk for aspiration pneumonia.

Cognitive and Motor Impairment. Like other antipsychotic agents, brexpiprazole potentially may impair judgment, thinking, or motor skills. In short-term major depressive disorder studies, somnolence (including sedation and hypersomnia) was reported in 4% of patients receiving brexpiprazole with an antidepressant compared with 1% of patients receiving placebo with an antidepressant. In short-term, placebo-controlled schizophrenia studies, somnolence (including sedation and hypersomnia) was reported in 5% of patients receiving brexpiprazole compared with 3% of placebo recipients. (See Advice to Patients.)

Specific Populations **Pregnancy.** There are no adequate and well-controlled studies to date of brexpiprazole use in pregnant women. In animals, brexpiprazole was not teratogenic but increased perinatal death in pups at dosages much higher than the maximum recommended human dosage.

Neonates exposed to antipsychotic agents during the third trimester of pregnancy are at risk for extrapyramidal and/or withdrawal symptoms following delivery. Symptoms reported to date have included agitation, hypertonia, hypotonia, tremor, somnolence, respiratory distress, and feeding disorder. Neonates exhibiting such symptoms should be monitored. The complications have varied in severity; some neonates recovered within hours to days without specific treatment while others have required intensive care unit support and prolonged hospitalization. For further information on extrapyramidal and withdrawal symptoms in neonates, see Cautions: Pregnancy, Fertility, and Lactation, in the Phenothiazines General Statement 28:16.08.24.

National Pregnancy Registry for Atypical Antipsychotics: 866-961-2388 and http://womensmentalhealth.org/clinical-and-research-programs/pregnancyregistry/atypicalantipsychotic/.

Lactation. It is not known whether brexpiprazole is distributed into milk in humans. The drug is distributed into milk in rats. The effects of brexpiprazole on nursing infants and on milk production also are unknown. The benefits of brexpiprazole therapy to the woman as well as the benefits of breast-feeding to the infant should be weighed against the potential risk to the infant resulting from exposure to the drug or from the underlying maternal condition.

Pediatric Use. Safety and efficacy of brexpiprazole in pediatric patients have not been established.

FDA warns that a greater risk of suicidal thinking or behavior (suicidality) occurred during the first few months of antidepressant treatment compared with placebo in children and adolescents with major depressive disorder, obsessive-compulsive disorder (OCD), or other psychiatric disorders based on pooled analyses of 24 short-term, placebo-controlled trials of 9 antidepressant drugs (SSRIs and other antidepressants). However, a later meta-analysis of 27 placebo-controlled trials of 9 antidepressants (SSRIs and others) in patients younger than 19 years of age with major depressive disorder, OCD, or non-OCD anxiety disorders suggests that the benefits of antidepressant therapy in treating these conditions may outweigh the risks of suicidal behavior or suicidal ideation. No suicides occurred in these pediatric trials. These findings should be carefully considered when assessing potential benefits and risks of brexpiprazole in a child or adolescent for any clinical use. (See Worsening of Depression and Suicidality Risk under Warnings/Precautions: Warnings, in Cautions.)

Geriatric Use. Clinical trials of the efficacy of brexpiprazole did not include any patients 65 years of age and older to determine whether they respond differently than younger adults. In a safety, tolerability, and pharmacokinetics study in geriatric patients (70–85 years of age) with major depressive disorder, the pharmacokinetics of brexpiprazole were similar to those observed in younger adults.

The manufacturer of brexpiprazole states that dosage selection for geriatric patients should be cautious, usually starting at the lower end of the dosage range, reflecting the greater incidence of decreased hepatic, renal, and cardiac function and concomitant illness and other drug therapy in this population.

Geriatric patients with dementia-related psychosis treated with antipsychotic agents are at an increased risk of death. In addition, an increased incidence of adverse cerebrovascular events (cerebrovascular accidents and transient ischemic attacks), including fatalities, has been observed in geriatric patients with dementia-related psychosis treated with certain atypical antipsychotic agents (aripiprazole, olanzapine, risperidone) in placebo-controlled studies. Brexpiprazole is *not* approved for the treatment of patients with dementia-related psychosis (see Increased Mortality in Geriatric Patients with Dementia-related Psychosis under Warnings/Precautions: Warnings, in Cautions and see Dysphagia under Warnings/Precautions: Other Warnings and Precautions, in Cautions). For additional information on the use of antipsychotic agents in the management of dementia-related psychosis, see Geriatric Considerations under Uses: Psychotic Disorders, in the Phenothiazines General Statement 28:16.08.24.

In pooled data analyses, a *reduced* risk of suicidality was observed in adults 65 years of age or older with antidepressant therapy compared with placebo. (See Worsening of Depression and Suicidality Risk under Warnings/Precautions: Warnings, in Cautions.)

Hepatic Impairment. Brexpiprazole is extensively metabolized in the liver. In individuals with mild, moderate, or severe hepatic impairment, brexpiprazole exposures were 26, 73, or 4% higher, respectively, than those in patients with normal hepatic function. Because greater exposure to the drug may increase the risk of adverse effects, a reduction in the maximum recommended dosage of brexpiprazole is recommended for patients with moderate or severe hepatic impairment (Child-Pugh score of 7 or higher). (See Dosage and Administration: Special Populations.)

Renal Impairment. Following a single 3-mg dose, brexpiprazole exposure was 72% higher in patients with severe renal impairment than in patients with normal renal function. In a population pharmacokinetic analysis, brexpiprazole exposures were similar between patients with mild renal impairment and those with normal renal function but exposure to the drug was 71% higher in patients with moderate renal impairment. Because greater exposure to the drug may increase the risk of adverse effects, a reduction in the maximum recommended dosage of brexpiprazole is recommended in patients with moderate or severe renal impairment (creatinine clearance less than 60 mL/minute) or end-stage renal disease. (See Dosage and Administration: Special Populations.)

Hemodialysis is not expected to affect plasma concentrations of brexpiprazole because the drug is highly bound to plasma proteins.

Poor CYP2D6 Metabolizers. Because higher concentrations of brexpiprazole have been observed in poor metabolizers of cytochrome P-450 (CYP) isoenzyme 2D6 than in extensive metabolizers, dosage adjustment of the drug is recommended in patients known to be poor metabolizers of CYP2D6. Approximately 8% of Caucasians and 3–8% of Blacks/African Americans cannot metabolize CYP2D6 substrates and are classified as poor CYP2D6 metabolizers. (See Hepatic Microsomal Enzyme Considerations under Dosage and Administration: Special Populations.)

■ **Common Adverse Effects** Adverse effects occurring in 2% or more of patients receiving brexpiprazole as adjunctive therapy for major depressive disorder and at a higher frequency than reported with placebo include akathisia, headache, weight gain, extrapyramidal symptoms (excluding akathisia), somnolence, nasopharyngitis, tremor, anxiety, increased appetite, dizziness, fatigue, restlessness, constipation, and decreased blood cortisol concentration. Akathisia and restlessness were found to be dose related in placebo-controlled studies.

Adverse effects occurring in 2% or more of patients receiving brexpiprazole for treatment of schizophrenia and at a higher frequency than reported with placebo include akathisia, extrapyramidal symptoms (excluding akathisia), weight gain, diarrhea, dyspepsia, tremor, increased serum creatine kinase (CK, creatine phosphokinase, CPK) concentrations, and sedation.

Drug Interactions

Brexpiprazole is metabolized principally by cytochrome P-450 (CYP) isoenzymes 3A4 and 2D6.

In vitro studies indicate that brexpiprazole and its principal major metabolite, DM-3411, are not potent inhibitors and/or inducers of CYP isoenzymes 1A2, 2A6, 2B6, 2C8, 2C9, 2C19, 2D6, 2E1, or 3A4/5.

In vitro studies indicate that brexpiprazole and its principal metabolite, DM-3411, are not clinically relevant substrates or inhibitors of the efflux transporters P-glycoprotein (P-gp) and breast cancer resistance protein (BCRP), organic anion transport proteins (OATP) 1B1 and 1B3, organic anion transporter 3 (OAT3), organic cation transporter 2 (OCT2), and multidrug and toxic compound extrusion (MATE) 1 and MATE2K.

■ **Drugs Affecting Hepatic Microsomal Enzymes** Clinically important pharmacokinetic interactions with brexpiprazole are possible with drugs that inhibit or induce CYP3A4 or CYP2D6.

Inhibitors of CYP3A4 Concomitant use of brexpiprazole with potent inhibitors of CYP3A4 (e.g., clarithromycin, itraconazole, ketoconazole) may result in substantially increased systemic exposure (area under the concentration-time curve [AUC]) of brexpiprazole. When the potent CYP3A4 inhibitor ketoconazole was administered concomitantly with brexpiprazole (single 2-mg dose), peak plasma concentrations and AUC of brexpiprazole were increased by approximately 1.2-fold and twofold, respectively.

Brexpiprazole dosage should be reduced by 50% of the usual dosage when used concurrently with potent CYP3A4 inhibitors. When the potent CYP3A4 inhibitor is withdrawn from combined therapy, the original brexpiprazole dosage may be resumed. Brexpiprazole dosage should be reduced to 25% of the usual dosage when used concurrently with moderate or potent CYP3A4 inhibitors in patients who are poor metabolizers of CYP2D6. In patients taking moderate or potent CYP3A4 inhibitors (e.g., clarithromycin, fluconazole, itraconazole) *and* moderate or potent CYP2D6 inhibitors (e.g., duloxetine, paroxetine, quinidine), brexpiprazole dosage also should be reduced to 25% of the usual dosage. Brexpiprazole dosage should be increased back to the original dosage when the CYP2D6 and CYP3A4 inhibitors are discontinued. (See Hepatic Microsomal Enzyme Considerations under Dosage and Administration: Special Populations.)

Ketoconazole. Concomitant administration of ketoconazole, a potent CYP3A4 inhibitor, and brexpiprazole (single 2-mg dose) increased peak plasma concentrations and AUC of brexpiprazole by approximately 1.2-fold and twofold, respectively, compared with administration of brexpiprazole alone. Brexpiprazole dosage should be reduced by 50% when used concurrently with ketoconazole.

Inhibitors of CYP2D6 Concomitant use of brexpiprazole with potent CYP2D6 inhibitors (e.g., fluoxetine, paroxetine, quinidine) may result in substantially increased systemic exposure to brexpiprazole. Brexpiprazole dosage should be reduced by 50% when used concurrently with potent CYP2D6 inhibitors. This dosage reduction is not necessary in patient receiving brexpiprazole for adjunctive treatment of major depressive disorder because CYP considerations have been taken into account for the general dosage recommendations. In patients taking moderate or potent CYP3A4 inhibitors (e.g., clarithromycin, fluconazole, itraconazole) *and* moderate or potent CYP2D6 inhibitors (e.g., duloxetine, paroxetine, quinidine), brexpiprazole dosage should be reduced to 25% of the usual dosage. Brexpiprazole dosage should be increased back to the original dosage when the CYP2D6 and CYP3A4 inhibitors are discontinued. (See Hepatic Microsomal Enzyme Considerations under Dosage and Administration: Special Populations.)

Quinidine. Concomitant administration of quinidine, a potent CYP2D6 inhibitor, and brexpiprazole (single 2-mg dose) increased peak plasma concentration and AUC of brexpiprazole by approximately 1.1- and 1.9-fold, respectively, compared with administration of brexpiprazole alone. Except when used in the adjunctive treatment of major depressive disorder, brexpiprazole dosage should be reduced by 50% when used concurrently with quinidine.

Inducers of CYP3A4 Concomitant use of brexpiprazole with potent CYP3A4 inducers (e.g., rifampin, St. John's wort [*Hypericum perforatum*]) may result in substantially decreased systemic exposure of brexpiprazole. The usual brexpiprazole dosage should therefore be doubled over 1–2 weeks during concurrent therapy with potent CYP3A4 inducers; further dosage adjustment should be based on clinical response. If the potent CYP3A4 inducer is discontinued, the brexpiprazole dosage should be reduced back to the original dosage over 1–2 weeks. (See Hepatic Microsomal Enzyme Considerations under Dosage and Administration: Special Populations.)

Rifampin. Concomitant administration of rifampin, a potent CYP3A4 inducer, and brexpiprazole (single 4-mg dose) decreased peak serum concentration and AUC of brexpiprazole by 40 and 73%, respectively. Brexpiprazole dosage should be doubled when used concomitantly with potent CYP3A4 inducers. (See Hepatic Microsomal Enzyme Considerations under Dosage and Administration: Special Populations.)

■ **Drugs Metabolized by Hepatic Microsomal Enzymes** The manufacturer states that no dosage adjustments are necessary if brexpiprazole is used concomitantly with substrates of CYP isoenzymes 3A4, 2B6, or 2D6.

Bupropion Concomitant administration of brexpiprazole (2 mg daily for 11 days) with the CYP2B6 substrate bupropion did not substantially affect the pharmacokinetics of bupropion.

Dextromethorphan Concomitant administration of brexpiprazole (2 mg daily for 11 days) with the CYP2D6 substrate dextromethorphan did not substantially affect the metabolism of dextromethorphan.

Lovastatin Concomitant administration of brexpiprazole (2 mg daily for 11 days) with the CYP3A4 substrate lovastatin did not substantially affect the pharmacokinetics of lovastatin.

■ **Drugs Affecting Gastric pH** Concomitant administration of brexpiprazole (single 4-mg dose) with omeprazole did not have a clinically important effect on the pharmacokinetics of brexpiprazole.

Drugs that increase gastric pH (e.g., antacids, histamine H_2-receptor antagonists, proton-pump inhibitors) are not expected to substantially affect the absorption of brexpiprazole following oral administration; therefore, dosage adjustment of brexpiprazole is not necessary during concomitant use of such drugs.

■ **Hypotensive Agents** Because patients receiving brexpiprazole are at increased risk of orthostatic hypotension and syncope, monitoring of orthostatic vital signs is recommended in patients concomitantly receiving antihypertensive agents. (See Orthostatic Hypotension and Syncope under Warnings/Precautions: Other Warnings and Precautions, in Cautions and also see Advice to Patients.)

■ **Protein-bound Drugs** Based on the results of in vitro studies, brexpiprazole protein binding does not appear to be affected by concurrent administration of other highly protein-bound drugs such as diazepam, digitoxin (no longer commercially available in the US), or warfarin. Therefore, clinically important drug interactions based on protein binding displacement appear to be unlikely with brexpiprazole.

■ **Anticholinergic Agents** Potential pharmacologic interaction (possible disruption of body temperature regulation); brexpiprazole should be used with caution in patients concurrently receiving drugs with anticholinergic activity. (See Body Temperature Dysregulation under Warnings/Precautions: Other Warnings and Precautions, in Cautions.)

■ **Fexofenadine** Concomitant administration of brexpiprazole (2 mg daily for 11 days) with the P-gp substrate fexofenadine did not affect the pharmacokinetics of fexofenadine. No dosage adjustment is necessary when brexpiprazole is used concomitantly with fexofenadine.

■ **Rosuvastatin** Concomitant administration of brexpiprazole (2 mg daily for 11 days) with the BCRP substrate rosuvastatin did not affect the pharmacokinetics of rosuvastatin. No dosage adjustment is necessary when brexpiprazole is used concomitantly with rosuvastatin.

■ **Ticlopidine** Concomitant administration of brexpiprazole (single 2-mg dose) with the potent CYP2B6 inhibitor ticlopidine did not affect the pharmacokinetics of brexpiprazole. No dosage adjustment is necessary when brexpiprazole is used concomitantly with ticlopidine or other CYP2B6 inhibitors.

Description

Brexpiprazole is considered an atypical or second-generation antipsychotic agent; the drug is structurally similar to aripiprazole. The exact mechanism of action of brexpiprazole in major depressive disorder and schizophrenia has not been fully elucidated but is thought to be mediated through a combination of partial agonist activity at dopamine type 2 (D_2) and serotonin type 1A (5-HT_{1A}) receptors and antagonist activity at serotonin type 2A (5-HT_{2A}) receptors.

Brexpiprazole, like aripiprazole, differs from many other atypical antipsychotic agents (which primarily antagonize D_2 receptors) because it is a D_2 partial agonist; these drugs also are partial agonists at 5-HT_{1A} receptors and antagonists at 5-HT_{2A} receptors. Compared with aripiprazole, brexpiprazole appears to have lower intrinsic activity at D_2 receptors and higher activity at 5-HT_{1A} and 5-HT_{1B} receptors and demonstrates stronger antagonism at 5-HT_{2A} receptors. Brexpiprazole also is a partial agonist at D_3 receptors and an antagonist at 5-HT_{2B}, 5-HT_7, and α_{1A}-, α_{1B}-, α_{1D}-, and α_{2C}-adrenergic receptors. It has been suggested that the lower activity of brexpiprazole compared with aripiprazole at D_2 receptors may reduce the potential for certain D_2 partial agonist-mediated adverse effects (e.g., akathisia, insomnia, restlessness, nausea). In addition, brexpiprazole exhibits moderate affinity for histamine (H_1) receptors, which are associated with sedation, and very low affinity for muscarinic (M_1) receptors.

Following oral administration of brexpiprazole tablets, peak plasma concentrations of the drug occur within 4 hours. Administration of the tablets with a high-fat meal does not substantially affect peak plasma concentration or systemic exposure of brexpiprazole. The absolute oral bioavailability of brexpiprazole tablets is 95%. Steady-state plasma concentrations of the drug are achieved within 10–12 days. Higher concentrations of brexpiprazole have been observed in poor metabolizers of cytochrome P-450 (CYP) isoenzyme 2D6 compared with extensive CYP2D6 metabolizers. (See Hepatic Microsomal Enzyme Considerations under Dosage and Administration: Special Populations.) Brexpiprazole has a large volume of distribution, which suggests extravascular distribution, and the drug is highly bound (greater than 99%) to plasma proteins (albumin and α_1-acid glycoprotein). The drug is extensively metabolized, principally by CYP3A4 and CYP2D6, to its principal metabolite, DM-3411. DM-3411 does not appear to contribute to the therapeutic effects of brexpiprazole. The elimination half-lives of brexpiprazole and DM-3411 are approximately 91 and 86 hours, respectively. Following administration of a single radiolabeled dose of brexpiprazole, approximately 46 and 25% of the dose is recovered in feces and urine (approximately 14% and less than 1% excreted unchanged), respectively.

Advice to Patients

Importance of providing a copy of written patient information (medication guide) each time brexpiprazole is dispensed. Importance of advising patients to read the patient information before taking brexpiprazole and each time the prescription is refilled.

Importance of advising patients that brexpiprazole tablets may be taken with or without food. Importance of also advising patients of the importance of following dosage escalation instructions.

Importance of advising patients and caregivers that geriatric patients with dementia-related psychosis treated with antipsychotic agents are at an increased risk of death. Patients and caregivers also should be informed that brexpiprazole is *not* approved for treating geriatric patients with dementia-related psychosis.

Risk of suicidality; importance of patients, family, and caregivers being alert to and immediately reporting emergence of suicidality, worsening depression, manic or hypomanic symptoms, irritability, agitation, or unusual changes in behavior, especially during the first few months of therapy or during periods of dosage adjustment. (See Worsening of Depression and Suicidality Risk under Warnings/Precautions: Warnings, in Cautions.)

Importance of informing patients and caregivers about the risk of neuroleptic malignant syndrome (NMS); importance of immediately contacting clinician or seeking emergency medical attention if signs and symptoms of this rare but potentially life-threatening syndrome develop (e.g., high fever, muscle stiffness, sweating, fast or irregular heart beat, change in blood pressure, confusion, kidney damage).

Importance of advising patients about the signs and symptoms of tardive dyskinesia. Importance of contacting a healthcare professional if abnormal muscle movements occur.

Importance of informing patients and caregivers about the risk of metabolic changes (e.g., hyperglycemia and diabetes mellitus, dyslipidemia, weight gain) with brexpiprazole and the need for specific monitoring for such changes during therapy. Importance of patients and caregivers being aware of the symptoms of hyperglycemia (e.g., increased thirst, increased urination, increased appetite, weakness) and monitoring all patients receiving brexpiprazole for these symptoms. Importance of informing patients who are diagnosed with diabetes or those with risk factors for diabetes (e.g., obesity, family history of diabetes) that they should have their blood glucose monitored at the beginning of and periodically during brexpiprazole therapy. Importance of informing patients that clinical monitoring of weight is recommended during brexpiprazole therapy.

Risk of leukopenia, neutropenia, and agranulocytosis. Importance of advising patients with a preexisting low leukocyte count or a history of drug-induced leukopenia/neutropenia that they should have their complete blood cell (CBC) count monitored during brexpiprazole therapy.

Importance of informing patients about the risk of orthostatic hypotension and syncope, especially when initiating or reinitiating treatment or increasing the dosage.

Importance of avoiding overheating or dehydration.

Because somnolence and impairment of judgment, thinking, or motor skills may be associated with brexpiprazole, patients should be cautioned about performing activities requiring mental alertness, such as driving or operating hazardous machinery, while taking brexpiprazole until they gain experience with the drug's effects.

Importance of informing clinicians of existing or contemplated concomitant therapy, including prescription and OTC drugs or herbal supplements (see Drug Interactions), as well as any concomitant illnesses (e.g., cardiovascular disease, diabetes mellitus, seizures).

Importance of women informing clinicians if they are or plan to become pregnant or plan to breast-feed. Importance of clinicians informing patients about the benefits and risks of taking antipsychotics during pregnancy, and encouraging enrollment in the pregnancy registry (see Pregnancy under Warnings/Precautions: Specific Populations, in Cautions). Importance of advising patients not to stop taking brexpiprazole if they become pregnant without consulting their clinician; abruptly stopping antipsychotic agents may cause complications.

Importance of informing patients of other important precautionary information. (See Cautions.)

Overview® (see Users Guide). For additional information on this drug until a more detailed monograph is developed and published, the manufacturer's labeling should be consulted. It is *essential* that the manufacturer's labeling be consulted for more detailed information on usual cautions, precautions, contraindications, potential drug interactions, laboratory test interferences, and acute toxicity.

Preparations

Excipients in commercially available drug preparations may have clinically important effects in some individuals; consult specific product labeling for details.

Brexpiprazole

Oral		
Tablets	0.25 mg	**Rexulti®**, Otsuka (also promoted by Lundbeck)
	0.5 mg	**Rexulti®**, Otsuka (also promoted by Lundbeck)
	1 mg	**Rexulti®**, Otsuka (also promoted by Lundbeck)
	2 mg	**Rexulti®**, Otsuka (also promoted by Lundbeck)
	3 mg	**Rexulti®**, Otsuka (also promoted by Lundbeck)
	4 mg	**Rexulti®**, Otsuka (also promoted by Lundbeck)

Selected Revisions June 2017,

Cariprazine Hydrochloride

■ Cariprazine hydrochloride is considered an atypical or second-generation antipsychotic agent.

Uses

■ **Psychotic Disorders** Drug therapy is integral to the management of acute psychotic episodes in patients with schizophrenia and generally is required for long-term stabilization to sustain symptom remission or control and to minimize the risk of relapse. Antipsychotic agents are the principal class of drugs used for the management of all phases of schizophrenia. Patient response and tolerance to antipsychotic agents are variable, and patients who do not respond to or tolerate one drug may be successfully treated with an agent from a different class or with a different adverse effect profile.

Schizophrenia Cariprazine hydrochloride is an atypical antipsychotic that is administered orally in the treatment of schizophrenia. Schizophrenia is a major psychotic disorder that frequently has devastating effects on various aspects of the patient's life and carries a high risk of suicide and other life-threatening behaviors. Manifestations of schizophrenia involve multiple psychologic processes, including perception (e.g., hallucinations), ideation, reality testing (e.g., delusions), emotion (e.g., flatness, inappropriate affect), thought processes (e.g., loose associations), behavior (e.g., catatonia, disorganization), attention, concentration, motivation (e.g., avolition, impaired intention and planning), and judgment. The principal manifestations of this disorder usually are described in terms of positive and negative (deficit) symptoms and, more recently, disorganized symptoms. Positive symptoms include hallucinations, delusions, bizarre behavior, hostility, uncooperativeness, and paranoid ideation, while negative symptoms include restricted range and intensity of emotional expression (affective flattening), reduced thought and speech productivity (alogia), anhedonia, apathy, and decreased initiation of goal-directed behavior (avolition). Disorganized symptoms include disorganized speech (thought disorder) and behavior and poor attention.

Short-term efficacy of cariprazine monotherapy in the treatment of schizophrenia has been established in 3 randomized, multicenter, double-blind, placebo-controlled studies of 6 weeks' duration (studies 1, 2, and 3) in adults who met DSM-IV-TR criteria for schizophrenia and were experiencing an acute exacerbation of psychotic symptoms. The primary and secondary efficacy end points in these studies were the change from baseline to week 6 on the Positive and Negative Syndrome Scale (PANSS) total score and the Clinical Global Impressions-Severity (CGI-S) score, respectively. Studies 1 and 2 included an active control arm (risperidone and aripiprazole, respectively) to assess assay sensitivity. Study 1 evaluated 3 fixed dosages of cariprazine (1.5, 3, or 4.5 mg daily), study 2 evaluated 2 fixed dosages of cariprazine (3 or 6 mg daily), and study 3 evaluated flexible dosages of cariprazine in the range of 3–6 or 6–9 mg daily. In all 3 studies, cariprazine was found to be more effective than placebo in improving the PANSS total score and CGI-S score at week 6. Antipsychotic efficacy was demonstrated at cariprazine dosages ranging from 1.5–9 mg daily, and a modest dose-response relationship for efficacy was observed. However, there was a dose-related increase in certain adverse effects, particularly at dosages above 6 mg daily; therefore, the manufacturer states that the maximum recommended dosage of cariprazine for the treatment of schizophrenia is 6 mg daily. An examination of population subgroups did not reveal any clear evidence of differential responsiveness to the drug based on age (there were few patients over 55 years of age), gender, or race.

The American Psychiatric Association (APA) considers most atypical antipsychotic agents first-line drugs for the management of the acute phase of schizophrenia (including first psychotic episodes), principally because of the decreased risk of adverse extrapyramidal effects and tardive dyskinesia, with the understanding that the relative advantages, disadvantages, and cost-effectiveness of conventional and atypical antipsychotic agents remain controversial. The APA states that, with the possible exception of clozapine for the management of treatment-resistant symptoms, there currently is no definitive evidence that one atypical antipsychotic agent will have superior efficacy compared with another agent in the class, although meaningful differences in response may be observed in individual patients. Conventional antipsychotic agents also may be an appropriate first-line option for some patients, including those who have been treated successfully in the past with or who prefer conventional agents. The choice of an antipsychotic agent should be individualized, considering past response to therapy, current symptomatology, concurrent medical conditions, other medications and treatments, adverse effect profile, and the patient's preference for a specific drug, including route of administration.

For additional information on the symptomatic management of schizophrenia, including treatment recommendations, see Schizophrenia and Other Psychotic Disorders under Uses: Psychotic Disorders, in the Phenothiazines General Statement 28:16.08.24.

■ **Bipolar Disorder** Cariprazine hydrochloride is used orally for the acute treatment of manic or mixed episodes associated with bipolar I disorder.

Efficacy of cariprazine in the acute treatment of bipolar mania was established in 3 double-blind, placebo-controlled studies of 3 weeks' duration (studies 1, 2, and 3) in adults who met DSM-IV-TR criteria for bipolar I disorder with manic or mixed episodes with or without psychotic features. The principal rating instrument used for assessing psychiatric signs and symptoms in these studies was the Young Mania Rating Scale (YMRS), an 11-item clinician-rated scale traditionally used to assess the degree of manic symptomatology in a range from 0 (no manic features) to 60 (maximum score). The main secondary rating instrument used in these trials was the CGI-S scale. The primary and secondary end points in these studies was the change from baseline to the end of week 3 on the YMRS and the CGI-S scores, respectively.

Study 1 evaluated flexible dosages of cariprazine in the ranges of 3–6 and 6–12 mg daily; studies 2 and 3 evaluated flexible dosages of cariprazine in the range of 3–12 mg daily. In all 3 studies, cariprazine was found to be more effective than placebo on the primary and secondary end points. Efficacy was demonstrated at daily cariprazine dosages ranging from 3–12 mg; however, no additional benefit was demonstrated at dosages above 6 mg daily and there was a dose-related increase in certain adverse effects. Therefore, the maximum recommended dosage of cariprazine in the acute treatment of manic or mixed episodes associated with bipolar I disorder is 6 mg daily. An examination of population subgroups did not reveal any clear evidence of differential responsiveness to the drug based on age (there were few patients over 55 years of age), gender, or race.

Dosage and Administration

■ **Administration** Cariprazine hydrochloride is commercially available as capsules, which are administered orally once daily without regard to meals. (See Description.)

■ **Dosage** Dosage of cariprazine hydrochloride is expressed in terms of cariprazine.

Because of the long half-life of cariprazine and its active metabolites, changes in dosage will not be fully reflected in plasma concentrations for several weeks (see Description). Therefore, patients receiving the drug should be monitored for adverse effects and clinical response for several weeks after initiation of therapy and after each dosage change. In addition, plasma concentrations of cariprazine and its active metabolites may not be immediately reflected in patients' clinical symptoms following discontinuance of the drug. Plasma concentrations of cariprazine and its active metabolites will decrease by 50% in approximately 1 week.

There are no systematically collected data to specifically address switching patients from cariprazine to other antipsychotic agents or concerning concomitant administration of cariprazine with other antipsychotic agents.

Schizophrenia For the management of schizophrenia in adults, the recommended dosage range of cariprazine is 1.5–6 mg orally once daily. Therapy should be initiated at 1.5 mg once daily and may be increased to 3 mg once daily on day 2. Based on clinical response and tolerability, further dosage adjustments can be made in increments of 1.5 or 3 mg once daily. The maximum recommended dosage of cariprazine is 6 mg daily. In short-term controlled studies, cariprazine dosages exceeding 6 mg daily did not provide increased efficacy sufficient to outweigh the risk of dose-related adverse effects.

The American Psychiatric Association (APA) states that prudent long-term treatment options in patients with schizophrenia with remitted first or multiple episodes include either indefinite maintenance therapy or gradual discontinuance of the antipsychotic agent with close follow-up and a plan to reinstitute treatment upon symptom recurrence. Discontinuance of antipsychotic therapy should be considered only after a period of at least 1 year of symptom remission or optimal response while receiving the antipsychotic agent. In patients who have had multiple previous psychotic episodes or 2 psychotic episodes within 5 years, indefinite maintenance antipsychotic treatment is recommended.

Bipolar Disorder For the acute treatment of manic or mixed episodes associated with bipolar I disorder in adults, the recommended dosage range of cariprazine is 3–6 mg orally once daily. Therapy should be initiated at 1.5 mg once daily and increased to 3 mg once daily on day 2. Based on clinical response and tolerability, further dosage adjustments can be made in increments of 1.5 or 3 mg once daily. The maximum recommended dosage of cariprazine is 6 mg daily. In short-term controlled studies, cariprazine dosages exceeding 6 mg daily did not provide increased efficacy sufficient to outweigh the risk of dose-related adverse effects.

■ **Special Populations** Dosage adjustment is not necessary in patients with mild to moderate renal impairment (creatinine clearance of 30 mL/minute or more). Cariprazine has not been studied in patients with severe renal impairment (creatinine clearance less than 30 mL/minute); use of the drug is not recommended in this patient population. (See Renal Impairment under Warnings/Precautions: Specific Populations, in Cautions.)

Dosage adjustment is not necessary in patients with mild to moderate hepatic impairment (Child-Pugh score 5–9). Cariprazine is not recommended in patients with severe hepatic impairment (Child-Pugh score 10–15); the drug has not been studied in this patient population. (See Hepatic Impairment under Warnings/Precautions: Specific Populations, in Cautions.)

In geriatric patients, the manufacturer states that dosage selection of cariprazine should be cautious, usually starting at the lower end of the recommended dosage range, reflecting the greater frequency of decreased hepatic, renal, and cardiac function; concomitant illnesses; and other drug therapy in this population. (See Geriatric Use under Warnings/Precautions: Specific Populations, in Cautions.)

Dosage adjustment is not required based on gender, race, or smoking status.

In patients receiving a stable dosage of cariprazine and in whom a potent inhibitor of cytochrome P-450 (CYP) isoenzyme 3A4 (e.g., itraconazole, ketoconazole) will be added to therapy, cariprazine dosage should be reduced to 50% of the current dosage. For patients taking 4.5 mg of cariprazine daily, the dosage should be reduced to 1.5 or 3 mg daily; for patients taking 1.5 mg daily, the dosing frequency should be reduced to every other day. Similarly, if cariprazine is initiated in patients already receiving a potent CYP3A4 inhibitor, the recommended initial dosage of cariprazine is 1.5 mg daily on days 1 and 3 (skipping day 2). From day 4 onward, the cariprazine dosage should be 1.5 mg daily; then, the dosage should be subsequently increased up to a maximum dosage of 3 mg daily. When the potent CYP3A4 inhibitor is withdrawn from combined therapy, the cariprazine dosage may need to be increased. (See Drug Interactions: Drugs Affecting Hepatic Microsomal Enzymes.)

Concomitant use of cariprazine and CYP3A4 inducers has not been evaluated and is not recommended. (See Drug Interactions: Drugs Affecting Hepatic Microsomal Enzymes.)

CYP2D6 poor metabolizer status does not have a clinically important effect on the pharmacokinetics of cariprazine and its metabolites; therefore, dosage adjustment is unlikely to be necessary in patients who are poor metabolizers of CYP2D6 substrates.

Cautions

■ **Contraindications** Known hypersensitivity to cariprazine. Hypersensitivity reactions, including rash, pruritus, urticaria, and manifestations of possible angioedema (e.g., swollen tongue, lip swelling, facial edema and swelling, pharyngeal edema), have been reported in patients receiving cariprazine.

■ **Warnings/Precautions** ***Warnings*** **Increased Mortality in Geriatric Patients with Dementia-related Psychosis.** Geriatric patients with dementia-related psychosis treated with antipsychotic drugs are at an increased risk of death. Analyses of 17 placebo-controlled trials (modal duration of 10 weeks) revealed a 1.6- to 1.7-fold increase in mortality among geriatric patients who were mainly receiving atypical antipsychotic drugs (i.e., aripiprazole, olanzapine, quetiapine, risperidone) compared with that observed in patients receiving placebo. Over the course of a typical 10-week controlled trial, the rate of death in drug-treated patients was about 4.5% compared with a rate of about 2.6% in the placebo group. Although the causes of death were varied, most of the deaths appeared to be either cardiovascular (e.g., heart failure, sudden death) or infectious (e.g., pneumonia) in nature. Observational studies suggest that, similar to atypical antipsychotics, treatment with conventional (first-generation) antipsychotics may increase mortality; the extent to which the findings of increased mortality in observational studies may be attributed to the antipsychotic drug as opposed to some characteristic(s) of the patients remains unclear. The manufacturer states that cariprazine is *not* approved for the treatment of patients with dementia-related psychosis. (See Adverse Cerebrovascular Events, including Stroke, in Geriatric Patients with Dementia-related Psychosis and see Dysphagia under Warnings/Precautions: Other Warnings and Precautions, in Cautions, and also see Geriatric Use under Warnings/Precautions: Specific Populations, in Cautions.)

Other Warnings and Precautions **Adverse Cerebrovascular Events, including Stroke, in Geriatric Patients with Dementia-related Psychosis.** An increased incidence of adverse cerebrovascular events (cerebrovascular accidents and transient ischemic attacks), including fatalities, has been observed in geriatric patients with dementia-related psychosis treated with certain atypical antipsychotic agents (aripiprazole, olanzapine, risperidone) in placebo-controlled studies. The manufacturer states that cariprazine is *not* approved for the treatment of patients with dementia-related psychosis. (See Increased Mortality in Geriatric Patients with Dementia-related Psychosis under Warnings/Precautions: Warnings, and also see Geriatric Use under Warnings/Precautions: Specific Populations, in Cautions.)

Neuroleptic Malignant Syndrome. Neuroleptic malignant syndrome (NMS), a potentially fatal syndrome requiring immediate discontinuance of the drug and intensive symptomatic treatment, has been reported in patients receiving antipsychotic agents. (See Advice to Patients.) For additional information on NMS, see Neuroleptic Malignant Syndrome under Cautions: Nervous System Effects, in the Phenothiazines General Statement 28:16.08.24.

Tardive Dyskinesia. Because use of antipsychotic agents, including cariprazine, may be associated with tardive dyskinesia (a syndrome of potentially irreversible, involuntary, dyskinetic movements), cariprazine should be prescribed in a manner that is most likely to minimize the occurrence of this syndrome. Chronic antipsychotic treatment generally should be reserved for patients who suffer from a chronic illness that is known to respond to antipsychotic agents, and for whom alternative, equally effective, but potentially less harmful treatments are not available or appropriate. In patients who do require chronic treatment, the lowest dosage and the shortest duration of treatment producing a satisfactory clinical response should be sought, and the need for continued treatment should be reassessed periodically.

The American Psychiatric Association (APA) recommends that patients receiving atypical antipsychotic agents be assessed clinically for abnormal involuntary movements every 12 months and that patients considered to be at increased risk for tardive dyskinesia be assessed every 6 months. If signs and symptoms of tardive dyskinesia appear in a cariprazine-treated patient, cariprazine discontinuance should be considered; however, some patients may require continued treatment with the drug despite the presence of the syndrome. For additional information on tardive dyskinesia, see Tardive Dyskinesia under Cautions: Nervous System Effects, in the Phenothiazines General Statement 28:16.08.24.

Late-occurring Adverse Effects. Adverse effects may first appear several weeks after initiation of cariprazine therapy, probably because plasma concentrations of cariprazine and its principal metabolites accumulate over time (see Description). Therefore, the incidence of adverse effects reported with cariprazine in short-term clinical trials may not reflect the incidence after longer-term exposure to the drug. Patients should therefore be monitored for adverse effects, including adverse extrapyramidal effects and akathisia, for several weeks after initiation of cariprazine therapy and after each dosage increase. (See Dosage and Administration: Dosage.)

Metabolic Changes. Atypical antipsychotic agents have been associated with metabolic changes, including hyperglycemia and diabetes mellitus, dyslipidemia, and body weight gain. While all of these drugs produce some metabolic changes, each drug has its own specific risk profile. (See Hyperglycemia and Diabetes Mellitus, see Dyslipidemia, and also see Weight Gain under Warnings/Precautions: Other Warnings and Precautions, in Cautions.)

Hyperglycemia and Diabetes Mellitus. Hyperglycemia, sometimes severe and associated with ketoacidosis, hyperosmolar coma, or death, has been reported in patients receiving atypical antipsychotic agents. In short-term controlled trials in patients with schizophrenia or bipolar mania, clinically important differences between cariprazine and placebo in the proportion of patients with shifts from normal or borderline to high fasting glucose concentrations were not observed. In longer-term, open-label studies, 4% of cariprazine-treated patients experienced a shift from normal to elevated (6.5% or higher) glycosylated hemoglobin (hemoglobin A_{1c}; HbA_{1c}) concentrations.

The manufacturer states that patients should undergo fasting blood glucose testing before or soon after initiation of cariprazine and periodically during long-term therapy.

Dyslipidemia. Undesirable changes in lipid parameters have been observed in patients treated with some atypical antipsychotic agents; however, cariprazine generally does not appear to adversely affect the lipid profile in patients receiving short-term therapy with the drug. In short-term, placebo-controlled studies in patients with schizophrenia or bipolar mania, clinically important differences between cariprazine and placebo in the proportion of patients with shifts in fasting total cholesterol, low-density lipoprotein (LDL)-cholesterol, high-density lipoprotein (HDL)-cholesterol, and triglyceride concentrations were not observed.

The manufacturer recommends baseline and periodic follow-up lipid evaluations in patients receiving cariprazine therapy.

Weight Gain. Weight gain has been observed with atypical antipsychotic therapy, including cariprazine. Mean weight gain during short-term studies in patients receiving cariprazine for schizophrenia or bipolar mania was 0.5–1 kg compared with 0.2–0.3 kg in those receiving placebo. In the 6-week schizophrenia studies, 8 and 17% of patients receiving cariprazine daily dosages of 1.5–6 mg and 9–12 mg, respectively, gained 7% or more of their baseline body weight compared with 5% of placebo recipients. In longer-term, uncontrolled trials with cariprazine in schizophrenia, mean weight gain from baseline at 12, 24, and 48 weeks was 1.2, 1.7, and 2.5 kg, respectively.

The manufacturer recommends baseline and frequent monitoring of weight in patients receiving cariprazine.

Leukopenia, Neutropenia, and Agranulocytosis. Leukopenia and neutropenia have been reported with antipsychotic agents, including cariprazine. Agranulocytosis (including fatal cases) also has been reported with other antipsychotic agents.

Possible risk factors for leukopenia and neutropenia include preexisting low leukocyte or absolute neutrophil count (ANC) and a history of drug-induced leukopenia or neutropenia. Patients with a preexisting low leukocyte count or a history of drug-induced leukopenia or neutropenia should have their complete blood count monitored frequently during the first few months of therapy. Cariprazine should be discontinued at the first sign of a clinically important decline in leukocyte count in the absence of other causative factors.

Patients with neutropenia should be carefully monitored for fever or other signs or symptoms of infection and promptly treated if such signs and symptoms occur. In patients with severe neutropenia (ANC less than 1000/mm^3), cariprazine should be discontinued and the leukocyte count monitored until recovery occurs. Lithium reportedly has been used successfully in the treatment of several cases of leukopenia associated with aripiprazole, clozapine, and some other drugs; however, further clinical experience is needed to confirm these anecdotal findings.

Orthostatic Hypotension and Syncope. Atypical antipsychotic agents can cause orthostatic hypotension and syncope. The risk is usually the greatest during initial dosage titration and when dosage is increased. In clinical trials with cariprazine, the incidence of symptomatic orthostatic hypotension was infrequent and was not higher in cariprazine-treated patients compared with those receiving placebo; syncope was not observed in patients receiving the drug.

Orthostatic vital signs should be monitored in patients receiving cariprazine who are susceptible to hypotension (e.g., geriatric patients, patients with dehydration or hypovolemia, patients concomitantly receiving antihypertensive therapy), patients with cardiovascular disease (e.g., history of myocardial infarction, ischemic heart disease, heart failure, or conduction abnormalities), and patients with cerebrovascular disease.

Falls. Cariprazine therapy may cause somnolence, postural hypotension, and motor and sensory instability, which may lead to falls; as a consequence, fractures or other injuries may occur. For patients with diseases, conditions, or other drugs that could exacerbate these effects, fall risk assessments should be completed when initiating antipsychotic treatment and periodically during long-term antipsychotic therapy.

Seizures. As with other antipsychotic agents, cariprazine may cause seizures. The risk of seizures is greatest in patients with a history of seizures or with conditions that lower the seizure threshold; such conditions may be more prevalent in older patients.

Cognitive and Motor Impairment. Like other antipsychotic agents, cariprazine potentially may impair judgment, thinking, or motor skills. In short-term schizophrenia trials, somnolence (including hypersomnia and sedation) was reported in 7% of patients receiving cariprazine compared with 6% of patients receiving placebo. In short-term bipolar mania clinical trials, somnolence was reported in 8% of patients receiving cariprazine compared with 4% of placebo recipients. (See Advice to Patients.)

Body Temperature Dysregulation. Disruption of the body's ability to reduce core body temperature has been attributed to antipsychotic agents. The manufacturer recommends appropriate caution when cariprazine is used in patients who will be experiencing conditions that may contribute to an elevation in core body temperature (e.g., strenuous exercise, extreme heat, dehydration, concomitant use of agents with anticholinergic activity). (See Advice to Patients.)

Dysphagia. Esophageal dysmotility and aspiration have been associated with the use of antipsychotic agents. Dysphagia has been reported in patients receiving cariprazine. Cariprazine and other antipsychotic agents should be used with caution in patients at risk for aspiration.

Specific Populations **Pregnancy.** There are no adequate and well-controlled studies to date of cariprazine use in pregnant women. Fetal developmental toxicity (including reduced body weight, skeletal and external malformations, lower pup survival, and developmental delays) was observed when cariprazine was administered to pregnant rats at dosages 0.2–3.5 times the maximum recommended human dosage.

Neonates exposed to antipsychotic agents during the third trimester of pregnancy are at risk for extrapyramidal and/or withdrawal symptoms following delivery. Symptoms reported to date have included agitation, hypertonia, hypotonia, tardive dyskinetic-like symptoms, tremor, somnolence, respiratory distress, and feeding disorder. Neonates exhibiting such symptoms should be monitored. The complications have varied in severity; some neonates recovered within hours to days without specific treatment while others have required intensive care unit support and prolonged hospitalization.

National Pregnancy Registry for Atypical Antipsychotics: 866-961-2388 and http://womensmentalhealth.org/clinical-and-research-programs/pregnancyregistry/atypicalantipsychotic/.

Lactation. It is not known whether cariprazine is distributed into milk in humans. The drug is distributed into milk in rats. The effects of the drug on breastfed infants or on milk production are not known. The benefits of cariprazine therapy to the woman as well as the benefits of breast-feeding to the infant should be weighed against the potential risk of infant exposure to the drug or from the underlying maternal condition.

Pediatric Use. Safety and effectiveness of cariprazine in pediatric patients have not been established. The manufacturer states that pediatric clinical studies with cariprazine have not been conducted to date.

Geriatric Use. Clinical trial experience with cariprazine in the treatment of schizophrenia and bipolar mania did not include sufficient numbers of patients 65 years of age and older to determine whether geriatric patients respond differently than younger adults.

Age did not have a clinically important effect on the pharmacokinetics of cariprazine and its principal metabolites (desmethyl cariprazine [DCAR] and didesmethyl cariprazine [DDCAR]). The manufacturer states that dosage selection in geriatric patients should be cautious, usually starting at the lower end of the dosage range, reflecting the greater incidence of decreased hepatic, renal, and cardiac function; concomitant illnesses; and other drug therapy in this population.

Geriatric patients with dementia-related psychosis treated with cariprazine are at an increased risk of death compared with those treated with placebo. In addition, an increased incidence of adverse cerebrovascular events (cerebrovascular accidents and transient ischemic attacks), including fatalities, has been observed in geriatric patients with dementia-related psychosis treated with certain atypical antipsychotic agents (aripiprazole, olanzapine, risperidone) in placebo-controlled studies. The manufacturer of cariprazine states that the drug is *not* approved for the treatment of patients with dementia-related psychosis (see Increased Mortality in Geriatric Patients with Dementia-related Psychosis under Warnings/Precautions: Warnings, in Cautions and see Dysphagia under Warnings/Precautions: Other Warnings and Precautions, in Cautions). For additional information on the use of antipsychotic agents in the management of dementia-related psychosis, see Geriatric Considerations under Uses: Psychotic Disorders, in the Phenothiazines General Statement 28:16.08.24.

Hepatic Impairment. Following single or multiple doses of cariprazine in individuals with mild or moderate hepatic impairment (Child-Pugh score 5–9), cariprazine exposure was approximately 25% higher and exposure to the drug's principal active metabolites, DCAR and DDCAR, was approximately 45% lower than in individuals with normal hepatic function. Dosage adjustment of cariprazine is not necessary in patients with mild to moderate hepatic impairment.

Cariprazine has not been studied in patients with severe hepatic impairment (Child-Pugh score 10–15), and use of the drug is not recommended in such patients.

Renal Impairment. Cariprazine and its principal active metabolites are minimally excreted in urine. Pharmacokinetic analyses indicate no substantial relationship between clearance of the drug and its metabolites and creatinine clearance. Dosage adjustment is not necessary for patients with mild to moderate renal impairment (creatinine clearance of 30 mL/minute or more). Cariprazine has not been studied in patients with severe renal impairment (creatinine clearance less than 30 mL/minute), and use of the drug is not recommended in such patients.

■ **Common Adverse Effects** Adverse effects occurring in 5% or more of patients receiving cariprazine for schizophrenia and at a frequency at least twice that reported with placebo in short-term clinical studies include extrapyramidal symptoms (e.g., parkinsonism, dystonia, dyskinesia, tardive dyskinesia) and akathisia.

Adverse effects occurring in 5% or more of patients receiving cariprazine for bipolar mania and at a frequency at least twice that reported with placebo in short-term clinical studies include extrapyramidal symptoms (e.g., parkinsonism, dystonia, dyskinesia, tardive dyskinesia), akathisia, dyspepsia, vomiting, somnolence, and restlessness.

Drug Interactions

Cariprazine is metabolized primarily by cytochrome P-450 (CYP) isoenzyme 3A4 and, to a lesser extent, CYP2D6 to its major active metabolites, desmethyl cariprazine (DCAR) and didesmethyl cariprazine (DDCAR). (See Description.)

In vitro studies indicate that cariprazine and its major active metabolites are not substrates of P-glycoprotein (P-gp), organic anion transport proteins (OATP) 1B1 and 1B3, or breast cancer resistance protein (BCRP).

In vitro studies indicate that cariprazine and its major active metabolites are weak inhibitors of CYP isoenzymes 1A2, 2A6, 2C9, 2C19, 2D6, 2E1, and 3A4 and do not induce CYP1A2 and CYP3A4. Cariprazine and its major active metabolites possess little or no inhibitory effects on OATP1B1, OATP1B3, BCRP, organic cation transporter (OCT) 2, and organic anion transporters (OAT) 1 and 3 in vitro. Clinically important interactions between cariprazine and substrates of these enzymes or transporters are unlikely.

Cariprazine's major active metabolites possess little or no inhibitory effects on P-gp; however, cariprazine probably inhibits P-gp.

■ **Drugs Affecting Hepatic Microsomal Enzymes** Clinically important pharmacokinetic interactions with cariprazine and its active metabolites DCAR and DDCAR are possible with drugs that inhibit or induce CYP3A4. CYP2D6 inhibitors are not expected to substantially affect the pharmacokinetics of cariprazine or its active metabolites.

CYP3A4 Inhibitors Concomitant use of cariprazine with a potent CYP3A4 inhibitor (e.g., itraconazole, ketoconazole) may result in increased systemic exposure to cariprazine and its major active metabolite, DDCAR. Cariprazine dosage should therefore be reduced when used concurrently with a potent CYP3A4 inhibitor. (See Dosage and Administration: Special Populations.)

The effect of moderate CYP3A4 inhibitors on the pharmacokinetics of cariprazine and its metabolites has not been studied to date.

Ketoconazole. Concomitant administration of ketoconazole (400 mg daily; a potent CYP3A4 inhibitor) and cariprazine (0.5 mg daily) increased peak plasma concentrations and AUC of cariprazine by approximately 3.5-fold and fourfold, respectively; increased peak concentrations and AUC of DDCAR by about 1.5-fold; and decreased peak concentrations and AUC of DCAR by about one-third.

CYP3A4 Inducers CYP3A4 is responsible for the formation and elimination of the active metabolites of cariprazine (see Description). The effect of CYP3A4 inducers on the pharmacokinetics of cariprazine and its active metabolites has not been studied to date, and the net effect is not known. Therefore, concomitant use of cariprazine with a CYP3A4 inducer (e.g., carbamazepine, rifampin) is not recommended.

CYP2D6 Inhibitors Based on observations in CYP2D6 poor metabolizers, CYP2D6 inhibitors are not likely to substantially affect the pharmacokinetics of cariprazine, DCAR, or DDCAR.

■ **Anticholinergic Agents** Potential pharmacologic interaction (possible disruption of body temperature regulation); use cariprazine with caution in patients concurrently receiving drugs with anticholinergic activity. (See Body Temperature Dysregulation under Warnings/Precautions: Other Warnings and Precautions, in Cautions.)

■ **Hypotensive Agents** The manufacturer states that patients receiving cariprazine may be at increased risk of orthostatic hypotension and syncope. Therefore, monitoring of orthostatic vital signs is recommended in patients receiving cariprazine and antihypertensive agents concomitantly. (See Orthostatic Hypotension and Syncope under Warnings/Precautions: Other Warnings and Precautions, in Cautions and see also Advice to Patients.)

■ **Smoking** Cariprazine is not a substrate for CYP1A2; therefore, smoking should not alter the pharmacokinetics of the drug. Dosage adjustment of cariprazine in patients who smoke is not necessary.

Description

Cariprazine hydrochloride is considered an atypical or second-generation antipsychotic agent. The exact mechanism of action of cariprazine in schizophrenia and bipolar mania has not been fully elucidated but may be mediated through a combination of partial agonist activity at central dopamine type 2 (D_2) and serotonin type 1 (5-hydroxytryptamine [5-HT_{1A}]) receptors and antagonist activity at serotonin type 2 (5-HT_{2A}) receptors.

Cariprazine acts as a partial agonist at D_2 and D_3 receptors with high binding affinity and at 5-HT_{1A} receptors in vitro. Cariprazine's partial agonist activity at D_2 receptors is similar to that of aripiprazole (another atypical antipsychotic agent with D_2 partial agonist activity) but cariprazine has shown approximately threefold to tenfold higher binding affinity at D_3 receptors compared with D_2 receptors; the clinical implications of the D_3-receptor selectivity are not known. In addition, cariprazine is a partial agonist at 5-HT_{1A} receptors; an antagonist at 5-HT_{2A} and 5-HT_{2B} receptors; and exhibits moderate to low binding affinity for histamine (H_1) receptors, lower binding affinity for 5-HT_{2C} and α_{1A}-adrenergic receptors than aripiprazole, and no appreciable affinity for muscarinic receptors.

The pharmacologic activity of cariprazine is thought to be mediated by cariprazine and its 2 principal active metabolites, desmethyl cariprazine (DCAR) and didesmethyl cariprazine (DDCAR). DCAR and DDCAR, which pharmacologically are as potent as cariprazine, are present in mean plasma concentrations that are approximately 30 and 400% of cariprazine plasma concentrations at the end of 12 weeks, respectively. Therefore, at steady state, DDCAR is the major active moiety circulating in plasma; in a pharmacokinetic study, DDCAR accounted for about 70% of the total activity after 27 days of dosing.

Following oral administration of cariprazine capsules, peak plasma concentrations of cariprazine occur in approximately 3–6 hours. Administration of a single dose of cariprazine with a high-fat meal does not substantially affect peak plasma concentration or systemic exposure of cariprazine or DCAR. Steady-state mean plasma concentrations of cariprazine and DCAR are achieved within 1–2 weeks. Steady-state plasma concentrations of DDCAR appear to approach steady state within about 4–8 weeks; however, the time varies and some patients did not reach steady-state DDCAR concentrations after 12 weeks of treatment. Cariprazine and its main metabolites are highly bound (91–97%) to plasma proteins. Cariprazine is extensively metabolized by cytochrome P-450 (CYP) isoenzyme 3A4 and, to a lesser extent, by CYP2D6 to DCAR and DDCAR. DCAR is further metabolized to DDCAR by CYP3A4 and CYP2D6; DDCAR is then metabolized by CYP3A4 to a hydroxylated metabolite. Following administration of cariprazine 12.5 mg daily for 27 days, approximately 21% of the daily dose is recovered in urine, with approximately 1.2% of the dose excreted in urine as unchanged cariprazine. The elimination half-lives of cariprazine and DDCAR are estimated to be 2–4 days and approximately 1–3 weeks, respectively. Following discontinuance of cariprazine, mean plasma concentrations of cariprazine and DCAR decrease by 50% in about 1 day and mean plasma concentrations of DDCAR decrease by about 50% in 1 week. CYP2D6 poor metabolizer status does not appear to affect the pharmacokinetics of cariprazine and its metabolites.

Advice to Patients

Importance of advising patients and caregivers that geriatric patients with dementia-related psychosis treated with antipsychotic agents are at an increased risk of death. Patients and caregivers also should be informed that cariprazine is *not* approved for treating geriatric patients with dementia-related psychosis.

Importance of advising patients that cariprazine hydrochloride capsules can be taken with or without food. Importance of advising patients to follow the dosage titration instructions for the drug.

Importance of informing patients and caregivers about the risk of neuroleptic malignant syndrome (NMS), a rare but potentially life-threatening syndrome that can cause high fever, stiff muscles, sweating, fast or irregular heart beat, change in blood pressure, confusion, and kidney damage. Importance of immediately contacting clinician if signs and symptoms of this syndrome develop.

Importance of informing patients of the signs and symptoms of tardive dyskinesia. Importance of advising patients to report any abnormal movements to a healthcare professional.

Importance of informing patients and caregivers about the risk of metabolic changes (e.g., hyperglycemia and diabetes mellitus, dyslipidemia, weight gain) with cariprazine and the need for specific monitoring, including blood glucose, lipids, and weight, for such changes during therapy. Importance of patients and caregivers being aware of the symptoms of hyperglycemia and diabetes mellitus (e.g., increased thirst, increased urination, increased appetite, weakness).

Risk of leukopenia/neutropenia. Importance of advising patients with a preexisting low leukocyte count or a history of drug-induced leukopenia/neutropenia that they should have their complete blood count (CBC) monitored during cariprazine therapy.

Importance of informing patients about the risk of orthostatic hypotension and syncope, especially when initiating or reinitiating treatment or increasing the dosage.

Because somnolence and impairment of judgment, thinking, or motor skills may be associated with cariprazine, patients should be cautioned about performing activities requiring mental alertness, such as driving or operating hazardous machinery, while taking the drug until they gain experience with the drug's effects.

Importance of avoiding overheating or dehydration.

Importance of informing clinicians of existing or contemplated concomitant therapy, including prescription (see Drug Interactions) and OTC drugs or herbal supplements, as well as any concomitant illnesses (e.g., cardiovascular disease, diabetes mellitus, seizures).

Importance of women informing clinicians if they are or plan to become pregnant or plan to breast-feed. Importance of clinicians informing patients about the benefits and risks of taking antipsychotics during pregnancy (see Pregnancy under Warnings/Precautions: Specific Populations, in Cautions). Importance of advising patients not to stop taking cariprazine if they become pregnant without consulting their clinician; abruptly stopping antipsychotic agents may cause complications.

Importance of informing patients of other important precautionary information. (See Cautions.)

Overview® (see Users Guide). For additional information on this drug until a more detailed monograph is developed and published, the manufacturer's labeling should be consulted. It is *essential* that the manufacturer's labeling be consulted for more detailed information on usual cautions, precautions, contraindications, potential drug interactions, laboratory test interferences, and acute toxicity.

Preparations

Excipients in commercially available drug preparations may have clinically important effects in some individuals; consult specific product labeling for details.

Cariprazine Hydrochloride

Oral		
Capsules	1.5 mg (of cariprazine)	**Vraylar®**, Allergan
	3 mg (of cariprazine)	**Vraylar®**, Allergan
	4.5 mg (of cariprazine)	**Vraylar®**, Allergan
	6 mg (of cariprazine)	**Vraylar®**, Allergan
Titration Pack	1 Capsule, 1.5 mg (of cariprazine) (Vraylar®) 6 Capsules, 3 mg (of cariprazine) (Vraylar®)	**Vraylar® Titration Pack,** Allergan

cloZAPine

■ Clozapine has been referred to as an atypical or second-generation antipsychotic agent.

REMS

FDA approved a shared REMS for clozapine. The REMS may consist of the following: elements to assure safe use and implementation system. See the FDA REMS page (https://www.accessdata.fda.gov/scripts/cder/rems/index.cfm). Also see Restricted Distribution Program under Dosage and Administration: Administration.

Uses

■ **Psychotic Disorders** Clozapine is used for the symptomatic management of psychotic disorders (e.g., schizophrenia). Drug therapy is integral to the management of acute psychotic episodes in patients with schizophrenia and generally is required for long-term stabilization to sustain symptom remission or control and to minimize the risk of relapse. Antipsychotic agents are the principal class of drugs used for the management of all phases of schizophrenia. Patient response and tolerance to antipsychotic agents are variable, and patients who do not respond to or tolerate one drug may be successfully treated with an agent from a different class or with a different adverse effect profile.

Clozapine has been shown to be an effective, relatively rapid-acting, broad-spectrum antipsychotic agent in both uncontrolled and controlled studies of patients with schizophrenia. In these studies, improvement in manifestations of schizophrenia was based on the results of various psychiatric rating scales, principally the Brief Psychiatric Rating Scale (BPRS) that assesses factors such as anergy, thought disturbance, activation, hostility/suspiciousness, and anxiety/depression. In clinical studies, clozapine improved both positive (florid symptomatology such as hallucinations, conceptual disorganization, and suspiciousness) and negative ("deficit" symptomatology such as emotional withdrawal, motor retardation, blunted affect, and disorientation) manifestations of schizophrenia; conventional (typical) antipsychotic agents appear to have lesser effects on negative manifestations of the disorder. In comparative studies, clozapine was at least as effective as, or more effective than several conventional antipsychotic agents, including chlorpromazine, haloperidol, perphenazine, or trifluoperazine.

Unlike conventional antipsychotic agents, however, clozapine generally does not induce extrapyramidal effects and has not been clearly implicated as a causative agent in tardive dyskinesia.

While the risks of adverse neurologic effects with long-term clozapine therapy remain to be fully elucidated, other adverse effects, including some potentially serious effects (e.g., severe neutropenia, seizures), may occur more frequently with clozapine therapy. Consequently, the manufacturers and most clinicians state that use of clozapine should be reserved for patients with severe disease that fails to respond adequately to other antipsychotic therapy. The American Psychiatric Association (APA) recommends that a trial of clozapine be considered in patients with schizophrenia who fail to respond or experience a partial or suboptimal response to adequate trials of 2 antipsychotic agents (including at least one second-generation [atypical] antipsychotic), in patients with a history of chronic and persistent suicidal ideation and behavior that has not responded to other treatments, and in patients with persistent hostility and aggression.

Treatment-resistant Schizophrenia Clozapine is used for the management of schizophrenia in severely ill patients who fail to respond adequately to standard antipsychotic therapy. Because of the risk of severe neutropenia and seizures associated with its use, clozapine should be used only in patients who have failed to respond adequately to standard antipsychotic treatment. (See Severe Neutropenia under Cautions: Hematologic Effects and also under Cautions: Precautions and Contraindications.)

Schizophrenia is a major psychotic disorder that frequently has devastating effects on various aspects of the patient's life and carries a high risk of suicide and other life-threatening behaviors. Manifestations of schizophrenia involve multiple psychologic processes, including perception (e.g., hallucinations), ideation, reality testing (e.g., delusions), emotion (e.g., flatness, inappropriate affect), thought processes (e.g., loose associations), behavior (e.g., catatonia, disorganization), attention, concentration, motivation (e.g., avolition, impaired intention and planning), and judgment. The principal manifestations of this disorder usually are described in terms of positive and negative (deficit) symptoms, and more recently, disorganized symptoms. Positive symptoms include hallucinations, delusions, bizarre behavior, hostility, uncooperativeness, and paranoid ideation, while negative symptoms include restricted range and intensity of emotional expression (affective flattening), reduced thought and speech productivity (alogia), anhedonia, apathy, and decreased initiation of goal-directed behavior (avolition). Disorganized symptoms include disorganized speech (thought disorder) and behavior and poor attention.

Evidence from both retrospective and controlled prospective studies indicates that clozapine is effective in many patients who fail to respond adequately to other antipsychotic therapy and/or in whom such therapy produces intolerable adverse effects. In a controlled, comparative study in patients with at least moderately severe schizophrenia whose disease was refractory to at least 3 antipsychotic agents from at least 2 different chemical classes during the past 5 years, an adequate clinical response (a 20% or greater decrease in total BPRS score and either a posttreatment Clinical Global Impressions [CGI] scale rating of mildly ill or a posttreatment BPRS score of 35 or less) was noted after 1–6 weeks of therapy in 30% of patients receiving clozapine (mean maximum dosage exceeding 600 mg daily) compared with 4% of patients receiving chlorpromazine (mean maximum dosage exceeding 1200 mg daily) plus benztropine. In addition, clozapine was substantially more effective than chlorpromazine plus benztropine in improving both positive and negative manifestations of schizophrenia. In this study, resistance to antipsychotic treatment prior to entry into the clozapine/chlorpromazine comparative phase was confirmed by a 6-week trial of haloperidol (mean dosage of 61 mg daily) combined with benztropine. This study provides evidence from both categorical and continuous measures not only of clozapine's efficacy as an antipsychotic agent but also of its superiority over conventional antipsychotic drug therapy in a well-defined group of antipsychotic-resistant patients. Similar 6-week response rates in treatment-resistant schizophrenia have been reported in other studies with the drug. Clinically important improvement in quality of life and social functioning, including deinstitutionalization, interpersonal relationships, and ability to hold a job or attend school, also have been reported following initiation of clozapine therapy in patients with antipsychotic-resistant schizophrenia.

For additional information on the symptomatic management of schizophrenia, including treatment recommendations, see Schizophrenia and Other Psychotic Disorders under Uses: Psychotic Disorders, in the Phenothiazines General Statement 28:16.08.24.

Pediatric Considerations. Although the manufacturers state that the safety and efficacy of clozapine in pediatric patients have not been established, the drug has been successfully used for the management of childhood-onset schizophrenia in a limited number of treatment-resistant children and adolescents†. While the lower risk of extrapyramidal adverse effects and tardive dyskinesia during treatment with atypical antipsychotic agents such as clozapine compared with conventional antipsychotic agents represents an advantage in the treatment of childhood-onset schizophrenia, concerns regarding serious adverse effects (e.g., neutropenia, seizures) associated with clozapine limit its use in clinical practice. (See Cautions: Pediatric Precautions.) Therefore, the American Academy of Child and Adolescent Psychiatry (AACAP) states that clozapine is not considered a first-line agent, and should be reserved for treatment-refractory patients who have failed to respond to adequate therapeutic trials (i.e., use of sufficient dosages over a period of 6 weeks) of at least 2 other first-line antipsychotic agents. For additional information on the symptomatic management of childhood-onset schizophrenia, see Pediatric Considerations under Psychotic Disorders: Schizophrenia, in Uses in the Phenothiazines General Statement 28:16.08.24.

In one randomized, double-blind, clinical study conducted by the National Institute of Mental Health (NIMH), a limited number of children and adolescents (mean: 14 years of age) with childhood-onset schizophrenia (i.e., development of the disorder by 12 years of age or younger) who were intolerant and/or nonresponsive to at least 2 different antipsychotic agents were treated with either clozapine (up to 525 mg daily; mean final dosage 176 mg daily) or haloperidol (up to 27 mg daily; mean final dosage 16 mg daily) for 6 weeks. In this study, children and adolescents receiving clozapine had substantially greater reductions in both positive and negative symptoms of schizophrenia than those receiving haloperidol. Additional follow-up of these patients over a 2-year period indicated that, as reported in adults, maximal antipsychotic effects in schizophrenic children and adolescents may not be evident until after 6–9 months of clozapine therapy. For most children and adolescents in the study, clozapine improved interpersonal functioning and enabled a return to a less restrictive setting. However, mild to moderate neutropenia occurred in 24% of the patients, and 29% required therapy with an anticonvulsant.

Suicide Risk Reduction in Schizophrenia and Schizoaffective Disorder Clozapine is used to reduce the risk of recurrent suicidal behavior in patients with schizophrenia or schizoaffective disorder who are judged to be at chronic risk for such behavior, based on history and recent clinical state. Efficacy of clozapine for this indication has been established in a multicenter, randomized, open-label clinical study (the International Suicide Prevention Trial [InterSePT]) of 2 years' duration comparing clozapine and olanzapine in patients with schizophrenia (62%) or schizoaffective disorder (38%) who were judged to be at risk for recurrent suicidal behavior. These patients either had attempted suicide or had been hospitalized to prevent a suicide attempt within the 3 years prior to their baseline evaluation or had demonstrated moderate-to-severe suicidal ideation with a depressive component or command hallucinations to do self-harm within 1 week prior to their baseline evaluation. Treatment resistance (i.e., resistance to standard antipsychotic drug therapies) was not a requirement for inclusion in this study, and only 27% of the total patient population was identified as being treatment resistant at baseline.

In the InterSePT study, patients who received flexible dosages of clozapine (mean dosage: 274.2 mg daily) for approximately 2 years had a 26% reduction in their risk for suicide attempts or hospitalization to prevent suicide compared with those who received flexible dosages of olanzapine (mean dosage: 16.6 mg daily); the treatment-resistant status of patients was not predictive of response to clozapine or olanzapine. The cumulative probability of experiencing a suicide attempt, including a completed suicide, or hospitalization due to imminent suicide risk (including increased level of surveillance for suicidal behavior for patients already hospitalized) also was lower for patients receiving clozapine (24%) than for those receiving olanzapine (32%) at year 2. In addition, patients receiving clozapine had a statistically significant longer delay in the time to recurrent suicidal behavior than those receiving olanzapine. These results, however, may have been confounded by extensive use of other treatments to reduce the suicide risk, including concomitant psychotropic agents (84% with antipsychotics; 65% with anxiolytics; 53% with antidepressants; 28% with mood stabilizers), hospitalization, and psychotherapy, the contributions of which to clozapine's efficacy are unknown.

Some clinicians state that methodologic problems (e.g., lack of actively suicidal patients in the study, possible bias and unblinding of suicide monitoring board members during the study, use of concomitant psychotropic agents) associated with the InterSePT study limit definitive conclusions about the efficacy of clozapine for prevention of suicide in patients with schizophrenia or schizoaffective disorder. The FDA advises clinicians to interpret the results of the InterSePT study only as evidence of the efficacy of clozapine in delaying time to recurrent suicidal behavior, and not as efficacy of the drug for treatment of suicidal behaviors or as a demonstration of the superior efficacy of clozapine over olanzapine. However, the APA states that, based on the available evidence from the InterSePT study, clozapine should be preferentially considered for schizophrenia patients with a history of chronic and persistent suicidal ideation and behaviors. Decisions to initiate clozapine therapy or switch patients from other antipsychotics to clozapine, therefore, should be individualized. In addition, safety and efficacy of clozapine in actively suicidal patients have yet to be determined.

■ **Parkinsonian Syndrome** Clozapine has been used in a limited number of patients with advanced, idiopathic parkinsonian syndrome for the management of dopaminomimetic psychosis† associated with antiparkinsonian drug therapy, but adverse effects such as sedation, confusion, and increased parkinsonian manifestations may limit the benefit of clozapine therapy in these patients. Attempts to relieve antiparkinsonian drug-induced delusions, paranoia, and hallucinations by reduction of antiparkinsonian drug dosage or administration of typical antipsychotic agents often aggravate parkinsonian symptoms. Limited data suggest that administration of clozapine in dosages of 6.25–400 mg daily can improve psychotic symptoms within a few days, reportedly without exacerbating parkinsonian manifestations. However, in a controlled study in a limited number of patients receiving clozapine dosages up to 250 mg daily, exacerbation of parkinsonian manifestations and development of delirium occurred frequently despite prevention of antiparkinsonian drug-induced deterioration of psychosis; it has been suggested that rapid clozapine dosage escalation may have contributed to the observed negative effect on parkinsonian manifestations and delirium. Clozapine dosages of 100–250 mg daily reportedly have been associated with hypersalivation, hypophonia, bradykinesia, and considerable sedation in patients with idiopathic parkinsonian syndrome, and withdrawal of clozapine therapy or a decrease in dosage also has exacerbated parkinsonian manifestations. Some clinicians suggest that the dosage of clozapine required to treat drug-induced dopaminomimetic psychosis may be substantially less than that required for treatment of psychosis in young, otherwise healthy individuals and that clozapine therapy should be initiated at low dosages (e.g., 6.25–50 mg daily) with cautious upward titration (e.g., to a maximum of 100–200 mg daily). Other clinicians have suggested that clozapine be used only as a last resort in patients with drug-induced dopaminomimetic psychosis.

Dosage and Administration

■ **Administration** Clozapine is administered orally without regard to meals; administration in divided doses may help minimize the risk of certain adverse effects. If daytime sleepiness occurs during therapy, bedtime administration may be helpful. The orally disintegrating tablets and conventional tablets of clozapine are bioequivalent; the oral suspension and conventional tablets of the drug also are bioequivalent. Clozapine also has been administered IM†, but a parenteral preparation currently is not commercially available in the US.

Prior to initiating clozapine therapy, a baseline complete blood cell (CBC) count, including the absolute neutrophil count (ANC), must be obtained to ensure the presence of a normal baseline neutrophil count and for later comparisons. In the general population, the baseline ANC must be at least 1500/mm^3 before clozapine therapy can be initiated. In patients with documented benign ethnic neutropenia (BEN), the baseline ANC must be at least 1000/mm^3 in order to be eligible for clozapine therapy. Regular ANC monitoring is required during clozapine therapy because of the risk of severe neutropenia associated with the drug. (See Severe Neutropenia under Cautions: Hematologic Effects.)

Patients receiving clozapine orally disintegrating tablets (e.g., FazaClo®) should be instructed not to remove a tablet from the blister until just prior to dosing. The tablet should not be pushed through the foil; instead, the foil blister backing should be peeled from the blister. The tablet should then be gently removed and immediately placed on the tongue, where it rapidly disintegrates in saliva, and then subsequently swallowed with or without liquid, or the tablet can be chewed as desired.

Clozapine oral suspension (Versacloz®) should be shaken for 10 seconds prior to each use. The bottle adapter and calibrated oral dosing syringe supplied by the manufacturer should be used to administer the suspension. After withdrawing the appropriate dose into the calibrated oral dosing syringe, the dose should be administered directly into the patient's mouth; clozapine oral suspension should not be stored in the syringe for later use.

Restricted Distribution Program Because of the risk of severe neutropenia, clozapine is available only through a restricted distribution program, the Clozapine REMS program. As of October 12, 2015, all previous clozapine registries, which had been maintained individually by each manufacturer of clozapine, were replaced by the Clozapine REMS program. Under this single, shared program, only ANC is used to monitor patients for clozapine-induced neutropenia; white blood cell (WBC) count, which previously also was required, was considered to be less relevant for monitoring neutropenia and is no longer required. In addition, ANC thresholds for clozapine treatment interruption were lowered from the previous clozapine registry requirements. Furthermore, the shared Clozapine REMS program established lower acceptable ANC levels for patients with documented benign ethnic neutropenia (BEN) and discontinued the National Non-Rechallenge Master File, allowing patients who previously were ineligible to receive clozapine due to low ANC or WBC count to be treated with the drug. (See Severe Neutropenia under Cautions: Hematologic Effects.)

Prescribers and pharmacies must be certified with the Clozapine REMS program; to be certified, physicians or an authorized representative of a pharmacy must enroll and complete training before they can prescribe or dispense clozapine, respectively. Certified prescribers must enroll patients in the Clozapine REMS program and report patients' ANC values according to the recommended monitoring guidelines. Pharmacies that are certified to dispense clozapine must train their staff members to verify that the prescriber is certified and the patient is enrolled in the program, and must verify that the ANC is current and acceptable for each patient or that continued treatment has been authorized by the prescriber before dispensing the drug to the patient. For additional information and to enroll in the program, clinicians, patients, and caregivers may visit the Clozapine REMS program website at http://www.clozapinerems.com or contact 844-267-8678.

■ **Dosage** Cautious dosage titration and administration of clozapine in divided doses are necessary to minimize the risk of certain adverse effects such as orthostatic hypotension, bradycardia, syncope, seizures, and sedation. (See Cautions: Nervous System Effects and also see Cautions: Cardiovascular Effects.)

Treatment-resistant Schizophrenia **Adult Dosage.** For the management of treatment-resistant schizophrenia, the usual initial adult dosage of clozapine is 12.5 mg given orally once or twice daily. If the drug is well tolerated, dosage may be increased in increments of 25–50 mg daily over a 2-week period until a target dosage of 300–450 mg daily (administered in divided doses) is achieved. Subsequent dosage increases can be made once or twice weekly in increments of up to 100 mg. The manufacturers state that use of a low initial daily dosage, a gradual titration schedule, and administration of the drug in divided doses are necessary to minimize the risks of orthostatic hypotension, bradycardia, syncope, seizures, and sedation. (See Cautions: Nervous System Effects and also see Cautions: Cardiovascular Effects.)

Daily administration of clozapine in divided doses should continue until an effective and tolerable dosage is reached, usually within 2–5 weeks. Although many patients may respond adequately to dosages between 200–600 mg daily, a dosage of 600–900 mg daily may be required in some patients. In the multicenter study that provides the principal support for the effectiveness of clozapine in patients resistant to standard antipsychotic therapy, the maximum dosage of clozapine was 900 mg daily, which was given in 3 divided doses. The mean and median clozapine dosages in this study both were approximately 600 mg daily. Although some clinicians suggest that dosages exceeding 450–500 mg daily have not been shown to be associated with increased therapeutic benefit, others state that added response is observed at higher dosages in some patients and stress the need for individualized therapy. The manufacturers and most clinicians recommend that the maximum daily dosage of clozapine not exceed 900 mg. Because of the possibility that high dosages of clozapine may be associated with an increased risk of adverse reactions, particularly seizures, patients generally should be given adequate time to respond to a given dosage before dosage escalation is considered.

Pediatric Dosage. The dosage of clozapine for the management of schizophrenia in children and adolescents† has not been established. However, the National Institute of Mental Health (NIMH) protocol used an initial dosage of 6.25–25 mg given orally daily depending on the patient's weight. Dosages could be increased in this study every 3–4 days by 1–2 times the initial dose on an individual basis up to a maximum of 525 mg daily.

Duration of Therapy. While some clinicians state that clozapine therapy should be continued for longer than 6 weeks only in patients who exhibit substantial benefit within this period, others state that even less than substantial degrees of benefit may warrant continued therapy and that an adequate trial of clozapine may require at least 12 weeks (e.g., at daily dosages of 200–600 mg daily) or possibly 5–9 months or longer unless clinical deterioration or intolerable or potentially serious toxicity precludes it. The manufacturers state that patients who respond to clozapine therapy generally should continue to receive maintenance treatment with the drug at their effective dosage beyond the acute episode. Extended therapy in patients failing to show an acceptable response to clozapine generally should be avoided because of the substantial, continuing risks of neutropenia and seizures. (See Severe Neutropenia under Cautions: Hematologic Effects and also see Seizures under Cautions: Nervous System Effects.)

The American Psychiatric Association (APA) states that prudent long-term treatment options in patients with schizophrenia with remitted first or multiple episodes include either indefinite maintenance therapy or gradual discontinuance of the antipsychotic agent with close follow-up and a plan to reinstitute treatment upon symptom recurrence. Discontinuance of antipsychotic therapy should be considered only after a period of at least 1 year of symptom remission or optimal response while receiving the antipsychotic agent. In patients who have had multiple previous psychotic episodes or 2 psychotic episodes within 5 years, indefinite maintenance antipsychotic treatment is recommended.

Suicide Risk Reduction For suicide risk reduction in schizophrenia and schizoaffective disorder, the usual initial adult dosage of clozapine is 12.5 mg given orally once or twice daily. If the drug is well tolerated, dosage may be increased in increments of 25–50 mg daily over a 2-week period until a target dosage of 300–450 mg daily (administered in divided doses) is achieved. Subsequent dosage increases can be made once or twice weekly in increments of up to 100 mg. The manufacturers state that use of a low initial daily dosage, a gradual titration schedule, and administration of the drug in divided doses are necessary to minimize the risks of orthostatic hypotension, bradycardia, syncope, seizures, and sedation. (See Cautions: Nervous System Effects and also see Cautions: Cardiovascular Effects.) In the multicenter InterSePT study that provides the principal support for the effectiveness of clozapine for suicide risk reduction, mean dosage was about 300 mg daily (range: 12.5–900 mg daily).

The manufacturers state that patients who respond to clozapine therapy generally should continue to receive maintenance treatment with the drug at their effective dosage beyond the acute episode; efficacy of clozapine for this indication was demonstrated over a 2-year treatment period in the InterSePT study.

Discontinuance of Therapy In the event of planned discontinuance of clozapine therapy, gradual reduction in dosage over a 1- to 2-week period is recommended if there is no evidence of moderate to severe neutropenia. However, if abrupt discontinuance of therapy is required because of moderate to severe neutropenia, ANC should be monitored according to the neutropenia monitoring recommendations. If abrupt discontinuance of clozapine is required for reasons unrelated to neutropenia, continuation of the existing ANC monitoring schedule is recommended; patients in the general population should be monitored until their ANC is in the normal range (i.e., at least 1500/mm^3) while patients with BEN should be monitored until their ANC is at least 1000/mm^3 or above their baseline. Additional ANC monitoring is necessary in any patient reporting onset of fever (temperature of 38.5°C or greater) during the 2 weeks after clozapine discontinuance. (See Severe Neutropenia under Cautions: Hematologic Effects.) Patients should be observed carefully for recurrence of psychotic symptoms and symptoms related to cholinergic rebound such as profuse sweating, headache, nausea, vomiting, and diarrhea. Sudden withdrawal from clozapine therapy can lead to rapid decompensation and rebound psychosis. (See Other Nervous System Effects under Cautions: Nervous System Effects.)

Reinitiation of Therapy If clozapine therapy is restarted in patients who have had even brief interruptions (i.e., 2 days or more since the last dose) in therapy, dosage generally should be titrated as with initial therapy (i.e., starting with 12.5 mg once or twice daily) to minimize the risk of hypotension, bradycardia, and syncope. If this dosage is well tolerated, dosage may be titrated back to the previous therapeutic dosage more quickly than recommended during initial treatment.

For clozapine treatment interruptions of less than 30 days in patients with normal ANC values, the same ANC monitoring schedule as before the treatment interruption may be continued. If clozapine treatment is interrupted for 30 days or more, the ANC monitoring schedule must be restarted as with initial therapy. (See Severe Neutropenia under Cautions: Hematologic Effects.)

Patients who develop severe neutropenia (ANC less than 500/mm^3) during clozapine therapy generally should not be restarted on the drug unless the clinician determines that the benefits of the drug outweigh the risks. (See Severe Neutropenia under Cautions: Hematologic Effects.)

■ **Dosage in Renal and Hepatic Impairment or Poor CYP2D6 Metabolizers** Although the pharmacokinetics of clozapine have not been specifically studied in patients with renal or hepatic impairment, increased plasma clozapine concentrations are possible in such patients since the drug is almost completely metabolized and then excreted. The manufacturers state that dosage reduction may be necessary in patients with substantial impairment of renal or hepatic function.

The manufacturers state that dosage reduction of clozapine also may be necessary in patients who are known poor metabolizers of cytochrome P-450 isoenzyme 2D6 (CYP2D6).

Cautions

Although clozapine differs chemically from the phenothiazines, the drug may be capable of producing many of the toxic manifestations of phenothiazine derivatives. Not all adverse effects of the phenothiazines have been reported with clozapine, but the possibility that they may occur should be considered. Adverse effects of clozapine and the phenothiazines are numerous and may involve nearly all organ systems. Although these effects usually are reversible when dosage is reduced or the drug is discontinued, some effects may be irreversible and, rarely, fatal. In some patients, unexpected death associated with antipsychotic therapy has been attributed to cardiac arrest or asphyxia resulting from failure of the gag reflex. (See Cautions: Cardiovascular Effects.) In other cases, the cause of death could not be determined or definitely attributed to antipsychotic drug therapy. An increased risk of death has been observed in geriatric patients with dementia-related psychoses receiving antipsychotic agents. (See Cautions: Geriatric Precautions.)

The most frequent adverse effects of clozapine involve the central and autonomic nervous systems (e.g., drowsiness or sedation, hypersalivation) and the cardiovascular system (e.g., tachycardia, orthostatic hypotension, syncope). While the frequency and severity of some adverse effects (e.g., extrapyramidal reactions, tardive dyskinesia) appear to be less with clozapine than with other antipsychotic agents, other potentially serious adverse effects (e.g., severe neutropenia, seizures) may occur more frequently with clozapine therapy, and the potential risks and benefits should be evaluated carefully whenever therapy with the drug is considered. Because of the risk of severe clozapine-associated neutropenia, which may lead to serious and potentially fatal infections, clozapine is available only through a restricted distribution program that ensures appropriate monitoring of absolute neutrophil count (ANC). (See REMS and also see Severe Neutropenia under Cautions: Hematologic Effects.)

■ **Hematologic Effects** ***Severe Neutropenia*** Clozapine has been associated with neutropenia (i.e., a low absolute neutrophil count [ANC]) which can, when severe, increase the risk of serious and potentially fatal infections. Previously, the terms "severe leukopenia," "severe granulocytopenia," and "agranulocytosis" were used in the clozapine prescribing information (labeling) to describe this hematologic effect; however, to improve and standardize understanding, these terms have been replaced with "severe neutropenia" throughout the labeling for the drug. The ANC is usually available as a component of the complete blood count (CBC), including differential, and is considered more clinically relevant for drug-induced neutropenia than the white blood cell (WBC) count. Severe neutropenia is defined as an ANC value of less than 500/mm^3 and occurs in a small percentage of patients receiving clozapine therapy.

Previously described agranulocytosis, which was defined as an ANC less than 500/mm^3 and characterized by leukopenia (WBC count less than 2000/mm^3) and relative lymphopenia, has been reported to have an estimated cumulative incidence of 1–2% after 1 year of clozapine therapy, as compared with an estimated incidence of 0.1–1% for phenothiazine-induced agranulocytosis. Some evidence has suggested that the incidence of clozapine-induced agranulocytosis is at least 10 times greater than the incidence associated with other antipsychotic agents, although it also has been suggested that the incidence of clozapine-induced agranulocytosis may be no higher than that associated with phenothiazines.

The precise mechanism by which clozapine induces neutropenia is not known and is not dose-dependent, but both immunologic and toxic mechanisms (including a direct myelotoxic effect of the drug and/or its metabolites) have been implicated. Some evidence suggests that granulocyte antibodies may be involved.

Identified risk factors for clozapine-induced neutropenia or agranulocytosis include advanced age, female gender, and African-American and Asian ethnicity; pediatric patients also are at an increased risk. Results of genetic typing indicate that genetic factors marked by a major histocompatibility complex haplotype (HLA-B38, DR4, DQw3) may be associated with the susceptibility of certain Jewish patients with schizophrenia to develop agranulocytosis when treated with clozapine; the incidence of some phenotypes common among Ashkenazi Jews has been found to be greatly increased in patients with clozapine-induced agranulocytosis.

The risk of clozapine-induced neutropenia appears to be greatest during the first 18 weeks of therapy and declines thereafter. However, rare cases of neutropenia or agranulocytosis have been reported after several years of treatment with the drug.

Benign ethnic neutropenia (BEN) is a condition observed in certain ethnic groups whose average ANC values are lower than standard laboratory ranges for neutrophils. BEN has an approximate prevalence of 25–50% in individuals of African descent and also is observed in some Middle Eastern ethnic groups and in other non-Caucasian ethnic groups with darker skin; the condition is more common in men than women. Patients with BEN have normal hematopoietic stem cell numbers and myeloid maturation, are healthy, and do not suffer from repeated or severe infections. Such patients are not at increased risk for developing clozapine-induced neutropenia. BEN may be diagnosed by repeated low ANC measurements (less than 1500/mm^3 and usually 1000/mm^3 or below) for several months without identifiable causes of the neutropenia. Additional evaluation may be necessary in some patients to determine whether their baseline neutropenia is caused by BEN. Consultation with a hematologist should be considered in patients with low baseline ANC values before initiating or during clozapine therapy, if necessary. Patients with documented BEN have different ANC monitoring and treatment recommendations during clozapine therapy than the general population because of their lower baseline ANC levels. (See Table 2.)

Because of the risk of severe neutropenia associated with clozapine use, patients must have a baseline CBC and ANC performed before initiation of therapy and regular ANC monitoring during treatment with the drug. (See Restricted Distribution Program under Dosage and Administration: Administration.) Clozapine therapy should not be initiated if baseline ANC is less than 1500/mm^3 (or less than 1000/mm^3 in patients with documented BEN).

When initiating clozapine therapy, ANC must be monitored every week for the first 6 months of therapy and then every 2 weeks for the next 6 months if ANC values remain in the normal range. If ANC values continue to be maintained in the normal range after an additional 6 months (i.e., following 12 months of continuous treatment), the frequency of monitoring may be reduced to once every 4 weeks thereafter. If clozapine treatment is interrupted for 30 days or longer, the initial ANC monitoring schedule should be restarted beginning with once-weekly ANC monitoring.

See Tables 1 and 2 for clozapine treatment recommendations based on ANC monitoring in the general patient population and in patients with BEN, respectively.

For hospice patients (i.e., patients who are terminally ill with an estimated life expectancy of 6 months or less) receiving clozapine therapy, the ANC monitoring frequency may be reduced by the clinician to once every 6 months, after a discussion with the patient and caregiver. Treatment decisions in such individuals should weigh the importance of ANC monitoring in the context of the need to control psychiatric symptoms and the patient's terminal illness.

Table 1. Clozapine Treatment Recommendations based on ANC Monitoring in the General Patient Population

ANC Value	Treatment Recommendations	Frequency of ANC Monitoring
Normal range (ANC ≥1500/mm^3)	Initiate treatment If treatment interrupted <30 days, continue monitoring as before If treatment interrupted ≥30 days, monitor as if new patient	Weekly from initiation to 6 months Every 2 weeks from 6–12 months Monthly after 12 months
Discontinuance for reasons other than neutropenia	See Discontinuance of Therapy under Dosage and Administration: Dosage	
Mild neutropenia (ANC 1000–1499/mm^3)[a]	Continue treatment	3 times weekly until ANC ≥1500/mm^3 When ANC ≥1500/mm^3, return to patient's last normal range ANC monitoring interval, if clinically appropriate
Moderate neutropenia (ANC 500–999/mm^3)[a]	Recommend hematology consultation Interrupt treatment for suspected clozapine-induced neutropenia Resume treatment once ANC ≥1000/mm^3	Daily until ANC ≥1000/mm^3 3 times weekly until ANC ≥1500/mm^3 When ANC ≥1500/mm^3, monitor weekly for 4 weeks, then return to the patient's last normal range ANC monitoring interval, if clinically appropriate
Severe neutropenia (ANC <500/mm^3)[a]	Recommend hematology consultation Interrupt treatment for suspected clozapine-induced neutropenia Do not rechallenge unless prescriber determines benefits outweigh risks	Daily until ANC ≥1000/mm^3 3 times weekly until ANC ≥1500/mm^3 If patient rechallenged, resume treatment and monitor as new patient under normal range monitoring once ANC ≥1500/mm^3

[a] Confirm all *initial* reports of ANC <1500/mm^3 with a repeat ANC measurement within 24 hours.

Table 2. Clozapine Treatment Recommendations based on ANC Monitoring in Patients with Benign Ethnic Neutropenia (BEN)

ANC Value	Treatment Recommendations	Frequency of ANC Monitoring
Normal BEN range (established ANC baseline ≥1000/mm^3)	Obtain ≥2 baseline ANC values before initiating treatment If treatment interrupted <30 days, continue monitoring as before If treatment interrupted ≥30 days, monitor as if new patient	Weekly from initiation to 6 months Every 2 weeks from 6–12 months Monthly after 12 months
Discontinuance of treatment for reasons other than neutropenia	See Discontinuance of Therapy under Dosage and Administration: Dosage	
BEN neutropenia (ANC 500–999/mm^3)[a]	Recommend hematology consultation Continue treatment	3 times weekly until ANC ≥1000/mm^3 or at patient's known baseline When ANC ≥1000/mm^3 or at patient's known baseline, monitor weekly for 4 weeks, then return to the patient's last normal BEN range ANC monitoring interval, if clinically appropriate
BEN severe neutropenia (ANC <500/mm^3)[a]	Recommend hematology consultation Interrupt treatment for suspected clozapine-induced neutropenia Do not rechallenge unless prescriber determines benefits outweigh risks	Daily until ANC ≥500/mm^3 3 times weekly until ANC at or above patient's baseline If patient rechallenged, resume treatment as a new patient under normal range monitoring once ANC ≥1000/mm^3 or at patient's baseline

[a] Confirm all *initial* reports of ANC <1500/mm^3 with a repeat ANC measurement within 24 hours.

If a patient develops fever (temperature of 38.5°C or higher) during therapy, clozapine should be interrupted and an ANC should be obtained. Fever is often the first sign of neutropenic infection. If fever occurs in any patient with an ANC value less than 1000/mm^3, the patient should be appropriately evaluated (see Tables 1 and 2) and treated for infection. A hematology consultation should be considered in all clozapine-treated patients with fever or neutropenia.

Although some clinicians have suggested that body temperature be measured at least once daily for the first 18 weeks of clozapine therapy, others state that such monitoring is not an adequate means of assessing infection in clozapine-treated patients because of the drug's pharmacologic potential for causing temperature elevation (see Cautions: Fever). Patients receiving clozapine should be advised to immediately report the appearance of lethargy, weakness, fever, sore throat, or any other potential manifestations of infection.

Supportive therapy with biosynthetic hematopoietic agents, including filgrastim, a recombinant human granulocyte colony-stimulating factor (G-CSF), and sargramostim, a recombinant human granulocyte-macrophage colony-stimulating factor (GM-CSF), has been effective in a limited number of patients with clozapine-induced neutropenia and agranulocytosis. Consultation with a hematologist and infectious disease expert is recommended.

Lithium has been used successfully in the treatment of clozapine-induced neutropenia or to facilitate initiation of therapy or rechallenge† with the drug in a limited number of patients, including in some patients with BEN. However, lithium should be used concurrently with clozapine with caution because, in addition to the possible increased risk of NMS and seizures, the drug can mask the development or delay the detection of severe neutropenia and other blood dyscrasias. (See Drug Interactions: Other CNS-active Agents.)

When neutropenia is diagnosed and clozapine therapy is discontinued, patients usually recover in 7–28 days. Most of these patients require further antipsychotic therapy because of a recurrence of psychotic symptoms. (See Other Nervous System Effects under Cautions: Nervous System Effects.) Since there appears to be no cross-sensitivity between clozapine and other antipsychotics in terms of hematologic toxicity, other antipsychotic drugs generally may be used without causing further hematologic complications in patients who develop clozapine-induced neutropenia. Patients who develop severe clozapine-induced neutropenia generally should *not* be rechallenged with clozapine. However, for some patients who have no acceptable alternatives to clozapine, the risk of serious psychiatric illness from discontinuing treatment may outweigh the risk of severe neutropenia upon rechallenge; in such cases, consultation with a hematology specialist may be helpful in deciding whether to rechallenge a patient with clozapine.

Eosinophilia Eosinophilia (defined as blood eosinophil count exceeding 700/mm^3) has been reported in approximately 1% of patients who received clozapine therapy in clinical trials. Clozapine-associated eosinophilia usually occurs during the first month of therapy and has been associated with myocarditis, pancreatitis, hepatitis, colitis, and/or nephritis in some patients. Such organ involvement could be consistent with drug reaction with eosinophilia and systemic symptoms (DRESS; also known as multiorgan hypersensitivity or drug-induced hypersensitivity syndrome).

The manufacturers state that if eosinophilia develops during clozapine therapy, the patient should be evaluated promptly for signs and symptoms of systemic reactions such as rash or other allergic symptoms, myocarditis, or other organ-specific disease associated with eosinophilia. If clozapine-associated systemic disease is suspected, the drug should be immediately discontinued. If a cause of eosinophilia unrelated to clozapine is identified (e.g., asthma, allergies, collagen vascular disease, parasitic infections, specific neoplasms), the underlying cause should be treated and clozapine therapy may be continued.

Clozapine-associated eosinophilia also has occurred without organ involvement and can resolve without intervention. In such cases, clozapine therapy may be continued with careful monitoring. If the patient's total eosinophil count continues to increase over several weeks in the absence of organ involvement, the decision whether to interrupt clozapine therapy and rechallenge after the eosinophil count decreases should be made based on the overall clinical assessment, in consultation with an internist or hematologist. There have been reports of successful rechallenge after discontinuance of clozapine without recurrence of eosinophilia.

Other Hematologic Effects Other hematologic effects reported with clozapine therapy include leukopenia/decreased WBC count and neutropenia, which has been reported in 3% of patients. Other clozapine-induced hematologic effects reportedly include basophilia and a substantial reduction in B cells. Elevated hemoglobin/hematocrit, elevated erythrocyte sedimentation rate (ESR), sepsis, thrombocytosis, and thrombocytopenia have been reported in patients receiving clozapine during postmarketing surveillance; however, a causal relationship to the drug has not been established.

■ **Nervous System Effects** ***Seizures*** Clozapine lowers the seizure threshold and can cause EEG changes, including the occurrence of spike and wave complexes. Seizures reportedly occurred in approximately 3.5% of patients exposed to the drug during clinical trials in the US (cumulative annual incidence of approximately 5%). In contrast, a seizure incidence of approximately 1% has been reported in patients treated with other antipsychotic agents. The risk of seizures with clozapine therapy is dose related, with a reported incidence of approximately 0.6–2% at dosages less than 300 mg daily, 1.4–5% at 300–600 mg daily, and 5–14% at high dosages (600–900 mg daily). Clozapine-induced seizures may be associated with rapid dosage escalations, particularly in patients receiving concomitant therapy with drugs that may cause increased plasma concentrations of clozapine. (See Seizures under Cautions: Precautions and Contraindications.)

One patient receiving clozapine experienced a generalized tonic-clonic (grand mal) seizure following accidental ingestion of an extra dose (total dose ingested within 24 hours: 1050 mg); the same patient had another seizure several weeks later, 2 hours after a usual 450-mg morning dose. Results of plasma clozapine determinations obtained at the time of the seizures revealed plasma clozapine concentrations of approximately 2000 ng/mL in each case. Another patient who had been taking clozapine for 27 months had a generalized tonic-clonic seizure following an apparent intentional overdosage (total dose ingested within 24 hours: approximately 3 g), after which the patient made an uneventful recovery. One hour after the seizure, the patient's plasma clozapine concentration was 1313 ng/mL.

Discontinuance of clozapine therapy, at least temporarily, should be seriously considered in patients who experience seizures while receiving the drug; however, some clinicians state that reduced clozapine dosage and/or, occasionally, addition of anticonvulsant therapy may adequately ameliorate this effect. If clozapine therapy is to be continued in such patients, many clinicians recommend obtaining additional informed consent from the patient. In patients in whom clozapine is withheld, it has been suggested that therapy with the drug can be reinitiated at one-half the previous dosage. Clozapine dosage may then be increased gradually, if clinically indicated, and the need for concomitant anticonvulsant therapy should be considered. Some clinicians recommend that patients who have experienced a clozapine-induced seizure *not* be given clozapine dosages exceeding 600 mg daily unless the results of an EEG performed prior to the anticipated dosage increase are normal; others suggest addition of anticonvulsant therapy and/or consultation with a neurologist in managing such patients. In patients with preexisting seizure disorders who are treated concomitantly with certain anticonvulsants and clozapine, the anticonvulsant dosage may need to be increased. (See Drug Interactions: Drugs Affecting Hepatic Microsomal Enzymes.)

Extrapyramidal Reactions In contrast to some other antipsychotic agents, clozapine has little or no potential for causing certain acute extrapyramidal effects (e.g., dystonias). Such effects, when they occur, have been limited principally to tremor, restlessness, rigidity, and akathisia. In addition, marked or total remission of such manifestations induced by other antipsychotics has occurred during treatment with clozapine in some patients.

One case of clozapine-associated tardive dystonia (blepharospasm) has been reported; the patient's symptoms in this case were alleviated by discontinuance of clozapine and initiation of clonazepam therapy.

Neuroleptic Malignant Syndrome Neuroleptic malignant syndrome (NMS), a potentially fatal syndrome, has been reported in patients receiving antipsychotic agents, including clozapine. NMS attributable to clozapine therapy alone has been reported in some patients, and there also have been reports of NMS in patients treated concomitantly with clozapine and lithium or other CNS drugs; some clinicians suggest that NMS may be more likely to occur when clozapine or other antipsychotic agents are used concomitantly with lithium. Manifestations of NMS (e.g., muscle rigidity, hyperpyrexia, tachycardia, increased serum creatine kinase [CK, creatine phosphokinase, CPK], diaphoresis, somnolence), all of which may not occur in all patients with the condition, have occurred in a few patients treated with clozapine alone or combined with lithium or carbamazepine; resolution of the syndrome occurred following discontinuance of clozapine. However, clozapine also has been used successfully and apparently without recurrence of NMS in at least one patient who developed the syndrome while receiving chlorpromazine. Atypical presentations of NMS (e.g., absence of or lessened rigidity, absence of fever) also have been reported in some patients receiving clozapine.

The diagnostic evaluation of patients with NMS is complicated. In arriving at a diagnosis, serious medical illnesses (e.g., severe neutropenia, infection) and extrapyramidal symptoms must be excluded. Other important considerations in the differential diagnosis include central anticholinergic toxicity, heat stroke, drug fever, and primary CNS pathology.

The management of NMS should include immediate discontinuance of antipsychotic agents and other drugs not considered essential to concurrent therapy, intensive symptomatic treatment and medical monitoring, and treatment of any concomitant serious medical conditions for which specific treatments are available. There currently is no specific drug therapy for NMS, although dantrolene, bromocriptine, amantadine, and benzodiazepines have been used in a limited number of patients. If a patient requires antipsychotic therapy following recovery from NMS, the potential reintroduction of drug therapy should be carefully considered. In addition, such patients should be carefully monitored since NMS may recur. For additional information on NMS, including treatment, see Neuroleptic Malignant Syndrome under Cautions: Nervous System Effects, in the Phenothiazines General Statement 28:16.08.24.

Tardive Dyskinesia Use of antipsychotic agents, including clozapine, may be associated with tardive dyskinesia, a syndrome of potentially irreversible, involuntary, dyskinetic movements. However, clozapine is considered less likely to cause tardive dyskinesia than many other antipsychotic agents, and dyskinetic movements in some patients have reportedly improved with clozapine therapy.

The risk of developing tardive dyskinesia and the likelihood that it will become irreversible are believed to increase as the duration of treatment and the total cumulative dose of antipsychotic drugs administered to the patient increase. However, the syndrome can develop following relatively brief treatment periods at low dosages. Management of tardive dyskinesia generally consists of gradual discontinuance of the precipitating antipsychotic agent when possible, reducing the dosage of the first-generation (conventional) antipsychotic agent or switching to a second-generation (atypical) antipsychotic agent, or switching to clozapine therapy. The syndrome may remit, partially or completely, if antipsychotic therapy is discontinued. However, antipsychotic therapy itself may suppress or partially suppress the signs and symptoms of the syndrome and thereby may possibly mask the underlying process. The effect that such symptomatic suppression has upon the long-term course of tardive dyskinesia is unknown. Vesicular monoamine transporter 2 (VMAT2) inhibitors (e.g., deutetrabenazine, valbenazine tosylate) have been shown to be effective in reducing symptoms of tardive dyskinesia in controlled clinical studies and may allow some patients to continue receiving antipsychotic therapy. (See Deutetrabenazine 28:56 and Valbenazine Tosylate 28:56.)

Clozapine should be prescribed in a manner that is most likely to minimize the occurrence of this syndrome. In patients who do require chronic treatment, the lowest dosage and the shortest duration of treatment producing a satisfactory clinical response should be sought, and the need for continued treatment should be reassessed periodically.

The American Psychiatric Association (APA) currently recommends that patients receiving atypical antipsychotic agents be assessed clinically for abnormal involuntary movements every 12 months and that patients considered to be at increased risk for tardive dyskinesia be assessed every 6 months. If signs and symptoms of tardive dyskinesia appear in a clozapine-treated patient, clozapine discontinuance should be considered; however, some patients may require continued treatment with the drug despite the presence of the syndrome.

For additional information on tardive dyskinesia, including manifestations and treatment, see Tardive Dyskinesia under Cautions: Nervous System Effects, in the Phenothiazines General Statement 28:16.08.24.

Other Nervous System Effects Drowsiness and/or sedation occurs frequently in patients receiving clozapine. (See Effects on Sleep under Pharmacology: Nervous System Effects.) Somnolence reportedly occurred in 46% of patients receiving clozapine in the International Suicide Prevention Trial (InterSePT) compared with 25% of those receiving olanzapine. The sedative-hypnotic effect of clozapine is most pronounced initially, diminishes after 1–4 weeks, and then generally, but not always, disappears during continued therapy. Daytime sleepiness may be minimized by administration of clozapine at bedtime. (See Dosage and Administration and also see Cognitive and Motor Impairment under Cautions: Precautions and Contraindications.)

Dizziness and vertigo, headache, syncope, disturbed sleep (e.g., insomnia) or nightmares, hypokinesia or akinesia, and agitation have been reported with clozapine therapy. In the InterSePT study, dizziness (excluding vertigo) and insomnia reportedly occurred in 27 and 20% of patients receiving clozapine, respectively, compared with 12 and 33% of those receiving olanzapine, respectively. Clozapine also may cause confusion or delirium, which may be related to central anticholinergic effects and has been ameliorated in some cases by IV administration of physostigmine. Depression, fatigue, hyperkinesia, weakness or lethargy, and slurred speech also have been reported.

Delirium, abnormal EEG, myoclonus, paresthesia, possible cataplexy, status epilepticus, obsessive-compulsive symptoms, and post-discontinuation cholinergic rebound reactions have been reported in patients receiving clozapine during postmarketing surveillance; however, a causal relationship to the drug has not been established.

Abrupt discontinuance of clozapine (e.g., because of hematologic toxicity or other medical condition) may result in recurrence of psychotic symptoms or behavior, including autism, auditory hallucinations, suicide attempts, development of parkinsonian symptoms, anxiety, insomnia, delusions, and violent behavior. It has been suggested that this "rebound psychosis" may result, at least in part, from clozapine-induced supersensitivity of mesolimbic dopamine receptors (see Behavioral Effects in Animals under Pharmacology: Nervous System Effects) and that the essential feature of this phenomenon appears to be recurrence of positive symptoms of schizophrenia. Patients who develop rebound psychosis following discontinuance of clozapine may improve with initiation of other antipsychotic therapy; however, clozapine generally should *not* be reinstituted in patients in whom severe neutropenia has occurred. (See Cautions: Hematologic Effects.)

■ **Fever** Fever or transient temperature elevations exceeding 38°C generally have been reported in 5% or more of patients receiving clozapine. The peak incidence of fever occurs within the first 3 weeks of therapy, usually between days 5–20 of treatment. Fever generally is benign and self-limiting, responds to supportive measures, and usually diminishes within a few (4–8) days despite continued clozapine therapy; however, it may necessitate discontinuance of the drug. Fever occasionally may be associated with an increase or decrease in WBC count. Clozapine therapy should be interrupted as a precautionary measure; an ANC should be obtained in any patient who develops fever (38.5°C or higher) during treatment, and patients should be evaluated for severe neutropenia or infection. In addition, ANC should be monitored in any patient who develops fever within 2 weeks after discontinuance of clozapine. (See Cautions: Hematologic Effects.) Neuroleptic malignant syndrome also must be considered. (See Neuroleptic Malignant Syndrome under Cautions: Nervous System Effects.)

The mechanism of clozapine-induced fever (other than that occurring secondary to some other factor such as infection) is not yet known. It may result from the drug's pronounced anticholinergic activity (see Anticholinergic Effects under Pharmacology: Nervous System Effects) or a direct effect on the hypothalamic thermoregulatory center. Clozapine-induced hyperthermia may be a hypersensitivity reaction, a common mechanism underlying drug fevers. It has been suggested that decreasing the dosage of clozapine and then gradually increasing it to the previous level may reverse the hyperthermia and not be accompanied by a recurrence of elevated temperature; however, recurrence is possible despite such dosage adjustment.

■ Cardiovascular Effects ***Myocarditis and Cardiomyopathy*** Myocarditis and cardiomyopathy, which are sometimes fatal, have been reported in patients receiving clozapine. Myocarditis most frequently presents within the first 2 months of clozapine treatment. Symptoms of clozapine-associated cardiomyopathy generally occur later than clozapine-associated myocarditis, usually after 8 weeks of treatment. However, myocarditis and cardiomyopathy can occur at any time during clozapine therapy. Overt manifestations of heart failure commonly are preceded by nonspecific flu-like symptoms (e.g., malaise, myalgia, pleuritic chest pain, low-grade fever). Typical laboratory findings include elevated troponin I or T concentrations, elevated CK-MB concentrations, peripheral eosinophilia, and elevated C-reactive protein (CRP) concentrations. Left ventricular dysfunction may be evident in cardiac imaging studies (e.g., electrocardiogram [ECG], radionucleotide studies, cardiac catheterization) and cardiac silhouette enlargement may be seen in chest radiographs.

The possibility of myocarditis or cardiomyopathy should be considered in patients receiving clozapine who present with chest pain, dyspnea, persistent tachycardia at rest, palpitations, fever, flu-like symptoms, hypotension, or other manifestations of heart failure or ECG changes associated with these conditions (e.g., low voltages, ST-T wave abnormalities, arrhythmias, right axis deviation, poor R wave progression). If myocarditis or cardiomyopathy is suspected, clozapine therapy should be discontinued and a cardiac evaluation should be obtained. Patients with a history of clozapine-associated myocarditis or cardiomyopathy generally should not be rechallenged with the drug. However, if the benefit of clozapine treatment is determined to outweigh the potential risks of recurrent myocarditis or cardiomyopathy, the clinician may consider rechallenge with the drug in consultation with a cardiologist, following a complete cardiac evaluation, and with close monitoring.

Thromboembolic Effects Deep-vein thrombosis and pulmonary embolism have been reported in patients receiving clozapine. Although a causal relationship between clozapine and these adverse effects has not been established, the possibility of pulmonary embolism should be considered in patients presenting with deep-vein thrombosis, acute dyspnea, chest pain, or respiratory symptomatology. (See Thromboembolic Events under Cautions: Precautions and Contraindications.)

Blood Pressure Effects Hypotension and hypertension reportedly occur in less than 10% of patients receiving clozapine. When they occur, changes in blood pressure, principally reductions in systolic pressure, appear soon after initiation of clozapine therapy and may be associated with rapid dosage increases. A decrease in arterial blood pressure below 90 mm Hg was reported in 18% of male patients and 33% of female patients receiving clozapine in one retrospective study. Hypotension may result from clozapine's antiadrenergic effects (see Adrenergic Effects under Pharmacology: Nervous System Effects). However, tolerance to the hypotensive effects of clozapine often develops with continued therapy.

Orthostatic hypotension, bradycardia, syncope, and cardiac arrest have been reported, particularly during initial titration or rapid escalation of clozapine dosage. Rarely (approximately 1 case per 3000 patients), orthostatic hypotension has been accompanied by profound collapse and respiratory and/or cardiac arrest in patients receiving initial doses as low as 12.5 mg. Such reactions, which are sometimes fatal, are consistent with neurally-mediated reflex bradycardia. In some cases when collapse and cardiac and/or respiratory arrest developed during initial therapy, benzodiazepines or other psychotropic agents were used concomitantly, suggesting a possible adverse interaction between clozapine and these agents. (See Benzodiazepines under Drug Interactions: CNS Depressants.)

The risk of orthostatic hypotension may be reduced by initiating clozapine therapy at lower dosages, followed by gradual increases, and administration in divided doses. (See Dosage and Administration: Dosage.) If hypotension occurs, dosage reduction of clozapine may be considered. In some cases, withholding the drug for 24 hours and then restarting at a lower dosage has been accomplished without recurrence of orthostatic hypotension. If clozapine therapy is temporarily interrupted (i.e., for 2 or more days), the manufacturers recommend that the drug be reinitiated at a lower dosage (12.5 mg once or twice daily).

Prolongation of QT Interval Prolongation of the QT interval, torsades de pointes and other life-threatening ventricular arrhythmias, cardiac arrest, and sudden death have occurred in patients receiving clozapine. Patients at particular risk for these serious cardiovascular reactions include those with a history of QT-interval prolongation, long QT syndrome, family history of long QT syndrome or sudden cardiac death, significant cardiac arrhythmia, recent myocardial infarction, and uncompensated heart failure and those concurrently receiving other drugs that prolong the QT interval or inhibit the metabolism of clozapine. (See Drug Interactions: Drugs that Prolong the QT Interval and see also Drug Interactions: Drugs Affecting Hepatic Microsomal Enzymes.) Electrolyte abnormalities such as hypokalemia and hypomagnesemia also increase the risk of QT-interval prolongation.

Prior to initiating clozapine therapy, a careful physical examination should be performed and a medical and concomitant medication history should be obtained. A baseline ECG and serum chemistry panel should also be considered before initiating clozapine therapy. Clozapine should be discontinued if the corrected QT (QT_c) interval exceeds 500 msec. Clozapine should also be discontinued and a cardiac evaluation performed in patients who experience symptoms consistent with torsades de pointes or other arrhythmias (e.g., syncope, presyncope, dizziness, palpitations).

Baseline serum potassium and magnesium concentrations should be determined and electrolyte abnormalities, if present, should be corrected prior to initiating clozapine therapy. In addition, serum electrolytes should be periodically monitored during clozapine therapy.

Other Cardiovascular Effects Tachycardia, which may persist throughout therapy in some cases, reportedly has been observed in up to 25% of patients receiving clozapine in clinical studies.

Postexercise decreases in left ventricular output, which may indicate left ventricular failure, have been reported in patients receiving clozapine. Although a causal relationship has not been established, atrial or ventricular fibrillation, ventricular tachycardia, and myocardial infarction also have been reported during postmarketing surveillance in patients receiving the drug.

■ Autonomic Nervous System Effects Adverse autonomic nervous system effects occur in more than 5% of patients receiving clozapine. Dry mouth occurs frequently, but hypersalivation, an apparently paradoxical effect considering the drug's potent anticholinergic activity, is more common. (See Cautions: GI Effects.)

Other autonomic nervous system effects of clozapine include hyperhidrosis, decreased sweating, and visual disturbances. Increased salivation occurred in 31%, dry mouth and sweating in 6%, and visual disturbances in 5% of patients receiving clozapine in controlled clinical trials.

■ Hepatic Effects Transient increases in liver function test results, including serum aminotransferases (transaminases), LDH, and alkaline phosphatase, may occur with clozapine therapy. Clozapine-induced changes in liver function test results may be more pronounced than those with other tricyclic antipsychotic agents. Clozapine causes slight liver hyperplasia in rats; hyperplasia was reversible and no histologic changes were detectable. Clozapine occasionally causes slight elevations of bilirubin concentration. Cholestasis, hepatitis, jaundice, hepatotoxicity, hepatic steatosis, hepatic necrosis, hepatic fibrosis, hepatic cirrhosis, liver injury (hepatic, cholestatic, and mixed), and liver failure have been reported in patients receiving clozapine during postmarketing surveillance; however, a causal relationship to the drug has not been established.

■ Endocrine and Metabolic Effects Atypical antipsychotic agents have been associated with metabolic changes, including hyperglycemia, dyslipidemia, and weight gain. Such metabolic changes may be associated with increased cardiovascular and cerebrovascular risk.

Weight Gain Weight gain has been observed with antipsychotic therapy. Clozapine may cause increased appetite, polyphagia, and weight gain in a substantial proportion (approximately one-third) of patients. Some clinicians suggest that the potential for weight gain with clozapine therapy may be similar to that with other antipsychotic therapy; others state that they have observed greater weight gain with clozapine in some patients. In the 2-year InterSePT trial, weight gain reportedly occurred in 31% of patients receiving clozapine compared with 56% of those receiving olanzapine. Some clozapine-treated patients reportedly have gained up to 1 kg weekly for 6 weeks. Pooled data from 11 clinical studies in patients with schizophrenia indicate that 35% of clozapine-treated patients (median duration of exposure 609 days), 46% of olanzapine-treated patients (median duration of exposure 728 days), and 8% of chlorpromazine-treated patients (median duration of exposure 42 days) gained 7% or more of their baseline body weight.

Weight gain may result from the drug's serotonergic-, histaminergic-, and adrenergic-blocking properties. Weight gain has been reported to be a problem for some patients during long-term therapy with clozapine and may be a major cause of outpatient noncompliance. Some clinicians suggest using exercise and active measures (e.g., dietary counseling) to control dietary intake in clozapine-treated patients.

Hyperglycemia and Diabetes Mellitus Hyperglycemia, sometimes severe and associated with ketoacidosis, hyperosmolar coma, or death, has been reported in patients receiving certain atypical antipsychotic agents, including clozapine. While confounding factors such as an increased background risk of diabetes mellitus in patients with schizophrenia and the increasing incidence of diabetes mellitus in the general population make it difficult to establish with certainty the relationship between use of agents in this drug class and glucose abnormalities, epidemiologic studies suggest an increased risk of treatment-emergent hyperglycemia-related adverse events in patients treated with the atypical antipsychotic agents included in the studies (e.g., clozapine, olanzapine, quetiapine, risperidone). (See Cautions: Precautions and Contraindications.)

Precise risk estimates for hyperglycemia-related adverse events in patients treated with atypical antipsychotics currently are not available. While some evidence suggests that the risk for diabetes may be greater with some atypical antipsychotics (e.g., clozapine, olanzapine) than with others (e.g., quetiapine, risperidone) in the class, available data are conflicting and insufficient to provide reliable estimates of relative risk associated with use of the various atypical antipsychotics.

In an analysis of 5 clinical studies in patients with schizophrenia (median treatment duration of 42 days), clozapine was associated with a greater average increase in fasting glucose concentrations compared with chlorpromazine (11 mg/dL versus 4 mg/dL, respectively). A greater proportion of patients receiving clozapine experienced shifts in fasting glucose concentrations from normal (less than 100 mg/dL) to high (126 mg/dL or higher) and from borderline (100–125 mg/dL) to high (126 mg/dL or higher) compared with those receiving chlorpromazine. Shifts in fasting glucose concentrations from normal to high were observed in 27 or 10%, and from borderline to high in 42 or 28% of patients receiving clozapine or chlorpromazine, respectively.

Dyslipidemia Like some other antipsychotic agents, clozapine therapy has been associated with undesirable changes in lipid parameters, including elevations in serum cholesterol and triglyceride concentrations.

In a pooled analysis of 10 clinical studies in adults with schizophrenia, the mean increase in total cholesterol concentrations was 13 or 15 mg/dL in patients receiving clozapine or chlorpromazine, respectively, and in a pooled analysis of 2 studies in adults with schizophrenia, the mean increase in fasting triglyceride concentrations in clozapine-treated patients was 71 mg/dL (54%) compared with 39 mg/dL (35%) in chlorpromazine-treated patients. In these studies, the median duration of exposure was 45 or 38 days for clozapine or chlorpromazine, respectively; specific data on high-density lipoprotein (HDL)- or low-density lipoprotein (LDL)-cholesterol were not collected. An increase in serum total cholesterol concentrations (random or fasting) of 40 mg/dL or higher occurred in 33 or 25%, and increases in fasting serum triglyceride concentrations of 50 mg/dL or higher occurred in 50 or 43% of adults receiving clozapine or chlorpromazine, respectively. In addition, a greater proportion of patients receiving clozapine experienced an increase in serum total cholesterol concentrations from normal (below 200 mg/dL) to high (240 mg/dL or higher) or from borderline (200–239 mg/dL) to high (240 mg/dL or higher) compared with those receiving chlorpromazine.

The manufacturers recommend clinical monitoring, including baseline and periodic follow-up lipid evaluations, in patients receiving clozapine.

Hyperprolactinemia Clozapine causes little or no elevation in serum prolactin concentrations. The drug has been reported to cause only a brief, transient elevation of prolactin concentration. (See Pharmacology: Neuroendocrine Effects.) Therefore, prolactin-dependent adverse effects such as galactorrhea and amenorrhea usually are not associated with clozapine therapy.

Other Endocrine and Metabolic Effects Hyperuricemia, hyponatremia, weight loss, and pseudopheochromocytoma also have been reported in patients receiving clozapine during postmarketing surveillance, although a causal relationship to the drug has not been established.

Small decreases in protein-bound iodine or thyroxine concentrations have been reported in some patients receiving clozapine, but these values remained within normal limits.

■ GI Effects Increased salivation may occur in approximately one-third of patients receiving clozapine; in some studies, hypersalivation was reported in up to 75–85% of clozapine-treated patients. In the InterSePT trial, increased salivation reportedly occurred in 48% of patients receiving clozapine compared with 6% of those receiving olanzapine. Salivation may be profuse, very fluid, and particularly troublesome during sleep because of decreased swallowing. Since clozapine exhibits intrinsic anticholinergic properties, hypersalivation is an unexpected paradoxical effect. A muscle-relaxant effect of the drug may contribute to hypersalivation, but the cause has not been fully elucidated. Difficulty in swallowing has been reported in a few clozapine-treated patients, and it has been suggested that the drug may cause esophageal dysfunction, which may contribute to or exacerbate the nocturnal hypersalivation associated with clozapine therapy. Some clozapine-treated patients develop tolerance to increased salivation within a few weeks. Nonpharmacologic interventions such as the use of a towel on the pillow at night may help reduce the discomfort associated with clozapine-associated hypersalivation during sleep. Occasionally, hypersalivation may be ameliorated by reduction of clozapine dosage or cautious use of a peripherally acting anticholinergic drug; however, some clinicians generally advise against the use of anticholinergic therapy for this adverse effect because of possible potentiation of clozapine's anticholinergic activity. (See Anticholinergic Toxicity under Cautions: Precautions and Contraindications.)

Other GI effects associated with clozapine therapy include constipation, diarrhea, nausea and vomiting, dyspepsia or heartburn, and abdominal discomfort; some of these effects have been reported in more than 5% of patients. Constipation, nausea, vomiting, and dyspepsia reportedly occurred in 14–25% of patients receiving clozapine in the InterSePT trial compared with 8–10% of those receiving olanzapine. Although some clinicians advocate the use of metoclopramide (e.g., in doses less than 30 mg daily) for the treatment of clozapine-induced nausea, other clinicians suggest that metoclopramide or other dopamine antagonists not be used or be used with extreme caution for the treatment of clozapine-induced nausea because of their potential for causing parkinsonian manifestations and tardive dyskinesia.

Although a causal relationship to the drug has not been established, acute pancreatitis, dysphagia, salivary gland swelling, and colitis also have been reported in patients receiving clozapine during postmarketing surveillance.

■ Genitourinary Effects Genitourinary effects reported with clozapine therapy include polyuria, enuresis, and impotence. Acute interstitial nephritis, renal failure, nocturnal enuresis, priapism, and retrograde ejaculation also have been reported with clozapine therapy during postmarketing surveillance, although a causal relationship to the drug has not been established.

■ Respiratory Effects Although a causal relationship to the drug has not been established, aspiration, pleural effusion, and pneumonia and lower respiratory tract infection have been reported with clozapine therapy during postmarketing surveillance.

Respiratory depression or failure, including arrest requiring resuscitation, also has been reported in patients receiving clozapine, usually at initiation of therapy and particularly in patients receiving concomitant benzodiazepine therapy or in those with a history of recent benzodiazepine use. Some evidence indicates that the incidence of respiratory arrest and vascular collapse is about 1–2% of patients receiving clozapine concomitantly with a benzodiazepine. For additional precautionary information about this potential effect, see Benzodiazepines under Drug Interactions: CNS Depressants.

■ Dermatologic and Sensitivity Reactions Rash has been reported in 2% of patients receiving clozapine.

Hypersensitivity reactions, including photosensitivity, vasculitis, erythema multiforme, skin pigmentation disorder, and Stevens-Johnson syndrome, have been reported with clozapine during postmarketing surveillance; however, a causal relationship to the drug has not been established.

■ Other Adverse Effects Myasthenic syndrome, rhabdomyolysis, systemic lupus erythematosus, angioedema, periorbital edema, leukocytoclastic vasculitis, and angle-closure (narrow angle) glaucoma have been reported with clozapine during postmarketing surveillance, although a causal relationship to the drug has not been established.

■ Precautions and Contraindications Clozapine shares many of the toxic potentials of other antipsychotic agents (e.g., phenothiazines), and the usual precautions associated with therapy with these agents should be observed. (See Cautions, in the Phenothiazines General Statement 28:16.08.24.)

Cognitive and Motor Impairment Because of clozapine's sedative effects and because the drug potentially may impair cognitive and motor performance, clozapine-treated patients should be cautioned about operating hazardous machinery, including driving a motor vehicle, until they are reasonably certain that the drug does not adversely affect them. Because such effects may be dose-related, a reduction in clozapine dosage should be considered if they occur.

Fever During clozapine therapy, patients may experience transient temperature elevations exceeding 38°C, with the peak incidence within the first 3 weeks of therapy. (See Cautions: Fever.) While this fever generally is benign and self-limiting, it may necessitate discontinuance of therapy. Occasionally, there may be an associated increase or decrease in leukocyte count.

Clozapine therapy should be interrupted as a precautionary measure and an ANC obtained in any patient who develops fever (38.5°C or higher) during treatment; patients should be carefully evaluated to rule out severe neutropenia or infection. In addition, ANC should be monitored in any patient who develops fever within 2 weeks after discontinuance of clozapine. In the presence of high fever, the possibility of neuroleptic malignant syndrome also must be considered. (See Neuroleptic Malignant Syndrome under Cautions: Nervous System Effects.)

Anticholinergic Toxicity Clozapine has potent anticholinergic activity, and therapy with the drug may result in CNS and peripheral anticholinergic toxicity. Clozapine should therefore be used with caution in individuals whose condition may be aggravated by anticholinergic effects (e.g., patients with prostatic hypertrophy, urinary retention, angle-closure [narrow-angle] glaucoma) and in those who are concurrently receiving other drugs with anticholinergic effects. (See Drug Interactions: Drugs with Anticholinergic Activity.)

Clozapine therapy has been associated with varying degrees of impairment of intestinal peristalsis, ranging from constipation to intestinal obstruction, fecal impaction, and paralytic ileus, that rarely have been fatal. The manufacturers state that constipation may be treated initially by maintaining adequate hydration and with appropriate supportive therapy such as bulk-forming laxatives. Consultation with a gastroenterologist is recommended in more severe cases.

Thromboembolic Events Pulmonary embolism and deep-vein thrombosis have been reported with clozapine therapy. The possibility of pulmonary embolism should be considered in patients presenting with deep-vein thrombosis, acute dyspnea, chest pain, or other respiratory signs and symptoms.

Individuals with Phenylketonuria Individuals with phenylketonuria (i.e., homozygous genetic deficiency of phenylalanine hydroxylase) and other individuals who must restrict their intake of phenylalanine should be warned that clozapine orally disintegrating tablets contain aspartame, which is metabolized in the GI tract to phenylalanine following oral administration; the respective manufacturer's labeling should be consulted for specific information regarding aspartame content of individual preparations and dosage strengths.

Neuroleptic Malignant Syndrome Neuroleptic malignant syndrome (NMS), a potentially fatal syndrome requiring immediate discontinuance of the drug and intensive symptomatic treatment, has been reported in patients receiving antipsychotic agents, including clozapine. If a patient requires antipsychotic therapy following recovery from NMS, the potential reintroduction of drug therapy should be carefully considered. If antipsychotic therapy is reintroduced, the dosage generally should be increased gradually, and an antipsychotic agent other than the agent believed to have precipitated NMS generally should be chosen. In addition, such patients should be carefully monitored since recurrences of NMS have been reported. (See Neuroleptic Malignant Syndrome under Cautions: Nervous System Effects.) For additional information on NMS, see Neuroleptic Malignant Syndrome under Cautions: Nervous System Effects, in the Phenothiazines General Statement 28:16.08.24.

Metabolic Effects Atypical antipsychotic agents are associated with metabolic changes that may increase cardiovascular and cerebrovascular risk (e.g., hyperglycemia, dyslipidemia, weight gain). While all atypical antipsychotics produce some metabolic changes, each drug has its own specific risk profile.

Hyperglycemia, sometimes severe and associated with ketoacidosis, hyperosmolar coma, or death, has been reported in patients receiving atypical antipsychotic agents, including clozapine. The manufacturers state that patients with preexisting diabetes mellitus in whom therapy with an atypical antipsychotic is initiated should be closely monitored for worsening glycemic control; those with risk factors for diabetes (e.g., obesity, family history of diabetes) should undergo fasting blood glucose testing upon therapy initiation and periodically throughout treatment. Any patient who develops manifestations of hyperglycemia (e.g., polydipsia, polyphagia, polyuria, weakness) during treatment with an atypical antipsychotic should undergo fasting blood glucose testing. In some cases, patients who developed hyperglycemia while receiving an atypical antipsychotic have required continuance of antidiabetic treatment despite discontinuance of the suspect drug; in other cases, hyperglycemia resolved with discontinuance of the antipsychotic.

Various experts have developed additional recommendations for the management of diabetes risks in patients receiving atypical antipsychotics; these include initial screening measures and regular monitoring (e.g., determination of diabetes risk factors; BMI determination using weight and height; waist circumference; blood pressure; fasting blood glucose; hemoglobin A_{1c} [HbA_{1c}]; fasting lipid profile), as well as provision of patient education and referral to clinicians experienced in the treatment of diabetes, when appropriate. Although some clinicians state that a switch from one atypical antipsychotic agent to another that has not been associated with substantial weight gain or diabetes should be considered in patients who experience weight gain (equal to or exceeding 5% of baseline body weight) or develop worsening glycemia or dyslipidemia at any time during therapy, such recommendations are controversial because differences in risk of developing diabetes associated with use of the different atypical antipsychotics remain to be fully established. Many clinicians consider antipsychotic efficacy the most important factor when making treatment decisions and suggest that detrimental effects of switching from a beneficial treatment regimen also should be considered in addition to any potential for exacerbation or development of medical conditions (e.g., diabetes). Decisions to alter drug therapy should be made on an individual basis, weighing the potential risks and benefits of the particular drug in each patient. (See Hyperglycemia and Diabetes Mellitus under Cautions: Endocrine and Metabolic Effects.)

Because undesirable changes in serum lipids have been observed with clozapine therapy, the manufacturers recommend appropriate clinical monitoring, including baseline and periodic follow-up lipid evaluations, in all patients receiving the drug. (See Dyslipidemia under Cautions: Endocrine and Metabolic Effects.)

Clozapine therapy may result in weight gain. Patients receiving the drug should be advised that weight gain has occurred during clozapine treatment. The manufacturers recommend clinical monitoring of weight in patients receiving the drug. (See Weight Gain under Cautions: Endocrine and Metabolic Effects.)

Orthostatic Hypotension, Bradycardia, and Syncope Orthostatic hypotension, bradycardia, syncope, and cardiac arrest can occur with clozapine therapy; these effects are more likely to occur during initial titration of the drug, particularly with rapid dose escalation, but may even occur with the first dose at clozapine dosages as low as 12.5 mg. The risk of orthostatic hypotension may be reduced by initiating therapy at lower dosages, followed by gradual increases, and administration in divided doses. (See Dosage and Administration: Dosage.) If hypotension occurs, dosage reduction of clozapine may be considered. Patients should be informed of the risk of orthostatic hypotension associated with use of clozapine, especially during the period of initial dosage titration. In addition, if clozapine therapy has been discontinued for more than 2 days, patients should be advised to contact their clinician for dosing instructions. (See Reinitiation of Therapy under Dosage: Psychotic Disorders, in Dosage and Administration.)

Clozapine should be used with particular caution in patients with known cardiovascular disease (history of myocardial infarction or ischemia, heart failure, or conduction abnormalities), cerebrovascular disease, or conditions that would predispose to hypotension (e.g., dehydration, hypovolemia, concomitant antihypertensive therapy). (See Blood Pressure Effects under Cautions: Cardiovascular Effects.)

Geriatric Patients with Dementia-related Psychosis Geriatric patients with dementia-related psychosis treated with antipsychotic drugs are at increased risk of death compared with patients receiving placebo.

An increased risk of adverse cerebrovascular events (e.g., stroke, transient ischemic attack), including fatalities, has been observed in geriatric patients with dementia-related psychosis treated with some atypical antipsychotic agents. Clozapine should therefore be used with caution in patients with risk factors for stroke.

The manufacturer states that clozapine is *not* approved for the treatment of patients with dementia-related psychosis. (See Cautions: Geriatric Precautions.)

Myocarditis and Cardiomyopathy Because myocarditis and cardiomyopathy, which are sometimes fatal, have been reported in patients treated with clozapine, signs and symptoms suggestive of these reactions, including chest pain, dyspnea, persistent tachycardia at rest, palpitations, fever, flu-like symptoms, hypotension, other manifestations of heart failure, or ECG changes, should alert the clinician to perform further investigations. If the diagnosis of myocarditis or cardiomyopathy is confirmed, clozapine therapy should be discontinued and generally should *not* be reinitiated unless the benefit to the patient clearly outweighs the potential risk of recurrent myocarditis or cardiomyopathy. (See Myocarditis and Cardiomyopathy under Cautions: Cardiovascular Effects.)

Seizures Generalized tonic-clonic (grand mal) seizures have occurred in patients receiving clozapine, particularly in patients receiving high dosages (greater than 600 mg daily) and/or in whom plasma clozapine concentrations were elevated. (See Seizures under Cautions: Nervous System Effects.) Clozapine should be used with caution in patients with a history of seizure disorders or other risk factors predisposing to seizures (e.g., history of head trauma or other preexisting CNS pathology, concomitant use of other drugs that lower the seizure threshold, history of alcohol abuse). Because of the substantial risk of seizures associated with clozapine use, patients should be advised not to engage in any activity where sudden loss of consciousness could cause serious risk to themselves or others (e.g., driving an automobile, operating complex machinery, swimming, climbing).

Severe Neutropenia Because of the risk of severe neutropenia, which can lead to serious and potentially fatal infections, clozapine therapy should be reserved for use in patients who have failed to respond adequately to standard antipsychotic therapy. Patients should be warned of this risk and informed that clozapine is only available through the Clozapine REMS program that ensures baseline and periodic monitoring of neutrophil counts. (See REMS and also see Cautions: Hematologic Effects.) In addition, patients receiving clozapine therapy should be advised to immediately report the development of flu-like symptoms, fever, lethargy, malaise, weakness, mucous membrane ulceration, skin, pharyngeal, vaginal, urinary, or pulmonary infection, or any other potential manifestation of infection. Patients who develop severe neutropenia (ANC less than 500/mm^3) while receiving clozapine generally should *not* be rechallenged with the drug. However, for some patients who have no acceptable alternatives to clozapine, the risk of serious psychiatric illness from discontinuing treatment may outweigh the risk of severe neutropenia upon rechallenge; in such cases, consultation with a hematology specialist may be helpful in deciding whether to rechallenge a patient with clozapine.

It is not known whether concurrent use of other drugs known to cause neutropenia increases the risk or severity of clozapine-induced neutropenia. (See Drug Interactions: Other Drugs Associated with Neutropenia.)

Other Precautions and Contraindications Clozapine is contraindicated in patients with a history of serious hypersensitivity to clozapine (e.g., photosensitivity, vasculitis, erythema multiforme, Stevens-Johnson syndrome) or any ingredient in the formulation. (See Cautions: Dermatologic and Sensitivity Reactions.)

■ **Pediatric Precautions** The manufacturers state that the safety and efficacy of clozapine in pediatric patients have not been established. However, clozapine has been used in a limited number of children and adolescents with treatment-refractory schizophrenia (see Pediatric Considerations under Psychotic Disorders: Treatment-resistant Schizophrenia, in Uses) and results of at least one randomized, double-blind clinical study indicate that adverse hematologic effects were a major concern for children and adolescents receiving clozapine†. Although no cases of agranulocytosis occurred in this study, 24% of these children and adolescents experienced mild to moderate neutropenia during 2 years of follow-up compared with an estimated cumulative risk of 1.5–2% of developing neutropenia in adults. The precise mechanism by which clozapine induces agranulocytosis is not known, but a higher concentration of the metabolite norclozapine, which has been associated with hematopoietic toxicity in children and adolescents receiving clozapine, has been suggested as a possible reason for the increased risk in this age group. As with adult patients, adjunctive lithium has been used successfully in the management of clozapine-induced neutropenia in pediatric patients with schizophrenia†.

In addition to adverse hematologic effects, clinically important seizure activity (e.g., epileptiform spikes, myoclonus, tonic-clonic seizures) also has been reported in children and adolescents with no previous history of epilepsy who received clozapine. In some cases, EEG abnormalities were associated with clinical deterioration (i.e., increased aggression, psychosis, irritability). Because some children and adolescents responded behaviorally to reduced dosages of clozapine and the addition of an anticonvulsant (e.g., valproate), it has been suggested that the EEG may be a sensitive indicator of clozapine toxicity in children as well as in adults.

■ **Geriatric Precautions** Clinical studies of clozapine did not include sufficient numbers of patients 65 years of age and older to determine whether geriatric patients respond differently than younger patients. Because geriatric patients may be at increased risk for certain cardiovascular (e.g., orthostatic hypotension, tachycardia) and anticholinergic effects of the drug (e.g., constipation, urinary retention in the presence of prostatic hypertrophy), clozapine should be used cautiously in this age group. In addition, geriatric patients generally are more sensitive than younger patients to drugs that affect the CNS. Data from clinical studies indicate that the incidence of tardive dyskinesia appears to be highest among geriatric patients, especially women. In general, dosage should be titrated carefully in geriatric patients, usually initiating therapy at the low end of the dosage range; the greater frequency of decreased hepatic, renal, and/or cardiac function and of concomitant disease and drug therapy observed in the elderly also should be considered.

Geriatric patients with dementia-related psychosis treated with antipsychotic drugs are at an increased risk of death compared with patients receiving placebo. Analyses of 17 placebo-controlled trials (modal duration of 10 weeks) revealed an approximate 1.6- to 1.7- fold increase in mortality among geriatric patients receiving atypical antipsychotic drugs (i.e., aripiprazole, olanzapine, quetiapine, risperidone) compared with that observed in patients receiving placebo. Over the course of a typical 10-week controlled trial, the rate of death in drug-treated patients was about 4.5% compared with a rate of about 2.6% in the placebo group. Although the causes of death were varied, most of the deaths appeared to be either cardiovascular (e.g., heart failure, sudden death) or infectious (e.g., pneumonia) in nature. Observational studies suggest that, similar to atypical antipsychotics, treatment with conventional (first-generation) antipsychotics may increase mortality; the extent to which the findings of increased mortality in observational studies may be attributed to the antipsychotic drug as opposed to some characteristic(s) of the patients remains unclear. Clozapine is not approved for the treatment of patients with dementia-related psychosis.

An increased risk of adverse cerebrovascular events has been observed in patients with dementia treated with some atypical antipsychotic agents. The mechanism for this increased risk is not known. The manufacturers state that an increased risk cannot be excluded for other antipsychotics, including clozapine, or other patient populations. Clozapine should therefore be used with caution in patients with risk factors for stroke.

■ **Mutagenicity and Carcinogenicity** Clozapine did not exhibit carcinogenic potential in long-term studies in mice and rats receiving dosages up to 0.3 and 0.4 times the maximum recommended human dosage on a mg/m^2 basis, respectively. Clozapine also did not exhibit genotoxic or mutagenic effects when assayed in appropriate bacterial and mammalian tests.

■ **Pregnancy, Fertility, and Lactation** Reproduction studies in rats and rabbits using clozapine dosages up to 0.4 and 0.9 times the maximum recommended human dosage on a mg/m^2 basis, respectively, have not revealed evidence of harm to the fetus.

Neonates exposed to antipsychotic agents, including clozapine, during the third trimester of pregnancy are at risk for extrapyramidal and/or withdrawal symptoms following delivery. There have been reports of agitation, hypertonia, hypotonia, tardive dyskinetic-like symptoms, tremor, somnolence, respiratory distress, and feeding disorder in these neonates. The majority of cases were also confounded by other factors, including concomitant use of other drugs known to be associated with withdrawal symptoms, prematurity, congenital malformations, and obstetrical and perinatal complications; however, some cases suggested that neonatal extrapyramidal and withdrawal symptoms may occur with exposure to antipsychotic agents alone. Some of the cases described time of symptom onset, which ranged from birth to one month after birth. Any neonate exhibiting extrapyramidal or withdrawal symptoms following in utero exposure to antipsychotic agents should be monitored. Symptoms were self-limiting in some neonates but varied in severity; some infants required intensive care unit support and prolonged hospitalization. For further information on extrapyramidal and withdrawal symptoms in neonates, see Cautions: Pregnancy, Fertility, and Lactation, in the Phenothiazines General Statement 28:16.08.24.

The manufacturers state that there are no adequate and well-controlled studies to date using clozapine in pregnant women, and the drug should be used during pregnancy only when clearly needed. Women should be advised to notify their clinician if they become pregnant or plan to become pregnant during therapy with the drug. In addition, clinicians should advise women of childbearing potential about the benefits and risks of using antipsychotic agents during pregnancy. Patients should also be advised not to stop taking their antipsychotic agent if they become pregnant without first consulting with their clinician, since abruptly discontinuing the drugs can cause clinically important complications.

Reproduction studies in rats using clozapine dosages up to 0.4 times the maximum recommended human dosage on a mg/m^2 basis have not revealed impaired fertility.

Clozapine is distributed into milk in humans. Because of the potential for serious adverse reactions to clozapine in nursing infants, a decision should be made whether to discontinue nursing or the drug, taking into account the importance of the drug to the woman.

Drug Interactions

■ **Drugs Affecting Hepatic Microsomal Enzymes** Clozapine is a substrate for many cytochrome P-450 (CYP) isoenzymes, in particular 1A2, 2D6, and 3A4. Concomitant use of clozapine with drugs that inhibit CYP1A2, CYP2D6, or CYP3A4 may result in increased plasma concentrations of clozapine. When used concomitantly with *potent* CYP1A2 inhibitors (e.g., ciprofloxacin, enoxacin [no longer commercially available in the US], fluvoxamine), clozapine dosage should be reduced to one-third of the original dosage. The dosage should be increased back to the original dosage when the potent CYP1A2 inhibitor is discontinued. When used concomitantly with moderate or weak CYP1A2 inhibitors (e.g., oral contraceptives, caffeine) or inhibitors of CYP2D6 or CYP3A4 (e.g., bupropion, cimetidine, duloxetine, erythromycin, escitalopram, fluoxetine, paroxetine, quinidine, sertraline, terbinafine), patients should be monitored for adverse effects and dosage reduction of clozapine should be considered, if necessary. If a moderate or weak CYP1A2 inhibitor or a CYP2D6 or CYP3A4 inhibitor is discontinued during clozapine therapy, patients should be monitored for decreased efficacy of clozapine and an increase in clozapine dosage may be necessary.

Conversely, concomitant use of clozapine with drugs or substances that induce CYP1A2 (e.g., tobacco smoke) or CYP3A4 (e.g., carbamazepine, phenytoin, rifampin, St. John's wort [*Hypericum perforatum*]) may result in decreased plasma concentrations of clozapine. The manufacturers state that concomitant use of a potent CYP3A4 inducer with clozapine is not recommended; however, if concomitant use cannot be avoided, patients should be monitored for decreased efficacy of clozapine and consideration should be given to increasing the dosage of clozapine, if necessary. If clozapine is used concomitantly with a moderate or weak CYP1A2 inducer (e.g., tobacco smoke), patients should be monitored for decreased efficacy of clozapine and an increase in clozapine dosage may be necessary. Likewise, if a CYP1A2 or CYP3A4 inducer is discontinued during clozapine therapy, patients should be monitored for possible adverse effects and dosage reduction of clozapine should be considered, if necessary.

Phenytoin Substantial reductions in plasma clozapine concentrations and exacerbation of psychosis have been reported in patients receiving concomitant therapy with clozapine and phenytoin. In 2 patients stabilized for 1–2 weeks on a given dosage of clozapine, addition of phenytoin for prevention of clozapine-induced seizures resulted in a 65–85% decrease in steady-state plasma clozapine concentrations. Control of psychotic manifestations was regained in both patients by gradually increasing the clozapine dosage.

Because phenytoin is a potent inducer of CYP3A4, the manufacturers of clozapine state that concomitant use of these drugs generally is not recommended. However, if concomitant use of clozapine and phenytoin is necessary, patients should be monitored for decreased efficacy of clozapine and consideration should be given to increasing the dosage of clozapine, if necessary. Likewise, if phenytoin is discontinued during clozapine therapy, patients should be monitored for possible adverse effects and dosage reduction of clozapine should be considered, if necessary.

Carbamazepine Concomitant use of clozapine and carbamazepine has been shown to decrease clozapine concentrations by about 40–50%. In addition, neuroleptic malignant syndrome has been reported rarely with clozapine therapy alone and during concomitant therapy with carbamazepine. (See Neuroleptic Malignant Syndrome under Cautions: Nervous System Effects.) Because carbamazepine is a potent inducer of CYP3A4, the manufacturers of clozapine state that concomitant use of these agents generally is not recommended. However, if concomitant use of clozapine and carbamazepine is necessary, patients should be monitored for decreased efficacy of clozapine and consideration should be given to increasing the dosage of clozapine if necessary. Likewise, if carbamazepine is discontinued during clozapine therapy, dosage reduction of clozapine should be considered.

Selective Serotonin-reuptake Inhibitors Concomitant use of clozapine with certain selective serotonin-reuptake inhibitors (SSRIs), including escitalopram, fluoxetine, fluvoxamine, paroxetine, and sertraline, can increase plasma concentrations of clozapine due to inhibition of clozapine metabolism by SSRIs. Modest (less than twofold) elevations in plasma clozapine concentrations have been reported in patients receiving clozapine concomitantly with certain SSRIs (i.e., fluoxetine, paroxetine, sertraline).

Substantial (threefold) increases in trough plasma clozapine concentrations have occurred in patients receiving concomitant therapy with clozapine and the potent CYP1A2 inhibitor fluvoxamine. Clozapine dosage should be reduced to one-third of the usual dosage when used concomitantly with fluvoxamine and should be increased back to the original dosage if fluvoxamine is discontinued.

■ **Drugs Metabolized by Hepatic Microsomal Enzymes** Clozapine may increase systemic exposure of other drugs metabolized by CYP2D6 (e.g., some antidepressants, phenothiazines, carbamazepine, class Ic antiarrhythmics [e.g., encainide, flecainide, propafenone]). Caution should be exercised when such drugs are used concomitantly with clozapine. The manufacturers state that dosage reduction of the CYP2D6 substrate may be necessary.

■ **Other Drugs Associated with Neutropenia** It is not known whether concurrent use of other drugs known to cause neutropenia increases the risk or severity of clozapine-induced neutropenia. The manufacturers of clozapine currently state that there is no strong scientific rationale to avoid clozapine treatment in patients concurrently treated with such drugs. However, if clozapine is used in patients concurrently receiving other drugs known to cause neutropenia (e.g., some antineoplastic agents), the manufacturers state that closer monitoring than usually recommended should be considered and, in patients concomitantly receiving antineoplastic agents, the treating oncologist should be consulted.

■ **Drugs Affecting the Seizure Threshold** Clozapine may lower the seizure threshold and is associated with dose-related increases in the risk of seizures (see Seizures under Cautions: Nervous System Effects). Therefore, the manufacturers state that clozapine should be used with caution in patients receiving concomitant therapy with other agents that lower the seizure threshold. In addition, caution is advised in patients in whom alcohol abuse is a concern.

■ **CNS Depressants** ***Benzodiazepines*** Severe hypotension (including absence of measurable blood pressure), respiratory or cardiac arrest, and loss of consciousness have been reported in several patients who received clozapine concomitantly with or following benzodiazepine (i.e., flurazepam, lorazepam, diazepam) therapy. Such effects occurred following administration of 12.5–150 mg of clozapine concurrently with or within 24 hours of the benzodiazepine, but patients generally have recovered within a few minutes to hours, usually spontaneously; the reactions usually developed on the first or second day of clozapine therapy. Although a causal relationship has not been established and such effects also have been observed in clozapine-treated patients who were not receiving a benzodiazepine concomitantly (see Cautions: Cardiovascular Effects), death resulting from respiratory arrest reportedly has occurred in at least one patient receiving clozapine concomitantly with a benzodiazepine. An increased incidence of dizziness and sedation and greater increases in liver enzyme test results also have been reported with this drug combination.

■ **Other CNS-active Agents** Although a causal relationship has not been established, at least one death has been reported with concomitant clozapine and haloperidol therapy. A 31-year-old woman with schizophrenia developed respiratory arrest, became comatose, and died 4 days after receiving 10 mg of haloperidol orally and a single 100-mg dose of clozapine IM. The patient had been maintained on oral clozapine 200 mg daily for 2 years and also had received smaller doses of haloperidol concomitantly with clozapine therapy without unusual adverse effect.

Neuroleptic malignant syndrome has been reported rarely with clozapine therapy alone and during concomitant therapy with clozapine and carbamazepine, lithium, or other CNS-active agents. (See Neuroleptic Malignant Syndrome under Cautions: Nervous System Effects.)

Concomitant use of clozapine and lithium may also increase the risk of seizures.

■ **Drugs that Prolong the QT Interval** Because of additive effects on QT-interval prolongation, clozapine should be used with caution in patients receiving other drugs known to prolong the QT interval, including class Ia antiarrhythmics (e.g., quinidine, procainamide), class III antiarrhythmics (e.g., amiodarone, sotalol), certain antipsychotic agents (e.g., chlorpromazine, haloperidol, iloperidone, mesoridazine [no longer commercially available in the US], pimozide, risperidone, thioridazine, ziprasidone), some anti-infective agents (e.g., erythromycin, gatifloxacin, moxifloxacin, sparfloxacin [no longer commercially available in the US]), and other drugs (e.g., dolasetron mesylate, droperidol, halofantrine [no longer commercially available in the US], levomethadyl acetate [no longer commercially available in the US], mefloquine, methadone, pentamidine, probucol [no longer commercially available in the US], tacrolimus). (See Prolongation of QT Interval under Cautions: Cardiovascular Effects.)

■ **Drugs with Anticholinergic Activity** Clozapine has potent anticholinergic effects and therefore should be used with caution in patients concurrently receiving other drugs with anticholinergic activity. (See Anticholinergic Toxicity under Cautions: Precautions and Contraindications.)

■ **Hypotensive Agents** Clozapine may be additive with or potentiate the actions of hypotensive agents; the drug should be used with particular caution in patients receiving concomitant antihypertensive therapy.

■ **Smoking** Smoking tobacco products (e.g., cigarettes) moderately induces CYP1A2, and may substantially reduce plasma clozapine concentrations. Limited data indicate that plasma clozapine concentrations following a given dose in smokers average 60–82% of those in nonsmokers. The manufacturers state that if clozapine is used in smokers, patients should be monitored for decreased efficacy of clozapine and consideration should be given to increasing the dosage, if necessary. Likewise, if smoking is discontinued during clozapine therapy, patients should be monitored for possible adverse effects and dosage reduction of clozapine should be considered, if necessary.

Acute Toxicity

■ **Pathogenesis** Acute toxicity studies in animals revealed that the LD_{50}s for clozapine administered orally, IV, or intraperitoneally are approximately 145–325, 58–61, and 90 mg/kg, respectively.

Although the acute lethal dose of clozapine in humans remains to be established, fatal overdoses with the drug generally have been associated with doses exceeding 2.5 g. However, there also have been reports of patients surviving overdoses that substantially exceeded 4 g of the drug.

■ **Manifestations** In general, overdosage of clozapine may be expected to produce effects that are extensions of the drug's pharmacologic and adverse effects. The most commonly reported signs and symptoms of clozapine overdosage have been altered states of consciousness and CNS depression (e.g., sedation, delirium, coma), tachycardia, hypotension, respiratory depression or failure, and hypersalivation. Seizures, cardiac arrhythmias, and aspiration pneumonia also have occurred with overdosage of clozapine in some patients. (See Seizures under Cautions: Nervous System Effects.)

A 24-year-old woman who ingested 2 g in excess of her prescribed daily dosage (i.e., total ingestion approximately 3 g within a 24-hour period) had a tonic-clonic (grand mal) seizure; her plasma clozapine concentration 1 hour after the seizure (1313 ng/mL) was 500 ng/mL higher than usual, but she recovered uneventfully. In a 50-year-old woman who ingested 1 g of clozapine, the only manifestations were confusion and hallucinations lasting about 48 hours. A 26-year-old man who ingested approximately 3 g of clozapine became drowsy, agitated, and disoriented; he also had visual hallucinations, dysarthria, tachycardia, and hypersalivation. The patient was treated with gastric lavage and also received diazepam, digitalis, and anti-infectives, but continued to exhibit manifestations of severe central anticholinergic toxicity. Administration of physostigmine salicylate 2 mg by slow IV injection resulted in improvement in the patient's mental status within minutes; however, symptoms recurred after approximately 1 hour. Symptoms finally remitted 18–24 hours later with no further treatment.

■ **Treatment** Treatment of clozapine overdosage generally requires symptomatic and supportive care, including monitoring of cardiac and vital signs. There is no specific antidote for the management of clozapine overdosage.

The manufacturers recommend establishing and maintaining an airway and ensuring adequate ventilation and oxygenation. Electrolyte and acid-base balance should be monitored and adjusted accordingly. Peritoneal dialysis or hemodialysis is of limited value in the treatment of clozapine overdosage because the drug is almost totally bound to serum proteins. While physostigmine salicylate may be useful as adjunctive treatment if severe anticholinergic toxicity is present, the drug should *not* be used routinely because of its potential adverse effects.

In managing clozapine overdosage, the clinician should consider the possibility of multiple drug involvement.

Chronic Toxicity

Chronic toxicity studies in mice, rats, dogs, and monkeys have revealed no specific organ toxicity. After 1 year of treatment with clozapine, a brown discoloration caused by increased lipopigment was observed in various organs in rats; this change normally appears with increasing age. Discoloration was noted in the thyroid, brain, liver, kidney, heart, spleen, and skeletal muscle of rats, but such increased pigmentation was not associated with deleterious changes. The liver did show slight, dose-dependent changes, including centrolobular vacuolation, hepatocyte swelling, and increased weight.

Pharmacology

Clozapine is a dibenzodiazepine-derivative antipsychotic agent. Clozapine shares some of the pharmacologic actions of other antipsychotic agents and has been described as an atypical or second-generation antipsychotic agent since many of its CNS effects differ from those of conventional (first-generation) agents (e.g., butyrophenones, phenothiazines). In fact, these apparent differences in actions on neostriatal dopaminergic receptors have led some investigators to question the importance of the dopaminergic system in mediating the therapeutic effects of neuroleptic drugs. The exact mechanism of antipsychotic action of clozapine has not been fully elucidated, but appears to be mediated through a combination of antagonist activity at dopamine type 2 (D_2) and serotonin type 2A (5-hydroxytryptamine [$5\text{-}HT_{2A}$]) receptors. Clozapine also acts as an antagonist at adrenergic, cholinergic, histaminergic, and other dopaminergic and serotonergic receptors.

■ **Nervous System Effects** Although the precise mechanism of action of antipsychotic drugs has not been fully elucidated, current data suggest that the therapeutic effects of atypical antipsychotic agents involve antagonism of dopaminergic and serotonergic systems in the CNS. In animals, classic neuroleptic agents increase muscle tone or induce postural abnormalities (catalepsy), antagonize stereotyped behaviors induced by the dopamine agonists apomorphine and amphetamine, accelerate dopamine turnover in various areas of the brain, increase serum prolactin concentrations, and produce dopamine receptor hypersensitivity on repeated administration. These effects, many of which have been attributed to blockade of dopamine receptors in the neostriatum, form the basis for the hypothesis that idiopathic psychoses result from overactivity of dopamine in neostriatal and mesolimbic systems.

Unlike typical antipsychotic agents, clozapine exerts relatively weak antidopaminergic action within the neostriatum and has a low propensity to produce extrapyramidal effects or stimulate prolactin secretion. While some studies have demonstrated that relatively high doses of clozapine suppress the conditioned avoidance response in animals, which is a characteristic of typical antipsychotic agents, this response is not completely blocked by clozapine, and tolerance to this effect develops rapidly with repeated dosing, suggesting that it is not specifically related to clozapine's antipsychotic action. Further research is needed to elucidate fully clozapine's antipsychotic action in terms of the drug's serotonergic, adrenergic, muscarinic, and peptidergic effects and their influences on functional alterations in dopamine receptor systems.

Antidopaminergic Effects The therapeutic effects of antipsychotic drugs are thought to be mediated by dopaminergic blockade in the mesolimbic and mesocortical areas of the CNS, while antidopaminergic effects in the neostriatum appear to be associated with extrapyramidal effects. Several (at least 5) different types or subtypes of dopamine receptors have been identified in animals and humans. The relative densities of these receptors and their distribution and function vary for different neuroanatomical regions, and clozapine's unique effects may be secondary to regionally specific receptor interactions and/or other effects on dopaminergic neurons. Results obtained from receptor binding, behavioral, metabolic, and electrophysiologic studies of clozapine as well as the apparently low incidence of extrapyramidal effects associated with clozapine therapy suggest that the drug is more active in the mesolimbic than the neostriatal dopaminergic system. Results of some studies suggest that clozapine is more effective in increasing dopamine turnover and release in the nucleus accumbens or olfactory tubercle than in the neostriatum with acute administration and that it reduces dopamine release in the accumbens but not in the neostriatum during prolonged administration, which suggests preferential effects on dopaminergic function in the limbic system. However, conflicting data (i.e., no preferential limbic effects) also have been reported with both acute and repeated administration of the drug, which may reflect differences in analytical techniques, regional differences in drug distribution or receptor affinity, or other variables.

Some evidence suggests that the effects of clozapine on dopamine metabolism in the neostriatum are dose related; unlike typical antipsychotic drugs, clozapine appears to increase striatal dopamine turnover only at supratherapeutic doses. Single high doses (80 mg/kg intraperitoneally) of clozapine in rats interfere with dopaminergic transmission by blocking postsynaptic dopamine receptors and causing a compensatory increase in dopaminergic neuronal firing, while lower doses retard dopamine release. Clozapine appears to increase striatal dopamine content when given either in single high doses or repeated low doses, and low doses of the drug reportedly decrease the degradation of dopamine to 3-methoxy-4-hydroxyphenylacetic acid (homovanillic acid, HVA) in the neostriatum. In a rodent model of tardive dyskinesia, single low doses (up to 1.2 mg/kg intraperitoneally) of clozapine suppressed ketamine-induced linguopharyngeal movements, which resemble symptoms of tardive dyskinesia (e.g., tongue protrusions, retrusions, and swallows), by 15–75% compared with baseline measures. At clozapine doses of 4.8 mg/kg or higher, clozapine caused total suppression of these movements, and duration of suppression became dose dependent. Since suppression of abnormal linguopharyngeal movements occurred at doses substantially lower than those reported to alter dopamine turnover, it has been suggested that doses of the drug lower than those required for antipsychotic activity may be useful for treating antipsychotic-induced tardive dyskinesia.

Current evidence suggests that the clinical potency and antipsychotic efficacy of both typical and atypical antipsychotic drugs generally are related to their affinity for and blockade of central dopamine D_2 receptors; however, antagonism at D_2 receptors does not appear to account fully for the antipsychotic effects of clozapine.

In in vitro studies, clozapine is a comparatively weak antagonist at D_2 receptors. Clozapine's affinity for the D_2 receptor on a weight basis reportedly is approximately one-third (33%) that of loxapine, one-tenth (10%) that of chlorpromazine, and one-fiftieth (2%) that of haloperidol. In oral dosages of 300 mg daily, clozapine produces a 40–65% occupancy of D_1 and D_2 receptors. During long-term clozapine therapy, the relative occupancy of D_1 receptors may become greater than that of D_2 receptors, or the long-term effects of the drug on D_2 receptors may be antagonized by its nondopaminergic properties. Although the in vitro affinity of clozapine for D_1 and D_2 receptors in brain tissue of animals appears to be similar, the drug's in vivo effects in many animals resemble those of D_1receptor-specific antagonists. Compared with typical antipsychotic agents, clozapine shows greater affinity for and appears to produce greater blockade of neostriatal dopamine D_1 receptors; other data suggest that clozapine preferentially but not selectively antagonizes D_1 receptor-mediated functions. At clinically effective dosages, however, the drug produces comparable blockade of D_1 and D_2 receptors and less D_2 blockade than typical antipsychotic drugs. Long-term administration of clozapine leads to a 35–50% "up-regulation" of D_1 receptors, which is comparable to that observed with administration of selective D_1 antagonists; however, the number of D_2 receptors is not changed, possibly because the proportion of occupied receptors required to elicit a response is less for D_1 than for D_2 receptors. Limited evidence suggests that D_1 receptors may exist either coupled to adenylate cyclase or in uncoupled form. Clozapine appears to be a potent, competitive inhibitor of dopamine-stimulated adenylate cyclase in vitro, and the adenylate cyclase-coupled state of the D_1 receptor binds clozapine with high affinity; in contrast, typical antipsychotic agents bind preferentially to the uncoupled D_1 receptor.

Although their role in eliciting the pharmacologic effects of antipsychotic agents remains to be fully elucidated, dopamine D_3, D_4, and D_5 receptors also have been identified; clozapine appears to have a much higher affinity for the D_4 receptor than for D_2 or D_3 receptors. Current information on D_3-receptor affinity for antipsychotic drugs suggests that most antipsychotics probably bind to both D_2 and D_3 receptors, although with higher affinity to D_2 receptors; however, the magnitude of the difference in D_3- versus D_2-receptor binding is much less with atypical antipsychotics such as clozapine, suggesting that effects on D_3 receptors may play a more important role in the pharmacologic actions of atypical versus typical antipsychotic drugs. The high affinity of the D_4 receptor for clozapine and its preferential distribution in cortical and limbic areas in animals may explain, in part, the relative lack of tardive dyskinesia and extrapyramidal effects during clozapine therapy. The cloning of a gene for a neuron-specific dopamine D_5 receptor, which binds antipsychotic drugs with similar affinity as the D_1 receptor but has a tenfold higher affinity for dopamine, also has been reported.

Clozapine's clinical potency appears to be twice that of chlorpromazine on a weight basis, although the drug demonstrates considerably weaker D_2-receptor binding affinity than chlorpromazine and appears to be much less potent in elevating dopamine metabolite concentrations in the brain. Clozapine produces a more potent blockade of central serotonergic, adrenergic, histamine H_1, and muscarinic receptors than typical antipsychotic agents; also, long-term administration of clozapine enhances striatal D_1-receptor function in animals and results in "down-regulation" of cortical, type 2 serotonergic (5-HT_2) receptors, suggesting that an interaction between these central neurotransmitter systems may be important for the drug's antipsychotic efficacy. Antagonism at cholinergic and α_1-adrenergic receptors in the mesolimbic system, compensating for dopaminergic blockade in the neostriatum, may explain the apparent selectivity and low incidence of extrapyramidal effects seen with clozapine. The amygdala also may be a site of action for clozapine, since repeated administration of the drug selectively induces supersensitivity to locally applied dopamine in the amygdala, and amygdaloid neurons are excited by clozapine but generally unresponsive to other antipsychotic agents (e.g., haloperidol).

Further studies are needed to elucidate the mechanism of clozapine's antipsychotic effects in various areas of the CNS.

Neurophysiologic Effects In vitro and in vivo electrophysiologic studies in animals demonstrate different sensitivities of various brain areas to clozapine-mediated postsynaptic receptor blockade. While clozapine increases firing rates of both nigrostriatal (A9 pathway) and mesolimbic (A10 pathway) dopaminergic neurons after acute administration, only mesolimbic dopaminergic neurons exhibit prolonged depolarization blockade following repeated exposure to the drug. Repeated administration of typical antipsychotic agents (e.g., haloperidol) concomitantly with an anticholinergic agent (trihexyphenidyl) or an α_1-adrenergic blocking drug (prazosin) mimicked these selective effects of clozapine on mesolimbic versus nigrostriatal dopaminergic neurons, suggesting that α_1-adrenergic blocking and/or anticholinergic effects may be responsible, in part, for the differential effects of clozapine in these midbrain areas. Some evidence suggests that the nucleus accumbens has greater sensitivity for clozapine than do other regions, which may explain why the drug appears to produce depolarization blockade of dopaminergic neurons only in the mesolimbic area. However, some studies have shown that neurons in the neostriatum also may be responsive to clozapine. Clozapine reportedly produces an increase in dopamine metabolites in the neostriatum comparable to or even greater than that in the nucleus accumbens. Demonstrable dopamine-receptor supersensitivity in both striatal and limbic forebrain regions also has been reported with prolonged clozapine administration. Therefore, it has been suggested that there may be a dissociation between the effects of clozapine on synthesis and metabolism of dopamine within nigrostriatal neurons and the drug's effects on neuronal firing rate and dopamine release.

Adrenergic Effects Clozapine has adrenergic-blocking activity, which may be partially responsible for the sedation, muscle relaxation, and cardiac effects observed in patients receiving the drug. (See Cautions: Cardiovascular Effects.) Although the drug appears to have relatively weak α-adrenergic blocking effects compared with typical antipsychotic drugs such as chlorpromazine, clozapine's in vitro affinity (relative to dopamine D_2-receptor affinity) for α_1- and α_2-adrenergic receptors is much higher than that of conventional antipsychotics, including chlorpromazine, haloperidol, loxapine, and thioridazine. Clozapine increases the number and sensitivity of α_1-adrenergic, but not dopamine D_2, receptors. The turnover rate of epinephrine and norepinephrine also may be increased by clozapine, but to a lesser extent than that of dopamine. Substantial increases in plasma norepinephrine concentrations, which decreased following discontinuance of the drug but remained above basal levels, have been noted in both schizophrenic and healthy individuals receiving clozapine; such increases may be the result of feedback mechanisms activated by adrenergic blockade.

Clozapine's central α_1-adrenergic blocking activity also may be responsible for the dose-related hypothermia observed in mice given the drug. Clozapine also induces ataxia and blocks amphetamine-induced hyperactivity in mice, although repeated administration of the drug results in almost complete tolerance to these effects. It has been suggested that clozapine's α_1-adrenergic blocking properties may, in part, mediate its differential effects on midbrain dopamine receptors and be responsible for its relative lack of extrapyramidal effects. However, the clinical importance of the drug's α_1-adrenergic effects has not been fully elucidated.

Anticholinergic Effects Clozapine possesses potent anticholinergic activity in vitro; the drug's affinity for muscarinic receptors substantially exceeds that of other antipsychotic agents (e.g., 39–50 times greater than that of chlorpromazine and 100 times that of loxapine) and may be similar to that of tricyclic antidepressants and antimuscarinic antiparkinsonian agents (e.g., benztropine, trihexyphenidyl). It has been suggested that clozapine's anticholinergic effects may be more potent centrally than peripherally and that adverse anticholinergic effects generally are not dose limiting; however, peripheral anticholinergic effects such as dry mouth are common and may be troublesome. Clozapine-induced delirium, which reportedly has occurred with rapid dosage escalation, has been reversed by physostigmine; this suggests that clozapine has central antimuscarinic activity. Some evidence also suggests that clozapine's anticholinergic properties may counteract the effects of dopamine receptor blockade in the neostriatum and thus prevent extrapyramidal reactions. Limited data suggest that the propensity of antipsychotic drugs to cause extrapyramidal effects varies inversely with anticholinergic potency and antimuscarinic activity; however, the relatively potent anticholinergic activity of clozapine does not appear to account adequately for its atypical actions.

Serotonergic Effects It has been suggested that schizophrenia may involve a dysregulation of serotonin- and dopamine-mediated neurotransmission, and clozapine may at least partially restore a normal balance of neurotransmitter function, possibly through serotonergic regulation of dopaminergic tone. Clozapine blocks central type 2A serotonergic (5-HT_{2A}) receptors; the drug also antagonizes central and peripheral type 3 serotonergic (5-HT_3) receptors. Long-term and acute administration of clozapine has produced down-regulation of 5-HT_2 receptors in the frontal cortex and neostriatum of male rats; single or repeated daily injections of clozapine also reduced the number of cortical 5-HT_2 receptors but did not change receptor affinity. In contrast to effects caused by typical antipsychotic agents, an increase in brain tryptophan, serotonin, and 5-hydroxyindoleacetic acid (5-HIAA) concentrations generally has been reported with clozapine administration in animals. It has been suggested that these effects might contribute to the pronounced sedative effects of clozapine, although increases in blood serotonin concentrations occurring during clozapine treatment in humans have been inconsistent and variable. (See Effects on Sleep under Pharmacology: Nervous System Effects.) Clozapine's serotonergic effects also reportedly may contribute to the drug's efficacy against negative symptoms of schizophrenia and to the weight gain observed during clozapine therapy. (See Cautions: Endocrine and Metabolic Effects.)

Effects on Other Central Neurotransmitters Clozapine appears to have important activity on the metabolism of γ-aminobutyric acid (GABA), which has inhibitory effects on dopaminergic neurons. In contrast to the effects of typical antipsychotic drugs, clozapine apparently augments GABA turnover in both the neostriatum and nucleus accumbens. Increases in neostriatal GABA turnover and release may attenuate extrapyramidal reactions, while a similar action in the nucleus accumbens may be related to antipsychotic efficacy.

Clozapine appears to have central histamine H_1-receptor blocking activity; such activity reportedly may be associated with sedation, hypotension, and weight gain. The drug's affinity (relative to dopamine D_2-receptor affinity) for histamine H_1-receptors is approximately 30 times that of chlorpromazine and 4 times that of loxapine.

Behavioral Effects in Animals Studies of the effects of clozapine on animal behavior routinely used to detect antipsychotic activity support its classification as an atypical antipsychotic drug. Such studies suggest that the neostriatum is relatively unresponsive to clozapine. Since the drug does not induce catalepsy or inhibit apomorphine-induced stereotypy, which are thought to be mediated principally by the nigrostriatal dopamine system, clozapine's antipsychotic activity appears to result from the drug's activity in other areas. Clozapine also does not block amphetamine-induced hyperactivity or apomorphine-induced emesis in animals as the typical antipsychotic agents do. Long-term administration of clozapine causes supersensitization of behaviors mediated by mesolimbic dopaminergic pathways (e.g., dopamine-induced locomotion) but not those mediated via neostriatal systems (e.g., dopamine-induced stereotypy). Long-term administration of clozapine in male rats caused a marked supersensitivity (of the same magnitude and duration as that of haloperidol) in the mesolimbic but not the nigrostriatal system. It has been suggested that supersensitivity of mesolimbic dopamine receptors may be associated with the apparent rebound psychosis that has been reported following clozapine therapy. (See Cautions: Other Nervous System Effects.)

EEG Effects Clozapine may produce dose-related changes in the EEG, including increased discharge patterns similar to those associated with seizure disorders, and may lower the seizure threshold; seizures have occurred in patients receiving the drug, particularly with high dosages (greater than 600 mg daily), rapid dosage increases, and/or in the presence of high plasma concentrations. (See Seizures in Cautions: Nervous System Effects.) Some EEG changes associated with clozapine administration are atypical of those generally seen with other antipsychotic agents, resembling more closely those produced by antidepressants. Clozapine increases beta-, delta-, and theta-band amplitudes and slows dominant alpha frequencies in clinical EEG studies. However, in patients with severe, treatment-resistant schizophrenia, increases in delta and theta band frequencies are more pronounced with clozapine than with haloperidol or chlorpromazine therapy, a finding that appears to parallel the drugs' relative antiserotonergic, antihistaminic, and anticholinergic activities. Enhanced EEG synchronization, paroxysmal sharp-wave activity, and spike and wave complexes also may develop during clozapine therapy. Clozapine-induced EEG changes generally appear soon after initiation of the drug and return to baseline upon cessation of therapy. In one study, the EEG showed slight general changes or slight diffuse slowing in 75% of patients receiving clozapine; in another study, clozapine caused marked EEG changes, including a slowing of basal activity, in 5% of patients.

Effects on Sleep Clozapine causes a shift in the sleep-wake pattern toward dozing in animals, with marked reductions in both slow-wave and paradoxical sleep times. However, tolerance to the drug's sedative effect usually occurs, although slowly in some patients, during continuous administration of clozapine. In a controlled study of short-term (3-day) administration in healthy young men, clozapine in dosages of 25 mg nightly substantially increased total sleep time on the first night of administration, but the duration of sleep returned to baseline by the third night. Clozapine did not substantially affect the time spent in stage 1, 2, 3, or slow-wave sleep, nor did it affect latency to the rapid eye movement (REM) period or the percentage of time spent in REM sleep. However, the percentage of time spent in stage 4 sleep was reduced substantially on the second and third nights of drug administration, while a variety of REM indices were increased on the third night of the study.

In a few patients receiving clozapine dosages of 150–800 mg daily, REM sleep increased to 85–100% of total sleep time after several days of drug therapy, with the onset of REM sleep occurring almost immediately after patients fell asleep. Intensification of dream activity also has been reported during clozapine therapy. Some clinicians have suggested that a correlation may exist between increases in body temperature and REM sleep and clozapine-induced improvement in psychosis. Cataplexy has been reported in some patients receiving clozapine.

■ Neuroendocrine Effects In contrast to typical antipsychotic drugs, clozapine therapy in usual dosages generally produces little or no elevation of prolactin concentration in humans. Administration of clozapine to rats has produced a transient, dose-related increase in prolactin concentrations that is of much shorter duration than that caused by other antipsychotic agents. Prolactin normally is inhibited by dopamine released from tuberoinfundibular (TIDA) neurons into the pituitary portal circulation. In rats, clozapine acutely increases the activity of TIDA neurons, which inhibit the release of prolactin; activation of TIDA neurons may be mediated by an enhanced release of neurotensin. Clozapine's effect on prolactin appears to be transient, possibly because the drug appears to dissociate from dopamine receptors more rapidly than typical antipsychotic agents and is therefore eliminated from the brain more rapidly.

Clozapine has an effect on corticotropin (ACTH) and corticosterone, possibly through its effects on dopamine metabolism in the hypothalamus. Short-term administration of clozapine (cumulative dose: 200 mg) to a few patients with schizophrenia resulted in marked inhibition of apomorphine-induced somatotropin (growth hormone) response, suggesting that clozapine may block the dopamine receptors responsible for eliciting this response. In contrast to typical antipsychotic agents, clozapine decreases or has no effect on basal cortisol levels. Clozapine markedly increases corticosterone concentrations in a dose-dependent fashion; other antipsychotic agents appear to increase corticosterone concentrations only at doses producing substantial D_2-receptor blockade. Clozapine-induced stimulation of corticosterone secretion may result from stimulation, rather than blockade, of dopamine receptors, but the exact mechanism has not been fully elucidated.

■ Other Effects Clozapine produced a dose-dependent delay in initiation of copulation in male rats, which may be related to blockade of mesolimbic dopamine receptors; however, the drug had no effect on copulatory behavior once the behavior had started. Fertility in male and female rats reportedly is not adversely affected by clozapine. (See Cautions: Pregnancy, Fertility, and Lactation.)

In animals, even small oral doses of clozapine cause ptosis, relaxation, and a reduction in spontaneous activity, effects that are consistent with the drug's sedative activity. Inhibition of locomotor activity induced by clozapine diminishes with repeated administration. With increasing doses of the drug, reactions to acoustic and tactile stimuli decline, and disturbances in equilibrium have been reported. Clozapine also inhibits isolation-induced aggression in mice at doses lower than those affecting motor function, suggesting a specific antiaggressive effect.

Studies in animals suggest that clozapine has a weak and variable diuretic effect; the clinical importance of this effect has not been established. In both rats and dogs, low doses of clozapine tend to increase the elimination of water and electrolytes, while higher doses are associated with increases in potassium excretion and sodium retention.

Pharmacokinetics

■ Absorption Clozapine is rapidly and almost completely absorbed following oral administration. However, because of extensive hepatic first-pass metabolism, only about 27–50% of an orally administered dose reaches systemic circulation unchanged. Some, but not all, evidence suggests that clozapine may exhibit nonlinear, dose-dependent pharmacokinetics, with oral bioavailability being approximately 30% less following a single 75-mg dose than at steady state following multiple dosing. GI absorption appears to occur principally in the small intestine and is approximately 90–95% complete within 3.5 hours after an oral dose. Food does not appear to have a clinically important effect on the rate or extent of GI absorption of the drug when given as conventional tablets. Administration of clozapine orally disintegrating tablets or oral suspension with a high-fat meal decreases peak plasma concentrations of clozapine by about 20%, but does not affect area under the plasma concentration-time curve (AUC). The differences in peak plasma concentrations are not considered clinically important; therefore, the manufacturers state that clozapine (as conventional tablets, orally disintegrating tablets, or oral suspension) can be taken without regard to meals.

The relative oral bioavailability of clozapine has been shown to be equivalent following administration of 25-mg and 100-mg conventional tablets; commercially available clozapine oral suspension and conventional tablets and orally disintegrating tablets and conventional tablets also are bioequivalent.

Following oral administration of a single 25- or 100-mg oral dose of clozapine as tablets in healthy adults, the drug is detectable in plasma within 25 minutes, and peak plasma clozapine concentrations occur at about 1.5 hours. Peak plasma concentrations may be delayed with higher single doses and with multiple dosing of the drug. In a multiple-dose study, peak plasma clozapine concentrations at steady state averaged 319 ng/mL (range: 102–771 ng/mL) and occurred on average at 2.5 hours (range: 1–6 hours) after a dose with 100 mg twice daily as conventional tablets; minimum plasma concentrations at steady state averaged 122 ng/mL (range: 41–343 ng/mL). Steady-state plasma concentrations ranging from 200–600 ng/mL generally are achieved with oral dosages of 300 mg daily, and steady-state peak plasma concentrations generally occur within 2–4 hours after a dose. Steady-state plasma concentrations of clozapine are achieved after 7–10 days of continuous dosing.

Following multiple-dose administration of clozapine orally disintegrating tablets at a dosage of 100 mg twice daily in adults, peak plasma clozapine concentrations at steady state averaged 413 ng/mL (range: 132–854 ng/mL) and occurred on average at 2.3 hours (range: 1–6 hours). Minimum plasma concentrations at steady state in this study averaged 168 ng/mL (range: 45–574 ng/mL). Following multiple-dose administration of clozapine oral suspension at a dosage of 100–800 mg once daily, peak plasma clozapine concentrations at steady state averaged 275 ng/mL (range: 105–723 ng/mL) and occurred on average at 2.2 hours (range: 1–3.5 hours). Minimum plasma concentrations at steady state in this study averaged 75 ng/mL (range: 11–198 ng/mL).

Considerable interindividual variation in plasma clozapine concentrations has been observed in patients receiving the drug, and some patients may exhibit either extremely high or extremely low plasma concentrations with a given dosage. Such variability may be particularly likely at relatively high dosages (e.g., 400 mg daily) of the drug. In one study, a sixfold interindividual variation in steady-state plasma clozapine concentration was observed in patients receiving such dosages. In addition, considerable intraindividual variation, particularly from week to week, may occur in some patients. However, substantial intraindividual variations in pharmacokinetic parameters typically are not observed from day to day. Although the interindividual variability in plasma clozapine concentrations is consistent with that reported for other antipsychotic drugs and may be secondary to differences in absorption, distribution, metabolism, or clearance of the drug, further study is needed to clarify whether such variation results principally from variable pharmacokinetics or other variables.

There is some evidence that interindividual differences in pharmacokinetic parameters for clozapine may result, at least in part, from nonlinear, dose-dependent pharmacokinetics of the drug. However, a linear dose-concentration relationship also has been reported. Results of a study in patients with chronic schizophrenia revealed a correlation between oral clozapine dosages of 100–800 mg daily and steady-state plasma concentrations of the drug. In addition, linearly dose-proportional changes in area under the plasma concentration-time curve (AUC) and in peak and trough plasma concentrations have been observed with oral dosages of 37.5, 75, and 150 mg twice daily in other studies.

Because clozapine is a substrate for many cytochrome P-450 (CYP) isoenzymes, including CYP1A2, CYP2D6, and CYP3A4, patients with poor-metabolizer phenotypes of CYP2D6 may have higher plasma clozapine concentrations at usual dosages. In addition, smokers appear to achieve plasma clozapine concentrations that are approximately 60–80% of those achieved by nonsmokers following oral administration of the drug, due to induction of CYP1A2 activity by tobacco smoke. (See Drug Interactions: Smoking.) There also is limited evidence that gender may affect plasma clozapine concentrations, with concentrations being somewhat reduced, perhaps by as much as 20–30%, in males compared with females. In addition, smoking has a greater effect on clozapine plasma concentrations in men than in women, although this difference could result simply from gender differences in smoking behavior. Plasma concentrations may be increased in geriatric individuals compared with relatively young (e.g., 18–35 years old) individuals, possibly secondary to age-related decreases in hepatic elimination of clozapine.

Pharmacologic effects of clozapine (e.g., sedation) reportedly are apparent within 15 minutes and become clinically important within 1–6 hours. The duration of action of clozapine reportedly ranges from 4–12 hours following a single oral dose. In one study in patients with schizophrenia, the sedative effect was apparent within hours of the first dose of the drug and was maximal within 7 days. (See Effects on Sleep under Pharmacology: Nervous System Effects.) However, antipsychotic activity generally is delayed for one to several weeks after initiation of clozapine therapy, and maximal activity may require several months of therapy with the drug.

Correlations between steady-state plasma concentrations of clozapine and therapeutic efficacy have not been established, and some evidence suggests that the degree of clinical improvement is independent of plasma concentrations ranging from 100–800 ng/mL. However, it also has been suggested that serum clozapine concentrations less than 600 ng/mL may be adequate for therapeutic effect in most patients. Results of one study of 29 patients treated with clozapine 400 mg daily for 4 weeks showed that patients were most likely to respond to therapy when their plasma clozapine concentrations were at least 350 ng/mL and/or when plasma concentrations of clozapine plus norclozapine (an active metabolite) totaled at least 450 ng/mL. Further study is needed to determine whether nonresponding patients with plasma clozapine concentrations less than 350 ng/mL will benefit from increasing their dosage in an attempt to achieve higher concentrations.

■ **Distribution** Distribution of clozapine into human body tissues is rapid and extensive; distribution of metabolites of the drug also appears to be extensive. In mice and rats, clozapine distributes principally into the lung, spleen, liver, kidney, gallbladder, and brain, achieving concentrations in these tissues up to 50 times those in blood. At 8 hours after IV injection, clozapine was still detectable in these organs but not in blood. There is limited evidence in animals that clozapine and its metabolites may be preferentially retained in the lungs by an energy-dependent, carrier-mediated process and by cellular binding. Evidence in animals also suggests that competition between clozapine and other drugs (e.g., chlorpromazine, imipramine, certain tetracycline antibiotics) for pulmonary binding sites may potentially affect plasma and tissue concentrations of clozapine, but the clinical importance, if any, of such an effect has not been established.

The volume of distribution of clozapine has been reported to be approximately 4.65 L/kg. In one study, the volume of distribution at steady state averaged 1.6 L/kg (range: 0.4–3.6 L/kg) in schizophrenic patients. Because the volume of distribution of clozapine is smaller than that of other antipsychotic agents, it has been suggested that clozapine is less sequestered in tissues than the other drugs. Clozapine is approximately 97% bound to serum proteins.

Results of receptor-binding studies in monkeys indicate that clozapine rapidly crosses the blood-brain barrier following IV injection. The highest brain uptake of the drug was in the striatum in these animals; lesser concentrations were achieved in the thalamus and mesencephalon, although they exceeded those in the cerebellum. The pharmacokinetic characteristics of the drug in the CNS paralleled those in plasma in these monkeys, with an elimination half-life from CNS of about 5 hours. Evidence from other animal studies indicates that CNS concentrations of the drug exceed those in blood. Distribution of the drug into the CNS in humans has not been characterized.

Clozapine reportedly is present in low concentrations in the placenta in animals; information on placental transfer of the drug in humans currently is unavailable. Clozapine distributes into human milk. (See Cautions: Pregnancy, Fertility, and Lactation.)

■ **Elimination** The decline of plasma clozapine concentrations in humans is biphasic. The elimination half-life of clozapine following a single 75-mg oral dose reportedly averages 8 hours (range: 4–12 hours); that after a 100-mg oral dose appears to be similar. The elimination half-life of clozapine at steady state following administration of 100 mg twice daily reportedly averages 12 hours (range: 4–66 hours). The rapid elimination phase may represent redistribution and is followed by a slower apparent mean terminal elimination half-life of 10.3–38 hours. Although a study comparing single and multiple dosing of clozapine demonstrated an increase in elimination half-life with multiple dosing, other evidence suggests this finding is not attributable to concentration-dependent pharmacokinetics.

Clozapine is almost completely metabolized in the liver prior to excretion by many CYP isoenzymes, particularly CYP1A2, CYP2D6, and CYP3A4. Clozapine may undergo *N*-demethylation, *N*-oxidation, 3′-carbon oxidation, epoxidation of the chlorine-containing aromatic ring, substitution of chlorine by hydroxyl or thiomethyl groups, and sulfur oxidation. A glucuronide metabolite, tentatively identified as a quaternary ammonium *N*-glucuronide of clozapine, also has been identified. Metabolism of clozapine may occur by one or more of these routes.

The rate of formation and biologic activity of clozapine metabolites have not been fully elucidated. The desmethyl metabolite of clozapine (norclozapine) has limited activity while the hydroxylated and *N*-oxide derivatives are inactive. The *N*-oxide and desmethyl derivatives are found in urine and plasma of humans in a proportion of 2:1.

Approximately 32% of a single oral dose of clozapine is found in plasma as the parent compound after 3 hours, 20% in 8 hours, and 10% up to 48 hours following the dose. Only limited amounts (approximately 2–5%) of unchanged drug are detected in urine and feces. Approximately 50% of an administered dose is excreted in urine and 30% in feces; maximum fecal excretion has been estimated at 38%. Approximately 46% of an oral dose of clozapine is excreted in urine within 120 hours.

Total plasma and blood clearance of clozapine reportedly average 217 and 250 mL/minute, respectively, but show considerable interindividual variation.

Chemistry and Stability

■ **Chemistry** Clozapine is a dibenzodiazepine-derivative antipsychotic agent. The drug is a piperazine-substituted tricyclic antipsychotic agent that is structurally similar to loxapine but that differs pharmacologically from this and other currently available antipsychotic agents (e.g., phenothiazines, butyrophenones). Because of these pharmacologic differences, clozapine is considered an atypical or second-generation antipsychotic agent.

While the structure-activity relationships of phenothiazine antipsychotic agents have been well described, these relationships for heterocyclic antipsychotic agents, including clozapine, have not been as fully characterized. Generally, the unsubstituted benzene ring seems to be important for interactions at dopamine receptors, while the chloro-substituted benzene ring seems more important for action at muscarinic receptors. In addition, an open carbon side chain replacing the piperazine moiety of clozapine generally leads to loss of activity.

Clozapine differs structurally from most currently available antipsychotic agents by the presence of a seven- rather than a six-membered central ring and the spatial relationship between the piperazine moiety and the chloro-substituted benzene ring. The core tricyclic ring system of clozapine is nonplanar and allows the piperazine moiety limited freedom of rotation.

Clozapine differs structurally from loxapine by the presence of a diazepine rather than an oxazepine central ring in the tricyclic nucleus and by the presence of a chlorine atom at position 8 rather than 2 of the tricyclic nucleus. The presence of a chlorine atom at position 8 of the tricyclic nucleus of clozapine appears to be associated with its distinct pharmacologic profile and may be responsible for the drug's antimuscarinic activity.

Clozapine occurs as a yellow, crystalline powder and is very slightly soluble in water.

■ **Stability** Commercially available conventional clozapine tablets should be stored in tight containers at a controlled room temperature of 20–25°C and not exceeding 30°C. Clozapine orally disintegrating tablets (e.g., FazaClo®) should be stored in their original package at a controlled room temperature of 20–25°C, but may be exposed to temperatures ranging from 15–30°C. The orally disintegrating tablets should be protected from moisture. Clozapine oral suspension (e.g., Versacloz®) should be stored at a controlled room temperature of 20–25°C, but may be exposed to temperatures ranging from 15–30°C; the oral suspension should be protected from light and should not be refrigerated or frozen. The oral suspension is stable for 100 days after initial bottle opening.

Preparations

Clozapine is available only through a shared REMS program, the Clozapine REMS program, which ensures appropriate monitoring and management of patients with severe neutropenia. (See REMS.)

Excipients in commercially available drug preparations may have clinically important effects in some individuals; consult specific product labeling for details.

cloZAPine

Oral		
Suspension	50 mg/mL	Versacloz®, Jazz
Tablets	25 mg*	cloZAPine Tablets (scored)
		Clozaril® (scored), HLS
	50 mg*	cloZAPine Tablets (scored)
	100 mg*	cloZAPine Tablets (scored)
		Clozaril® (scored), HLS
	200 mg*	cloZAPine Tablets (scored)
Tablets, orally disintegrating	12.5 mg*	FazaClo®, Jazz
	25 mg*	FazaClo®, Jazz
	100 mg*	FazaClo®, Jazz
	150 mg*	FazaClo®, Jazz
	200 mg*	FazaClo®, Jazz

*available from one or more manufacturer, distributor, and/or repackager by generic (nonproprietary) name

†Use is not currently included in the labeling approved by the US Food and Drug Administration

Iloperidone

Zomaril

■ Iloperidone is considered an atypical or second-generation antipsychotic agent.

Uses

■ **Psychotic Disorders** Drug therapy is integral to the management of acute psychotic episodes in patients with schizophrenia and generally is required for long-term stabilization to sustain symptom remission or control and to minimize the risk of relapse. Antipsychotic agents are the principal class of drugs used for the management of all phases of schizophrenia. Patient response and tolerance to antipsychotic agents are variable, and patients who do not respond to or tolerate one drug may be successfully treated with an agent from a different class or with a different adverse effect profile.

Schizophrenia Iloperidone is an atypical antipsychotic that is administered orally in the treatment of schizophrenia. Schizophrenia is a major psychotic disorder that frequently has devastating effects on various aspects of the patient's life and carries a high risk of suicide and other life-threatening behaviors. Manifestations of schizophrenia involve multiple psychologic processes, including perception (e.g., hallucinations), ideation, reality testing (e.g., delusions), emotion (e.g., flatness, inappropriate affect), thought processes (e.g., loose associations), behavior (e.g., catatonia, disorganization), attention, concentration, motivation (e.g., avolition, impaired intention and planning), and judgment. The principal manifestations of this disorder usually are described in terms of positive and negative (deficit) symptoms and, more recently, disorganized symptoms. Positive symptoms include hallucinations, delusions, bizarre behavior, hostility, uncooperativeness, and paranoid ideation, while negative symptoms include restricted range and intensity of emotional expression (affective flattening), reduced thought and speech productivity (alogia), anhedonia, apathy, and decreased initiation of goal-directed behavior (avolition). Disorganized symptoms include disorganized speech (thought disorder) and behavior and poor attention.

Short-term efficacy of oral iloperidone in the acute management of schizophrenia was supported by 2 placebo- and active comparator-controlled clinical studies of 4 and 6 weeks' duration in adults who met DSM-III/IV criteria for schizophrenia. The studies primarily used the Positive and Negative Syndrome Scale (PANSS) or the Brief Psychiatric Rating Scale (BPRS) to assess the effects of drug treatment in improving the clinical manifestations of schizophrenia. Patients enrolled in the 6-week study were randomized to receive one of two iloperidone dosage ranges (12–16 or 20–24 mg daily) with an initial 1-week titration period, the active control risperidone (6–8 mg daily), or placebo. At study end point, both dosage ranges of iloperidone were found to be superior to placebo as assessed by the change from baseline in the BPRS total score. Risperidone appeared to be superior to iloperidone within the first 2 weeks of this study, which may be due at least in part to the drug's more rapid dosage titration. Patients enrolled in the 4-week study were randomized to receive iloperidone (24 mg daily), ziprasidone (160 mg daily), or placebo for 3 weeks following a 1-week titration period. At study end point, iloperidone 24 mg daily was found to be superior to placebo as assessed by the change from baseline in the PANSS total score. Iloperidone appeared to have similar efficacy as the active control drug, ziprasidone, which also needed a slow titration period to reach the target dosage.

In a longer-term study, iloperidone was found to be effective in delaying the time to relapse in adults who met DSM-IV criteria for schizophrenia and who had been stabilized on iloperidone dosages of up to 24 mg daily. In this study, 303 outpatients with schizophrenia who remained stable following 12 weeks of open-label treatment with flexible dosages of iloperidone (8–24 mg daily given as twice-daily doses) entered a double-blind, relapse prevention phase in which they were randomized to receive placebo or to continue receiving their current iloperidone dosage for up to 26 weeks. Based on results from an interim analysis that demonstrated maintenance efficacy of iloperidone, the study was stopped early. These interim results, which were later confirmed by the final analysis, showed that iloperidone-treated patients (modal dosage of 12 mg daily) experienced a substantially longer time to relapse or impending relapse than those receiving placebo (mean time to relapse of 139 and 71 days, respectively). Approximately 20% of the iloperidone-treated patients experienced a relapse compared with about 63% of those receiving placebo. In addition, a pooled analysis of three 1-year studies in patients with schizophrenia or schizoaffective disorder has shown iloperidone (4–16 mg daily) to be effective for up to 1 year (with similar efficacy as haloperidol) in preventing relapse and to be generally well tolerated in such patients. The manufacturer states that the need for continued therapy with iloperidone should be reassessed periodically. (See Dosage and Administration: Dosage.)

When deciding among the alternative treatments available for schizophrenia, the manufacturer states that the clinician should consider that iloperidone is associated with prolongation of the corrected QT (QT_c) interval. (See Prolongation of QT Interval under Warnings/Precautions: Other Warnings and Precautions, in Cautions.) Prolongation of the QT_c interval with some other drugs has been associated with the ability to cause torsades de pointes-type arrhythmia (a potentially fatal polymorphic ventricular tachycardia that can result in sudden death). In many cases, consideration of this risk would lead to the conclusion that other drugs should be tried first. It is not yet known whether iloperidone will cause torsades de pointes or increase the rate of sudden death.

Because iloperidone must be titrated to achieve an effective dosage, symptom control may be more delayed during the first 1–2 weeks of therapy compared with some other antipsychotic agents that do not require a similar titration period. (See Dosage and Administration: Dosage.) Clinicians should keep this delay in mind when selecting an antipsychotic agent for the acute treatment of schizophrenia.

Preliminary evidence suggests that several genetic markers may help to predict the clinical response and tolerability of iloperidone in patients with schizophrenia; additional pharmacogenetic studies are under way to further investigate the potential use of such markers to optimize individualized antipsychotic therapy.

The American Psychiatric Association (APA) considers most atypical antipsychotic agents first-line drugs for the management of the acute phase of schizophrenia (including first psychotic episodes), principally because of the decreased risk of adverse extrapyramidal effects and tardive dyskinesia, with the understanding that the relative advantages, disadvantages, and cost-effectiveness of conventional and atypical antipsychotic agents remain controversial. The APA states that, with the possible exception of clozapine for the management of treatment-resistant symptoms, there currently is no definitive evidence that one atypical antipsychotic agent will have superior efficacy compared with another agent in the class, although meaningful differences in response may be observed in individual patients. Conventional antipsychotic agents also may be an appropriate first-line option for some patients, including those who have been treated successfully in the past with or who prefer conventional agents. The choice of an antipsychotic agent should be individualized, considering past response to therapy, current symptomatology, concurrent medical conditions, other medications and treatments, adverse effect profile, and the patient's preference for a specific drug, including route of administration.

For additional information on the symptomatic management of schizophrenia, including treatment recommendations and results of the Clinical Antipsychotic Trials of Intervention Effectiveness (CATIE) research program, see Schizophrenia and Other Psychotic Disorders under Uses: Psychotic Disorders, in the Phenothiazines General Statement 28:16.08.24.

Dosage and Administration

■ **Administration** Iloperidone is commercially available as tablets, which are administered orally twice daily without regard to meals. However, adverse effects may be minimized when the drug is taken with food. A parenteral formulation of iloperidone currently is not commercially available.

■ **Dosage** ***Schizophrenia*** Iloperidone must be titrated slowly from a low initial dosage to avoid orthostatic hypotension due to its α_1-adrenergic blocking activity. (See Orthostatic Hypotension and Syncope under Warnings/Precautions: Other Warnings and Precautions, in Cautions.)

For the management of schizophrenia in adults, the manufacturer recommends an initial iloperidone dosage of 1 mg given orally twice daily. Dosage increases to reach the recommended target dosage range of 6–12 mg given twice daily (total dosage of 12–24 mg daily) may then be made with daily dosage adjustments not to exceed 2 mg twice daily (4 mg daily) (e.g., 2, 4, 6, 8, 10, and 12 mg twice daily on days 2, 3, 4, 5, 6, and 7, respectively). In short-term clinical studies, iloperidone's efficacy was demonstrated in a dosage range of 6–12 mg given twice daily. The maximum recommended iloperidone dosage is 12 mg given twice daily (total dosage of 24 mg daily); dosages exceeding 24 mg daily have not been systematically evaluated in clinical trials.

Clinicians should be aware that patients need to be titrated to an effective dosage of iloperidone; therefore, symptom control may be delayed during the first 1–2 weeks of therapy compared with some other antipsychotic agents that do not require similar titration. Clinicians should also be aware that some adverse effects associated with iloperidone are dose related.

In a longer-term clinical study, maintenance therapy with iloperidone (in total dosages of up to 24 mg daily) has been shown to be effective in delaying time to relapse in adults who were stabilized on the drug. In addition, in a pooled analysis of 3 long-term (one-year) studies, iloperidone (4–16 mg daily) was found to be effective in preventing relapse in patients with schizophrenia or schizoaffective disorder and was generally well tolerated. The manufacturer states that the need for continued therapy should be reassessed periodically.

The American Psychiatric Association (APA) states that prudent long-term treatment options in patients with schizophrenia with remitted first or multiple episodes include either indefinite maintenance therapy or gradual discontinuance of the antipsychotic agent with close follow-up and a plan to reinstitute treatment upon symptom recurrence. Discontinuance of antipsychotic therapy should be considered only after a period of at least 1 year of symptom remission or optimal response while receiving the antipsychotic agent. In patients who have had multiple previous psychotic episodes or 2 psychotic episodes within 5 years, indefinite maintenance antipsychotic treatment is recommended.

Although there are no data to specifically address reinitiation of iloperidone therapy following a treatment interruption, the manufacturer recommends that the usual titration schedule be followed whenever patients have had a period off therapy of more than 3 days.

■ **Special Populations** Routine dosage adjustment of iloperidone is not necessary in patients with renal impairment.

Dosage adjustment of iloperidone is not necessary in patients with mild hepatic impairment. Dosage reduction may be required in patients with moderate hepatic impairment, if clinically indicated. Iloperidone is *not* recommended in patients with severe hepatic impairment. (See Hepatic Impairment under Warnings/Precautions: Specific Populations, in Cautions.)

Routine dosage adjustment is not necessary in geriatric patients. Dosage adjustment also is not necessary based on gender or race.

Iloperidone dosage should be reduced by 50% when administered concurrently with potent cytochrome P-450 (CYP) isoenzyme 2D6 inhibitors (e.g., fluoxetine, paroxetine) or potent CYP3A4 inhibitors (e.g., clarithromycin, itraconazole, ketoconazole). When the CYP2D6 or CYP3A4 inhibitor is withdrawn from combined therapy, the previous iloperidone dosage may be resumed. Iloperidone dosage should also be reduced by about 50% when given in combination with both a CYP2D6 and CYP3A4 inhibitor. (See Drug Interactions.)

Iloperidone dosage should be reduced by 50% in poor CYP2D6 metabolizers, since poor metabolizers of CYP2D6 have a higher exposure to iloperidone than extensive metabolizers (see Description). Laboratory tests are available to identify poor CYP2D6 metabolizers.

Cautions

■ **Contraindications** Iloperidone is contraindicated in patients with known hypersensitivity to iloperidone or any components in the formulation. Anaphylaxis, angioedema, and other hypersensitivity reactions (including throat tightness; oropharyngeal swelling; swelling of the face, lips, mouth, and tongue; urticaria; rash; and pruritus) have been reported in patients receiving iloperidone.

■ **Warnings/Precautions** ***Warnings*** **Increased Mortality in Geriatric Patients with Dementia-related Psychosis.** Antipsychotic agents increase the all-cause risk of death in geriatric patients with dementia-related psychosis. Analyses of 17 dementia-related psychosis placebo-controlled trials (modal duration of 10 weeks) revealed an approximate 1.6- to 1.7-fold increase in mortality among geriatric patients receiving mainly atypical antipsychotic agents (i.e., aripiprazole, olanzapine, quetiapine, risperidone) compared with that observed in patients receiving placebo. Over the course of a typical 10-week controlled trial, the rate of death in drug-treated patients was about 4.5% compared with a rate of about 2.6% in the placebo group. Although the causes of death were varied, most of the deaths appeared to be either cardiovascular (e.g., heart failure, sudden death) or infectious (e.g., pneumonia) in nature. The manufacturer states that iloperidone is *not* approved for the treatment of patients with dementia-related psychosis. (See Adverse Cerebrovascular Events, including Stroke, in Geriatric Patients with Dementia-related Psychosis and see Dysphagia under Warnings/Precautions: Other Warnings and Precautions, in Cautions and also see Geriatric Use under Warnings/Precautions: Specific Populations, in Cautions.)

Other Warnings and Precautions **Adverse Cerebrovascular Events, including Stroke, in Geriatric Patients with Dementia-related Psychosis.** An increased incidence of adverse cerebrovascular events (cerebrovascular accidents and transient ischemic attacks), including fatalities, has been observed in geriatric patients with dementia-related psychosis treated with certain atypical antipsychotic agents (aripiprazole, olanzapine, risperidone) in placebo-controlled studies. The manufacturer states that iloperidone is *not* approved for the treatment of patients with dementia-related psychosis. (See Increased Mortality in Geriatric Patients with Dementia-related Psychosis under Warnings/Precautions: Warnings, and also see Geriatric Use under Warnings/Precautions: Specific Populations, in Cautions.)

Prolongation of QT Interval. In patients with schizophrenia or schizoaffective disorder, iloperidone was associated with corrected QT (QT_c)-interval prolongation of 2.9, 3.9, and 9.1 msec at total daily dosages of 4–8, 10–16, and 20–24 mg, respectively. The effect of iloperidone on the QT interval was increased by the presence of cytochrome P-450 (CYP) isoenzyme 2D6 inhibition (paroxetine) or CYP3A4 inhibition (ketoconazole); under conditions of both CYP2D6 and CYP3A4 inhibition, iloperidone 12 mg twice daily was associated with a mean QT_c (Fridericia's formula) increase from baseline of about 19 msec. (See Ketoconazole, Itraconazole, and Other CYP3A4 Inhibitors and also see Paroxetine under Drug Interactions.) No cases of torsades de pointes or other severe cardiac arrhythmias were observed during the premarketing clinical trial program.

The manufacturer states that iloperidone should be avoided in patients concurrently receiving other drugs known to prolong the QT_c interval (see Drug Interactions: Drugs that Prolong QT Interval). The manufacturer also states that iloperidone should be avoided in patients with a known genetic susceptibility to congenital QT-interval prolongation and in those with a history of cardiac arrhythmias.

Certain circumstances may increase the risk of torsades de pointes and/or sudden death in association with drugs that prolong the QT_c interval, including bradycardia, hypokalemia or hypomagnesemia, concomitant use of other drugs that prolong the QT_c interval, presence of congenital prolongation of the QT interval, recent acute myocardial infarction, and/or uncompensated heart failure.

The manufacturer advises caution when using iloperidone concurrently with drugs that inhibit iloperidone's metabolism and in patients with reduced activity of CYP2D6 (see Special Populations under Dosage and Administration, see Drug Interactions, and also see Description).

The manufacturer recommends that patients being considered for iloperidone therapy who are at risk for substantial electrolyte (i.e., potassium, magnesium) disturbances have baseline serum potassium and magnesium measurements with periodic monitoring. Hypokalemia and/or hypomagnesemia may increase the risk of QT-interval prolongation and cardiac arrhythmias. Iloperidone should be avoided in patients with a history of substantial cardiovascular illness (e.g., QT-interval prolongation, recent acute myocardial infarction, uncompensated heart failure, cardiac arrhythmia). Iloperidone therapy should be discontinued in patients with persistent QT_c interval measurements exceeding 500 msec. Further evaluation, including cardiac monitoring, is recommended during iloperidone therapy in patients who experience symptoms that could indicate the occurrence of cardiac arrhythmias (e.g., dizziness, palpitations, syncope).

Neuroleptic Malignant Syndrome. Neuroleptic malignant syndrome (NMS), a potentially fatal syndrome requiring immediate discontinuance of the drug and intensive symptomatic treatment, has been reported in patients receiving antipsychotic agents, including iloperidone. (See Advice to Patients.) For additional information on NMS, see Neuroleptic Malignant Syndrome under Cautions: Nervous System Effects, in the Phenothiazines General Statement 28:16.08.24.

Tardive Dyskinesia. Because use of antipsychotic agents may be associated with tardive dyskinesia (a syndrome of potentially irreversible, involuntary, dyskinetic movements), iloperidone should be prescribed in a manner that is most likely to minimize the occurrence of this syndrome. Chronic antipsychotic treatment generally should be reserved for patients who suffer from a chronic illness that is known to respond to antipsychotic agents, and for whom alternative, equally effective, but potentially less harmful treatments are not available or appropriate. In patients who do require chronic treatment, the smallest dosage and the shortest duration of treatment producing a satisfactory clinical response should be sought, and the need for continued treatment should be reassessed periodically.

The American Psychiatric Association (APA) currently recommends that patients receiving atypical antipsychotic agents be assessed clinically for abnormal involuntary movements every 12 months and that patients considered to be at increased risk for tardive dyskinesia be assessed every 6 months. If signs and symptoms of tardive dyskinesia appear in an iloperidone-treated patient, iloperidone discontinuance should be considered; however, some patients may require continued treatment with the drug despite the presence of the syndrome. For additional information on tardive dyskinesia, see Tardive Dyskinesia under Cautions: Nervous System Effects, in the Phenothiazines General Statement 28:16.08.24.

Metabolic Changes. Atypical antipsychotic agents have been associated with metabolic changes, including hyperglycemia and diabetes mellitus, dyslipidemia, and body weight gain. While all of these drugs produce some metabolic changes, each drug has its own specific risk profile. (See Hyperglycemia and Diabetes Mellitus, see Dyslipidemia, and also see Weight Gain under Warnings/Precautions: Other Warnings and Precautions, in Cautions.)

Hyperglycemia and Diabetes Mellitus. Hyperglycemia, sometimes severe and associated with ketoacidosis, hyperosmolar coma, or death, has been reported in patients receiving atypical antipsychotic agents, including iloperidone. In a short-term controlled trial in patients with schizophrenia, 10.7% of iloperidone-treated patients and 2.5% of those receiving placebo experienced a shift from normal to high fasting glucose concentrations. While confounding factors such as an increased background risk of diabetes mellitus in patients with schizophrenia and the increasing incidence of diabetes mellitus in the general population make it difficult to establish with certainty the relationship between use of agents in this drug class and glucose abnormalities, epidemiologic studies (which did not include iloperidone) suggest an increased risk of treatment-emergent hyperglycemia-related adverse events in patients treated with the atypical antipsychotic agents included in the studies (e.g., clozapine, olanzapine, quetiapine, risperidone).

Patients with preexisting diabetes mellitus in whom therapy with an atypical antipsychotic is initiated should be periodically monitored for worsening of glucose control; those with risk factors for diabetes (e.g., obesity, family history of diabetes) should undergo fasting blood glucose testing upon therapy initiation and periodically throughout treatment. All patients treated with atypical antipsychotics should be monitored for symptoms of hyperglycemia (including polydipsia, polyuria, polyphagia, and weakness) during therapy, and any patient who develops such symptoms should undergo fasting blood glucose testing. (See Advice to Patients.) In some cases, patients who developed hyperglycemia while receiving an atypical antipsychotic have required continuance of antidiabetic treatment despite discontinuance of the atypical antipsychotic; in other cases, hyperglycemia resolved with discontinuance of the antipsychotic.

For further information on managing the risk of hyperglycemia and diabetes mellitus associated with atypical antipsychotic agents, see Hyperglycemia and Diabetes Mellitus under Cautions: Precautions and Contraindications, in Clozapine 28:16.08.04.

Dyslipidemia. Undesirable changes in lipid parameters have been observed in patients treated with atypical antipsychotic agents. In a short-term study in adults with schizophrenia, patients receiving iloperidone in a fixed dosage of 24 mg daily had a mean increase from baseline in fasting lipid concentrations of approximately 8.2 mg/dL in total cholesterol, 9 mg/dL in low-density lipoprotein (LDL)-cholesterol, and 0.55 mg/dL in high-density lipoprotein (HDL)-cholesterol and a mean decrease of 0.83 mg/dL in fasting triglycerides.

Weight Gain. Weight gain has been observed with use of atypical antipsychotics, including iloperidone. Based on pooled data from short-term clinical studies, the proportion of patients experiencing a weight gain of 7% or more of their baseline body weight was 12% for iloperidone 10–16 mg daily and 18% for iloperidone 20–24 mg daily compared with 4% for placebo recipients. In all short- and long-term studies, the overall mean weight gain in iloperidone-treated patients was 2.1 kg.

Clinical monitoring of weight is recommended in patients receiving iloperidone.

Seizures. In short-term clinical trials, seizures occurred in 0.1% of patients treated with iloperidone compared with 0.3% of patients receiving placebo. As with other antipsychotic agents, iloperidone should be used with caution in patients with a history of seizures or with conditions that may lower the seizure threshold; conditions that lower the seizure threshold may be more prevalent in patients 65 years of age or older.

Orthostatic Hypotension and Syncope. Orthostatic hypotension associated with dizziness, tachycardia, and syncope may occur during iloperidone therapy, particularly when treatment with the drug is initiated or reinitiated or the dosage is increased, because of the drug's α_1-adrenergic blocking activity. In short-term clinical trials where the dosage was increased slowly as recommended, syncope was reported in 0.4% of patients receiving iloperidone compared with 0.2% of placebo recipients. Orthostatic hypotension was reported in 5% of patients receiving 20–24 mg of iloperidone daily, 3% of patients receiving 10–16 mg of iloperidone daily, and 1% of patients given placebo. More rapid dosage titration would be expected to increase the incidence of orthostatic hypotension and syncope. (See Dosage and Administration: Dosage.)

Iloperidone should be used with caution in patients with known cardiovascular disease (e.g., heart failure, history of myocardial infarction, ischemic heart disease, conduction abnormalities), cerebrovascular disease, or conditions that would predispose patients to hypotension (e.g., dehydration, hypovolemia, concomitant antihypertensive therapy). Consideration should be given to monitoring orthostatic vital signs in iloperidone-treated patients who are susceptible to hypotension.

Falls. Iloperidone therapy may cause somnolence, postural hypotension, and motor and sensory instability, which may lead to falls; as a consequence, fractures or other injuries may occur. For patients with diseases or conditions or those receiving other drugs that could exacerbate these effects, fall risk assessments should be completed when initiating antipsychotic treatment and repeated periodically during long-term antipsychotic therapy.

Leukopenia, Neutropenia, and Agranulocytosis. In clinical trial and/or post-marketing experience, leukopenia and neutropenia have been temporally related to antipsychotic agents. Agranulocytosis (including fatal cases) also has been reported with other antipsychotic agents.

Possible risk factors for leukopenia and neutropenia include preexisting low leukocyte count and a history of drug-induced leukopenia or neutropenia. Patients with a preexisting low leukocyte count or a history of drug-induced leukopenia or neutropenia should have their complete blood count monitored frequently during the first few months of therapy. Iloperidone should be discontinued at the first sign of a decline in leukocyte count in the absence of other causative factors.

Patients with neutropenia should be carefully monitored for fever or other signs or symptoms of infection and promptly treated if such signs and symptoms occur. In patients with severe neutropenia (absolute neutrophil count [ANC] less than 1000/mm^3), iloperidone should be discontinued and the leukocyte count monitored until recovery occurs. Lithium has reportedly been used successfully in the treatment of several cases of leukopenia associated with aripiprazole, clozapine, and some other drugs; however, further clinical experience is needed to confirm these anecdotal findings.

Hyperprolactinemia. Similar to other antipsychotic agents and drugs with dopamine D_2 antagonistic activity, iloperidone can elevate plasma prolactin concentrations, which may persist during chronic use of the drug. In a short-term (4-week) trial, plasma prolactin concentrations increased an average of 2.6 ng/mL from baseline to study end point in iloperidone-treated patients (24 mg daily) compared with a decrease of 6.3 ng/mL in the placebo group; elevated prolactin concentrations were observed in 26% of patients receiving iloperidone compared with 12% of patients receiving placebo in this study. In short-term trials, iloperidone was associated with relatively modest elevations in prolactin concentrations compared with some other antipsychotic agents (e.g., first-generation antipsychotics including haloperidol, risperidone).

Clinical disturbances such as galactorrhea, amenorrhea, gynecomastia, and impotence have been associated with prolactin-elevating drugs. In a pooled analysis of iloperidone clinical trials, including longer-term trials, gynecomastia was reported in 2 males (0.1% of iloperidone-treated patients) compared with 0% of those receiving placebo, and galactorrhea was reported in 8 females (0.2% of iloperidone-treated patients) compared with 3 females (0.5%) receiving placebo. In addition, chronic hyperprolactinemia associated with hypogonadism may lead to decreased bone density in both female and male patients.

If iloperidone therapy is considered for a patient with previously detected breast cancer, clinicians should consider that approximately one-third of human breast cancers are prolactin-dependent in vitro.

Body Temperature Regulation. Disruption of the body's ability to reduce core body temperature has been attributed to antipsychotic agents. The manufacturer recommends appropriate caution when iloperidone is used in patients who will be experiencing conditions that may contribute to an elevation in core body temperature (e.g., strenuous exercise, extreme heat, concomitant use of agents with anticholinergic activity, dehydration).

Dysphagia. Esophageal dysmotility and aspiration have been associated with the use of antipsychotic agents. Aspiration pneumonia is a common cause of morbidity and mortality in geriatric patients. Iloperidone and other antipsychotic agents should be used with caution in patients at risk for aspiration pneumonia. (See Increased Mortality in Geriatric Patients with Dementia-related Psychosis under Warnings/Precautions: Warnings, in Cautions.)

Suicide. There is an attendant risk of suicide in patients with psychotic illnesses; high-risk patients should be closely supervised. Iloperidone should be prescribed in the smallest quantity consistent with good patient management to reduce the risk of overdosage.

Priapism. Priapism may occur with iloperidone therapy; 3 cases of priapism were reported in the premarketing program. Drugs with α-adrenergic blocking activity have been reported to cause priapism, and iloperidone shares this pharmacologic activity. Severe priapism may require surgical intervention.

Cognitive and Motor Impairment. Like other antipsychotic agents, iloperidone potentially may impair judgment, thinking, or motor skills. In short-term, placebo-controlled clinical trials, somnolence (including sedation) was reported in 11.9% of adults receiving iloperidone dosages of at least 10 mg daily compared with 5.3% of those receiving placebo. (See Advice to Patients.)

Specific Populations **Pregnancy.** *Pregnancy registry:* A pregnancy exposure registry has been established to monitor pregnancy outcomes in women exposed to iloperidone during pregnancy. For more information, clinicians may contact the National Pregnancy Registry for Atypical Antipsychotics at 866-961-2388 or visit http://womensmentalhealth.org/clinical-and-research-programs/pregnancyregistry/.

Risk summary: Limited data are available regarding use of iloperidone in pregnant women and are not sufficient to inform a drug-associated risk for major birth defects and miscarriage. The drug was not teratogenic when administered orally to pregnant rats during organogenesis at dosages up to 26 times the maximum recommended human dosage (MRHD) of 24 mg daily on a mg/m^2 basis. However, iloperidone prolonged the duration of pregnancy and parturition, increased still births and early intrauterine deaths, increased the incidence of developmental delays, and decreased postpartum pup survival. Iloperidone was not teratogenic when administered orally to pregnant rabbits during organogenesis at dosages up to 20 times the MRHD on a mg/m^2 basis. However, the drug increased early intrauterine deaths and decreased fetal viability at term at the highest dosage, which also was a maternally toxic dosage. The background risk of major birth defects and miscarriage for the indicated population is unknown. In the US general population, the estimated background risk of major birth defects and miscarriage in clinically recognized pregnancies is 2–4% and 15–20%, respectively.

Fetal/Neonatal adverse reactions: Neonates exposed to antipsychotic agents during the third trimester of pregnancy are at risk for extrapyramidal and/or withdrawal symptoms following delivery. Symptoms reported to date have included agitation, hypertonia, hypotonia, tardive dyskinetic-like symptoms, tremor, somnolence, respiratory distress, and feeding disorder. The symptoms have varied in severity; some neonates recovered within hours to days without specific treatment while others have required prolonged hospitalization. Neonates should be monitored for extrapyramidal and/or withdrawal symptoms and managed appropriately if symptoms occur.

Lactation. Iloperidone is distributed into milk in rats. It is not known whether iloperidone and/or its metabolites distribute into milk in humans. The effects of the drug on breastfed infants or on milk production also are not known. Because of the potential for serious adverse reactions in breastfed infants, the manufacturer recommends that women receiving iloperidone not breast-feed.

Pediatric Use. Safety and effectiveness of iloperidone in pediatric and adolescent patients have not been established.

Geriatric Use. Clinical trial experience with iloperidone in patients with schizophrenia who are 65 years of age or older is insufficient to determine whether they respond differently than younger adults. In premarketing clinical studies, 0.5% of 3210 iloperidone-treated patients were 65 years of age or older and no patients were 75 years of age or older.

Geriatric patients with dementia-related psychosis treated with iloperidone are at an increased risk of death compared with those receiving placebo. In addition, an increased incidence of adverse cerebrovascular events (cerebrovascular accidents and transient ischemic attacks), including fatalities, has been observed in geriatric patients with dementia-related psychosis treated with certain atypical antipsychotic agents (aripiprazole, olanzapine, risperidone) in placebo-controlled studies. The manufacturer states that the safety and efficacy of iloperidone in the treatment of dementia-related psychosis have not been established and that the drug is *not* approved for the treatment of patients with dementia-related psychosis. (See Increased Mortality in Geriatric Patients with Dementia-related Psychosis under Warnings/Precautions: Warnings, in Cautions and also see Cerebrovascular Adverse Events, including Stroke, in Geriatric Patients with Dementia-related Psychosis and Dysphagia under Warnings/Precautions: Other Warnings and Precautions, in Cautions). For additional information on the use of antipsychotic agents in the management of dementia-related psychosis, see Geriatric Considerations under Uses: Psychotic Disorders, in the Phenothiazines General Statement 28:16.08.24.

Hepatic Impairment. In a single-dose study evaluating the pharmacokinetics of iloperidone in patients with mild hepatic impairment, the pharmacokinetic profiles of iloperidone and its P88 and P95 metabolites (total or unbound) were not substantially altered. However, in subjects with moderate hepatic impairment, exposure to the P88 metabolite (unbound) was substantially higher (by twofold) and more variable compared with healthy individuals. (See Dosage and Administration: Special Populations.)

Iloperidone has not been studied in patients with severe hepatic impairment, and use of the drug in such patients is *not* recommended.

Renal Impairment. Because iloperidone is highly metabolized with less than 1% of the drug excreted unchanged, renal impairment is unlikely to substantially alter the pharmacokinetics of the drug. Following a single 3-mg dose, renal impairment (creatinine clearance <30 mL/minute) had minimal effect on peak plasma concentrations of iloperidone and its P88 and P95 metabolites. Area under the plasma concentration-time curve ($AUC_{0-\infty}$) was increased by 24% for iloperidone, decreased by 6% for P88, and increased by 52% for P95 in individuals with renal impairment. Routine dosage adjustment is not necessary in patients with renal impairment.

■ **Common Adverse Effects** Adverse effects occurring in clinical trials in 5% or more of patients receiving short-term iloperidone therapy for schizophrenia (for at least one iloperidone dosage studied) and at a frequency at least twice that reported among patients receiving placebo include dizziness, somnolence or sedation, fatigue, dry mouth, nasal congestion, tachycardia, orthostatic hypotension, and weight gain.

Drug Interactions

Iloperidone is metabolized principally by cytochrome P-450 (CYP) isoenzymes 3A4 and 2D6.

Iloperidone is not a substrate for CYP isoenzymes 1A1, 1A2, 2A6, 2B6, 2C8, 2C9, 2C19, or 2E1.

Iloperidone and its active metabolite P88 are not substrates of P-glycoprotein (P-gp). Iloperidone is a weak P-gp inhibitor.

■ **Drugs Affecting Hepatic Microsomal Enzymes** Inhibitors of CYP3A4 (e.g., clarithromycin, itraconazole, ketoconazole) or CYP2D6 (e.g., fluoxetine, paroxetine) may reduce clearance of iloperidone resulting in increased plasma concentrations of the drug. (See Dosage and Administration: Special Populations, see Drug Interactions: Fluoxetine and Other CYP2D6 Inhibitors, see Drug Interactions: Ketoconazole, Itraconazole, and Other CYP3A4 Inhibitors, and also see Drug Interactions: Paroxetine.)

Pharmacokinetic interactions with inhibitors or inducers of CYP isoenzymes 1A1, 1A2, 2A6, 2B6, 2C8, 2C9, 2C19, or 2E1 are unlikely since iloperidone is not a substrate for these isoenzymes.

■ **Drugs Metabolized by Hepatic Microsomal Enzymes** Clinically important pharmacokinetic interactions with substrates of CYP isoenzymes 1A1, 1A2, 2A6, 2B6, 2C8, 2C9, 2C19, 2E1, 3A4, or 3A5 are considered unlikely.

Pharmacokinetic interactions with substrates of CYP2D6 also are unlikely. (See Drug Interactions: Dextromethorphan and Other CYP2D6 Substrates.)

■ **Anticholinergic Agents** Because disruption of body temperature regulation is possible, iloperidone should be used with caution in patients concurrently receiving drugs with anticholinergic activity. (See Body Temperature Regulation under Warnings/Precautions: Other Warnings and Precautions, in Cautions.)

■ **Drugs that Prolong QT Interval** Because of additive effects on QT-interval prolongation, concomitant use of iloperidone with other drugs known to prolong the corrected QT (QT_c) interval, including class IA antiarrhythmics (e.g., procainamide, quinidine), class III antiarrhythmics (e.g., amiodarone, sotalol), some antipsychotic agents (e.g., chlorpromazine, thioridazine, haloperidol, asenapine, olanzapine, paliperidone, pimozide, quetiapine, ziprasidone), some anti-infective agents (e.g., gatifloxacin, moxifloxacin), and other drugs (e.g., levomethadyl acetate [no longer commercially available in the US], methadone, pentamidine, tetrabenazine), should be avoided. (See Prolongation of QT Interval under Warnings/Precautions: Other Warnings and Precautions, in Cautions.)

■ **Other CNS Agents or Alcohol** Concomitant use of iloperidone with other CNS agents or alcohol may produce additive CNS effects. Caution is advised when iloperidone and other CNS agents are used concomitantly; use of alcohol during iloperidone therapy should be avoided.

■ **Hypotensive Agents** Because of its α_1-adrenergic blocking activity and potential to cause orthostatic hypotension and syncope, the manufacturer recommends that iloperidone be used with caution in patients receiving antihypertensive agents and other drugs that can cause hypotension; monitoring of orthostatic vital signs should be considered in such patients. (See Orthostatic Hypotension and Syncope under Warnings/Precautions: Other Warnings and Precautions, in Cautions and also see Advice to Patients.)

■ **Dextromethorphan and Other CYP2D6 Substrates** Concomitant single-dose administration of iloperidone (3 mg) with dextromethorphan (80 mg), a CYP2D6 substrate, resulted in a 17% increase in total exposure and a 26% increase in peak plasma concentration of dextromethorphan in healthy individuals. The manufacturer states that an interaction between iloperidone and other CYP2D6 substrates is unlikely.

■ **Fluoxetine and Other CYP2D6 Inhibitors** Concomitant administration of fluoxetine (20 mg twice daily for 21 days), a potent inhibitor of CYP2D6, with a single 3-mg dose of iloperidone in healthy individuals classified as extensive CYP2D6 metabolizers increased the area under the concentration–time curve (AUC) of iloperidone and its P88 metabolite by approximately twofold to threefold and decreased the AUC of iloperidone's P95 metabolite by 50%. A single 3-mg dose of iloperidone had no effect on the pharmacokinetics of fluoxetine (20 mg twice daily). The manufacturer advises caution and states that the dosage of iloperidone should be reduced by 50% when given in combination with fluoxetine. When fluoxetine is withdrawn from combined therapy, the iloperidone dosage should be returned to the previous dosage. (See Dosage and Administration: Special Populations.)

The manufacturer states that other potent CYP2D6 inhibitors would be expected to have similar effects as fluoxetine and therefore advises caution and appropriate iloperidone dosage reduction. When the CYP2D6 inhibitor is withdrawn from combined therapy, the iloperidone dosage may then be returned to the previous level. (See Drug Interactions: Paroxetine.)

■ **Ketoconazole, Itraconazole, and Other CYP3A4 Inhibitors** Concomitant administration of ketoconazole (200 mg twice daily for 4 days), a potent CYP3A4 inhibitor, with a single 3-mg iloperidone dose in healthy individuals increased the AUC of iloperidone and its P88 and P95 metabolites by 57, 55, and 35%, respectively. The manufacturer therefore advises caution and recommends that the iloperidone dosage be reduced by about 50% when concurrently administered with itraconazole, ketoconazole, or other potent inhibitors of CYP3A4 (e.g., clarithromycin). When the CYP3A4 inhibitor is withdrawn from combined therapy, the iloperidone dosage should be increased to the previous dosage. (See Dosage and Administration: Special Populations.)

Concomitant administration of iloperidone with weaker CYP3A4 inhibitors (e.g., erythromycin, grapefruit juice) has not been studied.

Concomitant administration of both ketoconazole (200 mg twice daily) and paroxetine (20 mg once daily for 10 days) with iloperidone (8 or 12 mg twice daily) in patients with schizophrenia increased steady-state plasma iloperidone and P88 concentrations by 1.4-fold and decreased steady-state plasma P95 concentrations by 1.4-fold. Therefore, concurrent administration of iloperidone with inhibitors of both of its metabolic pathways did not add to the effect observed when either inhibitor was given alone. The manufacturer advises caution and states that iloperidone dosage should be reduced by about 50% when given in combination with both a CYP2D6 and CYP3A4 inhibitor. (See Dosage and Administration: Special Populations.)

Concomitant administration of paroxetine (20 mg daily) and ketoconazole (200 mg twice daily) with iloperidone (12 mg twice daily) resulted in a mean increase in corrected QT (QT_c) interval of about 19 msec compared with baseline. (See Prolongation of QT Interval under Warnings/Precautions: Other Warnings and Precautions, in Cautions.)

■ **Midazolam and other CYP3A4 Substrates** In patients with schizophrenia, concomitant administration of iloperidone (up to 10 mg twice daily for 14 days) and midazolam, a CYP3A4 substrate, resulted in a less than 50% increase in total exposure of midazolam at iloperidone steady state and had no effect on peak plasma concentrations of midazolam. The manufacturer therefore states that interactions between iloperidone and other CYP3A4 substrates are unlikely.

■ **Paroxetine** Concomitant administration of paroxetine (20 mg daily for 5–8 days), a potent inhibitor of CYP2D6, with multiple doses of iloperidone (8 or 12 mg twice daily) in patients with schizophrenia increased mean steady-state peak plasma concentrations of iloperidone and its P88 metabolite by about 1.6-fold and decreased mean steady-state peak concentrations of its P95 metabolite by 50%. The manufacturer advises caution and recommends that the iloperidone dosage be reduced by 50% when given concurrently with paroxetine. When paroxetine is withdrawn from combined therapy, the iloperidone dosage should be returned to the previous dosage. (See Dosage and Administration: Special Populations.) A similar effect is expected to occur with concomitant administration of other potent CYP2D6 inhibitors.

Concomitant administration of both paroxetine (20 mg once daily for 10 days) and ketoconazole (200 mg twice daily) with iloperidone (8 or 12 mg twice daily) in patients with schizophrenia increased steady-state plasma iloperidone and P88 concentrations by 1.4-fold and decreased steady-state P95 concentrations by 1.4-fold. Therefore, concurrent administration of iloperidone with inhibitors of both of its metabolic pathways did not add to the effect observed when either inhibitor was given alone. The manufacturer advises caution and states that the iloperidone dosage should be reduced by about 50% when given in combination with both a CYP2D6 and CYP3A4 inhibitor. (See Dosage and Administration: Special Populations.)

Concomitant administration of paroxetine (20 mg daily) and ketoconazole (200 mg twice daily) with iloperidone (12 mg twice daily) resulted in a mean increase in corrected QT (QT_c) interval of about 19 msec compared with baseline. (See Prolongation of QT Interval under Warnings/Precautions: Other Warnings and Precautions, in Cautions.)

■ **Smoking** Iloperidone is not a substrate for CYP1A2 in vitro; therefore, smoking should not alter the pharmacokinetics of the drug.

Description

Iloperidone is a piperidinyl-benzisoxazole derivative structurally related to risperidone; the drug has been referred to as an atypical or second-generation antipsychotic agent. Although the exact mechanism of action of iloperidone is unknown, it has been suggested that the efficacy of iloperidone is mediated through a combination of antagonist activity at central dopamine type 2 (D_2) and serotonin type 2 (5-hydroxytryptamine [5-HT_2]) receptors.

Iloperidone acts as an antagonist with high binding affinity for 5-HT_{2A}, D_2 and D_3, and α_1-adrenergic receptors. The drug has moderate affinity for D_4, 5-HT_6, and 5-HT_7 receptors and low affinity for 5-HT_{1A}, D_1, and histamine H_1 receptors. Iloperidone possesses no appreciable affinity for muscarinic cholinergic receptors. Iloperidone has 2 main metabolites, P88 and P95; the affinity of the P88 metabolite is generally equal to or less than that of the parent compound while the P95 metabolite demonstrates affinity for 5-HT_{2A} and α_{1A}-, α_{1B}-, α_{1D}-, and α_{2C}-adrenergic receptors.

Iloperidone is well absorbed following oral administration of the tablets, with peak plasma concentrations occurring within 2–4 hours. Steady-state plasma concentrations of iloperidone and its two main metabolites, P88 and P95, are reached within 3–4 days. At therapeutic concentrations, iloperidone and its metabolites (P88 and P95) are approximately 97 and 92% bound to plasma proteins, respectively. Iloperidone is primarily metabolized by carbonyl reduction, cytochrome P-450 (CYP) isoenzyme 2D6-mediated hydroxylation, and CYP3A4-mediated *O*-demethylation; the drug's two principal metabolites, P88 and P95, undergo further oxidation and/or conjugation with glucuronic acid. The P88 metabolite penetrates the CNS and is thought to contribute to the drug's antipsychotic activity whereas the P95 metabolite does not readily penetrate the CNS and primarily contributes to the adverse effect profile of the drug. The mean elimination half-lives of iloperidone, P88, and P95 are 18, 26, and 23 hours, respectively, in extensive metabolizers of CYP2D6 and 33, 37, and 31 hours, respectively, in poor metabolizers of CYP2D6. (See Dosage and Administration: Special Populations.) The majority of radiolabeled iloperidone was recovered in the urine (mean of 58.2 and 45.1% in extensive and poor metabolizers of CYP2D6, respectively), with feces accounting for 19.9% (extensive metabolizers) and 22.1% (poor metabolizers) of the radiolabeled dose.

Advice to Patients

Importance of advising patients and caregivers that geriatric patients with dementia-related psychosis treated with antipsychotic agents are at an increased risk of death. Patients and caregivers also should be informed that iloperidone is *not* approved for treating geriatric patients with dementia-related psychosis.

Importance of patients immediately informing their clinician if they feel faint, lose consciousness, or have heart palpitations. Importance of counseling patients not to take iloperidone with other drugs that prolong the QT interval. Patients should be instructed to inform clinicians that they are taking iloperidone before any new drug is taken. (See Prolongation of QT Interval under Warnings/Precautions: Other Warnings and Precautions, in Cautions and also see Drug Interactions: Drugs that Prolong QT Interval.)

Importance of informing patients and caregivers about the risk of neuroleptic malignant syndrome (NMS), a rare but potentially life-threatening syndrome that can cause high fever, muscle stiffness, sweating, fast or irregular heart beat, change in blood pressure, confusion, and kidney damage.

Importance of informing patients about the risk of metabolic changes (e.g., hyperglycemia and diabetes mellitus, weight gain) with iloperidone and the need for specific monitoring for such changes during therapy. Importance of patients being aware of the symptoms of hyperglycemia (e.g., increased thirst, increased urination, increased appetite, weakness). Importance of informing patients who are diagnosed with diabetes or those with risk factors for diabetes (e.g., obesity, family history of diabetes) that they should have their blood glucose monitored at the beginning of and periodically during iloperidone therapy. Importance of informing patients that clinical monitoring of weight is recommended during iloperidone therapy

Importance of informing patients about the risk of orthostatic hypotension, especially when initiating or reinitiating treatment or increasing the dosage.

Because somnolence and impairment of judgment, thinking, or motor skills may be associated with iloperidone, patients should be cautioned about performing activities requiring mental alertness, such as driving or operating hazardous machinery, while taking iloperidone until they gain experience with the drug's effects.

Importance of avoiding alcohol during iloperidone therapy.

Importance of avoiding overheating or dehydration.

Importance of informing clinicians of existing or contemplated concomitant therapy, including prescription and OTC drugs, dietary supplements, and/or herbal products, since there is a potential for adverse drug interactions (see Drug Interactions). Importance of also informing clinicians about any concomitant illnesses (e.g., cardiovascular disease, diabetes mellitus, seizures).

Importance of women informing clinicians if they are or plan to become pregnant or plan to breast-feed. Importance of clinicians informing patients about the benefits and risks of taking antipsychotics during pregnancy, including that third trimester use of iloperidone may cause extrapyramidal and/or withdrawal symptoms in neonates, and about the pregnancy exposure registry (see Pregnancy under Warnings/Precautions: Specific Populations, in Cautions). Importance of advising patients not to stop taking iloperidone if they become pregnant without consulting their clinician; abruptly stopping antipsychotic agents may cause complications. Importance of advising patients not to breast-feed during iloperidone therapy.

Importance of informing patients of other important precautionary information. (See Cautions.)

Overview® (see Users Guide). For additional information on this drug until a more detailed monograph is developed and published, the manufacturer's labeling should be consulted. It is *essential* that the manufacturer's labeling be consulted for more detailed information on usual cautions, precautions, contraindications, potential drug interactions, laboratory test interferences, and acute toxicity.

Preparations

Excipients in commercially available drug preparations may have clinically important effects in some individuals; consult specific product labeling for details.

Iloperidone

Oral		
Tablets	1 mg	**Fanapt®**, Vanda
	2 mg	**Fanapt®**, Vanda
	4 mg	**Fanapt®**, Vanda
	6 mg	**Fanapt®**, Vanda
	8 mg	**Fanapt®**, Vanda
	10 mg	**Fanapt®**, Vanda
	12 mg	**Fanapt®**, Vanda
Titration Pack	2 Tablets, Iloperidone 1 mg (Fanapt®) 2 Tablets, Iloperidone 2 mg (Fanapt®) 2 Tablets, Iloperidone 4 mg (Fanapt®) 2 Tablets, Iloperidone 6 mg (Fanapt®)	**Fanapt® Titration Pack,** Vanda

Lurasidone Hydrochloride

■ Lurasidone hydrochloride is considered an atypical or second-generation antipsychotic agent.

Uses

■ **Psychotic Disorders** Drug therapy is integral to the management of acute psychotic episodes in patients with schizophrenia and generally is required for long-term stabilization to sustain symptom remission or control and to minimize the risk of relapse. Antipsychotic agents are the principal class of drugs used for the management of all phases of schizophrenia. Patient response and tolerance to antipsychotic agents are variable, and patients who do not respond to or tolerate one drug may be successfully treated with an agent from a different class or with a different adverse effect profile.

Schizophrenia Lurasidone hydrochloride is an atypical antipsychotic that is administered orally in the acute treatment of schizophrenia in adults. Schizophrenia is a major psychotic disorder that frequently has devastating effects on various aspects of the patient's life and carries a high risk of suicide and other life-threatening behaviors. Manifestations of schizophrenia involve multiple psychologic processes, including perception (e.g., hallucinations), ideation, reality testing (e.g., delusions), emotion (e.g., flatness, inappropriate affect), thought processes (e.g., loose associations), behavior (e.g., catatonia, disorganization), attention, concentration, motivation (e.g., avolition, impaired intention and planning), and judgment. The principal manifestations of this disorder usually are described in terms of positive and negative (deficit) symptoms and, more recently, disorganized symptoms. Positive symptoms include hallucinations, delusions, bizarre behavior, hostility, uncooperativeness, and paranoid ideation, while negative symptoms include restricted range and intensity of emotional expression (affective flattening), reduced thought and speech productivity (alogia), anhedonia, apathy, and decreased initiation of goal-directed behavior (avolition). Disorganized symptoms include disorganized speech (thought disorder) and behavior and poor attention.

The short-term efficacy of oral lurasidone in the acute management of schizophrenia was supported in 5 placebo-controlled, fixed-dose clinical trials of 6 weeks' duration in adults who met DSM-IV criteria for schizophrenia. Two of these studies included an active-control arm (olanzapine or extended-release quetiapine) to assess assay sensitivity. The studies used either the Positive and Negative Syndrome Scale (PANSS) or the Brief Psychiatric Rating Scale derived (BPRSd) and the Clinical Global Impression severity scale (CGI-S) to assess the effects of drug treatment in improving clinical manifestations of schizophrenia. Studies 1 and 3 both evaluated 2 fixed dosages of lurasidone hydrochloride (40 or 120 mg daily), study 2 evaluated a fixed dosage of 80 mg daily, study 4 evaluated 3 fixed dosages (40, 80, or 120 mg daily), and study 5 evaluated 2 fixed dosages of the drug (80 or 160 mg daily). In all 5 studies, lurasidone was found to be more effective than placebo; however, in study 4 only the 80-mg daily dosage of lurasidone hydrochloride was found to be more effective than placebo, and neither 40 mg nor 120 mg could be distinguished from placebo. Thus, the efficacy of 40-, 80-, 120-, and 160-mg daily dosages of lurasidone hydrochloride was established in these studies as assessed by the change from baseline in the PANSS or BPRSd total scores and the CGI-S. An examination of population subgroups did not reveal any clear evidence of differential responsiveness to the drug based on age, gender, or race.

The manufacturer states that if lurasidone is used for extended periods (i.e., longer than 6 weeks) in the treatment of schizophrenia, the long-term usefulness of the drug should be reassessed periodically on an individualized basis. (See Dosage and Administration: Dosage.)

The American Psychiatric Association (APA) considers most atypical antipsychotic agents first-line drugs for the management of the acute phase of schizophrenia (including first psychotic episodes), principally because of the decreased risk of adverse extrapyramidal effects and tardive dyskinesia, with the understanding that the relative advantages, disadvantages, and cost-effectiveness of conventional and atypical antipsychotic agents remain controversial. The APA states that, with the possible exception of clozapine for the management of treatment-resistant symptoms, there currently is no definitive evidence that one atypical antipsychotic agent will have superior efficacy compared with another agent in the class, although meaningful differences in response may be observed in individual patients. Conventional antipsychotic agents also may be an appropriate first-line option for some patients, including those who have been treated successfully in the past with or who prefer conventional agents. The choice of an antipsychotic agent should be individualized, considering past response to therapy, current symptomatology, concurrent medical conditions, other medications and treatments, adverse effect profile, and the patient's preference for a specific drug, including route of administration.

For additional information on the symptomatic management of schizophrenia, including treatment recommendations and results of the Clinical Antipsychotic Trials of Intervention Effectiveness (CATIE) research program, see Schizophrenia and Other Psychotic Disorders under Uses: Psychotic Disorders, in the Phenothiazines General Statement 28:16.08.24.

■ **Bipolar Disorder** ***Depressive Episodes Associated with Bipolar Disorder*** Lurasidone hydrochloride is used orally as monotherapy or adjunctive therapy with lithium or valproate for the treatment of major depressive episodes associated with bipolar I disorder (bipolar depression) in adults.

The short-term efficacy of lurasidone monotherapy in the treatment of depressive episodes associated with bipolar I disorder was established in a randomized, double-blind, placebo-controlled, multicenter study of 6 weeks' duration in adults who met DSM-IV-TR criteria for major depressive episodes associated with bipolar I disorder, with or without rapid cycling and without psychotic features. The primary and key secondary end points were the change from baseline to week 6 on the Montgomery-Asberg Depression Rating Scale (MADRS) and the Clinical Global Impressions-Bipolar-Severity of Illness scale (CGI-BP-S) scores, respectively. Patients were randomized to receive lower-dose lurasidone hydrochloride (flexible dosage range of 20–60 mg daily), higher-dose lurasidone hydrochloride (flexible dosage range of 80–120 mg daily), or placebo. Lurasidone substantially reduced MADRS and CGI-BP-S scores at week 6 of therapy in both lurasidone dosage groups compared with placebo. The higher-dose range (80–120 mg daily) of lurasidone hydrochloride was not found to be more effective, on average, than the lower-dose regimen in this study.

The short-term efficacy of lurasidone as adjunctive therapy with lithium or valproate in the treatment of depressive episodes associated with bipolar I disorder was established in a randomized, double-blind, placebo-controlled, multicenter study of 6 weeks' duration in adults who met DSM-IV-TR criteria for major depressive episodes associated with bipolar I disorder, with or without rapid cycling and without psychotic features. Patients who remained symptomatic after lithium or valproate therapy were randomized to receive flexible-dose lurasidone hydrochloride (20–120 mg daily) or placebo. The primary end point was the change from baseline to week 6 in the MADRS score, and the secondary end point was the change from baseline to week 6 in the CGI-BP-S score. Lurasidone given as adjunctive therapy with lithium or valproate substantially reduced MADRS and CGI-BP-S scores at week 6 of therapy compared with placebo.

Clinical experience with lurasidone indicates that the drug is less likely to cause weight gain and to adversely affect metabolic parameters than some other atypical antipsychotic agents (e.g., olanzapine, quetiapine) that are used in the treatment of bipolar depression. Therefore, lurasidone may be a suitable alternative treatment for patients with bipolar depression who are at higher risk of metabolic abnormalities (e.g., those with diabetes mellitus or hyperlipidemia).

The manufacturer states that the efficacy of lurasidone for longer-term use (i.e., longer than 6 weeks) in bipolar depression has not been established in controlled studies. If lurasidone is used for extended periods, the long-term usefulness of the drug should be periodically reassessed on an individualized basis. (See Dosage and Administration: Dosage.)

The manufacturer states that the efficacy of lurasidone in the treatment of mania associated with bipolar disorder† has not been established.

For further information on the management of bipolar disorder, see Uses: Bipolar Disorder, in Lithium Salts 28:28.

Dosage and Administration

■ **Administration** Lurasidone hydrochloride is commercially available as tablets, which are administered orally once daily, usually in the morning or evening, and should be taken with food (containing at least 350 calories) to increase absorption. Food increases peak concentrations and areas under the plasma concentration-time curve (AUC) of lurasidone threefold and twofold, respectively; however, lurasidone exposure was not affected as meal size was increased from 350 to 1000 calories and was independent of meal fat content. Lurasidone was administered with food in the controlled clinical studies.

Patients receiving lurasidone should be monitored for possible worsening of depression, suicidality, or unusual changes in behavior, especially at the beginning of therapy or during periods of dosage adjustments. (See Worsening of Depression and Suicidality Risk under Warnings/Precautions: Warnings, in Cautions.)

■ **Dosage** Dosage of lurasidone hydrochloride is expressed in terms of the hydrochloride salt.

Schizophrenia For the acute management of schizophrenia in adults, the recommended initial dosage of lurasidone hydrochloride is 40 mg orally once daily. Initial dosage titration is not required. Dosages ranging from 40–160 mg daily were effective in 6-week controlled trials. The maximum recommended dosage of lurasidone hydrochloride for the treatment of schizophrenia is 160 mg daily.

The manufacturer states that efficacy of lurasidone in schizophrenia beyond 6 weeks has not been established in controlled studies. If lurasidone is used for an extended period, the long-term usefulness of the drug for the individual patient should be reassessed periodically.

The American Psychiatric Association (APA) states that prudent long-term treatment options in patients with schizophrenia with remitted first or multiple episodes include either indefinite maintenance therapy or gradual discontinuance of the antipsychotic agent with close follow-up and a plan to reinstitute treatment upon symptom recurrence. Discontinuance of antipsychotic therapy should be considered only after a period of at least 1 year of symptom remission or optimal response while receiving the antipsychotic agent. In patients who have had multiple previous psychotic episodes or 2 psychotic episodes within 5 years, indefinite maintenance antipsychotic treatment is recommended.

Depressive Episodes Associated with Bipolar Disorder For the management of depressive episodes associated with bipolar I disorder in adults, either as monotherapy or as adjunctive therapy with lithium or valproate, the recommended initial dosage of lurasidone hydrochloride is 20 mg orally once daily. Initial dosage titration is not required. Dosages ranging from 20–120 mg daily as monotherapy or as adjunctive therapy with lithium or valproate were effective in 6-week controlled studies. In the monotherapy study, the higher dosage range (80–120 mg daily) did not provide additional efficacy, on average, over the lower dosage range (20–60 mg daily). The maximum recommended dosage of lurasidone hydrochloride for the treatment of bipolar depression, either as monotherapy or as adjunctive therapy with lithium or valproate, is 120 mg daily.

The manufacturer states that efficacy of lurasidone in bipolar depression beyond 6 weeks has not been established in controlled studies. If lurasidone is used for an extended period, the long-term usefulness of the drug for the individual patient should be reassessed periodically.

■ **Special Populations** The manufacturer recommends dosage adjustment in patients with moderate (creatinine clearance from 30 to less than 50 mL/minute) or severe renal impairment (creatinine clearance less than 30 mL/minute). The recommended initial lurasidone hydrochloride dosage in these patients is 20 mg daily. The maximum recommended dosage in patients with moderate or severe renal impairment is 80 mg daily. The manufacturer makes no specific dosage recommendations for patients with mild renal impairment. (See Renal Impairment under Warnings/Precautions: Specific Populations, in Cautions.)

The manufacturer recommends dosage adjustment in patients with moderate (Child-Pugh score 7–9) or severe hepatic impairment (Child-Pugh score 10–15). The recommended initial lurasidone hydrochloride dosage in these patients is 20 mg daily. The manufacturer states that lurasidone hydrochloride dosage in patients with moderate hepatic impairment should not exceed 80 mg daily and that dosage should not exceed 40 mg daily in patients with severe hepatic impairment. The manufacturer makes no specific dosage recommendations for patients with mild hepatic impairment. (See Hepatic Impairment under Warnings/Precautions: Specific Populations, in Cautions.)

In patients receiving lurasidone and in whom a moderate inhibitor of cytochrome P-450 (CYP) isoenzyme 3A4 (e.g., atazanavir, diltiazem, erythromycin, fluconazole, verapamil) will be added to therapy, the lurasidone dosage should be reduced to 50% of the original dosage. Similarly, in patients receiving a moderate CYP3A4 inhibitor in whom lurasidone hydrochloride is initiated, the recommended initial dosage of lurasidone hydrochloride is 20 mg daily and the maximum recommended dosage is 80 mg daily. If lurasidone is used concurrently with a moderate CYP3A4 inducer, it may be necessary to increase the lurasidone dosage after chronic therapy (i.e., 7 days or more) with the CYP3A4 inducer. Lurasidone should *not* be given concurrently with potent CYP3A4 inhibitors (e.g., clarithromycin, ketoconazole, ritonavir, voriconazole) or potent CYP3A4 inducers (e.g., carbamazepine, phenytoin, rifampin, St. John's wort [*Hypericum perforatum*]). (See Cautions: Contraindications and also see Drug Interactions.)

The manufacturer states that is not known whether dosage adjustment is necessary in geriatric patients on the basis of age alone. (See Geriatric Use under Warnings/Precautions: Specific Populations, in Cautions.)

Dosage adjustment is not recommended based on gender or race.

Cautions

■ **Contraindications** Known hypersensitivity to lurasidone hydrochloride or any components in the formulation. Angioedema has been reported.

Concurrent use of potent cytochrome P-450 (CYP) isoenzyme 3A4 inhibitors (e.g., clarithromycin, ketoconazole, ritonavir, voriconazole) or potent CYP3A4 inducers (e.g., carbamazepine, phenytoin, rifampin, St. John's wort [*Hypericum perforatum*]). (See Drug Interactions.)

■ **Warnings/Precautions** ***Warnings*** **Increased Mortality in Geriatric Patients with Dementia-related Psychosis.** Geriatric patients with dementia-related psychosis treated with antipsychotic drugs are at an increased risk of death. Analyses of 17 placebo-controlled trials (modal duration of 10 weeks) revealed a 1.6- to 1.7-fold increase in mortality among geriatric patients who were mainly receiving atypical antipsychotic drugs (i.e., aripiprazole, olanzapine, quetiapine, risperidone) compared with that observed in patients receiving placebo. Over the course of a typical 10-week controlled trial, the rate of death in drug-treated patients was about 4.5% compared with a rate of about 2.6% in the placebo group. Although the causes of death were varied, most of the deaths appeared to be either cardiovascular (e.g., heart failure, sudden death) or infectious (e.g., pneumonia) in nature. Observational studies suggest that, similar to atypical antipsychotics, treatment with conventional (first-generation) antipsychotics may increase mortality; the extent to which the findings of increased mortality in observational studies may be attributed to the antipsychotic drug as opposed to some characteristic(s) of the patients remains unclear. The manufacturer states that lurasidone is *not* approved for the treatment of patients with dementia-related psychosis. (See Adverse Cerebrovascular Events, including Stroke, in Geriatric Patients with Dementia-related Psychosis and see Dysphagia under Warnings/Precautions: Other Warnings and Precautions, in Cautions, and also see Geriatric Use under Warnings/Precautions: Specific Populations, in Cautions.)

Worsening of Depression and Suicidality Risk. Worsening of depression and/or the emergence of suicidal ideation and behavior (suicidality) or unusual changes in behavior may occur in both adult and pediatric (see Pediatric Use under Warnings/Precautions: Specific Populations, in Cautions) patients with major depressive disorder or other psychiatric disorders, whether or not they are taking antidepressants. This risk may persist until clinically important remission occurs. Suicide is a known risk of depression and certain other psychiatric disorders, and these disorders themselves are the strongest predictors of suicide. However, there has been a long-standing concern that antidepressants may have a role in inducing worsening of depression and the emergence of suicidality in certain patients during the early phases of treatment. Pooled analyses of short-term, placebo-controlled studies of antidepressants (i.e., selective serotonin-reuptake inhibitors [SSRIs] and other antidepressants) have shown an increased risk of suicidality in children, adolescents, and young adults (18–24 years of age) with major depressive disorder and other psychiatric disorders. An increased suicidality risk was not demonstrated with antidepressants compared with placebo in adults older than 24 years of age, and a reduced risk was observed in adults 65 years of age or older.

The US Food and Drug Administration (FDA) recommends that all patients being treated with antidepressants for any indication be appropriately monitored and closely observed for clinical worsening, suicidality, and unusual changes in behavior, particularly during initiation of therapy (i.e., the first few months) and during periods of dosage adjustments. Families and caregivers of patients being treated with antidepressants for major depressive disorder or other indications, both psychiatric and nonpsychiatric, also should be advised to monitor patients on a daily basis for the emergence of agitation, irritability, or unusual changes in behavior as well as the emergence of suicidality, and to report such symptoms immediately to a health-care provider.

Although a causal relationship between the emergence of symptoms such as anxiety, agitation, panic attacks, insomnia, irritability, hostility, aggressiveness, impulsivity, akathisia, hypomania, and/or mania and either the worsening of depression and/or the emergence of suicidal impulses has not been established, there is concern that such symptoms may represent precursors to emerging suicidality. Consequently, consideration should be given to changing the therapeutic regimen or discontinuing therapy in patients whose depression is persistently worse or in patients experiencing emergent suicidality or symptoms that might be precursors to worsening depression or suicidality, particularly if such manifestations are severe, abrupt in onset, or were not part of the patient's presenting symptoms. FDA also recommends that the drugs be prescribed in the smallest quantity consistent with good patient management, in order to reduce the risk of overdosage.

Sensitivity Reactions Rash and pruritus have been reported frequently and angioedema has been reported rarely in patients receiving lurasidone. (See Contraindications under Cautions.)

Other Warnings and Precautions **Adverse Cerebrovascular Events, including Stroke, in Geriatric Patients with Dementia-related Psychosis.** An increased incidence of adverse cerebrovascular events (cerebrovascular accidents and transient ischemic attacks), including fatalities, has been observed in geriatric patients with dementia-related psychosis treated with certain atypical antipsychotic agents (aripiprazole, olanzapine, risperidone) in placebo-controlled studies. The manufacturer states that lurasidone is *not* approved for the treatment of patients with dementia-related psychosis. (See Increased Mortality in Geriatric Patients with Dementia-related Psychosis under Warnings/Precautions: Warnings, and also see Geriatric Use under Warnings/Precautions: Specific Populations, in Cautions.)

Neuroleptic Malignant Syndrome. Neuroleptic malignant syndrome (NMS), a potentially fatal syndrome requiring immediate discontinuance of the drug and intensive symptomatic treatment, has been reported in patients receiving antipsychotic agents, including lurasidone. (See Advice to Patients.) For additional information on NMS, see Neuroleptic Malignant Syndrome under Cautions: Nervous System Effects, in the Phenothiazines General Statement 28:16.08.24.

Tardive Dyskinesia. Because use of antipsychotic agents, including lurasidone, may be associated with tardive dyskinesia (a syndrome of potentially irreversible, involuntary, dyskinetic movements), lurasidone should be prescribed in a manner that is most likely to minimize the occurrence of this syndrome. Chronic antipsychotic treatment generally should be reserved for patients who suffer from a chronic illness that is known to respond to antipsychotic agents, and for whom alternative, equally effective, but potentially less harmful treatments are not available or appropriate. In patients who do require chronic treatment, the lowest dosage and the shortest duration of treatment producing a satisfactory clinical response should be sought, and the need for continued treatment should be reassessed periodically.

The American Psychiatric Association (APA) currently recommends that patients receiving atypical antipsychotic agents be assessed clinically for abnormal involuntary movements every 12 months and that patients considered to be at increased risk for tardive dyskinesia be assessed every 6 months. If signs and symptoms of tardive dyskinesia appear in a lurasidone-treated patient, lurasidone discontinuance should be considered; however, some patients may require continued treatment with the drug despite the presence of the syndrome. For additional information on tardive dyskinesia, see Tardive Dyskinesia under Cautions: Nervous System Effects, in the Phenothiazines General Statement 28:16.08.24.

Metabolic Changes. Atypical antipsychotic agents have been associated with metabolic changes that may increase cardiovascular and cerebrovascular risk, including hyperglycemia, dyslipidemia, and body weight gain. While all of these drugs produce some metabolic changes, each drug has its own specific risk profile. (See Hyperglycemia and Diabetes Mellitus, see Dyslipidemia, and also see Weight Gain under Warnings/Precautions: Other Warnings and Precautions, in Cautions.)

Hyperglycemia and Diabetes Mellitus. Hyperglycemia, sometimes severe and associated with ketoacidosis, hyperosmolar coma, or death, has been reported in patients receiving atypical antipsychotic agents. In short- and longer-term clinical trials in patients with schizophrenia or bipolar depression, clinically important differences between lurasidone and placebo in mean change from baseline to end point in serum glucose concentrations were not observed. While confounding factors such as an increased background risk of diabetes mellitus in patients with schizophrenia and the increasing incidence of diabetes mellitus in the general population make it difficult to establish with certainty the relationship between use of agents in this drug class and glucose abnormalities, epidemiologic studies (which did not include lurasidone) suggest an increased risk of treatment-emergent hyperglycemia-related adverse events in patients treated with the atypical antipsychotic agents included in the studies (e.g., clozapine, olanzapine, quetiapine, risperidone). It remains to be determined whether lurasidone also is associated with this increased risk.

Precise risk estimates for hyperglycemia-related adverse events in patients treated with atypical antipsychotics currently are not available. While some evidence suggests that the risk for diabetes may be greater with some atypical antipsychotics (e.g., clozapine, olanzapine) than with others (e.g., aripiprazole, asenapine, iloperidone, lurasidone, quetiapine, risperidone, ziprasidone) in the class, available data are conflicting and insufficient to provide reliable estimates of relative risk associated with use of the various atypical antipsychotics.

The manufacturers of atypical antipsychotic agents state that patients with preexisting diabetes mellitus in whom therapy with an atypical antipsychotic is initiated should be periodically monitored for worsening of glucose control; those with risk factors for diabetes (e.g., obesity, family history of diabetes) should undergo fasting blood glucose testing upon therapy initiation and periodically throughout treatment. Any patient who develops manifestations of hyperglycemia (including polydipsia, polyuria, polyphagia, and weakness) during treatment with an atypical antipsychotic should undergo fasting blood glucose testing. (See Advice to Patients.) In some cases, patients who developed hyperglycemia while receiving an atypical antipsychotic have required continuance of antidiabetic treatment despite discontinuance of the suspect drug; in other cases, hyperglycemia resolved with discontinuance of the antipsychotic.

For further information on managing the risk of hyperglycemia and diabetes mellitus associated with atypical antipsychotic agents, see Hyperglycemia and Diabetes Mellitus under Cautions: Precautions and Contraindications, in Clozapine 28:16.08.04.

Dyslipidemia. Undesirable changes in lipid parameters have been observed in patients treated with some atypical antipsychotic agents; however, lurasidone generally does not appear to adversely affect the lipid profile in patients receiving the drug. In a between-group comparison of pooled data from short-term, placebo-controlled studies, there were no clinically important changes in mean fasting total cholesterol and triglyceride concentrations from baseline to end point in the lurasidone-treated patients. In uncontrolled, longer-term schizophrenia studies, lurasidone was associated with decreases from baseline in mean total cholesterol and triglyceride concentrations of 3.8 and 15.1 mg/dL at week 24, 3.1 and 4.8 mg/dL at week 36, and 2.5 and 6.9 mg/dL at week 52, respectively. In an uncontrolled, longer-term bipolar depression study, lurasidone monotherapy was associated with decreases from baseline in mean total cholesterol and triglyceride concentrations of 0.5 and 1 mg/dL at week 24, respectively. In an uncontrolled, longer-term bipolar depression study of lurasidone given as adjunctive therapy with lithium or valproate, lurasidone was associated with a decrease in mean total cholesterol concentrations of 0.9 mg/dL and a mean increase in triglyceride concentrations of 5.3 mg/dL at week 24.

Weight Gain. Weight gain has been observed with atypical antipsychotic therapy. Although lurasidone generally appears to be associated with minimal weight gain and less weight gain than some other atypical antipsychotic agents (e.g., olanzapine, quetiapine, risperidone), the manufacturer recommends clinical monitoring of weight in patients receiving the drug.

Differences in mean weight gain between lurasidone-treated patients and placebo recipients were reported in short-term schizophrenia clinical studies. A mean weight gain of 0.43 kg was reported in lurasidone-treated patients compared with a loss of 0.02 kg in those receiving placebo; 4.8% of lurasidone-treated patients gained 7% or more of their baseline body weight compared with 3.3% of those receiving placebo. During uncontrolled, longer-term schizophrenia studies, lurasidone therapy was associated with a mean weight loss of 0.69 kg at week 24, 0.59 kg at week 36, and 0.73 kg at week 52.

The mean weight gain during a short-term study in patients receiving lurasidone as monotherapy for bipolar depression was 0.29 kg compared with a loss of 0.04 kg in those receiving placebo; 2.4% of lurasidone-treated patients gained 7% or more of their baseline body weight compared with 0.7% of those receiving placebo. During an uncontrolled, longer-term extension of this study, lurasidone monotherapy was associated with a mean weight loss of 0.02 kg at week 24. In the short-term studies of lurasidone as adjunctive therapy with lithium or valproate, lurasidone was associated with a mean weight gain of 0.11 kg compared with a gain of 0.16 kg in those receiving placebo. During an uncontrolled, longer-term bipolar depression study, lurasidone, given as adjunctive therapy with lithium or valproate, was associated with a mean weight gain of 1.28 kg at week 24.

For additional information on metabolic effects associated with atypical antipsychotic agents, see Hyperglycemia and Diabetes Mellitus under Warnings/Precautions: Other Warnings and Precautions, in Cautions.

Hyperprolactinemia. Similar to other antipsychotic agents and drugs with dopamine D_2 antagonistic activity, lurasidone can elevate serum prolactin concentrations.

In short-term schizophrenia clinical trials, the median change from baseline to end point in prolactin concentrations for lurasidone-treated patients was an increase of 0.4 ng/mL compared with a decrease of 1.9 ng/mL in the placebo group. The proportion of patients with prolactin elevations 5 or more times the upper limit of normal was 2.8% for lurasidone-treated patients compared with 1% for placebo recipients. In short-term bipolar depression trials, the median increase from baseline to end point in prolactin concentrations was 1.7 and 3.5 ng/mL in the lower- and higher-dosage lurasidone monotherapy groups, respectively, compared with an increase of 0.3 ng/mL in the placebo group. In the clinical study of lurasidone as adjunctive therapy with lithium or valproate, the median increase in prolactin was 2.8 ng/mL in the lurasidone-treated patients compared with no change in the placebo recipients. The increase in prolactin was generally greater in female patients than male patients. Clinical disturbances such as galactorrhea, amenorrhea, gynecomastia, and impotence have been associated with prolactin-elevating drugs. In addition, chronic hyperprolactinemia associated with hypogonadism may lead to decreased bone density in both female and male patients.

If lurasidone therapy is considered in a patient with previously detected breast cancer, clinicians should consider that approximately one-third of human breast cancers are prolactin-dependent in vitro.

Leukopenia, Neutropenia, and Agranulocytosis. In clinical trial and/or postmarketing experience, leukopenia and neutropenia have been temporally related to antipsychotic agents, including lurasidone. Agranulocytosis (including fatal cases) also has been reported with other antipsychotic agents.

Possible risk factors for leukopenia and neutropenia include preexisting low leukocyte count and a history of drug-induced leukopenia and neutropenia. Patients with a preexisting low leukocyte count or a history of drug-induced leukopenia or neutropenia should have their complete blood count monitored frequently during the first few months of therapy. Lurasidone should be discontinued at the first sign of a decline in leukocyte count in the absence of other causative factors.

Patients with neutropenia should be carefully monitored for fever or other signs or symptoms of infection and promptly treated if such signs and symptoms occur. In patients with severe neutropenia (absolute neutrophil count [ANC] less than 1000/mm³), lurasidone should be discontinued and the leukocyte count monitored until recovery occurs. Lithium reportedly has been used successfully in the treatment of several cases of leukopenia associated with aripiprazole, clozapine, and some other drugs; however, further clinical experience is needed to confirm these anecdotal findings.

Orthostatic Hypotension and Syncope. Orthostatic hypotension, dizziness, lightheadedness, tachycardia or bradycardia, and syncope may occur during lurasidone therapy in some patients, particularly early in treatment and when dosage is increased, perhaps because of the drug's α_1-adrenergic blocking activity. Patients at increased risk of these adverse reactions or of developing complications from hypotension include those with dehydration, hypovolemia, a history of cardiovascular disease (e.g., heart failure, myocardial infarction, ischemic heart disease, conduction abnormalities), or a history of cerebrovascular disease, as well as patients receiving concomitant antihypertensive therapy and those who are antipsychotic-naive.

In short-term schizophrenia trials, orthostatic hypotension was reported as an adverse event in 0.3% of patients receiving lurasidone compared with 0.1% of placebo recipients, and syncope was reported in 0.1% of patients receiving lurasidone compared with none of the placebo recipients. Orthostatic hypotension, as assessed by vital signs, was reported in 0.8, 2.1, 1.7, and 0.8% of patients receiving lurasidone hydrochloride 40, 80, 120, and 160 mg daily, respectively, compared with 0.7% of patients receiving placebo in short-term schizophrenia trials.

There were no reports of orthostatic hypotension or syncope as adverse events in short-term bipolar depression clinical trials. Orthostatic hypotension, as assessed by vital signs, occurred in 0.6–1.1% of lurasidone-treated patients compared with 0–0.9% of the placebo recipients in these trials.

The manufacturer recommends considering use of a lower initial lurasidone dosage and more gradual dosage titration in patients with a history of cardiovascular disease (e.g., heart failure, history of myocardial infarction, ischemic heart disease, conduction abnormalities) or cerebrovascular disease or with conditions that would predispose patients to hypotension (e.g., dehydration, hypovolemia, concomitant antihypertensive therapy) and in antipsychotic-naive patients. In addition, orthostatic vital signs should be monitored in such patients.

Seizures. In short-term schizophrenia trials, seizures occurred in 0.1% of patients receiving lurasidone compared with 0.1% of patients receiving placebo. There were no reports of seizures or convulsions in lurasidone-treated patients in short-term bipolar depression trials.

As with other antipsychotic agents, lurasidone should be used with caution in patients with a history of seizures or with conditions that lower the seizure threshold (e.g., dementia of the Alzheimer's type); conditions that lower the seizure threshold may be more prevalent in patients 65 years of age or older.

Cognitive and Motor Impairment. Like other antipsychotic agents, lurasidone potentially may impair judgment, thinking, or motor skills. In short-term, placebo-controlled schizophrenia trials, somnolence (including hypersomnia, hypersomnolence, and sedation) was reported in 17% of patients receiving lurasidone compared with 7.1% of placebo recipients. In a short-term bipolar depression trial, somnolence was reported in 7.3 and 13.8% of patients who received lower-dose (20–60 mg daily) and higher-dose (80–120 mg daily) lurasidone hydrochloride monotherapy, respectively, compared with 6.5% of placebo recipients. Frequency of somnolence was found to be dose related in the monotherapy study. (See Advice to Patients.)

Body Temperature Regulation. Disruption of the body's ability to reduce core body temperature has been attributed to antipsychotic agents. The manufacturer recommends appropriate caution when lurasidone is used in patients who will be experiencing conditions that may contribute to an elevation in core body temperature (e.g., strenuous exercise, extreme heat, concomitant use of agents with anticholinergic activity, dehydration). (See Advice to Patients.)

Suicide. There is an attendant risk of suicide in patients with psychotic illnesses; high-risk patients should be closely supervised. Lurasidone should be prescribed in the smallest quantity consistent with good patient management to reduce the risk of overdosage.

Activation of Mania/Hypomania. Antidepressants can increase the risk of developing manic or hypomanic episodes, particularly in patients with bipolar disorder. Manic or hypomanic episodes were reported in less than 1% of patients receiving lurasidone and in less than 1% of patients receiving placebo in the bipolar depression monotherapy and adjunctive therapy studies. Patients should be monitored for the emergence of manic or hypomanic episodes during lurasidone therapy.

Dysphagia. Esophageal dysmotility and aspiration have been associated with the use of antipsychotic agents. Aspiration pneumonia is a common cause of morbidity and mortality in geriatric patients, particularly in those with advanced Alzheimer's dementia. Lurasidone is *not* approved for the treatment of patients with dementia-related psychosis and should be used with caution in patients at risk for aspiration pneumonia. (See Increased Mortality in Geriatric Patients with Dementia-related Psychosis under Warnings/Precautions: Warnings, in Cautions.)

Neurologic Adverse Reactions in Patients with Parkinsonian Syndrome or Dementia with Lewy Bodies. Patients with parkinsonian syndrome or dementia with Lewy bodies reportedly have an increased sensitivity to antipsychotic agents. Clinical manifestations of this increased sensitivity have been reported to include confusion, obtundation, postural instability with frequent falls, extrapyramidal symptoms, and features consistent with NMS. For additional information on extrapyramidal adverse effects and NMS, see Cautions: Nervous System Effects, in the Phenothiazines General Statement 28:16.08.24.

Specific Populations **Pregnancy.** Category B. (See Users Guide.)

Neonates exposed to antipsychotic agents during the third trimester of pregnancy are at risk for extrapyramidal and/or withdrawal symptoms following delivery. Symptoms reported to date have included agitation, hypertonia, hypotonia, tardive dyskinetic-like symptoms, tremor, somnolence, respiratory distress, and feeding disorder. Neonates exhibiting such symptoms should be monitored. The complications have varied in severity; some neonates recovered within hours to days without specific treatment while others have required intensive care unit support and prolonged hospitalization.

The effect of lurasidone on labor and delivery is unknown.

Lactation. Lurasidone is distributed into milk in rats. It is not known whether lurasidone and/or its metabolites are distributed into milk in humans. Because of the potential for serious adverse reactions to lurasidone in nursing infants, the manufacturer states that a decision should be made whether to discontinue nursing or lurasidone, taking into consideration the risk of drug discontinuance to the woman.

Pediatric Use. Safety and effectiveness of lurasidone in pediatric patients have not been established.

FDA warns that a greater risk of suicidal thinking or behavior (suicidality) occurred during the first few months of antidepressant treatment compared with placebo in children and adolescents with major depressive disorder, obsessive-compulsive disorder (OCD), or other psychiatric disorders based on pooled analyses of 24 short-term, placebo-controlled trials of 9 antidepressant drugs (SSRIs and other antidepressants). However, a later meta-analysis of 27 placebo-controlled trials of 9 antidepressants (SSRIs and others) in patients younger than 19 years of age with major depressive disorder, OCD, or non-OCD anxiety disorders suggests that the benefits of antidepressant therapy in treating these conditions may outweigh the risks of suicidal behavior or suicidal ideation. No suicides occurred in these pediatric trials. These findings should be carefully considered when assessing potential benefits and risks of lurasidone in a child or adolescent for any clinical use. (See Worsening of Depression and Suicidality Risk under Warnings/Precautions: Warnings, in Cautions.)

Geriatric Use. Clinical trial experience with lurasidone in patients with schizophrenia who are 65 years of age and older is insufficient to determine whether they respond differently than younger adults.

In geriatric patients (65–85 years of age) with psychosis, serum lurasidone concentrations were similar to those observed in younger adults. The manufacturer states that it is unknown whether dosage adjustment is necessary in geriatric patients on the basis of age alone.

Geriatric patients with dementia-related psychosis treated with lurasidone are at an increased risk of death compared with those treated with placebo. In addition, an increased incidence of adverse cerebrovascular events (cerebrovascular accidents and transient ischemic attacks), including fatalities, has been observed in geriatric patients with dementia-related psychosis treated with certain atypical antipsychotic agents (aripiprazole, olanzapine, risperidone) in placebo-controlled studies. The manufacturer states that lurasidone is *not* approved for the treatment of patients with dementia-related psychosis (see Increased Mortality in Geriatric Patients with Dementia-related Psychosis under Warnings/Precautions: Warnings, in Cautions and see also Adverse Cerebrovascular Events, including Stroke, in Geriatric Patients with Dementia-related Psychosis and see Dysphagia under Warnings/Precautions: Other Warnings and Precautions, in Cautions). For additional information on the use of antipsychotic agents in the management of dementia-related psychosis, see Geriatric Considerations under Uses: Psychotic Disorders, in the Phenothiazines General Statement 28:16.08.24.

In pooled data analyses, a *reduced* risk of suicidality was observed in adults 65 years of age or older with antidepressant therapy compared with placebo. (See Worsening of Depression and Suicidality Risk under Warnings/Precautions: Warnings, in Cautions.)

Hepatic Impairment. In a single-dose study, mean areas under the serum concentration-time curve (AUCs) of lurasidone were 1.5, 1.7, and 3 times higher in individuals with mild (Child-Pugh score 5–6), moderate (Child-Pugh score 7–9), and severe hepatic impairment (Child-Pugh score 10–15), respectively, compared with values in healthy matched individuals. Mean peak serum concentrations of lurasidone were 1.3, 1.2, and 1.3 times higher for patients with mild, moderate, and severe hepatic impairment, respectively, compared with values for healthy matched individuals. Dosage adjustment is recommended for patients with moderate or severe hepatic impairment. (See Dosage and Administration: Special Populations.)

Renal Impairment. After administration of a single 40-mg dose of lurasidone hydrochloride to patients with mild, moderate, or severe renal impairment, mean peak serum concentrations increased by 40, 92, and 54%, respectively, and mean AUCs increased by 53%, 91%, and twofold, respectively, compared with healthy matched individuals. Dosage adjustment is recommended for patients with moderate or severe renal impairment (creatinine clearance from 10 to less than 50 mL/minute). (See Dosage and Administration: Special Populations.)

■ **Common Adverse Effects** Adverse effects occurring in 5% or more of patients receiving lurasidone for schizophrenia and at a frequency at least twice that reported with placebo include somnolence (including hypersomnia, hypersomnolence, and sedation), akathisia, extrapyramidal symptoms (including parkinsonian symptoms and dyskinesia), and nausea. Akathisia and extrapyramidal symptoms were found to be dose related in these studies.

Adverse effects occurring in 5% or more of patients receiving lurasidone for bipolar depression as monotherapy or as adjunctive therapy with lithium or valproate and at a frequency at least twice that reported with placebo include somnolence (including hypersomnia, hypersomnolence, and sedation), akathisia, nausea, extrapyramidal symptoms (including parkinsonian symptoms and dyskinesia), vomiting, diarrhea, and anxiety. Nausea, somnolence, akathisia, and extrapyramidal symptoms were found to be dose related in the monotherapy study.

Drug Interactions

■ **Drugs Affecting or Metabolized by Hepatic Microsomal Enzymes** ***CYP3A4 Inhibitors and Inducers*** Lurasidone is predominantly metabolized by cytochrome P-450 (CYP) isoenzyme 3A4. Pharmacokinetic interactions of lurasidone with potent and moderate inhibitors or potent inducers of CYP3A4 have been observed.

Lurasidone should not be used in combination with potent inhibitors (e.g., clarithromycin, ketoconazole, ritonavir, voriconazole) or potent inducers (e.g., carbamazepine, phenytoin, rifampin, St. John's wort [*Hypericum perforatum*]) of CYP3A4. (See Contraindications and also see Drug Interactions: Ketoconazole and Drug Interactions: Rifampin.) Lurasidone dosage should be adjusted when used concurrently with moderate CYP3A4 inhibitors (e.g., atazanavir, diltiazem, erythromycin, fluconazole, verapamil). (See Dosage and Administration: Special Populations and also see Drug Interactions: Diltiazem.)

If lurasidone is used concurrently with a moderate CYP3A4 inducer, an increase in lurasidone dosage may be necessary after chronic therapy (i.e., 7 days or more) with the CYP3A4 inducer.

Inhibitors and Inducers of Other CYP Isoenzymes Lurasidone is not a substrate of CYP isoenzymes 1A1, 1A2, 2A6, 4A11, 2B6, 2C8, 2C9, 2C19, 2D6, or 2E1; therefore, clinically important pharmacokinetic interactions between lurasidone and drugs that are either inhibitors or inducers of these enzymes are unlikely.

■ **Anticholinergic Agents** Potential pharmacologic interaction (possible disruption of body temperature regulation); use lurasidone with caution in patients concurrently receiving drugs with anticholinergic activity. (See Body Temperature Regulation under Warnings/Precautions: Other Warnings and Precautions, in Cautions.)

■ **CNS Agents or Alcohol** Potential pharmacologic interaction (additive CNS effects). Use with caution with other CNS agents and avoid use of alcohol during lurasidone therapy.

■ **Digoxin** Concomitant administration of lurasidone hydrochloride (120 mg daily at steady state) with a single 0.25-mg dose of digoxin, a P-glycoprotein substrate, increased peak plasma concentrations and areas under the serum concentration-time curve (AUCs) of digoxin by approximately 9 and 13%, respectively. Digoxin dosage adjustment is not required in patients receiving these drugs concurrently.

■ **Diltiazem** Concomitant administration of diltiazem (240 mg daily for 5 days), a moderate CYP3A4 inhibitor, and lurasidone hydrochloride (single 20-mg dose) increased peak serum lurasidone concentrations and AUCs by 2.1 and 2.2 times, respectively, compared with administration of lurasidone alone. If diltiazem is initiated in patients receiving lurasidone, the manufacturer states that lurasidone dosage should be reduced to 50% of the original dosage. If lurasidone is initiated in patients receiving diltiazem, the manufacturer recommends that lurasidone hydrochloride therapy be initiated at 20 mg daily and that dosage not exceed 80 mg daily.

■ **Grapefruit** Grapefruit and grapefruit juice should be avoided in patients receiving lurasidone since they may inhibit CYP3A4 and increase plasma concentrations of lurasidone. (See Advice to Patients.)

■ **Hypotensive Agents** Because of its α_1-adrenergic blocking activity, the manufacturer states that patients receiving lurasidone may be at increased risk of orthostatic hypotension and syncope and related adverse effects. A lower initial dosage of lurasidone and more gradual dosage titration should therefore be considered in patients concomitantly receiving antihypertensive agents; in addition, monitoring of orthostatic vital signs is recommended in such patients. (See Orthostatic Hypotension and Syncope under Warnings/Precautions: Other Warnings and Precautions, in Cautions and also see Advice to Patients.)

■ **Ketoconazole** Concomitant administration of ketoconazole (400 mg daily), a potent CYP3A4 inhibitor, and lurasidone hydrochloride (single 10-mg dose) increased peak serum concentrations and AUCs of lurasidone by 6.8 and 9.3 times, respectively, compared with administration of lurasidone alone. Ketoconazole should therefore not be used concurrently with lurasidone.

■ **Lithium** Concomitant administration of lithium (600 mg twice daily for 8 days) and lurasidone hydrochloride (120 mg daily for 8 days) decreased peak serum lurasidone concentrations by 8% and increased lurasidone AUC by 7% compared with lurasidone administration alone; these changes were not considered clinically important. In bipolar depression studies evaluating lurasidone and adjunctive lithium therapy, there was no evidence of additive CNS toxicity in patients receiving lurasidone and lithium in combination. Lurasidone dosage adjustment is not required in patients receiving lithium concurrently. In addition, lithium dosage adjustment is not necessary during concurrent use of lurasidone.

■ **Midazolam** Concomitant administration of lurasidone hydrochloride (120 mg daily at steady state) with a single 5-mg dose of midazolam, a CYP3A4 substrate, increased peak plasma concentrations and AUCs of midazolam by approximately 21 and 44%, respectively. Midazolam dosage adjustment is not required in patients receiving lurasidone concurrently.

■ **Oral Contraceptives** Concomitant administration of lurasidone hydrochloride (40 mg daily at steady state) with an oral contraceptive containing ethinyl estradiol and norgestimate resulted in equivalent peak plasma concentrations and AUCs of ethinyl estradiol and norgestimate relative to oral contraceptive administration alone. Sex hormone binding globulin concentrations also were not substantially affected by concurrent administration of the drugs. Oral contraceptive dosage adjustment is not required in patients receiving lurasidone concurrently.

■ **Rifampin** Concomitant administration of rifampin (600 mg daily for 8 days), a strong CYP3A4 inducer, and lurasidone hydrochloride (single 40-mg dose) decreased peak serum lurasidone concentrations and AUCs by approximately 85 and 82%, respectively. Rifampin should not be concurrently administered with lurasidone.

■ **Smoking** Lurasidone is not a substrate for CYP1A2 in vitro; therefore, smoking should not alter the pharmacokinetics of the drug.

■ **St. John's Wort** Lurasidone should not be used concurrently with St. John's wort (*Hypericum perforatum*), a potent inducer of CYP3A4.

■ **Valproate** The manufacturer states that a dedicated drug interaction study has not been conducted with lurasidone and valproate. However, pharmacokinetic data obtained from the bipolar depression studies indicate that valproate concentrations are not affected by concomitant use of lurasidone, and that lurasidone concentrations are not affected by concomitant use of valproate. Therefore, dosage adjustments are not required in patients receiving valproate and lurasidone concurrently.

Description

Lurasidone is a benzisothiazol-derivative antipsychotic agent and has been referred to as an atypical or second-generation antipsychotic agent. Lurasidone has also been described as an azapirone derivative. Although the exact mechanism of action of lurasidone in schizophrenia and bipolar depression is unknown, it has been suggested that the efficacy of lurasidone is mediated through a combination of antagonist activity at central dopamine type 2 (D_2) and serotonin type 2 (5-hydroxytryptamine [5-HT_{2A}]) receptors.

Lurasidone is an antagonist that exhibits high affinity for D_2, 5-HT_{2A}, and 5-HT_7 receptors and moderate affinity for α_{2C}-adrenergic receptors in vitro. The drug acts as a partial agonist at 5-HT_{1A} receptors and is an antagonist at α_{2A}-adrenergic receptors in vitro. Lurasidone exhibits weak affinity for α_1-adrenergic receptors and little or no affinity for histamine (H_1) receptors and muscarinic (M_1) receptors.

Lurasidone is rapidly absorbed following oral administration and reaches peak serum concentrations within about 1–3 hours. Approximately 9–19% of an administered dose is absorbed orally. Steady-state concentrations of the drug are achieved within 7 days. Lurasidone is highly bound (99.8%) to serum proteins, including albumin and α_1-acid glycoprotein. The drug is metabolized mainly via CYP3A4. The major biotransformation pathways are oxidative *N*-dealkylation, hydroxylation of the norbornane ring, and *S*-oxidation. Lurasidone is metabolized into 2 active metabolites (ID-14283 and ID-14326) and 2 major inactive metabolites (ID-20219 and ID-20220). Following administration of a single radiolabeled dose of lurasidone, approximately 80 and 9% of the dose is excreted in feces and urine, respectively.

Advice to Patients

Importance of providing a copy of written patient information (medication guide) each time lurasidone hydrochloride is dispensed. Importance of advising patients to read the patient information before taking lurasidone and each time the prescription is refilled.

Importance of advising patients and caregivers that geriatric patients with dementia-related psychosis treated with antipsychotic agents are at an increased risk of death. Patients and caregivers also should be informed that lurasidone is *not* approved for treating geriatric patients with dementia-related psychosis.

Risk of suicidality and activation of mania or hypomania; importance of patients, family, and caregivers being alert to and immediately reporting emergence of suicidality, worsening depression, manic or hypomanic symptoms, irritability, agitation, or unusual changes in behavior, especially during the first few months of therapy or during periods of dosage adjustment. (See Worsening of Depression and Suicidality Risk under Warnings/Precautions: Warnings, in Cautions.)

Importance of informing patients and caregivers about the risk of neuroleptic malignant syndrome (NMS), a rare but potentially life-threatening syndrome that can cause high fever, stiff muscles, sweating, fast or irregular heart beat, change in blood pressure, confusion, and kidney damage.

Importance of informing patients and caregivers about the risk of metabolic changes (e.g., hyperglycemia and diabetes mellitus, dyslipidemia, weight gain, cardiovascular reactions) with lurasidone and the need for specific monitoring for such changes during therapy. Importance of patients and caregivers being aware of the symptoms of hyperglycemia and diabetes mellitus (e.g., increased thirst, increased urination, increased appetite, weakness) and monitoring all patients receiving lurasidone for these symptoms. Importance of informing patients who are diagnosed with diabetes or those with risk factors for diabetes (e.g., obesity, family history of diabetes) that they should have their blood glucose monitored at the beginning of and periodically during lurasidone therapy; patients who develop symptoms of hyperglycemia during therapy should have their blood glucose assessed. Importance of informing patients that clinical monitoring of weight is recommended during lurasidone therapy.

Importance of informing patients about the risk of orthostatic hypotension, especially when initiating or reinitiating treatment or increasing the dosage.

Risk of leukopenia/neutropenia. Importance of advising patients with a preexisting low leukocyte count or a history of drug-induced leukopenia/neutropenia that they should have their complete blood cell (CBC) count monitored during lurasidone therapy.

Because somnolence (i.e., sleepiness, drowsiness) may be associated with lurasidone, patients should be cautioned about performing activities requiring mental alertness, such as driving or operating hazardous machinery, while taking lurasidone until they gain experience with the drug's effects.

Importance of avoiding eating grapefruit or drinking grapefruit juice during lurasidone therapy, since they can affect lurasidone concentrations in the blood.

Importance of avoiding alcohol during lurasidone therapy.

Importance of clinicians informing patients in whom chronic lurasidone use is contemplated about the risk of a movement problem called tardive dyskinesia. Importance of informing patients to report any muscle movements that cannot be stopped to a healthcare professional.

Importance of informing clinicians of existing or contemplated concomitant therapy, including prescription (see Drug Interactions) and OTC drugs or herbal supplements, as well as any concomitant illnesses (e.g., cardiovascular disease, diabetes mellitus, seizures).

Importance of women informing clinicians if they are or plan to become pregnant or plan to breast-feed. Importance of clinicians informing patients about the benefits and risks of taking antipsychotics during pregnancy (see Pregnancy under Warnings/Precautions: Specific Populations, in Cautions). Importance of advising patients not to stop taking lurasidone if they become pregnant without consulting their clinician; abruptly stopping antipsychotic agents may cause complications. Importance of advising patients not to breast-feed during lurasidone therapy.

Importance of avoiding overheating and dehydration.

Importance of informing patients of other important precautionary information. (See Cautions.)

Overview® (see Users Guide). For additional information on this drug until a more detailed monograph is developed and published, the manufacturer's labeling should be consulted. It is *essential* that the manufacturer's labeling be consulted for more detailed information on usual cautions, precautions, contraindications, potential drug interactions, laboratory test interferences, and acute toxicity.

Preparations

Excipients in commercially available drug preparations may have clinically important effects in some individuals; consult specific product labeling for details.

Lurasidone Hydrochloride

Oral		
Tablets, film-coated	20 mg	**Latuda®**, Sunovion
	40 mg	**Latuda®**, Sunovion
	60 mg	**Latuda®**, Sunovion
	80 mg	**Latuda®**, Sunovion
	120 mg	**Latuda®**, Sunovion

†Use is not currently included in the labeling approved by the US Food and Drug Administration

OLANZapine

Olanzapine Embonate

■ Olanzapine is considered an atypical or second-generation antipsychotic agent.

REMS

FDA approved a REMS for olanzapine to ensure that the benefits outweigh the risks. The REMS may apply to one or more preparations of olanzapine and consists of the following: medication guide, elements to assure safe use, communication plan, and implementation system. See the FDA REMS page (https://www.accessdata.fda.gov/scripts/cder/rems/index.cfm).

Uses

Olanzapine is used orally for the symptomatic management of psychotic disorders (e.g., schizophrenia) in adults and adolescents 13–17 years of age. In addition, oral olanzapine is used alone in adults and adolescents 13–17 years of age or in conjunction with lithium or valproate in adults for the management of acute manic or mixed episodes associated with bipolar I disorder; the drug also is used for longer-term maintenance monotherapy in patients with this disorder. Short-acting olanzapine injection is used IM for the management of acute agitation in patients with bipolar disorder or schizophrenia. Long-acting olanzapine pamoate injection is used IM for the management of schizophrenia in adults.

Olanzapine is used orally in combination with fluoxetine for the treatment of acute depressive episodes associated with bipolar I disorder in adults and pediatric patients 10–17 years of age. The drug also is used orally in combination with fluoxetine for the acute and maintenance therapy of treatment-resistant depression.

Olanzapine has been used orally in combination with other antiemetic agents for the prevention of nausea and vomiting associated with highly emetogenic cancer chemotherapy†, including high-dose cisplatin therapy in adults. The drug also has been used as rescue antiemetic therapy in patients with breakthrough cancer chemotherapy-induced nausea and vomiting†.

■ **Psychotic Disorders** Olanzapine is used orally and parenterally for the symptomatic management of psychotic disorders (e.g., schizophrenia). Drug therapy is integral to the management of acute psychotic episodes in patients with schizophrenia and generally is required for long-term stabilization to sustain symptom remission or control and to minimize the risk of relapse. Antipsychotic agents are the principal class of drugs used for the management of all phases of schizophrenia. Patient response and tolerance to antipsychotic agents are variable, and patients who do not respond to or tolerate one drug may be successfully treated with an agent from a different class or with a different adverse effect profile.

Schizophrenia Olanzapine is used orally for the management of schizophrenia in adults and adolescents from 13 to 17 years of age. The long-acting pamoate ester of olanzapine is used parenterally for the management of schizophrenia in adults. Schizophrenia is a major psychotic disorder that frequently has devastating effects on various aspects of the patient's life and carries a high risk of suicide and other life-threatening behaviors. Manifestations of schizophrenia involve multiple psychologic processes, including perception (e.g., hallucinations), ideation, reality testing (e.g., delusions), emotion (e.g., flatness, inappropriate affect), thought processes (e.g., loose associations), behavior (e.g., catatonia, disorganization), attention, concentration, motivation (e.g., avolition, impaired intention and planning), and judgment. The principal manifestations of this disorder usually are described in terms of positive and negative (deficit) symptoms, and more recently, disorganized symptoms. Positive symptoms include hallucinations, delusions, bizarre behavior, hostility, uncooperativeness, and paranoid ideation, while negative symptoms include restricted range and intensity of emotional expression (affective flattening), reduced thought and speech productivity (alogia), anhedonia, apathy, and decreased initiation of goal-directed behavior (avolition). Disorganized symptoms include disorganized speech (thought disorder) and behavior and poor attention.

The American Psychiatric Association (APA) considers most atypical antipsychotic agents (e.g., olanzapine, aripiprazole, quetiapine, risperidone, ziprasidone) first-line drugs for the management of the acute phase of schizophrenia (including first psychotic episodes), principally because of the decreased risk of adverse extrapyramidal effects and tardive dyskinesia, with the understanding that the relative advantages, disadvantages, and cost-effectiveness of conventional (first-generation) and atypical antipsychotic agents remain controversial. The APA states that, with the possible exception of clozapine for the management of treatment-resistant symptoms, there currently is no definitive evidence that one atypical antipsychotic agent will have superior efficacy compared with another agent in the class, although meaningful differences in response may be observed in individual patients. Conventional antipsychotic agents may be considered first-line in patients who have been treated successfully in the past with or who prefer conventional agents. The choice of an antipsychotic agent should be individualized, considering past response to therapy, adverse effect profile (including the patient's experience of subjective effects such as dysphoria), and the patient's preference for a specific drug, including route of administration.

To compare the long-term effectiveness and tolerability of older, first-generation antipsychotic agents (i.e., perphenazine) with those of newer, atypical antipsychotic agents (i.e., olanzapine, quetiapine, risperidone, ziprasidone), a double-blind, multicenter study (the first phase of Clinical Antipsychotic Trials of Intervention Effectiveness [CATIE]) was sponsored by the National Institute of Mental Health. More than 1400 patients with schizophrenia received one of these antipsychotics for up to 18 months or until therapy was discontinued for any reason. Patients with tardive dyskinesia could enroll in this trial; however, the randomization scheme prevented their assignment to the perphenazine group. The primary outcome measure in this study was the discontinuance of treatment for any cause; this measure was selected because discontinuing or switching an antipsychotic agent occurs frequently and is an important problem in the management of schizophrenia. In addition, this measure integrates the patient's and clinician's judgments concerning efficacy, safety, and tolerability into a more comprehensive measure of effectiveness reflecting therapeutic benefits in relation to adverse effects. Overall, 74% of patients in this study discontinued their medication before receiving the full 18 months of therapy because of inadequate efficacy, intolerable adverse effects, or for other reasons, suggesting substantial limitations in the long-term clinical effectiveness of currently available antipsychotic agents. Olanzapine appeared to be more effective than the other drugs evaluated in this study with a lower (64%) discontinuance rate and a lower rate of hospitalization for exacerbation of schizophrenia, while no significant differences between the effectiveness of the conventional agent, perphenazine, and the other second-generation agents studied were observed (discontinuance rates were 75, 82, 74, and 79% for perphenazine, quetiapine, risperidone, and ziprasidone, respectively). The time to discontinuance of therapy for any cause was found to be longer in the olanzapine group than in the quetiapine, risperidone, perphenazine, and ziprasidone groups in this study; however, the differences between the olanzapine and perphenazine groups and between the olanzapine and ziprasidone groups did not achieve statistical significance. Although there were no significant differences in the time until discontinuance of therapy because of drug intolerance among the drugs studied, the incidences of discontinuance for certain adverse effects differed among the drugs with olanzapine discontinued more frequently because of weight gain or metabolic effects (e.g., increases in glycosylated hemoglobin [hemoglobin A_{1c}; HbA_{1c}], cholesterol, and triglycerides) and perphenazine discontinued more frequently because of adverse extrapyramidal effects.

An open, multicenter, randomized, controlled trial comparing the relative long-term effectiveness (over a 1-year period) of a group of first-generation antipsychotic agents (e.g., chlorpromazine, flupentixol [not commercially available in the US], flupentixol decanoate [not commercially available in the US], fluphenazine decanoate, haloperidol, haloperidol decanoate, loxapine, methotrimeprazine [no longer commercially available in the US], pipothiazine palmitate [not commercially available in the US], sulpiride [not commercially available in the US], trifluoperazine, zuclopenthixol [not commercially available in the US], zuclopenthixol decanoate [not commercially available in the US]) with a group of second-generation antipsychotic agents other than clozapine (e.g., olanzapine, amisulpride [not commercially available in the US], quetiapine, risperidone, zotepine [not commercially available in the US]) in patients with schizophrenia was conducted throughout the United Kingdom by the National Health Service. In the Cost Utility of the Latest Antipsychotic Drugs in Schizophrenia Study (CUtLASS 1), the primary outcome measure was the Quality of Life Scale score, and secondary outcome measures included symptom improvement, adverse effects, patient satisfaction, and costs of health care. Patients in the first-generation antipsychotic group demonstrated a trend toward greater improvements in the Quality of Life Scale and symptom improvements scores in this study. In addition, the patients studied did not report a clear preference for either group of drugs and costs of health care in the 2 groups were found to be similar.

Emerging data from the first phase of the pivotal CATIE trial and the CUtLASS 1 trial suggest that newer, atypical antipsychotics may not provide clinically important advantages over older, first-generation antipsychotics in patients with chronic schizophrenia and that several factors, including adequacy of symptom relief, tolerability of adverse effects, and cost of therapy, may influence a patient's ability and willingness to remain on long-term antipsychotic medication. In addition, these results suggest that it may often be necessary to try 2 or more different antipsychotic agents in an individual patient in order to provide optimal therapeutic benefit with an acceptable adverse effect profile.

In a randomized, double-blind, second phase trial, patients with schizophrenia who had discontinued an atypical antipsychotic agent during the first phase of the CATIE trial were reassigned to treatment with a different atypical antipsychotic agent (olanzapine, quetiapine, risperidone, or ziprasidone). Similarly to the first phase of the CATIE trial, efficacy and tolerability in this second phase study were principally measured by time until drug discontinuance for any reason. The time until antipsychotic treatment was discontinued was longer for patients receiving risperidone and olanzapine than for those receiving quetiapine and ziprasidone (median: 7, 6.3, 4, and 2.8 months, respectively). Among patients who discontinued their prior antipsychotic agent because of lack of efficacy, olanzapine was found to be more effective than quetiapine and ziprasidone, while risperidone was more effective than quetiapine.

In another study that was part of the second phase of the CATIE investigation, schizophrenic patients who had discontinued treatment with olanzapine, quetiapine, risperidone, or ziprasidone during the first phase of the CATIE investigation, principally because of inadequate efficacy, were randomized to receive open-label clozapine therapy or blinded treatment with another atypical antipsychotic agent not previously received in the trial. Clozapine was found to be more effective in this study than switching to another atypical antipsychotic agent. Patients receiving clozapine also were found to be less likely to discontinue treatment for any reason than patients receiving quetiapine or risperidone. In addition, the clozapine-treated patients were less likely to discontinue therapy because of an inadequate clinical response than were patients receiving the other atypical antipsychotic agents.

Pending further data clarifying the relative effectiveness and tolerability of first- and second-generation antipsychotics in the treatment of schizophrenia, many clinicians recommend that the choice of an antipsychotic agent be carefully individualized taking into consideration the clinical efficacy and adverse effect profile (including the risk for extrapyramidal effects, weight gain, and adverse metabolic effects) of the antipsychotic agent as well as the individual patient's risk factors; the patient's previous experience of subjective effects such as dysphoria; the patient's preference for and willingness to take (i.e., compliance) a specific drug, including route of administration; and the relative cost of therapy. Olanzapine and clozapine may be reasonable alternatives in any patient with schizophrenia who has not achieved a full clinical remission with other antipsychotic agents; however, the risk of adverse metabolic effects with both drugs necessitates dietary and exercise counseling before therapy is initiated, monitoring during drug therapy, and possible discontinuance of therapy if these effects become troublesome during therapy. Additional analyses from data generated by the CATIE trial addressing other schizophrenia treatment-related issues such as quality of life and predictors of response are ongoing.

Atypical antipsychotic agents, including olanzapine, generally appear less likely to induce adverse extrapyramidal effects and tardive dyskinesia than conventional, first-generation antipsychotic agents. In addition, stabilization of or improvement in tardive dyskinesia associated with conventional antipsychotic agents has been reported in some patients when they have been switched to second-generation antipsychotic therapy, including olanzapine. Therefore, the APA and some clinicians recommend that atypical antipsychotic agents be considered in patients with schizophrenia who have experienced tardive dyskinesia associated with conventional antipsychotic agents.

For additional information on the symptomatic management of schizophrenia, see Schizophrenia and Other Psychotic Disorders under Uses: Psychotic Disorders, in the Phenothiazines General Statement 28:16.08.24.

The efficacy of oral olanzapine for the management of psychotic disorders in adults has been established in hospital settings by 2 placebo-controlled studies of 6 weeks' duration in patients who met the DSM-III-R criteria for schizophrenia. In these and several other studies, improvement in manifestations of schizophrenia was based principally on the results of various psychiatric rating scales, including the Brief Psychiatric Rating Scale (BPRS) that assesses factors such as anergy, thought disturbances, activation, hostility/suspiciousness, and anxiety/depression; the Scale for the Assessment of Negative Symptoms (SANS); the Positive and Negative Symptoms Scale (PANSS); and the Clinical Global Impression (CGI).

In the first 6-week, placebo-controlled study, olanzapine was given in a fixed dosage of 1 or 10 mg once daily. Results indicated that the 10-mg, but not the 1-mg, once-daily dosage was more effective than placebo in improving the scores on the PANSS total (also on the extracted BPRS total), the BPRS psychosis cluster, the PANSS Negative subscale, and the CGI Severity assessments. Results of the second 6-week, placebo-controlled study, which evaluated 3 fixed dosage ranges (5 ± 2.5 mg once daily, 10 ± 2.5 mg once daily, and 15 ± 2.5 mg once daily), found that the 2 highest dosages (actual mean dosages were 12 and 16 mg once daily, respectively) were more effective than placebo in reducing the BPRS total score, BPRS psychosis cluster, and CGI severity score; the highest dosage also was superior to placebo on the SANS. There appeared to be no therapeutic advantage for the higher dosage of olanzapine compared with the medium dosage in this study. No race- or gender-related differences in outcome were noted in either of these studies.

The efficacy of oral olanzapine for long-term use (i.e., longer than 6 weeks) in schizophrenia has been established in one controlled study in adults, and the drug has been used in some other patients for prolonged periods (e.g., reportedly up to 1 year) without apparent loss of clinical effect. In the long-term clinical trial, adult outpatients who predominantly met DSM-IV criteria for schizophrenia and who remained stable on olanzapine therapy during an open-label treatment phase lasting at least 8 weeks were randomized to continue receiving their current olanzapine dosage (ranging from 10–20 mg daily) or to receive placebo. Although the follow-up period to observe patients for relapse, which was defined in terms of increases in BPRS positive symptoms or hospitalization, initially was planned for 12 months, criteria were met for stopping the trial early because of an excess of placebo relapses compared with olanzapine relapses. In addition, olanzapine was found to be superior to placebo on prolonging time to relapse, which was the primary outcome measure in this study. Therefore, olanzapine was more effective than placebo at maintaining efficacy in schizophrenic patients stabilized for approximately 8 weeks and followed for an observation period of up to 8 months. If oral olanzapine is used for extended periods, the need for continued therapy should be reassessed periodically.

The short-term efficacy of long-acting IM olanzapine pamoate in schizophrenia has been established in a randomized, double-blind, placebo-controlled, multicenter study of 8 weeks' duration in 404 adults who were experiencing acute psychotic symptoms and met DSM-IV or DSM-IV-TR criteria for schizophrenia. Patients were randomized to receive IM injections of olanzapine pamoate (Zyprexa® Relprevv) in dosages of 210 mg (of olanzapine) every 2 weeks, 405 mg every 4 weeks, or 300 mg every 2 weeks or placebo every 2 weeks. Patients were discontinued from their previous antipsychotic regimen and underwent a washout period lasting 2–7 days. Supplementation with oral antipsychotics was not allowed throughout the study. The primary efficacy measure in this study was the change from baseline to end point in the total PANSS score (the mean baseline total PANSS score was 101). Total PANSS scores showed improvement from baseline to end point with each dosage of olanzapine pamoate compared with placebo. At week 8, PANSS total scores decreased by a mean of 22.5, 22.6, or 26.3 points in patients receiving IM olanzapine pamoate 210 mg every 2 weeks, 405 mg every 4 weeks, or 300 mg every 2 weeks, respectively, compared with a mean decrease of 8.5 points in patients receiving placebo. There were no substantial differences in efficacy among the 3 olanzapine pamoate dosage groups at the study end point. The onset of antipsychotic efficacy for the long-acting olanzapine pamoate injection was evident within the first week of treatment. The manufacturer states that the effectiveness of olanzapine pamoate injection in the treatment of schizophrenia also is supported by the established effectiveness of orally administered olanzapine.

Efficacy of long-acting IM olanzapine pamoate for long-term use (i.e., longer than 8 weeks) in the maintenance treatment of schizophrenia has been established in a randomized, double-blind, multicenter study in 1065 adults. Adult outpatients with schizophrenia who had remained stable on oral olanzapine therapy during an open-label treatment phase lasting 4–8 weeks were randomized to continue receiving their current olanzapine dosage orally (10, 15, or 20 mg daily) or to receive long-acting IM olanzapine pamoate (Zyprexa® Relprevv) in a low-dosage regimen (150 mg [of olanzapine] every 2 weeks), a medium-dosage regimen (405 mg every 4 weeks), or a high-dosage regimen (300 mg every 2 weeks), or a very low reference dosage regimen (45 mg every 4 weeks) for 24 weeks in the double-blind maintenance phase. No supplementation with oral antipsychotics was allowed throughout the study. The primary efficacy measure was time to exacerbation of symptoms of schizophrenia, which was defined as either increases in BPRS positive symptoms or hospitalization. IM olanzapine pamoate was found to be effective in the maintenance treatment of schizophrenia for up to 24 weeks and IM olanzapine pamoate dosage regimens of 150 mg every 2 weeks, 405 mg every 4 weeks, or 300 mg every 2 weeks were found to be superior to 45 mg every 4 weeks. Olanzapine pamoate generally demonstrated a similar safety profile to oral olanzapine with the exception of injection-related adverse effects. If IM olanzapine pamoate injection is used for extended periods, the need for continued therapy should be reassessed periodically.

Parenteral antipsychotic therapy with a long-acting IM preparation may be particularly useful in patients with schizophrenia and a history of poor compliance. In addition, long-acting antipsychotic preparations may be useful in patients with suspected GI malabsorption or variable GI absorption of the drug. The principal disadvantage of long-acting parenteral antipsychotics is the inability to terminate the drug's action when severe adverse reactions occur. The manufacturer of Zyprexa® Relprevv recommends that patients first receive oral olanzapine therapy to establish tolerability of the drug before long-acting IM olanzapine pamoate is used. Long-acting IM olanzapine pamoate may be most useful in schizophrenic patients who respond well to oral olanzapine therapy and for whom a depot antipsychotic can improve compliance.

Olanzapine has been shown to be an effective, relatively rapid-acting, broad-spectrum antipsychotic agent in both controlled and uncontrolled studies of patients with schizophrenia. Like other second-generation antipsychotic agents, olanzapine appears to improve both positive (florid symptomatology such as hallucinations, conceptual disorganization, and suspiciousness) and negative ("deficit" symptomatology such as emotional withdrawal, motor retardation, blunted affect, and disorientation) manifestations of schizophrenia; conventional antipsychotic agents may have lesser effects on negative manifestations of the disorder. Some evidence also suggests that atypical antipsychotic agents may be more effective in treating cognitive and mood symptoms as well as global psychopathology than conventional antipsychotic agents, but this is controversial and remains to be fully established. In addition, some patients with schizophrenia who have been stabilized on long-term conventional antipsychotic therapy have demonstrated further improvement following a switch to an atypical antipsychotic agent.

Results from one comparative study in adults suggest that oral olanzapine dosages of 7.5–17.5 mg daily may be as effective as oral haloperidol dosages of 10–20 mg daily in reducing positive symptoms of schizophrenia, while oral olanzapine dosages of 12.5–17.5 mg daily may be more effective than oral haloperidol dosages of 10–20 mg daily in reducing negative symptoms of schizophrenia. A randomized, controlled trial comparing the long-term (i.e., 1 year) effectiveness and cost of olanzapine and haloperidol therapy in patients with schizophrenia or schizoaffective disorder did not reveal any important advantage of olanzapine compared with haloperidol on measures of compliance, symptom improvement, adverse extrapyramidal effects, overall quality of life, and cost; olanzapine also was more frequently associated with weight gain. However, olanzapine therapy was associated with reduced akathisia, less tardive dyskinesia in a secondary analysis, and small but significant improvements in measures of memory and motor function compared with haloperidol. In other comparative studies, olanzapine usually was found to be at least as effective as or more effective than haloperidol and several other atypical antipsychotic agents, including quetiapine, risperidone, and ziprasidone. In a comparative, double-blind trial conducted in patients with schizophrenia or schizoaffective disorder, both olanzapine and risperidone were found to be effective and well tolerated, although greater reductions in the severity of positive and affective symptoms were noted in the risperidone-treated patients compared with those receiving olanzapine.

Olanzapine also has been studied in patients with treatment-refractory schizophrenia (i.e., patients who have demonstrated an inadequate response to prior antipsychotic therapy) in both open and comparative clinical trials. In an open trial of 6 weeks' duration, olanzapine (15–25 mg daily) was found to be effective and well tolerated in adult patients with treatment-refractory schizophrenia with 36% responding to the drug. In a double-blind trial of 8 weeks' duration, although olanzapine (25 mg daily) was found to be as effective as chlorpromazine (1.2 g daily with benztropine), the total amount of improvement with either drug was modest; olanzapine was better tolerated than chlorpromazine. In a double-blind trial of 14 weeks' duration comparing efficacy and safety of several atypical antipsychotics (olanzapine, clozapine, and risperidone) with each other and with haloperidol, olanzapine (mean dosage of approximately 30 mg daily) and clozapine produced greater clinical improvement in global psychopathology and negative symptoms than haloperidol (mean dosage of approximately 26 mg daily) in patients with chronic schizophrenia or schizoaffective disorder, but the effects of atypical antipsychotic agents were considered small and of limited clinical importance. In another study using the manufacturer's clinical trial database to retrospectively identify treatment-resistant schizophrenic patients, olanzapine (mean dosage of approximately 11 mg daily) was found to be more effective than haloperidol therapy (mean dosage of approximately 10 mg daily) in improving positive, negative, and mood symptoms and produced fewer extrapyramidal effects. The results of clinical trials to date suggest that olanzapine may be somewhat less effective than or similarly effective to clozapine in the management of resistant schizophrenia patients. Clozapine generally appears to be more effective in the management of treatment-refractory schizophrenia than most first-generation and other second-generation antipsychotic agents and may produce greater improvement in negative symptoms of schizophrenia than other antipsychotic agents; however, tolerability concerns (e.g., hematologic toxicity, hypotension, dizziness, sedation) limit its use in many patients. Although higher olanzapine dosages (i.e., up to 60 mg daily) have been used in some patients with treatment-resistant schizophrenia, it remains to be established whether higher dosages of the drug result in improved efficacy in such patients, and higher dosages may increase the risk of extrapyramidal and other adverse effects.

Like some other atypical antipsychotic agents (e.g., clozapine, risperidone), olanzapine therapy appears to reduce the risk of violent behavior in patients with schizophrenia. Although the precise mechanism(s) for the antiaggressive effects are not known, improved compliance with atypical antipsychotic agents may play a role.

Olanzapine also has been used with a variety of adjunctive agents, including other antipsychotic agents, antidepressants (including selective serotonin-reuptake inhibitors such as fluoxetine and fluvoxamine), valproate (e.g., divalproex sodium, valproic acid, valproate sodium), and topiramate, in some patients with treatment-refractory schizophrenia, inadequate response to antipsychotic therapy, or acute exacerbations of schizophrenia in both controlled and uncontrolled trials. Further controlled trials of olanzapine combined with these agents are necessary to more clearly determine the potential risks and benefits of such combined therapy.

Pediatric Considerations. Olanzapine is used orally for the management of schizophrenia in adolescents 13 to 17 years of age. Clinicians treating pediatric patients with schizophrenia should be aware that pediatric schizophrenia is a serious mental disorder; however, its diagnosis can be challenging. Symptom profiles in such patients can be variable. Therefore, it is recommended that drug therapy for pediatric schizophrenia be initiated only after a thorough diagnostic evaluation has been performed and careful consideration given to the risks associated with medication treatment. Medication treatment should only be part of a total treatment program that often includes psychological, educational, and social interventions.

When deciding among the alternative treatments available for adolescents with schizophrenia, clinicians should consider the increased potential for weight gain and dyslipidemia in adolescents treated with olanzapine (as compared with adults). Clinicians also should consider the potential long-term risks when prescribing olanzapine to adolescents; in many cases, this may lead them to consider prescribing other drugs first in adolescent patients. (See Cautions: Endocrine and Metabolic Effects, Cautions: Precautions and Contraindications, and see also Cautions: Pediatric Precautions.)

The short-term efficacy and tolerability of oral olanzapine in 107 adolescent inpatients and outpatients 13–17 years of age with schizophrenia were established in a randomized, double-blind, placebo-controlled, multicenter trial of 6 weeks' duration in which olanzapine was given in a flexible dosage range of 2.5–20 mg once daily. The principal rating instrument used for assessing psychiatric signs and symptoms in this trial was the Anchored Version of the BPRS for Children (BPRS-C) total score. Olanzapine (mean modal dosage: 12.5 mg daily; mean dosage: 11.1 mg daily) was found to be more effective than placebo in treating adolescents with schizophrenia, since the olanzapine-treated adolescents had a substantially greater mean reduction in the BPRS-C total score compared with those receiving placebo. However, weight gain and hyperprolactinemia occurred more often in patients receiving olanzapine compared with those receiving placebo.

Olanzapine has been successfully used orally for the management of childhood-onset schizophrenia in a limited number of children† and other adolescents. However, the manufacturers state that the safety and effectiveness of the drug in children younger than 13 years of age have not been established.

Although there is no body of evidence available to determine how long adolescent patients treated with oral olanzapine should be maintained on the drug, the manufacturer states that such efficacy can be extrapolated from adult data in addition to comparisons of olanzapine pharmacokinetic parameters in adult and adolescent patients. If olanzapine is used for an extended period, the continued need for maintenance therapy should be reassessed periodically.

Based on the observed efficacy and tolerability of atypical antipsychotics in adults and the available clinical experience in pediatric patients, the American Academy of Child and Adolescent Psychiatry (AACAP) currently states that the use of atypical antipsychotic agents in children and adolescents with schizophrenia is justified, and many clinicians consider atypical antipsychotic agents, with the exception of clozapine, among the drugs of first choice in the management of childhood-onset schizophrenia. However, well-controlled studies are necessary to more clearly establish the efficacy and safety of atypical antipsychotics in pediatric patients, particularly during long-term therapy. For additional information on the symptomatic management of childhood-onset schizophrenia, see Pediatric Considerations under Psychotic Disorders: Schizophrenia, in Uses in the Phenothiazines General Statement 28:16.08.24.

Acute Agitation. Short-acting olanzapine injection (e.g., Zyprexa® IntraMuscular) is used IM for the management of acute agitation in adult patients with schizophrenia for whom treatment with olanzapine is appropriate and who require an IM antipsychotic agent for rapid control of behaviors that interfere with diagnosis and care (e.g., threatening behaviors, escalating or urgently distressing behavior, self-exhausting behavior). According to DSM-IV, psychomotor agitation is excessive motor activity associated with a feeling of inner tension. The efficacy of IM olanzapine for the management of acute agitation in patients with schizophrenia was established in 2 short-term (single-day), placebo-controlled trials in hospital settings; an active comparator treatment arm using haloperidol injection was included in both studies. The patients in this study exhibited a level of agitation that met or exceeded a threshold score of 14 on the 5 items comprising the Positive and Negative Syndrome Scale (PANSS) Excited Component (i.e., poor impulse control, tension, hostility, uncooperativeness, and excitement items) with at least one individual item score of 4 ("moderate") or greater using a 1–7 scoring system, where scores of 1 or 7 indicate absent or extreme agitation, respectively. The primary measure used for assessing efficacy in managing agitation in these trials was the change from baseline in the PANSS Excited Component at 2 hours post-injection. Patients could receive up to 3 injections of IM olanzapine; however, patients could not receive the second injection until after the initial 2-hour period when the primary efficacy measure was assessed.

In the first placebo-controlled trial, short-acting IM olanzapine was given in fixed single doses of 2.5, 5, 7.5, or 10 mg in agitated hospitalized patients with schizophrenia. All 4 IM olanzapine doses were found to be statistically superior to placebo in reducing the PANSS Excited Component score at 2 hours following injection; however, the effect was larger and more consistent for the 3 highest doses studied. There were no significant differences in efficacy noted for the 7.5- and 10-mg doses compared with the 5-mg dose in this study. In the second placebo-controlled trial in agitated patients with schizophrenia, a fixed, 10-mg dose of short-acting IM olanzapine was evaluated and found to be superior to placebo on the PANSS Excited Component at 2 hours following injection. An analysis of these 2 controlled studies as well as an additional controlled study conducted in agitated patients with bipolar mania for possible age-, race-, or gender-related effects on treatment outcome did not suggest any difference in efficacy based on these patient characteristics.

■ Bipolar Disorder

Oral olanzapine is used alone in adults and adolescents 13–17 years of age or in conjunction with lithium or valproate in adults for the acute management of manic or mixed episodes associated with bipolar I disorder; the drug also is used orally for longer-term maintenance monotherapy in adults and adolescents 13–17 years of age with this disorder. In addition, oral olanzapine is used in combination with fluoxetine hydrochloride for the treatment of acute depressive episodes associated with bipolar I disorder in adults and pediatric patients 10–17 years of age. According to DSM-IV criteria, manic episodes are distinct periods lasting 1 week or longer (or less than 1 week if hospitalization is required) of abnormally and persistently elevated, expansive, or irritable mood accompanied by at least 3 (or 4 if the mood is only irritability) of the following 7 symptoms: grandiosity, reduced need for sleep, pressure of speech, flight of ideas, distractability, increased goal-directed activity (either socially, at work or school, or sexually) or psychomotor agitation, and engaging in high-risk behavior (e.g., unrestrained buying sprees, sexual indiscretions, foolish business investments).

For the initial management of less severe manic or mixed episodes in patients with bipolar disorder, current APA recommendations state that monotherapy with lithium, valproate (e.g., valproate sodium, valproic acid, divalproex), or an antipsychotic such as olanzapine may be adequate. For more severe manic or mixed episodes, combination therapy with an antipsychotic and lithium or valproate is recommended as first-line therapy. For further information on the management of bipolar disorder, see Uses: Bipolar Disorder, in Lithium Salts 28:28.

Acute Treatment of Manic or Mixed Episodes

Efficacy of oral olanzapine monotherapy in the acute treatment of manic or mixed episodes in adults has been demonstrated in 2 short-term (i.e., 3 or 4 weeks' duration), randomized, double-blind, placebo-controlled, parallel-group trials in patients who met DSM-IV criteria for bipolar I disorder (with or without a rapid-cycling course) and who met diagnostic criteria for an acute manic or mixed episode (with or without psychotic features). Olanzapine was given in an initial dosage of 10 mg once daily in the 3-week trial and 15 mg once daily in the 4-week trial; the dosage was subsequently adjusted within the range of 5–20 mg once daily in both of these trials. The principal rating instrument used for assessing manic symptoms in these trials was the Y-MRS score, an 11-item clinician-rated scale traditionally used to assess the degree of manic symptomatology (e.g., irritability, disruptive/aggressive behavior, sleep, elevated mood, speech, increased activity, sexual interest, language/thought disorder, thought content, appearance, insight) in a range from 0 (no manic features) to 60 (maximum score). All patients were hospitalized at the onset of these trials, but some patients were allowed to continue the studies on an outpatient basis after 1 week of hospitalization if their Clinical Global Impressions-Bipolar Version of severity of illness (CGI-BP) mania score was no greater than 3 (mild) and they had at least a 50% reduction in their Young Mania Rating Scale (Y-MRS) scores. In the 3- and 4-week placebo-controlled trials, approximately 49–65% of patients receiving 5–20 mg of olanzapine once daily achieved a 50% or greater improvement in Y-MRS total score from baseline compared with approximately 24–43% of those who received placebo. In addition, unlike therapy with typical antipsychotic agents, patients receiving olanzapine in these clinical studies did not experience a worsening in depressive symptoms (defined as an increase in the Hamilton Psychiatric Rating Scale for Depression-21 item [HAMD-21] score of at least 3 points) compared with those receiving placebo. In another 3-week, placebo-controlled trial that was designed identically to the first 3-week trial and was conducted simultaneously, olanzapine demonstrated a similar treatment difference in reduction of the Y-MRS total score but was not found to be superior to placebo on this outcome measure, possibly due to sample size and site variability.

Data from one limited comparative study suggest that oral olanzapine dosages of 10 mg daily may be as effective as lithium carbonate dosages of 400 mg twice daily in the treatment of manic episodes in adults with bipolar disorder. In a randomized, double-blind trial of 3 weeks' duration comparing olanzapine (5–20 mg daily) and divalproex sodium therapy in hospitalized adults with bipolar disorder experiencing acute manic or mixed episodes, olanzapine therapy was found to produce greater improvement in Y-MRS total scores, which was the primary efficacy measure in this trial. In addition, a substantially greater proportion of patients in the olanzapine group achieved remission compared with the divalproex group. In a randomized, double-blind study of 12 weeks' duration comparing olanzapine and divalproex sodium in patients with bipolar I disorder hospitalized for acute mania, the drugs were found to be equally effective although divalproex sodium was somewhat better tolerated than olanzapine.

Combined Therapy Efficacy of oral olanzapine when used in combination with lithium or valproate in the short-term treatment of acute manic or mixed episodes has been demonstrated in 2 randomized, double-blind, placebo-controlled studies of 6 weeks' duration in adult patients who met the DSM-IV criteria for bipolar I disorder (with or without a rapid-cycling course) and who met diagnostic criteria for an acute manic or mixed episode (with or without psychotic features). In these studies, patients with bipolar disorder experiencing manic or mixed episodes (Y-MRS scores of 16 or greater) who had not responded to at least 2 weeks of lithium or divalproex sodium monotherapy despite adequate plasma drug concentrations (in a therapeutic range of 0.6–1.2 mEq/L for lithium or 50–125 mcg/mL of valproate for divalproex sodium) were randomized to receive either olanzapine (initial dosage of 10 mg once daily; range: 5–20 mg once daily) or placebo, in combination with their original therapy. Addition of olanzapine to lithium or divalproex sodium was shown to be superior to continued monotherapy with lithium or divalproex sodium in the reduction of Y-MRS total score in both of these studies.

The manufacturer states that efficacy of adjunctive therapy with olanzapine for longer-term use (i.e., longer than 6 weeks) in patients with bipolar I disorder has not been systematically evaluated in controlled trials.

Maintenance Monotherapy of Bipolar Disorder Oral olanzapine is used for maintenance monotherapy in adults and adolescent patients 13–17 years of age with bipolar I disorder. The long-term efficacy of oral olanzapine as maintenance monotherapy in adults with bipolar disorder has been demonstrated in a double-blind, placebo-controlled trial and in double-blind comparative trials. In the placebo-controlled study, adult patients who met DSM-IV criteria for bipolar I disorder and experienced manic or mixed episodes and who had responded during an initial open-label treatment phase to oral olanzapine therapy (5–20 mg daily) for an average of about 2 weeks were randomized either to continue olanzapine at the same dosage or to receive placebo for up to 48 weeks and were observed for relapse. Response during the open-label phase was defined as a reduction in the Y-MRS total score of 12 or more and in the 21-item Hamilton Depression Rating Scale (HAM-D 21) of 8 or more; relapse during the double-blind phase of the study was defined as an increase in the Y-MRS or HAM-D 21 total score to 15 or more or being hospitalized for either mania or depression. Approximately 50% of the patients in the olanzapine group had discontinued therapy by day 59, and approximately 50% of the patients in the placebo group had discontinued placebo by day 23 of the double-blind phase. A longer time until relapse was observed in the patients receiving olanzapine compared with those receiving placebo (median of 174 and 22 days, respectively, for relapse into any mood episode) during the randomized phase of this study. The relapse rate also was significantly lower in the olanzapine group (approximately 47%) than in the placebo group (approximately 80%). If olanzapine is used for extended periods, the need for continued therapy should be reassessed periodically.

In a double-blind, 52-week trial comparing olanzapine and lithium maintenance therapy in adults with bipolar disorder, olanzapine was found to be significantly more effective than lithium in preventing relapses and recurrences of manic and mixed episodes following initial stabilization with combined olanzapine and lithium therapy. Olanzapine and lithium demonstrated comparable efficacy in preventing relapses and recurrences of depression in this study. In a retrospective analysis from this trial, patients were subcategorized into illness stage (early, intermediate, or later) based on the number of prior manic or mixed episodes they had experienced. The rates of relapse or recurrence of manic or mixed episodes were approximately 2 and 26%, 13 and 24%, and 24 and 33% for olanzapine and lithium in the early, intermediate, and later stage groups of bipolar patients, respectively; no substantial treatment effect for treatment or illness stage for depressive relapse or recurrence was observed. Because olanzapine was associated with a lower rate of relapse or recurrence of manic and mixed episodes in early-stage patients, it was suggested that the drug may be particularly effective early in the course of bipolar disorder.

In a double-blind, 47-week trial comparing monotherapy with olanzapine or divalproex sodium in adults with bipolar disorder experiencing manic or mixed episodes, mean improvement in Y-MRS scores was greater for olanzapine-treated patients. In addition, the median time to symptomatic mania remission was shorter for patients receiving olanzapine compared with those receiving divalproex sodium (14 days vs. 62 days, respectively). However, no significant differences in the rates of symptomatic mania remission and symptomatic relapse into mania or depression between the olanzapine- and divalproex-treated patients were observed in this study. In a double-blind, 18-month, relapse prevention trial comparing the efficacy of combined olanzapine plus lithium or valproate therapy with lithium or valproate therapy alone in patients with bipolar disorder, more sustained symptomatic remission (163 days vs 42 days, respectively) occurred in the group receiving combined olanzapine plus lithium or valproate therapy than in the group receiving lithium or valproate therapy alone.

Rapid-Cycling Bipolar Disorder In an analysis of pooled data from several trials comparing the clinical response to olanzapine therapy in rapid-cycling and non-rapid-cycling adult patients with bipolar disorder, relative clinical response to olanzapine was found to be similar in the 2 groups, although earlier responses were observed in the rapid-cycling group of patients, and long-term outcomes were more favorable in the non-rapid-cycling group. Rapid-cycling patients were found to be less likely to achieve an initial symptomatic remission, more likely to experience recurrences, especially of depression, and had more hospitalizations and suicide attempts than non-rapid-cycling patients in this study.

Depressive Episodes Associated with Bipolar Disorder Oral olanzapine is used in combination with fluoxetine for the treatment of acute depressive episodes associated with bipolar I disorder in adults and pediatric patients 10–17 years of age. In 2 randomized, double-blind studies of 8 weeks' duration comparing a fixed combination of olanzapine and fluoxetine hydrochloride (Symbyax®) with olanzapine monotherapy and placebo in adults, the fixed combination (given in flexible daily dosages of 6 mg olanzapine with 25 or 50 mg of fluoxetine or 12 mg of olanzapine with 50 mg of fluoxetine) was more effective than olanzapine monotherapy (5–20 mg daily) or placebo in improvement in depressive symptoms as assessed by the Montgomery-Asberg Depression Rating Scale (MADRS). Although the manufacturer states that efficacy beyond 8 weeks' duration remains to be established, patients have received the fixed combination for up to 24 weeks in clinical trials. Clinicians who elect to extend therapy beyond 8 weeks should reevaluate the risks and benefits of continued therapy periodically.

The manufacturers state that olanzapine monotherapy is not indicated for the treatment of depressive episodes associated with bipolar I disorder.

Pediatric Considerations Oral olanzapine is used as monotherapy in adolescents 13–17 years of age for the acute management of manic or mixed episodes associated with bipolar I disorder; the drug also is used orally for longer-term maintenance monotherapy in patients with this disorder. Oral olanzapine in combination with fluoxetine is used for the treatment of acute depressive episodes associated with bipolar I disorder in pediatric patients 10–17 years of age. When treating pediatric patients with bipolar I disorder, clinicians should be aware that pediatric bipolar I disorder is a serious mental disorder; however, its diagnosis can be challenging. Pediatric patients with bipolar disorder may have variable patterns of periodicity of manic or mixed symptoms. Therefore, it is recommended that drug therapy for pediatric bipolar disorder be initiated only after a thorough diagnostic evaluation has been performed and careful consideration given to the risks associated with medication treatment. Medication treatment should only be part of a total treatment program that often includes psychological, educational, and social interventions.

When deciding among the alternative treatments available for adolescents with bipolar disorder, clinicians should consider the increased potential for weight gain and dyslipidemia in adolescents receiving olanzapine (as compared with adults). Clinicians also should consider the potential long-term risks when prescribing olanzapine to adolescents; in many cases, this may lead them to consider prescribing other drugs first in adolescent patients. (See Cautions: Endocrine and Metabolic Effects, Cautions: Precautions and Contraindications, and see also Cautions: Pediatric Precautions.)

The short-term efficacy of oral olanzapine monotherapy in the acute treatment of bipolar I disorder in adolescents 13–17 years of age was established in a randomized, multicenter, double-blind, placebo-controlled trial of 3 weeks' duration in 161 patients who met DSM-IV-TR criteria for manic or mixed episodes associated with bipolar I disorder (with or without psychotic features). In this flexible-dosage trial, outpatients and inpatients were randomized to receive either olanzapine 2.5–20 mg daily (mean modal dosage of 10.7 mg daily; mean dosage of 8.9 mg daily) or placebo. Olanzapine was found to be more effective than placebo as demonstrated by substantially greater reduction in the total score on the Adolescent Structured Y-MRS, which was the primary efficacy measure in this study. However, the olanzapine-treated adolescents had substantially greater weight gain and elevations in serum transaminases, prolactin, fasting glucose, fasting total cholesterol, and uric acid compared with those receiving placebo.

The efficacy and safety of oral olanzapine in combination with fluoxetine hydrochloride for the acute treatment of depressive episodes associated with bipolar I disorder in pediatric patients 10–17 years of age were established in a randomized, double-blind, placebo-controlled trial of 8 weeks' duration in 255 patients who met the DSM-IV-TR criteria for bipolar I disorder, depressed episode. Patients randomized to receive olanzapine and fluoxetine were initially given 3 mg of olanzapine with 25 mg of fluoxetine and force-titrated to the maximum dosage of 12 mg of olanzapine with 50 mg of fluoxetine over 2 weeks; after 2 weeks, patients received flexible dosages of olanzapine 6–12 mg with fluoxetine 25–50 mg daily. At week 8, olanzapine in combination with fluoxetine was found to be substantially more effective than placebo in reducing the Children's Depression Rating Scale-Revised (CDRS-R) total score, which was the primary efficacy measure in this study. The average daily dosage was 7.7 mg of olanzapine and 37.6 mg of fluoxetine. The pediatric patients who received olanzapine in combination with fluoxetine had substantially greater weight gain and elevations in serum transaminases, serum lipids, and prolactin compared with those receiving placebo. The recommended initial dosage of the olanzapine/fluoxetine combination is lower in children and adolescents than in adults. In addition, the manufacturer states that flexible dosing is recommended in such patients instead of the forced-titration dosing initially used in this study. (See Bipolar Disorder under Dosage: Oral Dosage, in Dosage and Administration.)

Although there is no body of evidence available to determine how long adolescent patients with bipolar disorder treated with olanzapine should be maintained on the drug, the manufacturer states that such efficacy can be extrapolated from adult data in addition to comparisons of olanzapine pharmacokinetic parameters in adult and adolescent patients. If olanzapine is used for an extended period, the continued need for maintenance therapy should be reassessed periodically.

Based on the observed efficacy and tolerability of mood stabilizers and atypical antipsychotic agents in clinical trials in adults and the available clinical experience in pediatric patients, the American Academy of Child and Adolescent Psychiatry (AACAP) currently states that mood stabilizers (e.g., lithium, valproic acid, carbamazepine) and atypical antipsychotics (e.g., olanzapine, aripiprazole, risperidone, quetiapine, ziprasidone) are among drugs of first choice in the acute management of pediatric patients with bipolar I disorder experiencing manic or mixed episodes with or without psychosis. Additional controlled studies are necessary to more clearly establish the efficacy and safety of atypical antipsychotics in pediatric patients with bipolar disorder, particularly during long-term therapy.

Acute Agitation Short-acting olanzapine injection (e.g., Zyprexa® IntraMuscular) is used IM for the management of acute agitation in patients with bipolar I disorder for whom treatment with olanzapine is appropriate and who require an IM antipsychotic agent for rapid control of behaviors that interfere with their diagnosis and care (e.g., threatening behaviors, escalating or urgently distressing behavior, self-exhausting behavior). According to DSM-IV, psychomotor agitation is excessive motor activity associated with a feeling of inner tension.

The efficacy of short-acting IM olanzapine for the management of acute agitation in adults with bipolar mania was established in a short-term (single-day), double-blind, placebo-controlled trial in agitated, hospitalized patients who met the DSM-IV criteria for bipolar I disorder and who displayed an acute manic or mixed episode with or without psychotic features. The patients in this study exhibited a level of agitation that met or exceeded a threshold score of 14 on the 5 items comprising the Positive and Negative Syndrome Scale (PANSS) Excited Component (i.e., poor impulse control, tension, hostility, uncooperativeness, and excitement items) with at least one individual item score of 4 ("moderate") or greater using a 1–7 scoring system where scores of 1 or 7 indicate absent or extreme agitation, respectively. An active comparator treatment arm using IM lorazepam was included in this study. The primary measure used for assessing efficacy in managing agitation in this trial was the change from baseline in the PANSS Excited Component at 2 hours post-injection of a fixed, 10-mg IM dose of olanzapine. Patients in this study could receive up to 3 injections of IM olanzapine; however, patients could not receive the second injection until after the initial 2-hour period when the efficacy was assessed. IM olanzapine was found to be statistically superior to placebo in reducing the PANSS Excited Component score at 2 hours and at 24 hours following the initial injection. An analysis of this study as well as 2 additional controlled studies conducted in agitated patients with schizophrenia for possible age-, race-, or gender-related effects on treatment outcome did not suggest any difference in efficacy based on these patient characteristics.

■ **Treatment-resistant Depression** Oral olanzapine is used in combination with fluoxetine hydrochloride for the acute and maintenance therapy of treatment-resistant depression (i.e., major depressive disorder in patients who do not respond to 2 separate trials of different antidepressants of adequate dosage and duration in the current episode).

The efficacy and safety of oral olanzapine in combination with fluoxetine for the acute treatment of treatment-resistant depression were demonstrated in 3 clinical studies conducted in 579 adults 18–85 years of age. Daily dosages evaluated in these studies ranged from 6–18 mg of olanzapine and 25–50 mg of fluoxetine. In the first study, efficacy of the fixed combination of olanzapine and fluoxetine (Symbyax®) was evaluated in 300 patients who met DSM-IV criteria for major depressive disorder and did not respond to 2 different antidepressants after at least 6 weeks at or above the minimally effective labeled dosage in their current episode. Patients enrolled in this study entered an open-label fluoxetine lead-in phase in which the nonresponders were randomized to receive the fixed combination of olanzapine and fluoxetine, olanzapine alone, or fluoxetine alone for 8 weeks. The fixed combination of olanzapine and fluoxetine was flexibly dosed between 6–18 mg of olanzapine daily; all patients received 50 mg of fluoxetine daily. A substantially greater reduction in mean total MADRS scores from baseline to end point was observed in patients receiving olanzapine in fixed combination with fluoxetine compared with those receiving either fluoxetine or olanzapine alone. A second, smaller study with the same treatment-resistant depressed patient population also demonstrated a substantially greater reduction in MADRS scores in patients treated with the fixed combination compared with patients receiving fluoxetine or olanzapine monotherapy (when analyzed with change in MADRS score as the outcome measure). A third study demonstrated a substantially greater reduction in total MADRS scores in patients receiving the fixed combination of olanzapine and fluoxetine compared with those treated with fluoxetine or olanzapine alone, when data were analyzed in a subpopulation of 251 depressed patients who met the definition of treatment resistance (patients who had not responded to 2 antidepressants of adequate dosage and duration in the current episode).

The efficacy of oral olanzapine in combination with fluoxetine in the maintenance therapy of treatment-resistant depression was demonstrated in a 47-week study in 892 adults (18–65 years of age) who met DSM-IV criteria for major depressive disorder and did not respond to 2 different antidepressants after at least 6 weeks at or above the minimally effective labeled dosage in their current episode. Daily dosages evaluated in these studies ranged from 6–18 mg of olanzapine and 25–50 mg of fluoxetine. Patients were initially treated with open-label olanzapine and fluoxetine in fixed combination (Symbyax®). Patients who responded to and were stabilized on the fixed combination over approximately 20 weeks were randomized to continue receiving fixed-combination olanzapine and fluoxetine treatment or to receive fluoxetine alone for another 27 weeks. A total of 15.8% of patients receiving olanzapine and fluoxetine in fixed combination relapsed compared with 31.8% of patients receiving fluoxetine monotherapy; this difference was statistically significant. In addition, patients who continued to receive olanzapine and fluoxetine in fixed combination experienced a substantially longer time to relapse over the 27-week period compared with those receiving fluoxetine alone. If combined olanzapine and fluoxetine therapy is used for an extended period, the continued need for maintenance therapy should be reassessed periodically.

The manufacturer states that olanzapine monotherapy is not indicated for the treatment of treatment-resistant depression.

■ **Cancer Chemotherapy-induced Nausea and Vomiting** Olanzapine has been used orally in combination with other antiemetic agents for the prevention of acute and delayed nausea and vomiting associated with highly emetogenic cancer chemotherapy†, including high-dose cisplatin therapy. The drug also has been used as rescue therapy in patients with breakthrough cancer chemotherapy-induced nausea and vomiting†.

To prevent chemotherapy-induced nausea and vomiting associated with chemotherapy regimens with a high emetic risk (i.e., incidence of emesis exceeds 90% if no antiemetics are administered) in adults, the American Society of Clinical Oncology (ASCO) currently recommends a 4-drug antiemetic regimen consisting of a neurokinin 1 (NK_1) receptor antagonist (e.g., aprepitant, fosaprepitant, netupitant [in fixed combination with palonosetron], rolapitant), a type 3 serotonin ($5\text{-}HT_3$) receptor antagonist (e.g., dolasetron, granisetron, ondansetron, palonosetron, ramosetron [not commercially available in the US], tropisetron [not commercially available in the US]), dexamethasone, and olanzapine. If the fixed combination of netupitant and palonosetron is used as an NK_1 receptor antagonist, use of an additional $5\text{-}HT_3$ receptor antagonist is not necessary. For adults receiving carboplatin with a target area under the plasma concentration-time curve (AUC) of 4 mg/mL per minute or more, ASCO recommends a 3-drug antiemetic regimen consisting of an NK_1 receptor antagonist, a $5\text{-}HT_3$ receptor antagonist, and dexamethasone. For adults receiving other chemotherapy of moderate emetic risk (i.e., incidence of emesis without antiemetics exceeds 30% but does not exceed 90%), excluding carboplatin with a target AUC of 4 mg/mL per minute or more, ASCO recommends a 2-drug antiemetic regimen consisting of a $5\text{-}HT_3$ receptor antagonist and dexamethasone. Because of the limited clinical experience with oral olanzapine in adults receiving moderately emetogenic chemotherapy, ASCO states that olanzapine is not recommended for routine prophylaxis in such patients. For adults receiving chemotherapy regimens with a low emetic risk (i.e., incidence of emesis without antiemetics exceeds 10% but does not exceed 30%), ASCO recommends a single dose of either a $5\text{-}HT_3$ receptor antagonist or dexamethasone alone on the first day of chemotherapy. Routine antiemetic prophylaxis is not necessary in adults receiving chemotherapy with a minimal antiemetic risk (i.e., incidence of emesis is less than 10% without antiemetics).

For patients with breakthrough chemotherapy-induced nausea or vomiting, ASCO recommends that clinicians reevaluate emetic risk, disease status, concomitant medical conditions, and concurrent medications and determine whether the best antiemetic regimen is being provided for the emetic risk. Adults who experience nausea and vomiting despite optimal antiemetic prophylaxis and who have not received olanzapine prophylactically should be offered olanzapine in addition to continuing the standard antiemetic regimen. Adults who experience nausea or vomiting despite optimal antiemetic prophylaxis and who have already received olanzapine may be offered a drug from a different class such as an NK_1 receptor antagonist, lorazepam or alprazolam, a dopamine receptor antagonist (e.g., metoclopramide), dronabinol, or nabilone in addition to continuing the standard antiemetic regimen.

Clinical Experience Efficacy of oral olanzapine for the prevention of nausea and vomiting associated with cancer chemotherapy was established in a randomized, double-blind, phase 3 study comparing olanzapine with placebo, in combination with an NK_1 receptor antagonist (either IV fosaprepitant or oral aprepitant), a 5-HT_3 receptor antagonist (e.g., oral or IV granisetron, oral or IV ondansetron, IV palonosetron), and oral dexamethasone, in 380 adults receiving highly emetogenic chemotherapy (cisplatin-containing regimens or anthracycline plus cyclophosphamide). Patients received olanzapine 10 mg or matching placebo orally once daily on days 1 through 4. The proportion of patients who experienced no chemotherapy-induced nausea was substantially higher with olanzapine than with placebo during the early assessment period (0–24 hours after chemotherapy; 74 versus 45%, respectively), the later assessment period (25–120 hours after chemotherapy; 42 versus 25%, respectively), and the overall period (0–120 hours after chemotherapy; 37 versus 22%, respectively). The proportion of patients with a complete response (no emetic episodes and no use of rescue medication) was also substantially higher in patients receiving olanzapine than in those receiving placebo in all 3 assessment periods (86 versus 65%, 67 versus 52%, and 64 versus 41% during the early, later, and overall assessment periods, respectively). Olanzapine was generally well tolerated and no serious adverse reactions to the drug were reported in this study; however, olanzapine-treated patients experienced more drowsiness on day 2 following chemotherapy than at baseline. The sedation generally resolved on days 3, 4, and 5 despite continued administration of olanzapine on days 3 and 4.

Efficacy of antiemetic prophylactic regimens including oral olanzapine and antiemetic regimens not including olanzapine was compared in a meta-analysis of 10 randomized controlled trials in patients receiving either highly or moderately emetogenic chemotherapy. Six of these studies included patients receiving only highly emetogenic chemotherapy and 4 studies included patients receiving either highly emetogenic or moderately emetogenic chemotherapy. Antiemetic regimens containing olanzapine were found to be statistically superior in 5 of 6 end points and clinically superior in 4 of 6 end points compared with antiemetic regimens not containing olanzapine in this meta-analysis.

In a randomized, multicenter, double-blind, phase 2, dose-finding study, efficacy and safety of 2 olanzapine dosage regimens (5 mg or 10 mg orally once daily on days 1 through 4) used in combination with standard antiemetic prophylaxis (e.g., aprepitant or fosaprepitant, palonosetron, and dexamethasone) for the prevention of nausea and vomiting associated with cancer chemotherapy were compared in 153 adults with malignant solid tumors who were receiving highly emetogenic chemotherapy with cisplatin. The primary end point in this study was complete response (no emesis and no use of rescue medications) in the delayed phase (24–120 hours after the start of cisplatin therapy). Both dosages of olanzapine produced a significant improvement in delayed emesis; complete response rates in the delayed phase were 85.7 and 77.6% in the 5- and 10-mg olanzapine dosage groups, respectively. Somnolence was the most commonly reported adverse effect in this study and occurred in 45.5 and 53.3% of patients in the 5- and 10-mg olanzapine dosage groups, respectively.

Olanzapine has been shown to be an effective rescue antiemetic in patients who develop breakthrough chemotherapy-induced nausea and vomiting despite having received optimal antiemetic prophylaxis. In a randomized, double-blind, phase 3 study, efficacy and safety of orally administered olanzapine and metoclopramide for the treatment of breakthrough chemotherapy-induced nausea and vomiting were compared in chemotherapy-naive adults receiving highly emetogenic chemotherapy (cisplatin or doxorubicin and cyclophosphamide) who did not receive antiemetic prophylaxis with olanzapine. All patients had initially received guideline-directed antiemetic prophylaxis with fosaprepitant, palonosetron, and dexamethasone. Of 276 enrolled patients, 112 developed breakthrough nausea and vomiting and were randomized to receive olanzapine (10 mg orally once daily for 3 days) or metoclopramide (10 mg orally 3 times daily for 3 days); 108 of these patients were evaluable. Patients were monitored for emesis and nausea for 72 hours after receiving olanzapine or metoclopramide. During the 72-hour observation period after the breakthrough nausea and vomiting occurred, 70% of the olanzapine-treated patients had no emesis compared with 31% of the metoclopramide-treated patients and 68% of the olanzapine-treated patients had no nausea compared with 23% of the metoclopramide-treated patients. Olanzapine was found to be significantly better than metoclopramide in controlling breakthrough nausea and vomiting in patients receiving highly emetogenic chemotherapy. No grade 3 or 4 toxicities occurred with either olanzapine or metoclopramide.

Dosage and Administration

■ **Reconstitution and Administration** Olanzapine is administered orally or by IM injection. Olanzapine pamoate is administered only by IM injection.

Restricted Distribution Because of the risk of post-injection delirium/sedation syndrome (PDSS), extended-release olanzapine pamoate injection is available only under a restricted distribution program, the Zyprexa® Relprevv Patient Care Program. Zyprexa® Relprevv must not be dispensed directly to a patient. For a patient to receive treatment, the prescriber, healthcare facility, patient, and pharmacy must all be enrolled in the Patient Care Program. Clinicians may contact 877-772-9390 for additional information and to enroll in the Zyprexa® Relprevv Patient Care Program or consult the manufacturer's website (https://www.zyprexarelprevvprogram.com).

Oral Administration Olanzapine conventional tablets, orally disintegrating tablets, and capsules (in fixed combination with fluoxetine hydrochloride) are administered orally. Since food does not appear to affect GI absorption of olanzapine, the drug generally can be administered as conventional tablets or orally disintegrating tablets without regard to meals. In patients who experience persistent or troublesome daytime sedation during oral olanzapine therapy for psychiatric indications (e.g., psychotic disorders, bipolar disorder, treatment-resistant depression), administration of the daily dosage in the evening at bedtime may be helpful.

Patients receiving olanzapine orally disintegrating tablets should be instructed not to remove a tablet from the blister until just prior to dosing. The tablet should not be pushed through the foil. With dry hands, the blister backing should be peeled completely off the blister. The tablet should then be gently removed and immediately placed on the tongue, where it rapidly disintegrates in saliva, and then subsequently swallowed with or without liquid.

The fixed combination capsules of olanzapine with fluoxetine hydrochloride (e.g., Symbyax®) are administered once daily in the evening. Although the manufacturer states that food has no appreciable effect on absorption of either drug when administered alone, absorption of the drugs when administered as the fixed combination with food has not been studied.

Dispensing and Administration Precautions Because of similarities in spelling, dosage intervals (once daily), and tablet strengths (5 and 10 mg) of Zyprexa® (olanzapine) and Zyrtec® (cetirizine hydrochloride, an antihistamine), extra care should be exercised in ensuring the accuracy of prescriptions for these drugs. (See Cautions: Precautions and Contraindications.)

IM Administration *Clinicians should be aware that there are 2 IM formulations of olanzapine with different indications and dosing schedules; the short-acting, immediate-release formulation (e.g., Zyprexa IntraMuscular®; 10 mg per vial) is used for agitation associated with schizophrenia and bipolar mania and should not be confused with Zyprexa® Relprevv, a long-acting formulation (available in 210-, 300-, and 405-mg vial strengths) used for the treatment of schizophrenia.*

Short-acting Olanzapine Injection for Acute Agitation associated with Bipolar Disorder or Schizophrenia Commercially available short-acting olanzapine for injection (e.g., Zyprexa® IntraMuscular) must be reconstituted prior to administration by adding 2.1 mL of sterile water for injection to single-dose vials labeled as containing 10 mg of olanzapine to provide a solution containing approximately 5 mg/mL. Other solutions should not be used to reconstitute olanzapine for injection.

Following reconstitution, olanzapine for injection should be used immediately (within 1 hour). If necessary, the reconstituted solution may be stored for up to 1 hour at 20–25°C; after 1 hour, any unused portion should be discarded. Olanzapine for injection should be inspected visually for particulate matter and discoloration prior to administration whenever solution and container permit.

Olanzapine for injection is administered only by IM injection and should *not* be administered IV or subcutaneously. The drug should be injected slowly, deep into the muscle mass.

Extended-release Olanzapine Pamoate Injection for Schizophrenia The manufacturer states that tolerability with oral olanzapine therapy should be established prior to initiating IM therapy with extended-release olanzapine pamoate (Zyprexa® Relprevv).

Because of the risk of post-injection delirium/sedation syndrome (PDSS), Zyprexa® Relprevv must be administered in a registered healthcare facility (e.g., hospital, clinic, residential treatment center, community healthcare center) with ready access to emergency response services. The medication guide should be provided to the patient or legal guardian prior to each injection. After each injection, patients should be continuously monitored at the healthcare facility for at least 3 hours by a healthcare professional. Patients should be alert, oriented, and absent of any signs and symptoms of PDSS prior to being released. All patients receiving an IM injection of olanzapine pamoate must be accompanied to their destination upon leaving the facility.

Patients should not drive or operate heavy machinery for the remainder of the day following the injection. Patients should be advised to be vigilant for the symptoms of PDSS and to obtain medical assistance if needed. Close medical supervision and monitoring should be instituted in a facility capable of resuscitation if PDSS is suspected in any patient. (See Post-injection Delirium/Sedation Syndrome under Cautions: Nervous System Effects and also under Cautions: Precautions and Contraindications and see also Acute Toxicity.)

Extended-release olanzapine pamoate injection is administered only by deep IM injection into the gluteal area and should *not* be administered IV or subcutaneously. The injection should be administered by a healthcare professional every 2–4 weeks.

Olanzapine pamoate is commercially available as the Zyprexa® Relprevv Convenience Kit, which contains 2 single-use vials, needles, and a syringe; one of the vials contains olanzapine pamoate powder for suspension and the other vial contains diluent. Olanzapine pamoate powder for suspension must be reconstituted using only the diluent provided in the convenience kit prior to IM administration; other diluents should not be substituted. Reconstitution and administration instructions included in the kit should be closely followed, and the suspension should be administered within 24 hours of mixing. Reconstituted olanzapine pamoate suspension remains stable for up to 24 hours in the vial. However, if the suspension is not used immediately, the vial should be shaken vigorously to resuspend the drug.

The manufacturer recommends that gloves are used while reconstituting olanzapine pamoate powder for suspension since it may be irritating to the skin. If contact is made with skin, the affected area should be flushed with water.

Following insertion of the needle into the gluteal muscle for the IM injection, the healthcare professional should aspirate for several seconds to ensure that no blood is drawn into the syringe. If blood appears in the syringe, the dose should not be injected; the needle should be withdrawn and the syringe and dose discarded. A new convenience kit should be used for the new dose of olanzapine pamoate with a new syringe and needle. Following IM administration, the injection site should not be massaged.

■ Dosage

Olanzapine is commercially available as the base and as the pamoate salt; the dosage of olanzapine pamoate is expressed in terms of olanzapine.

Conventional olanzapine tablets and orally disintegrating tablets of the drug are bioequivalent. However, IM administration of a 5-mg dose of the commercially available short-acting olanzapine injection results in a maximum plasma olanzapine concentration that is about fivefold higher than that resulting from a 5-mg oral dose of the drug.

Dosage of olanzapine for psychiatric indications (e.g., psychotic disorders, bipolar disorder, treatment-resistant depression) must be adjusted carefully according to individual requirements and response, using the lowest possible effective dosage.

Oral Dosage

Schizophrenia. For the management of schizophrenia in adults, the recommended initial oral dosage of olanzapine is 5–10 mg daily, usually given as a single daily dose. Dosage may be increased by 5 mg daily within several days, to a target dosage of 10 mg daily. Because steady-state plasma concentrations of olanzapine may not be attained for approximately 7 days at a given dosage, subsequent dosage adjustments generally should be made at intervals of not less than 7 days, usually in increments or decrements of 5 mg once daily.

An initial adult olanzapine oral dosage of 5 mg daily is recommended in debilitated patients, in those predisposed to hypotension, in those who may be particularly sensitive to the effects of olanzapine, or in those who might metabolize olanzapine slowly (e.g., nonsmoking female patients who are 65 years of age or older). The manufacturers state that the presence of factors that might decrease the clearance or increase the pharmacodynamic response to olanzapine should lead to consideration of a lower initial dosage in all geriatric patients.

While a relationship between dosage and antipsychotic effect has not been established, the effective oral dosage of olanzapine in clinical studies in adults generally ranged from 10–15 mg daily. The manufacturers state that increasing olanzapine dosages beyond 10 mg daily usually does not result in additional therapeutic effect and recommend that such increases generally should occur only after the patient's clinical status has been assessed. In addition, the manufacturers state that olanzapine is not indicated for use in dosages exceeding 20 mg daily. However, olanzapine occasionally has been used in controlled and uncontrolled trials and in individual patients in dosages of up to 40 mg daily; dosages of up to 60 mg daily have been used in some patients with treatment-resistant schizophrenia. It remains to be established whether higher dosages of the drug are safe and result in improved efficacy in such patients. Some clinicians state that olanzapine dosages of up to 30 mg daily may produce further clinical improvement in schizophrenia patients who did not respond adequately to dosages of up to 20 mg daily; however, they recommend that caution be exercised when dosage of the drug exceeds 40 mg daily because of the potential for serious adverse effects (e.g., extrapyramidal reactions, excitement, metabolic changes, weight gain, cardiovascular complications).

For the management of schizophrenia in adolescents 13–17 years of age, the recommended initial oral dosage of olanzapine is 2.5 or 5 mg daily given as a single daily dose, and the recommended target dosage is 10 mg daily. When dosage adjustments are necessary, dosage increments or decrements of 2.5 or 5 mg daily are recommended. In clinical trials, efficacy of the drug in adolescents with schizophrenia was demonstrated based on a flexible dosage range of 2.5–20 mg daily, with a mean modal dosage of 12.5 mg daily (mean dosage of 11.1 mg daily). The manufacturer states that the safety and effectiveness of dosages exceeding 20 mg daily have not been evaluated in clinical trials.

The optimum duration of olanzapine therapy currently is not known, but maintenance therapy with antipsychotic agents is well established. The effectiveness of oral olanzapine given in a daily dosage of 10–20 mg in maintaining treatment response in adult schizophrenic patients who had been stable on olanzapine for approximately 8 weeks and were then followed for relapse has been demonstrated in a placebo-controlled study. If olanzapine is used for an extended period in adults, the long-term usefulness of the drug for the individual patient should be reassessed periodically.

Although there is no body of evidence available to determine how long adolescent patients treated with olanzapine should be maintained on the drug, the manufacturer states that such efficacy can be extrapolated from adult data in addition to comparisons of olanzapine pharmacokinetic parameters in adult and adolescent patients. Adolescent patients responding to olanzapine therapy should continue to receive the drug beyond the acute response, but at the lowest effective dosage, and the need for continued maintenance therapy with the drug should be reassessed periodically.

The American Psychiatric Association (APA) states that prudent long-term treatment options in adult patients with schizophrenia with remitted first episodes or multiple episodes include either indefinite maintenance therapy or gradual discontinuance of the antipsychotic agent with close follow-up and a plan to reinstitute treatment upon symptom recurrence. Discontinuance of antipsychotic therapy should be considered only after a period of at least 1 year of symptom remission or optimal response while receiving the antipsychotic agent. In patients who have had multiple previous psychotic episodes or 2 psychotic episodes within 5 years, indefinite maintenance antipsychotic treatment is recommended.

Bipolar Disorder. As monotherapy for the management of acute manic or mixed episodes associated with bipolar I disorder in adults, the usual initial oral dosage of olanzapine is 10 or 15 mg daily, given as a single dose. When dosage adjustments are necessary, the manufacturer recommends that dosage increments or decrements of 5 mg daily be made at intervals of not less than 24 hours, reflecting the procedures in the placebo-controlled trials. The effective dosage of olanzapine in short-term clinical studies generally has ranged from 5–20 mg daily. Safety of dosages exceeding 20 mg daily has not been established.

As monotherapy for the management of acute manic or mixed episodes associated with bipolar I disorder in adolescents 13–17 years of age, the recommended initial oral dosage of olanzapine is 2.5 or 5 mg daily, given as a single dose, with a target dosage of 10 mg daily. When dosage adjustments are necessary, the manufacturer recommends dosage increments or decrements of 2.5 or 5 mg daily. In short-term clinical trials, efficacy was demonstrated in a dosage range of 2.5–20 mg daily, with a mean modal dosage of 10.7 mg daily (average dosage of 8.9 mg daily). The manufacturer states that the safety and effectiveness of dosages exceeding 20 mg daily have not been evaluated in clinical trials.

When administered in conjunction with lithium or valproate for the management of acute manic or mixed episodes associated with bipolar I disorder in adults, the recommended initial oral dosage of olanzapine is 10 mg once daily. The effective dosage of olanzapine as adjunctive therapy for up to 6 weeks in clinical studies generally ranged from 5–20 mg daily. Safety of dosages exceeding 20 mg daily has not been established in clinical trials.

When used in fixed combination with fluoxetine hydrochloride (e.g., as the fixed combination Symbyax®) for acute depressive episodes in adults with bipolar disorder, olanzapine is administered once daily in the evening, usually initiating therapy with a dosage of 6 mg of olanzapine and 25 mg of fluoxetine. An initial dosage of 3 or 6 mg of olanzapine in fixed combination with 25 mg of fluoxetine should be used in patients with a predisposition to hypotensive reactions, patients with hepatic impairment, or those with factors that may slow metabolism of the drugs(s) (e.g., female gender, geriatric age, nonsmoking status); when indicated, dosage should be escalated with caution. In other patients, dosage can be increased according to patient response and tolerance as indicated. In clinical trials in adults, antidepressant efficacy was demonstrated at olanzapine dosages ranging from 6–12 mg daily and fluoxetine dosages ranging from 25–50 mg daily. Dosages exceeding 18 mg of olanzapine and 75 mg of fluoxetine daily have not been evaluated in clinical studies.

When used in conjunction with fluoxetine (as individual components of olanzapine and fluoxetine hydrochloride rather than the fixed-combination preparation) for acute depressive episodes in adults with bipolar disorder, olanzapine is administered once daily in the evening, usually initiating therapy with a dosage of 5 mg of olanzapine and 20 mg of fluoxetine. Dosage adjustments, if indicated, may be made based on efficacy and tolerability within the dosage ranges of olanzapine 5–12.5 mg daily and fluoxetine 20–50 mg daily. An initial dosage of 2.5–5 mg of olanzapine and 20 mg of fluoxetine should be used in patients with a predisposition to hypotensive reactions, patients with hepatic impairment, those with factors that may slow metabolism of the drugs(s) (e.g., female gender, geriatric age, nonsmoking status), or those who may be pharmacodynamically sensitive to olanzapine; when indicated, dosage adjustments should be made with caution in these patients. Dosages exceeding 18 mg of olanzapine and 75 mg of fluoxetine daily have not been evaluated in clinical studies.

The safety and efficacy of olanzapine and fluoxetine in combination (given as the individual components) were determined in clinical trials that supported the approval of Symbyax® (the fixed combination of olanzapine and fluoxetine). Dosage of the fixed-combination preparation ranges from olanzapine 3–12 mg and fluoxetine 25–50 mg daily. The following table provides the appropriate individual component dosages of olanzapine and fluoxetine compared with the fixed-combination preparation. If dosage adjustments are indicated, they should be made with the individual components according to efficacy and tolerability.

Table 1. Approximate Dosage Correspondence between Olanzapine in Fixed Combination with Fluoxetine (e.g., Symbyax®) and Combined Olanzapine (e.g., Zyprexa®) and Fluoxetine Therapy (Given Individually).

For fixed-combination dosages of:	Use in combination:	
	Olanzapine (mg/day)	Fluoxetine (mg/day)
3 mg olanzapine/25 mg fluoxetine	2.5	20
6 mg olanzapine/25 mg fluoxetine	5	20
12 mg olanzapine/25 mg fluoxetine	10 + 2.5	20
6 mg olanzapine/50 mg fluoxetine	5	40 + 10
12 mg olanzapine/50 mg fluoxetine	10 + 2.5	40 + 10

When used in fixed combination with fluoxetine hydrochloride (e.g., as the fixed combination Symbyax®) for acute depressive episodes in children and adolescents 10–17 years of age with bipolar disorder, olanzapine is administered once daily in the evening, usually initiating therapy with a dosage of 3 mg of olanzapine and 25 mg of fluoxetine. Dosage can then be adjusted to a target dosage within the FDA-labeled dosage range of olanzapine 6–12 mg daily and fluoxetine 25–50 mg daily. Concurrent administration of dosages exceeding 12 mg of olanzapine and 50 mg of fluoxetine daily has not been evaluated in pediatric clinical studies.

When used in conjunction with fluoxetine hydrochloride (as individual components of olanzapine and fluoxetine rather than the fixed-combination preparation) for acute depressive episodes in children and adolescents 10–17 years of age with bipolar disorder, olanzapine is administered once daily in the evening, usually initiating therapy with a dosage of 2.5 mg of olanzapine and 20 mg of fluoxetine. Dosage adjustments, if indicated, may be made based on efficacy and tolerability. Concurrent administration of dosages exceeding 12 mg of olanzapine and 50 mg of fluoxetine daily has not been evaluated in pediatric clinical studies.

The long-term efficacy of oral olanzapine (dosage range: 5–20 mg daily) for maintenance monotherapy in adults with bipolar disorder has been demonstrated in a double-blind, placebo-controlled trial of 52 weeks' duration and in comparative studies of 47–52 weeks' duration. The mean modal dosage of olanzapine in the placebo-controlled study was 12.5 mg daily. The manufacturer states that patients receiving oral olanzapine for extended periods should be reassessed periodically to determine the need for continued therapy.

Although the efficacy of oral olanzapine for maintenance treatment of adolescents with bipolar disorder has not been evaluated, the manufacturer states that such efficacy can be extrapolated from adult data in addition to comparisons of olanzapine pharmacokinetic parameters in adult and adolescent patients. If olanzapine is used for an extended period, the need for maintenance therapy should be reassessed periodically.

Although the manufacturer states that efficacy of the fixed combination of olanzapine and fluoxetine beyond 8 weeks' duration remains to be established, patients have received the fixed combination for up to 24 weeks in clinical trials. Clinicians who elect to use the fixed combination for extended periods should periodically reevaluate the long-term risks and benefits of the drug for the individual patient.

Treatment-resistant Depression. When used in fixed combination with fluoxetine hydrochloride (e.g., as the fixed combination Symbyax®) for the acute and maintenance treatment of treatment-resistant depression in adults, olanzapine is administered once daily in the evening, usually initiating therapy with a dosage of 6 mg of olanzapine and 25 mg of fluoxetine. An initial dosage of 3 or 6 mg of olanzapine in fixed combination with 25 mg of fluoxetine should be used in patients with a predisposition to hypotensive reactions, patients with hepatic impairment, or those with factors that may slow metabolism of the drugs(s) (e.g., female gender, geriatric age, nonsmoking status); when indicated, dosage should be escalated with caution. In other patients, dosage can be increased according to patient response and tolerance as indicated. In clinical trials in adults, antidepressant efficacy was demonstrated at olanzapine dosages ranging from 6–18 mg daily and fluoxetine dosages ranging from 25–50 mg daily. Dosages exceeding 18 mg of olanzapine and 75 mg of fluoxetine daily have not been evaluated in clinical studies. Clinicians who elect to use the fixed combination for extended periods should periodically reevaluate the long-term risks and benefits of the drug for the individual patient.

When used in conjunction with fluoxetine hydrochloride (as individual components of olanzapine and fluoxetine rather than the fixed-combination preparation) for the acute and maintenance treatment of treatment-resistant depression in adults, olanzapine is administered once daily in the evening, usually initiating therapy with a dosage of 5 mg of olanzapine and 20 mg of fluoxetine. Dosage adjustments, if indicated, may be made based on efficacy and tolerability within the dosage ranges of olanzapine 5–20 mg and fluoxetine 20–50 mg daily. An initial dosage of 2.5–5 mg of olanzapine and 20 mg of fluoxetine should be used in patients with a predisposition to hypotensive reactions, patients with hepatic impairment, those with factors that may slow metabolism of the drugs(s) (e.g., female gender, geriatric age, nonsmoking status), or those who may be pharmacodynamically sensitive to olanzapine; when indicated, dosage adjustment should be made with caution in these patients. Dosages exceeding 18 mg of olanzapine and 75 mg of fluoxetine daily have not been evaluated in clinical studies. Clinicians who elect to use the combination for extended periods should periodically reevaluate the long-term risks and benefits of the drug for the individual patient.

The safety and efficacy of olanzapine and fluoxetine in combination (given as the individual components) were determined in clinical trials that supported the approval of Symbyax® (the fixed combination of olanzapine and fluoxetine). Dosage of the fixed-combination preparation ranges from olanzapine 3–12 mg and fluoxetine 25–50 mg daily. Table 1 provides the appropriate individual component dosages of olanzapine and fluoxetine compared with the fixed-combination preparation. If dosage adjustments are indicated, they should be made with the individual components according to efficacy and tolerability.

Cancer Chemotherapy-induced Nausea and Vomiting. For the prevention of acute and delayed nausea and vomiting associated with highly emetogenic cancer chemotherapy† in adults, the American Society of Clinical Oncology (ASCO) currently recommends an oral olanzapine dosage of 10 mg once daily on the first day of chemotherapy (day 1) and then 10 mg once daily on days 2–4 of chemotherapy. Olanzapine usually has been administered as part of a 4-drug combination antiemetic regimen that includes a neurokinin 1 (NK_1) receptor antagonist, a 5-HT_3 receptor antagonist, and dexamethasone. This is the same dosage regimen that was used in the pivotal clinical study evaluating olanzapine as an antiemetic in patients receiving highly emetogenic chemotherapy. There is some evidence that 5-mg once-daily doses of olanzapine may be as effective as 10-mg once-daily doses in preventing chemotherapy-induced nausea and vomiting and reduce the risk of sedation observed with 10-mg once-daily doses; additional controlled studies are needed to determine the optimal dosing of olanzapine in prophylactic antiemetic regimens.

For the treatment of breakthrough nausea and vomiting† despite optimal antiemetic prophylaxis in adults receiving cancer chemotherapy, olanzapine has been given orally in a dosage of 10 mg orally once daily for 3 days in a pivotal clinical study. (See Uses: Cancer Chemotherapy-induced Nausea and Vomiting.)

IM Dosage **Immediate-release Olanzapine Injection for Acute Agitation associated with Bipolar Disorder or Schizophrenia.** For the prompt control of acute agitation in patients with schizophrenia or bipolar mania, the recommended initial adult IM dose of olanzapine injection (e.g., Zyprexa® IntraMuscular) is 10 mg given as a single dose. A lower initial IM dose (2.5, 5, or 7.5 mg) may be considered when clinically warranted. In clinical trials, the efficacy of IM olanzapine for controlling agitation in patients with schizophrenia or bipolar mania has been demonstrated in a dosage range of 2.5–10 mg.

If agitation necessitating additional IM doses of olanzapine persists following the initial dose, subsequent single doses of up to 10 mg may be given. However, the manufacturer states that the efficacy of repeated doses of IM olanzapine in agitated patients has not been systematically evaluated in controlled clinical trials. In addition, the safety of IM dosages exceeding 30 mg daily or of 10-mg IM doses given more frequently than 2 hours after the initial dose and 4 hours after the second dose has not been evaluated in clinical trials.

Maximal dosing of IM olanzapine (e.g., 3 doses of 10 mg administered 2–4 hours apart) may be associated with a substantial risk of clinically important orthostatic hypotension. Patients who experience drowsiness or dizziness after the IM injection should remain recumbent until an examination indicates that they are not experiencing orthostatic hypotension, bradycardia, and/or hypoventilation. (See Orthostatic Hypotension under Cautions: Precautions and Contraindications.)

If ongoing olanzapine therapy is clinically indicated, the manufacturer states that oral olanzapine may be initiated in a dosage range of 5–20 mg daily as soon as clinically appropriate. In one controlled study evaluating IM olanzapine in acutely agitated patients, patients initially received 1–3 IM injections of olanzapine 10 mg and were then switched to oral olanzapine therapy in dosages ranging from 5–20 mg daily for a period of 4 days.

A lower initial IM olanzapine dose of 5 mg may be considered for geriatric patients or when other clinical factors warrant. In addition, a lower IM dose of 2.5 mg per injection should be considered for patients who are debilitated, who may be predisposed to hypotensive reactions, or who may be more sensitive to the pharmacodynamic effects of olanzapine.

Extended-release Olanzapine Pamoate Injectable Suspension for Schizophrenia. The manufacturer recommends that patients first receive oral olanzapine to establish tolerability of the drug before the extended-release olanzapine pamoate injection is used IM.

The clinical efficacy of extended-release olanzapine pamoate injectable suspension (Zyprexa® Relprevv) in adults has been demonstrated within the dosage range of 150–300 mg administered every 2 weeks and with 405 mg administered every 4 weeks.

For the management of schizophrenia in *patients established on oral olanzapine 10 mg daily*, the recommended initial IM dosage of extended-release olanzapine pamoate is 210 mg administered every 2 weeks or 405 mg administered every 4 weeks during the first 8 weeks of therapy. Following the initial 8 weeks, the recommended maintenance dosage of olanzapine pamoate is 150 mg given every 2 weeks or 300 mg given every 4 weeks.

In *patients established on oral olanzapine 15 mg daily*, the recommended initial IM dosage of extended-release olanzapine pamoate is 300 mg administered every 2 weeks for the first 8 weeks of therapy. Following the initial 8 weeks, the recommended maintenance dosage of olanzapine pamoate is 210 mg given every 2 weeks or 405 mg given every 4 weeks.

In *patients established on oral olanzapine 20 mg daily*, the recommended initial and maintenance IM dosage of extended-release olanzapine pamoate is 300 mg administered every 2 weeks.

The manufacturer states that extended-release olanzapine pamoate IM dosages exceeding 405 mg every 4 weeks or 300 mg every 2 weeks have not been evaluated in clinical trials.

A lower initial IM olanzapine pamoate dosage of 150 mg every 4 weeks is recommended in patients who are debilitated, who may be predisposed to hypotensive reactions, who exhibit a combination of factors that may result in slower metabolism of olanzapine (e.g., nonsmoking female patients 65 years of age or older), or who may be more sensitive to the pharmacodynamic effects of the drug.

Although no controlled studies have been conducted to determine the optimum duration of extended-release olanzapine pamoate therapy in patients with stabilized schizophrenia, the long-term efficacy of the drug has been demonstrated over a 24-week period. In addition, long-term use of oral olanzapine has been shown to be effective in maintaining treatment response in patients with schizophrenia. If olanzapine pamoate is used for an extended period, the need for continued treatment should be reassessed periodically.

The manufacturer states that there are no systematically collected data to specifically address how to switch patients with schizophrenia receiving other antipsychotic agents to extended-release IM olanzapine pamoate therapy.

■ **Dosage in Renal and Hepatic Impairment** The manufacturer states that because only minimal amounts of olanzapine (about 7%) are excreted in urine and because the pharmacokinetics of olanzapine appear not to be altered in patients with renal or hepatic impairment, dosage adjustment is not necessary in such patients.

The manufacturer states that the extended-release IM formulation of olanzapine pamoate (Zyprexa® Relprevv) has not been specifically studied in patients with renal and/or hepatic impairment.

Cautions

■ **Adverse Effects** The adverse effect profile of olanzapine generally is similar to that of other atypical (second-generation) antipsychotic agents (e.g., aripiprazole, clozapine, quetiapine, risperidone, ziprasidone). Although olanzapine differs chemically from the phenothiazines, the drug also may be capable of producing many of the toxic manifestations of phenothiazine derivatives. (See Cautions in the Phenothiazines General Statement 28:16.08.24.) Not all adverse effects of the phenothiazines have been reported with olanzapine, but the possibility that they may occur should be considered. Adverse effects of olanzapine, other atypical antipsychotics, and the phenothiazines are numerous and may involve nearly all body organ systems.

In controlled studies in adults, the most common adverse effects occurring more frequently in patients receiving oral olanzapine for schizophrenia or bipolar mania than in those receiving placebo included central and autonomic nervous system effects such as somnolence, asthenia, dry mouth, dizziness, tremor, personality disorder, and akathisia; cardiovascular system effects such as postural hypotension; GI effects such as constipation, dyspepsia, and increased appetite; and weight gain. There was no clear relationship between the incidence of adverse events and dosage in patients receiving oral olanzapine for schizophrenia in placebo-controlled trials except for certain extrapyramidal symptoms, asthenia or fatigue, dry mouth, nausea, somnolence, tremor, weight gain, and elevated prolactin concentrations. Discontinuance of olanzapine therapy was required in 5% of adult patients with schizophrenia compared with 6% for placebo in controlled trials; however, discontinuance because of increased serum ALT (SGPT) concentrations was required in 2% of the olanzapine-treated patients compared with none of those receiving placebo, and this adverse effect was considered to be drug related. Similar between olanzapine and placebo discontinuance rates were observed in the controlled trials for oral olanzapine for bipolar mania (2% for olanzapine and 2% for placebo) and IM olanzapine for acute agitation (0.4% for IM olanzapine and 0% for placebo).

Adverse effects occurring in 5% or more of adult patients with schizophrenia receiving oral olanzapine in short-term clinical studies and with an incidence of at least twice that of placebo included dizziness (11%), constipation (9%), personality disorder (i.e., nonaggressive objectionable behavior; 8%), weight gain (6%), postural hypotension (5%), and akathisia (5%).

Adverse effects occurring in 6% or more of adult patients with acute mania associated with bipolar disorder receiving oral olanzapine in clinical studies and with an incidence of at least twice that of placebo included somnolence (35%), dry mouth (22%), dizziness (18%), asthenia (15%), constipation (11%), dyspepsia (11%), increased appetite (6%), and tremor (6%).

When oral olanzapine was used in conjunction with lithium or divalproex sodium for treatment of acute mania associated with bipolar disorder in adults, adverse effects occurring in 5% or more of patients in clinical studies and with an incidence of at least twice that of placebo included dry mouth (32%), weight gain (26%), increased appetite (24%), dizziness (14%), back pain (8%), constipation (8%), speech disorder (7%), increased salivation (6%), amnesia (5%), and paresthesia (5%).

Adverse effects occurring in 5% or more of adolescents (13–17 years of age) with schizophrenia or bipolar disorder receiving oral olanzapine in short-term, placebo-controlled clinical studies and with an incidence of at least twice that of placebo included sedation (39–48%), weight gain (29–31%), headache (17%), increased appetite (17–29%), dizziness (7–8%), abdominal pain (6%), pain in extremities (5–6%), fatigue (3–14%), and dry mouth (4–7%).

When short-acting IM olanzapine was used for the management of acute agitation in short-term clinical studies, somnolence was the only adverse effect that occurred in 5% or more of patients with schizophrenia or bipolar mania and with an incidence at least twice that of placebo (6% and 3%, respectively).

When extended-release olanzapine pamoate injection was used IM in adults with schizophrenia in a short-term, placebo-controlled clinical study, adverse effects occurring in 5% or more of patients and more frequently than with placebo included headache (13–18%), sedation (8–13%), weight gain (5–7%), cough (3–9%), diarrhea (2–7%), back pain (3–5%), nausea (4–5%), somnolence (1–6%), dry mouth (2–6%), nasopharyngitis (1–6%), increased appetite (1–6%), and vomiting (1–6%).

■ **Nervous System Effects** ***Seizures*** Seizures occurred in about 0.9% of adult patients receiving oral olanzapine in controlled clinical trials during premarketing testing. During premarketing testing of extended-release olanzapine pamoate IM injection, seizures occurred in 0.15% of adult patients. Confounding factors that may have contributed to the occurrence of seizures were present in many of these cases.

Myoclonic status reportedly occurred shortly after initiation of olanzapine in one patient with probable dementia of the Alzheimer's type (Alzheimer's disease) who was concurrently receiving citalopram and donepezil; the myoclonic jerks in this patient coincided with EEG changes indicative of seizure activity (spikes and polyspike/wave complexes), and the seizures subsided following discontinuance of olanzapine. A new-onset seizure also reportedly occurred in an adult female patient upon the addition of quetiapine to maintenance therapy with olanzapine and following discontinuance of clonazepam therapy. In addition, an apparent lowering of seizure threshold occurred in at least 2 epileptic patients who experienced increased seizure activity following initiation of olanzapine therapy that resolved upon discontinuance of the drug. Fatal status epilepticus also has been reported in a patient who had been receiving olanzapine therapy for 5 months.

Olanzapine should be administered with caution to patients with a history of seizures or conditions known to lower the seizure threshold (e.g., dementia of the Alzheimer's type); conditions that lower the seizure threshold may be more prevalent in patients 65 years of age or older.

Extrapyramidal Reactions Like other atypical antipsychotic agents, olanzapine has a low potential for causing certain adverse extrapyramidal effects (e.g., dystonias). Results from controlled clinical trials suggest that extrapyramidal reactions associated with olanzapine therapy are dose related.

Tremor was reported in about 4% of patients receiving oral olanzapine and in about 1% of patients receiving short-acting IM olanzapine in controlled clinical trials; the incidence of tremor appears to be dose related. In addition, akathisia occurred in about 3% of patients receiving oral olanzapine and in less than 1% of patients receiving short-acting IM olanzapine; hypertonia occurred in about 3% of patients receiving oral olanzapine in short-term controlled clinical trials. Oculogyric crisis also has been reported in a patient receiving olanzapine, lithium, and paroxetine concurrently. (See Drug Interactions: Other CNS-Active Agents and Alcohol.)

Neuroleptic Malignant Syndrome Neuroleptic malignant syndrome (NMS), a potentially fatal symptom complex, has been reported in patients receiving antipsychotic agents, including olanzapine. Clinical manifestations of NMS generally include hyperpyrexia, muscle rigidity, altered mental status, and evidence of autonomic instability (irregular pulse or blood pressure, tachycardia, diaphoresis, and cardiac arrhythmias). Additional signs of NMS may include increased serum creatine kinase (CK, creatine phosphokinase, CPK), myoglobinuria (rhabdomyolysis), and acute renal failure. NMS attributable to olanzapine therapy alone has been reported in some patients, and there also have been reports of NMS in olanzapine-treated patients concomitantly receiving other drugs, including antipsychotic agents, antidepressants, lithium, or valproate. Extrapyramidal reactions were present in approximately two-thirds of the olanzapine-treated patients diagnosed with NMS. Atypical presentations of NMS (e.g., absence of or lessened rigidity, presenting as fever of unknown origin) and less severe presentations of NMS also have been reported in some patients receiving olanzapine or other atypical antipsychotic agents.

The diagnostic evaluation of patients with NMS is complicated. In arriving at a diagnosis, serious medical illnesses (e.g., pneumonia, systemic infection) and untreated or inadequately treated extrapyramidal signs and symptoms must be excluded. In addition, clinical features of NMS and serotonin syndrome sometimes overlap, and it has been suggested that these 2 syndromes may share certain underlying pathophysiologic mechanisms. Other important considerations in the differential diagnosis include central anticholinergic toxicity, heat stroke, drug fever, and primary CNS pathology.

The management of NMS should include immediate discontinuance of antipsychotic agents and other drugs not considered essential to concurrent therapy, intensive symptomatic treatment and medical monitoring, and treatment of any concomitant serious medical problems for which specific treatments are available. There currently is no specific drug therapy for NMS, although dantrolene, bromocriptine, amantadine, and benzodiazepines have been used in a limited number of patients. If a patient requires antipsychotic therapy following recovery from NMS, the potential reintroduction of drug therapy after several weeks should be carefully considered. If antipsychotic therapy is reintroduced, the dosage generally should be increased gradually and an antipsychotic agent other than the agent believed to have precipitated NMS generally is chosen. In addition, tolerability with oral olanzapine should be established prior to initiating treatment with extended-release IM olanzapine pamoate. Such patients should be carefully monitored since recurrences of NMS have been reported in some patients. For additional information on NMS, see Neuroleptic Malignant Syndrome under Cautions: Nervous System Effects, in the Phenothiazines General Statement 28:16.08.24.

Tardive Dyskinesia Use of antipsychotic agents may be associated with tardive dyskinesia, a syndrome of potentially irreversible, involuntary, dyskinetic movements. Although the incidence of tardive dyskinesia appears to be highest among geriatric individuals, particularly geriatric females, it is not possible to reliably predict at the beginning of antipsychotic therapy which patients are likely to develop this syndrome. Tardive dyskinesia has been reported in less than 1% of patients receiving olanzapine therapy. Although the manufacturer states that it is not yet known whether antipsychotic agents differ in their potential to cause tardive dyskinesia, available evidence suggests that the risk appears to be substantially less with second-generation antipsychotic agents, including olanzapine, than with conventional, first-generation antipsychotic agents. Analyses from controlled, long-term trials have found an approximately 12-fold lower risk of tardive dyskinesia with olanzapine therapy compared with haloperidol therapy. In addition, stabilization of or improvement in tardive dyskinesia associated with conventional antipsychotic agents has been reported in some patients when they have been switched to second-generation antipsychotic therapy, including olanzapine. However, a transient increase in dyskinetic movements (sometimes referred to as withdrawal-emergent dyskinesia) occasionally may occur when a patient is switched from a first-generation to a second-generation antipsychotic agent or upon dosage reduction of an antipsychotic agent.

The risk of developing tardive dyskinesia and the likelihood that it will become irreversible are believed to increase as the duration of treatment and the total cumulative dose of antipsychotic drugs administered to the patient increase. However, the syndrome can develop, although much less commonly, following relatively brief treatment periods at low dosages or may even arise after discontinuance of treatment.

Management of tardive dyskinesia generally consists of gradual discontinuance of the precipitating antipsychotic agent when possible, reducing the dosage of the first-generation (conventional) antipsychotic agent or switching to a second-generation (atypical) antipsychotic agent, or switching to clozapine therapy. The syndrome may remit, partially or completely, if antipsychotic therapy is discontinued. However, antipsychotic therapy itself may suppress or partially suppress the signs and symptoms of the syndrome and thereby may possibly mask the underlying process. The effect that such symptomatic suppression has upon the long-term course of tardive dyskinesia is unknown. Vesicular monoamine transporter 2 (VMAT2) inhibitors (e.g., deutetrabenazine, valbenazine tosylate) have been shown to be effective in reducing symptoms of tardive dyskinesia in controlled clinical studies and may allow some patients to continue receiving antipsychotic therapy. (See Deutetrabenazine 28:56 and Valbenazine Tosylate 28:56.) There also is some evidence that vitamin E administration may reduce the risk of development of tardive dyskinesia; therefore, the American Psychiatric Association (APA) currently states that patients receiving antipsychotic agents may be advised to take 400–800 units of vitamin E daily for prophylaxis. (See Cautions in Vitamin E 88:20.)

Olanzapine should be prescribed in a manner that is most likely to minimize the occurrence of tardive dyskinesia. Chronic antipsychotic treatment generally should be reserved for patients who suffer from a chronic illness that is known to respond to antipsychotic agents, and for whom alternative, equally effective, but potentially less harmful treatments are not available or appropriate. In patients who do require chronic treatment, the smallest dosage and the shortest duration of treatment producing a satisfactory clinical response should be sought, and the need for continued treatment should be reassessed periodically.

The APA currently recommends that all patients receiving second-generation antipsychotic agents be assessed clinically for abnormal involuntary movements every 12 months and that patients considered to be at increased risk for tardive dyskinesia be assessed every 6 months. If signs and symptoms of tardive dyskinesia appear in a patient receiving olanzapine, drug discontinuance or a reduction in dosage should be considered. However, some patients may require treatment with olanzapine or another antipsychotic agent despite the presence of the syndrome.

For additional information on tardive dyskinesia, including manifestations and treatment, see Tardive Dyskinesia under Cautions: Nervous System Effects, in the Phenothiazines General Statement 28:16.08.24.

Post-injection Delirium/Sedation Syndrome During premarketing studies of extended-release olanzapine pamoate (Zyprexa® Relprevv), adverse events that presented with signs and symptoms consistent with olanzapine overdosage, particularly sedation (ranging from mild in severity to coma) and/or delirium, were reported following injection of the drug. Such cases of post-injection delirium/sedation syndrome (PDSS) occurred in less than 0.1% of injections and in approximately 2% of patients who received injections for up to 46 months. These events were correlated with an unintentional rapid increase in serum olanzapine concentrations to supratherapeutic ranges in some cases. Although a rapid and greater than expected increase in serum olanzapine concentrations has been noted in some patients with these adverse events, the precise mechanism by which the drug was unintentionally introduced into the bloodstream in these cases is not known.

Clinical signs and symptoms of PDSS include dizziness, confusion, disorientation, malaise, slurred speech, altered gait, ambulation difficulties, weakness, agitation, extrapyramidal symptoms, hypertension, convulsions, and reduced levels of consciousness ranging from mild sedation to coma. The time after injection to PDSS in most reported cases ranged from soon after the injection to greater than 3 hours after the injection; patients had largely recovered by 72 hours. Because the risk of PDSS is the same at each injection, the risk per patient is cumulative (i.e., the risk increases with the number of injections). (See Post-injection Delirium/Sedation Syndrome under Cautions: Precautions and Contraindications and see also Acute Toxicity.)

Other Nervous System Effects Somnolence or sedation, which usually appears to be moderate in severity compared with other antipsychotic agents and dose related, is among the most common adverse effects of olanzapine, occurring in approximately 29% of adults and 44% of adolescents receiving oral olanzapine in controlled clinical trials. In addition, sedation-related adverse events (defined as hypersomnia, lethargy, sedation, and somnolence) occurred more often in adolescents compared with adults. Sedation occurred in 8% of patients receiving extended-release olanzapine pamoate injection, and somnolence and sedation resulted in discontinuance of the drug in 0.6% of patients in the premarketing database. Somnolence associated with olanzapine and other antipsychotic agents generally is most pronounced during early therapy, since most patients develop some tolerance to the sedating effects with continued administration. Although sedation can have therapeutic benefits in some cases, persistent daytime drowsiness and increased sleep time can become troublesome in some patients and necessitate a lower dosage or evening administration of oral olanzapine. (See Reconstitution and Administration under Dosage and Administration, Cognitive and Motor Impairment under Cautions: Precautions and Contraindications, and see also Effects on Sleep under Pharmacology: Nervous System Effects.)

Insomnia occurred in about 12%, dizziness in about 11%, asthenia in about 10%, and abnormal gait in about 6% of adult patients receiving oral olanzapine in short-term controlled clinical trials. The incidence of asthenia appears to be dose related. In addition, articulation impairment was reported in about 2% of patients receiving oral olanzapine in short-term, controlled clinical trials.

Ataxia, decreased libido, dysarthria, stupor, and suicide attempt have been reported in 1% or less of patients receiving oral olanzapine in clinical trials.

In short-term (i.e., 24-hour), controlled clinical trials of short-acting IM olanzapine for acute agitation in adults, somnolence occurred in approximately 6%, dizziness in approximately 4%, and asthenia in about 2% of the patients.

■ **Cardiovascular Effects** ***Hemodynamic Effects*** Oral olanzapine may produce orthostatic hypotension that may be associated with dizziness, tachycardia, bradycardia, and, in some patients, syncope, particularly during the initial period of dosage titration. These adverse hemodynamic effects probably are due to the drug's α_1-adrenergic blocking activity. In short-term, controlled clinical trials of oral olanzapine in adults, postural hypotension and tachycardia occurred in approximately 3% and hypertension occurred in approximately 2% of patients. In an analysis of vital sign data from 41 clinical trials conducted with oral olanzapine in adults, orthostatic hypotension was reported in 20% or more of patients. Vasodilatation has been reported in 1% or less of patients treated with oral olanzapine; this adverse effect has not been definitely attributed to the drug.

Hypotension, bradycardia with or without hypotension, tachycardia, and syncope also were reported during the clinical trials with short-acting IM olanzapine. In an open trial in nonagitated patients with schizophrenia designed to evaluate the safety and tolerability of a dosage regimen of three 10-mg IM doses of olanzapine administered 4 hours apart, approximately one-third of the patients experienced a substantial orthostatic decrease in systolic blood pressure (i.e., decrease of 30 mm Hg or more).

Syncope was reported in 0.6% of olanzapine-treated patients in phase 2 and 3 clinical trials of oral olanzapine, and in 0.3% of patients receiving short-acting IM olanzapine in the acute agitation clinical trials. In phase 1 trials of olanzapine, 3 healthy volunteers experienced hypotension, bradycardia, and sinus pauses of up to 6 seconds that spontaneously resolved; 2 of these cases occurred in association with short-acting IM olanzapine and one case involved oral olanzapine. In short-term, controlled clinical trials for short-acting IM olanzapine for acute agitation, hypotension occurred in approximately 2% and postural hypotension occurred in approximately 1% of patients. Syncope has been reported in 1% or less of patients receiving short-acting IM olanzapine in clinical trials. The manufacturer states that the risk for this sequence of hypotension, bradycardia, and sinus pause may be greater in nonpsychiatric patients compared with psychiatric patients, who may be more adapted to certain pharmacologic effects of psychotropic agents. Long-acting IM olanzapine pamoate also may cause orthostatic hypotension associated with dizziness, tachycardia, bradycardia, and syncope (in some cases). Syncope-related adverse effects have been reported in 0.1% of patients receiving long-acting IM olanzapine pamoate in clinical trials. (See Dosage and Administration and see also Orthostatic Hypotension, under Cautions: Precautions and Contraindications.)

ECG Effects Pooled analyses from controlled clinical trials in adults as well as in adolescents did not reveal significant differences in the proportions of oral olanzapine-treated patients experiencing potentially important ECG changes, including QT, QT_c (Fridericia corrected), and PR intervals. Oral olanzapine was associated with a mean increase in heart rate of 2.4 beats/minute in adults and a mean increase of 6.3 beats/minute in adolescents compared with no change and a mean decrease of 5.1 beats/minute, respectively, among patients who received placebo in controlled trials. A comparison of extended-release IM olanzapine pamoate and oral olanzapine (in the 24-week study) did not reveal substantial differences in ECG changes between these formulations.

The manufacturer states that the tendency to cause tachycardia may be related to olanzapine's potential for inducing orthostatic changes in blood pressure.

Like some other antipsychotic agents, olanzapine has been associated with prolongation of the QT_c interval in some patients and there is some evidence that higher dosages of the drug may increase the risk of QT_c-interval prolongation; however, the clinical relevance of these findings remains to be established.

Other Cardiovascular Effects In short-term, controlled clinical trials for oral olanzapine, chest pain occurred in approximately 3% of patients. Cerebrovascular accident has been reported in 1% or less of patients.

Venous thromboembolic effects, including pulmonary embolism and deep venous thrombosis, have been reported in patients receiving olanzapine during postmarketing surveillance.

■ **Hepatic Effects** During premarketing clinical trials, oral olanzapine therapy was associated with asymptomatic elevations in serum aminotransferase (transaminase) concentrations, including elevations in serum concentrations of ALT (SGPT), AST (SGOT), and γ-glutamyltransferase (GGT). Clinically important ALT elevations 3 or more times the upper limit of the normal range were observed in 5% (77 of 1426) of adult patients exposed to olanzapine in placebo-controlled clinical studies; none of these patients experienced jaundice. ALT elevations 5 or more times the upper limit of the normal range were observed in 2% (29 of 1438) of adult patients treated with olanzapine. ALT values returned to normal, or were decreasing, at last follow-up in the majority of patients who either continued olanzapine therapy or discontinued the drug. None of the patients with elevated ALT values experienced jaundice, liver failure, or met the criteria for Hy's rule. Within the larger premarketing database of about 2400 adult patients with baseline ALT values of 90 IU/L or less, the incidence of ALT elevation exceeding 200 IU/L was 2% (50 of 2381 patients). None of these patients experienced jaundice or other symptoms attributable to hepatic impairment, and most had transient changes that tended to normalize while olanzapine therapy was continued. (See Hepatic Effects under Cautions: Precautions and Contraindications.)

Changes in serum transaminase concentrations observed with extended-release IM olanzapine pamoate are similar to those reported with oral olanzapine. In placebo-controlled studies of the extended-release IM formulation, clinically important ALT elevations 3 or more times the upper limit of normal were observed in 2.7% (8 of 291) of adult patients exposed to the drug compared with 3.2% (3 of 94) of placebo recipients; none of these patients experienced jaundice. In 3 of the patients, transaminase concentrations returned to normal despite continuing IM olanzapine pamoate therapy; in the other 5 patients transaminase concentrations decreased but remained about the normal range at the end of therapy. Within the larger premarketing database of 1886 patients with baseline ALT values of 90 IU/L or less, the incidence of ALT elevation exceeding 200 IU/L was 0.8%. None of these patients experienced jaundice or other symptoms attributable to hepatic impairment, and most had transient changes that tended to normalize while olanzapine pamoate IM therapy was continued. (See Hepatic Effects under Cautions: Precautions and Contraindications.)

In clinical studies with oral olanzapine, adolescents were more likely to have greater increases in serum transaminase concentrations compared with adults. In placebo-controlled monotherapy studies, clinically important ALT elevations (3 or more times the upper limit of the normal range) were observed in 12% (22 of 192) of adolescent patients exposed to olanzapine. ALT elevations 5 or more times the upper limit of the normal range were observed in 4% (8 of 192) of adolescent patients treated with olanzapine. ALT values returned to normal, or were decreasing, at last follow-up in the majority of adolescent patients who either continued olanzapine therapy or discontinued the drug. None of the adolescents with elevated ALT values experienced jaundice, liver failure, or met the criteria for Hy's rule.

Hepatitis and jaundice have rarely been reported in patients receiving different formulations of olanzapine during postmarketing experience, as well as very rare cases of cholestatic or mixed hepatic injury. In addition, fatty deposit in the liver has been reported in less than 0.1% of patients receiving oral olanzapine in short-term clinical trials, although a causal relationship to the drug remains to be established.

■ **Endocrine and Metabolic Effects** Atypical antipsychotic agents have been associated with metabolic changes, including hyperglycemia, dyslipidemia, and weight gain. Such metabolic changes may be associated with increased cardiovascular and cerebrovascular risk.

Weight Gain Like some conventional (first-generation) and atypical (second-generation) antipsychotic agents, olanzapine therapy may result in weight gain. In placebo-controlled studies of 6 weeks' duration in adults, weight gain occurred in approximately 6% of patients receiving oral olanzapine, and increased appetite occurred in 6% of patients receiving oral olanzapine in short-term controlled trials. In an analysis of 13 placebo-controlled monotherapy studies, adult patients receiving olanzapine gained an average of 2.6 kg compared with an average loss of 0.3 kg in those receiving placebo (with a median exposure of 6 weeks); 22.2% of the olanzapine-treated patients gained 7% or more of their baseline weight compared with 3% of placebo recipients (with a median exposure to event of 8 weeks). Dose group differences with regard to weight gain have been noted in a short-term, controlled study comparing fixed oral dosages of olanzapine in adults with schizophrenia or schizoaffective disorder; the mean baseline to end point increase in weight was 1.9 kg in patients receiving 10 mg of olanzapine daily, 2.3 kg in those receiving 20 mg daily, and 3 kg in those receiving 40 mg daily, with substantial differences between 10 and 40 mg daily. Discontinuance of olanzapine therapy because of weight gain occurred in 0.2% of olanzapine-treated patients compared with none of the placebo recipients. During long-term studies (at least 48 weeks' duration) with olanzapine in adults, mean weight gain was 5.6 kg (median exposure of 573 days); 64% of olanzapine-treated patients gained 7% or more of their baseline weight, 32% gained 15% or more of their baseline weight, and 12% gained 25% or more of their baseline weight.

In olanzapine-treated adolescent patients, both the magnitude of weight gain and the proportion of patients who had clinically significant weight gain were greater than in adult patients with comparable exposures. In short-term, placebo-controlled studies in adolescent patients with schizophrenia or bipolar disorder, weight gain occurred in approximately 30% of adolescents and increased appetite occurred in approximately 24% of adolescents receiving oral olanzapine. In 4 short-term, placebo-controlled monotherapy studies, adolescents receiving olanzapine gained an average of 4.6 kg compared with an average loss of 0.3 kg in those receiving placebo (with a median exposure of 3 weeks); 40.6% of the olanzapine-treated patients gained 7% or more of their baseline weight compared with 9.8% of placebo recipients (with median exposures to event of 4 and 8 weeks, respectively). Of the olanzapine-treated adolescents, 7.1% gained 15% or more of their baseline body weight compared with 2.7% of the placebo recipients (with median exposures to event of 19 and 8 weeks, respectively). In placebo-controlled studies of olanzapine therapy in adolescents, discontinuance due to weight gain occurred in 1% of olanzapine-treated patients compared with none of the placebo recipients. During long-term studies (at least 24 weeks' duration) in adolescents, the average weight gain was 11.2 kg (with a median exposure of 201 days). The percentages of adolescents who gained at least 7, 15, or 25% of their baseline body weight with long-term exposure were 89, 55, and 29%, respectively. Among adolescent patients, average weight gain according to baseline BMI category was 11.5, 12.1, and 12.7 kg for normal, overweight, and obese adolescents, respectively. Discontinuance because of weight gain occurred in 2.2% of olanzapine-treated adolescents following at least 24 weeks of olanzapine exposure.

In a 24-week, randomized, double-blind, fixed-dosage study that compared 3 different extended-release olanzapine pamoate IM dosage regimens in adult patients with schizophrenia, average weight gains of 0.7, 0.9, and 1.7 kg occurred in those receiving 150 mg of olanzapine every 2 weeks, 405 mg every 4 weeks, and 300 mg every 2 weeks, respectively.

Although the precise mechanism(s) remains to be clearly established, weight gain may result at least in part from the drug's serotonergic-, histaminergic-, and adrenergic-blocking properties. Weight gain has been reported to be troublesome for some patients during long-term therapy with atypical antipsychotics, particularly olanzapine and clozapine, and may be an important cause of outpatient noncompliance. Some clinicians suggest regular physical exercise and nutritional counseling in the prevention and treatment of weight gain associated with these drugs. There currently are no well established pharmacologic treatments for antipsychotic agent-induced weight gain; however, a number of drugs, including amantadine, bupropion, histamine H_2-receptor antagonists (e.g., nizatidine), orlistat, metformin, and topiramate, have been used with limited success to date. Because the potential risk of adverse effects in patients receiving these drugs may outweigh their possible weight-reducing effects in some cases, routine use of pharmacologic therapy currently is not recommended by most clinicians, although individual patients may benefit. Additional controlled studies are needed to more clearly determine the optimum management of antipsychotic-associated weight gain during long-term therapy with these drugs.

Hyperglycemia and Diabetes Mellitus Hyperglycemia, sometimes severe and associated with ketoacidosis, hyperosmolar coma, or death, has been reported in patients receiving atypical antipsychotic agents, including olanzapine. While confounding factors such as an increased background risk of diabetes mellitus in patients with schizophrenia and the increasing incidence of diabetes mellitus in the general population make it difficult to establish with certainty the relationship between use of agents in this drug class and glucose abnormalities, epidemiologic studies suggest an increased risk of treatment-emergent hyperglycemia-related adverse events in patients treated with atypical antipsychotic agents. (See Hyperglycemia and Diabetes Mellitus under Cautions: Precautions and Contraindications.)

Precise risk estimates for hyperglycemia-related adverse events in patients treated with atypical antipsychotics currently are not available. While relative risk estimates are inconsistent, the association between atypical antipsychotics and increases in glucose concentrations appears to fall on a continuum, and olanzapine appears to have a greater association with hyperglycemia than some other atypical antipsychotic agents (e.g., quetiapine, risperidone).

In the first phase of Clinical Antipsychotic Trials of Intervention Effectiveness (CATIE), the mean increase in serum glucose concentration (fasting and non-fasting samples) from baseline to the average of the 2 highest serum concentrations was 15 mg/dL in olanzapine-treated adult patients (median exposure of about 9 months). In a study in healthy individuals, subjects who received olanzapine for 3 weeks had a mean increase in fasting blood glucose of 2.3 mg/dL compared with baseline; the subjects who received placebo had a mean increase in fasting blood glucose of 0.34 mg/dL compared with baseline.

In an analysis of 5 placebo-controlled monotherapy studies in adults with a median treatment duration of about 3 weeks, olanzapine was associated with a greater average increase in fasting glucose concentrations compared with placebo (2.76 mg/dL versus 0.17 mg/dL, respectively). The difference in mean changes between olanzapine and placebo was greater in patients with evidence of glucose dysregulation at baseline (e.g., patients diagnosed with diabetes mellitus or related adverse reactions, patients treated with antidiabetic agents, patients with a random baseline glucose concentration of 200 mg/dL or more and/or a baseline fasting glucose level of 126 mg/dL). Olanzapine-treated patients had a mean glycosylated hemoglobin (hemoglobin A_{1c} [HbA_{1c}]) concentration increase from baseline of 0.04% (median exposure: 21 days) compared with a mean HbA_{1c} decrease of 0.06% in placebo-treated individuals (median exposure of 17 days). In an analysis of 8 placebo-controlled studies (median treatment exposure of 4–5 weeks), 6.1% of olanzapine-treated subjects had treatment-emergent glycosuria compared with 2.8% of those receiving placebo. In adults receiving olanzapine monotherapy for at least 48 weeks, fasting glucose concentrations changed from normal (less than 100 mg/dL) to high (126 mg/dL or higher) and from borderline (between 100 and less than 126 mg/dL) to high (126 mg/dL or higher) in 12.8% and 26% of the patients, respectively. The mean change in fasting glucose for patients exposed to at least 48 weeks of olanzapine therapy was 4.2 mg/dL. In analyses of patients who completed 9–12 months of olanzapine therapy, the average change in fasting and nonfasting glucose concentrations continued to increase over time.

Although increases in fasting glucose concentrations were similar in adolescents and adults treated with olanzapine, the difference in these values between the olanzapine and placebo groups was greater in adolescents than in adults. In an analysis of 3 short-term, placebo-controlled olanzapine monotherapy studies of 3 or 6 weeks' duration in adolescent patients, olanzapine was associated with a greater mean change from baseline in fasting glucose concentrations compared with placebo (an increase of 2.68 mg/dL versus a decrease of 2.59 mg/dL, respectively). The average increase in fasting glucose concentrations for adolescents exposed to at least 24 weeks of olanzapine therapy was 3.1 mg/dL. In adolescents receiving olanzapine monotherapy for at least 24 weeks, fasting glucose concentrations changed from normal (less than 100 mg/dL) to high (126 mg/dL or higher) and from borderline (between 100 and less than 126 mg/dL) to high (126 mg/dL or higher) in 0.9% and 23.1% of the patients, respectively.

Diabetic coma and diabetic ketoacidosis have been reported in olanzapine-treated patients during postmarketing surveillance.

Dyslipidemia Like some other antipsychotic agents, particularly clozapine, olanzapine therapy has been associated with undesirable changes in lipid parameters, including elevations in serum triglyceride and cholesterol concentrations. Clinically important, and sometimes very high (greater than 500 mg/dL), elevations in triglyceride concentrations have been observed with olanzapine therapy. Modest average increases in total cholesterol concentrations also have occurred with olanzapine use.

In an analysis of 5 placebo-controlled olanzapine monotherapy studies of up to 12 weeks' duration in adults, olanzapine-treated patients had increases from baseline in mean fasting serum total cholesterol, low-density lipoprotein (LDL)-cholesterol, and triglyceride concentrations of 5.3 mg/dL, 3 mg/dL, and 20.8 mg/dL, respectively, compared with decreases from baseline in mean fasting total cholesterol, LDL-cholesterol, and triglyceride concentrations of 6.1 mg/dL, 4.3 mg/dL, and 10.7 mg/dL for patients receiving placebo. For fasting high-density lipoprotein (HDL)-cholesterol, no clinically important differences were observed between olanzapine-treated patients and patients receiving placebo. Mean increases in fasting lipid values (total cholesterol, LDL-cholesterol, and triglycerides) were greater in patients without evidence of lipid dysregulation at baseline (defined as patients diagnosed with dyslipidemia or related adverse reactions, patients receiving antilipemic agents, or patients with high baseline lipid levels). In long-term studies (at least 48 weeks) in adults, patients had increases from baseline in mean fasting serum total cholesterol, LDL-cholesterol, and triglyceride concentrations of 5.6 mg/dL, 2.5 mg/dL, and 18.7 mg/dL, respectively, and a mean decrease in fasting HDL-cholesterol of 0.16 mg/dL. In an analysis of patients who completed 12 months of therapy, the mean nonfasting total cholesterol concentration did not increase further after approximately 4–6 months. In adult monotherapy studies, fasting serum triglyceride increases of 50 mg/dL or more occurred in approximately 61% of patients, fasting total cholesterol increases of 40 mg/dL or more occurred in approximately 33% of patients, and fasting LDL-cholesterol increases of 30 mg/dL or more occurred in approximately 40% of patients. In the first phase of the CATIE program, the mean increase in serum triglyceride concentrations in patients receiving olanzapine was 40.5 mg/dL (median exposure of about 9 months) and the mean increase in total cholesterol was 9.4 mg/dL.

In clinical studies, increases in fasting serum total cholesterol, LDL-cholesterol, and triglyceride concentrations were generally greater in adolescents than in adults treated with olanzapine. In an analysis of 3 placebo-controlled olanzapine monotherapy studies in adolescent patients, increases from baseline in mean fasting total cholesterol, LDL-cholesterol, and triglyceride concentrations of approximately 13 mg/dL, 7 mg/dL, and 28 mg/dL, respectively, occurred in adolescents receiving olanzapine compared with increases from baseline in mean fasting total cholesterol and LDL cholesterol of 1.3 mg/dL and 1 mg/dL and a decrease in triglycerides of 1.1 mg/dL in adolescents receiving placebo. For fasting HDL-cholesterol, no clinically important differences were observed between adolescents receiving olanzapine compared with adolescents receiving placebo. Adolescents receiving olanzapine monotherapy for at least 24 weeks had increases from baseline in mean fasting total cholesterol, LDL-cholesterol, and triglyceride concentrations of 5.5 mg/dL, 5.4 mg/dL, and 20.5 mg/dL, respectively, and a mean decrease in fasting HDL-cholesterol of 4.5 mg/dL. In adolescent monotherapy studies, fasting serum triglyceride increases of 50 mg/dL or more occurred in approximately 46% of adolescents, fasting total cholesterol increases of 40 mg/dL or more occurred in approximately 15% of patients, and fasting LDL-cholesterol increases of 30 mg/dL or more occurred in approximately 22% of patients.

Cholesterol concentrations of 240 mg/dL or higher and triglyceride concentrations of 1000 mg/dL or higher have been reported rarely during postmarketing surveillance.

The manufacturer recommends clinical monitoring, including baseline and periodic follow-up lipid evaluations, in all patients receiving olanzapine. In addition, some clinicians recommend that lipid profiles be monitored at baseline and periodically (e.g., every 3–6 months) in all patients receiving long-term therapy with atypical antipsychotic agents. There is some evidence from a study in individuals with developmental disabilities that the risk of dyslipidemia in patients receiving atypical antipsychotic agents may be minimized or avoided by careful monitoring, dietary management, and suitable physical activity. In patients who develop persistent and clinically important dyslipidemia during olanzapine therapy, nondrug therapies and measures (e.g., dietary management, weight control, an appropriate program of physical activity) and drug therapy (e.g., antilipemic agents) may be helpful. Consideration also may be given to switching to an alternative antipsychotic agent that is less frequently associated with dyslipidemia (such as aripiprazole, risperidone, or ziprasidone).

Hyperprolactinemia As with other drugs that antagonize dopamine D_2 receptors, olanzapine can elevate serum prolactin concentrations, and the elevation may persist during chronic administration of the drug. However, in contrast to conventional (first-generation) antipsychotic agents and similar to many other atypical antipsychotic agents, olanzapine therapy in usual dosages generally produces transient elevations in serum prolactin concentrations in humans. It has been suggested that the more transient effect of atypical antipsychotic agents on prolactin may be because these drugs appear to dissociate from dopamine receptors more rapidly than conventional antipsychotic agents.

In placebo-controlled studies with olanzapine (up to 12 weeks) in adults, changes from normal to high serum prolactin concentrations were observed in 30% of olanzapine-treated adults compared with 10.5% of adults receiving placebo. In a pooled analysis from clinical studies involving 8136 adults treated with olanzapine, potentially associated clinical manifestations of hyperprolactinemia included menstrual-related events (2% of females), sexual function-related events (2% of females and males), and breast-related events (0.7% of females and 0.2% of males).

Adolescents treated with olanzapine had a higher incidence of elevated prolactin concentrations compared with adults; the incidence of galactorrhea and gynecomastia also was higher in adolescents compared with adults. In placebo-controlled olanzapine monotherapy studies of up to 6 weeks' duration in adolescent patients with schizophrenia or bipolar disorder, changes from normal to high serum prolactin concentrations were observed in 47% of olanzapine-treated patients compared with 7% of those receiving placebo. In a pooled analysis from clinical trials that included 454 olanzapine-treated adolescents, potentially associated clinical manifestations included menstrual-related events (1% of females), sexual function-related events (0.7% of females and males), and breast-related events (2% of females and 2% of males).

In premarketing studies with extended-release IM olanzapine pamoate, substantial differences in prolactin concentrations have been observed in patients receiving different dosage regimens of the drug.

Olanzapine is considered by many experts to be relatively low to moderate among antipsychotic agents in its potential for inducing hyperprolactinemia in adults, and it has been recommended along with other prolactin-sparing atypical antipsychotics (e.g., aripiprazole, clozapine, quetiapine, ziprasidone) in patients with schizophrenia who are at risk of hyperprolactinemia. Although clinical disturbances such as galactorrhea, amenorrhea, gynecomastia, and impotence have been associated with prolactin-elevating drugs, the clinical importance of elevated prolactin concentrations is unknown for most patients.

Like other drugs that increase prolactin, an increase in mammary gland neoplasia was observed in olanzapine carcinogenicity studies conducted in mice and rats. However, neither clinical studies nor epidemiologic studies have demonstrated an association between chronic administration of dopamine antagonists and tumorigenesis in humans; the available evidence is considered too limited to be conclusive. (See Hyperprolactinemia under Cautions: Precautions and Contraindications and see also Cautions: Mutagenicity and Carcinogenicity.) In patients who develop elevated prolactin concentrations during antipsychotic therapy, some clinicians recommend reducing the dosage of the current antipsychotic agent or switching to a more prolactin-sparing antipsychotic agent (e.g., aripiprazole, clozapine, quetiapine, ziprasidone). Dopamine receptor agonists (e.g., bromocriptine) also may be helpful, and estrogen replacement therapy may be considered in hypoestrogenic female patients.

Other Endocrine and Metabolic Effects Peripheral edema has been reported in approximately 3% of adult patients receiving oral olanzapine in short-term clinical trials; increased serum alkaline phosphatase concentrations have been reported in at least 1% of patients. Bilirubinemia and hypoproteinemia have been reported in 1% or less of patients receiving oral olanzapine in short-term trials.

Increased serum creatine phosphokinase concentrations have been reported in less than 1% of patients receiving IM olanzapine in short-term clinical trials; however, a causal relationship remains to be established.

■ **GI Effects** Dryness of the mouth and constipation both occurred in about 9%, dyspepsia in about 7%, vomiting in about 4%, and increased appetite in about 3% of adult patients receiving oral olanzapine in short-term controlled clinical trials.

Nausea (4–5%), vomiting (1–6%), dry mouth (2–6%), diarrhea (2–7%), and increased appetite (1–6%) occurred in adult patients receiving extended-release IM olanzapine pamoate therapy in a short-term controlled clinical trial.

Nausea has been reported in less than 1% of patients receiving short-acting IM olanzapine in clinical trials.

Tongue edema has been reported in 1% or less of oral olanzapine-treated patients. Ileus and intestinal obstruction have been reported in less than 0.1% of patients receiving oral olanzapine in short-term clinical trials.

■ **Respiratory Effects** Rhinitis occurred in about 7%, increased cough in about 6%, and pharyngitis in about 4% of adult patients receiving oral olanzapine in short-term controlled clinical trials. Dyspnea has been reported in at least 1% of patients receiving oral olanzapine in short-term clinical trials. Epistaxis has been reported in 1% or less of olanzapine-treated patients. In addition, dyspnea and hyperventilation, which appeared to be dose related, have been reported together in a patient treated with oral olanzapine.

Lung edema has been reported in less than 0.1% of adult patients receiving oral olanzapine; however, a causal relationship to the drug has not been clearly established. Respiratory failure developed in a geriatric individual with chronic lung disease who was receiving olanzapine therapy; although not clearly established, it was suggested that the respiratory failure was due at least in part to the sedative effect of the drug.

■ **Dermatologic and Sensitivity Reactions** Alopecia and photosensitivity reaction have been reported in 1% or less of olanzapine-treated adults. Allergic/hypersensitivity reactions (e.g., anaphylactoid reaction, angioedema, pruritus, urticaria, rash) also have been reported during postmarketing surveillance of olanzapine. In addition, a case of Guillain-Barré syndrome associated with an apparent hypersensitivity reaction to olanzapine (manifested as rash and hepatic impairment) has been reported in at least one olanzapine-treated patient; the symptoms of the reaction gradually improved in this patient following discontinuance of the drug and plasma exchange.

Eruptive xanthomas, which are associated with hyperlipidemia, have occurred in several patients receiving olanzapine therapy. Leukocytoclastic vasculitis also has been reported in a geriatric patient receiving olanzapine and warfarin concurrently; the vasculitis improved following discontinuance of olanzapine in this patient but recurred when the drug was subsequently reintroduced.

Drug Reaction with Eosinophilia and Systemic Symptoms Drug reaction with eosinophilia and systemic symptoms (DRESS; also known as multiorgan hypersensitivity and hypersensitivity syndrome), a rare and serious dermatologic reaction, has been reported in patients receiving olanzapine. DRESS, which can be fatal in up to 10% of cases, consists of a combination of 3 or more of the following manifestations: cutaneous reaction (e.g., rash, exfoliative dermatitis), eosinophilia, fever, lymphadenopathy, and one or more systemic complications such as hepatitis, myocarditis, pericarditis, pancreatitis, nephritis, and pneumonitis. DRESS may start as a rash that can spread all over the body and include fever, lymphadenopathy, facial swelling, and injury to organs (including the liver, kidneys, lungs, heart, or pancreas) and possibly death.

FDA has identified 23 cases of DRESS, including one fatal case, associated with olanzapine use worldwide that were reported to its adverse event reporting system between 1996 and May 10, 2016. The median time to onset of symptoms in these cases was 19 days after initiation of olanzapine therapy and the median duration of olanzapine therapy was 2 months. The median reported olanzapine dosage was 20 mg daily; however, DRESS has been reported at olanzapine dosages as low as 5 mg daily. The 22 non-fatal cases all reported serious outcomes, including 18 that required hospitalization. Complete resolution of symptoms was reported in 9 cases after discontinuance of olanzapine. In one case, symptoms of DRESS recurred after reinitiation of the drug. In the fatal case, death was attributed to acute cardiac failure related to olanzapine; during hospitalization, the patient had an initial episode of DRESS, followed by a recurrence of DRESS. However, the patient in this case was taking multiple other drugs that may have contributed to death.

A published case report describes a severe and generalized pruritic eruption, fever, eosinophilia, and toxic hepatitis that developed in an adult male patient 60 days after beginning olanzapine therapy. The manifestations of DRESS/hypersensitivity syndrome in this patient improved following discontinuance of the drug, and skin and liver biopsy results suggested that the syndrome was caused by olanzapine. Another case of DRESS/hypersensitivity syndrome, which was manifested as rash, edema, generalized lymphadenopathy, hepatomegaly, eosinophilia, fever, and cough and confirmed by patch testing, was reported in an olanzapine-treated patient. (See Drug Reaction with Eosinophilia and Systemic Symptoms under Cautions: Precautions and Contraindications.)

■ **Local Effects** Pain at the injection site has been reported in at least 1% of patients receiving short-acting IM olanzapine in controlled clinical trials.

Injection site reactions were reported in 3.6% of patients receiving extended-release olanzapine pamoate IM in a short-term, placebo-controlled clinical trial, which included pain at the injection site, buttock pain, injection site mass, induration, and injection site induration. Pain at the injection site was reported most frequently (in 2.3% of patients). The injection site reactions were generally mild to moderate in severity, and none of the affected patients discontinued therapy because of the reactions.

■ **Genitourinary Effects** Urinary incontinence has been reported in approximately 2% of adult patients receiving oral olanzapine in short-term controlled clinical trials, although a causal relationship to the drug remains to be established. Amenorrhea, breast pain, decreased menstruation, increased menstruation, menorrhagia, metrorrhagia, lactation disorder, and gynecomastia have been reported in 1% or less of olanzapine-treated patients.

Impotence, polyuria, urinary frequency, urinary retention, urinary urgency, and impaired urination have been reported in 1% or less of adult patients receiving oral olanzapine in short-term clinical trials.

Priapism has been reported in several male patients and at least one case of clitoral priapism has been reported in a female patient. The α-adrenergic blocking effect of olanzapine appears to be responsible for this rare but potentially serious adverse effect requiring immediate medical attention to prevent long-term consequences such as erectile dysfunction.

■ **Musculoskeletal Effects** Joint pain, back pain, and extremity (other than joint) pain have been reported in 5% of adult patients receiving oral olanzapine in short-term controlled clinical trials. Osteoporosis has been reported in less than 0.1% of patients receiving oral olanzapine. Rhabdomyolysis also has been reported rarely in olanzapine-treated patients and may be seen as one of the clinical features of NMS. (See Neuroleptic Malignant Syndrome in Cautions: Nervous System Effects.)

■ **Ocular Effects** Amblyopia has been reported in 3% of adult patients receiving oral olanzapine in short-term clinical trials. Accommodation abnormality and dry eyes have been reported in 1% or less of oral olanzapine-treated patients. In addition, mydriasis has been reported in less than 0.1% of patients receiving oral olanzapine.

■ **Hematologic Effects** In clinical trial and/or postmarketing experience, leukopenia and neutropenia temporally related to antipsychotic agents, including olanzapine, have been reported. Agranulocytosis also has been reported.

Possible risk factors for leukopenia and neutropenia include a preexisting low leukocyte count and a history of drug-induced leukopenia or neutropenia. Therefore, patients with a history of clinically important low leukocyte count or drug-induced leukopenia and/or neutropenia should have their complete blood count monitored frequently during the first few months of olanzapine therapy. Discontinuance of olanzapine should be considered at the first sign of a clinically important decline in leukocyte count in the absence of other causative factors.

Patients with clinically significant neutropenia should be carefully monitored for fever or other signs or symptoms of infection and promptly treated if such signs or symptoms occur. In patients with severe neutropenia (absolute neutrophil count [ANC] less than 1000/mm^3), olanzapine should be discontinued and the leukocyte count monitored until recovery occurs.

Lithium reportedly has been used successfully in the treatment of several cases of leukopenia and neutropenia associated with aripiprazole, clozapine, olanzapine, and some other drugs; however, further clinical experience is needed to confirm these anecdotal findings.

Ecchymosis has been reported in 5% of adult patients receiving oral olanzapine in short-term clinical trials; however, a causal relationship to the drug remains to be established. Leukopenia and thrombocytopenia have been reported in less than 1% of patients receiving oral olanzapine. During premarketing clinical trials, asymptomatic elevation of the eosinophil count was reported in approximately 0.3% of patients receiving oral olanzapine.

■ **Other Adverse Effects** Accidental injury has been reported in approximately 12% of adult patients, and fever has been reported in approximately 6% of adult patients receiving oral olanzapine in short-term clinical trials. Chills and facial edema have been reported in 1% or less of oral olanzapine-treated patients. In addition, chills accompanied by fever, hangover effect, and sudden death have been reported in less than 0.1% of patients receiving oral olanzapine; however, a causal relationship to the drug has not been clearly established. Discontinuation reaction (diaphoresis, nausea, or vomiting) also has been reported during postmarketing surveillance of olanzapine.

Pancreatitis, which has been fatal in some cases, has occurred rarely in patients receiving atypical antipsychotic agents, including olanzapine, clozapine, and risperidone. In most of these cases, pancreatitis developed within 6 months of initiation of atypical antipsychotic therapy. Although the precise mechanism for this effect remains to be established, it has been suggested that it may be due at least in part to the adverse metabolic effects associated with these drugs.

■ **Precautions and Contraindications** Olanzapine shares many of the toxic potentials of other antipsychotic agents (e.g., other atypical antipsychotic agents, phenothiazines), and the usual precautions associated with therapy with these agents should be observed. (See Cautions in the Phenothiazines General Statement 28:16.08.24.)

When olanzapine is used in combination with fluoxetine, the usual cautions, precautions, and contraindications associated with fluoxetine must be considered in addition to those associated with olanzapine.

Laboratory Test Monitoring The manufacturer recommends fasting blood glucose testing and lipid profile determinations at the beginning of olanzapine therapy and periodically during treatment with the drug. (See Cautions: Endocrine and Metabolic Effects and see also Dyslipidemia and Hyperglycemia and Diabetes Mellitus under Cautions: Precautions and Contraindications.)

Hyperprolactinemia Similar to other antipsychotic agents, olanzapine can cause elevated serum prolactin concentrations, which may persist during chronic use of the drug. (See Hyperprolactinemia under Cautions: Endocrine and Metabolic Effects.) Clinical disturbances such as galactorrhea, amenorrhea, gynecomastia, and impotence have been associated with prolactin-elevating drugs. In addition, chronic hyperprolactinemia associated with hypogonadism may lead to decreased bone density.

If olanzapine therapy is considered in a patient with previously detected breast cancer, clinicians should consider that approximately one-third of human breast cancers are prolactin-dependent in vitro.

Cognitive and Motor Impairment Dose-related somnolence occurred in 26% of patients receiving oral olanzapine compared with 15% of those receiving placebo, and resulted in discontinuance of the drug in 0.4% of the patients in the premarketing database. Sedation occurred in 8% of patients receiving extended-release olanzapine pamoate injection; somnolence and sedation resulted in discontinuance of the drug in 0.6% of patients in the premarketing database.

Because of olanzapine's sedative effects and because the drug potentially may impair judgment, thinking, and motor skills, olanzapine-treated patients should be cautioned about operating hazardous machinery, including driving a motor vehicle, until they are reasonably certain that the drug does not adversely affect them. In addition, because of the risk of post-injection delirium/sedation syndrome, patients receiving extended-release olanzapine pamoate injection should not drive or operate heavy machinery for the remainder of the day after each injection.

Seizures Although seizures occurred in about 0.9% of patients receiving oral olanzapine in controlled clinical trials and in 0.15% of patients receiving extended-release olanzapine pamoate injection during premarketing testing, it should be noted that confounding factors that may have contributed to the occurrence of seizures were present in many of these cases. Olanzapine should be administered with caution to patients with a history of seizures, patients with conditions known to lower the seizure threshold (e.g., dementia of the Alzheimer's type), and during concurrent therapy with drugs that may lower the seizure threshold.

Body Temperature Regulation Because disruption of the body's ability to reduce core body temperature has been associated with the use of antipsychotic agents, caution is advised when olanzapine is administered in patients exposed to conditions that may contribute to an elevation in core body temperature. Such conditions include strenuous exercise, exposure to extreme heat, concomitant use of drugs with anticholinergic activity, or dehydration. Patients receiving olanzapine should be advised regarding appropriate precautions to avoid overheating and dehydration. Patients also should be advised to contact their clinician immediately if they become severely ill and have some or all of the symptoms of dehydration, including sweating too much or not at all, dry mouth, feeling very hot or thirsty, and unable to produce urine.

Hepatic Effects Because clinically important serum ALT elevations (3 or more times the upper limit of the normal range) were observed in adults and adolescents exposed to oral olanzapine and adults exposed to extended-release IM olanzapine pamoate in placebo-controlled clinical studies, the manufacturer states that olanzapine should be used with caution in patients with signs and symptoms of hepatic impairment, in patients with preexisting conditions associated with limited hepatic functional reserve, and in patients who are being treated concurrently with potentially hepatotoxic drugs.

Drug Reaction with Eosinophilia and Systemic Symptoms Drug reaction with eosinophilia and systemic symptoms (DRESS; also known as multiorgan hypersensitivity and hypersensitivity syndrome) has been reported in olanzapine-treated patients. (See Drug Reaction with Eosinophilia and Systemic Symptoms under Cautions: Dermatologic and Sensitivity Reactions.) Patients receiving olanzapine should be informed about the risk of DRESS and advised to seek immediate medical care if symptoms suggestive of DRESS, including rash, fever, facial swelling, and/or lymphadenopathy, occur. There currently is no specific treatment for DRESS. Management of the syndrome involves early recognition, immediate discontinuance of olanzapine if DRESS is suspected, and initiation of supportive care. Corticosteroid therapy also should be considered in cases of DRESS with extensive organ involvement.

Individuals with Phenylketonuria Individuals with phenylketonuria (i.e., homozygous genetic deficiency of phenylalanine hydroxylase) and other individuals who must restrict their intake of phenylalanine should be warned that olanzapine orally disintegrating tablets contain aspartame (e.g., NutraSweet®), which is metabolized in the GI tract to provide phenylalanine following oral administration; the respective manufacturer's labeling should be consulted for specific information regarding phenylalanine content of individual preparations and dosage strengths.

Dysphagia Esophageal dysmotility and aspiration have been associated with the use of antipsychotic agents. Aspiration pneumonia is a common cause of morbidity and mortality in patients with advanced Alzheimer's disease. The manufacturer states that olanzapine is *not* approved for the treatment of Alzheimer's disease.

Patients with Concomitant Illness Clinical experience with olanzapine in patients with certain concurrent systemic diseases is limited. Olanzapine has demonstrated anticholinergic activity in vitro and constipation, dryness of the mouth, and tachycardia, possibly related to the drug's anticholinergic effects, have occurred in premarketing clinical trials. Although these adverse effects did not often result in drug discontinuance, the manufacturer states that olanzapine should be used with caution in patients with clinically important prostatic hypertrophy, angle-closure glaucoma, or a history of paralytic ileus or related conditions.

Olanzapine has not been adequately evaluated in patients with a recent history of myocardial infarction or unstable cardiovascular disease to date and patients with these conditions were excluded from premarketing clinical trials. Because of the risk of orthostatic hypotension associated with olanzapine, the manufacturer states that the drug should be used with caution in patients with cardiovascular disease. (See Cautions: Cardiovascular Effects and see also Orthostatic Hypotension under Cautions: Precautions and Contraindications.)

Concomitant Medication or Alcohol Use Because of the potential for adverse drug interactions, the manufacturer recommends that patients receiving olanzapine be advised to notify their clinician if they are taking or plan to take other olanzapine-containing preparations (e.g., Symbyax® [an olanzapine/fluoxetine combination]). Patients receiving olanzapine should also be advised to inform their clinician if they are taking, plan to take, or have stopped taking any prescription or nonprescription (over-the-counter) medications, including herbal supplements. The manufacturer also recommends that patients be advised to avoid alcohol while receiving the drug. (See Drug Interactions.)

Tardive Dyskinesia Because use of antipsychotic agents may be associated with tardive dyskinesia, a syndrome of potentially irreversible, involuntary, dyskinetic movements, olanzapine should be prescribed in a manner that is most likely to minimize the occurrence of this syndrome. Chronic antipsychotic treatment generally should be reserved for patients who suffer from a chronic illness that is known to respond to antipsychotic agents, and for whom alternative, equally effective, but potentially less harmful treatments are not available or appropriate. In patients who do require chronic treatment, the smallest dosage and the shortest duration of treatment producing a satisfactory clinical response should be sought, and the need for continued treatment should be reassessed periodically.

The APA currently recommends that patients receiving second-generation antipsychotic agents be assessed clinically for abnormal involuntary movements every 12 months and that patients considered to be at increased risk for tardive dyskinesia be assessed every 6 months. (See Tardive Dyskinesia under Cautions: Nervous System Effects.)

Falls Olanzapine therapy may cause somnolence, postural hypotension, and motor and sensory instability, which may lead to falls; as a consequence, fractures or other injuries may occur. For patients with diseases or conditions or receiving other drugs that could exacerbate these effects, fall risk assessments should be completed when initiating antipsychotic treatment and periodically during long-term therapy.

Dispensing and Administration Precautions Because of similarities in spelling, dosage intervals (once daily), and tablet strengths (5 and 10 mg) of Zyprexa® (the trade name for olanzapine) and Zyrtec® (the trade name for cetirizine hydrochloride, an antihistamine), several dispensing or prescribing errors have been reported to the manufacturer of Zyprexa®. These medication errors may result in unnecessary adverse events or a potential relapse in patients with schizophrenia or bipolar disorder. Therefore, the manufacturer of Zyprexa® cautions that extra care should be exercised in ensuring the accuracy of written prescriptions for Zyprexa® and Zyrtec® such as printing both the proprietary (brand) and nonproprietary (generic) names on all prescriptions for these drugs. The manufacturer also recommends that pharmacists assess various measures of avoiding dispensing errors and implement them as appropriate (e.g., placing drugs with similar names apart from one another on pharmacy shelves, patient counseling).

Leukopenia, Neutropenia, and Agranulocytosis In clinical trial and/or postmarketing experience, leukopenia and neutropenia temporally related to antipsychotic agents, including olanzapine, have been reported; agranulocytosis also has been reported.

Because possible risk factors for leukopenia and neutropenia include a preexisting low leukocyte count and a history of drug-induced leukopenia and neutropenia, the manufacturer states that patients with a history of clinically important low leukocyte count or drug-induced leukopenia and/or neutropenia should have their complete blood count monitored frequently during the first few months of olanzapine therapy. Discontinuance of olanzapine should be considered at the first sign of a clinically important decline in leukocyte count in the absence of other causative factors.

Patients with clinically significant neutropenia should be carefully monitored for fever or other signs or symptoms of infection and promptly treated if such signs or symptoms occur. In patients with severe neutropenia (absolute neutrophil count [ANC] less than 1000/mm^3), olanzapine should be discontinued and the leukocyte count monitored until recovery occurs. (See Cautions: Hematologic Effects.)

Orthostatic Hypotension Orthostatic hypotension associated with dizziness, tachycardia, bradycardia, and/or syncope, particularly during the initial dosage titration period, has been reported in patients receiving oral olanzapine therapy. The risk of orthostatic hypotension and syncope may be minimized by initiating therapy with a dosage of 5 mg orally once daily. A more gradual titration to the target dosage should be considered if hypotension occurs. Patients should be cautioned about the risk of orthostatic hypotension, particularly during the initial dosage titration period and if the drug is given concurrently with drugs that may potentiate the orthostatic effect of olanzapine, including diazepam, or alcohol. Patients should be advised to change positions carefully to help prevent orthostatic hypotension and to lie down if they feel dizzy or faint until they feel better. Patients also should be advised to contact their clinician if they experience any of the following signs and symptoms associated with orthostatic hypotension: dizziness, fast or slow heart beat, or fainting.

Hypotension, bradycardia with or without hypotension, tachycardia, and syncope have been reported in patients receiving short-acting IM olanzapine. The use of maximum recommended dosages of IM olanzapine (i.e., 3 doses of 10 mg each given IM 2–4 hours apart) may be associated with a substantial risk of clinically important orthostatic hypotension. Patients who experience drowsiness or dizziness after the IM injection should remain recumbent until an examination indicates that they are not experiencing orthostatic hypotension, bradycardia, and/or hypoventilation. Patients requiring additional IM injections of olanzapine should be assessed for orthostatic hypotension prior to administration of any subsequent doses. Administration of additional IM doses to patients with clinically important postural change in blood pressure is not recommended.

Extended-release IM olanzapine pamoate therapy also may cause orthostatic hypotension associated with dizziness, tachycardia, bradycardia, and, in some cases, syncope.

The manufacturer states that olanzapine should be used with particular caution in patients with known cardiovascular disease (e.g., history of myocardial infarction or ischemia, heart failure, conduction abnormalities), cerebrovascular disease, and/or other conditions that would predispose patients to hypotension (e.g., dehydration, hypovolemia, concomitant antihypertensive therapy) where the occurrence of syncope, hypotension, and/or bradycardia might put the patient at increased risk. The manufacturer also states that the drug should be used with caution in patients receiving other drugs that can induce hypotension, bradycardia, or respiratory and CNS depression. (See Drug Interactions.) In such patients who have never taken oral olanzapine, tolerability should be established with oral olanzapine before initiating extended-release IM olanzapine pamoate therapy.

Concurrent administration of short-acting IM olanzapine and parenteral benzodiazepines is not recommended due to the potential for excessive sedation and cardiorespiratory depression. If use of short-acting IM olanzapine in combination with parenteral benzodiazepine therapy is considered, careful evaluation of the patient's clinical status for excessive sedation and cardiorespiratory depression is recommended.

Weight Gain Olanzapine therapy may result in weight gain. In olanzapine-treated adolescent patients, both the magnitude of weight gain and the proportion of patients who had clinically important weight gain were greater compared with adult patients with comparable exposures. (See Endocrine and Metabolic Effects under Cautions and see also Cautions: Pediatric Precautions.)

The potential consequences of weight gain should be considered in adults and adolescents prior to starting olanzapine therapy. All patients receiving the drug should be advised that weight gain has occurred during olanzapine treatment and receive regular monitoring of their weight.

Dyslipidemia Because undesirable changes in serum lipids have been observed with olanzapine therapy in both adults and adolescents, the manufacturer recommends appropriate clinical monitoring, including baseline and periodic follow-up lipid evaluations, in all patients receiving the drug. (See Endocrine and Metabolic Effects under Cautions and see also Cautions: Pediatric Precautions.)

Hyperglycemia and Diabetes Mellitus Because hyperglycemia, sometimes severe and associated with ketoacidosis, hyperosmolar coma, or death, has been reported in patients receiving atypical antipsychotic agents, including olanzapine, the manufacturer states that clinicians should consider the risks and benefits when prescribing olanzapine to adult and adolescent patients with an established diagnosis of diabetes mellitus or in those having borderline increased blood glucose concentrations (i.e., fasting values of 100–126 mg/dL or nonfasting values of 140–200 mg/dL). The manufacturer recommends that all patients beginning olanzapine therapy undergo fasting blood glucose testing upon therapy initiation and periodically during treatment. The manufacturer also recommends that all patients receiving olanzapine be regularly monitored for worsening of glucose control. Any patient who develops manifestations of hyperglycemia (e.g., polydipsia, polyphagia, polyuria, weakness) during treatment with an atypical antipsychotic should undergo fasting blood glucose testing. In some cases, patients who developed hyperglycemia while receiving an atypical antipsychotic have required continuance of antidiabetic treatment despite discontinuance of the suspect drug; in other cases, hyperglycemia resolved with discontinuance of the antipsychotic or with continuance of both the suspect drug and initiation of antidiabetic treatment.

Various experts have developed additional recommendations for the management of diabetes risks in patients receiving atypical antipsychotics; these include initial screening measures and regular monitoring (e.g., determination of diabetes risk factors; BMI determination using weight and height; waist circumference; blood pressure; fasting blood glucose; HbA_{1c}; fasting lipid profile), as well as provision of patient education and referral to clinicians experienced in the treatment of diabetes, when appropriate. Although some clinicians state that a switch from one atypical antipsychotic agent to another that has not been associated with substantial weight gain or diabetes should be considered in patients who experience weight gain (equal to or exceeding 5% of baseline body weight) or develop worsening glycemia or dyslipidemia at any time during therapy, such recommendations are controversial because differences in risk of developing diabetes associated with use of the different atypical antipsychotics remain to be fully established. Many clinicians consider antipsychotic efficacy the most important factor when making treatment decisions and suggest that detrimental effects of switching from a beneficial treatment regimen also should be considered in addition to any potential for exacerbation or development of medical conditions (e.g., diabetes). Decisions to alter drug therapy should be made on an individual basis, weighing the potential risks and benefits of the particular drug in each patient.

Neuroleptic Malignant Syndrome Neuroleptic malignant syndrome (NMS), a potentially fatal syndrome requiring immediate discontinuance of the drug and intensive symptomatic treatment, has been reported in patients receiving antipsychotic agents, including olanzapine. If a patient requires antipsychotic therapy following recovery from NMS, the potential reintroduction of drug therapy should be carefully considered. If antipsychotic therapy is reintroduced, the dosage generally should be increased gradually, and an antipsychotic agent other than the agent believed to have precipitated NMS generally should be chosen. In addition, such patients should be carefully monitored since recurrences of NMS have been reported in some patients. (See Neuroleptic Malignant Syndrome under Cautions: Nervous System Effects.)

Suicide Because the possibility of a suicide attempt is inherent in patients with schizophrenia and bipolar disorder, close supervision of high-risk patients is recommended during olanzapine therapy. The manufacturer recommends that the drug be prescribed in the smallest quantity consistent with good patient management to reduce the risk of overdosage.

Geriatric Patients with Dementia-related Psychosis Geriatric patients with dementia-related psychosis treated with antipsychotic drugs are at increased risk of death compared with patients receiving placebo. Analyses of 17 placebo-controlled trials (modal duration of 10 weeks) revealed an approximate 1.6- to 1.7-fold increase in mortality among geriatric patients receiving atypical antipsychotic drugs (i.e., aripiprazole, olanzapine, quetiapine, risperidone) compared with that observed in patients receiving placebo. Over the course of a typical 10-week controlled trial, the rate of death in drug-treated patients was about 4.5% compared with a rate of about 2.6% in the placebo group. Although the causes of death were varied, most of the deaths appeared to be either cardiovascular (e.g., heart failure, sudden death) or infectious (e.g., pneumonia) in nature. Observational studies suggest that, similar to atypical antipsychotics, treatment with conventional (first-generation) antipsychotics may increase mortality; the extent to which the findings of increased mortality in observational studies may be attributed to the antipsychotic drug as opposed to some characteristic(s) of the patients remains unclear. In placebo-controlled trials of geriatric patients with dementia-associated psychosis, the incidence of death was significantly greater in olanzapine-treated patients than in those receiving placebo (3.5 versus 1.5%, respectively).

Adverse cerebrovascular events (e.g., stroke, transient ischemic attack), including fatalities, have been reported in clinical trials of olanzapine in geriatric patients with dementia-related psychosis. In placebo-controlled studies, a significantly higher incidence of adverse cerebrovascular events was observed in olanzapine-treated patients compared with those receiving placebo.

The manufacturer states that olanzapine is *not* approved for the treatment of patients with dementia-related psychosis. (See Cautions: Geriatric Precautions.)

Post-injection Delirium/Sedation Syndrome Clinicians should discuss the potential risk of post-injection delirium/sedation syndrome (PDSS) with patients each time they prescribe and administer extended-release olanzapine pamoate injection (Zyprexa® Relprevv). (See Post-injection Delirium/Sedation Syndrome under Cautions: Nervous System Effects.)

Patients should be advised not to drive or operate heavy machinery for the remainder of the day following each injection, and should be vigilant for symptoms of PDSS and able to obtain medical assistance if needed. If PDSS is suspected, close medical supervision and monitoring should be instituted in a facility capable of resuscitation. For additional information concerning the pathogenesis, clinical manifestations, and management of possible PDSS and other types of olanzapine overdosage, see Acute Toxicity.

In March 2015, FDA concluded a review of 2 unexplained deaths that occurred 3–4 days after the patients received an appropriate dose of long-acting olanzapine pamoate injection (Zyprexa® Relprevv), which is well beyond the 3-hour post-injection monitoring period required under the current REMS program. Both patients were found to have very high blood concentrations of olanzapine after death. High doses of olanzapine can cause delirium, cardiopulmonary arrest, cardiac arrhythmias, and reduced levels of consciousness, ranging from sedation to coma. The review suggested that much of the drug level increase could have occurred after death. It is unclear whether the patients in these 2 cases died from PDSS; FDA states that the results of their review were inconclusive, and that the possibility that the deaths were caused by rapid but delayed entry of the drug into the bloodstream following IM injection could not be excluded. In clinical trials, cases of PDSS were observed within 3 hours of administration of olanzapine pamoate; however, no deaths were reported. If therapy with extended-release olanzapine pamoate is initiated or continued in patients, the FDA recommends that clinicians continue to follow the REMS requirements as well as the recommendations in the prescribing information for Zyprexa® Relprevv. The FDA states that patients should not discontinue therapy with extended-release olanzapine pamoate injection without consulting their clinician. (See Extended-release Olanzapine Pamoate Injection for Schizophrenia under Dosage and Administration: Reconstitution and Administration.)

Contraindications The manufacturer states that there are no contraindications associated with oral or short-acting IM olanzapine monotherapy.

When olanzapine is used in combination with fluoxetine, the usual contraindications associated with fluoxetine must be considered.

When olanzapine is used as adjunctive therapy with lithium or valproate, the manufacturer advises clinicians to refer to prescribing information for those other drugs.

The manufacturer states that there are no contraindications associated with use of the long-acting IM formulation of olanzapine pamoate.

■ Pediatric Precautions The safety and effectiveness of oral olanzapine in the treatment of schizophrenia and manic or mixed episodes associated with bipolar I disorder were established in short-term clinical trials in adolescents (13–17 years of age). Use of oral olanzapine in such adolescents is supported by evidence from adequate and well-controlled clinical trials in which 268 adolescents received olanzapine in a dosage range of 2.5–20 mg daily. The recommended initial dosage for adolescents is lower than that for adults (see Dosage and Administration: Dosage). Compared with adults in clinical trials, adolescents were likely to gain more weight, experience increased sedation, and have greater increases in serum concentrations of total cholesterol, triglycerides, LDL-cholesterol, prolactin, and hepatic transaminases. (See Pediatric Considerations under Psychotic Disorders: Schizophrenia in Uses, Pediatric Considerations under Bipolar Disorder in Uses, and Cautions.)

When deciding among the alternative treatments available for adolescents with schizophrenia or bipolar disorder, clinicians should consider the increased potential for weight gain and dyslipidemia with olanzapine in adolescents as compared with adults. Clinicians also should consider the potential long-term risks when prescribing olanzapine to adolescents; in many cases, this may lead them to consider prescribing other drugs first in such patients.

Adolescent patients and/or their caregivers should be advised that adolescent patients receiving olanzapine are likely to gain more weight and to develop sedation, dyslipidemia, higher prolactin elevations, and more elevated serum aminotransferase concentrations compared with adults. Adolescent patients and/or their caregivers also should be advised about the potential long-term risks associated with olanzapine therapy and that the risks may lead them to consider other drugs first.

Pediatric patients with schizophrenia or bipolar disorder should be advised that olanzapine is indicated as an integral part of a total treatment program that may include other measures (e.g., psychological, educational, social) for patients with the disorder. In addition, pediatric patients should be informed that atypical antipsychotic agents are not intended for use in pediatric patients who exhibit symptoms secondary to environmental factors and/or other primary psychiatric disorders. Appropriate educational placement is essential and psychosocial intervention is often helpful. The decision whether to prescribe atypical antipsychotic medication in pediatric patients with schizophrenia or bipolar disorder will depend upon the clinician's assessment of the chronicity and severity of the patient's symptoms.

Because adolescents receiving olanzapine are more likely to gain more weight and experience other metabolic problems compared with adults receiving the drug (see Cautions: Endocrine and Metabolic Effects), the American Academy of Child and Adolescent Psychiatry (AACAP) currently recommends that pediatric patients receiving atypical antipsychotic agents for the management of bipolar disorder have baseline body mass index (BMI), waist circumference, blood pressure, fasting glucose, and fasting lipid parameters determined at baseline. The AACAP also recommends that the BMI be followed monthly for the initial 3 months of therapy and then every 3 months thereafter. In addition, these experts recommend that blood pressure, fasting glucose, and lipid parameters be assessed after 3 months of therapy and then annually thereafter. (See Cautions: Precautions and Contraindications.)

The manufacturer states that safety and efficacy of oral olanzapine for the treatment of schizophrenia or manic or mixed episodes associated with bipolar I disorder in children and adolescents younger than 13 years of age have not been established. However, the drug has been used in a limited number of children and other adolescents with childhood-onset schizophrenia (see Pediatric Considerations under Psychotic Disorders: Schizophrenia, in Uses).

The safety and efficacy of oral olanzapine in combination with fluoxetine for the treatment of acute depressive episodes associated with bipolar I disorder were established in a short-term clinical trial in pediatric patients 10–17 years of age. Use of oral olanzapine and fluoxetine in such children and adolescents is supported by evidence from a well-controlled clinical trial in which 255 pediatric patients received olanzapine in a dosage range of 3–12 mg daily. The recommended initial dosage of olanzapine in combination with fluoxetine for adolescents is lower than that for adults (see Dosage and Administration: Dosage).

The manufacturer states that the safety and efficacy of oral olanzapine in combination with fluoxetine for the treatment of treatment-resistant depression have not been established in patients younger than 18 years of age.

The manufacturer states that the safety and efficacy of oral olanzapine in combination with fluoxetine have not been established in pediatric patients younger than 10 years of age.

Oral olanzapine also has been effective and well tolerated in a limited number of children† and adolescents with pervasive developmental disorder, including autistic disorder†. Additional controlled and longer-term studies are needed to confirm these initial findings and to evaluate the relative benefits and risks of olanzapine therapy in such patients.

The manufacturer states that the safety and efficacy of short-acting IM olanzapine have not been established in patients younger than 18 years of age.

The manufacturer states that the safety and efficacy of extended-release olanzapine pamoate IM injection in patients younger than 18 years of age have not been established.

■ Geriatric Precautions In premarketing clinical studies with oral olanzapine, 11% (263 of 2500) of the patients were 65 years of age or older. Clinical experience in patients with schizophrenia generally has not revealed differences in tolerability of oral olanzapine in geriatric patients compared with younger adults.

The first phase of the large-scale Clinical Antipsychotic Trials of Intervention Effectiveness—Alzheimer's Disease (CATIE-AD) trial was designed to evaluate the overall effectiveness of atypical antipsychotic agents in the treatment of psychosis, aggression, and agitation associated with Alzheimer's disease. Patients in this multicenter, double-blind, placebo-controlled trial were randomized to receive either olanzapine, quetiapine, risperidone, or placebo for up to 36 weeks; the principal outcomes were the time from initial treatment until discontinuance of treatment for any reason and the number of patients with at least minimum improvement on the Clinical Global Impression of Change (CGIC) Scale at 12 weeks. No statistically significant differences were found among the 4 groups with regard to the time until discontinuation of treatment for any reason; patients remained on olanzapine, quetiapine, risperidone, and placebo for median times of approximately 8, 5, 7, and 8 weeks, respectively. In addition, no significant differences in CGIC Scale improvements were noted. However, patients receiving atypical antipsychotic therapy reportedly experienced more frequent adverse effects (e.g., drowsiness, weight gain, adverse extrapyramidal effects, confusion, and psychotic symptoms) compared with those receiving placebo. The authors stated that these results indicate that the overall therapeutic benefit of atypical antipsychotics in patients with Alzheimer's disease may be offset by the potential risk of adverse effects.

Studies in patients with dementia-related psychosis have suggested that oral olanzapine may have a different tolerability profile in patients 65 years of age or older with this condition compared with younger patients with schizophrenia. Geriatric patients with dementia-related psychosis receiving antipsychotic agents, including olanzapine, are at an increased risk of death compared with that among patients receiving placebo. Analyses of 17 placebo-controlled trials (average duration of 10 weeks) revealed an approximate 1.6- to 1.7-fold increase in mortality among geriatric patients receiving atypical antipsychotic drugs (i.e., olanzapine, aripiprazole, quetiapine, risperidone) compared with that in patients receiving placebo. Over the course of a typical 10-week controlled trial, the rate of death in drug-treated patients was about 4.5% compared with a rate of about 2.6% in the placebo group. Although the causes of death were varied, most of the deaths appeared to be either cardiovascular (e.g., heart failure, sudden death) or infectious (e.g., pneumonia) in nature.

In placebo-controlled trials with oral olanzapine in geriatric individuals with dementia-related psychosis, an increased incidence of death also was observed; the incidence of death in olanzapine-treated patients was significantly higher than in patients receiving placebo (3.5% and 1.5%, respectively). In addition, a significantly higher incidence of adverse cerebrovascular events (e.g., stroke, transient ischemic attack), including fatalities, was observed in patients receiving olanzapine compared with those receiving placebo in these trials. In 5 placebo-controlled studies of olanzapine in geriatric individuals with dementia-related psychosis, certain treatment-emergent adverse effects, including falls, somnolence, peripheral edema, abnormal gait, urinary incontinence, lethargy, increased weight, asthenia, pyrexia, pneumonia, dry mouth, and visual hallucinations, occurred in at least 2% of the patients and the incidence was significantly higher than in patients receiving placebo. Discontinuance of therapy because of adverse effects occurred in a significantly higher number of olanzapine-treated patients than in those receiving placebo (13% and 7%, respectively) in these studies.

The manufacturer states that olanzapine is *not* approved for the treatment of patients with dementia-related psychosis. Some clinicians recommend that the potential risks, therapeutic benefits, and individual needs of patients be carefully considered prior to prescribing olanzapine and other atypical antipsychotic agents for the management of behavioral problems associated with Alzheimer's disease. For additional information on the use of antipsychotic agents in the management of dementia-related psychosis, see Geriatric Considerations under Uses: Psychotic Disorders, in the Phenothiazines General Statement 28:16.08.24.

The manufacturer states that the presence of factors that might decrease the clearance of or increase the pharmacodynamic response to olanzapine should lead to consideration of a lower initial dosage of the drug in geriatric patients.

Clinical studies of olanzapine in combination with fluoxetine did not include sufficient numbers of patients 65 years of age or older to determine whether they respond differently than younger patients.

Clinical studies of extended-release IM olanzapine pamoate did not include sufficient numbers of patients 65 years of age or older to determine whether they respond differently than younger patients.

■ Mutagenicity and Carcinogenicity Olanzapine did not exhibit genotoxic potential in the Ames reverse mutation test, in vivo micronucleus mutation test in mice, the chromosomal aberration test in Chinese hamster ovary cells, unscheduled DNA synthesis test in rat hepatocytes, induction of forward mutation test in mouse lymphoma cells, or in vivo sister chromatid exchange test in bone marrow of Chinese hamsters.

In oral carcinogenicity studies conducted in mice, olanzapine was administered in 2 studies of 78-weeks' duration at dosages of 3, 10, and 30 mg/kg initially then reduced to 20 mg/kg daily (equivalent to 0.8–5 times the maximum recommended human daily oral dosage on a mg/m^2 basis) and 0.25, 2, and 8 mg/kg daily (equivalent to 0.06–2 times the maximum recommended human daily oral dosage on a mg/m^2 basis). In oral carcinogenicity studies conducted in rats, olanzapine was administered for 2 years at dosages of 0.25, 1, 2.5, and 4 mg/kg daily in males (equivalent to 0.13–2 times the maximum recommended human daily oral dosage on a mg/m^2 basis) and 0.25, 1, 4, and 8 mg/kg daily in females (equivalent to 0.13–4 times the maximum recommended human daily oral dosage on a mg/m^2 basis). An increased incidence of liver hemangiomas and hemangiosarcomas was observed in one mouse study in female mice receiving 8 mg/kg of the drug daily (equivalent to 2 times the maximum recommended human daily oral dosage on a mg/m^2 basis). The incidence of these tumors was not increased in another study in female mice receiving 10 or 30 mg/kg (later reduced to 20 mg/kg) of olanzapine daily (equivalent to 2–5 times the maximum recommended human daily oral dosage on a mg/m^2 basis); in this study, there was a high incidence of early mortalities in males in the 30 mg/kg (later reduced to 20 mg/kg) daily group. The incidence of mammary gland adenomas and adenocarcinomas was increased in female mice receiving 2 mg/kg or more of olanzapine daily and in female rats receiving 4 mg/kg or more of the drug daily (equivalent to 0.5 and 2 times the maximum recommended human daily oral dosage on a mg/m^2 basis, respectively).

Antipsychotic agents have been shown to chronically elevate prolactin concentrations in rodents. Serum prolactin concentrations were not measured during the olanzapine carcinogenicity studies; however, measurements during subchronic toxicity studies demonstrated that olanzapine administration produced up to a fourfold increase in serum prolactin concentrations in rats receiving the same dosages used in the carcinogenicity study. In addition, an increase in mammary gland neoplasms has been observed in rodents following chronic administration of other antipsychotic agents and generally is considered to be prolactin-mediated. However, the clinical importance in humans of this finding of prolactin-mediated endocrine tumors in rodents is unknown.

■ Pregnancy, Fertility, and Lactation ***Pregnancy*** Limited experience to date with olanzapine administration during pregnancy has been encouraging and has not revealed evidence of any obvious teratogenic risks; however, additional cases of olanzapine exposure during pregnancy need to be evaluated to more fully determine the relative safety of olanzapine and other antipsychotic agents when administered during pregnancy. The manufacturer states that there have been 7 pregnancies reported during clinical trials with olanzapine, including 2 resulting in normal births, one resulting in neonatal death due to a cardiovascular defect, 3 therapeutic abortions, and one spontaneous abortion. In a separate compilation of pregnancy exposures to olanzapine reported to the manufacturer during clinical trials and from spontaneous reports worldwide, outcomes were available from 23 prospectively collected, olanzapine-exposed pregnancies. Spontaneous abortion occurred in 13% of these pregnancies, stillbirth in 5%, major malformations in 0%, and prematurity in 5%; these rates were all within the range of normal historical control rates. In 11 retrospectively collected, olanzapine-exposed pregnancies, there was one case of dysplastic kidney, one case of Down's syndrome, and one case of heart murmur and sudden infant death syndrome at 2 months of age. In another study, the majority of women with schizophrenia receiving atypical antipsychotic agents were found to be overweight and to have reduced folate intake and low serum folate concentrations, which may increase the potential risk of neural tube defects. In a prospective, comparative trial assessing pregnancy outcome in women receiving atypical antipsychotic agents (olanzapine, clozapine, risperidone, and quetiapine) during pregnancy, atypical antipsychotics did not appear to be associated with an increased risk of major congenital malformations. In addition, several case reports have described healthy infants born to women without complications despite prenatal exposure to olanzapine.

Neonates exposed to antipsychotic agents, including olanzapine, during the third trimester of pregnancy are at risk for extrapyramidal and/or withdrawal symptoms following delivery. There have been reports of agitation, hypertonia, hypotonia, tardive dyskinetic-like symptoms, tremor, somnolence, respiratory distress, and feeding disorder in these neonates. The majority of cases were also confounded by other factors, including concomitant use of other drugs known to be associated with withdrawal symptoms, prematurity, congenital malformations, and obstetrical and perinatal complications; however, some cases suggested that neonatal extrapyramidal and withdrawal symptoms may occur with exposure to antipsychotic agents alone. Some of the cases described time of symptom onset, which ranged from birth to one month after birth. Any neonate exhibiting extrapyramidal or withdrawal symptoms following in utero exposure to antipsychotic agents should be monitored. Symptoms were self-limiting in some neonates but varied in severity; some infants required intensive care unit support and prolonged hospitalization. For further information on extrapyramidal and withdrawal symptoms in neonates, see Cautions: Pregnancy, Fertility, and Lactation, in the Phenothiazines General Statement 28:16.08.24.

The manufacturer and some clinicians state that there are no adequate and well-controlled studies to date using olanzapine in pregnant women, and the drug should be used during pregnancy only when the potential benefits justify the potential risks to the fetus. Women should be advised to notify their clinician if they become pregnant or plan to become pregnant during therapy with the drug. In addition, clinicians should advise women of childbearing potential about the benefits and risks of using antipsychotic agents during pregnancy. Patients should also be advised not to stop taking their antipsychotic agent if they become pregnant without first consulting with their clinician, since abruptly discontinuing the drugs can cause clinically important complications.

Parturition in rats was not affected by olanzapine. The effect of olanzapine on labor and delivery is unknown.

In oral reproduction studies in rats receiving dosages of up to 18 mg/kg daily and in rabbits at dosages of up to 30 mg/kg daily (equivalent to 9 and 30 times the maximum recommended human daily oral dosage on a mg/m^2 basis, respectively), no evidence of teratogenicity was observed. In an oral rat teratology study, early resorptions and increased numbers of nonviable fetuses were observed at a dosage of 18 mg/kg daily (9 times the maximum recommended human daily oral dosage on a mg/m^2 basis), and gestation was prolonged at a dosage of 10 mg/kg daily (equivalent to 5 times the maximum recommended human daily oral dosage on a mg/m^2 basis). In an oral rabbit teratology study, fetal toxicity, which was manifested as increased resorptions and decreased fetal weight, occurred at a maternally toxic dosage of 30 mg/kg daily (equivalent to 30 times the maximum recommended human daily oral dosage on a mg/m^2 basis).

Fertility In an oral fertility and reproductive performance study in rats, male mating performance, but not fertility, was impaired at an olanzapine dosage of 22.4 mg/kg daily, and female fertility was decreased at a dosage of 3 mg/kg daily (equivalent to 11 and 1.5 times the maximum recommended human daily oral dosage on a mg/m^2 basis, respectively). Discontinuance of olanzapine administration reversed the effects on male mating performance. In a female rat fertility study, the precoital period was increased, and the mating index reduced at a dosage of 5 mg/kg daily (equivalent to 2.5 times the maximum recommended human daily oral dosage on a mg/m^2 basis). Diestrus was prolonged and estrus was delayed at a dosage of 1.1 mg/kg daily (equivalent to 0.6 times the maximum recommended human daily oral dosage on a mg/m^2 basis).

Lactation Olanzapine is distributed into milk. The mean dosage received by an infant at steady state is estimated to be about 1.8% of the maternal dosage. The manufacturer recommends that women receiving olanzapine not breast-feed.

Drug Interactions

■ Drugs Affecting Hepatic Microsomal Enzymes Olanzapine is a substrate for cytochrome P-450 (CYP) isoenzyme 1A2 and concomitant administration of drugs that induce CYP1A2 or glucuronyl transferase enzymes (e.g., carbamazepine, omeprazole, rifampin) may cause an increase in olanzapine clearance. Inhibitors of CYP1A2 (e.g., fluvoxamine) could potentially decrease olanzapine clearance. Although olanzapine is metabolized by multiple enzyme systems, induction or inhibition of a single enzyme may appreciably alter olanzapine clearance. Therefore, an increase or decrease in olanzapine dosage may be necessary during concomitant administration of olanzapine with specific drugs that induce or inhibit olanzapine metabolism, respectively.

Carbamazepine Carbamazepine therapy (200 mg twice daily for 2 weeks) causes an approximately 50% increase in the clearance of a single, 10-mg dose of olanzapine. The manufacturer of olanzapine states that higher dosages of carbamazepine may cause an even greater increase in olanzapine clearance. Increased clearance of olanzapine probably is caused by carbamazepine-induced induction of CYP1A2 activity.

Selective Serotonin-reuptake Inhibitors Concomitant administration of fluoxetine (60 mg as a single dose or 60 mg daily for 8 days) with a single 5-mg dose of oral olanzapine caused a small increase in peak plasma olanzapine concentrations (averaging 16%) and a small decrease (averaging 16%) in olanzapine clearance in one study; the elimination half-life was not substantially affected. A similar decrease in olanzapine clearance of 14% was observed in another study with concomitant administration of olanzapine doses of 6 or 12 mg and fluoxetine doses of 25 mg or more. Fluoxetine is an inhibitor of CYP2D6, and thereby may affect a minor metabolic pathway for olanzapine. Although the changes in pharmacokinetics are statistically significant when olanzapine and fluoxetine are given concurrently, the changes are unlikely to be clinically important in comparison to the overall variability observed between individuals; therefore, routine dosage adjustment is not recommended.

Fluvoxamine, a CYP1A2 inhibitor, has been shown to decrease the clearance of olanzapine, which is metabolized by CYP1A2; there is some evidence that fluvoxamine-induced CYP1A2 inhibition is dose dependent. In one pharmacokinetic study, peak plasma olanzapine concentrations increased by an average of 54 and 77% and area under the plasma concentration-time curve (AUC) increased by an average of 52 and 108% in female nonsmokers and male smokers, respectively, when fluvoxamine and olanzapine were administered concomitantly. Symptoms of olanzapine toxicity also have been reported in at least one patient during combined therapy. The manufacturer and some clinicians state that a lower olanzapine dosage should therefore be considered in patients receiving concomitant treatment with fluvoxamine. Preliminary data indicate that concurrent fluvoxamine administration may potentially be used to therapeutic advantage by reducing the daily dosage of olanzapine and thereby the cost of therapy; further controlled studies are needed to more fully evaluate this approach. Although combined therapy with olanzapine and fluvoxamine generally has been well tolerated and may be associated with clinical benefit, some clinicians recommend that caution be exercised and monitoring of plasma olanzapine concentrations be considered in patients receiving these drugs concurrently.

Preliminary results from a therapeutic drug monitoring service suggest that concurrent administration of sertraline and olanzapine does not substantially affect the pharmacokinetics of olanzapine.

Warfarin Concomitant administration of a single 20-mg dose of warfarin (which has a potential CYP2C9 interaction) and a single oral 10-mg dose of olanzapine did not substantially alter the pharmacokinetics of olanzapine.

■ **Drugs Metabolized by Hepatic Microsomal Enzymes** In vitro studies utilizing human liver microsomes suggest that olanzapine has little potential to inhibit metabolism of CYP1A2, CYP2C9, CYP2C19, CYP2D6, and CYP3A substrates. Therefore, clinically important drug interactions between olanzapine and drugs metabolized by these isoenzymes are considered unlikely.

■ **Anticholinergic Agents** Because of the potential for disruption of body temperature regulation, olanzapine should be used with caution in patients concurrently receiving other drugs with anticholinergic activity. (See Body Temperature Regulation under Cautions: Precautions and Contraindications.)

■ **Levodopa and Dopamine Agonists** Olanzapine may antagonize the effects of levodopa and dopamine agonists.

■ **Lamotrigine** In a multiple-dose study in healthy individuals, the pharmacokinetics of olanzapine and lamotrigine were not substantially affected when the drugs were administered concomitantly. In another multiple-dose study conducted in healthy volunteers, olanzapine did not substantially alter lamotrigine pharmacokinetics when the drugs were administered concurrently. However, the time to reach maximal plasma concentrations of lamotrigine was substantially prolonged in this study, possibly because of olanzapine's anticholinergic activity. The tolerability of this combination was found to be similar to that of olanzapine alone, with mild sedative effects reported in some patients receiving the drugs concurrently. Although routine dosage adjustment does not appear to be necessary when olanzapine and lamotrigine are given concurrently, adjustment in lamotrigine dosage may be necessary in some patients for therapeutic reasons when olanzapine therapy is initiated or discontinued. In addition, careful monitoring of patients receiving high dosages of olanzapine and lamotrigine has been recommended by some clinicians.

■ **Other CNS-Active Agents and Alcohol** Because of the prominent CNS actions of olanzapine, the manufacturer states that caution should be exercised when olanzapine is administered concomitantly with other centrally acting drugs and alcohol. The manufacturer also states that concomitant use of olanzapine with CNS agents that are associated with hypotension (e.g., diazepam) may potentiate the orthostatic hypotension associated with olanzapine.

Benzodiazepines Because of the prominent CNS actions of olanzapine, the manufacturer states that caution should be exercised when olanzapine is administered concomitantly with benzodiazepines. The manufacturer also states that concomitant use of olanzapine and diazepam or other benzodiazepines that are associated with hypotension may potentiate the orthostatic hypotension associated with olanzapine. However, administration of multiple doses of olanzapine did not substantially alter the pharmacokinetics of diazepam or its active metabolite *N*-desmethyldiazepam.

The pharmacokinetics of olanzapine, unconjugated lorazepam, and total lorazepam were not substantially affected when IM lorazepam (2 mg) was administered 1 hour after IM olanzapine (5 mg); however, increased somnolence was observed with this combination. Hypotension also has been reported when short-acting IM olanzapine and IM lorazepam have been administered concurrently. The manufacturer of olanzapine therefore states that concurrent use of short-acting IM olanzapine in conjunction with parenteral benzodiazepines is not recommended due to the potential for excessive sedation and cardiorespiratory depression.

Tricyclic Antidepressants Administration of single doses of olanzapine did not substantially affect the pharmacokinetics of imipramine or its active metabolite desipramine.

Lithium Multiple doses of oral olanzapine (10 mg for 8 days) did not affect the pharmacokinetics of a single dose of lithium. Although combined olanzapine and lithium therapy generally has been well tolerated in controlled clinical studies, rare cases of apparent lithium toxicity and adverse extrapyramidal effects, including oculogyric crisis, have been reported in patients receiving these drugs concurrently; the mechanism(s) for this potential drug interaction remains to be established. The manufacturer of olanzapine states that lithium dosage adjustment is not necessary during concurrent olanzapine administration.

Valproic Acid In vitro studies using human liver microsomes indicated that olanzapine has little potential to inhibit the major metabolic pathway (glucuronidation) of valproic acid. In addition, valproic acid has little potential effect on the metabolism of olanzapine in vitro. In a pharmacokinetic study, olanzapine administration (10 mg daily for 2 weeks) did not affect the steady-state plasma concentrations of valproic acid. However, substantially decreased plasma olanzapine concentrations have been reported in several patients following initiation of valproate in patients already receiving oral olanzapine; it was suggested that induction of the hepatic enzymes responsible for olanzapine's metabolism by valproate may have been responsible for these findings. Further studies are needed to determine whether a pharmacokinetic interaction exists between olanzapine and valproic acid since these drugs are frequently used in combination in clinical practice. The manufacturer of olanzapine currently states that routine dosage adjustment of valproic acid is not necessary during concurrent olanzapine administration.

Alcohol In a pharmacokinetic study, concomitant administration of a single dose of alcohol did not substantially alter the steady-state pharmacokinetics of olanzapine (given in dosages of up to 10 mg daily). However, concomitant use of olanzapine with alcohol potentiated the orthostatic hypotension associated with olanzapine. The manufacturer therefore states that alcohol should be avoided during olanzapine therapy.

■ **Hypotensive Agents** Olanzapine therapy potentially may enhance the effects of certain hypotensive agents during concurrent use. In addition, the administration of dopamine, epinephrine, and/or other sympathomimetic agents with β-agonist activity should be avoided in the treatment of olanzapine-induced hypotension, since such stimulation may worsen hypotension in the presence of olanzapine-induced α-blockade. (See Acute Toxicity: Treatment.)

■ **Antacids or Cimetidine** In pharmacokinetic studies, single doses of cimetidine (800 mg) or aluminum- and magnesium-containing antacids (30 mL) did not substantially affect the oral bioavailability of a single, 7.5-mg dose of olanzapine.

■ **Activated Charcoal** Concurrent administration of activated charcoal (1 g) reduced peak plasma concentrations and the AUC of a single, 7.5-mg oral dose of olanzapine by approximately 60%. Since peak plasma concentrations are not usually obtained until about 6 hours after oral administration, activated charcoal may be useful in the management of olanzapine intoxication. (See Acute Toxicity: Treatment.)

■ **Smoking** The manufacturer states that the clearance of olanzapine in smokers is approximately 40% higher than in nonsmokers. Therefore, plasma olanzapine concentrations generally are lower in smokers than in nonsmokers receiving the drug. Adverse extrapyramidal effects have been reported in one olanzapine-treated patient after a reduction in cigarette smoking, while worsened delusions, hostility, and aggressive behavior have been reported in another olanzapine-treated patient following a marked increase in smoking (i.e., an increase from 12 up to 80 cigarettes per day). Although the precise mechanism(s) for this interaction has not been clearly established, it has been suggested that induction of the CYP isoenzymes, particularly 1A2, by smoke constituents may be responsible at least in part for the reduced plasma olanzapine concentrations observed in smokers compared with nonsmokers.

Although the manufacturer states that routine dosage adjustment is not recommended in patients who smoke while receiving olanzapine, some clinicians recommend that patients treated with olanzapine should be monitored with regard to their smoking consumption and that dosage adjustment be considered in patients who have reduced or increased their smoking and/or who are not responding adequately or who are experiencing dose-related adverse reactions to the drug. In addition, monitoring of plasma olanzapine concentrations may be helpful in patients who smoke and have other factors associated with substantial alterations in metabolism of olanzapine (e.g., geriatric patients, women, concurrent fluvoxamine administration).

■ **Other Drugs** Multiple doses of olanzapine did not substantially alter the pharmacokinetics of theophylline or its metabolites.

Multiple doses of olanzapine did not substantially affect the pharmacokinetics of biperiden.

Acute Toxicity

■ **Pathogenesis and Manifestations** The acute lethal dose of olanzapine in humans remains to be established. However, the toxic and lethal doses of olanzapine and other atypical antipsychotic agents appear to be highly variable and depend on concurrent administration of other drugs or toxic substances, patient age and habituation, and the time from exposure until treatment is initiated; pediatric and/or nonhabituated patients appear to be more sensitive to the toxic effects of these drugs.

During premarketing clinical studies of extended-release olanzapine pamoate (Zyprexa® Relprevv), adverse events that presented with signs and symptoms consistent with olanzapine overdosage, particularly sedation (ranging from mild in severity to coma) and/or delirium, were reported following IM injection of the drug. Such cases of post-injection delirium/sedation syndrome (PDSS) occurred in less than 0.1% of injections and in approximately 2% of patients who received injections for up to 46 months. These events were correlated with an unintentional rapid increase in serum olanzapine concentrations to supratherapeutic ranges in some cases. Although a rapid and greater than expected increase in serum olanzapine concentrations has been noted in some patients with these adverse events, the precise mechanism by which the drug was unintentionally introduced into the bloodstream in these cases is not known. Clinical signs and symptoms of PDSS include dizziness, confusion, disorientation, malaise, slurred speech, altered gait, ambulation difficulties, weakness, agitation, extrapyramidal symptoms, hypertension, convulsion, and reduced levels of consciousness ranging from mild sedation to coma. The time after injection to PDSS in the reported cases ranged from soon after the injection to greater than 3 hours after the injection. The majority of patients required hospitalization, and supportive care, including intubation, was necessary in several cases. All patients had largely recovered by 72 hours. Because the risk of PDSS is the same at each injection, the risk per patient is cumulative (i.e., the risk increases with the number of injections). (See Post-injection Delirium/Sedation Syndrome under Cautions: Nervous System Effects and also under Cautions: Precautions and Contraindications.)

In postmarketing reports of overdosage with oral olanzapine alone, symptoms have been reported in the majority of cases. Following acute overdosage of oral olanzapine or other atypical antipsychotic agents, toxic effects usually begin within 1–2 hours and maximal toxic effects usually are seen 4–6 hours following acute ingestion. In general, overdosage of olanzapine may be expected to produce effects that are extensions of its pharmacologic and adverse effects. The most commonly reported manifestations of olanzapine overdosage and those that have occurred in 10% or more of symptomatic patients following postmarketing overdosage reports with olanzapine alone are agitation and/or aggressiveness, dysarthria, tachycardia, anticholinergic syndrome, miosis, various extrapyramidal symptoms, jerking and myoclonus, hypersalivation, and reduced level of consciousness ranging in severity from sedation to coma. Less commonly reported but potentially medically serious events included aspiration, cardiopulmonary arrest, cardiac arrhythmias (e.g., supraventricular tachycardia), delirium, possible neuroleptic malignant syndrome, respiratory depression and/or arrest, convulsions, hypertension, and hypotension (including orthostatic hypotension); one patient experienced sinus pause with spontaneous resumption of normal rhythm. Fatalities in association with overdosage of oral olanzapine alone have been reported. In one such case, the amount of acutely ingested oral olanzapine was reported to be possibly as low as 450 mg of oral olanzapine; however, in another case, a patient reportedly survived an acute ingestion of approximately 2 g of oral olanzapine.

In some cases of acute olanzapine intoxication, rapid fluctuation in mental status (i.e., between sedation and agitation or agitation despite sedation) has been reported. In addition, olanzapine overdosage may resemble opiate overdosage because CNS depression and miosis sometimes are observed. Increased creatine kinase (CK, creatine phosphokinase, CPK) concentrations also have occurred following acute olanzapine overdosage. Cardiac arrhythmias, persistent choreoathetosis, nonconvulsive status epilepticus, hypersalivation, and coma occurred in an adult following an intentional ingestion estimated to be 750 mg of olanzapine; both coma and choreoathetosis persisted until the patient's death 8 weeks later.

The toxic effects of olanzapine and other atypical antipsychotic agents in pediatric patients appear to be similar to those seen in adults. In young children, marked CNS depression and anticholinergic delirium have occurred following ingestion of 7.5–15 mg of olanzapine (equivalent to 0.5–1 mg/kg). In an adolescent who ingested 275 mg of olanzapine and had an extremely high serum olanzapine concentration (1503 ng/mL), somnolence, agitation, and extrapyramidal symptoms developed initially, but the patient recovered without complications. A 400-mg olanzapine overdosage in another adolescent reportedly produced severe respiratory depression requiring intubation and mechanical ventilation; the patient recovered after 3 days. In addition, polyuria and other signs suggesting possible diabetes insipidus, including hypoosmolar urine, normoosmolar plasma, and increased serum sodium concentrations, have been reported in one adolescent following an overdosage of olanzapine and prazepam (a benzodiazepine; not commercially available in the US).

■ **Treatment** Clinicians should be aware that post-injection delirium/sedation syndrome (PDSS) may occur with any IM injection of extended-release olanzapine pamoate (Zyprexa® Relprevv). Signs and symptoms consistent with olanzapine overdosage have been observed in such cases, and access to emergency response services must be readily available for safe use.

Management of olanzapine overdosage generally involves symptomatic and supportive care, including continuous cardiovascular and respiratory monitoring and ensuring IV access. Cardiovascular monitoring should be initiated immediately and should include continuous ECG monitoring to detect possible arrhythmias. There is no specific antidote for olanzapine intoxication. In managing olanzapine overdosage, the clinician should consider the possibility of multiple drug intoxication.

The manufacturer and many clinicians recommend establishing and maintaining an airway and ensuring adequate ventilation and oxygenation, which may include intubation. Gastric lavage (following intubation, if the patient is unconscious) and/or activated charcoal, which may be used with sorbitol, should be considered. (See Drug Interactions: Activated Charcoal.) The possibility that obtundation, seizures, or dystonic reaction of the head and neck following olanzapine overdosage may create a risk of aspiration with induction of emesis should be considered.

Hypotension and circulatory collapse, if present, should be treated with appropriate measures, such as Trendelenburg's position, IV fluids, and/or sympathomimetic agents (e.g., norepinephrine, phenylephrine). However, dopamine, epinephrine, and/or other sympathomimetic agents with β-adrenergic agonist activity should be avoided, since such stimulation may worsen hypotension in the presence of olanzapine-induced α-adrenergic blockade. Tachycardia associated with olanzapine intoxication usually does not require specific therapy. Atrial and ventricular arrhythmias and conduction disturbances should be treated with appropriate measures; sodium bicarbonate may be helpful if QRS-interval prolongation is present. Seizures following olanzapine overdosage may be treated initially with a benzodiazepine followed by barbiturates, if necessary. Acute extrapyramidal reactions should be treated with anticholinergic agents (e.g., diphenhydramine, benztropine).

Physostigmine salicylate or benzodiazepine therapy may be useful in the management of severe agitation and delirium in patients with severe anticholinergic toxicity and a narrow QRS complex on their ECG. Physostigmine has been used successfully in the treatment of anticholinergic toxicity associated with overdosages of olanzapine or clozapine, another atypical antipsychotic agent. However, experience with physostigmine in the management of atypical antipsychotic overdosage is limited, and some clinicians recommend that the drug be used only by experienced clinicians and in cases in which the potential therapeutic benefit outweighs the potential risks.

Resolution of toxic effects following atypical antipsychotic intoxication generally occurs within 12–48 hours following acute overdosage, although it has taken up to 6 days. Patients should remain under close medical supervision and monitoring until fully recovered.

Hemodialysis has not been shown to be useful for enhancing elimination of olanzapine in acute overdosage. Clinical experience with other enhanced elimination techniques, including multiple-dose activated charcoal, hemoperfusion, forced diuresis, and urinary alkalinization, is lacking; however, these treatments also are unlikely to be beneficial following olanzapine overdosage because of the drug's large volume of distribution and extensive protein binding.

Chronic Toxicity

In animal studies prospectively designed to assess abuse and dependence potential, olanzapine was shown to produce acute CNS depressive effects but little or no potential for abuse or physical dependence in rats administered oral doses up to 15 times the maximum recommended human daily oral dosage (20 mg) and rhesus monkeys administered oral doses up to 8 times the maximum recommended human daily oral dosage on a mg/m² basis. Olanzapine has not been systematically evaluated in humans to date for its potential for abuse, tolerance, or physical dependence. While clinical trials did not reveal any tendency for drug-seeking behavior, these observations were not systematic, and it is not possible to predict on the basis of this limited experience the extent to which a CNS-active drug will be misused, diverted, and/or abused once marketed. Consequently, patients should be evaluated carefully for a history of drug abuse, and such patients should be observed closely for signs of misuse or abuse of olanzapine (e.g., development of tolerance, increases in dose, drug-seeking behavior).

Pharmacology

Olanzapine is a thienobenzodiazepine-derivative antipsychotic agent. The drug shares some of the pharmacologic actions of other antipsychotic agents and has been described as an atypical or second-generation antipsychotic agent. Like other atypical or second-generation antipsychotics (e.g., aripiprazole, asenapine, clozapine, quetiapine, risperidone, ziprasidone), olanzapine is less likely to cause adverse extrapyramidal effects and tardive dyskinesia than conventional (first-generation) antipsychotic agents, and is effective in the treatment of positive, negative, and depressive manifestations of schizophrenia.

■ **Nervous System Effects** The exact mechanism of antipsychotic action of olanzapine and other atypical antipsychotic agents has not been fully elucidated but appears to be more complex than that of conventional, first-generation antipsychotic agents and may involve central antagonism at serotonin type 2 (5-hydroxytryptamine [5-HT_{2A}, 5-HT_{2C}]), type 3 (5-HT_3), and type 6 (5-HT_6) and dopamine receptors.

The exact mechanism(s) of action of olanzapine in the treatment of acute manic or mixed episodes associated with bipolar disorder is not fully known. However, it has been suggested that the ability of olanzapine to block and downregulate 5-HT_{2A} receptors may play a role in its antimanic activity. In addition, olanzapine's mood-stabilizing action may be caused at least in part by antagonism of D_2 receptors. Further studies are needed to more clearly elucidate the potential mechanism(s) of the drug's antimanic activity.

Although not clearly established, the efficacy of IM olanzapine in the treatment of acute agitation appears to be due at least in part to its distinct calming effects rather than solely to nonspecific sedation.

Antidopaminergic Effects The therapeutic effects of antipsychotic drugs are thought to be mediated by dopaminergic blockade in the mesolimbic and mesocortical areas of the CNS, while antidopaminergic effects in the neostriatum appear to be associated with extrapyramidal effects. The relatively low incidence of extrapyramidal effects associated with olanzapine therapy suggests that the drug is more active in the mesolimbic than the neostriatal dopaminergic system.

Several (at least 5) different types or subtypes of dopamine receptors have been identified in animals or humans. The relative densities of these receptors and their distribution and function vary for different neuroanatomical regions, and olanzapine's effects may be secondary to regionally specific receptor interactions and/or other effects on dopaminergic neurons. Current evidence suggests that the clinical potency and antipsychotic efficacy of both typical and atypical antipsychotic drugs generally are related at least in part to their affinity for and blockade of central dopamine D_2 receptors. Some studies suggest that clinically effective dosages of most antipsychotic agents result in occupation of between 60 and 80% of central dopamine D_2 receptors. However, antagonism at D_2 receptors does not appear to account fully for the antipsychotic effects of olanzapine. In vivo and in vitro studies have demonstrated that olanzapine is a comparatively weak antagonist at D_2 receptors. Although their role in eliciting the pharmacologic effects of antipsychotic agents remains to be fully elucidated, dopamine D_3, D_4, and D_5 receptors also have been identified. Olanzapine may have a higher affinity for D_4 receptors than for D_2 or D_3 receptors. K_I values of olanzapine for dopamine D_{1-4} receptors range from 11–31 nM.

Atypical antipsychotic agents generally have demonstrated relatively loose binding to dopamine D_2 receptors. Compared with typical antipsychotic agents, atypical antipsychotics appear to have faster dissociation rates from and lower affinity for dopamine D_2 receptors, which may result in fewer adverse extrapyramidal effects and less risk of elevated prolactin concentrations; however, further studies are needed to confirm these initial findings.

Serotonergic Effects It has been suggested that schizophrenia may involve a dysregulation of serotonin- and/or dopamine-mediated neurotransmission, and olanzapine may at least partially restore a normal balance of neurotransmitter function, possibly through serotonergic modulation of dopaminergic tone. Olanzapine blocks serotonin type 2 (5-hydroxytryptamine [5-

HT_{2A} and $5\text{-}HT_{2C}$; K_I of 4 and 11 nM, respectively]), type 3 ($5\text{-}HT_3$; K_I of 57 nM), and type 6 ($5\text{-}HT_6$; K_I of 5 nM) receptors.

Anticholinergic Effects Olanzapine blocks muscarinic cholinergic receptors and has demonstrated moderate affinity for all 5 muscarinic receptor subtypes (K_I values for $M_{1\text{-}5}$ were 73, 96, 132, 32, and 48 nM, respectively). Anticholinergic activity in antipsychotic agents may contribute to certain adverse anticholinergic events associated with these drugs but also may help reduce the risk of adverse extrapyramidal reactions.

Effects on Other Central Neurotransmitters Antagonism at receptors other than dopamine and $5\text{-}HT_2$ receptors may produce some of the therapeutic and adverse effects associated with olanzapine. Olanzapine exhibits α_1-adrenergic blocking activity (K_I of 19 nM), which may explain the occasional orthostatic hypotension associated with the drug. In addition, olanzapine blocks histamine H_1 receptors (K_I of 7 nM), which may explain the sedative effects associated with the drug; affinity for H_2 and H_3 receptors appears to be low.

Olanzapine demonstrated weak binding affinity (K_I exceeding 10 μM) for β-adrenergic, γ-aminobutyric acid (GABA), and benzodiazepine receptors; the drug also has little or no affinity for opiate receptors.

Neurophysiologic Effects In vivo electrophysiologic studies demonstrate different sensitivities of various brain areas to antipsychotic-mediated postsynaptic receptor blockade. While conventional antipsychotics generally reduce spontaneous firing activity in both the mesolimbic (A10) and nigrostriatal regions (A9), chronic administration of atypical antipsychotics generally reduces the number of spontaneously active dopaminergic neurons in the mesolimbic region but not in the nigrostriatal region. Although not clearly established, it has been suggested that the ability to decrease A10 but not A9 neurons is associated clinically with a low potential to cause adverse extrapyramidal reactions and tardive dyskinesia. Olanzapine has demonstrated such mesolimbic selectivity in the in vivo studies conducted to date.

Cognitive Effects in Humans Clinical experience suggests that second-generation antipsychotics, including olanzapine, improve cognition in patients with schizophrenia and that there may be differences between these drugs in their effects on neurocognitive functioning. In an initial clinical trial evaluating the short-term effects of atypical antipsychotic agents on cognitive function, olanzapine-treated schizophrenic patients demonstrated improved learning and memory, verbal fluency, and executive function. In a controlled clinical trial evaluating the neurocognitive effects of olanzapine, clozapine, risperidone, and haloperidol in patients with treatment-resistant schizophrenia or schizoaffective disorder, global neurocognitive function improved with olanzapine and risperidone treatment, and these improvements were found to be superior to those seen with haloperidol. Patients treated with olanzapine exhibited improvement in the general and attention domains but not more than that observed with the other antipsychotic agents. In another controlled trial, patients with schizophrenia receiving long-term (1 year) therapy with olanzapine demonstrated improved results on a general cognition index compared with those receiving haloperidol and risperidone. Neurocognition also improved in olanzapine- and risperidone-treated schizophrenic and schizoaffective patients receiving the drug for 1 year in another controlled study; improvements in executive function, learning and memory, processing speed, attention and vigilance, verbal working memory, and motor function were reported. The clinical relevance of these cognitive findings in the management of schizophrenia remains to be determined and requires further study.

EEG Effects Olanzapine may cause EEG changes. In one study, olanzapine-induced EEG slowing to a lesser extent than clozapine in patients with schizophrenia and did not appear to substantially alter epileptiform activity in most of the patients studied; further studies are needed to determine whether olanzapine can affect the seizure threshold. Similarly, a comparative study found that epileptiform activity did not increase during olanzapine therapy; however, EEG slowing and other nonspecific EEG changes did occur more frequently in olanzapine-treated patients than in those receiving certain other antipsychotic agents. In another study that was retrospective in design, EEG changes occurred more frequently in patients receiving olanzapine or clozapine than in those receiving typical antipsychotic agents, quetiapine, or risperidone. In a study in patients with schizophrenia, olanzapine therapy was associated with increased rates of slow waves, sharp waves, and paroxysmal slow wave discharges on EEG recordings in the patients evaluated; however, spike- and sharp-slow-wave complexes that indicate seizure risk were not observed in this study.

Seizures have been reported rarely in olanzapine-treated patients but confounding factors were present in most of these cases. Further studies and postmarketing surveillance are needed to determine whether olanzapine can affect the seizure threshold and to evaluate the clinical relevance of the observed EEG findings in patients receiving the drug.

Effects on Sleep The available evidence suggests that atypical antipsychotics, including olanzapine, clozapine, and risperidone, substantially increase total sleep time and stage 2 sleep; both olanzapine and risperidone also have been shown to enhance slow-wave sleep. Olanzapine's beneficial effects on sleep quality are thought to be mediated principally via type 2 serotonergic ($5\text{-}HT_2$) receptors.

In a controlled study, administration of single evening doses of olanzapine (5 or 10 mg orally) in healthy individuals significantly increased slow-wave sleep in a dose-related manner; sleep continuity measures and subjective sleep quality also increased significantly. Single 10-mg doses of the drug also suppressed rapid eye movement (REM) sleep and increased REM sleep latency in this study. In another study in healthy males and females, single 10-mg oral doses of olanzapine also were found to increase slow-wave sleep but preserved the normal structure of sleep; these effects were more prominent in females than in males.

During subchronic administration of olanzapine (15–20 mg) in patients with schizophrenia with predominantly negative symptoms in an uncontrolled study, parameters of sleep efficiency improved and delta sleep and REM sleep increased. Acute olanzapine administration (10 mg orally) in schizophrenic patients improved sleep continuity variables and total sleep time in another study; the principal changes observed in sleep architecture were a reduction in stage 1 sleep, a significant enhancement in stage 2 and delta sleep, and an increase in REM density. In a study comparing the effect of aging on the improvement of subjective sleep quality in patients with schizophrenia receiving atypical antipsychotic agents, including olanzapine, the proportion of patients experiencing improved subjective sleep quality was significantly higher in geriatric patients than in middle-aged patients.

■ **Neuroendocrine Effects** In contrast to conventional (first-generation) antipsychotic agents and similar to many other atypical antipsychotic agents, olanzapine therapy in usual dosages generally produces transient elevations in serum prolactin concentrations in humans. This prolactin-elevating effect appears to be mediated by dopamine blockade. The effect of atypical antipsychotic agents on prolactin generally appears to be transient, possibly because the drugs appear to dissociate from dopamine receptors more rapidly than conventional antipsychotic agents.

■ **Antiemetic Effects** Although the precise mechanism of olanzapine's antiemetic action has not been clearly established, its inhibitory activity at multiple dopaminergic and serotonergic receptors, particularly the D_2, $5\text{-}HT_{2C}$, and $5\text{-}HT_3$ receptors that may be involved in nausea and vomiting, may play a role in the drug's efficacy in both the prevention and rescue therapy of chemotherapy-induced nausea and vomiting†.

Pharmacokinetics

■ **Absorption** Olanzapine is well absorbed following oral administration. However, because of extensive first-pass metabolism, only about 60% of an orally administered dose reaches systemic circulation unchanged. Olanzapine exhibits linear and dose-proportional pharmacokinetics when given orally within the clinical dosage range. Food does not appear to affect the rate or the extent of GI absorption of the drug. The relative oral bioavailability of olanzapine has been shown to be equivalent following administration of the conventional and orally disintegrating tablets of the drug.

When olanzapine and fluoxetine hydrochloride are administered as the fixed-combination oral capsules, the pharmacokinetic characteristics of the drugs are expected to resemble those of the individual components; olanzapine pharmacokinetics are slightly altered when administered with fluoxetine, but the effects were not deemed to be clinically important. (See Selective Serotonin-reuptake Inhibitors under Drug Interactions: Drugs Affecting Hepatic Microsomal Enzymes.)

Following oral administration, peak plasma olanzapine concentrations occur in approximately 6 hours (range: 5–8 hours). Steady-state plasma concentrations of olanzapine are achieved after approximately 7 days of continuous dosing and are approximately twice those observed following single-dose administration.

Following IM administration of short-acting olanzapine injection (Zyprexa® IntraMuscular), olanzapine is rapidly absorbed with peak plasma olanzapine concentrations occurring within 15–45 minutes. In one pharmacokinetic study performed in healthy individuals, a single 5-mg IM dose of olanzapine produced peak plasma concentrations that were an average of approximately fivefold higher than the peak plasma concentrations produced following a single 5-mg oral dose of the drug. In this study, the areas under the plasma concentration-time curve (AUCs) achieved following IM and oral administration of the same dose of the drug were similar. Olanzapine exhibits linear pharmacokinetics when given IM within the clinical dosage range. Preliminary evidence suggests that the onset of antipsychotic action following IM administration of the drug is evident within 24 hours but may be observed as early as 2 hours after IM administration.

Following deep IM gluteal administration of extended-release olanzapine pamoate injection (Zyprexa® Relprevv), slow dissolution of the pamoate ester (which is practically insoluble) results in prolonged plasma olanzapine concentrations over a period of weeks to months. An IM injection every 2 or 4 weeks provides plasma olanzapine concentrations that are similar to those achieved with daily doses of oral olanzapine. Steady-state plasma concentrations achieved with extended-release olanzapine pamoate injection in IM dosages of 150–405 mg every 2 or 4 weeks are within the range achieved with oral olanzapine dosages of 5–20 mg daily. Plasma olanzapine concentrations generally reach a peak within the first week following each injection.

Plasma olanzapine concentrations may vary between individuals according to gender, smoking status, and age. There is limited evidence that gender may affect plasma olanzapine concentrations, with concentrations being somewhat higher, perhaps by as much as 30–40%, in females compared with males. Plasma concentrations of olanzapine also may be increased in geriatric individuals compared with younger individuals, possibly as a result of age-related decreases in hepatic elimination of the drug. Data from one limited study in children and adolescents 10–18 years of age with schizophrenia found that plasma olanzapine concentrations among adolescents were within the range reported in nonsmoking adult patients with schizophrenia. However, the manufacturer states that most adolescents (i.e., 13–17 years of age) in clinical studies were nonsmokers and had a lower average body weight, which resulted in higher average olanzapine exposure compared with adults. In vivo studies have shown that exposures to olanzapine are similar among Japanese, Chinese, and Caucasian individuals, particularly after normalization for body weight differences.

The therapeutic range for plasma olanzapine concentrations and the relationship of plasma concentration to clinical response and toxicity have not been clearly established; however, acutely ill schizophrenic patients with 24-hour post-dose plasma olanzapine concentrations of 9.3 ng/mL or higher in one study or 12-hour post-dose concentrations of 23.2 ng/mL or higher in another study appeared to have a better clinical response to therapy than patients with lower plasma concentrations.

■ **Distribution** Distribution of olanzapine, a highly lipophilic drug, into human body tissues is extensive.

The manufacturer states that the volume of distribution of olanzapine has been reported to be approximately 1000 L. In pharmacokinetic studies in healthy individuals, the apparent volume of distribution of the drug averaged 1150 L and ranged from 660 to 1790 L for the fifth to 95th percentiles. Olanzapine is 93% bound to plasma proteins over the concentration range of 7–1100 ng/mL, principally to albumin and α_1-acid glycoprotein.

Olanzapine and its glucuronide metabolite have been shown to cross the placenta in humans. Placental transfer of olanzapine also has been shown to occur in rat pups.

Olanzapine is distributed into milk. The manufacturer states that in a study in lactating, healthy women, the average infant dose of olanzapine at steady-state was estimated to be approximately 1.8% of the maternal olanzapine dose. In a separate study that evaluated the extent of infant exposure to olanzapine in 7 breastfeeding women who had been receiving 5–20 mg of olanzapine daily for periods ranging from 19–395 days, median and maximum relative infant doses of 1 and 1.2%, respectively, were observed. Olanzapine was not detected in the plasma of the breast-fed infants, and adverse effects possibly related to olanzapine exposure were not reported in the infants in this study. In addition, peak milk concentrations were achieved a median of 5.2 hours later than the corresponding maximal maternal plasma concentrations. In a case report, a relative infant dose of approximately 4% was estimated in one woman after 4 and 10 days (estimated to be at steady state) of olanzapine therapy at a dosage of 20 mg daily based on measurements of drug concentration in serum and in expressed breast milk. (See Cautions: Pregnancy, Fertility, and Lactation.)

■ **Elimination** Although the exact metabolic fate has not been clearly established, it appears that olanzapine is extensively metabolized. Following a single oral dose of radiolabeled olanzapine, 7% of the dose was recovered in urine as unchanged drug. Approximately 57 and 30% of the dose was recovered in the urine and feces, respectively. In plasma, olanzapine accounted for only 12% of the AUC for total radioactivity, suggesting substantial exposure to metabolites. After multiple doses of olanzapine, the principal circulating metabolites are the 10-*N*-glucuronide, which is present at steady state at 44% of the plasma concentration of the parent drug, and 4′-*N*-desmethyl olanzapine, which is present at steady state at 31% of the plasma concentration of olanzapine. Both of these metabolites lack pharmacologic activity at the concentrations observed.

Direct glucuronidation and cytochrome P-450 (CYP)-mediated oxidation are the principal pathways for olanzapine metabolism. In vitro studies suggest that the CYP isoenzymes 1A2 and 2D6 and the flavin-containing monooxygenase system are involved in the oxidation of olanzapine. However, CYP2D6-mediated oxidation appears to be a minor metabolic pathway for olanzapine in vivo since the clearance of the drug is not reduced in individuals deficient in this enzyme.

Following oral administration, olanzapine has an elimination half-life ranging from 21 to 54 hours for the fifth to 95th percentiles of individual values with a mean of 30 hours. Following IM administration of short-acting olanzapine injection (Zyprexa® IntraMuscular), the half-life and metabolic profile of olanzapine were similar to those observed with oral administration. Following IM administration of extended-release olanzapine pamoate injection (Zyprexa® Relprevv), the elimination half-life is approximately 30 days. Therefore, exposure to olanzapine may persist for months after a single extended-release IM injection of the drug.

The apparent plasma clearance of olanzapine ranges from 12 to 47 L/hour (mean: 25 L/hour).

The clearance of olanzapine in smokers is approximately 40% higher than in nonsmokers. (See Drug Interactions: Smoking.)

The clearance of olanzapine in females may be reduced by approximately 30% compared with males.

In a single-dose pharmacokinetic study, the elimination half-life of orally administered olanzapine was 1.5 times longer in healthy geriatric individuals 65 years of age or older than in healthy younger adults. (See Dosage and Administration: Dosage and see also Cautions: Geriatric Precautions.)

In one pharmacokinetic study conducted in a limited number of children and adolescents 10–18 years of age with schizophrenia who were treated with oral olanzapine, the apparent plasma clearance at steady-state averaged 9.6 L/hr, which was approximately half of the clearance values reported in adult studies but similar to clearance values reported in nonsmoking male and female schizophrenic patients. The elimination half-life averaged 37.2 hours in this same study. (See Dosage and Administration: Dosage and see also Cautions: Pediatric Precautions.)

The combined effects of age, smoking, and gender could result in substantial pharmacokinetic differences in populations. The clearance in younger, smoking adult male patients may be 3 times higher than that in geriatric, nonsmoking females. Dosage adjustment may be necessary in patients who exhibit a combination of factors that may result in slower metabolism of olanzapine. (See Dosage and Administration: Dosage.)

Because olanzapine is extensively metabolized before excretion and only 7% of the drug is excreted unchanged, renal impairment alone is unlikely to substantially alter the pharmacokinetics of olanzapine. The pharmacokinetics of olanzapine were similar in patients with severe renal impairment and healthy individuals, suggesting that dosage adjustment based upon the degree of renal impairment is not necessary. The effect of renal impairment on the elimination of olanzapine's metabolites has not been evaluated to date.

Although the presence of hepatic impairment would be expected to reduce the clearance of olanzapine, a pharmacokinetic study evaluating the effect of impaired hepatic function in individuals with clinically important cirrhosis (Child-Pugh classification A and B) revealed little effect on the pharmacokinetics of olanzapine.

Olanzapine is not appreciably removed by hemodialysis, probably due to its large volume of distribution and extensive protein binding. Clinical experience with other enhanced elimination techniques, including multiple-dose activated charcoal, hemoperfusion, forced diuresis, and urinary alkalinization, is lacking; however, these treatments are unlikely to be beneficial following olanzapine overdosage because of the drug's large volume of distribution and extensive protein binding.

Chemistry and Stability

■ **Chemistry** Olanzapine is a thienobenzodiazepine-derivative antipsychotic agent. The drug is considered an atypical or second-generation antipsychotic agent. Olanzapine is structurally similar to clozapine.

Olanzapine occurs as a yellow crystalline solid that is practically insoluble in water.

Olanzapine for injection (short-acting) contains lactose monohydrate and tartaric acid; hydrochloric acid and/or sodium hydroxide may have been added to adjust pH. When olanzapine for injection is reconstituted as directed, the resulting solution should appear clear and yellow.

■ **Stability** Commercially available olanzapine conventional tablets, orally disintegrating tablets, and short-acting olanzapine for IM injection should be stored at a controlled room temperature of 20–25°C but may be exposed to temperatures ranging from 15–30°C. Olanzapine orally disintegrating tablets should be stored in their original sealed blister. The conventional and orally disintegrating tablets should be protected from light and moisture and olanzapine for injection should be protected from light and freezing. Extended-release olanzapine pamoate for IM injection should be stored at room temperature (not to exceed 30°C).

Following reconstitution, olanzapine for injection (short-acting) may be stored at a controlled room temperature of 20–25°C for up to 1 hour if necessary, but immediate use is preferred.

Following reconstitution, extended-release olanzapine pamoate injection suspension may be stored at room temperature for 24 hours. The vial should be agitated immediately prior to withdrawal of the suspension.

Olanzapine orally disintegrating tablets contain aspartame (e.g., NutraSweet®). (See Individuals with Phenylketonuria, under Cautions: Precautions and Contraindications.)

Olanzapine for IM injection (short-acting) should not be combined with diazepam injection in a syringe because precipitation occurs when these drugs are mixed. Olanzapine for IM injection also should not be combined in a syringe with haloperidol injection because the resulting pH has been shown to degrade olanzapine over time. In addition, lorazepam injection should not be used to reconstitute olanzapine for injection since this delays reconstitution time. Specialized references should be consulted for additional specific compatibility information.

Preparations

Long-acting IM olanzapine pamoate (Zyprexa® Relprevv) is available only through a restricted distribution program. (See Restricted Distribution under Dosage and Administration: Reconstitution and Administration.)

Excipients in commercially available drug preparations may have clinically important effects in some individuals; consult specific product labeling for details.

OLANZapine

Oral		
Tablets, film-coated	2.5 mg*	**ZyPREXA**®, Lilly
	5 mg*	**ZyPREXA**®, Lilly
	7.5 mg*	**ZyPREXA**®, Lilly
	10 mg*	**ZyPREXA**®, Lilly
	15 mg*	**ZyPREXA**®, Lilly
	20 mg*	**ZyPREXA**®, Lilly

Tablets, orally disintegrating	5 mg*	**ZyPREXA® Zydis®**, Lilly
	10 mg*	**ZyPREXA® Zydis®**, Lilly
	15 mg*	**ZyPREXA® Zydis®**, Lilly
	20 mg*	**ZyPREXA® Zydis®**, Lilly
Parenteral		
For injection, for IM use only	10 mg*	**ZyPREXA® IntraMuscular**, Lilly

*available from one or more manufacturer, distributor, and/or repackager by generic (nonproprietary) name

OLANZapine Combinations

Oral		
Capsules	3 mg with Fluoxetine Hydrochloride 25 mg (of fluoxetine)*	**Symbyax®**, Lilly
	6 mg with Fluoxetine Hydrochloride 25 mg (of fluoxetine)*	**Symbyax®**, Lilly
	6 mg with Fluoxetine Hydrochloride 50 mg (of fluoxetine)*	**Symbyax®**, Lilly
	12 mg with Fluoxetine Hydrochloride 25 mg (of fluoxetine)*	**Symbyax®**, Lilly
	12 mg with Fluoxetine Hydrochloride 50 mg (of fluoxetine)*	**Symbyax®**, Lilly

*available from one or more manufacturer, distributor, and/or repackager by generic (nonproprietary) name

OLANZapine Pamoate

Parenteral		
For injectable suspension, extended-release, for IM use only	210 mg (of olanzapine)	**ZyPREXA® Relprevv®** (available as a convenience kit containing single-use vial, needles, syringe, and diluent), Lilly
	300 mg (of olanzapine)	**ZyPREXA® Relprevv®** (available as a convenience kit containing single-use vial, needles, syringe, and diluent), Lilly
	405 mg (of olanzapine)	**ZyPREXA® Relprevv®** (available as a convenience kit containing single-use vial, needles, syringe, and diluent), Lilly

†Use is not currently included in the labeling approved by the US Food and Drug Administration

Paliperidone

9-Hydroxyrisperidone

■ Paliperidone is considered an atypical or second-generation antipsychotic agent.

Uses

■ **Psychotic Disorders** Paliperidone is used for the symptomatic management of psychotic disorders (e.g., schizophrenia). Drug therapy is integral to the management of acute psychotic episodes in patients with schizophrenia and generally is required for long-term stabilization to sustain symptom remission or control and to minimize the risk of relapse. Antipsychotic agents are the principal class of drugs used for the management of all phases of schizophrenia. Patient response and tolerance to antipsychotic agents are variable, and patients who do not respond to or tolerate one drug may be successfully treated with an agent from a different class or with a different adverse effect profile.

Schizophrenia Paliperidone is used orally for the acute and maintenance treatment of schizophrenia in adults and adolescents 12–17 years of age. Schizophrenia is a major psychotic disorder that frequently has devastating effects on various aspects of the patient's life and carries a high risk of suicide and other life-threatening behaviors. Manifestations of schizophrenia involve multiple psychologic processes, including perception (e.g., hallucinations), ideation, reality testing (e.g., delusions), emotion (e.g., flatness, inappropriate affect), thought processes (e.g., loose associations), behavior (e.g., catatonia, disorganization), attention, concentration, motivation (e.g., avolition, impaired intention and planning), and judgment. The principal manifestations of this disorder usually are described in terms of positive and negative (deficit) symptoms, and more recently, disorganized symptoms. Positive symptoms include hallucinations, delusions, bizarre behavior, hostility, uncooperativeness, and paranoid ideation, while negative symptoms include restricted range and intensity of emotional expression (affective flattening), reduced thought and speech productivity (alogia), anhedonia, apathy, and decreased initiation of goal-directed behavior (avolition). Disorganized symptoms include disorganized speech (thought disorder) and behavior and poor attention.

The short-term efficacy of paliperidone in the acute treatment of schizophrenia in adults was established in 3 placebo-controlled and active comparator (olanzapine)-controlled, fixed-dose clinical trials of 6 weeks' duration in 1665 adult patients with schizophrenia. In these 3 studies, patients receiving paliperidone (3–15 mg daily as extended-release tablets) demonstrated substantially greater improvement in the Positive and Negative Syndrome Scale (PANSS) than did patients receiving placebo. The mean effects at all dosages (3, 6, 9, 12, and 15 mg daily) were fairly similar, although higher dosages produced numerically superior results. Paliperidone also was found to be superior to placebo in improving scores on the Personal and Social Performance (PSP) scale in these trials.

In a longer-term study, adult outpatients with schizophrenia who had clinically responded to oral paliperidone and who had received a stable fixed dosage of the drug for 2 weeks entered a 6-week, open-label, stabilization phase where they received a paliperidone dosage from 3–15 mg once daily as extended-release tablets. After the stabilization phase, patients were randomized in a double-blind manner to either continue receiving paliperidone at their stable dosage or to receive placebo until they experienced a relapse of schizophrenia symptoms. The median treatment exposure during this double-blind phase was 45 days for extended-release paliperidone and 29 days for placebo; the mean paliperidone dosage was approximately 11 mg daily throughout the phases of this trial. An interim analysis of the data showed a significantly longer time to relapse in the paliperidone-treated patients compared with those receiving placebo. In addition, 25% of the paliperidone-treated patients experienced a relapse of schizophrenia symptoms compared with 53% of those receiving placebo. The study was stopped early because maintenance of efficacy was demonstrated. If paliperidone is used for extended periods, the need for continued therapy should be reassessed periodically on an individualized basis. (See Dosage and Administration: Dosage.)

Short-term efficacy and safety of oral paliperidone in the acute treatment of schizophrenia in adolescents 12–17 years of age were established in a double-blind, placebo-controlled trial of 6 weeks' duration in 201 patients who met DSM-IV criteria for schizophrenia. The trial used a fixed-dosage, weight-based treatment group design over a dosage range of 1.5–12 mg once daily given as extended-release tablets. Patients were randomized to one of 4 treatment groups: a placebo group or a low-dosage (1.5 mg daily for all body weights), medium-dosage (3 or 6 mg daily depending on body weight), or high-dosage group (6 or 12 mg daily depending on body weight). Efficacy was evaluated using the PANSS. The study demonstrated the overall efficacy of paliperidone in adolescents with schizophrenia receiving dosages ranging from 3–12 mg once daily. However, no clear improvement in efficacy was observed at the higher dosages studied (i.e., 6 mg daily for adolescents weighing less than 51 kg and 12 mg daily for adolescents weighing 51 kg or more). Tolerability was adequate within the 3–12 mg daily dosage range; however, adverse effects were dose related. Longer-term efficacy and safety of extended-release paliperidone in adolescent patients with schizophrenia are currently being evaluated in clinical studies.

The American Psychiatric Association (APA) considers most atypical antipsychotic agents first-line drugs for the management of the acute phase of schizophrenia (including first psychotic episodes), principally because of the decreased risk of adverse extrapyramidal effects and tardive dyskinesia, with the understanding that the relative advantages, disadvantages, and cost-effectiveness of conventional and atypical antipsychotic agents remain controversial. The APA states that, with the possible exception of clozapine for the management of treatment-resistant symptoms, there currently is no definitive evidence that one atypical antipsychotic agent will have superior efficacy compared with another agent in the class, although meaningful differences in response may be observed in individual patients. Conventional antipsychotic agents may be considered first-line therapy in patients who have been treated successfully in the past with or who prefer conventional agents. The choice of an antipsychotic agent should be individualized, considering past response to therapy, adverse effect profile (including the patient's experience of subjective effects such as dysphoria), and the patient's preference for a specific drug, including route of administration.

For additional information on the symptomatic management of schizophrenia, including treatment recommendations and results of the Clinical Antipsychotic Trials of Intervention Effectiveness (CATIE) research program, see Schizophrenia and Other Psychotic Disorders under Uses: Psychotic Disorders, in the Phenothiazines General Statement 28:16.08.24.

■ **Schizoaffective Disorder** Paliperidone is used orally for the treatment of schizoaffective disorder as monotherapy and as an adjunct to mood stabilizers and/or antidepressant therapy in adults.

The acute efficacy of paliperidone in the treatment of schizoaffective disorder was principally established in 2 international, double-blind, placebo-controlled trials of 6 weeks' duration in nonelderly adults. Patients enrolled in these trials met DSM-IV criteria for schizoaffective disorder, had a PANSS total score of at least 60, and had prominent mood symptoms (confirmed by a score of at least 16 on the Young Mania Rating Scale [YMRS] and/or Hamilton Rating Scale for Depression [HRSD]). The patients in these trials included individuals with schizoaffective disorder bipolar and depressive types. In the first trial, efficacy was assessed in 211 patients who received flexible dosages of paliperidone (3–12 mg once daily as extended-release tablets). In the second trial, efficacy was assessed in 203 patients who were assigned to one of two different dosages of paliperidone: 6 mg with the option to reduce to 3 mg once daily or 12 mg with the option to reduce to 9 mg once daily. In both studies, patients received paliperidone either as monotherapy (55%) or as an adjunct to mood stabilizers and/or antidepressants (45%). The most commonly used mood stabilizers in the studies were valproic acid and lithium and the most commonly used antidepressants were selective serotonin-reuptake inhibitors and selective serotonin- and norepinephrine-reuptake inhibitors. Efficacy was principally evaluated using the PANSS; as secondary outcomes, mood symptoms were evaluated using the Hamilton Depression Rating Scale (HAM-D-21) and YMRS. The paliperidone-treated patients in the flexible-dose study (mean modal dosage of 8.6 mg daily) and the higher dosage group of paliperidone in the 2-dosage-level study were each found to be superior to placebo (as measured by the PANSS). The lower dosage group of paliperidone in the 2-dosage-level study (6 mg with option to reduce to 3 mg once daily) was not found to be substantially different from placebo (as measured by the PANSS). Improvements in mood symptoms (as measured by the HAM-D-21 and YMRS) also were observed in the studies.

In an analysis of both placebo-controlled studies in schizoaffective disorder, paliperidone improved the symptoms of schizoaffective disorder at the study end points when administered either as monotherapy or as an adjunct to mood stabilizers and/or antidepressants. An examination of population subgroups did not reveal evidence of differential responsiveness based on gender, age, or geographic region. There were insufficient data to explore differential effects based on race.

Dosage and Administration

■ **Administration** Paliperidone extended-release tablets are administered orally once daily, usually in the morning, with or without food.

Paliperidone extended-release tablets should be swallowed whole with fluids and should *not* be chewed, divided, or crushed. Patients should be advised *not* to become concerned if they notice a tablet-like substance in their stools; this is normal since the tablet is designed to remain intact and slowly release the drug from a nonabsorbable shell during passage through the GI tract.

■ **Dosage** ***Schizophrenia*** For the management of schizophrenia in adults, the usual recommended initial dosage of paliperidone is 6 mg orally once daily in the morning; initial dosage titration is not required. Although it remains to be systematically evaluated whether dosages exceeding 6 mg once daily provide additional clinical benefit, a general trend for greater clinical effects with higher dosages has been observed. However, the potential for increased clinical efficacy at higher dosages must be weighed against the potential for a dose-related increase in adverse effects. Some patients may benefit from higher dosages of up to 12 mg once daily, while a lower dosage of 3 mg once daily may be sufficient for other patients. The manufacturer states that increases beyond a dosage level of 6 mg once daily should be made only after clinical reassessment and generally should be made at intervals of more than 5 days. When dosage increases are necessary, increments of 3 mg daily are recommended. The maximum recommended dosage in adults is 12 mg once daily.

For the management of schizophrenia in adolescents 12–17 years of age, the usual recommended initial dosage of paliperidone is 3 mg (regardless of body weight) orally once daily in the morning; initial dosage titration is not required. The manufacturer states that dosage increases, if considered necessary, should be made only after clinical reassessment and should made in increments of 3 mg daily at intervals of more than 5 days. The recommended adolescent dosage range for patients weighing less than 51 kg is 3–6 mg once daily and for those weighing 51 kg or more is 3–12 mg once daily. However, clinicians should consider that, in the adolescent schizophrenia study, there was no clear improvement in efficacy at the higher paliperidone dosage studied (i.e., 6 mg once daily for adolescents weighing less than 51 kg and 12 mg once daily for adolescents weighing 51 kg or more) while adverse effects were found to be dose related. The maximum recommended adolescent dosage is 6 mg once daily for adolescents weighing less than 51 kg and 12 mg once daily for adolescents weighing 51 kg or more.

The optimum duration of oral paliperidone therapy in patients with schizophrenia currently is not known, but maintenance therapy with paliperidone 3–15 mg daily as extended-release tablets has been shown to be effective in preventing relapse in adults. Patients responding to paliperidone therapy should continue to receive the drug as long as clinically necessary and tolerated but at the lowest possible effective dosage, and the need for continued therapy with the drug should be reassessed periodically. The American Psychiatric Association (APA) states that prudent long-term treatment options in patients with schizophrenia with remitted first- or multiple-episodes include either indefinite maintenance therapy or gradual discontinuance of the antipsychotic agent with close follow-up and a plan to reinstitute treatment upon symptom recurrence. Discontinuance of antipsychotic therapy should be considered only after a period of at least 1 year of symptom remission or optimal response while receiving the antipsychotic agent. In patients who have had multiple previous psychotic episodes or 2 psychotic episodes within 5 years, indefinite maintenance antipsychotic treatment is recommended.

Schizoaffective Disorder The recommended initial and target dosage of paliperidone for the treatment of schizoaffective disorder in adults in 6 mg orally once daily. Initial dosage titration is not required. However, some patients may benefit from lower or higher dosages within the recommended dosage range of 3–12 mg once daily. Although a general trend for greater clinical effects with higher dosages has been observed, the potential for increased clinical efficacy must be weighed against the potential for a dose-related increase in adverse effects. Dosage adjustment, if necessary, should occur only after clinical reassessment and generally should be made at intervals of more than 4 days. When dosage increases are necessary, increments of 3 mg daily are recommended. The maximum recommended adult dosage is 12 mg once daily.

■ **Special Populations** The manufacturer states that the dosage of paliperidone must be individualized according to the patient's renal function status. In patients with mild renal impairment (creatinine clearance of 50–79 mL/minute), the recommended initial oral dosage of paliperidone is 3 mg once daily. The dosage may then be increased up to a maximum of 6 mg once daily based on clinical response and tolerability. In patients with moderate to severe renal impairment (creatinine clearance of 10–49 mL/minute), the recommended initial dosage of paliperidone is 1.5 mg once daily, which may be increased up to a maximum of 3 mg once daily after clinical reassessment. Use in patients with a creatinine clearance below 10 mL/minute is not recommended since paliperidone has not been studied in such patients. (See Renal Impairment under Warnings/Precautions: Specific Populations, in Cautions.)

Dosage adjustment is not necessary in patients with mild to moderate hepatic impairment (Child-Pugh class A and B). Paliperidone has not been studied in patients with severe hepatic impairment. (See Hepatic Impairment under Warnings/Precautions: Specific Populations, in Cautions.)

Because geriatric patients may have reduced renal function, dosage adjustment may be required based on renal function status. Geriatric patients with normal renal function generally may receive the same dosage recommended for younger adults with normal renal function. In geriatric patients with moderate or severe renal impairment, the maximum recommended paliperidone dosage is 3 mg once daily. (See Renal Impairment under Warnings/Precautions: Specific Populations, in Cautions.)

No dosage adjustment is necessary based on race, gender, or smoking status (see Drug Interactions: Smoking).

Cautions

■ **Contraindications** Hypersensitivity reactions, including anaphylactic reactions and angioedema, have been observed in patients receiving risperidone or paliperidone. Paliperidone is therefore contraindicated in patients with a known hypersensitivity to paliperidone, risperidone, or any ingredient in the paliperidone formulation.

■ **Warnings/Precautions** ***Warnings*** **Increased Mortality in Geriatric Patients with Dementia-related Psychosis.** Geriatric patients with dementia-related psychosis treated with antipsychotic drugs appear to be at an increased risk of death. Analysis of 17 placebo-controlled trials (modal duration of 10 weeks) revealed an approximate 1.6- to 1.7-fold increase in mortality among geriatric patients receiving atypical antipsychotic drugs (i.e., aripiprazole, olanzapine, quetiapine, risperidone) compared with that observed in patients receiving placebo. Over the course of a typical 10-week controlled trial, the rate of death in drug-treated patients was about 4.5% compared with a rate of about 2.6% in the placebo group. Although the causes of death were varied, most of the deaths appeared to be either cardiovascular (e.g., heart failure, sudden death) or infectious (e.g., pneumonia) in nature. Observational studies suggest that, similar to atypical antipsychotics, treatment with conventional (first-generation) antipsychotics may increase mortality; the extent to which the findings of increased mortality in observational studies may be attributed to the antipsychotic drug as opposed to some characteristic(s) of the patients remains unclear. The manufacturer states that paliperidone is *not* approved for the treatment of patients with dementia-related psychosis. (See Adverse Cerebrovascular Events, including Stroke, in Geriatric Patients with Dementia-related Psychosis under Warnings/Precautions: Other Warnings and Precautions, in Cautions, Dysphagia under Warnings/Precautions: Other Warnings and Precautions, in Cautions, and also see Geriatric Use under Warnings/Precautions: Specific Populations, in Cautions.)

Sensitivity Reactions Hypersensitivity reactions, including anaphylactic reactions and angioedema, have been observed in patients receiving risperidone or paliperidone. (See Contraindications under Cautions.)

Other Warnings and Precautions **Adverse Cerebrovascular Events, including Stroke, in Geriatric Patients with Dementia-related Psychosis.** An increased incidence of adverse cerebrovascular events (cerebrovascular accidents and transient ischemic attacks), including fatalities, has been observed in geriatric patients with dementia-related psychosis treated with certain atypical antipsychotic agents (aripiprazole, olanzapine, risperidone) in placebo-controlled studies. The manufacturer states that paliperidone is *not* approved for the treatment of patients with dementia-related psychosis. (See Increased Mortality in Geriatric Patients with Dementia-related Psychosis under Warnings/Precautions: Warnings and also see Geriatric Use under Warnings/Precautions: Specific Populations, in Cautions.)

Neuroleptic Malignant Syndrome. Neuroleptic malignant syndrome (NMS), a potentially fatal syndrome requiring immediate discontinuance of the drug and intensive symptomatic treatment, has been reported in patients receiving antipsychotic agents, including paliperidone. (See Advice to Patients.) For additional information on NMS, see Neuroleptic Malignant Syndrome under Cautions: Nervous System Effects, in the Phenothiazines General Statement 28:16.08.24.

Prolongation of QT Interval. Paliperidone causes a modest increase in the corrected QT (QT_c) interval. The risk of torsades de pointes in association with drugs that prolong the QT_c interval may be increased in patients with bradycardia, hypokalemia, or hypomagnesemia; patients receiving other drugs that prolong the QT_c interval; and in those with congenital prolongation of the QT interval. Therefore, the manufacturer states that paliperidone should be avoided in patients concurrently receiving other drugs known to prolong the QT_c interval, patients with congenital long QT syndrome, and those with a history of cardiac arrhythmias. (See Drug Interactions: Drugs that Prolong QT Interval.)

Tardive Dyskinesia. Because use of antipsychotic agents may be associated with tardive dyskinesia (a syndrome of potentially irreversible, involuntary, dyskinetic movements), paliperidone should be prescribed in a manner that is most likely to minimize the occurrence of this syndrome. Chronic antipsychotic treatment generally should be reserved for patients who suffer from a chronic illness that is known to respond to antipsychotic agents, and for whom alternative, equally effective, but potentially less harmful treatments are not available or appropriate. In patients who do require chronic treatment, the lowest dosage and the shortest duration of treatment producing a satisfactory clinical response should be sought, and the need for continued treatment should be reassessed periodically.

The American Psychiatric Association (APA) currently recommends that patients receiving atypical antipsychotic agents be assessed clinically for abnormal involuntary movements every 12 months and that patients considered to be at increased risk for tardive dyskinesia be assessed every 6 months. If signs and symptoms of tardive dyskinesia appear in a paliperidone-treated patient, paliperidone discontinuance should be considered; however, some patients may require continued treatment with the drug despite the presence of the syndrome. For additional information on tardive dyskinesia, see Tardive Dyskinesia under Cautions: Nervous System Effects, in the Phenothiazines General Statement 28:16.08.24.

Metabolic Changes. Atypical antipsychotic agents have been associated with metabolic changes that may increase cardiovascular and cerebrovascular risk, including hyperglycemia, dyslipidemia, and body weight gain. While all of these drugs produce some metabolic changes, each drug has its own specific risk profile. (See Hyperglycemia and Diabetes Mellitus, see Dyslipidemia, and also see Weight Gain under Warnings/Precautions: Other Warnings and Precautions, in Cautions.)

Hyperglycemia and Diabetes Mellitus. Hyperglycemia and diabetes mellitus, sometimes severe and associated with ketoacidosis, hyperosmolar coma, or death, have been reported in patients treated with all atypical antipsychotic agents. These cases were mainly seen in postmarketing clinical use and epidemiologic studies, not in clinical trials, and there have been few reports of hyperglycemia or diabetes mellitus in paliperidone-treated patients to date. While confounding factors such as an increased background risk of diabetes mellitus in patients with schizophrenia and the increasing incidence of diabetes mellitus in the general population make it difficult to establish with certainty the relationship between use of agents in this drug class and glucose abnormalities, epidemiologic studies (which did not include paliperidone) suggest an increased risk of treatment-emergent hyperglycemia-related adverse events in patients treated with atypical antipsychotic agents. It remains to be determined whether paliperidone also is associated with this increased risk.

The manufacturers of atypical antipsychotic agents state that patients with preexisting diabetes mellitus in whom therapy with an atypical antipsychotic is initiated should be closely monitored for worsening of glucose control; those with risk factors for diabetes (e.g., obesity, family history of diabetes) should undergo fasting blood glucose testing upon therapy initiation and periodically throughout treatment. Any patient who develops manifestations of hyperglycemia (including polydipsia, polyuria, polyphagia, and weakness) during treatment with an atypical antipsychotic should undergo fasting blood glucose testing. (See Advice to Patients.) In some cases, patients who developed hyperglycemia while receiving an atypical antipsychotic have required continuance of antidiabetic treatment despite discontinuance of the suspect drug; in other cases, hyperglycemia resolved with discontinuance of the antipsychotic.

For further information on managing the risk of hyperglycemia and diabetes mellitus associated with atypical antipsychotic agents, see Hyperglycemia and Diabetes Mellitus under Cautions: Precautions and Contraindications, in Clozapine 28:16.08.04.

Dyslipidemia. Undesirable changes in lipid parameters have been observed in patients treated with some atypical antipsychotics. Data from short- and longer-term clinical studies suggest that the risk of developing clinically important dyslipidemia during paliperidone therapy is minimal.

Weight Gain. Weight gain has been observed with atypical antipsychotic therapy. Monitoring of weight is recommended in patients receiving paliperidone and other atypical antipsychotic agents. (See Pediatric Use under Warnings/Precautions: Specific Populations, in Cautions.)

Hyperprolactinemia. Similar to other antipsychotic agents and drugs with dopamine D_2 antagonistic activity, paliperidone can elevate serum prolactin concentrations. Paliperidone's prolactin-elevating effect is similar to that seen with risperidone, which appears to be associated with a higher level of prolactin elevation than other currently available antipsychotic agents. Clinical disturbances such as galactorrhea, amenorrhea, gynecomastia, and impotence have been associated with prolactin-elevating drugs. In addition, chronic hyperprolactinemia associated with hypogonadism may lead to decreased bone density in both female and male patients.

If paliperidone therapy is considered in a patient with previously detected breast cancer, clinicians should consider that approximately one-third of human breast cancers are prolactin-dependent in vitro.

Potential for GI Obstruction. As with other nondeformable material, extended-release paliperidone tablets do not appreciably change in shape in the GI tract. Therefore, extended-release tablets of the drug generally should not be administered to patients with severe, preexisting GI narrowing (either pathologic or iatrogenic). Rare cases of obstructive symptoms in patients with known strictures have been reported in association with the ingestion of drugs in nondeformable, controlled-release formulations. Because of the extended-release design of paliperidone tablets, the drug should only be used in patients who are able to swallow the tablet whole.

Decreased bioavailability of paliperidone extended-release tablets would be expected in patients with a decreased GI transit time (e.g., those with diarrhea) while an increased bioavailability would be expected in patients with an increased GI transit time (e.g., those with GI neuropathy, diabetic gastroparesis, or due to other causes). Such changes in bioavailability are more likely when changes in transit time occur in the upper GI tract.

Orthostatic Hypotension and Syncope. Orthostatic hypotension and syncope may occur during paliperidone therapy in some patients, particularly early in treatment, perhaps because of the drug's α_1-adrenergic blocking activity. Syncope occurred in about 0.8% of patients receiving paliperidone in controlled clinical trials.

Paliperidone should be used with caution in patients with known cardiovascular disease (e.g., heart failure, history of myocardial infarction, ischemic heart disease, conduction abnormalities), cerebrovascular disease, or conditions that would predispose patients to hypotension (e.g., dehydration, hypovolemia, concomitant antihypertensive therapy) and in antipsychotic-naive patients. Consideration should be given to monitoring orthostatic vital signs in paliperidone-treated patients who are susceptible to hypotension (e.g., geriatric patients).

Leukopenia, Neutropenia, and Agranulocytosis. In clinical trial and/or postmarketing experience, leukopenia and neutropenia have been temporally related to antipsychotic agents, including paliperidone. Agranulocytosis also has been reported with antipsychotic agents.

Possible risk factors for leukopenia and neutropenia include preexisting low leukocyte count and a history of drug-induced leukopenia and neutropenia. Patients with a preexisting low leukocyte count or a history of drug-induced leukopenia or neutropenia should have their complete blood count monitored frequently during the first few months of therapy. Paliperidone should be discontinued at the first sign of a decline in leukocyte count in the absence of other causative factors.

Patients with clinically important neutropenia should be carefully monitored for fever or other signs or symptoms of infection and promptly treated if such signs and symptoms occur. In patients with severe neutropenia (absolute neutrophil count [ANC] less than 1000/mm³), paliperidone should be discontinued and the leukocyte count monitored until recovery occurs. Lithium reportedly has been used successfully in the treatment of several cases of leukopenia associated with aripiprazole, clozapine, and some other drugs; however, further clinical experience is needed to confirm these anecdotal findings.

Cognitive and Motor Impairment. Like other antipsychotic agents, paliperidone potentially may impair judgment, thinking, or motor skills. In short-term, placebo-controlled trials in adults with schizophrenia, somnolence (including hypersomnia, hypersomnolence, and sedation) was reported in 6–11% of patients receiving the drug. The frequency of somnolence appears to be dose related. (See Advice to Patients.)

Seizures. Seizures have occurred in approximately 0.2% of patients with schizophrenia receiving paliperidone in premarketing clinical studies. As with other antipsychotic agents, paliperidone should be used with caution in patients with a history of seizures or with other conditions that may lower the seizure threshold (e.g., dementia of the Alzheimer's type); conditions that lower the seizure threshold may be more prevalent in patients 65 years of age or older.

Dysphagia. Esophageal dysmotility and aspiration have been associated with the use of antipsychotic agents. Aspiration pneumonia is a common cause of morbidity and mortality in geriatric patients, particularly in those with advanced Alzheimer's dementia. Paliperidone is *not* approved for the treatment of patients with dementia-related psychosis and should be used with caution in patients at risk for aspiration pneumonia. (See Increased Mortality in Geriatric Patients with Dementia-related Psychosis under Warnings/Precautions: Warnings, in Cautions.)

Suicide. There is an attendant risk of suicide in patients with psychotic illnesses; high-risk patients should be closely supervised. Paliperidone should be prescribed in the smallest quantity consistent with good patient management to reduce the risk of overdosage.

Priapism. Drugs possessing α-adrenergic blocking activity have been reported to cause priapism. Priapism has been reported in paliperidone-treated patients during postmarketing surveillance. Severe priapism may require surgical intervention.

Thrombotic Thrombocytopenic Purpura. Thrombotic thrombocytopenic purpura (TTP) has not been reported in clinical trials of paliperidone. TTP has been reported in association with risperidone therapy; however, the relationship of this adverse event to risperidone is unknown.

Body Temperature Regulation. Disruption of the body's ability to reduce core body temperature has been attributed to antipsychotic agents. The manufacturer recommends appropriate caution when paliperidone is used in patients who will be experiencing conditions that may contribute to an elevation in core body temperature (e.g., strenuous exercise, extreme heat, concomitant use of agents with anticholinergic activity, dehydration).

Antiemetic Effect. Antiemetic effects were observed in preclinical studies with paliperidone; these effects also may occur in humans and mask signs of overdosage of other drugs or obscure cause of vomiting in various disorders (e.g., intestinal obstruction, Reye's syndrome, brain tumor).

Concomitant Illnesses. Clinical experience with paliperidone in patients with certain concomitant illnesses is limited.

Patients with parkinsonian syndrome or dementia with Lewy bodies who receive antipsychotics reportedly have an increased sensitivity to antipsychotic agents. Clinical manifestations of this increased sensitivity have been reported to include confusion, obtundation, postural instability with frequent falls, extrapyramidal symptoms, and features consistent with NMS. For additional information on extrapyramidal adverse effects and NMS, see Cautions: Nervous System Effects, in the Phenothiazines General Statement 28:16.08.24.

Paliperidone has not been adequately evaluated in patients with a recent history of myocardial infarction or unstable cardiovascular disease to date and patients with these conditions were excluded from premarketing clinical trials. Because of the risk of orthostatic hypotension associated with paliperidone, the manufacturer states that the drug should be used with caution in patients with known cardiovascular disease. (See Orthostatic Hypotension and Syncope under Warnings/Precautions: Other Warnings and Precautions, in Cautions.)

Laboratory Test Monitoring. No specific laboratory tests are recommended in patients receiving paliperidone.

Specific Populations **Pregnancy.** Category C. (See Users Guide.)

Neonates exposed to antipsychotic agents during the third trimester of pregnancy are at risk for extrapyramidal and/or withdrawal symptoms following delivery. Symptoms reported to date have included agitation, hypertonia, hypotonia, tardive dyskinetic-like symptoms, tremor, somnolence, respiratory distress, and feeding disorder. Neonates exhibiting such symptoms should be monitored. The complications have varied in severity; some neonates recovered within hours to days without specific treatment while others have required intensive care unit support and prolonged hospitalization. For further information on extrapyramidal and withdrawal symptoms in neonates, see Cautions: Pregnancy, Fertility, and Lactation, in the Phenothiazines General Statement 28:16.08.24.

Lactation. Paliperidone is distributed into milk in humans. The benefits of breastfeeding should be weighed against the unknown risks of infant exposure to the drug.

Pediatric Use. Safety and efficacy of oral paliperidone in the treatment of schizophrenia in adolescents 12–17 years of age have been established in a double-blind, placebo-controlled study of 6 weeks' duration.

Safety and efficacy of oral paliperidone in the treatment of schizophrenia have not been established in pediatric patients younger than 12 years of age.

Safety and efficacy of oral paliperidone in the treatment of schizoaffective disorder have not been established in pediatric patients younger than 18 years of age.

Weight gain has been associated with atypical antipsychotic use and monitoring of weight is recommended. However, in paliperidone-treated adolescents, weight gain should be assessed against that expected with normal growth. Weight gain in adolescents receiving paliperidone in an open-label, long-term study was not considered clinically substantial when compared with normative data.

The manufacturer states that the long-term effects of paliperidone on growth and sexual maturation have not been fully evaluated in children and adolescents.

Geriatric Use. In clinical studies, approximately 7% of nearly 1800 patients were 65 years of age or older. In addition, the short-term efficacy and safety of paliperidone have been demonstrated in a placebo-controlled trial of 6 weeks' duration in 114 geriatric patients with schizophrenia. While no substantial differences in efficacy or safety relative to younger adults were observed in these studies or in other clinical experience with the drug, increased sensitivity cannot be ruled out.

Because geriatric patients may have reduced renal function, dosage adjustment may be required based on renal function status; consider monitoring renal function. (See Dosage and Administration: Special Populations.)

Geriatric patients with dementia-related psychosis treated with atypical antipsychotic drugs appear to be at an increased risk of death compared with that among patients receiving placebo. Paliperidone is *not* approved for the treatment of dementia-related psychosis. (See Increased Mortality in Geriatric Patients with Dementia-related Psychosis under Warnings/Precautions: Warnings, in Cautions.)

Hepatic Impairment. Patients with moderate hepatic impairment (Child-Pugh class B) exhibited similar plasma concentrations of free paliperidone as healthy individuals, although total paliperidone exposure decreased because of decreased protein binding. Dosage adjustment is not necessary in patients with mild to moderate hepatic impairment (Child-Pugh class A and B). The effect of severe hepatic impairment on paliperidone pharmacokinetics is not known. (See Dosage and Administration: Special Populations.)

Renal Impairment. Clearance decreased by an average of 32, 64, and 71% in patients with mild, moderate, and severe renal impairment, respectively. Dosage adjustment is recommended in patients with renal impairment. (See Dosage and Administration: Special Populations.)

■ **Common Adverse Effects** Adverse effects reported in 5% or more of adults receiving paliperidone for schizophrenia and at a frequency at least twice that reported with placebo include extrapyramidal symptoms, tachycardia, and akathisia.

Adverse effects reported in 5% or more of adolescents receiving paliperidone for schizophrenia and at a frequency at least twice that reported with placebo include somnolence, extrapyramidal symptoms (e.g., akathisia, tremor, dystonia, cogwheel rigidity), anxiety, increased weight, and tachycardia.

Adverse effects reported in 5% or more of adults receiving paliperidone for schizoaffective disorder and at a frequency at least twice that reported with placebo include extrapyramidal symptoms, somnolence, dyspepsia, constipation, increased weight, and nasopharyngitis.

Drug Interactions

■ **Drugs Affecting Hepatic Microsomal Enzymes** Inhibitors or inducers of cytochrome P-450 (CYP) isoenzymes 2D6, 3A4, 1A2, 2A6, 2C9, and 2C19: pharmacokinetic interaction unlikely.

■ **Drugs Metabolized by Hepatic Microsomal Enzymes** Substrates of CYP1A2, CYP2A6, CYP2C8/9/10, CYP2D6, CYP2E1, CYP3A4, or CYP3A5: pharmacokinetic interaction unlikely.

■ **Drugs Inhibiting P-glycoprotein Transport System** At therapeutic concentrations, paliperidone did not inhibit P-glycoprotein; clinically relevant interactions unlikely.

■ **Drugs that Prolong QT Interval** Potential pharmacologic interaction (additive effect on QT-interval prolongation); avoid concomitant use of other drugs known to prolong the QT interval (e.g., amiodarone, quinidine, procainamide, sotalol, other Class Ia and III antiarrhythmics, chlorpromazine, thioridazine, gatifloxacin, moxifloxacin). (See Prolongation of QT Interval under Warnings/Precautions: Other Warnings and Precautions, in Cautions.)

■ **Alcohol** Potential pharmacologic interaction (additive CNS effects). Avoid alcoholic beverages during paliperidone therapy.

■ **Other CNS Agents** Potential pharmacologic interaction (additive CNS effects). Use with caution.

■ **Anticholinergic Agents** Potential pharmacologic interaction (possible disruption of body temperature regulation); use paliperidone with caution in patients concurrently receiving drugs with anticholinergic activity. (See Body Temperature Regulation under Warnings/Precautions: Other Warnings and Precautions, in Cautions.)

■ **Carbamazepine** Concurrent administration of carbamazepine and paliperidone decreased mean steady-state peak plasma concentrations and area under the concentration-time curves (AUCs) of paliperidone by approximately 37%. The manufacturer recommends reevaluating the dosage of paliperidone upon initiation of carbamazepine and increasing it, if necessary, based on clinical assessment. Upon discontinuance of carbamazepine, the dosage of paliperidone should also be reevaluated and decreased, if necessary.

■ **Hypotensive Agents** Because of its α_1-adrenergic blocking activity and potential to cause hypotension, the manufacturer recommends that paliperidone be used with caution in patients receiving antihypertensive agents; monitoring of orthostatic vital signs should be considered in such patients. (See Orthostatic Hypotension and Syncope under Warnings/Precautions: Other Warnings and Precautions, in Cautions and also see Advice to Patients.)

■ **Levodopa and Dopamine Agonists** Potential pharmacologic interaction (antagonistic effects).

■ **Lithium** A pharmacokinetic interaction between paliperidone and lithium is unlikely.

■ **Paroxetine** Concomitant administration of paroxetine (20 mg daily) and a single dose of paliperidone (3 mg as extended-release tablets) caused a small, clinically insignificant increase in paliperidone AUCs compared with paliperidone administration alone. Therefore, dosage adjustment of paliperidone is not necessary.

■ **Protein-bound Drugs** Pharmacokinetic interaction unlikely.

■ **Risperidone** Concurrent use of paliperidone with risperidone has not been studied to date. However, because paliperidone is the principal active metabolite of risperidone, consideration should be given to additive paliperidone exposure if risperidone and paliperidone are concomitantly administered.

■ **Valproate** Concurrent administration of a single dose of paliperidone (12 mg) and divalproex sodium extended-release tablets (two 500-mg tablets once daily) resulted in an approximate 50% increase in peak plasma concentrations and AUCs of paliperidone. The manufacturer states that paliperidone dosage reduction should be considered when valproate is concomitantly administered with paliperidone.

■ **Smoking** Pharmacokinetic interaction unlikely. Dosage adjustment in patients who smoke is not necessary.

Description

Paliperidone is a benzisoxazole-derivative antipsychotic agent that differs chemically from other currently available first-generation (typical) antipsychotic agents (e.g., butyrophenones, phenothiazines) and has been referred to as an atypical or second-generation antipsychotic agent. The drug is the major active metabolite of risperidone, another atypical antipsychotic agent.

The exact mechanism of paliperidone's antipsychotic action, like that of other antipsychotic agents, has not been fully elucidated, but may involve antagonism of central dopamine type 2 (D_2) and serotonin type 2 (5-hydroxytryptamine [5-HT_{2A}]) receptors. Antagonism at α_1- and α_2-adrenergic and histamine (H_1) receptors may contribute to other therapeutic and adverse effects observed with the drug. Paliperidone possesses no affinity for cholinergic muscarinic and β_1- and β_2-adrenergic receptors.

In vitro studies have suggested a role for cytochrome P-450 (CYP) isoenzymes 2D6 and 3A4 in the metabolism of paliperidone; however, the results of in vivo studies indicate that these isoenzymes play a limited role in the overall elimination of the drug from the body.

Approximately 80% and 11% of a single 1-mg oral dose of radiolabeled, immediate-release paliperidone is recovered in urine and feces, respectively, within 1 week. About 59% of the administered dose is recovered as unchanged drug in urine and 32% is recovered as metabolites. Following single-dose oral administration as extended-release tablets, paliperidone appears to have a mean terminal elimination half-life of about 23 hours.

Advice to Patients

Importance of advising patients and caregivers that geriatric patients with dementia-related psychosis treated with antipsychotic agents are at an increased risk of death. Patients and caregivers also should be informed that paliperidone is *not* approved for treating geriatric patients with dementia-related psychosis.

Importance of informing patients about the risk of orthostatic hypotension, especially when initiating or reinitiating treatment or increasing the dosage. Importance of advising patients who experience dizziness or fainting during therapy to get up slowly when sitting or lying down.

Because somnolence and impairment of judgment, thinking, or motor skills may be associated with paliperidone, patients should be cautioned about driving, operating machinery, or performing hazardous tasks while taking paliperidone until they gain experience with the drug's effects. Importance of avoiding alcohol during paliperidone therapy.

Importance of patients being aware of the symptoms of hyperglycemia and diabetes mellitus (e.g., increased thirst, increased urination, increased appetite, weakness). Importance of informing patients who are diagnosed with diabetes, those with risk factors for diabetes, and those who develop hyperglycemic symptoms during treatment that they should have their blood glucose monitored at the beginning of and periodically during paliperidone therapy.

Risk of weight gain. Importance of patients being aware that they should have their weight monitored regularly during therapy.

Risk of leukopenia/neutropenia. Importance of advising patients with a preexisting low leukocyte count or a history of drug-induced leukopenia/neutropenia that they should have their complete blood cell (CBC) count monitored during paliperidone therapy.

Importance of informing patients and caregivers about the risk of neuroleptic malignant syndrome (NMS), a rare but potentially life-threatening syndrome that can cause high fever, stiff muscles, sweating, fast or irregular heart beat, change in blood pressure, confusion, and kidney damage.

Importance of clinicians informing patients in whom chronic paliperidone use is contemplated about the risk of tardive dyskinesia. Importance of informing patients to report any muscle movements that cannot be stopped to a health-care professional.

Importance of informing clinicians of existing or contemplated concomitant therapy, including prescription (see Drug Interactions: Drugs that Prolong QT Interval) and OTC drugs, dietary supplements, and/or herbal products, as well as any concomitant illnesses (e.g., cardiovascular disease, diabetes mellitus, seizures).

Importance of women informing clinicians if they are or plan to become pregnant or plan to breast-feed. Importance of clinicians informing patients about the benefits and risks of taking antipsychotics during pregnancy (see Pregnancy under Warnings/Precautions: Specific Populations, in Cautions). Importance of advising patients not to stop taking paliperidone if they become pregnant without consulting their clinician; abruptly stopping antipsychotic agents may cause complications.

Importance of avoiding overheating or dehydration.

Importance of informing patients that paliperidone extended-release tablets should be swallowed whole with the aid of liquids, and should not be chewed, divided or crushed. Patients should not be concerned if they notice a tablet-like substance in their stool.

Importance of informing patients of other important precautionary information. (See Cautions.)

Overview® (see Users Guide). For additional information on this drug until a more detailed monograph is developed and published, the manufacturer's labeling should be consulted. It is *essential* that the manufacturer's labeling be consulted for more detailed information on usual cautions, precautions, contraindications, potential drug interactions, laboratory test interferences, and acute toxicity.

Preparations

Excipients in commercially available drug preparations may have clinically important effects in some individuals; consult specific product labeling for details.

Paliperidone

Oral		
Tablets, extended-release	1.5 mg	**Invega®**, Janssen
	3 mg	**Invega®**, Janssen
	6 mg	**Invega®**, Janssen
	9 mg	**Invega®**, Janssen

Pimavanserin Tartrate

■ Pimavanserin tartrate is an atypical antipsychotic agent.

Uses

■ **Parkinson's Disease Psychosis** Pimavanserin is used for the management of hallucinations and delusions associated with Parkinson's disease psychosis. Because antipsychotic drugs have been associated with an increased risk of death in geriatric patients with dementia-related psychosis, pimavanserin should *not* be used for the treatment of dementia-related psychosis not related to the hallucinations and delusions associated with Parkinson's disease psychosis. (See Increased Mortality in Geriatric Patients with Dementia-related Psychosis under Warnings/Precautions: Warnings, in Cautions.)

Efficacy of pimavanserin for the management of hallucinations and delusions associated with Parkinson's disease psychosis was established in a 6-week, randomized, placebo-controlled study that included 199 adults (mean age of 72 years) with Parkinson's disease psychosis. For inclusion in the study, patients were required to have established Parkinson's disease for at least one year and psychotic symptoms (hallucinations and/or delusions) that developed after the diagnosis of Parkinson's disease and were severe and frequent enough to require treatment with an antipsychotic agent. Patients also were required to have a Mini-Mental State Examination (MMSE) score of 21 or greater and no delirium at study entry. Use of other antipsychotic agents was not permitted during the study, but drugs used for the management of Parkinson's disease (at stable dosages) were allowed; the majority (99%) of patients were receiving dopaminergic drugs at baseline and throughout the study. Patients were randomized to receive pimavanserin 34 mg or placebo once daily. The primary outcome measure was evaluated in terms of the Parkinson's disease-adapted Scale for the Assessment of Positive Symptoms (SAPS-PD), a 9-item scale used to assess symptoms and severity of hallucinations and delusions. Total scores on the SAPS-PD range from 0–45, with higher scores indicating greater severity of illness and a negative change in score reflecting improvement. Because treatment of psychosis in patients with Parkinson's disease can potentially worsen motor symptoms associated with the disease, a secondary outcome of this study assessed the patient's underlying symptoms of Parkinson's disease using the Unified Parkinson's Disease Rating Scale (UPDRS) parts II (evaluating activities of daily living) and III (evaluating motor symptoms).

Pimavanserin was substantially more effective than placebo in decreasing the frequency and/or severity of hallucinations and delusions in patients with Parkinson's disease psychosis as assessed by independent blinded raters using the SAPS-PD scale; the placebo-subtracted difference in SAS-PD score for patients receiving pimavanserin was −3.06. Pimavanserin demonstrated an effect on both the hallucinations and delusions components of the SAPS-PD. In a post-hoc analysis, complete response (defined as no hallucinations or delusions) was achieved in 14% of patients receiving pimavanserin compared with 1% of those receiving placebo. Pimavanserin did not worsen motor function in this study based on a similar change in UPDRS score from baseline to 6 weeks in patients receiving pimavanserin and those receiving placebo.

Dosage and Administration

■ **Administration** Pimavanserin is administered orally without regard to food.

■ **Dosage** Dosage of pimavanserin tartrate is expressed in terms of pimavanserin.

For the management of hallucinations and delusions associated with Parkinson's disease psychosis, the recommended dosage of pimavanserin is 34 mg (two 17-mg tablets) once daily without dosage titration.

Dosage Modification for Concomitant Use with Cytochrome P-450 (CYP) 3A4 Inhibitors and Inducers **Potent Inhibitors of CYP3A4.** If used concomitantly with a potent inhibitor of CYP3A4, dosage of pimavanserin should be reduced to 17 mg once daily.

Potent Inducers of CYP3A4. If used concomitantly with a potent inducer of CYP3A4, patients should be monitored for reduced efficacy of pimavanserin; an increase in pimavanserin dosage may be required.

■ **Special Populations** Pimavanserin has not been evaluated in patients with hepatic impairment. (See Hepatic Impairment under Warnings/Precautions: Specific Populations, in Cautions.)

Dosage adjustment is not necessary in patients with mild to moderate renal impairment (creatinine clearance of 30 mL/minute or greater). Pimavanserin has not been evaluated in those with severe renal impairment (creatinine clearance less than 30 mL/minute). (See Renal Impairment under Warnings/Precautions: Specific Populations, in Cautions.)

The manufacturer states that dosage adjustment is not required based on age, gender, ethnicity, and weight.

No dosage adjustment is necessary in geriatric patients.

Cautions

■ **Contraindications** The manufacturer states that there are no contraindications to the use of pimavanserin.

■ **Warnings/Precautions** ***Warnings*** **Increased Mortality in Geriatric Patients with Dementia-related Psychosis.** Geriatric patients with dementia-related psychosis treated with antipsychotic drugs are at an increased risk of death. Analyses of 17 placebo-controlled trials (modal duration of 10 weeks) revealed a 1.6- to 1.7-fold increase in mortality among geriatric patients receiving atypical antipsychotic drugs (i.e., aripiprazole, olanzapine, quetiapine, risperidone) compared with that observed in patients receiving placebo. Over the course of a typical 10-week controlled trial, the rate of death in drug-treated patients was about 4.5% compared with a rate of about 2.6% in the placebo group. Although the causes of death were varied, most of the deaths appeared to be either cardiovascular (e.g., heart failure, sudden death) or infectious (e.g., pneumonia) in nature. Pimavanserin is *not* approved for the management of patients with dementia-related psychosis not related to the hallucinations and delusions associated with Parkinson's disease psychosis.

Other Warnings and Precautions **QT Interval Prolongation.** Pimavanserin is known to prolong the QT interval. Pharmacokinetic and pharmacodynamic analyses suggest that the prolongation occurs in a concentration-dependent manner.

Use of pimavanserin should be avoided in patients with known QT interval prolongation and in those who are receiving drugs known to prolong the QT interval (e.g., class IA and III antiarrhythmic agents). (See Drug Interactions: Drugs that Prolong the QT Interval.) Pimavanserin also should be avoided in patients with a history of cardiac arrhythmias or other conditions that may increase the risk of torsades de pointes and/or sudden death (e.g., symptomatic bradycardia, hypokalemia or hypomagnesemia).

Specific Populations **Pregnancy.** There are no available data on use of pimavanserin in pregnant women. Reproduction studies in rats and rabbits revealed no teratogenic effects when pimavanserin was administered orally during the period of organogenesis at doses up to 10 or 12 times the maximum recommended human dose. However, maternal toxicity and reduced pup survival and body weight were observed when the drug was administered to pregnant rats during pregnancy and lactation at doses 2 times the maximum recommended human dose.

Lactation. It is not known whether pimavanserin is distributed into human milk or if the drug has any effect on milk production or the nursing infant. The known benefits of breast-feeding should be considered along with the importance of pimavanserin to the woman and any potential adverse effects on the breast-fed infant from either the drug or underlying maternal condition.

Pediatric Use. Safety and efficacy of pimavanserin have not been established in pediatric patients.

Geriatric Use. In placebo-controlled studies evaluating pimavanserin in patients with Parkinson's disease psychosis, 49% of patients were 65–75 years of age and 31% were older than 75 years of age. In the pooled population of patients enrolled in these studies, 27% had Mini-Mental State Examination (MMSE) scores of 21–24 and 73% of patients had scores of 25 or greater. No clinically important differences in safety or efficacy were noted between these 2 groups. (See Increased Mortality in Geriatric Patients with Dementia-related Psychosis under Warnings/Precautions: Warnings, in Cautions.)

Hepatic Impairment. Pimavanserin has not been evaluated in patients with hepatic impairment and is not recommended in this patient population.

Renal Impairment. A population pharmacokinetic analysis indicated that exposure of pimavanserin in patients with mild to moderate renal impairment was similar to that in patients with normal renal function. Pimavanserin has not been evaluated in patients with severe renal impairment and is not recommended in this patient population.

■ **Common Adverse Effects** Adverse effects reported in 2% or more of patients receiving pimavanserin in clinical studies and more frequently than with placebo include nausea, peripheral edema, confusional state, hallucinations (visual, auditory, tactile, and somatic), constipation, and gait disturbance.

Drug Interactions

Pimavanserin is metabolized principally by cytochrome P-450 (CYP) isoenzymes 3A4 and 3A5. CYP3A4 is the main enzyme responsible for biotransformation of the drug to its major active metabolite (AC-279). In vitro studies indicate that pimavanserin does not cause clinically important inhibition or induction of CYP3A4. The active metabolite does not appear to induce CYP3A to a clinically important extent and is not expected to cause induction of any other CYP enzymes. Neither pimavanserin nor its active metabolite inhibits any of the major hepatic and intestinal human CYP isoenzymes involved in drug metabolism (CYP1A2, 2B6, 2C8, 2C9, 2C19, 2D6, and 3A4).

In vitro studies indicate that pimavanserin is not a substrate for the efflux transporters P-glycoprotein (P-gp) and breast cancer resistance protein (BCRP) or organic anion transport proteins (OATP) 1B1 and 1B3.

■ **Drugs Affecting Hepatic Microsomal Enzymes** ***Potent Inhibitors of CYP3A4*** Concomitant use of pimavanserin and potent inhibitors of CYP3A4 (e.g., clarithromycin, indinavir, itraconazole, ketoconazole) may increase exposure of pimavanserin. When used concomitantly with a potent CYP3A4 inhibitor, dosage of pimavanserin should be reduced to 17 mg once daily.

Potent Inducers of CYP3A4 Concomitant use of pimavanserin and potent inducers of CYP3A4 (e.g., carbamazepine, phenytoin, rifampin, St. John's wort [*Hypericum perforatum*]) may decrease exposure of pimavanserin and potentially reduce the drug's efficacy. Patients receiving such concomitant therapy should be monitored for reduced efficacy of pimavanserin; an increase in dosage of pimavanserin may be required.

■ **Drugs that Prolong the QT Interval** Concomitant use of pimavanserin and drugs known to prolong the QT interval including class IA (e.g., disopyramide, procainamide, quinidine) and class III (e.g., amiodarone, sotalol) antiarrhythmic agents, certain antipsychotic agents (e.g., chlorpromazine, thioridazine, ziprasidone), and certain anti-infective agents (e.g., gatifloxacin, moxifloxacin) should be avoided. Such concomitant therapy may cause a potential additive effect on QT interval prolongation and increase the risk of cardiac arrhythmias. (See QT Interval Prolongation under Warnings/Precautions: Other Warnings and Precautions, in Cautions.)

■ **Carbidopa/Levodopa** No dosage adjustment of carbidopa/levodopa is necessary when used concomitantly with pimavanserin based on pharmacokinetic studies.

■ **Ketoconazole** Ketoconazole (a potent CYP3A4 inhibitor) increased peak plasma concentration and area under the concentration-time curve (AUC) of pimavanserin by 1.5- and 3-fold, respectively. Dosage of pimavanserin should be reduced to 17 mg once daily when used concomitantly with ketoconazole.

Description

The exact mechanism of action of pimavanserin in the management of hallucinations and delusions associated with Parkinson's disease psychosis has not yet been determined. However, the effects of the drug are thought to be mediated by its inverse agonist and antagonist activity at serotonin type 2A (5-HT_{2A}) receptors and, to a lesser extent, at 5-HT_{2C} receptors. Studies have shown that the delusions and hallucinations associated with Parkinson's disease psychosis may be linked to alterations in the serotonin system. Pimavanserin exhibits potent inverse agonist activity at 5-HT_{2A} receptors and lesser affinity for 5-HT_{2C} receptors; the drug has no appreciable affinity for 5-HT_{2B}, dopaminergic, muscarinic, histaminergic, or adrenergic receptors. Pimavanserin is structurally and pharmacologically distinct from other atypical antipsychotic agents; a distinguishing feature is the drug's relative lack of dopamine-blocking activity.

Pimavanserin is extensively absorbed following oral administration. Relative bioavailability of the drug (tablet to solution) is approximately 99.7%. The median time to peak plasma concentration of pimavanserin is 6 hours (range 4–24 hours). When administered with a high-fat meal, peak plasma concentration of pimavanserin decreases by approximately 9%, while area under the concentration-time curve (AUC) increases by 8%. Pimavanserin exhibits dose-proportional pharmacokinetics following administration of single oral doses (range 17–255 mg). The drug is extensively (approximately 95%) bound to plasma proteins. The pharmacokinetics of pimavanserin do not appear to be affected by age, gender, ethnicity, or weight.

Pimavanserin is metabolized principally by cytochrome P-450 (CYP) 3A4/5, and to a lesser extent by CYP2D6, CYP2J2, and various other CYP and flavin-containing monooxygenase isoenzymes. CYP3A4 is the principal isoenzyme involved in the formation of the major active metabolite of pimavanserin (AC-279). The mean plasma half-lives of pimavanserin and its active metabolite are approximately 57 and 200 hours, respectively. Approximately 0.6% of a radiolabeled dose of pimavanserin is excreted in urine as unchanged drug, and 1.5% is eliminated in feces after 10 days. Less than 1% of the administered dose of pimavanserin and its active metabolite are recovered in urine.

Advice to Patients

Importance of advising patients and caregivers that geriatric patients with dementia-related psychosis treated with antipsychotic agents are at an increased risk of death. Patients and caregivers also should be informed that pimavanserin is *not* approved for the management of patients with dementia-related psychosis not related to the hallucinations and delusions associated with Parkinson's disease psychosis.

Importance of informing clinicians of existing or contemplated therapy, including prescription and OTC drugs, as well as any concomitant illnesses.

Importance of women informing clinicians if they are or plan to become pregnant or plan to breast-feed.

Importance of informing patients of other important precautionary information. (See Cautions.)

Overview® (see Users Guide). For additional information on this drug until a more detailed monograph is developed and published, the manufacturer's labeling should be consulted. It is *essential* that the manufacturer's labeling be consulted for more detailed information on usual cautions, precautions, contraindications, potential drug interactions, laboratory test interferences, and acute toxicity.

Preparations

Excipients in commercially available drug preparations may have clinically important effects in some individuals; consult specific product labeling for details.

Pimavanserin Tartrate

Oral		
Tablets, film-coated	17 mg (of pimavanserin)	**Nuplazid®**, Acadia

QUEtiapine Fumarate

■ Quetiapine fumarate is considered an atypical or second-generation antipsychotic agent.

Uses

■ **Psychotic Disorders** Quetiapine fumarate is used for the symptomatic management of psychotic disorders (e.g., schizophrenia). Drug therapy is integral to the management of acute psychotic episodes in patients with schizophrenia and generally is required for long-term stabilization to sustain symptom remission or control and to minimize the risk of relapse. Antipsychotic agents are the principal class of drugs used for the management of all phases of schizophrenia. Patient response and tolerance to antipsychotic agents are variable, and patients who do not respond to or tolerate one drug may be successfully treated with an agent from a different class or with a different adverse effect profile.

Schizophrenia Short-term efficacy of quetiapine for the management of schizophrenia has been established by placebo-controlled studies of 6 weeks' duration principally in hospitalized patients with schizophrenia. Schizophrenia is a major psychotic disorder that frequently has devastating effects on various aspects of the patient's life and carries a high risk of suicide and other life-threatening behaviors. Manifestations of schizophrenia involve multiple psychologic processes, including perception (e.g., hallucinations), ideation, reality testing (e.g., delusions), emotion (e.g., flatness, inappropriate affect), thought processes (e.g., loose associations), behavior (e.g., catatonia, disorganization), attention, concentration, motivation (e.g., avolition, impaired intention and planning), and judgment. The principal manifestations of this disorder usually are described in terms of positive and negative (deficit) symptoms, and more recently, disorganized symptoms. Positive symptoms include hallucinations, delusions, bizarre behavior, hostility, uncooperativeness, and paranoid ideation, while negative symptoms include restricted range and intensity of emotional expression (affective flattening), reduced thought and speech productivity (alogia), anhedonia, apathy, and decreased initiation of goal-directed behavior (avolition). Disorganized symptoms include disorganized speech (thought disorder) and behavior and poor attention.

In clinical studies in patients with schizophrenia, quetiapine was more effective than placebo in reducing the severity of symptoms associated with this disorder. Quetiapine appears to improve both positive and negative manifestations of schizophrenia. Results from comparative clinical studies and meta-analyses suggest that quetiapine is at least as effective as chlorpromazine or haloperidol in reducing positive and negative symptoms of schizophrenia.

The American Psychiatric Association (APA) considers certain atypical antipsychotic agents (i.e., quetiapine, aripiprazole, olanzapine, risperidone, ziprasidone) first-line drugs for the management of the acute phase of schizophrenia (including first psychotic episodes), principally because of the decreased risk of adverse extrapyramidal effects and tardive dyskinesia, with the understanding that the relative advantages, disadvantages, and cost-effectiveness of conventional and atypical antipsychotic agents remain controversial. The APA states that, with the possible exception of clozapine for the management of treatment-resistant symptoms, there currently is no definitive evidence that one atypical antipsychotic agent will have superior efficacy compared with another agent in the class, although meaningful differences in response may be observed in individual patients. Conventional antipsychotic agents may be considered first-line therapy in patients who have been treated successfully in the past with or who prefer conventional agents. The choice of an antipsychotic agent should be individualized, considering past response to therapy, adverse effect profile (including the patient's experience of subjective effects such as dysphoria), and the patient's preference for a specific drug, including route of administration.

Although the efficacy of quetiapine for long-term use has not been established in controlled studies, the manufacturer states that beneficial effects of the drug were maintained for up to 4 years in some patients during an open-label extension study in patients who achieved an initial response to treatment during double-blind clinical studies. If quetiapine is used for extended periods, the need for continued therapy should be reassessed periodically on an individualized basis. (See Dosage and Administration: Dosage.)

For additional information on the symptomatic management of schizophrenia, including treatment recommendations and results of the Clinical Antipsychotic Trials of Intervention Effectiveness (CATIE) research program, see Schizophrenia and Other Psychotic Disorders under Uses: Psychotic Disorders, in the Phenothiazines General Statement 28:16.08.24.

■ **Bipolar Disorder** Quetiapine is used alone or in conjunction with lithium or divalproex sodium for the management of acute manic episodes associated with bipolar I disorder. Efficacy of quetiapine monotherapy in the treatment of acute manic episodes has been demonstrated in 2 placebo-controlled studies of 12 weeks' duration in patients who met the DSM-IV criteria for bipolar disorder and who met diagnostic criteria for an acute manic episode (with or without psychotic features). Patients with rapid cycling and mixed episodes were excluded from these studies. The principal rating instrument used for assessing manic symptoms in these studies was the Young Mania Rating Scale (YMRS) score, an 11-item clinician rated scale traditionally used to assess the degree of manic symptomatology in a range from 0 (no manic features) to 60 (maximum score). In these studies, quetiapine was shown to be superior to placebo in reduction of the YMRS total score after 3 and 12 weeks of treatment.

Efficacy of quetiapine when used in combination with lithium or divalproex sodium in the management of acute manic episodes has been demonstrated in a placebo-controlled study of 3 weeks' duration in patients who met the DSM-IV criteria for bipolar I disorder with acute manic episodes (with or without psychotic features). Patients with rapid cycling and mixed episodes were excluded from enrollment and patients included in the study may or may not have received an adequate course of therapy with lithium or divalproex sodium prior to randomization. Quetiapine was shown to be superior to placebo when added to lithium or divalproex sodium alone in the reduction of YMRS total score. However, in a similarly designed study, quetiapine was associated with an improvement of YMRS scores but did not demonstrate superiority to placebo.

For the initial management of less severe manic or mixed episodes in patients with bipolar disorder, current APA recommendations state that monotherapy with lithium, valproate (e.g., valproate sodium, valproic acid, divalproex), or an antipsychotic (e.g., olanzapine) may be adequate. For more severe manic or mixed episodes, combination therapy with an antipsychotic and lithium or valproate is recommended as first-line therapy. For further information on the management of bipolar disorder, see Uses: Bipolar Disorder, in Lithium Salts 28:28.

Quetiapine also is used for the treatment of depressive episodes associated with bipolar disorder. Efficacy of quetiapine in the treatment of depressive episodes has been demonstrated in 2 randomized, double-blind, placebo-controlled studies of 8 weeks' duration in patients with bipolar I or II disorder (with or without a rapid cycling course). Patients in these studies received fixed daily quetiapine dosages of 300 or 600 mg once daily. The principal rating instrument used for assessing depressive symptoms in these studies was the Montgomery-Asberg Depression Rating Scale (MADRS), a 10-item clinician-rated scale with scores ranging from 0 to 60. In both studies, quetiapine was found to be superior to placebo in reduction of MADRS scores at week 8, with improvements in scores evident within one week of treatment. In addition, patients receiving 300 mg of quetiapine daily demonstrated significant improvements compared to placebo recipients in overall quality of life and satisfaction related to various areas of functioning.

Dosage and Administration

■ **Administration** Quetiapine fumarate is administered orally. While food reportedly can marginally increase the peak concentration and oral bioavailability of quetiapine, the drug generally can be administered without regard to meals.

Dispensing and Administration Precautions Because of similarity in spelling between Seroquel® (the trade name for quetiapine fumarate) and Serzone® (the former trade name for nefazodone hydrochloride, an antidepressant agent; no longer commercially available in the US under this trade name), dispensing errors have been reported to the US Food and Drug Administration (FDA) and the manufacturer of Seroquel® (AstraZeneca). According to the medication error reports, the overlapping strengths (100 and 200 mg), dosage forms (tablets), and dosing intervals (twice daily) and the fact that these 2 drugs were stored closely together in pharmacies also were critical in causing these errors. Therefore, extra care should be exercised in ensuring the accuracy of both oral and written prescriptions for Seroquel® and Serzone®. Although the Serzone brand was discontinued in June 2004, clinicians may continue to refer to nefazodone by the former brand name in prescribing. Some experts recommend that pharmacists assess the measures of avoiding dispensing errors and implement them as appropriate (e.g., by verifying all orders for these agents by spelling both the trade and generic names to prescribers, using computerized name alerts, attaching reminders to drug containers and pharmacy shelves, separating the drugs on pharmacy shelves, counseling patients). (See Dispensing and Administration Precautions under Warnings/Precautions: General Precautions in Cautions.)

■ **Dosage** Dosage of quetiapine fumarate is expressed in terms of quetiapine and must be carefully adjusted according to individual requirements and response, using the lowest possible effective dosage.

Higher maintenance dosages of quetiapine may be required in patients receiving the antipsychotic drug concomitantly with phenytoin or other hepatic enzyme-inducing agents (e.g., carbamazepine, barbiturates, rifampin, glucocorticoids), and an increase in the maintenance dosage of quetiapine may be required to reestablish efficacy in patients receiving such concomitant therapy. (See Drug Interactions: Drugs Affecting Hepatic Microsomal Enzymes and also Phenytoin.)

Patients receiving quetiapine should be monitored for possible worsening of depression, suicidality, or unusual changes in behavior, especially at the beginning of therapy or during periods of dosage adjustments. (See Worsening of Depression and Suicidality Risk under Warnings/Precautions: Warnings, in Cautions.)

The manufacturer states that if quetiapine therapy is reinitiated after a drug-free period of less than 1 week, dosage titration is not necessary. However, if quetiapine therapy is reinitiated after a drug-free period exceeding 1 week, dosage generally should be titrated as with initial therapy.

Schizophrenia For the management of schizophrenia, the recommended initial dosage of quetiapine in adults is 25 mg twice daily. Dosage may be increased in increments of 25–50 mg 2 or 3 times daily on the second or third day, as tolerated, to a target dosage of 300–400 mg daily in 2 or 3 divided doses by the fourth day. Because steady-state plasma concentrations of quetiapine may not be attained for 1–2 days at a given dosage, subsequent dosage adjustments generally should be made at intervals of not less than 2 days, usually in increments or decrements of 25–50 mg twice daily. Effective dosages of quetiapine in clinical trials generally ranged from 150–750 mg daily. While the manufacturer states that increasing quetiapine dosages beyond 300 mg daily usually does not result in additional therapeutic effect, dosages of 400–500 mg daily apparently have been required in some patients, and a dosage range of 300–800 mg daily has been recommended. Safety of quetiapine in dosages exceeding 800 mg daily has not been established.

The optimum duration of quetiapine therapy currently is not known, but the efficacy of maintenance therapy with antipsychotic agents used in the treatment of schizophrenia is well established. Patients responding to quetiapine therapy should continue to receive the drug as long as clinically necessary and tolerated but at the lowest possible effective dosage, and the need for continued therapy with the drug should be reassessed periodically. The American Psychiatric Association (APA) states that prudent long-term treatment options in patients with remitted first- or multiple-episodes include either indefinite maintenance therapy or gradual discontinuance of the antipsychotic agent with close follow-up and a plan to reinstitute treatment upon symptom recurrence. Discontinuance of antipsychotic therapy should be considered only after a period of at least 1 year of symptom remission or optimal response while receiving the antipsychotic agent. In patients who have had multiple previous psychotic episodes or 2 psychotic episodes within 5 years, indefinite maintenance antipsychotic treatment is recommended.

If antipsychotic therapy is to be discontinued in patients with schizophrenia, precautions should include slow, gradual dose reduction over many months, more frequent clinician visits, and use of early intervention strategies. Patients and their family and caregivers should be advised about early signs of relapse, and clinicians should collaborate with them to develop plans for action should they emerge. The treatment program should be designed to respond quickly to evidence of prodromal symptoms or behaviors or exacerbations of schizophrenic symptoms.

Bipolar Disorder For the management of depressive episodes associated with bipolar I or II disorder, the recommended dosage of quetiapine in adults is 50 mg administered once daily at bedtime on the first day of therapy. The dosage of quetiapine should then be increased to 100 mg once daily on the second day of therapy, 200 mg once daily on the third day of therapy, and 300 mg once daily on the fourth day of therapy. In clinical trials demonstrating clinical efficacy, quetiapine was given in a dosing schedule of 50, 100, 200, and 300 mg once daily on days 1–4, respectively; patients who received 600 mg daily received 400 mg daily on day 5 and 600 mg daily on day 8. Although antidepressant efficacy was demonstrated with quetiapine at dosages of 300 mg daily and 600 mg daily, no additional benefit was seen in the 600-mg daily group.

For the management of acute mania associated with bipolar I disorder (alone or in conjunction with lithium or divalproex sodium), the recommended initial dosage of quetiapine in adults is 100 mg daily, administered in 2 divided doses. The dosage of quetiapine should be increased in increments of up to 100 mg daily in 2 divided doses to 400 mg daily on the fourth day of therapy. Subsequent dosage adjustments up to 800 mg daily by the sixth day of therapy should be made in increments not exceeding 200 mg daily. Data indicate that most patients respond to 400–800 mg daily. The safety of quetiapine dosages exceeding 800 mg daily has not been established.

The APA states that for patients treated with an antipsychotic agent during an acute episode in bipolar disorder, the need for ongoing antipsychotic treatment should be reassessed upon entering the maintenance phase. The APA recommends that antipsychotics be slowly tapered and discontinued unless they are required to control persistent psychosis or provide prophylaxis against recurrence. While maintenance therapy with atypical antipsychotics may be considered, there currently is limited evidence regarding their efficacy in the maintenance phase compared with that of agents such as lithium or valproate. The manufacturer of quetiapine states that efficacy of the drug has not been systematically evaluated for more than 12 weeks as monotherapy of acute manic episodes associated with bipolar I disorder or for more than 3 weeks as combined therapy with divalproex or lithium. In addition, the manufacturer of quetiapine states that efficacy of the drug has not been systematically evaluated for more than 8 weeks in the management of depressive episodes in patients with bipolar I or II disorder. If quetiapine is used for extended periods, the need for continued therapy should be reassessed periodically on an individualized basis.

Switching to or Concomitant Use with Other Antipsychotic Agents The manufacturer states that there are no systematically collected data that specifically address switching from other antipsychotic agents to quetiapine or concerning concomitant use of quetiapine with other antipsychotic agents. Although abrupt discontinuance of the previous antipsychotic agent may be acceptable for some patients with schizophrenia, gradual discontinuance may be most appropriate for others. In all cases, the period of overlapping antipsychotic administration should be minimized. In patients being switched from long-acting (depot) parenteral antipsychotic therapy to oral quetiapine therapy, the first oral dose of quetiapine should be administered in place of the next scheduled dose of the long-acting preparation. The need for continuing existing drugs used for the symptomatic relief of extrapyramidal manifestations should be reevaluated periodically.

■ **Special Populations** The manufacturer states that because quetiapine is substantially metabolized in the liver and because the pharmacokinetics of quetiapine appear to be altered in patients with hepatic impairment, an initial dosage of 25 mg daily should be used in adults with hepatic impairment. The dosage should be increased by 25–50 mg daily according to clinical response and tolerability until an effective dosage is reached.

Although elimination of quetiapine was reduced in patients with severe renal impairment (e.g., creatinine clearance of 10–30 mL/minute), the plasma quetiapine concentrations were similar to those in patients with normal renal function; therefore, the manufacturer states that dosage adjustment is not necessary in such patients.

Geriatric or debilitated patients and patients predisposed to hypotension or in whom hypotension would pose a risk (e.g., patients with dehydration or hypovolemia, those receiving antihypertensive drugs, patients with known cardiovascular or cerebrovascular disease) should have a slower rate of dosage titration and should receive lower target dosages of quetiapine. The risk of orthostatic hypotension can be minimized by limiting the initial dosage of quetiapine to 25 mg twice daily. If orthostatic hypotension occurs during titration to the target dosage, the manufacturer recommends a return to the previous dosage in the titration schedule

Cautions

■ **Contraindications** The manufacturer states that there are no known contraindications to quetiapine use.

■ **Warnings/Precautions** ***Warnings*** **Increased Mortality in Geriatric Patients with Dementia-related Psychosis.** Geriatric patients with dementia-related psychosis treated with atypical antipsychotic drugs appear to be at an increased risk of death compared with that among patients receiving placebo. Analyses of 17 placebo-controlled trials (average duration of 10 weeks) revealed an approximate 1.6- to 1.7-fold increase in mortality among geriatric patients receiving atypical antipsychotic drugs (i.e., quetiapine, aripiprazole, olanzapine, risperidone) compared with that in patients receiving placebo. Over the course of a typical 10-week controlled trial, the rate of death in drug-treated patients was about 4.5% compared with a rate of about 2.6% in the placebo group. Although the causes of death were varied, most of the deaths appeared to be either cardiovascular (e.g., heart failure, sudden death) or infectious (e.g., pneumonia) in nature. The manufacturer states that quetiapine is not approved for the treatment of dementia-related psychosis. (See Dosage and Administration: Special Populations and also see Geriatric Use under Warnings/Precautions: Specific Populations, in Cautions.)

Worsening of Depression and Suicidality Risk. Worsening of depression and/or the emergence of suicidal ideation and behavior (suicidality) or unusual changes in behavior may occur in both adult and pediatric (see Pediatric Use under Warnings/Precautions: Specific Populations, in Cautions) patients with major depressive disorder or other psychiatric disorders, whether or not they are taking antidepressants. This risk may persist until clinically important remission occurs with therapy. Suicide is a known risk of depression and certain other psychiatric disorders, and these disorders themselves are the strongest predictors of suicide. However, there has been a long-standing concern that antidepressants may have a role in inducing worsening of depression and the emergence of suicidality in certain patients during the early phases of treatment. Pooled analyses of short-term, placebo-controlled studies of antidepressants (i.e., selective serotonin-reuptake inhibitors and other antidepressants) have shown an increased risk of suicidality in children, adolescents, and young adults (18–24 years of age) with major depressive disorder and other psychiatric disorders. An increased suicidality risk was not demonstrated with antidepressants compared to placebo in adults older than 24 years of age and a reduced risk was observed in adults 65 years of age or older.

The US Food and Drug Administration (FDA) recommends that all patients being treated with antidepressants for any indication be appropriately monitored and closely observed for clinical worsening, suicidality, and unusual changes in behavior, particularly during initiation of therapy (i.e., the first few months) and during periods of dosage adjustments. Families and caregivers of patients being treated with antidepressants for major depressive disorder or other indications, both psychiatric and nonpsychiatric, also should be advised to monitor patients on a daily basis for the emergence of agitation, irritability, or unusual changes in behavior as well as the emergence of suicidality, and to report such symptoms immediately to a health-care provider.

Although a causal relationship between the emergence of symptoms such as anxiety, agitation, panic attacks, insomnia, irritability, hostility, aggressiveness, impulsivity, akathisia, hypomania, and/or mania and either the worsening of depression and/or the emergence of suicidal impulses has not been established, there is concern that such symptoms may represent precursors to emerging suicidality. Consequently, consideration should be given to changing the therapeutic regimen or discontinuing therapy in patients whose depression is persistently worse or in patients experiencing emergent suicidality or symptoms that might be precursors to worsening depression or suicidality, particularly if such manifestations are severe, abrupt in onset, or were not part of the patient's presenting symptoms. FDA also recommends that the drugs be prescribed in the smallest quantity consistent with good patient management, in order to reduce the risk of overdosage.

Bipolar Disorder. It is generally believed (though not established in controlled trials) that treating a major depressive episode with an antidepressant alone may increase the likelihood of precipitating a mixed or manic episode in patients at risk for bipolar disorder. Therefore, patients should be adequately screened for bipolar disorder prior to initiating treatment with an antidepressant; such screening should include a detailed psychiatric history (e.g., family history of suicide, bipolar disorder, and depression). Quetiapine is approved for use in treating bipolar depression in adults. (See Bipolar Disorder under Uses.)

Neuroleptic Malignant Syndrome. Neuroleptic malignant syndrome (NMS), a potentially fatal syndrome requiring immediate discontinuance of the drug and intensive symptomatic treatment, has been reported in patients receiving antipsychotic agents, including quetiapine. (See Advice to Patients.) For additional information on NMS, see Neuroleptic Malignant Syndrome under Cautions: Nervous System Effects, in the Phenothiazines General Statement 28:16.08.24.

Tardive Dyskinesia. Use of antipsychotic agents, including quetiapine, may be associated with tardive dyskinesia, a syndrome of potentially irreversible, involuntary, dyskinetic movements. For additional information on tardive dyskinesia, see Tardive Dyskinesia under Cautions: Nervous System Effects, in the Phenothiazines General Statement 28:16.08.24.

Hyperglycemia and Diabetes Mellitus. Severe hyperglycemia, sometimes associated with ketoacidosis, hyperosmolar coma, or death, has been reported in patients receiving all atypical antipsychotic agents, including quetiapine. While confounding factors such as an increased background risk of diabetes mellitus in patients with schizophrenia and the increasing incidence of diabetes mellitus in the general population make it difficult to establish with certainty the relationship between use of agents in this drug class and glucose abnormalities, epidemiologic studies suggest an increased risk of treatment-emergent hyperglycemia-related adverse events in patients treated with the atypical antipsychotic agents included in the studies (e.g., quetiapine, clozapine, olanzapine, risperidone).

Precise risk estimates for hyperglycemia-related adverse events in patients treated with atypical antipsychotics currently are not available. While some evidence suggests that the risk for diabetes may be greater with some atypical antipsychotics (e.g., clozapine, olanzapine) than with others in the class (e.g., quetiapine, risperidone), available data are conflicting and insufficient to provide reliable estimates of relative risk associated with use of the various atypical antipsychotics.

The manufacturers of atypical antipsychotic agents state that patients with preexisting diabetes mellitus in whom therapy with an atypical antipsychotic is initiated should be closely monitored for worsening of glucose control; those with risk factors for diabetes (e.g., obesity, family history of diabetes) should undergo fasting blood glucose testing upon therapy initiation and periodically throughout treatment. Any patient who develops manifestations of hyperglycemia (e.g., polydipsia, polyphagia, polyuria, weakness) during treatment with an atypical antipsychotic should undergo fasting blood glucose testing. In some cases, patients who developed hyperglycemia while receiving an atypical antipsychotic have required continuance of antidiabetic treatment despite discontinuance of the suspect drug; in other cases, hyperglycemia resolved with discontinuance of the antipsychotic.

For further information on the risk of hyperglycemia and diabetes mellitus associated with atypical antipsychotic agents, see Cautions: Endocrine and Metabolic Effects and see also Hyperglycemia and Diabetes Mellitus under Cautions: Precautions and Contraindications, in Clozapine 28:16.08.04.

Sensitivity Reactions Contact dermatitis, maculopapular rash, and photosensitivity reactions were reported infrequently during clinical trials. Anaphylaxis and Stevens-Johnson syndrome have been reported during postmarketing surveillance.

General Precautions **Cardiovascular Effects.** Orthostatic hypotension with associated dizziness, tachycardia, and/or syncope, particularly during the initial dosage titration period, has been reported. The risk of orthostatic hypotension and syncope may be minimized by limiting initial dosage. (See Dosage and Administration: Special Populations.) Use with caution in patients with known cardiovascular (e.g., history of myocardial infarction or ischemia, heart failure, conduction abnormalities) or cerebrovascular disease and/or conditions that would predispose patients to hypotension (e.g., dehydration, hypovolemia, concomitant antihypertensive therapy).

Ocular Effects. The development of cataracts in association with quetiapine was observed in animal studies. Lens changes also have been reported in some patients receiving long-term quetiapine therapy, although a causal relationship has not been established. Because the possibility of lens changes cannot be excluded, the manufacturer recommends ophthalmologic examination of the lens by methods adequate to detect cataract formation (e.g., slit lamp exam) be performed at the initiation of quetiapine therapy, or shortly thereafter, and at 6-month intervals during chronic quetiapine therapy.

Nervous System Effects. Seizures occurred in 0.6% of patients receiving quetiapine in controlled clinical trials. Use with caution in patients with a history of seizures or with conditions known to lower the seizure threshold (e.g., dementia of the Alzheimer's type, geriatric patients).

Somnolence occurred in 16–18 or 34% of patients receiving quetiapine as monotherapy (for the treatment of schizophrenia or bipolar disorder) or in conjunction with lithium or divalproex sodium (for the treatment of bipolar disorder), respectively, during clinical studies compared with 4–11% of those receiving placebo.

Endocrine Effects. Dose-related decreases in total and free thyroxine (T4) of approximately 20% were observed in patients receiving quetiapine dosages at the higher end of the therapeutic dosage range during clinical studies. These decreases were maximal during the first 2–4 weeks of therapy and were maintained without adaptation or progression during more chronic therapy. Generally, these changes were not considered clinically important and were reversible upon discontinuance of quetiapine, regardless of duration of therapy. Increases in TSH were observed in about 0.4 or 12% of patients receiving quetiapine alone or in conjunction with lithium or divalproex sodium, respectively. In patients receiving quetiapine monotherapy, thyroid replacement therapy was necessary in some patients who experienced increases in TSH.

Although not observed in patients receiving quetiapine during clinical trials, increases in prolactin concentrations and associated increases in mammary gland neoplasia were reported in animal studies.

Metabolic Effects. During clinical studies, 23 or 21% of patients with schizophrenia or acute mania receiving quetiapine gained at least 7% of their baseline weight compared with 6–7% of those receiving placebo. In patients receiving quetiapine as adjunctive therapy for acute mania, 13% gained at least 7% of their baseline weight compared with 4% of those receiving placebo.

Increases from baseline in cholesterol and triglyceride concentrations of 11 and 17%, respectively, were reported in patients receiving quetiapine compared with slight decreases in patients receiving placebo in clinical studies in patients with schizophrenia. These changes were weakly related to increases in weight observed in patients receiving quetiapine. For additional information on metabolic effects, see Hyperglycemia and Diabetes Mellitus under Warnings/Precautions: Warnings, in Cautions.

Hepatic Effects. Asymptomatic, transient, and reversible increases in serum transaminases, principally ALT, have been reported in patients receiving quetiapine; these changes usually occurred within the first 3 weeks and resolved despite continued quetiapine therapy.

Priapism. Drugs possessing α-adrenergic blocking activity have been reported to cause priapism. One case of drug-induced priapism was reported in clinical studies of quetiapine. Severe priapism may require surgical intervention.

Body Temperature Regulation. Although not reported in clinical studies with quetiapine, disruption of the body's ability to reduce core body temperature has been associated with use of antipsychotic agents. The manufacturer recommends appropriate caution when quetiapine is used in patients who will be experiencing conditions that may contribute to an elevation in core body temperature (e.g., strenuous exercise, extreme heat, concomitant use of agents with anticholinergic activity, dehydration).

GI Effects. Esophageal dysmotility and aspiration have been associated with the use of antipsychotic agents. Use with caution in patients at risk for aspiration pneumonia (e.g., geriatric patients, those with advanced Alzheimer's dementia).

Suicide. Attendant risk with bipolar disorder and psychotic illnesses; closely supervise high-risk patients. In clinical studies in patients with bipolar depression, the incidence of treatment-emergent suicidal ideation or suicide attempt in quetiapine-treated patients was low (1.7–2.6%) and similar to that observed with placebo (2%). Prescribe in the smallest quantity consistent with good patient management to reduce the risk of overdosage. (See Worsening of Depression and Suicidality Risk under Warnings/Precautions: Warnings, in Cautions.)

Dispensing and Administration Precautions. Because of similarity in spelling between Seroquel® (the trade name for quetiapine fumarate) and Serzone® (the former trade name for nefazodone hydrochloride, an antidepressant agent; no longer commercially available in the US under this trade name), dispensing errors have been reported to the US Food and Drug Administration (FDA) and the manufacturer of Seroquel® (AstraZeneca). According to the medication error reports, the overlapping strengths (100 and 200 mg), dosage forms (tablets), and dosing intervals (twice daily) and the fact that these 2 drugs were stored closely together in pharmacies also were critical in causing these errors. These medication errors may be associated with adverse CNS (e.g., mental status deterioration, hallucination, paranoia, muscle weakness, lethargy, dizziness) and GI effects (e.g., nausea, vomiting, diarrhea). As of November 2001, 4 patients had required emergency room visits and 3 patients reportedly had been hospitalized because of dispensing errors involving these 2 agents. One female patient 25 years of age experienced fever and respiratory arrest after mistakenly taking Seroquel® for 3 days instead of taking Serzone®, and eventually died, although a causal relationship has not been established. FDA also is concerned that several patients unintentionally ingested Serzone® or Seroquel® for a prolonged period of time before the error was discovered. Therefore, extra care should be exercised in ensuring the accuracy of both oral and written prescriptions for Seroquel® and Serzone®. Although the Serzone brand was discontinued in June 2004, clinicians may continue to refer to nefazodone by the former brand name in prescribing. Some experts recommend that pharmacists assess the measures of avoiding dispensing errors and implement them as appropriate (e.g., by verifying all orders for these agents by spelling both the trade and generic names to prescribers, using computerized name alerts, attaching reminders to drug containers and pharmacy shelves, separating the drugs on pharmacy shelves, counseling patients).

Patients should be advised to question the dispensing pharmacist regarding any changes in the appearance of their prescription in terms of shape, color, or size of the tablets. Dispensing errors involving Seroquel® (quetiapine) and Serzone® (nefazodone) should be reported to the manufacturers or directly to the FDA MedWatch program by phone (800-FDA-1088), by fax (800-FDA-0178), by the Internet (http://www.fda.gov/Safety/MedWatch/default.htm), or by mail (FDA Safety Information and Adverse Event Reporting Program, FDA, 5600 Fishers Lane, Rockville, MD 20852-9787).

Specific Populations **Pregnancy.** Category C. (See Users Guide.)

Neonates exposed to antipsychotic agents during the third trimester of pregnancy are at risk for extrapyramidal and/or withdrawal symptoms following delivery. Symptoms reported to date have included agitation, hypertonia, hypotonia, tardive dyskinetic-like symptoms, tremor, somnolence, respiratory distress, and feeding disorder. Neonates exhibiting such symptoms should be monitored. The complications have varied in severity; some neonates recovered within hours to days without specific treatment, while others have required intensive care unit support and prolonged hospitalization. For further information on extrapyramidal and withdrawal symptoms in neonates, see Cautions: Pregnancy, Fertility, and Lactation, in the Phenothiazines General Statement 28:16.08.24.

The effect of quetiapine on labor and delivery is unknown.

Lactation. Quetiapine appears to be distributed into human milk in relatively small amounts. The manufacturer recommends that women receiving quetiapine not breast-feed.

Pediatric Use. Safety and efficacy not established in children younger than 18 years of age.

FDA warns that a greater risk of suicidal thinking or behavior (suicidality) occurred during first few months of antidepressant treatment (4%) compared with placebo (2%) in children and adolescents with major depressive disorder, obsessive-compulsive disorder (OCD), or other psychiatric disorders based on pooled analyses of 24 short-term, placebo-controlled trials of 9 antidepressant drugs (selective serotonin-reuptake inhibitors [SSRIs] and other antidepressants). However, a more recent meta-analysis of 27 placebo-controlled trials of 9 antidepressants (SSRIs and others) in patients younger than 19 years of age with major depressive disorder, OCD, or non-OCD anxiety disorders suggests that the benefits of antidepressant therapy in treating these conditions may outweigh the risks of suicidal behavior or suicidal ideation. No suicides occurred in these pediatric trials.

Carefully consider these findings when assessing potential benefits and risks of quetiapine in a child or adolescent for any clinical use. (See Worsening of Depression and Suicidality Risk under Warnings/Precautions: Warnings, in Cautions.)

Geriatric Use. In clinical studies, approximately 7% of 3400 patients were 65 years of age or older. While no substantial differences in safety relative to younger adults were observed, factors that decrease pharmacokinetic clearance, increase the pharmacodynamic response, or cause poorer tolerance (e.g., orthostasis) may be present in geriatric patients. (See Dosage and Administration: Special Populations and also see Increased Mortality in Geriatric Patients with Dementia-related Psychosis under Warnings/Precautions: Warnings, in Cautions.)

In pooled data analyses, a *reduced* risk of suicidality was observed in adults 65 years of age or older with antidepressant therapy compared with placebo. (See Worsening of Depression and Suicidality Risk under Warnings/Precautions: Warnings, in Cautions.)

Hepatic Impairment. Increased plasma concentrations expected in patients with hepatic impairment; dosage adjustment may be necessary. (See Dosage and Administration: Special Populations.)

Renal Impairment. Clearance may be decreased in patients with severe renal impairment, but dosage adjustment is not necessary.

■ **Common Adverse Effects** The most common adverse effects reported in 5% or more of patients receiving quetiapine therapy for schizophrenia or bipolar disorder and at a frequency twice that reported among patients receiving placebo in clinical trials include somnolence, sedation, asthenia, lethargy, dizziness, dry mouth, constipation, increased ALT, weight gain, dyspepsia, abdominal pain, postural hypotension, and pharyngitis.

Drug Interactions

■ **Drugs Affecting Hepatic Microsomal Enzymes** Inhibitors of cytochrome P-450 (CYP) isoenzyme 3A4 (e.g., erythromycin, fluconazole, itraconazole, ketoconazole): potential pharmacokinetic interaction (increased serum quetiapine concentrations). Use with caution.

Inducers of CYP3A4 (e.g., barbiturates, carbamazepine, glucocorticoids, phenytoin, rifampin): potential pharmacokinetic interaction (increased quetiapine metabolism and decreased serum quetiapine concentrations). Dosage adjustment may be necessary if these drugs are initiated or discontinued in patients receiving quetiapine. (See Drug Interactions: Phenytoin.)

■ **Drugs Metabolized by Hepatic Microsomal Enzymes** Substrates of CYP1A2, CYP3A4, CYP2C9, CYP2C19, or CYP2D6: pharmacokinetic interaction unlikely.

■ **Alcohol** Potential pharmacologic interaction (additive CNS effects). Avoid alcoholic beverages during quetiapine therapy.

■ **Anticholinergic Agents** Potential pharmacologic interaction (possible disruption of body temperature regulation); use quetiapine with caution in patients concurrently receiving drugs with anticholinergic activity. (See Body Temperature Regulation under Warnings/Precautions: General Precautions, in Cautions.)

■ **Cimetidine** Concomitant use of cimetidine (400 mg 3 times daily for 4 days) and quetiapine (150 mg 3 times daily) decreased mean clearance of quetiapine by 20%. However, dosage adjustment of quetiapine is not necessary.

■ **Divalproex** Potential pharmacokinetic interaction. Increased maximum plasma quetiapine concentrations, with no effect on extent of quetiapine absorption or mean clearance. Decreased maximum plasma valproic acid concentrations and extent of absorption (not clinically important).

■ **Fluoxetine, Haloperidol, Imipramine, Risperidone** No effect on steady-state pharmacokinetics of quetiapine observed.

■ **Hypotensive Agents** Potential pharmacologic interaction (additive hypotensive effects).

■ **Levodopa and Dopamine Agonists** Potential pharmacologic interaction (antagonistic effects).

■ **Lithium** No effect on steady-state lithium pharmacokinetics observed.

■ **Lorazepam** Potential pharmacokinetic interaction (decreased clearance of lorazepam). Concomitant use of quetiapine (250 mg 3 times daily) and lorazepam (single 2-mg dose) resulted in a 20% decrease in the mean clearance of lorazepam.

■ **Phenytoin** Concomitant use of quetiapine (250 mg 3 times daily) and phenytoin (100 mg 3 times daily) resulted in a fivefold increase in quetiapine clearance. An increase in quetiapine dosage may be required; caution advised if phenytoin is withdrawn and replaced with a noninducer of CYP3A4 (e.g., valproate).

■ **Thioridazine** Potential pharmacokinetic interaction (increased oral clearance of quetiapine).

■ **Other CNS Agents** Potential pharmacologic interaction (additive CNS effects). Use with caution.

■ **Smoking** Smoking does not affect the oral clearance of quetiapine.

Description

Quetiapine fumarate is a dibenzothiazepine-derivative antipsychotic agent. The drug is pharmacologically similar to clozapine, but differs pharmacologically from other currently available first-generation (typical) antipsychotic agents (e.g., phenothiazines, butyrophenones). Because of these pharmacologic differences, quetiapine is considered an atypical or second-generation antipsychotic agent.

The exact mechanism of quetiapine's antipsychotic action in schizophrenia and its mood stabilizing action in bipolar disorder has not been fully elucidated but may involve antagonism at serotonin type 1 (5-hydroxytryptamine [5-HT_{1A}]) and type 2 (5-HT_{2A}, 5-HT_{2C}) receptors, and at dopamine (D_1, D_2) receptors.

Current evidence suggests that the clinical potency and antipsychotic efficacy of both typical and atypical antipsychotic drugs generally are related to their affinity for and blockade of central dopamine D_2 receptors; however, antagonism at dopamine D_2 receptors does not appear to account fully for the antipsychotic effects of quetiapine. Results of in vivo and in vitro studies indicate that quetiapine is a comparatively weak antagonist at dopamine D_2 receptors. Receptor binding studies show quetiapine is a weak antagonist at D_1 receptors. Although their role in eliciting the pharmacologic effects of antipsychotic agents remains to be fully elucidated, dopamine D_3, D_4, and D_5 receptors also have been identified; quetiapine possesses no affinity for the dopamine D_4 receptor.

The therapeutic effects of antipsychotic drugs are thought to be mediated by dopaminergic blockade in the mesolimbic and mesocortical areas of the CNS, while antidopaminergic effects in the neostriatum appear to be associated with extrapyramidal effects. The apparently low incidence of extrapyramidal effects associated with quetiapine therapy suggests that the drug is more active in the mesolimbic than in the neostriatal dopaminergic system. In contrast to typical antipsychotic agents (e.g., chlorpromazine) but like other atypical antipsychotic drugs (e.g., clozapine), quetiapine does not cause sustained elevations in serum prolactin concentrations and therefore is unlikely to produce adverse effects such as amenorrhea, galactorrhea, and impotence.

Quetiapine exhibits α_1- and α_2-adrenergic blocking activity; blockade of α_1-adrenergic receptors may explain the occasional orthostatic hypotension associated with the drug. Quetiapine also blocks histamine H_1 receptors, which may explain the sedative effects associated with the drug. Quetiapine possesses little or no affinity for β-adrenergic, γ-aminobutyric acid (GABA), benzodiazepine, or muscarinic receptors.

Quetiapine is extensively metabolized in the liver principally via sulfoxidation and oxidation to inactive metabolites. In vitro studies suggest that the cytochrome P-450 (CYP) 3A4 isoenzyme is involved in the metabolism of quetiapine to the inactive sulfoxide metabolite, which is the principal metabolite. The mean terminal half-life of quetiapine is about 6 hours. Following oral administration of a single dose of quetiapine, approximately 73 and 20% of the dose is excreted in urine and feces, respectively; less than 1% of the dose is excreted unchanged. Based on in vitro studies, quetiapine and 9 of its metabolites do not appear likely to inhibit CYP isoenzymes 1A2, 3A4, 2C9, 2C19, or 2D6.

Advice to Patients

Risk of suicidality; importance of patients, family, and caregivers being alert to and immediately reporting emergence of suicidality, worsening depression, or unusual changes in behavior, especially during the first few months of therapy or during periods of dosage adjustment.

Importance of providing written patient information (medication guide) explaining risks of quetiapine each time the drug is dispensed.

Risk of orthostatic hypotension, especially during initial dosage titration and at times of reinitiation of therapy or increases in dosage.

Risk of somnolence and impairment of judgment, thinking, or motor skills; avoid driving, operating machinery, or performing hazardous tasks until effects on the individual are known.

Importance of avoiding alcohol during quetiapine therapy.

Importance of informing patients and caregivers about the risk of neuroleptic malignant syndrome (NMS), a rare but potentially life-threatening syndrome that can cause high fever, stiff muscles, sweating, fast or irregular heart beat, change in blood pressure, confusion, and kidney damage.

Importance of informing clinicians of existing or contemplated concomitant therapy, including prescription and OTC drugs, as well as any concomitant illnesses (e.g., diabetes mellitus).

Importance of women informing clinicians if they are or plan to become pregnant or plan to breast-feed. Importance of clinicians informing patients about the benefits and risks of taking antipsychotics during pregnancy (see Pregnancy under Warnings/Precautions: Specific Populations, in Cautions). Importance of advising patients not to stop taking quetiapine if they become pregnant without consulting their clinician; abruptly discontinuing antipsychotic agents may cause complications. Importance of advising patients not to breast-feed during quetiapine therapy.

Importance of avoiding overheating or dehydration.

Importance of informing patients of other important precautionary information. (See Cautions.)

Overview® (see Users Guide). For additional information on this drug until a more detailed monograph is developed and published, the manufacturer's labeling should be consulted. It is *essential* that the manufacturer's labeling be consulted for more detailed information on usual cautions, precautions, contraindications, potential drug interactions, laboratory test interferences, and acute toxicity.

Preparations

Excipients in commercially available drug preparations may have clinically important effects in some individuals; consult specific product labeling for details.

QUEtiapine Fumarate

Oral

Tablets, film-coated	25 mg (of quetiapine)	**SEROquel®**, AstraZeneca
	50 mg (of quetiapine)	**SEROquel®**, AstraZeneca
	100 mg (of quetiapine)	**SEROquel®**, AstraZeneca
	200 mg (of quetiapine)	**SEROquel®**, AstraZeneca
	300 mg (of quetiapine)	**SEROquel®**, AstraZeneca
	400 mg (of quetiapine)	**SEROquel®**, AstraZeneca

risperiDONE

■ Risperidone has been described as an atypical or second-generation antipsychotic agent.

Uses

■ **Psychotic Disorders** Risperidone is used orally and parenterally for the symptomatic management of psychotic disorders (e.g., schizophrenia). Drug therapy is integral to the management of acute psychotic episodes in patients with schizophrenia and generally is required for long-term stabilization to sustain symptom remission or control and to minimize the risk of relapse. Antipsychotic agents are the principal class of drugs used for the management of all phases of schizophrenia.

The American Psychiatric Association (APA) considers most atypical antipsychotic agents first-line drugs for the management of the acute phase of schizophrenia (including first psychotic episodes), principally because of the decreased risk of adverse extrapyramidal effects and tardive dyskinesia, with the understanding that the relative advantages, disadvantages, and cost-effectiveness of conventional and atypical antipsychotic agents remain controversial. The APA states that, with the possible exception of clozapine for the management of treatment-resistant symptoms, there currently is no definitive evidence that one atypical antipsychotic agent will have superior efficacy compared with another agent in the class, although meaningful differences in response may be observed in individual patients. Conventional antipsychotic agents also may be an appropriate first-line option for some patients, including those who have been treated successfully in the past with or who prefer conventional agents. The choice of an antipsychotic agent should be individualized, considering past response to therapy, current symptomatology, concurrent medical conditions, other medications and treatments, adverse effect profile, and the patient's preference for a specific drug, including route of administration. Patient response and tolerance to antipsychotic agents are variable, and patients who do not respond to or tolerate one drug may be successfully treated with an agent from a different class or with a different adverse effect profile.

Schizophrenia Risperidone is used orally for the treatment of schizophrenia in adults and adolescents 13–17 years of age and IM as an extended-release injection for the treatment of schizophrenia in adults. Schizophrenia is a major psychotic disorder that frequently has devastating effects on various aspects of the patient's life and carries a high risk of suicide and other life-threatening behaviors. Manifestations of schizophrenia involve multiple psychologic processes, including perception (e.g., hallucinations), ideation, reality testing (e.g., delusions), emotion (e.g., flatness, inappropriate affect), thought processes (e.g., loose associations), behavior (e.g., catatonia, disorganization), attention, concentration, motivation (e.g., avolition, impaired intention and planning), and judgment. The principal manifestations of this disorder usually are described in terms of positive and negative (deficit) symptoms, and more recently, disorganized symptoms. Positive symptoms include hallucinations, delusions, bizarre behavior, hostility, uncooperativeness, and paranoid ideation, while negative symptoms include restricted range and intensity of emotional expression (affective flattening), reduced thought and speech productivity (alogia), anhedonia, apathy, and decreased initiation of goal-directed behavior (avolition). Disorganized symptoms include disorganized speech (thought disorder) and behavior and poor attention.

Short-term efficacy of oral risperidone for the treatment of schizophrenia in adults was established in 4 controlled studies of 4–8 weeks' duration in patients who met DSM-III-R criteria for schizophrenia and who were hospitalized for psychotic symptoms. In these and other clinical studies conducted principally in patients with schizophrenia, oral risperidone was more effective than placebo and at least as effective as conventional (e.g., haloperidol, perphenazine) and certain atypical (e.g., olanzapine) antipsychotics in the treatment of schizophrenia. Data from limited clinical studies indicate that risperidone improves both positive and negative manifestations of schizophrenia, but that such improvements may not be substantially greater than those achieved by haloperidol, a conventional antipsychotic. In these studies, improvement in manifestations of schizophrenia was based on the results of various psychiatric rating scales, including the Brief Psychiatric Rating Scale (BPRS) that assesses factors such as anergy, thought disturbances, activation, hostility/suspiciousness, and anxiety/depression; the BPRS psychosis cluster that assesses factors such as conceptual disorganization, hallucinatory behavior, suspiciousness, and unusual thought content in actively psychotic schizophrenic patients; the Scale for the Assessment of Negative Symptoms (SANS); the Positive and Negative Syndrome Scale (PANSS); and the Clinical Global Impression (CGI) scale.

Long-term efficacy of oral risperidone for the treatment of schizophrenia was established in a randomized, double-blind study in 365 adult outpatients who met DSM-IV criteria for schizophrenia or schizoaffective disorder. Patients were randomized to receive either flexible dosages of risperidone (2–8 mg daily) or haloperidol (5–20 mg daily) for 1–2 years and observed for relapse. Patients receiving risperidone experienced a substantially longer time to relapse than those who received haloperidol. In this study, approximately 25% of patients who received usual dosages of risperidone had relapsed by the end of the study compared with approximately 40% of those receiving usual dosages of haloperidol.

Efficacy of oral risperidone for the treatment of schizophrenia in adolescents was demonstrated in 2 short-term, double-blind clinical trials of 6–8 weeks' duration in adolescent patients 13–17 years of age who met DSM-IV criteria for schizophrenia and were experiencing an acute episode of schizophrenia at the time of enrollment. In the first study, patients were randomized to receive flexible dosages of risperidone of 1–3 mg daily or 4–6 mg daily or placebo. In the second study, patients were randomized to receive either risperidone target dosages of 0.15–0.6 mg daily or 1.5–6 mg daily. The primary efficacy measure in both studies was the change in total PANSS score from baseline. In these studies, risperidone in the target dosage groups from 1–6 mg daily was found to be more effective than placebo in substantially reducing the total PANSS score; however, dosages higher than 3 mg daily did not demonstrate additional efficacy.

Efficacy of the extended-release IM formulation of risperidone (Risperdal® Consta®) in the treatment of schizophrenia in adults was established, in part, based on extrapolation of efficacy data from oral risperidone. In addition, efficacy of extended-release IM risperidone was established in a multicenter, placebo-controlled study of 12 weeks' duration in adult inpatients and outpatients who met DSM-IV criteria for schizophrenia. During the 1-week run-in period of this study, other oral antipsychotic agents were discontinued and all patients received oral risperidone therapy (initially, 2 mg daily and titrated up to 4 mg daily for at least 3 days). During the 12-week, double-blind phase, patients were randomized to receive IM injections of 25, 50, or 75 mg of extended-release risperidone or placebo every 2 weeks. Patients receiving extended-release IM injections of risperidone were also given oral risperidone (2 mg daily in the 25-mg group, 4 mg in the 50-mg group, and 6 mg in the 75-mg group) for 3 weeks following the first injection to provide therapeutic plasma concentrations of the drug until the main release phase of risperidone from the IM injection site had begun; patients who received placebo injections were given placebo tablets. The primary efficacy measure in this study was the change in total PANSS score from baseline to end point. Total PANSS scores demonstrated substantially greater improvement in the patients treated with each of the 3 IM dosages of extended-release risperidone (25, 50, and 75 mg every 2 weeks) compared with patients receiving placebo. Although there were no significant differences in treatment effects between the 3 dosage groups, the effect size for the 75-mg group was numerically less than that of the 50-mg group. Subgroup analyses did not reveal any differences in treatment outcomes based on age, race, or gender.

Efficacy of extended-release IM risperidone in the treatment of schizophrenia has not been evaluated in controlled clinical trials for longer than 12 weeks; however, oral risperidone has been shown to be effective in delaying time to relapse with longer-term use. If the extended-release IM injection of risperidone is used for extended periods, the long-term risks and benefits of the drug should be reassessed periodically on an individualized basis.

Parenteral antipsychotic therapy with a long-acting IM preparation may be particularly useful in patients with schizophrenia and a history of poor compliance. In addition, long-acting antipsychotic preparations may be useful in patients with suspected GI malabsorption or variable GI absorption of the drug. The principal disadvantage of long-acting parenteral antipsychotics is the inability to terminate the drug's action when severe adverse reactions occur.

The manufacturer of extended-release IM risperidone recommends that patients should first receive oral risperidone therapy to establish tolerability of the drug before the long-acting IM preparation is used.

For additional information on the symptomatic management of schizophrenia, including treatment recommendations and results of the Clinical Antipsychotic Trials of Intervention Effectiveness (CATIE) research program, see Schizophrenia and Other Psychotic Disorders under Uses: Psychotic Disorders, in the Phenothiazines General Statement 28:16.08.24.

Geriatric Considerations. Although risperidone has been studied for use in the management of psychosis and aggression in institutionalized geriatric patients with moderate to severe dementia of the Alzheimer's type† (Alzheimer's disease, presenile or senile dementia), vascular dementia†, or a combination of the 2 types of dementia (i.e., mixed dementia†), use of the drug in geriatric patients with dementia-related psychosis is associated with an increased risk of adverse cerebrovascular events. In randomized, placebo-controlled studies in nursing home residents with dementia, oral risperidone at a dosage of approximately 1 mg daily was more effective than placebo in decreasing psychotic and behavioral symptoms (e.g., aggression, agitation) of dementia, as assessed by the Behavioral Pathology in Alzheimer's Disease scale (BEHAVE-AD) and the Cohen-Mansfield Agitation Inventory (CMAI). However, evidence from these studies showed a significantly higher incidence of adverse cerebrovascular events such as stroke and transient ischemic attacks (TIAs) associated with risperidone therapy relative to placebo. In addition, geriatric patients with dementia-related psychosis treated with atypical antipsychotic agents are at an increased risk of death compared with that among patients receiving placebo. (See Cautions: Geriatric Precautions.) Risperidone is not approved for the treatment of dementia-related psychosis.

■ Bipolar Disorder

Risperidone is used orally as monotherapy for the treatment of acute manic and mixed episodes associated with bipolar I disorder in adults and adolescents 10–17 years of age, or in conjunction with lithium or valproate for the treatment of acute manic and mixed episodes associated with bipolar I disorder in adults. Risperidone as an extended-release injection is also used IM as monotherapy or adjunctive therapy with lithium or valproate for the maintenance treatment of bipolar I disorder in adults.

Efficacy of oral risperidone monotherapy in the treatment of acute manic and mixed episodes has been demonstrated in 2 placebo-controlled trials of 3 weeks' duration in adults who met the DSM-IV criteria for bipolar I disorder with acute manic or mixed episodes with or without psychotic features. The principal rating instrument used for assessing manic symptoms in these trials was the Young Mania Rating Scale (Y-MRS), an 11-item clinician-rated scale traditionally used to assess the degree of manic symptomatology in a range from 0 (no manic features) to 60 (maximum score). In the first 3-week, placebo-controlled trial, which was limited to patients with manic episodes, risperidone monotherapy was given at an initial dosage of 3 mg daily and subsequently in a flexible dosage ranging from 1–6 mg daily; the mean modal dosage was 4.1 mg daily. In the second 3-week, placebo-controlled trial, patients also were given an initial dosage of risperidone 3 mg daily and subsequently a flexible dosage ranging from 1–6 mg daily; the mean modal dosage was 5.6 mg daily. Risperidone was found to be superior to placebo in the reduction of the Y-MRS total score in both studies.

Efficacy of oral risperidone as monotherapy in the treatment of acute manic or mixed episodes associated with bipolar I disorder in children and adolescents 10–17 years of age was demonstrated in a 3-week, double-blind, placebo-controlled trial. The pediatric patients were randomized to receive 1 of 2 dosage ranges of risperidone or placebo. Risperidone was initiated at 0.25 mg daily and titrated to the maximum tolerated dosage within the target dosage ranges of 0.5–2.5 mg daily or 3–6 mg daily within 10 days. The principal rating instrument used for assessing manic symptoms in this trial was the Y-MRS. Both dosage ranges of risperidone were found to be substantially superior to placebo in reducing the Y-MRS total score; however, dosages exceeding 2.5 mg daily did not demonstrate greater efficacy than lower dosages of the drug (0.5–2.5 mg daily).

Efficacy of oral risperidone when used in conjunction with lithium or valproate in the treatment of acute manic or mixed episodes associated with bipolar I disorder has been demonstrated in one placebo-controlled trial of 3 weeks' duration in adults who met the DSM-IV criteria for bipolar I disorder (with or without a rapid cycling course) and who met diagnostic criteria for an acute manic or mixed episode (with or without psychotic features). In this study, inpatients and outpatients with bipolar disorder experiencing manic or mixed episodes who had not adequately responded to lithium or valproate monotherapy were randomized to receive risperidone, haloperidol, or placebo in conjunction with their original therapy. Risperidone therapy was given in an initial dosage of 2 mg daily and subsequently given in a flexible dosage ranging from 1–6 mg daily; the mean modal dosage was 3.8 mg daily. Lithium and valproate were given in conjunction with risperidone and plasma drug concentrations were maintained within therapeutic ranges of 0.6–1.4 mEq/L for lithium and 50–120 mcg/mL for valproate. Addition of risperidone to lithium or valproate was shown to be superior to continued monotherapy with lithium or valproate as assessed by reduction of Y-MRS total score.

In a second 3-week, placebo-controlled trial, inpatients and outpatients with bipolar mania receiving lithium, valproate (as divalproex), or carbamazepine therapy with inadequately controlled manic or mixed symptoms were randomized to receive oral risperidone or placebo in conjunction with their original therapy. Risperidone was given in a flexible dosage range of 1–6 mg daily, with an initial dosage of 2 mg daily; the mean modal dosage was 3.7 mg daily. Addition of risperidone to lithium, valproate, or carbamazepine therapy (with plasma drug concentrations maintained within therapeutic ranges of 0.6–1.4 mEq/L, 50–125 mcg/mL, or 4–12 mcg/mL, respectively) was not found to be superior to lithium, valproate, or carbamazepine given alone as assessed by reduction of the Y-MRS total score. A possible explanation for the failure of this trial was enzymatic induction of clearance of risperidone and its principal active metabolite, 9-hydroxyrisperidone, by carbamazepine in the subgroup of patients receiving combined therapy with these drugs, resulting in subtherapeutic plasma concentrations of risperidone and 9-hydroxyrisperidone.

Efficacy of the extended-release IM formulation of risperidone (Risperdal® Consta®) as monotherapy in the maintenance treatment of bipolar I disorder was established in a multicenter, placebo-controlled trial in adults who met the DSM-IV criteria for bipolar I disorder and who were either stable on their drug regimen or experiencing an acute manic or mixed episode. All patients in this study were treated with open-label extended-release IM risperidone therapy for 26 weeks. Patients received an initial risperidone dosage of 25 mg IM every 2 weeks; the dosage was increased to 37.5 or 50 mg or decreased to 12.5 mg every 2 weeks as clinically indicated; patients who maintained response at 26 weeks were randomized to double-blind treatment with either the same IM dosage of risperidone or placebo and then monitored for relapse. Time to relapse to any mood episode (the primary outcome variable) was substantially delayed in patients receiving extended-release IM risperidone therapy compared with placebo. The majority of relapses were caused by manic rather than depressive symptoms; based on patient history, patients enrolled in the study had more manic episodes than depressive episodes.

Efficacy of extended-release IM risperidone as adjunctive therapy with lithium or valproate in the maintenance treatment of bipolar I disorder was established in a multicenter, double-blind, placebo-controlled study in adults with bipolar I disorder treated with mood stabilizers (primarily lithium or valproate), antidepressants, and/or anxiolytics who had experienced at least 4 episodes of mood disorder requiring clinical intervention in the previous 12 months and at least 2 episodes in the previous 6 months. Following a 16-week, open-label treatment phase with extended-release IM risperidone (initial risperidone dosage of 25 mg every 2 weeks and increased to 37.5 or 50 mg or decreased to 12.5 mg, if necessary), patients who remained stable were randomized either to continue IM risperidone at the same dosage or to receive placebo for up to 52 weeks while continuing their usual treatment and were observed for relapse. Continuation of IM risperidone therapy in addition to mood stabilizers delayed time to relapse to any mood episode (depression, mania, hypomania, or mixed) compared with placebo; the relapses were approximately half depressive and half manic or mixed episodes in this study.

For the initial management of less severe manic or mixed episodes in patients with bipolar disorder, current APA recommendations state that monotherapy with lithium, valproate (e.g., valproate sodium, valproic acid, divalproex), or an antipsychotic such as olanzapine may be adequate. For more severe manic or mixed episodes, combined therapy with an antipsychotic and lithium or valproate is recommended as first-line therapy. For further information on the management of bipolar disorder, see Uses: Bipolar Disorder, in Lithium Salts 28:28.

The manufacturers state that clinicians who elect to use risperidone for extended periods should periodically reevaluate the long-term risks and benefits of the drug for the individual patient.

■ Autistic Disorder

Risperidone is used orally for the management of irritability associated with autistic disorder in children and adolescents, including symptoms of aggression towards others, deliberate self-injuriousness, temper tantrums, and quickly changing moods.

Short-term efficacy of oral risperidone in children and adolescents with autistic disorder was established in 2 placebo-controlled trials of 8 weeks' duration in 156 children and adolescents (aged 5–16 years) who met the DSM-IV criteria for autistic disorder. Over 90% of the patients in these 2 trials were under 12 years of age and the majority weighed over 20 kg (weight range: 16–104.3 kg). The principal rating instruments used for assessing efficacy in these trials were the Aberrant Behavior Checklist (ABC) and the Clinical Global Impression-Change (CGI-C) scale. The primary outcome measure in both trials was the change from baseline to endpoint in the Irritability subscale of the ABC (ABC-I), which measures the emotional and behavioral symptoms of autism, including aggression toward others, deliberate self-injuriousness, temper tantrums, and rapidly changing moods. The CGI-C rating at endpoint was a co-primary outcome measure in one of the studies.

In the first 8-week, placebo-controlled trial, children and adolescents 5–16 years of age with autistic disorder received twice-daily placebo or risperidone 0.5–3.5 mg daily on a weight-adjusted basis, starting at 0.25 mg daily or 0.5 mg daily if baseline weight was less than 20 kg or 20 kg or greater, respectively; dosage was then titrated according to clinical response. Risperidone (mean modal dosage of 1.9 mg/day; equivalent to 0.06 mg/kg daily) was found to substantially improve scores on the ABC-I subscale and the CGI-C scale compared with placebo in this study.

In the second 8-week, placebo-controlled trial, children and adolescents 5–12 years of age with autistic disorder were given an initial risperidone dosage of 0.01 mg/kg daily, which was then titrated up to 0.02–0.06 mg/kg daily based on clinical response. Risperidone (mean modal dosage of 0.05 mg/kg daily; equivalent to 1.4 mg daily) substantially improved scores on the ABC-I subscale compared with placebo.

A third clinical trial conducted in children and adolescents 5–17 years of age who met DSM-IV criteria for autistic disorder and who had associated irritability and related behavioral symptoms compared 2 weight-based, fixed dosages of oral risperidone (high-dose and low-dose). Over 77% of the enrolled patients were younger than 12 years of age (mean age: 9 years) and 88% of the patients were male. In this 6-week, multicenter, double-blind study, patients were randomized to receive high-dose risperidone (1.25 mg daily for patients weighing from 20 to up to 45 kg and 1.75 mg daily for patients weighing 45 kg or more), low-dose risperidone (0.125 mg daily for those weighing from 20 to up to 45 kg and 0.175 mg daily for those weighing 45 kg or more), or placebo; the doses were administered once daily in the morning or evening (if sedation occurred). The primary outcome measure in this study was the change from baseline to end point in the ABC-I subscale. Treatment with risperidone substantially improved ABC-I scores in the high-dose risperidone group but not in the low-dose group, compared with placebo.

The efficacy of oral risperidone for long-term use (i.e., longer than 8 weeks) in children and adolescents with autistic disorder has been demonstrated in an open-label extension of the first 8-week, placebo-controlled trial in which 63 patients received risperidone for 4 or 6 months (depending on whether they received risperidone or placebo in the double-blind study). During the open-label treatment period, patients were maintained on a mean modal risperidone dosage of 1.8–2.1 mg daily (equivalent to 0.05–0.07 mg/kg daily).

Children and adolescents who maintained their positive response to risperidone (defined as at least a 25% improvement on the ABC-I subscale and a CGI-C rating of much improved or very much improved) during the 4–6 month, open-label treatment period (average duration of therapy was 140 days) were randomized to receive either risperidone or placebo during an 8-week, double-blind withdrawal trial. A substantially lower relapse rate was observed in the risperidone group compared with the placebo group during the pre-planned interim analysis of data from this trial. Based on the interim analysis results, the study was terminated since a statistically significant effect on relapse prevention was demonstrated. Relapse was defined as at least a 25% worsening on the most recent assessment of the ABC-I subscale (in relation to baseline for the randomized withdrawal phase).

The manufacturers state that clinicians who elect to use risperidone in children and adolescents with autistic disorder for extended periods should periodically re-evaluate the long-term risks and benefits of the drug for the individual patient.

Although not curative, pharmacologic agents, such as risperidone, generally are used in children and adolescents with autistic disorder to reduce behavioral disturbances associated with autism and to help facilitate the child's or adolescent's adjustment and engagement in intensive, targeted educational interventions. In clinical studies, risperidone was not found to improve certain core symptoms of autism (e.g., language deficits, impaired social relatedness). However, the drug was more effective than placebo in improving scores on subscales for sensory motor behaviors, affectual reactions, and sensory responses in a controlled study. The possible risks, including clinically important weight gain, tardive dyskinesia, withdrawal dyskinesia, and other extrapyramidal reactions associated with the drug, should be considered. (See Cautions.)

Risperidone also has been used in a limited number of adults† for the treatment of autistic disorder and other pervasive developmental disorders.

Dosage and Administration

■ Administration

Risperidone is administered orally or by IM injection.

Oral Administration Risperidone is administered orally, either in a once-daily dose or in 2 equally divided doses daily. Since food reportedly does not affect the rate or extent of GI absorption, the drug can be administered without regard to meals. Some experts state that once-daily administration of risperidone may be sufficient in most patients receiving maintenance therapy because of the extended half-life of the drug's principal active metabolite (9-hydroxyrisperidone).

Because risperidone can cause orthostatic hypotension and syncope, twice-daily oral administration of the drug may be preferable in geriatric patients and patients with renal or hepatic impairment to minimize the risk of these adverse effects.

In pediatric patients receiving risperidone for the management of schizophrenia or bipolar mania who experience persistent somnolence, twice-daily administration may be helpful.

In children and adolescents receiving risperidone for the management of irritability associated with autistic disorder who experience persistent somnolence, administering the drug once daily at bedtime, twice-daily administration, or a reduction in dosage may be helpful.

Risperidone oral solution may be administered directly from the calibrated pipette provided by the manufacturer or mixed in a beverage prior to administration. The oral solution is compatible in the following beverages: water, coffee, orange juice, and low-fat milk; risperidone oral solution is *not* compatible in cola or tea.

Patients receiving risperidone orally disintegrating tablets should be instructed not to remove a tablet from the blister until just prior to dosing. The tablet should not be pushed through the foil, since this may damage the tablet. With dry hands, the blister backing should be peeled back to expose the tablet. The tablet should then be gently removed and immediately placed on the tongue, where it rapidly disintegrates (i.e., within seconds) in saliva, and then subsequently swallowed with or without liquid. Risperidone orally disintegrating tablets should not be divided or chewed.

IM Administration In patients who have never received oral risperidone, the manufacturer recommends that tolerability with oral risperidone therapy should be established prior to initiating IM therapy with extended-release risperidone (Risperdal® Consta®).

Risperidone extended-release injection is commercially available in a dose pack containing a vial of the drug in extended-release microspheres, a prefilled syringe containing 2 mL of diluent, a vial adapter device, and 2 safety needles for IM injection (one for deltoid and one for gluteal administration). Risperidone extended-release microspheres for injection must be reconstituted prior to administration using *only* the components of the dose pack supplied by the manufacturer. The dose pack should be allowed to sit at room temperature for at least 30 minutes before reconstitution; the dose pack should *not* be warmed any other way. Risperidone extended-release microspheres should be reconstituted using only the diluent in the prefilled syringe supplied by the manufacturer. The entire contents of the prefilled syringe should be injected into the vial, and the vial should be shaken vigorously while the plunger rod is held down with the thumb for at least 10 seconds to ensure a homogeneous suspension; the reconstituted suspension should appear uniform, thick, and milky. The manufacturer's prescribing information should be consulted for additional details on use of the components of the dose pack to reconstitute and administer risperidone injection. The manufacturer states that different dosage strengths of IM risperidone should not be combined in a single administration.

Following reconstitution, immediate use is necessary because the suspension will settle over time. Once the reconstituted suspension has been transferred to the syringe and the appropriate needle attached, the syringe should be vigorously shaken again to resuspend the drug just prior to the IM injection.

The entire contents of the vial should be administered by deep IM injection into either the deltoid muscle (using the 1-inch needle supplied by the manufacturer) or the upper outer quadrant of the gluteal area (using the 2-inch needle supplied by the manufacturer) every 2 weeks, alternating between the 2 arms or 2 buttocks, respectively. *Each injection should be administered by a health care professional.* IM injections at the same dosages into the deltoid and gluteal areas are bioequivalent and are, therefore, interchangeable. The injection should *not* be administered IV. In addition, care should be taken to avoid inadvertent injection into a blood vessel.

Dispensing and Administration Precautions The US Food and Drug Administration (FDA) alerted healthcare professionals and patients of medication error reports in which patients were given risperidone (Risperdal®) instead of ropinirole hydrochloride (Requip®, a nonergot-derivative dopamine receptor agonist) and vice versa. As of June 2011, the FDA had evaluated 226 wrong drug medication errors associated with confusion between these 2 drugs; all of the reports involved tablet formulations of the drugs. Several of these cases resulted in adverse effects (including confusion, lethargy, ataxia, hallucinations, tiredness, dizziness, tingling, numbness, and altered mental status) and some of the patients who took the wrong drug required hospitalization. The FDA has determined that the factors contributing to the confusion between these 2 products include similarities in both the trade (brand) and generic (nonproprietary) names, similarities in the container labels and carton packaging, illegible handwriting on the prescriptions, and overlapping product characteristics (such as drug strengths, dosage forms, and dosing intervals). It is also possible that the 2 products may be stocked close to one another on pharmacy shelves whether they are alphabeticized by brand or generic name. In addition, some generic manufacturers make both products. Healthcare professionals are therefore reminded to clearly print out or spell out the drug name on prescriptions and to make sure their patients know the name of their prescribed drug and the reason they are taking it.

■ Dosage

Schizophrenia **Oral Dosage.** Risperidone has a bell-shaped dose-response curve, with therapeutic efficacy of oral dosages of 12–16 mg daily lower than that of dosages of 4–8 mg daily in adults. Because dosage information contained in the manufacturers' labeling principally is derived from early clinical studies of the drug in patients not typical of the general population of patients treated in the community (i.e., in hospitalized, chronically ill schizophrenic patients accustomed to high-dose antipsychotic therapies), dosage of risperidone should be individualized according to the patient's response and tolerance. Clinicians also may consider consulting published protocols for specific dosage information, particularly in geriatric or younger patients, and in those experiencing their first psychotic episode.

The manufacturers' labeling states that the initial oral dosage of risperidone for the treatment of schizophrenia in adults is 2 mg daily (given as either 2 mg once daily or 1 mg twice daily). The dosage may be increased in increments of 1–2 mg daily at intervals of 24 hours or greater, as tolerated, up to a target dosage of 4–8 mg daily (administered once daily or in 2 equally divided doses). The manufacturers state that slower dosage titration may be appropriate in certain patients.

Evidence from open-labeled studies and clinical experience with the drug indicate that an initial dosage of 1–2 mg daily, with dosage increases in increments of 0.5–1 mg daily titrated over 6–7 days, as tolerated, to a target dosage of 4 mg daily may be appropriate for the management of schizophrenia in most otherwise healthy adult patients. Lower initial dosages (e.g., 1 mg daily) and slower dosage titrations to an initial target dosage of 2 mg daily may be appropriate for younger patients and in those being treated for their first psychotic episode; dosage may then be titrated up to 4 mg daily depending on clinical response at the lower dosage and adverse neurologic effects. Such patients appear to benefit optimally from a risperidone dosage of 1–3 mg daily. A substantial number of patients being treated for their first psychotic episode start to develop extrapyramidal symptoms once dosages are increased above 2 mg daily. Dosage reductions should be considered in any patient who develops extrapyramidal symptoms.

While antipsychotic efficacy has been established in clinical trials at oral risperidone dosages ranging from 4–16 mg daily, the manufacturers and some clinicians state that dosages exceeding 6 mg daily, when given in 2 divided doses, did not result in further improvement but were associated with increases in some adverse effects, including extrapyramidal manifestations. Therefore, the manufacturers state that dosages exceeding 6 mg (in 2 divided doses) daily generally are not recommended and those exceeding 16 mg daily have not been evaluated for safety. In a single study of once-daily dosing, efficacy results generally were stronger for 8 mg than for 4 mg.

For the treatment of schizophrenia in adolescents 13–17 years of age, the manufacturer recommends an initial oral risperidone dosage of 0.5 mg once daily in the morning or evening. Dosage adjustments may be made in increments of 0.5 or 1 mg daily at intervals of 24 hours or greater, as tolerated, up to the recommended dosage of 3 mg daily. While antipsychotic efficacy in adolescents has been demonstrated in clinical trials at oral dosages ranging from 1–6 mg daily, no additional benefit was observed with dosages exceeding 3 mg daily and higher dosages were associated with increased adverse effects. Dosages exceeding 6 mg daily in adolescents have not been evaluated in clinical studies. Pediatric patients who experience persistent somnolence may benefit from twice-daily administration of the drug in 2 equally divided doses.

The manufacturers state that there are no systematically collected data that specifically address switching from other antipsychotic agents to risperidone or concomitant administration with other antipsychotic agents. The first risperidone dose should be administered in place of the next scheduled parenteral antipsychotic dose in schizophrenic patients being switched from long-acting (depot) parenteral antipsychotic therapy to oral risperidone therapy.

The optimum duration of oral risperidone therapy currently is not known, but maintenance therapy with risperidone 2–8 mg daily has been shown to be effective in adults for up to 2 years. The manufacturers state that patients responding to risperidone therapy should generally continue to receive therapy at their effective dosage beyond the acute response. Patients should be reassessed periodically to determine the need for continued therapy with the drug. If risperidone therapy is reinitiated after a drug-free period, the manufacturers recommend that the appropriate recommended schedule of careful dosage titration be employed.

The American Psychiatric Association (APA) states that prudent long-term treatment options in adults with schizophrenia with remitted first episodes or multiple episodes include either indefinite maintenance therapy or gradual discontinuance of the antipsychotic agent with close follow-up and a plan to reinstitute treatment upon symptom recurrence. Discontinuance of antipsychotic therapy should be considered only after a period of at least 1 year of symptom remission or optimal response while receiving the antipsychotic agent. In patients who have had multiple previous psychotic episodes or 2 psychotic episodes within 5 years, indefinite maintenance antipsychotic treatment is recommended.

IM Dosage. For the management of schizophrenia in adults, the recommended dosage of extended-release risperidone injection is 25 mg administered by deep IM injection into the deltoid or gluteal area every 2 weeks. The manufacturer recommends that patients first receive oral risperidone to establish tolerability of the drug before the extended-release risperidone injection is used. To ensure that adequate plasma antipsychotic concentrations are maintained prior to the main release of risperidone from the injection site, therapy with oral risperidone or another oral antipsychotic agent (e.g., for patients being switched from other oral antipsychotic therapy to IM risperidone) should be given with the first IM injection of risperidone and continued for 3 weeks, then discontinued. The need for continuing any concomitant therapy for managing extrapyramidal manifestations should be periodically reevaluated.

Some patients not responding to the 25-mg dosage may benefit from increasing the IM dosage to 37.5 or 50 mg every 2 weeks. However, the dosage should not be increased more frequently than every 4 weeks, and clinical effects of the increased dosage should not be expected earlier than 3 weeks after the first injection of the higher dosage. The maximum IM dosage should not exceed 50 mg every 2 weeks since higher dosages were associated with an increased incidence of adverse effects, but no additional clinical benefit was observed.

In some patients, an initial risperidone dosage of 12.5 mg IM every 2 weeks and maintenance dosages as low as 12.5 mg every 2 weeks may be appropriate (e.g., patients with hepatic or renal impairment, patients who are receiving concurrent therapy with other drugs that increase plasma risperidone concentrations, patients with a history of poor tolerability to psychotropic drugs); however, efficacy of the 12.5 mg every 2 weeks dosage has not been evaluated in clinical trials.

Although no controlled studies have been conducted to establish the optimum duration of IM risperidone therapy in patients with schizophrenia, oral risperidone has been shown to be effective in delaying time to relapse with longer-term use. It is recommended that responding patients be continued on treatment with IM risperidone at the lowest dosage needed. Patients should periodically be reassessed to determine the need for continued treatment.

If therapy with IM risperidone is reinitiated after a drug-free period, oral risperidone (or another oral antipsychotic agent) should again be administered initially for supplementation.

Bipolar Disorder **Oral Dosage.** For the management of acute manic or mixed episodes associated with bipolar I disorder in adults, either as monotherapy or as adjunctive therapy with lithium or valproate, the recommended initial oral dosage of risperidone is 2–3 mg given once daily. Dosage may be increased or decreased by 1 mg daily at intervals of not less than 24 hours, reflecting the procedures in the placebo-controlled trials. In these trials, the short-term (i.e., 3-week) antimanic efficacy of risperidone was demonstrated in a flexible dosage ranging from 1 to 6 mg daily. Safety of dosages exceeding 6 mg daily has not been established.

For the treatment of acute manic or mixed episodes associated with bipolar I disorder in children and adolescents 10–17 years of age, the recommended initial oral dosage of risperidone is 0.5 mg given once daily in the morning or evening. Dosage adjustments may be made in increments of 0.5–1 mg at intervals of not less than 24 hours, as tolerated, up to a target dosage of 1–2.5 mg daily. While efficacy in pediatric patients with bipolar mania has been demonstrated in clinical trials at oral dosages ranging from 0.5–6 mg daily, no additional benefit was observed with dosages exceeding 2.5 mg daily and higher dosages were associated with increased adverse effects. Safety and efficacy of oral dosages exceeding 6 mg daily in children and adolescents have not been evaluated in clinical studies. Pediatric patients who experience persistent somnolence may benefit from twice-daily administration of the drug in 2 equally divided doses.

The optimum duration of risperidone therapy for bipolar disorder currently is not known. While it is generally agreed that pharmacologic treatment beyond an acute response in mania is desirable, both for maintenance of the initial response and for prevention of new manic episodes, there are no systematically obtained data to support the use of oral risperidone beyond 3 weeks. Therefore, the manufacturers state that clinicians who elect to use risperidone for extended periods should periodically reevaluate the long-term risks and benefits of the drug for the individual patient.

IM Dosage. For the maintenance treatment of bipolar I disorder in adults, either as monotherapy or as adjunctive therapy with lithium or valproate, the recommended dosage of extended-release risperidone injection is 25 mg administered by deep IM injection in the deltoid or gluteal area every 2 weeks. The manufacturer recommends that patients first receive oral risperidone to establish tolerability of the drug before the extended-release risperidone injection is used. To ensure that adequate therapeutic plasma concentrations are maintained prior to the main release of risperidone from the injection site, therapy with oral risperidone or another oral antipsychotic agent (e.g., for patients being switched from other oral antipsychotic therapy to IM risperidone) should be given with the first IM injection of risperidone and continued for 3 weeks, then discontinued. The need for continuing any concomitant therapy for managing extrapyramidal manifestations should be periodically reevaluated.

Some patients not responding to an initial IM risperidone dosage of 25 mg every 2 weeks may benefit from increasing the dosage to 37.5 or 50 mg every 2 weeks. However, the dosage should not be increased more frequently than every 4 weeks, and clinical effects of the increased dosage should not be expected earlier than 3 weeks after the first injection of the higher dosage. Safety and efficacy of IM dosages exceeding 50 mg every 2 weeks have not been evaluated in clinical trials of risperidone in the maintenance treatment of bipolar disorder.

In some patients, an initial dosage of 12.5 mg IM every 2 weeks may be appropriate (e.g., patients with hepatic or renal impairment, patients concurrently receiving drugs that increase plasma concentrations of risperidone, or patients with a history of poor tolerability to psychotropic drugs); however, efficacy of the 12.5-mg IM dosage has not been evaluated in clinical trials.

If therapy with IM risperidone is reinitiated after a drug-free period, oral risperidone (or another oral antipsychotic agent) should again be administered initially for supplementation.

The manufacturer states that clinicians who elect to use extended-release IM risperidone for extended periods should periodically reevaluate the long-term risks and benefits of the drug for the individual patient.

Autistic Disorder For the management of irritability associated with autistic disorder in children 5 years of age and older and adolescents, the recommended initial oral dosage of risperidone is 0.25 mg daily for patients weighing less than 20 kg and 0.5 mg daily for patients weighing 20 kg or more. The drug may be administered either once or twice daily. Patients experiencing persistent somnolence may benefit from a once-daily dosage administered at bedtime, administering half the daily dosage twice daily, or a reduction in dosage.

Dosage should be individualized according to clinical response and tolerability of the patient. After a minimum of 4 days following initiation of therapy, the dosage may be increased to the recommended dosage of 0.5 mg daily for patients weighing less than 20 kg and 1 mg daily for patients weighing 20 kg or more; this dosage should then be maintained for a minimum of 14 days. In patients not responding adequately, increases in dosage may be considered at intervals of 2 weeks or longer in increments of 0.25 mg daily for patients weighing less than 20 kg or 0.5 mg daily for patients weighing 20 kg or more. Dosages ranging from 0.5–3 mg daily were effective in clinical studies. Dosage data for children weighing less than 15 kg currently are lacking. In addition, safety and efficacy in pediatric patients younger than 5 years of age have not been established.

In the pivotal clinical trials, 90% of patients who responded to risperidone therapy (based on at least 25% improvement in the Irritability subscale of the Aberrant Behavior Checklist [ABC-I]) received dosages ranging from 0.5–2.5 mg daily. The maximum daily dosage in one of the trials, when the therapeutic effect reached a plateau, was 1 mg in patients weighing less than 20 kg, 2.5 mg in patients weighing 20 kg or more, and 3 mg in patients weighing more than 45 kg.

Once adequate clinical response has been achieved and maintained, a gradual reduction in dosage to achieve an optimal balance of efficacy and safety should be considered.

The manufacturers state that clinicians who elect to use risperidone in children and adolescents with autistic disorder for extended periods should periodically reevaluate the long-term risks and benefits of the drug for the individual patient.

Geriatric Patients and Others at Risk of Orthostatic Hypotension Like other α-adrenergic blocking agents, risperidone can induce orthostatic hypotension (e.g., manifested as dizziness, tachycardia, and occasionally syncope), particularly during initiation of oral therapy with the drug. The manufacturers and some clinicians state that the risk of this effect can be minimized by limiting the initial oral dosage of risperidone to 2 mg daily, given as a single daily dose or 1 mg twice daily, in otherwise healthy adults and to 0.5 mg twice daily in geriatric patients or patients with renal or hepatic impairment. However, other clinicians recommend initiating risperidone therapy at a dosage of 0.25 mg daily in geriatric patients and gradually increasing the dosage as tolerated. (See Cautions: Geriatric Precautions.) Most geriatric patients should not be maintained at an oral dosage exceeding 3 mg daily.

For geriatric patients with schizophrenia or bipolar disorder, the recommended IM risperidone dosage of the extended-release injection is 25 mg every 2 weeks. Oral risperidone (or another oral antipsychotic agent) should be given with the first risperidone extended-release injection and should be continued for 3 weeks to ensure that adequate therapeutic plasma concentrations are maintained prior to the main release phase of risperidone from the injection site.

Geriatric patients and patients with a predisposition to hypotensive reactions or for whom such reactions would pose a particular risk should be instructed in nonpharmacologic interventions that help reduce the occurrence of orthostatic hypotension (e.g., sitting on the edge of the bed for several minutes before attempting to stand in the morning, slowly rising from a seated position). These patients should avoid sodium depletion or dehydration and circumstances that accentuate hypotension (e.g., alcohol intake, high ambient temperature). Monitoring of orthostatic vital signs also should be considered.

Particular caution also is warranted in patients with known cardiovascular disease (e.g., history of myocardial infarction or ischemia, heart failure, conduction abnormalities), cerebrovascular disease, or conditions that would predispose to hypotension (e.g., dehydration, hypovolemia, concomitant antihypertensive therapy) and in those for whom such reactions would pose a risk, and cautious dosage titration and careful monitoring are necessary in such patients. Dosage reduction should be considered in any patient in whom hypotension develops.

■ **Dosage in Renal and Hepatic Impairment** Because elimination of risperidone may be reduced and the risk of adverse effects, particularly hypotension, increased in patients with renal impairment, oral risperidone therapy should be initiated at a reduced dosage of 0.5 mg twice daily in adults with severe renal impairment (creatinine clearance less than 30 mL/minute) and increased as necessary and tolerated in increments of 0.5 mg or less, administered twice daily; increases beyond a dosage level of 1.5 mg twice daily should be made at intervals of at least 7 days. Likewise, this reduced oral dosage should be employed in patients with severe hepatic impairment (Child-Pugh score 10–15) because of the risk of an increased free fraction of risperidone in such patients.

If IM risperidone is used for management of schizophrenia or bipolar disorder in adults with renal or hepatic impairment, the patient should be treated with titrated doses of oral risperidone prior to initiating treatment with the extended-release injection. The recommended starting oral risperidone dosage is 0.5 mg twice daily during the first week, which can be increased to 1 mg twice daily or 2 mg once daily during the second week. If a dosage of at least 2 mg daily of oral risperidone is well tolerated, an IM dosage of 25 mg of the extended-release injection can be administered every 2 weeks. Alternatively, such patients may receive an initial dosage of 12.5 mg IM every 2 weeks; however, efficacy of the 12.5-mg dosage has not been evaluated in clinical trials. Oral supplementation should be continued for 3 weeks after the first injection until the main release of risperidone from the injection site has begun. In some patients, slower titration may be medically appropriate.

■ **Dosage Adjustments for Specific Drug Interactions** Adjustment of risperidone dosage may be necessary in patients receiving concomitant therapy with cytochrome P-450 (CYP) enzyme inducers (e.g., carbamazepine, phenobarbital, phenytoin, rifampin) or CYP2D6 inhibitors (e.g., fluoxetine, paroxetine). When risperidone is used concomitantly with a CYP enzyme inducer (e.g., carbamazepine), the manufacturers recommend that the dosage of oral risperidone be increased, up to double the patient's usual dosage.

In patients receiving IM risperidone, an increase in the IM dosage or addition of oral risperidone may be considered when used concomitantly with a CYP enzyme inducer.

A decrease in the dosage of oral or IM risperidone may be necessary when the CYP enzyme inducer is discontinued.

When oral risperidone is used concomitantly with fluoxetine or paroxetine (CYP2D6 inhibitors), the manufacturers recommend decreasing the dosage of risperidone and not exceeding 8 mg daily in adults. If oral risperidone is initiated in patients receiving fluoxetine or paroxetine, risperidone should be titrated slowly. When fluoxetine or paroxetine is discontinued, an increase in the dosage of risperidone may be necessary.

If fluoxetine or paroxetine is initiated in patients receiving IM risperidone, a dosage reduction may be considered; dosage of IM risperidone may be reduced 2–4 weeks before initiating fluoxetine or paroxetine. If fluoxetine or paroxetine is initiated in patients receiving IM risperidone 25 mg every 2 weeks, the manufacturer recommends continuing 25 mg every 2 weeks; dosage reduction to 12.5 mg every 2 weeks or interruption of therapy may be necessary based on clinical judgment. In patients already receiving fluoxetine or paroxetine, IM risperidone may be initiated at a dosage of 12.5 mg every 2 weeks; however, efficacy of the 12.5-mg dosage has not been evaluated in clinical trials.

Cautions

Risperidone shares many of the toxic potentials of other antipsychotic agents (e.g., other atypical antipsychotic agents, phenothiazines), and the usual precautions associated with therapy with these agents should be observed. (See Cautions in the Phenothiazines General Statement 28:16.08.24.)

The most frequent adverse effects of oral risperidone reported in over 5% of patients who received the drug in clinical trials and with an incidence of at least twice that of those receiving placebo were parkinsonism, akathisia, dystonia, tremor, sedation, dizziness, anxiety, blurred vision, nausea, vomiting, upper abdominal pain, stomach discomfort, dyspepsia, diarrhea, salivary hypersecretion, constipation, dry mouth, increased appetite, weight gain, fatigue, rash, nasal congestion, upper respiratory tract infection, nasopharyngitis, and pharyngolaryngeal pain. Adverse effects associated with discontinuance of oral risperidone therapy in more than 1% of adults and/or more than 2% of pediatric patients were nausea, somnolence, sedation, vomiting, dizziness, and akathisia.

The most frequent adverse effects of oral risperidone reported in at least 5% of adult patients with schizophrenia who received the drug in 3 short-term (4–8 week) clinical studies and with an incidence of at least twice that of those who received placebo were nausea, parkinsonism, akathisia, sedation, and dizziness. Approximately 7% of adult patients receiving oral risperidone in placebo-controlled studies discontinued treatment because of adverse effects compared with 4% of those receiving placebo. Adverse effects associated with discontinuance of therapy in at least 2 risperidone-treated patients were dizziness, nausea, vomiting, parkinsonism, somnolence, dystonia, agitation, abdominal pain, orthostatic hypotension, and akathisia.

Adverse effects occurring in 5% or more of pediatric patients with schizophrenia receiving oral risperidone in a 6-week clinical study and with an incidence of at least twice that of those receiving placebo included salivary hypersecretion, sedation, parkinsonism, akathisia, dizziness, dystonia, and anxiety. Approximately 7% of pediatric patients receiving oral risperidone in the study discontinued treatment because of adverse effects compared with 4% of those receiving placebo. Adverse effects associated with discontinuance of therapy in more than one risperidone-treated patient included dizziness, somnolence, sedation, lethargy, anxiety, balance disorder, hypotension, and palpitation.

The most frequent adverse effects of oral risperidone reported in at least 5% of adult patients with bipolar mania who received the drug as monotherapy in placebo-controlled trials and with an incidence of at least twice that of those receiving placebo were nausea, parkinsonism, sedation, akathisia, tremor, and dystonia. In placebo-controlled trials of oral risperidone in conjunction with mood stabilizers, adverse effects reported in at least 5% of patients and with an incidence of at least twice that of those receiving placebo were parkinsonism, sedation, akathisia, dizziness, tremor, and pharyngolaryngeal pain. In placebo-controlled trials of risperidone monotherapy in adults, approximately 6% of patients receiving the drug discontinued therapy because of adverse effects compared with about 5% of those receiving placebo. Adverse effects associated with discontinuance of therapy in these studies included parkinsonism, lethargy, and dizziness.

Adverse effects reported in 5% or more of pediatric patients with bipolar mania receiving oral risperidone in a 3-week, placebo-controlled trial and with an incidence of at least twice that of those receiving placebo included blurred vision, upper abdominal pain, nausea, vomiting, diarrhea, dyspepsia, stomach discomfort, fatigue, increased appetite, sedation, dizziness, parkinsonism, dystonia, akathisia, anxiety, pharyngolaryngeal pain, and rash. In this study, 12% of pediatric patients receiving risperidone for bipolar mania discontinued treatment because of adverse effects compared with 7% of those receiving placebo. Adverse effects associated with discontinuance of therapy in at least one risperidone-treated patient were nausea, somnolence, sedation, and vomiting.

The most frequent adverse effects of oral risperidone reported in at least 5% of pediatric patients with irritability associated with autistic disorder who received the drug in 3 placebo-controlled trials and with an incidence of at least twice that of those receiving placebo were constipation, dry mouth, salivary hypersecretion, fatigue, nasopharyngitis, upper respiratory tract infection, weight gain, increased appetite, sedation, drooling, tremor, dizziness, parkinsonism, and nasal congestion. Sedation was the most frequent adverse effect in these trials, occurring in 63% of the risperidone-treated patients and in 15% of patients receiving placebo. (See Dosage and Administration: Administration and also see Cautions: Pediatric Precautions.)

The most frequent adverse effects associated with use of risperidone extended-release IM injection reported in at least 5% of adult patients with schizophrenia in clinical trials were headache, parkinsonism, dizziness, akathisia, fatigue, constipation, dyspepsia, sedation, weight gain, pain in extremity, and dry mouth. The most frequent adverse effects associated with the use of risperidone extended-release IM injection in adult patients with bipolar disorder were weight gain in the monotherapy study and tremor and parkinsonism in the adjunctive therapy study.

■ Nervous System Effects ***Tardive Dyskinesia*** Use of antipsychotic agents may be associated with tardive dyskinesia, a syndrome of potentially irreversible, involuntary, dyskinetic movements. In one open-label study, an annual incidence of tardive dyskinesia of 0.3% was reported in patients with schizophrenia who received approximately 8–9 mg of oral risperidone daily for at least 1 year. The risk of developing tardive dyskinesia and the likelihood that it will become irreversible appear to increase with the duration of therapy and cumulative dose of antipsychotic agents administered; however, the syndrome may occur, although much less frequently, after relatively short periods of treatment with low dosages.

Management of tardive dyskinesia generally consists of gradual discontinuance of the precipitating antipsychotic agent when possible, reducing the dosage of the first-generation (conventional) antipsychotic agent or switching to a second-generation (atypical) antipsychotic agent, or switching to clozapine therapy. The syndrome may remit, partially or completely, if antipsychotic therapy is discontinued. However, antipsychotic therapy itself may suppress or partially suppress the signs and symptoms of the syndrome and thereby may possibly mask the underlying process. The effect that such symptomatic suppression has upon the long-term course of tardive dyskinesia is unknown. Vesicular monoamine transporter 2 (VMAT2) inhibitors (e.g., deutetrabenazine, valbenazine tosylate) have been shown to be effective in reducing symptoms of tardive dyskinesia in controlled clinical studies and may allow some patients to continue receiving antipsychotic therapy. (See Deutetrabenazine 28:56 and Valbenazine Tosylate 28:56.)

Risperidone should be prescribed in a manner that is most likely to minimize the occurrence of tardive dyskinesia. Chronic antipsychotic treatment generally should be reserved for patients who suffer from a chronic illness that is known to respond to antipsychotic agents, and for whom alternative, equally effective, but potentially less harmful treatments are not available or appropriate. In patients who do require chronic treatment, the smallest dosage and the shortest duration of treatment producing a satisfactory clinical response should be sought, and the need for continued treatment should be reassessed periodically.

The American Psychiatric Association (APA) currently recommends that patients receiving atypical antipsychotic agents be assessed clinically for abnormal involuntary movements every 12 months and that patients considered to be at increased risk for tardive dyskinesia be assessed every 6 months. If signs and symptoms of tardive dyskinesia appear in a risperidone-treated patient, risperidone discontinuance should be considered; however, some patients may require continued treatment with the drug despite the presence of the syndrome.

For additional information on tardive dyskinesia, including manifestations and treatment, see Tardive Dyskinesia under Cautions: Nervous System Effects, in the Phenothiazines General Statement 28:16.08.24.

Extrapyramidal Reactions Extrapyramidal reactions occurred in 12–17% of adults with schizophrenia receiving oral risperidone dosages of 2–4 mg daily and in 20–35% of patients receiving dosages of 16 mg daily in clinical studies; these reactions appear to be dose related. At recommended therapeutic dosages of risperidone (4–8 mg daily) for schizophrenia, the severity of extrapyramidal reactions appears to be comparable to placebo and clozapine 400 mg daily, and substantially less than that associated with haloperidol 10 or 20 mg daily. Similarly, the severity of parkinsonian symptoms, as assessed on the parkinsonism subscale of the Extrapyramidal Symptom Rating Scale (ESRS), is also linearly related to risperidone dosages of 2–16 mg daily, with the incidence of parkinsonian symptoms at risperidone dosages of 6 mg daily or less comparable to that of placebo and substantially less than that seen with haloperidol dosages of 20 mg daily.

Neuroleptic Malignant Syndrome Neuroleptic malignant syndrome (NMS), a potentially fatal syndrome requiring immediate discontinuance of therapy and intensive symptomatic treatment, has been reported in patients receiving antipsychotic agents, including risperidone. For additional information on NMS, see Neuroleptic Malignant Syndrome under Nervous System Effects: Extrapyramidal Reactions in Cautions, in the Phenothiazines General Statement 28:16.08.24.

Other Nervous System Effects Dose-related somnolence is a commonly reported adverse effect associated with risperidone treatment. Approximately 41% of patients receiving 16 mg of oral risperidone daily and 16% of patients receiving placebo reported somnolence in a study utilizing a checklist to detect adverse events. Somnolence was reported in 5% of patients receiving extended-release IM risperidone in multiple-dose studies. (See Cautions: Pediatric Precautions.)

Insomnia and anxiety have been reported in 25–32 and 11–16%, respectively, of adult patients with schizophrenia receiving oral risperidone.

■ Cardiovascular Effects ***Orthostatic Hypotension*** Orthostatic hypotension associated with dizziness, tachycardia, and in some patients, syncope, especially during the initial dose-titration period, has been reported in patients receiving risperidone, probably reflecting the drug's α-adrenergic antagonistic properties. Syncope was reported in 0.2% of patients receiving oral risperidone in phase 2 and 3 studies in adults with schizophrenia and in 0.8% of patients receiving extended-release IM risperidone in multiple-dose studies.

Risperidone should be used with particular caution in patients with known cardiovascular disease (history of myocardial infarction or ischemia, heart failure, or conduction abnormalities), cerebrovascular disease, or conditions that would predispose to hypotension (e.g., dehydration, hypovolemia). Clinically important hypotension has been observed with concomitant use of oral risperidone and antihypertensive drug therapy.

The risk of orthostatic hypotension and syncope may be minimized by limiting initial oral risperidone dosages to 2 mg daily (given as 2 mg once daily or as 1 mg twice daily) in otherwise healthy adults and to 0.5 mg twice daily in geriatric patients and patients with renal or hepatic impairment. (See Dosage and Administration.) Monitoring of orthostatic vital signs should be considered in patients for whom orthostatic hypotension is of concern. Dosage reduction of risperidone should be considered if hypotension occurs.

Other Cardiovascular Effects Pooled analysis of results of placebo-controlled studies indicates that oral risperidone therapy generally is not associated with statistically significant changes in ECG parameters (e.g., PR, QT, or QT_c intervals) and heart rate. However, in short-term studies in adults with schizophrenia, higher oral dosages of risperidone (8–16 mg daily) were associated with a higher mean increase in heart rate of 4–6 beats per minute compared with placebo. In addition, sinus bradycardia, sinus tachycardia, atrioventricular (AV) block, and bundle branch block have been reported in patients receiving risperidone during clinical trials. Atrial fibrillation, cardiopulmonary arrest, QT interval prolongation, and sudden death also have been reported during postmarketing surveillance; however, a causal relationship to the drug has not been established.

■ Endocrine and Metabolic Effects Atypical antipsychotic agents have been associated with metabolic changes that may increase cardiovascular and cerebrovascular risk, including hyperglycemia, dyslipidemia, and body weight gain. While all of these drugs produce some metabolic changes, each drug has its own specific risk profile.

Hyperglycemia and Diabetes Mellitus Severe hyperglycemia, sometimes associated with ketoacidosis, hyperosmolar coma, or death, has been reported in patients receiving certain atypical antipsychotic agents, including risperidone. While confounding factors such as an increased background risk of diabetes mellitus in patients with schizophrenia and the increasing incidence of diabetes mellitus in the general population make it difficult to establish with certainty the relationship between use of agents in this drug class and glucose abnormalities, epidemiologic studies suggest an increased risk of treatment-emergent, hyperglycemia-related adverse events in patients treated with the atypical antipsychotic agents included in the studies (e.g., risperidone, clozapine, olanzapine, quetiapine).

Precise risk estimates for hyperglycemia-related adverse events in patients treated with atypical antipsychotics currently are not available. While some evidence suggests that the risk for diabetes may be greater with some atypical antipsychotics (e.g., clozapine, olanzapine) than with others (e.g., risperidone, quetiapine) in the class, available data are conflicting and insufficient to provide reliable estimates of relative risk associated with use of the various atypical antipsychotics. (See Cautions: Precautions and Contraindications.)

In a pooled analysis of short-term, placebo-controlled studies of 3–8 weeks' duration in adults with schizophrenia or bipolar disorder, risperidone was associated with a mean increase in random serum glucose concentrations of 0.6–0.8 mg/dL compared with a decrease of 1.4 mg/dL for placebo. During longer-term studies in adults, risperidone was associated with a mean increase in serum glucose of 2.8 mg/dL at week 24 and 4.1 mg/dL at week 48.

In children and adolescents receiving risperidone 0.5–6 mg daily for schizophrenia, bipolar disorder, or autistic disorder in short-term studies, the proportion of patients experiencing an increase in fasting serum glucose from below 100 mg/dL to 126 mg/dL or higher was 0.8% for risperidone-treated patients compared with 0% for placebo recipients. During longer-term studies in children and adolescents, risperidone was associated with a mean increase in fasting glucose of 5.2 mg/dL at week 24.

Diabetic coma and diabetic ketoacidosis (in patients with impaired glucose metabolism) have been reported in risperidone-treated patients.

Dyslipidemia Undesirable changes in lipid parameters have been observed in patients treated with atypical antipsychotics. In a pooled analysis of 7 short-term, placebo-controlled studies of 3–8 weeks' duration in adults receiving oral risperidone for schizophrenia or bipolar mania, random cholesterol concentrations increased from baseline by a mean of 6.9 and 1.8 mg/dL in patients receiving risperidone 1–8 mg and more than 8–16 mg daily, respectively, compared with 0.6 mg/dL in those receiving placebo. The proportion of patients with an increase in random cholesterol concentrations from below 200 mg/dL to 240 mg/dL or higher was 4.3% for those receiving risperidone 1–8 mg daily and 6.3% for those receiving more than 8–16 mg of risperidone daily compared with 2.7% for placebo recipients, and the proportion of risperidone-treated patients with an increase in triglyceride concentrations from below 500 mg/dL to 500 mg/dL or higher was 2.5–2.7% compared with 1.1% for placebo recipients. During longer-term studies of oral risperidone, therapy with the drug was associated with a mean increase in nonfasting cholesterol concentrations of 4.4 and 5.5 mg/dL at weeks 24 and 48, respectively, and a mean increase in nonfasting triglycerides of 19.9 mg/dL at week 24.

In children and adolescents receiving oral risperidone 0.5–6 mg daily for schizophrenia, bipolar mania, or autistic disorder in short-term studies, the proportion of risperidone-treated patients with an increase in fasting cholesterol concentrations from below 170 mg/dL to 200 mg/dL or higher was 3.8% compared with 2.4% for placebo recipients and the proportion of risperidone-treated patients with an increase in fasting triglyceride concentrations from below 150 mg/dL to 200 mg/dL or higher was 7.1% compared with 1.5% for placebo recipients. During longer-term studies in children and adolescents, oral risperidone was associated with a mean increase in fasting cholesterol and triglyceride concentrations of 2.1 and 6.8 mg/dL, respectively, at week 24.

Weight Gain Weight gain has been observed with atypical antipsychotic therapy. The manufacturers recommend clinical monitoring of weight in patients receiving risperidone.

In short-term clinical studies in adults with schizophrenia or bipolar mania, a mean weight gain from baseline of 0.7 and 2.2 kg was reported in patients receiving oral risperidone 1–8 mg and more than 8–16 mg daily, respectively, compared with a weight loss of 0.3 kg in those receiving placebo. The proportion of patients experiencing a weight gain of 7% or more of their baseline body weight was 8.7% for those receiving risperidone 1–8 mg daily and 20.9% for those receiving more than 8–16 mg of risperidone daily compared with 2.9% for placebo recipients. During longer-term studies of risperidone in adults, risperidone was associated with a mean weight gain of 4.3 kg at week 24 and 5.3 kg at week 48.

Hyperprolactinemia As with other drugs that antagonize dopamine D_2 receptors, risperidone can elevate serum prolactin concentrations, and the elevation may persist during chronic administration of the drug. Risperidone appears to be associated with a higher level of prolactin elevation than other antipsychotic agents. Elevated prolactin concentrations occur in children and adolescents as well as in adults receiving the drug. (See Cautions: Pediatric Precautions.) Clinical disturbances such as galactorrhea, amenorrhea, gynecomastia, and impotence have been associated with prolactin-elevating drugs. In addition, chronic hyperprolactinemia associated with hypogonadism may lead to decreased bone density in both female and male patients.

If risperidone therapy is considered in a patient with previously detected breast cancer, clinicians should consider that approximately one-third of human breast cancers are prolactin dependent in vitro.

Other Endocrine and Metabolic Effects Increased serum creatine kinase (CK, creatine phosphokinase, CPK) concentrations, decreased appetite, polydipsia, and anorexia have been reported during clinical trials in patients receiving risperidone. Although a causal relationship has not been established, inappropriate antidiuretic hormone secretion and water intoxication have been reported in patients receiving risperidone during postmarketing surveillance. Precocious puberty and pituitary adenomas also have been reported during postmarketing surveillance; however, a causal relationship remains to be established.

■ GI Effects Adverse GI effects that have been reported in 5% or more of patients receiving oral or IM risperidone in clinical studies include nausea, vomiting, upper abdominal pain, stomach discomfort, dyspepsia, diarrhea, salivary hypersecretion, constipation, dry mouth, and increased appetite. In addition, abdominal discomfort has been reported in 1% or more of patients receiving oral risperidone in clinical studies.

Other adverse GI effects reported during clinical trials with oral risperidone include dysphagia, fecaloma, fecal incontinence, gastritis, lip swelling, cheilitis, and aptyalism. Toothache and tongue spasm have been reported in patients treated with extended-release IM risperidone. Although a causal relationship to risperidone has not been established, dysgeusia, ileus, pancreatitis, and intestinal obstruction have been reported during postmarketing surveillance.

■ Respiratory Effects Nasal congestion, upper respiratory tract infection, nasopharyngitis, and pharyngolaryngeal pain were the most common adverse respiratory effects reported in more than 5% of patients receiving oral risperidone during clinical studies. In addition, cough and dyspnea have been reported in up to 2% of patients receiving risperidone in clinical studies. Wheezing, aspiration pneumonia, sinus congestion, dysphonia, productive cough, pulmonary congestion, rales, hyperventilation, and nasal edema also have been reported in patients receiving risperidone in clinical studies. Although a causal relationship to the drug has not been established, sleep apnea and pulmonary embolism have been reported during postmarketing surveillance.

■ Dermatologic Effects and Sensitivity Reactions Rash and dry skin have been reported in at least 2% of patients with schizophrenia receiving oral risperidone in clinical studies. In addition, erythema, skin discoloration, skin lesion, pruritus, acne, hyperkeratosis, and seborrheic dermatitis have been reported in clinical trials.

Although a causal relationship has not been established, hypersensitivity reactions, including anaphylaxis and anaphylactic reactions, angioedema, and alopecia, have been reported in patients receiving risperidone during postmarketing surveillance. (See Cautions: Precautions and Contraindications.)

■ Genitourinary Effects Urinary tract infection has been reported in 1% or more of adult patients with schizophrenia receiving oral risperidone in clinical trials. Adverse genitourinary effects reported in adult and pediatric patients receiving oral risperidone in clinical trials include enuresis, dysuria, pollakiuria, urinary incontinence, cystitis, irregular menstruation, amenorrhea, vaginal discharge, menstrual disorder, erectile dysfunction, retrograde ejaculation, ejaculation disorder, sexual dysfunction, and breast enlargement. Although a causal relationship has not been established, urinary retention has been reported in patients receiving risperidone during postmarketing surveillance.

Rare cases of priapism have been reported in risperidone-treated patients during postmarketing surveillance. Severe priapism may require surgical intervention.

■ Musculoskeletal Effects Back or chest pain, arthralgia, and pain in extremities have been reported in 1–4% of patients with schizophrenia receiving oral risperidone in clinical studies. In addition, joint stiffness, joint swelling, musculoskeletal chest pain, abnormal posture, myalgia, neck pain, muscular weakness, and rhabdomyolysis have been reported in patients receiving oral risperidone in clinical trials.

■ Hematologic Effects In clinical trial and/or postmarketing experience, leukopenia and neutropenia temporally related to antipsychotic agents, including risperidone, have been reported. Agranulocytosis also has been reported.

Possible risk factors for leukopenia and neutropenia include a preexisting low leukocyte count and a history of drug-induced leukopenia or neutropenia. Therefore, patients with a history of clinically important low leukocyte count or drug-induced leukopenia and/or neutropenia should have their complete blood count monitored frequently during the first few months of risperidone therapy. Discontinuance of risperidone should be considered at the first sign of a clinically important decline in leukocyte count in the absence of other causative factors.

Patients with clinically important neutropenia should be carefully monitored for fever or other signs or symptoms of infection and promptly treated if such signs or symptoms occur. In patients with severe neutropenia (absolute neutrophil count [ANC] less than $1000/mm^3$), risperidone should be discontinued and the leukocyte count monitored until recovery occurs. (See Cautions: Precautions and Contraindications.)

Lithium reportedly has been used successfully in the treatment of several cases of leukopenia and neutropenia associated with aripiprazole, clozapine, olanzapine, and some other drugs; however, further clinical experience is needed to confirm these anecdotal findings.

Anemia, granulocytopenia, eosinophilia, and epistaxis have been reported in patients receiving risperidone in clinical studies.

Thrombotic thrombocytopenic purpura occurred in at least one patient (a 28 year-old female patient) receiving risperidone in a large, open-labeled study. This patient experienced jaundice, fever, and bruising but eventually recovered after receiving plasmapheresis. The relationship of this adverse event to risperidone therapy is unknown.

■ Hepatic Effects Elevated ALT or aminotransferase concentrations have been reported in patients receiving oral risperidone in clinical studies. Although a causal relationship to the drug has not been established, jaundice also has been reported during postmarketing surveillance.

■ Ocular and Otic Effects Blurred vision has been reported in 1–3% of adults with schizophrenia or bipolar mania and in 4–7% of pediatric patients with bipolar disorder receiving oral risperidone in clinical studies. Ocular hyperemia, eye discharge, conjunctivitis, eye rolling, eyelid edema, eye swelling, eyelid margin crusting, dry eye, increased lacrimation, photophobia, glaucoma, and reduced visual acuity have been reported in patients receiving risperidone in clinical studies. Ear pain and tinnitus also have been reported in clinical studies with the drug.

Retinal artery occlusion has been reported in a patient treated with extended-release IM risperidone during postmarketing surveillance. This case occurred in the presence of abnormal arteriovenous anastomosis.

■ Precautions and Contraindications Atypical antipsychotic agents are associated with metabolic changes that may increase cardiovascular and cerebrovascular risk (e.g., hyperglycemia, dyslipidemia, weight gain). While all atypical antipsychotics produce some metabolic changes, each drug has its own specific risk profile.

Because hyperglycemia, sometimes severe and associated with ketoacidosis, hyperosmolar coma, or death, has been reported in patients receiving certain atypical antipsychotic agents, including risperidone, the manufacturers of atypical antipsychotic agents state that patients with preexisting diabetes mellitus in whom therapy with an atypical antipsychotic is initiated should be closely monitored for worsening of glucose control; those with risk factors for diabetes (e.g., obesity, family history of diabetes) should undergo fasting blood glucose testing upon therapy initiation and periodically throughout treatment. (See Cautions: Endocrine and Metabolic Effects.) Any patient who develops manifestations of hyperglycemia during treatment with an atypical antipsychotic should undergo fasting blood glucose testing. In some cases, patients who developed hyperglycemia while receiving an atypical antipsychotic have required continuance of antidiabetic treatment despite discontinuance of the antipsychotic; in other cases, hyperglycemia resolved with discontinuance of the suspect drug. For further information on the management of diabetes risks in patients receiving atypical antipsychotics, see Hyperglycemia and Diabetes Mellitus under Cautions: Precautions and Contraindications, in Clozapine 28:16.08.04.

Because of the possibility of orthostatic hypotension, caution should be observed in patients with known cardiovascular disease (e.g., history of myocardial infarction or ischemia, heart failure, conduction abnormalities), cerebrovascular disease (see Cautions: Geriatric Precautions), conditions that would predispose patients to hypotension (e.g., dehydration, hypovolemia), and patients receiving antihypertensive agents. Since patients with a recent history of myocardial infarction or unstable heart disease were excluded from premarketing clinical studies, clinicians should be aware that risperidone has not been evaluated or used to any appreciable extent in such patients. Patients receiving risperidone should be advised of the risk of orthostatic hypotension, especially during the period of initial dosage titration. (See Geriatric Patients and Others at Risk of Orthostatic Hypotension under Dosage and Administration: Dosage and see Cautions: Cardiovascular Effects.)

Clinical experience with IM risperidone therapy in patients with certain concomitant diseases is limited. The manufacturer of extended-release IM risperidone advises using the drug with caution in patients with altered metabolism or hemodynamics.

Patients with parkinsonian syndrome or dementia with Lewy bodies reportedly have an increased sensitivity to antipsychotic agents, including risperidone. Clinical manifestations of this increased sensitivity have been reported to include confusion, obtundation, postural instability with more frequent falls, extrapyramidal adverse effects, and clinical features consistent with neuroleptic malignant syndrome. For additional information on extrapyramidal adverse effects and neuroleptic malignant syndrome, see Cautions: Nervous System Effects, in the Phenothiazines General Statement 28:16.08.24.

Clearance of risperidone and its principal active metabolite, 9-hydroxyrisperidone, are decreased by 60% in patients with moderate to severe renal impairment (creatinine clearance 15–59 mL/minute), and free fraction of risperidone is increased by about 35% in patients with hepatic impairment. Therefore, lower initial dosages of oral risperidone should be used in patients with severe renal or hepatic impairment. (See Dosage and Administration: Dosage in Renal and Hepatic Impairment.)

Patients with a history of clinically important low leukocyte count or drug-induced leukopenia and/or neutropenia should have their complete blood count monitored frequently during the first few months of risperidone therapy. Patients with clinically important neutropenia should be carefully monitored for fever or other signs or symptoms of infection and promptly treated if such signs or symptoms occur. (See Cautions: Hematologic Effects.)

Individuals with phenylketonuria (i.e., homozygous genetic deficiency of phenylalanine hydroxylase) and other individuals who must restrict their intake of phenylalanine should be warned that risperidone orally disintegrating tablets contain aspartame (e.g., NutraSweet®), which is metabolized in the GI tract to provide phenylalanine following oral administration; the respective manufacturer's labeling should be consulted for specific information regarding phenylalanine content of individual preparations and dosage strengths.

Because seizures have occurred in 0.3% of patients receiving risperidone orally or IM in clinical studies, the drug should be administered with caution to patients with a history of seizures.

Esophageal dysmotility and aspiration have been associated with the use of antipsychotic agents, including risperidone. Because aspiration pneumonia is a common cause of morbidity and mortality in patients with advanced dementia of the Alzheimer's type, risperidone and other antipsychotic drugs should be used with caution in patients at risk for aspiration pneumonia.

Because disruption of the body's ability to regulate body temperature has been associated with the use of antipsychotic agents and because both hypothermia and hyperthermia have been associated with oral and extended-release IM risperidone therapy, the drug should be administered with caution in patients who will be exposed to temperature extremes.

Because risperidone has the potential to impair judgment, thinking, or motor skills, patients should be cautioned about operating hazardous machinery, including driving automobiles, until they are reasonably certain that risperidone therapy does not adversely affect them.

Risperidone has an antiemetic effect in animals; this effect also may occur in humans, and may mask manifestations of overdosage with certain drugs or may obscure the cause of vomiting in various disorders such as intestinal obstruction, Reye's syndrome, or brain tumor.

Osteodystrophy, renal tubular tumors, and adrenomedullary pheochromocytomas have been observed in rats following IM administration of extended-release risperidone; these findings were not observed previously with oral risperidone. The clinical relevance of these findings to humans is not known.

Because the possibility of a suicide attempt is inherent in patients with schizophrenia or bipolar disorder, close supervision of high-risk patients is recommended during risperidone therapy. Because extended-release IM risperidone is administered by a health care professional, suicide due to an overdose is unlikely.

Patients should be advised to inform their clinician if they are taking, or plan to take, any prescription or nonprescription drugs, or have any concomitant illnesses (e.g., diabetes mellitus). Patients also should be advised to avoid alcohol while taking risperidone.

Risperidone is contraindicated in patients with known hypersensitivity to the drug. (See Cautions: Dermatologic Effects and Sensitivity Reactions.)

■ **Pediatric Precautions** The safety and efficacy of risperidone in children younger than 13 years of age with schizophrenia or younger than 10 years of age with bipolar I disorder have not been established. Safety and efficacy of oral risperidone for the treatment of schizophrenia in adolescents 13–17 years of age were demonstrated in 2 short-term clinical trials in 417 patients. (See Schizophrenia under Uses: Psychotic Disorders.)

Efficacy and safety of risperidone for the treatment of acute manic or mixed episodes associated with bipolar I disorder in children and adolescents 10–17 years of age were demonstrated in a 3-week, placebo-controlled study in 169 patients. (See Uses: Bipolar Disorder.)

Efficacy and safety of the drug in the treatment of irritability associated with autistic disorder have been evaluated in 3 placebo-controlled trials of 6–8 weeks' duration in 252 children and adolescents 5–17 years of age. (See Uses: Autistic Disorder.) Additional safety information also was assessed from long-term studies in patients with schizophrenia or autistic disorder and from short- and long-term studies in more than 1200 pediatric patients with other psychiatric disorders who were of similar age and weight and who received similar risperidone dosages as patients treated for irritability associated with autistic disorder.

In clinical trials in 1885 children and adolescents treated with risperidone, 2 patients (0.1%) reportedly developed tardive dyskinesia, which resolved upon discontinuance of therapy. In addition, approximately 15% of children and adolescents receiving 0.5–2.5 mg daily dosages of risperidone developed withdrawal dyskinesia during the discontinuance phase of one long-term (6 month), open-label study.

In children and adolescents receiving oral risperidone 0.5–6 mg daily for schizophrenia, bipolar mania, autistic disorder, or other psychiatric disorders in short-term studies, approximately 33% of the risperidone-treated patients gained 7% or more of their baseline body weight compared with 7% of those receiving placebo; mean weight gain was 2 and 0.6 kg in the risperidone and placebo groups, respectively. During longer-term, open-label studies of risperidone in children and adolescents, risperidone was associated with a mean weight gain of 5.5 kg at week 24 and 8 kg at week 48.

In long-term, open-label trials in patients with autistic disorder or other psychiatric disorders, a mean body weight gain of 7.5 kg after 12 months of risperidone therapy was reported, which was higher than the normal expected weight gain (i.e., 3–3.5 kg per year adjusted for age, based on the US Centers for Disease Control and Prevention normative data). The majority of the weight increase occurred within the first 6 months of drug exposure. When treating pediatric patients with risperidone, the manufacturers recommend that weight gain should be assessed against that expected with normal growth.

Somnolence frequently occurred in placebo-controlled trials of oral risperidone in pediatric patients with autistic disorder. Most cases were mild to moderate in severity, occurred early during therapy (peak incidence during the first 2 weeks of therapy), and were transient (median duration of 16 days). Somnolence also was the most common adverse effect in clinical trials in children and adolescents with bipolar disorder as well as in schizophrenia clinical trials in adolescents; as in the autistic disorder trials, somnolence usually occurred early during therapy and was transient. Pediatric patients experiencing persistent somnolence may benefit from a change in dosage regimen. (See Dosage and Administration: Administration.)

Risperidone has been shown to elevate prolactin concentrations in children and adolescents as well as adults. In double-blind, placebo-controlled trials of up to 8 weeks' duration in children and adolescents 5–17 years of age, 49% of oral risperidone-treated patients had elevated prolactin concentrations compared with 2% of those receiving placebo. Similarly, in placebo-controlled trials in children and adolescents 10–17 years of age with bipolar disorder or adolescents 13–17 years of age with schizophrenia, 82–87% of risperidone-treated patients had elevated prolactin concentrations compared with 3–7% of placebo recipients. Increases in prolactin concentrations were dose dependent and generally greater in female than male patients across indications.

In clinical trials conducted in 1885 children and adolescents, galactorrhea and gynecomastia reportedly occurred in 0.8 and 2.3%, respectively, of risperidone-treated patients.

The manufacturers state that the long-term effects of risperidone on growth and sexual maturation have not been fully evaluated in children and adolescents.

■ **Geriatric Precautions** Clinical studies of oral risperidone for the management of schizophrenia did not include sufficient numbers of patients 65 years of age and older to determine whether geriatric patients respond differently than younger patients. Other clinical experience with oral risperidone has not identified differences in responses between geriatric and younger patients. However, serious adverse effects, including an increased risk of death, have been reported in geriatric patients receiving risperidone or other atypical antipsychotic agents in clinical trials in patients with dementia-related psychosis. Risperidone is not approved for the treatment of dementia-related psychosis. (See Geriatric Considerations in Uses: Psychotic Disorders.)

Geriatric patients with dementia-related psychosis treated with antipsychotic drugs are at an increased risk of death. Analyses of 17 placebo-controlled trials (modal duration of 10 weeks) revealed an approximate 1.6- to 1.7-fold increase in mortality among geriatric patients receiving atypical antipsychotic drugs (i.e., risperidone, aripiprazole, olanzapine, quetiapine) compared with that in patients receiving placebo. Over the course of a typical 10-week controlled trial, the rate of death in drug-treated patients was about 4.5% compared with a rate of about 2.6% in the placebo group. Although the causes of death were varied, most of the deaths appeared to be either cardiovascular (e.g., heart failure, sudden death) or infectious (e.g., pneumonia) in nature. Observational studies suggest that, similar to atypical antipsychotics, treatment with conventional (first-generation) antipsychotics may increase mortality; the extent to which the findings of increased mortality in observational studies may be attributed to the antipsychotic drug as opposed to some characteristic(s) of the patients remains unclear.

A higher incidence of mortality also was observed in geriatric patients with dementia-related psychosis receiving oral risperidone and furosemide concurrently in 2 out of 4 placebo-controlled trials when compared with that in patients receiving risperidone alone or placebo and furosemide concurrently. The pathologic mechanism for this finding remains to be established and no consistent pattern for the cause of death was observed.

Adverse cerebrovascular events (e.g., stroke, transient ischemic attack), some of which resulted in fatalities, have been reported in clinical studies of risperidone in geriatric patients (mean age 85 years; range: 73–97) with dementia-related psychosis.

Because of the greater frequency of decreased hepatic, renal, and/or cardiac function and of concomitant disease and drug therapy observed in geriatric patients, oral risperidone generally should be initiated at lower dosages in such patients. Although geriatric patients exhibit a greater tendency to orthostatic hypotension, the manufacturers state that its risk may be minimized by limiting the initial oral dosage to 0.5 mg twice daily followed by careful titration and close monitoring of orthostatic vital signs in patients for whom this is of concern. However, there is some evidence that even lower initial dosages and slower dosage titration are better tolerated in these patients. Therefore, some clinicians recommend initiating oral risperidone therapy at 0.25 mg daily, and gradually increasing dosages, as tolerated, to a dosage of 2 mg daily in these patients. Higher oral dosages (e.g., 3 or 4 mg daily) may be required in some patients, but are usually associated with greater incidence of extrapyramidal reactions. Most geriatric patients should *not* be maintained at an oral risperidone dosage exceeding 3 mg daily. (See Geriatric Patients and Others at Risk of Orthostatic Hypotension under Dosage and Administration: Dosage.)

No differences in the tolerability of extended-release IM risperidone were observed in an open-label study in otherwise healthy geriatric patients and younger patients with schizophrenia or schizoaffective disorder. Therefore, the manufacturer states that extended-release IM risperidone dosage recommendations for otherwise healthy geriatric patients are the same as for younger adults.

■ **Mutagenicity and Carcinogenicity** Risperidone did not exhibit mutagenic or clastogenic potential in the Ames gene mutation test, mouse lymphoma assay, in vitro rat hepatocyte DNA-repair assay, in vivo micronucleus test in mice, the sex-linked recessive lethal test in Drosophila, or the chromosomal aberration studies in human lymphocytes or Chinese hamster ovary cells.

Statistically significant increases in pituitary gland adenomas and mammary gland adenocarcinomas were observed in female mice receiving oral risperidone dosages of 0.63, 2.5, and 10 mg/kg (equivalent to approximately 2, 9, and 38 times the maximum recommended human dosage for schizophrenia on a mg/kg basis or 0.2, 0.75, and 3 times the maximum recommended human dosage on a mg/m^2 basis, respectively) for 18 months. In addition, statistically significant increases were observed in mammary gland adenocarcinomas in both male and female rats, and mammary gland neoplasms and endocrine pancreas adenomas in male rats receiving oral risperidone dosages of 0.63, 2.5, and 10 mg/kg (equivalent to approximately 2, 9, and 38 times the maximum recommended human dosage for schizophrenia on a mg/kg basis or 0.4, 1.5, and 6 times the maximum recommended human dosage on a mg/m^2 basis, respectively) for 25 months.

Although an increase in prolactin-mediated mammary, pituitary, and endocrine pancreas neoplasms has been found in rodents following long-term administration of other antipsychotic agents, no clinical or epidemiologic studies conducted to date have shown an association between long-term administration of antipsychotic drugs and tumorigenesis in humans; current evidence is considered too limited to be conclusive at this time. If risperidone therapy is considered in a patient with previously detected breast cancer, clinicians should consider that approximately one-third of human breast cancers are prolactin dependent in vitro.

■ **Pregnancy, Fertility, and Lactation** Reproductive studies in rats and rabbits using risperidone dosages of 0.4–6 times the maximum recommended human dosage on a mg/m^2 basis have not revealed evidence of fetal malformation. However, risperidone has been shown to cross the placenta in rats, and an increased rate of stillborn rat pups occurred at dosages 1.5 times higher than the maximum recommended human dosage on a mg/m^2 basis. In 3 reproductive studies in rats, there was an increase in pup deaths during the first 4 days of lactation at dosages 0.1–3 times the human dosage on a mg/m^2 basis. It is not known whether these deaths resulted from a direct effect on the fetuses or pups or to effects on the dams. In a separate reproductive study in rats, an increased number of pup deaths (at birth or by the day after birth) and a decrease in birth weight were observed in pups of dams treated with risperidone. Risperidone also appeared to impair maternal behavior, as evidenced by reduced weight gain and decreased survival (from day 1–4 of lactation) in pups born to control dams but reared by risperidone-treated dams.

Although there are no adequate and controlled studies to date in humans, one case of agenesis of the corpus callosum has been reported in an infant exposed to risperidone in utero; however, a causal relationship to risperidone therapy is unknown.

Neonates exposed to antipsychotic agents, including risperidone, during the third trimester of pregnancy are at risk for extrapyramidal and/or withdrawal symptoms following delivery. There have been reports of agitation, hypertonia, hypotonia, tardive dyskinetic-like symptoms, tremor, somnolence, respiratory distress, and feeding disorder in these neonates. The majority of cases were also confounded by other factors, including concomitant use of other drugs known to be associated with withdrawal symptoms, prematurity, congenital malformations, and obstetrical and perinatal complications; however, some cases suggested that neonatal extrapyramidal symptoms and withdrawal may occur with exposure to antipsychotic agents alone. Some of the cases described time of symptom onset, which ranged from birth to one month after birth. Any neonate exhibiting extrapyramidal or withdrawal symptoms following in utero exposure to antipsychotic agents should be monitored. Symptoms were self-limiting in some neonates but varied in severity; some infants required intensive care unit support and prolonged hospitalization. For further information on extrapyramidal and withdrawal symptoms in neonates, see Cautions: Pregnancy, Fertility, and Lactation, in the Phenothiazines General Statement 28:16.08.24.

Risperidone should be used during pregnancy only if the potential benefit justifies the potential risk to the fetus.

The effect of risperidone on labor and delivery in humans is unknown.

Oral risperidone (0.16–5 mg/kg) has been shown to impair mating, but not fertility, in Wistar rats in 3 reproductive studies at dosages 0.1–3 times the maximum recommended human dosage on a mg/m^2 basis. The effect appeared to be in females since impaired mating behavior was not noted in the mating and fertility study in which only males were treated. Sperm motility and concentration were decreased in beagles at dosages 0.6–10 times the maximum recommended human dosage on a mg/m^2 basis; dose-related decreases were also observed in serum testosterone concentrations at the same dosages. Serum testosterone and sperm parameters partially recovered but remained decreased after treatment was discontinued. A no-effect dosage was not found in these studies in either rats or dogs.

Risperidone and its principal active metabolite, 9-hydroxyrisperidone, are distributed into milk. Because of the potential for serious adverse reactions to risperidone in nursing infants, the manufacturers of oral risperidone state that a decision should be made whether to discontinue nursing or risperidone, taking into consideration the importance of the drug to the woman. The manufacturer of the long-acting risperidone injection states that women receiving IM risperidone should not breast-feed during treatment and for at least 12 weeks after the last injection.

Description

Risperidone is a benzisoxazole-derivative antipsychotic agent. The drug has been described as an atypical or second-generation antipsychotic agent. The principal active metabolite of risperidone, 9-hydroxyrisperidone, has similar pharmacologic activity to the parent drug and is commercially available as paliperidone (another atypical antipsychotic agent); the clinical effects of risperidone result from combined concentrations of risperidone and 9-hydroxyrisperidone. The exact mechanism of antipsychotic action of risperidone has not been fully elucidated but, like that of clozapine, may involve antagonism of central type 2 serotonergic (5-HT_2) receptors and central dopamine D_2 receptors. Antagonism at other receptors (e.g., α_1- and α_2-adrenergic receptors, histamine H_1 receptors) may contribute to other therapeutic and adverse effects of risperidone (e.g., orthostatic hypotension, somnolence). Risperidone exhibits low to moderate affinity for other serotonin receptor subtypes (e.g., $5HT_{1C}$, $5HT_{1A}$, $5HT_{1D}$), and weak affinity for dopamine D_1 receptors and the haloperidol-sensitive sigma site. The drug possesses no affinity for cholinergic muscarinic or β_1- and β_2-adrenergic receptors.

SumMon® (see Users Guide). For additional information on this drug until a more detailed monograph is developed and published, the manufacturer's labeling should be consulted. It is *essential* that the labeling be consulted for detailed information on the usual cautions, precautions, and contraindications concerning potential drug interactions and/or laboratory test interferences and for information on acute toxicity.

Preparations

Excipients in commercially available drug preparations may have clinically important effects in some individuals; consult specific product labeling for details.

risperiDONE

Oral		
Solution	1 mg/mL*	**RisperDAL®**, Janssen **risperiDONE Oral Solution**
Tablets	0.25 mg*	**RisperDAL®**, Janssen **risperiDONE Tablets**
	0.5 mg*	**RisperDAL®**, Janssen **risperiDONE Tablets**
	1 mg*	**RisperDAL®**, Janssen **risperiDONE Tablets**
	2 mg*	**RisperDAL®**, Janssen **risperiDONE Tablets**
	3 mg*	**RisperDAL®**, Janssen **risperiDONE Tablets**
	4 mg*	**RisperDAL®**, Janssen **risperiDONE Tablets**

Tablets, orally disintegrating	0.25 mg*	risperiDONE Orally Disintegrating Tablets
	0.5 mg*	RisperDAL® M-TAB®, Janssen
		risperiDONE Orally Disintegrating Tablets
	1 mg*	RisperDAL® M-TAB®, Janssen
		risperiDONE Orally Disintegrating Tablets
	2 mg*	RisperDAL® M-TAB®, Janssen
		risperiDONE Orally Disintegrating Tablets
	3 mg*	RisperDAL® M-TAB®, Janssen
		risperiDONE Orally Disintegrating Tablets
	4 mg*	RisperDAL® M-TAB®, Janssen
		risperiDONE Orally Disintegrating Tablets
Parenteral		
For injectable suspension, extended-release, for IM use	12.5 mg	RisperDAL® Consta® (available as dose pack containing a vial adapter device, 2 safety needles, and with 2-mL prefilled syringe diluent), Janssen
	25 mg	RisperDAL® Consta® (available as dose pack containing a vial adapter device, 2 safety needles, and with 2-mL prefilled syringe diluent), Janssen
	37.5 mg	RisperDAL® Consta® (available as dose pack containing a vial adapter device, 2 safety needles, and with 2-mL prefilled syringe diluent), Janssen
	50 mg	RisperDAL® Consta® (available as dose pack containing a vial adapter device, 2 safety needles, and with 2-mL prefilled syringe diluent), Janssen

*available from one or more manufacturer, distributor, and/or repackager by generic (nonproprietary) name

†Use is not currently included in the labeling approved by the US Food and Drug Administration

BUTYROPHENONES 28:16.08.08

Haloperidol

■ Haloperidol is a butyrophenone-derivative antipsychotic agent. The drug is considered a conventional or first-generation antipsychotic agent.

Uses

■ **Schizophrenia** Haloperidol is used orally and parenterally for the symptomatic management of psychotic disorders (i.e., schizophrenia). Drug therapy is integral to the management of acute psychotic episodes in patients with schizophrenia and generally is required for long-term stabilization to improve symptoms between episodes and to minimize the risk of recurrent acute episodes. Antipsychotic agents are the principal class of drugs used for the management of all phases of schizophrenia and generally are effective in all subtypes of the disorder and subgroups of patients. Conventional antipsychotic agents, such as haloperidol, generally are considered to exhibit similar efficacy in treating acute psychotic symptoms, although they vary in their potency and adverse effect profile. Haloperidol is a high-potency antipsychotic that has been shown to be effective in the management of acute and stable phases of schizophrenia, but is frequently associated with extrapyramidal reactions such as akathisia, dystonia, or parkinsonian symptoms, even at low dosages.

Results of short-term studies indicate that oral haloperidol is more effective than placebo and equally or less effective than atypical antipsychotics in the treatment of positive (e.g., delusions, hallucinations) and negative symptoms (e.g., withdrawal from social interaction, blunted emotional expression) of schizophrenia. However, in one clinical study, haloperidol was less effective than the atypical antipsychotic agent risperidone in preventing relapse in adult outpatients with clinically active schizophrenia or schizoaffective disorders who were assigned to receive either drug for a minimum of 1 year. In this study, approximately 40% of patients in the study who received usual dosages of haloperidol had relapsed by the end of the study compared with approximately 25% of those receiving usual dosages of risperidone.

Because atypical antipsychotics appear to be at least as effective in the treatment of positive symptoms and possibly more effective in the treatment of negative symptoms of schizophrenia and have fewer extrapyramidal reactions, some clinicians prefer use of atypical antipsychotics rather than conventional antipsychotics, such as haloperidol, for the management of schizophrenia, except in stable patients who have had good response to conventional antipsychotics without major adverse effects, in patients who require IM therapy, which is not yet available for some atypical antipsychotics, and for the acute management of aggression/violence in some patients, particularly those requiring long-acting (depot) parenteral preparations. However, patient response and tolerance to antipsychotic agents are variable, and patients who do not respond to or tolerate one drug may be successfully treated with an agent from a different class or with a different adverse effect profile.

The long-acting decanoate ester of haloperidol is used parenterally principally in patients requiring prolonged antipsychotic therapy (e.g., patients with chronic schizophrenic disorder). Parenteral antipsychotic therapy with a long-acting preparation may be particularly useful in patients with a history of poor compliance. In addition, long-acting antipsychotic preparations may be useful in patients with suspected GI malabsorption or variable GI absorption of the drug. The principal disadvantage of long-acting parenteral antipsychotics is the inability to terminate the drug's action when severe adverse reactions occur. Long-acting antipsychotic preparations should not be used in the acute management of severely agitated patients. Generally, patients should be stabilized on antipsychotic medication prior to conversion to haloperidol decanoate therapy and should have previously received and tolerated a shorter-acting haloperidol preparation so that the possibility of an unexpected adverse reaction that potentially could not be readily reversed following the decanoate can be minimized. For further information on the use of antipsychotic agents in the symptomatic treatment of schizophrenia, see Uses: Psychotic Disorders, in the Phenothiazines General Statement 28:16.08.24.

■ **Tourette's Syndrome** Haloperidol is used orally and parenterally for the control of tics and vocal utterances of Tourette's syndrome (Gilles de la Tourette's syndrome) in children and adults. Haloperidol generally has been considered the drug of choice for the management of Tourette's syndrome and pimozide has been an effective alternative in some patients who have an inadequate response to or do not tolerate haloperidol. Because limited data suggest that pimozide may be more effective than haloperidol in reducing tics and pimozide appears to be better tolerated than haloperidol, some clinicians and experts prefer the use of pimozide in patients with Tourette's syndrome.

In children with tic disorders (e.g., Tourette's syndrome) and comorbid attention deficit hyperactivity disorder† (ADHD) in whom stimulants alone cannot control tics, haloperidol may be used concomitantly with a stimulant.

■ **Delirium** Antipsychotic agents, mainly haloperidol, have been used in the management of delirium†.

General Considerations Delirium is principally a disturbance of consciousness, attention, cognition, and perception but also may affect sleep, psychomotor activity, and emotions. It is a common psychiatric illness among medically compromised patients, particularly hospitalized patients, and may be a harbinger of substantial morbidity and mortality.

Prevalence and Course The prevalence of delirium in hospitalized medically ill patients ranges from 10–30%; in those who are elderly, delirium ranges up to 40%. Up to 25% of hospitalized cancer patients and 30–40% of hospitalized patients with acquired immunodeficiency syndrome (AIDS) develop delirium. Up to about 50% of postoperative patients develop delirium, and up to 80% of terminally ill patients develop it near death. EEG abnormalities, mainly generalized slowing, have fairly good sensitivity for aiding in the diagnosis of delirium, but the absence of such changes does not rule out the diagnosis. Prodromal manifestations may progress to full-blown delirium over 1–3 days; the duration of delirium generally ranges from less than a week to more than 2 months, but typically does not exceed 10–12 days. Symptoms persist for up to 30 days or longer in up to 15% of patients, and frequently persist for longer than 1 month in geriatric patients. Although most patients recover fully, delirium may progress to stupor, coma, seizures, and death, particularly if untreated. Full recovery is less likely in geriatric patients and patients with AIDS, possibly because of underlying dementia in both populations.

Underlying general medical conditions associated with delirium include CNS disorders (e.g., head trauma, seizures, postictal state, vascular or degenerative disease), metabolic disorders (e.g., renal or hepatic failure, anemia, hypoxia, hypoglycemia, thiamine deficiency, endocrinopathy, fluid or electrolyte imbalance, acid-base imbalance), cardiopulmonary disorder (myocardial infarction, congestive heart failure, cardiac arrhythmia, shock, respiratory failure), and systemic illness (e.g., substance intoxication or withdrawal, infection, cancer, severe trauma, sensory deprivation, temperature dysregulation, postoperative state).

Management **Overview.** Clinicians should undertake an essential array of psychiatric management tasks designed to provide immediate interventions for urgent general medical conditions, identify and treat the etiology of delirium, ensure safety of the patient and others in contact with the patient, and improve the patient's functioning. Environmental (e.g., varying light levels in intensive care units to heighten awareness about time of day and reduce the perception of timelessness) and supportive interventions (e.g., to deal with disorientation, to assure the patient that manifestations are temporary and reversible and do not reflect a persistent psychiatric disorder) also generally are offered to patients with delirium† and are designed to reduce factors that may exacerbate delirium, to reorient patients, and to provide support. Patients may have life-threatening medical conditions that require therapeutic intervention even before a specific or definitive cause of the delirium is determined. The goal of diagnosis is to identify potentially reversible causes of delirium and prevent complications through prompt treatment of these specific disorders. Psychiatric management is essential and should be undertaken for all patients with delirium. Somatic interventions principally consist of drug therapy. The choice of somatic intervention will depend on the specific features of the patient's clinical condition, the underlying etiology of the delirium, and any associated comorbid conditions.

Drug Therapy. Antipsychotic agents often are the drugs of choice for the management of delirium†. Although other drugs (e.g., phenothiazines, droperidol) have been used, haloperidol generally is considered the antipsychotic of choice for most patients with delirium because of its relatively low risk of anticholinergic activity and of sedative and hypotensive effects. In addition, haloperidol has been studied most extensively, although few studies have used standardized definitions of delirium or reliable and valid delirium symptom rating measures to assess symptom severity before and after initiation of treatment. For drugs other than haloperidol, there have been no large, prospective studies that included a control. Evidence of efficacy for such alternative therapies, including second-generation antipsychotic agents (e.g., olanzapine, quetiapine, risperidone, ziprasidone), is principally from small case series, case reports, or open-label studies. In addition, interpretation of findings from many such case presentations is difficult because of use of nonstandardized delirium definitions and/or informal measures of delirium symptom severity. In general, evidence of the efficacy of antipsychotics, including haloperidol, in the management of delirium comes from numerous case reports and uncontrolled studies. However, evidence from a randomized, double-blind, comparator-drug controlled study (haloperidol, chlorpromazine, and lorazepam) in patients with AIDS that employed standardized clinical measures of delirium demonstrated clinical superiority of antipsychotic agents compared with benzodiazepines. Statistically significant improvement in the Delirium Rating Scale was evident after 2 days in patients receiving haloperidol or chlorpromazine but not in the lorazepam group (mean decreases in the score [i.e., improvement] were 8, 8.5, and 1, respectively). The symptomatic improvement in delirium occurred quickly among patients receiving antipsychotic therapy, usually before initiation of interventions directed at the medical etiologies of delirium.

Although various antipsychotic agents may be given orally, IM, or IV, IV administration is considered most effective in emergency situations or where oral access is limited. In addition, some evidence indicates that IV administration of antipsychotic agents may be associated with less severe extrapyramidal effects.

Special Precautions. Antipsychotic agents, particularly IV† haloperidol, used in the management of delirium have been associated with lengthening of the QT interval, possibly leading to atypical ventricular tachycardia (torsades de pointes), ventricular fibrillation, and sudden death. The manufacturer of Haldol® and the US Food and Drug Administration (FDA) state that although injectable haloperidol is approved *only* for IM injection and *not for IV administration*, there is considerable evidence from the medical literature that IV† administration of the drug is a relatively common, unlabeled ("off-label") clinical practice, principally for the treatment of severe agitation in intensive care units, and recommend ECG monitoring in any patient receiving the drug IV. Many clinicians also recommend that baseline and periodic or continuous ECG monitoring be performed with special attention paid to the length of the QT_c interval. Prolongation of the QT_c interval to greater than 450 msec or to greater than 15–25% over that in previous ECGs may warrant telemetry, a cardiology consultation, and dose reduction or discontinuance. Serum concentrations of magnesium and potassium also should be monitored at baseline and periodically in critically ill patients, especially those with baseline QT_c intervals of 440 msec or longer, those receiving other drugs known to increase the QT interval, and those who have electrolyte disorders. Limited evidence suggests that the incidence of torsades de pointes in patients receiving haloperidol IV is about 0.4–3.6%, but may increase to greater than 10% at relatively high IV doses (e.g., 35 mg or more over 24 hours). (See Cautions: Cardiovascular Effects and also see Cautions: Precautions and Contraindications.)

■ **Disruptive Behavior Disorder and Attention Deficit Hyperactivity Disorder** Haloperidol is used orally for the treatment of severe behavioral problems in children marked by combativeness and/or explosive hyperexcitable behavior (out of proportion to immediate provocations), and for the short-term treatment of hyperactive children who exhibit excessive motor activity with accompanying conduct disorders that are manifested as impulsive behavior, difficulty sustaining attention, aggression, mood lability, and/or poor frustration tolerance. However, the possible risks of tardive dyskinesia, withdrawal dyskinesia, and other extrapyramidal reactions should be considered. Some experts currently recommend use of haloperidol only for the treatment of comorbid tics in children with attention deficit hyperactivity disorder (ADHD). Some clinicians recommend routine administration of the Abnormal Involuntary Movement Scale (AIMS) to all children receiving antipsychotic agents.

■ **Nausea and Vomiting** Haloperidol also has been used in the prevention and control of severe nausea and vomiting† (e.g., cancer chemotherapy-induced emesis). Based on limited data, haloperidol appears to be as effective as phenothiazines in the prevention of cancer chemotherapy-induced emesis. Additional studies are required to determine the efficacy of haloperidol in the prevention and control of severe nausea and vomiting.

Dosage and Administration

■ **Administration** Haloperidol is administered orally. Haloperidol lactate is administered orally or by IM injection, and haloperidol decanoate is administered by IM injection. Pending accumulation of further data to establish safety and efficacy, IM administration of haloperidol lactate or decanoate in children is not recommended by the manufacturers. Haloperidol *lactate* also has been administered by IV injection† or infusion†. Haloperidol decanoate injection should *not* be administered IV.

Haloperidol decanoate should be administered by deep IM injection into the gluteal region using a 21-gauge needle. The manufacturers of haloperidol decanoate state that the maximum volume of haloperidol decanoate should not exceed 3 mL per IM injection site.

Haloperidol lactate and decanoate injections should be inspected visually for particulate matter and discoloration prior to administration whenever solution and container permit.

■ **Dosage** Dosage of haloperidol lactate and the decanoate is expressed in terms of haloperidol.

There is considerable interindividual variation in optimum dosage requirements of haloperidol, and dosage must be carefully adjusted according to individual requirements and response, using the lowest possible effective dosage. Dosage should be increased more gradually in children and in debilitated, emaciated, or geriatric patients. Because of the risk of adverse reactions associated with cumulative effects of butyrophenones, patients with a history of long-term therapy with haloperidol and/or other antipsychotic agents should be evaluated periodically to determine whether maintenance dosage could be decreased or drug therapy discontinued.

Oral Dosage For the symptomatic management of psychotic disorders or Tourette's disorder in adults with *moderate symptomatology and in geriatric or debilitated patients*, the manufacturers state that the usual initial oral dosage of haloperidol is 0.5–2 mg administered 2 or 3 times daily. To achieve prompt control, higher initial dosages may be required in some patients. Subsequent dosage should be carefully adjusted according to the patient's tolerance and therapeutic response. Dosage during prolonged maintenance therapy should be kept at the lowest effective level.

For the symptomatic management of psychotic disorders or Tourette's disorder in adults with *severe symptomatology and/or chronic or resistant disorders*, the manufacturers state that the usual initial oral dosage of haloperidol is 3–5 mg administered 2 or 3 times daily. To achieve prompt control, higher initial dosages may be required in some patients. Subsequent dosage should be carefully adjusted according to the patient's tolerance and therapeutic response. Dosage during prolonged maintenance therapy should be kept at the lowest effective level.

Similarly, the American Psychiatric Association (APA) recommends oral haloperidol dosages ranging from 5–20 mg daily in the treatment of adults with schizophrenia. The APA states that determining the optimal dosage of antipsychotic agents during the acute phase of schizophrenia is complicated because there usually is a delay between initiation of therapy and full therapeutic response. An initial response to antipsychotic therapy may take 2–4 weeks and up to 6 months or longer may be needed for a full or optimal response.

Patients who remain severely disturbed or inadequately controlled despite receiving recommended dosages of haloperidol may require dosage adjustment. Some manufacturers state that oral haloperidol dosages up to 100 mg daily may be necessary in some cases to achieve an optimal response. In addition, these manufacturers further state that haloperidol has been used infrequently in dosages exceeding 100 mg daily in severely resistant disorders in adults, but that the limited use has not demonstrated the safety of prolonged administration of such high dosages of the drug. However, extensive clinical experience suggests that higher-dosage haloperidol regimens (i.e., those exceeding 20–40 mg daily) are unlikely to be more effective or result in a faster clinical response in the majority of patients with schizophrenia, including in those with refractory or chronic schizophrenia, and supports the use of more moderate dosage regimens (i.e., from 4 mg daily up to 15–20 mg daily) in such patients. In addition, high-dosage haloperidol regimens are more likely to be associated with unacceptable short- and long-term adverse effects (see Cautions).

The usual initial oral dosage of haloperidol in children 3–12 years of age and weighing 15–40 kg is 0.5 mg daily given in 2 or 3 divided doses. Subsequent dosage may be increased by 0.5 mg daily at 5- to 7-day intervals, depending on the patient's tolerance and therapeutic response.

For the symptomatic management of psychotic disorders in children 3–12 years of age, the usual oral dosage range is 0.05–0.15 mg/kg daily given in 2 or 3 divided doses; however, severely disturbed psychotic children may require higher dosages. Dosage during prolonged maintenance therapy should be kept at the lowest possible effective level; once an adequate response has been achieved, dosage should be gradually reduced and subsequently adjusted according to the patient's therapeutic response and tolerance.

For the management of non-psychotic behavioral problems and for the control of Tourette's disorder in children 3–12 years of age, the usual oral dosage range is 0.05–0.075 mg/kg daily given in 2 or 3 divided doses. Unlike psychotic disorders for which prolonged therapy is usually required, non-psychotic or hyperactive behavioral problems in children may be acute, and short-term administration of haloperidol may be adequate. A maximum effective dosage of haloperidol for the management of behavioral problems in children has not been established; however, the manufacturers state that there is little evidence that improvement in behavior is further enhanced at dosages greater than 6 mg daily.

IM Dosage **Haloperidol Lactate.** For the prompt control of acutely agitated patients with moderately severe to very severe symptoms, the usual initial adult IM dose of haloperidol lactate is 2–5 mg (of haloperidol) given as a single dose. Depending on the response of the patient, this dose may be repeated as often as every hour; however, IM administration of haloperidol lactate every 4–8 hours may be adequate to control symptoms in some patients.

Oral therapy should replace short-acting parenteral therapy as soon as possible. Depending on the patient's clinical status, the first oral dose should be given within 12–24 hours following administration of the last parenteral dose of haloperidol lactate. Since bioavailability studies to establish bioequivalence between oral and parenteral dosage forms of haloperidol have not been conducted to date, the manufacturers suggest that the parenteral dosage administered during the preceding 24 hours be used for initial approximation of the total daily oral dosage required. Since this dosage is only an initial estimate, patients being switched from parenteral haloperidol lactate therapy to oral therapy should be closely monitored, particularly for clinical signs and symptoms of efficacy, sedation, and adverse effects, for the first several days following initiation of oral therapy. Subsequent dosage may be increased or decreased according to the patient's tolerance and therapeutic response, using the lowest possible effective dosage.

Haloperidol Decanoate. For patients requiring prolonged antipsychotic therapy (e.g., patients with chronic schizophrenic disorder), the long-acting haloperidol decanoate injection may be considered. If the decanoate is used, the patient's condition should initially be stabilized with an antipsychotic agent prior to attempting conversion to haloperidol decanoate. In addition, if the patient is receiving an antipsychotic agent other than haloperidol, it is recommended that the patient initially be converted to oral haloperidol therapy in order to minimize the risk of an unexpected adverse reaction to the drug, which might not be readily reversible following use of the decanoate.

The initial IM dose of haloperidol decanoate should be based on the patient's clinical history, physical condition, and response to previous antipsychotic therapy. To determine the minimum effective dosage, haloperidol decanoate therapy has been initiated at low initial doses and gradually titrated upward as necessary. A precise formula for converting from oral haloperidol to IM haloperidol decanoate dosage has not been established, but an initial adult dose 10–20 times the previous daily dose of oral haloperidol, not exceeding 100 mg (regardless of previous antipsychotic dosage requirements), is suggested, although limited clinical experience suggests that a lower initial dosage of the decanoate may be adequate. If conversion requires an initial dosage of haloperidol decanoate higher than 100 mg daily, such dosage should be administered in 2 injections (i.e., administering a maximum initial dose of 100 mg followed by the balance in 3–7 days). However, some clinicians have converted therapy to the decanoate using a higher initial dosage.

Lower initial IM dosages (e.g., 10–15 times the previous daily dose of oral haloperidol) and more gradual upward titration of haloperidol administered as the decanoate salt are recommended for patients who are geriatric, debilitated, or stabilized on low oral dosages (e.g., up to the equivalent of 10 mg daily of oral haloperidol). Higher initial IM dosages (e.g., 20 times the previous daily dosage of oral haloperidol) should be considered for patients who are stabilized on high oral dosages of antipsychotic agents, those who are at risk of relapse, and those who are tolerant to oral haloperidol, with downward titration on succeeding injections.

Haloperidol decanoate usually has been administered IM at monthly intervals (i.e., every 4 weeks), but individual response may dictate the need for adjusting the dosing interval as well as the dose.

The maintenance dosage of haloperidol decanoate must be individualized with upward or downward dosage titration based on clinical response. The usual adult maintenance IM dosage is 10–15 times the previous daily dosage of oral haloperidol for adult patients depending on the clinical response of the patient.

Close clinical observation is required during dosage titration in order to minimize the risk of overdosage and of emergence of psychotic manifestations prior to the next dose. If supplemental antipsychotic therapy is necessary during periods of dosage titration or for control of acute exacerbations of psychotic manifestations, a short-acting haloperidol preparation should be used. Experience with haloperidol decanoate dosages exceeding 450 mg (of haloperidol) monthly is limited.

IV Dosage **Haloperidol Lactate.** The optimum dosage of haloperidol (administered as haloperidol lactate) for the treatment of delirium has not been established. However, initiation of IV† haloperidol with dosages of 1–2 mg every 2–4 hours in adults has been suggested. Lower IV dosages (e.g., 0.25–0.5 mg every 4 hours) have been suggested for geriatric patients with delirium; severely agitated adults may require titration to higher dosages. Although single IV doses up to 50 mg or total daily dosages of 500 mg have been reported in adults, the risk of adverse effects, particularly prolongation of the QT interval and torsades de pointes, must be considered. (See Uses: Delirium and also see Cautions: Cardiovascular Effects and Cautions: Precautions and Contraindications.) Some evidence suggests that the risk of torsades de pointes increases at total daily dosages of 35–50 mg or more. In patients requiring multiple IV injections of the drug to control delirium (e.g., more than eight 10-mg doses in 24 hours or more than 10 mg/hour for more than 5 consecutive hours), consideration can be given to continuous IV infusion† of haloperidol; in such patients, an initial 10-mg dose followed by an infusion of 5–10 mg/hour has been suggested. If agitation persists, repeat 10-mg IV doses at 30-minute intervals, accompanied by a 5 mg/hour increase in the infusion rate, can be considered. ECG should be determined at baseline and periodically or continuously thereafter, with special attention paid to possible prolongation of the QT interval, and dosage should be reduced or the drug discontinued if clinically important QT prolongation (e.g., 15–25% or more over baseline) occurs or the QT_c exceeds 450 msec.

Cautions

Haloperidol shares the toxic potentials of phenothiazines, and the usual precautions of phenothiazine therapy should be observed. The overall incidence of adverse effects associated with haloperidol is similar to that associated with piperazine-derivative phenothiazines. (See Cautions in the Phenothiazines General Statement 28:16.08.24.)

Geriatric patients with dementia-related psychosis treated with antipsychotic agents are at an increased risk of mortality. (See Cautions: Geriatric Precautions.)

■ **Nervous System Effects** The most frequent adverse effects of haloperidol involve the CNS.

Extrapyramidal Reactions Extrapyramidal reactions occur frequently with haloperidol, especially during the first few days of therapy. In most patients, these reactions consist of parkinsonian symptoms (e.g., marked drowsiness and lethargy, drooling or hypersalivation, fixed stare), which are mild to moderate in severity and are usually reversible following discontinuance of the drug. Other adverse neuromuscular reactions have been reported less frequently, but are often more severe, and include feelings of motor restlessness (i.e., akathisia), tardive dystonia, and dystonic reactions (e.g., hyperreflexia, opisthotonos, oculogyric crisis, torticollis, trismus). Generally, the occurrence and severity of most extrapyramidal reactions are dose related, since they occur at relatively high dosages and disappear or become less severe following a reduction in dosage; however, severe extrapyramidal reactions have reportedly occurred at relatively low dosages. Most patients respond rapidly to treatment with an anticholinergic antiparkinsonian drug (e.g., benztropine, trihexyphenidyl). If persistent extrapyramidal reactions occur, haloperidol therapy may have to be discontinued.

Neuroleptic malignant syndrome (NMS) may occur in patients receiving haloperidol or other antipsychotic therapy. NMS is potentially fatal and requires immediate discontinuance of the drug and initiation of intensive symptomatic and supportive care. For additional information on NMS, see Extrapyramidal Reactions in Cautions: Nervous System Effects, in the Phenothiazines General Statement 28:16.08.24.

Tardive Dyskinesia Like other antipsychotic agents (e.g., phenothiazines), haloperidol has been associated with persistent dyskinesias. Tardive dyskinesia may occur in some patients during long-term administration of haloperidol or it may occur following discontinuance of the drug. The risk of developing tardive dyskinesia appears to be greater in geriatric patients receiving high dosages of the drug, especially females. The symptoms are persistent, and in some patients appear to be irreversible. Tardive dyskinesia is characterized by rhythmic involuntary movements of the tongue, face, mouth, or jaw (e.g., protrusion of the tongue, puffing of cheeks, chewing movements, puckering of the mouth), which sometimes may be accompanied by involuntary movements of the extremities and/or trunk. Although not clearly established, the risk of developing the syndrome and the likelihood that it will become irreversible may increase with the duration of therapy and total cumulative dose of antipsychotic agent(s) administered; however, the syndrome may occur, although much less frequently, after relatively short periods of treatment with low dosages.

Management of tardive dyskinesia generally consists of gradual discontinuance of the precipitating antipsychotic agent when possible, reducing the dosage of the first-generation (conventional) antipsychotic agent or switching to a second-generation (atypical) antipsychotic agent, or switching to clozapine therapy. The syndrome may partially or completely remit if antipsychotic agents are discontinued, although some patients may require many months for improvement. Tardive dyskinesia may be masked if antipsychotic therapy is reinstituted, dosage is increased, or therapy with another antipsychotic agent is initiated. The effect that masking of the symptoms may have on the long-term course of the syndrome is not known. Fine vermicular movement of the tongue may be an early sign of tardive dyskinesia; prompt discontinuance of haloperidol after this sign occurs may prevent development of the syndrome. Vesicular monoamine transporter 2 (VMAT2) inhibitors (e.g., deutetrabenazine, valbenazine tosylate) have been shown to be effective in reducing symptoms of tardive dyskinesia in controlled clinical studies and may allow some patients to continue receiving antipsychotic therapy. (See Deutetrabenazine 28:56 and Valbenazine Tosylate 28:56.) Antiparkinsonian agents do not alleviate and tend to exacerbate the symptoms of this syndrome.

In general, abrupt withdrawal of antipsychotic agents following short-term administration is not associated with adverse effects; however, transient dyskinetic signs have occurred following abrupt withdrawal in patients receiving prolonged maintenance therapy with haloperidol. In some patients, the dyskinetic movements are indistinguishable, except on the basis of their duration, from tardive dyskinesia. It is not known whether gradual withdrawal of antipsychotic agents reduces the incidence of withdrawal-emergent neurologic signs; however, if haloperidol therapy must be discontinued, gradual withdrawal of the drug is recommended, if possible, pending further accumulation of data.

For additional information on tardive dyskinesia, including manifestations and treatment, see Tardive Dyskinesia under Cautions: Nervous System Effects, in the Phenothiazines General Statement 28:16.08.24.

Other Nervous System Effects Tardive dystonia, not associated with tardive dyskinesia, has occurred in patients receiving haloperidol. Tardive dystonia is characterized by delayed onset of choreic or dystonic movements, often is persistent, and potentially can become irreversible.

Other adverse nervous system effects of haloperidol include insomnia, restlessness, anxiety, euphoria, agitation, drowsiness, depression, lethargy, headache, confusion, vertigo, and tonic-clonic seizures. Exacerbation of psychotic symptoms (including hallucinations and catatonic-like behavior), which may subside following discontinuance of therapy or treatment with anticholinergic agents, has also been reported.

Adverse anticholinergic effects of haloperidol include dry mouth (xerostomia), blurred vision, constipation, urinary retention, and diaphoresis. Priapism has also occurred.

■ **Hematologic Effects** Mild and usually transient leukopenia/neutropenia and leukocytosis have been reported in patients receiving antipsychotic agents, including haloperidol. Agranulocytosis (including fatal cases) has also been reported rarely in patients receiving haloperidol, but only when combined with other drugs. Possible risk factors for leukopenia and neutropenia include preexisting low leukocyte count and a history of drug-induced leukopenia or neutropenia. (See Cautions: Precautions and Contraindications.) Other adverse hematologic effects associated with haloperidol include anemia, minimal decreases in erythrocyte count, and a tendency toward lymphomonocytosis.

■ **Endocrine and Metabolic Effects** Moderate engorgement of the breast with lactation has occurred in some females receiving haloperidol. Galactorrhea, mastalgia, menstrual irregularities, gynecomastia, increased libido, impotence, hyperglycemia, hypoglycemia, and hyponatremia have also occurred in some patients. Antipsychotic agents increase serum prolactin concentrations. (See Cautions: Mutagenicity and Carcinogenicity.) Although not reported to date with haloperidol, the manufacturers caution that decreases in serum cholesterol concentration have occurred in patients receiving chemically related drugs.

■ **Cardiovascular Effects** Tachycardia, hypotension, hypertension, ECG changes (including those compatible with QT-interval prolongation and the polymorphous configuration of torsades de pointes), and sudden death have been reported in patients receiving haloperidol. The US Food and Drug Administration (FDA) states that there have been at least 28 case reports of QT-interval prolongation and torsades de pointes, including some that were fatal, in patients receiving the drug IV†. In addition, FDA states that case-control studies have demonstrated a dose-dependent relationship between IV haloperidol dosage and subsequent development of torsades de pointes. A postmarketing analysis of a worldwide safety database revealed 229 reports of QT-interval prolongation and torsades de pointes with oral or parenteral haloperidol; many of these cases were confounded by concomitant administration of drugs known to prolong the QT interval or medical conditions associated with QT-interval prolongation. The reports included 73 cases of torsades de pointes, 11 of which were fatal. In 8 out of 11 fatal cases, haloperidol was administered IV in various dosages. In another postmarketing analysis of adverse cardiovascular events associated with haloperidol decanoate, 13 cases of torsades de pointes, QT-interval prolongation, ventricular arrhythmias, and/or sudden death were identified.

FDA states that it is not possible to estimate the frequency with which QT-interval prolongation or torsades de pointes occurs following administration of haloperidol based on these case reports alone. However, use of higher than recommended doses of any haloperidol formulation and IV administration of the drug appear to be associated with an increased risk of these effects. Many of the reported cases of QT-interval prolongation and torsades de pointes have occurred in patients receiving relatively high dosages of IV haloperidol (e.g., exceeding 35 mg daily); however, such effects also have been reported in patients receiving lower IV dosages or oral therapy. Although cases of sudden death, torsades de pointes, and QT-interval prolongation have been reported even in the absence of predisposing factors, FDA, the manufacturer of Haldol®, and some clinicians state that particular caution is advised when using any formulation of haloperidol in patients who have other QT-interval prolonging conditions, including electrolyte imbalance (particularly hypokalemia and hypomagnesemia), underlying cardiac abnormalities, hypothyroidism, or familial long QT syndrome, or those who are concomitantly taking medications known to prolong the QT interval. (See Uses: Delirium, see Cautions: Precautions and Contraindications, and also see Acute Toxicity: Manifestations.) FDA states that clinicians should consider this cardiovascular risk information when making individual treatment decisions for their patients.

Cases of sudden and unexpected death have been reported in haloperidol-treated patients. The nature of the evidence makes it impossible to determine definitively what role, if any, haloperidol played in the outcome of the cases reported to date. Although the possibility that haloperidol played a causative role in these deaths cannot be excluded, it should be kept in mind that sudden and unexpected death may occur in psychotic patients when they remain untreated or when they are treated with other antipsychotic medications.

■ **Other Adverse Effects** Impaired liver function and/or jaundice, maculopapular and acneiform dermatologic reactions, photosensitivity, alopecia, anorexia, diarrhea, hypersalivation, dyspepsia, nausea, vomiting, cataracts, retinopathy, and visual disturbances have also been reported.

Hyperpyrexia and heat stroke, not associated with neuroleptic malignant syndrome (see Extrapyramidal Reactions in Cautions: Nervous System Effects), have been reported in some patients receiving haloperidol.

Laryngospasm, bronchospasm, and increased depth of respiration have occurred in patients receiving haloperidol. Bronchopneumonia, resulting in fatalities in some patients, has occurred following the use of antipsychotic agents, including haloperidol. It has been suggested that lethargy and decreased thirst, resulting from central inhibition, may cause dehydration, hemoconcentration, and reduced pulmonary ventilation.

Hyperammonemia following haloperidol treatment has been reported in at least one child with citrullinemia, an inherited disorder of ammonia excretion.

■ **Precautions and Contraindications** Haloperidol shares the toxic potentials of other antipsychotic agents (e.g., phenothiazines), and the usual precautions associated with therapy with these agents should be observed. (See Cautions in the Phenothiazines General Statement 28:16.08.24.)

Geriatric patients with dementia-related psychosis treated with antipsychotic agents are at an increased risk of mortality. (See Cautions: Geriatric Precautions.)

Patients should be warned that haloperidol may impair their ability to perform activities requiring mental alertness or physical coordination (e.g., operating machinery, driving a motor vehicle). Patients also should be warned that haloperidol may enhance their response to alcohol, barbiturates, or other CNS depressants.

Because of the possibility of transient hypotension and/or precipitation of angina, haloperidol should be used with caution in patients with severe cardiovascular disorders. If hypotension occurs, metaraminol, norepinephrine, or phenylephrine may be used; epinephrine should *not* be used since haloperidol causes a reversal of epinephrine's vasopressor effects and a further lowering of blood pressure.

Since haloperidol may lower the seizure threshold, the drug should be used with caution in patients receiving anticonvulsant agents and in those with a history of seizures or EEG abnormalities. Adequate anticonvulsant therapy should be maintained during administration of haloperidol.

The manufacturers state that haloperidol should be used with caution in patients with known allergies or with a history of allergic reactions to drugs.

When concomitant therapy with an antiparkinsonian drug is necessary to manage haloperidol-induced extrapyramidal symptoms, it may be necessary to continue the antiparkinsonian drug for a period of time after discontinuance of haloperidol in order to prevent emergence of these symptoms.

The manufacturers caution that when haloperidol is used to control mania in patients with bipolar disorder, there may be a rapid mood swing to depression.

Haloperidol should be used with caution in patients with thyrotoxicosis since severe neurotoxicity (e.g., rigidity, inability to walk or talk) may occur in these patients during therapy with an antipsychotic agent.

Cases of leukopenia and neutropenia have been reported in patients receiving antipsychotic agents, including haloperidol; agranulocytosis (including fatal cases) has also been reported. (See Cautions: Hematologic Effects.) Patients with a preexisting low leukocyte count or a history of drug-induced leukopenia or neutropenia should have their complete blood count monitored frequently during the first few months of therapy and haloperidol should be discontinued at the first sign of a decline in the leukocyte count in the absence of other causative factors. Haloperidol-treated patients with neutropenia should be carefully monitored for fever or other signs or symptoms of infection and be treated promptly should such signs and symptoms occur. Patients with severe neutropenia (absolute neutrophil count less than 1000/mm^3) should discontinue haloperidol and have their leukocyte count followed until recovery.

Care should be taken to avoid skin contact with haloperidol lactate oral solution and injection, since contact dermatitis has occurred rarely.

Cases of sudden death, QT-interval prolongation, and torsades de pointes have been reported in patients receiving haloperidol. (See Uses: Delirium and also see Cautions: Cardiovascular Effects.) Use of higher than recommended doses of any haloperidol formulation and IV† administration of the drug appear to be associated with an increased risk of QT-interval prolongation and torsades de pointes. Although these effects have been reported in the absence of predisposing factors, haloperidol should be used with particular caution in patients with other conditions that prolong the QT interval, including electrolyte imbalance (particularly hypokalemia and hypomagnesemia), underlying cardiac abnormalities, hypothyroidism, and familial long QT syndrome, as well as in those concurrently receiving other drugs known to prolong the QT interval. In addition, ECG monitoring is recommended whenever haloperidol is administered IV. (See Uses: Delirium.)

Haloperidol is contraindicated in patients with severe toxic CNS depression or in those who are comatose from any cause. Haloperidol also is contraindicated in patients who are hypersensitive to the drug and in those with parkinsonian syndrome.

■ **Pediatric Precautions** Safety and efficacy of haloperidol decanoate or lactate injection in children have not been established, and safety and efficacy of other haloperidol preparations in children younger than 3 years of age have not been established. Hyperammonemia was reported during postmarketing surveillance in a 5.5-year-old child with citrullinemia, an inherited disorder of ammonia excretion, following haloperidol therapy.

■ **Geriatric Precautions** Clinical studies of haloperidol did not include sufficient numbers of geriatric patients 65 years of age and older to determine whether this age group responds differently from younger adults. Other reported clinical experience has not consistently identified differences in responses between geriatric and younger patients. However, the prevalence of tardive dyskinesia appears to be highest among geriatric patients, particularly elderly women. In addition, the pharmacokinetics of haloperidol generally warrant the use of reduced dosages in geriatric patients. (See Dosage and Administration: Dosage.)

Geriatric patients with dementia-related psychosis treated with either conventional or atypical antipsychotic agents are at an increased risk of mortality. Analyses of 17 placebo-controlled trials (modal duration of 10 weeks) in geriatric patients mainly receiving atypical antipsychotic agents revealed an approximate 1.6- to 1.7-fold increase in mortality compared with that in patients receiving placebo. Over the course of a typical 10-week controlled trial, the rate of death in drug-treated patients was about 4.5% compared with a rate of about 2.6% in those receiving placebo. Although the causes of death were varied in these trials, most of the deaths appeared to be either cardiovascular (e.g., heart failure, sudden death) or infectious (e.g., pneumonia) in nature. Subsequently, 2 observational, epidemiologic studies have indicated that, similar to atypical antipsychotic agents, treatment with conventional antipsychotic agents may increase mortality; the causes of death were not reported in the first study, and cancer and cardiac disease were the causes of death with the highest relative risk in the second study. However, the extent to which these findings of increased mortality in observational studies may be attributed to the antipsychotic agent as opposed to certain patient characteristics remains unclear.

The US Food and Drug Administration (FDA) currently advises clinicians that antipsychotic agents, including haloperidol, are *not* FDA labeled for the treatment of dementia-related psychosis. The FDA further advises clinicians that no drugs currently are approved for the treatment of dementia-associated psychosis and that other management options should be considered in patients with this disorder. The decision whether to prescribe antipsychotic agents "off-label" in the treatment of dementia symptoms is left to the discretion of the clinician. Clinicians who prescribe antipsychotic agents for geriatric patients with dementia-related psychosis should discuss the increased mortality risk with patients, their families, and their caregivers. In addition, patients currently receiving antipsychotic agents for dementia-associated symptoms should not abruptly stop taking the drugs; caregivers and patients should discuss any possible concerns with their clinician. For additional information on the use of antipsychotic agents for dementia-associated psychosis and other behavioral disturbances, see Geriatric Considerations under Psychotic Disorders: Schizophrenia, see Other Psychoneurologic Disorders, in Uses, and also see Cautions: Geriatric Precautions, in the Phenothiazines General Statement 28:16.08.24.

■ **Mutagenicity and Carcinogenicity** Haloperidol did not exhibit mutagenic potential in the Ames test. Negative or inconsistent positive findings have been reported in in vitro and in vivo studies on the effects of conventional preparations of haloperidol on chromosome structure and number. However, the available cytogenetic evidence is considered too inconsistent to be conclusive at this time.

Although an increase in mammary neoplasms has been found in rodents following long-term administration of prolactin-stimulating antipsychotic agents, no clinical or epidemiologic studies conducted to date have shown an association between long-term administration of these drugs and mammary tumorigenesis in humans. Current evidence is considered too limited to be conclusive, and further study is needed to determine the clinical importance in most patients of elevated serum prolactin concentrations associated with antipsychotic agents. Since in vitro tests indicate that approximately one-third of human breast cancers are prolactin dependent, haloperidol should be used with caution in patients with previously detected breast cancer.

■ **Pregnancy, Fertility, and Lactation** Although there are no adequate and controlled studies to date in humans, 2 cases of limb malformations (e.g., phocomelia) have occurred in offspring of women who were given haloperidol concurrently with other potentially teratogenic drugs during the first trimester of pregnancy; these teratogenic effects have not been directly attributed to haloperidol. Haloperidol has been shown to be teratogenic and fetotoxic in animals at dosages 2–20 times the usual maximum human dosage.

Neonates exposed to antipsychotic agents, including haloperidol, during the third trimester of pregnancy are at risk for extrapyramidal and/or withdrawal symptoms following delivery. Symptoms reported in these neonates to date include agitation, hypertonia, hypotonia, tardive dyskinetic-like symptoms, tremor, somnolence, respiratory distress, and feeding disorder. Any neonate exhibiting extrapyramidal or withdrawal symptoms following in utero exposure to antipsychotic agents should be monitored. Symptoms were self-limiting in some neonates, but varied in severity; some infants required intensive care unit support and prolonged hospitalization. For further information on extrapyramidal and withdrawal symptoms in neonates, see Cautions: Pregnancy, Fertility, and Lactation, in the Phenothiazines General Statement 28:16.08.24.

Haloperidol should be used during pregnancy or in women likely to become pregnant only when the potential benefits justify the possible risks to the fetus.

The effect of haloperidol on fertility in humans is not known. Impotence, increased libido, priapism, and menstrual irregularities have occurred in some individuals during haloperidol therapy.

Haloperidol is distributed into milk. The manufacturers warn that nursing should not be undertaken by women receiving haloperidol.

Drug Interactions

■ **CNS Depressants** Haloperidol may be additive with, or may potentiate the action of, other CNS depressants such as opiates or other analgesics, barbiturates or other sedatives, anesthetics, or alcohol. When haloperidol is used concomitantly with other CNS depressants, caution should be used to avoid excessive sedation.

■ **Lithium** Although most patients receiving lithium and an antipsychotic agent (e.g., haloperidol, phenothiazines) concurrently do not develop unusual adverse effects, an acute encephalopathic syndrome occasionally has occurred, especially when high serum lithium concentrations were present. Patients receiving such combined therapy should be observed for evidence of adverse neurologic effects; treatment should be promptly discontinued if such signs or symptoms appear. (See Drug Interactions: Antipsychotic Agents, in the monograph on Lithium Salts 28:28.)

■ **Anticoagulants** Haloperidol has been reported to antagonize the anticoagulant activity of phenindione in one patient. Further study is needed to determine the clinical importance of this interaction.

■ **Rifampin** Concomitant oral therapy with rifampin and haloperidol in schizophrenic patients resulted in a mean 70% decrease in plasma haloperidol concentrations and decreased antipsychotic efficacy. Following discontinuance of rifampin in other schizophrenic patients treated with oral haloperidol, mean haloperidol concentrations increased 3.3-fold. Careful monitoring of clinical status and appropriate dosage adjustment are warranted whenever rifampin is initiated or discontinued in patients stabilized on haloperidol.

■ **Drugs with Anticholinergic Effects** The manufacturers caution that increases in intraocular pressure may occur in patients receiving anticholinergic drugs, including antiparkinsonian agents, concurrently with haloperidol.

■ **Drugs that Prolong QT Interval** Cases of QT-interval prolongation and torsades de pointes have been reported in patients receiving haloperidol. Patients receiving higher than recommended dosages of any haloperidol preparation and those receiving the drug IV appear to be at a higher risk of developing these adverse effects. (See Uses: Delirium and see also Cautions: Cardiovascular Effects.) Particular caution is advised when oral or parenteral haloperidol is used in patients concurrently receiving other drugs that prolong the QT interval.

■ **Methyldopa** Dementia has reportedly occurred in several patients who received haloperidol and methyldopa concomitantly. Although the clinical importance of this possible interaction has not been determined, patients should be carefully observed for adverse psychiatric symptoms if the drugs are used concurrently.

Acute Toxicity

■ **Manifestations** In general, overdosage of haloperidol may be expected to produce effects that are extensions of common adverse reactions; severe extrapyramidal reactions, hypotension, and sedation have been the principal effects reported. Coma with respiratory depression and hypotension (sometimes shock-like) may occur.

Substantial prolongation of the QT interval and atypical ventricular tachycardia (torsades de pointes) have occurred following haloperidol overdosage. The possibility of ECG changes associated with torsades de pointes should be considered following haloperidol overdosage, and ECG and vital signs should be monitored for signs of QT prolongation or dysrhythmias, continuing such monitoring until the ECG is normal.

Following accidental overdosage in a 2-year-old child, hypertension, rather than hypotension, reportedly occurred. Extrapyramidal reactions may consist of muscular weakness or rigidity and a generalized or localized tremor. Manifestations of overdosage with haloperidol decanoate injection may be prolonged.

■ **Treatment** Treatment of haloperidol overdosage generally involves symptomatic and supportive care. There is no specific antidote for haloperidol intoxication; however, anticholinergic or antiparkinsonian drugs may be useful in controlling extrapyramidal reactions associated with haloperidol overdosage.

Following acute ingestion of the drug, the stomach should be emptied by inducing emesis or by gastric lavage. If the patient is comatose, having seizures, or lacks the gag reflex, gastric lavage may be performed if an endotracheal tube with cuff inflated is in place to prevent aspiration of gastric contents. Activated charcoal should be administered after gastric lavage and/or emesis.

ECG and vital signs should be monitored, particularly for signs of QT prolongation or dysrhythmias. Severe arrhythmias should be treated with appropriate antiarrhythmic measures. Appropriate therapy should be instituted if hypotension or excessive sedation occurs; epinephrine should *not* be used (see Cautions: Precautions and Contraindications).

Pharmacology

The principal pharmacologic effects of haloperidol are similar to those of piperazine-derivative phenothiazines. The precise mechanism of antipsychotic action of haloperidol is unclear, but the drug appears to depress the CNS at the subcortical level of the brain, midbrain, and brain stem reticular formation. Haloperidol appears to inhibit the ascending reticular activating system of the brain stem (possibly through the caudate nucleus), thereby interrupting the impulse between the diencephalon and the cortex. The drug may antagonize the actions of glutamic acid within the extrapyramidal system. Inhibition of catecholamine receptors may also be important in the mode of action of haloperidol; the drug may also inhibit the reuptake of various neurotransmitters in the midbrain. Haloperidol appears to have strong central antidopaminergic and weak central anticholinergic activity. Like phenothiazines, haloperidol produces catalepsy and inhibits spontaneous motor activity and conditioned avoidance behaviors in animals. Haloperidol inhibits the central and peripheral effects of apomorphine, produces ganglionic blockade, and reduces affective responses. The precise mechanism of antiemetic action of haloperidol is unclear, but like some phenothiazines (e.g., chlorpromazine, prochlorperazine), haloperidol has been shown to directly affect the chemoreceptor trigger zone (CTZ), apparently by blocking dopamine receptors in the CTZ.

Like other dopamine receptor antagonists (e.g., phenothiazines), haloperidol may cause extrapyramidal reactions, and there appears to be a very narrow range between the effective therapeutic dosage for the management of acute psychotic disorders and that causing extrapyramidal symptoms.

Haloperidol produces less sedation, hypotension, and hypothermia than chlorpromazine.

Pharmacokinetics

■ **Absorption** Haloperidol is well absorbed from the GI tract following oral administration, but appears to undergo first-pass metabolism in the liver. Oral bioavailability of the drug has been reported to average 60%. The drug may undergo some enterohepatic circulation. Peak plasma concentrations of haloperidol occur within 2–6 hours following oral administration. Following IM administration of haloperidol lactate, peak plasma haloperidol concentrations occur within 10–20 minutes and peak pharmacologic action occurs within 30–45 minutes; in acutely agitated patients, control of psychotic manifestations may become apparent within 30–60 minutes, with substantial improvement often occurring within 2–3 hours. Haloperidol concentrations are detectable in plasma for several weeks following administration of a single dose of the drug.

Esterification of haloperidol results in slow and gradual release of haloperidol decanoate from fatty tissues, thus prolonging the duration of action; administration of the ester in a sesame oil vehicle further delays the rate of release. Following IM administration of haloperidol decanoate, plasma haloperidol concentrations are usually evident within 1 day and peak concentrations generally occur within about 6–7 days (range: 1–9 days). Steady-state plasma haloperidol concentrations are usually reached in approximately 3 months following once-monthly IM injection of the decanoate. In one group of patients receiving 20–400 mg monthly, data adjusted to 100-mg monthly doses suggested mean trough plasma haloperidol concentrations of 2 ng/mL after the first dose and of 4 ng/mL at steady state; accumulation during 24 months of therapy was not apparent. Within the usual dosage range, plasma haloperidol concentrations following IM administration of the decanoate are approximately proportional and linearly related to dosage; however, there is considerable interindividual and intraindividual variation in plasma concentrations attained with a given dosage.

■ **Distribution** Distribution of haloperidol into human body tissues and fluids has not been fully characterized. Following administration of haloperidol in animals, the drug is distributed mainly into the liver, with lower concentrations being distributed into the brain, lungs, kidneys, spleen, and heart.

Haloperidol is about 92% bound to plasma proteins.

Haloperidol is distributed into milk.

■ **Elimination** Although the exact metabolic fate has not been clearly established, it appears that haloperidol is principally metabolized in the liver. The drug appears to be metabolized principally by oxidative *N*-dealkylation of the piperidine nitrogen to form fluorophenylcarbonic acids and piperidine metabolites (which appear to be inactive), and by reduction of the butyrophenone carbonyl to the carbinol, forming hydroxyhaloperidol. Limited data suggest that the reduced metabolite, hydroxyhaloperidol, has some pharmacologic activity, although its activity appears to be less than that of haloperidol. Urinary metabolites in rats include *p*-fluorophenaceturic acid, *β-p*-fluorobenzoylpropionic acid, and several unidentified acids.

Haloperidol and its metabolites are excreted slowly in urine and feces. Approximately 40% of a single oral dose of haloperidol is excreted in urine within 5 days. About 15% of an oral dose of the drug is excreted in feces via biliary elimination. Small amounts of the drug are excreted for about 28 days following oral administration.

Following IM administration of haloperidol decanoate, the esterified compound is initially distributed into fatty tissue stores, from which the drug is then slowly and gradually released and subsequently undergoes hydrolysis by plasma and/or tissue esterases to form haloperidol and decanoic acid. Subsequent distribution, metabolism, and excretion of haloperidol appears to be similar to those of orally administered drug. Following IM administration of the decanoate, the drug has an apparent elimination half-life of approximately 3 weeks.

Chemistry and Stability

■ **Chemistry** Haloperidol is a butyrophenone-derivative antipsychotic agent. The drug is structurally similar to droperidol. Haloperidol is commercially available as the base, decanoic acid ester (decanoate), and lactate salt.

Haloperidol occurs as a white to faintly yellowish, amorphous or microcrystalline powder and has solubilities of less than 0.1 mg/mL in water and of approximately 16.7 mg/mL in alcohol at 25°C. The drug has a pK_a of 8.3.

Haloperidol decanoate occurs as a clear, light amber, oily liquid and is soluble in fixed oils (e.g., sesame oil) and in most organic solvents. The decanoate has a solubility of approximately 0.01 mg/mL in water. Haloperidol decanoate injection is commercially available as a sterile solution of the drug in sesame oil and contains benzyl alcohol as a preservative.

Haloperidol injection is prepared with the aid of lactic acid and contains the drug as the lactate salt; the injection is a sterile solution of the drug in water for injection. Commercially available injections are adjusted to pH 3–3.8 with lactic acid and also *may* contain parabens as preservatives. Haloperidol oral solution also is prepared with the aid of lactic acid and contains the drug as the lactate salt. The commercially available oral solution has a pH of 2.75–3.75.

■ **Stability** Commercially available haloperidol preparations should be stored in tight, light-resistant containers at controlled room temperature between 15–30°C; freezing of the oral solution and injections and refrigeration of the decanoate injection should be avoided.

Haloperidol lactate injection may be compatible with some drugs for a short period of time after mixing, but at least one manufacturer recommends that the lactate not be mixed with other drugs. Haloperidol decanoate injection is incompatible with sterile water for injection or sodium chloride injection and with other aqueous injections. Specialized references should be consulted for specific compatibility information.

Preparations

Excipients in commercially available drug preparations may have clinically important effects in some individuals; consult specific product labeling for details.

Haloperidol

Oral		
Tablets	0.5 mg*	**Haloperidol Tablets**
	1 mg*	**Haloperidol Tablets**
	2 mg*	**Haloperidol Tablets**
	5 mg*	**Haloperidol Tablets**
	10 mg*	**Haloperidol Tablets**
	20 mg*	**Haloperidol Tablets**

*available from one or more manufacturer, distributor, and/or repackager by generic (nonproprietary) name

Haloperidol Decanoate

Parenteral		
Injection, for IM use only	50 mg (of haloperidol) per mL*	**Haldol® Decanoate,** Ortho-McNeil-Janssen
		Haloperidol Decanoate Injection
	100 mg (of haloperidol) per mL*	**Haldol® Decanoate,** Ortho-McNeil-Janssen
		Haloperidol Decanoate Injection

*available from one or more manufacturer, distributor, and/or repackager by generic (nonproprietary) name

Haloperidol Lactate

Oral		
Solution	2 mg (of haloperidol) per mL*	**Haloperidol Lactate Oral Solution Concentrate**
Parenteral		
Injection	5 mg (of haloperidol) per mL*	**Haldol®,** Ortho-McNeil-Janssen
		Haloperidol Lactate Injection

*available from one or more manufacturer, distributor, and/or repackager by generic (nonproprietary) name

†Use is not currently included in the labeling approved by the US Food and Drug Administration

PHENOTHIAZINES 28:16.08.24

Phenothiazines General Statement

■ Phenothiazines are conventional (prototypical, first-generation) antipsychotic agents.

Uses

Phenothiazines mainly are used for the management of various psychoneurologic disorders and for the prevention and control of nausea and vomiting. The efficacy of individual phenothiazines varies in different neuropsychiatric and other conditions, and some phenothiazines are not used as antipsychotic agents. Promethazine is used as an antihistamine (see 4:04) and as a sedative (see 28:24.92) and thiethylperazine as an antiemetic. For further information, see the individual monographs on these derivatives.

■ **Psychotic Disorders** ***Schizophrenia and Other Psychotic Disorders*** Phenothiazines are used principally for the symptomatic management of psychotic disorders, especially those characterized by excessive psychomotor activity. The drugs produce substantial improvement in most schizophrenic patients. Phenothiazines are particularly effective in reducing hallucinations and motor and autonomic hyperactivity in patients with schizophrenic disorder; thought disorders, change in affect, and autism are also reduced during phenothiazine therapy. Patient response and tolerance to antipsychotic agents are variable, and patients who do not respond to or tolerate one drug may be successfully treated with an agent from a different class or with a different adverse effect profile.

General Considerations. Schizophrenia, a major psychotic disorder, is a chronic condition that frequently has devastating effects on various aspects of the patient's life and carries a high risk of suicide and other life-threatening behaviors. Manifestations of the disorder involve multiple psychologic processes, including perception (e.g., hallucinations), ideation, reality testing (e.g., delusions), emotion (e.g., flatness, inappropriate affect), thought processes (e.g., loose associations), behavior (e.g., catatonia, disorganization), attention, concentration, motivation (e.g., avolition, impaired intention and planning), and judgment. The behavioral and psychologic characteristics of schizophrenia are associated with a variety of impairments in social and occupational functioning. Although marked deterioration associated with impairments in multiple areas of functioning (e.g., learning, self-care, working, interpersonal relationships, living skills) can occur, the disorder is characterized by great interindividual heterogeneity and by intraindividual variability over time.

The principal manifestations of schizophrenia usually are described in terms of positive and negative (deficit) symptoms and, more recently, disorganized symptoms. Positive symptoms include hallucinations, delusions, bizarre behavior, hostility, uncooperativeness, and paranoid ideation, while negative symptoms include restricted range and intensity of emotional expression (affective flattening), reduced thought and speech productivity (alogia), anhedonia, apathy, and decreased initiation of goal-directed behavior (avolition). Disorganized symptoms include disorganized speech (thought disorder) and behavior and poor attention. Subtypes of schizophrenia include the paranoid, disorganized, catatonic, undifferentiated, and residual types.

Management of schizophrenia usually involves a variety of interventions (e.g., psychiatric management, psychosocial interventions, drug therapy, electroconvulsive therapy [ECT]) aimed at reducing or eliminating symptoms, maximizing quality of life and adaptive functioning, and enabling recovery by assisting patients in attaining personal life goals (e.g., in work, housing, relationships). The long-term outcome of schizophrenia varies along a continuum between reasonable recovery and complete incapacity. Most patients display exacerbations and remissions in the context of experiencing clinical deterioration, although approximately 10–15% of patients are free of further episodes after recovery from a first psychotic episode, and another 10–15% remain chronically severely psychotic.

Disease Phase Overview. Schizophrenia is a disorder that has been described as developing in phases, which have been characterized as premorbid, prodromal, and psychotic. The premorbid phase consists of a period of normal functioning, although certain events (e.g., complications in pregnancy and delivery during the prenatal and perinatal periods, trauma, family stress during childhood and adolescence) may contribute to the development of subsequent illness. During the prodromal phase, which lasts an average of 2–5 years, substantial functional impairment, nonspecific symptoms (e.g., sleep disturbance, anxiety, irritability, depressed mood, poor concentration, fatigue), and behavioral deficits (e.g., role functioning deterioration, social withdrawal) develop. Positive symptoms (e.g., perceptual abnormalities, ideas of reference, suspiciousness) occur late in the prodromal phase and signal the onset of impending psychosis. The onset of the first psychotic episode may be abrupt or insidious, and an average of 1–2 years passes between the first psychotic symptoms and the first adequate treatment in most Western countries. The psychotic phase progresses through an acute phase, a stabilization (or recovery) phase, and a stable phase.

During the acute phase of schizophrenia, patients generally exhibit florid psychotic features such as hallucinations and delusions (positive symptoms), formal thought disorder, and disorganized thinking and usually are unable to care for themselves properly. Negative symptoms also often increase in severity. Treatment during the acute phase of a psychotic exacerbation is aimed at preventing harm, controlling disturbed behavior, reducing the severity of psychosis and associated symptoms (e.g., agitation, aggression, negative symptoms, affective symptoms), determining and addressing the factors that led to the occurrence of the acute psychotic episode, effecting a rapid return to the best level of functioning, developing an alliance with the patient and family, formulating short- and long-term treatment plans, and connecting the patient with appropriate aftercare in the community.

During the stabilization (or recovery) phase, which refers to a period of 6–18 months after acute treatment and is characterized by decreasing severity of acute psychotic symptoms, therapy is aimed at sustaining symptom remission or control, minimizing stress, providing support to reduce the likelihood of relapse, enhancing the patient's adaptation to community life, facilitating the continued reduction in symptoms and consolidation of remission, and promoting the process of recovery.

Once symptoms become relatively stabilized, the disorder enters the stable phase. If symptoms are present during this period, they usually are consistent in magnitude and less severe than during the acute phase. Some patients may experience nonpsychotic symptoms such as tension, anxiety, depression, or insomnia during the stable phase. Treatment during the stable phase is aimed at sustaining symptom remission or control and maintaining or improving the patient's level of functioning and quality of life, while effectively treating symptoms, preventing relapse, and monitoring for and managing adverse effects.

Drug therapy is integral to the management of acute psychotic episodes in patients with schizophrenia and generally is required for long-term stabilization to sustain symptom remission or control and to minimize the risk of relapse. Antipsychotic agents are the principal class of drugs used for the management of all phases of schizophrenia. Adverse effects also are a critical aspect of antipsychotic therapy in the acute, stabilization, and maintenance phases of a psychotic exacerbation and are often a determining factor in choice of therapy, as well as a principal reason for drug discontinuance.

Acute Phase. For acute psychotic episodes in patients with schizophrenia, therapy with antipsychotic agents is indicated for almost all patients and should begin as soon as clinically feasible because exacerbations are associated with emotional distress, disruption to the patient's life, and a substantial risk of dangerous behaviors (i.e., to self, others, property). Delay of therapy may be reasonable in limited circumstances (e.g., for patients who require more extensive or prolonged diagnostic evaluation, who refuse drug therapy, or who may experience rapid recovery because substance use or acute stress reaction are thought to be potential causes of the symptom exacerbation). Before initiation of treatment with an antipsychotic agent, baseline laboratory studies may be indicated. In addition, it is important that clinicians assess the patient's ability to participate in drug therapy decisions and, as feasible, discuss the potential risks and benefits of the drug with the patient.

In patients with an acute psychotic episode who exhibit aggressive behaviors toward self, others, or objects, rapid initiation of emergency treatment is necessary. In such situations, existing therapeutic protocols of the emergency department, inpatient unit, or other acute treatment facility should be consulted. If a patient refuses drug therapy, emergency administration may be considered if allowed by state law. Use of short-acting parenteral formulations of antipsychotic agents (e.g., haloperidol, olanzapine, ziprasidone), with or without a parenteral benzodiazepine (e.g., lorazepam), may be considered in acutely agitated patients. Although patients may exhibit a dramatic calming response to an IM dose of a short-acting antipsychotic formulation, this calming effect on agitation should not be misinterpreted as a true antipsychotic effect, which may take several days or weeks of continued therapy to achieve. Rapidly dissolving (e.g., olanzapine, risperidone) or oral concentrate (e.g., haloperidol, risperidone) formulations of antipsychotic agents also may be used in acutely agitated patients.

In less emergent conditions in which the patient refuses drug therapy, the clinician may have limited options, but enlisting family members and psychotherapeutic interactions may be helpful in gaining patient acceptance of treatment. The use of advance directives to allow competent patients to state treatment preferences in the event of future decompensation or incapacity to make decisions should be encouraged, when available. In some cases, a judicial hearing may be necessary to seek permission to treat a patient who lacks capacity to make such decisions.

Short-term efficacy of antipsychotic drug therapy generally has been established by reductions in positive (e.g., hallucinations, delusions, bizarre behaviors) and negative (e.g., apathy, affective blunting, alogia, avolition) symptoms associated with schizophrenic psychosis over a 6- to 12-week treatment period; less clear is how such symptomatic improvement relates to improvements in patient functioning. Approximately 60% of patients treated with 6 weeks of conventional (first-generation) antipsychotic drug therapy for an acute episode exhibit symptomatic improvement to the point of complete remission or only mildly residual symptomatology, although 40% of patients continue to exhibit moderate to severe psychotic symptoms, including 8% of patients who show no improvement or worsening. A patient's prior history of response to antipsychotic therapy for an acute episode generally is a reliable predictor of response to a subsequent trial.

Long-term efficacy of antipsychotic agents generally has been established in terms of reductions in relapse (i.e., recurrence of acute episodes) or rehospitalization rates over a course of several years. More recently, long-term efficacy also has been measured in terms of quality of life, health services utilization, and social and vocational functioning. In addition, these outcome measures have been used to define level of patient recovery.

The choice of an antipsychotic agent should be individualized, taking into consideration past response to therapy, adverse effect profile (including the patient's experience of subjective effects such as dysphoria), and the patient's preference for a specific drug, including route of administration.

The American Psychiatric Association (APA) considers certain atypical (second-generation) antipsychotic agents (i.e., aripiprazole, olanzapine, quetiapine, risperidone, ziprasidone) first-line drugs for the management of the acute phase of schizophrenia (including first psychotic episodes), principally because of the decreased risk of adverse extrapyramidal effects and tardive dyskinesia, with the understanding that the relative advantages, disadvantages, and cost-effectiveness of conventional and atypical antipsychotic agents remain controversial. The APA states that, with the possible exception of clozapine for the management of treatment-resistant symptoms, there currently is no definitive evidence that one atypical antipsychotic agent will have superior efficacy compared with another agent in the class, although meaningful differences in response may be observed in individual patients. Conventional antipsychotic agents may be considered first-line in patients experiencing acute psychotic episodes who have been treated successfully in the past with, or who prefer, conventional agents.

To compare the long-term effectiveness and tolerability of older, first-generation antipsychotic agents (i.e., perphenazine) with those of newer, atypical antipsychotic agents (i.e., olanzapine, quetiapine, risperidone, ziprasidone), a double-blind, multicenter study (Clinical Antipsychotic Trials of Intervention Effectiveness; CATIE) was sponsored by the National Institute of Mental Health. More than 1400 patients with schizophrenia received one of the drugs for up to 18 months or until therapy was discontinued for any reason. Patients with tardive dyskinesia could enroll in this trial; however, the randomization scheme prevented their assignment to the perphenazine group. The primary outcome measure in this study was the discontinuance of treatment for any cause; this measure was selected because discontinuing or switching an antipsychotic agent occurs frequently and is an important problem in the management of schizophrenia. In addition, this measure integrates the patient's and clinician's judgments concerning efficacy, safety, and tolerability into a more comprehensive measure of effectiveness reflecting therapeutic benefits in relation to adverse effects. Overall, 74% of patients in this study discontinued their medication before receiving the full 18 months of therapy because of inadequate efficacy, intolerable adverse effects, or for other reasons, suggesting substantial limitations in the long-term clinical effectiveness of currently available antipsychotic agents. Olanzapine appeared to be slightly more effective than the other drugs evaluated in this study with a lower (64%) discontinuance rate and a lower rate of hospitalization for exacerbation of schizophrenia, while no significant differences between the effectiveness of the conventional agent, perphenazine, and the other second-generation agents studied were observed (discontinuance rates were 75, 82, 74, and 79% for perphenazine, quetiapine, risperidone, and ziprasidone, respectively). Although there were no significant differences in the time until discontinuance of therapy because of drug intolerance among the drugs studied, the incidences of discontinuance for certain adverse effects differed among the drugs with olanzapine discontinued more frequently because of weight gain or metabolic effects (e.g., increases in glycosylated hemoglobin, cholesterol, and triglycerides) and perphenazine discontinued more frequently because of adverse extrapyramidal effects.

Emerging data from the pivotal CATIE trial suggest that newer, atypical antipsychotics may not provide clinically important advantages over older, first-generation antipsychotics in patients with chronic schizophrenia and that several factors, including adequacy of symptom relief, tolerability of adverse effects, and cost of therapy, may influence a patient's ability and willingness to remain on long-term antipsychotic medication. In addition, these results suggest that it may often be necessary to try 2 or more different antipsychotic agents in an individual patient in order to provide optimal therapeutic benefit with an acceptable adverse effect profile.

Pending further data clarifying the relative effectiveness and tolerability of first- and second-generation antipsychotics in the treatment of schizophrenia, many clinicians recommend that the choice of an antipsychotic agent be carefully individualized taking into consideration the clinical efficacy and adverse effect profile (including the risk for extrapyramidal effects, weight gain, and adverse metabolic effects) of the antipsychotic agent as well as individual patient risk factors; the patient's previous experience of subjective effects such as dysphoria; the patient's preference for and willingness to take (i.e., compliance) a specific drug, including route of administration; and the relative cost of therapy. Clozapine and olanzapine may be reasonable alternatives in any patient with schizophrenia who has not achieved a full clinical remission with other antipsychotic agents; however, the risk of adverse metabolic effects with both drugs necessitates dietary and exercise counseling before therapy is initiated, monitoring during drug therapy, and possible discontinuance of therapy if these effects become troublesome during therapy. Additional analyses from data generated by the CATIE trial addressing other schizophrenia treatment-related issues such as cost-effectiveness of therapy, quality of life, and predictors of response are ongoing.

Some evidence suggests that atypical antipsychotic agents may have superior efficacy in treating cognitive, negative, and mood symptoms as well as global psychopathology, but this is controversial and remains to be fully established. Currently there is no definitive evidence that one atypical antipsychotic agent will have superior efficacy compared with another agent in the class, although clinically meaningful differences in response may be observed in individual patients.

Differences in risk of certain adverse effects are often predictable based on the potencies and receptor binding profiles of the various antipsychotic agents. When first-generation (conventional) antipsychotic agents are used, high-potency (e.g., haloperidol, fluphenazine) rather than conventional low-potency (e.g., chlorpromazine, thioridazine) antipsychotic agents often are selected initially despite their greater tendency to cause extrapyramidal reactions because their adverse effects often are easier to manage than the sedation, lethargy, and orthostatic hypotension associated with low-potency agents, and their dosage generally can be escalated more rapidly if necessary. However, a first-generation (conventional) antipsychotic agent of intermediate potency (e.g., loxapine, perphenazine) may be preferable in some patients, such as those who have difficulty tolerating extrapyramidal reactions (e.g., akathisia) from a high-potency agent and daytime drowsiness, dizziness, dry mouth, and constipation from a low-potency agent.

The route of administration that is preferred also should be considered in the selection of an antipsychotic agent. Although many patients prefer oral therapy, patients with recurrent relapses related to nonadherence or those who prefer injectable formulations are candidates for a long-acting injectable antipsychotic agent (e.g., fluphenazine decanoate, haloperidol decanoate, risperidone). In such patients, an oral formulation of the same antipsychotic agent is a logical choice for initial therapy during the acute phase of schizophrenia. Although the transition from an oral to a long-acting injectable formulation may begin during the acute phase, long-acting injectable agents usually are not initiated for acute psychotic episodes because steady-state plasma drug concentrations are not achieved for several months, and they are eliminated very slowly. However, in some circumstances (e.g., continued therapy with a long-acting injectable agent while temporarily supplementing it with an oral agent during an exacerbation of psychotic symptoms), a long-acting (depot) antipsychotic preparation may be useful during an acute psychotic episode.

When improvement is not observed in patients receiving an antipsychotic agent, nonadherence, rapid drug metabolism, or poor drug absorption should be considered. In patients receiving an antipsychotic agent with adequately described clinical pharmacokinetics (e.g., clozapine, haloperidol), measurement of plasma concentrations of the drug may be useful in determining whether the dosage is insufficient for efficacy or excessive and inducing adverse effects such as akathisia, agitation, or akinesia; whether the pharmacodynamics of the drug are affected by concurrent therapy with other drugs, young or old age, or comorbid condition; or whether adherence with therapy is inadequate. If nonadherence is suspected, behavioral tailoring (i.e., fitting medication administration into the patient's daily routine, psychotherapeutic techniques) may aid in the patient's understanding of the potential benefits of drug therapy. If surreptitious nonadherence (i.e., cheeking) is suspected, use of a liquid (e.g., clozapine, haloperidol, risperidone), rapidly disintegrating tablet (e.g., olanzapine, risperidone), or a short-acting IM formulation (e.g., haloperidol, ziprasidone) may be beneficial. In patients who do not respond to therapy despite adherence and adequate plasma concentrations of the drug, consideration should be given to alternative therapy. Increasing the dosage for a limited period (e.g., 2–4 weeks) can be attempted if tolerated by the patient. Failure of this alternative should lead to consideration of therapy with a different antipsychotic agent.

Adjunctive agents (e.g., benzodiazepines) are commonly added to antipsychotic drug therapy during the acute phase to treat comorbid conditions or associated symptoms (e.g., agitation, aggression, affective symptoms), to address sleep disturbances, or to treat adverse effects associated with antipsychotic agents. For patients with treatment-resistant schizophrenia or with persistent suicidal or aggressive behavior or hostility, a trial of clozapine should be considered, based on evidence of superior efficacy in such patients. Other than clozapine, limited options exist for many patients who have substantial residual symptoms even after optimization of antipsychotic monotherapy. Although efficacy data are limited, various augmentation strategies have been used, including addition of another antipsychotic agent or other psychoactive agents (e.g., anticonvulsants, benzodiazepines, glutamatergic agents, cholinergic agonists). ECT and cognitive behavior therapy techniques also may be useful in patients with treatment-resistant symptoms.

Because thioridazine and mesoridazine (no longer commercially available in the US) have the potential for substantial and possibly life-threatening proarrhythmic effects and can precipitate sudden death, use of these drugs is reserved for patients with schizophrenia whose disease fails to respond adequately to appropriate courses with at least 2 different antipsychotic agents, either because of insufficient efficacy or the inability to achieve an effective dosage due to intolerable adverse effects. (See Cautions: Arrhythmias and Associated Precautions and Contraindications, in Thioridazine 28:16.08.24.)

Stabilization Phase. In patients who have achieved an adequate therapeutic response and minimal adverse effects with a particular regimen, therapy with the same antipsychotic agent at the same dosage should be continued over the next 6 months. Therapy during the stabilization phase is empiric, both in terms of specific agent and dosage, and is based principally on the clinical observation that premature reduction of dosage or discontinuance of therapy may result in relatively rapid relapse. During the stabilization phase, assessment of ongoing adverse effects that may have developed during the acute phase also is essential, and drug therapy should be adjusted as necessary to minimize adverse effects that may lead to nonadherence and relapse.

Stable Phase. The efficacy of antipsychotic therapy in preventing relapse should be considered relative to the severity of adverse effects, and, as feasible, residual symptoms should be addressed in planning the long-term management of stabilized patients. The risk of relapse in patients in the stable phase of schizophrenia is reduced substantially with first-generation (conventional) antipsychotic agents but not eliminated completely (e.g., up to 25–30% may still experience relapse during the first year of therapy). Recent evidence suggests that use of second-generation (atypical) antipsychotics may result in greater efficacy in relapse prevention, although it currently is not known if other factors such as increased treatment adherence or reduced adverse effects contribute to this increase in efficacy.

During the stable phase of a psychotic episode, there currently is no reliable strategy to identify minimum effective antipsychotic dosages for prevention of relapse. However, clinicians should attempt to employ a dosage that minimizes adverse effects while remaining within the effective dosage range of the particular agent. In patients receiving first-generation (conventional) antipsychotic agents, therapy at a lower dosage (e.g., equivalent to 300–600 mg daily of chlorpromazine hydrochloride) may yield such benefits as improvement in adherence, better subjective state, and, possibly, better functioning. Evidence suggests that higher dosages (e.g., equivalent to a mean dosage of 5200 mg daily of chlorpromazine hydrochloride) usually are not more effective and increase the risk of subjectively intolerable adverse effects. However, potential advantages of a lower dosage should be considered relative to the somewhat greater risk of relapse and more frequent exacerbations of schizophrenic symptoms.

Some clinicians suggest that following management of an acute episode and patient stabilization, attempts be made to reduce the antipsychotic dosage by approximately 20% every 6 months until a minimum maintenance dosage is achieved; minimum maintenance dosages as low as 2.5 mg of oral fluphenazine hydrochloride or haloperidol daily, 50 mg of haloperidol decanoate every 4 weeks, or 5 mg of fluphenazine decanoate every 2 weeks have been suggested. Strategies in which dosage of a first-generation (conventional) antipsychotic agent is gradually reduced until completely discontinued during the stable phase, and drug therapy is reinitiated only intermittently to target symptom exacerbations and avert anticipated exacerbations may substantially increase the risk of relapse, and therefore are, not recommended.

Because most patients who develop schizophrenia are at very high risk for relapse in the absence of antipsychotic therapy, prudent long-term treatment options in patients with remitted first or multiple episodes include either indefinite maintenance therapy or gradual discontinuance of the antipsychotic agent with close follow-up and a plan to reinstitute treatment upon symptom recurrence. Discontinuance of antipsychotic therapy should be considered only after a period of at least 1 year of symptom remission or optimal response while receiving the antipsychotic agent. However, evidence suggests that continued drug therapy is associated with fewer relapses than targeted intermittent therapy and that intermittent treatment strategies may increase rather than decrease the risk of tardive dyskinesia. If antipsychotic therapy is to be discontinued, additional precautions should include slow, gradual dose reduction (e.g., 10% per month) over many months, more frequent visits, and use of early intervention strategies. Patients and their family and caregivers should be advised about early signs of relapse, and clinicians should collaborate with them to develop plans for action should such signs emerge.

In patients who have had multiple previous psychotic episodes or 2 psychotic episodes within 5 years, indefinite maintenance antipsychotic treatment is recommended, along with continued monitoring for manifestations of impending or actual relapse because risk of relapse in chronic schizophrenia, even in patients adherent to drug therapy, is approximately 30% per year. The treatment program should be designed to respond quickly to evidence of prodromal symptoms or behaviors or exacerbations of schizophrenic symptoms. Early use of supportive therapeutic techniques and a higher drug dose as indicated can be useful in reducing the likelihood of relapse and hospitalization. During prodromal episodes, more frequent treatment, monitoring, and support should be undertaken, and assertive outreach, including home visits, should be used when indicated.

In patients with schizophrenic disorder who have associated depression, phenothiazines may be given concomitantly with a tricyclic antidepressant (e.g., amitriptyline). A combination of a phenothiazine with a tricyclic antidepressant also may be used for the management of moderate to severe anxiety and depression associated with psychotic disorders, psychoneurosis, or chronic physical illness. Phenothiazines also have been used in combination with a monoamine oxidase (MAO) inhibitor in patients with depression accompanied by anxiety, agitation, or panic. Because of potentiation and a lowered margin of safety, combinations of psychotherapeutic agents should be used with caution and only in patients with severe disorders. When combination therapy is required, the commercially available preparations containing a phenothiazine in combination with an antidepressant should not be used to initiate therapy. Dosage should initially be adjusted by administering each drug separately. If it is determined that the optimum maintenance dosage corresponds to the ratio present in a commercially available combination, such a preparation may be used; however, when dosage adjustment is necessary, the drugs should be administered separately.

Pediatric Considerations. Schizophrenia in children and adolescents is classified according to the age at onset of symptoms. Schizophrenia developing in children prior to 13 years of age is referred to as very-early-onset schizophrenia or childhood-onset schizophrenia. Schizophrenia that develops in pediatric patients 13–18 years of age is referred to as early-onset schizophrenia. Very-early-onset schizophrenia is a poorly understood neurodevelopmental disorder, but data collected thus far from clinical studies, case reports, and clinical experience suggest that the pattern of response to antipsychotic agents in children and adolescents with schizophrenia is similar to that in adults. Because there are few published clinical studies in children and adolescents with schizophrenia, therapeutic recommendations for the management of schizophrenia mainly are based on extrapolation of demonstrated efficacy in adults and the likelihood that the disease course, pathophysiology, and drug activity are substantially similar between the 2 populations. The American Academy of Child and Adolescent Psychiatry (AACAP) states that many of the therapeutic recommendations for adult-onset schizophrenia are applicable for the treatment of children and adolescents with schizophrenia provided that developmental issues are addressed. The goal of therapy in early-onset or very-early-onset schizophrenia is to return the child to their premorbid level of functioning while also promoting the mastery of age-appropriate developmental tasks. Adequate treatment therefore requires a combination of drug therapy and psychosocial interventions, which may vary depending on the phase of illness.

As with treatment of adult-onset schizophrenia, antipsychotic agents are the principal class of drugs used for the management of all phases of schizophrenia in pediatric patients. Most clinical studies in children and adolescents with schizophrenia involved first-generation (conventional) antipsychotic agents (e.g., haloperidol, loxapine, thioridazine, thiothixene), and these agents are considered a reasonable choice for initial therapy. However, because of greater sensitivity of children to the sedative effects of low-potency antipsychotic agents (e.g., thioridazine), it has been suggested that high-potency antipsychotic agents (e.g., thiothixene), which are associated with less frequent sedation, may be preferred as initial therapy in some pediatric patients with schizophrenia. Second-generation (atypical) antipsychotic agents (e.g., olanzapine, risperidone) also may be appropriate for initial therapy in certain children and adolescents, but the role of these agents relative to conventional agents remains to be established, particularly regarding long-term safety and efficacy. Similar to treatment of schizophrenia in adults, the choice of an antipsychotic agent in children and adolescents with schizophrenia should be individualized, based on the agent's relative potency, potential adverse effects, and the patient's past response to therapy. Although the AACAP considers all antipsychotic agents (except clozapine) to have comparable antipsychotic effects, many clinicians consider atypical antipsychotic agents, with the exception of clozapine, the drugs of choice for the management of schizophrenia because such agents have been associated with a lower risk for extrapyramidal symptoms than conventional antipsychotic agents.

Because treatment resistance in adults with schizophrenia is associated with an earlier age of onset, children and adolescents who develop the disorder before age 18 may be less likely to respond adequately to either conventional or atypical antipsychotic agents than adults with the disorder. Clozapine currently is the only antipsychotic agent with clearly demonstrated efficacy in the management of treatment-refractory schizophrenia in adults. Results of one limited, double-blind, randomized clinical study indicate that clozapine (mean final dosage: 176 mg daily) is superior to haloperidol (mean final dosage: 16 mg daily) in reducing both positive and negative symptoms of schizophrenia in children and adolescents with very-early-onset treatment-resistant schizophrenia. As reported in adults, however, maximal antipsychotic effects in schizophrenic children and adolescents may not be evident until after 6–9 months of clozapine therapy. Clozapine is not considered a first-line agent because of its substantial potential for adverse effects and is recommended only in patients who have failed to respond to adequate therapeutic trials (i.e., use of sufficient dosages over a period of 4–6 weeks) of at least 2 other antipsychotic agents (at least one of which is an atypical antipsychotic) and/or have experienced substantial adverse effects (e.g., tardive dyskinesia) while receiving other antipsychotic agents. (See Uses: Psychotic Disorders, in Clozapine 28:16.08.04.)

Use of long-acting (depot) preparations also should be limited in children and adolescents with schizophrenia because these agents have not been adequately studied in this population and because of the risks of adverse effects associated with long-term exposure to these drugs. The AACAP currently does not recommend use of depot preparations in children with very-early-onset schizophrenia (i.e., development of the disorder before 13 years of age) and states that these preparations should only be considered in schizophrenic adolescents with documented chronic psychotic symptoms and a history of poor medication compliance.

Geriatric Considerations. In geriatric patients with schizophrenia, the approach to treatment is similar to that in younger adults, although age-related physiologic changes (e.g., reduced cardiac output, reduced glomerular filtration rate, possible reduction in hepatic metabolism, increased adipose content, receptor-site activity alterations, sensory deficits, cognitive impairment) may influence selection and dosage of an antipsychotic agent. Important considerations in selection of an antipsychotic agent in geriatric patients include the adverse effect profile, potential adverse interactions with the patient's current drug therapy or effects on concurrent physical illness, and the patient's previous response to the antipsychotic agent. The APA currently recommends second-generation (atypical) antipsychotic agents as first-line therapy in geriatric patients because of their substantially lower risk of extrapyramidal symptoms and tardive dyskinesia compared with first-generation (conventional) antipsychotic agents. However, geriatric patients, particularly those with reduced cardiac output, also may be more sensitive to some adverse effects associated with atypical agents (e.g., sedation, orthostatic hypotension, cardiac arrhythmia). The anticholinergic effects of antipsychotic agents also are a concern in geriatric patients because age-related decreases in cholinergic function may contribute to adverse effects such as urinary retention, confusion, and constipation or fecal impaction. Although weight gain associated with some antipsychotic agents may be beneficial in frail or malnourished geriatric patients, cardiovascular disease or osteoarthritis may be aggravated in patients with preexisting conditions. In addition, increased prolactin concentrations associated with antipsychotic agents may compromise bone-mineral density and increase osteoporosis in geriatric patients. (See Cautions: Precautions and Contraindications.)

Depression is common and may be functionally disruptive in geriatric patients with schizophrenia. In such patients, a variety of antidepressant agents have been added to the treatment regimen.

Psychotic symptoms, including delusions and hallucinations, and behavioral disturbances, including agitation and aggression, are common in patients with dementia (e.g., dementia of the Alzheimer's type). Antipsychotic agents are the only drugs currently available for the management of psychotic manifestations of dementia, and they are the most commonly used and best-studied drugs for the management of agitation in demented patients. However, the APA currently recommends that nonpharmacologic interventions be attempted before a trial of antipsychotic drug therapy and that the interventions attempted be guided by the patient's level of distress and the risk to the patient and caregiver. Antipsychotic drug therapy generally is reserved for patients who are distressed or when associated agitation, combativeness, or violent behavior places the patient or others in danger. Therapy for the management of psychosis and agitation associated with dementia should be reevaluated periodically to justify its continued use. There currently are limited data establishing efficacy of antipsychotic drug therapy for psychosis and agitation in demented patients beyond 8 weeks of follow-up, although clinical experience suggests that benefit extends for longer periods of treatment. The fact that psychosis and agitation may wax and wane or change in character as the dementing illness evolves should be considered and may prompt a modification or discontinuance of antipsychotic drug therapy.

The goal of therapy for the management of psychosis and agitation in patients with dementia is to decrease psychotic manifestations (e.g., paranoia, delusions, hallucinations) and associated or independent agitation, screaming, combativeness, and/or violence and thereby increase the comfort and safety of patients and their families and caregivers. Antipsychotic agents have been studied extensively for the management of psychosis and agitation in patients with dementia and current evidence indicates that the drugs can provide modest improvement in behavioral manifestations; some evidence suggests that antipsychotic efficacy may be better for psychosis than for other manifestations. The Clinical Antipsychotic Trials of Intervention Effectiveness—Alzheimer's Disease (CATIE-AD) effectiveness trial, which evaluated several atypical antipsychotics (olanzapine, quetiapine, and risperidone) in patients with Alzheimer's disease and psychosis or agitated behavior, found that these drugs were more effective for certain dementia-associated symptoms, including anger, aggression, and paranoid ideation, although their adverse effects may limit their clinical utility. Dropout rates in efficacy studies of antipsychotic agents have generally been high, both because of intolerable adverse effects and poor response. Antipsychotic efficacy appears to be similar among available agents and therefore the choice of agent should be based on adverse effect profile and other patient considerations; to minimize adverse effects, the lowest possible effective dosage should be used.

The US Food and Drug Administration (FDA) warns that geriatric patients with dementia-associated psychosis treated with conventional (first-generation) or atypical (second-generation) antipsychotic agents are at an increased risk of death. Analyses of 17 placebo-controlled trials (average duration of 10 weeks) revealed an approximate 1.6- to 1.7-fold increase in mortality among geriatric patients receiving atypical antipsychotic agents (i.e., aripiprazole, olanzapine, quetiapine, risperidone) compared with that in patients receiving placebo. Although the causes of death were varied, most of the deaths appeared to be either cardiovascular (e.g., heart failure, sudden death) or infectious (e.g., pneumonia) in nature. Because an increase in mortality was observed with atypical antipsychotics in all 3 chemical classes, this effect is considered to be related to the common pharmacologic effects of all atypical antipsychotic agents, including those that have not been specifically studied in patients with dementia. Subsequently, two observational, epidemiological studies have indicated that, similar to atypical antipsychotic agents, treatment with conventional antipsychotic agents in geriatric patients may increase mortality; the causes of death were not reported in the first study and cancer and cardiac disease were the causes of death with the highest relative risk in the second study. However, the extent to which these findings of increased mortality in observational studies may be attributed to the antipsychotic agent as opposed to certain patient characteristics remains unclear. FDA currently advises clinicians that antipsychotic agents are *not* approved for the treatment of dementia-related psychosis. The FDA further advises clinicians that no drugs currently are approved for the treatment of patients with dementia-associated psychosis and that other management options should be considered in such patients. The decision whether to prescribe antipsychotic agents "off-label" in the treatment of dementia symptoms is left to the discretion of the clinician. For additional information on the use of antipsychotic agents for dementia-associated psychosis and other behavioral disturbances, see Geriatric Precautions under Cautions.

For further information on the use of atypical antipsychotic agents in patients with dementia-associated psychosis, see the individual monographs in 28:16.08.04.

■ Delirium

Antipsychotic agents, including phenothiazines, are used in the management of delirium. Delirium is principally a disturbance of consciousness, attention, cognition, and perception but also may affect sleep, psychomotor activity, and emotions. It is a common psychiatric illness among medically compromised patients, particularly hospitalized patients, and may be a harbinger of substantial morbidity and mortality. The prevalence of delirium in hospitalized medically ill patients ranges from 10–30%; in those who are elderly, delirium ranges up to 40%. Up to 25% of hospitalized cancer patients and 30–40% of hospitalized patients with acquired immunodeficiency syndrome (AIDS) develop delirium. Up to about 50% of postoperative patients develop delirium, and up to 80% of terminally ill patients develop it near death. Prodromal manifestations may progress to full-blown delirium over 1–3 days; the duration of delirium generally ranges from less than a week to more than 2 months, but typically does not exceed 10–12 days. Symptoms persist for up to 30 days or longer in up to 15% of patients, and frequently persist for longer than 1 month in geriatric patients. Although most patients recover fully, delirium may progress to stupor, coma, seizures, and death, particularly if untreated. Full recovery is less likely in geriatric patients and patients with AIDS, possibly because of underlying dementia in both populations.

Underlying general medical conditions associated with delirium include CNS disorders (e.g., head trauma, seizures, postictal state, vascular or degenerative disease), metabolic disorders (e.g., renal or hepatic failure, anemia, hypoxia, hypoglycemia, thiamine deficiency, endocrinopathy, fluid or electrolyte imbalance, acid-base imbalance), cardiopulmonary disorder (myocardial infarction, congestive heart failure, cardiac arrhythmia, shock, respiratory failure), and systemic illness (e.g., substance intoxication or withdrawal, infection, cancer, severe trauma, sensory deprivation, temperature dysregulation, postoperative state). EEG abnormalities, mainly generalized slowing, have fairly good sensitivity for aiding in the diagnosis of delirium, but the absence of such changes does not rule out the diagnosis.

Clinicians should undertake an essential array of psychiatric management tasks designed to provide immediate interventions for urgent general medical conditions, identify and treat the etiology of delirium, ensure safety of the patient and others in contact with the patient, and improve the patient's functioning. Environmental (e.g., varying light levels in intensive care units to heighten awareness about time of day and reduce the perception of timelessness) and supportive interventions (e.g., to deal with disorientation, to assure the patient that manifestations are temporary and reversible and do not reflect a persistent psychiatric disorder) also generally are offered to patients with delirium and are designed to reduce factors that may exacerbate delirium, to reorient patients, and to provide support. Patients may have life-threatening medical conditions that require therapeutic intervention even before a specific or definitive cause of the delirium is determined. The goal of diagnosis is to identify potentially reversible causes of delirium and prevent complications through prompt treatment of these specific disorders. Psychiatric management is essential and should be undertaken for all patients with delirium. Somatic interventions principally consist of drug therapy. The choice of somatic intervention will depend on the specific features of the patient's clinical condition, the underlying etiology of the delirium, and any associated comorbid conditions.

Antipsychotic agents often are the drugs of choice for the management of delirium. Although phenothiazines have been used, haloperidol (a butyrophenone) generally is considered the antipsychotic of choice for most patients with delirium because of its relatively low risk of anticholinergic activity and of sedative and hypotensive effects. In addition, haloperidol has been studied most extensively, although few studies have used standardized definitions of delirium or reliable and valid delirium symptom rating measures to assess symptom severity before and after initiation of treatment. For drugs other than haloperidol, there have been no large, prospective studies that included a control. Evidence of efficacy for such alternative therapies, including for relatively new second-generation (atypical) antipsychotic agents (e.g., olanzapine, quetiapine, risperidone), is principally from small case series or case reports. In addition, interpretation of findings from many such case presentations is difficult because of use of nonstandardized delirium definitions and/or informal measures of delirium symptom severity. In general, evidence of the efficacy of antipsychotics, including haloperidol, in the management of delirium comes from numerous case reports and uncontrolled studies. However, evidence from a randomized, double-blind, comparator-drug controlled study (chlorpromazine, haloperidol, and lorazepam) in patients with AIDS that employed standardized clinical measures of delirium demonstrated clinical superiority of antipsychotic agents compared with benzodiazepines. Statistically significant improvement in the Delirium Rating Scale was evident after 2 days in patients receiving chlorpromazine or haloperidol but not in the lorazepam group (mean decreases in the score [i.e., improvement] were 8.5, 8, and 1, respectively). The symptomatic improvement in delirium occurred quickly among patients receiving antipsychotic therapy, usually before initiation of interventions directed at the medical etiologies of delirium.

Although various antipsychotic agents may be given orally, IM, or IV, IV administration is considered most effective in emergency situations or where oral access is limited. In addition, some evidence indicates that IV administration of antipsychotic agents may be associated with less severe extrapyramidal effects.

Because antipsychotic agents used in the management of delirium have been associated with lengthening of the QT interval, possibly leading to atypical ventricular tachycardia (torsades de pointes), ventricular fibrillation, and sudden death, baseline and periodic ECGs should be performed with special attention paid to the length of the QT_c interval. Prolongation of the QT_c interval to greater than 450 msec or to greater than 25% over that in previous ECGs may warrant telemetry, a cardiology consultation, and dose reduction or discontinuance. Serum concentrations of magnesium and potassium also should be monitored in critically ill patients, especially those with baseline QT_c intervals of 440 msec or longer, those receiving other drugs known to increase the QT interval, and those who have electrolyte disorders.

■ Other Psychoneurologic Disorders

Phenothiazines have been used for the management of the manic phase of bipolar disorder. Because antipsychotic agents (e.g., chlorpromazine) appear to be more effective than lithium in initially controlling the increased psychomotor activity of mania, many clinicians initiate treatment of acute mania with lithium and an antipsychotic agent. Once psychomotor activity has been controlled (usually within 3–7 days), the antipsychotic agent usually is tapered and lithium is continued to more specifically control disturbances of mood and ideation. Phenothiazines also have been used for the management of involutional, toxic, and senile psychoses.

Phenothiazines are used for the treatment of severe behavioral problems in children marked by combativeness and/or explosive hyperexcitable behavior (out of proportion to immediate provocations), and for the short-term treatment of hyperactive children who exhibit excessive motor activity with accompanying conduct disorders that are manifested as impulsivity, difficulty sustaining attention, aggression, mood lability, and/or poor frustration tolerance. However, the possible risks of tardive dyskinesia, withdrawal dyskinesia, and other extrapyramidal reactions associated with the drugs should be considered. Some clinicians recommend routine administration of the Abnormal Involuntary Movement Scale (AIMS) to all children receiving antipsychotic agents for this indication. In general, phenothiazines have not been shown to be effective for the management of behavioral complications in patients with mental retardation.

Some phenothiazines may be effective in controlling anxiety, tension, and agitation that occur in neuroses; however, the drugs may increase the severity of depression and do not appear to be effective in the treatment of patients with hysteria or obsessive-compulsive reactions. Further studies are needed to establish the efficacy of phenothiazines for their use in neuroses.

Phenothiazines have been used in the adjunctive treatment of alcohol dependence to reduce anxiety, tension, depression, and nausea and vomiting. Although phenothiazines have been used in the management of acute agitation associated with alcohol withdrawal, their efficacy has been equivocal; in addition, the safety of these drugs has been questioned in patients with alcoholic liver disease.

■ **Emesis** Phenothiazines are used for the prevention and control of severe nausea and vomiting of various etiologies. The drugs are effective in the management of postoperative nausea and vomiting, and that caused by toxins, radiation, various drugs including cytotoxic agents, or disease (e.g., uremia, cancer, protracted migraine). In general, phenothiazines are not effective in preventing vertigo or motion sickness, or for the management of emesis caused by the action of drugs on the nodose ganglion or locally on the GI tract. Safe use of phenothiazines for the prevention and treatment of nausea and vomiting of pregnancy has not been established, and the manufacturers recommend that the drugs be used during pregnancy only when the potential benefits justify the possible risks to the fetus; some phenothiazines are contraindicated during pregnancy. (See Pregnancy, Fertility, and Lactation: Pregnancy, in Cautions.)

■ **Other Uses** Some phenothiazines (e.g., chlorpromazine) are used for the treatment of intractable hiccups, acute intermittent porphyria, and as an adjunct in the treatment of tetanus.

Phenothiazines are also used to produce tranquilization and to reduce the incidence of nausea and vomiting in obstetrics and, in anesthesia and surgery, to reduce preoperative tension and anxiety, to permit smoother induction of anesthesia, to potentiate anesthetic agents (possibly lessening the danger of respiratory depression), and to reduce postoperative vomiting.

Some phenothiazines exert an antipruritic effect, especially in neurodermatitis and pruriginous eczema, and they may relieve psychogenic itching.

Dosage and Administration

■ **Administration** Phenothiazines may be administered orally, rectally, or by IM or IV injections; solutions of most phenothiazines are too irritating for subcutaneous injection. Phenothiazines should not be administered intra-arterially. IV administration of dilute solutions of phenothiazines may be accomplished by either fractional injection or slow infusion. IM injection should be made very slowly, deep into the upper outer quadrant of the gluteus maximus. IM injection of phenothiazines in geriatric patients who are thin or debilitated with reduced muscle mass should be avoided if possible because such injections may be painful, and absorption from the injection site may be erratic and unpredictable. Dilution of the commercially available injections with 0.9% sodium chloride injection or a local anesthetic such as 2% procaine hydrochloride injection and massaging the site of injection may help to reduce pain following IM administration. Because of the possibility of hypotension, patients should be in a supine position at the time of parenteral administration of a phenothiazine and should remain so for at least 30–60 minutes following completion of the injection or infusion.

■ **Dosage** There is a wide range of individual requirements for phenothiazine dosage, and dosage must be carefully adjusted according to individual requirements and response, using the lowest possible effective dosage. The initial dosage may be increased gradually according to the patient's tolerance and therapeutic response; dosage should be increased more gradually in debilitated, emaciated, or geriatric patients. After symptoms are controlled, dosage may be reduced gradually to a maintenance level. Weeks or months of treatment at optimum dosage levels may be necessary to produce maximum clinical improvement in patients with resistant mental and emotional disturbances. Relapses are less frequent when chronically ill patients are kept on a prolonged maintenance dosage. However, because of the risk of adverse reactions associated with cumulative effects of phenothiazines, patients with a history of long-term therapy with phenothiazines and/or other antipsychotic agents should be evaluated periodically to determine whether maintenance dosage could be decreased or drug therapy discontinued. Dosage should not be terminated abruptly in those patients receiving high dosage for prolonged periods of time. (See Other Nervous System Effects in Cautions: Nervous System Effects.)

Acute Psychotic Episodes Determination of the optimal dosage of an antipsychotic agent during an acute psychotic episode is complex because there usually is a delay between therapy initiation and full therapeutic response. An initial response to treatment may be apparent in 2–4 weeks, while a full or optimal response may take up to 6 months or longer. Generally, the optimal dosage of an antipsychotic agent is that which produces maximal therapeutic benefit and minimal adverse effects.

In recent years, studies have consistently found that modest doses of first-generation (conventional) antipsychotic agents (e.g., haloperidol dosages less than 10 mg daily or plasma haloperidol concentrations less than 18 ng/mL) are as effective or more effective than higher dosages; moderate dosages have been reported to improve comorbid depression, while higher dosages are associated with greater risk of extrapyramidal effects and dysphoria. For most patients receiving first-generation (conventional) antipsychotic agents, the optimal dosage occurs at the "EPS threshold," which is the dosage that will induce extrapyramidal effects but where minimal rigidity is observed upon physical examination of the patient. Atypical antipsychotic agents generally can be administered at dosages that are therapeutic but well below the EPS threshold.

Dosage should be titrated as quickly as tolerated to the target dosage, and unless uncomfortable adverse effects become evident, patients should be monitored for 2–4 weeks before further increasing dosage or changing to another antipsychotic agent. Rapid dosage escalation beyond the target dosage should be avoided because it may create a false impression of increased efficacy, and higher dosages may actually be detrimental.

Cautions

Adverse effects of phenothiazines are numerous and may involve almost all organ systems. Some adverse effects may be attributed to the actions of the drugs on the central and autonomic nervous systems, whereas others are hypersensitivity reactions. Although all adverse reactions have not been reported with each individual phenothiazine, the possibility that they may occur should be considered. Some adverse reactions may occur more frequently and/or with greater intensity in patients with certain medical conditions (e.g., severe hypotension in patients with pheochromocytoma or mitral insufficiency).

■ **Nervous System Effects** ***Extrapyramidal Reactions*** Extrapyramidal reactions may occur in patients receiving phenothiazines and are apparently mediated via blockade of central dopaminergic receptors involved in motor function. More than 60% of patients receiving acute therapy with phenothiazines or other antipsychotic drugs develop clinically important extrapyramidal reactions in one form or another; some patients may develop more than one form at the same time.

Extrapyramidal reactions can be divided into acute and chronic reactions. Acute extrapyramidal reactions are signs and symptoms that develop during the first days and weeks of phenothiazine or other antipsychotic agent administration, are dose related, and are reversible upon dosage reduction or discontinuance of the drug. However, severe extrapyramidal reactions have reportedly occurred even at relatively low dosages. Chronic extrapyramidal reactions are signs and symptoms that occur following months or years of therapy with phenothiazines or other antipsychotic drugs, are not clearly dose related, and may persist following drug discontinuance.

Acute extrapyramidal reactions produced by phenothiazines are classified into 3 major categories: dystonic reactions, feelings of motor restlessness (i.e., akathisia), and parkinsonian signs and symptoms. Chronic extrapyramidal reactions include tardive dyskinesia and tardive dystonia.

Dystonic reactions and feelings of motor restlessness occur most frequently in young patients, especially those with acute infections or severe dehydration, whereas parkinsonian signs and symptoms predominate in geriatric patients, especially those with brain damage. Dystonic reactions usually occur rather early during treatment, but the incidence of feelings of motor restlessness and parkinsonian signs and symptoms is greater after several weeks of therapy. Phenothiazines that are most effective as antiemetics and those that are the most potent on a weight basis have been associated with the greatest incidence of extrapyramidal reactions. In general, propylamino derivatives of phenothiazine are most likely to induce parkinsonian signs and symptoms, whereas propylpiperazine derivatives are most likely to cause dystonic reactions.

Dystonic reactions usually are sudden in onset, are dramatic in appearance, and may cause great distress to the patient but generally respond dramatically to treatment. The reactions are characterized by spastic contraction of discrete muscle groups and may include spasm of the neck muscles, sometimes progressing to acute, reversible torticollis; extensor rigidity of back muscles, sometimes progressing to opisthotonos; carpopedal spasm; trismus; mandibular tics; alteration of temporomandibular joint function; difficulty swallowing or talking; perioral spasms often with protrusion of the tongue; and oculogyric crisis. Dystonic reactions may be accompanied by profuse sweating, pallor, and fever. Risk factors include young age, male gender, use of high-potency agents, high doses, and IM administration. In most patients, acute dystonic reactions occur within 24–72 hours following initiation of therapy or an increase in dosage. Dystonic reactions usually subside within a few hours, and almost always within 24–48 hours following discontinuance of the drug. Most patients respond rapidly to treatment with an anticholinergic antiparkinsonian agent (e.g., benztropine, trihexyphenidyl) or with diphenhydramine. Short-term maintenance treatment with an oral anticholinergic antiparkinsonian agent may be used to prevent recurrence of acute dystonic reactions. If the dystonic symptoms are not controlled following administration of an antiparkinsonian agent or diphenhydramine, the etiology of the adverse neurologic effects should be reevaluated. In some patients, dystonic reactions (e.g., laryngospasm) can be dangerous and even life-threatening. Therefore, appropriate supportive therapy such as maintaining an adequate airway and hydration should be instituted, if necessary. If phenothiazine therapy is reinstituted, it should be at a reduced dosage; however, if dystonic reactions occur in children or pregnant women, the drug should not be reinstituted.

Feelings of motor restlessness (akathisia) consist of agitation, jitteriness, inability to sit still, tapping of feet, strong urge to move around (not associated with anxiety), and sometimes insomnia; akathisia also may sometimes include a psychic component that is similar to the patient's original neurotic or psychotic symptoms. Patients with akathisia typically complain of an inner sensation of restlessness and an irresistible urge to move various parts of their body. Akathisia often is extremely distressing to patients, is a frequent cause of noncompliance with therapy, and, if allowed to persist, can produce dysphoria and possibly even contribute to aggressive or suicidal behavior. Akathisia is manifest subjectively and objectively in up to 30% of patients receiving conventional antipsychotic agents. Akathisia appears to occur less commonly with low-potency first-generation (conventional) antipsychotic agents and even less frequently with atypical antipsychotic agents than with other first-generation antipsychotic agents; however, precise estimates of akathisia incidence with individual agents currently are not available.

In most cases, akathisia occurs within 2–3 days of therapy, although it can occur later (i.e., after several weeks). Diagnosis of phenothiazine-induced akathisia may be difficult since signs and symptoms may resemble dyskinesias, Huntington's chorea, or exacerbation of the patient's underlying condition. Signs and symptoms of akathisia may subside spontaneously; however, if they become troublesome, interventions include dosage reduction or switching to an atypical antipsychotic agent with less risk of akathisia. Concomitant administration of low-dose propranolol or a benzodiazepine is effective in decreasing symptoms of akathisia, but anticholinergic antiparkinsonian agents have limited efficacy.

Parkinsonian Manifestations. Phenothiazine-induced parkinsonian signs and symptoms include masklike facies, drooling or hypersalivation, tremors, pill-rolling motion of the fingers, cogwheel rigidity, postural abnormalities, shuffling gait, slow monotonous speech, and dysphagia. Akinesia or bradykinesia may also occur. Symptoms of phenothiazine-induced parkinsonism, particularly the cognitive and emotional features, should be carefully distinguished from the negative symptoms of schizophrenia. The first approach to treatment of parkinsonian signs and symptoms should be reduction in the phenothiazine dosage. If symptoms are not sufficiently improved after reduction in phenothiazine dosage, a switch to an atypical antipsychotic agent should be considered. Although anticholinergic antiparkinsonian agents or dopamine agonists (e.g., amantadine) often reduce the severity of parkinsonian symptoms, anticholinergic agents can cause anticholinergic adverse effects and dopamine agonists may exacerbate psychosis; thus, chronic use and excessive dosages of such agents should be minimized or avoided. In most patients, concomitant administration of an antiparkinsonian agent for a few weeks to 2 or 3 months is adequate.

Because of the high risk of acute extrapyramidal reactions in patients receiving phenothiazines and other antipsychotic drugs, the prophylactic use of anticholinergic antiparkinsonian agents may be considered. Although such prophylaxis has been shown to reduce the incidence of acute extrapyramidal adverse effects, routine prophylaxis with antiparkinsonian agents in *all* patients generally is not recommended because it may be clinically unnecessary and associated with bothersome adverse effects. However, minimizing uncomfortable, painful, and unnecessary adverse effects can contribute substantially to establishing a therapeutic alliance between the clinician and the patient. Some authorities recommend that prophylaxis be considered for patients with a previous history of acute extrapyramidal reactions and those receiving antipsychotic agents known to induce these effects (e.g., first-generation [conventional] antipsychotics, high-dose risperidone). In addition, young patients experiencing their first episode of schizophrenia also may be considered for prophylaxis with an anticholinergic antiparkinsonian agent since they are more likely to experience dystonic reactions. The continued need for prophylaxis should be reevaluated after the acute phase of treatment is complete and whenever the dosage of the antipsychotic agent is changed. If antipsychotic dosage is lowered, anticholinergic prophylaxis may no longer be necessary or may be given in a lower dosage. Patients who are very sensitive to adverse anticholinergic effects (e.g., dry mouth, blurred vision, constipation) may require lower dosages of the antiparkinsonian agent or a less potent drug (e.g., trihexyphenidyl, procyclidine hydrochloride).

Tardive Dyskinesia. Like other first-generation (conventional) antipsychotic agents, phenothiazines have been associated with persistent dyskinesias. The risk of tardive dyskinesia appears to be substantially less with second-generation (atypical) antipsychotics than with first-generation agents. Tardive dyskinesia may occur in some patients during long-term administration of the drugs or it may occur following discontinuance of the drugs. The risk of developing tardive dyskinesia appears to be greater in geriatric patients receiving high dosages of the drugs, especially females. Other possible risk factors include schizophrenia, presence of antipsychotic-induced parkinsonian symptoms, concurrent affective disorder, and concurrent medical conditions (such as diabetes mellitus). The symptoms are persistent and in some patients appear to be irreversible. Tardive dyskinesia is characterized by rhythmic involuntary movements of the tongue, face, mouth, or jaw (e.g., protrusion of the tongue, puffing of cheeks, chewing movements, puckering of the mouth), which sometimes may be accompanied by involuntary movements of the extremities. Although the majority of patients who develop tardive dyskinesia have mild symptoms, approximately 10% develop symptoms that are moderate to severe. Tardive dystonia, an often severe variant of tardive dyskinesia, is characterized by spastic muscle contractions and associated with severe distress and physical discomfort. Although not clearly established, the risk of developing tardive dyskinesia and the likelihood that it will become irreversible appear to increase with the duration of therapy and cumulative dose of antipsychotic agent(s) administered; however, the syndrome may occur, although much less frequently, after relatively short periods of treatment with low dosages. In addition, although continued therapy may increase the risk of persistence of tardive dyskinesia symptoms, the severity of tardive dyskinesia does not appear to increase over time in many patients receiving constant, moderate dosages. In clinical studies, intermittent, targeted treatment with a first-generation (conventional) antipsychotic agent was associated with an increased risk of tardive dyskinesia compared with that observed with maintenance antipsychotic treatment.

Some clinicians recommend that patients receiving antipsychotic agents for prolonged periods (for more than 4 weeks) be evaluated every 3 months or more often, depending on the frequency of visits, for signs or symptoms of tardive dyskinesia. If such signs or symptoms are present, clinicians should carefully evaluate the patient to rule out potential idiopathic causes of tardive dyskinesia. This evaluation should include a standard neurologic evaluation, a review of the patient's family medical history for neurologic disease (e.g., Huntington's disease), and appropriate laboratory tests. Once idiopathic causes of tardive dyskinesia have been ruled out, the patient may be considered to have tardive dyskinesia, and treatment options should be considered. Discontinuance of the phenothiazine should be considered only if the patient is in full remission or very stable with few residual positive symptoms or if the patient insists on discontinuing medication. Clinicians should consider the possibility that tardive dyskinesia may be masked if therapy is reinstituted, dosage is increased, or therapy with another antipsychotic agent is initiated. The effect that masking of the symptoms may have on the long-term course of the syndrome is unknown. Fine vermicular movement of the tongue may be an early sign of tardive dyskinesia; prompt evaluation and treatment if this sign occurs may help to prevent further development of the syndrome.

Management of tardive dyskinesia generally consists of gradual discontinuance of the precipitating antipsychotic agent when possible, reducing the dosage of the first-generation (conventional) antipsychotic agent or switching to a second-generation (atypical) antipsychotic agent, or switching to clozapine therapy. For example, the dosage of the phenothiazine could be reduced gradually (i.e., over 12 weeks) by 50%; frequently, this will produce a decrease or remission in the tardive dyskinesia. However, a temporary increase in symptoms upon withdrawal or dosage reduction also may occur in some patients. If withdrawal or dosage reduction does not produce substantial improvement in the tardive dyskinesia symptoms within 6–12 months, then the severity and degree of distress the symptoms cause the patient should be evaluated. If the symptoms are mild or do not cause the patient distress, then no further measures may be clinically necessary. However, treatment for tardive dyskinesia should be considered if the symptoms are severe or distressing to the patient.

Vesicular monoamine transporter 2 (VMAT2) inhibitors, including deutetrabenazine, tetrabenazine†, and valbenazine tosylate, have been shown to be effective in reducing symptoms of tardive dyskinesia in controlled clinical studies. Deutetrabenazine and valbenazine tosylate currently are indicated in the treatment of tardive dyskinesia. (See Deutetrabenazine 28:56 and Valbenazine Tosylate 28:56.) Although tetrabenazine, which is labeled for the treatment of chorea associated with Huntington's disease, had been considered a drug of choice by some clinicians for the management of moderate to severe tardive dyskinesia, the drug's short elimination half-life and dose-related adverse effect profile have limited the clinical use of the drug for tardive dyskinesia.

Although long-term prospective incidence studies are lacking, clozapine generally has been shown to improve the severity of dyskinetic movements compared with conventional antipsychotic agents in controlled short-term and long-term studies. Various other agents have been evaluated as possible treatment for tardive dyskinesia (e.g., amantadine†, benzodiazepines†, anticholinergic agents†, botulinum toxin†, calcium channel-blocking agents†, donepezil†, γ-aminobutyric acid agonists [baclofen, valproic acid]†, essential fatty acids, estrogen†, insulin†, lithium†, melatonin, propranolol†, pyridoxine), but their clinical efficacy remains unproven. Because some evidence suggests that vitamin E may decrease the risk of developing tardive dyskinesia and because there is a low risk of adverse effects associated with the drug, some clinicians recommend vitamin E (400–800 units daily) as prophylactic therapy.

Neuroleptic Malignant Syndrome Neuroleptic malignant syndrome (NMS) may occur in patients receiving phenothiazine or other antipsychotic therapy. NMS has been characterized by hyperthermia, severe extrapyramidal dysfunction (including severe hypertonicity of skeletal muscles), varying levels of consciousness (including stupor and coma), altered mental status (including catatonic reactions), and autonomic instability (including cardiovascular effects such as hypertension and tachycardia). Autonomic effects often include pallor, diaphoresis, alterations in blood pressure, tachycardia, and cardiac arrhythmias. Motor abnormalities often include akinesia and rigidity. Increased serum creatine kinase (CK, creatine phosphokinase, CPK) concentrations, rhabdomyolysis (evidenced by myoglobinuria), acute renal failure, and leukocytosis also may occur.

NMS appears to be a relatively uncommon adverse effect of phenothiazines, but the syndrome can be sudden and unpredictable in its onset, frequently is misdiagnosed, and can be fatal in 5–20% of cases if left untreated. The syndrome usually occurs early in the course of therapy with phenothiazines or other antipsychotics, often within 1 week after treatment is initiated or dosage is increased. NMS may not recur with rechallenge. The syndrome appears to occur more frequently in young men, and predisposing factors may include acute agitation, heat stress, physical illness, dehydration, concurrent organic brain disease or other neurologic disability, rapid escalation of dose, use of high-potency agents, and use of an intramuscular preparation. NMS appears to progress rapidly over 24–72 hours after initial manifestations occur, although a more insidious progression has also been described. When the syndrome is fatal, death generally occurs 3–30 days after onset and may result from cardiac arrhythmias, cardiovascular collapse, respiratory failure, thromboembolism, aspiration pneumonia, and/or rhabdomyolysis with acute renal failure.

Treatment of NMS includes immediate discontinuance of phenothiazine therapy and initiation of supportive and symptomatic therapy, including correction of fluid and electrolyte imbalances, cooling of the patient, maintenance of renal function, management of cardiovascular instability (e.g., stabilizing blood pressure), and prevention of respiratory complications. Some case series suggest that treatment with a dopamine agonist (e.g., bromocriptine, amantadine) or dantrolene may improve symptoms of NMS when compared with supportive treatment alone. Treatment with benzodiazepines (e.g., lorazepam) also may be helpful, based on the overlap in symptoms between catatonia and NMS. Electroconvulsive therapy (ECT) has been reported to improve symptoms in patients with severe and resistant NMS. Recovery generally occurs within 5–10 days after discontinuance of the phenothiazine, but may be substantially prolonged following discontinuance of long-acting depot preparations. Irreversible CNS damage may occur. Some clinicians suggest that, if psychotropic therapy is reinstituted following recovery, alternative therapies should be considered. If the benefit of antipsychotic therapy is thought to outweigh the risk, extreme caution and careful monitoring should be exercised and second-generation (atypical) or low-potency, first-generation (conventional) agents should be used with gradual increases in dosage, if possible. Additional experience is necessary, but the risk that NMS can recur *must* be considered.

Other Nervous System Effects Drowsiness, which is usually mild to moderate in severity, occurs frequently, particularly during the first weeks of therapy with some phenothiazines; however, tolerance to the sedative effect usually develops in most patients over a period of days or weeks during long-term administration. Although sedation is more common with low-potency, first-generation agents (such as chlorpromazine), it occurs to some extent with all phenothiazines. In agitated patients, the sedating effects of phenothiazines during initial therapy can be beneficial. However, sedation that persists during maintenance therapy and causes daytime drowsiness and increased sleep time can interfere with social, vocational, and recreational function. In such cases, a reduction in the daily dosage, administration of the entire daily dosage as one evening dose, or a switch to a less sedating (i.e., higher potency) phenothiazine or another antipsychotic agent can be helpful. Although there are no systematic data regarding specific pharmacologic interventions for sedation, some clinicians consider caffeine a relatively safe treatment option. Wakefulness-promoting agents (e.g., modafinil) also have been used to treat daytime drowsiness. Other adverse nervous system effects of phenothiazines include insomnia, restlessness, anxiety, euphoria, agitation, depression, weakness, headache, and cerebral edema.

Seizures may occur in patients receiving phenothiazines or other antipsychotic agents, particularly in patients with EEG abnormalities or a history of such disorders. Low-potency conventional antipsychotic agents and clozapine appear to be associated with the highest risk of seizures. The incidence of seizures is dose related and incidences generally are less than 1% for conventional antipsychotic agents when given in the usual recommended dosage range, although patients with a history of idiopathic or drug-induced seizures have an increased risk. If a patient receiving a phenothiazine or other antipsychotic agent (except clozapine) experiences a seizure, some authorities recommend the drug be withdrawn or the dosage reduced by 50% until a neurologic examination can be completed. Exacerbation of psychotic symptoms and catatonic-like behavior, which may subside following discontinuance of therapy or treatment with anticholinergic agents, also has been reported. Abnormality of the CSF proteins also has been reported.

Adverse anticholinergic effects of phenothiazines include dry mouth (xerostomia), blurred vision, mydriasis, constipation, obstipation, nausea, adynamic ileus, atonic colon, urinary retention, decreased sweating, and impotence (difficulty achieving and maintaining an erection). Dryness of the mouth may make retention of full dentures difficult. Although most anticholinergic adverse effects are mild and tolerable, these effects can be troublesome in older patients (e.g., older men with benign prostatic hypertrophy). The incidence and severity of adverse anticholinergic effects may be increased by concomitant administration of anticholinergic antiparkinsonian agents, antidepressants, and other drugs with marked anticholinergic activity. Adverse anticholinergic effects are usually dose related and may improve with dosage reduction or administration of the anticholinergic antiparkinsonian agent in divided doses. Parenteral physostigmine has been used to reverse the symptoms of anticholinergic delirium; however, it has resulted in serious adverse effects, including seizures, bronchospasm, and severe bradyarrhythmias, when given to patients with tricyclic antidepressant overdosage and other forms of anticholinergic toxicity. Therefore, most clinicians caution against the routine use of physostigmine in patients with anticholinergic manifestations.

Phenothiazines depress the hypothalamic mechanism for regulation of body temperature and, depending on the environmental temperature, may cause hyperthermia and heat prostration, or hypothermia and respiratory distress. Hypothermic collapse has been reported in patients swimming in cold water.

Phenothiazines are not associated with psychic dependence and do not produce tolerance or addiction; however, some symptoms resembling physical dependence such as gastritis, nausea and vomiting, dizziness, tremulousness, feeling of warmth or cold, sweating, tachycardia, headache, and insomnia have occurred following abrupt withdrawal in some patients receiving prolonged maintenance therapy with phenothiazines. These symptoms can usually be avoided, or their severity reduced, by gradual withdrawal of the drugs or by continuing concomitant anticholinergic antiparkinsonian agents for several weeks following discontinuance of phenothiazines.

■ **Cardiovascular Effects** Hypotension (including postural hypotension), tachycardia, increased pulse rate, syncope, and dizziness have occurred in patients receiving phenothiazines, especially with low-potency phenothiazines and following the first parenteral dose of a phenothiazine, but rarely after the first oral dose. These cardiovascular effects usually subside within 30–120 minutes; occasionally they may be more severe and prolonged, resulting in a shock-like syndrome. Tolerance to the hypotensive effects of the drugs usually develops. Marked hypotension occurs infrequently, and hypotension severe enough to cause fatal cardiac arrest has occurred rarely. Hypotension occurs most frequently when phenothiazines are given parenterally; therefore, patients should be in a supine position at the time of parenteral administration and should remain so for at least 30–60 minutes following completion of the injection or infusion. Patients who experience postural hypotension should be cautioned not to get up quickly and to obtain assistance when necessary. Hypotension may be a particular problem in patients with pheochromocytoma or mitral insufficiency, and severe hypotension has occurred with usual dosages in these patients. The management of antipsychotic-induced hypotension may include a variety of measures such as the use of support stockings, an increase in dietary salt intake, and/or fludrocortisone therapy. Severe hypotensive effects may be alleviated by the administration of norepinephrine or phenylephrine; epinephrine should *not* be used because phenothiazines cause a reversal of epinephrine's vasopressor effects and a further lowering of blood pressure.

Various ECG changes, including nonspecific, usually reversible, Q- and T-wave abnormalities have occurred in some patients receiving phenothiazines. (See Uses: Delirium.) ECG changes may resemble quinidine-like alterations or those induced by hypokalemia. Sudden death, apparently secondary to cardiac arrest, also has occurred.

Thioridazine and Mesoridazine Dose-related serious cardiac effects, including prolongation of the QT interval corrected for rate (QT_c), arrhythmias (e.g., atypical ventricular tachycardia [torsades de pointes]), and/or sudden death, have been reported in patients receiving thioridazine or mesoridazine (no longer commercially available in the US). A causal relationship to the drugs has not been established; however, since both drugs have been shown to prolong the QT_c interval, such relationships are possible.

Cardiotoxic effects may be associated with increased plasma concentrations of thioridazine and its metabolites (e.g., mesoridazine). Increased plasma concentrations of thioridazine are most likely to develop in patients with poor metabolizer phenotypes of the cytochrome P-450 (CYP) 2D6 isoenzyme and in patients receiving drugs known to inhibit the CYP2D6 isoenzyme (e.g., fluoxetine, paroxetine) or to reduce the clearance of thioridazine by other mechanisms (e.g., fluvoxamine, pindolol, propranolol). Patients with a history of cardiac arrhythmias and those with an underlying condition that might prolong the QT_c interval (e.g., hypokalemia, bradycardia, congenital prolongation of the QT interval) or who are receiving drugs that might prolong the QT_c interval also may be at increased risk of developing cardiac arrhythmias (e.g., torsades de pointes) and/or sudden death if thioridazine or mesoridazine were used. Therefore, the indications and circumstances for use of these drugs has been reduced substantially relative to other antipsychotic agents, and both thioridazine and mesoridazine are now contraindicated in a variety of patients because of such underlying risk factors of existing drug therapy. (See Cautions: Precautions and Contraindications.)

For further information on the cardiotoxic effects of thioridazine, see Cautions: Arrhythmias and Associated Precautions and Contraindications, in Thioridazine 28:16.08.24.

■ **Hematologic Effects** In clinical trial and/or postmarketing experience, leukopenia and neutropenia temporally related to antipsychotic agents have been reported. Agranulocytosis also has been reported.

Possible risk factors for leukopenia and neutropenia include a preexisting low leukocyte count and a history of drug-induced leukopenia or neutropenia. Therefore, patients with a history of clinically important low leukocyte count or drug-induced leukopenia and/or neutropenia should have their complete blood count monitored frequently during the first few months of antipsychotic agent therapy. Discontinuance of the antipsychotic agent should be considered at the first sign of a clinically important decline in leukocyte count in the absence of other causative factors.

Patients with clinically important neutropenia should be carefully monitored for fever or other signs or symptoms of infection and promptly treated if such signs or symptoms occur. In patients with severe neutropenia (absolute neutrophil count [ANC] less than 1000/mm^3), the antipsychotic agent should be discontinued and the leukocyte count monitored until recovery occurs.

Supportive therapy with biosynthetic hematopoietic agents, including filgrastim, a recombinant human granulocyte colony-stimulating factor (G-CSF), and sargramostim, a recombinant human granulocyte-macrophage colony-stimulating factor (GM-CSF), has been effective in a limited number of patients with clozapine- or chlorpromazine-induced neutropenia or agranulocytosis.

Lithium reportedly has been used successfully in the treatment of several cases of leukopenia and neutropenia associated with aripiprazole, clozapine, olanzapine, and some other drugs; however, further clinical experience is needed to confirm these anecdotal findings.

Other reported adverse hematologic effects of phenothiazines include eosinophilia; thrombocytopenia; aplastic anemia with pancytopenia, purpura, or granulocytopenia; and hemolytic anemia.

■ **Dermatologic Effects** Various dermatoses, often associated with pruritus and marked photosensitivity, may occur during treatment with phenothiazines. Photosensitivity occurs infrequently in patients receiving phenothiazines and other antipsychotic drugs and is most common with the low-potency phenothiazines. Patients should be instructed to avoid excessive sunlight and/or to apply sunscreen and wear protective clothing. Other adverse dermatologic effects include urticaria, erythema, eczema, and exfoliative dermatitis. In general, dermatologic reactions have been reported most frequently in patients receiving propylamino or alkylpiperidine derivatives of phenothiazine. Contact dermatitis, usually of the erythematous or eczematous type, has occurred rarely.

Long-term administration of high doses of phenothiazines may result in pigment depositions in various body tissues. Pigmentary changes of the skin are generally restricted to exposed areas of the body, and exposure to light appears to be a contributing factor. The skin is usually yellowish-brown, but pigmentary changes range from an almost imperceptible darkening of the skin to greyish-purple. In some patients, histologic examination has revealed a pigment that is a melanin-like complex and that usually occurs in the dermis. The pigment may also be widely distributed into the brain, heart, liver, kidneys, retina, and cornea. Pigmentation may fade following discontinuance of the drug. If pigmentary changes occur, it should be determined whether the potential benefits of continued therapy justify the possible risks, and whether therapy should be continued or withdrawn or dosage reduced.

■ **Ocular Effects** Ocular changes including deposition of fine particulate matter in the lens and cornea have been reported in patients receiving high doses of phenothiazines for prolonged periods of time. Pigmentary retinopathy and corneal opacities may occur during chronic therapy with the low-potency phenothiazines chlorpromazine and thioridazine, particularly at high dosages. Ocular changes reportedly occur more frequently than skin pigmentation and have occurred in patients with or without phenothiazine-induced skin pigmentation. In more advanced cases, star-shaped opacities may occur in the anterior portion of the lens. In extreme cases, visual impairment may occur. Epithelial keratopathy, lacrimation, and pigmentary retinopathy have also been reported. It has been suggested that ocular lesions may regress following discontinuance of phenothiazines. Although the precise cause of these adverse ocular effects is not known, exposure to light along with high dosage of phenothiazines and prolonged duration of therapy appear to be contributing factors. If ocular changes occur, it should be determined whether the potential benefits of continued phenothiazine therapy justify the possible risks, and whether therapy should be continued or withdrawn or dosage reduced.

■ **GI Effects** Adverse GI effects of phenothiazines include anorexia, dyspepsia, constipation, paralytic ileus, and, occasionally, diarrhea. The "oral syndrome" consisting of dryness of the mouth; diffuse redness of mucous membranes of the mouth; loosened dentures with or without vesicles in the mouth or on the tongue; denture stomatitis; cracking of the lips and corners of the mouth; white or black, hairy tongue or bald, beefy, red tongue; and thin, white pseudomembrane formation in the oral cavity has also been reported.

■ **Endocrine and Metabolic Effects** All first-generation (conventional) antipsychotic agents increase serum prolactin concentrations. (See Cautions: Carcinogenicity.) The resultant hyperprolactinemia may lead to galactorrhea in approximately 1–5% of patients and menstrual cycle changes (e.g., oligomenorrhea) in up to 20% of women. Mastalgia and gynecomastia also have occurred in some patients. A reduction in dosage may alleviate or decrease the severity of these adverse effects or drug therapy may be switched to an antipsychotic with less effect on prolactin (e.g., any atypical antipsychotic except risperidone). In patients with severe galactorrhea or in women with menstrual disturbances but in whom the antipsychotic dosage must be maintained, the administration of a low dosage of bromocriptine (2–10 mg daily) or amantadine may be helpful. Increased appetite, hyperglycemia, hypoglycemia, glycosuria, and high or prolonged glucose tolerance curves also have occurred in some patients.

Weight gain occurs with most antipsychotic agents, including in up to 40% of patients treated with the first-generation (conventional) antipsychotic agents, with the greatest risk associated with low-potency agents. Molindone appears less likely than other agents in this class to produce weight gain. Because weight loss is difficult for many patients, prevention of weight gain is important. In the event that clinically important weight gain occurs during therapy, diet and exercise interventions should be suggested. However, if the clinical benefit of the antipsychotic agent does not outweigh the potential health risks of weight gain (e.g., cardiovascular disease, hypertension, cancers, diabetes, osteoarthritis, sleep apnea), a trial of an antipsychotic with a lower weight-gain liability should be considered.

Phenothiazines may decrease urinary gonadotropin, estrogen, and progestin concentrations and decrease vasopressin and corticotropin secretion.

■ **Genitourinary Effects** Adverse effects on sexual function may occur in patients receiving phenothiazines and other antipsychotic agents. Erectile dysfunction appears to be the most common adverse effect in male patients, reportedly occurring in approximately 20–50% of men receiving first-generation (conventional) agents. Other effects include ejaculatory disturbances in men, including delayed or absent ejaculation, and loss of libido and anorgasmia in both men and women. In addition, certain drugs, including thioridazine and risperidone, have been associated with retrograde ejaculation. Priapism also had occurred during phenothiazine therapy. Although not clearly established, these effects appear to result principally from the α-adrenergic- and serotonergic-blocking effects of these drugs. A reduction in dosage or discontinuance of therapy usually results in improvement or elimination of these symptoms; in some patients, a switch to another agent may be helpful. There is some evidence that imipramine (25–50 mg daily at bedtime) may be helpful in treating retrograde ejaculation in thioridazine-treated patients. In patients in whom a reduction in dosage or switch to an alternative drug is not feasible, yohimbine or cyproheptadine therapy could be considered; psychoeducation also may help patients tolerate this bothersome but not clinically dangerous adverse effect.

■ **Sensitivity Reactions and Hepatic Effects** Sensitivity reactions and adverse hepatic effects including cholestatic jaundice, elevated hepatic enzyme concentrations, blood dyscrasias, dermatoses, and photosensitivity generally occur within the first few months after initiation of phenothiazine therapy, but occasionally they may occur following discontinuance of the drug.

Cholestatic jaundice usually occurs within 2–4 weeks after initiation of therapy in approximately 0.1–4% of all patients receiving phenothiazines. Jaundice may also occur in neonates whose mothers have received phenothiazines during pregnancy. Phenothiazine-induced jaundice resembles infectious hepatitis, with laboratory features of obstructive jaundice rather than parenchymal damage, and the clinician should be alert to the signs of cholestatic jaundice, including upper abdominal pain, nausea, yellow skin, influenza-like symptoms, rash, fever, and abnormal laboratory findings such as eosinophilia, bile in the urine, and elevated serum bilirubin, alkaline phosphatase, and transaminase concentrations. If signs of jaundice occur, the drug should be discontinued immediately. Weekly urine bilirubin tests during the first month of therapy may detect the reaction and warrant discontinuance of phenothiazine therapy. However, because antipsychotic-induced cholestatic jaundice occurs infrequently, other possible causes of jaundice should be ruled out before attributing the jaundice to the antipsychotic agent. Although fatalities are rare and clinical recovery from jaundice usually occurs within a few weeks following discontinuance of the drug in most patients, results of liver function tests and biopsies indicate that histopathologic changes may persist for longer periods, and chronic jaundice has been reported in some patients. There is *no* conclusive evidence that preexisting liver disease increases the susceptibility to phenothiazine-induced jaundice.

Laryngeal edema, laryngospasm, bronchospasm, angioedema, and anaphylactoid reactions have occurred in patients receiving phenothiazines.

Contact dermatitis, usually of the erythematous or eczematous type, has been reported in persons who come in contact with solutions of certain phenothiazine derivatives; care should be taken to avoid getting solutions of these drugs on the hands or clothing. Photosensitivity has occurred. Other dermatologic effects of phenothiazines may also be sensitivity reactions to the drugs. (See Cautions: Dermatologic Effects.)

■ **Other Adverse Effects** Hyperpyrexia, mild fever (following IM administration of large doses), diaphoresis, peripheral edema, and a systemic lupus erythematosus-like syndrome have occurred in patients receiving phenothiazines.

Sudden and unexpected deaths have occurred in patients receiving phenothiazines, especially during long-term administration of the drugs. In some patients, sudden death appeared to result from asphyxia (secondary to failure of the cough reflex) or cardiac arrest.

■ **Precautions and Contraindications** Because of the risk of inducing serious, potentially irreversible adverse effects (see Cautions: Nervous System Effects), the clinical need for phenothiazine and/or other antipsychotic therapy should be established, especially when prolonged therapy with the drugs is anticipated. The likelihood of some effects (e.g., tardive dyskinesia) becoming irreversible may increase with the duration of therapy and cumulative dose of antipsychotic agent(s) administered. Therefore, long-term therapy with antipsychotic drugs generally should be reserved for patients with a chronic disorder known to be responsive to these drugs and for which alternative, equally effective, but potentially less toxic therapy is not available or appropriate. In patients requiring long-term antipsychotic therapy, the smallest effective dosage and the shortest duration of therapy producing an adequate clinical response should be employed. The continued need for therapy should be assessed periodically. Because the risk of some of these effects may be increased in geriatric patients and because it is estimated that many geriatric patients residing in long-term care facilities are inappropriately prescribed antipsychotic therapy, it is important that the need for chronic therapy with the drugs be established in these patients. (See Geriatric Considerations under Psychotic Disorders: Schizophrenia and Other Psychotic Disorders, in Uses and see also Cautions: Geriatric Precautions.) Unless contraindicated, periodic efforts should be made in patients receiving long-term therapy to gradually reduce dosage and provide drug holidays and/or nondrug (e.g., behavioral) therapy in an attempt to discontinue antipsychotic drug therapy whenever clinically possible. Patients in whom long-term antipsychotic drug therapy is considered should be fully informed, if possible, about the risk of developing potentially irreversible adverse effects. Likewise, the decision to employ such therapy should be carefully considered by the patient (and/or the patient's family or guardians) and the physician if possible. The decision to inform the patient (and/or the patient's family or guardians) should take into account the clinical circumstances and the competency of the patient to understand the information.

Geriatric patients with dementia-related psychosis treated with antipsychotic agents are at an increased risk of mortality. (See Geriatric Considerations under Psychotic Disorders: Schizophrenia and Other Psychotic Disorders, in Uses and see also Cautions: Geriatric Precautions.)

Patients should be warned that phenothiazines may impair their ability to perform activities requiring mental alertness or physical coordination (e.g., operating machinery, driving a motor vehicle). Patients also should be warned that phenothiazines may enhance their response to alcohol, barbiturates, or other CNS depressants. Patients should also be warned to contact their physician if signs or symptoms of agranulocytosis such as sore throat or other signs of infection occur.

Phenothiazines and other antipsychotic agents may cause somnolence, postural hypotension, and motor and sensory instability, which may lead to falls; as a consequence, fractures or other injuries may occur. For patients with diseases or conditions or receiving other drugs that could exacerbate these effects, fall risk assessments should be completed when initiating antipsychotic treatment and periodically during long-term therapy.

Because of the risk of adverse cardiovascular effects, phenothiazines should be used with caution in patients with severe cardiovascular disorders. Low-potency agents (such as thioridazine), in particular, should be avoided in patients with symptomatic orthostatic hypotension, and the drugs, particularly thioridazine and mesoridazine (no longer commercially available in the US), also should be avoided in those with established cardiac disease, particularly prolongation of the QT interval or a history of cardiac arrhythmias. Phenothiazine-treated patients who experience postural hypotension should be cautioned not to get up quickly and to obtain assistance when necessary. The management of mild to moderate cases of hypotension may include a variety of measures such as the use of support stockings, an increase in dietary salt intake, and/or fludrocortisone therapy. If severe hypotension occurs, norepinephrine, metaraminol, or phenylephrine may be used; epinephrine or dopamine, should *not* be used since phenothiazines cause a reversal of these drugs' vasopressor effects and a further lowering of blood pressure.

Because phenothiazines may lower the seizure threshold, the drugs should be used with caution in patients with a history of seizures and in those receiving anticonvulsant agents. Adequate anticonvulsant therapy should be maintained during administration of phenothiazines. If a patient receiving a phenothiazine or another antipsychotic agent (except clozapine) experiences a seizure, some authorities recommend the drug be withdrawn or the dosage reduced by 50% until a neurologic examination can be completed. In patients with a history of substance abuse or dependence, clinicians should consider the possibility that phenothiazines and other antipsychotic agents can infrequently precipitate seizures during alcohol or benzodiazepine withdrawal.

Patients receiving prolonged phenothiazine therapy with moderate to high dosages should have periodic ophthalmologic examinations. (See Cautions: Ocular Effects.)

Phenothiazines should be used with caution in debilitated patients, in patients with hepatic or renal disease, and in patients with glaucoma or prostatic hypertrophy. There is some evidence that patients with a history of hepatic encephalopathy secondary to cirrhosis have an increased sensitivity to CNS effects (i.e., impaired cerebration, slowing of the EEG) of phenothiazines. Phenothiazines should be administered with caution to patients exposed to organophosphate insecticides.

Because phenothiazines depress the hypothalamic mechanism for regulation of body temperature, the drugs should also be administered with caution to patients exposed to extreme heat or cold; patients receiving phenothiazines should be advised that they are likely to have increased vulnerability when exposed to temperature extremes, possibly resulting in hyperthermia or hypothermia. Because of the CNS depressant effects of phenothiazines, the drugs should be used with caution in patients with chronic respiratory disorders such as severe asthma, emphysema, or acute respiratory tract infections. Because phenothiazines may suppress the cough reflex, aspiration of gastric contents is possible.

Phenothiazines should be used with caution in patients with hypocalcemia because these patients appear to be more susceptible to dystonic reactions.

When concomitant therapy with an anticholinergic antiparkinsonian drug is necessary to manage phenothiazine-induced extrapyramidal symptoms, it may be necessary to continue the antiparkinsonian drug for a period of time after discontinuance of phenothiazines in order to prevent emergence of these symptoms. The combined anticholinergic effects of the drugs should be considered.

Because neurologic reactions resulting from phenothiazine therapy may be similar to CNS signs and symptoms accompanying certain disorders such as encephalitis, Reye's syndrome, encephalopathy, meningitis, and tetanus, the diagnosis of these disorders may be obscured or the disease-associated signs and symptoms may be incorrectly diagnosed as drug induced.

It should be kept in mind that the antiemetic effect of phenothiazines may mask the signs of overdosage of toxic drugs (e.g., antineoplastic agents) or may obscure the cause of vomiting in various disorders such as intestinal obstruction, Reye's syndrome, or brain tumor.

Phenothiazines should be administered with caution and in reduced dosage to patients who have exhibited severe reactions to insulin or electroconvulsive therapy (ECT).

In general, patients who have demonstrated a hypersensitivity reaction (e.g., cholestatic jaundice) to any phenothiazine derivative should not be reexposed to another derivative, unless the potential benefits of phenothiazine therapy outweigh the possible risks.

Some commercially available preparations (i.e., tablets) of phenothiazines contain the dye tartrazine (FD&C yellow No. 5), which may cause allergic reactions including bronchial asthma in susceptible individuals. Although the incidence of tartrazine sensitivity is low, it frequently occurs in patients who are sensitive to aspirin.

Care should be taken to avoid skin contact with phenothiazine oral solutions and injections, since contact dermatitis has occurred rarely.

Phenothiazines are contraindicated in patients with severe toxic CNS depression or in those who are comatose from any cause. Phenothiazines also are contraindicated in patients with subcortical brain damage and in patients with bone marrow depression. Individual phenothiazines are contraindicated in patients who are hypersensitive to other phenothiazine derivatives unless the potential benefits outweigh the possible risks to the patient.

Because thioridazine and mesoridazine have been shown to prolong the QT interval corrected for rate (QT_c), which may be associated with life-threatening, proarrhythmic effects, concomitant use of these phenothiazines with drugs that prolong the QT_c interval is contraindicated. Use of these phenothiazines also is contraindicated in patients with underlying conditions (e.g., congenital long QT syndrome, history of arrhythmias) that might prolong the QT_c interval. In addition, thioridazine is contraindicated in patients receiving drugs that inhibit the cytochrome P-450 (CYP) 2D6 isoenzyme (e.g., fluoxetine, paroxetine) or reduce clearance of thioridazine by other mechanisms (e.g., fluvoxamine, pindolol, propranolol) and in those with poor metabolizer phenotypes of the CYP2D6 isoenzyme.

■ **Pediatric Precautions** Because children and adolescents may have substantial adverse effects that have yet to be identified, documentation of and monitoring for known adverse effects (e.g., extrapyramidal effects, weight gain) is required when phenothiazines are used in the management of childhood-onset schizophrenia. The risk of extrapyramidal adverse effects associated with antipsychotic agents, including phenothiazines, may be higher in children and adolescents than in adults. As many as 50% of children and adolescents who receive antipsychotic agents may experience some form of tardive or withdrawal dyskinesia. In addition, an analysis of published reports of neuroleptic malignant syndrome (NMS) in 77 children and adolescents who received antipsychotic agents showed that 9% of these patients died and another 20% had serious residual sequelae. Dopamine agonists (e.g., bromocriptine) and anticholinergic agents that are used to treat the syndrome in adults were effective in these children and adolescents, but dantrolene, a skeletal muscle relaxant, was not effective in these patients. However, these reports are not definitive and further studies are needed.

Phenothiazines should be used with caution in children with acute illnesses (e.g., varicella-zoster [chickenpox] infections, CNS infections, measles, gastroenteritis) or dehydration, since the incidence of extrapyramidal symptoms, especially dystonic reactions and akathisia, is increased in these patients.

Phenothiazines should not be used in children in conditions for which pediatric dosage has not been established. For specific recommendations regarding use of these drugs in children, see the individual monographs on phenothiazines in 28:16.08.24.

■ **Geriatric Precautions** Clinical studies of phenothiazines (e.g., perphenazine) generally did not include sufficient numbers of patients 65 years of age and older to determine whether geriatric patients respond differently than younger patients. Although other clinical experience has not revealed age-related differences in response or tolerance, drug dosage generally should be titrated carefully in geriatric patients, usually initiating therapy at the low end of the dosage range. The greater frequency of decreased hepatic function and of concomitant disease and drug therapy observed in the elderly also should be considered.

Geriatric patients appear to be particularly sensitive to adverse nervous system (e.g., tardive dyskinesia, parkinsonian signs and symptoms, akathisia, sedation), anticholinergic, and cardiovascular (e.g., orthostatic hypotension) effects of antipsychotic agents. Because the risk of falling and associated hip fracture in geriatric patients may be increased with use of antipsychotic agents, phenothiazine therapy should be initiated at reduced dosages and such patients observed closely.

Geriatric patients with dementia-related psychosis treated with either conventional (first-generation) or atypical (second-generation) antipsychotic agents are at an increased risk of mortality. Analyses of 17 placebo-controlled trials (average duration of 10 weeks) in geriatric patients mainly receiving atypical antipsychotic agents revealed an approximate 1.6- to 1.7-fold increase in mortality compared with that in patients receiving placebo. Over the course of a typical 10-week controlled trial, the rate of death in drug-treated patients was about 4.5% compared with a rate of about 2.6% in those receiving placebo. Although the causes of death were varied in these trials, most of the deaths appeared to be either cardiovascular (e.g., heart failure, sudden death) or infectious (e.g., pneumonia) in nature. Subsequently, two observational, epidemiological studies have indicated that, similar to atypical antipsychotic agents, treatment of geriatric patients with conventional antipsychotic agents may increase mortality; the causes of death were not reported in the first study and cancer and cardiac disease were the causes of death with the highest relative risk in the second study. However, the extent to which these findings of increased mortality in observational studies may be attributed to the antipsychotic agent as opposed to certain patient characteristics remains unclear. The US Food and Drug Administration (FDA) currently advises clinicians that antipsychotic agents are *not* approved for the treatment of dementia-related psychosis. The FDA further advises clinicians that no drugs currently are approved for the treatment of patients with dementia-associated psychosis and that other management options should be considered in such patients. The decision whether to prescribe antipsychotic agents "off-label" in the treatment of dementia symptoms is left to the discretion of the clinician. Clinicians who prescribe antipsychotic agents in geriatric patients with dementia-related psychosis should discuss the increased mortality risk with patients, their families, and their caregivers. In addition, patients currently receiving antipsychotic agents for dementia-associated symptoms should not abruptly stop taking the drugs; caregivers and patients should discuss any possible concerns with their clinician. For additional information on the use of antipsychotic agents for dementia-associated psychosis and other behavioral disturbances, see Geriatric Considerations under Psychotic Disorders: Schizophrenia and Other Psychotic Disorders, in Uses.

Geriatric patients with genetic deficiency of the cytochrome P-450 (CYP) 2D6 isoenzyme (i.e., those with the poor-metabolizer phenotype) appear to be at increased risk for drug-induced adverse effects when receiving usual dosages of phenothiazines that are metabolized principally via this pathway. In one study in 45 geriatric patients with dementia, the 5 patients who were prospectively identified as exhibiting the poor-metabolizer phenotype reported greater adverse effects during the first 10 days of perphenazine therapy than did the 40 patients exhibiting the extensive-metabolizer phenotype; thereafter, the adverse-effect profiles for the 2 groups tended to converge. One manufacturer of perphenazine states that phenotyping of geriatric patients prior to initiation of antipsychotic therapy may identify those at risk for adverse events. Some authorities also recommend that a comprehensive medical, psychiatric, and psychosocial examination be performed before prescribing antipsychotic agents in elderly patients. In addition, a baseline leukocyte count is useful in older patients treated with antipsychotic agents for the first time since these drugs, particularly phenothiazines, can lower the leukocyte count. (See Cautions: Hematologic Effects.) If the baseline leukocyte count is low or if the patient is receiving another drug that also may lower the leukocyte count, then a nonphenothiazine antipsychotic agent may be preferable.

■ **Mutagenicity and Carcinogenicity** Chromosomal aberrations in spermatocytes and abnormal sperm have been demonstrated in rodents treated with certain neuroleptic drugs.

Although an increase in mammary neoplasms has been found in rodents following long-term administration of prolactin-stimulating antipsychotic agents, no clinical or epidemiologic studies conducted to date have shown an association between long-term administration of these drugs and mammary tumorigenesis in humans. Current evidence is considered too limited to be conclusive, and further study is needed to determine the clinical importance in most patients of elevated serum prolactin concentrations associated with antipsychotic agents. Because in vitro tests indicate that approximately one-third of human breast cancers are prolactin dependent, phenothiazines should be used with caution in patients with previously detected breast cancer. Because clozapine causes only small, transient increases in prolactin concentrations (see Pharmacology: Neuroendocrine Effects, in Clozapine 28:16.08.04), it has been suggested that clozapine theoretically may be safer than other antipsychotic drugs for patients with schizophrenia who also are at high risk for or who have a history of breast cancer.

■ **Pregnancy, Fertility, and Lactation** Neonates exposed to antipsychotic agents, including phenothiazines, during the third trimester of pregnancy are at risk for extrapyramidal and/or withdrawal symptoms following delivery. On February 22, 2011, the US Food and Drug Administration (FDA) notified healthcare professionals that 69 cases of neonatal extrapyramidal symptoms or withdrawal have been identified with all antipsychotic agents in the Adverse Event Reporting System database through October 29, 2008. Symptoms reported in these cases included agitation, hypertonia, hypotonia, tardive dyskinetic-like symptoms, tremor, somnolence, respiratory distress, and feeding disorder. Because antipsychotic plasma concentrations were not provided, the FDA states it was not possible to determine whether the events resulted from antipsychotic toxicity or withdrawal. The majority of cases were also confounded by other factors, including concomitant use of other drugs associated with withdrawal symptoms (e.g., antidepressant agents, benzodiazepines, nonbenzodiazepine hypnotics, opiate agonists), prematurity, congenital malformations, and obstetric and perinatal complications (e.g., placental problems, preeclampsia). However, there were some cases that suggested neonatal extrapyramidal symptoms and withdrawal may occur with exposure to antipsychotic agents alone. Some of the cases described time of symptom onset, which ranged from birth to one month after birth. Any neonate exhibiting extrapyramidal or withdrawal symptoms following in utero exposure to antipsychotic agents should be monitored. Symptoms were self-limiting in some neonates but varied in severity; some infants required intensive care unit support and prolonged hospitalization. Drugs that have been used to treat suspected withdrawal reactions include phenobarbital and benzodiazepines.

Safety of phenothiazines during pregnancy has not been established. Animal reproduction studies have not been performed with most of the phenothiazines. It is not known whether phenothiazines can cause fetal harm when administered to pregnant women. Although several retrospective studies of infants born to women treated with a phenothiazine (e.g., chlorpromazine, trifluoperazine) have found no increased risk of adverse fetal effects associated with phenothiazine use, one study found an increased risk of malformations. In addition, prolonged jaundice, extrapyramidal symptoms, hyperreflexia, and hyporeflexia have occurred in some neonates born to women who were receiving phenothiazines during pregnancy. Phenothiazines should generally be used during pregnancy only when the potential benefits justify the possible risks to the fetus. Clinicians should advise women of childbearing potential about the benefits and risks of antipsychotic agent therapy during pregnancy. Patients should also be advised not to stop taking their antipsychotic agent if they become pregnant without first consulting with their clinician, since abruptly discontinuing the drugs can cause clinically important complications. In cases where antipsychotic agents must be used during pregnancy because the patient's psychosis places the mother and/or her fetus at substantial risk, some experts state that high-potency agents may be safer. In addition, the drug should be given in the lowest effective dosage and for as brief a period as possible and should be discontinued at least 5–10 days prior to anticipated delivery. Phenothiazines are generally contraindicated during the first trimester of pregnancy, particularly between weeks 6 and 10.

The effect of phenothiazines on fertility in humans is not known. Impotence, increased or decreased libido, inhibition of ejaculation, amenorrhea, and menstrual irregularities have occurred in some individuals during phenothiazine therapy.

Phenothiazines are distributed into milk. The manufacturers warn that nursing should not be undertaken by women receiving phenothiazines.

Drug Interactions

■ **CNS Depressants** Phenothiazines may be additive with, or may potentiate the action of, other CNS depressants such as opiates or other analgesics, barbiturates or other sedatives, general anesthetics, or alcohol. When phenothiazines are used concomitantly with other CNS depressants, caution should be used to avoid excessive sedation or CNS depression.

■ **Anticonvulsants** Because phenothiazines may lower the seizure threshold, dosage adjustment of anticonvulsant agents may be necessary when the drugs are used concomitantly. The CNS depressant effects of phenothiazines do *not* potentiate the anticonvulsant activity of anticonvulsants. Chlorpromazine reportedly has decreased the metabolism of phenytoin; if the drugs are used concomitantly, the patient should be closely monitored for phenytoin toxicity. Phenobarbital has been shown to increase urinary excretion and to decrease plasma concentrations of chlorpromazine. Although the clinical importance of this potential interaction has not been determined, the possibility that the therapeutic effects of chlorpromazine may be reduced during concurrent therapy with the drugs should be considered.

■ **Lithium** Although most patients receiving lithium and a phenothiazine antipsychotic agent concurrently do not develop unusual adverse effects, an acute encephalopathic syndrome occasionally has occurred, especially when high serum lithium concentrations were present. Patients receiving such combined therapy should be observed for evidence of adverse neurologic effects; treatment should be promptly discontinued if such signs or symptoms appear. (See Drug Interactions: Antipsychotic Agents, in the monograph on Lithium Salts 28:28.)

■ **Metrizamide** Animal studies suggest an increased risk of seizures when metrizamide (no longer commercially available in the US) is administered concurrently with drugs that lower the seizure threshold; however, the clinical importance of such an interaction has not been clearly established. The manufacturers have stated that phenothiazines should not be used in patients receiving metrizamide. Phenothiazines should be discontinued, if possible, at least 48 hours before and for at least 24–48 hours after administration of metrizamide. The manufacturers also stated that phenothiazines should not be used for the control of metrizamide-induced nausea and vomiting. However, if vomiting is severe, some clinicians believe that the benefit of a single dose of a phenothiazine may outweigh the low risk of seizures.

■ **Drugs Affecting Hepatic Microsomal Enzymes** Concomitant use of phenothiazines that are metabolized by the cytochrome P-450 (CYP) 2D6 isoenzyme (e.g., perphenazine, thioridazine) with drugs that inhibit the activity of CYP2D6 may increase plasma concentrations of the phenothiazine. (See Pharmacokinetics: Elimination.) Drugs that inhibit CYP2D6 activity include some of the tricyclic antidepressants and selective serotonin-reuptake inhibitors (e.g., fluoxetine, sertraline, paroxetine). Because thioridazine has been shown to prolong the QT interval corrected for rate (QT_c) in a dose-dependent manner, increased plasma concentrations of the drug may be expected to augment such prolongation and thus may increase the risk of serious, potentially fatal, cardiac arrhythmias (e.g., atypical ventricular tachycardia [torsades de pointes]). Therefore, concomitant use of thioridazine with drugs that inhibit the CYP2D6 isoenzyme is contraindicated. In patients receiving other phenothiazines (e.g., perphenazine), close monitoring is essential and dose reduction may be necessary to avoid toxicity if a drug that inhibits the activity of CYP2D6 is added to the existing drug regimen. In such patients, lower than usual dosages of either the phenothiazine or the other drug may be required.

■ **Other Drugs** The possibility that concomitant use of drugs that can reduce the clearance of thioridazine by other mechanisms (e.g., fluvoxamine, propranolol, pindolol) may result in accumulation of potentially cardiotoxic concentrations of this phenothiazine should be considered. The manufacturers of thioridazine state that concomitant use of thioridazine with such drugs is contraindicated. In addition, although specific drug interaction studies have not been performed to evaluate the concomitant use of thioridazine with drugs that prolong the QT_c interval, the manufacturers state that additive effects of such concomitant therapy on the QT_c interval can be expected and therefore such use is contraindicated. For additional information, see Drug Interactions in Thioridazine 28:16.08.24.

Laboratory Test Interferences

Urinary metabolites of phenothiazines may cause the urine to darken and result in false-positive test results for urobilinogen, amylase, uroporphyrins, porphobilinogens, and 5-hydroxyindolacetic acid. False-positive test results for phenylketonuria (PKU) may also occur during phenothiazine use.

False-positive pregnancy test (e.g., frog test, Gravindex®, HCG test, Pregnosticon®, UCG test) results have reportedly occurred in some patients receiving phenothiazines.

Acute Toxicity

■ **Manifestations** In general, overdosage of phenothiazines may be expected to produce effects that are extensions of common adverse reactions; severe extrapyramidal reactions, hypotension, and sedation have been the principal effects reported. CNS depression progressing to coma with areflexia or CNS stimulation with convulsions followed by respiratory depression may occur; patients with early or mild intoxication may experience drowsiness, restlessness, disorientation, confusion, and excitement. Other reported effects associated with acute phenothiazine overdosage have included shock (e.g., ECG changes and cardiac arrhythmias), increased QT and PR intervals, non-specific ST and T wave changes, bradycardia, sinus tachycardia, bilateral bundle branch block, atrioventricular block, ventricular tachycardia, ventricular fibrillation, torsades de pointes, myocardial depression, agitation, dry skin, nasal congestion, urinary retention, oliguria, uremia, blurred vision, hypothermia, hyperthermia, mydriasis, miosis, tremor, muscle twitching, spasm or rigidity, seizures, muscular hypotonia, constipation, ileus, dry mouth, vomiting, difficulty in swallowing or breathing, cyanosis, and respiratory and/or vasomotor collapse, and pulmonary edema, possibly with sudden apnea.

■ **Treatment** Treatment of phenothiazine overdosage generally involves symptomatic and supportive care. There is no specific antidote for phenothiazine intoxication; however, anticholinergic antiparkinsonian drugs may be useful in controlling extrapyramidal reactions associated with phenothiazine overdosage. Following acute ingestion of the drugs, the stomach should be emptied by gastric lavage and consideration also should be given to repeated doses of activated charcoal. If the patient is comatose, having seizures or a dystonic reaction, or lacks the gag reflex, gastric lavage may be performed if an endotracheal tube with cuff inflated is in place to prevent aspiration of gastric contents. Gastric lavage may be useful even several hours after the drug has been ingested, since GI motility may be greatly reduced following overdosage of phenothiazines. Induction of emesis should generally *not* be attempted, since a phenothiazine-induced dystonic reaction of the head or neck may result in aspiration of vomitus during emesis. Administration of a saline cathartic may be beneficial in enhancing evacuation of the drug from the GI tract.

Cardiovascular monitoring should begin immediately and should include continuous ECG monitoring to detect possible arrhythmias. Treatment may include correction of electrolyte abnormalities and acid-base balance, lidocaine, phenytoin, isoproterenol, ventricular pacing, and defibrillation. Antiarrhythmic agents that can prolong the QT interval (e.g., class IA [disopyramide, procainamide, quinidine] or III agents) should be *avoided* in treating overdosage-associated arrhythmias in which prolongation of QT_c is a manifestation. Appropriate therapy (IV fluids and a vasopressor) should be instituted if hypotension occurs; epinephrine, bretylium, or dopamine should *not* be used (see Cautions: Cardiovascular Effects). For the management of refractory hypotension, vasopressors such as phenylephrine, levarterenol, or metaraminol may be used. Appropriate therapy should be instituted if excessive sedation occurs; CNS stimulants that may cause seizures should be avoided. If seizures occur, treatment should not include barbiturates because these drugs may potentiate phenothiazine-induced respiratory depression. Hypothermia is common and sometimes difficult to control. In some patients with acute toxicity, exchange transfusions may be useful, but hemodialysis, forced diuresis, hemoperfusion, or manipulation of urine pH is of little value in enhancing elimination of phenothiazines.

Pharmacology

Phenothiazines are conventional (first-generation, prototypical) antipsychotic agents. The drugs also have been described as neuroleptic agents because of their ability to induce the neuroleptic syndrome (i.e., depressed initiative, decreased affect, disinterest in surroundings, suppression of complex behavior and spontaneous movements, decreased aggressiveness and impulsivity, decreased psychotic symptoms, extrapyramidal activity).

Phenothiazine, the structural prototype of the phenothiazines, has been used as a urinary tract antiseptic and as an anthelmintic; however, the toxicity of the drug in producing anemia, hepatitis, and skin reactions precludes its use in humans. Phenothiazine is still used as an anthelmintic in veterinary medicine and as an insecticide.

The development of phenothiazine derivatives as psychopharmacologic agents resulted from the observation that certain phenothiazine antihistaminic compounds produced sedation. In an attempt to enhance the sedative effects of these drugs, promethazine and chlorpromazine were synthesized.

Chlorpromazine is the pharmacologic prototype of the phenothiazines. The pharmacology of phenothiazines is complex, and because of their actions on the central and autonomic nervous systems, the drugs affect many different sites in the body. Although the actions of the various phenothiazines are generally similar, these drugs differ both quantitatively and qualitatively in the extent to which they produce specific pharmacologic effects.

■ **Nervous System Effects** In the CNS, phenothiazines act principally at the subcortical levels of the reticular formation, limbic system, and hypothalamus. Phenothiazines generally do not produce substantial cortical depression; however, there is minimal information on the specific effects of phenothiazines at the cortical level. Phenothiazines also act in the basal ganglia, exhibiting extrapyramidal effects.

The precise mechanism(s) of action, including antipsychotic action, of phenothiazines has not been determined, but may be principally related to antidopaminergic effects of the drugs. There is evidence to indicate that phenothiazines antagonize dopamine-mediated neurotransmission at the synapses. There is also some evidence that phenothiazines may block postsynaptic dopamine receptor sites. However, it has not been determined whether the antipsychotic effect of the drugs is causally related to their antidopaminergic effects. Phenothiazines also have peripheral and/or central antagonistic activity against α-adrenergic, serotonergic, histaminic (H_1-receptors), and muscarinic receptors. Phenothiazines also have some adrenergic activity, since they block the reuptake of monoamines at the presynaptic neuronal membrane, which tends to enhance neurotransmission. The effects of phenothiazines on the autonomic nervous system are complex and unpredictable because the drugs exhibit varying degrees of α-adrenergic blocking, muscarinic blocking, and adrenergic activity. The antipsychotic activity of phenothiazines may be related to any or all of these effects, but it has been suggested that the drugs' effects on dopamine are probably most important. It has also been suggested that effects of phenothiazines on other amines (e.g., γ-aminobutyric acid [GABA]) or peptides (e.g., substance P, endorphins) may contribute to their antipsychotic effect. Further study is needed to determine the role of central neuronal receptor antagonism and of effects on biochemical mediators in the antipsychotic action of the phenothiazines and other antipsychotic agents.

Phenothiazines produce varying degrees of sedation without hypnosis or anesthesia in normal and psychotic patients; however, the drugs potentiate the CNS depressant actions of sedatives, hypnotics, and anesthetics. (See Drug Interactions: CNS Depressants.) Tolerance to the sedative effects develops over a period of days or weeks during long-term therapy. Phenothiazines increase total sleep time, tend to normalize sleep disturbances in psychotic patients, and decrease rapid eye movement (REM) sleep. Phenothiazines may cause EEG changes, including a slowing of the EEG pattern and an increase in *theta*- and *delta*-wave activity. Some decrease in fast-wave and *alpha*-wave activity also occurs. Phenothiazines also may lower the seizure threshold and induce discharge patterns associated with seizure disorders; overt seizures may occur in patients with a history of seizure disorders or an underlying condition that predisposes the patient to seizure development.

Although the exact mechanism(s) of action has not been conclusively determined, phenothiazines have an antiemetic effect. The antiemetic activity may be mediated via a direct effect of the drugs on the medullary chemoreceptor trigger zone (CTZ), apparently by blocking dopamine receptors in the CTZ. Phenothiazines inhibit the central and peripheral effects of apomorphine and ergot alkaloids. Phenothiazines generally do not inhibit emesis caused by the action of drugs at the nodose ganglion or by local action on the GI tract.

In animals, phenothiazines inhibit conditioned avoidance behaviors and produce catalepsy. The drugs antagonize the behavioral effects mediated by amphetamines and other CNS stimulants. Like many other centrally acting agents, phenothiazines exhibit analgesic activity and potentiate the actions of analgesics.

Phenothiazines have a poikilothermic effect, interfering with temperature regulation in the hypothalamus; depending on environmental conditions, hypothermia or hyperthermia may occur.

Therapeutic dosages of phenothiazines have little effect on respiration; however, phenothiazines enhance the respiratory depression produced by other CNS depressants. (See Drug Interactions: CNS Depressants.)

The peripheral anticholinergic activity of phenothiazines is relatively weak; however, anticholinergic effects (e.g., dry mouth, blurred vision, urinary retention, constipation) have been associated with their use in some patients. (See Cautions: Nervous System Effects.)

■ **Cardiovascular Effects** The cardiovascular effects of phenothiazines are complex because the drugs exert both direct and indirect actions on the heart and vasculature. Phenothiazines exhibit peripheral α-adrenergic blocking activity and cause vasodilation. Following IV administration, the drugs cause orthostatic hypotension and reflex tachycardia; following oral administration, the drugs cause mild hypotension. (See Cautions: Precautions and Contraindications.) In addition, phenothiazines exert a negative inotropic effect at therapeutic dosages. The drugs may increase coronary blood flow as a result of an increase in heart rate.

Although phenothiazines do *not* appear to have clinically important antiarrhythmic properties at therapeutic dosages, transient antiarrhythmic effects have been observed in some patients at high concentrations. Antiarrhythmic effects may result from either a direct quinidine-like property or a local anesthetic effect of the drugs. Minimal ECG changes, including prolongation of the QT and PR intervals, blunting of T waves, and ST-segment depression, have occurred in some patients receiving phenothiazines. (See Cautions: Cardiovascular Effects.)

■ **Endocrine Effects** Phenothiazines may affect the endocrine system. Phenothiazines induce secretion of prolactin from the anterior pituitary by inhibiting dopamine receptors in the pituitary and hypothalamus. Elevated prolactin concentrations generally persist during long-term administration and may be associated with galactorrhea, menstrual cycle changes (e.g., oligomenorrhea, amenorrhea), and gynecomastia. In contrast to the phenothiazines and other typical antipsychotic drugs, clozapine generally produces little or no elevation of prolactin concentration at usual dosages in humans. (See Pharmacology: Neuroendocrine Effects, in Clozapine 28:16.08.04.)

Phenothiazines may decrease urinary concentrations of gonadotropin, estrogen, and progestins in some patients. Although the exact mechanism is not known, phenothiazines may decrease secretion of vasopressin and corticotropin.

■ **Other Effects** Phenothiazines may have anti-inflammatory and antipruritic effects, resulting from antagonism of various mediator substances (e.g., serotonin, histamine, bradykinin). At high concentrations, phenothiazines also have a membrane-stabilizing property, which can be manifested as a local anesthetic effect or as a direct quinidine-like effect on the heart.

Pharmacokinetics

■ **Absorption** Phenothiazines are generally well absorbed from the GI tract and from parenteral sites; however, absorption may be erratic, particularly following oral administration. Considerable interindividual variations in peak plasma concentrations have been reported. The variability may result from genetic differences in the rate of metabolism, biodegradation of the drug in the GI lumen, and/or metabolism of the drug during absorption (in the GI mucosa) and first pass through the liver. Plasma concentrations of some phenothiazine derivatives (e.g., perphenazine, thioridazine) that are metabolized by the cytochrome P-450 (CYP) microsomal enzyme system, particularly the CYP2D6 isoenzyme, may be elevated in patients with the poor-metabolizer phenotype. (See Pharmacokinetics: Elimination.) Such elevations may vary depending on the fraction of the drug that is metabolized by the CYP2D6 isoenzyme. Poor metabolizers may have an increased risk of adverse effects (e.g., cardiac toxicity) when receiving phenothiazines that are metabolized principally by CYP2D6. (See Drug Interactions: Drugs Affecting Hepatic Microsomal Enzymes.) Although not clearly established for all derivatives, some phenothiazines (e.g., chlorpromazine) and their metabolites undergo enterohepatic circulation. (See Pharmacokinetics: Elimination.)

Therapeutic ranges for plasma drug concentrations of phenothiazines and the relationship of plasma concentrations to clinical response and toxicity have not been clearly established.

■ **Distribution** Phenothiazines and their metabolites are distributed into most body tissues and fluids, with high concentrations being distributed into the brain, lungs, liver, kidneys, and spleen.

Phenothiazines are highly bound to plasma proteins.

Phenothiazines readily cross the placenta. It is not known if the drugs are distributed into milk; however, the size of the molecules and their ability to readily cross the blood-brain barrier suggest that the drugs would be distributed into milk.

■ **Elimination** Although the exact metabolic fate of phenothiazines has not been clearly established, the drugs are extensively metabolized, principally in the liver via hydroxylation, oxidation, demethylation, sulfoxide formation, and conjugation with glucuronic acid; metabolic alterations in the side chain also may occur. Some phenothiazine derivatives (e.g., perphenazine, thioridazine) are metabolized by the cytochrome P-450 (CYP) 2D6 isoenzyme, which is under genetic control. The ability to metabolize phenothiazines via CYP2D6 is associated with the ability to oxidatively metabolize debrisoquin. Approximately 7–10% of Caucasians and a low percentage of Asians have little or no ability to oxidatively metabolize debrisoquin and exhibit the poor-metabolizer phenotype. The percentage of extensive- and poor-metabolizer phenotypes among other populations has not been precisely determined. Individuals who extensively metabolize drugs via the CYP2D6 pathway exhibit the extensive-metabolizer phenotype, while those who have an impaired ability to metabolize the drugs by this pathway exhibit the poor-metabolizer phenotype. Individuals with the poor-metabolizer phenotype will metabolize phenothiazine derivatives (e.g., perphenazine, thioridazine) that are metabolized by CYP2D6 more slowly and will experience higher concentrations at usual dosages compared with those exhibiting the extensive-metabolizer phenotype. Because increased plasma concentrations of thioridazine may be expected to augment QT interval prolongation and thus may increase the risk of serious, potentially fatal, cardiac arrhythmias (e.g., atypical ventricular tachycardia [torsades de pointes]), use of the drug is contraindicated in patients with the poor-metabolizer phenotype.

Most metabolites of phenothiazines are pharmacologically inactive; however, certain metabolites (e.g., 7-hydroxychlorpromazine, mesoridazine) show moderate pharmacologic activity and may contribute to the action of the drugs. There is limited evidence to indicate that some phenothiazines (e.g., chlorpromazine) may induce their own metabolism.

Phenothiazines and their metabolites are excreted in urine and feces; the excretory patterns have not been fully characterized. The drugs are excreted in the feces via biliary elimination, principally as metabolites, and also appear to undergo enterohepatic circulation. Certain metabolites and unchanged drugs have been detected in urine in some patients for up to 6 months following discontinuance of therapy with a phenothiazine derivative.

Chemistry and Stability

■ **Chemistry** Phenothiazines are conventional (prototypical, first-generation) antipsychotic agents. Phenothiazine is the structural prototype of the phenothiazines. Phenothiazine derivatives differ by substitution of various alkylamino groups on the nitrogen atom at the 10 position of the basic phenothiazine nucleus, and may be classified on the basis of the substituent as follows:

ETHYLAMINO DERIVATIVES
ethopropazine
promethazine
propiomazine

PROPYLAMINO DERIVATIVES

chlorpromazine	triflupromazine
methotrimeprazine	trimeprazine
promazine	

PROPYLPIPERAZINE DERIVATIVES

acetophenazine	prochlorperazine
fluphenazine	thiethylperazine
perphenazine	trifluoperazine

ALKYLPIPERIDINE DERIVATIVES
thioridazine

MISCELLANEOUS ALKYL NITROGEN DERIVATIVES
methdilazine

The chemical group at the 10 position of the phenothiazine nucleus appears to determine the antipsychotic efficacy; compounds with 3 carbons between the 2 nitrogens have increased inhibitory effects on conditioned avoidance behaviors and enhanced α-adrenergic blocking activity, whereas compounds with 2 carbons between the nitrogens have predominantly antihistaminic activity. Substitution at the 2 position of the phenothiazine nucleus generally alters the potency and the incidence and/or severity of adverse effects associated with these drugs. The substituents at the 2 position of the phenothiazine nucleus have approximately the following order of relative potency: CF_3 > Cl > H approximately equal to OCH_3 approximately equal to $CONHNH_2$.

Phenothiazine derivatives are strong amines and have alkaline properties. These drugs usually are commercially available as salts of various acids and have a wide range of solubility in water and in alcohol.

■ **Stability** Commercially available preparations of phenothiazine derivatives should be stored in tight, light-resistant containers at a temperature less than 40°C, preferably between 15–30°C, unless otherwise specified by the manufacturer; freezing of the oral solutions and injections should be avoided. Slight yellowish discoloration of the oral solutions or injections will not affect potency or efficacy, but they should not be used if markedly discolored or if a precipitate is present. Oral solutions of phenothiazine derivatives should be dispensed in amber glass bottles.

Phenothiazine derivative injections are physically and/or chemically incompatible with some drugs, but the compatibility depends on several factors (e.g., concentrations of the drugs, specific diluents used, resulting pH, temperature). Specialized references should be consulted for specific compatibility information.

For further information on chemistry and stability, pharmacology, pharmacokinetics, uses, cautions, and dosage and administration of phenothiazine derivatives, see the individual monographs in 28:16.08.24.

†Use is not currently included in the labeling approved by the US Food and Drug Administration

chlorproMAZINE Hydrochloride

■ Chlorpromazine hydrochloride is a phenothiazine antipsychotic agent.

Uses

■ **Psychotic Disorders** Chlorpromazine hydrochloride is used for the symptomatic management of psychotic disorders. Drug therapy is integral to the management of acute psychotic episodes in patients with schizophrenia and generally is required for long-term stabilization to improve symptoms between episodes and to minimize the risk of recurrent acute episodes. Antipsychotic agents are the principal class of drugs used for the management of all phases of schizophrenia and generally are effective in all subtypes of the disorder and subgroups of patients. Patient response and tolerance to antipsychotic agents are variable, and patients who do not respond to or tolerate one drug may be successfully treated with an agent from a different class or with a different adverse effect profile. For additional information on the symptomatic management of schizophrenia, see Uses: Psychotic Disorders, in the Phenothiazines General Statement 28:16.08.24.

■ **Other Uses** Chlorpromazine is used for the prevention and treatment of nausea and vomiting; for relief of restlessness and apprehension before surgery; for acute intermittent porphyria; as an adjunct in the treatment of tetanus; for the symptomatic management of the manic phase of bipolar disorder; and for relief of intractable hiccups.

Chlorpromazine is also used for the treatment of severe behavioral problems in children marked by combativeness and/or explosive hyperexcitable behavior (out of proportion to immediate provocations), and for the short-term treatment of hyperactive children who exhibit excessive motor activity with accompanying conduct disorders that are manifested as impulsivity, difficulty sustaining attention, aggression, mood lability, and/or poor frustration tolerance. However, the possible risks of tardive dyskinesia, withdrawal dyskinesia, and other extrapyramidal reactions associated with the drug should be considered. Some clinicians recommend routine administration of the Abnormal Involuntary Movement Scale (AIMS) to all children receiving antipsychotic agents for this indication.

Chlorpromazine may be effective in controlling anxiety, tension, and agitation which occur in neuroses. Further studies are needed to establish the efficacy of the drug for this use.

Dosage and Administration

■ **Administration** Chlorpromazine hydrochloride may be administered orally, by deep IM or direct IV injection, or by IV infusion. Direct IV injection is intended for use only during surgery to control nausea and vomiting and in the adjunctive treatment of tetanus. IV infusion is only intended for use in the adjunctive treatment of intractable hiccups in adults. Subcutaneous administration of the drug is *not* recommended because of local irritation. Parenteral therapy should be reserved for recumbent patients; however, if cautions are taken to avoid orthostatic hypotension (i.e., patient remains recumbent for at least 30 minutes after injection), acutely agitated ambulatory patients may receive the drug IM.

For IM administration, injection should be made slowly, deep into a large muscle mass such as the upper outer quadrant of the gluteus maximus; if irritation at the IM injection site is a problem, the drug can be diluted with 0.9% sodium chloride injection or 2% procaine hydrochloride. For direct IV injection, chlorpromazine hydrochloride injection should be diluted with 0.9% sodium chloride injection to a concentration not exceeding 1 mg/mL and administered at a rate of 1 mg/minute in adults and 0.5 mg/minute in children. IV administration of undiluted chlorpromazine hydrochloride injection should be avoided. For IV infusion, chlorpromazine hydrochloride injection should be added to 500–1000 mL of 0.9% sodium chloride injection and administered slowly.

■ **Dosage** Dosage of chlorpromazine hydrochloride is expressed in terms of the hydrochloride salt.

The manufacturers state that the 100- and 200-mg tablets of chlorpromazine hydrochloride are intended for use in patients with severe neuropsychiatric conditions.

Dosage must be carefully adjusted according to individual requirements and response, using the lowest possible effective dosage. Dosage should be increased more gradually in debilitated, emaciated, or geriatric patients. Since geriatric patients may be more susceptible to hypotension and neuromuscular reactions, these patients should be observed closely; in general, dosages in the lower end of the range are sufficient for most geriatric patients. Because of the risk of adverse reactions associated with cumulative effects of phenothiazines, patients with a history of long-term therapy with chlorpromazine and/or other antipsychotic agents should be evaluated periodically to determine whether maintenance dosage should be decreased or drug therapy discontinued. Chlorpromazine should generally *not* be used in children younger than 6 months of age unless the condition to be treated is potentially life-threatening; dosage in this age group has not been established.

Psychotic Disorders and Excessive Anxiety, Tension, and Agitation **Adult Dosage.** For the symptomatic management of psychotic disorders in non-hospitalized patients with relatively mild symptomatology and for the management of excessive anxiety, tension, and agitation, the usual initial adult oral dosage of chlorpromazine hydrochloride is 30–75 mg daily given in 2–4 divided doses. For non-hospitalized patients with moderate to severe symptomatology, the usual initial adult oral dosage is 25 mg 3 times daily. After 1 or 2 days, dosage may be gradually increased twice weekly by 20–50 mg until symptoms are controlled. Although symptomatic relief may be seen in many patients during the first week of therapy, optimum therapeutic response may not occur for weeks or even months in some severely disturbed or symptomatic patients. Once an optimum dosage is achieved, this dosage should be continued for 2 weeks and then gradually reduced to the lowest possible effective dosage. In adult patients with excessive anxiety, tension, and agitation, the usual oral dosage during prolonged maintenance therapy is 200 mg daily; however, oral dosages up to 800 mg daily may be required in some patients (e.g., discharged psychiatric patients).

For prompt control of severe symptoms in non-hospitalized patients or in patients with anxiety, tension, and agitation, an IM chlorpromazine hydrochloride dose of 25 mg may be given initially; this dose may be repeated in 1 hour, if necessary. After the patient's symptoms are controlled, oral therapy should replace parenteral therapy at a dosage of 25–50 mg 3 times daily.

For the symptomatic management of psychotic disorders in hospitalized patients who are acutely agitated, manic, or disturbed, the usual initial adult IM dose of chlorpromazine hydrochloride is 25 mg. Additional IM doses of 25–50 mg may be given in 1 hour, if necessary. Subsequent IM dosage should be gradually increased over several days to a maximum of 400 mg every 4–6 hours until symptoms are controlled. Usually, patients become quiet and cooperative within 24–48 hours after initiation of therapy; oral therapy should replace parenteral therapy and dosage should be increased until the patient is calm. Oral dosages of 500 mg daily are generally sufficient in most patients. Although oral dosages greater than 2 g daily may be required in some patients, there is usually little therapeutic gain achieved by exceeding dosages of 1 g daily for extended periods. For hospitalized patients who are less acutely agitated, the usual initial adult oral dosage of chlorpromazine hydrochloride is 25 mg 3 times daily. Subsequent dosage should be gradually increased until optimum therapeutic response is obtained, but should usually not exceed 400 mg daily.

Pediatric Dosage. The usual initial oral dosage of chlorpromazine hydrochloride for the management of psychotic disorders and behavioral problems in children 6 months of age or older is 0.55 mg/kg every 4–6 hours as necessary.

The usual initial IM dosage of chlorpromazine hydrochloride for the management of psychotic disorders and behavioral problems in children 6 months of age or older is 0.55 mg/kg every 6–8 hours as necessary. Subsequent dosage may be gradually increased as necessary.

Higher dosages (50–100 mg daily) may be necessary in children with severe behavior disorders or psychotic conditions; older children may require 200 mg daily. There is little evidence that improvement in behavior in severely disturbed mentally retarded children is further enhanced at oral dosages greater than 500 mg daily. Maximum IM dosage of chlorpromazine hydrochloride in children younger than 5 years of age and in those weighing less than 22.7 kg is 40 mg daily; maximum IM dosage in children 5–12 years of age and weighing 22.7–45.5 kg should not exceed 75 mg daily, except in unmanageable patients.

Nausea and Vomiting **Adult Dosage.** For the prevention and treatment of nausea and vomiting in patients who can tolerate oral administration of the drug, the usual initial adult oral dosage of chlorpromazine hydrochloride is 10–25 mg every 4–6 hours as necessary; dosage may be increased if necessary. The usual adult rectal dosage for the prevention and control of nausea and vomiting is 100 mg every 6–8 hours as necessary; in some patients, 50 mg every 6–8 hours will be adequate. The usual initial adult IM dose of chlorpromazine hydrochloride for the control of nausea and vomiting is 25 mg. If hypotension does not occur, additional IM doses of 25–50 mg may be administered as necessary every 3–4 hours until symptoms subside; oral therapy should then replace parenteral therapy if necessary.

Pediatric Dosage. For the prevention and treatment of nausea and vomiting in children 6 months of age or older, the usual oral dosage of chlorpromazine hydrochloride is 0.55 mg/kg every 4–6 hours.

The usual initial IM dosage of chlorpromazine hydrochloride for the control of nausea and vomiting in these children is 0.55 mg/kg every 6–8 hours as necessary. Subsequent dosage should be carefully adjusted according to the severity of symptoms and the patient's response. Maximum IM dosage of chlorpromazine hydrochloride in children younger than 5 years of age and in those weighing less than 22.7 kg is 40 mg daily; maximum IM dosage in children 5–12 years of age and weighing 22.7–45.5 kg should not exceed 75 mg daily, except in severe cases.

Intermittent Porphyria For acute intermittent porphyria, the usual adult oral dosage of chlorpromazine hydrochloride is 25–50 mg 3 or 4 times daily. The usual adult IM dosage of chlorpromazine hydrochloride for acute intermittent porphyria is 25 mg 3 or 4 times daily. Oral therapy should replace parenteral therapy as soon as the patient can tolerate oral administration of the drug. Therapy can usually be discontinued after several weeks; however, maintenance therapy may be required in some patients.

Intractable Hiccups For relief of intractable hiccups, the usual adult oral dosage of chlorpromazine hydrochloride is 25–50 mg 3 or 4 times daily. If symptoms persist for 2–3 days, 25–50 mg may be given IM. If hiccups continue, 25–50 mg of the drug may be administered by slow IV infusion (see Dosage and Administration: Administration) with the patient in a supine position. Blood pressure should be closely monitored during IV administration of chlorpromazine.

Tetanus For adjunctive treatment of tetanus, the usual initial adult IM dosage of chlorpromazine hydrochloride is 25–50 mg 3 or 4 times daily, usually in conjunction with barbiturates. The usual adult direct IV dose of the drug is 25–50 mg. (See Dosage and Administration: Administration.) The usual IM or direct IV dosage of chlorpromazine hydrochloride for adjunctive treatment of tetanus in children 6 months of age or older is 0.55 mg/kg every 6–8 hours. Maximum parenteral dosage of chlorpromazine hydrochloride in children weighing less than 22.7 kg is 40 mg daily; maximum parenteral dosage in children weighing 22.7–45.5 kg should not exceed 75 mg daily, except in severe cases.

Surgery For relief of restlessness and apprehension before surgery, the usual adult oral dose of chlorpromazine hydrochloride is 25–50 mg given 2–3 hours before surgery. The usual adult IM dose is 12.5–25 mg given 1–2 hours before surgery. For relief of restlessness and apprehension before surgery in children 6 months of age or older, the usual oral or IM dose of chlorpromazine hydrochloride is 0.55 mg/kg administered 2–3 or 1–2 hours before surgery, respectively.

To control acute nausea and vomiting during surgery, the usual adult IM dose of chlorpromazine hydrochloride is 12.5 mg; this dose may be repeated in 30 minutes, if necessary and if hypotension does not occur. Alternatively during surgery in adults, fractional 2-mg doses may be given IV at 2-minute intervals up to a maximum total dose of 25 mg. To control acute nausea and vomiting during surgery in children 6 months of age or older, the usual IM dose of chlorpromazine hydrochloride is 0.275 mg/kg; this dose may be repeated in 30 minutes, if necessary and if hypotension does not occur. Alternatively during surgery in these children, fractional 1-mg doses may be given IV at 2-minute intervals up to a total dose of 0.275 mg/kg; if after 30 minutes it is necessary to readminister the drug and if hypotension does not occur, the fractional IV dosage regimen may be repeated.

Following surgery, the usual adult oral dosage of chlorpromazine hydrochloride is 10–25 mg every 4–6 hours as necessary. The usual adult IM dose of chlorpromazine hydrochloride following surgery is 12.5–25 mg; this dose may be repeated in 1 hour, if necessary and if hypotension does not occur. Following surgery in children 6 months of age or older, the usual initial oral or IM dose of chlorpromazine hydrochloride is 0.55 mg/kg. The initial oral dose may be repeated every 4–6 hours as needed; the initial IM dose may be repeated in 1 hour, if necessary and if hypotension does not occur.

Cautions

Chlorpromazine hydrochloride shares the toxic potentials of other phenothiazines, and the usual precautions of phenothiazine therapy should be observed. (See Cautions in the Phenothiazines General Statement 28:16.08.24.)

Geriatric patients with dementia-related psychosis treated with either conventional (first-generation) or atypical (second-generation) antipsychotic agents are at an increased risk of mortality. For additional information on the use of antipsychotic agents for dementia-associated psychosis and other behavioral disturbances, see Geriatric Considerations under Psychotic Disorders: Schizophrenia and Other Psychotic Disorders, in Uses and see Cautions: Geriatric Precautions, in the Phenothiazines General Statement 28:16.08.24.

Care should be taken to avoid skin contact with chlorpromazine hydrochloride injection, since contact dermatitis has occurred rarely.

Commercially available chlorpromazine hydrochloride injection contains sulfites that may cause allergic-type reactions, including anaphylaxis and life-threatening or less severe asthmatic episodes, in certain susceptible individuals. The overall prevalence of sulfite sensitivity in the general population is unknown but probably low; such sensitivity appears to occur more frequently in asthmatic than in nonasthmatic individuals.

Safety and efficacy of chlorpromazine in children younger than 6 months of age have not been established; the manufacturers recommend that the drug should generally *not* be used in these children unless the condition to be treated is potentially life-threatening. Chlorpromazine should not be used in conditions for which a pediatric dosage has not been established.

Pharmacology

The principal pharmacologic effects of chlorpromazine hydrochloride are similar to those of other propylamino derivatives of phenothiazine. Chlorpromazine has strong anticholinergic and sedative effects and moderate extrapyramidal effects. Chlorpromazine has strong antiemetic and adrenergic blocking activity and weak ganglionic blocking, antihistaminic, and antiserotonergic activity.

Pharmacokinetics

■ **Absorption** Chlorpromazine hydrochloride is rapidly absorbed from the GI tract and from parenteral sites of injection; however, following oral administration, the drug undergoes considerable metabolism during absorption (in the GI mucosa) and first pass through the liver. Although not clearly established in humans, chlorpromazine and its metabolites undergo enterohepatic circulation in animals. (See Pharmacokinetics: Elimination.)

Considerable interindividual variations in peak plasma concentrations have been reported with the same oral dose of chlorpromazine. The variability is thought to result from wide interindividual variation in bioavailability, apparently because of genetic differences in the rate of first-pass metabolism. As a result of first-pass metabolism, less chlorpromazine reaches systemic circulation as unchanged drug, and peak plasma chlorpromazine concentrations are much lower following oral administration than following IM administration.

Following oral administration of chlorpromazine hydrochloride in a tablet formulation, the onset of pharmacologic action occurs within 30–60 minutes; the duration of action is 4–6 hours.

The therapeutic range for plasma chlorpromazine concentrations and the relationship of plasma concentration to clinical response and toxicity have not been clearly established.

■ **Distribution** Chlorpromazine is widely distributed into most body tissues and fluids. Chlorpromazine crosses the blood-brain barrier, and concentrations of the drug in the brain are higher than those in plasma.

Chlorpromazine is 92–97% bound to plasma proteins, principally albumin, at plasma chlorpromazine concentrations of 0.01–1 mcg/mL.

Chlorpromazine and its metabolites cross the placenta and are distributed into milk.

■ **Elimination** Although the exact metabolic fate of chlorpromazine is not clearly established, the drug is extensively metabolized, principally in the liver and kidneys. About 10–12 metabolites which occur in humans in appreciable quantities have been identified. In addition to hydroxylation at positions 3 and 7 of the phenothiazine nucleus, the *N*-dimethylaminopropyl side chain of chlorpromazine undergoes demethylation and is also metabolized to an *N*-oxide. Two principal groups of metabolites have been found in urine. The unconjugated fraction, which represents approximately 20% of chlorpromazine and its metabolites excreted in urine, consists of unchanged drug, demonomethylchlorpromazine, dedimethylchlorpromazine, their sulfoxide metabolites, and chlorpromazine-*N*-oxide. The conjugated fraction, which represents approximately 80% of chlorpromazine and its metabolites excreted in urine, consists principally of *O*-glucuronides, with small amounts of ethereal sulfates of the mono- and dihydroxy-derivatives of chlorpromazine and their sulfoxide metabolites. The major metabolites found in urine are the monoglucuronide of *N*-dedimethylchlorpromazine and 7-hydroxychlorpromazine.

Following a single oral chlorpromazine dose of 120 mg/m^2 to 4 healthy men, less than 1% of the dose was excreted in urine as unchanged drug within 72 hours, with most urinary excretion of unchanged drug occurring within 6 hours. Following continuous oral administration of chlorpromazine to a limited number of psychiatric patients in a dosage ranging from 0.1–1.4 g daily, an average of 37% of the dose was excreted in urine, principally as metabolites. In blacks, a relatively high percentage of chlorpromazine is excreted in urine as unconjugated 7-hydroxychlorpromazine; however, in whites, this may be an indication of existing or developing hyperpigmentation of the skin.

Chemistry and Stability

■ **Chemistry** Chlorpromazine hydrochloride is a phenothiazine antipsychotic agent. The drug is a propylamino derivative of phenothiazine and is structurally similar to promazine, but differs from promazine in the substitution of a chlorine atom for hydrogen at the 2 position of the phenothiazine nucleus. Chlorpromazine is commercially available as the hydrochloride salt. Each 111 mg of chlorpromazine hydrochloride is approximately equivalent to 100 mg of chlorpromazine base.

Chlorpromazine occurs as a white, crystalline solid that has an amine odor and is practically insoluble in water and freely soluble in alcohol. Chlorpromazine hydrochloride occurs as a white or slightly creamy white, odorless, very bitter tasting, crystalline powder and has approximate solubilities of 1 g/mL in water and 667 mg/mL in alcohol at 25°C.

Chlorpromazine hydrochloride injection is a sterile solution of the drug in water for injection. The commercially available injection has a pH of 3–5 and may contain benzyl alcohol as a preservative, a sulfite(s), and other excipients.

■ **Stability** Chlorpromazine and its hydrochloride salt darken on prolonged exposure to light. Commercially available preparations of chlorpromazine hydrochloride should therefore be protected from light. Chlorpromazine hydrochloride tablets should be stored in well-closed, light-resistant containers at 20–25°C (excursions permitted to 15–30°C) and protected from moisture. Chlorpromazine hydrochloride injection should be stored at 20–25°C (excursions permitted to 15–30°C); freezing of the injection should be avoided. Slight yellowish discoloration of the injection will not affect potency or efficacy, but it should not be used if markedly discolored or if a precipitate is present. At the time of manufacture, air in the containers of the commercially available chlorpromazine hydrochloride injection is replaced with nitrogen to avoid oxidation. Oxidation of chlorpromazine hydrochloride occurs readily in alkaline media.

Chlorpromazine hydrochloride injection is physically and/or chemically incompatible with some drugs, but the compatibility depends on several factors (e.g., concentrations of the drugs, specific diluents used, resulting pH, temperature). Specialized references should be consulted for specific compatibility information.

For further information on chemistry and stability, pharmacology, pharmacokinetics, uses, cautions, acute toxicity, drug interactions, laboratory test interferences, and dosage and administration of chlorpromazine hydrochloride, see the Phenothiazines General Statement 28:16.08.24.

Preparations

Excipients in commercially available drug preparations may have clinically important effects in some individuals; consult specific product labeling for details.

chlorproMAZINE Hydrochloride

Oral		
Tablets	10 mg*	**chlorproMAZINE Hydrochloride Tablets**
	25 mg*	**chlorproMAZINE Hydrochloride Tablets**
	50 mg*	**chlorproMAZINE Hydrochloride Tablets**
	100 mg*	**chlorproMAZINE Hydrochloride Tablets**
	200 mg*	**chlorproMAZINE Hydrochloride Tablets**
Parenteral		
Injection	25 mg/mL*	**chlorproMAZINE Hydrochloride Injection,** Baxter

*available from one or more manufacturer, distributor, and/or repackager by generic (nonproprietary) name

Prochlorperazine
Prochlorperazine Edisylate
Prochlorperazine Maleate

■ Prochlorperazine is a phenothiazine antipsychotic agent. The drug is considered a conventional or first-generation antipsychotic agent.

Uses

■ **Psychotic Disorders** Prochlorperazine is used for the symptomatic management of psychotic disorders (i.e., schizophrenia). Drug therapy is integral to the management of acute psychotic episodes in patients with schizophrenia and generally is required for long-term stabilization to improve symptoms between episodes and to minimize the risk of recurrent acute episodes. Antipsychotic agents are the principal class of drugs used for the management of all phases of schizophrenia and generally are effective in all subtypes of the disorder and subgroups of patients. Patient response and tolerance to antipsychotic agents are variable, and patients who do not respond to or tolerate one drug may be successfully treated with an agent from a different class or with a different adverse effect profile. For additional information on the symptomatic management of schizophrenia, see Uses: Psychotic Disorders, in the Phenothiazines General Statement 28:16.08.24.

■ **Nonpsychotic Anxiety** Prochlorperazine also is used for the short-term management of nonpsychotic anxiety. Because of the risks of toxicity associated with its use, prochlorperazine should be used only as an alternative to other less toxic anxiolytic agents (e.g., benzodiazepines) in most patients. Since the efficacy of prochlorperazine in the management of nonpsychotic anxiety was established in patients with generalized anxiety disorder, it is not known if the drug will be useful for the management of other nonpsychotic conditions in which anxiety or manifestations that mimic anxiety are evident (e.g., physical illness, organic mental conditions, agitated depression, character pathologies).

■ **Other Uses** Prochlorperazine has not been shown to be effective for the management of behavioral complications in patients with mental retardation.

For the use of prochlorperazine as an antiemetic, see 56:22.08.

Dosage and Administration

■ **Administration** For psychiatric use, prochlorperazine edisylate is administered orally or by deep IM injection. Subcutaneous administration of the drug is *not* recommended because of local irritation. Prochlorperazine maleate is administered orally. Prochlorperazine is administered rectally. Prochlorperazine edisylate is also administered by direct IV injection or by IV infusion in the management of severe nausea and vomiting. (See 56:22.08.)

■ **Dosage** Dosage of prochlorperazine and its salts is expressed in terms of prochlorperazine. Dosage must be carefully adjusted according to individual requirements and response, using the lowest possible effective dosage. Dosage should be increased more gradually in debilitated, emaciated, or geriatric patients. Since geriatric patients may be more susceptible to hypotension and neuromuscular reactions, these patients should be observed closely; in general, dosages in the lower end of the range are sufficient for most geriatric patients. Because of the risk of adverse reactions associated with cumulative effects of phenothiazines, patients with a history of long-term therapy with prochlorperazine and/or other antipsychotic agents should be evaluated periodically to determine whether maintenance dosage could be decreased or drug therapy discontinued. Since children appear to be more prone to extrapyramidal reactions, even at moderate dosages, they should receive the lowest possible effective dosage, and parents should be instructed not to exceed the prescribed dosage.

Psychotic Disorders For the symptomatic management of psychotic disorders, including schizophrenia, in office patients and outpatients with relatively mild symptomatology, the usual adult oral dosage of prochlorperazine is 5 or 10 mg 3 or 4 times daily. For hospitalized or well-supervised patients with moderate to severe symptomatology, the usual initial adult oral dosage of prochlorperazine is 10 mg 3 or 4 times daily. Dosage is then gradually increased every 2 or 3 days until symptoms are controlled or adverse effects become troublesome. Although some patients exhibit optimum response with 50–75 mg daily, dosages up to 150 mg daily may be required in severely disturbed patients. The usual initial oral or rectal dosage of prochlorperazine for the management of psychotic disorders in children 2–12 years of age is 2.5 mg 2 or 3 times daily; total dosage should not exceed 10 mg during the first day. Dosage may then be increased according to the patient's therapeutic response and tolerance, but usually should not exceed 20 and 25 mg daily for children 2–5 and 6–12 years of age, respectively. Dosage for children younger than 2 years of age or those weighing less than 9 kg has not been established.

Symptomatic relief of psychotic disorders may be seen in many patients during the first 2 days of therapy; however, optimum antipsychotic effect usually requires prolonged administration of the drug.

For prompt control of severe psychotic symptoms, the usual adult IM dose of prochlorperazine is 10–20 mg. Although many patients respond shortly after the first dose, it may be necessary to repeat the initial dose every 1–4 hours to control symptoms in some patients. Generally, not more than 3 or 4 doses are required. If, in rare cases, prolonged parenteral therapy is needed, the usual adult IM dosage is 10–20 mg every 4–6 hours. After the patient's symptoms are controlled, oral therapy should replace parenteral therapy at the same dosage level or higher. For prompt control of severe psychotic symptoms, children younger than 12 years of age may be given 0.13 mg/kg IM. Generally, most pediatric patients respond after 1 dose, and oral therapy should replace parenteral therapy at the same dosage level or higher.

Nonpsychotic Anxiety For the short-term management of nonpsychotic anxiety, the usual adult oral dosage of prochlorperazine is 5 mg 3 or 4 times daily. Alternatively, a dosage of 15 mg (as the extended-release Spansule®) once daily upon arising or 10 mg (as the extended-release Spansule®) every 12 hours may be used. Dosage of prochlorperazine in the management of nonpsychotic anxiety should not exceed 20 mg daily nor should the drug be administered for longer than 12 weeks, since the use of higher dosages or longer periods of treatment may result in the development of persistent (and possibly irreversible) tardive dyskinesia.

Cautions

Prochlorperazine shares the toxic potentials of other phenothiazines, and the usual precautions of phenothiazine therapy should be observed. (See Cautions in the Phenothiazines General Statement 28:16.08.24.) The incidence of extrapyramidal reactions associated with prochlorperazine therapy appears to be relatively high in hospitalized psychiatric patients and in children. When preparations containing prochlorperazine maleate in combination with other drugs are administered, the cautions applicable to each ingredient should be considered.

Geriatric patients with dementia-related psychosis treated with either conventional (first-generation) or atypical (second-generation) antipsychotic agents are at an increased risk of mortality. For additional information on the use of antipsychotic agents for dementia-associated psychosis and other behavioral disturbances, see Geriatric Considerations under Psychotic Disorders: Schizophrenia and Other Psychotic Disorders, in Uses and see also Cautions: Geriatric Precautions, in the Phenothiazines General Statement 28:16.08.24.

Care should be taken to avoid skin contact with prochlorperazine edisylate oral solution or injection, since contact dermatitis has occurred rarely.

Safety and efficacy of prochlorperazine in children younger than 2 years of age or those weighing less than 9 kg have not been established.

Use of prochlorperazine should be avoided in children and adolescents with suspected Reye's syndrome, since the antiemetic and potential extrapyramidal effects produced by the drug may obscure the diagnosis of or be confused with the CNS signs of this condition; the drug is also hepatotoxic.

Prochlorperazine should not be used in children during surgery or in conditions for which pediatric dosage has not been established.

Pharmacology

The principal pharmacologic effects of prochlorperazine are similar to those of chlorpromazine. Prochlorperazine has weak anticholinergic effects, moderate sedative effects, and strong extrapyramidal effects. Prochlorperazine has strong antiemetic activity.

Chemistry and Stability

■ **Chemistry** Prochlorperazine is a phenothiazine antipsychotic agent. The drug is a propylpiperazine derivative of phenothiazine. Prochlorperazine is commercially available as the base, edisylate salt, and maleate salt. Each 7.5 mg of prochlorperazine edisylate or 8 mg of prochlorperazine maleate is approximately equivalent to 5 mg of prochlorperazine.

Prochlorperazine occurs as a clear, pale yellow, viscous liquid and is very slightly soluble in water and freely soluble in alcohol. Prochlorperazine edisylate occurs as a white to very light yellow, odorless, crystalline powder and has approximate solubilities of 500 mg/mL in water and 0.67 mg/mL in alcohol at 25°C. Prochlorperazine maleate occurs as a white to pale yellow, practically odorless, crystalline powder and is practically insoluble in water and has a solubility of approximately 0.83 mg/mL in alcohol at 25°C. Prochlorperazine edisylate injection is a sterile solution of the drug in water for injection. The commercially available injection has a pH of 4.2–6.2 and may contain benzyl alcohol as a preservative, and other excipients. The commercially available prochlorperazine edisylate oral solution has a pH of 4.5–5.

■ **Stability** Commercially available preparations of prochlorperazine should be stored in tight, light-resistant containers. Prochlorperazine edisylate oral solutions and injection, and prochlorperazine maleate tablets and extended-release capsules should be stored at a temperature less than 40°C, preferably between 15–30°C; freezing of the oral solutions and injection should be avoided. Prochlorperazine suppositories should be stored at a temperature less than 37°C. Prochlorperazine edisylate injection should be protected from light, which can cause discoloration; if discoloration occurs, the injection should be discarded.

Prochlorperazine edisylate injection is physically and/or chemically incompatible with some drugs, but the compatibility depends on several factors (e.g., concentrations of the drugs, specific diluents used, resulting pH, temperature). Specialized references should be consulted for specific compatibility information.

For further information on chemistry and stability, pharmacology, pharmacokinetics, uses, cautions, acute toxicity, drug interactions, labo-

ratory test interferences, and dosage and administration of prochlorperazine, see the Phenothiazines General Statement 28:16.08.24. For information on the use of prochlorperazine as an antiemetic, see 56:22.08.

Preparations

Excipients in commercially available drug preparations may have clinically important effects in some individuals; consult specific product labeling for details.

Prochlorperazine

Rectal		
Suppositories	2.5 mg	**Compazine®**, GlaxoSmithKline
	5 mg	**Compazine®**, GlaxoSmithKline
	25 mg*	**Compazine®**, GlaxoSmithKline
		Compro®, Paddock
		Prochlorperazine Suppositories

*available from one or more manufacturer, distributor, and/or repackager by generic (nonproprietary) name

Prochlorperazine Edisylate

Oral		
Solution	5 mg (of prochlorperazine) per 5 mL	**Compazine® Syrup**, GlaxoSmithKline
Parenteral		
Injection	5 mg (of prochlorperazine) per mL*	**Compazine®**, GlaxoSmithKline
		Prochlorperazine Edisylate Injection

*available from one or more manufacturer, distributor, and/or repackager by generic (nonproprietary) name

Prochlorperazine Maleate

Oral		
Capsules, extended-release	10 mg (of prochlorperazine)	**Compazine® Spansule®**, GlaxoSmithKline
	15 mg (of prochlorperazine)	**Compazine® Spansule®**, GlaxoSmithKline
Tablets, film-coated	5 mg (of prochlorperazine)*	**Compazine®**, GlaxoSmithKline
		Prochlorperazine Maleate Film-coated Tablets
	10 mg (of prochlorperazine)*	**Compazine®**, GlaxoSmithKline
		Prochlorperazine Maleate Film-coated Tablets

*available from one or more manufacturer, distributor, and/or repackager by generic (nonproprietary) name

ANTIPSYCHOTICS, MISCELLANEOUS 28:16.08.92

Pimozide

■ Pimozide is a diphenylbutylpiperidine-derivative antipsychotic agent. The drug is considered a conventional or first-generation antipsychotic agent.

Uses

■ **Tourette's Syndrome** Pimozide is used for suppression of motor and vocal tics of Tourette's syndrome (Gilles de la Tourette's syndrome).

Pimozide has been used concomitantly with a stimulant in children with tic disorders (e.g., Tourette's syndrome) and comorbid attention deficit hyperactivity disorder (ADHD)† in whom stimulants alone cannot control tics.

Overview Tourette's syndrome is a neurologic genetic disorder with a spectrum of neurobehavioral manifestations that may vary with time and fluctuate in severity and frequency of symptoms during the natural course of the disease. The diagnosis of Tourette's syndrome usually is based on a history and observation of tics often accompanied by behavioral disorders (e.g., ADHD, obsessive-compulsive disorder). Tics may be sudden, brief, intermittent, involuntary, or semivoluntary movements (motor tics) or sounds (phonic or vocal tics). For a diagnosis of Tourette's syndrome, the criteria established by the Tourette Syndrome Classification Study Group may be used. According to this classification, both multiple motor tics and one or more phonic tics must be present at some time during the disease (although not necessarily concurrently), and such tics must occur many times a day and nearly every day, or intermittently, throughout a period of more than 1 year. Motor and phonic tics must be witnessed directly by a reliable examiner some time during the disease or be recorded by video or cinematography. In addition, anatomical location, number, frequency, type, complexity, or severity of tics must undergo a change over time. Involuntary movements and sounds must not be explained by a medical condition other than Tourette's syndrome. Although the onset of the syndrome must occur in patients younger than 21 years of age, in most patients the disease is manifested by 11 years of age, usually beginning in children 2–15 years old. Generally, tics become more severe when patients reach the age of 10 years, and 50% of patients are free from tics by the time they reach the age of 18 years. Severity of tics usually decreases when reaching adulthood. These and other diagnostic criteria are designed to assist clinicians in reaching an accurate diagnosis (e.g., differentiating Tourette's syndrome from other tic disorders) and those investigating the genetic factors associated with the syndrome.

Therapeutic Considerations Initially, management of Tourette's syndrome should include proper education of patients, family members, and teachers in order to provide a proper environment (at home and in school) for children with the disease. Drug therapy usually is considered when symptoms of the disorder begin to interfere with the patient's activities of daily living (e.g., work, school, social activities). Because Tourette's syndrome is associated with a wide variety of neurologic and behavioral manifestations, drug therapy should be individualized and the most severe symptoms should be treated first. The goal in the management of tics is to relieve tic-related discomfort and embarrassment and to achieve a degree of control of tics that allows the patient to function as normally as possible. Dopamine receptor blocking agents are considered the most effective drugs for the management of tics, although only haloperidol and pimozide are approved by the US Food and Drug Administration (FDA) for the treatment of Tourette's syndrome. Haloperidol generally has been considered the drug of choice for the management of Tourette's syndrome and pimozide has been an effective alternative in some patients who have had an inadequate response to or did not tolerate haloperidol. Limited data suggest that pimozide may be more effective than haloperidol in reducing tics. Some clinicians, however, prefer other antipsychotic drugs including molindone, phenothiazines (e.g., fluphenazine, thioridazine, trifluoperazine), risperidone, thiothixene, or tiapride (not commercially available in the US). It is not known whether some other atypical antipsychotics (e.g., clozapine, olanzapine, quetiapine) are effective in the management of tics or other symptoms of Tourette's syndrome; however, limited data indicate that ziprasidone may decrease the severity of tics. Tetrabenazine, a drug that interferes with monoamine neurotransmitters and blocks dopamine receptors, has been effective for the management of tics and, unlike conventional antipsychotic agents, tetrabenazine does not appear to cause tardive dyskinesia. Although several other drugs (e.g., cannabinoids, clonazepam, pergolide, nicotine gum, nicotine transdermal system) have been shown to be effective in the management of tics, these agents have not been evaluated in well-designed, controlled studies. Focal motor and vocal tics have responded to injections of botulinum toxin in the affected muscles.

Pimozide is considered an orphan drug and is used for suppression of motor and vocal tics of Tourette's syndrome (Gilles de la Tourette's syndrome) in children and adults. The drug usually should be reserved for the treatment of those patients with Tourette's syndrome who have an inadequate response to, or who do not tolerate, conventional therapy (e.g., haloperidol) and whose development and/or daily life function is severely compromised by the presence of motor and vocal tics. Pimozide usually is *not* intended as a treatment of first choice for this syndrome, *nor* is it intended for suppression of tics that are only annoying or cosmetically troublesome.

Controlled studies in patients with Tourette's syndrome have shown that pimozide is effective in reducing the number of stimulated and unstimulated motor and vocal tics and the severity of associated symptomatology. Results of several studies suggest that pimozide is at least as effective as haloperidol in the management of Tourette's syndrome and may be associated with fewer and possibly less severe adverse effects, particularly sedation, in some patients. The long-term safety of pimozide in the management of this syndrome, however, remains to be determined, and additional well-controlled studies comparing pimozide and haloperidol are needed to assess their relative efficacy and safety. Haloperidol generally has been considered the drug of choice for the management of Tourette's syndrome, and pimozide has been an effective alternative in some patients who have an inadequate response to or do not tolerate haloperidol. Because limited data suggest that pimozide may be more effective than haloperidol in reducing tics and pimozide appears to be better tolerated than haloperidol, some clinicians and experts prefer the use of pimozide in patients with Tourette's syndrome. Limited data suggest that pimozide may be more effective than clonidine and that pimozide and penfluridol (not commercially available in the US) may have comparable efficacy in the management of Tourette's syndrome. Well-controlled clinical studies comparing the efficacy and safety of pimozide and other agents used in the management of Tourette's syndrome are needed.

Comorbid Conditions Patients with Tourette's syndrome often exhibit comorbid conditions (e.g., ADHD, obsessive-compulsive disorder). Although CNS stimulants, including amphetamines, have been reported to exacerbate motor and vocal tics in patients with Tourette's syndrome, results of several studies indicate that stimulants are effective in the management of ADHD in patients with Tourette's syndrome and the rate of tics is not increased in the majority of patients. In patients in whom the rate of tics increases, some experts recommend addition of an α-adrenergic agonist (e.g., clonidine, guanfacine), risperidone, pimozide, or haloperidol. Clonidine or guanfacine have been used in the management of ADHD. Although less effective than stimulants, clonidine and guanfacine do not increase the frequency or severity of tics. Tricyclic antidepressants (e.g., imipramine, nortriptyline) also may be used for the treatment of mild cases of ADHD and concomitant tics or Tourette's syndrome in patients who do not respond to or otherwise do not tolerate stimulants, in whom tics are exacerbated by stimulants, or those who develop clinically important depression.

In addition, there is a high incidence of obsessive-compulsive disorder in patients with Tourette's syndrome. Many clinicians recommend that patients with Tourette's syndrome and coexisting obsessive-compulsive disorder receive therapy with a selective serotonin-reuptake inhibitor or a selective serotonin- and norepinephrine-reuptake inhibitor (e.g., citalopram, fluoxetine, fluvoxamine, paroxetine, sertraline, venlafaxine) alone or, if needed, in combination with buspirone, clonazepam, lithium, or a dopamine receptor antagonist. In a limited number of patients, other drugs (e.g., clomipramine, risperidone) also have been effective in the management of this comorbid condition.

■ **Schizophrenia** Pimozide has been used for the symptomatic management of a variety of psychiatric illnesses†, principally schizophrenia†, but other agents generally are preferred.

Pimozide appears to be as effective as phenothiazines or haloperidol for the symptomatic management of schizophrenia†. The drug is effective in reducing hallucinations, thought disorders, change in affect, and autism. Pimozide also appears to be effective for the management of social adjustment problems, emotional withdrawal, motor retardation, apathy, and conceptual disorganization. Delusions, bizarre mannerisms, chronic paranoia, anxiety, guilt feelings, disorientation, and hostility also may be reduced during therapy with the drug. Pimozide should *not* be used for the management of schizophrenia in patients whose main manifestations include excitement, agitation, or hyperactivity, because the efficacy of the drug in these patients has not been established.

Pimozide also has been used for the symptomatic management of acute schizophrenic episodes†. Results of initial clinical studies were not encouraging, but subsequent uncontrolled clinical studies suggest that pimozide may be effective in the management of acute schizophrenic episodes when used at dosages substantially higher than those used for the management of schizophrenia. Limited data suggest that high-dose pimozide therapy may be as effective as haloperidol or phenothiazines; however, the frequency and severity of pimozide-induced extrapyramidal reactions are increased at high dosages. Pimozide currently is *not* recommended for the management of acute schizophrenic episodes. For further information on the symptomatic management of schizophrenia, see Uses: Psychotic Disorders, in the Phenothiazines General Statement 28:16.08.24.

■ **Mania** Pimozide has been used for the management of manic episodes† (mania) in patients with major affective disorders. Although limited data suggest that pimozide may be as effective as phenothiazines, the efficacy of the drug has not been clearly established, and pimozide currently is *not* recommended for the management of manic episodes.

■ **Behavioral Disorders** The efficacy of pimozide for the management of behavioral disorders in patients with mental retardation has not been established, but limited data suggest that the drug may reduce irritability, anxiety, and hyperactivity and improve social behavior in mentally retarded adolescents, without substantially affecting cognition or learning performance. Further controlled studies are needed.

■ **Dyskinesias** Pimozide has been used for the management of various dyskinesias†, including chronic progressive hereditary chorea (Huntington's chorea), acute chorea (Sydenham's chorea), tardive dyskinesia, and tardive dystonia; however, the usefulness of the drug for the management of dyskinesias is questionable because it has both dyskinesia-alleviating and dyskinesia-producing properties. Because pimozide tends to worsen parkinsonian symptoms, the drug should not be used for the management of levodopa-induced dyskinesias in patients with parkinsonian syndrome.

■ **Other Uses** Results of uncontrolled clinical studies suggest that pimozide may be useful for the management of phencyclidine-induced psychosis† or various personality disorders† (e.g., paranoid, schizoid, compulsive). Pimozide also has reportedly been beneficial in some patients for the management of pathologic jealousy†, erotomania†, and monosymptomatic hypochondriacal psychosis†, including delusions of parasitosis.

Although pimozide has been used in the treatment of anorexia nervosa†, use of the drug for this purpose does not appear to provide substantial benefit.

Dosage and Administration

■ **Administration** Pimozide is administered orally. The drug may usually be administered once daily but also may be given in divided doses, particularly if once-daily dosing is not well tolerated. Some clinicians recommend administration of the drug as a single dose at bedtime to minimize adverse effects.

■ **Dosage** When pimozide is used for suppression of motor and vocal tics in patients with Tourette's syndrome, the initial dosage of the drug should be low and dosage adjustments should be made gradually. Dosage of pimozide must be carefully adjusted to balance symptomatic relief and the suppression of tics against the adverse effects of the drug. Patients receiving pimozide should have an ECG performed before therapy with the drug is initiated and periodically thereafter, particularly during the period of dosage adjustment. (See Cautions: Precautions and Contraindications.)

Adult Dosage For the suppression of motor and vocal tics in adults with Tourette's syndrome, the usual initial dosage of pimozide is 1–2 mg daily. The manufacturer and some clinicians state that dosage may be increased every other day according to the patient's tolerance and therapeutic response. Because of pimozide's prolonged elimination half-life, other clinicians suggest that dosage be increased at longer intervals (e.g., every 5–7 days) until signs and symptoms of the disorder decrease by at least 70%, adverse effects occur without symptomatic benefit, or symptomatic benefit and adverse effects occur at the same time. If adverse effects are minimal and do not interfere with functioning (e.g., dry mouth, slight sedation) but adequate response has not been achieved, dosage should not be increased further until these adverse effects resolve. If adverse effects interfere with functioning but are not severe, dosage can be reduced by 1-mg increments at weekly intervals until such effects resolve. Dosage should be reduced by 50% immediately or the drug withheld if severe adverse effects occur. (See Cautions: Precautions and Contraindications.) Once serious adverse effects resolve, therapy can be reinstituted with more gradual titration, increasing dosage at intervals ranging from 7–30 days. Most patients are adequately treated with dosages less than 0.2 mg/kg daily or 10 mg daily, whichever is less, and the manufacturer recommends that these dosages not be exceeded.

Pediatric Dosage For the suppression of motor and vocal tics in children with Tourette's syndrome, the usual initial dosage of pimozide is 0.05 mg/kg daily, preferably at bedtime. The dose may be increased every third day to a maximum of 0.2 mg/kg or 10 mg per day. Reliable dose-response data for the effects of the drug on tic manifestations in children younger than 12 years of age are not available.

Dosage of pimozide during prolonged maintenance therapy should be kept at the lowest possible effective level. Once an adequate response has been achieved, periodic attempts (e.g., every 6–12 months) should be made to reduce dosage of the drug to determine whether the initial intensity and frequency of tics persist. When attempting to reduce the dosage of pimozide, consideration should be given to the possibility that observed increases of tic intensity and frequency may represent a transient, withdrawal-related phenomenon rather than a return of the syndrome's symptoms. Before concluding that an increase in tic manifestations is a function of the underlying disorder rather than a response to drug withdrawal, at least 1–2 weeks should be allowed to elapse. If pimozide therapy is to be discontinued, dosage of the drug should be gradually reduced.

Cautions

■ **Nervous System Effects** The most frequent and potentially severe adverse effects of pimozide involve the CNS.

Extrapyramidal Reactions Extrapyramidal reactions occur frequently with pimozide, especially during the first few days of therapy. In most patients, these reactions consist of parkinsonian symptoms (e.g., tremor, rigidity, akinesia) that are mild to moderate in severity and usually reversible following discontinuance of the drug. Dystonic reactions and feelings of motor restlessness (i.e., akathisia) occur less frequently. Generally, the occurrence and severity of most extrapyramidal reactions are dose related because they occur at relatively high dosages and disappear or become less severe following a reduction in dosage; however, severe extrapyramidal reactions have reportedly occurred at relatively low dosages. Extrapyramidal reactions appear to occur in about 10–15% of patients receiving usual dosages of pimozide. Administration of anticholinergic antiparkinsonian agents (e.g., benztropine, trihexyphenidyl) or diphenhydramine may be necessary to control parkinsonian extrapyramidal reactions. If persistent extrapyramidal reactions occur, pimozide therapy may have to be discontinued.

The most common dystonic reaction is torticollis, which generally is accompanied by orofacial symptoms and, in some instances, oculogyric crisis, as well as spasms of the face, tongue, and jaw. Trismus, dysarthria, muscle cramps, and athetoid movements have occurred occasionally.

Akathisia occurs relatively frequently in patients receiving pimozide, but usually can be managed by reducing the dosage of pimozide or by concomitant administration of an anticholinergic antiparkinsonian agent, diphenhydramine, a benzodiazepine, or propranolol.

Neuroleptic Malignant Syndrome Neuroleptic malignant syndrome (NMS), a potentially fatal symptom complex, has been reported in patients receiving antipsychotic agents, including pimozide. Clinical manifestations of NMS generally include hyperpyrexia, muscle rigidity, altered mental status (including catatonic signs), and evidence of autonomic instability (irregular pulse or blood pressure, tachycardia, diaphoresis, and cardiac arrhythmias). Additional signs of NMS may include increased serum creatine kinase (CK, creatine phosphokinase, CPK), myoglobinuria (rhabdomyolysis), and acute renal failure.

The diagnostic evaluation of patients with NMS is complicated. In arriving at a diagnosis, serious medical illnesses (e.g., pneumonia, systemic infection) and untreated or inadequately treated extrapyramidal signs and symptoms must be excluded. Other important considerations in the differential diagnosis include central anticholinergic toxicity, heat stroke, drug fever, and primary CNS pathology.

The management of NMS should include immediate discontinuance of antipsychotic agents and other drugs not considered essential to concurrent therapy, intensive symptomatic treatment and medical monitoring, and treatment of any concomitant serious medical problems for which specific treatments are available. If a patient requires antipsychotic therapy following recovery from NMS, the potential reintroduction of drug therapy should be carefully considered. In addition, such patients should be carefully monitored since recurrences of NMS have been reported. For additional information on NMS, see Neuroleptic Malignant Syndrome under Cautions: Nervous System Effects, in the Phenothiazines General Statement 28:16.08.24.

Hyperpyrexia, not associated with NMS, also has been reported in patients receiving other antipsychotic agents.

Tardive Dyskinesia Like other antipsychotic agents, pimozide has been associated with persistent dyskinesias. Tardive dyskinesia, a syndrome consisting of potentially irreversible, involuntary, dyskinetic movements, may occur in some patients during long-term administration of pimozide or possibly following discontinuance of the drug. Tardive dyskinesia is characterized by rhythmic involuntary movements of the tongue, face, mouth, or jaw (e.g., protrusion of the tongue, puffing of cheeks, chewing movements, puckering of the mouth), which sometimes may be accompanied by involuntary movements of the extremities and trunk. The risk of developing tardive dyskinesia appears to be greater in geriatric patients receiving high dosages of the drug, especially females. The symptoms are persistent and in some patients appear to be irreversible.

Although not clearly established, the risk of developing the syndrome and the likelihood that it will become irreversible may increase with the duration of therapy and total cumulative dose of antipsychotic agent(s) administered; however, the syndrome may occur, although much less frequently, after relatively short periods of treatment with low dosages. (See Cautions: Precautions and Contraindications.) For additional information on tardive dyskinesia, see Tardive Dyskinesia under Cautions: Nervous System Effects, in the Phenothiazines General Statement 28:16.08.24

Other Nervous System Effects Pimozide is generally considered to be relatively nonsedating compared with other antipsychotic agents, but sedation, lethargy, and/or drowsiness appear to be the most common adverse effects of the drug in patients with Tourette's syndrome. Other adverse nervous system effects of pimozide include insomnia, dizziness, excitement, agitation, nervousness, fainting, aggressiveness, irritability, anxiety, tension, headache, depression, decreased attentiveness, confusion, nightmares, hallucinations, phobia, impaired motivation, speech disorder, handwriting change, fatigue, weakness, transient affective disturbance, and aggravation of psychotic symptomatology. Rarely, pimozide has been associated with seizures, including tonic-clonic (grand mal) seizures, in patients without a previous history of seizure disorder.

Adverse anticholinergic effects of pimozide include dry mouth, blurred vision, difficulty with accommodation, urinary retention, constipation, and urinary and fecal incontinence.

■ **Cardiovascular Effects** Various ECG changes, such as prolongation of the QT (including QT_c) interval; flattening, notching, and inversion of the T wave; and appearance of U waves, have occurred in some patients receiving pimozide. The clinical importance of pimozide-induced ECG changes has not been clearly established, but some clinicians believe that the changes are comparable to those induced by phenothiazines. Sudden, unexpected deaths have occurred in some patients receiving high doses of the drug (i.e., exceeding 10 mg; in the range of 1 mg/kg) for conditions other than Tourette's syndrome or in patients receiving concomitant pimozide and clarithromycin. (See Drug Interactions: Drugs That Prolong the QT Interval and see also Drug Interactions: Drugs and Foods Affecting Hepatic Microsomal Enzymes.) A possible mechanism for these deaths is prolongation of the QT interval, predisposing the patients to ventricular arrhythmia. Patients receiving pimozide should have ECG evaluations before and periodically during therapy with the drug. (See Cautions: Precautions and Contraindications.)

Pimozide rarely may produce hypotension, orthostatic hypotension, hypertension, tachycardia, or palpitations. In some patients, particularly geriatric or debilitated patients, transient hypotension for several hours after administration of the drug has occurred.

■ **Endocrine and Metabolic Effects** Amenorrhea, dysmenorrhea, and mild galactorrhea have occurred in some patients receiving pimozide. Like other antipsychotic agents, pimozide increases serum prolactin concentrations. (See Cautions: Mutagenicity and Carcinogenicity.) Loss of libido, impotence, and weight gain or, more frequently, weight loss, have occurred in patients receiving pimozide.

■ **GI Effects** Adverse GI effects of pimozide include increased salivation, nausea, vomiting, anorexia, GI distress, diarrhea, constipation, and abdominal cramps or pain. Thirst, altered taste, gingival hyperplasia, and increased appetite also have been reported.

■ **Hematological Effects** In clinical trial and/or postmarketing experience, leukopenia, neutropenia, and agranulocytosis temporally related to antipsychotic agents have been reported. Possible risk factors for leukopenia and neutropenia include preexisting low leukocyte count and a history of drug-induced leukopenia or neutropenia. (See Cautions: Precautions and Contraindications.)

Hemolytic anemia also has occurred in pimozide-treated patients, although a causal relationship to the drug has not been established.

■ **Other Adverse Effects** Rash, urticaria, skin irritation, facial edema (may be severe), periorbital edema, sweating, cataracts, visual disturbances or sensitivity to light, chest pain, nocturia, and urinary frequency have been reported in patients receiving pimozide. Hyponatremia has occurred in patients receiving the drug following marketing approval.

The possibility that pimozide may cause other adverse effects reported with other antipsychotic agents should be considered. In addition, because clinical experience with pimozide for the management of Tourette's syndrome is limited, uncommon adverse effects may not have been detected to date.

■ **Precautions and Contraindications** Pimozide shares the toxic potentials of other antipsychotic agents (e.g., phenothiazines, butyrophenones), and the usual precautions associated with therapy with these agents should be observed. (See Cautions in the Phenothiazines General Statement 28:16.08.24.) Because treatment with pimozide exposes the patient to potentially serious risks, the decision to use the drug for the long-term management of Tourette's syndrome should be carefully considered by the patient (and/or the patient's family or guardians) and the physician. The use of pimozide for the management of Tourette's syndrome involves different considerations of risks and benefits than the use of other antipsychotic agents for other conditions. Because the goal of treatment is symptomatic improvement, the patient's view of the need for treatment and assessment of response are critical in evaluating the relative benefits and risks of pimozide therapy. Patients should be informed that pimozide has an adverse effect profile similar to that of other antipsychotic agents and that adverse effects associated with these agents may occur with pimozide.

Neuroleptic malignant syndrome (NMS), a potentially fatal syndrome requiring immediate discontinuance of the drug and intensive symptomatic treatment, has been reported in patients receiving antipsychotic agents, including pimozide. If a patient requires antipsychotic therapy following recovery from NMS, the potential reintroduction of drug therapy should be carefully considered. If antipsychotic therapy is reintroduced, the dosage generally should be increased gradually, and an antipsychotic agent other than the agent believed to have precipitated NMS generally should be chosen. In addition, such patients should be carefully monitored since recurrences of NMS have been reported. (See Neuroleptic Malignant Syndrome under Cautions: Nervous System Effects.)

Because of the likelihood that a proportion of patients receiving long-term therapy with an antipsychotic agent will develop tardive dyskinesia, patients in whom long-term pimozide therapy is considered should be fully informed, if possible, about the risk of developing this syndrome. The decision to inform the patient (and/or the patient's family or guardians) should take into account the clinical circumstances and the competency of the patient to understand the information. Pimozide should be prescribed in a manner that is most likely to minimize the occurrence of this syndrome. Chronic antipsychotic treatment generally should be reserved for patients who suffer from a chronic illness that is known to respond to antipsychotic agents, and for whom alternative, equally effective, but potentially less harmful treatments are not available or appropriate. In patients who do require chronic treatment, the smallest dosage and the shortest duration of treatment producing a satisfactory clinical response should be sought, and the need for continued treatment should be reassessed periodically. The American Psychiatric Association currently recommends that patients receiving first-generation antipsychotic agents be assessed clinically for abnormal involuntary movements every 6 months and that patients considered to be at increased risk for tardive dyskinesia be assessed every 3 months. (See Tardive Dyskinesia under Cautions: Nervous System Effects.)

Because sudden, unexpected deaths, which may be related to an effect of pimozide on the heart, have occurred in some patients receiving high doses of the drug (i.e., exceeding 10 mg; in the range of 1 mg/kg) for conditions other than Tourette's syndrome, an ECG should be performed before pimozide therapy is initiated and periodically thereafter, particularly during the period of dosage adjustment. Some clinicians recommend that a cardiologist be consulted before initiating therapy with the drug in patients with a baseline QT_c interval exceeding 440 ms. Patients should be instructed *not* to exceed the prescribed dosage and should be aware of the need for the initial ECG and follow-up ECGs during pimozide therapy. Prolongation of the QT_c interval (QT interval corrected for rate) to greater than 470 ms in children or 520 ms in adults, or more than 25% beyond the patient's pretreatment value, or the development of other T-wave abnormalities should be considered a basis for stopping further dosage increases and considering a dosage reduction. Dosage reduction also should be considered if bradycardia (less than 50 bpm) occurs. Some clinicians recommend that pimozide be withheld if T-wave inversion, U waves, or cardiac arrhythmia occurs and reinstituted only after ECG findings are normal. Because pimozide may cause ECG changes, the drug should be used with caution in patients with cardiovascular disorders. Because hypokalemia has been associated with ventricular arrhythmias, potassium insufficiency secondary to diuretics, diarrhea, or other causes should be corrected before pimozide therapy is initiated, and normal serum potassium concentrations should be maintained during pimozide therapy.

In clinical trial and/or postmarketing experience, leukopenia and neutropenia temporally related to antipsychotic agents have been reported; agranulocytosis also has been reported. Because possible risk factors for leukopenia and neutropenia include a preexisting low leukocyte count and a history of drug-induced leukopenia and neutropenia, the manufacturer states that patients with a history of clinically important low leukocyte count or drug-induced leukopenia and/or neutropenia should have their complete blood count monitored frequently during the first few months of therapy. Discontinuance of pimozide should be considered at the first sign of a clinically important decline in leukocyte count in the absence of other causative factors. Patients with clinically important neutropenia should be carefully monitored for fever or other signs or symptoms of infection and promptly treated if such signs or symptoms occur. In patients with severe neutropenia (absolute neutrophil count [ANC] less than 1000/mm^3), pimozide should be discontinued and the leukocyte count monitored until recovery occurs. (See Cautions: Hematologic Effects.)

The clinical importance is not known, but pimozide has produced a dose-related increase in benign pituitary tumors in female mice. (See Cautions: Mutagenicity and Carcinogenicity.) The tumorigenic potential of pimozide should be given careful consideration by the patient and physician in the decision to use the drug, especially if the patient is young and long-term therapy is anticipated.

Patients should be warned that pimozide may impair their ability to perform activities requiring mental alertness or physical coordination (e.g., operating machinery, driving a motor vehicle), especially during the first few days of therapy.

Because pimozide produces adverse anticholinergic effects, the drug should be used with caution in individuals whose conditions may be aggravated by anticholinergic activity.

Like other antipsychotic agents, pimozide should be used with caution in patients receiving anticonvulsant agents and in those with EEG abnormalities or a history of seizures because the drug may lower the seizure threshold. If necessary, adequate anticonvulsant therapy should be maintained during pimozide therapy.

Pimozide should be used with caution in patients with hepatic or renal impairment.

Because pimozide has an antiemetic effect, the drug should be used with caution when suppression of nausea and vomiting might obscure diagnosis of an underlying physical disorder.

Because increased plasma concentrations of pimozide have occurred following concomitant use of pimozide and sertraline, the manufacturers of pimozide and sertraline state that concomitant use of the drugs is contraindicated. In addition, increased plasma pimozide concentrations were observed during concurrent use with paroxetine. The manufacturers of paroxetine state that concomitant use of these drugs is contraindicated because of the narrow therapeutic index of pimozide and its known ability to prolong the QT interval. Because of the risk of QT-interval prolongation, concurrent use of either citalopram hydrobromide or escitalopram oxalate with pimozide is contraindicated. Concurrent use of pimozide and fluoxetine also is contraindicated because of the potential for adverse drug interactions or QT$_c$- interval prolongation. In addition, fluvoxamine should not be used concurrently with pimozide. (See Drug Interactions: Selective Serotonin-reuptake Inhibitors.)

Because pimozide prolongs the QT interval, the drug also is contraindicated in patients with congenital long QT syndrome or a history of cardiac arrhythmias, and in patients receiving other drugs that prolong the QT interval or that inhibit the metabolism of pimozide by inhibiting the cytochrome P-450 (CYP) 3A4 isoenzyme such as macrolide antibiotics (e.g., clarithromycin, erythromycin, azithromycin, dirithromycin, troleandomycin), azole antifungal agents (e.g., itraconazole, ketoconazole), protease inhibitors (e.g., boceprevir, indinavir, nelfinavir, ritonavir, saquinavir, telaprevir), nefazodone, or zileuton. (See Drug Interactions: Drugs That Prolong the QT Interval and see also Drug Interactions: Drugs and Foods Affecting Hepatic Microsomal Enzymes.)

Pimozide is contraindicated in the treatment of simple tics or tics other than those associated with Tourette's syndrome. Pimozide should not be used in patients receiving drugs that may cause motor and vocal tics (e.g., pemoline [no longer commercially available in the US], methylphenidate, amphetamines) until such drugs have been withdrawn to determine whether the drugs or Tourette's syndrome is responsible for the tics.

Pimozide is contraindicated in patients with known hypokalemia or hypomagnesemia.

Pimozide is contraindicated in patients with severe toxic CNS depression or in those who are comatose from any cause; patients with blood dyscrasias, depressive disorders, or parkinsonian syndrome; and in patients who are hypersensitive to the drug. It is not known whether cross-sensitivity exists among antipsychotic agents; however, pimozide should be used with particular caution in patients with known hypersensitivity to other antipsychotic agents.

■ **Pediatric Precautions** The onset of Tourette's syndrome usually occurs between the ages of 2 and 15 years, but data on the use and efficacy of pimozide in children younger than 12 years of age are limited. Further study is needed to fully evaluate the use and efficacy of the drug for Tourette's syndrome in this age group. Limited clinical evidence suggests that the safety profile of pimozide in children aged 2–12 years generally is comparable to that observed in older patients. Safety and efficacy of pimozide for the management of other conditions in children have not been evaluated, and use of the drug in children for any condition other than Tourette's syndrome is *not* recommended.

■ **Mutagenicity and Carcinogenicity** No evidence of pimozide-induced mutagenesis was seen in the Ames microbial mutagen test, the micronucleus test in rats, or the dominant lethal assay in mice.

No evidence of carcinogenesis was seen in rats receiving oral pimozide dosages up to 50 times the maximum recommended human dosage for 2 years; however, because of the limited number of rats surviving the study, the meaning of the results is unclear. Reversible gingival hyperplasia has occurred in dogs receiving oral pimozide dosages greater than 1.5 mg/kg daily (about 5 times the maximum recommended human dosage) for 12 months, and has occurred in at least one patient receiving the drug following marketing approval. Following oral administration of pimozide 0.62, 5, or 40 mg/kg daily for 18 months in mice, dose-related increases in the incidence of pituitary adenomas and mammary gland adenocarcinomas were observed in females. Pituitary changes at a dosage of 0.62 mg/kg daily were characterized as hyperplasia, while benign adenomas occurred at the higher dosages. The mechanism of pimozide-induced pituitary tumors in mice and the clinical importance of this finding are not known; however, the tumorigenic potential of pimozide should be given careful consideration by the patient and physician in the decision to use the drug, especially if the patient is young and long-term therapy is anticipated.

Although an increase in mammary neoplasms has been found in rodents following long-term administration of prolactin-stimulating antipsychotic agents, no clinical or epidemiologic studies conducted to date have shown an association between long-term administration of these drugs and mammary tumorigenesis in humans. Current evidence is considered too limited to be conclusive, and further study is needed to determine the clinical importance in most patients of elevated serum prolactin concentrations associated with antipsychotic agents. Because in vitro tests indicate that approximately one-third of human breast cancers are prolactin dependent, pimozide should be used with caution in patients with previously detected breast cancer.

■ **Pregnancy, Fertility, and Lactation** Reproduction studies in rats and rabbits using oral pimozide dosages up to 2.5 mg/kg daily (up to about 8 times the maximum recommended human dosage) have not revealed evidence of fetal malformation; however, in rats receiving oral pimozide dosages of 2.5 mg/kg daily or higher, a decreased pregnancy rate, increased fetal resorption, and retarded development of fetuses occurred. The observed effects may have resulted from delay or inhibition of implantation. In rabbits, dose-related maternotoxicity, mortality, decreased weight gain, and embryotoxicity, including increased fetal resorption, occurred.

Neonates exposed to antipsychotic agents during the third trimester of pregnancy are at risk for extrapyramidal and/or withdrawal symptoms following delivery. There have been reports of agitation, hypertonia, hypotonia, tardive dyskinetic-like symptoms, tremor, somnolence, respiratory distress, and feeding disorder in these neonates. The majority of cases were also confounded by other factors, including concomitant use of other drugs known to be associated with withdrawal symptoms, prematurity, congenital malformations, and obstetrical and perinatal complications; however, some cases suggested that neonatal extrapyramidal symptoms and withdrawal may occur with exposure to antipsychotic agents alone. Some of the cases described time of symptom onset, which ranged from birth to one month after birth. Any neonate exhibiting extrapyramidal or withdrawal symptoms following in utero exposure to antipsychotic agents should be monitored. Symptoms were self-limiting in some neonates but varied in severity; some infants required intensive care unit support and prolonged hospitalization. For further information on extrapyramidal and withdrawal symptoms in neonates, see Cautions: Pregnancy, Fertility, and Lactation, in the Phenothiazines General Statement 28:16.08.24.

Pimozide should be used during pregnancy only when the potential benefits justify the potential risks to the fetus. Women should be advised to notify their clinician if they become pregnant or plan to become pregnant during therapy with the drug. In addition, clinicians should advise women of childbearing potential about the benefits and risks of using antipsychotic agents during pregnancy. Patients should also be advised not to stop taking their antipsychotic agent if they become pregnant without first consulting with their clinician, since abruptly discontinuing the drugs can cause clinically important complications.

Reproduction studies in animals using oral pimozide were not adequate to fully assess potential effects of the drug on fertility. Female rats receiving oral pimozide dosages up to 2.5 mg/kg daily had prolonged estrus cycles.

It is not known whether pimozide is distributed into milk. Because of the potential for serious adverse reactions (e.g., tumorigenicity, unknown cardiovascular effects) to pimozide in nursing infants, a decision should be made whether to discontinue nursing or the drug, taking into account the importance of the drug to the woman.

Drug Interactions

■ **Selective Serotonin-reuptake Inhibitors** ***Citalopram*** In a controlled study, administration of a single 2-mg dose of pimozide in individuals receiving citalopram (40 mg once daily for 11 days) was associated with mean increases in the QT$_c$ interval of approximately 10 msec compared with pimozide given alone. Citalopram did not substantially affect the mean AUC or peak plasma concentrations of pimozide. The mechanism for this potential pharmacodynamic interaction is not known. Concomitant use of citalopram and pimozide is contraindicated.

Escitalopram In a controlled study, administration of a single 2-mg dose of pimozide in individuals receiving racemic citalopram (40 mg once daily for 11 days) was associated with mean increases in the QT$_c$ interval of approximately 10 msec compared with pimozide given alone. Racemic citalopram did not substantially affect the mean AUC or peak plasma concentrations of pimozide. Concurrent pimozide and escitalopram administration has not been specifically evaluated to date. Concomitant use of escitalopram and pimozide is contraindicated.

Fluoxetine Clinical studies evaluating pimozide and other antidepressants have demonstrated an increase in adverse drug interactions or QT$_c$ prolongation during combined therapy. In addition, rare case reports have suggested possible additive cardiovascular effects of pimozide and fluoxetine, resulting in bradycardia. Marked changes in mental status (e.g., stupor, inability to think clearly) and hypersalivation also were reported in one woman who received both drugs concurrently. Although a specific study evaluating concurrent pimozide and fluoxetine has not been performed to date, concurrent use of these drugs is contraindicated because of the potential for adverse drug interactions or QT_c prolongation.

Fluvoxamine Concomitant use of fluvoxamine is contraindicated in patients receiving pimozide, since fluvoxamine may inhibit the metabolism of pimozide and increase the potential for serious adverse cardiac effects.

Paroxetine In a controlled study, concurrent administration of single 2-mg doses of pimozide in healthy individuals receiving paroxetine (dosage titrated up to 60 mg daily) was associated with mean increases of 151 and 62% in the area under the plasma concentration-time curve (AUC) and peak plasma concentrations of pimozide, respectively, compared with pimozide given alone. The manufacturers of paroxetine state that concomitant use of paroxetine and pimozide is contraindicated because of the narrow therapeutic index of pimozide and its known ability to prolong the QT interval.

Sertraline Administration of a single 2-mg dose of pimozide in individuals receiving sertraline 200 mg daily has resulted in a mean increase of about 40% in pimozide AUC and peak plasma concentrations, but was not associated with changes in ECG parameters. The effect on QT interval and pharmacokinetic parameters of pimozide administered in higher doses (i.e., doses exceeding 2 mg) in combination with sertraline is as yet unknown. Concomitant use of sertraline and pimozide is contraindicated because of the low therapeutic index of pimozide and because the reported interaction between the 2 drugs occurred at a low dose of pimozide. The mechanism of this interaction is as yet unknown.

■ **Other CNS Agents** Pimozide may be additive with, or may potentiate the action of, other CNS depressants such as opiates or other analgesics, barbiturates or other sedatives, anxiolytics, or alcohol. When pimozide is used concomitantly with other CNS depressants, caution should be used to avoid excessive CNS depression.

■ **Drugs That Prolong the QT Interval** Because pimozide prolongs the QT interval, an additive effect on the QT interval might occur if the drug is administered with other agents that may prolong the QT interval such as phenothiazines, tricyclic antidepressants, or antiarrhythmic agents. Therefore, the manufacturer states that pimozide is contraindicated in patients receiving dofetilide, quinidine, sotalol, and other class IA and III antiarrhythmics; chlorpromazine, droperidol, mesoridazine (no longer commercially available in the US), and thioridazine; gatifloxacin, moxifloxacin, and sparfloxacin; halofantrine (licensed in the US but not commercially available); mefloquine; pentamidine; arsenic trioxide; levomethadyl acetate (no longer commercially available in the US); dolasetron mesylate; probucol (no longer commercially available in the US); tacrolimus; ziprasidone; and any other drugs that have demonstrated QT prolongation as one of their pharmacodynamic effects. (See Cautions: Cardiovascular Effects and see also Cautions: Precautions and Contraindications.)

■ **Drugs and Foods Affecting Hepatic Microsomal Enzymes** Prolongation of QT interval and, rarely, serious cardiovascular effects, including ventricular arrhythmias and death, have been reported in patients receiving drugs that inhibit the cytochrome P-450 (CYP) 3A4 isoenzyme such as macrolide antibiotics (e.g., clarithromycin, erythromycin, azithromycin, dirithromycin, troleandomycin), azole antifungal agents (e.g., itraconazole, ketoconazole), protease inhibitors (e.g., boceprevir, indinavir, nelfinavir, ritonavir, saquinavir, telaprevir), nefazodone, or zileuton concomitantly with pimozide. Macrolide antibiotics inhibit metabolism of pimozide, which may result in increased plasma concentrations of unchanged drug. Such alterations in pharmacokinetics of pimozide may be associated with prolongation of the QT and QT_c intervals, and, rarely, associated with ventricular arrhythmias. The manufacturer of pimozide states that concomitant administration of pimozide and macrolide antibiotics, azole antifungal agents, protease inhibitors, nefazodone, or zileuton is contraindicated.

Patients receiving pimozide should avoid grapefruit juice because it may inhibit drug metabolism by the CYP3A4 isoenzyme.

Because pimozide also may be metabolized by the CYP1A2 isoenzyme, the manufacturer states the theoretical potential for drug interactions with drugs that inhibit this enzyme system should be considered.

Acute Toxicity

■ **Pathogenesis** The acute lethal dose of pimozide in humans is not known. The oral LD_{50} of pimozide is 228, 5120, 188, and 40 mg/kg in mice, rats, guinea pigs, and dogs, respectively. The IV and subcutaneous LD_{50}s of pimozide are 11.1 and 40 mg/kg, respectively, for mice, and 5 and 40 mg/kg, respectively, for rats.

■ **Manifestations** In general, overdosage of pimozide may be expected to produce effects that are extensions of pharmacologic effects and adverse reactions, predominantly ECG abnormalities (including prolongation of the QT interval and torsades de pointes), severe extrapyramidal reactions, hypotension, seizures, and comatose state with respiratory depression.

A 17-year-old female who reportedly intentionally ingested 100 mg of pimozide and underwent gastric lavage (apparently no drug was recovered) had a complete and uneventful recovery except for slight tremor of the extremities that subsided within a few hours after ingestion. A 2½-year-old male who accidentally reportedly ingested 60 mg of pimozide exhibited mild extrapyramidal symptoms that subsequently subsided, and the patient recovered completely. Delayed-onset dystonia, hypotension, tachycardia, and drowsiness were reported in an 18-month-old female who ingested up to 6 mg (0.5 mg/kg) of pimozide; manifestations developed more than 12 hours after the accidental ingestion. The dystonia subsided over the following 12 hours while the drowsiness and tachycardia persisted for 40 hours. The child recovered fully without sequelae.

■ **Treatment** Treatment of pimozide overdosage generally involves symptomatic and supportive care, with ECG, blood pressure, and respiratory monitoring. There is no specific antidote for pimozide intoxication.

Following acute ingestion of the drug, the stomach should be emptied immediately, preferably by gastric lavage. If the patient is comatose, having seizures, or lacks the gag reflex, gastric lavage may be performed if an endotracheal tube with cuff inflated is in place to prevent aspiration of gastric contents. As in the case of phenothiazine overdosage, induction of emesis should generally *not* be attempted because a pimozide-induced dystonic reaction of the head or neck may result in aspiration of gastric contents during emesis; however, if the ingestion has only recently occurred (i.e., within an hour or so), induction of emesis may be considered. Following gastric lavage and/or emesis, activated charcoal should be administered. A patent airway should be established, using controlled or mechanically assisted respiration as necessary. ECG monitoring should be initiated immediately and continued until ECG parameters are within normal ranges. For hypotension or circulatory collapse, IV fluids, plasma, albumin, and/or vasopressor agents (e.g., norepinephrine) may be used. Epinephrine should *not* be used. For severe extrapyramidal reactions, anticholinergic antiparkinsonian agents or diphenhydramine should be administered. Because of the long elimination half-life of pimozide, patients should be observed for at least 4 days following acute ingestion of the drug. Clinicians should consider contacting a poison control center for additional information on the management of pimozide overdosage.

Pharmacology

The principal pharmacologic effects of pimozide are similar to those of haloperidol and, to a lesser extent, those of phenothiazines. In animal studies that are correlated with antipsychotic activity, pimozide is, on a weight basis, almost as potent as haloperidol and more potent than chlorpromazine following oral or subcutaneous administration.

■ **Nervous System Effects** In the CNS, pimozide has pharmacologic actions similar to those of haloperidol. The precise mechanism(s) of pimozide in suppressing motor and vocal tics in patients with Tourette's syndrome and its antipsychotic action have not been determined, but it may be related principally to the antidopaminergic effects of the drug. Although it has not been clearly established, most evidence suggests that pimozide is a selective dopamine-2 (D_2) receptor antagonist. Like butyrophenones (e.g., haloperidol), pimozide appears to predominantly block postsynaptic dopamine receptor sites, although the drug also may block presynaptic dopamine receptor sites. Blockade of dopamine receptors by pimozide may be accompanied by a series of secondary alterations in central dopamine metabolism and function that may contribute to the drug's therapeutic and adverse effects. Pimozide inhibits electrically induced dopamine release in brain tissue in vitro and increases synthesis and turnover of brain dopamine. Unlike most other currently available antipsychotic agents, pimozide appears to have little effect on catecholamines other than dopamine, although turnover of brain norepinephrine may be increased at high doses. Like other antipsychotic agents, however, pimozide has various effects on CNS receptor systems (e.g., γ-aminobutyric acid [GABA]) that are not fully characterized. Pimozide may decrease brain acetylcholine indirectly via its antidopaminergic effects, but such activity is considered relatively weak. Unlike haloperidol and chlorpromazine, the drug does not provide protection against a lethal dose of norepinephrine in rats.

Pimozide does not affect total sleep time or rapid eye movement (REM) sleep. The drug may cause EEG changes, including an increase in α-wave activity. Although not clearly established, pimozide may also lower the seizure threshold. The drug does not exhibit anticonvulsant activity in rats.

Although the exact mechanism(s) of action has not been elucidated, pimozide has an antiemetic effect. The antiemetic activity may be mediated via a direct effect of the drug on the medullary chemoreceptor trigger zone (CTZ), apparently by blocking dopamine receptors in the CTZ. Pimozide inhibits the central and peripheral effects of apomorphine.

Like haloperidol and phenothiazines, pimozide inhibits conditioned avoidance behaviors and produces catalepsy and ptosis in animals. The drug also antagonizes behavioral effects mediated by amphetamines in animals. In humans, pimozide antagonizes the euphoric response to amphetamines in amphetamine-dependent individuals, but apparently does not antagonize amphetamine-mediated behavioral effects in patients with schizophrenic disorder. Unlike many other centrally acting agents, pimozide does not appear to exhibit analgesic activity. The drug appears to exhibit anxiolytic activity in patients with chronic schizophrenic disorder who exhibit anxiety and in patients with various anxiety states.

In animals, pimozide does not substantially affect body temperature; however, the drug does inhibit apomorphine- and amphetamine-induced fever.

Pimozide exhibits some anticholinergic activity, although it is generally considered to be relatively weak compared with most other antipsychotic agents; however, anticholinergic effects (e.g., dry mouth, urinary retention, constipation) may occur during therapy with the drug.

■ **Cardiovascular Effects** Pimozide exhibits weak α-adrenergic blocking activity. The drug rarely may produce hypotension, orthostatic hypotension, hypertension, or tachycardia. Pimozide may also produce ECG changes, including prolongation of the QT interval; flattening, notching, and inversion of the T wave; and appearance of U waves. (See Cautions: Cardiovascular Effects.)

■ **Endocrine Effects** Pimozide induces secretion of prolactin from the anterior pituitary. The exact mechanism of increased prolactin secretion has not been determined, but it may be related principally to inhibition of dopamine receptors in the pituitary and hypothalamus.

■ **Other Effects** In vitro, pimozide exhibits weak antispasmodic effects, resulting from antagonism of various mediator substances (e.g., histamine, bradykinin, angiotensin). Pimozide also may inhibit transmembrane influx of extracellular calcium ions via slow calcium channels.

Pharmacokinetics

Limited information is available on the pharmacokinetics of pimozide.

■ **Absorption** Pimozide is slowly and variably absorbed from the GI tract following oral administration. Based on limited data, the drug appears to be at least 40–50% absorbed. Pimozide also appears to undergo extensive first-pass metabolism. It is not known whether food, disease, or concomitant administration of other drugs affects the absorption of pimozide.

Following oral administration of an individual dose of pimozide, peak plasma concentrations of the drug and its metabolites generally occur within 6–8 hours (range: 4–12 hours). Following oral administration of a single 6- or 24-mg dose in patients with chronic schizophrenic disorder, peak plasma pimozide concentrations of approximately 4 or 18–19 ng/mL, respectively, were attained. There are considerable interindividual variations in peak plasma concentrations and areas under the plasma concentration-time curves (AUCs) following single or multiple oral doses of pimozide. In a group of patients with chronic schizophrenic disorder receiving 2–10 mg of pimozide daily, steady-state serum concentrations of the drug varied considerably with specific dosages and ranged from undetectable (less than 1 ng/mL) to about 50 ng/mL. Because there is little correlation between plasma pimozide concentrations and clinical response, the clinical importance of interindividual variations is unclear. In a group of adults with acute schizophrenic disorder, a correlation between plasma pimozide concentration and dopamine receptor blocking activity, but not between clinical response and dopamine receptor blocking activity, was reported.

■ **Distribution** Distribution of pimozide into human body tissues and fluids has not been well characterized. Following subcutaneous administration in animals, pimozide is widely distributed, with highest concentrations attained in the liver, lungs, kidneys, and heart; the drug also is distributed into the brain, thymus, adrenals, thyroid, uterus, and ovaries, and apparently into bile. In animals, there is a direct relationship between the administered dose of pimozide and concentrations of the drug attained in the liver and brain. Following subcutaneous administration in animals, pimozide is widely distributed throughout the brain, principally as unchanged drug, with highest concentrations attained in the pituitary and caudate nucleus. The drug appeared to be selectively retained in the pituitary, caudate nucleus, chemoreceptor trigger zone (CTZ), floor of the third ventricle, lateral hypothalamus, and medulla. There was no correlation between concentrations of pimozide in the caudate nucleus and antagonism of effects mediated by amphetamine or apomorphine, but distribution of pimozide into nerve endings in the caudate nucleus was correlated with antagonism of these effects.

The extent of pimozide binding to plasma proteins is not known.

It is not known whether pimozide crosses the placenta or is distributed into milk.

■ **Elimination** Following multiple oral doses in patients with chronic schizophrenic disorder, the elimination half-life of pimozide averaged 55 hours. In one patient who developed a severe dystonic reaction, the elimination half-life of the drug was reportedly 154 hours.

The exact metabolic fate of pimozide is not clearly established, but the drug appears to undergo extensive first-pass metabolism. Pimozide is metabolized principally by oxidative *N*-dealkylation in the liver; this metabolism is catalyzed mainly by the cytochrome P-450 (CYP) 3A4 isoenzyme and, to a lesser extent, by cytochrome P-450 (CYP) isoenzyme 1A2. The major metabolites are 4,4-*bis*(4-fluorophenyl) butyric acid and 1-(4-piperidyl)-2-benzimidazolinone. The pharmacologic activity of these metabolites has not been determined; however, results of animal studies suggest that the metabolites of pimozide are inactive.

Pimozide and its metabolites are excreted principally in urine and, to a lesser extent, in feces. About 40% (range: 25–60%) of a single oral dose of the drug is excreted in urine and about 15% (range: 5–20%) in feces within 7 days; most urinary excretion occurs within 3–4 days, and most fecal excretion occurs within 3–6 days. Pimozide appears to be excreted in urine almost completely as metabolites, with probably less than 1% excreted as unchanged drug. Fecal excretion has not been well characterized, but pimozide appears to be excreted in feces mainly as unchanged drug and to a small extent as metabolites. It is not known whether fecal excretion of the drug and metabolites represents unabsorbed drug or drug excreted via biliary elimination. In animals, pimozide and its metabolites are excreted in feces following parenteral administration, apparently via biliary elimination.

It is not known if pimozide and/or its metabolites are removed by hemodialysis or peritoneal dialysis.

Chemistry and Stability

■ **Chemistry** Pimozide is a diphenylbutylpiperidine-derivative antipsychotic agent. The drug is structurally similar to butyrophenones (e.g., haloperidol). Pimozide occurs as a white microcrystalline powder and has solubilities of less than 0.01 mg/mL in water and approximately 7 mg/mL in alcohol at room temperature. The drug has a pK_a of 7.32.

■ **Stability** Pimozide tablets should be stored in tight, light-resistant containers at 25°C but may be exposed to temperatures ranging from 15–30°C.

Preparations

Excipients in commercially available drug preparations may have clinically important effects in some individuals; consult specific product labeling for details.

Pimozide

Oral		
Tablets	1 mg	**Orap®** (scored), Gate
	2 mg	**Orap®** (scored), Gate

†Use is not currently included in the labeling approved by the US Food and Drug Administration

Selected Revisions November 2011,

ANOREXIGENIC AGENTS AND RESPIRATORY AND CNS STIMULANTS 28:20

AMPHETAMINES 28:20.04

Amphetamines General Statement

■ Amphetamines exhibit pharmacologic actions that include CNS and respiratory stimulation and sympathomimetic effects.

Uses

Amphetamines are used as stimulants to decrease daytime sleepiness in the management of narcolepsy. Amphetamines also are used as adjuncts to psychological, educational, social, and other remedial measures in the treatment of attention-deficit/hyperactivity disorder (ADHD). Certain amphetamines also are used for the treatment of binge-eating disorder. In addition, certain amphetamines are used as adjuncts to caloric restriction and behavioral modification in the short-term treatment of exogenous obesity. However, short-term or intermittent therapy with anorexigenic drugs is unlikely to maintain a long-term benefit, and prolonged administration of amphetamines for the treatment of obesity is not recommended. Amphetamines, particularly methamphetamine, have been misused and abused for their CNS stimulatory effects.

■ **Narcolepsy** Amphetamines are used as stimulants to decrease daytime sleepiness in the management of narcolepsy. Amphetamines should not be used to combat fatigue or exhaustion or to replace sleep in normal individuals.

Amphetamines remain the mainstay of treatment for narcolepsy based on a long record of clinical experience. However, because most clinical trials have involved small numbers of patients, the risk-to-benefit remains to be further established.

In determining the most appropriate stimulant therapy for a given patient, clinicians should consider benefit-to-risk (including adverse effect profile), drug cost, convenience of administration, and cost of ongoing care (including the possible need for laboratory monitoring).

Patients who fail to respond to an adequate trial of stimulant drug therapy should be assessed carefully for other possible causes of excessive sleepiness such as insufficient sleep, inadequate sleep hygiene, circadian rhythm disorders, obstructive sleep apnea syndrome, or periodic limb movement disorder.

Tolerance to the clinical effects may develop with long-term therapy, particularly at high dosages.

Narcolepsy rarely occurs in children younger than 12 years of age, and the relative safety and efficacy of various stimulant drugs in this age group remains to be elucidated. Although amphetamines can be used for narcolepsy occurring in children, methylphenidate appears to be used most commonly based principally on extensive experience with the drug in pediatric patients with ADHD.

■ **Attention-Deficit/Hyperactivity Disorder** Amphetamines also are used as adjuncts to psychological, educational, social, and other remedial measures in the treatment of ADHD (hyperkinetic disorder, hyperkinetic syndrome of childhood, minimal brain dysfunction) in children, adolescents, and adults. Almost all studies comparing behavioral therapy versus stimulants alone have shown a much stronger therapeutic effect from stimulants than from behavioral therapy, and stimulants (e.g., methylphenidate, amphetamines) remain the drugs of choice for the management of ADHD. For a more detailed discussion on the management of ADHD, including the use of stimulants such as amphetamines, see Uses: Attention Deficit Hyperactivity Disorder, in Methylphenidate 28:20.32.

Few, if any, differences have been found between amphetamines (e.g., dextroamphetamine), methylphenidate, or pemoline (no longer commercially available in the US) or various dosage forms (short-, intermediate-, or long-acting formulations) of the drugs in short-term clinical studies in children with ADHD, and the choice of stimulant therapy should be individualized. Because hepatic toxicities have been associated with pemoline, some experts recommended its use *only* in patients who failed to respond to adequate trials of methylphenidate *and* an amphetamine, as well as adequate trials of second-line therapies (e.g., tricyclic antidepressants, bupropion). However, in 2005, the US Food and Drug Administration (FDA) determined that the risk of hepatic toxicity associated with the drug outweighs its benefits and the drug no longer is commercially available in the US.

Short-term and longer-term (up to 14 months' duration) studies have shown unequivocal beneficial effects of the stimulants on the defining core symptoms of ADHD (attention and concentration, activity, distractability, impulsivity) and associated aggressiveness during continued therapy with the drugs. Children who fail to show positive therapeutic effects or who experience intolerable adverse effects with one stimulant should be tried on an alternative stimulant since most such children will exhibit a positive response to alternative stimulants and current evidence from crossover studies supports the efficacy of different stimulants in the same child; likewise, children who fail an adequate trial of 2 stimulants should be tried on a third type or formulation of stimulant. However, stimulants usually do not normalize the entire spectrum of behavioral problems, and many children effectively treated with these drugs still manifest a higher level of some behavioral problems than children without ADHD or other behavioral disturbances. Although stimulants have been shown to remain effective over many years, long-term benefits remain to be established.

■ **Binge-Eating Disorder** Some amphetamines (e.g., lisdexamfetamine) are used in the treatment of binge-eating disorder. Controlled studies have demonstrated efficacy of lisdexamfetamine in reducing the mean number of binge days per week compared with placebo in adults with moderate to severe binge-eating disorder. **For additional information on the treatment of binge-eating disorder, see Uses: Binge-Eating Disorder, in Lisdexamfetamine Dimesylate 28:20.04.**

■ **Exogenous Obesity** Amphetamines also have been used as adjuncts to caloric restriction and behavioral modification in the short-term treatment of exogenous obesity. Amphetamine sulfate as a single-ingredient preparation is used for the treatment of exogenous obesity as a short-term (i.e., a few weeks) adjunct in a regimen of weight reduction based on caloric restriction in patients refractory to alternative therapy (e.g., repeated diets, group programs, other drugs). The anorexigenic effect of sympathomimetic compounds used in the treatment of obesity appears to be temporary, seldom lasting more than a few weeks, and tolerance may occur. To help bring about and maintain loss of weight, the patient must be taught to curtail overeating and to consume a suitable diet. Prolonged administration of amphetamines is not recommended; however, obesity usually is a chronic disease, and short-term or intermittent therapy with anorexigenic drugs is unlikely to maintain a long-term benefit and is not recommended. Other anorexigenic agents (e.g., amphetamine congeners such as phentermine) with better safety profiles, including reduced potentials for misuse and abuse, generally are preferred to prototype amphetamines for the management of obesity. In the past, it was suggested that combined† therapy with fenfluramine (an amphetamine congener that stimulates release of serotonin [5-HT] at synapses and selectively inhibits the reuptake of serotonin at the presynaptic serotonergic nerve endings resulting in increased postsynaptic concentrations of serotonin in the CNS) and phentermine (an amphetamine congener that inhibits uptake of norepinephrine and dopamine) may provide complementary anorexigenic effects; therefore, such combined† therapy had been used widely in the 1990s in the management of obesity. However, because accumulated data on adverse effects associated with the drugs, fenfluramine hydrochloride (Pondimin®) and its dextrorotatory isomer dexfenfluramine hydrochloride (Redux®) were withdrawn from the US market in 1997. (See Cautions.)

■ **Misuse and Abuse** Misuse and abuse of amphetamines, especially methamphetamine, for CNS stimulatory effects have experienced a resurgence. In large part, this resurgence has resulted from the relative ease with which methamphetamine can be synthesized clandestinely from readily available chemicals such as ephedrine or pseudoephedrine. (See Chronic Toxicity.) Recent restrictions (including enactment of the Comprehensive Methamphetamine Control Act of 1996, the Methamphetamine Anti-Proliferation Act [MAPA] of 2000, and the Combat Methamphetamine Epidemic Act of 2005) on the availability of these compounds are hoped to reverse this resurgence in misuse and abuse. For a more detailed discussion on methamphetamine abuse, see Uses: Misuse and Abuse, in Pseudoephedrine 12:12.12.

Dosage and Administration

■ **Administration** Amphetamines are administered orally. When used in the treatment of narcolepsy or attention-deficit/hyperactivity disorder, the initial dose is given in the morning or on awakening. When used in the treatment of binge-eating disorder, the daily dose should be given in the morning. Because of the potential for insomnia, when amphetamines are administered in divided doses, late evening doses should be avoided. When used as an anorexigenic, the dose is usually given 30–60 minutes before meals.

■ **Dosage** Since the effective dose varies considerably from patient to patient, initial doses of amphetamines should be small and dosage may be increased gradually as necessary. Amphetamines exhibit tachyphylaxis and dosage must be governed accordingly. In general, relatively smaller doses of dextroamphetamine salts may be given since dextroamphetamine possesses a stronger central action than does amphetamine.

Cautions

■ **Abuse Potential** CNS stimulants (e.g., amphetamines) have a high potential for abuse and dependence. The risk of abuse should be assessed prior to initiation of amphetamine therapy and patients should be monitored for signs of abuse and dependence during therapy.

■ **Valvulopathy and Pulmonary Hypertension** Temporal association between use of fenfluramine (Pondimin®) or dexfenfluramine (Redux®) and the development of unusual mitral, aortic, tricuspid, and/or pulmonary valvular (usually multivalvular) and echocardiographic abnormalities (that sometimes occurred concomitantly with pulmonary hypertension, occasionally required open heart surgery, and rarely were fatal) resulted in the withdrawal of these anorexigenic agents from the US market in 1997. While such information was based on limited clinical data that were difficult to evaluate fully, the manufacturer of fenfluramine and dexfenfluramine decided that it was prudent to withdraw these drugs from the market. Because of pharmacologic differences between these drugs and prototypical amphetamines, the importance of these findings to other anorexigenic agents currently is unclear.

The adverse effects associated with these drugs were based on postmarketing reports from the Mayo Clinic and other health-care facilities about heart valve disease occurring in patients who were receiving combined therapy with fenfluramine and phentermine for the management of obesity. As a result of these initial reports of valvulopathy, prior to the withdrawal from the market, the manufacturer had added a boxed warning to the labeling of fenfluramine and dexfenfluramine concerning heart valve disease reported with use of these drugs. Subsequently, an additional 28 cases of cardiac valvulopathy were reported to FDA, involving patients who had received phentermine in combination with fenfluramine or with dexfenfluramine or who had received monotherapy with dexfenfluramine or fenfluramine. Report of these additional cases coincided with final journal publication (*N Engl J Med*, August 28, 1997) of the earlier Mayo Clinic report and prompted FDA to issue an updated, stronger warning about the potential risks of combined fenfluramine and phentermine therapy or monotherapy with dexfenfluramine; the warning summarized these and other US cases that then totaled 82. At the time, FDA warned clinicians who chose to continue prescribing these drugs for obesity to limit such prescription to patients with substantial obesity.

Cardiovalvular Abnormalities Reports of abnormal heart valve findings, including echocardiographic features, dyspnea, chest pain, syncope, lower extremity edema, and/or new heart murmurs continued to accumulate during September 1997, and preliminary analysis by FDA of pooled data from several medical centers revealed abnormal echocardiographic findings in about 32% of 291 evaluated asymptomatic patients receiving fenfluramine or dexfenfluramine for up to 24 months, usually in combination with phentermine. Preliminary data suggest that the incidence of heart valve abnormalities may be higher in patients exposed to the anorexigenic agents for 6 months or longer when compared with those receiving the drugs for less than 6 months. In the pooled analysis, evidence of mild or more severe aortic regurgitation was present in 80 of the patients and that of moderate or more severe mitral regurgitation was present in 23 patients; aortic valve abnormalities of this severity reportedly are uncommon in the general population, occurring in about 5% of those not receiving these stimulants (placebo recipients) and in only about 1–2% of individuals younger than 50 years of age. While this analysis provided additional supportive evidence of a possible association between use of these anorexigenic agents and cardiac abnormalities, evaluation of the data has been difficult because of the absence of matched controls and pretreatment baseline data for the patients.

Subsequent data and analysis from several studies using matched controls have shown variable results when evaluating the estimated risk associated with the use of anorexigenic agents and abnormal heart valve findings. In one study, the prevalence of abnormal heart valve findings (as defined by FDA and the US Centers for Disease Control and Prevention [CDC] as at least mild aortic-valve or moderate mitral-valve insufficiency determined by an echocardiogram) was about 13, 25, or 26% in obese patients receiving dexfenfluramine (30 mg daily) alone, dexfenfluramine (30 mg daily) in combination with phentermine (30 mg daily), or fenfluramine (60–120 mg daily) in combination with phentermine (30 mg daily), respectively. Such valvulopathy reportedly only occurred in 1.3% of gender-, height-, age-, and weight-matched controls, thus indicating a substantially higher prevalence of abnormal heart valve findings in patients receiving the anorexigenic agents. Following modification of an ongoing randomized placebo-controlled study in obese patients originally designed to compare the efficacy and safety of conventional dexfenfluramine (15 mg twice daily) with those of extended-release dexfenfluramine (30 mg daily), valvulopathy (as defined by FDA) was reported in 6.9 or 4.5% of patients treated with dexfenfluramine (as conventional or extended-release preparations) or placebo, respectively, for a median of 2.5 months (the original study was terminated early) indicating an absolute difference of 2.4% between patients treated with the drug or placebo. In addition, results of a population-based follow-up study in obese patients receiving dexfenfluramine, fenfluramine, or phentermine and those of gender-, age-, and weight-matched controls also indicate an association between the anorexigenic agents and abnormal heart valve findings. The incidence of valvulopathy was zero cases per 10,000 in matched historical controls or in those who received phentermine while incidence of valvulopathy was 7.1 (0.071%) and 35 (0.35%) cases per 10,000 in patients who received either drug (dexfenfluramine or fenfluramine) for less than 4 months and for 4 months or longer, respectively. Patients diagnosed with heart valve abnormalities in this study received 15–60 or 60–120 mg of dexfenfluramine or fenfluramine, respectively.

In the population-based study, heart valve abnormalities were identified from clinical and echocardiographic findings from an electronic medical records database, and the higher-than-expected prevalence of valvular regurgitation occurring among anorexigenic agent users at the end of the follow-up was 1–2 times lower than that reported in the studies using FDA criteria for valvulopathy. It was suggested that such discordance may reflect the insensitivity of clinical evaluation in general practice in detecting mild to moderate valvular regurgitation. In addition, the use of echocardiographic findings that meet FDA criteria for valvulopathy may identify patients before the heart-valve abnormalities are clinically apparent. However, in the echocardiographic studies using placebo controls, the incidence of valvulopathy was in the range observed in echocardiographic studies of population samples, suggesting that the FDA criteria are reasonably specific and were applied in a consistent manner in the mentioned studies. In addition, analysis of the mentioned data provides further supportive evidence of the possible association between use of fenfluramine monotherapy, dexfenfluramine monotherapy, and combination of fenfluramine or dexfenfluramine with phentermine (but not with phentermine monotherapy) and cardiac abnormalities, especially in patients receiving long-term or high-dose administration of the drugs. However, such association may be less common than that suggested by the preliminary findings by FDA of pooled data from several medical centers in which abnormal echocardiographic findings occurred in about 32% of 291 evaluated asymptomatic patients receiving fenfluramine or dexfenfluramine for up to 24 months, usually in combination with phentermine. Subsequent studies have estimated a lower prevalence of such drug-related valvulopathy according to FDA criteria and identified age, dose, and duration of drug exposure as risk factors for the development of this abnormality. Very limited data indicate that cardiac valve abnormalities may regress in some patients.

Diagnostic Measures for Valvulopathy and Associated Precautions FDA and other experts recommend that patients who were receiving fenfluramine or dexfenfluramine therapy discontinue the drugs. While most patients could safely discontinue the drugs after such notification, gradual tapering of dosage (e.g., over 1–2 weeks) has been advisable in some patients; therefore, patients were advised to consult their clinician regarding specific instructions for discontinuing the drugs. In addition, because of the severity of these cardiac effects, the US Department of Health and Human Services (DHHS) issued in 1997 interim recommendations that were developed by FDA in conjunction with the CDC and the National Institutes of Health (NIH) (the National Heart, Lung, and Blood Institute and the National Institute of Diabetes and Digestive and Kidney Diseases) and in consultation with the American Heart Association (AHA), the American College of Cardiology (ACC), and the American Dental Association (ADA) for individuals who received fenfluramine or dexfenfluramine as monotherapy or in combination with other drugs (e.g., phentermine). These recommendations, based on data from patients who developed fenfluramine- or dexfenfluramine-associated heart valve disease, state that in order to determine whether heart valve abnormalities are present in individuals who were exposed to these drugs either alone or in combination therapy and to provide such patients with optimal care, a medical history and a cardiovascular examination should be performed in all patients who have received the anorexigenic drugs. In addition, an echocardiogram (ECHO) should be performed on all patients who received fenfluramine or dexfenfluramine either alone or in combination therapy for any period of time and who exhibit cardiopulmonary signs (e.g., new murmur) or symptoms (e.g., dyspnea) suggestive of heart valve disease. Echocardiographic examination also should be performed in patients in whom cardiac auscultation is not possible.

Patients with clinical and echocardiographic evidence of heart valve disease should undergo treatment and/or further testing based on the specific valve lesions. The DHHS also states that while the clinical importance of asymptomatic valvular regurgitation and the risk of developing bacterial endocarditis in such individuals is not known, clinicians should strongly consider performing an echocardiogram on all patients who have been exposed to the anorexigenic agents, regardless of whether they have developed signs and symptoms of heart valve disease, if they are about to undergo any invasive procedure for which anti-infective prophylaxis for the prevention of bacterial endocarditis is indicated by the current recommendations published by the AHA. In case of emergency procedures, when cardiac evaluation cannot be performed, empiric preventive antimicrobial therapy should be administered. Because of uncertainties about the described heart valve abnormalities (e.g., incidence of substantial heart valve abnormalities; which patients are at high or low risk for developing such abnormalities; whether such abnormalities are reversible upon discontinuance of the anorexigenic drugs; the optimal timing of follow-up echocardiograms to determine progression, regression, or stabilization of cardiac valve lesions), the DHHS states that clinicians should exercise their best judgment based on the individual patient's history and clinical and cardiac status to determine the need for additional echocardiographic follow-up. The DHHS anticipates that within 1 year sufficient data will become available to make further recommendations about such acquired valvular disease. Clinicians should continue to report to FDA at 800-332-1088 those patients with heart valve disease who have been exposed to fenfluramine, dexfenfluramine, phentermine, or any combination of these drugs.

Other Considerations for Valvulopathy FDA also issued an advisory to state boards of pharmacy alerting them to reports that a number of pharmacies in various parts of the country may have been extemporaneously compounding fenfluramine and dexfenfluramine preparations as a result of withdrawal of commercially manufactured products, and that the agency expected pharmacies to refrain from distributing such compounded preparations because of the serious health risks associated with use of these anorexigenics. As of mid-September 1997, recommendations concerning *phentermine* monotherapy for obesity were not affected by the recall and patients were not being advised to necessarily discontinue such therapy if indicated. However, manufacturers of the drug state that phentermine *only* should be used for short-term treatment (a few weeks) of exogenous obesity and the drug should *not* be used in combination with selective serotonin-reuptake inhibitor antidepressants (e.g., fluoxetine, sertraline, paroxetine, fluvoxamine) or monoamine oxidase [MAO] inhibitors). In addition, phentermine should *not* be used in combination with phendimetrazine tartrate since abnormal heart valve findings and primary pulmonary hypertension have been reported in some patients receiving phendimetrazine in combination with other anorexigenic agents (e.g., phentermine).

Mechanism of Cardiac Abnormalities The mechanism of these anorexigenic agent-associated adverse cardiac effects has not been elucidated. However, it has been suggested that the cardiac abnormalities may be related to serotonergic alterations induced by the drugs. Additional evidence purportedly supporting such a serotonin hypothesis includes the histopathologic similarity (e.g., plaque-like encasement of leaflets, chordal structures with a "stuck-on" appearance, intact valve architecture) between the anorexigenic valvulopathy observed in several patients who underwent cardiac surgery and the diseased valves observed in patients with carcinoid syndrome or in ergot toxicity. Although pulmonary hypertension has been reported in women who were found to have valvular regurgitation following fenfluramine or dexfenfluramine use, reversibility of valvular abnormalities also has been reported in some patients and the clinical course following discontinuance of the drugs remains to be elucidated.

Pulmonary Hypertension Pulmonary hypertension in the absence of documented valvulopathy also has been reported in patients receiving amphetamines and amphetamine congeners, including dexfenfluramine, fenfluramine, phendimetrazine, and/or phentermine. Further study is needed to identify the possible mechanisms of action and risk factors for developing such adverse effects. Animal evidence of serotonin depletion in the CNS with prolonged use of dexfenfluramine has raised additional unresolved concerns about the long-term safety of fenfluramine and dexfenfluramine.

■ **Peripheral Vascular Effects** Stimulants are associated with peripheral vascular disorders (e.g., Raynaud's phenomenon). Manifestations usually are intermittent and mild, but ulceration of the digits and/or breakdown of soft tissue may occur rarely. Peripheral vascular disorders have been reported during postmarketing experience in patients in all age groups receiving stimulants at therapeutic dosages and at various times throughout the treatment course. Manifestations generally improve following dosage reduction or drug discontinuance. Careful observation for digital changes is warranted during therapy with stimulants, and further clinical evaluation (e.g., referral to a rheumatologist) may be appropriate for certain patients.

■ **Serotonin Syndrome** Potentially life-threatening serotonin syndrome may occur when amphetamines are used concomitantly with other drugs that affect serotonergic neurotransmission, including MAO inhibitors, selective serotonin-reuptake inhibitors (SSRIs), selective serotonin- and norepinephrine-reuptake inhibitors (SNRIs), tricyclic antidepressants, 5-hydroxytryptamine (5-HT) type 1 receptor agonists ("triptans"), buspirone, fentanyl, lithium, tramadol, tryptophan, and St. John's wort *(Hypericum perforatum)*. Symptoms of serotonin syndrome may include mental status changes, autonomic instability, neuromuscular aberrations, seizures, and/or GI symptoms.

Serotonin syndrome also may occur when amphetamines and inhibitors of cytochrome P-450 (CYP) isoenzyme 2D6 are used concomitantly. Amphetamines and amphetamine derivatives are known to be metabolized to some degree by CYP2D6 and may show mild inhibition of CYP2D6 metabolism. The potential for a pharmacokinetic interaction exists, since such concomitant administration may increase amphetamine exposure, and thereby increase the risk of serotonin syndrome. **For further information on serotonin syndrome, including manifestations and management, see Serotonin Syndrome under Warnings/Precautions: Other Warnings and Precautions, in Cautions, in Lisdexamfetamine Dimesylate 28:20.04.**

■ **Other Adverse Effects** Adverse effects of amphetamines may include nervousness, insomnia, irritability, talkativeness, changes in libido, frequent or prolonged erections, dizziness, headaches, increased motor activity, chilliness, pallor or flushing, blurred vision, mydriasis, diplopia, difficulty with visual accommodation, and hyperexcitability. Exacerbation of motor or phonic tics, Tourette's syndrome, dyskinesia, dermatillomania, seizures, euphoria, dysphoria, emotional lability, impotence, alopecia, eosinophilic hepatitis, and rhabdomyolysis have been reported in patients receiving amphetamines. Psychotic episodes have occurred rarely in patients receiving amphetamines at recommended dosages. Psychologic disturbances have occurred in patients receiving anorexigenic agents combined with dietary restrictions. Paradoxical, increased depression or agitation in depressed patients receiving the drug are indications for discontinuing amphetamine drugs. Hypertension or hypotension, tachycardia, palpitation, or cardiac arrhythmias may occur in some patients. Cardiomyopathy, usually manifested as ventricular hypertrophy and/or congestive heart failure, has occurred in patients receiving amphetamines chronically (e.g., chronic abusers) and is potentially fatal; the cardiomyopathy is similar to adrenergic cardiomyopathies (e.g., that associated with pheochromocytoma). Sudden death, myocardial infarction (MI), and stroke have been reported in patients receiving amphetamines. GI disturbances consisting of nausea, vomiting, abdominal cramps, diarrhea or constipation, dryness of the mouth, bruxism, anorexia, weight loss, and dysgeusia (e.g., unpleasant or metallic taste) have also been reported. Dermatologic or hypersensitivity reactions (e.g., urticaria, rash, Stevens-Johnson syndrome, toxic epidermal necrolysis, angioedema, anaphylaxis) also have been reported. Tolerance to the drugs does occur.

■ Precautions and Contraindications *Psychiatric Precautions*

Aggressive behavior and hostility frequently are observed in children and adolescents with attention-deficit/hyperactivity disorder (ADHD) and have been reported in patients receiving drug therapy for the disorder. Although a causal relationship to stimulants has not been established, patients beginning treatment for ADHD should be monitored for the onset or worsening of aggressive behavior or hostility.

Psychotic or manic symptoms (e.g., hallucinations, delusional thinking, mania) have been reported in children and adolescents without prior history of psychotic illness or mania who received usual dosages of stimulants. In a pooled analysis of multiple short-term, placebo-controlled studies, such symptoms occurred in about 0.1% of patients receiving usual dosages of stimulants (i.e., amphetamine, methylphenidate) compared with 0% of those receiving placebo. If psychotic or manic symptoms occur during stimulant therapy, a causal relationship to stimulants should be considered, and discontinuance of therapy may be appropriate.

Amphetamines should be used with caution in the management of ADHD in patients with comorbid bipolar disorder because of the potential for precipitation of mixed or manic episodes in such patients. Prior to initiating amphetamine therapy, patients should be carefully screened to determine if they are at risk for bipolar disorder or for developing a manic episode; such screening should include a detailed psychiatric history (e.g., comorbid depressive symptoms or history of depressive symptoms; family history of suicide, bipolar disorder, or depression).

Stimulants may exacerbate symptoms of behavior disturbance and thought disorder (psychotomimetic effects) in psychotic patients, including those with schizophrenia, psychosis not otherwise specified, or manic episodes with psychosis.

Each time amphetamines are dispensed, a medication guide should be provided to the patient or caregiver, alerting them to the risks associated with stimulant therapy (e.g., adverse psychiatric effects, possible cardiovascular risks) and advising them of necessary precautions. (See Other Precautions and Contraindications under Cautions: Precautions and Contraindications.) Patients or caregivers should be instructed to inform clinicians of suicidal ideation or behaviors or any preexisting mental or psychiatric disorder. They also should be instructed to inform clinicians immediately if adverse psychiatric effects (e.g., hallucinations, delusional thinking, mania) occur during stimulant therapy.

The possibility of psychic dependence or addiction should be considered, particularly when amphetamines are administered to alcoholic patients or to those known to have been addicted to other drugs.

Abrupt withdrawal of an amphetamine following prolonged administration may unmask severe depression as well as the effects of chronic overactivity; paranoid and suicidal ideation, dysphoric mood (e.g., depression, irritability, anxiety), fatigue, insomnia or hypersomnia, psychomotor agitation, agoraphobia and disturbed sleep also may occur. Therefore, patients should be carefully supervised during withdrawal of the drug; long-term follow-up may be required since some manifestations (e.g., depression) may persist for prolonged periods.

Cardiovascular Precautions Stimulants cause modest increases in average blood pressure (i.e., by about 2–4 mm Hg) and heart rate (i.e., by about 3–6 bpm); larger increases may occur in some patients. Although modest increases would not be expected to have short-term sequelae, all patients should be monitored for larger changes in blood pressure and heart rate. Caution is advised in patients with underlying medical conditions that might be affected by increases in blood pressure or heart rate (e.g., hypertension, heart failure, recent MI, ventricular arrhythmia).

Serious cardiovascular events and sudden unexplained death have been associated with amphetamine abuse. In addition, although a causal relationship to stimulants has not been established, sudden unexplained death, stroke, and MI have been reported in adults receiving usual dosages of stimulants for the treatment of ADHD. Sudden unexplained death also has been reported in children and adolescents with underlying structural cardiac abnormalities or other serious cardiac conditions receiving usual dosages of stimulants. (See Cautions: Pediatric Precautions.) A very small number of cases of sudden unexplained death have been reported in children without structural cardiac abnormalities receiving amphetamine combinations (fixed-combination preparations containing dextroamphetamine sulfate, dextroamphetamine saccharate, amphetamine aspartate, and amphetamine sulfate); however, confounding factors were present in some of these incidents.

In February 2005, the Canadian drug regulatory agency suspended authorization for marketing of amphetamine combinations (Adderall XR®) based on postmarketing reports of serious cardiovascular events (e.g., stroke) and sudden unexplained death in patients receiving the drug. However, in October 2005, following review of the safety data by an independent expert panel, the agency reversed its previous decision, thereby allowing the manufacturer to market the drug in Canada. This change was based on the agency's acceptance of the panel's recommendations, which included revision of the cautionary information in the Canadian product labeling and enhanced postmarketing surveillance of all stimulants used in the treatment of ADHD.

In May 2006, following review of safety data on stimulants by 2 advisory committees, FDA directed manufacturers of ADHD stimulant preparations to revise the US product labeling to include stronger wording regarding serious adverse cardiovascular effects. According to revised US product labeling, children, adolescents, and adults who are being considered for stimulant therapy should undergo a thorough medical history review (including evaluation for family history of sudden death or ventricular arrhythmia) and physical examination to detect the presence of cardiac disease, and should receive further cardiac evaluation (e.g., ECG, echocardiogram) if initial findings suggest such disease. Stimulants generally should *not* be used in children, adolescents, or adults with known serious structural cardiac abnormalities, cardiomyopathy, serious heart rhythm abnormalities, coronary artery disease, or other serious cardiac conditions. Patients who develop exertional chest pain, unexplained syncope, or other manifestations suggestive of cardiac disease during stimulant therapy should undergo prompt cardiac evaluation.

In addition to stronger wording in the revised US product labeling, FDA, in February 2007, directed manufacturers of ADHD stimulant preparations to develop written patient information (a medication guide) to alert patients to possible cardiovascular risks and risks of adverse psychiatric effects associated with these drugs and to advise patients of necessary precautions. (See Other Precautions and Contraindications under Cautions: Precautions and Contraindications.) Patients and caregivers should be instructed to inform clinicians of preexisting cardiac or cardiovascular disease. They also should be instructed to inform clinicians immediately if adverse cardiovascular effects (e.g., chest pain, shortness of breath, fainting) occur during stimulant therapy.

Following release of the medication guide and revised US product labeling for stimulant drugs, the AHA issued additional recommendations regarding screening for cardiac conditions, selection of appropriate candidates for stimulant therapy, and monitoring for treatment-emergent cardiac conditions. In a recent scientific statement, the AHA recommends that, in addition to undergoing a thorough medical history review and physical examination, all children and adolescents being considered for stimulant therapy obtain a baseline ECG regardless of whether findings suggestive of cardiac disease are present. The AHA also recommends that an ECG, a thorough medical history review, and physical examination be obtained (if not already available) in children and adolescents currently receiving stimulants. In patients with a baseline ECG who currently are receiving stimulant therapy, the AHA states that a repeat ECG may be beneficial after the patient reaches 12 years of age or if symptoms suggestive of cardiac disease or a change in family history is reported. While sharing the AHA's goal of detecting silent but clinically important cardiac conditions, the American Academy of Pediatrics (AAP) does *not* support AHA's recommendation to obtain a baseline ECG before initiating stimulant therapy, noting that: (1) the incidence of sudden cardiac death in children and adolescents receiving therapy for ADHD is not higher than that in the general population; (2) there are no data indicating that stimulant therapy increases the risk of sudden cardiac death in patients with preexisting cardiac conditions; (3) there are no data indicating that routine ECG screening before initiation of therapy prevents sudden death; and (4) there is no cost-effectiveness analysis to justify ECG screening or special evaluations by pediatric cardiologists.

Results of one retrospective, case-control epidemiologic study showed that there may be an association between use of stimulant medications (amphetamine, dextroamphetamine, methamphetamine, methylphenidate, or their derivatives) and sudden unexplained death in healthy children and adolescents. (See Cautions: Pediatric Precautions.) Because of postmarketing reports and the results of this and other epidemiologic studies, FDA collaborated with the Agency for Healthcare Research and Quality (AHRQ) to sponsor 3 large, related, retrospective cohort studies using data from several health care claims databases to evaluate possible associations between ADHD drug use (stimulants, atomoxetine, and pemoline [no longer commercially available in the US]) and the following serious cardiovascular events: MI, stroke, and sudden cardiac death in children and young adults 2–24 years of age; MI and sudden cardiac death in adults 25–64 years of age; and stroke and the composite end point of stroke, MI, and sudden cardiac death in the same group of adults. None of the 3 studies (results of which were released in 2017) showed an association between serious cardiovascular events and current use of ADHD drugs, as compared with nonuse or as compared with former or remote use, although small increases in cardiovascular risk could not be excluded. The study in children and young adults included data for approximately 1.2 million patients and approximately 2.6 million patient-years of follow-up, including approximately 370,000 patient-years of current ADHD drug use, and found only 7 serious cardiovascular events (4 strokes, 3 sudden deaths) in current users of the drugs. The analyses in adults included data for approximately 440,000 patients, including approximately 150,000 current users of ADHD drugs; for the composite outcome of stroke, MI, and sudden cardiac death, there were approximately 107,000 patient-years of ADHD drug exposure and 234 such cardiovascular events in current users.

While the revised US product labeling states that stimulants generally should *not* be used in children, adolescents, or adults with known serious cardiac conditions, the AHA states that use of stimulants may be considered in children and adolescents with congenital heart disease that is not repaired, repaired but without current hemodynamic or arrhythmic concerns, or considered to be stable. In addition, the AHA states that, after considering or using other methods of treatment for ADHD, it is reasonable to use stimulants with caution and with careful monitoring in children and adolescents with cardiac conditions associated with sudden cardiac death (e.g., long- or short-QT syndrome, hypertrophic cardiomyopathy, Marfan syndrome, Wolff-Parkinson-White syndrome); a history of arrhythmias requiring resuscitation, cardioversion, defibrillation, or overdrive pacing; previous aborted sudden cardiac death; elevated heart rate and blood pressure; prolonged QT_c interval; or other clinically important arrhythmia not treated or controlled. However, if any of the aforementioned conditions or arrhythmias are diagnosed during stimulant therapy, the AHA recommends considering discontinuance of stimulant therapy until further testing and treatment can be obtained. If arrhythmias are treated and controlled, stimulant therapy may be reinitiated as appropriate.

Other Precautions and Contraindications The manufacturer's patient information (medication guide) should be provided to the patient or caregiver each time amphetamines are dispensed, and the clinician should discuss and answer questions about its contents (e.g., benefits and risks of stimulant therapy, appropriate use) as needed. The patient or caregiver should be instructed to read and understand the contents of the medication guide before initiating therapy and each time the prescription is refilled.

Patients or caregivers should be instructed to inform clinicians of preexisting illnesses or conditions (e.g., cardiac or cardiovascular disease, thyroid disease, glaucoma, suicidal ideation or behaviors, mental or psychiatric disorder, seizures, circulation problems in fingers and toes).

Patients should be warned that amphetamines may impair their ability to perform hazardous activities requiring mental alertness or physical coordination (e.g., operating machinery, driving a motor vehicle). Narcoleptic patients with severe sleepiness as a manifestation of their disease should be advised to avoid potentially dangerous activities at home and work and should not operate a motor vehicle until sleepiness is appropriately controlled by stimulant drug therapy.

Amphetamines should be administered with caution, if at all, to patients with hyperexcitability states or to those receiving drugs which may produce this effect. Amphetamines should also be used with caution in geriatric, debilitated, or asthenic patients or in those with psychopathic personalities or history of suicidal or homicidal tendencies.

Visual disturbances (difficulty with accommodation, blurred vision) have been reported in patients receiving stimulants.

There is some clinical evidence that stimulants may lower the seizure threshold in patients with a history of seizures, in those with prior EEG abnormalities but no history of seizures, and, very rarely, in those without a history of seizures and no prior evidence of EEG abnormalities. If seizures occur, stimulants should be discontinued.

Therapy with CNS stimulants may be associated with at least a temporary suppression of growth in children. (See Cautions: Pediatric Precautions.)

Large doses of amphetamines may cause fatigue, mental depression, an increase in blood pressure, cyanosis and respiratory failure, disorientation, hallucinations, seizures, and coma.

Phentermine should be discontinued in any patient who develops new, unexplained symptoms of dyspnea, angina, syncope, or edema of the lower extremities.

Amphetamines are contraindicated in patients with hyperthyroidism, advanced arteriosclerosis, agitated states, moderate to severe hypertension, symptomatic cardiovascular disease, glaucoma, or a history of drug abuse, and in those with a previous history of hypersensitivity or idiosyncrasy to sympathomimetic amines. Although amphetamines generally should not be used in patients with a history of drug abuse, some experts state that this is not an absolute contraindication, provided the patient can be monitored more carefully than would otherwise be indicated. Neurologic and circulatory reactions have been reported in patients who have received sympathomimetic amines concomitantly with MAO inhibitors, and fatalities have occurred. Amphetamines are contraindicated during or within 14 days of administration of MAO inhibitors. The drugs should not be used to prevent hypotension in patients who have undergone general anesthesia with drugs (cyclopropane, halothane) that sensitize the heart to the arrhythmia-producing potential of sympathomimetic amines.

■ **Pediatric Precautions** Amphetamines should not be used as anorexigenic agents in children younger than 12 years of age. Some manufacturers state that amphetamines should not be used in attention-deficit/hyperactivity disorder (ADHD) in children younger than 6 years of age, while others state that amphetamines should not be used in such disorder in children younger than 3 years of age. Lisdexamfetamine should not be used for the treatment of binge-eating disorder in pediatric patients younger than 18 years of age.

Aggressive behavior, hostility, and psychotic or manic symptoms (e.g., hallucinations, delusional thinking, mania) have been reported in children and adolescents receiving stimulants for the management of ADHD. (See Psychiatric Precautions under Cautions: Precautions and Contraindications.)

Sudden death has been reported in children and adolescents with structural cardiac abnormalities or other serious cardiac conditions receiving usual dosages of stimulants. Although a causal relationship to stimulants has not been established, and some serious cardiac conditions are independently associated with an increased risk of sudden death, stimulants generally should *not* be used in children or adolescents with known serious structural cardiac abnormalities, cardiomyopathy, serious heart rhythm abnormalities, or other serious cardiac conditions that may increase their vulnerability to the sympathomimetic effects of such drugs. Sudden unexplained death also has been reported in a small number of children without structural cardiac abnormalities receiving amphetamine combinations (fixed-combination preparations containing dextroamphetamine sulfate, dextroamphetamine saccharate, amphetamine aspartate, and amphetamine sulfate); however, confounding factors were present in some of these incidents. Results of one retrospective, case-control epidemiologic study suggested a possible association between use of stimulant medications (amphetamine, dextroamphetamine, methamphetamine, methylphenidate, or their derivatives) and sudden unexplained death in healthy children and adolescents. (See Cardiovascular Precautions under Cautions: Precautions and Contraindications.)

Prolonged administration of CNS stimulants to children with ADHD has been reported to cause at least a temporary suppression of normal weight and/or height patterns in some patients. Results of an analysis of weight and height patterns in children 7–13 years of age suggested that treatment with methylphenidate for up to 3 years was associated with a temporary slowing in growth rate (on average, height gain was suppressed by about 2 cm and weight gain was suppressed by 2.7 kg over 3 years), without evidence of growth rebound during this period of development. Published data are inadequate to determine whether long-term use of amphetamines may cause a similar suppression of growth; however, because appetite suppression and weight loss are common with stimulant therapy, and there is no apparent difference in their occurrence between amphetamine (e.g., dextroamphetamine) or methylphenidate therapy in children, it is anticipated that amphetamines, like methylphenidate, also cause temporary growth suppression. Therefore, the manufacturers of stimulant preparations state that growth should be monitored during therapy with stimulants, and children who are not growing or gaining height or weight as expected may require temporary discontinuance of therapy. Although concerns about potential dose-related growth delays in children have been raised, a prospective follow-up study into adulthood found no significant impairment in height achieved. In general, studies of stimulants in children have found little or no decrease in expected height, with any decrease in growth early in treatment being compensated for later on. Although drug holidays during summers have been suggested to minimize weight loss and other potential adverse effects, there currently are no data from controlled studies establishing whether such holidays are beneficial or associated with risks.

CNS stimulants, including amphetamines, have been reported to exacerbate motor and vocal tics and Tourette's disorder, and clinical evaluation for tics and Tourette's disorder in children and their families should precede use of the drugs. About 15–30% of children with ADHD experience tics while receiving stimulants, but such tics usually are transient. About half of children with ADHD have underlying Tourette's syndrome, and the effects of stimulants on tics are unpredictable; the presence or emergence of tics is not an absolute contraindication to stimulant therapy, and some evidence indicates that the incidence of tics is not increased with such therapy. In addition, clinical experience suggests that administration of amphetamines in psychotic children may exacerbate symptoms of behavior disturbance and thought disorder.

■ **Pregnancy and Lactation** Amphetamines may cause fetal harm. Amphetamines should be used during pregnancy only if the potential benefits justify the possible risks to the fetus. During pregnancy, it is questionable whether potential benefits from amphetamines outweigh potential risks.

Amphetamines may stimulate uterine contractions in pregnant women increasing the risk of premature delivery. Infants born to women dependent on amphetamines have an increased risk of prematurity, low birthweight, and withdrawal symptoms (e.g., dysphoria, lassitude, feeding difficulties, irritability, agitation, excessive drowsiness).

Amphetamines are distributed into milk in concentrations 2–8 times maternal blood concentrations. Large dosages of dextroamphetamine may interfere with milk production, especially in women whose lactation is not well established. Because of the potential for serious adverse effects in nursing infants, breast-feeding is not recommended during amphetamine therapy.

Acute Toxicity

■ **Pathogenesis** Despite the high toxicity and wide distribution of amphetamines, death occurs rarely following acute overdosage. There is a relatively large margin of safety between the amount of drug incorporated in a unit therapeutic dose and the lethal dose. In adults, 120 mg of amphetamine has caused death, but in one patient 200 mg produced only mild signs of peripheral sympathomimetic activity. Death usually is preceded by seizures and coma and usually results from cardiovascular collapse or from seizures.

■ **Manifestations** Overdose of an amphetamine may be manifested initially by cardiovascular symptoms including flushing or pallor, palpitation, tachypnea, tremor, labile pulse rate and blood pressure (hypertension or hypotension), cardiac arrhythmias (e.g., extrasystoles), heart block, circulatory collapse, and chest pain. Toxic doses of phenylisopropylamines produce marked and photosensitive mydriasis, profuse perspiration, and polypnea. Elevated environmental temperature and other environmental factors such as crowding or aggregation markedly increase the acute toxicity of amphetamines in experimental animals. Although comparable clinical data in humans are lacking, hyperpyrexia has been noted as a frequent and prominent sign of acute human intoxication. Rhabdomyolysis also has been associated with acute overdosage of amphetamines, and hyperpyrexia and/or rhabdomyolysis can result in associated complications. Mental disturbances such as confusion, delirium, belligerence, or acute psychoses with disorientation, delusions, and hallucinations may occur. Overdosage may be characterized by restlessness, vivid visual and auditory hallucinations, panic state, suicidal or homicidal tendencies, paranoid ideation, combativeness, loosening of associations, or changes in affect occurring in association with a clear sensorium. Fatigue and depression usually follow CNS stimulation. The psychotic syndrome may occur within 36–48 hours after ingestion of a single large dose of an amphetamine. In apparently hypersensitive individuals, psychosis may be produced by a single dose of 55–75 mg of dextroamphetamine. Overdose of an amphetamine also may be manifested by GI symptoms including nausea, vomiting, diarrhea, and abdominal cramps. After a single large oral dose, amphetamine is slowly excreted over a period of 5–7 days, suggesting the possibility that cumulative effects may occur with repeated administration of the drug. If the patient does not receive additional doses of the drug, the psychosis usually clears within about 1 week.

The toxic effects are more variable in children than in adults and acute toxicity in children has occurred over a wide range of dosage. In a 2-year-old child, 40–50 mg of dextroamphetamine produced toxicity even when 60–75 mg of phenobarbital were ingested at the same time. Another child, slightly older than 2 years of age, survived 115 mg of dextroamphetamine. Overdosage of amphetamines in children may be manifested by constant twisting and turning, purposeless movement, mumbling, and hyperirritability. Children may be in a tremulous state for up to 12 hours following ingestion of an overdosage of an amphetamine without having a seizure. In acute poisoning in a child, external stimuli precipitate increased hyperactivity. Overdosage in children may also produce confusion, delirium, hallucinations, carphology, panic state, and other acute psychotic syndromes. Children also may exhibit self-destructive behavior, such as head banging and mutilation of digits by biting, and violent, purposeless movements.

■ **Treatment** There is no specific antidote for amphetamine overdosage. Treatment of overdosage is symptomatic and includes administration of sedative drugs, preferably short-acting barbiturates, and isolation of the patient to avoid possible external stimuli. In the treatment of overdosage, general physiologic supportive measures should be immediately undertaken. Standard treatment for shock should be administered if necessary. Absorption of the drug should be delayed by use of a tourniquet and ice pack following injection or by emesis or gastric lavage if the drug has been ingested, and excretion may be hastened by acidification of the urine with ammonium chloride. Hypothermic measures may be used if necessary and if intracranial pressure rises, measures to combat cerebral edema and congestion should be used.

Chronic Toxicity

At normal dosage levels, administration of an amphetamine may produce tolerance within a few weeks. Prolonged use of an amphetamine may lead to habituation and possibly physical or psychic dependence. Amphetamines are abused by some users for their central exciting action and since these drugs temporarily lessen fatigue, they are frequently abused by persons in occupations requiring extremes of endurance, such as students, athletes, and drivers of motor vehicles. Some emotionally unstable individuals come to depend on the pleasant mental stimulation the drugs offer.

The symptoms of chronic abuse of amphetamines are similar to those of cocaine and consist of emotional lability, loss of appetite, somnolence, mental impairment, occupational deterioration, and a tendency to withdraw from social contacts. Chronic users of amphetamines exhibit continuous chewing or teeth-grinding movements, with rubbing of the tongue along the inside of the lower lip, frequently resulting in trauma and ulcers of the tongue and lip, and other choreoathetoid manifestations. Amphetamines are frequently used concurrently or alternately with alcohol or barbiturates. The average daily dose ingested by an abuser is equivalent to about 1–2 g of amphetamine. Prolonged use of high doses can elicit a syndrome that presents all characteristics of paranoid schizophrenia, including auditory and visual hallucinations and paranoid ideation. Rarely, prolonged use of amphetamine has caused aplastic anemia and fatal pancytopenia.

Because of the relative ease with which methamphetamine ("speed," "crystal," "crank," "go," "ice") can be synthesized clandestinely from commonly available chemicals such as ephedrine, pseudoephedrine, or phenylpropanolamine (see Uses: Misuse and Abuse in the respective monographs on these drugs in 12:12.12), misuse and abuse of amphetamines have experienced a resurgence in the US. Currently, methamphetamine is the most widely illegally manufactured, distributed, and abused amphetamine in the US, with an estimated 4 million Americans having abused the drug at least once. In addition, morbidity and mortality from methamphetamine abuse have increased substantially in the US since 1990, particularly in the West but also in the South and Midwest. From 1991 to 1994, the number of methamphetamine-related deaths reported by medical examiners in the US about tripled, with the number increasing by 850, 238, 144, and 113% in Phoenix, San Diego, San Francisco, and Los Angeles, respectively. Most decedents were 26–44 years of age, male, and white, and nearly all deaths involved methamphetamine taken in combination with at least one other drug, principally alcohol, heroin, or cocaine. Methamphetamine-related hospital emergency room visits more than tripled during this period, especially in Phoenix, Denver, Minneapolis/St. Paul, and Seattle but also in cities in the South and Midwest (e.g., Atlanta, St. Louis, Dallas). In some areas, the popularity of methamphetamine abuse exceeds that of cocaine. Contributing to the resurgence in abuse of methamphetamine are ready availability in many cities, relatively inexpensive cost, more immediate and sustained effect compared with cocaine or "crack" cocaine, and multiple routes of administration (injection, "snorting," ingestion, and smoking). In addition to the potential adverse effects directly attributable to methamphetamine, abuse of the drug also may be associated with indirect risks such as the development of human immunodeficiency virus (HIV) infection and acquired immunodeficiency syndrome (AIDS); in all regions of the US, sexually active bisexual and homosexual men were more likely than heterosexual men to report amphetamines as the principal parenteral drugs of abuse. Because of the regional variability in methamphetamine abuse in the US, local drug-abuse patterns should be evaluated for planning preventive and treatment services.

The addiction potential of amphetamines is subject to controversy. Most authorities agree that long-term therapy with amphetamine or one of its isomers is unlikely to produce addiction and that habituation or psychic dependence is caused by psychological factors which lead to abuse of the drug and not by any pharmacologic action. In one study, however, abrupt withdrawal of large doses of amphetamine caused a consistent increase in the percentage of the rhombencephalic phase of the EEG pattern during sleep. The percentage returns to normal levels when amphetamine is readministered and rises again when the drug is withheld. This phenomenon meets the usual criteria for a withdrawal symptom but does not alter the fact that abrupt discontinuation of sympathomimetic amines does not cause major physiological changes that would necessitate gradual reduction of the medication.

Pharmacology

The pharmacologic actions of amphetamines are qualitatively similar to those of ephedrine and include CNS and respiratory stimulation and sympathomimetic activity including pressor response, mydriasis, bronchodilation, and contraction of the urinary bladder sphincter. The effect of amphetamines on the motility of the GI tract is variable and unpredictable. On a weight basis, dextroamphetamine has a stronger CNS action and a lesser activity on the peripheral nervous system than does the racemic amphetamine. The CNS stimulating effect of dextroamphetamine is approximately twice that of amphetamine and about three or four times that of levamfetamine (no longer commercially available in the US). Levamfetamine is slightly more potent than dextroamphetamine in its cardiovascular effects. In healthy individuals, therapeutic doses of an amphetamine do not appreciably increase respiratory rate or minute volume, but when respiration is depressed by centrally acting drugs, an amphetamine stimulates respiration. The bronchodilating effect of amphetamines is less than that of ephedrine.

Amphetamines may superimpose psychic stimulation and excitability over fatigue, permitting a temporary increase in mental and physical activity. In healthy individuals, the drugs have not consistently facilitated improved mental performance and in some cases, nervousness produced by amphetamines is a distinct mental hazard. The most striking improvement caused by an amphetamine appears to occur when performance has been reduced by fatigue; such improvement may be due to alteration of unfavorable attitudes toward the task. Psychic stimulation produced by amphetamines is usually followed by depression and fatigue. Psychic effects depend on dose, mental state, and personality of the patient.

Theories of dysfunction in attention-deficit/hyperactivity disorder (ADHD) focus on the prefrontal cortex, which controls many executive functions (e.g., planning, impulse control). Stimulants have putative effects on central dopamine and norepinephrine pathways that are crucial in frontal lobe function. Stimulants act in the striatum by binding to the dopamine transporter, thus increasing synaptic dopamine. This effect may enhance functioning of executive control processes in the prefrontal cortex, ameliorating deficits in inhibitory control and working memory.

Amphetamines apparently produce an anorexigenic effect, leading to loss of weight. The mechanism of action of amphetamines on appetite suppression has not been elucidated. No primary effect on appetite has been demonstrated in humans and it has been postulated that anorexigenic effects of amphetamines are secondary to increased sympathetic activity resulting from amphetamine-induced release of norepinephrine and dopamine. In addition, amphetamines may cause a loss of acuity of smell and taste, which may contribute to the anorexigenic effect of the drugs. Amphetamines have little or no effect on the basal metabolic rate or on nitrogen excretion.

The anorexigenic effect of fenfluramine (no longer commercially available in the US) and dexfenfluramine (no longer commercially available in the US), amphetamine congeners, may have been associated with a different mechanism than those associated with amphetamines since the drugs appeared to stimulate release of serotonin (5-HT) at synapses and selectively inhibit the reuptake of serotonin at the presynaptic serotonergic nerve endings, which may have resulted in increased postsynaptic concentrations of serotonin in the CNS. In the past, it has been suggested that combined therapy with fenfluramine and phentermine (an amphetamine congener that inhibits uptake of norepinephrine and dopamine) may provide complementary anorexigenic effects; therefore, such combined therapy has been used in the management of obesity. However, because of accumulated data on adverse effects associated with the drugs, fenfluramine hydrochloride (Pondimin®) and its dextrorotatory isomer dexfenfluramine hydrochloride (Redux®) were withdrawn from the US market in 1997. (See Cautions.)

Pharmacokinetics

Amphetamines are readily absorbed from the GI tract and effects persist for 4–24 hours. Amphetamines are distributed into most body tissues with high concentrations occurring in the brain and CSF.

Amphetamine appears in the urine within about 3 hours following oral administration. Urinary excretion of the amphetamines is pH-dependent and excretion is enhanced in acidic urine. Following oral administration of racemic amphetamine to humans, approximately equal amounts of both isomers were excreted during the first 12 hours; after the first 12 hours, a continually decreasing proportion of the *d*-isomer was excreted. Following oral administration of a 70-mg radiolabeled dose of lisdexamfetamine (a prodrug of dextroamphetamine), 96% of the dose was recovered in the urine; of the recovered radioactivity, 42% of the dose was related to amphetamine, 25% to hippuric acid, and 2% to the parent drug. Dextroamphetamine and levamfetamine (no longer commercially available in the US) appear to have different metabolic fates, but the relationship between the fate of the drugs and their pharmacologic activity has not been determined. There are some data to indicate stereospecific metabolism of amphetamine and its isomers, but stereospecific urinary excretion appears unlikely.

Chemistry

Amphetamine is *d,l*-*α*-methylphenethylamine, an adrenergic agent of the phenylisopropylamine type. The levo- and dextroisomers, racemic amphetamine, and the salts of the isomers and of racemic amphetamine are used in medical practice. Amphetamine is a noncatechol, sympathomimetic amine and has a greater CNS stimulant activity than epinephrine and other catecholamines. Lisdexamfetamine dimesylate is a prodrug and has little, if any, pharmacologic activity until converted to dextroamphetamine in blood mainly via hydrolytic activity of erythrocytes.

Inactivation of sympathomimetic noncatecholamines largely depends on breakdown by monoamine oxidase and since substitution of an alkyl group for hydrogen on the *α*-carbon atom blocks enzymatic inactivation of the amino group, the duration of action of noncatecholamines (but not of catecholamines, which are inactivated largely by a different mechanism) is prolonged by *α*-substitution. The absence of a hydroxyl group on the aromatic ring of amphetamine reduces inactivation of the drug in the GI tract and the amphetamines are active following oral administration.

Amphetamines are subject to control under the Federal Controlled Substances Act of 1970.

For further information on the chemistry, pharmacology, pharmacokinetics, uses, cautions, drug interactions, and dosage and administration of amphetamines, see the individual monographs in 28:20.04.

†Use is not currently included in the labeling approved by the US Food and Drug Administration

Amphetamine

■ Amphetamine is a noncatechol, sympathomimetic amine with CNS-stimulating activity.

Uses

Amphetamine sulfate and amphetamine aspartate in fixed-combination preparations containing amphetamine aspartate, amphetamine sulfate, dextroamphetamine saccharate, and dextroamphetamine sulfate are used in the treatment of narcolepsy and as adjuncts to psychological, educational, social, and other remedial measures in the treatment of attention deficit hyperactivity disorder (ADHD).

■ Narcolepsy and Attention Deficit Hyperactivity Disorder

Amphetamine sulfate and amphetamine aspartate in fixed-combination preparations containing amphetamine aspartate, amphetamine sulfate, dextroamphetamine saccharate, and dextroamphetamine sulfate are used in the treatment of narcolepsy and as adjuncts to psychological, educational, social, and other remedial measures in the treatment of ADHD (hyperkinetic disorder, hyperkinetic syndrome of childhood, minimal brain dysfunction) in children, adolescents, and adults.

ADHD usually is characterized by developmentally inappropriate symptoms (e.g., moderate to severe distractibility, short attention span, hyperactivity, emotional lability, impulsivity). The final diagnosis of this disorder should not be made if these symptoms are of only comparatively recent origin. Nonlocalizing (soft) neurologic signs, learning disability, and abnormal EEG may or may not be present, and a diagnosis of CNS dysfunction may or may not be warranted. Drug therapy is not indicated in all children with ADHD, and such therapy should be considered only after a complete evaluation including medical history has been performed. The decision to use amphetamines should depend on the age of the child and the clinician's assessment of the severity and duration of symptoms and should not depend solely on one or more behavioral characteristics. When symptoms of ADHD are associated with acute stress reactions, use of amphetamines usually is not recommended. For a more detailed discussion on the management of ADHD, including the use of stimulants such as amphetamine, see Uses: Attention Deficit Hyperactivity Disorder, in Methylphenidate 28:20.32.

Dosage and Administration

■ Administration Amphetamine sulfate and amphetamine aspartate in fixed-combination preparations containing amphetamine aspartate, amphetamine sulfate, dextroamphetamine saccharate, and dextroamphetamine sulfate are administered orally. The commercially available extended-release capsules containing amphetamine sulfate and amphetamine aspartate in fixed-combination with dextroamphetamine saccharate and dextroamphetamine sulfate (Adderall® XR) may be swallowed intact with or without food or the entire contents of a capsule(s) may be sprinkled on a small amount of applesauce immediately prior to administration; subdividing the contents of a capsule is not recommended. The pellets contained in the capsules should not be chewed or crushed, and the sprinkle/food mixture must not be stored for use at a later time.

The initial dose of amphetamines (as conventional tablets or extended-release capsules) should be given on awakening; when amphetamines are administered as conventional tablets in divided doses (2 or 3), additional doses are given at intervals of 4–6 hours. Because of the potential for insomnia, administration of conventional tablets in the late evening or extended-release capsules in the afternoon should be avoided.

■ Dosage Dosage of amphetamines should be adjusted according to individual response and tolerance; the smallest dose required to produce the desired response should always be used.

Narcolepsy In the treatment of narcolepsy, the usual total dosage of amphetamines given in fixed-combination preparations containing amphetamine aspartate, amphetamine sulfate, dextroamphetamine saccharate, and dextroamphetamine sulfate is 5–60 mg daily, depending upon the patient's age and response, usually given in divided doses. In patients 12 years of age and older, the initial dosage is 10 mg daily; daily dosage is increased by 10 mg at weekly intervals until the optimum response is attained. Although narcolepsy seldom occurs in children younger than 12 years of age, such children also may receive dextroamphetamine alone. In patients 6–12 years of age, the recommended initial dosage is 5 mg daily; daily dosage is increased by 5 mg at weekly intervals until optimum response is attained. When intolerable adverse effects (e.g., insomnia, anorexia) occur, dosage should be reduced.

Attention Deficit Hyperactivity Disorder As an adjunct in the treatment of attention deficit hyperactivity disorder (ADHD) in children 6 years of age and older, the initial total dosage of amphetamines given in conventional fixed-combination preparations containing amphetamine aspartate, amphetamine sulfate, dextroamphetamine saccharate, and dextroamphetamine sulfate is 5 mg once or twice daily; the daily dosage is increased by 5 mg at weekly intervals until the optimum response is attained. Total daily dosage rarely should exceed 40 mg. In children 3–5 years of age, the initial dosage of amphetamines given in conventional fixed-combination preparations containing amphetamine aspartate, amphetamine sulfate, dextroamphetamine saccharate, and dextroamphetamine sulfate is 2.5 mg daily; the daily dosage is increased by 2.5 mg at weekly intervals until the optimum response is attained. When amphetamines are administered as conventional tablets in divided doses (2 or 3), additional doses are given at intervals of 4–6 hours.

Alternatively, in patients who are receiving drug therapy for ADHD for the first time or are being switched from therapy with another stimulant, amphetamine therapy may be initiated with extended-release capsules containing amphetamine aspartate, amphetamine sulfate, dextroamphetamine saccharate, and dextroamphetamine sulfate in fixed combination (Adderall® XR). In children 6–12 years of age, the initial dosage of amphetamines as extended-release capsules (Adderall® XR) is 10 mg once daily; daily dosage may be increased in increments of 5 or 10 mg at weekly intervals to a maximum dosage of 30 mg daily. Treatment may be initiated with a dosage of 5 mg once daily when, in the opinion of the clinician, a lower initial dosage is appropriate. In adolescents 13–17 years of age, the initial dosage of amphetamines as extended-release capsules (Adderall® XR) is 10 mg once daily. Dosage may be increased to 20 mg once daily after 1 week if symptoms are not adequately controlled. In adults who are receiving drug therapy for ADHD for the first time or are being switched from therapy with another drug, the recommended dosage of amphetamines as extended-release capsules (Adderall XR®) is 20 mg once daily. Although dosages of up to 60 mg daily (as extended-release capsules) have been used in adolescents 13–17 years of age and adults in clinical studies, there is no evidence that dosages exceeding 20 mg daily provide any additional benefit in these patients. When switching from conventional tablets (Adderall®) to extended-release capsules (Adderall® XR), the total daily dosage of amphetamines may remain the same but should be given once daily.

When possible, therapy should be interrupted occasionally to determine if there is a recurrence of behavioral symptoms sufficient to require continued treatment. Long-term use of conventional tablets or long-term use of extended-release capsules (i.e., more than 3 weeks in children or more than 4 weeks in adolescents or adults) has not been studied systematically. If conventional tablets or extended-release capsules are used for extended periods, the usefulness of the drug should be reevaluated periodically.

Chemistry and Stability

■ **Chemistry** Amphetamine, *d,l-α*-methylphenethylamine, occurs as a colorless, mobile liquid with an amine odor and is sparingly soluble in water (1:50) and soluble in alcohol. The base is volatile at room temperature and has been used as an inhalant but is no longer commercially available in the US. Amphetamine sulfate occurs as a white, odorless crystalline powder and has a slightly bitter taste. Amphetamine sulfate is freely soluble in water (1:9) and slightly soluble in alcohol (about 1:500). Amphetamine aspartate and amphetamine sulfate currently are commercially available in the US only as fixed-combination preparations containing amphetamine aspartate, amphetamine sulfate, dextroamphetamine saccharate, and dextroamphetamine sulfate.

■ **Stability** The fixed-combination conventional tablets or extended-release capsules containing amphetamine aspartate, amphetamine sulfate, dextroamphetamine saccharate, and dextroamphetamine sulfate should be stored in tight, light-resistant containers at 25°C but may be exposed to temperatures ranging from 15–30°C.

For further information on chemistry, pharmacology, pharmacokinetics, uses, cautions, chronic toxicity, acute toxicity, and dosage and administration of amphetamine and amphetamine sulfate, see the Amphetamines General Statement 28:20.04.

Preparations

Amphetamine sulfate preparations are subject to control under the Federal Controlled Substances Act of 1970 as schedule II (C-II) drugs.

Excipients in commercially available drug preparations may have clinically important effects in some individuals; consult specific product labeling for details.

Amphetamine Sulfate Combinations

Oral		
Capsules, extended-release	5 mg total amphetamine (as 1.25 mg, with Amphetamine Aspartate 1.25 mg, Dextroamphetamine Saccharate 1.25 mg, and Dextroamphetamine Sulfate 1.25 mg)	**Adderall XR**® (C-II), Shire
	10 mg total amphetamine (as 2.5 mg, with Amphetamine Aspartate 2.5 mg, Dextroamphetamine Saccharate 2.5 mg, and Dextroamphetamine Sulfate 2.5 mg)	**Adderall XR**® (C-II), Shire
	15 mg total amphetamine (as 3.75 mg, with Amphetamine Aspartate 3.75 mg, Dextroamphetamine Saccharate 3.75 mg, and Dextroamphetamine Sulfate 3.75 mg)	**Adderall XR**® (C-II), Shire
	20 mg total amphetamine (as 5 mg, with Amphetamine Aspartate 5 mg, Dextroamphetamine Saccharate 5 mg, and Dextroamphetamine Sulfate 5 mg)	**Adderall XR**® (C-II), Shire
	25 mg total amphetamine (as 6.25 mg, with Amphetamine Aspartate 6.25 mg, Dextroamphetamine Saccharate 6.25 mg, and Dextroamphetamine Sulfate 6.25 mg)	**Adderall XR**® (C-II), Shire
	30 mg total amphetamine (as 7.5 mg, with Amphetamine Aspartate 7.5 mg, Dextroamphetamine Saccharate 7.5 mg, and Dextroamphetamine Sulfate 7.5 mg)	**Adderall XR**® (C-II), Shire
Tablets	5 mg total amphetamine (as 1.25 mg, with Amphetamine Aspartate 1.25 mg, Dextroamphetamine Saccharate 1.25 mg, and Dextroamphetamine Sulfate 1.25 mg)*	**Adderall**® (C-II; double-scored), Shire **Dextroamphetamine Saccharate, Amphetamine Aspartate, Dextroamphetamine Sulfate, and Amphetamine Sulfate Tablets** (C-II; double-scored)
	7.5 mg total amphetamine (as 1.875 mg, with Amphetamine Aspartate 1.875 mg, Dextroamphetamine Saccharate 1.875 mg, and Dextroamphetamine Sulfate 1.875 mg)*	**Adderall**® (C-II; double-scored), Shire **Dextroamphetamine Saccharate, Amphetamine Aspartate, Dextroamphetamine Sulfate, and Amphetamine Sulfate Tablets** (C-II; double-scored)
	10 mg total amphetamine (as 2.5 mg, with Amphetamine Aspartate 2.5 mg, Dextroamphetamine Saccharate 2.5 mg, and Dextroamphetamine Sulfate 2.5 mg)*	**Adderall**® (C-II; double-scored), Shire **Dextroamphetamine Saccharate, Amphetamine Aspartate, Dextroamphetamine Sulfate, and Amphetamine Sulfate Tablets** (C-II; double-scored)
	12.5 mg total amphetamine (as 3.125 mg, with Amphetamine Aspartate 3.125 mg, Dextroamphetamine Saccharate 3.125 mg, and Dextroamphetamine Sulfate 3.125 mg)*	**Adderall**® (C-II; double-scored), Shire **Dextroamphetamine Saccharate, Amphetamine Aspartate, Dextroamphetamine Sulfate, and Amphetamine Sulfate Tablets** (C-II; double-scored)
	15 mg total amphetamine (as 3.75 mg, with Amphetamine Aspartate 3.75 mg, Dextroamphetamine Saccharate 3.75 mg, and Dextroamphetamine Sulfate 3.75 mg)*	**Adderall**® (C-II; double-scored), Shire **Dextroamphetamine Saccharate, Amphetamine Aspartate, Dextroamphetamine Sulfate, and Amphetamine Sulfate Tablets** (C-II; double-scored)
	20 mg total amphetamine (as 5 mg, with Amphetamine Aspartate 5 mg, Dextroamphetamine Saccharate 5 mg, and Dextroamphetamine Sulfate 5 mg)*	**Adderall**® (C-II; double-scored), Shire **Dextroamphetamine Saccharate, Amphetamine Aspartate, Dextroamphetamine Sulfate, and Amphetamine Sulfate Tablets** (C-II; double-scored)
	30 mg total amphetamine (as 7.5 mg, with Amphetamine Aspartate 7.5 mg, Dextroamphetamine Saccharate 7.5 mg, and Dextroamphetamine Sulfate 7.5 mg)*	**Adderall**® (C-II; double-scored), Shire **Dextroamphetamine Saccharate, Amphetamine Aspartate, Dextroamphetamine Sulfate, and Amphetamine Sulfate Tablets** (C-II; double-scored)

*available from one or more manufacturer, distributor, and/or repackager by generic (nonproprietary) name

Dextroamphetamine

■ Dextroamphetamine is the dextrorotatory isomer of amphetamine.

Uses

Dextroamphetamine sulfate alone and in fixed-combination preparations with dextroamphetamine saccharate, amphetamine aspartate, and amphetamine sulfate is used in the treatment of narcolepsy and as an adjunct to psychological, educational, social, and other remedial measures in the treatment of attention deficit hyperactivity disorder (ADHD).

■ **Narcolepsy and Attention Deficit Hyperactivity Disorder** Dextroamphetamine sulfate alone and in fixed-combination preparations with dextroamphetamine saccharate, amphetamine aspartate, and amphetamine sulfate is used in the treatment of narcolepsy and as an adjunct to psychological, educational, social, and other remedial measures in the treatment of ADHD (hyperkinetic disorder, hyperkinetic syndrome of childhood, minimal brain dysfunction) in children, adolescents, and adults.

ADHD usually is characterized by developmentally inappropriate symptoms (e.g., moderate to severe distractibility, short attention span, hyperactivity, emotional lability, impulsivity). The final diagnosis of this disorder should not be made if these symptoms are of only comparatively recent origin. Nonlocalizing (soft) neurologic signs, learning disability, and abnormal EEG may or may not be present, and a diagnosis of CNS dysfunction may or may not be warranted. Drug therapy is not indicated in all children with ADHD, and such therapy should be considered only after a complete evaluation including medical history has been performed. The decision to use amphetamines should depend on the age of the child and the clinician's assessment of the severity and duration of symptoms and should not depend solely on one or more behavioral characteristics. When symptoms of ADHD are associated with acute stress reactions, use of amphetamines usually is not recommended. For a more detailed discussion on the management of ADHD, including the use of stimulants such as dextroamphetamine, see Uses: Attention Deficit Hyperactivity Disorder, in Methylphenidate 28:20.32.

Dosage and Administration

■ Administration Preparations containing dextroamphetamine sulfate are administered orally. The commercially available extended-release capsules containing dextroamphetamine sulfate and dextroamphetamine saccharate in fixed-combination with amphetamine sulfate and amphetamine aspartate (Adderall XR®) may be swallowed intact with or without food or the entire contents of a capsule(s) may be sprinkled on a small amount of applesauce immediately prior to administration; subdividing the contents of a capsule is not recommended. The pellets contained in the capsules should not be chewed or crushed, and the sprinkle/food mixture must not be stored for use at a later time.

The initial dose of dextroamphetamine sulfate (alone or in fixed-combination preparations) is given on awakening; when the drug is given as conventional (short-acting) tablets in divided doses (2 or 3), additional doses are given at intervals of 4–6 hours. Because of the potential for insomnia, administration of dextroamphetamine sulfate conventional tablets (Dexedrine®), dextroamphetamine sulfate extended-release capsules (Dexedrine® Spansules®), or fixed-combination conventional tablets (Adderall®) in the late evening or administration of fixed-combination extended-release capsules (Adderall XR®) in the afternoon should be avoided.

■ Dosage Dosage of dextroamphetamines should be adjusted according to individual response and tolerance; the smallest dose required to produce the desired response should always be used.

Narcolepsy In the treatment of narcolepsy, the usual dosage of dextroamphetamine sulfate given alone or the total dosage of amphetamines given in fixed-combination preparations containing dextroamphetamine sulfate, dextroamphetamine saccharate, amphetamine aspartate, and amphetamine sulfate is 5–60 mg daily, depending upon the patient's age and response, usually given in divided doses. In patients 12 years of age and older, the initial dosage is 10 mg daily; daily dosage is increased by 10 mg at weekly intervals until the optimum response is attained. Although narcolepsy seldom occurs in children younger than 12 years of age, in pediatric patients 6–12 years of age, the recommended initial dosage of dextroamphetamine sulfate is 5 mg daily; daily dosage is increased by 5 mg at weekly intervals until the optimum response is attained. When intolerable adverse effects occur (e.g., insomnia, anorexia), dosage should be reduced. Dextroamphetamine sulfate extended-release capsules may be used for once-daily dosing whenever appropriate.

Attention Deficit Hyperactivity Disorder Dextroamphetamine sulfate dosage for the treatment of attention deficit hyperactivity disorder (ADHD) should be individualized based on patient response and tolerance. The first dosage that produces an observable response may not be the optimum dosage to improve function, and titration to higher dosages should continue in an attempt to achieve a better response. Such a strategy may require subsequent lowering of dosage when higher dosages produce adverse effects or no further clinical improvement. The best dosage for a given patient is the one that provides optimum therapeutic effects with minimal adverse effects. Dosing schedules also may vary, although there currently are no consistent controlled studies comparing alternative dosing schedules. Patients who require relief only during school may respond adequately to a 5-day (i.e., school day) regimen while those requiring relief at home and school may need a daily regimen throughout the week.

As an adjunct in the treatment of ADHD in children 6 years of age and older, the initial dosage of dextroamphetamine sulfate given in conventional (short-acting) preparations is 5 mg once or twice daily; daily dosage is increased by 5 mg at weekly intervals until the optimum response is attained. The usual dosage range is 5–15 mg twice daily or 5–10 mg 3 times daily. Total daily dosage rarely should exceed 40 mg. In children 3–5 years of age, the initial daily dosage is 2.5 mg; daily dosage is increased by 2.5 mg at weekly intervals until the optimum response is attained. When the drug is administered as conventional tablets in divided doses (2 or 3), additional doses are given at intervals of 4–6 hours. Dextroamphetamine sulfate extended-release capsules can be substituted for their respective conventional short-acting preparations if less frequent daily dosing is desirable.

Dextroamphetamine sulfate in fixed combination with other amphetamines (dextroamphetamine sulfate, dextroamphetamine saccharate, amphetamine aspartate, and amphetamine sulfate) also is used as an adjunct in the treatment of ADHD in children 6 years of age and older; the initial total dosage of amphetamines is 5 mg once or twice daily. The daily dosage is increased by 5 mg at weekly intervals until the optimum response is attained; total daily dosage rarely should exceed 40 mg. In children 3–5 years of age, the initial daily dosage is 2.5 mg; daily dosage is increased by 2.5 mg at weekly intervals until the optimum response is attained. The manufacturer recommends that the initial dose of dextroamphetamine sulfate in fixed combination with other amphetamines be given on awakening; additional doses (1 or 2) are given at intervals of 4–6 hours. The usual dosage for intermediate-acting preparations (e.g., Dexedrine® Spansules®, Adderall®) in children 6 years of age and older is 5–30 mg once daily or 5–15 mg twice daily.

Alternatively, in patients who are receiving drug therapy for ADHD for the first time or are being switched from therapy with another stimulant, dextroamphetamine therapy may be initiated with extended-release capsules containing dextroamphetamine sulfate in fixed-combination with dextroamphetamine saccharate, amphetamine aspartate, and amphetamine sulfate (Adderall XR®). In children 6–12 years of age, the initial dosage of total amphetamines as fixed-combination extended-release capsules (Adderall XR®) is 10 mg once daily; daily dosage may be increased in increments of 5 or 10 mg at weekly intervals to a maximum dosage of 30 mg daily. Treatment may be initiated with a dosage of 5 mg once daily when, in the opinion of the clinician, a lower initial dosage is appropriate. The usual dosage for such longer-acting preparations (e.g., Adderall XR®) is 10–30 mg daily. In adolescents 13–17 years of age, the initial dosage of total amphetamines as fixed-combination extended-release capsules (Adderall XR®) is 10 mg once daily. Dosage may be increased to 20 mg once daily after 1 week if symptoms are not adequately controlled. In adults who are receiving drug therapy for ADHD for the first time or are being switched from therapy with another drug, the recommended dosage of amphetamines as fixed-combination extended-release capsules (Adderall XR®) is 20 mg once daily. Although dosages of up to 60 mg daily (as fixed-combination extended-release capsules) have been used in adolescents 13–17 years of age and adults in clinical studies, there is no evidence that dosages exceeding 20 mg daily provide any additional benefit in these patients. When switching from fixed-combination conventional tablets (Adderall®) to fixed-combination extended-release capsules (Adderall XR®), the total daily dosage of amphetamines may remain the same but should be given once daily.

When possible, therapy should be interrupted occasionally to determine if there is a recurrence of behavioral symptoms sufficient to require continued treatment. Long-term use of fixed-combination extended-release capsules (i.e., more than 3 weeks in children or more than 4 weeks in adolescents or adults) has not been studied systematically. If fixed-combination extended-release capsules are used for extended periods, the usefulness of the drug should be periodically reevaluated.

Cautions

Dextroamphetamine shares the toxic potentials of amphetamines, and the usual cautions, precautions, and contraindications of amphetamine therapy should be observed. (See Cautions in the Amphetamines General Statement 28:20.04.)

Some commercially available preparations of dextroamphetamine (e.g., DextroStat®, Dexedrine® tablets) contain the dye tartrazine (FD&C yellow No. 5), which may cause allergic reactions including bronchial asthma in susceptible individuals. Although the incidence of tartrazine sensitivity is low, it frequently occurs in patients who are sensitive to aspirin.

Chemistry and Stability

■ Chemistry Dextroamphetamine is the dextrorotatory isomer of amphetamine. Dextroamphetamine sulfate occurs as a white, odorless, crystalline powder and has a bitter taste. Dextroamphetamine sulfate is freely soluble in water (about 1:10) and slightly soluble in alcohol (about 1:800). Dextroamphetamine sulfate also is commercially available as fixed-combination preparations with dextroamphetamine saccharate, amphetamine aspartate, and amphetamine sulfate.

■ Stability Preparations containing dextroamphetamine sulfate should be stored in tight, light-resistant containers at 15–30°C.

Preparations

Dextroamphetamine and dextroamphetamine sulfate preparations are subject to control under the Federal Controlled Substances Act of 1970 as schedule II (C-II) drugs.

Excipients in commercially available drug preparations may have clinically important effects in some individuals; consult specific product labeling for details.

Dextroamphetamine Sulfate

Oral		
Capsules, extended-release	5 mg*	**Dexedrine® Spansule®** (C-II), GlaxoSmithKline
		Dextroamphetamine Sulfate Capsules SR (C-II)
	10 mg*	**Dexedrine® Spansule®** (C-II), GlaxoSmithKline
		Dextroamphetamine Sulfate Capsules SR (C-II)
	15 mg*	**Dexedrine® Spansule®** (C-II), GlaxoSmithKline
		Dextroamphetamine Sulfate Capsules SR (C-II)
Tablets	5 mg*	**Dexedrine®** (C-II; scored), GlaxoSmithKline
		Dextroamphetamine Sulfate Tablets (C-II; scored)
		DextroStat® (C-II, scored), Shire
	10 mg*	**Dextroamphetamine Sulfate Tablets** (C-II; scored)
		DextroStat® (C-II; double-scored), Shire

*available from one or more manufacturer, distributor, and/or repackager by generic (nonproprietary) name

Dextroamphetamine Sulfate Combinations

Oral		
Capsules, extended-release	5 mg total amphetamine (as 1.25 mg with Amphetamine Sulfate 1.25 mg, Amphetamine Aspartate 1.25 mg, and Dextroamphetamine Saccharate 1.25 mg)	**Adderall XR**® (C-II), Shire
	10 mg total amphetamine (as 2.5 mg with Amphetamine Sulfate 2.5 mg, Amphetamine Aspartate 2.5 mg, and Dextroamphetamine Saccharate 2.5 mg)	**Adderall XR**® (C-II), Shire
	15 mg total amphetamine (as 3.75 mg with Amphetamine Sulfate 3.75 mg, Amphetamine Aspartate 3.75 mg, and Dextroamphetamine Saccharate 3.75 mg)	**Adderall XR**® (C-II), Shire
	20 mg total amphetamine (as 5 mg with Amphetamine Sulfate 5 mg, Amphetamine Aspartate 5 mg, and Dextroamphetamine Saccharate 5 mg)	**Adderall XR**® (C-II), Shire
	25 mg total amphetamine (as 6.25 mg with Amphetamine Sulfate 6.25 mg, Amphetamine Aspartate 6.25 mg, and Dextroamphetamine Saccharate 6.25 mg)	**Adderall XR**® (C-II), Shire
	30 mg total amphetamine (as 7.5 mg with Amphetamine Sulfate 7.5 mg, Amphetamine Aspartate 7.5 mg, and Dextroamphetamine Saccharate 7.5 mg)	**Adderall XR**® (C-II), Shire
Tablets	5 mg total amphetamine (as 1.25 mg with Amphetamine Aspartate 1.25 mg, Amphetamine Sulfate 1.25 mg, and Dextroamphetamine Saccharate 1.25 mg)*	**Adderall**® (C-II; double-scored), Shire **Dextroamphetamine Saccharate, Amphetamine Aspartate, Dextroamphetamine Sulfate, and Amphetamine Sulfate Tablets** (C-II; double-scored)
	7.5 mg total amphetamine (as 1.875 mg with Amphetamine Aspartate 1.875 mg, Amphetamine Sulfate 1.875 mg, and Dextroamphetamine Saccharate 1.875 mg)*	**Adderall**® (C-II; double-scored), Shire **Dextroamphetamine Saccharate, Amphetamine Aspartate, Dextroamphetamine Sulfate, and Amphetamine Sulfate Tablets** (C-II; double-scored)
	10 mg total amphetamine (as 2.5 mg with Amphetamine Aspartate 2.5 mg, Amphetamine Sulfate 2.5 mg, and Dextroamphetamine Saccharate 2.5 mg)*	**Adderall**® (C-II; double-scored), Shire **Dextroamphetamine Saccharate, Amphetamine Aspartate, Dextroamphetamine Sulfate, and Amphetamine Sulfate Tablets** (C-II; double-scored)
	12.5 mg total amphetamine (as 3.125 mg with Amphetamine Aspartate 3.125 mg, Amphetamine Sulfate 3.125 mg, and Dextroamphetamine Saccharate 3.125 mg)*	**Adderall**® (C-II; double-scored), Shire **Dextroamphetamine Saccharate, Amphetamine Aspartate, Dextroamphetamine Sulfate, and Amphetamine Sulfate Tablets** (C-II; double-scored)
	15 mg total amphetamine (as 3.75 mg with Amphetamine Aspartate 3.75 mg, Amphetamine Sulfate 3.75 mg, and Dextroamphetamine Saccharate 3.75 mg)*	**Adderall**® (C-II; double-scored), Shire **Dextroamphetamine Saccharate, Amphetamine Aspartate, Dextroamphetamine Sulfate, and Amphetamine Sulfate Tablets** (C-II; double-scored)
	20 mg total amphetamine (as 5 mg with Amphetamine Aspartate 5 mg, Amphetamine Sulfate 5 mg, and Dextroamphetamine Saccharate 5 mg)*	**Adderall**® (C-II; double-scored), Shire **Dextroamphetamine Saccharate, Amphetamine Aspartate, Dextroamphetamine Sulfate, and Amphetamine Sulfate Tablets** (C-II; double-scored)
	30 mg total amphetamine (as 7.5 mg with Amphetamine Aspartate 7.5 mg, Amphetamine Sulfate 7.5 mg, and Dextroamphetamine Saccharate 7.5 mg)*	**Adderall**® (C-II; double-scored), Shire **Dextroamphetamine Saccharate, Amphetamine Aspartate, Dextroamphetamine Sulfate and Amphetamine Sulfate Tablets** (C-II; double-scored)

*available from one or more manufacturer, distributor, and/or repackager by generic (nonproprietary) name

Selected Revisions December 2012,

Lisdexamfetamine Dimesylate

■ Prodrug of dextroamphetamine; noncatechol, sympathomimetic amine with CNS-stimulating activity.

Uses

■ **Attention-Deficit/Hyperactivity Disorder** Lisdexamfetamine dimesylate is used as an adjunct to psychological, educational, social, and other remedial measures in the treatment of attention-deficit/hyperactivity disorder (ADHD) (hyperkinetic disorder, hyperkinetic syndrome of childhood, minimal brain dysfunction). Safety and efficacy for this indication have been established in controlled clinical trials in children and adolescents 6 years of age or older and in adults.

Safety and efficacy of lisdexamfetamine dimesylate in the treatment of ADHD in children and adolescents 6 years of age or older have been evaluated in 5 short-term studies (3 in children 6–12 years of age, 1 in adolescents 13–17 years of age, and 1 in children and adolescents 6–17 years of age) and 1 randomized withdrawal study. Safety and efficacy of lisdexamfetamine dimesylate in adults with ADHD were evaluated in 2 short-term studies and 1 randomized withdrawal study.

In a short-term, randomized, double-blind, placebo-controlled parallel-group study in children 6–12 years of age with ADHD, improvement in symptom scores, as measured using the ADHD Rating Scale version IV (ADHD-RS-IV), the revised Conners' Parent Rating Scale (CPRS-R), and the Clinical Global Impression of Improvement (CGI-I) scale, from baseline to study end (4 weeks) was greater in children receiving lisdexamfetamine dimesylate titrated to a fixed, final dosage of 30, 50, or 70 mg daily than in those receiving placebo. Mean changes in symptom scores generally were similar for all 3 lisdexamfetamine dosage levels; however, changes in ADHD-RS-IV scores were numerically greater with the 70-mg dose than with the 30- and 50-mg doses. Symptom control in patients receiving the drug was maintained throughout the day up to 6 p.m.

In addition, 2 short-term, double-blind, placebo-controlled, crossover studies were conducted in children 6–12 years of age in an analog classroom environment using the Swanson, Kotkin, Agler, M-Flynn, and Pelham (SKAMP) deportment score (a measure of deportment problems leading to classroom disruptions) as the primary measure of efficacy. Both studies utilized a 3- or 4-week open-label, dose-optimization period followed by randomization to 1 week each of double-blind treatment with lisdexamfetamine dimesylate or placebo. One of the studies used an active comparator (extended-release mixed amphetamine salts [Adderall XR®] 10–30 mg daily) during dose-optimization and double-blind periods. In both studies, patients had substantially greater improvement in SKAMP deportment scores on day 7 of each treatment period while receiving lisdexamfetamine compared with placebo. This effect was observed at various intervals from 1.5–13 hours after dosing.

In a randomized, double-blind, controlled study in children and adolescents 6–17 years of age with ADHD, improvement in the ADHD-RS-IV score from baseline to study end (7 weeks) was greater in patients receiving lisdexamfetamine dimesylate (given as a flexible dosage of 30–70 mg daily during the first 4 weeks and as a fixed dosage from weeks 5–7) than in those receiving placebo.

Safety and efficacy of lisdexamfetamine in adolescents and adults with ADHD were evaluated in 2 similarly designed, double-blind, randomized, placebo-controlled studies of 4 weeks' duration in 314 adolescents 13–17 years of age and 420 adults 18–55 years of age who met DSM-IV-TR criteria for ADHD. In these parallel-group studies, patients were randomized to receive 30, 50, or 70 mg of lisdexamfetamine dimesylate daily or placebo. All patients receiving lisdexamfetamine initially received 30 mg daily for the first week, with subsequent dosage titrations occurring in 20-mg increments at weekly intervals for those randomized to receive 50 or 70 mg of the drug daily. The primary measure of efficacy in both studies was the ADHD Rating Scale (ADHD-RS) score. At study end point (4 weeks), patients randomized to receive lisdexamfetamine demonstrated significant improvements in ADHD symptoms compared with placebo recipients. Significant improvements in ADHD symptoms were evident within the first week of treatment in all lisdexamfetamine groups. In the adult study, patients randomized to receive lisdexamfetamine dimesylate 70 mg daily showed a greater reduction in ADHD-RS total score at weeks 3 and 4 compared with patients receiving lisdexamfetamine dimesylate 30 mg daily.

In a crossover study in adults 18–55 years of age conducted in a simulated workplace environment, patients entered a 4-week, open-label, dose-optimization period with lisdexamfetamine dimesylate initiated at 30 mg and titrated up to a maximum of 70 mg daily followed by randomization to receive 1 week each of treatment with lisdexamfetamine or placebo. The primary measure of efficacy was the Permanent Product Measure of Performance (PERMP) total score (a skill-adjusted math test that measures attention in ADHD) assessed on day 7 of each treatment period at various intervals from 2–14 hours after dosing. Patients had substantially greater improvement in PERMP total scores after the treatment period with lisdexamfetamine compared with placebo.

Efficacy of lisdexamfetamine dimesylate for maintenance therapy for ADHD was evaluated in 2 placebo-controlled, randomized withdrawal studies in children and adolescents 6–17 years of age and in adults 18–55 years of age with ADHD. In the pediatric study, patients who had demonstrated a clinical response to lisdexamfetamine during a 26-week, open-label, dose-optimization period were randomized to continue their lisdexamfetamine dosage or receive placebo during the 6-week, double-blind study period. In the adult study, patients who had received at least 6 months of lisdexamfetamine therapy and who maintained treatment response during a 3-week, open-label treatment period were randomized to continue their lisdexamfetamine dosage or receive placebo during the 6-week, double-blind study period. Treatment failure was defined as at least a 50% increase in ADHD-RS total score and at least a 2-point increase as measured using the Clinical Global Impression of Severity (CGI-S) scale; in both studies, substantially fewer patients receiving lisdexamfetamine (15.8 and 9% of pediatric and adult patients, respectively) experienced treatment failure than those receiving placebo (67.5 and 75% of pediatric and adult patients, respectively).

For further information on the management of ADHD, including the use of stimulants such as amphetamines, see Uses: Attention-Deficit/Hyperactivity Disorder in the Amphetamines General Statement 28:20.04, and also in Methylphenidate 28:20.32.

■ **Binge-Eating Disorder** Lisdexamfetamine dimesylate is used for the treatment of moderate to severe binge-eating disorder in adults. In controlled studies, treatment with lisdexamfetamine reduced the mean number of binge days per week compared with placebo.

Lisdexamfetamine dimesylate should *not* be used for weight loss; use of other sympathomimetic drugs for weight loss has been associated with serious adverse cardiovascular events. Efficacy and safety of the drug for treatment of obesity have not been established.

According to DSM-5 criteria, binge-eating disorder is characterized by recurrent episodes of binge eating (i.e., excessive food consumption during a discrete period of time, accompanied by a sense of lack of control) causing marked distress and occurring, on average, at least once per week for 3 months. Individuals with binge-eating disorder experience at least 3 of the following: eating much more rapidly than normal, eating until feeling uncomfortably full, eating large amounts of food when not feeling physically hungry, eating alone because of feeling embarrassed by how much one is eating, or feeling disgusted with onself, depressed, or very guilty afterward. Unlike bulimia nervosa, binge-eating disorder is not associated with recurrent and inappropriate compensatory behavior (e.g., purging, excessive exercise). DSM-5 describes binge-eating disorder as mild, moderate, severe, or extreme if the patient experiences 1–3, 4–7, 8–13, or 14 or more binge-eating episodes per week, respectively.

The efficacy of lisdexamfetamine dimesylate for the treatment of binge-eating disorder has been established in 2 randomized, double-blind, placebo-controlled studies of 12-weeks' duration in adults 18–55 years of age with moderate to severe binge-eating disorder (DSM-IV criteria). Because DSM-IV criteria did not define severity of disease, severity of binge-eating disorder in these studies was determined by the investigators; moderate to severe disorder was defined as having at least 3 binge days per week for 2 consecutive weeks prior to baseline and a baseline CGI-S score of 4 or greater. Patients were randomized to receive placebo or lisdexamfetamine; lisdexamfetamine dimesylate was initiated at 30 mg daily and increased to 50 mg daily after 1 week, with increases to 70 mg daily as tolerated and clinically indicated. In both studies, lisdexamfetamine was more effective than placebo in reducing the mean number of binge days per week from baseline to week 12. From a mean of 4.6–4.82 binge days per week at baseline, lisdexamfetamine-treated patients experienced an average of 1.35–1.66 fewer binge days per week by week 12 than those receiving placebo.

Dosage and Administration

■ **General** Patients should be assessed for the presence of cardiac disease prior to initiation of lisdexamfetamine therapy. (See Sudden Death and Serious Cardiovascular Events under Warnings/Precautions: Other Warnings and Precautions, in Cautions.)

In addition, the potential for abuse of CNS stimulants should be assessed prior to initiation of lisdexamfetamine therapy. (See Abuse Potential under Warnings/Precautions: Warnings, in Cautions.) After prescribing amphetamine therapy, prescription records should be carefully maintained, and patients should receive education regarding abuse of stimulants and be monitored for signs of abuse and overdose. The need for continued therapy with lisdexamfetamine should be reevaluated.

■ **Administration** ***Oral Administration*** Administer lisdexamfetamine dimesylate capsules or chewable tablets once daily in the morning without regard to meals. Because of potential for insomnia, avoid administering in the afternoon.

Capsules may be swallowed whole or may be opened and the entire contents mixed with water, orange juice, or yogurt until completely dispersed; resulting mixture should be administered immediately and *not* stored for use at a later time.

Do *not* subdivide capsule contents; do *not* administer a dose less than the entire contents of one capsule or one chewable tablet.

Chewable tablets should be chewed thoroughly before swallowing.

Lisdexamfetamine capsules can be substituted for chewable tablets on a mg-per-mg basis.

■ **Dosage** Available as lisdexamfetamine dimesylate; dosage expressed in terms of the salt.

Pediatric Patients **Attention-Deficit/Hyperactivity Disorder.** Children 6 years of age or older: Initially, 30 mg once daily; dosage may be adjusted in 10- or 20-mg increments at weekly intervals up to a maximum dosage of 70 mg daily.

If the initial 30-mg daily dosage is not tolerated, dosage can be decreased to 20 mg daily.

Adults **Attention-Deficit/Hyperactivity Disorder.** Initially, 30 mg once daily; dosage may be adjusted in 10- or 20-mg increments at weekly intervals up to a maximum dosage of 70 mg daily.

If the initial 30-mg daily dosage is not tolerated, dosage can be decreased to 20 mg daily.

Binge-Eating Disorder. Initially, 30 mg once daily. Dosage should be adjusted in 20-mg increments at weekly intervals to a target dosage of 50–70 mg daily. Dosages of 50 and 70 mg daily were effective in controlled trials. The maximum recommended dosage is 70 mg once daily.

Lisdexamfetamine therapy should be discontinued if binge eating does not improve.

■ **Special Populations** In patients with severe renal impairment (glomerular filtration rate [GFR] 15 to less than 30 mL/minute per 1.73 m^2), the maximum dosage of lisdexamfetamine dimesylate is 50 mg daily. In patients with end-stage renal disease (GFR less than 15 mL/minute per 1.73 m^2), the maximum recommended dosage is 30 mg daily.

Cautions

■ **Contraindications** Known hypersensitivity to amphetamines or any ingredient in the formulation of lisdexamfetamine dimesylate. Anaphylactic reactions, hypersensitivity, Stevens-Johnson syndrome, angioedema, and urticaria have been reported during postmarketing surveillance of lisdexamfetamine.

Concurrent or recent (i.e., within 14 days) therapy with a monoamine oxidase (MAO) inhibitor, including linezolid or IV methylene blue, since hypertensive crisis could result. (See Drug Interactions: MAO Inhibitors.)

■ **Warnings/Precautions** ***Warnings*** **Abuse Potential.** CNS stimulants (e.g., amphetamines, methylphenidate) have a high potential for abuse and dependence. The risk of abuse should be assessed prior to initiation of lisdexamfetamine and patients should be monitored for signs of abuse and dependence during therapy.

The possibility that family members may abuse the patient's medication should be considered.

Other Warnings and Precautions **Sudden Death and Serious Cardiovascular Events.** Sudden unexplained death, stroke, and myocardial infarction (MI) have been reported in adults with attention-deficit/hyperactivity disorder (ADHD) receiving usual dosages of stimulants; sudden death also has been reported in children and adolescents with structural cardiac abnormalities or other serious cardiac conditions receiving usual dosages of the drugs. A small number of cases of sudden unexplained death also has been reported in children without structural cardiac abnormalities receiving amphetamine combinations; however, confounding factors were present in some of these incidents. Postmarketing experience with lisdexamfetamine includes reports of cardiomyopathy and chest pain.

Results of one retrospective, case-control epidemiologic study showed a possible association between use of stimulant medications (amphetamine, dextroamphetamine, methamphetamine, methylphenidate, or their derivatives) and sudden unexplained death in healthy children and adolescents. (See Pediatric Use under Warnings/Precautions: Specific Populations, in Cautions.) Because of postmarketing reports and the results of this and other epidemiologic studies, FDA collaborated with the Agency for Healthcare Research and Quality (AHRQ) to sponsor 3 large, related, retrospective cohort studies using data from several health care claims databases to evaluate possible associations between ADHD drug use (stimulants, atomoxetine, and pemoline [no longer commercially available in the US]) and the following serious cardiovascular events: MI, stroke, and sudden cardiac death in children and young adults 2–24 years of age; MI and sudden cardiac death in adults 25–64 years of age; and stroke and the composite end point of stroke, MI, and sudden cardiac death in the same group of adults. None of the 3 studies showed an association between serious cardiovascular events and current use of ADHD drugs, as compared with nonuse or as compared with former or remote use, although small increases in cardiovascular risk could not be excluded. The study in children and young adults included data for approximately 1.2 million patients and approximately 2.6 million patient-years of follow-up, including approximately 370,000 patient-years of current ADHD drug use, and found only 7 serious cardiovascular events (4 strokes, 3 sudden deaths) in current users of the drugs. The analyses in adults included data for approximately 440,000 patients, including approximately 150,000 current users of ADHD drugs; for the composite outcome of stroke, MI, and sudden cardiac death, there were approximately 107,000 patient-years of ADHD drug exposure and 234 such cardiovascular events in current users.

A thorough medical history review (including evaluation for family history of sudden death or ventricular arrhythmia) *and* physical examination should be performed in all children, adolescents, and adults being considered for stimulant therapy, including lisdexamfetamine; if initial findings suggest presence of cardiac disease, further cardiac evaluation (e.g., ECG, echocardiogram) should be performed.

Use of CNS stimulants should be avoided in patients with known structural cardiac abnormalities, cardiomyopathy, serious arrhythmias, coronary artery disease, or other serious cardiac conditions.

Patients who develop exertional chest pain, unexplained syncope, arrhythmias, or other manifestations suggestive of cardiac disease during stimulant therapy should undergo prompt cardiac evaluation.

For further information on screening for cardiac conditions, selecting appropriate candidates for stimulant therapy, and monitoring for treatment-emergent cardiac conditions, see Cardiovascular Precautions under Cautions: Precautions and Contraindications, in the Amphetamines General Statement 28:20.04.

Effects on Blood Pressure and Heart Rate. Possible modest increases in average blood pressure (i.e., by about 2–4 mm Hg) and heart rate (i.e., by about 3–6 beats/minute); larger increases may occur. All patients should be monitored for potential hypertension and tachycardia.

Exacerbation or Precipitation of Psychotic Symptoms. May exacerbate symptoms of behavior disturbance and thought disorder in patients with preexisting psychotic disorder.

Psychotic symptoms (e.g., hallucinations, delusional thinking) may occur with usual dosages in children and adolescents without prior history of psychotic illness. If psychotic symptoms occur, consider causal relationship to stimulants, and discontinue therapy as appropriate.

Precipitation of Manic Symptoms. May precipitate mixed or manic episodes in patients with bipolar disorder. Prior to initiating therapy, patients should be screened for risk factors for developing a manic episode; screening should include a detailed psychiatric history (e.g., comorbid depressive symptoms or history of depressive symptoms; family history of suicide, bipolar disorder, or depression).

Manic symptoms may occur with usual dosages in children and adolescents without prior history of mania. If manic symptoms occur, consider causal relationship to stimulants, and discontinue therapy as appropriate.

Other Nervous System Effects. Amphetamines may impair the ability to engage in potentially hazardous activities (e.g., operating machinery or vehicles). Postmarketing experience with lisdexamfetamine includes reports of dyskinesia, tics, depression, dermatillomania, aggression, and seizures.

Growth Suppression. Long-term (i.e., exceeding 12 months) administration is expected to cause at least a temporary suppression of normal weight and/or height patterns in some children and adolescents. Dose-related weight loss has been reported in children and adolescents during 4 weeks of therapy with lisdexamfetamine.

Manufacturer recommends monitoring growth during treatment; patients not growing or gaining weight as expected may require temporary discontinuance of treatment. However, the American Academy of Pediatrics states that studies of stimulants in children found little or no decrease in expected height, with any decrease in growth early in treatment being compensated for later on.

Peripheral Vascular Effects. Stimulants, including lisdexamfetamine, are associated with peripheral vascular disorders, such as Raynaud's phenomenon. Manifestations usually are intermittent and mild, but ulceration of the digits and/or breakdown of soft tissue may occur rarely. Peripheral vascular disorders, including Raynaud's phenomenon, have been reported during postmarketing experience in patients in all age groups receiving stimulants at therapeutic dosages and at various times throughout the treatment course. Manifestations generally improve following dosage reduction or drug discontinuance. Careful observation for digital changes is warranted during therapy with stimulants, and further clinical evaluation (e.g., referral to a rheumatologist) may be appropriate for certain patients. (See Advice to Patients.)

Serotonin Syndrome. Potentially life-threatening serotonin syndrome may occur when amphetamines are used concomitantly with other drugs that affect serotonergic neurotransmission, including MAO inhibitors, selective serotonin-reuptake inhibitors (SSRIs), selective serotonin- and norepinephrine-reuptake inhibitors (SNRIs), tricyclic antidepressants, 5-hydroxytryptamine (5-HT) type 1 receptor agonists ("triptans"), buspirone, fentanyl, lithium, tramadol, tryptophan, and St. John's wort *(Hypericum perforatum)*. Symptoms of serotonin syndrome may include mental status changes (e.g., agitation, hallucinations, delirium, coma), autonomic instability (e.g., tachycardia, labile blood pressure, dizziness, diaphoresis, flushing, hyperthermia), neuromuscular aberrations (e.g., tremor, rigidity, myoclonus, hyperreflexia, incoordination), seizures, and/or GI symptoms (e.g., nausea, vomiting, diarrhea).

Serotonin syndrome also may occur when lisdexamfetamine and inhibitors of cytochrome P-450 [CYP] isoenzyme 2D6 are used concomitantly. Amphetamines and amphetamine derivatives are known to be metabolized to some degree by CYP2D6 and may show mild inhibition of CYP2D6 metabolism. The potential for a pharmacokinetic interaction exists, since such concomitant administration may increase the exposure of dextroamphetamine, the active metabolite of lisdexamfetamine, and thereby increase the risk of serotonin syndrome. In such clinical situations, alternative therapy should be considered with a non-serotonergic drug or a drug that does not inhibit CYP2D6. (See Drug Interactions: Drugs Affecting or Metabolized by Hepatic Microsomal Enzymes.)

Concomitant therapy with lisdexamfetamine and other serotonergic drugs or CYP2D6 inhibitors should only be used if the potential benefit justifies the risk. Concomitant use of lisdexamfetamine and MAO inhibitors is contraindicated. (See Cautions: Contraindications.) If symptoms of serotonin syndrome occur, therapy with lisdexamfetamine and any other concomitant serotonergic agents should be discontinued immediately and supportive therapy initiated. (See Drug Interactions: Serotonergic Drugs.)

Initiation of lisdexamfetamine therapy at lower dosages should be considered, if clinically warranted. Patients should be monitored for the emergence of serotonin syndrome during initiation of therapy or when dosage is increased. (See Advice to Patients.)

Visual Effects. Visual disturbances have been reported with stimulants. Postmarketing experience with lisdexamfetamine includes reports of mydriasis, diplopia, difficulty with visual accommodation, and blurred vision.

Hepatic Effects. Postmarketing experience with lisdexamfetamine includes reports of eosinophilic hepatitis.

GI Effects. Postmarketing experience with lisdexamfetamine includes reports of dysgeusia, bruxism, and constipation.

Musculoskeletal Effects. Postmarketing experience with lisdexamfetamine includes reports of rhabdomyolysis.

Alopecia. Postmarketing experience with lisdexamfetamine includes reports of alopecia.

Endocrine Effects. Postmarketing experience with lisdexamfetamine includes reports of changes in libido and frequent or prolonged erections.

Specific Populations **Pregnancy.** May cause fetal harm. Data are limited regarding use of lisdexamfetamine dimesylate in pregnant women. Amphetamines may stimulate uterine contractions in pregnant women increasing the risk of premature delivery. Infants born to amphetamine-dependent women have increased risk of prematurity and low birth weight; such infants should be monitored for withdrawal symptoms (e.g., feeding difficulties, irritability, agitation, excessive drowsiness).

In animals, lisdexamfetamine dimesylate had no effects on embryofetal morphology or survival when administered orally to rats and rabbits throughout the period of organogenesis. Prenatal and postnatal studies were not conducted specifically with lisdexamfetamine dimesylate. However, administration of amphetamine to pregnant rats during gestation and lactation resulted in decreased pup survival and body weight that correlated with developmental delays at clinically relevant dosages of amphetamine.

Lactation. Lisdexamfetamine (a prodrug of dextroamphetamine) is distributed into milk based on limited data with amphetamine. There are no reports of adverse effects on nursing infants. However, large dosages of dextroamphetamine may interfere with milk production, especially in women whose lactation is not well established. Because of the potential for serious adverse reactions to lisdexamfetamine in nursing infants, the manufacturer does not recommend breast-feeding during therapy.

Pediatric Use. Safety and efficacy of lisdexamfetamine for management of ADHD have not been established in children younger than 6 years of age.

Safety and efficacy of lisdexamfetamine for binge-eating disorder have not been established in pediatric patients younger than 18 years of age.

Psychotic (e.g., hallucinations, delusional thinking) or manic symptoms have been reported in children and adolescents receiving stimulants for management of ADHD. (See Exacerbation or Precipitation of Psychotic Symptoms and also see Precipitation of Manic Symptoms under Warnings/Precautions: Other Warnings and Precautions, in Cautions.)

Sudden death has been reported in children and adolescents with structural cardiac abnormalities or other serious cardiac conditions receiving usual dosages of stimulants. Sudden unexplained death also was reported in a small number of children without structural cardiac abnormalities receiving amphetamine combinations. Results of one retrospective, case-control epidemiologic study suggested a possible association between use of stimulant medications and sudden unexplained death in healthy children and adolescents. A more recent retrospective study in children and adolescents did not show an association between serious cardiovascular events and current use of drugs to treat ADHD compared with nonuse or former use, although small increases in cardiovascular risk could not be excluded. (See Sudden Death and Serious Cardiovascular Events under Warnings/Precautions: Other Warnings and Precautions, in Cautions.)

Long-term administration is expected to cause at least a temporary suppression of normal weight and/or height patterns in some children and adolescents. (See Growth Suppression under Warnings/Precautions: Other Warnings and Precautions, in Cautions.)

Geriatric Use. Clinical studies of lisdexamfetamine dimesylate did not include sufficient numbers of patients 65 years of age or older to determine whether geriatric patients respond differently than younger adults. While other reported clinical experience has not revealed differences in response between geriatric and younger adults, dosage selection in geriatric patients should generally start at the lower end of the dosage range, reflecting the greater frequency of decreased hepatic, renal, and/or cardiac function and of concomitant disease and drug therapy in such patients.

Hepatic Impairment. Not specifically studied in hepatic impairment.

Renal Impairment. Reduced clearance and increased exposure of dextroamphetamine have been observed in patients with severe renal impairment or end-stage renal disease compared with individuals with normal renal function. Dosage of lisdexamfetamine dimesylate should not exceed 50 mg daily in patients with severe renal impairment or 30 mg daily in patients with end-stage renal disease. (See Dosage and Administration: Special Populations.)

Dialysis does not substantially affect the clearance of dextroamphetamine.

■ **Common Adverse Effects** Adverse effects occurring in 5% or more of children, adolescents, or adults receiving lisdexamfetamine for ADHD and at a frequency at least twice that reported with placebo include anorexia, anxiety, decreased appetite, decreased weight, diarrhea, dizziness, dry mouth, irritability, insomnia, nausea, upper abdominal pain, and vomiting.

Adverse effects occurring in 5% or more of adults receiving lisdexamfetamine for binge-eating disorder and at a frequency at least twice that reported with placebo include dry mouth, insomnia, decreased appetite, increased heart rate, constipation, jittery feeling, and anxiety.

Drug Interactions

In one study, lisdexamfetamine did not inhibit cytochrome P-450 (CYP) isoenzymes 1A2, 2D6, or 3A, and may have minimally inhibited CYP2C19.

■ **Drugs Affecting or Metabolized by Hepatic Microsomal Enzymes** The prodrug lisdexamfetamine dimesylate is not metabolized by CYP isoenzymes before its conversion to dextroamphetamine; therefore, pharmacokinetic interactions are unlikely with drugs that inhibit or induce CYP isoenzymes. In one study, no clinically important changes in the pharmacokinetics of caffeine, dextromethorphan, or midazolam (substrates of CYP1A2, 2D6, and 3A, respectively) occurred when the drugs were administered concomitantly with lisdexamfetamine dimesylate (single 70-mg dose); minimal inhibition of CYP2C19 substrate metabolism was observed. The manufacturer states that lisdexamfetamine is unlikely to affect the pharmacokinetics of drugs metabolized by CYP isoenzymes 1A2 (e.g., duloxetine, melatonin, theophylline), 2D6 (e.g., atomoxetine, desipramine, venlafaxine), 2C19 (e.g., clobazam, lansoprazole, omeprazole), or 3A4 (e.g., midazolam, pimozide, simvastatin).

Pharmacokinetic interaction (increased exposure of dextroamphetamine) may occur when lisdexamfetamine is used concomitantly with inhibitors of CYP2D6 (e.g., fluoxetine, paroxetine, quinidine, ritonavir) and may increase the risk of serotonin syndrome. (See Serotonin Syndrome under Warnings/Precautions: Other Warnings and Precautions, in Cautions.)

■ **Urinary Acidifying Agents** Increased urinary excretion and decreased serum concentrations and efficacy of amphetamines may occur with concomitant use of urinary acidifying agents (ammonium chloride, ascorbic acid, methenamine salts, sodium acid phosphate, cranberry juice). Lisdexamfetamine dosage should be increased based on clinical response during such concomitant therapy.

■ **Urinary Alkalinizing Agents** Decreased urinary excretion and increased serum concentrations of amphetamines resulting in potentiation of action may occur with concomitant use of alkalinizing agents (carbonic anhydrase inhibitors, sodium bicarbonate, some thiazides). Concomitant use of lisdexamfetamine with urinary alkalinizing agents should be avoided.

■ **5-HT$_1$ Receptor Agonists ("Triptans")** Pharmacologic interaction (potentially life-threatening serotonin syndrome) may occur if lisdexamfetamine is used concomitantly with 5-hydroxytryptamine type 1 (5-HT$_1$) receptor agonists ("triptans"). Lisdexamfetamine and triptans should be used concomitantly only if the potential benefit justifies the risk. If concomitant use is clinically warranted, the patient should be observed carefully, particularly during treatment initiation or when dosage is increased. (See Serotonin Syndrome under Warnings/Precautions: Other Warnings and Precautions, in Cautions.)

■ **Guanfacine** No clinically important pharmacokinetic interactions were observed when guanfacine and lisdexamfetamine were used concomitantly. Dosage adjustment of either drug is not necessary.

■ **MAO Inhibitors** Concomitant use of monoamine oxidase (MAO) inhibitors and CNS stimulants can result in potentially life-threatening hypertensive crisis. Amphetamines are contraindicated in patients who are currently receiving or have recently (within 14 days) received an MAO inhibitor. (See Cautions: Contraindications.)

■ **Selective Serotonin-reuptake Inhibitors and Selective Serotonin- and Norepinephrine-reuptake Inhibitors** Potential pharmacologic interaction (potentially life-threatening serotonin syndrome) may occur when lisdexamfetamine is used concomitantly with selective serotonin-reuptake inhibitors (SSRIs) or selective serotonin- and norepinephrine-reuptake inhibitors (SNRIs). Lisdexamfetamine and SSRIs or SNRIs should be used concomitantly only if the potential benefit justifies the risk. (See Serotonin Syndrome under Warnings/Precautions: Other Warnings and Precautions, in Cautions.)

■ **Serotonergic Drugs** Potential pharmacologic interaction (potentially life-threatening serotonin syndrome) may occur with drugs affecting serotonergic neurotransmission, including buspirone, fentanyl, lithium, tramadol, tryptophan, and St. John's wort *(Hypericum perforatum)*. Lower dosages of lisdexamfetamine should be used during initiation of such concomitant therapy, and patients should be monitored for signs and symptoms of serotonin syndrome, especially when therapy is initiated or dosage is increased. If serotonin syndrome occurs, concomitant use of lisdexamfetamine and the serotonergic drug should be discontinued. (See Serotonin Syndrome under Warnings/Precautions: Other Warnings and Precautions, in Cautions.)

■ **Tricyclic Antidepressants** Enhanced activity of tricyclic antidepressants or sympathomimetic agents; desipramine or protriptyline may cause striking and sustained increases in the concentration of dextroamphetamine in the brain; cardiovascular effects can be potentiated. Patients receiving concomitant therapy with lisdexamfetamine and tricyclic antidepressants should be monitored frequently. Dosage of lisdexamfetamine should be adjusted or alternative therapy should be used based on clinical response.

Potential pharmacologic interaction (potentially life-threatening serotonin syndrome) may occur when lisdexamfetamine is used concomitantly with tricyclic antidepressants. Lisdexamfetamine and tricyclic antidepressants should be used concomitantly only if the potential benefit justifies the risk. (See Serotonin Syndrome under Warnings/Precautions: Other Warnings and Precautions, in Cautions.)

■ **Omeprazole** Concomitant use of omeprazole and lisdexamfetamine is not expected to have a clinically important effect on the pharmacokinetics of omeprazole. Dosage adjustment of either drug is not necessary.

■ **Venlafaxine** No clinically important pharmacokinetic interactions were observed when venlafaxine and lisdexamfetamine were used concomitantly; additive effects on blood pressure and heart rate have been reported. Dosage adjustment of either drug is not necessary. Monitoring of blood pressure and heart rate is recommended during concomitant therapy.

Description

Lisdexamfetamine, a prodrug of dextroamphetamine, is a CNS stimulant. Lisdexamfetamine is inactive until hydrolyzed in vivo to *l*-lysine, a naturally occurring essential amino acid, and dextroamphetamine, which is responsible for the drug's activity. For information on the pharmacology of amphetamines, see Pharmacology in the Amphetamines General Statement 28:20.04.

Lisdexamfetamine is rapidly absorbed from the GI tract; following oral administration, the onset of action occurs within 2 hours. Conversion of lisdexamfetamine to *l*-lysine and dextroamphetamine occurs mainly via hydrolytic activity of erythrocytes, which have a high capacity for this metabolism. Lisdexamfetamine is not metabolized by the cytochrome P-450 (CYP) enzyme system, and the ability of dextroamphetamine to inhibit this enzyme pathway has not been fully elucidated. The plasma half-lives of lisdexamfetamine and dextroamphetamine are less than 1 hour and 9.4–9.7 hours, respectively. Approximately 96% of a radiolabeled dose of lisdexamfetamine is excreted in urine, with the parent drug accounting for only about 2% of the recovered radioactivity.

Advice to Patients

Importance of providing patient or caregiver with a copy of the manufacturer's patient information (medication guide); discuss and answer questions about its contents as needed. Importance of advising patient or caregiver to read and understand contents of medication guide before initiating therapy and each time the prescription is refilled.

Importance of informing patients that lisdexamfetamine is a controlled substance that can be abused and can lead to dependence. Advise patients on proper storage and disposal of controlled substances.

Importance of taking the drug in the morning to minimize insomnia.

Risk of serious cardiovascular events (e.g., sudden death, myocardial infarction [MI], stroke, hypertension). Importance of patients immediately informing a clinician if they develop exertional chest pain, unexplained syncope, or other symptoms suggestive of cardiac disease.

Risk of increased blood pressure and heart rate; importance of advising patients to monitor blood pressure and heart rate during therapy.

Risk of psychiatric effects (e.g., psychosis, mania), even in patients without a history of such effects.

Risk of weight loss or decreased growth rate; importance of monitoring height and weight of pediatric patients during therapy.

Appetite suppression may occur. Giving the morning dose with a meal and providing a high-caloric drink or snack late in the evening when the stimulant effects have subsided may be helpful.

Importance of instructing patients about the potential for amphetamines to impair their ability to perform potentially hazardous activities, such as driving or operating heavy machinery.

Potential risk of peripheral vascular disorders, including Raynaud's phenomenon, and the associated signs and symptoms (e.g., numbness, coolness, pain, or changes in color [from pale to blue to red] in fingers or toes). Advise patients to report any new numbness, pain, skin color change, or sensitivity to temperature in fingers or toes and to immediately inform clinician if any signs of unexplained wounds appear on fingers or toes; further clinical evaluation may be appropriate.

Potential risk of serotonin syndrome with concomitant use of lisdexamfetamine and other serotonergic agents (e.g., buspirone, fentanyl, lithium, selective serotonin-reuptake inhibitors [SSRIs], selective serotonin- and norepinephrine-reuptake inhibitors [SNRIs], tramadol, tricyclic antidepressants, 5-hydroxytryptamine type 1 [5-HT$_1$] receptor agonists [triptans], tryptophan, and St. John's wort *[Hypericum perforatum]*) or drugs that impair metabolism of serotonin (e.g., MAO inhibitors), both those used to treat psychiatric disorders and others, such as the anti-infective agent linezolid. Importance of immediately contacting clinician if signs and/or symptoms of serotonin syndrome develop.

Importance of informing clinicians of existing or contemplated concomitant therapy, including prescription and OTC drugs, dietary supplements, and herbal products, as well as any concomitant illnesses/conditions (e.g., hypertension, cardiovascular disease, psychiatric disorders).

Importance of women informing clinicians if they are or plan to become pregnant.

Importance of advising women to avoid breast-feeding during therapy.

Importance of informing patients of other important precautionary information. (See Cautions.)

Overview® (see Users Guide). For additional information on this drug until a more detailed monograph is developed and published, the manufacturer's labeling should be consulted. It is *essential* that the manufacturer's labeling be consulted for more detailed information on usual cautions, precautions, contraindications, potential drug interactions, laboratory test interferences, and acute toxicity.

Preparations

Subject to control under the Federal Controlled Substances Act of 1970 as a schedule II (C-II) drug.

Excipients in commercially available drug preparations may have clinically important effects in some individuals; consult specific product labeling for details.

Lisdexamfetamine Dimesylate

Oral		
Capsules	10 mg	Vyvanse® (C-II), Shire
	20 mg	Vyvanse® (C-II), Shire
	30 mg	Vyvanse® (C-II), Shire
	40 mg	Vyvanse® (C-II), Shire
	50 mg	Vyvanse® (C-II), Shire
	60 mg	Vyvanse® (C-II), Shire
	70 mg	Vyvanse® (C-II), Shire
Tablets, chewable	10 mg	Vyvanse® (C-II), Shire
	20 mg	Vyvanse® (C-II), Shire
	30 mg	Vyvanse® (C-II), Shire
	40 mg	Vyvanse® (C-II), Shire
	50 mg	Vyvanse® (C-II), Shire
	60 mg	Vyvanse® (C-II), Shire

Methamphetamine Hydrochloride

Desoxyephedrine Hydrochloride

■ Methamphetamine hydrochloride, the dextrorotatory isomer of phenylmethylamine, has pharmacologic actions that are qualitatively similar to those of amphetamine and ephedrine.

Uses

Methamphetamine has been used as an adjunct to caloric restriction in the short-term (i.e., a few weeks) treatment of exogenous obesity. However, short-term or intermittent therapy with methamphetamine is unlikely to maintain a long-term benefit, and prolonged administration of methamphetamine for the treatment of obesity is not indicated. Methamphetamine also is used as an adjunct to psychological, educational, social, and other remedial measures in the treatment of attention deficit hyperactivity disorder (ADHD). Methamphetamine also has been misused and abused for its CNS stimulatory effects.

■ **Exogenous Obesity** Methamphetamine has been used as an adjunct to caloric restriction in the short-term (i.e., a few weeks) treatment of exogenous obesity. The anorexigenic effect of sympathomimetic compounds used in the treatment of obesity is temporary, seldom lasting more than a few weeks, and tolerance may occur. However, obesity usually is a chronic disease, and short-term or intermittent therapy with these drugs is unlikely to maintain a long-term benefit; therefore, short-term use of anorexigenic agents, including methamphetamine, is not recommended. Furthermore, prolonged administration of methamphetamine in the treatment of obesity is not indicated. (See Cautions: Precautions and Contraindications.) To help bring about and maintain loss of weight, the patient must be taught to curtail overeating and to consume a suitable diet. For further information on the treatment of exogenous obesity, see Uses: Exogenous Obesity, in the Amphetamines General Statement 28:20.04.

■ **Attention Deficit Hyperactivity Disorder** Methamphetamine also is used as an adjunct to psychological, educational, social, and other remedial measures in the treatment of ADHD (hyperkinetic disorder, hyperkinetic syndrome of childhood, minimal brain dysfunction) in children older than 6 years of age.

Methamphetamine should not be used to combat fatigue or exhaustion or to replace sleep in normal persons.

ADHD usually is characterized by developmentally inappropriate symptoms (e.g., moderate to severe distractibility, short attention span, hyperactivity, emotional lability, impulsivity). The final diagnosis of this disorder should not be made if these symptoms are of only comparatively recent origin. Nonlocalizing (soft) neurologic signs, learning disability, and abnormal EEG may or may not be present, and a diagnosis of CNS dysfunction may or may not be warranted. Drug therapy is not indicated in all children with ADHD, and such therapy should be considered only after a complete evaluation including medical history has been performed. The decision to use amphetamines should depend on the age of the child and the physician's assessment of the severity and duration of symptoms and should not depend solely on one or more behavioral characteristics. When symptoms of ADHD are associated with acute stress reactions, use of amphetamines usually is not recommended. For a more detailed discussion on the management of ADHD, including the use of stimulants such as methamphetamine, see Uses: Attention Deficit Hyperactivity Disorder, in Methylphenidate 28:20.32.

■ **Misuse and Abuse** Misuse and abuse of amphetamines, especially methamphetamine, for CNS stimulatory effects have experienced a resurgence. In large part, this resurgence has resulted from the relative ease with which methamphetamine can be synthesized clandestinely from readily available chemicals such as ephedrine, phenylpropanolamine (no longer commercially available in the US), or pseudoephedrine. (See Chronic Toxicity, in the Amphetamines General Statement 28:20.04.) Legal restrictions, including enactment of the US Comprehensive Methamphetamine Control Act of 1996 and later the Methamphetamine Anti-Proliferation Act of 2000 and the Combat Methamphetamine Epidemic Act of 2005, on the availability of these compounds have been enacted in an effort to reverse this resurgence in misuse and abuse.

Dosage and Administration

■ **Administration** Methamphetamine hydrochloride is administered orally. Because of the potential for insomnia, administration of methamphetamine in the late evening should be avoided.

■ **Dosage** Dosage and potency of methamphetamine hydrochloride are expressed in terms of the hydrochloride. (See Chemistry and Stability: Chemistry.)

Dosage of methamphetamine hydrochloride should be adjusted according to individual response and tolerance; the smallest dose required to produce the desired response should always be used.

Exogenous Obesity As an adjunct in the treatment of exogenous obesity, the usual adult dosage of methamphetamine hydrochloride is 2.5–5 mg 2 or 3 times daily, given one-half hour before meals. Treatment should not exceed a duration of a few weeks.

Attention Deficit Hyperactivity Disorder As an adjunct in the treatment of attention deficit hyperactivity disorder (ADHD) in children 6 years of age and older, the usual initial dosage of methamphetamine hydrochloride is 5 mg once or twice daily. Daily dosage may be increased by 5 mg at weekly intervals until an optimum clinical response is achieved. The usual effective dosage is 20–25 mg daily. The total daily dose may be given as conventional tablets in 2 divided doses daily.

When possible, therapy should be interrupted occasionally to determine if there is a recurrence of behavioral symptoms sufficient to require continued treatment.

Cautions

Methamphetamine shares the toxic potentials of amphetamines, and the usual cautions, precautions, and contraindications of amphetamine therapy should be observed. (See Cautions, in the Amphetamines General Statement 28:20.04.)

■ **Cardiovascular Effects** Sudden death, stroke, myocardial infarction, hypertension or hypotension, tachycardia, palpitation, or cardiac arrhythmias may occur in patients receiving stimulants, including methamphetamine. (See Cardiovascular Precautions under Cautions: Precautions and Contraindications, in the Amphetamines General Statement 28:20.04.) Fatal cardiorespiratory arrest has been reported following abuse or misuse of methamphetamine.

■ **Nervous System Effects** Adverse nervous system effects of methamphetamine may include nervousness, insomnia, irritability, talkativeness, dizziness, headache, blurred vision, mydriasis, dizziness, dysphoria, euphoria, tremor, restlessness and hyperexcitability. Rarely, psychotic episodes have occurred in patients receiving recommended dosages. The drug may also exacerbate motor and vocal tics and Tourette's disorder. Seizures, aggressive behavior, and hostility also have been reported with stimulants. (See Psychiatric Precautions under Cautions: Precautions and Contraindications, in the Amphetamines General Statement 28:20.04.)

■ **GI Effects** GI disturbances of methamphetamine may include nausea, vomiting, abdominal cramps, diarrhea or constipation, dryness of the mouth, anorexia, and unpleasant taste.

■ **Other Adverse Effects** Urticaria, impotence, and changes in libido may occur in patients receiving methamphetamine. Visual disturbances (difficulty with accommodation, blurred vision) have been reported with stimulants.

■ **Precautions and Contraindications** The manufacturer's patient information (medication guide) should be provided to the patient or caregiver each time methamphetamine is dispensed, and the clinician should discuss and answer questions about its contents (e.g., benefits and risks of stimulant therapy, appropriate use) as needed. The patient or caregiver also should be instructed to read and understand the contents of the medication guide before initiating therapy and each time the prescription is refilled.

Patients should be warned that methamphetamine may impair their ability to perform hazardous activities requiring mental alertness or physical coordination (e.g., operating machinery, driving a motor vehicle).

Methamphetamine should be administered with caution, if at all, to patients with hyperexcitability states or to those receiving drugs that may produce this effect. The drug also should be used with caution in geriatric, debilitated, mildly hypertensive, or asthenic patients or in those with psychopathic personalities or history of suicidal or homicidal tendencies.

Methamphetamine has a high potential for abuse. Misuse and/or abuse of methamphetamine have resulted in serious adverse cardiovascular effects and death, including fatal cardiorespiratory arrest. The possibility of psychic dependence or addiction should be kept in mind, particularly when methamphetamine is administered to alcoholic patients or to those known to have been addicted to other drugs. Administration of methamphetamine for prolonged periods of time in the treatment of obesity may lead to drug dependence and must be avoided. The possibility that methamphetamine may be obtained for nontherapeutic use and distributed to others should be considered, and the drug should be prescribed or dispensed sparingly. Abrupt withdrawal of methamphetamine following prolonged administration of high dosage may result in psychotic manifestations, lethargy, and depression, which may persist for some weeks.

Methamphetamine is contraindicated in patients with hyperthyroidism, advanced arteriosclerosis, glaucoma, moderate to severe hypertension, or symptomatic cardiovascular disease, and in those with a previous history of hypersensitivity or idiosyncrasy to sympathomimetic amines. The drug is also contraindicated in patients in agitated states or with a history of drug abuse and during or within 14 days of administration of monoamine oxidase inhibitors.

For additional information on the precautions and contraindications of methamphetamine and other amphetamines, see Cautions: Precautions and Contraindications, in the Amphetamines General Statement 28:20.04.

■ **Pediatric Precautions** Methamphetamine is not recommended for use as an anorexigenic agent in children younger than 12 years of age.

Therapy with CNS stimulants may be associated with at least a temporary suppression of growth in children. (See Cautions: Pediatric Precautions, in the Amphetamines General Statement 28:20.04.)

■ **Geriatric Precautions** Clinical studies of methamphetamine did not include sufficient numbers of patients 65 years of age and older to determine whether geriatric patients respond differently than younger patients. While other reported clinical experience has not revealed age-related differences in response, dosage selection for geriatric patients should be cautious, usually starting at the low end of the dosage range. The greater frequency of decreased hepatic, renal, and/or cardiac function and of concomitant disease or drug therapy observed in this population also should be considered.

■ **Pregnancy and Lactation** Methamphetamine has been shown to have teratogenic and embryocidal effects in mammals receiving doses exceeding the usual therapeutic human dosage. There are no adequate and controlled studies to date in pregnant women. Methamphetamine should not be used during pregnancy unless the potential benefits justify the possible risks to the fetus.

Amphetamines are distributed into milk. Therefore, nursing should be *avoided* during therapy with amphetamines.

Drug Interactions

■ **Antidepressants** Neurologic and circulatory reactions have been reported in patients who have received parenteral methamphetamine concomitantly with monoamine oxidase inhibitor drugs, and fatalities have occurred. Methamphetamine is therefore contraindicated during or within 14 days of administration of monoamine oxidase inhibitors.

Patients receiving concomitant therapy with tricyclic antidepressants and indirect-acting sympathomimetic amines (e.g., amphetamines) should be closely monitored, and dosage carefully adjusted.

■ **General Anesthetics** Methamphetamine should not be used to prevent hypotension in patients who have undergone general anesthesia with drugs (cyclopropane, halothane) that sensitize the heart to the arrhythmic action of sympathomimetic amines.

■ **Guanethidine** Methamphetamine may decrease the hypotensive effect of guanethidine (no longer commercially available in the US).

■ **Phenothiazines** Phenothiazines reportedly antagonize the CNS stimulant effect of amphetamines.

■ **Other Drugs** Insulin requirements in patients with diabetes mellitus may be decreased in association with the use of methamphetamine and the concomitant dietary regimen and weight loss; therefore, methamphetamine should be administered with caution in patients with diabetes mellitus.

Laboratory Test Interferences

Amphetamines may substantially increase plasma corticosteroid concentrations.

Pharmacology

The pharmacologic actions of methamphetamine are qualitatively similar to those of amphetamine and ephedrine and include CNS and respiratory stimulation, and sympathomimetic activity including pressor response, mydriasis, bronchodilation, and contraction of the urinary bladder sphincter. The drug depresses the motility of the GI tract. The CNS stimulating effect of methamphetamine is approximately equal to or greater than that of amphetamine but less than that of dextroamphetamine; the pressor effect of methamphetamine is less than that of amphetamine but greater than that of ephedrine. Small doses of methamphetamine have a pronounced effect on the CNS without substantial peripheral action, but in larger doses the drug produces a sustained rise in blood pressure resulting mainly from cardiac stimulation. Methamphetamine apparently produces an anorexigenic effect and loss of weight. As with other amphetamine derivatives, no primary effect on appetite has been demonstrated and it is probable that its anorexigenic effect is secondary to CNS stimulation.

Pharmacokinetics

Methamphetamine is readily absorbed from the GI tract and effects persist for 6–12 hours but may continue up to 24 hours after large doses.

Methamphetamine is metabolized in the liver by aromatic hydroxylation, *N*-dealkylation, and deamination; at least 7 metabolites have been identified in urine. The biologic half-life of methamphetamine reportedly is 4–5 hours. Methamphetamine is eliminated principally in urine. Urinary excretion of the drug is pH dependent, and excretion is enhanced in acidic urine. Following oral administration of methamphetamine hydrochloride, approximately 62% of the administered dose is excreted in urine within the first 24 hours, with metabolites and unchanged drug accounting for about two-thirds and one-third, respectively, of the recovered drug.

Chemistry and Stability

■ **Chemistry** Methamphetamine hydrochloride is the dextrorotatory isomer of phenylisopropylmethylamine. The drug occurs as white crystals or as a white, crystalline powder and is freely soluble in water (1:2) and in alcohol (1:3).

USP temporarily stated that potency of methamphetamine hydrochloride tablets should be expressed both in terms of the salt and the base ("active moiety"). However, USP recently reverted to its previous standard that potency be expressed *only* in terms of methamphetamine hydrochloride. Dosage currently continues to be expressed in terms of the salt. Therefore, care should be taken to avoid confusion between potencies that during a transitional period may be labeled as the salt and/or base and dosage of methamphetamine hydrochloride.

■ **Stability** Methamphetamine hydrochloride preparations should be stored in tight, light-resistant containers and at a temperature less than 30°C.

For further information on chemistry, pharmacology, pharmacokinetics, uses, cautions, chronic toxicity, acute toxicity, and dosage and administration of amphetamines, see the Amphetamines General Statement 28:20.04.

Preparations

Methamphetamine hydrochloride is subject to control under the Federal Controlled Substances Act of 1970 as a schedule II (C-II) drug.

Excipients in commercially available drug preparations may have clinically important effects in some individuals; consult specific product labeling for details.

Methamphetamine Hydrochloride

Oral

Tablets	5 mg	**Desoxyn®** (C-II), Ovation

ANOREXIGENIC AGENTS 28:20.08

SELECTIVE SEROTONIN RECEPTOR AGONISTS 28:20.08.32

Lorcaserin Hydrochloride

■ Lorcaserin hydrochloride, a selective serotonin type 2C (5-hydroxytryptamine [5-HT_{2C}]) receptor agonist, is an anorexigenic agent.

Uses

■ **Obesity** Lorcaserin is used as an adjunct to caloric restriction and increased physical activity in the chronic management of obesity. Appropriate candidates for lorcaserin therapy include patients who are obese (pretreatment body mass index [BMI] of 30 kg/m² or greater) or, in the presence of an underlying weight-related risk factor or disease (e.g., hypertension, type 2 diabetes mellitus, dyslipidemia), those who are overweight with a pretreatment BMI of 27 kg/m² or greater. Lorcaserin is indicated *only* for monotherapy in the management of obesity; safety and efficacy of the drug in combination with other products used to promote weight loss, including prescription drugs (e.g., phentermine), nonprescription (over-the-counter) drugs, and herbal preparations, have not been established.

Efficacy and safety of lorcaserin were evaluated in 3 randomized, double-blind, placebo-controlled studies of 1–2 years' duration in a total of 7794 patients who were obese (BMI of 30–45 kg/m²) or were overweight with a BMI of 27–29.9 kg/m² and at least one comorbid condition such as hypertension or dyslipidemia. All patients were given one-on-one instruction for a reduced-calorie diet and exercise counseling initially and every 4 weeks throughout the study. The primary measure of efficacy was weight loss at 1 year, as assessed by the proportion of patients achieving a reduction in body weight of at least 5%, the proportion achieving a reduction of at least 10%, and the mean weight change. Secondary measures of efficacy included changes in lipids, glycemic control, blood pressure, and quality of life. Approximately 34–50% of patients in the 3 studies discontinued treatment prior to completion of 1 year. The following results for 1 year of treatment are based on intention-to-treat analysis, with the last observation carried forward for imputation of missing data.

The Behavioral Modification and Lorcaserin for Overweight and Obesity Management (BLOOM) study evaluated lorcaserin hydrochloride 10 mg twice daily compared with placebo in 3182 patients over a 2-year period. Patients with type 2 diabetes mellitus were excluded from this study. The mean baseline body weight was 100 kg and mean BMI was 36.2 kg/m². At 1 year, more patients receiving lorcaserin had lost 5% or more (47.5%) or 10% or more (22.6%) of their baseline body weight compared with patients receiving placebo (20.3 or 7.7%, respectively). The mean reduction in body weight from baseline to 1 year was 5.8 or 2.2 kg in patients receiving lorcaserin or placebo, respectively. Following completion of 1 year of treatment, patients receiving lorcaserin were re-randomized in a 2:1 ratio to continue receiving lorcaserin or to switch to placebo, while patients receiving placebo continued to receive placebo during year 2. Among patients who received lorcaserin during year 1 and had weight loss of 5% or more at 1 year, the weight loss was maintained by a greater proportion of those who continued receiving the drug during year 2 compared with those who were reassigned to receive placebo (67.9 versus 50.3%).

In the Behavioral Modification and Lorcaserin Second Study of Obesity Management (BLOSSOM), 4008 patients were randomized to receive lorcaserin hydrochloride 10 mg once or twice daily or placebo for 1 year. Patients with type 2 diabetes mellitus were excluded from this study. The mean baseline body weight was 100.2 kg and mean BMI was 35.9 kg/m². Substantially more patients receiving twice-daily lorcaserin lost 5% or more of their baseline body weight compared with patients receiving once-daily lorcaserin or placebo (47.2 versus 40.2 or 25%, respectively). Similarly, more patients receiving twice-daily lorcaserin lost 10% or more of their baseline body weight compared with patients receiving once-daily lorcaserin or placebo (22.6 versus 17.4 or 9.7%, respectively). The mean reduction in body weight at 1 year was 5.8% in patients receiving twice-daily lorcaserin compared with 4.7% in those receiving once-daily lorcaserin and 2.8% in those receiving placebo. There were no substantial differences in observed changes in serum lipids or blood pressure between treatment groups at 1 year.

The Behavioral Modification and Lorcaserin for Obesity and Overweight Management in Diabetes Mellitus (BLOOM-DM) study evaluated lorcaserin hydrochloride 10 mg once or twice daily compared with placebo for 1 year in 604 patients with inadequately controlled type 2 diabetes mellitus (glycosylated hemoglobin [HbA_{1c}] of 7–10%). At baseline, the mean body weight was 103.6 kg, mean BMI was 36 kg/m², and mean HbA_{1c} was 8.1%. All patients were receiving metformin (91.5%), a sulfonylurea (50.4%), or both (41.9%) at the start of the study. Weight reduction was evident at 2 weeks and remained substantially greater throughout the study in patients receiving lorcaserin compared with those receiving placebo. Substantially more patients receiving lorcaserin once or twice daily lost 5% or more (44.7 or 37.5%, respectively) or 10% or more (18.1 or 16.3%, respectively) of their baseline body weight compared with patients receiving placebo (16.1 or 4.4% respectively). At 1 year, 52.2 or 50.4% of patients receiving lorcaserin once or twice daily, respectively, achieved HbA_{1c} of 7% or less compared with 26.3% of patients receiving placebo. The mean reduction in body weight from baseline to 1 year was 5 or 4.5% in those receiving lorcaserin once or twice daily, respectively, compared with 1.5% in those receiving placebo. However, changes in serum lipids and blood pressure generally were small and similar in the lorcaserin and placebo groups.

Patients in these studies who had not lost 5% or more of their baseline body weight by week 12 were unlikely to lose 5% or more of their body weight by 1 year.

The long-term effects of lorcaserin on the cardiovascular morbidity and mortality associated with obesity and safety and efficacy of the drug beyond 2 years of use have not been established.

Dosage and Administration

■ **Administration** Lorcaserin hydrochloride is administered orally without regard to meals.

■ **Dosage** Dosage of lorcaserin hydrochloride hemihydrate is expressed in terms of the anhydrous salt.

The recommended dosage of lorcaserin hydrochloride for chronic weight management in adults 18 years of age and older is 10 mg twice daily. Higher dosages are associated with a greater incidence of adverse reactions and should be avoided. The manufacturer states that lorcaserin should be discontinued if weight loss during the first 12 weeks of therapy is less than 5% of the patient's baseline body weight, since continued therapy with the drug is unlikely to be effective.

■ **Special Populations** No dosage adjustment is necessary in patients with mild renal impairment. In patients with moderate renal impairment, lorcaserin should be used with caution. Lorcaserin is not recommended in patients with severe renal impairment, including those with end-stage renal disease.

In patients with mild or moderate hepatic impairment, dosage adjustment is not necessary. Lorcaserin has not been studied in patients with severe hepatic impairment and should be used with caution in these patients.

Dosage adjustment based solely on age is not necessary in geriatric patients; geriatric patients with normal renal function may receive usual dosages of the drug. In addition, dosage adjustment is not recommended based on gender or race.

Cautions

■ **Contraindications** Lorcaserin is contraindicated in women who are pregnant. (See Pregnancy under Warnings/Precautions: Specific Populations, in Cautions.)

■ **Warnings/Precautions** ***Serotonin Syndrome or Neuroleptic Malignant Syndrome (NMS)-like Reactions*** Potentially life-threatening serotonin syndrome or neuroleptic malignant syndrome (NMS)-like reactions have been reported in patients receiving serotonergic drugs, including selective serotonin-reuptake inhibitors (SSRIs), selective serotonin- and norepinephrine-reuptake inhibitors (SNRIs), tricyclic antidepressants, bupropion, serotonin [5-hydroxytryptamine; 5-HT] type 1 receptor agonists ["triptans"]), dietary supplements (St. John's wort [*Hypericum perforatum*], tryptophan), drugs that impair the metabolism of serotonin (e.g., monoamine oxidase [MAO] inhibitors), dextromethorphan, lithium, tramadol, or antipsychotics or other dopamine antagonists, particularly when such drugs are used in combination. Manifestations of serotonin syndrome may include mental status changes (e.g., agitation, hallucinations, coma), autonomic instability (e.g., tachycardia, labile blood pressure, hyperthermia), neuromuscular aberrations (e.g., hyperreflexia, incoordination), and/or GI symptoms (e.g., nausea, vomiting, diarrhea). In its most severe form, serotonin syndrome may resemble NMS, which is characterized by hyperthermia, muscle rigidity, autonomic instability with possible rapid fluctuation in vital signs, and mental status changes. Because lorcaserin has serotonergic activity, patients receiving the drug should be monitored for possible emergence of manifestations of serotonin syndrome or NMS-like reactions.

Patients receiving SSRIs, SNRIs, bupropion, tricyclic antidepressants, or MAO inhibitors were excluded from clinical trials of lorcaserin; safety of lorcaserin when used concurrently with other serotonergic or antidopaminergic agents, including antipsychotic agents, or with drugs that impair metabolism of serotonin, including MAO inhibitors, has not been established. If concurrent therapy with lorcaserin and an agent that affects the serotonergic neurotransmitter system is clinically warranted, extreme caution should be used and the patient should be observed carefully, particularly during initiation of therapy and when dosage is increased.

If signs and symptoms of serotonin syndrome or NMS occur, treatment with lorcaserin and any concurrently administered serotonergic or antidopaminergic agents should be immediately discontinued and supportive and symptomatic treatment should be initiated.

Valvular Heart Disease Regurgitant cardiac valvular disease (primarily affecting mitral and/or aortic valves) has been reported in patients receiving serotonergic drugs with type 2B (5-hydroxytryptamine [$5\text{-}HT_{2B}$]) receptor agonist activity (e.g., fenfluramine, dexfenfluramine [both drugs no longer commercially available in the US]). (See Cautions: Valvulopathy and Pulmonary Hypertension, in the Amphetamines General Statement 28:20.04.) At therapeutic concentrations, lorcaserin is selective for $5\text{-}HT_{2C}$ receptors as compared with $5\text{-}HT_{2B}$ receptors (see Description). Analysis of pooled data from 3 clinical trials of lorcaserin indicated that echocardiographic evidence of new valvulopathy (i.e., mild or more severe aortic regurgitation and/or moderate or more severe mitral regurgitation) was present at 1 year of treatment in 2.4% of patients receiving lorcaserin and 2% of those receiving placebo (relative risk of 1.16; 95% confidence interval of 0.81–1.67); none of the patients had symptomatic valvular regurgitation.

Lorcaserin has not been studied in patients with congestive heart failure or hemodynamically important valvular heart disease. Preliminary data suggest that $5\text{-}HT_{2B}$ receptors may be overexpressed in patients with congestive heart failure; therefore, lorcaserin should be used with caution in patients with congestive heart failure.

Lorcaserin should not be used in combination with serotonergic and dopaminergic drugs that are potent $5\text{-}HT_{2B}$ receptor agonists and are known to increase the risk for cardiac valvulopathy (e.g., cabergoline).

If signs or symptoms of valvular heart disease, including dyspnea, dependent edema, congestive heart failure, or new cardiac murmur, develop in patients receiving lorcaserin, the patient should be evaluated and discontinuance of lorcaserin should be considered.

Cognitive Impairment Impairment of attention and memory has been reported in clinical trials in 1.9% of patients receiving lorcaserin and 0.5% of those receiving placebo. Confusion, somnolence, and fatigue also have been reported in clinical trials in patients receiving lorcaserin.

Psychiatric Effects Euphoria, hallucinations, and dissociation have occurred in patients receiving lorcaserin at supratherapeutic doses (see Dependence and Abuse Potential under Cautions: Warnings/Precautions). Dosage of lorcaserin hydrochloride should not exceed 10 mg twice daily.

Because certain centrally acting agents, including some such agents that promote weight loss, may be associated with emergence or worsening of depression or suicidal ideation, patients receiving lorcaserin should be monitored for the emergence or worsening of depression, suicidal thoughts or behavior (suicidality), and/or any unusual changes in mood or behavior. Lorcaserin should be discontinued in patients who experience suicidal thoughts or behaviors.

Hypoglycemia Weight loss may increase the risk of hypoglycemia in patients with type 2 diabetes mellitus who are receiving insulin and/or insulin secretagogues (e.g., sulfonylureas). In clinical trials, hypoglycemia was observed in 29.3% and was symptomatic in 7.4% of patients with type 2 diabetes mellitus treated with metformin and/or a sulfonylurea who were receiving lorcaserin at the recommended dosage.

In patients with type 2 diabetes mellitus, blood glucose concentrations should be monitored prior to and during lorcaserin therapy. Clinicians should consider reductions in dosage of concomitant non-glucose-dependent antidiabetic agents to minimize the risk of hypoglycemia. If hypoglycemia develops following initiation of lorcaserin therapy, appropriate changes should be made to the antidiabetic drug regimen.

Lorcaserin has not been studied in combination with insulin.

Priapism Priapism (painful erection exceeding 6 hours) is a possible effect of agonist activity at 5-HT_{2C} receptors. Because of the risk of irreversible penile tissue damage if priapism is not treated immediately, patients should be warned to immediately discontinue the drug and to seek medical attention if an erection persists for longer than 4 hours.

Lorcaserin should be used with caution in patients who have conditions that may predispose them to priapism (e.g., sickle cell anemia, multiple myeloma, leukemia) and in patients with anatomic deformation of the penis (e.g., angulation, cavernosal fibrosis, Peyronie's disease). Experience with concomitant use of lorcaserin and drugs indicated for the treatment of erectile dysfunction (e.g., phosphodiesterase type 5 [PDE5] inhibitors) is limited, and these drugs should be used concomitantly with caution.

Bradycardia In clinical trials of at least 1 year's duration, bradycardia was reported in 0.3% of patients receiving lorcaserin and 0.1% of those receiving placebo.

In patients without diabetes mellitus, the mean decrease in heart rate was 1.2 or 0.4 beats/minute in patients receiving lorcaserin or placebo, respectively; heart rate of less than 50 beats/minute was reported in 5.3% of patients receiving lorcaserin and 3.2% of those receiving placebo. In patients with type 2 diabetes mellitus, the mean decrease in heart rate was 2 or 0.4 beats/minute in patients receiving lorcaserin or placebo, respectively; heart rate of less than 50 beats/minute was reported in 3.6% of patients receiving lorcaserin and 2% of those receiving placebo.

Lorcaserin should be used with caution in patients with bradycardia or a history of heart block greater than first degree.

Hematologic Effects Decreases in leukocyte count (including leukopenia, lymphopenia, and neutropenia) and erythrocyte count (including anemia and decreases in hemoglobin and hematocrit) have been reported in patients receiving lorcaserin. Periodic monitoring of complete blood cell counts should be considered in patients receiving the drug.

Hyperprolactinemia Moderate elevations of prolactin concentrations have been reported in patients receiving lorcaserin in clinical trials of at least 1 year's duration. Prolactin concentration should be measured if signs and symptoms of prolactin excess, including galactorrhea and gynecomastia, are suspected.

Prolactinoma was reported during clinical trials in one patient receiving lorcaserin; a causal relationship to the drug has not been established.

Pulmonary Hypertension Pulmonary hypertension has been associated with certain centrally acting serotonergic anorexigenic agents (e.g., fenfluramine, dexfenfluramine [both drugs no longer commercially available in the US]); clinical trial experience with lorcaserin to date has been inadequate to determine if lorcaserin increases the risk for pulmonary hypertension.

Dependence and Abuse Potential In an abuse-potential study conducted in recreational drug abusers, administration of higher than recommended doses of lorcaserin hydrochloride (40 or 60 mg) was associated with hallucinations, sedation, and positive subjective assessments ("high," "good drug effects"), suggesting that the drug may produce psychic dependence; the incidence of euphoria following administration of lorcaserin hydrochloride 40 or 60 mg (19%) was similar to that following administration of zolpidem 15 or 30 mg. In addition, 16–19% of healthy individuals receiving lorcaserin hydrochloride 40 or 60 mg during short-term studies of the drug experienced euphoria. However, in clinical studies of 4 weeks' to 2 years' duration, euphoria or hallucinations occurred in less than 1% of obese patients receiving doses up to 40 mg.

The potential for lorcaserin to induce physical dependence, manifested as a withdrawal syndrome, has not been elucidated.

Specific Populations **Pregnancy.** Category X. (See Users Guide.) (See Cautions: Contraindications.)

Weight loss offers no potential benefit to pregnant women and may result in fetal harm. Maternal exposure to lorcaserin in late pregnancy in rats resulted in lower body weight in offspring, which persisted to adulthood. If lorcaserin is used during pregnancy or if the patient becomes pregnant while taking this drug, the patient should be apprised of the potential hazard of maternal weight loss to the fetus.

Lactation. It is not known whether lorcaserin is distributed into milk. Because many drugs are distributed into milk, a decision should be made whether to discontinue nursing or the drug, taking into account the importance of the drug to the woman.

Pediatric Use. Safety and efficacy of lorcaserin in patients younger than 18 years of age have not been established; use of lorcaserin is not recommended in pediatric patients.

Geriatric Use. In clinical trials of lorcaserin, 2.5% of patients were 65 years of age or older. Clinical studies of lorcaserin did not include sufficient numbers of patients 65 years of age and older to determine whether geriatric patients respond differently than younger adults. The possibility that some older patients may exhibit greater sensitivity to the drug cannot be ruled out. Because geriatric patients may have decreased renal function, use of lorcaserin in geriatric patients should be based on renal function.

Hepatic Impairment. In patients with mild (Child-Pugh score 5–6) or moderate (Child-Pugh score 7–9) hepatic impairment, peak plasma concentrations of lorcaserin were decreased by 7.8 or 14.3%, respectively, and exposure to the drug was increased by 22 or 30%, respectively, compared with patients with normal hepatic function. In patients with moderate hepatic impairment, half-life of lorcaserin was prolonged by 59%. Lorcaserin has not been studied in patients with severe hepatic impairment and should be used with caution in such patients.

Renal Impairment. In patients with impaired renal function, peak plasma concentrations of lorcaserin are decreased, while area under the concentration-time curve (AUC) is unchanged. Depending on the degree of renal impairment, exposure to the major circulating metabolite of lorcaserin (lorcaserin sulfamate [M1]) and the major urinary metabolite (*N*-carbamoyl glucuronide lorcaserin [M5]) may be altered. Exposure to M1 and M5 is increased by 1.7- and 1.5-fold, respectively, in patients with mild renal impairment (creatinine clearance of 50–80 mL/minute); by 2.3- and 2.5-fold, respectively, in patients with moderate renal impairment (creatinine clearance of 30–50 mL/minute); and by 10.5- and 5.1-fold, respectively, in patients with severe renal impairment (creatinine clearance less than 30 mL/minute). Lorcaserin and M1 are not removed by hemodialysis; approximately 18% of M5 is removed from the body by 4 hours of hemodialysis.

Lorcaserin should be used with caution in patients with moderate renal impairment and should not be used in patients with severe renal impairment, including those with end-stage renal disease.

■ **Common Adverse Effects** Adverse effects reported in more than 5% of nondiabetic patients receiving lorcaserin at the recommended dosage, and occurring more frequently than with placebo, include headache, dizziness, fatigue, nausea, dry mouth, and constipation.

Adverse effects reported in more than 5% of diabetic patients receiving lorcaserin at the recommended dosage, and occurring more frequently than with placebo, include hypoglycemia, headache, back pain, cough, and fatigue.

Drug Interactions

■ **Drugs Affecting Hepatic Microsomal Enzymes** In vitro studies indicate that lorcaserin is metabolized by multiple cytochrome P-450 (CYP) isoenzymes, including 1A1, 1A2, 2A6, 2B6, 2C19, 2D6, 2E1, and 3A4. Pharmacokinetic interactions mediated by CYP isoenzymes are unlikely since metabolism of lorcaserin does not appear to depend on any single metabolic pathway.

■ **Drugs Metabolized by Hepatic Microsomal Enzymes** Lorcaserin inhibits CYP2D6. Concomitant use of lorcaserin with CYP2D6 substrates may result in increased exposure to the CYP2D6 substrate drug; caution is advised when CYP2D6 substrates are used concomitantly with lorcaserin.

■ **Drugs Affecting Uridine Diphosphate-glucuronosyltransferase (UGT)** In vitro studies indicate that multiple UGT enzymes catalyze glucuronidation of lorcaserin. Therefore, inhibition of any single UGT enzyme is unlikely to substantially inhibit glucuronidation of lorcaserin.

■ **Serotonergic Drugs** Because of the theoretical potential for serotonin syndrome, extreme caution is advised when lorcaserin is used concomitantly with other serotonergic drugs, including serotonin type 1 (5-hydroxytryptamine [5-HT_1]) receptor agonists ("triptans"), monoamine oxidase (MAO) inhibitors (including linezolid), selective serotonin-reuptake inhibitors (SSRIs), selective serotonin- and norepinephrine-reuptake inhibitors (SNRIs), dextromethorphan, tricyclic antidepressants, bupropion, lithium, tramadol, tryptophan, and St. John's wort (*Hypericum perforatum*). (See Serotonin Syndrome or Neuroleptic Malignant Syndrome [NMS]-like Reactions under Cautions: Warnings/Precautions.)

■ **Dextromethorphan** Concomitant use of lorcaserin hydrochloride (10 mg twice daily for 4 days) with dextromethorphan in CYP2D6 extensive metabolizers increased peak dextromethorphan concentrations by approximately 76% and area under the plasma concentration-time curve (AUC) by approximately 100%.

Description

Lorcaserin hydrochloride, a selective serotonin type 2C (5-hydroxytryptamine [5-HT_{2C}]) receptor agonist, is an anorexigenic agent. The exact mechanism by which lorcaserin exerts its anorexigenic effect is unknown, but the drug appears to decrease food consumption and promote satiety by selectively activating 5-HT_{2C} receptors on pro-opiomelanocortin neurons located in the hypothalamus. Activation of 5-HT_{2C} receptors stimulates a precursor for α-melanocortin-stimulating hormone, which acts on melanocortin-4 receptors to decrease food intake. In overweight and obese patients, lorcaserin decreased energy intake without altering energy expenditure or respiratory quotient.

At the recommended daily dosage, lorcaserin selectively interacts with 5-HT_{2C} receptors as compared with 5-HT_{2A} and 5-HT_{2B} receptors, other 5-HT receptor subtypes, the 5-HT receptor transporter, and 5-HT reuptake sites. Potency of lorcaserin at 5-HT_{2C} receptors is approximately 14- and 60-fold greater than its potency at 5-HT_{2A} and 5-HT_{2B} receptors, respectively. Lorcaserin's affinity for 5-HT_{2C} receptors is approximately 7- and 11-fold greater than its affinity for 5-HT_{2A} and 5-HT_{2B} receptors, respectively. Lorcaserin does not appear to affect serotonin, norepinephrine, or dopamine release or uptake.

Lorcaserin is extensively metabolized in the liver by multiple enzymatic pathways; major metabolites of the drug lack serotonergic receptor activity. Lorcaserin sulfamate (M1) is the major circulating metabolite and *N*-carbamoyl glucuronide lorcaserin (M5) is the major metabolite in urine. Lorcaserin is excreted principally in urine (about 92% of an administered dose) as inactive metabolites. The plasma half-life of the drug is about 11 hours.

Advice to Patients

Importance of using lorcaserin in conjunction with a reduced-calorie diet and increased physical activity. If weight loss during the first 12 weeks of therapy is less than 5% of initial body weight, importance of discontinuing therapy since continued treatment is unlikely to be effective. Importance of not increasing dosage beyond the recommended dosage.

Importance of informing patients of potential risk of serotonin syndrome and neuroleptic malignant syndrome (NMS)-like reactions with concurrent use of lorcaserin and selective serotonin-reuptake inhibitors (SSRIs), selective serotonin- and norepinephrine-reuptake inhibitors (SNRIs), monoamine oxidase (MAO) inhibitors, 5-HT_1 receptor agonists (triptans), tramadol, tryptophan, St. John's wort, antipsychotic agents, or other serotonergic agents or dopamine antagonists. Importance of immediately contacting clinician if signs and symptoms of these syndromes (e.g., high fever, stiff muscles, sweating, fast or irregular heart beat, change in blood pressure, confusion, coordination problems, restlessness, nausea, vomiting, diarrhea) develop.

Importance of seeking medical attention if signs or symptoms of valvular heart disease, including dyspnea or dependent edema, develop.

Potential for lorcaserin to impair judgment, thinking, or motor skills; advise patient to avoid driving or operating hazardous machinery until the drug's effects on the individual are known.

Potential risk of suicidality; importance of patients being alert to and seeking medical attention in the event of suicidality, emergence or worsening of depression, or unusual changes in mood or behavior.

Importance of men discontinuing the drug and seeking immediate medical attention if an erection persists longer than 4 hours.

Importance of blood glucose monitoring in patients with type 2 diabetes mellitus treated with insulin and/or insulin secretagogues (e.g., sulfonylureas), since weight loss may increase the risk of hypoglycemia.

Importance of advising women of childbearing potential to avoid pregnancy and breast-feeding; importance of women informing clinicians if they are or plan to become pregnant or plan to breast-feed.

Importance of informing clinician of existing or contemplated concomitant therapy, including prescription and OTC drugs and dietary or herbal supplements, as well as any concomitant illnesses (e.g., cardiac disease, diabetes mellitus, conditions that may predispose to priapism).

Importance of informing patients of other important precautionary information. (See Cautions.)

Overview® (see Users Guide). For additional information on this drug until a more detailed monograph is developed and published, the manufacturer's labeling should be consulted. It is *essential* that the manufacturer's labeling be consulted for more detailed information on usual cautions, precautions, contraindications, potential drug interactions, laboratory test interferences, and acute toxicity.

Preparations

Lorcaserin is subject to control under the Federal Controlled Substances Act of 1970 as a schedule IV (C-IV) drug.

Excipients in commercially available drug preparations may have clinically important effects in some individuals; consult specific product labeling for details.

Lorcaserin Hydrochloride Hemihydrate

Oral

Tablets, film-coated	10 mg (of lorcaserin hydrochloride)	**Belviq®** (C-IV), Eisai

RESPIRATORY AND CNS STIMULANTS 28:20.32

Caffeine
Caffeine and Sodium Benzoate Injection
Caffeine Citrate

■ Caffeine is a xanthine-derivative CNS stimulant that occurs naturally in tea and coffee, but is prepared synthetically for commercial drug use.

Uses

■ **CNS Stimulation** Caffeine is used orally as a mild CNS stimulant to aid in staying awake and to restore mental alertness in fatigued patients.

Caffeine also is used orally in combination with antihistamines to overcome the sedative properties of the latter drugs, but the efficacy of caffeine and the dosage required have not been adequately established.

Caffeine and sodium benzoate injection has been used in conjunction with supportive measures to treat respiratory depression associated with overdosage of CNS depressant drugs (e.g., opiate analgesics, alcohol) and with electric shock. However, because of the questionable benefit and transient action, *most authorities believe caffeine and other analeptics should not be used in these conditions* and recommend other supportive therapy.

■ **Apnea of Prematurity** Caffeine citrate is used IV or orally in the short-term (10–12 days) treatment of apnea of prematurity in neonates who are between 28 and less than 33 weeks of gestational age. Caffeine is designated an orphan drug by the US Food and Drug Administration (FDA) for use in apnea in premature neonates.

The use of caffeine citrate in apnea of prematurity was established in a randomized, placebo-controlled clinical trial of the drug in premature neonates (gestational age 28 to less than 33 weeks) with apnea of prematurity (defined as having at least 6 episodes of apnea of greater than 20 seconds' duration in a 24-hour period with no other identifiable causes of apnea). A 20-mg/kg loading dose of caffeine citrate (10 mg/kg of caffeine) was administered IV, followed by a daily maintenance dose of 5 mg/kg of caffeine citrate (2.5 mg/kg of caffeine) IV or orally (generally via a feeding tube). Patients randomized to placebo were allowed to cross over to caffeine treatment if their apnea became uncontrolled during the double-blind phase of the trial; the study period lasted 10–12 days. The percentage of patients without apnea on the second day of treatment (i.e., 24–48 hours after the loading dose) was greater in the caffeine-treated patients compared with placebo-treated patients (26.7 versus 8.1%, respectively). The mean number of days with zero apnea events was 3 in the caffeine-treated group and 1.2 in the placebo group, while the mean number of days with a 50% reduction from baseline in apnea events was 6.8 in the caffeine-treated group and 4.6 in the placebo group. Serum caffeine concentrations ranged from 8–40 mcg/mL in treated patients; however, a therapeutic plasma concentration could not be determined from this clinical trial. In low-birthweight neonates, the drug has decreased the frequency of apneic episodes without any substantial effect on heart rate. Some clinicians recommend that when conservative measures (e.g., tactile stimulation, flotation on a waterbed) are ineffective in preventing severe, recurrent apnea in neonates, caffeine may be used as an alternative to mechanical ventilation†. The manufacturer states that the safety and efficacy of treatment with caffeine citrate in neonates with apnea of prematurity for longer than 10–12 days† have not been established. The manufacturer also states that use of caffeine citrate in the prevention of sudden infant death syndrome† (SIDS) or prior to extubation in mechanically ventilated neonates† also has not been established. Use of the combination preparation containing caffeine and sodium benzoate† in neonates is generally avoided because of the potential for sodium benzoate to produce kernicterus. (See Cautions: Pediatric Precautions.)

■ **Headache** Caffeine is used orally or rectally in combination with ergotamine tartrate to abort vascular headaches such as migraine and cluster headaches (histamine cephalalgia). There is conflicting evidence regarding the efficacy of this combination in the treatment of acute migraine attacks. Caffeine's cerebral vasoconstrictor effect is reportedly additive with that of ergotamine, but the results of one study suggest that the principal value of caffeine in this combination is related to its ability to increase GI absorption of ergotamine tartrate. Some clinicians question the value of the combination because caffeine may keep patients awake and sleep can contribute to the relief of migraine. (For further information on management and classification of migraine headache, see Vascular Headaches: General Principles in Migraine Therapy, under Uses in Sumatriptan 28:32.28.)

Caffeine is used orally alone and in combination with analgesics (e.g., acetaminophen, aspirin) for the treatment of headache. Some experts state that the combination of acetaminophen, aspirin, and caffeine is a reasonable first-line therapy for mild to moderate migraine attacks or for severe migraine attacks that have responded in the past to similar nonsteroidal anti-inflammatory agents (NSAIAs) or non-opiate analgesics. Caffeine exerts no intrinsic analgesic activity. Although analgesic-caffeine combinations have been reported to produce slightly more analgesia than analgesic agents alone and to have a beneficial effect on mood, which may be clinically important in some patients with headache, these results have not always been reproducible in well-controlled studies and additional studies are needed to determine the role, if any, of caffeine as an analgesic adjuvant.

Caffeine and sodium benzoate injection has been used for the symptomatic relief of headache following spinal puncture.

■ **Other Uses** Caffeine is used orally alone and in combination with other drugs (e.g., analgesics, diuretics) to relieve tension, fatigue, and fluid retention associated with menstruation. However, because caffeine's diuretic activity in patients with fluid retention is minimal, its usefulness in this condition is questionable.

Caffeine (30% in a topical hydrophilic base) has been used effectively alone or in combination with topical hydrocortisone in the topical treatment of atopic dermatitis†.

Caffeine also has been used in combination with ephedrine to promote weight loss in patients with exogenous obesity†. (See Uses: Misuse and Abuse, in Ephedrine 12:12.12.) It has been suggested that weight loss may be associated with increased energy expenditure (thermogenesis) and appetite suppression. However, the US Food and Drug Administration (FDA), which did not evaluate the efficacy of ephedrine dietary supplements in obesity therapy, has stated that such use of ephedrine may be associated with an unacceptable incidence of adverse effects. (See Misuse and Abuse: Dietary Supplements under Uses, in Ephedrine 12:12.12.)

Dosage and Administration

■ **Administration** Caffeine may be administered orally. Caffeine citrate is administered orally or by slow IV infusion using a syringe infusion pump. Caffeine and sodium benzoate injection may be administered by IM or slow IV injection; the drug has also been administered subcutaneously.

The preservative-free commercially available injection is for single use only, and any unused portion should be discarded. It is important that such oral solution be measured accurately (e.g., using a 1-mL or other appropriate syringe).

■ **Dosage** Some clinicians suggest that when used as a mild CNS stimulant to overcome fatigue, oral doses of 100–200 mg of anhydrous caffeine are required. The manufacturers state that adults and children 12 years of age or older may receive a dosage of 100–200 mg no more frequently than every 3–4 hours.

For the treatment of apnea of prematurity, commercially available caffeine citrate injection in a loading dose of 20 mg/kg (10 mg/kg when expressed in terms of anhydrous caffeine) is administered by slow IV infusion (i.e., over 30 minutes) using a syringe infusion pump. Beginning 24 hours after the loading dose, maintenance doses of caffeine citrate of 5 mg/kg (2.5 mg/kg when expressed as anhydrous caffeine) may be administered every 24 hours, either orally or via slow IV infusion (i.e., over 10 minutes) using a syringe infusion pump. The manufacturer states that the safety and efficacy of dosing periods exceeding 10–12 days have not been established. Other dosing regimens† for the treatment of apnea of prematurity have used caffeine doses (in terms of anhydrous caffeine) of 5–10 mg/kg, given IV, IM, or orally as a loading dose, and followed by 2.5–5 mg/kg, given IV, IM, or orally once daily. Maintenance dosage has been adjusted according to the patient's response and tolerance and plasma caffeine concentrations.

When caffeine citrate is used for the treatment of apnea of prematurity in infants with hepatic or renal impairment, serum concentrations of caffeine should be monitored and dosage adjusted to avoid toxicity.

Analeptic use of caffeine is strongly discouraged by most clinicians. However, the manufacturers of caffeine and sodium benzoate injection recommend IM, or in emergency respiratory failure, IV injection of 500 mg of the drug (about 250 mg of anhydrous caffeine) or a maximum single dose of 1 g (about 500 mg of anhydrous caffeine) for the treatment of respiratory depression associated with overdosage of CNS depressants, including opiate analgesics and alcohol, and with electric shock.

Some clinicians recommend that when caffeine and sodium benzoate injection is used in children for CNS stimulation†, an IM, IV, or subcutaneous dose of 8 mg/kg (about 4 mg of anhydrous caffeine per kg) (not to exceed 500 mg) or 250 mg/m^2 (about 125 mg of anhydrous caffeine per m^2) be given up to every 4 hours if necessary.

Cautions

■ **Adverse Effects** CNS stimulation and GI irritation usually occur with therapeutic dosages of caffeine. Adverse CNS effects, which are usually more severe in children than in adults, include insomnia, restlessness, nervousness, and mild delirium. Adverse GI effects include nausea, vomiting, and gastric irritation. Although chronic administration of caffeine in animals has been associated with gastric ulceration, such a causal relationship in humans has not been adequately established to date. Suppositories containing caffeine may produce rectal irritation. Large doses of caffeine may produce headache, excitement, agitation, a condition resembling anxiety neurosis, scintillating scotoma, hyperesthesia, tinnitus, muscle tremors or twitches, diuresis, tachycardia, extrasystoles, and possibly other cardiac arrhythmias.

Further CNS depression may occur when already depressed patients are too vigorously treated with caffeine and sodium benzoate.

In a placebo-controlled study, the most common adverse effects occurring more frequently in patients receiving caffeine citrate than in those receiving placebo included rash and feeding intolerance, each of which occurred in 8.7% of patients, and sepsis and necrotizing enterocolitis, each of which occurred in 4.3% of patients. In this same trial, accidental injury, hemorrhage, gastritis, GI hemorrhage, disseminated intravascular coagulation, acidosis, abnormal healing, cerebral hemorrhage, pulmonary edema, dyspnea, dry skin, skin breakdown, retinopathy of prematurity, and kidney failure each occurred in 2.2% of caffeine-treated patients. In addition, during the trial of caffeine citrate for the apnea of prematurity, 6 cases of necrotizing enterocolitis developed among the 85 neonates studied, 3 cases of which were fatal. Five of the 6 neonates had been randomized to treatment with or had been exposed to caffeine citrate. Adverse effects reported in the literature include CNS stimulation (i.e., irritability, restlessness, jitteriness), cardiovascular effects (i.e., tachycardia, increased left ventricular output, increased stroke volume), GI effects (i.e., increased gastric aspirate, GI intolerance), alterations in serum glucose (i.e., hyperglycemia or hypoglycemia), and renal effects (i.e., increased urine flow rate, increased creatinine clearance, increased sodium and calcium excretion).

Ingestion of large amounts of combinations containing aspirin, phenacetin, and caffeine (combinations containing phenacetin no longer are commercially available in the US) has been associated with analgesic nephropathy which is characterized by sterile pyuria, asymptomatic bacteriuria, pyelonephritis, papillary necrosis, interstitial fibrosis and nephritis, and increased excretion of renal tubular cells and erythrocytes. Caffeine's role in the etiology of this condition has not been conclusively established.

■ **Precautions and Contraindications** Because it has been suggested that caffeine may promote gastric ulceration, the drug should be used cautiously in patients with a history of peptic ulcer. Because of its suspected arrhythmogenic potential, it is generally recommended that caffeine be avoided in patients with symptomatic cardiac arrhythmias and/or palpitations and during the first several days to weeks after an acute myocardial infarction.

When *self-administered* as a mild CNS stimulant to overcome fatigue or drowsiness, caffeine is intended for occasional use only and should not be used as a substitute for sleep.

When preparations containing caffeine in combination with other drugs (see Preparations) are used, the cautions, precautions, and contraindications applicable to each ingredient should be considered.

Caffeine is contraindicated in patients with a history of hypersensitivity to the drug.

■ **Pediatric Precautions** Use of caffeine tablets for *self-medication* in children younger than 12 years of age is not recommended.

Adverse CNS effects of caffeine are usually more severe in children than in adults. (See Cautions: Adverse Effects.) The sodium benzoate component in caffeine and sodium benzoate injection reportedly produces kernicterus in neonates by uncoupling albumin-bilirubin binding. Long-term follow-up studies have not shown caffeine administration in premature neonates to affect adversely either neurologic development or growth parameters.

In neonates receiving caffeine citrate therapy, periodic monitoring of serum caffeine concentrations may be necessary to avoid toxicity. Prior to initiation of caffeine citrate therapy, baseline serum concentrations of caffeine should be measured in neonates previously treated with theophylline, since preterm neonates metabolize theophylline to caffeine. Similarly, baseline serum concentrations of caffeine should be measured in infants born to mothers who consumed caffeine prior to delivery since caffeine readily crosses the placenta. Serious toxicity has been reported when serum caffeine concentrations exceed 50 mcg/mL.

Because studies examining the pharmacokinetics of caffeine in neonates with renal or hepatic insufficiency have not been conducted, caffeine citrate should be administered with caution in premature neonates with impaired renal or hepatic function. Serum concentrations of caffeine should be monitored in these neonates, and dosage adjusted to avoid toxicity.

Few data exist on drug interactions with caffeine in premature neonates. Based on data in adults, lower doses of caffeine may be needed following concomitant use of drugs that are reported to decrease caffeine elimination (e.g., ketoconazole, cimetidine) and higher caffeine doses may be required following concomitant use of drugs that increase caffeine elimination (e.g., phenobarbital, phenytoin). Interconversion between caffeine and theophylline has been reported in premature neonates. The concurrent use of these drugs is not recommended. In healthy adults, concomitant administration of caffeine with ketoprofen resulted in decreased urinary volume; the clinical significance of this interaction in premature neonates is not known.

In clinical trials reported in the literature, cases of hypoglycemia and hyperglycemia have been reported in patients receiving caffeine; therefore, blood glucose concentration may need to be monitored periodically in neonates receiving caffeine citrate.

Although no cases of cardiac toxicity were reported in the placebo-controlled trial of caffeine citrate for the treatment of apnea of prematurity, caffeine has been shown to increase heart rate, left ventricular output, and stroke volume. Therefore, caffeine citrate should be used with caution in neonates with cardiovascular disease.

If signs of GI intolerance (e.g., abdominal distention, vomiting, bloody stools) or lethargy develops in premature neonates receiving caffeine citrate oral solution, a clinician should be consulted.

Because seizures have been reported in cases of caffeine overdose, caffeine citrate should be used with caution in neonates with seizure disorders.

The duration of treatment with caffeine citrate in neonates with apnea of prematurity was limited to 10–12 days in the placebo-controlled trial. The safety and efficacy of caffeine citrate for longer periods in this condition have not been established. If premature neonates receiving caffeine citrate oral solution continue to experience apnea events, dosage of the drug should not be increased without advice of a clinician. Safety and efficacy of caffeine citrate in the prevention of sudden infant death syndrome (SIDS) or prior to extubation in mechanically ventilated patients also have not been established.

Apnea of prematurity is a diagnosis of exclusion. Other causes of apnea (e.g., CNS disorders, primary lung disease, anemia, sepsis, metabolic disturbances, cardiovascular abnormalities, obstructive apnea) should be ruled out or treated appropriately prior to initiation of treatment with caffeine citrate.

During the placebo-controlled trial of caffeine citrate establishing efficacy in the US for apnea of prematurity, 6 cases of necrotizing enterocolitis developed among the 85 neonates studied, 3 cases of which were fatal. Five of the 6 neonates had been randomized to treatment with or had been exposed to caffeine citrate. Reports in the literature have raised the possibility of an association between the use of methylxanthines and the development of necrotizing enterocolitis, although a causal relationship between methylxanthine use and the development of necrotizing enterocolitis has not been established. Therefore, as with all premature neonates, patients being treated with caffeine citrate should be monitored carefully for the development of necrotizing enterocolitis.

■ **Mutagenicity and Carcinogenicity** Although clastogenicity and mutagenicity have been demonstrated in some in vitro and animal studies, most clinicians believe that these effects are not important in relation to the amounts of caffeine consumed by humans.

In a 2-year study in Sprague-Dawley rats, caffeine (as caffeine base) administered in drinking water was not carcinogenic in male rats at doses up to 102 mg/kg or in female rats at doses up to 170 mg/kg (approximately 2 and 4 times, respectively, the maximum IV loading dose for neonates on a mg/m^2 basis). In an 18-month study in C57BL/6 mice, no evidence of tumorigenicity was seen at dietary doses of up to 55 mg/kg (less than the maximum IV loading dose for neonates on a mg/m^2 basis).

Caffeine (as caffeine base) increased the sister chromatid exchange (SCE) SCE/cell metaphase (exposure time dependent) in an in vivo mouse metaphase analysis. Caffeine also potentiated the genotoxicity of known mutagens and enhanced the micronuclei formation fivefold in folate-deficient mice. However, caffeine did not increase chromosomal aberrations in in vitro Chinese hamster ovary (CHO) and human lymphocyte assays and was not mutagenic in an in vitro CHO/HGPRT gene mutation assay, except at cytotoxic concentrations. In addition, caffeine was not clastogenic in an in vivo mouse micronucleus assay.

Although it has been suggested that coffee consumption is associated with an increased risk of lower urinary tract, renal, and pancreatic cancers, most studies conducted to date have had methodologic flaws and there is currently no clear evidence that coffee consumption is causally related to an increased risk of these cancers.

■ **Pregnancy, Fertility, and Lactation** There are no adequate and well-controlled studies in pregnant women. In studies performed in adult animals, caffeine (as caffeine base) administered to pregnant mice as sustained-release pellets at 50 mg/kg (less than the maximum IV loading dose for neonates on a mg/m^2 basis) during the period of organogenesis caused a low incidence of cleft palate and exencephaly in fetuses. Based on data from a large retrospective epidemiologic study and from a large retrospective case-control study in humans, it appears that use of caffeine during pregnancy has little, if any, effect on the outcome of pregnancy. Although caffeine use during pregnancy does not appear to be associated with substantial risk, most clinicians recommend that pregnant women avoid or limit their consumption of foods, beverages, and drugs containing caffeine, since caffeine crosses the placenta.

Caffeine (as caffeine base) administered subcutaneously to male rats at 50 mg/kg daily (approximately equal to the maximum IV loading dose for neonates on a mg/m^2 basis) for 4 days prior to mating with untreated females caused decreased male reproductive performance in addition to causing embryotoxicity. In addition, long-term exposure to high oral doses of caffeine (3 g over 7 weeks) was toxic to rat testes as manifested by spermatogenic cell degeneration.

Caffeine is distributed into the milk of nursing women. Milk-to-plasma ratios of 0.5–0.76 have been reported. The amount of caffeine ingested from usual quantities of caffeinated beverages is considered compatible with breast-feeding; however, caffeine may accumulate in nursing infants following moderate to heavy maternal consumption of caffeine, resulting in irritability and poor sleeping patterns.

Drug Interactions

■ **Drugs Affecting or Metabolized by Hepatic Microsomal Enzymes** Caffeine is metabolized by the cytochrome P-450 (CYP) enzyme system, principally by isoenzyme 1A2. Therefore, caffeine has the potential to interact with drugs that are metabolized by CYP1A2 or with drugs that induce or inhibit this isoenzyme. (See Cautions: Pediatric Precautions.) Caffeine has been reported to increase its own metabolism.

■ ***β*-Adrenergic Agonists** Caffeine and other xanthines may enhance the cardiac inotropic effects of *β*-adrenergic stimulating agents.

■ **Disulfiram** When caffeine and disulfiram are administered concomitantly in healthy individuals or recovering alcohol-dependent patients, the total blood clearance of caffeine is substantially decreased and its elimination half-life is increased. The exact mechanism of the interaction is not known, but disulfiram may inhibit hepatic metabolism of caffeine. The clinical importance of the interaction has not been established, but the possibility that exaggerated or prolonged effects of caffeine might occur in patients receiving disulfiram who also ingest substantial quantities of coffee, tea, or other caffeine-containing beverages should be considered. Further studies are needed.

Laboratory Test Interferences

Caffeine produces false-positive elevations of serum urate as measured by the Bittner method. The drug also produces slight increases in urine levels of vanillylmandelic acid (VMA), catecholamines, and 5-hydroxyindoleacetic acid. Because high urine concentrations of VMA or catecholamines may result in false-positive diagnosis of pheochromocytoma or neuroblastoma, caffeine intake should be avoided during tests for these disorders.

Acute Toxicity

■ **Manifestations** Acute toxicity involving caffeine has been reported rarely. GI pain, mild delirium, insomnia, diuresis, dehydration, and fever commonly occur with overdosage. More serious symptoms of overdosage include cardiac arrhythmias and tonic-clonic seizures. In adults, IV doses of 57 mg/kg and oral doses of 18–50 g have been fatal. In one 5-year-old patient, death occurred following oral ingestion of approximately 3 g of caffeine.

Following overdose of caffeine citrate in preterm neonates, serum caffeine concentrations have ranged from approximately 24–350 mcg/mL. Signs and symptoms of caffeine overdose in premature neonates reported in the literature include fever, tachypnea, jitteriness, insomnia, fine tremor of the extremities, hypertonia, opisthotonos, tonic-clonic movements, nonpurposeful jaw and lip movements, vomiting, hyperglycemia, elevated BUN, and elevated total leukocyte concentration. Seizures also have been reported in cases of overdose. One case of caffeine overdose complicated by development of intraventricular hemorrhage and long-term neurologic sequelae has been reported. In another case of caffeine citrate overdosage, administration of caffeine citrate 600 mg (approximately 322 mg/kg) over 40 minutes was associated with tachycardia, ST-segment depression, respiratory distress, heart failure, gastric distension, acidosis, and severe extravasation burn with tissue necrosis at the peripheral infusion site. No deaths associated with caffeine overdose have been reported in premature neonates.

■ **Treatment** Treatment of caffeine overdose in premature neonates is mainly symptomatic and supportive. In acute oral caffeine overdosage, the stomach should be emptied immediately by inducing emesis or by lavage; activated charcoal may be administered; and supportive measures should be initiated. Serum caffeine concentrations have been shown to decrease following exchange transfusions. Administration of demulcents such as aluminum hydroxide gel may diminish GI irritation. Seizures may be treated with IV administration of diazepam or a barbiturate such as pentobarbital sodium.

Chronic Toxicity

Prolonged, high intake of caffeine may produce tolerance, habituation, and psychological dependence. Physical signs of withdrawal such as headaches, irritation, nervousness, anxiety, and dizziness may occur upon abrupt discontinuation of the stimulant.

Pharmacology

Caffeine is pharmacologically similar to the other xanthine drugs, theobromine and theophylline; however, these three agents differ in the intensity of their actions on various structures. Caffeine's CNS and skeletal muscle effects are greater than those of the other xanthines. In all other areas, theophylline has greater activity than caffeine, although some studies report that caffeine has a greater diuretic effect than theobromine. Caffeine competitively inhibits phosphodiesterase, the enzyme that degrades cyclic 3′,5′-adenosine monophosphate (AMP). Increased levels of intracellular cyclic AMP mediate most of caffeine's pharmacologic actions.

■ **CNS Effects** Caffeine stimulates all levels of the CNS. In oral doses of 100–200 mg, the drug stimulates the cerebral cortex producing a more rapid and clearer thought flow, wakefulness or arousal in fatigued patients, and improved psychomotor coordination. Caffeine's cortical effects are milder and of shorter duration than those of the amphetamines. In slightly larger doses, caffeine stimulates medullary vagal, vasomotor, and respiratory centers, promoting bradycardia, vasoconstriction, and increased respiratory rate. Tolerance to the CNS effects of caffeine may develop.

■ **Cardiovascular Effects** Caffeine produces a positive inotropic effect on the myocardium and a positive chronotropic effect at the sinoatrial node, causing transient increases in heart rate, force of contraction, cardiac output, and heart work. In doses of greater than 250 mg, the centrally mediated vagal effects of caffeine may be masked by increased sinus rates; tachycardia, extrasystoles, or possibly other major ventricular arrhythmias may result. The arrhythmogenic potential of caffeine remains to be fully evaluated.

Caffeine constricts cerebral vasculature. In contrast, the drug directly dilates peripheral blood vessels, decreasing peripheral vascular resistance. The effect of this decrease in peripheral vascular resistance (and possibly that of vagal cardiac stimulation) on blood pressure is offset by increased cardiac output (and possibly stimulation of the medullary vasomotor area). The overall effect of caffeine on heart rate and blood pressure depends on whether CNS or peripheral effects predominate. Generally, therapeutic doses of caffeine increase blood pressure only slightly, but in healthy individuals, chronic ingestion of caffeine has little or no effect on blood pressure, heart rate, plasma catecholamine concentrations, or plasma renin activity. Individuals with borderline hypertension do not appear to have an increased susceptibility to the pressor effects of caffeine or increased resistance to the tolerance to the cardiovascular effects that develops with prolonged administration.

■ **Other Effects** Caffeine stimulates voluntary skeletal muscle, increasing the force of contraction and decreasing muscular fatigue. The drug also stimulates gastric acid secretion from parietal cells. Caffeine increases renal blood flow and glomerular filtration rate and decreases proximal tubular reabsorption of sodium and water, resulting in mild diuresis; tolerance may develop to the diuretic effect.

Caffeine stimulates glycogenolysis and lipolysis, but increases in blood glucose and in plasma lipids are usually insignificant in normal patients.

Pharmacokinetics

■ **Absorption** Caffeine and citrated caffeine are well absorbed following oral administration. Absorption of caffeine following oral administration may be more rapid than that following IM injection of caffeine and sodium benzoate. Absorption following rectal administration of caffeine in suppositories may be slow and erratic. Absolute bioavailability of caffeine in preterm neonates has not been fully determined. Following oral administration of 100 mg of caffeine (as coffee), peak plasma concentrations of about 1.5–1.8 mcg/mL are reached after 50–75 minutes. After oral administration of 10 mg/kg caffeine to preterm neonates, the peak plasma concentration for caffeine ranged from 6–10 mg/L and the mean time to reach peak concentration ranged from 30 minutes to 2 hours. The time to reach peak plasma concentration was not affected by formula feeding.

■ **Distribution** Caffeine is rapidly distributed into body tissues, readily crossing the placenta and blood-brain barrier. Caffeine concentration in the CSF fluid of preterm neonates approximates the plasma concentration. The mean volume of distribution of caffeine in infants (0.8–0.9 L/kg) is slightly higher than that in adults (0.6 L/kg). Approximately 17–36% of the drug is bound to plasma proteins in adults. Plasma protein binding data are not available for neonates or infants. Caffeine has been shown to distribute into milk in a milk-to-plasma concentration ratio of 0.5–0.76.

■ **Elimination** Caffeine has a plasma half-life of 3–5 hours in adults. In one study, when administered to pregnant women prior to delivery, caffeine had a prolonged mean half-life of 80 hours in the neonates after delivery. In young infants, the elimination of caffeine is much slower than that in adults because of immature hepatic and/or renal function. Mean half-life and fraction excreted unchanged in urine of caffeine in infants have been shown to be related inversely to gestational/postconceptional age. In neonates, the half-life of caffeine is approximately 3–4 days, and the mean fraction excreted unchanged in urine is approximately 86% (within 6 days). By 9 months of age, the metabolism of caffeine approximates that seen in adults. Hepatic cytochrome P-450 (CYP) isoenzyme 1A2 is involved in caffeine enzymatic metabolism. In adults, the drug is rapidly metabolized in the liver to 1-methyluric acid, 1-methylxanthine, and 7-methylxanthine. Interconversion between caffeine and theophylline has been reported in preterm neonates; caffeine concentrations are approximately 25% of theophylline concentration following theophylline administration and approximately 3–8% of an administered dose of caffeine would be expected to convert to theophylline. Caffeine and its metabolites are excreted mainly by the kidneys; approximately 1% of a dose of caffeine is excreted unchanged in urine in adults.

Studies examining the pharmacokinetics of caffeine in neonates with renal or hepatic insufficiency have not been conducted.

Chemistry and Stability

■ **Chemistry** Caffeine, like theobromine and theophylline, is a xanthine derivative. Caffeine occurs naturally in tea and coffee, but is prepared synthetically for commercial drug use. Caffeine is present in amounts of about 100–150 mg/180 mL of brewed coffee; 60–80 mg/180 mL of instant coffee; 40–100 mg/180 mL of tea; and 17–55 mg/180 mL of cola beverage.

Caffeine occurs as a white powder or white, glistening needles that are usually matted together. The drug is odorless and has a bitter taste. Caffeine, which may contain one molecule of water or be anhydrous, is sparingly soluble in water and in alcohol. The hydrate effloresces in air.

Various synthetic mixtures of caffeine have been prepared to increase its solubility. The mixture of caffeine and sodium benzoate contains 45–52% anhydrous caffeine and occurs as a white powder with a slightly bitter taste. The mixture is freely soluble in water and soluble in alcohol. Caffeine and sodium benzoate injection has a pH of 6.5–8.5. Citrated caffeine is a white powder with a bitter taste, obtained by combining caffeine with citric acid. Citrated caffeine is freely soluble in water and soluble in alcohol and contains approximately 50% anhydrous caffeine. Commercially available caffeine citrate injection and oral solution have a pH of 4.7.

■ **Stability** Commercially available caffeine and sodium benzoate injection and caffeine citrate injection and oral solution should be stored at 15–30°C. The commercially available injections and oral solution should be inspected visually for particulate matter and discoloration prior to administration. Vials containing discolored solution or visible particulate matter should be discarded.

Based on compatibility studies, the commercially available caffeine citrate injection is chemically stable for 24 hours at room temperature when mixed with any of the following solutions: 5% dextrose injection; 50% dextrose injection; Intralipid® 20% emulsion; Aminosyn® 20% solution; dopamine hydrochloride injection (diluted to 0.6 mg/mL with 5% dextrose injection); calcium gluconate 10% injection; heparin sodium injection (diluted to 1 unit/mL with 5% dextrose injection); fentanyl citrate injection (diluted to 10 mcg/mL with 5% dextrose injection).

Preparations

Excipients in commercially available drug preparations may have clinically important effects in some individuals; consult specific product labeling for details.

Caffeine

Oral		
Tablets	100 mg*	**Caffeine Tablets**
	200 mg*	**Caffeine Tablets**
Tablets, film-coated	200 mg*	**Caffeine Film-coated Tablets**
		No Doz® Maximum Strength Caplets®, Novartis
		Vivarin®, GlaxoSmithKline

Caffeine also is commercially available in combination with analgesics, antacids, antihistamines, antipyretics, antitussives, belladonna alkaloids, diuretics, ergotamine tartrate, expectorants, nasal decongestants, skeletal muscle relaxants, sympathomimetics, and vitamins.

*available from one or more manufacturer, distributor, and/or repackager by generic (nonproprietary) name

Caffeine and Sodium Benzoate

Parenteral		
Injection	250 mg/mL (equivalent to caffeine anhydrous 125 mg/mL and sodium benzoate 125 mg/mL)*	**Caffeine and Sodium Benzoate Injection**

*available from one or more manufacturer, distributor, and/or repackager by generic (nonproprietary) name

Caffeine Citrate

Oral		
Solution	20 mg/mL (equivalent to 10 mg/mL caffeine anhydrous)*	**Cafcit®**, MeadJohnson
		Caffeine Citrate Oral Solution
Parenteral		
Injection	20 mg/mL (equivalent to 10 mg/mL caffeine anhydrous)*	**Cafcit®**, MeadJohnson
		Caffeine Citrate Injection
Powder*		

*available from one or more manufacturer, distributor, and/or repackager by generic (nonproprietary) name

†Use is not currently included in the labeling approved by the US Food and Drug Administration

Dexmethylphenidate Hydrochloride

■ Dexmethylphenidate hydrochloride, the *d-threo* enantiomer of racemic methylphenidate hydrochloride, is a CNS stimulant that has pharmacologic actions that are qualitatively similar to those of amphetamines.

Uses

Dexmethylphenidate hydrochloride is used alone or combined with behavioral treatment as an adjunct to psychological, educational, social, and other remedial measures in the treatment of attention deficit hyperactivity disorder (ADHD).

■ **Attention Deficit Hyperactivity Disorder** Dexmethylphenidate hydrochloride is used alone or combined with behavioral treatment as an adjunct to psychological, educational, social, and other remedial measures in the treatment of ADHD (hyperkinetic disorder, hyperkinetic syndrome of childhood, minimal brain dysfunction) in carefully selected children 6 years of age and older, adolescents, and adults.

Efficacy of dexmethylphenidate hydrochloride conventional tablets for this indication was established in 2 placebo-controlled clinical trials in patients 6–17 years of age who met DSM-IV criteria for ADHD. In the first controlled clinical trial, improvement in symptom scores from baseline to study end (4 weeks) was greater in children receiving dexmethylphenidate hydrochloride conventional tablets than in those receiving placebo. In the second trial, children who had responded to dexmethylphenidate hydrochloride as conventional tablets in a 6-week open-label trial were randomized to receive this formulation of the drug for an additional 2 weeks or to receive placebo. Treatment failure occurred in 63% of patients receiving placebo compared with 17% of those receiving dexmethylphenidate.

Efficacy of dexmethylphenidate hydrochloride extended-release tablets for this indication was established in clinical trials in children 6 years of age and older, adolescents, and adults who met DSM-IV criteria for ADHD. In a controlled clinical trial in pediatric patients 6–17 years of age, improvement in symptoms from baseline to study end (7 weeks) was greater in children receiving dexmethylphenidate hydrochloride extended-release capsules than in those receiving placebo. Because a limited number of adolescents were enrolled in the trial, data from the trial were insufficient to adequately assess efficacy of the extended-release capsules in adolescents; however, efficacy of dexmethylphenidate hydrochloride extended-release capsules in adolescents is supported by pharmacokinetic data and by evidence of the efficacy of conventional tablets of the drug in this population. In a controlled clinical trial in adults 18–60 years of age, improvement in signs and symptoms of ADHD from baseline to study end (5 weeks) was greater in adults receiving dexmethylphenidate hydrochloride extended-release capsules than in those receiving placebo.

For further information on the management of ADHD, see Uses: Attention Deficit Hyperactivity Disorder, in Methylphenidate Hydrochloride 28:20.32.

Dosage and Administration

■ Administration Dexmethylphenidate hydrochloride conventional tablets are administered orally twice daily without regard to meals; the manufacturer recommends that doses be administered at least 4 hours apart.

Dexmethylphenidate hydrochloride extended-release capsules are administered orally once daily in the morning, with or without food. The capsules should be swallowed intact and should *not* be crushed, chewed, or divided. Alternatively, the entire contents of the extended-release capsule(s) may be sprinkled onto a small amount (e.g., a spoonful) of applesauce immediately prior to administration. The entire sprinkle/applesauce mixture should be taken immediately and should not be stored for use at a later time.

■ Dosage The recommended initial dosage of dexmethylphenidate hydrochloride as conventional tablets in patients 6 years of age and older who currently are not receiving racemic methylphenidate or are receiving stimulants other than methylphenidate is 2.5 mg twice daily. In patients 6 years of age and older who are being transferred from racemic methylphenidate to dexmethylphenidate therapy, the initial dexmethylphenidate hydrochloride dosage is one-half the current methylphenidate hydrochloride dosage. Dosage of dexmethylphenidate hydrochloride may be increased by 2.5–5 mg daily at weekly intervals, up to a maximum dosage of 20 mg daily.

The recommended initial dosage of dexmethylphenidate hydrochloride as extended-release capsules in patients who currently are not receiving dexmethylphenidate or racemic methylphenidate or who are receiving stimulants other than methylphenidate is 5 mg once daily for pediatric patients 6 years of age and older or 10 mg once daily for adults. Patients currently receiving dexmethylphenidate hydrochloride conventional tablets may be switched to the extended-release capsules at the same total daily dosage. In patients being transferred from racemic methylphenidate to dexmethylphenidate therapy, the initial dexmethylphenidate hydrochloride dosage is one-half the current methylphenidate hydrochloride dosage. Dosage of dexmethylphenidate hydrochloride may be increased at weekly intervals in increments of 5 mg daily in pediatric patients or 10 mg daily in adults, up to a maximum dosage of 30 mg daily in pediatric patients or 40 mg daily in adults. In dose-response studies evaluating fixed dosages of 10–30 mg daily in pediatric patients or 20–40 mg daily in adults, all of the dosages within these ranges were more effective than placebo, but there was no clear evidence that the higher dosages within these ranges provided greater average benefits; however, adverse effects and drug discontinuance were dose related.

Dosage of dexmethylphenidate must be carefully adjusted according to individual requirements and response. The patient should be observed for a sufficient duration at a given dosage to ensure that maximum benefit has been achieved before dosage adjustment is considered. If a beneficial effect is not attained after appropriate dosage adjustment over a 1-month period, dexmethylphenidate therapy should be discontinued. If paradoxical aggravation of symptoms or other adverse effects occur during dexmethylphenidate therapy, dosage should be reduced or the drug discontinued if necessary.

The long-term efficacy (i.e., exceeding 6 weeks for conventional tablets or 7 weeks for extended-release capsules) has not been evaluated systematically in controlled studies; therefore, the long-term usefulness of the drug should be reevaluated periodically in patients receiving dexmethylphenidate for extended periods. In patients who have responded to dexmethylphenidate therapy, the drug should be discontinued periodically to assess the patient's condition; improvement may be maintained temporarily or permanently after the drug is discontinued. For children or adolescents whose symptoms are not severe outside the school setting, drug holidays may be attempted for all or part of the summer to assess continuing efficacy and need for such therapy as well as to minimize adverse effects.

■ Special Populations No special population dosage recommendations at this time.

Cautions

■ Contraindications Marked anxiety, tension, and agitation, since dexmethylphenidate may aggravate these symptoms. Glaucoma. Motor tics or a family history or a diagnosis of Tourette's syndrome; however, the American Academy of Pediatrics (AAP) states that the presence of tics before or during medical management of ADHD is *not* an absolute contraindication to stimulant drug use. (See the opening discussion in Cautions, in Methylphenidate Hydrochloride 28:20.32.) Recent (within 14 days) administration of monoamine oxidase (MAO) inhibitors, since hypertensive crisis could result.

Known hypersensitivity to dexmethylphenidate, methylphenidate, or any ingredient in the formulation.

■ Warnings/Precautions ***Warnings*** Dexmethylphenidate hydrochloride shares the toxic potentials of racemic methylphenidate, and the usual precautions of racemic methylphenidate therapy should be observed.

Abuse Potential. Marked tolerance and psychologic dependence with varying degrees of abnormal behavior can occur with chronic abuse of dexmethylphenidate. Psychotic episodes can occur, particularly with parenteral abuse. Dexmethylphenidate should be used with caution in patients with a history of drug or alcohol dependence. Caution also may be indicated in patients with comorbid conduct disorder or a chaotic family. If the risk of drug abuse by the patient or the patient's peers or family is considered high, a nonstimulant drug may be preferable.

Withdrawal. Withdrawal following chronic therapeutic use of dexmethylphenidate may unmask symptoms of the underlying disorder, which may require follow-up. Careful supervision is required during withdrawal from abusive use since severe depression may occur.

Sudden Death and Serious Cardiovascular Events. Although a causal relationship to stimulants has not been established, sudden unexplained death, stroke, and myocardial infarction have been reported in adults receiving usual dosages of stimulants for the treatment of ADHD. Sudden unexplained death also has been reported in children and adolescents with structural cardiac abnormalities or other serious cardiac conditions receiving usual dosages of CNS stimulants. Results of one retrospective, case-control epidemiologic study showed a possible association between use of stimulant medications (e.g., methylphenidate) and sudden unexplained death in healthy children and adolescents. (See Pediatric Use under Warnings/Precautions: Specific Populations, in Cautions.) Because of postmarketing reports and the results of this and other epidemiologic studies, the US Food and Drug Administration (FDA) collaborated with the Agency for Healthcare Research and Quality (AHRQ) to sponsor 3 large, related, retrospective cohort studies using data from several health care claims databases to evaluate possible associations between ADHD drug use (stimulants, atomoxetine, and pemoline [no longer commercially available in the US]) and the following serious cardiovascular events: myocardial infarction, stroke, and sudden cardiac death in children and young adults 2–24 years of age; myocardial infarction and sudden cardiac death in adults 25–64 years of age; and stroke and the composite end point of stroke, myocardial infarction, and sudden cardiac death in the same group of adults. None of the 3 studies showed an association between serious cardiovascular events and current use of ADHD drugs, as compared with nonuse or as compared with former or remote use, although small increases in cardiovascular risk could not be excluded. The study in children and young adults included data for approximately 1.2 million patients and approximately 2.6 million patient-years of follow-up, including approximately 370,000 patient-years of current ADHD drug use, and found only 7 serious cardiovascular events (4 strokes, 3 sudden deaths) in current users of the drugs. The analyses in adults included data for approximately 440,000 patients, including approximately 150,000 current users of ADHD drugs; for the composite outcome of stroke, myocardial infarction, and sudden cardiac death, there were approximately 107,000 patient-years of ADHD drug exposure and 234 such cardiovascular events in current users.

In a study of the effects of dexmethylphenidate hydrochloride (40 mg as extended-release capsules) on the QT interval in healthy individuals, clinically important changes in the QT interval corrected for heart rate (QT_c) were not observed.

Children, adolescents, and adults who are being considered for stimulant therapy should undergo a thorough medical history review (including evaluation for a family history of sudden death or ventricular arrhythmia) and physical examination to detect the presence of cardiac disease, and should receive further cardiac evaluation (e.g., ECG, echocardiogram) if initial findings suggest such disease. Although some serious cardiac conditions are independently associated with an increased risk of sudden death, CNS stimulants generally should *not* be used in children, adolescents, or adults with known serious structural cardiac abnormalities, cardiomyopathy, serious heart rhythm abnormalities, coronary artery disease, or other serious cardiac conditions. Patients who develop exertional chest pain, unexplained syncope, or other manifestations suggestive of cardiac disease during stimulant therapy should undergo prompt cardiac evaluation.

For further information on screening for cardiac conditions, selecting appropriate candidates for stimulant therapy, and monitoring for treatment-emergent cardiac conditions, see Cardiovascular Precautions under Cautions: Precautions and Contraindications, in the Amphetamines General Statement 28:20.04.

Effects on Blood Pressure and Heart Rate. Stimulants cause modest increases in average blood pressure (i.e., by about 2–4 mm Hg) and heart rate (i.e., by about 3–6 beats/minute); larger increases may occur in some patients. Although modest increases would not be expected to have short-term sequelae, all patients should be monitored for larger changes in blood pressure and heart rate. Caution is advised in patients with underlying medical conditions that might be affected by increases in blood pressure or heart rate (e.g., hypertension, heart failure, recent myocardial infarction, ventricular arrhythmia).

Psychiatric Effects. Stimulants may exacerbate symptoms of behavior disturbance and thought disorder in patients with a preexisting psychotic disorder.

Stimulants should be used with caution in the management of ADHD in patients with comorbid bipolar disorder because of the potential for precipitation of mixed or manic episodes in such patients. Prior to initiating stimulant therapy, patients with ADHD and comorbid depressive symptoms should be carefully screened to determine if they are at risk for bipolar disorder; such screening should include a detailed psychiatric history (e.g., family history of suicide, bipolar disorder, or depression).

Psychotic or manic symptoms (e.g., hallucinations, delusional thinking, mania) have been reported in children and adolescents without prior history of psychotic illness or mania who received usual dosages of stimulants. In a pooled analysis of multiple short-term, placebo-controlled studies, such symptoms occurred in about 0.1% of patients receiving usual dosages of stimulants (i.e., methylphenidate, amphetamine) compared with 0% of those receiving placebo. If psychotic or manic symptoms occur during stimulant therapy, a causal relationship to stimulants should be considered, and discontinuance of therapy may be appropriate.

Aggressive behavior and hostility frequently are observed in children and adolescents with ADHD and have been reported in patients receiving drug therapy for the disorder. Although a causal relationship to stimulants has not been established, patients beginning treatment for ADHD should be monitored for the onset or worsening of aggressive behavior or hostility.

Growth Suppression. Prolonged administration of stimulants in children with ADHD has been associated with at least a temporary suppression of normal weight and/or height patterns in some patients. Results of an analysis of weight and height patterns in children 7–13 years of age suggested that treatment with methylphenidate for up to 3 years was associated with a temporary slowing in growth rate (on average, height gain was suppressed by about 2 cm and weight gain was suppressed by 2.7 kg over 3 years), without evidence of growth rebound during this period of development. In a 7-week controlled study in children and adolescents, patients receiving placebo gained a mean of 0.4 kg, while those receiving dexmethylphenidate hydrochloride extended-release capsules *lost* a mean of 0.5 kg. Published data are inadequate to determine whether long-term use of amphetamines may cause similar suppression of growth; however, it is anticipated that amphetamines, like methylphenidate, also cause temporary growth suppression. Therefore, the manufacturers of stimulant preparations state that growth should be monitored during therapy with stimulants, and children who are not growing or gaining height or weight as expected may require temporary discontinuance of therapy. However, AAP states that studies of stimulants in children generally have found little or no decrease in expected height, with any decrease in growth early in treatment being compensated for later on. (See Cautions: GI and Growth Effects, in Methylphenidate Hydrochloride 28:20.32.)

Seizures. There is some clinical evidence that stimulants may lower the seizure threshold in patients with a history of seizures, in those with prior EEG abnormalities but no history of seizures, and, very rarely, in those without a history of seizures and no prior evidence of EEG abnormalities. One patient, without a history of seizure disorder, experienced a seizure while receiving dexmethylphenidate during a controlled clinical trial. If seizures occur, the drug should be discontinued.

Priapism. Prolonged and painful erections, in some cases requiring surgical intervention, have been reported in adult and pediatric patients receiving methylphenidate. Priapism has not been reported with drug initiation but rather has developed after patients have received the drug for some time, often occurring following an increase in dosage. Priapism also has occurred during temporary interruptions in therapy (e.g., drug holidays) or following drug discontinuance. If not treated immediately, priapism can lead to permanent penile damage. (See Advice to Patients.) FDA states that clinicians should be cautious if they consider switching patients from methylphenidate preparations because of this risk, since certain other alternative ADHD treatments (e.g., atomoxetine) also may cause priapism.

Peripheral Vascular Effects. Stimulants used to treat ADHD, including dexmethylphenidate, are associated with peripheral vascular disorders, including Raynaud's phenomenon. Manifestations usually are intermittent and mild, but ulceration of the digits and/or breakdown of soft tissue may occur rarely. Peripheral vascular disorders, including Raynaud's phenomenon, have been reported during postmarketing experience in patients in all age groups receiving stimulants at therapeutic dosages and at various times throughout the treatment course. Manifestations generally improve following dosage reduction or drug discontinuance. Careful observation for digital changes is warranted during ADHD stimulant therapy, and further clinical evaluation (e.g., referral to a rheumatologist) may be appropriate for certain patients.

Visual Effects. Visual disturbances (difficulty with accommodation, blurred vision) have been reported in patients receiving stimulants.

Sensitivity Reactions Hypersensitivity reactions, including angioedema and anaphylaxis, have been reported in patients receiving dexmethylphenidate.

General Precautions **Hematologic Monitoring.** The manufacturer recommends periodic monitoring of complete blood cell count (CBC), with differential, and platelet counts during prolonged therapy; however, AAP and many clinicians consider routine hematologic monitoring unnecessary in patients receiving recommended stimulants (e.g., methylphenidate, amphetamines) in the absence of clinical signs (e.g., fever, sore throat, unusual bleeding or bruising) suggestive of hematologic toxicity.

Specific Populations **Pregnancy.** Category C. (See Users Guide.)

Lactation. It is not known whether dexmethylphenidate is distributed into milk; caution is advised if the drug is used in nursing women. Limited data suggest that exclusively breast-fed infants receive about 0.2–0.7% of the maternal weight-adjusted dosage of racemic methylphenidate; in 4 case reports, milk concentrations of methylphenidate ranged from undetectable to 15.4 ng/mL in lactating women receiving the racemic drug at dosages of 35–80 mg daily.

Pediatric Use. Safety and efficacy of dexmethylphenidate have not been established in children younger than 6 years of age, and therefore the manufacturer states that the drug should not be used in this age group.

Therapy with stimulants may be associated with at least a temporary suppression of growth in children. (See Growth Suppression under Warnings/Precautions: Warnings, in Cautions.)

Sudden death has been reported in children and adolescents with structural cardiac abnormalities or other serious cardiac conditions receiving usual dosages of CNS stimulants. Results of one retrospective, case-control epidemiologic study suggested a possible association between use of stimulant medications and sudden unexplained death in healthy children and adolescents. (See Sudden Death and Serious Cardiovascular Events under Warnings/Precautions: Warnings, in Cautions.)

Renal Impairment. Safety and efficacy of dexmethylphenidate have not been established in patients with renal impairment.

Hepatic Impairment. Safety and efficacy of dexmethylphenidate have not been established in patients with hepatic impairment.

■ **Common Adverse Effects** Abdominal pain, fever, anorexia, and nausea each occurred in 5% or more of patients receiving dexmethylphenidate hydrochloride conventional tablets in clinical trials and were at least twice as frequent in patients receiving the drug as in those receiving placebo. Twitching (motor or vocal tics), anorexia, insomnia, and tachycardia each resulted in discontinuance of dexmethylphenidate hydrochloride conventional tablets in approximately 1% of patients.

Decreased appetite/anorexia, headache, dyspepsia, dry mouth, anxiety, insomnia, vomiting, and pharyngolaryngeal pain each occurred in 5% or more of patients receiving dexmethylphenidate hydrochloride extended-release capsules in clinical trials. Twitching (motor or vocal tics), anorexia, insomnia, and tachycardia each resulted in discontinuance of dexmethylphenidate hydrochloride extended-release capsules in approximately 1% of pediatric patients. In adults, insomnia, jittery feeling, anorexia, and anxiety each resulted in discontinuance of therapy in about 1–2% of patients.

Nervousness and insomnia are the most commonly reported adverse effects in patients receiving racemic methylphenidate preparations.

Drug Interactions

The possibility that drug interactions reported with racemic methylphenidate also could occur with dexmethylphenidate should be considered.

■ **Cardiovascular Agents** Potential pharmacologic interaction (increased hypertensive effects) with concomitant use of pressor agents and dexmethylphenidate; caution is advised. Pharmacodynamic interaction (decreased antihypertensive effect) reported with concomitant use of racemic methylphenidate and antihypertensive agents.

■ **Anticonvulsants** Potential pharmacokinetic interaction (decreased metabolism of anticonvulsant agent) with concomitant use of racemic methylphenidate and anticonvulsants (e.g., phenobarbital, phenytoin, primidone). Monitoring of plasma anticonvulsant concentrations is recommended when methylphenidate is initiated or discontinued in patients receiving anticonvulsants; adjustment of anticonvulsant dosage may be required.

■ **Anticoagulants** Potential pharmacokinetic interaction (decreased metabolism of anticoagulant) with concomitant use of racemic methylphenidate and coumarin anticoagulants. Monitoring of prothrombin time (PT)/international normalized ratio (INR) is recommended when methylphenidate is initiated or discontinued in patients receiving coumarin anticoagulants; adjustment of anticoagulant dosage may be required.

■ **Antidepressants** Pharmacologic interaction (possible hypertensive crisis) with monoamine oxidase (MAO) inhibitors. (See Cautions: Contraindications.) Pharmacokinetic interaction (decreased metabolism of antidepressant agent) reported with concomitant use of racemic methylphenidate and tricyclic antidepressants (e.g., imipramine, clomipramine, desipramine) or selective serotonin-reuptake inhibitors. Adjustment of antidepressant dosage may be required when methylphenidate is initiated or discontinued.

■ **Drugs Metabolized by Hepatic Microsomal Enzymes** Pharmacokinetic interaction is unlikely.

■ **Drugs Affecting GI pH** Studies to evaluate the effects of changes in gastric pH on the absorption of dexmethylphenidate hydrochloride administered as extended-release capsules have not been performed to date. However, the potential exists for a pharmacokinetic interaction (altered release of dexmethylphenidate hydrochloride) between Focalin® XR extended-release capsules and drugs that alter gastric pH (e.g., antacids, acid suppressants).

Description

Dexmethylphenidate hydrochloride, the more pharmacologically active (*d-threo*) enantiomer of racemic methylphenidate hydrochloride, is a CNS stimulant. The mechanism of action in the treatment of attention deficit hyperactivity disorder (ADHD) has not been determined.

Dexmethylphenidate hydrochloride is well absorbed following oral administration. Because of first-pass metabolism, mean absolute bioavailability is 22–25%. When dexmethylphenidate hydrochloride is administered orally as conventional tablets in fasting patients, peak plasma concentrations are achieved within 60–90 minutes after a dose. When the drug is administered as extended-release capsules (Focalin® XR), peak plasma concentrations are attained at 1.5 hours and again at 6.5 hours after a dose. Extended-release capsules are absorbed more slowly but to the same extent as conventional tablets. Plasma concentrations of dexmethylphenidate achieved following single-dose oral administration of dexmethylphenidate hydrochloride capsules are comparable to the dexmethylphenidate concentrations achieved following single-dose oral administration of racemic methylphenidate hydrochloride capsules at equimolar doses (twice the total mg amount of dexmethylphenidate hydrochloride). Dexmethylphenidate is metabolized principally by de-esterification to form *d*-ritalinic acid, which has little or no pharmacologic activity. In vitro studies indicate that the drug does not inhibit the cytochrome P-450 (CYP) enzyme system. The mean plasma elimination half-life of dexmethylphenidate is 2–3 hours in children or 2–4.5 hours in adults.

Dexmethylphenidate hydrochloride is commercially available as conventional tablets and extended-release capsules. Each bead-filled dexmethylphenidate hydrochloride extended-release capsule (Focalin® XR) contains one-half of the dose as immediate-release beads and one-half as enteric-coated, delayed-release beads, thus providing an immediate release of dexmethylphenidate hydrochloride followed by a second delayed release of the drug.

Advice to Patients

Importance of providing patient or caregiver with a copy of the manufacturer's patient information (medication guide); discuss and answer questions about its contents (e.g., benefits and risks of stimulant therapy, appropriate use) as needed. Importance of instructing the patient or caregiver to read and understand the contents of the medication guide before initiating therapy and each time the prescription is refilled.

Importance of informing patients that hypersensitivity reactions, including angioedema and anaphylaxis, have occurred in some patients receiving the drug.

Importance of informing clinicians immediately of any adverse cardiovascular (e.g., chest pain, shortness of breath, fainting) or psychiatric effects (e.g., hallucinations, delusional thinking, mania).

Importance of taking the drug exactly as prescribed.

Importance of not chewing or crushing the beads contained in the capsules and of not storing the sprinkle/food mixture for later use.

Importance of informing clinicians of existing or contemplated concomitant therapy, including prescription and OTC drugs and herbal supplements, as well as any concomitant illnesses/conditions (e.g., glaucoma, cardiac/cardiovascular disease, mental/psychiatric disorder, seizures, suicidal ideation or behaviors, history of substance abuse).

Importance of informing male patients and their caregivers about the signs and symptoms of priapism, stressing the need for immediate treatment if it occurs. Younger males, especially prepubertal males, may not recognize the problem or may be embarrassed to tell anyone if it occurs.

Importance of informing patients about the risk of peripheral vascular disorders, including Raynaud's phenomenon, and the associated signs and symptoms (e.g., feelings of numbness, coolness, or pain in fingers or toes; changes in color from pale to blue to red). Patients should be advised to report any new numbness, pain, skin color change, or sensitivity to temperature in fingers or toes to their clinician and to immediately contact their clinician if any signs of unexplained wounds appear on fingers or toes; further clinical evaluation may be appropriate.

Importance of women informing clinicians if they are or plan to become pregnant or plan to breast-feed.

Importance of informing patients of other important precautionary information. (See Cautions.)

Overview® (see Users Guide). For additional information on this drug until a more detailed monograph is developed and published, the manufacturer's labeling should be consulted. It is *essential* that the manufacturer's labeling be consulted for more detailed information on usual cautions, precautions, contraindications, potential drug interactions, laboratory test interferences, and acute toxicity.

Preparations

Dexmethylphenidate hydrochloride is subject to control under the Federal Controlled Substances Act of 1970 as a schedule II (C-II) drug.

Excipients in commercially available drug preparations may have clinically important effects in some individuals; consult specific product labeling for details.

Dexmethylphenidate Hydrochloride

Oral

Capsules, extended-release (containing beads)	5 mg (beads, delayed-release, enteric-coated extended-release 2.5 mg with immediate-release 2.5 mg)*	**Dexmethylphenidate Hydrochloride Extended-release Capsules** (C-II)
		Focalin® XR (C-II), Novartis
	10 mg (beads, delayed-release, enteric-coated extended-release 5 mg with immediate-release 5 mg)*	**Dexmethylphenidate Hydrochloride Extended-release Capsules** (C-II)
		Focalin® XR (C-II), Novartis
	15 mg (beads, delayed-release, enteric-coated extended-release 7.5 mg with immediate-release 7.5 mg)*	**Dexmethylphenidate Hydrochloride Extended-release Capsules** (C-II)
		Focalin® XR (C-II), Novartis
	20 mg (beads, delayed-release, enteric-coated extended-release 10 mg with immediate-release 10 mg)*	**Dexmethylphenidate Hydrochloride Extended-release Capsules** (C-II)
		Focalin® XR (C-II), Novartis
	25 mg (beads, delayed-release, enteric-coated extended-release 12.5 mg with immediate-release 12.5 mg)	**Focalin® XR** (C-II), Novartis
	30 mg (beads, delayed-release, enteric-coated extended-release 15 mg with immediate-release 15 mg)*	**Dexmethylphenidate Hydrochloride Extended-release Capsules** (C-II)
		Focalin® XR (C-II), Novartis
	35 mg (beads, delayed-release, enteric-coated extended-release 17.5 mg with immediate-release 17.5 mg)	**Focalin® XR** (C-II), Novartis
	40 mg (beads, delayed-release, enteric-coated extended-release 20 mg with immediate-release 20 mg)*	**Dexmethylphenidate Hydrochloride Extended-release Capsules** (C-II)
		Focalin® XR (C-II), Novartis
Tablets	2.5 mg*	**Dexmethylphenidate Hydrochloride Tablets** (C-II)
		Focalin® (C-II), Novartis
	5 mg*	**Dexmethylphenidate Hydrochloride Tablets** (C-II)
		Focalin® (C-II), Novartis
	10 mg*	**Dexmethylphenidate Hydrochloride Tablets** (C-II)
		Focalin® (C-II), Novartis

*available from one or more manufacturer, distributor, and/or repackager by generic (nonproprietary) name

Selected Revisions November 2015,

Methylphenidate Hydrochloride

Methylphenidylacetate Hydrochloride

■ Methylphenidate is a piperidine-derivative CNS stimulant that has pharmacologic actions that are qualitatively similar to those of amphetamines.

Uses

Methylphenidate is used alone or combined with behavioral treatment as an adjunct to psychological, educational, social, and other remedial measures in the treatment of attention deficit hyperactivity disorder (ADHD). Methylphenidate also is used in the symptomatic treatment of narcolepsy.

■ **Attention Deficit Hyperactivity Disorder** Methylphenidate is used alone or combined with behavioral treatment as an adjunct to psychological, educational, social, and other remedial measures in the treatment of ADHD (hyperkinetic disorder, hyperkinetic syndrome of childhood, minimal brain dysfunction) in carefully selected children 6 years of age and older, adolescents, and adults. Although long thought of as a childhood disorder, ADHD is now known to persist into adolescence and/or adulthood in some patients, and adults are increasingly being treated for ADHD. Adults maintaining only some of the manifestations of ADHD are considered by DSM-IV to have ADHD in partial remission. ADHD in adults also has been referred to as simply attention deficit disorder (ADD). Most evidence and experience on the treatment of ADHD has been in children. Almost all studies comparing behavioral therapy versus stimulants alone for ADHD have shown a much stronger therapeutic effect from stimulants than from behavioral therapy.

Diagnostic Considerations ADHD is one of the most commonly diagnosed neurobehavioral disorders of childhood, generally estimated as occurring in 3–12% of US school-age children, although wider ranges of prevalence have been reported. Within this range, reported prevalence rates generally are at the higher end for community samples versus school samples. ADHD also is one of the most prevalent chronic health conditions in school-aged children. Although ADHD has been reported more frequently in boys than in girls (ratio of boys versus girls varies between 3:1 to 9:1), this difference may be artifactual and decrease with age, being skewed in part to boys because of referral bias related to disruptive behavior since boys generally exhibit more hyperactive/impulsive symptoms and more conduct and oppositional symptoms than girls.

In addition, when DSM-IV rather than earlier criteria are used, more females have been diagnosed with the predominantly inattentive type.

The diagnosis of ADHD should be made using well-tested diagnostic interview methods; neuropsychologic and/or biologic tests are not recommended for routine clinical use, although they may be useful to researchers investigating links between symptoms and underlying attentional processes and brain functions.To help ensure an accurate diagnosis and decrease the variation in how the diagnosis is made, clinicians should employ DSM-IV criteria in the context of their clinical assessment to diagnose ADHD. However, given the lack of methods to confirm the diagnosis of ADHD through other means, clinicians must recognize the limitations of the DSM-IV definitions (e.g., most of the development and testing of DSM-IV occurred in children evaluated in psychiatric settings, there are no clear empiric data supporting the number of items required for the diagnosis, current criteria do not take into account gender differences nor developmental differences in behavior, behavioral characteristics remain subjective and may be interpreted differently). According to DSM-IV criteria, there are 3 subtypes of ADHD: the principally inattentive type (ADHD/I), the principally hyperactive-impulsive type (ADHD/HI), and the combined inattentive and hyperactive-impulsive type (ADHD/C).

There currently are *no* data establishing that ADHD results from brain malfunction. ADHD is a clinical diagnosis; while the diagnosis can be made reliably using interview methods, there currently is no independent valid test for ADHD nor have laboratory tests, physical examination findings, or general medical conditions been established as aiding in the clinical assessment of this disorder. Diagnostic methods employed in the clinical setting have been variable, and the frequency of diagnosis of ADHD varies widely among type of practitioner (primary care and developmental pediatricians, family physicians, child neurologists, psychologists, and psychiatrists). Pediatricians, family physicians, and psychiatrists tend to rely on parent rather than teacher input, and there is a general disconnect between developmental or educational (school-based) assessments and health-related (medical practice-based) services, including poor communication between diagnosticians and those who implement and monitor treatment in schools, and follow-up may be inadequate and fragmented. School-based clinics with a team approach that includes parents, teachers, school psychologists, and other mental health specialists may improve barriers to appropriate identification, evaluation, and intervention as well as access to assessment and treatment. Current formal diagnostic criteria for ADHD were designed principally for diagnosing this disorder in young children. However, the American Psychiatric Association (APA) and others (e.g., American Academy of Child and Adolescent Psychiatry [AACAP]) have developed diagnostic criteria (e.g., DSM-IV) for ADHD to ages extending through adulthood.

ADHD usually is characterized by developmentally inappropriate symptoms (e.g., moderate to severe distractability, short attention span, hyperactivity, emotional lability, impulsivity, carelessness, accident-proneness, irresponsibility, failure to complete tasks). The essential feature of ADHD is a persistent pattern of inattention and/or hyperactivity/impulsivity that is more frequent and severe than is observed in individuals with a comparable developmental level, and core symptoms include developmentally inappropriate levels of attention and concentration, activity, distractability, and impulsivity. Some hyperactive/impulsive or inattentive symptoms are present before 7 years of age, although many individuals are diagnosed after the symptoms have been present for many years. In most cases, ADHD becomes apparent (and thus comes to medical attention) during the first few years of grammar (grade) school. Some impairment from symptoms is present in at least 2 settings (e.g., at home, school, or work), and there is clear evidence of interference with developmentally appropriate social, academic, and/or occupational functioning. The final diagnosis of this disorder should not be made if these symptoms are of only comparatively recent origin.Nonlocalizing (soft) neurologic signs, learning disability, and abnormal EEG may or may not be present, and a diagnosis of CNS dysfunction may or may not be warranted.

Children with ADHD usually exhibit pronounced difficulties and impairment resulting from the disorder across multiple settings (at school, at home, with peers) as well as resultant long-term adverse effects on later academic, vocational, social-emotional, and psychiatric outcomes. Such children exhibit higher accident rates, and later in life, those with ADHD that is combined with conduct disorders exhibit drug abuse, antisocial behavior, and accidents of all sorts; for many individuals, the long-term effects of ADHD continue into adulthood. Individuals with a history of ADHD consume a disproportionate share of resources and attention from health-care services, the criminal justice system, schools, and other social services, and ADHD, often combined with coexisting conduct disorders, contributes to societal problems including violent crime and teenage pregnancy. Parents of children with ADHD, as with other behavioral disorders and chronic diseases, experience increased levels of parental frustration, marital discord, divorce, and costs for medical care that may not be covered by health insurance. Up to 80% of diagnosed hyperactive children continue to exhibit features of ADHD into adolescence and up to 65% into adulthood, and most experts consider it a chronic disorder that often seems to require ongoing treatment. As a result, ADHD represents a major public health problem with profound impact on individuals, families, schools, and society; however, because there currently are no established means for preventing this disorder, current efforts must be aimed at effectively identifying, diagnosing, and treating ADHD. Comorbid conditions are present in up to two-thirds of clinically referred children with ADHD, including high rates for oppositional defiant disorder, conduct disorder, mood disorders (e.g., depression), and anxiety disorders. Tourette's syndrome and chronic tic disorder also often are present, and speech and language delays are common.

Although some patients continue to experience the full range of ADHD symptoms into adulthood, the occurrence of adult-onset ADHD is unlikely; however, unrecognized cases of ADHD may not be diagnosed until adulthood. A clinical diagnosis of ADHD in adults, according to DSM-IV criteria, requires evidence of symptom onset before 7 years of age, persisting from childhood until the time of evaluation, and with distress and/or impairment in functioning occurring in more than one setting (e.g., home, work). Some symptoms of disinhibition may present differently in adults than children; the physical symptoms of hyperactivity in children may be replaced in adults with fidgetiness or an inner feeling of restlessness, difficulty relaxing, and a feeling of being chronically "on edge". The DMS-IV criteria also state that a diagnosis of ADHD in partial remission may be used for adults who no longer meet the full range of diagnostic criteria that was present in childhood, but still retain some of the manifestations that cause functional impairment. Confirmation of ADHD in previously undiagnosed adults may present challenges such as difficulty in obtaining a longitudinal history, poor insight and underestimation of the severity of symptoms and resulting impairment, and differentiation from other psychiatric conditions (e.g., bipolar disorder, depression, axis II personality disorders, learning disabilities, narcolepsy, undiagnosed borderline intellectual functioning). Rating scales such as the Wender Utah Rating Scale, Brown Attention-Deficit Disorder Scale for Adults, and the Conners Adult ADHD Rating Scale may be useful adjuncts to clinical assessment in confirming the diagnosis of ADHD in adults.

Therapeutic Considerations **Considerations in Choosing a Therapy.** The choice of therapeutic intervention(s) for ADHD will depend on comorbid conditions, specific target symptoms, and the strengths and weaknesses of the patient, family, school, and community. Parents, school personnel, and patients should be included in discussions of treatment options. A wide variety of treatments have been employed for the management of ADHD, including drug therapy with amphetamines and similar stimulants (e.g., methylphenidate, pemoline [no longer commercially available in the US]), psychotropic drugs (e.g., antidepressants such as desipramine or imipramine), and other drugs (e.g., atomoxetine, clonidine); psychosocial treatment; dietary management; herbal and homeopathic treatments; biofeedback; meditation; and perceptual stimulation/training. Drug therapy and psychosocial interventions have been the focus of research to date, and efficacy studies have focused principally on the combined-type of ADHD, meeting criteria for inattention and hyperactivity/impulsivity; most randomized trials have been of short duration (usually not exceeding 3 months), although a large, multicenter study with a treatment duration of 14 months recently was reported. Current evidence from these studies supports the efficacy of stimulants and psychosocial treatment; however, there are no well-designed, long-term studies employing these treatments beyond 14 months nor is there information on long-term outcomes of drug therapy on educational and occupational achievements, involvement with police, or other areas of social functioning. Results of 3 double-blind clinical studies in 416 children 6–12 years old with ADHD indicate that therapy with methylphenidate hydrochloride extended-release trilayer core tablets (Concerta®) was more effective than placebo in decreasing hyperactive-impulsive or inattentive symptoms based on evaluation by community school teachers using the Inattention/Overactivity with Aggression (IOWA) Conners scale. Stimulant drug therapy generally appears to be more effective than psychosocial therapy overall, including behavioral treatment that includes parent training, intensive child-focused treatment, and school-based interventions.

Drug therapy is not indicated in all children with ADHD, and such therapy should be considered only after a complete evaluation including medical history has been performed. The decision to use stimulants should depend on the age of the child and the physician's assessment of the severity and duration of symptoms and should not depend solely on one or more behavioral characteristics. The decision to initiate drug therapy is based on the diagnostic evidence of ADHD and persistent target symptoms that are sufficiently severe to cause functional impairment at school; functional impairment usually also is evident at home and with peers. The risks of drug therapy must be weighed carefully with the risks of the untreated disorder, and the expected benefits of drug therapy must be weighed relative to other treatment options. Drug therapy should *not* be used as a substitute for appropriate educational curricula, student-to-teacher ratios, or other environmental accommodations. When severe impulsivity, noncompliance, or aggression is present, the need to initiate drug therapy may be more urgent.

Stimulants. Stimulants (e.g., methylphenidate, amphetamines) remain the drugs of choice for the management of ADHD. Methylphenidate is the most extensively studied and frequently prescribed drug for the treatment of ADHD. Few, if any, differences have been found between methylphenidate, dextroamphetamine, or pemoline (no longer commercially available in the US) or various dosage forms (short-, intermediate, or long-acting formulations) of the drugs in short-term clinical studies in children with ADHD, and the choice of stimulant therapy should be individualized. However, because hepatic toxicities have been associated with pemoline, some experts recommended its use *only* in patients who failed to respond to adequate trials of methylphenidate *and* an amphetamine as well as adequate trials of second-line therapies (e.g., tricyclic antidepressants, bupropion). In 2005, the US Food and Drug Administration (FDA) determined that the risk of hepatic toxicity associated with the drug outweighs its benefits.

Short-term and longer-term (up to 14 months' duration) studies have shown unequivocal beneficial effects of the stimulants on the defining core symptoms of ADHD (attention and concentration, activity, distractability, impulsivity) and associated aggressiveness during continued therapy with the drugs. The response rate for any single stimulant drug in ADHD is about 70%, and at least 80% of children will respond to a single stimulant without major adverse effect if therapy is titrated carefully. Children who fail to show positive therapeutic effects or who experience intolerable adverse effects with one stimulant should be tried on an alternative stimulant since most such children will exhibit a positive response to alternative stimulants and current evidence from crossover studies supports the efficacy of different stimulants in the same child; likewise, children who fail an adequate trial of 2 stimulants, should be tried on a third type or formulation of stimulant. Another consideration for trials with alternative stimulants before resorting to a trial with an alternative therapeutic class is the fact that there currently is greater evidence for the safety and efficacy of stimulants in children with ADHD. However, stimulants usually do not normalize the entire spectrum of behavioral problems, and many children effectively treated with these drugs still manifest a higher level of some behavioral problems than children without ADHD or other behavior disturbances. In addition, titration of therapy may result in improvement in one area of functioning while eliciting no or even a detrimental effect in another area. Although stimulants have been shown to remain effective over many years, long-term benefits remain to be established.

Effects on attentional, academic, behavioral, and social domains exhibit substantial interindividual and intraindividual variation, and the principal disappointment with stimulant drug therapy has been the finding that despite improvement in core symptoms of ADHD, there is little consistent improvement in academic or social skills. Stimulants appear to be as effective in patients with ADHD and associated aggression as in those with pure ADHD. It currently is unclear whether patients with comorbid anxiety disorders respond as well to stimulants as other patients with ADHD; however, some evidence suggests that the emphasis for patients with comorbid anxiety should be on increased reliance on psychosocial interventions. For patients whose symptoms are not severe outside the school setting, drug holidays may be attempted for all or part of the summer to assess continuing efficacy and need for such therapy as well as to minimize adverse effects.

Although the abuse potential of stimulants such as amphetamines and methylphenidate is well established, there currently is no evidence that drug abuse is a major problem with properly monitored stimulant therapy for ADHD. In addition, while it has been suggested that the substantial increase in stimulant prescriptions for ADHD in recent years may pose societal risks, the threshold of drug availability that can lead to oversupply and resultant illicit use is unknown, and there is little evidence that current levels of stimulant production in the US have had a substantial effect on abuse. Drug abuse and cigarette smoking are associated with childhood ADHD, but there has been controversy whether therapy with stimulants increases or decreases the risk of abuse. Some evidence, including a pooled analysis of available prospective and retrospective studies that included information on stimulant use in children, adolescents, and adults with ADHD, indicates that stimulant use does not lead to an increased risk of substance experimentation, use, dependence, or abuse, and effective ADHD stimulant therapy actually may reduce the risk for subsequent drug and alcohol use disorders. Caution in prescribing stimulants may be indicated in patients with comorbid conduct disorder, preexisting dependency, or a chaotic family. If the risk of drug abuse by the patient or their peers or family is considered high, a nonstimulant drug may be preferable to methylphenidate or an amphetamine (e.g., dextroamphetamine).

Multimodal Therapy. Although multimodal therapy, integrating drug therapy with environmental, educational, psychotherapeutic, and school-based approaches, seems intuitively powerful and some studies and clinicians have suggested the superiority of such an approach versus drug therapy or psychosocial interventions, there currently is little evidence from well-designed studies substantiating this assertion, particularly outside a research setting. In addition, data from a large, well-designed study indicates that drug therapy employing systematic intensive monitoring methods over a period of about 1 year is superior to an intensive set of behavioral treatments on core ADHD symptoms; combined behavioral and drug therapy added little benefit overall but did result in greater improvements in social skills and was judged more favorably by parents and teachers. While it remains to be determined, however, whether the addition of behavioral therapy can improve functioning at reduced stimulant dosages, evidence from this study indicates significantly lower total daily dosages of methylphenidate during combined therapy compared with drug therapy alone.

Alternatives to Stimulants. For patients who are intolerant of or unresponsive to stimulants, various other drugs (e.g., tricyclic antidepressants, atomoxetine, bupropion, selective serotonin-reuptake inhibitors, clonidine, guanfacine) have proven useful in clinical practice. However, experience with such alternative drug therapy is far less extensive than with stimulants, and conclusions regarding relative efficacy currently cannot be made.

Most experts recommend use of a tricyclic antidepressant or bupropion for the treatment of ADHD in children who are nonresponsive or partial responders to adequate trials with at least 2 different stimulants.There currently are no data establishing that one of these alternative drugs is more efficacious than the other in the treatment of ADHD. Tricyclic antidepressants generally have been shown to be effective in the management of ADHD in children and adolescents, but are associated with a narrower margin of safety. In addition, although a causal relationship has not been established, several recent cases of sudden death in children receiving desipramine have raised concerns about the use of this tricyclic. (See Cautions: Pediatric Precautions in Desipramine 28:16.04.28.) Therefore, some experts no longer recommend use of desipramine for the treatment of ADHD in children. Tricyclic antidepressants appear to be less effective than stimulants in improving attentional and cognitive symptoms, but may be useful for impulsive or hyperactive behavior. Tricyclic antidepressant therapy may be indicated as second-line therapy in patients who do not respond to stimulants or who develop clinically important depression or otherwise do not tolerate the drugs; these antidepressants also may be useful for patients with tics or Tourette's disorder or in whom these conditions are exacerbated or not adequately controlled during stimulant therapy. Regardless of which tricyclic antidepressant is considered for use in the management of ADHD, the drugs should be used only if clearly indicated and with careful monitoring, including baseline and subsequent determinations of ECG and other parameters.

Atomoxetine, a selective norepinephrine-reuptake inhibitor, is used in the treatment of ADHD in children 6 years of age and older, adolescents, and adults. Efficacy of atomoxetine for this indication was established in short-term controlled clinical studies in children and adolescents 6–18 years of age and in adults who met DSM-IV criteria for ADHD; efficacy also was established in one longer-term (12 months) controlled clinical study in children and adolescents 6–15 years of age. In one of the short-term studies, atomoxetine and methylphenidate produced comparable results in the reduction of ADHD symptoms in children and adolescents; however, further evaluation in placebo-controlled clinical studies are needed to determine comparative efficacy and tolerance of atomoxetine and other therapies in the treatment of ADHD.

Therapeutic Considerations for Patients with Comorbid Conditions. Alternative drug therapies also may be used alone or in combination with stimulants in patients with ADHD and comorbid conditions (e.g., aggression, anxiety, depression, tic disorders) that are unresponsive to stimulants alone. For the management of anxiety or depression in children with ADHD, selective serotonin-reuptake inhibitors (SSRIs) are considered by some experts the drugs of choice usually to be used in combination with a stimulant. In one clinical study, combined use of methylphenidate and fluoxetine in 32 children with ADHD and a comorbid mood or conduct disorder resulted in marked improvement in school grades and behavior as rated by parents, with no serious adverse effects reported. However, some experts recommend a conservative approach to such combined use of these drugs because of suggestions of rare but potentially serious drug interactions between SSRIs and stimulants. (See Drug Interactions: Antidepressants.)

Some experts state that in the absence of contraindications, α-adrenergic agents (e.g., clonidine) are considered the drugs of choice for the treatment of tic disorders in children with ADHD who were intolerant of stimulants. Clonidine's use has been documented principally in children with ADHD and comorbid conditions, especially sleep disturbances. Antipsychotic agents (e.g., haloperidol, pimozide, risperidone) are recommended by some experts as alternative therapies.

For the management of comorbid intermittent explosive disorder in children with ADHD, mood stabilizing agents (e.g., lithium or valproic acid) are recommended as adjuncts to stimulant therapy. Clonidine, an α-adrenergic agonist, also has been used in the management of comorbid aggressive symptoms as an adjunct to methylphenidate therapy; however, this use is controversial and further study is needed to evaluate efficacy of such concomitant therapy and the potential risk of development of serious cardiovascular effects. Although carbamazepine has been widely used for the treatment of aggression in adults, its efficacy in children remains to be established. In one controlled study, use of the drug failed to reduce aggression in children. Further studies are needed to evaluate the relative role of carbamazepine in the treatment of intermittent explosive disorder in children with ADHD. In addition, some experts no longer recommend use of typical antipsychotic (neuroleptic) agents because of the possible risk of withdrawal and tardive dyskinesia. However, use of risperidone (an atypical antipsychotic agent) may be considered in severely aggressive children with ADHD in whom other treatments have failed.

Adolescents and Adults. Stimulants have been used effectively in the management of ADHD in adolescents and adults, but experience is far less extensive than in children and potential age-related differences in response remain to be elucidated. Children and adults appear to share a similar treatment-responsive, underlying disorder. Although reported rates of stimulant efficacy have varied widely in adults, this variation may have resulted from use of inadequate dosages, diagnostic differences, and/or high rates of comorbid disorders. Stimulants should be used cautiously in adults with comorbid substance abuse disorders.

■ **Narcolepsy** Methylphenidate is used in the symptomatic treatment of narcolepsy. Methylphenidate has been used with equivocal results in the treatment of apathetic or withdrawn senile behavior and mild depression, but the drug should not be used in the treatment of endogenous depression or agitated depressive states since anxiety may be aggravated.

Dosage and Administration

■ **Administration** Methylphenidate hydrochloride is administered orally. Methylphenidate is administered percutaneously by topical application of a transdermal system.

Oral Administration To avoid insomnia, the last daily dose of conventional (immediate-release) preparations should be given several hours before retiring.

Methylphenidate hydrochloride chewable tablets should be administered with a full glass (i.e., at least 240 mL [8 ounces]) of water or other fluid to avoid choking. (See Precautions and Contraindications Associated with Specific Methylphenidate Formulations under Cautions: Precautions and Contraindications.)

The extended-release tablets (Metadate® ER, Ritalin SR®; generics) and extended-release trilayer core tablets (Concerta®; generics) of methylphenidate hydrochloride should be swallowed intact and should *not* be crushed or chewed. The extended-release capsules (Aptensio XR®, Metadate® CD, Ritalin® LA; generics) may be swallowed intact or the entire contents of a capsule(s) may be sprinkled onto a small amount (e.g., one tablespoonful) of applesauce immediately prior to administration. The manufacturer of Ritalin® LA states that the capsule contents should not be mixed with warm applesauce because the release properties of the formulation could be affected. The sprinkle/applesauce mixture should be taken immediately; the sprinkle/applesauce mixture must not be stored for use at a later time. One manufacturer suggests that the patient should drink fluids immediately after swallowing the intact capsule or sprinkle/applesauce mixture. Subdividing the contents of a capsule is not recommended, and crushing or chewing of the extended-release capsule or the capsule contents should be avoided.

Patients receiving the extended-release capsules should be instructed to avoid consuming alcohol, since alcohol ingestion may result in more rapid release of the drug from these formulations. (See Pharmacokinetics: Absorption.)

Patients receiving methylphenidate hydrochloride extended-release trilayer core tablets (Concerta®; generics) should be instructed not to become concerned if they notice a tablet-like substance in their stools; this is normal since the tablet containing the drug is designed to remain intact and slowly release the drug from a nonabsorbable shell during passage through the GI tract. The manufacturer states that it is possible that the extended-release trilayer core tablets may be visible on abdominal radiographs under certain circumstances, particularly when digital enhancing techniques are utilized.

Methylphenidate hydrochloride powder for extended-release oral suspension (Quillivant XR®) must be reconstituted prior to dispensing. The bottle should be tapped until the powder flows freely, and then the bottle cap should be removed and 53, 105, 131, or 158 mL of water should be added to a bottle labeled as containing 300, 600, 750, or 900 mg, respectively, of the drug to provide an extended-release suspension containing 25 mg/5 mL. The bottle adapter should be inserted into the neck of the bottle and the bottle cap replaced. The suspension should then be shaken vigorously with a back and forth motion for at least 10 seconds. The bottle should be kept tightly closed and should be vigorously shaken for at least 10 seconds before each use. The bottle adapter and oral dosing dispenser supplied by the manufacturer should be used to administer the oral suspension. The adapter should remain in place as long as the bottle is in use (up to 4 months). A dose is dispensed by inserting the oral dosing dispenser into the adapter in the upright bottle and then inverting the bottle and withdrawing the appropriate dose into the oral dosing dispenser. The manufacturer's patient information should be consulted for more detailed information on administration of the extended-release oral suspension.

The manufacturers state that immediate-release preparations of methylphenidate hydrochloride (conventional tablets, chewable tablets, oral solution) preferably should be administered 30–45 minutes before meals and that Metadate® CD extended-release capsules should be administered before breakfast. The manufacturer states that administration of Ritalin® LA extended-release capsules relative to the timing and composition of meals may need to be individually adjusted. Methylphenidate hydrochloride extended-release trilayer core tablets, extended-release oral suspension, and Aptensio XR® extended-release capsules may be administered without regard to meals; however, the manufacturer recommends that Aptensio XR® extended-release capsules be administered in a consistent manner relative to food intake.

Transdermal Administration Patients receiving transdermal methylphenidate should be carefully instructed in the proper use and disposal of the transdermal system.

The methylphenidate transdermal system should be applied once daily in the morning, 2 hours before an effect is needed, and should be removed 9 hours after application. The system should be applied immediately after opening the package and removing the protective liner; the system should not be used if the package seal is broken. Transdermal systems should not be cut. After the transdermal system has been separated from the protective liner, the liner should be inspected to ensure that no adhesive (which contains the drug) has been transferred to the liner. The transdermal system should be discarded if adhesive transfer has occurred, if the transdermal system is torn or appears to be damaged, or if the transdermal system is difficult to separate from the liner. Only intact transdermal systems should be used. The adhesive side of the transdermal system should be placed on a clean, dry area of the hip that is not oily, damaged, or irritated; application of the transdermal system to the waistline or to areas under tight clothing should be avoided, since clothing may cause the system to rub off. The system should be pressed firmly in place with the palm of the hand for approximately 30 seconds, making sure that there is good contact with the skin, particularly around the edges of the system. Application sites should be alternated daily (e.g., opposite hip) if possible.

Topical preparations (e.g., corticosteroids or other creams; topical solutions, ointments, or emollients) should not be applied immediately prior to system application, since the effects of such preparations on system adhesion, methylphenidate absorption, or potential adverse effects of the corticosteroid are not known.

Exposure to water during bathing, swimming, or showering can affect adherence of the transdermal system to the skin. Transdermal systems should not be applied or re-applied with dressings, tape, or other common adhesives. If a system does not fully adhere to the skin upon application or becomes partially or fully dislodged during the intended period of use, it should be replaced with a new system applied at a different site, but the total wear time should not exceed 9 hours per day regardless of the number of transdermal systems used.

The transdermal system should be removed by slowly peeling it off the skin. If necessary, removal may be facilitated by gently applying an oil-based product (i.e., petroleum jelly, olive oil, mineral oil) to the edges of the transdermal system and gently working the oil underneath the edges. If any adhesive remains on the skin after the transdermal system has been removed, an oil-based product may be applied to the application site to gently loosen and remove any residual adhesive. In the unlikely event that a transdermal system remains tightly adhered to the skin despite these measures, the patient or caregiver should contact the patient's clinician or pharmacist. Nonmedical adhesive removers and acetone-based products (i.e., nail polish remover) should not be used to remove either the transdermal system or the adhesive.

After removal, used systems should be folded so that the adhesive side adheres to itself and then should be flushed down the toilet or disposed of in an appropriate lidded container. Any unused systems that are no longer needed should be removed from their packaging, separated from the protective liner, folded so that the adhesive side adheres to itself, and then flushed down the toilet or disposed of in an appropriate lidded container.

The manufacturer encourages parents to record on the administration chart included with each carton the time that each transdermal system was applied and removed. If a system was removed without the parent's or caregiver's knowledge, or if a system is missing from the tray, the parent or caregiver should be encouraged to ask the child when and how the system was removed.

■ Dosage

Dosage of methylphenidate hydrochloride must be carefully adjusted according to individual requirements and response. The extended-release tablets should not be used for initiating therapy nor until the daily dosage has been titrated using the conventional tablets; the extended-release tablets may be used and given at 8-hour intervals when the 8-hour dosage of the extended-release preparation corresponds to the titrated 8-hour dosage of the conventional tablets. Alternatively, dosage may be initiated with the methylphenidate hydrochloride extended-release capsules, extended-release oral suspension, or extended-release trilayer core tablets for patients who are not currently taking methylphenidate starting with the recommended initial dosage and increasing at approximately weekly intervals.

Patients receiving intermediate- or long-acting preparations also may require supplemental therapy with methylphenidate conventional tablets to increase the efficacy, particularly in the morning, or to extend the duration of therapeutic effects later in the day.

Attention Deficit Hyperactivity Disorder Methylphenidate hydrochloride dosage for the treatment of attention deficit hyperactivity disorder (ADHD) should be individualized based on patient response and tolerance. The first dosage that produces an observable response may not be the optimum dosage to improve function, and titration to higher dosages should continue in an attempt to achieve a better response. Such a strategy may require subsequent lowering of dosage when higher dosages produce adverse effects or no further clinical improvement. The best dosage for a given patient is the one that provides optimum therapeutic effects with minimal adverse effects. Dosing schedules also may vary, although there currently are no consistent controlled studies comparing alternative dosing schedules. Patients who require relief only during school may respond adequately to a 5-day (i.e., school day) regimen while those requiring relief at home and school may need a daily regimen throughout the week.

The optimum duration of treatment with methylphenidate has not been established; however, pharmacologic treatment may be required for extended periods. The long-term usefulness of the drug should be reevaluated periodically in patients receiving methylphenidate for extended periods. In patients who have responded to methylphenidate therapy, the drug should be discontinued periodically to assess the patient's condition; improvement may be maintained temporarily or permanently after the drug is discontinued.

Immediate-release Oral Preparations. As an adjunct in the treatment of ADHD in children 6 years of age and older, the usual initial dosage of methylphenidate hydrochloride as conventional (immediate-release) preparations is 5 mg before breakfast and lunch. Dosage may be increased by 5–10 mg daily at weekly intervals and can be administered in twice- or thrice-daily regimens. Although some clinicians have recommended weight-based dosing in children, dosage of methylphenidate, unlike most drugs, generally can be adjusted without regard to the child's weight. When weight-based dosing was employed, an initial dosage of 0.25 mg/kg daily was used. If adverse effects were not observed, the daily dose could be doubled each week until the optimum dosage of 2 mg/kg daily is reached.

Oral dosage in children generally ranges from 5–20 mg 2 or 3 times daily and should not exceed 60 mg daily. Although dosages for older adolescents and adults are similar to those for children, total daily dosages may be increased up to 65 mg since more doses are required to medicate these patients throughout a longer active day. Some clinicians have employed a regimen that included systematic intensive monitoring (referred to as "medical management") in the treatment of ADHD, and such a regimen was shown to be more effective than less intensively titrated and monitored regimens (referred to as "community management"). In the medical management regimen, methylphenidate dosage was titrated over a 28-day period via daily-switch titration involving 5 randomly ordered repeats each of placebo and 5-, 10-, 15-, or 20-mg (higher for children weighing more than 25 kg) daily dosages; each dose was repeated at breakfast and lunch, with a half dose (rounded to nearest 5 mg) given in the afternoon. Based on clinical assessment of response, a best dose was chosen for initial maintenance. In addition to the systematic dosage titration, patients underwent 30-minute monthly drug therapy assessment visits during maintenance. Pharmacotherapists could increase or decrease therapy during such visits by 10 mg daily. In general, patients received higher than typical dosages of the drug when this titration and monitoring method was employed. Dosage at the end of a 14-month study period averaged 37.7 mg daily administered in 3 unequally divided doses daily as noted above.

Children whose dosage is excessive or who are overly sensitive to the drug may become overfocused or appear dull or overly restricted; a dosage reduction may obviate such effects. Rarely, some children may experience psychotic reactions, mood disturbances, or hallucinations at relatively high dosages. If a beneficial effect is not attained after appropriate dosage adjustment over a one-month period, methylphenidate therapy should be discontinued.

Intermediate-acting Oral Preparations. Methylphenidate hydrochloride extended-release tablets (Metadate® ER, Ritalin–SR®; generics) may be used as an adjunct in the treatment of ADHD in children 6 years of age and older in patients whose ADHD symptoms are controlled with conventional methylphenidate hydrochloride tablets. The manufacturers suggest that extended-release methylphenidate hydrochloride tablets can be substituted for the conventional tablets at the nearest equivalent total daily dosage. For example, patients receiving 10 mg of conventional tablets in the morning and at noon can be switched to 20 mg of methylphenidate hydrochloride extended-release tablets administered once daily in the morning. In some patients, supplemental doses of a short-acting (conventional) preparation may be needed. The usual dosage of methylphenidate hydrochloride administered as an intermediate-acting oral preparation is 20–40 mg once daily or 40 mg in the morning and 20 mg in the early afternoon.

Long-acting Oral Preparations. Methylphenidate hydrochloride extended-release capsules (Aptensio XR®, Metadate® CD, Ritalin® LA; generics) or extended-release oral suspension (Quillivant XR®) may be used as an adjunct in the treatment of ADHD in children 6 years of age and older. The initial dosage of methylphenidate hydrochloride extended-release capsules is 20 mg once daily in the morning. Alternatively, when a lower initial daily dosage is appropriate, therapy may be initiated at a dosage of 10 mg once daily; the manufacturer of Aptensio XR® recommends that therapy be initiated at this lower dosage in all patients. Methylphenidate hydrochloride dosage may be increased by 10–20 mg daily at weekly intervals, until an optimum response is achieved or adverse effects are observed; the manufacturers of Aptensio XR® and Ritalin® LA recommend that dosage be increased at the slower rate of 10 mg daily at weekly intervals. The recommended initial dosage of methylphenidate hydrochloride extended-release oral suspension also is 20 mg once daily in the morning; dosage may be increased at weekly intervals in increments of 10–20 mg daily. Dosages of methylphenidate hydrochloride extended-release capsules or extended-release oral suspension exceeding 60 mg daily are not recommended.

Alternatively, as an adjunct in the treatment of ADHD, methylphenidate hydrochloride extended-release trilayer core tablets (Concerta®; generics) may be used. The usual initial dosage of the drug as extended-release trilayer core tablets in children and adolescents 6–17 years of age is 18 mg once daily in the morning; adults 18–65 years of age with ADHD may receive an initial dosage of 18 or 36 mg once daily in the morning. If adequate response does not occur, dosage may be increased at approximately weekly intervals in increments of 18 mg daily. The maximum dosage recommended by the manufacturer is 54 mg daily for children 6–12 years of age, 72 mg daily (not to exceed 2 mg/kg daily) for adolescents 13–17 years of age, and 72 mg daily for adults; however, some clinicians state that dosage in children 6–12 years of age may be increased to a maximum dosage of 72 mg daily.

Some clinicians state that patients currently receiving methylphenidate hydrochloride conventional tablets may be switched to Metadate® CD extended-release capsules. Patients being transferred from methylphenidate therapy using conventional tablets at a dosage of 10 mg twice daily can be switched to a dosage of 20 mg every morning as Metadate® CD extended-release capsules. Patients receiving methylphenidate hydrochloride therapy using conventional tablets at a dosage of 20 mg twice daily can be switched to a dosage of 40 mg every morning as Metadate® CD extended-release capsules.

The manufacturer of Ritalin® LA extended-release capsules states that patients receiving conventional or extended-release methylphenidate hydrochloride tablets may be switched to Ritalin® LA extended-release capsules. Patients being transferred from methylphenidate hydrochloride therapy using a conventional tablet at a dosage of 5 mg twice daily can be switched to a dosage of 10 mg every morning as Ritalin® LA extended-release capsules. Patients receiving methylphenidate hydrochloride therapy using a conventional tablet at a dosage of 10 mg twice daily or a 20-mg dosage of an extended-release tablet can be switched to a dosage of 20 mg every morning as Ritalin® LA extended-release capsules. Patients being transferred from methylphenidate hydrochloride therapy using a conventional tablet at a dosage of 15 mg twice daily can be switched to a dosage of 30 mg every morning as Ritalin® LA extended-release capsules. Patients receiving methylphenidate hydrochloride therapy using a conventional tablet at a dosage of 20 mg twice daily or a 40-mg dosage of an extended-release tablet can be switched to a dosage of 40 mg every morning as Ritalin® LA extended-release capsules. Patients being transferred from methylphenidate hydrochloride therapy using a conventional tablet at a dosage of 30 mg twice daily or a 60-mg dosage of an extended-release tablet can be switched to a dosage of 60 mg every morning as Ritalin® LA extended-release capsules. For other conventional or extended-release tablet regimens, the nearest daily dosage can be substituted based on clinical judgment.

The manufacturer of Concerta® extended-release methylphenidate hydrochloride trilayer core tablets states that patients receiving conventional methylphenidate hydrochloride preparations may be switched to Concerta® extended-release trilayer core tablets. Patients being transferred from methylphenidate hydrochloride therapy using a conventional formulation at a dosage of 5 mg 2 or 3 times daily can be switched to a dosage of 18 mg every morning as the extended-release trilayer core tablets. Patients receiving methylphenidate hydrochloride therapy using a conventional formulation at a dosage of 10 mg 2 or 3 times daily can be switched to 36 mg every morning of the methylphenidate hydrochloride extended-release trilayer core tablets. Patients receiving methylphenidate hydrochloride therapy using a conventional formulation at a dosage of 15 mg 2 or 3 times daily can be switched to 54 mg every morning as the extended-release trilayer core tablets, and those receiving a conventional formulation at a dosage of 20 mg 2 or 3 times daily can be switched to 72 mg every morning as the extended-release trilayer core tablets. The initial dosage of methylphenidate hydrochloride as extended-release trilayer core tablets in patients being switched from conventional tablets should not exceed 72 mg daily. A 27-mg extended-release trilayer core tablet also is available for patients who require a dosage in between 18 mg daily and 36 mg daily. For other conventional or extended-release tablet regimens, the nearest equivalent daily dosage can be substituted based on clinical judgment. Subsequent titration to higher or lower dosages may be necessary and should occur at approximately weekly intervals in increments or decrements of 18 mg daily, guided by the patient's clinical response and tolerance; however, the manufacturer states that daily dosages exceeding 54 mg daily in children 6–12 years of age, 72 mg daily (not to exceed 2 mg/kg daily) in adolescents, and 72 mg daily in adults are not recommended.

In some patients receiving long-acting methylphenidate preparations, supplemental doses of a short-acting (conventional) preparation may be needed.

Transdermal System. Dosage titration, final dosage, and wear time of the transdermal system should be individualized according to the needs and response of the patient.

The recommended initial dosage of methylphenidate in patients who are receiving the transdermal formulation as their initial methylphenidate regimen is 1 system delivering 10 mg/9 hours applied once daily. If adequate response is not achieved, dosage may be increased at weekly intervals by advancing to the next larger dosage system (i.e., a dosage system delivering 15 mg/9 hours applied once daily during week 2, followed by a dosage system delivering 20 mg/9 hours applied once daily during week 3, and then a dosage system delivering 30 mg/9 hours applied once daily during week 4).

Because differences in bioavailability exist between the methylphenidate transdermal system and other methylphenidate formulations, patients being transferred from therapy with other methylphenidate formulations to transdermal therapy with the drug should receive the same initial transdermal dosage and follow the same dosage titration schedule recommended for patients receiving transdermal methylphenidate as their initial methylphenidate regimen.

The methylphenidate transdermal system may be removed earlier than 9 hours if a shorter duration of effect is desired or if late-day adverse effects occur. If aggravation of symptoms or other adverse events occur, the dosage or wear time should be reduced, or, if necessary, the drug should be discontinued.

Narcolepsy In the treatment of narcolepsy, the usual oral adult dosage of methylphenidate hydrochloride is 10 mg 2 or 3 times daily, given 30–45 minutes before meals. Some patients may require 40–60 mg daily; in others, 10–15 mg daily may be adequate.

Cautions

Methylphenidate generally is well tolerated. Common adverse effects of the drug include nervous system (insomnia, delayed sleep onset, headache, nervousness, jitteriness, social withdrawal, anxiety, restlessness, affect lability, agitation, irritability, dizziness, vertigo, tremor), cardiovascular (increased blood pressure, increased heart rate, tachycardia, palpitations), GI (decreased appetite/anorexia, nausea, abdominal pain, dyspepsia, dry mouth, vomiting), and other (weight loss, blurred vision, hyperhidrosis, pyrexia) effects. Most adverse effects of methylphenidate can be managed successfully by adjustment in dosage and/or schedule. About 15–30% of children with ADHD experience tics while receiving stimulants such as methylphenidate, but such tics usually are transient. About half of children with ADHD have underlying Tourette's syndrome, and the effects of stimulants on tics are unpredictable; the presence or emergence of tics is not an absolute contraindication to stimulant therapy and some evidence indicates that the incidence of tics is not increased with such therapy.

In controlled studies in children and adolescents, adverse effects requiring discontinuance of therapy occurred in 0.6% of patients receiving extended-release trilayer core tablets and 1.9% of patients receiving placebo; the reasons for discontinuance of methylphenidate included depressed mood in one patient and headache and insomnia in another patient. In controlled studies in adults, adverse effects requiring discontinuance of therapy occurred in 6% of patients receiving extended-release trilayer core tablets and 3% of patients receiving placebo; the principal reasons for discontinuance of methylphenidate were anxiety, irritability, increased blood pressure, and nervousness (each occurring in 0.7–1.7% of patients). In open-label studies in children, adolescents, and adults, adverse effects requiring discontinuance of therapy occurred in 7% of patients receiving extended-release trilayer core tablets; the principal reasons for drug discontinuance were insomnia, irritability, anxiety, decreased appetite, and tics (each occurring in 0.6–1.2% of patients). Discontinuance of methylphenidate therapy also occurred in 2 patients (1%) receiving Metadate® CD extended-release capsules in controlled clinical trials, principally because of rash and pruritus in one patient and headache, abdominal pain, and dizziness in the other patient. In addition, discontinuance of methylphenidate therapy because of depression occurred in a child with ADHD (1.5%) receiving Ritalin® LA extended-release capsules in a double-blind controlled clinical trial. Discontinuance also occurred in 6 patients (3.7%) receiving the drug in this trial during the initial single-blind titration period; the reasons for discontinuance were anger (2 patients), hypomania, anxiety, depressed mood, fatigue, migraine, and lethargy. Discontinuance of methylphenidate therapy also occurred in 2 patients (4.4%) receiving Aptensio XR® extended-release capsules in controlled clinical trials; the reasons for discontinuance were insomnia in one patient and nausea and rapid heart rate in the other patient. In a 7-week controlled trial in children, adverse effects requiring discontinuance of therapy occurred in 7.1% of patients receiving transdermal methylphenidate and 1.2% of those receiving placebo; the most common reasons for discontinuance of transdermal methylphenidate therapy included application site reactions, headache, irritability, and tics. In a 7-week controlled trial in adolescents, adverse effects requiring discontinuance of therapy occurred in 5.5% of patients receiving transdermal methylphenidate and 2.8% of those receiving placebo; the most common reasons for discontinuance of transdermal methylphenidate therapy included application site reactions and decreased appetite/anorexia.

Loss of appetite, abdominal pain, weight loss during prolonged therapy, insomnia, and tachycardia may occur more frequently in children than in adults receiving methylphenidate.

■ Nervous System Effects The most frequent adverse effects of methylphenidate appear to be dose related and include nervousness and insomnia. Insomnia has been reported in 3% of children and adolescents with ADHD receiving methylphenidate hydrochloride extended-release trilayer core tablets, in 5% of children with ADHD receiving Metadate® CD extended-release capsules, in 10% of children and adolescents with ADHD receiving Aptensio XR® extended-release capsules, in about 3% of children with ADHD receiving Ritalin® LA extended-release capsules, and in 13% of children and 6% of adolescents with ADHD receiving the drug as a transdermal system in clinical trials. Nervousness and insomnia usually can be controlled by reducing dosage and not administering the drug in the afternoon or evening. Headache has been reported in 9–14% of children and adolescents with ADHD receiving methylphenidate hydrochloride extended-release trilayer core tablets, 11–12% of children or adolescents with ADHD receiving extended-release capsules of the drug, and 12–15% of children and adolescents receiving transdermal methylphenidate in clinical trials. Irritability has been reported in 7% of children and 11% of adolescents with ADHD receiving transdermal methylphenidate in clinical trials. Affect lability has been reported in 9% of children with ADHD receiving methylphenidate hydrochloride extended-release oral suspension in clinical trials. Affect lability (including emotionality and emotional sensitivity, instability, and lability) also has been reported in 6% of children with ADHD receiving methylphenidate as a transdermal system in clinical trials. Dizziness was reported in 2% of children and adolescents with ADHD receiving extended-release trilayer core tablets or Aptensio XR® extended-release capsules and in 6% of adolescents receiving transdermal methylphenidate in clinical trials. In 2 uncontrolled studies, the cumulative incidence of new-onset tics in children receiving methylphenidate hydrochloride extended-release trilayer core tablets was reported to be 9% after 27 months of treatment (first study) and 1% after up to 9 months of treatment (second study). Tics were reported in 7% of children with ADHD receiving methylphenidate as a transdermal system in clinical trials. Tics and initial insomnia each were reported in 2% of children receiving methylphenidate hydrochloride extended-release oral suspension in clinical trials.

Headache and insomnia were reported in 22 and 12%, respectively, and anxiety, dizziness, and irritability each were reported in 6–8% of adults with ADHD receiving methylphenidate hydrochloride extended-release trilayer core tablets in clinical trials. Other adverse nervous system effects reported in clinical trials in adults with ADHD receiving methylphenidate hydrochloride extended-release trilayer core tablets included initial insomnia, depressed mood, nervousness, restlessness, and tremor (each occurring in approximately 3–4% of patients) and agitation, aggression, depression, affect lability, confusional state, tension, vertigo, paresthesia, sedation, and tension headache (each occurring in approximately 1–2% of patients).

Toxic psychosis and Tourette's syndrome have been reported rarely in patients receiving methylphenidate. Neuroleptic malignant syndrome (NMS) also has been reported rarely in patients receiving methylphenidate; most of these patients also were receiving other drugs that have been associated with NMS. An NMS-like syndrome developed in one 10-year old boy (who had been receiving methylphenidate for about 18 months) 45 minutes after ingesting the first dose of venlafaxine. It is not known if such a reaction was associated with administration of either drug alone or if it represented a drug interaction between methylphenidate and venlafaxine or, alternatively, if the reaction was of unknown etiology.

Other adverse effects of methylphenidate include dyskinesia, drowsiness, psychomotor hyperactivity, lethargy, asthenia, fatigue, sleep disorder, somnolence, anger, hypervigilance, mood swings, panic attack, tearfulness, and aggressive behavior. Depression, anxiety, abnormal behavior, disorientation, hallucinations, mania, logorrhea, irritability, migraine, obsessive-compulsive disorder, suicidal behavior (including completed suicide), and seizures have been reported in patients receiving methylphenidate, but a causal relationship to the drug has not been definitely established.

■ GI and Growth Effects Abdominal pain and anorexia have been reported in 7 and 9%, respectively, of children with ADHD receiving Metadate® CD extended-release capsules in clinical trials. Anorexia also has been reported in about 3% of children with ADHD receiving Ritalin® LA extended-release capsules and in 5% of children with ADHD receiving methylphenidate as a transdermal system in controlled clinical trials. Decreased appetite has been reported in 5% of children and adolescents receiving Aptensio XR® extended-release capsules and in 2% of children receiving methylphenidate hydrochloride extended-release oral suspension in clinical trials. Upper abdominal pain has been reported in 8% of children and adolescents with ADHD receiving Aptensio XR® extended-release capsules and in 6% of children and adolescents with ADHD receiving methylphenidate hydrochloride extended-release trilayer core tablets in clinical trials. Abdominal pain, decreased appetite, and anorexia also have been reported in 5–7, 26, and 5%, respectively, of children and adolescents receiving transdermal methylphenidate in clinical trials.

Although appetite suppression and weight loss are common with stimulant therapy, there is no apparent difference in their occurrence between methylphenidate or amphetamine (e.g., dextroamphetamine) therapy in children. Results of one study suggest that prolonged methylphenidate hydrochloride therapy (30–40 mg daily) may cause suppression of normal weight gain in children. Results of an analysis of weight and height patterns in children 7–13 years of age suggested that treatment with methylphenidate for up to 3 years was associated with a temporary slowing in growth rate (on average, height gain was suppressed by about 2 cm and weight gain was suppressed by 2.7 kg over 3 years), without evidence of growth rebound during this period of development. Published data are inadequate to determine whether long-term use of amphetamines may cause similar suppression of growth; however, it is anticipated that amphetamines, like methylphenidate, also cause temporary growth suppression. Therefore, the manufacturers of stimulant preparations state that growth should be monitored during therapy with stimulants, and children who are not growing or gaining height or weight as expected may require temporary discontinuance of therapy. Although concerns about potential dose-related growth delays in children have been raised, a prospective follow-up study into adulthood found no significant impairment in height achieved. In general, studies of stimulants in children have found little or no decrease in expected height, with any decrease in growth early in treatment being compensated for later on. Although drug holidays during summers have been suggested to minimize weight loss and other potential adverse effects, there currently are no data from controlled studies establishing whether such holidays are beneficial or associated with risks.

Vomiting has been reported in 3% of children and adolescents with ADHD receiving methylphenidate hydrochloride extended-release trilayer core tablets in clinical trials. Nausea and vomiting each have been reported in 4% of children and adolescents with ADHD receiving Aptensio XR® extended-release capsules. Nausea and vomiting also were reported in 12 and 10%, respectively, of children and 10 and 3%, respectively, of adolescents with ADHD receiving methylphenidate as a transdermal system in clinical trials. Vomiting also has been reported in 2% of children receiving methylphenidate hydrochloride extended-release oral suspension. Other adverse GI effects of methylphenidate include weight loss during prolonged therapy and dryness of the throat. Weight loss has been reported in 9% of children and 6% of adolescents receiving transdermal methylphenidate in clinical trials. Thirst, abdominal discomfort, and diarrhea also have been reported in patients receiving methylphenidate.

Decreased appetite, dry mouth, nausea, and weight loss have been reported in 25, 14, 13, and 7%, respectively, of adults with ADHD receiving methylphenidate hydrochloride extended-release trilayer core tablets. Anorexia, bruxism, constipation, vomiting, and dyspepsia each were reported in 1–2% of adults with ADHD receiving methylphenidate hydrochloride extended-release trilayer core tablets.

■ Hepatic Effects Abnormal liver function, ranging from serum aminotransferase (transaminase) elevations to hepatic coma, has been reported in patients receiving methylphenidate, although a definite causal relationship has not been established. Hepatotoxicity was associated with methylphenidate therapy in at least one patient.

■ Dermatologic and Sensitivity Reactions Hypersensitivity reactions including rash, macular rash, urticaria, fever, arthralgia, exfoliative dermatitis, erythema multiforme with histopathologic findings of necrotizing vasculitis, and thrombocytopenic purpura may occur in patients receiving methylphenidate. Stevens-Johnson syndrome has been reported rarely. Fixed drug eruption, angioedema, anaphylactic reaction, auricular swelling, bullous conditions, pruritus, eruptions, and exanthemas have been reported in patients receiving methylphenidate, although a definite causal relationship has not been established. Erythema occurs in a majority of patients receiving methylphenidate as the transdermal system but generally causes minimal or no discomfort. Excoriation has been reported in 4% of children receiving methylphenidate hydrochloride extended-release oral suspension.

In an open-label study evaluating dermatologic reactions to methylphenidate transdermal system (9-hour wear time) in 305 children with ADHD, sensitization to methylphenidate (allergic contact dermatitis) was diagnosed and confirmed by patch testing in 1 child (0.3%). Sensitization was manifested by erythema and edema at application sites with concurrent urticarial lesions on the abdomen and legs; treatment with the transdermal system was discontinued and the child was not switched to oral methylphenidate therapy. No cases of systemic sensitization have been observed to date in clinical trials of the methylphenidate transdermal system. (See Precautions and Contraindications Associated with Specific Methylphenidate Formulations under Cautions: Precautions and Contraindications.)

Chemical leukoderma (permanent loss of pigmentation due to repeated exposure to specific chemical compounds) has been reported in patients receiving methylphenidate as the transdermal system. In most cases, depigmentation or hypopigmentation has been limited to application sites. However, a small number of patients have reported skin color changes on areas of the body where the transdermal system was never applied. Time to onset of chemical leukoderma following initiation of transdermal methylphenidate therapy has ranged from 2 months to 4 years, and the affected areas have ranged up to 8 inches in diameter. If loss of pigmentation occurs, transdermal methylphenidate should be discontinued and alternative therapy considered.

Other application site reactions, including bleeding, bruising, burn, burning, dermatitis, discharge, discoloration, discomfort, dryness, eczema, edema, erosion, excoriation, exfoliation, fissure, hyperpigmentation, induration, infection, inflammation, irritation, pain, papules, paresthesia, pruritus, rash, scab, swelling, ulcer, urticaria, vesicles, and warmth, have been reported in patients receiving transdermal methylphenidate, but a causal relationship to the drug has not been established.

Hyperhidrosis has been reported in 5% of adults with ADHD receiving methylphenidate hydrochloride extended-release trilayer core tablets in clinical trials.

Alopecia also has been reported in patients receiving methylphenidate, but a causal relationship to the drug has not been established.

■ **Hematologic Effects** Thrombocytopenia and/or easy bruisability, epistaxis, and gingival bleeding; leukopenia; anemia; pancytopenia; and eosinophilia have been reported rarely in patients receiving methylphenidate, but a causal relationship to the drug has not been definitely established. (See Other Precautions and Contraindications under Cautions: Precautions and Contraindications.)

■ **Cardiovascular Effects** Sudden death, stroke, myocardial infarction, angina, tachycardia, cardiac arrhythmias, palpitation, and increase or decrease in blood pressure and pulse rate may occur in patients receiving stimulants, including methylphenidate. (See Cardiovascular Precautions under Cautions: Precautions and Contraindications.) Tachycardia and palpitations were reported in 5 and 3%, respectively, of adults with ADHD receiving methylphenidate hydrochloride extended-release trilayer core tablets in clinical trials. Cerebral arteritis and/or occlusion, cerebrovascular vasculitis, cerebral hemorrhage, cardiac murmur, and hot flush also have been reported in patients receiving methylphenidate. Tachycardia was reported in 1% of children and adolescents with ADHD receiving transdermal methylphenidate in clinical trials. Cardiac arrest, bradycardia, extrasystole, supraventricular tachycardia, ventricular extrasystole, peripheral coldness, and reversible ischemic neurologic deficit have been reported in patients receiving methylphenidate, although a definite causal relationship has not been established.

Stimulants used to treat ADHD, including methylphenidate, are associated with peripheral vascular disorders, including Raynaud's phenomenon. Manifestations usually are intermittent and mild, but ulceration of the digits and/or breakdown of soft tissue may occur rarely. Peripheral vascular disorders, including Raynaud's phenomenon, have been reported during postmarketing experience in patients in all age groups receiving stimulants at therapeutic dosages and at various times throughout the treatment course. Manifestations generally improve following dosage reduction or drug discontinuance; however, further clinical evaluation (e.g., referral to a rheumatologist) may be appropriate for certain patients.

■ **Ocular Effects** Blurred vision has been reported in 2% of adults with ADHD receiving methylphenidate hydrochloride extended-release trilayer core tablets in clinical trials. Eye pain has been reported in 2% of children receiving methylphenidate hydrochloride extended-release oral suspension in clinical trials. Dry eye and difficulty with accommodation also have been reported in patients receiving methylphenidate. Diplopia, mydriasis, and visual disturbances or impairment have been reported in patients receiving methylphenidate, although a causal relationship to the drug has not been definitely established.

■ **Respiratory Effects** Nasal congestion and nasopharyngitis were reported in 6 and 5%, respectively, of children receiving methylphenidate as a transdermal system in clinical trials. Cough, nasopharyngitis, and oropharyngeal pain were each reported in 1–3% of children and adolescents receiving methylphenidate hydrochloride extended-release trilayer core tablets in clinical trials. Upper respiratory infection and oropharyngeal pain were each reported in 2% of adults with ADHD receiving methylphenidate hydrochloride extended-release trilayer core tablets in clinical trials. Dyspnea and sinusitis also have been reported in patients receiving methylphenidate.

■ **Other Adverse Effects** Pulmonary talc granulomata, superficial abscesses, other foreign body reactions, and eosinophilia have been reported in drug abusers who have dissolved methylphenidate hydrochloride tablets in water and injected the resulting solution.

Prolonged and painful erections, in some cases requiring surgical intervention, have been reported in adult and pediatric patients receiving methylphenidate. Priapism has not been reported with drug initiation but rather has developed after patients have received the drug for some time, often occurring following an increase in dosage. Priapism also has occurred during temporary interruptions in therapy (e.g., drug holidays) or following drug discontinuance. If not treated immediately, priapism can lead to permanent penile damage.

Changes in libido and erectile dysfunction have been reported in patients receiving methylphenidate. Decreased libido has been reported in approximately 2% of adults with ADHD receiving methylphenidate hydrochloride extended-release trilayer core tablets in clinical trials.

Motion sickness has been reported in 2% of children with ADHD receiving methylphenidate hydrochloride extended-release oral suspension in clinical trials. Pyrexia has been reported in 2% of children and adolescents with ADHD receiving methylphenidate hydrochloride extended-release trilayer core tablets in clinical trials. Muscle tightness has been reported in 2% of adults with ADHD receiving methylphenidate hydrochloride extended-release trilayer core tablets in clinical trials.

Rhabdomyolysis and muscle spasms have been reported in patients receiving methylphenidate. Arthralgia, myalgia, muscle twitching, hyperpyrexia, chest pain or discomfort, and scalp hair loss also have been reported, but a causal relationship to the drug has not been definitely established.

■ **Precautions and Contraindications** ***Psychiatric Precautions*** Aggressive behavior and hostility frequently are observed in children and adolescents with ADHD and have been reported in patients receiving drug therapy for the disorder. Although a causal relationship to stimulants has not been established, patients beginning treatment for ADHD should be monitored for the onset or worsening of aggressive behavior or hostility.

Psychotic or manic symptoms (e.g., hallucinations, delusional thinking, mania) have been reported in children and adolescents without prior history of psychotic illness or mania who received usual dosages of stimulants. In a pooled analysis of multiple short-term, placebo-controlled studies, such symptoms occurred in about 0.1% of patients receiving usual dosages of stimulants (i.e., methylphenidate, amphetamine) compared with 0% of those receiving placebo. If psychotic or manic symptoms occur during stimulant therapy, a causal relationship to stimulants should be considered, and discontinuance of therapy may be appropriate.

Stimulants should be used with caution in the management of ADHD in patients with comorbid bipolar disorder because of the potential for precipitation of mixed or manic episodes in such patients. Prior to initiating stimulant therapy, patients with ADHD and comorbid depressive symptoms should be carefully screened to determine if they are at risk for bipolar disorder; such screening should include a detailed psychiatric history (e.g., family history of suicide, bipolar disorder, or depression).

Stimulants may exacerbate symptoms of behavior disturbance and thought disorder in patients with a preexisting psychotic disorder.

Each time methylphenidate is dispensed, a medication guide should be provided to the patient or caregiver, alerting them to the risks associated with stimulant therapy (e.g., adverse psychiatric effects) and advising them of necessary precautions. (See Other Precautions and Contraindications under Cautions: Precautions and Contraindications.) Patients or caregivers should be instructed to inform clinicians of preexisting illnesses or conditions, including suicidal ideation or behaviors or mental or psychiatric disorders. They also should be instructed to inform clinicians immediately if adverse psychiatric effects (e.g., hallucinations, delusional thinking, mania) occur during stimulant therapy.

Cardiovascular Precautions Stimulants, including methylphenidate, cause modest increases in average blood pressure (i.e., by about 2–4 mm Hg) and heart rate (i.e., by about 3–6 beats/minute); larger increases may occur in some patients. Although modest increases would not be expected to have short-term sequelae, all patients should be monitored for larger changes in blood pressure and heart rate. Caution is advised in patients with underlying medical conditions that might be affected by increases in blood pressure or heart rate (e.g., hypertension, heart failure, recent myocardial infarction, ventricular arrhythmia).

Although a causal relationship to stimulants has not been established, sudden unexplained death, stroke, and myocardial infarction have been reported in adults receiving usual dosages of stimulants for the treatment of ADHD. Sudden unexplained death also has been reported in children and adolescents with structural cardiac abnormalities or other serious cardiac conditions receiving usual dosages of CNS stimulants. Results of one retrospective, case-control epidemiologic study showed that there may be an association between use of stimulant medications (e.g., methylphenidate) and sudden unexplained death in healthy children and adolescents. (See Cautions: Pediatric Precautions.) Because of postmarketing reports and the results of this and other epidemiologic studies, FDA collaborated with the Agency for Healthcare Research and Quality (AHRQ) to sponsor 3 large, related, retrospective cohort studies using data from several health care claims databases to evaluate possible associations between ADHD drug use (stimulants, atomoxetine, and pemoline [no longer commercially available in the US]) and the following serious cardiovascular events: myocardial infarction, stroke, and sudden cardiac death in children and young adults 2–24 years of age; myocardial infarction and sudden cardiac death in adults 25–64 years of age; and stroke and the composite end point of stroke, myocardial infarction, and sudden cardiac death in the same group of adults. None of the 3 studies showed an association between serious cardiovascular events and current use of ADHD drugs, as compared with nonuse or as compared with former or remote use, although small increases in cardiovascular risk could not be excluded. The study in children and young adults included data for approximately 1.2 million patients and approximately 2.6 million patient-years of follow-up, including approximately 370,000 patient-years of current ADHD drug use, and found only 7 serious cardiovascular events (4 strokes, 3 sudden deaths) in current users of the drugs. The analyses in adults included data for approximately 440,000 patients, including approximately 150,000 current users of ADHD drugs; for the composite outcome of stroke, myocardial infarction, and sudden cardiac death, there were approximately 107,000 patient-years of ADHD drug exposure and 234 such cardiovascular events in current users.

Children, adolescents, and adults who are being considered for stimulant therapy should undergo a thorough medical history review (including evaluation for a family history of sudden death or ventricular arrhythmia) and physical examination to detect the presence of cardiac disease, and should receive further cardiac evaluation (e.g., ECG, echocardiogram) if initial findings suggest such disease. Although some serious cardiac conditions are independently associated with an increased risk of sudden death, CNS stimulants generally should *not* be used in children, adolescents, or adults with known serious structural cardiac abnormalities, cardiomyopathy, serious heart rhythm abnormalities, coronary artery disease, or other serious cardiac conditions. Patients who develop exertional chest pain, unexplained syncope, or other manifestations suggestive of cardiac disease during stimulant therapy should undergo prompt cardiac evaluation.

Each time methylphenidate is dispensed, a medication guide should be provided to the patient or caregiver, alerting them to the risks associated with stimulant therapy (e.g., possible cardiovascular risks) and advising them of necessary precautions. (See Other Precautions and Contraindications under Cautions: Precautions and Contraindications.) Patients or caregivers should be instructed to inform clinicians of preexisting illnesses or conditions, including cardiac or cardiovascular disease. They also should be instructed to inform clinicians immediately if adverse cardiovascular effects (e.g., chest pain, shortness of breath, fainting) occur during stimulant therapy.

For further information on screening for cardiac conditions, selecting appropriate candidates for stimulant therapy, and monitoring for treatment-emergent cardiac conditions, see Cardiovascular Precautions under Cautions: Precautions and Contraindications, in the Amphetamines General Statement 28:20.04.

Precautions and Contraindications Associated with Specific Methylphenidate Formulations Administration of methylphenidate hydrochloride chewable tablets without adequate fluid may cause tablet contents to swell, resulting in blockage of the throat or esophagus and, possibly, choking. Therefore, chewable tablets should be taken with a full glass (i.e., at least 240 mL [8 ounces]) of water or other fluid and should *not* be administered in patients with difficulty swallowing. Patients should be advised to immediately seek medical attention if they experience chest pain, vomiting, or difficulty in swallowing or breathing following administration of the chewable tablets.

Individuals with phenylketonuria (i.e., homozygous genetic deficiency of phenylalanine hydroxylase) and other individuals who must restrict their intake of phenylalanine should be warned that each 2.5-, 5-, or 10-mg chewable tablet contains aspartame (NutraSweet®), which is metabolized in the GI tract to provide about 0.42, 0.84, or 1.68 mg, respectively, of phenylalanine following oral administration.

Methylphenidate hydrochloride extended-release capsules (Metadate® CD) contain sucrose and should not be used in patients with hereditary fructose intolerance, glucose-galactose malabsorption, or sucrase-isomaltase insufficiency.

Methylphenidate hydrochloride extended-release tablets (Metadate® ER) contain lactose and should not be used in patients with hereditary galactose intolerance, Lapp lactase deficiency, or glucose-galactose malabsorption.

Methylphenidate hydrochloride extended-release trilayer core tablets generally should not be used in patients with preexisting severe GI narrowing since obstruction may occur.

Patients receiving the methylphenidate transdermal system should be advised to avoid exposing the application site to direct external heat sources (e.g., hair dryers, heating pads, electric blankets, heated water beds) while wearing the transdermal system. Release of methylphenidate from the transdermal system is temperature dependent; release may increase more than twofold when the system is exposed to heat, and this may result in overdosage of the drug. (See Pharmacokinetics: Absorption.)

Use of the methylphenidate transdermal system may result in contact sensitization. Transdermal methylphenidate should be discontinued if contact sensitization is suspected (i.e., if erythema develops and is accompanied by evidence of a more intense local reaction [e.g., edema, papules, vesicles] that does not improve substantially within 48 hours or that spreads beyond the application site). Diagnosis of allergic contact dermatitis should be confirmed by appropriate diagnostic testing. Patients sensitized from use of the methylphenidate transdermal system may develop systemic sensitization or other systemic reactions if methylphenidate-containing products are administered via other routes (e.g., orally). Manifestations of systemic sensitization may include a flare-up of previous dermatitis or of prior positive patch test sites, or generalized skin eruptions in previously unaffected skin. Other systemic reactions may include headache, fever, malaise, arthralgia, diarrhea, or vomiting. Patients who develop contact sensitization to the methylphenidate transdermal system should be under close medical supervision if oral methylphenidate therapy is initiated. Some patients sensitized to methylphenidate by exposure to the methylphenidate transdermal system may not be able to receive methylphenidate in any form.

Patients receiving the methylphenidate transdermal system should be monitored for loss of skin pigmentation, especially at application sites, since chemical leukoderma has been reported in patients receiving this formulation. Patients should be advised to immediately report changes in skin color to their clinician.

Other Precautions and Contraindications The manufacturer's patient information (medication guide) should be provided to the patient or caregiver each time methylphenidate is dispensed, and the clinician should discuss and answer questions about its contents (e.g., benefits and risks of stimulant therapy, appropriate use) as needed. The patient or caregiver also should be instructed to read and understand the contents of the medication guide before initiating therapy and each time the prescription is refilled.

Patients or caregivers should be instructed to inform clinicians of preexisting illnesses or conditions (e.g., cardiac or cardiovascular disease, thyroid disease, glaucoma, suicidal ideation or behaviors, mental or psychiatric disorder, seizures, history of substance abuse).

The manufacturers recommend that laboratory tests, including periodic complete blood cell (with differential) and platelet counts, be performed periodically during prolonged methylphenidate hydrochloride therapy. However, the clinical rationale for this precaution has been questioned by some clinicians since adverse hematologic effects have occurred only rarely in patients receiving methylphenidate and a causal relationship to the drug has not been conclusively established in these cases. Most clinicians consider routine hematologic monitoring unnecessary in the absence of clinical signs (e.g., fever, sore throat, unusual bleeding or bruising) suggestive of possible hematologic toxicity, although some clinicians suggest annual hematologic monitoring in any patient receiving prolonged therapy with the drug. In addition, the American Academy of Pediatrics (AAP) states that routine hematologic, serologic, or ECG monitoring is *not* necessary during methylphenidate therapy.

If paradoxical aggravation of symptoms occurs during methylphenidate therapy, dosage should be reduced or the drug discontinued.

The risk of abuse should be assessed prior to initiation of therapy. Tolerance and psychological dependence with varying degrees of abnormal behavior have been reported in patients chronically taking large doses of methylphenidate. Frank psychotic episodes including hallucinosis can occur, particularly with parenteral abuse. The possibility of psychological or physical dependence should be considered, particularly when methylphenidate is administered to alcoholics, emotionally unstable patients, or those known to have been addicted to other drugs. The drug should be administered with caution to persons with a history of drug or alcohol dependence since such patients may increase dosage on their own initiative. Patients receiving the drug should be monitored for signs of abuse and dependence, and the need for continued therapy should be periodically reevaluated. Patients and/or their caregivers should be advised that methylphenidate is a drug of potential abuse and should be protected from theft or misuse. The drug should be disposed of properly when it is no longer needed. (See Chronic Toxicity.)

Abrupt withdrawal of methylphenidate following prolonged administration may unmask severe depression as well as the effects of chronic overactivity; paranoid and suicidal ideation, dysphoric mood (e.g., depression, irritability, anxiety), fatigue, insomnia or hypersomnia, psychomotor agitation, and disturbed sleep also may occur. Therefore, patients should be carefully supervised during withdrawal of the drug; long-term follow-up may be required since some manifestations (e.g., depression) may persist for prolonged periods.

Visual disturbances (difficulty with accommodation, blurred vision) have been reported in patients receiving stimulants, including methylphenidate.

Patients should be informed that stimulants may impair their ability to perform potentially hazardous tasks and advised to use caution when driving or operating machinery until they know how the drug affects them.

Methylphenidate may in rare instances cause prolonged and sometimes painful erections. If not treated immediately, priapism can lead to permanent penile damage. Clinicians should inform male patients and their caregivers about the signs and symptoms of priapism, stressing the need for immediate medical treatment if it occurs. Younger males, especially prepubertal males, may not recognize the problem or may be embarrassed to tell anyone if it occurs. FDA states that clinicians should be cautious if they consider switching patients from methylphenidate preparations because of this risk, since certain other alternative ADHD treatments (e.g., atomoxetine) also may cause priapism.

Because stimulants used to treat ADHD, including methylphenidate, are associated with peripheral vascular disorders, including Raynaud's phenomenon, careful observation for digital changes is warranted during stimulant therapy, and further clinical evaluation (e.g., referral to a rheumatologist) may be appropriate for certain patients. Patients should be informed about the risk of peripheral vascular disorders, including Raynaud's phenomenon, and the associated signs and symptoms (e.g., feelings of numbness, coolness, or pain in fingers or toes; changes in color from pale to blue to red). Patients should be advised to report any new numbness, pain, skin color change, or sensitivity to temperature in fingers or toes to their clinician and to immediately contact their clinician if any signs of unexplained wounds appear on fingers or toes.

Methylphenidate should be used with caution in patients with a history of seizures and/or EEG abnormalities. There is some clinical evidence that stimulants, including methylphenidate, may lower the seizure threshold in patients with a history of seizures, in those with prior EEG abnormalities in the absence of seizures, and, very rarely, in those without a history of seizures and no prior evidence of EEG abnormalities. Although safe concomitant use of methylphenidate and anticonvulsants has not been established, studies of methylphenidate use have not shown an increase in seizure frequency or severity when the stimulant was used in patients receiving appropriate anticonvulsant therapy. If seizures occur in patients receiving methylphenidate, the drug should be discontinued.

Therapy with CNS stimulants may be associated with at least a temporary suppression of growth in children. (See Cautions: GI and Growth Effects.)

Methylphenidate is contraindicated in patients with a history of marked anxiety, tension, and agitation, since the drug may aggravate these symptoms. Methylphenidate is also contraindicated in patients with glaucoma, in patients with motor tics or a family history or diagnosis of Tourette's syndrome, and in those known to be hypersensitive to the drug. However, AAP states that the presence of tics before or during medical management of ADHD is *not* an absolute contraindication to stimulant drug use. (See the opening discussion in Cautions.) Methylphenidate also is contraindicated during or within 14 days of administration of monoamine oxidase (MAO) inhibitors since hypertensive crisis could result. (See Drug Interactions: Antidepressants.)

■ **Pediatric Precautions** Although safety and efficacy of methylphenidate in children younger than 6 years of age have not been established, the drug has been used in several controlled clinical studies in preschool-aged children up to 6 years of age. Some studies reported higher rates of adverse effects, particularly with higher dosages, than had previously been reported in children 6 years of age and older and the adverse effects reported in preschool-aged children may be different than those reported in older children with ADHD. Some of the adverse behavioral effects reported in clinical studies in preschool-aged children receiving methylphenidate also were reported in those receiving placebo; some of these behaviors may actually improve in preschool-aged children receiving methylphenidate therapy. Other issues involved with the use of stimulants in children younger than 6 years of age are the lack of established dosage recommendations for this population. Additional study and experience are required to elucidate further the safety and efficacy of the drug in this age group.

Long-term administration of CNS stimulants has been associated with at least a temporary suppression of normal weight and/or height patterns in children; patients requiring long-term therapy with methylphenidate should be carefully monitored and the drug should be discontinued temporarily in children in whom suppression of normal growth or weight gain is observed. However, AAP states that studies of stimulants in children generally have found little or no decrease in expected height, with any decrease in growth early in treatment being compensated for later on. (See Cautions: GI and Growth Effects.)

Sudden death has been reported in children and adolescents with structural cardiac abnormalities or other serious cardiac conditions receiving usual dosages of CNS stimulants. Results of one retrospective, case-control epidemiologic study suggested a possible association between use of stimulant medications and sudden unexplained death in healthy children and adolescents. However, a subsequent large epidemiologic study found no evidence of increased risk of serious cardiovascular effects in children or young adults with ADHD receiving such therapy. (See Cardiovascular Precautions under Cautions: Precautions and Contraindications.)

■ **Pregnancy and Lactation** Although there are no adequate and controlled studies to date in humans, methylphenidate hydrochloride has been shown to have teratogenic effects in rabbits when given at dosages 100 and 40 times the recommended human dosage on a mg/kg or mg/m^2 basis, respectively. CNS stimulants, such as methylphenidate, can cause vasoconstriction and thereby decrease placental perfusion. No fetal and/or neonatal adverse reactions have been reported with the use of therapeutic doses of methylphenidate during pregnancy; however, premature delivery and low birth-weight infants have been reported in amphetamine-dependent women. Methylphenidate hydrochloride should be used during pregnancy only when the potential benefits justify the possible risks to the fetus.

Limited data suggest that breast-fed infants receive 0.2–0.7% of the maternal weight-adjusted dosage of methylphenidate; in 5 case reports, the milk-to-plasma ratio of the drug ranged from 1.1–2.7. Adverse effects on the breast-fed infant or on milk production have not been reported to date; however, any long-term neurodevelopmental effects are unknown. The developmental and health benefits of breast-feeding should be considered along with the importance of methylphenidate to the woman and any potential adverse effects on the breast-fed infant from either the drug or the underlying maternal condition. If a woman receiving methylphenidate breast-feeds, the infant should be monitored for adverse effects (e.g., agitation, anorexia, reduced weight gain).

Drug Interactions

■ **Drugs Affecting or Metabolized by Hepatic Microsomal Enzymes** Because methylphenidate is not metabolized by cytochrome P-450 (CYP) isoenzymes to a clinically important extent, inducers or inhibitors of CYP isoenzymes are not expected to substantially affect the pharmacokinetics of methylphenidate. The *d*- and *l*-enantiomers of methylphenidate do not inhibit CYP isoenzymes 1A2, 2C8, 2C9, 2C19, 2D6, 2E1, or 3A to a clinically important extent.

■ **Antidepressants** Because monoamine oxidase (MAO) inhibitors potentiate the pressor effects of sympathomimetic drugs, methylphenidate is contraindicated in patients currently receiving, or having recently received (i.e., within 2 weeks), MAO inhibitor therapy. The metabolism of tricyclic antidepressants (e.g., imipramine, clomipramine, desipramine) has been reported to be inhibited when these drugs are used in patients receiving methylphenidate. Some manufacturers state that the metabolism of selective serotonin-reuptake inhibitors (SSRIs) may be inhibited when methylphenidate is used concomitantly. Dosage reduction of tricyclic antidepressants and SSRIs may be required in patients receiving concomitant methylphenidate therapy.

■ **Cardiovascular Agents** Methylphenidate should be used with caution in patients receiving pressor agents. Methylphenidate may decrease the efficacy of antihypertensive agents.

■ **Other Drugs** The metabolism of coumarin anticoagulants and anticonvulsants (e.g., phenobarbital, phenytoin, primidone) has been reported to be inhibited when these drugs are administered in patients receiving methylphenidate. Although additional studies did not confirm the reported inhibition of metabolism of anticonvulsants and coumarin anticoagulants, the possibility that methylphenidate may raise the serum concentrations of these drugs to toxic concentrations necessitating a decrease in dosage should be considered. Additionally, metabolism of phenylbutazone (no longer commercially available in the US) has been reported to be inhibited when administered in patients receiving methylphenidate hydrochloride conventional or extended-release tablets. Dosage reduction of coumarin anticoagulants, anticonvulsants, or phenylbutazone may be required in patients receiving concomitant methylphenidate therapy. It may be necessary to monitor plasma drug concentrations (or, in the case of coumarin anticoagulants, prothrombin time [PT]) when methylphenidate is initiated or discontinued.

Studies to evaluate the effects of changes in gastric pH on the absorption of methylphenidate hydrochloride administered as extended-release capsules (Ritalin® LA) have not been performed to date; the manufacturer states that concurrent use of drugs that increase gastric pH (e.g., antacids, H_2-receptor antagonists) could potentially alter the release characteristics of the formulation.

Clearance of methylphenidate may be affected by urinary pH, either being increased with acidifying agents or decreased with alkalinizing agents; clinicians should consider these potential effects when methylphenidate is administered concomitantly with agents that alter urinary pH.

There is a risk of sudden blood pressure increases during surgery in patients receiving methylphenidate and halogenated anesthetics; some manufacturers state that methylphenidate should not be administered on the day of planned surgery.

Acute Toxicity

■ **Manifestations** Acute toxicity due to methylphenidate overdosage results in symptoms similar to those of acute amphetamine intoxication and may be manifested by cardiovascular symptoms including flushing, palpitation, hypertension, cardiac arrhythmias, and tachycardia. Mental disturbances such as confusion, delirium, euphoria, hallucinations, and toxic psychosis may also occur. Other symptoms of overdosage include agitation, headache, vomiting, dryness of mucous membranes, mydriasis, hyperpyrexia, sweating, tremors, hyperreflexia, muscle twitching, and seizures which may be followed by coma. Rhabdomyolysis also has been reported.

■ **Treatment** In the treatment of methylphenidate overdosage, general physiologic supportive measures, including maintenance of adequate circulation and respiratory exchange should be immediately instituted. The patient should be protected against self-injury and should be isolated to avoid possible external stimuli. In cases of overdosage involving transdermal methylphenidate, all transdermal systems of the drug should be removed immediately and the skin cleansed of any remaining adhesive; the potential for continued absorption of residual drug in the skin following system removal should be considered. If signs and symptoms of acute toxicity are not too severe and the patient is conscious, gastric contents may be evacuated following ingestion of oral dosage forms by induction of emesis or gastric lavage. In patients with severe intoxication, administration of a carefully titrated dose of a short-acting barbiturate may be required before beginning gastric lavage. External cooling procedures may be required for the treatment of hyperpyrexia. Effectiveness of peritoneal dialysis or extracorporeal hemodialysis for the treatment of methylphenidate overdosage has not been established.

Chronic Toxicity

CNS stimulants, including methylphenidate, have a high potential for abuse and dependence. Marked tolerance and psychological dependence with varying degrees of abnormal behavior can occur with chronic abuse. Psychotic episodes can occur, particularly with parenteral abuse. Signs and symptoms of CNS stimulant abuse include increased heart rate, respiratory rate, blood pressure, and/or sweating; dilated pupils; hyperactivity, restlessness, insomnia, loss of coordination, and tremors; flushed skin; decreased appetite; and vomiting and/or abdominal pain. Anxiety, psychosis, hostility, aggression, and suicidal or homicidal ideation also have been observed. Abuse of CNS stimulants by unintended routes of administration (e.g., chewing, snorting, or injecting the formulation) can result in overdosage and death.

Tolerance can occur during chronic therapy with methylphenidate, and physical dependence can occur. Withdrawal symptoms, including extreme fatigue and depression, can occur when CNS stimulants are discontinued abruptly following prolonged high-dosage administration. Careful supervision is required during withdrawal from abusive use since severe depression may occur. Withdrawal of methylphenidate following prolonged therapeutic administration may unmask symptoms of the underlying disorder, which may require follow-up.

The abuse potential of extended-release methylphenidate hydrochloride (Concerta®, formulated to provide 22% of the total dose for immediate release) compared with an immediate-release formulation of the drug was evaluated in 2 placebo-controlled studies in individuals with a history of recreational stimulant use. In both studies, responses on subjective measures suggestive of abuse potential were evaluated over an 8-hour period following single-dose oral administration. The first study evaluated abuse potential at 1 dose level for each formulation: 108 mg of extended-release methylphenidate hydrochloride and 60 mg of the immediate-release drug. In this study, both formulations of methylphenidate produced greater responses compared with placebo on 5 subjective measures of abuse potential; the 108-mg dose of extended-release methylphenidate hydrochloride produced variable responses on positive subjective measures that were either statistically indistinguishable from (on measures of abuse potential, drug liking, amphetamine, and morphine benzedrine group [euphoria]) or less than (on measure of stimulation-euphoria) responses produced by 60 mg of immediate-release methylphenidate hydrochloride. The second study evaluated abuse potential following single oral doses at 2 dose levels for each formulation: 54 or 108 mg of extended-release methylphenidate hydrochloride and 50 or 90 mg of the immediate-release drug. Both doses of both formulations produced greater responses compared with placebo on 2 primary scales of abuse potential (drug liking, euphoria). The 54-mg dose of extended-release methylphenidate hydrochloride produced lower subjective responses compared with the 50-mg immediate-release dose; the same pattern was observed for the 108-mg extended-release dose and the 90-mg immediate-release dose. Responses following the 108-mg extended-release dose and the 50-mg immediate-release dose were indistinguishable. Although these findings indicated a relatively lower response to the extended-release formulation compared with the immediate-release formulation following oral administration at roughly equivalent total doses, the relevance of these findings to abuse potential in the community is unknown.

Pharmacology

The pharmacologic actions of methylphenidate are qualitatively similar to those of the amphetamines and include CNS and respiratory stimulation and weak sympathomimetic activity. The mechanism of action involved in the central effect of methylphenidate has not been determined. The main sites of CNS action appear to be the cerebral cortex and subcortical structures including the thalamus; stimulation by methylphenidate causes an increase in motor activity, mental alertness, diminished sense of fatigue, brighter spirits, and mild euphoria. Methylphenidate apparently produces an anorexigenic effect. In usual therapeutic oral dosage, methylphenidate exhibits only moderate effects on the peripheral circulatory system. In a study of the effects of dexmethylphenidate (the pharmacologically active enantiomer of racemic methylphenidate) on the QT interval in healthy individuals, clinically important changes in the QT interval corrected for heart rate (QT_c) were not observed following administration of a single 40-mg dose of dexmethylphenidate hydrochloride as extended-release capsules.

Pharmacokinetics

■ **Absorption** Methylphenidate hydrochloride appears to be well absorbed from the GI tract; however, oral bioavailability of the drug is low (about 30%; range: 10–52%), which suggests substantial first-pass metabolism. Following oral administration of methylphenidate hydrochloride as conventional tablets, oral solution, or chewable tablets, peak plasma concentrations were attained at approximately 1–2 hours. Methylphenidate hydrochloride oral solution and chewable tablets are bioequivalent to methylphenidate hydrochloride conventional tablets.

Extended-release methylphenidate hydrochloride tablets are absorbed more slowly but to the same extent as the conventional tablets. Following oral administration of methylphenidate hydrochloride extended-release tablets (Methylin® ER, Ritalin-SR®) in children, peak plasma concentrations were attained at 4.7 hours.

After oral administration of methylphenidate hydrochloride 20 or 40 mg as Metadate® CD extended-release capsules in children, peak plasma concentrations were attained at 1.5 hours and again at 4.5 hours after a dose. In children, the mean peak plasma concentration and mean area under the plasma concentration-time curve (AUC) for methylphenidate were slightly lower following administration of 20 mg of the drug once daily as Metadate® CD extended-release capsules than following administration of 10 mg twice daily as conventional tablets. In children and adults, the relative bioavailability of Ritalin® LA extended-release capsules administered once daily is comparable to that of the conventional tablets administered twice daily 4 hours apart. The initial rate of absorption of methylphenidate hydrochloride and the time to first and second peak plasma concentrations were similar following administration of 40 mg of the drug once daily as Ritalin® LA extended-release capsules or 20 mg twice daily (given 4 hours apart) as conventional tablets, but greater interindividual variability and a smaller difference between peak and trough plasma concentrations (resulting from a lower second peak concentration and a higher minimum concentration between the 2 peak concentrations) were observed with the extended-release capsules.

Following oral administration of Aptensio XR® extended-release capsules in adults, peak plasma methylphenidate concentrations were attained at approximately 2 hours and again at approximately 8 hours after a dose. In adults, the relative bioavailability of Aptensio XR® extended-release capsules or the extended-release trilayer core tablets (Concerta®) of methylphenidate hydrochloride administered once daily is comparable to that of the conventional tablets administered 3 times daily. Following oral administration of the extended-release trilayer core tablets of methylphenidate hydrochloride in healthy adults, an initial peak plasma concentration is attained within 1 hour while peak plasma concentrations of about 3.7 ng/mL are achieved within approximately 6–10 hours.

Following oral administration of a single 60-mg dose of methylphenidate hydrochloride as extended-release oral suspension in the fasted state in healthy adults, peak plasma concentrations of *d*-methylphenidate (the more pharmacologically active isomer of the drug) were achieved at a median of 5 hours; bioavailability of the extended-release oral suspension (single 60-mg dose) relative to that of an immediate-release oral solution (given as two 30-mg doses 6 hours apart) was 95%.

Systemic absorption of methylphenidate from transdermal systems (Daytrana®) is a function of both the length of time the system is worn and the size of the system. In patients with ADHD, peak plasma concentrations of methylphenidate are achieved about 10 hours after single-dose transdermal application and 8 hours after repeated applications of transdermal systems worn for up to 9 hours. Following single-dose transdermal application in children and adolescents, there was an average delay of 2 hours before *d*-methylphenidate was detectable in the circulation; with repeated administration, low concentrations of the drug were detected earlier after application because of a carry-over effect. Application of the transdermal system to inflamed skin results in shorter time to peak plasma concentration (4 hours) and a threefold increase in peak plasma concentration and AUC compared with application to intact skin. When heat is applied to the transdermal system after application, time to peak plasma concentration occurs 0.5 hour earlier, and median peak plasma concentration and AUC are twofold and 2.5-fold higher, respectively, than those observed following application without heat. Application sites other than the hip can have different absorption characteristics and have not been adequately studied. Some data suggest that transdermal absorption of methylphenidate may be increased with repeated administration; on average, steady state is likely to be achieved by approximately day 14 of dosing.

Effects persist for 3–6 hours after oral administration of conventional tablets, about 3–8 hours after oral administration of certain extended-release tablets (e.g., Metadate® ER, Methylin® ER, Ritalin-SR®), and about 8–12 hours after oral administration of extended-release trilayer core tablets (Concerta®), extended-release capsules (e.g., Aptensio XR®, Metadate® CD, Ritalin® LA), and extended-release oral suspension (Quillivant XR®).

Because of substantially greater first-pass metabolism following oral compared with transdermal administration, a lower transdermal dose of methylphenidate may result in greater systemic exposure to *d*-methylphenidate (the more pharmacologically active isomer) than a higher (on a mg/kg basis) oral dose of the drug. Following repeated transdermal administration of methylphenidate, *l*-methylphenidate is systemically available; on average, systemic exposure to *l*-methylphenidate is 27–45% less than exposure to *d*-methylphenidate. Little, if any, *l*-methylphenidate is systemically available following oral administration of the drug.

In adults, administration of methylphenidate hydrochloride 20 mg as an oral solution with a high-fat meal delayed the peak plasma concentration by approximately 1 hour and increased the average peak plasma concentration and AUC for methylphenidate by 13 and 25%, respectively; the magnitude of increase in peak plasma concentration and AUC is similar between methylphenidate hydrochloride oral solution and conventional tablets. Administration of methylphenidate hydrochloride 20 mg as chewable tablets with a high-fat meal in adults delayed the time to peak plasma concentration by approximately 1 hour and increased the AUC by about 20%; the magnitude of food effect is comparable to that observed with conventional tablets.

Administration of methylphenidate hydrochloride 60 mg as an extended-release oral suspension (Quillivant XR®) in adults with a high-fat meal reduced the time to peak concentration of the drug by approximately 1 hour; peak plasma concentration and AUC were increased by approximately 28 and 19%, respectively, but these effects were not considered clinically important.

Administration of methylphenidate hydrochloride 40 mg as Metadate® CD extended-release capsules with a high-fat meal in adults delayed the first peak plasma concentration by approximately 1 hour and increased the average peak plasma concentration and AUC for methylphenidate by 30 and 17%, respectively. In a single-dose study in healthy adults, administration of Ritalin® LA extended-release capsules with a high-fat breakfast delayed the first and second peak plasma concentrations and decreased the second mean peak plasma concentration by 25% compared with administration in the fasting state. Administration of Aptensio XR® extended-release capsules with a high-fat meal decreased the second peak plasma concentration and increased the average peak concentration and AUC by about 28 and 19%, respectively; in clinical trials, this formulation of the drug was administered without regard to meals. The bioavailability of the extended-release capsules (i.e., Aptensio XR®, Metadate® CD, Ritalin® LA) was not affected by opening the capsules and sprinkling the contents onto applesauce.

In vitro studies evaluating the effect of alcohol on the release of methylphenidate hydrochloride from certain extended-release preparations of the drug indicated that 98 or 84% of the drug was released from Ritalin® LA 40-mg or Metadate® CD 60-mg extended-release capsules within the first hour at an alcohol concentration of 40%; at an alcohol concentration of up to 40%, 96% of the drug was released from Aptensio XR® 80-mg extended-release capsules within 2 hours. When similar studies were conducted with Concerta® 18-mg extended-release trilayer core tablets, drug release was not increased. The manufacturers state that these results are representative for the available strengths of the respective preparations.

■ **Distribution** The extent of methylphenidate distribution in humans is unknown. Methylphenidate is about 10–33% bound to plasma proteins.

■ **Elimination** Methylphenidate is metabolized primarily by de-esterification by carboxylesterase 1A1 to form α-phenylpiperidine acetic acid (ritalinic acid), which has little or no pharmacologic activity. Some data indicate that clearance of methylphenidate increases with increasing weight, suggesting that patients with higher body weight may have lower exposures to total methylphenidate at similar doses.

Following oral administration of methylphenidate hydrochloride conventional tablets in adults or children, the mean terminal elimination half-life was reported to be 3.5 or 2.5 hours, respectively. The mean terminal elimination half-life following oral administration of methylphenidate hydrochloride as an oral solution in adults is similar to that following administration of conventional tablets. The mean terminal half-life following oral administration of methylphenidate hydrochloride 20 mg as chewable tablets in adults is 3 hours, which is comparable to that following administration of conventional tablets. Following oral administration of methylphenidate hydrochloride conventional (5 mg 3 times daily) or extended-release trilayer core tablets (Concerta®) (18 mg once daily) in adults, the plasma elimination half-life reportedly is 3 or 3.5 hours, respectively. The mean half-life of methylphenidate following oral administration as Ritalin® LA extended-release capsules was 2.5 hours in children and 3.5 hours in adults.

Following oral administration of a single 20-mg dose of methylphenidate hydrochloride as Metadate® CD extended-release capsules in adults, the mean terminal half-life of the drug was reported to be 6.8 hours. Following oral administration of a single 80-mg dose of methylphenidate hydrochloride as Aptensio XR® extended release-capsules in adults, the half-life was 5 hours. Following oral administration of a single 60-mg dose of methylphenidate hydrochloride as an extended-release oral suspension, the mean terminal elimination half-life of *d*-methylphenidate was 5.6 hours in healthy adults.

The mean elimination half-life of methylphenidate following removal of the transdermal system in children and adolescents 6–17 years of age was approximately 4–5 hours for *d*-methylphenidate and 1.4–2.9 hours for *l*-methylphenidate.

Following oral administration of 20 mg of radiolabeled methylphenidate hydrochloride as conventional tablets, approximately 50, 80, and 95% of the dose was recovered as metabolites in urine within 6, 24, and 90 hours, respectively.

Chemistry and Stability

■ **Chemistry** Methylphenidate hydrochloride is a piperidine-derivative stimulant. The drug occurs as a fine, white, odorless, crystalline powder and is freely soluble in water and soluble in alcohol. Methylphenidate hydrochloride is commercially available as conventional tablets, chewable tablets, and an oral solution formulated for immediate release of the drug; extended-release tablets (Metadate® ER, Ritalin-SR®; generics) with an intermediate duration of action; and extended-release capsules (Aptensio XR®, Metadate® CD, Ritalin® LA; generics), extended-release trilayer core tablets (e.g., Concerta®; generics), and a powder for oral suspension formulated for extended release of the drug (Quillivant ER®) with a longer duration of action. Methylphenidate is commercially available as a transdermal system.

The commercially available methylphenidate hydrochloride extended-release capsules (Metadate® CD; generics) contain 30% of the dose in immediate-release pellets and 70% of the dose in extended-release pellets that slowly release methylphenidate. The commercially available methylphenidate hydrochloride extended-release capsules (Ritalin® LA) contain the drug in equal amounts in immediate- and extended-release pellets. The commercially available extended-release capsules (Aptensio XR®) contain multilayered pellets that are composed of an immediate-release layer containing approximately 40% of the dose and an extended-release layer containing approximately 60% of the dose.

The commercially available extended-release trilayer core tablets of methylphenidate hydrochloride (Concerta®; generics) contain the drug in an oral osmotic delivery system formulation. The osmotic delivery system consists of an osmotically active trilayer core (comprised of two layers containing the drug and a push layer containing osmotically active components) surrounded by a semipermeable membrane with an immediate-release drug overcoat and a laser-drilled delivery orifice. When exposed to water in the GI tract, the drug overcoat is solubilized providing an initial dose of methylphenidate; as water enters the formulation, the osmotic layer expands and the drug is pushed out the delivery orifice of the membrane into the GI tract at a controlled rate. The rate of methylphenidate delivery in the GI tract is independent of GI pH or the presence of food in the GI tract. The inert tablet ingredients remain intact and are eliminated in feces.

The powder for extended-release oral suspension contains approximately 20% immediate-release and 80% extended-release methylphenidate hydrochloride.

The commercially available transdermal system of methylphenidate consists of a laminate film backing layer, an adhesive layer containing the drug, and a protective liner attached to the adhesive surface. The methylphenidate dosage delivered is dependent on the size of the transdermal system and the length of time the system is worn.

■ **Stability** Methylphenidate hydrochloride tablets, extended-release tablets, extended-release trilayer core tablets (Concerta®), powder for extended-release oral suspension, extended-release capsules (Metadate® CD, Ritalin® LA) and methylphenidate transdermal systems should be stored at a controlled room temperature of 25°C, but may be exposed to temperatures ranging from 15–30°C. The transdermal systems should not be stored in a refrigerator or freezer. Methylphenidate hydrochloride oral solution, chewable tablets, and extended-release capsules (Aptensio XR®) should be stored at 20–25°C. Following reconstitution, oral extended-release suspensions of methylphenidate hydrochloride should be stored at 25°C, but may be exposed to temperatures ranging from 15–30°C, and any unused suspension should be discarded after 4 months.

Preparations

Methylphenidate hydrochloride is subject to control under the Federal Controlled Substances Act of 1970 as a schedule II (C-II) drug.

Excipients in commercially available drug preparations may have clinically important effects in some individuals; consult specific product labeling for details.

Methylphenidate

Topical		
Transdermal System	10 mg/9 hours (27.5 mg/12.5 cm²)	**Daytrana®** (C-II), Noven
	15 mg/9 hours (41.3 mg/18.75 cm²)	**Daytrana®** (C-II), Noven
	20 mg/9 hours (55 mg/25 cm²)	**Daytrana®** (C-II), Noven
	30 mg/9 hours (82.5 mg/37.5 cm²)	**Daytrana®** (C-II), Noven

Methylphenidate Hydrochloride

Oral		
Capsules, extended-release (containing beads)	10 mg (beads, extended-release 5 mg with 5 mg immediate-release)*	**Methylphenidate Hydrochloride Extended-release Capsules** (C-II) **Ritalin® LA** (C-II), Novartis
	10 mg (beads, extended-release 6 mg with 4 mg immediate-release)	**Aptensio XR®** (C-II), Rhodes
	10 mg (beads, extended-release 7 mg with 3 mg immediate-release)*	**Metadate® CD** (C-II), UCB **Methylphenidate Hydrochloride Extended-release Capsules** (C-II)
	15 mg (beads, extended-release 9 mg with 6 mg immediate-release)	**Aptensio XR®** (C-II), Rhodes
	20 mg (beads, extended-release 10 mg with 10 mg immediate-release)*	**Methylphenidate Hydrochloride Extended-release Capsules** (C-II) **Ritalin® LA** (C-II), Novartis
	20 mg (beads, extended-release 12 mg with 8 mg immediate-release)	**Aptensio XR®** (C-II), Rhodes
	20 mg (beads, extended-release 14 mg with 6 mg immediate-release)*	**Metadate® CD** (C-II), UCB **Methylphenidate Hydrochloride Extended-release Capsules** (C-II)
	30 mg (beads, extended-release 15 mg with 15 mg immediate-release)*	**Methylphenidate Hydrochloride Extended-release Capsules** (C-II) **Ritalin® LA** (C-II), Novartis
	30 mg (beads, extended-release 18 mg with 12 mg immediate-release)	**Aptensio XR®** (C-II), Rhodes
	30 mg (beads, extended-release 21 mg with 9 mg immediate-release)*	**Metadate® CD** (C-II), UCB **Methylphenidate Hydrochloride Extended-release Capsules** (C-II)

	40 mg (beads, extended-release 20 mg with 20 mg immediate-release)*	**Methylphenidate Hydrochloride Extended-release Capsules** (C-II)
		Ritalin® LA (C-II), Novartis
	40 mg (beads, extended-release 24 mg with 16 mg immediate-release)	**Aptensio XR®** (C-II), Rhodes
	40 mg (beads, extended-release 28 mg with 12 mg immediate-release)*	**Metadate® CD** (C-II), UCB
		Methylphenidate Hydrochloride Extended-release Capsules (C-II)
	50 mg (beads, extended-release 30 mg with 20 mg immediate-release)	**Aptensio XR®** (C-II), Rhodes
	50 mg (beads, extended-release 35 mg with 15 mg immediate-release)*	**Metadate® CD** (C-II), UCB
		Methylphenidate Hydrochloride Extended-release Capsules (C-II)
	60 mg (beads, extended-release 30 mg with 30 mg immediate-release)	**Ritalin® LA** (C-II), Novartis
	60 mg (beads, extended-release 36 mg with 24 mg immediate-release)	**Aptensio XR®** (C-II), Rhodes
	60 mg (beads, extended-release 42 mg with 18 mg immediate-release)*	**Metadate® CD** (C-II), UCB
		Methylphenidate Hydrochloride Extended-release Capsules (C-II)
For suspension, extended-release	25 mg (extended-release 20 mg with 5 mg immediate-release) per 5 mL	**Quillivant XR®** (C-II), Pfizer
Solution	5 mg/5 mL*	**Methylin®** (C-II), Shionogi
		Methylphenidate Hydrochloride Oral Solution (C-II)
	10 mg/5 mL*	**Methylin®** (C-II), Shionogi
		Methylphenidate Hydrochloride Oral Solution (C-II)
Tablets	5 mg*	**Methylphenidate Hydrochloride Tablets** (C-II)
		Ritalin® Hydrochloride (C-II), Novartis
	10 mg*	**Methylphenidate Hydrochloride Tablets** (C-II)
		Ritalin® Hydrochloride (C-II; scored), Novartis
	20 mg*	**Methylphenidate Hydrochloride Tablets** (C-II)
		Ritalin® Hydrochloride (C-II; scored), Novartis
Tablets, chewable	2.5 mg	**Methylin®** (C-II), Shionogi
	5 mg	**Methylin®** (C-II), Shionogi
	10 mg	**Methylin®** (C-II; scored), Shionogi
Tablets, extended-release	10 mg*	**Methylphenidate Hydrochloride Extended-release Tablets** (C-II)
	20 mg*	**Metadate® ER** (C-II), UCB
		Methylphenidate Hydrochloride Extended-release Tablets (C-II)
		Ritalin-SR® (C-II), Novartis
Tablets, extended-release core	18 mg (core 14 mg with 4 mg immediate-release)*	**Concerta®** (C-II), Janssen
		Methylphenidate Hydrochloride Extended-release Tablets (C-II)
	27 mg (core 21 mg with 6 mg immediate-release)*	**Concerta®** (C-II), Janssen
		Methylphenidate Hydrochloride Extended-release Tablets (C-II)
	36 mg (core 28 mg with 8 mg immediate-release)*	**Concerta®** (C-II), Janssen
		Methylphenidate Hydrochloride Extended-release Tablets (C-II)
	54 mg (core 42 mg with 12 mg immediate-release)*	**Concerta®** (C-II), Janssen
		Methylphenidate Hydrochloride Extended-release Tablets (C-II)

*available from one or more manufacturer, distributor, and/or repackager by generic (nonproprietary) name

WAKEFULNESS-PROMOTING AGENTS 28:20.80

Armodafinil

■ Armodafinil, the *R*-enantiomer of racemic modafinil, is a wakefulness-promoting agent.

Uses

Armodafinil is used orally to improve wakefulness in adults with excessive sleepiness associated with obstructive sleep apnea/hypopnea syndrome (OSAHS), narcolepsy, and shift work sleep disorder (SWSD). Careful attention to the diagnosis and treatment of the underlying sleep disorder is essential whenever armodafinil is used in patients with these conditions. (See Diagnosis of Sleep Disorders under Warnings/Precautions: General Precautions, in Cautions.)

Armodafinil is the *R*-enantiomer of racemic modafinil, which contains equal amounts of *R*-modafinil and *S*-modafinil. Both drugs are wakefulness-promoting agents and differ primarily in their pharmacokinetic profiles; armodafinil has a longer elimination half-life and produces higher plasma concentrations later in the waking day compared with modafinil on a milligram-to-milligram basis. There currently are no well controlled clinical studies directly comparing armodafinil and modafinil in OSAHS, narcolepsy, or SWSD. Further studies are needed to determine whether these pharmacokinetic differences affect armodafinil's clinical efficacy compared with modafinil.

■ **Obstructive Sleep Apnea/Hypopnea Syndrome** Armodafinil is used in the symptomatic treatment of OSAHS to improve wakefulness in adults with excessive sleepiness. The drug should be used as an adjunct to standard treatment(s) for the underlying obstruction (e.g., nasal continuous positive airway pressure [CPAP]). If CPAP is considered the treatment of choice for a patient with OSAHS, every effort should be made to optimize CPAP therapy for an adequate period of time prior to initiating armodafinil therapy. When armodafinil is used adjunctively with CPAP treatment, encouragement of and periodic assessment of CPAP compliance is necessary.

Efficacy of armodafinil as adjunctive therapy for reducing excessive sleepiness in patients with OSAHS was principally established in 2 similarly designed multicenter, placebo-controlled, double-blind, parallel-group studies of 12 weeks' duration. Both studies enrolled outpatients with a diagnosis of OSAHS according to criteria established by the International Classification of Sleep Disorders (ICSD), which also are consistent with DSM-IV criteria. These criteria include either excessive sleepiness or insomnia with frequent episodes of impaired breathing during sleep and associated features (e.g., loud snoring, morning headaches, dry mouth upon awakening) or excessive sleepiness or insomnia with polysomnography demonstrating one or more of the following: more than 5 obstructive apneic episodes (each greater than 10 seconds in duration) per hour of sleep, frequent arousals from sleep associated with the apneic episodes, bradytachycardia, or arterial oxygen desaturation in association with the apneic episodes. In addition, all patients had moderate to severe illness as indicated by a Clinical Global Impression of Severity of Illness (CGI-S) score of at least 4 and excessive sleepiness despite regular use of CPAP (based on a score of 10 or higher on the Epworth Sleepiness Scale [ESS]). Compliance with CPAP therapy, defined as CPAP use for 4 hours or more per night on at least 70% of the nights, was required and monitored throughout the studies.

In the first study, 395 patients were randomized to receive armodafinil 150 mg daily, armodafinil 250 mg daily, or placebo; in the second study, 263 patients were randomized to receive armodafinil 150 mg daily or placebo. Efficacy of armodafinil was principally evaluated by the sleep latency on the Maintenance of Wakefulness Test (MWT), an objective measure of the ability to remain awake for a defined period of time, and by the Clinical Global Impression of Change (CGI-C) Scale, an investigator-rated assessment of the patient's overall disease status. In both studies, armodafinil (at the 2 dosages studied) was found to be more effective than placebo in improving daytime wakefulness. In addition, a substantially greater proportion of armodafinil-treated patients showed improvement in overall clinical status compared with those receiving placebo as indicated by CGI-C scores. Both the 150- and 250-mg daily dosages of armodafinil produced similar clinical efficacy. Nighttime sleep as measured by polysomnography was not affected by use of armodafinil in either of these studies. However, there was a slight trend toward decreased CPAP use over time with armodafinil (mean reductions of 18 minutes in patients receiving armodafinil and 6 minutes in those receiving placebo).

Although the manufacturer states that the long-term efficacy (e.g., longer than 12 weeks) of armodafinil in patients with OSAHS has not been systematically evaluated in placebo-controlled studies, preliminary findings from a flexible-dosage, open-label extension study indicate that therapy for 12 months or longer is associated with sustained improvement in wakefulness in patients with this condition. The manufacturer states that when armodafinil is used for extended periods, the need for continued therapy should be reassessed periodically.

■ **Narcolepsy** Armodafinil is used to improve wakefulness in adults with excessive sleepiness associated with narcolepsy. Narcolepsy is a neurologic sleep disorder characterized by excessive daytime sleepiness and abnormal transitions into rapid eye movement (REM) sleep while awake. Other manifestations may include cataplexy (sudden and transient attacks of weakness), disrupted nocturnal sleep, hypnagogic hallucinations, and/or sleep paralysis.

Efficacy of armodafinil in reducing excessive sleepiness associated with narcolepsy was established in a 12-week double-blind, multicenter, placebo-controlled, parallel-group study in 196 adult outpatients who met the ICSD criteria for narcolepsy. Such criteria include either recurrent daytime naps or lapses into sleep that occur almost daily for at least 3 months, with sudden bilateral loss of postural muscle tone associated with intense emotion (cataplexy), or a complaint of excessive sleepiness or sudden muscle weakness with sleep paralysis, hypnagogic hallucinations, automatic behaviors, disrupted major sleep episode, and polysomnography demonstrating one of the following: sleep latency of less than 10 minutes or a REM sleep latency of less than 20 minutes and a mean sleep latency of less than 5 minutes on the Multiple Sleep Latency Test (MSLT) and 2 or more sleep onset REM periods; no other medical or mental disorders can account for these symptoms. Enrolled patients also were required to have a mean sleep latency of 6 minutes or less on the MSLT and a CGI-S score of at least 4 (moderately ill); the majority of patients enrolled in the study had marked or severe excessive daytime sleepiness. In this study, patients were randomized to receive armodafinil 150 mg, armodafinil 250 mg, or placebo once daily for 12 weeks. Both dosages of armodafinil were associated with substantially greater improvements in daytime wakefulness relative to placebo as measured by the MWT. In addition, the proportion of patients with at least minimal improvement in overall disease status (measured by the CGI-C Scale) was substantially greater for those who received armodafinil versus placebo at all time points in the study; about 71% of patients in the combined armodafinil treatment groups (150- and 250-mg daily groups) were rated as having an overall clinical improvement compared with 33% of those in the placebo group. Both dosages of armodafinil produced similar effects on the CGI-C outcome, but a greater magnitude of effect was seen on the MWT variable with the higher (250-mg daily) dosage. Both armodafinil dosages were also associated with significant improvements in memory, attention, and fatigue. Nighttime sleep as measured by polysomnography was not adversely affected by use of armodafinil in this study.

Although the manufacturer states that the long-term efficacy (e.g., longer than 12 weeks) of armodafinil in patients with narcolepsy has not been systematically evaluated in placebo-controlled studies to date, preliminary findings from a flexible-dosage, open-label extension study indicate that therapy for 12 months or longer is associated with sustained improvement in wakefulness in patients with this condition. The manufacturer states that when armodafinil is used for extended periods, the need for continued therapy should be reassessed periodically.

■ **Shift Work Sleep Disorder** Armodafinil is used in the symptomatic treatment of SWSD to improve wakefulness in adults with excessive sleepiness. Shift work sleep disorder is a subtype of circadian rhythm sleep disorder in which a nonstandard work schedule (e.g., late night, early morning, or rotating shift work) leads to development of sleep disturbances and impairment of alertness and performance while awake.

Efficacy of armodafinil in reducing excessive sleepiness associated with SWSD was demonstrated in a 12-week, multicenter, double-blind, placebo-controlled, parallel-group study in 254 adults with chronic SWSD (who met the ICSD criteria, which are consistent with DSM-IV criteria for circadian rhythm sleep disorder: shift work type). Such criteria require a primary complaint of excessive sleepiness or insomnia that is temporally associated with a work period (usually night work) that occurs during the habitual sleep phase or loss of a normal sleep-wake pattern (i.e., disturbed chronobiological rhythmicity) as demonstrated on polysomnography and the MSLT and that the manifestations are not accounted for by another medical or mental disorder and do not meet criteria for any other sleep disorder that produces insomnia or excessive sleepiness (e.g., time zone change [jet lag] syndrome). Not all patients engaged in shift work who complain of sleepiness meet the criteria for the diagnosis of SWSD; only patients who were symptomatic for at least 3 months were enrolled in this study. Patients enrolled in this study were also required to work a minimum of 5 night shifts per month, have excessive sleepiness at the time of their night shifts (MSLT score of 6 minutes or less), and have daytime insomnia documented by a daytime polysomnogram. Patients who were treated with armodafinil (150 mg daily before each work shift) demonstrated a significant prolongation of the time to sleep onset (as measured by the nighttime MSLT at the final visit) compared with those receiving placebo (mean sleep latency increased by 3 versus 0.4 minutes, respectively). In addition, a substantially greater proportion of armodafinil-treated patients showed an improvement in overall clinical status as measured by CGI-C scores compared with those who received placebo. Despite these improvements, a proportion of patients who received active treatment in this study continued to have residual sleepiness, suggesting that armodafinil 150 mg daily may not be equally effective in all patients with SWSD. (See Persistent Sleepiness under Warnings/Precautions: Warnings, in Cautions.) Use of armodafinil did not adversely affect daytime sleep variables (e.g., sleep latency, sleep duration, sleep-stage distribution) as measured by polysomnography in this study.

Although the manufacturer states that the long-term efficacy (e.g., longer than 12 weeks) of armodafinil in patients with SWSD has not been systematically evaluated in placebo-controlled studies to date, preliminary findings from a flexible-dosage, open-label extension study indicate that therapy for 12 months or longer is associated with sustained improvement in wakefulness in patients with this condition. The manufacturer states that when armodafinil is used for extended periods, the need for continued therapy should be reassessed periodically.

Dosage and Administration

■ **Administration** Armodafinil is administered orally. In patients with obstructive sleep apnea/hypopnea syndrome (OSAHS) or narcolepsy, armodafinil usually is administered once daily in the morning. In patients with shift work sleep disorder (SWSD), armodafinil should be taken approximately 1 hour prior to the start of their work shift.

The manufacturer makes no specific recommendations regarding administration of armodafinil with regard to meals. Although the effect of food on the overall bioavailability of armodafinil is considered minimal, time to reach peak plasma concentrations may be delayed by approximately 2–4 hours when the drug is administered with food and result in elevated plasma concentrations later than when the drug is administered without food. Such changes may potentially affect the onset and time course of armodafinil's pharmacologic effects.

■ **Dosage** The usual recommended dosage of armodafinil to improve wakefulness in adults and adolescents 17 years of age and older with excessive sleepiness associated with OSAHS or narcolepsy is 150 or 250 mg daily. Although dosages up to 250 mg daily have been well tolerated in patients with OSAHS, there is no consistent evidence indicating that this dosage provides additional clinical benefit beyond that provided by the 150-mg daily dosage.

The usual recommended dosage of armodafinil to improve wakefulness in adults and adolescents 17 years of age and older with SWSD is 150 mg daily.

Although the long-term efficacy (i.e., longer than 12 weeks) of armodafinil has not been systematically evaluated in controlled trials to date, the drug has demonstrated efficacy over a period of 12 months or more in maintaining wakefulness in patients with OSAHS, narcolepsy, or SWSD in an open-label extension study. Clinicians who elect to prescribe armodafinil for an extended period should periodically reevaluate the long-term usefulness of the drug for the individual patient.

■ **Special Populations** Dosage of armodafinil should be reduced in patients with severe hepatic impairment, with or without cirrhosis, because of the possibility of reduced clearance of the drug. (See Hepatic Impairment under Warnings/Precautions: Specific Populations, in Cautions.)

The manufacturer states that there is not sufficient information to determine the safety and efficacy of armodafinil dosing in patients with severe renal impairment. (See Renal Impairment under Warnings/Precautions: Specific Populations, in Cautions.)

Because elimination of armodafinil and its metabolites may be reduced with age in geriatric patients, consideration should be given to using dosages lower than the usual recommended dosages in this age group. (See Geriatric Use under Warnings/Precautions: Specific Populations, in Cautions.)

Cautions

■ **Contraindications** Known hypersensitivity to armodafinil, modafinil, or any ingredient in the formulation.

■ **Warnings/Precautions** *Warnings* **Serious Dermatologic Reactions.** Serious rash (including Stevens-Johnson syndrome [SJS]) requiring hospitalization and drug discontinuance has been reported in adults receiving armodafinil and in adults and pediatric patients receiving modafinil. Rare cases of serious or life-threatening rash, including SJS, toxic epidermal necrolysis (TEN), and drug rash with eosinophilia and systemic symptoms (DRESS), have been reported in adults and pediatric patients during worldwide postmarketing experience with modafinil. Severe rashes, including 1 case of possible SJS and 1 case of multi-organ hypersensitivity reaction also were observed in modafinil clinical trials in pediatric patients younger than 17 years of age; several of these cases were associated with fever and other abnormalities (e.g., vomiting, leukopenia). Because armodafinil is the *R*-enantiomer of racemic modafinil, the manufacturer states that a similar risk of serious rash in pediatric patients receiving armodafinil cannot be ruled out. Armodafinil is *not* FDA-labeled for use in pediatric patients for any indication. (See Pediatric Use under Warnings/Precautions: Specific Populations, in Cautions.)

No risk factors are known to predict the occurrence or severity of rash associated with armodafinil or modafinil. Nearly all the cases of serious rash occurred within 1–5 weeks following initiation of therapy with either drug; however, isolated cases have presented after prolonged treatment (e.g., 3 months) with modafinil. Accordingly, duration of therapy cannot be used to predict the potential risk associated with the first appearance of a rash. Although benign rashes also occur with armodafinil, it is not possible to predict which rashes will become serious; therefore, the drug should ordinarily be discontinued at the first sign of a rash unless the rash is clearly not drug related. (See Advice to Patients.) However, treatment discontinuance may not prevent a rash from becoming life-threatening or permanently disabling or disfiguring.

Angioedema and Anaphylactoid Reactions. One serious case of angioedema and 1 case of hypersensitivity (with rash, dysphagia, and bronchospasm) were reported among 1,595 patients treated with armodafinil in clinical studies. Patients should be advised to discontinue therapy and immediately report to their clinician any signs or symptoms suggestive of angioedema or anaphylaxis (e.g., swelling of face, eyes, lips, tongue, or larynx; difficulty swallowing or breathing; hoarseness). (See Advice to Patients.)

Multiorgan Hypersensitivity Reactions. Multiorgan hypersensitivity reactions, including at least one fatality during postmarketing experience, have been reported with modafinil. Because armodafinil is closely related to modafinil, a similar risk with armodafinil cannot be ruled out. The multiorgan hypersensitivity reactions occurred in close temporal association (median time to detection: 13 days; range: 4–33 days) with initiation of modafinil therapy. Although there have been only a limited number of cases reported to date, such reactions may result in hospitalization or be life-threatening. Although the clinical presentation of such reactions is variable, patients typically presented with fever and rash associated with other organ system involvement; other manifestations included myocarditis, hepatitis, liver function test abnormalities, hematologic abnormalities (e.g., eosinophilia, leukopenia, thrombocytopenia), pruritus, and asthenia. No risk factors are known to predict the risk of occurrence or severity of modafinil-associated multiorgan hypersensitivity reactions.

If a multiorgan hypersensitivity reaction is suspected, armodafinil should be discontinued. Although there are no reports of cross-sensitivity with other drugs that produce this syndrome, the potential for cross-sensitivity exists.

Persistent Sleepiness. Patients who have abnormal levels of sleepiness and are receiving armodafinil should be advised that the drug has been shown to improve, but *not* to eliminate, this abnormal tendency to fall asleep. (See Advice to Patients.)

All patients with excessive sleepiness, including those receiving armodafinil, should be frequently reassessed for their degree of sleepiness and, if appropriate, advised to avoid driving or any other potentially dangerous activity. Clinicians should be aware that patients may not acknowledge sleepiness or drowsiness until directly questioned about these symptoms during specific activities.

Psychiatric Effects. Adverse psychiatric effects have been reported in patients receiving modafinil. Because modafinil and armodafinil are closely related, the incidence and type of psychiatric effects are expected to be similar. Postmarketing adverse psychiatric effects associated with modafinil include mania, delusions, hallucinations, suicidal ideation, and aggression and have resulted in hospitalization in some cases. Many, but not all, of the patients had a prior psychiatric history. In the controlled clinical trial database for armodafinil, psychiatric symptoms requiring treatment discontinuance more often in armodafinil-treated patients than in placebo recipients included anxiety, agitation, nervousness, and irritability. Depression also required treatment discontinuance in controlled clinical trials more often in armodafinil-treated patients compared with those receiving placebo; 2 cases of suicidal ideation were observed in these trials.

The manufacturer states that armodafinil should be used with caution in patients with a history of psychosis, depression, or mania. Some clinicians also recommend careful monitoring of patients receiving therapy with armodafinil or other CNS stimulants for possible psychiatric effects. If psychiatric symptoms develop in patients receiving armodafinil, discontinuance of the drug should be considered. (See Advice to Patients.)

General Precautions

Diagnosis of Sleep Disorders. The manufacturer states that armodafinil should be used only in patients who have had a complete evaluation of their excessive sleepiness and in whom a diagnosis of narcolepsy, obstructive sleep apnea/hypopnea syndrome (OSAHS), and/or shift work sleep disorder (SWSD) has been made in accordance with the International Classification of Sleep Disorders (ICSD) or DSM diagnostic criteria. Such an evaluation usually consists of a complete history and physical examination, which may be supplemented with testing in a laboratory setting (e.g., polysomnography). Clinicians should be aware that some patients may have more than one sleep disorder contributing to their daytime sleepiness (e.g., OSAHS and SWSD concurrently in the same patient).

Continuous Positive Airway Pressure in OSAHS. In OSAHS, armodafinil is indicated as an adjunct to standard treatment(s) for the underlying obstruction. If continuous positive airway pressure (CPAP) is the treatment of choice for a patient, a maximal effort should be made to treat with CPAP for an adequate period of time prior to initiating armodafinil therapy. In clinical trials of armodafinil, there was a slight trend for reduced CPAP use over time in the armodafinil-treated patients compared with those receiving placebo. If armodafinil is used adjunctively with CPAP, the encouragement of and periodic assessment of CPAP compliance is necessary. (See Advice to Patients.)

Cognitive/Psychomotor Impairment. Although armodafinil has not been shown to cause functional impairment, the possibility that the drug, like any other drug affecting the CNS, may alter judgment, thinking, or motor skills should be considered. Patients should be cautioned about operating an automobile or other hazardous machinery until they are reasonably certain that armodafinil will not adversely affect their ability to engage in such activities.

Cardiovascular Effects. In clinical studies with modafinil, a few patients have experienced adverse cardiovascular effects such as chest pain, palpitations, dyspnea, and transient ischemic T-wave changes in association with mitral valve prolapse or left ventricular hypertrophy. The manufacturer recommends that armodafinil *not* be used in patients with a history of left ventricular hypertrophy or in patients with mitral valve prolapse who have experienced the mitral valve prolapse syndrome with previous use of CNS stimulants. Clinical manifestations of mitral valve prolapse syndrome include, but are not limited to, ischemic ECG changes, chest pain, or arrhythmia. If new onset of any of these symptoms occurs during armodafinil therapy, a cardiac evaluation should be considered.

Armodafinil should be used with caution in patients with a recent history of myocardial infarction or unstable angina since the drug has not been evaluated or used to any appreciable extent in such patients.

In short-term (i.e., 3 months or less) clinical studies, small average increases in mean systolic and diastolic blood pressure were observed in patients receiving armodafinil compared with placebo. In these studies, new or increased use of antihypertensive agents was observed in a slightly greater proportion of patients receiving armodafinil (2.9%) compared with those receiving placebo (1.8%). The manufacturer states that increased monitoring of blood pressure may be appropriate during armodafinil therapy.

Abuse and Misuse Potential. The abuse potential with armodafinil has not been specifically studied to date, but is expected to be similar to that of modafinil. Modafinil produces psychoactive and euphoric effects and alterations in mood, perception, thinking, and feelings similar to those observed with other CNS stimulants (e.g., amphetamines, methylphenidate). (See Description.) However, because of evidence indicating that the risk of abuse or misuse of modafinil is lower than that associated with CNS stimulants that are subject to control as schedule II drugs (e.g., amphetamine, methylphenidate), armodafinil and modafinil are subject to control as schedule IV drugs.

The manufacturer states that patients should be closely followed during armodafinil therapy for possible signs of misuse or abuse (e.g., incrementation of doses, drug-seeking behavior), particularly in those with a history of drug or stimulant abuse (e.g., amphetamine, cocaine, methylphenidate).

Contraceptive Precautions. Efficacy of hormonal contraceptives may be reduced during and for 1 month after discontinuance of armodafinil therapy. Patients using such contraceptives should be advised to use alternative or concomitant methods of contraception during these periods. (See Hormonal Contraceptives under Drug Interactions: Drugs Affecting or Metabolized by Hepatic Microsomal Enzymes and see Advice to Patients.)

Drug Interaction with Cyclosporine. Cyclosporine blood concentrations may be reduced when cyclosporine is given concurrently with armodafinil. (See Drug Interactions: Drugs Affecting or Metabolized by Hepatic Microsomal Enzymes.)

Specific Populations

Pregnancy. Category C. (See Users Guide.)

Women of childbearing potential should be advised of possible hormonal contraceptive failure (i.e., increased risk of pregnancy) during and for 1 month after armodafinil use. (See Contraceptive Precautions under Warnings/Precautions: General Precautions, under Cautions and see Advice to Patients.)

The effect of armodafinil on labor and delivery is unknown.

Lactation. It is not known whether armodafinil or its metabolites are distributed into milk. Caution should be exercised when armodafinil is used in nursing women.

Pediatric Use. Armodafinil is not approved for use in pediatric patients for *any* indication. Safety and efficacy of the drug have not been established in children younger than 17 years of age.

Modafinil, a drug closely related to armodafinil, has been studied in children and adolescents with attention deficit hyperactivity disorder (ADHD)† in several controlled trials; however, the drug currently is *not* approved for treating ADHD or for use in pediatric patients with any other condition. In a controlled study of 6 weeks' duration, 165 pediatric patients (5–17 years of age) with narcolepsy were treated with modafinil or placebo. The results did not demonstrate a statistically significant difference favoring modafinil over placebo in prolonging sleep latency (as measured by the Multiple Sleep Latency Test [MSLT]) or in perceptions of sleepiness (as determined by the Clinical Global Impression of Change [CGI-C] score).

Serious rashes, including erythema multiforme and Stevens-Johnson syndrome, have been associated with use of modafinil in pediatric patients. (See Serious Dermatologic Reactions under Warnings/Precautions: Warnings, in Cautions.)

Geriatric Use. Safety and efficacy of armodafinil have not been established in geriatric patients older than 65 years of age.

Elimination of armodafinil and its metabolites may be reduced in geriatric patients. Therefore, the manufacturer states that the use of reduced armodafinil dosages should be considered in geriatric patients. (See Dosage and Administration: Special Populations.)

Renal Impairment. There is inadequate information to determine safety and efficacy of armodafinil dosing in patients with severe renal impairment. In a single-dose study with racemic modafinil, severe chronic renal impairment (creatinine clearance of 20 mL/minute or less) did not substantially affect the pharmacokinetics of modafinil, but increased exposure to modafinil acid (a metabolite of the drug) by ninefold.

Hepatic Impairment. Information specific to armodafinil use in patients with hepatic impairment is not available. In patients with severe hepatic impairment and cirrhosis (Child-Pugh class B, B+, C, or C+) receiving modafinil, clearance of the drug was decreased by 60% and steady-state concentrations were doubled. Reduced dosages of armodafinil are therefore recommended in patients with severe hepatic impairment, with or without cirrhosis. (See Dosage and Administration: Special Populations.)

■ Common Adverse Effects

Adverse effects reported in 5% or more of patients receiving armodafinil in clinical trials and more frequently than with placebo include headache, nausea, dizziness, and insomnia. Although armodafinil generally was well tolerated, 7% of patients in placebo-controlled trials discontinued the drug because of adverse effects; the most frequent reason for drug discontinuance was headache (1% of patients).

Drug Interactions

■ **Drugs Affecting or Metabolized by Hepatic Microsomal Enzymes** Potent inducers (e.g., carbamazepine, phenobarbital, rifampin) or inhibitors (e.g., erythromycin, ketoconazole, itraconazole) of cytochrome P-450 (CYP) 3A isoenzymes can potentially alter plasma concentrations of armodafinil because of partial involvement of these enzymes in the drug's metabolism.

In vitro studies indicate that armodafinil is a weak inducer of CYP1A2 and possibly CYP3A, and a reversible inhibitor of CYP2C19. In vitro data also demonstrate that armodafinil is a substrate of the efflux transporter P-glycoprotein. In clinical interaction studies in healthy individuals, chronic administration of armodafinil moderately induced the activity of CYP3A4; therefore, dosage adjustments of CYP3A4/5 substrates (e.g., cyclosporine, ethinyl estradiol, midazolam, triazolam) may be necessary when such drugs are used concomitantly with armodafinil.

Because armodafinil was shown in healthy individuals to moderately inhibit CYP2C19 activity, reduced dosages of some drugs that are CYP2C19 substrates (e.g., clomipramine, diazepam, phenytoin, propranolol, omeprazole) and monitoring for toxicity may be necessary when such drugs are administered concomitantly with armodafinil.

Chronic administration of armodafinil did not affect the pharmacokinetics of caffeine (a probe substrate of CYP1A2 induction activity) in healthy individuals despite results of in vitro studies.

Cyclosporine Blood concentrations of cyclosporine (a CYP3A4/5 substrate) may be reduced when cyclosporine is given concomitantly with armodafinil, which may reduce the effectiveness of the immunosuppressive agent. Monitoring of cyclosporine concentrations and appropriate cyclosporine dosage adjustments should be considered when these drugs are used concomitantly.

Hormonal Contraceptives The possibility of decreased plasma concentrations of ethinyl estradiol secondary to induction of CYP3A4 by armodafinil resulting in decreased efficacy of hormonal contraceptives and possible contraceptive failure should be considered. Women of childbearing potential should be advised to use an alternative or concomitant method of contraception during and for 1 month following discontinuance of armodafinil therapy. (See Contraceptive Precautions under Warnings/Precautions: General Precautions, in Cautions and see Advice to Patients.)

Midazolam Following administration of single oral (5 mg) and IV (2 mg) doses of midazolam in healthy individuals receiving armodafinil 250 mg daily, systemic exposure to midazolam was reduced by approximately 32 and 17%, respectively. Concurrent administration of the drugs was generally well tolerated. Dosage adjustment of midazolam may be necessary when used concomitantly with armodafinil.

Omeprazole Concomitant administration of a single oral dose of armodafinil (400 mg) and omeprazole (40 mg), a CYP2C19 substrate, increased systemic exposure to omeprazole by approximately 40% compared with administration of omeprazole alone. Concurrent administration of the drugs was generally well tolerated. Dosage reduction of omeprazole and other CYP2C19 substrates may be necessary when these drugs are used concomitantly.

Tricyclic Antidepressants Because armodafinil appears to moderately inhibit CYP2C19 activity, the manufacturer states that a reduced dosage of clomipramine, a CYP2C19 substrate, and monitoring for toxicity may be necessary when clomipramine is administered concomitantly with armodafinil.

■ **Protein-bound Drugs** Because armodafinil is not highly bound to plasma proteins, a pharmacokinetic interaction with drugs that are highly protein bound is considered unlikely.

■ **Alcohol** Concomitant use of armodafinil with alcohol has not been evaluated and is not recommended.

■ **Amphetamines** Specific drug interaction studies have not been conducted with armodafinil and amphetamines; however, the manufacturer states that available drug interaction information with modafinil should also apply to armodafinil. In a single-dose study in healthy individuals, concomitant administration of a single 200-mg modafinil dose and a 10-mg dextroamphetamine dose did not produce a clinically important pharmacokinetic interaction with either drug. However, the absorption of modafinil was delayed by approximately 1 hour when these drugs were given concurrently in this study. In a subsequent study in healthy individuals, the steady-state pharmacokinetics of modafinil (200 mg daily for 7 days followed by 400 mg daily for 21 days) were not significantly affected by chronic administration of a 20-mg dose of dextroamphetamine given in the afternoon; the adverse event profile of these drugs administered concurrently was similar to that of modafinil alone.

■ **Caffeine** Chronic armodafinil administration (250 mg) did not affect the pharmacokinetics of caffeine, which is a probe substrate for CYP1A2 activity.

■ **Methylphenidate** Specific drug interaction studies have not been conducted with armodafinil and methylphenidate; however, the manufacturer states that available drug interaction information with modafinil should also apply to armodafinil. In a single-dose study in healthy individuals, concomitant administration of a single 200-mg dose of modafinil and a 40-mg dose of methylphenidate did not significantly alter the pharmacokinetics of either drug. GI absorption of modafinil was delayed by approximately 1 hour; however, the extent of absorption was not affected. In a multiple-dose study in healthy individuals, concomitant administration of methylphenidate 20 mg daily and modafinil (200 mg daily for 7 days followed by 400 mg daily for 21 days) did not significantly alter the pharmacokinetics of modafinil. Therefore, a clinically important pharmacokinetic interaction between these drugs seems unlikely.

■ **Monoamine Oxidase Inhibitors** One case of acute chorea, confusion, and hyperthermia (possibly related to serotonin syndrome) has been reported with concurrent modafinil and tranylcypromine administration. Because drug interaction studies have not been performed with monoamine oxidase (MAO) inhibitors and either armodafinil or modafinil, caution is advised when these drugs are administered concomitantly.

■ **Other CNS-active Drugs** Specific drug interaction studies have not been conducted with armodafinil and many CNS-active drugs; however, the manufacturer states that available drug interaction information with modafinil should also apply to armodafinil.

■ **Warfarin** In a study performed in healthy individuals, chronic administration of racemic modafinil did not substantially alter the single-dose pharmacokinetics of warfarin when compared with placebo. However, a potential pharmacodynamic interaction cannot be ruled out with multiple-dose administration. Pending further evaluation of this potential interaction, more frequent monitoring of prothrombin time and/or international normalized ratio (INR) is recommended whenever armodafinil and warfarin are given concurrently.

Description

Armodafinil is a non-amphetamine wakefulness-promoting agent. The drug is the *R*-enantiomer of modafinil, which is a racemic compound containing equal amounts of the *R*- and *S*- isomers. Both armodafinil and modafinil are benzhydrylsulfinylacetamides. Armodafinil is the longer-lasting *R*-isomer of modafinil, having a half-life approximately 3–4 times longer than that of *S*-modafinil. Both armodafinil and modafinil have similar pharmacologic properties; however, armodafinil has been shown to produce consistently higher plasma drug concentrations later in the day than modafinil. In a randomized controlled study in healthy male volunteers, administration of a single dose of armodafinil 200 mg produced comparable peak plasma concentrations but higher plasma drug concentrations 6–14 hours postdose compared with modafinil 200 mg; such findings were associated with longer wakefulness-promoting and attention-sustaining effects in individuals receiving armodafinil versus modafinil. Results of pooled analyses of pharmacokinetic data from several randomized studies in healthy individuals who received single or multiple doses of armodafinil or modafinil also demonstrated consistently higher plasma concentrations with armodafinil later in the dosing period relative to modafinil when the drugs were compared on a milligram-to-milligram basis. Further studies are needed to determine whether these pharmacokinetic differences result in an improved clinical response with armodafinil compared with modafinil.

The exact mechanism by which armodafinil and modafinil promote wakefulness is not known, but may involve activation of certain arousal centers of the brain (e.g., hypothalamus, prefrontal cortex, anterior cingulate cortex). At pharmacologically relevant concentrations, armodafinil does not bind to or inhibit certain receptors and enzymes, including those for serotonin, dopamine, adenosine, galanin, melatonin, melanocortin, orexin-1, orphanin, pituitary adenylate cyclase-activating polypeptide (PACAP) or benzodiazepines; transporters for γ-aminobutyric acid (GABA), serotonin, norepinephrine, or choline; or phosphodiesterase VI, catechol-O-methyl transferase (COMT), GABA transaminase, or tyrosine hydroxylase, potentially involved in the regulation of sleep and wakefulness. Unlike traditional sympathomimetic CNS stimulants, the manufacturer states that armodafinil does not appear to be a direct- or indirect-acting dopamine-receptor agonist, but has been shown in in vitro studies to bind to the dopamine transporter and inhibit dopamine reuptake. Such inhibitory effects have been associated with increased extracellular dopamine concentrations in animal models. Modafinil was also found to block dopamine transporters and increase dopamine concentrations in the human brain (including the nucleus accumbens) in one pilot study; such drugs generally have abuse potential. (See Abuse and Misuse Potential under Warnings/Precautions: General Precautions, in Cautions.) The stimulant effects of modafinil can be attenuated by the α_1-adrenergic receptor antagonist prazosin, but modafinil is inactive in other assay systems known to be responsive to α_1-adrenergic receptor agonists.

Armodafinil is classified under the Federal Controlled Substances Act as a schedule IV drug. Although the abuse potential of armodafinil has not been specifically evaluated, it is expected to be similar to that of modafinil. Like other CNS stimulants, modafinil is reinforcing in animals and produces psychoactive (e.g., alterations in mood and thinking), euphoric, and subjective effects typical of classic CNS stimulants (e.g., amphetamines, methylphenidate) in humans. Despite pharmacologic similarity to such stimulants, the physical or chemical properties of modafinil (e.g., not water soluble, decomposes in heat) may limit its abuse potential. In addition, there are substantial differences in relative potency between modafinil and schedule II CNS stimulants. These differences reduce the likelihood that modafinil could be abused by the parenteral, intranasal, or inhalation route, as are cocaine, methylphenidate, and amphetamine. Because of the lower potential for abuse, modafinil and armodafinil are subject to control as schedule IV rather than schedule II drugs. (See Abuse and Misuse Potential under Warnings/Precautions: General Precautions, in Cautions.)

The active component of Nuvigil® is armodafinil, which is the longer-acting enantiomer of modafinil. Armodafinil is readily absorbed following oral administration, with peak plasma concentrations occurring at approximately 2 hours in the fasted state. The effect of food on the overall bioavailability of armodafinil appears minimal, but time to achieve peak concentrations may be delayed by approximately 2–4 hours in the fed state. Armodafinil exhibits linear pharmacokinetics following administration of single or multiple oral doses of the drug over the dosage range of 50–400 mg. Steady-state plasma concentrations of armodafinil are achieved within 7 days of daily administration, and the mean elimination half-life of the drug is approximately 15 hours. Armodafinil undergoes hydrolytic deamidation, S-oxidation, and aromatic ring hydroxylation, with subsequent glucuronide conjugation of the hydroxylated products. The 2 principal metabolites (*R*-modafinil acid and modafinil sulfone) of armodafinil or modafinil do not appear to contribute to the CNS-activating properties of the parent compounds. Although the metabolic fate of armodafinil has not been specifically studied, racemic modafinil is mainly eliminated via metabolism, predominantly in the liver, with 80% of the drug excreted in urine and 1% in feces, mainly as metabolites.

Advice to Patients

Importance of reading patient information leaflet provided by the manufacturer prior to initiating therapy.

Importance of advising clinician of existing or contemplated therapy, including prescription and OTC drugs and/or herbal supplements, as well as any concomitant illnesses. Advise patient that it is prudent to avoid alcohol while taking armodafinil since combined use has not been studied.

Importance of advising patients about the potential increased risk of pregnancy in women taking hormonal contraceptives (including oral contraceptives, injectable or implantable contraceptives, transdermal systems, vaginal rings, and intrauterine devices) during and for 1 month after discontinuing armodafinil therapy; discuss use of alternative or concomitant methods of contraception with patient. (See Contraceptive Precautions under Warnings/Precautions: General Precautions, in Cautions.) Importance of informing clinician if patient is or plans to become pregnant or plans to breast-feed.

Risk of serious rash or serious allergic reaction. Importance of advising patient to immediately discontinue armodafinil and notify their clinician if they develop a rash or other manifestations of an allergic reaction (e.g., hives, mouth sores, blisters, peeling skin, difficulty swallowing or breathing, a related allergic phenomenon).

Risk of mental (psychiatric) symptoms. Importance of discontinuing armodafinil and informing clinician if depression, anxiety, hallucinations, mania, suicidal thoughts, aggression, or other psychiatric symptoms associated with psychosis or mania occur.

Risk of heart problems. Importance of discontinuing armodafinil and informing clinician if heart problems, including chest pain, occur.

Importance of advising patient that armodafinil may affect judgment, thinking, or motor skills. Importance of using caution when operating machinery or driving a motor vehicle until effects of the drug are known.

Importance of advising patient that armodafinil may improve, but not eliminate, the abnormal tendency to fall asleep. Advise against altering previous behavior with regard to potentially dangerous activities (e.g., driving, operating machinery) or other activities requiring appropriate levels of wakefulness until and unless armodafinil has been shown to produce levels of wakefulness that permit such activities. Patients should be advised that armodafinil is *not* a replacement for sleep.

Importance of continuing previously prescribed therapy (e.g., advising patients with obstructive sleep apnea/hypopnea syndrome [OSAHS] that armodafinil is used along with other medical therapies for this condition and that the drug is not a replacement for the continuous positive airway pressure [CPAP] machine). Importance of advising patients with OSAHS to continue using their CPAP machine while sleeping.

Importance of informing patient of other important precautionary information. (See Cautions.)

Overview (see Users Guide). For additional information until a more detailed monograph is developed and published, the manufacturer's labeling should be consulted. It is *essential* that the manufacturer's labeling be consulted for more detailed information on the usual cautions, precautions, and contraindications, potential drug interactions, laboratory test interferences, and acute toxicity.

Preparations

Armodafinil is subject to control under the Federal Controlled Substances Act of 1970 as a schedule IV (C-IV) drug.

Excipients in commercially available drug preparations may have clinically important effects in some individuals; consult specific product labeling for details.

Armodafinil

Oral

Tablets	50 mg	**Nuvigil**® (C-IV), Cephalon
	150 mg	**Nuvigil**® (C-IV), Cephalon
	250 mg	**Nuvigil**® (C-IV), Cephalon

†Use is not currently included in the labeling approved by the US Food and Drug Administration

Modafinil

■ Modafinil is a wakefulness-promoting agent that is structurally and pharmacologically distinct from most other currently available CNS stimulants. The drug is a 50:50 racemic mixture of the *R*- and *S*-enantiomers; the *R*-enantiomer of modafinil is also commercially available as armodafinil.

Uses

Modafinil is used orally to improve wakefulness in adults with excessive sleepiness associated with narcolepsy, obstructive sleep apnea/hypopnea syndrome (OSAHS), and shift work sleep disorder (SWSD). Careful attention to the diagnosis and treatment of the underlying sleep disorder is essential whenever modafinil is used in patients with these conditions. (See Diagnosis of Sleep Disorders under Warnings/Precautions: General Precautions, in Cautions.)

■ **Narcolepsy** Modafinil is used in the symptomatic treatment of narcolepsy to improve wakefulness in adults with excessive daytime sleepiness (EDS). Narcolepsy is a CNS disorder characterized by somnolence, often accompanied by sudden attacks of weakness (cataplexy) while awake and disrupted nocturnal sleep, and occasionally by hypnagogic hallucinations and/or sleep paralysis before falling asleep or awakening. The disorder involves dysregulation of wakefulness and sleep.

Efficacy of modafinil has been established in the US in 2 double-blind, multicenter, placebo-controlled clinical trials of 9 weeks' duration. In these and other clinical studies, modafinil 200 or 400 mg daily increased daytime wakefulness and alertness and decreased the number of daytime sleep episodes as determined by several objective (e.g., the Multiple Sleep Latency Test [MSLT], the Maintenance of Wakefulness Test [MWT], the Steer Clear Performance Test [SCPT]) and subjective (e.g., the Epworth Sleepiness Scale [ESS]) measures of sleepiness. Patients showed an enhanced ability to remain awake with both dosages relative to placebo at 3, 6, and 9 weeks, and at study end point (last post-baseline assessment while the patient was in the study) and also greater global improvement in overall disease status (measured by the Clinical Global Impression of Change [CGI-C]). However, despite the clinical improvement, mean objective and subjective measures of sleepiness did not completely normalize with modafinil therapy, with a degree of clinically important physiologic sleepiness persisting despite therapy. The percentage of patients exhibiting any degree of improvement in overall disease status on the CGI-C in the two 9-week studies establishing efficacy in the US was 60–72, 58–64, or 37–38% for the 400-mg regimen, 200-mg regimen, or placebo, respectively. The efficacy of the 2 modafinil dosage regimens was not shown to differ significantly in these studies.

Although the long-term efficacy of modafinil has not been established systematically beyond 9 weeks, improvements in overall disease status on the CGI-C and in subjective measures of sleepiness on the ESS were maintained in a 40-week open-label extension of one of the trials. In this open-label extension, the percentage of patients exhibiting improvement on the CGI-C ranged from 84% after 2 weeks of extension therapy to 91% after 40 weeks. The drug also was well tolerated for up to 40 weeks of therapy, with 11% of patients discontinuing modafinil because of adverse effects and 14% because of inadequate therapeutic effect. Although most patients enrolled in the 2 clinical trials establishing efficacy in the US had histories of cataplexy, those requiring anticataplectic therapy generally were excluded from enrollment. Therefore, current evidence of efficacy for modafinil is limited principally to effects on excessive daytime sleepiness. In one study in a limited number of patients, cataplexy was not affected by modafinil therapy.

Modafinil did not affect the initiation, maintenance, quality, or quantity of nighttime sleep and did not affect the ability to voluntarily sleep (nap) during the daytime. Like other CNS stimulants modafinil can alter mood, perception, thinking, and feelings and can cause psychoactive and euphoric effects. However, in clinical trials, there was no clinically important association between modafanil and the incidence of agitation in patients. In animals, modafinil is reinforcing; however, the somatic effects of the drug were comparable to those of caffeine and differed from those of amphetamine. Although current evidence indicates that the risk of abuse or misuse of modafinil is lower than that associated with some other CNS stimulants (e.g., amphetamines, methylphenidate), caution is recommended in patients with a history of drug or stimulant abuse. Withdrawal of modafinil has not been associated with any manifestations of dependency.

■ **Obstructive Sleep Apnea/Hypopnea Syndrome** Modafinil is used in the symptomatic treatment of OSAHS to improve wakefulness in adults with excessive sleepiness. The drug should be used as an adjunct to standard treatment(s) for the underlying obstruction (e.g., nasal continuous positive airway pressure [CPAP]). If CPAP is considered the treatment of choice for a patient with OSAHS, every effort should be made to optimize CPAP treatment for an adequate period of time prior to initiating modafinil therapy. When modafinil is used adjunctively with CPAP treatment, the encouragement of and periodic assessment of CPAP compliance is necessary.

Efficacy of modafinil in reducing excessive daytime sleepiness in patients with OSAHS was established principally in 2 multicenter, placebo-controlled clinical trials. In both of these studies, enrolled patients met the International Classification of Sleep Disorders (ICSD) criteria for OSAHS, which also are consistent with DSM-IV criteria. These criteria include either excessive sleepiness or insomnia with frequent episodes of impaired breathing during sleep and associated features (e.g., loud snoring, morning headaches, dry mouth upon awakening) or polysomnography demonstrating more than 5 obstructive apneic episodes (each greater than 10 seconds in duration) per hour of sleep and one or more of the following: frequent arousals from sleep associated with the apneic episodes; bradytachycardia; and arterial oxygen desaturation in association with the apneic episodes. In addition, all patients enrolled in these studies had excessive daytime sleepiness as demonstrated by a score of 10 or higher on the Epworth Sleepiness Scale (ESS) despite treatment with CPAP. Evidence that CPAP was effective in reducing the episodes of apnea/hypopnea also was required along with documentation of CPAP use.

In the first multicenter, placebo-controlled study, which was of 12 weeks' duration, patients were randomized to receive modafinil 200 mg daily, modafinil 400 mg daily, or placebo. The majority of patients (80%) in this study were fully compliant with CPAP (defined as CPAP use for more than 4 hours per night on more than 70% of nights); the remainder of patients were partially CPAP compliant (defined as CPAP use for less than 4 hours per night on more than 30% of nights). Efficacy of modafinil was principally evaluated by measurement of sleep latency as assessed by the Maintenance of Wakefulness Test (MWT) and change in the patient's overall disease status as measured by the Clinical Global Impression of Change (CGI-C) at week 12 or at the final visit. The modafinil-treated patients demonstrated a significant improvement in their ability to remain awake as measured by the MWT at the study end point and in their clinical condition as measured by the CGI-C compared with those receiving placebo. The 200- and 400-mg daily doses produced similar clinical efficacy in this study.

In the second multicenter, placebo-controlled study, which was of 4 weeks' duration, patients were randomized to receive either modafinil 400 mg daily or placebo. Documentation of regular CPAP use (for at least 4 hours each night on 70% of nights) was required for all patients. Efficacy in reducing daytime sleepiness was principally assessed by the change from baseline on the ESS at week 4 or the final visit. Patients who received modafinil demonstrated a significant reduction in their ESS score from baseline (mean scores reduced by 4.6) compared with patients receiving placebo (mean scores reduced by 2). In addition, the percentage of patients with normalized daytime sleepiness (ESS score less than 10) was significantly higher for the modafinil group than for those receiving placebo (51 and 27%, respectively). Nighttime sleep as measured by polysomnography was not affected by modafinil administration in these 2 studies.

The manufacturer states that the long-term efficacy (e.g., longer than 12 weeks) of modafinil in OSAHS has not been systematically evaluated in placebo-controlled studies to date. However, a 12-month, noncomparative extension phase of the 12-week, placebo-controlled trial in which patients received modafinil 200, 300, or 400 mg daily demonstrated substantial reductions in ESS scores compared with baseline following 3, 6, 9, and 12 months of therapy. When modafinil is used for extended periods, the need for continued therapy should be reassessed periodically.

■ Shift Work Sleep Disorder Modafinil is used in the symptomatic treatment of SWSD to improve wakefulness in adults with excessive sleepiness. Criteria of the International Classification of Sleep Disorders (ICSD-10) for chronic SWSD (which are consistent with DSM-IV criteria for circadian rhythm sleep disorder: shift work type) require a primary complaint of excessive sleepiness or insomnia that is temporally associated with a work period (usually night work) that occurs during the habitual sleep phase or loss of a normal sleep-wake pattern (i.e., disturbed chronobiological rhythmicity) as demonstrated on polysomnography and the Multiple Sleep Latency Test (MSLT) and that the manifestations are not accounted for by another medical or mental disorder and do not meet criteria for any other sleep disorder that produces insomnia or excessive sleepiness (e.g., time zone change [jet lag] syndrome).

Efficacy of modafinil for excessive sleepiness associated with SWSD was demonstrated in a 12-week, placebo-controlled trial in patients with chronic SWSD who were randomized to receive either modafinil 200 mg daily or placebo. Not all patients engaged in shift work who complain of sleepiness meet the criteria for the diagnosis of SWSD; only patients who were symptomatic for at least 3 months were enrolled in the trial. Patients enrolled in this trial also were required to work a minimum of 5 night shifts per month, have excessive sleepiness at the time of their night shifts (MSLT score of less than 6 minutes), and have daytime insomnia documented by a daytime polysomnogram. Patients who were treated with modafinil demonstrated a significant prolongation of the time to sleep onset compared with those receiving placebo as assessed by the nighttime MSLT; significant improvement in the Clinical Global Impression of Change (CGI-C) also was demonstrated in the modafinil group. Despite these improvements, patients receiving the drug in this study continued to have residual sleepiness and impaired performance at night. (See Persistent Sleepiness under Warnings/Precautions: Warnings, in Cautions.) Daytime sleep measured by polysomnography was not affected by modafinil administration.

The long-term efficacy (e.g., longer than 12 weeks) of modafinil in SWSD has not been systematically evaluated in placebo-controlled studies to date. When modafinil is used for extended periods, the need for continued therapy should be reassessed periodically.

Dosage and Administration

■ Administration Modafinil is administered orally. In patients with narcolepsy or obstructive sleep apnea/hypopnea syndrome (OSAHS), modafinil usually is administered once daily in the morning. The drug also has been administered in 2 divided doses daily for narcolepsy, in the morning and at noon†. In patients with shift work sleep disorder (SWSD), modafinil should be taken approximately 1 hour prior to the start of their work shift.

Although administration with food can delay GI absorption of modafinil by approximately 30 minutes, food does not affect the extent of absorption and the drug can be administered without regard to meals.

■ Dosage The usual recommended dosage of modafinil to improve wakefulness in adults with excessive sleepiness associated with narcolepsy, obstructive sleep apnea/hypopnea syndrome, or shift work sleep disorder is 200 mg daily. Although a dosage of 400 mg daily has been well tolerated, there is no consistent evidence indicating that this dosage provides additional clinical benefit beyond that provided by the 200-mg daily dosage.

■ Special Populations Hepatic impairment may result in decreased clearance of modafinil. The clearance of modafinil was decreased by 60% and the steady-state concentrations were doubled in patients with severe hepatic impairment and cirrhosis (Child stage B, B+, C, or C+); clinically, all had ascites and almost all were icteric. Therefore, modafinil dosage should be reduced to 100 mg daily (i.e., one-half the usual recommended dosage) in patients with severe hepatic impairment.

Current information is inadequate to make specific modafinil dosage recommendations for patients with severe renal impairment. In such patients (mean creatinine clearance of 16.6 mL/minute), a single 200-mg dose did not result in increased exposure to unchanged modafinil but did result in much higher exposure to modafinil acid, an inactive metabolite. While this metabolite does not appear to contribute to the CNS stimulant effects of modafinil, there is little information on the safety of increased concentrations of modafinil acid.

Because elimination of modafinil and its metabolites may be reduced with age in geriatric patients, consideration should be given to using lower than the usual recommended dosage in this age group. In addition, that possibility that geriatric patients may have decreased renal and/or hepatic function should be considered.

Cautions

■ Contraindications Known hypersensitivity to modafinil, armodafinil (the *R*-enantiomer of modafinil), or any ingredient in the formulation.

■ Warnings/Precautions ***Warnings*** **Serious Dermatologic Reactions.** Serious rash (including Stevens-Johnson syndrome) and hypersensitivity reactions requiring hospitalization and drug discontinuance have been reported in adult and pediatric patients receiving modafinil. The manufacturer states that modafinil is *not* approved for use in pediatric patients for any indication. (See Cautions: Pediatric Use.)

Rare cases of serious or life-threatening rash, including Stevens-Johnson syndrome (SJS), toxic epidermal necrolysis (TEN), and drug rash with eosinophilia and systemic symptoms (DRESS), have been reported during pediatric clinical trials and during postmarketing experience with modafinil in adults and pediatric patients worldwide; serious rashes were not reported during clinical trials in adults. No known risk factors predict the occurrence or the severity of rash. The majority of cases occurred within 1–5 weeks after initiation of therapy; however, isolated cases also have been reported after prolonged treatment (e.g., 3 months). Accordingly, duration of therapy cannot be used to predict the potential risk associated with the first appearance of a rash. Although benign rashes also occur with modafinil, it is not possible to predict which rashes will prove to be serious; therefore, the drug should ordinarily be discontinued at the first sign of rash unless the rash is clearly not drug related. (See Advice to Patients.) However, treatment discontinuance may not prevent a rash from becoming life-threatening or permanently disabling or disfiguring.

Angioedema and Anaphylactoid Reactions. Angioedema has been reported during postmarketing experience with modafinil. One serious case of angioedema and 1 case of hypersensitivity (with rash, dysphagia, and bronchospasm) were reported among 1,595 patients treated with armodafinil (the *R*-enantiomer of modafinil). No such cases were observed during clinical trials with modafinil. The manufacturer states that patients should be advised to discontinue therapy and immediately report to their clinician any signs or symptoms suggestive of angioedema or anaphylaxis (e.g., swelling of face, eyes, lips, tongue or larynx; difficulty swallowing or breathing; hoarseness). (See Advice to Patients.)

Multiorgan Hypersensitivity Reactions. Multiorgan hypersensitivity reactions, including at least one fatality, have been reported during postmarketing experience with modafinil. These reactions occurred in close temporal association (median time to detection: 13 days; range: 4–33 days) to initiation of modafinil therapy. Although reported in a limited number of patients, multiorgan hypersensitivity reactions may result in hospitalization or be life-threatening. There are no known factors to predict the risk of occurrence or severity of such reactions to modafinil. Signs and symptoms in the cases reported to date were diverse; however, patients typically presented with fever and rash associated with other organ system involvement. Other reported manifestations included myocarditis, hepatitis, liver function test abnormalities, hematological abnormalities (e.g., eosinophilia, leukopenia, thrombocytopenia), pruritus, and asthenia. However. the manufacturer states that multiorgan hypersensitivity reactions are variable in their clinical presentation and that other organ system signs and symptoms may occur.

If a multiorgan hypersensitivity reaction is suspected, modafinil should be discontinued. The manufacturer states that although there are no case reports indicating cross-sensitivity with other drugs that produce this syndrome, experience with other drugs associated with multiorgan hypersensitivity suggests that cross-sensitivity is a possibility.

Persistent Sleepiness. Modafinil is used in patients who have abnormal levels of sleepiness. In such patients, the drug has been shown to improve, but *not* to eliminate, this abnormal tendency to fall asleep. (See Advice to Patients.) All patients with excessive sleepiness, including those receiving modafinil, should be frequently reassessed for their degree of sleepiness and, if appropriate, advised to avoid driving or any other potentially dangerous activity. Clinicians also should be aware that patients may not acknowledge sleepiness or drowsiness until directly questioned about drowsiness or sleepiness during specific activities.

Psychiatric Effects. Adverse psychiatric effects have been reported in patients receiving modafinil. Postmarketing adverse psychiatric effects associated with the drug include mania, delusions, hallucinations, and suicidal ideation and have resulted in hospitalization in some cases, and aggression. In many, but not all, cases, patients had a prior psychiatric history. However, one healthy male developed ideas of reference, paranoid delusions, and auditory hallucinations in association with modafinil and sleep deprivation; there was no evidence of psychosis 36 hours after drug discontinuance. In controlled clinical trials in adults, psychiatric symptoms leading to drug discontinuance in at least 0.3% of patients and reported more frequently in modafinil-treated patients than placebo recipients included anxiety, nervousness, insomnia, confusion, agitation, and depression.

The manufacturer states that modafinil should be used with caution in patients with a history of psychosis, depression, or mania. The manufacturer also states that the possible emergence or exacerbation of psychiatric symptoms in patients treated with the drug should be considered. If adverse psychiatric effects develop in modafinil-treated patients, discontinuance of the drug should be considered. (See Advice to Patients.)

General Precautions

Diagnosis of Sleep Disorders. The manufacturer states that modafinil should be used only in patients who have had a complete evaluation of their excessive sleepiness and in whom a diagnosis of narcolepsy, obstructive sleep apnea/hypopnea syndrome (OSAHS), and/or shift work sleep disorder (SWSD) has been made in accordance with the International Classification of Sleep Disorders (ICSD) or DSM diagnostic criteria. Such an evaluation usually consists of a complete history and physical examination, which may be supplemented with testing in a laboratory setting (e.g., polysomnography). Clinicians should be aware that some patients may have more than one sleep disorder contributing to their daytime sleepiness (e.g., OSAHS and SWSD concurrently in the same patient).

Cognitive/Psychomotor Impairment. Although modafinil has not been shown to cause functional impairment, the possibility that the drug, like any other drug affecting the CNS, may alter judgment, thinking, or motor skills should be considered. Patients should be cautioned about operating an automobile or other hazardous machinery until they are reasonably certain that modafinil does not adversely affect their ability to engage in such activities.

Cardiovascular Effects. The manufacturer recommends that modafinil *not* be used in patients with a history of left ventricular hypertrophy or ischemic ECG changes, chest pain, arrhythmia, or other clinically important manifestation of mitral valve prolapse associated with CNS stimulant use. In clinical studies with modafinil, a few patients have exhibited manifestations such as chest pain, palpitations, dyspnea, and transient ischemic T-wave changes in association with mitral valve prolapse or left ventricular hypertrophy. If new onset of any of these cardiovascular symptoms occurs during modafinil therapy, the manufacturer states that a cardiac evaluation should be considered.

Modafinil should be used with caution in patients with a recent history of myocardial infarction or unstable angina since the drug has not been evaluated or used to any appreciable extent in such patients.

Periodic monitoring of blood pressure may be appropriate during modafinil therapy. No clinically important changes in mean systolic or diastolic blood pressure were observed in patients receiving modafinil in short-term (i.e., less than 3 months) clinical trials. However, a retrospective analysis indicated that new or increased use of hypotensive agents was required among a greater proportion of patients receiving modafinil (2.4%) than among those receiving placebo (0.7%) in these studies. When studies of patients with OSAHS were considered separately, the difference was increased, with 3.4 or 1.1% of patients receiving modafinil or placebo, respectively, requiring new or altered therapy with hypotensive agents.

Abuse and Misuse Potential. Patients should be followed closely during modafinil use for possible signs of misuse or abuse (e.g., incrementation of doses, drug-seeking behavior), especially those with a history of drug or stimulant abuse (e.g., amphetamine, cocaine, methylphenidate). Although modafinil can produce psychoactive and euphoric effects and feelings consistent with other CNS stimulants (e.g., amphetamines, methylphenidate), current evidence indicates that the risk of abuse or misuse of modafinil is lower than that associated with such CNS stimulants that are subject to control as schedule II drugs (e.g., amphetamine, methylphenidate). (See Description.) Therefore, modafinil is only subject to control as a schedule IV drug.

Contraceptive Precautions. Because efficacy of hormonal contraceptives may be reduced during and for 1 month after modafinil therapy, patients using such contraceptives should be advised to use alternative or concomitant nonhormonal contraceptive methods during these periods. (See Drug Interactions: Drugs Affecting Hepatic Microsomal Enzymes.)

Specific Populations

Pregnancy. Category C. (See Users Guide.) Provigil® Pregnancy Registry at 866-404-4106; registry information is also available on the website http://provigilpregnancyregistry.com.

Women of childbearing potential should be advised of possible hormonal contraceptive failure (i.e., increased risk of pregnancy) during and for 1 month after modafinil use. (See Drug Interactions.)

Lactation. It is not known whether modafinil or its metabolites are distributed into milk. Caution should be exercised when modafinil is used in nursing women.

Pediatric Use. Modafinil is not approved for use in pediatric patients for *any* indication, including attention deficit hyperactivity disorder (ADHA). The manufacturer states that safety and efficacy of the drug have not been established in children younger than 16 years of age.

In a controlled study of 6 weeks' duration, 165 pediatric patients (5–17 years of age) with narcolepsy were treated with modafinil or placebo. The results did not demonstrate a statistically significant difference favoring modafinil over placebo in prolonging sleep latency (as measured by the Multiple Sleep Latency Test [MSLT]) or in perceptions of sleepiness (as determined by the Clinical Global Impression of Change [CGI-C] score).

Serious rashes, including erythema multiforme major and Stevens-Johnson syndrome, have been associated with modafinil use in pediatric patients. In clinical trials in pediatric patients younger than 17 years of age, the incidence of rash resulting in drug discontinuance was 0.8% (13 cases out of 1,585); these cases included 1 case of possible Stevens-Johnson syndrome and 1 case of apparent multi-organ hypersensitivity reaction. Several cases were associated with fever and other abnormalities (e.g., vomiting, leukopenia). The median time to rash that resulted in drug discontinuance was 13 days. No such cases were observed among placebo recipients. (See Serious Dermatologic Reactions under Warnings/Precautions: Warnings, in Cautions.)

In controlled and open-label clinical trials, adverse CNS effects reported in modafinil-treated pediatric patients included Tourette's syndrome, insomnia, hostility, increased cataplexy, increased hypnagogic hallucinations, and suicidal ideation. Transient leukopenia, which resolved without medical intervention, also occurred. In the controlled clinical trial, dysmenorrhea occurred in 3 out of 38 girls 12 years of age or younger treated with modafinil compared with 0 out of 10 girls receiving placebo.

Geriatric Use. Safety and efficacy of modafinil have not been established in geriatric patients 65 years of age and older, although experience in a limited number of patients in this age group showed an adverse effect profile similar to that in younger patients. Reduced dosage should be considered. (See Dosage and Administration: Special Populations.)

Renal Impairment. Caution is advised if modafinil is used in patients with severe renal impairment. (See Dosage and Administration: Special Populations.)

Hepatic Impairment. Reduced dosage of modafinil is recommended if the drug is used in patients with severe hepatic impairment, with or without cirrhosis, because clearance of the drug is reduced in such patients. (See Dosage and Administration: Special Populations.)

■ Common Adverse Effects

Adverse effects occurring in 5% or more of patients receiving modafinil and more frequently than with placebo include headache, nausea, nervousness, rhinitis, diarrhea, back pain, anxiety, insomnia, dizziness, and dyspepsia. In placebo-controlled, phase III clinical trials, although adverse effects generally were mild to moderate and well tolerated, 8% of patients discontinued modafinil because of adverse effects, principally because of headache, nausea, anxiety, dizziness, insomnia, chest pain, and nervousness. In a Canadian trial, a 35-year-old obese narcoleptic male with a history of syncopal episodes experienced a 9-second episode of asystole after 27 days of modafinil 300 mg daily in divided doses.

Drug Interactions

■ Drugs Affecting Hepatic Microsomal Enzymes

Potent inducers (e.g., carbamazepine, phenobarbital, rifampin) or inhibitors (e.g., ketoconazole, itraconazole) of the cytochrome P-450 (CYP) isoenzyme 3A4 could alter the elimination of modafinil because of the partial involvement of this isoenzyme in modafinil's metabolism.

The possibility that modafinil might also induce its own metabolism (e.g., with chronic administration of relatively high [400 mg daily] dosages) also should be considered.

Modafinil has been shown to slightly induce CYP isoenzymes 1A2, 2B6, and 3A4 in a concentration-dependent manner. Although induction results from in vitro studies are not necessarily predictive of response in vivo, caution should be exercised if modafinil is administered in patients receiving drugs that are metabolized by these isoenzymes. The possibility of an interaction with the clearance (increased) of cyclosporine, hormonal contraceptives, and, to a lesser degree, theophylline should be considered.

In vitro studies have shown that modafinil has little or no capacity to inhibit major CYP isoenzymes except 2C19, which is reversibly inhibited at pharmacologically relevant concentrations. Therefore, the possibility of prolonged elimination of drugs that are largely eliminated via the CYP2C19 isoenzyme (e.g., diazepam, propranolol, phenytoin, *S*-mephenytoin) should be considered when modafinil is used concomitantly.

Clozapine

Elevated serum clozapine concentrations and resulting clozapine toxicity occurred in a patient receiving modafinil for clozapine-associated sedation. Although the precise mechanism is unclear, this interaction was thought to be caused by decreased clearance of clozapine (a CYP2C19 substrate). Pending further evaluation of this potential interaction, caution should be used whenever modafinil and clozapine are given concurrently; close monitoring of serum clozapine concentrations also is recommended.

Cyclosporine In at least one patient, blood cyclosporine concentrations were decreased by 50% after 1 month of therapy with modafinil 200 mg daily. This interaction was thought to be caused by increased metabolism of cyclosporine (a CYP3A4 substrate) since no other factor expected to affect the disposition of the drug had changed. Monitoring of cyclosporine concentrations and appropriate dosage adjustment should be considered when these drugs are used concomitantly.

Hormonal Contraceptives In female volunteers receiving long-term ethinyl estradiol therapy, administration of modafinil 200 mg daily for 7 days followed by 400 mg daily for an additional 21 days resulted in mean decreases of 11 and 18% in the peak concentrations and area under the plasma concentration-time curve (AUC), respectively, of ethinyl estradiol. No change in the elimination rate of ethinyl estradiol was observed in this study. The possibility of hormonal contraceptive failure secondary to induction of metabolism of the hormones by modafinil should be considered, and women of childbearing potential should be advised to use an alternative or concomitant nonhormonal contraceptive during and for 1 month after modafinil therapy.

Phenytoin Because phenytoin is a substrate for the CYP2C9 isoenzyme, patients receiving the anticonvulsant concomitantly with modafinil should be monitored for signs of phenytoin toxicity.

Triazolam Administration of a single dose of triazolam (0.125 mg) in female volunteers receiving modafinil 200 mg daily for 7 days followed by 400 mg daily for an additional 21 days resulted in mean decreases of 42 and 59% in the peak plasma concentrations and AUC, respectively, of triazolam and a decrease in its elimination half-life of approximately 1 hour. Dosage adjustment of triazolam may be necessary when these drugs are used concomitantly.

Tricyclic Antidepressants CYP2C19 provides an ancillary pathway for the metabolism of certain tricyclic antidepressants (e.g., clomipramine, desipramine) that are principally metabolized via the CYP2D6 isoenzyme. In patients treated with such tricyclics who are CYP2D6 deficient (i.e., those who are poor metabolizers of debrisoquin; 7–10% of the Caucasian population, similar or lower percentages of other populations), the dependency on CYP2C19 metabolism may be increased and concomitant modafinil therapy could increase serum concentrations of drugs metabolized by this isoenzyme. Therefore, clinicians should be aware that a reduction of tricyclic antidepressant dosage may be necessary during modafinil therapy.

Although concomitant administration of a single 50-mg clomipramine dose on the first of 3 days of modafinil 200 mg daily in healthy individuals did not appear to alter the pharmacokinetics of either drug, at least one patient with narcolepsy developed a dose-dependent and reversible increase in plasma concentrations of clomipramine and its active desmethyl metabolite following initiation of modafinil therapy. The patient was a phenotypic CYP2D6 poor metabolizer. Because clomipramine may be considered for concomitant therapy to manage manifestations of cataplexy in narcoleptic patients, the possibility of this metabolic interaction should be considered.

Warfarin In vitro evidence suggested that modafinil can suppress the expression of CYP2C9 activity in a concentration-dependent manner. In a subsequent clinical study performed in healthy individuals, chronic modafinil administration did not substantially alter the single-dose pharmacokinetics of warfarin when compared with placebo. However, pending further evaluation of this potential interaction, the manufacturer recommends more frequent monitoring of prothrombin time and/or international normalized ratio (INR) whenever modafinil and warfarin are given concurrently.

■ **Amphetamines** In a single-dose study in healthy individuals, concomitant administration of a single 200-mg modafinil dose and a 10-mg dextroamphetamine dose did not produce a clinically important pharmacokinetic interaction with either drug. However, the absorption of modafinil was delayed by approximately 1 hour when these drugs were given concurrently in this study. In a subsequent study in healthy individuals, the steady-state pharmacokinetics of modafinil (200 mg daily for 7 days followed by 400 mg daily for 21 days) were not significantly affected by chronic administration of a 20-mg dose of dextroamphetamine given in the afternoon; the adverse event profile of these drugs administered concurrently was similar to that of modafinil alone.

■ **Methylphenidate** In a single-dose study in healthy individuals, concomitant administration of a single 200-mg dose of modafinil and 40-mg dose of methylphenidate did not significantly alter the pharmacokinetics of either drug. GI absorption of modafinil was delayed by approximately 1 hour; however, the extent of absorption was not affected. In a multiple-dose study in healthy individuals, concomitant administration of methylphenidate 20 mg daily and modafinil (200 mg daily for 7 days followed by 400 mg daily for 21 days) did not significantly alter the pharmacokinetics of modafinil. Therefore, a clinically important pharmacokinetic interaction between these drugs seems unlikely.

■ **Monoamine Oxidase Inhibitors** One case of acute chorea, confusion, and hyperthermia (possibly related to serotonin syndrome) has been reported with concurrent modafinil and tranylcypromine administration. Because drug interaction studies have not been performed with monoamine oxidase (MAO) inhibitors and either armodafinil or modafinil, caution is advised when these drugs are administered concomitantly.

Description

Modafinil, a benzhydryl sulfinylacetamide derivative, is a CNS stimulant that is structurally and pharmacologically distinct from most other currently available CNS stimulants (e.g., amphetamines, caffeine, cocaine, methylphenidate). The drug is a 50:50 racemic mixture of the *R*- and *S*-enantiomers; the *R*-enantiomer of modafinil is also commercially available as armodafinil. Modafinil promotes vigilance and wakefulness and decreases the number of daytime sleep episodes associated with narcolepsy and obstructive sleep apnea/hypopnea syndrome and reduces the excessive sleepiness associated with shift work sleep disorder. Although the wakefulness-promoting effects of modafinil are comparable to those exhibited by amphetamines or methylphenidate, modafinil alters metabolic activity and increases neuronal activity in specific areas of the brain that control sleep/wakefulness and the biologic clock while amphetamines increase neuronal activity more widely throughout the brain, suggesting distinct mechanisms for modafinil and relatively high selectivity.

The exact mechanism(s) of action of modafinil is unknown, but animal studies have shown that the drug inhibits the release of γ-aminobutyric acid (GABA) and increases the release of glutamate from the cerebral cortex, hippocampus, nucleus acumbens, medial preoptic area, and posterior hypothalamus. GABA is an inhibitory neurotransmitter that acts as a CNS depressant while glutamate is an excitatory neurotransmitter. Modafinil does not appear to be an indirect- or direct-acting dopamine-receptor agonist nor to act as a sympathomimetic agent. Haloperidol, a dopamine-receptor antagonist, inhibits the wake-promoting activity of amphetamine but not the wake-promoting activity of modafinil.

The manufacturer states that modafinil does not appear to be a direct or indirect α_1-adrenergic agonist, as evidenced by lack of activity in assay systems known to be responsive to such agonists. However, the drug's stimulant effects (e.g., on wakefulness, locomotion, and the EEG) are antagonized by α_1-antagonists (e.g., prazosin, phenoxybenzamine), thus indicating that an intact central α_1-adrenergic system is necessary for modafanil's CNS activity. In addition, it has been suggested that the drug itself may stimulate central α_1-adrenergic activity (e.g., at the postsynaptic level). Modafinil does not appear to exhibit clinically important peripheral adrenergic activity, even at high doses. In animals, modafinil increased locomotor activity but did not increase dopamine activity; however, in vitro studies showed that modafinil binds to dopamine reuptake sites and increases extracellular dopamine concentrations. Modafinil was also found to block dopamine transporters and increase dopamine concentrations in the human brain (including the nucleus accumbens) in one pilot study; drugs with such activity generally are associated with abuse potential. (See Abuse and Misuse Potential under Warnings/Precautions: General Precautions, in Cautions.)

At usual pharmacologic concentrations, modafinil does not bind to certain norepinephrine, serotonin, dopamine, GABA, adenosine, histamine H_3, melatonin, or benzodiazepine receptors that regulate sleep and wakefulness. The drug also does not inhibit type B monoamine oxidase (MAO-B) or phosphodiesterase and does not alter plasma melatonin or cortisol hormone profiles, which may limit short-term adverse effects.

Although the effects, if any, of modafinil on blood pressure during long-term therapy remain to be elucidated, 300 mg (200 mg before breakfast and 100 mg before lunch) given on a single day in normotensive patients with obstructive sleep apnea did not appear to substantially affect blood pressure, although increases were noted relative to placebo under mental and physical stress tests.

Like other CNS stimulants, modafinil is reinforcing in animals and produces psychoactive (e.g., alterations in mood and thinking), euphoric, and subjective effects typical of classic psychomotor stimulants (e.g., amphetamines, methylphenidate) in humans. Despite this pharmacologic similarity to such stimulants, the chemical properties of modafinil (e.g., not water soluble, decomposes in heat) may limit its abuse potential. In addition, there are substantial relative potency differences between modafinil and CNS stimulants that are subject to control under the Federal Controlled Substances Act as schedule II drugs. These differences reduce the likelihood that modafinil could be abused by the parenteral, intranasal, or inhalation route, as are cocaine, methylphenidate, and amphetamine; therefore, modafinil is subject to control as a schedule IV rather than II drug.

With chronic dosing, modafinil induces its own metabolism via induction of the cytochrome P-450 (CYP) isoenzyme 3A4. Clearance of modafinil may be altered by other inducers (e.g., phenobarbital, carbamazepine, rifampin) or inhibitors (e.g., ketoconazole, itraconazole) of this isoenzyme. (See Drug Interactions.) Inhibition of the CYP isoenzymes 2C9 and 2C19 by modafinil results in several potential drug interactions (e.g., warfarin, phenytoin, diazepam, propranolol, clomipramine, desipramine). (See Drug Interactions.)

Advice to Patients

Importance of providing copy of written patient information (medication guide) each time modafinil is dispensed, and importance of reading this information prior to taking modafinil.

Importance of advising clinician of existing or contemplated therapy, including prescription and OTC drugs and/or herbal supplements, as well as any concomitant illnesses. Advise patient that it is prudent to avoid alcohol while taking modafinil since combined use has not been studied.

Importance of advising patients about the potential increased risk of pregnancy in women taking hormonal contraceptives (including oral contraceptives, injectable or implantable contraceptives, vaginal rings, and intrauterine devices) during and for 1 month after discontinuing modafinil therapy; discuss use of alternative or concomitant methods of contraception with patient. (See Contraceptive Precautions under Warnings/Precautions: General Precautions, in Cautions.) Importance of informing clinician if patient is or plans to become pregnant or plans to breast-feed. Importance of clinicians informing women about the existence of and encouraging enrollment in the Provigil® pregnancy registry (see Pregnancy under Warnings/Precautions: Specific Populations, in Cautions).

Risk of serious rash or serious allergic reaction. Importance of immediately discontinuing modafinil and seeking immediate medical attention if rash or other signs of allergic reaction occur (e.g., hives, mouth sores, blisters, peeling skin, difficulty swallowing or breathing, a related allergic phenomenon).

Risk of mental (psychiatric) symptoms. Importance of discontinuing modafinil and informing clinician if depression, anxiety, hallucinations, mania, suicidal thoughts, aggression, or other psychiatric symptoms associated with psychosis or mania occur.

Risk of heart problems. Importance of discontinuing modafinil and informing clinician if heart problems, including chest pain, occur.

Advise that modafinil may affect judgment, thinking, or motor skills. Importance of using caution when operating machinery or driving a motor vehicle until effects of the drug are known.

Advise that modafinil may improve, but not eliminate, the abnormal tendency to fall asleep. Advise against altering previous behavior with regard to potentially dangerous activities (e.g., driving, operating machinery, other activities requiring appropriate levels of wakefulness) until and unless modafinil has been shown to produce levels of wakefulness that permit such activities. Advise that modafinil is *not* a replacement for sleep.

Importance of continuing previously prescribed therapy (e.g., advising patients with obstructive sleep apnea/hypopnea syndrome [OSAHS] that modafinil is used along with other medical therapies for this condition and that the drug is not a replacement for the continuous positive airway pressure [CPAP] machine). Importance of advising patients with OSAHS to continue using their CPAP machine while sleeping.

Importance of informing patient of other important precautionary information. (See Cautions.)

Overview (see Users Guide). For additional information until a more detailed monograph is developed and published, the manufacturer's labeling should be consulted. It is *essential* that the manufacturer's labeling be consulted for more detailed information on the usual cautions, precautions, and contraindications, potential drug interactions, laboratory test interferences, and acute toxicity.

Preparations

Modafinil is subject to control under the Federal Controlled Substances Act of 1970 as a schedule IV (C-IV) drug.

Excipients in commercially available drug preparations may have clinically important effects in some individuals; consult specific product labeling for details.

Modafinil

Oral		
Tablets	100 mg	**Provigil**® (C-IV), Cephalon
	200 mg	**Provigil**® (C-IV; scored), Cephalon

†Use is not currently included in the labeling approved by the US Food and Drug Administration

ANXIOLYTICS, SEDATIVES, AND HYPNOTICS 28:24

BENZODIAZEPINES 28:24.08

Benzodiazepines General Statement

■ Benzodiazepines are used as anxiolytics, sedatives, hypnotics, anticonvulsants, and/or skeletal muscle relaxants.

Uses

Benzodiazepines are used for preoperative relief of anxiety and provision of sedation, light anesthesia, and anterograde amnesia of perioperative events; for procedural sedation; for continuous sedation in intubated and mechanically ventilated patients undergoing treatment in a critical care setting (e.g., intensive care unit [ICU]); for induction and maintenance of anesthesia; as hypnotics in the treatment of insomnia; for the management of agitation associated with acute alcohol withdrawal; and for the management of anxiety (e.g., generalized anxiety disorder, panic disorder). Benzodiazepines also are used as anticonvulsants and skeletal muscle relaxants. In addition, benzodiazepines have been used alone and as adjuncts to antipsychotic agents in the management of schizophrenia†. Generally, the drugs are not effective in the treatment of depressive reactions.

All benzodiazepines have similar actions, and their use is more a reflection of the way in which the drugs have been studied and the way the manufacturers promote their use than real differences between the drugs. In general, there is no evidence that any one benzodiazepine is more effective than another if an adequate dosage is given. However, pharmacokinetic and pharmacodynamic differences have influenced the therapeutic application of these drugs.

■ **Anxiety and Insomnia** Benzodiazepines are used for the management of anxiety disorders and insomnia. These drugs appear to have a tranquilizing effect on the CNS with no appreciable effect on the respiratory or cardiovascular systems. Most clinicians prefer benzodiazepines to barbiturates or meprobamate for the management of anxiety and tension and to other hypnotics such as barbiturates in the management of insomnia, because benzodiazepines have a relatively low abuse potential, produce less sedation with effective anxiolytic doses, and produce less toxicity with acute overdosage. In addition, benzodiazepines generally do not induce hepatic microsomal enzymes or produce substantial changes in prothrombin time or in oral anticoagulant dosage requirements. (See Drug Interactions.) For the symptomatic treatment of anxiety or insomnia in geriatric patients and patients with liver disease, some clinicians prefer lorazepam, oxazepam, or triazolam to other benzodiazepines or barbiturates because they have a relatively short elimination half-life even in patients with liver disease, and they do not have active metabolites.

Anxiety Disorders Benzodiazepines are used for the management of anxiety disorders, principally generalized anxiety disorder, and for the short-term relief of symptoms of anxiety or anxiety associated with depressive symptoms. Generalized anxiety disorder is characterized by unrealistic or excessive anxiety and worry (apprehensive expectation) about several life circumstances (e.g., misfortune of one's child; finances; academic, athletic, or social performance) for 6 months or longer, during which time such concerns are bothersome more often than not. When anxiety is present, it is accompanied by many signs of motor tension (e.g., trembling, twitching, shakiness, restlessness, easy fatigability), autonomic hyperactivity (e.g., shortness of breath, smothering sensation, tachycardia, palpitations, sweating, cold clammy hands, dry mouth, diarrhea, hot flushes), and vigilance and scanning (e.g., feeling keyed up or on edge, exaggerated startle response, trouble falling or staying asleep, difficulty concentrating or mind going blank because of anxiety). When such signs are associated with panic attacks, the patient may be suffering from panic disorder, which also can be treated effectively with benzodiazepines. Mild depressive symptoms commonly are associated with generalized anxiety disorder, and an associated and unrelated panic disorder or depressive disorder often is present.

In the management of anxiety disorders and anxiety symptoms, benzodiazepines are more effective than barbiturates or meprobamate. Anxiety or tension associated with the stress of everyday life usually does not require treatment with an anxiolytic. The efficacy of benzodiazepines for long-term use (i.e., longer than 4 months) as anxiolytics has not been evaluated. The need for continued therapy with benzodiazepines should be periodically reassessed.

Benzodiazepines (principally alprazolam and clonazepam, but also diazepam and lorazepam) have been used effectively in the management of panic disorder (an anxiety disorder), with or without agoraphobia. Panic disorder is characterized by recurrent, unexpected panic attacks (discrete periods of intense fear or discomfort), associated concern about having additional attacks, anxiety about the implications or consequences of the attacks, and/or a clinically important change in behavior related to the attacks. Panic attacks have a sudden onset, reach a peak effect rapidly (usually in 10 minutes or less), are associated with at least 4 characteristic symptoms, and often are accompanied by a feeling of imminent danger or impending doom and an urge to escape. Characteristic symptoms include palpitations, pounding heart, or tachycardia; sweating; trembling or shaking; dyspnea or smothering sensation; feeling of choking; chest pain or discomfort; nausea or abdominal distress; dizziness, unsteady feelings, lightheadedness, or faintness; derealization or depersonalization; fear of losing control or going crazy; fear of dying; paresthesias; and chills or hot flushes.

Efficacy of benzodiazepines in the management of panic disorder has been established mainly in short-term (for periods of 4–10 weeks) controlled studies, although the drugs have been used without apparent loss of efficacy for longer periods (e.g., 8–12 months or longer) in many patients. Benzodiazepines can reduce the number of spontaneous and situational panic attacks and associated anxiety, avoidance behavior, phobic fears, somatic manifestations, and secondary disability (e.g., interference with normal work or social activities). Although the drugs also can reduce depressive symptomatology in many patients with panic disorder, including those who are depressed or nondepressed, emergence of depressive symptomatology has occurred occasionally in such patients.

Following discontinuance of benzodiazepines, a relapse of the condition, including a rebound in panic attacks and anxiety, and/or the development of withdrawal frequently occurs. In one study despite gradual withdrawal over 4 weeks in patients receiving high-dose alprazolam therapy for 8 weeks, a rebound in panic attacks and anxiety occurred in 27 and 13% of patients, respectively, and a transient, mild to moderate withdrawal syndrome developed in 35% of patients, but both rebound effects and withdrawal manifestations subsided after 2 weeks. Additional study is needed to establish the optimum duration of benzodiazepine therapy in the management of panic disorder, and to determine the most appropriate method of tapered withdrawal of the drugs. The potential dependence liability of benzodiazepines should be considered in weighing the possible risks and benefits of therapy with the drugs in this condition.

Anxiety Associated with Myocardial Infarction Benzodiazepines (e.g., diazepam) have been used to relieve anxiety associated with acute myocardial infarction (MI); however, evidence suggests that these drugs are no more effective than placebo in managing anxiety and ischemic-type pain in patients with MI. Experts state that routine use of anxiolytics is neither necessary nor recommended in patients with acute MI. Morphine sulfate is considered the drug of choice for relief of pain and associated anxiety following acute MI. (See Uses in the Opiate Agonists General Statement 28:08.08.)

Insomnia Benzodiazepines generally are preferred to most other hypnotics for the management of insomnia because of their established short- and intermediate-term efficacy and relative safety. However, while experience with zolpidem and zaleplon is less extensive than that with benzodiazepines, these non-benzodiazepines may be preferred in some patients because of their relatively rapid onset of effect, short duration of action, and safety profile. Because of zaleplon's short half-life and benefit in decreasing sleep latency, it appears to be most useful for sleep initiation disorders. Eszopiclone also has a relatively rapid onset of effect and has an intermediate duration of action. Although eszopiclone has been evaluated in controlled clinical trials for periods up to 6 months in duration, experience with eszopiclone is less extensive than that with benzodiazepines and its role relative to other sedative and hypnotic agents remains to be fully established. Cost considerations also may factor into the choice of hypnotic.

While experience to date in the management of insomnia principally has been with estazolam, flurazepam, quazepam, temazepam, and triazolam, other benzodiazepines also can be used for insomnia. Flurazepam is the prototype benzodiazepine hypnotic, and most clinical studies have shown that the hypnotic efficacy of flurazepam is equal to or greater than that of other hypnotics such as barbiturates, chloral hydrate, or glutethimide, but the incidence of hangover or morning drowsiness is about the same for flurazepam as for other hypnotics. Sleep laboratory studies have demonstrated a carry-over effect for flurazepam (i.e., the drug is more effective on the second, third, and fourth nights of use than on the first night) because of accumulation of an active metabolite which has a long half-life. Also, when flurazepam is withdrawn, the effect continues on the first and sometimes the second night. Compared with nonbenzodiazepine hypnotics, benzodiazepines have shown continued efficacy when administered for at least 28 consecutive nights; however, the efficacy of prolonged use of benzodiazepines in patients with chronic insomnia has not been established.

The choice of a specific benzodiazepine must be individualized according to patient response and tolerance, taking into consideration pharmacokinetic and pharmacodynamic characteristics of the drug, patient age and other characteristics, and the underlying sleep disorder being treated. Benzodiazepines with a relatively short elimination half-life (e.g., triazolam) may be more likely to result in transient rebound insomnia after discontinuance and in pharmacodynamic tolerance and adaptation to the hypnotic effect after several weeks of therapy, with resultant diminished effectiveness during the end of each night's use (early morning insomnia) and, possibly, increased daytime anxiety. Benzodiazepines with a relatively long half-life (e.g., flurazepam, quazepam) may be more likely to result in residual daytime sedative effects and in impaired psychomotor and mental performance during continued therapy, although partial tolerance to these effects can occur. Differences in residual and cumulative CNS depressant effects may be particularly important in geriatric patients and in patients with potentially impaired elimination of the drugs and those whose job or lifestyle requires unimpaired intellectual or psychomotor function. Benzodiazepines with relatively slow GI absorption (e.g., temazepam) may be less effective in initial sleep induction; therefore, it has been suggested that the efficacy of such drugs may be diminished in patients whose principal symptom is initial difficulty in falling asleep (sleep-latency insomnia). Alterations in dosing (e.g., administering slowly absorbed drugs 1 or 2 hours before bedtime) may in part compensate for this delayed onset.

Treatment strategies for transient (insomnia of several days' duration related to minor situational stress), short-term (insomnia of several weeks' duration usually related to stress associated with work and/or family-life conditions such as job performance, job loss, bereavement, or illness), and long-term (insomnia of prolonged duration often associated with some underlying condition such as a psychiatric disorder, chronic drug and/or alcohol dependence, or other medical condition) insomnia will differ. For example, in the management of transient insomnia, use of relatively low-dose therapy with a relatively rapidly eliminated benzodiazepine for one to several nights may be preferred, unless sustained sedation is desired. For short-term insomnia, benzodiazepines are used as an adjunct to efforts aimed at improving sleep hygiene (e.g., avoidance of caffeine, alcohol, daytime naps, or retiring to bed too early), but therapy with the drugs generally should be limited to no more than several weeks, administering the drugs intermittently (e.g., skipping a nightly dose after one or two good nights' sleep) if possible; the choice of benzodiazepine should be individualized. Reevaluation of the patient's condition is recommended if continued hypnotic use exceeds 2–3 weeks, since sleep disturbance may be a presenting manifestation of an underlying physical and/or psychiatric disorder. Such underlying disorders also could result in worsening of insomnia or the emergence of new abnormalities of mentation or behavior; however, the possibility that such effects may be associated with benzodiazepine therapy itself also should be considered.

The management of long-term insomnia is more complex and depends in part on the presence of any identifiable underlying condition that is a contributing factor. The need for therapy with hypnotic drugs such as benzodiazepines may persist despite therapy aimed at treating the underlying condition; benzodiazepine therapy also may be useful in patients with no readily identifiable cause of the insomnia and usually is combined with psychological-behavioral therapies (e.g., relaxation techniques, sleep curtailment, stimulus control therapy) aimed at modifying negative conditioning related to sleep habits. If hypnotic drug therapy is employed, intermittent (e.g., every third night) therapy with a benzodiazepine having a relatively long elimination half-life has been suggested; efforts generally should be made to gradually discontinue such therapy after several months. Data from one study comparing the effects of triazolam and behavioral therapy on sleep latency in patients with persistent sleep-onset insomnia suggest that combined use of drug and behavioral therapies may offer both immediate relief and sustained effects upon drug discontinuance; however, behavioral therapy is a useful alternative to drug treatment and may be preferable, given its sustained effectiveness, particularly in individuals in whom use of hypnotic agents is problematic (e.g., individuals prone to drug abuse, pregnant or breast-feeding women). Referral to a sleep disorders clinic may be necessary for some patients.

Because of evidence from animal studies that the drugs can entrain circadian rhythms, benzodiazepines with a relatively short elimination half-life (e.g., triazolam) have been used for the prevention or short-term treatment of transient insomnia associated with sleep-wake schedule changes† (e.g., rapid travel across time zones ["jet lag"], rotating shift work). While such therapy may be useful in the management of sleep disorders associated with such schedule changes in some patients, the possibility that transient impairment of cognitive function (e.g., anterograde amnesia ["traveler's amnesia"]) may be induced by the drugs should be considered. (See Cautions: CNS Effects.)

Because benzodiazepines suppress stage 4 sleep, diazepam has been used effectively in some studies to prevent night terrors in adults.

■ **Procedural Sedation** Benzodiazepines (e.g., midazolam, diazepam) are used for procedural sedation, anxiolysis, and amnesia. Procedural sedation is a technique in which sedative and dissociative agents are administered with or without analgesics to allow patients to tolerate painful or unpleasant medical procedures; a depressed state of consciousness is intentionally induced while cardiorespiratory function is maintained. Because sedation is a continuum ranging from minimal sedation to general anesthesia, airway reflexes and cardiorespiratory function may be impaired if a deeper than intended level of sedation is produced. The appropriate level of sedation should be individualized according to the specific procedure and needs of the patient. Benzodiazepines are typically used to produce moderate to deep sedation for patients undergoing diagnostic or therapeutic procedures such as endoscopic procedures, radiologic procedures, coronary catheterization, coronary angiography, oncology procedures, and laceration repairs. Although these drugs can produce amnestic and sedative effects, they have no analgesic activity, and therefore, are usually administered in conjunction with an analgesic agent.

■ **Preoperative Sedation, Anxiolysis, and Amnesia** Benzodiazepines (e.g., lorazepam, midazolam, diazepam) are used preoperatively (prior to the induction of anesthesia) to relieve anxiety and produce sedation and anterograde amnesia. When used for this indication, benzodiazepines have been administered parenterally or orally. Benzodiazepines are particularly useful as a preoperative medication when relief of anxiety and diminished recall of events associated with the surgical procedure are desired. Studies have shown that diazepam, chlordiazepoxide hydrochloride (parenteral dosage form no longer commercially available in the US), or midazolam hydrochloride was as effective for preoperative sedation as opiate agonists or barbiturates and resulted in fewer undesirable effects, such as respiratory depression or hypotension. Because of midazolam's relatively rapid onset, short duration of effect, and improved local tolerance at the site of injection compared with other currently available parenteral benzodiazepines, some clinicians consider midazolam the benzodiazepine of choice for preoperative use associated with short surgical procedures.

■ **Sedation in Critical Care Settings** Benzodiazepines (e.g., lorazepam, midazolam, diazepam) are used for sedation of intubated and mechanically ventilated patients in a critical care setting (e.g., ICU). Midazolam has a quicker onset of action than lorazepam and is generally the preferred benzodiazepine for ICU sedation; lorazepam is used less frequently and diazepam is rarely used.

Sedative agents are administered in critically ill patients to reduce agitation and anxiety, and increase tolerance to invasive procedures (e.g., mechanical ventilation). The provision of adequate analgesia and other measures to ensure patient comfort is recommended before sedatives are administered. Sedative agents should be titrated to the desired level of sedation; in most cases, a light rather than deep level of sedation is recommended in critically ill, mechanically ventilated adults because of improved clinical outcomes that have been demonstrated (e.g., shortened duration of mechanical ventilation and reduced ICU length of stay). The depth and quality of sedation should be assessed using a validated and reliable assessment tool (e.g., Richmond Agitation-Sedation Scale [RASS], Sedation-Agitation Scale [SAS]).

Common sedative agents used in the ICU include benzodiazepines (e.g., lorazepam, midazolam), propofol, and dexmedetomidine. These agents appear to be similarly effective in providing adequate sedation in critically ill, mechanically ventilated adults. However, modest benefits with respect to other clinical outcomes (e.g., reduced duration of mechanical ventilation, shorter time to extubation, reduced risk of delirium) have been observed with the nonbenzodiazepine sedatives (dexmedetomidine and propofol) compared with benzodiazepines. Comparative studies have demonstrated a shorter time to light sedation and shorter time to extubation with propofol compared with benzodiazepines, and a shorter time to extubation and reduced risk of delirium with dexmedetomidine compared with benzodiazepines. In most of these studies, benzodiazepines were administered as a continuous IV infusion rather than as intermittent IV injections. In one study comparing dexmedetomidine and midazolam infusion in critically ill adults requiring mechanical ventilation and sedation for more than 24 hours (SEDCOM study), both drugs demonstrated a similar time within target sedation range; patients receiving dexmedetomidine experienced a higher incidence of bradycardia that resolved without intervention, while patients receiving midazolam experienced a higher incidence of tachycardia and hypertension requiring treatment. Because of the apparent advantages and an overall favorable benefit-to-risk profile, nonbenzodiazepine sedatives (dexmedetomidine or propofol) are generally preferred to benzodiazepines (midazolam or lorazepam) in mechanically ventilated, critically ill adults. This recommendation should be considered in the context of the specific clinical situation since benzodiazepines may still be preferred in certain situations (e.g., patients with anxiety, seizures, or alcohol or benzodiazepine withdrawal). When selecting an appropriate sedative agent, the patient's individual sedation goals should be considered in addition to specific drug-related (e.g., pharmacology, pharmacokinetics, adverse effects, availability, cost) and patient-related (e.g., comorbid conditions) factors.

Midazolam is more lipid soluble than lorazepam, possibly resulting in a quicker onset of sedation. Because lorazepam is more potent and is cleared more slowly than midazolam, emergence time from short-term sedation may be longer with lorazepam than with midazolam; however, comparative studies have suggested that midazolam is associated with greater variability and a longer time to awakening than lorazepam when used for prolonged sedation.

■ **Induction and Maintenance of Anesthesia** Midazolam is used IV for induction of general anesthesia prior to administration of other anesthetic agents; induction with the drug results in anxiolysis, anterograde amnesia, and dose-related hypnotic effects, but not analgesia. Midazolam also is used as a component of balanced anesthesia during short surgical procedures.

■ **Alcohol Withdrawal** Benzodiazepines (e.g., diazepam) are used in the management of acute alcohol withdrawal to relieve agitation and tremor and to prevent or to provide symptomatic relief of delirium tremens and hallucinations. It has not been proven that benzodiazepines prevent hallucinations or delirium tremens; however, some studies suggest that diazepam may shorten the duration and decrease the mortality of delirium tremens.

■ **Seizure Disorders** ***Status Epilepticus*** Benzodiazepines (e.g., lorazepam, midazolam, diazepam) are considered the initial drugs of choice for the management of status epilepticus because of their rapid onset of action, demonstrated efficacy, safety, and tolerability.

Status epilepticus is a medical emergency that must be treated promptly to reduce substantial morbidity and mortality. Initial treatment should include standard critical care and supportive therapy (e.g., blood pressure and respiratory support, oxygen, IV access, identification and correction of underlying causes), followed by administration of a benzodiazepine. Although IV lorazepam is generally preferred because of its longer duration of action, studies generally have not identified any substantial differences between IV lorazepam, IV diazepam, and IM midazolam in terms of seizure cessation, and experts consider these therapies to be equivalent first-line options. Selection of an appropriate benzodiazepine should be individualized based on local availability, route of administration, pharmacokinetics, cost, and other factors (e.g., treatment setting). To achieve a rapid therapeutic effect, IV administration of a benzodiazepine is preferred; however, administration via other routes (e.g., IM, rectal, intranasal, buccal) may be considered when IV administration is not possible (e.g., in the prehospital setting). If seizures continue after initial therapy with a benzodiazepine, a second-line anticonvulsant agent (e.g., IV fosphenytoin or phenytoin, IV valproate sodium, IV levetiracetam, IV phenobarbital) should be administered. If refractory status epilepticus occurs, continuous IV infusion of anticonvulsants, IV barbiturates, or general anesthetics may be necessary.

Early treatment with benzodiazepines in the prehospital setting can improve outcomes in patients with status epilepticus. Results of a placebo-controlled study in adults with out-of-hospital status epilepticus indicated that IV administration of benzodiazepines by paramedics was safe and effective in the management of this condition. Findings from this study indicated that both IV lorazepam and IV diazepam were more effective than placebo in controlling status epilepticus by the time of patient arrival in the emergency department. Because the need to establish IV access may delay administration of an IV benzodiazepine in the prehospital environment, use of other less invasive routes of administration may decrease the time to active treatment. Results of a randomized controlled study (RAMPART) indicate that IM administration of midazolam by paramedics in the prehospital setting may improve outcomes in patients with status epilepticus; in this study, 73% of patients who received IM midazolam achieved seizure resolution at the time of arrival in the emergency department compared with 63% of those who received IV lorazepam.

Other nonparenteral benzodiazepines that have been used for the treatment of status epilepticus include rectal diazepam, intranasal midazolam, and buccal midazolam; studies evaluating these benzodiazepines generally were conducted in the pediatric population. Potential limitations of these nonparenteral routes include difficulty with administration during an acute seizure episode, unpredictable absorption, and lack of commercially available dosage forms.

Other benzodiazepines such as clonazepam and chlordiazepoxide also have been evaluated for the treatment of status epilepticus, but are infrequently used due to the unavailability of a commercially available parenteral dosage form in the US.

Acute Repetitive Seizures or Seizure Clusters Rectal diazepam and midazolam nasal spray also are used for the acute management of intermittent stereotypic episodes of increased seizure activity (also referred to as serial, cyclic, cluster, breakthrough, or crescendo seizures; acute repetitive seizures), especially for out-of-hospital management. Acute repetitive seizures are exacerbations of an underlying seizure disorder that exhibit a pattern distinct from the patient's usual seizure pattern; the repetitive, periodic episodes often are predictable by the patient and caregivers according to a prodrome/aura, time of day when they originate, particular seizure type, and/or accompanying patient behavioral changes. Patients typically experience recovery between the repetitions; however, if untreated, acute repetitive seizures can evolve into more serious problems, including status epilepticus. The distinguishing features of these seizures are their predictability and pattern that differs from the underlying disorder rather than the actual seizure type; thus, while the pattern of presentation and patient and caregiver recognition are common features of the diagnosis, the actual seizure type can be different albeit definable for each individual patient. (See Uses and also see Rectal Dosage under Dosage and Administration: Dosage, in Diazepam 28:24.08.)

Midazolam also is administered intranasally for the acute management of seizures, including rescue therapy for prolonged, recurrent, or cyanotic seizures.

Adjunctive Therapy of Seizure Disorders Benzodiazepines have been used orally as adjuncts to other anticonvulsants in the prophylactic management of partial seizures with elementary symptomatology, including those with motor symptoms (e.g., Jacksonian seizures), partial seizures with complex symptomatology (psychomotor seizures), absence (petit mal) seizures, seizures associated with Lennox-Gastaut syndrome (petit mal variant epilepsy), and akinetic or myoclonic seizures that are refractory to other drugs. Clonazepam is used alone or with other drugs for the management of absence seizures, especially Lennox-Gastaut syndrome (petit mal variant epilepsy), and of akinetic or myoclonic seizures. (See Clonazepam 28:12.08.) Clobazam is used in combination with other anticonvulsants for the management of seizures associated with Lennox-Gastaut syndrome, and also has been used as adjunctive therapy for the management of other seizure disorders, which have sometimes been refractory, including partial, generalized, and myoclonic seizures†. (See Clobazam 28:12.08.) Tolerance often develops to the anticonvulsant effects of benzodiazepines, which can limit their usefulness in the long-term management of seizure disorders.

■ **Skeletal Muscle Spasticity** Benzodiazepines may be useful adjuncts to rest, physical therapy, analgesics, and other measures for the relief of discomfort associated with acute, painful musculoskeletal conditions. There is no convincing evidence that oral benzodiazepines are more effective than barbiturates or meprobamate in these conditions. Most studies indicate that diazepam is superior to other skeletal muscle relaxants (e.g., methocarbamol, carisoprodol) for relief of musculoskeletal pain; however, there is some evidence that diazepam is no more effective than aspirin or placebo. The benzodiazepines are useful in the short- and long-term management of skeletal muscle spasticity such as reflex spasm secondary to local pathology (e.g., trauma, inflammation), spasticity caused by upper motor neuron disorders (e.g., cerebral palsy, paraplegia), athetosis, stiff-man syndrome, strychnine poisoning, or tetanus. Diazepam is generally as effective as dantrolene sodium or baclofen for spasticity in patients with various upper motor neuron disorders. For the management of moderate muscle spasm in tetanus, parenteral diazepam in large doses may be adequate; however, in severe tetanus, neuromuscular blocking agents may be the drugs of choice. The value of diazepam in neonatal tetanus has not been established.

■ **Schizophrenia** Benzodiazepines have been used both as monotherapy for schizophrenia† and as adjuncts to antipsychotic drugs in the symptomatic management of schizophrenia, most commonly in acutely agitated patients during the acute phase of therapy, but also in patients who fail to respond sufficiently to an adequate trial of an antipsychotic agent alone. Schizophrenia is a major psychotic disorder that frequently has devastating effects on various aspects of the patient's life and carries a high risk of suicide and other life-threatening behaviors. Manifestations of schizophrenia involve multiple psychologic processes, including perception (e.g., hallucinations), ideation, reality testing (e.g., delusions), emotion (e.g., flatness, inappropriate affect), thought processes (e.g., loose associations), behavior (e.g., catatonia, disorganization), attention, concentration, motivation (e.g., avolition, impaired intention and planning), and judgment. The principal manifestations of this disorder usually are described in terms of positive and negative (deficit) symptoms, and, more recently, disorganized symptoms. Positive symptoms include hallucinations, delusions, bizarre behavior, hostility, uncooperativeness, and paranoid ideation, whereas negative symptoms include restricted range and intensity of emotional expression (affective flattening), reduced thought and speech productivity (alogia), anhedonia, and decreased initiation of goal-directed behavior (avolition). Disorganized symptoms include disorganized speech (thought disorder) and behavior and poor attention.

The American Psychiatric Association (APA) recommends that adjunctive benzodiazepine therapy be considered for patients with certain residual symptoms of schizophrenia and comorbid conditions during the acute and stable phases of therapy. The APA states that a benzodiazepine (e.g., lorazepam) may be helpful for the management of anxiety, agitation, and sleep disturbances that are often present during the acute phase of schizophrenia in patients receiving antipsychotic therapy. In addition, the APA states that benzodiazepines also may be helpful in the management of anxiety and insomnia during the stable phase of schizophrenia. Benzodiazepines (most commonly lorazepam, although clonazepam and oxazepam also have been used) also may be useful for the treatment of acute catatonic reactions†, whether associated with schizophrenia or other conditions.

Benzodiazepines, most commonly lorazepam or clonazepam, may be helpful in patients who experience akathisia† while receiving antipsychotic drugs. Because it may be difficult for clinicians to distinguish between akathisia related to antipsychotic drugs and psychomotor agitation associated with psychosis, the nonspecific effects of benzodiazepines on both akathisia and agitation may be useful; however, higher dosages of benzodiazepines usually are necessary in the management of psychotic agitation compared with akathisia. For additional information on the symptomatic management of schizophrenia, see Uses: Psychotic Disorders, in the Phenothiazines General Statement 28:16.08.04.

■ Cancer Chemotherapy-induced Nausea and Vomiting Benzodiazepines (e.g., alprazolam, lorazepam) have been used alone, but usually in combination with other drugs, such as 5-HT_3 receptor antagonists and/or corticosteroids, for the management of nausea and vomiting associated with emetogenic cancer chemotherapy†, including that associated with cisplatin. The antiemetic activity of benzodiazepines appears to be low, and their anxiolytic, sedative, and amnesic effects may account for beneficial effects in patients receiving emetogenic chemotherapy; the drugs appear to be most useful in reducing anticipatory and anxiety-related effects associated with administration of such chemotherapy. Various combinations of antiemetic agents have been used, and comparative efficacy is continually being evaluated. Because the management of *delayed* and *anticipatory* nausea and vomiting associated with emetogenic chemotherapy remains problematic, pending further elucidation of optimal regimens, some clinicians suggest antiemetic regimens that include one or more of the following drugs: aprepitant, a 5-HT_3 receptor antagonist (e.g., dolasetron, granisetron, ondansetron, palonosetron) for antiemetic activity, a corticosteroid (e.g., dexamethasone or methylprednisolone for antiemetic activity), metoclopramide (for antiemetic activity), and/or a benzodiazepine (e.g., alprazolam or lorazepam for anxiolytic, amnesic, and possibly antiemetic effects). However, aggressive antiemetic therapy during early courses of emetogenic chemotherapy is the best way to prevent anticipatory nausea and vomiting; behavior modification and hypnosis also may be useful.

■ Delirium Benzodiazepines, alone or combined with an antipsychotic agent, have been used in the management of delirium. However, the possibility that benzodiazepines may exacerbate symptoms of delirium in some patients and, when used alone, may be ineffective should be considered. Delirium is principally a disturbance of consciousness, attention, cognition, and perception but also may affect sleep, psychomotor activity, and emotions. It is a common psychiatric illness among medically compromised patients, particularly hospitalized patients, and may be a harbinger of substantial morbidity and mortality. Antipsychotic agents alone, usually haloperidol, often are considered the drugs of choice for the management of delirium (see Uses: Delirium, in Haloperidol 28:16.08.08).

There are few controlled studies that evaluated the efficacy of benzodiazepines as monotherapy for the management of delirium. Limited data suggest that benzodiazepines alone may be ineffective or at least less effective than antipsychotic agents for general cases of delirium. While there appears to be little evidence to support the use of benzodiazepine monotherapy for general delirium, the drugs may have advantages and therefore would be preferred for certain types of delirium. For example, benzodiazepines are the drugs of choice for the management of delirium associated with alcohol or benzodiazepine withdrawal. The drugs also may be useful when a drug that can raise the seizure threshold is needed (antipsychotic agents can decrease the seizure threshold) or when anticholinergic effects or akathisia associated with antipsychotic agents would seriously exacerbate the patient's condition.

There is some evidence that combined use of a benzodiazepine and antipsychotic agent may decrease certain adverse effects and improve efficacy in certain patients with delirium (e.g., those with AIDS, those severely ill with cancer). Results of several open studies suggested that combined therapy with IV haloperidol and IV lorazepam was more effective than IV haloperidol alone. During combined therapy, shorter duration of delirium and fewer extrapyramidal manifestations have been observed. If a benzodiazepine is used for the treatment of delirium, those with a short duration and no active metabolites (e.g., lorazepam) are preferred.

■ Drug-induced Cardiovascular Emergencies Benzodiazepines (e.g., diazepam, lorazepam) are used as adjuncts in the management of certain drug-induced cardiovascular emergencies†. If drug-induced cardiac arrest occurs, usual guidelines for advanced cardiovascular life support (ACLS) should be followed.

Cocaine-induced Acute Coronary Syndrome Benzodiazepines have been used adjunctively in patients with severe cardiovascular toxicity associated with cocaine overdose†. Experts state that administration of a benzodiazepine may be beneficial for cocaine-induced hypertension or chest discomfort.

■ Other Uses Parenteral diazepam also has been used to relieve agitation in the management of neonatal opiate withdrawal†.

Dosage and Administration

■ Administration Benzodiazepines are usually administered orally. When oral therapy is not feasible or when a rapid therapeutic effect is necessary, diazepam or lorazepam may be administered IV. Diazepam also may be given rectally. Midazolam hydrochloride is administered orally or by IM or IV injection and also has been administered intranasally† and intrabuccally†, and midazolam is administered intranasally. Although diazepam may also be given by deep IM injection, this route of administration is rarely justified because absorption of these drugs is slow and erratic. Chlordiazepoxide hydrochloride has also been given IV† and IM†; however, a parenteral dosage form of the drug is no longer commercially available in the US.

Concomitant oral administration of certain benzodiazepines (e.g., midazolam, triazolam) with grapefruit juice usually should be avoided since potentially clinically important increases in hemodynamic effects can result. (See Drug Interactions: Grapefruit Juice.)

■ Dosage Dosage of benzodiazepines must be carefully individualized, and the smallest effective dosage generally should be used (especially in geriatric or debilitated patients) to avoid oversedation. Sensitivity to the CNS depressant effects of the benzodiazepines differs among individual patients, and the patient's age, gender, physical or emotional status, and/or concurrent use of other drugs (including cigarette smoking) may alter the response.

Because of the episodic nature of anxiety, dosage may require frequent adjustments, and the drugs should generally be administered for a short period of time. The usefulness of the drug for each patient should be periodically reassessed. The effectiveness of benzodiazepines as anxiolytics for periods greater than 4 months or for panic disorder for periods greater than 4–10 weeks has not been established.

Because it is often difficult to predict how a patient will respond to a sedative agent, benzodiazepines used for procedural sedation should be titrated to effect.

The amount of time necessary for a particular benzodiazepine and its metabolites to reach steady-state plasma concentrations should be considered when dosage adjustments are made. (See Pharmacokinetics: Elimination.)

In patients who have received prolonged (e.g., for several months) benzodiazepine therapy, abrupt discontinuance of the drug should be avoided since manifestations of withdrawal, including rebound anxiety and insomnia, can be precipitated; if the drug is to be discontinued in such patients, it is recommended that dosage be gradually tapered. (See Chronic Toxicity.) It is particularly important that benzodiazepines *not* be discontinued abruptly in patients with a history of a seizure disorder to minimize the risk of precipitating seizures, seizure exacerbation, or status epilepticus. In addition, abrupt discontinuance of some benzodiazepines (e.g., those with a relatively short elimination half-life such as triazolam), even after relatively short periods of therapy (e.g., 1 week), can result in withdrawal effects such as rebound insomnia.

Cautions

Dose-dependent adverse CNS effects are common with the benzodiazepines. Many other adverse reactions have been reported with the drugs, but they are exceedingly rare.

■ CNS Effects Adverse CNS effects are an extension of the pharmacologic actions of benzodiazepines and include drowsiness, ataxia, fatigue, confusion, weakness, dizziness, vertigo, and syncope. Somnolence is the principal adverse effect associated with rectal diazepam administration, occurring in 13–33% of patients. Adverse CNS effects usually occur during the first few days of benzodiazepine therapy and may diminish with continued therapy or reduction in dosage. Geriatric or debilitated patients, children, and patients with liver disease or low serum albumin are most likely to experience these adverse CNS effects and generally should receive decreased initial dosages of the drugs. Benzodiazepines may produce prolonged CNS depression in neonates. Reversible dementia has been reported in geriatric patients after prolonged administration of benzodiazepines. Benzodiazepines with a relatively long elimination half-life may be more likely to cause residual daytime sedative effects and impaired psychomotor and mental performance during continued therapy, although partial tolerance to these effects can occur. Differences in residual and cumulative CNS depressant effects among benzodiazepines may be particularly important in geriatric patients and in patients with potentially impaired elimination of the drugs and those whose job or lifestyle requires unimpaired intellectual or psychomotor function. There is some evidence that ataxia and the risk of falling and associated hip fracture in geriatric patients is increased with use of benzodiazepines having a relatively long elimination half-life compared with use of those having a relatively short half-life. However, in several short-term studies in geriatric patients receiving quazepam, ataxia and morning hangover did not occur more frequently with the drug relative to placebo. Benzodiazepine therapy should be individualized and monitored closely in geriatric patients, and the need for continued therapy with the drugs should be determined periodically.

Amnesia Benzodiazepines can cause amnesic effects, principally anterograde amnesia, and the magnitude and duration of these effects may vary depending on the patient (e.g., age), drug, dosage, and route of administration. Immediate recall usually does not appear to be affected substantially. Some evidence suggests that amnesic effects may be particularly likely with midazolam, triazolam, and lorazepam, although other benzodiazepines also have been reported to cause such effects. Anterograde amnesia may be particularly disturbing with triazolam, especially when relatively high doses (e.g., 0.5 mg) are used. Anterograde amnesia ("traveler's amnesia") that occurred upon awakening and persisted for several hours has been reported in patients receiving triazolam for the prevention or treatment of insomnia associated with sleep-wake schedule changes (e.g., rapid travel across time zones ["jet lag"], rotating shift work); although behavior appeared normal in many of these patients (e.g., they performed what appeared to observers to be normal activities and they exhibited no apparent confusion or concern about memory at the time of amnesia), these patients subsequently had no recollection of the events that occurred during this period. Some of these patients consumed alcohol concomitantly, which also can cause anterograde amnesia. Similar anterograde amnesia has occurred in other patients receiving triazolam, and bizarre behavior has been associated with the period of amnesia in some patients. The risk of anterograde amnesia should be considered in patients receiving benzodiazepines, particularly when therapy with relatively high doses of triazolam is considered (e.g., for transient insomnia associated with sleep-wake schedule changes) or when the duration of drug effect is likely to exceed the intended period of sleep (e.g., when taken to induce sleep while traveling, such as during an airplane flight in which the patient will awake earlier than dissipation of hypnotic effects).

Behavioral Changes and Associated Effects Potentially serious behavioral changes and abnormal mentation occasionally have been associated with benzodiazepine use. Such effects include confusion, bizarre or abnormal behavior, agitation, hyperexcitability, auditory and visual hallucinations, paranoid ideation, panic, delirium, depersonalization, agitation, sleepwalking, and disinhibition manifested as aggression, excessive extroversion, and/or antisocial acts; in some cases, amnesia about the behavior may occur. Decreased inhibition may be similar to that associated with use of alcohol or other CNS depressants. Emergence or worsening of mental depression, including suicidal ideation, also has been associated with benzodiazepine use, principally in patients with preexisting depression. It appears that some of these behavioral effects may be dose related. There also is some epidemiologic and other evidence that the risk of some such behavioral effects may be increased with triazolam; however, a precise causal relationship rarely can be established with certainty.

There also is a potential risk of complex sleep-related behaviors such as sleep-driving (i.e., driving while not fully awake after ingesting a sedative-hypnotic drug, with no memory of the event), making phone calls, or preparing and eating food while asleep in patients receiving benzodiazepines.

An analysis of spontaneous reports of adverse effects received by the FDA for triazolam and temazepam from the date of marketing through 1985 revealed that the reporting rates for confusion, amnesia, abnormal or bizarre behavior, agitation, and hallucinations were substantially higher for triazolam. An updated aggregate analysis of spontaneous reports in the US for the first 7 years of marketing for each drug confirmed the higher frequency associated with triazolam compared with temazepam. While it could not be completely ruled out that some selection factors may have contributed to the differences in reporting rates, analysis of these data with adjustment for various factors suggested that a higher occurrence of these reactions existed for triazolam; a large epidemiologic study that follows up new users for adverse reactions and includes adjustment for potentially contributing factors would be required to determine the risk factors for adverse behavioral effects associated with these and other benzodiazepines.

Data from a limited number of patients suggest that individuals with borderline personality disorder, a history of violent or aggressive behavior, or a history of alcohol or drug abuse may be at increased risk for adverse behavioral effects with benzodiazepine use. Irritability, hostility, and intrusive thoughts have been reported in patients with posttraumatic stress disorder during discontinuance of alprazolam. While emergence of abnormalities in behavior and mentation or worsening of preexisting abnormalities may be the consequence of an underlying, possibly unrecognized, physical and/or psychiatric condition, it rarely can be determined with certainty whether such effects are drug induced, spontaneous in origin, or secondary to such underlying causes. Therefore, the emergence of any new behavioral sign or symptom of concern during benzodiazepine therapy requires careful and immediate evaluation.

Seizures When IV diazepam has been used to control absence status or Lennox-Gastaut syndrome status epilepticus, tonic status epilepticus has occurred. When oral benzodiazepines are used as adjuncts in the treatment of mixed epilepsy, increased frequency and/or severity of tonic-clonic seizures may occur, necessitating an increase in dosage of other anticonvulsants.

Abrupt withdrawal of diazepam therapy in patients with epilepsy may also result in a temporary increase in the frequency and/or severity of seizures. Changes in EEG patterns with characteristic low voltage, fast activity have been observed in some patients receiving benzodiazepines but are of no known importance. Withdrawal seizures also have been reported with alprazolam; in most cases, only a single seizure occurred, but multiple seizures and status epilepticus also have been reported. All anticonvulsants, including benzodiazepines, should be withdrawn gradually to minimize the risk of precipitating seizures, seizure exacerbation, or status epilepticus. (See Dosage and Administration: Dosage.)

Other CNS Effects Other adverse CNS effects of benzodiazepines include headache, vivid dreams, and dysarthria. Encephalopathy reportedly occurred in patients with renal failure receiving both diazepam and flurazepam. Extrapyramidal reactions, tremor, and oral buccal dyskinesia also have been reported. Abrupt withdrawal of benzodiazepines after use in the management of anxiety may lead to increased anxiety; rebound insomnia also has occurred following abrupt withdrawal of the drugs, particularly those with a relatively short elimination half-life. Withdrawal reactions also can be precipitated by dosage tapering and inadvertent dosage reduction (e.g., forgotten dose, admission to hospital). Such effects also can emerge in the early morning or between doses of benzodiazepines with a relatively short half-life.

Paradoxical CNS stimulation resulting in talkativeness, restlessness, anxiety, mania, euphoria, tremulousness, sleep disturbances, nightmares, excitement, hyperactivity, acute rage reactions, increased muscle spasticity, and hyperreflexia may occur, usually early in benzodiazepine therapy. Excitation is particularly likely to occur in psychiatric patients and in hyperactive aggressive children. Benzodiazepine therapy usually should be discontinued if CNS stimulation occurs.

The CNS depressant effect of benzodiazepines also can result in respiratory depression. (See Cautions: Respiratory and Cardiovascular Effects.)

■ Respiratory and Cardiovascular Effects Parenteral administration of benzodiazepines may produce apnea, hypotension, bradycardia, or cardiac arrest, particularly in geriatric or severely ill patients and in patients with limited pulmonary reserve or unstable cardiovascular status or if the drug is administered too rapidly IV. IV diazepam has reportedly caused ventricular premature complexes and other arrhythmias when used prior to cardioversion. Death has occurred rarely shortly after initiation of alprazolam therapy in patients with severe pulmonary disease. Respiratory depression and apnea have been reported infrequently with benzodiazepines in patients with compromised respiratory function.

Decreased gag reflex has been reported when IV diazepam was used prior to endoscopy. During peroral endoscopic procedures, coughing, depressed respiration, dyspnea, hyperventilation, laryngospasm, and pain in the throat or chest have been reported. Although the risk of respiratory depression may be greatest with rapid IV administration or large doses of the drugs, such depression also has been reported with rectal administration. Respiratory and cardiovascular depressant effects may be caused in part by the propylene glycol present in diazepam injection, a formulation that also has been administered rectally. In clinical studies with diazepam rectal gel, respiratory depressant effects (e.g., hypoventilation) occurred rarely.

Palpitation, tachycardia, shortness of breath, diaphoresis, and flushing also have been reported in patients receiving benzodiazepines.

■ GI and Hepatic Effects Adverse GI effects reported in patients receiving benzodiazepines include nausea and other GI complaints, hiccups, constipation, increased appetite, anorexia, weight gain or loss, dry mouth, increased salivation and bronchial secretions, swollen tongue, and bitter or metallic taste. Animals have developed esophageal dilation after very high doses of lorazepam for prolonged periods, and patients receiving this drug should be observed for the development of GI disease. Benzodiazepines may cause elevated serum AST (SGOT), ALT (SGPT), LDH, and alkaline phosphatase and total and direct serum bilirubin; jaundice has been reported.

Hepatitis and hepatic failure have been reported during postmarketing experience with alprazolam; however, a causal relationship to the drug has not been established.

In addition to typical benzodiazepine-associated adverse effects, rectal administration of diazepam gel may result in diarrhea and rarely rectal burning/pain.

■ Dermatologic and Sensitivity Reactions There is a potential risk of anaphylaxis and angioedema in patients receiving benzodiazepines; such reactions may occur as early as with the first dose of the drug. Urticaria, rash, pruritus, photosensitivity, immediate hypersensitivity reactions, hypotension, nonthrombocytopenic purpura, and edema may occur in patients receiving benzodiazepines. Paresthesia, Stevens-Johnson syndrome, and a lupus-like syndrome have been reported.

■ Local Effects IM administration of parenteral benzodiazepines (e.g., diazepam, lorazepam, or midazolam) may result in pain. Redness, burning, induration, or muscle stiffness also has been reported with IM administration of some benzodiazepines (e.g., lorazepam). IV administration of benzodiazepines may result in pain or thrombophlebitis. Intra-arterial administration of diazepam and other parenteral benzodiazepines has resulted in tissue necrosis. Adverse local effects associated with IM or IV administration occur less frequently and generally are less severe with midazolam than with other currently available parenteral benzodiazepines (e.g., diazepam).

■ Genitourinary and Renal Effects Increased or decreased libido, menstrual irregularities, failure to ovulate, hyperprolactinemia, gynecomastia, and galactorrhea have been reported in patients receiving benzodiazepines. Genitourinary complaints such as urinary retention, difficulty in micturition, and urinary incontinence have occurred. Alprazolam exhibits weak uricosuric activity. Transient decreases in renal function have occurred after IV administration of diazepam or midazolam, and abnormal renal function test results have been reported after oral benzodiazepines.

■ Musculoskeletal Effects Serum creatine kinase (CK, creatine phosphokinase, CPK) concentrations increase after IM injection of diazepam. Body joint pains and muscle cramps also have been reported.

■ Hematologic Effects A few cases of leukopenia (including neutropenia and granulocytopenia), agranulocytosis, aplastic anemia, hemolytic anemia, decreased hematocrit, eosinophilia, and leukocytosis have been attributed to benzodiazepine administration.

■ Ocular Effects Conjunctivitis and visual disturbances such as diplopia, nystagmus, and blurred vision have occurred in patients receiving benzodiazepines.

■ Precautions and Contraindications Concomitant use of benzodiazepines and opiate agonists or opiate partial agonists may result in profound sedation, respiratory depression, coma, and death. Concomitant use of such drugs should be reserved for patients in whom alternative treatment options are inadequate; the lowest effective dosages and shortest possible duration of concomitant therapy should be used, and the patient should be monitored closely for respiratory depression and sedation. Patients receiving benzodiazepines and/or their caregivers should be apprised of the risks associated with concomitant therapeutic or illicit use of benzodiazepines and opiates. (See Opiate Agonists and Opiate Partial Agonists under Drug Interactions: CNS Agents.)

Patients should be warned that benzodiazepines may impair ability to perform hazardous activities requiring mental alertness or physical coordination (e.g., operating machinery, driving a motor vehicle). There also is a potential risk of complex sleep-related behaviors such as sleep-driving (i.e., driving while not fully awake after ingesting a sedative-hypnotic drug, with no memory of the event), making phone calls, or preparing and eating food while asleep in patients receiving benzodiazepines. Patients also should be warned about possible effects on memory (anterograde amnesia) and to report promptly to their physician any behavioral or mental change, including disturbing thoughts and unusual manners of conduct, that develops during benzodiazepine therapy. (See Cautions: CNS Effects.) Benzodiazepines should be used with caution and large quantities of the drugs should not be prescribed for patients with suicidal tendencies or whose history indicates that they may increase dosage on their own initiative.

Because benzodiazepines may produce psychologic and physical dependence, patients should be advised to consult their clinician before increasing the dose of, or abruptly discontinuing, benzodiazepine therapy. (See Chronic Toxicity.)

Liver and kidney function tests and blood cell counts should be performed regularly during long-term therapy, and benzodiazepines should be administered with caution to patients with hepatic or renal disease.

Benzodiazepines should be used with caution in patients with chronic pulmonary insufficiency or sleep apnea. Facilities and age- and size-appropriate equipment for respiratory or cardiovascular assistance should be readily available whenever benzodiazepines are administered IV. The drugs should not be administered IV to patients in whom the hypnotic or hypotensive effects may be prolonged or intensified such as those with shock or coma, to patients with depressed respiration, or to those who have recently received other respiratory depressant drugs. Diazepam rectal gel should be used with caution in patients with compromised respiratory function associated with a concurrent disease process (e.g., asthma, pneumonia) or neurologic damage.

Benzodiazepines generally should not be used in patients with depressive neuroses or psychotic reactions in which anxiety is not prominent. Many benzodiazepines are contraindicated in patients with known hypersensitivity to the drugs. Because the frequency of suicide appears to be increased in untreated patients with panic disorder, and because panic disorder may be associated with primary and secondary major depressive disorders, the usual precautions of psychotropic therapy in depressed patients or those at risk for concealed suicidal ideation should be exercised during benzodiazepine therapy for panic disorder. According to most manufacturers of benzodiazepines, the drugs are contraindicated in patients with acute angle-closure glaucoma but may be administered to patients receiving appropriate treatment for open-angle glaucoma. However, the clinical rationale for this contraindication has been questioned since benzodiazepines do not have anticholinergic effects and do not increase intraocular pressure; only one case of increased intraocular pressure after use of a benzodiazepine and other drugs has been reported.

■ Pediatric Precautions FDA warns that repeated or prolonged use of general anesthetics and sedation drugs, including benzodiazepines such as lorazepam and midazolam, in children younger than 3 years of age or during the third trimester of pregnancy may affect brain development. Animal studies in multiple species, including nonhuman primates, have demonstrated that use for longer than 3 hours of anesthetic and sedation drugs that block *N*-methyl-D-aspartic acid (NMDA) receptors and/or potentiate γ-aminobutyric acid (GABA) activity leads to widespread neuronal and oligodendrocyte cell loss and alterations in synaptic morphology and neurogenesis in the brain, resulting in long-term deficits in cognition and behavior. Across animal species, vulnerability to these neurodevelopmental changes occurs during the period of rapid brain growth or synaptogenesis; this period is thought to correlate with the third trimester of pregnancy through the first year of life in humans, but may extend to approximately 3 years of age. The clinical relevance of these animal findings to humans is not known.

While some published evidence suggests that similar deficits in cognition and behavior may occur in children following repeated or prolonged exposure to anesthesia early in life, other studies have found no association between pediatric anesthesia exposure and long-term adverse neurodevelopmental outcomes. Most studies to date have had substantial limitations, and it is not clear whether the adverse neurodevelopmental outcomes observed in children were related to the drug or to other factors (e.g., surgery, underlying illness). There is some clinical evidence that a single, relatively brief exposure to general anesthesia in generally healthy children is unlikely to cause clinically detectable deficits in global cognitive function or serious behavioral disorders; however, further research is needed to fully characterize the effects of exposure to general anesthetics in early life, particularly for prolonged or repeated exposures and in more vulnerable populations (e.g., less healthy children).

Results from an observational study (the Pediatric Anesthesia Neurodevelopment Assessment [PANDA] study) and preliminary results from an ongoing multicenter, randomized trial (the General Anesthesia Compared to Spinal Anesthesia [GAS] trial) provide some evidence that a single, relatively brief exposure to general anesthesia in generally healthy children is unlikely to cause clinically detectable deficits in global cognitive function or serious behavioral disorders. The PANDA study compared global cognitive function (as measured by intelligence quotient [IQ] score) of children 8–15 years of age who had a single anesthesia exposure for elective inguinal hernia surgery before the age of 3 years with that of a biologically related sibling who had no anesthesia exposure before the age of 3 years. All of the children had a gestational age at birth of at least 36 weeks, and sibling pairs were within 3 years of being the same age. Children who underwent the elective procedure were mostly males (90%) and generally healthy. The mean duration of anesthesia was 84 minutes; 16% of those receiving anesthesia had exposures exceeding 2 hours. The study found no substantial difference in IQ score between children who had a single anesthesia exposure before the age of 3 years and their siblings who had not. The GAS trial was designed to compare neurodevelopmental outcomes in children who received general anesthesia with those in children who received awake regional (caudal and/or spinal) anesthesia for inguinal herniorrhaphy before they reached a postmenstrual age of 60 weeks (with a gestational age at birth of more than 26 weeks); the primary outcome was the Wechsler Preschool and Primary Scale of Intelligence Third Edition (WPPSI-III) Full Scale IQ at 5 years of age. In an interim analysis at the age of 2 years, no difference in composite cognitive score (as measured by the Bayley Scales of Infant and Toddler Development III) was detected between children who had received sevoflurane anesthesia of less than 1 hour's duration (median duration: 54 minutes) compared with those who had received awake regional anesthesia.

Anesthetic and sedation drugs are an essential component of care for children and pregnant women who require surgery or other procedures that cannot be delayed; no specific general anesthetic or sedation drug has been shown to be less likely to cause neurocognitive deficits than any other such drug. Pending further accumulation of data in humans from well-designed studies, decisions regarding the timing of elective procedures requiring anesthesia should take into consideration both the benefits of the procedure and the potential risks. When procedures requiring the use of general anesthetics or sedation drugs are considered for young children or pregnant women, clinicians should discuss with the patient, parent, or caregiver the benefits, risks (including potential risk of adverse neurodevelopmental effects), and appropriate timing and duration of the procedure. FDA states that procedures that are considered medically necessary should not be delayed or avoided.

■ Pregnancy and Lactation Benzodiazepines can cause fetal harm when administered to pregnant women. Results of retrospective studies suggest an increased risk of congenital malformations in infants of mothers who received benzodiazepines (e.g., chlordiazepoxide, diazepam) during the first trimester of pregnancy. An increase in fetal heart rate has occurred after diazepam use during labor. Hypoactivity, hypotonia, hypothermia, apnea, feeding problems, impaired metabolic response to cold stress, hyperbilirubinemia, and kernicterus have been reported in neonates born to mothers who received large doses of diazepam (generally greater than 30 mg) shortly before delivery. Infants of mothers who chronically ingested benzodiazepines during pregnancy have been reported to have withdrawal symptoms. Neonatal flaccidity, respiratory and feeding difficulties, and hypothermia have been reported in infants born to women who received benzodiazepines late in pregnancy. Since the use of anxiolytics is rarely urgent, their use during the first trimester of pregnancy should almost always be avoided. Benzodiazepines used solely as hypnotics (flurazepam, temazepam, triazolam) are contraindicated during pregnancy.

Although there is an association between anticonvulsant drug use in pregnant women with seizure disorders and an increased incidence of teratogenic effects in children born to such women, anticonvulsant therapy should not be discontinued in women in whom the drugs are administered to prevent seizures because of the strong possibility of precipitating status epilepticus and the attendant hypoxia and threat to life. In cases where the severity and frequency of the seizure disorder are such that removal of the anticonvulsant does not pose a serious threat to the patient, discontinuance of the drug may be considered prior to and during pregnancy. However, it cannot be said with confidence that even mild seizures do not pose some hazard to the developing embryo or fetus. In general, benzodiazepines should be considered for use as anticonvulsant therapy in women of childbearing potential, and more specifically during known pregnancy, only when the clinical situation warrants the risk to the fetus.

Based on animal data, repeated or prolonged use of general anesthetics and sedation drugs, including benzodiazepines such as lorazepam and midazolam, during the third trimester of pregnancy may result in adverse neurodevelopmental effects in the fetus. The clinical relevance of these animal findings to humans is not known; the potential risk of adverse neurodevelopmental effects should be considered and discussed with pregnant women undergoing procedures requiring general anesthetics and sedation drugs. (See Cautions: Pediatric Precautions.)

The possibility that a woman of childbearing potential may be pregnant at the time benzodiazepine therapy is initiated should be considered. Patients should be advised that if they become pregnant or intend to become pregnant during benzodiazepine therapy, they should communicate with their clinician about the desirability of discontinuing the drug.

Since many benzodiazepines are distributed into milk and because of the potential for adverse reactions from the drugs in nursing infants, a decision should be made whether to discontinue nursing or the drug, taking into account the importance of the drug to the woman.

Drug Interactions

■ **Drugs and Foods Affecting Hepatic Microsomal Enzymes** Some benzodiazepines (e.g., alprazolam, clobazam, diazepam, estazolam, midazolam, triazolam) are metabolized by cytochrome P-450 (CYP) isoenzymes, predominantly by CYP3A4 and/or CYP2C19. Clearance of these benzodiazepines may be reduced by drugs or foods that inhibit CYP3A4 (e.g., some azole antifungals, some macrolide antibiotics, HIV protease inhibitors, some calcium-channel blocking agents, some selective serotonin-reuptake inhibitors [SSRIs], nefazodone, grapefruit juice) or inhibit CYP2C19 (e.g., fluvoxamine, omeprazole, ticlopidine), possibly resulting in enhanced or prolonged benzodiazepine effects. Conversely, concomitant use of these benzodiazepines with drugs that induce CYP3A4 (e.g., carbamazepine, phenobarbital, phenytoin, rifampin) may decrease plasma concentrations of the benzodiazepines.

■ **Antihistamines** Concomitant administration of temazepam and diphenhydramine in a pregnant woman at the end of the third trimester has been associated with violent intrauterine fetal movements within several hours after maternal ingestion of the drugs; within 8 hours, the infant was delivered stillborn. Reproduction studies in rabbits have suggested that concomitant administration of these drugs markedly increases perinatal mortality; neonatal deaths were associated with increased irritability and seizures.

■ **Anti-infective Agents** ***Antifungal Agents*** Concomitant use of some benzodiazepines (e.g., alprazolam, clobazam, estazolam, midazolam, triazolam) with some azole antifungal agents (e.g., fluconazole, itraconazole, ketoconazole) may result in increased plasma concentrations and systemic exposure of these benzodiazepines. Following concomitant administration of oral midazolam with itraconazole or ketoconazole, large increases in the peak plasma concentration (up to 240 or 309%, respectively) and area under the serum concentration-time curve (AUC) (up to 980 or 1490%, respectively) of midazolam were observed. When alprazolam was given concomitantly with itraconazole or ketoconazole, increases of 2.7- or 4-fold, respectively, in the AUC of alprazolam were observed. In healthy adults receiving multiple doses of itraconazole (200 mg daily for 6 days), the elimination half-life of alprazolam was increased by 260% and AUC was increased by 270% following administration of a single 0.8-mg dose of alprazolam; substantial changes in psychomotor function (e.g., sleepiness) were also noted. Administration of a single 200-mg dose of itraconazole given 3, 12, or 24 hours prior to or simultaneously with a single 0.25-mg dose of triazolam increased the peak plasma concentration of triazolam by 140–180% and AUC of triazolam by 300–500%, depending on ingestion time of the dose, while the elimination half-life of triazolam was increased by 300%. When oral midazolam was administered concomitantly with fluconazole in healthy adults, the peak plasma concentration and AUC of midazolam were increased by 150 and 250%, respectively.

Alprazolam, estazolam, and triazolam are contraindicated in patients receiving concomitant therapy with potent CYP3A inhibitors such as ketoconazole and itraconazole; concomitant use of other azole antifungal agents that are considered potent CYP3A inhibitors is not recommended. Because of the potential for intense and prolonged sedation and respiratory depression, oral midazolam should be administered only when absolutely necessary and with extreme caution (e.g., with appropriate equipment and personnel available to respond to respiratory insufficiency) in patients receiving ketoconazole or itraconazole.

Antimycobacterial Agents **Isoniazid.** Concomitant use of isoniazid with triazolam has been shown to increase the peak plasma concentration and half-life of triazolam by 20 and 31%, respectively, and decrease clearance of triazolam by 42%. Caution is advised when triazolam or other benzodiazepines that are metabolized by the CYP3A isoenzyme (e.g., alprazolam, estazolam) are used concomitantly with isoniazid.

Antiretroviral Agents **HIV Protease Inhibitors.** Because of the potential for intense and prolonged sedation and respiratory depression, the manufacturers of HIV protease inhibitors (e.g., atazanavir, darunavir, fosamprenavir, indinavir, lopinavir/ritonavir, nelfinavir, ritonavir, saquinavir, tipranavir) state that concomitant use of these agents with midazolam or triazolam is contraindicated.

Concomitant use of HIV protease inhibitors (e.g., fosamprenavir, ritonavir, saquinavir) with certain other benzodiazepines (e.g., alprazolam, clorazepate, diazepam, flurazepam) also may result in increased concentrations of the benzodiazepine. While the clinical importance of the interaction is unknown, a reduction in dosage of the benzodiazepine may be needed.

Nonnucleoside Reverse Transcriptase Inhibitors. Concomitant use of efavirenz with midazolam or triazolam and of delavirdine with alprazolam, midazolam, or triazolam should be avoided because of the potential for the nonnucleoside reverse transcriptase inhibitor (NNRTI) to decrease metabolism of the benzodiazepine and result in intense or prolonged sedation or respiratory depression.

Macrolide Antibiotics Concomitant use of erythromycin decreases clearance of midazolam and triazolam and could increase the pharmacologic effects of these benzodiazepines. Available data also suggest that some macrolide antibiotics (i.e., erythromycin, clarithromycin) might interact with alprazolam. In addition, it might be anticipated that erythromycin could interfere with the metabolism of estazolam.

Patients receiving benzodiazepines that are metabolized by the CYP3A isoenzyme concomitantly with some macrolide antibiotics (i.e., erythromycin, clarithromycin) should be monitored closely; reduction in the benzodiazepine dosage may be necessary.

■ **Cardiovascular Agents** ***Amiodarone*** Although specific drug interaction studies are not available, concomitant use of amiodarone with some benzodiazepines (e.g., alprazolam, triazolam) may result in decreased metabolism of the benzodiazepine; caution is advised.

Calcium-channel Blocking Agents Concomitant use of diltiazem or verapamil with oral midazolam results in increased plasma midazolam concentrations and may lead to increased and prolonged sedation and respiratory depression. If midazolam is used concomitantly with diltiazem or verapamil, caution is advised and dosage reduction of midazolam may be necessary.

Although specific drug interaction studies are not available, clinically important decreases in the metabolism and clearance of other benzodiazepines metabolized by the CYP3A isoenzyme (e.g., alprazolam, estazolam, triazolam) may occur when these benzodiazepines are used concomitantly with some calcium-channel blocking agents (e.g., diltiazem, verapamil); caution is advised. Drug interactions also are possible when some benzodiazepines (e.g., alprazolam, estazolam, triazolam) are used concomitantly with nicardipine or nifedipine.

Digoxin Limited evidence suggests that diazepam may reduce the renal excretion of digoxin, resulting in an increased plasma half-life of the cardiac glycoside and possible digoxin toxicity. Digoxin toxicity has been reported in one geriatric patient who was receiving alprazolam and digoxin concurrently; serum digoxin concentrations increased threefold in this patient following initiation of alprazolam therapy, but returned to within normal limits following discontinuance of the benzodiazepine. Although the exact mechanism for the effect of benzodiazepines on the renal excretion of digoxin has not been clearly established, increased plasma protein binding of digoxin and/or an effect of benzodiazepines on the renal tubular transport of digoxin have been suggested. Pending further accumulation of data, serum digoxin concentrations should be monitored and patients should be carefully observed for signs and/or symptoms of digoxin toxicity during concomitant therapy with benzodiazepines and digoxin. Dosage reduction of digoxin may be necessary in some patients receiving concomitant therapy.

■ **CNS Agents** ***CNS Depressants*** Additive CNS depression may occur when benzodiazepines are administered concomitantly with other CNS depressants, including other anticonvulsants and alcohol. If benzodiazepines are used concomitantly with other depressant drugs, caution should be used to avoid overdosage. Patients receiving benzodiazepines should be advised to avoid alcohol.

Anticonvulsants In patients receiving clonazepam and phenytoin concurrently, plasma concentrations of phenytoin may decrease; patients receiving these drugs concurrently should be closely observed.

Concurrent administration of carbamazepine with alprazolam or clonazepam has been shown to increase the rate of metabolism and decrease plasma concentrations of these benzodiazepines. In one study, administration of a single 0.8-mg dose of alprazolam after 10 days of low-dose carbamazepine (300 mg daily) resulted in a 2.4-fold increase in oral clearance of alprazolam and decreased the elimination half-life of alprazolam from 17.1 hours to 7.7 hours.

Concomitant administration of oral midazolam with phenytoin or carbamazepine has been shown to decrease the peak plasma concentration and AUC of midazolam by about 93–94%.

In a limited number of healthy men, concurrent use of valproate (250 mg twice daily orally, for 3 days) with a single 2-mg IV dose of lorazepam reportedly decreased total clearance of lorazepam by 40% and increased plasma concentration of the benzodiazepine approximately twofold (that persisted for at least 12 hours after dosing) compared with administration of lorazepam alone. The dosage of lorazepam should be reduced by approximately 50% when administered concomitantly with valproate.

Antidepressants **Nefazodone.** Concomitant use of nefazodone with some benzodiazepines (e.g., alprazolam, triazolam) results in clinically important increases in plasma concentrations of the benzodiazepine. Concomitant use of triazolam and nefazodone should be avoided. If alprazolam is used concomitantly with nefazodone, caution is advised and reduction of the alprazolam dosage should be considered. Although specific drug interaction studies are not available, concomitant use of estazolam with nefazodone would be expected to increase plasma concentrations of estazolam.

Selective Serotonin-reuptake Inhibitors. Concomitant use of some SSRIs (e.g., fluoxetine, fluvoxamine) with alprazolam has been reported to decrease clearance and increase plasma concentrations of alprazolam and impair psychomotor performance. In one study, peak plasma concentrations of alprazolam were doubled, half-life of alprazolam was increased by 71%, and clearance of the drug was reduced by 49% when alprazolam was given concomitantly with fluvoxamine. When alprazolam was given concomitantly with fluoxetine, the peak plasma concentration and half-life of alprazolam were increased by 46 and 17%, respectively, and clearance of alprazolam was reduced by 21%. Caution is advised if fluvoxamine or fluoxetine is used concomitantly with alprazolam, midazolam, or triazolam. If fluvoxamine is used concomitantly with alprazolam, reduction of the alprazolam dosage also should be considered.

Although specific drug interaction studies are not available, concomitant use of estazolam with fluvoxamine would be expected to result in increased plasma concentrations of estazolam. In one study, concomitant use of estazolam (2 mg daily) and fluoxetine (20 mg twice daily) for 7 days did not appear to affect the peak plasma concentration or AUC of estazolam.

The clearance of diazepam was reduced by 65% and that of its active metabolite *N*-desmethyldiazepam could not be determined during concomitant administration with fluvoxamine in one study. Concomitant use of diazepam and fluvoxamine generally should be avoided.

The clearance of benzodiazepines that are metabolized by glucuronidation (e.g., lorazepam, oxazepam, temazepam) is unlikely to be affected by fluvoxamine.

In vitro studies suggest a possible interaction between triazolam and sertraline or paroxetine; caution is advised if these drugs are used concomitantly. Although in vitro data also suggest the possibility of an interaction between alprazolam and sertraline or paroxetine, no substantial changes in alprazolam pharmacokinetics were evident in one study involving multiple-dose administration of sertraline (50–150 mg daily) and single-dose administration of alprazolam (1 mg). Nonetheless, the manufacturers of alprazolam state that caution is advised when alprazolam is used concomitantly with sertraline or paroxetine.

Tricyclic Antidepressants. Although some studies showed no substantial alteration of tricyclic antidepressant plasma concentrations during simultaneous administration of benzodiazepines, one study indicated that the elimination half-life and steady-state plasma concentrations of amitriptyline may be increased in patients receiving diazepam. In addition, steady-state plasma concentrations of imipramine and desipramine reportedly were increased by 31 and 20%, respectively, in patients receiving these antidepressants concomitantly with alprazolam (up to 4 mg daily). The clinical importance of these possible interactions has not been determined. There have been reports of impaired motor function when tricyclic antidepressants were used with benzodiazepines, but these have not been confirmed and the drugs have often been administered concomitantly without adverse effects.

Antipsychotic Agents **Clozapine.** Severe hypotension (including absence of measurable blood pressure), respiratory or cardiac arrest, and loss of consciousness have been reported in several patients who received benzodiazepines (i.e., diazepam, flurazepam, lorazepam) concomitantly with or before clozapine therapy. Such effects occurred following administration of 12.5–150 mg of clozapine concurrently with or within 24 hours of the benzodiazepine, but patients generally have recovered within a few minutes to hours, usually spontaneously; the reactions usually developed on the first or second day of clozapine therapy. Although a causal relationship has not definitely been established and such effects also have been observed in clozapine-treated patients who were not receiving a benzodiazepine concomitantly, death resulting from respiratory arrest reportedly has rarely occurred when a benzodiazepine (e.g., lorazepam) was used concomitantly with clozapine. An increased incidence of dizziness and sedation and greater increases in liver enzyme test results also have been reported when benzodiazepines and clozapine were used concomitantly.

The manufacturers of lorazepam and clozapine recommend caution when clozapine is initiated in patients receiving benzodiazepine therapy. However, some clinicians advise that, pending further accumulation of data, greater precaution should be exercised. These clinicians recommend that because initial titration of clozapine may cause respiratory arrest requiring resuscitation, which may be potentiated by recent benzodiazepine therapy, these latter drugs should be discontinued for at least 1 week prior to initiating clozapine therapy.

Other Antipsychotic Agents. Respiratory depression, stupor, and/or hypotension have been reported rarely in patients receiving lorazepam concomitantly with loxapine. In addition, apnea, coma, bradycardia, arrhythmia, cardiac arrest, and death have occurred in patients receiving lorazepam and haloperidol concomitantly. The manufacturer of lorazepam states that lorazepam should be used with caution in patients receiving haloperidol or loxapine because concomitant administration of these drugs has not been evaluated systematically.

Opiate Agonists and Opiate Partial Agonists Concomitant use of benzodiazepines with opiate agonists or opiate partial agonists may result in profound sedation, respiratory depression, coma, and death. Epidemiologic studies have shown that a substantial proportion of fatal opiate overdoses involve the concurrent use of benzodiazepines.

Whenever possible, concomitant use of opiate agonists or partial agonists and benzodiazepines should be avoided. Opiate antitussive agents should be avoided in patients receiving benzodiazepines, and concomitant use of opiate analgesics and benzodiazepines should be reserved for patients in whom alternative treatment options are inadequate. (See Cautions: Precautions and Contraindications, in the Opiate Agonists General Statement 28:08.08.) If a decision is made to prescribe opiates and benzodiazepines concomitantly, the lowest effective dosages and shortest possible duration of concomitant therapy should be used, and the patient should be monitored closely for respiratory depression and sedation. If a benzodiazepine is required for any indication other than epilepsy in a patient receiving opiate therapy, the drug should be initiated at a lower dosage than indicated in the absence of opiate therapy and titrated based on clinical response. In patients receiving benzodiazepines, opiate analgesics should be initiated at a reduced dosage and titrated based on clinical response. Some experts state that consideration should be given to offering the opiate antagonist naloxone when opiates are prescribed for patients at increased risk of opiate overdosage, including those receiving benzodiazepines concomitantly.

■ **Cyclosporine** Although specific drug interaction studies are not available, concomitant use of cyclosporine with some benzodiazepines (e.g., alprazolam, triazolam) may result in decreased metabolism of the benzodiazepine; caution is advised.

■ **Disulfiram** Concurrent administration of disulfiram and benzodiazepines may result in inhibition of metabolism of some benzodiazepines. Disulfiram has reduced the plasma clearance and increased the plasma half-lives of chlordiazepoxide and diazepam during concomitant administration. It is likely that other benzodiazepines that undergo oxidative metabolism (e.g., alprazolam, clonazepam, clorazepate, estazolam, flurazepam, triazolam) would also interact with disulfiram. Benzodiazepines metabolized by glucuronide conjugation (e.g., lorazepam, oxazepam, temazepam) are probably not affected by disulfiram. Patients should be closely observed for evidence of enhanced benzodiazepine response during concomitant therapy with disulfiram; some patients may require reduction in benzodiazepine dosage.

■ **Ergot Alkaloids** Although specific drug interaction studies are not available, concomitant use of ergotamine with some benzodiazepines (e.g., alprazolam, triazolam) may result in decreased metabolism of the benzodiazepine; caution is advised.

■ **GI Drugs** ***Antacids*** Concurrent administration of chlordiazepoxide or diazepam with antacids such as aluminum and magnesium hydroxides may decrease the rate, but not the extent, of GI absorption of chlordiazepoxide or diazepam. Concurrent administration of antacids and clorazepate may decrease the rate and extent of conversion of the latter drug to desmethyldiazepam, and these drugs should not be given concurrently.

Cimetidine Concomitant administration of some benzodiazepines (e.g., alprazolam, chlordiazepoxide, clobazam, clorazepate, diazepam, midazolam, triazolam) and cimetidine may result in decreased benzodiazepine plasma clearance and increased plasma half-lives and concentrations of these benzodiazepines. Cimetidine reduces plasma clearance of benzodiazepines that undergo oxidative metabolism, apparently via inhibition of hepatic microsomal enzymes involved in oxidative metabolism. Consequently, the elimination of clonazepam, estazolam, and flurazepam may also be similarly affected by cimetidine. Benzodiazepines metabolized by conjugation with glucuronic acid (e.g., lorazepam, oxazepam, temazepam) do not appear to be affected by concomitant cimetidine therapy. Although an increased sedative effect has been observed in some patients receiving concomitant therapy with a benzodiazepine and cimetidine, the degree to which the pharmacologic response to the benzodiazepine may be increased is not well established. Benzodiazepine dosage reduction may be necessary in patients receiving concomitant therapy with cimetidine. Altered benzodiazepine response may occur following initiation or discontinuance of cimetidine therapy in patients receiving affected benzodiazepines.

Ranitidine There have been reports of increased systemic availability of benzodiazepines (e.g., oral midazolam, triazolam) when these benzodiazepines were administered concomitantly with ranitidine. The mechanism has not been fully elucidated.

■ **Grapefruit Juice** Concomitant oral administration of grapefruit juice with midazolam or triazolam has been reported to increase bioavailability of the drugs. The interaction between grapefruit juice and benzodiazepine bioavailability appears to result from inhibition, probably prehepatic, of the cytochrome P-450 enzyme system by some constituent(s) in the juice. Following oral administration of these benzodiazepines, such prehepatic inhibition of drug metabolism by grapefruit juice appears mainly to involve the CYP3A4 isoenzyme, principally within the small intestinal wall (e.g., in the jejunum), thus increasing systemic availability of these drugs. (See Grapefruit Juice under Drug Interactions: Drugs and Foods Affecting Hepatic Microsomal Enzymes, in Cyclosporine 92:44.)

■ **Hormonal Contraceptives** In a limited number of healthy women, concurrent use of an oral estrogen-progestin contraceptive (1 mg of norethindrone acetate and 50 mcg of ethinyl estradiol daily for at least 6 months) with a single 2-mg IV dose of lorazepam decreased half-life of lorazepam by 55% and increased volume of distribution by 50%, resulting in an almost 3.7-fold increase in total clearance of lorazepam. Dosage of lorazepam may need to be increased when administered to women receiving oral contraceptives.

Concomitant use of oral contraceptives with alprazolam or triazolam has been shown to decrease clearance of these benzodiazepines. In one study, the peak plasma concentration and elimination half-life of alprazolam were increased by 18 and 29%, respectively, and clearance of alprazolam was decreased by 22% when oral contraceptives were given concomitantly. Similar results were observed in a study with triazolam; the peak plasma concentration and elimination half-life of triazolam were increased by 6 and 16%, respectively, and clearance of triazolam was decreased by 32% when oral contraceptives were given concomitantly. Caution is advised when alprazolam or triazolam is used concomitantly with oral contraceptives.

Clobazam may reduce the efficacy of some hormonal contraceptives (e.g., oral or other hormonal contraceptives) that are metabolized by CYP3A4. Additional nonhormonal forms of contraception are recommended in women receiving hormonal contraceptives during clobazam therapy and for 28 days following discontinuance of the drug.

■ **Levodopa** A few levodopa-treated patients experienced decreased control of parkinsonian symptoms when chlordiazepoxide hydrochloride or diazepam was added to their therapeutic regimen. Therefore, benzodiazepines should be administered with caution to patients receiving levodopa.

■ **Probenecid** In a limited number of healthy adults, concurrent use of probenecid (500 mg every 6 hours) with a single 2-mg IV dose of lorazepam increased the half-life of lorazepam by 130% and decreased its clearance by 45%. Dosage of lorazepam should be reduced by 50% when administered concomitantly with probenecid.

■ **Scopolamine** An increased incidence of sedation, hallucinations, and irrational behavior has been reported in patients receiving lorazepam injection concomitantly with scopolamine. The manufacturer of lorazepam states that the benzodiazepine should be used with caution in patients receiving scopolamine, because concomitant administration of these drugs has not been evaluated systematically.

■ **Smoking** Cigarette smoking may decrease the sedative effects of usual doses of benzodiazepines. Clearance of benzodiazepines may be increased in smokers compared with nonsmokers. Plasma alprazolam concentrations reportedly are decreased by up to 50% in cigarette smokers compared with nonsmokers.

Laboratory Test Interferences

■ **Pregnancy Test** Chlordiazepoxide may cause a false-positive reaction in the Gravindex® pregnancy test.

■ **Tests for Urinary Steroids and Alkaloids** Chlordiazepoxide reportedly interferes with the Zimmerman reaction for urinary 17-ketosteroids, resulting in falsely elevated or decreased concentrations. Chlordiazepoxide and diazepam may interfere with urine alkaloids determined by the Frings thin layer chromatography procedure, resulting in falsely elevated readings.

■ **Tests for Urinary Glucose** False-negative reactions for glucose in the urine may occur in patients receiving diazepam when the test is performed with Clinistix® and Diastix®, but not with Tes-Tape®.

Acute Toxicity

■ **Manifestations** Benzodiazepine overdosage may result in somnolence, impaired coordination, slurred speech, confusion, coma, and diminished reflexes. Hypotension, seizures, respiratory depression, and apnea also may occur. Although cardiac arrest has been reported, death from overdosage of benzodiazepines in the absence of concurrent ingestion of alcohol or other CNS depressants is rare. Most patients recover rapidly.

■ **Treatment** Treatment of benzodiazepine intoxication consists of general supportive therapy. Flumazenil, a benzodiazepine antagonist, can be used in the management of benzodiazepine overdosage, but the drug is an adjunct to, not a substitute for, appropriate supportive and symptomatic therapy. (See Flumazenil 28:92.) The possibility that the antagonist could precipitate withdrawal (e.g., seizures) in benzodiazepine-dependent individuals should be considered.

If ingestion of the benzodiazepine is recent and the patient is fully conscious, emesis should be induced. If the patient is comatose, gastric lavage may be done if an endotracheal tube with cuff inflated is in place to prevent aspiration of gastric contents. Activated charcoal and a saline cathartic may be administered after gastric lavage and/or emesis to remove any remaining drug. Pulse, respiration, and blood pressure should be monitored and the patient should be closely observed. IV fluids should be administered and an adequate airway maintained. Hypotension may be controlled, if necessary, by IV administration of norepinephrine or metaraminol. Although some manufacturers recommend use of caffeine and sodium benzoate to combat CNS depression, most authorities believe caffeine and other analeptic agents should *not* be used, because these drugs have questionable benefit and transient action. Instead, administration of flumazenil, if indicated, generally would be preferred. Hemodialysis is not useful in the treatment of benzodiazepine overdosage.

Chronic Toxicity

Tolerance and psychologic and physical dependence may occur following prolonged use of benzodiazepines. The possibility that such effects also may occur following short-term use of benzodiazepines, particularly at high dosages, also should be considered. Symptoms of benzodiazepine dependence are similar to barbiturate dependence or chronic alcoholism and may include drowsiness, ataxia, slurred speech, and vertigo.

Sudden discontinuance of benzodiazepines in physically dependent patients (usually patients who have received excessive doses for an extended period of time but also occasionally with therapeutic dosages for relatively short periods) may produce severe withdrawal symptoms including anxiety, agitation, tension, dysphoria, anorexia, insomnia, sweating, vomiting, diarrhea, blurred vision, irritability, memory impairment, impaired concentrating ability, clouded sensorium, paresthesias, ataxia, tremors, muscle and abdominal cramps, heightened sensory perception, hallucinations, acute psychosis, decreased appetite/weight loss, and seizures which are clinically indistinguishable from tonic-clonic seizures. In addition, milder withdrawal symptoms such as dysphoria and insomnia have been reported following abrupt discontinuance of benzodiazepines in patients receiving therapeutic dosages for several months. It may be difficult to distinguish between withdrawal symptoms and those that are manifestations of illness return or rebound, although their management may differ. Because some benzodiazepines and their metabolites have long elimination half-lives, withdrawal symptoms may not occur until several days after the drugs have been discontinued.

Treatment of benzodiazepine physical dependence consists of cautious and gradual withdrawal of the drug using a dosage tapering schedule. Gradual dosage tapering is particularly important in patients with a seizure history. Occasionally, temporary reinstitution of benzodiazepine therapy at dosages adequate to suppress withdrawal symptoms may be necessary.

Pharmacology

The exact sites and mode of action of the benzodiazepines have not been fully elucidated, but the effects of the drugs appear to be mediated through the inhibitory neurotransmitter γ-aminobutyric acid (GABA). The drugs appear to act at the limbic, thalamic, and hypothalamic levels of the CNS, producing anxiolytic, sedative, hypnotic, skeletal muscle relaxant, and anticonvulsant effects. Benzodiazepines are capable of producing all levels of CNS depression—from mild sedation to hypnosis to coma.

Specific binding sites with high affinity for benzodiazepines have been detected in the CNS, and the affinity of these sites for the drugs is enhanced by both GABA and chloride. The sites and actions of benzodiazepines within the CNS appear to involve a macromolecular (oligomer or possibly a tetramer) complex ($GABA_A$-receptor-chloride ionophore complex) that includes $GABA_A$ receptors (GABA recognition sites), high-affinity benzodiazepine receptors, and chloride channels, although precise relationships between the sites of action of benzodiazepines and GABA-regulated (-gated) chloride channels remain to be more fully elucidated. Allosteric interactions of central benzodiazepine receptors with $GABA_A$ receptors and subsequent opening of chloride channels appear to be involved in eliciting the CNS effects of the drugs; the benzodiazepine receptors act as modulatory sites on the complex. Some evidence suggests that benzodiazepine receptor sites are heterogeneous, with at least 2 CNS subtypes (type 1 [BZ_1] and type 2 [BZ_2] benzodiazepine receptors) being described to date. While quazepam and 2-oxoquazepam (an active metabolite), like halazepam (another 1-*N*-trifluoroethyl derivative [no longer commercially available in the US]) but unlike other currently available benzodiazepines, exhibit relative selectivity for type 1 receptors (2-oxoquazepam is the most potent and selective of the three), the clinical importance, if any, of this finding remains to be established. Some evidence suggests that such selectivity may be responsible for the reduced ataxic effect of quazepam observed in animal studies; the possibility that the spectrum of other benzodiazepine-induced effects may be narrowed by such selectivity also has been suggested.

Clobazam, a 1,5-benzodiazepine, has been shown to have a broader spectrum of anticonvulsant activity and an improved adverse effect profile (e.g., less sedative effects) compared with the traditional 1,4-benzodiazepines (e.g., diazepam, lorazepam); these differences have been attributed to differences in binding affinity for the $GABA_A$ receptor. Because the active metabolite of clobazam, *N*-desmethylclobazam, is extensively metabolized by cytochrome P-450 (CYP) 2C19, genetic polymorphism of CYP2C19 can result in possible increased concentrations of the active metabolite. Systemic exposure to *N*-desmethylclobazam is approximately 3–5 and 2 times higher in poor (CYP2C19*2/*2) and intermediate (CYP2C19*1/*2) metabolizers of CYP2C19, respectively, than in extensive (CYP2C19*1/*1) metabolizers. The frequency of poor CYP2C19 metabolizers in the population varies widely depending on ethnic or racial background.

Anxiolytic and possibly paradoxical CNS stimulatory effects of benzodiazepines are postulated to result from release of previously suppressed responses (disinhibition). After usual doses of benzodiazepines for several days, the drugs cause a moderate decrease in rapid eye movement (REM) sleep. REM rebound does not occur when the drugs are withdrawn. Stage 3 and 4 sleep are markedly reduced by usual doses of the drugs; the clinical importance of these sleep stage alterations has not been established.

Benzodiazepines appear to produce skeletal muscle relaxation predominantly by inhibiting spinal polysynaptic afferent pathways, but the drugs may also inhibit monosynaptic afferent pathways. The drugs may inhibit monosynaptic and polysynaptic reflexes by acting as inhibitory neuronal transmitters or by blocking excitatory synaptic transmission. The drugs may also directly depress motor nerve and muscle function.

In animals, benzodiazepines protect against seizures induced by electrical stimulation and by pentylenetetrazol; benzodiazepines appear to act, at least partly, by augmenting presynaptic inhibition. The drugs suppress the spread of seizure activity but do not abolish the abnormal discharge from a focus in experimental models of epilepsy. In usual doses, benzodiazepines appear to have very little effect on the autonomic nervous system, respiration, or the cardiovascular system.

Pharmacokinetics

■ **Absorption** Benzodiazepines are generally well absorbed from the GI tract. Following IM administration of diazepam, absorption is slow and erratic. Absorption of lorazepam and midazolam hydrochloride after IM administration appears to be rapid and complete. Following oral administration of clorazepate dipotassium, it appears that most of the drug is rapidly decarboxylated in the GI tract and is absorbed as desmethyldiazepam (nordiazepam). The rate of decarboxylation of clorazepate decreases as gastric pH increases. Flurazepam undergoes first-pass metabolism in the liver, and plasma concentrations of the parent compound are minimal after oral administration. Plasma concentrations of the benzodiazepines and their metabolites (which in general are active) exhibit considerable interpatient variation, and therapeutic plasma concentrations are difficult to define.

Following oral administration of usual doses of flurazepam, onset of hypnotic action is 15–45 minutes, and the duration of action is 7–8 hours. In general, orally administered benzodiazepines produce anxiolytic, skeletal muscle relaxant, and anticonvulsant effects after the first dose; however, these effects may increase until steady-state plasma concentrations are achieved. After IV administration of single doses of diazepam or lorazepam, the onset of anticonvulsant, anxiolytic, or sedative action occurs in 1–5 minutes; after usual doses of IV diazepam, the duration of action is 15 minutes–1 hour, and after IV lorazepam, the duration of action is 12–24 hours. Following repeated doses of IV diazepam, prolonged duration of sedative action may occur, because of the presence of its long-acting metabolites. Following IV administration of usual doses of midazolam hydrochloride, the onset of sedative, anxiolytic, and amnesic action usually occurs within 1–5 minutes. The duration of action following IV administration of midazolam is usually less than 2 hours; however, the pharmacologic effects may persist up to 6 hours in some patients and the duration of action appears to be dose related. After IM administration, the onset of action of lorazepam is 15–30 minutes, and the duration of action is 12–24 hours. Following IM administration of midazolam hydrochloride, onset of action occurs within 5–15 minutes but may not be maximal until 20–60 minutes; the duration of action usually is about 2 hours (range: 1–6 hours).

Midazolam appears to be rapidly and well absorbed transmucosally following intrabuccal administration. The drug also appears to be rapidly and well absorbed transmucosally following intranasal administration; however, the effect of increased nasal discharge and mucus production on intranasal midazolam absorption is unknown, and breathing may discharge drugs that are administered intranasally.

Diazepam is rapidly and well absorbed systemically following rectal administration as a gel or solution (e.g., using parenteral formulations). Peak plasma or serum concentrations generally are achieved within 5–90 minutes following rectal administration of these formulations, with bioavailabilities averaging 80–102%. Diazepam is less predictably absorbed systemically following rectal administration as suppositories (e.g., bioavailability of 67–84%), exhibiting slow and variable absorption. When a single 15-mg dose was administered rectally as a commercially available viscous gel (Diastat®) in healthy adults pretreated with an enema to ensure an empty rectum, plasma diazepam concentrations exceeded 200 ng/mL within 15 minutes and reached an initial peak of 373 ng/mL at 45 minutes and a second peak of 447 ng/mL at approximately 70 minutes. The manufacturer states that peak plasma concentrations of the drug are achieved within 1.5 hours following rectal administration of the gel in adults. In the healthy adults who received a single 15-mg rectal dose of diazepam following pretreatment with an enema, the absolute systemic bioavailability averaged about 90% (range: 71–110%). Peak plasma concentrations of the desmethyl metabolite in these adults averaged 62 ng/mL and were achieved 68 hours after rectal administration; areas under the plasma concentration-time curve (AUCs) and peak plasma concentrations for this metabolite were similar with rectal or IV administration. The elimination half-lives for diazepam and desmethyldiazepam averaged about 45–46 and 71–99 hours, respectively, following rectal administration of the gel in healthy adults. The pharmacokinetics of diazepam rectal gel in pediatric patients have not been determined, although some evidence suggests that more rapid absorption may be likely.

Clobazam is rapidly and almost completely absorbed following oral administration; peak plasma concentrations of the drug are achieved within 0.5–4 hours after single- or multiple-dose administration. The main circulating metabolite, *N*-desmethylclobazam, is pharmacologically active with potency estimates ranging from one-fifth to equal potency of the parent drug; therefore, the active metabolite may contribute to the efficacy and tolerability of the drug. At therapeutic dosages, plasma concentrations of *N*-desmethylclobazam are approximately 3–5 times higher than those of clobazam.

■ **Distribution** Benzodiazepines are widely distributed into body tissues and cross the blood-brain barrier. Following IV administration of diazepam, there is an early, rapid decline in plasma concentrations of the drug, principally associated with distribution into the tissues. After IV administration of lorazepam, plasma concentrations decline less rapidly. Generally, benzodiazepines and their metabolites cross the placenta; the concentration of diazepam in the fetal circulation has been reported to be equal to or greater than maternal plasma drug concentrations. The drugs and their metabolites are distributed into milk.

Benzodiazepines and their metabolites are highly bound to plasma proteins.

■ **Elimination** Elimination half-lives ($t_{1/2}$s) of benzodiazepines and their metabolites exhibit wide interpatient variation. (See Table 1.)

Table 1. The $t_{1/2}$s of benzodiazepines and their major active metabolites in healthy individuals.

Drug ($t_{1/2}$ in hours)	Major Active Metabolites ($t_{1/2}$ in hours)
Alprazolam (11–15)	None
Chlordiazepoxide (5–30)	Demoxepam (14–95)
	Desmethylchlordiazepoxide (18)
	Desmethyldiazepam (30–200)
	Oxazepam (3–21)
Clobazam (36–42)	*N*-desmethylclobazam (71–82)
Clonazepam (18–50)	None
Clorazepate	Desmethyldiazepam (30–200)
	Oxazepam (3–21)
Diazepam (20–50)	Desmethyldiazepam (30–200)
	3-Hydroxydiazepam (5–20)
	Oxazepam (3–21)
Estazolam (10–24)	None
Flurazepam	Desalkylflurazepam (47–100)
	N-1-Hydroxyethylflurazepam (2–4)
Halazepam (14)	Desmethyldiazepam (30–200)
Lorazepam (10–20)	None
Midazolam (1–12.3)	1-Hydroxymethylmidazolam (1–1.3)
Oxazepam (3–21)	None
Quazepam (25–41)	2-Oxoquazepam (40)
	N-Desalkyl-2-oxoquazepam (70–75)
Temazepam (10–20)	None
Triazolam (1.6–5.4)	None

Geriatric patients and patients with liver disease may have prolonged elimination half-lives of all benzodiazepines and their metabolites, except possibly lorazepam, oxazepam, temazepam, and triazolam. However, limited data in healthy geriatric individuals (average age: 69 years) receiving single doses (0.125 or 0.25 mg) of triazolam indicate that values for peak plasma concentration and AUCs are increased and clearance decreased by an average of approximately 50% compared with values in younger adults (average age: 30 years). Evidence suggesting accumulation of triazolam (as determined by benzodiazepine receptor binding activity) with prolonged (i.e., 4 weeks) administration in geriatric individuals also has been reported. In premature and newborn infants, the half-lives of diazepam are longer than in adults and older children. Steady-state plasma concentrations of benzodiazepines and their metabolites are reached after administration of a fixed dosage for approximately 5 elimination half-lives. Plasma concentrations of metabolites with long half-lives may be greater than those of the unchanged drugs.

Benzodiazepines are metabolized in the liver. Lorazepam, oxazepam, temazepam, and the hydroxylated metabolites of chlordiazepoxide, clorazepate, diazepam, flurazepam, halazepam (no longer commercially available in the US), midazolam, quazepam, and triazolam are conjugated with glucuronic and/or sulfuric acid; these inactive conjugates are excreted principally in urine. Benzodiazepines are not appreciably removed by hemodialysis.

Chemistry

Alprazolam, chlordiazepoxide, clobazam (see 28:12.08), clonazepam (see 28:12.08), clorazepate, diazepam, estazolam, flurazepam, halazepam (no longer commercially available in the US), lorazepam, midazolam, oxazepam, quazepam, temazepam, and triazolam are benzodiazepines that are used as anxiolytics, sedatives, hypnotics, anticonvulsants, and/or skeletal muscle relaxants. Benzodiazepines are subject to control under the Federal Controlled Substances Act of 1970.

Benzodiazepines contain a benzene ring structure fused to a 7-membered diazepine ring. The classic benzodiazepines (e.g., chlordiazepoxide, clonazepam, diazepam, lorazepam) are referred to as 1,4-benzodiazepines because they contain nitrogen atoms at positions 1 and 4 on the diazepine ring. Clobazam, a 1,5-benzodiazepine, differs structurally from 1,4-benzodiazepines in that its nitrogen atoms are at positions 1 and 5 and a keto group occupies the 4 position on the diazepine ring; clobazam is the only 1,5-benzodiazepine that is currently used in clinical practice. Commercially available 1,4-benzodiazepines, except alprazolam, chlordiazepoxide, estazolam, midazolam, quazepam, and triazolam, have the same characteristic structure but differ in the substitutions at the R^1, R^3, R^7, and $R^{2'}$ positions.

■ **Comparative Structures of Benzodiazepines**

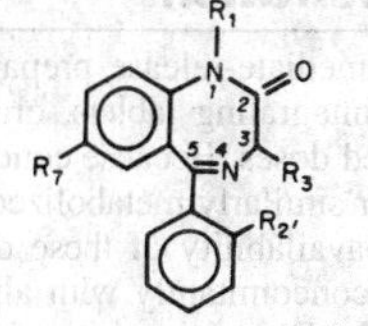

benzodiazepine nucleus

Table 2. Comparative structures of 1,4-benzodiazepines.

	R^1	R^3	R^7	$R^{2'}$
Clonazepam	-H	-H	$-NO_2$	-Cl
Clorazepate dipotassium	-H	-COOK	-Cl	-H
Diazepam	$-CH_3$	-H	-Cl	-H
Flurazepam	$-CH_2CH_2N(C_2H_5)_2$	-H	-Cl	-F
Halazepam	$-CH_2CF_3$	-H	-Cl	-H
Lorazepam	-H	-OH	-Cl	-Cl
Oxazepam	-H	-OH	-Cl	-H
Quazepam	$-CH_2CF_3$	-H	-Cl	-F
Temazepam	$-CH_3$	-OH	-Cl	-H

In chlordiazepoxide, a 1,4-benzodiazepine-4-oxide, a methylamino group replaces the ketone at the 2 position, and a chlorine atom is at R^7. In alprazolam, estazolam, and triazolam, triazolobenzodiazepines, a triazolo ring is formed by the addition of a ring to the benzodiazepine nucleus at the 1 and 2 positions, and a chlorine atom is at R^7; triazolam also has a chlorine atom at $R^{2'}$. In midazolam, an imidazobenzodiazepine, an imidazole ring fused at positions 1 and 2 of the benzodiazepine nucleus replaces the ketone at position 2 of the nucleus; midazolam has a fluorine atom at $R^{2'}$ and a chlorine atom at R^7. Quazepam, a 1,4-benzodiazepine-2-thione, has a sulfur atom rather than a ketone at position 2 of the nucleus; the drug also has a trifluoroethyl group at R^1, a fluorine atom at $R^{2'}$, and a chlorine atom at R^7. The presence of the trifluoroethyl group (1-*N*-trifluoroethyl derivative) distinguishes halazepam (no longer commercially available in the US) and quazepam from other currently available benzodiazepines and results in relative selectivity for type 1 (BZ_1) benzodiazepine receptors. (See Pharmacology.)

For further information on chemistry and stability, uses, cautions, and dosage and administration of benzodiazepines, see the individual monographs in 28:24.08. See also the Anticonvulsants General Statement 28:12, Clobazam 28:12.08, and Clonazepam 28:12.08.

†Use is not currently included in the labeling approved by the US Food and Drug Administration

ALPRAZolam

■ Alprazolam is a benzodiazepine.

Uses

■ **Anxiety Disorder** Alprazolam shares the actions of other benzodiazepines and is used for the management of anxiety disorders or for the short-term relief of symptoms of anxiety or anxiety associated with depressive symptoms. Anxiety or tension associated with the stress of everyday life usually does not require treatment with an anxiolytic. The efficacy of alprazolam for long-term use (i.e., longer than 4 months) has not been evaluated. The need for continued therapy with the drug should be periodically reassessed.

■ **Panic Disorder** Alprazolam is used in the management of panic disorder, with or without agoraphobia. Efficacy of alprazolam in the management of panic disorder has been established in short-term (for periods up to 4–10 weeks) controlled studies, although the drug has been used without apparent loss of efficacy for longer periods (e.g., 8 months or longer) in many patients. Following discontinuance of the drug, a relapse of the condition, including a rebound in panic attacks and anxiety, and/or the development of withdrawal frequently occurs. Additional study is needed to establish the optimum duration of alprazolam therapy in the management of panic disorder, and to determine the most appropriate method of tapered withdrawal of the drug.

The potential dependence liability of alprazolam should be considered in weighing the possible risks and benefits of therapy with the drug in this condition. Effective treatment of panic disorder with alprazolam often has required dosages exceeding 4 mg daily, and spontaneous reporting data suggest that the risk and severity of dependence is increased in patients receiving such dosages for prolonged periods (e.g., longer than 12 weeks). In 2 controlled studies of 6- to 8-weeks' duration in which the patient's ability to discontinue therapy was assessed, 7–29% of patients with panic disorder did not completely taper off of alprazolam therapy. In a controlled postmarketing study, the ability of patients with panic disorder to discontinue alprazolam therapy was reduced in those receiving dosages exceeding 4 mg daily but did not appear to differ between those receiving the drug for 3 months compared with those receiving the drug for 6 months.

Dosage and Administration

■ **Administration** Immediate-release preparations of alprazolam (i.e., conventional and orally disintegrating tablets, oral solution concentrate) are administered orally in divided doses. Because concomitant oral administration of grapefruit juice with other similarly metabolized benzodiazepines has been reported to increase the bioavailability of these drugs, caution is advised if grapefruit juice is ingested concomitantly with alprazolam. (See Drug Interactions: Grapefruit Juice under Drug Interactions in the Benzodiazepines General Statement 28:24.08.)

When alprazolam oral concentrate is used, the dose should be added to 30 mL or more of diluent (e.g., water, juices, carbonated or soda-like beverages) or to semi-solid foods (e.g., applesauce, pudding) just before administration.

The orally disintegrating tablets should be administered immediately after the tablet is removed from the container by the patient; if only half a tablet is administered, the unused portion should be discarded immediately since it may not remain stable. The orally disintegrating tablet should be removed with a dry hand and placed on the tongue, where it disintegrates rapidly in saliva, and then subsequently can be swallowed with or without water. Any cotton that is present in the container when initially opened should be discarded, and the container should be resealed tightly to prevent the introduction of moisture, which might cause tablet disintegration. Although peak plasma concentrations are achieved 15 minutes sooner when the orally disintegrating tablets are administered with water, the peak concentration and oral bioavailability are not affected by administration with water. Administration of the orally disintegrating tablets with a high-fat meal does not affect the extent of absorption but may delay and reduce peak plasma concentrations of the drug by about 2 hours and 25%, respectively. If the orally disintegrating tablets are used in the presence of conditions or in conjunction with drugs that increase gastric pH or cause dry mouth, disintegration or dissolution of the tablets might be slower, potentially resulting in reduced or slower absorption of alprazolam.

Alprazolam extended-release tablets are administered once daily, preferably in the morning. When the extended-release tablets are administered at night rather than in the morning, peak plasma concentrations are about 30% higher and occur about 1 hour sooner. The extended-release tablets should be swallowed whole and should *not* be chewed, crushed, or broken. The relative oral bioavailability of alprazolam when administered as extended-release tablets is 100% that of conventional (immediate-release) tablets; however, the rate of GI absorption is slower. The slower absorption rate results in a relatively constant plasma concentration of the drug that is maintained between 5–11 hours after dosing. Multiple-dose studies indicate that the metabolism and elimination of the drug are similar with the immediate- and extended-release tablets. Food affects the rate but not the extent of absorption of alprazolam extended-release tablets. Peak plasma concentrations are increased by 25% when alprazolam extended-release tablets are administered within 2 hours after a high-fat meal; time to peak plasma concentrations may be reduced by about one-third if the dose is administered immediately after a meal but may be increased by about one-third if administered 1 hour or more before a meal.

■ **Dosage** Dosage of alprazolam must be individualized, and the smallest effective dosage should be used (especially in geriatric or debilitated patients and in those with liver disease, low serum albumin, or obesity) to avoid oversedation. If early morning anxiety occurs or emergence of symptoms occurs between doses of an immediate-release preparation in patients previously stabilized, the need for dosage adjustment or maintenance of the same daily dosage but divided and administered at more frequent intervals should be considered.

Anxiety Disorders **Immediate-release Preparations.** Optimum dosage for the management of anxiety disorders has only been established for immediate-release preparations of alprazolam (i.e., conventional and orally disintegrating tablets, oral solution concentrate). The extended-release tablets currently are not labeled for use the management of anxiety disorders.

The usual initial adult dosage of immediate-release alprazolam for the management of anxiety disorders (other than panic disorder) or transient symptoms of anxiety is 0.25–0.5 mg 3 times daily. Dosage may be gradually increased at intervals of 3 or 4 days according to individual requirements and response to a maximum dosage of 4 mg daily, given in divided doses. In geriatric or debilitated patients, immediate-release alprazolam therapy for anxiety should be initiated with 0.25 mg 2 or 3 times daily; if adverse effects occur at this initial dosage, dosage should be decreased. If adverse effects do not occur at this initial dosage, dosage may be gradually increased if necessary according to individual tolerance and response.

When it is necessary to reduce the dosage or discontinue therapy with alprazolam, dosage of the drug should be reduced or withdrawn gradually to prevent the development of withdrawal symptoms. (See Cautions.) Although studies have not been performed to date to determine the optimal regimen for tapering alprazolam dosage, the manufacturer recommends that dosage of the drug be decreased by no more than 0.5 mg every 3 days. Some patients may require an even slower dosage reduction, and some clinicians suggest that more gradual tapering (e.g., decreasing by no more than 0.25 mg every 3–7 days) may be necessary in some patients to prevent symptom recurrence (for the condition being treated) and/or the development of manifestations of withdrawal.

Panic Disorder **Immediate-release Preparations.** For the management of panic disorder, therapy with immediate-release alprazolam (conventional or orally disintegrating tablets) generally should be initiated at a low dosage to minimize the risk of adverse effects. Dosage subsequently may be increased until an acceptable therapeutic response is achieved (e.g., substantial reduction in or elimination of panic attacks), intolerable adverse effects occur, or a maximum recommended dosage of 10 mg daily is achieved. Therapy with immediate-release alprazolam may be initiated in adults at a dosage of 0.5 mg 3 times daily and then increased as necessary at 3- or 4-day intervals in increments of no more than 1 mg daily. However, slower titration to dosages exceeding 4 mg daily may be advisable so that full expression of the pharmacodynamic effects with a given dosage can occur.

To minimize the risk of interdose symptom emergence, doses of the immediate-release preparation should be distributed as evenly as possible throughout waking hours on a 3- or 4-times-daily schedule. The optimum duration of therapy is not known, but a carefully supervised tapered discontinuance of therapy can be attempted after a period of extended freedom from attacks. Unfortunately, current evidence indicates that such tapered discontinuance often is difficult to achieve without recurrence of symptoms and/or manifestations of withdrawal.

Extended-release Tablets. For the management of panic disorder, the usual adult dosage range for alprazolam extended-release tablets is 3–6 mg once daily. Dosage should be individualized for maximum benefit. While a dosage of 3–6 mg daily will meet the needs of most patients with panic disorder, some patients will require higher dosages. In such cases, dosage should be increased cautiously to avoid adverse effects.

For most adults with panic disorder, therapy with alprazolam extended-release tablets may be initiated at a dosage of 0.5–1 mg once daily. Thereafter, dosage may be increased according to response at intervals of 3 or 4 days in increments not exceeding 1 mg daily. Slower dosage titration may be advisable to allow full expression of the pharmacodynamic effect of the extended-release tablets. Dosage generally should be increased until an acceptable therapeutic response is achieved, intolerance occurs, or a maximum dosage of 10 mg once daily is achieved.

In geriatric patients, in adults with advanced liver disease or another debilitating disease, and in those especially sensitive to the drug, the usual initial dosage of alprazolam extended-release tablets for the management of panic disorder is 0.5 mg once daily. If necessary, this dosage may be increased gradually according to patient response and tolerance as described for most adults.

Maintenance Therapy and Dosage Reduction. The following recommendations for maintenance dosage in adults with panic disorder apply to both immediate- and extended-release alprazolam preparations on a daily basis. However, the dosage should be divided as evenly as possible during waking hours on a 3- or 4-times daily schedule for immediate-release preparations whereas the dosage is given once daily, preferably in the morning, for extended-release tablets.

Patients being switched from immediate-release alprazolam therapy to the extended-release tablets can receive the same total daily dosage administered once daily rather than in divided doses. If the therapeutic response is not adequate after switching to the same dosage administered once daily, the dosage may be increased in the usual fashion.

Effective treatment of panic disorder with alprazolam often has required dosages exceeding 4 mg daily in adults. Dosage (as immediate-release preparations) generally has averaged 5–6 mg daily, but has ranged from 1–10 mg daily; about 20% of patients required maximum alprazolam dosages exceeding 7 mg daily, with about one-third of these requiring maximum dosages exceeding 9 mg daily. An alprazolam dosage of 3–6 mg daily as extended-release tablets generally has been effective, but dosage has ranged from 1–10 mg daily. Occasionally, a dosage of 10 mg daily has been required for adequate response.

For patients receiving dosages exceeding 4 mg daily, periodic reassessment and consideration of dosage reduction is recommended. In a controlled post-marketing dose-response study, patients receiving alprazolam at dosages exceeding 4 mg daily for 3 months were able to taper their daily maintenance dosage by 50% without apparent loss of clinical benefit.

Reduction of alprazolam dosage must be undertaken under close supervision and must be gradual. If significant withdrawal symptoms develop, the previous dosing schedule should be reinstituted and, only after stabilization, should a less rapid schedule of dosage tapering be attempted. Although not systematically evaluated, a reduction by 0.5 mg daily at 3-day intervals has been suggested, although more gradual reductions may be necessary in some patients. When this suggested tapering schedule was compared with a slower dosage taper, there was no difference in the proportion of patients able to completely discontinue alprazolam, but the slower tapering schedule was associated with fewer withdrawal symptoms. Some patients may prove resistant to all discontinuance regimens.

Cautions

Alprazolam shares the toxic potentials of the benzodiazepines, and the usual precautions of benzodiazepine administration should be observed. (See Cautions in the Benzodiazepines General Statement 28:24.08.)

Seizures, delirium, and withdrawal symptoms (similar to those reported following abrupt withdrawal of other benzodiazepines) have occurred in some patients following rapid dosage reduction and/or abrupt discontinuance of alprazolam. In most cases, only a single seizure occurred; however, multiple seizures and status epilepticus also have been reported and may be life-threatening. Withdrawal-related effects appearing after abrupt discontinuance of alprazolam have occurred from 18 hours to 3 days after the last dose of the drug. Seizures resulting from rapid dosage reduction or abrupt withdrawal of alprazolam have occurred in patients receiving usual or higher than recommended dosages of the drug for relatively short periods of time (from 1 week to 4 months). Seizures also have occurred occasionally in patients apparently tapering dosage gradually. The risk of seizures appears to be greatest 24–72 hours after discontinuance of alprazolam. The use of dosages exceeding 4 mg daily (e.g., those employed for panic disorder) and use of the drug for prolonged periods of time may be associated with an increased frequency and severity of withdrawal symptoms. When it is necessary to reduce the dosage or discontinue therapy with alprazolam, dosage of the drug should be reduced or withdrawn gradually. Patients should be advised not to discontinue the drug abruptly without consulting their physician.

Episodes of mania and hypomania have been reported in depressed patients receiving alprazolam.

The initial step in alprazolam metabolism is hydroxylation catalyzed by the hepatic cytochrome P-450 (CYP) 3A isoenzyme, and concomitant use of alprazolam with agents that inhibit the CYP3A isoenzyme may result in decreased alprazolam metabolism and clearance and increased plasma alprazolam concentrations. The manufacturers state that caution should be exercised and alprazolam dosage adjustment considered during concomitant use of the drug with some inhibitors of the CYP3A isoenzyme (e.g., nefazodone, fluvoxamine, cimetidine). Other CYP3A inhibitors (e.g., fluoxetine, diltiazem, macrolide antibiotics [i.e., clarithromycin, erythromycin], isoniazid, sertraline, paroxetine, grapefruit juice, amiodarone) may cause clinically important decreases in alprazolam metabolism and clearance and should be used with caution in patients receiving the drug. Concomitant use with some other drugs (propoxyphene, oral contraceptives, ergotamine, cyclosporine, nicardipine, nifedipine) may result in decreases in alprazolam metabolism and clearance; caution is advised if alprazolam is administered with one of these agents.

Concomitant use of alprazolam with delavirdine should be avoided because of the potential for delavirdine to decrease metabolism of alprazolam and result in intense or prolonged sedation or respiratory depression.

Because itraconazole and ketoconazole are very potent CYP3A isoenzyme inhibitors that can markedly decrease the metabolism and clearance of alprazolam, the manufacturers state that concomitant use of these drugs with alprazolam is contraindicated. In addition, concomitant use of alprazolam with other azole antifungal agents that are very potent inhibitors of CYP3A should be avoided.

For further information about potential drug interactions between benzodiazepines and drugs and foods affecting hepatic microsomal enzymes, see Drug Interactions in the Benzodiazepines General Statement 28:24.08.

■ **Pediatric Precautions** Safety and efficacy of alprazolam have not been established in children younger than 18 years of age.

■ **Geriatric Precautions** Clearance of alprazolam is reduced in geriatric patients, and geriatric patients may be particularly sensitive to the effects of benzodiazepines; therefore, the smallest effective dosage of alprazolam should be used in these patients to avoid oversedation and ataxia.

Chemistry and Stability

■ **Chemistry** Alprazolam is a benzodiazepine. Alprazolam occurs as a white to off-white, crystalline powder. The drug is insoluble in water and soluble in alcohol.

■ **Stability** Commercially available alprazolam tablets should be stored in tight, light-resistant containers at 15–30°C. Alprazolam extended-release tablets should be stored at 25°C, but may be exposed to temperatures ranging from 15–30°C. The orally disintegrating tablets should be stored in tight containers, protected from moisture, at 20–25°C, but may be exposed to temperatures ranging from 15–30°C; any unused half of a scored orally disintegrating tablet should be immediately discarded because it may not remain stable. (See Dosage and Administration: Administration.)

For further information on chemistry, pharmacology, pharmacokinetics, uses, cautions, chronic toxicity, acute toxicity, drug interactions, laboratory test interferences, and dosage and administration of alprazolam, see the Benzodiazepines General Statement 28:24.08.

Preparations

Alprazolam is subject to control under the Federal Controlled Substances Act of 1970 as a schedule IV (C-IV) drug.

Excipients in commercially available drug preparations may have clinically important effects in some individuals; consult specific product labeling for details.

ALPRAZolam

Oral		
Solution, concentrate	1 mg/mL	**ALPRAZolam Intensol®** (C-IV), Roxane
Tablets	0.25 mg*	**ALPRAZolam Tablets**
		Xanax® (C-IV; scored), Pfizer
	0.5 mg*	**ALPRAZolam Tablets**
		Xanax® (C-IV; scored), Pfizer
	1 mg*	**ALPRAZolam Tablets**
		Xanax® (C-IV; scored), Pfizer
	2 mg*	**ALPRAZolam Tablets**
		Xanax® (C-IV; multi-scored), Pfizer
Tablets, extended-release	0.5 mg*	**ALPRAZolam Extended-Release Tablets** (C-IV)
		Xanax XR® (C-IV), Pfizer
	1 mg*	**ALPRAZolam Extended-Release Tablets** (C-IV)
		Xanax XR® (C-IV), Pfizer

	2 mg*	**ALPRAZolam Extended-Release Tablets** (C-IV)
		Xanax XR® (C-IV), Pfizer
	3 mg*	**ALPRAZolam Extended-Release Tablets** (C-IV)
		Xanax XR® (C-IV), Pfizer
Tablets, orally disintegrating	0.25 mg	**Niravam®** (C-IV; scored), Schwarz
	0.5 mg	**Niravam®** (C-IV; scored), Schwarz
	1 mg	**Niravam®** (C-IV; scored), Schwarz
	2 mg	**Niravam®** (C-IV; scored), Schwarz

*available from one or more manufacturer, distributor, and/or repackager by generic (nonproprietary) name

chlordiazePOXIDE
chlordiazePOXIDE Hydrochloride

Librium

■ Chlordiazepoxide is a benzodiazepine.

Uses

■ **Anxiety Disorders, Preoperative Anxiolysis, and Alcohol Withdrawal** Chlordiazepoxide shares the actions of other benzodiazepines and is used for the management of anxiety disorders or for short-term relief of symptoms of anxiety, preoperatively to relieve anxiety and tension, and for the management of agitation associated with acute alcohol withdrawal. Anxiety or tension associated with the stress of everyday life usually does not require treatment with an anxiolytic. The efficacy of chlordiazepoxide for long-term use (i.e., for longer than 4 months) has not been established, and the need for continued therapy with the drug should be periodically reassessed.

Chlordiazepoxide hydrochloride, as the fixed-combination with amitriptyline, also has been used in the management of depression associated with severe anxiety.

■ **Peptic Ulcer Disease, Irritable Bowel Syndrome, Acute Enterocolitis** Chlordiazepoxide hydrochloride, as the fixed-combination with clidinium bromide, has been used as an adjunct in the treatment of peptic ulcer disease and in the treatment of functional disturbances of GI motility such as irritable bowel syndrome and acute enterocolitis. For further information on the treatment of these disorders, see Uses in Clidinium 12:08.08.

Dosage and Administration

■ **Administration** Chlordiazepoxide and its hydrochloride salt are usually administered orally in 3 or 4 doses daily. After dosage has been stabilized, most clinicians believe that the drug may be administered in 1 or 2 doses daily. Although chlordiazepoxide hydrochloride also has been administered parenterally†, a parenteral dosage form of the drug is no longer commercially available in the US.

■ **Dosage** On the basis of molecular weight, 89 mg of chlordiazepoxide is equivalent to 100 mg of chlordiazepoxide hydrochloride; however, the manufacturer of chlordiazepoxide base claims that chlordiazepoxide and its hydrochloride salt may be used interchangeably on a milligram-for-milligram basis.

Dosage must be individualized, and the smallest effective dosage should be used (especially in geriatric or debilitated patients and in those with liver disease or low serum albumin) to avoid oversedation.

Since chlordiazepoxide and its metabolites have long elimination half-lives, time to reach steady-state plasma concentrations should be considered when dosage adjustments are made.

Commercially available preparations containing chlordiazepoxide or its hydrochloride salt in fixed combination with an anticholinergic (clidinium) or an antidepressant (amitriptyline) generally should not be used as initial therapy in patients who require both drugs. Dosage should first be adjusted by administering each drug separately. If it is determined that the optimum maintenance dosage corresponds to the ratio in a commercial combination preparation, such a product may be used. When dosage adjustment is necessary, the drugs should be administered separately.

In patients who have received prolonged (e.g., for several months) chlordiazepoxide hydrochloride therapy, abrupt discontinuance of the drug should be avoided since manifestations of withdrawal can be precipitated; if the drug is to be discontinued in such patients, it is recommended that dosage be gradually tapered.

Adult Dosage **Anxiety Disorders.** For the management of mild to moderate anxiety, the usual adult oral dosage of chlordiazepoxide hydrochloride is 5–10 mg 3 or 4 times daily. For severe anxiety, 20–25 mg may be given orally 3 or 4 times daily.

Preoperative Anxiolysis. To relieve anxiety and tension preoperatively in adults, the manufacturer recommends that 5–10 mg of chlordiazepoxide hydrochloride be given orally 3 or 4 times daily for several days preceding surgery.

Acute Alcohol Withdrawal. For the management of agitation associated with acute alcohol withdrawal, the initial oral dose is 50–100 mg; doses are repeated until agitation is controlled.

The manufacturers state that in acute alcohol withdrawal, oral dosage should not exceed 300 mg daily; however, some clinicians have used chlordiazepoxide hydrochloride dosages of 600–800 mg daily to control symptoms without adverse effects. After agitation is controlled, the drug should be withdrawn slowly.

Peptic Ulcer Disease, Irritable Bowel Syndrome, Acute Enterocolitis. When chlordiazepoxide hydrochloride is used in fixed combination with clidinium bromide, the usual adult maintenance dosage of chlordiazepoxide hydrochloride is 5 or 10 mg given orally 3 or 4 times daily, administered before meals and at bedtime.

Pediatric Dosage Because of the unpredictable response of children to CNS drugs, chlordiazepoxide therapy should be initiated with the lowest dosage and increased as required.

Anxiety Disorders, Preoperative Anxiolysis, and Alcohol Withdrawal. The usual oral dosage of chlordiazepoxide hydrochloride in children older than 6 years of age is 5 mg 2–4 times daily; the initial dosage should not exceed 10 mg daily. If necessary, dosage for children may be increased to 10 mg 2 or 3 times daily. Alternatively, some clinicians have recommended a pediatric oral dosage of 0.5 mg/kg daily or 15 mg/m² daily, given in 3 or 4 divided doses.

Dosage in Geriatric or Debilitated Patients Geriatric or debilitated patients may receive 5 mg of chlordiazepoxide hydrochloride orally 2–4 times daily; the initial dose should not exceed 10 mg daily. When chlordiazepoxide hydrochloride is used in fixed combination with clidinium bromide, the recommended initial geriatric dosage of chlordiazepoxide hydrochloride is 10 mg daily, which may be increased gradually as needed and tolerated. (See Cautions: Geriatric Precautions.)

Cautions

■ **Precautions** Chlordiazepoxide shares the toxic potentials of the benzodiazepines, and the usual precautions of benzodiazepine administration should be observed. (See Cautions in the Benzodiazepines General Statement 28:24.08.) The precautions and contraindications associated with antimuscarinics or tricyclic antidepressants also should be considered when commercially available preparations containing chlordiazepoxide or its hydrochloride salt in fixed combination with clidinium or amitriptyline are used. (See Cautions in the Antimuscarinics/Antispasmodics General Statement 12:08.08 and also see Cautions in the Tricyclic Antidepressants General Statement 28:16.04.28.)

■ **Pediatric Precautions** Safety and efficacy of orally administered chlordiazepoxide or chlordiazepoxide hydrochloride in children younger than 6 years of age have not been established.

Safety and efficacy of the fixed-combination preparation containing chlordiazepoxide hydrochloride and clidinium bromide in pediatric patients have not been established.

■ **Geriatric Precautions** Although safety and efficacy of chlordiazepoxide in geriatric patients have not been studied specifically to date, one manufacturer states that geriatric adults may be especially prone to adverse effects such as drowsiness, ataxia, and confusion when receiving chlordiazepoxide hydrochloride in fixed combination with clidinium bromide. These adverse effects usually can be prevented by proper dosage adjustment. Therefore, it is recommended that the initial dosage of this combination in geriatric patients be selected carefully and gradually increased if needed and tolerated. However, these adverse effects occasionally have been observed in geriatric patients receiving the lower range of the usual dosage of this combination.

Chemistry and Stability

■ **Chemistry** Chlordiazepoxide is a benzodiazepine. Chlordiazepoxide occurs as a yellow, practically odorless, crystalline powder and has solubilities of less than 0.1 mg/mL in water and approximately 20 mg/mL in alcohol at 25°C. Chlordiazepoxide hydrochloride occurs as a white or practically white, odorless, crystalline powder and is soluble in water and in alcohol and slightly soluble in propylene glycol. Chlordiazepoxide has a pK_a of 4.8.

■ **Stability** Chlordiazepoxide tablets and chlordiazepoxide hydrochloride capsules must be protected from light.

For further information on chemistry, pharmacology, pharmacokinetics, uses, cautions, chronic toxicity, acute toxicity, drug interactions, laboratory test interferences, and dosage and administration of chlordiazepoxide, see the Benzodiazepines General Statement 28:24.08.

Preparations

Single-entity preparations of chlordiazepoxide and its hydrochloride salt and preparations containing the drug in combination with amitriptyline hydrochloride are subject to control under the Federal Controlled Substances Act of 1970 as schedule IV (C-IV) drugs.

Excipients in commercially available drug preparations may have clinically important effects in some individuals; consult specific product labeling for details.

chlordiazePOXIDE and Amitriptyline Hydrochloride

Oral

Tablets, film-coated	5 mg Chlordiazepoxide and Amitriptyline Hydrochloride 12.5 mg (of amitriptyline)*	**chlordiazePOXIDE and Amitriptyline Hydrochloride Tablets** (C-IV)
	10 mg Chlordiazepoxide and Amitriptyline Hydrochloride 25 mg (of amitriptyline)*	**chlordiazePOXIDE and Amitriptyline Hydrochloride Tablets** (C-IV)

*available from one or more manufacturer, distributor, and/or repackager by generic (nonproprietary) name

chlordiazePOXIDE Hydrochloride

Oral

Capsules	5 mg*	**chlordiazePOXIDE Hydrochloride Capsules** (C-IV)
	10 mg*	**chlordiazePOXIDE Hydrochloride Capsules** (C-IV)
	25 mg*	**chlordiazePOXIDE Hydrochloride Capsules** (C-IV)

*available from one or more manufacturer, distributor, and/or repackager by generic (nonproprietary) name

chlordiazePOXIDE Hydrochloride and Clidinium Bromide

Oral

Capsules	5 mg Chlordiazepoxide Hydrochloride and Clidinium Bromide 2.5 mg*	**chlordiazePOXIDE Hydrochloride and Clidinium Bromide Capsules**
		Librax®, Valeant

*available from one or more manufacturer, distributor, and/or repackager by generic (nonproprietary) name

diazePAM

■ Diazepam is a benzodiazepine. The drug has anticonvulsant, anxiolytic, sedative, and skeletal muscle relaxant properties.

Uses

■ **Anxiety Disorders, Preoperative or Preprocedural Anxiolysis, Alcohol Withdrawal, and Musculoskeletal Conditions** Diazepam is used for preoperative sedation, anxiolysis, and anterograde amnesia; for relief of anxiety and stress in patients undergoing procedures (e.g., endoscopic procedures, cardioversion); for the management of agitation associated with acute alcohol withdrawal; as an adjunct for the relief of acute, painful musculoskeletal conditions; to manage skeletal muscle spasticity such as reflex spasm secondary to local pathology (e.g., trauma, inflammation), spasticity caused by upper motor neuron disorders (e.g., cerebral palsy, paraplegia), athetosis, stiff-man syndrome, or tetanus; and for the management of anxiety disorders or for the short-term relief of symptoms of anxiety.

Anxiety or tension associated with the stress of everyday life usually does not require treatment with an anxiolytic. The efficacy of diazepam for long-term use (i.e., longer than 4 months) has not been evaluated. (See Uses in the Benzodiazepines General Statement 28:24.08.)

■ **Seizures** Diazepam also is used as an anticonvulsant. Diazepam is used parenterally (IV administration preferred) for the treatment of status epilepticus and severe recurrent convulsive seizures. Oral diazepam may be used for adjunctive therapy of seizure disorders; however, loss of response to the anticonvulsant effects of the drug often develops with prolonged use. Diazepam also may be administered rectally either as a commercially available gel (e.g., Diastat®) or using parenteral† formulations for the management of seizure disorders and status epilepticus.

Benzodiazepines are considered the initial drugs of choice for the management of status epilepticus because of their rapid onset of action, demonstrated efficacy, safety, and tolerability. (See Uses: Seizure Disorders, in the Benzodiazepines General Statement 28:24.08.) Although IV lorazepam is generally preferred because of its longer duration of action, there is also evidence supporting the use of IV diazepam and IM midazolam and experts consider these therapies to be equivalent first-line options. Selection of an appropriate agent should be individualized based on local availability, route of administration, pharmacokinetics, cost, and other factors (e.g., treatment setting). If seizures continue after initial therapy with a benzodiazepine, a second-line anticonvulsant agent (e.g., IV fosphenytoin or phenytoin, IV valproate sodium, IV levetiracetam, IV phenobarbital) should be administered. If refractory status epilepticus occurs, continuous IV infusion of anticonvulsants, IV barbiturates, or general anesthetics may be necessary. (See Status Epilepticus under Seizure Disorders: Principles of Anticonvulsant Drug Therapy, in the Anticonvulsants General Statement 28:12.)

To achieve a rapid therapeutic effect, IV administration of a benzodiazepine generally is preferred for the management of status epilepticus; however, administration via other routes (e.g., rectal) may be considered when IV administration is not possible (e.g., in a prehospital setting). Rectal administration of diazepam may be particularly useful for out-of-hospital management of status attacks (e.g., at home or school, during transport to an emergency room).

Rectal diazepam also may be used for the management of acute repetitive seizures (also referred to as serial, cyclic, cluster, breakthrough, or crescendo seizures), especially for out-of-hospital management. Acute repetitive seizures are exacerbations of an underlying seizure disorder that exhibit a pattern distinct from the patient's usual seizure pattern; the repetitive, periodic episodes often are predictable by the patient and caregivers according to a prodrome/aura, time of day when they originate, particular seizure type, and/or accompanying patient behavioral changes. Patients typically experience recovery between the repetitions; however, if untreated, acute repetitive seizures can evolve into more serious problems, including status epilepticus. The distinguishing features of these seizures are their predictability and pattern that differs from the underlying disorder rather than the actual seizure type; thus, while the pattern of presentation and patient and caregiver recognition are common features of the diagnosis, the actual seizure type can be different albeit definable for each individual patient. In the 2 clinical studies establishing efficacy of rectal diazepam for the management of acute repetitive seizures in adults and children 2 years of age and older, the drug was more effective than placebo in reducing seizure frequency and improving global assessment of treatment outcome as judged by caregivers (e.g., frequency and severity of seizures and patient tolerance of therapy). In these studies, the time to next seizure was prolonged in diazepam-treated patients relative to placebo, and about 55–62% of patients were seizure-free during the 12-hour observation period versus 20–34% for placebo recipients. In these studies, patients with a history of acute repetitive seizures that typically progressed to status epilepticus were excluded from study entry. Similar efficacy has been reported in other placebo-controlled and open-label studies. Although formal economic analyses have not been performed to date, patients treated with rectal diazepam out of the hospital required emergency medical treatment less commonly than did placebo recipients.

■ **Sedation in Critical Care Settings** Diazepam has been used for the sedation of intubated and mechanically ventilated patients in critical care settings† (e.g., intensive care unit [ICU]). Because of some modest clinical benefits (e.g., reduced duration of mechanical ventilation, shorter time to extubation, reduced risk of delirium) and an overall favorable benefit-to-risk profile, nonbenzodiazepine sedatives (dexmedetomidine or propofol) are generally preferred to benzodiazepines (midazolam or lorazepam) in mechanically ventilated, critically ill adults. If a benzodiazepine is required, midazolam or lorazepam generally is used; diazepam is rarely used for this indication. (See Uses: Sedation in Critical Care Settings, in the Benzodiazepines General Statement 28:24.08.)

■ **Drug-induced Cardiovascular Emergencies** Diazepam has been used adjunctively in the management of certain drug-induced cardiovascular emergencies† and cocaine-induced acute coronary syndrome†.

■ **Other Uses** Diazepam has been used orally to prevent night terrors†. Although not recommended by the manufacturer, parenteral diazepam is used to reduce the requirements for opiate analgesics and produce anterograde amnesia during labor and delivery†. The drug has been used parenterally to manage neonatal opiate withdrawal†.

Dosage and Administration

Diazepam is administered orally, by IV or IM injection, or rectally.

■ **Administration** ***Oral Administration*** Diazepam is administered orally as tablets or oral solution.

When diazepam oral concentrate solution is used, the dose should be diluted (e.g., with water, juice, carbonated or soda-like beverages) or mixed with semi-solid foods (e.g., applesauce, pudding) using only the calibrated dropper provided by the manufacturer. The liquid or food mixture should be stirred gently for a few seconds and then consumed immediately; the mixture should not be stored for future use.

Parenteral Administration When oral therapy is not feasible or when a rapid therapeutic effect is necessary, diazepam may be administered by slow IV injection at a rate not exceeding 5 mg/minute in adults and over a 3-minute period in children. When given IV, diazepam should be administered directly into a large vein to avoid thrombosis; if this is not feasible, the drug should be given into the tubing of a flowing IV solution as close as possible to the vein insertion. Small veins such as those of the wrist or the dorsum of the hand should not be used. Care should be taken to avoid intra-arterial administration or extravasation. Some clinicians have suggested IV administration of dilute solutions of the drug to avoid extravasation; however, the drug may precipitate when diluted and the manufacturers do not recommend this method of administration. (See Chemistry and Stability: Stability.)

Although diazepam may also be given by deep IM injection, this route of administration of the drug is rarely justified because absorption is slow and erratic.

Therapy with oral diazepam should replace parenteral administration as soon as possible.

Rectal Administration When diazepam is administered rectally, the drug may be given as a commercially available rectal gel via the delivery device (a plastic applicator with a flexible molded tip) provided by the manufacturer. Diazepam also has been administered rectally as the parenteral solution† via a syringe and rectally inserted tubing or via a lubricated tuberculin syringe (*without* a needle) inserted 4–5 cm into the rectum.

Diazepam rectal gel is commercially available in prefilled syringe applicators containing 2.5, 10, or 20 mg of diazepam. The 2.5-mg Diastat® applicator delivers a dose of 2.5 mg of diazepam; the 10-mg Diastat® AcuDial® applicator can be set to deliver a dose of 5, 7.5, or 10 mg of the drug; and the 20-mg Diastat® AcuDial® applicator can be set to deliver a dose of 12.5, 15, 17.5, or 20 mg of the drug. Both the 2.5- and 10-mg applicators are fitted with a plastic applicator tip that is 4.4 cm in length; the 20-mg applicator is fitted with an applicator tip that is 6 cm in length. The 4.4-cm rectal tip applicator generally is used for pediatric patients. Although dosage of diazepam rectal gel is calculated on a mg/kg basis by age, the actual dose administered is approximate and determined by rounding upward to the next available dose (i.e., the next multiple of 2.5 mg).

Prior to dispensing the Diastat® AcuDial® preparation, the pharmacist must dial in and lock the correct dose to be administered. While holding the barrel of the applicator in one hand, the pharmacist turns the cap of the applicator to select the dose. After confirming that the dose visible in the display window is correct, the pharmacist locks the dose by grasping the locking ring and pushing upward to lock both sides of the ring. Once the dose-locking ring on the device is engaged, a green "ready" band becomes visible at the base of the applicator. The process should be repeated for each applicator to be dispensed. Upon receiving the drug from the pharmacy, the patient or caregiver should verify that the prescribed dose is visible in the display window and that the green "ready" band is visible.

Caregivers should be instructed carefully in the use of diazepam rectal gel and should be given a copy of the administration instructions provided by the manufacturer. As soon as an episode of acute repetitive seizures is recognized, the caregiver should place the patient on their side so they won't fall and administer the prescribed dose of rectal diazepam. Before the prescribed dose is administered, the expiration date of the appropriate applicator(s) should be checked to ensure that it is in date; with the AcuDial® applicators, the visibility of the green "ready" band and the dose displayed in the display window also should be checked. The applicator is prepared for use by removing the protective cap from the syringe and ensuring that the seal pin is removed with the cap. The rectal applicator tip should be lubricated with the water-soluble lubricant (jelly) provided by the manufacturer and the patient should be turned so that they are resting on their side facing the caregiver; the patient's upper leg should be bent forward and the buttocks separated to expose the rectum. The lubricated applicator tip should then be inserted rectally until the rim of the syringe is snug against the rectal opening; once inserted, the plunger should be pushed slowly (counting aloud slowly to 3) until it stops (i.e., until the entire dose of the applicator has been expelled into the rectum). The caregiver should again count aloud slowly to 3 before removing the syringe from the rectum; to prevent leakage of the administered dose from the rectum, the buttocks should then be held together while again counting aloud slowly to 3. The patient should be left on their side facing the caregiver, the time the dose was given noted, and the patient observed. If bowel leakage occurs during rectal administration, it may be necessary to administer a supplemental dose. (See Dosage: Rectal Dosage, in Dosage and Administration.)

The rectal delivery system and all unused materials should be discarded in the garbage and *not* reused. Such disposal should be in a safe place away from children. Any diazepam rectal gel remaining in the AcuDial® applicator after use should be disposed of before the applicator is discarded. With the applicator tip pointed over the sink or toilet, the plunger should be pulled back and removed from the barrel of the syringe applicator and then replaced in the barrel and gently depressed until it stops, thereby forcing gel from the applicator tip into the sink or toilet. The toilet then should be flushed or the sink rinsed with water until gel is no longer visible. The applicator may then be discarded.

■ Dosage

Dosage of diazepam must be individualized, and the smallest effective dosage should be used (especially in geriatric or debilitated patients or in those with liver disease or low serum albumin) to avoid oversedation. The doses recommended by the manufacturers for IM and IV administration are identical. When parenteral diazepam is used with an opiate analgesic, the dosage of the opiate should be reduced by at least one-third and administered in small increments. Because of the unpredictable response of children to CNS drugs, diazepam therapy should be initiated with the lowest dosage and increased as required. Since diazepam and its metabolites have long elimination half-lives, time to reach steady-state plasma concentrations should be considered when dosage adjustments are made.

In patients who have received prolonged (e.g., for several months) diazepam therapy, abrupt discontinuance of the drug should be avoided since manifestations of withdrawal can be precipitated; if the drug is to be discontinued in such patients, it is recommended that dosage be gradually tapered. It is particularly important that the drugs *not* be discontinued abruptly in patients with a history of a seizure disorder since seizures may be precipitated.

Oral Dosage

Adult Dosage. For the management of anxiety or for adjunctive treatment of seizure disorders, the usual adult oral dosage of diazepam is 2–10 mg 2–4 times daily as tablets or oral solution.

For adjunctive treatment of skeletal muscle spasticity, the usual adult oral dosage of diazepam is 2–10 mg 3 or 4 times daily as tablets or oral solution.

For the management of acute alcohol withdrawal, the usual adult oral dosage of diazepam is 10 mg 3 or 4 times as tablets or oral solution during the first 24 hours, followed by 5 mg 3 or 4 times daily as needed.

In adults with night terrors†, 5–20 mg of diazepam has been administered orally as tablets or oral solution at bedtime.

The initial oral dosage of diazepam for geriatric or debilitated patients should be 2–2.5 mg once or twice daily as tablets or oral solution. Dosage should be adjusted gradually according to response and tolerance.

Pediatric Dosage. The manufacturers state that children 6 months of age or older may receive an initial oral diazepam dosage of 1–2.5 mg 3 or 4 times daily as tablets or oral solution. When used as a sedative or muscle relaxant in children, some clinicians recommend an oral diazepam dosage of 0.12–0.8 mg/kg daily in 3 or 4 divided doses. Dosage should be adjusted gradually according to response and tolerance.

As an adjunct in the management of epilepsy in children, 6–15 mg daily (and occasionally up to 30 mg daily) in divided doses as tablets or oral solution has been used by some clinicians.

Parenteral Dosage

Adult Dosage. If diazepam injection is used for rapid relief of acute anxiety, the usual adult IV or IM dose is 2–5 mg for moderate anxiety or 5–10 mg for severe anxiety. The dose may be repeated in 3–4 hours if necessary. Some clinicians recommend that the adult dosage should not exceed 30 mg within an 8-hour period.

For the management of acute alcohol withdrawal, the manufacturer states that the usual adult dose of diazepam is 10 mg administered IM or IV initially; some clinicians recommend an initial dose of up to 20 mg. If necessary, the manufacturer states that an additional dose of 5–10 mg may be administered in 3–4 hours if necessary. For acute alcohol withdrawal, some clinicians recommend 10 mg of diazepam IV initially, followed by 10 mg at 20- to 30-minute intervals until the patient is calm.

To relieve anxiety and stress and produce amnesia in adults undergoing cardioversion, 5–15 mg of diazepam may be given IV within 5–10 minutes prior to the procedure.

To reduce anxiety prior to endoscopy, diazepam is administered slowly IV immediately before the procedure; dosage is titrated to obtain the desired sedative response, such as slurring of speech. Generally, IV administration of up to 10 mg is adequate in adults, but up to 20 mg may be required especially if opiates are not given concomitantly. If IV administration is not feasible, 5–10 mg of diazepam may be given IM approximately 30 minutes prior to endoscopy in adults.

For preoperative sedation in adults, 10 mg of diazepam may be administered parenterally 1–2 hours prior to surgery. IM administration is preferred. Some clinicians have recommended a dose of up to 20 mg preoperatively.

For the treatment of skeletal muscle spasticity in adults, 5–10 mg may be administered IM or IV initially, and 3–4 hours later if necessary. For tetanus in adults, larger doses may be required; up to 20 mg has been given every 2–8 hours.

For the treatment of status epilepticus or severe recurrent convulsive seizures, the usual initial adult dose of diazepam is 5–10 mg administered IV. The initial dose may be repeated at 10- to 15-minute intervals, if necessary, until a maximum total dose of 30 mg has been given. If necessary, therapy with diazepam may be repeated in 2–4 hours, with consideration that residual active metabolites may persist following readministration. Although IV administration is preferred, diazepam may be given IM if IV administration is not possible.

To reduce the requirements for opiate analgesics and produce anterograde amnesia during labor and delivery†, the usual parenteral dosage of diazepam is 10–20 mg.

If diazepam is used for sedation in intubated and mechanically ventilated adults in critical care settings†, an IV loading dose of 5–10 mg, followed by intermittent diazepam injections of 0.03–0.1 mg/kg every 0.5–6 hours as needed is recommended by some experts. Dosage should be titrated to the desired level of sedation; in most cases, a light rather than deep level of sedation is recommended in critically ill, mechanically ventilated adults. The depth and quality of sedation should be assessed frequently using a validated and reliable assessment tool.

In geriatric or debilitated patients or in patients receiving other sedative drugs, lower parenteral diazepam doses (usually 2–5 mg) should be used, and dosage should be slowly increased if needed.

Pediatric Dosage. In pediatric patients, IV diazepam should be given slowly over a 3-minute period. The manufacturers recommend that the initial dose not exceed 0.25 mg/kg. The dose may be repeated after 15–30 minutes; if relief of symptoms is not obtained after a third dose, adjunctive therapy appropriate to the condition being treated is recommended.

For the treatment of status epilepticus or severe recurrent convulsant seizures in children 30 days to less than 5 years of age, the usual initial dose of diazepam is 0.2–0.5 mg administered slowly IV; this dose may be repeated every 2–5 minutes up to a maximum total dose of 5 mg. In children 5 years of age or older, the initial dose for the management of seizures is 1 mg administered slowly IV; this dose may be repeated every 2–5 minutes up to a maximum total dose of 10 mg. If necessary, the initial dose of diazepam may be repeated in 2–4 hours. Although IV administration is preferred, diazepam may be given IM if IV administration is not possible. Some clinicians prefer IV lorazepam because of its more prolonged duration of effect. If seizures continue with either diazepam or lorazepam, an additional long-acting anticonvulsant (e.g., IV phenytoin or fosphenytoin) generally is initiated.

For tetanus in children, the manufacturers recommend 1–2 mg of diazepam for infants older than 30 days to 5 years of age and 5–10 mg for children older than 5 years of age administered slowly IV or by IM injection. This dose may be repeated every 3–4 hours as needed.

In painful musculoskeletal conditions and spasticity including tetanus in children, some clinicians recommend diazepam 0.04–0.3 mg/kg IV every 2–4 hours; however, dosage generally should not exceed 0.6 mg/kg in an 8-hour period.

Although the manufacturers have not established pediatric dosage recommendations for preoperative sedation, some clinicians have recommended IM administration of 0.4 mg/kg of diazepam in children older than 2 years of age 1–2 hours prior to surgery.

For acute anxiety reactions in children, some clinicians recommend 0.04–0.2 mg/kg of diazepam IV; this dose may be repeated in 3–4 hours, but dosage should not exceed 0.6 mg/kg in an 8-hour period.

Although the safety and efficacy of parenteral diazepam in infants 30 days of age or younger have not been established, neonates with agitation due to opiate withdrawal have received 0.5–2 mg IM every 8 hours followed by gradual reduction in dosage.

Rectal Dosage When diazepam is administered rectally as the commercially available gel for the management of acute repetitive seizures, the dose should be individualized for maximum benefit. Children 2–5 years of age should receive 0.5 mg/kg and those 6–11 years of age should receive 0.3 mg/kg; adults and children 12 years of age and older should receive 0.2 mg/kg. These age-adjusted doses were based on the observation that diazepam clearance in children declines with age until about 12 years of age, at which time adult values are reached. The actual dose to be administered is determined by rounding up to the nearest commercially available dose (i.e., the next multiple of 2.5 mg). Using this method of rounded dosing, patients will receive 90–180% of the dose calculated on a weight and age basis. The safety of this dosing method has been established in clinical studies in adults and children 2 years of age and older. For geriatric or debilitated patients, the dose of the rectal gel should be adjusted downward to reduce the likelihood of ataxia and oversedation. The 2.5-mg applicator also may be used to provide a partial replacement dose (supplemental dose) for patients who partially expel the recommended dose within 5 minutes after administration.

If necessary for adequate seizure control, the usual age- and weight-adjusted dose of diazepam rectal gel may be repeated 4–12 hours after the initial dose. Although the usual dose was repeated a third time 8 hours after the second dose in adults in one clinical study, the additional dose resulted in increased sedation and appeared to negatively affect global caregiver assessment of treatment outcome; therefore, a third dose currently is not recommended by the manufacturer. Dosage should be adjusted periodically by the clinician to reflect changes in the patient's age and/or weight; the manufacturer recommends dosage reevaluation at 6-month intervals.

The manufacturer states that diazepam rectal gel is intended for use solely on an intermittent basis and therefore should be administered by caregivers outside the hospital no more frequently than one treatment course every 5 days nor more frequently than 5 treatment courses per month. In addition, chronic daily use of the rectal gel is not recommended because of the potential for development of tolerance to diazepam; chronic daily use may increase the frequency and/or severity of tonic-clonic seizures, requiring an increase in the dosage of concomitant chronic anticonvulsant therapy. In such cases, abrupt withdrawal of chronic diazepam also may be associated with a temporary increase in the frequency and/or severity of seizures.

Because caregivers will be responsible for recognizing seizure episodes suitable for treatment, making the decision to initiate treatment, administering the drug, monitoring the patient, and assessing the adequacy of response, a major component of the prescribing process is the careful instruction of these individuals. The clinician and caregiver must share a common explicit understanding of what constitutes a seizure episode (and/or the events, which may be nonconvulsive, presumed to herald their onset) that is appropriate for treatment, the timing of administration in relation to the onset of the episode, the mechanics of competently administering the drug, how and what to observe following administration, when to repeat a dose, and what would constitute an outcome requiring immediate and direct medical attention.

The caregiver should be instructed to contact the patient's clinician or seek other medical assistance if the seizure episode persists for longer than 15 minutes after administering the rectal gel (or as otherwise instructed), if the seizure behavior differs from other episodes, if the seizure frequency or severity or patient color or breathing is alarming, or if the patient is experiencing unusual or serious problems.

The patient's underlying seizure disorder should be stabilized with a standard chronic anticonvulsant drug regimen, and rectal diazepam should be used only as an adjunct to this regimen for characteristic breakthrough bouts of repetitive seizures.

When using the parenteral solution† of diazepam for rectal administration in the treatment of status epilepticus, a dose of 0.5 mg/kg (up to 20 mg) has been used in adults and children. Some clinicians state that a second dose of 0.25 mg/kg may be administered after 10 minutes if needed.

Cautions

Drowsiness, fatigue, muscle weakness, and ataxia are the most common adverse effects of diazepam. With parenteral therapy, local reactions (venous thrombosis, phlebitis) at the injection site are the most common adverse effects of the drug. For further information on adverse effects reported with benzodiazepines, see Cautions in the Benzodiazepines General Statement 28:24.08

■ **Precautions and Contraindications** Diazepam shares the toxic potentials of the benzodiazepines, and the usual precautions of benzodiazepine administration should be observed. (See Cautions in the Benzodiazepines General Statement 28:24.08.)

Parenterally administered diazepam may cause hypotension and/or respiratory depression, particularly if the drug is administered too rapidly IV. The drug should be administered slowly IV at a rate not exceeding 5 mg/minute in adults and over a 3-minute period in children; facilities and equipment for respiratory or cardiovascular assistance should be readily available.

The possibility that respiratory depression could occur with rectal administration of diazepam also should be considered, although the risk of its development probably is less than that with IV administration. The drug should be used with caution in patients with compromised respiratory function secondary to an underlying disease (e.g., asthma, pneumonia) or neurologic damage. Repeated rectal therapy at relatively short intervals by out-of-hospital caregivers should be avoided because of the possibility of life-threatening respiratory depression; the manufacturer recommends that out-of-hospital rectal diazepam therapy be repeated no more frequently than once during a 5-day period or 5 times monthly and that dosing be limited to 2 doses per treatment course. (See Dosage: Rectal Dosage, in Dosage and Administration.)

Diazepam is contraindicated in patients with known hypersensitivity to the drug. The manufacturers state that the drug is contraindicated in patients with acute angle-closure glaucoma but may be used with caution in patients with open-angle glaucoma who are receiving appropriate therapy. However, the clinical rationale for this contraindication has been questioned.

■ **Pediatric Precautions** Safety and efficacy of oral diazepam in infants younger than 6 months of age have not been established. Safety and efficacy of parenteral diazepam in infants 30 days of age or younger have not been established. Safety and efficacy of rectal diazepam have not been established via clinical studies in children younger than 2 years of age, and the manufacturer states that the rectal gel is not recommended for use in infants younger than 6 months of age.

Chemistry and Stability

■ **Chemistry** Diazepam is a benzodiazepine. Diazepam occurs as an off-white to yellow, practically odorless, crystalline powder. The drug is sparingly soluble in propylene glycol and has solubilities of approximately 3 mg/mL in water and 62.5 mg/mL in alcohol at 25°C. Diazepam has a pK_a of 3.4. Sodium benzoate and benzoic acid are added to the commercially available injection to adjust the pH to 6.2–6.9.

Diazepam rectal gel is commercially available as a nonsterile viscous gel formulated in an aqueous base that contains propylene glycol, alcohol (10%), hydroxypropyl methylcellulose, sodium benzoate, benzyl alcohol (1.5%), and benzoic acid. The rectal gel is clear to slightly yellow and has a pH of 6.5–7.2.

■ **Stability** Diazepam injection should be protected from light and stored at 15–30°C; freezing should be avoided. Diazepam tablets and extended-release capsules should be stored in tight, light-resistant containers at 15–30°C. Diazepam oral solution and oral concentrate solution should be stored at 20–25°C.

The manufacturers state that diazepam injection should not be mixed with other drugs or IV fluids. Although some studies indicate that diazepam injection may be compatible with various drugs and IV fluids (e.g., diluted to a concentration of 5 mg/50 mL to 5 mg/100 mL with 0.9% sodium chloride, 5% dextrose, Ringer's, or lactated Ringer's injection), compatibility may depend on several factors (e.g., the concentration of the drugs, resulting pH, temperature). Specialized references should be consulted for more specific compatibility information. The addition of diazepam injection to an IV infusion solution or plastic syringes may result in adsorption of diazepam to the plastic container and tubing.

Diazepam rectal gel should be stored at a controlled room temperature of 25° but may be exposed to temperatures ranging from 15–30°C.

For further information on chemistry, pharmacology, pharmacokinetics, uses, cautions, chronic toxicity, acute toxicity, drug interactions, laboratory test interferences, and dosage and administration of diazepam, see the Benzodiazepines General Statement 28:24.08.

Preparations

Diazepam is subject to control under the Federal Controlled Substances Act of 1970 as a schedule IV (C-IV) drug.

Excipients in commercially available drug preparations may have clinically important effects in some individuals; consult specific product labeling for details.

diazePAM

Oral		
Solution	5 mg/5 mL*	**diazePAM Solution** (C-IV)
Solution, concentrate	5 mg/mL*	**diazePAM Intensol**® (C-IV), West-ward
		diazePAM Solution Concentrate (C-IV)
Tablets	2 mg*	**diazePAM Tablets** (C-IV)
		Valium® (C-IV; scored), Genentech

	5 mg*	**diazePAM Tablets** (C-IV)
		Valium® (C-IV; scored), Genentech
	10 mg*	**diazePAM Tablets** (C-IV)
		Valium® (C-IV; scored), Genentech
Parenteral		
Injection	5 mg/mL*	**diazePAM Injection** (C-IV)
Rectal		
Gel	5 mg/mL (2.5, 10, and 20 mg)*	**Diastat**® **Rectal Delivery System** (C-IV; in prefilled applicators with pediatric universal or adult applicator tips), Valeant
		diazePAM Gel Rectal Delivery System (C-IV; in prefilled applicators with pediatric universal or adult applicator tips)

*available from one or more manufacturer, distributor, and/or repackager by generic (nonproprietary) name

†Use is not currently included in the labeling approved by the US Food and Drug Administration

LORazepam

■ Lorazepam is a benzodiazepine. The drug has anticonvulsant, anxiolytic, and sedative properties.

Uses

■ **Anxiety Disorders** Lorazepam is used for the management of anxiety disorders or for the short-term relief of symptoms of anxiety or anxiety associated with depressive symptoms. Anxiety or tension associated with the stress of everyday life usually does not require treatment with an anxiolytic. The efficacy of lorazepam for long-term use (i.e., longer than 4 months) has not been evaluated. The need for continued therapy with the drug should be periodically reassessed.

■ **Preoperative Sedation, Anxiolysis, and Amnesia** Lorazepam injection is used for preoperative sedation, anxiolysis, and anterograde amnesia. Administration of lorazepam is especially useful in patients with preoperative anxiety who prefer diminished recall of events associated with the day of surgery.

■ **Status Epilepticus** Lorazepam injection is used for the treatment of status epilepticus.

Benzodiazepines are considered the initial drugs of choice for the management of status epilepticus because of their rapid onset of action, demonstrated efficacy, safety, and tolerability. (See Uses: Seizure Disorders, in the Benzodiazepines General Statement 28:24.08.) Although IV lorazepam is generally preferred because of its longer duration of action, there is also evidence supporting the use of IV diazepam and IM midazolam and experts consider these therapies to be equivalent first-line options. Selection of an appropriate benzodiazepine should be individualized based on local availability, route of administration, pharmacokinetics, cost, and other factors (e.g., treatment setting). If seizures continue after initial therapy with a benzodiazepine, a second-line anticonvulsant agent (e.g., IV fosphenytoin or phenytoin, IV valproate sodium, IV levetiracetam, IV phenobarbital) should be administered. If refractory status epilepticus occurs, continuous IV infusion of anticonvulsants, IV barbiturates, or general anesthetics may be necessary. (See Status Epilepticus under Seizure Disorders: Principles of Anticonvulsant Drug Therapy, in the Anticonvulsants General Statement 28:12.)

Efficacy of IV lorazepam was established in 2 multicenter controlled trials in patients (mostly 18–65 years of age) with tonic-clonic status epilepticus, simple partial and complex partial status epilepticus, or absence status. The first study was a double-blind, randomized, active-control study that compared lorazepam 2 mg (with an additional 2-mg IV dose given if necessary) with diazepam 5 mg (with an additional 5-mg IV dose given if necessary). In this study, 80 or 57% of patients receiving lorazepam or diazepam, respectively, were considered responders, defined as the percentage of patients in whom seizures were terminated within 10 minutes after administration of the drug and who continued to be seizure-free for at least an additional 30 minutes. When an additional dose of study drug was administered to nonresponders, the overall response rate increased to 93% with lorazepam and 86% with diazepam. The second study was a double-blind, dose comparison trial; in this study, 61, 57, and 76% of patients receiving 1, 2, and 4 mg of lorazepam, respectively, were responders (as defined above).

Although IV lorazepam is often the preferred benzodiazepine for treatment of status epilepticus, the need to establish IV access may delay administration of the drug in the prehospital environment. Results of a randomized controlled study (RAMPART) indicate that IM administration of midazolam by paramedics in the prehospital setting may improve outcomes in patients with status epilepticus; in this study, 73% of patients who received IM midazolam achieved seizure resolution at the time of arrival in the emergency department compared with 63% of those who received IV lorazepam.

■ **Sedation in Critical Care Settings** Lorazepam, administered by intermittent injection or continuous IV infusion, has been used for sedation of intubated and mechanically ventilated adults and children in critical care settings† (e.g., intensive care unit [ICU]).

Sedative agents are administered in critically ill patients to reduce agitation and anxiety and increase tolerance to invasive procedures (e.g., mechanical ventilation). The provision of adequate analgesia and other measures to ensure patient comfort is recommended before sedatives are administered. Common sedative agents used in the ICU include benzodiazepines (e.g., midazolam, lorazepam), propofol, and dexmedetomidine. These agents appear to be similarly effective in providing adequate sedation in critically ill, mechanically ventilated adults. However, modest benefits in terms of other clinical outcomes (e.g., reduced duration of mechanical ventilation, shorter time to extubation, reduced risk of delirium) have been observed with the nonbenzodiazepine sedatives (dexmedetomidine and propofol) compared with benzodiazepines. (See Uses: Sedation in Critical Care Settings, in the Benzodiazepines General Statement 28:24.08.) Because of the apparent advantages and an overall favorable benefit-to-risk profile, experts state that nonbenzodiazepine sedatives (dexmedetomidine or propofol) may be preferred to benzodiazepines (midazolam or lorazepam) in mechanically ventilated, critically ill adults. This recommendation should be considered in the context of the specific clinical situation since benzodiazepines may still be preferred in certain situations (e.g., patients with anxiety, seizures, or alcohol or benzodiazepine withdrawal). When selecting an appropriate sedative agent, the patient's individual sedation goals should be considered in addition to specific drug-related (e.g., pharmacology, pharmacokinetics, adverse effects, availability, cost) and patient-related (e.g., comorbid conditions) factors.

Results of several clinical studies indicate that lorazepam is as effective as midazolam in terms of level of sedation, the time required to achieve adequate sedation, and usually, the number of daily dose adjustments. In one study, midazolam IV infusions required more frequent dosage adjustments to maintain the desired level of sedation than lorazepam. Studies comparing lorazepam and midazolam for prolonged use in ICU patients suggest greater variability and longer time to awakening with midazolam than with lorazepam. Because of lorazepam's slow onset of action, the drug is not effective for the treatment of acute agitation and midazolam is preferred for rapid sedation of the acutely agitated patient.

■ **Schizophrenia** Lorazepam also has been used in the management of schizophrenia and may be helpful for the management of anxiety, agitation, and sleep disturbances that are often present during the acute phase of schizophrenia in patients receiving antipsychotic therapy. In addition, the drug also has been used in patients who experience akathisia† while receiving antipsychotic drugs and for the treatment of acute catatonic reactions†, whether associated with schizophrenia or other conditions. (See Uses: Schizophrenia, in the Benzodiazepines General Statement 28:24.08.)

■ **Cancer Chemotherapy-induced Nausea and Vomiting** Lorazepam also has been used alone, but usually in combination with other drugs, such as 5-HT_3 receptor antagonists and/or corticosteroids, for the management of nausea and vomiting associated with emetogenic cancer chemotherapy†, including that associated with cisplatin. (See Uses: Cancer Chemotherapy-induced Nausea and Vomiting, in the Benzodiazepines General Statement 28:24.08.)

■ **Delirium** Lorazepam also has been used in the management of delirium.† Results of several open studies suggest that combined therapy with IV lorazepam and IV haloperidol was more effective than IV haloperidol alone, with a shorter duration of delirium during combined therapy and fewer extrapyramidal manifestations. If a benzodiazepine is used for the treatment of delirium, those with a short duration and no active metabolites (e.g., lorazepam) are preferred. (See Uses: Delirium, in the Benzodiazepines General Statement 28:24.08.)

■ **Drug-induced Cardiovascular Emergencies** Lorazepam has been used adjunctively in the management of certain drug-induced cardiovascular emergencies† and cocaine-induced acute coronary syndrome†.

Dosage and Administration

■ **Administration** Lorazepam is administered orally, IM, or by IV injection or IV infusion. *The drug should not be administered by intra-arterial injection since arteriospasm can occur, which may cause gangrene and possibly require amputation.*

Oral Administration Lorazepam is administered orally as tablets or oral solution.

Lorazepam oral concentrate solution should be mixed with a liquid (e.g., water, juices, carbonated or soda-like beverages) or semi-solid food (e.g., applesauce, pudding) just before administration using only the calibrated dropper provided by the manufacturer.

Parenteral Administration IM injections of lorazepam, administered as undiluted solutions, should be made deep into the muscle mass.

Lorazepam injection must be diluted with an equal volume of compatible diluent, such as sterile water for injection, 0.9% sodium chloride injection, or 5% dextrose injection, immediately prior to IV administration. Following dilution, the solution should be mixed thoroughly by gently inverting the container repeatedly until a homogenous solution is obtained; the solution should not be shaken vigorously. Solutions of lorazepam injection should *not* be used if they appear discolored or contain a precipitate.

Following dilution of the drug, lorazepam may be injected directly into a vein or into the tubing of a free-flowing compatible IV infusion (e.g., 0.9% sodium chloride, 5% dextrose). Injections should be administered slowly at a rate not exceeding 2 mg/minute. Direct IV injection with the drug should be made with repeated aspiration to ensure that none of the drug is injected intra-arterially and that perivascular extravasation does not occur.

Equipment necessary to maintain a patent airway and to support respiration and ventilation should be immediately available prior to administration of IV lorazepam. Vital signs should be monitored during IV infusion of the drug.

■ **Dosage** Dosage of lorazepam must be individualized, and the smallest effective dosage should be used (especially in geriatric or debilitated patients, in those with low serum albumin, and in patients currently receiving other CNS depressants) to avoid oversedation.

Anxiety Disorders The usual initial adult oral dosage of lorazepam for the symptomatic treatment of anxiety is 2–3 mg daily, divided in 2 or 3 doses; dosage should be adjusted if necessary and as tolerated. In geriatric or debilitated patients, lorazepam therapy should be initiated with 1–2 mg daily, divided in 2 or 3 doses; dosage should be adjusted if necessary and as tolerated. Dosage may range from 1–10 mg daily (usually 2–6 mg) in divided doses, with the largest single dose given at bedtime. For insomnia caused by anxiety or transient situational stress in adults, 2–4 mg of lorazepam is given as a single daily dose, usually at bedtime. In patients who have received prolonged (e.g., for several months) lorazepam therapy, abrupt discontinuance of the drug should be avoided since manifestations of withdrawal can be precipitated; if the drug is to be discontinued in such patients, it is recommended that dosage be gradually tapered.

Preoperative Sedation, Anxiolysis, and Amnesia For preoperative IM use in adults, the usual dose of lorazepam is 0.05 mg/kg administered by deep IM injection at least 2 hours prior to surgery. The IM dose should be individualized, but should not exceed 4 mg.

Alternatively, lorazepam may be administered IV for preoperative use. For preoperative IV use, the usual initial dose of lorazepam for sedation and relief of anxiety is 0.044 mg/kg (or up to 2 mg total, whichever is smaller) administered 15–20 minutes prior to surgery; this dose is sufficient for sedating most adults and generally should not be exceeded in patients older than 50 years of age. For those patients in whom increased lack of recall about perioperative events is considered beneficial, lorazepam doses up to 0.05 mg/kg (maximum total dose of 4 mg) may be administered IV.

Status Epilepticus For the management of status epilepticus, the usual dose of lorazepam in adults is 4 mg by slow IV injection (rate of 2 mg/minute); if seizures continue or recur after a 10- to 15-minute period of observation, an additional 4-mg dose of the drug may be administered. The manufacturer states that experience with administration of additional doses of lorazepam is limited. IM administration of lorazepam is not recommended for the treatment of status epilepticus because therapeutic plasma concentrations of the drug are not achieved as rapidly as with IV administration of the drug. However lorazepam may be given IM if IV access is not available.

For the management of status epilepticus in children†, IV doses of 0.05–0.1 mg/kg have been used.

Sedation in Critical Care Settings Dosage of sedative agents should be titrated to the desired level of sedation; in most cases, a light rather than deep level of sedation is recommended in critically ill mechanically ventilated adults because of improved clinical outcomes that have been demonstrated (e.g., shortened duration of mechanical ventilation, reduced ICU length of stay). The depth and quality of sedation should be assessed frequently using a validated and reliable assessment tool (e.g., Richmond Agitation-Sedation Scale [RASS], Sedation-Agitation Scale [SAS]).

If lorazepam is used for sedation in intubated and mechanically ventilated adults in critical care settings†, some experts recommend an IV loading dose of 0.02–0.04 mg/kg (not to exceed 2 mg); the loading dose should be followed by intermittent injections of 0.02–0.06 mg/kg every 2–6 hours as needed or a continuous IV infusion at a rate of 0.01–0.1 mg/kg per hour (not to exceed 10 mg/hour). The infusion rate should be titrated to the lowest effective dosage to provide the desired level of sedation. Frequent assessment of the patient's sedation requirements and tapering of the infusion rate may prevent prolonged sedative effects.

Although there is limited information available on the use of lorazepam for sedation in intubated and mechanically ventilated children in critical care settings†, some clinicians have suggested lorazepam dosages of 0.025–0.05 mg/kg (maximum initial dose of 2 mg) given as intermittent IV infusions every 2–4 hours in children 2 months of age or older. Alternatively, in these pediatric patients, lorazepam may be administered by a continuous IV infusion, at a rate of 0.025 mg/kg per hour (up to 2 mg/hour) which may be titrated as necessary or supplemented with rapid ("bolus") injections of the drug to provide the desired level of sedation. Because of wide interpatient variations in dosage requirements and low hepatic metabolic function, the initial lorazepam dose should be reduced by 50% in infants younger than 2 months of age.

Cancer Chemotherapy-induced Nausea and Vomiting For the management of nausea and vomiting associated with emetogenic cancer chemotherapy†, including that associated with cisplatin, adults have received 2.5 mg of lorazepam orally the evening before and just after initiation of chemotherapy. Alternatively, adults have received 1.5 mg/m^2 (usually up to a maximum dose of 3 mg) of lorazepam administered IV (usually over 5 minutes) 45 minutes before initiation of chemotherapy.

Delirium For the management of delirium† in combination with haloperidol, combined therapy can be initiated in adults with an IV haloperidol dose of 3 mg followed immediately with an IV lorazepam dose of 0.5–1 mg. Dosage of the drugs should then be adjusted according to patient response and tolerance. ECG should be determined at baseline and periodically because of the risk of QT prolongation with haloperidol therapy. (See Uses: Delirium and also see Dosage: IV Dosage, in Haloperidol 28:16.08.32.)

Dosage in Renal and Hepatic Impairment The manufacturer states that a dosage adjustment is *not* required in patients with impaired renal function for single doses of lorazepam injection; however, caution should be exercised with administration of multiple doses of lorazepam injection over a short period of time.

Since the pharmacokinetics of parenteral lorazepam do not appear to be altered in patients with hepatic impairment, dosage adjustment is not necessary in such patients. However, because oral lorazepam may exacerbate hepatic encephalopathy, dosage of oral lorazepam should be adjusted carefully in patients with severe hepatic insufficiency and lower than recommended dosages may be sufficient in these patients.

Cautions

Adverse effects reported with lorazepam are similar to those reported with other benzodiazepines. Changes in vital signs (e.g., respiratory rate, blood pressure) are the most frequent adverse effects associated with parenteral lorazepam administration. For further information on adverse effects reported with benzodiazepines, see Cautions in the Benzodiazepines General Statement 28:24.08. Flumazenil, a benzodiazepine antagonist, can be used in hospitalized patients as an adjunct, not a substitute for, proper management of lorazepam overdose. (See Flumazenil 28:92.)

■ **Precautions and Contraindications** Lorazepam shares the toxic potentials of the benzodiazepines, and the usual precautions of benzodiazepine administration should be observed. (See Cautions in the Benzodiazepines General Statement 28:24.08.)

Drugs that affect the CNS (e.g., phenothiazines, barbiturates, antidepressants, alcohol, scopolamine, monoamine oxidase inhibitors) may have additive CNS effects when used concomitantly with, or during the period of recovery from, lorazepam. Such combinations, or IV lorazepam used alone in higher than recommended doses, can produce excessive sedation which may result in partial airway obstruction. The manufacturer warns that scopolamine does *not* provide additional benefit when used concomitantly with lorazepam, but may increase sedation, hallucinations, and irrational behavior.

Concomitant use of benzodiazepines, including lorazepam, and opiate agonists or opiate partial agonists may result in profound sedation, respiratory depression, coma, and death. Patients receiving lorazepam and/or their caregivers should be apprised of the risks associated with concomitant therapeutic or illicit use of benzodiazepines and opiates. For further information on potential interactions with opiates, see Opiate Agonists and Opiate Partial Agonists under Drug Interactions: CNS Agents, in the Benzodiazepines General Statement 28:24.08.

When lorazepam is administered IV prior to regional or local anesthesia, especially at doses greater than 0.05 mg/kg or when opiate agonists or partial agonists are used concomitantly with recommended lorazepam doses, excessive sedation or drowsiness may occur; these effects may possibly interfere with patient cooperation in determining levels of anesthesia.

Lorazepam should be administered IV only in settings in which continuous monitoring of respiratory and cardiac function (i.e., pulse oximetry) is possible. Safety and efficacy of lorazepam may vary according to the dose administered and clinical status of the patient. Since lorazepam is capable of producing several levels of CNS depression—from mild to deep sedation, facilities, age- and size-appropriate equipment for bag/mask/valve ventilation and intubation, drugs, and skilled personnel necessary for ventilation and intubation, administration of oxygen, assisted or controlled respiration, airway management, and cardiovascular support should be immediately available whenever this drug is administered. Monitoring of vital signs also should continue during the recovery period. Lorazepam injection should be administered with extreme caution to geriatric or debilitated patients, and to patients with compromised pulmonary function (decreased reserve), since underventilation and/or hypoxic cardiac arrest may occur. For deeply sedated pediatric patients, a dedicated individual other than the clinician performing the procedure should monitor the patient throughout the procedure.

Lorazepam should only be used for the treatment of status epilepticus by clinicians experienced in the comprehensive management of the disease. Since these patients may be at increased risk of respiratory depression associated with administration of IV lorazepam, they require careful monitoring of respiratory rate and maintenance of an adequate, patent airway. Ventilatory support also may be needed in some patients. Because of the prolonged duration of action of lorazepam, it should be considered that the sedative effects of the drug (especially after multiple doses) may increase the impairment of consciousness observed in the postictal state.

The manufacturer warns that there is no evidence to date to support the use of lorazepam injection in patients with coma, shock, or acute alcohol intoxication. The manufacturer warns that there are insufficient data to support the use of lorazepam injection for outpatient endoscopic procedures; when these procedures are conducted in inpatients, adequate recovery room observation time is necessary and pharyngeal reflex activity should be minimized prior to the procedure by administering adequate topical or regional anesthesia.

Adverse effects associated with propylene glycol (e.g., lactic acidosis, hyperosmolality, hypotension) or polyethylene glycol (e.g., acute tubular necrosis) may occur in patients receiving lorazepam injection. Manifestations of toxicity are more likely to occur in patients with renal impairment and those receiving higher than recommended dosages, although total daily IV doses as low as 1 mg/kg also have been reported to cause propylene glycol toxicity.

Lorazepam injection is *not* recommended for use in patients with hepatic and/or renal failure, since the drug is most likely conjugated in the liver and since conjugated lorazepam is excreted via the kidneys. However, this does not preclude use of the drug in patients with mild to moderate hepatic or renal disease; in these patients, the lowest possible effective dose of lorazepam injection should be administered since the effects of the drug may be prolonged. The manufacturer states that administration of oral lorazepam may exacerbate hepatic encephalopathy and, therefore, the drug should be used with caution in patients with severe hepatic insufficiency and/or encephalopathy. Dosage of lorazepam should be adjusted carefully in patients with severe hepatic insufficiency; lower than recommended dosages may be sufficient in these patients. Because of the possibility of suicide in depressed patients, oral lorazepam should not be used in such patients without adequate antidepressant therapy.

Patients should be informed of the pharmacologic effects of lorazepam (e.g., sedation, relief of anxiety, lack of recall) and the duration of these effects (8 hours or longer) so that they may adequately perceive the risks and benefits of use of lorazepam injection. Patients should be warned that lorazepam injection may impair their ability to perform activities requiring mental alertness or physical coordination (e.g., operating machinery, driving a motor vehicle) for 24–48 hours following administration of the drug. Impaired performance may persist for longer periods in geriatric patients, in patients using other drugs concomitantly, and as a result of the stress of surgery or general condition of the patient. Patients also should be warned that premature ambulation (within 8 hours of receiving lorazepam injection) may result in injury from falling. Patients also should be warned that concomitant use of lorazepam with sedatives, opiate analgesics (opiate agonists or partial agonists), or tranquilizers may increase the extent and duration of impaired performance, may cause excessive sedation, and, rarely, may interfere with recall and recognition of events on the day of surgery and the following day. Patients should be advised to abstain from consumption of alcoholic beverages for 24–48 hours following administration of lorazepam injection.

Lorazepam is contraindicated in patients with known hypersensitivity to benzodiazepines or any ingredients in the formulation (i.e., polyethylene glycol, propylene glycol, or benzyl alcohol) and in patients with acute angle-closure glaucoma or sleep apnea syndrome. Lorazepam injection also is contraindicated in patients with severe respiratory insufficiency, except in those requiring relief of anxiety and/or diminished recall of events while being mechanically ventilated. In addition, the injection is contraindicated in premature infants because the formulation contains benzyl alcohol.

■ **Pediatric Precautions** Safety and efficacy of lorazepam tablets and oral concentrate solution in children younger than 12 years of age have not been established.

Safety and efficacy of lorazepam injection in pediatric patients younger than 18 years of age have not been established.

In several open label studies conducted in pediatric patients (neonates as young as a few hours up to adolescents 18 years of age), paradoxical excitation, characterized by tremors, agitation, euphoria, logorrhea, and brief episodes of visual hallucinations, was reported in 10–30% of children younger than 8 years of age. Seizures and myoclonus have been reported in pediatric patients (especially in very low birth-weight neonates) receiving lorazepam injection. Brief tonic-clonic seizures were reported in pediatric patients who received lorazepam for the management of atypical petit mal status epilepticus.

FDA warns that repeated or prolonged use of general anesthetics and sedation drugs, including lorazepam, in children younger than 3 years of age or during the third trimester of pregnancy may affect brain development. Animal studies in multiple species, including nonhuman primates, have demonstrated that use for longer than 3 hours of anesthetic and sedation drugs that block *N*-methyl-D-aspartic acid (NMDA) receptors and/or potentiate γ-aminobutyric acid (GABA) activity leads to widespread neuronal and oligodendrocyte cell loss and alterations in synaptic morphology and neurogenesis in the brain, resulting in long-term deficits in cognition and behavior. Across animal species, vulnerability to these neurodevelopmental changes occurs during the period of rapid brain growth or synaptogenesis; this period is thought to correlate with the third trimester of pregnancy through the first year of life in humans, but may extend to approximately 3 years of age. The clinical relevance of these animal findings to humans is not known. While some published evidence suggests that similar deficits in cognition and behavior may occur in children following repeated or prolonged exposure to anesthesia early in life, other studies have found no association between pediatric anesthesia exposure and long-term adverse neurodevelopmental outcomes. Most studies to date have had substantial limitations, and it is not clear whether the adverse neurodevelopmental outcomes observed in children were related to the drug or to other factors (e.g., surgery, underlying illness). There is some clinical evidence that a single, relatively brief exposure to general anesthesia in generally healthy children is unlikely to cause clinically detectable deficits in global cognitive function or serious behavioral disorders; however, further research is needed to fully characterize the effects of exposure to general anesthetics in early life, particularly for prolonged or repeated exposures and in more vulnerable populations (e.g., less healthy children). For further information, see Cautions: Pediatric Precautions, in the Benzodiazepines General Statement 28:24.08.

Anesthetic and sedation drugs are an essential component of care for children and pregnant women who require surgery or other procedures that cannot be delayed; no specific general anesthetic or sedation drug has been shown to be less likely to cause neurocognitive deficits than any other such drug. Pending further accumulation of data in humans from well-designed studies, decisions regarding the timing of elective procedures requiring anesthesia should take into consideration both the benefits of the procedure and the potential risks. When procedures requiring the use of general anesthetics or sedation drugs are considered for young children or pregnant women, clinicians should discuss with the patient, parent, or caregiver the benefits, risks (including potential risk of adverse neurodevelopmental effects), and appropriate timing and duration of the procedure. FDA states that procedures that are considered medically necessary should not be delayed or avoided.

Lorazepam injection contains benzyl alcohol, polyethylene glycol, and propylene glycol and some pediatric patients (particularly premature and low-birth weight infants or those receiving high doses of the injection) may be susceptible to adverse effects associated with these ingredients. Although a causal relationship has not been established, administration of injections preserved with benzyl alcohol has been associated with toxicity in neonates. Toxicity appears to have resulted from administration of large amounts (i.e., 100–400 mg/kg daily) of benzyl alcohol in these neonates. Exposure to such excessive amounts of benzyl alcohol has been associated with CNS depression, metabolic acidosis, gasping respirations, gradual neurological deterioration, seizures, intracranial hemorrhage, hematologic abnormalities, skin breakdown, hepatic and renal failure, hypotension, bradycardia, and cardiovascular collapse. Although use of drugs preserved with benzyl alcohol should be avoided in neonates whenever possible, the American Academy of Pediatrics (AAP) states that the presence of small amounts of the preservative in a commercially available injection should not proscribe its use when indicated in neonates.

In pediatric patients, propylene glycol present in high doses of lorazepam injections, has been associated with adverse effects, including CNS toxicity, seizures, intraventricular hemorrhage, unresponsiveness, tachypnea, tachycardia, and diaphoresis.

■ **Geriatric Precautions** Clinical trials of lorazepam did not include sufficient numbers of patients 65 years and older to determine whether they respond differently than younger adults. However, unless enhanced suppression of recall is desired, patients older than 50 years of age generally should not be given an initial parenteral lorazepam dose greater than 2 mg since excessive and prolonged sedation may occur.

No age-related differences in the pharmacokinetics of lorazepam have been identified; however, because of greater sensitivity and increased frequency of impaired hepatic or renal function in geriatric patients, the manufacturer suggests that patients in this age group receive initial dosages of the drug in the lower end of the usual range. (See Dosage and Administration: Dosage) Geriatric patients should be warned that lorazepam injection may cause excessive sedation for 6–8 hours or longer after surgery.

■ **Mutagenicity and Carcinogenicity** Studies to determine the mutagenic potential of lorazepam have not been performed. No evidence of carcinogenicity was observed in rats or mice during an 18-month study using oral lorazepam.

■ **Pregnancy, Fertility, and Lactation** Lorazepam may cause fetal toxicity when administered to pregnant women. An increased risk of congenital malformations associated with use of anxiolytic agents (i.e., chlordiazepoxide, diazepam, and/or meprobamate) during the first trimester of pregnancy has been suggested by several human studies. In humans, lorazepam and its glucuronide have been shown to cross the placenta (as determined from samples of umbilical cord blood). The drug has also been shown to cause various adverse fetal effects during reproduction studies in animals. Lorazepam injection should *not* be used during pregnancy. In addition, the manufacturer does *not* recommend preoperative use of the injection for obstetric procedures (e.g., cesarean section) or during labor and delivery, since safety of the injection has not been established in such procedures. Oral or injectable lorazepam should be used during pregnancy only in life-threatening situations or severe disease (e.g., status epilepticus) for which safer drugs cannot be used or are ineffective. The possibility that a woman of childbearing potential may be pregnant at the time lorazepam is initiated should be considered. When lorazepam is administered during pregnancy or if the patient becomes pregnant while receiving the drug, the patient should be advised of the potential hazard to the fetus and about the desirability of discontinuing lorazepam.

Based on animal data, repeated or prolonged use of general anesthetics and sedation drugs, including lorazepam, during the third trimester of pregnancy may result in adverse neurodevelopmental effects in the fetus. The clinical relevance of these animal findings to humans is not known; the potential risk of adverse neurodevelopmental effects should be considered and discussed with pregnant women undergoing procedures requiring general anesthetics and sedation drugs. (See Cautions: Pediatric Precautions.)

It is not known whether lorazepam affects fertility in humans. No evidence of impaired fertility was observed in rats following oral administration of lorazepam doses of 20 mg/kg. At doses of 40 mg/kg or more, there was evidence of fetal resorption and increased fetal loss in rabbits.

Lorazepam is distributed into milk. The potential exists that lorazepam can cause sedation or other adverse effects in nursing infants. The manufacturer of oral lorazepam states that the drug should not be administered to nursing women unless the potential benefits to the woman outweigh the possible risk to the infant. Nursing infants receiving oral lorazepam should be monitored for adverse effects (e.g., sedation, irritability). The manufacturer of lorazepam injection states that the drug should not be administered to nursing women because of possible adverse effects (e.g., sedation).

Chemistry and Stability

■ **Chemistry** Lorazepam is a benzodiazepine. Lorazepam occurs as a nearly white powder and is practically insoluble in water and slightly soluble in alcohol. The drug has pK_a values of 1.3 and 11.5. Lorazepam is commercially available as oral tablets, an oral concentrate solution, and an injection. The commercially available oral concentrate solution of lorazepam contains 0.6 g of polyethylene glycol 400 per mL of solution. The commercially available injection of lorazepam contains 0.18 mL of polyethylene glycol 400 in propylene glycol per mL of solution; benzyl alcohol 2% is added to the solution as a preservative.

■ **Stability** Lorazepam oral concentrate solution and lorazepam injection should be stored at 2–8°C and protected from light. Lorazepam tablets should be stored in well-closed containers at 25°C, but may be exposed to temperatures of 15–30°C.

The manufacturer states that lorazepam injection should be diluted prior to IV administration with an equal volume of compatible diluent, including 0.9% sodium chloride injection or 5% dextrose injection. Solutions of lorazepam should not be used if they are discolored or contain a precipitate.

For further information on chemistry, pharmacology, pharmacokinetics, uses, cautions, chronic toxicity, acute toxicity, drug interactions, laboratory test interferences, and dosage and administration of lorazepam, see the Benzodiazepines General Statement 28:24.08.

Preparations

Lorazepam is subject to control under the Federal Controlled Substances Act of 1970 as a schedule IV (C-IV) drug.

Excipients in commercially available drug preparations may have clinically important effects in some individuals; consult specific product labeling for details.

LORazepam

Oral		
For solution, concentrate	2 mg/mL*	**LORazepam Solution Concentrate** (C-IV)
Tablets	0.5 mg*	**Ativan**® (C-IV), Valeant
		LORazepam Tablets (C-IV)
	1 mg*	**Ativan**® (C-IV; scored), Valeant
		LORazepam Tablets (C-IV)
	2 mg*	**Ativan**® (C-IV; scored), Valeant
		LORazepam Tablets (C-IV)
Parenteral		
Injection	2 mg/mL*	**Ativan**® (C-IV), West-Ward
		LORazepam Injection (C-IV)
	4 mg/mL*	**Ativan**® (C-IV), West-Ward
		LORazepam Injection (C-IV)

*available from one or more manufacturer, distributor, and/or repackager by generic (nonproprietary) name

†Use is not currently included in the labeling approved by the US Food and Drug Administration

Midazolam Hydrochloride Midazolam

■ Midazolam is a benzodiazepine. The drug has anticonvulsant, anxiolytic, sedative/hypnotic, and amnestic properties.

Uses

■ **Preoperative Sedation, Anxiolysis, and Amnesia** Midazolam hydrochloride is used parenterally (IM or IV) or orally for preoperative sedation, anxiolysis, and anterograde amnesia. The drug should be used only in monitored settings (i.e., hospital or ambulatory care setting).

Like other benzodiazepines (e.g., lorazepam, diazepam), midazolam is particularly useful as a premedication when relief of anxiety and diminished recall of events associated with the surgical procedure are desired. In studies using memory recall tests, IM midazolam produced anterograde amnesia in 40–73% of adults and up to 85% of pediatric patients. The degree and duration of anterograde amnesia appear to be dose related and can vary based on concomitantly administered drugs.

IM administration of midazolam usually results in less irritation at the site of injection than some other agents commonly used for preoperative sedation, including hydroxyzine or diazepam. In addition, IM midazolam appears to produce a more rapid onset of sedative effects, more pronounced anxiolytic effects during the first hour following administration, and more pronounced anterograde amnesia when compared with IM hydroxyzine. Because of midazolam's relatively rapid onset, short duration of effect, and improved local tolerance at the site of injection compared with other currently available parenteral benzodiazepines, some clinicians consider midazolam the benzodiazepine of choice for preoperative use associated with short surgical procedures. Midazolam also is used IV for preoperative sedation and anxiolysis with good results.

Oral midazolam is commonly used as a premedication to reduce anxiety in pediatric patients undergoing surgery. Studies have demonstrated that children may be separated from their parents as early as 10 minutes after receiving the drug. Efficacy of oral midazolam as a premedicant to sedate and calm pediatric patients prior to the induction of general anesthesia was evaluated in a randomized, double-blind study in patients 6 months to less than 16 years of age with ASA physical status I, II, or III. In this study, more than 90% of patients receiving midazolam achieved satisfactory sedation and anxiolysis within 30 minutes post-treatment. Similarly high proportions of patients exhibited satisfactory ease of separation from their parent or guardian and were cooperative at the time of mask induction with nitrous oxide and halothane administration.

■ **Procedural Sedation** Midazolam hydrochloride is used IV or orally for procedural sedation, anxiolysis, and amnesia, either alone or in combination with other CNS depressants. The drug should be used only in monitored settings (i.e., hospital or ambulatory care setting). Midazolam produces amnestic and sedative effects, but no analgesia; therefore, the drug is usually administered in conjunction with an analgesic agent.

Procedural sedation is a technique in which sedative or dissociative agents are administered with or without analgesics to allow patients to tolerate painful or unpleasant medical procedures; a depressed state of consciousness is intentionally induced while cardiorespiratory function is maintained. Because sedation is a continuum ranging from minimal sedation to general anesthesia, airway reflexes and cardiorespiratory function may be impaired if a deeper than intended level of sedation is produced. The appropriate level of sedation should be individualized according to the specific procedure and needs of the patient.

Procedures for which midazolam sedation has been used include dental or minor surgical procedures; diagnostic, therapeutic, or endoscopic procedures such as upper GI endoscopy, bronchoscopy, or cystoscopy; cardiac catheterization; coronary angiography; oncology procedures; radiologic procedures (e.g., computerized tomography); and suture of lacerations. Like other benzodiazepines, midazolam is particularly useful for sedation when relief of anxiety and diminished recall of events associated with such procedures are desired.

Anterograde amnesia occurs within 1–5 minutes following IV administration of midazolam and generally persists for 20–40 minutes after IV injection of a single dose. However, onset and duration of action depend on many factors, including the dose of midazolam, rate of administration, and concurrently administered drugs. (See Pharmacokinetics: Absorption.) IV midazolam produced amnestic effects (i.e., no recall of endoscope withdrawal) in 82% of adults in endoscopy studies. In pediatric patients, impaired or no recall of events related to lumbar puncture, bone marrow aspiration, or an oncology procedure was observed in 88–91% of those who received IV midazolam.

Midazolam generally produces less pain and venous irritation (e.g., thrombophlebitis) at the site of IV injection than diazepam. In addition, IV midazolam may have a slightly more rapid onset of action and more pronounced anterograde amnestic effects when compared with IV diazepam. Although data are conflicting, there is some evidence that midazolam's duration of action following IV administration may be slightly shorter than that of diazepam, but further comparative studies are needed; the duration of action of midazolam is substantially shorter than that of IV lorazepam. Because of the drug's relatively rapid onset and short duration of action, pronounced amnesic effect, and improved local tolerance at the site of injection compared with other currently available parenteral benzodiazepines, some clinicians consider midazolam the benzodiazepine of choice for moderate sedation (formerly known as conscious sedation) prior to short procedures.

■ **Induction and Maintenance of Anesthesia** Midazolam hydrochloride is used IV for induction of general anesthesia prior to administration of other anesthetic agents. Induction with IV midazolam results in anxiolysis, anterograde amnesia, and dose-related hypnotic effects (progressing from sedation to loss of consciousness), but not analgesia. Midazolam also is used as a component of balanced anesthesia (e.g., nitrous oxide and oxygen) for maintenance of anesthesia during short surgical procedures.

There is substantial interpatient variation in induction time and in the dose of midazolam required for induction of anesthesia, especially in young patients and/or patients who have not received premedication with an opiate agonist. Premedication with an opiate agonist results in more rapid and reliable induction of anesthesia within a narrower midazolam dosage range, and smaller doses of midazolam generally are required. Midazolam should not be used alone for maintenance of anesthesia; the drug usually is given in conjunction with inhalation anesthetic agents, balanced anesthesia (e.g., nitrous oxide and oxygen), and/or opiate agonists (e.g., fentanyl). Concurrent use of an opiate agonist usually is necessary to maintain adequate anesthesia.

The benefits of midazolam include its pronounced anterograde amnestic effects and good patient acceptability. The incidence of postoperative emergence delirium, nausea, and vomiting is relatively low following midazolam administration as compared with other anesthetic agents. Because midazolam does not appear to increase intraocular pressure, the drug appears to be safe for use in patients undergoing surgery for ocular trauma. Use of midazolam in patients without underlying ocular disease may result in moderate reduction of intraocular pressure. Midazolam generally has been well tolerated in patients with ischemic heart disease, although mild to moderate alterations in cardiovascular function may occur. Severe hypotension has occurred, however, when midazolam was used with high-dose fentanyl anesthesia in patients undergoing coronary artery bypass grafting procedures. Limited data suggest that midazolam attenuates both the postoperative emergence delirium and the cardiovascular stimulation associated with the use of ketamine during surgery.

IV midazolam has historically been compared with IV thiopental for induction and maintenance of anesthesia, and was considered to be more favorable than thiopental in certain characteristics (e.g., more pronounced anterograde amnesia, more gradual induction of anesthesia, less need for adjuvant anesthetic agents), but not in others (e.g., did not induce anesthesia as rapidly or consistently, required a longer recovery period). However, thiopental is no longer commercially available in the US and its use has been largely replaced by propofol.

■ **Sedation in Critical Care Settings** Midazolam is used as a continuous IV infusion for sedation of intubated and mechanically ventilated patients in critical care settings (e.g., intensive care unit [ICU]).

Sedative agents are administered in critically ill patients to reduce agitation and anxiety, and increase tolerance to invasive procedures (e.g., mechanical ventilation). The provision of adequate analgesia and other measures to ensure patient comfort is recommended before sedatives are administered. Common sedative agents used in the ICU include benzodiazepines (e.g., midazolam, lorazepam), propofol, and dexmedetomidine. These agents appear to be similarly effective in providing adequate sedation in critically ill, mechanically ventilated adults. However, modest benefits with respect to other outcomes (e.g., reduced duration of mechanical ventilation, shorter time to extubation, reduced risk of delirium) have been observed with the nonbenzodiazepine sedatives (dexmedetomidine and propofol) compared with benzodiazepines. (See Uses: Sedation in Critical Care Settings, in the Benzodiazepines General Statement 28:24.08.) Because of the apparent advantages and an overall favorable benefit-to-risk profile, nonbenzodiazepine sedatives (dexmedetomidine or propofol) are generally preferred to benzodiazepines (midazolam or lorazepam) in mechanically ventilated critically ill adults. This recommendation should be considered in the context of the specific clinical situation since benzodiazepines may still be preferred in certain situations (e.g., patients with anxiety, seizures, or alcohol or benzodiazepine withdrawal). When selecting an appropriate sedative agent, the patient's individual sedation goals should be considered in addition to specific drug-related (e.g., pharmacology, pharmacokinetics, adverse effects, availability, cost) and patient-related (e.g., comorbid conditions) factors.

Results of several clinical studies indicate that midazolam is as effective as lorazepam in terms of level of sedation, the time required to achieve adequate sedation, and, usually, the number of daily dose adjustments. However, in one study, midazolam IV infusions did require more frequent dosage adjustments to maintain the desired level of sedation than did lorazepam. Because of the rapid onset and short duration of action of single doses of midazolam, some clinicians have recommended midazolam as one of the preferred drugs for sedation in acutely agitated patients in critical care settings. Studies comparing midazolam and lorazepam for prolonged use in ICU patients suggest greater variability and longer time to awakening with midazolam than with lorazepam.

■ **Seizure Disorders** ***Status Epilepticus*** Midazolam hydrochloride is used IM for the treatment of status epilepticus. While IM midazolam is FDA-labeled for use only in adults, the drug also has been used in pediatric patients† for the treatment of status epilepticus.

Benzodiazepines are considered the initial drugs of choice for the management of status epilepticus because of their rapid onset of action, demonstrated efficacy, safety, and tolerability. (See Uses: Seizure Disorders, in the Benzodiazepines General Statement 28:24.08.) Although IV lorazepam is generally preferred because of its longer duration of action, there is also evidence supporting the use of IV diazepam and IM midazolam and experts consider these therapies to be equivalent first-line options. Selection of an appropriate benzodiazepine should be individualized based on local availability, route of administration, pharmacokinetics, cost, and other factors (e.g., treatment setting). If seizures continue after initial therapy with a benzodiazepine, a second-line anticonvulsant agent (e.g., IV fosphenytoin or phenytoin, IV valproate sodium, IV levetiracetam, IV phenobarbital) should be administered. If refractory status epilepticus occurs, continuous IV infusion of anticonvulsants, IV barbiturates, or general anesthetics may be necessary. (See Status Epilepticus under Seizure Disorders: Principles of Anticonvulsant Drug Therapy, in the Anticonvulsants General Statement 28:12.)

Although IV administration of a benzodiazepine is the preferred method of treatment to achieve a rapid therapeutic effect in patients with status epilepticus, the need to establish IV access may delay administration of the drug in the prehospital environment. Results of a randomized controlled study (RAMPART) indicate that IM administration of midazolam by paramedics in the prehospital setting may improve outcomes in patients with status epilepticus; in this study, 73% of patients who received IM midazolam achieved seizure resolution at the time of arrival in the emergency department compared with 63% of those who received IV lorazepam.

Midazolam also has been administered by intranasal† and buccal† routes for treatment of status epilepticus; limitations of these routes include unpredictable absorption, difficulty with administration during an acute seizure episode, and lack of commercial availability.

Acute Repetitive Seizures or Seizure Clusters Midazolam nasal spray is used for the acute treatment of intermittent, stereotypic episodes of frequent seizure activity (i.e., seizure clusters, acute repetitive seizures) that are distinct from the patient's usual seizure pattern.

Efficacy of intranasal midazolam for this use has been established in a randomized, double-blind, placebo-controlled study in epileptic patients 12 years of age or older who were receiving a stable anticonvulsant regimen, but were experiencing intermittent seizure activity distinct from their usual seizure pattern. The primary efficacy end point (i.e., termination of seizures within 10 minutes after administration of study drug and absence of recurrence within 6 hours) was achieved in substantially more patients receiving intranasal midazolam than those receiving placebo. Patients who received midazolam also experienced a longer time to the next seizure than those who received placebo.

■ **Other Uses** Parenterally administered midazolam has been used in the management of acute agitation†.

Dosage and Administration

■ **Administration** Midazolam hydrochloride is administered orally, by IM or slow IV injection, or by IV infusion. Midazolam is administered intranasally. Midazolam also has been orally administered as the maleate salt†; however, midazolam maleate currently is not commercially available in the US.

Because serious and life-threatening adverse cardiorespiratory effects can occur during therapy with midazolam, provision should be made for monitoring, detecting, and correcting such effects in every patient in whom the drug is administered, regardless of age or health status. (See Cautions: Precautions and Contraindications.)

When IV or oral midazolam is used for sedation or anesthesia, the drug should be administered in a hospital or ambulatory care setting equipped to provide continuous monitoring of cardiorespiratory function. Resuscitative equipment, drugs, and personnel for airway and ventilation management should be immediately available. For deeply sedated pediatric patients, a dedicated individual other than the clinician performing the procedure should monitor the patient throughout the procedure.

When IM midazolam is used for status epilepticus, the drug should be administered in a monitored setting that allows for immediate access to resuscitative drugs, and the patient's cardiorespiratory function should be continuously monitored until stabilized.

When midazolam nasal spray is used, consideration should be given to administering the drug under the supervision of a healthcare professional.

Parenteral Administration **Midazolam Hydrochloride Injection for Sedation or Anesthesia.** Midazolam hydrochloride injection is administered IV or IM for sedation or anesthesia; the parenteral preparation should not be administered by any other route (e.g., intrathecal, intra-arterial).

For IV injection, midazolam hydrochloride is injected in incremental doses. The drug is a potent sedative that requires slow administration and individualized titration of dosage. The manufacturer states that the appropriate dose usually is injected over 2 or more minutes at intervals of at least 2 minutes for procedural sedation in healthy patients; incremental doses and the rate of IV injection should be reduced in patients 60 years of age and older, in debilitated patients, in patients with chronic disease states (e.g., congestive heart failure), and in patients with decreased pulmonary reserve, since such patients are at increased risk of underventilation, airway obstructions, and apnea, and the time to peak effect may be slower. For induction of anesthesia, the appropriate dose usually is injected over 20–30 seconds; supplemental doses may be given at 2-minute intervals. To facilitate dosage titration, midazolam hydrochloride injection containing 1 mg/mL (of midazolam) may be used, or the 1- or 5-mg/mL injection may be diluted with 0.9% sodium chloride injection or 5% dextrose injection. For procedural sedation, use of midazolam hydrochloride injection containing 1 mg/mL (of midazolam) is recommended to facilitate slow IV injection of the drug.

For continuous IV infusion, the 5-mg/mL (of midazolam) injection should be diluted to a concentration of 0.5 mg/mL with 0.9% sodium chloride injection or 5% dextrose injection.

IM injections of midazolam hydrochloride should be administered deep into a large muscle mass. Care should be taken to avoid intra-arterial injection or extravasation of the drug.

Midazolam Hydrochloride Injection for Status Epilepticus. Midazolam hydrochloride injection (Seizalam®) should be administered by IM injection into the mid-outer thigh (vastus lateralis muscle). Administration of the injection by a clinician who has adequate training in the recognition and management of status epilepticus is recommended.

Oral Administration Midazolam oral solution is intended for use in monitored settings (e.g., hospital or ambulatory care settings, including physician and dental offices) only, and is not intended for chronic or home use.

(See Cautions: Precautions and Contraindications.) For instruction on use of the special press-in bottle adapter and oral dispensers for administration of midazolam oral syrup, the manufacturer's labeling should be consulted. The drug should be administered from the individual oral dispenser directly into the child's mouth; the oral solution should *not* be mixed with any other liquid (e.g., grapefruit juice) prior to administration. Although the effect of food on absorption of the oral solution has not been determined, food intake generally is precluded prior to procedural sedation in pediatric patients.

Intranasal Administration Midazolam nasal spray is administered intranasally using a single-dose nasal spray unit supplied by the manufacturer. Each nasal spray unit delivers 5 mg of midazolam in 0.1 mL of solution. The intranasal preparation is commercially available in boxes of 2 nasal spray units; each unit is contained within an individual blister pack that should not be opened until ready to use. The nasal spray unit should not be tested or primed before use. The manufacturer's instructions should be consulted for additional information on use of the midazolam nasal spray.

■ Dosage

Midazolam is commercially available as midazolam or the hydrochloride salt; dosage is expressed in terms of midazolam. Midazolam is a potent sedative that requires individualized dosing.

When midazolam is used for sedation or anesthesia, dosage must be carefully adjusted according to individual requirements and response, age, body weight, physical and clinical status, underlying pathologic condition(s), type and amount of premedication or concomitant medication, and the nature and duration of the surgical or other procedure; however, individual response to the drug also may vary independent of these factors. Titration should be more gradual in patients 60 years of age and older for procedural sedation, in those 55 years of age and older for induction of anesthesia, and in patients with chronic debilitating diseases. Excessive doses or rapid or single large IV injections may result in respiratory depression and/or arrest, particularly in geriatric or debilitated patients and in patients receiving other cardiorespiratory depressants concomitantly. (See Cautions: Cardiorespiratory Effects.) The smallest effective dose should be used, especially in geriatric and/or debilitated patients.

It should be recognized that the depth of sedation/anxiolysis needed for pediatric patients depends on the type of procedure performed. For example, simple light sedation in the preoperative period is different from the deeper sedation required for a therapeutic or diagnostic procedure (e.g., endoscopy); therefore, there is a broad dosage range. For all pediatric patients, regardless of the indications for sedation/anxiolysis, it is vital to titrate the midazolam dose and the dose of other concomitant drugs slowly for the desired clinical effect. Unlike adults, pediatric patients generally receive increments of midazolam on a mg/kg basis; drug dose in obese pediatric patients should be calculated on the basis of ideal body weight. Pediatric patients generally require higher dosages of midazolam on a mg/kg basis than adults, and pediatric patients younger than 6 years of age generally require higher dosages on a mg/kg basis than older pediatric patients and may require closer monitoring.

When midazolam is used for sedation in geriatric patients, the initial dose should be reduced, since some degree of organ impairment frequently is present. Dosage requirements in this age group generally appear to decrease with increasing age, and the possibility of profound and/or prolonged effects should be considered in older and/or debilitated patients. Low doses of midazolam usually are required in high-risk surgical patients, debilitated patients, and geriatric patients when the drug is administered with or without premedication. (See Cautions: Geriatric Precautions.)

Preoperative Sedation, Anxiolysis, and Amnesia For preoperative sedation, anxiolysis, and amnesia in good-risk (e.g., ASA Physical Status I and II) *adults younger than 60 years of age*, the usual dose of midazolam is 0.07–0.08 mg/kg (about 5 mg) administered by IM injection approximately 30–60 minutes prior to surgery. The dosage must be individualized and reduced when IM midazolam is administered to patients with chronic obstructive pulmonary disease, other higher-risk surgical patients, patients 60 years of age or older, and patients who have received opiate agonists or other CNS depressants concomitantly. In a study in patients 60 years of age or older who did not receive concomitant opiate agonist therapy, IM doses of 2–3 mg (0.02–0.05 mg/kg) reportedly produced adequate sedation during the preoperative period; the manufacturer states that an IM midazolam dose of 1 mg may be sufficient in some geriatric patients if the anticipated intensity and duration of sedation are less critical. As with any potential respiratory depressant, such patients should be observed for signs of cardiorespiratory depression following administration of IM midazolam. Sedative effects usually are apparent within 15 minutes and peak at 30–60 minutes. Midazolam can be administered concomitantly with atropine sulfate, scopolamine hydrochloride, and/or reduced doses of opiate agonists. (See Chemistry and Stability: Stability.)

If IM midazolam is used for preoperative sedation in *non-neonatal pediatric patients*, the usual dose is 0.1–0.15 mg/kg; doses in this range usually are effective and do not prolong emergence from general anesthesia. Sedation after IM administration of midazolam is age and dose dependent; higher doses may result in deeper and more prolonged sedation. For more anxious patients, IM doses of up to 0.5 mg/kg have been used. The manufacturer states that the total IM dose usually does not exceed 10 mg, although this has not been systematically studied. If midazolam is administered with an opiate, the initial dose of each drug must be reduced. IM midazolam may be used to initially sedate pediatric patients in order to facilitate less traumatic insertion of an IV catheter for further dosage titration.

If IV midazolam is used for preoperative sedation in *non-neonatal pediatric patients*, the usual dose (as an intermittent injection) is age dependent; prolonged sedation and risk of hypoventilation may be associated with the higher doses in each recommended range. IV injections of midazolam should be administered over 2–3 minutes. It is essential to wait 2–3 minutes to fully evaluate the sedative effect before starting the procedure or administering a repeat dose. In *pediatric patients 6 months to 5 years of age*, an initial IV dose of 0.05–0.1 mg/kg is recommended; a total dose of up to 0.6 mg/kg may be required to reach the desired end point, but usually does not exceed a total of 6 mg. In *pediatric patients 6–12 years of age*, an initial IV dose of 0.025–0.05 mg/kg is recommended; a total dose of up to 0.4 mg/kg may be required to reach the desired end point, but usually does not exceed a total of 10 mg. *Pediatric patients 12–16 years of age* should be dosed as adults; although some patients in this age range may require higher than recommended adult doses, the total dose usually does not exceed 10 mg. In nonintubated pediatric patients younger than 6 months of age, limited dosing information is available. The manufacturer states that because it is uncertain when a patient transfers from a neonatal to pediatric physiology, dosing recommendations are unclear in nonintubated pediatric patients younger than 6 months of age. However, because such patients are vulnerable to airway obstruction and hypoventilation, titration of drug dose in small increments to clinical effect and careful monitoring are essential.

If oral midazolam is used for preoperative sedation in *pediatric patients 6 months to 16 years of age*, a single dose of 0.25–0.5 mg/kg is recommended, depending on the status of the patient and the desired effect, up to a maximum of 20 mg. In general, it is recommended that the dose be individualized and modified based on patient age, level of anxiety, concomitantly administered drugs, and medical need. Younger pediatric patients (e.g., 6 months to younger than 6 years of age) and less cooperative patients may require a higher than usual oral dose of up to 1 mg/kg (up to a maximum of 20 mg). A dose of 0.25 mg/kg may be sufficient for older children 6–16 years of age or for cooperative patients, especially if the anticipated intensity and duration of sedation are less critical. For pediatric patients with cardiac or respiratory compromise, other higher-risk surgical pediatric patients, and pediatric patients who have received concomitant opiates or other CNS depressants, an oral dose of 0.25 mg/kg should be considered. Use of the oral solution in children younger than 6 months of age has not been established.

Procedural Sedation For procedural sedation, midazolam may be administered by slow IV injection or as an oral solution before the procedure. In non-neonatal pediatric patients, IM midazolam may be used to initially sedate the patient in order to facilitate less traumatic insertion of an IV catheter for further dosage titration. The manufacturer of midazolam hydrochloride injection states that for peroral procedures (e.g., upper GI endoscopy, bronchoscopy), use of a topical anesthetic is generally recommended, and for bronchoscopy, use of an opiate analgesic for premedication also is generally recommended. For procedural sedation, premedication with an opiate agonist appears to produce less variable response to midazolam.

If IV midazolam is used for procedural sedation in healthy adults younger than 60 years of age, the manufacturer states that dosage should be titrated slowly to the desired effect (e.g., onset of slurred speech). The initial IV dose should not exceed 2.5 mg (administered over at least 2 minutes), although some patients may respond to as little as 1 mg of the drug. Patients 60 years of age or older and debilitated or chronically ill patients, and patients with decreased pulmonary reserve should receive 1–1.5 mg as an initial IV dose over a longer period of injection. The manufacturer recommends that not more than 1.5 mg over at least 2 minutes be administered as an initial dose in these patients. After waiting at least 2 minutes to fully evaluate the patient's clinical response, midazolam dosage may be further titrated in small increments if further sedative effect is required. Patients 60 years of age or older, chronically ill and/or debilitated patients, or patients with decreased pulmonary reserve should receive incremental doses of not more than 1 mg of midazolam. A total dose of up to 5 mg generally is adequate for procedural sedation in an average healthy adult younger than 60 years of age, and a total dose of up to 3.5 mg usually is adequate for patients 60 years of age or older, chronically ill and/or debilitated patients, and patients with decreased pulmonary reserve. If a thorough clinical evaluation clearly indicates a need for additional doses of midazolam to maintain the desired level of sedation, additional doses of the drug may be administered in increments of approximately 25% of the initial dose used to reach the first sedative end point. Some clinicians have recommended initiating dosing with 0.5–2 mg and repeating doses, as necessary, at 2- to 3-minute intervals up to a total dose of 0.1–0.15 mg/kg. In patients 60 years of age and older, these clinicians have recommended reducing midazolam dosage by 25% or more.

If IV midazolam is used concomitantly with an opiate agonist or other CNS depressant, dosage requirements of midazolam may be reduced by about 30% in healthy adults younger than 60 years of age and by at least 50% in patients 60 years of age or older, chronically ill and/or debilitated patients, and patients with decreased pulmonary reserve. Because the risk of underventilation or apnea is greatest in geriatric patients, patients with chronic debilitating disease, and patients with decreased pulmonary reserve, and because peak effect of the drug may occur later in these patients, increments in dose should be smaller, and the rate of injection should be slower.

If IM midazolam is used for procedural sedation in *non-neonatal pediatric patients*, the usual dose is 0.1–0.15 mg/kg. Sedation after IM administration of midazolam is age and dose dependent; higher doses may result in deeper and more prolonged sedation. For more anxious patients, IM doses of up to 0.5 mg/

kg have been used. The manufacturer states that the total IM dose usually does not exceed 10 mg, although this has not been systematically studied. If midazolam is administered with an opiate, the initial dose of each must be reduced.

If IV midazolam is used for procedural sedation in *non-neonatal pediatric patients*, the usual IV dose (as an intermittent injection) is age dependent; prolonged sedation and risk of hypoventilation may be associated with the higher doses in each recommended range. IV injections of midazolam should be administered over 2–3 minutes. It is essential to wait 2–3 minutes to fully evaluate the sedative effect before starting the procedure or administering a repeat dose. In *pediatric patients 6 months to 5 years of age*, an initial IV dose of 0.05–0.1 mg/kg is recommended; a total dose of up to 0.6 mg/kg may be required to reach the desired end point, but usually does not exceed a total of 6 mg. In *pediatric patients 6–12 years of age*, an initial IV dose of 0.025–0.05 mg/kg is recommended; a total dose of up to 0.4 mg/kg may be required to reach the desired end point, but usually does not exceed a total of 10 mg. *Pediatric patients 12–16 years of age* should be dosed as adults; although some patients in this age range may require higher than recommended adult doses, the total dose usually does not exceed 10 mg. In nonintubated pediatric patients younger than 6 months of age, limited dosing information is available. The manufacturer states that because it is uncertain when a patient transfers from a neonatal to pediatric physiology, dosing recommendations are unclear in nonintubated pediatric patients younger than 6 months of age. However, because such patients are vulnerable to airway obstruction and hypoventilation, titration of drug dose in small increments to clinical effect and careful monitoring are essential.

If oral midazolam is used for procedural sedation in *pediatric patients 6 months to 16 years of age*, a single dose of 0.25–0.5 mg/kg is recommended, depending on the status of the patient and the desired effect, up to a maximum of 20 mg. In general, it is recommended that the dose be individualized and modified based on patient age, level of anxiety, concomitantly administered drugs, and medical need. Younger pediatric patients (e.g., 6 months to younger than 6 years of age) and less cooperative patients may require a higher than usual oral dose of up to 1 mg/kg (up to a maximum of 20 mg). A dose of 0.25 mg/kg may be sufficient for older children 6–16 years of age or for cooperative patients, especially if the anticipated intensity and duration of sedation are less critical. For pediatric patients with cardiac or respiratory compromise, other higher-risk surgical pediatric patients, and pediatric patients who have received concomitant opiates or other CNS depressants, an oral dose of 0.25 mg/kg should be considered. Use of the oral solution in children younger than 6 months of age has not been established.

Induction and Maintenance of Anesthesia For induction of general anesthesia, midazolam should be administered prior to other anesthetic agents. Because individual response to midazolam is variable, especially when opiate agonist premedication is not used, dosage of midazolam should be titrated carefully to the desired clinical effect, taking into consideration the patient's age and clinical status. When midazolam is administered prior to other IV agents for induction of anesthesia, the initial dose of each of these agents may be substantially reduced, in some instances to as low as 25% of the usual initial dose of the individual agents.

For induction of general anesthesia prior to administration of other anesthetic agents, average adults younger than 55 years of age who have not received premedications usually require an initial midazolam dose of 0.3–0.35 mg/kg, administered IV over 20–30 seconds; approximately 2 minutes should be allowed for clinical effect. Some clinicians have suggested a lower initial dose (e.g., 0.2 mg/kg) in these adults. Supplemental doses of about 25% of the initial dose may be given as necessary to complete induction. Alternatively, induction of anesthesia may be completed with inhalation agents. Total IV induction doses of up to 0.6 mg/kg may be required in some resistant patients, but such doses may prolong recovery from anesthesia. Patients 55 years of age or older who have not been premedicated usually require lower induction doses of midazolam; the manufacturer recommends an initial IV induction dose of 0.3 mg/kg in these patients. Patients with severe systemic disease or other debilitation who have not been premedicated also usually require lower induction doses. Initial IV doses of 0.2–0.25 mg/kg usually are adequate in such patients, and doses as low as 0.15 mg/kg may be adequate for induction in some debilitated patients.

In premedicated patients, especially those who have received an opiate agonist, the usual IV induction dose of midazolam is 0.15–0.35 mg/kg. In premedicated adults younger than 55 years of age, the usual induction dose is 0.25 mg/kg administered IV over 20–30 seconds; about 2 minutes should be allowed for clinical effect. In premedicated, good-risk (e.g., ASA I and II) adults older than 55 years of age, an initial IV induction dose of 0.2 mg/kg is recommended by the manufacturer. In some premedicated patients with severe systemic disease or debilitation, an initial IV induction dose of 0.15 mg/kg may be sufficient.

For maintenance of anesthesia as a component of balanced anesthesia during surgical procedures, premedication with an opiate agonist is especially recommended. Midazolam may be administered in incremental IV doses of approximately 25% of the induction dose when lightening of anesthesia is evident and repeated, as necessary, to maintain the required level of anesthesia.

Sedation in Critical Care Settings Dosage of sedative agents should be titrated to the desired level of sedation; in most cases, a light rather than deep level of sedation is recommended in critically ill mechanically ventilated adults because of improved clinical outcomes that have been demonstrated (e.g., shortened duration of mechanical ventilation, reduced ICU length of stay). The depth and quality of sedation should be assessed frequently using a validated and reliable assessment tool (e.g., Richmond Agitation-Sedation Scale [RASS], Sedation-Agitation Scale [SAS]).

For sedation in intubated and mechanically ventilated adult patients in critical care settings (e.g., ICU), midazolam is administered as a continuous IV infusion. In adults, if a loading dose is necessary to initiate sedation rapidly, 0.01–0.05 mg/kg (approximately 0.5–4 mg for a typical adult) may be given slowly or infused over several minutes. This dose may be repeated at 10- to 15-minute intervals until adequate sedation is achieved. For maintenance of sedation in adults, the usual initial infusion rate is 0.02–0.1 mg/kg per hour (approximately 1–7 mg per hour). Higher loading or maintenance infusion rates occasionally may be required in some patients. The lowest recommended doses should be used in patients with residual effects from anesthetic drugs, or in those currently receiving other sedatives or opiates. Individual response to midazolam is variable and the infusion rate should be titrated to the desired level of sedation, taking into account the patient's age, clinical status, and current drugs. In general, midazolam should be infused at the lowest rate that produces the desired level of sedation. Assessment of sedation should be performed at regular intervals and the infusion rate adjusted up or down by 25–50% of the initial infusion rate to ensure adequate titration of the sedation level. Larger adjustments or even a small, incremental dose may be necessary if rapid changes in the level of sedation are required. In addition, the infusion rate should be decreased by 10–25% every few hours to find the minimum effective infusion rate. Finding the minimum effective infusion rate decreases the potential accumulation of midazolam and provides for the most rapid recovery once the infusion is terminated. Patients who exhibit agitation, hypertension, or tachycardia in response to noxious stimulation, but who are otherwise adequately sedated, may benefit from concomitant administration of an opioid analgesic; however, addition of an opiate generally will reduce the minimum effective midazolam infusion rate.

For sedation of intubated non-neonatal pediatric patients, midazolam generally is initiated with an IV loading dose of 0.05–0.2 mg/kg administered over at least 2–3 minutes; the drug should *not* be administered as a rapid IV injection. The loading dose may be followed by a continuous IV infusion to maintain the desired clinical effect. Based on pharmacokinetic parameters and clinical experience, continuous IV infusions of midazolam should be initiated at a rate of 0.06–0.12 mg/kg per hour (1–2 mcg/kg per minute). The infusion rate may be increased or decreased (generally by 25% of the initial or subsequent infusion rate) as required, or supplemental IV doses of midazolam may be administered to increase or maintain the desired effect. Frequent patient assessment at regular intervals using standard pain/sedation scales is recommended. Midazolam infusions have been used in pediatric patients whose trachea was intubated but who were allowed to breathe spontaneously; however, assisted ventilation is recommended for pediatric patients who are receiving other CNS depressants (e.g., opiates). Midazolam elimination may be delayed in patients receiving concomitant drugs (e.g., drugs interfering with midazolam metabolism), patients with hepatic dysfunction, patients with low cardiac output (especially those requiring inotropic support), and in neonates. Hypotension may be observed in patients who are critically ill, particularly those receiving opiates and/or if midazolam is administered rapidly. When initiating a midazolam infusion in pediatric patients who are hemodynamically compromised, the usual loading dose should be titrated in small increments and the patient monitored for hemodynamic instability (e.g., hypotension). These patients also are vulnerable to the respiratory depressant effects of midazolam and require careful monitoring of respiratory rate and oxygen saturation.

For sedation of intubated preterm neonates (i.e., born at less than 32 weeks' gestation) in critical care settings, midazolam generally is initiated as an IV infusion at a rate of 0.03 mg/kg per hour (0.5 mcg/kg per minute); for sedation of intubated neonates who were born after 32 weeks of gestation, midazolam is generally initiated as an IV infusion at a rate of 0.06 mg/kg per hour (1 mcg/kg per minute). IV loading doses should *not* be used in neonates; rather, the infusion may be administered more rapidly for the first several hours to establish therapeutic plasma drug concentrations. The infusion rate should be reassessed carefully and frequently, particularly after the first 24 hours, to administer the lowest possible effective dose and to reduce the potential for drug accumulation. This is particularly important because of the potential for adverse effects related to benzyl alcohol metabolism if not using the preservative-free formulation. (See Cautions: Pediatric Precautions.) Hypotension may be observed in critically ill neonates and in preterm and term neonates, especially in those receiving fentanyl and/or in patients in whom midazolam is administered rapidly. Because of an increased risk of apnea, extreme caution is advised when sedating a preterm or former preterm neonate whose trachea is not intubated.

Status Epilepticus For the treatment of status epilepticus in adults, the manufacturer recommends a single midazolam dose of 10 mg by IM injection. The manufacturer states that safety and efficacy of midazolam for the treatment of status epilepticus have not been established in pediatric patients. However, the drug has been used in pediatric patients†. Some clinicians recommend an IM midazolam dose of 10 mg for the treatment of status epilepticus in patients weighing more than 40 kg and a dose of 5 mg for those weighing 13–40 kg. Other clinicians have recommended a usual weight-based dose of 0.15–0.3 mg/kg in both children and adults.

Acute Repetitive Seizures or Seizure Clusters For the acute treatment of intermittent, stereotypic episodes of frequent seizure activity (e.g., seizure clusters, acute repetitive seizures), the recommended initial dose of intranasal midazolam in adults and pediatric patients 12 years of age or older is 1 spray (5 mg) into one nostril. An additional spray into the opposite nostril may be administered after 10 minutes if a response is not obtained with the first dose; however, a second dose should not be administered if the patient has difficulty breathing or excessive sedation that is uncharacteristic for the patient during a seizure cluster episode. No more than 2 doses should be used to treat a single seizure episode.

The manufacturer recommends that midazolam nasal spray be used to treat no more than one seizure episode every 3 days and no more than 5 seizure episodes a month.

Cautions

Adverse effects reported with midazolam are similar to those reported with other benzodiazepines. Changes in vital signs (e.g., respiratory rate, blood pressure, pulse rate) are the most frequent adverse effects associated with parenteral midazolam administration. For further information on adverse effects reported with benzodiazepines, see Cautions in the Benzodiazepines General Statement 28:24.08. The immediate availability of flumazenil, a specific benzodiazepine reversal agent, is highly recommended. (See Flumazenil 28:92.)

■ Cardiorespiratory Effects Midazolam can depress respiration. Relatively small doses, such as those used for preoperative sedation, usually do not substantially impair respiratory function; however, relatively large doses (e.g., more than 0.1–0.2 mg/kg) may substantially depress the ventilatory response to carbon dioxide (CO_2) stimulation. In addition, some patients (e.g., geriatric patients, patients with chronic obstructive pulmonary disease) may be predisposed to respiratory depression induced by midazolam.

Decreases in tidal volume and/or respiratory rate occur in about 23 or 11% of adults following IV or IM administration of midazolam, respectively. Apnea occurs in approximately 15% of adults receiving the drug parenterally. Desaturation or apnea has been reported in 4.6 or 2.8%, respectively, of pediatric patients receiving the drug IV. Hypoxia and laryngospasm were each reported in 2% of pediatric patients receiving the drug orally, and respiratory depression, rhonchi, airway obstruction, or upper airway obstruction was reported in 1% of these patients. Hypercarbia and stridor generally have been reported in less than 1% of patients receiving the drug orally. Serious, occasionally fatal, cardiorespiratory effects, including respiratory depression, apnea, respiratory arrest, and/or cardiac arrest, have occurred in patients receiving midazolam, particularly when the drug was used for procedural sedation. In some patients in whom midazolam-induced respiratory depression was not promptly recognized and effectively managed, hypoxic encephalopathy or death has resulted. Although many of the serious cardiorespiratory adverse effects reported to date have occurred in patients receiving excessive doses or rapid IV injection or infusion of midazolam, in geriatric or debilitated and/or higher-risk surgical patients, and in patients receiving other cardiorespiratory depressants concomitantly, some of these adverse reactions have occurred in younger, healthy patients, including those who did not receive concomitant drugs, and in patients receiving midazolam doses within the dosage range recommended by the manufacturer. Patients with chronic obstructive pulmonary disease appear to be particularly sensitive to the respiratory depressant effects of midazolam (e.g., impairment of the ventilatory response to CO_2), exhibiting more marked and prolonged depression than patients with healthy lungs.

Underventilation or apnea can result in potentially serious hypoxia and/or cardiac arrest unless effective countermeasures are initiated at the earliest sign of compromised respiration or ventilation. Early recognition and treatment of underventilation and apnea are necessary to avoid hypoxic cardiac arrest. Therefore, cardiorespiratory status should be monitored continuously during parenteral or oral midazolam use, dosage of the drug *must* be carefully individualized, and facilities and equipment for respiratory and ventilatory support should be readily available. (See Cautions: Precautions and Contraindications.) Concomitant administration of CNS depressants may increase the risk of underventilation and apnea and may prolong and/or exacerbate the effects of midazolam. (See Drug Interactions: CNS Depressants.) Use of supplemental oxygen should be considered when heavy sedation is anticipated or required.

Changes in systolic or diastolic blood pressure, principally decreases, and in heart rate are frequently associated with parenteral or oral administration of midazolam; however, in some cases, these effects may be associated with endotracheal intubation, changes in the depth of anesthesia, concomitantly administered drugs, and/or surgical manipulation rather than with midazolam itself. Hypotensive episodes requiring treatment have been reported rarely during or following diagnostic or surgical manipulation in patients receiving midazolam. Concomitant administration of an opiate agonist (e.g., as premedication for moderate sedation [formerly known as conscious sedation]) appears to increase the risk of severe hypotension associated with midazolam administration. Severe hypotensive effects may be alleviated by the judicious administration of IV fluids, repositioning the patient, and/or the cautious use of vasopressors. Induction of anesthesia with midazolam in patients with a relatively slow baseline heart rate (less than 65 beats/minute) is associated with a slight increase in heart rate, especially in patients receiving a β-adrenergic blocking agent for angina. However, use of midazolam in patients with a relatively fast baseline heart rate (greater than 85 beats/minute) appears to result in slight slowing of the heart rate.

Other adverse respiratory effects of midazolam include hiccups and coughing, which occur in up to 4 and 1% of patients, respectively, receiving the drug IV. Laryngospasm, bronchospasm, dyspnea, hyperventilation, wheezing, shallow respiration, airway obstruction, and tachypnea occur in less than 1% of patients, principally those receiving the drug IV.

Other adverse cardiovascular effects of midazolam include decreases in systemic vascular resistance, cardiac index, and stroke index. Bradycardia has been reported in up to 1% of pediatric patients receiving midazolam oral solution. Bigeminy, ventricular premature complexes, vasovagal episodes, tachycardia, and nodal rhythms reportedly occur in less than 1% of patients. Trigeminy also has been reported in patients receiving midazolam.

■ Nervous System Effects Adverse nervous system effects of midazolam generally are extensions of the pharmacologic actions of the drug; however, some reactions (e.g., agitation, involuntary movements) may be paradoxical in nature, manifestations of an underlying iatrogenic disorder (e.g., cerebral hypoxia), and/or associated with the surgical or other procedures employed. Paradoxical reactions have been reported in 2% of pediatric patients receiving the drug IV.

Excessive sedation, headache, and drowsiness occur in 1–2% of patients following parenteral administration of midazolam. Agitation, involuntary movements (e.g., tonic/clonic movements, muscle tremor), hyperactivity, and combativeness also have been reported. Such reactions may have resulted from inadequate or excessive doses of midazolam, improper administration of the drug, or cerebral hypoxia, or may have been paradoxical. (See Cautions: Precautions and Contraindications.) Agitation has been reported in 2% of pediatric patients receiving the drug orally. Seizure-like activity or nystagmus was reported in 1.1% of pediatric patients receiving the drug IV.

Other adverse nervous system effects that occur in less than 1% of patients receiving oral or IV midazolam include retrograde amnesia, euphoria, hallucinations, dysphoria, prolonged emergence from anesthesia, emergence delirium or agitation, dreaming during emergence, prolonged sedation, sleep disturbance, insomnia, nightmares, paresthesia, adverse behavior, mood swings, aggression, excitation, disinhibition, argumentativeness, nervousness, anxiety, restlessness, seizure-like activity, dysarthria, and athetoid movements. Confusion, grogginess, ataxia, dizziness, loss of balance or vertigo, lightheadedness, lethargy, yawning, faint feeling, weakness, slurred speech, blurred vision, strabismus, diplopia, and dysphonia have also been reported in less than 1% of patients.

Somnolence, headache, and dysarthria have been reported in 10, 4, and 2%, respectively, of patients receiving midazolam nasal spray.

Midazolam has reduced cerebral blood flow and oxygen consumption in animals and humans. In patients without intracranial pathology, induction of anesthesia with midazolam results in a moderate decrease in CSF pressure, similar to that occurring with thiopental (no longer commercially available in the US). There is some evidence that, in patients with normal intracranial pressure but decreased intracranial compliance who are undergoing intracranial surgery, induction of anesthesia with midazolam results in increased intracranial pressure during intubation similar to that occurring with thiopental.

■ GI Effects Nausea and/or vomiting occurs in 2–3% of adult patients receiving midazolam IV and in up to 4 or 8%, respectively, of pediatric patients receiving the drug orally. Acid taste, excessive salivation, gagging, drooling, and retching occur in less than 1% of patients. Other adverse GI effects include metallic taste, dry mouth, and constipation.

■ Sensitivity Reactions Hypersensitivity reactions reported in less than 1% of patients receiving midazolam include anaphylactoid reactions, urticaria, rash, and pruritus.

■ Local Effects Tenderness at the site of injection and pain during injection occur in 5–6% of patients receiving midazolam IV. Erythema and induration occur at the IV site in 2–3% of patients, and phlebitis occurs in less than 1%. Pain at the site of IM injection occurs in about 4% of patients, and local induration, erythema, and muscle stiffness occur in less than 1% of patients receiving midazolam IM. Adverse local effects associated with IM or IV administration occur less frequently and generally are less severe with midazolam than with other currently available parenteral benzodiazepines (e.g., diazepam).

Urticaria-like elevation at the injection site, swelling or feeling of burning, and warmth or coldness at the injection site occur in less than 1% of patients receiving midazolam parenterally, principally in those receiving the drug IV.

Nasal discomfort, throat irritation, rhinorrhea, and abnormal taste were reported in 9, 3, 3, and 2%, respectively, of patients receiving midazolam nasal spray.

■ Ocular Effects Adverse ocular effects occur in less than 1% of patients receiving parenteral midazolam, principally in those receiving the drug IV, and include blurred vision, diplopia, nystagmus, pinpoint pupils, cyclic movements of eyelids, visual disturbances, and focusing difficulty.

Increased lacrimation was reported in 2% of patients receiving midazolam nasal spray.

■ Other Adverse Effects Chills, toothache, blockage of ears, and hematoma occur in less than 1% of patients receiving midazolam parenterally, principally in those receiving the drug IV. Limited data suggest that administration of midazolam as an adjunct to anesthesia may result in transient decreases in renal blood flow and glomerular filtration rate.

■ Precautions and Contraindications Midazolam shares the toxic potentials of the benzodiazepines, and the usual precautions of benzodiazepine administration should be observed. (See Cautions in the Benzodiazepines General Statement 28:24.08.)

Concomitant use of benzodiazepines, including midazolam, and opiate agonists or opiate partial agonists may result in profound sedation, respiratory depression, coma, and death. Patients receiving midazolam and/or their caregivers should be apprised of the risks associated with concomitant therapeutic or illicit use of benzodiazepines and opiates. (See Opiate Agonists and Opiate Partial Agonists under Drug Interactions: CNS Depressants.)

Agitation, involuntary movements, hyperactivity, and/or combativeness may be signs of inadequate or excessive dosing, improper administration, or cerebral hypoxia or may be paradoxical. If such adverse reactions occur during midazolam therapy, the patient's response to each dose of midazolam as well as to any concomitantly administered drug, including local anesthetics, should be evaluated before proceeding.

Midazolam should be used with caution and dosage individualized carefully in patients with renal impairment, since the pharmacokinetics of the drug may be altered in such patients. Induction of anesthesia may occur more rapidly in patients with renal impairment, and recovery may be prolonged.

Although the clinical importance has not been determined, some clinicians state that midazolam should be used with caution and dosage individualized carefully in patients with congestive heart failure. Pharmacokinetics of the drug may be substantially altered in such patients (e.g., prolonged elimination half-life, increased volume of distribution, delayed onset of action secondary to prolonged circulation time).

Patients should be informed of the potentially profound pharmacologic effects of midazolam (e.g., sedation, relief of anxiety, lack of recall) and that the duration of these effects varies considerably among individuals, so that they may adequately perceive the risks and benefits of use of the drug. Patients should also be warned that midazolam may impair their ability to perform activities requiring mental alertness or physical coordination (e.g., operating machinery, driving a motor vehicle). The decision regarding when patients who have received midazolam can safely perform such activities must be individualized, especially when the patient received the drug as part of an outpatient procedure. Gross tests of recovery after awakening (e.g., orientation, ability to stand and walk, return to baseline Trieger competency) cannot be relied on alone to predict reaction time under stress. Patients should not operate a motor vehicle or hazardous machinery until the effects of the drug (e.g., drowsiness) have subsided or the day after anesthesia and surgery, whichever is longer. Impaired performance may persist for longer periods in geriatric patients, in patients using other drugs concomitantly, and secondary to the stress of surgery or general condition of the patient. For pediatric patients, particular care should be taken to ensure safe ambulation. Patients should be warned that concomitant use of midazolam with other CNS depressants may increase the extent and duration of impaired performance, cause excessive sedation, and interfere with recall and recognition of events on the day of surgery and the following day.

Some preparations of midazolam hydrochloride injection contain the preservative benzyl alcohol and should not be used in neonates and infants.

Midazolam is contraindicated in patients with known hypersensitivity to the drug. Midazolam oral solution also is contraindicated in patients allergic to cherries or to formulation excipients. Benzodiazepines can increase intraocular pressure in patients with glaucoma and some manufacturers state that the drug is contraindicated in patients with acute angle-closure glaucoma, but may be used in patients with open-angle glaucoma if they are receiving appropriate treatment. However, the clinical rationale for this contraindication has been questioned. The manufacturer of midazolam nasal spray states that patients with open-angle glaucoma may need an ophthalmologic evaluation following treatment with the drug.

Precautions Specific to the Use of Midazolam for Sedation or Anesthesia Midazolam should be administered orally or IV only in hospital or ambulatory-care settings, including physicians' or dentists' offices, in which continuous monitoring of respiratory and cardiac function (i.e., pulse oximetry) is possible. Safety and efficacy of midazolam may vary in patients as functions of the dose administered and clinical status of the patient. Midazolam is a potent sedative and requires slow administration and individualized titration of dosage. Since the drug is capable of producing several levels of CNS depression—from mild to deep sedation, facilities, age- and size-appropriate equipment for bag/mask/valve ventilation and intubation, drugs, and skilled personnel necessary for ventilation and intubation, administration of oxygen, assisted or controlled respiration, airway management, and cardiovascular support should be immediately available whenever midazolam is administered. The immediate availability of specific benzodiazepine reversal agent (e.g., flumazenil) is highly recommended when the drug is administered IV or orally. Pediatric and adult patients undergoing procedures involving the upper airway, such as upper endoscopy or dental care, are particularly vulnerable to episodes of desaturation and hypoventilation due to partial airway obstruction. The incidence of such adverse events is higher in patients undergoing procedures involving the airway without the protective effect of an endotracheal tube. Patients receiving midazolam should be monitored continuously for early signs of underventilation or apnea since hypoxia and/or cardiac arrest can occur unless effective countermeasures are undertaken immediately. Monitoring of vital signs also should continue during the recovery period. Because midazolam can depress respiration and because opiate agonists or other sedatives can potentiate this effect, midazolam should be administered as an induction agent only by individuals who are experienced in the use of general anesthesia and should be used for procedural sedation only in the presence of personnel experienced in early detection of underventilation, maintenance of an adequate airway, and respiratory support. For deeply sedated pediatric patients, a dedicated individual other than the clinician performing the procedure should monitor the patient throughout the procedure. In addition, the possibility that the procedure may obscure early recognition of potential complications (e.g., performance of endoscopy in diminished light which can make visual observation of the patient difficult) or may interfere with effective countermeasures (e.g., patient positioning during colonoscopy) should be considered.

Careful monitoring and individualization of dosing are essential when parenteral midazolam is used for sedation or anesthesia; dosage individualization is particularly important in certain patient populations (e.g., geriatric patients, patients with various underlying disease states [e.g., chronic obstructive pulmonary disease, renal failure, congestive heart failure], and patients receiving other CNS depressants).

Midazolam should not be administered parenterally to patients with shock or who are comatose or to patients with acute alcohol intoxication and accompanying depression of vital signs. Caution should be exercised if midazolam is administered IV to patients with uncompensated acute illnesses, including severe fluid or electrolyte imbalances. Sedation guidelines recommend a careful presedation history to determine how a patient's underlying medical condition or concomitant drugs may affect the response to sedation/analgesia, as well as a physical examination including a focused examination of the airway for abnormalities. Further recommendations include appropriate presedation fasting.

There have been limited reports of intra-arterial injection of midazolam; adverse effects have included local reactions as well as isolated reports of seizure activity in which no clear causal relationship was established. Precautions against unintended intra-arterial injection should be taken, and drug extravasation should be avoided.

Midazolam does not fully prevent the increase in intracranial pressure or the cardiovascular effects (e.g., increase in blood pressure and/or heart rate) associated with endotracheal intubation under light general anesthesia. Midazolam also does not appear to prevent the usual cardiovascular stimulatory effects associated with administration of some neuromuscular blocking agents (e.g., succinylcholine, pancuronium) or the increase in intracranial pressure associated with succinylcholine.

Patients receiving continuous IV infusion of midazolam in critical care settings over an extended period of time may experience symptoms of withdrawal following discontinuance.

Precautions Specific to the Use of Midazolam Nasal Spray If midazolam nasal spray is used in patients at risk of benzodiazepine-induced respiratory depression, it is recommended that the drug be administered under the supervision of a clinician.

The possibility of an increased risk of suicidality (suicidal behavior or ideation) should be considered in patients receiving midazolam nasal spray. An analysis of suicidality reports from 199 placebo-controlled studies found that patients receiving anticonvulsants for any indication had approximately twice the risk of suicidal behavior or ideation compared with those receiving placebo; the increased risk was observed as early as one week after beginning therapy and continued through 24 weeks. Although patients treated with an anticonvulsant for epilepsy, psychiatric disorders, and other conditions were all found to be at increased risk for suicidality when compared with those receiving placebo, the relative suicidality risk was higher for patients with epilepsy compared with those receiving anticonvulsants for other conditions. Clinicians should inform patients, their families, and caregivers of the potential for an increased risk of suicidality with anticonvulsant therapy; all patients currently receiving or beginning therapy with any anticonvulsant should be closely monitored for the emergence or worsening of suicidal thoughts or behavior or depression. (See Suicidality under Cautions: CNS Effects, in the Anticonvulsants General Statement 28:12.)

■ **Pediatric Precautions** The safety and efficacy of midazolam oral solution have not been established in pediatric patients younger than 6 months of age. Safety and efficacy of midazolam nasal spray have not been established in pediatric patients younger than 12 years of age.

Unlike adults, the dose of midazolam in pediatric patients is calculated on a mg/kg basis. As a group, pediatric patients require a higher parenteral dosage of midazolam on a mg/kg basis than do adults, and pediatric patients younger than 6 years of age generally require higher dosages on a mg/kg basis than do older pediatric patients and may require closer monitoring. In obese pediatric patients, the drug dose should be calculated on the basis of ideal body weight. When midazolam is administered in conjunction with opiates or other sedatives in the pediatric population, the potential for respiratory depression, airway obstruction, or hypoventilation is increased. Particular care should be taken to ensure safe ambulation of pediatric patients following sedation with midazolam. Clinicians who use this drug in pediatric patients should be aware of, and follow, accepted professional guidelines for pediatric sedation appropriate to the situation.

Higher-risk pediatric surgical patients may require lower midazolam doses, whether or not concomitant sedating drugs have been administered. Pediatric patients with cardiac or respiratory compromise may be unusually sensitive to the respiratory depressant effect of midazolam. Pediatric patients undergoing procedures involving the upper airway (e.g., upper endoscopy, dental care) are particularly vulnerable to episodes of desaturation and hypoventilation secondary to partial airway obstruction.

Because of reduced and/or immature organ function, neonates are vulnerable to profound and/or prolonged adverse respiratory effects of midazolam. The drug should not be administered by rapid IV injection in neonates. When administered as a rapid (i.e., over less than 2 minutes) IV injection in neonates, the drug has been associated with severe hypotension, particularly when coadministered with fentanyl. Likewise, severe hypotension has been observed in neonates receiving midazolam as a continuous infusion who then also received a rapid IV injection of fentanyl. Seizures also have been reported in neonates receiving midazolam as a rapid IV injection.

FDA warns that repeated or prolonged use of general anesthetics and sedation drugs, including midazolam, in children younger than 3 years of age or during the third trimester of pregnancy may affect brain development. Animal studies in multiple species, including nonhuman primates, have demonstrated that use for longer than 3 hours of anesthetic and sedation drugs that block *N*-methyl-D-aspartic acid (NMDA) receptors and/or potentiate γ-aminobutyric acid (GABA) activity leads to widespread neuronal and oligodendrocyte cell loss and alterations in synaptic morphology and neurogenesis in the brain, resulting in long-term deficits in cognition and behavior. Across animal species, vulnerability to these neurodevelopmental changes occurs during the period of rapid brain growth or synaptogenesis; this period is thought to correlate with the third trimester of pregnancy through the first year of life in humans, but may extend to approximately 3 years of age. The clinical relevance of these animal findings to humans is not known. While some published evidence suggests that similar deficits in cognition and behavior may occur in children following repeated or prolonged exposure to anesthesia early in life, other studies have found no association between pediatric anesthesia exposure and long-term adverse neurodevelopmental outcomes. Most studies to date have had substantial limitations, and it is not clear whether the adverse neurodevelopmental outcomes observed in children were related to the drug or to other factors (e.g., surgery, underlying illness). There is some clinical evidence that a single, relatively brief exposure to general anesthesia in generally healthy children is unlikely to cause clinically detectable deficits in global cognitive function or serious behavioral disorders; however, further research is needed to fully characterize the effects of exposure to general anesthetics in early life, particularly for prolonged or repeated exposures and in more vulnerable populations (e.g., less healthy children). For further information, see Cautions: Pediatric Precautions, in the Benzodiazepines General Statement 28:24.08.

Anesthetic and sedation drugs are an essential component of care for children and pregnant women who require surgery or other procedures that cannot be delayed; no specific general anesthetic or sedation drug has been shown to be less likely to cause neurocognitive deficits than any other such drug. Pending further accumulation of data in humans from well-designed studies, decisions regarding the timing of elective procedures requiring anesthesia should take into consideration both the benefits of the procedure and the potential risks. When procedures requiring the use of general anesthetics or sedation drugs are considered for young children or pregnant women, clinicians should discuss with the patient, parent, or caregiver the benefits, risks (including potential risk of adverse neurodevelopmental effects), and appropriate timing and duration of the procedure. FDA states that procedures that are considered medically necessary should not be delayed or avoided.

Midazolam hydrochloride injections containing benzyl alcohol should not be used in neonates or infants. Although a causal relationship has not been established, administration of injections preserved with benzyl alcohol has been associated with toxicity in neonates. Toxicity appears to have resulted from administration of large amounts (i.e., 100-400 mg/kg daily) of benzyl alcohol in these neonates. Exposure to such excessive amounts of benzyl alcohol has been associated with hypotension and metabolic acidosis in neonates, and an increased incidence of kernicterus, particularly in small, preterm infants. There have been reports of death, particularly in preterm infants, associated with exposure to excessive amounts of benzyl alcohol. Although use of drugs preserved with benzyl alcohol should be avoided in neonates whenever possible, the American Academy of Pediatrics (AAP) states that the presence of small amounts of the preservative in a commercially available injection should not proscribe its use when indicated in neonates. The amount of benzyl alcohol exposure from drugs usually is considered negligible compared with that from benzyl alcohol-containing flush solutions. Administration of high dosages of drugs containing this preservative, including midazolam hydrochloride, must take into account the total amount of benzyl alcohol administered. The recommended dosage range of midazolam for preterm and term infants includes amounts of benzyl alcohol well below that associated with toxicity; however, the amount of benzyl alcohol at which toxicity may occur is not known. If the patient requires more than the recommended midazolam dosages, or if other benzyl alcohol-containing preparations are to be used in the patient, the clinician must take into account the total daily metabolic load of benzyl alcohol from these sources.

■ Geriatric Precautions Because distribution of midazolam may be altered in geriatric patients and these patients may have decreased hepatic and/or renal function, the manufacturer of midazolam hydrochloride injection recommends that dosage of the drug be selected carefully in this age group. IV or IM dosage of midazolam should be reduced in geriatric or debilitated patients, particularly in those 70 years of age and older. (See Dosage and Administration: Dosage.) When IV midazolam is used for induction of anesthesia, time to recovery may be delayed in this population. In addition, rare fatalities (possibly associated with cardiorespiratory depression) have been reported in geriatric and/or high-risk surgical patients receiving IV or IM midazolam (often in combination with other CNS depressants [e.g., opiates]). (See Cautions: Cardiorespiratory Effects.)

The manufacturer of oral midazolam states that a safe dosing regimen has not been established in geriatric patients and that the drug should not be used in such patients until further information is available.

■ Mutagenicity and Carcinogenicity In vitro and in vivo microbial and mammalian test systems using midazolam have not revealed evidence of mutagenicity. No evidence of carcinogenic potential was seen in rats or mice receiving oral midazolam maleate dosages up to 9 mg/kg daily (about 25 times the recommended human dosage) for 24 months. However, an increased incidence of liver tumors was observed following oral administration of 80 mg/kg daily for 24 months in female mice, and an increased incidence of benign thyroid follicular cell tumors was observed following this dosage in male rats. The pathogenesis of induction of these tumors is not known. In addition, the relevance of these findings to usual use of midazolam in humans is not known, since these effects occurred after long-term administration of the drug in animals, whereas use in humans usually is short term.

■ Pregnancy, Fertility, and Lactation An increased risk of congenital malformations associated with the use of benzodiazepines (e.g., chlordiazepoxide, diazepam) during pregnancy has been suggested by several retrospective studies in humans. Midazolam has been shown to cross the placenta in humans. Reproduction studies in rabbits and rats using IV midazolam in doses up to 1.85 times the human induction dose have not revealed evidence of fetal malformation. If the drug is administered during pregnancy, the patient should be informed of the potential hazard to the fetus. Use of midazolam injection for obstetric procedures or during labor and delivery is not recommended, since such use has not been evaluated and use of other benzodiazepines during the last weeks of pregnancy has caused CNS depression in the neonate.

Based on animal data, repeated or prolonged use of general anesthetics and sedation drugs, including midazolam, during the third trimester of pregnancy may result in adverse neurodevelopmental effects in the fetus. The clinical relevance of these animal findings to humans is not known; the potential risk of adverse neurodevelopmental effects should be considered and discussed with pregnant women undergoing procedures requiring general anesthetics and sedation drugs. (See Cautions: Pediatric Precautions.)

No evidence of impaired fertility was observed in rats following oral administration of midazolam in doses producing exposures as high as 1.85 times the recommended human IV induction dose of 0.35 mg/kg.

Women who are pregnant while receiving midazolam nasal spray should be encouraged to enroll in the North American Antiepileptic Drug (NAAED) Pregnancy Registry at 888-233-2334 or http://www.aedpregnancyregistry.org.

Midazolam is distributed into milk in humans, and caution should be exercised when midazolam is administered to nursing women.

Drug Interactions

■ Drugs Affecting Hepatic Microsomal Enzymes Metabolism of midazolam is mediated by cytochrome P-450 (CYP) isoenzyme 3A4. Concomitant use of midazolam and drugs that inhibit CYP3A4 (e.g., erythromycin, diltiazem, verapamil, ketoconazole, fluconazole, itraconazole, HIV protease inhibitors) may result in clinically important increases in peak plasma concentrations and area under the plasma concentration-time curve (AUC) of midazolam; conversely, concomitant use of midazolam with drugs that induce CYP3A4 (e.g., rifampin, carbamazepine, phenytoin, phenobarbital) may result in clinically important decreases in peak plasma concentrations and AUC of midazolam. Caution should be observed if midazolam is administered concomitantly with these drugs and dosage adjustments may be necessary. The manufacturer states that oral midazolam should be used concomitantly with ketoconazole, itraconazole, or saquinavir only when absolutely necessary and with appropriate equipment and personnel available to respond to respiratory insufficiency.

Manufacturers of HIV protease inhibitors and the nonnucleoside reverse transcriptase inhibitors (NNRTIs) delavirdine and efavirenz state that concomitant use of midazolam with these antiretroviral agents is contraindicated; however, some experts state that a single midazolam dose can be used with caution for procedural sedation in monitored situations in patients receiving these antiretroviral agents.

■ Commonly Used Drugs During Anesthesia or Surgery Concomitant use of IV midazolam and IV fentanyl has resulted in severe hypotension in neonates. No adverse interactions have been observed when midazolam was administered concomitantly with other common premedications or drugs used during anesthesia or surgery (e.g., atropine, scopolamine, glycopyrrolate, diazepam, hydroxyzine, succinylcholine, nondepolarizing neuromuscular blocking agents, topical local anesthetics).

■ Anesthetic Agents Patients who have received midazolam as an induction agent may require reduced amounts of inhalation agents during maintenance of anesthesia.

The cardiovascular stimulatory effects and the postoperative emergence delirium usually associated with administration of ketamine appear to be antagonized, at least partially, by midazolam.

■ Anticonvulsants Concomitant administration of oral midazolam and phenytoin or carbamazepine has been shown to decrease peak plasma concentrations and AUC of midazolam by about 93–94%. Although not studied specifically, phenobarbital would be expected to have similar effects on the pharmacokinetics of midazolam.

■ **Antifungal Agents** Concomitant administration of oral midazolam in patients receiving ketoconazole or itraconazole has been shown to increase peak plasma concentrations of midazolam (by 309% or 80–240%, respectively) as a result of decreased plasma clearance. Because of the potential for intense and prolonged sedation and respiratory depression, midazolam oral solution should be coadministered with these drugs only if absolutely necessary and with appropriate equipment and personnel available to respond to respiratory insufficiency.

While fluconazole has been shown to increase peak plasma concentrations of midazolam by 150%, terbinafine does not appear to affect the pharmacokinetics of midazolam.

■ **Antimycobacterial Agents** Concomitant administration of oral midazolam and rifampin has been shown to decrease the peak plasma concentration of midazolam by 94% and the AUC of midazolam by 96%. Although not studied specifically, rifabutin would be expected to have similar effects on the pharmacokinetics of midazolam.

■ **Antiretroviral Agents** Large increases in peak plasma concentrations and AUC of midazolam (by about 235 and 514%, respectively) have been observed when saquinavir (1.2 g 3 times daily given as liquid-filled capsules [no longer commercially available in the US]) was administered concomitantly with oral midazolam. In one study, concomitant use of saquinavir (1.2 g 3 times daily for 5 days) with a single 0.05-mg/kg IV dose of midazolam decreased the clearance of midazolam by 56% and approximately doubled the half-life of the benzodiazepine. Because of the potential for intense and prolonged sedation and respiratory depression, the manufacturers of HIV protease inhibitors (e.g., atazanavir, darunavir, fosamprenavir, indinavir, lopinavir/ritonavir, nelfinavir, ritonavir, saquinavir, tipranavir) state that concomitant use of midazolam with HIV protease inhibitors is contraindicated. However, some experts state that a single midazolam dose can be used with caution for procedural sedation in a monitored situation in patients receiving HIV protease inhibitors.

The manufacturers of delavirdine and efavirenz state that concomitant use of these agents with midazolam should be avoided because of the potential for the NNRTI to decrease metabolism of midazolam and result in intense or prolonged sedation or respiratory depression. However, some clinicians state that a single midazolam dose can be used with caution for procedural sedation in a monitored situation in patients receiving delavirdine or efavirenz.

■ **Calcium-channel Blockers** Concomitant administration of oral midazolam and diltiazem or verapamil increased peak plasma concentrations of midazolam by 105 or 97%, respectively, and increased AUC of midazolam by 275 or 192%, respectively. In another study, half-life of midazolam was increased from 5 to 7 hours when the drug was administered in conjunction with diltiazem or verapamil.

Nifedipine does not appear to alter the pharmacokinetics of midazolam.

■ **CNS Depressants** Midazolam may potentiate the action of other CNS depressants, including opiate agonists or other analgesics, barbiturates or other sedatives, anesthetics, or alcohol, possibly resulting in respiratory depression and profound and/or prolonged underventilation or apnea. When midazolam is used concomitantly with a depressant drug, caution should be exercised and appropriate dosage adjustments should be made to avoid overdosage. (See Cautions: Precautions and Contraindications.)

The sedative effect of IV midazolam is potentiated by premedication with CNS depressants, especially opiates, barbiturates, or combined fentanyl and droperidol. Midazolam dosage should be adjusted according to the type and amount of premedication administered. (See Dosage and Administration: Dosage.)

Opiate Agonists and Opiate Partial Agonists Concomitant use of benzodiazepines, including midazolam, and opiate agonists or opiate partial agonists may result in profound sedation, respiratory depression, coma, and death. Opiate agonists can impair the ventilatory response to carbon dioxide (CO_2), and appear to increase the risk of hypotension and prolong the recovery period compared with midazolam alone. Severe hypotension, possibly secondary to increased venous pooling, has occurred when midazolam was used concomitantly with high-dose fentanyl. When concomitant therapy is required, the lowest effective dosages and shortest possible duration of concomitant therapy should be used, and the patient should be monitored closely for respiratory depression and sedation. Opiate antitussive agents should be avoided in patients receiving benzodiazepines, and concomitant use of opiate analgesics and benzodiazepines should be reserved for patients in whom alternative treatment options are inadequate. For further information on potential interactions between benzodiazepines and opiates, see Opiate Agonists and Opiate Partial Agonists under Drug Interactions: CNS Agents, in the Benzodiazepines General Statement 28:24.08.

■ **Grapefruit Juice** Concomitant administration of grapefruit juice with oral midazolam has been reported to increase bioavailability of the drug. Grapefruit juice does not appear to interfere with metabolism following IV administration of the drug. The interaction between grapefruit juice and the benzodiazepine bioavailability appears to result from inhibition, probably prehepatic, of the cytochrome P-450 enzyme system by some constituent(s) in the juice. Following oral administration of midazolam, such prehepatic inhibition of drug metabolism by grapefruit juice appears mainly to involve the CYP3A4 isoenzyme, principally within the small intestinal wall (e.g., in the jejunum), thus increasing systemic availability of these drugs. (See Grapefruit Juice under Drug Interactions: Drugs and Foods Affecting Hepatic Microsomal Enzymes, in Cyclosporine 92:44.) The manufacturer states that oral midazolam should not be taken in conjunction with grapefruit juice.

■ **Histamine H_2-Receptor Antagonists** The effects of concomitant administration of midazolam and cimetidine or ranitidine have not been fully elucidated. Orally administered cimetidine or ranitidine did not substantially alter the pharmacokinetics of either IV or oral midazolam in one study in healthy adults. However, in another study, plasma midazolam concentrations were increased by about 30% following oral administration of cimetidine, but not ranitidine, in healthy adults receiving midazolam IV. Oral bioavailability of midazolam may be increased by up to about 30% when cimetidine or ranitidine is given concomitantly, possibly secondary to a pH-dependent enhancement of gastric absorption of midazolam and/or a reduction in hepatic clearance of the drug. In another study, concomitant administration of oral midazolam and cimetidine (800–1200 mg up to 4 times daily) increased peak plasma concentrations and AUC of midazolam by 6–138 and 10–102%, respectively; and concomitant administration of oral midazolam and ranitidine (150 mg 2 or 3 times daily or 300 mg once daily) increased peak plasma concentrations and AUC of midazolam by 15–67 and 9–66%, respectively. If changes in the pharmacokinetics of midazolam occur during concomitant use with one of these histamine H_2-receptor antagonists, enhanced pharmacologic effects of midazolam may result. Pending further accumulation of data, patients receiving midazolam and cimetidine or ranitidine concomitantly should be observed carefully for signs of midazolam-induced CNS and respiratory depression, and dosage of midazolam reduced if necessary.

■ **Macrolide Antibiotics** Concomitant administration of midazolam and erythromycin may affect the pharmacokinetics of midazolam. In one study, concomitant use of erythromycin (500 mg 3 times daily for 1 week) with a single 0.05-mg/kg IV dose of midazolam doubled the half-life of midazolam and reportedly decreased clearance of the benzodiazepine. In another study in healthy individuals, pretreatment with erythromycin (500 mg 3 times daily for 6 days) reportedly increased peak plasma concentrations and AUC of oral midazolam following a single 15-mg oral dose of the benzodiazepine. Because increased plasma concentrations of midazolam may be associated with excessive sedative effects, some clinicians state that erythromycin should not be given to patients receiving midazolam, or alternatively, the dose of midazolam should be reduced in patients receiving the anti-infective.

While erythromycin has been shown to increase peak plasma concentrations and AUC of oral midazolam by about 170 and 281–341%, respectively, azithromycin does not appear to affect the pharmacokinetics of midazolam.

■ **Neuromuscular Blocking Agents** Midazolam and pancuronium have been used concomitantly in adults without any clinically important changes in dosage, onset, or duration. Midazolam does not cause a clinically important change in dosage, onset, or duration of a single intubating dose of succinylcholine.

■ **Quinupristin and Dalfopristin** Concomitant use of midazolam and quinupristin/dalfopristin may affect the pharmacokinetics of midazolam. In healthy individuals, concomitant administration of a single IV dose of midazolam with IV quinupristin/dalfopristin increased mean peak plasma concentrations and AUC of midazolam by 14 and 33%, respectively.

Acute Toxicity

■ **Pathogenesis** Limited information is available on the acute toxicity of midazolam in humans. The IV and oral LD_{50}s of midazolam have been reported to be about 86 and 760 mg/kg, respectively, in mice.

■ **Manifestations and Treatment** Overdosage of midazolam hydrochloride is likely to produce symptoms that are mainly extensions of the usual pharmacologic effects of benzodiazepines, such as sedation, somnolence, confusion, impaired coordination, diminished reflexes, coma, and alterations in vital signs. The manufacturer states that organ toxicity specific to midazolam overdosage would not be expected. Flumazenil, a benzodiazepine antagonist, can be used to completely or partially reverse midazolam-induced sedation when the drug is used for induction or maintenance of anesthesia or for diagnostic or therapeutic procedures. Flumazenil also can be used as an adjunct to symptomatic and supportive care in the management of midazolam overdosage. (See Flumazenil 28:92.)

The value of peritoneal dialysis, hemodialysis, forced diuresis, and/or hemoperfusion in the management of midazolam overdosage is not known. For further information on the clinical manifestations and management of midazolam toxicity, see Acute Toxicity in the Benzodiazepines General Statement 28:24.08.

Pharmacology

Midazolam shares the actions of other benzodiazepines. Although initial data indicated that the sedative potency of midazolam was about 1.5–2.5 times that of diazepam, clinical experience with the drug suggests that potency may be 3–4 times that of diazepam.

For further information on the pharmacology of midazolam hydrochloride, see the Benzodiazepines General Statement 28:24.08.

Pharmacokinetics

In studies described in the Pharmacokinetics section, midazolam was administered as the hydrochloride, maleate, or lactate salt; dosages and concentrations of the drug are expressed in terms of midazolam. Studies demonstrate that the pharmacokinetic properties of midazolam following administration of a single parenteral dose in pediatric patients aged 1 year and older are similar to those reported in adults.

■ **Absorption** Absorption of midazolam hydrochloride from IM injection sites is rapid and nearly complete (mean absolute bioavailability is greater than 90%). IM bioavailability of the lactate appears to be similar to or slightly less than that of the hydrochloride; however, any such difference does not appear to be clinically important. Pharmacologic effects of midazolam usually are apparent within 5–15 minutes but may not be maximal until 15–60 minutes following IM administration; the duration of action usually is about 2 hours (range: 1–6 hours). Peak plasma midazolam concentrations generally are attained within 30–45 minutes following IM administration. Following IM administration of a single 12.5-mg (of midazolam) dose of the hydrochloride in healthy adults, peak plasma midazolam concentrations of approximately 200 ng/mL (range: 88–269 ng/mL) are attained. Peak plasma concentrations of midazolam and 1-hydroxymethylmidazolam (an active metabolite) attained following IM injection are approximately 50% of those attained following IV injection of a dose.

Following IV administration of usual doses of midazolam hydrochloride, the onset of sedative, anxiolytic, and amnesic action usually occurs within 1–5 minutes. However, onset is affected by many factors, including total dose administered, rate of administration, patient age, serum albumin concentration, renal function, and the presence of other drugs. Induction of anesthesia usually occurs in about 1.5 minutes when opiate agonists are administered concurrently with midazolam and in 2–2.5 minutes when midazolam is administered without an opiate agonist or concurrently with other sedatives. Duration of action following IV administration is usually less than 2 hours; however, the pharmacologic effects may persist up to 6 hours in some patients, and the duration of action appears to be dose related. Limited data suggest that the onset may be more rapid and the duration prolonged in patients with chronic renal failure, probably secondary to decreased protein binding in these patients.

In one study in healthy adults who received a single 75-mcg/kg dose of midazolam IV over 1 minute, peak plasma concentrations of the drug averaged 323.8 ng/mL and plasma concentrations 0.25, 0.5, 1, 2, 4, 6, and 8 hours after the dose averaged 246.8, 206.8, 141.7, 84.2, 37.0, and 20.2 ng/mL, respectively. Following single IV doses, plasma concentrations of midazolam generally are 10–30 times higher than those of the principal metabolite, 1-hydroxymethylmidazolam.

Following intranasal administration of a single 5-mg dose of midazolam in healthy adults, peak plasma concentrations were obtained in approximately 17 minutes. Absolute bioavailability is approximately 44%. The onset of sedative and psychomotor impairment effects usually occurs within 10 minutes, while maximal effects are achieved within 30 minutes to 2 hours after a dose is administered.

Midazolam hydrochloride is absorbed rapidly from the GI tract, with maximum plasma concentrations usually occurring within 1–2 hours. Following oral administration, the drug undergoes substantial first-pass metabolism in the liver and intestine, with only about 40–50% (range: 28–72%) of an orally administered dose reaching systemic circulation unchanged. Pharmacologic effects of midazolam usually are apparent within 10–20 minutes following administration of midazolam oral solution in pediatric patients. In pharmacokinetic studies of pediatric patients (6 months to less than 16 years of age) receiving midazolam oral solution at doses of 250 mcg/kg, 500 mcg/kg, or 1 mg/kg, midazolam exhibited linear pharmacokinetics. The mean time to maximal plasma concentration in these patients ranged from 0.17–2.65 hours, and the absolute bioavailability of the drug was about 36%; bioavailability was not affected by pediatric age or weight. The effect of food on absorption of midazolam oral solution has not been studied; however, in adults receiving the drug as a 15-mg oral tablet, absorption was not affected by food.

A relationship between plasma midazolam concentrations and clinical effects has not been clearly established, and the manufacturer states that a direct relationship does not exist. However, some data suggest that sedation may be associated with plasma midazolam concentrations greater than 30–100 ng/mL. In one study, pronounced hypnotic effects (e.g., slurred speech, sleep with dreaming, nystagmus) were noted when plasma concentrations exceeded 100 ng/mL.

■ **Distribution** At physiologic pH, midazolam is highly lipophilic; however, the lipophilicity of the drug decreases with decreasing pH. (See Chemistry and Stability: Chemistry.) Following IV administration in humans, midazolam is rapidly and apparently widely distributed. The apparent volume of distribution of the drug in healthy adults reportedly averages 0.8–2.5 L/kg (range: 0.6–6.6 L/kg). Volume of distribution of midazolam appears to be 1.5–2 times higher in adults with chronic renal failure and 2–3 times higher in adults with congestive heart failure compared with healthy adults. In pediatric patients (6 months to younger than 16 years of age) receiving IV midazolam 0.15 mg/kg, the mean steady-state volume of distribution ranged from 1.24–2.02 L/kg.

Following IV administration of midazolam hydrochloride in animals, the drug is widely distributed, with highest concentrations occurring in liver, kidneys, lungs, fat, and heart. The drug crosses the blood-brain barrier and distributes into CSF in humans and animals. In animals, equilibration of midazolam between plasma and CSF occurs within a few minutes following IV administration, and CSF:plasma ratios of the drug are highly correlated with unbound midazolam once equilibrium is reached. Distribution of the drug into human lumbar CSF may be slow and erratic. Distribution of midazolam may be altered in geriatric patients.

In both adult and pediatric patients older than 1 year of age, approximately 94–97% of midazolam hydrochloride is bound to plasma proteins, mainly to serum albumin; protein binding of the drug is decreased in patients with chronic renal failure. In healthy individuals, the drug's principal metabolite, 1-hydroxymethylmidazolam, is 89% protein bound. The degree of protein binding appears to be independent of the plasma concentration of the drug.

Midazolam crosses the placenta and is distributed into amniotic fluid in animals and humans; however, placental transfer of drug appears to occur more slowly than with diazepam. In humans, measurable midazolam concentrations were achieved in maternal venous serum, umbilical venous serum, umbilical arterial serum, and amniotic fluid following a single 15-mg (of midazolam) oral or 50-mcg/kg (of midazolam) IM dose of the maleate given 15–60 minutes prior to cesarean section; both umbilical venous and umbilical arterial midazolam concentrations were lower than maternal concentrations. Midazolam reportedly is distributed into milk in humans. (See Cautions: Pregnancy, Fertility, and Lactation.)

■ **Elimination** Plasma midazolam concentrations appear to decline in a biphasic manner following IV administration. Following a single IV dose in healthy adults, the half-life of midazolam in the initial distribution phase ($t_{1/2\alpha}$) averages 6–20 minutes, and the half-life in the terminal elimination phase ($t_{1/2\beta}$) averages 1–4 hours (range: 1–12.3 hours). Limited data suggest that the half-life of midazolam may be prolonged in obese patients (presumably secondary to an increased volume of distribution), geriatric individuals, and patients with impaired hepatic function or with congestive heart failure. The half-life of midazolam is also reportedly prolonged in patients receiving the drug for induction of anesthesia associated with major surgical procedures. Elimination half-life does not appear to be altered substantially in patients with chronic renal failure. Mean elimination half-life ranged from 2.2–6.8 hours following single oral doses of 250 mcg/kg, 500 mcg/kg, and 1 mg/kg of midazolam oral solution in pediatric patients (6 months to younger than 16 years of age). Mean elimination half-life ranged from 2.9–4.5 hours in pediatric patients (6 months to less than 16 years of age) receiving IV midazolam 150 mcg/kg. In seriously ill neonates, the terminal elimination half-life is substantially prolonged (i.e., 6.5–12 hours). Following IM administration of midazolam 10 mg, elimination half-life of the drug was approximately 4 hours. Following intranasal administration of midazolam nasal spray, elimination half-life of the drug ranged from 2.1 to 6.2 hours.

Midazolam is metabolized extensively in the liver and intestine by cytochrome P-450 CYP3A4. The drug rapidly undergoes hydroxylation via hepatic microsomal enzymes to form 1-hydroxymethylmidazolam (α-hydroxymidazolam), the principal metabolite, and 4-hydroxymidazolam; a small portion of 1-hydroxymethylmidazolam is further hydroxylated to 1-hydroxymethyl-4-hydroxymidazolam (α,4-dihydroxymidazolam). These metabolites undergo rapid conjugation with glucuronic acid in the liver. Although the elimination half-life of the principal metabolite, 1-hydroxymethylmidazolam, is not clearly established, it is estimated to be about 60–80 minutes. The 1-hydroxymethyl and 4-hydroxy metabolites are reportedly pharmacologically active; potency of 1-hydroxymethylmidazolam appears to be similar to that of midazolam. The 1-hydroxymethyl-4-hydroxy metabolite appears to have little, if any, pharmacologic activity.

Midazolam is excreted in urine almost entirely as conjugated metabolites. Approximately 45–57% of an IV dose is excreted in urine as conjugated 1-hydroxymethylmidazolam, small amounts as conjugates of 4-hydroxymidazolam and 1-hydroxymethyl-4-hydroxymidazolam, and less than 0.03% as unchanged drug. In healthy adults who received a single 10-mg oral dose of radiolabeled midazolam, about 90% of the radioactivity was excreted in urine within 24 hours, principally (about 60–70% of a dose) as conjugated 1-hydroxymethylmidazolam. Approximately 2–10% of an oral dose is excreted in feces.

It is not known whether midazolam is removed by hemodialysis or peritoneal dialysis.

Following IV administration in healthy individuals and pediatric patients, total apparent plasma clearance of midazolam averages 2.5–12.8 mL/minute per kg. In seriously ill neonates, the clearance is reduced to 0.07–0.12 L/hr per kg; it cannot be determined whether these differences are because of age, immature organ function or metabolism, underlying illness, or debility. Total apparent plasma clearance of the drug reportedly is decreased in geriatric individuals but, in one study, such clearance was decreased substantially only in geriatric males. Total plasma clearance and volume of distribution of total (bound and unbound) midazolam are 1.5–2 times higher in patients with chronic renal failure compared with individuals with normal renal function, but these alterations are attributable to changes in protein binding of the drug and are not apparent when these pharmacokinetic parameters are determined for unbound midazolam. Although the effects of hepatic impairment on the elimination of midazolam have not been fully evaluated, preliminary data suggest that total apparent plasma clearance of the drug may be decreased in some patients with chronic liver disease. In a limited number of patients with congestive heart failure, total body clearance of midazolam appeared to remain unchanged following a single 5-mg IV dose, although elimination half-life and volume of distribution were increased twofold to threefold.

Chemistry and Stability

■ **Chemistry** Midazolam is a benzodiazepine. The drug is an imidazobenzodiazepine, differing structurally from other benzodiazepines by the presence of an imidazole ring fused at positions 1 and 2 of the benzodiazepine nucleus, which replaces the ketone at position 2 of the nucleus. The imidazole ring results in the ability of midazolam to readily form salts, which have increased aqueous solubility and stability to hydrolysis compared with other benzodiazepines. Presence of a methyl group at position 1 of the imidazole ring may result in increased susceptibility to metabolism. In acidic solutions, such as in the commercially available oral solution (pH 2.8–3.6) or parenteral injections (pH 3–4 in the 1 mg/mL solutions and pH 3–3.6 in the 5 mg/mL solutions), a pH-dependent equilibrium exists between midazolam and a ring-opened structure (the corresponding benzophenone) at position 4 of the benzodiazepine nucleus, resulting in up to 40 or 25% ring-opened forms for the oral solution or parenteral injections, respectively. At physiologic pH (5–8), under which midazolam is absorbed into the systemic circulation, the drug is almost (at least 99%) completely ring-closed, resulting in increased lipophilicity.

Midazolam occurs as a white to light yellow, crystalline powder. Midazolam is commercially available as the hydrochloride salt, which is formed *in situ*. The aqueous solubility of midazolam hydrochloride is pH dependent; the drug has solubilities of approximately 0.24, 1.09, 3.67, 10.3, or greater than 22 mg (of midazolam) per mL in water at pH 6.2, 5.1, 3.8, 3.4, or 2.8, respectively, at 25°C. Midazolam has a pK_a of 6.15. Midazolam also is commercially available as a solution for intranasal administration.

Midazolam hydrochloride injection is commercially available as a sterile solution for IM or IV administration. Hydrochloric acid and, if necessary, sodium hydroxide are added during manufacture of the injection to adjust the pH to about 3. The injection also contains disodium edetate and sodium chloride; some preparations also may contain benzyl alcohol. Commercially available midazolam hydrochloride oral solution is a red to purplish-red colored solution containing 2 mg/mL of the drug in a cherry-flavored vehicle. The pH of the oral solution has been adjusted to approximately 2.8–3.6 with hydrochloric acid. Commercially available midazolam nasal spray is a clear, colorless to yellowish colored solution; each 0.1 mL of solution contains 5 mg of midazolam.

■ **Stability** Midazolam hydrochloride injection should be stored at 20–25°C, but may be exposed to temperatures ranging from 15–30°C. The injection was physically stable when frozen for 3-day periods and allowed to thaw at room temperature. Preservative-free midazolam hydrochloride injection should be stored at 20–25°C. Midazolam oral solution should be stored at 20–25°C. Midazolam nasal spray should be stored at 20–25°C, but may be exposed to temperatures ranging from 15–30°C.

Midazolam hydrochloride injection is chemically and physically compatible with the following IV solutions: 5% dextrose, 0.9% sodium chloride, or lactated Ringer's. Midazolam hydrochloride injection that has been diluted to a final concentration of 0.5 mg or less per mL is stable for 24 hours in 5% dextrose or 0.9% sodium chloride injection and for 4 hours in lactated Ringer's injection when stored in glass or PVC containers at 25°C. When diluted and stored as recommended, it is not necessary to protect these solutions from light.

When admixed in the same syringe at room temperature, midazolam hydrochloride injection is reported to be physically compatible for at least 30 minutes with atropine sulfate, meperidine hydrochloride, morphine sulfate, or scopolamine hydrobromide, and for at least 8 hours with fentanyl citrate, glycopyrrolate, hydroxyzine hydrochloride, ketamine hydrochloride, nalbuphine hydrochloride, promethazine hydrochloride, or sufentanil citrate. Since the compatibility of these and other admixtures with midazolam hydrochloride injection depends on several factors (e.g., concentrations of the drugs, specific diluents used, resulting pH, temperature), specialized references should be consulted for specific information.

Preparations

Midazolam hydrochloride is subject to control under the Federal Controlled Substances Act of 1970 as a schedule IV (C-IV) drug.

Excipients in commercially available drug preparations may have clinically important effects in some individuals; consult specific product labeling for details.

Midazolam

Nasal		
Solution	5 mg/0.1 mL	**Nayzilam® Nasal Spray** (C-IV), UCB

Midazolam Hydrochloride

Oral		
Solution	2 mg (of midazolam) per mL*	**Midazolam Hydrochloride Syrup** (C-IV)
Parenteral		
Injection	1 mg (of midazolam) per mL*	**Midazolam Hydrochloride Injection** (C-IV)
	5 mg (of midazolam) per mL*	**Midazolam Hydrochloride Injection** (C-IV)
		Seizalam® (C-IV), Meridian

*available from one or more manufacturer, distributor, and/or repackager by generic (nonproprietary) name

†Use is not currently included in the labeling approved by the US Food and Drug Administration

Anxiolytics, Sedatives, and Hypnotics, Miscellaneous 28:24.92

busPIRone Hydrochloride

■ Buspirone hydrochloride is an anxiolytic agent.

Uses

■ **Anxiety Disorders** Buspirone is used for the management of anxiety disorders (anxiety and phobic neuroses) and for short-term relief of symptoms of anxiety. Anxiety or tension associated with the stress of everyday life usually does not require treatment with an anxiolytic. The efficacy of buspirone for long-term use (i.e., longer than 3–4 weeks) as an anxiolytic has not been established by controlled studies, but the drug has been used in some patients for substantially longer periods (e.g., 6–12 months) without apparent loss of clinical effect. If the drug is used for extended periods, the need for continued therapy should be reassessed periodically.

Generalized Anxiety Disorder Efficacy of buspirone has been established principally in outpatient settings for the management of generalized anxiety disorder in which anxiety was present for periods of 1 month up to 1 year (average symptom duration: 6 months) of continual duration. Generalized anxiety disorder is characterized principally by unrealistic or excessive anxiety and worry (apprehensive expectation) about 2 or more life circumstances (e.g., worry about possible misfortune to a child who is in no danger, worry about personal finances for no good reason, anxiety and worry about academic, athletic, and/or social performance). The disorder is manifested as symptoms of motor tension (e.g., trembling, twitching, shakiness, muscle tension, restlessness), autonomic hyperactivity (e.g., sweating, palpitation and/or tachycardia, dyspnea, dry mouth, dizziness, clammy hands, hot flushes [flashes]), and vigilance and scanning (e.g., hyperattentativeness, feeling keyed up or on edge, difficulty concentrating, insomnia, irritability). Although patients with generalized anxiety disorder may have another underlying mental disorder (axis I disorder), the focus of the anxiety and worry is unrelated to the latter disorder. In addition, symptoms of generalized anxiety disorder should not occur only during the course of a mood or psychotic disorder, nor should the anxiety be initiated and maintained by an underlying organic factor (e.g., hyperthyroidism, caffeine intoxication).

Controlled studies in patients with generalized anxiety disorder have shown that buspirone at usual dosages is as effective as usual dosages of benzodiazepines (e.g., alprazolam, clorazepate, diazepam, lorazepam) and more effective than placebo in reducing symptoms associated with anxiety. Limited evidence suggests that buspirone may be more effective for cognitive and interpersonal problems, including anger and hostility, associated with anxiety, while benzodiazepines may be more effective for somatic symptoms of anxiety. The drug also has been shown to reduce symptoms of anxiety in patients with coexisting depressive symptoms. Buspirone therapy generally is associated with fewer and less severe adverse CNS effects (e.g., sedation, psychomotor impairment) compared with benzodiazepines and appears to have little, if any, dependence liability. Because of these differences, buspirone may be preferred as initial therapy in some patients with generalized anxiety disorder. The drug may be particularly useful in patients in whom potential adverse effects of benzodiazepines would be of concern (e.g., patients whose work or life-style requires mental acuity, geriatric patients who may be particularly sensitive to the adverse CNS effects of benzodiazepines) and/or those in whom the abuse potential, dependence liability, and/or potential withdrawal associated with benzodiazepines are of concern. In addition, buspirone may be safer than benzodiazepines in those patients with anxiety disorders who, despite all warnings, are considered likely to combine anxiolytic therapy with CNS depressants and/or alcohol. (See Drug Interactions: Alcohol and also Other CNS Depressants.)

Depressive Symptoms. In addition to symptoms of anxiety, buspirone has reduced depressive symptoms in patients with generalized anxiety disorder, as determined using the Hamilton (HAM-D) or Raskin depression rating scale. Buspirone generally has been as effective as benzodiazepines in relieving symptoms of depression in these patients, although the drug may be less effective than benzodiazepines in relieving sleep disturbances. It has been suggested that improvement in depressive symptoms observed in these patients actually may reflect improvement in anxiety symptoms that are included in the depression rating scales rather than an antidepressant effect per se, and additional study is needed to determine whether the drug has clinically important antidepressant activity. Buspirone also has been used in combination with antidepressants in a limited number of patients with symptoms of both anxiety and depression.

Symptoms of Sexual Dysfunction. The efficacy of buspirone for the management of sexual dysfunction in patients with generalized anxiety disorder has not been established, but limited data suggest that the drug may improve sexual function in these patients. Although the improvement in sexual function paralleled improvement in anxiety in one study, other mechanisms may have been involved. Further study is needed to more fully elucidate the value of buspirone in these patients.

Other Anxiety Disorders Because buspirone may diminish anger and hostility and appears to be less likely than benzodiazepines to cause disinhibition, some clinicians suggest that buspirone may be preferred in patients with a history of aggression or in whom disinhibition has occurred during benzodiazepine therapy. Benzodiazepines may be preferred as initial therapy in patients with anxiety symptoms (e.g., insomnia, muscle tension) that might benefit from the sedative and/or muscle relaxant effects of these drugs. If buspirone is used in patients whose anxiety includes insomnia as a component, concomitant use of a sedative/hypnotic at bedtime may be necessary. Because buspirone may have a slower onset of action than some anxiolytics (e.g., diazepam) (see Dosage and Administration: Dosage), patients may become discouraged during initial therapy with the drug, particularly when buspirone is used for the short-term management of anxiety associated with severe stress.

The influence of previous, long-term benzodiazepine therapy on the anxiolytic response to buspirone remains to be fully elucidated, but response may be discouraging in some patients, possibly because buspirone has a slower onset of action and does not attenuate manifestations of benzodiazepine withdrawal. In addition, the anxiolytic expectations of some patients who previously have received long-term benzodiazepine therapy may differ considerably from the actual effects of buspirone therapy, which also could contribute to a discouraging response to buspirone in such patients. Because of the sometimes discouraging response to buspirone in such patients, some clinicians suggest that newly diagnosed patients and those with no previous benzodiazepine use may be optimal candidates for buspirone therapy.

Efficacy of buspirone in the management of panic attacks† or disorder† has not been established.

■ **Other Uses** Results of an uncontrolled study suggest that relatively high dosages of buspirone hydrochloride (i.e., usually 40–60 but up to 90 mg daily) may provide some reduction in depressive symptoms in patients with major depression† (nonmelancholic type), but not in patients whose major depression is of the melancholic type. Well-controlled studies, particularly those comparing buspirone with antidepressants, are necessary to determine whether buspirone has clinically important antidepressant activity.

Although buspirone exhibited some evidence of neuroleptic potential in several animal models and reportedly has produced transient antipsychotic effects when administered in large doses to patients with schizophrenia, the drug has no established antipsychotic activity in humans at usual dosages and should *not* be used in place of appropriate antipsychotic therapy when such therapy is indicated.

Because of buspirone's effects on dopamine receptors, the drug has been studied for potential therapeutic effects in patients with parkinsonian syndrome†. At dosages of 10–70 mg daily, buspirone provided no clinically important improvement or deterioration in a limited number of patients with parkinsonian syndrome who were receiving antiparkinsonian therapy (e.g., levodopa/carbidopa, bromocriptine) concomitantly. At higher dosages, however, some deterioration in parkinsonian manifestations (e.g., functional disability) was observed. Therefore, current evidence indicates that buspirone is not useful in the management of parkinsonian syndrome and may exacerbate the syndrome at relatively high dosages. The drug may be useful, however, as an anxiolytic in parkinsonian patients, provided high dosages are avoided.

Dosage and Administration

■ **Administration** Buspirone hydrochloride is administered orally. Concomitant administration of the drug with food can increase oral bioavailability of buspirone. Therefore, the manufacturer states that the drug should be given in a consistent manner relative to food intake. (See Drug Interactions: Food.)

The 15- and 30- mg tablets are provided as Dividose® tablets and are scored to be broken in 2 halves (each providing a dose of 7.5 and 15 mg, respectively, or in 3 thirds) (each providing a dose of 5 and 10 mg, respectively).

■ **Dosage** For the management of anxiety disorders, the usual initial adult dosage of buspirone hydrochloride is 10–15 mg daily, usually in 2 or 3 divided doses. Dosage is increased as necessary in increments of 5 mg daily every 2–4 days, according to the patient's response and tolerance. In clinical studies, most patients responded to maintenance dosages of 15–30 mg daily in 2 or 3 divided doses. Modification of the usual adult dosage does not appear necessary for geriatric patients. The manufacturer recommends that adult dosage not exceed 60 mg daily.

The manufacturer states that when buspirone is administered concomitantly with a potent CYP3A4 inhibitor, it should be administered at a low dosage (i.e., 2.5 mg once or twice daily) and that subsequent dosage adjustment of either drug should be based on clinical assessment. (See Drug Interactions: Drugs Affecting Microsomal Enzymes and see Dosage and Administration: Administration.)

Buspirone may have a slower onset of action than some anxiolytics (e.g., diazepam), and some patients may require motivation and education about the drug's effects during initial therapy to assure compliance. Symptomatic relief may occur during the first 2 weeks of buspirone therapy in some patients, but optimum anxiolytic effect usually requires at least 3–4 weeks of therapy; occasionally, 4–6 weeks may be required for optimum effect.

The efficacy of continued buspirone therapy for longer than 3–4 weeks has not been established by controlled studies. However, the drug has been used for longer periods (e.g., several months to a year) without unusual adverse effect or decreased efficacy in some patients. If buspirone is administered for longer than 3–4 weeks, the need for continued therapy should be reassessed periodically. Dosage during prolonged maintenance therapy should be kept at the lowest effective level; once an adequate response has been achieved, dosage should be reduced gradually and subsequently adjusted according to the patient's response and tolerance.

Discontinuance of benzodiazepines and some other anxiolytic agents has been associated with symptoms of withdrawal, and buspirone will not prevent the development of these symptoms. Therefore, it is important that therapy with such agents be withdrawn gradually in patients being switched to buspirone, particularly when therapy with one of these agents has been prolonged and/or when relatively high dosages were used.

■ **Dosage in Renal and Hepatic Impairment** The need for modification of buspirone hydrochloride dosage in patients with renal impairment has not been fully elucidated, and the drug should be used with caution in such patients. There is some evidence that the pharmacokinetics of buspirone and its active metabolite, 1-pyrimidinylpiperazine (1-PP), are not affected substantially in patients with mild to moderate renal impairment. (See Pharmacokinetics: Elimination) In anuric patients, however, accumulation of 1-PP may occur, and adjustment in buspirone hydrochloride dosage may be necessary. Some clinicians suggest that dosage of the drug be reduced by 25–50% in anuric patients. However, other clinicians state that because of the high interindividual and intraindividual variability in plasma concentrations of buspirone and 1-PP, it is difficult to make dosage adjustment recommendations for patients with renal impairment. Based on results from other studies, several clinicians state that because of the high interindividual and intraindividual variability in plasma buspirone concentrations, dosing recommendations for patients with renal impairment receiving buspirone cannot be made at this time. In addition, the manufacturer states that the drug is not recommended for use in patients with severe renal impairment. The need for supplemental doses during hemodialysis has not been determined, but such doses do not appear necessary since the drug does not appear to be removed substantially by hemodialysis.

Buspirone hydrochloride should be used with caution in patients with impaired hepatic function, and the need for reduced dosage should be considered. (See Pharmacokinetics: Elimination.) The manufacturer states that the drug is not recommended for use in patients with severe hepatic impairment.

Cautions

Buspirone generally is well tolerated. A causal relationship between many adverse reactions and the drug has not been established but cannot be excluded. In controlled studies, the incidence of some adverse effects was similar in patients receiving buspirone or placebo.

Nervous system effects (e.g., dizziness, headache, drowsiness, light-headedness) are the most common adverse effects of buspirone, but those secondary to CNS depression (e.g., sedation, psychomotor dysfunction) generally occur less frequently than with other currently available anxiolytics (e.g., benzodiazepines). In clinical studies, adverse reactions requiring discontinuance of buspirone therapy occurred in about 10% of patients and included nervous system effects (e.g., dizziness, insomnia, nervousness, drowsiness, light-headedness, headache, fatigue) and GI effects (e.g., nausea). There is some evidence that tolerance of buspirone's adverse effects (e.g., dizziness) may be slightly less in geriatric patients than in younger adults.

The incidence and severity of adverse reactions to buspirone relative to dosage and duration of therapy have not been fully characterized; however, adverse effects appear to occur more frequently at increasing dosages but generally appear to diminish with time during continued therapy. Because buspirone can bind to central dopamine receptors, the possibility exists that chronic therapy could result in adverse effects secondary to changes in dopamine-mediated neurologic function. (See Cautions: Nervous System Effects.) Although clinical experience to date has failed to reveal substantial evidence of such long-term effects at usual dosages, the possibility of risk cannot be ruled out and additional experience is needed to determine buspirone's potential for long-term sequelae.

■ **Nervous System Effects** The most frequent adverse effects associated with buspirone therapy are nervous system effects. In controlled studies, dizziness, drowsiness, and headache occurred in about 10% of patients; fatigue, nervousness, insomnia, and light-headedness occurred in about 5%; and excitement, depression, decreased concentration, nightmares/vivid dreams, anger/hostility, confusion, weakness, incoordination, paresthesia, numbness, and tremor occurred less frequently. In these studies, dizziness, headache, nervousness, light-headedness, paresthesia, and excitement occurred appreciably more frequently in patients receiving buspirone than in those receiving placebo. Insomnia and nervousness may become particularly evident at high dosages (e.g., 100 mg daily), and may be secondary to a dose-dependent stimulation of α-adrenergic (noradrenergic) cells of the locus ceruleus.

Buspirone is relatively nonsedating compared with other currently available anxiolytics (e.g., benzodiazepines), although sedative effects (e.g., drowsiness, lethargy, sedation) may become more prominent as dosage is increased (e.g., at dosages exceeding 20 mg daily). In addition, buspirone's sedative effects often are most apparent during initiation of therapy or upward titration of dosage and tend to decrease with time. However, the drug's CNS effects show interindividual variation and the potential for their development may not be predictable in a given patient. Adverse effects resulting from CNS and psychomotor depression (e.g., drowsiness, fatigue, mental depression, confusion, decreased concentration, incoordination, weakness) generally occur less frequently with buspirone than with benzodiazepines (e.g., clorazepate, diazepam, lorazepam), while dizziness, headache, nervousness, and paresthesia generally occur more frequently with buspirone.

Dream disturbances occur in at least 1% of patients receiving buspirone, but a causal relationship to the drug has not been established. Other adverse nervous system effects not directly attributed to the drug but occurring less frequently include depersonalization, dysphoria, noise intolerance, euphoria, fearfulness, loss of interest, dissociative reaction, hallucinations, suicidal ideation, and seizures. Claustrophobic feelings, cold intolerance, stupor, slurred speech, and psychosis occur rarely. Depression and increased appetite occasionally have emerged during chronic (i.e., 6 months or longer) therapy with the drug.

Buspirone's potential for causing acute and chronic changes in dopamine-mediated neurologic function (e.g., dystonia, parkinsonian-like manifestations, akathisia, tardive dyskinesia) has not been fully elucidated. Clinical experience to date suggests that the risk for such effects during buspirone therapy at usual anxiolytic dosages is minimal, and such experience has not revealed evidence of definitive extrapyramidal reactions directly attributable to the drug. However, akathisia, hypertonia, dystonia, tremor, involuntary movements, slowed reaction time, and rigid/stiff muscles reportedly have been associated with anxiolytic dosages of buspirone in a few patients. In addition, a syndrome of restlessness, appearing shortly after initiation of therapy with the drug, has been reported occasionally. This syndrome may have resulted from increased central α-adrenergic activity or from dopaminergic or other effects. In addition, extrapyramidal manifestations (e.g., akathisia, tremor, rigidity) also have occurred in at least one patient receiving a buspirone hydrochloride dosage substantially exceeding usual anxiolytic dosages. In a limited number of patients with parkinsonian syndrome, dosages of 10–70 mg daily caused no clinically important deterioration in manifestations of the syndrome, although some deterioration (e.g., in functional ability) was apparent at relatively high dosages (e.g., 90–100 mg daily). (See Uses: Other Uses.) Myoclonus, which may have been serotonergically mediated, also has been reported in at least one patient shortly after initiation of usual anxiolytic dosages of buspirone; the myoclonus resolved following discontinuance of the drug and administration of clonazepam.

Increased anxiety, agitation, and restlessness accompanied by pressured speech and racing thoughts occurred in several patients with panic disorder or generalized anxiety disorder who were receiving buspirone with tricyclic antidepressants and/or alprazolam; these manifestations resolved within 1–5 days following discontinuance of buspirone therapy. Hypomania also has been reported in a patient with bipolar disorder and symptoms of anxiety concurrently receiving buspirone, lithium, tranylcypromine, and alprazolam; symptoms of hypomania resolved within 3 days following discontinuance of buspirone therapy in this patient. Although the mechanism is unclear, it has been suggested that these reactions may have been caused by a buspirone-induced increase in dopaminergic or α-adrenergic activity, effects of the drug on 5-HT_1 receptors, and/or a possible drug interaction between buspirone and alprazolam.

■ **GI Effects** Nausea has been reported in 6–8% of patients receiving buspirone in controlled studies, occurring more frequently than with placebo. Adverse GI effects occurring in 1–5% of patients include dry mouth, abdominal/gastric distress, diarrhea, constipation, and vomiting. Flatulence, anorexia, increased appetite, salivation, irritable colon, and rectal bleedingoccur less frequently, and burning of the tongue occurs rarely, but these effects have not been directly attributed to the drug.

■ **Cardiovascular Effects** Tachycardia and/or palpitation have been reported in about 1–2% of patients receiving buspirone, and nonspecific chest pain has been reported in at least 1% of patients; however, these effects have occurred at a frequency not appreciably different from that occurring with placebo. Syncope, hypotension, and hypertension occur less frequently, and cerebrovascular accident, congestive heart failure, myocardial infarction, cardiomyopathy, and bradycardia occur rarely; a causal relationship to the drug also has not been established for these effects.

■ **Dermatologic Effects** Adverse dermatologic effects occur occasionally in patients receiving buspirone and include rash, edema, pruritus, flushing, easy bruisability, hair loss, dry skin, facial edema, and blisters. Acne and thinning of the nails occur rarely. A causal relationship to the drug for most of these dermatologic effects has not been established.

■ **Other Adverse Effects** Buspirone produces a dose-dependent stimulation of prolactin secretion (see Pharmacology: Neuroendocrine Effects); however, the clinical importance of the drug's effect on prolactin has not been fully determined. Menstrual irregularities (e.g., spotting, amenorrhea), galactorrhea, and thyroid abnormalities have occurred occasionally in patients receiving buspirone, but a causal relationship has not been established. Increased or decreased libido, delayed ejaculation, and impotence also have occurred occasionally in patients receiving the drug, but therapy with the drug also has improved sexual function in some patients with generalized anxiety disorder and associated sexual dysfunction. (See Uses: Anxiety Disorders.)

Blurred vision has been reported in 2% of the patients receiving buspirone in controlled studies. A causal relationship for most other adverse effects generally has not been established, although such effects have been reasonably associated with buspirone therapy. Tinnitus, sore throat, and nasal congestion occur occasionally in patients receiving the drug. Redness and itching of the eyes, conjunctivitis, and altered taste or smell also occur occasionally. Rarely, inner-ear abnormality, eye pain, photophobia, and pressure on the eyes have occurred.

Urinary frequency or hesitancy; dysuria; muscle aches/pain, cramps, spasm, and weakness; arthralgia; hyperventilation; dyspnea; and chest congestion occur occasionally in patients receiving buspirone. Fever, weight loss or gain, and increased serum aminotransferase (transaminase) concentrations (e.g., AST [SGOT], ALT [SGPT]) also have been reported occasionally. Rarely, pelvic inflammatory disease, enuresis, nocturia, epistaxis, alcohol abuse, bleeding disturbance, loss of voice, and hiccups have occurred in patients receiving the drug. Eosinophilia, leukopenia, and thrombocytopenia also have occurred rarely.

■ **Precautions and Contraindications** Although buspirone generally is less sedating than other currently available anxiolytics and does not produce substantial impairment of cognitive or psychomotor function at usual dosages, the CNS effects of buspirone exhibit interindividual variation and may not be predictable. Therefore, patients should be cautioned that buspirone may impair their ability to perform activities requiring mental alertness or physical coordination (e.g., operating machinery, driving a motor vehicle) and to avoid such activities until they experience how the drug affects them. While drug interaction studies indicate that buspirone does not increase substantially alcohol-induced impairment of motor and mental performance, patients should be advised that it would be prudent to avoid concomitant use. (See Drug Interactions: Alcohol.)

Buspirone does not exhibit cross-tolerance with benzodiazepines or other sedative/hypnotic drugs, and will not prevent symptoms of withdrawal that may occur following cessation of therapy with these drugs. Therefore, it is important that therapy with such drugs be withdrawn gradually in patients being switched to buspirone, particularly when therapy with one of these agents has been prolonged and/or when relatively high dosages were used. Rebound or withdrawal symptoms may occur over varying time periods, depending in part on the type of drug being discontinued and its elimination characteristics. Clinicians should be aware that the development of any combination of irritability, anxiety, agitation, insomnia, tremor, abdominal or muscle cramps, vomiting, sweating, flu-like symptoms without fever, or even seizures following initiation of buspirone therapy in patients previously receiving other anxiolytics and/or sedative/hypnotics may be manifestations of withdrawal from these drugs.

Because the potential risk of buspirone-induced changes in dopamine-mediated neurologic function, particularly those associated with long-term therapy, currently has not been elucidated, the possibility that such changes could occur in patients receiving the drug should be considered. (See Cautions: Nervous System Effects.)

In patients currently receiving a monoamine oxidase inhibitor, buspirone therapy should *not* be initiated. (See Drug Interactions: Psychotherapeutic Agents.)

Buspirone should be used with caution in patients with impaired renal function, since the drug and its metabolites are excreted principally by the kidneys. Buspirone also should be used with caution in patients with hepatic dysfunction. (See Dosage and Administration: Dosage in Renal and Hepatic Impairment.)

Buspirone has no established antipsychotic efficacy in humans at usual anxiolytic dosages, and the drug should not be used in place of appropriate antipsychotic therapy when such therapy is indicated.

Buspirone is contraindicated in patients who are hypersensitive to the drug.

■ **Pediatric Precautions** Safety and efficacy of buspirone in children younger than 18 years of age have not been established. Although safety and efficacy of buspirone in children have not been fully evaluated, the drug has been used in pediatric patients without unusual adverse effects. In 2 controlled studies in 559 pediatric patients 6–17 years of age with generalized anxiety disorder (GAD), no unexpected adverse effects were associated with buspirone; however, there was no difference in symptoms of GAD between those receiving buspirone 7.5–30 mg twice daily or placebo for 6 weeks. Long-term safety and efficacy of the drug in children younger than 18 years of age have not been evaluated.

■ **Geriatric Precautions** Results of a study in about 600 geriatric patients (mean age: 70.8 years) indicate that safety and efficacy of buspirone in geriatric patients appear to be similar to those of younger adults (mean age: 43.3 years); no age-related differences in the pharmacokinetics of buspirone were observed. Although postmarketing experience has not revealed differences in the incidence of adverse effects between geriatric patients and younger adults, the possibility that some older patients may exhibit increased sensitivity to the drug cannot be ruled out.

■ **Mutagenicity and Carcinogenicity** No evidence of buspirone-induced mutagenesis was seen in the Ames microbial mutagen test, with or without metabolic activation, or in the mouse lymphoma L5178Y/TK$^+$ cell test system, nor was DNA damage observed in Wi-38 human cells. No chromosomal aberrations or abnormalities were observed in bone marrow cells of mice given one or five daily doses of buspirone.

No evidence of carcinogenesis was observed after 24 months in rats receiving oral buspirone hydrochloride dosages up to 133 times the maximum recommended human dosage or after 18 months in mice receiving oral dosages up to 167 times the maximum recommended human dosage.

■ **Pregnancy, Fertility, and Lactation** Reproduction studies in rats and rabbits using oral buspirone hydrochloride dosages up to 30 times the maximum recommended human dosage have not revealed evidence of fetal abnormality or impaired fertility. There are no adequate and controlled studies to date using buspirone in pregnant women, and the drug should be used during pregnancy only when clearly needed.

The effect of buspirone on labor and delivery in women is not known, but no adverse effects were observed during reproduction studies in animals.

Although the extent of distribution of buspirone and its metabolites into human milk is not known, the drug and its metabolites are distributed into milk in rats. Therefore, the manufacturer recommends that the use of buspirone in nursing women be avoided whenever clinically possible.

Drug Interactions

■ **Psychotherapeutic Agents** Elevations in blood pressure have been observed in several patients receiving buspirone and a monoamine oxidase (MAO) inhibitor concomitantly; however, no adverse sequelae were associated with these elevations. In addition, buspirone may have been partially responsible for a case of serotonin syndrome that resulted in death of a patient receiving buspirone, fluoxetine, and an MAO inhibitor (tranylcypromine) concomitantly. Pending additional data, it currently is recommended that buspirone not be used concomitantly with an MAO inhibitor and that at least 10 days elapse following discontinuation of an MAO inhibitor and administration of buspirone.

In a patient with depression, generalized anxiety disorder, and panic attacks who was receiving concomitant buspirone and trazodone therapy, an increase in anxiety symptoms to a level comparable to that observed prior to buspirone therapy occurred when fluoxetine was added to the regimen. Although the mechanism of this possible interaction has not been established, it was suggested that fluoxetine may have either directly antagonized the therapeutic activity of buspirone or may have precipitated the anxiety symptoms through a separate mechanism. However, combined use of the drugs also has been reported to potentiate therapeutic efficacy in patients with obsessive compulsive disorder.

Concomitant administration of buspirone and trazodone has resulted in a threefold to sixfold elevation in serum ALT (SGPT) concentrations in a few patients. However, in a study designed to attempt to confirm these findings, concomitant administration of the drugs was *not* associated with an interactive effect on aminotransferases. The manufacturer states that current evidence suggests that buspirone and trazodone can be used concomitantly, provided that liver function is monitored.

Concomitant administration of buspirone and haloperidol has resulted in increased serum haloperidol concentrations. When oral buspirone hydrochloride 45 mg daily and oral haloperidol 5 mg daily were administered concomitantly in healthy adults, peak serum concentrations of haloperidol increased by about 30% and area under the serum concentration-time curve increased by 46%. Buspirone pharmacokinetics were not affected and the increase in haloperidol concentrations was not associated with a substantial increase in adverse haloperidol effects. It has been suggested that buspirone's effect on haloperidol concentrations may have resulted from competitive inhibition of oxidative dealkylation of haloperidol, since both drugs are metabolized principally via this pathway. The manufacturer states that the clinical importance of this interaction has not been established.

Concomitant administration of buspirone hydrochloride 45 mg daily and amitriptyline hydrochloride 75 mg daily in healthy adults did not result in substantial changes in steady-state amitriptyline or nortriptyline (an active metabolite) concentrations. In addition, no increase in amitriptyline-induced adverse effects was observed during concomitant use of the drugs.

Because the effects of concomitant use of buspirone and most other psychotherapeutic agents have not been studied to date, such use should be undertaken with caution.

■ **Protein-bound Drugs** Because buspirone is highly protein bound, it theoretically could be displaced from binding sites by, or could displace from binding sites, other protein-bound drugs. The manufacturer states that therapeutic concentrations of aspirin, desipramine, diazepam, flurazepam, ibuprofen, propranolol, thioridazine, and tolbutamide had only a limited effect on the extent of buspirone binding to plasma proteins. Although an in vitro study indicated that buspirone did not displace some highly protein bound drugs (e.g., phenytoin, propranolol, warfarin), it may displace less firmly bound drugs (e.g., digoxin). In an in vitro protein binding study, aspirin increased free plasma buspirone concentrations by 23%, while flurazepam decreased free plasma buspirone concentrations by 20%, but the in vivo effects of aspirin or flurazepam on free buspirone plasma concentrations, and their clinical importance, are unknown. Also, there has been 1 report of increased prothrombin time when buspirone was added to the drug regimen of a patient receiving warfarin, phenytoin, phenobarbital, digoxin, and levothyroxine (Synthroid®). However, the manufacturer states that the clinical importance of these changes is unknown.

■ **Drugs and Food Affecting Hepatic Microsomal Enzymes** In vitro, metabolism of buspirone has been shown to be mediated by the cytochrome P-450 (CYP) isoenzyme 3A4. Drugs (e.g., erythromycin, itraconazole, nefazodone) that inhibit this enzyme increase plasma concentrations of buspirone, and drugs (e.g., rifampin) that induce this enzyme decrease plasma concentrations of buspirone. Therefore, if buspirone is to be administered concomitantly with a drug that is a potent inhibitor of the CYP3A4 isoenzyme, a low buspirone dosage (e.g., 2.5 mg once or twice daily) is recommended, and subsequent dosage adjustment of either drug should be based on clinical assessment. Alternatively, when buspirone is used concomitantly with a drug that is a potent inducer of the CYP3A4 isoenzyme, dosage adjustment of buspirone may be necessary to maintain the anxiolytic effect.

Erythromycin In a study in healthy individuals, concomitant use of buspirone (10 mg daily) and erythromycin (1.5 g daily) increased peak plasma buspirone concentrations and area under the plasma concentration-time curve (AUC) by fivefold and sixfold, respectively, and was accompanied by an increased incidence of adverse effects attributable to buspirone. Therefore, the manufacturer states that if buspirone is administered concomitantly with erythromycin, a low buspirone dosage (e.g., 2.5 mg twice daily) is recommended, and subsequent dosage adjustment of either drug should be based on clinical assessment.

Itraconazole In a study in healthy individuals, concomitant administration of buspirone (10 mg daily) and itraconazole (200 mg daily) increased peak plasma buspirone concentrations and AUC 13- and 19-fold, respectively, and was accompanied by an increased incidence of adverse effects attributable to buspirone. Therefore, if buspirone is administered concomitantly with itraconazole, a low buspirone dosage (e.g., 2.5 mg once daily) is recommended by the manufacturer, and subsequent dosage adjustment of either drug should be based on clinical assessment.

Nefazodone In a steady-state pharmacokinetics study in healthy individuals, concomitant administration of buspirone (2.5 or 5 mg twice daily) and nefazodone (250 mg twice daily) increased peak plasma buspirone concentrations and AUC 20- and 50-fold, respectively, and substantially decreased buspirone metabolite 1-pyrimidinylpiperazine (1-PP) plasma concentrations by about 50%. Also, AUCs of nefazodone, hydroxynefazodone, and meta-chlorophenylpiperazine were increased by 23, 17, and 9%, respectively, and peak plasma concentrations of nefazodone and hydroxynefazodone were increased by 8 and 11%, in individuals receiving buspirone 5 mg twice daily with nefazodone. In addition, lightheadedness, asthenia, dizziness, and somnolence have been reported in patients receiving buspirone (5 mg twice daily) and nefazodone (250 mg twice daily); these adverse effects also have been reported when either drug was administered alone. Therefore, if buspirone is used concomitantly with nefazodone, a low buspirone dosage (e.g., 2.5 mg once daily) is recommended by the manufacturer, and subsequent dosage adjustment of either drug should be based on clinical assessment.

Calcium-Channel Blocking Agents In a small study in healthy individuals, concomitant administration of buspirone (10 mg as a single dose) with verapamil (80 mg 3 times daily) or diltiazem (60 mg 3 times daily) increased peak plasma concentrations of buspirone by 3.4 or 4-fold, respectively, and increased AUC of buspirone by 3.4- or 5.5-fold, respectively. Because of the increased potential for adverse effects during concomitant use of buspirone with verapamil or diltiazem, the manufacturer suggests that dosage adjustment may be necessary.

Rifampin Administration of a single 30-mg dose of buspirone to healthy individuals receiving rifampin (600 mg daily for 5 days) decreased peak plasma concentrations and AUC of buspirone by 83.7 and 89.6%, respectively. Decreased pharmacodynamic effects also were reported. The manufacturer of buspirone recommends that if the drug used concomitantly with rifampin, dosage adjustment of buspirone may be necessary to maintain anxiolytic effect.

Grapefruit Juice In healthy individuals, concomitant administration of buspirone (10 mg as a single dose) with double-strength grapefruit juice (200 mL administered 3 times daily for 2 days) increased the peak plasma concentration and AUC of the drug by 4.3- and 9.2-fold, respectively. Therefore, the manufacturer states that concomitant administration of buspirone with large quantities of grapefruit juice should be avoided.

■ **Cimetidine** Current limited evidence suggests that concomitant use of usual dosages of buspirone and cimetidine would be unlikely to result in a clinically important interaction. In a study in healthy adults, there was some evidence of cimetidine-induced changes in buspirone pharmacokinetics (e.g., shortened elimination half-life of buspirone, increased peak serum concentrations of buspirone (about 40%) and 1-pyrimidinylpiperazine [1-PP, an active metabolite of buspirone] increased time to achieve peak serum concentrations of buspirone [about twofold]) and an increase in certain adverse buspirone effects (e.g., light-headedness) during combined use, but such changes were not considered clinically important. Because of considerable interindividual and intraindividual differences in some buspirone pharmacokinetic parameters observed in this study and problems in study design, however, some clinicians state that firm conclusions regarding the possibility of a clinically important interaction between buspirone and cimetidine currently cannot be made. The drugs also have been used concomitantly without evidence of a clinically important interaction in patients with anxiety, but additional study is necessary.

■ **Food** Food may delay GI absorption of buspirone, thereby decreasing the extent of presystemic clearance of the drug (e.g., via first-pass metabolism in the liver) and increasing the amount of unchanged drug reaching systemic circulation. Following oral administration of a single 20-mg dose of buspirone hydrochloride with food, the area under the plasma concentration-time curve (AUC) and peak plasma concentration of unchanged buspirone increased by 84 and 116%, respectively, compared with administration in the fasted state, but the total amount of drug (changed and unchanged) in plasma was not affected. To minimize the variability in systemic exposure to buspirone, the manufacturer recommends that the drug should be given consistently with or without food.

■ **Alcohol** Buspirone does not appear to alter blood alcohol concentrations nor to potentiate substantially alcohol-induced impairment of psychomotor and cognitive performance, and actually may produce some improvement in such impairment. In addition, patients receiving buspirone and alcohol may be more aware of alcohol-induced impairment, when present, than those receiving benzodiazepines and alcohol. It should be recognized, however, that subjective adverse effects, including fatigue, drowsiness, and dizziness, have occurred in some patients during administration of buspirone alone, and that adverse CNS effects associated with buspirone in individual patients may be unpredictable. In a controlled study in healthy adults, buspirone did not enhance alcohol-induced psychomotor impairment (as determined by objective measures such as lateral-gaze nystagmus, body sway, and the Maddox wing test), and subjective effects associated with concomitant buspirone and alcohol use were similar to those with buspirone alone. In another study in patients with a history of moderate to low-heavy alcohol use, driving-related motor skill performance was better in those given a single dose of alcohol after receiving buspirone for 9 days than in those given alcohol after receiving placebo. Although results of drug interaction studies suggest that buspirone does not potentiate substantially alcohol-induced psychomotor and cognitive impairment, patients should be advised that it would be prudent to avoid concomitant use.

■ **Other CNS Depressants** Buspirone appears to interact minimally, if at all, with benzodiazepines. In a multiple-dose study, the addition of buspirone in patients receiving diazepam for 11 days did not substantially alter plasma diazepam concentrations measured on day 22 (11 days after initiating buspirone therapy), but corresponding plasma nordiazepam concentrations increased by approximately 20%. It is not known whether the increase in nordiazepam concentrations resulted from the relatively long time required for the metabolite to achieve steady-state plasma concentrations or from concomitant buspirone administration. In patients concurrently receiving buspirone and diazepam, mild adverse effects, including headache, nausea, dizziness, and muscle twitches, occurred but usually subsided within several days; however, such effects, except muscle twitches, appeared qualitatively similar to those associated with buspirone alone. Buspirone has potentiated the effects of diazepam on several tests of psychomotor function (e.g., the Maddox wing and letter cancellation tests) and has subjectively potentiated diazepam-induced sedation, but the drug also has counteracted diazepam-induced impairment of divided attention and learning acquisition; the combined effect of these drugs on psychomotor function did not appear to be more harmful than diazepam alone. Buspirone did not substantially alter the hypnotic or psychomotor effects of either flurazepam or triazolam when the drugs were administered concurrently in a limited number of patients, although a minimal decrease in card-sorting ability occurred in some patients. Although drug interaction studies suggest that buspirone does not potentiate benzodiazepine-induced CNS depression to a clinically important degree, the effects of combined therapy have not been fully evaluated to date. Pending further accumulation of data, benzodiazepines should be used with caution in patients receiving buspirone.

Data obtained from clinical studies indicate that other CNS depressants, including analgesics, antihistamines, and sedative/hypnotics, generally have little or no effect on the frequency or severity of adverse effects associated with buspirone. It should be recognized, however, that subjective adverse effects, including fatigue, drowsiness, and dizziness, have been reported in some patients receiving buspirone alone, and that adverse CNS effects associated with buspirone in individual patients may be unpredictable. Because the effects of concurrent administration have not been fully evaluated to date, caution should be exercised when buspirone and CNS depressants are administered concomitantly.

Acute Toxicity

Limited information is available on the acute toxicity of buspirone.

■ **Pathogenesis** The acute lethal dose of buspirone in humans is not known. The oral LD_{50} of the drug is 655, 196, 586, and 356 mg/kg in mice, rats, dogs, and monkeys, respectively.

■ **Manifestations** A few cases of overdosage of buspirone have been reported; usually, all patients had complete recovery and no fatalities have been reported after overdosage of buspirone alone. In general, overdosage of buspirone may be expected to produce effects that are mainly extensions of pharmacologic and adverse effects. In clinical pharmacology studies in healthy adults, nausea, vomiting, dizziness, drowsiness, miosis, and gastric distension predominated as oral dosage approached 375 mg daily.

■ **Treatment** There is no specific antidote for buspirone intoxication, and treatment of overdosage with the drug generally involves symptomatic and supportive care. Following acute ingestion of buspirone, the stomach should be emptied immediately by inducing emesis or by gastric lavage. If the patient is comatose, having seizures, or lacks the gag reflex, gastric lavage may be performed if an endotracheal tube with cuff inflated is in place to prevent aspiration of gastric contents. Pulse, blood pressure, and respiration should be monitored.

Chronic Toxicity

Buspirone appears to have little, if any, potential for tolerance or psychologic and/or physical dependence. In animal studies, there was no evidence of abuse potential or dependence liability. In studies in individuals with a history of recreational drug or chronic alcohol abuse, single 10-mg buspirone hydrochloride doses were neither euphoric nor dysphoric, and the drug's effects were indistinguishable from placebo. In addition, such individuals preferred methaqualone or diazepam to buspirone and experienced dysphoria and other unpleasant effects when single 40-mg buspirone hydrochloride doses were administered. Dysphoria also has occurred in healthy nonabusers during initiation of buspirone hydrochloride 20 mg daily. The dysphoric potential of buspirone and absence of euphoria observed in these individuals indicates that the drug has little, if any, abuse potential. However, it is difficult to predict from animal and human studies the extent to which a CNS-active drug like buspirone will be misused, diverted, and/or abused once it is marketed, and additional long-term experience is necessary to confirm findings of these studies.

There has been no substantial evidence to date of a withdrawal syndrome associated with sudden discontinuance of buspirone therapy. Discontinuance of the drug after 6 or 12 weeks of 5–20 mg daily in patients with anxiety disorders was not associated with manifestations suggestive of withdrawal. In addition, substantial evidence of rebound anxiety or withdrawal was not observed following abrupt discontinuance of buspirone therapy in patients with anxiety disorders receiving an average of 27 mg of the drug daily for 6 months, although manifestations of withdrawal occurred following discontinuance of 6 months of clorazepate dipotassium at an average dosage of 33 mg daily. There also was no evidence of resorting to a reserve supply of drug, intended to counter serious or intolerable symptoms, following abrupt discontinuance of buspirone, while 40% of patients receiving clorazepate required doses of the benzodiazepine following discontinuance.

Despite the absence of substantial evidence for abuse potential or dependence liability, clinicians should carefully evaluate patients for a history of substance abuse prior to initiating buspirone therapy. If buspirone is initiated in patients with a history of substance abuse, they should be monitored closely for signs of misuse or abuse of the drug (e.g., development of tolerance, use of increasing doses, drug-seeking behavior). In addition, it should be recognized that the potential for developing withdrawal following abrupt discontinuance of high dosages of buspirone hydrochloride (e.g., greater than 40 mg daily) or after prolonged therapy (e.g., longer than 6 months) has not been fully elucidated, and additional experience with chronic buspirone therapy is necessary.

Pharmacology

■ **Nervous System Effects** The principal pharmacologic effect of buspirone is anxiolysis. Buspirone has been described as an anxioselective drug since, unlike benzodiazepines, it has no anticonvulsant or muscle relaxantac-tivity, does not substantially impair psychomotor function, and has little sedative effect. Buspirone's anxiolytic potency is approximately equivalent to that of diazepam on a weight basis following oral administration.

The precise mechanism of buspirone's anxiolytic action is not known but appears to be complex and distinct from benzodiazepines, and probably involves several central neurotransmitter systems. Likewise, a variety of sites in the CNS have been postulated as contributing to the anxiolytic action of the drug. Because of the variety and location of the drug's effects on central neurotransmitter systems, including serotonergic, dopaminergic, cholinergic, and noradrenergic (α-adrenergic) systems, buspirone has been described as a midbrain modulator.

Buspirone has no appreciable affinity for the benzodiazepine receptor complex, nor does it inhibit or stimulate benzodiazepine binding at the receptor complex in vitro, although binding may be stimulated in vivo. Buspirone also does not appear to directly affect γ-aminobutyric acid (GABA) binding in vitro or in vivo. In vitro radioligand studies indicate that buspirone does not *directly* affect cholinergic (muscarinic), α-adrenergic, type 2 serotonergic (5-HT_2), β-adrenergic, histamine (H_1 or H_2), opiate, adenosine (A_1 or A_2), glutamate, or glycine receptors or uptake of dopamine, GABA, norepinephrine, or serotonin. The drug does exhibit high affinity for type 1 serotonergic (5-HT_1) receptors and moderate affinity for dopamine D_2 receptors in vitro.

Serotonergic Effects The contribution of the serotonergic system to anxiety has not been fully characterized, and the extent to which the anxiolytic action of buspirone might depend on this neurotransmitter system has not been fully elucidated. It has been suggested that serotonergic mechanisms may play a predominant role in the drug's anxiolytic activity; however, because of conflicting evidence, additional study is needed to establish the role of serotonergic receptors in mediating anxiolysis. The anticonflict effect of the drug has been shown to be reduced in serotonin-depleted animals. In addition, buspirone has been shown to inhibit spontaneous firing of serotonergic neurons in the dorsal raphe nucleus, an effect that also is exhibited by benzodiazepines and may be related to anxiolytic activity, and to inhibit stress-induced renin secretion that is mediated by serotonin.

Buspirone has a high affinity for 5-HT_1 receptors in the CNS, and appears to have a higher relative affinity for the 5-HT_{1A} site on this receptor than for the 5-HT_{1B} site. Buspirone appears to act as a partial agonist or mixed agonist/antagonist at this receptor, and there is some evidence to suggest that such activity may be associated with anxiolysis. Although buspirone has failed to induce the serotonin behavioral syndrome in some animal studies, the drug has exhibited agonist properties by inducing the syndrome in other studies that focused on 5-HT_1- rather than 5-HT_2-mediated behaviors; differences in methodology and interpretation and lack of insight regarding characterization of serotonin receptor subtypes and associated behaviors likely contributed to these discrepancies. It also has been suggested that agonist activity at the 5-HT_{1A} receptor may be associated with antidepressant activity.

Reports of buspirone's effects on serotonin metabolism have been conflicting. The drug has been reported to decrease or have no effect on striatal concentrations of serotonin and its principal metabolite, 5-hydroxyindoleacetic acid (5-HIAA), to decrease or have no effect on hippocampal serotonin and 5-HIAA concentrations, and to decrease serotonin but not 5-HIAA concentrations in the frontal cortex.

Dopaminergic Effects The effects of buspirone on the dopaminergic neurotransmitter system are complex and have not been clearly elucidated. The drug appears to possess mixed dopamine agonist and antagonist activities. Buspirone may act as an agonist at postsynaptic dopamine receptor sites and as an antagonist at both presynaptic autoreceptor and postsynaptic sites. The relative contribution of these effects to the anxiolytic activity and toxic potential of the drug has not been clearly established and requires additional study.

Buspirone has moderate affinity for dopamine D_2 receptors in the CNS. Unlike most antipsychotic agents, buspirone appears to preferentially block presynaptic dopamine autoreceptors rather than postsynaptic D_2 receptors in the striatum. The resultant buspirone-induced increases in dopamine metabolism and impulse formation, however, appear to resemble those of antipsychotic agents. The drug reportedly stimulates dopamine metabolism in a dose-related manner, and has increased striatal concentrations of the dopamine metabolites, 3-methoxy-4-hydroxyphenylacetic acid (homovanillic acid, HVA) and 3,4-dihydroxyphenylacetic acid (DOPAC). Buspirone also has been reported to increase tyrosine 3-monooxygenase (tyrosine hydroxylase) activity in the striatum but not in the frontal cortex, which appears to lack autoreceptors, and has blocked apomorphine-induced inhibition of this enzyme. Unlike benzodiazepines but like butyrophenones (e.g., haloperidol), buspirone enhances spontaneous firing of dopaminergic neurons. Such effects on dopamine metabolism and impulse flow are consistent with presynaptic autoreceptor blockade.

There is some evidence from animal studies that buspirone may act as an antagonist at postsynaptic D_2 receptors and potentially may possess antipsychotic activity; the drug has inhibited conditioned avoidance behavior, blocked apomorphine-induced stereotypy and emesis, and blocked amphetamine-induced stereotypy. However, unlike most antipsychotic agents, buspirone does not induce catalepsy in animals, indicating that the drug may not produce substantial postsynaptic D_2 blockade usually associated with antipsychotic activity. Although buspirone reportedly has produced transient antipsychotic effects when administered in large dosages (e.g., 600–2400 mg daily) to humans, the drug has no established clinical antipsychotic efficacy at usual anxiolytic dosages. The failure of buspirone to induce catalepsy in animal studies also suggests that the risk of drug-induced extrapyramidal reactions is minimal. No definitive extrapyramidal reactions have been attributed directly to buspirone therapy at usual anxiolytic dosages to date, although such reactions (e.g., akathisia, hypertonia, dystonia, tremor) reportedly have been associated with anxiolytic therapy with the drug in a few patients and also have occurred in at least one patient receiving a large dosage for potential antipsychotic effects. Unlike most antipsychotic agents, buspirone does not produce postsynaptic receptor supersensitivity following long-term therapy and has reversed such supersensitivity induced by antipsychotic agents; therefore, the drug appears unlikely to produce tardive dyskinesia. However, additional clinical experience is needed to determine buspirone's potential for inducing dopamine-mediated neurologic sequelae with long-term use. (See Cautions: Nervous System Effects and also Precautions and Contraindications.) Buspirone has been shown to produce a dose-dependent elevation in plasma prolactin concentrations (see Neuroendocrine Effects), possibly mediated by postsynaptic dopamine receptor blockade in the pituitary gland.

Buspirone appears to possess some dopamine agonist activity. Like apomorphine, buspirone produces weak turning behavior in lesioned animals and, like amantadine, potently reverses catalepsy induced by antipsychotic agents, suggesting that the drug has some dopamine agonist activity. Buspirone reportedly elevates plasma somatotropin (growth hormone) concentrations (see Neuroendocrine Effects), an effect possibly mediated by postsynaptic dopamine agonist activity in the hypothalamus.

Effects on GABA and the Benzodiazepine Receptor Complex Buspirone has no appreciable affinity for the GABA-benzodiazepine-chloride ionophore receptor complex, and does not appear to inhibit or stimulate binding of benzodiazepines at the receptor complex in vitro, although binding may be stimulated in vivo. It is not known whether the increase in in vivo benzodiazepine binding observed in some studies reflects a change in the number of binding sites or an increase in receptor affinity. Buspirone does not appear to directly affect GABA binding in vitro or in vivo, and does not influence uptake of GABA. Benzodiazepine antagonists do not appear to block the anticonflict action of buspirone, suggesting that the drug does not exert its anxiolytic effect by directly affecting benzodiazepine receptors.

Buspirone or an active metabolite may indirectly affect some component of the GABA-benzodiazepine-chloride ionophore receptor complex other than the benzodiazepine or GABA binding site, such as picrotoxin-sensitive chloride ionophore segments. It has been suggested that the drug may have a picrotoxin-like antagonistic effect on presynaptic GABA receptors, thereby enhancing GABA transmission; however, inhibitory effects of GABA on impulse flow do not appear to be altered by the drug. Further study is required to determine whether there is an association between buspirone's effects on the benzodiazepine receptor complex and the anticonflict and anxiolytic actions of the drug.

Adrenergic Effects Buspirone does not appear to have a direct effect on α_1-, α_2-, or β-adrenergic receptors in vitro, and has no apparent effect on biogenic amine uptake, including norepinephrine. The drug does, however, appear to exhibit weak central α-adrenergic blocking activity in vivo. Limited evidence suggests that 1-pyrimidinylpiperazine (1-PP), a metabolite of buspirone, possesses central and peripheral α_2-adrenergic blocking activity, which may contribute to the drug's anxiolytic and/or antidepressant effects. Unlike benzodiazepines, which inhibit spontaneous firing of noradrenergic neurons in the locus ceruleus and decrease norepinephrine metabolism in the brain, buspirone and its metabolite 1-PP enhance neuronal activity in the locus ceruleus and increase norepinephrine metabolism, suggesting that a reduction in locus ceruleus output is not a prerequisite for anxiolytic activity. It has been suggested that buspirone-induced facilitation of noradrenergic neuronal firing may contribute to alertness and alleviate any benzodiazepine-like impairment of psychomotor performance, thereby preserving arousal and attentional processes. The drug has been shown to decrease striatal concentrations of norepinephrine and to increase striatal concentrations of 3-methoxy-4-hydroxyethylenephenylglycol (MOPEG, MHPG), a major metabolite of norepinephrine. The drug does not appear to alter monoamine oxidase (MAO_A or MAO_B) activity.

Cholinergic Effects Buspirone does not appear to directly affect cholinergic receptors, but the drug's effects on the cholinergic neurotransmitter system and their relationship with the dopaminergic neurotransmitter system have not been fully elucidated to date. Like antipsychotic agents but unlike benzodiazepines, the drug decreases striatal concentrations of acetylcholine; the activity of acetylcholinesterase or choline acetyltransferase does not appear to be affected. There is some evidence that buspirone-induced decreases in acetylcholine concentrations may be dopaminergically mediated. The drug has enhanced the effects of cholinergic agonists on cholinergically induced catalepsy when administered at doses that decrease striatal acetylcholine concentrations. Buspirone does not protect against physostigmine-induced lethality in animals and appears to lack clinically important anticholinergic activity in humans.

Effects on Sleep Buspirone does not appear to possess clinically important sedative/hypnotic activity. At usual anxiolytic dosages, the drug does not appear to affect sleep (e.g., sleep pattern or efficiency, total wake time, number of awakenings) substantially in patients with mild or chronic insomnia but without underlying anxiety, although decreased total rapid eye movement (REM) time and increased REM onset time may occur. In anxious patients, buspirone may produce subjective improvement in quality of sleep, secondary to the drug's anxiolytic action, without accompanying hypnotic and/or sedative effects. In animals, buspirone has increased sleep latency and total sleep time while decreasing both REM and nonREM sleep. Although not clearly established, the increase in wakefulness and decrease in sleep observed in animals may be serotonergically mediated, since the drug has been shown to inhibit firing of serotonergic neurons in the dorsal raphe nucleus.

Other Nervous System Effects Unlike benzodiazepines, buspirone produces anxiolysis without causing substantial impairment of psychomotor function or sedation. In addition, buspirone lacks anticonvulsant activity and appears to have little effect on the EEG. The drug has increased fast-wave activity slightly at a dosage of 15 mg daily and decreased fast-wave activity at 30 mg daily, but these changes were not considered clinically important.

■ **Neuroendocrine Effects** Buspirone appears to cause a dose-related increase in prolactin secretion, possibly via postsynaptic dopamine receptor blockade in the pituitary gland. The drug has increased plasma prolactin concentrations at single oral doses ranging from 25–100 mg, but substantial alterations in prolactin secretion were not apparent at lower doses. Long-term oral administration of buspirone hydrochloride at a dosage of 30 mg daily also does not appear to be associated with substantial alterations in prolactin secretion.

Buspirone can increase plasma somatotropin (growth hormone) concentrations, an effect possibly mediated by postsynaptic dopamine agonist activity in the hypothalamus. Single 30- to 90-mg oral doses of the drug have been associated with substantial, although not dose-related, increases in somatotropin concentrations; substantial alterations were not apparent at lower doses. Long-term oral administration of buspirone hydrochloride dosages of 30 mg daily also does not appear to be associated with substantial alterations in plasma somatotropin concentrations.

■ **Cardiovascular Effects** Buspirone appears to cause minimal cardiovascular effects when administered at usual anxiolytic dosages. (See Cautions: Cardiovascular Effects.) Clinically important ECG changes and changes in vital signs generally do not occur during therapy with the drug. Tachycardia and/or palpitation and nonspecific chest pain have been reported in some patients receiving buspirone, although a causal relationship has not been established. Buspirone possesses only weak α_1-adrenergic blocking activity and therefore is not expected to cause clinically important hypotension. In addition, although limited evidence in animals receiving high doses of the drug suggests that buspirone may possess some peripheral vascular postsynaptic α_1-adrenergic agonist activity, clinically important cardiovascular effects do not appear likely at usual anxiolytic doses.

■ **Other Effects** Limited data from healthy adults receiving single, 10-mg oral doses suggest that buspirone does not substantially depress the ventilatory response to carbon dioxide (CO_2) stimulation; however, additional study is necessary to more fully determine the drug's effects on respiration.

Pharmacokinetics

The pharmacokinetics of buspirone hydrochloride have been studied in healthy adults, geriatric patients, and in patients with renal or hepatic impairment. Single- and multiple-dose studies of buspirone have not revealed gender- or age-related differences in the pharmacokinetics (e.g., area under the plasma-concentration time curve [AUC], peak plasma concentrations) of the drug. Pharmacokinetics of buspirone hydrochloride with respect to race have not been determined.

■ **Absorption** Buspirone hydrochloride is rapidly and almost completely absorbed from the GI tract. However, the drug undergoes extensive first-pass metabolism, with only about 4% (range: 1.5–13%) of a dose reaching systemic circulation unchanged following oral administration. The relative oral bioavailability of buspirone hydrochloride tablets reportedly is about 90% that of a solution of the drug; a lower relative bioavailability (i.e., 65%) has been reported for another tablet formulation of the drug that is *not* commercially available. Food may delay GI absorption of buspirone hydrochloride, thereby decreasing the extent of presystemic clearance of the drug and increasing the amount of unchanged buspirone reaching systemic circulation. (See Drug Interactions: Food.) Following multiple-dose administration of buspirone in patients with renal impairment (creatinine clearance of 10–70 mL/minute per 1.73 m^2), the steady-state AUC was increased fourfold compared with healthy adults (creatinine clearance of 80 mL/minute per 1.73 m^2 or more). Following multiple-dose administration in patients with hepatic impairment, steady-state AUC of buspirone was increased 13-fold compared with healthy adults. AUC and peak plasma concentration of unchanged buspirone are increased substantially in patients with liver cirrhosis, exceeding those achieved in healthy adults by about 16-fold in one study following a single, 20-mg oral dose.

Following oral administration of a single 20-mg dose in healthy individuals, peak plasma buspirone concentrations of 1–6 ng/mL occur within 40–90 minutes. Peak plasma concentrations of the drug averaged 0.9, 1.7, and 3.2 ng/mL following single oral doses of 10, 20, and 40 mg, respectively, in a study in healthy adults. Plasma concentrations of unchanged buspirone exhibit interindividual variation following oral administration of the drug but generally are low, averaging about 1% of the total plasma drug concentration in one study in fasting, healthy adults receiving single doses of the drug. Although it has been suggested that the drug exhibits nonlinear pharmacokinetics and that increasing and/or multiple doses may result in higher plasma concentrations than those predicted from single-dose studies, this interpretation of the drug's pharmacokinetics has been questioned. In addition, in a study in healthy adults, the relationship between plasma buspirone concentration and dose appeared to be linear at single oral doses ranging from 10–40 mg. Following oral administration of buspirone hydrochloride, the onset of anxiolytic activity may be apparent within the first 2 weeks of therapy, but optimum therapeutic effect usually requires at least 3–4 weeks; occasionally, 4–6 weeks may be required for optimum effect. The relationship, if any, between plasma buspirone and active metabolite concentrations and the therapeutic and/or toxic effects of the drug have not been established.

■ **Distribution** Distribution of buspirone into human body tissues and fluids has not been well characterized. Following IV administration in rats, buspirone is extensively distributed, achieving highest concentrations in lung, kidney, and adipose tissue, and lower concentrations in skeletal muscle, heart, liver, brain, and plasma. The concentration-time curve profiles of buspirone and its active metabolite 1-pyrimidinylpiperazine (1-PP) in brain almost parallel those in plasma after oral or IV administration, although 1-PP concentrations generally are higher in brain than in plasma, particularly following oral administration of the drug. In animals, 1-PP accumulates in the brain and reaches concentrations that are approximately 4–5 times higher than those in plasma. The apparent volume of distribution of buspirone in healthy adults reportedly averages 5.3 L/kg following a single IV dose.

Buspirone is approximately 86–95% bound to plasma proteins in vitro, mainly to albumin and, to a lesser extent, α_1-acid glycoprotein (α_1-AGP).

Buspirone and its metabolites are distributed into milk in animals. It is not known whether the drug distributes into milk in humans.

■ **Elimination** Following single oral doses of 10–40 mg in healthy adults, the elimination half-life of buspirone averages about 2–4 hours (range: 2–11 hours). The elimination half-life of the drug appears to be slightly longer in females than in males, although the clinical importance of this difference has not been established. The elimination half-life does not appear to be affected by increases in dose or by concomitant administration with food, but may be prolonged in patients with renal impairment, particularly those with anuria, and in patients with liver impairment, including those with cirrhosis. In a limited number of patients with mild to moderate renal impairment (creatinine clearances of 60 mL/minute or less per 1.73 m^2) or with anuria, the buspirone elimination half-life averaged 5.7 or 6.1 hours, respectively, while it averaged 4 hours in healthy individuals. Elimination half-life of the drug averaged 6.1 hours in a limited number of patients with liver cirrhosis following oral administration.

Buspirone is metabolized extensively in the liver, mainly via oxidation by the cytochrome P-450 (CYP) isoenzyme 3A4, to form several hydroxylated metabolites, including 5-hydroxybuspirone (5-HB) and 1-pyrimidinylpiperazine (1-PP). 5-Hydroxybuspirone is further oxidized to at least 2 additional hydroxy metabolites, which subsequently undergo conjugation. Following oral administration of a single 20-mg dose of buspirone hydrochloride in healthy adults, the elimination half-lives of 1-PP, 5-HB, and the glucuronide of 5-HB have been reported to average about 6.1, 4.8, and 3.2 hours, respectively.

The major pharmacologically active metabolite is 1-PP. In animals, 1-PP has about 20–25% of the anxiolytic activity of buspirone but is present in the brain in concentrations up to 15-to 30-fold greater than those of unchanged drug. In humans, however, blood concentrations of 1-PP remain relatively low even after chronic administration of buspirone, and the contribution of this metabolite to the pharmacologic and/or toxic effects of the drug has not been fully elucidated. In one study, blood 1-PP concentrations reportedly averaged 3 ng/mL during chronic oral administration and did not exceed 17 ng/mL, which is less than 0.5% of the 1-PP concentrations found in animals that were given large doses (50–200 mg/kg) of buspirone hydrochloride without exhibiting signs of toxicity. Unlike buspirone, 1-PP does not affect the dopaminergic system but does appear to possess some α_2-adrenergic blocking activity, which may contribute to buspirone's anxiolytic and/or antidepressant effects.

Buspirone and its metabolites are excreted principally in urine and, to a lesser extent, in feces. About 29–63% of a single oral dose of the drug is excreted in urine and about 18–38% in feces within 24 hours, mainly as metabolites. Buspirone appears to be excreted in urine almost completely as metabolites, with less than 0.1% of the total oral dose being excreted as unchanged drug. Fecal excretion of the drug appears to occur via biliary secretion.

Following IV administration in healthy adults, total body clearance of buspirone from plasma averaged approximately 28 mL/minute per kg. Limited data suggest that elimination of unchanged buspirone is not altered substantially in patients undergoing hemodialysis, although plasma concentrations and elimination half-life of 1-PP may be reduced. The reduced clearance of 1-PP observed in anuric patients with chronic renal failure appears to be only partly reversed by hemodialysis. It is not known whether buspirone and/or its metabolites are removed by peritoneal dialysis.

Chemistry and Stability

■ **Chemistry** Buspirone hydrochloride is an azaspirodecanedione-derivative anxiolytic agent. The drug also has been referred to as an arylpiperazine derivative. Buspirone differs structurally and pharmacologically from benzodiazepines, barbiturates, and other currently available anxiolytic agents. The heteroaryl piperazine nature of buspirone appears to be responsible for the drug's anxiolytic activity, serotonergic effects, and dopamine antagonist properties. Presence of the pyrimidinylpiperazine moiety as the heteroaryl component of buspirone's structure appears to be an important structural feature for the drug's anxiolytic activity and serotonergic effects, which may be related, and presence of this moiety also may contribute to the drug's relative lack of antipsychotic activity. Susceptibility of the drug to rapid and extensive 5-hydroxylation in vivo also may contribute to the relative lack of antipsychotic activity. Binding of the drug to dopamine receptors appears to depend on presence of the pyrimidinylpiperazine moiety, which can bind at several primary sites of the receptors, and on the azaspirodecanedione moiety, which can bind at a lipophilic accessory site of the receptors.

Buspirone hydrochloride occurs as a white, crystalline powder and has solubilities of greater than 865 mg/mL in water and approximately 20 mg/mL in alcohol at 25°C. The manufacturer states that the drug has pK_as of 1.22 and 7.32.

■ **Stability** Buspirone hydrochloride tablets should be stored in tight, light-resistant containers at a temperature less than 30°C and have an expiration date of 36 months following the date of manufacture.

Preparations

Excipients in commercially available drug preparations may have clinically important effects in some individuals; consult specific product labeling for details.

busPIRone Hydrochloride

Oral		
Tablets	5 mg*	**BuSpar®** (scored), Bristol-Myers Squibb
		busPIRone Hydrochloride Tablets (scored)
	7.5 mg*	**busPIRone Hydrochloride Tablets**
	10 mg*	**BuSpar®** (multi-scored), Bristol-Myers Squibb
		busPIRone Hydrochloride Tablets (scored)
	15 mg*	**BuSpar® Dividose** (scored), Bristol-Myers Squibb
		busPIRone Hydrochloride Tablets (multi-scored)
	30 mg*	**BuSpar® Dividose** (multi-scored), Bristol-Myers Squibb
		busPIRone Hydrochloride Tablets (multi-scored)

*available from one or more manufacturer, distributor, and/or repackager by generic (nonproprietary) name

†Use is not currently included in the labeling approved by the US Food and Drug Administration

Eszopiclone

■ Eszopiclone, the *S*-enantiomer of zopiclone (not commercially available in the US), is a sedative and hypnotic agent structurally unrelated to the benzodiazepines.

Uses

■ **Insomnia** Eszopiclone is used as a hypnotic agent in the management of transient and chronic insomnia. In controlled clinical studies, eszopiclone reportedly has been shown to have continued efficacy in decreasing sleep latency, improving sleep maintenance, and prolonging total sleep time when administered nightly for periods up to 6 months in duration.

Efficacy of eszopiclone for the management of transient insomnia was established in a controlled study in adults experiencing such insomnia during the first night in a sleep laboratory. In this study, 2- and 3-mg doses of eszopiclone were superior to placebo on the polysomnographic parameters of latency to persistent sleep (LPS) and wake time after sleep onset (WASO). Individuals receiving the 3-mg dose, but not those receiving the 2-mg dose, experienced substantially fewer awakenings than did individuals receiving placebo. Residual daytime psychomotor and/or cognitive impairment, as rated on a visual analog scale for morning sleepiness and assessed objectively using the Digit Symbol Substitution test (DSST), appeared to be minimal at eszopiclone doses of 3 mg or less. At such doses, sleep architecture (i.e., the percentage of time spent in each sleep stage) generally was preserved.

Efficacy of eszopiclone for the management of chronic insomnia was established in 5 controlled studies of up to 6 months' duration, including 3 studies in adults and 2 in geriatric patients. Results of these studies indicate that usual doses of eszopiclone (i.e., 2–3 mg in adults and 1–2 mg in geriatric patients) substantially decrease sleep latency; however, only the 3-mg dose in adults and the 2-mg dose in geriatric patients were superior to placebo on measures of sleep maintenance (e.g., WASO). Pharmacodynamic tolerance and adaptation to the hypnotic effect of eszopiclone were not observed during 6 months of therapy with the drug. Evidence to suggest, however, that such sleep improvements are maintained following discontinuance of eszopiclone is currently lacking. Consequently, some clinicians suggest that use of hypnotic agents in the management of chronic insomnia should be reserved for patients who do not respond to psychotherapy/behavioral therapies (e.g., relaxation techniques, sleep hygiene education, sleep curtailment, stimulus control therapy).

For additional information on the management of insomnia, see Uses: Anxiety and Insomnia, in the Benzodiazepines General Statement 28:24.08.

Dosage and Administration

■ **Administration** Eszopiclone is administered orally at bedtime. The drug should be taken immediately before retiring and only when the patient is able to get 7–8 hours of sleep before it is necessary to be active again.

Eszopiclone should not be administered with or immediately after a meal; administration with or immediately after a heavy, high-fat meal results in a decreased rate of absorption of eszopiclone and would be expected to decrease the drug's effect on sleep latency.

■ **Dosage** Dosage of eszopiclone should be individualized, and the lowest effective dosage should be used in all patient populations.

For the management of insomnia, the recommended initial adult dosage of eszopiclone is 1 mg immediately before bedtime. The recommended initial dosage is the same for women and men. If clinically indicated, dosage may be increased to 2 or 3 mg immediately before bedtime.

The dosage range of 2–3 mg has been shown to be effective in decreasing sleep latency and improving measures of sleep maintenance in adults younger than 65 years of age. However, in some patients, the 2- or 3-mg dose may produce higher morning blood concentrations of eszopiclone, resulting in an increased risk of next-day impairment of driving and other activities that require full alertness. (See CNS Depressant Effects and Next-day Impairment under Warnings/Precautions: Other Warnings and Precautions, in Cautions.) The adult dosage of eszopiclone should not exceed 3 mg immediately before bedtime.

■ **Special Populations** In geriatric or debilitated patients, the recommended initial dosage of eszopiclone is 1 mg immediately before bedtime. If clinically indicated, dosage may be increased to 2 mg immediately before bedtime. The dosage range of 1–2 mg has been shown to be effective in decreasing sleep latency and improving measures of sleep maintenance in geriatric patients. Dosage of eszopiclone in geriatric or debilitated patients should not exceed 2 mg immediately before bedtime.

In patients receiving a potent inhibitor of cytochrome P-450 (CYP) isoenzyme 3A4, dosage of eszopiclone should not exceed 2 mg immediately before bedtime. (See Inhibitors of CYP3A4 under Drug Interactions: Drugs Affecting Hepatic Microsomal Enzymes.)

Dosage adjustment is not necessary in patients with mild to moderate hepatic impairment. However, in patients with severe hepatic impairment, dosage of eszopiclone should not exceed 2 mg immediately before bedtime.

No eszopiclone dosage adjustment is necessary in patients with renal impairment.

Cautions

■ **Contraindications** Eszopiclone is contraindicated in patients who have previously experienced an episode of complex sleep behavior while taking eszopiclone, zaleplon, or zolpidem. (See Risk of Serious Injury and Death Resulting From Complex Sleep Behaviors under Warnings/Precautions: Warnings, in Cautions.)

Eszopiclone also is contraindicated in patients with known hypersensitivity (e.g., anaphylaxis, angioedema) to eszopiclone or any ingredient in the formulation.

■ **Warnings/Precautions** ***Warnings*** **Risk of Serious Injury and Death Resulting From Complex Sleep Behaviors.** Complex sleep behaviors in which patients engage in activities while they are not fully awake, sometimes resulting in serious injuries and/or death, have been reported rarely following use of the sedative and hypnotic agents eszopiclone, zaleplon, and zolpidem. Such behaviors may include sleepwalking, sleep driving (i.e., driving while not fully awake after ingesting a sedative-hypnotic drug, with no memory of the event), and engaging in other activities (e.g., making phone calls, preparing and eating food) while not fully awake. In April 2019, FDA issued a drug safety communication requiring that a boxed warning be added to the prescribing information and medication guides of these 3 drugs to alert clinicians and patients of this risk, as well as a contraindication to avoid use in patients who previously experienced an episode of complex sleep behavior with eszopiclone, zaleplon, or zolpidem.

FDA has identified 66 cases of complex sleep behaviors resulting in serious injuries or death in patients who took eszopiclone, zaleplon, or zolpidem that were reported to the FDA Adverse Event Reporting System (FAERS) database and/or in published literature between December 1992 and March 2018. Of the 66 cases, 20 were reported as resulting in fatal outcomes and 46 reported serious nonfatal injuries; in the nonfatal cases, patients usually did not remember experiencing these complex sleep behaviors. These cases included falls with serious injuries such as intracranial hemorrhages, vertebral fractures, and hip fractures as well as fatal falls, self-injuries, accidental overdoses, hypothermia, suicide attempts and apparent completed suicides, fatal motor vehicle collisions, gunshot wounds, carbon monoxide poisoning, drowning or near drowning, burns, and homicide. Most of the patients in these cases reported using zolpidem (about 92%) when they experienced the complex sleep behavior; the remaining patients took eszopiclone (about 5%) or zaleplon (about 3%), reflecting the higher number of zolpidem prescriptions that were dispensed over this period compared with eszopiclone and zaleplon. The underlying mechanisms by which these drugs cause complex sleep behaviors are not fully understood.

FDA states that serious injuries and fatalities from complex sleep behaviors have occurred in patients with and without a history of such behaviors and can occur even at the lowest recommended dosages and after just one dose of eszopiclone, zaleplon, and zolpidem. These behaviors can occur when these drugs are taken alone or when taken with alcohol or other CNS depressants. Patients should be warned about this risk and advised to discontinue taking these drugs if they experience an episode of complex sleep behavior. (See Cautions: Contraindications and see also Advice to Patients.)

Other Warnings and Precautions **Hypersensitivity Reactions.** Angioedema involving the tongue, glottis, or larynx has occurred rarely following initial or subsequent doses of sedative and hypnotic drugs, including eszopiclone; airway obstruction may occur and may be fatal. Other symptoms suggestive of anaphylaxis (e.g., dyspnea, throat closing, nausea, vomiting) also have occurred. Medical therapy in the emergency department has been required in some patients.

Patients who develop angioedema following treatment with eszopiclone should not be rechallenged with the drug.

CNS Depressant Effects and Next-day Impairment. CNS depressant effects (i.e., memory impairment, confusion) have been reported in patients receiving higher doses of eszopiclone. In clinical studies evaluating CNS depressant effects of eszopiclone doses of 2–3 mg in adults, memory impairment was reported in 1–1.3% of patients receiving eszopiclone compared with 0% of those receiving placebo, and confusion was reported in 3% of patients receiving eszopiclone compared with 0% of those receiving placebo. In clinical studies evaluating CNS depressant effects of eszopiclone 2 mg in geriatric patients, memory impairment was reported in 1.5% of patients receiving eszopiclone compared with 0% of those receiving placebo, and confusion was reported in 2.5% of patients receiving eszopiclone compared with 0% of those receiving placebo.

Next-day impairment of psychomotor function has been reported in patients receiving the 3-mg dose of eszopiclone. In a study in 91 healthy individuals, treatment with eszopiclone 3 mg at bedtime was associated with next-morning impairment of psychomotor function (i.e., ability to maintain a motor vehicle in the driving lane, working memory, motor coordination); such impairment was most severe at 7.5 hours postdose but was still present and potentially clinically meaningful at 11.5 hours postdose. Patients often were unaware of these impairments.

The risk of next-day psychomotor impairment is increased if eszopiclone is administered with less than 7–8 hours of sleep time remaining. The risk of next-day impairment also is increased if a higher than recommended dose of eszopiclone is administered or when eszopiclone is used concomitantly with other CNS depressants or with drugs capable of increasing eszopiclone concentrations.

To reduce the potential risk of next-day impairment, the manufacturer and FDA have lowered the recommended initial dosage of eszopiclone from 2 mg to 1 mg immediately before bedtime (see Dosage and Administration: Dosage). Women and men are equally susceptible to impairment from eszopiclone; therefore, the recommended initial dosage (1 mg immediately before bedtime) is the same for women and men. This lower initial dosage will result in less drug in the blood the next day. FDA states that patients currently receiving eszopiclone should continue therapy at the prescribed dosage and should contact their clinician to determine the most appropriate dosage. FDA is continuing to evaluate the risk of impaired mental alertness associated with other sedative and hypnotic drugs, including nonprescription (over-the-counter, OTC) preparations, and will update the public as new information becomes available. The agency states that nonprescription sedative and hypnotic drugs should not be considered safer than prescription drugs.

Patients receiving eszopiclone should be monitored for excessive CNS depressant effects; however, impairment may occur in the absence of symptoms and may not be reliably detected by ordinary clinical examination (i.e., formal psychomotor testing may be required). Patients receiving the 3-mg dose should be cautioned against driving or engaging in other activities that require complete mental alertness the day after use.

Concomitant use of eszopiclone with other CNS depressants (e.g., alcohol, benzodiazepines, opiates, tricyclic antidepressants) results in additive CNS depression. Concomitant use of eszopiclone with other sedative and hypnotic drugs, including OTC preparations used to treat insomnia (e.g., diphenhydramine, doxylamine succinate), at bedtime or in the middle of the night is not recommended. (See Drug Interactions: CNS Depressants.)

Adequate Patient Evaluation. Because sleep disturbances may be a manifestation of a physical and/or psychiatric disorder, symptomatic treatment of insomnia should be initiated only after careful evaluation of the patient. Failure of insomnia to remit after 7–10 days of eszopiclone therapy, worsening of insomnia, or emergence of new abnormal thinking or behavior may indicate the presence of an underlying psychiatric, physical, and/or medical condition that requires evaluation; patients should be reevaluated if insomnia persists after 7–10 days of therapy.

Abnormal Thinking and Behavioral Changes. Abnormal thinking and behavioral changes have been reported in patients receiving sedative and hypnotic drugs. Some of these changes are similar to manifestations of alcohol intoxication or effects associated with other CNS depressants and include decreased inhibition (e.g., aggressiveness and extroversion that seem out of character), bizarre behavior, agitation, depersonalization, and hallucinations. Amnesia and other neuropsychiatric symptoms may occur unpredictably. Worsening of depression and suicidal thoughts and actions (including completed suicides) have been reported in primarily depressed patients receiving sedative and hypnotic drugs.

Complex behaviors such as sleep-driving (i.e., driving while not fully awake after ingesting a sedative and hypnotic drug, with no memory of the event) have been reported in sedative and hypnotic drug-naive as well as in sedative and hypnotic drug-experienced patients. Although behaviors such as sleep-driving have occurred with eszopiclone alone at therapeutic dosages, the concomitant use of alcohol and other CNS depressants with eszopiclone or the use of eszopiclone at dosages exceeding the maximum recommended dosage appears to increase the risk of such behaviors. (See Risk of Serious Injury and Death Resulting From Complex Sleep Behaviors under Warnings/Precautions: Warnings, in Cautions.)

It can rarely be determined with certainty whether a particular instance of the abnormal behavior is drug induced, spontaneous, or results from an underlying psychiatric or physical disorder. Nevertheless, the emergence of any new behavioral sign or symptom of concern in patients receiving eszopiclone requires careful and immediate evaluation.

Withdrawal Effects. Manifestations of withdrawal have been reported following abrupt discontinuance or rapid reduction in dosage of sedative and hypnotic drugs. Clinical trials of eszopiclone did not reveal evidence of a serious withdrawal syndrome; however, anxiety, abnormal dreams, nausea, upset stomach, hyperesthesia, and neurosis were reported at an incidence of 2% or less after placebo substitution within 48 hours following the last dose of eszopiclone.

Rebound insomnia of 1 day's duration was noted in controlled trials of eszopiclone.

Abuse Potential. Studies using relatively high eszopiclone dosages (e.g., 2–4 times the maximum recommended hypnotic dosage) in individuals with a history of benzodiazepine abuse suggest that the abuse potential of eszopiclone is similar to that of benzodiazepines (e.g., diazepam); caution is advised in patients with a history of drug or alcohol abuse or a history of psychiatric disorders.

Tolerance. Pharmacodynamic tolerance and adaptation to the hypnotic effect of eszopiclone were not observed during studies of up to 6 months' duration.

Timing of Drug Doses. Ingesting eszopiclone while still up and about could result in adverse CNS effects such as short-term memory impairment, hallucinations, dizziness, and impaired coordination. Therefore, eszopiclone should be administered immediately before retiring. (See Dosage and Administration: Administration.)

Geriatric and/or Debilitated Patients. Geriatric and/or debilitated patients may be more sensitive to pharmacologic and adverse effects (e.g., impaired motor and/or cognitive performance) of sedative and hypnotic agents; reduction of the maximum dosage is recommended in such patients. (See Dosage and Administration: Special Populations.)

Concomitant Diseases. Experience in patients with concomitant disease is limited; eszopiclone should be used with caution in patients with diseases that may affect metabolism or hemodynamic responses.

Although respiratory depression was not reported in healthy individuals receiving doses 2.5-fold higher than the recommended dose, caution is advised in patients with impaired respiratory function.

Use in Patients with Depression. As with other sedative and hypnotic agents, eszopiclone should be used with caution in patients with depression. Suicidal tendencies may be present, and protective measures may be required. Intentional overdosage is more common in this patient population, and the least amount of drug feasible should be prescribed and dispensed at any one time to avoid such intentional overdosage.

Specific Populations **Pregnancy.** Category C. (See Users Guide.)

Lactation. It is not known whether eszopiclone is distributed into milk; however, racemic zopiclone is distributed into milk.

Pediatric Use. Safety and efficacy of eszopiclone have not been established in pediatric patients.

Eszopiclone has not been shown to be effective in the management of insomnia associated with attention deficit hyperactivity disorder (ADHD). In a 12-week controlled study in 483 pediatric patients (6–17 years of age) with insomnia associated with ADHD, eszopiclone (1, 2, or 3 mg at bedtime) did not decrease sleep latency as compared with placebo. In this study, the most frequent treatment-emergent adverse effects (compared with placebo) were psychiatric and nervous system effects, including dysgeusia (9 versus 1%), dizziness (6 versus 2%), hallucinations (2 versus 0%), and suicidal ideation (0.3 versus 0%). Discontinuance of therapy was required in 3% of patients receiving eszopiclone and in 2% of those receiving placebo.

Geriatric Use. In clinical studies, a total of 287 patients randomized to receive eszopiclone were 65 years of age or older (range: 65–86 years). The adverse effect profile of the 2-mg dose in geriatric patients (median age: 71 years) was similar to that observed in clinical trials of the drug in younger adults. However, patients 65 years of age or older had a longer elimination half-life and higher total systemic exposure to eszopiclone compared with younger adults. Reduction of the maximum dosage is recommended because of impaired motor and cognitive performance as well as increased sensitivity in geriatric patients. (See Dosage and Administration: Special Populations.)

Hepatic Impairment. Systemic exposure to eszopiclone is increased twofold in patients with severe hepatic impairment compared with healthy individuals.

Eszopiclone should be used with caution in patients with hepatic impairment. Dosage adjustment is not necessary in patients with mild to moderate hepatic impairment; however, reduction of the maximum dosage is recommended in those with severe hepatic impairment. (See Dosage and Administration: Special Populations.)

Renal Impairment. No dosage adjustment appears necessary in patients with renal impairment, since less than 10% of an oral dose of eszopiclone is excreted unchanged in urine.

■ **Common Adverse Effects** Adverse effects reported in 2% or more of adults younger than 65 years of age receiving eszopiclone (2- or 3-mg doses) and more frequently than with placebo include unpleasant taste, headache, somnolence, respiratory infection, dizziness, dry mouth, dyspepsia, nausea, nervousness, rash, depression, viral infection, anxiety, hallucinations, vomiting, confusion, decreased libido, dysmenorrhea, and gynecomastia.

Adverse effects reported in 2% or more of geriatric patients receiving eszopiclone (1- or 2-mg doses) and more frequently than with placebo include headache, unpleasant taste, dry mouth, dyspepsia, dizziness, pain, diarrhea, pruritus, neuralgia, abnormal dreams, urinary tract infection, accidental injuries, and nervousness.

Drug Interactions

Eszopiclone is metabolized principally by cytochrome P-450 (CYP) isoenzymes 3A4 and 2E1; the drug does not appear to inhibit CYP isoenzymes 1A2, 2A6, 2C9, 2C19, 2D6, 2E1, or 3A4. Eszopiclone is not expected to alter the clearance of drugs that are metabolized by common CYP isoenzymes.

■ **Drugs Affecting Hepatic Microsomal Enzymes** ***Inhibitors of CYP3A4*** Concomitant use of eszopiclone with inhibitors of CYP3A4 may result in increased systemic exposure to eszopiclone. When the potent CYP3A4 inhibitor ketoconazole (400 mg daily for 5 days) was administered concomitantly with eszopiclone (3 mg at bedtime), eszopiclone exposure, peak plasma concentration, and half-life were increased by 2.2-, 1.4-, and 1.3-fold, respectively.

If eszopiclone is used concomitantly with a potent CYP3A4 inhibitor (e.g., clarithromycin, itraconazole, ketoconazole, nefazodone, nelfinavir, ritonavir, troleandomycin), dosage of eszopiclone should not exceed 2 mg once daily immediately before bedtime.

Inducers of CYP3A4 Concomitant use of eszopiclone with inducers of CYP3A4 may result in decreased systemic exposure to and efficacy of eszopiclone. When zopiclone (not commercially available in the US) was administered concomitantly with the potent CYP3A4 inducer rifampin, exposure to zopiclone was decreased by 80%; a similar effect would be expected with eszopiclone.

■ **CNS-active Drugs** When eszopiclone (3 mg) was administered concomitantly with olanzapine (10 mg), no alteration in the pharmacokinetics of either drug was observed; however, a pharmacodynamic interaction (effect on psychomotor function, as manifested by a decrease in Digit Symbol Substitution test [DSST] scores) was noted.

When eszopiclone (single 3-mg dose) was administered concomitantly with paroxetine (20 mg daily for 7 days), no pharmacokinetic or pharmacodynamic interactions were observed; however, the possibility of a pharmacodynamic interaction between the drugs following long-term concomitant use cannot be ruled out.

■ **CNS Depressants** Concomitant use of eszopiclone with other CNS depressants (e.g., alcohol, benzodiazepines, opiates, sedatives and hypnotics, tricyclic antidepressants) may result in additive CNS depression. Concomitant use of alcohol with eszopiclone results in additive psychomotor impairment. Although no clinically important pharmacokinetic or pharmacodynamic interaction was observed following single-dose administration of eszopiclone 3 mg with lorazepam 2 mg, the possibility of a pharmacodynamic interaction between the drugs following long-term concomitant use cannot be ruled out.

Concomitant use of eszopiclone with alcohol should be avoided. Concurrent use of other sedative and hypnotic drugs used to treat insomnia (including OTC preparations such as diphenhydramine and doxylamine succinate) should also be avoided in patients receiving eszopiclone. When eszopiclone is used concomitantly with other CNS depressants, dosage reduction of eszopiclone and the CNS depressant may be necessary.

■ **Digoxin** The pharmacokinetics of digoxin were not affected following concomitant administration of eszopiclone (single 3-mg dose) with digoxin (0.5 mg twice daily for 1 day, followed by 0.25 mg daily for 6 days).

■ **Protein-bound Drugs** Because eszopiclone is not highly bound (52–59%) to plasma proteins, concomitant use of eszopiclone with highly protein-bound drugs is not expected to affect the free concentration of either drug.

■ **Warfarin** Concomitant administration of eszopiclone (3 mg daily for 5 days) with warfarin (single 25-mg dose) in healthy individuals did not affect the pharmacokinetics of *R*- or *S*-warfarin, nor were there any changes in the pharmacodynamic profile (prothrombin time).

Description

Eszopiclone, the *S*-enantiomer of zopiclone (not commercially available in the US), is a sedative and hypnotic agent that is structurally unrelated to benzodiazepines and other sedative and hypnotic agents that are commercially available in the US, including barbiturates, imidazopyridines (e.g., zolpidem), and pyrazolopyrimidines (e.g., zaleplon). Eszopiclone is pharmacologically similar to zaleplon and zolpidem; all of these agents have been shown to interact with the CNS γ-aminobutyric acid ($GABA_A$) receptor complex at binding domains located close to or allosterically coupled to benzodiazepine receptors. In vitro binding affinity of eszopiclone for benzodiazepine receptors is about 50 times that of the *R*-enantiomer of zopiclone. Preclinical data suggest that most, if not all, of the hypnotic effects of racemic zopiclone are attributable to the *S*-enantiomer. However, further studies are needed to determine whether these differences result in any clinical superiority of eszopiclone compared with zopiclone.

Eszopiclone is rapidly absorbed from the GI tract following oral administration. Eszopiclone has an intermediate duration of action (i.e., possesses a half-life of approximately 5–7 hours). Following oral administration, eszopiclone is extensively metabolized to several active and inactive metabolites via demethylation and oxidation by the cytochrome P-450 (CYP) 3A4 and 2E1 isoenzymes. Eszopiclone does not appear to have any inhibitory effect on CYP isoenzymes 1A2, 2A6, 2C9, 2C19, 2D6, 2E1, or 3A4.

Advice to Patients

Importance of advising patients to read the manufacturer's medication guide and instructions for use carefully prior to initiating therapy and each time the prescription is refilled.

Importance of taking eszopiclone immediately before retiring and only when able to get 7–8 hours of sleep before it is necessary to be active again.

Importance of taking eszopiclone only as prescribed (e.g., not with or immediately after a high-fat meal) and of not increasing the dose or duration of therapy unless otherwise instructed by a clinician.

Importance of not taking eszopiclone if alcohol has been consumed in the evening or before bedtime. Importance of avoiding concurrent use of other sedative and hypnotic drugs used to treat insomnia (including OTC preparations such as diphenhydramine or doxylamine succinate) or CNS depressants during eszopiclone therapy unless otherwise instructed by a clinician.

Importance of informing patients about the risk of complex sleep behaviors (e.g., sleepwalking, sleep driving, engaging in other activities while not fully awake) that, although rare, may result in serious injury or death. Such events can occur following just one dose of these drugs as well as after a longer duration of treatment. Importance of advising patients to discontinue taking eszopiclone and to notify a clinician immediately if an episode of complex sleep behavior occurs during therapy, even if it did not result in a serious injury.

Risk of next-day impairment, even when used as prescribed; impairment may be present despite feeling fully awake. In patients receiving the 3-mg dose, importance of avoiding driving or engaging in other activities that require complete mental alertness the day after use.

Risk of severe anaphylactic and anaphylactoid reactions; importance of immediately seeking medical attention if hypersensitivity reactions occur.

Risk of abnormal thinking and behavioral changes. Importance of contacting a clinician immediately if these adverse effects occur.

Importance of immediately reporting any suicidal thoughts.

Importance of informing clinicians of existing or contemplated concomitant therapy, including prescription and OTC drugs and herbal products, as well as concomitant or past illnesses (e.g., depression, substance abuse).

Importance of women informing clinicians if they are or plan to become pregnant or plan to breast-feed.

Importance of informing patients of other important precautionary information. (See Cautions.)

Overview® (see Users Guide). For additional information on this drug until a more detailed monograph is developed and published, the manufacturer's labeling should be consulted. It is *essential* that the manufacturer's labeling be consulted for more detailed information on usual cautions, precautions, contraindications, potential drug interactions, laboratory test interferences, and acute toxicity.

Preparations

Eszopiclone is subject to control under the Federal Controlled Substances Act of 1970 as a schedule IV (C-IV) drug.

Excipients in commercially available drug preparations may have clinically important effects in some individuals; consult specific product labeling for details.

Eszopiclone

Oral		
Tablets, film-coated	1 mg*	**Eszopiclone Tablets** (C-IV)
		Lunesta® (C-IV), Sunovion
	2 mg*	**Eszopiclone Tablets** (C-IV)
		Lunesta® (C-IV), Sunovion
	3 mg*	**Eszopiclone Tablets** (C-IV)
		Lunesta® (C-IV), Sunovion

*available from one or more manufacturer, distributor, and/or repackager by generic (nonproprietary) name

Selected Revisions October 2019,

hydrOXYzine Hydrochloride hydrOXYzine Pamoate

■ Hydroxyzine is a piperazine-derivative antihistamine.

Uses

Hydroxyzine is used for the symptomatic management of anxiety and tension associated with psychoneuroses and as an adjunct in patients with organic disease states who have associated anxiety; for the management of pruritus caused by allergic conditions such as chronic urticaria or atopic or contact dermatoses, and in histamine-mediated pruritus; and for its sedative effects before and after general anesthesia. The efficacy of hydroxyzine as an anxiolytic agent during long-term administration (i.e., longer than 4 months) has not been established; most clinicians believe that benzodiazepines, barbiturates, and meprobamate are more effective than hydroxyzine for anxiety. Patients with a history of long-term therapy with hydroxyzine should be evaluated periodically to determine the efficacy and need for further treatment. Hydroxyzine should not be used as the sole agent for the treatment of depression or psychoses.

Hydroxyzine has also been used for the management of agitation caused by acute alcohol withdrawal; to reduce opiate analgesic dosage; to control motion sickness; and to control nausea and vomiting of various etiologies (e.g., postoperative). Safe use of hydroxyzine for the prevention and treatment of nausea and vomiting of pregnancy has not been established, and the drug is contraindicated during early pregnancy.

Dosage and Administration

■ **Administration** Hydroxyzine hydrochloride and hydroxyzine pamoate are administered orally; hydroxyzine hydrochloride may also be administered by IM injection. Because severe adverse effects may occur, the drug must *not* be administered by subcutaneous, intra-arterial, or IV injection. (See Cautions: Local Effects.) Oral therapy should replace IM therapy as soon as possible.

For IM administration, the commercially available hydroxyzine injection is used without further dilution. The Z-track technique of injection may be used to prevent subcutaneous infiltration. For IM administration in adults, injection should be made preferably deep into the upper outer quadrant of the gluteus maximus or the midlateral thigh. The deltoid area should be used with caution and only if well developed, in order to avoid radial nerve injury. IM injections should *not* be made into the lower and mid-third of the upper arm. For IM administration in children, injections should be made preferably into the midlateral muscles of the thigh; in infants and small children, the periphery of the upper outer quadrant of the gluteus maximus should be used only when necessary (e.g., burn patients), in order to minimize the possibility of damage to the sciatic nerve.

■ **Dosage** Dosage of hydroxyzine hydrochloride or pamoate is expressed in terms of the hydrochloride. Dosage must be carefully adjusted according to individual requirements and response, using the lowest possible effective dosage.

For the symptomatic management of anxiety and tension associated with psychoneuroses and as an adjunct in patients with organic disease states who have associated anxiety, the usual adult oral dosage of hydroxyzine is 50–100 mg 4 times daily. The usual oral dosage of hydroxyzine for the symptomatic management of anxiety and tension associated with psychoneuroses and as an adjunct in organic disease states in children 6 years of age or older is 50–100 mg daily given in divided doses; for children younger than 6 years of age, the usual oral dosage is 50 mg daily given in divided doses.

For prompt control of acutely disturbed or hysterical patients and for the management of agitation caused by alcohol withdrawal, the usual adult IM dose of hydroxyzine is 50–100 mg. This dose may be repeated every 4–6 hours, as needed to control symptoms.

For the management of pruritus caused by allergic conditions such as chronic urticaria or atopic or contact dermatoses, and in histamine-mediated pruritus, the usual adult oral dosage of hydroxyzine is 25 mg 3 or 4 times daily. The usual oral dosage of hydroxyzine for the management of pruritus caused by allergic conditions in children 6 years of age or older is 50–100 mg daily given in divided doses; for children younger than 6 years of age, the usual oral dosage is 50 mg daily given in divided doses.

For sedation before and following general anesthesia, the usual adult dose of hydroxyzine is 50–100 mg orally or 25–100 mg IM. When used as a sedative before and following general anesthesia in children, the usual dose of hydroxyzine is 0.6 mg/kg orally or 1.1 mg/kg IM.

For control of nausea and vomiting (excluding nausea and vomiting of pregnancy), the usual initial IM dose of hydroxyzine is 25–100 mg in adults and 1.1 mg/kg in children. Subsequent dosage should be adjusted according to individual requirements and response.

For control of emesis, to permit reduction in opiate dosage, or to allay anxiety in prepartum and postpartum states, the usual initial adult IM dose of hydroxyzine is 25–100 mg. Subsequent dosage should be adjusted according to individual requirements and response.

For further information on chemistry and stability, pharmacology, pharmacokinetics, uses, cautions, acute toxicity, drug interactions, and dosage and administration of hydroxyzine, see the Antihistamines General Statement 4:00.

Cautions

Adverse reactions to hydroxyzine generally involve the CNS and are usually mild, transient, and reversible following discontinuance of the drug.

■ **Nervous System Effects** The most frequent adverse effects of hydroxyzine are drowsiness and dry mouth. Drowsiness usually diminishes with continued therapy or reduction in dosage. Other less frequent adverse nervous system effects of hydroxyzine include dizziness, ataxia, weakness, slurred speech, headache, agitation, and increased anxiety. Involuntary motor activity, including tremor and seizures, has occurred rarely, usually in patients receiving higher than recommended dosages of the drug.

■ **Local Effects** Marked local discomfort, sterile abscesses, erythema, local irritation, and tissue necrosis may occur at the site of IM injection, and marked localized subcutaneous tissue induration has been reported as a result of extravasation of the drug.

Following inadvertent intra-arterial injection of hydroxyzine hydrochloride, thrombosis and digital gangrene necessitating amputation have occurred. Phlebitis and hemolysis have been reported following IV administration of the drug. Following inadvertent subcutaneous administration of hydroxyzine hydrochloride, tissue necrosis, tissue slough, swelling, edema, petechial hemorrhage, and abscess have occurred.

■ **Other Adverse Effects** Other adverse effects that have been reported following administration of hydroxyzine include a bitter taste in the mouth, nausea, increased GI peristalsis, flushing, wheezing, and tightness of the chest.

■ **Precautions and Contraindications** Hydroxyzine shares the toxic potentials of the antihistamines, and the usual precautions of antihistamine therapy should be observed. (See Cautions in the Antihistamines General Statement 4:00.)

Because of the risk of adverse local effects, which may be severe (e.g., gangrene, thrombosis), IM administration of hydroxyzine should be performed with caution to avoid extravasation or inadvertent subcutaneous, IV, or intra-arterial injection.

Patients should be warned that hydroxyzine may impair their ability to perform activities requiring mental alertness or physical coordination (e.g., operating machinery, driving a motor vehicle). Patients also should be warned that hydroxyzine may enhance their response to alcohol, barbiturates, or other CNS depressants.

Hydroxyzine is contraindicated in patients who are hypersensitive to the drug.

■ **Pregnancy and Lactation** Although there are no adequate and controlled studies to date in humans, hydroxyzine has been shown to be teratogenic in mice, rats, and rabbits when given at dosages substantially greater than the therapeutic human dosage. Pending accumulation of further data regarding safety in pregnant women, hydroxyzine is contraindicated during early pregnancy.

It is not known whether hydroxyzine is distributed into milk. The manufacturers recommend that hydroxyzine not be given to nursing women.

Drug Interactions

■ **CNS Depressants** Hydroxyzine may be additive with, or may potentiate the action of, other CNS depressants such as opiates or other analgesics, barbiturates or other sedatives, anesthetics, or alcohol. When hydroxyzine is used concomitantly with other CNS depressants, caution should be used to avoid excessive sedation, and the manufacturers recommend that dosage of the CNS depressant be reduced by up to 50%.

■ **Anticholinergic Agents** Additive anticholinergic effects may occur when hydroxyzine is administered concomitantly with other anticholinergic agents.

■ **Epinephrine** Hydroxyzine has been shown to inhibit and reverse the vasopressor effect of epinephrine. If a vasopressor agent is required in patients receiving hydroxyzine, norepinephrine or metaraminol should be used; epinephrine should *not* be used.

Laboratory Test Interferences

Hydroxyzine has been reported to cause falsely elevated urinary concentrations of 17-hydroxycorticosteroids when the Porter-Silber reaction or the Glenn-Nelson method is used.

Acute Toxicity

Limited information is available on the acute toxicity of hydroxyzine. The acute lethal dose of hydroxyzine in humans is not known. In addition, there is no clearly defined relationship between plasma hydroxyzine concentration and severity of intoxication.

■ **Manifestations** In general, overdosage of hydroxyzine may be expected to produce effects that are extensions of common adverse reactions; excessive sedation has been the principal effect reported. Hypotension, although rare, may also occur.

■ **Treatment** Treatment of hydroxyzine overdosage generally involves symptomatic and supportive care; there is no specific antidote for hydroxyzine intoxication. Following acute ingestion of the drug, the stomach should be emptied immediately by inducing emesis or by gastric lavage. If the patient is comatose, having seizures, or lacks the gag reflex, gastric lavage may be performed if an endotracheal tube with cuff inflated is in place to prevent aspiration of gastric contents. Appropriate therapy should be instituted if hypotension or excessive sedation occurs. If hypotension occurs, it may be controlled with IV fluids and norepinephrine or metaraminol; epinephrine should *not* be used. Although one manufacturer states that caffeine and sodium benzoate may be used to counteract CNS depressant effects of the drug, most authorities believe caffeine and other analeptics should *not* be used in overdosage resulting from CNS depressants. Although hemodialysis or peritoneal dialysis is probably *not* effective in enhancing elimination of hydroxyzine, if other agents (e.g., barbiturates) have been ingested concomitantly, dialysis may be indicated.

Pharmacology

The principal pharmacologic effects of hydroxyzine are similar to those of other antihistamines. (See Pharmacology in the Antihistamines General Statement 4:00.)

■ **Nervous System Effects** Hydroxyzine has CNS depressant, anticholinergic, antispasmodic, and local anesthetic activity, in addition to antihistaminic effects. The drug also has sedative and antiemetic activity. The sedative and tranquilizing effects of hydroxyzine are thought to result principally from suppression of activity at subcortical levels of the CNS; the drug does not have cortical depressant activity. The precise mechanism of antiemetic and antimotion sickness actions of hydroxyzine are unclear, but appear to result, at least in part, from its central anticholinergic and CNS depressant properties.

Like many other centrally acting agents, hydroxyzine exhibits analgesic activity in a variety of analgesic test systems; this effect may be related to its sedative activity. Hydroxyzine also has primary skeletal muscle relaxant activity.

■ **GI Effects** Hydroxyzine does not appear to increase gastric secretions or acidity, and usually has mild antisecretory effects. The antispasmodic activity of hydroxyzine is apparently mediated through interference with the mechanism that responds to spasmogenic agents such as acetylcholine, histamine, and serotonin.

■ **Cardiovascular Effects** Although hydroxyzine does not appear to have clinically important antiarrhythmic properties, mild antiarrhythmic activity has been observed in some experimentally induced ventricular arrhythmias.

Therapeutic dosages of hydroxyzine produce only minimal effects on blood pressure; however, hypotension may occur following overdosage.

■ **Other Effects** Hydroxyzine has been shown to produce bronchodilation in healthy individuals and in patients with chronic obstructive pulmonary disease.

Pharmacokinetics

■ **Absorption** Hydroxyzine is rapidly absorbed from the GI tract following oral administration.

The onset of sedative action of hydroxyzine is 15–30 minutes following oral administration. Sedative effects persist for 4–6 hours following administration of a single dose. Hydroxyzine suppresses the inflammatory response (wheal and flare reaction) and pruritus for up to 4 days after intradermal skin tests with allergens and histamine.

The therapeutic range for plasma hydroxyzine concentrations and the relationship of plasma concentration to clinical response or toxicity have not been established.

■ **Distribution** Distribution of hydroxyzine into human body tissues and fluids has not been fully characterized. Following administration of hydroxyzine in animals, the drug is widely distributed into most body tissues and fluids with highest concentrations in the liver, lungs, spleen, kidneys, and adipose tissue. The drug is also distributed into bile in animals.

It is not known if hydroxyzine crosses the placenta or is distributed into milk.

■ **Elimination** Although the exact metabolic fate of hydroxyzine is not clearly established, it appears that the drug is completely metabolized, principally in the liver. In animals, hydroxyzine and its metabolites are excreted in feces via biliary elimination. The carboxylic acid metabolite of hydroxyzine, cetirizine (Zyrtec®, Pfizer), is a long-acting antihistamine. (See Cetirizine 4:08)

Chemistry and Stability

■ **Chemistry** Hydroxyzine is a piperazine-derivative antihistamine that is structurally similar to meclizine. Hydroxyzine is chemically unrelated to reserpine, meprobamate, benzodiazepines, or phenothiazines. Hydroxyzine is commercially available as the hydrochloride and pamoate salts.

Hydroxyzine hydrochloride occurs as a white, odorless powder and is very soluble in water and freely soluble in alcohol. The drug has pK_as of 2.6 and 7.0. Hydroxyzine hydrochloride injection is a sterile solution of the drug in water for injection. Sodium hydroxide is added during manufacture of the injection to adjust the pH to 3.5–6. The commercially available injection also contains benzyl alcohol as a preservative.

Hydroxyzine pamoate occurs as a light yellow, practically odorless powder and is practically insoluble in water and in alcohol. The commercially available hydroxyzine pamoate oral suspension has a pH of 4.5–7.

■ **Stability** Commercially available preparations of hydroxyzine should be stored in tight, light-resistant containers at a temperature less than 40°C, preferably at 15–30°C; freezing of the oral solution, oral suspension, or injection should be avoided.

Hydroxyzine hydrochloride injection is physically and/or chemically incompatible with some drugs, but the compatibility depends on several factors (e.g., concentrations of the drugs, specific diluents used, resulting pH, temperature). Specialized references should be consulted for specific compatibility information.

Preparations

Excipients in commercially available drug preparations may have clinically important effects in some individuals; consult specific product labeling for details.

hydrOXYzine Hydrochloride

Oral		
Solution	10 mg/5 mL*	**Atarax® Syrup**, Pfizer **Hydroxyzine Hydrochloride Oral Solution**
Tablets	10 mg*	**Atarax®**, Pfizer **Hydroxyzine Hydrochloride Tablets**
	25 mg*	**Atarax®**, Pfizer **Hydroxyzine Hydrochloride Tablets**
	50 mg*	**Atarax®**, Pfizer **Hydroxyzine Hydrochloride Tablets**
	100 mg	**Atarax®**, Pfizer
Tablets, film-coated	10 mg*	
	25 mg*	**Anx®** (scored), EconoMed **Hydroxyzine Hydrochloride Film-coated Tablets**
	50 mg*	
Parenteral		
Injection, for IM use only	25 mg/mL*	**Vistaril®**, Pfizer **Hydroxyzine Hydrochloride Injection**
	50 mg/mL*	**Vistaril®**, Pfizer **Hydroxyzine Hydrochloride Injection**

*available from one or more manufacturer, distributor, and/or repackager by generic (nonproprietary) name

hydrOXYzine Pamoate

Oral		
Capsules	equivalent to hydroxyzine hydrochloride 25 mg*	**Vistaril®**, Pfizer **Hydroxyzine Pamoate Capsules**
	equivalent to hydroxyzine hydrochloride 50 mg*	**Vistaril®**, Pfizer **Hydroxyzine Pamoate Capsules**
	equivalent to hydroxyzine hydrochloride 100 mg*	**Vistaril®**, Pfizer **Hydroxyzine Pamoate Capsules**
Suspension	equivalent to hydroxyzine hydrochloride 25 mg/5 mL	**Vistaril®** (with propylene glycol), Pfizer

*available from one or more manufacturer, distributor, and/or repackager by generic (nonproprietary) name

Selected Revisions January 2009,

Promethazine Hydrochloride

■ Promethazine hydrochloride is an ethylamino derivative of phenothiazine with potent sedative and antiemetic properties.

Uses

Promethazine is used for its sedative and antiemetic effects in surgery and obstetrics (during labor). The drug reduces preoperative tension and anxiety, facilitates sleep, and reduces postoperative nausea and vomiting. As a preanesthetic medication, promethazine is used in conjunction with reduced doses of an opiate analgesic and an atropine-like drug. Promethazine also may be used as a routine sedative and as an adjunct to analgesics for control of pain.

For the use of promethazine as an antihistamine and for the management of motion sickness, see Promethazine Hydrochloride 4:04 and also see the Phenothiazines General Statement 28:16.08.24.

Dosage and Administration

■ **Administration** Promethazine hydrochloride may be administered orally, rectally, or by deep IM injection. Promethazine hydrochloride also is administered by IV injection. However, because IV administration of the drug has been associated with severe tissue injury, including gangrene requiring amputation, the US Food and Drug Administration (FDA) states that deep IM injection is the preferred method for administration of promethazine hydrochloride injections. (See Cautions: Precautions and Contraindications.) If IV administration of promethazine hydrochloride is required, FDA states that the drug should be administered through the tubing of an IV infusion set that is known to be correctly functioning; FDA also states that the *maximum* rate of IV administration is 25 mg/minute, and the *maximum* concentration of the injection is 25 mg/mL. If the patient complains of pain at the injection site during presumed IV injection of the drug, the injection should immediately be stopped, and the possibility of intra-arterial placement of the needle or perivascular extravasation should be evaluated. Promethazine hydrochloride injection is commercially available in 2 strengths: 25 mg/mL and 50 mg/mL. FDA states that the preparation containing 50 mg/mL is for IM injection *only*; the preparation containing 25 mg/mL may be administered by IM or IV injection.

Because of the risk of severe tissue injury and amputations if promethazine hydrochloride is inadvertently administered intra-arterially or if extravasation were to occur, some medication safety experts (e.g., the Institute for Safe Medication Practices [ISMP]) recommend that parenteral administration of the drug be avoided and replaced by safer alternative therapies (e.g., a type 3 serotonin [$5\text{-}HT_3$] receptor antagonist such as ondansetron).

Subcutaneous or intra-arterial injection of promethazine hydrochloride is contraindicated.

Promethazine hydrochloride injections should be inspected visually for particulate matter and discoloration prior to administration whenever solution and container permit. The injection should be discarded if the solution is discolored or contains a precipitate.

■ **Dosage** Dosages of promethazine hydrochloride by the various routes of administration are identical.

For routine, preoperative or postoperative sedation or as an adjunct to analgesics for the control of pain, the usual adult dose of promethazine hydrochloride is 25–50 mg; children may receive 12.5–25 mg or 0.5–1.1 mg/kg.

When promethazine is used as an adjunct to opiate analgesics, dosage of the analgesic should usually be reduced.

In obstetrics, 50 mg of promethazine hydrochloride may be given to provide sedation during the early stage of labor. When labor is established, 25–75 mg may be given with a reduced therapeutic dose of an opiate agonist. Although additional doses are usually not required, the manufacturers state that 25- to 50-mg doses of promethazine may be repeated once or twice at 4-hour intervals if necessary. The maximum total dosage of promethazine during a 24-hour period of labor is 100 mg.

For the prevention and management of nausea and vomiting, the usual adult dose of promethazine hydrochloride is 12.5–25 mg; additional doses of 12.5–25 mg may be given every 4 hours if necessary. Children have been given 0.25–0.5 mg/kg or 7.5–15 mg/m^2 4–6 times daily for the treatment of nausea and vomiting. (See Cautions: Pediatric Precautions.)

Cautions

■ **Adverse Effects** Promethazine has adverse effects similar to those of other antihistamines and shares the toxic potentials of the phenothiazines; the usual precautions of antihistamine and phenothiazine therapy should be observed. (See Cautions in the Antihistamines General Statement 4:00 and in the Phenothiazines General Statement 28:16.08.24.) Although the risk of adverse reactions (e.g., blood dyscrasias, hepatotoxicity, reactivation of psychotic processes, tachycardia, cardiac arrest, endocrine disturbances, dermatologic disorders, ocular changes, hypersensitivity reactions) that have occurred during long-term administration of antipsychotic phenothiazines appears to be minimal, the possibility that such reactions could occur with prolonged administration of promethazine should be considered.

Adverse anticholinergic effects of promethazine include dryness of the mouth, blurring of vision and, rarely, dizziness. Confusion and disorientation also may occur. Extrapyramidal reactions may occur with high doses and usually subside with dosage reduction. Lassitude, fatigue, incoordination, tinnitus, diplopia, oculogyric crises, insomnia, excitation, nervousness, euphoria, hysteria, tremors, seizures, abnormal movements, nightmares, delirium, agitation, hallucinations, torticollis, tongue protrusion, oversedation, dystonic reactions, and catatonic-like states have been reported. Restlessness, akathisia, and, occasionally, marked irregular respiration have occurred. Neuroleptic malignant syndrome (NMS) also may occur. Patients with pain who have received inadequate or no analgesia have developed athetoid-like movements of the upper extremities following parenteral administration of promethazine. These symptoms usually disappeared when the pain was controlled.

Leukopenia, thrombocytopenia, thrombocytopenic purpura, and agranulocytosis have been reported in patients receiving promethazine.

Tachycardia, bradycardia, increased or decreased blood pressure, and faintness have occurred in patients receiving promethazine. Although rapid IV administration of promethazine may produce a transient fall in blood pressure, blood pressure usually is maintained or slightly elevated when the drug is given slowly. Venous thrombosis at the injection site also has been reported.

Promethazine has been associated with obstructive jaundice, which usually was reversible following discontinuance of the drug. Cholestatic jaundice, nausea, and vomiting have been reported in patients receiving promethazine. Photosensitivity has been reported and may be a contraindication to further promethazine therapy. Urticaria, dermatitis, asthma, dermatologic reactions, and angioedema also have occurred. Nasal stuffiness, respiratory depression (may be fatal), cardiac arrest, and apnea (may be fatal) also may occur.

Local Reactions Associated with Promethazine Hydrochloride Injection Severe chemical irritation and damage to tissues (e.g., burning, pain, erythema, swelling, severe spasm of distal vessels, thrombophlebitis, venous thrombosis, phlebitis, abscesses, tissue necrosis, gangrene) may occur with administration of promethazine injection regardless of the route of administration. Such irritation and damage also may result from perivascular extravasation, unintentional intra-arterial injection, and intraneuronal or perineuronal infiltration. Parenteral administration of promethazine may produce nerve damage (ranging from temporary sensory loss to palsies and paralysis) while injection near or into a nerve may result in permanent tissue damage. In some cases, surgical intervention (e.g., fasciotomy, skin graft, amputation) may be needed. (See Dosage and Administration: Administration and see also Cautions: Precautions and Contraindications.)

■ **Precautions and Contraindications** Promethazine has adverse effects similar to those of other antihistamines and shares the toxic potentials of the phenothiazines; the usual precautions of antihistamine and phenothiazine therapy should be observed. (See Cautions: Precautions and Contraindications in the Antihistamines General Statement 4:00 and in the Phenothiazines General Statement 28:16.08.24.)

Ambulatory patients should be warned that promethazine may impair their ability to perform hazardous tasks requiring mental alertness or physical coordination such as operating machinery or driving a motor vehicle. It should be kept in mind that the antiemetic effect of promethazine may obscure signs of overdosage of other drugs or of symptoms of conditions such as intestinal obstruction or brain tumor, and thereby interfere with diagnosis.

Promethazine should be used with caution in patients with cardiovascular disease or impaired liver function or patients who are having an asthmatic attack. Some manufacturers state that promethazine should be used cautiously in individuals with peptic ulcer. Some manufacturers also state that the drug should be used with caution in patients with acute or chronic respiratory impairment, particularly children, because the cough reflex may be suppressed. Promethazine should be used with caution, if at all, in patients with sleep apnea. (See Cautions: Pediatric Precautions.)

Some commercially available formulations of promethazine hydrochloride contain sulfites that may cause allergic-type reactions, including anaphylaxis and life-threatening or less severe asthmatic episodes, in certain susceptible individuals. The overall prevalence of sulfite sensitivity in the general population is unknown but probably low; such sensitivity appears to occur more frequently in asthmatic than in nonasthmatic individuals.

Because IV administration of the drug has been associated with severe tissue injury, including gangrene requiring amputation, the US Food and Drug Administration (FDA) states that deep IM injection is the preferred method for administration of promethazine hydrochloride injections. If IV administration of promethazine hydrochloride is required, extreme care should be exercised to avoid extravasation or inadvertent intra-arterial injection. (See Dosage and Administration: Administration and see Local Reactions Associated with Promethazine Hydrochloride Injection under Cautions: Adverse Effects.) If the patient complains of pain at the injection site during presumed IV injection of the drug, the injection should immediately be stopped, and the possibility of intra-arterial placement of the needle or perivascular extravasation should be evaluated. Clinicians should be alert for signs and symptoms of potential tissue injury, including burning or pain at the site of injection, phlebitis, swelling, and blistering, and patients should be informed that adverse effects may occur immediately (i.e., while receiving the injection) or may develop hours to days after an injection of promethazine. Although there are no proven successful treatment regimens for the management of extravasation or inadvertent intra-arterial injection of promethazine, sympathetic block and administration of heparin are commonly employed during the acute management.

Because of the risk of severe tissue injury and amputations if promethazine hydrochloride is inadvertently administered intra-arterially or if extravasation were to occur, some medication safety experts (e.g., the Institute for Safe Medication Practices [ISMP]) recommend that parenteral administration of the drug be avoided and replaced by safer alternative therapies (e.g., a type 3 serotonin [5-HT$_3$] receptor antagonist such as ondansetron).

FDA states that subcutaneous or intra-arterial administration of promethazine hydrochloride is contraindicated. Promethazine hydrochloride should *not* be administered intra-arterially, because chemical irritation may be severe and cause severe arteriospasm, possibly resulting in impairment of circulation and gangrene requiring amputation. Since promethazine discolors blood on contact, aspiration of dark blood at the site of injection does *not* rule out the possibility of intra-arterial placement of the needle.

Promethazine is contraindicated in patients who have exhibited hypersensitivity or idiosyncrasy to promethazine or other phenothiazines. Promethazine also is contraindicated in pediatric patients younger than 2 years of age because of risk of developing potentially fatal respiratory depression. (See Cautions: Pediatric Precautions.) In addition, the drug is contraindicated in patients who have received large doses of other CNS depressants and/or who are comatose. The manufacturers state that the drug is contraindicated for use in the treatment of lower respiratory tract symptoms (e.g., asthma). There is some evidence that epileptic patients may experience increased severity of seizures if treated with promethazine, and the drug may be contraindicated in these patients. Since increases in blood pressure may occur, promethazine should be administered with extreme caution, if at all, to patients in hypertensive crisis. Some manufacturers state that promethazine also is contraindicated in patients with bone marrow depression, angle-closure glaucoma, prostatic hypertrophy, stenosing peptic ulcer, pyloroduodenal obstruction, or bladder neck obstruction, although others state that the drug may be used with caution in such patients. Some experts do *not* recommend administering promethazine to pediatric patients who are vomiting, unless the vomiting is prolonged and there is a known cause. (See Cautions: Pediatric Precautions.)

■ **Pediatric Precautions** Because respiratory depression (sometimes fatal) has been reported in pediatric patients younger than 2 years of age receiving a wide range of weight-adjusted doses of promethazine during postmarketing surveillance, the drug is contraindicated in pediatric patients younger than 2 years of age.

Promethazine should be administered with caution in children 2 years of age and older because of possible respiratory depression and/or apnea that may be fatal. The lowest effective dose of the drug should be used. Concomitant use of promethazine with other respiratory depressant drugs should be avoided.

Children receiving promethazine should be supervised closely while performing hazardous activities such as bike riding. Adults responsible for the supervision of a child receiving promethazine should be warned that children may be at increased risk for experiencing CNS stimulant effects with antihistamines. Promethazine should not be used in vomiting of unknown etiology in children. The drug should not be used in acutely ill or dehydrated children or children with acute infections, since these patients have an increased susceptibility to dystonias. Use of promethazine also should be avoided in children with signs and symptoms that suggest Reye's syndrome, since the potential extrapyramidal effects produced by the drug may obscure the diagnosis of or be confused with the CNS signs and symptoms of this condition, and in children with signs and symptoms of other hepatic disease. Because promethazine may cause marked drowsiness that may be potentiated by other CNS depressants (e.g., sedatives, tranquilizers), promethazine should be used in children receiving one of these drugs only under the direction of a physician. Promethazine should not be used in children with asthma, liver disease, a seizure disorder, or glaucoma unless otherwise directed by a clinician.

Excessively high dosages of promethazine have caused sudden death in pediatric patients, although sleep apnea and sudden infant death syndrome (SIDS) have been reported in a number of infants and young children who were receiving usual dosages of promethazine or trimeprazine (no longer commercially available in the US). The relationship to the drugs and possible mechanism(s) of such effects have not been elucidated. In one study, the number but not the duration of central apneas during sleep was increased and obstructive apnea during sleep (accompanied by decreased heart rate and arterial oxygen pressure) developed in 4 healthy infants who were receiving 1 mg/kg of promethazine hydrochloride daily for 3 days. Promethazine should be used with caution in children with a history of sleep apnea, those with a family history of SIDS, and those who are less prone than usual to spontaneous arousal from sleep.

■ **Geriatric Precautions** Clinical studies of promethazine did not include sufficient numbers of patients 65 years of age and older to determine whether geriatric patients respond differently than younger patients. Although clinical experience generally has not revealed age-related differences in response to the drug, care should be taken in dosage selection of promethazine. Because of increased risk of sedative effects and confusion (associated with promethazine) and the greater frequency of decreased hepatic, renal, and/or cardiac function and of concomitant disease and drug therapy in geriatric patients, the manufacturers suggest that patients in this age group receive initial dosages of the drug in the lower end of the usual range.

■ **Mutagenicity and Carcinogenicity** Long-term animal studies to determine the carcinogenic potential of promethazine have not been performed to date. There was no evidence of promethazine-induced mutagenesis in the Ames microbial mutagen test. There are no human or other animal data concerning the carcinogenic or mutagenic potentials of the drug. For information on the carcinogenic potential of phenothiazines, see Cautions: Carcinogenicity, in the Phenothiazines General Statement 28:16.08.24.

■ **Pregnancy, Fertility, and Lactation** Safe use of promethazine during pregnancy (except during labor) with respect to possible adverse effects on fetal development has not been established. Although there are no adequate and controlled studies to date in humans, promethazine has not been shown to be teratogenic in rats receiving oral dosages of 6.25–12.5 mg/kg daily (about 2.1–4.2 times the maximum recommended human dosage, depending on the use of the drug). The drug has been shown to produce fetal mortality in rats receiving intraperitoneal dosages of 25 mg/kg daily. Antihistamines, including promethazine, have been fetocidal in rodents, but the pharmacologic effects of histamine in rodents differ from those in humans. Promethazine should be used during pregnancy only when the potential benefits justify the possible risks to the fetus.

There are no animal or human data concerning the effect of promethazine on fertility.

It is not known whether promethazine is distributed into milk. Because many drugs are distributed in human milk and because of the potential for serious adverse reactions to promethazine in nursing infants if it were distributed, a decision should be made whether to discontinue nursing or the drug, taking into account the importance of the drug to the woman.

Drug Interactions

■ **CNS Depressants** Promethazine hydrochloride is additive with or may potentiate the sedative action of opiates or other analgesics and other CNS depressants such as barbiturates or other sedatives, antihistamines, tranquilizers, or alcohol. When promethazine is used concomitantly with other depressant drugs, caution should be used to avoid overdosage. When promethazine is used concomitantly with barbiturates or narcotics, dosage of these drugs should be reduced by at least 50 or 25–50%, respectively.

■ **Epinephrine** Although reversal of the vasopressor effect of epinephrine has not been reported with promethazine, such possibility should be considered. If patients receiving promethazine require a vasopressor agent, norepinephrine or phenylephrine should be used; *epinephrine should not be used* because it may further decrease blood pressure in patients with partial adrenergic blockade.

■ **Anticholinergic Agents** Caution should be used during concomitant use of promethazine with drugs having anticholinergic properties.

■ **Monoamine Oxidase (MAO) Inhibitors** Increased incidence of extrapyramidal effects has been reported in patients receiving phenothiazines concomitantly with MAO inhibitors.

Laboratory Test Interferences

Promethazine may interfere with several immunologic urinary pregnancy tests. The drug may elicit a false-positive Gravindex® test and false-negative Prepurex® and Dap® test. Promethazine may interfere with blood grouping in the ABO system. The drug substantially alters the flare response in intradermal allergen tests.

Acute Toxicity

■ **Manifestations** In adults, overdosage of promethazine may range from mild depression of the CNS and cardiovascular system to profound hypotension, respiratory depression, seizures, deep sleep, unconsciousness, and sudden death. Hyperreflexia, hypertonia, ataxia, athetosis, and extensor-plantar reflexes (Babinski reflex) also may occur. In children, a paradoxical reaction characterized by hyperexcitability, abnormal movements, nightmares, and respiratory depression may occur. A 12-year-old patient who had taken 200 mg of the drug exhibited numbness and pain in the left leg, tactile hallucinations, extreme hyperesthesia and hyperalgesia, and sinus tachycardia.

■ **Treatment** For information on the treatment of promethazine overdosage, see Acute Toxicity: Treatment in the Phenothiazines General Statement 28:16.08.24.

Pharmacology

Promethazine is a phenothiazine derivative with potent sedative properties. Although the drug can produce either CNS stimulation or CNS depression, CNS depression manifested by sedation is more common with therapeutic doses of promethazine. The precise mechanism of the CNS effects of the drug is not known.

Promethazine also has antihistaminic, antiemetic, antimotion sickness, anticholinergic, and local anesthetic effects. Although it has been reported that the drug has slight antitussive activity, this may result from its anticholinergic and CNS depressant effects. In therapeutic doses, promethazine appears to have no substantial effect on the cardiovascular system. Although rapid IV administration of promethazine may produce a transient fall in blood pressure, blood pressure usually is maintained or slightly elevated when the drug is given slowly.

Pharmacokinetics

■ **Absorption** Promethazine is well absorbed from the GI tract and from parenteral sites. Plasma concentrations of promethazine required for sedative effects are unknown. The onset of sedative effects occurs within 20 minutes following oral, rectal, or IM administration, and within 3–5 minutes following IV administration. The duration of sedative effects varies but may range from 2–8 hours depending on the dose and route of administration.

■ **Distribution** Promethazine is widely distributed in body tissues. Compared with other organs, lower concentrations of the drug are found in the brain, but this concentration is higher than the plasma concentration. Promethazine has been reported to be 93% protein bound when determined by gas chromatography and as 76–80% bound when determined by high-performance liquid chromatography. Promethazine readily crosses the placenta. It is not known whether the drug is distributed into milk.

■ **Elimination** Promethazine is metabolized in the liver. The drug is excreted slowly in urine (mainly) and feces principally as inactive promethazine sulfoxide and glucuronides.

Chemistry and Stability

■ **Chemistry** Promethazine hydrochloride is an ethylamino derivative of phenothiazine and occurs as a racemic mixture. The drug occurs as a white to faint yellow, practically odorless, crystalline powder that slowly oxidizes and turns blue on prolonged exposure to air. Promethazine hydrochloride is very soluble in water and in hot dehydrated alcohol. Commercially available promethazine hydrochloride injection has a pH of 4–5.5. The pK_a of the drug is 9.1.

■ **Stability** Promethazine hydrochloride preparations should be protected from light. Promethazine hydrochloride oral solution and tablets should be stored in tight, light-resistant containers at 15–30 and 20–25°C, respectively, while the rectal suppositories should be stored in well-closed containers at 2–8°C. Freezing of the oral solution should be avoided. Following the date of manufacture, commercially available promethazine preparations have expiration dates of 2–5 years depending on the dosage form and manufacturer.

Promethazine hydrochloride injection should be stored in tight, light-resistant containers at 20–25°C, but may be exposed to temperatures ranging from 15–30°C. The injection should be discarded if the solution is discolored or contains a precipitate. Promethazine hydrochloride injection has been reported to be chemically incompatible with several drugs, especially those with an alkaline pH. However, the compatibility depends on several factors (e.g., concentration of the drugs, specific diluents used, resulting pH, temperature). Specialized references should be consulted for specific compatibility information.

Preparations

Excipients in commercially available drug preparations may have clinically important effects in some individuals; consult specific product labeling for details.

Promethazine Hydrochloride

Oral		
Solution	6.25 mg/5 mL*	**Promethazine Hydrochloride Syrup**
Tablets	12.5 mg*	**Phenergan®** (scored), Wyeth
		Promethazine Hydrochloride Tablets
	25 mg*	**Phenergan®** (scored), Wyeth
		Promethazine Hydrochloride Tablets
	50 mg*	**Phenergan®**, Wyeth
		Promethazine Hydrochloride Tablets

Parenteral		
Injection	25 mg/mL*	**Promethazine Hydrochloride Injection**
Injection, for IM use only	50 mg/mL*	**Promethazine Hydrochloride Injection**
Rectal		
Suppositories	12.5 mg*	**Phenadoz®**, Paddock
		Phenergan®, Wyeth
		Promethazine Hydrochloride Suppositories
	25 mg*	**Phenadoz®**, Paddock
		Phenergan®, Wyeth
		Promethazine Hydrochloride Suppositories
	50 mg*	**Phenergan®**, Wyeth
		Promethazine Hydrochloride Suppositories
		Promethegan®, G&W

*available from one or more manufacturer, distributor, and/or repackager by generic (nonproprietary) name

Promethazine Hydrochloride Combinations

Oral		
Solution	6.25 mg/5 mL with Phenylephrine Hydrochloride 5 mg/5 mL*	**Prometh® VC Syrup**, Actavis

*available from one or more manufacturer, distributor, and/or repackager by generic (nonproprietary) name

Ramelteon

■ Ramelteon, a melatonin receptor agonist, is a hypnotic agent.

Uses

■ **Insomnia** Ramelteon is used in the management of insomnia characterized by difficulty with sleep onset.

Efficacy of ramelteon in the management of transient insomnia was established in a randomized, double-blind, parallel-group study in healthy adults 18–64 years of age. In this study, an 8-mg (but not a 16-mg) dose of ramelteon was superior to placebo in decreasing mean sleep latency, as determined by polysomnography (PSG).

Efficacy of ramelteon in the management of chronic insomnia was established in 3 randomized, double-blind studies of up to 35 days' duration in patients with chronic insomnia persisting for at least 3 months. In the first study, patients 18–64 years of age were randomized to receive 8 or 16 mg of ramelteon or placebo at bedtime for 35 nights. PSG was performed during the first 2 nights of weeks 1, 3, and 5. At each of these time points, both the 8- and 16-mg doses of ramelteon were superior to placebo in decreasing mean sleep latency. In the second study (3-period crossover study), geriatric patients (65 years of age and older) were randomized to receive 4 or 8 mg of ramelteon or placebo for 2 consecutive nights, followed by a 5- to 12-day washout period between each treatment. Both the 4- and 8-mg doses of ramelteon were superior to placebo in decreasing mean sleep latency (as determined by PSG) in geriatric patients. The third study evaluated efficacy of ramelteon in geriatric patients by employing subjective efficacy measures (i.e., sleep diaries). In this study, treatment with 4 or 8 mg of ramelteon at bedtime for 35 consecutive nights was superior to placebo in decreasing subjective mean sleep latency. A similarly designed study in younger adults receiving 8- and 16-mg doses of the drug did not replicate these results.

Dosage and Administration

■ **Administration** Ramelteon is administered orally within 30 minutes of bedtime. The drug should not be administered with or immediately after a high-fat meal because of a potentially decreased rate of absorption. (See Description.)

■ **Dosage** The recommended adult dosage of ramelteon for the management of insomnia is 8 mg within 30 minutes of bedtime.

■ **Special Populations** No specific dosage recommendations for patients with hepatic impairment at this time. Ramelteon should be used with caution in patients with moderate hepatic impairment; the drug should *not* be used in those with severe hepatic impairment. (See Hepatic Impairment under Warnings/Precautions: Specific Populations, in Cautions.)

No dosage adjustment is necessary in patients with mild, moderate, or severe (i.e., creatinine clearance of 30 mL/minute or less) renal impairment or in those requiring chronic hemodialysis.

Cautions

■ **Contraindications** Hypersensitivity to ramelteon or any ingredient in the formulation.

■ **Warnings/Precautions** ***Warnings*** **Adequate Patient Evaluation.** Because sleep disturbances may be the principal manifestation of a physical and/or psychiatric disorder, symptomatic treatment of insomnia should be initiated only after careful evaluation of the patient. Failure of insomnia to remit after a reasonable treatment period may indicate the presence of an underlying psychiatric and/or medical condition requiring evaluation. Exacerbation of insomnia and/or emergence of new cognitive or behavioral abnormalities, which have been reported with ramelteon, also may indicate the presence of an underlying psychiatric or physical disorder that requires further patient evaluation. (See Psychiatric Effects under Warnings/Precautions: Major Toxicities, in Cautions.)

Complex Sleep-related Behaviors. There is a potential risk of complex sleep-related behaviors such as sleep-driving (i.e., driving while not fully awake after ingesting a sedative-hypnotic drug, with no memory of the event), making phone calls, or preparing and eating food while asleep.

Sensitivity Reactions There is a potential risk of anaphylaxis and angioedema in patients receiving ramelteon; such reactions may occur as early as with the first dose of the drug.

Major Toxicities **Psychiatric Effects.** Cognitive and behavioral changes have been reported with hypnotic agents, including ramelteon. In primarily depressed patients, exacerbation of depression and suicidal ideation have been reported following use of hypnotics. As with other sedative-hypnotics, emergence of new psychiatric abnormalities during ramelteon therapy requires evaluation.

Endocrine Effects. Increased prolactin concentrations have been reported in patients with chronic insomnia receiving ramelteon therapy (16 mg once daily for 6 months). Effects of intermittent or long-term ramelteon therapy on the human reproductive axis is not known.

Abnormal morning cortisol concentrations (resulting in abnormal corticotropin [ACTH] stimulation test results) were reported in 2 patients and prolactinoma was reported in 1 patient receiving long-term (up to 12 months) ramelteon therapy; a causal relationship to the drug has not been established.

If unexplained amenorrhea, galactorrhea, decreased libido, or fertility problems occur, consider evaluating prolactin or testosterone concentrations.

Abuse Potential and Dependence. No evidence of abuse potential was detected following administration of relatively high ramelteon doses (up to 20 times the recommended hypnotic dose) in patients with a history of drug (e.g., sedative-hypnotic, anxiolytic) abuse or dependence.

Ramelteon does not appear to produce physical dependence.

Withdrawal Effects. Studies employing subjective measures (e.g., questionnaires) did not reveal evidence of a withdrawal syndrome (including rebound insomnia) following discontinuance of long-term ramelteon therapy (4, 8, or 16 mg daily for up to 35 days).

Residual Effects. In a 35-night randomized study evaluating next-day residual effects of ramelteon, adult patients receiving 8 mg of the drug every night experienced reduced immediate/delayed memory recall and increased sluggishness, fatigue, and irritation at weeks 1 and 3 of treatment compared with those receiving placebo. However, next-day residual effects were not substantially different between ramelteon- and placebo-treated patients at week 5. A similar study in geriatric patients receiving 4 or 8 mg of ramelteon every night did not produce any substantial differences in measures of residual effects.

General Precautions **Long-term Safety.** Long-term safety of ramelteon was evaluated in a multicenter, open-label study of up to 1 year's duration in patients with chronic insomnia. In this study, treatment with 8 or 16 mg of ramelteon daily in geriatric patients or younger adults, respectively, for up to 1 year resulted in no clinically meaningful changes in laboratory parameters, endocrine tests, vital signs, ECG recordings, or intensity of menstrual bleeding over time. Furthermore, rebound insomnia, as determined by subjective sleep latency, was not observed following 1 year of therapy.

Concomitant Diseases. Ramelteon did not demonstrate a respiratory depressant effect in patients with mild to moderate chronic obstructive pulmonary disease (COPD). The effect of ramelteon in patients with severe COPD (e.g., those with elevated pCO_2, those requiring nocturnal oxygen therapy) has not been studied, and use in these patients is not recommended.

In studies in patients with mild to moderate obstructive sleep apnea, ramelteon did not produce differences in measures of apnea indices. However, the effect of ramelteon on severe obstructive sleep apnea has not been studied, and use in these patients is not recommended.

Specific Populations **Pregnancy.** Category C. (See Users Guide.) Ramelteon has no established use in labor or delivery.

Lactation. Distributed into milk in rats; not known whether ramelteon is distributed into human milk. Use in nursing women is not recommended.

Pediatric Use. Safety and efficacy of ramelteon have not been established in pediatric patients.

Geriatric Use. Increased exposure to ramelteon has been reported in geriatric patients. However, no substantial differences in safety and efficacy relative to younger adults have been observed.

Hepatic Impairment. Following administration of 16 mg of ramelteon daily for 7 days, exposure to the drug was increased by approximately fourfold in patients with mild hepatic impairment and more than tenfold in those with moderate hepatic impairment. The pharmacokinetics of ramelteon have not been evaluated in patients with severe hepatic impairment (Child-Pugh class C).

Use with caution in patients with moderate hepatic impairment; avoid use in those with severe hepatic impairment.

Renal Impairment. The pharmacokinetics of ramelteon were not altered in patients with renal impairment or in those requiring chronic hemodialysis. No dosage adjustment is necessary in such patients.

■ **Common Adverse Effects** Adverse effects reported in 2% or more of patients receiving ramelteon during clinical trials include headache, somnolence, fatigue, dizziness, nausea, exacerbation of insomnia, upper respiratory tract infection, diarrhea, myalgia, depression, dysgeusia, and arthralgia.

Drug Interactions

■ **Drugs Affecting Hepatic Microsomal Enzymes** Inhibitors of the cytochrome P-450 (CYP) 1A2 isoenzyme: Pharmacokinetic interaction observed during concomitant use with fluvoxamine (substantially increased ramelteon concentrations). Avoid concomitant use with fluvoxamine; caution if used concomitantly with less potent CYP1A2 inhibitors.

Inhibitors of CYP3A4 isoenzyme: Pharmacokinetic interaction observed during concomitant use with ketoconazole (increased concentrations of ramelteon and active metabolite). Caution if used concomitantly with ketoconazole or other potent inhibitors of CYP3A4.

Inhibitors of CYP2C9 isoenzyme: Pharmacokinetic interaction observed during concomitant use with fluconazole (increased concentrations of ramelteon and active metabolite). Caution if used concomitantly with fluconazole or other potent inhibitors of CYP2C9.

Inhibitors of CYP2D6 isoenzyme: Pharmacokinetic interaction with fluoxetine unlikely.

Inducers of CYP isoenzymes: Pharmacokinetic interaction observed during concomitant use with rifampin (decreased concentrations of ramelteon and active metabolite). Possibly reduced ramelteon efficacy when used concomitantly with potent CYP inducers such as rifampin.

■ **Drugs Metabolized by Hepatic Microsomal Enzymes** Substrates of CYP isoenzymes 1A2 (e.g., theophylline), 2C9 (e.g., warfarin), 2C19 (e.g., omeprazole), 2D6 (e.g., dextromethorphan), or 3A4 (e.g., midazolam): Pharmacokinetic interaction unlikely.

■ **Alcohol** Potential pharmacologic interaction (additive sedative effects). Avoid concomitant use with alcohol.

■ **Digoxin** Pharmacokinetic interaction unlikely.

■ **Warfarin** Pharmacokinetic interaction unlikely.

■ **Laboratory Test Interferences** In vitro data indicate that ramelteon does not elicit false-positive results for benzodiazepines, opiates, barbiturates, cocaine, cannabinoids, or amphetamines in 2 standard urine drug screening methods.

Description

Ramelteon, a melatonin receptor agonist, is a hypnotic agent. The drug exhibits high affinity for melatonin MT_1 and MT_2 receptors. The agonist activity of ramelteon at these receptors is thought to contribute to the drug's sleep-inducing properties, as stimulation of these receptors by endogenous melatonin is thought to be responsible for the regulation of circadian rhythm underlying the normal sleep-wake cycle. Ramelteon demonstrates lower selectivity for melatonin MT_3 receptors than for MT_1 and MT_2 receptors; the drug has no appreciable affinity for the gamma-aminobutyric acid (GABA) receptor complex or for receptors that bind neuropeptides, cytokines, serotonin, dopamine, norepinephrine, acetylcholine, or opiates.

Ramelteon is rapidly absorbed and undergoes extensive first-pass metabolism. Following oral administration in the fasting state, peak ramelteon concentrations occur at approximately 0.75 hours (range: 0.5–1.5 hours). Although total absorption of ramelteon is at least 84%, the absolute bioavailability is only 1.8% due to extensive first-pass metabolism. Administration with a high-fat meal delays GI absorption, reduces peak plasma concentration, and increases the area under the plasma-concentration time curve (AUC) of ramelteon. Ramelteon is extensively distributed to tissues; the drug is approximately 82% bound to human serum proteins (mainly [70%] albumin).

Ramelteon is metabolized by the cytochrome P-450 (CYP) microsomal enzyme system, principally by CYP1A2 and, to a lesser extent, by the CYP2C subfamily and by CYP3A4 to active (M-II) and inactive metabolites. The elimination half-life of ramelteon or M-II is 1–2.6 or 2–5 hours, respectively. Following oral administration of radiolabeled ramelteon, approximately 84% of the radioactivity is eliminated in urine and 4% is eliminated in feces, principally as metabolites.

Advice to Patients

Necessity of taking ramelteon within 30 minutes of bedtime and of limiting activities to only those necessary to prepare for bed. Avoid taking with or immediately after a high-fat meal.

Necessity of avoiding driving, operating machinery, or performing hazardous tasks after taking ramelteon. Importance of avoiding alcohol during therapy.

Importance of consulting a clinician if worsening insomnia or emergence of new behavioral manifestations occurs.

Importance of consulting a clinician if cessation of menses or galactorrhea (in women), decreased libido, or problems with fertility occur.

Importance of women informing clinicians if they are or plan to become pregnant or plan to breast-feed.

Importance of informing clinicians of existing or contemplated concomitant therapy, including prescription and OTC drugs, as well as any concomitant illnesses.

Importance of informing patients of other important precautionary information. (See Cautions.)

Overview® (see Users Guide). For additional information on this drug until a more detailed monograph is developed and published, the manufacturer's labeling should be consulted. It is *essential* that the manufacturer's labeling be consulted for more detailed information on usual cautions, precautions, contraindications, potential drug interactions, laboratory test interferences, and acute toxicity.

Preparations

Excipients in commercially available drug preparations may have clinically important effects in some individuals; consult specific product labeling for details.

Ramelteon

Oral

Tablets, film-coated	8 mg	Rozerem®, Takeda

Suvorexant

■ Suvorexant, a dual orexin-1 and orexin-2 receptor antagonist, is a hypnotic agent.

Uses

■ **Insomnia** Suvorexant is used as a hypnotic agent in the management of insomnia characterized by difficulty with sleep onset and/or sleep maintenance. In controlled clinical studies, suvorexant demonstrated efficacy in decreasing sleep latency and improving sleep maintenance when administered nightly for periods up to 3 months in duration.

Efficacy of suvorexant in the management of insomnia was established in 2 multicenter, randomized, double-blind, placebo-controlled, parallel-group studies of 3 months' duration (studies 1 and 2) and supported by a 1-month multicenter, randomized, double-blind, placebo-controlled, crossover study (study 3) in patients who met DSM-IV-TR criteria for primary insomnia.

In studies 1 and 2, which were similar in design, a total of 1260 patients received suvorexant (at doses of 20 mg in patients 18–64 years of age [mean age: 46 years] and 15 mg in patients 65 years of age and older [mean age: 71 years]) or placebo. Patients with sleep disorders other than primary insomnia, confounding neurologic disorders, current major affective or psychotic psychiatric illnesses, substance abuse, or unstable medical conditions were excluded. In both studies, suvorexant was superior to placebo on measures of sleep maintenance, as assessed by polysomnographic wake time after sleep onset (WASO) during the first night of use and at 1 and 3 months and as assessed subjectively as patient-reported total sleep time (sTST) during the first week of use and at 1 and 3 months. Suvorexant also was superior to placebo for decreasing sleep latency, as assessed by polysomnographic latency to persistent sleep (LPS) during the first night of use, at 1 month, and at 3 months (in study 1 only) and patient-reported time to sleep onset (sTSO) during the first week of use, at 1 month (in study 2 only), and at 3 months.

In these studies, the efficacy and safety of suvorexant at doses of 30 mg (in patients 65 years of age and older) and 40 mg (in patients 18–64 years of age) also were evaluated; while also effective in decreasing sleep latency and improving sleep maintenance, the higher doses were associated with substantially more adverse effects.

Study 3 included patients 18–64 years of age. In this study, 249 patients received placebo and 123 patients received suvorexant 10 or 20 mg; doses up to 80 mg also were studied. During the first night of use and at week 4 of treatment, suvorexant doses of 10 and 20 mg were superior to placebo on polysomnographic measures of sleep latency and sleep maintenance (i.e., LPS and WASO).

Suvorexant also was evaluated in a long-term safety study in 781 patients with primary insomnia. Although the study was designed to primarily assess safety of suvorexant, results indicate that the higher doses used in the study (40 mg in patients younger than 65 years of age and 30 mg in patients 65 years of age and older) were superior to placebo based on subjective measures of sleep latency and sleep maintenance (i.e., sTSO and sTST) at 1 month, and efficacy was maintained for periods of up to 12 months.

Dosage and Administration

■ **Administration** Suvorexant is administered orally no more than once per night, within 30 minutes of bedtime and at least 7 hours before the planned time of awakening.

Although suvorexant may be administered without regard to meals, administration with or immediately after a meal decreases the rate of drug absorption and may delay the onset of effect. (See Description.)

■ **Dosage** The smallest effective dosage of suvorexant should be used.

For the management of insomnia, the recommended adult dosage of suvorexant is 10 mg once daily. If the 10-mg dose is well tolerated but not effective, dosage may be increased but should not exceed 20 mg once daily.

In patients receiving a moderate inhibitor of cytochrome P-450 (CYP) isoenzyme 3A, the recommended initial dose of suvorexant is 5 mg and dosage generally should not exceed 10 mg once daily. Suvorexant is not recommended for use in patients receiving a potent CYP3A inhibitor. (See Inhibitors of CYP3A under Drug Interactions: Drugs Affecting Hepatic Microsomal Enzymes.)

When suvorexant is used with other CNS depressants, dosage adjustment of suvorexant and/or the concomitantly administered agent(s) may be necessary because of potentially additive effects. (See Drug Interactions: CNS Depressants.)

■ **Special Populations** No dosage adjustment is necessary in patients with mild to moderate hepatic impairment; however, suvorexant has not been adequately studied in patients with severe hepatic impairment and is not recommended for use in such patients.

No dosage adjustment is necessary in patients with renal impairment.

Adjustment of suvorexant dosage in geriatric patients is not necessary based solely on age.

Systemic exposure to suvorexant is greater in women compared with men, and in obese patients (body mass index [BMI] exceeding 30 kg/m^2) compared with patients who are not overweight (BMI 25 kg/m^2 or less). The manufacturer makes no specific dosage recommendation for obese patients. Dosage adjustment generally is not necessary based solely on gender; however, caution should be used when increasing dosage in obese women. (See Specific Populations under Cautions: Warnings/Precautions.)

Cautions

■ **Contraindications** Suvorexant is contraindicated in patients with narcolepsy. (See Description and also see Narcolepsy-like Events under Cautions: Warnings/Precautions.)

■ **Warnings/Precautions** ***CNS Depressant Effects and Next-day Impairment*** Suvorexant, like other hypnotic agents, has CNS depressant effects and may impair daytime wakefulness even when used as prescribed. Patients receiving suvorexant should be monitored for somnolence and CNS depressant effects; however, impairment may occur in the absence of symptoms and may not be reliably detected by ordinary clinical examination (i.e., formal psychomotor testing may be required). CNS depressant effects may persist for up to several days after discontinuance of suvorexant.

Suvorexant may impair the ability to drive a motor vehicle and may increase the risk of falling asleep while driving. In clinical trials in healthy adults, administration of suvorexant at bedtime (15 or 30 mg in individuals 65 years of age and older and 20 or 40 mg in individuals younger than 65 years of age) was associated with next-morning impairment of driving performance in individuals receiving a single 20- or 40-mg dose. In these trials, 5 individuals (1 geriatric and 4 younger women) discontinued their driving tests prematurely because of somnolence. Therefore, although tolerance or adaptation to some depressant effects may develop with daily use, patients receiving the 20-mg dose should be cautioned against driving or engaging in other activities that require complete mental alertness the day after use. Patients receiving lower doses of the drug also should be advised of the risk of driving impairment. If daytime somnolence develops in patients who drive, suvorexant should be discontinued or the dosage decreased.

Concomitant use of suvorexant with other CNS depressants (e.g., alcohol, benzodiazepines, opiates, tricyclic antidepressants) increases the risk of CNS depression. Dosage adjustment of suvorexant and/or other CNS depressants may be necessary if the drugs are used concomitantly. (See Drug Interactions: CNS Depressants.) Concomitant use of suvorexant with alcohol or other drugs to treat insomnia is not recommended.

The risk of next-day impairment is increased if suvorexant is administered with less than a full night of sleep remaining, if a higher than recommended dose of suvorexant is administered, or when suvorexant is used concomitantly with other CNS depressants or with drugs capable of increasing suvorexant concentrations. (See Inhibitors of CYP3A under Drug Interactions: Drugs Affecting Hepatic Microsomal Enzymes.)

Adequate Patient Evaluation Because sleep disturbances may be a manifestation of a physical and/or psychiatric disorder, symptomatic treatment of insomnia should be initiated only after careful evaluation of the patient. Failure of insomnia to remit after 7–10 days of suvorexant therapy, worsening of insomnia, or emergence of new abnormal thinking or behavior may indicate the presence of an underlying psychiatric, physical, and/or medical condition that requires evaluation.

Abnormal Thinking and Behavioral Changes Abnormal thinking and behavioral changes (e.g., amnesia, anxiety, hallucinations, other neuropsychiatric symptoms) have been reported in patients receiving hypnotic agents. Sleep-driving (i.e., driving while not fully awake after taking a hypnotic agent) and other complex behaviors (e.g., preparing and eating food, making phone calls, having sex) with no memory of the event have been reported in association with the use of hypnotic agents, in hypnotic agent-naive as well as in hypnotic agent-experienced patients. Concomitant use of alcohol and other CNS depressants with suvorexant may increase the risk of such behaviors. Discontinuance of suvorexant should be strongly considered in patients who report any complex sleep behavior.

Worsening of Depression and Suicidality Risk In clinical studies, a dose-dependent increase in suicidal ideation was observed in patients receiving suvorexant.

Worsening of depression and suicidal thoughts and actions (including completed suicides) have been reported in primarily depressed patients receiving sedative and hypnotic agents. Suicidal tendencies may be present, and protective measures may be required. Intentional overdosage is more common in this patient population, and the least amount of drug feasible should be prescribed and dispensed at any one time to avoid such intentional overdosage. Patients should be immediately evaluated if emergence of suicidality or any new behavioral abnormalities occurs during suvorexant therapy.

Patients with Compromised Respiratory Function Effects of suvorexant on respiratory function should be considered if the drug is used in patients with compromised respiratory function.

In a randomized, placebo-controlled crossover study in 26 patients with mild to moderate obstructive sleep apnea (OSA), suvorexant 40 mg given nightly was associated with a small increase in the average number of episodes of apnea and hypopnea per hour of sleep (mean apnea/hypopnea index [AHI] treatment difference of 2.7 for suvorexant compared with placebo) after 4 nights of use; however, substantial interindividual and intraindividual variation was observed and clinically meaningful respiratory depressant effects in patients with OSA cannot be excluded. Effects of suvorexant on respiratory function in patients with severe OSA have not been established.

In a randomized, placebo-controlled crossover study in 25 patients with mild to moderate chronic obstructive pulmonary disease (COPD), suvorexant (30 mg in geriatric individuals and 40 mg in nongeriatric individuals) had no effect on oxygen saturation after 1 and 4 nights of use. However, substantial interindividual and intraindividual variation was observed and clinically meaningful respiratory depressant effects in patients with COPD cannot be excluded. Effects of suvorexant on respiratory function in patients with severe COPD have not been established.

Single suvorexant doses of up to 150 mg did not have a respiratory depressant effect as measured by oxygen saturation in healthy individuals with normal respiratory function.

Narcolepsy-like Events Sleep paralysis (inability to move or speak for up to several minutes during sleep-wake transition) and hypnagogic/hypnopompic hallucinations, including disturbing perceptions, have been reported in patients receiving suvorexant. In addition, dosage-dependent symptoms similar to mild cataplexy (e.g., periods of leg weakness lasting from seconds to a few minutes) may occur at night and/or during the day and may not be associated with an identified triggering event (e.g., laughter, surprise). Patients should be informed of the possibility of these effects. (See Description.)

Abuse Potential and Dependence In an abuse-potential study conducted in recreational drug users, administration of higher than recommended doses of suvorexant (40–150 mg) produced subjective responses (e.g., "drug liking") similar to those produced by higher doses of zolpidem tartrate (15–30 mg), a schedule IV (C-IV) hypnotic agent. Because patients with a history of drug or alcohol abuse or addiction are at increased risk for abuse of and addiction to suvorexant, such patients should be monitored carefully when receiving the drug. Suvorexant is subject to control under the Federal Controlled Substances Act of 1970 as a schedule IV drug.

In clinical studies of 3 months' duration, there was no clear evidence of rebound insomnia following discontinuance of suvorexant. In addition, clinical studies of the drug provided no evidence of physical dependence with prolonged use, and no withdrawal symptoms were reported following drug discontinuance.

Specific Populations **Pregnancy.** Category C. (See Users Guide.)

Lactation. Suvorexant and a hydroxyl metabolite are distributed into milk in rats; it is not known whether the drug is distributed into human milk. Because many drugs are distributed into human milk, caution should be exercised when suvorexant is administered to a nursing woman.

Pediatric Use. Safety and efficacy of suvorexant have not been established in pediatric patients.

Geriatric Use. In clinical studies, 46% of patients who received suvorexant were 65 years of age and older, while 9% were 75 years of age and older. No substantial differences in safety and efficacy relative to younger adults were observed at recommended dosages of the drug.

In a small, randomized, double-blind, placebo-controlled crossover trial in healthy geriatric individuals 65–80 years of age, administration of a single 30-mg dose of suvorexant at bedtime resulted in impairment of balance (body sway area) compared with placebo when individuals were awakened 90 minutes after the dose. In this study, memory impairment was not observed when individuals were awakened 4 hours after the dose.

Hepatic Impairment. Following a single dose of suvorexant, systemic exposure to the drug in patients with moderate hepatic impairment (Child-Pugh score of 7–9) was similar to that in healthy individuals, even though the half-life of the drug was longer (19 versus 15 hours) in patients with moderate hepatic impairment; therefore, no dosage adjustment is necessary in patients with mild or moderate hepatic impairment. Suvorexant has not been studied in patients with severe hepatic impairment and use of the drug in such patients is not recommended.

Renal Impairment. In a pharmacokinetic study, systemic exposure to suvorexant in patients with severe renal impairment (creatinine clearance 30 mL/minute or less) was similar to that in healthy individuals. Therefore, dosage adjustment is not necessary in patients with renal impairment.

Gender. Systemic exposure to suvorexant is greater in women than in men. Peak plasma concentration and area under the concentration-time curve (AUC) are increased by 9 and 17%, respectively, in women compared with men following a 40-mg dose of suvorexant. At 9 hours after a dose, mean plasma concentrations of suvorexant are 5% higher in women than in men. In clinical studies, efficacy appeared to be similar in men and women; however, at doses of 15 or 20 mg, somnolence, headache, abnormal dreams, dry mouth, cough, and upper respiratory infection occurred in women at an incidence of at least twice that in men. Dosage adjustment generally is not necessary based solely on gender; however, caution should be used when increasing dosage in obese women. (See Dosage and Administration: Special Populations.)

Obesity. Clearance of suvorexant is decreased in patients with higher body mass index (BMI). Peak plasma concentration and systemic exposure are 17 and 31% higher, respectively, in obese patients (BMI exceeding 30 kg/m^2) compared with patients who are not overweight (BMI 25 kg/m^2 or less). Mean plasma concentrations at 9 hours after a 20-mg dose of suvorexant are 15% higher in obese patients than patients who are not overweight. In obese women, peak plasma concentration and AUC are increased by 25 and 46%, respectively, compared with nonobese women. The manufacturer makes no specific dosage recommendation for obese patients; however, caution should be used when increasing dosage in obese women. (See Dosage and Administration: Special Populations.)

■ **Common Adverse Effects** Adverse effects occurring in 2% or more of patients receiving suvorexant (at doses of 15 or 20 mg in geriatric or nongeriatric adults, respectively) for up to 3 months and more frequently with the drug than with placebo include somnolence, headache, dizziness, abnormal dreams, cough, diarrhea, dry mouth, and upper respiratory tract infection.

Drug Interactions

Suvorexant is metabolized principally by cytochrome P-450 (CYP) isoenzyme 3A and, to a lesser extent, by CYP2C19. In vitro studies suggest that suvorexant may potentially inhibit CYP3A isoenzymes and intestinal P-glycoprotein (P-gp). The drug does not appear to inhibit CYP isoenzymes 1A2, 2B6, 2C8, 2C9, 2C19, or 2D6 and is not expected to cause clinically important inhibition of organic anion-transporting polypeptide (OATP) 1B1, breast cancer resistance protein (BCRP), or organic cation transporter (OCT) 2.

■ **Drugs Affecting Hepatic Microsomal Enzymes** ***Inhibitors of CYP3A*** Concomitant use of suvorexant with a potent CYP3A inhibitor (e.g., boceprevir, clarithromycin, conivaptan, indinavir, itraconazole, ketoconazole, nefazodone, nelfinavir, posaconazole, ritonavir, saquinavir, telithromycin) is not recommended, as suvorexant exposure may be substantially increased.

If suvorexant is used concomitantly with a moderate CYP3A inhibitor (e.g., aprepitant, atazanavir, ciprofloxacin, diltiazem, erythromycin, fluconazole, fosamprenavir, grapefruit juice, imatinib, verapamil), the recommended initial dose of suvorexant is 5 mg; dosage may be increased if the 5-mg dose is not effective, but generally should not exceed 10 mg once daily.

Diltiazem. Concomitant administration of suvorexant (single 20-mg dose) and the moderate CYP3A inhibitor diltiazem hydrochloride (240 mg as an extended-release preparation daily for 6 days) increased the area under the concentration-time curve (AUC) of suvorexant by approximately twofold.

Ketoconazole. Concomitant administration of suvorexant (single 4-mg dose) and the potent CYP3A inhibitor ketoconazole (400 mg daily for 11 days) increased the AUC of suvorexant by approximately threefold.

Inducers of CYP3A Concomitant use of suvorexant with a potent CYP3A inducer (e.g., carbamazepine, phenytoin, rifampin) may result in substantially decreased systemic exposure to suvorexant and decreased hypnotic efficacy. The manufacturer states that the maximum recommended dosage of 20 mg once daily should not be exceeded in patients receiving concomitant therapy with potent CYP3A inducers.

Rifampin. Concomitant administration of suvorexant (single 40-mg dose) and the potent CYP3A inducer rifampin (600 mg daily for 17 days) resulted in a substantial (approximately 88%) decrease in the AUC of suvorexant.

■ **Drugs Metabolized by Hepatic Microsomal Enzymes** ***Midazolam*** No clinically important changes in exposure to midazolam (a CYP3A substrate) occurred when midazolam (single oral 2-mg dose) was administered concomitantly with suvorexant (single- or multiple-dose administration of suvorexant 80 mg). No dosage adjustment is necessary when suvorexant is used concomitantly with midazolam.

Warfarin Concomitant administration of suvorexant (40 mg daily for 20 days) with the CYP2C9 substrate warfarin sodium (single 30-mg dose) did not affect the pharmacokinetics of *R*- or *S*-warfarin. No dosage adjustment is necessary when suvorexant is used concomitantly with warfarin.

■ **CNS Depressants** Concomitant use of suvorexant with other CNS depressants (e.g., alcohol, benzodiazepines, opiates, tricyclic antidepressants) may result in additive CNS depression. When suvorexant is used concomitantly with other CNS depressant drugs, dosage reduction of suvorexant and/or the CNS depressant may be necessary. Concomitant use of suvorexant with other hypnotic agents is not recommended.

Alcohol An additive effect on psychomotor impairment was observed following single-dose administration of suvorexant 40 mg with alcohol 0.7 g/kg; no clinically important pharmacokinetic interaction was observed. The manufacturer therefore recommends that suvorexant not be taken if alcohol was consumed that evening or before bedtime.

■ **Digoxin** Concomitant administration of suvorexant (40 mg daily for 11 days) and digoxin (single 0.5-mg dose) resulted in slight increases in digoxin peak plasma concentration and AUC (increases of 21 and 27%, respectively) via inhibition of P-gp. The manufacturer of suvorexant recommends monitoring of digoxin concentrations as clinically indicated when the drugs are used concomitantly.

■ **Oral Contraceptives** Concomitant administration of suvorexant (40 mg daily for 18 days) and a single dose of an oral estrogen-progestin combination contraceptive containing ethinyl estradiol 35 mcg and norgestimate 0.25 mg did not have a clinically important effect on the pharmacokinetics of ethinyl estradiol or norelgestromin, the active metabolite of norgestimate. No dosage adjustment is necessary when suvorexant is used concomitantly with ethinyl estradiol and norgestimate.

■ **Paroxetine** Concomitant administration of suvorexant (single 40-mg dose) and paroxetine (20 mg daily) in healthy individuals did not have a clinically important effect on the pharmacokinetics or pharmacodynamics (psychomotor performance) of either drug.

Description

Suvorexant, a dual orexin-1 and orexin-2 receptor antagonist, is a hypnotic agent structurally unrelated to benzodiazepines and other hypnotic agents, including eszopiclone, ramelteon, zaleplon, and zolpidem. Orexin (also known as hypocretin) receptors located in the brain promote and maintain wakefulness; these receptors are activated by the binding of orexin A and B, neuropeptides produced in the lateral hypothalamus. Loss of orexin-producing neurons and the resulting absence of orexin circulating in the CSF are associated with narcolepsy with cataplexy in humans. (See Cautions: Contraindications.) Suvorexant binds with high affinity to orexin-1 and orexin-2 receptors; blockade of these receptors is thought to suppress the wake drive and promote sleep.

Following oral administration in the fasting state, the median time to peak plasma concentration is approximately 2 hours (range: 0.5–6 hours). Administration of suvorexant with a high-fat meal prolongs time to peak plasma concentration by approximately 1.5 hours; peak plasma concentration and area under the plasma concentration-time curve (AUC) are not substantially affected. (See Dosage and Administration: Administration.) Suvorexant is highly bound (more than 99%) to plasma proteins. Suvorexant is metabolized by the cytochrome P-450 (CYP) microsomal enzyme system, principally by CYP3A and, to a lesser extent, by CYP2C19; the major circulating metabolite is a hydroxy derivative that is not expected to be pharmacologically active. The elimination half-life of suvorexant is approximately 12 hours. Following oral administration of radiolabeled suvorexant, approximately 66% of the dose is eliminated in feces and 23% is eliminated in urine.

Advice to Patients

Importance of advising patients to read the manufacturer's medication guide prior to initiating therapy and each time the prescription is refilled.

Importance of taking suvorexant only once per night within 30 minutes of going to bed and only when able to stay in bed for at least 7 hours before it is necessary to be active again. Importance of advising patients that taking suvorexant with or immediately after a meal may delay its effect.

Importance of taking suvorexant only as prescribed and of not increasing the dose unless otherwise instructed by a clinician.

Importance of not taking suvorexant if alcohol has been consumed in the evening or before bedtime.

Importance of avoiding activities requiring complete mental alertness or physical coordination (e.g., driving a motor vehicle) for at least 8 hours after a dose.

Risk of next-day impairment. In patients receiving the 20-mg dose, importance of avoiding driving or engaging in other activities that require complete mental alertness the day after use.

Risk of abnormal thinking, behavioral changes, sleep-walking, sleep-driving, and other complex behaviors (e.g., preparing and eating food, making phone calls, having sex) while not fully awake. Importance of contacting a clinician immediately if these adverse effects occur.

Importance of patients being alert to and immediately reporting emergence or worsening of depression or suicidality and any unusual changes in thoughts or behavior.

Importance of patients being aware that vivid hallucinations or an inability to move or talk for several minutes (sleep paralysis) may occur while going to sleep or waking up and that temporary leg weakness (cataplexy-like symptoms) may occur during the day or night.

Importance of women informing clinicians if they are or plan to become pregnant or plan to breast-feed.

Importance of informing clinicians of existing or contemplated concomitant therapy, including prescription and OTC drugs and dietary or herbal supplements, as well as any concomitant or past illnesses (e.g., depression, substance abuse).

Importance of informing patients of other important precautionary information. (See Cautions.)

Overview® (see Users Guide). For additional information on this drug until a more detailed monograph is developed and published, the manufacturer's labeling should be consulted. It is *essential* that the manufacturer's labeling be consulted for more detailed information on usual cautions, precautions, contraindications, potential drug interactions, laboratory test interferences, and acute toxicity.

Preparations

Suvorexant is subject to control under the Federal Controlled Substances Act of 1970 as a schedule IV (C-IV) drug.

Excipients in commercially available drug preparations may have clinically important effects in some individuals; consult specific product labeling for details.

Suvorexant

Oral		
Tablets, film-coated	5 mg	**Belsomra®**, Merck
	10 mg	**Belsomra®**, Merck
	15 mg	**Belsomra®**, Merck
	20 mg	**Belsomra®**, Merck

Zaleplon

■ Zaleplon, a pyrazolopyrimidine derivative, is a sedative and hypnotic agent structurally unrelated to the benzodiazepines and other sedative-hypnotic agents.

Uses

■ **Insomnia** Zaleplon is used in the short-term management of insomnia. Zaleplon has been shown to decrease sleep latency with repeated use for periods up to 30 days in duration. Because of the drug's short half-life, clinical studies have focused on decreasing sleep latency. The drug has not been shown to substantially increase total sleep time or decrease the number of awakenings, and therefore appears to be most useful for sleep initiation disorders.

Efficacy of zaleplon for the treatment of transient insomnia was established in a controlled study in adults experiencing such insomnia during the first night in a sleep laboratory; a 10-mg but not a 5-mg dose of zaleplon was superior to placebo in this patient population. Efficacy for the treatment of chronic insomnia in adults was established in 9 controlled studies of 1–35 days' duration. The 10- and 20-mg doses of zaleplon were superior to placebo in decreasing sleep latency; some studies demonstrated efficacy versus placebo throughout the study, while others had a substantial number of placebo responders resulting in only 2 days' duration of superior efficacy for zaleplon. Although both the 10- and 20-mg doses were effective, the therapeutic effect was greater and more consistent with the 20-mg dose, and the 5-mg dose was less consistently effective. In one study, 10-mg doses of zaleplon were shown to have continued efficacy when administered for at least 30 consecutive nights. However, patients who require sedative-hypnotic therapy for longer than 2–3 weeks should be evaluated for the presence of an underlying psychiatric and/or medical condition. Insomnia often is the primary or first symptom of an unrecognized psychiatric and/or physical disorder.

Efficacy for the treatment of chronic initial insomnia in geriatric patients was established in 3 controlled studies of 2–14 days' duration in which 5- and 10-mg doses were shown to be superior to placebo in decreasing sleep latency.

Dosage and Administration

■ **General** ***Administration*** Zaleplon is administered orally without regard to meals, although administration with a high-fat meal should be avoided because of a potential decreased rate of drug absorption. Such delay in GI absorption could result in decreased efficacy on sleep latency.

Because of its rapid onset of action, zaleplon should be taken immediately before retiring when the patient is ready to go to sleep or after the patient has already gone to bed but has experienced difficulty falling asleep. Patients should be advised that zaleplon should only be used in circumstances where they are able to get at least 4 hours of sleep, since less prolonged sleep (e.g., for an overnight flight of less than 4 hours' duration) could result in amnesic episodes.

Dosage Dosage of zaleplon should be individualized. The lowest effective dosage of the drug should be used in all patient populations.

The recommended initial dosage of zaleplon for the management of insomnia in most adults younger than 65 years of age is 10 mg immediately before bedtime or after unsuccessfully attempting to sleep. Although the risk of certain adverse effects appears to be dose dependent, 20-mg doses have been shown to be adequately tolerated and may be considered in most such adults who do not respond adequately to lower doses. Doses exceeding 20 mg have not been adequately studied and are not recommended by the manufacturer.

■ **Special Populations** For certain low-weight nongeriatric adults as well as for geriatric adults 65 years of age and older and debilitated patients, 5-mg doses of zaleplon may be sufficient. Doses exceeding 10 mg are not recommended in these populations.

Japanese adults demonstrated pharmacokinetic parameter differences that potentially could be explained by differences in body weight or hepatic enzyme activity.

Patients with mild to moderate hepatic impairment, or those receiving cimetidine concomitantly, should receive the 5-mg zaleplon dosage since drug clearance is reduced in these populations. Zaleplon is not recommended for use in patients with severe hepatic impairment.

No zaleplon dosage adjustment is necessary in patients with mild to moderate renal impairment; zaleplon has not been adequately studied in patients with severe renal impairment.

Cautions

■ **Contraindications** Zaleplon is contraindicated in patients with hypersensitivity to zaleplon or any ingredient in the formulation.

Zaleplon is contraindicated in patients who have previously experienced an episode of complex sleep behavior while taking eszopiclone, zaleplon, or zolpidem. (See Risk of Serious Injury and Death Resulting From Complex Sleep Behaviors under Warnings/Precautions: Warnings, in Cautions.)

■ **Warnings/Precautions** ***Warnings*** **Risk of Serious Injury and Death Resulting From Complex Sleep Behaviors.** Complex sleep behaviors in which patients engage in activities while they are not fully awake, sometimes resulting in serious injuries and/or death, have been reported rarely following use of the sedative and hypnotic agents eszopiclone, zaleplon, and zolpidem. Such behaviors may include sleepwalking, sleep driving (i.e., driving while not fully awake after ingesting a sedative-hypnotic drug, with no memory of the event), and engaging in other activities (e.g., making phone calls, preparing and eating food) while not fully awake. In April 2019, FDA issued a drug safety communication requiring that a boxed warning be added to the prescribing information of these 3 drugs to alert clinicians and patients of this risk, as well as a contraindication to avoid use in patients who previously experienced an episode of complex sleep behavior with eszopiclone, zaleplon, or zolpidem.

FDA has identified 66 cases of complex sleep behaviors resulting in serious injuries or death in patients who took eszopiclone, zaleplon, or zolpidem that were reported to the FDA Adverse Event Reporting System (FAERS) database and/or in published literature between December 1992 and March 2018. Of the 66 cases, 20 were reported as resulting in fatal outcomes and 46 reported serious nonfatal injuries; in the nonfatal cases, patients usually did not remember experiencing these complex sleep behaviors. These cases included falls with serious injuries such as intracranial hemorrhages, vertebral fractures, and hip fractures as well as fatal falls, self-injuries, accidental overdoses, hypothermia, suicide attempts and apparent completed suicides, fatal motor vehicle collisions, gunshot wounds, carbon monoxide poisoning, drowning or near drowning, burns, and homicide. Most of the patients in these cases reported using zolpidem (about 92%) when they experienced the complex sleep behavior; the remaining patients took eszopiclone (about 5%) or zaleplon (about 3%), reflecting the higher number of zolpidem prescriptions that were dispensed over this period compared with eszopiclone and zaleplon. The underlying mechanisms by which these drugs cause complex sleep behaviors are not fully understood.

FDA states that serious injuries and fatalities resulting from complex sleep behaviors have occurred in patients with and without a history of such behaviors and can occur even at the lowest recommended dosages and after just one dose of eszopiclone, zaleplon, and zolpidem. These behaviors can occur when these drugs are taken alone or when taken with alcohol or other CNS depressants. Patients should be warned about this risk and advised to discontinue taking these drugs if they experience an episode of complex sleep behavior. (See Cautions: Contraindications and see also Advice to Patients.)

Other Warnings and Precautions **Adequate Patient Evaluation.** Since sleep disturbances may be a manifestation of a physical and/or psychiatric disorder, symptomatic treatment of insomnia should be initiated only after careful evaluation of the patient. The failure of insomnia to remit after 7–10 days of therapy may indicate the presence of an underlying psychiatric and/or medical condition requiring evaluation.

Sensitivity Reactions. Rare cases of angioedema involving the tongue, glottis, or larynx have been reported in patients receiving their first or subsequent doses of sedatives-hypnotics, including zaleplon. Some patients have experienced additional symptoms such as dyspnea, closing of the throat, or nausea and vomiting that suggest anaphylaxis. Some of these patients have required medical treatment in an emergency department. If angioedema involves the tongue, glottis, or larynx, airway obstruction may occur, which could be fatal. Patients who develop angioedema following treatment with zaleplon should not be rechallenged with the drug.

Some formulations of zaleplon may contain the dye tartrazine (FD&C yellow No. 5), which may cause allergic reactions including bronchial asthma in susceptible individuals. Although the incidence of tartrazine sensitivity is low, it frequently occurs in patients who are sensitive to aspirin.

Psychiatric Effects. Sedative-hypnotic agents are associated with numerous abnormal thought and behavioral processes (e.g., decreased inhibition, agitation, hallucinations, depersonalization, amnesia, depression/suicidal ideation); many are similar to manifestations of alcohol intoxication. Studies demonstrate short-term amnesic effects with zaleplon. Because of rapid clearance of the drug, amnesic effects peak at 1 hour after dosing, dissipate as early as 2 hours in some cases, and usually are gone within 3–4 hours; however, next-day memory impairment may occasionally occur and is dose dependent. As with other sedative-hypnotics, emergence of new psychiatric abnormalities during zaleplon therapy requires evaluation. (See Cautions: Precautions and Contraindications, in Zolpidem Tartrate 28:24.92.)

Abuse Potential. Studies using relatively high zaleplon doses (2.5–7.5 times the recommended hypnotic dose) suggest abuse potential similar to benzodiazepine and related hypnotics; the drug should be used with caution in patients with a history of drug or alcohol dependence or abuse.

Tolerance. No manifestations of tolerance for the therapeutic effects of zaleplon occurred during studies of 4 weeks' duration.

Dependence. Physical dependence results in the manifestation of withdrawal symptoms (e.g., rebound insomnia, anxiety) upon rapid dose decrease or abrupt discontinuance of many sedative-hypnotics, including zaleplon. Rebound insomnia of 1 day's duration was noted in controlled and open-label studies, principally in patients receiving the 20-mg dose of zaleplon. Although premarketing studies did not reveal evidence of a withdrawal syndrome other than such mild rebound insomnia, studies to date do not provide a reliable estimate of the incidence of dependence with zaleplon; in addition, at least 2 cases of seizure (one with a seizure history) have been reported.

Monitor patients closely during zaleplon discontinuance, as other sedative-hypnotics have manifested withdrawal symptoms such as seizures, vomiting, and abdominal cramps and experience with zaleplon to date is limited. Moreover, very short-acting hypnotics such as zaleplon may potentially demonstrate between-dose withdrawal symptoms, although no substantial clinical evidence of this phenomenon exists to date for zaleplon.

Timing of Drug Doses. Ingesting zaleplon while still up and about could result in adverse CNS effects such as short-term memory impairment, hallucinations, dizziness, and impaired coordination. Therefore, administer immediately before retiring or after experiencing difficulty falling asleep. (See Dosage under Dosage and Administration: General.)

Geriatric or Debilitated Patients. Potential increased sensitivity to pharmacologic and adverse effects of hypnotic agents; use with caution and monitor such patients closely. (See Dosage and Administration: Special Populations.)

Concomitant Illness. Experience is limited in patients with concomitant illnesses; zaleplon should be used with caution in patients with diseases or conditions that may affect metabolism or hemodynamic responses.

In general, sedative-hypnotic agents have the potential to depress respiration. Although no reports of respiratory depression have been noted with recommended zaleplon doses in studies to date (including in patients with obstructive sleep apnea or chronic obstructive pulmonary disease [COPD]), patients with impaired respiratory function due to preexisting illness should be monitored carefully during zaleplon therapy.

Hepatic and Renal Disease. See Warnings/Precautions: Specific Populations.

Use in Patients with Depression. As with other sedative-hypnotic agents, zaleplon should be used with caution in patients with signs or symptoms of depression. Suicidal tendencies may be present in such patients and protective measures may be required. Intentional overdosage is more common in this patient population, and the least amount of drug that is feasible should be prescribed for the patient at any one time.

Specific Populations **Pregnancy.** There are no studies of zaleplon in pregnant women to date. The manufacturer does not recommend use in this population, and there is no established use of the drug in labor and delivery.

Lactation. Zaleplon is distributed in milk. Since the effects of zaleplon on nursing infants are not known but even small amounts might be potentially important, the manufacturer does not recommend use in nursing women.

Pediatric Use. Safety and efficacy not established in pediatric patients younger than 18 years of age.

Geriatric Use. Patients 65 years of age and older may be more sensitive to pharmacologic and adverse effects of sedative-hypnotic agents; initial and maximum dose reduction recommended. (See Dosage and Administration: Special Populations.)

Hepatic Impairment. Dosage reduction recommended for mild to moderate impairment; zaleplon use is not recommended in patients with severe impairment. (See Dosage and Administration: Special Populations.)

Renal Impairment. Dosage adjustment is not necessary in mild to moderate renal impairment; zaleplon has not been adequately studied in patients with severe renal impairment.

■ **Common Adverse Effects** Adverse effects occurring in 1% or more of patients and more frequently than placebo at 20-mg zaleplon doses include headache, asthenia, dizziness, nausea, abdominal pain, somnolence, myalgia, amnesia, confusion, dysmenorrhea, ocular pain, paresthesia, malaise, anorexia, depersonalization, hyperesthesia, hypertonia, tremor, abnormal vision, hyperacusis, parosmia, photosensitivity reaction, colitis, peripheral edema, hallucinations, vertigo, epistaxis, and ear pain. Impairment of memory and psychomotor function was no longer present after 3–4 hours in clinical studies to date.

Drug Interactions

■ **Protein-bound Drugs** Zaleplon is not highly bound to plasma proteins; therefore, the disposition of zaleplon is not expected to be sensitive to alterations in protein binding. In addition, administration of zaleplon in patients receiving a highly protein-bound drug is not expected to cause a transient increase in free (unbound) concentration of the highly protein-bound drug.

■ **Alcohol** Potential pharmacodynamic interaction with alcohol: additive CNS effects. Alcohol should be avoided during zaleplon therapy.

■ **Other CNS Depressants** Potential pharmacodynamic interaction with other CNS depressants such as imipramine, thioridazine, and diphenhydramine; anesthetics; anticonvulsants; antihistamines; sedatives and hypnotics; and opiates: may result in additive CNS effects.

Concomitant use of sedative and hypnotic drugs used to treat insomnia (including OTC preparations such as diphenhydramine and doxylamine succinate) should be avoided in patients receiving zaleplon.

Dosage adjustment may be necessary during concurrent use of other CNS depressants.

■ **Cytochrome P-450 Isoenzyme 3A4 Inducers** Potential pharmacokinetic interaction with cytochrome P-450 isoenzyme 3A4 inducers such as rifampin, phenytoin, carbamazepine, and phenobarbital: may result in decreased efficacy of zaleplon.

■ **Cytochrome P-450 Isoenzyme 3A4 Inhibitors** Pharmacokinetic interaction unlikely.

■ **Cimetidine** Potential pharmacokinetic (CYP3A4 and aldehyde oxidase inhibition) interaction; initial zaleplon dose reduction to 5 mg recommended. (See Dosage and Administration: Special Populations.)

■ **Diphenhydramine** Pharmacokinetic (aldehyde oxidase inhibition) interaction unlikely; possible additive pharmacodynamic (CNS depressant) effect. (See Drug Interactions: Other CNS Depressants.)

■ **Digoxin** Administration of zaleplon (10 mg) did not affect the pharmacokinetic or pharmacodynamic profile of digoxin (375 mcg once daily for 8 days).

■ **Ibuprofen** Pharmacokinetic interaction unlikely.

■ **Warfarin** Pharmacokinetic or pharmacodynamic (prothrombin time) interactions unlikely.

Description

Zaleplon, a pyrazolopyrimidine derivative, is a sedative and hypnotic agent structurally unrelated to the benzodiazepines and other sedative-hypnotic agents. Pharmacologically and pharmacokinetically, zaleplon is similar to zolpidem; both are hypnotic agents with short half-lives, and both have been shown to interact with the CNS γ-aminobutyric acid ($GABA_A$)-receptor-chloride ionophore complex at benzodiazepine (BZ) omega-1 (BZ_1, o_1) receptors. In contrast, some benzodiazepines nonselectively activate central BZ_1 (o_1) and BZ_2 (o_2) receptors as well as peripheral BZ_3 (o_3) receptors, resulting in nonspecific pharmacologic actions.

Zaleplon is extensively metabolized, principally by aldehyde oxidase, and to a lesser extent by the cytochrome P-450 (CYP) isoenzyme 3A4. Zaleplon generally appears to be absorbed and eliminated more rapidly than zolpidem.

Advice to Patients

Importance of advising patients to read the manufacturer's medication guide prior to initiating zaleplon therapy and each time the prescription is refilled.

Necessity to administer zaleplon immediately before retiring, or after attempting to fall asleep, and only when able to get 4 or more hours of sleep before it is necessary to be active again. To optimize efficacy, avoid taking with or immediately after a high-fat meal.

Advise to take zaleplon only as prescribed and not to increase the dose or duration of therapy unless otherwise instructed by a clinician.

Importance of informing patients about the risk of complex sleep behaviors (e.g., sleepwalking, sleep driving, engaging in other activities while not fully awake) that, although rare, may result in serious injury or death. Such events can occur following just one dose of these drugs as well as after a longer duration of treatment. Importance of advising patients to discontinue taking zaleplon and to notify a clinician immediately if an episode of complex sleep behavior occurs during therapy, even if it did not result in a serious injury.

Necessity of exercising caution when operating machinery or performing hazardous tasks while using zaleplon; importance of avoidance of alcohol and concurrent use of other sedative and hypnotic drugs used to treat insomnia (including OTC preparations such as diphenhydramine or doxylamine succinate) or CNS depressants during zaleplon therapy unless otherwise instructed by a clinician.

Importance of identifying and reporting to clinicians any potential adverse effects, such as memory impairment, dependence/withdrawal symptoms after multiple dosing, behavioral abnormalities, or tolerance potential. Advise of possibility of rebound insomnia for 1 or 2 nights after discontinuing zaleplon.

Importance of informing clinicians of existing or contemplated concomitant therapy, including prescription and OTC drugs and dietary or herbal supplements, as well as any concomitant illnesses (e.g., psychiatric disorders including depression or suicidality, history of drug or alcohol abuse or addiction, kidney or liver disease, lung disease or breathing difficulty).

Importance of women informing clinicians if they are or plan to become pregnant or plan to breast-feed.

Importance of informing patients of other important precautionary information. (See Cautions.)

Overview (see Users Guide). For additional information until a more detailed monograph is developed and published, the manufacturer's labeling should be consulted. It is *essential* that the manufacturer's labeling be consulted for more detailed information on usual cautions, precautions, contraindications, potential drug interactions, laboratory test interferences, and acute toxicity.

Preparations

Zaleplon is subject to control under the Federal Controlled Substances Act of 1970 as a schedule IV (C-IV) drug.

Excipients in commercially available drug preparations may have clinically important effects in some individuals; consult specific product labeling for details.

Zaleplon

Oral		
Capsules	5 mg*	**Sonata**® (C-IV), Pfizer
		Zaleplon Capsules (C-IV)
	10 mg*	**Sonata**® (C-IV), Pfizer
		Zaleplon Capsules (C-IV)

*available from one or more manufacturer, distributor, and/or repackager by generic (nonproprietary) name

Zolpidem Tartrate

■ Zolpidem tartrate, a type A γ-aminobutyric acid ($GABA_A$)-receptor agonist of the imidazopyridine class, is a sedative and hypnotic agent structurally unrelated to the benzodiazepines and other sedative and hypnotic agents.

Uses

Zolpidem tartrate as conventional tablets, oral spray, or sublingual tablets (Edluar®) is used as a hypnotic agent in the short-term management of insomnia characterized by difficulties with sleep initiation. Because zolpidem has a short half-life, the drug may be of particular benefit in the initiation of sleep (i.e., decreasing sleep latency). In controlled clinical studies of 4–5 weeks' duration, the drug reportedly has been effective in decreasing sleep latency for periods up to 35 days in duration.

Zolpidem tartrate as extended-release tablets is used in the management of insomnia characterized by difficulty with sleep onset or sleep maintenance. However, zolpidem tartrate extended-release tablets may not be an appropriate treatment choice for patients (men or women) with insomnia who need to drive or perform activities that require full alertness the next morning (see Cognitive and Psychomotor Impairment under Cautions: Precautions and Contraindications and also Next-day Impairment under Cautions: Nervous System Effects). In two 3-week, randomized, double-blind, placebo-controlled clinical trials in patients with chronic primary insomnia, zolpidem tartrate given as extended-release tablets improved sleep induction (as measured by latency to persistent sleep [LPS]) and sleep maintenance (as measured by wake time after sleep onset [WASO]). In one study in adults 18–64 years of age, zolpidem tartrate 12.5 mg as extended-release tablets at bedtime decreased WASO for the first 7 hours during the first 2 nights of use and for the first 5 hours after 2 weeks of treatment. In a similarly designed study in patients 65 years of age or older, a 6.25-mg dosage of the drug decreased WASO for the first 6 hours during the first 2 nights of use and for the first 4 hours after 2 weeks of treatment. In both studies, the drug decreased LPS during the first 2 nights of use and after 2 weeks of treatment and improved wakefulness at the end of the night (both measured by polysomnographic recordings) compared with placebo, and the drug was rated by patients as superior to placebo on a global impressions measure after 2 nights and after 3 weeks of use. In a 24-week, randomized, double-blind, placebo-controlled clinical trial in adults 18–64 years of age with chronic primary insomnia, zolpidem tartrate 12.5-mg extended-release tablets administered as needed 3–7 nights per week were superior to placebo on a patient-rated global impressions measure and on specific patient-reported parameters for sleep induction and maintenance; no substantial increase in frequency of drug use over time was observed.

Zolpidem tartrate as sublingual tablets (Intermezzo®) is used as needed for the management of insomnia when middle-of-the-night awakening is followed by difficulty returning to sleep. The drug should be used in this manner *only* when 4 or more hours remain before the patient plans to awaken. In 2 randomized, double-blind, placebo-controlled clinical trials in patients with primary insomnia characterized by difficulty returning to sleep after a middle-of-the-night awakening, sublingual zolpidem tartrate improved sleep latency (as measured by polysomnography and patient-estimated reports) after middle-of-the-night awakening compared with placebo. In one crossover study, adults 19–64 years of age received each of 3 treatments (a 1.75- or 3.5-mg dose of zolpidem tartrate sublingual tablets or placebo) after a scheduled middle-of-the-night awakening on 2 consecutive nights in a sleep laboratory; the effect on sleep latency was similar for women receiving a 1.75-mg dose and men receiving a 3.5-mg dose. In the second study, adults 18–64 years of age received a 3.5-mg dose of zolpidem tartrate sublingual tablets or placebo on an as-needed basis over 4 weeks in an outpatient setting when the patient had difficulty returning to sleep after awakening in the middle of the night, provided at least 4 hours remained before the patient planned to awaken.

The choice of hypnotic agent must be individualized based on patient tolerance and response, taking into consideration pharmacokinetic and pharmacodynamic characteristics of the drug, patient age and other characteristics, and the underlying sleep disorder being treated.

Hypnotics with a relatively short half-life may be more likely to result in transient rebound insomnia after discontinuance and in pharmacodynamic tolerance and adaptation to the hypnotic effect, with resultant diminished effectiveness during the end of each night's use (early morning insomnia) and, possibly, increased daytime anxiety. However, despite zolpidem's short half-life, the manufacturer states that increased wakefulness during the last third of the night and objective evidence of rebound insomnia following discontinuance of zolpidem tartrate as conventional tablets have not been observed in clinical trials to date, although there was subjective evidence of impaired sleep on the first posttreatment night in geriatric patients receiving zolpidem tartrate as conventional tablets in doses that exceeded the recommended geriatric dose of 5 mg. Rebound insomnia was observed in two 3-week clinical trials on the first night after abrupt discontinuance of zolpidem tartrate as extended-release tablets, but there was no worsening compared with baseline on the second night. In a 24-week clinical trial evaluating zolpidem tartrate extended-release tablets administered as needed 3–7 nights per week, a rebound effect was observed within the first month for total sleep time, but not for WASO, during the first night that the drug was not used; however, no further rebound insomnia was observed after the first month or after final treatment discontinuance.

In addition, hypnotics with relatively short half-lives may be less likely to result in residual daytime sedative effects and in impaired psychomotor and mental performance during continued therapy. Residual daytime sedative effects of zolpidem were evaluated in several placebo-controlled studies in healthy adults and in geriatric individuals. A small but statistically significant decrease in performance (determined by the Digit Symbol Substitution test [DSST]) was observed in some adults and geriatric individuals receiving zolpidem tartrate as conventional tablets compared with those receiving placebo. Several studies of zolpidem tartrate as conventional tablets in adults with insomnia found no evidence of residual daytime sedative effects, determined by DSST, the Multiple Sleep Latency Test (MSLT), and patient rating of alertness. In studies of zolpidem tartrate extended-release tablets (given at recommended doses) in adult and geriatric patients, neurocognitive tests performed 8 hours after a dose and patient reports of sedation revealed no evidence of decreased performance or next-day residual effects. However, during the 3-week clinical trials evaluating the extended-release tablets, next-day somnolence was reported by 15 or 2% of adults receiving zolpidem or placebo, respectively, and by 6 or 5% of geriatric patients receiving zolpidem or placebo, respectively. In the 24-week clinical trial, the overall incidence of next-day somnolence was 5.7 or 2% in patients receiving zolpidem tartrate as extended-release tablets or placebo, respectively. The minimal effect of zolpidem on sleep stages at usual hypnotic dosages may offer a therapeutic advantage. However, the fact that zolpidem has minimal anxiolytic and muscle relaxant properties at usual hypnotic doses also should be considered. Blood concentrations of zolpidem may be high enough in some patients on the morning after use to impair performance of activities that require alertness, including driving, and the US Food and Drug Administration (FDA) states that all drugs used in the management of insomnia can impair driving and performance of activities that require alertness on the morning after use. For additional information, see Next-day Impairment under Cautions: Nervous System Effects and also Cognitive and Psychomotor Impairment under Cautions: Precautions and Contraindications.

Additional experience is needed to elucidate more fully the comparative efficacy and safety of zolpidem and benzodiazepines. For additional information on the management of insomnia, see Uses: Anxiety and Insomnia, in the Benzodiazepines General Statement 28:24.08.

Dosage and Administration

■ **Administration** Zolpidem tartrate is administered orally (as conventional tablets, extended-release tablets, or an oral solution using a metered-dose spray pump) or sublingually (as sublingual tablets).

Oral Administration Zolpidem tartrate is administered orally at bedtime. Zolpidem tartrate should be taken only once per night immediately before bedtime and at least 7–8 hours before the planned time of awakening; patients should be advised of the importance of only taking the drug at such time. In addition, because food can reduce both the rate and extent of GI absorption of zolpidem tartrate, the drug should not be administered with or immediately after a meal in order to facilitate the onset of sleep.

Zolpidem tartrate extended-release tablets are commercially available as a coated bilayer formulation in which a portion of the labeled dose is contained in an immediate-release layer and the remaining portion is contained in a layer that slowly releases the drug. Following oral administration, the extended-release tablets exhibit biphasic absorption with a rapid initial absorption that is similar to that of immediate-release (conventional) tablets and extended absorption exceeding 3 hours after administration.

Zolpidem tartrate extended-release tablets should be swallowed whole and should *not* be divided, crushed, or chewed.

The manufacturer's instructions for patients should be consulted for detailed information on use of zolpidem tartrate oral spray. Prior to initial use, the spray pump must be primed by actuating 5 sprays while pointing the spray opening away from the patient's face and other individuals. If the oral spray has not been used for 14 days or longer, the pump must be primed again by actuating 1 spray. To administer the drug, the patient should hold the container upright with the spray opening pointed directly into the mouth, then fully press down on the pump to ensure that a full dose of the drug is sprayed directly into the mouth over the tongue. Based on the indicated dose of zolpidem tartrate, the appropriate number of sprays of the drug should be administered. Zolpidem tartrate oral spray delivers 5 mg of zolpidem tartrate per metered spray.

The commercially available zolpidem tartrate oral spray delivers about 60 metered sprays per 8.2-g container after 5 initial priming actuations. The total number of available doses is dependent on the number of sprays per dose (1 or 2 actuations) and the frequency of priming. Zolpidem tartrate oral spray should be discarded when the labeled number of actuations (60 sprays) have been used. The manufacturer states that there are no special requirements for cleaning and maintaining the zolpidem tartrate oral spray pump.

Sublingual Administration Zolpidem tartrate is administered sublingually.

Zolpidem tartrate 5- and 10-mg sublingual tablets (Edluar®) should be taken only once per night immediately before bedtime and at least 7–8 hours before the planned time of awakening; patients should be advised of the importance of only taking the drug at such time. The tablet should be placed under the tongue, where it will disintegrate. The tablet should not be swallowed or administered with water. In addition, because food can reduce both the rate and extent of absorption of zolpidem tartrate, the drug should not be administered with or immediately after a meal in order to facilitate the onset of sleep.

Zolpidem tartrate 1.75- and 3.5-mg sublingual tablets (Intermezzo®) should be taken in bed, only once per night as needed if a middle-of-the-night awakening is followed by difficulty returning to sleep, and only if at least 4 hours remain before the planned time of awakening; patients should be advised of the importance of only taking the drug at such time. The tablet should be placed under the tongue and allowed to disintegrate completely before swallowing. The tablet should not be swallowed whole. In addition, because food can reduce both the rate and extent of absorption of zolpidem tartrate, the drug should not be administered with or immediately after a meal for optimal effect. The tablet should be removed from the pouch just prior to administration.

■ **Dosage** The lowest effective dosage of zolpidem tartrate should be used.

Because manifestations of withdrawal have been reported following abrupt discontinuance or rapid reduction in dosage of zolpidem, patients should be monitored for tolerance, abuse, and dependence. (See Tolerance, Dependence, and Abuse under Cautions: Precautions and Contraindications.) There also is evidence that abrupt discontinuance of sedative and hypnotic drugs, including zolpidem tartrate, may result in rebound insomnia, which usually persists for 1 or 2 nights; this effect may occur with some sedative and hypnotic drugs even after relatively short periods of therapy (e.g., 1 week). Therefore, some clinicians suggest that gradual dosage reduction (e.g., over several nights) be considered when discontinuing therapy, since the development of rebound insomnia can perpetuate continued use of hypnotics in patients with insomnia.

Oral Dosage For the management of insomnia characterized by difficulties with sleep initiation, the recommended initial dose of zolpidem tartrate as an oral immediate-release preparation (conventional tablets or oral spray) is 5 mg in women and either 5 or 10 mg in men. For the management of insomnia characterized by difficulty with sleep initiation or sleep maintenance, the recommended initial dose of zolpidem tartrate as extended-release tablets is 6.25 mg in women and either 6.25 or 12.5 mg in men. The lower doses (5 or 6.25 mg) should be effective in most women and many men. However, if the 5-mg dose of immediate-release zolpidem tartrate is not effective in men or women, the dose may be increased to 10 mg. If the 6.25-mg dose of extended-release zolpidem tartrate is not effective in men or women, the dose may be increased to 12.5 mg. In some patients, higher morning blood concentrations following use of a 10-mg dose of immediate-release zolpidem tartrate or a 12.5-mg dose of extended-release zolpidem tartrate increase the risk of next-day impairment of driving and other activities that require full alertness. (See Next-day Impairment under Cautions: Nervous System Effects and also Cognitive and Psychomotor Impairment under Cautions: Precautions and Contraindications.) Total dosage should not exceed 10 mg of immediate-release zolpidem tartrate or 12.5 mg of extended-release zolpidem tartrate given once daily immediately before bedtime. The recommended initial doses of zolpidem tartrate for women and men differ because clearance of the drug is slower in women. (See Special Populations under Pharmacokinetics: Elimination.)

In geriatric or debilitated patients, the recommended bedtime dosage of zolpidem tartrate is 5 mg as an immediate-release preparation or 6.25 mg as extended-release tablets given once daily immediately before bedtime.

When oral formulations of zolpidem tartrate are used concomitantly with other CNS depressants, dosage adjustment of zolpidem and the concomitantly administered agent(s) may be necessary because of potentially additive effects. (See Cognitive and Psychomotor Impairment under Cautions: Precautions and Contraindications.)

Sublingual Dosage For the short-term management of insomnia characterized by difficulties with sleep initiation, the recommended initial dose of zolpidem tartrate sublingual tablets (Edluar®) is 5 mg for women and either 5 or 10 mg for men. The 5-mg dose should be effective in most women and many men. However, if the 5-mg dose is not effective in men or women, the dose may be increased to 10 mg. In some patients, higher morning blood concentrations following use of a 10-mg dose increase the risk of next-day impairment of driving and other activities that require full alertness. (See Next-day Impairment under Cautions: Nervous System Effects and also Cognitive and Psychomotor Impairment under Cautions: Precautions and Contraindications.) Total dosage should not exceed 10 mg given once daily immediately before bedtime. The recommended initial doses of zolpidem tartrate for women and men differ because clearance of the drug is slower in women. (See Special Populations under Pharmacokinetics: Elimination.) In geriatric or debilitated patients, the recommended sublingual dose of zolpidem tartrate for management of insomnia characterized by difficulties with sleep initiation is 5 mg once daily immediately before bedtime. When zolpidem tartrate sublingual tablets (Edluar®) are used concomitantly with other CNS depressants, dosage adjustment of zolpidem and the concomitantly administered agent(s) may be necessary because of potentially additive effects. (See Cognitive and Psychomotor Impairment under Cautions: Precautions and Contraindications.)

For as-needed use in the management of insomnia when middle-of-the-night awakening is followed by difficulty returning to sleep, the recommended and maximum dose of zolpidem tartrate sublingual tablets (Intermezzo®) is 1.75 mg for women and 3.5 mg for men. The recommended doses for women and men differ because clearance of the drug is slower in women. (See Special Populations under Pharmacokinetics: Elimination and also Next-day Impairment under Cautions: Nervous System Effects.) In men and women older than 65 years of age, the recommended sublingual dosage of zolpidem tartrate for middle-of-the-night awakening is 1.75 mg taken only once per night if needed. In men and women receiving other CNS depressants concomitantly, the recommended sublingual dose of zolpidem tartrate for middle-of-the-night awakening is 1.75 mg; dosage adjustment of the concomitant CNS depressant may be necessary because of potentially additive effects. (See Cognitive and Psychomotor Impairment under Cautions: Precautions and Contraindications.)

■ **Dosage in Renal and Hepatic Impairment** Elimination of zolpidem tartrate is prolonged in patients with hepatic impairment. For the management of insomnia characterized by difficulties with sleep initiation in patients with hepatic impairment, the recommended dosage of zolpidem tartrate as an immediate-release preparation (conventional tablets, oral spray, sublingual tablets) is 5 mg once daily immediately before bedtime. For the management of insomnia characterized by difficulty with sleep initiation or sleep maintenance in patients with hepatic impairment, the recommended dosage of zolpidem tartrate as extended-release tablets is 6.25 mg once daily immediately before bedtime. For use in the management of insomnia when middle-of-the-night awakening is followed by difficulty returning to sleep, the recommended sublingual dosage of zolpidem tartrate in patients with hepatic impairment is 1.75 mg once per night if needed.

The manufacturers and some clinicians state that dosage adjustment is not necessary in patients with renal impairment. Other clinicians, however, state that the possibility that dosage reduction may be needed for patients with renal disease should be considered because of slower zolpidem elimination rates and other pharmacokinetic alterations observed in nondialyzed patients with chronic renal disease and in patients undergoing periodic dialysis.

Cautions

Zolpidem tartrate conventional tablets generally are well tolerated at recommended doses (i.e., up to 10 mg). Adverse effects of the drug tend to be dose related, particularly in geriatric patients and at doses exceeding those recommended. (See Cautions: Geriatric Precautions.) The most common adverse effects of zolpidem tartrate as conventional tablets, including those that most frequently require discontinuance of the drug, involve the nervous system and GI tract. In controlled clinical trials of short-term (up to 10 days) treatment with recommended doses of zolpidem tartrate conventional tablets, the most frequent adverse effects and those that were substantially more frequent with the drug than with placebo were drowsiness, dizziness, and diarrhea, which occurred in 2, 1, and 1% of patients, respectively. In controlled clinical trials of prolonged therapy (4–5 weeks) with recommended doses of zolpidem tartrate conventional tablets, the most frequent adverse effects and those that were substantially more frequent with the drug than with placebo were dizziness and drugged feelings, which occurred in 5 and 3% of patients, respectively. The frequencies of many adverse nervous system and GI effects were similar to those of placebo in clinical trials of the drug at recommended doses. Adverse effects have required discontinuance of zolpidem tartrate as conventional tablets in approximately 4% of patients overall in worldwide clinical trials at doses ranging from 1–90 mg. These adverse effects included daytime drowsiness, headache, amnesia, dizziness, vertigo, falls, nausea, and vomiting.

Adverse effects of zolpidem tartrate as extended-release tablets also tend to be dose related, particularly for certain adverse nervous system and GI effects. The most common adverse effects of zolpidem tartrate as extended-release tablets, including those that most frequently require discontinuance of the drug, involve the nervous system. In 3-week controlled clinical trials of zolpidem tartrate administered as extended-release tablets at recommended doses, the most frequent adverse effects were headache, next-day somnolence, and dizziness, which occurred in 19, 15, and 12% of adults, respectively, and in 14, 6, and 8% of geriatric patients, respectively. In a 24-week clinical trial of zolpidem tartrate administered as extended-release tablets, the most frequent adverse effects were consistent with those reported in the 3-week clinical trials, except for a higher incidence of anxiety (6.3%). Adverse effects have required discontinuance of zolpidem tartrate when given as extended-release tablets at recommended doses in approximately 3.5% of patients in the 3-week clinical trials and 8.5% of patients in the 24-week clinical trial; the adverse effects most frequently associated with discontinuance of the drug were somnolence, which required discontinuance in 1% of patients in the 3-week clinical trials, and anxiety (anxiety, restlessness, or agitation) and depression (depression, major depression, or depressed mood), which each required discontinuance in 1.5% of patients in the 24-week clinical trial. The manufacturers state that adverse effects reported at frequencies of less than 1% in clinical trials of zolpidem tartrate extended-release tablets do not appear to differ substantially from those seen in studies with the conventional tablets.

The incidence of adverse effects in patients receiving zolpidem tartrate 1.75 mg as sublingual tablets on 2 consecutive nights in a sleep laboratory study was similar to the incidence observed in patients receiving 3.5-mg sublingual doses as needed after middle-of-the-night awakenings in a 4-week outpatient study. The most frequent adverse effects in patients receiving zolpidem tartrate as 1.75- or 3.5-mg sublingual tablets were headache, fatigue, and nausea.

■ **Nervous System Effects** Headache, drowsiness or somnolence (i.e., drowsiness and drugged feeling), and dizziness were the most frequent adverse nervous system effects of zolpidem tartrate in clinical trials, and among the most frequent adverse effects requiring discontinuance of the drug. Headache occurred in 7% of patients receiving short-term (up to 10 days) treatment with recommended doses of zolpidem tartrate conventional tablets, 19% of adults and 14% of geriatric patients receiving recommended doses of zolpidem tartrate extended-release tablets in clinical trials of 3 weeks' duration, 3% of patients receiving as-needed therapy with zolpidem tartrate 3.5-mg sublingual tablets in an outpatient study of 4 weeks' duration, and 1–22% of patients receiving placebo. Headache has required discontinuance of zolpidem tartrate conventional tablets in about 0.4–0.5% of patients. Drowsiness occurred in 2 or 8% of patients receiving short-term or prolonged (4–5 weeks) treatment, respectively, with recommended doses of zolpidem tartrate conventional tablets and in 5% of those receiving placebo. Drowsiness has required discontinuance of zolpidem tartrate conventional tablets in about 0.5–1.1% of patients. Somnolence occurred in 15% of adults and 6% of geriatric patients receiving recommended doses of zolpidem tartrate extended-release tablets and in 2–5% of those receiving placebo. Somnolence has required discontinuance of zolpidem tartrate extended-release tablets in about 1% of patients in clinical trials of 3 weeks' duration. Dizziness occurred in 1 or 5% of patients receiving short-term or prolonged treatment, respectively, with recommended doses of zolpidem tartrate conventional tablets; 12% of adults and 8% of geriatric patients receiving recommended doses of zolpidem tartrate extended-release tablets; and 1–5% of those receiving placebo. Dizziness has required discontinuance of therapy in about 0.4–0.8% of patients receiving zolpidem tartrate conventional tablets.

Lethargy and drugged feeling occurred in 3% of patients receiving prolonged therapy (4–5 weeks) with recommended doses of zolpidem tartrate conventional tablets in clinical trials, and lethargy occurred in 1% of patients receiving placebo. Drugged feeling was one of the most frequent adverse effects of short-term treatment with zolpidem tartrate conventional tablets. Lightheadedness and depression occurred in 2% of patients receiving prolonged therapy with recommended doses of zolpidem tartrate conventional tablets and 1% of patients receiving placebo. Depression also occurred in 1–2% of patients receiving recommended doses of zolpidem tartrate extended-release tablets.

Amnesia, sleep disorder, and abnormal dreams occurred in 1% of patients receiving prolonged therapy (4–5 weeks) with recommended doses of zolpidem tartrate conventional tablets. Memory disorders (i.e., memory impairment, amnesia, anterograde amnesia) occurred in 1–3% of patients receiving recommended doses of zolpidem tartrate extended-release tablets. Anxiety occurred in 2–3% of patients receiving recommended doses of zolpidem tartrate extended-release tablets and in 2% of those receiving placebo.

Ataxia, asthenia, disorientation, euphoria, balance disorder, and vertigo have been reported in 1–3% of adults receiving recommended doses of zolpidem tartrate extended-release tablets, and disorientation occurred in 2% of placebo-treated patients. Ataxia, asthenia, confusion, euphoria, headache, insomnia, and vertigo have been reported in more than 1% of patients receiving zolpidem tartrate as conventional tablets. Agitation, anxiety, decreased cognition, detached feeling, difficulty concentrating, dysarthria, emotional lability, fatigue, hallucination, hypoesthesia, illusion, malaise, migraine, nervousness, paresthesia, sleeping (after daytime dosing), speech disorder, stupor, increased sweating, and tremor have been reported in 0.1–1% of patients receiving zolpidem tartrate as conventional tablets. Hallucinations, fatigue, disturbance in attention, hypoesthesia, and psychomotor retardation each have been reported in 2–4% of adults receiving recommended doses of zolpidem tartrate extended-release tablets, and fatigue and hypoesthesia have been reported in 1–2% of placebo-treated patients. Psychomotor retardation also has been reported in 2% of geriatric patients receiving recommended doses of zolpidem tartrate extended-release tablets. Appetite disorder, binge eating, paresthesia, depersonalization, disinhibition, mood swings, and stress symptoms each occurred in 1% of adults receiving recommended doses of zolpidem tartrate extended-release tablets. Apathy, burning sensation, postural dizziness, involuntary muscle contractions, paresthesia, and tremor each occurred in 1% of geriatric patients receiving recommended doses of zolpidem tartrate extended-release tablets. Fatigue has been reported in 1% of patients receiving zolpidem tartrate as 3.5-mg sublingual tablets and in none of those receiving placebo. Abnormal gait, abnormal thinking, aggressive reaction, apathy, increased appetite, decreased libido, delusion, dementia, depersonalization, dysphasia, feeling strange, hypokinesia, hypotonia, hysteria, intoxicated feeling, manic reaction, neuralgia, neuritis, neuropathy, neurosis, pain, panic attacks, paresis, personality disorder, somnambulism, suicide attempts, tetany, and yawning have been reported in less than 0.1% of patients receiving zolpidem tartrate as conventional tablets. Psychotic reactions also have been reported rarely in patients receiving zolpidem tartrate as conventional tablets.

Abnormal thinking and behavioral changes have been reported in patients receiving sedative and hypnotic drugs, including zolpidem. Some of these changes included decreased inhibition (e.g., aggressiveness and extroversion that seemed out of character), bizarre behavior, agitation, depersonalization, and visual and auditory hallucinations. Amnesia, anxiety, and other neuropsychiatric symptoms also may occur. (See Mood, Thought, and Behavioral Changes under Cautions: Precautions and Contraindications.)

Complex sleep behaviors such as sleepwalking, sleep driving (i.e., driving while not fully awake after ingesting a sedative-hypnotic drug, with no memory of the event), and engaging in other activities (e.g., making phone calls, preparing and eating food) while not fully awake after ingesting a prescription sedative and hypnotic drug, with no memory of the event, have been reported in sedative and hypnotic drug-naive patients as well as in sedative and hypnotic drug-experienced patients. Such complex sleep behaviors can result in serious injury and/or death. These behaviors appear to be more common with eszopiclone, zaleplon, and zolpidem. Although behaviors such as sleep-driving have occurred with zolpidem alone at therapeutic dosages, the concomitant use of alcohol and other CNS depressants with zolpidem or the use of zolpidem at dosages exceeding the maximum recommended dosage appears to increase the risk of such behaviors. Zolpidem should be discontinued in patients who experience a complex sleep behavior. (See Risk of Serious Injury and Death Resulting From Complex Sleep Behaviors under Cautions: Precautions and Contraindications.)

Although no consistent objective evidence for anterograde amnesia was found in controlled studies in adults receiving zolpidem tartrate as conventional tablets, results of one study indicate that the day following administration of 10- and 20-mg doses of zolpidem tartrate conventional tablets, substantial memory loss was reported regarding information presented to these individuals during periods of maximal sedative effect (i.e., 90 minutes after administration of zolpidem). In addition, although there is subjective evidence for anterograde amnesia occurring in association with zolpidem tartrate as conventional tablets (predominantly at doses exceeding 10 mg), limited studies involving objective measures of memory yielded little evidence for memory impairment following administration of the drug.

Next-day Impairment Driving simulation and laboratory studies indicate that blood zolpidem concentrations exceeding approximately 50 ng/mL appear to be capable of impairing driving performance to a degree that increases the risk of a motor vehicle accident. The risk for next-morning impairment is highest for patients receiving extended-release preparations of the drug. In addition, women appear to be more susceptible to this risk because clearance of zolpidem is slower in women than in men. In pharmacokinetic studies evaluating 10-mg doses of immediate-release zolpidem tartrate (i.e., conventional tablet or bioequivalent preparations) in approximately 250 men and 250 women, zolpidem concentrations measured approximately 8 hours after a dose exceeded 50 ng/mL in 15% of women and 3% of men; results of 3 concentration measurements in women and 1 concentration measurement in men were at least 90 ng/mL. In pharmacokinetic studies evaluating 12.5-mg doses of extended-release zolpidem tartrate, zolpidem concentrations measured approximately 8 hours after a dose exceeded 50 ng/mL in 33% of women and 25% of men, and were at least 100 ng/mL in about 5% of patients. In studies evaluating 6.25-mg doses of extended-release zolpidem tartrate, zolpidem concentrations measured approximately 8 hours after a dose were 50 ng/mL or higher in about 15% of nongeriatric women, 5% of nongeriatric men, and 10% of both geriatric men and women. Because of these findings, currently recommended bedtime doses of zolpidem tartrate (see Dosage and Administration: Dosage) are lower than the original labeled doses, and all patients (including both men and women) receiving zolpidem should be cautioned about the risks of next-morning impairment for activities (e.g., driving) that require complete mental alertness. (See Cognitive and Psychomotor Impairment under Cautions: Precautions and Contraindications.)

The effect of middle-of-the-night sublingual administration of zolpidem tartrate on next-morning driving performance has been evaluated in a randomized, double-blind, placebo- and active-controlled crossover study in healthy individuals. In this study, individuals received a 3.5-mg sublingual dose of zolpidem tartrate 3 or 4 hours before driving, placebo, or an active control 9 hours before driving. When the driving test began 3 hours after the zolpidem dose, impairment (as measured by a standard test of road tracking precision ["weaving"]) was significantly worse than during the placebo test period, and testing was terminated for one individual (a 23-year-old woman) because of somnolence. When the driving test began 4 hours after the zolpidem dose, results were numerically worse than during the placebo period, but statistical significance was not established. Blood concentrations of zolpidem were not measured. However, the manufacturer states that the estimated zolpidem concentration in individuals with worse driving performance during the zolpidem test period is considered to present a risk for driving impairment. In some women, zolpidem concentrations remain at or sometimes considerably higher than this concentration for 4 or more hours after a 3.5-mg sublingual dose of the drug; therefore, the recommended dose of zolpidem tartrate for management of middle-of-the-night awakening in women is 1.75 mg (see Sublingual Dosage under Dosage and Administration: Dosage). Because a small adverse effect on road tracking precision may remain 4 hours after a 1.75-mg dose in women or a 3.5-mg dose in men, potential impairment of driving performance at these recommended dosages cannot be completely excluded.

■ **GI Effects** Diarrhea was one of the most frequent adverse effects of short-term (up to 10 days) treatment with recommended doses of zolpidem tartrate conventional tablets in clinical trials, occurring in 1% of patients. Diarrhea occurred in 3% of patients receiving prolonged therapy (4–5 weeks) with recommended doses of zolpidem tartrate conventional tablets in clinical trials and in 2% of those receiving placebo. Frequent bowel movements occurred in 1% of adults receiving recommended doses of zolpidem tartrate extended-release tablets. Nausea occurred in more than 1% of patients receiving zolpidem tartrate as conventional tablets, 7% of adults receiving recommended doses of zolpidem tartrate extended-release tablets, 1% of patients receiving zolpidem tartrate as 3.5-mg sublingual tablets, and 1–4% of patients receiving placebo. Dry mouth occurred in 3% of patients receiving prolonged therapy with recommended doses of zolpidem tartrate conventional tablets in clinical trials and in 1% of those receiving placebo. Dry throat or throat irritation occurred in 1% of patients receiving recommended doses of zolpidem tartrate extended-release tablets. Nausea was one of the most frequent adverse effects requiring discontinuance of zolpidem tartrate as conventional tablets in clinical trials, with 0.5–0.6% of patients discontinuing therapy. Vomiting occurred in 0.1–1% of patients receiving zolpidem tartrate as conventional tablets and in 1% of patients receiving recommended doses of zolpidem tartrate extended-release tablets; however, it was one of the most frequent adverse effects requiring discontinuance of zolpidem tartrate conventional tablets in clinical trials, with 0.5% of patients discontinuing therapy.

Constipation occurred in 2% of patients receiving prolonged therapy with recommended doses of zolpidem tartrate conventional tablets in clinical trials and in 1% of those receiving placebo. Constipation occurred in 2% of adults receiving recommended doses of zolpidem tartrate extended-release tablets. Abdominal pain occurred in 2% of patients receiving prolonged therapy with recommended doses of zolpidem tartrate conventional tablets in clinical trials and in 2% of those receiving placebo. Abdominal discomfort, abdominal tenderness, gastroesophageal reflux disease (GERD), and gastroenteritis each occurred in 1% of adults receiving recommended doses of zolpidem tartrate extended-release tablets. Dyspepsia and hiccups have been reported in more than 1% of patients receiving zolpidem tartrate as conventional tablets. Flatulence has occurred in 1% of geriatric patients receiving recommended doses of zolpidem tartrate extended-release tablets. Anorexia, constipation, dysphagia, flatulence, gastroenteritis, and taste perversion have been reported in 0.1–1% of patients, and altered or increased saliva, enteritis, eructation, esophagospasm, gastritis, hemorrhoids, intestinal obstruction, rectal hemorrhage, tenesmus, and dental caries have been reported in less than 0.1% of patients receiving zolpidem tartrate as conventional tablets.

■ **Musculoskeletal Effects** Myalgia has been reported in more than 1% of patients receiving zolpidem tartrate as conventional tablets and in 4% of adults receiving recommended doses of zolpidem tartrate extended-release tablets. Arthralgia has been reported in more than 1% of patients receiving zolpidem tartrate as conventional tablets and in 2% of geriatric patients receiving recommended doses of zolpidem tartrate extended-release tablets. Back pain occurred in 3% of patients receiving prolonged therapy with recommended doses of zolpidem tartrate conventional tablets, 4% of adults receiving recommended doses of zolpidem tartrate extended-release tablets, and 2–3% of those receiving placebo. Neck pain occurred in 1–2% of patients receiving recommended doses of zolpidem tartrate extended-release tablets. Muscle cramps occurred in 2% of geriatric patients receiving recommended doses of zolpidem tartrate extended-release tablets. Arthritis and leg cramps have been reported in 0.1–1% of patients, and arthrosis, muscle weakness, sciatica, tendinitis, and restless legs have been reported in less than 0.1% of patients receiving zolpidem tartrate as conventional tablets.

■ **Respiratory Effects** Sinusitis and pharyngitis occurred in 3–4% of patients receiving prolonged therapy (4–5 weeks) with recommended doses of zolpidem tartrate conventional tablets in clinical trials, frequencies slightly higher than those reported in individuals receiving placebo. Nasopharyngitis occurred in 6% of geriatric patients receiving recommended doses of zolpidem tartrate extended-release tablets and in 4% of those receiving placebo. Upper and lower respiratory tract infections each occurred in more than 1% of patients receiving zolpidem tartrate as conventional tablets and in 1% of geriatric patients receiving recommended doses of zolpidem tartrate extended-release tablets. Bronchitis, coughing, dyspnea, and rhinitis have been reported in 0.1–1% of patients, and bronchospasm, epistaxis, hypoxia, laryngitis, pneumonia, and respiratory depression have been reported in less than 0.1% of patients receiving zolpidem tartrate as conventional tablets.

■ **Cardiovascular Effects** Palpitation was reported in 2% of patients receiving prolonged therapy (4–5 weeks) with recommended doses of zolpidem tartrate conventional tablets and in 2% of geriatric patients receiving recommended doses of zolpidem tartrate extended-release tablets. Increased blood pressure occurred in 1% of adults receiving recommended doses of zolpidem tartrate extended-release tablets. Cerebrovascular disorder, hypertension, postural hypotension, edema, chest pain, syncope, and tachycardia have been reported in 0.1–1% of patients, and angina pectoris, arrhythmia, arteritis, circulatory failure, extrasystoles, flushing, hypotension, aggravated hypertension, myocardial infarction, phlebitis, pulmonary embolism, pulmonary or facial edema, varicose veins, and ventricular tachycardia have been reported in less than 0.1% of patients receiving zolpidem tartrate as conventional tablets.

■ **Dermatologic and Sensitivity Reactions** Rash occurred in 2% of patients receiving prolonged therapy (4–5 weeks) with recommended doses of zolpidem tartrate conventional tablets, and rash and urticaria each occurred in 1% of patients receiving recommended doses of zolpidem tartrate extended-release tablets. Skin wrinkling occurred in 1% of adults receiving recommended doses of zolpidem tartrate extended-release tablets. Pruritus has been reported in 0.1–1% of patients and acne, bullous eruption, dermatitis, furunculosis, injection-site inflammation, and urticaria have been reported in less than 0.1% of patients receiving zolpidem tartrate as conventional tablets.

Allergy occurred in 4% of patients receiving prolonged therapy (4–5 weeks) with recommended doses of zolpidem tartrate conventional tablets in clinical trials and in 1% of those receiving placebo. Allergic reaction, aggravated allergy, photosensitivity reaction, and anaphylactic shock have been reported in less than 0.1% of patients receiving zolpidem tartrate as conventional tablets.

Angioedema involving the tongue, glottis, or larynx has been reported following initial or subsequent doses of sedative and hypnotic drugs, including zolpidem. Some patients have experienced additional symptoms (e.g., dyspnea, closing of the throat, nausea and vomiting) suggestive of anaphylaxis, and some individuals have required medical treatment in an emergency department. (See Cautions: Precautions and Contraindications.)

■ **Local Effects** The effect of chronic daily administration of zolpidem tartrate oral spray on oral tissue has not been established; however, in a pharmacokinetic study in healthy individuals, examination of the oral mucosa following administration of single doses of the oral spray did not reveal evidence of irritation. The effect of chronic daily administration of zolpidem tartrate 5- and 10-mg sublingual tablets on oral tissue has been evaluated in an open-label study of 60 days' duration in 60 patients with insomnia; transient sublingual erythema and transient paresthesia of the tongue each occurred in one patient.

■ **Genitourinary and Renal Effects** Urinary tract infection occurred in more than 1% of patients receiving zolpidem tartrate conventional tablets. Dysuria and vulvovaginal dryness each occurred in 1% of geriatric patients receiving recommended doses of zolpidem tartrate extended-release tablets. Menorrhagia occurred in 1% of adults receiving recommended doses of zolpidem tartrate extended-release tablets. Cystitis, menstrual disorder, urinary incontinence, and vaginitis have been reported in 0.1–1% of patients, and increased BUN, acute renal failure, dysuria, micturition frequency, nocturia, polyuria, pyelonephritis, renal pain, urinary retention, and impotence have been reported in less than 0.1% of patients receiving zolpidem tartrate as conventional tablets.

■ **Ocular and Otic Effects** Visual disturbance, eye redness, blurred vision, altered visual depth perception, and asthenopia occurred in 1–3% of patients receiving recommended doses of zolpidem tartrate extended-release tablets. Diplopia and abnormal vision were reported in more than 1% of patients; eye irritation, ocular pain, and scleritis were reported in 0.1–1% of patients; and abnormal accommodation, conjunctivitis, corneal ulceration, glaucoma, abnormal lacrimation, periorbital edema, and photopsia were reported in less than 0.1% of patients receiving zolpidem tartrate as conventional tablets.

Tinnitus and labyrinthitis each have been reported in 1% of adults and otitis externa has been reported in 1% of geriatric patients receiving recommended doses of zolpidem tartrate extended-release tablets. Tinnitus has been reported in 0.1–1% of patients, and otitis externa and otitis media have been reported in less than 0.1% of patients receiving zolpidem tartrate as conventional tablets.

■ **Hepatic Effects** Increased serum concentrations of ALT (SGPT) and abnormal liver function test results have been reported in 0.1–1% of patients, and bilirubinemia, increased serum concentrations of AST (SGOT), and increased serum alkaline phosphatase have been reported in less than 0.1% of patients receiving zolpidem tartrate as conventional tablets.

■ **Hematologic Effects** Increased erythrocyte sedimentation rate, anemia, hyperhemoglobinemia, leukopenia, lymphadenopathy, macrocytic anemia, purpura, and thrombosis have been reported in less than 0.1% of patients receiving zolpidem tartrate as conventional tablets.

■ **Other Adverse Effects** Influenza was reported in 3% of adults receiving recommended doses of zolpidem tartrate extended-release tablets in clinical trials. Flu-like symptoms occurred in 2% of patients receiving prolonged therapy (4–5 weeks) with recommended doses of zolpidem tartrate conventional tablets and in 1% of geriatric patients receiving recommended doses of zolpidem tartrate extended-release tablets. Infection occurred in 0.1–1% of patients receiving zolpidem tartrate as conventional tablets. Chest discomfort, increased body temperature, contusion, and exposure to poisonous plant each occurred in 1% of adults and pyrexia and neck injury each occurred in 1% of geriatric patients receiving recommended doses of zolpidem tartrate extended-release tablets. Falling, fever, hyperglycemia, pallor, thirst, and trauma have been reported in 0.1–1% of patients, and hot flushes, rigors, parosmia, increased drug tolerance, abscess, herpes simplex, herpes zoster, breast fibroadenosis, breast neoplasm, breast pain, gout, hypercholesterolemia, hyperlipidemia, and weight decrease have been reported in less than 0.1% of patients receiving zolpidem tartrate as conventional tablets.

■ Precautions and Contraindications Patients and their families should be advised of the benefits and risks of zolpidem therapy. Patients should be instructed about the proper use of zolpidem and that the drug should be taken only as prescribed. Patients should be given a copy of the medication guide provided by the manufacturer, and the contents of this information should be discussed with every patient prior to initiation of therapy. Patients should be instructed to read the medication guide prior to initiation of therapy and each time the prescription is refilled.

Cognitive and Psychomotor Impairment Zolpidem, like other sedative and hypnotic drugs, has CNS depressant effects and may impair daytime function in some patients even when used as prescribed. (See Next-day Impairment under Cautions: Nervous System Effects.) To decrease the potential risk of next-day impairment, clinicians should prescribe and patients should take the smallest effective dose of zolpidem capable of managing the patient's insomnia. Bedtime dosages of zolpidem that currently are recommended by the manufacturers and the US Food and Drug Administration (FDA) (see Dosage and Administration: Dosage) are lower than the original labeled dosages; the dosage reductions were prompted by concerns about excessively high concentrations of the drug in some patients on the morning after use and the attendant risks of next-day psychomotor impairment. Patients receiving zolpidem should be monitored for excessive CNS depressant effects; however, impairment may occur in the absence of symptoms and may not be reliably detected by ordinary clinical examination (i.e., formal psychomotor testing may be required). Concomitant use of zolpidem with other CNS depressants (e.g., alcohol, benzodiazepines, opiates, tricyclic antidepressants) increases the risk of additive CNS depression, and reductions in dosage of zolpidem and any concomitant CNS depressants may be necessary. Patients taking zolpidem should be advised of the importance of not consuming alcohol in the evening or before bedtime. The use of zolpidem with other sedative and hypnotic drugs (including other zolpidem-containing preparations and OTC preparations used to treat insomnia [e.g., diphenhydramine, doxylamine succinate]) at bedtime or in the middle of the night also is not recommended. (See Drug Interactions: CNS Depressants.)

The risk of next-day psychomotor impairment, including impaired driving, is increased if zolpidem preparations intended for bedtime administration (e.g., conventional tablets, extended-release tablets, oral spray, 5- or 10-mg sublingual tablets) are administered with less than 7–8 hours of sleep time remaining or if zolpidem preparations intended for middle-of-the-night administration (e.g., 1.75- or 3.5-mg sublingual tablets) are administered with less than 4 hours of sleep time remaining. The risk of next-day impairment also is increased if a higher than recommended dose of zolpidem is administered or when zolpidem is used concomitantly with other CNS depressants or with drugs capable of increasing zolpidem concentrations. Women appear to be more susceptible to next-day psychomotor impairment because zolpidem clearance is slower in women than in men. (See Special Populations under Pharmacokinetics: Elimination.) Patients receiving zolpidem should be cautioned against driving a motor vehicle or performing other activities requiring complete mental alertness if the drug is taken in any of the aforementioned circumstances.

Administration of zolpidem as extended-release tablets also increases the risk of next-day impairment and may impair daytime function in some patients even when used as prescribed. Concomitant use of extended-release zolpidem with other CNS depressants, including daytime use of CNS depressants, results in additive effects; reduced dosages of extended-release zolpidem and any concomitant CNS depressants should be considered. Zolpidem tartrate extended-release tablets may not be an appropriate treatment choice for patients who need to drive or perform activities that require full alertness the next morning. While pharmacodynamic tolerance or adaptation to some adverse CNS depressant effects of extended-release zolpidem may develop, concentrations of the drug may remain high enough the next day to impair performance of these activities.

All patients (men and women) receiving zolpidem should be informed of the potential for next-day impairment, that the risk is increased if dosing instructions are not carefully followed, and that impairment may be present despite feeling fully awake. Patients receiving zolpidem tartrate immediate-release preparations intended for bedtime administration (e.g., conventional tablets, oral spray, 5- or 10-mg sublingual tablets) should be advised to wait at least 8 hours after administering zolpidem before driving or engaging in other activities requiring full mental alertness, and those receiving zolpidem tartrate preparations intended for middle-of-the-night administration (e.g., 1.75- or 3.5-mg sublingual tablets) should be advised to wait at least 4 hours and until they feel fully awake before engaging in such activities. Patients receiving zolpidem tartrate extended-release tablets should be cautioned against driving a motor vehicle or performing other activities requiring complete mental alertness on the day after using the drug. Patients should be advised not to use zolpidem if they have consumed alcohol that evening or before bedtime.

Adequate Patient Evaluation Because sleep disturbances may be a manifestation of a physical and/or psychiatric disorder, symptomatic treatment of insomnia should be initiated only after careful evaluation of the patient. The failure of insomnia to remit after 7–10 days of zolpidem therapy may indicate the presence of an underlying psychiatric and/or medical condition that should be evaluated. Prolonged use of hypnotics (e.g., for longer than 2–3 weeks) usually is not indicated and should be undertaken only on further evaluation of the patient. Worsening of insomnia or emergence of new thinking or behavioral abnormalities during therapy with sedative and hypnotic drugs, including zolpidem, may be the consequence of an unrecognized psychiatric or physical disorder.

Risk of Serious Injury and Death Resulting From Complex Sleep Behaviors Serious injuries and/or death resulting from complex sleep behaviors can occur following use of the sedative and hypnotic agents eszopiclone, zaleplon, and zolpidem. Such behaviors may include sleepwalking, sleep driving, and engaging in other activities while not fully awake and have occurred in patients with and without a history of such behaviors. In April 2019, the FDA issued a drug safety communication requiring that a boxed warning be added to the labeling of these drugs to alert clinicians and patients of this risk.

Complex sleep behaviors in which patients engage in activities while they are not fully awake, sometimes resulting in serious injuries and/or death, have been reported rarely following use of eszopiclone, zaleplon, and zolpidem. Such behaviors may include sleepwalking, sleep driving (i.e., driving while not fully awake after ingesting a sedative-hypnotic drug, with no memory of the event), and engaging in other activities (e.g., making phone calls, preparing and eating food) while not fully awake. In addition to the boxed warning, FDA required addition of a contraindication to the prescribing information to avoid use in patients who previously experienced an episode of complex sleep behavior with eszopiclone, zaleplon, or zolpidem.

FDA has identified 66 cases of complex sleep behaviors resulting in serious injuries or death in patients who took eszopiclone, zaleplon, or zolpidem that were reported to the FDA Adverse Event Reporting System (FAERS) database and/or in published literature between December 1992 and March 2018. Of the 66 cases, 20 were reported as resulting in fatal outcomes and 46 reported serious nonfatal injuries; in the nonfatal cases, patients usually did not remember experiencing these complex sleep behaviors. These cases included falls with serious injuries such as intracranial hemorrhages, vertebral fractures, and hip fractures as well as fatal falls, self-injuries, accidental overdoses, hypothermia, suicide attempts and apparent completed suicides, fatal motor vehicle collisions, gunshot wounds, carbon monoxide poisoning, drowning or near drowning, burns, and homicide. Most of the patients in these cases reported using zolpidem (about 92%) when they experienced the complex sleep behavior; the remaining patients took eszopiclone (about 5%) or zaleplon (about 3%), reflecting the higher number of zolpidem prescriptions that were dispensed over this period compared with eszopiclone and zaleplon. The underlying mechanisms by which these drugs cause complex sleep behaviors are not fully understood.

FDA states that serious injuries and fatalities from complex sleep behaviors have occurred in patients with and without a history of such behaviors and can occur even at the lowest recommended dosages and after just one dose of eszopiclone, zaleplon, and zolpidem. These behaviors can occur when these drugs are taken alone or when taken with alcohol or other CNS depressants. Patients should be warned about this risk and advised to discontinue taking these drugs if they experience an episode of complex sleep behavior.

Mood, Thought, and Behavioral Changes Abnormal thinking and behavioral changes have been reported in patients receiving sedative and hypnotic drugs, including zolpidem. (See Cautions: CNS Effects, in the Benzodiazepines General Statement 28:24.08.) In addition, complex behaviors such as sleep-driving (i.e., driving while not fully awake after ingesting a sedative and hypnotic drug, with no memory of the event), making phone calls, preparing and eating food, or having sex have been reported in patients who were not fully awake after receiving zolpidem. (See Risk of Serious Injury and Death Resulting from Complex Sleep Behaviors under Cautions: Precautions and Contraindications.) Decreased inhibition (e.g., aggressiveness and extroversion that seem out of character), bizarre behavior, agitation, depersonalization, and visual and auditory hallucinations also have been associated with use of these drugs; amnesia, anxiety, and other neuropsychiatric symptoms also may occur. Therefore, the emergence of any new behavioral sign or symptom of concern in patients receiving zolpidem requires careful and immediate evaluation. Patients should be advised of the potential risk of abnormal thinking and behavioral changes, and to immediately inform their clinician if any such changes occur.

In primarily depressed patients receiving treatment with sedative and hypnotic drugs, worsening of depression and suicidal thoughts and actions (including completed suicides) have been reported. Suicidal tendencies may be present in such patients, and protective measures may be required. Intentional overdosage is more common in this patient population; therefore, the least amount of zolpidem that is feasible should be prescribed for such patients at any one time. Patients should be advised to immediately inform their clinician if any suicidal thoughts occur.

Respiratory Depression Although clinical studies did not reveal respiratory depressant effects following 10-mg doses of zolpidem tartrate in healthy individuals or in patients with mild-to-moderate chronic obstructive pulmonary disease (COPD), decreased oxygen saturation was observed in patients with mild-to-moderate sleep apnea. Respiratory insufficiency has been reported during postmarketing experience in patients receiving 10-mg doses of zolpidem tartrate, most of whom had preexisting respiratory impairment. Since sedative and hypnotic drugs have the capacity to depress respiratory drive, the drug should be used with caution in patients with compromised respiratory function. The risk of respiratory depression should be considered prior to use of zolpidem in patients with respiratory impairment, including those with sleep apnea or myasthenia gravis.

Tolerance, Dependence, and Abuse Because manifestations of withdrawal have been reported following abrupt discontinuance or rapid reduction in dosage of zolpidem, patients should be monitored for tolerance, abuse, and dependence. Withdrawal symptoms associated with sedative and hypnotic drugs range from mild dysphoria and insomnia to a withdrawal syndrome that may include abdominal and muscle cramps, vomiting, sweating, tremors, and seizures. In clinical trials with zolpidem in the US, manifestations of uncomplicated sedative and hypnotic withdrawal, including fatigue, nausea, flushing, lightheadedness, uncontrolled crying, emesis, stomach cramps, panic attack, nervousness, and abdominal discomfort, were reported after placebo substitution within 48 hours following the last dose of the drug. These adverse events occurred in 1% or less of patients. Available data cannot provide a reliable estimate of the frequency, if any, of dependency during therapy with recommended dosages of zolpidem. Studies of abuse potential in former drug abusers found that the effects of single 40-mg doses of zolpidem tartrate and 20-mg doses of diazepam were similar but not identical, while the effects of a 10-mg dose of zolpidem tartrate were difficult to distinguish from those of placebo. Because patients with a history of addiction to or abuse of drugs or alcohol are at increased risk for misuse or abuse of or addiction to zolpidem, such patients should be monitored carefully when receiving zolpidem or any other hypnotic drug. Patients should be advised not to increase the dosage of zolpidem and to inform their clinician if the drug is not effective.

Other Precautions and Contraindications Angioedema involving the tongue, glottis, or larynx has been reported following initial or subsequent doses of sedative and hypnotic drugs, including zolpidem, and may result in airway obstruction and death. Anaphylaxis also has occurred. Patients who develop angioedema following treatment with zolpidem should not be rechallenged with the drug. Patients should be informed of the potential risk of severe anaphylactic and anaphylactoid reactions, informed of the signs and symptoms of such reactions, and advised to immediately seek medical attention if such reactions occur.

Because elimination of zolpidem is prolonged in patients with hepatic impairment, reduced doses of the drug should be used in patients with hepatic impairment. (See Dosage and Administration: Dosage in Renal and Hepatic Impairment.) The manufacturers and some clinicians state that dosage adjustment is not necessary in patients with renal impairment. Other clinicians, however, state that the possibility that dosage reduction may be needed for patients with renal disease should be considered because of slower zolpidem elimination rates and other pharmacokinetic alterations observed in nondialyzed patients with chronic renal disease and in patients undergoing periodic dialysis.

Zolpidem is contraindicated in patients who have experienced an episode of complex sleep behavior while taking eszopiclone, zaleplon, or zolpidem. (See Risk of Serious Injury and Death Resulting From Complex Sleep Behaviors under Cautions: Precautions and Contraindications.)

Zolpidem tartrate is contraindicated in patients with known hypersensitivity to the drug.

■ **Pediatric Precautions** Zolpidem tartrate is not recommended for use in pediatric patients. Safety and efficacy of the drug have not been established in pediatric patients younger than 18 years of age. In an 8-week clinical study in pediatric patients (6–17 years of age) with insomnia associated with attention deficit hyperactivity disorder (ADHD), zolpidem tartrate (0.25 mg/kg administered as an oral solution at bedtime) did not appear to decrease sleep latency as compared with placebo. In this study, the most frequent treatment-emergent adverse effects (compared with placebo) were nervous system effects, including dizziness (23.5 versus 1.5%), headache (12.5 versus 9.2%), and hallucinations (7 versus 0%).

■ **Geriatric Precautions** Safety and efficacy of zolpidem for the treatment of insomnia in geriatric patients have been evaluated in controlled, double-blind studies. Geriatric or debilitated patients may be particularly sensitive to the effects of zolpidem. Adverse effects of the drug tend to be dose related, particularly in geriatric patients. In addition, peak plasma zolpidem concentrations, elimination half-life, and area under the plasma concentration-time curve (AUC) are increased substantially in geriatric patients compared with younger adults receiving zolpidem tartrate as conventional tablets.

In placebo-controlled clinical trials in geriatric patients receiving zolpidem tartrate doses of 10 mg or less (as conventional tablets), the most frequent adverse effects were dizziness, drowsiness, and diarrhea. Dizziness, drowsiness, or diarrhea was reported in 3, 5, or 3% of patients receiving the drug, respectively, while such adverse effects occurred in 0, 2, or 1% of patients receiving placebo, respectively. In placebo-controlled clinical trials in geriatric patients receiving zolpidem tartrate 6.25 mg as extended-release tablets, the most frequent adverse effects were headache, dizziness, and next-day somnolence. Headache, dizziness, or next-day somnolence was reported in 14, 8, or 6% of patients receiving the drug, respectively, while such adverse effects occurred in 11, 3, or 5% of patients receiving placebo, respectively. In clinical trials performed outside the US, involving approximately 2000 patients, falls were reported in about 1.5% of patients (93% of those being 70 years of age or older); 82% of the patients 70 years of age or older who experienced falls received zolpidem tartrate doses exceeding 10 mg (as conventional tablets). In these clinical trials, confusion was reported in 1.2% of patients (75% of those being 70 years of age or older); 78% of the patients 70 years of age or older who experienced confusion were receiving doses exceeding 10 mg (as conventional tablets).

The manufacturers recommend that zolpidem dosage be reduced in geriatric and/or debilitated patients to minimize adverse effects related to impaired motor and/or cognitive performance and unusual sensitivity to sedative and hypnotic drugs. (See Dosage and Administration: Dosage.) Sedatives may cause confusion and oversedation in geriatric patients; geriatric patients should be observed closely.

■ **Mutagenicity and Carcinogenicity** Zolpidem was not mutagenic when tested in vitro in bacterial reverse mutation, mouse lymphoma, and chromosomal aberration assays or in vivo in the mouse micronucleus assay.

Carcinogenicity studies in animals were performed using zolpidem rather than zolpidem tartrate; dosages in these studies are expressed in terms of the base. Studies to determine the carcinogenic potential of zolpidem were performed in mice and rats receiving oral dosages of 4, 18, and 80 mg/kg daily for 2 years. In mice, these dosages were approximately 2.5, 10, and 50 times, respectively, the maximum recommended human dosage (MRHD) of zolpidem tartrate as conventional tablets (10 mg daily) on a mg/m^2 basis. In rats, these dosages were approximately 5, 20, and 100 times, respectively, the MRHD of zolpidem tartrate as conventional tablets on a mg/m^2 basis. No evidence of carcinogenic potential was observed in mice. In rats, renal tumors (lipoma, liposarcoma) were observed at the mid- and high-dosage levels.

■ **Pregnancy, Fertility, and Lactation** There are no adequate and well-controlled studies to date evaluating zolpidem tartrate in pregnant women, and the drug should be used during pregnancy only if the potential benefits justify the possible risks to the fetus. Studies in children to assess the effects of prenatal exposure to zolpidem have not been conducted; however, severe neonatal respiratory depression has been reported when zolpidem was used at the end of pregnancy, particularly when used concomitantly with other CNS depressants. In addition, children born to women receiving sedative or hypnotic drugs may be at risk for withdrawal symptoms during the postnatal period. Neonatal flaccidity also has been reported in infants whose mothers received sedative or hypnotic drugs during pregnancy. Zolpidem has no established use in labor and delivery.

Reproduction studies in animals were performed using zolpidem rather than zolpidem tartrate; dosages are expressed in terms of the base. Administration of zolpidem to pregnant rats and rabbits resulted in adverse effects on offspring development at dosages exceeding the maximum recommended human dosage (MRHD) of zolpidem tartrate as conventional tablets (10 mg daily); however, teratogenicity was not observed. When zolpidem was administered at oral dosages of 4, 20, and 100 mg/kg daily to pregnant rats during the period of organogenesis, dose-related decreases in fetal skull ossification occurred at all but the lowest dosage (4 mg/kg daily, which is approximately 5 times the MRHD of zolpidem tartrate as conventional tablets on a mg/m^2 basis). In addition, administration of zolpidem to rats at oral dosages of 4, 20, and 100 mg/kg daily during the latter part of pregnancy and throughout lactation decreased offspring growth and survival at all but the lowest dosage. In rabbits receiving zolpidem during organogenesis at oral dosages of 1, 4, and 16 mg/kg daily, increased embryofetal death and incomplete fetal skeletal ossification occurred at the highest dosage studied. The no-effect dosage for embryofetal toxicity in rabbits is approximately 10 times the MRHD of zolpidem tartrate as conventional tablets on a mg/m^2 basis.

Oral administration of zolpidem at dosages of 4, 20, and 100 mg/kg daily to rats prior to and during mating, and continuing in females through postpartum day 25, resulted in irregular estrus cycles and prolonged precoital intervals at the highest dosage studied. The no-effect dosage for these findings is approximately 24 times the MRHD of zolpidem tartrate as conventional tablets on a mg/m^2 basis. There was no evidence of impaired fertility at any dosage studied.

Zolpidem is distributed into milk in small amounts in humans. The effect, if any, of zolpidem on the nursing infant is not known. Caution should be exercised when zolpidem is used in nursing women, and infants should be monitored closely for increased sedation, lethargy, and changes in feeding habits.

Drug Interactions

Zolpidem is metabolized principally by cytochrome P-450 (CYP) isoenzyme 3A4 and, to a lesser extent, by CYP1A2 and CYP2D6.

■ **Drugs Affecting Hepatic Microsomal Enzymes** Some drugs that inhibit CYP3A may increase systemic exposure to zolpidem. (See Drug Interactions: Ketoconazole.) The effect of inhibitors of other CYP isoenzymes on the pharmacokinetics (e.g., systemic exposure) of zolpidem is not known.

■ **CNS Depressants** Concomitant use of zolpidem with other CNS depressants (e.g., alcohol, benzodiazepines, opiates, sedating antihistamines, tricyclic antidepressants) increases the risk of CNS depression. (See Cognitive and Psychomotor Impairment under Cautions: Precautions and Contraindications.)

Concomitant use of alcohol with zolpidem results in an additive adverse effect on psychomotor performance. Patients should be advised of the importance of not taking zolpidem after consuming alcohol in the evening or before bedtime.

When zolpidem is used concomitantly with other CNS depressants, dosage adjustments of zolpidem and the concomitant CNS depressant may be necessary because of potentially additive effects. (See Dosage and Administration: Dosage.) Concomitant use of zolpidem with other sedative and hypnotic drugs (including other zolpidem-containing preparations and OTC preparations used to treat insomnia [e.g., diphenhydramine, doxylamine succinate]) at bedtime or in the middle of the night is not recommended.

■ **Chlorpromazine** Pharmacokinetic interactions have not been observed during concomitant use of zolpidem and chlorpromazine; however, additive effects in reducing alertness and psychomotor performance have been observed.

■ **Cimetidine** Cimetidine does not appear to affect the pharmacokinetics or pharmacodynamics of zolpidem.

■ **Digoxin** Zolpidem had no effect on digoxin pharmacokinetics in healthy individuals.

■ **Fluoxetine** Clinically important pharmacokinetic or pharmacodynamic interactions have not been observed when zolpidem was used concomitantly with fluoxetine in healthy individuals. In healthy men, concomitant use of fluoxetine (20 mg once daily for 17 days) with zolpidem tartrate (single 10-mg dose) resulted in no clinically important changes in the pharmacokinetics of zolpidem or fluoxetine, and no substantial changes in performance on psychomotor tests were observed. In healthy women, concomitant use of fluoxetine (20 mg once daily for 30 days) with zolpidem tartrate (10 mg once daily for 5 days) increased the half-life of zolpidem by 17%, but there was no evidence of additive effects on psychomotor function.

■ **Haloperidol** Haloperidol does not appear to affect the pharmacokinetics or pharmacodynamics of zolpidem. However, the lack of an interaction following single-dose administration does not predict the absence of an effect following chronic administration.

■ **Imipramine** Concomitant use of zolpidem and imipramine has been associated with a 20% decrease in peak plasma concentrations of imipramine; although other pharmacokinetic interactions have not been observed, an additive effect in reducing alertness has been observed during concomitant use.

■ **Itraconazole** Concomitant use of the potent CYP3A4 inhibitor itraconazole (200 mg once daily for 4 days) with zolpidem tartrate (single 10-mg dose) in healthy individuals increased the area under the serum concentration-time curve (AUC) of zolpidem by 34% but did not substantially alter patient ratings of drowsiness, performance on psychomotor tests, or postural sway compared with zolpidem alone.

■ **Ketoconazole** Concomitant use of the potent CYP3A4 inhibitor ketoconazole (200 mg twice daily for 2 days) with zolpidem tartrate (single 5-mg dose) increased the peak plasma concentration, AUC, and elimination half-life of zolpidem by 30, 70, and 30%, respectively, and also increased pharmacodynamic effects of zolpidem. Because concomitant use may increase the hypnotic effects of zolpidem, a lower dose of zolpidem should be considered when the drug is used concomitantly with ketoconazole.

■ **Ranitidine** Ranitidine does not appear to affect the pharmacokinetics or pharmacodynamics of zolpidem.

■ **Rifampin** Rifampin, a potent CYP3A4 inducer, substantially reduces systemic exposure to and pharmacodynamic effects of zolpidem. Concomitant use with rifampin may decrease the hypnotic efficacy of zolpidem. In healthy women, concomitant use of zolpidem tartrate (single 20-mg dose) and rifampin (600 mg once daily for 5 days) reduced AUC, peak plasma concentration, and half-life of zolpidem by 73, 58, and 36%, respectively; substantial reductions in the effects of zolpidem on psychomotor performance also were observed.

■ **Sertraline** Concomitant use of zolpidem and sertraline increases systemic exposure to zolpidem and may increase the pharmacodynamic effects of zolpidem, potentially resulting in earlier hypnotic onset and greater hypnotic effect. When zolpidem tartrate (10 mg daily at bedtime for 5 days) was used concomitantly with sertraline (50 mg daily in the morning for 17 days) in healthy women, peak plasma concentration of zolpidem was increased by 43% and time to peak plasma concentration of zolpidem was decreased by 53%. Zolpidem did not appear to have clinically important effects on the pharmacokinetics of sertraline or *N*-desmethylsertraline.

■ **Warfarin** Zolpidem did not appear to affect prothrombin time (PT) when used concomitantly with warfarin in healthy individuals.

Pharmacokinetics

■ **Absorption** ***Bioavailability*** Conventional tablets: Zolpidem is rapidly absorbed from the GI tract following oral administration as conventional tablets, with peak plasma concentrations attained in about 1.6 hours. Absolute bioavailability is about 70%.

Extended-release tablets: The extended-release tablets exhibit biphasic absorption characteristics; there is rapid initial absorption following oral administration (similar to conventional tablets), but with extended plasma concentrations beyond 3 hours after administration. Peak plasma concentrations are attained in about 1.5 hours.

Oral spray: The oral spray is bioequivalent to conventional tablets. Zolpidem is rapidly absorbed from the oral mucosa and GI tract, with peak plasma concentrations attained in about 0.9 hours.

Sublingual tablets (Edluar®): The sublingual tablets are bioequivalent to conventional tablets with respect to peak plasma concentration and area under the concentration-time curve (AUC). Like conventional tablets, the sublingual tablets result in a pharmacokinetic profile characterized by rapid absorption. Peak plasma concentrations are attained in approximately 82 minutes.

Sublingual tablets (Intermezzo®): The sublingual tablets disintegrate in the sublingual cavity following administration and the drug is rapidly absorbed in both men and women, with peak plasma concentrations attained in about 35–75 minutes.

Food Conventional tablets: Food decreases AUC by 15%, decreases peak plasma concentration by 25%, and prolongs time to peak plasma concentration by 60%.

Extended-release tablets: Food decreases AUC by 23%, decreases peak plasma concentration by 30%, and prolongs time to peak plasma concentration by about 2 hours (from 2 hours to 4 hours).

Oral spray: Food decreases AUC by 27%, decreases peak plasma concentration by 58%, and prolongs time to peak plasma concentration by 225% (from 0.8 hours to 2.6 hours).

Sublingual tablets (Edluar®): Food decreases AUC by 20%, decreases peak plasma concentration by 31%, and prolongs time to peak plasma concentration by 28% (from 82 minutes to 105 minutes).

Sublingual tablets (Intermezzo®): Food decreases AUC by 19%, decreases peak plasma concentration by 42%, and prolongs time to peak plasma concentration to nearly 3 hours.

Plasma Concentrations Driving simulation and laboratory studies indicate that zolpidem blood concentrations exceeding approximately 50 ng/mL appear to be capable of impairing driving to a degree that increases the risk of a motor vehicle accident. (See Next-day Impairment under Cautions: Nervous System Effects.)

Special Populations In women receiving zolpidem tartrate as an immediate-release formulation, peak plasma concentration and AUC of zolpidem are approximately 45% higher than values attained in men receiving the same dose. In women receiving zolpidem tartrate as extended-release tablets, peak plasma concentration and AUC of zolpidem are approximately 50 and 75% higher, respectively, than values attained in men receiving the same dose. Zolpidem concentrations measured 6–12 hours after administration of zolpidem tartrate as extended-release tablets are 2–3 times higher in women compared with men. (See Special Populations under Pharmacokinetics: Elimination.)

In geriatric individuals receiving zolpidem tartrate as conventional tablets, peak plasma concentration and AUC are increased by 50 and 64%, respectively, compared with younger adults receiving the same dose. In geriatric individuals receiving a 3.5-mg dose of zolpidem tartrate as sublingual tablets, peak plasma concentration and AUC are increased by 34 and 30%, respectively, compared with younger adults receiving the same dose; likewise, peak plasma concentration and AUC are consistently higher in geriatric individuals receiving a 1.75-mg dose than in younger adults receiving a 1.75-mg dose, but are consistently lower in geriatric individuals receiving a 1.75-mg dose than in younger adults receiving a 3.5-mg dose.

In patients with chronic hepatic impairment receiving zolpidem tartrate as conventional tablets, peak plasma concentration and AUC are 2 and 5 times higher, respectively, than in healthy individuals. Zolpidem tartrate extended-release tablets have not been studied to date in patients with hepatic impairment.

■ **Distribution** ***Extent*** Zolpidem is distributed into milk in small amounts.

Plasma Protein Binding Zolpidem is approximately 92–93% bound to plasma proteins.

■ **Elimination** ***Metabolism*** Zolpidem is metabolized in the liver via oxidation and hydroxylation, principally by cytochrome P-450 (CYP) isoenzyme 3A4 and, to a lesser extent, by CYP1A2 and CYP2D6, to form inactive metabolites.

Elimination Route Zolpidem is excreted principally in urine as inactive metabolites.

Half-life The half-life of zolpidem is approximately 2.5–3 hours.

Special Populations Zolpidem is eliminated more slowly in women than in men. Lower doses are recommended for women since use of the same dose in women and men would result in greater drug exposure and increased susceptibility to next-day impairment in women. In the geriatric population, clearance of zolpidem is similar in men and women and dosage is not gender specific. (See Special Populations under Pharmacokinetics: Absorption; see Next-day Impairment under Cautions: Nervous System Effects; and see Dosage and Administration: Dosage.)

In geriatric patients receiving zolpidem tartrate as conventional or extended-release tablets, the half-life of the drug is 2.9 hours. In geriatric patients receiving the drug as conventional tablets, the half-life reportedly is increased by 32% compared with younger adults; in those receiving the drug as sublingual tablets (Intermezzo®), the half-life reportedly is unchanged compared with younger adults.

In patients with cirrhosis receiving zolpidem tartrate as conventional tablets, half-life is about 9.9 hours. Zolpidem tartrate extended-release tablets have not been studied to date in patients with hepatic impairment.

In nondialyzed patients with chronic renal disease and in patients undergoing periodic dialysis, slower elimination rates have been reported with IV zolpidem (not commercially available in the US). No substantial pharmacokinetic alterations have been reported with oral zolpidem in patients with end-stage renal failure undergoing hemodialysis. Zolpidem tartrate extended-release tablets have not been studied to date in patients with renal impairment.

Zolpidem is not removed by hemodialysis.

Description

Zolpidem tartrate, a type A γ-aminobutyric acid ($GABA_A$)-receptor agonist of the imidazopyridine class, is a sedative and hypnotic agent. Although zolpidem is structurally unrelated to the benzodiazepines and other sedative and hypnotic agents, it shares some of the pharmacologic properties of benzodiazepines and has been shown to interact with the CNS GABA-benzodiazepine-chloride ionophore receptor complex. Unlike some benzodiazepines, which nonselectively bind to and activate central type 1 (BZ_1) and 2 (BZ_2) benzodiazepine receptors, as well as peripheral type 3 (BZ_3) receptors, resulting in nonspecific pharmacologic actions, zolpidem reportedly may bind preferentially to BZ_1 receptors with a high affinity ratio of the α_1/α_5 subunits. Such selectivity of zolpidem for the BZ_1 receptor is not absolute, but may account for the decreased muscle relaxant, anxiolytic, and anticonvulsant effects compared with benzodiazepines observed in certain animals and also may explain the preservation of deep (stages 3 and 4) sleep at hypnotic doses in humans. Such selectivity reportedly also may result in reduced abuse potential and tolerance development as well as in only minor effects on duration of sleep stages compared with benzodiazepines. However, some in vivo data from an animal (mouse) model have not confirmed such selectivity, and other data suggest that pharmacologic and toxicologic selectivity of zolpidem may be dose and species dependent. In addition, changes in sleep EEG observed with zolpidem are similar to those associated with benzodiazepines. Although some evidence suggests that the risk of residual daytime sedative effects and impairment of psychomotor and mental performance is minimal with zolpidem at usual dosages, blood concentrations of the drug may be high enough in some patients on the morning after use to impair performance of activities that require alertness, including driving. The US Food and Drug Administration (FDA) states that all drugs used in the management of insomnia can impair driving and performance of activities that require alertness on the morning after use. (See Next-day Impairment under Cautions: Nervous System Effects and also Cognitive and Psychomotor Impairment under Cautions: Precautions and Contraindications.) For additional information on benzodiazepines, see Pharmacology, in the Benzodiazepines General Statement 28:24.08.

Preparations

Zolpidem is subject to control under the Federal Controlled Substances Act of 1970 as a schedule IV (C-IV) drug.

Excipients in commercially available drug preparations may have clinically important effects in some individuals; consult specific product labeling for details.

Zolpidem Tartrate

Oral		
Solution	5 mg/metered spray	**Zolpimist**® (C-IV), ECR
Tablets, extended-release, film-coated	6.25 mg*	**Ambien CR**® (C-IV), Sanofi-Aventis
		Zolpidem Tartrate Extended-release Tablets (C-IV)
	12.5 mg*	**Ambien CR**® (C-IV), Sanofi-Aventis
		Zolpidem Tartrate Extended-release Tablets (C-IV)
Tablets, film-coated	5 mg*	**Ambien**® (C-IV), Sanofi-Aventis
		Zolpidem Tartrate Tablets (C-IV)
	10 mg*	**Ambien**® (C-IV), Sanofi-Aventis
		Zolpidem Tartrate Tablets (C-IV)
Sublingual		
Tablets	1.75 mg*	**Intermezzo**® (C-IV), Purdue
		Zolpidem Tartrate Sublingual Tablets (C-IV)
	3.5 mg*	**Intermezzo**® (C-IV), Purdue
		Zolpidem Tartrate Sublingual Tablets (C-IV)
	5 mg*	**Edluar**® (C-IV), Meda
		Zolpidem Tartrate Sublingual Tablets (C-IV)
	10 mg*	**Edluar**® (C-IV), Meda
		Zolpidem Tartrate Sublingual Tablets (C-IV)

*available from one or more manufacturer, distributor, and/or repackager by generic (nonproprietary) name

ANTIMANIC AGENTS 28:28

Lithium Salts

■ Lithium salts are antimanic agents.

Uses

Lithium salts are used in the treatment of a variety of psychiatric disorders but are most commonly used in the treatment of affective (mood) disorders. Currently, lithium salts are principally used in the treatment of bipolar disorder, particularly in the treatment of acute manic or mixed episodes in patients with bipolar 1 or bipolar 2 disorder. In addition, maintenance therapy with lithium salts has been shown to prevent or diminish the intensity of subsequent manic episodes in patients with bipolar disorder with a history of mania.

Lithium salts also are used in the prophylaxis and treatment of major depressive disorder† (unipolar depression).

■ **Bipolar Disorder** ***Diagnostic Considerations*** Affective disorders currently are categorized as either bipolar (manic-depressive) or unipolar (depressive). A diagnosis of bipolar disorder is made if the patient has ever had a manic or hypomanic episode; otherwise, the criteria for bipolar depression and unipolar (major) depression are identical. According to DSM-IV-TR criteria, manic episodes are distinct periods lasting 1 week or longer (or less than 1 week if hospitalization is required) of abnormally and persistently elevated, expansive, or irritable mood accompanied by at least 3 (or 4 if the mood is only irritability) of the following 7 symptoms: inflated self-esteem or grandiosity, reduced need for sleep, pressure of speech, flight of ideas, distractibility, increased goal-directed activity (either socially, at work or school, or sexually) or psychomotor agitation, and engaging in high risk behavior (e.g., unrestrained buying sprees, sexual indiscretions, foolish business investments). In addition, to meet the criteria for manic episodes, the mood disturbances must be sufficiently severe that they cause marked impairment in occupational functioning, usual social activities, or relationships with others; they may necessitate hospitalization to prevent harm to self or others; and may be accompanied by psychotic features.

According to DSM-IV-TR criteria, bipolar disorder can be classified as bipolar 1 disorder, bipolar 2 disorder, cyclothymia, or bipolar disorder not otherwise specified. Bipolar 1 disorder is characterized by the occurrence of one or more manic episodes or mixed episodes. In addition, patients with bipolar I disorder often have had previous depressive episodes and most patients will have subsequent episodes that can be either manic or depressive. Hypomanic and mixed episodes also may occur in bipolar I disorder as well as substantial subthreshold mood lability between episodes. Bipolar 1 disorder is further characterized according to whether the patient is experiencing a first manic episode (which is classified as single manic episode) or whether the most recent episode is manic, hypomanic, depressive, mixed (concurrent or rapidly alternating manic and depressive features), or unspecified.

Patients meeting DSM-IV-TR criteria for bipolar 2 disorder have a history of one or more major depressive episodes accompanied by at least one hypomanic episode. However, patients with bipolar 2 disorder should not have had a previous manic or mixed episode.

Some patients with bipolar disorder may exhibit evidence of mood lability, hypomania, and depressive symptoms but fail to meet the diagnostic criteria for any specific bipolar disorder. This condition is called bipolar disorder not otherwise specified according to DSM-IV-TR criteria.

Cyclothymic disorder (cyclothymia) may be diagnosed in patients who have never experienced a manic, mixed, or major depressive episode but who have experienced numerous periods of depressive as well as hypomanic symptoms for at least 2 years in adults or 1 year in children, with no symptom-free period lasting longer than 2 months.

Bipolar 1 or 2 disorder may be diagnosed as rapid-cycling if the patient has 4 or more mood disturbances within a single year that meet DSM-IV-TR criteria for a major depressive, mixed, manic, or hypomanic episode. These episodes are demarcated either by a partial or full remission for at least 2 months or a switch to an episode of the opposite nature (e.g., from a major depressive to a manic episode). Rapid-cycling bipolar disorder is sometimes associated with certain medical conditions (e.g., hypothyroidism) or drug or substance abuse. Certain drugs, such as antidepressants, also may contribute to rapid cycling, particularly in patients who are not receiving a mood-stabilizing agent (e.g., lithium, carbamazepine, valproic acid).

Considerations in Choosing Therapy for Manic and Mixed Episodes Although there presently is no cure for bipolar disorder, treatment may decrease the associated morbidity and mortality. The principal aim of acute treatment for patients with bipolar disorder experiencing a manic or mixed episode is to control the symptoms to allow a return to normal levels of psychosocial functioning. The rapid control of certain symptoms (e.g., agitation, aggression, impulsivity) may be particularly important for the safety of the patient and others.

A variety of drugs currently are available for the treatment of acute manic and mixed episodes, including mood-stabilizing agents, olanzapine and other antipsychotics, and benzodiazepines. In bipolar disorder, drugs generally are considered mood stabilizers if they provide relief from acute episodes of mania or depression or prevent such episodes from recurring and they do not worsen depression or mania or lead to increased cycling. Lithium salts, valproic acid or divalproex, carbamazepine, and some other anticonvulsants (e.g., oxcarbazepine, lamotrigine, gabapentin) have been used clinically as mood stabilizers in bipolar disorder. However, the American Psychiatric Association (APA) states that there is no consensus on the definitions of "mood stabilizers" and does not use this term in its most recent guidelines for the treatment of bipolar disorder.

For the initial management of less severe manic or mixed episodes in patients with bipolar disorder, monotherapy with lithium, valproate (e.g., sodium valproate, valproic acid, divalproex), or an antipsychotic agent such as olanzapine may be adequate. For more severe manic or mixed episodes, many experts recommend combination therapy involving lithium plus an antipsychotic or valproate plus an antipsychotic for first-line therapy. Some clinicians state that divalproex may be preferable to valproic acid in the treatment of bipolar disorder because of its more favorable adverse effect profile. Some experts recommend that carbamazepine or oxcarbazepine be used as alternatives to lithium or valproate therapy for patients who do not respond adequately to or who cannot tolerate other first-line therapies.

Bipolar patients experiencing manic or mixed episodes with psychotic features or psychosis often require therapy with an antipsychotic agent. Antipsychotic agents also are commonly used in the treatment of manic or mixed episodes in patients with bipolar disorder to control psychotic symptoms and for sedation. Some evidence indicates that certain atypical antipsychotic agents also possess mood-stabilizing properties and may therefore help to control depressive and manic episodes. When an antipsychotic agent is clinically indicated in patients with bipolar disorder, some experts recommend the use of atypical antipsychotics (e.g., olanzapine, risperidone) over conventional antipsychotic agents (e.g., chlorpromazine, haloperidol) because of their more favorable adverse effect profile and possible mood-stabilizing activity.

Short-term adjunctive therapy with a benzodiazepine (e.g., lorazepam, clonazepam) during manic episodes may be helpful for sedation and to help restore sleep in patients experiencing acute manic or mixed episodes. Some experts currently prefer high-potency benzodiazepines instead of antipsychotics in the management of acute manic episodes to avoid the risk of tardive dyskinesia and other adverse extrapyramidal effects associated with antipsychotic agents. However, benzodiazepines should be used with caution in bipolar patients with a history of substance abuse because of their addictive potential.

In bipolar patients who experience an acute manic or mixed episode while receiving antidepressant therapy, many experts recommend that the antidepressant be tapered and discontinued, if possible. If psychosocial therapy is used, this treatment should be combined with pharmacotherapy.

In patients with mixed episodes, many clinicians recommend valproate (valproic acid or divalproex) or carbamazepine rather than lithium as initial first-line therapy. In patients with dysphoric mania, combined divalproex and olanzapine currently is recommended by some clinicians.

In patients who experience a manic or mixed episode (i.e., a "breakthrough" episode) while receiving maintenance therapy, some experts recommend that the dosage(s) of the current medication be optimized as an initial approach (e.g., ensuring that plasma drug concentrations are within the therapeutic range). In addition, an antipsychotic agent may be added or reinitiated. Severely ill or agitated patients also may require short-term therapy with a benzodiazepine. When first-line therapy given at optimal dosages fails to control the symptoms, another first-line drug may be added to the regimen.Alternatively, carbamazepine or oxcarbazepine may be added instead of a first-line agent and an antipsychotic agent may be added in patients not already receiving one. In addition, changing to a different antipsychotic agent occasionally may be helpful.

In patients with refractory manic episodes, some experts recommend a trial of therapy with the antipsychotic clozapine. Electroconvulsive therapy (ECT) also may be considered in patients with particularly severe or treatment-resistant mania and in patients who prefer ECT in consultation with their clinician. ECT also has been recommended by some experts in patients experiencing mixed episodes or in patients who develop severe mania during pregnancy.

Lithium Therapy for Acute Manic and Mixed Episodes Extensive clinical experience and data from randomized, controlled studies have shown lithium to be effective in the treatment of acute mania and the acute manic phase of mixed bipolar disorder. Based on data from 5 controlled clinical trials, lithium appears to be more effective than placebo in the treatment of acute manic and mixed episodes. Data from these studies indicate that about 70% of patients receiving lithium display at least a partial reduction of manic symptoms.

Based on data from several controlled clinical trials, lithium appears to be more effective than chlorpromazine in the treatment of acute mania. The percentage of patients achieving a complete or partial remission of a manic episode and the degree to which manic symptomatology is reduced are greater in patients treated with lithium than in those treated with chlorpromazine. Lithium is particularly effective in reducing affective and ideational signs and symptoms of mania, especially elation, grandiosity, feelings of persecution, flight of ideas, expansiveness, irritability, manipulativeness, anxiousness, and other manic behavior. Signs and symptoms of hyperactivity associated with mania, including sleep disturbances, pressured speech, increased motor activity, assaultive or threatening behavior, and distractability are reduced to a lesser extent. Because antipsychotic agents appear to be more effective than lithium in initially controlling the increased psychomotor activity of mania, many clinicians initiate treatment of acute mania with lithium or valproate (e.g., valproic acid, valproate sodium, divalproex) and an antipsychotic agent. Once psychomotor activity has been controlled (usually within 3–7 days), the antipsychotic agent usually is tapered and lithium or valproate therapy is continued to more specifically control disturbances of mood and ideation.

Considerations in Choosing Therapy for Depressive Episodes

In patients with bipolar disorder experiencing a depressive episode, many experts recommend that therapy with either lithium or lamotrigine be initiated as first-line therapy. Antidepressant monotherapy and therapy with tricyclic antidepressants generally should be avoided in such cases because of the possibility of inducing rapid cycling of symptoms. Alternatively, some clinicians recommend initiation of combination therapy with lithium and an antidepressant, particularly in patients with more severe depressive episodes. Psychotherapy (interpersonal therapy and cognitive behavior therapy) may be useful as an adjunct to pharmacotherapy.In patients with life-threatening inanition, suicidality, or psychosis, ECT may be considered. ECT may also may be helpful for managing severe depressive episodes during pregnancy.

In bipolar patients who suffer from a breakthrough depressive episode despite maintenance therapy, many experts recommend optimizing the dosages of the current medication as an initial step. For acute depressive episodes in bipolar disorder patients not responding adequately to first-line interventions at optimal dosages, some experts recommend the addition of a selective serotonin-reuptake inhibitor (e.g., paroxetine), bupropion, venlafaxine, lamotrigine, or a monoamine oxidase (MAO) inhibitor. When an antidepressant is indicated in patients with bipolar depression, nonsedating antidepressants (i.e., bupropion, selective serotonin-reuptake inhibitors, MAO inhibitors) usually are preferred. ECT should be considered in bipolar patients with severe or treatment-resistant depression or in those with depression accompanied by psychotic or catatonic features.

Because the likelihood of antidepressant therapy precipitating a switch into a hypomanic or manic episode may be somewhat lower in patients with type 2 bipolar disorder than in patients with type 1 bipolar disorder, many clinicians choose to initiate antidepressant therapy earlier in patients with bipolar 2 disorder. Depressive episodes accompanied by psychotic features usually require adjunctive antipsychotic therapy.

Considerations in Choosing Therapy for Rapid Cycling According to DSM-IV-TR criteria, rapid cycling refers to the occurrence of 4 or more mood-related disturbances within a single year that meet criteria for a major depressive, mixed, manic, or hypomanic episode. These episodes are demarcated either by partial or full remission for at least 2 months or a switch to an episode of the opposite nature (e.g., from a major depressive to a manic episode). Initially, many experts advise that any concurrent medical condition that may contribute to rapid cycling, such as hypothyroidism or drug or alcohol abuse, be identified and treated.Certain drugs, such as antidepressants, also may contribute to rapid cycling in bipolar disorder, particularly in patients not receiving other therapy such as lithium, carbamazepine, or valproic acid. Therefore, the need for continued antidepressant therapy should be reassessed in rapid-cycling patients and antidepressant therapy should be gradually discontinued, if possible.

The initial therapy in bipolar patients who experience rapid cycling usually includes lithium or valproate (e.g., valproate sodium, valproic acid, divalproex). Alternatively, lamotrigine may be used. In many patients, combination therapy (e.g., with 2 first-line agents or a combination of a first-line agent with an atypical antipsychotic) is required to adequately treat rapid cycling. Recent evidence suggests that atypical antipsychotic agents (e.g., olanzapine, clozapine) combined with mood stabilizers, such as valproic acid and/or lithium, may be effective in rapid cycling patients.

Considerations in Choosing Maintenance Therapy Following treatment of an acute episode, patients with bipolar disorder remain at high risk of relapse. Therefore, following a single manic episode, maintenance therapy is recommended by many experts. The principal goals of maintenance therapy are relapse prevention, reduction of subthreshold symptoms, and reduction of suicide risk. Other aims of maintenance therapy include reduction in cycling frequency, reduction of mood instability, and improvement in overall functioning.

The choice of a maintenance regimen for initial therapy should be individualized and take into consideration illness severity, associated clinical features (e.g., rapid cycling, psychosis), and patient preference. Clinical experience to date indicates that either lithium or valproate (e.g., valproate sodium, valproic acid, divalproex) should be considered for first-line maintenance therapy in bipolar disorder; possible alternatives include lamotrigine, carbamazepine, or oxcarbazepine. If one of these agents was used to achieve remission from the most recent manic or depressive episode, many experts advise that it generally should be continued. Maintenance ECT therapy also should be considered in patients whose acute episode responded to ECT.

In patients who received an antipsychotic agent during the preceding acute episode, the need for continued antipsychotic therapy should be reassessed during the maintenance phase of therapy. Many experts recommend that antipsychotic therapy be tapered and discontinued unless needed for control of persisting psychotic symptoms or to prevent recurrence of such symptoms. Although maintenance therapy with atypical antipsychotic agents also may be considered, their efficacy as maintenance therapy compared with lithium or valproate has yet to be fully established. Patients with bipolar disorder are also likely to benefit from psychosocial interventions, including psychotherapy, during the maintenance phase.

Patients who continue to experience subthreshold symptoms or breakthrough episodes may require the addition of another mood-stabilizing maintenance agent (lithium or valproate), an atypical antipsychotic agent, or an antidepressant. Currently, data to support one combination over another are insufficient. Maintenance sessions of ECT also may be considered in patients whose acute episode responded to ECT.

Maintenance Therapy with Lithium Lithium is effective in preventing or attenuating recurrences of bipolar episodes when used for long-term maintenance treatment of bipolar affective disorder. In patients with bipolar disorder, the drug is more effective at preventing signs and symptoms of mania than those of depression.

Approximately 65–90% of patients with bipolar disorder will have relapses if left untreated. During long-term lithium therapy, less than 40% of patients with bipolar disorder relapse during the first 2 years of therapy. The decision to initiate long-term prophylaxis with lithium in such patients is based on the history of recurrence of signs and symptoms.

Suicide Considerations Patients with bipolar disorder are at high risk for suicide. Among the phases of bipolar disorder, depression is associated with the highest risk of suicide, followed by mixed episodes and the presence of psychotic symptoms, with episodes of mania being the least frequently associated with suicide. All patients with bipolar disorder should therefore be carefully evaluated to assess suicidal risk.

Long-term lithium therapy has been associated with a reduction in suicidal risk in patients with bipolar disorder. However, it has not been clearly established whether this reflects possible anti-impulsivity properties in addition to lithium's established mood-stabilizing activity. Lithium also may reduce the greater mortality risk observed among bipolar disorder patients from causes other than suicide. It remains to be established whether other drugs used as maintenance therapy such as valproic and carbamazepine also may prolong survival in patients with bipolar disorder.

■ Major Depression Lithium appears to be an effective antidepressant in some acutely depressed patients†. Depressive symptomatology, including feelings of hopelessness, worthlessness, and guilt; psychomotor retardation; weight loss; early awakening; and suicidal ideation, often improves during treatment with lithium. The acute antidepressant effect of lithium is more likely to occur in patients with bipolar disorder than in patients with major depression. In acutely depressed patients, complete or partial response occurs in 60–80% of patients treated with the drug. In controlled studies in acutely depressed patients, the antidepressant effect of lithium was about equal to that of tricyclic antidepressants; however, in one study imipramine was more effective than lithium. Because the effectiveness of other antidepressants (e.g., tricyclic antidepressants) in the treatment of acute depression is better established, and because lithium may worsen depressive symptoms in some patients, most clinicians reserve a trial of lithium therapy for those depressed patients who fail to respond to other antidepressants.

Based on data from several controlled studies, lithium appears to be more effective than placebo at reducing the rate of relapse in patients with recurrent depression† (recurrent unipolar affective disorder). Lithium also appears to be at least as effective as tricyclic antidepressants at reducing the number of depressive episodes in such patients. Although lithium appears to be effective in the prophylactic treatment of recurrent depression, only a small number of patients have been studied. Some clinicians believe that these studies justify the long-term use of lithium in recurrent depression; however, most clinicians believe that additional comparative studies are needed to determine the efficacy of lithium in the prophylactic treatment of recurrent depression.

■ Schizoaffective and Schizophrenic Disorders In patients with schizoaffective disorder† or schizophrenia†, lithium has been used with varying results. In patients with mildly active schizoaffective disorder in which the affective component predominates, lithium appears to be as effective as chlorpromazine. Such patients often show improvement in mannerisms, posturing, excitement, cooperation, and thought disorders during lithium therapy. In the treatment of patients with highly active schizoaffective disorder in which the schizophrenic component predominates, lithium appears to be less effective than chlorpromazine. In these patients, lithium alone generally fails to adequately control hostile, excited behavior. In patients with schizophrenia, lithium has demonstrated limited effectiveness when given as monotherapy and has caused worsening of the disorder in some cases.

Most clinicians consider antipsychotic agents to be the treatment of choice in patients with schizoaffective disorder or schizophrenia. The addition of lithium to a regimen containing an antipsychotic agent may be beneficial in some patients such as those with predominantly affective signs and symptoms who fail to respond to an antipsychotic agent alone, especially when acute episodes are of recent onset (e.g., less than 6 months). The American Psychiatric Association (APA) states that lithium has limited efficacy when used alone in the treatment of schizophrenia and is less effective than antipsychotic agents when used as monotherapy in patients with this condition. Earlier studies suggested that when added to antipsychotic agents in patients with schizophrenia, lithium increased overall efficacy and improved negative symptoms in particular. Other early studies indicated that lithium was beneficial in schizophrenic patients with prominent affective symptoms and in patients with schizoaffective disorder. However, more recent studies evaluating combined antipsychotic agent and lithium therapy have not confirmed those earlier findings and suggest that adjunctive therapy with lithium is not more effective than antipsychotics used alone in schizophrenia. The addition of relatively low doses of lithium over an 8-week period to an existing antipsychotic regimen improved anxiety but did not improve other symptoms in one placebo-controlled study. In another placebo-controlled study, the addition of lithium did not result in clinical improvement in schizophrenic patients who had not responded to 6 months of fluphenazine decanoate therapy. Although controlled studies of lithium combined with atypical antipsychotic agents are lacking, some of the newer antipsychotic agents have demonstrated antidepressant, anxiolytic, and mood stabilizing activity; therefore, the potential value of combined therapy with these agents and lithium may be limited.

When lithium and antipsychotic agents are used in combination, the APA states that lithium generally is added to the antipsychotic drug that the patient is already receiving after the patient has received an adequate trial but has reached a plateau in the level of clinical response and residual symptoms persist. The APA recommends that the dosage of lithium be adjusted so that serum lithium concentrations in the range of 0.8–1.2 mEq/L are achieved. Response to lithium therapy usually is evident soon after initiating therapy, and a trial of 3–4 weeks of lithium therapy usually is sufficient to determine effectiveness; however, clinical improvement may require 3 months or longer in some cases. In addition to monitoring for the usual adverse effects associated with lithium therapy, clinicians should carefully monitor patients for possible adverse drug interactions with the antipsychotic agent (e.g., adverse extrapyramidal effects, confusion, disorientation, and other signs of neuroleptic malignant syndrome), particularly during the early stage of combined therapy. For further information on the symptomatic management of schizophrenia, see Uses: Psychotic Disorders in the Phenothiazines General Statement 28:16.08.24.

■ Disorders of Impulse Control Lithium has been used successfully in the treatment of impulsive-aggressive behavior in a small number of adults with disorders of impulse control†. Lithium reduced temper outbursts, impulsive antisocial behavior, and the number of assaultive acts. Further studies are needed to confirm the usefulness of the drug in these patients.

■ Psychiatric Disorders in Children Lithium has been used to treat children with apparent mixed bipolar disorder symptomatology†, hyperactivity with psychotic or neurotic components†, or aggressive behavior† or aggressive outbursts† associated with attention-deficit hyperactivity disorder (ADHD). Although children with violent and aggressive behavior who do not have an underlying affective disorder may respond to lithium, children with a definite affective disorder are more likely to respond to the drug. Late-adolescent patients who have mixed bipolar disorder and a parent with a lithium-responsive mixed bipolar disorder are most likely to respond to lithium. Although lithium appears to be useful in children with mixed bipolar disorder†, emotionally unstable character disorder†, depression†, or aggressiveness†, data are too limited to support routine use of the drug in these children. When lithium is used in the treatment of these disorders after an adequate trial with more conservative therapy, the duration of lithium therapy should be short (i.e., not greater than 6 months) and continued only in the presence of unequivocal response to the drug.

■ Alcohol Dependence Although early studies reported limited evidence of improved outcomes in patients with or without depression who received lithium for the management of alcohol dependence†, evidence from a large, randomized, double-blind, placebo-controlled study sponsored by the Department of Veterans Affairs indicated that lithium was not an effective treatment for alcohol dependence in either depressed or nondepressed alcoholics. In this study, clinical outcome measurements such as abstinence rates, number of days of drinking, number of alcohol-related hospitalizations, change in severity of alcoholism, and change in severity of depression in alcoholics who received lithium were comparable to those of alcoholics who received placebo. Unlike previous studies, the Department of Veterans Affairs Cooperative Study was large enough to have sufficient statistical power to detect a medium-effect size difference between the efficacy of lithium and placebo. This study also was controlled for comorbidity; alcoholics with antisocial personality disorder and major psychiatric illnesses other than nonpsychotic depression were excluded from the study.

■ Neutropenia and Anemia Lithium has been used to treat neutropenia† or anemia† secondary to a variety of causes. Only in patients with antineoplastic drug-induced neutropenia have well-controlled studies of lithium therapy been reported.

In a limited number of patients with neutropenia secondary to myelosuppressive antineoplastic chemotherapy regimens, the addition of lithium to the regimen has decreased the number of days neutropenia is present, decreased the frequency of absolute neutrophil counts less than 500/mm^3, and increased the neutrophil count at its nadir. The number of hospitalizations related to infection or fever and the number of infection-related deaths also have been reduced when lithium was added to a myelosuppressive antineoplastic chemotherapy regimen. There is no evidence to date that lithium increases the response of the underlying neoplastic disease to chemotherapy.

Patients receiving antineoplastic chemotherapy often are debilitated and generally are more susceptible to the adverse effects of lithium. Therefore, the benefit-to-risk ratio of lithium therapy in these patients remains to be established. Some clinicians recommend short-term lithium therapy when a patient has had severe neutropenic episodes during previous courses of chemotherapy or when a patient is undergoing treatment with combination chemotherapy known to be severely myelosuppressive.

Lithium has limited efficacy in the treatment of patients with congenital, idiopathic, or cyclic neutropenias†; Felty's syndrome†; or aplastic anemia†. In these patients, lithium has inconsistently increased leukocyte and/or erythrocyte counts. Most clinicians do not recommend routine use of lithium in these conditions since the efficacy of the drug has been limited and studies to date have not been adequately controlled.

■ **Other Uses** Lithium has been used in the treatment of hyperthyroidism†; however, because of its adverse effects, other treatments (e.g., radioactive iodine, surgery, propylthiouracil, methimazole) currently are preferred. Lithium also has been used to prolong the presence of radioactivity in the thyroid gland in patients receiving radioactive iodine†; however, use of the drug for this purpose requires further study.

Although lithium previously was considered one of the therapies of choice in the treatment of the syndrome of inappropriate secretion of antidiuretic hormone† (SIADH), it generally has been replaced with other more effective and/or less toxic therapies (e.g., demeclocycline).

Dosage and Administration

■ **General Dosage and Administration** Lithium salts are administered orally, preferably with meals. Extended-release preparations should be swallowed intact and should *not* be chewed, crushed, or halved. Although there may be minor differences in bioavailability of commercially available lithium preparations, data do not support the use of one preparation over another. The choice of preparation usually is based on expense and patient preference. Lithium citrate oral solution may be useful in patients unable to swallow capsules or tablets; 5 mL of a commercially available solution contains about 8 mEq of lithium and is approximately equivalent to 300 mg of lithium carbonate.

Careful monitoring of serum lithium concentrations and clinical status of the patient is mandatory and patients should be carefully instructed in the safe use of the drug. The precautions and contraindications associated with lithium use should be reviewed carefully before initiating therapy. (See Cautions: Precautions and Contraindications.)

Serum lithium concentrations generally should be monitored twice weekly during initiation of the acute phase of therapy and until the serum concentration and clinical condition of the patient have been stabilized. Thereafter, serum concentrations should be monitored at least every 2 months in most patients. In patients whose affective disorder is not improving or in whom adverse effects are occurring, serum lithium concentrations should be monitored more frequently (e.g., weekly). There is wide interindividual variation in the dosage needed to achieve a given serum lithium concentration and in the serum lithium concentration needed to achieve therapeutic response. The established therapeutic range of serum lithium concentrations is based on correlations determined with monitoring of steady-state concentrations in the morning 12 hours after a dose in patients receiving a divided daily dosing regimen. Therefore, serum lithium concentrations should be determined at consistent times as close as possible to the twelfth hour after a dose. The manufacturers suggest that steady-state serum lithium concentrations be determined immediately before the next dose (i.e., 8–12 hours after the previous lithium dose). Total reliance must not be placed on serum lithium concentrations alone; accurate patient evaluation requires both careful clinical and laboratory evaluation. Dosage should be reduced and serum lithium concentration determined when a patient exhibits signs and symptoms of adverse nervous system, GI, or renal effects.

Although lithium has a long serum half-life and could be given in a single daily dose, the drug usually is given in divided doses because single daily doses often produce more frequent adverse effects (e.g., nausea, diarrhea). Several preliminary studies, however, indicate that the incidence of polyuria may be lower in patients receiving single daily doses rather than divided doses. Twice-daily dosing of conventional or extended-release preparations is sufficient for most patients. When adverse GI or nervous system effects occur, they may be minimized or prevented by giving the drug as conventional preparations in 3 or 4 divided doses. When lithium is used during pregnancy (see Cautions: Pregnancy, Fertility, and Lactation), some clinicians recommend dividing the total daily dose of conventional preparations into 3–5 doses to avoid exposing the fetus to high peak serum concentrations of the drug.

■ **Dosage for Acute Episodes** Serum lithium concentrations of 1–1.2 mEq/L are usually required during acute affective episodes. Although higher serum lithium concentrations may be required in some patients, *the serum concentration should not exceed 1.5 mEq/L during the acute treatment phase.* If manifestations of lithium toxicity occur, the drug should be temporarily discontinued for 24–48 hours, then resumed at a lower dosage.

Adult Dosage During acute episodes of an affective disorder, the manufacturers recommend an initial lithium dosage of 1.8 g daily as conventional capsules or tablets of lithium carbonate, given in 3 or 4 divided doses, or 30 mL (about 48 mEq of lithium) of lithium citrate oral solution daily, given in 3 divided doses. Alternatively, the usual initial dosage of lithium carbonate of 1.8 g daily may be administered as extended-release tablets of lithium carbonate, given in 2 or 3 divided doses. However, because long-term compliance may be affected by a patient's initial experience with the drug, some clinicians recommend that lower initial dosages of lithium be used (e.g., 900 mg of lithium carbonate daily or less), especially in geriatric patients, in an attempt to minimize initial adverse effects, and then dosage be titrated slowly to achieve therapeutic serum lithium concentrations. Dosage must be individualized according to serum lithium concentrations, patient tolerance, and clinical response. The manufacturers state that serum lithium concentrations should be determined twice weekly during the acute phase of therapy and until the serum concentration and clinical condition of the patient have been stabilized. However, some clinicians recommend more frequent monitoring of serum lithium concentrations (e.g., before and after each dosage increase), particularly if a rapid dosage increase is necessary (e.g., in the treatment of acute mania) or if toxicity is suspected. Following resolution of acute manic signs and symptoms, many patients will not tolerate serum lithium concentrations of 1–1.2 mEq/L, and dosage reduction with appropriate patient monitoring is usually necessary.

Pediatric Dosage Although the usual dosage of lithium salts for acute episodes in children† has not been established, lithium carbonate dosages of 15–20 mg/kg (about 0.4–0.5 mEq/kg) daily or equivalent lithium citrate dosages have been given in 2 or 3 divided doses to children 11 years of age or younger. However, the usual adult dosage should not be exceeded. When lithium salts are used in children, dosage should be adjusted according to serum lithium concentrations, patient tolerance, and clinical response. Dosages for children 12 years of age and older usually are the same of those of adults.

■ **Maintenance Dosage** Maintenance dosage of lithium should be based on serum lithium concentrations noted during the acute phase of therapy and on steady-state serum lithium concentrations determined 12 hours after a dose. Manufacturers recommend maintaining steady-state serum lithium concentrations at 0.6–1.2 mEq/L, using the minimum effective dosage that produces serum concentrations in this range, while avoiding excessive adverse effects. Geriatric patients often can be maintained with dosages that produce serum concentrations at the lower end of this range. During maintenance therapy, serum lithium concentrations are generally determined at least every 2 months in patients whose disease is well controlled.

Adult Dosage The usual adult maintenance dosage is 900 mg to 1.2 g daily of lithium carbonate as conventional tablets or capsules, given in 3 or 4 divided doses, or 15–20 mL of lithium citrate oral solution (about 24–32 mEq) daily, given in 3 or 4 divided doses. Alternatively, the usual maintenance dosage of lithium carbonate of 900 mg to 1.2 g daily may be administered as extended-release tablets, given in 2 or 3 divided doses. This dosage generally provides serum lithium concentrations of 0.6–1.2 mEq/L. Maintenance dosage usually should not exceed 2.4 g of lithium carbonate (65 mEq) daily.

Pediatric Dosage The usual maintenance dosage of lithium salts in children† has not been established. When lithium salts are used in children†, dosage should be adjusted according to serum lithium concentrations, patient tolerance, and clinical response.

Cautions

Adverse reactions to lithium generally involve the CNS, GI tract, and kidneys. These adverse reactions usually are dose-dependent and generally occur at 12-hour steady-state serum lithium concentrations greater than 1–1.3 mEq/L; however, adverse CNS effects have occurred at serum concentrations less than 1 mEq/L, especially in children and geriatric patients. Other adverse effects, particularly GI effects, have been related to high peak serum concentrations of lithium.

■ **Nervous System and Neuromuscular Effects** Mild adverse CNS and neuromuscular effects initially occur in about 40–50% of patients receiving lithium. Lethargy, fatigue, muscle weakness, and tremor occur most frequently. As many as 40% of patients receiving lithium initially complain of headache, minor memory impairment and mental confusion, and/or a slightly decreased ability to concentrate.

Hand tremor occurs in about 45–50% of patients during initiation of lithium therapy and is usually benign. The tremor is a fine, rapid intention tremor, which generally resolves during continued therapy with the drug. After 1 year of lithium therapy, less than 10% of patients exhibit tremor. A coarsening of the tremor or its spread to other parts of the body may indicate lithium intoxication. Although hand tremor usually occurs early in the course of therapy, it can occur at any time and may be aggravated by anxiety, caffeine, or thyrotoxicosis. Most patients do not find lithium-induced tremor particularly troublesome. For those who do, a reduction in lithium dosage or low doses of a β-adrenergic blocking agent (e.g., propranolol) may be beneficial. The tremor is not responsive to antimuscarinic or other antiparkinsonian drugs.

Transient muscle weakness occurs in about 30% of lithium-treated patients; after 1 year of lithium therapy, about 1% of lithium-treated patients complain of muscle weakness. Similarly, fatigue, lethargy, dulled senses, and ataxia occur early in therapy but seem to resolve after 2–3 weeks of therapy. Dysarthria and aphasia also have been reported.

Muscle hyperirritability (including fasciculations, twitching, clonic movements of limbs), hyperactive deep tendon reflexes, hypertonia (hypertonicity), and choreoathetoid movements occur in less than 15% of patients receiving lithium. Cogwheel rigidity occurs in about 5% of patients. In one study, cogwheel rigidity reportedly occurred in 75% of patients receiving lithium; however, persistent concentrations of antipsychotic agents may have accounted for the higher incidence of cogwheel rigidity noted in these patients. Lithium-induced cogwheel rigidity generally is mild to moderate. Although it rarely may be associated with other extrapyramidal signs, lithium-induced cogwheel rigidity does not respond to antiparkinsonian agents.

Blackout spells, giddiness, dizziness, vertigo, disturbances in accommodation, somnolence and tendency to sleep, stupor, coma, restlessness, psychomotor retardation, acute dystonia, down-beat nystagmus, centrally mediated incontinence of urine and feces, and worsening of organic brain syndrome have occurred during lithium therapy. In one study, vertigo and disturbances in accommodation occurred in 15 and 10% of patients receiving the drug, respectively. Asterixis has occurred in at least one patient.

Pseudotumor cerebri (with increased intracranial pressure and papilledema) has occurred in patients receiving lithium. If undetected, this condition may result in enlargement of the blind spot, constriction of visual fields, and/or eventual blindness resulting from optic atrophy. If pseudotumor cerebri occurs during lithium therapy, the drug should be discontinued, if clinically possible. Papilledema with no evidence of increased intracranial pressure has also been reported.

Seizures and localizing neurologic findings have occurred in patients receiving lithium. Seizures generally are associated with toxic serum lithium concentrations and/or other signs of lithium neurotoxicity, but seizures also have occurred when lithium concentrations were within the therapeutic range. In one study, there was an increased frequency of lithium-induced seizures in patients with temporal-lobe epilepsy. Various EEG changes, including diffuse slowing, widening of frequency spectrum, and potentiation and disorganization of background rhythm, also have been reported. (See Pharmacology: Nervous System Effects.)

■ **GI Effects** Adverse GI effects occur frequently during initiation of lithium therapy but tend to be mild and reversible. Nausea, anorexia, epigastric bloating, diarrhea, vomiting, or abdominal pain occur in about 10–30% of patients. These adverse GI effects usually resolve during continued therapy and are present in 1–10% of patients after 1–2 years of therapy. These effects often are related to high peak serum lithium concentrations and are alleviated by taking the drug with meals, dividing dosage, or using an extended-release preparation. Some patients report a reduction in adverse GI effects when switched from one conventional capsule or tablet preparation to another.

Dry mouth occurs in about 20–50% of patients receiving lithium and is related to lithium-induced polyuria. Dysgeusia and sialorrhea also have been reported. An increased frequency of dental caries has been reported in patients treated with lithium, but this effect is probably related to increased consumption of sugar-containing fluids by patients with lithium-induced polydipsia. Contact stomatitis has occurred in at least one patient and was attributed to the formulation of the preparation.

■ **Renal Effects** Nephrogenic diabetes insipidus manifested as polyuria and polydipsia occurs in about 30–50% of lithium-treated patients, usually develops shortly after starting lithium therapy, and persists in about 10–25% of treated patients after 1–2 years of therapy. Polydipsia is largely a consequence of polyuria; both usually are well tolerated in most patients. Polyuria rarely is associated with serum electrolyte abnormalities, weight loss, or other signs and symptoms of dehydration; however, these effects may occur in patients who develop severe diabetes insipidus during lithium therapy. Many patients actually respond to polyuria with weight gain, probably because of increased consumption of high-calorie fluids. Although polyuria is a persistent and sometimes progressive finding in patients treated with lithium, it usually is reversible within 1 year after discontinuance of the drug; irreversible diabetes insipidus occurs rarely. Polyuria has been treated with lithium dosage reduction and/or with thiazide diuretics or amiloride (See Drug Interactions: Diuretics.)

Nonspecific nephron atrophy characterized by glomerular sclerosis, tubular atrophy, interstitial fibrosis, and urinary casts has been observed in patients treated with lithium. The tubular lesions are limited mainly to the distal convoluted tubule and collecting ducts. Sclerosis of 10–20% of glomeruli has been noted in some patients. These nonspecific changes have not been associated with a decrease in renal function. Although available data do not support a causal relationship between these findings and lithium therapy, studies of large numbers of patients receiving the drug for many years have not been conducted. In several trials using appropriate controls, there was no difference in the frequency of abnormal renal findings in pretreatment and posttreatment patients. However, cellular pleomorphism in the distal renal tubule has been associated with a decrease in renal-concentrating ability. Albuminuria and glycosuria also have occurred.

Modest decreases in glomerular filtration rate occasionally occur in patients receiving long-term lithium therapy; however, a causal relationship has not yet been established. Oliguric renal failure, reported in a few intoxicated patients, probably is not a direct renal effect of lithium but is related to circulatory collapse that may accompany lithium intoxication. (See Chronic Toxicity: Manifestations.)

Distal renal tubular acidosis of the incomplete type has occurred in some patients receiving lithium, but it does not appear to be clinically important unless these patients are stressed by an acid load. Most patients receiving lithium show a normal urine acidification response.

■ **Endocrine Effects** In therapeutic concentrations, lithium causes clinically evident hypothyroidism in about 1–4% of patients receiving the drug. These patients may require supplemental thyroid therapy. Symptoms of hypothyroidism may vary from mild to severe myxedema and may occur within weeks to years after initiating lithium therapy; rarely, hypothyroidism may persist after discontinuance of the drug. In addition, about 5% of lithium-treated patients develop goiters, resulting from stimulation of the thyroid gland by an indirect lithium-induced increase in thyrotropin release. Goiters may develop even in the absence of hypothyroidism in some patients receiving lithium. Lithium-induced goiters usually are diffuse and nontender and often so small as to be noticed only on palpation. Many patients have only laboratory evidence of hypothyroidism, including decreased serum concentrations of thyroxine (T_4) and triiodothyronine (T_3) and increased radioactive iodine uptake. Even in patients whose baseline serum thyrotropin concentrations are within normal limits, an exaggerated thyrotropin response to IV protirelin often occurs. Geriatric patients and patients with antithyroglobulin antibody, a prior history of Graves' disease or Hashimoto's thyroiditis, or those receiving iodine may be more likely to develop hypothyroidism during lithium therapy. Paradoxically, a few cases of hyperthyroidism have been reported.

Mild asymptomatic primary hyperparathyroidism has occurred during long-term lithium therapy and, rarely, may persist after discontinuance of the drug. (See Pharmacology: Endocrine Effects.)

Transient hyperglycemia has occurred rarely in patients receiving lithium.

■ **Cardiovascular Effects** Benign, reversible ECG T-wave depression occurs in 20–30% of patients receiving lithium. Isoelectricity or inversion of T waves also may occur. Reversible sinus node dysfunction (e.g., sinus bradycardia, sinoatrial block), atrioventricular (AV) node dissociation with AV block and junctional rhythms, and ventricular premature depolarizations occur rarely at therapeutic and toxic serum lithium concentrations. Syncope has occurred in patients with lithium-induced nodal dysfunction. In contrast, lithium also has been found to reduce the frequency of preexisting atrial premature depolarizations and supraventricular tachycardia.

Mild to moderate pretibial edema has occurred in a few patients during lithium therapy and appears to be associated with high sodium intake (more than 170 mEq/day). The edema has responded to spironolactone. Edematous swelling of the wrists also has occurred.

Other cardiovascular effects, including hypotension and cardiovascular collapse, have been noted during severe lithium intoxication and probably are not direct effects of the drug. Peripheral circulatory collapse also has been reported. Cardiomyopathy with associated myocardial and thyroid fibrosis was reported in one patient receiving lithium, amitriptyline, and potassium iodide.

Signs and symptoms resembling Raynaud's disease, which included painful discoloration of fingers and toes and coldness of the extremities, occurred in some patients within 1 day after initiating lithium therapy. The mechanism of this effect is not known; recovery occurred following discontinuance of the drug.

■ **Dermatologic Effects** Adverse dermatologic effects occur in about 1% of patients receiving lithium and rarely necessitate discontinuance of the drug. Acneiform eruptions and folliculitis appear to occur most frequently. Lithium-induced acneiform eruptions usually involve the face, neck, axilla, groin, and breast. The papules may become confluent or may subside spontaneously. Temporary discontinuance of the drug usually results in resolution of the eruption. Lithium-induced folliculitis resembles keratosis pilaris, is asymptomatic and usually limited to the extensor surfaces of the extremities, and often remits spontaneously. Pruritic maculopapular rashes occur rarely and usually remit with dosage reduction or discontinuance of lithium.

Lithium-induced or -exacerbated psoriasis has occurred occasionally; it is unclear whether a causal relationship to the drug exists. Alopecia, drying and thinning of the hair, xerosis cutis, anesthesia of the skin, cutaneous ulcers, exfoliative dermatitis, and lupus erythematosus-like rash also have occurred.

■ **Hematologic Effects** Most patients receiving lithium develop a reversible leukocytosis, with leukocyte counts of 10,000–15,000/mm³. Increases in erythrocyte and platelet counts are less frequently observed.

Lithium has been associated with the development of leukemia (see Cautions: Mutagenicity and Carcinogenicity), but a causal relationship to the drug has not been established. Aplastic anemia has been reported in at least one patient receiving lithium. Positive serum titers for antinuclear antibodies (ANA) have occurred during lithium therapy, but patients with positive serum ANA titers usually were receiving other drugs in addition to lithium.

■ **Other Adverse Effects** Other adverse effects associated with lithium therapy include weight loss or excessive weight gain (which may be associated with polyuria, see Cautions: Renal Effects), transient scotomata, exophthalmos, and generalized discomfort.

■ **Precautions and Contraindications** Since lithium toxicity is closely related to serum lithium concentrations and may occur at doses closely associated with therapeutic serum concentrations, monitoring of serum lithium concentrations and the clinical status of the patient is necessary in all patients receiving the drug. Lithium dosing should be monitored carefully when a patient's initial manic symptoms begin to subside, since the patient's ability to tolerate high serum lithium concentrations decreases as these symptoms resolve. (See Dosage and Administration: Dosage for Acute Episodes.)

Patients receiving lithium should be carefully instructed to avoid dehydration and to report polyuria and any prolonged vomiting, diarrhea, or fever to their physician. Patients should maintain their usual fluid (2.5–3 L/day) and sodium intake, and supplement these in the event of fever (e.g., during infections), vomiting, or diarrhea. A temporary reduction in dosage or discontinuance of the drug also may be required in these patients. Lithium should be used cautiously in patients whose sodium intake is restricted; in these patients, sodium intake should be stabilized and lithium dosage carefully titrated to avoid increased serum lithium concentrations that may occur with sodium depletion.

Outpatients and their families should be warned that the patient must discontinue lithium therapy immediately and consult a physician if signs of lithium intoxication such as muscle twitching, tremor, mild ataxia, drowsiness, muscle weakness, diarrhea, or vomiting occur. Patients also should be warned that lithium may impair their ability to perform activities requiring mental alertness or physical coordination (e.g., operating machinery, driving a motor vehicle).

Because nonspecific nephron atrophy has occurred in patients receiving lithium, many clinicians recommend a thorough assessment of renal function before initiating therapy. Many clinicians recommend that measurement of 24-hour creatinine clearance, renal-concentrating ability, and a urinalysis should ideally be performed in all patients prior to initiating therapy. Many clinicians also recommend that renal function be evaluated every 2–3 months for the first 6 months, then every 6–12 months during therapy or whenever clinically indicated. If progressive or sudden changes in renal function, even within the normal range, occur during lithium therapy, the need for therapy with the drug should be reevaluated.

Lithium should be used cautiously in patients with preexisting cardiovascular or thyroid disease. Patients with underlying cardiovascular disease should be observed carefully for signs and symptoms of arrhythmia (including periodic ECG determinations), and serum lithium concentrations should be kept within the therapeutic range since nodal arrhythmias may occur. Patients with underlying hypothyroidism should have thyroid function (T_3, T_4, and TSH concentrations) evaluated yearly and be given supplemental thyroid therapy when needed.

Lithium should be used with caution in geriatric patients since they appear to be more susceptible to adverse effects of the drug (e.g., adverse nervous system and neuromuscular effects), even at therapeutic serum concentrations. Because geriatric patients are more prone than younger patients to developing lithium-induced goiter and clinical hypothyroidism, some clinicians recommend that thyroid function tests be performed every 6–12 months in these patients. In addition, because of decreased renal function, geriatric patients are more likely to develop lithium intoxication subsequent to accumulation of the drug.

Although most patients receiving lithium and an antipsychotic agent (e.g., haloperidol, phenothiazines) concurrently do not develop unusual adverse effects, an acute encephalopathic syndrome (consisting of confusion, disorientation, adverse extrapyramidal effects, and possibly neuroleptic malignant syndrome) occasionally has occurred, especially when high serum lithium concentrations were present and associated with dehydration. Patients receiving such combined therapy should be observed for evidence of adverse neurologic effects; treatment should be promptly discontinued if such signs or symptoms appear. (See Drug Interactions: Antipsychotic Agents.)

Lithium generally should not be used in patients with severe renal or cardiovascular disease or severe dehydration, sodium depletion, or debilitation since the risk of toxicity is increased in these patients. If the psychiatric indication is life-threatening and other forms of therapy are contraindicated or ineffective, lithium may be used with extreme caution in these patients; if lithium therapy is initiated in these patients, the patient should be hospitalized, serum lithium concentration should be monitored carefully, and dosage should be adjusted as necessary. Although the manufacturers caution against the concurrent use of lithium and a diuretic, when combined therapy is necessary, some clinicians recommend that the usual dosage of lithium initially be reduced by about 50%, the patient and serum lithium concentrations be monitored carefully, and lithium dosage be adjusted as necessary. (See Drug Interactions: Diuretics.)

■ **Pediatric Precautions** Safety and efficacy of lithium therapy in children younger than 12 years of age have not been established; however, the drug has been used in this age group when benefits were thought to outweigh risks. Transient acute dystonia and hyperreflexia occurred in a 15-kg child who ingested 300 mg of lithium carbonate.

■ **Geriatric Precautions** Clinical studies of lithium carbonate as extended-release tablets did not include sufficient numbers of patients 65 years of age and older to determine whether geriatric patients respond differently than younger patients. While clinical experience with lithium therapy generally has not revealed age-related differences in response to the drug, care should be taken in dosage selection of lithium. Because of the greater frequency of decreased hepatic, renal, and/or cardiac function and of concomitant disease and drug therapy in geriatric patients, patients in this age group should receive initial dosages of the drug in the lower end of the usual range. Lithium is substantially excreted by the kidneys and the risk of severe adverse reactions to the drug may be increased in patients with impaired renal function. Because geriatric patients may have decreased renal function, renal function should be monitored and dosage adjusted accordingly.

■ **Mutagenicity and Carcinogenicity** It is not known if lithium is mutagenic or carcinogenic.

An increased number of chromosomal breaks, gaps, and satellite associations, as well as a reduced percentage of replicating cells were found in one study of lithium-containing leukocyte cultures. Similar findings were not found in 2 other in vitro studies. Mice inoculated with viable sarcoma cells have shown an earlier incidence of tumor development but no change in tumor size when treated with lithium. The number and growth of induced mammary tumors in rats have not been increased by lithium.

There have been occasional reports of lithium-induced hematologic neoplasms (e.g., acute leukemia), but a causal relationship to the drug has not been established. Studies have shown no changes in blast and mature neutrophil counts in patients with various blood dyscrasias who were receiving lithium. One study found the incidence of leukemia not to be increased in a group of manic-depressive patients receiving chronic lithium therapy.

■ **Pregnancy, Fertility, and Lactation** Lithium can cause fetal toxicity when administered to pregnant women, but potential benefits may be acceptable in certain conditions despite the possible risks to the fetus. Lithium should be used during pregnancy only in life-threatening situations or severe disease for which safer drugs cannot be used or are ineffective. When lithium is administered during pregnancy or if the patient becomes pregnant while receiving the drug, the patient should be informed of the potential hazard to the fetus. When possible, lithium should be withdrawn for at least the first trimester unless it is determined that this would seriously endanger the mother. Women of childbearing age receiving lithium should be counseled about methods of birth control.

When lithium is used during pregnancy, serum lithium concentrations should be carefully monitored and dosage adjusted if necessary since renal clearance of the drug and distribution of the drug into erythrocytes may be increased during pregnancy. Pregnant women receiving lithium may have subtherapeutic serum lithium concentrations if dosage of the drug is not increased during pregnancy. Immediately postpartum, renal clearance of lithium may decrease to pre-pregnancy levels; therefore, to decrease the risk of postpartum lithium intoxication, dosage of the drug should be reduced 1 week before parturition or when labor begins.

Lithium has caused various teratogenic effects in submammalian species and cleft palates in mice. Studies in rats, rabbits, and monkeys have shown no evidence of lithium-induced teratology.

Data from lithium birth registries suggest that the drug may increase the incidence of cardiac and other anomalies, especially Ebstein's anomaly (distorted tricuspid valve with secondary dilation of the right ventricular outflow tract). Atrial septal defect, patent foramen ovale, and right ventricular conduction delay also have occurred. Other reported fetal cardiovascular abnormalities included mitral atresia, coarctation of the aorta, ventricular septal defect, tricuspid atresia, patent ductus arteriosus, and dextrocardia. Down's syndrome, clubfoot, meningomyelocele, transient hypothyroidism with goiter, and transient nephrogenic diabetes insipidus also have been reported. Lithium-exposed neonates also have presented briefly with muscular hypotonia (floppy infant syndrome) and apneic spells. A 5-year follow-up study of children without apparent congenital abnormalities who were born to women treated with lithium found no increase in the frequency of physical or mental abnormalities in these children compared with matched controls (i.e., siblings during whose pregnancy the mother did not take lithium).

The effect of lithium on fertility in humans is not known. Erective impotence has been noted by a few men receiving the drug. Lithium has had adverse effects on nidation in rats and on embryo viability in mice. In vitro metabolism of rat testes and human spermatozoa also have been observed.

Lithium is distributed into milk. (See Pharmacokinetics: Distribution.) Because of the potential for serious adverse reactions from lithium in nursing infants, a decision generally should be made to discontinue nursing or the drug, taking into account the importance of the drug to the woman.

Drug Interactions

■ **Diuretics** In general, the concomitant use of lithium and diuretics should be avoided. In those cases where concomitant use is necessary, extreme caution is advised because diuretic-induced sodium loss may reduce the renal clearance of lithium and increase the risk of lithium toxicity. When such combinations are used, the lithium dosage may need to be decreased and more frequent monitoring of serum lithium concentrations is recommended.

Thiazide diuretics, sometimes used in combination with lithium to reduce lithium-induced polyuria, will reduce renal lithium clearance within several days. The reduced lithium clearance has resulted in increased serum lithium concentrations and several cases of lithium intoxication. When thiazide diuretics are used to treat lithium-induced polyuria, most clinicians recommend reducing lithium dosage by about 50% and carefully monitoring serum lithium concentrations. Other diuretics that enhance sodium excretion (e.g., furosemide, spironolactone) also may reduce renal clearance of lithium; however, this effect does not occur consistently and lithium clearance often is increased initially. Urea also has increased renal clearance of lithium. Amiloride does not appear to substantially affect lithium pharmacokinetics in most patients. (See Drug Interactions: Lithium, in Amiloride Hydrochloride 40:28.10.)

■ **Antipsychotic Agents** Numerous pharmacokinetic and clinical interactions have been reported between phenothiazines and lithium. Phenothiazines have been shown to increase erythrocyte lithium concentrations and to increase renal clearance of lithium. Lithium has been reported to decrease serum chlorpromazine concentrations. The clinical result of these pharmacokinetic interactions is unpredictable; therefore, patients receiving lithium and a phenothiazine should be monitored for altered response to either drug. In addition, an acute encephalopathic syndrome (toxic-confusional state) consisting of confusion, disorientation, extrapyramidal adverse effects, and possibly neuroleptic malignant syndrome occasionally has been reported in patients receiving lithium and antipsychotic agents concurrently, particularly in dehydrated patients with high serum lithium concentrations. Therefore, patients receiving combined therapy should be observed for evidence of adverse neurologic effects (e.g., adverse extrapyramidal effects, confusion, disorientation, and other signs of neuroleptic malignant syndrome), particularly during the early stage of combined therapy. Nausea and vomiting, which are occasionally signs of lithium intoxication, may be masked by the antiemetic effect of some phenothiazines when used concurrently.

Occasionally, patients have developed acute encephalopathic syndromes or extrapyramidal reactions when concurrently using lithium and an antipsychotic agent (e.g., haloperidol, phenothiazines). Irreversible brain damage, parkinsonian movements, and dyskinesias have resulted. Although a causal relationship has not been established and most patients can receive the drugs concurrently without adverse effect, caution is advised. Patients receiving such combined therapy should be monitored for adverse neurologic effects, especially when large dosages of lithium and an antipsychotic agent are used; combined therapy should be promptly discontinued if such signs or symptoms appear.

■ **Nonsteroidal Anti-inflammatory Agents** Indomethacin, mefenamic acid, phenylbutazone, piroxicam, and ibuprofen have been reported to increase serum lithium concentrations by 30–60%, resulting in lithium toxicity in some cases. These nonsteroidal anti-inflammatory agents (NSAIAs) appear to decrease renal clearance of lithium. There is evidence that other NSAIAs, including selective inhibitors of cyclooxygenase-2 (COX-2), have the same effect. In one clinical study, mean steady-state plasma lithium concentrations increased approximately 17% in healthy individuals who received lithium (450 mg twice daily) in conjunction with celecoxib (200 mg twice daily) compared with those who received lithium alone. When these agents are started or discontinued in a patient receiving lithium, serum lithium concentrations should be closely monitored and the patient should be observed for signs and symptoms of lithium intoxication. Appropriate adjustment in lithium dosage may be required when therapy with the NSAIA is discontinued.

■ **Anticonvulsants** Adverse neurologic effects have occurred in patients receiving lithium concurrently with carbamazepine or phenytoin. Concurrent use of lithium and phenytoin also has resulted in increased serum lithium concentrations in at least one patient; however, the clinical importance of this effect has not been determined and further substantiation of this interaction is required.

■ **Angiotensin-converting Enzyme Inhibitors** Concomitant administration of lithium and an ACE inhibitor (e.g., captopril, enalapril, lisinopril) may result in elevated plasma lithium concentrations and has resulted in several cases of lithium intoxication. Consequently, at least one manufacturer of lithium and some clinicians recommend that such concomitant use of these agents be avoided, particularly in geriatric patients or in those with congestive heart failure, renal insufficiency, or volume depletion. The mechanism of this interaction is not known, but it has been postulated that dehydration and loss of sodium may decrease excretion of lithium. Moderate renal insufficiency (serum creatinine of 2.2 mg/dL) or acute renal failure also has occurred in some patients receiving an ACE inhibitor concomitantly with lithium. (See Drug Interactions: Lithium, in Enalapril 24:32.04.) If lithium is used with an ACE inhibitor, the dosage of lithium may need to be reduced and serum lithium concentrations should be carefully monitored.

■ **Calcium-channel Blocking Agents** Serum lithium concentrations may decrease following initiation of verapamil in patients stabilized on lithium therapy. In a patient with bipolar disorder whose lithium dosage had been stabilized for several years, manic symptoms emerged and serum lithium concentrations decreased to subtherapeutic levels within 1 month after initiating 320 mg of verapamil hydrochloride daily, requiring an increase in lithium carbonate dosage from 900–1200 mg daily to 1800–2100 mg daily. Serum lithium concentrations also decreased in another patient and urinary excretion of the cation increased.

Although the mechanism of this interaction currently is not known, serum lithium concentrations and the patient should be monitored closely and lithium dosage adjusted accordingly when verapamil is initiated or discontinued in patients receiving lithium therapy.

There also is some evidence that calcium-channel blocking agents may potentiate the toxic effects of lithium; neurotoxicity (e.g., ataxia, choreoathetosis, tremors, tinnitus), adverse GI effects (e.g., nausea, vomiting, diarrhea), and bradycardia have been reported in patients receiving lithium concomitantly with a calcium-channel blocking agent. When 240 mg of verapamil hydrochloride daily was initiated for potential antimanic effects in a patient whose bipolar disorder was inadequately controlled with a therapeutic dosage of lithium, bipolar disorder was controlled within 1 week after initiating combined therapy, but manifestations of neurotoxicity occurred 2 days later despite therapeutic serum lithium concentrations. Neurotoxicity subsided within 2 days following discontinuance of verapamil but recurred when the patient was rechallenged with verapamil in an attempt to regain control of the bipolar disorder. Verapamil did not appear to affect the pharmacokinetics of lithium in this patient. The mechanism of this interaction is not known, but a similar interaction has been described in a patient receiving lithium and diltiazem concomitantly. Calcium-channel blocking agents appear to share some of the neuropharmacologic effects of lithium, and combined therapy with the drugs may potentiate neurotoxicity. Pending further accumulation of data, verapamil and possibly other calcium-channel blocking agents should be used concomitantly with lithium cautiously.

■ **Selective Serotonin-Reuptake Inhibitors** Adverse effects possibly associated with increased serum lithium concentrations, lithium toxicity, and/or serotonin syndrome (e.g., absence seizures, agitation, ataxia, confusion, diarrhea, dizziness, dysarthria, stiffness of the extremities, tremor) have been reported in patients receiving lithium concomitantly with selective serotonin-reuptake inhibitors (SSRIs). In addition, concomitant use of lithium and fluoxetine has resulted in both increased and decreased serum lithium concentrations; therefore, patients receiving such combined therapy should be monitored closely. Lithium appears to have some serotonergic activity and serotonin syndrome has been reported following initiation of lithium therapy in patients receiving SSRIs such as fluoxetine or paroxetine. For further information on serotonin syndrome, including manifestations and treatment, see Serotonin Syndrome under Drug Interactions: Drugs Associated with Serotonin Syndrome, in Fluoxetine Hydrochloride 28:16.04.20. The clinical importance of this potential interaction remains to be determined and further substantiation is required; however, caution should be exercised when lithium and serotonin reuptake-inhibitors are used concurrently.

■ **Neuromuscular Blocking Agents** Lithium has been reported to prolong the latency of neuromuscular blockade induced by succinylcholine or pancuronium. In limited clinical studies, however, no prolongation of neuromuscular blockade was noted in patients receiving electroconvulsive therapy, succinylcholine, and lithium concurrently. Patients receiving neuromuscular blocking agents should have lithium temporarily withdrawn during their use or should be carefully monitored if lithium is continued.

■ **Iodides** Concurrent use of lithium salts and iodides may result in an additive or synergistic hypothyroid effect. Lithium carbonate and potassium iodide have produced hypothyroidism in several patients when used concurrently. A lithium salt and potassium iodide generally should not be used concomitantly; when the drugs are used together, the patient should be monitored closely for signs and symptoms of hypothyroidism.

■ **Sodium** Changes in sodium intake in patients receiving lithium may alter the renal elimination of lithium. The renal clearance of lithium may be increased or decreased by as much as 30–50% by increased or decreased sodium intake, respectively. Patients should be advised to avoid substantial changes in their sodium intake. (See Cautions: Precautions and Contraindications.) When drugs with a high sodium content (e.g., antacids) are used concomitantly with lithium, serum lithium concentrations should be monitored.

■ **Electroconvulsive Therapy** Acute neurotoxicity with prominent delirium has occurred in patients receiving lithium and electroconvulsive therapy (ECT) concurrently. Some clinicians recommend decreasing lithium dosage or withdrawing the drug 2 days prior to ECT.

■ **Metronidazole** Initiation of short-term metronidazole therapy in patients stabilized on a relatively high dosage of lithium has been reported to increase serum lithium concentrations, resulting in signs of lithium toxicity in several patients; in some cases, signs of renal damage (e.g., persistent elevations in serum creatinine concentration, hypernatremia, abnormally dilute urine) were present. Pending further accumulation of data, caution should be exercised and frequent monitoring of serum lithium concentrations should be performed when metronidazole and lithium are administered concurrently.

■ **β-Adrenergic Blocking Agents** Although β-adrenergic blocking agents have been used to suppress lithium-induced tremor, the absence of tremor may make lithium intoxication more difficult to diagnose. Therefore, patients should be monitored for other signs and symptoms of lithium intoxication when the drugs are used concomitantly.

■ **Alkalinizing Agents** Urinary alkalinizing agents such as sodium bicarbonate may increase renal excretion of lithium, and a higher dosage of lithium may be required in patients receiving these agents concomitantly.

■ **Methyldopa** Symptoms of lithium intoxication, including confusion, disorientation, hand tremor, and slurred speech, have been reported occasionally when methyldopa was administered in patients already receiving lithium. Although plasma lithium concentrations were reported to be within the therapeutic range in some of the published cases, increased lithium concentrations have also been reported during concurrent administration of methyldopa. The possible mechanism for this interaction remains to be established. Pending further experience with this combination, some clinicians recommend that patients receiving lithium and methyldopa should be closely monitored for signs of lithium toxicity and that consideration should be given to the use of alternative antihypertensive agents in patients receiving lithium.

■ **Tetracycline** Tetracycline reportedly increased serum lithium concentrations when the 2 drugs were used concurrently in one patient; however, the clinical importance of this effect has not been determined.

■ **Diazepam** Profound hypothermia has been reported in one patient taking lithium and diazepam concurrently; however, widespread use of this combination without unusual adverse effects indicates that it is safe in most patients.

■ **Opiate Analgesics** Lithium reportedly interferes with opiate-induced euphoria and diminishes the analgesic effect of opiates (narcotic analgesics).

■ **Other Drugs** Decreased serum lithium concentrations as a result of increased urinary lithium excretion may occur when lithium is used concomitantly with acetazolamide or xanthine derivatives (e.g., aminophylline).

Hyperkinetic movements and tardive dyskinesia have been reported when lithium was used concomitantly with baclofen or a monoamine oxidase (MAO) inhibitor, respectively.

Acute Toxicity

Since the pathophysiology, manifestations, and treatment of acute lithium intoxication are similar to those of chronic lithium intoxication, the Chronic Toxicity section should be consulted for additional information.

■ **Pathogenesis** Acute lithium intoxication occurs as the result of ingestion of a single toxic dose. The acute lethal dose of lithium varies but is generally associated with a dose that produces serum lithium concentrations greater than 3.5 mEq/L 12 hours after ingestion.

■ **Manifestations** In individuals not previously receiving the drug, acute ingestion of a single massive dose of lithium may produce only vomiting and diarrhea usually within 1 hour of ingestion. Manifestations associated with chronic lithium intoxication also may occur. A transient syndrome of acute dystonia and hyperreflexia has been reported in a 15-kg child following ingestion of 300 mg of lithium carbonate. Death has occurred in adults who ingested single 10- to 60-g doses of lithium. However, some patients who ingested a single 6-g dose of lithium have had no signs of lithium intoxication.

■ **Treatment** In acute overdosage, the stomach should be emptied immediately by inducing emesis or by gastric lavage. If the patient is comatose, having seizures, or lacks the gag reflex, gastric lavage may be performed if an endotracheal tube with cuff inflated is in place to prevent aspiration of gastric contents. Following induction of emesis or gastric lavage, the treatment described for chronic intoxication generally should be followed. (See Chronic Toxicity: Treatment.)

Chronic Toxicity

■ **Pathogenesis** Chronic lithium intoxication, when it occurs, generally results from high dosages, prolonged therapy with high dosages, or changes in lithium pharmacokinetics. The main contributing factor to the development of chronic intoxication often is water loss, which may result from fever, decreased fluid or food intake during acute manic or depressive episodes, diuretics, abnormal GI conditions (e.g., nausea, diarrhea, vomiting), or pyelonephritis. Geriatric patients also are more prone to develop chronic lithium intoxication.

Although there is no clearly defined relationship between serum lithium concentration and severity of intoxication, the serum concentration 12 hours after the last dose may roughly predict severity of intoxication. Serum lithium concentrations of 1.5–2.5 mEq/L often indicate slight to moderate intoxication; concentrations of 2.5–3.5 mEq/L often indicate severe intoxication; and concentrations greater than 3.5 mEq/L often indicate potentially lethal intoxication. In addition to the serum lithium concentration, the severity of lithium intoxication depends on the length of time the serum concentration remains in the toxic range. *It is important to promptly recognize the signs and symptoms of lithium intoxication and to initiate treatment if necessary.*

■ **Manifestations** Initial manifestations of lithium intoxication often involve the nervous system and include drowsiness, confusion, giddiness, apathy, coarse hand tremor, and dysarthria. Occasionally, GI symptoms are seen (e.g., decreased appetite, nausea, vomiting, diarrhea). Muscle rigidity or fasciculations, slight ataxia, tinnitus, increased lethargy, increased deep tendon reflexes, blurred vision, and vertical nystagmus usually follow; photophobia also has occurred. Lithium intoxication can progress to impaired consciousness, increasing fasciculations and ataxia, coarse and irregular limb tremors, choreoathetoid movements, cogwheel rigidity, and other focal neurologic signs. Coma, twitching, coarse contractions of muscles, generalized tonic-clonic seizures, cardiovascular collapse with oliguria and anuria, and death may ensue. Arrhythmias, electrocardiographic widening of the QRS interval, inverted T waves, and myocardial infarction also have occurred. The clinical course of lithium intoxication is quite variable; patients may present with any of the above signs and symptoms.

Approximately 70–80% of lithium-intoxicated patients fully recover. Persistent sequelae, including dementia, ataxia, polyuria, dysarthria, spasticity, nystagmus, and tremor, have occurred in about 10% of intoxications. Death has occurred in 10–25% of reported lithium intoxications.

■ **Treatment** There is no specific antidote for lithium intoxication. Treatment of lithium intoxication is principally supportive and depends on the patient's clinical condition and serum lithium concentration. Early symptoms of milder lithium intoxication (e.g., diarrhea, vomiting, drowsiness, muscular weakness, lack of coordination) usually respond to dosage reduction or temporary discontinuance of the drug and correction of fluid and electrolyte abnormalities. When intoxication is more severe, the patient generally should be hospitalized and provided intensive, supportive care, including infection prophylaxis and regular chest X-rays. Discontinuance of lithium and any concurrently administered diuretic is essential.

IV infusion of 0.9% sodium chloride injection is begun when lithium intoxication is thought to be secondary to total body depletion of sodium. Rapid administration of large volumes of IV solutions, or IV administration of potassium or a diuretic apparently provides no additional benefit. Although diuretics (e.g., furosemide, mannitol, urea), carbonic anhydrase inhibitors, and xanthine derivatives (e.g., aminophylline) may increase lithium clearance. The increased clearance is insufficient to be useful in treating intoxication. Because dehydration resulting in sodium and lithium retention may also occur when these agents are used, these agents are not recommended for the treatment of lithium intoxication.

Hemodialysis is the only reliable method of rapidly removing excess lithium in patients who manifest lithium intoxication and/or who cannot excrete lithium. Because lithium is not metabolized and is only excreted renally, patients with chronic renal failure should undergo hemodialysis following potentially toxic exposures to lithium. In addition, patients with acute lithium intoxication who were not previously receiving the drug should undergo hemodialysis regardless of their clinical status if their serum lithium concentration equals or exceeds 4 mEq/L. These patients will not be able to excrete lithium in time to prevent a clinically important amount from entering the CNS and causing severe and potentially permanent neurologic toxicity. Because patients with an acute on chronic overdosage or chronic overdosage of lithium already have a body burden of the drug, a serum lithium concentration of 2.5 mEq/L or greater and moderate-to-severe neurologic toxicity are reasonable indications for hemodialysis. Hemodialysis for 8–12 hours is also recommended when fluid or electrolyte abnormalities are unresponsive to supportive treatment; when creatinine clearance or urine output decreases substantially; or when serum lithium concentration is not reduced by at least 20% in 6 hours. Serum lithium concentrations usually rebound within 5–8 hours after hemodialysis because of redistribution of the drug, often necessitating repeated courses of hemodialysis. The goal of hemodialysis is to produce a serum lithium concentration less than 1 mEq/L 8 hours after hemodialysis is completed. Although intermittent hemodialysis usually is performed in severe cases of lithum intoxication, continuous venovenous hemodialysis has also been successfully used in several patients in order to more slowly remove lithium from the body in hemodynamically unstable patients and to avoid postdialysis rebound elevations in lithium levels. Peritoneal dialysis is less effective at removing lithium and is used only when hemodialysis is not possible.

Pharmacology

Lithium has numerous pharmacologic effects. Although traces of lithium are found in animal tissues, lithium has no known physiologic function. Although the mechanisms of action have not been fully elucidated, lithium, as a monovalent cation, competes with other monovalent and divalent cations (potassium, sodium, calcium, magnesium) at cellular sites in body tissues, including the following: at cell membranes, where lithium passes readily through sodium channels and, at high concentrations, blocks potassium channels; at cellular binding sites sensitive to changes in cation concentration; at the level of cellular proteins sensitive to usual cation concentrations; and at cellular carrier-binding and transport sites for monovalent and divalent cations.

Lithium also interacts with a number of cyclic adenosine monophosphate (AMP) second-messenger cellular processes, including those regulated by polypeptide hormones. By inhibiting adenylate cyclase, lithium reduces intracellular concentrations of cyclic AMP. To a lesser extent, lithium also reduces plasma concentrations of cyclic guanosine monophosphate (cGMP).

■ **Nervous System Effects** Lithium has antimanic and antidepressant effects. Because of the complexity of the CNS, the exact mechanism(s) of these effects is unknown. Univalent and divalent cations appear to be critical to the synthesis, storage, release, and reuptake of central monoamine neurotransmitters, including indoleamines (e.g., serotonin) and catecholamines. These neurotransmitters appear to be involved in the pathogenesis of mania and depression.

Evidence suggests that dopamine and norepinephrine may be involved in the pathogenesis of mania. In animals, brain tissue lithium concentrations of 1–10 mEq/L inhibit depolarization-provoked and calcium-dependent release of norepinephrine, dopamine, and serotonin from nerve terminals and synapses. Lithium only minimally affects catecholamine-sensitive adenylate cyclase activity or the binding of ligands to adrenergic receptors in the CNS. Turnover of norepinephrine in the CNS is initially increased with lithium therapy, but the increased turnover does not persist with prolonged administration. Lithium may block the development of supersensitive dopamine receptors in the CNS of manic patients. Lithium blocks some of the behavioral manifestations of mania (e.g., euphoria, hyperactivity, talkativeness, decrease in sleep, increase in libido) induced by drugs (e.g., amphetamines, cocaine) that produce functional increases in CNS dopamine concentrations.

Serotonin may play a role in the pathogenesis of depressive episodes. Serotonin is present in low concentrations in the CNS of some patients with bipolar affective disorders. Animal studies have shown that lithium increases the concentrations of serotonin metabolites (e.g., 5-hydroxyindoleacetic acid) and decreases hemispheric asymmetry of serotonin and other indoleamines. Lithium is thought to increase neuronal tryptophan uptake and serotonin synthesis by decreasing the affinity of tryptophan hydroxylase for tryptophan at low tryptophan concentrations.

In healthy individuals, lithium has been shown to increase lethargy and lassitude, decrease clearheadedness, and cause deficits in cognitive motor tasks. Lithium also produces small but consistent delays in sleep-wake circadian rhythm and decreases rapid eye movement (REM) sleep, increases delta-wave sleep, and normalizes the sleep of some depressed patients. Lithium may cause benign EEG changes, including diffuse slowing and increased amplitude of alpha waves with an increase in beta-wave activity as alpha rhythm diminishes. In some patients, lithium has produced changes similar to those induced by electroconvulsive therapy (ECT), including marked epileptiform discharge; these effects generally are associated with toxic serum lithium concentrations and/or other signs of lithium neurotoxicity, but also have occurred when lithium concentrations were within the therapeutic range.

■ **Hematologic Effects** Lithium produces neutrophilia and may also increase erythrocyte and platelet counts and decrease lymphocyte counts; however, the latter 3 effects appear to occur less consistently than neutrophilia.

The hematologic effects of lithium appear to be related to its effect on the pluripotent stem cell of the myeloid series. Although there probably are many modifiers of stem-cell production, the monocyte appears to be the key modifier involved in the effect of lithium on the stem cell. Lithium stimulates the production of colony-stimulating factor by monocytes. Colony-stimulating factor in turn stimulates production of neutrophils by the pluripotent stem cell and, to a lesser extent, production of erythrocytes, platelets, and macrophages. The increase in colony-stimulating factor is related to the action of lithium on cyclic nucleotides.

Lithium causes a true increase in neutrophil production and survival time and in granulocyte marrow reserve; neutrophilia does not result from demargination. Neutrophilia is seen generally within 3–7 days after lithium therapy is initiated and occurs at serum lithium concentrations of 0.5–1 mEq/L; the effect rapidly reverses (within 1–2 weeks) when the drug is discontinued. Data from one in vitro study indicate that the effect of lithium on neutrophil production is apparently transient when stem cells are severely depleted, since increases in neutrophil counts were not seen after 4 weeks. Although some studies indicate that lithium produces neutrophilia at the expense of neutrophil function, most studies have shown no effect of the drug on phagocytosis, chemotaxis, adherence, or bactericidal activity of neutrophils. Although not clearly established, lithium may enhance lymphocyte activity.

■ **Renal Effects** Lithium causes alterations in renal function and often produces a mild nephrogenic diabetes insipidus manifested as polyuria. The drug decreases renal-concentrating ability and water reabsorption and initially increases sodium and potassium excretion. Some of these effects are overcome by counteracting physiologic mechanisms, while others may persist. Glomerular filtration rate may be slightly decreased in patients receiving prolonged lithium therapy.

A decrease in renal-concentrating ability occurs in 30–50% of patients shortly after starting lithium therapy and persists in about 25% of treated patients after 1–2 years of lithium therapy. The decrease in renal-concentrating ability is usually reversible following discontinuance of the drug; however, in one study, this effect persisted in more than 50% of patients 1 year after discontinuing lithium therapy. Lithium-induced polyuria results from a major disturbance in the water conservation system and a minor disturbance in the thirst regulatory system. Although a central mechanism for lithium-induced diabetes insipidus has been described in one patient, most evidence indicates that the impairment of renal-concentrating ability is nephrogenic, since lithium inhibits vasopressin-induced adenylate cyclase activity. In most patients with lithium-induced nephrogenic diabetes insipidus, plasma vasopressin concentrations usually are elevated and urine osmolality is reduced. Lithium-induced diabetes insipidus has been inhibited by increased urinary potassium or hydrogen ion concentrations, and by thiazide diuretics, triamterene, or amiloride.

The effects of lithium on serum and urinary electrolytes are variable and time and dose related. Lithium initially increases sodium and potassium excretion and urine volume; after 2–3 days, excretion of these electrolytes is reduced, probably because of a feedback increase in aldosterone. Sodium and potassium excretion return to pretreatment levels within 1 week of continuous therapy. Overall, lithium generally does not affect sodium reabsorption in the ascending limb of the loop of Henle or in the distal renal tubule; free water clearance is unchanged even in the presence of lithium-induced polyuria. However, high serum concentrations of lithium have been associated with increased renin release and resultant inhibition of sodium reabsorption in the proximal and distal renal tubules and collecting ducts.

■ **Endocrine Effects** Lithium has various effects on the thyroid gland, but its principal effect is to block the release of thyroxine (T_4) and triiodothyronine (T_3) mediated by thyrotropin. This results in a decrease in circulating T_4 and T_3 concentrations and a feedback increase in serum thyrotropin concentration. Lithium also inhibits thyrotropin-stimulated adenylate cyclase activity and thyrotropin-induced release of thyroidal iodine 131, decreases intrathyroidal iodothyronine-iodotyrosine ratios, and inhibits colloid droplet formation.

Long-term lithium therapy may alter calcium, magnesium, and parathyroid hormone homeostasis; these alterations may cause a mild asymptomatic primary hyperparathyroidism. Lithium may cause slight increases in serum calcium (total), magnesium, and parathyroid hormone concentrations and a decrease in serum phosphate concentration. Lithium may also cause slight alterations in bone mineral metabolism.

Lithium has varying effects on carbohydrate metabolism. Increased and decreased glucose tolerance and decreased sensitivity to insulin have been observed. It is unclear whether these are direct effects of lithium or are related to changes in the course of the underlying psychiatric disorder.

In animals, lithium decreases hepatic cholesterol and fatty acid synthesis.

■ **Cardiovascular Effects** In patients with therapeutic serum lithium concentrations, reversible ECG T-wave depression occurs frequently. T-wave inversion occurs rarely. Resting or exercise-induced ST-segment abnormalities have not been observed. Arrhythmias have occurred rarely. (See Cautions: Cardiovascular Effects.)

The cardiac effects of lithium may result partly from displacement of potassium from intracellular myocardial sites by lithium; this displacement may result in a slow, partial depletion of intracellular potassium.

■ **GI Effects** Lithium reduces intestinal absorption of glucose and water, probably by incompletely substituting for sodium in a sodium-dependent transport mechanism at the intestinal mucosa. These actions may be responsible for the osmotic diarrhea and other adverse GI effects that frequently occur during initiation of lithium therapy.

Pharmacokinetics

■ **Absorption** Lithium is readily absorbed from the GI tract. Food does not appear to affect the bioavailability of lithium. Although lithium carbonate capsules show a slightly longer dissolution time than do tablets, differences in the disintegration and dissolution properties of various preparations do not appear to be clinically important. Conventional lithium carbonate capsules and tablets are 95–100% absorbed. Extended-release lithium carbonate tablets are 60–90% absorbed, and lithium citrate oral solutions are essentially 100% absorbed.

Absorption from conventional lithium carbonate tablets and capsules is usually complete within 1–6 hours with peak serum lithium concentrations usually occurring within 0.5–3 hours. Following oral administration of a single 300-mg dose of lithium carbonate to fasting adults, peak serum lithium concentrations of 0.4–0.5 and 0.4–0.9 mEq/L have been reported for conventional tablets and capsules, respectively. Absorption of lithium carbonate from extended-release tablets is both delayed and prolonged, with peak serum lithium concentrations occurring within 4–12 hours. Oral solutions of lithium citrate are the most rapidly absorbed, with peak serum lithium concentrations usually occurring within 15–60 minutes. Following oral administration to fasting patients of single doses of lithium citrate solution equivalent in lithium content to 600 mg and 0.9–1 g of lithium carbonate, peak serum lithium concentrations of about 0.7 and 1 mEq/L, respectively, have been reported.

During the first 6–10 hours after dosing, serum lithium concentrations fluctuate depending on the absorption of the drug and tissue distribution. Therefore, the 12-hour steady-state serum lithium concentration is used by most clinicians for monitoring serum concentrations; this concentration shows a high intraindividual (but not interindividual) reproducibility. Steady-state serum lithium concentrations of 0.4–1.3 mEq/L are considered necessary for therapeutic effect in the treatment of affective and schizoaffective disorders. At 12- to 16-hour steady-state serum concentrations of less than 0.4 mEq/L, about 60% of lithium-responsive patients with bipolar disorder relapse, compared with about 15% relapse at concentrations of 0.4–0.59 mEq/L and about 20% relapse at concentrations of 0.6–1 mEq/L. Steady-state serum lithium concentrations of 1–1.4 mEq/L usually are required for an acute antimanic effect. Onset of the acute antimanic effect of lithium usually occurs within 5–7 days; full therapeutic effect often requires 10–21 days. The likelihood of toxicity increases substantially at steady-state serum lithium concentrations of 1.5 mEq/L or greater, but some patients who are sensitive to the effects of lithium may develop toxicity at serum concentrations less than 1 mEq/L. Salivary lithium concentrations have been used by some clinicians to monitor lithium therapy, but most clinicians have not found this method practical. (See Pharmacokinetics: Distribution.)

■ **Distribution** Lithium is widely distributed into most body tissues and fluids. Lithium is initially distributed into extracellular fluid and then gradually accumulates in varying degrees in tissues. The drug is rapidly distributed into thyroid, bone, and brain tissue; concentrations in these tissues often are 50% greater than simultaneous serum concentrations. Lithium is distributed more slowly and less completely into heart, lung, kidney, and muscle; concentrations in these tissues approximate those in serum. Lithium concentrations in CSF and liver usually are 30–50% of simultaneous serum concentrations.

Lithium also distributes into saliva. The ratio of serum-to-mixed saliva lithium concentrations shows considerable interindividual variation, but once steady-state is achieved there is little intraindividual variation. Steady-state mixed saliva lithium concentrations are generally 2- to 3-fold greater than concurrent serum concentrations.

Lithium distributes into erythrocytes against an electrochemical potential gradient, drawn by an oppositely directed sodium ion gradient. The ratio of the lithium concentration in erythrocytes to that in serum shows wide interindividual variation but less intraindividual variation. Steady-state lithium concentrations in erythrocytes may range from 30–90% of concurrent serum concentrations but usually are 50% or less. The ratio has been shown to be slightly higher in women (especially during pregnancy), in patients with bipolar illness compared with patients with unipolar illness, and in patients with affective illness in remission compared with those in acute stages; however, the clinical importance of these findings is unknown. Distribution of lithium into erythrocytes also may depend partially on genetic factors.

Lithium initially distributes into an apparent volume that is about 25–40% of body weight, and later into a volume that is equal to that of total body water. Steady-state and initial apparent distribution volumes of about 0.7–1 L/kg and 0.3–0.4 L/kg, respectively, have been reported. Geriatric patients may have slightly smaller volumes of distribution, while individuals younger than 30 years of age may have slightly larger volumes of distribution. Lithium is not bound to plasma proteins.

Lithium freely crosses the placenta; maternal and fetal serum concentrations are approximately equal. The milk of nursing women contains lithium concentrations that are approximately 33–50% of those in serum.

■ **Elimination** Serum concentrations of lithium appear to decline in a biphasic manner. In patients with normal renal function, an initial half-life ($t_{1/2\alpha}$) of 0.8–1.2 hours and a terminal half-life ($t_{1/2\beta}$) of 20–27 hours have been observed following single-dose administration of lithium. Patients receiving lithium for more than 1 year had terminal half-lives of 2.4 days in one study. In geriatric patients and patients with impaired renal function, serum half-lives of 36 and 40–50 hours, respectively, have been reported.

Lithium is not metabolized; it is excreted almost entirely in the urine. About

80% of the lithium that is filtered by the renal glomeruli is reabsorbed in the proximal renal tubules. Thus, renal plasma clearance of lithium is about 20% of the glomerular filtration rate or about 20–40 mL/minute. Geriatric patients may have lower, and younger patients and pregnant women may have higher, renal clearances. Proximal tubular reabsorption of lithium occurs against electrical and concentration gradients that do not distinguish between sodium and lithium. Lithium clearance can be increased or decreased by as much as 30–50% by sodium loading or depletion, respectively. Sodium depletion generally has a greater effect than does sodium loading. Several drugs (e.g., thiazide diuretics, aminophylline, urea) have been shown to increase or decrease renal clearance of lithium. Polyuria and potassium chloride administration do not increase renal clearance of lithium. Beyond the proximal tubule, lithium reabsorption is minimal. For this reason, most diuretics do not enhance renal lithium clearance. (See Drug Interactions: Diuretics.)

Approximately 95–99% of a single dose of lithium is excreted in urine. Small amounts may be excreted in feces as unabsorbed drug or in sweat. In patients with normal renal function, about 30–70% of a single dose is excreted in urine within 6–12 hours and 50–80% within 24 hours; the remainder is excreted slowly over 10–14 days. Lithium is readily removed by hemodialysis with reported clearances of about 50–90 mL/minute; however, the amount of lithium removed during hemodialysis depends of several factors (e.g., type of coil used, dialysis flow-rate). The drug is removed less readily by peritoneal dialysis, with reported clearances of 13–15 mL/minute. Because of slow equilibration between intracellular and extracellular fluid compartments, rebound increases in serum lithium concentration frequently occur 5–8 hours after dialysis.

Chemistry and Stability

■ **Chemistry** Lithium salts are antimanic agents. Lithium is a monovalent cation belonging to the group of alkali metals, but it also shares some of the chemical properties of calcium and magnesium. Lithium is commercially available as the carbonate and citrate salts.

Lithium Carbonate Lithium carbonate occurs as a white, granular powder that has a slight saline taste. The drug is sparingly soluble in water, very slightly soluble in alcohol, and dissolves, with effervescence, in dilute mineral acids. Each gram of lithium carbonate contains 27 mEq of lithium.

Lithium Citrate Lithium citrate occurs as a tetrahydrate, white, somewhat deliquescent, crystalline powder that has a slight saline taste. The drug is very soluble in water and practically insoluble in alcohol. Each gram of anhydrous lithium citrate contains approximately 14.3 mEq of lithium. Lithium citrate oral solution is prepared from lithium citrate or lithium hydroxide to which an excess of citric acid has been added. The oral solution has a pH of 4–5.

■ **Stability** ***Lithium Carbonate*** Lithium carbonate conventional tablets, extended-release tablets, and capsules should be stored in well-closed containers at 15–30°C. When stored as directed, commercially available lithium carbonate extended-release tablets (Lithobid®) have an expiration date of 18 months following the date of manufacture.

Lithium Citrate Lithium citrate oral solution should be stored in tight containers at 15–30°C.

Preparations

Excipients in commercially available drug preparations may have clinically important effects in some individuals; consult specific product labeling for details.

Lithium Carbonate

Oral		
Capsules	150 mg (4.06 mEq of lithium)*	**Lithium Carbonate Capsules**
	300 mg (8.12 mEq of lithium)*	**Eskalith®**, GlaxoSmithKline **Lithium Carbonate Capsules**
	600 mg (16.24 mEq of lithium)*	**Lithium Carbonate Capsules,** Roxane
Tablets	300 mg (8.12 mEq of lithium)	**Lithium Carbonate Tablets** (scored)
Tablets, extended-release	450 mg (12.18 mEq of lithium)*	**Eskalith CR®** (scored), GlaxoSmithKline **Lithium Carbonate Extended-release Tablets**
Tablets, extended-release, film-coated	300 mg (8.12 mEq of lithium)*	**Lithobid® Slow-release,** JDS Pharma **Lithium Carbonate Extended-release Film-coated Tablets**

*available from one or more manufacturer, distributor, and/or repackager by generic (nonproprietary) name

Lithium Citrate

Oral		
Solution	8 mEq (of lithium) per 5 mL	**Lithium Citrate Syrup**

†Use is not currently included in the labeling approved by the US Food and Drug Administration

ANTIMIGRAINE AGENTS 28:32

CALCITONIN GENE-RELATED PEPTIDE (CGRP) ANTAGONISTS 28:32.12

Erenumab-aooe

■ Erenumab, a recombinant fully human immunoglobulin G_2 (IgG_2) monoclonal antibody that inhibits calcitonin gene-related peptide (CGRP) receptor function, is an antimigraine agent.

Uses

■ **Preventive Treatment of Migraine** Erenumab-aooe is used for the preventive treatment of migraine. In clinical studies, erenumab prophylaxis substantially reduced monthly migraine days and acute antimigraine agent-use days in patients with episodic or chronic migraine when compared with placebo.

Efficacy and safety of erenumab for the preventive treatment of migraine have been established in 3 randomized, double-blind, placebo-controlled, multicenter studies in adults with a history of migraine, with or without aura, according to the International Classification of Headache Disorders, Third Edition (ICHD-3) diagnostic criteria. Two studies included patients with episodic migraine (4–14 migraine days per month) and another study included patients with chronic migraine (at least 15 headache days per month with at least 8 migraine days per month). The median age of patients in these studies was 42–43 years; the majority of patients were female (83–85%) and white (89–94%). All of the studies excluded patients with medication overuse headache (study 3 excluded those with medication overuse headache caused by opiates only) and patients with recent (within 12 months) cardiovascular or cerebrovascular events (i.e., myocardial infarction, stroke, transient ischemic attacks, unstable angina, coronary artery bypass surgery or other revascularization procedures). In all 3 studies, patients received treatment with erenumab-aooe or placebo, and were permitted to use acute headache treatments including antimigraine agents (e.g., serotonin type 1 [$5\text{-}HT_1$]-selective receptor agonists [triptans], ergotamine derivatives) and nonsteroidal anti-inflammatory agents (NSAIAs) as needed during the study. Concomitant preventive antimigraine treatment was permitted in the episodic migraine studies (studies 1 and 2). The primary measure of efficacy in these studies was the change from baseline in mean monthly migraine days. Secondary end points included the proportion of patients achieving at least a 50% reduction in mean migraine days per month and the number of acute antimigraine agent-use days per month. In the episodic migraine studies (studies 1 and 2), a patient-reported outcome, the mean monthly Migraine Physical Function Impact Diary (MPFID) score, also was assessed. The MPFID records the impact of migraine on everyday activities and physical impairment using an electronic diary administered daily and is calculated as a monthly score averaged over 28 days; reductions from baseline in MPFID scores indicate improvement.

In study 1 (STRIVE), adults with a history of episodic migraine were randomized to receive erenumab-aooe 70 mg, erenumab-aooe 140 mg, or placebo subcutaneously every month for 6 months; primary and secondary efficacy end points were assessed as the change from baseline to months 4 through 6. A total of 955 patients underwent randomization and 90% completed the study. Erenumab-aooe treatment substantially reduced monthly migraine days compared with placebo; from a mean baseline of approximately 8 migraine days per month, treatment with erenumab-aooe 70 or 140 mg reduced monthly migraine days by 3.2 or 3.7 days, respectively, compared with a reduction of 1.8 days in patients receiving placebo. At least a 50% reduction in mean migraine days per month was achieved in a substantially greater proportion of patients receiving erenumab-aooe 70 or 140 mg (43.3 or 50%, respectively) compared with placebo (26.6%), and the mean number of acute antimigraine agent-use days per month was reduced by 1.1 or 1.6 days in patients receiving erenumab-aooe 70 or 140 mg, respectively, compared with 0.2 days in placebo recipients. In addition, mean monthly MPFID scores for everyday activity and physical impairment were substantially reduced in patients treated with erenumab-aooe 70 or 140 mg compared with placebo.

In study 2 (ARISE), adults with a history of episodic migraine were randomized to receive erenumab-aooe 70 mg or placebo subcutaneously every month for 3 months; primary and secondary end points were assessed at month 3 in this study. A total of 577 patients underwent randomization and 95% completed the study. From a mean baseline of approximately 8 migraine days per month, treatment with erenumab-aooe 70 mg reduced monthly migraine days by 2.9 days compared with a reduction of 1.8 days in patients receiving placebo. At least a 50% reduction in mean migraine days per month was achieved in a substantially greater proportion of patients receiving erenumab-aooe 70 mg compared with placebo (39.7 and 29.5%, respectively), and the mean number of acute antimigraine agent-use days per month was reduced by 1.2 days in patients receiving erenumab-aooe 70 mg compared with 0.6 days in placebo recipients. The mean monthly MPFID scores for everyday activity and physical impairment in patients receiving erenumab-aooe 70 mg did not differ substantially from those receiving placebo in this study.

In study 3, adults with a history of chronic migraine were randomized to receive erenumab-aooe 70 mg, erenumab-aooe 140 mg, or placebo subcutaneously every month for 3 months; primary and secondary efficacy end points were assessed at month 3. A total of 667 patients underwent randomization and 95% completed the study. From a mean baseline migraine frequency of approximately 18 migraine days per month, treatment with erenumab-aooe 70 or 140 mg reduced monthly migraine days by 6.6 days compared with a reduction of 4.2 days in patients receiving placebo. At least a 50% reduction in mean migraine days per month was achieved in a substantially greater proportion of patients receiving erenumab-aooe 70 or 140 mg (39.9 or 41.2%, respectively) compared with placebo (23.5%), and the mean number of acute antimigraine agent-use days per month was reduced by 3.5 or 4.1 days in patients receiving erenumab-aooe 70 or 140 mg, respectively, compared with 1.6 days in placebo recipients.

Post hoc analysis of studies 1 and 3 using weekly migraine days as a measure of efficacy indicate that a reduction in migraine days may be observed as early as the first week of treatment in patients with episodic or chronic migraine. In a long-term, open-label extension of a phase 2 study in patients with episodic migraine, 80% of enrolled patients completed 1 year of treatment with erenumab-aooe 70 mg once monthly; reductions from baseline in monthly migraine days and acute antimigraine agent-use days were sustained over at least 1 year of treatment with erenumab-aooe. Additional studies to evaluate long-term efficacy and safety of erenumab-aooe are needed.

The American Headache Society (AHS) states that erenumab and other calcitonin gene-related peptide (CGRP) antagonists offer a number of advantages over some oral migraine preventive therapies, including no need for dosage escalation, rapid onset of therapeutic activity (within days to weeks), demonstrated efficacy in patients with migraine after prior preventive treatments have failed as well as in those concurrently receiving oral preventive treatments, minimal risk of adverse drug interactions, and favorable overall tolerability profiles. However, because of the relatively high cost of CGRP antagonists compared with other preventive therapies, the AHS recommends that CGRP antagonists be considered for use only in patients with migraine who are unable to tolerate oral preventive therapies and/or who have an inadequate response to a 6-week trial of at least 2 oral preventive therapies (e.g., topiramate, valproate, β-adrenergic blocking agents, tricyclic antidepressants, selective serotonin- and norepinephrine-reuptake inhibitors). Like other commercially available antimigraine agents, erenumab is unlikely to make patients completely free of migraines, but substantial reductions in migraine frequency were observed in controlled clinical trials.

Dosage and Administration

■ **Administration** Erenumab-aooe is administered by subcutaneous injection only. Erenumab-aooe injection is commercially available in single-dose prefilled auto-injectors (i.e., injection pens) and single-dose prefilled syringes, which both contain 70 or 140 mg of the drug. Both the auto-injectors and syringes are intended for patient *self-administration.*

Prior to use, patients and/or caregivers should receive proper training on how to prepare and administer erenumab-aooe using the single-dose prefilled auto-injectors or single-dose prefilled syringes, including aseptic technique. The manufacturer's labeling should be consulted for detailed instructions regarding subcutaneous administration of the drug using the prefilled auto-injectors or syringes.

Erenumab-aooe should be administered subcutaneously into the abdomen, thigh, or outer area of the upper arm; injections within 2 inches of the navel should be avoided. The upper arm should only be used if someone other than the patient (e.g., caregiver, healthcare professional) is administering the injection. Injection into areas where the skin is tender, bruised, erythematous, or indurated should be avoided.

Some packaging components of erenumab-aooe contain dry natural rubber, which may cause allergic reactions in individuals sensitive to latex. (See Latex Sensitivity under Warnings/Precautions: Sensitivity Reactions, in Cautions and see also Advice to Patients.)

Prefilled auto-injectors and syringes of erenumab-aooe should be stored at 2–8°C in the original carton to protect from light until time of use. The auto-injectors and syringes may be stored at room temperature up to 25°C in the original carton for up to 7 days. If the auto-injectors or syringes are stored at room temperature for more than 7 days, they should be discarded. The prefilled auto-injectors and syringes should *not* be frozen or shaken.

Prior to subcutaneous administration, prefilled auto-injectors and syringes of erenumab-aooe should be removed from their carton and allowed to sit at room temperature for at least 30 minutes; exposure to direct sunlight should be avoided. The auto-injectors and syringes should not be warmed by using a heat source (e.g., microwave, hot water). Prior to administration, the solution should be inspected visually for particulate matter and discoloration; the prefilled auto-injector or syringe should not be used if the solution is cloudy or discolored or contains flakes or particles. The prefilled auto-injectors and syringes are intended for single-use only; any unused portions should be discarded.

■ **Dosage** For the preventive treatment of migraine in adults, the recommended dosage of erenumab-aooe is 70 mg once monthly by subcutaneous injection. A higher dosage of 140 mg subcutaneously once monthly may be considered in some patients. There does not appear to be a need for dosage titration with erenumab-aooe; therapy may be initiated with either the 70- or 140-mg dose.

If a dose of erenumab-aooe is missed, the missed dose should be administered as soon as possible. Subsequent doses may then be scheduled monthly from the date of the last administered dose.

The risk of adverse drug interactions with erenumab appears to be minimal. (See Drug Interactions.) When initiating therapy with erenumab or another calcitonin gene-related peptide (CGRP) antagonist in a patient who is already receiving a preventive treatment for migraine, the American Headache Society (AHS) recommends adding the CGRP antagonist to the existing antimigraine regimen and not making other changes until the clinical efficacy of the CGRP antagonist is determined.

Patients who respond to erenumab therapy usually respond following the first 3 monthly subcutaneous injections. Therefore, the AHS recommends assessing the clinical efficacy of erenumab after 3 months of treatment and continuing therapy only if treatment benefits have been observed with the drug by that time.

■ **Special Populations** The manufacturer makes no specific dosage recommendations for patients with hepatic or renal impairment. (See Specific Populations under Cautions: Warnings/Precautions.)

Dosage should be selected carefully in geriatric patients, usually starting at the low end of the dosage range. (See Geriatric Use under Warnings/Precautions: Specific Populations, in Cautions.)

Cautions

■ **Contraindications** Erenumab is contraindicated in patients with serious hypersensitivity to erenumab or to any excipient in the formulation. Reactions have included anaphylaxis and angioedema. (See Sensitivity Reactions under Cautions: Warnings/Precautions.)

■ **Warnings/Precautions** ***Sensitivity Reactions*** **Hypersensitivity Reactions.** Hypersensitivity reactions, including rash, angioedema, and anaphylaxis, have been reported in patients receiving erenumab during postmarketing experience. Most of the hypersensitivity reactions reported to date were not serious and occurred within hours of administration; however, some reactions occurred more than one week following administration.

If a serious or severe hypersensitivity reaction occurs, administration of erenumab should be discontinued and appropriate therapy should be initiated. (See Cautions: Contraindications and see also Advice to Patients.)

Latex Sensitivity. Some packaging components (e.g., needle shield within cap of the prefilled auto-injector, needle cap of the prefilled syringe) of erenumab-aooe injection contain dry natural rubber (a derivative of latex), which may cause allergic reactions in individuals sensitive to latex. Some individuals may be hypersensitive to natural latex proteins found in a wide range of medical devices, including such packaging components, and the level of sensitivity may vary depending on the form of natural rubber present; rarely, hypersensitivity reactions to natural latex proteins have been fatal.

Immunogenicity As with all therapeutic proteins, there is a potential for immunogenicity with erenumab therapy. In controlled clinical studies, anti-erenumab antibodies were detected in 6.2 or 2.6% of patients who received subcutaneous injections of the drug at dosages of 70 or 140 mg once monthly, respectively. Anti-erenumab antibodies with neutralizing activity were detected in 0.26% of patients who received the 70-mg dosage and in none of the patients who received the 140-mg dosage. Although available data do not demonstrate an effect of anti-erenumab antibody development on the efficacy or safety of erenumab, the data are too limited to make definitive conclusions.

Specific Populations **Pregnancy.** There are no adequate data to date on the developmental risk associated with the use of erenumab in pregnant women. Animal studies in pregnant monkeys administered erenumab-aooe subcutaneously at dosages resulting in systemic exposures approximately 20 times the exposure from the maximum recommended human dosage (140 mg monthly) throughout gestation have not revealed evidence of harm to the offspring.

The estimated rates of major birth defects and miscarriage among deliveries to women with migraine (2.2–2.9 and 17%, respectively) are similar to rates reported in women without migraine. Clinicians should be aware that published data suggest that women with migraine may be at increased risk of preeclampsia during pregnancy.

Lactation. It is not known whether erenumab is distributed into human milk. The effects of the drug on the breast-fed infant or on milk production also are unknown. The manufacturer states that the developmental and health benefits of breast-feeding should be considered along with the mother's clinical need for erenumab and any potential adverse effects on the breast-fed infant from the drug or from the underlying maternal condition.

Pediatric Use. The manufacturer states that the safety and efficacy of erenumab-aooe have not been established in pediatric patients younger than 18 years of age.

Pending further clinical experience with the use of CGRP antagonists in pediatric patients, the Pediatric and Adolescent Headache special interest group of the American Headache Society (AHS) recommends that CGRP antagonists (e.g., erenumab, fremanezumab, galcanezumab) should be considered mainly for use in postpubertal adolescents† with relatively frequent migraines (i.e., 8 or more headache days per month) who have moderate to severe disability associated with migraine (e.g., PedMIDAS score of 30 or more) and in whom at least 2 preventive therapies (including pharmacologic and non-pharmacologic therapies and dietary supplements) have failed. For younger pediatric patients† with severe chronic migraine that is refractory to multiple preventive therapies, these experts recommend that CGRP antagonists be considered only in carefully selected patients with close monitoring (e.g., pubertal status, bone health, linear growth, weight, body mass index [BMI], infectious complications).

Geriatric Use. Clinical trials of erenumab did not include sufficient numbers of patients 65 years of age or older to determine whether they respond differently than younger adults. The manufacturer recommends cautious dosage selection in geriatric patients, usually starting at the low end of the dosage range, taking into consideration the greater frequency of decreased hepatic, renal, and/or cardiac function and other concomitant disease and drug therapy in this population.

Hepatic Impairment. Formal pharmacokinetic studies of erenumab have not been conducted in patients with hepatic impairment. Hepatic impairment is not expected to affect pharmacokinetics of the drug.

Renal Impairment. Renal impairment is not expected to affect the pharmacokinetics of erenumab. Formal pharmacokinetic studies of the drug have not been conducted in patients with renal impairment. Analysis of population pharmacokinetic data indicates that the pharmacokinetics of erenumab are not influenced by mild or moderate renal impairment. Erenumab has not been evaluated in patients with severe renal impairment (estimated glomerular filtration rate [eGFR] less than 30 mL/minute per 1.73 m^2).

■ **Common Adverse Effects** Adverse effects reported in 3% or more of patients receiving erenumab-aooe for migraine in placebo-controlled clinical studies and more frequently than with placebo include injection site reactions (e.g., pain, erythema, pruritus), which were usually mild and transient in nature, and constipation.

Drug Interactions

The risk of clinically important drug interactions with erenumab appears to be minimal. Erenumab is not metabolized by cytochrome P-450 (CYP) isoenzymes. In addition, erenumab is unlikely to have an effect on drug-metabolizing enzymes or drug transporters. Therefore, pharmacokinetic interactions with drugs affecting or metabolized by CYP enzymes or substrates of various drug transport systems are not expected.

■ **Oral Contraceptives** Concomitant administration of erenumab-aooe (single 140-mg subcutaneous dose) and an oral contraceptive containing ethinyl estradiol and norgestimate in healthy females did not affect the pharmacokinetics of the oral contraceptive.

■ **Sumatriptan** In a double-blind, placebo-controlled study, concomitant administration of erenumab-aooe (single 140-mg IV† dose) and sumatriptan (two 6-mg subcutaneous doses given 1 hour apart) in healthy individuals did not affect the pharmacokinetics of sumatriptan. Concomitant administration of erenumab-aooe and sumatriptan also did not increase mean arterial pressure and resting blood pressure any more than sumatriptan administered alone. In addition, administration of erenumab-aooe alone does not appear to affect resting blood pressure. Concomitant administration of erenumab-aooe and sumatriptan generally appears to be well tolerated.

Description

Erenumab is a fully human immunoglobulin G_2 (IgG_2) monoclonal antibody that binds to the calcitonin gene-related peptide (CGRP) receptor and antagonizes CGRP receptor function. The drug is produced using recombinant DNA technology in Chinese hamster ovary cells.

CGRP is a potent vasodilator and pain-signaling neuropeptide that has been associated with migraine pathophysiology. CGRP and its receptors are located at sites that are relevant to migraine development such as the trigeminal neurons and are also widely distributed throughout the CNS and peripheral nervous system as well as in non-neuronal tissues throughout the body.

Increased serum CGRP concentrations have been observed in individuals during acute migraine attacks (with or without aura) and IV infusion of CGRP has been shown to induce migraines in patients with a history of migraines. Erenumab potently and selectively binds to the extracellular binding site of the CGRP receptor thereby competitively blocking its interaction with CGRP. Because of its large molecular size, erenumab is unlikely to cross the blood-brain barrier and probably antagonizes CGRP receptor function peripherally rather than centrally within the nervous system.

Erenumab exhibits nonlinear pharmacokinetics due to binding to the CGRP receptor. However, at clinically relevant dosages (70–140 mg by subcutaneous injection once monthly), pharmacokinetics of the drug are predominantly linear because of saturation of binding to the CGRP receptor. Following a single subcutaneous dose of 70 or 140 mg in healthy adults, peak serum erenumab concentrations are attained in approximately 6 days. Following once-monthly subcutaneous administration of erenumab-aooe in migraine patients, steady-state trough serum concentrations of the drug are approached in 3 months; systemic accumulation of the drug is less than twofold. The estimated absolute bioavailability following a single subcutaneous dose of 70 or 140 mg is 82%. Antimigraine effects of erenumab usually are evident following 1–3 monthly subcutaneous injections of the drug in responding patients. At low concentrations, erenumab is predominantly eliminated through saturable binding to the CGRP receptor while at higher concentrations, elimination of the drug is principally through a nonspecific, nonsaturable proteolytic pathway. The effective half-life of erenumab-aooe is 28 days.

The pharmacokinetics of erenumab-aooe are not affected by age, sex, race, or subtypes of migraine spectrum (e.g., episodic or chronic migraine).

Advice to Patients

Importance of advising patients to read the manufacturer's patient information and instructions for use.

Importance of providing guidance to patients and/or caregivers on proper subcutaneous administration of erenumab-aooe, including the use of aseptic technique, and use of the single-dose prefilled auto-injectors or syringes. Importance of instructing patients and/or caregivers to read and follow the instructions for use each time they use erenumab-aooe.

If a dose of erenumab-aooe is missed, the missed dose should be administered as soon as possible. Subsequent doses may then be scheduled monthly from the date of the last administered dose.

Some packaging components of erenumab-aooe (e.g., needle shield within cap of the prefilled auto-injector; needle cap of the prefilled syringe) contain dry natural rubber (a derivative of latex), which may cause allergic reactions in individuals sensitive to latex. Importance of alerting clinician if allergy to rubber or latex exists.

Importance of advising patients to seek immediate medical attention if they experience any symptoms of serious or severe hypersensitivity reactions.

Importance of informing clinicians of existing or contemplated concomitant therapy, including prescription and OTC drugs and dietary or herbal supplements, as well as any concomitant illnesses.

Importance of women informing clinicians if they are or plan to become pregnant or plan to breast-feed. (See Pregnancy under Warnings/Precautions: Specific Populations, in Cautions.)

Importance of informing patients of other important precautionary information. (See Cautions.)

Overview® (see Users Guide). For additional information on this drug until a more detailed monograph is developed and published, the manufacturer's labeling should be consulted. It is *essential* that the manufacturer's labeling be consulted for more detailed information on usual cautions, precautions, contraindications, potential drug interactions, laboratory test interferences, and acute toxicity.

Preparations

Excipients in commercially available drug preparations may have clinically important effects in some individuals; consult specific product labeling for details.

Erenumab-aooe

Parenteral

Injection, for subcutaneous use only	70 mg/1 mL	**Aimovig®** (available as single-dose prefilled auto-injectors [SureClick®] and single-dose prefilled syringes), Amgen(comarketed with Novartis)
	140 mg/1 mL	**Aimovig®** (available as single-dose prefilled auto-injectors [SureClick®] and single-dose prefilled syringes), Amgen(comarketed with Novartis)

†Use is not currently included in the labeling approved by the US Food and Drug Administration

Fremanezumab-vfrm

■ Fremanezumab, a recombinant fully humanized immunoglobulin G_{2a} (IgG_{2a}) monoclonal antibody that inhibits calcitonin gene-related peptide (CGRP) receptor function, is an antimigraine agent.

Uses

■ **Preventive Treatment of Migraine** Fremanezumab-vfrm is used for the preventive treatment of migraine. In clinical studies, fremanezumab prophylaxis substantially reduced the monthly average number of migraine or headache days and acute antimigraine agent- or headache medication-use days in patients with episodic or chronic migraine compared with placebo.

Efficacy and safety of fremanezumab for the preventive treatment of migraine have been established in 2 randomized, double-blind, placebo-controlled, multicenter studies (studies 1 and 2) in adults with a history of migraine according to the International Classification of Headache Disorders, third edition, beta version (ICHD-3 beta) diagnostic criteria. Study 1 included patients with episodic migraine (fewer than 15 headache days per month with at least 4 days fulfilling ICHD-3 beta criteria for migraine with or without aura, probable migraine, or use of selective serotonin type 1 [5-hydroxytryptamine type 1; 5-HT_1] receptor agonists [triptans] or ergotamine derivatives) and study 2 included patients with chronic migraine (at least 15 headache days per month with at least 8 days fulfilling ICHD-3 beta criteria for migraine with or without aura or use of triptans or ergotamine derivatives).

Patients in both clinical studies received treatment with fremanezumab or placebo; concomitant use of a single preventive antimigraine agent (e.g., β-adrenergic blocking agents, tricyclic antidepressants, anticonvulsants) was permitted in a subset of 21% of patients in both studies. In addition, patients were allowed to use acute antimigraine agents and headache medication during both studies. The median age of patients in these studies was 41–43 years; the majority of patients were female (85–88%) and Caucasian (77–84%). The studies excluded patients with a history of clinically important cardiovascular disease, vascular ischemia, or thromboembolic events.

In study 1, patients with a history of episodic migraine were randomized to receive subcutaneous injections of fremanezumab-vfrm 225 mg once monthly, a single fremanezumab-vfrm 675-mg dose (to represent an intended quarterly, or every 3 month, dose), or placebo once monthly for 3 months. The primary efficacy end point was the mean change from baseline in the monthly average number of migraine days over the 3-month treatment period after the first dose. Secondary end points included the proportion of patients achieving at least a 50% reduction in the monthly average number of migraine days over the 3-month treatment period, the mean change from baseline in the monthly average number of acute headache medication-use days over the 3-month period, and the mean change from baseline in the number of migraine days during the first month of treatment. A total of 875 patients underwent randomization and 791 (90%) of those patients completed the study.

Results of study 1 showed that fremanezumab treatment substantially reduced monthly migraine days compared with placebo; from a mean baseline of approximately 9 migraine days per month, treatment with fremanezumab-vfrm 225 mg monthly or 675 mg quarterly reduced monthly migraine days by 3.7 or 3.4 days, respectively, compared with a reduction of 2.2 days with placebo. Treatment benefit with both dosages of fremanezumab-vfrm was observed by the first month of treatment and continued throughout the 3-month treatment period. At least a 50% reduction in the monthly average number of migraine days was achieved in a substantially greater proportion of patients receiving fremanezumab-vfrm 225 mg monthly or 675 mg quarterly (47.7 or 44.4%, respectively) compared with those receiving placebo (27.9%), and the mean number of acute headache medication-use days per month was reduced by 3 or 2.9 days in patients who received fremanezumab-vfrm 225 mg monthly or 675 mg quarterly, respectively, compared with 1.6 days in placebo recipients.

In study 2, 1130 patients with a history of chronic migraine were randomized to receive subcutaneous injections of fremanezumab-vfrm 225 mg once monthly (with an initial 675-mg loading dose), a single fremanezumab-vfrm 675-mg dose (to represent an intended quarterly, or every 3 month, dose), or placebo once monthly for 3 months. The primary efficacy end point was the mean change from baseline in the monthly average number of headache days of at least moderate severity over the 3-month treatment period. Secondary end points included the mean change from baseline in the monthly average number of migraine days over the 3-month treatment period, the proportion of patients achieving at least a 50% reduction in the monthly average number of headache days of at least moderate severity over the 3-month treatment period, the mean change from baseline in the monthly average number of acute headache medication-use days over 3 months, and the mean change from baseline in the number of headache days of at least moderate severity during the first month of treatment.

Results of study 2 showed that from a mean baseline frequency of approximately 13 headache days per month, treatment with fremanezumab-vfrm 225 mg monthly or 675 mg quarterly reduced the monthly average number of headache days of at least moderate severity by 4.6 or 4.3 days, respectively, compared with a reduction of 2.5 days with placebo. Treatment benefit with both dosages of fremanezumab-vfrm was observed by the first month of treatment and continued throughout the 3-month treatment period. In addition, monthly migraine days were reduced by approximately 5 days in patients receiving either dosage of fremanezumab-vfrm compared with 3.2 days in patients receiving placebo. At least a 50% reduction in monthly average number of headache days of at least moderate severity was achieved in a substantially greater proportion of patients receiving fremanezumab-vfrm 225 mg monthly or 675 mg quarterly (40.8 or 37.6%, respectively) compared with those receiving placebo (18.1%), and the mean number of acute headache medication-use days per month was reduced by 4.2 or 3.7 days in patients who received fremanezumab-vfrm 225 mg monthly or 675 mg quarterly, respectively, compared with 1.9 days in placebo recipients.

The American Headache Society (AHS) states that fremanezumab and other calcitonin gene-related peptide (CGRP) antagonists offer a number of advantages over some oral migraine preventive therapies, including no need for dosage escalation, rapid onset of therapeutic activity (within days to weeks), demonstrated efficacy in patients with migraine in whom prior preventive treatments have failed as well as in those concurrently receiving oral preventive treatments, minimal risk of adverse drug interactions, and favorable overall tolerability profiles. However, because of the relatively high cost of CGRP antagonists compared with other preventive therapies, the AHS recommends that CGRP antagonists be considered for use only in patients with migraine who are unable to tolerate oral preventive therapies and/or who have had an inadequate response to a 6-week trial of at least 2 oral preventive therapies (e.g., topiramate, valproate, β-adrenergic blocking agents, tricyclic antidepressants, selective serotonin- and norepinephrine-reuptake inhibitors). Like other commercially available antimigraine agents, fremanezumab is unlikely to make patients completely free of migraines, but substantial reductions in migraine frequency were observed in controlled clinical trials.

Dosage and Administration

■ Administration Fremanezumab-vfrm is administered by subcutaneous injection only. Fremanezumab-vfrm injection is commercially available in single-use prefilled syringes containing 225 mg of the drug in 1.5 mL of solution. The drug may be administered by healthcare professionals or caregivers and/or *self-administered.*

Prior to use, patients and/or caregivers should receive proper training on how to prepare and administer fremanezumab-vfrm using the single-use prefilled syringes, including aseptic technique. The manufacturer's labeling should be consulted for detailed instructions regarding subcutaneous administration of the drug using the prefilled syringes.

Fremanezumab-vfrm should be administered subcutaneously into the abdomen, anterior thigh, or back of the upper arm; injections within 2 inches of the navel, knee, or groin should be avoided. Multiple injections of the drug (i.e., to administer a 675-mg dose) may be administered at the same body site, but not at the exact location of the previous injection. Fremanezumab-vfrm should not be administered concomitantly with other parenteral drugs at the same injection site. Injection into areas where the skin is tender, bruised, erythematous, or indurated should be avoided.

Prefilled syringes of fremanezumab-vfrm should be stored at 2–8°C in the original outer carton to protect from light. The syringes may be stored at room temperature up to 25°C in the original carton for up to 24 hours; the syringes should not be returned to the refrigerator after storage at room temperature. If the syringes are stored at room temperature for 24 hours or more, they should be discarded. The prefilled syringes should *not* be frozen, shaken, or exposed to extreme heat or direct sunlight.

Prior to subcutaneous administration, prefilled syringes of fremanezumab-vfrm should be removed from the refrigerator and allowed to sit at room temperature for 30 minutes protected from direct sunlight. The syringes should not be warmed by using a heat source (e.g., microwave, hot water). Prior to administration, the solution should be inspected visually for particulate matter and discoloration; the syringe should not be used if the solution is cloudy or discolored or contains particles. The prefilled syringes are intended for single use only and should be discarded after use.

■ Dosage For the preventive treatment of migraine in adults, the recommended dosage of fremanezumab-vfrm is 225 mg once monthly *or* 675 mg every 3 months (quarterly) by subcutaneous injection. The 675-mg dose should be administered as 3 consecutive subcutaneous injections of 225 mg each. (See Dosage and Administration: Administration.) There does not appear to be a need for dosage titration with fremanezumab-vfrm; therapy may be initiated with either the 225-mg monthly dose or the 675-mg quarterly dose.

When switching dosage regimens, the first dose of the new dosage regimen should be administered on the next scheduled date of administration.

If a dose of fremanezumab-vfrm is missed, the missed dose should be administered as soon as possible. Subsequent doses may then be scheduled monthly (225-mg doses) or every 3 months (675-mg doses) from the date of the last administered dose.

The risk of adverse drug interactions with fremanezumab appears to be minimal. (See Drug Interactions.) When initiating therapy with fremanezumab or another calcitonin gene-related peptide (CGRP) antagonist in a patient who is already receiving a preventive treatment for migraine, the American Headache Society (AHS) recommends adding the CGRP antagonist to the existing antimigraine regimen and not making other changes until the clinical efficacy of the CGRP antagonist is determined.

Patients who respond to CGRP antagonist therapy usually respond following the first 3 subcutaneous injections. Therefore, the AHS recommends assessing the clinical efficacy of fremanezumab after 3 months (if using the monthly dosage regimen) or 6 months (if using the quarterly dosage regimen) of treatment and continuing therapy only if treatment benefits have been observed with the drug by that time.

■ Special Populations The manufacturer makes no specific dosage recommendations for patients with hepatic or renal impairment. (See Specific Populations under Cautions: Warnings/Precautions.)

The manufacturer makes no specific dosage recommendations for geriatric patients.

The manufacturer states that no dosage adjustments are necessary based on age, race, sex, body weight, or body mass index (BMI).

Cautions

■ Contraindications Fremanezumab is contraindicated in patients with serious hypersensitivity to fremanezumab or to any excipients in the formulation. (See Sensitivity Reactions under Cautions: Warnings/Precautions.)

■ Warnings/Precautions ***Sensitivity Reactions*** Hypersensitivity reactions, including rash, pruritus, drug hypersensitivity, and urticaria, have been reported in patients receiving fremanezumab in clinical trials. Most of the hypersensitivity reactions were mild to moderate in severity, but some led to discontinuance of the drug or required corticosteroid therapy. Most reactions occurred within hours to one month after administration.

If a hypersensitivity reaction occurs during fremanezumab therapy, discontinuance of the drug should be considered and appropriate medical therapy initiated. (See Cautions: Contraindications and see also Advice to Patients.)

The manufacturer states that the prefilled syringe cap for fremanezumab-vfrm injection is *not* made with natural rubber latex.

Immunogenicity As with all therapeutic proteins, there is a potential for immunogenicity with fremanezumab therapy. In placebo-controlled clinical studies of 3 months' duration, anti-fremanezumab antibodies were detected in 6 of 1701 patients (0.4%) who received the drug. Anti-fremanezumab antibodies with neutralizing activity were detected in one of these patients at day 84 of treatment. In an ongoing long-term, open-label study, anti-fremanezumab antibodies were detected in 30 of 1888 patients (1.6%); over half of these patients (about 57%) had anti-fremanezumab antibodies with neutralizing activity. Although available data do not demonstrate an effect of anti-fremanezumab antibody development on the efficacy or safety of fremanezumab, the data currently are too limited to make definitive conclusions.

Specific Populations **Pregnancy.** There are no adequate data to date on the developmental risk associated with the use of fremanezumab in pregnant women. The manufacturer states that the long elimination half-life of fremanezumab should be considered if the drug is used in women who are pregnant or plan to become pregnant during therapy. (See Description.) Animal studies in pregnant rats and rabbits administered fremanezumab subcutaneously at dosages resulting in systemic exposures up to approximately 2–3 times the exposure from the maximum recommended human dosage (675 mg) did not adversely affect the development of the offspring.

The estimated rates of major birth defects and miscarriage among deliveries to women with migraine (2.2–2.9 and 17%, respectively) are similar to rates reported in women without migraine. Clinicians should be aware that published data suggest that women with migraine may be at increased risk of preeclampsia during pregnancy.

Lactation. It is not known whether fremanezumab is distributed into human milk. The effects of the drug on breast-fed infants and on milk production also are unknown. The manufacturer states that the developmental and health benefits of breast-feeding should be considered along with the mother's clinical need for fremanezumab and any potential adverse effects on the breast-fed infant from the drug or from the underlying maternal condition.

Pediatric Use. The manufacturer states that the safety and efficacy of fremanezumab have not been established in pediatric patients.

Pending further clinical experience with the use of calcitonin gene-related peptide (CGRP) antagonists in pediatric patients, the Pediatric and Adolescent Headache special interest group of the American Headache Society (AHS) recommends that CGRP antagonists (e.g., erenumab, fremanezumab, galcanezumab) should be considered mainly for use in postpubertal adolescents† with relatively frequent migraines (i.e., 8 or more headache days per month) who have moderate to severe disability associated with migraine (e.g., PedMIDAS score of 30 or more) and in whom at least 2 preventive therapies (including pharmacologic and nonpharmacologic therapies and dietary supplements) have failed. For younger pediatric patients† with severe chronic migraine that is refractory to multiple preventive therapies, these experts recommend that CGRP antagonists be considered only in carefully selected patients with close monitoring (e.g., pubertal status, bone health, linear growth, weight, body mass index [BMI], infectious complications).

Geriatric Use. Clinical trials of fremanezumab did not include sufficient numbers of patients 65 years of age or older to determine whether they respond differently than younger adults.

Hepatic Impairment. Hepatic impairment is not expected to substantially affect the pharmacokinetics of fremanezumab. Formal pharmacokinetic studies of fremanezumab have not been conducted in patients with hepatic impairment. Population pharmacokinetic analysis from clinical studies with the drug did not reveal a difference in the pharmacokinetics of fremanezumab in patients with mild hepatic impairment compared with those with normal hepatic function. Only 4 patients with moderate hepatic impairment and no patients with severe hepatic impairment were enrolled in clinical studies with the drug.

Renal Impairment. Because of its large molecular size, renal excretion of intact fremanezumab is unlikely. Therefore, renal impairment is not expected to substantially affect pharmacokinetics of the drug. Formal pharmacokinetic studies of fremanezumab have not been conducted in patients with renal impairment.

■ **Common Adverse Effects** Adverse effects reported in 5% or more of patients receiving fremanezumab-vfrm for preventive treatment of migraine in clinical studies and more frequently than with placebo include injection site reactions (e.g., pain, induration, erythema), most of which were mild to moderate in severity and self-limited.

Drug Interactions

Formal drug interaction studies with fremanezumab have not been conducted to date. The risk of clinically important drug interactions with the drug appears to be minimal. Fremanezumab is not metabolized by cytochrome P-450 (CYP) enzymes. In addition, fremanezumab, a monoclonal antibody, is unlikely to affect drug-metabolizing enzymes or drug transport systems. Therefore, pharmacokinetic interactions with drugs affecting or metabolized by CYP enzymes or substrates of various drug transport systems are not expected.

■ **Antimigraine Agents** Population pharmacokinetic modeling suggests that other antimigraine agents, including acute (i.e., analgesics, selective serotonin type 1 [5-hydroxytryptamine type 1; 5-HT_1] receptor agonists [triptans], ergotamine derivatives) and preventive agents, do not affect systemic exposure of fremanezumab.

In post hoc analyses from 2 controlled studies evaluating fremanezumab as add-on preventive therapy in patients receiving stable dosages of preventive migraine treatments (e.g., β-adrenergic blocking agents, calcium-channel blocking agents, gabapentin, topiramate, valproate, tricyclic and other antidepressants), fremanezumab did not appear to adversely interact with other migraine preventive treatments and could be initiated without requiring other migraine preventive treatments to be gradually titrated then discontinued first. (See Dosage and Administration: Dosage.)

Description

Fremanezumab is a fully humanized immunoglobulin G_{2a} (IgG_{2a}) delta/kappa monoclonal antibody that binds to the calcitonin gene-related peptide (CGRP) ligand and blocks its binding with the CGRP receptor. The drug is produced using recombinant DNA technology in Chinese hamster ovary cells.

CGRP is a potent vasodilator and pain-signaling neuropeptide that has been associated with migraine pathophysiology. CGRP and its receptors are located at sites that are relevant to migraine development such as the trigeminal neurons and are also widely distributed throughout the central and peripheral nervous systems as well as in nonneuronal tissues throughout the body.

Increased serum CGRP concentrations have been observed in individuals during acute migraine attacks (with or without aura) and IV infusion of CGRP has been shown to induce migraines in patients with a history of migraines. Fremanezumab binds to the CGRP ligand and blocks its interaction with the CGRP receptor. Because of its large molecular size, fremanezumab is unlikely to cross the blood-brain barrier and probably antagonizes CGRP function peripherally rather than centrally within the nervous system.

The pharmacokinetics of fremanezumab in patients with migraine are similar to those reported in healthy individuals. Following single subcutaneous doses of 225, 675, or 900 mg in healthy adults, median time to peak plasma concentrations is 5–7 days. Steady-state concentrations are achieved in approximately 6 months following multiple doses; median systemic accumulation is approximately 2.3- or 1.2-fold following 225-mg once-monthly or 675-mg quarterly dosage regimens, respectively. Pharmacokinetics of fremanezumab are dose proportional over a subcutaneous dose range of 225–900 mg. Antimigraine effects of CGRP antagonists, including fremanezumab, usually are evident following 1–3 monthly subcutaneous injections or 1–2 quarterly subcutaneous injections in responding patients. Similar to other monoclonal antibodies, metabolism of fremanezumab is mediated by proteolytic degradation into small peptides and amino acids. The elimination half-life of the drug is approximately 31 days.

The pharmacokinetics of fremanezumab-vfrm are not substantially affected by age, sex, race (including between Japanese and Caucasian healthy individuals), body weight, or body mass index (BMI).

Advice to Patients

Importance of advising patients and/or caregivers to read the manufacturer's patient information and to read and follow the instructions for use each time they use fremanezumab.

Importance of providing guidance to patients and/or caregivers on proper subcutaneous administration of fremanezumab-vfrm, including the use of aseptic technique and how to use the single-dose prefilled syringes.

Importance of informing patients receiving the 675-mg dose that the dose should be administered as 3 consecutive injections of 225 mg each.

If a dose of fremanezumab-vfrm is missed, the missed dose should be administered as soon as possible. Subsequent doses may then be scheduled monthly or quarterly from the date of the last administered dose.

Importance of informing patients of possible signs and symptoms of hypersensitivity reactions (e.g., rash, pruritus, urticaria), which can occur within hours and up to 1 month after administration of fremanezumab. Patients should immediately contact their healthcare provider if signs or symptoms of a hypersensitivity reaction occur.

Importance of informing clinicians of existing or contemplated concomitant therapy, including prescription and OTC drugs and dietary or herbal supplements, as well as any concomitant illnesses.

Importance of women informing clinicians if they are or plan to become pregnant or plan to breast-feed. (See Pregnancy under Warnings/Precautions: Specific Populations, in Cautions.)

Importance of informing patients of other important precautionary information. (See Cautions.)

Overview® (see Users Guide). For additional information on this drug until a more detailed monograph is developed and published, the manufacturer's labeling should be consulted. It is *essential* that the manufacturer's labeling be consulted for more detailed information on usual cautions, precautions, contraindications, potential drug interactions, laboratory test interferences, and acute toxicity.

Preparations

Excipients in commercially available drug preparations may have clinically important effects in some individuals; consult specific product labeling for details.

Fremanezumab-vfrm

Parenteral

Injection, for subcutaneous use only	225 mg/1.5 mL	**Ajovy®** (available as single-dose prefilled syringes), Teva

†Use is not currently included in the labeling approved by the US Food and Drug Administration

Galcanezumab-gnlm

■ Galcanezumab-gnlm, a recombinant humanized immunoglobulin G_4 (IgG_4) monoclonal antibody that inhibits calcitonin gene-related peptide (CGRP) function, is an antimigraine agent.

Uses

■ Preventive Treatment of Migraine Galcanezumab-gnlm is used for the preventive treatment of migraine. In clinical studies, galcanezumab prophylaxis substantially reduced monthly migraine days in patients with episodic or chronic migraine and reduced acute antimigraine agent-use days in patients with episodic migraine when compared with placebo.

Efficacy and safety of galcanezumab for the preventive treatment of migraine have been established in 3 randomized, double-blind, placebo-controlled, multicenter studies in adults with a history of migraine, with or without aura, according to the International Classification of Headache Disorders, third edition, beta version (ICHD-3 beta) diagnostic criteria. Two studies of 6 months' duration included adults with episodic migraine (4–14 migraine days per month) and another study of 3 months' duration included adults with chronic migraine (at least 15 headache days per month with at least 8 migraine days per month). In all 3 studies, patients received treatment with galcanezumab-gnlm 120 mg (with an initial 240-mg loading dose), galcanezumab-gnlm 240 mg, or placebo given subcutaneously every month, and were permitted to use acute headache treatments, including antimigraine agents (e.g., selective serotonin type 1 [5-hydroxytryptamine type 1; 5-HT_1] receptor agonists [triptans], ergotamine derivatives), nonsteroidal anti-inflammatory agents (NSAIAs), and acetaminophen, as needed during the studies. The studies excluded patients who failed to respond to adequate trials of 3 or more migraine preventive treatments, patients with ECG abnormalities indicating risk for acute cardiovascular events, and those with a recent history (within 6 months) of cardiovascular or cerebrovascular events (i.e., stroke, myocardial infarction [MI], unstable angina, percutaneous coronary intervention, coronary artery bypass grafting, deep-vein thrombosis [DVT], pulmonary embolism). The episodic migraine studies (EVOLVE-1 and -2) also excluded patients with medication overuse headache. Patients in EVOLVE-1 and -2 were not permitted to receive other preventive migraine treatments concurrently or within 30 days of the study baseline period, while concomitant use of stable dosages of either propranolol or topiramate as preventive antimigraine therapy was permitted in the chronic migraine study (REGAIN).

The primary measure of efficacy in these studies was the mean change from baseline in monthly migraine days over the 6-month treatment period. Secondary end points included response rates (i.e., the proportion of patients achieving at least 50, 75, and 100% reductions in mean migraine days per month) and the mean change from baseline in the number of migraine days per month on which any acute headache medication was taken. A patient-reported outcome, the Migraine-Specific Quality of Life Questionnaire (MSQ) Role Function-Restrictive domain score that indicates the impact of migraine on daily activities, also was assessed. Higher MSQ scores (scaled from 0 to 100) indicate less impact of migraine on daily activities.

In the episodic migraine studies (EVOLVE-1 and -2), a total of 1773 adults with episodic migraine underwent randomization and 1448 (82%) of the adults completed the 6-month, double-blind treatment phase. From a mean baseline of approximately 9 migraine days per month in these studies, monthly migraine days were reduced by 4.7 and 4.3 days, respectively, in patients who received galcanezumab 120 mg once monthly compared with a reduction of 2.8 and 2.3 days, respectively, in patients receiving placebo. Reductions in monthly migraine days were evident within the first month of galcanezumab treatment and were sustained throughout 6 months of treatment. Substantially greater proportions of patients receiving galcanezumab-gnlm 120 mg once monthly achieved at least 50, 75, or 100% reductions in mean migraine days per month compared with those receiving placebo, and the mean number of migraine days per month that acute headache medication was taken was reduced by 4 and 3.7 days in EVOLVE-1 and -2, respectively, in patients receiving galcanezumab compared with 2.2 and 1.9 days, respectively, in placebo recipients. In addition, the MSQ Role Function-Restrictive domain scores were substantially improved in patients treated with galcanezumab-gnlm 120 mg once monthly compared with placebo. The 240-mg monthly dosage of galcanezumab-gnlm did not demonstrate additional clinical benefit compared with the 120-mg monthly dosage in these studies.

In the chronic migraine study (REGAIN), 1113 adults with chronic migraine underwent randomization and 1037 (93%) of the adults completed the 3-month, double-blind treatment phase. From a mean baseline migraine frequency of approximately 19 migraine days per month, treatment with galcanezumab-gnlm 120 mg once monthly reduced monthly migraine days by 4.8 compared with a reduction of 2.7 days in patients receiving placebo. Reductions in monthly migraine days were evident in the first month of treatment with galcanezumab and were sustained through 3 months of treatment. At least a 50% reduction in mean migraine days per month was achieved in a substantially greater proportion of patients receiving galcanezumab-gnlm 120 mg compared with placebo (28 versus 15%, respectively). Treatment with the 240-mg monthly dosage did not demonstrate additional benefit over the 120-mg monthly dosage.

Galcanezumab also was evaluated in a long-term, open-label, multicenter safety study in adults with migraine. A total of 270 patients with episodic or chronic migraine were enrolled (135 patients each received galcanezumab-gnlm 120 mg [with initial 240-mg loading dose] or 240 mg monthly by subcutaneous injection) and approximately 78% of those patients completed the 12-month treatment phase in the study. Although the primary objective of this study was to assess the long-term safety and tolerability of the drug, galcanezumab therapy was associated with reductions in monthly migraine days and acute antimigraine or headache agent-use days. Efficacy was observed as early as the first month of treatment and was sustained throughout the 12-month treatment period. This study demonstrated no substantial differences in efficacy between the 120- and 240-mg monthly dosages of the drug.

The American Headache Society (AHS) states that galcanezumab and other calcitonin gene-related peptide (CGRP) antagonists offer a number of advantages over some oral migraine preventive therapies, including no need for dosage escalation, rapid onset of therapeutic activity (within days to weeks), demonstrated efficacy in patients with migraine after prior preventive treatments have failed as well as in those concurrently receiving oral preventive treatments, minimal risk of adverse drug interactions, and favorable overall tolerability profiles. However, because of the relatively high cost of CGRP antagonists compared with other preventive therapies, the AHS recommends that CGRP antagonists be considered for use only in patients with migraine who are unable to tolerate oral preventive therapies and/or who have had an inadequate response to a 6-week trial of at least 2 oral preventive therapies (e.g., topiramate, valproate, β-adrenergic blocking agents, tricyclic antidepressants, selective serotonin- and norepinephrine-reuptake inhibitors). Like other commercially available antimigraine agents, galcanezumab is unlikely to make patients completely free of migraines, but substantial reductions in migraine frequency were observed in clinical trials.

■ Treatment of Episodic Cluster Headache Galcanezumab-gnlm is used for the treatment of episodic cluster headache. In the principal efficacy study, galcanezumab treatment substantially reduced weekly cluster headache attack frequency in patients with episodic cluster headache compared with placebo.

Cluster headache is a type of headache that produces extreme pain and is highly debilitating. The headaches usually occur in clusters, often at the same time of day (commonly in the overnight hours), and last for several weeks or months (i.e., cluster periods or bouts) separated by remission periods lasting months or years in patients with episodic cluster headache. In patients with chronic cluster headache, attacks occur for one year or longer without remission or with remission periods lasting less than 3 months. Cluster headache attacks are characterized by unilateral pain, which may be orbital, supraorbital, temporal, or in any combination of these areas; attacks usually last between 15 minutes and 3 hours and occur from once every day to up to 8 times daily. Cluster headache pain may be accompanied by a variety of clinical manifestations, which may include ipsilateral conjunctival injection or lacrimation, rhinorrhea and/or nasal congestion, miosis, ptosis and/or eyelid edema, forehead and facial sweating, and/or restlessness or agitation. Age of onset of cluster headache is usually 20–40 years, and the condition is 3 times more common in men than women. Diagnosis of cluster headache is often delayed in the US, and the incidence of suicidality in affected patients is substantial (occurring in 55% of patients).

Efficacy of galcanezumab for the treatment of episodic cluster headache has been established in a randomized, double-blind, placebo-controlled study of 8 weeks' duration in adults with episodic cluster headache according to the ICHD-3 beta diagnostic criteria. Patients enrolled in the study had a maximum of 8 cluster headache attacks each day, a minimum of 1 attack every other day, and at least 4 attacks during the prospective 7-day baseline period. Patients were randomized to receive either once-monthly subcutaneous injections of galcanezumab-gnlm 300 mg or placebo, and were permitted to use certain acute/abortive cluster headache treatments during the study, including triptans, acetaminophen, NSAIAs, and oxygen. Patients receiving other treatments intended to reduce the frequency of cluster headache attacks, patients with medication overuse headache, and patients with ECG abnormalities consistent with an acute cardiovascular event or conduction delay or a recent history (within 6 months) of cardiovascular or cerebrovascular events (i.e., MI, unstable angina, percutaneous coronary intervention, coronary artery bypass grafting, DVT, pulmonary embolism) were excluded from the study. Patients with a history of stroke, intracranial or carotid aneurysm, intracranial hemorrhage, or vasospastic angina; clinical evidence of peripheral vascular disease; or Raynaud's disease also were excluded.

The primary efficacy end point in the study was the mean change from baseline in weekly cluster headache attack frequency from weeks 1 to 3, and a secondary end point was the proportion of patients who achieved a response (defined as a reduction from baseline of at least 50% in weekly cluster headache attack frequency) at week 3. Out of 106 patients who were randomized and treated, 90 patients completed the 8-week, double-blind phase of the study. During the 3-week period, patients taking galcanezumab experienced 8.7 fewer weekly cluster headache attacks than they did at baseline, compared with 5.2 fewer attacks for patients receiving placebo; 71.4% of patients taking galcanezumab were responders at week 3 compared with 52.6% of those receiving placebo. Although study enrollment was stopped before reaching the planned sample size due to the low number of patients entering an active cluster bout during the screening period, available data were sufficient for analysis of the primary and secondary end points. Larger and longer-term studies are needed to better determine the durability of response and safety profile of galcanezumab in patients with episodic cluster headache.

Dosage and Administration

■ **Administration** Galcanezumab-gnlm is administered by subcutaneous injection only. Galcanezumab-gnlm injection is commercially available in single-dose prefilled auto-injectors (i.e., injection pens), which contain 120 mg of the drug, and single-dose prefilled syringes, which contain either 100 or 120 mg of the drug. Both formulations of the drug are intended for patient *self-administration.*

Prior to use, patients and/or caregivers should receive proper training on how to prepare and administer galcanezumab-gnlm using the single-dose prefilled auto-injectors or syringes, including aseptic technique. The manufacturer's labeling should be consulted for detailed instructions regarding subcutaneous administration of the drug.

Galcanezumab-gnlm should be administered subcutaneously into the abdomen, anterior thigh, back of the upper arm, or buttocks; injections within 2 inches of the navel, knee, or groin should be avoided. The back of the upper arm or buttocks may be used if someone other than the patient is administering the injection (e.g., caregiver, healthcare professional). Multiple injections of the drug (i.e., the initial loading dose for preventive treatment of migraine consisting of 2 injections and the dose for treatment of episodic cluster headache consisting of 3 injections) may be administered at separate locations at the same body site. Injection into areas where the skin is tender, bruised, erythematous, or indurated should be avoided.

Prefilled auto-injectors and syringes of galcanezumab-gnlm should be stored at 2–8°C in the original carton to protect from light until time of use. These formulations of the drug may be stored at room temperature up to 30°C in the original carton for up to 7 days; they should not be returned to the refrigerator after storage at room temperature for longer than 1 hour. The prefilled auto-injectors and syringes should *not* be frozen or shaken. If the auto-injectors or syringes are stored at room temperature for more than 7 days or are frozen or shaken vigorously (i.e., shaking beyond the normal vibration, shaking, or bumping that occurs during typical transport activities), they should be discarded. If galcanezumab-gnlm prefilled auto-injectors or syringes are exposed to conditions outside of the recommended storage and handling conditions, the manufacturer may be able to provide further information regarding stability and product quality assessment; patients or healthcare professionals may contact the manufacturer by calling 800-545-5979.

Prior to subcutaneous administration, prefilled auto-injectors and syringes of galcanezumab-gnlm should be removed from their carton and allowed to sit at room temperature for 30 minutes; exposure to direct sunlight should be avoided. The auto-injectors and syringes should not be warmed by using a heat source (e.g., microwave, hot water). Prior to administration, the solution should be inspected visually for particulate matter and discoloration; the prefilled auto-injector or syringe should not be used if the solution is cloudy or discolored or contains particles. The prefilled auto-injectors and syringes are intended for single use only and should be discarded after use.

■ **Dosage** ***Preventive Treatment of Migraine*** For the preventive treatment of migraine in adults, therapy with galcanezumab-gnlm should be initiated with a one-time loading dose of 240 mg (administered as 2 consecutive subcutaneous injections of 120 mg each) followed by monthly doses of 120 mg by subcutaneous injection. In clinical studies, a higher dosage of galcanezumab-gnlm (240 mg once monthly) did not demonstrate additional clinical benefit over the recommended dosage (120 mg once monthly).

If a dose of galcanezumab is missed, the missed dose should be administered as soon as possible. Subsequent doses may then be scheduled monthly from the date of the last administered dose.

The risk of adverse drug interactions with galcanezumab appears to be minimal. (See Drug Interactions.) When initiating therapy with galcanezumab or another calcitonin gene-related peptide (CGRP) antagonist in a patient who is already receiving a preventive treatment for migraine, the American Headache Society (AHS) recommends adding the CGRP antagonist to the existing antimigraine regimen and not making other changes until the clinical efficacy of the CGRP antagonist is determined.

Patients who respond to CGRP antagonist therapy usually respond following the first 3 subcutaneous injections. Therefore, the AHS recommends assessing the clinical efficacy of galcanezumab after 3 months of treatment and continuing therapy only if treatment benefits have been observed with the drug by that time.

Treatment of Episodic Cluster Headache For the treatment of episodic cluster headache in adults, the recommended dosage of galcanezumab-gnlm is 300 mg (administered as 3 consecutive subcutaneous injections of 100 mg each) at the onset of the cluster period and then monthly until the end of the cluster period.

If a dose of galcanezumab is missed, the missed dose should be administered as soon as possible. Subsequent doses may then be scheduled monthly from the date of the last administered dose until the end of the cluster period.

■ **Special Populations** The manufacturer makes no specific dosage recommendations for geriatric patients or patients with hepatic or renal impairment. (See Specific Populations under Cautions: Warnings/Precautions.)

Cautions

■ **Contraindications** Galcanezumab is contraindicated in patients with serious hypersensitivity to the drug or to any of the excipients in the formulation. (See Sensitivity Reactions under Cautions: Warnings/Precautions.)

■ **Warnings/Precautions** ***Sensitivity Reactions*** Hypersensitivity reactions, including rash, urticaria, and dyspnea, have been reported in patients receiving galcanezumab in clinical trials. Hypersensitivity reactions may occur days after administration of galcanezumab and may be prolonged.

If a serious or severe hypersensitivity reaction occurs during galcanezumab therapy, the drug should be discontinued and appropriate medical therapy initiated. (See Cautions: Contraindications and see also Advice to Patients.)

The manufacturer states that the prefilled auto-injectors and syringes of galcanezumab-gnlm are *not* made with natural rubber latex.

Immunogenicity As with all therapeutic proteins, there is a potential for immunogenicity with galcanezumab therapy. In controlled clinical studies of up to 6 months' duration, anti-galcanezumab antibodies were detected in 33 of 688 patients (4.8%) who received galcanezumab once monthly; anti-galcanezumab antibodies with neutralizing activity were detected in 32 of the 33 patients (97%). In an open-label study of 12 months' duration, anti-galcanezumab antibodies were detected in up to 12.5% of galcanezumab-treated patients, most of whom had anti-galcanezumab antibodies with neutralizing activity. Although available data do not demonstrate an effect of anti-galcanezumab antibody development on the pharmacokinetics, efficacy, or safety of the drug, the data are too limited to make definitive conclusions.

Specific Populations **Pregnancy.** There are no adequate data on the developmental risk associated with the use of galcanezumab in pregnant women. Animal studies in pregnant rats and rabbits administered galcanezumab subcutaneously throughout the period of organogenesis or to rats throughout pregnancy at systemic exposures greater than those expected clinically have not revealed evidence of harm to the offspring.

The estimated rate of major birth defects and miscarriage among deliveries to women with migraine (2.2–2.9 and 17%, respectively) are similar to rates reported in women without migraine. Clinicians should be aware that published data suggest that women with migraine may be at an increased risk of vascular complications such as preeclampsia during pregnancy. The long elimination half-life of galcanezumab should be considered if the drug is used in women who are pregnant or plan to become pregnant during therapy. (See Description.)

Lactation. It is not known whether galcanezumab is distributed into human milk. The effects of the drug on the breast-fed infant or on milk production also are unknown. The manufacturer states that the developmental and health benefits of breast-feeding should be considered along with the mother's clinical need for galcanezumab and any potential adverse effects on the breast-fed infant from the drug or from the underlying maternal condition.

Pediatric Use. The manufacturer states that the safety and efficacy of galcanezumab have not been established in pediatric patients. A clinical study to evaluate the efficacy and safety of galcanezumab in the preventive treatment of episodic migraine in pediatric patients 6–17 years of age† is currently under way.

Pending further clinical experience with the use of calcitonin gene-related peptide (CGRP) antagonists in pediatric patients, the Pediatric and Adolescent Headache special interest group of the American Headache Society (AHS) recommends that CGRP antagonists (e.g., erenumab, fremanezumab, galcanezumab) should be considered mainly for use in postpubertal adolescents† with relatively frequent migraines (i.e., 8 or more headache days per month) who have moderate to severe disability associated with migraine (e.g., PedMIDAS score of 30 or more) and in whom at least 2 preventive therapies (including pharmacologic and nonpharmacologic therapies and dietary supplements) have failed. For younger pediatric patients† with severe chronic migraine that is refractory to multiple preventive therapies, these experts recommend that CGRP antagonists be considered only in carefully selected patients with close monitoring (e.g., pubertal status, bone health, linear growth, weight, body mass index [BMI], infectious complications).

Geriatric Use. Clinical trials of galcanezumab did not include sufficient numbers of patients 65 years of age or older to determine whether they respond differently than younger adults.

Hepatic Impairment. Hepatic impairment is not expected to affect pharmacokinetics of galcanezumab. Formal pharmacokinetic studies of the drug have not been conducted in patients with hepatic impairment. Analysis of population pharmacokinetic data indicates that clearance of galcanezumab is not substantially influenced by serum bilirubin concentration (an indirect marker of hepatic function).

Renal Impairment. Renal impairment is not expected to affect pharmacokinetics of galcanezumab. Formal pharmacokinetic studies of the drug have not been conducted in patients with renal impairment. Analysis of population pharmacokinetic data indicates that creatinine clearance does not affect the pharmacokinetics of galcanezumab in patients with mild or moderate renal impairment. Galcanezumab has not been evaluated in patients with severe renal impairment (creatinine clearance less than 30 mL/minute).

■ **Common Adverse Effects** Adverse effects reported in 2% or more of patients receiving galcanezumab for the preventive treatment of migraine in clinical studies and at least 2% more frequently than with placebo include injection site reactions (e.g., pain, erythema, pruritus, swelling), which were usually mild to moderate in severity and resolved within a few days to 2 weeks.

The manufacturer states that the tolerability profile of galcanezumab in patients with episodic cluster headache is consistent with the tolerability profile observed in migraine patients.

Drug Interactions

Formal drug interaction studies with galcanezumab have not been conducted to date. The risk of clinically important drug interactions with galcanezumab appears to be minimal. Galcanezumab is not metabolized by cytochrome P-450 (CYP) enzymes. In addition galcanezumab, a monoclonal antibody, is not likely to be affected by drug transport systems. Therefore, pharmacokinetic interactions with drugs affecting or metabolized by CYP enzymes or substrates of various drug transport systems are not expected.

Description

Galcanezumab is a humanized immunoglobulin G_4 (IgG_4) monoclonal antibody that binds to the calcitonin gene-related peptide (CGRP) ligand and blocks its binding with the CGRP receptor. The drug is produced using recombinant DNA technology in Chinese hamster ovary cells.

CGRP is a potent vasodilator and pain-signaling neuropeptide that has been associated with migraine pathophysiology. CGRP and its receptors are located at sites that are relevant to migraine development such as the trigeminal neurons and are also widely distributed throughout the central and peripheral nervous systems as well as in nonneuronal tissues throughout the body.

Increased serum CGRP concentrations have been observed in individuals during acute migraine attacks (with or without aura) and IV infusion of CGRP has been shown to induce migraines in patients with a history of migraines. Galcanezumab binds to the CGRP ligand and blocks its interaction with the CGRP receptor. Animal studies indicate possible limited distribution of galcanezumab into the CNS and cerebrospinal fluid. Because of their large molecular size, however, CGRP antagonists are considered unlikely to cross the blood-brain barrier in substantial amounts and probably antagonize CGRP function peripherally rather than centrally within the nervous system.

The pharmacokinetics of galcanezumab appear to be similar in healthy individuals, patients with episodic or chronic migraine, and patients with episodic cluster headache. The drug exhibits linear and dose-proportional pharmacokinetics over a dosage range of 1–600 mg when given by subcutaneous injection. Following a 240-mg loading dose given subcutaneously, steady-state concentrations of galcanezumab are achieved after the first dose. When 300 mg of the drug is given subcutaneously once monthly, steady-state concentrations are achieved following the fourth dose. Peak plasma concentrations occur approximately 5 days following subcutaneous doses of galcanezumab. Antimigraine effects of CGRP antagonists, including galcanezumab, usually are evident following 1–3 monthly subcutaneous injections of the drug in responding patients. Galcanezumab is expected to be degraded into small peptides and amino acids via catabolic pathways in the same manner as endogenous IgG. The elimination half-life of galcanezumab is approximately 27 days.

Population pharmacokinetic analysis indicates that the pharmacokinetics of galcanezumab are not affected by age, sex, race, subtypes of migraine spectrum (e.g., episodic or chronic migraine), or headache diagnosis (e.g., migraine, episodic cluster headache). Body weight does not have a clinically important effect on the pharmacokinetics of the drug.

Advice to Patients

Importance of advising patients to read the manufacturer's patient information and to read and follow the instructions for use each time they use galcanezumab.

Importance of providing guidance to patients and/or caregivers on proper subcutaneous administration of galcanezumab, including the use of aseptic technique and how to use the single-dose prefilled syringes or auto-injectors.

If a dose of galcanezumab for the preventive treatment of migraine is missed, the missed dose should be administered as soon as possible. Subsequent doses may then be scheduled monthly from the date of the last administered dose.

If a dose of galcanezumab for the treatment of episodic cluster headache is missed, the missed dose should be administered as soon as possible. If the cluster headache period has not yet ended, subsequent doses may then be scheduled monthly from the date of the last administered dose.

Importance of informing patients of possible signs and symptoms of hypersensitivity reactions (e.g., rash, urticaria, dyspnea), which can occur days after administration and may be prolonged. Patients should seek immediate medical attention if symptoms of a serious or severe hypersensitivity reaction occur.

Importance of informing clinicians of existing or contemplated concomitant therapy, including prescription and OTC drugs and dietary or herbal supplements, as well as any concomitant illnesses.

Importance of women informing clinicians if they are or plan to become pregnant or plan to breast-feed. (See Pregnancy under Warnings/Precautions: Specific Populations, in Cautions.)

Importance of informing patients of other important precautionary information. (See Cautions.)

Overview® (see Users Guide). For additional information on this drug until a more detailed monograph is developed and published, the manufacturer's labeling should be consulted. It is *essential* that the manufacturer's labeling be consulted for more detailed information on usual cautions, precautions, contraindications, potential drug interactions, laboratory test interferences, and acute toxicity.

Preparations

Excipients in commercially available drug preparations may have clinically important effects in some individuals; consult specific product labeling for details.

Galcanezumab-gnlm

Parenteral		
Injection, for subcutaneous use only	100 mg/1 mL	**Emgality®** (available as single-dose prefilled syringes), Lilly
	120 mg/1 mL	**Emgality®** (available as single-dose prefilled auto-injectors [pens] and single-dose prefilled syringes), Lilly

†Use is not currently included in the labeling approved by the US Food and Drug Administration

SELECTIVE SEROTONIN AGONISTS 28:32.28

Eletriptan Hydrobromide

■ Eletriptan hydrobromide is a selective agonist of serotonin (5-hydroxytryptamine; 5-HT) type 1B and 1D receptors ("triptan").

Uses

■ **Vascular Headaches** *Migraine* Eletriptan hydrobromide is used for the acute treatment of attacks of migraine with or without aura in adults. The manufacturer states that eletriptan should *not* be used for the management of hemiplegic or basilar migraine or for the *prophylaxis* of migraine. Safety and efficacy have not been established for the management of cluster headaches.

Efficacy of eletriptan administered at the recommended dosage of 20 or 40 mg has been evaluated for the acute treatment of migraine attacks in several randomized, placebo-controlled studies in adult outpatients with moderate to severe headaches. In these studies, 47–54 or 54–65% of patients receiving eletriptan 20 or 40 mg, respectively, achieved a response (mild to no pain) 2 hours after treatment, compared with 19–40% of patients receiving placebo. The drug also relieved manifestations of migraine other than headache (including nausea, photophobia, and phonophobia) and reduced the need for supplemental migraine therapy.

Eletriptan appears to be at least as effective as oral sumatriptan in alleviating the pain associated with migraine 2 hours after treatment. In several comparative studies, response rates 2 hours after treatment were substantially higher in patients receiving eletriptan 40 mg (64–67%) than in patients receiving sumatriptan 50 mg (50%) or 100 mg (53–59%). In another study, similar response rates were reported for eletriptan 20 or 40 mg (54 or 65%, respectively) and sumatriptan 100 mg (55%). In all comparative studies to date, sumatriptan tablets were encapsulated for the purpose of blinding, while eletriptan tablets were not. The encapsulated sumatriptan formulations were reportedly bioequivalent to conventional sumatriptan tablets; however, in another study, encapsulation of sumatriptan delayed absorption of the drug during the first 2 hours after dosing compared with conventional sumatriptan tablets. Results of a pooled analysis suggest that headache response rates 2 hours after treatment may be lower with eletriptan 20 mg than with sumatriptan 100 mg.

The US Headache Consortium considers $5\text{-}HT_{1B/1D}$ receptor agonists (e.g., eletriptan) an appropriate treatment choice for the acute management of moderate to severe migraine headaches in patients without contraindications to these drugs and recommends use of $5H\text{-}T_{1B/1D}$ receptor agonists, dihydroergotamine, or ergotamine in patients with more severe migraine attacks as well as in patients in whom previous therapy with nonsteroidal anti-inflammatory agents (NSAIAs) or fixed-combination preparations such as acetaminophen, aspirin, and caffeine has been ineffective.

For further information on management and classification of migraine headache, see Vascular Headaches: General Principles in Migraine Therapy, under Uses in Sumatriptan 28:32.28.

Dosage and Administration

■ **General** Eletriptan hydrobromide is administered orally without regard to meals. Dosage of eletriptan hydrobromide is expressed in terms of eletriptan.

■ **Vascular Headaches** *Migraine* For the acute treatment of migraine attacks with or without aura in adults, single oral eletriptan doses of 20 or 40 mg were effective in clinical studies, although the 40-mg dose was effective in a greater proportion of patients. Because individuals vary in their response to eletriptan, dosage selection should be individualized. In clinical studies, doses exceeding 40 mg were effective but were associated with an increased risk of adverse effects. The maximum single dose of eletriptan should not exceed 40 mg.

If headache recurs following an initial dose, additional doses of eletriptan may be administered at intervals of not less than 2 hours, up to a maximum adult dosage of 80 mg in any 24-hour period. However, additional doses of eletriptan are unlikely to provide benefit in patients who do not respond to the first dose of the drug for the same headache. The safety of treating an average of more than 3 headaches per 30-day period has not been established.

■ **Special Populations** Use of eletriptan is contraindicated in patients with severe hepatic impairment. The manufacturer states that dosage adjustment is not necessary in mild to moderate hepatic impairment.

Cautions

■ **Contraindications** Known or suspected ischemic heart disease (e.g., angina pectoris, myocardial infarction, silent ischemia), coronary vasospasm (e.g., Prinzmetal variant angina), uncontrolled hypertension, other serious underlying cardiovascular disease, cerebrovascular syndromes (e.g., stroke syndrome, transient ischemic attacks), peripheral vascular disease, or ischemic bowel disease. Basilar or hemiplegic migraine. Treatment within the previous 24 hours with another 5-HT_1 receptor agonist or with an ergot alkaloid (e.g., ergotamine, dihydroergotamine, methysergide [no longer commercially available in the US]). Severe hepatic impairment (Child-Pugh grade C). Known hypersensitivity to eletriptan or any ingredient in the formulation.

■ **Warnings/Precautions** ***Careful Diagnosis of Migraine*** Eletriptan should be used only in patients in whom a clear diagnosis of migraine has been established. Care should be taken to exclude other potentially serious neurologic disorders before eletriptan is administered to patients not previously diagnosed with migraine or to patients who present with atypical symptoms.

Interactions with CYP3A4 Inhibitors Eletriptan should not be used within at least 72 hours of treatment with potent inhibitors of the cytochrome P-450 (CYP) 3A4 isoenzyme (e.g., ketoconazole, itraconazole, nefazodone, troleandomycin, clarithromycin, ritonavir, nelfinavir). (See Drug Interactions: Drugs Affecting Hepatic Microsomal Enzymes.)

Cardiac Effects Serious cardiac events, including acute myocardial infarction and fatal or life-threatening cardiac rhythm disturbances (e.g., ventricular tachycardia or fibrillation), have occurred within a few hours following administration of 5-HT_1 receptor agonists. Myocardial ischemia/infarction or coronary vasospasm (e.g., Prinzmetal variant angina) may occur even in patients without a history of coronary artery disease. Use of eletriptan is contraindicated in patients with ischemic or vasospastic heart disease. (See Cautions: Contraindications.) Therapy with 5-HT_1 receptor agonists should be discontinued if disturbances in cardiac rhythm occur.

Although sensations of tightness, pain, pressure, and heaviness in the precordium, throat, neck, and jaw occur frequently following administration of 5-HT_1 receptor agonists, these sensations usually are noncardiac in origin. However, the manufacturer states that patients experiencing symptoms suggestive of angina after receiving eletriptan should be evaluated for the presence of coronary artery disease or predisposition to Prinzmetal variant angina before receiving additional doses of the drug. If administration of eletriptan is resumed and such symptoms recur, electrocardiographic evaluation should be performed.

Patients with multiple cardiovascular risk factors (e.g., postmenopausal women; men older than 40 years of age; patients with risk factors such as hypertension, hypercholesterolemia, smoking, obesity, diabetes, or family history of coronary artery disease) who have not previously received therapy with a 5-HT_1 receptor agonist should undergo cardiovascular evaluation prior to initiation of 5-HT_1 receptor agonist therapy. If the evaluation provides evidence of coronary artery disease or coronary artery vasospasm, the drug should not be administered. For patients with a satisfactory cardiovascular evaluation, the manufacturer states that consideration should be given to administration of the first dose in a medically supervised setting with electrocardiographic monitoring performed immediately following administration of the dose. Periodic cardiovascular evaluation is recommended for patients with risk factors for coronary artery disease who are receiving intermittent long-term therapy with 5-HT_1 receptor agonists, including eletriptan.

For further information on the systematic approach to administering 5-HT_1 receptor agonists in patients with risk factors for the development of coronary artery disease, see Cautions: Precautions and Contraindications, in Sumatriptan 28:32.28.

Cerebrovascular Effects Cerebral or subarachnoid hemorrhage and stroke, sometimes fatal, have occurred in patients receiving 5-HT_1 receptor agonists. In a number of cases, it appears possible that the cerebrovascular event was the primary event, and the 5-HT_1 receptor agonist was administered in the mistaken belief that the patient's symptoms were caused by a migraine attack. Patients with migraine may be at increased risk for certain cerebrovascular events (e.g., stroke, hemorrhage, transient ischemic attack). Therapy with 5-HT_1 receptor agonists should be discontinued in patients experiencing a cerebrovascular event. (See Cautions: Contraindications.)

Other Cardiovascular or Vasospastic Effects Noncoronary vasospastic reactions, including peripheral vascular ischemia, GI ischemia and infarction (presenting with abdominal pain and bloody diarrhea), splenic infarction, and Raynaud's syndrome, have been reported in patients receiving 5-HT_1 receptor agonists. (See Cautions: Contraindications.) Transient or permanent blindness and partial vision loss also have been reported in patients receiving 5-HT_1 receptor agonists, although visual disorders may occur as manifestations of migraine attacks. Patients experiencing signs or symptoms suggestive of vasospastic reactions following administration of any 5-HT_1 receptor agonist should be evaluated to rule out vasospastic reactions before receiving additional doses of eletriptan.

Substantial increases in blood pressure, including hypertensive crisis with acute impairment of organ systems, have been reported rarely following administration of 5-HT_1 receptor agonists in patients with or without a history of hypertension. (See Cautions: Contraindications.) Transient increases in blood pressure have been observed following administration of eletriptan doses of 60 mg or greater and may be more pronounced in patients with renal impairment and geriatric patients.

Increases (18%) in mean pulmonary arterial pressure have been observed following administration of another 5-HT_1 receptor agonist to patients with suspected coronary artery disease who were undergoing cardiac catheterization.

Serotonin Syndrome Potentially life-threatening serotonin syndrome has been reported in patients receiving 5-HT_1 receptor agonists, particularly in those receiving concomitant therapy with selective serotonin-reuptake inhibitors (SSRIs) or selective serotonin- and norepinephrine-reuptake inhibitors (SNRIs). Serotonin syndrome also may occur in patients receiving 5-HT_1 receptor agonists concomitantly with monoamine oxidase (MAO) inhibitors or tricyclic antidepressants. Symptoms of serotonin syndrome may include mental status changes (e.g., agitation, hallucinations, coma), autonomic instability (e.g., tachycardia, labile blood pressure, hyperthermia), neuromuscular aberrations (e.g., hyperreflexia, incoordination), and/or GI symptoms (e.g., nausea, vomiting, diarrhea). If concurrent therapy with a 5-HT_1 receptor agonist and an SSRI or SNRI is clinically warranted, the patient should be observed carefully, particularly during initiation of therapy, when dosage is increased, or when another serotonergic agent is initiated. If manifestations of serotonin syndrome occur, treatment with eletriptan and any concurrently administered serotonergic agents should be discontinued and supportive and symptomatic treatment should be initiated.

Medication Overuse Headache Excessive use of drugs indicated for the management of acute migraine attacks (e.g., use of 5-HT_1 receptor agonists, ergotamine, opiates, or certain analgesic combinations on a regular basis for 10 or more days per month) may result in migraine-like daily headaches or a marked increase in the frequency of migraine attacks. Detoxification, including withdrawal of the overused drugs; treatment of withdrawal symptoms (which often include transient worsening of headaches); and consideration of prophylactic therapy for migraine attacks may be necessary.

Sensitivity Reactions Serious allergic reactions, including angioedema, have been reported in patients receiving eletriptan.

Ocular Effects Accumulation of eletriptan and/or its metabolites in melanin-rich tissues (such as the eye) may occur over time, resulting in potential toxicity in these tissues with extended use.

Specific Populations **Pregnancy.** Category C. (See Users Guide.)

Lactation. Eletriptan is distributed into human milk. Caution is advised if used in nursing women.

Pediatric Use. Safety and efficacy have not been established in children younger than 18 years of age. Eletriptan is not recommended for use in patients younger than 18 years of age.

Geriatric Use. Pharmacokinetic profile in patients 65 years of age and older is similar to that in younger adults, although half-life was increased in geriatric patients during clinical trials. No substantial differences in efficacy or safety relative to younger adults have been observed; however, there is limited clinical experience in patients 65 years of age or older. Increases in blood pressure may be more pronounced in geriatric patients.

Hepatic Impairment. Peak plasma concentrations and area under the plasma concentration-time curve (AUC) of eletriptan were increased 18 and 34%, respectively, in patients with mild to moderate hepatic impairment. Eletriptan has not been studied in patients with severe hepatic impairment; use in such patients is contraindicated.

■ **Common Adverse Effects** Adverse effects occurring in 2% or more of patients receiving eletriptan include asthenia, headache, nausea, paresthesia, dizziness, somnolence, dry mouth, flushing or feeling of warmth, pain/pressure sensations (i.e., chest pain [tightness/pressure], abdominal pain/discomfort/stomach pain/cramps/pressure), dyspepsia, and dysphagia (i.e., throat tightness, difficulty swallowing).

Drug Interactions

■ **Drugs Affecting Hepatic Microsomal Enzymes** Because in vitro studies have shown that eletriptan is metabolized via the cytochrome P-450 (CYP) isoenzyme 3A4, concomitant use with drugs that inhibit this enzyme (e.g., fluconazole, ketoconazole, itraconazole, nefazodone, troleandomycin, clarithromycin, ritonavir, nelfinavir) may increase peak plasma concentrations and area under the plasma concentration-time curve (AUC) of the drug. Administration of eletriptan within 72 hours of drugs with demonstrated potent CYP3A4 inhibition is not recommended.

In vitro studies of human liver microsomes indicate that eletriptan has little potential to inhibit or induce CYP isoenzymes 1A2, 2C9, 2E1, or 3A4; pharmacokinetic interaction is unlikely. The manufacturer states that while eletriptan has an effect on the isoenzyme CYP2D6 at high drug concentrations, such an effect should not interfere with metabolism of other drugs when eletriptan is used at recommended dosages.

■ **Ergot Alkaloids and Other 5-HT_1 Receptor Agonists** Potential pharmacologic interaction (additive vasospastic effects) when eletriptan is used concomitantly with ergot alkaloids (e.g., ergotamine, dihydroergotamine, methysergide [no longer commercially available in the US]) or other 5-HT_1 receptor agonists. Use within 24 hours is contraindicated.

■ **Monoamine Oxidase (MAO) Inhibitors** Pharmacokinetic interaction is unlikely.

■ **Propranolol** Potential pharmacokinetic interaction (increases in the maximum plasma concentrations and AUC of eletriptan); no dosage adjustment is required.

■ **Selective Serotonin-reuptake Inhibitors and Selective Serotonin- and Norepinephrine-reuptake Inhibitors** Potential pharmacologic interaction (potentially life-threatening serotonin syndrome). If concomitant use is clinically warranted, the patient should be observed carefully, particularly during treatment initiation, when dosage is increased, or when another serotonergic agent is initiated. (See Serotonin Syndrome under Cautions: Warnings/Precautions.)

Description

Eletriptan hydrobromide is a selective agonist of serotonin (5-hydroxytryptamine; 5-HT) type 1B and 1D receptors. Eletriptan is structurally and pharmacologically related to other selective 5-$HT_{1B/1D}$ receptor agonists (e.g., almotriptan, frovatriptan, naratriptan, rizatriptan, sumatriptan, zolmitriptan). Because the mechanisms involved in the pathogenesis of migraine are not clearly understood, the precise mechanism of action of 5-HT_1 receptor agonists in the management of migraine has yet to be established. However, current data suggest that 5-HT_1 receptor agonists, including eletriptan, may ameliorate migraine through selective constriction of certain intracranial blood vessels, inhibition of neuropeptide release, and/or reduced transmission in the trigeminal pain pathway.

Eletriptan is well absorbed following oral administration. Peak plasma concentrations are achieved in approximately 1.5 and 2 hours in healthy adults and patients with moderate to severe migraine, respectively.

In vitro, eletriptan is metabolized principally by cytochrome P-450 (CYP) isoenzyme 3A4. Since plasma concentrations of the *N*-demethylated metabolite, the only active metabolite identified for eletriptan, generally are only about 10–20% of the parent drug, the metabolite does not appear to contribute substantially to the overall effect of the parent drug. The elimination half-life of eletriptan is approximately 4 hours. Renal clearance accounts for about 10% of total clearance of eletriptan.

Advice to Patients

Risk of dizziness or fatigue.

Risk of serious cardiovascular or cerebrovascular events (e.g., myocardial infarction, stroke) or other vasospastic reactions. Importance of seeking medical care if symptoms of such reactions (e.g., shortness of breath, weakness, slurring of speech, sudden or severe abdominal pain, difficulty in seeing, or tightness, pain, pressure, or heaviness in chest, throat, jaw, or neck) occur after taking eletriptan and of *not* taking eletriptan again until evaluated by clinician.

Importance of adhering to prescribed directions for use. Provide copy of manufacturer's patient information.

Overuse of drugs indicated for the management of acute migraine attacks may exacerbate headaches; importance of recording headache frequency and drug use to monitor effectiveness of treatment.

Importance of informing clinician of existing or contemplated concomitant therapy, including prescription and OTC drugs and herbal supplements, as well as any concomitant illnesses (e.g., cardiovascular disease).

Importance of informing patients of risk of serotonin syndrome, particularly with concurrent use of eletriptan and a selective serotonin-reuptake inhibitor (SSRI) or selective serotonin- and norepinephrine-reuptake inhibitor (SNRI). Importance of seeking immediate medical attention if symptoms of serotonin syndrome develop.

Importance of women informing clinicians if they are or plan to become pregnant or plan to breast-feed.

Importance of informing patients of other important precautionary information. (See Cautions.)

Overview® (see Users Guide). For additional information on this drug until a more detailed monograph is developed and published, the manufacturer's labeling should be consulted. It is *essential* that the manufacturer's labeling be consulted for more detailed information on usual cautions, precautions, contraindications, potential drug interactions, laboratory test interferences, and acute toxicity.

Preparations

Excipients in commercially available drug preparations may have clinically important effects in some individuals; consult specific product labeling for details.

Eletriptan Hydrobromide

Oral		
Tablets, film-coated	20 mg (of eletriptan)	Relpax®, Pfizer
	40 mg (of eletriptan)	Relpax®, Pfizer

Naratriptan Hydrochloride

■ Naratriptan hydrochloride is a selective agonist of serotonin (5-hydroxytryptamine; 5-HT) type 1B and 1D receptors ("triptan").

Uses

■ **Vascular Headaches** ***Migraine*** Naratriptan hydrochloride is used for the acute treatment of attacks of migraine with or without aura in adults. The manufacturer states that naratriptan should *not* be used for the management of hemiplegic or basilar migraine or for the *prophylaxis* of migraine. Safety and efficacy have not been established for the management of cluster headaches.

Efficacy of naratriptan administered at the recommended dosage of 1 or 2.5 mg has been evaluated for the acute treatment of migraine attacks in several randomized, placebo-controlled studies in adult outpatients with moderate to severe headaches. In these studies, 50–54 or 60–66% of patients receiving naratriptan 1 or 2.5 mg, respectively, achieved a response (mild or no headache pain) 4 hours after treatment, compared with 27–34% of patients receiving placebo. The drug also relieved manifestations of migraine other than headache (including nausea, photophobia, and phonophobia) and reduced the need for supplemental migraine therapy.

The US Headache Consortium considers 5-$HT_{1B/1D}$ receptor agonists (e.g., naratriptan) an appropriate treatment choice for the acute management of moderate to severe migraine headaches in patients without contraindications to these drugs and recommends use of 5-$HT_{1B/1D}$ receptor agonists, dihydroergotamine, or ergotamine in patients with more severe migraine attacks as well as in patients in whom previous therapy with nonsteroidal anti-inflammatory agents (NSAIAs) or fixed-combination preparations such as acetaminophen, aspirin, and caffeine has been ineffective.

For further information on management and classification of migraine headache, see Vascular Headaches: General Principles in Migraine Therapy, under Uses in Sumatriptan 28:32.28.

Dosage and Administration

■ **General** Naratriptan hydrochloride is administered orally. Dosage of naratriptan hydrochloride is expressed in terms of naratriptan.

Vascular Headaches **Migraine.** For the acute treatment of migraine attacks with or without aura in adults, single oral naratriptan doses of 1 or 2.5 mg were effective in clinical studies, although the 2.5-mg dose was effective in a greater proportion of patients. Because individuals vary in their response to naratriptan, dosage selection should be individualized, weighing the possible benefit of the 2.5-mg dose with the potential for an increased risk of adverse effects.

If headache recurs or only a partial response is achieved following an initial dose, the dose may be repeated once after 4 hours. However, following failure of a given attack of migraine to respond to the first dose of naratriptan, the diagnosis of migraine should be reconsidered prior to administration of a second dose. The maximum dosage of naratriptan to be administered in any 24-hour period is 5 mg. The safety of treating an average of more than 4 headaches per 30-day period has not been established.

■ **Special Populations** For patients with mild or moderate renal or hepatic impairment, the manufacturer recommends a maximum dosage of 2.5 mg of naratriptan per 24-hour period and consideration of a reduced initial dosage. Use of naratriptan is contraindicated in patients with severe renal or hepatic impairment. (See Cautions: Contraindications.)

Cautions

■ **Contraindications** Known or suspected ischemic heart disease (e.g., angina pectoris, myocardial infarction, silent ischemia), coronary vasospasm (e.g., Prinzmetal variant angina), uncontrolled hypertension, other serious underlying cardiovascular disease, cerebrovascular syndromes (e.g., stroke syndrome, transient ischemic attacks), peripheral vascular disease, or ischemic bowel disease.

Severe renal impairment (e.g., creatinine clearance less than 15 mL/minute) or severe hepatic impairment (e.g., Child-Pugh grade C).

Basilar or hemiplegic migraine. Treatment within the previous 24 hours with another 5-HT_1 receptor agonist or with an ergot alkaloid (e.g., ergotamine, dihydroergotamine, methysergide [no longer commercially available in the US]).

Known hypersensitivity to naratriptan or any ingredient in the formulation.

■ **Warnings/Precautions** ***Careful Diagnosis of Migraine*** Naratriptan should be used only in patients in whom a clear diagnosis of migraine has been established. Following failure of a given attack of migraine to respond to the first dose of naratriptan, the diagnosis of migraine should be reconsidered prior to administration of a second dose. Care should be taken to exclude other potentially serious neurologic disorders before naratriptan is administered to patients not previously diagnosed with migraine or to patients who present with atypical symptoms.

Cardiac Effects Serious cardiac events, including acute myocardial infarction and fatal or life-threatening cardiac rhythm disturbances (e.g., ventricular tachycardia or fibrillation), have occurred within a few hours following administration of 5-HT_1 receptor agonists. Myocardial ischemia/infarction or coronary vasospasm (e.g., Prinzmetal variant angina) may occur even in patients without a history of coronary artery disease. Use of naratriptan is contraindicated in patients with ischemic or vasospastic heart disease. (See Cautions: Contraindications.) Therapy with 5-HT_1 receptor agonists should be discontinued if disturbances in cardiac rhythm occur.

Although sensations of tightness, pain, pressure, and heaviness in the precordium, throat, neck, and jaw occur frequently following administration of 5-HT_1 receptor agonists, these sensations usually are noncardiac in origin. However, the manufacturer states that patients experiencing symptoms suggestive of angina after receiving naratriptan should be evaluated for the presence of coronary artery disease or predisposition to Prinzmetal variant angina before receiving additional doses of the drug. If administration of naratriptan is resumed and such symptoms recur, electrocardiographic evaluation should be performed.

Patients with multiple cardiovascular risk factors (e.g., postmenopausal women; men older than 40 years of age; patients with risk factors such as hypertension, hypercholesterolemia, smoking, obesity, diabetes, or family history of coronary artery disease) who have not previously received therapy with a 5-HT_1 receptor agonist should undergo cardiovascular evaluation prior to initiation of 5-HT_1 receptor agonist therapy. If the evaluation provides evidence of coronary artery disease or coronary artery vasospasm, the drug should not be administered. For patients with a satisfactory cardiovascular evaluation, the manufacturer states that consideration should be given to administration of the first dose in a medically supervised setting with electrocardiographic monitoring performed immediately following administration of the dose. Periodic cardiovascular evaluation is recommended for patients with risk factors for coronary artery disease who are receiving intermittent long-term therapy with 5-HT_1 receptor agonists.

For further information on the systematic approach to administering 5-HT_1 receptor agonists in patients with risk factors for the development of coronary artery disease, see Cautions: Precautions and Contraindications, in Sumatriptan 28:32.28.

Cerebrovascular Effects Cerebral or subarachnoid hemorrhage and stroke, sometimes fatal, have occurred in patients receiving 5-HT_1 receptor agonists. In a number of cases, it appears possible that the cerebrovascular event was the primary event, and the 5-HT_1 receptor agonist was administered in the mistaken belief that the patient's symptoms were caused by a migraine attack. Patients with migraine may be at increased risk for certain cerebrovascular events (e.g., stroke, hemorrhage, transient ischemic attack). Therapy with 5-HT_1 receptor agonists should be discontinued in patients experiencing a cerebrovascular event. (See Cautions: Contraindications.)

Other Cardiovascular or Vasospastic Effects Noncoronary vasospastic reactions, including peripheral vascular ischemia, GI ischemia and infarction (presenting with abdominal pain and bloody diarrhea), splenic infarction, and Raynaud's syndrome, have been reported in patients receiving 5-HT_1 receptor agonists, including naratriptan. (See Cautions: Contraindications.) Transient or permanent blindness and partial vision loss also have been reported in patients receiving 5-HT_1 receptor agonists, although visual disorders may occur as manifestations of migraine attacks. Patients experiencing signs or symptoms suggestive of vasospastic reactions following administration of any 5-HT_1 receptor agonist should be evaluated to rule out vasospastic reactions before receiving additional doses of naratriptan.

Substantial increases in blood pressure, including hypertensive crisis with acute impairment of organ systems, have been reported rarely following administration of 5-HT_1 receptor agonists in patients with or without a history of hypertension. (See Cautions: Contraindications.) Increases in blood pressure have been observed following administration of naratriptan and may be more pronounced in geriatric patients and patients with hypertension.

Increases in mean pulmonary arterial pressure and mean aortic pressure following naratriptan administration have been observed in patients with suspected coronary artery disease who were undergoing cardiac catheterization.

Serotonin Syndrome Potentially life-threatening serotonin syndrome has been reported in patients receiving 5-HT_1 receptor agonists, particularly in those receiving concomitant therapy with selective serotonin-reuptake inhibitors (SSRIs) or selective serotonin- and norepinephrine-reuptake inhibitors (SNRIs). Serotonin syndrome also may occur in patients receiving 5-HT_1 receptor agonists concomitantly with monoamine oxidase (MAO) inhibitors or tricyclic antidepressants. Symptoms of serotonin syndrome may include mental status changes (e.g., agitation, hallucinations, coma), autonomic instability (e.g., tachycardia, labile blood pressure, hyperthermia), neuromuscular aberrations (e.g., hyperreflexia, incoordination), and/or GI symptoms (e.g., nausea, vomiting, diarrhea). If concurrent therapy with a 5-HT_1 receptor agonist and an SSRI or SNRI is clinically warranted, the patient should be observed carefully, particularly during initiation of therapy, when dosage is increased, or when another serotonergic agent is initiated. If manifestations of serotonin syndrome occur, treatment with naratriptan and any concurrently administered serotonergic agents should be discontinued and supportive and symptomatic treatment should be initiated.

Sensitivity Reactions Hypersensitivity reactions, including anaphylaxis or anaphylactoid reactions, may occur in patients receiving naratriptan; such reactions may be life-threatening or fatal.

Medication Overuse Headache Excessive use of drugs indicated for the management of acute migraine attacks (e.g., use of 5-HT_1 receptor agonists, ergotamine, opiates, or certain analgesic combinations on a regular basis for 10 or more days per month) may result in migraine-like daily headaches or a marked increase in the frequency of migraine attacks. Detoxification, including withdrawal of the overused drugs; treatment of withdrawal symptoms (which often include transient worsening of headaches); and consideration of prophylactic therapy for migraine attacks may be necessary.

Specific Populations **Pregnancy.** Category C. (See Users Guide.)

Lactation. Naratriptan and/or its metabolites are distributed into milk in rats. Caution is advised if used in nursing women.

Pediatric Use. Safety and efficacy have not been established in children younger than 18 years of age.

Geriatric Use. Use in geriatric patients is not recommended. There is a greater frequency of coronary artery disease in this patient population. The risk of adverse effects may be increased in those with renal or hepatic impairment. Increases in blood pressure may be more pronounced in geriatric patients.

Renal and Hepatic Impairment. Clearance of naratriptan is reduced approximately 50% in patients with moderate renal impairment (creatinine clearance of 18–39 mL/minute) and 30% in patients with moderate hepatic impairment (Child-Pugh grade A or B). Naratriptan should be used with caution in such patients; dosage adjustment is recommended. (See Dosage and Administration: Special Populations.) Use is contraindicated in patients with severe renal or hepatic impairment. (See Cautions: Contraindications.)

■ **Common Adverse Effects** Adverse effects occurring in 2% or more of patients receiving naratriptan include paresthesia, nausea, dizziness, drowsiness, malaise/fatigue, and throat/neck symptoms (e.g., pain, pressure).

Drug Interactions

■ **Ergot Alkaloids and Other 5-HT_1 Receptor Agonists** Potential pharmacologic interaction (additive vasospastic effects) when naratriptan is used concomitantly with ergot alkaloids (e.g., dihydroergotamine, ergotamine, methysergide [no longer commercially available in the US]) or 5-HT_1 receptor agonists. Use within 24 hours is contraindicated.

■ **Selective Serotonin-reuptake Inhibitors and Selective Serotonin- and Norepinephrine-reuptake Inhibitors** Potential pharmacologic interaction (potentially life-threatening serotonin syndrome). If concomitant use is clinically warranted, the patient should be observed carefully, particularly during treatment initiation, when dosage is increased, or when another serotonergic agent is initiated. (See Serotonin Syndrome under Cautions: Warnings/Precautions.)

■ **Oral Contraceptives** Potential pharmacokinetic interaction (decreased clearance and volume of distribution, resulting in slightly increased concentrations of naratriptan).

Description

Naratriptan hydrochloride is a selective agonist of serotonin (5-hydroxytryptamine; 5-HT) type 1B and 1D receptors. Naratriptan is structurally and pharmacologically related to other selective 5-$HT_{1B/1D}$ receptor agonists (e.g., almotriptan, eletriptan, frovatriptan, rizatriptan, sumatriptan, zolmitriptan). Because the mechanisms involved in the pathogenesis of migraine are not clearly understood, the precise mechanism of action of 5-HT_1 receptor agonists in the management of migraine has yet to be established. However, current data suggest that 5-HT_1 receptor agonists, including naratriptan, may ameliorate migraine through selective constriction of certain intracranial blood vessels, inhibition of neuropeptide release, and reduced transmission in the trigeminal pain pathway.

Naratriptan is eliminated principally in urine, with approximately 50% of an administered dose excreted as unchanged drug and 30% as metabolites. In vitro, naratriptan is metabolized by a wide range of cytochrome P-450 (CYP) isoenzymes to numerous inactive metabolites.

Advice to Patients

Importance of informing clinicians of any atypical migraine symptoms.

Risk of serious cardiovascular or cerebrovascular events (e.g., myocardial infarction, stroke) or other vasospastic reactions. Importance of seeking medical care if symptoms of such reactions (e.g., shortness of breath, weakness, slurring of speech, sudden or severe abdominal pain, difficulty in seeing, or tightness, pain, pressure, or heaviness in chest, throat, jaw, or neck) occur after taking naratriptan and of *not* taking naratriptan again until evaluated by clinician.

Importance of adhering to prescribed directions for use. Provide copy of manufacturer's patient information.

Overuse of drugs indicated for the management of acute migraine attacks may exacerbate headaches; importance of recording headache frequency and drug use to monitor effectiveness of treatment.

Importance of informing clinician of existing or contemplated concomitant therapy, including prescription and OTC drugs and herbal supplements, as well as any concomitant illnesses (e.g., cardiovascular disease).

Importance of informing patients of risk of serotonin syndrome, particularly with concurrent use of naratriptan and a selective serotonin-reuptake inhibitor (SSRI) or selective serotonin- and norepinephrine-reuptake inhibitor (SNRI). Importance of seeking immediate medical attention if symptoms of serotonin syndrome develop.

Importance of women informing clinicians if they are or plan to become pregnant or plan to breast-feed.

Importance of informing patients of other important precautionary information. (See Cautions.)

Overview® (see Users Guide). For additional information on this drug until a more detailed monograph is developed and published, the manufacturer's labeling should be consulted. It is *essential* that the manufacturer's labeling be consulted for more detailed information on usual cautions, precautions, contraindications, potential drug interactions, laboratory test interferences, and acute toxicity.

Preparations

Excipients in commercially available drug preparations may have clinically important effects in some individuals; consult specific product labeling for details.

Naratriptan Hydrochloride

Oral		
Tablets, film-coated	1 mg (of naratriptan)*	Amerge®, GlaxoSmithKline
		Naratriptan Hydrochloride Tablets
	2.5 mg (of naratriptan)*	Amerge®, GlaxoSmithKline
		Naratriptan Hydrochloride Tablets

*available from one or more manufacturer, distributor, and/or repackager by generic (nonproprietary) name

Rizatriptan Benzoate

■ Rizatriptan benzoate is a selective agonist of serotonin (5-hydroxytryptamine; 5-HT) type 1B and 1D receptors ("triptan").

Uses

■ **Vascular Headaches** ***Migraine*** Rizatriptan benzoate is used for the acute treatment of attacks of migraine with or without aura in adults and pediatric patients 6–17 years of age. The manufacturer states that rizatriptan should *not* be used for the management of hemiplegic or basilar migraine or for the *prophylaxis* of migraine. Safety and efficacy have not been established for the management of cluster headaches.

The current indication for rizatriptan in adults is based principally on the results of 4 randomized, placebo-controlled studies of rizatriptan conventional tablets and 2 similarly designed studies of rizatriptan orally disintegrating tablets in adults with moderate to severe headaches. In these studies, substantially more patients receiving single doses of rizatriptan 5 or 10 mg achieved a response (mild or no headache pain) 2 hours after treatment compared with patients receiving placebo. Rizatriptan also relieved manifestations of migraine other than headache (including nausea, photophobia, and phonophobia), reduced the need for supplemental migraine therapy, and improved functional ability. Limited data from studies of up to one year's duration suggest that intermittent rizatriptan has remained effective throughout subsequent migraine attacks. Data from several comparative studies indicate that rizatriptan is at least as effective as oral sumatriptan in alleviating the pain associated with migraine 2 hours after treatment.

Efficacy of rizatriptan in pediatric patients has been established in a randomized double-blind, placebo-controlled study of the orally disintegrating tablets in pediatric patients 6–17 years of age (mean age: 13 years) with moderate to severe migraine headaches. Patients enrolled in the study had at least a 6-month history of migraine attacks with or without aura and an inadequate response to nonsteroidal anti-inflammatory agents (NSAIAs) and acetaminophen. In this study, substantially more patients receiving rizatriptan (5 mg in those weighing at least 20 kg but less than 40 kg and 10 mg in those weighing 40 kg or more) achieved a response (no headache pain) 2 hours after treatment compared with patients receiving placebo; however, the frequency of migraine-associated symptoms (i.e., nausea, photophobia, phonophobia) at 2 hours after treatment was similar in those receiving rizatriptan and those receiving placebo.

The US Headache Consortium considers 5-$HT_{1B/1D}$ receptor agonists (e.g., rizatriptan) an appropriate treatment choice for the acute management of moderate to severe migraine headaches in patients without contraindications to these drugs and recommends use of 5-$HT_{1B/1D}$ receptor agonists, dihydroergotamine, or ergotamine in patients with more severe migraine attacks as well as in patients in whom previous therapy with nonsteroidal anti-inflammatory agents or fixed-combination preparations such as acetaminophen, aspirin, and caffeine has been ineffective. For further information on management and classification of migraine headache, see Vascular Headaches: General Principles in Migraine Therapy, under Uses in Sumatriptan 28:32.28.

Dosage and Administration

■ **Administration** Rizatriptan benzoate is administered orally without regard to meals.

The rizatriptan orally disintegrating tablet is packaged in a blister in an aluminum pouch. The blister should not be removed from the aluminum pouch until just prior to administration. With dry hands, the blister package should be peeled open and the tablet placed on the tongue to dissolve and be swallowed with saliva. Administration with liquid is not necessary.

■ **Dosage** Dosage of rizatriptan benzoate is expressed in terms of rizatriptan.

Vascular Headaches **Adult Dosage.** For the acute treatment of migraine attacks with or without aura in adults, the recommended initial oral dose of rizatriptan is a single dose of 5 or 10 mg. Single oral doses of 5 or 10 mg (conventional tablets or orally disintegrating tablets) were effective in clinical studies, although the 10-mg dose may provide a greater effect than the 5-mg dose. However, the 10-mg dose also may be associated with an increased risk of adverse effects.

Although efficacy of a second dose or subsequent doses has not been established in placebo-controlled trials, if the migraine headache recurs, a second dose of rizatriptan may be administered 2 hours after the first dose. The maximum dosage administered in any 24-hour period should not exceed 30 mg. The safety of treating an average of more than 4 headaches per 30-day period has not been established.

Pediatric Dosage. For the acute treatment of migraine attacks with or without aura in pediatric patients 6–17 years of age, the recommended dose of rizatriptan is a single dose of 5 mg in patients weighing less than 40 kg or 10 mg in those weighing 40 kg or more. Efficacy and safety of more than one dose within any 24-hour period have not been established in pediatric patients.

■ **Special Populations** Dosage selection for geriatric patients should be cautious, usually starting at the low end of the dosage range, and reflect the greater frequency of decreased hepatic, renal, or cardiac function and of concomitant disease or other drug therapy in such patients.

Cautions

■ **Contraindications** Ischemic heart disease (e.g., angina pectoris, history of myocardial infarction, documented silent ischemia), coronary artery vasospasm (e.g., Prinzmetal variant angina), uncontrolled hypertension, or other serious underlying cardiovascular disease. History of stroke or transient ischemic attack, peripheral vascular disease, or ischemic bowel disease. Basilar or hemiplegic migraine. Treatment within the previous 24 hours with another 5-HT_1 receptor agonist or with an ergot alkaloid (e.g., ergotamine, dihydroergotamine, methysergide [no longer commercially available in the US]). Concurrent or recent (within 2 weeks) treatment with a monoamine oxidase-A (MAO-A) inhibitor. Known hypersensitivity to rizatriptan or any ingredient in the formulation.

■ **Warnings/Precautions** ***Careful Diagnosis of Migraine*** Rizatriptan should be used only in patients in whom a clear diagnosis of migraine has been established. If the first attack of migraine treated with rizatriptan fails to respond to the drug, the diagnosis of migraine should be reconsidered before rizatriptan is administered to treat subsequent attacks. Care should be taken to exclude other potentially serious neurologic disorders before rizatriptan is administered to patients not previously diagnosed with migraine or to patients who present with atypical symptoms.

Cardiac Effects Serious cardiac events, including acute myocardial infarction and fatal or life-threatening cardiac rhythm disturbances (e.g., ventricular tachycardia or fibrillation), have occurred within a few hours following administration of 5-HT_1 receptor agonists. Myocardial ischemia/infarction or coronary vasospasm (e.g., Prinzmetal variant angina) may occur even in patients without a history of coronary artery disease. Use of rizatriptan is contraindicated in patients with ischemic or vasospastic heart disease. (See Cautions: Contraindications.) The drug should be discontinued if disturbances in cardiac rhythm occur.

Although sensations of tightness, pain, pressure, and heaviness in the precordium, throat, neck, and jaw occur frequently following administration of 5-HT_1 receptor agonists, these sensations usually are noncardiac in origin. The manufacturer states that a cardiovascular evaluation should be performed if a cardiac origin is suspected.

Patients with multiple cardiovascular risk factors (e.g., postmenopausal women; men older than 40 years of age; patients with risk factors such as hypertension, hypercholesterolemia, smoking, obesity, diabetes, or family history of coronary artery disease) who have not previously received therapy with a 5-HT_1 receptor agonist should undergo cardiovascular evaluation prior to initiation of 5-HT_1 receptor agonist therapy. If the evaluation provides evidence of coronary artery disease or coronary artery vasospasm, the drug should not be administered. For patients with a satisfactory cardiovascular evaluation, the manufacturer states that consideration should be given to administration of the first dose in a medically supervised setting with electrocardiographic monitoring performed immediately following administration of the dose. Periodic cardiovascular evaluation is recommended for patients with risk factors for coronary artery disease who are receiving intermittent long-term therapy with 5-HT_1 receptor agonists.

For further information on the systematic approach to administering 5-HT_1 receptor agonists in patients with risk factors for the development of coronary artery disease, see Cautions: Precautions and Contraindications, in Sumatriptan 28:32.28.

Cerebrovascular Effects Cerebral or subarachnoid hemorrhage and stroke, sometimes fatal, have occurred in patients receiving 5-HT_1 receptor agonists. In a number of cases, it appears possible that the cerebrovascular event was the primary event, and the 5-HT_1 receptor agonist was administered in the mistaken belief that the patient's symptoms were caused by a migraine attack. Patients with migraine may be at increased risk for certain cerebrovascular events (e.g., stroke, hemorrhage, transient ischemic attack). Rizatriptan should be discontinued in patients experiencing a cerebrovascular event. (See Cautions: Contraindications.)

Other Cardiovascular or Vasospastic Effects Noncoronary vasospastic reactions, including peripheral vascular ischemia, GI ischemia and infarction (presenting with abdominal pain and bloody diarrhea), splenic infarction, and Raynaud's syndrome, have been reported in patients receiving 5-HT_1 receptor agonists, including rizatriptan. (See Cautions: Contraindications.) Transient or permanent blindness and partial vision loss also have been reported in patients receiving 5-HT_1 receptor agonists, although visual disorders may occur as manifestations of migraine attacks. Patients experiencing signs or symptoms suggestive of vasospastic reactions following administration of any 5-HT_1 receptor agonist should be evaluated to rule out vasospastic reactions before receiving additional doses of rizatriptan.

Substantial increases in blood pressure, including hypertensive crisis with acute impairment of organ systems, have been reported rarely following administration of 5-HT_1 receptor agonists in patients with or without a history of hypertension. (See Cautions: Contraindications.) In young, otherwise healthy, adult patients who received the maximum recommended rizatriptan dosage (10 mg every 2 hours for 3 doses), slight increases in blood pressure of approximately 2–3 mm Hg were observed.

Serotonin Syndrome Potentially life-threatening serotonin syndrome has been reported in patients receiving 5-HT_1 receptor agonists, particularly in those receiving concomitant therapy with selective serotonin-reuptake inhibitors (SSRIs) or selective serotonin- and norepinephrine-reuptake inhibitors (SNRIs). Serotonin syndrome also may occur in patients receiving 5-HT_1 receptor agonists concomitantly with MAO inhibitors or tricyclic antidepressants. Symptoms of serotonin syndrome may include mental status changes (e.g., agitation, hallucinations, coma), autonomic instability (e.g., tachycardia, labile blood pressure, hyperthermia), neuromuscular aberrations (e.g., hyperreflexia, incoordination), and/or GI symptoms (e.g., nausea, vomiting, diarrhea). If concurrent therapy with a 5-HT_1 receptor agonist and an SSRI or SNRI is clinically warranted, the patient should be observed carefully, particularly during initiation of therapy, when dosage is increased, or when another serotonergic agent is initiated. If manifestations of serotonin syndrome occur, treatment with rizatriptan and any concurrently administered serotonergic agents should be discontinued and supportive and symptomatic treatment should be initiated.

Medication Overuse Headache Excessive use of drugs indicated for the management of acute migraine attacks (e.g., use of 5-HT_1 receptor agonists, ergotamine, opiates, or certain analgesic combinations on a regular basis for 10 or more days per month) may result in migraine-like daily headaches or a marked increase in the frequency of migraine attacks. Detoxification, including withdrawal of the overused drugs; treatment of withdrawal symptoms (which often include transient worsening of headaches); and consideration of prophylactic therapy for migraine attacks may be necessary.

Sensitivity Reactions Hypersensitivity reactions (e.g., angioedema, anaphylaxis, wheezing, toxic epidermal necrolysis) have been reported in patients receiving rizatriptan.

Phenylketonuria Individuals who must restrict their intake of phenylalanine should be warned that each 5- or 10-mg Maxalt-MLT® orally disintegrating tablet contains aspartame, which is metabolized in the GI tract to provide 1.1 or 2.1 mg of phenylalanine, respectively, following oral administration. Maxalt® conventional tablets do not contain aspartame.

Generic preparations of rizatriptan also may contain aspartame; the manufacturer's prescribing information should be consulted.

Specific Populations **Pregnancy.** Category C. (See Users Guide.) The manufacturer has established a pregnancy registry to facilitate assessment of fetal outcomes in women who received rizatriptan during pregnancy. Clinicians are encouraged to report prenatal exposures to rizatriptan by calling 800-986-8999.

Lactation. Rizatriptan is distributed into milk in rats. Caution is advised if used in nursing women.

Pediatric Use. Safety and efficacy have not been established in children younger than 6 years of age. Adverse effects in pediatric patients are expected to be similar to those reported in adults.

Geriatric Use. Pharmacokinetic profile is similar to that in younger adults. Clinical studies of rizatriptan did not include sufficient numbers of patients 65 years of age and older to determine whether they respond differently than younger patients. While other clinical experience has not revealed age-related differences in response, dosage should be selected with caution in geriatric patients.

Renal Impairment. Exposure to rizatriptan is increased approximately 44% in patients undergoing hemodialysis.

Hepatic Impairment. Plasma concentrations of rizatriptan are increased approximately 30% in patients with moderate hepatic impairment. Rizatriptan has not been studied in patients with severe hepatic impairment.

■ **Common Adverse Effects** Adverse effects occurring in 2% or more of adults receiving rizatriptan and occurring more frequently with rizatriptan than with placebo include pain/pressure sensations (i.e., chest pain [tightness/pressure, heaviness], pain/tightness/pressure in neck/throat/jaw, regional pain [tightness/pressure/heaviness], pain at location not specified), asthenia/fatigue, dizziness, headache, somnolence, dry mouth, nausea, and paresthesia.

Drug Interactions

■ **Ergot Alkaloids and Other 5-HT_1 Receptor Agonists** Potential pharmacologic interaction (additive vasospastic effects) when rizatriptan is used concomitantly with ergot alkaloids (e.g., ergotamine, dihydroergotamine, methysergide [no longer commercially available in the US]) and other 5-HT_1 receptor agonists. Use within 24 hours is contraindicated.

■ **Monoamine Oxidase (MAO) Inhibitors** Potential pharmacokinetic interaction (increased systemic exposure to rizatriptan and active *N*-monodesmethyl metabolite) with MAO-A inhibitors. (See Description.) Use within 2 weeks of MAO-A inhibitor therapy is contraindicated.

■ **Metoprolol and Nadolol** Pharmacokinetic interaction is unlikely; no dosage adjustment is necessary.

■ **Oral Contraceptives** Pharmacokinetic interaction is unlikely.

■ **Propranolol** Potential pharmacokinetic interaction (increased plasma concentrations of rizatriptan). When rizatriptan and propranolol are used concomitantly in adults, the maximum recommended rizatriptan dosage is 5 mg per single dose and 3 doses (maximum total dosage of 15 mg) per 24-hour period. Pediatric patients who weigh 40 kg or more may receive a single 5-mg dose of rizatriptan concomitantly with propranolol; only one 5-mg dose should be administered in any 24-hour period. Rizatriptan and propranolol should not be used concomitantly in pediatric patients who weigh less than 40 kg.

■ **Selective Serotonin-reuptake Inhibitors and Selective Serotonin- and Norepinephrine-reuptake Inhibitors** Potential pharmacologic interaction (potentially life-threatening serotonin syndrome). If concomitant use is clinically warranted, the patient should be observed carefully, particularly during treatment initiation, when dosage is increased, or when another serotonergic agent is initiated. (See Serotonin Syndrome under Cautions: Warnings/Precautions.)

A study in healthy individuals showed no effect of paroxetine on rizatriptan's safety profile or plasma concentrations of rizatriptan and its active *N*-monodesmethyl metabolite.

Description

Rizatriptan benzoate is a selective agonist of serotonin (5-hydroxytryptamine; 5-HT) type 1B and 1D receptors. Rizatriptan is structurally and pharmacologically related to other selective 5-$HT_{1B/1D}$ receptor agonists (e.g., almotriptan, eletriptan, frovatriptan, naratriptan, sumatriptan, zolmitriptan). Because the mechanisms involved in the pathogenesis of migraine are not clearly understood, the precise mechanism of 5-HT_1 receptor agonists in the management of migraine has yet to be established. However, current data suggest that 5-HT_1 receptor agonists, including rizatriptan, may ameliorate migraine through selective constriction of certain intracranial blood vessels, inhibition of neuropeptide release, and reduced transmission in the trigeminal pain pathway.

Rizatriptan is metabolized principally via oxidative deamination by monoamine oxidase-A (MAO-A) to an inactive indole acetic acid metabolite. Other minor metabolites, including an N-monodesmethyl derivative with 5-$HT_{1B/1D}$ receptor activity similar to that of rizatriptan, have been identified. Rizatriptan is eliminated principally in urine, with approximately 14% of an administered dose excreted as unchanged drug and 51% as the indole acetic acid metabolite.

Advice to Patients

Risk of dizziness or somnolence; importance of exercising caution when driving or operating machinery.

Risk of serious cardiovascular or cerebrovascular events (e.g., myocardial infarction, stroke) or other vasospastic reactions. Importance of seeking medical care if symptoms of such reactions (e.g., shortness of breath, weakness, slurring of speech, sudden or severe abdominal pain, difficulty in seeing, or tightness, pain, pressure or heaviness in the chest, throat, neck, or jaw) occur after taking rizatriptan and of *not* taking rizatriptan again until evaluated by a clinician.

Importance of adhering to prescribed directions for use. Provide copy of manufacturer's patient information.

For patients taking rizatriptan orally disintegrating tablets, importance of not removing the blister from the outer pouch until just before administering dose; importance of opening blister pack with dry hands and of placing tablet on tongue to dissolve and be swallowed with saliva.

Importance of informing clinician of existing or contemplated concomitant therapy, including prescription and OTC drugs and herbal supplements, as well as any concomitant illnesses (e.g., cardiovascular disease).

Importance of informing patients of risk of serotonin syndrome, particularly with concurrent use of rizatriptan and a selective serotonin-reuptake inhibitor (SSRI) or selective serotonin- and norepinephrine-reuptake inhibitor (SNRI). Importance of seeking immediate medical attention if symptoms of serotonin syndrome develop.

Overuse of drugs indicated for the management of acute migraine attacks may exacerbate headaches; importance of recording headache frequency and drug use to monitor effectiveness of treatment.

Importance of informing patients with phenylketonuria that rizatriptan orally disintegrating tablets contain aspartame.

Importance of women informing clinicians if they are or plan to become pregnant or plan to breast-feed.

Importance of informing patients of other important precautionary information. (See Cautions.)

Overview® (see Users Guide). For additional information on this drug until a more detailed monograph is developed and published, the manufacturer's labeling should be consulted. It is *essential* that the manufacturer's labeling be consulted for more detailed information on usual cautions, precautions, contraindications, potential drug interactions, laboratory test interferences, and acute toxicity.

Preparations

Excipients in commercially available drug preparations may have clinically important effects in some individuals; consult specific product labeling for details.

Rizatriptan Benzoate

Oral		
Tablets, film-coated	5 mg (of rizatriptan)*	Maxalt®, Merck Rizatriptan Benzoate Tablets
	10 mg (of rizatriptan)*	Maxalt®, Merck Rizatriptan Benzoate Tablets
Tablets, orally disintegrating	5 mg (of rizatriptan)*	Maxalt®-MLT, Merck Rizatriptan Benzoate Orally Disintegrating Tablets
	10 mg (of rizatriptan)*	Maxalt®-MLT, Merck Rizatriptan Benzoate Orally Disintegrating Tablets

*available from one or more manufacturer, distributor, and/or repackager by generic (nonproprietary) name

SUMAtriptan

■ Sumatriptan is a selective agonist of vascular serotonin (5-hydroxytryptamine; 5-HT) type 1B and 1D receptors ("triptan").

Uses

■ **Vascular Headaches** Sumatriptan is used orally, by subcutaneous injection, or intranasally for the acute management of attacks of migraine with aura (also called classic migraine) or migraine without aura (also called common migraine) and by subcutaneous injection for the acute management of cluster headache episodes. Sumatriptan should be used only in patients in whom a clear diagnosis of migraine or cluster headache has been established. The manufacturers and some clinicians state that the drug is *not* to be used for the management of hemiplegic or basilar migraine or for *prophylaxis* of migraine or cluster headache. In patients with a history of migraine or cluster headache who present with atypical symptoms (e.g., ataxia, vertigo, tinnitus, mental status changes, visual field cuts/ blindness, paresthesia, hemiparesis), care should be taken to exclude other potentially serious neurologic conditions (e.g., cerebrovascular accident, subarachnoid hemorrhage) before initiation of sumatriptan therapy. (See Cautions: Precautions and Contraindications.)

General Principles in Migraine Therapy Drug therapy in the management of migraine headache must be individualized and adjusted based on the severity and frequency of attacks, response to therapy (single or multiple drugs), and tolerance to drug-induced adverse effects. Important considerations in the choice of drug therapy include the wide range in severity of the attacks, considerable interindividual variation in response and tolerance, toxic potentials of the drugs, presence of concomitant illness (e.g., cardiovascular disease, uncontrolled hypertension) or pregnancy, potential tolerance to the therapeutic effects of the drugs, the potential for abuse and misuse of the drugs, and cost. Decisions regarding drug therapy in the management of migraine headache should be weighed carefully (e.g., do the headaches threaten to disrupt the patient's normal functioning), particularly when potentially toxic, habituating, and/or potent drugs are considered. Although the benefit of therapy may principally be pain relief, the long-term goals of therapy are to prevent or reduce the frequency and severity of attacks, reduce the disability associated with migraine headaches, improve quality of life, avoid escalation of antimigraine drug therapy, and educate and enable patients to manage their illness. Management also should include appropriate nondrug therapy such as lifestyle modification, avoidance of precipitating factors, and behavioral and/or psychologic therapy. Although the pathogenesis of migraine headache has not been fully elucidated (see Pharmacology), it is known that avoidance of certain triggering factors such as alcohol (e.g., red wine), certain foods or food additives (e.g., chocolate, certain cheeses, monosodium glutamate, nitrates), irregular eating habits, irregular sleep, and acute changes in stress level as well as proper management of other factors such as travel across time zones, high-altitude barometric pressure changes, and association with the menstrual cycle may be useful in the management of migraine attacks. The possible presence of other types of headaches (e.g., tension-type, cluster) should be evaluated.

Although migraine headache is common (about 15–18% of women and 6% of men in the general population suffer migraine attacks), the condition is underrecognized and undertreated probably because of the lack of biologic markers to confirm the diagnosis. About two-thirds of patients with migraine headache experience infrequent attacks (e.g., 1 or 2 per year), with the remainder experiencing one or more migraine attacks each month. Over 80% of migraine sufferers experience some degree of headache-associated disability. For a diagnosis of migraine without aura (also called common migraine) or with aura (also called classic migraine), the criteria established by the International Headache Society (IHS) usually are used. According to IHS, migraine without aura is an idiopathic, recurring headache disorder manifested by untreated or unsuccessfully treated attacks lasting 4–72 hours and characterized by unilateral, pulsating headache of moderate to severe intensity that may disrupt routine physical activity and is associated with nausea, vomiting, photophobia, and/or phonophobia and worsens with movement; some experts also consider osmophobia a diagnostic criterion. Migraine with aura is characterized by the same manifestations as migraine without aura, but it also is accompanied before or during the attack by neurologic manifestations (e.g., visual disturbance) indicating focal cerebral cortical and/or brain stem dysfunction.

Acute Attacks. Because patients may experience a wide spectrum of severity in migraine attacks with variable effects on functioning, multiple appropriate therapies for attacks of differing severity generally are made available to the patient. The goals of acute migraine therapy are as follows: provide rapid and consistent relief of migraine attacks without recurrence; restore the patient's ability to function; minimize the use of back-up and rescue medications (i.e., drugs used at home when other therapies fail); optimize self-care and reduce subsequent use of medical resources; be cost-effective for overall management; and relieve the headache while minimizing or avoiding adverse effects of therapy. To meet these goals, some experts recommend use of selective 5-HT_1 receptor agonists, dihydroergotamine, or ergotamine in patients with moderate or severe migraine or in those with mild to moderate headaches that respond poorly to nonsteroidal anti-inflammatory agents (NSAIAs) or fixed-combination analgesics such as those containing aspirin, acetaminophen, and caffeine. Failure to promptly use an effective treatment may increase pain, disability, and the impact of the headache. Patients should be advised, however, that excessive use of some of these drugs (e.g., ergotamine [but not dihydroergotamine], opiates, selective 5-HT_1 analgesics [including fixed combinations containing butalbital, caffeine, or isometheptene]) may cause rebound headache. Medical attention (including hospitalization) may be necessary for detoxification from drug overuse or abuse. Because nausea is one of the most aversive and disabling symptoms of migraine attacks, selection of nonoral routes of administration and/or use of antiemetics is recommended in patients in whom nausea and/or vomiting are prominent early symptoms of migraine attacks. Antiemetics should not be restricted to patients who are vomiting or likely to vomit. In some patients, concomitant therapy with an antiemetic and an oral antimigraine drug may be appropriate. In addition, some experts state that IV metoclopramide may be considered as monotherapy for relief of migraine pain.

Some clinicians recommend that mild migraine headache (patient's normal activities are minimally disrupted; headache usually lasts for 4–8 hours and may be accompanied by nausea) be treated with an NSAIA (e.g., aspirin, ibuprofen, indomethacin, naproxen sodium) or combined acetaminophen, aspirin, and caffeine. In addition to these analgesics, an antiemetic (e.g., dimenhydrinate, metoclopramide, prochlorperazine), mild vasoconstrictor (e.g., isometheptene), or sedative-hypnotic may be beneficial.

For the management of moderate migraine headache (patient's normal activities are moderately disrupted; headache may last for more than 4 hours and up to about 24 hours and may be accompanied by nausea and vomiting), many clinicians recommend an oral NSAIA either given alone or in fixed combination with acetaminophen, an opiate analgesic (e.g., codeine), a barbiturate (e.g., butalbital), and/or caffeine. However, because of the risk of dependency and misuse or abuse, some clinicians recommend that use of opiate analgesics and barbiturates be reserved for patients with infrequent migraine headaches, for those who do not respond to other drugs, and when the sedative effects of the drugs will not put the patient at risk and the abuse potential has been addressed. In addition, many clinicians state that moderate migraine headache can be treated with a 5-HT_1 selective (e.g., almotriptan, frovatriptan, naratriptan, rizatriptan, sumatriptan [given orally, subcutaneously, or intranasally], zolmitriptan) or nonselective (e.g., dihydroergotamine [given parenterally or intranasally], or possibly ergotamine [given alone or in fixed combination with caffeine and/or a barbiturate]) receptor agonist. Parenteral dihydroergotamine or 5-HT_1 selective receptor agonists are particularly useful in patients with rapid onset of migraine, and parenteral and intranasal preparations of these drugs may be particularly useful in those unable to take oral drugs because of severe nausea and/or vomiting. Many moderate headaches may respond to an NSAIA alone; combinations of an NSAIA or acetaminophen with an opiate or barbiturate may be useful for attacks not responding to initial therapy or if vasoconstrictors are not tolerated. Although the role of ergotamine has been questioned (e.g., because of toxicity profile [including severe nausea and vomiting], rebound effect), some patients continue to find the drug useful, particularly when combined with an antiemetic.

For the initial management of severe migraine headache (patient's normal activities are severely disrupted; headache generally lasts for longer than 12 hours and usually is accompanied by nausea, and vomiting occasionally may occur), many clinicians recommend dihydroergotamine (given parenterally or intranasally) or a 5-HT_1 selective receptor agonist, including almotriptan (given orally), frovatriptan (given orally), naratriptan (given orally), rizatriptan (given orally), zolmitriptan (given orally), or sumatriptan (given orally, subcutaneously, or intranasally). Alternatively, a phenothiazine (e.g., chlorpromazine given IM, IV, or rectally) may be used; if pain is not relieved, a parenteral NSAIA (e.g., ketorolac given IM) or a corticosteroid (e.g., dexamethasone given IV) may be considered. *Self-administration* of rescue medications (e.g., butorphanol nasal solution, parenteral opiates) in a home setting also should be considered for patients with severe migraine attacks that do not respond adequately to other treatments once the drugs' abuse potential has been addressed. Although rescue medications often do not completely eliminate pain and return patients to normal functioning, they permit the patient to achieve relief without the discomfort and expense of an office or emergency department visit.

For the management of ultra-severe migraine attacks, including status migrainosus (patient's normal activities are severely disrupted for more than 72 hours) that are accompanied by vomiting, it is recommended that patients be rehydrated initially, which should be followed by administration of dihydroergotamine (given IV every 8 hours for 24 hours), and each dose should be preceded by a dose of metoclopramide to prevent nausea. Some clinicians state, however, that IV dihydroergotamine should be reserved for patients who do not respond to any other drug therapy, including 5-HT_1 selective receptor agonists. Alternatively, for ultra-severe migraine attacks, an IV phenothiazine (e.g., chlorpromazine, prochlorperazine) may be given alone or in combination with a parenteral corticosteroid (e.g., dexamethasone, methylprednisolone) and/or an opiate agonist (e.g., meperidine). Parenteral opiate-agonist therapy generally is considered a last resort because of the risks of dependence, tolerance, and associated adverse effects.

Prophylaxis of Chronic Attacks. Previously accepted recommendations for prophylaxis of chronic migraine attacks principally focused on patients who had 2 or more attacks per month. Such recommendations have been described by some experts as being arbitrary and as failing to account for individual patient needs or other migraine characteristics. Therefore, prophylactic therapy currently can be considered in patients with recurring migraine attacks when, in the opinion of the patient and despite acute therapy, the attacks substantially interfere with daily routines; in patients in whom the frequency of migraine attacks and resultant reliance on acute therapy would increase the potential for drug-induced (rebound) headache; in patients in whom acute therapy is ineffective, contraindicated, or not tolerated; in patients who prefer prophylactic therapy; and in those with uncommon migraine conditions, including hemiplegic migraine, basilar migraine, migraine with prolonged aura, or migrainous infarction (to prevent neurologic damage). The goals of prophylactic therapy are to decrease the frequency, severity, and duration of migraine attacks and the disability associated with such attacks; improve responsiveness of acute attacks to therapy; and improve patient functioning. For prevention of migraine headache, a β-adrenergic blocking agent (e.g., atenolol, metoprolol, nadolol, propranolol, timolol), calcium-channel blocking agent (e.g., verapamil), tricyclic antidepressant (e.g., amitriptyline), anticonvulsant (e.g., valproate sodium), high-dose riboflavin (e.g., 400 mg daily), or NSAIA (e.g., naproxen sodium) may be used. However, analysis of clinical studies in which these agents were used for prophylaxis of chronic migraine attacks has shown that efficacy and safety of individual agents, even within the same class of drugs, may exhibit substantial interpatient variation.

Although most studies of drugs used for prophylaxis of migraine attacks are limited by poor study design and/or interpretation of study findings, analysis of these studies by the US Headache Consortium suggests that drugs with medium to high efficacy, good strength of evidence, and mild to moderate adverse effects include amitriptyline, divalproex sodium, propranolol, and timolol. Comparative studies have demonstrated few clinically important differences in efficacy among these agents. Agents with lower efficacy or limited strength of clinical evidence, and mild to moderate adverse effects include aspirin (alone), atenolol, fenoprofen, flurbiprofen, fluoxetine, gabapentin, guanfacine, ketoprofen, magnesium, mefenamic acid, metoprolol, nadolol, naproxen/naproxen sodium, nimodipine, riboflavin, and verapamil. While clinical efficacy has not been established in controlled studies for bupropion, cyproheptadine, diltiazem, doxepin, fluvoxamine, ibuprofen, imipramine, mirtazepine, nortriptyline, paroxetine, protriptyline, sertraline, tiagabine, topiramate, trazodone, or venlafaxine, experts consider these agents efficacious based on consensus and clinical experience. Experts consider phenelzine to be efficacious based on consensus and clinical experience, but the drug has adverse effects that are of concern to some experts. Similarly, methysergide (no longer commercially available in the US) has medium to high efficacy for prophylaxis of migraine attacks, but its usefulness is limited by reports of retroperitoneal and retropleural fibrosis associated with long-term (principally uninterrupted) therapy. Evidence from clinical studies indicate that efficacy of agents such as acebutolol, carbamazepine, clomipramine, clonazepam, clonidine, indomethacin, lamotrigine, nabumetone, nicardipine, nifedipine, and pindolol is comparable to that of placebo for prophylaxis of migraine attacks in patients with chronic migraine.

Experts from the US Headache Consortium currently recommend that the choice of an initial agent for prophylaxis of migraine attacks be individualized, taking into account concomitant illness (e.g., stroke, myocardial infarction, Raynaud's syndrome, seizure disorder, affective or anxiety disorders). Such experts recommend use of drugs that are effective for both the concomitant illness and migraine prophylaxis whenever possible.

Some clinicians recommend that drug therapy for migraine prophylaxis be initiated as monotherapy at a low dosage and then titrated upward as tolerated to a maximum effective dosage; such therapy should be given for several months and then withdrawn slowly to prevent rebound headaches. If initial drug therapy is not effective, a combination of drugs may be used.

Selection of an agent for prophylaxis of migraine attacks in women who are or may become pregnant should take into account the teratogenic potential of such agents. If drug therapy for migraine prophylaxis is absolutely necessary, some experts state that the prophylactic agent with the lowest risk of adverse effects to the fetus should be used.

Use of Sumatriptan in Migraine Sumatriptan provides rapid relief of migraine headache and generally is well tolerated when appropriate precautions regarding patient selection are employed. (See Cautions: Precautions and Contraindications.) The drug also relieves manifestations of migraine other than headache (including nausea, vomiting, photophobia, and phonophobia), decreases the need for supplemental analgesic therapy, and improves functional ability. Few comparative studies evaluating the efficacy and safety of sumatriptan relative to other antimigraine therapies have been performed to date. However, available evidence suggests that sumatriptan is at least as effective as current therapies for migraine (e.g., ergot alkaloids, oral analgesics) and generally provides more rapid headache relief and return to normal functioning than these therapies but may be associated more frequently with headache recurrence. Although cost considerations and concerns about the potential for headache recurrence may favor the use of other antimigraine agents (e.g., dihydroergotamine) over subcutaneous sumatriptan, effective self-management of migraine through patient self-administration of sumatriptan may be cost-effective if associated with a reduced need for hospital visits. While clinical studies directly comparing subcutaneous versus oral therapy with sumatriptan in patients with migraine have not been performed, response to oral sumatriptan therapy occurs later and generally is somewhat less than that with subcutaneous therapy. Therefore, subcutaneous therapy with the drug may be particularly advantageous in patients with severe migraine headache in whom the most rapid onset of action is desirable and/or in those who have appreciable nausea and vomiting associated with migraine; oral sumatriptan therapy should be less costly and may be useful in patients who are unable to tolerate subcutaneous sumatriptan, unwilling or unable to self-administer the injection, or who have relatively less severe migraine symptoms.

The efficacy of sumatriptan in alleviating established migraine attacks does not appear to be influenced by type of migraine (i.e., with or without aura), duration of the attack, timing of the attack (e.g., early morning, menstruation-associated), concomitant use of non-ergot-alkaloid drugs for migraine prophylaxis (e.g., β-blockers, calcium-channel blockers, tricyclic antidepressants), or by patient gender or age. Unlike other antimigraine drugs (e.g., ergotamine), sumatriptan has been effective even when given late in the attack. However, subsequent doses of sumatriptan in patients not responding adequately to an initial dose generally have not provided additional benefit.

Most controlled clinical studies of sumatriptan therapy involved patients who had migraine with aura or migraine without aura as defined by criteria established by the Headache Classification Committee of the International Headache Society (IHS). However, while a clear diagnosis of migraine is recommended before initiation of sumatriptan therapy, some evidence suggests that response to sumatriptan may be similar in patients not meeting strict IHS criteria for migraine. The efficacy of therapy for migraine in controlled studies generally was evaluated in terms of a reduction in headache severity as rated by the patient (i.e., a reduction in pain from severe or moderately severe to mild or absent using a 4-point scale). In placebo-controlled clinical studies, approximately 70–88% of patients receiving a single 6-mg subcutaneous dose of sumatriptan attained relief of migraine headache within 1–2 hours compared with 18–39% of placebo recipients; at 2 hours, 48–65% of sumatriptan-treated patients were pain free. Relief of migraine headache generally begins as early as 10 minutes following subcutaneous administration of sumatriptan and is maximal at 2 hours. Smaller doses (less than 6 mg) of sumatriptan also may be effective in relieving migraine, although the proportion of patients obtaining adequate relief is reduced and the time to obtain relief is greater. Subcutaneous doses exceeding 6 mg (e.g., 8 mg) do not appear to provide additional therapeutic benefit and are associated with a greater incidence of adverse effects.

Onset of relief of migraine symptoms with oral sumatriptan therapy is slower than that with subcutaneous administration of the drug, generally occurring 0.5–3 hours after single oral doses of 25–100 mg; maximum pain relief is attained within 3–6 hours. In clinical trials, 50–73% of patients receiving sumatriptan in single oral doses of 25–300 mg obtained relief of headache pain (defined as no pain or only mild pain) within 2 hours compared with 10–33% of patients receiving placebo; 65–78% of patients receiving sumatriptan reported relief of pain at 4 hours. The proportion of patients obtaining relief from single oral doses of sumatriptan appears to be greater with doses of 50 or 100 mg than with 25 mg; however, doses of 100 mg do not appear to provide greater benefit than doses of 50 mg.

In 2 controlled clinical studies in adults with moderate to severe migraine headache, efficacy of a single oral dose of sumatriptan 85 mg given in fixed combination with naproxen sodium 500 mg was compared with that of placebo and of each drug given in the same dosage as monotherapy. In these studies, a greater proportion of patients receiving combined therapy with sumatriptan and naproxen (57–65%) obtained relief of headache pain (defined as mild or no pain) within 2 hours of treatment compared with those receiving sumatriptan alone (50–55%) or placebo (28–29%). In addition, a greater proportion of patients receiving sumatriptan and naproxen (23–25%) remained free of headache pain without the use of rescue therapy through 24 hours after treatment compared with those receiving sumatriptan or naproxen monotherapy (14–16 or 10%, respectively) or placebo (7–8%). Combined therapy with sumatriptan and naproxen also relieved manifestations of migraine other than headache (including nausea, photophobia, and phonophobia).

Since migraine is a chronic, recurrent condition, successful therapy may require long-term, intermittent use of sumatriptan. In several controlled studies of 6–24 months' duration in patients with migraine, intermittent sumatriptan has remained effective throughout subsequent attacks. Among patients receiving oral sumatriptan during 9 migraine attacks, approximately 14% of patients responded during all 9 migraine episodes, 24% responded during 8 of 9 attacks, and 62% responded during 7 of 9 attacks. Among patients in a controlled study who were treated for 4 migraine attacks (3 with subcutaneous sumatriptan and one with placebo), 73% of patients responded to therapy during all 3 sumatriptan-treated attacks, 89% responded in at least 2 of 3 such attacks, and 93% responded in at least 1 of 3 such attacks; only 7% of patients receiving sumatriptan therapy did not respond at all. Data from long-term (1 year) uncontrolled studies suggest that oral sumatriptan was effective in 82–86% of patients and in 55% of all attacks treated. Patients who received subcutaneous or oral sumatriptan treated a median of 18 and 22 attacks per year, respectively, and used a mean of 1.4 injections or 1.9 tablets per attack. The mean number of doses used was similar in patients with frequent (more than 30) and infrequent (less than 10) attacks.

Data from comparative trials suggest that sumatriptan is at least as effective as current antimigraine therapies (e.g., ergot alkaloids, oral analgesics) and generally provides more rapid headache relief than these therapies. In a double-blind, controlled study in patients with migraine, subcutaneous therapy with sumatriptan was associated with headache relief and improvement in functional ability in a greater proportion of patients than was dihydroergotamine at 1 hour (78 versus 57%, respectively) and 2 hours (85 versus 73%, respectively) following the dose; headache relief and functional ability at 3 and 4 hours were similar with both drugs. However, the rate of headache recurrence within 24 hours after treatment was approximately 2.5 times as great with sumatriptan as with dihydroergotamine (45 versus 18%, respectively). In another placebo-controlled, comparative study, 66% of patients receiving oral sumatriptan (100 mg) obtained pain relief (reduction in headache intensity from severe or moderate to mild or none) at 2 hours compared with 48% of patients receiving the combination of ergotamine tartrate 2 mg and caffeine 200 mg (Cafergot®). The onset of headache relief was more rapid with sumatriptan therapy, although more patients reported recurrence of migraine within 48 hours with sumatriptan; the incidence of adverse effects with both therapies was similar. In another controlled study in patients who treated up to 3 migraine attacks during a 3-month period either with oral sumatriptan (100 mg) or with oral aspirin (900 mg) and metoclopramide hydrochloride (10 mg), the proportion of patients who had pain relief at 2 hours during the initial attack (the primary end point) with sumatriptan versus aspirin and metoclopramide was similar (56 versus 45%, respectively), although sumatriptan was more effective than aspirin and metoclopramide during attack 2 (58 versus 36%, respectively, of patients with pain relief) and attack 3 (65 versus 34%, respectively, of patients with pain relief). In addition, sumatriptan therapy was associated with a reduced need for supplemental analgesics and greater incidence of improvement in functional ability than aspirin and metoclopramide therapy. Relief of nausea, vomiting, photophobia, and phonophobia was similar for both therapies, while the incidence of adverse effects, which usually were mild to moderate in intensity and transient, was higher with sumatriptan.

Recurrence of migraine within 24 hours after successful treatment of the initial migraine attack occurs in up to about 60% or up to about 40% of patients receiving initial therapy with subcutaneous or oral sumatriptan, respectively. The high rate of recurrent migraine with sumatriptan may be related to the short half-life of sumatriptan or the reversibility of the drug's binding to 5-HT receptors; however, in some cases, apparent repeat attacks of migraine may have been the result of breakthrough of the suppressed but ongoing original attack. Recurrent migraine has been characterized as resolution followed by return of headache within the typical 4–72 hours of a migraine attack without recurrence of aura or other premigraine symptoms. Recurrence of migraine appears to be more common with sumatriptan therapy than with ergotamine, dihydroergotamine, combined therapy with aspirin and metoclopramide, or placebo. The median time to headache recurrence has been reported to be approximately 9–13 hours in patients receiving sumatriptan subcutaneously and 14–24 hours in patients receiving the oral drug. Data from a limited number of controlled studies and clinical experience in patients treated for 3–12 episodes of migraine with oral or subcutaneous sumatriptan indicate that the incidence of migraine recurrence decreases as the number of successfully treated migraine attacks increases. An additional dose of oral sumatriptan appears to be more effective than placebo in treating recurrent migraine after successful treatment of the initial attack; 65–81% of patients receiving oral sumatriptan (100 mg) for the treatment of a recurrent headache following initial use of oral or subcutaneous sumatriptan experience relief of headache pain. However, the benefit or safety of administering a second dose of subcutaneous or oral sumatriptan in patients who have not responded to an *initial* dose has not been demonstrated conclusively in controlled studies.

While most patients with migraine respond to initial subcutaneous or oral doses of sumatriptan, some patients do not experience relief; exacerbation of migraine has been reported in a few patients. Although administration of a second subcutaneous dose of sumatriptan generally does not provide relief of ongoing migraine headache in patients not responding to an initial subcutaneous dose for that attack, data from several studies in which multiple doses of subcutaneous or oral sumatriptan were administered over several episodes of migraine indicate that patients who fail to respond to therapy for one episode may respond to sumatriptan during subsequent episodes; only 5–7% of patients are consistent nonresponders.

Data from several long-term (1–2 year) studies suggest that subcutaneous or oral therapy with sumatriptan does not alter the frequency of migraine attacks. However, some case reports and data from uncontrolled and/or post-marketing surveillance studies indicate an increased frequency of initial or recurrent migraine attacks in some patients taking sumatriptan. In some patients with a history of frequent migraines or dependence on other antimigraine drugs, such as analgesics or ergot-alkaloid-containing compounds, this increased frequency of migraine attacks has been associated with inappropriate use/misuse of the drug. (See Cautions: Precautions and Contraindications.) The contribution of sumatriptan to the increased frequency of migraine headaches in such patients has not been established.

Intranasal administration of sumatriptan is more effective than placebo in relieving migraine headache. In double-blind, controlled studies in patients with migraine, headache relief (defined as reduction in pain from moderate or severe to mild or none) at 2 hours following the dose occurred in approximately 55–75% of patients receiving intranasal sumatriptan (20 mg) versus about 25–36% of those receiving placebo; associated nausea, vomiting, photophobia, and functional disability also were improved in sumatriptan-treated patients. Smaller doses (5 or 10 mg) also may be effective, although in several studies the proportion of patients obtaining relief was reduced. Although sumatriptan has been given IV† in patients with acute migraine attacks, this route of administration has been associated with a high incidence of adverse effects (probably because of the rapid increase in plasma drug concentrations associated with such administration); the manufacturers and most clinicians state that the drug should *not* be given IV. (See Cautions: Precautions and Contraindications.)

The manufacturers state that sumatriptan is not to be used for prophylaxis of migraine headache†, and prophylactic use of the drug following successful treatment of an initial attack has produced equivocal results. In one study, routine addition of a second oral dose of sumatriptan (100 mg) 2 hours after successful treatment of the initial migraine episode did not influence the frequency or time to recurrence of subsequent attacks. However, in another study, routine administration of a single oral dose of sumatriptan (100 mg) 4 hours after successful treatment with a subcutaneous dose of the drug (6 mg) delayed recurrence of the migraine attack.

Cluster Headache Sumatriptan also is used subcutaneously for the acute management of cluster headache episodes; *oral* therapy with sumatriptan is unlikely to be beneficial because of its slower onset of action and is *not* indicated in the management of cluster headache. Cluster headache occurs principally in older men and is characterized by brief, unilateral, extremely intense headaches occurring up to 8 times daily and generally accompanied by ipsilateral manifestations of autonomic dysfunction, such as lacrimation, conjunctival injection, and rhinorrhea. Management of cluster headaches is difficult since the onset of action of many therapies often is delayed beyond the duration of the attack. Inhalation of 100% oxygen, rectal or sublingual ergotamine, or parenteral dihydroergotamine typically has been used effectively to treat cluster headache; intranasal administration of lidocaine, cocaine, or capsaicin also has been used with some success in treating acute attacks. Oral agents (e.g., ergot alkaloids, analgesics, oral sumatriptan) generally have not been effective in treating these brief headaches, as the onset of action of these drugs is too slow.

While comparative studies with oxygen and/or oral analgesic therapy have not been performed, subcutaneous sumatriptan may be particularly useful in patients with cluster headache because of its ease of administration compared with oxygen and its rapid onset of action compared with oral analgesics. In 2 placebo-controlled studies in which patients were treated for up to 3 consecutive cluster headache attacks, headache improvement (as indicated by a reduction in headache pain to mild or no pain) occurred within 15 minutes in about 75% of patients receiving subcutaneous sumatriptan (6 mg) compared with 26–35% of patients receiving placebo. Amelioration of autonomic manifestations associated with cluster headache, such as nasal congestion, rhinorrhea, lacrimation, miosis, ptosis, photophobia, and periorbital edema, also has been reported with subcutaneous sumatriptan therapy. In the 2 placebo-controlled studies, conjunctival injection persisted in 36–38 or 60–74% of patients 15 minutes after receiving subcutaneous sumatriptan or placebo, respectively. Approximately 14% of patients receiving subcutaneous sumatriptan and 38–49% of patients receiving placebo in these studies required supplemental therapy with oxygen 15 minutes after administration of the study drug. Use of higher subcutaneous doses of sumatriptan (12 mg) does not appear to increase the response rate in patients with cluster headache; in fact, lower subcutaneous doses (e.g., 3 mg) reportedly may be effective in the management of acute cluster headache episodes.

Although an increased frequency of cluster headache attacks has been reported in some patients receiving sumatriptan in uncontrolled studies, such increases in attack frequency generally have been transient (lasting up to a few weeks) and may have been related in part to withdrawal of prophylactic antimigraine medication prior to initiation of sumatriptan therapy. Limited data based on long-term (e.g., up to 3 months) experience with the drug in patients with cluster headache suggest that tolerance to the effects of sumatriptan does not develop with such use; at least one patient used a total of 480 injections (6 mg each) of the drug over an 11-month period with reportedly consistent efficacy. Sumatriptan therapy is not associated with an increase in early recurrence of cluster headache and has little effect on the incidence of subsequent episodes (i.e., those occurring from 2–24 hours after the first cluster headache). In a controlled study, prophylactic† administration of oral sumatriptan (100 mg 3 times daily for 7 days) did not reduce the number, severity, or duration of subsequent cluster headache attacks in patients who responded successfully to a single 6-mg subcutaneous dose of the drug for the first cluster attack of a series. Patients with a history of more than 2 cluster headaches per day may require prophylactic therapy in addition to the use of sumatriptan for the management of acute breakthrough cluster attacks, as 12 mg (two 6-mg injections) is the maximum recommended daily subcutaneous dose of sumatriptan.

Sumatriptan has been used with some success in a limited number of patients with chronic paroxysmal hemicrania†, a rare, variant form of cluster headache. Sumatriptan also has been used in at least one patient with short-lasting, unilateral, neuralgiform headache with conjunctival injection and tearing (SUNCT)†, a possible variant of cluster headache characterized by brief (30–60 seconds), recurrent episodes of intense pain. In this patient, sumatriptan therapy was associated with relief of pain and limited relief of accompanying manifestations (e.g., conjunctival injection, Horner's syndrome, lacrimation).

■ **Other Types of Headache** Sumatriptan has been used subcutaneously or orally in a limited number of patients with chronic tension-type headache†, acute post-traumatic (e.g., post-dural puncture) headache†, drug-induced headache† (e.g., in combination with amitriptyline and dexamethasone), or high-altitude headache†. In a limited number of patients receiving sumatriptan subcutaneously for the treatment of postdural puncture headache†, a complication of spinal anesthesia and unintentional dural puncture during attempted epidural anesthesia, the onset of pain relief and the potential for headache recurrence was similar to that reported in patients with migraine. Additional study and experience are required to elucidate the safety and efficacy of sumatriptan therapy in these conditions.

■ **Other Uses** Sumatriptan has been used in a few patients with intractable cyclic vomiting†, which appears to share some common pathogenesis to migraine, and in the management of adverse events (e.g., perioperative migraine, severe anesthesia-associated vomiting) associated with general anesthesia† in patients with a history of migraine. The safety and efficacy of sumatriptan therapy in these conditions require further evaluation.

Dosage and Administration

■ **Administration** Sumatriptan succinate is administered orally. The drug also can be administered parenterally but *only* by subcutaneous injection. Sumatriptan also can be administered intranasally. *Sumatriptan should not be given IV because of the potential risk of inducing coronary vasospasm.* (See Cautions: Precautions and Contraindications.) Sumatriptan has been administered as an iontophoretic transdermal system; however, the manufacturer voluntarily suspended marketing of the formulation because of reports of serious application site reactions. (See Cautions: Local Effects.)

The manufacturer states that tablets containing sumatriptan succinate in fixed combination with naproxen sodium may be administered without regard to meals. The fixed-combination tablets should not be split, crushed, or chewed.

Autoinjection devices are available for subcutaneous administration of sumatriptan to facilitate *self-administration* of the drug by patients for whom the commercially available doses of 4 or 6 mg are deemed appropriate. An injection pen is available for use with prefilled cartridges labeled as containing 4 or 6 mg of sumatriptan; the needles that accompany this device penetrate approximately 5–6 mm (¼ inch). In addition, a prefilled, single-use injection pen labeled as containing 6 mg of sumatriptan (also with ¼-inch projection of the needle following activation of the device) is available. Patients using these devices should be instructed to use injection sites with adequate skin and subcutaneous thickness to accommodate the length of the needle (e.g., lateral thigh, upper arm); care should be taken to avoid IM or IV administration. A prefilled needleless device for subcutaneous administration that is labeled as containing 6 mg of sumatriptan also is available; patients using this device should be instructed to use sites on the abdomen (avoiding the 2-inch area around the umbilicus) or thigh with adequate subcutaneous thickness to accommodate penetration of the injection solution into the subcutaneous space; use of administration sites on the upper arm should be avoided since the delivered dose may be suboptimal. Patients should be given adequate instructions by their clinician, as well as the written instructions supplied with the autoinjection device, before they self-administer sumatriptan injection for the first time.

The patient information provided by the manufacturer should be consulted for directions on intranasal administration of sumatriptan.

Consideration should be given to administering the *initial* dose of sumatriptan under medical supervision in patients with multiple risk factors for cardiovascular disease (e.g., postmenopausal women, men older than 40 years of age, smokers, patients with hypertension, hypercholesterolemia, obesity, diabetes mellitus, or a family history of coronary artery disease) but who have had a satisfactory cardiovascular evaluation. Electrocardiographic evaluation during the interval immediately after administration of sumatriptan should be considered in these patients since cardiac ischemia can occur in the absence of symptoms.

If a patient does not respond to the first dose of sumatriptan for a given attack, the diagnosis of migraine or cluster headache should be reconfirmed before administration of subsequent doses.

Although sumatriptan generally is effective at whatever stage of a migraine attack it is administered, it is advisable to initiate therapy with the drug as soon as possible after the onset of an attack so that the patient may experience maximum relief.

■ **Dosage** Dosage of sumatriptan succinate is expressed in terms of sumatriptan.

Subcutaneous Dosage For the symptomatic treatment of acute attacks of migraine with aura (also called classic migraine) or migraine without aura (also called common migraine) or cluster headache, the maximum single adult subcutaneous dose of sumatriptan recommended by the manufacturers is 6 mg given as a single injection. Smaller subcutaneous doses of the drug may also prove effective for the symptomatic treatment of migraine, although the proportion of patients obtaining adequate relief is decreased and the time to attain that relief is greater. In patients in whom dose-limiting adverse effects occur following a single 6-mg dose of sumatriptan, lower doses (e.g., 1–5 mg) of the drug may be given. The manufacturers state that efficacy of doses lower than 6 mg have not been established for the treatment of cluster headache; however, some patients may derive benefit from such doses (e.g., 3 mg). In patients receiving doses other than 4 or 6 mg, only the single-dose vials containing 6 mg/0.5 mL should be used to provide the desired dose.

If the patient fails to respond to an initial 6-mg subcutaneous dose of sumatriptan for the symptomatic treatment of migraine, additional subcutaneous or oral doses are unlikely to provide benefit. However, following successful treatment with an initial subcutaneous dose, a second 6-mg subcutaneous dose or additional oral doses of sumatriptan (see following section on oral dosage) may be given if manifestations of migraine recur. The manufacturers state that the maximum subcutaneous dosage of sumatriptan to be administered in any 24-hour period is 12 mg (i.e., two 6-mg injections); doses should be given at least 1 hour apart.

Oral Dosage For the management of acute migraine pain and associated symptoms, single oral sumatriptan doses of 25, 50, or 100 mg were effective in adults in clinical studies. Available evidence suggests that oral doses of 50 or 100 mg may provide greater benefit than 25 mg, but doses of 100 mg do not provide substantially greater relief than doses of 50 mg. Because individuals may vary in their response to oral sumatriptan, dosage selection should be individualized, weighing the possible benefit of higher doses with the potential for an increased risk of adverse effects. The maximum recommended single oral dose is 100 mg. If a satisfactory response has not been obtained within 2 hours following the initial dose, a second oral dose of up to 100 mg may be given. If headache recurs, additional oral doses of sumatriptan may be taken at intervals of not less than 2 hours up to a maximum oral dosage of 200 mg daily. If headache recurs following an initial *subcutaneous* dose of sumatriptan, additional *oral* doses may be given at intervals of not less than 2 hours (up to a maximum *oral* dosage of 100 mg daily). Oral sumatriptan dosages of up to 300 mg daily have been given, administered either as a single 300-mg dose or as 3 single doses of 100 mg each given at intervals of not less than 2 hours. However, while these doses generally have been well tolerated, there is no evidence that such doses afford greater relief than the recommended dose, and these high doses are associated with an increased incidence of adverse effects. The safety of treating an average of more than 4 headaches per 30-day period has not been established.

When sumatriptan is used in fixed combination with naproxen sodium for the acute management of migraine attacks in adults, the recommended dosage of sumatriptan is 85 mg (given in fixed combination with naproxen sodium 500 mg) as a single dose. Efficacy of more than 1 dose has not been established. If a second dose is administered, an interval of at least 2 hours should elapse between the first and second doses. No more than 2 doses (total sumatriptan dosage of 170 mg) should be administered in any 24-hour period. The safety of treating an average of more than 5 headaches per 30-day period has not been established.

Intranasal Dosage For the management of acute migraine pain and associated symptoms, single intranasal sumatriptan doses of 5, 10, or 20 mg were effective in adults in clinical studies, although the 20-mg dose was effective in a greater proportion of patients. Individuals vary in their response to intranasal sumatriptan, and the choice of dose in this range should be individualized, weighing the possible benefit of the 20-mg dose with the potential for an increased risk of adverse effects. A 5- or 20-mg dose is administered into one nostril using the corresponding single-use nasal spray; if a 10-mg dose is used, it is administered by spraying a 5-mg dose into each nostril. Single doses exceeding 20 mg do not provide greater benefit.

If the headache returns, the dose of intranasal sumatriptan may be repeated once after 2 hours, not to exceed 40 mg daily. The safety of treating an average of more than 4 headaches per 30-day period has not been established.

■ **Dosage in Renal and Hepatic Impairment** Although the effect of renal impairment on the pharmacokinetics of sumatriptan has not been evaluated, little clinical effect would be expected since the drug is largely inactivated metabolically.

The liver plays an important role in the presystemic clearance of orally administered sumatriptan. Accordingly, the bioavailability of sumatriptan following oral administration may be increased markedly in patients with liver disease. (See Pharmacokinetics: Elimination.) If *oral* sumatriptan therapy is considered in patients with hepatic impairment, the manufacturers state that the maximum single dose generally should not exceed 50 mg. Fixed-combination tablets containing sumatriptan 85 mg and naproxen sodium 500 mg should not be used in patients with hepatic impairment since sumatriptan dosage cannot be appropriately adjusted. Sumatriptan is contraindicated in patients with severe hepatic impairment.

Cautions

Sumatriptan generally is well tolerated when given in recommended dosage. Most adverse effects associated with sumatriptan are well defined, transient, and mild to moderate in intensity, although serious adverse events (e.g., coronary artery vasospasm, transient myocardial ischemia, myocardial infarction, ventricular tachycardia, ventricular fibrillation, stroke, subarachnoid hemorrhage) have been reported rarely. Adverse effects associated with the drug usually occur within 1 hour after subcutaneous or oral administration of sumatriptan and generally resolve within 10–30 minutes (subcutaneous) or 1 hour (oral). The incidence of adverse effects associated with sumatriptan generally remains unchanged or decreases with repeated use of the drug. However, the incidence of adverse effects appears to increase with higher than recommended doses of the drug. In addition, the overall incidence of adverse effects among patients receiving sumatriptan injection for the treatment of cluster headache is lower than that in patients being treated with the drug for migraine.

The most frequently reported adverse effects associated with subcutaneous sumatriptan succinate therapy are injection site reaction (e.g., minor pain, edema, tingling at the site of injection, stinging/burning, bruising, bleeding, transient erythema); tingling; dizziness or vertigo; sensations of warmth, heat, or burning; sensations of heaviness, pressure, or tightness; flushing; and numbness. Common adverse effects reported in patients receiving oral sumatriptan for the treatment of migraine or cluster headache include malaise or fatigue, nausea or vomiting, dizziness or vertigo, tingling, nasal discomfort, atypical sensations (e.g., sensations of warmth or cold, paresthesia), and sensations of pain, heaviness, pressure, or tightness. Since some adverse effects noted with sumatriptan therapy (e.g., nausea or gastric symptoms, tingling, photophobia, visual disturbances, headache, numbness, neck pain, drowsiness/sedation, asthenia, fatigue) also are symptoms associated with migraine attacks and/or the postdromal period, it may be difficult to distinguish the effects of underlying disease processes from drug-induced effects. The most frequently reported adverse effects associated with intranasal sumatriptan include disturbances of taste, nausea or vomiting, throat discomfort, and disease or discomfort of nasal cavity or sinuses. For adverse effects reported with sumatriptan therapy in the Cautions section, a causal relationship to the drug has not always been established. In addition, the incidence of adverse effects reported in clinical trials may not predict precisely the likelihood of encountering these effects under usual medical practice where patient characteristics and other factors differ from those prevailing in the trials.

■ Local Effects

Pooled data from controlled studies indicate that the most frequently reported adverse effect associated with subcutaneous sumatriptan succinate therapy is injection site reaction, consisting of minor pain, edema, induration, swelling, contusions, subcutaneous bleeding, stinging or tingling at the site of injection, burning, and/or transient erythema. Lipoatrophy (depression in the skin) or lipohypertrophy (enlargement or thickening of tissue) has been reported in less than 0.1% of patients receiving the drug subcutaneously. Injection site reactions occurred in 59% of patients receiving the drug by subcutaneous injection in controlled trials; in some studies, this effect occurred with less frequency in patients using a needle-based autoinjector to administer the drug. In one uncontrolled study, bruising, pain, and hemorrhage each occurred in 6–16% of patients receiving sumatriptan via a needle-based autoinjector. In studies comparing the safety and tolerability of subcutaneous administration of sumatriptan using a needleless device versus needle-based injection, local reactions (minor bleeding, swelling, erythema, and bruising at the administration site) occurred more frequently immediately after administration via the needleless system; however, most such reactions resolved spontaneously and differences between the 2 administration techniques had largely disappeared by 8 hours (for bleeding and bruising) or 24 hours (for swelling and erythema) after the dose.

Nasal and/or throat irritation were reported in approximately 5% of patients receiving 5-, 10-, or 20-mg doses of intranasal sumatriptan on 1 or 2 occasions in controlled clinical studies. Transient irritative symptoms (e.g., burning, numbness, paresthesia, discharge, pain or soreness) were reported to be severe in about 1% of patients receiving intranasal sumatriptan; these symptoms generally resolved in less than 2 hours. Limited examination of the nose and throat did not reveal clinically noticeable injury in these patients. In addition, an increased incidence of local irritation has not been observed in patients receiving intranasal sumatriptan repeatedly for up to 1 year. However, epithelial hyperplasia (with and without keratinization) and squamous metaplasia were observed in the larynx of rats receiving inhaled sumatriptan daily for 1 month at dosages as low as one-half the maximum daily human exposure (based on dose per surface area of nasal cavity). In addition, evidence of epithelial hyperplasia, focal squamous metaplasia, granulomata, bronchitis, and fibrosing alveolitis was observed in the respiratory and nasal mucosa in dogs administered various formulations of sumatriptan by intranasal instillation daily for up to 13 weeks, at exposure rates of 2–4 times the maximum daily human exposure (based on dose per surface area of nasal cavity). The changes observed in both species are not considered to be signs of preneoplastic or neoplastic transformation. Local effects on nasal and respiratory tissues after chronic, repeated intranasal administration of sumatriptan have not been studied in animals or humans.

Burns and scarring have been reported at the application site of sumatriptan iontophoretic transdermal system (Zecuity®). Reactions have included severe erythema, cracked skin, blistering or welts, burns or scars, skin discoloration, severe pain, pruritus, and burning sensation. Although many cases resolved within hours to weeks, some reactions, typically skin discoloration, were unresolved after several months. Because of these serious application site reactions, the manufacturer voluntarily suspended marketing of the formulation.

■ Nervous System Effects

Atypical sensations are the most commonly reported adverse nervous system effects of sumatriptan, occurring in up to 42% of patients receiving sumatriptan in controlled trials. Atypical sensations include sensations of warmth, heat, burning, cold, tingling, or numbness; paresthesia; pressure sensation or feelings of heaviness or tightness; and/or strange feeling. The incidence of these sensations varies, ranging from 0.4–14% of patients receiving sumatriptan.

Although sumatriptan distributes poorly into the CNS, adverse CNS effects have been reported in patients receiving the drug. Dizziness/vertigo has been reported in up to 12% of patients receiving subcutaneous sumatriptan in clinical trials. In addition, agitation, anxiety, drowsiness/sedation, headache, and malaise/fatigue have been reported in up to 3% of patients receiving sumatriptan in controlled trials. Severe rebound migraine headache, which occurred upon withdrawal of sumatriptan therapy and persisted for a few days, has been reported in several patients inappropriately taking sumatriptan on a daily basis for headache prophylaxis. Other adverse nervous system effects occurring in up to 1% of patients receiving sumatriptan therapy include aggressiveness, apathy, bradylogia, chills, cluster headache, confusion, depression, detachment, difficulties in concentration,disturbance of smell, drug abuse, dysarthria, dysesthesia, dysphoria, dystonia, emotional disturbance, euphoria, facial pain, facial paralysis, hallucinations, heat sensitivity, hyperesthesia, hysteria, incoordination, increased alertness, increased intracranial pressure, intoxication, lacrimation, memory disturbance, monoplegia/diplegia, motor dysfunction, myoclonia, neuralgia, neurotic disorders, panic disorder, paralysis, personality change, phobia, phonophobia/photophobia, psychomotor disorders, radiculopathy, restlessness, rigidity, seizures, sensations of lightness, "serotonin agonist effect" or serotonin syndrome, shivering, sleep disturbance, stress, suicide, syncope, transient hemiplegia, tremor, twitching, unsteadiness, speech disturbance, voice disturbance, and yawning. Although some patients who experienced seizures had a history of seizures or conditions predisposing to seizures, other patients had no apparent predisposing factors.

■ Cardiovascular Effects

The most common adverse cardiovascular effect associated with subcutaneous administration of sumatriptan is flushing, which has been reported in 7% of patients receiving the drug by this route in placebo-controlled trials. Flushing has been reported infrequently in patients receiving the drug intranasally or orally. Chest discomfort/pain, pressure, or tightness occurred in up to 5% of patients receiving subcutaneous sumatriptan in controlled trials; these adverse effects have been reported in up to 2% of patients receiving intranasal or oral sumatriptan. In patients experiencing chest pain while receiving subcutaneous sumatriptan therapy, onset of pain was within 1–60 minutes after injection of the drug, and the duration of chest pain was 2 minutes to 12 hours. In some patients, chest pain was severe and accompanied by other manifestations such as paresthesia or numbness; nausea; syncope; flushing; anxiety; diaphoresis; pain radiating into shoulders, neck, or throat; dyspnea; palpitation; bronchospasm; decreases in heart rate and blood pressure; and fatigue. Several patients receiving subcutaneous sumatriptan in controlled trials experienced chest pain/pressure and paresthesia that was severe enough to necessitate discontinuance of the drug; upon rechallenge, some patients developed similar reactions.

Chest, jaw, throat, and/or neck tightness, pain, pressure, and heaviness are relatively common in patients receiving subcutaneous sumatriptan and have been reported following use of oral or intranasal sumatriptan, but usually are noncardiac in origin. Data from patients who participated in clinical trials with subcutaneous or oral sumatriptan indicate that 8 of more than 1900 patients receiving subcutaneous sumatriptan and 2 of 6348 patients receiving the drug orally may have developed coronary vasospasm shortly after receiving the drug. In addition, data from patients who participated in clinical trials with intranasal sumatriptan indicate that 1 of approximately 4000 patients receiving the drug experienced asymptomatic subendocardial infarction, possibly secondary to coronary vasospasm. Coronary vasospasm may result in myocardial ischemia or infarction or Prinzmetal variant angina. Serious adverse cardiac effects reported within a few hours following administration of subcutaneous or oral sumatriptan include acute myocardial infarction, life-threatening or fatal disturbances of cardiac rhythm, and death. Cardiac arrhythmias/ECG abnormalities associated with chest pain, coronary artery disease, or myocardial ischemia in patients receiving sumatriptan include ST-wave changes, ventricular fibrillation or tachycardia, abnormal T waves, abnormal Q waves, and sinus bradycardia or atrial fibrillation. Some of these events occurred in patients without known coronary artery disease and may represent sequelae of coronary artery vasospasm. Sumatriptan may cause coronary artery vasospasm even in patients without a history of coronary artery disease.

Other arrhythmias or ECG abnormalities reported infrequently in patients receiving sumatriptan therapy include bradycardia, tachycardia, nonspecific ST or T wave changes, prolongation of PR or QT_c intervals, abnormal P waves with nodal rhythm, QRS/T-axis deviations, nonsustained ventricular premature complexes, isolated junctional ectopic beats, atrial ectopic beats, and delayed activation of the right ventricle.

Transient increases in systolic and/or diastolic blood pressure have been observed in patients receiving sumatriptan. Increases of 2–6 mm Hg in diastolic pressure have been noted after oral administration of the drug in some but not in other studies. Increases or decreases in blood pressure have been reported in up to 1% of patients receiving subcutaneous sumatriptan; hypertensive episodes, including hypertensive crises, have occurred on rare occasions in patients with or without a history of hypertension who were receiving the drug.

Other adverse cardiovascular effects reported in up to 1% of patients receiving sumatriptan include edema, abdominal aortic aneurysm, angina, atherosclerosis, cardiomyopathy, cerebral ischemia, cerebrovascular lesion, heart block, increased heart rate, pallor, palpitation, peripheral cyanosis, phlebitis, pulmonary embolism, pulsating sensations, Raynaud's syndrome, retinal artery occlusion, syncope, temporal arteritis, thrombosis, transient myocardial ischemia, and vasodilation.

Impairment or death attributed to stroke, cerebral hemorrhage, cerebral infarction, CNS vasculitis, subarachnoid hemorrhage, and other cerebrovascular events have been reported in patients treated with oral or subcutaneous sumatriptan. In some of these patients, sumatriptan was used to treat severe, atypical headaches thought to be migraine but actually secondary to an evolving neurologic lesion (e.g., cerebrovascular accident, subarachnoid hemorrhage). Patients with migraine may be at increased risk for the development of certain cerebrovascular events (e.g., stroke, hemorrhage, transient ischemic attack, aphasia, or hemiparesis).

■ **GI Effects** Dysgeusia/taste disturbance has occurred in approximately 14–25% of patients receiving intranasal sumatriptan compared with 1.7% of those receiving placebo in controlled trials. Dysgeusia/taste disturbance also has been reported with oral sumatriptan therapy; this adverse effect appears to be minimized with the currently available film-coated tablets. In addition, nausea and vomiting have been reported in up to 14% of patients receiving sumatriptan for the treatment of migraine. The incidence of nausea and vomiting was greater among patients receiving the drug subcutaneously for cluster headache than for the treatment of migraine. However, nausea and vomiting also are symptoms associated with migraine attacks and/or the postdromal period, and it may be difficult to distinguish the effects of underlying disease processes from drug-induced effects.

Other adverse GI effects reported in up to 5% of patients receiving sumatriptan include abdominal discomfort, abdominal distention, colitis or ischemic colitis, constipation, dental pain, diarrhea, dyspeptic symptoms, dysphagia, flatulence/eructation, gallstone, gastric symptoms (e.g., pain, pressure), gastritis, gastroenteritis, gastroesophageal reflux, GI hemorrhage, hematemesis, hypersalivation, intestinal obstruction, jaw discomfort, melena, orolingual disorders (e.g., burning or numbness of tongue, discomfort, swallowing disorders, dry mouth), oral itching and irritation, pancreatitis, peptic ulcer, rectal bleeding, retching, salivary gland swelling, and xerostomia. Changes in esophageal motility also have been reported in patients receiving high doses (16 mg) of subcutaneous sumatriptan, and some clinicians suggest that chest pain occurring in the absence of cardiac manifestations may be related to changes in esophageal motility. (See Pharmacology: Other Effects.)

■ **Musculoskeletal Effects** Neck pain/stiffness and weakness have been reported in up to 5% of patients receiving sumatriptan in controlled trials. Neck stiffness was severe enough in at least one patient receiving the drug to necessitate discontinuance. Myalgia has been reported in up to 2% of patients receiving sumatriptan in controlled clinical trials.

Other adverse musculoskeletal effects reported in patients receiving sumatriptan include acquired musculoskeletal deformity, arthritis, articular rheumatitis, backache, swelling of the extremities, intervertebral disc disorder, muscle atrophy, muscle cramps, muscle stiffness, muscle tightness, the need to flex calf muscles, muscle tiredness/rigidity, muscle weakness, musculoskeletal inflammation, tetany, difficulty walking, and various joint disturbances (e.g., arthralgia, edema, pain, stiffness).

■ **Dermatologic and Sensitivity Reactions** Hypersensitivity reactions, including allergic vasculitis, rash, urticaria, pruritus, erythema, wheal and flare at injection site, shortness of breath, angioedema, hypertension, increased heart rate, pallor, hyperventilation, diaphoresis, shock, and anaphylaxis or anaphylactoid reactions have occurred rarely in patients receiving sumatriptan. Hypersensitivity reactions to sumatriptan can be life-threatening or fatal. At least one patient receiving subcutaneous sumatriptan in a controlled trial discontinued therapy as a result of moderate urticaria; this patient also had a history of intolerance to ergotamine. In general, hypersensitivity reactions are more likely to occur in individuals with a history of sensitivity to multiple allergens.

Other adverse dermatologic or sensitivity reactions associated with sumatriptan include dry/scaly skin, eczema, exacerbation of sunburn, peeling of skin, photosensitivity, seborrheic dermatitis, skin eruptions, nodules, skin tenderness, tightness/wrinkling of skin, sweating, and facial swelling.

■ **Respiratory Effects** Discomfort of the nasal cavity/sinuses or throat has been reported in up to 4% of patients receiving sumatriptan in controlled trials; several of these patients discontinued therapy after moderate to severe throat tightness/discomfort. Dyspnea or hyperventilation has been reported in up to 1% of patients receiving sumatriptan. Upon rechallenge, some patients again experienced dyspnea. Bronchospasm has been reported in at least 1% of patients with or without a history of asthma receiving sumatriptan; the incidence of bronchospasm among patients with cluster headaches appears to be greater than the incidence among those with migraine receiving the drug subcutaneously. Influenza, diseases of the upper and lower respiratory tract, hiccups, asthma, bronchitis, and cough have been reported in up to 1% of patients receiving sumatriptan.

■ **Renal and Genitourinary Effects** Adverse renal effects reported in up to 1% of patients receiving sumatriptan include acute renal failure, bladder inflammation, dysuria, hematuria, increased urination, micturition disorders, urethritis, urinary infections, and urinary frequency.

Adverse genitourinary effects reported in up to 1% of patients receiving sumatriptan include abnormal menstrual cycle, abortion, disorders of the breast (e.g., tenderness, nipple discharge,) dysmenorrhea, endometriosis, inflammation of fallopian tubes, intermenstrual bleeding, and menstruation or menstrual cycle symptoms.

■ **Ocular Effects** Vision alteration/disturbance, ocular irritation, accommodation disorders, conjunctivitis, disorders of sclera, external ocular muscle disorders, keratitis, lacrimation, blindness/low vision, miosis, mydriasis, and ocular edema, hemorrhage, itching, pain, or swelling have been reported in up to 1% of patients receiving sumatriptan in clinical studies. In addition, ischemic optic neuropathy, retinal artery occlusion, retinal vein thrombosis, and vision loss have been reported during postmarketing surveillance. Transient or permanent blindness and substantial partial vision loss have been reported very rarely with sumatriptan use. (Vision disorders also may be part of a migraine attack.)

Corneal opacities and defects in the corneal epithelium have been noted in dogs receiving sumatriptan. Defects in the corneal epithelium were evident in a 60-week study. Corneal opacities were noted after 1 month of treatment in dogs receiving oral sumatriptan 2 mg/kg daily (representing about 5, 22, or 3 times the human exposure after a 100-mg oral, 20-mg intranasal, or 6-mg subcutaneous dose, respectively). Changes in corneal appearance were evident in dogs receiving intranasal sumatriptan on the first day of dosing and at a dosage representing 0.5 or 2 times the human exposure after a 100-mg oral or 20-mg intranasal dose, respectively, on a mg/m² basis. Results of studies in rats given a single subcutaneous (0.5 mg/kg) dose of radiolabeled sumatriptan suggest that sumatriptan and its metabolites bind to melanin in the eye (as indicated by an ocular elimination half-life of 15 days); the clinical importance of this binding is unknown.

■ **Otic Effects** Adverse otic effects reported in up to 1% of patients receiving sumatriptan include ear infection, external otitis, feeling of fullness in the ears, hearing disturbances (e.g., increased sensitivity to noise, hearing loss), Ménière's disease, otalgia, and tinnitus. In addition, deafness has been reported during postmarketing surveillance.

■ **Endocrine and Metabolic Effects** Adverse endocrine and metabolic effects reported in up to 1% of patients receiving sumatriptan in clinical studies include elevations in thyrotropin (TSH), endocrine cysts, lumps, or masses, fluid disturbances (e.g., retention), galactorrhea, hyperglycemia, hypoglycemia, hypothyroidism, thirst, hunger, increased/decreased appetite, and weight gain/loss.

■ **Hematologic Effects** Anemia, elevated platelet count and lymphadenopathy, have been reported in up to 1% of patients receiving sumatriptan. In addition, hemolytic anemia, pancytopenia, and thrombocytopenia have been reported during postmarketing surveillance.

■ **Other Adverse Effects** Other adverse effects reported in up to 1% of patients receiving sumatriptan include diaphoresis, fever, overdose, and pituitary neoplasm.

■ **Precautions and Contraindications** Because sumatriptan rarely can cause potentially serious or life-threatening adverse effects, the manufacturers caution that the drug should be used subcutaneously only in patients in whom a clear diagnosis of migraine or cluster headache has been established, and the drug should be used orally or intranasally only in patients with a clear diagnosis of migraine. If the first attack of migraine treated with sumatriptan fails to respond to the drug, the diagnosis of migraine should be reconsidered before sumatriptan is administered to treat subsequent attacks. In patients not previously diagnosed with migraine attacks and in those with a history of migraine or cluster headache who present with atypical symptoms, care should be taken to exclude other potentially serious neurologic conditions (e.g., cerebrovascular accident, subarachnoid hemorrhage) before initiation of sumatriptan therapy. Patients with a history of migraine may be at increased risk of certain cerebrovascular events (e.g., stroke, hemorrhage, transient ischemic attack).

Patients should be cautioned about potential misuse (e.g., for prophylaxis) of sumatriptan for vascular headache. Patients also should be cautioned against frequent use/misuse of sumatriptan, since abuse of sumatriptan has resulted in rebound headache in patients with a history of analgesic or ergot alkaloid abuse. Patients should be encouraged to record headache frequency and drug use so that the effectiveness of treatment may be monitored. Excessive use of drugs indicated for the management of acute migraine attacks (e.g., use of 5-HT_1 receptor agonists, ergotamine, opiates, or certain analgesic combinations on a regular basis for 10 or more days per month) may result in migraine-like daily headaches or a marked increase in the frequency of migraine attacks. Detoxification, including withdrawal of the overused drugs; treatment of withdrawal symptoms (which often include transient worsening of headaches); and consideration of prophylactic therapy for migraine attacks may be necessary.

Because sumatriptan can cause somnolence and dizziness, patients should be advised to avoid performing hazardous activities that require mental alertness (e.g., operating machinery, driving a motor vehicle) if such effects occur.

Because there have been rare reports of seizure following administration of sumatriptan, the drug should be used with caution in patients with a history of seizure disorders or conditions associated with a lowered seizure threshold.

Because substantial increases in blood pressure, including hypertensive crisis with acute impairment of organ systems, have been reported rarely in patients with or without a history of hypertension, sumatriptan is contraindicated in patients with uncontrolled hypertension. Sumatriptan should be used with caution in patients with controlled hypertension, and blood pressure should be monitored in all patients receiving the drug.

Sumatriptan should be used with caution in patients with diseases that may alter the absorption, metabolism, or excretion of the drug, such as impaired renal or hepatic function. (See Dosage and Administration: Dosage in Renal and Hepatic Impairment.)

When sumatriptan is used in fixed combination with naproxen sodium, the cautions, precautions, and contraindications associated with naproxen must be considered in addition to those associated with sumatriptan.

Cases of potentially life-threatening serotonin syndrome have been reported in patients receiving 5-HT_1 receptor agonists, particularly in those receiving concomitant therapy with selective serotonin-reuptake inhibitors (SSRIs) or selective serotonin- and norepinephrine-reuptake inhibitors (SNRIs). Serotonin syndrome also may occur in patients receiving 5-HT_1 receptor agonists concomitantly with monoamine oxidase (MAO) inhibitors or tricyclic antidepressants. Symptoms of serotonin syndrome may include mental status changes (e.g., agitation, hallucinations, coma), autonomic instability (e.g., tachycardia, labile blood pressure, hyperthermia), neuromuscular aberrations (e.g., hyperreflexia, incoordination), and/or GI symptoms (e.g., nausea, vomiting, diarrhea). If concurrent therapy with a 5-HT_1 receptor agonist and an SSRI or SNRI is clinically warranted, the patient should be observed carefully, particularly during initiation of therapy, when dosage is increased, or when another serotonergic agent is initiated. (See Drug Interactions: Selective Serotonin-reuptake Inhibitors and Selective Serotonin- and Norepinephrine-reuptake Inhibitors.) If manifestations of serotonin syndrome occur, treatment with sumatriptan and any concurrently administered serotonergic agents should be discontinued and supportive and symptomatic treatment should be initiated. Patients receiving sumatriptan should be cautioned about the risk of serotonin syndrome, particularly with concomitant use of SSRIs, SNRIs, MAO inhibitors, or tricyclic antidepressants, and they should be instructed to report symptoms suggestive of serotonin syndrome to their clinician immediately.

Because sumatriptan has the potential to cause vasospasm, the drug is contraindicated in patients with ischemic heart disease (angina pectoris, history of myocardial infarction, or documented silent ischemia), coronary artery vasospasm (e.g., Prinzmetal variant angina), history of stroke or transient ischemic attack, peripheral vascular disease, or ischemic bowel disease. Patients who experience signs or symptoms suggestive of angina following sumatriptan administration should be evaluated for the presence of coronary artery disease or a predisposition to Prinzmetal variant angina before receiving additional doses of the drug and should be monitored electrocardiographically if dosing is resumed and similar symptoms recur. Similarly, patients who experience symptoms or signs suggestive of noncoronary vasospastic reactions (e.g., manifestations of peripheral vascular ischemia, GI vascular ischemia or infarction, splenic infarction, or Raynaud's syndrome) following administration of any 5-HT_1 receptor agonist should be evaluated to rule out vasospastic reactions before receiving additional doses of sumatriptan. Although sensations of tightness, pain, pressure, and heaviness in the precordium, throat, neck, and jaw commonly occur after administration of sumatriptan, these sensations usually are noncardiac in origin; however, a cardiac evaluation should be performed if the patient is at high cardiac risk. Patients receiving sumatriptan should be advised of the importance of seeking medical care if symptoms of vasospastic reactions (e.g., shortness of breath; weakness; slurring of speech; sudden or severe abdominal pain; difficulty in seeing; tightness, pain, pressure, or heaviness in the chest, throat, neck, or jaw) occur following administration of sumatriptan and to *not* take sumatriptan again until they are evaluated by a clinician.

Patients with multiple cardiovascular risk factors (e.g., postmenopausal women; men older than 40 years of age; patients with risk factors such as hypertension, hypercholesterolemia, obesity, diabetes, smoking, or family history of coronary artery disease) who have not previously received therapy with a 5-HT_1 receptor agonist should undergo cardiovascular evaluation prior to initiation of sumatriptan therapy. (In addition to these recognized risk factors contributing to the development of coronary vasospasm, history of migraine also may be a possible risk factor in that migraine may be part of a generalized vasospastic disorder predisposing to the development of cardiomyopathy.) If the cardiovascular evaluation provides evidence of coronary artery disease or coronary artery vasospasm, the drug should not be administered. For patients with risk factors for coronary artery disease who nevertheless have completed a satisfactory cardiovascular evaluation, consideration should be given to administering the initial dose of sumatriptan under medical supervision (e.g., in the clinician's office). Because myocardial ischemia can occur in the absence of clinical symptoms, clinicians should consider obtaining an ECG immediately following the initial dose of sumatriptan in these patients. Patients with risk factors for the development of coronary artery disease should undergo periodic cardiovascular evaluation while receiving intermittent long-term sumatriptan therapy. If symptoms of angina occur after sumatriptan administration, electrocardiographic evaluation should be used to identify possible ischemic changes associated with coronary artery disease or a predisposition to Prinzmetal variant angina before sumatriptan therapy is continued. IV nitroglycerin has been shown to reverse mild coronary artery vasoconstriction that was associated with subcutaneous sumatriptan therapy in patients with suspected coronary artery disease.

Because the incidence of adverse effects and the risk of precipitating coronary vasospasm increases with IV administration, sumatriptan should *not* be administered IV.

If life-threatening disturbances of cardiac rhythm (e.g., ventricular tachycardia or fibrillation) occur, therapy with sumatriptan should be discontinued. Sumatriptan is contraindicated in patients with Wolff-Parkinson-White syndrome or arrhythmias associated with other cardiac accessory conduction pathway disorders.

Concomitant use of sumatriptan and MAO-A inhibitor therapy or use of sumatriptan within 2 weeks of discontinuance of MAO-A inhibitor therapy is contraindicated because of the potential of these drugs to substantially increase systemic exposure to sumatriptan. (See Drug Interactions: Monoamine Oxidase Inhibitors.) In addition, use of sumatriptan within 24 hours of treatment with ergot alkaloids (e.g., ergotamine, dihydroergotamine, methysergide [no longer commercially available in the US]) or another 5-HT_1 receptor agonist is contraindicated. (See Drug Interactions: Ergot Alkaloids.)

Sumatriptan is contraindicated in patients with hemiplegic or basilar migraine.

Sumatriptan also is contraindicated in patients with severe hepatic impairment and/or known hypersensitivity to sumatriptan or any of its components. Patients should be advised to discontinue use of sumatriptan and contact their clinician immediately if they experience symptoms suggestive of hypersensitivity to the drug, such as shortness of breath, wheezing, palpitations, swelling of the eyelids, face or lips, rash, or urticaria.

■ **Pediatric Precautions** The manufacturers state that safety and efficacy of sumatriptan in those younger than 18 years of age have not been established.

Available data from placebo-controlled clinical trials have failed to establish the efficacy of oral sumatriptan (25–100 mg) or intranasal sumatriptan (5–20 mg) for the treatment of migraine in adolescents 12–17 years of age†. Adverse effects observed in adolescents who received sumatriptan in clinical trials were similar in nature to those reported in clinical trials in adults; the incidence of all adverse effects in adolescents appears to be both dose and age dependent, with younger patients reporting adverse effects more commonly than older adolescents. Serious adverse effects, including effects similar in nature to those rarely reported in adults (including stroke, loss of vision, and death), have been reported during postmarketing surveillance in children following use of sumatriptan. Myocardial infarction reportedly occurred in one 14-year-old boy within 1 day of receiving oral sumatriptan. Because there are insufficient data to determine the incidence of serious adverse effects in pediatric patients receiving sumatriptan, use of the drug in patients younger than 18 years of age is not recommended by the manufacturers.

■ **Geriatric Precautions** Clinical trials of sumatriptan injection did not include sufficient numbers of patients 65 years of age and older to determine whether geriatric patients respond differently than younger adults. While other clinical experience has not revealed age-related differences in response, dosage selection generally should be cautious in geriatric patients, usually starting at the low end of the dosage range. The greater frequency of decreased hepatic, renal, and/or cardiac function and of concomitant disease and drug therapy observed in the elderly also should be considered. Increases in blood pressure may be more pronounced in geriatric patients than in younger adults. Because advanced age is a risk factor for coronary artery disease, geriatric patients with additional cardiovascular risk factors should undergo a cardiovascular evaluation prior to receiving sumatriptan. (See Cautions: Precautions and Contraindications.)

■ **Mutagenicity and Carcinogenicity** Sumatriptan did not exhibit evidence of mutagenicity in vitro in gene mutation assays (i.e., the Ames microbial mutagen test and the V-79/HGPRT assay in Chinese hamster cells) with or without metabolic activation. No increase in chromosomal aberrations was observed in the in vitro human lymphocyte assay or in the in vivo rat micronucleus assay.

No evidence of carcinogenicity was demonstrated in a 78-week study in mice given oral sumatriptan dosages representing up to 40 or 110 times, respectively, the exposure in humans receiving the maximum recommended single dose of 100 mg orally or 6 mg subcutaneously. In addition, no evidence of carcinogenicity was seen in rats given dosages representing 15 or 260 times, respectively, the exposure in humans receiving the maximum recommended single dose of 100 mg orally or 6 mg subcutaneously on a mg/m^2 basis for 104 weeks.

■ **Pregnancy, Fertility, and Lactation** There are no adequate and well-controlled studies evaluating the use of sumatriptan in pregnant women. Although a causal relationship to the drug has not been definitely established, agenesis of the corpus callosum has been reported in an infant whose mother received oral sumatriptan at week 4 and 6 of pregnancy. Sumatriptan should be used during pregnancy only if the potential benefit justifies the risk to the fetus.

Sumatriptan has been associated with fetal abnormalities and embryo and fetal mortality in animals. Embryolethality was noted in pregnant rabbits given IV sumatriptan throughout the period of organogenesis in daily doses at or close to those producing maternal toxicity, representing systemic exposures less than the maximum recommended daily subcutaneous dosage in humans of 12 mg (on a mg/m² basis). The mechanism of the embryolethality is not known. This effect was not seen in pregnant rats given IV sumatriptan throughout organogenesis at dosages representing approximately 10 times the maximum recommended daily subcutaneous human dosage of 12 mg (on a mg/m² basis) or in pregnant rats given subcutaneous sumatriptan prior to and throughout pregnancy. In pregnant rabbits, oral sumatriptan dosages of 100 mg/kg daily (representing 18 times the maximum single human oral dose of 100 mg on a mg/m² basis) throughout the period of organogenesis produced embryolethality and maternotoxicity; these effects were not observed at oral sumatriptan dosages of 50 mg/kg daily. No fetal effects were observed in rats receiving 50 mg/kg daily (representing 5 times the maximum single oral human dose of 100 mg on a mg/m² basis).

Sumatriptan has been shown to be teratogenic in pregnant rats given long-term oral sumatriptan dosages of 500 mg/kg daily (representing 50 times the maximum single human oral dose of 100 mg on a mg/m² basis); an increased incidence of a syndrome of malformations (short tail/short body and vertebral disorganization) was observed in these animals. Sumatriptan was associated with an increased incidence of cervicothoracic vascular defects and skeletal abnormalities in fetuses of rabbits receiving oral dosages greater than 15 mg/kg daily (representing 3 times the maximum single human oral dose of 100 mg on a mg/m² basis); these effects were not observed at lower dosages. Blood vessel abnormalities (cervicothoracic and umbilical) occurred in offspring of pregnant rats given oral dosages of 250 mg/kg daily or greater (representing 25 times the maximum single human oral dose of 100 mg on a mg/m² basis); these effects were not observed at oral dosages of approximately 60 mg/kg daily or less (representing 6 times the maximum single human oral dose of 100 mg on a mg/m² basis). In a study in rats dosed daily with subcutaneous sumatriptan prior to and throughout pregnancy, there was no evidence of teratogenicity.

Oral sumatriptan produced a decrease in pup survival between birth and postnatal day 4 when administered to pregnant rats at dosages of 250 mg/kg daily or higher (representing 25 times the maximum single human oral dose of 100 mg on a mg/m² basis) during the period of organogenesis; pups were not affected when dams were given 60 mg/kg daily (representing 6 times the maximum single human dose of 100 mg on a mg/m² basis). In rats given oral dosages of 1000 mg/kg daily (representing 100 times the maximum single human oral dose of 100 mg on a mg/m² basis) from gestational day 17 through postnatal day 21, decreased pup survival was found at postnatal days 2, 4, and 20; pups were not affected when dams were given 100 mg/kg of sumatriptan daily.

Reproduction studies in rats given subcutaneous sumatriptan at a dosage representing 100 times the maximum recommended single subcutaneous human dose of 6 mg (on a mg/m² basis) prior to and during the mating period have shown no evidence of impaired fertility. However, similar reproduction studies in rats given oral dosages of 50 and 500 mg/kg daily prior to and during mating revealed evidence of drug-induced decreases in mating ability; no effects on fertility were observed at oral doses representing half the maximum recommended single oral dose of 100 mg or 8 times the maximum recommended single subcutaneous dose of 6 mg in humans (on a mg/m² basis). Whether mating impairment is related to sumatriptan in females or males has not been determined.

Sumatriptan is distributed into breast milk following administration of the drug to lactating animals or nursing women. (See Pharmacokinetics: Distribution.) Some manufacturers state that caution is advised when sumatriptan is administered to nursing women. It has been suggested that exposure of the infant to the limited amount of drug distributed into milk following a single 6-mg subcutaneous dose could be minimized by expressing and discarding all milk for 8 hours after the dose. The manufacturers recommend minimizing infant exposure to sumatriptan by avoiding breast-feeding for 12 hours after receiving the drug as oral tablets or nasal spray.

Drug Interactions

■ **Monoamine Oxidase Inhibitors** Because of the important role of monoamine oxidase (MAO), particularly the A isoenzyme (MAO-A), in the presystemic clearance of sumatriptan, concomitant therapy with MAO-A inhibitors may decrease sumatriptan clearance and increase half-life and blood concentrations of the drug. In healthy women receiving sumatriptan subcutaneously, pretreatment with an MAO-A inhibitor resulted in a 40% increase in the half-life of sumatriptan, a decrease in plasma clearance, and a twofold increase in area under the plasma concentration-time curve (AUC). In one small study, pretreatment with an MAO-A inhibitor resulted in an approximately sevenfold increase in systemic exposure to sumatriptan following administration of a single 25-mg oral dose of the drug. In contrast, pretreatment with an MAO-B inhibitor does not have an appreciable effect on the metabolism of sumatriptan. The manufacturer states that although studies of this interaction have not been performed with intranasal sumatriptan, the effects of an MAO-A inhibitor on intranasal sumatriptan bioavailability would be expected to be greater than those seen with subcutaneous sumatriptan but less than those seen with the oral drug, since only swallowed drug would be subject to first-pass effects. Concurrent use of sumatriptan and MAO-A inhibitors or use of sumatriptan within 2 weeks of discontinuance of MAO-A inhibitor therapy is contraindicated.

■ **Ergot Alkaloids** Because ergot alkaloids (e.g., ergotamine, dihydroergotamine, methysergide [no longer commercially available in the US]) have been reported to cause prolonged vasospastic reactions and the vasoconstrictor effects of these drugs may be additive to those of sumatriptan, the manufacturers state that use of ergot alkaloids and sumatriptan within 24 hours of each other is contraindicated. However, in a placebo-controlled study in patients with a history of migraine who were receiving dihydroergotamine prophylaxis, no clinical evidence of a drug interaction was observed when subcutaneous sumatriptan was used to treat breakthrough migraine attacks.

■ **Selective Serotonin-reuptake Inhibitors and Selective Serotonin- and Norepinephrine-reuptake Inhibitors** Cases of potentially life-threatening serotonin syndrome have been reported during concurrent therapy with 5-HT_1 receptor agonists and selective serotonin-reuptake inhibitors (SSRIs) or selective serotonin- and norepinephrine-reuptake inhibitors (SNRIs). Symptoms of serotonin syndrome may include mental status changes (e.g., agitation, hallucinations, coma), autonomic instability (e.g., tachycardia, labile blood pressure, hyperthermia), neuromuscular aberrations (e.g., hyperreflexia, incoordination), and/or GI symptoms (e.g., nausea, vomiting, diarrhea). If concurrent therapy with a 5-HT_1 receptor agonist and an SSRI or SNRI is clinically warranted, the patient should be observed carefully, particularly during initiation of therapy, when dosage is increased, or when another serotonergic agent is initiated. In addition, patients receiving such concomitant therapy should be advised of potential drug interaction symptoms (e.g., weakness, progressive agitation, tingling, incoordination, chest pain, dyspnea) and be instructed to report such symptoms to their clinician immediately.

Oral or subcutaneous sumatriptan and serotonin reuptake inhibitors were used concomitantly in some clinical studies without unusual adverse effects. However, an increase in the frequency of migraine attacks and a decrease in the effectiveness of sumatriptan in relieving migraine headache have been reported in a patient receiving subcutaneous injections of sumatriptan intermittently while undergoing fluoxetine therapy.

■ **Protein-bound Drugs** The effect of sumatriptan on the protein binding of other drugs has not been evaluated but would be expected to be minor because of the low-level protein binding of sumatriptan.

■ **Acetaminophen** In patients with migraine, pretreatment with oral sumatriptan followed by administration of oral acetaminophen delayed the absorption of acetaminophen, although the extent of acetaminophen absorption over 8 hours was not affected. Since IV sumatriptan has been shown to delay gastric emptying time in healthy individuals, it has been suggested that delayed absorption of acetaminophen following pretreatment with oral sumatriptan may be the result of a delay in gastric emptying time.

■ **Alcohol** In a limited number of healthy individuals, administration of alcohol (0.8 mg/kg) 30 minutes prior to oral sumatriptan (200 mg) did not affect the pharmacokinetics (e.g., peak plasma concentration, time to peak plasma concentration, area under the plasma concentration-time curve, half-life) of the drug.

■ **Topical Vasoconstrictors** Topical application of xylometazoline to the nasal mucosa 15 minutes prior to an intranasal sumatriptan dose of 20 mg reportedly did not affect the pharmacokinetics of sumatriptan.

■ **Other Drugs** Retrospective evaluation of phase III clinical trials in which certain drugs used for migraine prophylaxis, such as verapamil, amitriptyline, or propranolol, were used concomitantly with sumatriptan did not indicate any effect of such concomitant therapy on the efficacy of sumatriptan. Pretreatment with propranolol (80 mg twice daily for 7 days) did not alter the pharmacokinetics (e.g., plasma concentrations, time to peak plasma concentration, half-life) or pharmacodynamics (as determined by changes in heart rate and blood pressure) of oral sumatriptan given as a single 300-mg dose.

Laboratory Test Interferences

Sumatriptan is not known to interfere with commonly employed clinical laboratory tests.

Acute Toxicity

No gross overdoses in clinical practice have been reported. Single oral or intranasal doses of 140–300 or up to 40 mg, respectively, have been administered to patients with migraine, and single oral or intranasal doses of 140–400 or up to 40 mg, respectively, have been administered to healthy individuals, without clinically important adverse effects. However, coronary vasospasm has been observed after IV administration of usual doses of sumatriptan. (See Cautions: Precautions and Contraindications.) Based on studies in animals given high doses of sumatriptan (0.1 g/kg in dogs and 2 g/kg in rats), overdosage with the drug may be expected to cause seizures, tremor, inactivity, ptosis, erythema of the extremities, reduced respiratory rate, cyanosis, ataxia, mydriasis, salivation, lacrimation, injection site reactions (desquamation, hair loss, scab formation), and paralysis. Since the elimination half-life of sumatriptan is about 2–2.5 hours, monitoring of patients after overdosage should continue while symptoms persist or for at least 10–12 hours.

The effect of hemodialysis or peritoneal dialysis on serum concentrations of sumatriptan is not known.

Chronic Toxicity

Currently available data from long-term and/or postmarketing surveillance studies suggest that subcutaneous or oral sumatriptan use is not associated with dose escalation or withdrawal symptoms in patients using the drug as recommended for acute treatment of migraine or cluster headache attacks. However, misuse of sumatriptan (e.g., daily use as prophylaxis) has been reported in a few patients receiving the drug orally or subcutaneously for migraine headache, most of whom had a history of analgesic or ergot alkaloid abuse. Some clinicians state that frequent (e.g., daily) use of sumatriptan may be associated with rebound headache; overuse of sumatriptan has been reported to sustain ergotamine-induced headache, with the addition of superimposed migraine-like episodes, in at least one patient. Patients should be cautioned against frequent use/misuse of sumatriptan for headache prophylaxis. (See Cautions: Precautions and Contraindications.)

Pharmacology

Sumatriptan is a selective agonist of vascular serotonin (5-hydroxytryptamine; 5-HT) type 1B and 1D receptors. The mechanisms involved in the pathogenesis of migraine and cluster headache are not clearly understood; consequently, the precise mechanism of action of sumatriptan in the management of these disorders has not been established. However, current data suggest that sumatriptan may ameliorate migraine and cluster headache through selective constriction of certain large cranial blood vessels and/or inhibition of neurogenic inflammatory processes in the CNS. While some features of migraine clearly reflect effects on cerebral blood vessels, neurogenic mechanisms involving activation of the trigeminovascular system also have been implicated; current evidence suggests that both mechanisms may be involved.

No single pathogenic mechanism has been identified to explain the various manifestations of cluster headache, although several pathophysiologic abnormalities that appear to involve direct or indirect activation of the trigeminovascular and cranial parasympathetic nervous systems have been identified in patients with this disorder. It has been suggested that the neuroendocrinologic abnormalities associated with cluster headache may indicate dysfunction of the "biologic clock" in the hypothalamus.

Although sumatriptan therapy has been associated with adverse CNS effects such as drowsiness, sedation, fatigue, dizziness, and vertigo, available evidence from animal studies indicates that the drug penetrates the blood-brain barrier poorly; therefore, it has been suggested that disruption of the blood-brain barrier may occur during migraine attacks. However, since sumatriptan also decreases migraine-associated nausea and vomiting, a more likely hypothesis is that sumatriptan acts on areas of the brain not protected by the blood-brain barrier (e.g., the circumventricular organs, the chemoreceptor trigger zone).

Indirect evidence suggests that serotonin is involved in the pathogenesis of migraine because of observed correlations between the physiologic effects of serotonin, which include vasoconstriction, and the clinical features of migraine. Serotonin levels in platelets within the vascular system have been shown to increase before, and decrease rapidly during, a migraine attack. In addition, increases in the urinary excretion of 5-hydroxyindoleacetic acid (5-HIAA), a major metabolite of serotonin, have been found in patients with migraine, suggesting rapid degradation of serotonin during migraine attacks. Both spontaneous migraine and that induced by reserpine, a drug that depletes serotonin stores, are ameliorated by IV administration of serotonin. However, clinical use of serotonin is precluded by adverse effects such as nausea, syncope, hyperpnea, peripheral vasoconstriction, and paresthesia.

Sumatriptan and other currently available drugs that are effective for acute migraine, including dihydroergotamine and ergotamine, have binding affinity for serotonin type 1 (5-HT_1) receptors, particularly the 5-HT_{1D} (also called 5-$HT_{1D\alpha}$) and 5-HT_{1B} (also called 5-$HT_{1D\beta}$) subtypes located on trigeminal sensory neurons innervating dural blood vessels. The 5-HT_{1B} and 5-HT_{1D} receptors function as autoreceptors, activation of which leads to inhibition of firing of serotonin neurons and a reduction in the synthesis and release of serotonin. Upon binding to these 5-HT_1 receptor subtypes, sumatriptan inhibits adenylate cyclase activity via regulatory G proteins, increases intracellular calcium, and affects other intracellular events that lead to vasoconstriction and inhibition of sensory nociceptive (trigeminal) nerve firing and vasoactive neuropeptide release. Sumatriptan has the highest affinity for the 5-HT_{1D} receptor, the most common serotonin receptor subtype in the brain, and a 2- to 17-fold lower affinity for 5-HT_{1A} receptors; agonist activity at 5-HT_{1A} and other serotonin receptors may be responsible for some of the adverse effects noted with administration of serotonin or serotonergic antimigraine drugs (e.g., ergotamine, dihydroergotamine). Sumatriptan has essentially no affinity for (based on standard radioligand binding assays) nor pharmacologic activity at other serotonin receptors (e.g., 5-HT_2, 5-HT_3) or at receptors of the dopamine$_1$, dopamine$_2$, muscarinic, histamine, benzodiazepine, or α_1-, α_2-, or β-adrenergic type.

■ **Cerebrovascular Effects** Some evidence suggests that migraine may be caused by initial vasoconstriction of cerebral vessels, opening of arteriovenous anastomoses, and diversion of blood from capillary beds; these vascular changes may result in ischemia and hypoxia, vasodilation of intracranial and scalp vessels, and extravasation of plasma proteins into the dura mater. Sumatriptan and ergot alkaloids appear to exert their therapeutic effects in migraine by reducing blood flow to anastomoses and redirecting flow to capillary beds. Sumatriptan selectively constricts certain large cranial blood vessels (e.g., as indicated by a selective increase in blood flow velocity in the internal carotid and middle cerebral arteries) and arteriovenous anastomoses in the carotid circulation that become inflamed and dilated during a migraine attack. These vasoconstrictor effects occur apparently without compromising blood flow in the cerebral or extracerebral circulation. It has been suggested that the vasoconstriction observed following administration of sumatriptan may be related in part to a direct action on vascular smooth muscle.

Sumatriptan inhibits activation of the trigeminovascular system and associated release of vasoactive neuropeptides (i.e., substance P, neurokinin A, calcitonin gene-related peptide [CGRP]) from trigeminal nerve terminals, thereby preventing subsequent vasodilation, inflammation, and plasma extravasation from dural blood vessels. Sumatriptan also has been shown to reduce the ultrastructural changes resulting from trigeminal sensory nerve stimulation in the dura mater, such as vesiculation, vacuolation, microvillus projections within the endothelium of postcapillary venules, platelet aggregation and adhesion, and mast cell degranulation.

In cluster headache, activation of trigeminal nerves and the parasympathetic nervous system leads to frontotemporal vasodilation, neuroinflammation, and venous stasis; these effects may be manifested as nasal congestion, rhinorrhea, lacrimation, abnormal sweating, and/or periorbital edema. Limited data currently suggest that sumatriptan, like oxygen, may alleviate cluster headache attacks through normalization of elevated CGRP concentrations in cranial venous blood; such normalization of CGRP levels reflects termination of activity in the trigeminovascular system. In addition, vasoconstriction following administration of sumatriptan may be related in part to a return of firing of sympathetic nerve fibers following a decrease in neuroinflammation.

Although sumatriptan does not appear to have a direct analgesic effect, the drug inhibits firing of sensory nociceptive nerves in the trigeminovascular system that may be involved in central pain modulatory mechanisms (as indicated by inhibition of *c-fos* protein expression, an indicator of neuronal activation).

■ **Cardiovascular Effects** Sumatriptan has shown modest vasoconstrictor effects on the coronary, pulmonary, and systemic circulation in in vitro studies in animals and in most studies in humans, but these effects are much less potent than those of ergot alkaloids. In vitro studies of human diseased and normal coronary artery rings and angiographic evidence in patients undergoing coronary arteriography indicate that sumatriptan causes relatively weak contractions of coronary arteries compared with the effects of serotonin or ergotamine. Although coronary vasospasm and myocardial ischemia or infarction have been reported in a few patients receiving sumatriptan, most of these patients had risk factors predictive of coronary artery disease, and use of the drug may have been contraindicated in some of these cases. (See Cautions: Precautions and Contraindications.) It has been suggested that the presence of atherosclerosis and/or associated changes in the function of vasoactive factors (e.g., substance P, nitric oxide, thromboxane A) in damaged coronary artery endothelium may result in enhanced sensitivity of the coronary vessels to the vasoconstrictor effects of sumatriptan in patients with coronary artery disease.

Sumatriptan selectively reduces carotid arterial blood flow and/or constricts carotid arteriovenous anastomoses in anesthetized animals without appreciable effects on arterial blood pressure or total peripheral resistance. The drug produces contraction of vascular smooth muscle in vitro in saphenous veins in dogs and humans, but such contractions are weaker than those produced by serotonin or ergot alkaloids (e.g., methysergide). Administration of sumatriptan in healthy individuals did not appreciably increase arterial resistance (as measured by decreases in mean toe-arm systolic blood pressure gradients) in small peripheral arteries of the leg. Increases in systolic and diastolic blood pressure noted in patients receiving sumatriptan in clinical studies generally have been small and transient and have not been accompanied by appreciable changes in heart rate; however, clinically important increases in blood pressure, including hypertensive crisis with acute impairment of organ systems, have been reported rarely with sumatriptan therapy in patients with or without a history of hypertension. (See Cautions: Cardiovascular Effects.)

■ **Hormonal and Metabolic Effects** Limited data in healthy individuals indicate that subcutaneous administration of sumatriptan may increase plasma somatotropin (growth hormone), corticotropin (ACTH), and β-endorphin concentrations through stimulation of serotonin (possibly 5-HT_{1D}) receptors on the pituitary gland, which is not protected by the blood-brain barrier. The effect of sumatriptan on the hypothalamic-pituitary-adrenal (HPA) axis has not been studied in patients with migraine. Limited data in healthy individuals suggest that stimulation of corticotropin secretion by sumatriptan may be accompanied by increased secretion of cortisol; however, increased cortisol concentrations have not been consistently demonstrated with single-dose subcutaneous or oral administration of sumatriptan. Secretion of other pituitary hormones, such as prolactin, luteinizing hormone (LH), or follicle-stimulating hormone (FSH, follitropin), does not appear to be affected in healthy individuals receiving subcutaneous sumatriptan (6 mg); however, increases in thyrotropin (TSH) have been reported rarely in patients receiving the drug.

■ **Other Effects** Sumatriptan has been shown to prolong GI transit time following IV administration in healthy individuals. In addition, large subcutaneous doses of sumatriptan (16 mg) increase esophageal motility (as measured by increases in the frequency, strength, and duration of repetitive peristaltic contractions upon swallowing). It has been suggested that some instances of chest pain reported in patients receiving sumatriptan in clinical trials may have been attributable to increased esophageal motility, which may itself be associated with chest pain, rather than to cardiac problems. (See Cautions: Cardiovascular Effects.)

Clinical experience with sumatriptan in patients with migraine suggests that the drug has no appreciable effect on respiratory rate. Bronchospasm has been reported with sumatriptan therapy, but a causal relationship between asthmatic symptoms and sumatriptan or an increase in adverse effects in asthmatic patients receiving the drug has not been established. (See Cautions: Respiratory Effects.)

Pharmacokinetics

In all studies described in the Pharmacokinetics section, sumatriptan was administered as the base (nasal spray) or as the succinate salt (oral tablets or injection); dosages and concentrations of the drug are expressed in terms of sumatriptan. Most of the early pharmacokinetic studies of oral sumatriptan used a dispersible formulation of the drug rather than the currently marketed film-coated tablet; the dispersible tablet is bioequivalent to the film-coated tablet.

The pharmacokinetics of sumatriptan do not appear to be altered by patient age or gender. Limited data suggest that the systemic clearance and peak plasma concentrations of sumatriptan are similar in black and white healthy individuals.

■ **Absorption** Sumatriptan is rapidly absorbed following subcutaneous or oral administration; oral absorption appears to occur in the small intestine. The drug also is absorbed rapidly following intranasal administration. The bioavailability of sumatriptan given subcutaneously is almost complete, averaging about 97% of that obtained with IV administration of the drug. The bioavailability of sumatriptan following oral or intranasal administration averages only about 15 or 17%, respectively, principally because of presystemic metabolism of the drug and in part because of incomplete absorption. The area under the plasma concentration-time curve (AUC) and peak serum concentration of sumatriptan increase linearly with single subcutaneous doses of 1–16 mg. The extent of sumatriptan absorption (AUC) also is dose-proportional following single oral doses of 25–200 mg; however, peak plasma concentrations after a 100-mg oral dose of sumatriptan are approximately 25% less than those predicted from a 25-mg oral dose. Interindividual variability in the absorption of sumatriptan after oral administration results in multiple peaks in plasma concentration, possibly because of differences in the rates of gastric emptying, small-bowel transit, and/or presystemic metabolism; however, 75–80% of the final peak plasma concentration is reached within 45 minutes after dosing. Administration of higher than recommended single oral doses of sumatriptan (i.e., 200–400 mg) is associated with a decrease in the rate of absorption. Following oral administration of sumatriptan 85 mg in fixed combination with naproxen sodium 500 mg, the AUC of sumatriptan was similar to that achieved following oral administration of sumatriptan 100 mg alone.

Food does not appreciably affect the oral bioavailability of sumatriptan but prolongs the time to peak concentration. In healthy individuals, oral administration of sumatriptan 100 mg with a high-fat meal increased AUC and peak plasma concentrations by 12 and 15%, respectively, compared with administration in the fasted state. Following oral administration of the fixed combination of sumatriptan 85 mg and naproxen sodium 500 mg with food, the time to peak sumatriptan concentration was delayed slightly (by about 0.6 hour), but bioavailability of sumatriptan was not appreciably affected. Oral absorption of the drug does not appear to be affected appreciably by gastric stasis that may occur during a migraine attack; however, the time to peak concentration is prolonged by about 30 minutes. The pharmacokinetics of sumatriptan following subcutaneous injection or following oral administration in fixed combination with naproxen sodium reportedly are similar during migraine attacks and pain-free periods. Absorption of subcutaneous sumatriptan is not affected by race or gender.

Peak plasma sumatriptan concentrations after administration of a single 6-mg subcutaneous dose of the drug in healthy individuals reportedly have ranged from 55–108 ng/mL at 5–20 minutes after the dose. Peak plasma sumatriptan concentrations averaged about 75 ng/mL and median time to peak concentration was 12 minutes in healthy men receiving a single 6-mg subcutaneous dose of the drug by manual injection in the deltoid area. Following subcutaneous injection of a single 6-mg dose into the thigh in these individuals, peak plasma sumatriptan concentrations averaged 61 ng/mL with manual injection of the drug and 52 ng/mL when a needle-based autoinjection device was used. In this study, the time to peak plasma concentration and the amount of drug absorbed were not affected by injection site or technique. When a single 6-mg dose of sumatriptan was administered subcutaneously via a needleless delivery device at sites on the thigh or abdomen, peak plasma concentrations averaged 72 or 79 ng/mL, respectively, and the time to peak plasma concentration was 12 minutes; administration using this technique at sites on the upper arm may result in delivery of a suboptimal dose.

Peak plasma concentrations of 27–137 ng/mL have been reported 0.5–5 hours after administration of a single 100-mg oral dose in healthy individuals and patients with migraine. After a single 25- or 50-mg oral dose, peak plasma sumatriptan concentrations averaged 18 or 31 ng/mL, respectively, at 0.5–3 hours, while a single 100-mg oral dose of sumatriptan produced peak plasma drug concentrations averaging 51 ng/mL approximately 2–2.5 hours after drug administration. Following oral administration of sumatriptan 85 mg in fixed combination with naproxen sodium 500 mg, peak plasma concentrations of sumatriptan were similar to those achieved following oral administration of sumatriptan 100 mg, and the median time to peak plasma sumatriptan concentrations was about 1 hour (versus 1.5 hours with oral sumatriptan alone).

In a randomized, controlled study in patients with migraine receiving sumatriptan 10, 20, or 40 mg intranasally in one or both nostrils, peak plasma sumatriptan concentrations averaged 7.7–8.7, 11.8–12.4, or 20.1–21.7 ng/mL at 0.8, 1, or 1.8 hours, respectively, following the dose. The possible contribution of oral absorption of the drug to sumatriptan plasma concentrations as a result of swallowing the intranasal dose has not been determined.

The onset of action of sumatriptan in patients with migraine or cluster headaches correlates well with peak plasma drug concentrations. Plasma sumatriptan concentrations associated with therapeutic effects in patients with migraine have ranged from 8–66 ng/mL with subcutaneous therapy and from 18–60 ng/mL with oral sumatriptan. In controlled clinical studies in patients with moderate to severe migraine headache pain, onset of pain relief following subcutaneous injection of sumatriptan usually occurred within 10–34 minutes, maximum relief was achieved within 1–2 hours, and pain relief persisted for 9–24 hours in some patients. In patients with cluster headache, the onset of pain relief following subcutaneous injection of sumatriptan generally occurs within 4–7 minutes, with resolution of the headache shortly thereafter. Onset of relief of migraine symptoms with oral sumatriptan therapy generally occurs 1–3 hours after single oral doses of 25–100 mg, with maximum pain relief attained within 3–6 hours. Although the delayed onset of action of oral versus subcutaneous sumatriptan may result from slower absorption, a small decrease in oral bioavailability of the drug also has been reported during migraine attacks. Compared with subcutaneous sumatriptan, the prolonged absorption observed with oral administration may lead to sustained plasma drug concentrations that delay recurrences of headache. (See Uses: Vascular Headaches.) However, administration of a second oral dose of sumatriptan 2 hours after the first dose during a migraine attack does not influence the development of recurrences, and factors other than pharmacokinetic alterations may contribute to the development of recurrent migraine attacks.

In patients with migraine who received sumatriptan 10, 20, or 40 mg intranasally, the onset of headache relief occurred within 30 minutes following the dose.

■ **Distribution** After subcutaneous administration, sumatriptan is rapidly and widely distributed into body tissues, with an apparent volume of distribution of 2.4 L/kg. Following IV administration of radiolabeled sumatriptan in rats, the drug was detected in the liver, small intestine, and kidney within 10 minutes. Sumatriptan is approximately 14–21% bound to plasma proteins over a concentration range of 10–1000 ng/mL.

Sumatriptan, like exogenously administered serotonin, does not cross the blood-brain barrier in appreciable amounts in animals; however, the occurrence of adverse effects such as transient drowsiness, sedation, dizziness, vertigo, and fatigue with sumatriptan therapy in humans suggests that the drug may have access to the CNS.

In vitro studies in isolated, perfused human placenta suggest that only small amounts of sumatriptan cross the placenta by passive transport.

Sumatriptan is distributed into milk in humans and animals; in animals, sumatriptan concentrations are eightfold higher than concurrent maternal plasma concentrations. In a limited number of healthy lactating women, the total recovery of sumatriptan in breast milk averaged 0.24% of a single 6-mg subcutaneous dose, corresponding to an average infant exposure of 3.5% of the maternal dose on a weight-adjusted basis.

Results of studies in rats given a single subcutaneous (0.5 mg/kg) dose of radiolabeled sumatriptan suggest that sumatriptan and its metabolites bind to melanin in the eye (as indicated by an ocular elimination half-life of 15 days); the clinical importance of this binding is unknown.

■ **Elimination** Following single subcutaneous (6 mg) or oral (50–100 mg) doses of sumatriptan in healthy individuals, the terminal elimination half-life of the drug is 1.5–2.6 hours. Following single-dose oral administration of large doses of sumatriptan (300–400 mg) or repeated administration of smaller doses (100 mg), a second terminal elimination phase has been observed but not characterized. The prolonged elimination half-life with multiple dosing or administration of large single doses may indicate enterohepatic recycling or prolonged oral absorption and does not appear to affect substantially the disposition of the drug. Most of a dose of sumatriptan is excreted within 10–24 hours. Following intranasal administration of sumatriptan, the elimination half-life reportedly is about 2 hours.

Metabolism is the principal clearance process for sumatriptan. Sumatriptan is metabolized in the liver and possibly in the GI tract and is eliminated in urine and feces. In vitro studies suggest that sumatriptan is metabolized by monoamine oxidase (MAO), principally the A isoenzyme (MAO-A); inhibitors of this enzyme may increase systemic exposure to sumatriptan. (See Drug Interactions: Monoamine Oxidase Inhibitors.)

The principal metabolite of sumatriptan is its inactive indole acetic acid analog, which is formed by oxidative *N*-deamination of the *N*-dimethyl side chain. The indole acetic acid metabolite of sumatriptan achieves plasma concentrations 6–7 times higher than those of sumatriptan but has a half-life similar to that of the parent compound, suggesting that clearance of this metabolite is formation-rate limited. Other minor metabolites of sumatriptan, an ester glucuronide of the indole acetic acid derivative and an indole ethyl alcohol derivative, also have been identified.

Data in a limited number of patients with hepatic impairment indicate that the area under plasma concentration-time curve (AUC) and peak concentration of sumatriptan increase by 70%, and time to peak plasma concentration occurs 40 minutes earlier compared with such values in healthy individuals receiving a single 50-mg oral dose of sumatriptan. When sumatriptan was administered by subcutaneous injection, the pharmacokinetic profile of the drug in patients with moderate hepatic impairment was similar to that in healthy individuals. The pharmacokinetics of sumatriptan following subcutaneous injection have not been elucidated in patients with severe hepatic impairment. (See Dosage and Administration: Dosage in Renal and Hepatic Impairment.)

Sumatriptan is excreted in urine via glomerular filtration and tubular secretion, but renal plasma clearance accounts for only 22% of the systemic clearance of 1176–1200 mL/minute. Since the major route of elimination is by metabolism in the liver, reduction of renal elimination is unlikely to be clinically important. Following subcutaneous administration of a single 6-mg dose of sumatriptan, approximately 22 and 38–53% of the dose is excreted in urine as unchanged drug and as the indole acetic acid metabolite, respectively. Approximately 0.6 and 3.3% of the sumatriptan dose is excreted in feces as unchanged sumatriptan and as the indole acetic acid metabolite, respectively, after subcutaneous administration.

Following administration of a single oral radiolabeled dose of sumatriptan (200 mg) in healthy individuals, 37–40 and 57–60% of the dose is excreted in feces and urine, respectively. Only 3 and 9% of the dose of radiolabeled sumatriptan is excreted unchanged in urine and feces, respectively, after oral administration. Urinary and fecal recovery of sumatriptan metabolites average 46 and 11% of the administered dose, respectively. It is not known whether sumatriptan metabolites excreted in feces are the metabolic product of MAO enzymes present in the GI tract or are derived from biliary excretion.

Chemistry and Stability

■ Chemistry Sumatriptan is a selective agonist of vascular serotonin (5-hydroxytryptamine; 5-HT) type 1B and 1D receptors. Sumatriptan is structurally and pharmacologically related to serotonin, differing structurally from serotonin principally by the substitution of methane sulfonamide for the alcohol group on the indole ring of serotonin.

Sumatriptan and sumatriptan succinate occur as white to off-white powders and are freely soluble in water and in 0.9% sodium chloride. The drug reportedly has pK_as of 4.21 and 5.67 (succinic acid), 9.63 (tertiary amine group), and 12 or greater (sulfonamide group).

Sumatriptan succinate is commercially available as a clear, colorless to pale yellow, sterile, nonpyrogenic solution for subcutaneous injection and as tablets for oral administration. Each 0.5 mL of the 8-mg/mL injection contains 4 mg of sumatriptan and 3.8 mg of sodium chloride. Each 0.5 mL of the 12-mg/mL injection contains 6 mg of sumatriptan and 3.5 mg of sodium chloride. The commercially available injection has a pH of approximately 4.2–5.3 and an osmolality of 291 mOsm/kg. Commercially available sumatriptan tablets contain 35, 70, or 140 mg of sumatriptan succinate equivalent to 25, 50 or 100 mg, respectively, of sumatriptan.

Sumatriptan nasal spray is commercially available as aqueous buffered solutions in single-use delivery devices. The solutions have a pH of approximately 5.5 and osmolalities of 372 and 742 mOsm/kg for the 5 and 20 mg per 0.1 mL single-use doses, respectively.

■ Stability Sumatriptan succinate injection in cartridges and vials, sumatriptan succinate tablets, and sumatriptan nasal spray should be stored at 2–30°C; the injection should be protected from light. The fixed-combination tablets containing sumatriptan succinate and naproxen sodium should be stored in the original container with the desiccant packet at 25°C but may be exposed to temperatures ranging from 15–30°C; the fixed-combination tablets should not be repackaged. Sumatriptan succinate prefilled, single-use injection pens should be protected from light and stored at 25°C but may be exposed to temperatures ranging from 15–30°C; refrigeration should be avoided. Sumatriptan succinate prefilled, single-use needleless devices should be stored at 20–25°C but may be exposed to temperatures ranging from 15–30°C; freezing should be avoided.

Preparations

Excipients in commercially available drug preparations may have clinically important effects in some individuals; consult specific product labeling for details.

SUMAtriptan

Nasal		
Solution	5 mg/0.1 mL*	**Imitrex® Nasal Spray**, GlaxoSmithKline
		SUMAtriptan Nasal Spray
	20 mg/0.1 mL*	**Imitrex® Nasal Spray**, GlaxoSmithKline
		SUMAtriptan Nasal Spray

*available from one or more manufacturer, distributor, and/or repackager by generic (nonproprietary) name

SUMAtriptan Succinate

Oral		
Tablets, film-coated	25 mg (of sumatriptan)*	**Imitrex®**, GlaxoSmithKline
		SUMAtriptan Succinate Tablets
	50 mg (of sumatriptan)*	**Imitrex®**, GlaxoSmithKline
		SUMAtriptan Succinate Tablets
	100 mg (of sumatriptan)*	**Imitrex®**, GlaxoSmithKline
		SUMAtriptan Succinate Tablets
Parenteral		
Injection, for subcutaneous use only	4 mg (of sumatriptan) per 0.5 mL*	**Imitrex®** (available in 0.5-mL unit-of-use injection-pen cartridges), GlaxoSmithKline
		SUMAtriptan Succinate Injection (available in 0.5-mL unit-of-use injection-pen cartridges)
	6 mg (of sumatriptan) per 0.5 mL*	**Alsuma®** (available in prefilled disposable single-use 0.5-mL injection pen), Pfizer
		Imitrex® (available in 0.5-mL unit-of-use injection-pen cartridges and as 0.5-mL single-dose vials), GlaxoSmithKline
		SUMAtriptan Succinate Injection (available in 0.5-mL unit-of-use injection-pen cartridges and as 0.5-mL single-dose vials)
		Sumavel® (available in prefilled disposable single-use 0.5-mL needleless delivery device), Zogenix

*available from one or more manufacturer, distributor, and/or repackager by generic (nonproprietary) name

SUMAtriptan Succinate Combinations

Oral		
Tablets, film-coated	85 mg (of sumatriptan) with 500 mg Naproxen Sodium	**Treximet®**, GlaxoSmithKline

†Use is not currently included in the labeling approved by the US Food and Drug Administration

Selected Revisions November 2017,

ZOLMitriptan

■ Zolmitriptan is a selective agonist of serotonin (5-hydroxytryptamine; 5-HT) type 1B and 1D receptors ("triptan").

Uses

■ Vascular Headaches ***Migraine*** Zolmitriptan is used orally or intranasally for the acute treatment of attacks of migraine with or without aura in adults. The manufacturer states that zolmitriptan should not be used for the management of hemiplegic or basilar migraine or for the *prophylaxis* of migraine. Safety and efficacy have not been established for the management of cluster headaches.

Efficacy of zolmitriptan administered orally at dosages of 1, 2.5, or 5 mg has been evaluated for the acute treatment of migraine attacks in several randomized, placebo-controlled studies in adults with moderate to severe headaches. In these studies, substantially more patients receiving zolmitriptan achieved a response (mild or no headache pain) 2 hours after treatment than those receiving placebo. In dose-ranging studies, 65 or 60–67% of patients receiving zolmitriptan 2.5 or 5 mg, respectively, achieved a response 2 hours after treatment, compared with 27–50% of patients receiving zolmitriptan 1 mg; headache response at 2 hours in patients receiving zolmitriptan 2.5 mg did not differ substantially from that observed in patients receiving zolmitriptan 5 mg. The drug also relieved manifestations of migraine other than headache (including nausea, photophobia, and phonophobia) and reduced the need for supplemental migraine therapy. In long-term (6–12 months) open-label studies, intermittent zolmitriptan remained effective during subsequent migraine attacks.

Efficacy of zolmitriptan administered intranasally has been evaluated for the acute treatment of migraine attacks in a randomized, placebo-controlled study in adults with moderate to severe headaches. In this study, substantially more patients receiving zolmitriptan intranasally at a dosage of 5 mg achieved a response (mild or no headache pain) 2 hours after treatment than those receiving placebo (69 versus 31%, respectively). The drug also relieved manifestations of migraine other than headache (including nausea, photophobia, and phonophobia) and reduced the need for supplemental migraine therapy. Interim analysis of a similarly designed study supported these findings and showed that substantially more patients receiving intranasally administered zolmitriptan achieved a response 2 hours after treatment than those receiving placebo (70 versus 47%, respectively).

Limited data suggest that 2.5 or 5 mg of oral zolmitriptan is at least as effective as 25 or 50 mg of oral sumatriptan in alleviating the pain associated with migraine 2 hours after treatment.

The US Headache Consortium considers $5\text{-HT}_{1B/1D}$ receptor agonists (e.g., zolmitriptan) an appropriate treatment choice for the acute management of moderate to severe migraine headaches in patients without contraindications to these drugs and recommends use of $5\text{-HT}_{1B/1D}$ receptor agonists, dihydroergotamine, or ergotamine in patients with more severe migraine attacks as well as in patients in whom previous therapy with nonsteroidal anti-inflammatory agents (NSAIAs) or fixed-combination preparations such as acetaminophen, aspirin, and caffeine has been ineffective.

For further information on management and classification of migraine headache, see Vascular Headaches: General Principles in Migraine Therapy, under Uses in Sumatriptan 28:32.28.

Dosage and Administration

■ **General** Zolmitriptan is administered orally as conventional or orally disintegrating tablets without regard to meals. Zolmitriptan also can be administered intranasally.

Patients receiving zolmitriptan orally disintegrating tablets should be instructed not to remove a tablet from the blister package until just prior to dosing. The blister should then be peeled open, and the tablet placed on the tongue, where it will dissolve and be swallowed with saliva; administration with liquid is not necessary.

The patient information provided by the manufacturer should be consulted for directions on intranasal administration of zolmitriptan.

For the acute treatment of migraine attacks with or without aura in adults, the recommended initial oral dose of zolmitriptan is a single dose of 1.25 or 2.5 mg. The maximum recommended single oral dose of the drug is 5 mg. Single oral zolmitriptan doses of 1 (not commercially available in the US), 2.5, or 5 mg were effective in clinical studies, although the 2.5- and 5-mg doses were effective in a greater proportion of patients. The 5-mg dose provided little additional benefit compared with the 2.5-mg dose but was associated with an increased risk of adverse effects. A dose of 1.25 mg can be achieved by manually breaking the scored 2.5-mg conventional tablet in half. However, the manufacturer states that orally disintegrating tablets are not scored and should *not* be broken.

If the headache has not resolved by 2 hours following an initial oral dose of zolmitriptan, or if it recurs after transient improvement, the dose may be repeated after at least 2 hours. However, in patients who fail to respond to an initial dose, a diagnosis of migraine should be reconsidered prior to administration of a second oral dose . The maximum dosage of zolmitriptan to be administered orally in any 24-hour period is 10 mg. The safety of treating an average of more than 3 headaches with oral zolmitriptan per 30-day period has not been established.

For the acute treatment of migraine attacks with or without aura in adults, a single intranasal zolmitriptan dose of 5 mg was effective in adults in controlled clinical studies. A 5-mg dose is administered into one nostril using the single-use nasal spray. If the headache returns, a single 5-mg dose may be repeated after 2 hours; however, the efficacy of a second dose has not been established in controlled clinical studies. A diagnosis of migraine should be reconsidered prior to administration of a second intranasal dose in patients who fail to respond to an initial dose. The maximum dosage of zolmitriptan to be administered intranasally in any 24-hour period is 10 mg (i.e., 2 sprays). A dose of less than 5 mg can be achieved only with use of oral formulations of the drug. Because individuals may vary in their response to zolmitriptan nasal spray, the choice of dose and route of administration must be made on an individual basis. The safety of treating an average of more than 4 headaches with intranasal zolmitriptan per 30-day period has not been established.

■ **Special Populations** When zolmitriptan is used in patients with moderate to severe hepatic impairment, an oral dose of 1.25 mg is recommended. In patients with severe hepatic impairment, the maximum dosage to be administered orally in any 24-hour period is 5 mg. A dose of 1.25 mg can be achieved by manually breaking the scored 2.5-mg conventional tablet in half. Because the orally disintegrating tablets are not scored and should *not* be broken, use of this formulation in patients with moderate to severe hepatic impairment is not recommended. Because systemic exposure is similar following oral or intranasal administration, dosage adjustments with oral and intranasal formulations should be similar; however, recommended doses for patients with hepatic impairment can be achieved only with use of conventional oral formulations.

Dosage selection for geriatric patients should be cautious, usually starting at the low end of the dosage range, and reflect the greater frequency of decreased hepatic, renal, or cardiac function and of concomitant disease or other drug therapy in such patients.

Cautions

■ **Contraindications** Ischemic heart disease (e.g., angina pectoris, myocardial infarction, silent ischemia), coronary vasospasm (e.g., Prinzmetal variant angina), Wolff-Parkinson-White syndrome or cardiac arrhythmias associated with other accessory pathway conduction disorders, uncontrolled hypertension, other serious underlying cardiovascular disease, history of stroke or transient ischemic attack, peripheral vascular disease, or ischemic bowel disease. Basilar or hemiplegic migraine. Treatment within the previous 24 hours with another 5-HT_1 receptor agonist or with an ergot alkaloid (e.g., ergotamine, dihydroergotamine, methysergide [no longer commercially available in the US]). Concurrent or recent (within 2 weeks) treatment with a monoamine oxidase-A (MAO-A) inhibitor. Known hypersensitivity to zolmitriptan or any ingredient in the formulation.

■ **Warnings/Precautions** ***Careful Diagnosis of Migraine*** Zolmitriptan should be used only in patients in whom a clear diagnosis of migraine has been established. If the first attack of migraine treated with zolmitriptan fails to respond to the drug, the diagnosis of migraine should be reconsidered before zolmitriptan is administered to treat subsequent attacks. Care should be taken to exclude other potentially serious neurologic disorders before zolmitriptan is administered to patients not previously diagnosed with migraine or to patients who present with atypical symptoms.

Cardiac Effects Serious cardiac events, including acute myocardial infarction and fatal or life-threatening cardiac rhythm disturbances (e.g., ventricular tachycardia or fibrillation), have occurred within a few hours following administration of 5-HT_1 receptor agonists. Myocardial ischemia/infarction or coronary vasospasm (e.g., Prinzmetal variant angina) may occur even in patients without a history of coronary artery disease. Use of zolmitriptan is contraindicated in patients with ischemic or vasospastic heart disease. The drug should be discontinued if disturbances in cardiac rhythm occur. (See Cautions: Contraindications.)

Although sensations of tightness, pain, pressure, and heaviness in the precordium, throat, neck, and jaw occur frequently following administration of 5-HT_1 receptor agonists, these sensations usually are noncardiac in origin. However, the manufacturer states that a cardiovascular evaluation should be performed if the patient is at high cardiac risk.

Patients with multiple cardiovascular risk factors (e.g., postmenopausal women; men older than 40 years of age; patients with risk factors such as hypertension, hypercholesterolemia, smoking, obesity, diabetes, or family history of coronary artery disease) who have not previously received therapy with a 5-HT_1 receptor agonist should undergo cardiovascular evaluation prior to initiation of 5-HT_1 receptor agonist therapy. If the evaluation provides evidence of coronary artery disease or coronary artery vasospasm, the drug should not be administered. For patients with a satisfactory cardiovascular evaluation, the manufacturer states that consideration should be given to administration of the first dose in a medically supervised setting with electrocardiographic monitoring performed immediately following administration of the dose. Periodic cardiovascular evaluation is recommended for patients with risk factors for coronary artery disease who are receiving intermittent long-term therapy with 5-HT_1 receptor agonists.

For further information on the systematic approach to administering 5-HT_1 receptor agonists in patients with risk factors for the development of coronary artery disease, see Cautions: Precautions and Contraindications, in Sumatriptan 28:32.28.

Cerebrovascular Effects Cerebral or subarachnoid hemorrhage and stroke, sometimes fatal, have occurred in patients receiving 5-HT_1 receptor agonists. In a number of cases, it appears possible that the cerebrovascular event was the primary event, and the 5-HT_1 receptor agonist was administered in the mistaken belief that the patient's symptoms were caused by a migraine attack. Patients with migraine may be at increased risk for certain cerebrovascular events (e.g., stroke, hemorrhage, transient ischemic attack). Therapy with 5-HT_1 receptor agonists should be discontinued in patients experiencing a cerebrovascular event. (See Cautions: Contraindications.)

Other Cardiovascular or Vasospastic Effects Noncoronary vasospastic reactions, including peripheral vascular ischemia, GI ischemia and infarction (presenting with abdominal pain and bloody diarrhea), splenic infarction, and Raynaud's syndrome, have been reported in patients receiving 5-HT_1 receptor agonists, including zolmitriptan. (See Cautions: Contraindications.) Transient or permanent blindness and partial vision loss also have been reported very rarely in patients receiving 5-HT_1 receptor agonists, although visual disorders may occur as manifestations of migraine attacks. Patients experiencing signs or symptoms suggestive of vasospastic reactions following administration of any 5-HT_1 receptor agonist should be evaluated to rule out vasospastic reactions before receiving additional doses of zolmitriptan.

Substantial increases in blood pressure, including hypertensive crisis with acute impairment of organ systems, have been reported rarely following administration of 5-HT_1 receptor agonists in patients with or without a history of hypertension. (See Cautions: Contraindications.) Blood pressure should be monitored in all patients receiving zolmitriptan. In healthy individuals receiving zolmitriptan 5 mg, increases in systolic and diastolic blood pressure of 1 and 5 mm Hg, respectively, were observed. However, substantial increases in blood pressure have been observed in patients with moderate to severe hepatic disease. (See Hepatic Impairment under Warnings/Precautions: Specific Populations, in Cautions.)

Increases in mean pulmonary arterial pressure have been observed following administration of another 5-HT_1 receptor agonist to patients with suspected coronary artery disease who were undergoing cardiac catheterization.

Serotonin Syndrome Potentially life-threatening serotonin syndrome has been reported in patients receiving 5-HT_1 receptor agonists, particularly in those receiving concomitant therapy with selective serotonin-reuptake inhibitors (SSRIs) or selective serotonin- and norepinephrine-reuptake inhibitors (SNRIs). Serotonin syndrome also may occur in patients receiving 5-HT_1 receptor agonists concomitantly with MAO inhibitors or tricyclic antidepressants. Symptoms of serotonin syndrome may include mental status changes (e.g., agitation, hallucinations, coma), autonomic instability (e.g., tachycardia, labile blood pressure, hyperthermia), neuromuscular aberrations (e.g., hyperreflexia, incoordination), and/or GI symptoms (e.g., nausea, vomiting, diarrhea). If concurrent therapy with a 5-HT_1 receptor agonist and an SSRI or SNRI is clinically warranted, the patient should be observed carefully, particularly during initiation of therapy, when dosage is increased, or when another serotonergic agent is initiated. If manifestations of serotonin syndrome occur, treatment with zolmitriptan and any concurrently administered serotonergic agents should be discontinued and supportive and symptomatic treatment should be initiated.

Medication Overuse Headache Excessive use of drugs indicated for the management of acute migraine attacks (e.g., use of 5-HT_1 receptor agonists, ergotamine, opiates, or certain analgesic combinations on a regular basis for

10 or more days per month) may result in migraine-like daily headaches or a marked increase in the frequency of migraine attacks. Detoxification, including withdrawal of the overused drugs; treatment of withdrawal symptoms (which often include transient worsening of headaches); and consideration of prophylactic therapy for migraine attacks may be necessary.

Sensitivity Reactions Hypersensitivity reactions (e.g., angioedema, anaphylaxis) have been reported in patients receiving zolmitriptan.

Ocular Effects Accumulation of zolmitriptan and/or its metabolites in melanin-rich tissues (such as the eye) may occur over time, resulting in potential toxicity in these tissues with extended use.

Phenylketonuria Individuals with phenylketonuria (i.e., homozygous genetic deficiency of phenylalanine hydroxylase) and other individuals who must restrict their intake of phenylalanine should be warned that each zolmitriptan 2.5- or 5-mg orally disintegrating tablet contains aspartame, which is metabolized in the GI tract to provide 2.81 or 5.62 mg of phenylalanine, respectively, following oral administration. Zolmitriptan conventional tablets do not contain aspartame.

Specific Populations **Pregnancy.** Category C. (See Users Guide.)

Lactation. Zolmitriptan is distributed into milk in rats. It is not known whether zolmitriptan is distributed into milk in humans. A decision should be made whether to discontinue nursing or the drug, taking into account the importance of the drug to the woman.

Pediatric Use. Safety and efficacy of zolmitriptan have not been established in children younger than 18 years of age. Randomized, placebo-controlled studies in adolescents 12–17 years of age with migraine headaches failed to demonstrate efficacy of the drug. Adverse effects reported in adolescents were similar to those reported in adults. Serious adverse events have been reported during postmarketing experience in a limited number of pediatric patients receiving 5-HT_1 receptor agonists, including zolmitriptan. Zolmitriptan has not been studied in children younger than 12 years of age,

Geriatric Use. Experience in patients 65 years of age and older is insufficient to determine whether they respond differently than younger adults; dosage in geriatric patients should be selected with caution.

Pharmacokinetic profile of zolmitriptan in geriatric patients is similar to that in younger adults.

Hepatic Impairment. Peak plasma concentrations, time to achieve peak plasma concentrations, and area under the plasma concentration-time curve (AUC) of zolmitriptan reportedly were 1.5-, 2-, and 3-fold higher, respectively, in patients with severe hepatic impairment receiving orally administered zolmitriptan compared with healthy individuals. The effect of hepatic impairment on the pharmacokinetics of intranasally administered zolmitriptan has not been evaluated. Substantial elevation of blood pressure (increase in systolic and/or diastolic blood pressure of 20–80 mm Hg) was observed in some patients with moderate to severe hepatic impairment following a 10-mg dose of zolmitriptan. The drug should be used with caution in patients with moderate to severe hepatic impairment; dosage adjustment is recommended in such patients. (See Dosage and Administration: Special Populations.)

Renal Impairment. Clearance of zolmitriptan reportedly was reduced by 25% in patients with severe renal impairment (creatinine clearance of 5–25 mL/minute) receiving orally administered zolmitriptan; no substantial change in clearance was observed in patients with moderate renal impairment (creatinine clearance of 26–50 mL/minute). The effect of renal impairment on the pharmacokinetics of intranasally administered zolmitriptan has not been evaluated.

■ **Common Adverse Effects** Adverse effects occurring in 2% or more of patients receiving orally administered zolmitriptan and more frequently (by at least 2 percentage points) with zolmitriptan than with placebo include dizziness, paresthesia, neck/throat/jaw/chest symptoms (e.g., pain, tightness, pressure, heaviness), other sensations of heaviness/pressure/tightness, nausea, somnolence, warm or cold sensation, asthenia, dry mouth, dyspepsia, dysphagia, vertigo, and sweating.

Adverse effects occurring in 2% or more of patients receiving intranasal zolmitriptan and more frequently with zolmitriptan than with placebo include paresthesia, hyperesthesia, unusual taste, throat pain, pain of specified location, nausea, somnolence, disorder or discomfort of the nasal cavity, asthenia, tightness of the throat, and dry mouth.

Drug Interactions

■ **Acetaminophen** Potential pharmacokinetic interaction (increased time to peak plasma concentrations of acetaminophen).

■ **Cimetidine** Potential pharmacokinetic interaction (approximately two-fold increase in half-life of and systemic exposure to zolmitriptan and its active metabolite). When zolmitriptan and cimetidine are used concomitantly, the maximum recommended single dose of zolmitriptan is 2.5 mg and the total dosage administered in any 24-hour period should not exceed 5 mg.

■ **Ergot Alkaloids and Other 5-HT_1 Receptor Agonists** Potential pharmacologic interaction (additive vasospastic effects) when zolmitriptan is used concomitantly with ergot alkaloids (e.g., ergotamine, dihydroergotamine, methysergide [no longer commercially available in the US]) and other 5-$HT_{1B/1D}$ receptor agonists. Use of oral or intranasal zolmitriptan within 24 hours is contraindicated.

■ **Metoclopramide** A single 10-mg dose of metoclopramide did not alter the pharmacokinetics of zolmitriptan or its metabolites.

■ **Monoamine Oxidase (MAO) Inhibitors** Potential pharmacokinetic interaction (increased plasma concentrations of zolmitriptan and its active metabolite) with MAO-A inhibitors. (See Description.) Selegiline, a selective MAO-B inhibitor, did not alter the pharmacokinetics of zolmitriptan or its active metabolite. Use of oral or intranasal zolmitriptan within 2 weeks of MAO-A inhibitor therapy is contraindicated.

■ **Oral Contraceptives** Potential pharmacokinetic interaction (increased plasma concentrations of zolmitriptan; possible delay in achieving peak zolmitriptan concentrations).

■ **Propranolol** Potential pharmacokinetic interaction (increased plasma concentrations of zolmitriptan).

■ **Selective Serotonin-reuptake Inhibitors and Selective Serotonin- and Norepinephrine-reuptake Inhibitors** Potential pharmacologic interaction (potentially life-threatening serotonin syndrome). If concomitant use is clinically warranted, the patient should be observed carefully, particularly during treatment initiation, when dosage is increased, or when another serotonergic agent is initiated. (See Serotonin Syndrome under Cautions: Warnings/Precautions.)

Pretreatment with oral fluoxetine (20 mg daily for 4 weeks) did not alter the pharmacokinetic profile or effect on blood pressure of a single 10-mg dose of zolmitriptan.

■ **Topical Vasoconstrictors** Topical application of xylometazoline to the nasal mucosa 30 minutes prior to an intranasal zolmitriptan dose did not alter the pharmacokinetics of zolmitriptan.

Description

Zolmitriptan is a selective agonist of serotonin (5-hydroxytryptamine; 5-HT) type 1B and 1D receptors. Zolmitriptan is structurally and pharmacologically related to other selective 5-$HT_{1B/1D}$ receptor agonists (e.g., almotriptan, eletriptan, frovatriptan, naratriptan, rizatriptan, sumatriptan). Because the mechanisms involved in the pathogenesis of migraine are not clearly understood, the precise mechanism of action of 5-HT_1 receptor agonists in the management of migraine has yet to be established. However, current data suggest that 5-HT_1 receptor agonists, including zolmitriptan, may ameliorate migraine through selective constriction of certain intracranial blood vessels, inhibition of neuropeptide release, and/or reduced transmission in the trigeminal pain pathway.

Zolmitriptan undergoes hepatic metabolism to form 3 principal metabolites, including *N*-desmethyl zolmitriptan, which exhibits 5-$HT_{1B/1D}$ potency that is 2–6 times that of the parent drug and which may contribute substantially to the observed effects of zolmitriptan. The other principal metabolites (*N*-oxide and indole acetic acid derivatives) are inactive. In vitro studies suggest that formation of *N*-desmethyl zolmitriptan may depend on cytochrome P-450 (CYP) isoenzyme 1A2, while monoamine oxidase-A (MAO-A) appears to be responsible for further metabolism of this metabolite. Following oral administration of a single dose of radiolabeled zolmitriptan, 65 and 30% of the dose is recovered in urine and feces, respectively, as unchanged drug and metabolites. Approximately 8% of the dose is recovered in urine as unchanged zolmitriptan, while the indole acetic acid, *N*-oxide, and *N*-desmethyl metabolites account for about 31, 7, and 4% of the dose recovered in urine, respectively. Zolmitriptan and its active metabolite have elimination half-lives of approximately 3 hours in healthy individuals following oral or intranasal administration.

Advice to Patients

Risk of serious cardiovascular or cerebrovascular events (e.g., myocardial infarction, stroke) or other vasospastic reactions. Importance of seeking medical care if symptoms of such reactions (e.g., shortness of breath, weakness, slurring of speech, sudden or severe abdominal pain, difficulty in seeing, or tightness, pain, pressure, or heaviness in the chest, throat, neck, or jaw) occur after taking zolmitriptan and of *not* taking zolmitriptan again until evaluated by a clinician.

Importance of adhering to prescribed directions for use. Importance of reading manufacturer's patient information before initial use and each time the prescription is refilled.

Importance of informing patients of risk of serotonin syndrome, particularly with concurrent use of zolmitriptan and a selective serotonin-reuptake inhibitor (SSRI) or selective serotonin- and norepinephrine-reuptake inhibitor (SNRI). Importance of seeking immediate medical attention if symptoms of serotonin syndrome develop.

Overuse of drugs indicated for the management of acute migraine attacks may exacerbate headaches; importance of recording headache frequency and drug use to monitor effectiveness of treatment.

For patients taking zolmitriptan orally disintegrating tablets, importance of not removing a tablet from the blister package until just before administering a dose; importance of peeling blister open and placing tablet on tongue to dissolve and be swallowed with saliva. Orally disintegrating tablets should not be broken.

Importance of informing patients with phenylketonuria that zolmitriptan orally disintegrating tablets contain aspartame.

For patients using zolmitriptan nasal spray, importance of not spraying nasal solution into the eyes.

Importance of informing clinicians of existing or contemplated concomitant therapy, including prescription and OTC drugs, dietary supplements, and herbal supplements, as well as any concomitant illnesses (e.g., cardiovascular disease).

Importance of women informing clinicians if they are or plan to become pregnant or plan to breast-feed.

Importance of informing patients of other important precautionary information. (See Cautions.)

Overview® (see Users Guide). For additional information on this drug until a more detailed monograph is developed and published, the manufacturer's labeling should be consulted. It is *essential* that the manufacturer's labeling be consulted for more detailed information on usual cautions, precautions, contraindications, potential drug interactions, laboratory test interferences, and acute toxicity.

Preparations

Excipients in commercially available drug preparations may have clinically important effects in some individuals; consult specific product labeling for details.

ZOLMitriptan

Nasal		
Solution	5 mg/0.1 mL	**Zomig® Nasal Spray,** AstraZeneca
Oral		
Tablets, film-coated	2.5 mg	**Zomig®** (scored), AstraZeneca
	5 mg	**Zomig®**, AstraZeneca
Tablets, orally disintegrating	2.5 mg	**Zomig-ZMT®**, AstraZeneca
	5 mg	**Zomig-ZMT®**, AstraZeneca

ANTIPARKINSONIAN AGENTS 28:36

ADAMANTANES 28:36.04

Amantadine Hydrochloride

Adamantanamine Hydrochloride

■ Amantadine hydrochloride is a synthetic adamantane derivative that is used in the treatment of parkinsonian syndrome and drug-induced extrapyramidal reactions, and in the prevention and symptomatic treatment of influenza caused by A influenza virus strains.

Uses

■ **Parkinsonian Syndrome and Drug-induced Extrapyramidal Effects** Amantadine hydrochloride is used in the symptomatic treatment of all forms of parkinsonian syndrome including the postencephalitic, idiopathic, and arteriosclerotic types and for the relief of parkinsonian signs and symptoms of carbon monoxide poisoning and antipsychotic agent-induced (e.g., phenothiazines) extrapyramidal effects. There is no evidence that the drug alters the course of parkinsonian syndrome. Amantadine is less effective than levodopa in the treatment of parkinsonian syndrome. Although amantadine's efficacy in comparison to anticholinergic antiparkinsonian agents has not been definitely established, results of several studies suggest that amantadine is at least as effective as the anticholinergic agents. Similarly, in studies in patients with phenothiazine-induced parkinsonian signs and symptoms, amantadine was at least as effective in decreasing extrapyramidal symptoms as benztropine mesylate or trihexyphenidyl hydrochloride. Amantadine may be especially useful in the treatment of drug-induced extrapyramidal symptoms when drugs with anticholinergic properties should be avoided (e.g., in patients with glaucoma or urinary retention).

Amantadine has been reported to produce objective or subjective improvement in extrapyramidal symptoms, including akinesia, rigidity, tremor, salivation, gait disturbances, and total functional disability, in approximately one-half of the patients treated. Subjective responses such as a sense of well-being or elevation of mood have also been reported. Improvement in extrapyramidal symptoms is apparent within 4–48 hours following initiation of amantadine therapy, and optimum results are achieved within 2 weeks to 3 months. A definite correlation between the degree of improvement and the age or sex of the patient and duration or severity of disease has not been determined. Sustained improvement may last up to 30 months; however, some patients experience a reduction in benefit after 1–3 months of amantadine therapy. In some patients, benefits may be regained by increasing dosage or by discontinuing the drug for several weeks and then resuming therapy.

Addition of amantadine to a therapeutic regimen of anticholinergic antiparkinsonian agents (e.g., benztropine mesylate, trihexyphenidyl hydrochloride, or procyclidine hydrochloride) has produced further improvement. Concomitant administration of amantadine and levodopa has resulted in a greater reduction in parkinsonian symptoms than occurred with amantadine alone. Combined therapy with amantadine and levodopa has been reported to be more effective than levodopa alone in patients who cannot tolerate large doses of levodopa; however, the addition of amantadine to levodopa therapy does not usually provide significant additional benefit when patients are already receiving full therapeutic doses of levodopa.

■ **Other Uses** Amantadine has been used in the treatment of spastic pseudosclerosis† (Jakob-Creutzfeldt disease) with some success, although exacerbations of the disease have occurred in some patients. There is no evidence that the drug is effective in the treatment of mental depression†, Huntington's chorea†, essential tremor†, tardive dyskinesia†, or other neurologic diseases†.

For information on the use of amantadine in the prophylaxis and symptomatic treatment of influenza A virus infections, see Amantadine Hydrochloride 8:18.04.

Dosage and Administration

■ **Administration** Amantadine hydrochloride is administered orally. It has been suggested that if insomnia occurs, the last daily dose should be taken several hours before retiring.

■ **Dosage** The usual dosage of amantadine may need to be reduced in patients with congestive heart failure, peripheral edema, orthostatic hypotension, or impaired renal function.

In the treatment of all forms of parkinsonian syndrome including the postencephalitic, idiopathic, and arteriosclerotic types and for the relief of parkinsonian signs and symptoms of carbon monoxide poisoning or antipsychotic agent-induced (e.g., phenothiazines) extrapyramidal effects, the usual dosage of amantadine in patients without recognized renal disease is 100 mg twice daily. When patients are receiving other antiparkinsonian drugs or have other serious illnesses, the initial dosage is 100 mg daily. The onset of action of amantadine usually occurs within 48 hours. After 1–2 weeks, dosage may be increased to 100 mg twice daily, if necessary. Occasionally, patients with drug-induced extrapyramidal reactions whose responses are not optimal with a dosage of 200 mg daily may benefit from a dosage increase to 300 mg daily in divided doses, and patients with parkinsonian syndrome may benefit from a dosage increase up to 400 mg daily in divided doses. However, patients receiving more than 200 mg daily should be supervised closely by their physicians. In one study, increasing the daily dose from 200 mg to 400 mg increased the severity of adverse effects without significantly increasing beneficial effects.

Since renal function normally declines with age and amantadine-induced adverse effects have been reported more frequently in geriatric patients, patients 65 years of age or older without recognized renal disease should receive a reduced dosage of 100 mg daily to minimize the risk of toxicity.

Patients with parkinsonian syndrome who derive benefit from amantadine occasionally experience a decrease in effectiveness after a few months of therapy. If loss of effectiveness occurs, benefit may be regained by increasing the dosage to 300 mg daily. Alternatively, temporary discontinuation of the drug for several weeks, followed by reinstitution of amantadine therapy may result in regained benefit in some patients. The use of other antiparkinson drugs may be necessary. If amantadine and levodopa therapy are initiated concurrently, the manufacturer of amantadine recommends that amantadine dosage be continued at 100 mg once or twice daily while the daily dosage of levodopa is gradually increased to optimal benefit.

■ **Dosage in Renal Impairment** In patients with renal impairment, amantadine dosage should be carefully adjusted and some clinicians recommend that blood concentrations of the drug be monitored frequently. One manufacturer recommends that patients with creatinine clearances of 15–50 mL/minute per 1.73 m^2 receive 200 mg of amantadine on the first day, followed by 100-mg maintenance doses given once daily in patients with creatinine clearances of 30–50 mL/minute per 1.73 m^2 or once every other day in those with creatinine clearances of 15–29 mL/minute per 1.73 m^2. This manufacturer recommends that patients with creatinine clearances less than 15 mL/minute per 1.73 m^2 and hemodialysis patients receive 200 mg of amantadine every 7 days.

Cautions

■ **Nervous System Effects** Many of the adverse effects of amantadine hydrochloride are manifested as CNS or psychic disturbances which are reversible, usually dose related, and may appear within a few hours or days after initiation of amantadine therapy or after an increase in drug dosage. Dizziness (lightheadedness), insomnia, nervousness, anxiety, and impaired concentration are among the most frequent adverse effects of amantadine and have been reported in 5–10% of healthy, young adults receiving usual dosage of the drug (200 mg daily). However, limited data suggest that the incidence of adverse CNS effects may be lower in adults receiving a lower dosage of the drug. These adverse effects are usually mild, but may be more disturbing for geriatric patients than for younger patients. Symptoms generally diminish or cease soon after amantadine is discontinued; in some patients, symptoms subside after the first week of continued therapy with the drug. Irritability, depression, ataxia, confusion, somnolence, abnormal dreams, agitation, fatigue, headache, and hallucinations have been reported in 1–5% and psychosis, abnormal thinking, amnesia, hyperkinesia, weakness, and slurred speech have been reported in 1% or less of patients receiving amantadine. In addition, euphoria, forgetfulness, a sense of drunkenness or detachment, drowsiness, coma, stupor, delirium, hypokinesia, delusions, aggressive behavior, paranoid reaction, manic reaction, involuntary muscle contractions, gait abnormalities, paresthesia, EEG changes, tremor, and, rarely, lingual facial dyskinesia or seizures have been reported. Patients with active seizure disorders appear to be at risk of an increased frequency of seizures during amantadine therapy. Seizures also have been reported in patients with renal impairment and in geriatric individuals.

Suicide attempts (resulting in death in some patients) have been reported rarely in patients receiving amantadine, many of whom received short courses of the drug for influenza prophylaxis or treatment. The manufacturer states that the incidence and pathophysiology of these suicide attempts are not known. Suicide ideation or attempts have been reported in patients both with or without a prior history of psychiatric disorders. Amantadine can exacerbate mental status in patients with a history of psychiatric disorders or substance abuse. Patients with suicidal tendencies may exhibit abnormal mental states including disorientation, confusion, depression, personality changes, agitation, aggressive behavior, hallucinations, paranoia, other psychotic reactions, somnolence, or insomnia. Because of the possibility of serious adverse effects, amantadine should be administered with caution to patients receiving drugs with CNS activity and in those in whom potential risks outweigh benefits of therapy with the drug. Since intentional overdosage with amantadine has been reported in some patients, the least amount of drug feasible should be prescribed.

Sporadic cases of possible neuroleptic malignant syndrome (NMS) have been reported in patients receiving amantadine and were associated with dosage reduction or withdrawal of the drug. NMS is potentially fatal and requires immediate initiation of intensive symptomatic and supportive care. For additional information on NMS, see Extrapyramidal Reactions in Cautions: Nervous System Effects in the Phenothiazines General Statement 28:16.08.24.

■ **Livedo Reticularis** Livedo reticularis is a frequent adverse effect in patients receiving amantadine for treatment of parkinsonian syndrome. Livedo reticularis occurs mainly in the legs and diminishes when the legs are elevated. Livedo reticularis has been reported in 1–5% of patients, generally appears within 1 month to 1 year following initiation of amantadine therapy, and subsides within a few weeks to several months after discontinuance of the drug. In one study, livedo reticularis tended to fade or change into brown spots with prolonged amantadine therapy. It has been suggested that, in many instances, this adverse effect is actually an accentuation of preexisting, minor livedo reticularis and is a result of abnormal capillary permeability associated with peripheral vasoconstriction with lowering of skin temperature and decreased peripheral blood flow, and/or amantadine's depletion of catecholamines in peripheral nerve endings. Peripheral edema may precede or accompany livedo reticularis and may require dosage reduction or discontinuance of amantadine. The edema does not appear to be associated with an increase in total body water or sodium retention; it also may result from increased vascular permeability in cutaneous tissues.

■ **GI Effects** Nausea is one of the most frequent adverse effects of amantadine and has been reported in 5–10% of patients receiving the usual dosage of the drug. Anorexia, constipation, and dry mouth have been reported in 1–5% and vomiting has been reported in up to 1% of patients receiving amantadine. Abdominal discomfort or dysphagia has also been reported.

■ **Other Adverse Effects** Orthostatic hypotension and peripheral edema have been reported in 1–5% and congestive heart failure, urinary retention, decreased libido, dyspnea, rash, and visual disturbances (e.g., punctate subepithelial or other corneal opacity, decreased visual acuity), corneal edema, light sensitivity, and optic nerve palsy have been reported in up to 1% of patients receiving amantadine. Other adverse effects that have been reported rarely include leukopenia, neutropenia, eczematoid dermatitis, photosensitization, oculogyric episodes, and increased frequency of urination. Cardiac arrest, arrhythmias (including malignant arrhythmias), hypotension, tachycardia, acute respiratory failure, pulmonary edema, tachypnea, keratitis, mydriasis, allergic reactions (including anaphylactic reactions), edema, and fever have occurred in patients receiving amantadine. Leukocytosis, pruritus, and diaphoresis also have occurred in patients receiving amantadine. Reversible elevations of serum liver enzyme concentrations have been reported in some patients receiving amantadine.

■ **Precautions and Contraindications** Amantadine should be administered with caution in patients with liver disease or a history of recurrent eczematoid dermatitis, uncontrolled psychosis or severe psychoneurosis, epilepsy or other seizures, and in those receiving drugs with CNS activity. Patients with a history of seizures should be observed closely for possible increased seizure activity. Because of possible CNS effects or visual disturbances, patients receiving amantadine should be warned that the drug may impair ability to perform hazardous activities requiring mental alertness or physical coordination such as operating machinery or driving a motor vehicle. Because amantadine may cause mydriasis, the drug should not be used in patients with untreated angle-closure glaucoma. Amantadine should be used with caution and dosage of the drug may need careful adjustment in patients with renal impairment, congestive heart failure, peripheral edema, or orthostatic hypotension. Dosage of the drug should be reduced in patients with active seizure disorders and in geriatric patients 65 years of age or older. Geriatric patients with cerebrovascular disease and/or renal impairment should be observed particularly closely for signs of amantadine toxicity. Patients who respond to amantadine should resume normal activities gradually and with caution, especially if other underlying conditions such as osteoporosis or phlebothrombosis are present.

Amantadine should not be abruptly discontinued in patients with parkinsonian syndrome because some patients have experienced exacerbations of parkinsonian symptoms within 24 hours after discontinuance of the drug. A few patients have developed parkinsonian crises, manifested as confusion, marked increase in rigidity, urinary retention, and bulbar palsy, within 3 days after abrupt discontinuance of the drug, even in the absence of apparent clinical improvement with amantadine therapy. In patients receiving concomitant levodopa-amantadine therapy, continued levodopa administration may not compensate fully for the withdrawal of amantadine.

Because possible neuroleptic malignant syndrome was reported in patients receiving amantadine and was associated with a dosage reduction or withdrawal of the drug, patients, especially those receiving antipsychotic agents, should be observed closely when the dosage of amantadine is reduced or the drug is discontinued.

Amantadine is contraindicated in patients with known hypersensitivity to the drug.

■ **Pediatric Precautions** Safety and efficacy of amantadine in children younger than 1 year of age have not been established. When used in children, amantadine has caused CNS symptoms which resolved when the drug was discontinued. An increased incidence of seizures has been reported in children with an underlying seizure disorder receiving amantadine.

■ **Mutagenicity and Carcinogenicity** Amantadine was not mutagenic in the Ames microbial test using *Salmonella typhimurium* or a mammalian mutagen assay using Chinese hamster ovary cells when the tests were performed with or without metabolic activation. In addition, there was no evidence of chromosome damage in an in vitro test using freshly derived and stimulated human peripheral blood lymphocytes (with or without metabolic activation) or an in vivo mouse bone marrow micronucleus test (140–550 mg/kg; estimated human equivalent dosage of 11.7–45.8 mg/kg based on body surface area conversion).

Long-term animal studies have not been performed to evaluate the carcinogenic potential of amantadine.

■ **Pregnancy, Fertility, and Lactation** Amantadine hydrochloride has been reported to be embryotoxic/teratogenic in rats when administered in dosages of 50 and 100 mg/kg daily (1.5 and 3 times, respectively, the maximum recommended human dosage on a mg/m^2 basis), but not when administered in a dosage of 37 mg/kg daily (the maximum recommended human dosage on a mg/m^2 basis). One woman with a movement disorder similar to parkinsonian syndrome who may have been treated with amantadine hydrochloride (100 mg daily) during the first trimester of pregnancy delivered a child with a complex cardiovascular lesion (single ventricle and pulmonary atresia) that may have been caused by the drug. Fallot and tibial hemimelia (normal karyotype) were reported in an infant exposed to oral amantadine hydrochloride during the first trimester of pregnancy (100 mg daily for 7 days during week 6 and 7 of gestation). There are no adequate and well-controlled studies using amantadine in pregnant women, and the drug should be used during pregnancy only when the potential benefits outweigh the possible risks to the fetus.

In a rat reproduction study involving 3 litters, fertility was slightly impaired when amantadine hydrochloride was administered to both males and females in a dosage of 32 mg/kg daily (the maximum recommended human dosage on a mg/m^2 basis). Fertility was not affected when the drug was given in a dosage of 10 mg/kg daily (0.3 times the maximum recommended human dosage on a mg/m^2 basis); intermediate doses were not tested.

In one instance, failure was reported during human in vitro fertilization (IVF) when the sperm donor ingested amantadine 2 weeks before and during the IVF cycle.

Because amantadine is distributed into milk, the drug should not be used in nursing women.

Drug Interactions

■ **Drugs with Anticholinergic Activity** Concomitant use of amantadine and an anticholinergic antiparkinson agent may provide additional benefit in patients who experience only marginal benefit with either agent alone. However, administration of amantadine in patients receiving drugs with anticholinergic activity may result in increased adverse anticholinergic effects. When amantadine is administered to patients already near the limit of tolerance for anticholinergic agents, atropinism with nocturnal confusion and hallucinations may gradually develop. It has been suggested that the dosage of the anticholinergic agent be reduced prior to the initiation of amantadine therapy or that the dose of either drug be reduced if atropine-like adverse effects appear.

Although concomitant administration of amantadine and thioridazine has been reported to worsen tremor in geriatric patients with Parkinson's disease, it is not known whether a similar effect would occur with other phenothiazines.

■ **Influenza Virus Vaccine** Amantandine hydrochloride does not interfere with the antibody response to influenza virus vaccine and may be given concomitantly with the vaccine.

■ **CNS Stimulants** To avoid the possibility of additive CNS stimulant effects, amantadine should be administered with caution to patients receiving other CNS stimulant drugs.

■ **Other Drugs** Concomitant administration of amantadine (100 mg 3 times daily) and a combination preparation containing triamterene and hydrochlorothiazide (co-triamterzide) in a 61-year-old man with Parkinson's disease resulted in increased plasma concentrations of amantadine; however, it is not known which component of the combination preparation may have been responsible for the interaction or whether related drugs would produce a similar effect.

Concomitant administration of quinidine or quinine with amantadine may reduce the renal clearance of amantadine.

Toxic delirium has occurred following initiation of co-trimoxazole in at least one patient who had been stabilized on amantadine; rapid resolution occurred following discontinuance of the drugs.

Acute Toxicity

■ **Manifestations** Fatalities have been reported following overdosage of amantadine. The lowest reported acute lethal dose of the drug has been 1 g.

Acute overdosage of amantadine has resulted in cardiac dysfunction (e.g., arrhythmia, tachycardia, hypertension); pulmonary edema and respiratory distress (including adult respiratory distress syndrome [ARDS]); renal dysfunction (e.g., increased BUN, decreased creatinine clearance, renal insufficiency); or CNS toxicity (e.g., insomnia, anxiety, aggressive behavior, hypertonia, hyperkinesia, tremor, confusion, disorientation, depersonalization, fear, delirium, hallucinations, psychotic reactions, lethargy, somnolence, coma). Hyperthermia has occurred with amantadine overdosage. In addition, seizures may be exacerbated in patients with prior history of seizure disorders.

One patient who ingested 2.8 g of amantadine hydrochloride developed urinary retention; mild, mixed acid-base disturbances; slightly dilated pupils which contracted minimally to light; and an acute toxic psychosis manifested as disorientation, confusion, visual hallucinations, and aggressive behavior. Another patient who ingested 2.5 g became comatose and developed cardiopulmonary arrest several hours after the ingestion. Although the arrest was successfully treated, during the arrest and subsequent 48 hours, ventricular tachyarrhythmias manifested as atypical ventricular tachycardia (torsades de pointes) and ventricular fibrillation occurred; therapy with adrenergic agents, particularly dopamine, appeared to exacerbate the ventricular tachyarrhythmias. The patient subsequently died of aspiration pneumonia and respiratory distress.

■ **Treatment** There is no specific antidote for overdosage of amantadine. If overdosage of amantadine is recent, prompt gastric lavage or induction of emesis is indicated. General supportive measures (including establishment of adequate respiratory exchange by maintenance of adequate airway, control of respiration and oxygen administration) should be instituted and cardiovascular status, blood pressure, pulse, respiration, temperature, serum electrolytes, urinary output, and urine pH should be monitored. Fluids should be forced and, if necessary, given IV. Acidifying agents may be administered to increase the rate of amantadine excretion; only minimal amounts of amantadine are removed by hemodialysis. If there is no record of recent voiding, catheterization should be done. The patient should be observed for hyperactivity and seizures; if required, sedatives and anticonvulsant therapy should be administered. Slow IV administration of physostigmine 1- and 2-mg doses at 1- to 2-hour intervals in one adult and 0.5-mg doses at 5- to 10-minute intervals (to a maximum of 2 mg/hour) in a child has been effective in the management of CNS toxicity caused by amantadine. The patient also should be observed for the possible development of arrhythmias and hypotension; if required, appropriate antiarrhythmic and antihypotensive therapy should be administered. Electrocardiographic monitoring may be necessary since malignant tachyarrhythmias can occur following amantadine overdosage. Caution should be employed when using adrenergic agents to maintain blood pressure and heart rate, since these agents may further predispose the patient to the development of serious ventricular tachyarrhythmias.

Pharmacology

The exact mechanism of action of amantadine hydrochloride in the treatment of parkinsonian syndrome and drug-induced extrapyramidal reactions is not known but appears to be unrelated to its activity in the prophylaxis and symptomatic treatment of influenza A virus infections. Amantadine does not have any appreciable anticholinergic activity; the drug probably exerts a potentiating effect on catecholaminergic, including dopaminergic, neurotransmission in the CNS. In one study, amantadine hydrochloride given IV to dogs reportedly caused release of catecholamines from peripheral nerve storage sites; a similar mechanism for the drug's central activity was proposed. It has been postulated that amantadine causes release of dopamine from synaptosomes; however, this may occur only following doses higher than those employed clinically. There is some evidence that amantadine, in usual therapeutic concentrations, may exert its antiparkinsonian activity by blocking the reuptake of dopamine into presynaptic neurons, thus causing accumulation of dopamine in the presynaptic clefts of dopaminergic neurons in the basal ganglia. In addition, the drug may cause direct stimulation of postsynaptic receptors.

Pharmacokinetics

■ **Absorption** Amantadine hydrochloride is well absorbed from the GI tract. Mean peak blood amantadine concentrations of 0.3 mcg/mL have been reported to occur 1–4 hours after an oral dose of amantadine hydrochloride 2.5 mg/kg. Following oral administration of a single 100-mg capsule of amantadine hydrochloride, mean peak plasma concentrations of 0.22 mcg/mL occurred within 3.3 hours. Following oral administration of a single 100-mg dose of amantadine hydrochloride as the oral solution, peak plasma concentrations averaged 0.24 mcg/mL and were achieved within 2–4 hours. Peak plasma concentrations averaged 0.47 mcg/mL in individuals receiving amantadine hydrochloride oral solution 100 mg twice daily for 15 days. Following oral administration of amantadine hydrochloride 200 mg as a tablet in fasting adults 19–27 years of age or fasting geriatric individuals 60–70 years of age, peak plasma concentrations averaged 0.51 or 0.8 mcg/mL, respectively. While peak plasma concentrations are directly related to amantadine hydrochloride dose up to a dosage of 200 mg daily, dosages exceeding 200 mg daily may result in a greater than proportional increase in peak plasma concentration. In a small number of patients who received 300 mg of amantadine hydrochloride daily (200 mg in the morning and 100 mg in the afternoon), steady-state blood concentrations of 0.68–1.01 mcg/mL were reached after 4–5 days of therapy. In healthy young adults receiving 25, 100, or 150 mg twice daily, steady-state trough plasma concentrations averaged 0.11, 0.3, or 0.59 mcg/mL, respectively.

Plasma amantadine concentrations in geriatric patients receiving the drug in a dosage of 100 mg daily reportedly approximate those attained in younger adults receiving the drug in a dosage of 200 mg daily; it is not known whether this occurs because of normal decline in renal function or other age-related factors. In one study, 3 patients with severe renal impairment showed symptoms of toxicity and elevated steady-state blood concentrations (2.5–4.4 mcg/mL) following 200 mg of amantadine hydrochloride daily. One metabolite, acetylamantadine, has been detected in plasma in less than 50% of individuals receiving a single amantadine hydrochloride 200-mg dose. In those individuals with detectable plasma acetylamantadine, concentration of the metabolite represented up to 80% of the concurrent amantadine concentration.

■ **Distribution** Distribution of amantadine hydrochloride into body tissues and fluids has not been fully characterized.

In animals, amantadine is distributed into heart, lung, liver, kidney, and spleen. In a study in mice, lung tissue concentrations of amantadine were much higher than blood concentrations.

Following oral administration, amantadine is distributed into nasal secretions in concentrations that are lower than plasma concentrations. Following oral administration of a single 200-mg dose of amantadine hydrochloride in healthy young and geriatric adults, amantadine concentrations in nasal secretions or plasma averaged 0.15 mcg/g or 0.58 mcg/mL at 1 hour, 0.28 mcg/g or 51 mcg/mL at 4 hours, and 0.39 mcg/g or 0.45 mcg/mL at 8 hours. A substantial proportion of amantadine appears to distribute into erythrocytes, with an erythrocyte to plasma ratio of 2.7 reported in men with normal renal function and 1.4 in men with substantial renal impairment. In one patient, the CSF concentration of amantadine was approximately one-half the blood concentration. Amantadine distributes into human breast milk.

The volume of distribution following IV administration of amantadine reportedly is 3–8 L/kg. Amantadine is about 67% bound to plasma proteins over a concentration range of 0.1–2 mcg/mL.

■ **Elimination** The elimination half-life of amantadine has been variously reported as 9–37 hours, with an average of 24 hours or less. Clearance of amantadine is reduced, plasma concentrations of the drug are increased, and elimination half-life may be prolonged in healthy geriatric adults compared with healthy young adults. A half-life of 29 hours (range: 20–41 hours) has been reported in geriatric men 60–76 years of age. In addition, the half-life of amantadine is prolonged at least twofold to threefold in patients with impaired renal function (i.e., creatinine clearance less than 40 mL/minute per 1.73 m^2). In one study, the half-life ranged from 18.5–81.3 hours in patients with creatinine clearances of 13.7–43.1 mL/minute per 1.73 m^2 and averaged 8.3 days (range: 7–10.3 days) in patients undergoing chronic hemodialysis.

While amantadine principally is excreted unchanged in urine by glomerular filtration and tubular secretion, at least 8 metabolites have been identified in urine. Amantadine undergoes *N*-acetylation, and about 5–15% of an absorbed dose is excreted in urine as acetylamantadine. Whether this metabolic pathway is affected by acetylator phenotype remains to be determined. The clinical importance of amantadine metabolites is unknown. Acidification of urine increases the rate of amantadine excretion, and administration of urine-acidifying drugs may increase amantadine elimination from the body. Amantadine is only minimally removed by hemodialysis. In patients with renal failure who received a single 300-mg oral dose of amantadine hydrochloride, only 5% or less of the dose was removed into the dialysate following a 4-hour period of hemodialysis.

Chemistry and Stability

■ **Chemistry** Amantadine hydrochloride is a synthetic adamantane derivative (a symmetric tricyclic amine) that is used in the treatment of parkinsonian syndrome and drug-induced extrapyramidal reactions, and in the prevention and symptomatic treatment of influenza caused by A influenza virus strains. (See Amantadine Hydrochloride 8:18.04.) Amantadine hydrochloride is structurally unrelated to other antiparkinsonian agents.

Amantadine hydrochloride occurs as a white or practically white, crystalline powder which has a bitter taste and has solubilities of approximately 400 mg/mL in water and 200 mg/mL in alcohol at 25°C. Amantadine hydrochloride has a pK_a of 9.

■ **Stability** Commercially available amantadine hydrochloride tablets and capsules should be stored in tight containers at a controlled room temperature of 25°C; limited exposure to temperatures of 15–30°C is permitted. Amantadine hydrochloride oral solution should be stored in tight containers at a controlled room temperature of 25°C; limited exposure to temperatures of 15–30°C is permitted, and freezing should be avoided.

Preparations

Excipients in commercially available drug preparations may have clinically important effects in some individuals; consult specific product labeling for details.

Amantadine Hydrochloride

Oral		
Capsules	100 mg*	Amantadine Hydrochloride Capsules
Solution	50 mg/5 mL*	Amantadine Hydrochloride Solution
Tablets	100 mg*	Amantadine Hydrochloride Tablets
		Symmetrel®, Endo

*available from one or more manufacturer, distributor, and/or repackager by generic (nonproprietary) name

†Use is not currently included in the labeling approved by the US Food and Drug Administration

ANTICHOLINERGIC AGENTS 28:36.08

Benztropine Mesylate

■ Benztropine mesylate is an antimuscarinic antiparkinsonian agent.

Uses

Benztropine mesylate is used for the adjunctive treatment of all forms of parkinsonian syndrome including the postencephalitic, idiopathic, and arteriosclerotic types. Benztropine is also used for the relief of parkinsonian signs and symptoms of antipsychotic agent-induced (e.g., phenothiazines) extrapyramidal reactions except tardive dyskinesia. Benztropine may be used alone or in conjunction with other antiparkinsonian drugs. Geriatric patients who do not tolerate cerebral-stimulating agents may respond to benztropine.

Dosage and Administration

■ **Administration** Benztropine mesylate is administered orally or by IM injection. Parenteral administration should be reserved for patients who cannot take oral medication or for emergency situations, such as acute dystonic reactions, when rapid response is desired. Although benztropine may also be administered IV, the manufacturer states that there is no clinically important difference in onset between IM or IV injection; therefore, IV administration of the drug is rarely necessary.

■ **Dosage** ***Parkinsonian Syndrome*** Dosage of benztropine mesylate should be individualized according to the age and weight of the patient and the type of parkinsonian syndrome being treated. Geriatric patients or those with less than average body weight generally cannot tolerate high dosages of the drug.

For the adjunctive treatment of arteriosclerotic, idiopathic, or postencephalitic parkinsonian syndrome, the usual adult oral or parenteral dosage of benztropine mesylate is 1–2 mg daily (range: 0.5–6 mg daily). Benztropine therapy should be initiated at low dosages and gradually increased by 0.5-mg increments at 5- or 6-day intervals to a maximum dosage of 6 mg daily or until optimum symptomatic relief is obtained. For the arteriosclerotic and idiopathic types of parkinsonian syndrome, patients should be started on a single daily dose of 0.5–1 mg at bedtime. The dosage is then increased in increments of 0.5 mg every few days until the optimum tolerated dosage is reached. The increments may be added to the single daily dose or given as separate doses up to 4 times daily. Sometimes a single dose of 2 mg, usually given at bedtime, is sufficient to control symptoms for 24 hours. Younger patients with postencephalitic parkinsonian syndrome may tolerate larger initial doses and may require 2 mg 2 or 3 times daily for maintenance therapy. Older patients may be controlled with 1 or 2 mg daily.

Periodic dosage adjustment may be required in patients receiving benztropine with levodopa or a combination of levodopa and carbidopa to maintain optimum symptomatic relief. When benztropine is given to replace or supplement other antiparkinsonian drugs, the change should be gradual, with the dosage of the previous medication reduced as the dosage of benztropine is increased.

Drug-Induced Extrapyramidal Reactions For the symptomatic relief of antipsychotic agent-induced extrapyramidal reactions (except tardive dyskinesia), the recommended oral or parenteral dosage of benztropine mesylate is 1–4 mg once or twice daily. Dosage must be individualized according to the patient's response and tolerance. For the symptomatic relief of extrapyramidal disorders that develop shortly after initiation of antipsychotic (e.g., phenothiazines) therapy, 1–2 mg 2 or 3 times daily usually provides relief within 1 or 2 days. Since acute extrapyramidal symptoms are generally transient, the need for benztropine should be reevaluated after 1–2 weeks of therapy.

For the relief of an acute dystonic reaction, 1–2 mg of benztropine mesylate may be given IV, followed by 1–2 mg orally twice daily to prevent recurrence.

Cautions

■ **Adverse Effects** Adverse reactions to benztropine are mainly extensions of its anticholinergic (see Cautions: Adverse Effects, in the Antimuscarinics/Antispasmodics General Statement 12:08.08) and antihistaminic effects. Dryness of the mouth, blurred vision, mydriasis, nausea, nervousness, tachycardia, or skin rash may occur. In high dosage or in particularly susceptible patients, mental confusion and excitement, weakness and inability to move certain muscle groups, and, occasionally, urinary retention and/or difficulty in urination may result. Constipation, numbness of the extremities, listlessness, depression, vomiting, paralytic ileus, hyperthermia, fever, heat stroke, and visual hallucinations have also been reported. Adjustment of dosage will usually overcome most adverse effects of benztropine, but in the event of severe reactions, such as excitement or vomiting, the drug should be withdrawn and later resumed at a lower dosage.

■ **Precautions and Contraindications** Benztropine should be used with caution or may be contraindicated in patients with conditions in which anticholinergic effects are undesirable. The usual precautions and contraindications associated with antimuscarinics should be observed with benztropine. For a complete discussion of the precautions and contraindications associated with antimuscarinics,see Cautions: Precautions and Contraindications, in the Antimuscarinics/Antispasmodics General Statement 12:08.08.

Since benztropine has cumulative effects, continuous supervision of patients receiving the drug is advised, especially for those with a tendency toward tachycardia, or with prostatic hypertrophy. Patients with mental disorders receiving benztropine for control of drug-induced extrapyramidal effects should also be carefully observed, especially at the beginning of therapy or during dosage adjustment, since worsening of mental symptoms or toxic psychosis can occur.

Patients receiving benztropine concomitantly with phenothiazines or other drugs with anticholinergic effects should be warned to promptly report any adverse GI effects, since paralytic ileus, sometimes fatal, has occurred during concomitant therapy with these drugs.

Benztropine should not be used in patients with tardive dyskinesia, since the drug generally does not relieve signs and symptoms of this condition and may aggravate them. Benztropine is also contraindicated in patients with hypersensitivity to the drug or other components of the tablet or parenteral preparation.

■ **Pediatric Precautions** Benztropine is contraindicated in children younger than 3 years of age and should be used with caution in older children because of the drug's adverse anticholinergic effects.

■ **Pregnancy** Safe use of benztropine during pregnancy has not been established.

Drug Interactions

Concomitant administration of benztropine with other drugs having anticholinergic effects may increase the risk of adverse anticholinergic effects. Concomitant administration of an anticholinergic antiparkinsonian agent (e.g., benztropine) with phenothiazines and/or tricyclic antidepressants may cause paralytic ileus, hyperthermia, or heat intolerance, effects that occasionally have been fatal. Patients who are receiving benztropine concomitantly with phenothiazines, haloperidol, or other drugs with anticholinergic or antidopaminergic activity should notify their clinicians promptly if adverse GI effects, fever, or heat intolerance occurs.

Pharmacology

The anticholinergic effect of benztropine is about equal to that of atropine. The antihistaminic activity of benztropine is similar to that of pyrilamine maleate. Benztropine does not produce as much central stimulation as does trihexyphenidyl. The effects of the drug are cumulative and may not be evident until 2 or 3 days after treatment is begun.

Chemistry and Stability

■ **Chemistry** Benztropine mesylate is a synthetic, tertiary amine antimuscarinic antiparkinsonian agent. The drug resembles both atropine and diphenhydramine in chemical structure and exhibits anticholinergic, antihistaminic, and local anesthetic properties. Benztropine mesylate occurs as a white, odorless, slightly hygroscopic, crystalline powder and is very soluble in water and freely soluble in alcohol. Benztropine mesylate injection has a pH of 5–8.

■ **Stability** Benztropine mesylate tablets should be stored in well-closed containers. Benztropine mesylate tablets and injection should be stored at a temperature less than 40°C, preferably between 15–30°C; freezing of the injection should be avoided.

For further information on pharmacology, cautions, acute toxicity, and drug interactions of benztropine, see the Antimuscarinics/Antispasmodics General Statement 12:08.08.

Preparations

Excipients in commercially available drug preparations may have clinically important effects in some individuals; consult specific product labeling for details.

Benztropine Mesylate

Oral		
Tablets	0.5 mg*	**Benztropine Mesylate Tablets**
	1 mg*	**Benztropine Mesylate Tablets**
	2 mg*	**Benztropine Mesylate Tablets**
Parenteral		
Injection	1 mg/mL	**Cogentin®**, Ovation

*available from one or more manufacturer, distributor, and/or repackager by generic (nonproprietary) name

Selected Revisions January 2009,

CATECHOL-*O*-METHYLTRANSFERASE (COMT) INHIBITORS 28:36.12

Entacapone

■ Entacapone is a selective and reversible inhibitor of catechol-*O*-methyltransferase (COMT); concomitant administration of entacapone with levodopa and a decarboxylase inhibitor (e.g., carbidopa) results in increased and more sustained plasma levodopa concentrations compared with administration of levodopa and a decarboxylase inhibitor.

Uses

■ **Parkinsonian Syndrome** Entacapone is used as an adjunct to levodopa-carbidopa in the symptomatic treatment of idiopathic parkinsonian syndrome in patients who experience manifestations of end-of-dose "wearing-off." Efficacy of entacapone as an adjunct to levodopa for the management of parkinsonian syndrome has been established in 3 randomized, double-blind, placebo-controlled studies of up to 24 weeks' duration in patients receiving levodopa in combination with a decarboxylase inhibitor (i.e., benserazide, carbidopa). In 2 of these studies, participation was limited to patients who exhibited end-of-dose motor fluctuations in response to levodopa (i.e., fluctuating response with "off" phenomena); patients in the third study were not required to exhibit end-of-dose fluctuations for enrollment. In the first 2 studies, daily "on" time increased by 1–1.5 hours with entacapone therapy compared with minimal changes (0.1–0.4 hours) in patients receiving placebo. In the third study, slight but insignificant improvements in "on" time were observed in the subgroup of patients with "off" phenomena. When manifestations of parkinsonian syndrome were assessed using parts of the Unified Parkinson's Disease Rating Scale (UPDRS), substantial improvements were observed in the total score and in UPDRS subscales II (activities of daily living) and III (motor functioning) in all 3 studies. No substantial improvement was observed using subscale I (mentation). In the first 2 studies, the investigator's global assessment also improved, and the mean daily dosage of levodopa was decreased substantially in patients receiving entacapone. No substantial changes occurred in levodopa dosage or global percent improved in patients enrolled in the third study. Although patients in the third study were not required to have been experiencing motor fluctuations, the drug has not been evaluated systematically in patients who do not experience such fluctuations.

For additional information on the management of parkinsonian syndrome, see Uses: Parkinsonian Syndrome, in Levodopa/Carbidopa 28:92.

Dosage and Administration

■ **General** Entacapone is administered orally without regard to meals.

The recommended dosage is 200 mg administered with each levodopa-carbidopa dose up to a maximum of 8 times daily (1.6 g daily). Clinical experience with dosages exceeding 1.6 g daily is limited. Entacapone should be administered only in conjunction with levodopa-carbidopa.

To optimize patient response, reductions in the daily levodopa dosage or frequency of administration may be necessary. In clinical studies, most patients (58%) who were receiving 800 mg or more of levodopa daily or who had moderate or severe dyskinesias before initiating entacapone therapy required a reduction in levodopa dosage; the average reduction in daily levodopa dosage was about 25%.

Entacapone can be administered with conventional tablets, orally disintegrating tablets, or extended-release preparations of levodopa-carbidopa or as a fixed-combination preparation containing levodopa, carbidopa, and entacapone (Stalevo®).

The fixed-combination preparation containing levodopa, carbidopa, and entacapone (Stalevo®) generally is used in patients receiving stable dosages of levodopa, carbidopa, and entacapone equivalent to those in the combination preparation, but also may be used in certain patients receiving stable dosages of levodopa and carbidopa equivalent to the dosages in the fixed-combination preparation when a decision has been made to add entacapone to the regimen. Tablets containing the fixed combination of levodopa, carbidopa, and entacapone should not be divided, and only one tablet should be administered per dosing interval. Because there is limited clinical experience with entacapone dosages exceeding 1.6 g daily, the maximum dosage of fixed-combination preparations containing levodopa 50–150 mg, carbidopa 12.5–37.5 mg, and entacapone 200 mg (Stalevo® 50, 75, 100, 125, and 150) is 8 tablets daily. Because there is limited clinical experience with carbidopa dosages exceeding 300 mg daily, maximum dosage of the fixed-combination preparation containing levodopa 200 mg, carbidopa 50 mg, and entacapone 200 mg (Stalevo® 200) is 6 tablets daily.

For patients transferring from therapy with levodopa-carbidopa and entacapone (as separate preparations) to the fixed-combination preparation, recommendations are available for transferring patients currently receiving levodopa-carbidopa preparations containing a 1:4 ratio of carbidopa to levodopa. Patients receiving entacapone 200 mg with each dose of levodopa-carbidopa (e.g., conventional tablet preparation containing 100 mg of levodopa and 25 mg of carbidopa) can be switched to the corresponding strength of the fixed-combination preparation containing levodopa, carbidopa, and entacapone (Stalevo®). The manufacturer states that there is no experience to date in transferring patients currently receiving entacapone together with extended-release preparations of levodopa-carbidopa or levodopa-carbidopa preparations containing a 1:10 ratio of carbidopa to levodopa to the fixed-combination preparation.

For patients initiating entacapone therapy, recommendations regarding use of the fixed-combination preparation should be individualized according to the current levodopa dosage and the presence of dyskinesias. For patients treated with levodopa-carbidopa conventional tablets who are receiving more than 600 mg of levodopa daily or who have a history of moderate or severe dyskinesias before initiation of entacapone therapy, dosage should first be adjusted by administering levodopa-carbidopa (1:4 ratio) and entacapone as separate preparations. If it is determined that optimum maintenance dosages of levodopa, carbidopa, and entacapone correspond to the doses in the commercial combination product, the fixed-combination preparation (Stalevo®) may be used. For patients receiving levodopa dosages of 600 mg or less daily (conventional tablets, 1:4 ratio) and who do not have dyskinesias, an attempt can be made to initiate therapy with the fixed-combination preparation. The initial dosage of the fixed-combination preparation of levodopa, carbidopa, and entacapone should provide the same dosage of levodopa and carbidopa that the patient currently is taking. However, a reduction in the dosage of levodopa-carbidopa or entacapone may be necessary. Because dosage of levodopa, carbidopa, or entacapone cannot be adjusted individually using the fixed-combination preparation, administration of levodopa-carbidopa and entacapone as separate preparations may be necessary.

■ **Special Populations** Entacapone should be administered with caution in patients with biliary obstruction because biliary excretion is the principal route of elimination of the drug. Based on limited data, pharmacokinetics may be altered in patients with hepatic failure, and the drug should be used with caution in such patients. The effects of liver disease on the pharmacokinetics of entacapone following long-term therapy in conjunction with levodopa and carbidopa have not been evaluated to date.

Pharmacokinetics of entacapone were not affected by age or renal impairment, and dosage adjustment is *not* necessary for patients with renal impairment *nor* for geriatric patients. The manufacturer makes no special population (e.g., hepatic impairment) dosage recommendations at this time.

Cautions

■ **Contraindications** Known hypersensitivity to entacapone or any ingredient in the formulation.

■ **Warnings/Precautions** ***Warnings*** **Monoamine Oxidase Inhibitors.** Because monoamine oxidase (MAO) and catechol-*O*-methyltransferase (COMT) are the 2 major enzyme systems involved in the metabolism of catecholamines, the possibility exists that concomitant use of entacapone and a nonselective MAO inhibitor (e.g., phenelzine, tranylcypromine) could result in inhibition of the principal pathways involved in the metabolism of catecholamines. Therefore, patients ordinarily should not be treated concomitantly with entacapone and a nonselective MAO inhibitor. However, entacapone can be used concomitantly with a selective MAO-B inhibitor (e.g., selegiline).

Drugs Metabolized by COMT. Concomitant use of entacapone and drugs known to be metabolized by COMT (e.g., bitolterol [no longer commercially available in the US], dobutamine, dopamine, epinephrine, isoetharine, isoproterenol, methyldopa, norepinephrine) may result in increased heart rate, arrhythmias, and excessive changes in blood pressure regardless of the route of administration (including inhalation). The manufacturer of entacapone includes apomorphine in this list of drugs. However, data from in vivo studies indicate that apomorphine is not metabolized by COMT.

Potential Risk of Prostate Cancer. In 2010, the US Food and Drug Administration (FDA) notified healthcare professionals and patients about the results of a long-term, randomized, controlled study (Stalevo Reduction in Dyskinesia Evaluation in Parkinson's Disease [STRIDE-PD]) suggesting an increased risk of prostate cancer in patients receiving combined therapy with levodopa, carbidopa, and entacapone (administered as the fixed-combination preparation

Stalevo®) compared with those receiving a conventional levodopa-carbidopa formulation. The STRIDE-PD study, which was conducted over 4 years in more than 700 patients requiring initiation of levodopa therapy for early parkinsonian syndrome, was designed to evaluate the time to onset of dyskinesias in patients initiating such therapy with levodopa, carbidopa, and entacapone compared with those initiating therapy with levodopa-carbidopa. A higher incidence of prostate cancer was observed among patients receiving levodopa, carbidopa, and entacapone compared with those receiving levodopa-carbidopa (3.7 versus 0.9%, respectively). Patients received the combined regimen of levodopa, carbidopa, and entacapone for an average of 664 days (range: 148–949 days) prior to the diagnosis of prostate cancer. While previous controlled studies evaluating entacapone as an adjunct to levodopa-carbidopa in patients with parkinsonian syndrome have not found an increased risk of prostate cancer, most of these trials were of shorter duration (e.g., less than 1 year) than the STRIDE-PD trial.

FDA subsequently required that the manufacturer conduct a study to further evaluate this potential risk. FDA also studied this issue independently using data from the Department of Veterans Affairs health care system. Based on these additional studies, FDA announced in August 2019 that the agency had concluded that entacapone use is not associated with an increased risk of prostate cancer. As a result, FDA's recommendations for using entacapone will remain the same in the prescribing information. Health care professionals should follow standard prostate cancer screening recommendations for patients.

Major Toxicities **Cardiovascular Effects.** Entacapone enhances levodopa availability and therefore may be expected to increase the occurrence of orthostatic hypotension or syncope when administered with levodopa/carbidopa. However, in clinical studies, the incidence of orthostatic hypotension or syncope was similar in patients receiving entacapone or placebo.

Findings from an FDA-conducted meta-analysis, which combined cardiovascular-related findings from 15 clinical trials, suggested an increased risk of cardiovascular events (i.e., myocardial infarction, stroke, cardiovascular death) with entacapone. In the meta-analysis, patients who received combined therapy with levodopa, carbidopa, and entacapone had a small but statistically significant increase in the risk of cardiovascular events compared with those who received levodopa-carbidopa, raising concerns about entacapone (the drug component lacking in the comparator regimen). However, the increased risk was driven largely by results of a single trial (STRIDE-PD), and subsequent analysis of the available data found no evidence to support such an association. Results of 2 additional analyses that were conducted using data from Medicare or a commercial insurance database showed no increased risk of cardiovascular events (myocardial infarction, stroke, death) with entacapone compared with other antiparkinsonian agents. Based on this information, FDA believes that the cardiovascular findings from the previous meta-analysis were due to chance and do not represent a true risk associated with entacapone.

GI Effects. Diarrhea was reported in 10% of patients receiving entacapone in clinical studies, and about 2% of patients required discontinuance of the drug because of diarrhea. Diarrhea generally was of mild to moderate intensity, but severe diarrhea, which required hospitalization, may occur rarely. Diarrhea generally occurs during the first 4–12 weeks of entacapone therapy, but may occur as early as the first week or as late as several months following initiation of entacapone therapy. Diarrhea generally resolved following discontinuance of the drug.

Hallucinations. Hallucinations were reported in about 4% of patients receiving entacapone or placebo in clinical studies and resulted in hospitalization in 1 or 0.3% of patients, respectively.

Dyskinesia. Entacapone may potentiate the adverse dopaminergic effects of levodopa and may cause or exacerbate dyskinesias. Although decreasing the dosage of levodopa may ameliorate the dyskinesias, many patients in placebo-controlled studies continued to experience frequent dyskinesias despite a reduction in levodopa dosage. Discontinuance of therapy because of dyskinesia was required in 2 or 1% of patients receiving entacapone or placebo, respectively.

Rhabdomyolysis. Severe rhabdomyolysis has been reported rarely in patients receiving entacapone. Because of the complex nature of these adverse events, the role of the drug, if any, remains to be determined.

Nervous System and Muscular Effects. A symptom complex resembling neuroleptic malignant syndrome (NMS; elevated temperature, muscular rigidity, altered consciousness, elevated CPK) has been reported in association with abrupt withdrawal or dosage lowering of other dopaminergic agents. Similar episodes have been reported in association with entacapone, although limited information is available on dosage adjustments in these patients and a causal relationship to the drug has not been established. No such manifestations were reported following the abrupt withdrawal or dosage reduction of entacapone during clinical studies of the drug. (See Warnings/Precautions: General Precautions, in Cautions.)

Respiratory Effects. Retroperitoneal fibrosis, pulmonary infiltrates, pleural effusion, and thickening of the pleura have been reported in a few patients treated with ergot-derivative dopamine receptor agonists (e.g., bromocriptine, pergolide). Although these adverse effects presumably are related to the ergoline structure of these compounds, the possibility exists that nonergot-derived drugs that increase dopaminergic activity such as entacapone may induce similar pulmonary changes. Pulmonary fibrosis occurred in 4 patients receiving entacapone in clinical studies for 7–17 months; these patients also were receiving an ergot-derivative dopamine-receptor agonist (i.e., bromocriptine, pergolide).

General Precautions Whenever the fixed-combination preparation containing levodopa, carbidopa, and entacapone (Stalevo®) is used, the precautions and contraindications associated with all the drugs in the preparation must be considered.

Withdrawal of Therapy. If entacapone therapy is discontinued, the patient should be closely monitored and adjustments made, if necessary, in the dosage of dopaminergic therapy. Although tapering the dosage of entacapone has not been systematically evaluated, the manufacturer recommends the slow withdrawal of the drug if the decision to discontinue treatment is made. If a patient experiences hyperpyrexia or severe rigidity following discontinuance of entacapone, the possibility that the patient is experiencing a symptom complex resembling the neuroleptic malignant syndrome should be considered in the differential diagnosis.

Melanoma. Data from epidemiologic studies indicate that patients with parkinsonian syndrome have a twofold to approximately sixfold greater risk of developing melanoma than the general population. It is unclear whether this increased risk is due to parkinsonian syndrome or other factors (e.g., drugs used to treat the disease). Because of these findings, patients and clinicians should monitor for melanoma on a frequent and regular basis. The manufacturer recommends that dermatologic examinations be performed periodically by qualified clinicians (e.g., dermatologists).

Intense Urges. Intense urges (e.g., urge to gamble, increased sexual urges, other intense urges) and inability to control these urges have been reported in some patients receiving antiparkinsonian agents that increase central dopaminergic tone (including entacapone). Although a causal relationship has not been established, these urges stopped in some cases when dosage was reduced or the drug was discontinued. Clinicians should ask patients whether they have developed new or increased gambling urges, sexual urges, or other urges while receiving entacapone and should advise them of the importance of reporting such urges. If a patient develops such urges while receiving entacapone, consideration should be given to reducing the dosage or discontinuing the drug.

Specific Populations **Pregnancy.** Category C. (See Users Guide.)

Lactation. Entacapone is distributed into milk in rats; caution if used in nursing women.

Pediatric Use. Not indicated.

Geriatric Use. No substantial differences in safety or pharmacokinetics relative to younger adults.

Hepatic Impairment. Use with caution.

Biliary Obstruction. Use with caution.

■ **Common Adverse Effects** Adverse effects occurring in 1% or more of patients receiving entacapone and more frequently than placebo include dyskinesia, nausea, hyperkinesia, diarrhea, urine discoloration, hypokinesia, dizziness, abdominal pain, constipation, fatigue, vomiting, back pain, dry mouth, dyspnea, increased sweating, anxiety, somnolence, dyspepsia, flatulence, purpura, asthenia, taste perversion, agitation, gastritis, GI disorder, and bacterial infection. Adverse effects resulting in discontinuance include psychiatric reasons, diarrhea, dyskinesia/hyperkinesia, nausea, abdominal pain, and aggravation of parkinsonian syndrome.

Drug Interactions

■ **Levodopa** Pharmacokinetic interaction (increased plasma concentration of levodopa, improved therapeutic and adverse effect profile of levodopa). (See Warnings/Precautions: Major Toxicities, in Cautions.)

■ **Drugs Metabolized by Catechol-*O*-methyltransferase** Potential pharmacokinetic interaction with drugs metabolized by catechol-*O*-methyltransferase (COMT) (e.g., dopamine, epinephrine, isoproterenol). (See Warnings/Precautions: Warnings, in Cautions.)

■ **Drugs Affecting Hepatic Microsomal Enzymes** Pharmacokinetic interaction unlikely.

■ **Monoamine Oxidase Inhibitors** Potential pharmacologic interaction (inhibits catecholamine metabolism) with nonselective monoamine oxidase (MAO) inhibitors (e.g., phenelzine, tranylcypromine). (See Warnings: Monoamine Oxidase Inhibitors, in Cautions: Warnings/Precautions.) Pharmacologic interaction unlikely with selective MAO-B inhibitors (e.g., selegiline).

■ **Drugs Interfering with Biliary Excretion, Glucuronidation, and Intestinal β-Glucuronidase** Potential pharmacokinetic interaction (decreased entacapone excretion) with drugs interfering with biliary excretion, glucuronidation, and intestinal β-glucuronidase (e.g., cholestyramine, probenecid, some anti-infectives [e.g., ampicillin, chloramphenicol, erythromycin, rifampin]).

■ **Protein-bound Drugs** Pharmacokinetic interaction unlikely. In vitro studies of entacapone have shown no binding displacement with drugs such as diazepam, phenylbutazone, salicylic acid, or warfarin.

■ **Imipramine** Pharmacologic interaction unlikely.

■ **CNS Depressants** Potential pharmacologic interaction (additive sedative effects).

Description

Entacapone is a selective and reversible inhibitor of catechol-*O*-methyltransferase (COMT) that is structurally and pharmacologically related to tolcapone. The drugs are nitrocatechols and are chemically and pharmacologically unrelated to other currently available antiparkinsonian agents (e.g., levodopa, carbidopa, ergot- and nonergot-derivative dopamine-receptor agonists, the selective monoamine oxidase [MAO]-B inhibitor selegiline hydrochloride). However, unlike tolcapone, entacapone has not been associated with hepatotoxicity (e.g., drug-induced hepatitis, fatal liver failure). In humans, entacapone inhibits the COMT enzyme in peripheral tissues. The effects of the drug on central COMT activity in humans have not been studied. For information on COMT, see Pharmacology in Tolcapone 28:36.12.

Concomitant administration of entacapone with levodopa and a decarboxylase inhibitor (e.g., carbidopa) results in increased and more sustained plasma levodopa concentrations compared with administration of levodopa and a decarboxylase inhibitor. Sustained levodopa concentrations presumably result in more consistent dopaminergic stimulation, resulting in greater reduction in the manifestations of parkinsonian syndrome. Entacapone lacks antiparkinsonian activity when administered alone.

Entacapone is almost completely metabolized prior to excretion with only 0.2% of a dose excreted unchanged in urine. The main metabolic pathway is isomerization followed by glucuronidation to an inactive conjugate. Biliary excretion apparently is the principal route of elimination of the drug and its metabolites.

Advice to Patients

Importance of not discontinuing entacapone abruptly and of taking only as prescribed.

Necessity of exercising caution when driving or operating machinery when entacapone is initiated. Caution when taking other CNS depressants.

Advise that entacapone may cause a change in the color of their urine (a brownish orange discoloration); not clinically important.

Advise that hallucinations, nausea, and increased dyskinesia can occur.

Importance of informing clinicians of existing or contemplated concomitant therapy, including prescription and OTC drugs.

Importance of asking patients whether they have developed any new or increased gambling urges, sexual urges, or other urges while receiving entacapone and of advising them of the importance of reporting such urges.

Importance of frequent monitoring for melanoma and periodic dermatologic examinations performed by a dermatologist.

Importance of women informing clinicians if they are or plan to become pregnant or plan to breast-feed.

Advise not to rise rapidly after prolonged sitting or lying down, especially during the first few weeks of entacapone therapy.

Importance of informing patients of other important precautionary information. (See Cautions.)

Overview (see Users Guide). For additional information until a more detailed monograph is developed and published, the manufacturer's labeling should be consulted. It is *essential* that the manufacturer's labeling be consulted for more detailed information on usual cautions, precautions, contraindications, potential drug interactions, laboratory test interferences, and acute toxicity.

Preparations

Excipients in commercially available drug preparations may have clinically important effects in some individuals; consult specific product labeling for details.

Entacapone

Oral		
Tablets, film-coated	200 mg	Comtan®, Novartis

Entacapone Combinations

Oral		
Tablets, film-coated	200 mg with Carbidopa 12.5 mg (of anhydrous carbidopa) and Levodopa 50 mg	Stalevo®, Novartis
	200 mg with Carbidopa 18.75 mg (of anhydrous carbidopa) and Levodopa 75 mg	Stalevo®, Novartis
	200 mg with Carbidopa 25 mg (of anhydrous carbidopa) and Levodopa 100 mg	Stalevo®, Novartis
	200 mg with Carbidopa 31.25 mg (of anhydrous carbidopa) and Levodopa 125 mg	Stalevo®, Novartis
	200 mg with Carbidopa 37.5 mg (of anhydrous carbidopa) and Levodopa 150 mg	Stalevo®, Novartis
	200 mg with Carbidopa 50 mg (of anhydrous carbidopa) and Levodopa 200 mg	Stalevo®, Novartis

Tolcapone

■ Tolcapone is a reversible catechol-*O*-methyltransferase (COMT) inhibitor; concomitant administration of tolcapone with levodopa and a decarboxylase inhibitor results in more sustained plasma levodopa concentrations compared with administration of levodopa and a decarboxylase inhibitor.

Uses

■ **Parkinsonian Syndrome** Tolcapone is used as an adjunct to levodopa/carbidopa therapy for the symptomatic treatment of parkinsonian syndrome. Because of the risk of potentially fatal, acute fulminant liver failure, tolcapone generally should be reserved for patients with parkinsonian syndrome receiving levodopa/carbidopa who are experiencing symptom fluctuations and are not responding adequately to other adjunctive therapies (e.g., ergot- and nonergot-derivative dopamine receptor agonists, selegiline hydrochloride) or are not candidates for these adjunctive therapies. Tolcapone therapy should not be initiated until the risks of therapy have been discussed with the patient and the patient has provided written informed consent. (See Cautions: Precautions and Contraindications.) Following initiation of tolcapone therapy, symptomatic improvement generally is evident within 3 weeks. Because of the risk of liver injury in patients receiving tolcapone, the drug should be discontinued in patients who fail to show substantial clinical benefit (symptomatic improvement) within 3 weeks of initiating tolcapone therapy. (See Cautions: Hepatic Effects.)

Levodopa currently is the most effective drug for relieving the manifestations of parkinsonian syndrome. However, the effectiveness of levodopa decreases substantially after the third year of treatment, and about 50% of patients develop motor response fluctuations after 5 years of treatment. Several types of motor fluctuations including a return of parkinsonian manifestations toward the end of an interdose period ("off" effect) may occur in some patients during long-term levodopa therapy. While the mechanisms underlying the changes in response to levodopa have not been fully elucidated, the "off" effect may be related to the pharmacokinetics of levodopa and its short plasma elimination half-life. The short half-life of levodopa is a result of rapid absorption and rapid metabolism by enzymatic decarboxylation and *O*-methylation.

Several strategies have been evaluated and/or used to optimize the pharmacokinetics of levodopa. One widely employed strategy is administration of levodopa in combination with a decarboxylase inhibitor. Concomitant administration of a decarboxylase inhibitor (e.g., carbidopa) with levodopa increases the bioavailability of levodopa, but does not increase plasma half-life. Catechol-*O*-methyltransferase (COMT) inhibitors (e.g., tolcapone) provide another strategy to optimize the pharmacokinetics of levodopa.

Tolcapone enhances the clinical efficacy of levodopa by increasing the area under the plasma concentration-time curve (AUC) and half-life of levodopa without increasing the peak plasma concentration. Pharmacokinetic alterations associated with tolcapone may be preferred to increasing the levodopa dosage, since increasing the levodopa dosage results in increased peak plasma levodopa concentrations and increased incidence of dyskinesia and other potential toxicities as well as in potentially greater peak-trough fluctuations. While extended-release preparations of levodopa/carbidopa slow absorption and may result in decreased peak-trough fluctuations when dosed appropriately, these preparations also result in less predictable time to peak plasma levodopa concentrations and reduced bioavailability of levodopa and have not resulted in substantially different incidences of motor complications compared with conventional preparations in some studies; it has been suggested that more frequent dosing of extended-release preparations, particularly when combined with a COMT inhibitor, may improve therapeutic benefit.

Efficacy of tolcapone as an adjunct to levodopa for the management of parkinsonian syndrome has been established in several randomized, placebo controlled studies of up to 12 months' duration in patients receiving levodopa in combination with a decarboxylase inhibitor (e.g., carbidopa). Tolcapone has been evaluated in patients who exhibited predictable end-of-dose motor fluctuations in response to levodopa (i.e., fluctuating response with "off" phenomena) and in patients with early parkinsonian syndrome whose response to levodopa was stable (nonfluctuating). In studies in patients with "off" phenomena, the primary efficacy index was change between baseline and month 3 in the amount of time in a 16-hour day spent "on" (period of good functioning) and "off" (period of poor functioning) as measured using self rating charts. In addition, improvement in manifestations of parkinsonian syndrome was assessed using parts of the Unified Parkinson's Disease Rating Scale (UPDRS), a Global Assessment of Change (IGA), the Sickness Impact Profile (SIP), and changes in levodopa dosage. In patients with early parkinsonian syndrome whose response to levodopa was stable, the primary efficacy index was the UPDRS subset II (activities of daily living). Improvement in manifestations of parkinsonian syndrome was also assessed using UPDRS subset III (motor functioning), SIP scores, and changes in levodopa dosage.

Results of clinical studies indicate that tolcapone enhances the efficacy of levodopa. In placebo-controlled studies in patients who were experiencing a deteriorating response to levodopa, tolcapone reduced the severity of "off" motor fluctuations, allowed a reduction in levodopa dosage, and improved overall clinical status. In placebo-controlled studies in North American and European patients whose levodopa therapy was complicated by "off" phenomena, therapy with tolcapone 200 mg 3 times daily was associated with a decrease in "off" time of 1.6–3 hours and an increase in "on" time of 1.7–2.9 hours.

Clinically important changes in "on/off" time in North American patients receiving tolcapone 100 mg 3 times daily were not observed; however, a decrease in "off" time of 2 hours and an increase in "on" time of 1.7 hours occurred in European patients receiving tolcapone 100 mg 3 times daily. Response to tolcapone in terms of changes in "off" time in patients receiving levodopa as levodopa/carbidopa conventional tablets could not be distinguished from that in patients receiving levodopa/carbidopa extended-release tablets; however, the study was not specifically designed to assess potential differences between the levodopa/carbidopa formulations. While further study is needed to establish safety and efficacy of tolcapone during long-term therapy, improvement in "off" phenomena observed at 3 months was maintained throughout the study (i.e., at 9–12 months).

In these studies, maintenance dosage of levodopa was reduced in patients receiving tolcapone. The mean total daily levodopa dosage decreased 166 mg from the baseline dose of 788 mg in North American patients receiving tolcapone 100 mg 3 times daily for 3 months, and 207 mg from a baseline of 865 mg in North American patients receiving tolcapone 200 mg 3 times daily. The mean total daily levodopa dosage decreased 109 mg from the baseline dose of 667 mg in European patients receiving tolcapone 100 mg 3 times daily for 3 months, and 122 mg from a baseline of 675 mg in European patients receiving tolcapone 200 mg 3 times daily. In addition, 3 months of therapy with tolcapone 100 or 200 mg 3 times daily resulted in an overall improvement as measured by IGA in 70–71 or 78–91% of patients, respectively. Improvement in the UPDRS subscale III (motor functioning) and total SIP scores was seen in European patients receiving tolcapone 200 mg 3 times daily; however, substantial improvement in UPDRS subscale II (activities in daily living), UPDRS subscale III, and total SIP scores was not observed in North American patients receiving either tolcapone dosage or in European patients receiving tolcapone 100 mg 3 times daily. While both dosages of tolcapone were equally effective in terms of changes in "on-off" time in European patients, changes in "on-off" time in North American patients and UPDRS and SIP scores in European patients suggest that tolcapone 200 mg 3 times daily is more effective than 100 mg 3 times daily. Because the 200-mg dose is not as well tolerated as the 100-mg dose, the higher dosage should be reserved for patients who do not respond adequately to the lower dosage.

Only limited information is available on the efficacy of tolcapone versus other antiparkinsonian agents. In one comparative study, tolcapone (200 mg 3 times daily) was as effective or more effective than bromocriptine (mean final dose of 22.4 mg daily) in increasing "on" time and decreasing "off" time in patients whose levodopa therapy was complicated by "off" phenomena.

While the precise role of tolcapone in the management of patients with advanced parkinsonian syndrome remains to be determined, strategies to be considered in patients whose therapy is complicated by suboptimal peak response, "off" phenomena, or unpredictable "on-off" response include addition of tolcapone to levodopa therapy. However, because of the risk of potentially fatal, acute fulminant liver failure, tolcapone generally should be reserved for patients receiving levodopa/carbidopa who are experiencing symptom fluctuations and are not responding adequately to other adjunctive therapies (i.e., ergot- and nonergot-derivative dopamine receptor agonists, selegiline hydrochloride) or are not candidates for these adjunctive therapies.

In placebo-controlled studies in levodopa-treated patients with early parkinsonian syndrome, addition of tolcapone 100 or 200 mg 3 times daily for 6 months was associated with a substantial reduction in UPDRS activity of daily living and motor scores, and a reduction in mean daily levodopa dosage of 21–32 mg from a baseline of 370–381 mg. The effect of tolcapone on activities of daily living was evident after 1–2 weeks of therapy; continued improvement occurred during the first 6 weeks, and was greatest in those with the most severe impairment at baseline. Improvement in quality of life was maintained throughout the study (i.e., 12 months). While both dosages appear to be equally effective in improving clinical status in stable patients with early parkinsonian syndrome, fewer patients receiving the 200-mg dose of tolcapone developed levodopa-associated motor fluctuation than those receiving placebo.

Although the role of tolcapone in the management of early parkinsonian syndrome has not been established, benefits (more consistent levodopa concentrations, reduced risk of motor complications) associated with use of tolcapone in such patients must be weighed against the risk of liver injury associated with the drug.

Initially, it had been hoped that the long-term benefits of tolcapone therapy might be greatest if therapy were initiated early in the course of parkinsonian syndrome before motor complications of levodopa had developed or become established; however, reports of severe hepatotoxicity have resulted in a far more cautious and conservative approach to tolcapone therapy.

For additional information on the management of parkinsonian syndrome, see Uses: Parkinsonian Syndrome, in Levodopa 28:92.

Dosage and Administration

Because of the risk of potentially fatal, acute fulminant liver failure, tolcapone generally should be reserved for patients with parkinsonian syndrome receiving levodopa/carbidopa who are experiencing symptom fluctuations and are not responding adequately to other adjunctive therapies (e.g., ergot- and nonergot-derivative dopamine receptor agonists, selegiline hydrochloride) or are not candidates for these adjunctive therapies. Following initiation of tolcapone therapy, symptomatic improvement generally is evident within 3 weeks. Because of the risk of liver injury in patients receiving tolcapone, the drug should be discontinued in patients who do not experience symptomatic improvement within 3 weeks of initiating tolcapone therapy. Tolcapone therapy should not be initiated in patients with clinical evidence of active liver disease, or ALT (SGPT) or AST (SGOT) concentrations exceeding the upper limit of normal, or any other evidence of hepatocellular dysfunction. Tolcapone therapy generally should not be reintroduced in a patient who previously experienced tolcapone-associated hepatic injury. Tolcapone should be used with caution in patients with severe dystonia or dyskinesia.

■ **Administration** Tolcapone is administered orally in 3 equally divided doses daily. Although food may reduce the bioavailability of tolcapone (e.g., by 10–20%), the manufacturer states that the drug can be taken without regard to meals. In clinical studies, the first dose of the day of tolcapone was administered together with the first dose of the day of levodopa/carbidopa; subsequent doses of tolcapone are administered 6 and 12 hours later. Tolcapone can be administered with conventional or extended-release preparations of levodopa/carbidopa.

Tolcapone therapy should not be initiated until the risks of therapy have been discussed with the patient and the patient has provided written informed consent.

■ **Dosage** For the management of parkinsonian syndrome, tolcapone is given in conjunction with levodopa/carbidopa. To optimize patient response, reductions in the daily levodopa/carbidopa dosage may be necessary. In clinical studies, most patients (70%) who were receiving more than 600 mg of levodopa daily or who had moderate to severe dyskinesias before initiating tolcapone therapy required a reduction in levodopa dosage; the average reduction in daily levodopa dosage was about 30%.

The usual initial dosage of tolcapone is 100 mg 3 times daily. In clinical studies, increases in liver function test results (i.e., ALT) occurred more frequently in patients receiving tolcapone 200 mg 3 times daily than in those receiving 100 mg 3 times daily. Whether the risk of fulminant hepatic failure is increased in patients receiving the higher dosage is not known; however, the manufacturer states that it is prudent to reserve the higher dosage of 200 mg 3 times daily for situations when the anticipated incremental benefit is justified. If a patient fails to show the expected clinical benefit while receiving tolcapone 200 mg 3 times daily for 3 weeks, the drug should be discontinued.

■ **Dosage in Renal Impairment** The manufacturer states that dosage adjustment is not required in patients with mild to moderate renal impairment (creatinine clearance exceeding 30 mL/minute). The safety of tolcapone in patients with creatinine clearance less than 25 mL/minute has not been evaluated.

■ **Discontinuance of Tolcapone Therapy** Like dopaminergic drugs, discontinuance of tolcapone or abrupt reduction in dosage may lead to reemergence of the signs and symptoms of parkinsonian syndrome or a symptom complex resembling neuroleptic malignant syndrome (e.g., hyperpyrexia and confusion). If tolcapone therapy is discontinued, the patient should be closely monitored and adjustments made, if needed, in the dosage of dopaminergic therapy. If a patient experiences hyperpyrexia or severe rigidity following discontinuance of tolcapone, the possibility that the patient is experiencing a symptom complex resembling neuroleptic malignant syndrome should be considered in the differential diagnosis. Tapering the dosage of tolcapone has not been systematically evaluated. Reducing the frequency of administration to twice or once daily prior to discontinuing may not prevent these events, since the duration of COMT inhibition associated with tolcapone therapy is 5–6 hours or longer.

Cautions

Information on the safety of tolcapone has been obtained principally from clinical studies in patients experiencing a deteriorating response to levodopa and in patients with early parkinsonian syndrome whose response to levodopa was stable. While tolcapone generally is well tolerated, cases of serious and potentially fatal adverse effects (e.g., severe hepatocellular injury) have been reported during postmarketing surveillance. (See Cautions: Precautions and Contraindications.)

The most frequent adverse effects reported in patients receiving tolcapone in clinical studies included dyskinesia, dystonia, nausea, anorexia, sleep disturbances/insomnia, orthostatic instability, muscle cramping, excessive dreaming, and somnolence; these effects are dopaminergic effects associated with levodopa therapy. The most frequent adverse nondopaminergic effect reported in patients receiving tolcapone was diarrhea. Discontinuance of tolcapone therapy was required in about 16% of patients in clinical studies, principally because of diarrhea.

■ **Hepatic Effects** Severe hepatocellular injury, including fulminant liver failure resulting in death, has been reported during postmarketing surveillance. As of May 2005, 3 cases of fatal fulminant hepatic failure have been reported from more than 40,000 patient-years of worldwide use. The 3 cases of fatal fulminant hepatic failure occurred during the first 6 months of tolcapone therapy. This incidence may be 10- to 100-fold higher than the background incidence in the general population. While these figures provide an estimate of the increased risk of severe hepatocellular injury associated with tolcapone therapy, a more precise determination of risk cannot be made because of possible underreporting of the number of tolcapone-treated patients who experienced adverse hepatic effects and uncertainty in the base rate of hepatic failure in individuals in the same age group and with the same health profile as the patients who received tolcapone.

Elevations in the results of one or more liver function test results have occurred in patients receiving tolcapone in phase III clinical studies, and required discontinuance of therapy in 0.3% of those receiving tolcapone 100 mg 3 times daily and in 1.7% of those receiving tolcapone 200 mg 3 times daily. Increases in liver function test results have been reported more frequently in women than men (5 versus 2%), and were accompanied by diarrhea in about one-third of patients. Increases in serum concentrations in ALT (SGPT) or AST (SGOT) (more than 3 times the upper limit of normal) occurred in 1 or 3% of patients receiving tolcapone 100 or 200 mg 3 times daily in clinical studies. Substantial increases in serum concentrations of ALT or AST (more than 8 times the upper limit of normal) occurred in 0.3 or 0.7% of patients receiving tolcapone 100 or 200 mg 3 times daily.

Most cases of elevated liver function test results occurred 6 weeks to 6 months following initiation of tolcapone therapy; enzyme concentrations generally returned to baseline within 1–3 months in about 50% of patients in clinical studies who continued tolcapone therapy and within 2–3 weeks up to 1–2 months in patients who discontinued tolcapone. However, the patient's condition also can deteriorate rapidly and result in death despite discontinuance of the drug. (See Cautions: Precautions and Contraindications.) Liver biopsy findings in fulminant cases of hepatitis with tolcapone have included severe centrolobular necrosis and lobular inflammatory infiltrate consisting mainly of plasma cells and eosinophilia; hepatic changes may not be visible on ultrasound.

■ **GI Effects** Diarrhea has been reported in 16–18% of patients receiving tolcapone in clinical studies, and 6% of patients required discontinuance of the drug because of diarrhea. Discontinuance of tolcapone was related to the severity of diarrhea, with 8, 40, or 70% of those with mild, moderate, or severe diarrhea discontinuing the drug. While diarrhea generally was of mild to moderate intensity, severe diarrhea occurred in 3–4% of patients and resulted in hospitalization in 0.7 or 1.7% of patients receiving tolcapone 100 or 200 mg 3 times daily. Diarrhea generally occurs during the first 6–12 weeks of tolcapone therapy, but may occur as early as 2 weeks or as late as several months following initiation of tolcapone therapy. Diarrhea frequently is associated with anorexia, is dose-related, and resolves with continuing therapy or following discontinuance of tolcapone.

Nausea, which likely is a dopaminergic effect (secondary to tolcapone-induced increases in levodopa concentrations) and generally occurs during the first 3 months of therapy, was reported in 30–35% of patients receiving tolcapone in clinical studies. Anorexia, vomiting, constipation, abdominal pain, xerostomia, dyspepsia, or flatulence was reported in 19–23, 8–10, 6–8, 5–6, 5–6, 3–4, or 2–4%, respectively, of patients receiving tolcapone in clinical studies. While a causal relationship to the drug has not been established, taste alteration, tooth disorder, or weight loss occurred in at least 1% of patients receiving tolcapone, and dysphagia, GI hemorrhage, gastroenteritis, mouth ulceration, increased salivation, abnormal stools, esophagitis, cholelithiasis, colitis, tongue disorder, or rectal disorder occurred in 0.1–1% of patients. Cholecystitis, duodenal ulcer, GI carcinoma, or stomach atony occurred in less than 0.1% of patients.

■ **Nervous System and Muscular Effects** Addition of tolcapone may exacerbate levodopa-associated dyskinesias, especially in patients already experiencing dyskinesias. This effect, which was reported in 42 or 51% of patients receiving tolcapone 100 or 200 mg 3 times daily in clinical studies, usually occurs within 24 hours after initiating tolcapone therapy and is controlled by reducing the levodopa dosage 20–30%. However, some patients continue to experience frequent dyskinesias after reduction in the levodopa dosage. Discontinuance of tolcapone because of dyskinesia was required in 0.3 or 1% of patients receiving tolcapone 100 or 200 mg 3 times daily.

Dystonia, muscle cramping, hyperkinesia, hypokinesia, or hypertonia was reported in 19–22, 17–18, 2–3, 1–3, or 1%, respectively, of patients receiving tolcapone in clinical studies. Dystonia has been reported more frequently in patients younger than 75 years of age than in older patients.

Numerous CNS and psychiatric disturbances may occur in patients receiving tolcapone in conjunction with levodopa, and many are likely to be the result of increased levodopa concentrations and CNS bioavailability induced by tolcapone. Hallucinations have been reported in 8–10% of patients receiving tolcapone in clinical studies, required hospitalization in up to 1.7% of patients, and resulted in discontinuance of the drug in 1–1.4% of patients. Hallucinations generally present within the first 2 weeks of tolcapone therapy, are commonly accompanied by confusion and to a lesser extent insomnia and excessive dreaming, and occur more frequently in patients 75 years of age or older than in younger patients. Experience from clinical studies indicates that tolcapone-associated hallucinations may be responsive to levodopa dosage reduction; patients whose hallucinations resolved had a mean levodopa dosage reduction from baseline (i.e., onset of hallucinations) of 175–200 mg daily (20–25%). Sleep disturbances/insomnia, excessive dreaming, somnolence, confusion, dizziness, or headache has been reported in 24–25, 16–21, 14–18, 10–11, 6–13, or 10–11%, respectively, of patients receiving tolcapone in clinical studies. Somnolence was reported more frequently in women than men. Most of these effects presumably result from increased dopaminergic effects.

Adverse nervous system effects occurring in 1–3% of patients include paresthesia, stiffness, arthritis, agitation, irritability, mental deficiency, hyperactivity, panic reaction, or euphoria. While a causal relationship has not been established, mental depression, hypesthesia, tremor, speech disorder, vertigo, emotional disorder, myalgia, arthralgia, limb pain, anxiety, paresis, lethargy, asthenia, or abnormal gait has been reported in at least 1% of tolcapone- treated patients, and migraine headache, neuralgia, amnesia, extrapyramidal syndrome, hostility, increased or decreased libido, manic reactions, nervousness, paranoid reaction, cerebral ischemia, cerebrovascular accident, delusions, neuropathy, apathy, choreoathetosis, myoclonus, psychosis, abnormal thinking, twitching, tenosynovitis, arthrosis, or joint disorder has occurred in 0.1–1% of patients. Antisocial reaction, delirium, encephalopathy, hemiplegia, or meningitis has occurred in less than 0.1% of patients.

Neuroleptic malignant syndrome has occurred in patients receiving psychotherapeutic agents and in patients with parkinsonian syndrome during withdrawal of dopaminergic agents (i.e., levodopa, amantadine, bromocriptine). In clinical studies, a symptom complex resembling neuroleptic malignant syndrome (elevated temperature, muscular rigidity, altered consciousness) in association with abrupt withdraw or lowering of the dosage of tolcapone occurred in 4 patients. Creatine kinase (CK, creatine phosphokinase, CPK) values were increased in 3 patients; one patient died, and the other patients recovered over 2–6 weeks. There also have been rare postmarketing reports of this symptom complex; however, the role of tolcapone in these events remains to be determined since they were of a complicated nature and involved concomitant administration of other drugs that affect brain monoaminergic (i.e., nonselective MAO inhibitors, tricyclic antidepressants, selective serotonin- reuptake inhibitors) and anticholinergic systems.

Severe rhabdomyolysis, including multiorgan system failure progressing to death in one patient, has been reported in a few patients receiving tolcapone. Because of the complex nature of these adverse events, the role of tolcapone, if any, in severe rhabdomyolysis has not been determined. While severe prolonged motor activity including dyskinesia may be associated with the development of rhabdomyolysis, some cases have included fever, alteration of consciousness, and muscular rigidity and resembled neuroleptic malignant syndrome.

■ **Cardiovascular Effects** Orthostatic instability occurs frequently in parkinsonian patients receiving dopaminergic agents, including levodopa. In clinical studies, orthostatic instability occurred more frequently in patients receiving tolcapone in combination with levodopa and a decarboxylase inhibitor than in patients receiving levodopa and a decarboxylase inhibitor (17 versus 14%). While the mechanism of this increased incidence has not been fully elucidated, such an increase would be expected because tolcapone increases the bioavailability of levodopa. Orthostatic hypotension was documented in 13–14% of patients receiving tolcapone in clinical studies; however, it was usually asymptomatic and only 4–5% of tolcapone-treated patients reported orthostatic symptoms. While patients (including those randomized to placebo therapy) with orthostatic instability at baseline were more likely than patients without symptoms to experience orthostatic hypotension, therapy with a dopamine agonist or selegiline hydrochloride at baseline did not appear to increase the incidence of orthostatic hypotension in patients receiving tolcapone. About 0.7% of patients receiving tolcapone in clinical studies discontinued the drug because of adverse effects related to hypotension.

Syncope has occurred in 4–5% of patients receiving tolcapone in clinical studies. Syncope was reported more frequently in patients (including those randomized to placebo) who had an episode of documented hypotension than in those who did not have an episode of documented hypotension. Falls or loss of balance occurred in 4–6 or 2–3% of patients receiving tolcapone in clinical studies.

Adverse cardiovascular effects reported in 1–3% of patients receiving tolcapone in clinical studies included chest pain, hypotension, or chest discomfort. While a causal relationship has not been established, peripheral edema or palpitations have occurred in at least 1% of patients receiving tolcapone, and hypertension, vasodilation, angina pectoris, heart failure, atrial fibrillation, tachycardia, aortic stenosis, arrhythmia, arteriospasm, bradycardia, cerebral hemorrhage, coronary artery disorder, heart arrest, myocardial infarction, myocardial ischemia, or pulmonary embolus has occurred in 0.1–1% of patients. Arteriosclerosis, cardiovascular disorder, pericardial effusion, or thrombosis has occurred in less than 0.1% of patients.

■ **Respiratory Effects** Upper respiratory tract infection, dyspnea, or sinus congestion has been reported in 5–7, 3, or 1–2%, respectively, of patients receiving tolcapone in clinical studies. Pneumonia, sinusitis, bronchitis, or pharyngitis has occurred in at least 1% of patients receiving tolcapone, and increased cough, rhinitis, asthma, epistaxis, hyperventilation, laryngitis, or hiccup has occurred in 0.1–1% of patients. Apnea, hypoxia, or lung edema has occurred in less than 0.1% of patients; however, these adverse effects have not been directly attributed to the drug.

Retroperitoneal fibrosis, pulmonary infiltrates, pleural effusion, and thickening of the pleura have been reported in a few patients receiving ergot-derivative dopamine receptor agonists (e.g., bromocriptine, pergolide). In most reported cases, these pulmonary changes slowly reverted to normal following discontinuance of the ergot-derivative dopamine receptor agonist; however, complete resolution did not always occur. While these pulmonary changes presumably are related to the ergoline structure of bromocriptine or pergolide, the possibility exists that non-ergot derived drugs that increase dopaminergic activity such as tolcapone may induce similar pulmonary changes. Pleural effusion occurred in 3 patients and pulmonary fibrosis occurred in 1 patient in clinical studies evaluating tolcapone; these patients also were receiving an ergot-derivative dopamine-receptor agonist (i.e., bromocriptine, pergolide) and had a history of cardiac disease or pulmonary pathology (i.e., nonmalignant lung lesion).

■ **Genitourinary Effects** Urinary tract infection, urine discoloration (i.e., increased yellow color attributed to tolcapone metabolites), micturition disorder, or uterine tumor has occurred in 5, 2–7, 1–2, or 1% of patients receiving tolcapone. Although not directly attributable to tolcapone, micturition frequency, urinary incontinence, or impotence has been reported in at least 1% of tolcapone-treated patients, and prostatic disorder, dysuria, nocturia, polyuria, urinary retention, urinary tract disorder, renal calculus, prostatic carcinoma, oliguria, uterine atony, uterine disorder, or vaginitis has been reported in 0.1–1% of patients. Bladder calculus, ovarian carcinoma, or uterine hemorrhage has been reported in less than 0.1% of patients.

Hematuria occurred in 4–5% of patients receiving tolcapone in placebo-controlled studies, and microscopically confirmed hematuria was reported in 2% of patients receiving the drug in US placebo-controlled studies. While the etiology of the increased incidence of hematuria in tolcapone-treated patients remains to be determined, the increased incidence was not attributed to urinary tract infection or oral anticoagulant therapy.

Rats given tolcapone in a dosage equivalent to 6 times or more of the recommended human dosage for 1 or 2 years developed a high incidence of proximal tubule cell damage consisting of degeneration, single cell necrosis, hyperplasia, karyocytomegaly and atypical nuclei. These effects were not accompanied by changes in clinical chemistry parameters, and currently there is no established method for monitoring the possible occurrence of these types of lesions in humans. While it has been suggested that these toxic renal effects may result from a species-specific mechanism, experiments to confirm such a theory have not been conducted.

■ **Dermatologic and Sensitivity Reactions** Increased sweating has occurred in 4–7% of patients receiving tolcapone in clinical studies; dermal bleeding, skin tumor, or alopecia has been reported in 1% of patients. Rash has occurred in at least 1% of tolcapone-treated patients, and allergic reaction, herpes zoster, pruritus, seborrhea, skin discoloration, eczema, erythema multiforme, skin disorder, cellulitis, furunculosis, herpes simplex, facial edema, or urticaria has occurred in 0.1–1% of patients; however, these adverse effects have not been directly attributed to the drug.

■ **Otic and Ocular Effects** While not directly attributed to tolcapone, otic or ocular effects reported in at least 1% of tolcapone-treated patients include cataract, inflamed eye, blurred vision, or tinnitus; those occurring in 0.1–1% of patients include diplopia, ear pain, ocular hemorrhage, ocular pain, lacrimation disorder, otitis media, or parosmia. Glaucoma has occurred in less than 0.1% of tolcapone-treated patients.

■ **Other Adverse Effects** Fatigue or influenza has occurred in 3–7 or 3–4% of tolcapone-treated patients and neck pain, burning, malaise, or fever has occurred in 1–2% of patients. Fractures, flank pain, accidental injury, or infection has occurred in at least 1% of patients receiving tolcapone, and hernia, pain, bacterial infection, fungal infection, viral infection, chills, breast carcinoma, carcinoma, neoplasm, abscess, edema, hypercholesteremia, thirst, dehydration, anemia, or diabetes mellitus has occurred in 0.1–1% of patients; these adverse effects have not been directly attributed to tolcapone. Other events not directly attributable to the drug include surgical procedure. Death has been reported in less than 0.1% of tolcapone-treated patients in clinical studies.

Studies in rats and monkeys given tolcapone have not revealed any potential for physical or psychologic dependence. While clinical studies have not revealed any evidence of potential for abuse, systematic studies in humans designed to evaluate abuse potential have not been performed.

■ **Precautions and Contraindications** Therapy with tolcapone should not be initiated until the clinician has fully explained the risks of such therapy and the patient (or his representative) has provided written informed consent.

Hepatotoxic Risk Because of the risk of potentially fatal, acute fulminant liver failure, tolcapone generally should be reserved for patients with parkinsonian syndrome receiving levodopa/carbidopa who are experiencing symptom fluctuations and are not responding adequately to other adjunctive therapies (e.g., ergot- and nonergot-derivative dopamine receptor agonists, selegiline hydrochloride) or are not candidates for these adjunctive therapies. Following initiation of tolcapone therapy, symptomatic improvement generally is evident within 3 weeks. Because of the risk of hepatic injury in patients receiving tolcapone and the normal time course of tolcapone response, the drug should be discontinued in patients who do not experience symptomatic improvement within 3 weeks of initiating tolcapone therapy. Tolcapone therapy should not be initiated in patients with clinical evidence of active liver disease, ALT (SGPT) or AST (SGOT) concentrations exceeding the upper limit of normal, or any other evidence of hepatocellular dysfunction. In addition, tolcapone therapy should be discontinued if ALT or AST concentrations increase to more than 2 times the upper limit of normal or if clinical manifestations suggest the onset of hepatic failure (e.g., persistent nausea, fatigue, lethargy, anorexia, jaundice, dark urine, pruritus, upper right quadrant tenderness).

Patients who develop evidence of hepatocellular injury while receiving tolcapone and in whom such therapy is discontinued for any reason may be at increased risk for hepatic injury if tolcapone is reintroduced. Accordingly, such patients ordinarily should not be considered for retreatment with the drug.

Patients receiving tolcapone should be monitored for evidence of emergent liver injury. In addition, patients should be advised of the clinical manifestations that suggest the onset of hepatic injury such as clay-colored stools, jaundice, fatigue, loss of appetite, and lethargy. If signs or symptoms suggestive of hepatic failure occur, patients should be advised to contact their clinician immediately.

Because tolcapone therapy has been associated with alterations in some liver function laboratory test results, liver enzymes (i.e., serum AST, ALT) should be evaluated at baseline, every 2–4 weeks during the first 6 months of therapy, and then as often as is clinically indicated. If the dose of tolcapone is increased to 200 mg 3 times daily, serum AST and ALT should be determined prior to increasing the dosage and then at the same frequency as that recommended when therapy is initiated.

While a program of frequent laboratory monitoring for evidence of hepatocellular injury is considered essential, whether periodic monitoring of liver enzymes will prevent the occurrence of fulminant tolcapone-induced liver failure is not known. Frequent monitoring is considered important since early detection of drug-induced hepatic injury along with immediate discontinuance of the suspect drug is believed to enhance the likelihood for recovery.

Other Precautions and Contraindications Catechol-*O*-methyltransferase (COMT) and monoamine oxidase (MAO) are the 2 principal enzymes involved in the metabolism of catecholamines. Because the possibility exists that concomitant administration of tolcapone and a nonselective MAO inhibitor (e.g., phenelzine, tranylcypromine) would result in inhibition of the principal pathways involved in the metabolism of catecholamines, administration of tolcapone with a nonselective MAO inhibitor should be avoided. However, tolcapone can be administered concomitantly with a selective inhibitor of MAO-B (e.g., selegiline hydrochloride). (See Drug Interactions: MAO Inhibitors.)

Tolcapone may exacerbate levodopa-associated adverse effects in some patients, presumably by increasing dopaminergic activity; many of these adverse effects can be mitigated by reducing the levodopa dosage. Patients should be advised that they may develop orthostatic hypotension with or without symptoms such as dizziness, nausea, syncope, and sweating. The manufacturer states that patients should be cautioned against rising rapidly after prolonged sitting or lying down, especially during the first few weeks of tolcapone therapy. Patients should be informed that hallucinations can occur with tolcapone therapy. Patients also should be advised that tolcapone may cause somnolence and that they should not drive a car or operate other complex machinery until they have gained sufficient experience with the drug to determine whether it has adverse effects on their mental and/or motor performance. In addition, the possibility of additive sedative effects should be considered in patients receiving other CNS depressants concomitantly with tolcapone.

Patients experiencing persistent diarrhea should be evaluated by appropriate clinical and laboratory studies, including fecal occult blood studies. Patients receiving tolcapone should be advised that they may experience nausea, especially during the *first 3 months of therapy.

Tolcapone should be used with caution in patients with dystonia or dyskinesia. Tolcapone also should be used with caution in patients with severe renal failure.

Tolcapone is contraindicated in patients with liver disease, those in whom tolcapone was discontinued because of evidence of tolcapone-induced hepatocellular injury, and those with known hypersensitivity to the drug or any ingredient in the formulation. Tolcapone also is contraindicated in patients with a history of nontraumatic rhabdomyolysis, or drug-related hyperpyrexia and confusion.

■ **Pediatric Precautions** The manufacturer states that there is no identified potential use of tolcapone in pediatric patients. Therefore, safety and efficacy of the drug in children have not been determined.

■ **Geriatric Precautions** Safety and efficacy of tolcapone in geriatric patients have not been studied specifically to date; however, parkinsonian syndrome, for which safety and efficacy have been established, occurs principally in patients older than 50 years of age. Experience in clinical studies suggests that patients 75 years of age or older are more likely to develop hallucinations but less likely to develop dystonia than younger patients. Pharmacokinetic studies have not revealed age-related differences in the pharmacokinetics of tolcapone.

■ **Mutagenicity and Carcinogenicity** Tolcapone was not mutagenic in the Ames test, the in vitro V79/HPRT gene mutation assay, or the unscheduled DNA synthesis assay. Tolcapone was clastogenic in the in vitro mouse lymphoma/thymidine kinase assay in the presence of metabolic activation; however, tolcapone was not clastogenic in an in vitro chromosomal aberration assay in cultured human lymphocytes or in an in vivo micronucleus assay in mice.

There was no evidence of carcinogenicity in male or female mice given oral tolcapone dosages of 100, 300, or 800 mg/kg daily (equivalent to 0.8, 1.6, or 4 times the human exposure based on area under the plasma concentration-time curve [AUC] at a dosage of 600 mg daily) for 80–95 weeks.

The carcinogenic potential of tolcapone has been evaluated in rats given oral dosages of 50, 250, or 450 mg/kg daily (equivalent in male rats to 1, 6.3, or 13 times the human exposure based on AUC at a dosage of 600 mg daily and in female rats to 1.7, 11.8, or 26.4 times human exposure) for 104 weeks. An increased incidence of uterine adenocarcinomas was observed in female rats at exposure levels equivalent to 26.4 times human exposure.

While exposure equivalent to one times the human exposure in male rats or 1.7 in female rats were not associated with renal tumors, renal tubular cell adenomas occurred at middle and high doses in female rats and tubular cell carcinomas occurred in middle and high doses in male rats and high doses in female rats. Minimal to marked damage to the renal tubules, characterized by proximal tubule cell degeneration, single cell necrosis, hyperplasia, and karyocytomegaly, occurred at doses associated with renal tumors. Renal tubule damage, characterized by proximal tubule cell degeneration and presence of atypical nuclei, were observed in rats receiving oral tolcapone dosages of 150 or 450 mg/kg daily for 1 year; in addition, adenocarcinoma was reported in one male rat receiving tolcapone 450 mg/kg daily. These histopathologic changes suggest that the renal tumor formation might be secondary to chronic cell damage and sustained repair; however, further study is needed to define this relationship. The clinical importance of these findings in rats to humans remains to be determined. The carcinogenic potential of tolcapone in combination with levodopa/carbidopa has not been examined.

■ **Pregnancy, Fertility, and Lactation** Reproductive studies in rats or rabbits given oral tolcapone dosages up to 300 or 400 mg/kg daily (5.7 or 15 times the 600-mg daily dose on a mg/m^2 basis) during organogenesis did not reveal teratogenic effects. However, an increased rate of abortion occurred in rabbits given tolcapone 100 mg/kg daily (3.7 times the 600-mg daily dose on a mg/m^2 basis), and maternal toxicity (i.e., decreased weight gain, death) occurred in rats given 300 mg/kg daily and in rabbits given 400 mg/kg daily. Decreased litter size and impaired growth and learning performance in female pups was observed in reproductive studies in female rats given tolcapone 250–150 mg/kg daily (4.8–2.9 times the 600-mg daily dose on a mg/m^2 basis; dose reduced from 250 mg/kg daily to 150 mg/kg daily during late gestation because of high rate of maternal toxicity) during the last part of gestation and during lactation.

Tolcapone is administered in conjunction with levodopa/carbidopa; levodopa/carbidopa cause visceral and skeletal malformations in rabbits. An increased incidence of fetal malformations (i.e., principally external and skeletal digit defects) was observed in rabbits given tolcapone 100 mg/kg daily (plasma exposure 0.5 times the expected human exposure based on AUC) in combination with levodopa 80 mg/kg daily (plasma exposure 6 times the expected human exposure) and carbidopa 20 mg/kg daily throughout organogenesis compared with rabbits given levodopa/carbidopa. In embryo/fetal development studies, fetal body weights were reduced in offspring of rats given tolcapone 10, 30, or 50 mg/kg daily (at least 0.5 times the expected human exposure) in combination with levodopa 120 mg/kg daily (at least 21 times the expected human exposure) and carbidopa 30 mg/kg daily or levodopa/carbidopa alone, but not in offspring of rats given tolcapone 50 mg/kg daily (1.4 times the expected human exposure). While tolcapone does not appear to be teratogenic in animals, there are no adequate and controlled studies to date in humans. Tolcapone should only be used during pregnancy when the potential benefits justify the possible risks to the fetus. Because tolcapone is used in conjunction with levodopa/carbidopa (which cause skeletal malformations in animals), patients should notify their clinician if they are or intend to become pregnant while receiving tolcapone in combination with levodopa/carbidopa.

Reproductive studies in rats using tolcapone dosages up to 300 mg/kg daily (5.7 times the human dose on a mg/m^2 basis) have not revealed evidence of impaired fertility or changes in general reproductive performance.

Because it is not known whether tolcapone is distributed into human milk, the drug should be used with caution in nursing women. Patients should be advised to notify their physician if they are nursing an infant or intend to nurse an infant.

Drug Interactions

■ **Levodopa and Other Catecholamines** Tolcapone alters the pharmacokinetics of levodopa (i.e., increases the area under the plasma concentration-time curve and half-life) and enhances the clinical efficacy of levodopa. (See Pharmacology.) Thus, this interaction is used for therapeutic effect.

While tolcapone may influence the pharmacokinetics of drugs metabolized by catechol-*O*-methyltransferase (COMT), tolcapone does not alter the pharmacokinetics of carbidopa. Although the effect of tolcapone on other drugs metabolized by COMT (i.e., methyldopa, dobutamine, apomorphine, isoproterenol) has not been evaluated, a dosage reduction in these drugs should be considered if they are administered in conjunction with tolcapone.

■ **Drugs Undergoing Microsomal Enzyme-mediated Metabolism** The manufacturer of tolcapone states that clinically important drug interactions involving tolcapone and drugs metabolized by microsomal cytochrome P-450 isoenzymes CYP2C9 and CYP2D6 are not expected to occur. Results from in vitro studies that assessed the potential for tolcapone to interact with cytochrome P-450 isoenzymes did not reveal important interactions with substrates for CYP2A6 (warfarin), CYP1A2 (caffeine), CYP3A4 (cyclosporine, midazolam, terfenadine), CYP2C19 (*S*-mephenytoin), or CYP2D6 (desipramine).

In in vivo studies, tolcapone did not alter the pharmacokinetics of desipramine or tolbutamide (a substrate for CYP2C9). The possibility that tolcapone may affect the metabolism of warfarin via CYP2C9 should be considered. (See Drug Interactions: Anticoagulants.)

■ **Anticoagulants** Tolcapone has affinity for CYP2C9, the isoenzyme involved in the metabolism of *S*-warfarin. While not studied specifically, concomitant administration of tolcapone and warfarin may result in increased plasma concentration of the anticoagulant. Because warfarin has a narrow therapeutic index, prothrombin time, preferably using the international normalized ratio (INR), should be determined frequently and appropriate dosage adjustments made in patients receiving concomitant tolcapone.

■ **Protein-bound Drugs** In in vitro studies, tolcapone 50 mcg/mL did not displace therapeutic concentrations of warfarin (0.5–7.2 mcg/mL), phenytoin (4–38.7 mcg/mL), tolbutamide (24.5–96.1 mcg/mL) or digitoxin (9–27 mcg/mL) from binding sites.

■ **Monoamine Oxidase Inhibitors** Because the possibility exists that concomitant administration of tolcapone and a nonselective MAO inhibitor (e.g., phenelzine, tranylcypromine) could result in inhibition of the principal pathways involved in the metabolism of catecholamines, administration of tolcapone with a nonselective MAO inhibitor should be avoided. However, tolcapone can be administered concomitantly with a selective inhibitor of MAO-B (i.e., selegiline).

The adverse effect profile associated with regimens that include tolcapone, levodopa/carbidopa, and selegiline is similar to that associated with regimens that do not include selegiline.

■ **CNS Depressants** The possibility of additive sedative effects should be considered in patients receiving CNS depressants concomitantly with tolcapone.

■ **Other Drugs Affecting the CNS or Cholinergic System** Caution is advised if tolcapone is administered with other drugs that affect brain monoaminergic (i.e., nonselective MAO inhibitors, tricyclic antidepressants, selective serotonin- reuptake inhibitors) or anticholinergic systems since a symptom complex resembling neuroleptic malignant syndrome has been reported in patients receiving such combinations.

Tolcapone does not appear to alter the tolerability of ephedrine (i.e., hemodynamic parameters or plasma catecholamine concentrations at rest or during exercise), and these drugs can be administered concomitantly. Because regimens that include tolcapone, levodopa/carbidopa, and desipramine are not tolerated as well as regimens that do not include desipramine, caution is advised if desipramine is used in patients with parkinsonian syndrome receiving tolcapone and levodopa/carbidopa.

Acute Toxicity

■ **Manifestations** Based on animal data, the threshold for the lethal plasma concentration of tolcapone in humans is predicted to exceed 100 mcg/mL. The highest dosage of tolcapone, with or without levodopa/carbidopa, evaluated in healthy geriatric individuals has been 800 mg 3 times daily for 1 week; peak plasma tolcapone concentrations in elderly individuals receiving this dosage averaged 30 mcg/mL. Nausea, vomiting, and dizziness occurred in these patients and were more pronounced in patients receiving tolcapone in combination with levodopa/carbidopa than in those receiving tolcapone alone.

Respiratory difficulties were observed in rats receiving high oral (i.e., gavage) or IV doses of the drug and in dogs receiving IV tolcapone.

■ **Treatment** The manufacturer recommends that, in the event of tolcapone overdosage, supportive and symptomatic treatment should be initiated and the patient hospitalized. Hemodialysis is unlikely to remove substantial amounts of tolcapone from the body, and this procedure should not be relied on to enhance elimination of the drug.

Pharmacology

Tolcapone is a selective, potent, peripheral and to a lesser extent central, reversible inhibitor of catechol-*O*-methyltransferase (COMT). Although tolcapone produces beneficial effects in levodopa-treated patients with parkinsonian syndrome, the drug lacks antiparkinsonian activity when administered alone.

COMT is an enzyme that catalyzes the transfer of a methyl group from *S*-adenosyl-L-methionine to a phenol group of a substrate containing a catechol structure. Physiologic substrates of COMT include dopa, catecholamines (dopamine, epinephrine, norepinephrine), their hydroxylated metabolites, catechol estrogens, and ascorbic acid. COMT, along with monoamine oxidase, plays a role in the metabolic transformation of dopamine, epinephrine, and norepinephrine. While COMT is found in many organs and tissues including neuronal tissues (especially glial cells), erythrocytes, the GI tract, heart, lung, adipose tissue, smooth and skeletal muscle, reproductive organs, and skin, the highest activity is present in the liver and kidney.

Levodopa currently is the most effective drug for relieving manifestations of parkinsonian syndrome; however, duration of response is limited. One approach for improving the effect of levodopa is to prevent its degradation by metabolizing enzymes. Following oral administration of levodopa, about 70% of a dose undergoes enzymatic decarboxylation and about 10% is *O*-methylated by COMT. When levodopa is administered concomitantly with a decarboxylase inhibitor (e.g., carbidopa), COMT is the major enzyme catalyzing the metabolism of levodopa to 3-methoxy-4-hydroxy-L-phenylalanine (3-OMD).

While the precise mechanism of action of tolcapone remains to be determined, the drug is believed to act principally by inhibiting COMT and altering the plasma pharmacokinetics of levodopa. Concomitant administration of tolcapone with levodopa and a decarboxylase inhibitor results in more sustained plasma levodopa concentrations compared with administration of levodopa and a decarboxylase inhibitor. The principal effect of tolcapone is inhibition of COMT in *peripheral* tissues; secondarily, the reductions in circulating 3-OMD that result from decreased peripheral metabolism of levodopa may increase distribution of levodopa into the CNS by reducing the competitive substrate (i.e., 3-OMD) for transport mechanisms. Sustained levodopa concentrations presumably result in more consistent dopaminergic stimulation, resulting in greater reduction in the manifestations of parkinsonian syndrome. In addition, fluctuations in plasma levodopa concentrations cause dopamine receptors in the striatum to be exposed to alternating high and low concentrations of dopamine; under physiologic conditions, (e.g., in healthy individuals), stimulation of these receptors would be tonic (continuous). Pulsatile stimulation of dopamine receptors resulting from levodopa fluctuations is believed to induce post-synaptic changes that result in the development of motor fluctuations and dyskinesia in parkinsonian patients receiving long-term levodopa therapy. In addition, the decrease in striatal dopamine terminals that occurs with parkinsonian disease progression results in a diminished capacity of these terminals to buffer plasma levodopa fluctuations. Compared with administration of levodopa/carbidopa, administration of tolcapone in combination with levodopa/carbidopa increases the levodopa area under the plasma concentration-time curve (AUC) twofold, increases the terminal elimination half-life of levodopa from 2 hours (conventional tablets) to 3.5 hours, but does not increase the peak plasma levodopa concentration or change the time to peak plasma concentration, resulting in more stable plasma concentrations of levodopa. This stabilization in plasma levodopa concentrations combined with increased central bioavailability of levodopa (secondary to reductions in 3-OMD as a competitive substrate for central distribution) results in enhanced and smoother availability of levodopa to the CNS.

The effect of tolcapone on the pharmacokinetics of levodopa is evident with the initial tolcapone dose and is maintained throughout long-term therapy. Dose response studies in healthy individuals and patients with parkinsonian syndrome indicate that optimum effect on the pharmacokinetics of levodopa (i.e., an increase in AUC and half-life without an increase in peak plasma concentration) occurs with a tolcapone dose of 100–200 mg. Studies to date indicate that the effects of tolcapone on the pharmacokinetics of levodopa in healthy individuals are similar to those in patients with parkinsonian syndrome.

Complications such as motor fluctuations that occur with long-term levodopa therapy may be related to the peripheral conversion of levodopa to 3-OMD; this metabolite may compete with levodopa for transport across the GI membrane and blood-brain barrier. While the importance of competition between levodopa and 3-OMD remains to be determined, tolcapone's inhibition of COMT increases peripheral and central availability of levodopa and prevents biotransformation to 3-OMD. Peak plasma concentrations and AUC values for 3-OMD are substantially lower in individuals receiving tolcapone in conjunction with levodopa/carbidopa compared with individuals receiving levodopa/carbidopa. In one study in healthy individuals 55–75 years of age receiving tolcapone in conjunction with levodopa/carbidopa, the AUC for 3-OMD decreased about 80%.

In addition to its effect on the pharmacokinetics of levodopa, tolcapone is expected to reduce utilization of *S*-adenosyl-L-methionine, a compound that reportedly has a therapeutic effect in mental depression. Tolcapone's potential to reduce metabolic degradation of dopamine in the striatum also may contribute to the drug's activity. However, the CNS effect of tolcapone appears to be minimal and clinically unimportant since the drug lacks antiparkinsonian effects when administered as monotherapy.

Tolcapone reversibly inhibits human erythrocyte COMT. Measurement of erythrocyte COMT activity is a sensitive and precise method of estimating COMT activity in the liver, kidney, and lung. Inhibition of COMT activity is related to plasma tolcapone concentrations over a dosage range of 5–400 mg. Following oral administration of a single oral 200-mg dose of tolcapone in healthy individuals, maximum inhibition of erythrocyte COMT activity was achieved within 1 hour and exceeded 80%; inhibitory activity persisted for 16–24 hours. Following oral administration of tolcapone 200 mg 3 times daily for 7 days in healthy individuals, maximum erythrocyte COMT inhibition was about 80% and erythrocyte COMT inhibition at trough tolcapone concentrations was 30–45%. In vivo studies indicate that tolcapone inhibits brain COMT activity.

Tolcapone does not affect monoamine oxidase, hydroxy-indole-*O*-methyltransferase, histamine-*N*-methyltransferase, or phenyl-ethanolamine-*N*-methyltransferase activities. Tolcapone does not interact with α- or β-adrenergic, serotonergic, or cholinergic receptors.

Pharmacokinetics

Tolcapone exhibits linear pharmacokinetics, which are independent of levodopa/carbidopa coadministration, over the dosage range of 50–400 mg. Pharmacokinetic studies have not revealed gender-, age-, or weight-related differences in the pharmacokinetics of tolcapone. In addition, there has been no evidence of race-related differences in the pharmacokinetics of the drug in white, black, and Japanese individuals. Analysis of population pharmacokinetic data from clinical trials indicates that renal function does not alter the pharmacokinetics of tolcapone in individuals with creatinine clearance of 30–130 mL/minute. Although the pharmacokinetics of tolcapone have been studied in clinical studies in patients with moderate non-cirrhotic liver impairment (ALT [SGPT] concentrations at least 2 times the upper limit of normal, alkaline phosphatase concentrations at least 1.5 times the upper limit of normal, γ-glutamyltransferase [GGT, γ-glutamyltranspeptidase, GGTP] concentrations outside the normal range) and in patients with moderate cirrhotic liver disease (Child-Pugh class B), tolcapone therapy should not be initiated in patients with clinical evidence of active liver disease, or two ALT (SGPT) or AST (SGOT) values exceeding the upper limit of normal, or any other evidence of hepatocellular dysfunction. In addition, tolcapone therapy should be discontinued if ALT or AST concentrations exceed the upper limit of normal or if clinical signs and symptoms suggest the onset of hepatic failure.

In healthy individuals, reversible inhibition of erythrocyte COMT activity following oral administration of tolcapone has been shown to be closely related to plasma concentrations of the drug. Maximum COMT inhibition following a single 200-mg oral dose averages greater than 80%, while inhibition with trough plasma tolcapone concentrations during multiple dosing (200 mg 3 times daily) is 30–45%.

■ **Absorption** Tolcapone is rapidly absorbed from the GI tract, with peak plasma concentrations generally occurring within 2 hours following single oral doses of 5–800 mg. The absolute bioavailability following oral administration is about 65–68%. When tolcapone is administered with food (within 1 hour before or 2 hours after a meal), bioavailability is reduced 10–20% compared with administration in the fasting state.

In one study in healthy individuals 55–75 years of age, oral administration of a single dose of tolcapone 100 or 200 mg produced peak plasma concentrations of 2.8 or 5.9 mcg/mL, respectively. Following oral administration of tolcapone 100 or 200 mg 3 times daily for 7 days in healthy individuals 55–75 years of age, peak plasma tolcapone concentrations were 3.5 or 6.4 mcg/mL, respectively; in individuals receiving either tolcapone dosage, trough concentrations on day 8 were essentially the same as levels on day 2. Oral administration of tolcapone 100 or 200 mg 3 times daily is not associated with accumulation of tolcapone. The extent of absorption (i.e., AUC) is proportional to dose in individuals receiving single oral tolcapone doses of 5–800 mg.

In clinical studies in a limited number of patients with moderate cirrhotic liver disease (Child-Pugh class B), plasma concentrations of unbound tolcapone were increased less than twofold compared with concentrations in individuals with normal hepatic function or non-cirrhotic liver disease.

■ **Distribution** Distribution of tolcapone into body tissues and fluids has not been fully characterized. The volume of distribution of tolcapone at steady-state is 9 L. The volume of distribution of unbound tolcapone reportedly was reduced almost 50% in clinical studies in patients with moderate cirrhotic liver disease (Child-Pugh class B). While tolcapone is not widely distributed, the drug is distributed into brain tissue.

Tolcapone is more than 99.9% bound to plasma proteins, principally serum albumin, over a concentration range of 0.32–210 mcg/mL.

It is not known whether tolcapone is distributed into human milk; however, the drug is distributed into milk in rats.

■ **Elimination** Tolcapone is extensively metabolized by a variety of mechanisms. The principal metabolic pathway identified involves glucuronidation. In addition, tolcapone is metabolized by catechol-*O*-methyltransferase (COMT) to 3-*O*-methyltolcapone. Tolcapone also undergoes hydroxylation of the methyl group resulting in a primary alcohol, which is then oxidized to the carboxylic acid. In vitro data indicate that cytochrome P-450 isoenyzmes CYP3A4 and CYP2A6 catalyze the oxidation to the carboxylic acid. Tolcapone also is reduced to an amine, which subsequently is *N*-acetylated.

Tolcapone is a low-extraction ratio drug (0.15) with a systemic clearance of 7 L/hour. The terminal elimination half-life of tolcapone at recommended dosages is 2–3 hours. While the terminal elimination half-life of catechol-3-*O*-methyltolcapone is 30–60 hours, the metabolite does not appear to accumulate with multiple-dosing because tolcapone inhibits COMT. Clearance of unbound tolcapone was reduced almost 50% in clinical studies in patients with moderate cirrhotic liver disease (Child-Pugh class B).

About 13% of an oral dose of tolcapone is excreted in the urine as the glucuronide metabolite, 2% as the carboxylic acid metabolite, and less than 0.5% as unchanged drug. While the glucuronide conjugate is excreted principally in urine, this metabolite also undergoes biliary excretion. Following oral administration of radiolabeled tolcapone, about 60% of a labeled dose is excreted in urine and 40% is excreted in feces.

Chemistry and Stability

■ **Chemistry** Tolcapone, a reversible catechol-*O*-methyltransferase (COMT) inhibitor, is a nitrocatechol. Tolcapone differs chemically and pharmacologically from currently available antiparkinsonian agents (e.g., levodopa, carbidopa, ergot- and nonergot- derivative dopamine receptor agonists, the selective monoamine oxidase [MAO]-B inhibitor selegiline hydrochloride).

Tolcapone occurs as a yellow, nonhygroscopic, crystalline compound.

■ **Stability** Commercially available tolcapone tablets should be stored in tight containers at a controlled room temperature of 20–25°C.

Preparations

Excipients in commercially available drug preparations may have clinically important effects in some individuals; consult specific product labeling for details.

Tolcapone

Oral

Tablets, film-coated	100 mg	**Tasmar®**, Valeant
	200 mg	**Tasmar®**, Valeant

DOPAMINE PRECURSORS 28:36.16

Levodopa
l-3-Hydroxytyrosine, L-Dopa

Carbidopa
α-Methyldopa Hydrazine

■ Levodopa is the levorotatory isomer of dihydroxyphenylalanine and the metabolic precursor of dopamine, and carbidopa is a decarboxylase inhibitor that inhibits the peripheral decarboxylation of levodopa to dopamine.

Uses

■ **Parkinsonian Syndrome** Levodopa is used in the symptomatic treatment of parkinsonian syndrome (e.g., parkinsonism, idiopathic Parkinson disease [paralysis agitans]); the drug also is used in the symptomatic treatment of parkinsonian syndrome resulting from encephalitis (postencephalitic parkinsonism), carbon monoxide intoxication, or manganese intoxication.

Levodopa (in combination with carbidopa) currently is the most effective drug for relieving the motor symptoms of parkinsonian syndrome and is considered by many clinicians to be the drug of choice for this use. Levodopa completely or partially relieves akinesia, rigidity, and tremor in about 80% of patients treated, and improves functional ability and other secondary motor manifestations such as those affecting gait, postural stability, facial expression, swallowing, speech, and handwriting. Levodopa also may be useful in the management of other symptoms of parkinsonian syndrome including dysphagia, sialorrhea, and seborrhea. Levodopa therapy often produces a general alerting response, increased vigor, and a sense of well-being. However, the effectiveness of levodopa tends to decrease over time and most patients develop motor complications such as motor fluctuations (e.g., end-of-dose failure, "on-off" phenomenon, akinesia) and dyskinesias (drug-induced involuntary movements) with long-term use. (See Cautions: Nervous System and Muscular Effects.) Strategies for reducing the risk of motor complications include adjusting the dosage of levodopa or adding other antiparkinsonian agents such as a dopamine agonist (e.g., pramipexole, ropinirole, rotigotine), selective monoamine oxidase (MAO)-B inhibitor (e.g., rasagiline, safinamide, selegiline), catechol-*O*-methyltransferase (COMT) inhibitor (entacapone, tolcapone), or amantadine; the goal of adjunctive therapy is to improve motor fluctuations without exacerbating dyskinesia. Another strategy to reduce the risk of motor complications and to improve long-term outcome in patients receiving levodopa is to initiate symptomatic therapy with other antiparkinsonian agents first and then add levodopa when these other therapies no longer provide adequate symptom control. This delayed approach is often used in younger patients who have a higher risk of developing motor complications and a longer life expectancy. Levodopa generally is used for initial therapy in individuals older than 70 years of age (since these individuals are less likely than younger individuals to develop levodopa-related motor complications and because of concerns about cognitive dysfunction), in patients with cognitive impairment, and in those with severe disease. Treatment must be individualized; factors to consider when selecting a drug for the initial symptomatic management of parkinsonian syndrome include patient age, cognitive status, disease severity, and cost.

Carbidopa, a decarboxylation inhibitor, is used in conjunction with levodopa to inhibit the decarboxylation of peripheral levodopa and increase the amount of levodopa available for transport to the brain. Concomitant administration of levodopa and carbidopa generally decreases levodopa dosage requirements by 70–80%, reduces the incidence of levodopa-induced nausea and vomiting, allows a more rapid dosage titration, and may provide a smoother response to levodopa. Certain patients who responded poorly to levodopa alone (no longer commercially available in the US as a single-entity preparation) have improved when carbidopa and levodopa were administered concomitantly; however, patients with markedly irregular "on-off" responses to levodopa (see Cautions: Nervous System and Muscular Effects) usually have not benefited from combination therapy. Carbidopa has no therapeutic effect when given alone to patients with parkinsonian syndrome and should be used only in conjunction with levodopa. Combination preparations containing levodopa in fixed combinations with carbidopa are commercially available. Carbidopa is also available alone from the manufacturer for use in conjunction with the combination preparations in patients who do not have adequate reduction in nausea and vomiting with the fixed-dosage preparations.

In the treatment of parkinsonian syndrome, levodopa-carbidopa therapy may be used in combination with selective MAO-B inhibitors (e.g., rasagiline, safinamide, selegiline), dopamine agonists (e.g., pramipexole, ropinirole, rotigotine), amantadine, antihistamines (e.g., diphenhydramine), or anticholinergic agents (e.g., benztropine, trihexyphenidyl). When used as adjunctive therapy to levodopa in patients with advanced parkinsonian syndrome, MAO-B inhibitors and dopamine agonists can reduce motor fluctuations and permit the use of lower dosages of levodopa. Although anticholinergics may be useful for controlling tremor and drooling, the adverse effects of these drugs may limit their use. When levodopa is administered with an anticholinergic agent, the dosage of each drug may need to be reduced. (See Drug Interactions: Anticholinergic Agents.) Combined therapy with amantadine and levodopa has been reported to be more effective than levodopa alone in some patients who cannot tolerate large dosages of levodopa; however, the addition of amantadine does not usually provide substantial additional benefit when patients are already receiving full therapeutic dosages of levodopa.

Levodopa-carbidopa also may be used in conjunction with a COMT inhibitor (i.e., entacapone, tolcapone) for the symptomatic treatment of idiopathic parkinsonian syndrome. Concomitant administration of entacapone or tolcapone with levodopa-carbidopa enhances the efficacy of levodopa in patients with motor fluctuations and in those with stable responses to levodopa. However, tolcapone therapy has been associated with severe hepatocellular injury in some patients. Because of the risk of potentially fatal, acute fulminant liver failure, tolcapone generally should be reserved for patients receiving levodopa who are experiencing symptom fluctuations and are not responding adequately to other adjunctive therapies. Some clinicians consider entacapone the COMT inhibitor of choice. For additional information on such combined therapy, see Tolcapone 28:36.12.

Levodopa may be useful in the management of reserpine-induced parkinsonian symptoms; however, levodopa is not effective in controlling extrapyramidal effects induced by antipsychotic agents such as phenothiazines or butyrophenones.

■ **Other Uses** Although levodopa is not effective in the management of extrapyramidal effects induced by antipsychotic agents and is not generally useful in the management of other neurologic diseases, the drug may be of some benefit in conditions in which marked akinesia is present. Levodopa is not useful in the treatment of mental disorders.

Dosage and Administration

■ **Administration** Levodopa and carbidopa are administered orally.

Levodopa and carbidopa are commercially available as fixed-combination conventional tablets, orally disintegrating tablets, extended-release tablets, and extended-release capsules. Levodopa-carbidopa conventional tablets and orally disintegrating tablets contain a 1:4 or 1:10 ratio of carbidopa to levodopa. Levodopa-carbidopa extended-release tablets and capsules contain a 1:4 ratio of carbidopa to levodopa. Levodopa and carbidopa also are commercially available in fixed combination with entacapone (Stalevo®) in a tablet preparation containing a 1:4 ratio of carbidopa to levodopa combined with 200 mg of entacapone. Carbidopa also is commercially available as single-entity conventional tablets; levodopa no longer is commercially available in the US as a single-entity preparation.

In patients with moderate to severe motor fluctuations, better global improvement may be achieved in some patients when extended-release rather than conventional preparations of levodopa-carbidopa are used. However, in clinical studies, such patients receiving the extended-release tablets did not experience *quantitatively* significant reductions in "off" time compared with conventional preparations. In patients without motor fluctuations, the preparations were comparably effective but less frequent dosing was required with the extended-release preparation. In a study in patients receiving the extended-release capsule formulation of levodopa-carbidopa, "off" time was improved with the extended-release preparation compared with the immediate-release preparation.

Extended-release tablets of levodopa-carbidopa can be administered as whole or halved tablets, but these should be swallowed intact and not chewed or crushed. Patients should be advised that the extended-release tablets are designed to release the drugs over a 4- to 6-hour period and of the importance of taking the drug at regular intervals according to the prescribed schedule. Patients also should be advised that the onset of effect with the morning dose of extended-release tablets occasionally may be delayed up to 1 hour compared with that experienced with conventional tablets.

Extended-release levodopa-carbidopa capsules should be swallowed whole without chewing, dividing, or crushing. Patients with difficulty swallowing may open the capsules and sprinkle the entire contents on a small amount of applesauce (e.g., 1–2 tablespoons); the mixture should be administered immediately and not stored for later use.

Patients receiving levodopa-carbidopa orally disintegrating tablets should be instructed to gently remove a tablet from the bottle with dry hands just prior to administration. The tablet should then be immediately placed on the tongue to dissolve (usually within seconds) and be swallowed with saliva; administration with liquid is not necessary.

The fixed-combination preparation containing levodopa, carbidopa, and entacapone (Stalevo®) generally is used in patients receiving stable dosages of levodopa, carbidopa, and entacapone equivalent to those in the combination preparation. The fixed-combination preparation containing levodopa, carbidopa, and entacapone also may be used in certain patients receiving stable dosages of levodopa and carbidopa equivalent to those in the fixed-combination preparation when a decision has been made to add entacapone to the regimen. (See Levodopa, Carbidopa, and Entacapone Fixed Combination, under Dosage: Parkinsonian Syndrome, in Dosage and Administration.) Tablets containing levodopa, carbidopa, and entacapone in fixed combination (Stalevo®) should not be divided, and only one tablet should be administered per dosing interval.

Patients should be cautioned not to alter the prescribed dosage regimen and not to add any additional antiparkinsonian therapy, including other levodopa-carbidopa preparations, without first consulting their clinician.

Whenever a general anesthetic is required, levodopa may be continued as long as the patient is able to take fluids and medication orally. If therapy is interrupted, the patient should be observed for neuroleptic malignant syndrome and the usual daily dose may be given as soon as the patient can take oral medication.

■ **Dosage** ***Parkinsonian Syndrome*** Dosage of levodopa-carbidopa must be carefully adjusted according to individual requirements, response, and tolerance. Because patients receiving carbidopa dosages lower than 70–100 mg daily are likely to experience levodopa-induced nausea and vomiting, the minimum recommended daily dosage of carbidopa is 70–100 mg.

Because parkinsonian syndrome is progressive, the patient's clinical condition should be evaluated periodically and therapy adjusted as necessary.

Because of the risk of precipitating a symptom complex resembling neuroleptic malignant syndrome, patients should be observed closely if levodopa dosage is reduced abruptly or the drug is discontinued. (See Cautions: Precautions and Contraindications.)

Immediate-release Levodopa-Carbidopa Preparations. When levodopa-carbidopa therapy is initiated using an immediate-release combination preparation (i.e., conventional tablets, orally disintegrating tablets), therapy usually is initiated with a preparation containing 100 mg of levodopa and 25 mg of carbidopa. When a preparation containing 100 mg of levodopa and 25 mg of carbidopa is used, the usual initial dosage is 1 tablet 3 times daily and dosage may be increased by 1 tablet every 1 or 2 days until a maximum dosage of 8 tablets daily (800 mg of levodopa and 200 mg of carbidopa) is reached or adverse effects prevent further increases or necessitate discontinuance of therapy. If an immediate-release combination preparation containing 100 mg of levodopa with 10 mg of carbidopa is used, therapy usually is initiated with 1 tablet 3 or 4 times daily; however, this dosage will not provide an adequate amount of carbidopa for many patients. Dosage may be increased by 1 tablet every 1 or 2 days until a maximum dosage of 8 tablets daily (800 mg of levodopa and 80 mg of carbidopa) is reached or adverse effects prevent further increases or necessitate discontinuance of therapy. If the patient requires a higher dosage of levodopa, an immediate-release combination preparation containing 250 mg of levodopa with 25 mg of carbidopa should be used, and if necessary, dosage increased by one-half or 1 tablet every 1 or 2 days until a maximum dosage of 8 tablets daily (2 g of levodopa and 200 mg of carbidopa) is reached.

Maintenance levodopa-carbidopa therapy should be individualized and adjusted according to the desired therapeutic response. Patients receiving maintenance therapy with levodopa-carbidopa should receive at least 70–100 mg of carbidopa daily, since peripheral aromatic L-amino acid decarboxylase is saturated at this dosage and patients receiving a lower daily dosage of carbidopa are likely to experience nausea and vomiting. Patients who require a low dosage of levodopa (e.g., less than 700 mg daily) will receive doses of carbidopa that will not saturate peripheral aromatic L-amino acid decarboxylase when the combination preparation containing a 1:10 ratio of carbidopa to levodopa is used. Therefore, if nausea and vomiting occur in patients receiving an immediate-release combination preparation containing 100 mg of levodopa with 10 mg of carbidopa, one tablet of an immediate-release preparation containing 100 mg of levodopa with 25 mg of carbidopa may be substituted for one tablet of the preparation containing 100 mg of levodopa with 10 mg of carbidopa. If additional carbidopa is still required, carbidopa dosage may be supplemented by giving a 25-mg dose of carbidopa to these patients with each first daily dose of levodopa-carbidopa and 12.5-mg or 25-mg doses of carbidopa with each subsequent dose of levodopa-carbidopa. If patients require higher dosages of levodopa while receiving an immediate-release combination preparation containing 100 mg of levodopa with 10 or 25 mg of carbidopa, a combination preparation containing 250 mg of levodopa with 25 mg of carbidopa should be used. Patients receiving an immediate-release combination preparation containing 250 mg of levodopa with 25 mg of carbidopa who require additional carbidopa may receive 25-mg doses of carbidopa with any dose of levodopa-carbidopa as required for optimum therapeutic response. Because experience with carbidopa daily dosages greater than 200 mg is limited, dosage of carbidopa should not exceed 200 mg daily.

Extended-release Levodopa-Carbidopa Tablets. If extended-release tablets of levodopa-carbidopa are used, it should be recognized that this formulation is less bioavailable than immediate-release preparations (i.e., conventional tablets, orally disintegrating tablets) and that increased daily dosage may be required to achieve the same level of symptomatic relief provided by immediate-release preparations. Dosage should be individualized based on patient tolerance and clinical response.

Patients being transferred from an immediate-release levodopa-carbidopa preparation should receive an initial dosage of the extended-release tablets that provides approximately 10% *more* levodopa daily than they previously were receiving with the immediate-release preparation. In some patients, up to 30% *more* levodopa daily may be required initially depending on clinical response.

For patients in whom levodopa therapy is initiated with extended-release levodopa-carbidopa tablets (i.e., those not being switched from existing levodopa therapy), an initial dosage of levodopa 200 mg with carbidopa 50 mg twice daily usually is sufficient. Initial dosage in such patients should not be given at intervals of less than 6 hours.

Following initiation of therapy with the extended-release levodopa-carbidopa tablets, doses and/or dosing intervals can be increased or decreased carefully according to patient tolerance and clinical response. Most patients are treated adequately with levodopa 400 mg to 1.6 g daily and carbidopa 100–400 mg daily as extended-release tablets, administered in divided doses at intervals ranging from 4–8 hours while awake. Higher dosages (levodopa 2.4 g and carbidopa 600 mg) and shorter intervals (less than 4 hours) have been used with the extended-release tablets but usually are not recommended. If the dosing interval is shorter than 4 hours and/or the divided doses are not equal, it is recommended that the smaller doses be given at the end of the day. Dosage of the extended-release tablets generally should be adjusted no more frequently than at 3-day intervals. Some patients with advanced disease may benefit from the addition of doses of a conventional preparation of levodopa-carbidopa during brief periods of the day when additional levodopa is needed for symptomatic control.

Extended-release Levodopa-Carbidopa Capsules. The extended-release capsule formulation of levodopa-carbidopa is less bioavailable than immediate-release preparations (i.e., conventional tablets, orally disintegrating tablets) and increased daily dosages generally are required to achieve the same level of symptomatic relief provided by immediate-release preparations. Dosage should be individualized based on patient tolerance and clinical response.

Dosages of the extended-release capsule formulation of levodopa-carbidopa are not directly interchangeable with dosages of other levodopa-carbidopa preparations. The manufacturer's prescribing information should be consulted for recommended dosage conversions in patients transferring from therapy with immediate-release levodopa-carbidopa preparations to the extended-release capsules. Following conversion, dose and/or dosing intervals can be increased or decreased as necessary based on patient tolerance and clinical response.

If extended-release capsules of levodopa-carbidopa are used in treatment-naive patients (i.e., those not being switched from existing levodopa-carbidopa therapy), the recommended initial dosage is levodopa 95 mg and carbidopa 23.75 mg administered 3 times daily for the first 3 days. Dosage may be increased to levodopa 145 mg and carbidopa 36.25 mg 3 times daily on the fourth day of treatment. Thereafter, dosage may be increased based on patient tolerance and clinical response up to a maximum recommended dosage of levodopa 390 mg and carbidopa 97.5 mg 3 times daily; if needed, dosing frequency may be increased to a maximum of 5 times daily. Patients should be maintained on the lowest possible dosage necessary to achieve adequate symptom control while minimizing adverse effects. The manufacturer recommends a maximum daily dose of levodopa 2.45 g and carbidopa 612.5 mg when using the extended-release capsules.

Levodopa, Carbidopa, and Entacapone Fixed Combination. For patients transferring from therapy with levodopa-carbidopa to the fixed-combination preparation containing levodopa, carbidopa, and entacapone (Stalevo®), recommendations are available for transferring patients currently receiving levodopa-carbidopa preparations containing a 1:4 ratio of carbidopa to levodopa. Patients receiving entacapone 200 mg with each dose of levodopa-carbidopa (e.g., conventional preparation containing 100 mg of levodopa and 25 mg of carbidopa) can be switched to the corresponding strength of the fixed-combination preparation containing levodopa, carbidopa, and entacapone. The manufacturer states that there is no experience to date in transferring patients currently receiving entacapone together with extended-release preparations of levodopa-carbidopa or levodopa-carbidopa preparations containing a 1:10 ratio of carbidopa to levodopa to the fixed-combination preparation Stalevo®.

For patients initiating entacapone therapy, recommendations regarding use of the fixed-combination preparation Stalevo® should be individualized according to the current levodopa dosage and the presence of dyskinesias. Patients treated with levodopa-carbidopa conventional tablets who are receiving more than 600 mg of levodopa daily or have a history of moderate or severe dyskinesias before initiation of entacapone therapy are likely to require a reduction in levodopa dosage. In such patients, dosage should first be adjusted by administering levodopa-carbidopa (1:4 ratio) and entacapone as separate preparations. If it is determined that optimum maintenance dosages of levodopa, carbidopa, and entacapone correspond to the doses in the commercial combination product, the fixed-combination preparation containing levodopa, carbidopa, and entacapone (Stalevo®) may be used. For patients receiving levodopa dosages of 600 mg or less daily (conventional tablets, 1:4 ratio) and who do not have dyskinesias, an attempt can be made to initiate entacapone therapy with the fixed-combination preparation containing levodopa, carbidopa, and entacapone. The initial dosage of the fixed-combination preparation of levodopa, carbidopa, and entacapone should provide the same dosage of levodopa and carbidopa that the patient currently is taking. However, a reduction in the dosage of levodopa-carbidopa or entacapone may be necessary. Because dosage of levodopa, carbidopa, or entacapone cannot be adjusted individually using the fixed-combination preparation, administration of levodopa-carbidopa and entacapone as separate preparations may be necessary.

Because there is limited clinical experience with entacapone dosages exceeding 1.6 g daily, the maximum recommended dosage of fixed-combination preparations containing levodopa 50–150 mg, carbidopa 12.5–37.5 mg, and entacapone 200 mg (Stalevo® 50, 75, 100, 125, and 150) is 8 tablets daily. Because there is limited clinical experience with carbidopa dosages exceeding 300 mg daily, the maximum recommended dosage of the fixed-combination preparation containing levodopa 200 mg, carbidopa 50 mg, and entacapone 200 mg (Stalevo® 200) is 6 tablets daily.

Cautions

Adverse effects occur in most patients who receive levodopa (with or without carbidopa). Adverse effects of levodopa are numerous and are usually dose dependent and reversible. The incidence of levodopa-induced nausea and vomiting is generally less when carbidopa is used in conjunction with the drug. However, concomitant administration of carbidopa does not decrease adverse reactions resulting from the central effects of levodopa and in fact some CNS effects may occur at lower dosage and more rapidly during therapy with levodopa-carbidopa combinations than with levodopa alone. The adverse effect profile reported with levodopa and carbidopa administered as extended-release tablets is comparable to that with conventional oral preparations.

Whenever the fixed-combination preparation containing levodopa, carbidopa, and entacapone (Stalevo®) is used, consideration should be given to the possible adverse effects reported with the individual components.

■ Nervous System and Muscular Effects The most common adverse effects of levodopa are dyskinesias including choreiform, dystonic, dyskinetic, and other involuntary movements. Involuntary movements occur in about 50% of patients on long-term therapy and may consist of grimacing, bruxism, gnawing, chewing, twisting and protrusion of the tongue, rhythmic opening and closing of the mouth, bobbing and wave-like motions of the head with or without gesticulation, slow rhythmic movements of the neck, hands or feet, jerky movements of the shoulder or pelvic girdle, and opisthotonos or ballismus. Intermittent myoclonic body jerks during sleep, ataxia, increased hand tremor, and muscle twitching and blepharospasm (which may be an early sign of excessive dosage) may also occur. Dyskinesias usually are dose related and may require reduction of dosage. They do not usually occur in nonparkinsonian patients such as those with chronic manganese intoxication. Because carbidopa allows more levodopa to reach the brain, dyskinesias may occur at lower dosages and more rapidly when levodopa is used in conjunction with carbidopa than when levodopa is used alone.

Several types of motor fluctuations also may occur in patients receiving long-term levodopa therapy. In one form, a gradual return of parkinsonian symptoms may occur toward the end of an inter-dose period. This can be minimized by more frequent administration of the drug. In the "on-off" phenomenon, a sudden loss of effectiveness with an abrupt onset of akinesia ("off" effect) which may last from 1 minute to an hour followed by an equally sudden return of effectiveness ("on" effect) may occur many times daily. This occasionally can be minimized by increasing the number of doses per day. Akinesia paradoxica ("start hesitation"), a sudden hypotonic freezing in which the patient frequently falls because he becomes akinetic just as he starts to walk, may be relieved by reducing the dosage of levodopa. Although the cause of these episodes has not been precisely determined, it appears that they may result from a combination of progression of the disease and excessive levodopa dosage.

Numerous mild to severe CNS and psychiatric disturbances may be produced by levodopa and may include decreased attention span, memory loss, insouciance, nervousness, anxiety, agitation, restlessness, confusion, insomnia, vivid dreams, nightmares, daytime somnolence, euphoria, malaise, fatigue, pathologic gambling, increased libido (including hypersexuality), and symptoms related to impulse control. Hallucinations and abnormal thoughts or behavior (e.g., paranoia, confusion, psychotic disorder, delusions, delirium, psychotic-like behavior, disorientation, aggressive behavior) have been reported in some patients receiving dopaminergic drugs. Hallucinations generally present soon after initiation of levodopa therapy and may be alleviated by reducing dosage of the drug. Serious psychiatric disturbances requiring reduction of dosage or complete withdrawal of levodopa have included severe mental depression with or without suicidal tendencies, dementia, toxic delirium, paranoid delusions, hallucinations, and hypomania with inappropriate or excessive sexual behavior. Severe psychotic episodes are most likely to occur in patients with a history of mental disorders. Levodopa promotes release of pituitary growth hormone which may potentiate the cerebral effects of the drug.

A symptom complex resembling neuroleptic malignant syndrome also has been reported in patients who abruptly discontinue or reduce dosage of levodopa. (See Cautions: Precautions and Contraindications.)

■ GI Effects Nausea, vomiting, and anorexia (which may be accompanied by weight loss) occur frequently in patients receiving levodopa. Adverse GI effects of levodopa generally occur early in therapy while dosage is being increased and may be relieved by temporary reduction of dosage or administration of the drug with food. Other adverse GI effects which have been reported less frequently include duodenal ulcer, GI bleeding, constipation, diarrhea, epigastric and abdominal distress and pain, flatulence, hiccups, sialorrhea, dry mouth, dysphagia, change in taste sensation (including bitter taste), burning of the tongue, and trismus.

■ Cardiovascular Effects Orthostatic hypotension occurs frequently following therapeutic doses of levodopa; however, it is usually asymptomatic and tolerance usually develops within a few months.

Cardiac irregularities occur infrequently with levodopa and may include palpitation, sinus tachycardia, ventricular tachycardia or extrasystole, atrial flutter or fibrillation, or block of atrioventricular conduction. Other reported adverse cardiovascular effects of levodopa include flushing and hypertension.

Cardiac ischemic events have been reported in clinical studies using the extended-release fixed-combination capsule preparation containing levodopa and carbidopa.

■ Other Adverse Effects Adverse respiratory effects of levodopa include episodic hyperventilation, bizarre breathing patterns, hoarseness, and excessive nasal discharge. Adverse reactions affecting the urinary tract include urinary frequency, retention, incontinence, and dark urine. Adverse ocular effects include blurred vision, diplopia, mydriasis or miosis, widening of the palpebral fissures, activation of latent Horner's syndrome, and oculogyric crises. However, levodopa has been reported to reduce the incidence and severity of oculogyric crises in some patients with postencephalitic parkinsonian syndrome. Rarely, phlebitis, leukopenia, hemolytic or nonhemolytic anemia, thrombocytopenia, agranulocytosis, and decreased hemoglobin and hematocrit have occurred. If leukopenia occurs during levodopa therapy, the drug should be discontinued, at least temporarily.

Other adverse effects reported to occur in patients receiving levodopa include muscle cramps, a sense of stimulation, headache, weakness, numbness, increased sweating, dark sweat or other body fluids (e.g., saliva), pigmentation of the skin and teeth, rash, hot flashes, postmenopausal bleeding, weight gain or loss, priapism, edema, and alopecia. The development or exacerbation of malignant melanoma has been reported rarely in patients receiving levodopa therapy; however, a causal relationship to the drug has not been fully established to date.

Transient elevations in serum alkaline phosphatase, AST (SGOT), ALT (SGPT), LDH, bilirubin, and BUN concentrations may occur in patients receiving levodopa therapy. Serum concentrations of BUN, creatinine, and uric acid may be lower when levodopa is used in conjunction with carbidopa than when levodopa is used alone. Rarely, positive direct antiglobulin (Coombs') test results have been reported during prolonged therapy with levodopa.

Development of a scleroderma-like illness, manifested by proximal muscle weakness, pain and swelling of the hands and feet, a pruritic rash, and weight loss, has been reported in one patient receiving carbidopa and oxitriptan (L-5HTP) for the treatment of intention myoclonus. Although the exact pathogenetic mechanism of this adverse effect has not been determined, it has been suggested that a simultaneous increase in blood serotonin concentration and an enzyme defect producing an increase in serum kynurenine (a metabolite of tryptophan) concentration, which result from the combined use of carbidopa and oxitriptan, are responsible for the occurrence of this scleroderma-like illness.

■ Precautions and Contraindications Levodopa should be used with extreme caution, if at all, in patients with a history of myocardial infarction who have residual atrial, nodal, or ventricular arrhythmias. When levodopa therapy is initiated in these patients, intensive coronary care facilities should be immediately available. Levodopa also should be administered with caution to patients with severe cardiovascular, pulmonary (e.g., bronchial asthma), renal, hepatic, or endocrine disease.

Levodopa should be administered with caution to patients with a history of active peptic ulcer because there is a possibility that levodopa may cause upper GI hemorrhage in such patients.

Since levodopa may cause psychiatric changes, the drug generally should not be used in patients with major psychotic disorders. Patients should be cautioned about the possibility of developing hallucinations and instructed to notify a clinician promptly should these manifestations occur.

Patients should be observed closely when levodopa dosage is reduced abruptly or the drug is discontinued, especially in patients receiving an antipsychotic agent concomitantly, since a symptom complex resembling neuroleptic malignant syndrome has occurred following abrupt withdrawal of antiparkinsonian agents. The symptom complex may include muscular rigidity, elevated body temperature, mental changes, diaphoresis, tachycardia, tachypnea, and/or increased serum creatine kinase (CK, creatine phosphokinase, CPK) concentrations.

Patients receiving dopaminergic agents have reported falling asleep while engaged in activities of daily living, including operating a motor vehicle (which has sometimes resulted in accidents). Although many patients reported somnolence while receiving dopaminergic agents, some patients did not perceive warning signs, such as excessive drowsiness, and believed they were alert prior to the episode of falling asleep. Falling asleep while engaged in such activities usually occurs in a setting of preexisting somnolence, although some patients may not give such a history. Patients may not acknowledge drowsiness or sleepiness until directly questioned about these adverse effects during specific activities. Prior to initiating levodopa-carbidopa therapy, patients should be advised of the potential to develop drowsiness and specifically asked about any factors that may increase the risk of somnolence (e.g., concomitant use of sedating drugs, presence of sleep disorders). Patients should be continually reassessed for drowsiness or sleepiness during therapy, especially since some of the episodes of falling asleep occur well after starting treatment. Patients receiving therapy with dopaminergic agents, including levodopa, must be informed of this risk and advised to exercise caution when driving or operating machinery. Patients should be advised that they must refrain from driving or operating machinery if they experience somnolence and/or an episode of sudden sleep onset. If a patient develops daytime sleepiness or episodes of falling asleep during activities that require active participation (e.g., driving a motor vehicle, conversations, eating), discontinuance of levodopa-carbidopa therapy should be considered. If a decision is made to continue therapy, the patient should be advised not to drive and to avoid other potentially dangerous activities. There is insufficient information to establish whether dosage reduction will eliminate episodes of falling asleep while engaged in activities of daily living.

Data from epidemiologic studies indicate that patients with parkinsonian syndrome have a twofold to approximately sixfold greater risk of developing melanoma than the general population. It is unclear whether this increased risk is due to parkinsonian syndrome or other factors (e.g., drugs used to treat the disease). Because of these findings, patients should be monitored for melanoma on a frequent and regular basis. The manufacturer recommends that dermatologic examinations be performed periodically by qualified clinicians (e.g., dermatologists).

Intense urges (e.g., urge to gamble, increased sexual urges, other intense urges) and inability to control these urges have been reported in some patients receiving antiparkinsonian agents that increase central dopaminergic tone (including levodopa-carbidopa). Although a causal relationship has not been established, these urges stopped in some cases when dosage was reduced or the drug was discontinued. Clinicians should ask patients whether they have developed new or increased gambling urges, sexual urges, or other urges while receiving levodopa-carbidopa and should advise them of the importance of reporting such urges. If a patient develops such urges while receiving levodopa-carbidopa, consideration should be given to reducing the dosage or discontinuing the drug.

Geriatric patients who respond to levodopa should resume normal activity gradually and with caution because increased mobility may lead to fractures, particularly if an underlying condition such as osteoporosis is present. Diabetic patients should be closely monitored during levodopa therapy because the drug may adversely affect control of blood glucose.

Individuals with phenylketonuria (i.e., homozygous genetic deficiency of phenylalanine hydroxylase) and other individuals who must restrict their intake of phenylalanine should be warned that levodopa-carbidopa orally disintegrating tablets contain aspartame (NutraSweet®), which is metabolized in the GI tract to provide phenylalanine following oral administration.

When the fixed-combination preparation containing levodopa, carbidopa, and entacapone (Stalevo®) is used, the precautions and contraindications associated with all the drugs in the formulation must be considered.

Patients should be advised of the possibility that dark color (red, brown, black) may appear in saliva, urine, or sweat after ingestion of levodopa-carbidopa, and that garments may become discolored.

Periodic evaluations of hepatic, hematopoietic, cardiovascular, and renal function should be performed in all patients receiving extended levodopa therapy. Because some patients receiving levodopa have experienced abnormal bleeding episodes following prostatectomy, it has been recommended that hematologic studies be performed during the postoperative evaluation of all patients receiving the drug. Levodopa is contraindicated in patients receiving nonselective monoamine oxidase inhibitors (e.g., phenelzine, tranylcypromine). (See Drug Interactions: Psychotherapeutic Agents.) Levodopa and carbidopa are contraindicated in patients with known hypersensitivity to the drugs and in patients with angle-closure glaucoma. Levodopa-carbidopa may be administered with caution to patients with chronic open-angle glaucoma if intraocular pressure is monitored and remains well controlled.

■ Pediatric Precautions Safety and efficacy of levodopa with carbidopa in patients younger than 18 years of age have not been established.

■ Pregnancy and Lactation Safe use of levodopa or carbidopa during pregnancy has not been established. Reproduction studies in rodents using levodopa in daily dosages greater than 200 mg/kg have shown adverse effects on fetal and postnatal growth and viability, and studies in rabbits using the drug alone or in conjunction with carbidopa have shown visceral and skeletal malformations. Levodopa should be administered to pregnant women or women who might become pregnant only when the benefits to the mother outweigh the possible risks to the mother and fetus.

Levodopa is distributed into human milk. Carbidopa is distributed into milk in rats; it is not known whether carbidopa is distributed into human milk. Levodopa-carbidopa should be used with caution in nursing women.

Drug Interactions

■ Psychotherapeutic Agents Nonselective monoamine oxidase (MAO) inhibitors (e.g., phenelzine, tranylcypromine) should not be administered concomitantly with levodopa-carbidopa because hypertensive crises may result. Therapy with these monoamine oxidase inhibitors must be discontinued at least 2 weeks prior to initiation of levodopa-carbidopa therapy. Levodopa may be administered concomitantly with a selective inhibitor of MAO-B (e.g., selegiline). However, concomitant use of levodopa-carbidopa and selegiline may be associated with severe orthostatic hypotension not attributable to levodopa-carbidopa alone.

Tricyclic antidepressants may be administered to patients receiving levodopa; however, tricyclic antidepressants can augment postural hypotension and possibly interfere with absorption of levodopa by delaying gastric emptying and retarding delivery of levodopa to intestinal absorption sites. In addition, other adverse reactions, including hypertension and dyskinesia, have been reported rarely when the drugs were used concomitantly. Although the clinical importance of these interactions has not been established, the possibility that they may occur should be considered.

Antipsychotic agents (e.g., phenothiazines, butyrophenones, risperidone) may antagonize the therapeutic effects of levodopa; patients receiving these drugs concomitantly should be observed for loss of therapeutic response to levodopa. A few levodopa-treated patients have experienced decreased control of parkinsonian symptoms when chlordiazepoxide hydrochloride or diazepam was added to their therapeutic regimen. For this reason, these drugs and probably other benzodiazepines should be administered with caution to patients receiving levodopa.

■ Pyridoxine Administration of 10–25 mg of pyridoxine hydrochloride (vitamin B_6) may cause a rapid reversal of antiparkinsonian effects of levodopa when levodopa is used alone. Concomitant administration of carbidopa with levodopa prevents the reversal of levodopa effects caused by pyridoxine.

■ Anticholinergic Agents Anticholinergic agents may act synergistically with levodopa to decrease tremor in the management of parkinsonian syndrome and this interaction is often used to therapeutic advantage; however, anticholinergic agents can exacerbate abnormal involuntary movements. In addition, these drugs (particularly in high dosage) may diminish the beneficial effects of levodopa by delaying its absorption thus increasing gastric metabolism of the drug. At least theoretically, this could result in levodopa toxicity when anticholinergic therapy is stopped.

■ Hypotensive Agents Levodopa should be used with caution in patients receiving hypotensive agents. If used concomitantly, the hypotensive effect of levodopa may necessitate dosage reduction of these drugs. In addition, methyldopa (like carbidopa) is a decarboxylase inhibitor and can cause toxic CNS effects such as psychosis if administered concomitantly with levodopa.

■ Other Drugs Several patients have experienced decreased therapeutic response to levodopa when papaverine was added to their therapeutic regimen of levodopa-carbidopa. It has been suggested that papaverine should not be administered to patients receiving levodopa.

Phenytoin administration has substantially interfered with the therapeutic effects of levodopa in several patients receiving levodopa for the treatment of idiopathic parkinsonian syndrome or chronic manganese intoxication. It has been suggested that it is inadvisable to add phenytoin to therapeutic regimens containing levodopa.

Although metoclopramide-induced increases in gastric emptying may enhance the bioavailability of levodopa, metoclopramide can exacerbate parkinsonian symptoms secondary to its antagonistic effects on dopamine receptors.

Iron salts have been reported to decrease the bioavailability of levodopa and carbidopa, and should be administered concomitantly with caution.

Isoniazid may antagonize the therapeutic effects of levodopa and should be used with caution during levodopa therapy; patient should be observed for loss of therapeutic response to levodopa.

Concomitant use of levodopa and dopamine-depleting agents (reserpine, tetrabenazine) or other drugs known to deplete monoamine stores is not recommended.

Laboratory Test Interferences

Elevated protein-bound iodine concentrations have been reported during levodopa therapy but were apparently caused by an iodine dye used to color the levodopa capsules used in the study. Elevation of serum and urinary uric acid concentrations have been noted during levodopa therapy when colorimetric test methods were used. Levodopa administration does not affect uric acid determinations utilizing uricase.

Levodopa can produce false-positive reactions for urinary glucose in tests based on cupric sulfate reagent (Benedict's reagent or Clinitest® tablets) and false-negative reactions in tests using glucose oxidase (Clinistix®, Tes-Tape®). An accurate measurement of urinary glucose may be obtained if the paper strip is only partially immersed in the urine so that the paper strip can act as an ascending chromatographic system; the top portion of the paper will give a true color change for glucose. False-positive reactions for urine ketones have been reported in patients receiving levodopa when the test was performed with sodium nitroprusside reagent (Acetest®, Ketostix®, Labstix®). In urine screening tests for phenylketonuria, the urine of patients receiving levodopa turned a black-brown color on addition of ferric chloride solution thus interfering with the test.

Patients receiving levodopa have also shown falsely elevated urinary catecholamine concentrations as measured by the Hingerty method. Although levodopa administration results in small increases in urinary VMA excretion, urinary VMA as measured by the Pisano method may be falsely decreased in patients receiving the drug.

Acute Toxicity

Levodopa overdosage should be treated symptomatically. Immediate gastric lavage, maintenance of an adequate airway, and judicious administration of IV fluids is indicated. ECG monitoring and careful observation of the patient for development of cardiac arrhythmias are imperative. Antiarrhythmic therapy should be given if necessary. The value of hemodialysis in the management of levodopa overdosage is not known. The usefulness of pyridoxine administration in levodopa overdosage has not been established, but pyridoxine is not effective in reversing the actions of levodopa-carbidopa combination.

Pharmacology

Levodopa penetrates the CNS and is enzymatically converted to dopamine in the basal ganglia. There is considerable evidence that symptoms of parkinsonian syndrome, regardless of the cause of the syndrome, are related to depletion of dopamine in the corpus striatum, and levodopa is believed to act principally by increasing dopamine concentration in the brain. In addition, other metabolites of levodopa may contribute to the drug's antiparkinsonian activity. Dysregulation of brain serotonin activity may also occur.

Concurrent administration of a decarboxylase inhibitor such as carbidopa inhibits the peripheral decarboxylation of levodopa by aromatic L-amino acid decarboxylase without affecting the metabolism of the drug within the CNS. Thus, more levodopa is available for transport to the brain. Carbidopa, in doses that effectively inhibit peripheral decarboxylation of levodopa, has little effect on the CNS, cardiovascular system, or GI system. Carbidopa also inhibits peripheral decarboxylation of oxitriptan (L-5-hydroxytryptophan, L-5HTP) to serotonin (5-hydroxytryptamine) by aromatic L-amino acid decarboxylase. Thus, more oxitriptan is available for transport to the brain.

Pharmacokinetics

■ **Absorption** Although substantial amounts of levodopa are metabolized in the lumen of the stomach and intestines, the drug is considered rapidly and well absorbed from the GI tract. GI absorption of levodopa from conventional preparations is slower and peak plasma concentrations are lower when the drug is ingested with food. Absorption of the drug from conventional tablet preparations may be particularly impaired in patients receiving a high-protein diet, since levodopa competes with certain amino acids for GI transport mechanisms. In one study in patients with parkinsonian syndrome receiving 3–8 g of levodopa daily as a conventional tablet preparation with food, average plasma concentrations of levodopa were approximately 1 mcg/mL with a range of 0.2–2.8 mcg/mL. However, considerable variation in plasma concentrations has been reported among patients and in the same patient on different occasions. The relationship of plasma levodopa concentrations to clinical effects has not been established.

Conventional and orally disintegrating tablets of levodopa-carbidopa are formulated to begin releasing the drugs within 30 minutes of administration. Administration of levodopa and carbidopa as orally disintegrating tablets reportedly results in pharmacokinetic values similar to values observed with the conventional tablet preparation.

Oral bioavailability of levodopa from extended-release tablets of the combination is reduced and peak plasma concentrations are delayed compared with those from conventional tablet preparations; however, there is considerably less fluctuation in plasma levodopa concentrations between doses with the extended-release tablets. Food increases the extent of GI absorption and peak plasma levodopa concentration achieved by about 50 and 25%, respectively, following a single oral dose as extended-release tablets. In healthy geriatric individuals 56–67 years of age, the mean time to peak plasma levodopa concentration was 2 or 0.5 hours with single doses of extended-release or conventional tablet preparations of the combination, respectively, and the peak concentration achieved with the extended-release tablets was 35% of that achieved with conventional tablet preparations. Bioavailability of levodopa from the oral extended-release tablets was about 70–75% of that from conventional tablet preparations of the combination or IV levodopa in this age group. However, in young adults, the bioavailability from oral extended-release tablets of the combination was 44% of that of IV levodopa. Oral bioavailability and peak plasma levodopa concentrations are comparable following single doses and thrice-daily doses (at steady state) of extended-release tablets in geriatric individuals. In addition, mean trough plasma concentrations of levodopa at steady state with extended-release tablets were about twice those with conventional oral preparations.

The extended-release capsule formulation of levodopa-carbidopa consists of both immediate-release and extended-release components. Following oral administration of the extended-release capsules, an initial rapid increase in plasma levodopa concentrations is observed, followed by sustained plasma concentrations for about 4–5 hours; lower peak to trough fluctuation is observed at steady state with the extended-release capsules compared with immediate-release levodopa-carbidopa preparations. The bioavailability of levodopa from extended-release levodopa-carbidopa capsules is approximately 70% relative to immediate-release preparations. Peak levodopa concentrations achieved with the extended-release capsules is 30% of that achieved with immediate-release preparations when given in comparable doses.

Therapeutic response to levodopa usually consists of short-duration improvement (occurring after each dose and disappearing within 5 hours) and long-duration improvement (occurring with prolonged therapy and not subsiding during the 10-hour period following the last dose at night and the first morning dose). The long-duration response usually does not disappear until 3–5 days after levodopa is discontinued.

About 40–70% of a dose of carbidopa is absorbed following oral administration. Although levodopa does not appear to enhance the absorption of carbidopa, carbidopa may enhance the absorption of levodopa by suppressing the metabolism of levodopa in the GI tract. Plasma levodopa concentrations are increased when carbidopa and levodopa are administered concomitantly, principally because of inhibition by carbidopa of the peripheral metabolism of levodopa. (See Pharmacokinetics: Elimination.)

■ **Distribution** Levodopa is widely distributed into most body tissues and the total volume of distribution is about 65% of body weight. There is considerable uptake of levodopa by the pancreas, liver, GI tract, salivary glands, kidneys, and skin. Probably less than 1% of absorbed levodopa penetrates the CNS and only a small amount enters the brain.

Levodopa is approximately 10–30% bound to plasma proteins.

Carbidopa is also widely distributed into most body tissues; however, it does not cross the blood-brain barrier. Carbidopa crosses the placenta and is distributed into milk.

At a concentration of 1 mcg/mL, about 36% of carbidopa is bound to plasma proteins.

■ **Elimination** The plasma half-life of levodopa is approximately 1 hour. The plasma half-life of carbidopa is 1–2 hours. When levodopa and carbidopa are administered concurrently, the plasma half-life of levodopa is increased to about 1.5–2 hours. When levodopa and carbidopa are administered with entacapone or tolcapone, (catechol-*O*-methyltransferase COMT inhibitors), the plasma half-life of levodopa is increased to 1.3–2 or 3.5 hours respectively. Because administration as extended-release tablets results in prolonged release and absorption of levodopa from the GI tract, the apparent half-life of levodopa may be prolonged with this formulation compared with conventional tablet formulations.

Substantial amounts of levodopa are metabolized in the lumen of the stomach and intestines and on first pass through the liver. There is some evidence that the metabolism of levodopa is accelerated during prolonged therapy, possibly secondary to enzyme induction. Most absorbed levodopa is decarboxylated to dopamine; more than 95% of the drug is decarboxylated peripherally by aromatic L-amino acid decarboxylase, a widely distributed enzyme. Carbidopa inhibits only the peripheral decarboxylation of levodopa since, like dopamine, carbidopa does not cross the blood-brain barrier. Peripheral aromatic L-amino acid decarboxylase is saturated by daily doses of 70–100 mg of carbidopa. Small amounts of levodopa are metabolized to norepinephrine, epinephrine, and 3-methoxytyramine. A small quantity of levodopa is methylated to 3-*O*-methyldopa; this metabolite is present in plasma and accumulates in the CNS because of its long half-life. The importance of these minor metabolites has not yet been determined, but 3-*O*-methyldopa does not appear to relieve parkinsonian symptoms. Dopamine is further metabolized to 3,4-dihydroxyphenylacetic acid (DOPAC) and 3-methoxy-4-hydroxyphenylacetic acid (homovanillic acid, HVA) and excreted in urine. HVA, DOPAC, and dopamine are the metabolites of levodopa present in CSF. Carbidopa is not extensively metabolized; about 30% of an oral dose of carbidopa is excreted in urine unchanged within 24 hours.

About 80–85% of a dose of radiolabeled levodopa is excreted in urine within 24 hours. DOPAC and HVA account for about 50% and HVA has been reported to account for 13–42% of an ingested dose. Small amounts of the drug are excreted in urine as vanillylmandelic acid (VMA), 3-*O*-methyldopa, and norepinephrine. Less than 1% of a dose of levodopa is excreted in urine unchanged. When carbidopa and levodopa are administered concurrently, the urinary excretion of dopamine, DOPAC, and HVA is substantially diminished, and the amount of unchanged levodopa excreted in urine has been reported to be increased to 6%.

Chemistry and Stability

■ **Chemistry**

Levodopa Levodopa is the levorotatory isomer of dihydroxyphenylalanine and the metabolic precursor of dopamine. The drug is used in the treatment of parkinsonian syndrome. Levodopa is commercially available in combination with carbidopa. Levodopa also is commercially available as a fixed-combination preparation containing levodopa, carbidopa, and entacapone (Stalevo®). Levodopa occurs as a white to off-white, odorless, crystalline powder and is slightly soluble in water and insoluble in alcohol.

Extended-release tablets of levodopa and carbidopa (Sinemet® CR) contain the drugs in a polymeric-based delivery system that controls the release of the drugs over an approximately 4- to 6-hour period by slowly eroding in the GI tract.

Carbidopa Carbidopa is a decarboxylase inhibitor which inhibits decarboxylation of levodopa to dopamine. Carbidopa is commercially available in combination with levodopa and is also available alone from the manufacturer. Carbidopa occurs as a white to creamy white, odorless or practically odorless powder and is slightly soluble in water and practically insoluble in alcohol. Although carbidopa is commercially available as the monohydrate, potency is described in terms of anhydrous carbidopa.

■ **Stability** Levodopa is rapidly oxidized and darkens in the presence of moisture; the color change indicates loss of potency. Commercially available preparations containing levodopa and carbidopa should be protected from exposure to light, moisture, and excessive heat. Tablets containing levodopa and carbidopa should be stored at a temperature of 25°C but many be exposed briefly to temperatures ranging from 15–30°C. Extended-release tablets of the drugs should be stored at a temperature of less than 30°C.

Preparations

Excipients in commercially available drug preparations may have clinically important effects in some individuals; consult specific product labeling for details.

Carbidopa

Oral

Tablets	25 mg (of anhydrous carbidopa)*	**Carbidopa Tablets**
		Lodosyn® (scored), Valeant

*available from one or more manufacturer, distributor, and/or repackager by generic (nonproprietary) name

Carbidopa-Levodopa (Co-careldopa)

Oral

Capsules, extended-release	Carbidopa 23.75 mg (of anhydrous carbidopa) and Levodopa 95 mg	**Rytary**®, Impax
	Carbidopa 36.25 mg (of anhydours carbidopa) and Levodopa 145 mg	**Rytary**®, Impax
	Carbidopa 48.75 mg (of anhydrous carbidopa) and Levodopa 195 mg	**Rytary**®, Impax
	Carbidopa 61.25 mg (of anhydrous carbidopa) and Levodopa 245 mg	**Rytary**®, Impax

Tablets	Carbidopa 10 mg (of anhydrous carbidopa) and Levodopa 100 mg*	**Carbidopa and Levodopa Tablets**
		Sinemet®, Merck
	Carbidopa 25 mg (of anhydrous carbidopa) and Levodopa 100 mg*	**Carbidopa and Levodopa Tablets**
		Sinemet®, Merck
	Carbidopa 25 mg (of anhydrous carbidopa) and Levodopa 250 mg*	**Carbidopa and Levodopa Tablets**
		Sinemet®, Merck
Tablets, extended-release	Carbidopa 50 mg (of anhydrous carbidopa) and Levodopa 200 mg*	**Carbidopa and Levodopa Extended-release Tablets**
		Sinemet® CR, Merck
	Carbidopa 25 mg (of anhydrous carbidopa) and Levodopa 100 mg*	**Carbidopa and Levodopa Extended-release Tablets**
		Sinemet® CR, Merck
Tablets, orally disintegrating	Carbidopa 10 mg (of anhydrous carbidopa) and Levodopa 100 mg*	**Carbidopa and Levodopa Orally-disintegrating Tablets**
	Carbidopa 25 mg (of anhydrous carbidopa) and Levodopa 100 mg*	**Carbidopa and Levodopa Orally-disintegrating Tablets**
	Cabridopa 25 mg (of anhydrous carbidopa) and Levodopa 250 mg*	**Carbidopa and Levodopa Orally-disintegrating Tablets**

*available from one or more manufacturer, distributor, and/or repackager by generic (nonproprietary) name

Other Carbidopa Combinations

Oral

Tablets, film-coated	Carbidopa 12.5 mg (of anhydrous carbidopa) Entacapone 200 mg and Levodopa 50 mg	**Stalevo®**, Novartis
	Carbidopa 18.75 mg (of anhydrous carbidopa) Entacapone 200 mg and Levodopa 75 mg	**Stalevo®**, Novartis
	Carbidopa 25 mg (of anhydrous carbidopa) Entacapone 200 mg and Levodopa 100 mg	**Stalevo®**, Novartis
	Carbidopa 31.25 mg (of anhydrous carbidopa) Entacapone 200 mg and Levodopa 125 mg	**Stalevo®**, Novartis
	Carbidopa 37.5 mg (of anhydrous carbidopa) Entacapone 200 mg and Levodopa 150 mg	**Stalevo®**, Novartis
	Carbidopa 50 mg (of anhydrous carbidopa) Entacapone 200 mg and Levodopa 200 mg	**Stalevo®**, Novartis

DOPAMINE RECEPTOR AGONISTS 28:36.20

ERGOT-DERIVATIVE DOPAMINE RECEPTOR AGONISTS 28:36.20.04

Bromocriptine Mesylate

Bromocryptine, Brom-ergocryptine, 2-Bromoergocryptine, 2-Br-α-ergocryptine

■ Bromocriptine mesylate, an ergot-derivative dopamine receptor agonist and a prolactin inhibitor, is an antiparkinsonian agent and also causes sustained suppression of somatropin (growth hormone) secretion in acromegaly.

Uses

■ **Hyperprolactinemic Disorders** Bromocriptine is used in males and females for the treatment of dysfunctions associated with hyperprolactinemia including amenorrhea, with or without galactorrhea; hypogonadism; and infertility. The drug is used in patients with prolactin-secreting adenomas (e.g., prolactinoma), including macroadenomas; this tumor may be the basic underlying endocrinopathy contributing to dysfunctions associated with hyperprolactinemia. The drug has decreased tumor size in both males and females with macroadenomas and may be used to reduce tumor size prior to surgery in patients undergoing excision of the tumor (adenectomy).

Amenorrhea and Galactorrhea Bromocriptine mesylate is used for the short-term treatment of amenorrhea and/or galactorrhea associated with hyperprolactinemia of various etiologies. Bromocriptine reduces serum prolactin concentrations in patients with prolactin-secreting adenomas; however, use of the drug in these patients does not obviate the need for radiotherapy or surgery when indicated. Although bromocriptine may be effective in restoring menses in some patients with prolactin-secreting tumors and may decrease tumor growth during pregnancy in patients who have had partial surgical tumor removal, the risks associated with the use of the drug in these patients should be considered. (See Cautions: Pregnancy and Lactation and also Carcinogenicity.) Bromocriptine is not effective in patients with ovarian failure or inadequate concentrations of gonadotropin. Bromocriptine is not indicated in patients with normal prolactin concentrations although it is effective in the treatment of amenorrhea and/or galactorrhea in some of these patients. Treatment with bromocriptine mesylate is not curative. Following discontinuance of bromocriptine therapy, the recurrence rate of amenorrhea and/or galactorrhea is 70–80%.

Male Hypogonadism and Galactorrhea Bromocriptine has been used effectively in hyperprolactinemic males with prolactin-secreting adenomas (e.g., prolactinoma) and adequate concentrations of testosterone to treat hypogonadism and galactorrhea which persisted following radiation therapy or surgery. Recent studies indicate that bromocriptine therapy, in addition to relieving symptoms of the disease, also results in a reduction in the size of prolactin-secreting adenomas in most patients. Some clinicians suggest that bromocriptine may be the treatment of choice for hyperprolactinemic males with large tumors (macroadenomas).

Female Infertility Bromocriptine is used to induce ovulation in appropriately selected anovulatory women desiring pregnancy. Although the manufacturer states that bromocriptine is indicated in the treatment of female infertility associated with hyperprolactinemia in the absence of a demonstrable pituitary tumor, some clinicians state that bromocriptine is the treatment of choice to restore fertility in selected patients with prolactin-secreting adenomas. Bromocriptine restores ovulation without ovarian hyperstimulation and the risk of multiple ovulations with resulting plural gestations. However, bromocriptine probably should be reserved for patients who are not responsive to clomiphene, menotropins with chorionic gonadotropin, or estrogens. In some anovulatory women requiring concomitant treatment with 100–150 mg of clomiphene citrate and chorionic gonadotropin to induce ovulation, bromocriptine and a lower dosage of clomiphene have been used effectively to induce ovulation.

■ **Parkinsonian Syndrome** Bromocriptine is used for the treatment of idiopathic or postencephalitic parkinsonian syndrome.

Dopamine receptor agonists (bromocriptine mesylate, pramipexole dihydrochloride, pergolide mesylate, ropinirole hydrochloride) are used as adjuncts to levodopa for the symptomatic management of parkinsonian syndrome in patients with advanced disease. Dopamine receptor agonists also are used as monotherapy for the initial symptomatic management of parkinsonian syndrome. Levodopa currently is the most effective drug for relieving the symptoms of parkinsonian syndrome and traditionally has been considered the drug of choice for the initial symptomatic management of idiopathic parkinsonian syndrome. However, long-term administration of levodopa is associated with motor complications. One strategy to reduce the risk of motor complications and to improve long-term outcome is to initiate symptomatic therapy with a dopamine receptor agonist and to add levodopa as supplemental therapy when dopamine receptor agonist monotherapy no longer provides adequate symptom control. However, clinical studies evaluating this strategy are limited both in number and duration, and it remains to be determined whether initiating therapy with a dopamine receptor agonist rather than levodopa results in a more favorable long-term outcome. Factors to consider when choosing an agent for the initial symptomatic management of idiopathic parkinsonian syndrome include patient age, cognitive status, disease severity, and cost. Most clinicians would use levodopa for initial therapy in individuals older than 70 years of age since these individuals are less likely than younger individuals to develop levodopa-related motor complications and because of concerns about cognitive dysfunction, in patients with cognitive impairment, and in those with severe disease. A dopamine receptor agonist may be preferred for initial therapy in patients 70 years of age or younger.

In controlled, double-blind studies in patients receiving optimum treatment of parkinsonian syndrome which included levodopa therapy, addition of bromocriptine allowed a gradual reduction in levodopa (with or without carbidopa) dosage. When used in conjunction with levodopa (alone or with a peripheral decarboxylase inhibitor), bromocriptine may provide additional therapeutic benefits in patients who are currently maintained on optimal dosages of levodopa, patients who are beginning to develop tolerance to levodopa, and patients who are experiencing "end-of-dose failure" on levodopa therapy. In several controlled studies, bromocriptine was as effective as levodopa (with or without carbidopa) when bromocriptine was substituted for levodopa in patients who were well controlled on levodopa therapy. Patients unresponsive to levodopa are poor candidates for bromocriptine therapy. Data are insufficient to evaluate the potential benefits of bromocriptine in patients with newly diagnosed parkinsonian syndrome. A higher incidence of adverse effects (e.g., nausea, hallucinations, confusion, hypotension) have been reported in patients receiving bromocriptine than in patients receiving levodopa and carbidopa; however, bromocriptine has a longer duration of action and causes the "on-off" phenomenon less often than does levodopa. Bromocriptine may be useful in patients who are unable to tolerate levodopa's adverse effects or when levodopa is ineffective; however, continued efficacy of bromocriptine for more than 2 years has not been established and long-term or high-dose bromocriptine therapy has caused adverse effects such as erythromelalgia and psychosis. (See Cautions: Nervous System Effects.) Further study is required to determine the precise role of bromocriptine in the treatment of parkinsonian syndrome and to establish safety and efficacy of the drug during long-term administration.

■ **Acromegaly** Bromocriptine is used in the treatment of acromegaly. Although bromocriptine is not effective in all patients with acromegaly, the drug has reduced growth hormone concentrations in some patients. Reduction in growth hormone concentrations in these patients is associated with abolition of excessive sweating, reduction in soft tissue thickening, improvement in facial features, improvement in glucose tolerance, and reduction in urinary hydroxyproline excretion. However, further studies are required to determine the long-term effectiveness of bromocriptine in the treatment of acromegaly and to determine which patients may respond to the drug.

■ **Other Uses** Although bromocriptine had been used to prevent lactation after stillbirth or abortion or when breast-feeding was contraindicated or the mother elected not to breast-feed†, such use has been controversial (e.g., because of the low incidence of substantial painful engorgement, cost considerations, efficacy of appropriate supportive therapy, and concerns about potentially fatal toxicity) despite efficacy of the drug in inhibiting lactogenesis and the subsequent development of secretion, congestion, and engorgement. In addition, such use of bromocriptine no longer is recommended because of the risks of serious adverse effects (e.g., hypertension, seizures, myocardial infarction, cerebrovascular accidents, which may be fatal) nor is it included in the current US labeling for the drug. In 1994, the US Food and Drug Administration (FDA) proposed formally to withdraw approval of this indication based on accumulating reports of potentially fatal, serious adverse effects. The manufacturer of the drug (Sandoz) subsequently agreed voluntarily to withdraw the mentioned use for lactation prevention from their labeling, and FDA's approval withdrawal was finalized in February 1995. Although the absolute incidence and relative risk of associated serious effects remain to be clearly defined, the decision of FDA to seek withdrawal was based, in part, on conclusions by FDAs Fertility and Maternal Health Drugs Advisory Committee that the possible risks of serious adverse effects outweigh the limited benefits associated with the use of bromocriptine in postpartum breast engorgement, a temporary condition, that can be managed by more conservative treatments (e.g., cold packs, compression bandages, analgesics).

Bromocriptine has been used to relieve premenstrual breast symptoms† (e.g., swelling, discomfort, discharge), edema†, weight gain†, migraine headache†, and changes in mood†.

Bromocriptine has been used to restore fertility† in oligospermic men without hyperprolactinemia. Unlike traditional therapy with fluoxymesterone, testosterone, or chorionic gonadotropin, bromocriptine may increase sperm counts both during and after treatment. However, unless these patients are unresponsive to traditional drug therapy, bromocriptine should not be used since safety and efficacy of the drug for the management of this condition have not been established.

Bromocriptine has been used with some success in the treatment of neuroleptic malignant syndrome† (NMS) associated with neuroleptic drug therapy (e.g., haloperidol, fluphenazine). In a limited number of patients, bromocriptine has relieved extrapyramidal reactions, hyperthermia, and hypertension associated with NMS.

In a limited number of patients, bromocriptine has been used effectively in the management of Cushing's disease† or chronic hepatic encephalopathy†.

Bromocriptine is not effective in the management of Huntington's chorea.

Dosage and Administration

■ **Administration** Bromocriptine mesylate is administered orally with food.

■ **Dosage** Dosage of bromocriptine mesylate is expressed in terms of bromocriptine. Dosage of bromocriptine should be individualized and carefully adjusted, using frequent evaluation during dosage adjustment and employing the lowest possible effective dosage. A temporary reduction in dosage or discontinuance of the drug may occasionally be necessary in patients who develop intolerable adverse effects.

When bromocriptine therapy is discontinued (e.g., during pregnancy) in patients receiving the drug for hyperprolactinemic disorders, the patient should be carefully monitored for signs and symptoms of tumor development or progression. (See Cautions: Carcinogenicity.) Patients receiving bromocriptine for the treatment of macroadenoma should be warned to *not* discontinue the drug unless otherwise directed by their physician, since such discontinuance could result in rapid regrowth of the tumor and recurrence of symptoms.

The safety of bromocriptine dosages exceeding 100 mg daily has not been established.

Hyperprolactinemic Disorders The usual initial adult dosage of bromocriptine for the treatment of dysfunctions associated with hyperprolactinemia such as amenorrhea, galactorrhea, hypogonadism, and/or infertility in males and females is 1.25 or 2.5 mg daily. Dosage may be increased in increments of 2.5 mg daily at 3- to 7-day intervals as tolerated until the desired therapeutic response is achieved. The usual therapeutic dosage in these patients is 5–7.5 mg daily but ranges from 2.5–15 mg daily. Up to 30 mg daily has been required in some patients with amenorrhea and/or galactorrhea. For the treatment of hypogonadism in hyperprolactinemic males, dosages up to 40 mg daily have occasionally been used.

To reduce the possibility of prolonged exposure to bromocriptine in an unsuspected pregnancy during initial therapy with the drug in women in whom one of the goals of therapy is successful pregnancy, a mechanical contraceptive should be used in conjunction with bromocriptine therapy until normal ovulatory menstrual cycles have been restored. Contraception can then be discontinued. If menstruation does not occur within 3 days of the expected date, bromocriptine should be discontinued and a pregnancy test performed. Women not desiring pregnancy and women with large adenomas should use a mechanical contraceptive throughout bromocriptine therapy. (See Cautions: Carcinogenicity.)

Parkinsonian Syndrome For the treatment of parkinsonian syndrome, bromocriptine therapy is initiated at a low dosage and increased slowly until the maximum therapeutic response is achieved. The usual initial adult dosage of bromocriptine for the treatment of parkinsonian syndrome is 1.25 mg twice daily. In patients receiving levodopa, therapy with the drug should be continued, if possible, during initiation of bromocriptine therapy. Assessments of the patient's therapeutic response are generally made at 2-week intervals to ensure that the lowest effective dosage is not exceeded. If necessary, dosage may be increased by 2.5 mg daily every 14–28 days. If levodopa dosage must be decreased because of adverse effects, daily dosage of bromocriptine may be increased gradually in 2. 5-mg increments. The manufacturer states that safety of bromocriptine in dosages greater than 100 mg daily has not been established.

Acromegaly To reduce growth hormone concentrations in adults with acromegaly, the usual initial bromocriptine dosage is 1.25 or 2.5 mg daily at bedtime for 3 days. Dosage may be increased in increments of 1.25 or 2.5 mg daily at 3- to 7-day intervals until the desired therapeutic effect is achieved. The usual therapeutic dosage in these patients is 20–30 mg daily; the manufacturer states that dosage should not exceed 100 mg daily. Dosages of 20–60 mg of bromocriptine have been administered daily in divided doses.

Serum growth hormone concentrations should be determined monthly, and bromocriptine dosage should be adjusted based on the reduction in these concentrations and the patient's clinical response. If an adequate response is not apparent after a brief trial with the drug and/or dosage adjustment and clinical evaluation, discontinuance of bromocriptine should be considered. Bromocriptine therapy should be withdrawn annually in patients undergoing radiation therapy of the pituitary to determine if continued therapy with the drug and/or radiation is necessary. Usually, a 4- to 8-week period is adequate; if signs and/or symptoms of acromegaly recur or growth hormone concentrations increase during this period, the disease process is probably still active and additional bromocriptine therapy should be considered.

Other Uses Premenstrual symptoms† have been treated with 2.5–7.5 mg of bromocriptine twice daily from the tenth day of the menstrual cycle until onset of menstruation.

For the treatment of neuroleptic malignant syndrome† (NMS) associated with neuroleptic drug therapy (e.g., haloperidol, fluphenazine), 2.5–5 mg of bromocriptine has been given 2–6 times daily.

For the treatment of Cushing's disease†, 1.25–2.5 mg of bromocriptine has been given 2–4 times daily. For the treatment of chronic hepatic encephalopathy†, the initial dosage of bromocriptine was 1.25 mg daily followed by increases of 1.25 mg daily every third day up to a total maintenance dosage of 15 mg daily.

Cautions

The incidence of adverse effects associated with bromocriptine mesylate therapy is quite high, especially at the beginning of treatment and with dosages greater than 20 mg daily. Adverse effects are usually mild to moderate and can be minimized by starting with small doses, increasing dosage gradually to effective levels, and administering the drug with food and in the evening. Generally, adverse effects are decreased when dosage is reduced and then increased more gradually, although treatment with bromocriptine may have to be discontinued in a few patients because of adverse effects. Healthy individuals seem to be the most sensitive to adverse effects, while patients with hyperprolactinemia and acromegaly are not as sensitive, and women immediately postpartum experience minimal adverse effects. About 70% of patients receiving the drug for hyperprolactinemic disorders experience adverse effects; discontinuance of the drug was necessary in 5% of such patients.

■ **GI Effects** Nausea occurs frequently in patients receiving bromocriptine. Nausea has been reported in about 50 or 20% of patients receiving the drug for hyperprolactinemic disorders or acromegaly, respectively. Vomiting, anorexia, abdominal cramps or discomfort, epigastric pain, indigestion or dyspepsia, constipation during long-term use, or diarrhea occurs less frequently. These adverse GI effects may be relieved by temporary reduction of dosage or administration of the drug with food. Dysphagia has occurred occasionally in patients receiving the drug for parkinsonian syndrome. Some patients receiving bromocriptine have developed peptic ulcer, possibly as a result of increased gastric acid secretion; GI hemorrhage has also been reported.

■ **Nervous System Effects** Adverse nervous system effects of bromocriptine include headache, migraine, dizziness, drowsiness, fatigue, insomnia, lightheadedness, faintness, fainting, and sedation. Headache or dizziness occurs in about 20 or less than 2% of patients receiving the drug for hyperprolactinemic disorders or acromegaly, respectively. Confusion, hallucinations, delusions (usually paranoid), nightmares, and erythromelalgia may occur, especially in patients with parkinsonian syndrome receiving long-term and/or high-dose (100 mg or greater daily) bromocriptine therapy; these adverse effects are usually reversible 2–3 weeks after the drug is discontinued and are generally more severe and persist longer than with levodopa. Patients with parkinsonian syndrome have also experienced abnormal involuntary movements, "on-off" phenomenon, asthenia, ataxia, mental depression, epileptiform seizure, anxiety, nervousness, and paresthesia. Mania also has been reported in several patients without parkinsonian syndrome receiving bromocriptine; after the drug was discontinued, mania was treated successfully with haloperidol. Patients receiving the drug for acromegaly have also experienced decreased sleep requirements, visual hallucinations, lassitude, sluggishness, paresthesia, vertigo, delusional psychosis, paranoia, heavy headedness, and tingling of the ears.

One patient receiving bromocriptine experienced a relapse of severe depression with suicidal thoughts and another developed anxiety and extreme agitation; these effects are similar to those seen with levodopa and are probably caused by dopamine receptor stimulation. Therefore, bromocriptine may be contraindicated in patients with preexisting psychiatric disorders.

CSF rhinorrhea has occurred in a few patients receiving bromocriptine for the treatment of large prolactinomas. CSF rhinorrhea occurs rarely, mainly in patients who previously underwent transsphenoidal surgery and/or radiation therapy and who were receiving the drug for tumor recurrence. CSF rhinorrhea may also occur in patients with previously untreated prolactinoma that extends into the sphenoid sinus.

Seizures and stroke have been associated rarely with bromocriptine therapy for suppression of postpartum lactation (see Cautions: Cardiovascular Effects); however, the drug no longer is labeled for such use in the US. (See Uses: Other Uses)

■ **Cardiovascular Effects** A persistent hypotensive effect commonly accompanies bromocriptine mesylate treatment, and the drug may produce postural hypotension, syncope, and severe prolonged hypotension or shock. Exacerbation of angina may occur. Other adverse cardiovascular effects reported include palpitation, arrhythmia, ventricular tachycardia, bradycardia, and erythematous and edematous ankles and feet. Cold-induced vasospasm with pallor of fingers and toes has been reported in patients receiving 20–60 mg of bromocriptine daily; when the drug was discontinued, vasospasm was reversed and pain did not occur during recovery. Exacerbation of Raynaud's syndrome and decreased tolerance to cold have also occurred. The drug's vasodilating action on renal arteries may produce diuresis in some patients. Very high dosages of bromocriptine (100 mg daily) may cause cardiac dysrhythmia. One patient receiving 35 mg of bromocriptine daily for 8 weeks developed paroxysmal breathlessness and acute left ventricular failure associated with atrial flutter-fibrillation; sinus rhythm returned within 24 hours following discontinuance of the drug.

Decreases in blood pressure (20 mm Hg or greater systolic and 10 mm Hg or greater diastolic) have occurred at least once during the first 3 days postpartum in about 30% of women receiving bromocriptine for suppression of postpartum lactation (no longer included as a labeled use in the US); the hypotensive effect is usually transient. Occasionally, supine systolic blood pressure has decreased by as much as 50–60 mm Hg in these women. Since decreases in blood pressure are common during the puerperium independent of drug therapy, many but not all of these decreases may have not been drug related. Fainting during the puerperium also has occurred rarely and may have been related to the drug.

Hypertension (sometimes developing with initiation of therapy but often during the second week); seizures (mean onset about 7 days postpartum but up to 2 weeks in some patients), with or without hypertension, occasionally presenting as status epilepticus; potentially fatal cerebrovascular accident (stroke) (mean onset about 13 days postpartum), principally in postpartum women whose prenatal and obstetric courses were uncomplicated; and acute myocardial infarction have occurred rarely in women receiving the drug for postpartum lactation. Some of these women had toxemia of pregnancy (including postpartum eclampsia) and some (including at least one fatality) received concomitant therapy with other ergot alkaloids or other drugs that can increase blood pressure. Accumulating reports of such adverse effects when the drug was used for postpartum lactation prevention include 31 cases of stoke, 9 of which were fatal, and 63 cases of seizures; no other potential cause for stroke or seizures could be identified in 40% of these cases. While the absolute incidence and relative risk (the ratio of the incidence of these bromocriptine-associated effects to the background of such effects occurring in the postpartum period in women *not* receiving the drug) remain to be clearly defined, FDA's Fertility and Maternal Health Drugs Advisory Committee concluded that the possibility of serious adverse effects associated with use of bromocriptine for postpartum lactation prevention outweighs the limited benefits of such therapy.

Many postpartum patients who developed stroke and/or seizures in associated with bromocriptine therapy complained of constant and often progressively severe headaches hours to days prior to the acute event. Some such patients also developed prodromal visual disturbances (blurred vision and transient cortical blindness). At least one case of stroke was associated with sagittal sinus thrombosis, and another was associated with cerebral and cerebellar vasculitis. At least one case of acute myocardial infarction was associated with unexplained disseminated intravascular thrombosis, and another was associated with concomitant use of another ergot alkaloid. Most of the women who developed hypertension became normotensive only after discontinuance of therapy with the drug; in 2 patients who were rechallenged, hypertension recurred in one and remained elevated during the entire week of rechallenge. Seizures also resolved following discontinuance of bromocriptine. Although spontaneous, late-onset postpartum hypertension or eclampsia has been reported in women not receiving bromocriptine, it is unlikely that all cases associated with bromocriptine therapy were due to chance alone. In addition, postpartum hypertension or eclampsia as an adverse effect with other ergot alkaloids has been well documented.

Although there currently is no conclusive evidence of an interaction between bromocriptine and other ergot alkaloids, concomitant use of the drugs is not recommended. Particular caution is indicated in patients who recently have received other drugs that can alter blood pressure, and bromocriptine should *not* be used in patients with uncontrolled hypertension or toxemia of pregnancy. Because the risks of serious adverse effects (e.g., hypertensive crisis, seizures, stroke) outweigh the limited benefits of bromocriptine therapy for the prevention of postpartum lactation, such use no longer is recommended. (See Uses: Other Uses.) However, if bromocriptine were used for the prevention of lactation, therapy with the drug should not be initiated until postpartum vital signs have stabilized and no sooner than 4 hours after parturition. Periodic monitoring of blood pressure, especially during the first weeks of bromocriptine therapy and particularly during the postpartum period, is prudent. Bromocriptine therapy should be discontinued immediately and the patient evaluated promptly if hypertension; severe, progressive, or unremitting headache (with or without visual disturbances); or evidence of CNS toxicity develops; in addition, patients should be advised to discontinue the drug and seek prompt medical attention if any of these manifestations occurs. FDA states that similar hypertensive crises have not been reported with other drugs used to suppress lactation to date; however, reporting bias may contribute to this difference. Acute myocardial infarction also has occurred in at least one patient not receiving the drug for the prevention of lactation.

■ **Other Adverse Effects** Other reported adverse effects of bromocriptine include leg cramps, dry mouth, metallic taste, anorexia, burning discomfort of the eyes, blepharospasm, diplopia or other visual disturbances, nasal congestion, rash, mottling of the skin, facial pallor, and urticaria. Hair loss, vasovagal attack, muscle cramps, and potentiation of the effects of alcohol have also occurred rarely in patients with acromegaly.

Pulmonary infiltrates, pleural effusion, and thickening of the pleura have been reported in a few patients receiving bromocriptine in dosages ranging from 20–100 mg daily for 6–36 months. In most reported cases in which bromocriptine therapy was discontinued, these pulmonary changes slowly reverted towards normal. Shortness of breath has been reported rarely. Retroperitoneal fibrosis also has been reported in a few patients receiving bromocriptine in dosages ranging from 30–140 mg daily for 2–10 years.

Signs and symptoms of ergotism such as tingling of fingers, cold feet, numbness, muscle cramps of feet and legs, or exacerbation of Raynaud's syndrome have been reported rarely in patients receiving bromocriptine for the treatment of parkinsonian syndrome. Urinary frequency, urinary incontinence, and urinary retention have also been reported rarely in these patients.

Bromocriptine therapy has caused transient increases in serum concentrations of AST (SGOT), ALT (SGPT), γ-glutamyl transferase (γ-glutamyltranspeptidase, GGT, GGTP), creatine kinase (CK, creatine phosphokinase, CPK), alkaline phosphatase, uric acid, and BUN.

■ **Precautions and Contraindications** Blood pressure should be monitored periodically in all patients receiving bromocriptine, especially during the first few days of therapy with the drug. Particular care should be exercised in patients receiving other hypotensive drugs concomitantly. Decreases in blood pressure frequently have been reported during the puerperium independent of drug therapy, and some women have developed bromocriptine-induced hypotension or, rarely, hypertension, including hypertensive crisis. (See Cautions: Cardiovascular Effects.) Because of the risk of this and other potentially serious adverse effects, which may be fatal, use of bromocriptine for the prevention of postpartum lactation no longer is recommended.

Patients should be warned that bromocriptine may impair their ability to perform activities requiring mental alertness or physical coordination (e.g., operating machinery, driving a motor vehicle).

Hepatic, hematopoietic, cardiovascular, and renal function should be evaluated periodically in patients receiving prolonged therapy with bromocriptine, as in the treatment of parkinsonian syndrome. The safety of long-term bromocriptine therapy for periods longer than 2 years at dosages used in the treatment of parkinsonian syndrome has not been established. Since high dosages of bromocriptine may be associated with confusion and mental disturbances, the drug should be used with caution in patients with parkinsonian syndrome who manifest mild degrees of dementia. Bromocriptine therapy, alone or combined with levodopa, has been associated with visual or auditory hallucinations in patients receiving the drug(s) for parkinsonian syndrome; hallucinations usually resolve following dosage reduction, but discontinuance of bromocriptine may occasionally be necessary. Rarely, after high dosages, hallucinations may persist for several weeks following discontinuance of the drug.

Bromocriptine should be used with caution in patients with impaired liver or renal function, since safety and efficacy of the drug in these patients have not been definitely established. Dosage of bromocriptine may have to be reduced in patients with impaired liver function.

Bromocriptine should also be used with caution in patients, particularly those with parkinsonian syndrome, who have a history of myocardial infarction and a residual atrial, nodal, or ventricular arrhythmia.

The relative efficacy of bromocriptine therapy versus surgery in preserving the visual fields in patients with hyperprolactinemic disorders is not known. Patients with rapidly progressing visual field loss should be evaluated by a neurosurgeon.

Patients receiving bromocriptine for hyperprolactinemic disorders associated with macroadenomas and those who have undergone transsphenoidal surgery should be advised to report to their physician any persistent, watery nasal discharge that occurs during therapy with the drug, since this may be a sign of CSF rhinorrhea. (See Cautions: Nervous System Effects.)

Patients receiving long-term (e.g., 6–36 months), high-dose (e.g., 20–100 mg daily) bromocriptine therapy should be observed for pulmonary changes such as infiltrates, effusion, and thickening of the pleura since these effects have occasionally occurred.

Patients with acromegaly should be monitored for cold-induced digital vasospasm during bromocriptine therapy. Vasospasm usually resolves following a reduction in dosage and may be prevented by keeping the fingers warm. Patients with acromegaly should also be monitored for signs and symptoms of peptic ulcer during bromocriptine therapy; such signs and symptoms should be thoroughly evaluated and appropriate therapy instituted if necessary. GI bleeding from peptic ulcers, sometimes fatal, has occurred during therapy with the drug in patients with acromegaly, but bromocriptine has not been shown to increase the incidence of peptic ulcer in these patients.

Patients with hyperprolactinemic amenorrhea-galactorrhea and infertility should undergo complete evaluation of the pituitary, including radiographs and posterior-anterior and lateral tomography, to rule out the possibility of a pituitary tumor before treatment with bromocriptine is initiated.

Since bromocriptine may restore fertility and pregnancy may subsequently occur, women receiving the drug who do not desire pregnancy should use mechanical contraceptive measures; estrogen-progestin contraceptives are contraindicated since they may cause amenorrhea-galactorrhea. The manufacturer recommends that a pregnancy test be performed every 4 weeks in amenorrheic women and, once menses are reinstated, whenever a menstrual period is missed. If pregnancy occurs during bromocriptine therapy, the drug should be discontinued immediately. (See Cautions: Pregnancy and Lactation.)

Bromocriptine is contraindicated in patients with uncontrolled hypertension or toxemia of pregnancy and in those who are sensitive to any ergot alkaloid.

■ **Pediatric Precautions** Safety and efficacy of bromocriptine mesylate have not been established in children younger than 15 years of age.

■ **Carcinogenicity** Because the natural history of growth hormone-secreting tumors is not known, patients with acromegaly should be carefully monitored for tumor expansion during bromocriptine therapy; if evidence of tumor expansion occurs, the drug should be discontinued and alternative therapies considered. Possible tumor expansion has occurred during bromocriptine therapy in these patients.

Women with hyperprolactinemic disorders who become pregnant and subsequently discontinue bromocriptine therapy during pregnancy may develop enlargement of a previously undetected or existing prolactin-secreting tumor when therapy with the drug is suspended. These women should be monitored closely throughout pregnancy for signs and symptoms of tumor progression. Women not seeking pregnancy or those with large adenomas should be advised to use contraceptive measures, other than estrogen-progestin contraceptives, during bromocriptine therapy. Careful evaluation of the pituitary to detect the presence of a prolactin-secreting tumor is essential prior to initiating bromocriptine therapy in hyperprolactinemic women with amenorrhea-galactorrhea and hypogonadism (infertility), since one of the goals of bromocriptine therapy in these women often is successful pregnancy.

Rapid tumor regrowth occurs in most patients with known macroadenoma following discontinuance of bromocriptine therapy.

■ **Pregnancy and Lactation** Recent studies indicate that the incidence of spontaneous abortions and adverse effects in infants born to mothers who were receiving bromocriptine therapy at conception does not appear to exceed that generally reported for such occurrences in the population at large. Most of these women received the drug during the first 2–3 weeks of pregnancy, although some received the drug for up to 3 months and several throughout pregnancy. Use of bromocriptine to reduce serum prolactin concentrations and prevent possible pituitary tumor expansion has been reported in some women during the last week of pregnancy. Nevertheless, bromocriptine should be discontinued immediately if pregnancy occurs during therapy and the patient should be carefully observed throughout the pregnancy, including regular checks of the visual field. In pregnant women with underlying prolactin-secreting pituitary tumors, sudden enlargement of the tumors as a result of an increase in pituitary size which normally occurs during pregnancy may cause optic nerve compression, visual impairment, and even blindness, which usually disappear after delivery; diabetes insipidus and possible pituitary apoplexy also may occur.

In pregnant women receiving bromocriptine, fetal prolactin (but not growth hormone) concentrations are suppressed; concentrations of prolactin in amniotic fluid are not affected. Prolactin concentrations return to normal in these infants after birth. Cervical incompetence and premature delivery have been reported after bromocriptine therapy in pregnant women, but a direct correlation with the drug's use has not been established.

Since bromocriptine interferes with lactation, the drug should not be administered to women who elect to breast-feed.

Drug Interactions

Effectiveness of bromocriptine mesylate in reducing serum prolactin concentrations is inhibited by drugs which increase prolactin concentrations, including amitriptyline, butyrophenones, imipramine, methyldopa, phenothiazines, and reserpine; therefore, the dosage of bromocriptine may have to be increased in patients receiving these drugs.

Administration of bromocriptine mesylate especially in high dosage, may result in decreased alcohol tolerance, and patients should be cautioned to limit alcohol intake while receiving bromocriptine.

There may be an additive neurologic effect of bromocriptine and levodopa in patients with parkinsonian syndrome which may be used to therapeutic advantage, enabling a reduction of levodopa dosage.

Additive hypotensive effects may occur in patients receiving bromocriptine mesylate and antihypertensive agents. Careful adjustment of antihypertensive dosage may be necessary when these drugs are used concomitantly. Although there currently is no conclusive evidence of an interaction between bromocriptine and other ergot alkaloids, concomitant use of the drugs is not recommended since potentially severe adverse effects (e.g., hypertension, myocardial infarction) have occurred when the drugs were used together. (See Cautions: Cardiovascular Effects.)

Acute Toxicity

Overdosage of bromocriptine may cause nausea, vomiting, and severe hypotension. Treatment of bromocriptine overdosage consists of emptying the stomach by aspiration and lavage and administration of IV fluids to treat hypotension.

Pharmacology

Bromocriptine reduces serum prolactin concentrations by inhibiting release of prolactin from the anterior pituitary gland by a direct effect on the pituitary and/or by stimulating postsynaptic dopamine receptors in the hypothalamus to release prolactin-inhibitory factor via a complicated catecholamine pathway. Bromocriptine substantially reduces high serum prolactin concentrations and thereby restores ovulation and ovarian function in amenorrheic women and suppresses puerperal or nonpuerperal lactation in women with adequate gonadotropin concentrations and ovarian function. In some patients, menses is initiated by bromocriptine despite continued hyperprolactinemia, which may indicate that the drug stimulates the release of hypothalamic luteinizing hormone releasing factor. Bromocriptine may also act directly on dopaminergic receptors in the ovary to restore ovulation. Although the mechanism is not clear, bromocriptine also suppresses galactorrhea and initiates menses in amenorrheic women with normal serum prolactin concentrations. Bromocriptine reduces serum prolactin concentrations in males with normal or increased serum prolactin concentrations.

The time required for resumption of menses or ovulation and suppression of galactorrhea is increased in patients with reduced gonadotropin response to luteinizing hormone releasing factor and is increased with increased duration of amenorrhea or galactorrhea prior to therapy, but is not related to either pretreatment serum prolactin concentrations or degree of prolactin suppression by bromocriptine. Restoration of ovulatory menses usually occurs prior to complete cessation of galactorrhea, although suppression of galactorrhea may occur within a few days. The average time for alleviation of amenorrhea is 6–8 weeks but may range from a few days to 24 weeks. The delay in onset of menses results from the time required for the endometrium to develop to a mature secretory phase. It appears that women who have been amenorrheic for more than 4 years may have late resumption of menses during therapy with bromocriptine. In most patients with galactorrhea, at least a 75% reduction in secretion is usually observed after 7–12 weeks of bromocriptine therapy; however, in some patients, complete cessation of secretion fails to occur even after 24 weeks. Degree of suppression of galactorrhea is dependent on the degree of stimulation of the mammary tissue prior to therapy. Tolerance to the prolactin-lowering effects of bromocriptine mesylate during long-term treatment apparently does not occur. In most hyperprolactinemic patients, serum prolactin rapidly increases to pretreatment values within 1–6 weeks following discontinuance of the drug; amenorrhea returns within 4–24 weeks and galactorrhea within 2–12 weeks.

Bromocriptine may decrease the rate of growth of prolactin-dependent pituitary adenomas. Bromocriptine transiently increases growth hormone secretion in individuals with normal growth hormone concentrations but paradoxically causes sustained suppression of growth hormone secretion in some patients with acromegaly. Following discontinuance of bromocriptine therapy in patients with acromegaly, plasma growth hormone concentrations return to pretreatment concentrations within 2 weeks. Bromocriptine does not affect the release of any other anterior pituitary hormones.

Bromocriptine activates dopaminergic receptors in the neostriatum of the CNS, which may aid in the treatment of parkinsonian syndrome. Dysregulation of brain serotonin activity may also occur. Improvement in the signs of parkinsonian syndrome may occur within 30–90 minutes following administration of a single dose of bromocriptine and is maximal within approximately 2 hours. Tolerance apparently does not develop to the neurologic effects. Bromocriptine has been reported to substantially reduce blood pressure in hypertensive and normotensive patients, possibly because of its dopaminergic effects. In some patients, renal sodium excretion may increase slightly, perhaps as a result of an action of the drug on dopamine receptors in the kidneys. Peripheral vasoconstriction may occur with large doses of bromocriptine. The drug does not have an oxytocic effect.

Pharmacokinetics

■ **Absorption** Studies with radiolabeled bromocriptine mesylate have shown that approximately 28% of an oral dose of the drug is absorbed from the GI tract following oral administration; however, because of a substantial first-pass effect, only 6% of the dose reaches systemic circulation unchanged. Following oral administration of 3 mg of tritium-labeled bromocriptine in one study, the drug and its metabolites appeared in plasma in 10 minutes and maximum mean plasma concentrations were attained in about 1–1.5 hours. With fixed dosage, there are large interindividual variations in plasma concentrations. Plasma concentrations required for prolactin-lowering and antiparkinsonian effects are not known. Following oral administration of 2.5 mg of radiolabeled bromocriptine, peak plasma concentrations of unchanged drug and its metabolites range from 4–6 ng/mL.

Following oral administration of a single 1.25- to 5-mg dose of bromocriptine, serum prolactin decreases within 2 hours, is maximally decreased at 8 hours, and is still decreased at 24 hours. Maximum obtainable reduction of serum prolactin in hyperprolactinemic patients usually occurs within the first 4 weeks of bromocriptine therapy. A single oral dose of 2.5 mg of bromocriptine substantially reduces plasma growth hormone concentrations in patients with acromegaly within 1–2 hours and decreased concentrations persist for at least 4–5 hours.

■ **Distribution** Bromocriptine and/or its metabolites do not distribute appreciably into erythrocytes. In vitro studies have found that bromocriptine is 90–96% bound to serum albumin.

■ **Elimination** In one study, the elimination half-life of bromocriptine following a 3-mg oral dose of the drug was 4–4.5 hours for the initial phase and 45–50 hours for the terminal phase.

Bromocriptine mesylate is completely metabolized in the liver, principally by hydrolysis of the amide bond to produce lysergic acid and a peptide fragment. The metabolites apparently are not pharmacologically active or toxic. Bromocriptine and its metabolites are excreted principally in feces via biliary elimination; approximately 2.5–5.5% of a single dose is excreted in urine. Within 5 days, about 85% of a dose is excreted in feces.

Chemistry and Stability

■ **Chemistry** Bromocriptine mesylate, a semisynthetic derivative of the ergotoxin group of ergot alkaloids, is a dopamine receptor agonist and a prolactin inhibitor. Bromocriptine mesylate occurs as a yellowish-white crystalline powder and is very slightly soluble in water and sparingly soluble in alcohol.

■ **Stability** Bromocriptine mesylate tablets and capsules should be stored in tight, light-resistant containers at a temperature less than 25°C.

Preparations

Excipients in commercially available drug preparations may have clinically important effects in some individuals; consult specific product labeling for details.

Bromocriptine Mesylate

Oral

Capsules	5 mg (of bromocriptine)*	**Bromocriptine Mesylate Tablets** **Parlodel®**, Novartis
Tablets	2.5 mg (of bromocriptine)*	**Bromocriptine Mesylate Tablets** **Parlodel® SnapTabs®** (scored), Novartis

*available from one or more manufacturer, distributor, and/or repackager by generic (nonproprietary) name

†Use is not currently included in the labeling approved by the US Food and Drug Administration

Selected Revisions October 2009,

Cabergoline

■ Cabergoline is an ergot-derivative dopamine receptor agonist and prolactin inhibitor.

Uses

■ **Hyperprolactinemic Disorders** Cabergoline is used in the treatment of hyperprolactinemic disorders due to prolactinoma (prolactin-secreting adenomas) or idiopathic hyperprolactinemia. The drug suppresses prolactin secretion, restores gonadal function, and reduces the size of prolactinomas.

Cabergoline is at least as effective as bromocriptine in normalizing serum prolactin concentrations and restoring gonadal function in women with hyperprolactinemic amenorrhea. Fewer adverse effects, especially adverse GI effects, were reported in cabergoline-treated women than in bromocriptine-treated women. Bromocriptine is preferred when restoration of fertility is the goal of therapy; this recommendation is based on the safety record of bromocriptine in pregnant women.

■ **Parkinsonian Syndrome** Cabergoline has been used for the symptomatic management of parkinsonian syndrome†.

Cabergoline has been used as monotherapy for the initial symptomatic management of parkinsonian syndrome†. Most clinicians would use levodopa for initial therapy in individuals >70 years of age (less likely than younger individuals to develop levodopa-related motor complications and because of concerns about cognitive dysfunction), in patients with cognitive impairment, and in those with severe disease. A dopamine receptor agonist may be preferred for initial therapy in patients 70 years of age or younger.

Cabergoline has been used as an adjunct to levodopa for the symptomatic management of parkinsonian syndrome† in patients with advanced disease.

Dosage and Administration

■ **Administration** ***Oral Administration*** Administer orally without regard to meals.

Hyperprolactinemic disorders: Administer twice weekly.

Parkinsonian syndrome: Administer once daily.

■ **Dosage** ***Adults*** **Hyperprolactinemic Disorders.** *Oral:*

Initiate at low dosage and increase slowly (at intervals of at least 4 weeks) until therapeutic response is achieved.

Initially, 0.25 mg twice weekly; increase in increments of 0.25 mg twice weekly up to 1 mg twice weekly. Base dosage adjustments on serum prolactin concentrations; use lowest effective dosage.

Consider decreasing the dosage if normal serum prolactin concentrations maintained for 24 months and size of tumor decreased by at least 50%; periodically monitor to determine whether retreatment is needed. Some patients (e.g., those with microadenomas) may be able to discontinue the drug; discontinuance in those with macroadenomas should be undertaken with extreme caution. The manufacturer states that efficacy beyond 24 months not established.

Parkinsonian Syndrome†. *Oral:*

Initiate at low dosage and increase slowly (at intervals of 7- or 14-days) until the maximum therapeutic response is achieved.

2–6 mg daily has been used.

Therapy has been initiated with 1 mg once daily, then increased in increments of 0.5–1 mg at 7- or 14-day intervals until control of symptoms obtained.

When cabergoline is used as an adjunct to levodopa, the levodopa dosage may be decreased gradually as tolerated.

When therapy with a dopamine receptor agonist is discontinued, the drug is discontinued gradually.

Prescribing Limits: Adults **Hyperprolactinemic Disorders.** *Oral:*

Dosages >1 mg twice weekly have not been systematically evaluated.

■ **Special Populations** ***Hepatic Impairment*** No specific dosage recommendations at this time; use with caution in patients with severe hepatic impairment. (See Cautions: Hepatic Impairment.)

Renal Impairment No specific dosage recommendations at this time.

Geriatric Patients Select dosage carefully; start at low dosage.(See Cautions: Geriatric Use.)

Cautions

■ **Contraindications** Known hypersensitivity to cabergoline or other ergot derivatives.

Uncontrolled hypertension.

■ **Warnings/Precautions** ***Warnings*** **Hypertension during Pregnancy.** Should not be used in patients with pregnancy-induced hypertension (e.g., preeclampsia, eclampsia) unless potential benefits outweigh possible risks.

Fibrotic Effects. Pleural effusion, pulmonary fibrosis, and cardiac valvulopathy reported. Signs and symptoms have improved after discontinuance.

Use with caution in patients with history of, or current signs and/or symptoms of, respiratory or cardiac disorders linked to fibrotic tissue.

General Precautions When used for parkinsonian syndrome, observe the usual precautions associated with dopamine receptor agonist therapy in this patient population. Usual dosage for parkinsonian syndrome exceeds dosage used for hyperprolactinemia.

Symptomatic Hypotension. Orthostatic hypotension reported, especially if initial doses exceeding 1 mg are used. Exercise care in patients currently receiving drugs known to lower blood pressure.

Postpartum Breast Engorgement. Not indicated for the inhibition or suppression of lactation. Hypertension, cerebrovascular accidents, and seizures reported rarely when another dopamine receptor agonist (i.e., bromocriptine) was used for this indication.

Specific Populations **Pregnancy.** Category B. (See Cautions: Hypertension during Pregnancy.) (See Users Guide.)

Lactation. Not known whether cabergoline is distributed into milk; drug is expected to interfere with lactation. Discontinue nursing or the drug.

Pediatric Use. Safety and efficacy not established.

Geriatric Use. Insufficient experience from clinical studies to determine whether patients 65 years of age or older respond differently than younger adults. Other clinical experience has not identified age-related differences in responses.

Select dosage carefully, generally initiating therapy at low dosage. Consider the greater frequency of decreased hepatic, renal, or cardiac function and of concomitant disease or drug therapy in geriatric patients.

Hepatic Impairment. Cabergoline is extensively metabolized in liver; use with caution and monitor carefully.

■ **Common Adverse Effects** Patients with hyperprolactinemia: Nausea, constipation, abdominal pain, headache, dizziness, asthenia, fatigue, somnolence.

Patients with parkinsonian syndrome: Dyskinesia, hallucinations, confusion, peripheral edema.

Drug Interactions

■ **Dopamine Antagonists (e.g., phenothiazines, butyrophenones, thioxanthenes, metoclopramide)** Possible reduced efficacy of cabergoline. Generally should not be used concomitantly.

■ **Levodopa** Additive therapeutic and/or adverse (e.g., dyskinesia) effects. Consider a reduction in levodopa dosage when cabergoline is added to levodopa therapy.

Description

Cabergoline, a long-acting dopamine receptor agonist, has high binding affinity for dopamine D_2 receptors and lesser affinity for D_1, α_1- and α_2-adrenergic, and serotonin (5-HT_1 and 5-HT_2) receptors.

Cabergoline reduces serum prolactin concentrations by inhibiting release of prolactin from the anterior pituitary gland. This effect on hypothalamic/pituitary function attributed to the drug's agonist activity at D_2 receptors.

Advice to Patients

Potential for hypotension.

Importance of patients informing clinicians if cough or dyspnea develops.

Importance of women informing clinicians if they are or plan to become pregnant or plan to breast-feed.

Importance of informing clinicians of existing or contemplated concomitant therapy, including prescription and OTC drugs, as well as any concomitant illnesses (e.g., respiratory or cardiac disorders associated with fibrosis).

Importance of informing patients of other important precautionary information. (See Cautions.)

Overview® (see Users Guide). For additional information on this drug until a more detailed monograph is developed and published, the manufacturer's labeling should be consulted. It is *essential* that the manufacturer's labeling be consulted for more detailed information on usual cautions, precautions, contraindications, potential drug interactions, laboratory test interferences, and acute toxicity.

Preparations

Excipients in commercially available drug preparations may have clinically important effects in some individuals; consult specific product labeling for details.

Cabergoline

Oral		
Tablets	0.5 mg*	Dostinex® (scored), Pfizer Cabergoline Tablets

*available from one or more manufacturer, distributor, and/or repackager by generic (nonproprietary) name

†Use is not currently included in the labeling approved by the US Food and Drug Administration

NONERGOT-DERIVATIVE DOPAMINE RECEPTOR AGONISTS 28:36.20.08

Apomorphine Hydrochloride

■ Apomorphine hydrochloride is a nonergot-derivative dopamine receptor agonist.

Uses

■ **Hypomobility Episodes Associated with Parkinson's Disease** Apomorphine hydrochloride is used for the acute, intermittent management of episodes of hypomobility (i.e., "off" episodes, including both end-of-dose "wearing off" and unpredictable "on-off" episodes) associated with advanced Parkinson's disease. Apomorphine is designated an orphan drug by the US Food and Drug Administration (FDA) for this use.

Efficacy of apomorphine hydrochloride for this indication has been established in 3 randomized, controlled studies in patients with advanced Parkinson's disease (average duration of illness: 11.3 years) who had received levodopa and at least one other agent, usually an oral dopamine receptor agonist. One of the three studies was conducted in patients who did not have prior exposure to apomorphine and two were conducted in patients who had received apomorphine therapy for at least 3 months immediately prior to study enrollment. In these studies, the primary efficacy measurement was change in part III (motor performance) of the Unified Parkinson's Disease Rating Scale (UPDRS). Use of apomorphine was associated with a substantial reduction in the UPDRS motor score in all 3 studies. In the randomized study conducted in patients who did not have prior exposure to apomorphine, use of apomorphine was associated with a 62% improvement in UPDRS score; in addition, apomorphine aborted 95% of "off" episodes during 4 weeks of therapy.

Following subcutaneous administration, apomorphine generally has an onset of action of 10–20 minutes and a duration of action of about 60 minutes. Clinical response has been maintained for up to 5 years in some studies.

■ **Acute Poisoning** Apomorphine hydrochloride (adult dose: 5–6 mg administered subcutaneously) was formerly used to induce vomiting in the early management of acute oral drug overdosage and in certain cases of oral poisoning.

Dosage and Administration

■ **Administration** Apomorphine hydrochloride is administered by subcutaneous injection using a dosing pen. Injections may be made into the abdomen, thigh, or upper arm; injections sites should be rotated.

Apomorphine hydrochloride should *not* be given IV because of the possibility of serious adverse effects (e.g., thrombosis, pulmonary embolism).

To minimize nausea and/or vomiting associated with apomorphine therapy, an antiemetic (i.e., trimethobenzamide hydrochloride 300 mg orally 3 times daily) should be administered beginning 3 days prior to initiation of apomorphine therapy and continuing for the first 2 months of apomorphine therapy or until tolerance develops. However, antiemetic agents that selectively inhibit type 3 serotonergic receptors (5-HT_3; e.g., dolasetron, granisetron, ondansetron, palonosetron) or dopamine receptors (e.g., metoclopramide, phenothiazines) should not be used. (See Drug Interactions.)

■ **Dosage** Dosage of apomorphine hydrochloride must be individualized according to the patient's response and tolerance.

The manufacturer states that apomorphine hydrochloride dosing instructions for the patient or their caregiver should always be expressed in mL because the dose is expressed on the dosing pen in terms of mL.

Hypomobility Episodes Associated with Parkinson's Disease

The dose of apomorphine hydrochloride must be titrated based on efficacy and tolerance. An initial test dose of 0.2 mL (2 mg) of apomorphine hydrochloride should be administered in a medical setting where blood pressure can be closely monitored by a health-care provider; this test dose should be administered while the patient is experiencing an "off" episode. Induction of an "off" episode can be facilitated by withholding the patient's antiparkinsonian agents overnight. Both supine and standing blood pressures should be measured prior to and at 20, 40, and 60 minutes after administration of the test dose. Patients who develop clinically important orthostatic hypotension in response to the initial 0.2-mL (2-mg) test dose should not be considered candidates for apomorphine therapy. If the 0.2-mL (2-mg) dose is effective and well tolerated, this dose may be used on an as-needed, outpatient basis to reverse "off" episodes; if necessary, doses can be increased in 0.1-mL (1-mg) increments every few days on an outpatient basis.

For patients who tolerate but do not respond to the initial 0.2-mL (2-mg) test dose, a second test dose of 0.4 mL (4 mg) may be administered at the next observed "off" period, but no sooner than 2 hours after the initial test dose. Both supine and standing blood pressures should be measured prior to and at 20, 40, and 60 minutes after administration of the test dose. If this dose is effective and well tolerated, a 0.3-mL (3-mg) dose may be used on an as-needed, outpatient basis to reverse "off" episodes. If necessary, the dose can be increased in 0.1-mL (1-mg) increments every few days on an outpatient basis.

If the patient responds to but does not tolerate an apomorphine hydrochloride test dose of 0.4 mL (4-mg), a third test dose of 0.3 mL (3 mg) may be administered during a separate "off" period, but no sooner than 2 hours after the 0.4-mL (4-mg) test dose. Both supine and standing blood pressures should be measured prior to and at 20, 40, and 60 minutes after administration of the test dose. If the 0.3-mL (3-mg) dose is well tolerated and effective, a 0.2-mL (2-mg) dose may be used on an as-needed, outpatient basis to reverse "off" episodes. If the 0.2-mL (2-mg) dose is tolerated, the dose can be increased, if necessary, to 0.3 mL (3 mg) after a few days. In such a patient, the dose ordinarily should not be increased to 0.4 mL (4 mg) on an outpatient basis.

In clinical trials of apomorphine hydrochloride in patients with moderate to severe Parkinson's disease, most patients responded to doses of 0.3–0.6 mL (3–6 mg); average frequency of dosing was 3 times daily. Doses exceeding 0.6 mL (6 mg) have not been shown to result in additional therapeutic effect and are not recommended by the manufacturer. In addition, there is limited experience with administration of more than 5 doses per day or total daily doses exceeding 2 mL (20 mg).

Safety and efficacy of a second dose of apomorphine hydrochloride during the same hypomobility episode in patients who did not respond to the initial dose have not been established. Therefore, no more than one dose of apomorphine hydrochloride should be administered for the treatment of a single "off" episode.

If apomorphine therapy has been interrupted for more than one week and reinitiation of the drug is not contraindicated, therapy should be reinitiated at a dose of 0.2 mL (2 mg) and gradually titrated to effect.

■ **Special Populations** The manufacturer recommends an initial test dose and subsequent starting dose of 0.1 mL (1 mg) in patients with mild or moderate renal impairment.

No special recommendations for patients with hepatic impairment at this time. (See Cautions: Hepatic Impairment.)

Cautions

■ **Contraindications** Concomitant use with selective 5-HT_3 receptor antagonists (e.g., alosetron, dolasetron, granisetron, ondansetron, palonosetron). (See Drug Interactions.)

Known hypersensitivity to apomorphine hydrochloride or any ingredient in the formulation (e.g., sodium metabisulfite).

■ **Warnings/Precautions** ***Warnings*** **Administration.** Serious adverse events (thrombus formation, pulmonary embolism) have occurred following IV administration of apomorphine. Intravascular thrombosis, believed to be secondary to the formation of apomorphine crystals and requiring cardiothoracic surgical intervention, has been reported in at least 3 patients receiving IV apomorphine.

Nausea and Vomiting. Severe nausea and vomiting can be expected with recommended doses of apomorphine and concomitant use of an antiemetic is recommended. (See Dosage and Administration: Administration.) Almost all patients who participated in clinical trials in the US received trimethobenzamide; antiemetics other than trimethobenzamide were not evaluated in these trials. Concomitant use with antiemetics that selectively inhibit 5-HT_3 receptors is contraindicated and concomitant use with antiemetics that inhibit dopamine receptors should be avoided. (See Drug Interactions.)

Symptomatic Hypotension. Orthostatic hypotension, hypotension, and/or syncope were reported in approximately 11% of patients receiving apomorphine in clinical studies; these adverse effects were observed during initiation of apomorphine therapy as well as during long-term treatment. Whether hypotension contributes to other adverse events (e.g., falls) is unknown. (See Warnings/Precautions: Nervous System and Muscular Effects.)

Prolongation of QT Interval. Possible prolonged QT interval; however, apomorphine hydrochloride doses of 6 mg or less are associated with minimal increases in QT_c interval.

Use with caution in patients with congenital or known prolongation of the QT interval, those with clinically important bradycardia or uncorrected hypokalemia or hypomagnesemia, and those receiving concomitant therapy with drugs that prolong the QT_c interval.

Nervous System and Muscular Effects. Patients with Parkinson's disease are at risk of falling as a result of underlying postural instability and autonomic instability. In addition, patients may be at increased risk of falling as a result of the simultaneous effects of apomorphine on blood pressure and mobility. In clinical trials, 30% of patients had events that could be considered falls and about 5% of patients had falls that were considered serious.

A symptom complex resembling the neuroleptic malignant syndrome (NMS; elevated temperature, muscular rigidity, altered consciousness, autonomic instability) has been reported in association with abrupt withdrawal, dosage lowering, or changes in antiparkinsonian therapy.

Hallucinations. Hallucinations were reported in about 14% of patients receiving apomorphine in clinical studies and resulted in discontinuance of the drug in 1% of patients.

Sudden Sleep Episodes. Patients receiving apomorphine have reported falling asleep while engaged in activities of daily living. Although somnolence is commonly associated with apomorphine, these patients perceived no warning signs and believed they were alert immediately prior to the event.

Many experts believe that falling asleep while engaged in activities of daily living always occurs in a setting of preexisting somnolence although patients may not give such a history. Therefore, it is recommended that clinicians continually reassess patients for drowsiness or sleepiness especially because some incidents of sudden sleep onset occurred well after the start of apomorphine therapy. Clinicians also should be aware that patients may not acknowledge drowsiness or sleepiness until directly questioned about such adverse effects during specific activities. Prior to initiation of therapy, patients should be advised of the possibility that they may develop drowsiness and asked about any factors that may increase the risk of somnolence during apomorphine therapy (e.g., concomitant sedating drugs, the presence of sleep disorders). If a patient develops clinically important daytime sleepiness or episodes of falling asleep during activities that require active participation (e.g., conversations, eating), apomorphine generally should be discontinued. If a decision is made to continue the drug, patients should be advised not to drive and to avoid other potentially dangerous activities. The manufacturer states that there is insufficient information to establish whether dosage reduction will eliminate episodes of falling asleep while engaged in activities of daily living.

Cardiovascular Effects. Angina, myocardial infarction, cardiac arrest, and/or sudden death have been reported in 4% of patients receiving apomorphine. Angina and myocardial infarction occurred in some patients in close proximity to apomorphine dosing (within 2 hours); cardiac arrest and sudden death occurred at times unrelated to dosing in some patients.

Apomorphine may exacerbate coronary and cerebral ischemia as a result of its effect on blood pressure. The drug should be used with extreme caution in patients with known cardiovascular and cerebrovascular disease.If patients develop signs and symptoms of coronary or cerebral ischemia, the continued use of apomorphine should be carefully evaluated.

Injection Site Reactions. Injection site reactions, including bruising, granuloma, and pruritus, were reported in 26% of patients in clinical studies.

Abuse and Misuse Potential. Hypersexuality and increased erections can occur and have been associated with abuse of apomorphine. Escalation of apomorphine dose beyond the prescribed frequency has been reported in patients who attempt to avoid all symptoms of an "off" episode. Patients should be closely followed for excessive use (e.g., use out of proportion to motor signs).

Sensitivity Reactions The commercially available formulation of apomorphine hydrochloride injection contains sodium metabisulfite, which can cause serious allergic-type reactions in certain susceptible individuals. The overall prevalence of sulfite sensitivity in the general population is probably low, but in susceptible individuals, exposure to sulfites can result in acute bronchospasm or, less frequently, life-threatening anaphylaxis. Sulfite sensitivity appears to occur more frequently in asthmatic than in nonasthmatic individuals.

General Precautions **Dyskinesia.** Apomorphine may cause or exacerbate dyskinesias. Dyskinesia or worsening of dyskinesia was reported in 24% of patients and resulted in discontinuance of the drug in 2% of patients in clinical studies.

Cardiorespiratory Fibrosis and Fibrotic Complications. Retroperitoneal fibrosis, pulmonary infiltrates, pleural effusion, pleural thickening, and cardiac valvulopathy reported in a few patients treated with ergot-derivative dopamine receptor agonists. Although these adverse effects presumably are related to the ergoline structure of these compounds, the possibility exists that nonergot-derived drugs that increase dopaminergic activity such as apomorphine may induce similar changes.

Priapism. May cause prolonged painful erections. Severe priapism may require surgical intervention.

Ocular Effects. Retinal degeneration has been observed in albino rats given dopamine agonists for prolonged periods (generally during 2-year carcinogenicity studies) and in rats exposed to high-intensity light given these agents for shorter periods; however, retinal degeneration was not observed in a 2-year carcinogenicity study in albino mice or in rats or monkeys given these agents for 1 year. Apomorphine has not been evaluated in carcinogenicity studies; however, apomorphine is expected to cause similar ocular effects in animals. Although the clinical importance of these findings has not been established, the presumed mechanism of action of the effect may be applicable to all vertebrates (e.g., disk shedding).

Specific Populations **Pregnancy.** Category C. (See Users Guide.)

Lactation. Not known whether apomorphine is distributed into milk. Potential risk in nursing infants. Discontinue nursing or the drug, taking into account the importance of the drug to the women.

Pediatric Use. Safety and efficacy for hypermobility episodes not established in pediatric patients.

Geriatric Use. Increased incidence of confusion, hallucinations, serious adverse events (life-threatening events or events resulting in hospitalization and/or increased disability), falls, cardiovascular events, respiratory disorders, and GI events in geriatric individuals relative to younger adults.

Hepatic Impairment. Systemic exposure to apomorphine is increased in patients with mild to moderate hepatic impairment; use with caution. Apomorphine has not been evaluated systematically in patients with severe hepatic impairment.

Renal Impairment. The initial dose of apomorphine hydrochloride should be reduced in patients with mild to moderate renal impairment. (See Dosage and Administration: Special Populations.) Apomorphine has not been evaluated systematically in patients with severe renal impairment. Studies have not been conducted in patients undergoing dialysis.

■ **Common Adverse Effects** Common adverse effects include yawning, dyskinesias, nausea and/or vomiting, somnolence, dizziness, rhinorrhea, hallucinations, edema, chest pain, increased sweating, flushing, and pallor.

Drug Interactions

■ **Drugs that Prolong QT Interval** Potential pharmacologic interaction (additive effect on QT interval prolongation). (See Warnings: Prolongation of QT Interval.)

■ **Drugs Affecting or Metabolized by Hepatic Microsomal Enzymes** Pharmacokinetic interactions are unlikely.

■ **5-HT_3 Receptor Antagonists** Potential pharmacologic interaction (profound hypotension and loss of consciousness). Concomitant use contraindicated.

■ **Dopamine Antagonists** Potential pharmacologic interaction (reduced efficacy of apomorphine) when apomorphine is used with certain antipsychotic agents (e.g., phenothiazines, butyrophenones, thioxanthenes) or metoclopramide.

Patients with major psychosis receiving certain antipsychotic agents (e.g., phenothiazines, butyrophenones, thioxanthenes) should receive dopamine agonists only if benefit outweighs risk.

■ **Hypotensive Agents and Vasodilators** Potential pharmacologic interaction (additive hypotensive effects); use with caution.

Hypotension, myocardial infarction, pneumonia, serious falls, and bone and joint injuries reported more frequently in patients receiving concomitant antihypertensive drugs or vasodilators. The mechanism underlying many of these events is unknown, but may be associated with hypotension. (See Warnings: Symptomatic Hypotension.)

■ **CNS Depressants** Potential pharmacologic interaction (additive sedative and hypotensive effects) with alcohol. Potential pharmacologic interaction with CNS depressants (additive sedative effects).

■ **Levodopa/Carbidopa** Potential pharmacologic interaction (additive neurologic effect; used to therapeutic advantage in the management of "off" episodes). Pharmacokinetic interaction unlikely.

■ **Catechol-*O*-Methyltransferase (COMT) Inhibitors** Pharmacokinetic interaction unlikely. The manufacturer of entacapone advises caution if the drug is used concomitantly with apomorphine.

Description

Apomorphine hydrochloride is a nonergot-derivative dopamine receptor agonist that is structurally and pharmacologically related to dopamine. In in vitro studies, apomorphine hydrochloride demonstrated a higher affinity for the dopamine D_4 receptor than for dopamine D_2, D_3, or D_5 receptors. Apomorphine hydrochloride binds with moderate affinity to α-adrenergic (α_{1D}, α_{2B}, α_{2C}) receptors but has little or no affinity for dopamine D_1 receptors, serotonergic (5-HT_{1A}, 5-HT_{2A}, 5-HT_{2B}, 5-HT_{2C}) receptors, β_1- or β_2-adrenergic receptors, or histamine H_1 receptors.

The exact mechanism of action of apomorphine hydrochloride in the treatment of Parkinson's disease has not been fully elucidated but may involve stimulation of postsynaptic dopamine D_2 receptors within the caudate-putamen in the brain. Apomorphine has been shown to improve motor function in an animal model of Parkinson's disease. In particular, apomorphine attenuates the motor deficits associated with neurotoxin (1-methyl-4-phenyl-1,2,3,6-tetrahydropyridine ([MPTP])-induced lesions in the ascending nigrostriatal dopaminergic pathway in primates.

Routes of apomorphine metabolism in humans are not known. Potential metabolic routes include sulfation, *N*-demethylation, glucuronidation, and oxidation. Apomorphine undergoes rapid auto-oxidation in vitro. Cytochrome P-450 (CYP) enzymes play a minor role in the metabolism of apomorphine. In vitro studies have suggested that apomorphine may be metabolized by COMT. Data from in vivo studies indicate that apomorphine is not metabolized by COMT.

Advice to Patients

Importance of taking apomorphine only as prescribed.

Importance of instructing patient and/or caregiver regarding proper dosage and administration of apomorphine, including detailed instruction in the use of the dosing pen, in patients whose clinician has determined that the drug can safely and effectively be self-administered in the patient's home by the patient, family member, or other responsible caregiver.

Advise that hallucinations, hypotension, and other adverse effects (e.g., injection site reactions) may occur.

Risk of postural hypotension with or without dizziness, nausea, syncope, or sweating. Advise not to rise rapidly after prolonged sitting or lying down, especially during the first few weeks of therapy.

Risk of somnolence and the possibility of falling asleep during activities of daily living; necessity of exercising caution when driving or operating machinery.

Importance of informing clinicians if increased somnolence or new episodes of falling asleep during activities of daily living (e.g., watching television, riding in a car as a passenger) occur at any time during apomorphine therapy. Patients should not drive or participate in potentially dangerous activities until their clinician has been notified.

Importance of women informing clinicians if they are or plan to become pregnant or plan to breast-feed.

Importance of informing clinicians of existing or contemplated concomitant therapy, including prescription and OTC drugs, as well as any concomitant illnesses.

Importance of informing patients of other important precautionary information. (See Cautions.)

Overview® (see Users Guide). For additional information on this drug until a more detailed monograph is developed and published, the manufacturer's labeling should be consulted. It is *essential* that the manufacturer's labeling be consulted for more detailed information on usual cautions, precautions, contraindications, potential drug interactions, laboratory test interferences, and acute toxicity.

Preparations

Excipients in commercially available drug preparations may have clinically important effects in some individuals; consult specific product labeling for details.

Apomorphine Hydrochloride (Hemihydrate)

Parenteral		
Injection, for subcutaneous use only	10 mg/mL	Apokyn® (in cartridges), Mylan

Selected Revisions October 2007, © Copyright, August 2004, American Society of Health-System Pharmacists, Inc.

Pramipexole Dihydrochloride

■ Pramipexole dihydrochloride is a nonergot-derivative dopamine receptor agonist.

Uses

■ **Parkinsonian Syndrome** Pramipexole dihydrochloride is used for the symptomatic management of idiopathic parkinsonian syndrome.

Dopamine receptor agonists (bromocriptine mesylate, pramipexole dihydrochloride, pergolide mesylate, ropinirole hydrochloride) are used as adjuncts to levodopa for the symptomatic management of parkinsonian syndrome in patients with advanced disease. Dopamine receptor agonists also are used as monotherapy for the initial symptomatic management of parkinsonian syndrome. Levodopa currently is the most effective drug for relieving the symptoms of parkinsonian syndrome and traditionally has been considered the drug of choice for the initial symptomatic management of idiopathic parkinsonian syndrome. However, long-term administration of levodopa is associated with motor complications. One strategy to reduce the risk of motor complications and to improve long-term outcome is to initiate symptomatic therapy with a dopamine receptor agonist and to add levodopa as supplemental therapy when dopamine receptor agonist monotherapy no longer provides adequate symptom control. However, clinical studies evaluating this strategy are limited both in number and duration, and it remains to be determined whether initiating therapy with a dopamine receptor agonist rather than levodopa results in a more favorable long-term outcome. Factors to consider when choosing an agent for the initial symptomatic management of idiopathic parkinsonian syndrome include patient age, cognitive status, disease severity, and cost. Most clinicians would use levodopa for initial therapy in individuals older than 70 years of age (since these individuals are less likely than younger individuals to develop levodopa-related motor complications and because of concerns about cognitive dysfunction), in patients with cognitive impairment, and in those with severe disease. A dopamine receptor agonist may be preferred for initial therapy in patients 70 years of age or younger.

Efficacy of pramipexole for the management of idiopathic parkinsonian syndrome has been established in several placebo-controlled studies of up to 6 months' duration in patients with early parkinsonian syndrome receiving no concomitant levodopa therapy, and in patients with advanced parkinsonian syndrome who were receiving levodopa therapy concomitantly. In these studies, improvement in manifestations of parkinsonian syndrome was assessed principally using the Unified Parkinson's Disease Rating Scale (UPDRS), a 4-part rating scale intended to evaluate mentation, activities of daily living, motor performance, and complications of therapy.

Pramipexole appears to improve activities of daily living as well as motor manifestations of parkinsonian syndrome, such as tremor, rigidity, bradykinesia, and postural stability. In a limited number of clinical studies in patients with early parkinsonian syndrome, pramipexole was more effective than placebo in reducing the severity of symptoms associated with this disorder. In a study in patients with early (less than 7 years' duration) parkinsonian syndrome, 10 weeks of therapy with pramipexole resulted in an average 20% improvement in total UPDRS scores compared with placebo (score of 5.9–7 versus 0.9 units, respectively). In this study, concomitant therapy with amantadine, selegiline, or anticholinergic drugs, but not levodopa or other dopamine receptor agonists, was allowed.

In placebo-controlled clinical studies in patients with advanced parkinsonian syndrome who were receiving concomitant levodopa therapy, pramipexole reduced the severity of symptoms associated with this disorder and allowed a reduction in levodopa dosage. In patients with advanced parkinsonian syndrome who were experiencing "on-off" phenomena (i.e., a deteriorating response to levodopa therapy), pramipexole was more effective than placebo in reducing "off" time (as measured by the activities of daily living portion of the UPDRS). In one study, the duration of "off" time with pramipexole or placebo was reduced by an average of 31 or 7%, respectively, while the severity of "off" time was reduced by 17 or 5%, respectively. Further study is required to establish safety and efficacy of pramipexole during long-term administration and to determine the long-term effect of the drug on disability in parkinsonian syndrome.

In 2 controlled studies of up to 33 weeks' duration in patients with early or advanced parkinsonian syndrome, pramipexole dihydrochloride extended-release tablets (given once daily) were more effective than placebo and as effective as conventional tablets of the drug (given 3 times daily) in improving activities of daily living and motor manifestations of the disease (as assessed by the UPDRS); tolerability of the 2 pramipexole formulations was similar. In another study in patients with early parkinsonian syndrome, about 81% of patients who were switched overnight from conventional tablets of pramipexole given 3 times daily to extended-release tablets of the drug given once daily at the same total daily dosage required no dosage adjustment following the change in therapy; about 84% of patients were successfully switched to the extended-release formulation with or without a change in dosage.

Sudden, irresistible attacks of sleep that resemble narcolepsy have been reported in patients treated with pramipexole. Patients receiving a dopamine receptor agonist (e.g., pramipexole, ropinirole) have reported falling asleep while engaged in activities of daily living, including business meetings, telephone calls, and operating a motor vehicle, which occasionally resulted in accidents. Although many of these patients reported somnolence while receiving pramipexole or ropinirole, some perceived no warning signs (e.g., excessive drowsiness) and believed that they were alert immediately prior to the event. Some of these events have been reported as late as 1 year after initiation of therapy with the drug. Spontaneous postmarketing reports indicate that patients with a previous history of sleep disorders (e.g., somnolence) or who were taking multiple drugs known to cause sedation may be at an increased risk of experiencing sudden sleep onset. Although such sleep attacks may occur more frequently at higher dosages of pramipexole, they may occur at any dosage. Although the incidence of somnolence with pramipexole dihydrochloride at a dosage of 1.5 mg daily was comparable to that reported with placebo, somnolence is a common adverse effect in patients receiving the drug at dosages exceeding 1.5 mg daily.

Many experts believe that falling asleep while engaged in activities of daily living always occurs in a setting of preexisting somnolence, although patients may not give such a history. Therefore, it is recommended that clinicians continually reassess patients for drowsiness or sleepiness especially since some incidents of sudden sleep onset occurred well after the start of pramipexole therapy. Clinicians also should be aware that patients may not acknowledge drowsiness or sleepiness until directly questioned about such adverse effects during specific activities. In addition, patients should be asked about any factors that may increase the risk of somnolence during pramipexole therapy (e.g., concomitant sedating drugs, the presence of sleep disorders, concomitant drugs that increase pramipexole plasma concentrations [e.g., cimetidine]). If a patient develops clinically important daytime sleepiness or episodes of falling asleep during activities that require active participation (e.g., conversations, eating), pramipexole generally should be discontinued. If a decision is made to continue the drug, patients should be advised not to drive and to avoid other potentially dangerous activities. While dose reduction clearly reduces the degree of somnolence, the manufacturer states that there is insufficient information to establish that dose reduction will eliminate episodes of falling asleep while engaged in activities of daily living.

Patients should be informed that hallucinations can occur with pramipexole therapy; geriatric patients are at increased risk for this adverse effect. Patients also should be advised that pramipexole may cause somnolence and that they should not drive a car or operate other complex machinery until they have gained sufficient experience with the drug to determine whether it has adverse effects on their mental and/or motor performance. In addition, the possibility of additive sedative effects should be considered in patients receiving other CNS depressants concomitantly with pramipexole.

■ **Restless Legs Syndrome** Pramipexole dihydrochloride is used for the symptomatic management of moderate-to-severe primary restless legs syndrome (Ekbom syndrome). Restless legs syndrome is a sensorimotor disorder characterized by a distressing urge to move the legs accompanied by sensations deep in the limbs that have been described as twitching, pulling, and sometimes painful. These symptoms are present at rest, especially in the evening and at night, and are relieved by movement. Some clinicians consider a dopamine receptor agonist (e.g., pramipexole) the drug of choice for patients with symptoms that occur nightly.

Efficacy of pramipexole for this indication has been established in 4 randomized, double-blind, placebo-controlled studies in patients with primary moderate-to-severe restless legs syndrome (defined in most of the studies as a score exceeding 15 on the International Restless Legs Syndrome [IRLS] scale and a history of symptoms of restless legs syndrome at least 2 or 3 days per week for at least the past 3 months). Patients were excluded from these studies if they had restless legs syndrome associated with other conditions, such as renal failure, anemia, or pregnancy. Pramipexole dihydrochloride was administered in dosages ranging from 0.125–0.75 mg daily (administered 2–3 hours before bedtime), and response was assessed using the IRLS scale and the Clinical Global Impression-Improvement (CGI-I) scale. Two studies evaluated fixed dosages of the drug, one study evaluated flexible dosages, and one study evaluated time to treatment failure following discontinuance of the drug. The 4 studies together included about 1000 patients.

The 3-week, placebo-controlled, fixed-dosage study evaluated 4 dosages of pramipexole dihydrochloride (0.125, 0.25, 0.5, and 0.75 mg once daily); each treatment group in this dose-finding study included about 20 patients. The results indicated that a dosage of 0.5 mg daily generally was superior to 0.25 mg daily, but there were no significant differences in response between the 0.125-mg dosage and placebo or between the 0.5- and 0.75-mg dosages. Three of these dosage levels (0.25, 0.5, and 0.75 mg once daily) were evaluated in a larger 12-week, placebo-controlled, fixed-dosage study in 344 patients. At 12 weeks, the mean improvement in IRLS score was greater in patients receiving pramipexole than in those receiving placebo, but improvement was similar across all 3 pramipexole dosages. In addition, 74.7, 67.9, or 72.9% of patients receiving pramipexole dihydrochloride 0.25, 0.5, or 0.75 mg once daily, respectively, were described as responders (defined as being much improved or very much improved) on the CGI-I scale, compared with 51.2% of those receiving placebo. Although all 3 dosage levels were superior to placebo in this study, there was no clear evidence of a dose-response relationship across the 3 dosage groups.

In the flexible-dosage study, 345 patients were randomized in a 2:1 ratio to receive pramipexole dihydrochloride (median dosage of 0.35 mg daily; range: 0.125–0.75 mg daily) or placebo for 6 weeks. At 6 weeks, the mean improvement in IRLS score was greater in patients receiving pramipexole than in those receiving placebo; in addition, 62.9% of patients receiving pramipexole compared with 32.5% of those receiving placebo were described as responders (defined as being much improved or very much improved) on the CGI-I scale.

In the randomized drug withdrawal study, 147 patients who had achieved a sustained response after 6 months of open-label pramipexole therapy were randomized to receive continued pramipexole therapy or placebo. Following 12 weeks of follow-up, approximately 85% of patients switched to placebo experienced treatment failure, compared with approximately 21% of those who continued receiving pramipexole. Most of the treatment failures occurred within 10 days of randomization.

Augmentation of the symptoms of restless legs syndrome may occur in patients receiving therapy for this disorder; augmentation can take the form of onset of symptoms earlier in the day, increase in symptoms, or extension of symptoms to other extremities. In a 26-week clinical trial in patients with restless legs syndrome, augmentation was reported more frequently in patients receiving pramipexole dihydrochloride (up to 0.75 mg once daily) compared with those receiving placebo (12% versus 9%), and the incidence of augmentation increased with increasing duration of treatment. Patients receiving pramipexole also were more likely than placebo recipients to report a rebound in symptoms of the disorder when treatment was discontinued abruptly (10% versus 2%); the worsening of symptoms generally was considered mild. The incidence, severity, and appropriate management of augmentation and/or rebound in patients receiving long-term therapy with pramipexole have not been adequately evaluated in controlled clinical trials to date.

In clinical trials evaluating pramipexole for the symptomatic management of restless legs syndrome, somnolence was reported in 6% of patients receiving the drug at dosages of 0.25–0.75 mg daily and in 3% of placebo recipients.

Dosage and Administration

■ **Administration** Pramipexole dihydrochloride is administered orally. For the management of parkinsonian syndrome, pramipexole dihydrochloride is administered as conventional tablets in 3 equally divided doses daily or as extended-release tablets given once daily. When used for the management of restless legs syndrome, the drug is administered as conventional tablets given once daily 2–3 hours before bedtime.

Pramipexole dihydrochloride extended-release tablets should be swallowed whole and should not be chewed, crushed, or divided.

Administration of pramipexole dihydrochloride conventional tablets with food decreases the rate, but not the extent, of absorption; time to peak concentration is delayed by about 1 hour. Administration of the extended-release tablets with food increases peak plasma concentrations by approximately 20% and delays time to peak concentration by approximately 2 hours, but does not affect the extent of exposure. Therefore, pramipexole dihydrochloride conventional or extended-release tablets may be administered without regard to meals. Patients in whom pramipexole causes nausea should be advised that taking the drug with food may reduce the occurrence of this adverse effect.

■ **Dosage** The manufacturer states that safety and efficacy of pramipexole in children have not been established.

Dosage of pramipexole dihydrochloride is calculated in terms of the monohydrated form of this salt.

Pramipexole therapy is initiated at a low dosage and then titrated slowly based on response and tolerability. Increases in blood pressure and heart rate have been observed in healthy individuals when dosage was titrated up to 4.5 mg daily more quickly (i.e., every 3 days) than is recommended.

Use of dopamine agonists in patients with parkinsonian syndrome or restless legs syndrome ordinarily requires careful monitoring for manifestations of orthostatic hypotension, especially during dosage escalation, since these drugs appear to impair systemic regulation of blood pressure. In addition, patients with parkinsonian syndrome generally have a reduced capacity to respond to an orthostatic challenge. In clinical trials in patients with parkinsonian syndrome, symptomatic orthostatic hypotension occurred in 3% of patients receiving extended-release pramipexole and 1% of those receiving placebo. However, unexpectedly, the reported incidence of clinically important orthostatic hypotension with pramipexole as conventional tablets did not differ from that with placebo in clinical trials in patients with parkinsonian syndrome, although the incidence of postural hypotension increased in a dose-dependent manner over the dosage range of 1.5–6 mg daily. The manufacturer states that patients with either parkinsonian syndrome or restless legs syndrome should be cautioned about rising rapidly after sitting or lying down, especially if they have been in a seated or recumbent position for prolonged periods and/or if they are just beginning pramipexole therapy.

Patients treated with pramipexole have reported falling asleep while engaged in activities of daily living, including operating a motor vehicle, which sometimes resulted in accidents. (See Uses: Parkinsonian Syndrome for associated precautions.)

Intense urges and compulsive behaviors (e.g., urge to gamble, increased sexual urges, binge eating, uncontrolled spending, other intense urges) and inability to control these urges have been reported in some patients receiving agents that increase central dopaminergic tone (including pramipexole). Although a causal relationship has not been established, these urges stopped in some cases when dosage was reduced or the drug was discontinued. Clinicians should ask patients whether they have developed new or increased gambling urges, sexual urges, uncontrolled spending, or other urges while receiving pramipexole and should advise them of the importance of reporting such urges. If a patient develops such urges while receiving pramipexole, consideration should be given to reducing the dosage or discontinuing the drug.

Parkinsonian Syndrome For the management of idiopathic parkinsonian syndrome, therapy with pramipexole dihydrochloride (as conventional tablets) is initiated at a low dosage and increased slowly (at intervals of not less than 5–7 days) until the maximum therapeutic response is achieved. The usual initial dosage of pramipexole dihydrochloride is 0.125 mg 3 times daily (total of 0.375 mg daily) the first week, then 0.25 mg 3 times daily (total of 0.75 mg daily) the second week, 0.5 mg 3 times daily (total of 1.5 mg daily) the third week, 0.75 mg 3 times daily (total of 2.25 mg daily) the fourth week, 1 mg 3 times daily (total of 3 mg daily) the fifth week, 1.25 mg 3 times daily (total of 3.75 mg daily) the sixth week, and 1.5 mg 3 times daily (total of 4.5 mg daily) the seventh week.

When pramipexole dihydrochloride extended-release tablets are used for the management of idiopathic parkinsonian syndrome, therapy is initiated at a dosage of 0.375 mg once daily and increased slowly (at intervals of not less than 5–7 days). Based on response and tolerability (assessed after the patient has received each dosage for 5 or more days), dosage may be increased to 0.75 mg once daily and then in increments of 0.75 mg, up to a maximum recommended dosage of 4.5 mg once daily. Dosages exceeding 4.5 mg daily have not been evaluated in clinical trials. If therapy is interrupted for a substantial period of time, retitration of dosage may be warranted.

Because equivalent daily dosages of pramipexole dihydrochloride conventional tablets (administered 3 times daily) and extended-release tablets (administered once daily) result in comparable peak and trough plasma concentrations and systemic exposure over 24 hours, patients may be switched overnight from the conventional tablets to the extended-release tablets at the same total daily dosage. However, because some patients may require dosage adjustment, patients being switched between the 2 formulations should be monitored to determine if dosage adjustment is necessary.

The dosage of pramipexole dihydrochloride must be continually reevaluated and changed according to the needs of the patient in a constant effort to find a dosage schedule that provides maximum relief of symptoms with minimum adverse effects. In a fixed-dose study in patients with early parkinsonian syndrome, pramipexole dihydrochloride dosages exceeding 1.5 mg daily (i.e., 3, 4.5, or 6 mg daily as conventional tablets) were not associated with additional therapeutic benefit. However, as the dosage increased over the range from 1.5 mg to 6 mg daily, the incidence of postural hypotension, nausea, constipation, somnolence, and amnesia also increased. For pramipexole dosages exceeding 3 mg daily, the frequency of these events generally was twofold greater than with placebo. Specific relationships between dose and either therapeutic response or frequency of adverse effects have not been established for the extended-release formulation.

In clinical studies, pramipexole dihydrochloride 1.5–4.5 mg daily in 3 equally divided doses has been effective and well tolerated when administered with or without concomitant levodopa therapy (approximately 800 mg daily). Since concomitant therapy with pramipexole and levodopa may result in additive therapeutic and/or adverse (e.g., dyskinesia) effects, a reduction in levodopa dosage should be considered when pramipexole is added to levodopa therapy. In a controlled study in patients with advanced parkinsonian syndrome, the dosage of levodopa was reduced by an average of 27% from baseline with concomitant pramipexole therapy.

Although not reported in clinical trials with pramipexole, a symptom complex resembling neuroleptic malignant syndrome (e.g., elevated temperature, muscular rigidity, altered consciousness, autonomic instability) has been reported in association with rapid dosage reduction, withdrawal of, or changes in antiparkinsonian therapy. The manufacturer recommends that discontinuance of pramipexole therapy in patients with parkinsonian syndrome take place over a period of 1 week. However, in some studies, abrupt discontinuance of the drug (as conventional tablets) has been uneventful.

Restless Legs Syndrome The usual initial dosage of pramipexole dihydrochloride (as conventional tablets) for the management of restless legs syndrome in adults is 0.125 mg given once daily 2–3 hours before bedtime. If symptomatic relief with the initial dosage is inadequate, dosage may be increased at intervals of 4–7 days to 0.25 mg daily and then to 0.5 mg daily. Although some patients received a dosage of 0.75 mg daily during long-term open-label treatment with the drug, there is no evidence in patients with restless legs syndrome that a dosage of 0.75 mg daily provides additional benefit compared with a dosage of 0.5 mg daily.

Pramipexole dihydrochloride (administered at dosages of up to 0.75 mg once daily) was discontinued without a taper in clinical trials in patients with restless legs syndrome. However, in a 26-week clinical trial, patients receiving the drug at dosages of up to 0.75 mg daily were more likely than placebo recipients to report a rebound in symptoms of restless legs syndrome when treatment was discontinued abruptly. (See Uses: Restless Legs Syndrome.)

■ **Dosage in Renal and Hepatic Impairment** When pramipexole dihydrochloride is used for the management of idiopathic parkinsonian syndrome in patients with impaired renal function, dosage and/or frequency of administration must be modified in response to the degree of impairment.

When conventional tablets of pramipexole dihydrochloride are used for the management of idiopathic parkinsonian syndrome in patients with creatinine clearances of 60 mL/minute or greater, the usual dosage of pramipexole dihydrochloride (0.125 mg 3 times daily in an ascending dosage schedule up to a maximum dosage of 1.5 mg 3 times daily) is recommended. (See Parkinsonian Syndrome under Dosage and Administration: Dosage.) Patients with creatinine clearances of 35–59 mL/minute should receive an initial pramipexole dihydrochloride dosage (as conventional tablets) of 0.125 mg *twice* daily (up to a maximum dosage of 1.5 mg *twice* daily), and those with creatinine clearances of 15–34 mL/minute should receive 0.125 mg *once* daily (up to a maximum dosage of 1.5 mg *once* daily). Safety and efficacy of pramipexole dihydrochloride (as conventional tablets) have not been evaluated systematically in patients with creatinine clearances of less than 15 mL/minute or in those undergoing hemodialysis, and the manufacturer currently makes no specific recommendation for dosage adjustment in such patients.

When extended-release tablets of pramipexole dihydrochloride are used for the management of idiopathic parkinsonian syndrome in patients with creatinine clearances exceeding 50 mL/minute, the usual dosage of pramipexole dihydrochloride is recommended. (See Parkinsonian Syndrome under Dosage and Administration: Dosage.) In patients with creatinine clearances of 30–50 mL/minute, treatment with the extended-release tablets should be initiated with an *every-other-day* dosing schedule; response and tolerability should be carefully assessed before increasing to daily dosing after one week and before any further dosage titration. Dosage may be titrated no more frequently than once weekly in increments of 0.375 mg, up to a maximum dosage of 2.25 mg once daily. Extended-release tablets of the drug have not been studied in patients with creatinine clearances of less than 30 mL/minute or in those undergoing hemodialysis, and are not recommended for use in these patients.

When conventional tablets of pramipexole dihydrochloride are used for the management of restless legs syndrome in patients with creatinine clearances of 20–60 mL/minute, the interval between dosage adjustments should be increased to 14 days.

The effect of hepatic impairment on the pharmacokinetics of pramipexole has not been evaluated to date, and the manufacturer currently makes no specific recommendation for dosage adjustment in patients with hepatic impairment. Because pramipexole is eliminated mainly (90%) as unchanged drug in the urine, hepatic impairment would not be expected to substantially affect pramipexole elimination.

Description

Pramipexole dihydrochloride, a synthetic benzothiazolamine derivative, is a nonergot-derivative dopamine receptor agonist. In in vitro binding studies, pramipexole demonstrated high binding specificity for and intrinsic activity at dopamine D_2 receptors compared with other dopamine receptor agonists (e.g., bromocriptine, pergolide), having a higher affinity for the D_3 receptor subtype than for the D_2 or D_4 subtypes. Pramipexole binds with moderate affinity to α_2-adrenergic receptors but has little or no affinity for α_1- or β-adrenergic, acetylcholine, dopamine D_1, or serotonin (5-hydroxytryptamine [5-HT]) receptors.

The exact mechanism(s) of action of pramipexole in the management of parkinsonian syndrome has not been fully elucidated. There is considerable evidence that manifestations of parkinsonian syndrome, regardless of the cause of the syndrome, are related to depletion of dopamine in the corpus striatum. While levodopa is believed to act principally by increasing dopamine concentration in the brain, pramipexole appears to act by directly stimulating postsynaptic dopamine receptors in the corpus striatum.

The exact mechanism(s) of action of pramipexole in the management of restless legs syndrome remains to be determined. While the etiology of restless legs syndrome is unclear, dopaminergic systems appear to be involved.

SumMon® (see Users Guide). For additional information on this drug until a more detailed monograph is developed and published, the manufacturer's labeling should be consulted. It is *essential* that the labeling be consulted for detailed information on the usual cautions, precautions, and contraindications.

Preparations

Excipients in commercially available drug preparations may have clinically important effects in some individuals; consult specific product labeling for details.

Pramipexole Dihydrochloride

Oral		
Tablets	0.125 mg	**Mirapex®**, Boehringer Ingelheim
	0.25 mg	**Mirapex®** (scored), Boehringer Ingelheim
	0.5 mg	**Mirapex®** (scored), Boehringer Ingelheim

	0.75 mg	**Mirapex®**, Boehringer Ingelheim
	1 mg	**Mirapex®** (scored), Boehringer Ingelheim
	1.5 mg	**Mirapex®** (scored), Boehringer Ingelheim
Tablets, extended-release	0.375 mg	**Mirapex ER®**, Boehringer Ingelheim
	0.75 mg	**Mirapex ER®**, Boehringer Ingelheim
	1.5 mg	**Mirapex ER®**, Boehringer Ingelheim
	2.25 mg	**Mirapex ER®**, Boehringer Ingelheim
	3 mg	**Mirapex ER®**, Boehringer Ingelheim
	3.75 mg	**Mirapex ER®**, Boehringer Ingelheim
	4.5 mg	**Mirapex ER®**, Boehringer Ingelheim

rOPINIRole Hydrochloride

■ Ropinirole hydrochloride is a nonergot-derivative dopamine receptor agonist.

Uses

■ **Parkinsonian Syndrome** Ropinirole hydrochloride is used for the symptomatic management of idiopathic parkinsonian syndrome.

Dopamine receptor agonists (bromocriptine mesylate, pramipexole dihydrochloride, pergolide mesylate, ropinirole hydrochloride) are used as adjuncts to levodopa for the symptomatic management of parkinsonian syndrome in patients with advanced disease. Dopamine receptor agonists also are used as monotherapy for the initial symptomatic management of parkinsonian syndrome. Levodopa currently is the most effective drug for relieving the symptoms of parkinsonian syndrome and traditionally has been considered the drug of choice for the initial symptomatic management of idiopathic parkinsonian syndrome. However, long-term administration of levodopa is associated with motor complications. One strategy to reduce the risk of motor complications and to improve long-term outcome is to initiate symptomatic therapy with a dopamine receptor agonist and to add levodopa as supplemental therapy when dopamine receptor agonist monotherapy no longer provides adequate symptom control. However, clinical studies evaluating this strategy are limited both in number and duration, and it remains to be determined whether initiating therapy with a dopamine receptor agonist rather than levodopa results in a more favorable long-term outcome. Factors to consider when choosing an agent for the initial symptomatic management of idiopathic parkinsonian syndrome include patient age, cognitive status, disease severity, and cost. Most clinicians would use levodopa for initial therapy in individuals older than 70 years of age (since these individuals are less likely than younger individuals to develop levodopa-related motor complications and because of concerns about cognitive dysfunction), in patients with cognitive impairment, and in those with severe disease. A dopamine receptor agonist may be preferred for initial therapy in patients 70 years of age or younger.

Efficacy of ropinirole for the management of parkinsonian syndrome has been established in several placebo-controlled studies of up to 6 months' duration in patients with early (approximately 2 years' duration) parkinsonian syndrome receiving no concomitant levodopa therapy, and in patients with advanced parkinsonian syndrome who were receiving levodopa therapy concomitantly. In these studies, improvement in manifestations of parkinsonian syndrome was assessed principally using the Unified Parkinson's Disease Rating Scale (UPDRS), a 4-part rating scale intended to evaluate mentation, activities of daily living, motor performance, and complications of therapy.

Ropinirole appears to improve activities of daily living as well as motor manifestations of parkinsonian syndrome, such as tremor, rigidity, bradykinesia, and postural stability. In clinical studies in patients with early parkinsonian syndrome, ropinirole was more effective than placebo in reducing the severity of symptoms associated with this disorder. In a study in patients with early parkinsonian syndrome, clinical response (defined as improvement of at least 30% in UPDRS motor score) occurred in 71% of patients receiving ropinirole (mean daily dosage: 7.4 mg) compared with 41% of patients receiving placebo for 12 weeks. In addition, improvement from baseline in the UPDRS motor score averaged 43% in ropinirole-treated patients versus 21% with placebo. In this study, concomitant therapy with amantadine, selegiline, or anticholinergic drugs, but not levodopa or other dopamine receptor agonists, was allowed. In another placebo-controlled study in patients with early parkinsonian syndrome, 47% of patients receiving ropinirole (mean daily dosage: 15.7 mg on an intent-to-treat basis) responded to therapy (defined as improvement of at least 30% in UPDRS motor score) compared with 20% of those receiving placebo; average UPDRS motor score improved by 22–24% with ropinirole therapy and worsened by 3–4% in the placebo group. In this study, addition of levodopa therapy for symptomatic relief was required in 29% of patients treated with placebo versus 11% of those receiving ropinirole.

In placebo-controlled clinical studies in patients with advanced parkinsonian syndrome who were receiving concomitant levodopa therapy, ropinirole reduced the severity of symptoms associated with this disorder and allowed a reduction in levodopa dosage. In patients with advanced parkinsonian syndrome who were experiencing "on-off" phenomena (i.e., a deteriorating response to levodopa therapy), ropinirole was more effective than placebo in reducing "off" time. In a study in patients with advanced (mean disease duration: 9 years) parkinsonian syndrome, average daily "off" time was reduced from a baseline value of 6.4 hours to 4.9 hours following 6 months of therapy with ropinirole, while "off" time with placebo averaged 7.3 hours at baseline and 6.4 hours after 6 months. In another study in patients with advanced parkinsonian syndrome not optimally controlled with levodopa therapy, "off" time was reduced by at least 30% in 65 versus 39% of patients (on an intent-to-treat basis) treated with ropinirole versus placebo, respectively, for 12 weeks.

A preliminary report of a long-term (approximately 3 years' duration), comparative study in patients with early parkinsonian syndrome receiving ropinirole or bromocriptine (with supplemental levodopa therapy in some patients) indicated clinically important improvements in UPDRS motor score and activities of daily living (ADL) score with either therapy, although functional status (as measured by the ADL score) was more improved in ropinirole-treated patients at the end of the study. Further study is required to establish safety and efficacy of ropinirole during long-term administration and to determine the long-term effect of the drug on disability in parkinsonian syndrome.

Patients receiving a dopamine receptor agonist (e.g., pramipexole, ropinirole) have reported falling asleep while engaged in activities of daily living, including business meetings, telephone calls, and operating a motor vehicle, which occasionally resulted in accidents. Although many of these patients reported somnolence while receiving pramipexole or ropinirole, some perceived no warning signs (e.g., excessive drowsiness) and believed that they were alert immediately prior to the event. Some of these events have been reported as late as 1 year after initiation of therapy with the drug.

Many experts believe that falling asleep while engaged in activities of daily living always occurs in a setting of preexisting somnolence, although patients may not give such a history. Therefore, it is recommended that clinicians continually reassess patients for drowsiness or sleepiness especially since some incidents of sudden sleep onset occurred well after the start of dopamine receptor agonist therapy. Clinicians also should be aware that patients may not acknowledge drowsiness or sleepiness until directly questioned about such adverse effects during specific activities. In addition, patients should be asked about any factors that may increase the risk of somnolence during ropinirole therapy (e.g., concomitant sedating drugs, the presence of sleep disorders [other than restless legs syndrome], concomitant drugs that increase ropinirole plasma concentrations [e.g., ciprofloxacin]). If a patient develops clinically important daytime sleepiness or episodes of falling asleep during activities that require active participation (e.g., conversations, eating), ropinirole generally should be discontinued. If a decision is made to continue the drug, patients should be advised not to drive and to avoid other potentially dangerous activities. The manufacturers state that there is insufficient information to establish that dose reduction will eliminate episodes of falling asleep while engaged in activities of daily living.

Patients should be informed that hallucinations can occur with ropinirole therapy; geriatric patients are at increased risk for this adverse effect. Patients also should be advised that ropinirole may cause somnolence and that they should not drive a car or operate other complex machinery until they have gained sufficient experience with the drug to determine whether it has adverse effects on their mental and/or motor performance. In addition, the possibility of additive sedative effects should be considered in patients receiving other CNS depressants concomitantly with ropinirole.

■ **Restless Legs Syndrome** Ropinirole is used for the symptomatic management of moderate-to-severe primary restless legs syndrome (Ekbom syndrome). Restless legs syndrome is a sensorimotor disorder characterized by a distressing urge to move the legs accompanied by sensations deep in the limbs that have been described as twitching, pulling, and sometimes painful. These symptoms are present at rest, especially in the evening and at night, and are relieved by movement. Some clinicians consider a dopamine receptor agonist (e.g., ropinirole) the drug of choice for patients with symptoms that occur nightly.

Efficacy of ropinirole for this indication has been established in 3 randomized, placebo-controlled studies in patients with moderate-to-severe restless legs syndrome (score of at least 15 on the International Restless Legs Syndrome [IRLS] scale and a history of symptoms of restless legs syndrome on at least 15 nights per month). Patients were excluded from these studies if they had restless legs syndrome associated with end-stage renal failure, anemia, or pregnancy. Ropinirole was initiated at a dosage of 0.25 mg once daily (given 1–3 hours before bedtime) and increased over 7 weeks to a maximum dosage of 4 mg once daily; the average dosage after 7 weeks of therapy was 2 mg once daily. The primary end point of these studies was the mean change in IRLS score from baseline to week 12. The Clinical Global Impression-Global Improvement (CGI-I) scale was used to assess general improvement. At week 12, the mean improvement in IRLS score in patients receiving ropinirole was greater than that in patients receiving placebo. In addition, 73.3, 53.4, and

59.5% of patients receiving ropinirole in the 3 studies were described as responders (defined as being much improved or very much improved) on the CGI-I scale compared with 56.5, 40.9, and 39.6%, respectively, of patients receiving placebo. Ropinirole therapy was associated with greater improvement in sleep and quality-of-life scores than placebo. Improvement was observed in ropinirole-treated patients as early as week 1. Efficacy has been maintained over 36 weeks in patients who continued to receive ropinirole.

Use of dopamine receptor agonists in patients with restless legs syndrome can result in end-of-dose rebound (i.e., worsening of symptoms in the early morning hours). Long-term use of dopamine receptor agonists in patients with restless legs syndrome has been associated with augmentation of the symptoms of restless legs syndrome; augmentation can take the form of onset of symptoms earlier in the day, increase in symptoms, or extension of symptoms from the legs to the arms or trunk. Because patients with rebound restless legs syndrome or augmentation were excluded from clinical studies that evaluated efficacy of ropinirole and the duration of these studies was not long enough to evaluate the incidence of these events, the incidence and appropriate management of rebound and/or augmentation in patients receiving long-term therapy with ropinirole have not been evaluated in controlled clinical studies.

The reported incidence of somnolence is lower in patients receiving ropinirole for restless legs syndrome (12%) than in those receiving the drug for parkinsonian syndrome (up to 40%). (See Uses: Parkinsonian Syndrome.)

Dosage and Administration

■ **Administration** Ropinirole hydrochloride is administered orally. For the management of parkinsonian syndrome, ropinirole is administered in 3 equally divided doses daily. For the management of restless legs syndrome, ropinirole is administered once daily, 1–3 hours before bedtime. Ropinirole may be administered without regard to meals. Patients in whom ropinirole causes nausea should be advised that taking the drug with food may reduce the occurrence of this adverse effect. If the patient skips a dose of ropinirole, a double dose should not be taken to make up for the missed dose.

Dispensing and Administration Precautions The US Food and Drug Administration (FDA) alerted healthcare professionals and patients of medication error reports in which patients were given risperidone (Risperdal®), an antipsychotic agent, instead of ropinirole hydrochloride (Requip®) and vice versa. As of June 2011, the FDA had evaluated 226 wrong drug medication errors associated with confusion between these 2 drugs; all of the reports involved tablet formulations of the drugs. Several of these cases resulted in adverse effects (including confusion, lethargy, ataxia, hallucinations, tiredness, dizziness, tingling, numbness, and altered mental status) and some of the patients who took the wrong drug required hospitalization. The FDA has determined that the factors contributing to the confusion between these 2 products include similarities in both the trade (brand) and generic (nonproprietary) names, similarities in the container labels and carton packaging, illegible handwriting on the prescriptions, and overlapping product characteristics (such as drug strengths, dosage forms, and dosing intervals). It is also possible that the 2 products may be stocked close to one another on pharmacy shelves whether they are alphabetized by brand or generic name. In addition, some generic manufacturers make both products. Healthcare professionals are therefore reminded to clearly print out or spell out the drug name on prescriptions and to make sure their patients know the name of their prescribed drug and the reason they are taking it.

■ **Dosage** The manufacturers state that the safety and efficacy of ropinirole hydrochloride in pediatric patients have not been established.

Dosage of ropinirole hydrochloride is expressed in terms of ropinirole.

Because the dosage of ropinirole is titrated to clinical response, routine dosage adjustment based solely on age is not necessary in geriatric adults.

If ropinirole therapy is interrupted for a substantial period of time, retitration of therapy, beginning at the usual recommended initial dosage, may be warranted.

Parkinsonian Syndrome For the management of parkinsonian syndrome, therapy with ropinirole is initiated at a low dosage and increased slowly until the maximum therapeutic response is achieved. The usual initial dosage of ropinirole is 0.25 mg 3 times daily (total of 0.75 mg daily) the first week, then 0.5 mg 3 times daily (total of 1.5 mg daily) the second week, 0.75 mg 3 times daily (total of 2.25 mg daily) the third week, and 1 mg 3 times daily (total of 3 mg daily) the fourth week. After the fourth week, the daily dosage may be increased by 1.5 mg daily each week up to 9 mg daily, and then by up to 3 mg daily each week to a total daily dosage of 24 mg. Dosages exceeding 24 mg daily have not been evaluated in clinical trials. As with other dopamine agonists, the dosage of ropinirole must be reevaluated and adjusted according to the needs of the patient in a constant effort to find a dosage schedule that provides maximum relief of symptoms with minimum adverse effects.

In clinical studies in patients with parkinsonian syndrome, ropinirole 0.25–8 mg daily in 3 equally divided doses has been effective and well tolerated when administered with or without concomitant levodopa therapy. Since concomitant therapy with ropinirole and levodopa may result in additive therapeutic and/or adverse (e.g., dyskinesia) effects, a reduction in levodopa dosage should be considered when ropinirole is added to levodopa therapy. In a controlled study in patients with advanced parkinsonian syndrome, the dosage of levodopa initially was reduced by an average of 31% from baseline with concomitant ropinirole therapy.

Although not reported in clinical trials with ropinirole, a symptom complex resembling neuroleptic malignant syndrome (e.g., NMS; elevated temperature, muscular rigidity, altered consciousness, autonomic instability) has been reported in association with rapid dosage reduction of, withdrawal of, or changes in antiparkinsonian therapy. The manufacturers recommend that in patients with parkinsonian syndrome, discontinuance of ropinirole therapy take place gradually over a period of 1 week. Frequency of administration of ropinirole should be reduced from 3 times daily to twice daily for 4 days, then to once daily for the next 3 days, before complete discontinuance of the drug. In clinical trials in patients with restless legs syndrome, ropinirole, given at dosages of up to 4 mg once daily, was discontinued without a taper.

Use of dopamine agonists in patients with parkinsonian syndrome ordinarily requires careful monitoring for manifestations of orthostatic hypotension, especially during dosage escalation, since these drugs appear to impair systemic regulation of blood pressure. Syncope, sometimes associated with bradycardia, has been reported in clinical trials of ropinirole in patients with early (without concomitant levodopa) or advanced (with concomitant levodopa) parkinsonian syndrome; these episodes generally occurred more than 4 weeks after initiation of therapy and in association with a recent increase in ropinirole dosage. Patients with parkinsonian syndrome generally have a reduced capacity to respond to an orthostatic challenge; therefore, the manufacturers state that patients should be cautioned about rising rapidly after sitting or lying down, especially if they have been in a seated or recumbent position for prolonged periods and/or if they are just beginning ropinirole therapy.

Restless Legs Syndrome For the management of restless legs syndrome, therapy with ropinirole is initiated at a low dosage and increased slowly until the maximum therapeutic response is achieved. The usual initial dosage of ropinirole is 0.25 mg daily for 2 days, then 0.5 mg once daily for 5 days (days 3–7), and then 1 mg daily for 1 week (week 2). After the second week, the daily dosage may be increased by 0.5 mg daily each week up to a dosage of 3 mg daily at week 6, with a final increase to 4 mg daily at week 7.

■ **Dosage in Renal and Hepatic Impairment** Adjustment in ropinirole dosage is not necessary in patients with creatinine clearances of 30–50 mL/minute. The use of ropinirole has not been evaluated in patients with severe renal impairment or in those undergoing hemodialysis, and the manufacturers currently make no specific recommendation for dosage adjustment in such patients. However, because of the large apparent volume of distribution (7.5 L/kg) of ropinirole, removal of substantial amounts of the drug by hemodialysis is unlikely.

Clearance of ropinirole may be reduced, and plasma ropinirole concentrations increased, in patients with hepatic impairment. The manufacturers state that the drug should be used with caution in patients with hepatic impairment but make no specific recommendations for dosage adjustment in such patients.

Description

Ropinirole hydrochloride, a dipropylaminoethyl indolone derivative, is a nonergot-derivative dopamine receptor agonist. In vitro binding studies, ropinirole demonstrated high binding specificity for and intrinsic activity at dopamine D_2 receptors compared with other dopamine receptor agonists (e.g., bromocriptine, pergolide), having a higher affinity for the D_3 subtype than for the D_2 or D_4 subtypes. Ropinirole binds with moderate affinity to opiate receptors but has little or no affinity for α_1-, α_2-, or β-adrenergic; dopamine D_1; benzodiazepine; γ-aminobutyric acid (GABA); serotonin type 1 (5-hydroxytryptamine [5-HT_1]); serotonin type 2 (5-HT_2); or muscarinic receptors.

The exact mechanism(s) of action of ropinirole in the management of parkinsonian syndrome has not been fully elucidated. There is considerable evidence that manifestations of parkinsonian syndrome, regardless of the cause of the syndrome, are related to depletion of dopamine in the corpus striatum. While levodopa is believed to act principally by increasing dopamine concentrations in the brain, ropinirole appears to act by directly stimulating postsynaptic dopamine receptors in the corpus striatum.

The mechanism(s) of action of ropinirole in the management of restless legs syndrome remains to be determined. While the etiology of restless legs syndrome is unclear, dopaminergic systems appear to be involved.

SumMon® (see Users Guide). For additional information on this drug until a more detailed monograph is developed and published, the manufacturer's labeling should be consulted. It is *essential* that the labeling be consulted for detailed information on the usual cautions, precautions, and contraindications.

Preparations

Excipients in commercially available drug preparations may have clinically important effects in some individuals; consult specific product labeling for details.

rOPINIRole Hydrochloride

Oral		
Tablets, film-coated	0.25 mg (of ropinirole)	**Requip® Tiltab®**, GlaxoSmithKline
		rOPINIRole Hydrochloride Tablets
	0.5 mg (of ropinirole)*	**Requip® Tiltab®**, GlaxoSmithKline
		rOPINIRole Hydrochloride Tablets

1 mg (of ropinirole)*	**Requip® Tiltab®**, GlaxoSmithKline
	rOPINIRole Hydrochloride Tablets
2 mg (of ropinirole)*	**Requip® Tiltab®**, GlaxoSmithKline
	rOPINIRole Hydrochloride Tablets
3 mg (of ropinirole)*	**Requip® Tiltab®**, GlaxoSmithKline
	rOPINIRole Hydrochloride Tablets
4 mg (of ropinirole)*	**Requip® Tiltab®**, GlaxoSmithKline
	rOPINIRole Hydrochloride Tablets
5 mg (of ropinirole)*	**Requip® Tiltab®**, GlaxoSmithKline
	rOPINIRole Hydrochloride Tablets

*available from one or more manufacturer, distributor, and/or repackager by generic (nonproprietary) name

Rotigotine

■ Rotigotine is a nonergot-derivative dopamine receptor agonist.

Uses

■ **Parkinsonian Syndrome** Transdermal rotigotine is used for the symptomatic management of idiopathic parkinsonian syndrome.

Efficacy of transdermal rotigotine for the symptomatic management of idiopathic parkinsonian syndrome has principally been established in 5 randomized, double-blind, placebo-controlled studies conducted in the US and abroad; 3 of the studies enrolled patients with early parkinsonian syndrome not receiving concomitant levodopa therapy and 2 studies enrolled patients with advanced parkinsonian syndrome who were receiving levodopa therapy concomitantly. Patients in these studies underwent a weekly titration of their rotigotine transdermal system (Neupro®) dosage in increments of 2 mg/24 hours to either the randomized dosage or the optimal dosage (depending on the individual trial design); dosage reduction (i.e., in decrements of 2 mg/24 hours) was permitted for intolerable adverse effects. In the studies in patients with early parkinsonian syndrome, improvement in manifestations of parkinsonian syndrome was assessed principally using the Unified Parkinson's Disease Rating Scale (UPDRS), parts II and III; these parts of the 4-part rating scale evaluate activities of daily living (ADL) and motor performance, respectively. In studies in patients with advanced parkinsonian syndrome (with levodopa), the primary efficacy measurement was the time spent in the "off" state (emergence of parkinsonian symptoms) based on 24-hour home diaries.

In the 3 clinical studies evaluating transdermal rotigotine in patients with early parkinsonian syndrome, enrolled patients had limited or no prior exposure to levodopa, and patients receiving selegiline, anticholinergic agents, or amantadine must have received a stable dosage and been able to maintain that dosage for the duration of the study. The first study was a multinational dose-response study in which 316 patients with early parkinsonian syndrome received one of 4 fixed dosages of transdermal rotigotine (2 mg/24 hours, 4 mg/24 hours, 6 mg/24 hours, or 8 mg/24 hours) or placebo patches for a 7-week maintenance period after an initial 4-week titration period; downward titration of dosage was performed during a final week. Transdermal rotigotine was substantially more effective than placebo in improving motor performance and activities of daily living at the 3 highest dosages in this study; the 6 mg/24 hours and 8 mg/24 hours dosages had a similar effect (as measured by mean change in combined scores from parts II and III of the UPDRS).

In the second study, which was flexible-dosage in design and conducted in the US and Canada, 277 patients with early parkinsonian syndrome were assigned in a 2:1 ratio to receive either transdermal rotigotine (2 mg/24 hours, 4 mg/24 hours, or 6 mg/24 hours) or placebo for up to 28 weeks. Approximately 90% of the patients randomized to transdermal rotigotine in this study achieved a maximal transdermal rotigotine dosage of 6 mg/24 hours, and 70% of the patients were able to remain on this dosage for most of the maintenance phase. Clinical response (defined as improvement of at least 20% in UPDRS scores [parts II and III]) occurred in 48% of patients receiving transdermal rotigotine (mean daily dosage: 5.7 mg/24 hours) compared with 19% of patients receiving placebo. Mean decrease from baseline to the end of treatment in the combined UPDRS score (parts II and III) was 4 in the patients receiving transdermal rotigotine in this study. An open-label extension of this trial demonstrated the long-term safety and tolerability of transdermal rotigotine in patients with early parkinsonian syndrome; patients received an optimal dosage (mean dosage at the end of treatment was 7.2 mg/24 hours) for up to 6 years.

The third study in patients with early parkinsonian syndrome was a placebo- and active comparator-controlled multinational study in which 561 patients with early parkinsonian syndrome were randomized to receive either transdermal rotigotine, oral ropinirole, or placebo for up to approximately 39 weeks. The mean daily dosage of transdermal rotigotine was just under 8 mg/24 hours, and approximately 90% of the patients achieved the maximal dosage of 8 mg/24 hours in this study. The mean decrease from baseline to the end of treatment in the combined UPDRS score (parts II and III) was 6.8 in the patients receiving transdermal rotigotine, and 52% of patients receiving transdermal rotigotine responded to therapy (defined as improvement of at least 20% in UPDRS parts II and III score) compared with 68% of those receiving ropinirole and 30% of those receiving placebo.

In patients with advanced parkinsonian syndrome experiencing "on-off" phenomena despite optimal dosages of levodopa, transdermal rotigotine was more effective than placebo in reducing "off" time. In a study conducted in 351 patients with advanced parkinsonian syndrome (at least 3 years since diagnosis) receiving levodopa, patients were randomized to receive transdermal rotigotine 8 mg/24 hours, transdermal rotigotine 12 mg/24 hours, or placebo for 24 weeks (followed by a downward titration period over a final week). Patients receiving transdermal rotigotine experienced a mean decrease in "off" time from baseline to end of treatment of 2.7 and 2.1 hours with rotigotine 8 mg/24 hours and rotigotine 12 mg/24 hours, respectively, compared with 0.9 hours with placebo.

In a double-blind, placebo- and active-controlled study of 6 months' duration conducted in 506 patients with advanced parkinsonian syndrome (mean time since diagnosis of approximately 8–9 years), transdermal rotigotine (mean dosage: approximately 13 mg/24 hours; range: 4–16 mg/24 hours) was more effective than placebo and non-inferior to oral pramipexole in reducing "off" time. The mean decrease in daily "off" time from baseline to the end of treatment was 2.5 and 2.8 hours for patients receiving rotigotine and pramipexole, respectively, compared with 0.9 hours in patients receiving placebo. Onset of treatment benefit was noted as early as the first week of treatment. In addition, patients receiving either transdermal rotigotine or pramipexole had substantially greater responder rates (proportion of patients with at least 30% reduction in absolute "off" time per day) compared with placebo (59.7, 67, and 35% for patients receiving rotigotine, pramipexole, and placebo, respectively).

For additional information on treatment options in parkinsonian syndrome, see Uses: Parkinsonian Syndrome, in Levodopa/Carbidopa 28:36.16.

■ **Restless Legs Syndrome** Transdermal rotigotine is used for the symptomatic management of moderate-to-severe primary restless legs syndrome (RLS; also called Willis-Ekbom disease). Restless legs syndrome is a sensorimotor disorder characterized by a distressing urge to move the legs accompanied by sensations deep in the limbs that have been described as twitching, pulling, and sometimes painful. These symptoms are present at rest, especially in the evening and at night, and are relieved by movement. Nonergot-derivative dopamine receptor agonists (e.g., pramipexole, ropinirole, transdermal rotigotine) are generally considered among the drugs of first choice for treating patients with restless legs syndrome.

Efficacy of transdermal rotigotine in the management of restless legs syndrome has mainly been established in 2 fixed-dose, randomized, double-blind, placebo-controlled trials with maintenance periods of 6 months' duration in patients with moderate-to-severe restless legs syndrome (sum score of at least 15 on the International Restless Legs Syndrome [IRLS] rating scale and score of at least 4 on the Clinical Global Impressions [CGI] Item 1 assessment [severity of symptoms]). The 2 outcome measures used to assess efficacy of treatment as co-primary efficacy endpoints were the IRLS scale and the Clinical Global Impression-Improvement (CGI-I) scale.

In the first clinical study, 505 patients with moderate-to-severe restless legs syndrome were randomized to receive placebo or transdermal rotigotine in one of 4 dosages (0.5 mg/24 hours, 1 mg/24 hours, 2 mg/24 hours, or 3 mg/24 hours following a 4-week dosage titration period) for a 6-month maintenance period. The mean decrease from baseline in the IRLS sum score was 11.1, 11.2, 13.5, and 14.2 for transdermal rotigotine dosages of 0.5 mg/24 hours, 1 mg/24 hours, 2 mg/24 hours, and 3 mg/24 hours, respectively, compared with 9 for placebo. The mean decrease from baseline in the CGI Item 1 score was 1.8, 1.7, 2.1, and 2.3 for transdermal dosages of rotigotine of 0.5 mg/24 hours, 1 mg/24 hours, 2 mg/24 hours, and 3 mg/24 hours, respectively, compared with 1.4 for placebo. On both of these co-primary efficacy measures, transdermal rotigotine dosages of 2 mg/24 hours and 3 mg/24 hours were substantially more effective in alleviating restless legs syndrome symptoms than placebo. In addition, 60 and 67% of patients receiving transdermal rotigotine 2 mg/24 hours and 3 mg/24 hours, respectively, were considered responders (defined as 50% or greater score reduction) on the IRLS scale compared with 37.4% of patients receiving placebo. On the CGI Item 1 scale, 52.6 and 59.7% of patients receiving transdermal rotigotine 2 mg/24 hours and 3 mg/24 hours, respectively, were described as responders (defined as 50% or greater score reduction) compared with 30.3% of patients receiving placebo. Onset of treatment benefit was observed with the 1 mg/24 hours dosage, and efficacy of the drug was maintained throughout the 6-month treatment period.

In the second study, 458 patients with moderate-to-severe restless legs syndrome were randomized to receive transdermal rotigotine (1 mg/24 hours, 2 mg/24 hours, or 3 mg/24 hours following a 3-week titration period) or placebo for a 6-month maintenance period. The mean changes in IRLS and CGI scores were substantially improved in patients receiving rotigotine compared with patients receiving placebo. The mean decrease from baseline in the IRLS sum score was 13.7, 16.2, and 16.8 for transdermal rotigotine dosages of 1 mg/24 hours, 2 mg/24 hours, and 3 mg/24 hours, respectively, compared with 8.6 for placebo. The mean decrease from baseline in the CGI Item 1 score was 2, 2.4, and 2.5 for transdermal rotigotine dosages of 1 mg/24 hours, 2 mg/24 hours, and 3 mg/24 hours, respectively, compared with 1.3 for placebo. In this study, 51.8, 57.8, and 55.4% of patients receiving transdermal rotigotine 1 mg/24 hours, 2 mg/24 hours, and 3 mg/24 hours, respectively, were considered responders (defined as 50% or greater score reduction) on the IRLS scale compared with 25.4% of patients receiving placebo. On the CGI Item 1 scale, 50.9, 53.2, and 61.6% of patients receiving transdermal rotigotine 1 mg/24 hours, 2 mg/24 hours, and 3 mg/24 hours, respectively, were considered responders (defined as 50% or greater score reduction) compared with 31.6% of patients receiving placebo. Improvement was observed in rotigotine-treated patients as early as week 1 and was stable during the 6-month maintenance period.

In an open-label extension study, transdermal rotigotine therapy (in dosages up to 4 mg/24 hours) in patients with moderate-to-severe restless legs syndrome was well tolerated after 1 year of treatment and provided sustained efficacy at a stable dosage for up to 5 years.

Long-term use of dopaminergic agents in patients with restless legs syndrome has been associated with augmentation of the symptoms of restless legs syndrome; augmentation can take the form of onset of symptoms earlier in the day, an increase in symptom severity, or extension of symptoms from the legs to the arms, trunk, or head. In a retrospective analysis, the risk of clinically important augmentation with transdermal rotigotine was found to be low in patients treated with the drug for up to 18 months. (See Augmentation and Rebound in Restless Legs Syndrome under Cautions: Warnings/Precautions.)

Dosage and Administration

■ **Administration** Rotigotine is administered percutaneously by topical application of a transdermal system (Neupro®). The transdermal system (patch) should be applied once daily at a convenient time for the patient during the day or night, but should be applied at approximately the same time each day.

Because rotigotine is administered transdermally, food is not expected to affect absorption of the drug, and the transdermal system may be applied without regard to meals.

Patients should be carefully instructed in the proper use and disposal of the rotigotine transdermal system and advised to read the patient information, including the instructions for use, before starting therapy and each time the drug is refilled.

The rotigotine transdermal system should be applied immediately after removal from its pouch and removal of the protective liner. The transdermal system should be applied to clean, dry, intact healthy skin on the front of the abdomen, thigh, hip, flank, shoulder, or upper arm by firmly pressing the system with the palm of the hand for 30 seconds with the adhesive side touching the skin to ensure good contact, particularly around the edges. The application site should not be oily, irritated, or damaged. In addition, application to areas where the transdermal system could be rubbed by tight clothing or under a waistband and skin folds should be avoided.

If application of the transdermal system to a hairy area is necessary, the area at the application site should be shaved at least 3 days prior to application. Creams, lotions, oils, ointments, or powders should not be applied to the skin where the transdermal system will be placed.

The application site for the rotigotine transdermal system should be moved on a daily basis (i.e., from the right side to the left side, from the upper body to the lower body). The transdermal system should not be applied to the same application site more often than once every 14 days. (See Application Site Reactions under Cautions: Warnings/Precautions.)

Each rotigotine transdermal system should be worn continuously for 24 hours. If a transdermal system should inadvertently come off during the period of use or if a patient forgets to change the patch, a new system should be applied for the remainder of the day; the patient should then change the patch the following day according to their regular time schedule. Patients who experience difficulty with patch adhesion should be advised that they may tape the edges of the system in place with bandage tape.

After handling a rotigotine transdermal system, patients should wash their hands to remove any drug; patients also should avoid touching their eyes or other objects prior to handwashing.

Because the backing layer of the rotigotine transdermal system contains aluminum, the patch should be removed prior to magnetic resonance imaging (MRI) or cardioversion to avoid skin burns.

■ **Dosage** The rotigotine transdermal system (Neupro®) is labeled in terms of the approximate rate of drug delivery per 24 hours.

The prescribed dosage of transdermal rotigotine may be achieved using either single or multiple patches of the drug.

Parkinsonian Syndrome For the management of *early* parkinsonian syndrome in adults, transdermal rotigotine therapy should be initiated at a dosage of 2 mg/24 hours. Based on individual patient response and tolerability, the dosage may be increased weekly by 2 mg/24 hours, if tolerated and if additional therapeutic effect is needed. In clinical studies, the lowest effective dosage was 4 mg/24 hours. The maximum recommended dosage for early parkinsonian syndrome is 6 mg/24 hours.

For management of *advanced* parkinsonian syndrome in adults, transdermal rotigotine therapy may be initiated at a dosage of 4 mg/24 hours. Based on individual patient response and tolerability, the dosage may be increased weekly by 2 mg/24 hours, if tolerated and if additional therapeutic effect is needed. The recommended dosage for advanced parkinsonian syndrome is 8 mg/24 hours.

When discontinuing treatment with transdermal rotigotine in patients with parkinsonian syndrome, the daily dosage should be reduced by a maximum of 2 mg/24 hours with a dosage reduction preferably every other day, until complete withdrawal of the drug is achieved. (See Withdrawal-emergent Hyperpyrexia and Confusion under Cautions: Warnings/Precautions.)

Restless Legs Syndrome For the management of restless legs syndrome in adults, transdermal rotigotine therapy should be initiated at a dosage of 1 mg/24 hours. Based on individual patient response and tolerability, the dosage may be increased weekly by 1 mg/24 hours, if tolerated and if additional therapeutic effect is needed. The lowest effective dosage is 1 mg/24 hours. The maximum recommended dosage is 3 mg/24 hours.

When discontinuing treatment with transdermal rotigotine in patients with restless legs syndrome, the daily dosage should be reduced by 1 mg/24 hours with a dosage reduction preferably every other day, until complete withdrawal of the drug is achieved. (See Augmentation and Rebound in Restless Legs Syndrome and also see Withdrawal-emergent Hyperpyrexia and Confusion under Cautions: Warnings/Precautions.)

■ **Special Populations** Dosage adjustment is not necessary in patients with mild to severe renal impairment, including in those receiving hemodialysis. (See Renal Impairment under Warnings/Precautions: Specific Populations, in Cautions.)

No dosage adjustment is necessary for patients with moderate hepatic impairment. Rotigotine has not been studied in patients with severe hepatic impairment; the manufacturer does not provide specific dosage recommendations for such patients. (See Hepatic Impairment under Warnings/Precautions: Specific Populations, in Cautions.)

The manufacturer does not provide specific dosage recommendations for geriatric patients. (See Geriatric Use under Warnings/Precautions: Specific Populations, in Cautions.)

Dosage adjustment is not necessary based on race, weight, or gender.

Cautions

■ **Contraindications** Rotigotine is contraindicated in patients who are hypersensitive to the drug or to any components in the transdermal administration system.

■ **Warnings/Precautions** ***Patient Monitoring for Adverse Reactions*** Patients receiving transdermal rotigotine should be monitored for possible adverse reactions described throughout the Cautions: Warnings/Precautions section. If any of these adverse reactions develops, dosage reduction or discontinuance of therapy may be beneficial.

Sulfite Sensitivity Rotigotine transdermal system (Neupro®) contains sodium metabisulfite, a sulfite that may cause allergic-type reactions (including anaphylactic symptoms and life-threatening or less severe asthmatic episodes) in certain susceptible individuals. The overall prevalence of sulfite sensitivity in the general population is unknown and probably low; however, such sensitivity appears to occur more often in asthmatic than in nonasthmatic individuals.

Falling Asleep During Activities of Daily Living and Somnolence Falling asleep while engaged in activities of daily living, including operating a motor vehicle (which has sometimes resulted in accidents), has been reported in patients with early or advanced parkinsonian syndrome and in patients with restless legs syndrome treated with transdermal rotigotine. Although many patients reported somnolence while receiving transdermal rotigotine, some patients did not perceive warning signs, such as excessive drowsiness, and believed they were alert prior to the episode of falling asleep. Some of the cases were reported as late as 1 year after initiation of transdermal rotigotine therapy. In clinical trials of restless legs syndrome, sleep attacks were reported in 2% of patients receiving the highest recommended dosage of transdermal rotigotine (3 mg/24 hours) but in none of the placebo recipients. Many experts believe that falling asleep while engaged in such activities always occurs in a setting of preexisting somnolence, although patients may not give such a history.

Somnolence commonly occurs in patients receiving transdermal rotigotine. However, patients may not acknowledge drowsiness or sleepiness until directly questioned about such adverse effects during specific activities. The possibility of additive sedative effects should be considered in patients taking alcohol or other CNS depressants concomitantly with rotigotine. (See Drug Interactions: Alcohol and other CNS Depressants.)

Clinicians should advise patients receiving transdermal rotigotine to exercise caution while driving, operating other machinery, or working at heights.

Before beginning transdermal rotigotine, patients should be advised of the potential to develop drowsiness and specifically asked about any factors that may increase the risk of somnolence (e.g., concomitant use of sedating drugs, the presence of sleep disorders). Patients receiving transdermal rotigotine should be continually reassessed for drowsiness or sleepiness during therapy, especially since some of the episodes of falling asleep occur well after starting treatment. If a patient develops daytime sleepiness or episodes of falling asleep during activities that require active participation (e.g., conversations, eating), rotigotine generally should be discontinued. If a decision is made to continue therapy, the patient should be advised not to drive and to avoid other potentially dangerous activities. There is insufficient information to establish whether dosage reduction will eliminate episodes of falling asleep while engaged in activities of daily living. (See Advice to Patients.)

Hallucinations/Psychotic-like Behavior An increased risk of hallucinations, which is dose related, has been observed in patients with advanced parkinsonian syndrome treated with transdermal rotigotine. Hallucinations were reported in approximately 7 and 3% of patients with advanced parkinsonian syndrome receiving transdermal rotigotine 8 mg/24 hours and placebo, respectively, and resulted in discontinuance of the drug (mainly during the dose titration period) in 3 and 1% of patients receiving transdermal rotigotine 8 mg/24 hours and placebo, respectively.

Other new or worsening mental status and behavioral changes, which can be severe and include psychotic-like behavior, have been reported during transdermal rotigotine therapy or after initiating therapy or increasing the dosage of the drug. Geriatric patients are at a higher risk for such changes than younger patients with parkinsonian syndrome. Such abnormal thinking and behavior may consist of one or more of the following manifestations: paranoid ideation, delusions, hallucinations, confusion, psychotic-like behavior, disorientation, aggressive behavior, agitation, and delirium. Other drugs used in the treatment of parkinsonian syndrome can produce similar effects on thinking and behavior.

Because of the risk of exacerbating psychosis, rotigotine should not ordinarily be used in patients with a major psychotic disorder. In addition, concomitant use of rotigotine with antipsychotic agents may exacerbate parkinsonian symptoms and result in decreased efficacy of transdermal rotigotine therapy.

If hallucinations or psychotic-like behavior occurs, a reduction in transdermal rotigotine dosage or discontinuance of therapy may be beneficial.

Symptomatic Hypotension and Syncope Transdermal rotigotine and other dopamine agonists appear to impair systemic regulation of blood pressure, resulting in postural/orthostatic hypotension, particularly during dosage escalation. Patients with parkinsonian syndrome generally have a reduced capacity to respond to orthostatic challenge. Syncope also has been reported in patients receiving dopamine agonists.

Mild to moderate decreases in systolic and diastolic blood pressure occurred more frequently in patients with early or advanced parkinsonian syndrome or restless legs syndrome receiving the highest recommended dosage of transdermal rotigotine. More severe decreases in systolic blood pressure (greater than 40 mm Hg) and in diastolic blood pressure (20 mm Hg or greater) occurred more frequently in patients with early or advanced parkinsonian syndrome during blood pressure measurements when supine, standing, and/or changing from a supine to standing position.

The manufacturer states that the increased risk for symptomatic hypotension and decreases in blood pressure occurred in a setting in which the dosage of transdermal rotigotine was very carefully titrated; in addition, patients with clinically relevant cardiovascular disease or symptomatic orthostatic hypotension were excluded from the clinical study. The increased risk for clinically significant decreases in blood pressure or orthostatic hypotension was observed especially during the dosage titration period.

The manufacturer states that transdermal rotigotine should be used with caution in patients with severe cardiovascular disease. In addition, patients with parkinsonian syndrome or restless legs syndrome receiving transdermal rotigotine and/or other dopamine agonists should be carefully monitored for signs and symptoms of orthostatic hypotension, particularly during dosage escalation. Patients receiving the drug should be informed of the risk of orthostatic hypotension and possible syncope during therapy. (See Advice to Patients.)

If orthostatic hypotension or syncope occurs during transdermal rotigotine therapy, reducing the dosage or discontinuing the drug may be beneficial.

Impulse Control/Compulsive Behaviors Intense urges and compulsive behaviors (e.g., urge to gamble, increased sexual urges, uncontrolled spending, binge eating, other intense urges) and inability to control these urges have been reported in some patients receiving one or more agents that increase central dopaminergic tone and that are generally used for the treatment of parkinsonian syndrome, including transdermal rotigotine. Although a causal relationship has not been established, these urges stopped in some cases when the dosage was reduced or the drug was discontinued. Because patients may not recognize these behaviors as abnormal, clinicians should ask patients whether they have developed new or increased gambling urges, sexual urges, uncontrolled spending, or other urges while receiving transdermal rotigotine and should advise them of the importance of reporting such urges. If a patient develops such urges while receiving rotigotine, consideration should be given to reducing the dosage or discontinuing the drug.

Elevation of Blood Pressure and Heart Rate Moderate to severe increases in blood pressure while supine and/or standing have been reported in patients receiving transdermal rotigotine. Patients with advanced parkinsonian syndrome had a 2% increased risk for systolic blood pressure exceeding 180 mm Hg and a 4% increased risk for diastolic blood pressure exceeding 105 mm Hg compared with patients receiving placebo. Patients with restless legs syndrome had a 4% increased risk of diastolic blood pressure exceeding 105 mm Hg compared with patients receiving placebo.

Mild to moderate increases in blood pressure (increase in systolic or diastolic blood pressure of 20 or 10 mm Hg or more, respectively) occurred more frequently in all patients (i.e., those with early or advanced parkinsonian syndrome or restless legs syndrome) receiving the highest recommended dosage of transdermal rotigotine compared with those receiving placebo. These increases in blood pressure were observed when supine, standing, and changing from supine to standing position. More severe increases in blood pressure (increase in systolic or diastolic blood pressure of greater than 40 or 20 mm Hg or more, respectively) also occurred in patients with early or advanced parkinsonian syndrome or with restless legs syndrome during measurements taken when supine, standing, and/or changing from supine to standing position. Patients with advanced parkinsonian syndrome or restless legs syndrome receiving the highest recommended dosage of transdermal rotigotine had an increased risk for hypertension compared with patients receiving placebo.

Some patients receiving transdermal rotigotine had a moderately increased heart rate (exceeding 100 beats per minute) while supine and/or standing. Patients with advanced parkinsonian syndrome or restless legs syndrome had a 2 or 5% increased risk of elevated heart rate, respectively.

The possibility of blood pressure and heart rate elevations should be considered when treating patients with cardiovascular disease with transdermal rotigotine. If elevations of blood pressure and/or heart rate occur, reducing the transdermal rotigotine dosage or discontinuing the drug may be beneficial.

Weight Gain and Fluid Retention Patients receiving the highest recommended transdermal rotigotine dosage for early parkinsonian syndrome had a higher incidence of substantial weight gain (more than 10% of baseline weight) than patients receiving placebo (2 vs 0%, respectively). Patients receiving the highest recommended transdermal rotigotine dosage for advanced parkinsonian syndrome also had a higher incidence of substantial weight gain than patients receiving placebo (9 vs 1%, respectively). Weight gain was frequently associated with the development of peripheral edema in patients with parkinsonian syndrome, suggesting that the drug may cause substantial fluid retention in some patients with parkinsonian syndrome. Although weight gain usually was well tolerated in clinical studies, it may cause greater difficulty in patients who are especially vulnerable to the negative consequences of fluid retention, such as those with significant congestive heart failure or renal insufficiency.

The treatment difference incidence for peripheral edema in patients receiving the highest recommended dosage of transdermal rotigotine was 1% for early parkinsonian syndrome and 8% for advanced parkinsonian syndrome. These treatment differences increased further when transdermal rotigotine was administered at dosages above the highest recommended dosages.

Dyskinesia and Concurrent Levodopa Therapy Transdermal rotigotine may potentiate the adverse dopaminergic effects of levodopa and may cause and/or exacerbate preexisting dyskinesia. In a clinical study in patients with advanced parkinsonian syndrome, dyskinesia was reported in 14% of patients receiving transdermal rotigotine (8 mg/24 hours) and levodopa compared with 7% of those receiving placebo and levodopa; the incidence of dyskinesia was found to be dose related. An increased risk of drug discontinuance because of dyskinesia also was observed in patients receiving the highest recommended transdermal rotigotine dosage in conjunction with levodopa in this study (3 versus 0% in the placebo groups). (See Drug Interactions: Levodopa/Carbidopa.)

Application Site Reactions Dose-dependent application site reactions (e.g., localized erythema, edema, or pruritus limited to the patch area) have been reported in patients receiving transdermal rotigotine. The treatment difference incidence (transdermal rotigotine incidence minus placebo incidence) for the highest recommended rotigotine dosage compared with placebo was 15, 23, and 39% for patients with early parkinsonian syndrome, advanced parkinsonian syndrome, and restless legs syndrome, respectively. Application site reactions were severe enough to result in drug discontinuance in 3, 2, and 12% of patients with early parkinsonian syndrome, advanced parkinsonian syndrome, and restless legs syndrome, respectively, receiving the highest recommended transdermal rotigotine dosage.

Most application site reactions were mild or moderate in severity and did not result in dosage reduction. Generalized (nonapplication site) skin reactions (e.g., allergic rash [including erythematous, maculopapular rash, or pruritus]) have been reported less frequently than application site reactions.

Daily rotation of transdermal rotigotine application sites has been shown to reduce the incidence of application site reactions. (See Dosage and Administration: Administration.) If a patient reports a persistent application site reaction (i.e., lasting for more than a few days), an increase in severity, or a skin reaction spreading outside the application site, the potential risks and benefits of continued therapy should be evaluated in the individual patient. If a generalized skin reaction associated with the use of transdermal rotigotine is observed, therapy should be discontinued.

Melanoma Data from epidemiologic studies indicate that patients with parkinsonian syndrome have an approximately sixfold greater risk of developing melanoma than the general population. It is unclear whether this increased risk is due to parkinsonian syndrome or other factors (e.g., drugs used to treat the disease). Because of these findings, patients and clinicians should monitor for melanoma on a frequent and regular basis when using transdermal rotigotine for any indication. The manufacturer states that periodic skin examinations should ideally be performed by qualified clinicians (e.g., dermatologists).

Augmentation and Rebound in Restless Legs Syndrome Augmentation is a worsening of restless legs syndrome symptoms during treatment, leading to an increase in overall symptom severity or earlier time of symptom onset each day compared with before initiation of therapy. Dopaminergic drugs, including rotigotine, may result in augmentation. A retrospective analysis of data from several clinical trials suggests that the risk of augmentation with transdermal rotigotine is relatively low for up to 18 months; augmentation was observed in 9.7% of the patients treated with transdermal rotigotine and was clinically relevant in 2.9% of the patients.

Rebound, an exacerbation of restless legs syndrome symptoms, is considered to be an end-of-dose effect, which is related to the half-life of the therapeutic agent. Discontinuance or wearing off of dopaminergic medications can result in rebound.

Magnetic Resonance Imaging and Cardioversion Because the backing layer of the rotigotine transdermal system contains aluminum, the patch should be removed prior to magnetic resonance imaging (MRI) or cardioversion to avoid skin burns.

Heat Application Although the effect of heat application to the rotigotine transdermal system has not been specifically studied, heat application has been shown to increase drug absorption several fold with transdermal formulations of other drugs. Clinicians should advise patients to avoid exposing the application site to external sources of direct heat, such as heating pads or electric blankets, heat lamps, saunas, hot baths, hot tubs, heated water beds, hair dryers, and prolonged direct sunlight. (See Advice to Patients.)

Withdrawal-emergent Hyperpyrexia and Confusion A symptom complex resembling neuroleptic malignant syndrome (NMS; characterized by elevated temperature, muscular rigidity, altered consciousness, rhabdomyolysis, and/or autonomic instability), with no other obvious cause, has been reported in association with rapid dosage reduction, withdrawal of, or changes in antiparkinsonian therapy. The manufacturer therefore recommends that the dosage of transdermal rotigotine be tapered when discontinuing therapy as a preventative measure. (See Dosage and Administration: Dosage.)

Fibrotic Complications Fibrotic complications, including retroperitoneal fibrosis, pulmonary infiltrates, pleural effusion, pleural thickening, pericarditis, and/or cardiac valvulopathy (which may be accompanied by clinically important regurgitation), have been reported in some patients treated with ergot-derivative dopamine agonists (e.g., bromocriptine, cabergoline, pergolide [no longer commercially available in the US]). These complications may resolve when the drug is discontinued; however, complete resolution does not always occur. These adverse effects are believed to be related to the ergoline structure of these compounds. Data are limited for fibrotic complications other than cardiac valvulopathy, and it is not known whether nonergot-derivative dopamine agonists (e.g., pramipexole, ropinirole, rotigotine) can also cause such fibrotic reactions.

Binding to Melanin Binding to melanin-containing tissues (e.g., eyes) was noted in the pigmented rat and monkey after a single dose of rotigotine. However, the binding to melanin slowly cleared over a 14-day observation period. Similar binding to melanin has been reported with other dopamine agonists.

Specific Populations **Pregnancy.** Category C. (See Users Guide.)

Lactation. Because rotigotine decreases prolactin secretion, the drug is expected to inhibit lactation.

Rotigotine and/or its metabolites are distributed into milk in rats; it is not known whether rotigotine is distributed into human milk. Because many drugs are distributed into human milk, caution is advised if the drug is administered in nursing women.

Pediatric Use. Safety and efficacy of rotigotine in pediatric patients have not been established for any indication. In addition, the pharmacokinetics of rotigotine in pediatric patients younger than 18 years of age have not been evaluated.

Geriatric Use. Of the patients with parkinsonian syndrome receiving transdermal rotigotine in clinical studies, approximately 50% were 65 years of age or older and approximately 11% were 75 years of age or older. Of the patients with restless legs syndrome receiving transdermal rotigotine in clinical studies, 26% were 65 years of age or older. No overall differences in safety or efficacy were observed between these geriatric patients and younger individuals. Other clinical experience has not revealed age-related differences in response; however, the possibility of greater sensitivity in some geriatric patients cannot be ruled out.

Geriatric patients with parkinsonian syndrome are at increased risk for hallucinations and other psychotic-like changes during therapy with dopaminergic agents. (See Hallucinations/Psychotic-like Behavior under Cautions: Warnings/Precautions.)

Plasma concentrations of rotigotine in healthy individuals and patients 65–80 years of age were similar to those in younger adults (approximately 40–64 years of age) receiving the same transdermal dosage of the drug. The manufacturer states that rotigotine exposures in older geriatric patients (exceeding 80 years of age) have not been studied, but may be higher because of the skin changes that occur with aging.

Hepatic Impairment. In patients with moderate hepatic impairment (Child-Pugh class B), there were no relevant changes in rotigotine plasma concentrations. No dosage adjustment is necessary in patients with moderate hepatic impairment.

The effects of severe hepatic impairment on the pharmacokinetics of rotigotine have not been evaluated.

Renal Impairment. In individuals with mild (creatinine clearance of 50 to less than 80 mL/minute) to severe renal impairment (creatinine clearance of less than 30 mL/minute), including in those with end-stage renal disease (creatinine clearance of less than 15 mL/minute) requiring dialysis, there were no relevant changes in rotigotine plasma concentrations compared with values in healthy individuals. In individuals with severe renal impairment (creatinine clearance of 15 to less than 30 mL/minute) not receiving dialysis, exposure to conjugated rotigotine metabolites was doubled. Dosage adjustment of transdermal rotigotine is not necessary in patients with any degree of renal impairment, including in those receiving dialysis.

■ **Common Adverse Effects** In patients with early parkinsonian syndrome (not receiving concomitant levodopa), the most common adverse reactions (incidence at least 5% higher with rotigotine than that reported with placebo) were nausea, vomiting, somnolence, application site reactions, dizziness, anorexia, hyperhidrosis, insomnia, headache, fatigue, anxiety, peripheral edema, and dyspepsia.

In patients with advanced parkinsonian syndrome (receiving concomitant levodopa), the most common adverse reactions (incidence at least 5% higher with rotigotine than that reported with placebo) were application site reactions, nausea, dyskinesia, dizziness, peripheral edema, insomnia, and hallucinations.

In patients with restless legs syndrome, the most common adverse reactions (incidence at least 5% higher with rotigotine than that reported with placebo) were application site reactions, nausea, somnolence, headache, and insomnia.

Drug Interactions

Multiple cytochrome P-450 (CYP) isoenzymes are capable of catalyzing the metabolism of rotigotine. If an individual CYP isoenzyme is inhibited, other isoenzymes can catalyze rotigotine metabolism. In addition, rotigotine is metabolized by multiple sulfotransferases and 2 uridine diphosphate-glucuronosyltransferases (UGT1A9 and UGT2B15); therefore, it is unlikely that inhibition of any one metabolic pathway would substantially alter rotigotine concentrations.

■ **Drugs Affecting or Metabolized by Hepatic Microsomal Enzymes** In vitro studies indicate that there is no risk for inhibition of CYP isoenzymes 1A2-, 2C9-, and 3A4-catalyzed metabolism of other drugs and a low risk of inhibition of CYP2C19- and CYP2D6-catalyzed metabolism of other drugs at therapeutic rotigotine concentrations. Pharmacokinetic interactions mediated by CYP isoenzymes are unlikely since metabolism of rotigotine does not depend on any single metabolic pathway. If an individual CYP isoenzyme is inhibited, other isoenzymes can catalyze rotigotine metabolism.

In vitro, there is no indication of induction of CYP isoenzymes 1A2, 2B6, 2C9, 2C19, and 3A4. Therefore, inducers of these CYP isoenzymes are unlikely to substantially affect rotigotine concentrations.

■ **Drugs Affecting Uridine Diphosphate-glucuronosyltransferase (UGT)** Rotigotine is metabolized by multiple pathways, including by 2 UGT enzymes (UGT1A9 and UGT2B15); therefore, it is unlikely that inhibition of any one metabolic pathway would substantially alter rotigotine concentrations.

■ **Alcohol and other CNS Depressants** Alcohol and other CNS depressants (e.g., sedatives, anxiolytics, antidepressants, antipsychotics, opiate analgesics) may increase the risk of additive effects, including somnolence and falling asleep during activities of daily living, in patients receiving transdermal rotigotine, and should therefore be used concomitantly with caution. (See Falling Asleep During Activities of Daily Living and Somnolence under Cautions: Warnings/Precautions.)

■ **Cimetidine** Concurrent administration of transdermal rotigotine (up to 4 mg/24 hours) and cimetidine (400 mg twice daily), an inhibitor of CYP1A2, CYP2C19, CYP2D6, and CYP3A4, in healthy individuals did not alter the steady-state pharmacokinetics of rotigotine.

■ **Digoxin** Rotigotine did not influence P-glycoprotein-mediated transport of digoxin; therefore, rotigotine is not expected to alter the pharmacokinetics of digoxin.

■ **Dopamine Agonists** Transdermal rotigotine may potentiate the therapeutic and/or adverse dopaminergic effects (including dyskinesia) of other dopamine agonists used in the treatment of parkinsonian syndrome and restless legs syndrome. (See Dyskinesia and Concurrent Levodopa Therapy under Cautions: Warnings/Precautions and also see Drug Interactions: Levodopa/Carbidopa.)

■ **Dopamine Antagonists** Dopamine antagonists (e.g., antipsychotic agents, metoclopramide) may diminish the effectiveness of rotigotine.

■ **Hormonal Contraceptives** Concurrent administration of transdermal rotigotine (3 mg/24 hours) did not substantially affect the pharmacodynamics or pharmacokinetics of an oral estrogen-progestin combination contraceptive (ethinyl estradiol 0.03 mg with 0.15 mg levonorgestrel) in healthy females. Possible interactions with rotigotine and other forms of hormonal contraceptives have not been evaluated to date.

■ **Levodopa/Carbidopa** Concurrent oral administration of levodopa/carbidopa (100/25 mg twice daily) and transdermal rotigotine (4 mg/24 hours) in patients with restless legs syndrome had no effect on the steady-state pharmacokinetics of any of the drugs. Transdermal rotigotine may potentiate the therapeutic effects of levodopa as well as its adverse dopaminergic effects (including dyskinesia). (See Dyskinesia and Concurrent Levodopa Therapy under Cautions: Warnings/Precautions.)

■ **Omeprazole** Concurrent administration of oral omeprazole (40 mg daily), a selective CYP2C19 inhibitor, and transdermal rotigotine (4 mg/24 hours) had no effect on the steady-state pharmacokinetics of rotigotine in healthy individuals.

■ **Warfarin** No potential for displacement of warfarin by rotigotine (and vice versa) from their respective human serum albumin binding sites was detected in vitro.

Description

Rotigotine is a nonergot-derivative dopamine receptor agonist. In in vitro studies, rotigotine demonstrated binding specificity for and intrinsic activity at dopamine D_1, D_2, D_3, D_4, and D_5 receptors, with the highest affinity for the D_3 dopamine receptor subtype. Rotigotine has antagonistic effects at α_{2B}-adrenergic receptors and agonistic effects at serotonin type 1A (5-hydroxytryptamine [5-HT_{1A}]) receptors, but no activity on 5-HT_{2B} receptors.

The exact mechanism(s) of action of rotigotine in the management of parkinsonian syndrome has not been fully elucidated. However, the drug appears to act by stimulating dopamine receptors (D_3, D_2, and D_1) in the caudate putamen of the brain.

The precise mechanism(s) of action of rotigotine in the management of restless legs syndrome is unknown, but appears to be related to its ability to stimulate dopamine receptors.

Following topical application, the rotigotine transdermal system releases an average of approximately 45% of the rotigotine from the system within 24 hours. When single doses of 8 mg/24 hours were applied to the trunk, there was an average lag time of approximately 3 hours (range: 1–8 hours) until the drug was detected in plasma. Peak rotigotine concentrations typically occur 15–18 hours postdose, but can occur from 4–27 hours postdose. However, there is no characteristic peak concentration observed. Steady-state plasma concentrations of rotigotine were observed within 2–3 days of daily dosing when administered to healthy individuals in a 14-day study. Because rotigotine is administered transdermally, food should not affect absorption. In a study in patients with early parkinsonian syndrome receiving transdermal rotigotine, relative bioavailability at steady state by application site ranged from less than 1% (abdomen versus hip) to 46% (shoulder versus thigh), with shoulder application showing higher bioavailability. In a study in healthy males, absolute bioavailability of the drug when applied as a transdermal system was 37%. Rotigotine is approximately 92% bound to human plasma proteins in vitro and 89.5% bound in vivo. Rotigotine is extensively metabolized by conjugation and *N*-dealkylation. Multiple cytochrome P-450 (CYP) isoenzymes, sulfotransferases, and 2 uridine diphosphate-glucuronosyltransferases (UGT1A9 and UGT2B15) are capable of catalyzing the metabolism of rotigotine. Approximately 71 and 23% of a single IV dose of rotigotine is excreted in urine and feces, respectively, as metabolites over 9 days; less than 1% of the dose is excreted as unchanged drug in urine. The major metabolites found in urine include rotigotine sulfate, rotigotine glucuronide, *N*-despropyl-rotigotine sulfate, and *N*-desthienylethyl-rotigotine sulfate. Following removal of the transdermal system, elimination of the drug was biphasic with an initial half-life of 3 hours and a terminal half-life of 5–7 hours.

Advice to Patients

Importance of reading the manufacturer's patient information before beginning transdermal rotigotine therapy and each time the drug is dispensed.

Importance of using the rotigotine transdermal system (patch) as prescribed. Importance of instructing patients to wear the system continuously for 24 hours. Advise patients to remove the patch after 24 hours and immediately apply a new one. If a patient forgets to change a patch, they should be advised to apply a new patch as soon as possible and then replace it at the usual time the following day.

Risk of severe allergic reactions. Rotigotine transdermal system (Neupro®) contains sodium metabisulfite, which is a sulfite that can cause severe allergic-type reactions (including anaphylactic symptoms and life threatening or less severe asthmatic episodes) in certain susceptible individuals. An allergy to sulfites is not the same as an allergy to sulfa drugs. Individuals with asthma are more likely to be allergic to sulfites. Patients should be advised to immediately remove the patch and seek immediate medical attention if they experience swelling of the lips or tongue, chest pain, and/or difficulty breathing or swallowing.

Importance of advising patients of the potential for sedating effects, including somnolence and the possibility of falling asleep without feeling drowsy or without warning while engaged in activities of daily living. Patients should avoid driving or engaging in other potentially dangerous activities until the effects on the individual are known. Importance of advising patients that if increased somnolence or new episodes of falling asleep during activities of daily living (e.g., watching television, passenger in a car) occur at any time during therapy, they should not drive or participate in potentially dangerous activities until they have contacted their clinician. Patients should not drive, operate machinery, or work at heights during treatment if they have previously experienced somnolence and/or have fallen asleep without warning prior to use of rotigotine. Patients should inform their clinician if they take any medications that make them drowsy before starting transdermal rotigotine therapy.

Importance of informing patients that hallucinations or other psychotic-like behavior can occur during therapy, particularly in geriatric patients with parkinsonian syndrome.

Importance of advising patients of risk of symptomatic (e.g., dizziness, nausea, sweating) or asymptomatic orthostatic hypotension and syncope during therapy, particularly during initial therapy and following an increase in dosage. Patients should avoid rising rapidly after sitting or lying down, especially if they have been in a seated or recumbent position for prolonged periods and/or if they are just beginning transdermal rotigotine therapy. Patients should be advised to contact their clinician if they experience any signs or symptoms of lowered blood pressure during therapy.

Risk of increased blood pressure or exacerbation of hypertension and increased heart rate.

Importance of asking patients whether they have developed any new or increased urges or compulsive behaviors (e.g., gambling urges, sexual urges, uncontrolled spending, binge eating) while receiving transdermal rotigotine and of advising them of the importance of reporting such urges.

Risk of weight gain and fluid retention, which may manifest as peripheral edema. Patients should be advised to contact their clinician if they experience swelling or fluid retention, especially in the ankles or legs, or have an unusually fast increase in weight.

Risk of new onset or exacerbation of dyskinesia.

Importance of informing patients that application site reactions can occur with transdermal rotigotine and that the application site should be rotated on a daily basis. The patch should not be applied to the same application site more often than once every 14 days. Patients should report persistent application site reactions (lasting more than a few days), increases in severity, or skin reactions that spread outside the application site. If there is a skin rash or irritation from the transdermal system, direct sunlight on the area should be avoided until the skin heals; such exposure may lead to changes in skin color.

Importance of advising patients with parkinsonian syndrome that they are at higher risk of developing melanoma. Advise patients to monitor for melanoma frequently and on a regular basis when using transdermal rotigotine for any indication.

Importance of informing patients that transdermal rotigotine may cause restless legs symptoms to have an earlier onset during the day or become worse.

Importance of informing patients to remove the rotigotine patch before undergoing magnetic resonance imaging (MRI) or cardioversion to avoid possible skin burns.

Importance of advising patients about the potential for heat application to increase rotigotine absorption from the patch. Patients should be instructed to avoid applying external heat sources (e.g., heating pads, electric blankets, heat lamps, saunas, hot baths, hot tubs, heated water beds, hair dryers) to the transdermal system and to avoid direct sun exposure of the transdermal system.

Importance of informing patients that transdermal rotigotine may cause nausea, vomiting, and general GI distress (i.e., dyspepsia, abdominal discomfort). Nausea and vomiting may occur more frequently during initial therapy and may require dosage adjustment.

Importance of following recommended procedure for administration, removal, and disposal of rotigotine transdermal systems and of reviewing the instruction sheet provided by the manufacturer.

Importance of patient (or individual assisting the patient) thoroughly washing hands with soap and water after handling the rotigotine transdermal system (e.g., initial application, removal) and to wash the application site thoroughly after removing the system.

Importance of proper transdermal system disposal, including keeping it out of the reach of children or pets.

Importance of informing clinicians of existing or contemplated concomitant therapy, including prescription (e.g., CNS depressants including sedatives, antidepressants, and antipsychotics) and OTC drugs and herbal supplements, as well as any concomitant illnesses.

Importance of women informing clinicians if they are or plan to become pregnant or plan to breast-feed.

Importance of informing patients of other important precautionary information. (See Cautions.)

Overview® (see Users Guide). For additional information on this drug until a more detailed monograph is developed and published, the manufacturer's labeling should be consulted. It is *essential* that the manufacturer's labeling be consulted for more detailed information on usual cautions, precautions, contraindications, potential drug interactions, laboratory test interferences, and acute toxicity.

Preparations

Excipients in commercially available drug preparations may have clinically important effects in some individuals; consult specific product labeling for details.

Rotigotine

Topical

Transdermal System	1 mg/24 hours (2.25 mg/5 cm²)	**Neupro®**, UCB
	2 mg/24 hours (4.5 mg/10 cm²)	**Neupro®**, UCB
	3 mg/24 hours (6.75 mg/15 cm²)	**Neupro®**, UCB
	4 mg/24 hours (9 mg/20 cm²)	**Neupro®**, UCB
	6 mg/24 hours (13.5 mg/30 cm²)	**Neupro®**, UCB
	8 mg/24 hours (18 mg/40 cm²)	**Neupro®**, UCB

FIBROMYALGIA AGENTS 28:40

Milnacipran Hydrochloride

Dalcipran, Ixel

■ Milnacipran hydrochloride is a selective serotonin- and norepinephrine-reuptake inhibitor (SNRI). The drug is a fibromyalgia agent.

Uses

■ **Fibromyalgia** Milnacipran hydrochloride is used for the management of fibromyalgia in adults.

Fibromyalgia, which is estimated to affect from 2–4% of the population in the US, is a complex syndrome associated with chronic widespread musculoskeletal pain and a reduced pain threshold, with hyperalgesia and allodynia (pain-related behavior in response to normally innocuous stimuli). Some associated clinical features include fatigue, depression and other mood disorders, anxiety, sleep disturbances, headache (including migraine), changes in bowel habits (including irritable bowel syndrome), diffuse abdominal pain, and urinary frequency.

The American College of Rheumatology (ACR) initially published criteria for the classification of fibromyalgia in 1990, which included a history of widespread pain for at least 3 months and the presence of pain in at least 11 of 18 specific tender point sites. In 2010, the ACR developed new diagnostic criteria for fibromyalgia that no longer included tender point counts and focused more on patient symptoms, including use of a widespread pain index (WPI) and symptom severity (SS) scale. According to the 2010 diagnostic criteria, a diagnosis of fibromyalgia can be made if a patient has a WPI of 7 or greater and SS scale score of 5 or greater *or* a WPI of 3–6 and SS scale score of 9 or greater; symptoms must have been present at a similar level for at least 3 months and the patient should not have a disorder that would otherwise explain the pain. Due to the complex nature of the fibromyalgia syndrome, optimal treatment often requires a combination of nonpharmacologic therapy (e.g., cognitive behavioral therapy, education, exercise and other forms of physical therapy) and pharmacologic therapy (e.g., selective serotonin-reuptake inhibitors [SSRIs], SNRIs, tricyclic antidepressants, other agents [e.g., pregabalin], topical and systemic analgesics).

Efficacy of milnacipran for the management of fibromyalgia has principally been established in 2 double-blind, placebo-controlled, multicenter studies conducted in the US in 2084 adults with a diagnosis of fibromyalgia based on the 1990 ACR criteria. Approximately 35% of the patients in these studies had a history of depression. Study 1 was of 6 months' duration and study 2 was of 3 months' duration; both studies compared total daily milnacipran hydrochloride dosages of 100 mg and 200 mg with placebo. In these studies, a larger proportion of patients treated with milnacipran than those treated with placebo experienced a simultaneous reduction in pain from baseline of at least 30% on the visual analog scale (VAS) and rated themselves as much improved or very much improved on the Patient Global Impression of Change (PGIC) scale. In addition, a larger proportion of patients treated with milnacipran met the criteria for treatment response as measured by the composite endpoint that concurrently evaluated improvement in pain (VAS), physical function (Short Form-36 Physical Component Summary), and the PGIC. In both studies, some patients who rated themselves as much or very much improved experienced a decrease in pain as early as week 1 of treatment with a stable milnacipran dosage, and the pain reduction persisted throughout the studies. Neither study demonstrated an additional therapeutic benefit of 200 mg of milnacipran hydrochloride daily compared with 100 mg daily.

A multicenter, randomized, blinded extension of study 1, which was of 6 months' duration, subsequently demonstrated that continuing milnacipran therapy (100 or 200 mg daily) for an additional 6 months provides sustained efficacy for up to 1 year and generally is well tolerated in patients with fibromyalgia.

Fatigue is one of the core symptoms associated with fibromyalgia and affects patients both physically and mentally. In a pooled analysis of 3 randomized, placebo-controlled clinical trials of milnacipran (100 or 200 mg daily) in patients with fibromyalgia, milnacipran-treated patients experienced substantial and clinically important reductions in fatigue as measured by the Multidimensional Fatigue Inventory (MFI; a scale that assesses physical, mental, and psychosocial aspects of fatigue). The improvement in fatigue observed in the milnacipran-treated patients could not be completely attributed to indirect effects of the drug on pain reduction.

■ **Major Depressive Disorder** Although milnacipran has been used in the treatment of major depressive disorder† and is approved for treating depression in some countries outside the US, this indication is *not* an FDA-labeled use. Levomilnacipran hydrochloride (Fetzima®), the 1*S*,2*R*-enantiomer of milnacipran, is labeled by the FDA for the treatment of major depressive disorder.

There are insufficient data, to date, to determine if the efficacy and tolerability of milnacipran as an antidepressant are superior, inferior, or equal to that of other antidepressant agents for the acute phase treatment of major depressive disorder. However, some studies indicate improved tolerability with milnacipran when compared with tricyclic antidepressants.

Dosage and Administration

■ **Administration** Milnacipran hydrochloride is administered orally twice daily in divided doses without regard to meals; however, taking the drug with food may improve tolerability.

The manufacturer states that at least 2 weeks must elapse between discontinuance of a monoamine oxidase (MAO) inhibitor intended to treat psychiatric disorders and initiation of milnacipran therapy and that at least 5 days must elapse between discontinuance of milnacipran and initiation of MAO inhibitor therapy intended to treat psychiatric disorders. (See Contraindications, Serotonin Syndrome under Warnings/Precautions: Other Warnings and Precautions, in Cautions, and Drug Interactions: Monoamine Oxidase Inhibitors.)

Patients receiving milnacipran for any indication should be monitored appropriately and observed closely for clinical worsening, suicidality, and unusual changes in behavior, particularly during initial therapy or following any change (increase or decrease) in dosage. (See Worsening of Depression and Suicidality Risk under Warnings/Precautions: Warnings, in Cautions.)

■ **Dosage** Dosage of milnacipran hydrochloride is expressed in terms of the salt.

Fibromyalgia For the management of fibromyalgia in adults, the recommended maintenance dosage of milnacipran hydrochloride is 100 mg daily (given as 50 mg twice daily). The manufacturer states that the dosage should be titrated based on efficacy and tolerability, beginning with 12.5 mg administered once on the first day of therapy, 25 mg daily (given as 12.5 mg twice daily) on days 2 and 3, and 50 mg daily (given as 25 mg twice daily) on days 4 through 7. After day 7, the usual maintenance dosage of 100 mg daily (given as 50 mg twice daily) should be given. Based upon individual patient response, the dosage may be increased to 200 mg daily (given as 100 mg twice daily). Safety and efficacy of milnacipran hydrochloride dosages above 200 mg daily have not been evaluated.

Discontinuance of Therapy Because withdrawal effects may occur, abrupt discontinuance of milnacipran should be avoided after extended use. When milnacipran therapy is discontinued, dosage should be tapered gradually and the patient monitored to reduce the risk of withdrawal symptoms. If intolerable symptoms occur following dosage reduction or upon discontinuance of treatment, reinstitution of milnacipran therapy at the previously prescribed dosage may be considered until symptoms abate. Clinicians may resume dosage reductions at that time but at a more gradual rate. (See Withdrawal of Therapy under Warnings/Precautions: Other Warnings and Precautions, in Cautions.)

■ **Special Populations** Dosage adjustment is not necessary in patients with mild renal impairment. Milnacipran should be used with caution in patients with moderate renal impairment. In patients with severe renal impairment (creatinine clearance of 5–29 mL/minute), the usual maintenance dosage should be reduced by 50% to 50 mg daily (given as 25 mg twice daily). Based on individual patient response, the dosage may be increased to 100 mg daily (given as 50 mg twice daily). Milnacipran is *not* recommended in patients with end-stage renal disease.

Dosage adjustment is not necessary in patients with hepatic impairment. However, the drug should be used with caution in patients with severe hepatic impairment. In addition, the manufacturer states that milnacipran generally should not be prescribed to patients with substantial alcohol use or evidence of chronic hepatic disease. (See Hepatic Effects under Warnings/Precautions: Other Warnings and Precautions, in Cautions and also see Specific Populations under Cautions: Warnings/Precautions.)

The manufacturer does not recommend routine dosage adjustment in geriatric patients; however, possible age-related decreases in renal function should be considered. Dosage adjustment is necessary in geriatric patients with severely impaired renal function.

Dosage adjustment based on gender is not necessary.

Cautions

■ **Contraindications** Concurrent or recent (i.e., within 2 weeks) therapy with a monoamine oxidase (MAO) inhibitor intended to treat psychiatric disorders. Use of an MAO inhibitor intended to treat psychiatric disorders within 5 days of milnacipran discontinuance. (See Serotonin Syndrome under Warnings/Precautions: Other Warnings and Precautions, in Cautions and also see Drug Interactions: Monoamine Oxidase Inhibitors.)

Initiation of milnacipran therapy in patients receiving MAO inhibitors such as linezolid or IV methylene blue. (See Drug Interactions: Linezolid and also see Drug Interactions: Methylene Blue.)

■ **Warnings/Precautions** ***Warnings*** **Worsening of Depression and Suicidality Risk.** Milnacipran is a selective serotonin- and norepinephrine-reuptake inhibitor (SNRI) and is similar to some drugs used for the treatment of depression and other psychiatric disorders.

Worsening of depression and/or the emergence of suicidal ideation and behavior (suicidality) or unusual changes in behavior may occur in both adult and pediatric (see Pediatric Use under Cautions: Specific Populations) patients with major depressive disorder or other psychiatric disorders, whether or not they are taking antidepressants. This risk may persist until clinically important remission occurs. Suicide is a known risk of depression and certain other psychiatric disorders, and these disorders themselves are the strongest predictors of suicide. However, there has been a long-standing concern that antidepressants, including drugs that inhibit the reuptake of norepinephrine and/or serotonin, may have a role in inducing worsening of depression and the emergence of suicidality in certain patients during the early phases of treatment. Pooled analyses of short-term, placebo-controlled studies of antidepressants (i.e., selective serotonin-reuptake inhibitors [SSRIs] and other antidepressants) have shown an increased risk of suicidality in children, adolescents, and young adults (18–24 years of age) with major depressive disorder and other psychiatric disorders. An increased suicidality risk was not demonstrated with antidepressants compared with placebo in adults older than 24 years of age and a reduced risk was observed in adults 65 years of age or older.

In controlled trials of adults with fibromyalgia, the incidence of suicidal ideation among patients with a history of depression at treatment initiation was 0% in patients receiving milnacipran 100 mg daily, 1.3% in patients receiving milnacipran 200 mg daily, and 0.5% in patients receiving placebo. No suicides occurred in the short-term or longer-term (up to 1 year) fibromyalgia trials.

All patients being treated with drugs inhibiting the reuptake of norepinephrine and/or serotonin for any indication should be appropriately monitored and closely observed for clinical worsening, suicidality, and unusual changes in behavior, particularly during initiation of therapy (i.e., the first few months) and during periods of dosage adjustments. Families and caregivers of such patients also should be advised to monitor patients on a daily basis for the emergence of agitation, irritability, or unusual changes in behavior as well as the emergence of suicidality, and to report such symptoms immediately to a health-care provider.

Although a causal relationship between the emergence of symptoms such as anxiety, agitation, panic attacks, insomnia, irritability, hostility, aggressiveness, impulsivity, akathisia, hypomania, and/or mania and either the worsening of depression and/or the emergence of suicidal impulses has not been established, there is concern that such symptoms may represent precursors to emerging suicidality. Consequently, consideration should be given to changing the therapeutic regimen or discontinuing therapy in patients who may experience worsening depressive symptoms or who are experiencing emergent suicidality or symptoms that might be precursors to worsening depression or suicidality, particularly if such manifestations are severe, abrupt in onset, or were not part of the patient's presenting symptoms. The manufacturer also recommends that milnacipran be prescribed in the smallest quantity consistent with good patient management, in order to reduce the risk of overdosage.

Other Warnings and Precautions **Serotonin Syndrome.** Potentially life-threatening serotonin syndrome has been reported with SSRIs and SNRIs, including milnacipran, when used alone, but particularly with concurrent use of other serotonergic drugs (including serotonin [5-hydroxytryptamine; 5-HT] type 1 receptor agonists ["triptans"], tricyclic antidepressants, buspirone, fentanyl, lithium, tramadol, tryptophan, St. John's wort [*Hypericum perforatum*]) and with drugs that impair the metabolism of serotonin (particularly MAO inhibitors, both those used to treat psychiatric disorders and others, such as linezolid and methylene blue). Manifestations of serotonin syndrome may include mental status changes (e.g., agitation, hallucinations, delirium, coma), autonomic instability (e.g., tachycardia, labile blood pressure, dizziness, diaphoresis, flushing, hyperthermia), neuromuscular symptoms (e.g., tremor, rigidity, myoclonus, hyperreflexia, incoordination), seizures, and/or GI symptoms (e.g., nausea, vomiting, diarrhea). Patients receiving milnacipran should be monitored for the development of serotonin syndrome.

Concurrent or recent (i.e., within 2 weeks) therapy with MAO inhibitors intended to treat psychiatric disorders is contraindicated. Use of an MAO inhibitor intended to treat psychiatric disorders within 5 days of milnacipran discontinuance also is contraindicated. (See Contraindications and also see Drug Interactions: Monoamine Oxidase Inhibitors.) Milnacipran also should not be initiated in patients who are being treated with other MAO inhibitors such as linezolid or IV methylene blue. (See Drug Interactions: Linezolid and also see Drug Interactions: Methylene Blue.)

If concurrent therapy with milnacipran and other serotonergic drugs is clinically warranted, the patient should be made aware of the potential increased risk for serotonin syndrome, particularly during initiation of therapy or when dosage is increased. (See Drug Interactions.)

If manifestations of serotonin syndrome occur, treatment with milnacipran and any concurrently administered serotonergic agents should be immediately discontinued and supportive and symptomatic treatment initiated.

For further information on serotonin syndrome, including manifestations and treatment, see Drug Interactions: Serotonergic Drugs, in Fluoxetine Hydrochloride 28:16.04.20.

Elevated Blood Pressure. SNRIs, including milnacipran, have been associated with increases in blood pressure. In a double-blind, placebo-controlled ambulatory blood pressure monitoring study conducted in 321 patients with fibromyalgia, a greater percentage of milnacipran-treated patients who were normotensive at baseline had a hypertensive blood pressure measurement at weeks 4 (50 mg twice daily steady-state visit) and 7 (100 mg twice daily steady-state visit) compared with those who received placebo (17.7% versus 3.7% and 14.3% versus 0% at weeks 4 and 7, respectively). Mean 24-hour systolic and diastolic blood pressure increased by 5–6 mm Hg and 4–6 mm Hg, respectively, following 4–6 weeks of milnacipran therapy. Increases in blood pressure were similar between milnacipran-treated patients who were hypertensive at baseline and those who were normotensive at baseline.

Similar patterns of treatment-emergent blood pressure elevations were observed in phase 3 and clinical pharmacology studies with milnacipran. In controlled studies in fibromyalgia, approximately twice as many milnacipran-treated patients (about 17–20%) who were not hypertensive at baseline became hypertensive by the end of the study compared with patients receiving placebo (approximately 7%). In addition, a greater percentage of milnacipran-treated patients who were hypertensive at baseline experienced increases in systolic and diastolic blood pressure of more than 15 and 10 mm Hg, respectively, compared with placebo recipients.

Sustained increases in blood pressure also have been reported. In controlled fibromyalgia studies, sustained increases in systolic and diastolic blood pressure occurred in 6–9 and 10–13% of milnacipran-treated patients, respectively, compared with 2 and 4% of placebo recipients, respectively. Sustained blood pressure increases may have adverse consequences in patients receiving the drug. Some cases of elevated blood pressure requiring immediate treatment have been reported with milnacipran.

Concurrent use of milnacipran with other drugs that increase blood pressure and heart rate has not been evaluated, and the manufacturer recommends that such combinations be used with caution. (See Drug Interactions: Epinephrine and Norepinephrine and also see Drug Interactions: Drugs that Increase Blood Pressure and Heart Rate.)

Effects of milnacipran on blood pressure in patients with clinically important hypertension or cardiovascular disease have not been systematically evaluated; the drug should be used with caution in such patients.

The manufacturer states that preexisting hypertension and other cardiovascular disease should be treated before initiating milnacipran therapy. In addition, blood pressure should be measured prior to initiating milnacipran and then periodically throughout treatment. For patients who experience a sustained increase in blood pressure during milnacipran therapy, the dosage should be reduced or the drug discontinued, if clinically warranted.

Elevated Heart Rate. SNRIs, including milnacipran, have been associated with increases in heart rate. In a double-blind, placebo-controlled ambulatory blood pressure monitoring study, patients with fibromyalgia who were normotensive at baseline had a mean increase in 24-hour heart rate of 13 beats per minute at week 4 (50 mg twice daily steady-state visit) and also at week 7 (100 mg twice daily steady-state visit).

In clinical trials, relative to placebo, milnacipran was associated with similar mean increases in heart rate of approximately 7–8 beats per minute. Increases in heart rate of at least 20 beats per minute were reported in 8% of milnacipran-treated patients compared with 0.3% of placebo recipients.

Concurrent use of milnacipran with other drugs that increase blood pressure and heart rate has not been evaluated, and the manufacturer recommends that such combinations be used with caution. (See Drug Interactions: Epinephrine and Norepinephrine and also see Drug Interactions: Drugs that Increase Blood Pressure and Heart Rate.)

Milnacipran has not been systematically evaluated in patients with cardiac rhythm disorders.

The manufacturer states that preexisting tachyarrhythmias and other cardiovascular disease should be treated before initiating milnacipran therapy. In addition, heart rate should be measured prior to initiating milnacipran and periodically throughout treatment. For patients who experience a sustained increase in heart rate during milnacipran therapy, the dosage should be reduced or the drug discontinued, if clinically warranted.

Seizures. Milnacipran has not been systematically evaluated in patients with seizure disorders. Seizures were not reported during clinical trials of milnacipran for fibromyalgia; however, seizures have been reported infrequently in patients receiving the drug for other conditions. The manufacturer states that milnacipran should be used with caution in patients with a history of a seizure disorder.

Hepatic Effects. In fibromyalgia clinical trials, mild elevations in serum ALT (SGPT) or AST (SGOT) concentrations were reported more frequently in milnacipran-treated patients (6–7% and 3–5%, respectively) than in those receiving placebo (3 and 2%, respectively). An elevation in ALT of more than 5 times the upper limit of normal but not exceeding 10 times the upper limit of normal was reported in one patient who received the drug (0.2%). Increases in serum bilirubin concentrations reported in these trials were not found to be clinically significant.

Cases of elevated serum transaminase concentrations and severe hepatic injury, including fulminant hepatitis, have been reported during foreign post-marketing surveillance. In the cases of severe hepatic injury, there were significant underlying clinical conditions and/or concomitant use of multiple medications.

Milnacipran should be discontinued in any patient who develops jaundice or other evidence of hepatic dysfunction; therapy should not be resumed unless another cause for the hepatic dysfunction can be established.

Milnacipran should not ordinarily be prescribed to patients with a history of substantial alcohol consumption or evidence of chronic hepatic disease. (See Concomitant Use with Alcohol under Warnings/Precautions: Other Warnings and Precautions, in Cautions.)

Withdrawal of Therapy. Withdrawal symptoms have been observed in clinical trials following discontinuance of milnacipran, other SNRIs, and SSRIs; there also have been spontaneous reports of adverse effects indicative of withdrawal and physical dependence during marketing of these drugs, particularly when discontinuance was abrupt. These withdrawal effects include dysphoric mood, irritability, agitation, dizziness, sensory disturbances (e.g., paresthesias, such as electric shock sensations), anxiety, confusion, headache, lethargy, emotional lability, insomnia, hypomania, tinnitus, and seizures. While these events generally are self-limiting, there have been severe cases.

Patients should be monitored for possible withdrawal symptoms when discontinuing milnacipran therapy. A gradual reduction in dosage rather than abrupt cessation is recommended after extended use. If intolerable symptoms occur following dosage reduction or discontinuance of milnacipran, reinstituting the previously prescribed dosage until symptoms abate may be considered; subsequently, resuming dosage reductions at a more gradual rate may be considered. (See Dosage and Administration: Dosage.)

Hyponatremia/Syndrome of Inappropriate Antidiuretic Hormone Secretion. Treatment with SSRIs and SNRIs, including milnacipran, may result in hyponatremia. In many cases, hyponatremia appears to be due to the syndrome of inappropriate antidiuretic hormone secretion (SIADH). Cases with serum sodium concentrations lower than 110 mmol/L have been reported. Geriatric individuals and patients receiving diuretics or who are otherwise volume depleted may be at greater risk of developing hyponatremia. Signs and symptoms of hyponatremia include headache, difficulty concentrating, memory impairment, confusion, weakness, and unsteadiness, which may lead to falls; more severe and/or acute cases have been associated with hallucinations, syncope, seizures, coma, respiratory arrest, and death. Drug discontinuance should be considered in patients with symptomatic hyponatremia.

Abnormal Bleeding. SSRIs and SNRIs, including milnacipran, may increase the risk of bleeding events. Concurrent use of aspirin, nonsteroidal anti-inflammatory agents (NSAIAs), warfarin, and other anticoagulants may add to this risk. Case reports and epidemiologic studies have demonstrated an association between the use of drugs that interfere with serotonin reuptake and the occurrence of GI bleeding. Bleeding events related to SSRI and SNRI use have ranged from ecchymoses, hematomas, epistaxis, and petechiae to life-threatening hemorrhages. The manufacturer recommends that patients be advised of the risk of bleeding associated with the concomitant use of milnacipran and aspirin or other NSAIAs, warfarin, or other drugs that affect coagulation. (See Drug Interactions: Drugs Affecting Hemostasis.)

Activation of Mania/Hypomania. Activation of mania or hypomania was not reported in clinical trials evaluating milnacipran for fibromyalgia; however, patients with a current major depressive episode were excluded from participating in those trials. Activation of mania and hypomania have been reported in patients with mood disorders treated with other similar drugs for major depressive disorder. Milnacipran should be used with caution in patients with a history of mania.

Patients with History of Dysuria. Because of their noradrenergic effect, SNRIs, including milnacipran, may affect urethral resistance and micturition. In controlled fibromyalgia trials, dysuria occurred in 1% of milnacipran-treated patients compared with 0.5% of those receiving placebo. The manufacturer recommends exercising caution if milnacipran is used in patients with a history of dysuria, particularly in males with prostatic hypertrophy, prostatitis, and other lower urinary tract obstructive disorders. Male patients are more likely to experience adverse genitourinary effects, such as dysuria and urinary retention; they may also experience testicular pain or ejaculation disorders.

Angle-closure Glaucoma. The pupillary dilation (mydriasis) that occurs following the use of SNRIs, including milnacipran, may trigger an acute attack of angle-closure glaucoma (narrow-angle glaucoma) in patients with anatomically narrow angles who do not have a patent iridectomy. (See Advice to Patients.)

Concomitant Use with Alcohol. In clinical trials, more milnacipran-treated patients developed elevated serum transaminases than did those receiving placebo. Because it is possible that milnacipran may aggravate preexisting hepatic disease, the drug should not be prescribed to patients with substantial alcohol consumption or evidence of chronic hepatic disease. (See Hepatic Effects under Warnings/Precautions: Other Warnings and Precautions, in Cautions.)

Specific Populations

Pregnancy. Category C. (See Users Guide.)

The Savella Pregnancy Registry may be contacted at 877-643-3010 (for clinicians and patients); registry information also is available on the website http://www.savellapregnancyregistry.com or by e-mail at pregnancyregistries2@INCResearch.com.

Some neonates exposed to SNRIs or SSRIs late in the third trimester of pregnancy have developed complications, which have sometimes been severe and required prolonged hospitalization, respiratory support, enteral nutrition, and other forms of supportive care in special-care nurseries. Such complications may arise immediately upon delivery and usually last several days or up to 2–4 weeks. Clinical findings reported to date in the neonates have included respiratory distress, cyanosis, apnea, seizures, temperature instability or fever, feeding difficulty, dehydration, excessive weight loss, vomiting, hypoglycemia, hypotonia, hypertonia, hyperreflexia, tremor, jitteriness, irritability, lethargy, reduced or lack of reaction to pain stimuli, and constant crying. These clinical features appear to be consistent with either a direct toxic effect of the SNRI or SSRI or, possibly, a drug withdrawal syndrome. In some cases, the clinical picture was consistent with serotonin syndrome (see Serotonin Syndrome under Warnings/Precautions, in Cautions).

Lactation. Milnacipran is distributed into human milk. In a pharmacokinetic study in lactating women given a single, 50-mg dose of the drug, the maximum estimated daily infant dose from breast milk was 5% of the maternal dose based on peak plasma concentrations. In most patients, peak concentrations of milnacipran in breast milk occurred within 4 hours after the maternal dose. Because data regarding infant exposure to milnacipran are limited, caution should be exercised when milnacipran is administered to a nursing woman.

Pediatric Use. The manufacturer states that safety and effectiveness of milnacipran in pediatric patients younger than 18 years of age with fibromyalgia have not been established and that the drug is *not* recommended for use in such patients. Fibromyalgia in children and adolescents has not been as well studied as in adults to date; however, the syndrome appeared to be characterized by diffuse pain and sleep disturbances in one pediatric patient series.

Milnacipran is an SNRI and is similar to some drugs used for the treatment of depression and other psychiatric disorders. FDA warns that a greater risk of suicidal thinking or behavior (suicidality) occurred during the first few months of antidepressant treatment compared with placebo in children and adolescents with major depressive disorder, obsessive-compulsive disorder (OCD), or other psychiatric disorders based on pooled analyses of 24 short-term, placebo-controlled trials of 9 antidepressant drugs (SSRIs and other antidepressants). However, a more recent meta-analysis of 27 placebo-controlled trials of 9 antidepressants (SSRIs and others) in patients younger than 19 years of age with major depressive disorder, OCD, or non-OCD anxiety disorders suggests that the benefits of antidepressant therapy in treating these conditions may outweigh the risks of suicidal behavior or suicidal ideation. No suicides occurred in these pediatric trials.

These findings should be carefully considered when assessing potential benefits and risks of milnacipran in a child or adolescent for any clinical use. (See Worsening of Depression and Suicidality Risk under Warnings/Precautions: Warnings, in Cautions.)

Geriatric Use. In controlled trials of milnacipran, 402 patients were 60 years of age or older; no overall differences in efficacy or safety were observed between these patients and younger adults.

Because milnacipran and its metabolites are eliminated principally by renal excretion and because of expected decreases in renal function with increasing age, renal function should be considered prior to using the drug in geriatric patients. (See Dosage and Administration: Special Populations.)

SSRIs and SNRIs, including milnacipran, have been associated with clinically important hyponatremia in geriatric patients, who may be at greater risk for this adverse effect. (See Hyponatremia/Syndrome of Inappropriate Antidiuretic Hormone Secretion under Warnings/Precautions: Other Warnings and Precautions, in Cautions.)

In pooled data analyses, a *reduced* risk of suicidality was observed in adults 65 years of age or older with antidepressant therapy compared with placebo. (See Worsening of Depression and Suicidality Risk under Warnings/Precautions: Warnings, in Cautions.)

Hepatic Impairment. Pharmacokinetics of milnacipran are not substantially affected by mild to moderate hepatic impairment. However, patients with severe hepatic impairment had 31% higher area under the plasma concentration-time curve (AUC) and 55% longer elimination half-lives compared with healthy individuals. Milnacipran should be used with caution in patients with severe hepatic impairment. (See Dosage and Administration: Special Populations.)

Renal Impairment. The elimination half-life of milnacipran is increased in patients with renal impairment compared with healthy individuals. The drug should be used with caution in patients with moderate renal impairment. Dosage adjustment is necessary in patients with severe renal impairment (creatinine clearance of 5–29 mL/minute). (See Dosage and Administration: Special Populations.)

■ **Common Adverse Effects** Adverse effects reported in at least 5% of patients with fibromyalgia receiving milnacipran and at an incidence greater than that reported with placebo in controlled studies include nausea, vomiting, constipation, headache, insomnia, dizziness, hot flushes, hyperhidrosis, palpitations, increased heart rate, hypertension, dry mouth, and migraine.

Drug Interactions

In vitro and in vivo studies suggest that milnacipran is unlikely to be involved in clinically important pharmacokinetic drug interactions.

■ **Drugs Metabolized by Hepatic Microsomal Enzymes** Milnacipran generally does not inhibit cytochrome P-450 (CYP) isoenzymes 1A2, 2A6, 2B6, 2C8, 2C9, 2C19, 2D6, 2E1, or 3A4 in vitro, nor does it induce CYP isoenzymes 1A2, 2B6, 2C8, 2C9, 2C19, or 3A4/5 in vitro.

■ **Drugs Affecting Hepatic Microsomal Enzymes** Milnacipran undergoes minimal CYP-related metabolism.

Inhibitors or inducers of CYP isoenzymes: clinically important pharmacokinetic interaction is unlikely.

■ **Drugs Affecting Hemostasis** Altered anticoagulant effects, including increased bleeding, have been reported when SSRIs or SNRIs were administered concurrently with warfarin.

Steady-state milnacipran (200 mg daily) did not affect the pharmacokinetics or pharmacodynamics (assessed by measurement of prothrombin international normalized ratio [INR]) of a single 25-mg dose of warfarin. Warfarin did not affect the pharmacokinetics of milnacipran.

The risk of bleeding may be increased if milnacipran is used concurrently with aspirin or other nonsteroidal anti-inflammatory agents (NSAIAs). Patients should be advised of the risk of bleeding associated with the concomitant use of milnacipran and aspirin or other NSAIAs, warfarin, or other drugs that affect coagulation.

■ **CNS-active Drugs** Because of the CNS effects of milnacipran, use caution when administered concurrently with other centrally-acting drugs, including those with a similar mechanism of action.

■ **Monoamine Oxidase Inhibitors** Concomitant use of SSRIs and SNRIs (e.g., milnacipran) and monoamine oxidase (MAO) inhibitors is associated with a risk of serious, sometimes fatal, serotonin syndrome. Concomitant use of MAO inhibitors intended to treat psychiatric disorders with milnacipran is contraindicated. In addition, at least 2 weeks should elapse between discontinuance of an MAO inhibitor intended to treat psychiatric disorders and initiation of milnacipran and at least 5 days should elapse between discontinuance of milnacipran and initiation of an MAO inhibitor intended to treat psychiatric disorders. (See Contraindications and also see Serotonin Syndrome under Warnings/Precautions: Other Warnings and Precautions, in Cautions.)

■ **Serotonergic Drugs** Concomitant use of milnacipran and other serotonergic drugs, including selective serotonin-reuptake inhibitors (SSRIs), selective serotonin- and norepinephrine-reuptake inhibitors (SNRIs), serotonin (5-hydroxytryptamine; 5-HT) type 1 receptor agonists ("triptans"), tricyclic antidepressants, buspirone, fentanyl, lithium, tramadol, tryptophan, and St. John's wort (*Hypericum perforatum*), is associated with a risk of serious, sometimes fatal, serotonin syndrome. If concomitant use of milnacipran and other serotonergic drugs is clinically warranted, patients should be advised of the increased risk for serotonin syndrome, particularly during treatment initiation and dosage increases (see Advice to Patients). If serotonin syndrome manifestations occur, treatment with milnacipran and any concurrently administered serotonergic agents should be discontinued immediately and supportive and symptomatic treatment should be initiated. (See Serotonin Syndrome under Warnings/Precautions: Other Warnings and Precautions, in Cautions.)

Clomipramine Switching from clomipramine (75 mg once daily) to milnacipran (100 mg daily) without a washout period did not result in clinically important changes in the pharmacokinetics of milnacipran. However, because an increase in adverse effects (e.g., euphoria, postural hypotension) was observed after switching from clomipramine to milnacipran therapy, the manufacturer of milnacipran recommends monitoring patients during the treatment switch.

Fluoxetine Switching patients from fluoxetine (20 mg once daily) to milnacipran (100 mg daily) without a washout period did not substantially affect the pharmacokinetics of milnacipran.

Lithium Multiple-dose administration of milnacipran (100 mg daily) did not affect the pharmacokinetics of lithium.

■ **Drugs that Increase Blood Pressure and Heart Rate** Concurrent use of milnacipran with other drugs that increase blood pressure and heart rate has not been evaluated; such combinations should be used with caution.

■ **Alcohol** Because milnacipran may possibly aggravate preexisting hepatic disease, the drug should not be prescribed to patients with substantial alcohol consumption or evidence of chronic hepatic disease. (See Hepatic Effects under Warnings/Precautions: Other Warnings and Precautions, in Cautions.)

■ **Carbamazepine** Carbamazepine (200 mg twice daily) given concomitantly with milnacipran (100 mg daily) did not result in clinically important changes in the pharmacokinetics of milnacipran. The pharmacokinetics of carbamazepine or its epoxide metabolite also were not substantially affected during concomitant milnacipran administration.

■ **Clonidine** Because milnacipran inhibits norepinephrine reuptake, concurrent administration with clonidine may inhibit clonidine's antihypertensive effect.

■ **Digoxin** Concomitant milnacipran and digoxin administration may be associated with potentiation of adverse hemodynamic effects. Postural hypotension and tachycardia have been reported in patients receiving combined milnacipran and IV digoxin (1 mg). The manufacturer of milnacipran therefore recommends avoiding combined milnacipran and IV digoxin therapy.

There was no pharmacokinetic interaction between milnacipran (200 mg daily) and digoxin (200 mcg daily given as Lanoxicaps®) following multiple-dose oral administration to healthy individuals.

■ **Diuretics** Concomitant use of milnacipran and diuretics may increase the risk of hyponatremia. (See Hyponatremia/Syndrome of Inappropriate Antidiuretic Hormone Secretion under Warnings/Precautions: Other Warnings and Precautions, in Cautions.)

■ **Epinephrine and Norepinephrine** Because milnacipran inhibits norepinephrine reuptake, concurrent administration with epinephrine or norepinephrine may be associated with paroxysmal hypertension and possible cardiac arrhythmias.

■ **Linezolid** Linezolid, an anti-infective agent that is also a reversible MAO inhibitor, has been associated with drug interactions resulting in serotonin syndrome, including some associated with SSRIs and SNRIs. Because of this potential risk, linezolid generally should not be used in patients receiving serotonergic drugs such as milnacipran. However, the manufacturer of milnacipran and the US Food and Drug Administration (FDA) state that certain life-threatening or urgent situations may necessitate immediate linezolid treatment in a patient receiving a serotonergic drug such as milnacipran. In such emergency situations, the availability of alternative anti-infectives should be considered and the benefits of linezolid should be weighed against the risk of serotonin syndrome. If linezolid is indicated in such emergency situations, milnacipran must be immediately discontinued and the patient monitored for symptoms of CNS toxicity for 5 days or until 24 hours after the last linezolid dose, whichever comes first. Treatment with milnacipran may be resumed 24 hours after the last linezolid dose.

Treatment with milnacipran should not be initiated in a patient receiving linezolid. In patients who require more urgent treatment of a psychiatric condition, other interventions, including hospitalization, should be considered. Milnacipran may be started 24 hours after the last linezolid dose. (See Contraindications and also see Serotonin Syndrome under Warnings/Precautions: Other Warnings and Precautions, in Cautions.)

■ **Lorazepam** There was no pharmacokinetic interaction between a single dose of milnacipran 50 mg and lorazepam 1.5 mg.

■ **Methylene Blue** Methylene blue, a potent and reversible inhibitor of MAO-A, has been associated with drug interactions resulting in serotonin syndrome, including some associated with SSRIs and SNRIs. Most of these cases occurred when methylene blue (1–8 mg/kg IV) was used as a diagnostic (visualizing) dye† during parathyroid surgery; it is unclear whether there is a risk of serotonin syndrome when methylene blue is administered by other routes or in lower IV doses in patients receiving serotonergic drugs. Because of this potential risk, methylene blue generally should not be used in patients receiving serotonergic drugs such as milnacipran. However, the manufacturer of milnacipran and the FDA state that certain life-threatening or urgent situations may necessitate immediate IV methylene blue use in a patient receiving a serotonergic drug such as milnacipran. In such emergency situations, the availability of alternative interventions should be considered and the benefits of methylene blue should be weighed against the risk of serotonin syndrome. If methylene blue is indicated in such emergency situations, milnacipran must be immediately discontinued and the patient monitored for symptoms of CNS toxicity for 5 days or until 24 hours after the last methylene blue dose, whichever comes first. Treatment with milnacipran may be resumed 24 hours after the last methylene blue dose.

Treatment with milnacipran should not be initiated in a patient receiving IV methylene blue. In patients who require more urgent treatment of a psychiatric condition, other interventions, including hospitalization, should be considered. Milnacipran may be started 24 hours after the last IV methylene blue dose. (See Contraindications and also see Serotonin Syndrome under Warnings/Precautions: Other Warnings and Precautions, in Cautions.)

The manufacturer of milnacipran states that the risk of administering methylene blue by non-IV routes (e.g., oral tablets, local injection) or in IV doses much lower than 1 mg/kg in patients receiving milnacipran is unclear. Clinicians should be aware of the possibility of the emergent symptoms of serotonin syndrome with concomitant use.

■ **Pregabalin** Concomitant administration of milnacipran (50 mg twice daily) and pregabalin (150 mg twice daily) did not have a clinically important effect on the steady-state pharmacokinetics of either drug. In an open-label study, the addition of milnacipran to pregabalin therapy in patients with fibromyalgia was generally well tolerated and did not appear to exacerbate adverse effects associated with either drug.

Description

Milnacipran hydrochloride is a selective serotonin- and norepinephrine-reuptake inhibitor (SNRI). The drug is pharmacologically related to duloxetine, desvenlafaxine, and venlafaxine. Milnacipran is a racemic mixture of the 1*S*,2*R* and 1*R*,2*S* enantiomers; the more active 1*S*,2*R* enantiomer of milnacipran, levomilnacipran, is used in the treatment of major depressive disorder.

The exact mechanisms of the central pain inhibitory action of milnacipran hydrochloride and its ability to improve the symptoms of fibromyalgia have not been fully elucidated, but appear to be related to the drug's inhibitory effect on the reuptake of both serotonin and norepinephrine. Like other SNRIs, milnacipran has demonstrated antidepressant activity in clinical studies, presumably also due to potentiation of serotonergic and noradrenergic activity in the CNS. The drug inhibits the reuptake of norepinephrine with approximately threefold greater potency than serotonin in vitro without directly affecting the uptake of dopamine or other neurotransmitters. Milnacipran hydrochloride has not demonstrated substantial affinity for serotonergic (5-HT_{1-7}), α- and β-adrenergic, muscarinic (M_{1-5}), histaminergic (H_{1-4}), dopaminergic (D_{1-5}), opiate, benzodiazepine, and γ-aminobutyric acid (GABA) receptors in vitro. The drug does not inhibit the activity of human monoamine oxidases (MAO-A and MAO-B) or acetylcholinesterase.

Milnacipran hydrochloride is principally metabolized via glucuronide conjugation and, to a lesser extent, *N*-dealkylation. The drug generally does not inhibit the cytochrome P-450 (CYP) 1A2, 2A6, 2C9, 2C19, 2D6, 2E1, and 3A4 isoenzymes and does not induce the CYP1A2, 2B6, 2C8, 2C9, 2C19, or 3A4/5 isoenzymes. The drug exhibits a low degree of protein binding (13%) and has a mean elimination half-life of approximately 6–8 hours. Milnacipran and its metabolites are eliminated principally (90%) by renal excretion. Following administration of a single radiolabeled dose of milnacipran hydrochloride, approximately 55% of the dose is eliminated unchanged in urine, approximately 17% is eliminated as the *l*-milnacipran carbamoyl-O-glucuronide, approximately 2% as the *d*-milnacipran carbamoyl-O-glucuronide, and approximately 8% as the *N*-desmethyl milnacipran metabolite.

Advice to Patients

Importance of providing copy of written patient information (medication guide) each time milnacipran hydrochloride is dispensed. Importance of advising patients to read the patient information before taking milnacipran and each time the prescription is refilled.

Risk of suicidality; importance of patients, family, and caregivers being alert to and immediately reporting emergence of suicidality, worsening depression, or unusual changes in behavior, especially during the first few months of therapy or during periods of dosage adjustment. (See Worsening of Depression and Suicidality Risk under Warnings/Precautions: Warnings, in Cautions.)

Importance of informing patients of potential risk of serotonin syndrome, particularly with concurrent use of milnacipran and other serotonergic agents, including 5-HT_1 receptor agonists (triptans), tricyclic antidepressants, buspirone, fentanyl, lithium, tramadol, tryptophan, and St. John's wort (*Hypericum perforatum*), and with drugs that impair serotonin metabolism, particularly monoamine oxidase (MAO) inhibitors, both those used to treat psychiatric disorders and others (e.g., linezolid). Importance of immediately contacting clinician if manifestations of serotonin syndrome develop (e.g., restlessness, hallucinations, delirium, loss of coordination, tachycardia, increased body temperature, sweating, muscle stiffness, labile blood pressure, diarrhea, coma, nausea, vomiting, confusion).

Importance of instructing patients not to take milnacipran with an MAO inhibitor or within 14 days of stopping an MAO inhibitor, and to allow 5 days after stopping milnacipran before starting therapy with an MAO inhibitor.

Possible increased risk of hepatotoxicity in patients with a history of substantial alcohol use. Importance of advising patients to discuss their alcohol intake with their clinician prior to initiating milnacipran therapy. (See Hepatic Effects under Warnings/Precautions: Other Warnings and Precautions and also see Drug Interactions: Alcohol.)

Risk of increased blood pressure and heart rate; importance of advising patients that their blood pressure and heart rate should be measured prior to initiating milnacipran and periodically during therapy.

Risk that milnacipran may diminish mental and physical capacities necessary to drive motor vehicles or operate machinery; importance of cautioning patients about not operating machinery or driving motor vehicles until patients are reasonably certain that milnacipran therapy does not adversely affect their ability to engage in such activities.

Importance of advising patients not to stop taking milnacipran without first talking with their clinician. Importance of patients being aware that discontinuance effects may occur when stopping milnacipran, especially with abrupt discontinuance of the drug.

If a dose of milnacipran is missed, importance of advising patients that the missed dose should be skipped and the next dose should be taken at the regularly scheduled time.

Importance of informing patients that if they receive diuretics, are otherwise volume depleted, or are elderly, that they may be at greater risk of developing hyponatremia during milnacipran therapy.

Importance of advising patients that milnacipran can cause mild pupillary dilation, which can lead to an episode of angle-closure glaucoma in susceptible individuals. Possible symptoms include eye pain, vision changes, and swelling or redness in or around the eye. Preexisting glaucoma is almost always open-angle glaucoma since angle-closure glaucoma can be treated definitively with iridectomy when diagnosed; open-angle glaucoma is not a risk factor for angle-closure glaucoma. Patients may wish to be examined to determine whether they are susceptible to angle-closure glaucoma and have a prophylactic procedure (e.g., iridectomy) if they are susceptible.

Importance of women informing clinicians if they are or plan to become pregnant or plan to breast-feed. Importance of clinicians informing women about the existence of and encouraging enrollment in the Savella Pregnancy Registry (see Pregnancy under Warnings/Precautions: Specific Populations, in Cautions).

Importance of informing clinicians of existing or contemplated concomitant therapy, including prescription and OTC drugs or herbal supplements, as well as any concomitant illnesses (e.g., cardiovascular disease, liver disease, glaucoma) or personal or family history of suicidality or bipolar disorder. Importance of advising patients about the risk of bleeding associated with concomitant use of milnacipran with aspirin or other nonsteroidal anti-inflammatory agents, warfarin, or other drugs that affect coagulation.

Importance of informing patients of other important precautionary information. (See Cautions.)

Overview® (see Users Guide). For additional information on this drug until a more detailed monograph is developed and published, the manufacturer's labeling should be consulted. It is *essential* that the manufacturer's labeling be consulted for more detailed information on usual cautions, precautions, contraindications, potential drug interactions, laboratory test interferences, and acute toxicity.

Preparations

Excipients in commercially available drug preparations may have clinically important effects in some individuals; consult specific product labeling for details.

Milnacipran Hydrochloride

Oral		
Titration Pack	5 Tablets, film-coated, Milnacipran Hydrochloride 12.5 mg (Savella®)	Savella® Titration Pack (available as blister package for first month of therapy), Forest
	8 Tablets, film-coated, Milnacipran Hydrochloride 25 mg (Savella®)	
	42 Tablets, film-coated, Milnacipran Hydrochloride 50 mg (Savella®)	
Tablets, film-coated	12.5 mg	Savella®, Forest
	25 mg	Savella®, Forest
	50 mg	Savella®, Forest
	100 mg	Savella®, Forest

†Use is not currently included in the labeling approved by the US Food and Drug Administration

Vesicular Monoamine Transporter 2 (VMAT2) Inhibitors 28:56

Deutetrabenazine

■ Deutetrabenazine, a vesicular monoamine transporter 2 (VMAT2) inhibitor, is a monoamine-depleting agent. The drug is a deuterium-substituted derivative of tetrabenazine.

Uses

■ **Huntington's Chorea** Deutetrabenazine is used in the treatment of chorea associated with Huntington's disease. The drug has been designated an orphan drug by FDA for the treatment of Huntington's disease.

Efficacy of deutetrabenazine in the management of chorea associated with Huntington's disease was established primarily in a randomized, double-blind, placebo-controlled, multicenter study in 90 ambulatory adults with manifest chorea associated with Huntington's disease. The treatment duration in this study was 12 weeks, and included an 8-week dosage titration period followed by a 4-week maintenance period and a 1-week washout period. Deutetrabenazine therapy was initiated at a dosage of 6 mg daily and then titrated in 6-mg increments every week until satisfactory control of chorea was achieved or intolerable adverse effects occurred, up to a maximum dosage of 48 mg daily. The mean deutetrabenazine dosage after titration was approximately 40 mg daily. The primary measure of efficacy was the Total Maximal Chorea (TMC) score, an item from the Unified Huntington's Disease Rating Scale that totals maximal chorea scores for 7 regions of the body. From baseline to the 4-week maintenance period, the TMC score (average of the scores obtained at weeks 9 and 12) was substantially reduced in deutetrabenazine-treated patients compared with those who received placebo (a reduction of approximately 4.4 units compared with a reduction of approximately 1.9 units, respectively). In addition, in both patient- and physician-rated global impression of change scales, a substantially greater percentage of patients receiving deutetrabenazine achieved treatment success (i.e., a rating of their symptoms as "much improved" or "very much improved") compared with those who received placebo. Following discontinuance of therapy, TMC scores in both groups of patients returned to pretreatment baseline values following the 1-week washout period in this study.

Although no direct, comparative studies between deutetrabenazine and tetrabenazine have been conducted to date, an analysis of the similarly designed, principal phase 3 efficacy studies of both drugs in patients with Huntington's disease suggested that deutetrabenazine is associated with a lower risk of moderate to severe adverse effects than tetrabenazine. The rate of dosage reduction or drug discontinuance due to adverse effects also was lower in the deutetrabenazine study than in the tetrabenazine study. In addition to an apparently lower risk of adverse effects with deutetrabenazine compared with tetrabenazine, deutetrabenazine may be given twice daily compared with 3 times daily for most patients receiving tetrabenazine. These clinical differences appear to be related to the different pharmacokinetic profiles of deutetrabenazine and tetrabenazine (see Description).

■ **Tardive Dyskinesia** Deutetrabenazine is used for the treatment of tardive dyskinesia.

Tardive dyskinesia is a hyperkinetic movement disorder characterized by stereotypical, repetitive, involuntary movements in the oral-facial region (e.g., lip smacking or pursing, movement and/or protrusion of the tongue, chewing movements); symptoms can range from mild to severe and can be socially and functionally disabling in some patients. Involvement of the trunk, extremities, and respiratory system occurs less commonly and can affect balance, speech, and breathing. The syndrome can develop with prolonged use of antidopaminergic drugs, particularly conventional or first-generation antipsychotic agents and metoclopramide; symptoms of tardive dyskinesia typically persist for years or decades. The risk of developing tardive dyskinesia appears to be greater in geriatric patients and women (particularly postmenopausal women); other risk factors include the use of higher dosages and longer duration of antidopaminergic drug exposure, presence of antipsychotic-induced parkinsonian symptoms, concurrent affective disorder, presence of negative schizophrenia symptoms, alcohol and drug abuse, and certain concurrent medical conditions (such as diabetes mellitus).

Management of tardive dyskinesia generally includes gradual discontinuance of the precipitating drug or reducing its dosage, if possible; switching from a conventional or first-generation antipsychotic agent to an atypical or second-generation antipsychotic agent; or switching to clozapine therapy. For additional information on tardive dyskinesia, including manifestations and treatment, see Tardive Dyskinesia under Cautions: Nervous System Effects, in the Phenothiazines General Statement 28:16.08.24.

Efficacy of deutetrabenazine in the management of tardive dyskinesia was established in 2 randomized, double-blind, placebo-controlled, multicenter studies of 12 weeks' duration conducted in 335 ambulatory adults with tardive dyskinesia caused by dopamine receptor antagonists (the AIM-TD and ARM-TD studies). In both of these studies, deutetrabenazine-treated patients experienced greater improvement in tardive dyskinesia symptoms compared with those who received placebo. Patients in both studies had a diagnosis of tardive dyskinesia for at least 3 months prior to screening with a score of at least 6 on the Abnormal Involuntary Movement Scale (AIMS) and a history of antidopaminergic drug exposure for at least 3 months (or at least 1 month in patients 60 years of age and older). In both of these studies, 62% of patients had schizophrenia or schizoaffective disorder and 33% had a mood disorder; 64% of patients were concurrently receiving atypical antipsychotics, 12% were receiving first-generation or combination antipsychotic therapy, and 24% were not receiving any antipsychotic therapy. Patients with suicidal ideation or behavior within 6 months of screening and those with untreated or undertreated psychiatric conditions were excluded from the studies. The primary measure of efficacy for assessing tardive dyskinesia was the AIMS dyskinesia total score, a subset of items 1–7 of the 12-item AIMS that assesses the severity of involuntary movements across body regions; the primary efficacy endpoint in both studies was the change in AIMS total score from baseline to week 12. AIMS scores were verified by expert central reviewers blinded to treatment assignment, visit number, investigation site, and recording date via video recording.

AIM-TD was a fixed-dose study; patients were randomized in a 1:1:1:1 ratio to receive fixed deutetrabenazine target dosages of 12, 24, or 36 mg daily or placebo. Deutetrabenazine was initiated at a dosage of 12 mg daily (administered as 6 mg twice daily) and then increased in 6-mg increments at weekly intervals over 4 weeks until the target dosage was reached; the target dosage was then maintained for 8 weeks followed by a 1-week washout period. From baseline to week 12, the mean AIMS dyskinesia total score significantly improved in patients receiving deutetrabenazine 24 or 36 mg daily but not in those receiving deutetrabenazine 12 mg daily or placebo; the improvement was evident by week 2 and maintained throughout the treatment period.

ARM-TD was a flexible-dose study; deutetrabenazine was initiated at a dosage of 12 mg daily (administered as 6 mg twice daily) and then could be increased in 6-mg increments at weekly intervals over 6 weeks until satisfactory control of dyskinesia was achieved, intolerable adverse effects occurred, or a maximum dosage of 48 mg daily was reached; the individualized dosage was maintained for another 6 weeks followed by a 1-week washout period. From baseline to week 12, the mean AIMS dyskinesia total score significantly improved in patients receiving deutetrabenazine compared with patients receiving placebo. The average deutetrabenazine dosage after titration was 38.8 mg daily, and the dosage remained stable (38.3 mg) through week 12.

■ **Tourette's Syndrome** Deutetrabenazine has been used for the symptomatic management of Tourette's syndrome (Gilles de la Tourette's syndrome)† in a limited number of patients (see Pediatric Use under Warnings/Precautions: Specific Populations, in Cautions). The drug has been designated an orphan drug by FDA for the treatment of Tourette's syndrome in pediatric patients.

Dosage and Administration

■ **General** ***Restricted Distribution*** Deutetrabenazine is available only through a specialty pharmacy program called Shared Solutions®. Patients and clinicians may consult Shared Solutions® for specific availability information at http://www.sharedsolutions.com/ or at 800-887-8100.

■ **Administration** Deutetrabenazine is administered orally with food. The tablets should be swallowed whole and *not* chewed, crushed, or broken.

Total daily dosages less than 12 mg are administered once daily; total daily dosages of 12 mg or higher should be administered in 2 divided doses.

Patients with Huntington's disease receiving deutetrabenazine should be observed closely for clinical worsening or emergence of depression, suicidal thoughts or behavior (suicidality), or unusual changes in behavior. (See Depression and Suicidality in Patients with Huntington's Disease under Warnings/Precautions: Warnings, in Cautions.)

In patients at risk for QT-interval prolongation, the QT interval should be monitored before and after increasing the total deutetrabenazine dosage above 24 mg daily. (See Prolongation of QT Interval under Warnings/Precautions: Other Warnings and Precautions, in Cautions.)

The manufacturer states that at least 14 days must elapse between discontinuance of a monoamine oxidase (MAO) inhibitor and initiation of deutetrabenazine; in addition, at least 20 days must elapse between discontinuance of reserpine and initiation of deutetrabenazine. (See Cautions: Contraindications.)

■ **Dosage** Dosage of deutetrabenazine should be individualized based on efficacy (i.e., reduction of chorea or tardive dyskinesia) and tolerability.

Huntington's Chorea In patients not currently receiving tetrabenazine, the recommended initial dosage of deutetrabenazine for the management of chorea associated with Huntington's disease in adults is 6 mg once daily. Dosage may be increased in 6-mg increments at weekly intervals up to the maximum recommended dosage of 48 mg daily. Daily dosages of 12 mg or higher should be administered in 2 divided doses.

If deutetrabenazine therapy is interrupted for more than 1 week, the drug should be retitrated (i.e., starting with 6 mg once daily). Following treatment interruptions of less than 1 week, treatment can be resumed at the previous maintenance dosage without titration.

Treatment with deutetrabenazine may be discontinued without tapering the dosage.

Tardive Dyskinesia In patients not currently receiving tetrabenazine, the recommended initial dosage of deutetrabenazine for the treatment of tardive dyskinesia in adults is 12 mg daily administered in 2 divided doses (6 mg twice daily). Dosage may be increased in 6-mg increments at weekly intervals up to the maximum recommended dosage of 48 mg daily. Daily dosages of 12 mg or higher should be administered in 2 divided doses.

If deutetrabenazine therapy is interrupted for more than 1 week, the drug should be retitrated (i.e., starting with 12 mg daily administered in 2 divided doses). Following treatment interruptions of less than 1 week, treatment can be resumed at the previous maintenance dosage without titration.

Treatment with deutetrabenazine may be discontinued without tapering the dosage.

Transferring Patients from Tetrabenazine to Deutetrabenazine When transferring patients from tetrabenazine to deutetrabenazine therapy, the manufacturer states that tetrabenazine should be discontinued and deutetrabenazine initiated the following day. The recommended initial dosage of deutetrabenazine should be based on the current total daily dosage of tetrabenazine (see Table 1). After switching to deutetrabenazine therapy, dosage of the drug may be adjusted at weekly intervals.

Table 1. Initial Dosage Recommendations for Adults Being Transferred from Tetrabenazine to Deutetrabenazine Therapy.

Current Tetrabenazine Daily Dosage	Initial Deutetrabenazine Dosage Regimen
12.5 mg	6 mg once daily
25 mg	6 mg twice daily
37.5 mg	9 mg twice daily
50 mg	12 mg twice daily
62.5 mg	15 mg twice daily
75 mg	18 mg twice daily
87.5 mg	21 mg twice daily
100 mg	24 mg twice daily

■ **Special Populations** Deutetrabenazine is contraindicated in patients with hepatic impairment. (See Hepatic Impairment under Warnings/Precautions: Specific Populations, in Cautions.)

The manufacturer makes no specific dosage recommendations for deutetrabenazine in patients with renal impairment. The drug has not been evaluated in such patients.

The manufacturer states that the dosage of deutetrabenazine should be selected with caution in geriatric patients, usually beginning with the lower end of the dosage range, because of the greater frequency of decreased hepatic, renal, and/or cardiac function and of concomitant disease or other drug therapy in such patients.

Hepatic Microsomal Enzyme Considerations In patients who are known poor metabolizers of cytochrome P-450 (CYP) isoenzyme 2D6 substrates, the maximum recommended daily dosage of deutetrabenazine is 36 mg and the maximum recommended single dose is 18 mg.

If deutetrabenazine is used concurrently with potent CYP2D6 inhibitors (e.g., bupropion, fluoxetine, paroxetine, quinidine), the maximum recommended daily dosage of deutetrabenazine is 36 mg and the maximum recommended single dose is 18 mg. (See Drug Interactions: Drugs Affecting Hepatic Microsomal Enzymes.)

Cautions

■ **Contraindications** Patients with Huntington's disease who are suicidal or have untreated or inadequately treated depression. (See Depression and Suicidality in Patients with Huntington's Disease under Warnings/Precautions: Warnings, in Cautions.)

Hepatic impairment. (See Hepatic Impairment under Warnings/Precautions: Specific Populations, in Cautions.)

Concomitant therapy with reserpine. At least 20 days should elapse between discontinuance of reserpine and initiation of deutetrabenazine. (See Drug Interactions: Reserpine.)

Concomitant therapy with a monoamine oxidase (MAO) inhibitor. At least 14 days should elapse between discontinuance of an MAO inhibitor and initiation of deutetrabenazine. (See Drug Interactions: Monoamine Oxidase Inhibitors.)

Concomitant therapy with tetrabenazine or valbenazine. (See Drug Interactions: Tetrabenazine and Valbenazine.)

■ Warnings/Precautions

Warnings

Depression and Suicidality in Patients with Huntington's Disease. Patients with Huntington's disease are at an increased risk for depression and suicidal ideation or behavior (suicidality). Deutetrabenazine may increase this risk. In the principal efficacy study evaluating deutetrabenazine in Huntington's disease, depression and suicidal ideation were reported in 4 and 2% of deutetrabenazine-treated patients, respectively, compared with none of the patients receiving placebo. No suicide attempts or completed suicides were reported.

Clinicians considering the use of deutetrabenazine in patients with Huntington's disease must balance the risks of depression and suicidality with the clinical need for treatment of chorea. Patients with Huntington's disease receiving deutetrabenazine should be closely monitored for the emergence or worsening of depression, suicidality, or unusual changes in behavior. In addition, patients and their caregivers and families should be informed of the risk of depression and suicidality and instructed to promptly report any behaviors of concern to the treating clinician. Patients with Huntington's disease who express suicidal ideation require immediate evaluation. If depression or suicidality does not resolve, discontinuance of deutetrabenazine should be considered.

Particular caution should be exercised in treating patients with a history of depression or prior suicide attempts or ideation, which are increased in patients with Huntington's disease. Deutetrabenazine is contraindicated in patients with Huntington's disease who are suicidal or have untreated or inadequately treated depression.

Other Warnings and Precautions

Clinical Worsening and Adverse Effects in Patients with Huntington's Disease. Huntington's disease is a progressive disorder characterized by changes in mood, cognition, chorea, rigidity, and functional capacity over time. Vesicular monoamine transporter 2 (VMAT2) inhibitors, including deutetrabenazine, may cause worsening in mood, cognition, rigidity, and functional capacity.

Clinicians should periodically reevaluate the need for deutetrabenazine in individual patients by assessing its effect on chorea and possible adverse effects, including sedation or somnolence, depression and suicidality, parkinsonism, akathisia, restlessness, and cognitive decline. Distinguishing between drug-induced adverse effects and progression of the underlying disease may be difficult; decreasing the dosage of deutetrabenazine or discontinuing the drug may help the clinician to distinguish between these two possibilities. Underlying chorea also may improve over time in some patients, which may decrease the need for deutetrabenazine.

Prolongation of QT Interval. Deutetrabenazine may prolong the QT interval. In a double-blind, placebo-controlled, crossover study in healthy individuals, a single 24-mg dose of deutetrabenazine caused an approximately 4.5-msec mean increase in the corrected QT (QT_c) interval. In a similar study, a single 50-mg dose of tetrabenazine (a closely related VMAT2 inhibitor) caused a mean increase of approximately 8 msec in the QT_c interval. Effects on the QT interval at higher exposures to deutetrabenazine or tetrabenazine or their metabolites have not been evaluated.

Clinically important QT-interval prolongation with deutetrabenazine may occur in patients who are poor metabolizers of the cytochrome P-450 (CYP) isoenzyme 2D6 or those who are concurrently receiving a potent CYP2D6 inhibitor; dosage reduction may be necessary in such patients. (See Hepatic Microsomal Enzyme Considerations under Dosage: Special Populations, in Dosage and Administration and see also Drug Interactions: Drugs Affecting Hepatic Microsomal Enzymes.)

The risk of torsades de pointes and/or sudden death in association with drugs that prolong the QT_c interval may be increased in certain circumstances, including patients with bradycardia, hypokalemia, or hypomagnesemia; patients receiving other drugs that prolong the QT_c interval; and those with congenital long QT syndrome. Therefore, the manufacturer states that deutetrabenazine should be avoided in patients with congenital long QT syndrome and in those with a history of cardiac arrhythmias. In patients requiring deutetrabenazine dosages above 24 mg daily and who are concurrently receiving other drugs known to prolong the QT_c interval, the manufacturer recommends assessing the QT_c interval before and after increasing the dosage of deutetrabenazine or other drugs known to prolong the QT_c interval. (See Drug Interactions: Drugs that Prolong QT Interval.)

Neuroleptic Malignant Syndrome. Neuroleptic malignant syndrome (NMS), a potentially fatal syndrome, has been reported with drugs that reduce dopaminergic transmission. Although NMS has not been reported in patients receiving deutetrabenazine, the syndrome has been reported in patients receiving tetrabenazine (a closely related VMAT2 inhibitor). Clinicians should be aware of the manifestations of NMS, including hyperpyrexia, muscle rigidity, altered mental status, and autonomic instability (e.g., irregular heart rate, labile blood pressure, tachycardia, diaphoresis, cardiac arrhythmias). Other signs may include increased serum creatine kinase (CK, creatine phosphokinase, CPK) concentrations, myoglobinuria, rhabdomyolysis, and acute renal failure. Management of NMS should include immediate discontinuance of deutetrabenazine, intensive symptomatic treatment and medical monitoring, and treatment of any serious concomitant medical conditions for which specific treatments are available. Recurrence of NMS has been reported; if deutetrabenazine is required following recovery from NMS, the patient should be monitored for signs of recurrence.

For additional information on NMS, see Neuroleptic Malignant Syndrome under Cautions: Nervous System Effects, in the Phenothiazines General Statement 28:16.08.24.

Akathisia, Agitation, and Restlessness. Deutetrabenazine can increase the risk of akathisia, agitation, and restlessness in patients with Huntington's disease or tardive dyskinesia. In patients with Huntington's disease, akathisia, agitation, or restlessness was reported in 4% of deutetrabenazine-treated patients compared with 2% of patients receiving placebo. In patients with tardive dyskinesia, these adverse effects were reported in 2% of deutetrabenazine-treated patients compared with 1% of patients receiving placebo.

Patients receiving deutetrabenazine should be monitored for the presence of akathisia as well as for signs and symptoms of restlessness and agitation since they may indicate developing akathisia. If a patient develops akathisia, the dosage of deutetrabenazine should be reduced; discontinuance of the drug may be necessary in some patients.

Parkinsonism in Patients with Huntington's Disease. Deutetrabenazine may cause parkinsonism in patients with Huntington's disease. Because rigidity can develop as part of the underlying disease process in Huntington's disease, it may be difficult to distinguish between this drug-induced adverse effect and possible disease progression. Drug-induced parkinsonism potentially can cause more functional disability than untreated chorea for some patients with Huntington's disease. If parkinsonism develops during deutetrabenazine therapy, the dosage of deutetrabenazine should be reduced; discontinuance of the drug may be necessary in some patients.

Sedation and Somnolence. Sedation is a common dose-limiting adverse effect of deutetrabenazine. In the principal efficacy study in patients with Huntington's disease, somnolence and fatigue were reported in 11 and 9% of patients receiving the drug, respectively. Deutetrabenazine may impair cognitive and/or motor skills required to perform tasks such as driving or operating complex machinery. (See Advice to Patients.)

Hyperprolactinemia. Although prolactin concentrations were not evaluated in the deutetrabenazine clinical development program, elevated prolactin concentrations have been observed with tetrabenazine, a closely related VMAT2 inhibitor. Peak plasma prolactin concentrations increased four- to fivefold following a single 25-mg tetrabenazine dose in healthy individuals. Although amenorrhea, galactorrhea, gynecomastia, and impotence have been associated with elevated prolactin concentrations, the clinical importance of such elevations for most patients is unknown.

If deutetrabenazine therapy is considered for a patient with previously detected breast cancer, clinicians should consider that approximately one-third of human breast cancers are prolactin dependent in vitro. In addition, chronic hyperprolactinemia (although not evaluated in the deutetrabenazine or tetrabenazine clinical development programs) has been associated with low estrogen concentrations and an increased risk of osteoporosis. If symptomatic hyperprolactinemia is suspected during deutetrabenazine therapy, appropriate laboratory testing should be performed and discontinuance of the drug should be considered.

Binding to Melanin-containing Tissues. Deutetrabenazine and/or its metabolites bind to melanin-containing tissues, which may result in accumulation and possible toxicity with long-term use. The clinical importance of the drug's binding to these tissues is unknown; ophthalmologic monitoring in clinical studies was inadequate to exclude the possibility of injury after long-term drug exposure. Although the manufacturer does not make specific recommendations for periodic ophthalmologic monitoring during deutetrabenazine therapy, the manufacturer states that clinicians should be aware of possible long-term ophthalmologic effects in patients receiving the drug.

Specific Populations

Pregnancy. The manufacturer states that there are no adequate data regarding the developmental risk associated with the use of deutetrabenazine in pregnant women. Reproduction studies revealed no clear adverse effect on embryofetal development when deutetrabenazine was administered orally during the period of organogenesis to rats at dosages up to 6 times the maximum recommended human dosage. However, when tetrabenazine (a closely related VMAT2 inhibitor) was administered to rats throughout pregnancy and lactation, increased stillbirths, reduced pup survival, and delayed pup maturation were observed.

Lactation. It is not known whether deutetrabenazine or its metabolites are distributed into milk in humans. The effects of deutetrabenazine or its metabolites on nursing infants and on milk production also are unknown. The developmental and health benefits of breast-feeding to the infant should be considered along with the mother's clinical need for deutetrabenazine and any potential adverse effects on the breast-fed infant from the drug or from the underlying maternal condition.

Pediatric Use. The manufacturer states that the safety and efficacy of deutetrabenazine in pediatric patients have not been established.

Deutetrabenazine has been used in a limited number of adolescents with tics associated with Tourette's syndrome†. In a short-term, open-label study in 23 adolescents 12–18 years of age, the drug improved tic severity and appeared to be well tolerated. (See Uses: Tourette's Syndrome.)

Geriatric Use. Clinical studies of deutetrabenazine did not include sufficient numbers of patients 65 years of age and older to determine whether geriatric patients respond differently than younger adults. Other clinical experience with deutetrabenazine has not identified differences in responses between geriatric and younger adult patients.

Because of the greater frequency of decreased hepatic, renal, and/or cardiac function and of concomitant disease and drug therapy in geriatric patients, the manufacturer recommends that dosage selection of deutetrabenazine in geriatric patients should be cautious, usually beginning with the lower end of the dosage range.

Renal Impairment. The pharmacokinetics of deutetrabenazine have not been evaluated to date in patients with renal impairment.

Hepatic Impairment. Pharmacokinetics of deutetrabenazine have not been evaluated in patients with hepatic impairment; however, in a clinical study of tetrabenazine (a closely related VMAT2 inhibitor) in patients with hepatic impairment, substantially increased exposure of tetrabenazine and its active metabolites was observed. The clinical importance of this increased exposure of tetrabenazine and its metabolites is unknown. Because of the potential for serious adverse reactions, the manufacturer states that deutetrabenazine is contraindicated in patients with hepatic impairment.

Poor CYP2D6 Metabolizers. Increased exposure of deutetrabenazine's active metabolites (deuterated α-dihydrotetrabenazine [deuterated α-HTBZ] and deuterated β-dihydrotetrabenazine [deuterated β-HTBZ]) is expected in patients who are poor metabolizers of cytochrome P-450 (CYP) isoenzyme 2D6 substrates; in such patients the maximum recommended daily dosage of deutetrabenazine is 36 mg and the maximum recommended single dose is 18 mg.

■ Common Adverse Effects Adverse effects occurring in 4% or more of patients receiving deutetrabenazine in the principal efficacy study in patients with Huntington's disease and at a higher frequency than reported with placebo include somnolence, diarrhea, dry mouth, fatigue, urinary tract infection, insomnia, anxiety, constipation, and contusion.

Adverse effects occurring in 2% or more of patients receiving deutetrabenazine in the principal efficacy studies in patients with tardive dyskinesia and at a higher frequency than reported with placebo include nasopharyngitis, insomnia, somnolence, fatigue, depression or dysthymic disorder, anxiety, diarrhea, dry mouth, and akathisia, agitation, or restlessness.

Drug Interactions

Drug interaction studies evaluating the effect of deutetrabenazine or its active metabolites (deuterated α-dihydrotetrabenazine [deuterated α-HTBZ] and deuterated β-dihydrotetrabenazine [deuterated β-HTBZ]) on cytochrome P-450 (CYP) isoenzymes or P-glycoprotein (P-gp) have not been conducted to date. In vitro studies indicate that other metabolites of deutetrabenazine (M1 and M4) are not expected to cause clinically important drug interactions.

Tetrabenazine, a closely related VMAT2 inhibitor, and its active metabolites (α-HTBZ and β-HTBZ) do not substantially inhibit CYP isoenzymes 1A2, 2B6, 2C8, 2C9, 2C19, 2D6, 2E1, or 3A, nor do they substantially induce CYP isoenzymes 1A2, 2B6, 2C8, 2C9, 2C19, or 3A4 in vitro. Neither tetrabenazine nor its active metabolites are likely to be substrates or inhibitors of P-gp at clinically relevant concentrations.

Deutetrabenazine's active metabolites (deuterated α-HTBZ and deuterated β-HTBZ) are substrates of CYP2D6.

■ Drugs Affecting Hepatic Microsomal Enzymes Concomitant use of deutetrabenazine with potent inhibitors of CYP2D6 (e.g., bupropion, fluoxetine, paroxetine, quinidine) can result in decreased clearance and substantially increased exposure of deutetrabenazine's active metabolites, deuterated α-HTBZ and deuterated β-HTBZ. When the potent CYP2D6 inhibitor paroxetine (20 mg daily for 8 days) was administered concomitantly with deutetrabenazine (single 22.5-mg dose) in healthy individuals, peak plasma concentrations of deuterated α-HTBZ and deuterated β-HTBZ increased 1.2- and 2.2-fold, and area under the plasma concentration-time curve (AUC) increased 1.9- and 6.5-fold, respectively; total combined AUC of deuterated α-HTBZ and deuterated β-HTBZ increased approximately threefold.

Dosage reduction of deutetrabenazine may be required when the drug is used concomitantly with potent CYP2D6 inhibitors. During concurrent use with potent CYP2D6 inhibitors, the maximum recommended daily dosage of deutetrabenazine is 36 mg and the maximum recommended single dose is 18 mg. The effect of moderate or weak CYP2D6 inhibitors (e.g., amiodarone, duloxetine, sertraline, terbinafine) on the pharmacokinetics of deutetrabenazine and its metabolites has not been evaluated.

■ Drugs that Prolong QT Interval Clinically important QT-interval prolongation may occur if deutetrabenazine is used concomitantly with other drugs known to prolong the corrected QT (QT_c) interval, including some antipsychotic agents (e.g., chlorpromazine, haloperidol, thioridazine, ziprasidone), antibiotics (e.g., moxifloxacin), and class Ia (e.g., quinidine, procainamide) and class III antiarrhythmics (e.g., amiodarone, sotalol). In patients receiving such concomitant therapy, the QT_c interval should be assessed before and after deutetrabenazine dosage increases above 24 mg daily or dosage increases of other concurrently administered drugs known to prolong the QT_c interval. (See Prolongation of QT Interval under Warnings/Precautions: Other Warnings and Precautions, in Cautions.)

■ Alcohol and Other CNS Depressants Additive CNS depressant effects (e.g., worsening of sedation and somnolence) may occur when deutetrabenazine is used concomitantly with alcohol or other CNS depressants.

■ Antipsychotic Agents and Other Dopamine Antagonists The manufacturer states that the risk of certain adverse effects associated with deutetrabenazine (e.g., QT_c-interval prolongation, parkinsonism, akathisia, neuroleptic malignant syndrome [NMS]) may be increased with concomitant use of deutetrabenazine and dopamine antagonists, including antipsychotic agents. (See Drug Interactions: Drugs that Prolong QT Interval.)

■ Monoamine Oxidase Inhibitors Because of the potential for antagonistic effects and increased toxicity, concomitant use of deutetrabenazine with a monoamine oxidase (MAO) inhibitor is contraindicated. At least 14 days should elapse between discontinuance of MAO inhibitor therapy and initiation of deutetrabenazine.

■ Reserpine Concomitant use of deutetrabenazine and reserpine (an irreversible VMAT2 inhibitor with a long duration of effect) may result in deutetrabenazine overdosage and major serotonin and norepinephrine depletion in the CNS. Concomitant use of deutetrabenazine with reserpine is therefore contraindicated. Clinicians should wait for signs of chorea or dyskinesia to reemerge after discontinuing reserpine before initiating deutetrabenazine therapy. At least 20 days should elapse after reserpine discontinuance prior to initiating deutetrabenazine therapy.

■ Tetrabenazine and Valbenazine Concomitant use of deutetrabenazine and the related VMAT2 inhibitors tetrabenazine and valbenazine is contraindicated. In patients switching from tetrabenazine therapy, deutetrabenazine may be initiated the following day after discontinuance of tetrabenazine. (See Transferring Patients from Tetrabenazine to Deutetrabenazine under Dosage and Administration: Dosage.)

Description

Deutetrabenazine, a vesicular monoamine transporter 2 (VMAT2) inhibitor, is a monoamine-depleting agent. The drug is a deuterium-substituted analog of tetrabenazine; deuterium, a nontoxic, naturally occurring isotope of hydrogen with a higher relative mass, forms a stronger bond with carbon molecules that hinders metabolism by cytochrome P-450 isoenzymes. Deuterium substitution results in deutetrabenazine active metabolites that have a longer elimination half-life, higher area under the concentration-time curve (AUC), and lower peak plasma concentrations than those achieved with an equivalent dose of tetrabenazine.

Patients with Huntington's disease appear to exhibit oversensitivity to dopamine stimulation, resulting in choreic movements. Although the exact mechanism by which deutetrabenazine exerts its effects in the treatment of tardive dyskinesia and chorea in patients with Huntington's disease has not been fully elucidated, the drug, like tetrabenazine, selectively and reversibly inhibits VMAT2-mediated uptake of monoamine neurotransmitters (e.g., dopamine, norepinephrine, serotonin, histamine) into presynaptic vesicles in the CNS; monoamines not transported into synaptic vesicles are degraded by monoamine oxidase (MAO), resulting in depleted monoamine stores in nerve terminals. Like tetrabenazine, deutetrabenazine and its active metabolites preferentially affect dopaminergic neurotransmission in the CNS over adrenergic, serotonergic, and histaminergic neurotransmission at clinically relevant plasma concentrations.

Following oral administration, deutetrabenazine is rapidly and extensively metabolized, mainly by carbonyl reductase, to the active metabolites deuterated α-dihydrotetrabenazine (deuterated α-HTBZ) and deuterated β-dihydrotetrabenazine (deuterated β-HTBZ); plasma concentrations of the parent drug are generally undetectable. Peak plasma concentrations of deuterated α-HTBZ and deuterated β-HTBZ occur within 3–4 hours following oral administration of the drug; administration with food increases peak plasma concentrations of deuterated α-HTBZ and deuterated β-HTBZ by approximately 50%, but has no effect on the AUC. The drug distributes rapidly into the CNS, with highest and lowest concentrations occurring in the striatum and cortex, respectively. Deuterated α-HTBZ and deuterated β-HTBZ are metabolized primarily by CYP2D6 with minor contributions by CYP isoenzymes 1A2 and 3A4/5 to form several minor metabolites. Approximately 75–86 and 8–11% of a deutetrabenazine dose is eliminated in urine and feces, respectively, with less than 10% eliminated as unchanged deuterated α-HTBZ and deuterated β-HTBZ. The half-life of deuterated α-HTBZ and deuterated β-HTBZ combined is approximately 9–10 hours.

Advice to Patients

Importance of advising patients and their caregivers to read the manufacturer's patient information (medication guide).

Importance of informing patients that deutetrabenazine should be taken with food and that the tablets should be swallowed whole and not chewed, crushed, or broken.

Risk of depression, worsening of depression, and suicidality in patients with Huntington's disease; importance of immediately notifying clinicians of emergence of suicidality, emergence or worsening of depression, suicidality, or unusual changes in behavior in such patients.

Risk of corrected QT (QT_c)-interval prolongation. Importance of patients immediately notifying clinicians if they feel faint, lose consciousness, or experience heart palpitations. Importance of patients advising clinicians that they are taking deutetrabenazine before any new drug is taken.

Risk of sedation and somnolence. Importance of advising patients to exercise caution or avoid engaging in activities requiring mental alertness and coordination such as operating a motor vehicle or other dangerous machinery until they are receiving a maintenance dosage of deutetrabenazine and the effects of the drug on the individual are known.

Importance of informing patients that concomitant use of alcohol or other CNS depressants may worsen the sedative effects of deutetrabenazine.

Importance of informing clinicians of existing or contemplated concomitant therapy, including prescription and OTC drugs or herbal supplements (see Drug Interactions), as well as any concomitant illnesses (e.g., depression or other psychiatric disorders, liver disease, arrhythmias).

Importance of women informing clinicians if they are or plan to become pregnant or plan to breast-feed.

Importance of informing patients of other important precautionary information. (See Cautions.)

Overview® (see Users Guide). For additional information on this drug until a more detailed monograph is developed and published, the manufacturer's labeling should be consulted. It is *essential* that the manufacturer's labeling be consulted for more detailed information on usual cautions, precautions, contraindications, potential drug interactions, laboratory test interferences, and acute toxicity.

Preparations

Distribution of deutetrabenazine is restricted. (See Restricted Distribution under Dosage and Administration: General.)

Excipients in commercially available drug preparations may have clinically important effects in some individuals; consult specific product labeling for details.

Deutetrabenazine

Oral		
Tablets, coated	6 mg	**Austedo®**, Teva
	9 mg	**Austedo®**, Teva
	12 mg	**Austedo®**, Teva

†Use is not currently included in the labeling approved by the US Food and Drug Administration

Valbenazine Tosylate

■ Valbenazine tosylate, a vesicular monoamine transporter 2 (VMAT2) inhibitor, is a monoamine-depleting agent.

Uses

■ **Tardive Dyskinesia** Valbenazine tosylate is used for the treatment of tardive dyskinesia.

Tardive dyskinesia is a hyperkinetic movement disorder characterized by stereotypical, repetitive, involuntary movements in the oral-facial region (e.g., lip smacking or pursing, movement and/or protrusion of the tongue, chewing movements); symptoms can range from mild to severe and can be socially and functionally disabling. Involvement of the trunk, extremities, and respiratory system occurs less commonly and can affect balance, speech, and breathing. The syndrome can develop with prolonged use of antidopaminergic drugs, particularly conventional or first-generation antipsychotic agents and metoclopramide; symptoms of tardive dyskinesia typically persist for years or decades. The risk of developing tardive dyskinesia appears to be greater in geriatric patients and women (particularly postmenopausal women); other risk factors include the use of higher dosages and longer duration of antidopaminergic drug exposure, presence of antipsychotic-induced parkinsonian symptoms, concurrent affective disorder, presence of negative schizophrenia symptoms, alcohol and drug abuse, and certain concurrent medical conditions (such as diabetes mellitus).

Management of tardive dyskinesia generally includes gradual discontinuance of the precipitating drug or reducing its dosage, if possible; switching from a conventional or first-generation antipsychotic agent to an atypical or second-generation antipsychotic agent; or switching to clozapine therapy. For additional information on tardive dyskinesia, including manifestations and treatment, see Tardive Dyskinesia under Cautions: Nervous System Effects, in the Phenothiazines General Statement 28:16.08.24.

Efficacy of valbenazine in the management tardive dyskinesia was established primarily in a randomized, double-blind, phase 3 study (KINECT 3), which consisted of an initial 6-week, placebo-controlled phase followed by a 42-week extension phase, in 234 adults with moderate or severe tardive dyskinesia. Patients in this study met DSM-IV criteria for schizophrenia, schizoaffective disorder, or a mood disorder and had a diagnosis of tardive dyskinesia for at least 3 months prior to screening. In this study, 66% of patients had schizophrenia or schizoaffective disorder, and 34% had a mood disorder; 70% of patients were concurrently receiving atypical antipsychotics, 14% were receiving first-generation or combination antipsychotic therapy, and 16% were not receiving any antipsychotic therapy. Patients considered to be at risk for suicidal or violent behavior and those with unstable psychiatric symptoms were excluded from the study. Patients were initially randomized to receive fixed valbenazine dosages of 40 or 80 mg once daily or placebo for 6 weeks. Following the 6-week, placebo-controlled phase, patients receiving placebo were re-randomized to receive valbenazine 40 or 80 mg once daily in a 42-week extension phase followed by a 4-week washout period. Patients originally randomized to valbenazine continued to receive the drug at the randomized dosage. The primary measure of efficacy for assessing tardive dyskinesia in this study was the Abnormal Involuntary Movement Scale (AIMS) dyskinesia total score, a subset of items 1–7 of the 12-item AIMS that assesses the severity of involuntary moments across body regions. The AIMS was scored by expert central reviewers blinded to subject identification, treatment assignment, and visit number via video recording.

From baseline to week 6, the mean AIMS dyskinesia total score substantially improved in patients receiving valbenazine 80 mg daily compared with patients receiving placebo. Patients receiving the 40-mg dosage also experienced improvement in AIMS dyskinesia total scores; however, the difference was not statistically significant compared with placebo. No substantial difference in mean Clinical Global Impression of Change-Tardive Dyskinesia (CGI-TD) score was observed between either valbenazine dosage group and placebo at week 6. Improvement in mean AIMS dyskinesia total score was observed by week 2 and maintained throughout the 42-week extension period. Following discontinuance of therapy, mean AIMS dyskinesia total scores in both dosage groups returned toward baseline values during the 4-week washout period.

Dosage and Administration

■ **General** ***Restricted Distribution*** Valbenazine tosylate is available only through a specialty pharmacy. Patients and clinicians may contact the INBRACE® Support Program at 844-647-3992 or visit http://inbracesupportprogram.com for further information.

■ **Administration** Valbenazine tosylate capsules are administered orally once daily without regard to meals. (See Description.)

In the principal efficacy study, patients who had received antipsychotic agents continued to receive the antipsychotic treatment regimen they had been stabilized on during valbenazine therapy.

■ **Dosage** Dosage of valbenazine tosylate is expressed in terms of valbenazine.

Tardive Dyskinesia For the treatment of tardive dyskinesia in adults, the recommended initial dosage of valbenazine is 40 mg once daily. After 1 week, the dosage should be increased to the recommended dosage of 80 mg once daily. Continuing therapy at a dosage of 40 mg daily may be considered in some patients.

Continued valbenazine therapy appears to be necessary in patients with tardive dyskinesia; symptoms recur following discontinuance of the drug.

■ **Special Populations** In patients with moderate or severe hepatic impairment (Child-Pugh score of 7–15), the recommended dosage is 40 mg once daily. The manufacturer makes no specific dosage recommendations for patients with mild hepatic impairment.

Dosage adjustment is not necessary in patients with mild to moderate renal impairment (creatinine clearance 30–90 mL/minute). The manufacturer states that valbenazine is not recommended in patients with severe renal impairment (creatinine clearance less than 30 mL/minute).

The manufacturer states that no dosage adjustment is necessary in geriatric patients.

Hepatic Microsomal Enzyme Considerations Dosage adjustments of valbenazine are recommended in patients who are known poor metabolizers of cytochrome P-450 (CYP) isoenzyme 2D6 substrates and in patients concomitantly receiving potent CYP3A4 and/or CYP2D6 inhibitors.

In patients who are known poor metabolizers of CYP2D6, dosage reduction of valbenazine should be considered based on tolerability. (See Poor CYP2D6 Metabolizers under Warnings/Precautions: Specific Populations, in Cautions.)

If valbenazine is used concurrently with potent CYP2D6 inhibitors, valbenazine dosage reduction should be considered based on tolerability. (See Inhibitors of CYP2D6 under Drug Interactions: Drugs Affecting Hepatic Microsomal Enzymes.)

Valbenazine dosage should be reduced to 40 mg once daily when used concurrently with potent CYP3A4 inhibitors. (See Inhibitors of CYP3A4 under Drug Interactions: Drugs Affecting Hepatic Microsomal Enzymes.)

Concomitant use of valbenazine and potent CYP3A4 inducers is not recommended. (See Inducers of CYP3A4 under Drug Interactions: Drugs Affecting Hepatic Microsomal Enzymes.)

Cautions

■ **Contraindications** The manufacturer states there are no known contraindications to the use of valbenazine tosylate.

■ **Warnings/Precautions** ***Somnolence*** Valbenazine can cause somnolence and may impair cognitive and/or physical abilities required to perform potentially hazardous tasks such as driving or operating machinery. (See Advice to Patients.) In several short-term, placebo-controlled trials, somnolence (including fatigue and sedation) was reported in 10.9% of patients receiving valbenazine compared with 4.2% of placebo recipients.

Prolongation of QT Interval Valbenazine therapy may prolong the QT interval; however, the degree of QT-interval prolongation is not clinically important at drug concentrations expected with recommended dosing. Higher than expected plasma concentrations of valbenazine and/or its active metabolite and clinically important QT-interval prolongation may occur in poor metabolizers of cytochrome P-450 (CYP) isoenzyme 2D6 and in patients concurrently receiving a potent CYP2D6 or CYP3A4 inhibitor. Dosage reduction may therefore be required in patients who are poor metabolizers of CYP2D6 or in those concurrently receiving a potent CYP2D6 inhibitor. In patients concurrently receiving a potent CYP3A4 inhibitor, valbenazine dosage should be reduced to 40 mg once daily. (See Hepatic Microsomal Enzyme Considerations under Dosage: Special Populations, in Dosage and Administration and also see Drug Interactions: Drugs Affecting Hepatic Microsomal Enzymes.)

The manufacturer states that valbenazine should be avoided in patients with congenital long QT syndrome or with cardiac arrhythmias associated with a prolonged QT interval. In patients at increased risk of QT-interval prolongation, the QT interval should be assessed prior to increasing the dosage of valbenazine.

Specific Populations **Pregnancy.** The limited available data regarding valbenazine use in pregnant women are insufficient to inform a drug-associated risk. Reproduction studies in animals revealed no malformations when valbenazine was administered orally during the period of organogenesis in rats and rabbits at dosages up to 1.8 and 24 times the maximum recommended human dosage, respectively. However, increased stillbirths and reduced postnatal pup survival were observed when the drug was administered to pregnant rats during organogenesis and lactation at dosages less than the maximum recommended human dosage. Pregnant women should be advised of the potential risk to the fetus.

Lactation. Valbenazine and its metabolites are distributed into milk in rats at concentrations higher than those in maternal plasma; it is not known whether the drug and/or its metabolites distribute into human milk. The effects of valbenazine on nursing infants and on milk production also are not known. Because increased perinatal mortality has been observed in exposed fetuses and pups in animal studies, the manufacturer recommends that women not breast-feed while receiving valbenazine and for 5 days after discontinuance of the drug.

Pediatric Use. Safety and efficacy of valbenazine in pediatric patients have not been established. Tardive dyskinesia rarely occurs in pediatric patients since prolonged antipsychotic therapy usually is needed to cause the condition.

Geriatric Use. In controlled clinical trials of valbenazine, 16% of patients were 65 years of age or older. Safety and efficacy of valbenazine in geriatric patients in these studies were similar to those observed in younger adults. The manufacturer states that dosage adjustment is not necessary in geriatric patients.

Hepatic Impairment. In patients with mild hepatic impairment, peak plasma concentrations and the area under the concentration-time curve (AUC) of valbenazine and its active metabolite are increased less than 1.5-fold; the manufacturer makes no specific dosage recommendations for such patients.

Peak plasma concentrations and AUCs of valbenazine and its active metabolite are increased by up to 2.5- and 3.4-fold, respectively, in patients with moderate or severe hepatic impairment (Child-Pugh score of 7–15); dosage reduction is recommended in such patients. (See Dosage and Administration: Special Populations.)

Renal Impairment. Valbenazine does not undergo primary renal clearance. Dosage adjustment of the drug is not necessary in patients with mild to moderate renal impairment (creatinine clearance 30–90 mL/minute). Use of valbenazine is not recommended in patients with severe renal impairment (creatinine clearance less than 30 mL/minute).

Poor CYP2D6 Metabolizers. Because increased exposure (peak plasma concentration and AUC) of valbenazine's active metabolite is expected in patients who are poor metabolizers of CYP2D6, dosage reduction of valbenazine should be considered in such patients. Increased exposure of the active metabolite may increase the risk of exposure-related adverse effects. (See Hepatic Microsomal Enzyme Considerations under Dosage and Administration: Special Populations.)

■ **Common Adverse Effects** Adverse effects occurring in 2% or more of patients receiving valbenazine in short-term tardive dyskinesia clinical trials and at a higher frequency than reported with placebo include somnolence (including fatigue and sedation), anticholinergic effects (including dry mouth, constipation, attention disturbance, blurred vision, and urinary retention), balance disorders (including falls, gait disturbances, and dizziness), headache, akathisia/restlessness, vomiting, nausea, and arthralgia.

Drug Interactions

Valbenazine is metabolized in part by cytochrome P-450 (CYP) isoenzyme 3A4/5; further biotransformation of the active metabolite is mediated in part by CYP2D6. (See Description.)

In vitro studies indicate that valbenazine and its active metabolite do not inhibit CYP isoenzymes 1A2, 2B6, 2C8, 2C9, 2C19, 2E1, or 3A4/5, nor induce CYP isoenzymes 1A2, 2B6, or 3A4/5 at clinically relevant concentrations.

Valbenazine and its active metabolite are unlikely to inhibit breast cancer resistance protein (BCRP), organic anion transporters (OAT) 1 and OAT3, organic cation transporter (OCT) 2, or organic anion transport proteins (OATP) 1B1 and OATP1B3 at clinically relevant concentrations. Valbenazine inhibits intestinal P-glycoprotein (P-gp).

■ **Drugs Affecting Hepatic Microsomal Enzymes** ***Inhibitors of CYP3A4*** Concomitant use of valbenazine with potent inhibitors of CYP3A4 (e.g., clarithromycin, itraconazole, ketoconazole) may increase exposure of valbenazine and its active metabolite and increase the risk of adverse effects. When the potent CYP3A4 inhibitor ketoconazole was administered concomitantly with valbenazine in healthy individuals, exposures of valbenazine and its active metabolite increased approximately twofold.

Valbenazine dosage should be reduced to 40 mg once daily when used concurrently with potent CYP3A4 inhibitors.

Dosage reduction of valbenazine is not necessary when used concomitantly with weak or moderate CYP3A4 inhibitors.

Inducers of CYP3A4 Concomitant use of valbenazine and potent CYP3A4 inducers (e.g., carbamazepine, phenytoin, rifampin, St. John's wort [*Hypericum perforatum*]) may decrease exposure of valbenazine and its active metabolite and potentially reduce the drug's efficacy. When the potent CYP3A4 inducer rifampin was administered concomitantly with valbenazine in healthy individuals, exposures of valbenazine and its active metabolite were decreased by approximately 70–80%. Concomitant use of valbenazine and potent CYP3A4 inducers is therefore not recommended.

Inhibitors of CYP2D6 Concomitant use of valbenazine with potent inhibitors of CYP2D6 (e.g., fluoxetine, paroxetine, quinidine) may increase the exposure of valbenazine's active metabolite and increase the risk of adverse effects. Dosage reduction of valbenazine based on tolerability should be considered if valbenazine is used concurrently with potent CYP2D6 inhibitors.

■ **Drugs Metabolized by Hepatic Microsomal Enzymes** The manufacturer states that clinically important pharmacokinetic interactions are unlikely and that dosage adjustment of the concurrently administered drug is not necessary when valbenazine is used concurrently with substrates of CYP isoenzymes 1A2, 2B6, 2C8, 2C9, 2C19, 2E1, or 3A4/5.

No clinically important pharmacokinetic interaction was observed when valbenazine was administered with midazolam (a CYP3A4 substrate).

■ **Digoxin** Concomitant use of valbenazine and digoxin resulted in approximately twofold and 1.5-fold increases in peak plasma concentration and the area under the concentration-time curve (AUC) of digoxin, respectively, because of inhibition of intestinal P-glycoprotein. Increased digoxin exposure may increase the risk of exposure-related adverse effects. If digoxin and valbenazine are used concomitantly, serum digoxin concentrations should be monitored and digoxin dosage adjusted, if necessary.

■ **Monoamine Oxidase Inhibitors** Concomitant use of valbenazine and monoamine oxidase (MAO) inhibitors (e.g., isocarboxazid, phenelzine, selegiline, tranylcypromine) may increase the concentration of monoamine neurotransmitters in synapses, potentially leading to an increased risk of adverse reactions such as serotonin syndrome. In addition, valbenazine's efficacy may be reduced. Concomitant use of valbenazine and MAO inhibitors should therefore be avoided.

Description

Valbenazine tosylate, a vesicular monoamine transporter 2 (VMAT2) inhibitor, is a monoamine-depleting agent. Valbenazine is a valine ester prodrug of (+)-α-dihydrotetrabenazine ([+]-α-HTBZ), which also is one of the active metabolites of tetrabenazine. Of the 4 tetrabenazine metabolite isomers, (+)-α-HTBZ has the highest binding affinity and selectivity for VMAT2.

Although the exact mechanism of action of valbenazine in the treatment of tardive dyskinesia has not been fully elucidated, the drug selectively and reversibly inhibits VMAT2, a transporter that regulates the uptake of monoamines (e.g., dopamine, norepinephrine, serotonin, histamine) from the cytoplasm to the synaptic vesicles for storage and release in the CNS. Monoamines not transported into synaptic vesicles are rapidly degraded by monoamine oxidase (MAO), resulting in depleted monoamine stores in nerve terminals.

Valbenazine and its (+)-α-HTBZ metabolite have no appreciable binding affinity for VMAT1 or for dopaminergic (including D_2), serotonergic (including 5-HT_{2B}), adrenergic, histaminergic, or muscarinic receptors.

Following oral administration of valbenazine tosylate capsules, the drug undergoes ester hydrolysis to form the major active metabolite, (+)-α-HTBZ. Peak plasma concentrations of valbenazine and (+)-α-HTBZ occur in 30–60 minutes and 4–8 hours, respectively. The absolute oral bioavailability of valbenazine is approximately 49%. Steady-state plasma concentrations of valbenazine are achieved within 1 week. Administration of the capsules with a high-fat meal decreases peak plasma concentration and AUC of valbenazine by approximately 47 and 13%, respectively; peak plasma concentration and AUC of (+)-α-HTBZ are not substantially affected. In addition to undergoing ester hydrolysis to the major active metabolite (+)-α-HTBZ, valbenazine is metabolized by cytochrome P-450 (CYP) isoenzyme 3A4/5 to other metabolites, including NBI-136110. (+)-α-HTBZ is further metabolized in part by CYP2D6. The parent drug and NBI-136110 also inhibit VMAT2 but have approximately 40- to 65-fold lower binding affinity than (+)-α-HTBZ. Valbenazine is highly bound (greater than 99%) to plasma proteins while its active metabolite is approximately 64% protein bound. In rats, valbenazine can bind to melanin-containing structures of the eye such as the uveal tract; the clinical relevance of this observation is not known. Following administration of a single radiolabeled dose of valbenazine, approximately 60 and 30% of the dose is recovered in urine and feces, respectively. Less than 2% of the dose is excreted as unchanged valbenazine or its active metabolite. The half-lives of valbenazine and (+)-α-HTBZ are both 15–22 hours.

Advice to Patients

Importance of advising patients to read the manufacturer's patient information.

Risk of somnolence. Importance of advising patients to exercise caution or avoid engaging in activities requiring mental alertness and coordination such as operating a motor vehicle or other dangerous machinery until the effects of the drug on the individual are known.

Risk of QT-interval prolongation. Importance of informing clinicians immediately if abnormal heartbeat, palpitations, shortness of breath, feelings of dizziness or faintness, or loss of consciousness occurs.

Importance of women informing clinicians if they are or plan to become pregnant or plan to breast-feed. Apprise patient of potential risk to the fetus if used during pregnancy. Importance of advising women to avoid breast-feeding while receiving valbenazine and for 5 days after discontinuance of the drug.

Importance of informing clinicians of existing or contemplated concomitant therapy, including prescription and OTC drugs or herbal supplements (see Drug Interactions), as well as any concomitant illnesses (e.g., liver or kidney disease, cardiovascular disease, arrhythmias).

Importance of informing patients of other important precautionary information. (See Cautions.)

Overview® (see Users Guide). For additional information on this drug until a more detailed monograph is developed and published, the manufacturer's labeling should be consulted. It is *essential* that the manufacturer's labeling be consulted for more detailed information on usual cautions, precautions, contraindications, potential drug interactions, laboratory test interferences, and acute toxicity.

Preparations

Distribution of valbenazine tosylate is restricted. (See Restricted Distribution under Dosage and Administration: General.)

Excipients in commercially available drug preparations may have clinically important effects in some individuals; consult specific product labeling for details.

Valbenazine Tosylate

Oral		
Capsules	40 mg (of valbenazine)	**Ingrezza®**, Neurocrine

CENTRAL NERVOUS SYSTEM AGENTS, MISCELLANEOUS 28:92

Atomoxetine Hydrochloride

■ Atomoxetine is a selective norepinephrine-reuptake inhibitor.

Uses

Atomoxetine hydrochloride is used as an adjunct to psychological, educational, social, and other remedial measures in the treatment of attention-deficit hyperactivity disorder (ADHD).

■ **Attention Deficit Hyperactivity Disorder** Atomoxetine hydrochloride is used as an adjunct to psychological, educational, social, and other remedial measures in the treatment of ADHD (hyperkinetic disorder, hyperkinetic syndrome of childhood, minimal brain dysfunction) in adults and children 6 years of age and older. Efficacy of the drug for this indication was established in short-term (6–9 weeks) controlled clinical studies in children and adolescents 6–18 years of age and also in 10-week controlled clinical studies in adults who met DSM-IV criteria for ADHD. Efficacy of atomoxetine in the treatment of ADHD also was established in one longer-term (12 months) controlled clinical study in children and adolescents 6–15 years of age.

In controlled clinical studies in children 7–13 years of age with ADHD, therapy with atomoxetine (mean final dosage of 1.6 mg/kg daily, administered in 2 divided doses in the morning and late afternoon for 9 weeks) was more effective than placebo in decreasing inattention and hyperactive/impulsive symptoms, as measured by the ADHD Rating Scale-IV-Parent Version (ADHDRS), Clinical Global Impressions-ADHD-Severity (CGI-ADHD-S), and Conners Parent Rating Scale-Revised: Short Form (CPRS-R:S). In another controlled clinical study in children and adolescents 6–16 years of age with ADHD, therapy with atomoxetine (mean final dosage of 1.3 mg/kg once daily in the morning for 6 weeks) was more effective than placebo in decreasing inattention and hyperactive/impulsive symptoms, as measured by the ADHDRS, Conners Parent Rating Scale, and Conners Teacher Rating Scale.

In a randomized, placebo-controlled, dose-response study with atomoxetine (0.5, 1.2, or 1.8 mg/kg daily, administered in 2 divided doses in the morning and late afternoon for 8 weeks) in children and adolescents 8–18 years of age with ADHD, therapy with atomoxetine 1.2 or 1.8 mg/kg daily was more effective than placebo in decreasing inattention and hyperactive/impulsive symptoms, as measured by the ADHDRS, and improving social and family functioning, as measured by the Child Health Questionnaire (CHQ). Patients receiving atomoxetine 0.5 mg/kg daily exhibited responses intermediate to those observed in patients receiving placebo or atomoxetine at higher dosages (1.2 or 1.8 mg/kg daily), but no differences in response were observed between patients receiving dosages of 1.2 versus 1.8 mg/kg daily.

In an open-label, multicenter study in boys 7–15 years of age and girls 7–9 years of age with ADHD, therapy with atomoxetine (up to 2 mg/kg daily, administered in 2 divided doses in the morning and late afternoon) or methylphenidate (up to 60 mg daily, administered once daily or in 2 or 3 divided doses) for 10 weeks produced similar results in the reduction of ADHD symptoms; however, double-blind clinical studies are needed to establish the comparative efficacy and tolerance of these therapies.

In a randomized, double-blind, placebo-controlled maintenance study, 604 children and adolescents 6–15 years of age with ADHD initially received open-label atomoxetine (1.2–1.8 mg/kg daily in 2 divided doses) for 10 weeks. Patients who responded to therapy during the open-label phase were randomized at week 12 to receive either atomoxetine (at the same dosage) or placebo for an additional 9 months. At study end point, relapse (defined as an increase in ADHDRS total score to 90% of baseline score *and* an increase of 2 or more points on the CGI-S scale) occurred in fewer patients receiving atomoxetine compared with those receiving placebo (22 versus 38%). When the more sensitive secondary definition of relapse (an increase in ADHDRS total score to 50% of baseline score *and* an increase of 2 or more points on the CGI-S scale) was used, the relapse rate also was substantially lower in atomoxetine-treated patients (28%) than in placebo-treated patients (48%). In addition, patients who continued receiving atomoxetine experienced a longer time to relapse and achieved superior psychosocial functioning compared to those receiving placebo.

In controlled clinical studies in adults with ADHD, therapy with atomoxetine (mean final dosage of 95 mg daily, administered in 2 equally divided doses in the morning and late afternoon/early evening for 10 weeks) was more effective than placebo in decreasing inattention and hyperactive/impulsive symptoms, as measured by the Conners Adult ADHD Rating Scale (CAARS).

Dosage and Administration

■ **Administration** Atomoxetine hydrochloride may be administered orally once daily in the morning or in 2 equally divided doses in the morning and late afternoon/early evening. The drug may be administered without regard to meals.

The manufacturer states that atomoxetine is an ocular irritant; therefore, the capsules should be swallowed whole and should not be broken or opened, nor should the capsule contents be sprinkled on food.

■ **Dosage** Dosage of atomoxetine hydrochloride is expressed in terms of atomoxetine.

The usual initial dosage of atomoxetine in adults or in children and adolescents weighing more than 70 kg is 40 mg daily; dosage may be increased after a minimum of 3 days to a target dosage of approximately 80 mg daily. If an optimum response has not been achieved after 2–4 additional weeks of therapy, dosage may be increased to a maximum of 100 mg daily; dosages exceeding 100 mg daily have not been shown in clinical trials to result in additional therapeutic benefit. In adults or in children and adolescents weighing more than 70 kg, if atomoxetine is used concomitantly with potent inhibitors of the cytochrome P-450 2D6 (CYP2D6) isoenzyme (e.g., paroxetine, fluoxetine, quinidine) or in patients with poor metabolizer phenotypes of the CYP2D6 isoenzyme, the initial atomoxetine dosage should be 40 mg daily and dosage should be increased to the usual target dosage of 80 mg daily only if ADHD symptoms fail to improve after 4 weeks of therapy and the initial dosage is well tolerated. The maximum recommended dosage of atomoxetine in adults or in children and adolescents weighing more than 70 kg is 100 mg daily. The safety of single doses exceeding 120 mg and total daily dosages exceeding 150 mg has not been established.

The usual initial dosage of atomoxetine in children and adolescents weighing 70 kg or less is approximately 0.5 mg/kg daily; dosage may be increased after a minimum of 3 days to a target dosage of approximately 1.2 mg/kg daily. In children and adolescents weighing 70 kg or less, if atomoxetine is used concomitantly with potent CYP2D6 inhibitors (e.g., paroxetine, fluoxetine, quinidine) or in patients with poor metabolizer phenotypes of the CYP2D6 isoenzyme, the initial atomoxetine dosage should be 0.5 mg/kg daily and dosage should be increased to the usual target dosage of 1.2 mg/kg daily only if ADHD symptoms fail to improve after 4 weeks of therapy and the initial dosage is well tolerated. Daily dosage of atomoxetine in children and adolescents weighing 70 kg or less should not exceed 100 mg or 1.4 mg/kg, whichever is less; dosages exceeding 1.2 mg/kg daily have not been shown in clinical trials to result in additional therapeutic benefit.

Because the effectiveness of atomoxetine for long-term use (i.e., more than 12 months in children and adolescents 6–15 years of age, more than 9 weeks in those 16–18 years of age, and more than 10 weeks in adults) has not been established, patients receiving atomoxetine for extended periods should be periodically reevaluated to assess the long-term usefulness of the drug.

Atomoxetine may be discontinued without tapering the dosage.

■ **Special Populations** The manufacturer recommends that usual initial and target dosages of atomoxetine be reduced by 50% in patients with moderate hepatic impairment (Child-Pugh class B) and by 75% in those with severe hepatic impairment (Child-Pugh class C).

Cautions

■ **Contraindications** Known hypersensitivity to atomoxetine or any ingredient in the formulation.

The manufacturer states that atomoxetine is contraindicated in patients currently receiving or having recently received (i.e., within 2 weeks) monoamine oxidase (MAO) inhibitor therapy. In addition, at least 2 weeks should elapse after discontinuing atomoxetine before initiating MAO inhibitor therapy. Severe, potentially fatal, reactions (including hyperthermia, rigidity, myoclonus, autonomic instability with possible rapid fluctuations of vital signs, and mental status changes that include extreme agitation progressing to delirium and coma) have been reported in patients receiving other drugs that affect brain monoamine concentrations concomitantly with MAO inhibitor therapy.

The manufacturer also states that atomoxetine should not be used in patients with angle-closure glaucoma, since the drug was associated with an increased risk of mydriasis in some patients during controlled clinical trials.

■ **Warnings/Precautions** ***Warnings*** **Suicidality Risk.** Atomoxetine may increase the risk of suicidal ideation in children and adolescents with attention deficit hyperactivity disorder (ADHD). (See Pediatric Use under Warnings/Precautions: Specific Populations, in Cautions.) Pediatric patients should be closely monitored for clinical worsening, suicidality (suicidal ideation or behaviors), or unusual changes in behavior, particularly during the first few months after initiation of therapy and during periods of dosage adjustments. Monitoring should include daily observation by family members and caregivers and frequent contact with the prescribing clinician, particularly if the patient's behavior changes or is a concern. The manufacturer recommends face-to-face contact between clinicians and patients or their family members or caregivers at least weekly during the first 4 weeks of therapy and then every other week for the next 4 weeks, with subsequent face-to-face contact at 12 weeks and as clinically indicated thereafter; additional contact via telephone may be appropriate between visits.

Discontinuance of therapy should be considered in patients with emergent suicidality or manifestations that may be precursors to emerging suicidality (e.g., anxiety, agitation, panic attacks, insomnia, irritability, hostility, aggressiveness, impulsivity, akathisia, hypomania, mania), particularly if such manifestations are severe or abrupt in onset or were not part of the patient's presenting symptoms.

Sensitivity Reactions Allergic reactions, including angioedema, urticaria, and rash, have been reported rarely in patients receiving atomoxetine.

Other Warnings and Precautions **Severe Hepatic Injury.** Severe hepatic injury was reported during postmarketing surveillance in 2 patients (an adolescent and an adult) who had received atomoxetine for several months. In one patient, hepatic injury was manifested by increased hepatic enzymes (up to 40 times the upper limit of normal [ULN]) and jaundice (bilirubin up to 12 times the ULN); manifestations recurred upon rechallenge with atomoxetine and resolved upon discontinuance of the drug, providing evidence that the hepatic injury was caused by atomoxetine. Both patients recovered and did not require liver transplantation. However, the manufacturer notes that severe drug-related hepatic injury may progress to acute hepatic failure resulting in death or requiring liver transplantation in a small percentage of patients. The actual incidence of hepatic injury in patients receiving atomoxetine is unknown because of possible underreporting of postmarketing adverse effects.

Adverse hepatic effects may occur several months after initiation of atomoxetine, and laboratory abnormalities may continue to worsen for several weeks after discontinuance of the drug. Hepatic enzyme concentrations should be determined after the first manifestation of hepatic dysfunction (e.g., pruritus, dark urine, jaundice, right upper quadrant tenderness, unexplained flu-like symptoms) in patients receiving atomoxetine. Atomoxetine should be discontinued in patients with jaundice or laboratory evidence of hepatic injury, and therapy with the drug should *not* be reinitiated in such patients.

Sudden Death and Serious Cardiovascular Events. Although a causal relationship to atomoxetine has not been established, sudden unexplained death, stroke, and myocardial infarction have been reported in adults receiving usual dosages of atomoxetine for the treatment of ADHD. Sudden unexplained death also has been reported in children and adolescents with structural cardiac abnormalities or other serious cardiac conditions receiving usual dosages of atomoxetine. Children, adolescents, and adults who are being considered for atomoxetine therapy should undergo a thorough medical history review (including evaluation for a family history of sudden death or ventricular arrhythmia) and physical examination to detect the presence of cardiac disease, and should receive further cardiac evaluation (e.g., ECG, echocardiogram) if initial findings suggest such disease. Although some serious cardiac conditions are independently associated with an increased risk of sudden death, atomoxetine generally should *not* be used in children, adolescents, or adults with known serious structural cardiac abnormalities, cardiomyopathy, serious heart rhythm abnormalities, coronary artery disease, or other serious cardiac conditions. Patients who develop exertional chest pain, unexplained syncope, or other manifestations suggestive of cardiac disease during atomoxetine therapy should undergo prompt cardiac evaluation.

For further information on screening for cardiac conditions, selecting appropriate candidates for stimulant therapy, and monitoring for treatment-emergent cardiac conditions, see Cardiovascular Precautions under Cautions: Precautions and Contraindications, in the Amphetamines General Statement 28:20.04.

Psychiatric Effects. Atomoxetine should be used with caution in the management of ADHD in patients with comorbid bipolar disorder because of the potential for precipitation of mixed or manic episodes in such patients. Prior to initiating atomoxetine therapy, patients with ADHD and comorbid depressive symptoms should be carefully screened to determine if they are at risk for bipolar disorder; such screening should include a detailed psychiatric history (e.g., family history of suicide, bipolar disorder, or depression).

Psychotic or manic symptoms (e.g., hallucinations, delusional thinking, mania) have been reported in children and adolescents without prior history of psychotic illness or mania who received usual dosages of atomoxetine. In a pooled analysis of multiple short-term, placebo-controlled studies, such symptoms occurred in about 0.2% of patients receiving usual dosages of atomoxetine compared with 0% of those receiving placebo. If psychotic or manic symptoms occur, a causal relationship to atomoxetine should be considered, and discontinuance of therapy may be appropriate.

Cardiovascular Effects. Increased blood pressure and heart rate were reported in children, adolescents, and adults receiving atomoxetine in controlled clinical studies. The drug should be used with caution in patients with hypertension, tachycardia, or cardiovascular or cerebrovascular disease that might be affected by increases in blood pressure or heart rate. Blood pressure and pulse rate should be measured before initiation of atomoxetine, following any increase in dosage, and periodically during therapy.

Orthostatic hypotension and syncope also were reported in patients receiving atomoxetine in controlled clinical studies. The drug should be used with caution in patients with conditions that would predispose them to hypotension.

Peripheral Vascular Effects. Exacerbation or precipitation of Raynaud's phenomenon was reported during postmarketing surveillance in patients receiving atomoxetine.

Genitourinary Effects. Urinary retention and urinary hesitation were reported in adults receiving atomoxetine in controlled clinical studies.

Growth Effects. Temporary suppression of normal weight and height patterns has been observed in pediatric patients receiving atomoxetine therapy. Gains in weight and height generally lag behind predicted population values for about the first 9–12 months of therapy; however, weight and height gains rebound with continued treatment. Similar growth patterns have been observed regardless of metabolizer phenotype (poor or extensive metabolizer of the drug) or pubertal status upon initiation of treatment. The manufacturer states that growth should be monitored in patients receiving therapy with atomoxetine.

Children and adolescents 6–18 years of age receiving atomoxetine for up to 9 weeks in controlled clinical studies had an average weight loss of 0.4 kg compared with an average weight gain of 1.5 kg in those receiving placebo for the same time period; similar rates of weight loss have been reported in other controlled clinical studies with the drug. In one clinical trial, decreases in body weight of at least 3.5% occurred in 7–29% of patients receiving atomoxetine at various dosages, compared with 1.3% of patients receiving placebo. However, in patients receiving atomoxetine for 3 years, weight increased by an average of 17.9 kg (0.5 kg more than predicted by baseline data) and height increased by an average of 19.4 cm (0.4 cm less than predicted by baseline data) at 3 years. Gain in height stabilized at about 12 months.

Behavioral Effects. Aggressive behavior and hostility frequently are observed in pediatric patients with ADHD and have been reported in patients receiving drug therapy (including atomoxetine) for the disorder. In controlled clinical studies in pediatric patients, aggressive behavior or hostility was reported slightly (overall risk ratio of 1.33), but not significantly, more frequently in those receiving atomoxetine compared with those receiving placebo. Patients beginning treatment for ADHD should be monitored for the onset or worsening of aggressive behavior or hostility.

Priapism. Priapism was reported rarely during postmarketing surveillance in pediatric and adult patients receiving atomoxetine; if priapism is suspected, prompt medical attention is required. (See Advice to Patients.)

Tics. In a controlled study, atomoxetine did not worsen tics in patients with ADHD and comorbid Tourette's disorder.

Specific Populations **Pregnancy.** Category C. (See Users Guide.)

Lactation. Atomoxetine and/or its metabolites are distributed into milk in rats; it is not known whether the drug is distributed into milk in humans. Therefore, atomoxetine should be used with caution in nursing women.

Pediatric Use. Safety and efficacy of atomoxetine have not been established in children younger than 6 years of age.

Atomoxetine may increase the risk of suicidal ideation in children and adolescents with ADHD. In a pooled analysis of 12 short-term controlled clinical studies in pediatric patients with ADHD (11 studies) or enuresis (1 study), the risk of suicidal ideation was about 0.4% in those receiving atomoxetine versus 0% in those receiving placebo. One child receiving the drug attempted suicide; no completed suicides were reported. All events representing suicidal behavior or thinking occurred in children 12 years of age or younger and occurred during the first month of therapy. It is not known whether the risk of suicidal ideation in pediatric patients extends to long-term use of the drug. A similar analysis of data from adults with ADHD or major depressive disorder found no increased risk of suicidal ideation or behavior in those receiving atomoxetine. The potential risks of suicidality should be weighed against the clinical need for the drug prior to initiating atomoxetine therapy in children or adolescents. (See Suicidality Risk under Warnings/Precautions: Warnings, in Cautions.)

Sudden death has been reported in children and adolescents with structural cardiac abnormalities or other serious cardiac conditions receiving usual dosages of stimulants. (See Sudden Death and Serious Cardiovascular Events under Warnings/Precautions: Other Warnings and Precautions, in Cautions.)

Temporary suppression of normal weight and/or height patterns has been reported during the first 9–12 months of atomoxetine therapy; however, weight and height gains have rebounded with continued treatment. (See Growth Effects under Warnings/Precautions: Other Warnings and Precautions, in Cautions.) The growth of pediatric patients receiving atomoxetine should be monitored.

Geriatric Use. Safety and efficacy of atomoxetine have not been established in geriatric patients.

Hepatic Impairment. Systemic exposure to atomoxetine concentrations is increased twofold in patients with moderate hepatic impairment (Child-Pugh class B) and fourfold in those with severe hepatic impairment (Child-Pugh class C). (See Dosage and Administration: Special Populations.)

■ **Common Adverse Effects** Abdominal pain, decreased appetite, vomiting, somnolence, nausea, fatigue, irritability, and dizziness each occurred in 5% or more of children and adolescents receiving atomoxetine in controlled clinical studies and were at least twice as frequent in patients receiving the drug as in those receiving placebo. Dry mouth, nausea, insomnia, decreased appetite, constipation, fatigue, erectile dysfunction, hot flush, urinary disorders (urinary hesitation, urinary retention), and dysmenorrhea each occurred in 5% or more of adults receiving atomoxetine in controlled clinical studies and were at least twice as frequent in patients receiving the drug as in those receiving placebo.

Drug Interactions

■ **Drugs Affecting Hepatic Microsomal Enzymes** Potential pharmacokinetic interaction (decreased metabolism of atomoxetine) when atomoxetine is used concomitantly with drugs that inhibit the activity of the cytochrome P-450 2D6 (CYP2D6) isoenzyme. Inhibitors of CYP2D6 may increase plasma concentrations of atomoxetine in patients with the extensive-metabolizer phenotype to such an extent that plasma concentrations of the drug are similar to those achieved in poor metabolizers. When atomoxetine is used concomitantly with potent CYP2D6 inhibitors (e.g., paroxetine, fluoxetine, quinidine), or in patients with poor-metabolizer phenotypes of the CYP2D6 isoenzyme, the manufacturer states that dosage adjustment of atomoxetine should be considered. (See Dosage and Administration: Dosage.) However, in vitro studies suggest that concomitant use of atomoxetine with CYP2D6 inhibitors will not increase plasma concentrations of atomoxetine in patients with the poor-metabolizer phenotype.

■ **Drugs Metabolized by Hepatic Microsomal Enzymes** Pharmacokinetic interaction unlikely; evidence to date suggests that atomoxetine does not cause clinically important inhibition or induction of cytochrome P-450 enzymes, including CYP1A2, CYP3A, CYP2D6, and CYP2C9.

■ **GI Drugs** No important pharmacokinetic interactions reported with drugs that increase gastric pH (e.g., antacids containing magnesium hydroxide and aluminum hydroxide, omeprazole).

■ **Protein-bound Drugs** Pharmacokinetic interaction unlikely. In vitro studies indicate that atomoxetine is not displaced from binding sites by, and does not displace from binding sites, other highly protein-bound drugs (e.g., warfarin, aspirin, phenytoin, diazepam) in therapeutic concentrations.

■ **Alcohol** No change in the intoxicating effects of alcohol when alcohol was ingested by individuals receiving atomoxetine.

■ **β-Adrenergic Agonists** Potential pharmacologic interaction (increased cardiovascular effects [e.g., increased heart rate and blood pressure]) when atomoxetine is used concomitantly with oral or parenteral β_2-adrenergic agonists (e.g., albuterol). Use with caution.

■ **Cardiovascular Agents** Potential pharmacologic interaction (increased hypertensive effects) with concomitant use of pressor agents (e.g., dopamine, dobutamine) and atomoxetine. Use with caution.

■ **Methylphenidate** No increase in cardiovascular effects with concomitant use of methylphenidate and atomoxetine relative to use of methylphenidate alone.

■ **Monoamine Oxidase Inhibitors** Potential pharmacologic interaction (inhibition of catecholamine metabolism). (See Cautions: Contraindications.)

Description

Atomoxetine is a selective norepinephrine-reuptake inhibitor. Atomoxetine is not considered a stimulant and also is structurally unrelated to other agents used for the treatment of attention deficit hyperactivity disorder (ADHD). The exact mechanism(s) of action of atomoxetine in the management of ADHD has not been fully elucidated but, based on in vitro studies, appears to be related to selective inhibition of the presynaptic norepinephrine transporter; the drug appears to have minimal affinity for other noradrenergic receptors or for other neurotransmitter transporters or receptors.

Atomoxetine is readily absorbed following oral administration. The drug is approximately 98% bound to plasma proteins, principally albumin, at therapeutic concentrations. Atomoxetine is metabolized principally via oxidation by the cytochrome P-450 2D6 (CYP2D6) isoenzyme and subsequent glucuronidation. Individuals who extensively metabolize atomoxetine via the CYP2D6 pathway exhibit the extensive-metabolizer phenotype, while those who have an impaired ability to metabolize the drug by this pathway exhibit the poor-metabolizer phenotype. In patients with the poor-metabolizer phenotype (about 7% of Caucasians and 2% of African-Americans), metabolic clearance of atomoxetine may be decreased; a fivefold increase in peak plasma concentrations of atomoxetine and a tenfold increase in area under the plasma concentration-time curve (AUC) have been reported in individuals with the poor-metabolizer phenotype relative to those with the extensive-metabolizer phenotype. The mean elimination half-life of atomoxetine is 5.2 or 21.6 hours in extensive or poor metabolizers, respectively. Atomoxetine does not inhibit or induce CYP2D6.

Advice to Patients

Importance of providing patient or caregiver with a copy of the manufacturer's patient information (medication guide); discuss and answer questions about its contents (e.g., benefits and risks of atomoxetine therapy, appropriate use) as needed. Importance of instructing the patient or caregiver to read and understand the contents of the medication guide before initiating therapy and each time the prescription is refilled.

Risk of suicidal thinking. Importance of patients, caregivers, and family members immediately informing clinician if clinical worsening, anxiety, agitation, panic attacks, insomnia, irritability, aggressive behaviors, hostility, impulsivity, restlessness, mania, depression, suicidal ideation or behaviors, or unusual changes in behavior occur, particularly during the first few months after initiation of therapy or following dosage adjustments.

Patients and/or caregivers should be advised that hepatic dysfunction may develop rarely. Importance of informing clinician immediately if symptoms of hepatic injury occur (e.g., pruritus, jaundice, dark urine, upper right-sided abdominal tenderness, unexplained flu-like symptoms).

Importance of informing clinician immediately if adverse cardiovascular effects (e.g., chest pain, shortness of breath, fainting) occur.

Importance of informing clinician immediately if precipitation of psychotic (e.g., hallucinations, delusional thinking) or manic symptoms occurs.

Importance of exercising caution when driving or operating machinery until the effects of the drug on the individual are known.

Risk of priapism. Importance of seeking immediate medical attention if an erection persists for more than 4 hours.

Importance of taking atomoxetine exactly as prescribed. If a patient misses a dose of the drug, the missed dose should be taken as soon as it is remembered, but the amount of atomoxetine taken within a 24-hour period should not exceed the prescribed total daily dosage of the drug.

Importance of advising patient and/or caregivers that atomoxetine capsules should not be opened because the drug is an ocular irritant; if eye contact occurs, flush the affected eye(s) with water immediately, obtain medical advice, and wash hands and potentially contaminated surfaces as soon as possible.

Importance of informing clinician of any history of physical or mental disorders (e.g., cardiovascular disease, liver disease, depression).

Importance of women informing clinicians if they are or plan to become pregnant or plan to breast-feed.

Importance of informing clinicians of existing or contemplated concomitant therapy, including prescription and OTC drugs, dietary supplements, and herbal products, as well as any concomitant illnesses/conditions (e.g., glaucoma, suicidal ideation or behaviors, cardiac/cardiovascular disease, mental/psychiatric disorder, hepatic disease).

Importance of informing patients and/or caregivers of other important precautionary information. (See Cautions.)

Overview® (see Users Guide). For additional information on this drug until a more detailed monograph is developed and published, the manufacturer's labeling should be consulted. It is *essential* that the manufacturer's labeling be consulted for more detailed information on usual cautions, precautions, contraindications, potential drug interactions, laboratory test interferences, and acute toxicity.

Preparations

Excipients in commercially available drug preparations may have clinically important effects in some individuals; consult specific product labeling for details.

Atomoxetine Hydrochloride

Oral

Capsules	10 mg (of atomoxetine)	**Strattera®**, Lilly
	18 mg (of atomoxetine)	**Strattera®**, Lilly
	25 mg (of atomoxetine)	**Strattera®**, Lilly
	40 mg (of atomoxetine)	**Strattera®**, Lilly
	60 mg (of atomoxetine)	**Strattera®**, Lilly
	80 mg (of atomoxetine)	**Strattera®**, Lilly
	100 mg (of atomoxetine)	**Strattera®**, Lilly

Flumazenil

■ Flumazenil, a 1,4-imidazobenzodiazepine derivative, is a benzodiazepine antagonist.

Uses

Flumazenil is used in adults for the complete or partial reversal of benzodiazepine-induced sedation when benzodiazepines are used for induction or maintenance of general anesthesia or for diagnostic or therapeutic procedures (i.e., conscious sedation) and for the management of benzodiazepine intoxication. Flumazenil also is used in children 1–17 years of age for the reversal of benzodiazepine-induced sedation when benzodiazepines are used for diagnostic or therapeutic procedures. The manufacturer states that the safety and efficacy of flumazenil have *not* been established in pediatric patients for reversal of benzodiazepine-induced sedation when benzodiazepines are used for induction of general anesthesia, for the management of benzodiazepine intoxication, nor for the resuscitation of neonates. (See Special Populations: Pediatric Use.)

■ **Reversal of General Anesthesia** Flumazenil has been shown to be effective in reversing sedation and restoring psychomotor function in adults who received midazolam for induction or maintenance of general anesthesia. Efficacy was established in 4 clinical studies in adults who received 5–80 mg of midazolam alone or in conjunction with skeletal muscle relaxants, nitrous oxide, regional or local anesthetics, opiates, and/or inhalational anesthetics. A 0. 2-mg dose of flumazenil was administered, followed by additional 0. 2-mg doses as needed to reach a complete response (up to a maximum of 1 mg). In these studies, 81% of patients became completely alert or remained only slightly drowsy following total flumazenil doses of 0.4–0.6 mg (36%) or 0.8–1 mg (64%). However, resedation occurred in 10–15% of patients who responded to flumazenil. (See Warnings: Resedation.) Flumazenil failed to restore memory completely as tested by picture recall. In addition, flumazenil was not as effective in the reversal of sedation in patients who received multiple anesthetic agents in addition to benzodiazepines.

■ **Reversal of Conscious Sedation** Flumazenil has been shown to be effective in reversing the sedative and psychomotor effects of benzodiazepines when these drugs are used for diagnostic or therapeutic procedures but was less effective in completely and consistently reversing benzodiazepine-induced amnesia. Efficacy was established in 4 clinical studies in adults who received an average of 30 mg of diazepam or 10 mg of midazolam for sedation (with or without an opiate) for both inpatient and outpatient diagnostic or surgical procedures. Flumazenil was administered as an initial dose of 0.4 mg (2 doses of 0.2 mg each), with additional 0. 2-mg doses administered as needed to achieve complete awakening, up to a maximum of 1 mg. In these studies, 78% of patients receiving flumazenil achieved complete consciousness, but approximately 50% of these patients required 2–3 additional doses of the drug in order to achieve this level of consciousness. In addition, while most patients remained alert throughout the 3-hour postprocedure observation period, resedation occurred in 3–9% of these patients.

Pediatric Considerations The safety and efficacy of flumazenil for the reversal of benzodiazepine-induced conscious sedation have been established in children 1 year of age and older. In one uncontrolled clinical trial involving 107 children 1–17 years of age who had received midazolam for conscious sedation, flumazenil was administered at doses of 0.01 mg/kg (maximum of 0.2 mg) up to a maximum of 5 doses or a total dose of 1 mg. In this study, 56% of the children achieved complete consciousness within 10 minutes of flumazenil administration, but 51% of them required the maximum number of doses of the drug allowed for initial treatment in order to achieve this level of consciousness. In addition, approximately 12% of the patients (all of whom were 1–5 years of age) who achieved complete consciousness following flumazenil administration experienced resedation within 19–50 minutes of initial administration of the drug. Episodes of resedation were reversed by additional doses of flumazenil. However, the manufacturer states that the safety and efficacy of repeated flumazenil administration in pediatric patients experiencing resedation have *not* been established.

■ **Benzodiazepine Overdosage** Flumazenil is used in adults for the management of benzodiazepine overdosage. The drug is an adjunct to, not a replacement for, appropriate supportive and symptomatic measures (e.g., ventilatory and circulatory support) in the management of benzodiazepine overdosage. Because patients admitted to hospitals for drug overdoses may have ingested multiple substances and/or are being treated for concomitant illnesses (e.g., depression, substance abuse), the presence of contraindications or precautions, which may limit the use of flumazenil therapy, should be considered. (See Contraindications under Warnings/Precautions, in Cautions.) Flumazenil has no known benefit other than reversal of benzodiazepine-induced sedation in seriously ill patients with multiple-drug overdosage, and the drug should *not* be used in cases where seizures (from any cause) are likely. In addition, the manufacturer warns that flumazenil should *not* be used in patients with serious cyclic depressant overdosage. (See Drug Interactions: Cyclic Antidepressants.) For information on the pathogenesis, manifestations, and treatment of benzodiazepine overdosage, see Acute Toxicity in the Benzodiazepines General Statement 28:24.08.

Efficacy of flumazenil has been established in 2 studies in patients who were presumed to have taken an overdose of a benzodiazepine, either alone or in combination with a variety of other agents. In these studies, of patients who were proven to have taken a benzodiazepine, 80% of those who received flumazenil responded with an improvement in level of consciousness. Of those who responded to flumazenil, 75% responded to a total dose of 1–3 mg. However, reversal of sedation was associated with an increased frequency of symptoms of CNS excitation, and 1–3% of patients who received flumazenil were treated for agitation or anxiety.

■ **Other Uses** The manufacturer states that the safety and efficacy of flumazenil for the treatment of benzodiazepine dependence or for the management of protracted benzodiazepine abstinence syndrome have not been established and therefore such use currently is not recommended.

Dosage and Administration

■ **General** Flumazenil is administered by rapid (over 15–30 seconds) IV injection through a freely flowing IV infusion into a large vein. Because of the risk of local irritation, the drug is recommended for IV use only, and extravasation into perivascular tissues should be avoided. Patients should have a secure airway and established IV access prior to administration of the drug.

While flumazenil dosages exceeding the minimally effective dose may be tolerated by most adults, such dosages can complicate the management of patients who are physically dependent on benzodiazepines or in whom the therapeutic benefit of the drugs is needed (e.g., for seizure control in cyclic antidepressant overdosage). Therefore, flumazenil dosage should be titrated carefully using the smallest effective dosage. Currently recommended flumazenil dosing regimens involve multiple small doses rather than large bolus doses in order to provide better control of sedation reversal while minimizing the risk of adverse effects.

Reversal of General Anesthesia and Conscious Sedation in Adults When flumazenil is used to reverse benzodiazepine-induced sedative effects after anesthesia or conscious sedation in adults, the usual initial dose is 0.2 mg given IV over 15 seconds; if the desired consciousness level is not achieved after waiting 45 seconds, additional 0.2-mg doses may be administered at 1-minute intervals until an adequate response is achieved or a maximum of 4 additional doses is administered (i.e., maximum cumulative dose of 1 mg during an initial 5-minute dosing period). If resedation occurs, the initial dosing regimen (i.e., up to 1 mg given in divided 0.2-mg doses at 1-minute intervals) may be repeated no more frequently than every 20 minutes up to a maximum of 3 mg in any 1-hour period. In certain high risk patients (consult the manufacturer's labeling), it may be necessary to reduce the dose and/or increase the interval between doses to longer than 1 minute. Most patients respond to cumulative flumazenil doses of 0.6–1 mg, but individual requirements may vary considerably depending on the dose and duration of effect of the benzodiazepine administered and patient characteristics. In clinical situations where resedation is not yet apparent but must be prevented, the initial dosing regimen can be repeated at 30 and possibly repeated at 60 minutes despite the current absence of manifestations of recurrence.

Reversal of Conscious Sedation in Children When flumazenil is used in children to reverse benzodiazepine-induced sedative effects after conscious sedation, the usual initial dose is 0.01 mg/kg (up to 0.2 mg) given IV over 15 seconds; if the desired consciousness level is not achieved after waiting 45 seconds, additional 0.01-mg/kg (up to 0.2 mg) doses may be administered at 1-minute intervals until an adequate response is achieved or a maximum of 4 additional doses is administered (i.e., maximum cumulative dose of 0.05 mg/kg or 1 mg, whichever is lower). In the pediatric clinical trial of flumazenil, a mean total dose of 0.65 mg (range: 0.08–1 mg) was administered to children 1–17 years of age with approximately 50% of children requiring the maximum of 5 injections. The safety and efficacy of repeated flumazenil administration in pediatric patients experiencing resedation have not been established.

Management of Benzodiazepine Overdosage in Adults When flumazenil is used for known or suspected benzodiazepine overdosage in adults, the usual initial dose is 0.2 mg given IV over 30 seconds; if the desired consciousness level is not achieved after waiting 30 seconds, an additional 0.3-mg dose may be administered over 30 seconds. If an adequate response still is not achieved, further additional 0.5-mg doses may be administered over 30 seconds at 1-minute intervals up to a cumulative dose of 3 mg. Most patients respond to cumulative flumazenil doses of 1–3 mg, and cumulative doses exceeding 3 mg have not been shown reproducibly to provide additional benefit. However, some patients who exhibit a partial response after a 3-mg cumulative dose rarely may require additional doses up to a total of 5 mg. If no response is observed within 5 minutes after administration of an initial 5-mg cumulative dose of flumazenil, the major cause of sedation may not be a benzodiazepine and additional flumazenil doses likely will provide little if any beneficial effect. If resedation occurs, the initial dosing regimen (i.e., up to 1 mg given in divided 0.5-mg doses at 1-minute intervals) may be repeated no more frequently than every 20 minutes up to a maximum dose of 3 mg in any 1-hour period.

■ **Special Populations** Patients with hepatic impairment have decreased clearance of flumazenil. While the initial dose of flumazenil for reversal of benzodiazepine effects is not affected, repeat doses of the drug should be reduced in size or frequency in patients with hepatic impairment.

Cautions

■ **Contraindications** Flumazenil is contraindicated in patients receiving a benzodiazepine for control of a potentially life-threatening condition (e.g., control of intracranial pressure or status epilepticus) and in those exhibiting manifestations of serious cyclic antidepressant overdosage. (See Warnings: Seizures.) Flumazenil also is contraindicated in patients with known hypersensitivity to the drug or benzodiazepines.

■ **Warnings/Precautions** ***Warnings*** **Seizures.** Use of flumazenil for the reversal of benzodiazepine effects may be associated with the onset of seizures in certain high-risk patients. Seizures are most frequent in patients who have been receiving benzodiazepines for long-term sedation or in patients with manifestations of serious cyclic antidepressant overdose. Other risk factors for seizures following flumazenil administration include major sedative-hypnotic drug withdrawal, recent therapy with repeated doses of parenteral benzodiazepines, myoclonic jerking or seizure activity prior to flumazenil administration in overdose cases, or concurrent cyclic antidepressant poisoning. Most convulsions associated with flumazenil administration require treatment, and have been successfully managed with anticonvulsants such as phenytoin, barbiturates, or benzodiazepines. However, if benzodiazepines are used to treat flumazenil-associated seizures, higher dosages than usual may be required.

Hypoventilation. The manufacturer states that the efficacy of flumazenil in reversing benzodiazepine-induced hypoventilation has not been established, and the drug may not fully reverse postoperative airway problems or ventilatory insufficiency associated with benzodiazepine administration. In addition, even if initial efficacy is observed, the ventilatory effects of flumazenil may subside prior to those of the benzodiazepine; therefore, facilities and equipment for immediate ventilatory support should be readily available for any patient receiving the drug. In patients with serious pulmonary disease who experience serious benzodiazepine-induced respiratory depression, primary therapy should be appropriate ventilatory support rather than flumazenil therapy.

General Precautions **Return of Sedation.** Resedation may occur in patients who have responded to flumazenil. Resedation is most likely to occur in cases where a large single or cumulative dose of a benzodiazepine (e.g., midazolam dosages exceeding 10 mg) has been administered in the course of a long procedure (e.g., longer than 60 minutes) along with neuromuscular blocking agents and multiple anesthetic agents and least likely to occur in cases where flumazenil is administered to reverse a low dose of a short-acting benzodiazepine (less than 10 mg of midazolam). In clinical studies, resedation was observed in 1–3% of adults and in about 12% of children. Therefore, patients should be carefully monitored for an adequate period of time (i.e., up to 2 hours) based on the dose and duration of effect of the benzodiazepine employed for signs of resedation, respiratory depression, or other residual benzodiazepine effects. Although the safety and efficacy of repeated flumazenil administration in pediatric patients experiencing resedation have not been established, repeated doses of flumazenil may be administered to adult patients when necessary. (See Dosage and Administration: Dosage.)

Withdrawal Reactions. Flumazenil may precipitate dose-dependent manifestations of withdrawal in patients with established physical dependence on benzodiazepines. An acute withdrawal syndrome characterized by dizziness, mild confusion, emotional lability, agitation (with signs and symptoms of anxiety), and mild sensory distortions has occurred in adults receiving flumazenil, particularly at doses above 1 mg. However, such reactions rarely required treatment other than reassurance and were usually short-lived. When treatment was necessary, patients were successfully treated with usual doses of barbiturates, benzodiazepines, or other sedative agents. Because benzodiazepine tolerance and dependence is frequently observed in patients with alcoholism and other drug dependencies, clinicians should assume that flumazenil administration may complicate the management of withdrawal syndromes for alcohol, barbiturates, and cross-tolerant sedatives. Seizures also may occur following flumazenil administration in patients with established physical dependence on benzodiazepines. (See Warnings: Seizures.)

Intensive Care Setting. The manufacturer states that use of flumazenil in an intensive care setting to define CNS depression as being benzodiazepine induced is *not* recommended because of the risk of precipitating potentially serious manifestations of withdrawal (e.g., seizures) in cases of unrecognized benzodiazepine dependence and because of the prognostic uncertainty of failure to respond to flumazenil in cases confounded by a metabolic disorder, traumatic injury, effects of other drugs, or any other factor not associated with benzodiazepine-receptor occupancy.

Head Injury. Because flumazenil may precipitate seizures or alter cerebral blood flow in patients receiving benzodiazepines, the drug should be used with caution and only by clinicians who are prepared to manage such complications in patients with head injury.

Panic Disorders. Flumazenil has been reported to provoke panic attacks in patients with a history of panic disorder.

Pulmonary Disease. Because the efficacy of flumazenil in reversing benzodiazepine-induced alterations in ventilatory drive has not been established, the primary treatment of patients with serious lung disease who experience serious respiratory depression secondary to benzodiazepines should be appropriate ventilatory support (see Warnings: Hypoventilation) rather than the administration of flumazenil.

Cardiovascular Disease. Use of flumazenil alone had no clinically important effects on cardiovascular parameters when administered to patients with stable ischemic heart disease to reverse the effects of benzodiazepines.

Specific Populations **Pregnancy.** Category C. (See Users Guide.) Use during labor and delivery is not recommended since the effects of flumazenil on the neonate are not known.

Lactation. It is not known whether flumazenil is distributed in milk. Caution is advised if the drug is administered in nursing women.

Pediatric Use. Safety and efficacy of flumazenil in the reversal of conscious sedation in infants younger than 1 year of age have not been established. In addition, the manufacturer states that safety and efficacy of flumazenil, including the potential risks, benefits, and appropriate dosages, have not been established for the management of benzodiazepine overdosage, for neonatal resuscitation, nor for the reversal of sedation when benzodiazepines are used for induction of general anesthesia. However, published anecdotal reports discussing the use of flumazenil in pediatric patients for these indications have reported similar safety profiles and dosing guidelines to those described for the reversal of conscious sedation. The risks associated with flumazenil use in the adult population also apply to pediatric patients. (See Cautions: Warnings/Precautions.)

Geriatric Use. No substantial differences in safety or efficacy relative to younger adults, but increased sensitivity to flumazenil cannot be ruled out.

■ **Common Adverse Effects** Adverse effects occurring in 3–9% of patients receiving flumazenil include dizziness, injection site pain, increased sweating, headache, and abnormal or blurred vision. In addition, serious adverse effects such as cardiac arrhythmias (e.g., junctional or ventricular tachycardias), seizures, and deaths have occurred. Most deaths occurred in patients with serious underlying disease or in patients who had ingested large amounts of non-benzodiazepine drugs (usually cyclic antidepressants) as part of an overdose. (See Warnings: Seizures in Cautions.)

Drug Interactions

■ **Cyclic Antidepressants** Potential pharmacodynamic interactions. (See Warnings: Seizures.) Flumazenil should *not* be used in patients exhibiting manifestations of serious concurrent cyclic antidepressant overdosage, such as motor abnormalities (e.g., twitching, rigidity, focal seizures), arrhythmias (e.g., wide QRS complexes, ventricular arrhythmias, heart block), anticholinergic effects (e.g., mydriasis, dry mucosa, hypoperistalsis), or cardiovascular collapse. In such cases, the patient should be managed with ventilatory and circulatory supportive measures as needed until the signs of antidepressant toxicity have subsided. For information on the pathogenesis, manifestations, and treatment of cyclic antidepressant overdosage, see Acute Toxicity in the Tricyclic Antidepressants General Statement 28:16.04.28.

■ **Benzodiazepines** Pharmacokinetic interaction unlikely. However, flumazenil may precipitate dose-dependent manifestations of withdrawal in patients with established physical dependence on benzodiazepines.

■ **Other Drugs** Interactions of flumazenil with CNS depressants other than benzodiazepines have not been studied. However, no deleterious interactions have been observed when flumazenil was administered after opiates, inhalational anesthetics, skeletal muscle relaxants, or muscle relaxant antagonists administered in conjunction with sedation or anesthesia. Flumazenil should not be administered until the effects of neuromuscular blockade have been fully reversed.

Description

Flumazenil, a 1,4-imidazobenzodiazepine derivative, is a benzodiazepine antagonist. Flumazenil antagonizes the CNS effects (e.g., sedation, impaired recall, psychomotor impairment, respiratory depression) of benzodiazepines by competitively inhibiting the activity of the drugs at the benzodiazepine recognition site on the γ-aminobutyric acid (GABA)/benzodiazepine receptor complex. Reversal of benzodiazepine-induced effects usually is evident within 1–2 minutes following completion of IV injection of flumazenil, with an 80% response occurring within 3 minutes, and the peak effect occurring at 6–10 minutes. The duration and degree of reversal of benzodiazepine-induced effects appear to be related to the dose and plasma concentrations of flumazenil. However, because the elimination half-life of flumazenil (0.7–1.3 hours) is shorter than that of benzodiazepines, repeat doses of the drug may be needed to prevent resedation. The half-life of flumazenil appears to be shorter (averaging 40 minutes; range: 20–75 minutes) and more variable in children 1–17 years of age compared with that of adults.

Flumazenil is extensively metabolized in the liver with less than 1% of an administered dose excreted unchanged in urine. Ingestion of food during an IV infusion of the drug results in a 50% increase in clearance, most likely because of the increased hepatic blood flow that accompanies a meal.

Advice to Patients

Impairment of memory and judgment may occur. Importance of avoiding activities that require complete alertness, and not operating hazardous machinery or a motor vehicle until at least 18–24 hours after discharge and it is certain that no residual sedative effects of the benzodiazepine remain. Importance of avoiding alcohol or nonprescription drugs for 18–24 hours following flumazenil administration or in the presence of persistent benzodiazepine effects.

Importance of informing clinicians of existing or contemplated concomitant therapy, including prescription and OTC drugs.

Importance of women informing clinicians if they are or plan to become pregnant or to breast-feed.

Overview® (see Users Guide). For additional information on this drug until a more detailed monograph is developed and published, the manufacturer's labeling should be consulted. Is is *essential* that the manufacturer's labeling be consulted for more detailed information on usual uses, cautions, precautions, contraindications, potential drug interactions, laboratory test interferences, and acute toxicity.

Preparations

Excipients in commercially available drug preparations may have clinically important effects in some individuals; consult specific product labeling for details.

Flumazenil

Parenteral		
Injection, for IV use	0.1 mg/mL (0.5 and 1 mg)*	**Flumazenil Injection**
		Romazicon®, Roche

*available from one or more manufacturer, distributor, and/or repackager by generic (nonproprietary) name

Selected Revisions January 2009,

Memantine Hydrochloride

■ Memantine hydrochloride is an *N*-methyl-D-aspartate (NMDA) receptor antagonist.

Uses

■ **Alzheimer's Disease** Memantine hydrochloride is used for the palliative treatment of moderate to severe dementia of the Alzheimer's type (Alzheimer's disease). The current indication is based principally on 2 short-term (24 or 28 weeks) randomized, controlled clinical studies in adults (50–93 years of age) with a diagnosis of probable Alzheimer's disease that was moderate to severe. In both studies, patients treated with memantine hydrochloride received an initial dosage of 5 mg once daily, with weekly increases in increments of 5 mg daily until a dosage of 20 mg daily (10 mg twice daily) was reached. Patients enrolled in the 24-week study had received donepezil hydrochloride (a reversible acetylcholinesterase inhibitor) for at least 6 months (at a stable dosage for the preceding 3 months) and continued to receive donezepil hydrochloride in addition to either memantine hydrochloride or placebo during the study period. Various instruments were used to assess efficacy. In both studies, changes from baseline in cognitive performance were assessed using the Severe Impairment Battery (SIB) scale. Changes from baseline in overall daily function and overall clinical effects (including information from caregivers) were assessed using the modified Alzheimer's disease Cooperative Study Activities of Daily Living inventory (ADCS-ADL) and the Clinician's Interview Based Impression of Change (CIBIC plus), respectively. In both studies, patients receiving memantine hydrochloride experienced less deterioration in cognitive and daily function than patients receiving placebo. In the 24-week study, patients receiving memantine experienced less decline in CIBIC plus scores than patients receiving placebo; however, while improvements in CIBIC plus scores were observed in patients receiving memantine in the 28-week study, the difference from placebo (intent-to-treat analysis) was not statistically significant. In an unpublished 24-week open-label extension of the 28-week trial, improvement relative to the projected rate of continued decline in cognition, daily function, and overall clinical impression of change was observed in patients who were switched from placebo to memantine.

A third randomized, controlled clinical study of 12 weeks' duration was conducted in nursing home patients with severe dementia (Alzheimer's disease or vascular dementia). In patients randomized to receive memantine hydrochloride, therapy was initiated at a dosage of 5 mg once daily and increased to 10 mg once daily after one week. In this study, daily function was assessed using the care dependency subscale of the Behavioral Rating Scale for Geriatric Patients (BGP), and overall clinical effects were assessed using the Clinical Global Impression of Change scale (CGI-C); cognitive function was not evaluated. In a subset of patients diagnosed as having Alzheimer's disease, memantine hydrochloride was more effective than placebo, as assessed by changes from baseline in both the BGP and CGI-C scales.

Dosage and Administration

■ **Administration** Memantine hydrochloride is administered orally (as a tablet or oral solution) without regard to meals. Memantine hydrochloride tablets and oral solution are equivalent on a mg-per-mg basis. The oral solution should be administered using the dosing device with oral syringe provided by the manufacturer, referring to the accompanying patient information for instructions. Memantine hydrochloride oral solution should not be mixed with any other liquid.

■ **Dosage** The recommended initial adult dosage of memantine hydrochloride is 5 mg once daily. The dosage of memantine hydrochloride shown to be effective in clinical trials and the recommended target dosage is 20 mg daily, given in 2 divided doses (10 mg twice daily). Dosage should be increased to the target dosage in increments of 5 mg daily at intervals of not less than 1 week. Following initiation of therapy at a dosage of 5 mg once daily, dosage should be increased to 10 mg daily (5 mg twice daily), with subsequent increases to 15 mg daily (5 mg and 10 mg as separate doses) and then to 20 mg daily (10 mg twice daily).

■ **Special Populations** No dosage adjustment is needed in patients with mild to moderate renal impairment. However, in patients with severe renal impairment (i.e., creatinine clearance of 5–29 mL/minute), a target dosage of 5 mg twice daily is recommended. Creatinine clearance may be estimated using the following formulas:

$$Ccr\ male = \frac{(140 - age) \times weight}{72 \times serum\ creatinine}$$

$$Ccr\ female = 0.85 \times Ccr\ male$$

where age is in years, weight is in kg, and serum creatinine is in mg/dL.

Cautions

■ **Contraindications** Known hypersensitivity to memantine hydrochloride or any ingredient in the formulation.

■ **Warnings/Precautions** ***General Precautions*** **Seizures.** Memantine has not been systematically evaluated in patients with a seizure disorder. In clinical studies, seizures occurred in 0.2% of patients receiving memantine and in 0.5% of patients receiving placebo.

Urinary Excretion. Conditions that increase urinary pH (e.g., dietary changes [e.g., from a high-protein to a vegetarian diet], concomitant use of drugs that alkalinize urine [e.g., carbonic anhydrase inhibitors, sodium bicarbonate], renal tubular acidosis, severe urinary tract infections) may decrease elimination of memantine, resulting in increased plasma memantine concentrations; use with caution under such conditions.

Specific Populations **Pregnancy.** Category B. (See Users Guide.)

Lactation. Not known whether memantine is distributed into human milk. However, since many drugs are distributed into human milk, caution is advised if memantine is administered in nursing women.

Pediatric Use. Safety and efficacy not established in children.

Geriatric Use. Clinical studies have been conducted principally in older patients since dementia of the Alzheimer's type occurs mainly in an older patient population. Memantine pharmacokinetics were similar in elderly patients and younger adults.

Hepatic Impairment. Although pharmacokinetics have not been evaluated in patients with hepatic impairment, only a modest effect on clearance would be expected.

Renal Impairment. The area under the plasma concentration-time curve AUC was increased by 4, 60, or 115% in individuals with mild (creatinine clearance exceeding 50 but less than 80 mL/minute), moderate (creatinine clearance 30–49 mL/minute), or severe (creatinine clearance 5–29 mL/minute) renal impairment, respectively. Terminal elimination half-life was increased by 18, 41, or 95% in those with mild, moderate, or severe renal impairment, respectively. Dosage adjustment is recommended in patients with severe renal impairment, but not in those with mild or moderate renal impairment. (See Dosage and Administration: Special Populations.)

■ **Common Adverse Effects** Adverse effects occurring in 2% or more of patients receiving memantine in clinical studies and more frequently than with placebo include dizziness (7%), confusion (6%), headache (6%), constipation (5%), cough (4%), hypertension (4%), back pain (3%), hallucination (3%), pain (3%), somnolence (3%), vomiting (3%), dyspnea (2%), and fatigue (2%).

Drug Interactions

■ **Drugs Affecting Hepatic Microsomal Enzymes** Inhibitors or inducers of cytochrome P-450 (CYP) system; pharmacokinetic interaction unlikely.

■ **Drugs Metabolized by Hepatic Microsomal Enzymes** Minimal inhibition of CYP isoenzymes 1A2, 2A6, 2C9, 2D6, 2E1, or 3A4 by memantine observed in vitro. No induction of CYP isoenzymes 1A2, 2C9, 2E1, or 3A4/5 observed in vitro at concentrations exceeding those associated with therapeutic efficacy. Pharmacokinetic interaction unlikely.

■ **Protein-bound Drugs** Because plasma protein binding of memantine is low (45%), a pharmacokinetic interaction with drugs that are highly protein bound (e.g., digoxin, warfarin) is unlikely.

■ **Drugs Secreted by Renal Tubular Cationic Transport** Potential pharmacokinetic interaction (altered plasma concentrations of both drugs) when memantine is used with drugs secreted by the same renal cationic system (e.g., cimetidine, hydrochlorothiazide, metformin, nicotine, quinidine, ranitidine, triamterene). However, concomitant use of memantine with a fixed combination of hydrochlorothiazide and triamterene did not affect bioavailability of either memantine or triamterene, and maximum plasma concentrations and area under the plasma concentration-time curve (AUC) of hydrochlorothiazide decreased by only 20%. In addition, concomitant use of memantine with a fixed combination of glyburide and metformin hydrochloride did not affect the pharmacokinetics of memantine, metformin, or glyburide, and the hypoglycemic effects of the glyburide-metformin combination were not affected.

■ **Alkalinizing Agents** Potential decreased memantine clearance with resulting increases in adverse effects when the drug is used concomitantly with agents that increase urine pH (e.g., carbonic anhydrase inhibitors, sodium bicarbonate). Use with caution. Memantine clearance was decreased by approximately 80% at alkaline urine conditions (i.e., pH 8).

■ **Cholinesterase Inhibitors** Concomitant use of memantine with the acetylcholinesterase inhibitor donepezil did not affect the pharmacokinetics of either drug or substantially alter acetylcholinesterase inhibition by donepezil. In a 24-week clinical study in patients with moderate to severe Alzheimer's disease, adverse effects observed with combination therapy with memantine and donepezil were similar to those observed with donepezil alone. In vitro and animal studies indicate that memantine does not affect the reversible inhibition of acetylcholinesterase produced by donepezil, galantamine, or tacrine.

■ ***N*-Methyl-D-aspartate (NMDA) Antagonists** Concomitant use of memantine hydrochloride with other NMDA antagonists (e.g., amantadine, ketamine, dextromethorphan) has not been systematically evaluated. Use with caution.

Description

Memantine hydrochloride is a low- to moderate-affinity, noncompetitive *N*-methyl-D-aspartate (NMDA) receptor antagonist that binds preferentially to NMDA receptor-operated cation channels. The drug differs structurally and pharmacologically from other currently available agents used for the palliative treatment of Alzheimer's disease.

Memantine is thought to act by blocking the actions of glutamate, the principal excitatory neurotransmitter in the CNS. The effects of glutamate are mediated by different receptor types, including NMDA receptors, which play a role in physiologic processes such as learning and memory formation. Persistent activation of NMDA receptors by glutamate has been implicated as a possible cause of neurodegeneration in various types of dementia, including dementia of the Alzheimer's type (Alzheimer's disease), and is thought to contribute to the symptomatology of Alzheimer's disease. In vitro studies have shown that β-amyloid, which accumulates to form amyloid plaques in patients with Alzheimer's disease, increases the release of glutamate upon neuronal depolarization, supporting a role for pathologic NMDA receptor activation in the disease. It has been postulated that low- to moderate-affinity NMDA receptor antagonists may prevent glutamate-induced neurotoxicity without interfering with the physiologic processes mediated by the activation of NMDA receptors. However, there currently is no evidence that memantine prevents or slows neurodegeneration in patients with Alzheimer's disease.

In addition to exhibiting antagonist activity at the NMDA receptor, memantine exhibits antagonist activity at the type 3 serotonergic (5-HT_3) receptor with a potency that appears to be similar to that at the NMDA receptor. Memantine also blocks the nicotinic acetylcholine receptor with a potency of about one-sixth to one-tenth that at the NMDA receptor. Memantine exhibits little or no affinity for γ-aminobutyric acid (GABA), benzodiazepine, dopamine, adrenergic, histamine, or glycine receptors or for voltage-dependent calcium, sodium, or potassium channels.

Memantine hydrochloride is well absorbed following oral administration, with peak plasma concentrations achieved in about 3–7 hours. Memantine is eliminated principally in urine, with approximately 57–82% of an administered dose excreted as unchanged drug; the remainder of the dose is converted to metabolites that exhibit minimal NMDA receptor antagonist activity. The hepatic microsomal cytochrome P-450 (CYP) isoenzyme system does not play a substantial role in the metabolism of memantine. The terminal elimination half-life of memantine is approximately 60–80 hours.

Advice to Patients

Importance of instructing caregiver regarding proper administration (twice daily for dosages exceeding 5 mg daily) and dosage escalation (minimal interval of 1 week between dosage increases).

Importance of instructing patients and/or caregivers in proper use of the oral syringe and dosing device provided with the oral solution. Ensure that patients and/or caregivers are aware of the patient instruction sheet that is enclosed with the solution. Oral solution should not be mixed with any other liquids. Advise that questions about administration should be directed to their pharmacist or clinician.

Importance of informing clinician of existing or contemplated concomitant therapy, including prescription and OTC drugs, as well as any concomitant illnesses.

Importance of women informing clinicians if they are or plan to become pregnant or plan to breast-feed.

Importance of informing patients of other important precautionary information. (See Cautions.)

Overview® (see Users Guide). For additional information on this drug until a more detailed monograph is developed and published, the manufacturer's labeling should be consulted. It is *essential* that the manufacturer's labeling be consulted for more detailed information on usual cautions, precautions, contraindications, potential drug interactions, laboratory test interferences, and acute toxicity.

Preparations

Excipients in commercially available drug preparations may have clinically important effects in some individuals; consult specific product labeling for details.

Memantine Hydrochloride

Oral		
Solution	10 mg/5 mL	**Namenda®**, Forest
Tablets, film-coated	5 mg	**Namenda®**, Forest
	10 mg	**Namenda®**, Forest
	5 mg (28 tablets) and 10 mg (21 tablets)	**Namenda® Titration Pak**, Forest

Selected Revisions November 2014,

36:00 Diagnostic Agents*

36:04 Adrenocortical Insufficiency
Cosyntropin§

36:06 Allergenic Extracts

36:08 Amyloidosis

36:10 Appendicitis

36:12 Blood Volume

36:16 Brucellosis

36:18 Cardiac Function
Indocyanine Green§
Regadenoson§

36:24 Circulation Time

36:26 Diabetes Mellitus

36:28 Diphtheria

36:30 Drug Hypersensitivity

36:32 Fungi
Coccidioidin§
Histoplasmin§

36:34 Gallbladder Function
Sincalide§

36:36 Gastric Function

36:38 Intestinal Absorption

36:40 Kidney Function
Aminohippurate§
Indigotindisulfonate§
Mannitol§

36:44 Liver Function
Indocyanine Green§

36:46 Lymphatic System

36:48 Lymphogranuloma Venereum

36:52 Mumps
Mumps Skin Test Antigen§

36:56 Myasthenia Gravis
Edrophonium§
see also:
Neostigmine 12:04

36:58 Ocular Disorders

36:60 Thyroid Function
Thyrotropin Alfa§

36:61 Pancreatic Function
Secretin§

36:62 Phenylketonuria

36:64 Pheochromocytoma

36:66 Pituitary Function
Arginine§
Metyrapone§

36:68 Roentgenographic and Other Imaging Agents

36:70 Respiratory Function

36:72 Scarlet Fever

36:76 Sweating

36:78 Trichinosis

36:84 Tuberculosis
Tuberculin§

36:88 Urine and Feces Contents
36:88.12 Ketones*
36:88.20 Occult Blood*
36:88.24 pH*
36:88.28 Protein*
36:88.40 Sugar*

§ Omitted from the print version of *AHFS Drug Information*® because of space limitations. This monograph is available on the *AHFS Drug Information*® website, http://ahfsdruginformation.com. Username: ahfs2020; Password: ASHP94498.
* Please see the full *AHFS Pharmacologic-Therapeutic Classification*© on p. viii. Many drugs may have more than one possible *AHFS* classification.

40:00 ELECTROLYTIC, CALORIC, AND WATER BALANCE*

§ Omitted from the print version of *AHFS Drug Information*® because of space limitations. This monograph is available on the *AHFS Drug Information*® website, http://ahfsdruginformation.com. Username: ahfs2020; Password: ASHP94498.
* Please see the full AHFS Pharmacologic-Therapeutic Classification© on p. viii. Not all classes are used in the printed edition.

ELECTROLYTIC, CALORIC, AND WATER BALANCE 40:00

ACIDIFYING AGENTS 40:04

Ammonium Chloride

■ Ammonium chloride is an acidifying agent.

Uses

Ammonium chloride is used as a systemic acidifier in patients with metabolic alkalosis resulting from chloride loss following vomiting, gastric suction, gastric fistula drainage, and pyloric stenosis. Ammonium chloride also has been used in the treatment of diuretic-induced chloride depletion. A solution containing isotonic or hypotonic sodium chloride with potassium chloride usually has been more effective than ammonium chloride in hypokalemic patients. Ammonium chloride also has been used to treat alkalosis resulting from excessive use of alkalinizing drugs.

Ammonium chloride has been used in a variety of conditions to induce incipient acidosis for the purpose of promoting diuresis, particularly in edematous conditions associated with hypochloremia. Ammonium chloride had limited value as a diuretic when used alone because of its limited period of effectiveness, but the drug has been useful when administered alone or in combination with a xanthine diuretic (e.g., caffeine, pamabrom) for *short-term* therapy to relieve temporary water-weight gain, edema, bloating, and/or full feeling associated with premenstrual and menstrual periods. Ammonium chloride also has been used for its diuretic effect in Ménière's syndrome.

Ammonium chloride also has been used to increase the solubility of calcium and phosphate ions in the management of patients with phosphatic calculi in the urinary tract and to increase calcium inization in alkalotic tetany. The drug also has been used in the treatment of lead poisoning to solubilize calcium and facilitate excretion of the lead-calcium complex; but more effective treatments (e.g., edetate calcium disodium, dimercaprol) are currently available. Ammonium chloride also has been used in the treatment of bromism.

Ammonium chloride also has been used as an adjunct in the treatment of urinary tract infections when a low urinary pH is desired. During therapy with methenamine salts, ammonium chloride is used to acidify the urine to ensure the dissociation of formaldehyde from methenamine. Some clinicians, however, discourage the use of the drug in this manner because of the occurrence of concurrent systemic acidosis; acidosis can be avoided by administering other acidifying agents such as ascorbic acid.

Ammonium chloride also has been used as an expectorant, usually in combination with other expectorants and cough mixtures.

Dosage and Administration

■ **Administration** As an acidifying agent, ammonium chloride is administered by slow IV infusion. Ammonium chloride has been administered orally as an acidifying agent and as a diuretic; however, an oral dosage form of the drug is no longer commercially available in the US. Solutions of the drug should *not* be administered subcutaneously, intraperitoneally, or rectally. The 26.75% for injection concentrate *must* be diluted in 0.9% sodium chloride injection prior to administration. A dilute solution may be prepared by adding 100 or 200 mEq of ammonium chloride (20 or 40 mL of the 26.75% injection) to 500 or 1000 mL of 0.9% sodium chloride injection. For IV infusion, the dilute solution should be administered at a rate not exceeding 5 mL/minute in adults.

■ **Dosage** For the treatment of metabolic alkalosis, ammonium chloride usually is administered by IV infusion. Dosage of the drug depends on the severity of the alkalosis and the tolerance of the patient. Dosage may be determined on the basis of the patient's carbon dioxide combining power. Each gram of ammonium chloride will reduce the carbon dioxide combining power of a 70-kg adult by about 1.1 volume %, or 16 mg/kg will lower the carbon dioxide combining power by 1 volume %. Alternatively, in the absence of edema or hyponatremia, dosage may be calculated on the basis of chloride deficit by the following formula:

mEq of chloride ion (as ammonium chloride) = (chloride deficit in mEq/L × (0.2 × body weight in kg)

Approximately one-half the calculated volume of ammonium chloride solution should be administered; the carbon dioxide combining power should be rechecked and necessity for further treatment determined. IV solutions of ammonium chloride should be administered very slowly to avoid ammonia toxicity. (See Cautions: Other Adverse Effects.)

Cautions

■ **Metabolic and Electrolyte Effects** Large doses of ammonium chloride may cause metabolic acidosis secondary to hyperchloremia, especially in patients with impaired renal function. Acidosis or electrolyte loss resulting from ammonium chloride therapy may be treated with IV sodium bicarbonate or sodium lactate. Potassium depletion has been reported during ammonium chloride therapy and potassium gluconate may be administered orally if hypokalemia results.

■ **Local Effects** Adverse local effects, including pain and irritation, have occurred at the site of injection or along the venous route following rapid IV administration of ammonium chloride. These local effects may be decreased by administering the drug slowly during IV infusion.

■ **Other Adverse Effects** Other adverse effects of excessive ammonium chloride dosage include rash, headache, hyperventilation, bradycardia, progressive drowsiness, mental confusion, and phases of excitement alternating with coma. Calcium-deficient tetany, hyperglycemia, glycosuria, twitching, hyperreflexia, and EEG abnormalities have also been reported. Most of these adverse effects are secondary to ammonia toxicity resulting from inability of the liver to convert the ammonium ion to urea. Because rapid IV injection may increase the likelihood of ammonia toxicity, IV infusions of ammonium chloride should be administered slowly to permit metabolism of ammonium ions by the liver.

■ **Precautions and Contraindications** Patients receiving ammonium chloride should be closely monitored for signs and symptoms of ammonia toxicity such as pallor, sweating, irregular breathing, vomiting, bradycardia, cardiac arrhythmias, local or generalized twitching, asterixis, tonic seizures, and coma.

Prior to IV infusion of ammonium chloride and during therapy, the carbon dioxide combining power of the patient's serum should be monitored to avoid serious acidosis.

Ammonium chloride should be administered with caution to patients with pulmonary insufficiency or cardiac edema. The drug should not be used in patients with primary respiratory acidosis and high total carbon dioxide and buffer base.

Sustained correction of hypochloremia cannot be achieved by administering ammonium chloride alone in patients with secondary metabolic alkalosis resulting from intracellular potassium depletion; concomitant administration of potassium chloride is necessary in such patients.

In patients with severe renal dysfunction, ammonium chloride should not be used alone when metabolic alkalosis secondary to vomiting of hydrochloric acid is accompanied by substantial sodium loss. In such patients, sodium chloride repletion, alone or in combination with ammonium chloride, may be necessary to correct both sodium and chloride depletion.

Ammonium chloride should not be administered to patients with severe hepatic dysfunction, since ammonia toxicity may occur in these patients.

■ **Pediatric Precautions** Safety and efficacy of ammonium chloride concentrate for injection in children have not been established.

■ **Pregnancy** Animal reproduction studies have not been performed with ammonium chloride. It is not known whether ammonium chloride can cause fetal harm when administered to pregnant women. Ammonium chloride should be used during pregnancy only when clearly needed.

Pharmacology

The acid-forming properties of ammonium chloride result from dissociation of the salt to an ammonium cation and a chloride anion. In patients with normal hepatic function, the ammonium cation is converted to urea by the liver and a hydrogen cation is released which reacts with a bicarbonate ion to form water and carbon dioxide. The chloride anion combines with fixed bases in the extracellular fluid, thereby reducing the alkaline reserve of the body. The net result is the displacement of bicarbonate ions by chloride anions:

$$2\ NH_4^+ + 2\ Cl^- + 2\ HCO_3^- \rightarrow CO(NH_2)_2 + CO_2 + 3\ H_2O + 2\ Cl^-$$

The displacement of bicarbonate by chloride alters the bicarbonate:carbonic acid ratio of the body and acidosis results.

The increased chloride concentration in the extracellular fluid produces an increased load to the renal tubules and appreciable amounts of chloride anions escape reabsorption. These anions are excreted along with cations and water. Sodium is the principal cation excreted; however, potassium excretion may also be increased to some degree. By increasing the excretion of both extracellular electrolytes and water, ammonium chloride causes a net loss of extracellular fluid and promotes the mobilization of edema fluid. A diuretic response occurs in both normal and edematous patients. The diuretic effect of ammonium chloride is generally overridden by compensatory renal effects within 3 days of continuous therapy with the drug. (See Pharmacokinetics.)

Although the safety and efficacy of ammonium chloride as an expectorant have not been established, it has been suggested that the drug may act as an expectorant by reflex stimulation of bronchial mucous glands resulting from irritation of gastric mucosa following oral administration of the drug. However, an oral dosage form of ammonium chloride is no longer commercially available in the US.

Pharmacokinetics

Following oral administration, ammonium chloride is rapidly absorbed from the GI tract, complete absorption occurring within 3–6 hours. However, an oral dosage form of ammonium chloride is no longer commercially available in the US. The drug is metabolized in the liver to form urea and hydrochloric acid. (See Pharmacology.) If ammonium chloride is administered for only 3 or 4 days at a time, it usually produces a mild asymptomatic acidosis. However, if it is given continuously, particularly to patients with renal impairment, it may cause severe metabolic acidosis. The kidney usually compensates for sodium loss by elaborating ammonia through the deamination of amino acids, secreting hydrogen cations in exchange for sodium cations, and thereby excreting chloride anions in combination with ammonium cations. This compensatory effect reaches its peak within about 3 days, at which time ammonium chloride will be eliminated by the kidneys as rapidly as it is ingested. Once this balance occurs, the drug is no longer effective as a diuretic.

Chemistry and Stability

■ **Chemistry** Ammonium chloride is an acid-forming salt. Ammonium chloride occurs as colorless crystals or a white, fine or coarse, crystalline powder. The drug has a cool, saline taste and is somewhat hygroscopic. Ammonium chloride is freely soluble in water (1:3) and sparingly soluble in alcohol (1:100). Aqueous solutions of ammonium chloride have a salty taste which can be masked by raspberry, cherry, or other acidic syrups.

Each gram of ammonium chloride contains 18.7 mEq each of ammonium and chloride ions. The 26.75% concentrate for injection contains ammonium chloride 5.35 g/20 mL or 5 mEq each of ammonium and chloride ions per mL; the 26.75% concentrate for injection has a calculated osmolarity of 10.018 mOsm/mL. Following dilution of 20 mL of the 26.75% concentrate for injection in 500 mL of 0.9% sodium chloride injection, the resultant dilution contains 200 mEq of ammonium and 354 mEq of chloride ions per liter.

Ammonium chloride concentrate for injection (26.75%) contains disodium edetate as a stabilizer. Hydrochloric acid may be added during the manufacture of the 26.75% concentrate for injection to adjust the pH to 5.

■ **Stability** Ammonium chloride for injection concentrate should be stored at a temperature of 40°C or less; freezing should be avoided. Concentrated solutions of ammonium chloride may crystallize when exposed to low temperatures. If crystallization occurs, the concentrate for injection should be warmed to room temperature in a water bath prior to use.

Ammonium chloride is incompatible with alkalies and their carbonates and with lead and silver salts. Explosive mixtures may result if ammonium chloride is compounded with potassium chlorate or other strong oxidizing agents.

Preparations

Excipients in commercially available drug preparations may have clinically important effects in some individuals; consult specific product labeling for details.

Ammonium Chloride

Parenteral

For injection, concentrate	26.75% (5 mEq of NH_4^+ and Cl^- per mL)*	**Ammonium Chloride Injection**

*available from one or more manufacturer, distributor, and/or repackager by generic (nonproprietary) name

ALKALINIZING AGENTS 40:08

Citrates

Shohl's Solution

■ Citrates (i.e., potassium citrate and citric acid, sodium citrate, sodium citrate and citric acid, tricitrates) are alkalinizing agents.

Uses

■ **Alkalinizing Alternatives to Sodium Bicarbonate** Administration of sodium citrate and other citrate preparations appears to be associated with formation of bicarbonate; therefore, the drugs are used as alkalinizing agents.

Oral citrate solutions, including potassium citrate and citric acid, sodium citrate and citric acid, and tricitrates, are used as alkalinizing agents in conditions where long-term maintenance of an alkaline urine is desirable and in the management of chronic metabolic acidosis associated with conditions such as chronic renal insufficiency or renal tubular acidosis.

Selection of a specific preparation may in part be determined by the potassium and sodium contents. Preparations containing sodium citrate and citric acid are especially useful when administration of potassium salts is undesirable or contraindicated, while those containing potassium citrate and citric acid are used when administration of sodium salts is undesirable or contraindicated. Unlike sodium bicarbonate solution, these preparations are generally considered highly palatable and pleasant tasting, and may be particularly useful as an alkalinizing agent in patients who do not tolerate the taste of sodium bicarbonate oral solution.

■ **Adjuvant in Gout Therapy** Potassium citrate and citric acid oral solution and tricitrates oral solution are used as adjuvant therapy to uricosuric agents in gout therapy.

■ **Prevention of Milk Curdling** Sodium citrate has been used to alter cow's milk so that large hard curds are not formed in the stomach of feeding infants†.

Dosage and Administration

■ **Administration** Citrate preparations (i.e., potassium citrate and citric acid, sodium citrate, sodium citrate and citric acid, tricitrates) are administered orally. Oral citrate solutions should be diluted with adequate amounts of water prior to administration to minimize the risk of GI complications, and followed by additional water after administration; palatability may be enhanced by chilling the solution before administration. For reconstitution of potassium citrate and citric acid for oral solution in single-dose packets, the contents of one packet should be mixed thoroughly with at least 180 mL of cool water or juice prior to administration and followed by additional water or juice after administration. Oral citrate solutions should preferably be taken after meals to avoid the saline laxative effect of the drug.

■ **Dosage** ***Potassium Citrate and Citric Acid*** The usual adult dosage of potassium citrate and citric acid solution is 15–30 mL after meals and at bedtime. The usual dosage of potassium citrate and citric acid solution in children is 5–15 mL after meals and at bedtime. The usual adult dosage of potassium citrate and citric acid for oral solution is one single-dose packet (containing 3300 mg of potassium citrate monohydrate and 1002 mg of citric acid monohydrate), reconstituted as directed 4 times daily, after meals and at bedtime. The single-dose packets of potassium citrate and citric acid for oral solution are not recommended for pediatric use, since dosage for these patients can be more easily regulated with the commercially available oral solution. Dosage should be individualized according to the patient's tolerance and response.

Sodium Citrate The usual adult dosage of sodium citrate as an alkalinizing agent is 1–2 g every 2–4 hours as necessary.

To prevent formation of large curds in the stomach of feeding infants, 100 mg of sodium citrate has been added to each 30 mL of cow's milk.

Sodium Citrate and Citric Acid The usual adult dosage of sodium citrate and citric acid solution is 10–30 mL, diluted in 30–90 mL of water, after meals and at bedtime. The usual dosage of sodium citrate and citric acid solution in children 2 years of age or older is 5–15 mL of solution, diluted in 30–90 mL of water, after meals and at bedtime. A clinician should be consulted for use of the drug in children younger than 2 years of age. Dosage should be individualized according to the patient's tolerance and response.

Sodium citrate and citric acid may be used as a buffer to maintain an approximate pH in various extemporaneous formulations. Addition of the following concentration of the drugs should generally produce a solution buffered to the approximate pH listed:

Table 1. Citrate Buffer

pH	Citric Acid Monohydrate g/L	Sodium Citrate Dihydrate g/L
2.5	64.4	7.8
3.0	57.4	17.6
3.5	47.6	31.4
4.0	40.6	41.2
4.5	30.8	54.9
5.0	19.6	70.6
5.5	9.8	84.3
6.0	4.2	92.1
6.5	1.8	95.6

Adapted from Schumacher GE. Buffer formulations. *Am J Hosp Pharm.* 1966; 23:628-9.

Tricitrates The usual adult dosage of tricitrates solution is 15–30 mL diluted in water 4 times daily, after meals and at bedtime. The usual dosage of tricitrates solution in children is 5–15 mL 4 times daily, after meals and at bedtime. Dosage should be individualized according to the patient's tolerance and response.

Cautions

■ **Adverse Effects** Oral citrate preparations generally are well tolerated when given in the usual dosages to patients with normal renal function and urine output. Excessive doses of sodium-containing formulations may cause metabolic alkalosis, especially in patients with renal dysfunction or hypocalcemia. Large doses also may cause tetany or depression of the heart associated with decreasing ionized calcium concentrations. Large doses of potassium-containing formulations may cause hyperkalemia and alkalosis, particularly in patients with impaired renal function. Listlessness, weakness, mental confusion, and paresthesia of the extremities may be associated with hyperkalemia. Oral citrate preparations may have a saline laxative effect when administered orally.

■ **Precautions and Contraindications** To avoid complications, the clinical condition of the patient should be evaluated and laboratory determinations (e.g., serum electrolytes, acid-base balance) obtained periodically during therapy with oral citrate preparations, especially in patients with renal disorders. Patients with renal impairment are at risk of developing hypernatremia or alkalosis in the presence of hypocalcemia.

Sodium-containing citrate preparations should be used with caution in patients with low urine output unless the patient is closely supervised during therapy. Citrate preparations containing sodium should be used with extreme caution in patients with congestive heart failure, hypertension, renal dysfunction, peripheral or pulmonary edema, or toxemia of pregnancy. Citrate preparations containing potassium should be used with extreme caution in patients in whom excessive potassium may have a deleterious effect.

Sodium citrate and citric acid oral solution (Cytra-2, Bicitra®) is contraindicated in patients receiving a sodium-restricted diet and in those with severe renal impairment. Tricitrates oral solution is contraindicated in patients with severe renal impairment with azotemia or oliguria, untreated Addison's disease, or severe myocardial damage. Sodium citrate and citric acid (Oracit®) is contraindicated in patients with severe renal impairment, oliguria or azotemia, untreated Addison's disease, adynamia episodica hereditaria, acute dehydration, heat cramps, anuria, severe myocardial damage, and hyperkalemia. Potassium citrate and citric acid oral solution and potassium citrate and citric acid for oral solution are also contraindicated in patients with adynamia episodica hereditaria, acute dehydration, heat cramps, anuria, severe myocardial damage, or hyperkalemia (from any cause).

■ **Pregnancy and Lactation** Controlled studies to date in pregnant women receiving potassium citrate have not shown a risk to the fetus in the first trimester of pregnancy and there is no evidence of risk in subsequent trimesters.

It is not known whether potassium citrate is distributed into milk. Because potassium freely distributes into and out of milk, use of potassium citrate by a nursing woman with normal plasma potassium concentrations should have no adverse effect on the nursing infant; milk potassium concentrations may be increased in hyperkalemic women.

Drug Interactions

■ **Antacids** Concomitant use of citrate preparations and aluminum-containing antacids may increase GI absorption of aluminum. In patients with chronic kidney disease who require aluminum-containing phosphate binders, concomitant use of citrate preparations should be avoided because of the risk of aluminum absorption and potential toxicity with concomitant use. Sodium bicarbonate may be an alternative to citrates if aluminum-containing phosphate binders are required.

■ **Cardiac Glycosides** The potential for toxicity exists in patients receiving cardiac glycosides concomitantly with citrate preparations.

■ **Drugs Affecting the Renin-Angiotensin-Aldosterone System** Concomitant use of potassium-containing citrate preparations with an angiotensin converting-enzyme (ACE) inhibitor or mineralocorticoid (aldosterone) receptor antagonist (e.g., eplerenone, spironolactone) may increase serum potassium concentrations and increase the risk of hyperkalemia and associated toxicity.

■ **Drugs Increasing Serum Potassium Concentrations** Concomitant administration of potassium-containing citrate preparations with potassium-sparing diuretics (e.g., amiloride, triamterene) or potassium-containing agents may increase serum potassium concentrations and increase the risk of hyperkalemia and associated toxicity.

■ **Drugs with pH-dependent Urinary Excretion** Alkalinization of the urine with citrates may enhance urinary excretion and decrease therapeutic and toxic effects of salicylates. (For further information on the effects of alkalinizing agents on salicylate pharmacokinetics, see Drug Interactions: Acidifying and Alkalinizing Agents and also see Pharmacokinetics: Elimination, in the Salicylates General Statement 28:08.04.24.) Alkalinization of the urine with citrates also may enhance urinary excretion of chlorpropamide and lithium.

Alkalinization of the urine with citrates may decrease urinary excretion of amphetamines, pseudoephedrine, and quinidine and increase serum concentrations of these drugs. Dosage reduction of pseudoephedrine may be necessary. Concomitant use of amphetamines and citrates should be avoided, especially in patients with amphetamine overdosage, since toxicity will be prolonged. If citrate therapy is initiated or discontinued in a patient receiving a stable quinidine dosage regimen, ECGs and serum quinidine concentrations should be monitored.

Pharmacology

Citrates (i.e., potassium citrate and citric acid, sodium citrate, sodium citrate and citric acid, tricitrates) are alkalinizing agents. Metabolism of these drugs appears to be associated with formation of bicarbonate. Citrates are extensively metabolized, and less than 5% of an oral dose is excreted in urine unchanged.

Sodium citrate has anticoagulant activity. Sodium citrate prevents the clotting of blood by forming an undissociated calcium citrate complex, making calcium unavailable to the clotting mechanism. Anticoagulant sodium citrate solution, when added to blood, prevents the clotting of blood and the crenation or swelling of cells. The sterile solution is used as an anticoagulant for banked blood for transfusion and to prepare citrated human plasma and blood for fractionation.

Sodium citrate prevents the curdling of milk by rennin, and has been used for this purpose to alter cow's milk so that large hard curds are not formed in the stomach of feeding infants.

Chemistry and Stability

■ **Chemistry** Citrates (i.e., potassium citrate and citric acid, sodium citrate, sodium citrate and citric acid, tricitrates) are alkalinizing agents.

Citric Acid Citric acid occurs as colorless, translucent crystals or as a white, granular to fine, crystalline powder. The drug is odorless or practically odorless and has a strongly acidic taste. Citric acid may occur as the anhydrous form or may contain 1 molecule of water; concentration is expressed in terms of anhydrous citric acid. Citric acid is very soluble in water and freely soluble in alcohol.

Potassium Citrate Potassium citrate occurs as transparent crystals or as a white, granular powder. The drug is odorless and has a cooling, saline taste. Potassium citrate may occur as the anhydrous form or may contain 1 molecule of water; concentration is expressed in terms of anhydrous potassium citrate. The drug is freely soluble in water and almost insoluble in alcohol.

Potassium Citrate and Citric Acid for Oral Solution Potassium citrate and citric acid for oral solution contains potassium citrate and citric acid in a sugar-free base. Each single-dose packet contains 3300 mg of potassium citrate monohydrate and 1002 mg of citric acid monohydrate and when reconstituted as directed, each single-dose packet provides 2 mEq of potassium, which is equivalent to 2 mEq of bicarbonate. Each packet of potassium citrate and citric acid for oral solution is equivalent to 15 mL of the potassium citrate and citric acid oral solution.

Potassium Citrate and Citric Acid Oral Solution Potassium citrate and citric acid oral solution is a solution of potassium citrate and citric acid in a suitable aqueous medium. Each 100 mL of potassium citrate and citric acid oral solution contains 7.55–8.35 g of potassium, 12.18–13.46 g of citrate (equivalent to 20.9–23.1 g of potassium citrate monohydrate), and 6.34–7.02 g of citric acid monohydrate. Each mL of potassium citrate and citric acid oral solution contains about 2 mEq of potassium and provides approximately 2 mEq of bicarbonate. Potassium citrate and citric acid oral solution has a pH of 4.9–5.4.

Sodium Citrate Sodium citrate occurs as colorless crystals or as a white, crystalline powder. Sodium citrate may occur as the anhydrous form or may contain 2 molecules of hydration; concentration is expressed in terms of anhydrous sodium citrate. The hydrous form of the drug is freely soluble in water, very soluble in boiling water, and insoluble in alcohol.

Sodium Citrate and Citric Acid Oral Solution Sodium citrate and citric acid oral solution is a solution of sodium citrate and citric acid in a suitable aqueous medium and occurs as a clear solution having the color of any added preservative or flavoring agent. Each 100 mL of sodium citrate and citric acid oral solution contains 2.23–2.46 g of sodium, 6.11–6.75 g of citrate (equivalent to 9.5–10.5 g of sodium citrate dihydrate), and 6.34–7.02 g of citric acid monohydrate. Each mL of sodium citrate and citric acid oral solution contains about 1 mEq of sodium and provides approximately 1 mEq of bicarbonate. Sodium citrate and citric acid oral solution has a pH of 4–4.4.

Tricitrates Oral Solution Tricitrates oral solution is a solution of citric acid, potassium citrate, and sodium citrate in a suitable aqueous medium. Each 100 mL of tricitrates oral solution contains 6.34–7.02 g of citric acid monohydrate, 12.20–13.48 g of citrate as potassium citrate and sodium citrate, 3.78–4.18 g of potassium (equivalent to 10.45–11.55 g of potassium citrate monohydrate), and 2.23–2.46 g of sodium (equivalent to 9.5–10.5 g of sodium citrate dihydrate. Each mL of tricitrates oral solution contains about 1 mEq each of potassium and sodium and provides approximately 2 mEq of bicarbonate. Tricitrates oral solution has a pH of 4.9–5.4.

■ **Stability** ***Citric Acid*** The hydrous form of citric acid is efflorescent in dry air.

Potassium Citrate Potassium citrate is deliquescent when exposed to moist air.

Potassium Citrate and Citric Acid for Oral Solution Potassium citrate and citric acid for oral solution should be protected from excessive heat and freezing.

Potassium Citrate and Citric Acid Oral Solution Potassium citrate and citric acid oral solution should be stored in tight, light-resistant container at 20–25°C and protected from excessive heat and freezing.

Sodium Citrate and Citric Acid Oral Solution Sodium citrate and citric acid oral solution generally should be stored in tight containers and protected from freezing or excessive heat. The manufacturer's labeling should be consulted for specific storage recommendations.

Tricitrates Oral Solution Tricitrates oral solution should be stored in tight container at 20–25°C and protected from excessive heat and freezing.

Preparations

Excipients in commercially available drug preparations may have clinically important effects in some individuals; consult specific product labeling for details.

Potassium Citrate and Citric Acid

Oral		
For solution	Potassium Citrate Monohydrate 3300 mg and Citric Acid Monohydrate 1002 mg per packet	**Cytra-K Crystals,** Cypress
Solution	Potassium Citrate Monohydrate 1100 mg/5 mL and Citric Acid Monohydrate 334 mg/5 mL*	**Cytra-K,** Cypress **Potassium Citrate Monohydrate and Citric Acid Monohydrate Solution**

*available from one or more manufacturer, distributor, and/or repackager by generic (nonproprietary) name

Sodium Citrate

Powder

Sodium Citrate and Citric Acid

Oral		
Solution (Shohl's Solution)	Hydrous Sodium Citrate 490 mg/5 mL and Citric Acid 640 mg/5 mL	**Oracit®,** Carolina Medical
	Sodium Citrate Dihydrate 500 mg (321.5 mg of citrate) per 5 mL and Citric Acid Monohydrate 334 mg/5 mL	**Bicitra®,** Ortho-McNeil **Cytra-2,** Cypress

Tricitrates

Oral		
Solution	Citric Acid Monohydrate 334 mg/5 mL, Potassium Citrate Monohydrate 550 mg/5 mL, and Sodium Citrate Dihydrate 500 mg (321.5 mg of citrate) per 5 mL*	**Citric Acid Monohydrate, Potassium Citrate Monohydrate, and Sodium Citrate Dihydrate Solution** **Cytra-3 Syrup,** Cypress

*available from one or more manufacturer, distributor, and/or repackager by generic (nonproprietary) name

†Use is not currently included in the labeling approved by the US Food and Drug Administration

Sodium Bicarbonate

Baking Soda, Sodium Acid Carbonate, Sodium Hydrogen Carbonate

■ Sodium bicarbonate is an alkalinizing agent.

Uses

■ **Overview** Sodium bicarbonate is used as an alkalinizing agent in the treatment of metabolic acidosis. Sodium bicarbonate also is used to increase urinary pH in order to increase the solubility of certain weak acids (e.g., cystine, sulfonamides, uric acid) or in the treatment of hemolytic reactions requiring alkalinization of the urine to diminish the nephrotoxic effects of blood pigments. In addition, the drug is used in the treatment of severe diarrhea accompanied by substantial GI bicarbonate loss.

■ **Acidosis** Sodium bicarbonate is used in the treatment of metabolic acidosis associated with many conditions including severe renal disease (e.g., renal tubular acidosis), uncontrolled diabetes (ketoacidosis), extracorporeal circulation of the blood, cardiac arrest, circulatory insufficiency caused by shock or severe dehydration, ureterosigmoidostomy, lactic acidosis, alcoholic ketoacidosis, use of carbonic anhydrase inhibitors, and ammonium chloride administration. In metabolic acidosis, the principal disturbance is a loss of proton acceptors (e.g., loss of bicarbonate during severe diarrhea) or accumulation of an acid load (e.g., ketoacidosis, lactic acidosis, renal tubular acidosis).

Mild acidosis may have minimal clinical importance and require no corrective therapy; physiologic compensatory mechanisms may be adequate to correct the disorder. When the underlying cause can be treated effectively in more severe acidosis, there is often no need to specifically treat the acid-base disorder. Generally, administration of sodium bicarbonate is not necessary unless the acidosis is severe (e.g., arterial pH less than 7.1–7.2 or plasma bicarbonate concentration of 8 mEq/L or less) or the underlying cause of the acidosis cannot be determined and/or corrected.

When specific alkalinizing therapy is necessary, complete correction of the acidosis with an alkalinizing agent is usually not necessary, and may be hazardous, since metabolic alkalosis can be precipitated. Generally, the goal of alkalinizing therapy is to correct the acid-base disturbance toward normal and allow physiologic compensatory mechanisms to complete the correction, if possible. Sodium bicarbonate is generally considered the alkalinizing agent of choice for oral or parenteral therapy. When sodium bicarbonate is used in the treatment of metabolic acidosis, the acid-base status of the patient must be monitored frequently and dosage modified according to response; the bicarbonate deficit can only be estimated, and no more than 50% of the calculated deficit should be replaced initially in patients whose compensatory mechanisms are expected to contribute to correction of the acidosis.

■ **Diabetic Ketoacidosis** The specific role of sodium bicarbonate therapy in the treatment of diabetic ketoacidosis has not been established. Because correction of the underlying metabolic disorder generally results in correction of acid-base abnormalities and because of the potential risks of sodium bicarbonate therapy in the treatment of this disorder, administration of sodium bicarbonate is generally reserved for the treatment of severe acidosis (e.g., arterial pH less than 7–7.15 or serum bicarbonate concentration of 8 mEq/L or less). Rapid correction of acidosis with sodium bicarbonate in patients with diabetic ketoacidosis may cause hypokalemia, paradoxical acidosis in CSF since carbon dioxide diffuses more rapidly into CSF than does bicarbonate, and lactic acidosis since increased pH increases hemoglobin-oxygen affinity which, when combined with erythrocyte 2,3-diphosphoglycerate (2,3-DPG) deficiency in these patients, results in peripheral tissue hypoxia. However, the benefits and risks of sodium bicarbonate therapy in ketoacidosis have not been fully determined, and additional controlled studies of the safety and efficacy of the drug are necessary. Generally, when sodium bicarbonate is used in the treatment of diabetic ketoacidosis, the acidosis should only be partially corrected (e.g., to an arterial pH of about 7.2) to avoid rebound metabolic alkalosis as ketones are metabolized.

■ **Advanced Cardiovascular Life Support** The American Heart Association (AHA) guidelines for cardiopulmonary resuscitation (CPR) and emergency cardiovascular care state that IV sodium bicarbonate is not recommended for *routine* use during cardiac arrest. There are only limited data that support therapy with buffers during cardiac arrest, and routine administration of sodium bicarbonate has not been reported to improve outcomes of resuscitation. There is no evidence indicating that sodium bicarbonate improves the likelihood of defibrillation or survival rates in animals with ventricular fibrillation and cardiac arrest. In addition, the drug potentially may have detrimental effects (e.g., compromised coronary perfusion pressure [CPP] caused by reduction of systemic vascular resistance; paradoxical intracellular acidosis caused by production of carbon dioxide that freely diffuses into myocardial and cerebral cells and may depress function, especially in ischemic myocardium; shift in the oxyhemoglobin saturation curve, inhibiting release of oxygen; induction of hyperosmolarity and hypernatremia; adverse effects secondary to extracellular alkalosis; exacerbation of central venous acidosis; inactivation of concomitantly administered catecholamines).

Restoration of oxygen content with appropriate ventilation with oxygen, support of some tissue perfusion and cardiac output with good chest compressions, then rapid return of spontaneous circulation (ROSC), are the mainstays of restoring acid-base balance during cardiac arrest. By ensuring adequate alveolar ventilation, a major component of depressed pH (respiratory acidosis) during cardiac arrest generally can be managed without sodium bicarbonate. Sodium bicarbonate may be useful in some resuscitation situations (e.g., preexisting metabolic acidosis, hyperkalemia, tricyclic antidepressant overdosage). In addition, some experts state that sodium bicarbonate may be considered in the treatment of ventricular arrhythmias associated with cocaine toxicity in addition to standard treatments.

It must be kept in mind that administration of sodium bicarbonate is followed by release of carbon dioxide, which requires adequate alveolar ventilation to assure continued excretion of this source of potential acid. Thus, the importance of adequate alveolar ventilation in the control of pH must be emphasized, as well as the need for repeated arterial determination of blood pH and Pa_{co_2}, if possible. Whenever possible, sodium bicarbonate therapy should be guided by the bicarbonate concentration or calculated base deficit obtained from blood gas analysis or laboratory measurement. To minimize the risk of iatrogenically induced alkalosis, complete correction of the base deficit should not be attempted. Some experts state that other non-carbon dioxide generating buffers (e.g., tromethamine) have shown a potential to minimize some adverse effects of sodium bicarbonate (e.g., carbon dioxide generation, hyperosmolarity, hypernatremia, hypoglycemia, intracellular acidosis, myocardial acidosis, overshoot alkalosis) when used in certain resuscitation situations; however, clinical experience is limited and outcome studies are lacking.

■ **Antacid Therapy** **For the use of sodium bicarbonate as an antacid, see Antacids 56:04.**

Dosage and Administration

■ **Administration** Sodium bicarbonate is administered by IV infusion. Sodium bicarbonate may be administered by rapid IV injection when initial immediate administration of the drug is considered necessary (e.g., during cardiac arrest). The drug also may be administered orally in the treatment of mild to moderately severe acidosis, in conditions (e.g., chronic renal failure) requiring prolonged therapy with an alkalinizing agent, and in conditions in which IV administration of the drug is not necessary (e.g., alkalinization of the urine). The drug has also been administered by subcutaneous injection if diluted to isotonicity (1.5% sodium bicarbonate solution). Extravasation of hypertonic sodium bicarbonate injections must be avoided. (See Cautions: Adverse Effects.) Sodium bicarbonate also has been administered by intraosseous (IO) injection† in the setting of pediatric advanced life support (PALS); onset of action and systemic concentrations are comparable to those achieved with venous administration. However, acid-base balance analysis may be inaccurate after administration of sodium bicarbonate via the IO cannula.

In neonates and children younger than 2 years of age, hypertonic sodium bicarbonate injections generally should be administered by slow IV infusion of a 4.2% solution up to 8 mEq/kg daily. (See Cautions: Pediatric Precautions.)

■ **Dosage** Dosage of sodium bicarbonate injection is determined by severity of the acidosis, appropriate laboratory determinations, and the patient's age, weight, and clinical condition. Frequent laboratory determinations and clinical evaluation of the patient are essential during therapy with sodium bicarbonate, especially during prolonged therapy, to monitor changes in fluid and electrolyte and acid-base balance.

Generally, full correction of bicarbonate deficit should not be attempted during the first 24 hours of sodium bicarbonate therapy, since this may result in precipitation of metabolic alkalosis because of delayed physiologic compensatory mechanisms. When total carbon dioxide content is returned to normal or beyond within the first day of therapy, substantially alkaline values for blood pH and subsequent adverse effects are likely to occur. When initial, rapid administration of the drug is considered necessary, it is generally recommended that no more than 33–50% of the calculated bicarbonate requirements be administered initially. Several methods for estimating bicarbonate requirements in patients with metabolic acidosis have been suggested; specialized references on fluid and electrolyte and acid-base balance should be consulted for specific recommendations.

Sodium bicarbonate is not recommended for *routine* use in advanced cardiovascular life support (ACLS) during cardiac arrest (see Uses: Advanced Cardiovascular Life Support); however, if the drug is used in certain resuscitation situations (e.g., preexisting metabolic acidosis, hyperkalemia, tricyclic antidepressant overdosage), an IV dose of 1 mEq/kg is usually given initially in adults. Whenever possible, dosage of sodium bicarbonate should be guided by the bicarbonate concentration or by the calculated base deficit obtained from blood gas analysis or laboratory measurement. Complete correction of the base deficit is not recommended to minimize the risk of alkalosis. For the management of cardiac arrest due to hyperkalemia in adults, 50 mEq of sodium bicarbonate has been administered IV over 5 minutes as adjunctive therapy to other standard ACLS measures.

If sodium bicarbonate is used for pediatric resuscitation, the guidelines for pediatric advanced life support (PALS) recommend a pediatric dose of 1 mEq/kg, administered slowly by IV or IO† injection. If blood gas tensions and pH measurements are available, subsequent doses should be determined by the following equation:

$$\text{mEq NaHCO}_3 = 0.3 \times \text{bodyweight (in kg)} \times \text{base deficit (in mEq/L)}$$

In less urgent forms of metabolic acidosis, a 2–5 mEq/kg dose of sodium bicarbonate may be administered to older children or adults as a 4- to 8-hour IV infusion. Subsequent doses should be determined by the response of the patient and appropriate laboratory determinations. Sodium bicarbonate therapy should be planned in a stepwise manner, since the degree of response following a given dose is not always predictable. Generally, the dose and frequency of administration should be reduced after severe symptoms have improved.

For the treatment of ventricular arrhythmias associated with cocaine toxicity in pediatric patients, 1–2 mEq/kg of IV sodium bicarbonate has been administered.

Although the specific role of sodium bicarbonate therapy in the treatment of diabetic ketoacidosis has not been established (see Uses: Diabetic Ketoacidosis), when IV sodium bicarbonate is administered, the acidosis should only partially be corrected, generally to an arterial pH of about 7.2, in order to avoid rebound alkalosis.

For the treatment of acidosis associated with chronic renal failure, oral sodium bicarbonate therapy is generally initiated when plasma bicarbonate concentration is less than 15 mEq/L. Therapy is usually initiated in adults with an oral sodium bicarbonate dosage of 20–36 mEq daily, given in divided doses. Dosage is then titrated to provide a plasma bicarbonate concentration of about 18–20 mEq/L. Because of the sodium content of sodium bicarbonate, the fluid and electrolyte balance of the patient must be carefully monitored during therapy with the drug. To relieve symptoms and prevent or stabilize renal failure and osteomalacia in patients with renal tubular acidosis, higher dosages of sodium bicarbonate are necessary. In adults with distal (type 1) renal tubular acidosis, an initial oral dosage of 0.5–2 mEq/kg daily, given in 4 or 5 divided doses, has been suggested. Dosage is titrated until hypercalciuria and acidosis are controlled, and according to the response and tolerance of the patient. Alternatively, an adult dosage of 48–72 mEq (about 4–6 g) daily has been suggested. Higher dosages are generally required in patients with proximal (type 2) renal tubular acidosis; oral dosages of 4–10 mEq/kg daily, given in divided doses, have been suggested.

The usual oral dosage of sodium bicarbonate for alkalinization of urine in adults is 48 mEq (4 g) initially, followed by 12–24 mEq (1–2 g) every 4 hours. Dosages of 30–48 mEq (2.5–4 g) every 4 hours, up to 192 mEq (16 g) daily, may be required in some patients. Dosage should be individually titrated to maintain the desired urinary pH. For alkalinization of urine in children, an oral dosage of 1–10 mEq (84–840 mg) per kg daily, adjusted according to response, has been suggested.

Cautions

■ Adverse Effects Gastric distention and flatulence may occur when sodium bicarbonate is administered orally. Inadvertent extravasation of hypertonic solutions of sodium bicarbonate has reportedly caused chemical cellulitis because of their alkalinity, subsequently resulting in tissue necrosis, ulceration, and/or sloughing at the site of injection. One manufacturer recommends that extravasation be treated by elevating the affected area, applying warm compresses to the site, and locally injecting lidocaine or hyaluronidase.

Sodium bicarbonate, when given in large doses or to patients with renal insufficiency, may cause metabolic alkalosis. Metabolic alkalosis may be accompanied by hyperirritability or tetany. The manufacturers recommend that severe bicarbonate-induced alkalosis be treated with a parenteral calcium salt (e.g., calcium gluconate) and/or an acidifying agent (e.g., ammonium chloride). In patients with ketoacidosis, rapid alkalinization with sodium bicarbonate may reportedly result in clouding of consciousness, cerebral dysfunction, obtundation, seizures, and peripheral tissue hypoxia and lactic acidosis.

Sodium and water retention and edema may occur during sodium bicarbonate therapy, especially when the drug is given in large doses or to patients with renal insufficiency, congestive heart failure, or those predisposed to sodium retention and edema. Sodium and water overload may result in hypernatremia and hyperosmolality. Severe hyperosmolal states may develop during cardiopulmonary resuscitation when excessive doses of sodium bicarbonate are administered. (See Pharmacology.)

■ Precautions and Contraindications Generally, the goal of alkalinizing therapy is to correct the acid-base disturbance while avoiding overdosage and resultant metabolic alkalosis.

Sodium bicarbonate should be used with extreme caution in patients with congestive heart failure or other edematous or sodium-retaining conditions; in patients with renal insufficiency, especially those with severe insufficiency such as oliguria or anuria; and in patients receiving corticosteroids or corticotropin, since each gram of sodium bicarbonate contains about 12 mEq of sodium. (For the sodium content of commercially available injections, see Chemistry and Stability: Chemistry.) IV administration of sodium bicarbonate may cause fluid and/or solute overload resulting in dilution of serum electrolytes, overhydration, congestive conditions, or pulmonary edema. The risk of dilutional conditions is inversely proportional to the electrolyte concentration administered, and the risk of solute overload and resultant congestive conditions with peripheral and/or pulmonary edema is directly proportional to the electrolyte concentration administered.

Potassium depletion may predispose to metabolic alkalosis and coexistent hypocalcemia may result in tetany and carpopedal spasm as the plasma pH increases. To minimize the risks of preexisting hypokalemia and/or hypocalcemia, these electrolyte disturbances should be corrected prior to initiation of, or concomitantly with, sodium bicarbonate therapy.

Sodium bicarbonate is generally contraindicated in patients with metabolic or respiratory alkalosis, in patients with hypocalcemia in whom alkalosis may induce tetany, in patients with excessive chloride loss from vomiting or continuous GI suctioning, and in patients at risk of developing diuretic-induced hypochloremic alkalosis. Sodium bicarbonate should not be used orally as an antidote in the treatment of acute ingestion of strong mineral acids, since carbon dioxide gas forms during neutralization and may cause gastric distention and possible rupture. Some experts state that non-lipid soluble drugs (e.g., sodium bicarbonate) may injure the airway and should not be administered via the endotracheal route.

■ Pediatric Precautions One manufacturer cautions that rapid injection (10 mL/minute) of hypertonic sodium bicarbonate solutions in neonates and children younger than 2 years of age may produce hypernatremia, decreased CSF pressure, and possible intracranial hemorrhage. It is recommended that the rate of IV administration in these children not exceed 8 mEq/kg daily and that slow IV administration of a 4.2% solution may be preferred. In emergencies such as cardiac arrest, the risk of rapid infusion of the drug in these children must be weighed against the potential for death from acidosis.

■ Pregnancy Animal reproduction studies have not been performed with sodium bicarbonate. It is also not known whether sodium bicarbonate can cause fetal harm when administered to pregnant women. Sodium bicarbonate should be used during pregnancy only when clearly needed.

Pharmacology

Sodium bicarbonate is an alkalinizing agent which dissociates to provide bicarbonate ion.

Bicarbonate is the conjugate base component of the principal extracellular buffer in the body, the bicarbonate:carbonic acid buffer. Various metabolic processes in the body either generate or consume hydrogen ions. Despite the dynamic nature of these processes, the hydrogen ion concentration in plasma and interstitial fluid is maintained at an almost constant level between 38–42 nmole/L (pH 7.37–7.42). The acid-base balance is maintained by 3 interacting mechanisms: buffers, regulation of carbonic acid concentration by the pulmonary system, and renal excretion of acid or base.

In body fluids, there are many buffers, including hemoglobin, proteins, and phosphates; however, the principal extracellular buffer is the bicarbonate:carbonic acid buffer. At a given pH, the ratio of bicarbonate:carbonic acid is constant. At pH 7.4, the bicarbonate:carbonic acid ratio is 20:1. Although buffers are most efficient when the ratio is 1, the unique characteristics of the bicarbonate:carbonic acid buffer make it highly effective even at a ratio of 20:1. In a solution such as plasma, all buffers are in equilibrium with the same hydrogen ion concentration and with each other. Thus, assessment of any one of these buffers (e.g., bicarbonate:carbonic acid) is reflective of the hydrogen ion concentration of the entire solution and the ratios of conjugate base to undissociated acid for all buffers. The bicarbonate:carbonic acid buffer is the only buffer in the body whose component concentrations can be varied independently by physiologic regulatory mechanisms. The bicarbonate buffer is extremely effective in buffering fixed acids and bases since changes in its components can be compensated by physiologic mechanisms such as formation and excretion of high concentrations of carbon dioxide, regulation by the pulmonary system of carbon dioxide concentration in body fluids, and generation or excretion by the kidney of substantial amounts of bicarbonate. Since carbonic acid is readily converted to or from carbon dioxide gas, its concentration is responsive to changes in alveolar Pco_2 and can be readily altered by changes in pulmonary ventilation.

Carbonic acid and dissolved carbon dioxide constitute the weak acid component and bicarbonate is the conjugate base component in the bicarbonate:carbonic acid buffer. The bicarbonate:carbonic acid buffer can be expressed as the following form of the Henderson-Hasselbalch equation:

$$pH = 6.1 + \log \frac{[HCO_3^-]}{[H_2CO_3] + [\text{dissolved } CO_2]}$$

At equilibrium, the amount of dissolved carbon dioxide in plasma greatly exceeds that of carbonic acid. Thus, measurement of carbon dioxide is used to determine the concentration of the weak acid component of the buffer. Since the concentration of dissolved carbon dioxide in plasma (liquid phase) is in equilibrium with alveolar carbon dioxide (gas phase), the concentration of carbon dioxide in plasma can be calculated from the partial pressure of carbon dioxide using the following equation:

$$CO_2 \text{ (mmol/L)} = 0.03 \times Pco_2 \text{ (mm Hg)}$$

and the Henderson-Hasselbalch equation can be expressed as follows:

$$pH = 6.1 + \log \frac{[HCO_3^-]}{0.03 \times P_{CO_2}}$$

Changes in the concentration of either component of the buffer can cause a decrease or increase in pH. Administration of sodium bicarbonate will increase the plasma bicarbonate concentration and possibly increase plasma pH; however, pH is usually maintained within the normal range, since compensatory mechanisms such as increased glomerular filtration and decreased tubular reabsorption of bicarbonate in the kidneys will rapidly decrease the plasma concentration of bicarbonate and restore the bicarbonate:carbonic acid ratio. Although metabolic alkalosis may result from IV infusion or ingestion of large amounts of sodium bicarbonate, renal mechanisms for increasing bicarbonate excretion are usually adequate to compensate for the acid-base imbalance. Primary acid-base disturbances (i.e., respiratory acidosis or alkalosis and metabolic acidosis or alkalosis) result from an initial change in one of the components of the bicarbonate:carbonic acid buffer. Generally, compensatory physiologic mechanisms and correction of the underlying cause of the disturbance are sufficient to restore acid-base balance. Occasionally, when acidemia is severe or plasma bicarbonate concentration is severely depleted, administration of sodium bicarbonate may be necessary to restore acid-base balance in patients with metabolic or respiratory acidosis. However, administration of sodium bicarbonate in these patients may result in metabolic alkalosis.

Changes in acid-base balance also stimulate compensatory ion-exchange mechanisms. Cations such as potassium and sodium can exchange for extracellular hydrogen ions. When the extracellular hydrogen ion concentration increases, as in acidosis, there is a redistribution of potassium ions from intracellular to extracellular fluid. Administration of sodium bicarbonate, by decreasing pH, can cause a redistribution of potassium ions into cells in patients with acidosis.

Since sodium bicarbonate provides bicarbonate which is readily excreted in urine, administration of the drug will increase urinary pH in patients with normal renal function. Alkalinizing the urine can increase the solubility of certain weak acids (e.g., cystine, uric acid) and can increase the ionization and urinary excretion of lipid-soluble organic acids (e.g., phenobarbital, salicylates) that are reabsorbed in the kidney via diffusion of the un-ionized species.

Sodium bicarbonate has a potent antacid action. Each gram of sodium bicarbonate has an in vitro neutralizing capacity of about 12 mEq of acid. For a discussion on sodium bicarbonate's antacid action, see Antacids 56:04.

Chemistry and Stability

■ **Chemistry** Sodium bicarbonate is an alkalinizing agent. Sodium bicarbonate occurs as a white, crystalline powder which has a saline and slightly alkaline taste. The drug is soluble in water and insoluble in alcohol. Aqueous solutions of sodium bicarbonate, when freshly prepared, are alkaline to litmus; alkalinity increases as the solutions stand, are agitated, or are heated. Each 84 mg or 1 g of sodium bicarbonate contains 1 or about 12 mEq, respectively, each of sodium and bicarbonate ions.

Sodium bicarbonate injections are sterile solutions of the drug in water for injection. Carbon dioxide may be added during the manufacture of the injection to adjust the pH to 7–8.5. An 8.4% solution contains 1 mEq each of sodium and bicarbonate ions per mL and has a calculated osmolarity of 2000 mOsm/L. A 7.5% solution contains 0.892 mEq/mL each of sodium and bicarbonate ions and has a calculated osmolarity of 1786 mOsm/L. A 5% solution contains 0.595 mEq each of sodium and bicarbonate ions per mL and has a calculated osmolarity of 1190–1203 mOsm/L. A 4.2% solution contains 0.5 mEq each of sodium and bicarbonate ions per mL and has a calculated osmolarity of 1000 mOsm/L. Sodium bicarbonate is also available as a 4% small volume parenteral additive solution (Neut®) which provides 2.4 mEq each of sodium and bicarbonate ions per 5 mL and is used to increase the pH of acidic infusion solutions.

A 1.5% solution of sodium bicarbonate is isotonic. A 1.5% sodium bicarbonate solution can be prepared by diluting each mL of an 8.4, 7.5, or 4.2% solution of the drug with 4.6, 4, or 1.8 mL of sterile water for injection, respectively.

■ **Stability** Sodium bicarbonate tablets and effervescent tablets should be stored in tightly closed containers at a temperature less than 40°C, preferably between 15–30°C. Sodium bicarbonate injection should be stored at a temperature less than 40°C, preferably between 15–30°C; freezing should be avoided.

Sodium bicarbonate is stable in dry air, but slowly decomposes into sodium carbonate, carbon dioxide, and water in moist air. When heated, sodium bicarbonate loses water and carbon dioxide and is converted into sodium carbonate. Solutions of sodium carbonate are much more alkaline than sodium bicarbonate; since sodium carbonate may be formed when the dry salt or its solutions are sterilized with heat, the pH of heat-sterilized solutions or of solutions prepared from heat-sterilized powder should be determined prior to use. When sodium bicarbonate is combined with acids in aqueous solutions, a vigorous evolution of carbon dioxide gas occurs; the liberated carbon dioxide bubbles through the solution resulting in effervescence. In the dry state, sodium bicarbonate and acids do not react.

Sodium bicarbonate is physically and/or chemically incompatible with many drugs including acids, acidic salts, and many alkaloidal salts, but the compatibility depends on several factors (e.g., concentrations of the drugs, specific diluent used, resulting pH, temperature). Sodium bicarbonate injection should not be admixed with solutions containing calcium salts, except where compatibility has been specifically established, since haze formation or precipitation may result from such combinations. Also, sodium bicarbonate should not be admixed with or administered in the same IV line as catecholamines (e.g., epinephrine) because sodium bicarbonate may inactivate simultaneously administered catecholamines. Specialized references should be consulted for specific compatibility information.

Preparations

Excipients in commercially available drug preparations may have clinically important effects in some individuals; consult specific product labeling for details.

Sodium Bicarbonate

Oral		
Powder*		**Arm & Hammer® Baking Soda,** Church & Dwight
Tablets	325 mg*	**Soda Mint,** CMC
		Sodium Bicarbonate Tablets
	650 mg*	
Parenteral		
Injection	4.2% (0.5 mEq/mL) (2.5 or 5 mEq)*	**Sodium Bicarbonate Injection**
	5% (0.595 mEq/mL) (297.5 mEq)*	**Sodium Bicarbonate Injection**
	7.5% (0.892 mEq/mL) (8.92 or 44.6 mEq)*	**Sodium Bicarbonate Injection**
	8.4% (1 mEq/mL) (10 or 50 mEq)*	**Sodium Bicarbonate Injection**
Injection, for preparation of IV admixtures	7.5% (0.892 mEq/mL) (178.4 mEq) pharmacy bulk package	**Sodium Bicarbonate Injection MaxiVial®,** Abraxis
Solution, sterile, to adjust pH of injections	4% (0.48 mEq/mL) (2.4 mEq)	**Neut®,** Hospira
	4.2% (0.5 mEq/mL) (2.5 mEq)*	**Sodium Bicarbonate Additive Solution**

*available from one or more manufacturer, distributor, and/or repackager by generic (nonproprietary) name

†Use is not currently included in the labeling approved by the US Food and Drug Administration

AMMONIA DETOXICANTS 40:10

Lactulose

■ Lactulose, a synthetic derivative of lactose, is an ammonia detoxicant.

Uses

■ **Portal-Systemic Encephalopathy** Lactulose is used as an adjunct to protein restriction and supportive therapy for the prevention and treatment of portal-systemic encephalopathy (PSE) including hepatic pre-coma and coma. Lactulose has been useful in the management of PSE resulting from surgical portacaval shunts or from chronic hepatic diseases such as cirrhosis. In patients with PSE, lactulose therapy reduces the blood ammonia concentration and this is usually accompanied by substantial improvement in the mental state of the patient and improved EEG tracings. Many patients are able to tolerate increased dietary protein during lactulose therapy. The drug does not, however, alter the course of the underlying liver disease. Therefore, use of lactulose in the treatment of PSE does not obviate treatment of underlying liver disease, nor preclude other measures used in the treatment of PSE.

A good clinical response has been achieved in 75–85% of PSE patients receiving lactulose therapy. Because lactulose is relatively nontoxic, it is a valuable alternative to antibiotics such as neomycin, especially when prolonged therapy is required or when neomycin is contraindicated. Some well-controlled comparative studies have shown that the efficacy of lactulose is superior to that of laxative controls (such as magnesium sulfate or sorbitol) and about equal to that of neomycin in the treatment of acute and chronic PSE. Some patients who had previously failed to respond to neomycin and dietary protein restriction responded to lactulose therapy. Conversely, other patients responded better to neomycin than to lactulose.

Since neomycin destroys bacteria and lactulose requires bacterial degradation for its effectiveness, concomitant therapy with these agents is theoretically counterproductive. (See Drug Interactions: Anti-infective Agents.) It appears, however, that lactulose remains active when administered with neomycin and, in fact, there is some evidence that concomitant therapy with lactulose and neomycin may be more effective than either drug alone. Some clinicians recommend neomycin for acute episodes of PSE and lactulose for the long-term management of chronic PSE.

Lactulose is not useful in the management of non-nitrogenous types of encephalopathy such as those induced by drugs or metabolic or electrolyte disturbances. Lactulose therapy is not effective in the treatment of coma associated with infectious hepatitis or other acute disorders of the liver. In a case of hyperammonemia, which was apparently caused by an inborn error of metabolism, lactulose therapy was ineffective.

■ **Constipation** Lactulose is useful as a laxative in the treatment of chronic constipation in adults and geriatric patients. The drug has been used in the treatment of chronic constipation in children†; however, the manufacturers state that safety and efficacy of lactulose for the treatment of chronic constipation in children have not been established. Lactulose has also been used to restore regular bowel movements in hemorrhoidectomy patients†. Following a barium meal examination, the drug has been used to induce bowel evacuation in geriatric patients with colonic retention of barium and severe constipation†. Although lactulose is effective in the treatment of chronic constipation, its superiority to conventional laxatives has not been established.

Dosage and Administration

■ **Reconstitution and Administration** Lactulose is usually administered orally. The sweet taste of lactulose solution, which may be unpleasant to some patients, can be minimized by diluting the solution with water, fruit juice, or milk or administering it in food such as desserts. When lactulose solution is administered via a gastric tube, it should be well diluted to prevent induction of vomiting and the possibility of aspiration pneumonia.

Lactulose may also be administered rectally to adults with portal-systemic encephalopathy (PSE) during stages of hepatic pre-coma or coma when the possibility of aspiration exists, or when necessary endoscopic or intubation procedures interfere with oral administration.

For oral administration, lactulose powder should be reconstituted by dissolving the contents of a packet labeled as containing 10 or 20 g of the drug in approximately 120 mL of water.

■ **Dosage** Each 15 mL of commercially available lactulose solution provides approximately 10 g of the drug; corresponding doses provided by 2.5, 5, 7.5, 10, 30, 40, 45, 90, 150, and 300 mL of the commercial solution are approximately 1.67, 3.3, 5, 6.67, 20, 27, 30, 60, 100, and 200 g, respectively. Following reconstitution of the oral powder as directed, a 10 or 20 g dose is provided by the total volume.

Portal-Systemic Encephalopathy For the prevention and treatment of PSE in adults, the usual initial oral dosage of lactulose is 20–30 g 3 or 4 times daily. Dosage is then adjusted every 1–2 days as necessary to produce 2 or 3 soft stools daily. Some clinicians recommend that dosage be adjusted according to the acidity of the colonic contents by measuring stool pH (with indicator paper) at the start of therapy and adjusting the dosage until stool pH is about 5. This pH is usually achieved when the patient has 2 or 3 soft stools daily during lactulose therapy. For most adults, lactulose dosage is usually 60–100 g daily, although some patients may require higher dosage.

In the management of acute episodes of PSE in adults, 20–30 g may be given orally at 1- to 2-hour intervals to induce rapid laxation. When the laxative effect has been achieved, the dose of lactulose is reduced to the amount required to produce 2 or 3 soft stools daily. When lactulose is administered in the treatment of PSE, improvement in the clinical condition of the patient usually occurs within 1–3 days. Continuous long-term therapy with lactulose may decrease the severity and prevent the recurrence of PSE.

Based on limited information, the initial oral dosage of lactulose for the prevention and treatment of PSE in infants is 1.67–6.67 g daily given in divided doses. In older children and adolescents, the total daily dose of lactulose suggested by the manufacturers is 27–60 g. Dosage is adjusted every 1–2 days as necessary to produce 2–3 soft stools daily. If the initial dose of lactulose produces diarrhea, the dose should be reduced immediately; if diarrhea persists, the drug should be discontinued.

When lactulose is used rectally in the treatment of PSE to reverse hepatic coma in adults, 200 g is diluted with 700 mL of water or 0.9% sodium chloride solution; the diluted solution is administered rectally via a rectal balloon catheter and retained for 30–60 minutes. Lactulose retention enemas may be administered every 4–6 hours; if the enema is retained for less than 30 minutes, it may be repeated immediately. In some patients, reversal of hepatic coma may occur within 2 hours of the first enema. Before discontinuance of lactulose retention enemas, recommended oral dosages of the drug should be started. Cleansing enemas containing soapsuds or other alkaline agents should not be used concomitantly with lactulose enemas.

Constipation For the treatment of chronic constipation in adults, the usual initial dosage of lactulose is 10–20 g daily. Dosage may be increased to 40 g daily if necessary. Following oral lactulose administration, 24–48 hours may be required to restore normal bowel movements.

For the treatment of chronic constipation in children†, lactulose dosages of least 5 g daily, usually given as a single dose after breakfast, have been used. When lactulose was used to restore bowel movements in hemorrhoidectomy patients†, a 10-g dose was given twice during the day before surgery and twice daily for 5 days postoperatively. To induce bowel evacuation in geriatric patients with colonic retention of barium and severe constipation following a barium meal examination†, lactulose dosages of 3.3–6.7 g twice daily for 1–4 weeks have been used.

Cautions

■ **Adverse Effects** During the first few days of therapy, lactulose frequently produces gaseous distention, belching, flatulence, borborygmi, and/or abdominal discomfort such as cramping. These adverse effects usually subside with continued therapy, but dosage reduction may be required. Diarrhea indicates overdosage and responds to dosage reduction. Potential complications of diarrhea include fluid loss, hypokalemia, and hypernatremia. Infants receiving lactulose may develop dehydration and hyponatremia. Nausea and vomiting have been reported infrequently in patients receiving the drug.

■ **Precautions and Contraindications** In the treatment of PSE, it is important to remember that the serious underlying liver disease may produce complications such as electrolyte disturbances (e.g., hypokalemia) which require additional therapy. In addition, if diarrhea occurs it may severely deplete fluids and potassium and may intensify symptoms of PSE. For these reasons, some clinicians recommend periodic determinations of serum potassium concentrations during long-term treatment with lactulose.

Lactulose solution should be administered with caution to patients who may require electrocautery procedures during proctoscopy or colonoscopy, since the drug can cause accumulation of hydrogen gas in high concentrations which in the presence of an electrical spark may theoretically result in an explosive reaction. Although this reaction has not been reported to date, patients receiving lactulose therapy should have a thorough bowel cleansing with a nonfermentable solution prior to these procedures. In addition, insufflation of carbon dioxide may be used but is probably an unnecessary measure.

If an unusual diarrheal condition occurs during lactulose therapy, patients should contact their physician. Geriatric, debilitated patients who receive lactulose for more than 6 months should have serum electrolytes (e.g., potassium, chloride, carbon dioxide) measured periodically during therapy.

Since lactulose solution contains some free lactose and galactose, the drug should be used with caution in patients with diabetes mellitus and is contraindicated in patients who require a low-galactose diet.

Laxatives should not be administered with lactulose. (See Drug Interactions: Laxatives.)

■ **Pediatric Precautions** Limited information on the use of lactulose for prevention and treatment of PSE in young children and adolescents is available. Safety and efficacy of the drug for the treatment of chronic constipation in children have not been established.

■ **Mutagenicity and Carcinogenicity** Data on the long-term mutagenic potential of lactulose in animals or humans and on the long-term carcinogenic potential in humans are not available. Administration of lactulose solution in concentrations of 3 and 10% v/w in the diet of mice for 18 months did not produce evidence of carcinogenicity.

■ **Pregnancy, Fertility, and Lactation** Use of lactulose during pregnancy has not been studied in humans. Reproduction studies in rats, mice, and rabbits receiving oral lactulose doses up to 6 times the usual human oral dose have not revealed evidence of harm to the fetus. Lactulose should be used during pregnancy only when clearly needed.

Reproduction studies in rats, mice, and rabbits using oral lactulose dosages of up to 4 or 8 g/kg (6 or 12 mL/kg) daily did not reveal evidence of impaired fertility.

It is not known if lactulose is distributed into milk. The drug should be used with caution in nursing women.

Drug Interactions

■ **Laxatives** Additional laxatives should not be administered with lactulose solution, especially when lactulose therapy is initiated, because the loose stools produced may be falsely interpreted as an indication that adequate dosage of lactulose has been achieved.

■ **Anti-infective Agents** Theoretically, orally administered neomycin and possibly other anti-infective agents, when administered concurrently with lactulose, could eliminate colonic bacteria that are necessary to metabolize lactulose and thereby prevent acidification of the contents of the colon. Limited data obtained from experiments in healthy individuals tend to support the theoretical incompatibility of these agents. There is, however, evidence that lactulose remains active when administered with neomycin to patients with PSE. In addition, there have been reports that concomitant therapy with lactulose and neomycin may be more effective than either drug alone in the treatment of PSE. Therefore, until there is conclusive evidence that concurrent administration of lactulose and neomycin or other oral anti-infective agents is efficacious, patients receiving lactulose and an oral anti-infective agent should be closely monitored for possible inadequate response to lactulose.

■ **Antacids** Results of limited studies in rats and humans suggest that nonabsorbable antacids administered concomitantly with lactulose may inhibit the desired decrease in fecal pH in the colon. The potential lack of desired effect of lactulose should be considered before a nonabsorbable antacid is administered concomitantly with lactulose.

Acute Toxicity

No information is available on the acute overdosage of lactulose in humans. The oral LD_{50} of the drug is 48.8 mL/kg in mice and greater than 30 mL/kg in rats. Overdosage of lactulose presumably would be manifested by abdominal cramps and diarrhea (which could result in severe fluid and electrolyte depletion), and treatment would consist of fluid and electrolyte replacement, as required.

Pharmacology

In patients with portal-systemic encephalopathy (PSE), lactulose causes a decrease in blood ammonia concentration and reduces the degree of PSE. Although the mechanism of action of lactulose has not been clearly defined, it appears to be associated primarily with the metabolism of the sugar in the lower intestinal tract. The breakdown of lactulose to organic acids (i.e., lactic acid and small amounts of formic and acetic acids) by the saccharolytic bacteria in the colon acidifies the contents of the colon. In patients with PSE who respond to lactulose, a decrease in fecal pH occurs. Acidification of colon contents inhibits the nonionic diffusion of ammonia from the colon into the blood. In addition, since the contents of the colon are more acidic than is blood, ammonia (NH_3) can diffuse from the blood into the colon. In the acidic colon, ammonia is converted to ammonium ions (NH_4^+) thereby preventing its absorption. In a similar manner, the absorption of amines (which may also contribute to the development of PSE) may also be reduced. Finally the cathartic action of lactulose (which is probably caused by the osmotic effect of the organic acid metabolites of the drug) expels the trapped ammonium ions and possibly other nitrogenous substances from the colon. The osmotic effect of the organic acid metabolites of lactulose causes an increase in water content of the stool and a softening of the stool; this effect on the stool may not be seen for 24–48 hours after administration of the drug. In patients with chronic constipation, the drug increases the number of bowel movements per day and the number of days when bowel movements occur.

Pharmacokinetics

Following oral administration, less than 3% of a dose of lactulose is absorbed from the small intestine. Absorbed lactulose is not metabolized and is excreted in the urine unchanged within 24 hours. Unabsorbed lactulose reaches the colon unchanged where it is metabolized by bacteria to form lactic acid and small amounts of acetic and formic acids. The bacteria normally present in the colon which are capable of metabolizing lactulose include *Lactobacilli, Bacteroides, Escherichia coli,* and *Clostridia,* but not *Proteus mirabilis, Enterococcus faecalis* (formerly *Streptococcus faecalis*), *Salmonella,* or *Shigella.* Only negligible amounts of lactulose or its metabolites are absorbed from the colon.

Chemistry and Stability

■ **Chemistry** Lactulose, a disaccharide sugar containing one molecule of galactose and one molecule of fructose, is a synthetic derivative of lactose. Lactulose occurs as a white powder or crystals and is very soluble in water and very slightly soluble in alcohol.

Each 10 g of lactulose powder for oral solution also contains a combined total of 0.3 g of galactose and lactose. Following reconstitution of the powder as directed, resultant solutions are colorless to slightly pale yellow and have a pH of 3–7. Commercially available lactulose solutions (which also contain galactose, lactose, and other sugars) are pale yellow to yellow, sweet, viscous liquids. Sodium hydroxide is added to the commercially available solutions to adjust pH when necessary; the pH of the solutions is 2.5–6.5.

■ **Stability** Lactulose powder and solutions should be stored at 15–30°C; freezing of the solutions should be avoided. Although heat causes cloudiness, and heat and light cause darkening of the solutions, the manufacturers state that these changes do not indicate loss of potency. Prolonged exposure to freezing temperatures may cause lactulose solutions to become semisolid and too viscous to pour; viscosity returns to normal following warming to room temperature. Lactulose solutions have an expiration date of 2 years following the date of manufacture.

Preparations

Excipients in commercially available drug preparations may have clinically important effects in some individuals; consult specific product labeling for details.

Lactulose

Oral		
For solution	10 g/packet*	**Kristalose®**, Mylan (also promoted by Cumberland)
		Lactulose for Oral Solution
	20 g/packet*	**Kristalose®**, Mylan (also promoted by Cumberland)
		Lactulose for Oral Solution
Solution	3.33 g/5 mL*	**Constilac® Syrup**, Alra
		Constulose®, Actavis
		Evalose® Syrup, Teva
		Lactulose Oral Solution
Oral or Rectal		
Solution	3.33 g/5 mL*	**Cholac® Syrup**, Alra
		Enulose®, Actavis
		Generlac®, Morton Grove
		Heptalac®, Teva
		Lactulose Oral or Rectal Solution

*available from one or more manufacturer, distributor, and/or repackager by generic (nonproprietary) name

†Use is not currently included in the labeling approved by the US Food and Drug Administration

REPLACEMENT PREPARATIONS 40:12

Calcium Salts

■ Calcium salts are used as a source of calcium, an essential nutrient cation.

Uses

Calcium salts are used as a source of calcium cation for the treatment or prevention of calcium depletion in patients in whom dietary measures are inadequate. Conditions that may be associated with calcium deficiency include hypoparathyroidism, achlorhydria, chronic diarrhea, vitamin D deficiency, steatorrhea, sprue, pregnancy and lactation, menopause, pancreatitis, renal failure, alkalosis, and hyperphosphatemia. Administration of certain drugs (e.g., some diuretics, anticonvulsants) may sometimes result in hypocalcemia which may warrant calcium replacement therapy. Calcium should be administered in long-term electrolyte replacement regimens and is also recommended for the routine prophylaxis of hypocalcemia during transfusions with citrated blood. Administration of calcium salts should not preclude the use of other measures intended to correct the underlying cause of calcium depletion.

■ **Dietary Requirements** Since 1941, the Institute of Medicine's (IOM) Food and Nutrition Board of the National Academy of Sciences (NAS) has developed guidelines for adequate dietary intake of essential nutrients. Nutrient recommendations are issued through Dietary Reference Intakes (DRIs), which are a set of reference values that can be used for planning and assessing diets for healthy populations and for many other purposes. DRIs for calcium include the Estimated Average Requirement (EAR), Recommended Dietary Allowance (RDA), Adequate Intake (AI), and Tolerable Upper Intake Level (UL). DRIs apply to the healthy general population and consider nutrient levels needed to prevent deficiency as well as those associated with disease risk reduction. The current methods for establishing DRIs differ from those used in the past and incorporate increased understanding of both population and individual nutrient needs. The EAR is the nutrient intake value that is estimated to meet the nutrient needs of 50% of individuals in a particular life-stage and gender group. The RDA, which is derived from the EAR, currently is defined as the estimated daily dietary intake level that is sufficient to meet the nutrient requirements of 97.5% of the population's requirements. The RDA for a given nutrient, in a prescriptive sense, is the *goal* for dietary intake in individuals. If data are insufficient to establish an RDA for a given life-stage group, the AI may be used instead. AIs are based on observed or experimentally determined approximations of the average nutrient intake, by a defined population or subgroup, that appears to sustain a defined nutritional state (e.g., usual circulating nutrient levels, nutrient levels for normal growth).

The previous NAS report from 1997 was unable to establish EARs and RDAs for calcium because of inadequate data attributed in part to uncertainties in the methods used in calcium balance studies, the lack of concordance between observational and experimental data, and the lack of longitudinal data to verify the association between calcium intake, calcium retention, and bone loss. Since then, emerging data from large-scale randomized controlled studies and more recent calcium balance studies have allowed for estimation of EARs and RDAs in all life stage groups except for infants.

The principal goal of maintaining an adequate intake of calcium in the US and Canada is to support the development and preservation of bone mass at a level sufficient to prevent fractures associated with osteopenia or osteoporosis in later life and of other calcified tissues (e.g., teeth), although other biologic roles for calcium and related nutrients (e.g., fluoride, magnesium, phosphorus) have been considered in establishing DRIs. Lifelong intake of adequate calcium is necessary for good bone health at any age. Although some evidence indicates an inverse relationship between calcium intake and blood pressure and that increased calcium intake can reduce blood pressure in certain healthy individuals and some hypertensive patients, there currently is no rationale for recommending calcium supplementation solely to reduce blood pressure; the importance of maintaining adequate calcium intake should be emphasized though, since potential secondary benefits on blood pressure may result.

Adequate intakes of calcium can be accomplished through changes in food consumption behaviors, consumption of nutrient-fortified foodstuffs, use of dietary supplements, or a combination of these. In the US and Canada, calcium principally is obtained from dairy products. Other principal sources include fruits, vegetables, and grain products. In addition, many healthy individuals take dietary supplements containing calcium.

For specific information on currently recommended dietary reference intakes for calcium, see Dosage and Administration: Dosage.

■ **Parenteral Preparations** Calcium salts are administered IV to treat acute hypocalcemic tetany secondary to renal failure, hypoparathyroidism, premature delivery, and/or maternal diabetes mellitus in infants, and poisoning with magnesium, oxalic acid, radiophosphorus, carbon tetrachloride, fluoride, phosphate, strontium, or radium. Some experts state that administration of calcium also may be useful in the treatment of β-adrenergic blocking agent toxicity in patients with shock refractory to other treatment measures.

IV calcium gluconate is considered by most clinicians to be the salt of choice for the treatment of acute hypocalcemia. In some situations (e.g., critically ill children with hypocalcemia), calcium chloride may be preferred because it can provide a greater increase in ionized calcium concentrations. Some clinicians believe that calcium chloride is the calcium salt of choice for the prevention of hypocalcemia during transfusions with citrated blood. In addition to being irritating, however, the chloride salt is acidifying and generally should not be used when acidosis coincides with hypocalcemia (e.g., renal failure).

Calcium salts have been used IV as adjunctive therapy to reduce spasms in renal†, biliary†, intestinal†, or lead colic. Calcium salts also have been used IV as adjuncts to relieve muscle cramps in the treatment of insect bites or stings (e.g., black widow spider) or to decrease capillary permeability in sensitivity reactions characterized by urticaria or angioedema† and in allergic conditions, including nonthrombocytopenic purpura, dermatitis herpetiformis, drug-induced pruritus, hay fever†, and asthma†.

The calcium glycerophosphate and calcium lactate fixed-combination injection is used IM to increase serum calcium concentrations.

Calcium infusions ("calcium challenge") are used to diagnose the Zollinger-Ellison syndrome† and medullary thyroid carcinoma†. In addition, calcium salt injections are used to antagonize neuromuscular blockade† resulting from the use of aminoglycoside antibiotics (e.g., gentamicin, kanamycin, neomycin) with or without agents possessing neuromuscular blocking properties (e.g., gallamine triethiodide).

Advanced Cardiovascular Life Support Because of the lack of demonstrated benefit and potential for detrimental effects, the American Heart Association (AHA) guidelines for cardiopulmonary resuscitation (CPR) and emergency cardiovascular care currently state that calcium should not be used routinely for advanced cardiovascular life support (ACLS) during cardiac arrest in adults and pediatric patients unless there is documented hypocalcemia, calcium-channel blocker toxicity, hypermagnesemia, or hyperkalemia. When used in this setting, experts state that either calcium chloride or calcium gluconate may be administered.

■ **Oral Preparations** Oral calcium therapy may be used for the treatment of osteoporosis, osteomalacia, chronic hypoparathyroidism, rickets, latent tetany, and hypocalcemia secondary to the administration of anticonvulsant drugs. Calcium salts are also used orally in the adjunctive treatment of myasthenia gravis and the Eaton-Lambert syndrome, and as supplemental therapy for pregnant, postmenopausal, or nursing women. In general, any of the oral calcium salts may be used for chronic replacement therapy.

Although some evidence from early trials suggested a beneficial effect of calcium supplementation on preeclampsia, a more recent, large, well-designed study did *not* confirm a beneficial effect of calcium supplementation in preventing preeclampsia during pregnancy. In this study, supplemental administration of calcium (2 g of elemental calcium daily) beginning during the 13th–21st week and continued for the remainder of pregnancy did not prevent preeclampsia, pregnancy-associated hypertension, or adverse perinatal outcomes in healthy nulliparous women. However, these findings do not obviate adequate dietary calcium intake during pregnancy nor do they address whether adequate or increased calcium intake can affect blood pressure favorably in pregnant women.

Calcium acetate or carbonate is considered to be the salt of choice in patients with chronic renal failure. In addition to providing a source of calcium, calcium acetate or carbonate sequesters phosphate in the intestine by forming insoluble phosphates that are excreted fecally, thus reducing serum phosphate concentrations and secondary hyperparathyroidism; calcium carbonate also partially corrects metabolic acidosis which may occur in patients with chronic renal failure. Because of the risk of aluminum accumulation and resultant neurotoxic and osteomalacic effects, most clinicians no longer use aluminum hydroxide to inhibit phosphorus absorption; instead calcium acetate or carbonate and/or non-calcium-, non-aluminum-, non-magnesium-containing phosphate binders (e.g., lanthanum carbonate, sevelamer hydrochloride) currently are used. Therapeutic measures to control hyperphosphatemia in patients with chronic renal disease include reduction in dietary intake of phosphates, inhibition of intestinal phosphate absorption, and removal via dialysis. In individuals with moderate to severe renal impairment (i.e., glomerular filtration rate of 15–59 mL/minute per 1.73 m^2), calcium carbonate or acetate may be used to sequester phosphates in the intestine if serum phosphorus or parathyroid hormone (PTH) concentrations are not controlled through dietary restrictions and/or vitamin D therapy. In patients with chronic renal failure, reductions in serum phosphate through dietary restrictions and dialysis generally are insufficient, and inhibition of intestinal phosphate absorption usually is necessary. In these individuals, either a calcium-containing phosphate binder or a non-calcium-, non-aluminum-, non-magnesium-containing phosphate binder may be used as primary therapy. Some experts state that dialysis patients who remain hyperphosphatemic despite treatment with either calcium-based phosphate binders or non-calcium-, non-aluminum-, non-magnesium-containing phosphate binders should receive both types of phosphate binders in combination. Non-calcium-containing phosphate binders are preferred in dialysis patients with severe vascular and/or other soft-tissue calcification. Calcium-containing phosphate binders should not be used in dialysis patients who are hypercalcemic or whose plasma PTH concentrations are less than 150 pg/mL on 2 consecutive measurements. Use of aluminum-containing phosphate binders should be limited to short periods of time (e.g., a single 4-week course) in patients with difficult-to-control serum phosphorus concentrations (e.g., concentrations exceeding 7 mg/dL).

When taken with meals, calcium acetate or carbonate can contribute to controlling hyperphosphatemia in patients with chronic renal failure by binding to and inhibiting absorption of phosphates in the GI tract. Caution should be observed in patients undergoing chronic hemodialysis to prevent hypophosphatemia. Patients with end-stage renal failure may develop hypercalcemia when calcium is administered with meals; therefore, other calcium supplementation should not be given concomitantly when calcium salts are used to control hyperphosphatemia in such patients. Progressive hypercalcemia secondary to overdose of calcium salts in patients with chronic renal disease can occur and may require emergency treatment measures. Chronic hypercalcemia also may lead to vascular and other soft-tissue calcification. Therefore, periodic (e.g., twice weekly) monitoring of calcium concentrations is recommended during the initial dose adjustment period in patients with chronic renal failure. One manufacturer recommends that the serum calcium times phosphate (Ca×P) product should not exceed 66. Radiographic evaluation of a suspected anatomic region for early soft-tissue calcification may be useful.

Vitamin D analogs may be administered concomitantly with oral calcium salts for the treatment of chronic hypocalcemia, especially when caused by vitamin D deficiency.

Calcium chloride, an acid-forming salt, has been used to promote diuresis but, because it is irritating and loses effectiveness after a few days, it is rarely used for this effect.

For the use of calcium carbonate as an antacid, see Antacids 56:04.

Osteoporosis Calcium salts (e.g., calcium carbonate, calcium citrate) are used as supplements for the prevention and treatment of osteoporosis in patients whose dietary intake of calcium is insufficient.

A principal long-term consequence of inadequate calcium intake is osteoporosis, which is characterized by reduced bone mass, increased bone fragility, and increased fracture risk. Reduced absorption of calcium causes declines in circulating ionized calcium concentrations, which induce increased parathyroid hormone (PTH) synthesis and release. PTH then acts to restore circulating calcium concentrations to normal levels by promoting the reabsorption of calcium in the distal renal tubule, by indirectly increasing intestinal absorption secondary to stimulation of activated vitamin D synthesis, and by inducing bone resorption. Thus, while circulating calcium concentrations can be maintained at normal levels during calcium deprivation, it is at the expense of skeletal mass.

Adequate intake of calcium and vitamin D (which increases absorption of calcium) is universally recommended for all individuals to diminish age-related bone loss and prevent osteoporosis. Controlled clinical studies have demonstrated that the combination of calcium and vitamin D can reduce fracture risk. In addition to lifestyle modifications (e.g., regular weight-bearing exercise, avoidance of excessive alcohol and tobacco use), the National Osteoporosis Foundation recommends a calcium intake of 1 g daily in men 50–70 years of age, and an intake of 1.2 g daily in women 51 years of age or older and men 71 years of age or older. There is no evidence to suggest that increasing intake above these amounts will provide any additional benefit on bone strength; excess calcium intake has been linked to increased risks of kidney stones, cardiovascular disease, and stroke. It is important to also ensure sufficient calcium and vitamin D intake in children and younger adults to prevent the development of osteoporosis. (See Uses: Dietary Requirements.) If adequate calcium cannot be obtained from diet, calcium supplements are recommended.

Glucocorticoid-induced Osteoporosis The American College of Rheumatology (ACR) recommends optimizing dietary intake of calcium (1–1.2 g daily) and vitamin D (600–800 units daily) for the prevention of glucocorticoid-induced osteoporosis in all patients receiving long-term glucocorticoid therapy (defined as a daily dosage equivalent to 2.5 mg of prednisone or greater for at least 3 months). Because of concerns about potential harms (e.g., adverse cardiovascular effects), ACR states that additional study is needed to determine the potential benefits versus risks of calcium and vitamin D supplementation in patients receiving glucocorticoids. For additional information on the prevention and treatment of glucocorticoid-induced osteoporosis, see Cautions: Musculoskeletal Effects, in the Corticosteroids General Statement 68:04.

Dosage and Administration

■ **Administration** The acetate, carbonate, citrate, gluconate, lactate, and phosphate salts of calcium are administered orally. It has been recommended that most oral calcium supplements be administered 1–1.5 hours after meals or with a demulcent (e.g., milk). However, calcium carbonate powder (i.e., CAL CARB-HD®) should generally be administered with meals, since the manufacturer recommends mixing the powder with food for administration. Calcium salts used to bind dietary phosphate in patients with end-stage renal disease should be administered with meals (e.g., 10–15 minutes before, or during, the meal).

Calcium chloride and calcium gluconate may be administered IV. Calcium chloride also may be administered by intraosseous (IO) injection† in the setting of pediatric resuscitation; onset of action and systemic concentrations are comparable to those achieved with venous administration. Parenteral calcium salts may be administered in large volume IV infusion fluids.

IV calcium injections must be administered slowly at a rate not exceeding 0.7–1.8 mEq/minute, and the injection should be stopped if the patient complains of discomfort. Following IV injection, the patient should remain recumbent for a short time. Close monitoring of serum calcium concentrations is essential during IV administration of calcium. *Calcium chloride should not be injected IM or into subcutaneous or perivascular tissue, since severe necrosis and sloughing may occur.* Although other calcium salts may cause mild to severe local reactions, they are generally less irritating than calcium chloride. (See Cautions.) The fixed combination of calcium glycerophosphate and calcium lactate is injected IM. Although some manufacturers previously stated that calcium gluconate could be injected IM when IV administration was not possible, manufacturers of calcium gluconate currently state that the drug should not be injected IM or into subcutaneous tissue because of the potential for severe local reactions. In children, calcium salts should not be administered through scalp veins. Oral administration of calcium supplements or calcium-rich foods should replace parenteral calcium therapy as soon as possible.

The interaction of calcium and phosphate in parenteral nutrition solutions is a complex phenomenon; various factors have been identified as playing a role in the solubility or precipitation of a given combination. Calcium salts are conditionally compatible with phosphate in parenteral nutrition solutions; incompatibility is dependent on a solubility and concentration phenomenon and is not entirely predictable. Precipitation may occur during compounding or at some time after compounding is completed. Specialized references should be consulted for specific compatibility information.

■ **Dosage** Dosage of the oral calcium supplements is usually expressed in grams or mg of elemental calcium and depends on the requirements of the individual patient. Dosage of parenteral calcium replacements is usually expressed as mEq of calcium and depends on individual patient requirements. One mEq of elemental calcium is equivalent to 20 mg. See Table 1 for the approximate calcium content of the various calcium salts.

Table 1.

Calcium Salt	Calcium Content
calcium acetate	253 mg (12.7 mEq) per g
calcium carbonate	400 mg (20 mEq) per g
calcium chloride	270 mg (13.5 mEq) per g
calcium citrate	211 mg (10.6 mEq) per g
calcium gluceptate	82 mg (4.1 mEq) per g
calcium gluconate	90 mg (4.5 mEq) per g
calcium glycerophosphate	191 mg (9.6 mEq) per g
calcium lactate	130 mg (6.5 mEq) per g
calcium phosphate dibasic anhydrous	290 mg (14.5 mEq) per g
calcium phosphate dibasic dihydrate	230 mg (11.5 mEq) per g
calcium phosphate tribasic	400 mg (20 mEq) per g

Oral calcium supplements usually are administered in 3 or 4 divided doses daily. Optimum calcium absorption may require supplemental vitamin D in individuals with inadequate vitamin D intake, those with impaired renal activation of the vitamin, or those not receiving adequate exposure to sunlight.

Dietary and Replacement Requirements Because of insufficient data to establish estimated average requirements (EARs) in infants younger than 1 year of age, the National Academy of Sciences (NAS) has developed adequate intakes (AIs) for calcium in this population (see Uses: Dietary Requirements). Calcium requirements in infants are presumed to be met by human milk; thus, AIs developed for this age group are principally based on mean intake data from infants receiving human milk. The AI recommended for healthy **infants up to 6 months of age** is 200 mg daily and for **infants 6–12 months of age** is 260 mg daily (taking into account additional intake of calcium from food).

In **children and adolescents 1–18 years of age**, the recommended dietary reference intake values for calcium are determined based on levels required to support bone accretion and calcium retention. Using this approach, the EAR of elemental calcium currently recommended by the NAS for healthy children 1–3, 4–8, or 9–18 years of age is 500, 800, or 1100 mg daily, respectively, and the Recommended Dietary Allowance (RDA) for these respective age groups is 700, 1000, and 1300 mg daily. Many chronic illnesses that affect children are associated with abnormalities in calcium metabolism and bone mineralization, and special consideration should be given for different calcium requirements in such children; some such diseases include juvenile rheumatologic conditions, renal disease, liver failure, and certain endocrine disorders, including type 1 (insulin-dependent) diabetes mellitus.

The goal of calcium intake in **adults 19–50 years of age** is to promote bone maintenance and neutral calcium balance. Based on a series of controlled calcium balance studies in this age group, NAS recommends an EAR of 800 mg daily and an RDA of 1 g daily.

Calcium intake in **adults 51–70 years of age** is principally focused on lessening the degree of bone loss that manifests during later stages of adulthood. Because of menopause, the natural process of bone loss occurs earlier for women than for men. Findings from the Women's Health Initiative (WHI) study revealed modest improvements in BMD and risk of fractures in women 50–79 years of age who received daily supplementation with 1 g calcium plus 400 units vitamin D; however, these results should be interpreted cautiously because of possible confounding factors (e.g., concomitant use of hormone replacement therapy). While considering these limitations, NAS states that the emerging evidence indicates that a somewhat higher intake of calcium may be justified in postmenopausal women 51–70 years of age compared with similarly aged men. In men 51–70 years of age, the recommended EAR for calcium is 800 mg daily and the RDA is 1 g daily; in women 51–70 years of age, the recommended EAR for calcium is 1 g daily and the recommended RDA is 1.2 g daily.

Bone loss and resulting risk of fractures are the predominant concerns when developing calcium intake recommendations in **adults older than 70 years of age.** However, a dose-response relationship for calcium and fracture risk has not been established and calcium balance studies are lacking in this age group. Given these limitations, NAS recommends the same calcium requirements in adults older than 70 years of age as for those recommended in postmenopausal women (EAR of 1 g daily and RDA of 1.2 g daily).

Because of adaptive maternal responses to fetal calcium needs (e.g., changes in calciotropic hormones and resultant enhanced calcium absorption) and the fact that the maternal skeleton does not appear to act as a reservoir for fetal calcium needs, calcium requirements are not increased during pregnancy. Randomized controlled studies have not demonstrated any additional benefits to the mother or fetus from increased intake of calcium during pregnancy. Therefore, the usual calcium recommendations that are appropriate for age in nonpregnant women should be used in pregnant women. Likewise, there is no evidence that calcium requirements are increased during lactation and the same calcium intake recommendations are given for lactating as for nonlactating women. Physiologic changes occur naturally in maternal bone during and after lactation to provide the infant with calcium without impairing maternal bone mass, and increased calcium intake does not appear to alter this process.

Calcium replacement requirements can be estimated by clinical condition and/or serum calcium determinations. Prophylactic administration of calcium supplements may be necessary in some patients in order to maintain serum calcium above 9 mg/dL. The average adult oral dosage of elemental calcium for prevention of hypocalcemia is about 1 g daily, and the usual oral dosage for treatment of calcium depletion is 1–2 g or more daily. In children, the usual supplemental dosage of elemental calcium is 45–65 mg/kg daily. In neonatal hypocalcemia, the daily dosage of elemental calcium is 50–150 mg/kg and should not exceed 1 g.

Calcium gluconate is usually administered IV as a 10% solution and calcium chloride as a 2–10% solution. The manufacturers state that the usual initial IV dose of calcium for prompt elevation of serum calcium is 2.3–14 mEq for adults, 0.93–2.3 mEq for children, and less than 0.93 mEq for infants. It has been recommended that these doses be repeated every 1–3 days depending on the patient's response. Alternatively, one manufacturer recommends a pediatric IV dose of 0.272 mEq of calcium per kg, up to a maximum total daily dosage of 1.36–13.6 mEq, in the treatment of hypocalcemic disorders. For the treatment of hypocalcemic tetany, 4.5–16 mEq doses of calcium may be administered IV to adults until therapeutic response occurs. In children with hypocalcemic tetany, 0.5–0.7 mEq/kg may be administered IV 3 or 4 times daily or until tetany is controlled. Neonatal tetany may be treated with divided doses totaling about 2.4 mEq/kg daily.

The usual adult IM dosage of the calcium glycerophosphate and calcium lactate fixed-combination preparation given to increase serum calcium concentrations is 0.8 mEq of calcium 1–4 times weekly or as directed by a clinician.

Advanced Cardiovascular Life Support **Adult Dosage.** If calcium administration is necessary during cardiac arrest, an IV dose of 0.109–0.218 mEq/kg (repeated as necessary) using calcium chloride has been recommended. Alternatively, adults have been given IV calcium doses of 7–14 mEq using calcium chloride. However, routine administration of calcium in patients with cardiac arrest is not recommended. (See Advanced Cardiovascular Life Support under Uses: Parenteral Preparations.)

Pediatric Dosage. If administration of calcium is indicated for the treatment of hypocalcemia, calcium-channel blocker overdosage, hypermagnesemia, or hyperkalemia during pediatric resuscitation, experts recommend a pediatric IV or IO† calcium dose of 0.272 mEq/kg using calcium chloride. In critically ill children, calcium chloride may provide a greater increase in ionized calcium than calcium gluconate. The appropriate dose should be administered by slow IV or IO† injection.

Other Dosages When calcium acetate is used orally to control hyperphosphatemia in adults with chronic renal failure, the recommended initial dosage is 1.334 g of calcium acetate (338 mg of calcium) with each meal. Dosage may be increased gradually according to serum phosphate concentrations, provided hypercalcemia does not occur. The manufacturer states that most patients require about 2–2.67 g (about 500–680 mg of calcium) with each meal. However, some experts state that the dosage of calcium provided by calcium-containing phosphate binders should not exceed 1.5 g daily and that the total calcium intake (including dietary calcium) should not exceed 2 g daily. These experts state that dialysis patients who remain hyperphosphatemic despite such therapy should receive a calcium-containing phosphate binder in combination with a non-calcium-, non-aluminum-, non-magnesium-containing phosphate binder. The manufacturer recommends that serum calcium concentrations be monitored twice weekly during initiation of calcium acetate therapy and subsequent dosage adjustment; serum phosphorus concentrations also should be monitored periodically. If hypercalcemia occurs, dosage should be reduced or the salt should be withheld. If severe hypercalcemia occurs, specific measures (e.g., hemodialysis) for the management of overdosage may be necessary. Patients should be advised of the importance of dosage compliance, adherence to instructions about diet, and avoidance of concomitant use of antacids or other preparations containing clinically important concentrations of calcium. Patients also should be advised of potential manifestations of hypercalcemia.

For the treatment of hyperkalemia with secondary cardiac toxicity, 2.25–14 mEq of calcium may be administered IV while monitoring the ECG. Doses may be repeated after 1–2 minutes if necessary.

Magnesium intoxication in adults is treated initially with 7 mEq of IV calcium; subsequent doses should be adjusted according to patient response. Alternatively, for the treatment of hypermagnesemia in adults, an IV calcium dose of 6.8–13.6 mEq using 10% calcium chloride (5–10 mL) has been administered, and repeated as necessary.

For the treatment of drug-induced cardiovascular emergencies associated with calcium-channel blocking agent toxicity in pediatric patients, an IV calcium dose of 0.272 mEq/kg using 10% calcium chloride (0.2 mL/kg) has been administered over 5–10 minutes; if a beneficial effect was observed, an IV calcium infusion of 0.27-0.68 mEq/kg per hour using calcium chloride has been administered. Ionized calcium concentrations should be monitored to prevent hypercalcemia.

Calcium is also administered IV during exchange transfusions in neonates in a dosage of 0.45 mEq of calcium after every 100 mL of citrated blood exchanged. In adults receiving transfusions of citrated blood, about 1.35 mEq of calcium should be administered IV concurrently with each 100 mL of citrated blood.

In the calcium infusion test†, calcium is given IV in a dosage of 0.25 mEq/kg per hour for a 3-hour period; serum gastrin concentrations are determined 30 minutes before the infusion, at the start of the infusion, and at 30-minute intervals thereafter for 4 hours. In most patients with Zollinger-Ellison syndrome, preinfusion serum gastrin concentrations increase by more than 50% or by greater than 500 pg/mL during the infusion. In the diagnosis of medullary thyroid carcinoma†, about 7 mEq of calcium is given IV over 5–10 minutes. In patients with medullary thyroid carcinoma, plasma calcitonin concentrations are elevated above normal basal concentrations.

Cautions

■ **Local Effects** Calcium salts are irritating to tissue when administered by IM or subcutaneous injection and cause mild to severe local reactions including burning, necrosis and sloughing of tissue, cellulitis, and soft tissue calcification; venous irritation may occur with IV administration. When injected IV, calcium salts should be administered slowly through a small needle into a large vein to avoid too rapid an increase in serum calcium and extravasation of calcium solution into the surrounding tissue with resultant necrosis. Patients may complain of tingling sensations, a sense of oppression or heat waves, and a calcium or chalky taste following IV administration of calcium salts.

■ **Cardiovascular Effects** Rapid IV injection of calcium salts may cause vasodilation, decreased blood pressure, bradycardia, cardiac arrhythmias, syncope, and cardiac arrest.

■ **GI Effects** Orally administered calcium salts may be irritating to the GI tract. Calcium salts also may cause constipation. Calcium chloride, by any route of administration, produces more irritation than the other calcium salts and has been reported to cause GI hemorrhage when taken orally.

■ **Hypercalcemia** Hypercalcemia is rarely produced by administration of calcium alone, but may occur when large doses are given to patients with chronic renal failure. Since hypercalcemia may be more dangerous than hypocalcemia, overtreatment of hypocalcemia should be avoided. Mild hypercalcemia may be asymptomatic or manifest as constipation, anorexia, nausea, and vomiting, with mental changes such as confusion, delirium, stupor, and coma becoming evident as the degree of hypercalcemia increases. Mild hypercalcemia usually is readily controlled by reducing calcium intake (e.g., decreasing the dose of or avoiding supplemental calcium); more severe hypercalcemia may require specific management (e.g., hemodialysis). In dialysis patients with chronic renal failure receiving calcium salts, adjustments in calcium concentrations in the dialysate may be necessary to reduce the risk of hypercalcemia. The long-term effect of chronic calcium administration (e.g., in patients with chronic renal failure receiving calcium salts to control hyperphosphatemia) on progression of vascular or soft-tissue calcification is not known.

■ **Renal Calculi** Because the principal constituents of most renal calculi (kidney stones) are calcium salts, a high dietary intake of calcium has long been suspected as contributing to the risk of renal calculi, and restriction of calcium intake (i.e., low-calcium diets) had long been considered a reasonable measure in an attempt to prevent calculi formation in patients with idiopathic hypocalciuria. However, recent evidence from studies in men 40–75 years of age with no history of kidney stones and in women 34–59 years of age participating in the Nurses'; Health Study I indicates that high dietary intake of calcium actually decreases the risk of symptomatic renal calculi, while intake of supplemental calcium may increase the risk of symptomatic stones. High calcium intake can reduce urinary oxalate excretion, which is thought to lower the risk of renal calculi. In addition, dietary calcium can reduce the GI absorption of oxalate. Therefore, differences in calculi risk between high dietary calcium intake and calcium supplementation may be associated in part with differences in the timing of calcium ingestion relative to oxalate consumption or with other factors present in dairy products (the principal source of dietary calcium) that are not present in supplements.

■ **Precautions and Contraindications** Frequent determinations of serum calcium concentrations should be performed, and serum calcium concentrations should be maintained at 9–10.4 mg/dL (4.5–5.2 mEq/L). Some clinicians prefer to maintain serum calcium at slightly lower concentrations. Serum calcium concentrations usually should not be allowed to exceed 12 mg/dL. Administration of calcium in patients who have received transfusions of citrated blood may result in higher than normal total serum calcium concentrations. In these patients, however, most of the excess calcium is bound to citrate and is inactive; therefore, serious toxicity usually does not result. Although determinations of urine calcium have been advised, they are generally unreliable and hypercalciuria can occur in the presence of hypocalcemia. Some clinicians recommend forcing fluids to produce increased urine volume and thus prevent the formation of renal stones in patients with hypercalciuria. When hypercalcemia occurs, discontinuance of the drug is usually sufficient to return serum calcium concentrations to normal.

Calcium salts should be used cautiously, if at all, in patients with sarcoidosis, renal or cardiac disease, and in patients receiving cardiac glycosides. (See Drug Interactions: Cardiac Glycosides.) Calcium salts are contraindicated in patients with ventricular fibrillation or hypercalcemia. IV administration of calcium is contraindicated when serum calcium concentrations are above normal.

Drug Interactions

■ **Bisphosphonates** Concomitant administration of calcium salts with bisphosphonates (e.g., alendronate, etidronate, ibandronate, risedronate) may reduce absorption of the bisphosphonate from the GI tract. To minimize this effect, the drugs should be administered at separate times.

■ **Cardiac Glycosides** The inotropic and toxic effects of cardiac glycosides and calcium are synergistic and arrhythmias may occur if these drugs are given together (particularly when calcium is given IV). IV administration of calcium should be avoided in patients receiving cardiac glycosides, particularly if digoxin toxicity is suspected; if necessary, calcium should be given slowly in small amounts.

■ **Iron Preparations** Concomitant administration of calcium salts and oral iron preparations may result in reduced absorption of iron. Patients should be advised to take the drugs at different times, whenever possible.

■ **Levothyroxine** Calcium carbonate may form an insoluble chelate with levothyroxine, resulting in decreased levothyroxine absorption and increased serum thyrotropin concentrations. To minimize or prevent this interaction, oral levothyroxine sodium should be administered at least 4 hours apart from calcium carbonate.

■ **Quinolones** Concomitant administration of calcium salts and some fluoroquinolones (e.g., ciprofloxacin) may reduce oral bioavailability of the fluoroquinolone. For further information, including any specific instructions regarding timing of drug administration when concomitant use is necessary, see the individual monographs for quinolones in 8:12.18.

■ **Tetracyclines** Calcium complexes tetracycline antibiotics rendering them inactive; the 2 drugs should not be given at the same time orally nor should they be mixed for parenteral administration.

For further information on drug interactions with calcium salts, see Drug Interactions in Antacids 56:04.

Laboratory Test Interferences

Transient elevations of plasma 11-hydroxycorticosteroid concentrations (Glenn-Nelson technique) may occur when IV calcium is administered, but concentrations return to control values after 1 hour. In addition, IV calcium salts can produce false-negative values for serum and urinary magnesium as measured by the Titan yellow method.

Pharmacology

Calcium is essential for maintenance of the functional integrity of nervous, muscular, and skeletal systems and cell-membrane and capillary permeability. The cation is an important activator in many enzymatic reactions and is essential to a number of physiologic processes including transmission of nerve impulses; contraction of cardiac, smooth, and skeletal muscles; renal function; respiration; and blood coagulation. Calcium also plays regulatory roles in the release and storage of neurotransmitters and hormones, in the uptake and binding of amino acids, and in cyanocobalamin (vitamin B_{12}) absorption and gastrin secretion. There is evidence indicating an inverse relationship between calcium intake and blood pressure and that calcium supplementation may be associated with a reduction in blood pressure in healthy young adults and healthy pregnant women and in some patients with hypertension; however, further study is needed to evaluate further the role of calcium in blood pressure regulation.

Calcium accounts for 1–2% of adult body weight, and more than 99% of total body calcium is found in bone and teeth. Calcium also is present in blood, extracellular fluid, muscle, and other tissues where it has roles in mediating vascular contraction and vasodilation, muscle contraction, nerve transmission, and glandular secretion. Calcium is present in bone mainly as hydroxyapatite, with bone mineral content representing about 40% of bone weight. Bone is a dynamic tissue that constantly undergoes osteoclastic bone resorption and osteoblastic bone formation, with a portion of bone being remodeled (reabsorbed and replaced with new bone) each year. Formation exceeds resorption in growing children, is balanced with resorption in healthy adults, and lags behind resorption after menopause and with aging in both genders. The rate of cortical (compact) bone remodeling can be as high as 50% annually in young children and is about 5% annually in adults; trabecular (cancellous) bone remodeling is about fivefold that of cortical remodeling in adults. In addition to serving as a structural support for the body, the skeleton also serves as a reservoir for calcium. Although both exercise and calcium intake influence bone mass, it currently is unclear whether calcium intake influences the degree of benefit on bone derived from exercise.

Conditions associated with reduced concentrations of circulating estrogen alter calcium homeostasis. Exercise-induced amenorrhea results in reduced calcium retention and lower bone mass, and anorexia-induced amenorrhea results in reduced net calcium absorption, increased urinary calcium excretion, and a reduced rate of bone formation, when compared with eumenorrheic women. Decreased estrogen production at menopause is associated with accelerated bone loss, particularly from the lumbar spine, for about 5 years, during which time skeletal mass loss averages about 3% per year. Reduced estrogen concentrations are associated with reduced calcium absorption efficiency and increased bone turnover rates. While it is unclear whether the principal effect of estrogens on calcium is at the skeletal or intestinal level, examination of the skeletal response to calcium supplementation in premenopausal and early postmenopausal women indicates that increased calcium intake will not prevent the rapid trabecular bone loss that occurs during the first 5 years after menopause and that the calcium intake requirement for women does not appear to change acutely with menopause. Calcium responsiveness of cortical bone appears to depend less on menopausal status than does that of trabecular bone. Calcium requirements in vegetarians may be increased because of the negative effects of oxalate and phytate (present in high concentrations in vegetarian diets) on calcium bioavailability. Because lactose-intolerant individuals often avoid consumption of dairy products, the principal source of calcium in the US and Canada, they may be calcium deficient; however, there is no evidence to indicate that lactose intolerance influences the calcium requirement per se, although it may negatively influence calcium intake.

Pharmacokinetics

■ **Absorption** Calcium is absorbed from the GI tract by active transport and passive diffusion. Calcium is actively absorbed in the duodenum and proximal jejunum and, to a lesser extent, in the more distal segments of the small intestine. The degree of absorption depends on a number of factors; calcium is never completely absorbed from the intestine. For absorption to occur, calcium must be in a soluble, ionized form. The efficiency of intestinal calcium absorption may be increased when calcium intake is reduced and during pregnancy and lactation when calcium requirements are higher than normal. However, when hypocalcemia is caused by deficiency of either parathyroid hormone or vitamin D, calcium absorption decreases. As serum calcium concentration rises, negative feedback control by parathyroid hormone results in decreased calcium absorption. Vitamin D, in its activated forms, is required for calcium absorption and increases the capability of the absorptive mechanisms. Active transport of calcium into enterocytes and out on the serosal side of the intestinal mucosa depends on the action of activated vitamin D (1,25-dihydroxyvitamin D) and its intestinal receptors; this mechanism accounts for most of the calcium absorption from the GI tract at low and moderate intake levels. Calcium also diffuses passively between intestinal mucosal cells, depending on the luminal:serosal concentration gradient of the ion; the importance of passive diffusion increases with high calcium intakes. An acidic intestinal pH is necessary for ionization of calcium; thus an alkaline pH impedes absorption.

Oral bioavailability of calcium from nonfood sources and supplements depends on intestinal pH, the presence or absence of a meal, and the dose. When a 250-mg dose of calcium is administered with a standardized breakfast, average oral bioavailability in adults ranges from 25–35% with various salts; under the same conditions, absorption from milk was about 29%. Calcium absorption is decreased in the absence of a meal. The extent of calcium absorption from supplements is greatest when calcium is taken in doses of 500 mg or less.

Fractional calcium absorption varies with age, being highest during infancy (about 60%), declining to about 28% in prepubertal children, and rising again during early puberty (about 34%); fractional absorption remains at about 25% in young adults, although it increases during the last 2 trimesters of pregnancy. With aging, fractional absorption declines, decreasing on average by 0.21% annually in postmenopausal women. Similar declines also appear to occur with aging in men.

Absorption is retarded by certain anions (e.g., oxalates, phytates, sulfates) and by fatty acids which precipitate or complex calcium ions; however, an intestinal pH of 5–7 facilitates maximal dissolution and dissociation of these complexes. As a result, calcium may be poorly absorbed from foods rich in oxalic acid (e.g., spinach, sweet potatoes, rhubarb, beans) or phytic acid (e.g., unleavened bread, raw beans, seeds, nuts, grains, soy isolates). Although soybeans contain high concentrations of phytic acid, calcium absorption is relatively high from this food. Glucocorticoids and low serum concentrations of calcitonin may depress the absorption of calcium. Calcium absorption is decreased in patients with certain disease states such as achlorhydria, renal osteodystrophy, steatorrhea, or uremia.

IM or IV administered calcium salts are absorbed directly into the blood stream. Following IV injection of calcium salts, serum calcium concentrations increase almost immediately and may return to previous values in 30 minutes to 2 hours.

■ **Distribution** Following absorption, calcium first enters the extracellular fluid and is then rapidly incorporated into skeletal tissue. Bone formation, however, is not stimulated by administration of calcium. Bone contains 99% of the body's calcium; the remaining 1% is distributed equally between the intracellular and extracellular fluids.

Normal total serum calcium concentrations range from 9–10.4 mg/dL (4.5–5.2 mEq/L), but only ionized calcium is physiologically active. Serum calcium concentrations are not necessarily accurate indications of total body calcium; total body calcium may be decreased in the presence of hypercalcemia, and hypocalcemia can occur even though total body calcium is increased. Of the total serum calcium concentration, 50% is in the ionic form and 5% is complexed by phosphates, citrates, and other anions. Approximately 45% of the serum calcium is bound to plasma proteins; for a change in serum albumin of 1 g/dL, the serum calcium concentration may change about 0.8 mg/dL (0.04 mEq/dL). Hyperproteinemia is associated with increased total serum calcium concentrations; in hypoproteinemia, total serum calcium concentrations decrease. Acidosis results in increased concentrations of ionic calcium, while alkalosis promotes a decrease in the ionic serum calcium concentration.

CSF concentrations of calcium are about 50% of serum calcium concentrations and tend to reflect ionized serum calcium concentrations. Calcium crosses the placenta and reaches higher concentrations in fetal blood than in maternal blood. Calcium is distributed into milk.

■ **Elimination** Calcium is excreted mainly in the feces and consists of unabsorbed calcium and that secreted via bile and pancreatic juice into the lumen of the GI tract. Most of the calcium filtered by renal glomeruli is reabsorbed in the ascending limb of the loop of Henle and proximal and distal convoluted tubules. Only small amounts of the cation are excreted in urine. Parathyroid hormone, vitamin D, and thiazide diuretics decrease urinary excretion of calcium, whereas other diuretics, calcitonin, and growth hormone promote renal excretion of the cation. Urinary excretion of calcium decreases with reduction of ionic serum calcium concentrations but is proportionately increased as serum ionized calcium concentrations increase. In healthy adults on a regular diet, urinary excretion of calcium may be as high as 250–300 mg daily. With low calcium diets, urinary excretion usually does not exceed 150 mg daily. Urinary excretion of calcium decreases during pregnancy and in the early stages of renal failure. Urinary excretion of calcium decreases with aging, possibly because of age-related decreases in intestinal calcium absorption efficiency and an associated decrease in filtered calcium load. Endogenous fecal calcium excretion does not change appreciably with aging. Calcium is also excreted by the sweat glands.

Chemistry and Stability

■ **Chemistry** Calcium is an essential nutrient cation, and calcium salts are used for the prevention or treatment of calcium depletion. For oral administration, the acetate, carbonate, citrate, gluconate, lactate, and phosphate salts of calcium are available as single ingredients and/or as components of combination products. The chloride, gluconate, and a combination of the glycerophosphate and lactate salts are available as injections.

Calcium chloride is freely soluble, and calcium lactate and calcium acetate are soluble in water. Calcium gluconate and calcium glycerophosphate are sparingly soluble, and the carbonate and phosphate salts of calcium are insoluble in water. Calcium chloride is deliquescent, and calcium lactate is somewhat efflorescent. Calcium gluconate injection may contain small amounts of calcium d-saccharate or other calcium salts as stabilizers and has a pH of 6–8.2. Calcium chloride injection has a pH of 5.5–7.5 and calcium glycerophosphate-calcium lactate injection has a pH of about 7.

■ **Stability** The interaction of calcium and phosphate in parenteral nutrition solutions is a well-documented, but complex, phenomenon (see Dosage and Administration: Administration). Calcium injections have been reported to be incompatible with IV solutions containing various drugs. Published data are too varied and/or limited to permit generalizations, and specialized references should be consulted for specific compatibility information.

Preparations

Excipients in commercially available drug preparations may have clinically important effects in some individuals; consult specific product labeling for details.

Calcium Acetate

Powder		**Calcium Acetate Powder**
Oral		
Capsules	667 mg (169 mg calcium; 8.45 mEq of Ca++)*	**Calcium Acetate Capsules**
		PhosLo® GelCaps, Fresenius

*available from one or more manufacturer, distributor, and/or repackager by generic (nonproprietary) name

Calcium Carbonate, Precipitated

Powder		**Calcium Carbonate, Precipitated Powder**
Oral		
Capsules	1.25 g (500 mg calcium)	**Calci-Mix®,** Watson
Capsules, liquid-filled	600 mg (240 mg of calcium)	**Liqui-Cal® Softgels®,** Advanced Nutritional Technology
Suspension	1.25 g (500 mg calcium) per 5 mL*	**Calcium Carbonate Suspension**
Tablets	650 mg (260 mg calcium)*	**Calcium Carbonate Tablets**
	1.25 g (500 mg calcium)*	**Calcium Carbonate Tablets** (scored)
		Os-Cal® 500, GlaxoSmithKline
Tablets, chewable	420 mg (168 mg calcium)	**Titralac®,** 3M
	500 mg (200 mg calcium)	**Chooz®,** Insight
	750 mg (300 mg calcium)	**Tums E-X® 750,** GlaxoSmithKline
	850 mg (340 mg calcium)	**Alka-Mints®,** Bayer
	1 g (400 mg calcium)	**Tums® Ultra 1000,** GlaxoSmithKline

	1.25 g (500 mg calcium)*	**Calci-Chew®**, Watson
		Calcium Carbonate Chewable Tablets
		Os-Cal® 500, GlaxoSmithKline
Tablets, film-coated	1.5 g (600 mg calcium)*	**Calcium Carbonate Tablets**
		Caltrate® 600, Wyeth

*available from one or more manufacturer, distributor, and/or repackager by generic (nonproprietary) name

Calcium Carbonate, Precipitated, Combinations

Oral		
Pieces, chewable	1.25 g (500 mg calcium) with Cholecalciferol 100 units and Phytonadione 40 mcg	**Viactiv® Soft Calcium Chews**, McNeil
Tablets	Calcium Carbonate 240 mg with Calcium Gluconate 240 mg, Calcium Lactate 240 mg, (152.8 mg calcium) and Cholecalciferol 100 units	**Calcet®**, Mission
	1.25 g (500 mg calcium) with Cholecalciferol 200 units	**Os-Cal® 500+D**, GlaxoSmithKline
	1.5 g (600 mg calcium) with Cholecalciferol 125 units*	**Calcium Carbonate, Precipitated, and Cholecalciterol Tablets**
	1.5 g (600 mg calcium) with Cholecalciferol 280 units*	**Calcium Carbonate, Precipitated, and Cholecalciterol Tablets**
		Healthy Woman® (scored), Personal Products
Tablets, film-coated	1.5 g (600 mg calcium) with Cholecalciferol 400 units	**Caltrate® 600 + Vitamin D**, Wyeth

*available from one or more manufacturer, distributor, and/or repackager by generic (nonproprietary) name

Calcium Chloride

Powder		
		Calcium Chloride Powder
Parenteral		
Injection	10% (1.36–1.4 mEq of Ca^{++} and Cl^- per mL)*	**Calcium Chloride Injection**

*available from one or more manufacturer, distributor, and/or repackager by generic (nonproprietary) name

Calcium Citrate

Oral		
Tablets	950 mg (200 mg calcium)	**Citracal®**, Bayer

Calcium Citrate Combinations

Oral		
Tablets	1.5 g (315 mg calcium) with Cholecalciferol 250 units	**Citracal® + D Caplets®**, Bayer

Calcium Gluceptate

Powder		
		Calcium Gluceptate Powder

Calcium Gluconate

Powder		
		Calcium Gluconate Powder
Oral		
Tablets	500 mg (45 mg calcium)*	**Calcium Gluconate Tablets**
	650 mg (58.5 mg calcium)*	**Calcium Gluconate Tablets**
	1 g (90 mg calcium)*	**Calcium Gluconate Tablets**
Parenteral		
Injection	10% (0.45–0.48 mEq of Ca^{++} per mL provided by calcium gluconate and other calcium salt stabilizers)*	**Calcium Gluconate Injection**
Injection, for preparation of IV admixtures	10% (0.45–0.48 mEq of Ca^{++} per mL provided by calcium gluconate and calcium saccharate or other calcium salts stabilizers) pharmacy bulk package*	**Calcium Gluconate Injection**

*available from one or more manufacturer, distributor, and/or repackager by generic (nonproprietary) name

Calcium Glycerophosphate

Powder		
		Calcium Glycerophosphate Powder

Calcium Glycerophosphate and Calcium Lactate

Parenteral		
Injection	0.08 mEq of Ca^{++} (provided by calcium glycerophosphate 5 mg and calcium lactate 5 mg) per mL	**Calphosan®**, Glenwood

Calcium Lactate

Powder		
		Calcium Lactate Powder
Oral		
Tablets	325 mg (42.25 mg calcium)*	**Calcium Lactate Tablets**
	650 mg (84.5 mg calcium)*	**Calcium Lactate Tablets**

*available from one or more manufacturer, distributor, and/or repackager by generic (nonproprietary) name

Calcium Phosphate Dibasic

Powder		
		Calcium Phosphate Dibasic Powder

Calcium Phosphate Tribasic

Powder		
		Calcium Phosphate Tribasic Powder
Oral		
Tablets, film-coated	1.5652 g (600 mg calcium)	**Posture®** (scored), Inverness

Calcium Phosphate Tribasic Combinations

Oral		
Tablets, film-coated	1.5652 g (600 mg calcium) with Cholecalciferol 125 units	**Posture-D®** (scored), Inverness

Calcium salts are also commercially available in combination with vitamins, minerals, electrolytes, and antacids.

†Use is not currently included in the labeling approved by the US Food and Drug Administration

Hetastarch

Hydroxyethyl Starch, HES

■ Hetastarch, a nonprotein synthetic colloid, is a plasma volume expander.

Uses

■ **Hypovolemia** Hetastarch solutions are used for plasma volume expansion in the treatment of hypovolemia associated with elective surgery; safety of hetastarch in the treatment of hypovolemia in situations other than elective surgery has not been established. Hetastarch should not be used as a substitute for whole blood or plasma.

Plasma volume expansion produced by hetastarch solutions is comparable to that of albumin. For additional information on use of colloids in the treatment of hypovolemia, see Uses in Albumin Human 16:00.

■ **Leukapheresis** Solutions containing 6% hetastarch in 0.9% sodium chloride injection are used as an adjunct in leukapheresis to enhance the yield of granulocytes by centrifugal means. The solution containing 6% hetastarch in lactated electrolyte injection, however, is *not* indicated for such use.

■ **Other Uses** Hetastarch has been used as a cryoprotective agent for the long-term storage of whole blood†.

Dosage and Administration

■ **Administration** Hetastarch solutions are administered by IV infusion.

When used as an adjunct in leukapheresis, 6% hetastarch in 0.9% sodium chloride injection should be thoroughly mixed with a citrate anticoagulant prior to IV infusion. (See Dosage and Administration: Dosage.) Hetastarch volumes of 500–560 mL are compatible with citrate concentrations up to 2.5% for 24 hours at room temperature. The safety and compatibility of additives other than citrate have not been established.

Because 6% hetastarch in lactated electrolyte injection contains calcium, it should not be administered simultaneously with blood through the same administration set due to the potential risk of coagulation.

Hetastarch solutions contain no preservatives and are intended for single use only; partially used containers of the drug should be discarded.

Hetastarch solutions should be stored at room temperature (25°C); brief exposure to temperatures up to 40°C does not adversely affect the preparation. Hetastarch solutions should not be frozen or exposed to excessive heat.

■ **Dosage** When hetastarch is used for the treatment of hypovolemia, total dosage and rate of infusion depend on the amount of blood or plasma lost, the resultant hemoconcentration, and the patient's age, weight, and clinical condition. The usual adult dose of hetastarch is 30–60 g (500–1000 mL of 6% hetastarch in 0.9% sodium chloride injection or 6% hetastarch in lactated electrolyte injection). Hetastarch doses up to 90 g (1500 mL) have been used during surgery, generally without a need for blood or blood products. The manufacturers state that daily dosages exceeding 1.2 g/kg (20 mL/kg) or 90 g (1500 mL) usually are not required; however, such dosages have been used when severe blood loss has occurred (e.g., in postoperative or trauma patients), although generally only in conjunction with the administration of blood and blood products.

When used as an adjunct in leukapheresis, a citrate anticoagulant should be added to 250–700 mL of 6% hetastarch in 0.9% sodium chloride injection and mixed thoroughly. The resultant solution should be aseptically added to the input line of the centrifugation apparatus and infused at a ratio of 1:8 to 1:13 to venous whole blood.

■ **Special Populations** There are no specific dosage recommendations for geriatric patients; however, because of the greater frequency of decreased renal function in these patients, dosage should be selected with caution. (See Geriatric Use and also see Renal Impairment under Warnings/Precautions: Specific Populations, in Cautions.)

Cautions

■ **Contraindications** Hydroxyethyl starch (HES) preparations, including hetastarch, are contraindicated in critically ill adult patients, including those with sepsis, because of the increased risk of mortality and renal replacement therapy in such patients. (See Increased Mortality and Severe Renal Injury under Warnings/Precautions: Warnings, in Cautions.) HES preparations also are contraindicated in patients with severe liver disease, preexisting coagulation or bleeding disorders, and/or clinical conditions that may be exacerbated by volume overload (e.g., congestive heart failure, renal disease with oliguria or anuria not related to hypovolemia). The drug also is contraindicated in patients with known hypersensitivity to HES.

Because 6% hetastarch in lactated electrolyte injection contains lactate, the solution is contraindicated in the treatment of lactic acidosis.

■ **Warnings/Precautions** ***Warnings*** **Increased Mortality and Severe Renal Injury.** Increased mortality and/or severe renal injury requiring renal replacement therapy have been reported in critically ill adults, including patients with sepsis, receiving various preparations of HES. Data from randomized controlled trials in critically ill adults receiving lower-molecular-weight HES preparations (e.g., 6% hydroxyethyl starch 130/0.4) indicate that increased mortality and/or severe renal injury occurred within the recommended dosage range for HES (30–90 g [500–1500 mL] daily). Although the increased risks were reported principally with lower-molecular-weight HES preparations, such safety results may be applicable to higher-molecular-weight HES (e.g., 6% hydroxyethyl starch 450/0.7) because of similarities in chemical structure and mechanism of action, and also because lower- and higher-molecular-weight HES preparations are both metabolized by α-amylase into similar smaller fragments that may be associated with renal toxicity. Data from several meta-analyses and observational studies evaluating various preparations of HES confirmed the increased risk of mortality and/or severe renal injury in critically ill adults. Based on the reported evidence, the US Food and Drug Administration (FDA) considers the increased risk of mortality and renal injury requiring renal replacement therapy in critically ill adults, including those with sepsis, to be class effects of HES.

No evidence of renal injury was noted in a review of randomized controlled trials in which HES preparations were administered in the operating room to adult and pediatric patients who were undergoing surgery and were monitored for a short period of time (less than 7 days). Possible explanations for the lack of observed toxicity in these surgical populations include low exposure to HES in a relatively healthier population, requirement for post-administration follow-up monitoring, and/or other unknown factors.

Because of the increased risk of mortality and severe renal injury, HES solutions are contraindicated in critically ill adults, including those with sepsis. HES solutions should be avoided in patients with preexisting renal dysfunction. Use of HES should be discontinued at the first sign of renal injury. Because the need for renal replacement therapy has been reported up to 90 days after administration of HES, renal function should be monitored for at least 90 days in hospitalized patients receiving HES. (See Advice to Patients.)

Sensitivity Reactions **Hypersensitivity Reactions.** Life-threatening anaphylactic or anaphylactoid reactions (e.g., rash, erythema multiforme, urticaria, pruritus, angioedema, facial and periorbital edema, chills, flushing, severe hypotension, tachycardia, bradycardia, ventricular fibrillation, cardiac arrest, wheezing, shortness of breath, stridor, tachypnea, cough, chest pain, noncardiac pulmonary edema, laryngeal edema, bronchospasm, restlessness, fever, sneezing) have been reported rarely in patients receiving hetastarch; death has occurred, but a causal relationship to the drug has not been established. Hypersensitivity reactions can occur after discontinuance of hetastarch.

Hetastarch is made from corn starch; the drug should be used with caution in patients with known allergy to corn because such patients may also exhibit sensitivity to hetastarch.

If a hypersensitivity reaction occurs, hetastarch should be discontinued immediately and appropriate treatment and supportive measures should be initiated and continued until symptoms have resolved.

Other Warnings and Precautions **Hemodilution and Circulatory Overload.** Substantial hemodilution may occur following administration of hetastarch volumes exceeding 25% of blood volume in less than 24 hours. Slight decreases in platelet counts and hemoglobin concentrations have occurred as a result of the volume-expanding effects of hetastarch and the collection of platelets and erythrocytes in donors undergoing repeated leukapheresis procedures. Hemoglobin concentration usually returns to normal within 24 hours. Hemodilution by hetastarch may also result in 24-hour reductions in concentrations of total protein, albumin, calcium, and fibrinogen; these reductions are not considered clinically relevant.

The risk of circulatory overload is largely dependent on clinical circumstances; however, use of hetastarch doses exceeding 1.2 g/kg (20 mL/kg) within 24 hours may substantially increase such risk.

Excessive hemodilution and circulatory overload should be avoided, particularly in patients at risk of congestive heart failure or pulmonary edema. If excessive hemodilution occurs, administration of blood or blood products (e.g., packed red blood cells, platelets, fresh frozen plasma) should be considered.

Hematologic Effects and Coagulopathy. Administration of large volumes of hetastarch may transiently alter the coagulation mechanism (due to hemodilution and direct inhibition of factor VIII). Transient prolongation of prothrombin time (PT), activated partial thromboplastin time (aPTT), clotting time, and bleeding time may occur. Large volumes of hetastarch solution may decrease hematocrit and dilute plasma proteins. Bleeding, anemia (secondary to hemodilution and/or factor VIII deficiency), and coagulopathy (including rare cases of disseminated intravascular coagulation and hemolysis) have been reported. Increased risk of coagulation abnormalities and bleeding is associated with higher hetastarch doses. (See Patient Evaluation and Laboratory Monitoring under Warnings/Precautions: Other Warnings and Precautions, in Cautions.)

The safety of prolonged use (i.e., over several days) of hetastarch has not been established in situations other than leukapheresis. Prolonged use of the drug has been associated with coagulation abnormalities in conjunction with an acquired, reversible von Willebrand-like syndrome and/or factor VIII deficiency. Replacement therapy should be considered if severe factor VIII deficiency or von Willebrand disease occurs. Coagulopathy may take several days to resolve. Certain conditions appear to be associated with substantial risk during chronic use of hetastarch. Clinically important bleeding may occur in patients with subarachnoid hemorrhage receiving hetastarch repeatedly over a number of days for the prevention of cerebral vasospasm; severe intracranial bleeding resulting in cerebral herniation and death has been reported in at least one patient receiving 6% hetastarch in 0.9% sodium chloride injection. Therefore, it currently is recommended that hetastarch *not* be used for the management of cerebral vasospasm associated with subarachnoid hemorrhage or for conditions other than leukapheresis that necessitate repeated use of the drug over several days. In addition, some clinicians suggest that use of hetastarch be avoided in all neurosurgical patients, since prevention of intracranial hemorrhage in such patients is critical.

Increased bleeding has been reported in patients undergoing open heart surgery in association with cardiopulmonary bypass receiving HES solutions; such excess bleeding occurred irrespective of the molecular weight or molar substitution of the HES preparation and, therefore, is considered by FDA to be a class effect of HES. The coagulation status of patients undergoing open heart surgery in association with cardiopulmonary bypass should be monitored. 6% Hetastarch in 0.9% sodium chloride injection should not be used as a cardiac bypass pump prime, during cardiopulmonary bypass, or in the immediate period after discontinuance of the pump. Use of HES should be discontinued at the first sign of coagulopathy.

Hepatic Effects. Elevated indirect serum bilirubin concentrations have been reported in 2 of 20 healthy individuals who received multiple infusions of 6% hetastarch in 0.9% sodium chloride injection; however, total bilirubin concentrations remained within normal limits. Indirect bilirubin concentrations returned to normal within 96 hours after the final infusion. The importance of these elevations is not known; however, hetastarch should be used with caution in patients with a history of liver disease.

Liver function should be monitored in patients receiving HES preparations, including hetastarch.

Hetastarch and other HES preparations are contraindicated in patients with severe liver disease.

Pancreatic Effects. Transient increases in amylase concentrations may occur following administration of hetastarch; elevated serum amylase concentrations may persist for longer periods in patients with renal impairment. There is no association of the increased amylase concentration with pancreatitis, but this effect limits the use of serum amylase concentrations as an aid in the diagnosis of pancreatitis for up to 3–5 days after hetastarch administration.

Hetastarch has not been shown to increase serum lipase concentrations.

Electrolyte and Other Components of Hetastarch Preparations. Solutions containing 6% hetastarch in 0.9% sodium chloride injection contain sodium; at least one manufacturer states that preparations containing sodium should be used with caution in patients receiving concomitant therapy with drugs affecting electrolyte balance (e.g., corticosteroids, corticotropin). Such preparations should be used with extreme caution, if at all, in patients with edema with sodium retention.

The solution containing 6% hetastarch in lactated electrolyte injection contains dextrose and various electrolytes (e.g., lactate, potassium, sodium). Therefore, the preparation should be used with caution in patients with known subclinical or overt diabetes mellitus, patients with cardiac disease (particularly those receiving digoxin), and patients receiving concomitant therapy with drugs affecting electrolyte balance (e.g., corticosteroids, corticotropin). The preparation should be used with extreme caution in patients with metabolic or respiratory alkalosis and in patients with conditions that result in increased concentrations or impaired utilization of lactate ions (e.g., severe hepatic impairment). The solution containing 6% hetastarch in lactated electrolyte injection also should be used with extreme caution, if at all, in patients with hyperkalemia, potassium retention, or edema with sodium retention.

Patient Evaluation and Laboratory Monitoring. When used for treatment of hypovolemia, the patient's vital signs, fluid balance, electrolyte concentrations, acid-base balance, hemoglobin, hematocrit, platelet count, PT, and aPTT should be closely monitored.

When used as an adjunct in leukapheresis, regular and frequent clinical evaluation and complete blood cell counts (CBCs) are necessary. Additional laboratory determinations (i.e., total leukocyte and platelet counts, leukocyte differential count, hemoglobin, hematocrit, PT, and aPTT) should be considered if the frequency of leukapheresis exceeds the guidelines for whole blood donation.

Specific Populations **Pregnancy.** Category C. (See Users Guide.)

Lactation. It is not known whether hetastarch is distributed into milk in humans. Caution is advised if the drug is administered to nursing women.

Pediatric Use. Safety and efficacy of hetastarch have not been established in pediatric patients. However, in a small double-blind study in which a limited number of pediatric patients (1–15.5 years of age) were randomized to receive either hetastarch (i.e., 6% hetastarch in 0.9% sodium chloride injection) or albumin as a postoperative volume expander during the first 24 hours after surgery for repair of congenital heart disease, no differences in coagulation parameters or amount of required replacement fluids were found between pediatric patients receiving 1.2 g/kg (20 mL/kg) or less of hetastarch compared with those receiving albumin. However, an increase in PT was observed among patients receiving more than 1.2 g/kg of hetastarch.

Geriatric Use. In clinical trials of 6% hetastarch in lactated electrolyte injection, 30% of patients were 65 years of age or older, and 12% were 70 years of age or older. Experience with 6% hetastarch in 0.9% sodium chloride injection has not revealed overall differences in response relative to younger adults, but increased sensitivity in some older individuals cannot be ruled out.

Because hetastarch is primarily excreted by the kidneys and geriatric patients are more likely to have decreased renal function, caution should be exercised in dosage selection, and renal function should be monitored for at least 90 days in hospitalized patients receiving HES. (See Increased Mortality and Severe Renal Injury under Warnings/Precautions: Warnings and also see Renal Impairment under Warnings/Precautions: Specific Populations, in Cautions.)

Hepatic Impairment. Hetastarch should be used with caution in patients with a history of liver disease. (See Hepatic Effects under Warnings/Precautions: Other Warnings and Precautions, in Cautions.) Liver function should be monitored in patients receiving HES preparations, including hetastarch. (See Hepatic Effects under Warnings/Precautions: Other Warnings and Precautions, in Cautions.)

Hetastarch and other HES preparations are contraindicated in patients with severe liver disease.

Because of the lactate component in 6% hetastarch in lactated electrolyte injection, the preparation should be used with extreme caution in patients with severe hepatic impairment. (See Electrolyte and Other Components of Hetastarch Preparations under Warnings/Precautions: Other Warnings and Precautions, in Cautions.)

Renal Impairment. The manufacturers and FDA state that HES solutions, including hetastarch, should be avoided in patients with preexisting renal impairment. (See Increased Mortality and Severe Renal Injury under Warnings/Precautions: Warnings, in Cautions.) Hetastarch is contraindicated in patients with renal disease with oliguria or anuria not related to hypovolemia. (See Cautions: Contraindications.)

Limited data suggest that in the presence of renal glomerular damage, larger molecules of hetastarch can leak into urine and elevate the specific gravity, which can obscure the diagnosis of renal failure.

■ **Common Adverse Effects** Adverse effects reported in patients receiving hetastarch include hypersensitivity reactions, coagulopathy, hemodilution, circulatory overload, metabolic acidosis, congestive heart failure, pulmonary edema, bleeding, vomiting, peripheral edema, submaxillary and parotid glandular enlargement, mild influenza-like symptoms, headache, and muscle pain.

Drug Interactions

■ **Drugs Affecting Coagulation** Because hetastarch may alter the coagulation mechanism, the drug should be used with caution in patients receiving drugs that affect the coagulation system.

■ **Drugs Affecting Electrolyte Balance** Because of the electrolyte components in hetastarch preparations, at least one manufacturer states that hetastarch should be used with caution in patients receiving concomitant therapy with drugs that affect electrolyte balance (e.g., corticosteroids, corticotropin).

Description

Hetastarch, a hydroxyethyl starch (HES), is a synthetic colloid derived from a waxy starch composed mainly of amylopectin. Hydroxyethyl ether groups are introduced into glucose units of the starch, and the resultant material is hydrolyzed to yield a product with a molecular weight suitable for use as a plasma volume expander and for use in leukapheresis to promote erythrocyte sedimentation and thereby enhance granulocyte yield. Hetastarch resembles glycogen, and the polymerized D-glucose units in the hetastarch polymer are primarily joined by α-1-4-glycosidic linkages with occasional α-1-6 linkages. Hetastarch is characterized by its molecular weight and molar substitution. The average molecular weight of hetastarch is approximately 600 (6% hetastarch in 0.9% sodium chloride injection [Hespan®]) or 670 (6% hetastarch in lactated electrolyte injection [Hextend®]); while the average molecular weight of hetastarch ranges from 450–800, at least 80% of the polymers have molecular weights ranging from 200–2600. The molar substitution of hetastarch is approximately 0.75 (i.e., there are 75 hydroxyethyl groups per 100 glucose units). Hetastarch is commercially available as premixed solutions containing 6 g of hetastarch per 100 mL of 0.9% sodium chloride injection (e.g., Hespan®) or lactated electrolyte injection (Hextend®). Hespan® and Hextend® are designated as 6% HES 450/0.7.

Hetastarch exhibits colloidal oncotic effects. The drug retains intravascular fluid, resulting in plasma volume expansion. The degree of plasma volume expansion and improvement in hemodynamic state depend on the intravascular status of the patient. Plasma volume expansion produced by hetastarch is comparable to that of albumin human 5% solution. Maximum plasma volume expansion in hypovolemic patients is reached within a few minutes after the end of infusion; the extent and duration of the expansion in plasma volume vary with the volume of solution infused and depend on the preadministration plasma volume, the distribution of hetastarch through body water, and the rate of renal clearance of the drug. Following IV infusion, plasma volume expansion diminishes over 24–36 hours. In hypovolemic patients, hetastarch causes a temporary increase in arterial and venous pressures, cardiac index, stroke work index, and pulmonary wedge pressure. When added to whole blood, 6% hetastarch in 0.9% sodium chloride injection increases the erythrocyte sedimentation rate.

Hetastarch is not completely metabolized. The hydroxyethyl group is not cleaved during metabolism but remains intact and attached to glucose units when excreted; therefore, metabolism of hetastarch does not produce substantial amounts of glucose. Hetastarch is primarily excreted by the kidneys; molecules with a molecular weight of less than 50 are rapidly excreted, while larger molecules are retained for varying periods depending on their size and ease of breakdown. Following IV infusion of a single 30-g (500-mL) dose of 6% hetastarch in 0.9% sodium chloride injection, about 33% of the dose is excreted in urine within 24 hours. Although excretion of hetastarch is variable, intravascular concentration of the drug decreases to less than 10% of the total administered dose within 2 weeks following IV infusion. Biliary excretion of hetastarch accounts for less than 1% of the dose. Hetastarch is not removed by hemodialysis; it is not known whether hetastarch is removed by other extracorporeal elimination techniques.

Each liter of 6% hetastarch in 0.9% sodium chloride injection provides 154 mEq each of sodium and chloride. Each liter of 6% hetastarch in lactated electrolyte injection provides 143 mEq of sodium, 124 mEq of chloride, 28 mEq of lactate, 5 mEq of calcium, 3 mEq of potassium, and 0.9 mEq of magnesium; the electrolyte content of 6% hetastarch in lactated electrolyte injection resembles that of the principal ionic constituents of normal plasma. Commercially available hetastarch solutions have a pH of approximately 5.9 and a calculated osmolarity of approximately 307–309 mOsm/L.

Advice to Patients

Risk of severe kidney damage. Importance of immediately reporting signs and symptoms suggestive of kidney damage (e.g., change in frequency, volume, or color of urine; blood in urine; difficulty in urinating; swelling of the legs, ankles, feet, face, or hands; unusual weakness or fatigue; nausea and vomiting; shortness of breath).

Importance of informing clinicians of existing or contemplated concomitant therapy, including prescription and OTC drugs and herbal supplements, as well as any concomitant illnesses (e.g., congestive heart failure, liver disease, renal impairment).

Importance of women informing clinicians if they are or plan to become pregnant or plan to breast-feed.

Importance of informing patients of other important precautionary information. (See Cautions.)

Overview® (see Users Guide). For additional information on this drug until a more detailed monograph is developed and published, the manufacturer's labeling should be consulted. It is *essential* that the manufacturer's labeling be consulted for more detailed information on usual cautions, precautions, contraindications, potential drug interactions, laboratory test interferences, and acute toxicity.

Preparations

Excipients in commercially available drug preparations may have clinically important effects in some individuals; consult specific product labeling for details.

Hetastarch in Sodium Chloride

Parenteral

Injection, for IV infusion only	6% Hetastarch in 0.9% Sodium Chloride*	**Hespan®**, Braun **6% Hetastarch in 0.9% Sodium Chloride Injection**

*available from one or more manufacturer, distributor, and/or repackager by generic (nonproprietary) name

Hetastarch in Lactated Electrolyte Injection

Parenteral

Injection, for IV infusion only	6% Hetastarch in Lactated Electrolyte Injection	**Hextend®**, Hospira

†Use is not currently included in the labeling approved by the US Food and Drug Administration

Selected Revisions April 2014, © Copyright, July 1973, American Society of Health-System Pharmacists, Inc.

Hydroxyethyl Starch 130/0.4

■ Hydroxyethyl starch 130/0.4 (tetrastarch), a third-generation hydroxyethyl starch (HES), is a nonprotein synthetic colloid that is used as a plasma volume expander.

Uses

■ **Hypovolemia** Hydroxyethyl starch 130/0.4 solution is used for prevention or treatment of hypovolemia. It is not a substitute for red blood cells or coagulation factors in plasma.

Safety and efficacy of hydroxyethyl starch 130/0.4 have been evaluated in controlled studies in adult and pediatric patients undergoing various types of surgery (i.e., orthopedic, urologic, cardiac) that required prevention (i.e., autologous blood donation, acute normovolemic hemodilution, hypervolemic hemodilution before cardiac surgery) or treatment of hypovolemia. Safety and efficacy of the drug also have been evaluated in adults in the intensive care unit (ICU).

Hydroxyethyl starch 130/0.4 has been shown to be as effective as hetastarch for intraoperative volume replacement in adults undergoing major elective orthopedic surgery. In a double-blind, multicenter study, 100 adults (24–93 years of age) undergoing major elective orthopedic surgery (primarily of the hip and spine) were randomized in a 1:1 ratio to receive either 6% hydroxyethyl starch 130/0.4 in 0.9% sodium chloride injection or 6% hetastarch in 0.9% sodium chloride injection by IV infusion intraoperatively. The primary efficacy end point was the total volume of colloid solution required for intraoperative volume replacement. In this study, the mean volume required for intraoperative volume replacement was similar between hydroxyethyl starch 130/0.4 and hetastarch (1613 versus 1584 mL). In addition, no substantial difference was observed between the 2 treatment groups with respect to secondary efficacy end points (i.e., hemodynamic stability, body temperature, hemodynamic parameters, blood pressure, central venous pressure, heart rate, fibrinogen concentration, platelet count). Data from exploratory safety analyses suggest that adverse effects on coagulation parameters (i.e., reduction in concentrations of factor VIII and von Willebrand factor to below the lower limit of normal) may be less pronounced in patients receiving hydroxyethyl starch 130/0.4 compared with those receiving hetastarch; however, such safety data should be interpreted with caution, and additional study is needed to confirm these results.

Safety and efficacy of hydroxyethyl starch 130/0.4 for the treatment of hypovolemia have been evaluated in patients with severe sepsis. (See Cautions: Contraindications.) In a double-blind, multicenter study (CRYSTMAS study), 196 adults with severe sepsis were randomized to receive either 6% hydroxyethyl starch 130/0.4 in 0.9% sodium chloride injection or 0.9% sodium chloride injection by IV infusion for up to 4 days for the treatment of hypovolemia. The primary efficacy end point was the volume of solution required to achieve initial hemodynamic stabilization. In this study, the mean volume required to achieve initial hemodynamic stabilization was lower for hydroxyethyl starch 130/0.4 compared with 0.9% sodium chloride injection (1379 versus 1709 mL). In addition, initial hemodynamic stabilization was achieved slightly more quickly in patients receiving hydroxyethyl starch 130/0.4 (11.8 versus 14.3 hours, respectively), although the difference was not statistically significant. The number of treatment-emergent serious adverse events and the number of treatment-emergent serious adverse events leading to death were higher in patients receiving hydroxyethyl starch 130/0.4 compared with those receiving 0.9% sodium chloride injection (53 versus 44 and 38 versus 32, respectively). Although acute kidney injury scores were similar between the two groups, more patients receiving hydroxyethyl starch 130/0.4 required renal replacement therapy over the first 7 days following treatment (17 versus 8 patients) and during the 90-day observation period (21 versus 11 patients) compared with those receiving 0.9% sodium chloride injection; the mean duration of renal replacement therapy was 9.1 days in patients receiving hydroxyethyl starch 130/0.4 compared with 4.3 days in patients receiving 0.9% sodium chloride injection.

Data from a large study in patients admitted to the ICU suggested that use of hydroxyethyl starch 130/0.4 does not provide any mortality benefit over 0.9% sodium chloride injection. In this randomized, controlled study (CHEST study), a heterogeneous population of 7000 adults (including septic, trauma, and postoperative patients) admitted to the ICU was randomized to receive either 6% hydroxyethyl starch 130/0.4 in 0.9% sodium chloride injection or 0.9% sodium chloride injection by IV infusion for fluid resuscitation until ICU discharge, death, or 90 days after randomization. The primary efficacy end point was death within 90 days; secondary end points included acute kidney injury and requirement for renal replacement therapy. Results of this study indicate no substantial difference in the mortality rate at 90 days between patients receiving hydroxyethyl starch 130/0.4 and those receiving 0.9% sodium chloride injection (18 versus 17%). While use of hydroxyethyl starch 130/0.4 was associated with administration of lower volumes of resuscitation fluid, renal replacement therapy was required in more patients receiving hydroxyethyl starch 130/0.4 compared with those receiving 0.9% sodium chloride injection (7 versus 5.8%). Use of hydroxyethyl starch 130/0.4 also was associated with increased use of blood products and an increased incidence of adverse effects, particularly pruritus and rash.

Because of the increased risk of mortality and severe renal injury, hydroxyethyl starch 130/0.4 solution is contraindicated in critically ill adults, including those with sepsis. (See Cautions: Contraindications and also see Increased Mortality and Severe Renal Injury under Warnings/Precautions: Warnings, in Cautions.)

Dosage and Administration

■ **General** In patients with severe dehydration, the manufacturer recommends that a crystalloid solution be given prior to administration of hydroxyethyl starch 130/0.4 solution. In general, a sufficient volume of fluid should be administered to avoid dehydration.

■ **Administration** Hydroxyethyl starch 130/0.4 in 0.9% sodium chloride injection is administered by IV infusion.

The rate of infusion of hydroxyethyl starch 130/0.4 solution depends on the amount of blood lost, the hemodynamic status of the patient, and the resultant hemoconcentration (i.e., dilution effect of the drug). The initial 10–20 mL of the solution should be infused slowly, and the patient should be closely observed for possible anaphylactoid reactions. The infusion should be discontinued if an adverse reaction occurs.

Hydroxyethyl starch 130/0.4 solution can be administered repeatedly over several days; however, the manufacturer recommends that administration sets be changed at least once every 24 hours.

The solution containing hydroxyethyl starch 130/0.4 in 0.9% sodium chloride injection is intended for single use only; unused portions of the drug should be discarded.

Hydroxyethyl starch 130/0.4 solution should be stored at 15–25°C and should not be frozen.

■ **Dosage** The daily dosage of hydroxyethyl starch 130/0.4 solution depends on the amount of blood lost, the hemodynamic status of the patient, and the resultant hemoconcentration (i.e., dilution effect of the drug).

For prevention or treatment of hypovolemia in adult and pediatric patients older than 12 years of age, the manufacturer recommends a hydroxyethyl starch 130/0.4 dosage of up to 3 g/kg (50 mL/kg of 6% hydroxyethyl starch 130/0.4 in 0.9% sodium chloride injection) daily. In clinical studies, a daily dosage of 30–270 g (500–4500 mL of 6% hydroxyethyl starch 130/0.4 in 0.9% sodium chloride injection) has been used perioperatively in surgical patients, and a cumulative dose of 360–3960 g (6–66 L of 6% hydroxyethyl starch 130/0.4 in 0.9% sodium chloride injection) has been used in intensive-care-unit (ICU) patients following traumatic brain injury.

When used for prevention or treatment of hypovolemia in pediatric patients younger than 12 years of age, dosage of hydroxyethyl starch 130/0.4 should be individualized based on the colloid needs of the patient, taking into account the patient's disease state and hemodynamic and hydration status. The manufacturer recommends a hydroxyethyl starch 130/0.4 dosage of up to 3 g/kg (50 mL/kg of 6% hydroxyethyl starch 130/0.4 in 0.9% sodium chloride injection) daily in all pediatric age groups. However, in clinical studies, infants younger than 2 years of age received a mean dose of 0.96 g/kg (16 mL/kg), and children 2–12 years of age received a mean dose of 2.2 g/kg (36 mL/kg).

■ **Special Populations** There are no specific dosage recommendations for geriatric patients; however, because of the greater frequency of decreased renal function in these patients, dosage should be selected with caution. (See Geriatric Use and also see Renal Impairment under Warnings/Precautions: Specific Populations, in Cautions.)

Dosage should be adjusted in patients with cardiac insufficiency. (See Hemodilution under Warnings/Precautions: Other Warnings and Precautions, in Cautions.)

Cautions

■ **Contraindications** Hydroxyethyl starch 130/0.4 is contraindicated in critically ill adult patients, including those with sepsis, because of the increased risk of mortality and renal replacement therapy in such patients. (See Increased Mortality and Severe Renal Injury under Warnings/Precautions: Warnings, in Cautions.)Hydroxyethyl starch 130/0.4 also is contraindicated in patients with severe liver disease, volume overload, preexisting coagulation or bleeding disorders, renal failure with oliguria or anuria not related to hypovolemia, severe hypernatremia, severe hyperchloremia, or intracranial bleeding, and in patients undergoing dialysis. The drug also is contraindicated in patients with known hypersensitivity to hydroxyethyl starch (HES).

■ **Warnings/Precautions** ***Warnings*** **Increased Mortality and Severe Renal Injury.** Increased mortality and/or severe renal injury requiring renal replacement therapy have been reported in critically ill adults, including patients with sepsis, receiving various preparations of HES. (See Uses: Hypovolemia.) Data from randomized controlled trials in critically ill adults receiving lower-molecular-weight HES preparations (e.g., 6% hydroxyethyl starch 130/0.4) indicate that increased mortality and/or severe renal injury occurred within the recommended dosage range for HES (30–90 g [500–1500 mL] daily). Although the increased risks were reported principally with lower-molecular-weight HES preparations, such safety results may be applicable to higher-molecular-weight HES (e.g., 6% hydroxyethyl starch 450/0.7) because of similarities in chemical structure and mechanism of action, and also because lower- and higher-molecular-weight HES preparations are both metabolized by α-amylase into similar smaller fragments that may be associated with renal toxicity. Data from several meta-analyses and observational studies evaluating various preparations of HES confirmed the increased risk of mortality and/or severe renal injury in critically ill adults. Based on the reported evidence, the US Food and Drug Administration (FDA) considers the increased risk of mortality and severe renal injury requiring renal replacement therapy in critically ill adults, including those with sepsis, to be class effects of HES.

No evidence of renal injury was noted in a review of randomized controlled trials in which HES preparations were administered in the operating room to adult and pediatric patients who were undergoing surgery and were monitored for a short period of time (less than 7 days). Possible explanations for the lack of observed toxicity in these surgical populations include low exposure to HES in a relatively healthier population, requirement for post-administration follow-up monitoring, and/or other unknown factors.

Because of the increased risk of mortality and severe renal injury, HES solutions are contraindicated in critically ill adults, including those with sepsis. HES solutions should be avoided in patients with preexisting renal dysfunction. Use of HES should be discontinued at the first sign of renal injury. Because the need for renal replacement therapy has been reported up to 90 days after administration of HES, renal function should be monitored for at least 90 days in hospitalized patients receiving HES. (See Advice to Patients.)

Sensitivity Reactions **Hypersensitivity Reactions.** Hypersensitivity reactions, including anaphylactic and anaphylactoid reactions (e.g., mild influenza-like symptoms, bradycardia, tachycardia, bronchospasm, noncardiac pulmonary edema), have been reported very rarely in patients receiving hydroxyethyl starch 130/0.4.

If a hypersensitivity reaction occurs, hydroxyethyl starch 130/0.4 should be discontinued immediately, and appropriate treatment and supportive measures should be initiated and continued until symptoms have resolved.

Other Warnings and Precautions **Hemodilution.** Hemodilution, resulting in dilution of blood components (e.g., coagulation factors, other plasma proteins) and decreased hematocrit, has been reported in patients receiving hydroxyethyl starch 130/0.4. (See Hematologic Effects and Coagulopathy under Warnings/Precautions: Other Warnings and Precautions, in Cautions.)Fluid overload should be avoided. Fluid status of the patient and rate of infusion of hydroxyethyl starch 130/0.4 should be regularly assessed during treatment, particularly in patients with cardiac insufficiency. (See Dosage and Administration: Special Populations.)

Hematologic Effects and Coagulopathy. Administration of high dosages of hydroxyethyl starch 130/0.4 may result in decreased concentrations of coagulation factors, other plasma proteins, and hematocrit. Depending on the dosage administered, disturbances of blood coagulation beyond hemodilution effects can occur rarely. Coagulation parameters should be monitored in patients receiving prolonged therapy or as clinically indicated.

Increased bleeding has been reported in patients undergoing open heart surgery in association with cardiopulmonary bypass who received HES solutions; such excess bleeding occurred irrespective of the molecular weight or molar substitution of the HES preparation, and, therefore, is considered by FDA to be a class effect of HES. The coagulation status of patients undergoing open heart surgery in association with cardiopulmonary bypass should be monitored. Use of HES should be discontinued at the first sign of coagulopathy.

Pancreatic Effects. Transient elevations in serum amylase concentrations may occur following administration of hydroxyethyl starch 130/0.4. Such elevations can obscure the diagnosis of pancreatitis.

Cardiovascular Effects. Hypotension, shock, and circulatory collapse have been reported very rarely in patients receiving hydroxyethyl starch 130/0.4. A causal relationship to the drug has not been established.

Patient Evaluation and Laboratory Monitoring. Fluid balance, electrolyte concentrations, renal function, acid-base balance, and coagulation parameters should be monitored in patients receiving prolonged therapy or as clinically indicated. Liver function should be monitored in patients receiving hydroxyethyl starch 130/0.4.

Specific Populations **Pregnancy.** Category C. (See Users Guide.)

Lactation. It is not known whether hydroxyethyl starch 130/0.4 is distributed into milk in humans. Caution is advised if the drug is administered to nursing women.

Pediatric Use. Safety and efficacy of hydroxyethyl starch 130/0.4 have been evaluated in a limited number of infants younger than 2 years of age undergoing elective surgery and in children 2–12 years of age undergoing cardiac surgery. Use of hydroxyethyl starch 130/0.4 in adolescents older than 12 years of age is supported by evidence from well-controlled studies in adults. (See Dosage and Administration: Dosage.)

Geriatric Use. In clinical studies of hydroxyethyl starch 130/0.4, 32% of patients were 65 years of age or older and 7% were 75 years of age or older. No overall differences in safety or efficacy were observed between geriatric and younger patients, but increased sensitivity in some older individuals cannot be ruled out.

Because hydroxyethyl starch 130/0.4 is principally eliminated by the kidneys, and geriatric patients are more likely to have decreased renal function, caution should be exercised in dosage selection, and renal function should be monitored for at least 90 days in hospitalized patients receiving HES. (See Increased Mortality and Severe Renal Injury under Warnings/Precautions: Warnings and also see Renal Impairment under Warnings/Precautions: Specific Populations, in Cautions.)

Hepatic Impairment. The effects of hepatic impairment on the pharmacokinetics of hydroxyethyl starch 130/0.4 have not been evaluated.

Liver function should be monitored in patients receiving hydroxyethyl starch 130/0.4. Hydroxyethyl starch 130/0.4 is contraindicated in patients with severe liver disease.

Renal Impairment. Following IV administration of a single 500-mL dose of 6% hydroxyethyl starch 130/0.4 in 0.9% sodium chloride injection in individuals with creatinine clearance less than 50 mL/minute, the area under the plasma concentration-time curve (AUC) of hydroxyethyl starch 130/0.4 increased by 73% and clearance decreased by 42% compared with values in individuals with creatinine clearance exceeding 50 mL/minute. However, the terminal half-life and peak hydroxyethyl starch concentration were not affected by renal impairment. Plasma concentrations of hydroxyethyl starch 130/0.4 returned to baseline levels at 24 hours postinfusion.

Hydroxyethyl starch 130/0.4 has not been studied in patients undergoing hemodialysis.

Hydroxyethyl starch 130/0.4 is principally excreted by the kidneys, and the risk of adverse reactions to the drug may be greater in patients with renal impairment. Because severe renal injury requiring renal replacement therapy has been reported in critically ill adults receiving various preparations of HES, the manufacturer and FDA state that HES solutions, including hydroxyethyl starch 130/0.4, should be avoided in patients with preexisting renal impairment. (See Increased Mortality and Severe Renal Injury under Warnings/Precautions: Warnings, in Cautions.) Hydroxyethyl starch 130/0.4 is contraindicated in patients with renal failure with oliguria or anuria not related to hypovolemia; the drug also is contraindicated in patients undergoing dialysis. (See Cautions: Contraindications.)

■ **Common Adverse Effects** Adverse effects reported in 1% or more of patients receiving hydroxyethyl starch 130/0.4 include pruritus, increased serum amylase concentrations, and hemodilution (resulting in decreased concentrations of coagulation factors, other plasma proteins, and hematocrit). (See Hemodilution and also see Hematologic Effects and Coagulopathy under Warnings/Precautions: Other Warnings and Precautions, in Cautions.)

Drug Interactions

There are no known interactions between hydroxyethyl starch 130/0.4 and other drugs or nutritional preparations. Safety and compatibility of hydroxyethyl starch 130/0.4 when administered with other additives have not been established.

Description

Hydroxyethyl starch 130/0.4 (tetrastarch), a third-generation hydroxyethyl starch (HES), is a synthetic colloid derived from thin boiling waxy corn starch composed mainly of highly-branched amylopectin. Hydroxyethyl groups are introduced into glucose units of the starch to yield a product with a molecular weight suitable for use as a plasma volume expander. The polymerized glucose units of the hydroxyethyl starch polymer are primarily joined by α-1-4-glycosidic linkages with occasional α-1-6 linkages.

Hydroxyethyl starch 130/0.4 is characterized by its concentration, molecular weight, and molar substitution. At a concentration of 6%, hydroxyethyl starch 130/0.4 solution is iso-oncotic in vivo and will expand circulating blood volume by an amount approximately equal to the volume infused. The average molecular weight of hydroxyethyl starch 130/0.4 is approximately 130 (range: 110–150). The molar substitution of hydroxyethyl starch 130/0.4 is 0.4 (i.e., there are on average 4 hydroxyethyl groups per 10 glucose units) (range: 0.38–0.45). Hydroxyethyl starch 130/0.4 is designated as 6% HES 130/0.4.

Hydroxyethyl starch 130/0.4 exhibits colloidal oncotic effects, resulting in plasma volume expansion. Plasma volume expansion produced by hydroxyethyl starch 130/0.4 is comparable to that of hetastarch. Following isovolemic exchange of blood with 500 mL of hydroxyethyl starch 130/0.4 in healthy individuals, blood volume is maintained for at least 6 hours.

Hydroxyethyl starch 130/0.4 has a lower molecular weight and molar substitution compared with first- or second-generation HES preparations (e.g., hetastarch) and is, therefore, more rapidly metabolized and cleared from the body. Following IV infusion of a single 500-mL dose of 6% hydroxyethyl starch 130/0.4 in 0.9% sodium chloride injection in healthy individuals, plasma concentrations of the drug remain at 75% of peak concentration at 30 minutes postinfusion, decrease to 14% at 6 hours postinfusion, and return to baseline at 24 hours postinfusion. The mean in vivo molecular weight of hydroxyethyl starch 130/0.4 in plasma is 70–80 immediately following infusion and remains above the renal threshold (60–70) throughout the treatment period. The elimination half-life of hydroxyethyl starch 130/0.4 in healthy individuals is 12 hours. Hydroxyethyl starch 130/0.4 is principally excreted by the kidneys; molecules smaller than the renal threshold are readily and rapidly excreted in urine, while larger molecules are metabolized by plasma α-amylase before being excreted in urine. Following IV administration of a single 500-mL dose, approximately 62% of the drug is excreted as hydroxyethyl starch molecules in urine within 72 hours.

The pharmacokinetics of hydroxyethyl starch 130/0.4 are similar following single- and multiple-dose administration. No substantial plasma accumulation was observed following daily administration of 500 mL of a 10% solution containing hydroxyethyl starch 130/0.4 (not commercially available in the US) for 10 days. Approximately 70% of the drug was excreted as hydroxyethyl starch molecules in urine within 72 hours.

Hydroxyethyl starch 130/0.4 is commercially available as a premixed solution containing 6 g hydroxyethyl starch 130/0.4 per 100 mL of 0.9% sodium chloride injection. Each liter of 6% hydroxyethyl starch 130/0.4 in 0.9% sodium chloride injection provides 154 mEq each of sodium and chloride. The commercially available solution of 6% hydroxyethyl starch 130/0.4 in 0.9% sodium chloride injection has a pH of 4–5.5 and a calculated osmolarity of 308 mOsm/L.

Advice to Patients

Risk of severe kidney damage. Importance of immediately reporting signs and symptoms suggestive of kidney damage (e.g., change in frequency, volume, or color of urine; blood in urine; difficulty in urinating; swelling of the legs, ankles, feet, face, or hands; unusual weakness or fatigue; nausea and vomiting; shortness of breath).

Importance of informing clinicians of existing or contemplated concomitant therapy, including prescription and OTC drugs and dietary or herbal supplements, as well as any concomitant illnesses (e.g., congestive heart failure, liver disease, renal impairment).

Importance of women informing clinicians if they are or plan to become pregnant or plan to breast-feed.

Importance of informing patients of other important precautionary information. (See Cautions.)

Overview® (see Users Guide). For additional information on this drug until a more detailed monograph is developed and published, the manufacturer's labeling should be consulted. It is *essential* that the manufacturer's labeling be consulted for more detailed information on usual cautions, precautions, contraindications, potential drug interactions, laboratory test interferences, and acute toxicity.

Preparations

Excipients in commercially available drug preparations may have clinically important effects in some individuals; consult specific product labeling for details.

Hydroxyethyl Starch 130/0.4 Injection

Parenteral		
Injection, for IV infusion only	6% Hydroxyethyl Starch 130/0.4 in 0.9% Sodium Chloride Injection	Voluven®, Fresenius Kabi

Potassium Supplements

■ Potassium supplements are used as a source of potassium, an essential nutrient cation.

Uses

■ **Potassium Depletion** Potassium supplements are used as a source of potassium cation for treatment or prevention of potassium depletion in patients in whom dietary measures are inadequate. Conditions which may indicate or result in potassium deficiency include vomiting, diarrhea, drainage of GI fluids, hyperadrenalism, malnutrition, debilitation, prolonged negative nitrogen balance, prolonged parenteral alimentation without addition of potassium, dialysis, metabolic alkalosis, metabolic or diabetic acidosis, GI tract abnormalities which result in poor absorption, certain renal diseases, and familial periodic paralysis characterized by hypokalemia. Potassium should be included in long-term electrolyte replacement regimens and has been recommended for routine prophylactic administration following surgery after adequate urine flow has been established. Administration of certain drugs including thiazide diuretics, carbonic anhydrase inhibitors, furosemide, ethacrynic acid, some corticosteroids, corticotropin, aminosalicylic acid, and amphotericin B may sometimes result in potassium depletion which may warrant potassium replacement therapy. Ingestion of potassium-rich foods and/or use of potassium-containing salt substitutes may prevent potassium depletion in patients receiving potassium-depleting drugs; however, judicious prophylactic administration of potassium may be advisable in selected patients during prolonged diuretic or corticosteroid therapy, especially if they are digitalized.

Potassium chloride is usually the salt of choice in the treatment of potassium depletion, since the chloride ion is required to correct hypochloremia which frequently accompanies potassium deficiency. In addition, hypochloremia may develop if the citrate, bicarbonate, gluconate, or another alkalinizing salt of potassium is administered, particularly in conjunction with chloride-restricted diets. In the rare instances in which metabolic acidosis exists concurrently with potassium depletion (e.g., renal tubular acidosis), alkalinizing salts of potassium are preferred.

■ **Hypertension** Inadequate dietary intake of potassium may play an important role in the development of hypertension, and high dietary intake of potassium (e.g., with supplementation) may protect against the development of high blood pressure and improve blood pressure control in patients with hypertension. Epidemiologic studies have suggested that a lower sodium-potassium ratio may result in a lower risk of cardiovascular disease as compared with that observed with a reduction of sodium or increase in potassium alone. Most experts currently recommend enhanced intake of potassium (3.5–5 g daily) as part of lifestyle modifications for hypertensive patients, unless contraindicated by chronic kidney disease (CKD) or use of drugs that reduce potassium excretion. (See Cautions: Precautions and Contraindications.) Potassium supplementation is recommended particularly in those unable to adequately reduce their sodium intake. Adequate intake of potassium also should be considered as a means of preventing the development of hypertension. Food sources high in potassium such as fruits and vegetables preferably should be used instead of potassium supplements. In pooled analysis of data from 33 randomized controlled trials in which potassium supplementation was the only difference between intervention and control groups, such supplementation was associated with a reduction in mean systolic blood pressure of 3.11 mm Hg and a reduction in mean diastolic blood pressure of 1.97 mm Hg. The effects of potassium supplementation appeared to be particularly evident in patients exposed to high sodium intake.

■ **Other Uses** Potassium salts may be used cautiously to abolish arrhythmias of cardiac glycoside toxicity precipitated by a loss of potassium. It has been reported that elevation of plasma potassium concentrations by 0.5–1.5 mEq/L or to the upper limits of normal may be useful in the management of tachyarrhythmias following cardiac surgery. This regimen should not be used in patients with atrioventricular block, however, since potassium may further impair nodal conduction.

Limited data suggest that potassium may be useful in the treatment of thallium poisoning; however, such treatment is limited by the amount of thallium that can be released into the blood without worsening cerebral symptoms.

Dosage and Administration

■ **Administration** The acetate, bicarbonate, chloride, citrate, and gluconate salts of potassium are administered orally. Potassium chloride, potassium acetate, and potassium phosphate may be administered by slow IV infusion. Rarely, potassium-containing injections are given by hypodermoclysis, in which case potassium concentrations should not exceed 10 mEq/L in order to avoid local pain. Whenever possible, potassium supplements should be given orally since the relatively slow absorption from the GI tract prevents sudden, large increases in plasma potassium concentrations. Oral potassium supplements should preferably be administered as liquid with or after meals with a full glass of water or fruit juice to minimize the possibility of GI irritation and a saline cathartic effect. Enteric-coated (no longer commercially available in the US) and wax matrix tablets must be swallowed and not allowed to dissolve in the mouth. Other commercially available oral dosage forms of potassium should be dissolved and/or diluted and administered according to the instructions of the manufacturer.

Potassium for injection concentrates must be diluted with a compatible IV solution prior to administration. Diluted solutions of potassium acetate, potassium chloride, and potassium phosphate for injection concentrates *must* be administered slowly. Potassium injections should generally be administered only in patients with adequate urine flow. In dehydrated patients, 1 liter of potassium-free fluid should be administered prior to initiating potassium therapy. Generally, potassium concentrations in IV fluids should not exceed 40 mEq/L and the rate of administration should not exceed 20 mEq/hour. However, higher potassium concentrations (e.g., 60–80 mEq/L) administered more rapidly occasionally may be needed initially in cases of severe hypokalemia and associated cardiac arrhythmias or for the management of diabetic ketoacidosis or the diuretic phase of acute renal failure. Local vascular intolerance may limit the ability to administer such concentrated solutions. In such cases, use of a large vein with a relatively high blood flow (e.g., femoral vein) or splitting and administering the dose in less concentrated solutions via 2 veins simultaneously can be considered. Administration of such concentrated potassium solutions via a subclavian, jugular, or right atrial catheter should be *avoided* since local potassium concentrations achieved in the heart may be high and potentially cardiotoxic. The ECG should be monitored closely when the rate of IV potassium administration exceeds 20 mEq/hour. Peaking of the T wave or other ECG changes associated with hyperkalemia (see Cautions: Hyperkalemia) indicate that the rate of potassium infusion is excessive and should be reduced.

Viaflex® Plus containers of potassium chloride injections should be checked for minute leaks by firmly squeezing the bag. The injection should be discarded if the container seal is not intact or leaks are found or if the solution is cloudy or contains a precipitate. The injection in plastic containers should not be used in series connections with other plastic containers, since such use could result in air embolism from residual air being drawn from the primary container before administration of fluid from the secondary container is complete.

Oral administration of potassium supplements or ingestion of potassium-rich foods should replace IV potassium therapy as soon as possible.

■ **Dosage** Dosage of potassium supplements is usually expressed as mEq of potassium and depends on the requirements of the individual patient. The normal adult daily requirement and the usual dietary intake of potassium is 40–80 mEq; infants may require 2–3 mEq/kg or 40 mEq/m^2 daily. Potassium replacement requirements can be estimated only by initial clinical condition and response, ECG monitoring, and/or plasma potassium determinations. Prophylactic administration of potassium supplements may be necessary in some patients in order to maintain plasma potassium concentration above 3.0 mEq/L. The average oral dosage of potassium supplements for the prevention of hypokalemia is about 20 mEq daily, and the usual oral dosage of potassium for the treatment of potassium depletion is 40–100 mEq or more daily. However, it is important to remember that dosage must be individualized for each patient. Forty mEq of potassium is provided by approximately:

3.9 g of potassium acetate
4.0 g of potassium bicarbonate
3.0 g of potassium chloride
4.3 g of potassium citrate
9.4 g of potassium gluconate
5.4 g of monobasic potassium phosphate
3.5 g of dibasic potassium phosphate

Oral potassium supplements are usually administered in 2–4 doses daily. To avoid serious hyperkalemia, replacement of potassium deficits must be undertaken gradually usually over a 3- to 7-day period depending on the severity of the deficit. Potassium dosage for adults should usually not exceed 150 mEq daily, and the dosage for young children should not exceed 3 mEq/kg daily. Close monitoring of the ECG and plasma potassium concentrations is essential during IV administration of potassium.

Cautions

■ GI and Other Local Effects Adverse effects of potassium salts may include nausea, vomiting, diarrhea, flatulence, and abdominal pain or discomfort. Small bowel ulcerations have been reported following administration of enteric-coated potassium chloride tablets (no longer commercially available in the US). Ulcerations have been accompanied by stenosis, hemorrhage, obstruction, and perforation; surgery is frequently required and deaths have been reported. A few cases of small bowel ulceration, stricture, and perforation have been associated with wax matrix formulations of potassium chloride. Esophageal ulceration and stricture have occurred in patients with esophageal compression associated with an enlarged left atrium, and mouth ulceration occurred when a patient sucked rather than swallowed the wax matrix tablets. Following release of the drug from wax matrix tablets, the expended wax matrix is not absorbed systemically and may be detected in feces. Numerous wax matrices accumulated in a patient with partial obstruction of the lower bowel causing an impaction. To date, the incidence of GI lesions (ulceration, stricture, and perforation) with wax matrix tablets appears to be much lower than with enteric-coated (no longer commercially available in the US) tablets (less than 1 per 100,000 patient-years vs 40–50 per 100,000 patient-years). Extended-release tablets containing coated potassium chloride crystals are also formulated to minimize the likelihood of the drug causing GI lesions, but the frequency of GI lesions with these tablets currently is not known. Like enteric-coated tablets (no longer commercially available in the US), the wax matrix tablets and extended-release tablets containing coated crystals of the drug should be administered with caution and should be discontinued immediately if abdominal pain, distention, severe vomiting, or GI bleeding occurs. (See Cautions: Precautions and Contraindications.) Some authorities question the use of any potassium tablet, since use of dilute liquid preparations of potassium minimizes the risk of GI complications.

Pain at the site of injection and phlebitis may occur during IV administration of solutions containing 30 mEq or more potassium per liter.

■ Hyperkalemia Hyperkalemia is the most common and serious hazard of potassium therapy. Since an exact measurement of potassium deficiency is not usually possible, potassium supplements should be administered slowly and with caution. The presence of adequate renal function must be confirmed, and frequent observations of the clinical status of the patient and periodic ECGs and/or determinations of plasma potassium concentrations should be made. ECG changes are probably the most important indicator of potassium toxicity and include tall, peaked T waves, depression of the ST segment, disappearance of the P wave, prolongation of the QT interval, and widening and slurring of the QRS complex. Clinical signs and symptoms of potassium overdosage include paresthesia of the extremities, listlessness, mental confusion, weakness or heaviness of the legs, flaccid paralysis, cold skin, gray pallor, peripheral vascular collapse with fall in blood pressure, cardiac arrhythmias, and heart block. Extremely high plasma potassium concentrations (8–11 mEq/L) may cause death from cardiac depression, arrhythmias, or arrest. It has been suggested that hyperkalemia may decrease the excitability of the myocardium to electrical stimulation resulting in the possibility that the myocardium may not respond to implanted pacemakers.

Except in the presence of severe renal impairment, hyperkalemia is not likely to result from oral administration or from slow IV administration of dilute solutions of potassium. Nonetheless, hyperkalemia can occur from therapeutic doses of potassium salts and, when detected, must be treated immediately since lethal plasma potassium concentrations can be reached within a few hours. Hyperkalemia may result from rapid IV administration of potassium solutions. Hyperkalemia has occurred following addition of concentrated potassium chloride solutions to infusions from a hanging flexible plastic container, apparently as a result of pooling of the concentrated potassium solution at the base of the container and infusion of undiluted solution. Squeezing the container did not facilitate mixing but tended to pump the concentrated solution into the infusion chamber. Mixing of the solutions can be achieved if the plastic container is inverted during the addition of potassium solutions and subsequently agitated and/or kneaded.

Treatment of hyperkalemia depends on its severity and various regimens have been recommended. It must be kept in mind that rapid lowering of plasma potassium concentrations in digitalized patients can cause cardiac glycoside toxicity. Administration of potassium-rich foods and drugs and potassium-sparing diuretics must be discontinued. In patients with severe hyperkalemia, measures which facilitate shift of potassium into cells, such as administration of sodium bicarbonate, a calcium salt, and/or dextrose with or without insulin, have been recommended. In patients with plasma potassium concentrations greater than 6.5 mEq/L, IV infusion of 40–160 mEq of sodium bicarbonate over a 5-minute period has been recommended. This dose may be repeated after 10–15 minutes if ECG abnormalities persist. Dextrose therapy usually consists of IV infusion of 300–500 mL of 10–25% dextrose injection containing 5–10 units of insulin per 20 grams of dextrose over a 1-hour period. Some clinicians report that dextrose is less reliable and does not produce effects as rapidly as does sodium bicarbonate. In addition, studies indicate that the addition of insulin to an infusion solution results in adsorption of insulin to the glass and tubing. For this reason, it has been recommended that insulin be given as a separate injection. Patients whose ECGs show absent P waves or a broad QRS complex and who are *not* receiving cardiac glycosides should immediately be given 0.5–1 g (5–10 mL of a 10% solution) of calcium gluconate or another calcium salt IV over a 2-minute period (with continuous ECG monitoring) to antagonize the cardiotoxic effects of potassium. If ECG abnormalities persist, repeated doses of the calcium salt may be given, allowing 1–2 minutes between doses. When hyperkalemia is associated with water loss, administration of potassium-free fluids may be useful to decrease plasma potassium concentrations.

When the ECG approaches normal, efforts should be directed toward removal of excess potassium from the body. Some adsorption and/or exchange of potassium may be accomplished by administration of sodium polystyrene sulfonate orally or as a retention enema. Hemodialysis or peritoneal dialysis will reduce plasma potassium concentrations and may be required in patients with renal insufficiency. Administration of large doses of sodium chloride has been recommended to increase urinary excretion of potassium in patients with functional kidneys. Other drugs which have been used in an effort to reduce plasma potassium concentrations include testosterone to promote anabolism, and desoxycorticosterone acetate in patients with adrenal insufficiency who have adequate renal function.

■ Precautions and Contraindications Potassium supplements should be administered with caution in patients with cardiac disease. These drugs may intensify symptoms of myotonia congenita. Potassium supplements should not be administered to patients receiving potassium-sparing drugs such as amiloride, spironolactone, and triamterene. Potassium should generally not be given in the immediate postoperative period until urine flow is established. In patients with renal impairment, its use must be carefully controlled by frequent determinations of plasma potassium concentrations.

Because intestinal and gastric ulceration and bleeding have occurred with extended-release potassium chloride preparations, these dosage forms of the drug should be reserved for patients who cannot tolerate or refuse to take liquid or effervescent potassium preparations or for those in whom there is a problem of compliance with these latter dosage forms. If abdominal pain, distension, severe vomiting, or GI bleeding occurs in patients receiving an extended-release preparation, the drug should be discontinued immediately and the possibility of intestinal obstruction or perforation considered. Because Micro-K® LS contains docusate sodium as a dispersing agent, minor changes in consistency of feces may commonly occur; these changes are generally well tolerated. However, rarely, patients may experience diarrhea and cramping or abdominal pain. Patients with severe or chronic diarrhea or who are dehydrated generally should not receive supplemental potassium therapy using Micro-K® LS.

Some preparations of potassium contain the dye tartrazine (FD&C yellow No. 5), which may cause allergic reactions including bronchial asthma in susceptible individuals. Although the incidence of tartrazine sensitivity is low, it frequently occurs in patients who are sensitive to aspirin.

Potassium supplements are contraindicated in patients with severe renal impairment with oliguria, anuria, or azotemia; untreated chronic adrenocortical insufficiency (Addison's disease); the hyperkalemic form of familial periodic paralysis or other hyperkalemias; acute dehydration; heat cramps; or extensive tissue breakdown such as severe burns. Wax matrix formulations of potassium chloride should not be administered to patients with esophageal compression caused by an enlarged left atrium; a liquid preparation of potassium should be used in these patients. Solid oral dosage forms of potassium supplements are contraindicated in patients in whom there is a structural, pathological (e.g., diabetic gastroparesis), and/or pharmacologic (e.g., induced by anticholinergic agents) cause for arrest or delay in passage of the dosage form through the GI tract; an oral liquid preparation of potassium should be used in these patients.

Pharmacology

Potassium is the major cation of intracellular fluid and is essential for maintenance of acid-base balance, isotonicity, and electrodynamic characteristics of the cell. Potassium is an important activator in many enzymatic reactions and is essential to a number of physiologic processes including transmission of nerve impulses; contraction of cardiac, smooth, and skeletal muscles; gastric secretion; renal function; tissue synthesis; and carbohydrate metabolism.

Pharmacokinetics

■ **Absorption** Potassium salts are well absorbed from the GI tract. Enteric-coated potassium chloride tablets (no longer commercially available in the US) pass through the stomach releasing the drug in the small intestine and may produce dangerously high, localized concentrations of potassium chloride. Ingestion of sugar-coated tablets containing potassium chloride imbedded in a wax matrix (e.g., Kaon-Cl®, Slow-K®) produces a slow release of the drug. The wax matrix and potassium chloride crystals are blended so that the salt can be slowly leached from the tablet by GI fluids, and thus the potassium chloride is gradually released over a large segment of the intestine. Compared to liquid preparations, absorption of potassium from a single dose in these wax matrix formulations is somewhat delayed, probably because of the time required for dissolution of the drug. However, when potassium chloride is administered chronically, the bioavailability of potassium from the wax matrix preparations appears to be similar to that of liquid preparations of the drug. Dangerously high, localized concentrations of potassium chloride are not likely to occur with this dosage form unless blockage of passage of the tablet through the GI tract occurs. Similarly, extended-release granules for suspension and tablets containing coated potassium chloride crystals produce a slow release of the drug and minimize the likelihood of high, localized concentrations in the GI tract.

■ **Distribution** Potassium first enters the extracellular fluid and is then actively transported into the cells where its concentration is up to 40 times that outside the cell. Dextrose, insulin, and oxygen facilitate movement of potassium into cells. In healthy adults, plasma potassium concentrations generally range from 3.5–5 mEq/L. Plasma concentrations up to 7.7 mEq/L may be normal in neonates. Plasma potassium concentrations, however, are not necessarily accurate indications of cellular potassium concentrations; cellular deficits can occur without decreases in plasma potassium concentrations and hypokalemia may occur without substantial depletion of cellular potassium. Changes in extracellular fluid pH produce reciprocal effects on plasma potassium concentrations. A change of 0.1 unit in plasma pH has been reported to produce an inverse change of 0.6 mEq/L in plasma potassium concentration. Potassium concentrations in gastric and intestinal secretions are higher than plasma concentrations, and diarrheal fluid may contain up to 60 mEq/L.

■ **Elimination** Potassium is excreted mainly by the kidneys. The cation is filtered by the glomeruli, reabsorbed in the proximal tubule, and secreted in the distal tubule, the site of sodium-potassium exchange. Tubular secretion of potassium is also influenced by chloride ion concentration, hydrogen ion exchange, acid-base equilibrium, and adrenal hormones. Healthy patients on potassium-free diets usually excrete 40–50 mEq of potassium daily. Surgery and/or tissue injury result in increased urinary excretion of potassium which may continue for several days. Postoperative patients or patients under stress of disease with normal kidneys may excrete up to 80–90 mEq of potassium daily, even though they are not receiving any potassium. Small amounts of potassium may be excreted via the skin and intestinal tract, but most of the potassium excreted into the intestine is later reabsorbed.

Chemistry and Stability

■ **Chemistry** Potassium supplements are used in the prevention or treatment of potassium depletion. For oral administration, the acetate, bicarbonate, chloride, citrate, and gluconate salts of potassium are available as single ingredients and/or components of combination products. Potassium acetate, potassium chloride, and potassium phosphate are available as concentrates for injection that must be diluted prior to IV administration (for injection concentrate). In addition, potassium chloride is a component of several multiple electrolyte IV infusion fluids. The salts used as potassium supplements are very soluble or freely soluble in water. Potassium chloride for injection concentrate has a pH of 4–8, potassium acetate for injection concentrate has a pH of 7.1–7.7, and potassium phosphates for injection concentrate has a pH of 7–7.8.

■ **Stability** Some commercially available injections of potassium chloride are provided in Viaflex® Plus containers. Viaflex® Plus plastic containers are fabricated from specially formulated polyvinyl chloride (PL 146® plastic). The amount of water that can permeate from inside the container into the overwrap is insufficient to substantially affect the solution. Solutions in contact with the plastic can leach out some of its chemical components in very small amounts (e.g., bis(2-ethylhexyl)phthalate [BEHP, DEHP] in up to 5 ppm) within the expiration period of the injection; however, safety of the plastic has been confirmed in tests in animals according to USP biological tests for plastic containers as well as by tissue culture toxicity studies.

Potassium chloride, potassium acetate, and potassium phosphates concentrates for injection have been reported to be physically incompatible with IV solutions containing various drugs. Published data are too varied and/or limited to permit generalizations, and specialized references should be consulted for specific compatibility information.

Preparations

Excipients in commercially available drug preparations may have clinically important effects in some individuals; consult specific product labeling for details.

Potassium Acetate

Parenteral		
For injection concentrate	2 mEq of K^+/mL and CH_3COO^-/mL*	**Potassium Acetate Injection**
	2 mEq of K^+/mL and CH_3COO^-/mL pharmacy bulk package*	**Potassium Acetate Injection** **Potassium Acetate Injection MaxiVial®**, Abraxis
	4 mEq of K^+/mL and CH_3COO^-/mL*	**Potassium Acetate Injection**

*available from one or more manufacturer, distributor, and/or repackager by generic (nonproprietary) name

Potassium Bicarbonate

Oral		
Tablets, for solution	6.5 mEq of K^+	**Quic-K®**, Western Research
	25 mEq of K^+*	**K+ Care® Effervescent Tablets,** Alra **K-Lyte® Effervescent Tablets,** Bristol-Myers Squibb **Klor-Con®/EF,** Upsher-Smith **Potassium Bicarbonate Effervescent Tablets**

*available from one or more manufacturer, distributor, and/or repackager by generic (nonproprietary) name

Potassium Chloride

Oral		
Capsules, extended-release	8 mEq of K^+ and Cl^-*	**Micro-K®**, Ther-Rx **Potassium Chloride Extended-Release Capsules**
	10 mEq of K^+ and Cl^-*	**Micro-K®**, Ther-Rx **Potassium Chloride Extended-Release Capsules**
For solution	20 mEq of K^+ and Cl^- per packet*	**K+ Care®**, Alra **K-Lor®**, Abbott **Kay Ciel®**, Forest **Klor-Con® Powder,** Upsher-Smith **Potassium Chloride for Oral Solution**
	25 mEq of K^+ and Cl^- per packet	**Klor-Con®/25 Powder,** Upsher-Smith
Solution	6.7 mEq of K^+/5 mL and Cl^-/5 mL*	**Kaochlor® 10%,** Savage **Kay Ciel®**, Forest **Potassium Chloride Oral Solution**
	10 mEq of K^+/5 mL and Cl^-/5 mL*	**Potassium Chloride Oral Solution** **Rum-K®**, Fleming
	13.3 mEq of K^+/5 mL and Cl^-/5 mL*	**Kaon-Cl® 20% Elixir,** Savage **Potassium Chloride Oral Solution**
Tablets, extended-release	8 mEq of K^+ and Cl^-*	**Potassium Chloride Extended-Release Tablets** **Slow-K®**, Novartis
	10 mEq of K^+ and Cl^-	**Kaon-Cl-10®**, Savage
Tablets, extended-release (containing coated potassium chloride crystals)	10 mEq of K^+ and Cl^-	**K-Dur® 10,** Key
	20 mEq of K^+ and Cl^-	**K-Dur® 20** (scored), Key
Tablets, extended-release, film-coated	8 mEq of K^+ and Cl^-*	**K+ 8®**, Alra **Klor-Con® 8,** Upsher-Smith **Potassium Chloride Extended-Release Tablets**
	10 mEq of K^+ and Cl^-*	**K+ 10®**, Alra **Klor-Con® 10,** Upsher-Smith **Klotrix®**, Bristol-Myers Squibb **K-Tab® Filmtab®**, Abbott **Potassium Chloride Extended-Release Tablets**
Tablets, film-coated	2.5 mEq of K^+ and Cl^-*	**Potassium Chloride Tablets**
	10 mEq K^+ and Cl^-*	**Potassium Chloride Tablets**

Parenteral		
For injection concentrate	1.5 mEq of K^+ and Cl^- per mL*	**Potassium Chloride for Injection Concentrate**
	2 mEq of K^+ and Cl^- per mL*	**Potassium Chloride for Injection Concentrate**
	2 mEq of K^+ and Cl^- per mL pharmacy bulk package*	**Potassium Chloride for Injection Concentrate**
For injection concentrate, for IV infusion	0.1 mEq of K^+ and Cl^- per mL (10 mEq)*	**Potassium Chloride for Injection Concentrate**
		Potassium Chloride Injection Highly Concentrated (Viaflex®), Baxter
	0.2 mEq of K^+ and Cl^- per mL (10 and 20 mEq)*	**Potassium Chloride Injection Highly Concentrated** (Viaflex®), Baxter
	0.3 mEq of K^+ and Cl^- per mL (30 mEq)*	**Potassium Chloride Injection Highly Concentrated** (Viaflex®), Baxter
	0.4 mEq of K^+ and Cl^- per mL (20 and 40 mEq)*	**Potassium Chloride Injection Highly Concentrated** (Viaflex®), Baxter

*available from one or more manufacturer, distributor, and/or repackager by generic (nonproprietary) name

Potassium Chloride in Dextrose Injection

Parenteral		
Injection, for IV infusion only	10 mEq of K^+ per L in 5% Dextrose*	**10 mEq/L Potassium Chloride in 5% Dextrose Injection** (Viaflex®), Baxter
	20 mEq of K^+ per L in 5% Dextrose*	**20 mEq/L Potassium Chloride in 5% Dextrose Injection** (Viaflex®), Baxter
		20 mEq/L 0.15% Potassium Chloride in 5% Dextrose Injection
	30 mEq of K^+ per L in 5% Dextrose*	**30 mEq/L Potassium Chloride in 5% Dextrose Injection** (Viaflex®), Baxter
		30 mEq/L 0.224% Potassium Chloride in 5% Dextrose Injection
	40 mEq of K^+ per L in 5% Dextrose*	**40 mEq/L Potassium Chloride in 5% Dextrose Injection** (Viaflex®), Baxter
		40 mEq 0.3% Potassium Chloride in 5% Dextrose Injection

*available from one or more manufacturer, distributor, and/or repackager by generic (nonproprietary) name

Potassium Chloride in Sodium Chloride Injection

Parenteral		
Injection, for IV infusion only	20 mEq of K^+ per L in 0.9% Sodium Chloride*	**20 mEq/L Potassium Chloride in 0.9% Sodium Chloride Injection** (Viaflex®), Baxter
		20 mEq/L 0.15% Potassium Chloride in 0.9% Sodium Chloride Injection
	40 mEq of K^+ per L in 0.9% Sodium Chloride*	**40 mEq/L Potassium Chloride in 0.9% Sodium Chloride Injection** (Viaflex®), Baxter
		40 mEq/L 0.3% Potassium Chloride in 0.9% Sodium Chloride Injection

*available from one or more manufacturer, distributor, and/or repackager by generic (nonproprietary) name

Potassium Chloride in Dextrose and Lactated Ringer's Injection

Parenteral		
Injection, for IV infusion only	20 mEq of K^+ per L in 5% Dextrose and Lactated Ringer's*	**20 mEq/L Potassium Chloride in 5% Dextrose and Lactated Ringer's Injection** (Viaflex®), Baxter
		20 mEq/L 0.15% Potassium Chloride in 5% Dextrose and Lactated Ringer's Injection
	40 mEq of K^+ per L in 5% Dextrose and Lactated Ringer's*	**40 mEq/L Potassium Chloride in 5% Dextrose and Lactated Ringer's Injection** (Viaflex®), Baxter
		40 mEq/L 0.3% Potassium Chloride in 5% Dextrose and Lactated Ringer's Injection

*available from one or more manufacturer, distributor, and/or repackager by generic (nonproprietary) name

Potassium Chloride in Dextrose and Sodium Chloride Injection

Parenteral		
Injection, for IV infusion only	10 mEq of K^+ per L in 5% Dextrose and 0.2–0.225% Sodium Chloride*	**10 mEq/L Potassium Chloride in 5% Dextrose and 0.2% Sodium Chloride Injection** (Viaflex®), Baxter
		10 mEq/L 0.075% Potassium Chloride in 5% Dextrose and 0.2% Sodium Chloride Injection
		10 mEq/L 0.075% Potassium Chloride in 5% Dextrose and 0.225% Sodium Chloride Injection
	10 mEq of K^+ per L in 5% Dextrose and 0.3–0.33% Sodium Chloride*	**10 mEq/L (0.075%) Potassium Chloride in 5% Dextrose and 0.3% Sodium Chloride Injection**
		10 mEq/L Potassium Chloride in 5% Dextrose and 0.33% Sodium Chloride Injection (Viaflex®), Baxter
	10 mEq of K^+ per L in 5% Dextrose and 0.45% Sodium Chloride*	**10 mEq/L Potassium Chloride in 5% Dextrose and 0.45% Sodium Chloride Injection** (Viaflex®), Baxter
		10 mEq/L 0.075% Potassium Chloride in 5% Dextrose and 0.45% Sodium Chloride Injection
	20 mEq of K^+ per L in 5% Dextrose and 0.2–0.225% Sodium Chloride*	**20 mEq/L Potassium Chloride in 5% Dextrose and 0.2% Sodium Chloride Injection** (Viaflex®), Baxter
		20 mEq/L 0.15% Potassium Chloride in 5% Dextrose and 0.225% Sodium Chloride Injection
		0.15% 20 mEq/L Potassium Chloride in 5% Dextrose and 0.2% Sodium Chloride Injection
	20 mEq K^+ per L in 5% Dextrose and 0.3–0.33% Sodium Chloride*	**20 mEq/L Potassium Chloride in 5% Dextrose and 0.33% Sodium Chloride Injection** (Viaflex®), Baxter
		20 mEq/L 0.15% Potassium Chloride in 5% Dextrose and 0.3% Sodium Chloride Injection
	20 mEq of K^+ per L in 5% Dextrose and 0.45% Sodium Chloride*	**20 mEq Potassium Chloride in 5% Dextrose and 0.45% Sodium Chloride Injection** (Viaflex®), Baxter
		20 mEq/L 0.15% Potassium Chloride in 5% Dextrose and 0.45% Sodium Chloride Injection
	20 mEq of K^+ per L in 5% Dextrose and 0.9% Sodium Chloride*	**20 mEq/L Potassium Chloride in 5% Dextrose and 0.9% Sodium Chloride Injection** (Viaflex®), Baxter
		20 mEq 0.15% Potassium Chloride in 5% Dextrose and 0.9% Sodium Chloride Injection
	20 mEq of K^+ per L in 10% Dextrose and 0.2% Sodium Chloride*	**0.15% 20 mEq/L Potassium Chloride in 10% Dextrose and 0.2% Sodium Chloride Injection**
	30 mEq of K^+ per L in 5% Dextrose and 0.2–0.225% Sodium Chloride*	**30 mEq/L Potassium Chloride in 5% Dextrose and 0.2% Sodium Chloride Injection** (Viaflex®), Baxter
		30 mEq/L 0.224% Potassium Chloride in 5% Dextrose and 0.225% Sodium Chloride Injection
		0.22% 30 mEq/L Potassium Chloride in 5% Dextrose and 0.2% Sodium Chloride Injection
	30 mEq of K^+ per L in 5% Dextrose and 0.3–0.33% Sodium Chloride*	**30 mEq/L Potassium Chloride in 5% Dextrose and 0.33% Sodium Chloride Injection** (Viaflex®), Baxter
		30 mEq/L 0.224% Potassium Chloride in 5% Dextrose and 0.3% Sodium Chloride Injection

	30 mEq of K^+ per L in 5% Dextrose and 0.45% Sodium Chloride*	**30 mEq/L Potassium Chloride in 5% Dextrose and 0.45% Sodium Chloride Injection** (Viaflex®), Baxter
		30 mEq/L 0.224% Potassium Chloride in 5% Dextrose and 0.45% Sodium Chloride Injection
		0.22% 30 mEq/L Potassium Chloride in 5% Dextrose and 0.45% Sodium Chloride Injection
	40 mEq of K^+ per L in 5% Dextrose and 0.2–0.225% Sodium Chloride*	**40 mEq/L Potassium Chloride in 5% Dextrose and 0.2% Sodium Chloride Injection** (Viaflex®), Baxter
		40 mEq/L 0.3% Potassium Chloride in 5% Dextrose and 0.225% Sodium Chloride Injection
		0.3% 40 mEq/L Potassium Chloride in 5% Dextrose and 0.2% Sodium Chloride Injection
	40 mEq of K^+ per L in 5% Dextrose and 0.3–0.33% Sodium Chloride*	**40 mEq/L Potassium Chloride in 5% Dextrose and 0.33% Sodium Chloride Injection**
		40 mEq/L 0.3% Potassium Chloride in 5% Dextrose and 0.3% Sodium Chloride Injection
	40 mEq of K^+ per L in 5% Dextrose and 0.45% Sodium Chloride*	**40 mEq/L Potassium Chloride in 5% Dextrose and 0.45% Sodium Chloride Injection** (Viaflex®), Baxter
		40 mEq/L 0.3% Potassium Chloride in 5% Dextrose and 0.45% Sodium Chloride Injection
	40 mEq of K^+ per L in 5% Dextrose and 0.9% Sodium Chloride*	**40 mEq/L Potassium Chloride in 5% Dextrose and 0.9% Sodium Chloride Injection** (Viaflex®), Baxter

*available from one or more manufacturer, distributor, and/or repackager by generic (nonproprietary) name

Potassium Chloride in Water

Parenteral		
Injection, for IV infusion only	0.1 mEq per mL (10 mEq)*	**Potassium Chloride in Water for Injection (Premixed)** (LifeCare®), Hospira
	0.2 mEq per mL (10 and 20 mEq)*	**Potassium Chloride in Water for Injection (Premixed)** (LifeCare®), Hospira
	0.3 mEq per mL (30 mEq)*	**Chloride in Water for Injection (Premixed)** (LifeCare®), Hospira
	0.4 mEq per mL (20 and 40 mEq)*	**Potassium Chloride in Water for Injection (Premixed)** (LifeCare®), Hospira

*available from one or more manufacturer, distributor, and/or repackager by generic (nonproprietary) name

Potassium Gluconate

Oral		
Elixir	6.7 mEq of K^+ per 5 mL*	**Kaon® Elixir,** Savage
		Potassium Gluconate Elixir
Tablets	2 mEq of K^+*	**Glu-K®,** Western Research
		Potassium Gluconate Tablets

*available from one or more manufacturer, distributor, and/or repackager by generic (nonproprietary) name

Potassium Acetate, Potassium Bicarbonate, and Potassium Citrate

Oral		
Solution	15 mEq of K^+ (provided by potassium acetate 500 mg, potassium bicarbonate 500 mg, and potassium citrate 500 mg) per 5 mL	**Tri-K®,** Century

Potassium Bicarbonate and Potassium Chloride

Oral		
Tablets, for solution	25 mEq of K^+ and Cl^- (provided by potassium bicarbonate 0.5 g and potassium chloride 1.5 g)*	**Potassium Bicarbonate and Potassium Chloride Effervescent Tablets**
	25 mEq of K^+ and Cl^- (provided by potassium bicarbonate 0.5 g, potassium chloride 1.5 g, and lysine hydrochloride 0.91 g)	**K-Lyte/CL® Effervescent Tablets,** Bristol-Myers Squibb
		Potassium Bicarbonate and Potassium Chloride Effervescent Tablets
	50 mEq of K^+ and Cl^- (provided by potassium bicarbonate 2 g, potassium chloride 2.24 g, and lysine hydrochloride 3.65 g)	**K-Lyte/CL® 50 Effervescent Tablets,** Bristol-Myers Squibb
		Potassium Bicarbonate and Potassium Chloride Effervescent Tablets

*available from one or more manufacturer, distributor, and/or repackager by generic (nonproprietary) name

Potassium Bicarbonate and Potassium Citrate

Oral		
Tablets, for solution	50 mEq of K^+ (provided by potassium bicarbonate 2.5 g and potassium citrate 2.7 g)	**K-Lyte® DS Effervescent Tablets,** Bristol-Myers Squibb

Potassium Citrate and Potassium Gluconate

Oral		
Solution	6.7 mEq of K^+ (provided by potassium citrate 0.17 g and potassium gluconate 1.17 g) per 5 mL	**Twin-K®,** Boots

Potassium Phosphates

Parenteral		
For injection concentrate	4.4 mEq of K^+ and 3 mM of P (provided by potassium phosphate dibasic 236 mg and potassium phosphate monobasic 224 mg) per mL*	**Potassium Phosphates Injection**
	4.4 mEq of K^+ and 3 mM of P (provided by potassium phosphate dibasic 236 mg and potassium phosphate monobasic 224 mg) per mL pharmacy bulk package*	**Potassium Phosphates Injection**

*available from one or more manufacturer, distributor, and/or repackager by generic (nonproprietary) name

ION-REMOVING AGENTS 40:18

POTASSIUM-REMOVING AGENTS 40:18.18

Patiromer Sorbitex Calcium

■ Patiromer sorbitex calcium, which consists of patiromer, a nonabsorbed cation-exchange polymer, and a calcium-sorbitol counterion, is used for the removal of excess potassium.

Uses

■ **Hyperkalemia** Patiromer sorbitex calcium is used in the treatment of hyperkalemia. Patiromer has been shown to decrease elevated serum potassium concentrations and to reduce the recurrence of hyperkalemia in patients with chronic kidney disease who are receiving drugs that inhibit the renin-angiotensin-aldosterone system. Because of the delayed onset of action of patiromer, the drug is not used as an emergency treatment for life-threatening hyperkalemia.

Efficacy of patiromer was established in a 2-part single-blind study that consisted of a 4-week single-group treatment phase followed by an 8-week, randomized, placebo-controlled withdrawal phase. Patients with stage 3 or 4 chronic kidney disease who were hyperkalemic with serum potassium concentrations of 5.1 to less than 6.5 mEq/L and who were receiving stable dosages of at least one drug that inhibits the renin-angiotensin-aldosterone system (i.e., angiotensin-converting enzyme [ACE] inhibitor, angiotensin II receptor antagonist, aldosterone antagonist) were included in the study. The mean patient age was 64 years and most patients were male (58%) and Caucasian (98%); approximately 97% of patients had hypertension, 57% had type 2 diabetes mellitus, and 42% had heart failure.

In the initial phase of the study, 243 patients received patiromer. Initial dosage of the drug was based on baseline serum potassium concentration; patients with mild or moderate-to-severe hyperkalemia (baseline serum potassium concentration of 5.1 to less than 5.5 mEq/L or 5.5 to less than 6.5 mEq/L, respectively) received an initial patiromer dosage of 8.4 or 16.8 g daily, respectively, in 2 divided doses. Dosage was adjusted based on serum potassium concentration on day 3 and at weeks 1, 2, and 3 to achieve and maintain concentrations in the target range of 3.8 to less than 5.1 mEq/L. The mean patiromer dosage was 13 or 21 g daily in patients with mild or moderate-to-severe hyperkalemia, respectively. The mean reduction in serum potassium concentration from baseline to week 4 was 1.01 mEq/L; 76% of patients had serum potassium concentrations within the target range at week 4.

The randomized placebo-controlled withdrawal phase included 107 patients with moderate-to-severe hyperkalemia at study entry whose serum potassium concentration was in the target range at the end of the initial study phase, and who were still receiving drugs that inhibit the renin-angiotensin-aldosterone system. Patients randomized to continue patiromer therapy received the same dosage they were receiving at the end of the initial study phase. For those who received patiromer, the mean dosage was 21 g daily at the beginning of and during the withdrawal phase. The primary end point of the randomized withdrawal phase was change in serum potassium concentration from the start of the withdrawal phase to the earliest visit at which the patient's serum potassium concentration was outside the range of 3.8 to less than 5.5 mEq/L, or to week 4 of the withdrawal phase if the patient's serum potassium concentration remained in range. Serum potassium concentration increased by a median of 0.72 mEq/L in patients who were switched to placebo but was unchanged in patients who continued receiving patiromer. A greater proportion of patients who received placebo had a serum potassium concentration of 5.1 mEq/L or greater (91 versus 43%) or 5.5 mEq/L or greater (60 versus 15%) at any time during the withdrawal phase compared with those who received patiromer.

Efficacy of patiromer in reducing serum potassium concentration is maintained with continued use. In a phase 2, open-label, dose-ranging study in 304 hyperkalemic patients with chronic kidney disease and type 2 diabetes mellitus who were receiving drugs that inhibit the renin-angiotensin-aldosterone system, the effect of patiromer on serum potassium concentration was maintained during continued therapy for periods of up to 52 weeks. The mean patiromer dosage during the study was 14 g daily in patients with a baseline serum potassium concentration of greater than 5 to 5.5 mEq/L who received an initial dosage of 8.4 g daily in 2 divided doses and was 20 g daily in those with a baseline serum potassium concentration of greater than 5.5 to 6 mEq/L who received an initial dosage of 16.8 g daily in 2 divided doses.

Dosage and Administration

■ **Administration** Patiromer sorbitex calcium should be administered at least 3 hours before or 3 hours after other oral drugs. (See Drug Interactions: Effects on GI Absorption of Drugs.)

Patiromer is administered orally without regard to food. Patiromer should not be heated (e.g., in a microwave) or added to heated foods or liquids.

Patiromer should not be taken in its dry form. The powder should be mixed with water immediately prior to administration to form an oral suspension. The entire contents of the packet(s) containing patiromer should be emptied into a glass or cup containing 40 mL of water. The mixture should be stirred and then an additional 40 mL of water should be added to the suspension. The suspension should again be stirred thoroughly and more water may be added to achieve the desired consistency. The suspension should be administered immediately after preparation. If powder remains in the glass after initial administration, more water should be added and the mixture should be stirred and then administered immediately; this should be repeated, as needed, until the entire dose is administered.

■ **Dosage** Dosage of patiromer sorbitex calcium is expressed in terms of patiromer.

The recommended initial adult dosage of patiromer is 8.4 g once daily. Serum potassium concentration should be monitored, and the dosage of patiromer may be increased (in 8.4-g increments at intervals of 1 week or longer, up to a maximum dosage of 25.2 g once daily) or reduced based on the serum potassium concentration and desired target range.

■ **Special Populations** Dosage adjustments are not necessary in patients with renal impairment.

Cautions

■ **Contraindications** Patiromer is contraindicated in patients with known hypersensitivity to the drug or to any ingredient in the formulation.

■ **Warnings/Precautions** ***Worsening of GI Motility Disorders*** Patients with a history of bowel obstruction or major GI surgery, severe GI disorders, or swallowing disorders were excluded from clinical studies evaluating patiromer. Use of patiromer should be avoided in patients with severe constipation, bowel obstruction, or fecal impaction, including abnormal postoperative bowel motility disorders, because the drug may not be effective and may worsen GI conditions.

Hypomagnesemia Hypomagnesemia was reported in 5.3% of patients receiving patiromer in clinical studies. Patiromer binds to magnesium in the colon, which can lead to hypomagnesemia. Serum magnesium concentrations should be monitored in patients receiving patiromer, and magnesium supplementation should be considered in those with low serum magnesium concentrations.

Specific Populations **Pregnancy.** Patiromer is not expected to cause fetal harm when administered to pregnant women because the drug is not absorbed systemically following oral administration.

Lactation. Breast-feeding is not expected to result in risk to infants of patiromer-treated women because the drug is not absorbed systemically following oral administration.

Pediatric Use. Safety and efficacy of patiromer have not been established in pediatric patients.

Geriatric Use. In clinical studies of patiromer, 60% of patients receiving the drug were 65 years of age or older, while 20% were 75 years of age or older. No overall differences in efficacy were observed between geriatric patients and younger adults. However, adverse GI effects were reported more frequently in those 65 years of age or older compared with younger patients.

Renal Impairment. In clinical studies of patiromer, 93% of patients receiving the drug had chronic kidney disease. No dosage adjustments are necessary in patients with renal impairment.

■ **Common Adverse Effects** Adverse effects reported in 2% or more of patients receiving patiromer include constipation, hypomagnesemia, diarrhea, nausea, abdominal discomfort, and flatulence.

Drug Interactions

■ **Effects on GI Absorption of Drugs** In vitro binding studies have shown that patiromer binds to approximately 50% of the oral drugs tested; in clinical interaction studies, concomitant oral administration with patiromer altered the bioavailability of some of these drugs. Clinically meaningful in vitro binding (i.e., 30% or more) was not observed between patiromer and allopurinol, amoxicillin, apixaban, aspirin, atorvastatin, cephalexin, digoxin, glipizide, lisinopril, phenytoin, riboflavin, rivaroxaban, spironolactone, or valsartan. Although clinically meaningful in vitro binding was observed between patiromer and amlodipine, cinacalcet, clopidogrel, furosemide, lithium, metoprolol, trimethoprim, verapamil, and warfarin, studies in healthy individuals indicated that systemic exposure to these drugs was not affected by concomitant oral administration with patiromer. Decreased systemic exposure to ciprofloxacin, levothyroxine, and metformin was observed when these oral drugs were administered concomitantly with patiromer but not when the administration times were separated by 3 hours. Since binding of patiromer to other concomitantly administered oral drugs could reduce GI absorption of the drugs and result in loss of efficacy when administration times are close to those of patiromer, other oral agents should be administered at least 3 hours before or 3 hours following administration of patiromer.

Description

Patiromer sorbitex calcium, which consists of patiromer, a nonabsorbed cation-exchange polymer, and a calcium-sorbitol counterion, is used for the removal of excess potassium. The drug increases fecal potassium excretion via binding of potassium in the lumen of the GI tract, which decreases the concentration of free potassium in the GI lumen and, consequently, reduces serum potassium concentrations. Animal studies indicate that orally administered patiromer is not absorbed systemically and is excreted in feces.

In an open-label study in patients with chronic kidney disease and hyperkalemia (mean baseline serum potassium concentration of 5.9 mEq/L), serum potassium concentrations were reduced by 0.2 and 0.8 mEq/L at 7 and 48 hours, respectively, following initiation of therapy with patiromer (16.8 g daily in divided doses for 2 days); potassium concentrations remained stable for 24 hours after the last dose and then began to increase. Following twice-daily dosing, maximum (steady-state) effects on serum potassium concentration are attained in approximately 7–14 days.

In healthy individuals, patiromer produced a dose-dependent increase in fecal potassium excretion with a corresponding dose-dependent decrease in urinary potassium excretion, resulting in no change in serum potassium concentrations, when administered at dosages up to 50.4 g daily in 3 divided doses for 8 days. Substantial increases in mean daily fecal potassium excretion with concomitant decreases in mean daily urinary potassium excretion also were observed in healthy individuals receiving patiromer 25.2 g daily for 6 days; fecal and urinary potassium excretion were similar whether the drug was administered as a single daily dose or in 2 or 3 divided doses daily. Mean patiromer dosage and effects of the drug on serum potassium concentration are similar whether patiromer is administered with or without food.

Advice to Patients

Importance of informing patients who are taking other oral drugs to administer these drugs at least 3 hours before or 3 hours after administration of patiromer.

Importance of informing patients that patiromer may be administered without regard to food and that patients should adhere to their prescribed diets.

Importance of preparing each dose immediately before administration according to the manufacturer's instructions. Importance of advising patients that patiromer should not be heated (e.g., in a microwave) or added to heated foods or liquids and that the drug should not be taken in its dry form.

Importance of women informing clinicians if they are or plan to become pregnant or plan to breast-feed.

Importance of informing clinicians of existing or contemplated concomitant therapy, including prescription and OTC drugs, as well as any concomitant illnesses.

Importance of informing patients of other important precautionary information. (See Cautions.)

Overview® (see Users Guide). For additional information on this drug until a more detailed monograph is developed and published, the manufacturer's labeling should be consulted. It is *essential* that the manufacturer's labeling be consulted for more detailed information on usual cautions, precautions, contraindications, potential drug interactions, laboratory test interferences, and acute toxicity.

Preparations

Excipients in commercially available drug preparations may have clinically important effects in some individuals; consult specific product labeling for details.

Patiromer Sorbitex Calcium

Oral		
For suspension	8.4 g (of patiromer) per packet	**Veltassa®**, Relypsa
	16.8 g (of patiromer) per packet	**Veltassa®**, Relypsa
	25.2 g (of patiromer) per packet	**Veltassa®**, Relypsa

Sodium Polystyrene Sulfonate

Kayexalate

■ Sodium polystyrene sulfonate is a sulfonated cation-exchange resin that is used for the removal of excess potassium.

Uses

■ **Hyperkalemia** Sodium polystyrene sulfonate is used in the treatment of hyperkalemia. The drug aids in the removal of excess potassium from the body and should be considered an adjunct to other measures such as restriction of electrolyte intake, control of acidosis, and a high caloric diet. Before therapy is instituted, the cause of hyperkalemia should be determined and eliminated if possible. Because the action of the resin is slow, sodium polystyrene sulfonate alone may be insufficient (effective lowering of serum potassium may occur within hours to days) to rapidly correct severe hyperkalemia, including that associated with states of rapid tissue breakdown (e.g., burns, renal failure). Treatments that facilitate shift of potassium into cells, such as administration of sodium bicarbonate and/or dextrose (with or without insulin), and/or other treatments (e.g., a calcium salt) are indicated in patients with hyperkalemia evidenced by conduction defects (widening of the QRS complex) or arrhythmias. If hyperkalemia is severe, other definitive measures, including dialysis, should be considered. Sodium polystyrene sulfonate is most useful when hyperkalemia is not life-threatening or when other measures have reduced the dangers of hyperkalemia. The drug should not be used as an emergency treatment for life-threatening hyperkalemia.

Dosage and Administration

■ **Reconstitution and Administration** Sodium polystyrene sulfonate is administered orally or rectally.

Oral Administration Oral administration of sodium polystyrene sulfonate should be separated from oral administration of other drugs by at least 3 hours, and the separation time should be increased to 6 hours for patients with gastroparesis. (See Drug Interactions: Effects on GI Absorption of Drugs.)

When sodium polystyrene sulfonate is administered orally, each 1 g of the powdered resin should be reconstituted in 3–4 mL of water or a syrup and given as a suspension; usually 20–100 mL of fluid is used. Alternatively, the resin may be administered orally as a commercially available suspension. The suspension should be shaken well prior to administration. Sodium polystyrene sulfonate suspension also may be introduced into the stomach via a tube or the powdered resin or suspension may be mixed with the patient's food. The drug should *not* be mixed with foods or liquids that contain a large amount of potassium such as bananas or orange juice. Full precautions to prevent aspiration (e.g., placing and keeping the patient in an upright position during administration) should be observed.

Rectal Administration When sodium polystyrene sulfonate is administered rectally as a retention enema, each dose of the powdered resin is administered in 100–200 mL of an aqueous vehicle, such as 1% methylcellulose, 10% dextrose, or water, which has been warmed to body temperature. Although a somewhat thicker suspension may be used, care should be taken that a paste, which would greatly reduce the exchange surface and be particularly ineffective if deposited in the rectal ampulla, is not formed. Alternatively, 120–200 mL of a commercially available suspension may be administered as a retention enema, after the suspension has been warmed to body temperature. The suspension should be shaken well prior to administration. After an initial cleansing enema, a soft, large (French 28) rubber tube should be inserted about 20 cm into the rectum, with the tip well into the sigmoid colon, and taped in place. The extemporaneously prepared suspension of the resin, kept in suspension by stirring, or the commercially available suspension is then administered rectally by gravity feed. The tube may then be flushed with 50–100 mL of fluid, clamped, and left in place. If back leakage occurs, the hips should be elevated on pillows or a knee-chest position assumed. The suspension is retained in the colon for at least 30–60 minutes or for several hours if possible, after which the colon is irrigated with a non-sodium-containing solution at body temperature to remove the resin. Returns should be drained constantly through a Y-tube connection. Care should be taken to ensure that adequate volumes of non-sodium-containing cleansing enemas are administered. Approximately 2 L of irrigating solution may be needed to adequately flush out the resin. Proper removal of the resin is particularly important if sorbitol is used (administration of sorbitol is not recommended). Some clinicians believe that the preferred method of rectal administration is to place the resin in a sealed dialysis bag and insert the bag into the rectum.

■ **Dosage** ***Hyperkalemia*** The dosage and duration of sodium polystyrene sulfonate therapy must be individualized and depend on daily assessment of total body potassium. (See Cautions: Precautions and Contraindications.)

The usual adult oral dosage of sodium polystyrene sulfonate is 15 g (approximately 4 level teaspoonfuls of the powder or 60 mL of the commercially available suspension) 1–4 times daily (average 15–60 g daily).

Sodium polystyrene sulfonate may also be given rectally as a retention enema (see Rectal Administration, in Dosage and Administration: Reconstitution and Administration) in adult doses of 30–50 g (120–200 mL of the commercially available suspension) every 6 hours.

Reduced dosage is recommended in infants and small children. Pediatric dosage may be based on the fact that 1 g of the resin binds approximately 1 mEq of potassium. Oral administration is contraindicated in neonates. Some manufacturers also state that rectal administration is contraindicated in neonates and premature infants. (See Cautions: Pediatric Precautions.)

Cautions

■ **GI Effects** Sodium polystyrene sulfonate may cause some degree of gastric irritation. Anorexia, nausea, vomiting, and constipation may occur, especially if large doses are given. Large doses of the drug may cause fecal impaction, especially in geriatric patients. If clinically important constipation occurs, therapy with sodium polystyrene sulfonate should be discontinued until normal bowel movements resume; administration of magnesium hydroxide laxatives or sorbitol is not recommended. (See Drug Interactions.) Occasionally, the resin causes diarrhea.

Intestinal necrosis, which may be fatal, and other serious adverse GI events (bleeding, ischemic colitis, perforation) have been reported in patients receiving sodium polystyrene sulfonate. Most cases have occurred in patients receiving sorbitol concomitantly; many of the patients had risk factors for adverse GI events (e.g., prematurity, history of intestinal disease or surgery, hypovolemia, renal insufficiency or failure). (See Cautions: Precautions and Contraindications.) Although a causal relationship to the resin and/or sorbitol has not been established, some clinicians have suggested that studies in uremic rats implicate sorbitol rather than sodium polystyrene sulfonate as being principally responsible for intestinal necrosis. However, the occurrence of GI injury in patients receiving sodium polystyrene sulfonate without sorbitol and the presence of sodium polystyrene sulfonate crystals in injured segments of the GI tract have led others to suggest that the resin itself may be pathogenic.

In a systematic review of 58 cases of adverse GI events associated with sodium polystyrene sulfonate use, 71% of patients received the resin in combination with sorbitol, and 77% received the resin orally; 71% of patients had a history of chronic kidney disease or end-stage renal disease requiring dialysis, 16% had undergone prior solid organ transplantation, and 28% had undergone a recent surgical procedure. The colon was the most common site of injury (76% of patients); injuries in more proximal segments of the GI tract often were accompanied by colonic injury. Histolopathologic examination of GI specimens revealed transmural necrosis in 62% and ulceration in 48% of patients; sodium polystyrene sulfonate crystals were detected in injured segments of the GI tract in 90% of patients. Common presenting symptoms included abdominal pain and distension, GI bleeding, nausea and vomiting, and diarrhea; the median time from initiation of therapy to onset of symptoms was 2 days. The mortality rate in this series of patients was 33%, with 94% of the deaths occurring in patients with evidence of colonic necrosis.

■ **Electrolyte Effects** Hypokalemia and clinically important sodium retention may occur in patients receiving sodium polystyrene sulfonate therapy. Since the cation-exchange action of sodium polystyrene sulfonate is not totally selective for potassium, increased excretion of other cations occurs. (See Pharmacology.) Hypocalcemia and other electrolyte disturbances may occur.

■ **Pulmonary Effects** Acute bronchitis and bronchopneumonia following aspiration of sodium polystyrene sulfonate particles have been reported.

■ **Precautions and Contraindications** Patients receiving sodium polystyrene sulfonate should be monitored for electrolyte (e.g., calcium, magnesium, potassium) abnormalities. Serum potassium concentrations should be determined frequently within each 24-hour period during therapy; the duration of treatment with the resin must be determined individually for each patient. Because intracellular potassium deficiency is not always reflected by serum potassium concentrations, electrocardiograms and the clinical condition of the patient also should be closely monitored. ECG abnormalities seen with hypokalemia include lengthened QT intervals; widened, flat, or inverted T waves; and prominent U waves. Cardiac abnormalities, including premature atrial, nodal, or ventricular contractions and supraventricular and ventricular tachycardias, may also occur. Early signs of severe hypokalemia include a pattern of irritable confusion, delayed thought processes, and muscle cramps. Marked hypokalemia can also be manifested by severe muscle weakness and occasionally frank paralysis. The risk of precipitating hypokalemia-induced cardiotoxic effects of cardiac glycosides should be considered when sodium polystyrene sulfonate is administered to patients receiving these glycosides.

Because of the potential for intestinal necrosis and other serious adverse

GI events (bleeding, ischemic colitis, perforation), sodium polystyrene sulfonate should be used only in patients with normal bowel function. Use of the drug should be avoided in patients at risk for developing constipation or impaction (e.g., those with a history of fecal impaction, chronic constipation, inflammatory bowel disease, ischemic colitis, vascular intestinal atherosclerosis, previous bowel resection, or bowel obstruction) and in postoperative patients who have not had a bowel movement following surgery. Because most of the reported cases of intestinal necrosis or other serious adverse GI events occurred in patients who received sorbitol concomitantly with sodium polystyrene sulfonate, concomitant administration of sorbitol is not recommended. Most commercially available suspensions of sodium polystyrene sulfonate have been reformulated without sorbitol; however, preparations in a 33% sorbitol vehicle remain commercially available. Therapy with sodium polystyrene sulfonate should be discontinued if constipation occurs.

Precautions (e.g., placing and keeping the patient in an upright position during oral administration) should be taken to prevent aspiration. Patients with an impaired gag reflex, altered level of consciousness, or predisposition to regurgitation may be at an increased risk of aspirating sodium polystyrene sulfonate following oral administration.

Because administration of sodium polystyrene sulfonate may represent a clinically important sodium load (see Chemistry and Stability: Chemistry), the resin should be administered cautiously to patients whose sodium intake must be restricted, such as those with heart failure, hypertension, or edema. In these patients, compensatory restriction of sodium intake from other sources may be indicated.

In vitro studies have shown that sodium polystyrene sulfonate can bind to other drugs, which may decrease the extent of absorption of these drugs following concomitant oral administration. Other oral drugs should be administered at least 3 hours before or 3 hours after oral administration of sodium polystyrene sulfonate, and the separation time should be increased to 6 hours for patients with gastroparesis. (See Drug Interactions: Effects on GI Absorption of Drugs.)

Sodium polystyrene sulfonate is contraindicated in patients with hypokalemia, those with obstructive bowel disease, and those with known hypersensitivity to sodium polystyrene sulfonate resins. The drug also is contraindicated in neonates with decreased gut motility. Oral administration of sodium polystyrene sulfonate is contraindicated in neonates; some manufacturers state that use of the drug (oral or rectal administration) is contraindicated in neonates and premature infants. (See Cautions: Pediatric Precautions.)

■ **Pediatric Precautions** Efficacy of sodium polystyrene sulfonate in pediatric patients has not been established.

Sodium polystyrene sulfonate is contraindicated in neonates with reduced gut motility. Premature or low-birthweight infants may have an increased risk of adverse GI effects (e.g., intestinal necrosis) with sodium polystyrene sulfonate use. Some manufacturers state that use of the drug is contraindicated in premature infants.

Oral administration of sodium polystyrene sulfonate is contraindicated in neonates. The drug should be administered rectally in children and neonates with particular caution, since excessive dosages or inadequate dilution may result in impaction of the resin; care should be taken to ensure an adequate volume of non-sodium-containing cleansing enemas after rectal administration. Some manufacturers state that rectal administration is contraindicated in neonates.

■ **Geriatric Precautions** Large doses of sodium polystyrene sulfonate may cause fecal impaction in geriatric patients.

■ **Pregnancy and Lactation** Animal reproduction studies have not been performed with sodium polystyrene sulfonate. Sodium polystyrene sulfonate is not absorbed systemically following oral or rectal administration, and use in pregnant women is not expected to result in fetal risk.

Breast-feeding is not expected to result in risk to infants of sodium polystyrene sulfonate-treated women because the drug is not absorbed systemically.

Drug Interactions

■ **Effects on GI Absorption of Drugs** In vitro studies have shown that sodium polystyrene sulfonate may bind to other drugs (e.g., amlodipine, amoxicillin, furosemide, metoprolol, phenytoin, warfarin). Binding of sodium polystyrene sulfonate to other oral drugs could reduce GI absorption of the concomitantly administered agents and result in loss of efficacy when administration times are close to those of sodium polystyrene sulfonate. Therefore, other oral drugs should be administered at least 3 hours before or 3 hours after oral administration of sodium polystyrene sulfonate. Patients with gastroparesis or other conditions resulting in delayed gastric emptying may require a 6-hour separation. FDA states that the recommended spacing interval is based on the expected time for either sodium polystyrene sulfonate or the other drug to pass through the stomach. Clinical response and/or blood concentrations of the drugs should be monitored whenever possible. The manufacturers state that sodium polystyrene sulfonate may decrease absorption of lithium and thyroxine.

■ **Antacids and Laxatives** Sodium polystyrene sulfonate, when given orally with cation-donating antacids and laxatives such as magnesium hydroxide or calcium carbonate, has been reported to cause metabolic alkalosis in patients with renal disease. Magnesium hydroxide and calcium carbonate neutralize gastric hydrochloric acid and form the ionizable compounds magnesium chloride and calcium chloride. Upon entry into the small intestine, the magnesium and calcium ions react with bicarbonate and form magnesium carbonate and calcium carbonate, both of which are insoluble. However, sodium polystyrene sulfonate prevents this reaction by binding with the magnesium and calcium before they react with bicarbonate. This results in a loss of hydrogen ions from the stomach without a loss of bicarbonate ions from the intestine and, subsequently, in metabolic alkalosis. Rectal use of sodium polystyrene sulfonate may avoid this reaction.

In one study in patients with renal impairment (i.e., creatinine clearance ranging from 10–60 mL/minute), increases in plasma CO_2 concentration and in plasma and urinary pH were reported following concomitant use of sodium polystyrene sulfonate and calcium- or magnesium-containing antacids. Severe systemic alkalosis and a tonic-clonic seizure reportedly occurred in one patient with chronic hypocalcemia secondary to renal failure who received magnesium hydroxide and sodium polystyrene sulfonate concomitantly. In one patient with impaired renal function and chronic metabolic acidosis, the systemic alkalosis produced by concomitant use of sodium polystyrene sulfonate and magnesium hydroxide was used to therapeutic advantage.

Simultaneous oral administration of cation-donating antacids and laxatives with sodium polystyrene sulfonate may also reduce the resin's potassium exchange capability. Although there are no controlled studies to date, some clinicians have observed resistance to the potassium-lowering effect of sodium polystyrene sulfonate in hyperkalemic patients receiving magnesium hydroxide; response to sodium polystyrene sulfonate was reportedly restored when magnesium hydroxide was discontinued.

One case of small bowel obstruction resulting from aluminum hydroxide concretion has been reported to be associated with concurrent sodium polystyrene sulfonate therapy. However, the patient was receiving 720–1440 mL of aluminum hydroxide gel per day, and intestinal obstruction has been reported to occur with doses of aluminum hydroxide gel as low as 120 mL per day without concurrent administration of the resin.

Sodium polystyrene sulfonate and calcium- or magnesium-containing antacids or laxatives should be used with caution, especially in patients with renal impairment. The manufacturer warns that magnesium hydroxide should not be used as a laxative for the treatment of sodium polystyrene sulfonate-induced constipation.

■ **Sorbitol** Concomitant use of sorbitol with sodium polystyrene sulfonate may result in intestinal necrosis and is not recommended. (See Cautions: GI Effects and Cautions: Precautions and Contraindications.)

■ **Cardiac Glycosides** Sodium polystyrene sulfonate-induced hypokalemia may increase toxic effects of cardiac glycosides on the heart (e.g., ventricular arrhythmias, AV nodal dissociation).

Pharmacology

Sodium polystyrene sulfonate is a cation-exchange resin that releases sodium in exchange for other cations. Following oral administration, sodium is released from the resin in exchange for hydrogen ions in the acidic environment of the stomach. As the resin passes through the intestines, hydrogen cations exchange with those cations that are in greater concentrations and the cationically modified resin is excreted in the feces. Because of the relatively high concentration of potassium present in the large intestine, conversion of the resin to the potassium form occurs principally at this site. Following rectal administration of sodium polystyrene sulfonate, sodium ions are partially released from the resin in exchange for other cations present. In clinical use, much of the exchange capacity of sodium polystyrene sulfonate is utilized for cations other than potassium such as calcium, magnesium, iron, organic cations, lipids, steroids, and proteins. Thus, although 1 g of the resin has an in vitro exchange capacity of about 3.1 mEq of potassium, an in vivo exchange capacity greater than 1 mEq of potassium per g of resin is not likely.

Chemistry and Stability

■ **Chemistry** Sodium polystyrene sulfonate is a sulfonated cation-exchange resin prepared in the sodium phase and used for the removal of excess potassium. Each gram of the resin has an in vitro exchange capacity of about 3.1 mEq (range: 2.81–3.45 mEq) of potassium. Sodium polystyrene sulfonate occurs as a cream to light brown, fine powder that is odorless and tasteless and is insoluble in water. Each gram of the powdered resin contains approximately 4.1 mEq of sodium.

Sodium polystyrene sulfonate is commercially available as the powder or as a suspension. The commercially available suspension is an amber-colored, cherry-flavored suspension of the resin; the vehicle contains purified water, propylene glycol, magnesium aluminum silicate, sucralose, citric acid, flavoring agent, and parabens as a preservative. Each 100 mL of the commercially available suspension contains 25 g of sodium polystyrene sulfonate and 114 mEq of sodium. The drug also remains available as a light brown, cherry-flavored suspension in a 33% sorbitol vehicle that contains alcohol, purified water, propylene glycol, magnesium aluminum silicate, sodium saccharin, flavoring agent, and parabens as a preservative. (See Drug Interactions: Sorbitol.)

■ **Stability** Sodium polystyrene sulfonate powder and commercially available suspensions should be stored in well-closed containers at a temperature of 20–25°C, but some preparations may be exposed to temperatures ranging from 15–30°C. If repackaged, the commercially available suspensions should be refrigerated and used within 14 days of repackaging.

Sodium polystyrene sulfonate should not be heated because changes in the exchange properties of the resin may occur. The manufacturers of the powdered resin state that extemporaneous suspensions of the resin should be freshly prepared and should not be stored for more than 24 hours. However, an extemporaneously prepared 25% suspension of the powdered resin in water using a combination of 0.5% carboxymethylcellulose and 0.3% magnesium aluminum silicate as suspending agents was reportedly stable (i.e., easily redispersed, minimal sedimentation) for at least 30 days.

Preparations

Excipients in commercially available drug preparations may have clinically important effects in some individuals; consult specific product labeling for details.

Sodium Polystyrene Sulfonate

Oral or Rectal		
Powder, for suspension		Kionex®, Perrigo
		Sodium Polystyrene Sulfonate Powder
Suspension	1.25 g/5 mL*	Kionex®, Perrigo
		Sodium Polystyrene Sulfonate Suspension
		SPS®, CMP

*available from one or more manufacturer, distributor, and/or repackager by generic (nonproprietary) name

Selected Revisions November 2018,

Sodium Zirconium Cyclosilicate

ZS-9

■ Sodium zirconium cyclosilicate, a nonabsorbed cation-exchange crystalline compound, is used for the removal of excess potassium.

Uses

■ **Hyperkalemia** Sodium zirconium cyclosilicate is used in the treatment of hyperkalemia. Because of its delayed onset of action, the manufacturer states that the drug should not be used as an emergency treatment for life-threatening hyperkalemia.

The current indication for sodium zirconium cyclosilicate is based principally on the results of 3 studies demonstrating efficacy of the drug in reducing elevated serum potassium concentrations and maintaining normal serum potassium concentrations in patients with hyperkalemia. Approximately 60–68% of patients in these studies had chronic kidney disease, 62–66% had diabetes mellitus, 10–38% had heart failure, and 67–70% were receiving therapy with a drug that inhibits the renin-angiotensin-aldosterone system. The first study was a randomized, double-blind, placebo-controlled dose-ranging study that consisted of 2 phases (an initial 48-hour acute treatment phase followed by a 12-day maintenance phase). In the acute treatment phase, 753 adults with hyperkalemia (mean baseline serum potassium concentration 5.3 mEq/L, range: 5–6.5 mEq/L) were randomized to receive sodium zirconium cyclosilicate (1.25, 2.5, 5, or 10 g) or placebo 3 times daily for 48 hours. The primary efficacy end point was the exponential rate of change in mean serum potassium concentration during the first 48 hours of treatment; patients receiving sodium zirconium cyclosilicate 2.5, 5, or 10 g 3 times daily demonstrated substantial reductions in serum potassium concentrations from baseline (mean reductions of 0.16, 0.21, or 0.3%, respectively) compared with those receiving placebo (mean reduction of 0.09%). Corresponding dose-dependent absolute reductions in mean serum potassium concentrations at 48 hours in the 2.5-, 5-, and 10-g sodium zirconium cyclosilicate groups were 0.5, 0.5, and 0.7 mEq/L, respectively, with a greater response to the drug demonstrated in patients with higher baseline serum potassium concentrations. At the end of the initial treatment period, patients who achieved normokalemia (serum potassium concentration of 3.5–5 mEq/L) were continued into the subsequent 12-day maintenance phase; patients who had been receiving sodium zirconium cyclosilicate were re-randomized to receive either their original sodium zirconium cyclosilicate dose or placebo once daily, and patients who had been receiving placebo were re-randomized to receive sodium zirconium cyclosilicate 1.25 or 2.5 g once daily. The 5- and 10-g once-daily dosages of sodium zirconium cyclosilicate were substantially more effective than placebo in maintaining normokalemia.

The second study (Hyperkalemia Randomized Intervention Multidose ZS-9 Maintenance Study; HARMONIZE) consisted of an acute open-label treatment phase followed by a 1-month randomized, double-blind, placebo-controlled withdrawal phase. In the open-label phase, 258 adults with hyperkalemia (mean baseline serum potassium concentration 5.6 mEq/L, range: 5.1–7.4 mEq/L) received 10 g of sodium zirconium cyclosilicate 3 times daily for 48 hours; the absolute mean reduction in serum potassium concentration during this period was 1.1 mEq/L. At the end of the open-label treatment period, 92% of the patients achieved normokalemia and were subsequently randomized to receive sodium zirconium cyclosilicate (5, 10, or 15 g) or placebo once daily for 28 days in the double-blind withdrawal portion of the study. Dosage reductions were permitted for patients with serum potassium concentrations between 3 and 3.4 mEq/L. The primary efficacy end point was the mean serum potassium concentration during days 8–29. Serum potassium concentrations were maintained in the normal range with all dosages of sodium zirconium cyclosilicate compared with placebo; the mean serum potassium concentration in patients receiving 5, 10, or 15 g of sodium zirconium cyclosilicate daily was 4.8, 4.5, or 4.4 mEq/L, respectively, compared with a mean serum potassium concentration of 5.1 mEq/L in the placebo group. More patients receiving sodium zirconium cyclosilicate (approximately 80–94%) had mean serum potassium concentrations in the normal range compared with patients receiving placebo (46%). In a subgroup analysis of patients with heart failure, mean serum potassium concentrations achieved with sodium zirconium cyclosilicate were comparable to those observed in the overall study population despite continued renin-angiotensin-aldosterone system inhibitor use in 60% of the patients. Patients who completed the HARMONIZE study had the option to continue treatment with sodium zirconium cyclosilicate in an open-label extension study for up to 11 months; the drug effectively maintained mean serum potassium concentrations within the normal range during continued therapy.

The third study evaluated long-term (12-month) efficacy and safety of sodium zirconium cyclosilicate in 751 adults with hyperkalemia (mean baseline serum potassium concentration 5.6 mEq/L). In the acute treatment phase, patients received 10 g of sodium zirconium cyclosilicate 3 times daily for 24–72 hours depending on their baseline potassium concentration. Approximately 99% of the patients achieved normokalemia within 72 hours and were entered into the maintenance phase. In the maintenance phase, patients received an initial sodium zirconium cyclosilicate dosage of 5 g once daily; dosage was subsequently adjusted within the range of 5 g every other day to 15 g once daily based on serum potassium concentrations, and therapy was continued for up to 12 months. The treatment effect of sodium zirconium cyclosilicate on serum potassium concentrations was maintained with continued therapy.

Efficacy of sodium zirconium cyclosilicate generally was consistent among various subgroups of patients that were evaluated in these studies, including patients with chronic kidney disease, heart failure, diabetes mellitus, and those receiving renin-angiotensin-aldosterone system inhibitor therapy. In addition, subgroup analysis of patients with severe hyperkalemia (serum potassium concentration of at least 6 mEq/L) indicated that the drug rapidly and substantially reduced serum potassium concentrations as early as 1 hour after administration of a single 10-g dose. The median time to serum potassium concentration less than 6 mEq/L was 1.07 hours and the median time to serum potassium concentration of 5.5 mEq/L or less was 4 hours in these patients.

Dosage and Administration

■ **Reconstitution and Administration** Sodium zirconium cyclosilicate is administered orally as a suspension.

The suspension generally should be administered at least 2 hours before or 2 hours after other oral drugs. (See Drug Interactions: Drugs that Exhibit pH-dependent Solubility.)

Sodium zirconium cyclosilicate powder should be mixed with water immediately prior to administration to form an oral suspension. To reconstitute the powder, the entire contents of the packet(s) containing sodium zirconium cyclosilicate should be emptied into a glass containing approximately 45 mL of water, or more if desired. The mixture should be stirred thoroughly and administered immediately. If any powder remains in the glass after initial administration, more water should be added and the mixture should be stirred and then administered immediately; this procedure should be repeated, as needed, until the entire dose is administered.

■ **Dosage** The recommended adult dosage of sodium zirconium cyclosilicate for the initial treatment of hyperkalemia is 10 g 3 times daily for up to 48 hours.

For continued maintenance treatment of hyperkalemia, the recommended adult dosage of sodium zirconium cyclosilicate is 10 g once daily. Serum potassium concentrations should be monitored and dosage should be adjusted accordingly. Dosage may be increased (in 5-g increments at intervals of 1 week or longer) or decreased, or therapy may be discontinued based on the patient's serum potassium concentration and desired target range. The recommended maintenance dosage range of sodium zirconium cyclosilicate is 5 g every other day to 15 g once daily.

■ **Special Populations** The manufacturer makes no specific dosage recommendations for geriatric patients or patients with hepatic or renal impairment.

Cautions

■ **Contraindications** The manufacturer states that there are no known contraindications to the use of sodium zirconium cyclosilicate.

■ **Warnings/Precautions** ***Worsening of GI Motility Disorders*** Sodium zirconium cyclosilicate has not been studied in patients with severe constipation, bowel obstruction, or fecal impaction, including abnormal post-operative bowel motility disorders. Use of sodium zirconium cyclosilicate should be avoided in such patients because the drug may not be effective and may worsen GI conditions.

Edema Each 5-g dose of sodium zirconium cyclosilicate contains approximately 400 mg of sodium; therefore, edema can occur if sodium is absorbed from the preparation. In clinical trials, edema was generally mild to moderate in severity and was more commonly observed in patients treated with higher dosages of sodium zirconium cyclosilicate (i.e., 15 g once daily). In placebo-controlled trials of 28 days' duration, edema was reported in 4.4, 5.9, or 16.1% of patients receiving sodium zirconium cyclosilicate 5, 10, or 15 g daily, respectively, compared with 2.4% of those receiving placebo. In longer-term, uncontrolled trials in which most patients were maintained on dosages less than 15 g once daily, edema was reported in 8–11% of patients.

Patients receiving sodium zirconium cyclosilicate, especially those who should restrict their sodium intake or have conditions predisposing them to fluid overload (e.g., heart failure, renal disease), should be monitored for signs of edema. Patients should be advised to reduce dietary sodium intake, and dosage of concomitant diuretics should be increased as needed.

Specific Populations **Pregnancy.** Because sodium zirconium cyclosilicate is not absorbed systemically following oral administration, use of the drug during pregnancy is not expected to result in fetal exposure.

Lactation. Breast-feeding is not expected to result in infant exposure to sodium zirconium cyclosilicate because the drug is not systemically absorbed following oral administration.

Pediatric Use. Safety and efficacy of sodium zirconium cyclosilicate have not been established in pediatric patients.

Geriatric Use. In clinical studies of sodium zirconium cyclosilicate, 58% of patients receiving the drug were 65 years of age or older and 25% were 75 years of age or older. No overall differences were observed between geriatric patients and younger adults.

Renal Impairment. Approximately 60–68% of patients in clinical studies of sodium zirconium cyclosilicate had chronic kidney disease. Patients with renal disease are prone to fluid overload and may be at greater risk of edema during therapy with the drug. (See Edema under Cautions: Warnings/Precautions.)

■ **Common Adverse Effects** Adverse effects reported in 4% or more of patients receiving sodium zirconium cyclosilicate in clinical studies include edema and hypokalemia.

Drug Interactions

■ **Drugs that Exhibit pH-dependent Solubility** Sodium zirconium cyclosilicate can cause transient increases in gastric pH and affect the solubility (and consequent bioavailability) of certain pH-dependent drugs. Increased plasma concentrations of weakly acidic drugs (e.g., atorvastatin, furosemide, warfarin) and decreased plasma concentrations of weakly basic drugs (e.g., dabigatran) have been observed following concomitant administration with sodium zirconium cyclosilicate. Because such interactions can potentially affect many drugs, the manufacturer states that administration of sodium zirconium cyclosilicate generally should be separated (by at least 2 hours) from the administration of other oral drugs unless it has been determined that the other drug does *not* exhibit pH-dependent solubility. (See Advice to Patients.)

■ **Drugs that Inhibit the Renin-angiotensin-aldosterone System** Concomitant use of sodium zirconium cyclosilicate and drugs that inhibit the renin-angiotensin-aldosterone system did not alter the pharmacokinetics of the renin-angiotensin-aldosterone system inhibitor.

No interaction was observed in vitro between sodium zirconium cyclosilicate and captopril, lisinopril, or quinapril.

Although an interaction was observed in vitro, concomitant use of sodium zirconium cyclosilicate and losartan in healthy volunteers did not result in any changes in losartan exposure.

■ **Allopurinol** No interaction was observed in vitro between sodium zirconium cyclosilicate and allopurinol.

■ **Amlodipine** Concomitant use of amlodipine and sodium zirconium cyclosilicate did not substantially alter peak plasma concentrations and area under the plasma concentration-time curve (AUC) of amlodipine.

■ **Anticoagulants** ***Apixaban*** No interaction was observed in vitro between sodium zirconium cyclosilicate and apixaban.

Dabigatran Concomitant use of dabigatran, a weakly basic drug, and sodium zirconium cyclosilicate in healthy volunteers decreased peak plasma concentrations and AUC of dabigatran, likely due to the effect of sodium zirconium cyclosilicate on gastric pH and the pH-dependent solubility of dabigatran. (See Drug Interactions: Drugs that Exhibit pH-dependent Solubility.)

Warfarin Concomitant use of warfarin, a weakly acidic drug, and sodium zirconium cyclosilicate in healthy volunteers increased peak plasma concentrations of *R*- and *S*-warfarin by about 38%, likely due to the effect of sodium zirconium cyclosilicate on gastric pH and the pH-dependent solubility of warfarin. (See Drug Interactions: Drugs that Exhibit pH-dependent Solubility.)

■ **Antidiabetic Agents** ***Glipizide*** Although an interaction was observed in vitro, concomitant use of glipizide and sodium zirconium cyclosilicate in healthy volunteers did not result in any changes in glipizide exposure.

Metformin No interaction was observed in vitro between sodium zirconium cyclosilicate and metformin.

■ **Antiplatelet Agents** ***Aspirin*** No interaction was observed in vitro between sodium zirconium cyclosilicate and aspirin.

Clopidogrel Concomitant use of clopidogrel and sodium zirconium cyclosilicate in healthy volunteers increased systemic exposure of clopidogrel but did not substantially alter peak plasma concentrations of the drug.

Ticagrelor No interaction was observed in vitro between sodium zirconium cyclosilicate and ticagrelor.

■ **Atorvastatin** Concomitant use of atorvastatin, a weakly acidic drug, and sodium zirconium cyclosilicate in healthy volunteers increased peak plasma concentrations of atorvastatin by 69%, likely due to the effect of sodium zirconium cyclosilicate on gastric pH and the pH-dependent solubility of atorvastatin. (See Drug Interactions: Drugs that Exhibit pH-dependent Solubility.)

■ **Cyclosporine** No interaction was observed in vitro between sodium zirconium cyclosilicate and cyclosporine.

■ **Digoxin** No interaction was observed in vitro between sodium zirconium cyclosilicate and digoxin.

■ **Diuretics** ***Furosemide*** Concomitant use of furosemide, a weakly acidic drug, and sodium zirconium cyclosilicate in healthy volunteers increased peak plasma concentrations of furosemide by 66%, likely due to the effect of sodium zirconium cyclosilicate on gastric pH and the pH-dependent solubility of furosemide. (See Drug Interactions: Drugs that Exhibit pH-dependent Solubility.)

Spironolactone No interaction was observed in vitro between sodium zirconium cyclosilicate and spironolactone.

■ **Ethinyl Estradiol** No interaction was observed in vitro between sodium zirconium cyclosilicate and ethinyl estradiol.

■ **Levothyroxine** Although an interaction was observed in vitro, concomitant use of levothyroxine and sodium zirconium cyclosilicate in healthy volunteers did not result in any changes in levothyroxine exposure.

■ **Lithium** Concomitant use of lithium and sodium zirconium cyclosilicate decreased the potassium exchange capacity of sodium zirconium cyclosilicate by 12%. This interaction was attributed to the similarity in size between lithium and potassium ions.

■ **Magnesium** No interaction was observed in vitro between sodium zirconium cyclosilicate and magnesium.

■ **Phenytoin** No interaction was observed in vitro between sodium zirconium cyclosilicate and phenytoin.

■ **Prednisone** No interaction was observed in vitro between sodium zirconium cyclosilicate and prednisone.

■ **Propranolol** No interaction was observed in vitro between sodium zirconium cyclosilicate and propranolol.

Description

Sodium zirconium cyclosilicate is a highly selective inorganic cation-exchange crystalline compound that preferentially captures potassium in exchange for hydrogen (i.e., protons) and sodium. Sodium zirconium cyclosilicate binds potassium throughout the intestinal tract (including potassium in food), reducing the concentration of free potassium in the GI lumen, increasing fecal potassium excretion, and consequently reducing serum potassium concentrations. The drug's high specificity for potassium has been attributed to the chemical composition and diameter of the micropores contained in the zirconium silicate crystal structure, which mimic the action of physiologic potassium channels. The potassium-binding capacity of sodium zirconium cyclosilicate is 9.3 times that of sodium polystyrene sulfonate. In vitro, sodium zirconium cyclosilicate has a high affinity for potassium ions, even in the presence of other cations (e.g., calcium, magnesium). Sodium zirconium cyclosilicate is more than 25 times more selective for potassium than for calcium and magnesium. Compared with nonselective organic exchange resins that exert their function in the colon, the stable crystal structure of sodium zirconium cyclosilicate allows for binding of potassium throughout the entire lumen of the GI tract, including the acidic conditions of the duodenum. Sodium zirconium cyclosilicate is insoluble and does not absorb water within the GI tract.

Pharmacodynamic studies of sodium zirconium cyclosilicate have demonstrated efficient uptake and removal of potassium ions. In simulations performed in intestinal fluid, initial rapid uptake of potassium occurred within 5 minutes of administration, followed by a slower re-equilibration phase over a period of 20–100 minutes depending on the pH of the intestinal fluid and potassium concentration. When administered at dosages of 5 or 10 g daily for 4 days in healthy individuals, sodium zirconium cyclosilicate produced dose-dependent increases in fecal potassium excretion and corresponding decreases in urinary potassium excretion and serum potassium concentrations. The potassium-lowering effect of sodium zirconium cyclosilicate is rapid in patients with hyperkalemia; in patients receiving a dosage of 10 g 3 times daily for up to 48 hours, reductions in serum potassium concentration were observed within 1 hour after administration of the first dose and continued to decline over the 48-hour treatment period. The degree of reduction was greater in patients with higher potassium concentrations at baseline. Serum potassium concentrations increased in patients who did not continue maintenance treatment. Sodium zirconium cyclosilicate causes mild, dose-dependent increases in serum bicarbonate concentrations. Mild increases in urinary pH and reductions in blood urea nitrogen (BUN) also have been observed, which have been attributed to the binding of ammonium to sodium zirconium cyclosilicate. The clinical importance of these physiologic effects is not known.

Sodium zirconium cyclosilicate is neither systemically absorbed nor metabolized; in vivo mass balance studies demonstrated 99% fecal recovery of the drug in rats.

Advice to Patients

Importance of instructing patients regarding proper preparation and administration of sodium zirconium cyclosilicate, including the importance of taking the full dose.

Importance of informing patients who are taking other oral drugs to administer these drugs at least 2 hours before or 2 hours after administration of sodium zirconium cyclosilicate.

Risk of edema. Importance of advising patients that reduced dietary sodium intake may be required.

Importance of women informing clinicians if they are or plan to become pregnant or plan to breast-feed.

Importance of informing clinicians of existing or contemplated concomitant therapy, including prescription and OTC drugs, as well as any concomitant illnesses.

Importance of informing patients of other important precautionary information. (See Cautions.)

Overview® (see Users Guide). For additional information on this drug until a more detailed monograph is developed and published, the manufacturer's labeling should be consulted. It is *essential* that the manufacturer's labeling be consulted for more detailed information on usual cautions, precautions, contraindications, potential drug interactions, laboratory test interferences, and acute toxicity.

Preparations

Excipients in commercially available drug preparations may have clinically important effects in some individuals; consult specific product labeling for details.

Sodium Zirconium Cyclosilicate

Oral		
Powder, for suspension	5 g per packet	Lokelma®, AstraZeneca
	10 g per packet	Lokelma®, AstraZeneca

DIURETICS 40:28

LOOP DIURETICS 40:28.08

Bumetanide

■ Bumetanide is a sulfonamide loop-type diuretic and antihypertensive agent.

Uses

■ **Edema** Bumetanide is used for the management of edema associated with heart failure or hepatic or renal disease (including nephrotic syndrome). The drug may be effective in some patients whose condition is unresponsive or refractory to other diuretics. In a limited number of patients, approximately 60% of those with edema refractory to other diuretic therapy showed an improved diuretic response with bumetanide. Patients who had received 80–160 mg of furosemide daily with little or no diuretic response showed a marked diuresis with 2–6 mg of bumetanide daily; however, in some of these patients, improvement observed during initial therapy did not continue during maintenance therapy with bumetanide. Further study is needed to determine the role of bumetanide in the management of edema refractory to other diuretics.

Careful etiologic diagnosis should precede the use of any diuretic. Because the potent diuretic effect of loop diuretics may result in severe electrolyte imbalance and excessive fluid loss, hospitalization of the patient during initiation of therapy is advisable, especially for patients with hepatic cirrhosis and ascites or chronic renal failure. In prolonged diuretic therapy, intermittent use of the loop diuretics for only a few days each week may be advisable.

Heart Failure Bumetanide is effective for the short- and long-term management of edema associated with heart failure. In addition to decreasing edema, the drug relieves other signs and symptoms of heart failure such as dyspnea, rales, and hepatomegaly. Bumetanide appears to be as effective as furosemide in reducing edema, body weight, abdominal girth, rales, hepatomegaly, blood pressure, and heart rate in patients with heart failure.

Most experts state that all patients with symptomatic heart failure who have evidence for, or a history of, fluid retention generally should receive diuretic therapy in conjunction with moderate sodium restriction, an agent to inhibit the renin-angiotensin-aldosterone-aldosterone (RAA) system (e.g., angiotensin-converting enzyme [ACE] inhibitor, angiotensin II receptor antagonist, angiotensin receptor-neprilysin inhibitor [ARNI]), a β-adrenergic blocking agent (β-blocker), and in selected patients, an aldosterone antagonist. Some experts state that because of limited and inconsistent data, it is difficult to make precise recommendations regarding daily sodium intake and whether it should vary with respect to the type of heart failure (e.g., reduced versus preserved ejection fraction), disease severity (e.g., New York Heart Association [NYHA] class), heart failure-related comorbidities (e.g., renal dysfunction), or other patient characteristics (e.g., age, race). The American College of Cardiology Foundation (ACCF) and American Heart Association (AHA) state that limiting sodium intake to 1.5 g daily in patients with ACCF/AHA stage A or B heart failure may be reasonable. While data currently are lacking to support recommendation of a specific level of sodium intake in patients with ACCF/AHA stage C or D heart failure, ACCF and AHA state that limiting sodium intake to some degree (e.g., less than 3 g daily) in such patients may be considered for symptom improvement. Diuretics play a key role in the management of heart failure because they produce symptomatic benefits more rapidly than any other drugs, relieving pulmonary and peripheral edema within hours or days compared with weeks or months for cardiac glycosides, ACE inhibitors, or β-blockers. However, since there are no long-term studies of diuretic therapy in patients with heart failure, the effects of diuretics on morbidity and mortality in such patients are not known. Although there are patients with heart failure who do not exhibit fluid retention in the absence of diuretic therapy and even may develop severe volume depletion with low doses of diuretics, such patients are rare and the unique pathophysiologic mechanisms regulating their fluid and electrolyte balance have not been elucidated.

Most experts state that loop diuretics (e.g., bumetanide, ethacrynic acid, furosemide, torsemide) are the diuretics of choice for most patients with heart failure. However, thiazides may be preferred in some patients with concomitant hypertension because of their sustained antihypertensive effects. If resistance to diuretics occurs, IV administration of a diuretic or concomitant use of 2 or more diuretics (e.g., a loop diuretic and metolazone, a loop diuretic and a thiazide diuretic) may be necessary; alternatively, short-term administration of a drug that increases blood flow (e.g., a positive inotropic agent such as dopamine) may be necessary. ACCF and AHA state that IV loop diuretics should be administered promptly to all hospitalized heart failure patients with substantial fluid overload to reduce morbidity. In addition, ACCF and AHA state that low-dose dopamine infusions may be considered in combination with loop diuretics to augment diuresis and preserve renal function and renal blood flow in patients with acute decompensated heart failure, although data are conflicting and additional study and experience are needed. For additional information, see Heart Failure under Uses: Edema, in the Thiazides General Statement 40:28.20.

Hepatic Disease Bumetanide is used for the short- and long-term management of edema and ascites associated with hepatic disease (e.g., cirrhosis). Short-term administration of 2–4 mg of bumetanide daily or long-term administration of up to 6 mg daily has produced appreciable diuretic and natriuretic effects without substantial serum electrolyte disturbance in some patients with this condition. Patients with hepatic ascites reportedly have responded to an initial bumetanide dosage of 1 mg daily with weight loss averaging about 0.6 kg daily and a marked increase in urinary volume and natriuresis. The major complications observed during bumetanide therapy in these patients included hypokalemia and hyponatremia; however, electrolyte disturbances are commonly observed in patients with severe hepatic disease who are receiving diuretic therapy. Some patients developed encephalopathy during bumetanide administration. (See Cautions: Hepatic Effects.)

Bumetanide appears to be as effective as furosemide in reducing body weight and in causing diuresis and increased urinary excretion of sodium, potassium, and chloride in patients with hepatic cirrhosis and ascites. Following IV administration, single 0.5-mg doses of bumetanide were as effective as 20-mg doses of furosemide in patients with refractory ascites.

In most clinical studies in patients with hepatic cirrhosis and ascites, patients received concomitant therapy with bumetanide and potassium salts or potassium-sparing diuretics to prevent hypokalemia.

Renal Disease Bumetanide is used for the management of edema in patients with impaired renal function. In patients with severe renal impairment (i.e., GFR less than 10 mL/minute), high dosages of the drug may be needed to produce an adequate diuretic response. (See Dosage in Renal and Hepatic Impairment in Dosage and Administration.)

Bumetanide (1–10 mg orally daily) appears to be as effective as furosemide (40–400 mg orally daily) in reducing edema, body weight, and abdominal girth in patients with edema secondary to renal disease. However, in one study, substantial reductions in body weight, edema, and mean arterial pressure were observed in patients with severe renal impairment who received oral bumetanide dosages of 1–18 mg daily but not in those who received oral furosemide dosages of 20–480 mg daily.

Oral bumetanide dosages of 2–6 mg daily appear to be as effective as oral furosemide dosages of 40–160 mg daily in reducing edema in patients with nephrotic syndrome; however, in some patients with nephrotic syndrome and moderately impaired renal function (i.e., creatinine clearance of 4–34 mL/minute), a decreased response compared with that of patients with nephrotic syndrome and normal renal function has been reported.

Other Edematous Conditions Bumetanide has been used for the management of postoperative† or premenstrual edema† and edema associated with disseminated carcinoma†.

■ **Hypertension** Bumetanide has been used alone or in combination with other classes of antihypertensive agents for the management of hypertension†, especially when complicated by heart failure, acute pulmonary edema, or renal disease. Because of established clinical benefits (e.g., reductions in overall mortality and in adverse cardiovascular, cerebrovascular, and renal outcomes), current evidence-based practice guidelines for the management of hypertension in adults generally recommend the use of drugs from 4 classes of antihypertensive agents (ACE inhibitors, angiotensin II receptor antagonists, calcium-channel blockers, and thiazide diuretics). (See Uses: Hypertension in Adults, in the Thiazides General Statement 40:28.20.) However, some experts state that loop diuretics (e.g., furosemide, bumetanide, torsemide) are preferred over thiazides in patients with moderate to severe chronic kidney disease (CKD) or symptomatic heart failure. Loop diuretics may be particularly useful in patients with heart failure and reduced left ventricular ejection fraction (LVEF) who have evidence of fluid retention; however, some experts state that thiazide diuretics my be considered in hypertensive patients with heart failure and mild fluid retention because of their more persistent antihypertensive effect.

For further information on the role of diuretics in antihypertensive drug therapy and information on overall principles and expert recommendations for treatment of hypertension, see Uses: Hypertension in Adults and also see Uses: Hypertension in Pediatric Patients, in the Thiazides General Statement 40:28.20.

■ **Other Uses** Bumetanide has been used to enhance the elimination of drugs or toxic substances following intoxication. Like furosemide, bumetanide has been used as an adjunct in forced alkaline diuresis to enhance salicylate elimination following acute aspirin intoxication. (See Measures to Enhance Salicylate Elimination in Acute Toxicity: Treatment, in the Salicylates General Statement 28:08.04.24.) IV bumetanide and IV sodium bicarbonate have reportedly produced a more rapid decrease in blood salicylate concentration compared with parenteral fluid therapy alone.

Dosage and Administration

■ **Administration** ***Oral Administration*** Bumetanide is usually administered orally as a single daily dose in the morning. Bumetanide may also be given by intermittent administration on alternate days or on 3 or 4 consecutive days alternating with drug-free periods of 1 or 2 days. For optimum therapeutic effect in some patients, it may be necessary to administer bumetanide in 2 divided doses in the morning and evening. Administration of bumetanide in 2 divided doses daily has been reported to be more effective in increasing urinary sodium output and urinary volume than administration of the drug as a single daily dose, and the evening dose appeared to have a greater diuretic effect than the morning dose. Therefore, some clinicians suggest that, when the drug is administered once daily, it may be preferable to administer the dose in the evening. Further study is needed to determine the optimum dosage schedule for oral bumetanide administration.

Parenteral Administration When the patient is unable to take oral medication or GI absorption is impaired, bumetanide may be administered by IM or IV injection or by IV infusion. Parenteral administration of bumetanide should be replaced by oral therapy as soon as possible. Bumetanide injection should be inspected visually for particulate matter and discoloration prior to administration.

For IV injection, bumetanide should be given slowly over a period of 1–2 minutes. For IV infusion, bumetanide injection should be diluted in 5% dextrose, 0.9% sodium chloride, or lactated Ringer's injection. IV infusions should be freshly prepared and used within 24 hours.

■ **Dosage** Dosage of bumetanide should be adjusted according to individual requirements and response. Since the diuretic response following oral or parenteral administration is similar, bumetanide dosage is identical for oral, IV, or IM administration. For the management of fluid retention (e.g., edema) associated with heart failure, experts state that diuretics should be administered at a dosage sufficient to achieve optimal volume status and relieve congestion without inducing an excessively rapid reduction in intravascular volume, which could result in hypotension, renal dysfunction, or both. The manufacturer states that, in furosemide-allergic patients, bumetanide may be substituted for furosemide at approximately a 1:40 ratio since cross-sensitivity between the drugs does not appear to occur; however, some clinicians question the safety of bumetanide administration in furosemide-sensitive patients. (See Cautions: Precautions and Contraindications.)

Edema **Oral Dosage.** For the management of edema, the usual initial adult oral dosage of bumetanide recommended by the manufacturers is 0.5–2 mg daily. If the diuretic response to an initial dose of the drug is inadequate, repeated doses may be given at 4- to 5-hour intervals until the desired response is obtained or a maximum dosage of 10 mg daily is reached. For maintenance therapy, the effective dose of bumetanide may be administered intermittently. For the management of fluid retention (e.g., edema) associated with heart failure, some experts recommend initiating bumetanide at a low dosage (e.g., 0.5–1 mg once or twice daily) and increasing the dosage (maximum of 10 mg daily) until urine output increases and weight decreases, generally by 0.5–1 kg daily. (See Dosage and Administration: Administration.)

Parenteral Dosage. The usual initial adult IV or IM dose of bumetanide for the management of edema is 0.5–1 mg. In patients with inadequate response to the initial parenteral dose of bumetanide, repeated doses may be given at 2- to 3-hour intervals until the desired diuretic response is obtained or a maximum dosage of 10 mg daily is reached.

Hypertension **Oral Dosage.** For the management of hypertension† in adults, the usual oral dosage of bumetanide is 0.5–2 mg daily, administered in 2 divided doses.

Monitoring and Blood Pressure Treatment Goals. The patient's renal function and electrolytes should be assessed 2–4 weeks after initiation of diuretic therapy. Blood pressure should be monitored regularly (i.e., monthly) during therapy and dosage of the antihypertensive drug adjusted until blood pressure is controlled. If an adequate blood pressure response is not achieved, the dosage may be increased or another antihypertensive agent with demonstrated benefit and preferably with a complementary mechanism of action (e.g., angiotensin-converting enzyme [ACE] inhibitor, angiotensin II receptor antagonist, calcium-channel blocker) may be added; if target blood pressure is still not achieved, a third drug may be added. (See Uses: Hypertension in Adults, in the Thiazides General Statement 40:28.20.) In patients who develop unacceptable adverse effects with bumetanide, the drug should be discontinued and another antihypertensive agent from a different pharmacologic class should be initiated.

The goal of hypertension management and prevention is to achieve and maintain optimal control of blood pressure. However, the optimum blood pressure threshold for initiating antihypertensive drug therapy and specific treatment goals remain controversial. A 2017 multidisciplinary hypertension guideline from the American College of Cardiology (ACC), American Heart Association (AHA), and a number of other professional organizations generally recommends a blood pressure goal of less than 130/80 mm Hg in all adults, regardless of comorbidities or level of atherosclerotic cardiovascular disease (ASCVD) risk. Many patients will require at least 2 drugs from different pharmacologic classes to achieve this blood pressure goal; the potential benefits of hypertension management and drug cost, adverse effects, and risks associated with the use of multiple antihypertensive drugs also should be considered when deciding a patient's blood pressure treatment goal.

For additional information on target levels of blood pressure and on monitoring therapy in the management of hypertension, see Blood Pressure Monitoring and Treatment Goals under Dosage: Hypertension, in Dosage and Administration in the Thiazides General Statement 40:28.20.

Pediatric Dosage Although the manufacturer states that safety and efficacy have not been established, dosages of 0.015 mg/kg on alternate days to 0.1 mg/kg daily have been used safely and effectively in a limited number of children with heart failure†. For information on overall principles for treatment of hypertension and overall expert recommendations for such disease in pediatric patients, see Uses: Hypertension in Pediatric Patients, in the Thiazides General Statement 40:28.20.

■ **Dosage in Renal and Hepatic Impairment** Although the manufacturer recommends that maximum oral or parenteral dosage of bumetanide not exceed 10 mg daily, oral or IV dosages up to 20 mg daily have been administered to patients with impaired renal function for the management of edema. Single-dose studies have shown that IV doses greater than 2 mg are needed to achieve a diuretic response in patients with creatinine clearances less than 5 mL/minute.

In patients with impaired hepatic function, bumetanide dosage should be kept to a minimum; if bumetanide dosage must be increased in these patients, it should be adjusted carefully.

Cautions

Adverse effects occurring frequently during bumetanide therapy include muscle cramps, dizziness, hypotension, headache, nausea, and encephalopathy; these adverse effects may be related to bumetanide. The manufacturer states that one or more of these adverse effects occurs in 4.1% of bumetanide-treated patients. Laboratory test alterations, including electrolyte, hematologic, renal, and hepatic abnormalities, occur in approximately 49% of patients receiving the drug. Many of the adverse effects associated with bumetanide therapy may be caused by diuresis or the underlying disease being treated.

■ **Fluid, Electrolyte, Cardiovascular, and Renal Effects** Bumetanide may produce profound diuresis resulting in fluid and electrolyte depletion. Fluid and electrolyte depletion is more likely to occur with excessive doses or too frequent administration of the drug or in those with restricted sodium intake.

Too vigorous diuresis may result in profound water loss and dehydration, especially in geriatric patients. The resultant hypovolemia may lead to circulatory collapse or thromboembolic episodes such as vascular thromboses and/or emboli. Pronounced reductions in plasma volume associated with rapid or excessive diuresis may also result in an abrupt fall in glomerular filtration rate, as evidenced by increased BUN and serum creatinine concentration. Hypotension reportedly occurs in less than 1% of patients receiving bumetanide. Orthostatic hypotension has occurred during concomitant therapy with other hypotensive agents.

Hypokalemia and hypochloremia reportedly occur in about 15% of patients receiving bumetanide and hyponatremia occurs in about 10% of patients. Hypophosphatemia and hypocalcemia have been reported less frequently. Potassium depletion is particularly likely to occur in patients with hyperaldosteronism with normal renal function, hepatic cirrhosis and ascites, potassium-losing renal diseases, or certain diarrheal conditions and may require particular attention in patients with heart failure receiving cardiac glycosides and diuretics, those with a history of ventricular arrhythmias, and those with other conditions in which hypokalemia is considered to represent a risk. Prevention of hypokalemia is particularly important in these patients. Diuretic-induced hypokalemia and hypochloremia may result in metabolic alkalosis, especially in patients with other losses of potassium and chloride secondary to vomiting, diarrhea, GI drainage, excessive sweating, paracentesis, or potassium-losing renal diseases. Metabolic alkalosis, with increased serum bicarbonate concentration and changes in total CO_2 content, has been reported in patients receiving bumetanide. Sudden changes in electrolyte balance may precipitate hepatic encephalopathy and coma in patients with hepatic cirrhosis and ascites. Supplemental therapy with potassium chloride or potassium-sparing diuretics (e.g., spironolactone) may be necessary for the prevention of hypokalemia and/or metabolic alkalosis in some patients. Diuretics also have shown to increase urinary excretion of magnesium, which may result in hypomagnesemia.

Other adverse cardiovascular effects of bumetanide include ECG changes and chest pain.

Hyperuricemia has been reported in about 20% of patients receiving bumetanide; however, most reported cases to date have been asymptomatic. Gouty arthritis has occurred in at least one patient receiving the drug. Serum uric acid concentrations have returned to pretreatment levels in some patients during continued therapy with the drug. Serum uric acid concentrations have increased to more than 12 mg/dL in a few patients receiving bumetanide but have returned to within normal limits following discontinuance of the drug.

Reversible azotemia and increased serum creatinine concentration have been reported in 10% or less of bumetanide-treated patients. These adverse renal effects are especially likely to occur in patients with impaired renal function and appear to be associated with dehydration. Decreased creatinine clearance reportedly has been observed in less than 1% of patients receiving the drug. Bumetanide-induced renal failure has occurred rarely. Although acute interstitial nephritis has been reported rarely with furosemide, there are no reports to date of this adverse renal effect with bumetanide.

■ **Otic Effects** Ototoxicity has been reported in cats, dogs, and guinea pigs receiving bumetanide. On a weight basis, the ototoxic potential of bumetanide in these animals was 5–6 times greater than that of furosemide; however, the relative ototoxic potential of bumetanide at equivalent diuretic dosages was 0.11–0.16 times that of furosemide, since bumetanide has about 40–60 times the diuretic potency of furosemide. The likelihood of serum bumetanide concentrations achieving a level necessary to produce ototoxicity in humans is small; however, the possibility of bumetanide-induced ototoxicity must be considered following IV administration of the drug, especially at high dosages, after too rapid administration, in patients with impaired renal function, and/or in patients receiving other ototoxic drugs (e.g., aminoglycosides). (See Drug Interactions: Ototoxic Drugs.) Impaired hearing and otic discomfort have reportedly occurred rarely in patients receiving bumetanide. Combined data from comparative studies indicate that the frequency of drug-related hearing loss based on audiometric testing was 1.1% in patients receiving oral bumetanide dosages of 0.5–18 mg daily and 6.4% in patients receiving oral furosemide dosages of 20–640 mg daily. In addition, there are reports of furosemide-induced ototoxicity that improved following substitution of bumetanide therapy.

■ **Metabolic Effects** Although changes in plasma insulin, glucagon, or growth hormone concentration or in glucose tolerance generally have not been observed to date in patients receiving bumetanide, the possibility that the drug may adversely affect glucose metabolism should be considered. Hyperglycemia has reportedly occurred in about 7% of patients receiving the drug. Although comparative differences have not been fully determined, the frequency of bumetanide-induced hyperglycemia has been reported to be lower than that of furosemide. Bumetanide has also been associated with glycosuria and proteinuria in less than 1% of patients. The drug has been associated with decreased glucose tolerance without glycosuria in at least one patient. In general, diabetic control has not been adversely affected in patients with diabetes mellitus who were receiving bumetanide for the management of edema.

Diuretics, including bumetanide, can increase serum total cholesterol concentrations in some patients; increases in low-density lipoprotein cholesterol and/or very low-density lipoprotein cholesterol subfractions appear to be principally responsible for these increases.

■ **Musculoskeletal Effects** Adverse musculoskeletal effects reportedly occurring in about 1% or less of patients receiving bumetanide include muscle cramps, arthritic pain, musculoskeletal pain, muscle stiffness and tenderness, and asterixis. Musculoskeletal pain (sometimes severe) generally develops about 4 hours following oral administration or 1–2 hours following IV administration of the drug and persists for about 6–12 hours. In most patients, musculoskeletal pain is more severe in the extremities. The development of musculoskeletal pain appears to be a dose-related effect but varies among individuals. Some clinicians suggest that bumetanide-induced musculoskeletal pain may be related to electrolyte disturbances.

■ **Nervous System Effects** Adverse nervous system effects occurring in 1% or less of patients receiving bumetanide include dizziness, headache, weakness, vertigo, and fatigue.

■ **Hepatic Effects** Adverse hepatic effects of bumetanide include alteration of liver function test results and encephalopathy (in patients with preexisting hepatic disease). Increased total serum bilirubin, serum LDH, AST (SGOT), ALT (SGPT), or alkaline phosphatase concentration and increased or decreased cholesterol concentration have occurred in 1% or less of patients receiving bumetanide. Although these adverse hepatic effects have been associated with bumetanide, a causal relationship to the drug has not been established.

■ **Hematologic Effects** Adverse hematologic effects of bumetanide reportedly occurring in less than 1% of patients include increased or decreased hemoglobin concentration, prothrombin time, or hematocrit. Thrombocytopenia, increased or decreased leukocyte count, and changes in the differential leukocyte count, including eosinophilia, have occurred rarely. Bumetanide-induced leukopenia and thrombocytopenia have usually been transient and not associated with serious adverse systemic effects; however, one patient developed purpura alone and another developed purpura, epistaxis, and intestinal hemorrhage which proved fatal. Although the development of blood dyscrasias has been associated with bumetanide, a causal relationship to the drug has not been established.

■ **GI Effects** Adverse GI effects reportedly occurring in less than 1% of patients receiving bumetanide include nausea, abdominal pain, vomiting, xerostomia, dyspepsia, diarrhea, and stomach cramps.

■ **Dermatologic Effects** Adverse dermatologic effects reportedly occurring rarely in patients receiving bumetanide include pruritus, urticaria, and rash. The drug has been associated with Stevens-Johnson syndrome in at least one patient; a causal relationship to bumetanide has been suggested since the condition resolved following discontinuance of the drug.

■ **Other Adverse Effects** Premature ejaculation, erectile impotence, and nipple tenderness have occurred rarely in patients receiving bumetanide. Bumetanide has been associated with the development of mammary tenderness or gynecomastia in a few patients; however, a causal relationship to the drug has not been established and some of these patients were receiving concomitant therapy with spironolactone.

Other adverse effects of bumetanide include sweating, hyperventilation, and increased or decreased serum protein concentrations.

■ **Precautions and Contraindications** Bumetanide is a potent diuretic that may produce profound diuresis with fluid and electrolyte depletion, especially when administered at high dosages or for prolonged periods. Patients receiving bumetanide should be carefully observed for signs of electrolyte depletion, especially hypokalemia. Patients should be informed of the signs and symptoms of electrolyte imbalance and instructed to report to their physician if weakness, dizziness, fatigue, faintness, mental confusion, lassitude, muscle cramps, headache, paresthesia, thirst, anorexia, nausea, and/or vomiting occur. Excessive fluid and electrolyte loss may be minimized by monitoring the patient carefully and by initiating therapy with small doses, adjusting dosage carefully, and using an intermittent dosage schedule if possible. Careful monitoring, including hospitalization during initiation of therapy, and dosage adjustment are especially important in patients with hepatic cirrhosis and ascites.

Serum potassium concentration should be measured periodically during therapy with bumetanide. Supplemental therapy with potassium chloride or potassium-sparing diuretics may be used if necessary to prevent or treat hypokalemia and/or metabolic alkalosis. Prevention of hypokalemia is particularly important for patients with heart failure receiving cardiac glycosides and diuretics or for those with hepatic cirrhosis and ascites, hyperaldosteronism with normal renal function, potassium-losing renal diseases, certain diarrheal conditions, or other conditions (e.g., history of ventricular arrhythmias) in which hypokalemia is considered to represent a risk. Periodic determination of other serum electrolyte concentrations is recommended for patients receiving therapy at high dosages or for prolonged periods, especially in those with restricted sodium intake. Administration of bumetanide at high dosages or for prolonged periods may cause profound water loss, electrolyte depletion, dehydration, or hypovolemia and circulatory collapse with the possibility of vascular thrombosis and embolism, especially in geriatric patients. If excessive diuresis and/or electrolyte abnormalities occur, the drug should be withdrawn or dosage reduced until homeostasis is restored. Electrolyte abnormalities should be corrected by appropriate measures.

Bumetanide should be used with caution in patients with hepatic cirrhosis and ascites, since sudden alterations in fluid and electrolyte balance may precipitate hepatic encephalopathy and/or coma. Bumetanide administration in these patients should be initiated at low dosages in a hospital setting with careful monitoring of the patient's fluid and electrolyte balance and clinical status. Supplemental therapy with potassium chloride or potassium-sparing diuretics may be used to prevent hypokalemia and metabolic alkalosis in these patients.

Although changes in plasma insulin, glucagon, or growth hormone concentration or in glucose tolerance generally have not been observed during therapy with bumetanide, the possibility of an adverse effect on glucose metabolism cannot be excluded. Blood glucose concentration should be determined periodically, especially in patients with known or suspected (e.g., marginally impaired glucose tolerance) diabetes mellitus.

Patients receiving bumetanide should be observed carefully for the development of blood dyscrasias (especially thrombocytopenia), liver damage, or idiosyncratic reactions which have been reported occasionally during therapy with the drug.

Although bumetanide's potential for producing ototoxicity is small compared with furosemide, the possibility of bumetanide-induced ototoxicity must be considered following IV administration of the drug, especially at high dosages, after too rapid administration, in patients with impaired renal function, and/or in patients receiving other ototoxic drugs.

Bumetanide should be used with extreme caution, if at all, in patients who are allergic to sulfonamides, since these patients may show hypersensitivity to bumetanide. Although the manufacturer states that bumetanide does not appear to exhibit cross-sensitivity in patients allergic to furosemide, the drugs are structurally similar and some clinicians believe that there is insufficient evidence to support a lack of cross-sensitivity. Bumetanide is contraindicated in patients with known hypersensitivity to the drug.

Bumetanide is contraindicated in patients with anuria. Although bumetanide may be used to produce diuresis in patients with impaired renal function, the drug is contraindicated for further use when marked increases in BUN or serum creatinine concentration or oliguria occur during treatment of progressive renal disease. In patients with hepatic coma or severe electrolyte depletion, bumetanide therapy should not be instituted until the basic condition is improved or corrected.

■ **Pediatric Precautions** Safety and efficacy of bumetanide in children younger than 18 years of age have not been established. Bumetanide has been used effectively as a diuretic for up to 40 weeks in a limited number of infants ranging from 2 weeks to 7 months of age who had congenital heart disease and heart failure†. However, in vitro studies using pooled serum from critically ill neonates have shown substantial displacement of bilirubin from albumin by bumetanide. (See Pharmacokinetics: Distribution.) Therefore, bumetanide should be used with caution in critically ill or jaundiced neonates who are at risk for kernicterus. In addition, the elimination of bumetanide appears to be slower in neonates than in adults, possibly because of immature renal and hepatobiliary functions. (See Pharmacokinetics: Elimination.) For information on overall principles and expert recommendations for treatment of hypertension in pediatric patients, see Uses: Hypertension in Pediatric Patients, in the Thiazides General Statement 40:28.20.

■ **Mutagenicity and Carcinogenicity** It is not known whether bumetanide is mutagenic or carcinogenic in humans. Bumetanide did not produce mutagenic activity in various strains of *Salmonella typhimurium* when tested with or without metabolic activation. Following oral administration of bumetanide, an increased number of mammary tumors was observed in female rats receiving 2000 times the maximum recommended human dosage for 18 months; however, these findings could not be duplicated when the study was repeated with the same dosage.

■ **Pregnancy, Fertility, and Lactation** Limited clinical experience with bumetanide in pregnant women to date has not revealed evidence of harm to the fetus; however, the possibility of adverse fetal effects cannot be excluded. Bumetanide should be used during pregnancy only when the potential benefits justify the possible risks to the fetus.

Although there are no adequate and controlled studies to date in humans, bumetanide has been shown to have a slight embryocidal effect in rats when given at a dosage 3400 times the maximum recommended human dosage; evidence of moderate growth retardation and delayed ossification of sternebrae in fetal offspring and maternal weight loss also occurred. Fetotoxic effects were not observed in rats when bumetanide was administered at 1000–2000 times the maximum recommended human dosage. Reproduction studies in mice using dosages up to 3400 times the maximum recommended human dosage have not revealed evidence of teratogenic or embryocidal effects. Bumetanide was not teratogenic in hamsters following oral administration of 0.5 mg/kg daily (17 times the maximum recommended human dosage) or in mice or rats at IV dosages up to 140 times the maximum recommended human dosage. A dose-related decrease in litter size and increase in fetal resorption rate occurred in rabbits receiving oral dosages of 0.1 and 0.3 mg/kg daily (3.4 and 10 times the maximum recommended human dosage, respectively); a slight embryocidal effect occurred in those receiving 0.1 mg/kg daily, and an increased frequency of delayed ossification of the sternebrae also occurred in those receiving 0.3 mg/kg daily. Adverse fetal effects were not observed in rabbits receiving 0.03 mg/kg daily.

The effect of bumetanide on fertility in humans is not known. Reproduction studies in rats using bumetanide dosages of 10, 30, 60, or 100 mg/kg daily showed a slightly decreased rate of pregnancy; however, the differences were small and not statistically significant.

Since it is not known if bumetanide is distributed into milk, the manufacturer cautions that nursing should not be undertaken in women receiving the drug.

Drug Interactions

■ **Diuretics** Concomitant administration of bumetanide and most other diuretics results in enhanced diuretic and natriuretic effects. Spironolactone, triamterene, or amiloride hydrochloride may reduce the potassium loss resulting from bumetanide therapy; this effect has been used to therapeutic advantage.

■ **Drugs Affected by or Causing Potassium Depletion** In patients receiving a cardiac glycoside (e.g., digoxin), electrolyte disturbances produced by bumetanide (principally hypokalemia but also hypomagnesemia) predispose the patient to digitalis toxicity; possibly fatal cardiac arrhythmias may result. Therefore, it is particularly important that hypokalemia be prevented in patients receiving bumetanide and a cardiac glycoside concomitantly. Periodic electrolyte determinations should be performed in patients receiving a cardiac glycoside and bumetanide, and correction of hypokalemia undertaken if warranted. Bumetanide does not affect serum digoxin concentrations or renal excretion of digoxin when the drugs are used concomitantly.

Like furosemide, bumetanide potentially can cause prolonged neuromuscular blockade in patients receiving nondepolarizing neuromuscular blocking agents (e.g., tubocurarine chloride, gallamine triethiodide [no longer commercially available in the US]), presumably because of potassium depletion or decreased urinary excretion of the muscle relaxant. Although there are no reports to date of prolonged neuromuscular blockade during concomitant administration of bumetanide and nondepolarizing neuromuscular blocking agents, the possibility of this drug interaction should be considered.

Some drugs such as corticosteroids, corticotropin, and amphotericin B also cause potassium loss, and severe potassium depletion may occur when one of these drugs is administered during bumetanide therapy.

■ **Lithium** Renal clearance of lithium is apparently decreased in patients receiving diuretics, and lithium toxicity may result. Bumetanide and lithium should generally not be given together. If concomitant therapy is necessary, serum lithium concentrations should be monitored carefully and dosage adjusted accordingly.

■ **Hypotensive Agents** The antihypertensive effect of hypotensive agents may be enhanced during concomitant bumetanide administration. This effect is usually used to therapeutic advantage; however, orthostatic hypotension may result. Dosage of the hypotensive agent, and possibly both drugs, should be reduced when bumetanide is added to an existing antihypertensive regimen.

■ **Indomethacin** Indomethacin may reduce the diuretic and natriuretic effects of bumetanide. The mechanism(s) of these interactions has not been established but has been attributed to indomethacin-induced inhibition of prostaglandin synthesis which may result in fluid retention and/or changes in vascular resistance. Indomethacin also inhibits the bumetanide-induced increase in plasma renin activity. Although the clinical importance of these interactions has not been determined, the manufacturer states that concomitant therapy with bumetanide and indomethacin is not recommended. However, some clinicians suggest that, if concomitant therapy is necessary, an increase in bumetanide dosage may overcome an indomethacin-induced decrease in diuretic activity.

■ **Probenecid** Probenecid may reduce the diuretic and natriuretic effects of bumetanide. Probenecid may also inhibit the bumetanide-induced increase in plasma renin activity. The mechanism(s) of these interactions does not appear to result from direct inhibition of sodium excretion but probably involves inhibition by probenecid of the renal tubular secretion of bumetanide. Although the clinical importance of these interactions has not been determined, the manufacturer recommends that probenecid not be administered concomitantly with bumetanide.

■ **Ototoxic Drugs** Concomitant parenteral administration of bumetanide and aminoglycoside antibiotics or other ototoxic drugs (e.g., cisplatin) may result in increased risk of ototoxicity, especially in patients with impaired renal function. Although potentiation of aminoglycoside-induced ototoxicity with bumetanide has not been reported to date in humans, permanent changes in cochlear activity have occurred following administration of bumetanide in animals pretreated with kanamycin. Concomitant parenteral administration of bumetanide and aminoglycoside antibiotics should be avoided, except in life-threatening conditions.

■ **Nephrotoxic Drugs** Although there is no clinical experience to date with concomitant administration of bumetanide and nephrotoxic agents, concomitant use of these drugs should be avoided since bumetanide may enhance the nephrotoxic effects.

■ **Anticoagulants** Bumetanide does not appear to affect the plasma prothrombin activity or the metabolism of oral anticoagulants (e.g., warfarin). In 2 studies in healthy individuals, no substantial differences in prothrombin time or in plasma concentration or half-life of warfarin were observed when a single dose of warfarin (40–65 mg) was administered alone or concomitantly with 1 or 2 mg of bumetanide daily.

Acute Toxicity

■ **Pathogenesis** The LD_{50} of bumetanide following IV administration has been reported to be 330 mg/kg in mice and 70 mg/kg in rabbits. The oral LD_{50} of the drug in rabbits has been reported to be 350 mg/kg. However, mice and rats have survived oral doses of 2000 mg/kg in one study and 6000 mg/kg in another study.

■ **Manifestations** Overdosage of bumetanide may result in acute, profound water loss, volume and electrolyte depletion, and hypovolemia and circulatory collapse with a possibility of vascular thrombosis and embolism. Electrolyte depletion may be manifested as weakness, dizziness, mental confusion, anorexia, lethargy, vomiting, and cramps.

Following intraperitoneal administration of 300 mg/kg of bumetanide to mice, ataxia, reduced muscle tone, tremors, and seizures occurred and persisted for 1 day. In dogs receiving 0.5 mg/kg of the drug IV, leg muscle fasciculations, opisthotonos, and trismus occurred and were present from 10 seconds to 2 minutes followed by complete recovery.

■ **Treatment** In acute bumetanide overdose, supportive and symptomatic treatment consisting of fluid and electrolyte replacement should be initiated. Urinary output and serum and urinary electrolyte concentrations should be carefully monitored.

Pharmacology

The pharmacologic effects of bumetanide are similar to those of furosemide.

■ **Renal Effects** Bumetanide acts directly on the ascending limb of the loop of Henle to inhibit sodium and chloride reabsorption. Although the exact mechanism(s) of action has not been established, bumetanide decreases electrolyte reabsorption by inhibiting the active chloride and, possibly, sodium transport systems in the ascending limb of the loop of Henle. Bumetanide may interfere with renal cyclic 3′,5′-adenosine monophosphate (cAMP) activity or with binding of cAMP to renal tissue. Inhibition of cAMP-dependent protein kinase or sodium-potassium adenosine triphosphatase (ATPase), an enzyme with high activity in the ascending limb of the loop of Henle, may be involved. Unlike ethacrynic acid, bumetanide does not bind sulfhydryl groups of renal cellular proteins. Bumetanide also appears to inhibit electrolyte reabsorption in the proximal renal tubule. Since phosphate and bicarbonate reabsorption occur mainly in the proximal tubule, phosphaturia and increased bicarbonate excretion during bumetanide-induced diuresis are indicative of this additional effect. Inhibition of electrolyte reabsorption in the proximal tubule may result from inhibition of sodium phosphate-linked transport, but is apparently not related to inhibition of carbonic anhydrase activity. Bumetanide indirectly increases potassium secretion in the distal renal tubule secondary to an increased sodium load in the tubule; the drug does not appear to have a direct effect on electrolyte reabsorption in the distal tubule. The drug is not an aldosterone antagonist. Although bumetanide reportedly has about 40 times the diuretic activity of furosemide on a weight basis, the relative potency may vary when different dosages and/or routes of administration are compared.

Bumetanide increases urinary excretion of sodium, chloride, potassium, hydrogen, calcium, magnesium, and ammonium; excretion of phosphate and bicarbonate may also be increased. The chloruretic effect of the drug is greater than its natriuretic effect and its effect on urinary calcium and magnesium excretion is less than that on sodium excretion. Although urinary excretion of calcium and magnesium is initially (4–6 hours after administration) increased, retention of these electrolytes subsequently occurs and no substantial net loss of calcium or magnesium is observed over a 24-hour period. Bumetanide-induced increases in urinary excretion of hydrogen and ammonium ions are generally associated with little or no effect on urinary pH; however, in one study, urinary pH decreased from 6.1 to 5.1 following administration of the drug. The drug decreases free water clearance in humans during hydration and tubular free water reabsorption during hydropenia. The decrease in free water clearance results from inhibition of electrolyte reabsorption and active transport at the ascending limb of the loop of Henle.

Bumetanide decreases uric acid excretion and increases serum uric acid concentration. Hyperuricemia has been reported in some patients receiving the drug. (See Cautions: Renal Effects.) The overall decrease in uric acid excretion appears to be less than that attributed to therapeutically equivalent doses of furosemide.

Bumetanide produces renal vascular dilation and substantially increases renal blood flow. Maximum increases in renal blood flow have ranged from 30–40% during bumetanide therapy. In animals, the drug causes redistribution of renal blood flow to the midcortical and juxtamedullary regions of the kidney. Increased urinary prostaglandin E concentrations have been observed in bumetanide-treated animals. It has been suggested that the drug's effect on renal prostaglandin activity may result in changes in renal hemodynamics. Although the effect of bumetanide on prostaglandin activity in humans has not been determined, the drug's effects on renal blood flow and renal cortical redistribution in animals are inhibited by prior treatment with a prostaglandin synthetase inhibitor (e.g., indomethacin). (See Drug Interactions: Indomethacin.) Bumetanide has a variable effect on glomerular filtration rate (GFR) in humans.

Bumetanide produces variable but substantial increases in plasma renin activity (PRA). In one study in healthy adults, increased PRA was observed 1 hour after bumetanide administration and persisted for up to 12 hours.

■ Cardiovascular Effects Bumetanide may produce hypotensive effects resulting from decreased plasma volume. Substantial reductions in blood pressure and in body weight have been observed in patients with hypertensive cardiovascular disease and heart failure who received the drug. Reductions in mean pulmonary venous pressure, left ventricular end-diastolic pressure (LVEDP), mean pulmonary artery pressure, and mean right atrial pressure have also been observed in patients with valvular heart disease receiving bumetanide; pulmonary and systemic arteriolar resistance were slightly reduced. Following administration of the drug in patients with coronary artery disease, reductions in cardiac output, cardiac index, stroke volume, stroke index, and in diastolic pressures (beginning, mean, and end) have occurred.

■ Metabolic Effects There is conflicting evidence to date on bumetanide's effect on carbohydrate metabolism. In healthy individuals receiving the drug, changes in plasma insulin, glucagon, or growth hormone concentration or in glucose tolerance generally have not been observed. However, hyperglycemia reportedly has occurred in some patients receiving the drug. (See Cautions: Metabolic Effects.) Diuretic-induced hyperglycemia may result from potassium depletion which has been associated with impaired insulin secretion. In one study in healthy individuals, a single 1-mg IV dose of bumetanide did not alter insulin response to IV glucose or the rate of decrease in blood glucose concentration. In individuals with impaired glucose tolerance (chemical, latent, or borderline diabetes mellitus), 1 mg of the drug daily for 10 days did not impair glucose tolerance further. When the effects of bumetanide and furosemide on oral glucose tolerance and insulin response to glucose were compared in another study, similar effects on carbohydrate metabolism were observed in bumetanide- and in furosemide-treated patients. Further study is needed to fully characterize the effects of bumetanide on carbohydrate metabolism; however, the drug does not appear to be associated with consistent or clinically important changes in blood glucose concentration.

Pharmacokinetics

■ Absorption Bumetanide is rapidly and almost completely absorbed from the GI tract. In several studies in healthy individuals, at least 85–95% of a single oral dose of the drug was absorbed; however, in one study, the bioavailability of bumetanide tablets reportedly was only 72%. The oral bioavailability of the drug in patients with impaired renal or hepatic function does not appear to differ substantially from that in healthy individuals. Limited data suggest that food may delay the absorption of oral bumetanide. The drug appears to be completely absorbed following IM administration.

Following oral administration, bumetanide appears in plasma within 15–20 minutes and peak plasma concentrations of the drug generally occur within 0.5–2 hours. Following oral administration of a single 1-mg dose of the drug in healthy adults, peak plasma or serum bumetanide concentrations have reportedly averaged 31–48 ng/mL; after a single 2-mg dose in one study, the peak plasma concentration averaged 73 ng/mL.

Bumetanide-induced diuresis begins within 30–60 minutes following oral administration, about 40 minutes following IM administration, and within a few minutes following IV administration; peak diuretic activity generally occurs within 1–2 hours following oral or IM administration and within 15–30 minutes after IV administration. Diuresis is generally complete within 4 hours following oral or IM administration of 1–2 mg of the drug; however, diuretic activity may persist for up to 5–6 hours, particularly when doses greater than 2 mg are used. Following IV administration, diuresis generally persists for 2–3 hours.

■ Distribution Distribution of bumetanide into human body tissues and fluids has not been fully characterized. Following IV administration of bumetanide in dogs, highest concentrations of the drug were observed in kidney, liver, and plasma, with lowest concentrations in heart, lung, muscle, and adipose tissue; bumetanide showed 3 times the affinity for renal tissue compared with that of furosemide. Following IV administration of bumetanide in healthy adults, the steady-state volume of distribution (V_{ss}) has been reported to range from 9.45–19.7 L and the volume of distribution of the central compartment (V_c) has been reported to range from 3.26–5.84 L. Following IV administration of bumetanide in neonates, the mean volume of distribution has been reported to range from 0.26–0.38 L/kg. V_{ss} may be decreased in patients with hepatic impairment. V_{ss} may be increased in patients with renal impairment. In one study in patients with varying degrees of renal dysfunction, V_{ss}, but not V_c, was increased compared with that of individuals with normal renal function (V_{ss}: 22 versus 17 L).

Approximately 94–97% of bumetanide is bound to plasma proteins in vitro. In vivo, approximately 92.6 or 96% of the drug is bound to plasma proteins based on Sephadex batch or ultrafiltration method, respectively. Protein binding may be decreased in patients with renal impairment; binding appears to be correlated with plasma albumin concentration in these patients. In one study, when bumetanide or furosemide was added to pooled human serum (adult or neonatal) in equimolar concentrations, bumetanide's displacement of bilirubin from albumin-binding sites was equivalent to that of furosemide in adult serum but less than that of furosemide in neonatal cord serum. In addition, results of an vitro study of pooled serum from critically ill neonates indicate that serum concentrations of free (unbound) bilirubin increased in a linear manner at bumetanide concentrations of 0.5–50 mcg/mL; however, such a correlation was not observed at bumetanide concentrations of 0.25 mcg/mL. Bumetanide does not appear to bind to erythrocytes.

Bumetanide and its metabolites are distributed into bile. Following oral administration of radiolabeled bumetanide in one patient with a biliary T tube in place, 1.8% of the dose was distributed into bile as unchanged drug and 12.6% as metabolites.

It is not known whether bumetanide crosses the blood-brain barrier or the placenta or is distributed into milk.

■ Elimination Plasma concentrations of bumetanide have generally been reported to decline in a monophasic or biphasic manner; however, studies using sensitive assay methods indicate that plasma concentrations may decline in a triphasic manner following IV administration.

Following oral administration, the terminal elimination half-life of bumetanide reportedly ranges from 1–1.5 hours in healthy adults. Following IV administration in adults with normal renal and hepatic function, the half-life in the initial phase ($t_{1/2\alpha}$) averages 5–6.9 minutes, the half-life in the secondary phase ($t_{1/2\beta}$) averages 46–47 minutes, and the half-life in the terminal phase ($t_{1/2\gamma}$) averages 3.1–3.4 hours. Serum concentrations of bumetanide may be higher and the terminal elimination half-life prolonged in patients with impaired renal and/or hepatic function. In neonates and infants, the elimination of bumetanide appears to be slower than in older pediatric patients and adults, possibly because of immature renal and hepatobiliary functions. The mean serum elimination half-life of bumetanide reportedly is 2.5 and 1.5 hours in infants younger than 2 months of age and in those 2–6 months of age, respectively. In addition, limited data indicate that the apparent half-life of the drug may be prolonged to about 6 hours (with a range up to 15 hours) in premature or full-term neonates with respiratory disorders receiving IV bumetanide.

Total body clearance of bumetanide from plasma reportedly averages 120–250 mL/minute in adults with normal renal and hepatic function; renal clearance of the drug is about 50–65% of the total body clearance. Total body clearance of bumetanide is decreased in patients with impaired renal function, with or without concomitant hepatic impairment; in patients with only renal impairment, nonrenal clearance of the drug is about 90% or more of the total body clearance. Clearance also may be decreased in neonates and infants possibly, because of immature renal and hepatobiliary functions. In neonates with volume overload, mean serum clearance of bumetanide reportedly was about 2.2 and 3.8 mL/minute per kg in those younger than 2 months of age and 2–6 months of age, respectively. In addition, limited data indicate that serum clearance of the drug may be decreased to about 0.2–1.1 mL/minute per kg in premature or full-term neonates with respiratory disorders receiving IV bumetanide.

Bumetanide is partially metabolized in the liver to at least 5 metabolites. Metabolism apparently occurs only by oxidation of the *N*-butyl side chain of the bumetanide molecule; the phenyl ring structures do not appear to be metabolized. Hydroxylation occurs at each carbon of the *N*-butyl side chain. The major urinary metabolite is the 3′-alcohol derivative. The major metabolite excreted in bile and/or feces is the 2′-alcohol derivative. Minor metabolites include the 4′-alcohol, *N*-desbutyl, and 3′-acid derivatives. Bumetanide metabolites in urine and bile are present as conjugates, principally glucuronide conjugates. Conjugates of the drug and its metabolites do not appear in feces.

Bumetanide and its metabolites are excreted principally in urine. Renal excretion of the drug appears to occur mainly via glomerular filtration; tubular secretion may also occur. Following oral or IV administration in healthy adults, about 80% of a dose is excreted in urine and 10–20% in feces within 48 hours; about 50% of a dose is excreted unchanged in urine. Bumetanide is excreted in feces almost completely as metabolites, apparently via biliary elimination; less than 2% of a dose is excreted unchanged in feces within 48 hours. Following IV administration of radiolabeled bumetanide in one study in patients with varying degrees of renal dysfunction, about 25% of a dose was excreted in urine within 48 hours and about 40% (range: 4–94%) was excreted in feces within 7 days.

Chemistry and Stability

■ **Chemistry** Bumetanide is a sulfonamide-type, loop diuretic. The drug is a derivative of metanilamide and is structurally related to furosemide. Bumetanide differs structurally from furosemide by the presence of 4-phenoxy and 5-butylamino substituents.

Bumetanide occurs as a practically white, crystalline powder with a slightly bitter taste. The drug has solubilities of 0.1 mg/mL in water and 30.6 mg/mL in alcohol at 25°C. Bumetanide has pK_as of 0.3, 4, and 10. Commercially available bumetanide injection is a sterile solution of the drug containing 0.85% sodium chloride and 0.4% ammonium acetate as buffers, 1% benzyl alcohol as a preservative, and 0.01% disodium edetate. Sodium hydroxide is added during the manufacture of the injection to adjust the pH to 6.8–7.8.

■ **Stability** Bumetanide is photosensitive and will discolor when exposed to light. Commercially available preparations of bumetanide should be protected from light and stored at 15–30°C. Bumetanide tablets should be stored in tight, light-resistant containers. The commercially available tablets are stable for 5 years and the injection is stable for 3 years after the date of manufacture.

Bumetanide injection is reportedly stable at a pH of 4–10. Substantial adsorption of the drug to glass or PVC containers reportedly does not occur. Bumetanide injection is physically and chemically compatible in glass and PVC containers with the following IV solutions: 5% dextrose, 0.9% sodium chloride, or lactated Ringer's injection. Bumetanide injection that has been diluted with one of these compatible IV solutions should be used within 24 hours after preparation.

Preparations

Excipients in commercially available drug preparations may have clinically important effects in some individuals; consult specific product labeling for details.

Bumetanide

Oral		
Tablets	0.5 mg*	**Bumetanide Tablets**
	1 mg*	**Bumetanide Tablets**
	2 mg*	**Bumetanide Tablets**
Parenteral		
Injection	0.25 mg/mL*	**Bumetanide Injection**

*available from one or more manufacturer, distributor, and/or repackager by generic (nonproprietary) name

†Use is not currently included in the labeling approved by the US Food and Drug Administration

Selected Revisions April 2019,

Furosemide

Frusemide

■ Furosemide is a sulfonamide, loop-type diuretic and antihypertensive agent.

Uses

■ **Edema** Furosemide is used in the management of edema associated with heart failure, nephrotic syndrome, and hepatic cirrhosis. IV furosemide also may be used as an adjunct in the treatment of acute pulmonary edema.

Careful etiologic diagnosis should precede the use of any diuretic. Because the potent diuretic effect of furosemide may result in severe electrolyte imbalance and excessive fluid loss, hospitalization of the patient during initiation of therapy is advisable, especially for patients with hepatic cirrhosis and ascites or chronic renal failure. In prolonged diuretic therapy, intermittent use of the drug for only a few days each week may be advisable. Furosemide may be administered cautiously for additive effect with most other diuretics; however, since furosemide and other loop diuretics (e.g., ethacrynic acid) act in a similar manner, there is no rationale for using these drugs together.

Heart Failure Furosemide is used in the management of edema associated with heart failure. Most experts state that all patients with symptomatic heart failure who have evidence for, or a history of, fluid retention generally should receive diuretic therapy in conjunction with moderate sodium restriction, an agent to inhibit the renin-angiotensin-aldosterone (RAA) system (e.g., angiotensin-converting enzyme [ACE] inhibitor, angiotensin II receptor antagonist, angiotensin receptor-neprilysin inhibitor [ARNI]), a β-adrenergic blocking agent (β-blocker), and in selected patients, an aldosterone antagonist. Some experts state that because of limited and inconsistent data, it is difficult to make precise recommendations regarding daily sodium intake and whether it should vary with respect to the type of heart failure (e.g., reduced versus preserved ejection fraction), disease severity (e.g., New York Heart Association [NYHA] class), heart failure-related comorbidities (e.g., renal dysfunction), or other patient characteristics (e.g., age, race). The American College of Cardiology Foundation (ACCF) and American Heart Association (AHA) state that limiting sodium intake to 1.5 g daily in patients with ACCF/AHA stage A or B heart failure may be reasonable. While data currently are lacking to support recommendation of a specific level of sodium intake in patients with ACCF/AHA stage C or D heart failure, ACCF and AHA state that limiting sodium intake to some degree (e.g., less than 3 g daily) in such patients may be considered for symptom improvement.

Diuretics play a key role in the management of heart failure because they produce symptomatic benefits more rapidly than any other drugs, relieving pulmonary and peripheral edema within hours or days compared with weeks or months for cardiac glycosides, ACE inhibitors, or β-blockers. However, since there are no long-term studies of diuretic therapy in patients with heart failure, the effects of diuretics on morbidity and mortality in such patients are not known. Although there are patients with heart failure who do not exhibit fluid retention in the absence of diuretic therapy and even may develop severe volume depletion with low doses of diuretics, such patients are rare and the unique pathophysiologic mechanisms regulating their fluid and electrolyte balance have not been elucidated.

Most experts state that loop diuretics (e.g., bumetanide, ethacrynic acid, furosemide, torsemide) are the diuretics of choice for most patients with heart failure. If resistance to diuretics occurs, IV administration of a diuretic or concomitant use of 2 or more diuretics (e.g., a loop diuretic and metolazone, a loop diuretic and a thiazide diuretic) may be necessary; alternatively, short-term administration of a drug that increases blood flow (e.g., a positive inotropic agent such as dopamine) may be necessary. ACCF and AHA state that IV loop diuretics should be administered promptly to all hospitalized heart failure patients with substantial fluid overload to reduce morbidity. In addition, ACCF and AHA state that low-dose dopamine infusions may be considered in combination with loop diuretics to augment diuresis and preserve renal function and renal blood flow in patients with acute decompensated heart failure, although data are conflicting and additional study and experience are needed. For additional information, see Heart Failure under Uses: Edema, in the Thiazides General Statement 40:28.20.

Pulmonary Disease Furosemide may be administered IV as an adjunct in the treatment of acute pulmonary edema; however, the drug should be used cautiously when pulmonary edema is a complication of cardiogenic shock associated with acute myocardial infarction because diuretic-induced hypovolemia may reduce cardiac output.

Hepatic and Renal Disease Furosemide also may be used cautiously in the management of edema associated with the nephrotic syndrome and in patients with hepatic cirrhosis, but such edema is frequently refractory to treatment. When metabolic alkalosis may be anticipated, a potassium-rich diet, potassium supplements, or potassium-sparing diuretics may be necessary before and during furosemide therapy to mitigate or prevent hypokalemia in cirrhotic, nephrotic, or digitalized patients. (See Cautions: Fluid, Electrolyte, Cardiovascular, and Renal Effects.)

Large oral or IV doses of furosemide have been employed as an adjunct to other therapy, including peritoneal dialysis or hemodialysis, in patients with acute or chronic renal failure. In some patients, the use of furosemide may delay the need for dialysis, increase the intervals between dialyses, shorten the period of hospitalization, or permit a slightly more liberal fluid intake.

■ **Hypertension** Furosemide may be used alone or in combination with other classes of antihypertensive agents for the management of hypertension, especially when complicated by heart failure or renal disease. Because of established clinical benefits (e.g., reductions in overall mortality and in adverse cardiovascular, cerebrovascular, and renal outcomes), current evidence-based practice guidelines for the management of hypertension in adults generally recommend the use of drugs from 4 classes of antihypertensive agents (ACE inhibitors, angiotensin II receptor antagonists, calcium-channel blockers, and thiazide diuretics). (See Uses: Hypertension in Adults, in the Thiazides General Statement 40:28.20) However, some experts state that loop diuretics (e.g., bumetanide, furosemide, torsemide) are preferred over thiazides in patients with moderate to severe chronic kidney disease (CKD) or symptomatic heart failure. Loop diuretics may be particularly useful in patients with heart failure and reduced left ventricular ejection fraction (LVEF) who have evidence of fluid retention; however, some experts state that thiazide diuretics may be considered in hypertensive patients with heart failure and mild fluid retention because of their more persistent antihypertensive effect.

In most patients, hypertension not controllable by thiazides alone probably will not respond adequately to furosemide alone.

For information on antihypertensive therapy for patients with chronic kidney disease or heart failure, see Chronic Kidney Disease and also see Heart Failure under Hypertension in Adults: Considerations for Drug Therapy in

Patients with Underlying Cardiovascular and Other Risk Factors, in Uses in the Thiazides General Statement 40:28.20.

For further information on the role of diuretics in antihypertensive therapy and information on overall principles and expert recommendations for treatment of hypertension, see Uses: Hypertension in Adults and also see Uses: Hypertension in Pediatric Patients, in the Thiazides General Statement 40:28.20.

Hypertensive Crises IV furosemide has been found useful as an adjunct to hypotensive agents in the treatment of hypertensive crises†, especially when associated with acute pulmonary edema or renal failure. In addition to producing a rapid diuresis, furosemide enhances the effects of other hypotensive drugs and counteracts the sodium retention caused by some of these agents.

■ **Other Uses** Furosemide has been used IV alone or with 0.9% sodium chloride injection or sodium sulfate to increase renal excretion of calcium in patients with hypercalcemia†. Oral furosemide has been suggested for maintenance.

Dosage and Administration

■ **Administration** Furosemide usually is administered orally. Furosemide injection in which the drug is present as the sodium salt (see Chemistry and Stability: Chemistry) may be given by IM or IV injection when a rapid onset of diuresis is desired or the patient is unable to take oral medication.

The manufacturers suggest that when oral furosemide therapy is indicated, infants and children should receive furosemide oral solution, because of ease of administration and dosage flexibility.

IV injections of furosemide should be given slowly over 1–2 minutes. Parenteral administration of furosemide should be replaced by oral therapy as soon as possible. If high-dose parenteral furosemide therapy is necessary, the manufacturer recommends that the drug be administered as a controlled infusion at a rate not exceeding 4 mg/minute in adults. For IV infusion, furosemide should be diluted with an infusion solution of 0.9% sodium chloride, lactated Ringer's, or 5% dextrose, adjusting the pH to greater than 5.5 when necessary. (See Chemistry and Stability: Stability.) One investigator recommended that 1-g doses should be infused over at least a 3-hour period in order to prevent ototoxicity.

■ **Dosage** Dosage of furosemide injection, in which the drug is present as the sodium salt (see Chemistry and Stability: Chemistry), is expressed in terms of furosemide. Furosemide dosage must be adjusted according to the patient's requirements and response. If furosemide is added to the regimen of a patient stabilized on a potent hypotensive agent, the dosage of the hypotensive agent and possibly both drugs should initially be reduced in order to avoid severe hypotension.

For the management of fluid retention (e.g., edema) associated with heart failure, experts state that diuretics should be administered at a dosage sufficient to achieve optimal volume status and relieve congestion without inducing an excessively rapid reduction in intravascular volume, which could result in hypotension, renal dysfunction, or both.

When high-dose furosemide infusions are used, dosage should be individualized according to patient response, titrating the dosage to gain maximum therapeutic effect while using the lowest possible effective dosage; the patient should be closely observed during therapy.

Edema **Oral Dosage.** The usual initial adult oral dose of furosemide for the management of edema is 20–80 mg given as a single dose, preferably in the morning. In adults who do not respond, the second and each succeeding oral dose may be increased in 20- to 40-mg increments every 6–8 hours until the desired diuretic response (including weight loss) is obtained. The effective dose may be given once or twice daily thereafter, or, in some cases, by intermittent administration on 2–4 consecutive days each week. For maintenance, dosage may be reduced in some patients. Adult oral dosage of furosemide may be carefully titrated up to 600 mg daily in severely edematous patients.

For the management of fluid retention (e.g., edema) associated with heart failure, some experts recommend initiating furosemide at a low dosage (e.g., 20–40 mg once or twice daily) and increasing the dosage (maximum of 600 mg daily) until urine output increases and weight decreases, generally by 0.5–1 kg daily.

For infants and children, the usual initial oral dose of furosemide for the management of edema is 2 mg/kg administered as a single dose. If necessary, dosage may be increased in increments of 1 or 2 mg/kg every 6–8 hours to maximum individual doses of 6 mg/kg; however, it usually is not necessary to exceed individual doses of 4 mg/kg or a dosing frequency of once or twice daily. For maintenance, the minimum effective dosage should be employed.

Parenteral Dosage. As a diuretic, the usual adult IM or IV dose is 20–40 mg given as a single injection. In adults who do not respond to the initial parenteral dose of furosemide, the second and each succeeding dose may be increased in 20-mg increments and given not more often than every 2 hours until the desired diuretic response is obtained. The effective single dose may then be given once or twice daily.

For the management of acute pulmonary edema in adults, 40 mg of furosemide may be slowly injected IV over 1–2 minutes. If the initial adult dose does not produce a satisfactory response within 1 hour, the dose may be increased to 80 mg IV given over 1–2 minutes. In adults with hypertensive crises†, who have normal renal function, 40–80 mg of furosemide (administered concomitantly with other hypotensive agents) may be given IV over 1–2 minutes; in patients with reduced renal function higher does may be required.

For infants and children, the usual initial IV or IM dose of furosemide for the management of acute pulmonary edema or edema associated with heart failure or renal disease† is 1 mg/kg. If necessary for resistant forms of edema, the initial dose may be increased by 1 mg/kg no more often than every 2 hours until the desired effect has been obtained. Adequate response usually is obtained with individual parenteral doses of 1 mg/kg, but occasionally individual doses of 2 mg/kg may be required. Maximum individual parenteral doses recommended by the manufacturer for infants and children are 6 mg/kg; however, the potential risks associated with large parenteral doses of the drug should be considered and the patient should be monitored closely.

Literature reports suggest that the recommended maximum dosage of furosemide injection for respiratory distress syndrome (RDS) in premature neonates less than 31 weeks postconception age (gestational age at birth plus postnatal age) should not exceed 1 mg/kg in 24 hours. (See Cautions: Pediatric Precautions.)

Large doses of furosemide have been administered orally or IV to adults with acute or chronic renal failure. One investigator recommends beginning therapy in adults with 80 mg of furosemide orally daily and increasing dosage in increments of 80–120 mg daily until the desired effect is achieved. When immediate diuresis is needed, an initial adult dose of 320–400 mg orally daily has been suggested. Some patients have received as much as 4 g orally daily†. Initial IV doses have ranged from 100 mg to 2 g in adults. In some studies, the initial IV doses were doubled at 2- to 24-hour intervals until the desired effect was attained. The highest IV dosage of furosemide was 6 g daily.

Hypertension **Adult Dosage.** The manufacturer states that the usual adult oral dosage of furosemide for the management of hypertension is 40 mg twice daily initially and for maintenance. If a satisfactory lowering of blood pressure does not occur, dosage can be increased gradually. Careful monitoring of blood pressure is essential when furosemide is used alone or in combination with other hypotensive agents, especially during initial therapy. If a satisfactory lowering of blood pressure does not occur when 40 mg is administered orally twice daily, the manufacturer recommends adding other antihypertensive agents rather than increasing the dosage of furosemide. Some experts state that the usual oral antihypertensive dosage of furosemide for adults is 20–80 mg daily given in 2 divided doses.

Monitoring and Blood Pressure Treatment Goals. The patient's renal function and electrolytes should be assessed 2–4 weeks after initiation of diuretic therapy. Blood pressure should be monitored regularly (i.e., monthly) during therapy and dosage of the antihypertensive drug adjusted until blood pressure is controlled. If an adequate blood pressure response is not achieved, the dosage may be increased or another antihypertensive agent with demonstrated benefit and preferably with a complementary mechanism of action (e.g., angiotensin-converting enzyme [ACE] inhibitor, angiotensin II receptor antagonist, calcium-channel blocker) may be added; if target blood pressure is still not achieved, a third drug may be added. (See Uses: Hypertension in Adults, in the Thiazides General Statement 40:28.20.) In patients who develop unacceptable adverse effects with furosemide, the drug should be discontinued and another antihypertensive agent from a different pharmacologic class should be initiated.

The goal of hypertension management and prevention is to achieve and maintain optimal control of blood pressure. However, the optimum blood pressure threshold for initiating antihypertensive drug therapy and specific treatment goals remain controversial. A 2017 multidisciplinary hypertension guideline from the American College of Cardiology (ACC), American Heart Association (AHA), and a number of other professional organizations generally recommends a blood pressure goal of less than 130/80 mm Hg in all adults, regardless of comorbidities or level of atherosclerotic cardiovascular disease (ASCVD) risk. Many patients will require at least 2 drugs from different pharmacologic classes to achieve this blood pressure goal; the potential benefits of hypertension management and drug cost, adverse effects, and risks associated with the use of multiple antihypertensive drugs also should be considered when deciding a patient's blood pressure treatment goal.

For additional information on target levels of blood pressure and on monitoring therapy in the management of hypertension, see Blood Pressure Monitoring and Treatment Goals under Dosage: Hypertension, in Dosage and Administration in the Thiazides General Statement 40:28.20.

Pediatric Dosage. For the management of hypertension in children†, some experts have recommended an initial oral dosage of 0.5–2 mg/kg administered once or twice daily. Such experts have suggested that dosage may be increased as necessary up to 6 mg/kg daily. For information on overall principles and expert recommendations for treatment of hypertension in pediatric patients, see Uses: Hypertension in Pediatric Patients in the Thiazides General Statement 40:28.20.

Other In the treatment of hypercalcemia†, adults have been given 80–100 mg of furosemide IV at intervals of 1–2 hours. In one study, total IV dosage ranged from 160 mg to 3.2 g. Slight elevations of blood calcium concentration have been treated with 120 mg of oral furosemide daily.

Dosage in Renal Impairment Large doses of furosemide have been administered orally or IV to adults with acute or chronic renal failure. One investigator recommends beginning therapy in adults with 80 mg of furosemide orally daily and increasing dosage in increments of 80–120 mg daily until the desired effect is achieved. When immediate diuresis is needed, an initial adult dose of 320–400 mg orally daily has been suggested. Some patients have received as much as 4 g orally daily†. Initial IV doses have ranged from 100 mg to 2 g in adults. In some studies, the initial IV doses were doubled at 2- to 24-hour intervals until the desired effect was attained. The highest IV dosage of furosemide was 6 g daily.

Cautions

■ **Fluid, Electrolyte, Cardiovascular, and Renal Effects** Furosemide may produce profound diuresis resulting in fluid and electrolyte depletion. Fluid and electrolyte depletion are especially likely to occur when large doses are given and/or in patients with restricted sodium intake.

Too vigorous diuresis, as evidenced by rapid and excessive weight loss, may induce orthostatic hypotension or acute hypotensive episodes, and the patient's blood pressure should be closely monitored. Excessive dehydration is most likely to occur in geriatric patients and/or patients with chronic cardiac disease treated with prolonged sodium restriction or those receiving sympatholytic agents. The resultant hypovolemia may cause hemoconcentration, which could lead to circulatory collapse or thromboembolic episodes such as possibly fatal vascular thromboses and/or emboli. Pronounced reductions in plasma volume associated with rapid or excessive diuresis may also result in an abrupt fall in glomerular filtration rate and renal blood flow, which may be restored by replacement of fluid loss. Rarely, sudden death from cardiac arrest has been reported following IV or IM administration of furosemide.

Potassium depletion occurs frequently in patients with secondary hyperaldosteronism which may be associated with cirrhosis or nephrosis and is particularly important in cirrhotic, nephrotic, or digitalized patients. Hypokalemia and hypochloremia may result in metabolic alkalosis, especially in patients with other losses of potassium and chloride due to vomiting, diarrhea, GI drainage, excessive sweating, paracentesis, or potassium-losing renal diseases. In patients with cor pulmonale, alkalosis may cause compensatory respiratory depression. Intermittent administration of furosemide and/or ingestion of potassium-rich foods or administration of a potassium-sparing diuretic may reduce or prevent potassium depletion. However, potassium supplements may be necessary in patients whose serum potassium concentration is less than approximately 3 mEq/L or those receiving digitalis glycosides. To prevent hypokalemic and hypochloremic alkalosis, potassium chloride supplementation should be used. Furosemide increases calcium excretion; rarely, tetany has been reported. Magnesium depletion may also occur.

Furosemide may cause a transient rise in BUN which is usually readily reversible upon withdrawal of the drug. Elevated BUN is especially likely to occur in patients with chronic renal disease. Hyperuricemia may result from furosemide administration and rarely gout has been precipitated; patients with a history of gout or elevated serum uric acid concentrations should be observed closely during therapy. However, large IV doses of furosemide may cause temporary uricosuria. Elevations of BUN and uric acid concentrations may be associated with dehydration, which should be avoided, particularly in patients with renal insufficiency. Allergic interstitial nephritis leading to reversible renal failure has been attributed to furosemide. Blood ammonia concentrations may be increased, especially in patients with preexisting elevations of blood ammonia.

Chronic administration of furosemide 50 mg/kg in rats has caused renal tubular degeneration. Calcification and scarring of the renal parenchyma has occurred in dogs receiving 10 mg/kg for 6 months.

■ **Otic Effects** Tinnitus, reversible or permanent hearing impairment, or reversible deafness have occurred, usually following rapid IV or IM administration of furosemide in doses greatly exceeding the usual therapeutic dose of 20–40 mg. Otic effects are most likely to occur in patients with severe impairment of renal function and/or in patients receiving other ototoxic drugs (e.g., aminoglycosides). (See Drug Interactions: Other Drugs.) It has been postulated that administering furosemide by slow IV infusion rather than as a bolus may reduce the ototoxic effects of the drug by preventing high peak plasma concentrations; if high-dose parenteral furosemide therapy is necessary in patients with severely impaired renal function, the manufacturers recommend that the drug be infused in adults at a rate not exceeding 4 mg/minute.

■ **GI Effects** Adverse GI effects of furosemide include nausea, anorexia, oral and gastric irritation, vomiting, cramping, diarrhea, and constipation. Because furosemide oral solutions contain sorbitol, they may cause diarrhea, especially in children, when high dosages are administered. In children, mild to moderate abdominal pain has been reported after furosemide was administered IV. In addition, rare occurrences of sweet taste have been reported, but a causal relationship to the drug has not been established.

■ **Metabolic Effects** Furosemide may produce hyperglycemia and glycosuria, possibly as a result of hypokalemia, in patients with predisposition to diabetes. Rarely, precipitation of diabetes mellitus has been reported.

Diuretics, including furosemide, can increase serum total cholesterol concentrations in some patients; increases in low-density lipoprotein (LDL)-cholesterol and/or very low-density lipoprotein (VLDL)-cholesterol subfractions appear to be principally responsible for these increases. In addition, the ratio of serum total cholesterol to high-density lipoprotein (HDL)-cholesterol has been increased in some patients in whom total serum cholesterol did not appear to be elevated. Increases in serum triglyceride concentrations also can occur.

■ **Nervous System Effects** Adverse nervous system effects of furosemide include dizziness, lightheadedness, vertigo, headache, xanthopsia, blurred vision, and paresthesias.

■ **Hematologic Effects** Anemia, hemolytic anemia, leukopenia, neutropenia, and thrombocytopenia have occurred in patients receiving furosemide. In addition, rare cases of agranulocytosis and aplastic anemia have been reported.

■ **Dermatologic and Sensitivity Reactions** Adverse dermatologic and/or hypersensitivity reactions to furosemide include purpura, photosensitivity, rash, urticaria, pruritus, exfoliative dermatitis, erythema multiforme, interstitial nephritis, and necrotizing angiitis (vasculitis, cutaneous vasculitis). Patients with known sulfonamide sensitivity may show allergic reactions to furosemide. Anaphylaxis, manifested as urticaria, angioedema, and hypotension, occurred within 5 minutes after IV administration of furosemide in at least one patient; subsequent intradermal skin testing showed sensitivity to furosemide and other sulfonamides.

■ **Local Effects** Transient pain at the injection site has been reported after IM administration of furosemide. Thrombophlebitis has occurred with IV administration.

■ **Other Adverse Effects** Other adverse effects of furosemide include increased perspiration, weakness, fever, restlessness, muscle spasm, urinary bladder spasm, and urinary frequency. A few cases of flank and loin pain have been reported in adults receiving oral furosemide, possibly resulting from calyceal dilation, increased bladder pressure, or spasms caused by formation of calcium-containing crystals in the urine. Intrahepatic cholestatic jaundice and pancreatitis have also occurred in patients receiving furosemide. Furosemide may possibly exacerbate or activate systemic lupus erythematosus.

■ **Precautions and Contraindications** Patients receiving furosemide must be carefully observed for signs of hypovolemia, hyponatremia, hypokalemia, hypocalcemia, hypochloremia, and hypomagnesemia. Patients should be informed of the signs and symptoms of electrolyte imbalance and instructed to report to their physicians if weakness, dizziness, fatigue, faintness, mental confusion, lassitude, muscle cramps, headache, paresthesia, thirst, anorexia, nausea, and/or vomiting occur. Excessive fluid and electrolyte loss may be minimized by initiating therapy with small doses, careful dosage adjustment, using an intermittent dosage schedule if possible, and monitoring the patient's weight. To prevent hyponatremia and hypochloremia, intake of sodium may be liberalized in most patients; however, patients with cirrhosis usually require at least moderate sodium restriction while on diuretic therapy. Determinations of serum electrolytes, BUN, and carbon dioxide should be performed early in therapy with furosemide and periodically thereafter. If excessive diuresis and/or electrolyte abnormalities occur, the drug should be withdrawn or dosage reduced until homeostasis is restored. Electrolyte abnormalities should be corrected by appropriate measures.

Furosemide should be used with caution in patients with hepatic cirrhosis because rapid alterations in fluid and electrolyte balance may precipitate hepatic precoma or coma.

Periodic blood studies and liver function tests should be performed in patients receiving furosemide, especially in those on prolonged therapy.

Urine and blood glucose concentration determinations should be made periodically in diabetics and suspected latent diabetics receiving furosemide.

Furosemide therapy during the first few weeks of life in premature neonates reportedly may increase the risk of persistent patent ductus arteriosus (PDA), possibly through a prostaglandin E (PGE)-mediated process.

Furosemide is contraindicated in patients with anuria. The drug is contraindicated for further use if increasing azotemia and/or oliguria occur during the treatment of severe, progressive renal disease. In patients with hepatic coma or electrolyte depletion, therapy should not be instituted until the basic condition is improved or corrected. Furosemide is also contraindicated in patients with a history of hypersensitivity to the drug.

■ **Pediatric Precautions** In premature neonates with respiratory distress syndrome (RDS), diuretic therapy with furosemide during the first weeks of life may increase the risk of persistent patent ductus arteriosus (PDA), an effect that may be mediated by prostaglandins, presumably of the E series. Hearing loss has been reported in neonates receiving furosemide. Ototoxicity may be associated with elevated plasma concentrations of furosemide secondary to renal immaturity in these patients. Therefore, the manufacturers state that parenteral furosemide dosages should not exceed 1 mg/kg per 24 hours in premature neonates with less than 31 weeks postconception age (gestational age at birth plus postnatal age), because higher dosages may be associated with potentially toxic plasma concentrations of the drug.

■ **Pregnancy, Fertility, and Lactation** In reproduction studies in mice, rats, and rabbits, administration of furosemide caused unexplained abortions and maternal and fetal deaths. In addition, an increased incidence of hydronephrosis occurred in fetuses of animals treated with the drug. There are no adequate and well controlled studies in pregnant women. Furosemide should be used during pregnancy only when the potential benefits justify the possible risks to the fetus.

Reproduction studies in male and female rats using furosemide dosages of 100 mg/kg daily (the maximum effective diuretic dosage in rats and 8 times the maximum human dosage of 600 mg daily) have not revealed evidence of impaired fertility.

Since furosemide is distributed into milk, the manufacturers recommend that nursing be discontinued if administration of the drug is necessary.

Drug Interactions

■ **Diuretics** Concomitant administration of furosemide and most other diuretics results in enhanced effects, and furosemide should be administered in reduced dosage when the drug is added to an existing diuretic regimen. Spironolactone, triamterene, or amiloride hydrochloride may reduce the potassium loss resulting from furosemide therapy; this effect has been used to therapeutic advantage.

■ **Drugs Affected by or Causing Potassium Depletion** In patients receiving cardiac glycosides, electrolyte disturbances produced by furosemide (principally hypokalemia but also hypomagnesemia) predispose the patient to glycoside toxicity. Possibly fatal cardiac arrhythmias may result. Periodic electrolyte determinations should be performed in patients receiving a cardiac glycoside and furosemide, and correction of hypokalemia undertaken if warranted. (See Cautions: Fluid, Electrolyte, Cardiovascular, and Renal Effects.)

Furosemide reportedly causes prolonged neuromuscular blockade in patients receiving nondepolarizing neuromuscular blocking agents (e.g., tubocurarine chloride, gallamine triethiodide [no longer commercially available in the US]), presumably because of potassium depletion or decreased urinary excretion of the muscle relaxant. Furosemide may also cause decreased arterial responsiveness to pressor amines. Orally administered furosemide should be discontinued 1 week, and parenterally administered furosemide 2 days, prior to elective surgery.

Some drugs such as corticosteroids, corticotropin, and amphotericin B also cause potassium loss, and severe potassium depletion may occur when one of these drugs is administered during furosemide therapy.

■ **Lithium** Renal clearance of lithium is apparently decreased in patients receiving diuretics, and lithium toxicity may result. Furosemide and lithium should generally not be given together. If concomitant therapy is necessary, the patient should be hospitalized. Serum lithium concentrations should be monitored carefully and dosage adjusted accordingly.

■ **Antidiabetic Agents** Administration of furosemide to diabetic patients may interfere with the hypoglycemic effect of insulin or oral antidiabetic agents, possibly as a result of hypokalemia. Patients should be observed for possible decrease of diabetic control. If correction of the potassium deficit does not restore control, dosage adjustments of the antidiabetic agent may be needed.

■ **Hypotensive Agents** The antihypertensive effect of hypotensive agents may be enhanced when given concomitantly with furosemide. This effect is usually used to therapeutic advantage; however, orthostatic hypotension may result. Dosage of the hypotensive agent, and possibly both drugs, should be reduced when furosemide is added to an existing regimen.

■ **Indomethacin** In some patients, indomethacin may reduce the natriuretic and hypotensive effects of furosemide. The mechanism(s) of these interactions is uncertain but has been attributed to indomethacin-induced inhibition of prostaglandin synthesis which may result in fluid retention and/or changes in vascular resistance. The clinical importance of these interactions has not been established; however, when indomethacin and furosemide are administered concurrently, patients should be observed closely to determine if the desired diuretic and/or hypotensive effect is obtained. When evaluating plasma renin activity in hypertensive patients, it should be kept in mind that indomethacin blocks the furosemide-induced increase in plasma renin activity.

■ **Ototoxic Drugs** Concomitant administration of furosemide and aminoglycoside antibiotics or other ototoxic drugs may result in increased incidence of ototoxicity and concomitant use of these drugs should be avoided. In addition, the possibility that IV furosemide may increase aminoglycoside toxicity by altering serum and tissue concentrations of the antibiotic should be considered. It has been proposed, but not proven, that furosemide may enhance the nephrotoxicity of neomycin.

■ **Nonsteroidal Anti-inflammatory Agents** Furosemide and salicylates reportedly have competitive renal excretory sites and, therefore, patients receiving high doses of salicylates with furosemide may experience salicylate toxicity at lower dosage than usual. Concomitant administration of furosemide and aspirin reportedly has been associated with a transient reduction in creatinine clearance in a few patients with chronic renal insufficiency. Weight gain and increases in BUN, serum creatinine, and serum potassium concentrations also have been reported in patients receiving furosemide in combination with other nonsteroidal anti-inflammatory agents (NSAIAs).

■ **Anticonvulsants** In one study, epileptic patients receiving chronic anticonvulsant therapy had a reduced diuretic response to furosemide as compared to controls. All of the epileptic patients were receiving phenytoin sodium and phenobarbital and some were also receiving other anticonvulsants. It has been postulated that renal sensitivity to furosemide is diminished by these drugs.

■ **Chloral Hydrate** A reaction characterized by diaphoresis, flushes, variable blood pressure including hypertension, and uneasiness has been reported in some patients with acute myocardial infarction and heart failure who received furosemide IV within 24 hours after administration of an oral hypnotic dose of chloral hydrate (no longer commercially available in the US). Therefore, it may be preferable to use an alternate hypnotic drug (e.g., a benzodiazepine) in patients who require IV furosemide.

■ **Probenecid or Sulfinpyrazone** It has been suggested that furosemide, by increasing serum uric acid concentrations, may interfere with the uricosuric effects of probenecid or sulfinpyrazone. Serum uric acid concentrations should be monitored in patients receiving both drugs, and dosage of the uricosuric drug should be increased if necessary.

Pharmacology

The pharmacologic effects of furosemide are similar to those of ethacrynic acid. The exact mode of action of furosemide has not been clearly defined; in contrast to ethacrynic acid, it does not bind sulfhydryl groups of renal cellular proteins. Furosemide inhibits the reabsorption of electrolytes in the ascending limb of the loop of Henle. The drug also decreases reabsorption of sodium and chloride and increases potassium excretion in the distal renal tubule and exerts a direct effect on electrolyte transport at the proximal tubule. Furosemide does not inhibit carbonic anhydrase and is not an aldosterone antagonist.

Furosemide diuresis results in enhanced excretion of sodium, chloride, potassium, hydrogen, calcium, magnesium, ammonium, bicarbonate, and possibly phosphate. Chloride excretion exceeds that of sodium. In studies in patients with normal renal function, the diuretic response was similar following oral or IV administration of equal doses of furosemide. In one study in uremic patients, however, diuresis and urinary excretion of sodium and potassium were greater after IV administration of furosemide than after equal oral doses. Excessive losses of potassium, hydrogen, and chloride may result in metabolic alkalosis. Urinary pH usually falls after administration of furosemide; however, increased bicarbonate excretion in some patients may temporarily raise urinary pH. Low doses of furosemide promote uric acid retention while large IV doses may cause temporary uricosuria. Maximum diuresis and electrolyte loss is greater with furosemide than with the thiazides or most other diuretics except ethacrynic acid. Like the thiazide diuretics and ethacrynic acid, the effectiveness of furosemide is independent of the acid-base balance of the patient.

Furosemide has some renal vasodilator effect; renal vascular resistance decreases and renal blood flow increases following administration of the drug. A temporary but substantial increase in glomerular filtration rate, as well as decreased peripheral vascular resistance and increased peripheral venous capacitance, has been reported following IV administration of furosemide in patients with heart failure associated with acute myocardial infarction. The renal and peripheral vascular effects may contribute toward the beneficial effects of the drug in these patients, as a decrease in left ventricular filling pressure occurs before the onset of substantial diuresis. In addition, IV administration of furosemide in patients with heart failure results in a decrease in plasma volume, increased hematocrit, and a fall in mean arterial pressure associated with increased cardiac output and decreased peripheral resistance. When large doses of furosemide are administered to patients with chronic renal insufficiency, glomerular filtration rate may be increased temporarily. A fall in renal blood flow and glomerular filtration rate may occur if excessive drug-induced diuresis results in a reduction in plasma volume.

As with other diuretics, a hypotensive effect may result from decreased plasma volume in patients receiving furosemide. However, the drug has been reported to produce only mild decreases in the supine systolic blood pressure and in the erect systolic and diastolic blood pressures when administered alone in the recommended oral dosage.

Furosemide appears to have less effect on carbohydrate metabolism and blood glucose concentrations than do the thiazides; however, the drug may cause elevations of blood glucose, glycosuria, and alterations in glucose tolerance possibly as a result of hypokalemia.

Pharmacokinetics

■ **Absorption** In one study in patients with normal renal function, approximately 60% of a single 80-mg oral dose of furosemide was absorbed from the GI tract. When administered to fasting adults in this dosage, the drug appeared in the serum within 10 minutes, reached a peak concentration of 2.3 mcg/mL in 60–70 minutes, and was almost completely cleared from the serum in 4 hours. When the same dose was given after a meal, the serum concentration of furosemide increased slowly to a peak of about 1 mcg/mL after 2 hours and similar concentrations were present 4 hours after ingestion. However, a similar diuretic response occurred regardless of whether the drug was given with food or to fasting patients. In another study, the rate and extent of absorption varied considerably when 1 g of furosemide was given orally to uremic patients. An average of 76% of a dose was absorbed, and peak plasma concentrations were achieved within 2–9 hours (average 4.4 hours). Serum concentrations required to produce maximum diuresis are not known, and it has been reported that the magnitude of response does not correlate with either the peak or the mean serum concentrations.

The diuretic effect of orally administered furosemide is apparent within 30 minutes to 1 hour and is maximal in the first or second hour. The duration of action is usually 6–8 hours. The maximum hypotensive effect may not be apparent until several days after furosemide therapy is begun. After IV administration of furosemide, diuresis occurs within 5 minutes, reaches a maximum within 20–60 minutes, and persists for approximately 2 hours. After IM administration, peak plasma concentrations are attained within 30 minutes; onset of diuresis occurs somewhat later than after IV administration. In patients with severely impaired renal function, the diuretic response may be prolonged.

■ **Distribution** Only limited information is available on the distribution of furosemide. The drug crosses the placenta and is distributed into milk.

Furosemide is approximately 95% bound to plasma proteins in both normal and azotemic patients.

■ **Elimination** Plasma concentrations of furosemide decline in a biphasic manner. Various investigators have reported a wide range of elimination half-lives for furosemide. In one study, the elimination half-life averaged about 30 minutes in healthy patients who received 20–120 mg of the drug IV. In another study, the elimination half-life averaged 9.7 hours in patients with advanced renal failure who received 1 g of furosemide IV. The elimination half-life was more prolonged in 1 patient with concomitant liver disease.

In patients with normal renal function, a small amount of furosemide is metabolized in the liver to the defurfurylated derivative, 4-chloro-5-sulfamoylanthranilic acid. Furosemide and its metabolite are rapidly excreted in urine by glomerular filtration and by secretion from the proximal tubule. In patients with normal renal function, approximately 50% of an oral dose and 80% of an IV or IM dose are excreted in urine within 24 hours; 69–97% of these amounts is excreted in the first 4 hours. The remainder of the drug is eliminated by nonrenal mechanisms including degradation in the liver and excretion of unchanged drug in the feces. In patients with marked renal impairment without liver disease, nonrenal clearance of furosemide is increased so that up to 98% of the drug is removed from the plasma within 24 hours. One patient with uremia and hepatic cirrhosis eliminated only 58% of an IV dose in 24 hours. Furosemide is not removed by hemodialysis.

Chemistry and Stability

■ **Chemistry** Furosemide is a sulfonamide-type, loop diuretic. The drug occurs as a white to slightly yellow, odorless, crystalline powder with a pK_a of 3.9. Furosemide is insoluble in dilute acids, practically insoluble in water, sparingly soluble in alcohol, and freely soluble in alkali hydroxides.

Furosemide injection, a nonpyrogenic, sterile solution of the drug, contains the sodium salt of furosemide which is formed *in situ* by the addition of sodium hydroxide during the manufacturing process. The injection contains 0.162 mEq of sodium per mL and has a pH of 8–9.3.

■ **Stability** Furosemide injection should be stored at a temperature of 15–30°C and protected from light; injections having a yellow color should not be used. Exposure of furosemide tablets to light may cause discoloration; discolored tablets should not be dispensed. Furosemide tablets should be stored and dispensed in well-closed, light-resistant containers at a controlled room temperature of 15–30°C.. Commercially available 40-mg furosemide tablets have an expiration date of 5 years and the commercially available injection has an expiration date 42 months following the date of manufacture. The 20-mg tablets do not have a specific expiration dating period. Furosemide oral solutions should be stored at 15–30°C and protected from light and freezing; once opened, unused portions of the oral solution should be discarded after the time period recommended by the manufacturer.

Furosemide injection usually can be mixed with weakly alkaline and neutral solutions having a pH of 7–10, such as 0.9% sodium chloride injection or Ringer's injection, and with some weakly acidic solutions having a low buffer capacity. The injection should *not* be mixed with strongly acidic solutions (i.e., pH less than 5.5), such as those containing ascorbic acid, tetracycline, epinephrine, or norepinephrine, because furosemide may be precipitated. In addition, furosemide may precipitate at pH less than 7 and should not be used with certain drugs (e.g., amrinone, ciprofloxacin, labetalol, milrinone). Other drugs which should not be mixed with furosemide injection include most salts of organic bases including local anesthetics, alkaloids, antihistamines, hypnotics, meperidine, and morphine. Specialized references should be consulted for specific compatibility information.

Preparations

Excipients in commercially available drug preparations may have clinically important effects in some individuals; consult specific product labeling for details.

Furosemide

Oral		
Solution	40 mg/5 mL*	**Furosemide Solution**
	10 mg/mL*	**Furosemide Solution**
Tablets	20 mg*	**Furosemide Tablets**
		Lasix®, Sanofi-Aventis
	40 mg*	**Furosemide Tablets**
		Lasix® (scored), Sanofi-Aventis
	80 mg*	**Furosemide Tablets**
		Lasix®, Sanofi-Aventis
Parenteral		
Injection	10 mg/mL*	**Furosemide Injection**

*available from one or more manufacturer, distributor, and/or repackager by generic (nonproprietary) name

†Use is not currently included in the labeling approved by the US Food and Drug Administration

Torsemide

Torasemide

■ Torsemide is a sulfonamide, loop-type diuretic and antihypertensive agent.

Uses

■ **Edema** Torsemide is used for the management of edema associated with heart failure or hepatic or renal disease. Most experts state that all patients with symptomatic heart failure who have evidence for, or a history of, fluid retention generally should receive diuretic therapy in conjunction with moderate sodium restriction, an agent to inhibit the renin-angiotensin-aldosterone (RAA) system (e.g., angiotensin-converting enzyme [ACE] inhibitor, angiotensin II receptor antagonist, angiotensin receptor-neprilysin inhibitor [ARNI]), a β-adrenergic blocking agent (β-blocker), and in selected patients, an aldosterone antagonist. For additional information on the use of loop diuretics in the management of edema associated with heart failure, see Heart Failure under Uses: Edema, in Bumetanide, Ethacrynic Acid, and Furosemide 40:28.08.

■ **Hypertension** Torsemide is used alone or in combination with other classes of antihypertensive agents for the management of hypertension. Because of established clinical benefits (e.g., reductions in overall mortality and in adverse cardiovascular, cerebrovascular, and renal outcomes), current evidence-based practice guidelines for the management of hypertension in adults generally recommend the use of drugs from 4 classes of antihypertensive agents (ACE inhibitors, angiotensin II receptor antagonists, calcium-channel blockers, and thiazide diuretics). (See Uses: Hypertension in Adults, in the Thiazides General Statement 40:28.20.) However, some experts state that loop diuretics (e.g., bumetanide, furosemide, torsemide) are preferred over thiazides in patients with moderate to severe chronic kidney disease (CKD) or symptomatic heart failure. Loop diuretics may be particularly useful in patients with heart failure and reduced left ventricular ejection fraction (LVEF) who have evidence of fluid retention; however, some experts state that thiazide diuretics may be considered in hypertensive patients with heart failure and mild fluid retention because of their more persistent antihypertensive effect.

For further information on the role of diuretics in antihypertensive drug therapy and information on overall principles and expert recommendations for treatment of hypertension, see Uses: Hypertension in Adults, and also see Uses: Hypertension in Pediatric Patients, in the Thiazides General Statement 40:28.20.

Dosage and Administration

■ **Administration** Torsemide usually is administered orally. Food decreases the rate but not the extent of GI absorption, and the manufacturers state that the drug may be administered without regard to meals.

Torsemide also may be given by IV injection when a rapid onset of diuresis is desired or when oral therapy is not practical. IV injections of torsemide should be administered slowly over 2 minutes ("bolus"); alternatively, the drug may be administered as a continuous IV infusion.

If torsemide injection is administered through an IV line, it is recommended that the IV line be flushed with 0.9% sodium chloride injection before and after the drug is administered. Because the pH of torsemide injection exceeds 8.3, flushing is necessary to avoid potential incompatibilities that may result from differences in pH.

For administration of torsemide as a continuous IV infusion, 200 mg of the drug may be diluted in 250 mL of 5% dextrose or 0.9% sodium chloride injection or in 500 mL of 0.45% sodium chloride injection; alternatively, 50 mg of torsemide may be diluted in 500 mL of 5% dextrose, 0.9% sodium chloride injection, or 0.45% sodium chloride injection. Following dilution in these solutions in plastic containers, the drug is stable for up to 24 hours at room temperature.

■ **Dosage** The manufacturers state that since oral and IV doses of torsemide are therapeutically equivalent, torsemide dosage is identical for oral or IV administration.

For the management of fluid retention (e.g., edema) associated with heart failure, experts state that diuretics should be administered at a dosage sufficient to achieve optimal volume status and relieve congestion without inducing an excessively rapid reduction in intravascular volume, which could result in hypotension, renal dysfunction, or both.

Safety and efficacy of torsemide in children have not been established.

Edema For the management of edema associated with heart failure, the usual initial adult oral or IV dosage of torsemide is 10–20 mg daily, given as a single dose. If the diuretic response is inadequate, dosage can be titrated upward by approximately doubling the daily dose until the desired response is attained. The manufacturers state that single doses exceeding 200 mg have not been adequately studied. Some experts recommend initiating torsemide at a low dosage (10–20 mg once daily) and increasing the dosage (maximum of 200 mg daily) until urine output increases and weight decreases, generally by 0.5–1 kg daily.

Hypertension For the management of hypertension, the usual initial adult dosage of torsemide recommended by the manufacturers is 5 mg once daily. If a satisfactory lowering of blood pressure does not occur within 4–6 weeks, dosage of torsemide may be increased to 10 mg once daily. Some experts state that the usual dosage of torsemide is 5–10 mg once daily. If a satisfactory lowering of blood pressure does not occur when 10 mg is administered daily, other antihypertensive agents should be added to the regimen.

Monitoring and Blood Pressure Treatment Goals. The patient's renal function and electrolytes should be assessed 2–4 weeks after initiation of diuretic therapy. Blood pressure should be monitored regularly (i.e., monthly) during therapy and dosage of the antihypertensive drug adjusted until blood pressure is controlled. If an adequate blood pressure response is not achieved, the dosage may be increased or another antihypertensive agent with demonstrated benefit and preferably with a complementary mechanism of action (e.g., angiotensin-converting enzyme [ACE] inhibitor, angiotensin II receptor antagonist, calcium-channel blocker) may be added; if target blood pressure is still not achieved, a third drug may be added. (See Uses: Hypertension in Adults, in the Thiazides General Statement 40:28.20.) In patients who develop unacceptable adverse effects with torsemide, the drug should be discontinued and another antihypertensive agent from a different pharmacologic class should be initiated.

The goal of hypertension management and prevention is to achieve and maintain optimal control of blood pressure. However, the optimum blood pressure threshold for initiating antihypertensive drug therapy and specific treatment goals remain controversial. A 2017 multidisciplinary hypertension guideline from the American College of Cardiology (ACC), American Heart Association (AHA), and a number of other professional organizations generally recommends a blood pressure goal of less than 130/80 mm Hg in all adults, regardless of comorbidities or level of atherosclerotic cardiovascular disease (ASCVD) risk. Many patients will require at least 2 drugs from different pharmacologic classes to achieve this blood pressure goal; the potential benefits of hypertension management and drug cost, adverse effects, and risks associated with the use of multiple antihypertensive drugs also should be considered when deciding a patient's blood pressure treatment goal.

For additional information on target levels of blood pressure and on monitoring therapy, see Blood Pressure Monitoring and Treatment Goals under Dosage: Hypertension, in Dosage and Administration in the Thiazides General Statement 40:28.20.

■ **Dosage in Renal and Hepatic Impairment** For the management of edema in patients with chronic renal failure, the usual initial adult oral or IV dosage of torsemide is 20 mg daily, given as a single dose. If the diuretic response is inadequate, dosage may be titrated upward by doubling the dose until desired response is attained. However, the manufacturers state that single doses exceeding 200 mg or chronic use in patients with renal impairment have not been adequately studied.

For the management of edema in patients with hepatic cirrhosis, torsemide is administered concomitantly with an aldosterone antagonist or a potassium-sparing diuretic; the usual initial adult oral or IV dosage of torsemide is 5–10 mg daily, given as a single dose. If the diuretic response to this initial dosage is inadequate, dosage may be titrated upward by doubling the dose until the desired response is attained. Single doses exceeding 40 mg have not been adequately studied in patients with hepatic cirrhosis.

Description

Torsemide is a sulfonamide-type, loop diuretic.

SumMon® (see Users Guide). For additional information on this drug until a more detailed monograph is developed and published, the manufacturer's labeling should be consulted. It is *essential* that the labeling be consulted for detailed information on the usual cautions, precautions, and contraindications.

Preparations

Excipients in commercially available drug preparations may have clinically important effects in some individuals; consult specific product labeling for details.

Torsemide

Oral		
Tablets 5 mg*		**Demadex®**, Roche
		Torsemide Tablets
10 mg*		**Demadex®** (scored), Roche
		Torsemide Tablets
20 mg*		**Demadex®** (scored), Roche
		Torsemide Tablets
100 mg*		**Demadex®** (scored), Roche
		Torsemide Tablets
Parenteral		
Injection, for IV use	10 mg/mL*	**Torsemide Injection**

*available from one or more manufacturer, distributor, and/or repackager by generic (nonproprietary) name

OSMOTIC DIURETICS 40:28.12

Mannitol

■ Mannitol is an osmotic diuretic.

Uses

■ **Oliguric Acute Renal Failure** In conjunction with adequate replacement of water and electrolytes and maintenance of normal blood pressure, mannitol is used to promote diuresis for the prevention and/or treatment of the oliguric phase of acute renal failure which may occur after massive hemorrhage, trauma, shock, burns, transfusion reactions caused by mismatched blood, or major surgery. The drug may prevent or reverse acute functional renal failure before there is evidence of tubular necrosis or multiple vascular thrombosis; however, mannitol has no effect and may be harmful if used after tubular necrosis and irreversible renal failure become established.

Mannitol has been used during cardiovascular surgical procedures, including open heart surgery and surgery to correct aortic aneurysms. Use of the drug may prevent hemoglobin buildup during cardiopulmonary bypass procedures. Mannitol has been used to protect renal function in patients with poor renal function undergoing various surgical procedures such as nephrolithotomy or renal artery surgery; however, the drug does not permit prolonging the time of occlusion and renal ischemia during renovascular reconstructive surgery. The drug has also been recommended for use during abdominal surgery or other major surgery, especially in jaundiced patients who appear to be particularly susceptible to postoperative renal failure. In one study, mannitol prevented azotemia, but not systemic acidosis, caused by amphotericin B in 4 patients being treated for systemic fungal infections following kidney transplantation.

■ **Reduction of Intracranial Pressure** Mannitol is used prior to and during neurosurgery to reduce greatly increased intracranial pressure and for the treatment of cerebral edema. The drug is especially indicated when there is evidence of herniation and developing brainstem compression. A rebound increase in intracranial pressure may occur approximately 12 hours after osmotic diuresis is employed; however, this occurs less frequently with mannitol than with urea. Mannitol is also useful for the early treatment of cerebral edema in patients with diabetic ketoacidosis or in patients in hypoglycemic coma who fail to respond to increases in blood glucose concentrations. Mannitol has also been used to reduce edema in the traumatized area of the spinal cord prior to corrective surgery.

■ **Reduction of Intraocular Pressure** Mannitol is used to reduce elevated intraocular pressure when the pressure cannot be lowered by other means. The drug is especially useful for treating acute episodes of angle-closure, absolute, or secondary glaucoma and for lowering intraocular pressure prior to intraocular surgery. Mannitol may be of value in those cases of cataract extraction in which vitreous loss is likely. Unlike urea, mannitol does not penetrate the eye and may be used when irritation is present.

■ **Other Uses** Mannitol is used alone or with other diuretics such as furosemide or ethacrynic acid to promote the urinary excretion of toxins such as aspirin or other salicylates, some barbiturates, bromides, or imipramine as an adjunct to usual treatment regimens in patients with severe intoxications. Continuous infusion of mannitol in some cases of drug poisoning has reduced the period of unconsciousness and maintained urine flow. Renal lesions caused by inhalation or ingestion of carbon tetrachloride may possibly be prevented by early treatment with mannitol. Unlike many other diuretics, mannitol increases the urinary excretion of lithium and may be useful for the treatment of lithium intoxication. The drug has also been used to promote excretion of uric acid and prevent hyperuricemia and/or uric acid nephropathy in patients who develop uricemia following chemotherapy or radiation therapy for leukemia or lymphoma. Concomitant administration of sodium bicarbonate may be needed to alkalinize the urine in the treatment of salicylate or barbiturate poisonings or uricemia. Mannitol has also been found useful in treating carbon monoxide poisoning and ethylene glycol intoxication.

There is limited evidence that mannitol may be useful in the management of ciguatera fish poisoning, but additional study and experience are necessary. Although the mechanism(s) of action is not known, the drug appeared to reverse neurologic and neurosensory manifestations of such poisoning as well as GI manifestations in a limited number of patients. No specific antidote for ciguatera fish poisoning has been identified to date, and treatment remains supportive and symptomatic; therefore, pending further accumulation of data, some clinicians suggest that use of mannitol (e.g., 1 g/kg by IV infusion) be considered for initial therapy, combined with other supportive therapy as necessary, in patients with clinically important manifestations of such poisoning.

Mannitol has been used alone or in conjunction with other diuretics to promote diuresis for the supportive treatment of edema and ascites of nephrotic, cirrhotic, or cardiac origin. The drug may also be useful to relieve the symptoms and congestion of pulmonary edema caused by bronchopneumonia. Mannitol may be indicated when thiazides or other diuretics that act by inhibiting transport mechanisms fail because of decreased glomerular filtration rate caused by shock, dehydration, or trauma or when further depression of renal function produced by other diuretics is contraindicated. However, mannitol diuresis offers only symptomatic relief of edema and is independent of and has no effect on the underlying disease process. IV therapy with mannitol is impractical for the treatment of chronic edema. Use of the drug requires larger volumes of fluid to be administered than do other osmotic diuretics; however, unlike dextrose, it is not contraindicated for use in diabetic patients and it causes less local irritation and necrosis than does urea.

Mannitol is also used as an irrigating solution in transurethral prostatic resection. Use of the drug minimizes the hemolytic effects of water, the entrance of hemolyzed blood into the circulation, and the resulting hemoglobinemia which is considered a major factor in producing serious renal complications. In addition, mannitol has been administered IV before, during and after transurethral prostatectomy to maintain urine output, promote rapid excretion of absorbed irrigants, and reduce the need for postoperative irrigation.

Mannitol has been administered by intra-amniotic instillation in attempts to terminate pregnancy; however, the drug has been reported to have a high failure rate and therefore to be unreliable for this purpose.

For the use of mannitol to measure glomerular filtration rate, see Mannitol 36:40.

Dosage and Administration

■ **Administration** Mannitol injections are administered by IV infusion. An administration set with a filter should be used for infusion of injections containing 20% or more, since mannitol crystals may be present. For transurethral prostatic resection, mannitol irrigation solutions are instilled into the bladder via an indwelling urethral catheter.

■ **Dosage** The dosage, concentration of solution, and rate of administration of mannitol vary with the condition being treated and the patient's fluid requirements, urinary output, and response to the drug.

Test Dose Patients with marked oliguria or suspected inadequate renal function should receive a dose of about 0.2 g/kg or 12.5 g as a 15 or 20% solution infused over a period of 3–5 minutes to test renal response before mannitol therapy is initiated. A response is considered adequate if at least 30–50 mL of urine per hour is excreted over the next 2–3 hours. If an adequate response is not attained, a second test dose may be given. If a satisfactory response is not obtained after the second test dose, the patient should be re-evaluated and mannitol should not be used.

Oliguric Acute Renal Failure For the prevention of oliguria or acute renal failure, 50–100 g of mannitol may be given. Generally, a concentrated solution of the drug is given initially followed by a 5 or 10% solution. When used prophylactically in surgical procedures, administration of the drug may be initiated before or immediately following surgery and may be continued postoperatively. When mannitol was used to reduce nephrotoxicity caused by amphotericin B, 12.5 g of mannitol was administered immediately before and after each dose of amphotericin B. For the treatment of oliguria, 100 g of mannitol is usually given as a 15 or 20% solution over 90 minutes to several hours.

Reduction of Intracranial or Intraocular Pressure To reduce intracranial pressure and brain mass, and to lower elevated intraocular pressure, the usual dose of mannitol is 1.5–2 g/kg administered as a 15, 20, or 25% solution over a period of 30–60 minutes. Some clinicians have recommended as little as 1 g or as much as 3.2 g/kg to lower intraocular pressure. When used preoperatively, the drug should be administered 1–1.5 hours prior to surgery in order to achieve maximum reduction of pressure before surgery.

Other Parenteral Uses To promote diuresis in the adjunctive treatment of severe drug intoxications, various mannitol regimens have been used. In general, a urinary output of at least 100 mL/hour, but preferably 500 mL/hour, and a positive fluid balance of 1–2 L should be maintained. Some clinicians recommend an initial loading dose of 25 g, followed by infusion of a solution at a rate that will maintain a urinary output of at least 100 mL/hour. In barbiturate poisoning, an initial dose of 0.5 g/kg, followed by administration of a 5 or 10% solution at a rate to maintain the desired urine output, has been recommended. Alternatively, it has been recommended that 1 L of a 10% solution be given during the first hour. Urine volume and pH should be measured and cumulative fluid balance calculated at the end of the first hour and subsequent 2-hour periods. If positive fluid balance remains at 1–2 L, another liter of 10% mannitol may be given over the next 2 hours. If positive fluid balance falls below 1 L, mannitol should be replaced with 1 L of ⅙ *M* sodium lactate over the next 2 hours (if urine pH is less than 7) or 1 L of 0.9% sodium chloride over 2 hours (if urine pH is greater than 7). If the positive fluid balance is more than 2 L, 10% mannitol may be given at the slowest possible rate. IV administration of furosemide was recommended if the positive fluid balance exceeded 2.5 L. For the treatment of uricemia, 50 g/m^2 has been given in 24 hours.

As a diuretic for the adjunctive treatment of edema and ascites, 100 g of mannitol may be infused as a 10–20% solution over a period of 2–6 hours.

Transurethral Prostatic Resection Solutions containing 2.5–5% mannitol are used as irrigating solutions in transurethral prostatic resection. One limited study indicates that mannitol concentrations of at least 3.5% are necessary to prevent hemolysis.

Pediatric Dosage Mannitol dosage requirements for patients 12 years of age and younger have not been established. However, some clinicians have suggested the following dosages for pediatric patients. In oliguria or anuria, a test dose of 0.2 g/kg or 6 g/m^2 may be given as a single dose over 3–5 minutes. For therapeutic purposes, 2 g/kg or 60 g/m^2 may be given. For the treatment of edema and ascites, this dose may be given as a 15 or 20% solution over 2–6 hours. To reduce cerebral or ocular edema, the dose may be given as a 15 or 20% solution over 30–60 minutes. For the treatment of intoxications, the drug may be given as a 5 or 10% solution as needed.

Cautions

■ **Effects on Fluids and Electrolytes** The most severe adverse effects encountered during mannitol therapy are fluid and electrolyte imbalance. Accumulation of mannitol caused by inadequate urinary output or to rapid administration of large doses may result in overexpansion of extracellular fluid. The resulting circulatory overload may result in pulmonary edema, signs and symptoms of water intoxication, and fulminating congestive heart failure, especially in patients with diminished cardiac reserve. Overhydration may be corrected by hemodialysis or administration of a potent diuretic (e.g., furosemide).

Electrolyte imbalance, in some cases severe enough to alter acid-base balance or depress respiration, may result from mannitol-induced diuresis. Hyponatremia or hypernatremia and hypokalemia or hyperkalemia may occur. The shift of sodium-free intracellular fluid into extracellular spaces may result in dilutional lowering of serum sodium concentrations and may cause hyponatremia or aggravate preexisting hyponatremia. Hyponatremia may be accompanied by tremor or seizures and may result in death. Loss of water in excess of sodium, as may occur during prolonged therapy with mannitol, may result in hypernatremia and hyperosmolality. A natriuretic agent such as a thiazide may be administered concomitantly if this occurs.

■ **Nervous System Effects** Symptoms of CNS toxicity have occurred in 3 patients with acute renal failure who received 25 g of mannitol every 12 hours for at least 36 hours. When large doses of mannitol are administered, especially in the presence of acidosis, the drug may cross the blood-brain barrier and interfere with the ability of the brain to maintain CSF pH. Cerebral dessication may also occur, and the mechanisms that protect the brain from the effects of systemic acidosis may be disrupted. CNS damage may result, and death has occurred in patients with organic CNS disease who received mannitol.

■ **Other Adverse Effects** Other adverse effects that have occurred during mannitol therapy include acidosis, dryness of the mouth, thirst, urinary retention, headache, blurred vision, uricosuria, nausea, vomiting, rhinitis, arm pain, backache, thrombophlebitis, chills, dizziness, urticaria, hypotension, hypertension, tachycardia, fever, transient muscle rigidity, and angina-like chest pain.

Vacuolar nephrosis, possibly irreversible, has occurred during administration of mannitol. Reversible, acute oligoanuric renal failure has occurred in several patients with normal pretreatment renal function who received large IV dosages (400–900 g daily) of mannitol for the reduction of intracranial or intraocular pressure; the mechanism of this effect has not been fully elucidated. Urine output and glomerular filtration rate declined abruptly in these patients but returned toward or exceeded normal within several days after discontinuance of mannitol; one patient underwent ultrafiltration and hemodialysis.

Extravasation of mannitol should be avoided, since local edema and skin necrosis may result. In a patient with a history of allergies, mannitol caused a severe allergic reaction and anaphylaxis which responded to treatment with epinephrine hydrochloride. Intraocular hemorrhage has also occurred but could not be definitely attributed to mannitol.

■ **Precautions and Contraindications** Mannitol should not be administered until the adequacy of the patient's renal function and urine flow has been established. A test dose may be employed for this purpose. (See Dosage and Administration: Dosage.) In patients with shock with oliguria and rising BUN, mannitol should not be administered until fluids, plasma, blood, and electrolytes have been replaced. The cardiovascular status of the patient should also be carefully evaluated prior to mannitol administration.

Renal function, urine output, fluid balance, serum sodium and potassium concentrations, and central venous pressure should be monitored during mannitol administration. If urine output continues to decline, the patient's clinical status should be reviewed and mannitol discontinued if necessary. If central venous pressure rises or there is any other evidence of circulatory overload, the infusion should be slowed or stopped. Fluid administration should not exceed 1 L/day in excess of urinary output. The sustained diuresis caused by mannitol may obscure and intensify inadequate hydration or hypovolemia. Tissue dehydration may occur, especially when urine output is less than 40 mL/minute, and may lead to coma. Hypovolemia reduces glomerular filtration rate and enhances the reabsorption of sodium and water, thus promoting oliguria. In addition, preexisting hemoconcentration may be intensified.

Mannitol is not a substitute for fluid and electrolyte therapy, and homeostasis should be maintained by hydration and electrolyte therapy. Volume and electrolyte depletion may be prevented or treated by administering dilute mannitol solutions with sodium chloride added or by alternating each liter of mannitol solution with a liter of sodium chloride injection to which 40 mEq of potassium chloride has been added. If the threat of renal shutdown exists, potassium supplementation should be administered subsequent to, but not concomitantly with, mannitol.

Mannitol is contraindicated in patients with well established anuria caused by severe renal disease or impaired renal function who do not respond to a test dose. (See Dosage and Administration: Dosage.) The drug is also contraindicated in patients with severe pulmonary congestion, frank pulmonary edema, severe congestive heart disease, severe dehydration, metabolic edema associated with capillary fragility or membrane permeability and not due to renal, cardiac or hepatic disease, or active intracranial bleeding except during craniotomy. Mannitol is contraindicated for further use when progressive renal disease or dysfunction, including increasing oliguria and azotemia, or progressive heart failure or pulmonary congestion occur after institution of mannitol therapy. Electrolyte-free mannitol solutions should not be given concomitantly with blood. If blood must be given simultaneously with mannitol, at least 20 mEq of sodium chloride should be added to each liter of mannitol solution to avoid pseudoagglutination.

■ **Pregnancy and Fertility** Animal reproduction studies have not been performed with mannitol. It is also not known whether mannitol can caused fetal harm when administered to pregnant women. Mannitol should be used during pregnancy only when clearly needed.

It is not known whether mannitol affects fertility in humans.

Drug Interactions

Because mannitol increases urinary excretion of lithium, patients being treated with lithium should be observed for possible impairment of response to that drug if they receive mannitol.

Laboratory Test Interferences

In addition to alterations in laboratory test values resulting from mannitol-induced electrolyte changes, the drug may affect the results of other tests. Determinations of inorganic phosphorus blood concentrations are interfered with by use of the drug; values may be increased or decreased. Mannitol will also interfere with laboratory determinations of blood ethylene glycol concentrations, because both substances are oxidized to an aldehyde during the test procedure.

Pharmacology

IV administration of mannitol induces diuresis mainly by elevating the osmotic pressure of the glomerular filtrate to such an extent that the tubular reabsorption of water and solutes is hindered. For mannitol to be effective, enough renal blood flow and glomerular filtration must exist to enable the drug to reach the tubules. Increased renal blood flow resulting from dilation of vascular segments between the renal artery and glomeruli, lowered renal vascular resistance, and reduced blood viscosity may also contribute to the diuretic effect of the drug. Mannitol promotes the excretion of sodium; however, proportionately more water than sodium is excreted. Excretion of potassium, chloride, calcium, phosphorus, lithium, magnesium, urea, and uric acid is also increased during mannitol-induced diuresis. The drug protects the kidneys from nephrotoxins by preventing toxins from becoming concentrated in the tubular fluid.

Mannitol may prevent or reverse acute functional renal failure by reversing the acute reductions in renal blood flow, glomerular filtration rate, urine flow, and sodium excretion which may occur after trauma. However, the drug must exert its effect before decreases in filtration rate and renal blood flow produce tubular damage, interstitial edema, and/or diffuse ischemia.

The osmotic effect of mannitol causes water to be drawn from cells to extracellular fluid and from erythrocytes cells to plasma. As a result, extracellular fluid volume, plasma volume, and circulation time are increased and extracellular stores of sodium are diluted. Cellular dehydration may result. Plasma pH is decreased. Erythrocyte volume becomes more concentrated and hematocrit is decreased. The fluid shifts caused by the drug result in reduction of cerebral edema by a reduction in brain mass and in the lowering of elevated CSF pressure. However, a rebound increase in intracranial pressure may occur approximately 12 hours after the administration of mannitol. Fluids are also withdrawn from the anterior chamber of the eye, resulting in a reduction of elevated intraocular pressure.

When administered orally, mannitol causes profound osmotic diarrhea, resulting in a loss of fluid, sodium, and potassium. Serum sodium concentrations are increased, but serum potassium and blood urea concentrations are reduced.

Pharmacokinetics

■ **Absorption** Although mannitol has been thought not to be absorbed when administered orally, one study revealed that about 17% of an oral dose of radiolabeled drug was excreted unchanged in urine.

Diuresis may occur within 1–3 hours after IV administration of mannitol. Lowering of elevated intraocular pressure occurs within 30–60 minutes and persists for 4–6 hours. Elevated CSF pressure may be reduced within 15 minutes after starting an infusion of mannitol, and the effect may last for 3–8 hours after the infusion is stopped.

■ **Distribution** When administered IV, mannitol remains confined to the extracellular compartment. The drug does not cross the blood-brain barrier unless very high concentrations are present in the plasma or the patient has acidosis. Unlike urea, mannitol does not penetrate the eye.

■ **Elimination** Mannitol is metabolized only very slightly, if at all, to glycogen in the liver. The drug is freely filtered by the glomeruli, with less than 10% tubular reabsorption; it is not secreted by tubular cells. The elimination half-life in adults is about 100 minutes. Approximately 80% of a 100-g dose is excreted unchanged in urine within 3 hours. When large dose are given as in forced diuresis, retention of the drug may occur. In the presence of renal disease in which glomerular function is impaired or in conditions that impair small vessel circulation, such as congestive heart failure, cirrhosis with ascitic accumulation, shock, or dehydration, mannitol clearance is lower than normal.

Chemistry and Stability

■ **Chemistry** Mannitol, a hexahydroxy alcohol chemically related to mannose, is an osmotic diuretic. Mannitol occurs as a white, crystalline powder or free-flowing granules with a sweet taste. The drug is very slightly soluble in alcohol and has a solubility of approximately 182 mg/mL in water at 25°C. Commercially available mannitol injections have a pH of 4.5–7.

The approximate osmolarities of mannitol solutions are as follows:

% Mannitol	mOsm/L
5	275
10	550
15	825
20	1100
25	1375

■ **Stability** Mannitol solutions should be stored at 15–30°C and protected from freezing. Solutions of mannitol are chemically stable but, in concentrations of 15% and more, mannitol may crystallize when exposed to low temperatures. If crystallization occurs, the solution should be autoclaved or warmed by immersing the container in hot water (approximately 60°C) and periodically shaking vigorously. The solution should be cooled to body temperature before administration. If all crystals cannot be completely dissolved, the solution should not be used. The addition of potassium or sodium chloride to mannitol solutions of 20% concentration or greater may cause precipitation of mannitol. Mannitol should not be added to whole blood for transfusion.

Preparations

Excipients in commercially available drug preparations may have clinically important effects in some individuals; consult specific product labeling for details.

Mannitol

Powder

Parenteral

Injection	5%*	**Mannitol Injection**
		Osmitrol®, Baxter
	10%*	**Mannitol Injection**
		Osmitrol®, Baxter
	15%*	**Mannitol Injection**
		Osmitrol®, Baxter
	20%*	**Mannitol Injection**
		Osmitrol®, Baxter
	25%*	**Mannitol Injection**

*available from one or more manufacturer, distributor, and/or repackager by generic (nonproprietary) name

Mannitol Combinations

Urogenital

Solution	0.54% with Sorbitol 2.7%*	**Sorbitol-Mannitol Irrigating Solution**

*available from one or more manufacturer, distributor, and/or repackager by generic (nonproprietary) name

POTASSIUM-SPARING DIURETICS 40:28.16

Triamterene

■ Triamterene is a potassium-sparing diuretic.

Uses

■ **Edema** Triamterene is used in the management of edema associated with heart failure, cirrhosis of the liver, or the nephrotic syndrome, as well as in the management of steroid-induced edema, idiopathic edema, and edema caused by secondary hyperaldosteronism. Careful etiologic diagnosis should precede the use of any diuretic. Triamterene should not be used alone as initial therapy in severe heart failure since its maximum therapeutic effect may occur slowly. However, it may be used in combined initial therapy with more effective, rapidly acting diuretics such as thiazides, chlorthalidone, furosemide, or ethacrynic acid or after rapid initial diuresis has been achieved by other means.

Triamterene may be particularly useful in patients excreting excessive amounts of potassium (especially those who cannot tolerate potassium supplements) and for those in whom potassium loss could be detrimental, such as digitalized patients or those with myasthenia gravis. Triamterene promotes increased diuresis when patients prove resistant or only partially responsive to thiazides or other diuretics because of secondary hyperaldosteronism. Unlike spironolactone, the effectiveness of triamterene is independent of aldosterone concentrations; therefore, triamterene may be effective in some patients unresponsive to spironolactone. Although triamterene is effective alone, its chief value lies in combined therapy with other diuretics that act at different sites in the nephron. Some patients resistant to triamterene alone may respond to combined therapy with a thiazide diuretic, furosemide, ethacrynic acid, or chlorthalidone. Triamterene decreases potassium excretion caused by kaliuretic diuretics.

Heart Failure Triamterene generally is used concomitantly with other more effective, rapidly acting diuretics (e.g., thiazides, chlorthalidone, loop diuretics) in the management of edema associated with heart failure. Most experts state that all patients with symptomatic heart failure who have evidence for, or a history of, fluid retention generally should receive diuretic therapy in conjunction with moderate sodium restriction, an agent to inhibit the renin-angiotensin-aldosterone (RAA) system (e.g., angiotensin-converting enzyme [ACE] inhibitor, angiotensin II receptor antagonist, angiotensin receptor-neprilysin inhibitor [ARNI]), a β-adrenergic blocking agent (β-blocker) and in selected patients, an aldosterone antagonist. Some experts state that because of limited and inconsistent data, it is difficult to make precise recommendations regarding daily sodium intake and whether it should vary with respect to the type of heart failure (e.g., reduced versus preserved ejection fraction), disease severity (e.g., New York Heart Association [NYHA] class), heart failure-related comorbidities (e.g., renal dysfunction), or other patient characteristics (e.g., age, race). The American College of Cardiology Foundation (ACCF) and American Heart Association (AHA) state that limiting sodium intake to 1.5 g daily in patients with ACCF/AHA stage A or B heart failure may be reasonable. While data currently are lacking to support recommendation of a specific level of sodium intake in patients with ACCF/AHA stage C or D heart failure, ACCF and AHA state that limiting sodium intake to some degree (e.g., less than 3 g daily) in such patients may be considered for symptom improvement.

Diuretics play a key role in the management of heart failure because they produce symptomatic benefits more rapidly than any other drugs, relieving pulmonary and peripheral edema within hours or days compared with weeks or months for cardiac glycosides, ACE inhibitors, or β-blockers. However, since there are no long-term studies of diuretic therapy in patients with heart failure, the effects of diuretics on morbidity and mortality in such patients are not known. Although there are patients with heart failure who do not exhibit fluid retention in the absence of diuretic therapy and even may develop severe volume depletion with low doses of diuretics, such patients are rare and the unique pathophysiologic mechanisms regulating their fluid and electrolyte balance have not been elucidated.

Most experts state that loop diuretics (e.g., bumetanide, ethacrynic acid, furosemide, torsemide) are the diuretics of choice for most patients with heart failure. However, thiazides may be preferred in some patients with concomitant hypertension because of their sustained antihypertensive effects. For additional information, see Heart Failure under Uses: Edema in the Thiazides General Statement 40:28.20.

■ **Hypertension** Triamterene has been used in the management of hypertension†. However, because of established clinical benefits (e.g., reductions in overall mortality and in adverse cardiovascular, cerebrovascular, and renal outcomes), current evidence-based practice guidelines for the management of hypertension in adults generally recommend the use of drugs from 4 classes of antihypertensive agents (ACE inhibitors, angiotensin II receptor antagonists, calcium-channel blockers, and thiazide diuretics). (See Uses: Hypertension in Adults, in the Thiazides General Statement 40:28.20.) Triamterene alone has little if any hypotensive effect; however, it may be used with another diuretic (e.g., hydrochlorothiazide) or a hypotensive agent in the management of mild to moderate hypertension. In the management of hypertension, triamterene is used principally in patients with diuretic-induced hypokalemia or to prevent hypokalemia in patients receiving diuretics and at risk of this adverse effect. Potassium-sparing diuretics should be avoided in patients with substantial renal insufficiency.

For additional information on overall principles and expert recommendations for treatment of hypertension, see Uses: Hypertension in Adults and also see Uses: Hypertension in Pediatric Patients, in the Thiazides General Statement 40:28.20.

Dosage and Administration

■ **Administration** Triamterene is administered orally. Triamterene has been administered IV†, but the poor solubility of the drug and acidity of the solutions make administration by this route extremely difficult and a parenteral dosage form currently is not available in the US.

■ **Dosage** Dosage of triamterene should be individualized according to the patient's requirements and response. It has been theorized that abrupt withdrawal of triamterene may result in rebound kaliuresis; therefore, the drug should be withdrawn gradually. Experts state that diuretics should be administered at a dosage sufficient to achieve optimal volume status and relieve congestion without inducing an excessively rapid reduction in intravascular volume, which could result in hypotension, renal dysfunction, or both.

Triamterene Therapy **Edema.** The usual initial adult dosage of triamterene in the management of edema is 100 mg twice daily after meals. Once edema is controlled, most patients can be maintained on 100 mg daily or every other day. Dosage should not exceed 300 mg daily. When triamterene is used in combination with other diuretics, the initial dosage of each drug should be lowered and adjusted to individual requirements and tolerance.

For the management of fluid retention (e.g., edema) associated with heart failure, some experts recommend initiating triamterene at a low dosage (e.g., 50–75 mg twice daily) and increasing the dosage (maximum of 200 mg daily) until urine output increases and weight decreases, generally by 0.5–1 kg daily.

Hypertension. When triamterene is used in the management of hypertension† in adults (usually in combination with a kaliuretic diuretic), some experts state that the usual dosage range is 50–100 mg daily given as a single dose or in 2 divided doses.

The patient's renal function and electrolytes should be assessed 2–4 weeks after initiation of diuretic therapy. Blood pressure should be monitored regularly (i.e., monthly) during therapy and dosage of the antihypertensive drug adjusted until blood pressure is controlled. If an adequate blood pressure response is not achieved, the dosage may be increased or another antihypertensive agent with demonstrated benefit and preferably with a complementary mechanism of action (e.g., angiotensin-converting enzyme [ACE] inhibitor, angiotensin II receptor antagonist, calcium-channel blocker) may be added; if target blood pressure is still not achieved, a third drug may be added. (See Uses: Hypertension.) In patients who develop unacceptable adverse effects with triamterene, the drug should be discontinued and another antihypertensive agent from a different pharmacologic class should be initiated.

The goal of hypertension management and prevention is to achieve and maintain optimal control of blood pressure. However, the optimum blood pressure threshold for initiating antihypertensive drug therapy and specific treatment goals remain controversial. A 2017 multidisciplinary hypertension guideline from the American College of Cardiology (ACC), American Heart Association (AHA), and a number of other professional organizations generally recommends a blood pressure goal of less than 130/80 mm Hg in all adults, regardless of comorbidities or level of atherosclerotic cardiovascular disease (ASCVD) risk. Many patients will require at least 2 drugs from different pharmacologic classes to achieve this blood pressure goal; the potential benefits of hypertension management and drug cost, adverse effects, and risks associated with the use of multiple antihypertensive drugs also should be considered when deciding a patient's blood pressure treatment goal.

For additional information on target levels of blood pressure and on monitoring therapy in the management of hypertension, see Blood Pressure Monitoring and Treatment Goals under Dosage: Hypertension, in Dosage and Administration in the Thiazides General Statement 40:28.20.

Triamterene/Hydrochlorothiazide Fixed-combination Therapy Commercially available preparations containing triamterene and hydrochlorothiazide in fixed combination generally should not be used as initial therapy, except in patients in whom the clinical consequences of potential thiazide-induced hypokalemia represent an important risk (e.g., patients receiving cardiac glycosides or patients with cardiac arrhythmias).

When Dyazide®, Maxzide® or Maxzide®-25 mg, or therapeutically equivalent formulations of the combination are used, the manufacturers state that the usual adult dosage in terms of triamterene is 37.5–75 mg once daily with appropriate monitoring of serum potassium concentrations. Patients who become hypokalemic while receiving hydrochlorothiazide 25 or 50 mg daily may be switched to a fixed-combination preparation containing triamterene in combination with the equivalent hydrochlorothiazide dosage. In patients who require hydrochlorothiazide and in whom hypokalemia cannot be risked, therapy with the fixed combination may be initiated at a triamterene dosage of 37.5 mg daily (with hydrochlorothiazide 25 mg daily). The manufacturers state that clinical experience with the fixed-combination tablets suggests that the risk of electrolyte imbalance and renal dysfunction may be increased when triamterene 75 mg daily (with hydrochlorothiazide 50 mg daily) is administered in 2 divided doses rather than as a single daily dose. The manufacturers also state that there is no clinical experience to date with dosages of these more bioavailable formulations exceeding 75 mg of triamterene and 50 mg of hydrochlorothiazide daily. (See Pharmacokinetics: Absorption.)

Pediatric Dosage The safety and efficacy of triamterene in children† have not been established; however, some clinicians suggest an initial dosage of 4 mg/kg daily or 115 mg/m² daily, given in two divided doses after meals. If necessary, dosage may be increased to 6 mg/kg daily; however, pediatric dosage should not exceed 300 mg daily. Dosage should be reduced if triamterene is used with other diuretics.

If triamterene is used for the management of hypertension in children†, some experts have recommended an initial triamterene dosage of 1–2 mg/kg daily given in 2 divided doses. Such experts have suggested that dosage may be increased as necessary up to 3–4 mg/kg (maximum 300 mg) daily given in 2 divided doses. For information on overall principles and expert recommendations for treatment of hypertension in pediatric patients, see Uses: Hypertension in Pediatric Patients, in the Thiazides General Statement 40:28.20.

Cautions

■ **Adverse Effects** In general, adverse effects of triamterene are mild and respond to withdrawal of the drug. The most serious adverse effect of triamterene therapy is electrolyte imbalance, mainly hyperkalemia (serum potassium concentrations may exceed 5.5 mEq/L), especially in patients with renal insufficiency or diabetes, geriatric or severely ill patients, or those receiving prolonged therapy with large doses. Hyperkalemia may be associated with cardiac irregularities. At least 3 fatal cases of hyperkalemia have been reported in patients receiving triamterene and a thiazide diuretic; however, 2 of these patients were also receiving spironolactone which may have contributed to the hyperkalemia.

Potassium loss has been reported during triamterene therapy in some patients with hepatic cirrhosis and may result in signs and symptoms of hepatic coma or precoma. Serum potassium concentrations should be closely monitored in patients with hepatic cirrhosis and potassium supplementation administered if required.

Diuretics increase urinary sodium excretion and decrease physical signs of fluid retention in patients with heart failure. Results of short-term studies in patients with heart failure indicate that diuretic therapy is associated with a reduction in jugular venous pressures, pulmonary congestion, ascites, peripheral edema, and body weight within a few days of initiating such therapy. In addition, diuretics may improve cardiac function, symptoms, and exercise tolerance in these patients. However, since there are no long-term studies of diuretic therapy in patients with heart failure, the effects of diuretics on morbidity and mortality are not known. Nevertheless, most long-term studies of therapeutic interventions for heart failure have been in patients receiving diuretic therapy. Diuretics should *not* be used as monotherapy in patients with heart failure even if symptoms of fluid overload (e.g., peripheral edema, pulmonary congestion) are well controlled, because diuretics alone do not prevent progression of heart failure.

Depending on the dosage employed, diuretics may alter the efficacy and safety of concomitantly used drugs in heart failure, and therefore diuretic dosage should be selected carefully. Excessive diuretic dosages may lead to volume depletion, which can increase the risk of hypotension in patients receiving angiotensin-converting enzyme (ACE) inhibitors or vasodilators and renal insufficiency in patients receiving ACE inhibitors or angiotensin II receptor antagonists. Inadequate diuretic dosages may lead to fluid retention, which can decrease the response to ACE inhibitors and increase the risk of β-adrenergic blocking agent (β-blocker) therapy. Patients with mild heart failure may respond favorably to low doses of diuretics, since absorption of diuretics from the GI tract is rapid and the drugs are distributed rapidly to the renal tubules in such patients; however, as heart failure advances, absorption of the drugs may be delayed because of bowel edema or intestinal hypoperfusion, and distribution may be impaired because of decreases in renal perfusion and function. Therefore, dosage of diuretics usually needs to be increased with progression of heart failure; eventually, patients may become resistant to even high dosages of diuretic therapy. If resistance to diuretics occurs, IV administration of a diuretic or concomitant use of 2 or more diuretics (e.g., a loop diuretic and metolazone, a loop diuretic and a thiazide diuretic) may be necessary, or alternatively, short-term administration of a drug that increases blood flow (e.g., a positive inotropic agent such as dopamine) may be necessary. ACCF and AHA state that IV loop diuretics should be administered promptly to all hospitalized heart failure patients with substantial fluid overload to reduce morbidity. ACCF and AHA state that low-dose dopamine infusions may be considered in combination with loop diuretics to augment diuresis and preserve renal function and renal blood flow in patients with acute decompensated heart failure, although data are conflicting and additional study and experience are needed.

Most experts state that the diuretics of choice for most patients with heart failure usually are loop diuretics (e.g., bumetanide, ethacrynic acid, furosemide, torsemide), especially in those with renal impairment or substantial fluid retention, since loop diuretics increase sodium excretion to 20–25% of the filtered load of sodium, enhance free water clearance, and maintain their efficacy unless renal function is severely impaired (e.g., creatinine clearance less than 5 mL/minute). In contrast, thiazide diuretics increase fractional sodium excretion to only 5–10% of the filtered load, tend to decrease free water clearance, and lose their efficacy in patients with moderate renal impairment (e.g., creatinine clearance less than 30 mL/minute). Thiazides may be preferred in some patients with concomitant hypertension because of their sustained effects. If electrolyte imbalance(s) occurs during diuretic therapy for heart failure, the patient should be treated aggressively (preferably with low doses of a potassium-sparing diuretic instead of potassium or magnesium supplements) and diuresis should be continued. In patients who develop azotemia or hypotension before therapeutic goals are achieved, consideration to decreasing the rate of diuresis may be made, but diuretic therapy should continue until fluid retention is eliminated, provided that decreases in blood pressure remain asymptomatic; excessive concern about hypotension and azotemia may result in suboptimal diuretic therapy leading to refractory edema.

Once fluid retention has resolved in patients with heart failure, diuretic therapy should be maintained to prevent recurrence of fluid retention. Ideally, diuretic therapy should be adjusted according to changes in body weight (as an indicator of fluid retention) rather than maintained at a fixed dose.

Sodium depletion may occur when triamterene is administered to markedly edematous patients whose sodium chloride intake is restricted. Magnesium depletion may also occur, especially if triamterene is used concomitantly with another diuretic such as a thiazide which also increases excretion of magnesium. Serum chloride may be increased and serum bicarbonate decreased during triamterene therapy, resulting in decreased alkali reserve with the possibility of metabolic acidosis. Slight alkalinization of the urine may occur.

Increased BUN concentration caused by decreased glomerular filtration rate has been reported during therapy with triamterene. However, a rise in BUN concentration seldom occurs with intermittent (every other day) therapy and is reversible upon withdrawal of the drug. Serum creatinine concentration may be moderately increased during administration of triamterene but returns to pretreatment levels in 7–14 days after the drug is discontinued. Serum uric acid concentrations may be increased, especially in patients with gouty arthritis.

Megaloblastic anemia has occurred in patients with alcoholic cirrhosis receiving triamterene.

Renal colic occurred in one patient receiving triamterene and hydrochlorothiazide who had a previously asymptomatic partial urinary tract obstruction. Triamterene has occasionally caused nephrolithiasis. Renal calculi have been composed of triamterene and/or its metabolites (i.e., 6-*p*-hydroxytriamterene and its sulfate) alone, but apparently in a protein matrix, or combined with other usual calculus components (e.g., calcium oxalate monohydrate and dihydrate, uric acid, hydroxylapatite). Triamterene usually appears as the nucleus of the calculus as a central amorphous deposit around which calcium oxalate monohydrate or dihydrate or uric acid is deposited. Triamterene has reportedly caused acute interstitial nephritis in one patient.

Other adverse effects of triamterene include nausea, vomiting, diarrhea, or other GI disturbances. Nausea may be minimized by giving the drug after meals; however, nausea and vomiting may also be symptoms of electrolyte imbalance. Dizziness, hypotension, weakness, headache, muscle cramps, dry mouth, anaphylaxis, photosensitivity, rash, and blood dyscrasias such as granulocytopenia and eosinophilia have also been attributed to use of the drug.

■ Precautions and Contraindications When triamterene is used as a fixed-combination preparation that includes hydrochlorothiazide, the cautions, precautions, and contraindications associated with thiazide diuretics must be considered in addition to those associated with triamterene.

Patients receiving prolonged triamterene therapy should be monitored for signs of electrolyte imbalance, especially those with heart failure, renal disease, or cirrhosis of the liver. It is particularly important that serum potassium concentrations be checked periodically, especially in geriatric, cirrhotic, or diabetic patients; in patients with impaired renal function; or when there is a change in dosage of triamterene. If hyperkalemia occurs, the drug should be discontinued. Periodic BUN and serum creatinine determinations should be performed, especially in patients with suspected or confirmed renal insufficiency.

Potassium supplementation in the form of potassium salts, a high potassium diet, or salt substitutes should not be given to patients receiving triamterene alone. When triamterene is added to other diuretic therapy or when patients are switched to triamterene from other diuretics, potassium supplementation should be discontinued. Patients receiving triamterene concomitantly with a thiazide or other diuretic that promotes potassium excretion (kaliuretic diuretic) should receive dietary potassium supplements only if they develop hypokalemia or their dietary intake of potassium is markedly impaired. It has been theorized that abrupt withdrawal of triamterene after intense or prolonged therapy may result in a rebound kaliuresis; therefore, the drug should be discontinued gradually.

Although a causal relationship has not been established between the drug and megaloblastic anemia, triamterene should be used with caution in pregnant women and in patients with alcohol dependence since these patients may have reduced stores of folate. Periodic blood studies should be performed in cirrhotic patients with splenomegaly as they are subject to marked hematologic variations; such patients also should be observed for exacerbation of underlying hepatic disease.

Triamterene should be used with caution in patients with impaired hepatic function. Diuretic therapy in such patients should be initiated while the patient is hospitalized, because rapid alterations in fluid and electrolyte balance may precipitate hepatic coma. Patients receiving the drug should be observed for signs of liver damage, blood dyscrasias, or other idiosyncratic reactions. Triamterene should be administered cautiously to patients with impaired renal function. Although the manufacturer states that triamterene should be used with caution in patients with a history of renal calculi, some clinicians recommend that the drug not be used in these patients because of the risk of triamterene nephrolithiasis. If a patient passes a urinary calculus during triamterene therapy, the drug should be discontinued and the calculus analyzed for the presence of triamterene and/or its metabolites. (See Cautions: Adverse Effects.)

Triamterene should be administered with caution to patients with diabetes mellitus and should be given only to those diabetic patients whose blood glucose concentration is well controlled. The drug does not appear to be diabetogenic or to alter carbohydrate metabolism; however, diabetic patients appear to be more sensitive to changes in serum potassium concentrations than are nondiabetics. Elevations of serum potassium concentrations are exacerbated by administration of large quantities of glucose; therefore, comatose diabetic patients receiving triamterene therapy should not be tested for hypoglycemia by IV administration of dextrose.

Potassium-conserving therapy should generally be avoided in severely ill patients in whom respiratory or metabolic acidosis may occur; acidosis may result in rapid increases in serum potassium concentrations. If potassium-conserving therapy (e.g., triamterene) is used, frequent assessment of acid-base balance and serum electrolytes should be performed.

Triamterene is contraindicated in patients with severe or progressive kidney disease, severe hepatic disease, preexisting or drug-induced hyperkalemia, or hypersensitivity to the drug. Triamterene should also not be used in patients who develop hyperkalemia while receiving the drug.

■ **Pediatric Precautions** Safety and efficacy of triamterene in children have not been established. For information on overall principles and expert recommendations for treatment of hypertension in pediatric patients, see Uses: Hypertension in Pediatric Patients, in the Thiazides General Statement 40:28.20.

■ **Mutagenicity and Carcinogenicity** Studies to determine the mutagenic and carcinogenic potentials of triamterene currently are not available.

■ **Pregnancy, Fertility, and Lactation** There are no adequate and well-controlled studies using triamterene in pregnant women, and the drug should be used during pregnancy only when the potential benefits justify the possible risks (these include adverse effects reported in adults) to the fetus.

Reproduction studies in rats using triamterene doses up to 30 times the human dose have not revealed evidence of harm to the fetus or impaired fertility. The drug has been shown to cross the placental barrier and appear in the cord blood of ewes; similar distribution may occur in humans.

Since triamterene has been shown to distribute into milk in animals and may distribute into human milk, the drug should not be used in nursing women. If use of triamterene is deemed essential, nursing should be discontinued.

Drug Interactions

■ **Potassium-sparing Agents** Triamterene should not be used concurrently with another potassium-sparing agent (e.g., amiloride, spironolactone), since concomitant therapy with these drugs may increase the risk of hyperkalemia compared with triamterene alone. At least 2 deaths have been reported in patients receiving triamterene and spironolactone concurrently; in one patient, recommended dosages were exceeded and, in the other patient, serum electrolytes were not closely monitored.

Potassium-sparing diuretics should be used with caution and serum potassium should be determined frequently in patients receiving an angiotensin-converting enzyme (ACE) inhibitor (e.g., captopril, enalapril), since concomitant administration with an ACE inhibitor may increase the risk of hyperkalemia. Dosage of triamterene should be reduced or the drug should be discontinued as necessary. Patients with renal impairment may be at increased risk of hyperkalemia.

■ **Potassium-containing Preparations** Concurrent administration of triamterene with potassium supplements, potassium-containing medications (e.g., parenteral penicillin G potassium), or other substances containing potassium (e.g., salt substitutes, low-salt milk) may increase the risk of hyperkalemia as compared with triamterene alone, and such combined use is contraindicated.

■ **Nonsteroidal Anti-inflammatory Agents** Concomitant use of triamterene and indomethacin has adversely affected renal function. In one study, concomitant administration of indomethacin and triamterene to 4 healthy adults resulted in a 60–70% decrease in creatinine clearance in 2 individuals; renal function returned to normal within 2 weeks after both drugs were discontinued. When the drugs were given separately, triamterene caused no consistent change in renal function; indomethacin induced an average 10% decrease in creatinine clearance. Acute anuric renal failure occurred within 2 days after concomitant use of indomethacin and triamterene in a 79-year-old woman with compensated heart failure. BUN and serum creatinine concentrations increased to 102 and 10.2 mg/dL, respectively, 5 days after discontinuance of the drugs in this woman, and subsequently returned toward normal over 2 months; anuria persisted for 11 days after discontinuance of the drugs. Although the mechanism of this interaction was not determined, it has been postulated that indomethacin may inhibit triamterene-stimulated synthesis of renal prostaglandins that mediate an adaptive mechanism for renal blood flow preservation in response to triamterene-mediated renal vasoconstriction. The manufacturer of indomethacin recommends that the combination of indomethacin and triamterene not be used. Triamterene should be used with caution in patients receiving other nonsteroidal anti-inflammatory agents.

■ **Angiotensin-converting Enzyme Inhibitors** Potassium-sparing diuretics (e.g., triamterene) should be used with caution and serum potassium should be determined frequently in patients receiving an ACE inhibitor (e.g., enalapril), since hyperkalemia may occur. Potassium-sparing diuretics should be used with great caution, if at all, in patients receiving an ACE inhibitor (e.g., enalapril) for heart failure. Potassium-sparing diuretics should be discontinued or their dosage reduced as necessary in patients receiving an ACE inhibitor. (See Drug Interactions: Drugs Increasing Serum Potassium Concentration in Enalapril 24:32.04.)

■ **Other Drugs** Although triamterene alone does not consistently cause hypotension, lowering of blood pressure may occur, especially when it is used with hypotensive agents.

Diuretics including triamterene, generally should not be used concurrently with lithium since diuretics reduce renal lithium clearance and may increase the risk of lithium toxicity. (See Lithium Salts 28:28.)

Laboratory Test Interferences

A pale blue fluorescence may be produced in urine of patients receiving triamterene which may interfere with methods of enzyme assay that depend on fluorometry, such as determinations of lactic dehydrogenase activity. Triamterene interferes with the fluorometric assay of quinidine as the two drugs have similar fluorescence spectra.

Acute Toxicity

■ **Pathogenesis** The amount of triamterene ingested as a single dose that would usually be associated with symptoms of overdosage or would likely be life-threatening is not known. The oral LD_{50} of the drug in mice is 380 mg/kg.

■ **Manifestations** Overdosage of triamterene may cause electrolyte imbalance, especially hyperkalemia. Nausea, vomiting, other GI disturbances, and weakness may also occur. Hypotension may also result, especially when the drug is used concomitantly with hydrochlorothiazide or other diuretics or hypotensive agents.

■ **Treatment** Severe hypotension may be alleviated by administration of pressor agents such as norepinephrine. Immediate gastric lavage or emesis should be induced in conscious patients. Careful evaluation of the electrolyte pattern and fluid balance should be made and corrective therapy initiated if indicated. Although triamterene is relatively highly protein bound, dialysis may be of some benefit.

Pharmacology

Like amiloride, triamterene acts directly on the distal renal tubule of the nephron to depress reabsorption of sodium and excretion of potassium and hydrogen which are stimulated at that site by aldosterone. Triamterene is a potassium-sparing diuretic that does not competitively inhibit aldosterone, and its activity is independent of aldosterone concentrations. Triamterene does not inhibit carbonic anhydrase.

Administration of triamterene increases excretion of sodium, calcium, magnesium, and bicarbonate. Excretion of chloride is increased but not always in proportion to sodium excretion; slightly more sodium than chloride is excreted. Excretion of potassium is usually reduced; however, slight potassium loss was reported in one study in some patients with cirrhosis and ascites. Serum concentrations of potassium and chloride are usually increased, and serum bicarbonate is consistently decreased during triamterene therapy. Triamterene may cause decreased alkali reserve with the possibility of metabolic acidosis. Urinary pH is increased slightly.

Glomerular filtration rate is reduced during daily but not during intermittent administration of the drug, suggesting a reversible effect on renal blood flow. Cardiac output is decreased. In contrast to other diuretics, triamterene does not appear to inhibit excretion of uric acid; however, serum uric acid concentrations may be elevated in some patients, especially those predisposed to gouty arthritis. Triamterene has been reported to inhibit dehydrofolate reductase in vitro; however, in vivo interference with folic acid utilization has not been demonstrated.

Triamterene alone has little if any hypotensive effect. The drug does not appear to be diabetogenic or to alter carbohydrate metabolism.

Pharmacokinetics

■ **Absorption** Triamterene is rapidly absorbed from the GI tract; however, the degree of absorption varies in different individuals. Diuresis usually occurs within 2–4 hours and diminishes in approximately 7–9 hours after oral administration of the drug, although the total duration of action may be 24 hours or longer. The maximum therapeutic effect may not occur until after several days of therapy. Peak plasma concentrations of 0.05–0.28 mcg/mL are achieved within 2–4 hours following administration of a 100- to 200-mg single oral dose.

Oral bioavailability of hydrochlorothiazide from the original formulation (no longer commercially available) of Dyazide® capsules was about 50–65% that from Maxzide® tablets or single-entity tablets or solutions of the drug. In one crossover study in a limited number of healthy adults receiving single doses of the drug, the mean hydrochlorothiazide dose recovered in urine within 72 hours was about 30% for the original formulation of Dyazide® capsules and about 60% for Maxzide® or single-entity tablets of the drug. In 1995, Dyazide® capsules were reformulated to improve the oral bioavailability of triamterene and hydrochlorothiazide. The oral bioavailabilities of triamterene and hydrochlorothiazide from the reformulated Dyazide® capsules now are comparable to those of aqueous suspensions of the individual drugs, averaging 85 and 82%, respectively, for the new formulation and 100 and 100%, respectively, for the suspensions. In addition, intraindividual variation in bioavailability from the reformulated Dyazide® capsules was reduced by about 40% compared with the original formulation. The manufacturer states that the reformulated Dyazide® capsules also are bioequivalent to single-entity 25-mg hydrochlorothiazide tablets and 37.5-mg triamterene capsules. Administration of reformulated Dyazide® with a high-fat meal in healthy adults increased the average bioavailabilities of triamterene by about 67%, 6-*p*-hydroxytriamterene by about 50%, and hydrochlorothiazide by about 17% and the peak concentrations of triamterene and its *p*-hydroxy metabolite and delayed the absorption of the active drugs by up to 2 hours.

■ **Distribution** In animals, triamterene has been detected in the brain, heart, ocular fluid, fat, liver, and skeletal muscles. The drug is distributed into bile. Approximately 67% of the drug in the plasma is bound to proteins. Triamterene crosses the placenta in animals. No human data are available indicating whether triamterene appears in the milk of nursing women; however, animal studies have demonstrated the presence of very small amounts of the drug in breast milk.

■ **Elimination** The plasma half-life of triamterene is 100–150 minutes. The metabolic and excretory fate of triamterene has not been fully determined.

The drug is reportedly metabolized to 6-*p*-hydroxytriamterene and its sulfate conjugate. Triamterene is excreted in urine as unchanged drug and metabolites. In one study in healthy males, the urinary excretion of 6-*p*-hydroxytriamterene was up to 3 times that of unchanged drug. Limited data indicate that the renal clearances of triamterene, hydroxytriamterene sulfate, and hydrochlorothiazide are reduced in geriatric patients receiving combined triamterene and hydrochlorothiazide therapy, principally as a result of age-related reductions in renal function.

Chemistry and Stability

■ **Chemistry** Triamterene is a pteridine derivative, potassium-sparing diuretic that is structurally related to folic acid. Triamterene occurs as a yellow, odorless, crystalline powder and is practically insoluble in water and very slightly soluble in alcohol. The drug has a pK_a of 6.2.

■ **Stability** Triamterene capsules should be stored in tight, light-resistant containers at a temperature less than 40°C, preferably between 15–30°C.

Preparations

Excipients in commercially available drug preparations may have clinically important effects in some individuals; consult specific product labeling for details.

Triamterene

Oral		
Capsules	50 mg	**Dyrenium®**, WellSpring
	100 mg	**Dyrenium®**, WellSpring

Triamterene and Hydrochlorothiazide (Co-triamterzide)

Oral		
Capsules	37.5 mg Triamterene and Hydrochlorothiazide 25 mg*	**Dyazide®**, GlaxoSmithKline
		Triamterene and Hydrochlorothiazide Capsules
Tablets	37.5 mg Triamterene and Hydrochlorothiazide 25 mg*	**Maxzide®-25** (scored), Mylan
		Triamterene and Hydrochlorothiazide Tablets
	75 mg Triamterene and Hydrochlorothiazide 50 mg*	**Maxzide®** (scored), Mylan
		Triamterene and Hydrochlorothiazide Tablets

*available from one or more manufacturer, distributor, and/or repackager by generic (nonproprietary) name

†Use is not currently included in the labeling approved by the US Food and Drug Administration

THIAZIDE DIURETICS 40:28.20

Thiazides General Statement

■ Thiazides are diuretics and antihypertensive agents.

Uses

■ **Edema** Thiazide diuretics are used in the management of edema resulting from a number of causes; however, careful etiologic diagnosis should precede the use of any diuretic. There are no substantial differences in the clinical effects or toxicity of comparable dosages of the thiazides or thiazide-like diuretics except that metolazone may be more effective than other thiazide-like diuretics in the management of edema in patients with impaired renal function. Determination of the specific agent to be used is, therefore, usually determined by factors such as cost and patient convenience.

Heart Failure **Clinical Role.** Thiazides are used in the management of edema associated with heart failure. Most experts state that all patients with symptomatic heart failure who have evidence for, or a history of, fluid retention generally should receive diuretic therapy in conjunction with moderate sodium restriction, an agent to inhibit the renin-angiotensin-aldosterone (RAA) system (e.g., angiotensin-converting enzyme [ACE] inhibitor, angiotensin II receptor antagonist, angiotensin receptor-neprilysin inhibitor [ARNI]), a β-adrenergic blocking agent (β-blocker), and in selected patients, an aldosterone antagonist. Some experts state that because of limited and inconsistent data, it is difficult to make precise recommendations regarding daily sodium intake and whether it should vary with respect to the type of heart failure (e.g., reduced versus preserved ejection fraction), disease severity (e.g., New York Heart Association [NYHA] class), heart failure-related comorbidities (e.g., renal dysfunction), or other patient characteristics (e.g., age, race). The American College of Cardiology Foundation (ACCF) and American Heart Association (AHA) state that limiting sodium intake to 1.5 g daily in patients with ACCF/AHA stage A or B heart failure may be reasonable. While data currently are lacking to support recommendation of a specific level of sodium intake in patients with ACCF/AHA stage C or D heart failure, ACCF and AHA state that limiting sodium intake to some degree (e.g., less than 3 g daily) in such patients may be considered for symptom improvement.

Diuretics play a key role in the management of heart failure because they produce symptomatic benefits more rapidly than any other drugs, relieving pulmonary and peripheral edema within hours or days compared with weeks or months for cardiac glycosides, ACE inhibitors, or β-blockers. However, since there are no long-term studies of diuretic therapy in patients with heart failure, the effects of diuretics on morbidity and mortality in such patients are not known. Although there are patients with heart failure who do not exhibit fluid retention in the absence of diuretic therapy and even may develop severe volume depletion with low doses of diuretics, such patients are rare and the unique pathophysiologic mechanisms regulating their fluid and electrolyte balance have not been elucidated.

Most experts state that loop diuretics (e.g., bumetanide, ethacrynic acid, furosemide, torsemide) are the diuretics of choice for most patients with heart failure, especially in those with renal impairment or substantial fluid retention, since loop diuretics increase sodium excretion to 20–25% of the filtered load of sodium, enhance free water clearance, and maintain their efficacy unless renal function is severely impaired (e.g., creatinine clearance less than 5 mL/minute). In contrast, thiazide diuretics increase fractional sodium excretion to only 5–10% of the filtered load, tend to decrease free water clearance, and lose their efficacy in patients with moderate renal impairment (e.g., creatinine clearance less than 30 mL/minute). However, thiazides may be preferred in some patients with concomitant hypertension because of their sustained antihypertensive effects. In patients who develop azotemia or hypotension before therapeutic goals are achieved, consideration to decreasing the rate of diuresis may be made, but diuretic therapy should continue until fluid retention is eliminated, provided that decreases in blood pressure remain asymptomatic; excessive concern about hypotension and azotemia may result in suboptimal diuretic therapy leading to refractory edema.

Efficacy. Diuretics increase urinary sodium excretion and decrease physical signs of fluid retention in patients with heart failure. Results of short-term studies in patients with heart failure indicate that diuretic therapy is associated with a reduction in jugular venous pressures, pulmonary congestion, ascites, peripheral edema, and body weight within a few days of initiating such therapy. In addition, diuretics may improve cardiac function, symptoms, and exercise tolerance in these patients. However, since there are no long-term studies of diuretic therapy in patients with heart failure, the effects of diuretics on morbidity and mortality are not known. Nevertheless, most long-term studies of therapeutic interventions for heart failure have been in patients receiving diuretic therapy. Diuretics should *not* be used as monotherapy in patients with heart failure even if symptoms of fluid overload (e.g., peripheral edema, pulmonary congestion) are well controlled, because diuretics alone do not prevent progression of heart failure.

Dosing Considerations. Depending on the dosage employed, diuretics may alter the efficacy and safety of concomitantly used drugs in heart failure, and therefore diuretic dosage should be selected carefully. Excessive diuretic dosages may lead to volume depletion, which can increase the risk of hypotension in patients receiving ACE inhibitors or vasodilators and renal insufficiency in patients receiving ACE inhibitors or angiotensin II receptor antagonists. Inadequate diuretic dosages may lead to fluid retention, which can decrease the response to ACE inhibitors and increase the risk of β-blocker therapy. Patients with mild heart failure may respond favorably to low doses of diuretics, since absorption of diuretics from the GI tract is rapid and the drugs are distributed rapidly to the renal tubules in such patients; however, as heart failure advances, absorption of the drugs may be delayed because of bowel edema or intestinal hypoperfusion, and distribution may be impaired because of decreases in renal perfusion and function. Therefore, dosage of diuretics usually needs to be increased with progression of heart failure; eventually, patients may become resistant to even high dosages of diuretics. If resistance to diuretics occurs, IV administration of a diuretic or concomitant use of 2 or more diuretics (e.g., a loop diuretic and metolazone, a loop diuretic and a thiazide diuretic) may be necessary, or alternatively, short-term administration of a drug that increases blood flow (e.g., a positive inotropic agent such as dopamine) may be necessary. ACCF and AHA state that IV loop diuretics should be administered promptly to all hospitalized heart failure patients with substantial fluid overload to reduce morbidity. In addition, ACCF and AHA state that low-dose dopamine infusions may be considered in combination with loop diuretics to augment diuresis and preserve renal function and renal blood flow in patients with acute decompensated heart failure, although data are conflicting and additional study and experience are needed.

Maintenance Therapy. Once fluid retention has resolved in patients with heart failure, diuretic therapy should be maintained to prevent recurrence of fluid retention. Ideally, diuretic therapy should be adjusted according to changes in body weight (as an indicator of fluid retention) rather than maintained at a fixed dosage. Diuretics also should be continued in patients with comorbid conditions (e.g., hypertension) where ongoing therapy with the drugs is indicated.

Other Edematous Conditions In edema secondary to nephrotic syndrome, thiazides may be useful if the patient fails to respond to corticosteroid therapy. Edema secondary to nephrotic syndrome is more likely to become refractory to therapy than edema associated with heart failure, and more potent diuretics may be required. Other forms of edema caused by renal disease and edema caused by corticosteroids and estrogens also may be relatively resistant to treatment with the thiazides. Thiazides and thiazide-like diuretics (with the exception of metolazone) are ineffective in patients with serum creatinine or BUN concentrations greater than about twice normal. Some clinicians state that thiazides are ineffective in patients with a glomerular filtration rate (GFR) of less than 15–25 mL/minute, whereas others suggest that use of a more potent diuretic should be considered whenever the GFR is less than 50 mL/minute.

Edema associated with pregnancy generally responds well to thiazides except when caused by renal disease. Hypertension during pregnancy also responds well, but preeclampsia and eclampsia may require more potent diuretics. The routine use of thiazides is contraindicated in pregnant women with mild edema who are otherwise healthy.

■ **Hypertension in Adults** Thiazide diuretics are used alone or in combination with other classes of antihypertensive agents in the management of all stages of hypertension.

Current evidence-based practice guidelines for the management of hypertension in adults generally recommend the use of drugs from 4 classes of antihypertensive agents (ACE inhibitors, angiotensin II receptor antagonists, calcium-channel blockers, and thiazide diuretics); data from clinical outcome trials indicate that lowering blood pressure with any of these drug classes can reduce the complications of hypertension and provide similar cardiovascular protection. However, recommendations for initial drug selection and use in specific patient populations may vary across these expert guidelines. This variability is due, in part, to differences in the guideline development process and the types of studies (e.g., randomized controlled studies only versus a range of studies with different study designs) included in the evidence reviews. Ultimately, choice of antihypertensive therapy should be individualized, considering the clinical characteristics of the patient (e.g., age, ethnicity/race, comorbid conditions, cardiovascular risk factors) as well as drug-related factors (e.g., ease of administration, availability, adverse effects, costs).

Thiazide diuretics historically have been considered the drugs of choice for most patients with uncomplicated hypertension because of their established benefits, cost, and favorable adverse effects profile. However, current evidence indicates no overall differences in clinical outcomes between thiazide diuretics and other classes of antihypertensive drugs, including calcium-channel blockers, ACE inhibitors, and angiotensin II receptor antagonists. While there may be individual differences with respect to specific outcomes, these antihypertensive drug classes all generally produce comparable effects on overall mortality and cardiovascular, cerebrovascular, and renal outcomes. Because many patients eventually will need drugs from 2 or more antihypertensive classes, experts generally state that the emphasis should be placed on achieving appropriate blood pressure control rather than on identifying a preferred drug to achieve that control.

Disease Overview Worldwide, hypertension is the most common modifiable risk factor for cardiovascular events and mortality. The lifetime risk of developing hypertension in the US exceeds 80%, with higher rates observed among African Americans and Hispanics compared with whites or Asians. The systolic blood pressure (SBP) and diastolic blood pressure (DBP) values defined as hypertension (see Blood Pressure Classification under Uses: Hypertension in Adults) in a 2017 multidisciplinary guideline of the American College of Cardiology (ACC), AHA, and a number of other professional organizations (subsequently referred to as the 2017 ACC/AHA hypertension guideline in this monograph) are lower than those defined in the Seventh Report of the Joint National Committee on Prevention, Detection, Evaluation, and Treatment of High Blood Pressure (JNC 7) guidelines, which results in an increase of approximately 14% in the prevalence of hypertension in the US. However, this change in definition results in only a 2% increase in the percentage of patients requiring antihypertensive drug therapy because nonpharmacologic treatment is recommended for most adults now classified by the 2017 ACC/AHA hypertension guideline as hypertensive who would *not* meet the JNC 7 definition of hypertension. Among US adults receiving antihypertensive drugs, approximately 53% have inadequately controlled blood pressure according to current ACC/AHA treatment goals.

Cardiovascular and Renal Sequelae. The principal goal of preventing and treating hypertension is to reduce the risk of cardiovascular and renal morbidity and mortality, including target organ damage. The relationship between blood pressure and cardiovascular disease is continuous, consistent, and independent of other risk factors. It is important that very high blood pressure be managed promptly to reduce the risk of target organ damage. The higher the blood pressure, the more likely the development of myocardial infarction (MI), heart failure, stroke, and renal disease. For adults 40–70 years of age, each 20-mm Hg increment in SBP or 10-mm Hg increment in DBP doubles the risk of developing cardiovascular disease across the entire blood pressure range of 115/75 to 185/115 mm Hg. For those older than 50 years of age, SBP is a much more important risk factor for developing cardiovascular disease than is DBP. The rapidity with which treatment is required depends on the patient's clinical presentation (presence of new or worsening target organ damage) and the presence or absence of cardiovascular complications; the 2017 ACC/AHA hypertension guideline states that treatment of very high blood pressure should be initiated within 1 week.

Blood Pressure Classification Accurate blood pressure measurement is essential for the proper diagnosis and management of hypertension. Error in measuring blood pressure is a major cause of inadequate blood pressure control and may lead to overtreatment. Because a patient's blood pressure may vary in an unpredictable fashion, a single blood pressure measurement is not sufficient for clinical decision-making. An average of 2 or 3 blood pressure measurements obtained on 2–3 separate occasions using proper technique should be used to minimize random error and provide a more accurate blood pressure reading. Out-of-office blood pressure measurements may be useful for confirming and managing hypertension. The 2017 ACC/AHA hypertension guideline document (available on the ACC and AHA websites) should be consulted for key steps on properly measuring blood pressure.

According to the 2017 ACC/AHA hypertension guideline, blood pressure in adults is classified into 4 categories: normal, elevated, stage 1 hypertension, and stage 2 hypertension. (See Table 1.) The 2017 ACC/AHA hypertension guideline lowers the blood pressure threshold used to define hypertension in the US; previous hypertension guidelines (JNC 7) considered adults with SBP of 120–139 mm Hg or DBP of 80–89 mm Hg to have prehypertension, those with SBP of 140–159 mm Hg or DBP of 90–99 mm Hg to have stage 1 hypertension, and those with SBP of 160 mm Hg or higher or DBP of 100 mm Hg or higher to have stage 2 hypertension. The blood pressure definitions in the 2017 ACC/AHA hypertension guideline are based upon data from studies evaluating the association between SBP/DBP and cardiovascular risk and the benefits of blood pressure reduction. Individuals with SBP and DBP in 2 different categories should be designated as being in the higher blood pressure category.

Table 1. ACC/AHA Blood Pressure Classification in Adults[ab]

Category	SBP (mm Hg)		DBP (mm Hg)
Normal	<120	and	<80
Elevated	120–129	and	<80
Hypertension, Stage 1	130–139	or	80–89
Hypertension, Stage 2	≥140	or	≥90

[a] Source: Whelton PK, Carey RM, Aronow WS et al. 2017 ACC/AHA/AAPA/ABC/ACPM/AGS/APhA/ASH/ASPC/NMA/PCNA guideline for the prevention, detection, evaluation, and management of high blood pressure in adults: a report of the American College of Cardiology/American Heart Association Task Force on Clinical Practice Guidelines. *Hypertension*. 2018;71:e13-115.

[b] Individuals with SBP and DBP in 2 different categories (e.g., elevated SBP and normal DBP) should be designated as being in the higher blood pressure category (i.e., elevated BP).

The blood pressure thresholds used to define hypertension, when to initiate drug therapy, and the ideal target blood pressure values remain controversial. The 2017 ACC/AHA hypertension guideline recommends a blood pressure goal of less than 130/80 mm Hg in all adults who have confirmed hypertension and known cardiovascular disease or a 10-year atherosclerotic cardiovascular disease (ASCVD) event risk of 10% or higher; the ACC/AHA guideline also states that this blood pressure goal is reasonable to attempt to achieve in adults with confirmed hypertension who do *not* have increased cardiovascular risk. The lower blood pressure values used to define hypertension and the lower target blood pressure goals outlined in the 2017 ACC/AHA hypertension guideline are based on clinical studies demonstrating a substantial reduction in the composite end point of major cardiovascular disease events and the combination of fatal and nonfatal stroke when a lower SBP/DBP value (i.e., 130/80 mm Hg) was used to define hypertension. These lower target blood pressure goals also are based upon clinical studies demonstrating continuing reduction of cardiovascular risk at progressively lower levels of SBP. A linear relationship has been demonstrated between cardiovascular risk and blood pressure even at low blood pressures (e.g., 120–124 mm Hg SBP). The 2017 ACC/AHA hypertension guideline recommends estimating a patient's ASCVD risk using the ACC/AHA Pooled Cohort equations (available online at http://tools.acc.org/ASCVD-Risk-Estimator), which are based on a variety of factors including age, race, gender, cholesterol levels, statin use, blood pressure, treatment for hypertension, history of diabetes mellitus, smoking status, and aspirin use. While the 2017 ACC/AHA hypertension guideline has lowered the threshold for *diagnosing* hypertension in adults, the threshold for *initiating drug therapy* has only been lowered for those patients who are at high risk of cardiovascular disease. Clinicians who support the 2017 ACC/AHA hypertension guideline believe that these recommendations have the potential to increase hypertension awareness, encourage lifestyle modification, and focus antihypertensive drug initiation and intensification in those adults at high risk for cardiovascular disease.

The lower blood pressure goals advocated in the 2017 ACC/AHA hypertension guideline have been questioned by some clinicians who have concerns regarding the guideline's use of extrapolated observational data, the lack of generalizability of some of the randomized trials (e.g., SPRINT) used to support the guideline, the difficulty of establishing accurate representative blood pressure values in typical clinical practice settings, and the accuracy of the cardiovascular risk calculator used in the guideline. Some clinicians state the lower blood pressure threshold used to define hypertension in the 2017 ACC/AHA hypertension guideline is not fully supported by clinical data, and these clinicians have expressed concerns about the possible harms (e.g., adverse effects of antihypertensive therapy) associated with classifying more patients as being hypertensive. Some clinicians also state that using this guideline, a large number of young, low-risk patients would need to be treated in order to observe a clinical benefit, while other clinicians state that the estimated gains in life expectancy attributable to long-term use of blood pressure-lowering drugs are correspondingly greater in this patient population.

Treatment Benefits In clinical trials, antihypertensive therapy has been found to reduce the risk of developing stroke by about 34–40%, MI by about 20–25%, and heart failure by more than 50%. In a randomized, controlled study (SPRINT) that included hypertensive patients without diabetes mellitus who had a high risk of cardiovascular disease, intensive SBP lowering of approximately 15 mm Hg was associated with a 25% reduction in cardiovascular disease events and a 27% reduction in all-cause mortality. However, the exclusion of patients with diabetes mellitus, prior stroke, and those younger than 50 years of age may decrease the generalizability of these findings. Some experts estimate that if the SBP goals of the 2017 ACC/AHA hypertension guideline are achieved, major cardiovascular disease events may be reduced by an additional 340,000 and total deaths by an additional 156,000 compared with implementation of the JNC 8 expert panel guideline goals but these benefits may be accompanied by an increase in the frequency of adverse events. While there was no overall difference in the occurrence of serious adverse events in patients receiving intensive therapy for blood pressure control (SBP target of less than 120 mm Hg) compared with those receiving less intense control (SBP target of less than 140 mm Hg) in the SPRINT study, hypotension, syncope, electrolyte abnormalities, and acute kidney injury or acute renal failure occurred in substantially more patients receiving intensive therapy.

Clinical Benefits of Thiazides in Hypertension. The Antihypertensive and Lipid-Lowering Treatment to Prevent Heart Attack Trial (ALLHAT), which compared the long-term cardiovascular morbidity and mortality benefit of chlorthalidone (a thiazide-like diuretic), amlodipine (a long-acting dihydropyridine calcium-channel blocker), and lisinopril (an ACE inhibitor), supports the clinical benefits of thiazides in the management of hypertension.

ALLHAT provides strong evidence that usual dosages of chlorthalidone, amlodipine, and lisinopril are comparably effective in providing important cardiovascular benefit in a broad population of patients with stage 1 or 2 hypertension at risk for coronary heart disease, but apparent differences in certain secondary outcomes were observed. After a mean follow-up of 4.9 years, an intent-to-treat analysis revealed no difference in the primary outcome of combined fatal coronary heart disease or nonfatal myocardial infarction among the treatments. Compared with chlorthalidone, the relative risks for the primary outcome were 0.98 for amlodipine and 0.99 for lisinopril. In addition, all-cause mortality, a secondary outcome, did not differ among the treatments.

Chlorthalidone was superior to amlodipine (by 25%) in preventing heart failure overall and also for hospitalized or fatal cases, although the drugs were comparably effective in preventing overall cardiovascular disease. Subgroup analysis (age [younger than 65 years vs 65 years or older], race [black vs nonblack], gender, underlying diabetes mellitus status) revealed no subgroup differences in outcomes between amlodipine and chlorthalidone therapy. Unlike some previously reported evidence with short-acting calcium-channel blockers (see Cautions: Precautions and Contraindications, in Diltiazem 24:28.92 and Cautions in Nifedipine 24:28.08), ALLHAT revealed no evidence of excess coronary heart disease associated with long-acting calcium-channel blocker therapy.

Chlorthalidone also was superior to lisinopril in preventing aggregate cardiovascular events, principally stroke, heart failure, angina, and the need for coronary revascularization. Much of the superiority in reducing these events may be attributable to the greater antihypertensive effect of chlorthalidone (i.e., an overall difference of 2–4 mm Hg in SBP) compared with that of lisinopril. In addition, chlorthalidone was better tolerated than lisinopril.

In ALLHAT, an α-blocker (doxazosin) treatment arm was terminated prematurely after an interim analysis indicated that use of doxazosin in high-risk (at least 2 risk factors for coronary heart disease) hypertensive patients 55 years of age and older was associated with a higher risk of stroke and incidence of combined cardiovascular disease events. (See Uses: Hypertension, in Doxazosin 24:20.)

Post hoc analysis of ALLHAT directly comparing cardiovascular and other outcomes in patients receiving amlodipine versus those receiving lisinopril revealed no difference in the primary outcome of combined fatal coronary heart disease or nonfatal MI between patients receiving the ACE inhibitor and those receiving the calcium-channel blocker. However, patients receiving lisinopril were at higher risk for stroke, combined cardiovascular disease, GI bleeding, and angioedema, while those receiving amlodipine were at higher risk of developing heart failure. ALLHAT investigators suggested that the observed differences in cardiovascular outcome may be attributable, at least in part, to the greater antihypertensive effect of amlodipine compared with that of lisinopril, especially in women and black patients.

Subgroup analysis for race-related effects revealed no difference in the primary outcome of combined fatal coronary heart disease or nonfatal MI among the treatments in both black and nonblack patients. However, substantial race-related effects were observed in the incidence of secondary outcomes (e.g., stroke, combined cardiovascular disease events, heart failure). Compared with chlorthalidone, the relative risk for lisinopril was 1.4 or 1 (in black or nonblack patients, respectively) for stroke and 1.19 or 1.06 (in black or nonblack patients, respectively) for combined cardiovascular disease events. When amlodipine was compared with chlorthalidone, the only race-related difference observed was in the incidence of heart failure; the relative risk was 1.46 or 1.32 (in black or nonblack patients, respectively). The relative risk for heart failure in black patients versus nonblack patients receiving lisinopril was not considered to be statistically significant, and the overall relative risk for both groups was 1.19. In addition, after 4 years, in each treatment group, blood pressure reductions were greater in nonblack than in black patients; about 68 or 60% of nonblack or black patients, respectively, achieved a SBP/DBP of less than 140/90 mm Hg. In nonblack patients receiving chlorthalidone, amlodipine, or lisinopril 69, 69, or 67% achieved the mentioned blood pressure, respectively, while in black patients receiving chlorthalidone, amlodipine, or lisinopril 63, 60, or 54% achieved such blood pressure, respectively.

Based on cost and other considerations (e.g., differences in secondary outcomes, differences in patient tolerance), ALLHAT provides compelling evidence that thiazides, in particular the long-acting drug chlorthalidone, should be considered as one of the initial drugs of choice in most patients with hypertension. ALLHAT did not include a first-line β-blocker treatment arm.

General Considerations for Initial and Maintenance Antihypertensive Therapy **Nonpharmacologic Therapy.** Nonpharmacologic measures (i.e., lifestyle/behavioral modifications) that are effective in lowering blood pressure include weight reduction (for those who are overweight or obese), dietary changes to include foods such as fruits, vegetables, whole grains, and low-fat dairy products that are rich in potassium, calcium, magnesium, and fiber (i.e., adoption of the Dietary Approaches to Stop Hypertension [DASH] eating plan), sodium reduction, increased physical activity, and moderation of alcohol intake. Such lifestyle/behavioral modifications, including smoking cessation, enhance antihypertensive drug efficacy and decrease cardiovascular risk and remain an indispensable part of the management of hypertension. Lifestyle/behavioral modifications without antihypertensive drug therapy are recommended for individuals classified by the 2017 ACC/AHA hypertension guideline as having elevated blood pressure (SBP 120–129 mm Hg and DBP less than 80 mm Hg) and in those with stage 1 hypertension (SBP 130–139 mm Hg or DBP 80–89 mm Hg) who do *not* have preexisting cardiovascular disease or an estimated 10-year ASCVD risk of 10% or greater.

Initiation of Drug Therapy. Drug therapy in the management of hypertension must be individualized and adjusted based on the degree of blood pressure elevation while also considering cardiovascular risk factors. Drug therapy generally is reserved for patients who respond inadequately to nondrug therapies or in whom the degree of blood pressure elevation or coexisting risk factors, especially increased cardiovascular risk, require more prompt or aggressive therapy; however, the optimum blood pressure threshold for initiating antihypertensive drug therapy and specific treatment goals remain controversial. Recommendations generally are based on specific blood pressure levels shown in clinical studies to produce clinical benefits and can therefore vary depending on the studies selected for review.

The 2017 ACC/AHA hypertension guideline and many experts currently state that the treatment of hypertension should be based not only on blood pressure values but also on patients' cardiovascular risk factors. For *secondary prevention* of recurrent cardiovascular disease events in adults with clinical cardiovascular disease or for *primary prevention* in adults with an estimated 10-year ASCVD risk of 10% or higher, the 2017 ACC/AHA hypertension guideline recommends initiation of antihypertensive drug therapy in conjunction with lifestyle/behavioral modifications at an average SBP of 130 mm Hg or an average DBP of 80 mm Hg or higher. For *primary prevention* of cardiovascular disease events in adults with a low (less than 10%) estimated 10-year risk of ASCVD, the 2017 ACC/AHA hypertension guideline recommends initiation of antihypertensive drug therapy in conjunction with lifestyle/behavioral modifications at an SBP of 140 mm Hg or higher or a DBP of 90 mm Hg or higher. After initiation of antihypertensive drug therapy, regardless of the ASCVD risk, the 2017 ACC/AHA hypertension guideline generally recommends a blood pressure goal of less than 130/80 mm Hg in all adults. In addition, an SBP goal of less than 130 mm Hg also is recommended for noninstitutionalized ambulatory patients 65 years of age or older. While these blood pressure goals are lower than those recommended for most patients in previous guidelines, they are based upon clinical studies demonstrating continuing reduction of cardiovascular risk at progressively lower levels of SBP.

Most data indicate that patients with a higher cardiovascular risk will benefit the most from tighter blood pressure control; however, some experts state this treatment goal also may be beneficial in those at lower cardiovascular risk. Other clinicians believe that the benefits of such blood pressure lowering do not outweigh the risks in those patients considered to be at lower risk of cardiovascular disease and that reclassifying individuals formerly considered to have prehypertension as having hypertension may potentially lead to use of drug therapy in such patients without consideration of cardiovascular risk. Previous hypertension guidelines, such as those from the JNC 8 expert panel, generally recommended initiation of antihypertensive treatment in patients with an SBP of at least 140 mm Hg or DBP of at least 90 mm Hg, targeted a blood pressure goal of less than 140/90 mm Hg regardless of cardiovascular risk, and used higher SBP thresholds and targets in geriatric patients. Some clinicians continue to support the target blood pressures recommended by the JNC 8 expert panel because of concerns that such recommendations in the 2017 ACC/AHA hypertension guideline are based on extrapolation of data from the high-risk population in the SPRINT study to a lower-risk population. Also, because more than 90% of patients in SPRINT were already receiving antihypertensive drugs at baseline, data are lacking on the effects of *initiating* drug therapy at a lower blood pressure threshold (130/80 mm Hg) in patients at high risk of cardiovascular disease. The potential benefits of hypertension management and drug cost, adverse effects, and risks associated with the use of multiple antihypertensive drugs should be considered when deciding a patient's blood pressure treatment goal.

The 2017 ACC/AHA hypertension guideline recommends an ASCVD risk assessment for all adults with hypertension; however, experts state that it can be assumed that patients with hypertension and diabetes mellitus or chronic kidney disease (CKD) are at high risk for cardiovascular disease and that antihypertensive drug therapy should be initiated in these patients at a blood pressure of 130/80 mm Hg or higher. The 2017 ACC/AHA hypertension guideline also recommends a blood pressure goal of less than 130/80 mm Hg in patients with hypertension and diabetes mellitus or CKD. These recommendations are based on a systematic review of high-quality evidence from randomized controlled trials, meta-analyses, and post hoc analyses that have demonstrated substantial reductions in the risk of important clinical outcomes (e.g., cardiovascular events) regardless of comorbid conditions or age when SBP is lowered to less than 130 mm Hg. However, some clinicians have questioned the generalizability of findings from some of the trials (e.g., SPRINT) used to support the 2017 ACC/AHA hypertension guideline. For example, SPRINT included adults (mean age: 68 years) *without* diabetes mellitus who were at high risk of cardiovascular disease. While benefits of intensive blood pressure control were observed in this patient population, some clinicians have questioned whether these findings apply to younger patients who have a low risk of cardiovascular disease. In patients with CKD in the SPRINT trial, intensive blood pressure management (achieving a mean SBP of approximately 122 mm Hg compared with 136 mm Hg with standard treatment) provided a similar beneficial reduction in the composite cardiovascular disease primary outcome and all-cause mortality as in the full patient cohort. Because most patients with CKD die from cardiovascular complications, the findings of this study further support a lower blood pressure target of less than 130/80 mm Hg.

Data are lacking to determine the ideal blood pressure goal in patients with hypertension and diabetes mellitus; also, studies evaluating the benefits of intensive blood pressure control in patients with diabetes mellitus have provided conflicting results. Clinical studies reviewed for the 2017 ACC/AHA hypertension guideline have shown similar quantitative benefits from blood pressure lowering in hypertensive patients with or without diabetes mellitus. In a randomized, controlled study (ACCORD-BP) that compared a higher (SBP less than 140 mm Hg) versus lower (SBP less than 120 mm Hg) blood pressure goal in patients with diabetes mellitus, there was no difference in the incidence of cardiovascular outcomes (e.g., composite outcome of cardiovascular death, nonfatal MI, and nonfatal stroke). However, some experts state that this study was underpowered to detect a difference between the 2 treatment groups and that the factorial design of the study complicated interpretation of the results. Although SPRINT did not include patients with diabetes mellitus, patients in this study with prediabetes demonstrated a similar cardiovascular benefit from intensive treatment of blood pressure as normoglycemic patients. A meta-analysis of data from ACCORD and SPRINT suggests that the findings of both studies are consistent and that patients with diabetes mellitus benefit from more intensive blood pressure control. These data support the 2017 ACC/AHA hypertension guideline recommendation of a blood pressure treatment goal of less than 130/80 mm Hg in patients with hypertension and diabetes mellitus. Alternatively, the American Diabetes Association (ADA) recommends a blood pressure goal of less than 140/90 mm Hg in patients with diabetes mellitus. The ADA states that a lower blood pressure goal (e.g., less than 130/80 mm Hg) may be appropriate for patients with a high risk of cardiovascular disease and diabetes mellitus if it can be achieved without undue treatment burden.

Further study is needed to more clearly define optimum blood pressure goals in patients with hypertension, particularly in high-risk groups (e.g., patients with diabetes mellitus, cardiovascular disease, or cerebrovascular disease; black patients); when determining appropriate blood pressure goals, individual risks and benefits should be considered in addition to the evidence from clinical studies.

Choice of Initial Drug Therapy. In current hypertension management guidelines, thiazide diuretics are recommended as one of several preferred drugs for the initial treatment of hypertension. Results of clinical trials (e.g., ALLHAT) indicate that thiazide diuretics appear to prevent cardiovascular complications associated with hypertension as effectively as ACE inhibitors or calcium-channel blockers and better than β-blockers. (See Clinical Benefits of Thiazides in Hypertension under Hypertension in Adults: Treatment Benefits, in Uses.) These findings, in addition to cost and other considerations, have prompted some experts in the past to recommend thiazides as the initial drugs of choice in most patients with hypertension. ACC/AHA and most experts currently recommend selection of the initial antihypertensive agent from among several preferred drug classes that have been shown to reduce clinical events. The 2017 ACC/AHA hypertension guideline states that a thiazide or thiazide-like diuretic (preferably chlorthalidone), ACE inhibitor, angiotensin II receptor antagonist, or calcium-channel blocker are all acceptable choices for initial antihypertensive drug therapy in the general population of nonblack patients, including those with diabetes mellitus; drugs from any of these classes generally produce similar benefits in terms of overall mortality and cardiovascular, cerebrovascular, and renal outcomes. In black patients, including those with diabetes mellitus, the initial drug choice should include a thiazide diuretic or calcium-channel blocker. Because many patients eventually will need more than one antihypertensive drug to achieve blood pressure control, any of the recommended drug classes may be considered for add-on therapy.

In patients with hypertension and compelling indications (e.g., CKD with albuminuria [urine albumin 300 mg/day or greater, or urine albumin:creatinine ratio of 300 mg/g or equivalent in the first morning void]), angiotensin II receptor antagonists are usually considered an alternative for ACE inhibitor-intolerant patients. (See Chronic Kidney Disease under Hypertension in Adults: Considerations for Drug Therapy in Patients with Underlying Cardiovascular and Other Risk Factors, in Uses.) However, data indicate no difference in efficacy between ACE inhibitors and angiotensin II receptor antagonists with regard to blood pressure lowering and clinical outcomes (i.e., all-cause mortality, cardiovascular mortality, MI, heart failure, stroke, and end-stage renal disease). Adverse events (e.g., cough, angioedema) leading to drug discontinuance occur more frequently with ACE inhibitor therapy than with angiotensin II receptor antagonist therapy. Because of similar efficacy and a lower frequency of adverse effects, some experts believe that angiotensin II receptor antagonists should be used instead of an ACE inhibitor for the treatment of hypertension or hypertension with certain compelling indications.

Most guidelines no longer recommend β-blockers as first-line therapy for hypertension because of the lack of established superiority over other recommended drug classes and evidence from at least one study demonstrating that they may be less effective than angiotensin II receptor antagonists in preventing cardiovascular death, MI, or stroke. However, therapy with a β-blocker may still be considered in some patients with a compelling indication such as ischemic heart disease, history of MI, or heart failure.

Experts state that in patients with stage 1 hypertension (especially the elderly, those with a history of hypotension, or those who have experienced adverse drug effects), it is reasonable to initiate drug therapy using the stepped-care approach in which one drug is initiated and titrated and other drugs are added sequentially to achieve the target blood pressure. Although some patients can begin treatment with a single antihypertensive agent, starting with 2 drugs in different pharmacologic classes (either as separate agents or in a fixed-dose combination) is recommended in patients with stage 2 hypertension and an average blood pressure more than 20/10 mm Hg above their target blood pressure. Such combined therapy may increase the likelihood of achieving goal blood pressure in a more timely fashion, but also may increase the risk of adverse effects (e.g., orthostatic hypotension) in some patients (e.g., elderly). Drug regimens with complementary activity, where a second antihypertensive agent is used to block compensatory responses to the first agent or affect a different pressor mechanism, can result in additive blood pressure lowering and are preferred. Drug combinations that have similar mechanisms of action or clinical effects (e.g., the combination of an ACE inhibitor and an angiotensin II receptor antagonist) generally should be avoided. Many patients who begin therapy with a single antihypertensive agent will subsequently require at least 2 drugs from different pharmacologic classes to achieve their blood pressure goal. Experts state that other patient-specific factors, such as age, concurrent medications, drug adherence, drug interactions, the overall treatment regimen, cost, and comorbidities, also should be considered when deciding on an antihypertensive drug regimen. For any stage of hypertension, antihypertensive drug dosages should be adjusted and/or other agents substituted or added until goal blood pressure is achieved. (See Follow-up and Maintenance Drug Therapy under Hypertension in Adults: General Considerations for Initial and Maintenance Antihypertensive Therapy, in Uses.)

Follow-up and Maintenance Drug Therapy. Several strategies are used for the titration and combination of antihypertensive drugs; these strategies, which are generally based on those used in randomized controlled studies, include maximizing the dosage of the first drug before adding a second drug, adding a second drug before achieving maximum dosage of the initial drug, or initiating therapy with 2 drugs simultaneously (either as separate preparations or as a fixed-dose combination). Combined use of an ACE inhibitor and angiotensin II receptor antagonist should be avoided because of the potential risk of adverse renal effects. After initiating a new or adjusted antihypertensive drug regimen, patients should have their blood pressure reevaluated monthly until adequate blood pressure control is achieved. Effective blood pressure control can be achieved in most hypertensive patients, but many will ultimately require therapy with 2 or more antihypertensive drugs. In addition to measuring blood pressure, clinicians should evaluate patients for orthostatic hypotension, adverse drug effects, adherence to drug therapy and lifestyle modifications, and the need for drug dosage adjustments. Laboratory testing such as electrolytes and renal function status and other assessments of target organ damage also should be performed.

Considerations for Drug Therapy in Patients with Underlying Cardiovascular and Other Risk Factors Drug therapy in patients with hypertension and underlying cardiovascular or other risk factors should be carefully individualized based on the underlying disease(s), concomitant drugs, tolerance to drug-induced adverse effects, and blood pressure goal.

The following table lists compelling indications for which certain antihypertensive drug classes are recommended. The drug selections recommended for these compelling indications are based on favorable outcome data from clinical trials and existing expert guidelines; the specific drug classes that are included in the table are meant to be considered, but not necessarily all administered at the same time in an individual patient. For additional information on the management of hypertension in patients with compelling indications, individual expert clinical guidelines should be consulted.

Table 2. Compelling Indications for Drug Classes based on Comorbid Conditions

Compelling Indication[a]	Recommended Drugs					
	Diuretics	β-Blockers	ACE Inhibitors	Angiotensin II Receptor Antagonists	Calcium-channel Blockers	Aldosterone Antagonists[b]
Heart failure	x	x	x	x		x
Post-MI		x	x	x		x
Ischemic heart disease		x	x	x	x	
Diabetes mellitus[c]			x	x		
Chronic kidney disease[d]			x	x		
Recurrent stroke prevention	x		x	x		

[a] Compelling indications for antihypertensive drugs are based on benefits from outcome studies or existing clinical guidelines; the compelling indication is managed in parallel with hypertension.

[b] e.g., eplerenone, spironolactone

[c] The 2017 ACC/AHA hypertension guideline states that in adults with diabetes mellitus and hypertension who do not have albuminuria, all first-line classes of antihypertensive agents (i.e., thiazide diuretics, ACE inhibitors, angiotensin II receptor antagonists, calcium-channel blockers) are useful and effective; ACE inhibitors (or angiotensin II receptor antagonists if intolerant of ACE inhibitors) are preferred in patients with albuminuria.

[d] The 2017 ACC/AHA hypertension guideline states that adults with hypertension and stage 1 or 2 CKD without albuminuria can be treated with any of the first-line classes of antihypertensive agents (i.e., thiazide diuretics, ACE inhibitors, angiotensin II antagonists, and calcium-channel blockers); use of ACE inhibitor or angiotensin II receptor antagonist may be reasonable in those with hypertension and stage 1 or 2 CKD with albuminuria or stage 3 CKD.

Ischemic Heart Disease. Adequate control of blood pressure in patients with ischemic heart disease substantially reduces cardiovascular morbidity and mortality (e.g., stroke, coronary events, death). The 2017 ACC/AHA hypertension guideline recommends initiating antihypertensive drug therapy in patients with stable ischemic heart disease who have a blood pressure of 130/80 mm Hg or higher; alternatively, other experts recommend initiating antihypertensive drug therapy in patients with coronary artery disease who have a blood pressure of 140/90 mm Hg or higher, including in those with stable ischemic heart disease. The selection of an appropriate antihypertensive agent should be based on individual patient characteristics, but may include ACE inhibitors and/or β-blockers, with the addition of other drugs such as thiazide diuretics or calcium-channel blockers as necessary to achieve blood pressure goals. Many experts recommend the use of ACE inhibitors in hypertensive patients with stable ischemic heart disease because of the cardioprotective benefits of these drugs; angiotensin II receptor antagonists are recommended as an alternative if ACE inhibitors are not tolerated or are contraindicated. Because of the demonstrated mortality benefit of β-blockers following MI, these drugs should be administered in all patients who have survived an MI. Aldosterone receptor antagonists are also recommended to reduce morbidity and mortality following an acute MI in patients with reduced left ventricular ejection fraction (LVEF) (40% or less) who develop symptoms of heart failure or have a history of diabetes mellitus.

Heart Failure. Thiazide diuretics may be considered in hypertensive patients with heart failure and mild fluid retention. ACCF, AHA, and the Heart Failure Society of America (HFSA) also recommend the addition of an aldosterone antagonist (i.e., spironolactone or eplerenone) in selected patients with chronic heart failure and reduced LVEF who are already receiving an agent to inhibit the renin-angiotensin system (e.g., ACE inhibitor, angiotensin II receptor antagonist) and a β-blocker. The 2017 ACC/AHA hypertension guideline states that diuretics should be used to control hypertension in patients with heart failure with preserved ejection fraction who have symptoms of volume overload.

Diabetes Mellitus. The presence of diabetes mellitus increases the risk of coronary events by twofold in men and fourfold in women, and observational studies suggest that the risk of cardiovascular disease is approximately twice as high in hypertensive patients with diabetes mellitus as in nondiabetic hypertensive patients. Epidemiologic data indicate that SBP and DBP exceeding 115 and 75 mm Hg, respectively, are associated with increased cardiovascular event rates and mortality in patients with diabetes mellitus. Data are lacking to determine the ideal blood pressure goal in patients with hypertension and diabetes mellitus. Some randomized clinical studies have shown benefit from lowering SBP to less than 140 mm Hg and DBP to less than 80 mm Hg in patients with diabetes mellitus and hypertension, while other data indicate that lower blood pressure targets (e.g., less than 130/80 mm Hg) provide additional benefits. (See General Considerations for Initial and Maintenance Antihypertensive Therapy under Uses: Hypertension in Adults.) Results of several studies indicate that adequate control of blood pressure in patients with type 2 diabetes mellitus reduces the development or progression of complications of diabetes (e.g., diabetes-related death, stroke, heart failure, microvascular disease).

The ADA recommends lifestyle/behavioral modification in adults with diabetes mellitus who have elevated blood pressure (i.e., higher than 120/80 mm Hg); if blood pressure is higher than 140/90 mm Hg, the ADA recommends prompt initiation of drug therapy in addition to these nondrug interventions. However, other experts recommend initiating drug therapy at a blood pressure of 130/80 mm Hg or higher in addition to nondrug interventions in such patients.

Experts state that initial treatment of hypertension in adults with diabetes mellitus and hypertension should include any of the usual first-line agents (thiazide diuretics, ACE inhibitors, angiotensin II receptor antagonists, calcium-channel blockers). In adults with diabetes mellitus, hypertension, and albuminuria, treatment with an ACE inhibitor or angiotensin II receptor antagonist may be considered to reduce the progression of kidney disease. In the absence of albuminuria, the risk of progressive kidney disease is low, and ACE inhibitors and angiotensin II receptor antagonists have not demonstrated superior cardioprotection when compared with other first-line agents. Most patients with diabetes mellitus will require 2 or more antihypertensive agents to achieve blood pressure control.

Chronic Kidney Disease. Hypertensive patients with CKD (GFR less than 60 mL/minute per 1.73 m² or kidney damage for 3 or more months) usually will require more than one antihypertensive agent to reach target blood pressure. Use of ACE inhibitors or angiotensin II receptor antagonists may be reasonable in patients with diabetic or nondiabetic CKD (stage 1 or 2 with albuminuria or stage 3 or higher); these drugs have been shown to slow the progression of kidney disease. Evidence of a renoprotective benefit is strongest in those with higher levels of albuminuria. Increases in serum creatinine (up to 30%) may be observed as a result of a decrease in intraglomerular pressure and concurrent reduction in GFR. The 2017 ACC/AHA hypertension guideline states that in patients with less severe kidney disease (i.e., stage 1 or 2 CKD without albuminuria), any of the first-line antihypertensive agents (e.g., thiazide diuretics, ACE inhibitors, angiotensin II receptor antagonists, calcium-channel blockers) can be used for the initial treatment of hypertension. Diuretics also may be useful in the management of CKD, and may potentiate the effects of ACE inhibitors, angiotensin II receptor antagonists, and other antihypertensive agents when used in combination. Thiazides are not effective in patients with advanced renal impairment (e.g., GFR less than 30 mL/minute per 1.73 m², serum creatinine 1.5 mg/dL or greater); loop diuretics should be used instead in such patients.

Cerebrovascular Disease. Some experts recommend a blood pressure goal of less than 140/90 mm Hg in patients with ischemic stroke or transient ischemic attack (TIA), while others state that a blood pressure goal of less than 130/80 mm Hg may be reasonable. The 2017 ACC/AHA hypertension guideline states that adults not previously treated for hypertension who experience a stroke or TIA and who have an established blood pressure of 140/90 mm Hg or higher should receive antihypertensive therapy a few days after the event to reduce the risk of recurrent stroke or other vascular events. In patients with a recent lacunar stroke, experts suggest that an SBP goal of 130 mm Hg may be reasonable based on results of a randomized open-label study (the Secondary Prevention of Small Subcortical Strokes [SPS3] trial). Although experts state that the optimal choice of drug for the management of hypertension in patients with a previous TIA or ischemic stroke is uncertain, available data indicate that a thiazide diuretic, ACE inhibitor, angiotensin II receptor antagonist, or the combination of a thiazide diuretic and an ACE inhibitor may be effective. Administration of an ACE inhibitor in combination with a thiazide diuretic has been shown to lower rates of recurrent stroke.

Other Special Considerations for Antihypertensive Drug Therapy

Race. Most patients with hypertension, especially black patients, will require at least 2 antihypertensive drugs to achieve adequate blood pressure control. In general, black hypertensive patients tend to respond better to monotherapy with thiazide diuretics or calcium-channel blockers than to monotherapy with ACE inhibitors, angiotensin II receptor antagonists, or β-blockers. In a prespecified subgroup analysis of the ALLHAT study, a thiazide-like diuretic was more effective than an ACE inhibitor in improving cerebrovascular and cardiovascular outcomes in black patients; when compared with a calcium-channel blocker, the ACE inhibitor was less effective in reducing blood pressure and was associated with a 51% higher rate of stroke. However, the combination of an ACE inhibitor or an angiotensin II receptor antagonist with a calcium-channel blocker or thiazide diuretic produces similar blood pressure lowering in black patients as in other racial groups. In addition, some experts state that when use of ACE inhibitors, angiotensin II receptor antagonists, or β-blockers is indicated in hypertensive patients with underlying cardiovascular or other risk factors, these indications should be applied equally to black hypertensive patients. (See Considerations for Drug Therapy in Patients with Underlying Cardiovascular and Other Risk Factors under Uses: Hypertension in Adults.)

Advanced Age. Antihypertensive drugs recommended for initial therapy in geriatric patients, including those with isolated systolic hypertension, generally are the same as those recommended for younger patients. US guidelines have provided inconsistent recommendations regarding the optimal target SBP in geriatric patients. While some experts have recommended a higher blood pressure threshold for initiating treatment (e.g., 150/90 mm Hg) and a higher target blood pressure (less than 150/90 mm Hg) for older patients, the 2017 ACC / AHA hypertension guideline generally recommends the same blood pressure treatment lowering goal in patients regardless of age. The recommendation of higher blood pressure goals in geriatric patients was based on studies providing moderate to strong evidence that lowering blood pressure to less than 150/90 mm Hg in individuals 60 years of age or older was associated with clinical benefits (i.e., reduction in incidence of stroke, heart failure, and coronary heart disease) and some evidence, albeit less compelling, that an SBP goal of less than 140 mm Hg provided no additional benefit over a higher SBP goal (e.g., 140–160 mm Hg) in this age group. The 2017 ACC/AHA hypertension guideline recommendation that patients 65 years of age and older generally should have the same target SBP goal of younger adults (less than 130 mm Hg) is supported by data from several large, randomized, controlled studies demonstrating that more intensive blood pressure control results in lower rates of cardiovascular disease in patients older than 65, 75, and 80 years of age and does not exacerbate orthostatic hypotension or increase the risk of injurious falls. However, elderly patients should be carefully monitored for orthostatic hypotension while they are receiving antihypertensive drugs, especially when 2 agents are initiated simultaneously. Some experts state that it can be assumed that most adults 65 years of age or older with hypertension have a 10-year ASCVD risk of at least 10%, which places these individuals in the higher-risk category that requires initiation of antihypertensive drugs at an SBP of 130 mm Hg or higher. In geriatric patients with hypertension, multiple comorbidities, and a limited life expectancy, clinical judgment and patient preference should be used to determine the intensity of blood pressure lowering and the choice of antihypertensive drugs.

In several controlled studies, thiazide diuretics alone or in combination with other antihypertensive agents have been shown to reduce morbidity and mortality effectively in patients 50 years of age or older, including those with isolated systolic hypertension. Antihypertensive therapy initiated with a calcium-channel blocker also has been shown to reduce cardiovascular morbidity in older patients with isolated systolic hypertension. Although some experts state that diuretics or calcium-channel blockers may be preferred in geriatric patients, ACE inhibitors and angiotensin II receptor antagonists also have shown beneficial effects and may be considered in this population. Results of a prospective, randomized, open-label study in about 6000 hypertensive patients 65–84 years of age (the Second Australian National Blood Pressure trial) have demonstrated that initiation of therapy with ACE inhibitors may result in slightly better outcomes (concerning cardiovascular events), particularly in men, than those associated with diuretics.

Thiazides may be preferred in patients with osteoporosis. Limited data suggest that thiazide therapy may have a secondary beneficial effect in geriatric patients of reducing the risk of osteoporosis secondary to the drugs' effect on calcium homeostasis and bone mineralization.

Elevated Uric Acid and Gout. Hyperuricemia is common in patients with untreated hypertension and thiazides can increase serum uric acid concentrations. Thiazides generally should be avoided or used with caution in patients with a history of gout unless the patient is on uric acid-lowering therapy. (See Cautions: Electrolyte, Fluid, and Renal Effects.)

■ Hypertension in Pediatric Patients

Disease Overview Clinical studies have shown that elevated blood pressure during childhood increases the risk of adult hypertension and metabolic syndrome. Additionally, children with hypertension are likely to experience accelerated vascular aging. Because the long-term health risks in hypertensive children and adolescents may be substantial, it is important that clinical measures be taken to reduce such risks and optimize health outcomes.

Primary hypertension is now the predominant form of hypertension seen in children and adolescents in the US. The general characteristics of a child with primary hypertension include older age (6 years of age or older), family history of hypertension, and excess body weight (overweight or obese). An extensive evaluation for secondary causes of hypertension is not needed in such patients or in those without physical examination findings suggestive of a secondary cause.

Secondary hypertension is more common in children than in adults. The most common secondary causes of hypertension in children are renal and renovascular diseases. Hypertension secondary to a renal cause should be strongly considered in hypertensive children, particularly in those younger than 6 years of age.

Obesity and other Risk Factors. Pediatric patients with primary hypertension frequently are overweight; the rate of hypertension increases with increasing body mass index (BMI) percentile. In addition, obesity in children with hypertension may be accompanied by other cardiometabolic risk factors (e.g., dyslipidemia, disordered glucose metabolism) that may affect blood pressure. Poor diet, inactivity, and obesity contribute to pediatric hypertension and lipid disorders. Children with other chronic conditions such as sleep-disordered breathing, CKD, and those born preterm also are more likely to have hypertension.

Blood Pressure Classification The current definition of hypertension in children and adolescents is based on the normative distribution of blood pressure (auscultatory measurements) in healthy, normal-weight children. According to a 2017 clinical practice guideline of the American Academy of Pediatrics (AAP), normal blood pressure in patients 1 to less than 13 years of age is defined as an SBP and DBP that are less than in the 90th percentile for gender, age, and height, and hypertension is defined as an average SBP and/or DBP that is at least in the 95th percentile on at least 3 separate occasions. An ambulatory blood pressure monitor should be used to confirm a diagnosis of hypertension; however, for technical reasons, ambulatory monitoring may need to be limited to those who can tolerate the procedure and those for whom reference data are available. In patients 1 to less than 13 years of age, elevated blood pressure is defined as blood pressure levels that range from the 90th percentile or 120/80 mm Hg (whichever is lower) to less than the 95th percentile, stage 1 hypertension is defined as blood pressure levels that range from the 95th percentile to less than 12 mm Hg above 95th percentile (or 130/80–139/89 mm Hg, whichever is lower), and stage 2 hypertension is defined as blood pressure levels of at least 12 mm Hg above the 95th percentile (or at least 140/90 mm Hg, whichever is lower). For patients 13 years of age or older, hypertension is defined using the same blood pressure values as those recommended by ACC and AHA for adults (see Table 1). Using data from the 2001–2016 National Health and Nutrition Examination Survey (NHANES), the US Centers for Disease Control and Prevention (CDC) has estimated that approximately 800,000 individuals 12–19 years of age would be newly classified as having hypertension according to the 2017 ACC/AHA hypertension guidelines.

Considerations for Initial and Maintenance Antihypertensive Therapy The overall goals for the treatment of pediatric hypertension include achieving a blood pressure that reduces both the risk of childhood target organ damage and the risk of hypertension and cardiovascular disease in adulthood. Lifestyle/behavioral modifications that include weight reduction (for those who are overweight or obese), dietary changes, and increased physical activity are strongly encouraged in pediatric patients to limit or prevent future or excess increases in blood pressure. Data from clinical studies suggest that the relationship between diet, physical activity, and blood pressure in childhood is similar to that observed in adults.

When a pediatric patient has been diagnosed with hypertension (blood pressure being in the 95th percentile or greater), management decisions should be determined by the degree or severity of hypertension. The treatment goal for most children and adolescents treated with antihypertensive drugs and lifestyle/behavior modifications is a reduction in blood pressure to less than in the 90th percentile or less than 130/80 mm Hg. While previous guidelines have recommended a goal blood pressure less than in the 95th percentile, some evidence suggests that markers of target organ damage can be detected among children with blood pressure greater than in the 90th percentile (or greater than 120/80 mm Hg). Because hypertension is a known risk factor for the progression of CKD, a target 24-hour mean arterial pressure (MAP) less than the 50th percentile by ambulatory blood pressure monitoring is recommended in children and adolescents with hypertension and CKD to reduce the rate of decline in kidney function.

Choice of Initial Drug Therapy. Drug therapy in the management of hypertension must be individualized and adjusted based on the degree of blood pressure elevation and other patient- and drug-related factors. Drug therapy generally is reserved for pediatric patients who inadequately respond to nondrug therapies or in whom the degree of blood pressure elevation or coexisting risk factors require more prompt or aggressive therapy. Some experts recommend antihypertensive drug therapy in all pediatric patients with symptomatic hypertension, those with secondary hypertension without a clearly modifiable factor (e.g., obesity), those with persistent hypertension who fail to respond to lifestyle/behavioral modifications (especially those with an abnormal echocardiogram), and those with diabetes mellitus or CKD.

For initial drug therapy, many experts recommend use of a single antihypertensive drug (e.g., an ACE inhibitor, an angiotensin II receptor antagonist, a long-acting calcium-channel blocker, a thiazide diuretic) given at the low end of the dosing range. Because black patients may not have a robust response to an ACE inhibitor, a higher initial dosage of an ACE inhibitor may be considered in such patients; alternatively, therapy may be initiated with a thiazide diuretic or long-acting calcium-channel blocker. Clinical studies comparing the effectiveness of different antihypertensive agents in children are lacking; however, a few studies have demonstrated no clinically important differences in the degree of blood pressure lowering among drugs. It is recommended that hypertensive pediatric patients with underlying or concurrent medical conditions receive specific classes of hypotensive agents (e.g., use of ACE inhibitors or angiotensin II receptor antagonists in children with diabetes, proteinuria, or CKD). For further information on drug therapy in patients with underlying or concurrent medical conditions, see Considerations for Drug Therapy in Patients with Underlying Cardiovascular and Other Risk Factors under Uses: Hypertension in Adults.

For additional information on the management of hypertension in children, the AAP Clinical Practice Guideline for Screening and Management of High Blood Pressure in Children and Adolescents may be consulted at https://www.aap.org.

Follow-up and Maintenance Drug Therapy. In pediatric patients who fail to respond adequately to initial therapy with a single drug (i.e., a thiazide diuretic, an ACE inhibitor, an angiotensin II receptor antagonist, a long-acting calcium-channel blocker), dosage of the initial drug therapy may be increased every 2–4 weeks until the desired blood pressure goal is achieved or the maximum recommended dosage is attained or tolerated; an antihypertensive agent from another class (preferably an agent having complementary mechanism of action with the initial drug) may then be added.

Although the dosage of antihypertensive drugs may be increased every 2–4 weeks based on home blood pressure measurements, the patient should be evaluated every 4–6 weeks by a clinician until blood pressure has normalized. After the patient's blood pressure is at goal, the patient may be evaluated less frequently (i.e., every 3–4 months). Pediatric hypertensive patients also should be periodically monitored for target organ damage and adverse effects while emphasizing nonpharmacologic measures and the importance of drug therapy adherence.

■ Diabetes Insipidus

Thiazides have been widely used in the treatment of diabetes insipidus†. The drugs are effective in both the neurohypophyseal and nephrogenic forms of the disease, decreasing urine volume by up to 50%. Thiazides are particularly useful in nephrogenic diabetes insipidus, since this form of the disease is unresponsive to vasopressin or lypressin and chlorpropamide. Thiazides are also useful in patients who are allergic or refractory to vasopressin or lypressin and have been used in combination with one of these hormones and a low-salt diet in patients who excrete an exceptionally large volume of urine.

■ **Other Uses** Thiazide diuretics have been used with success in the prophylaxis of renal calculus formation associated with hypercalciuria† and in the treatment of the electrolyte disturbances associated with renal tubular acidosis†.

Dosage and Administration

■ **Administration** Thiazides are administered orally. Chlorothiazide sodium is administered IV; however, the IV route should be reserved for emergency situations or when patients are unable to take the drug orally.

■ **Dosage** Dosage of the thiazides should be adjusted according to the patient's requirements and response. The response of the patient depends on factors such as the nature and degree of the disease, state of hydration, cardiac output, physical activity, diet, and concurrent administration of other drugs. Therapy should be adjusted to attain the maximum therapeutic effect at minimum dosage. Dosage among the individual thiazides varies greatly; however, the maximum diuretic response is approximately equal with all agents.

Maintenance therapy with thiazides may be intermittent, such as administration of the drug on alternate days or once daily 3–5 days a week to minimize electrolyte imbalances. In hypertensive patients, however, a decrease in hypotensive effect often occurs during intermittent therapy, except when agents with a very long duration of action (e.g., chlorthalidone, a thiazide-like diuretic) are used. If the response is reduced when intermittent therapy is instituted, the drug should be given more frequently and alternate measures should be used to minimize electrolyte disturbances.

Edema In the management of severe edema, a large thiazide dosage may be administered until fluid retention is resolved, then a lower maintenance dosage may be instituted. Large initial dosages generally are not necessary in other conditions.

For the management of fluid retention (e.g., edema) associated with heart failure, experts state that diuretics should be administered at a dosage sufficient to achieve optimal volume status and relieve congestion without inducing an excessively rapid reduction in intravascular volume, which could result in hypotension, renal dysfunction, or both.

Hypertension Chlorthalidone dosages of 12.5–25 mg once daily or hydrochlorothiazide dosages of 25–50 mg once daily have been shown to provide optimal benefit in patients with hypertension; the effectiveness of lower dosages is unknown or has been shown to be less effective in clinical studies. The usual dosages of other thiazide or thiazide-like diuretics for the treatment of hypertension include indapamide 1.25–2.5 mg once daily and metolazone 2.5–5 mg once daily.

The patient's renal function and electrolytes should be assessed 2–4 weeks after initiation of diuretic therapy. Blood pressure should be monitored regularly (i.e., monthly) during therapy and dosage of the antihypertensive drug adjusted until blood pressure is controlled. If an adequate blood pressure response is not achieved with thiazide monotherapy, the dosage may be increased or another antihypertensive agent with demonstrated benefit (e.g., angiotensin-converting enzyme [ACE] inhibitor, angiotensin II receptor antagonist, calcium-channel blocking agent) and preferably with a complementary mechanism of action may be added; if target blood pressure is still not achieved, a third drug may be added. (See Uses: Hypertension in Adults.) In patients who develop unacceptable adverse effects with a thiazide, the drug should be discontinued and another antihypertensive agent from a different pharmacologic class should be initiated.

Blood Pressure Monitoring and Treatment Goals. Blood pressure monitoring using an out-of-office (home [self-monitored]) or ambulatory method (using a device that measures blood pressure over a 24-hour period) as an adjunct to in-office monitoring generally is recommended to provide a more reliable assessment of blood pressure; studies suggest that out-of-office blood pressure may be a better predictor of hypertension-induced organ damage and cardiovascular risk than office blood pressure. Periodic determination of blood pressure in both the morning and evening (before taking the morning or evening dose) is useful in monitoring daytime control and ensuring that the surge in blood pressure that occurs with arising has been modulated adequately. Occasionally, particularly in geriatric patients and those with orthostatic symptoms, monitoring should include blood pressure determinations in both the seated position and, to recognize possible postural hypotension, after standing quietly for 2–5 minutes.

Once antihypertensive drug therapy has been initiated, dosage generally is adjusted at approximately monthly intervals if blood pressure control is inadequate at a given dosage; additional drugs may need to be added to an antihypertensive drug regimen to achieve adequate blood pressure control. Once blood pressure has been stabilized, follow-up visits generally can be scheduled at 3- to 6-month intervals, depending on patient status.

The goal of hypertension management and prevention is to achieve and maintain optimal control of blood pressure. However, the optimum blood pressure threshold for initiating antihypertensive drug therapy and specific treatment goals remain controversial. While other hypertension guidelines have based target blood pressure goals on age and comorbidities, the 2017 ACC/AHA hypertension guideline incorporates underlying cardiovascular risk into decision making regarding treatment and generally recommends the same target blood pressure (i.e., less than 130/80 mm Hg) for all adults. Many patients will require at least 2 drugs from different pharmacologic classes to achieve this blood pressure goal; the potential benefits of hypertension management and drug cost, adverse effects, and risks associated with the use of multiple antihypertensive drugs also should be considered when deciding a patient's blood pressure treatment goal. (See General Considerations for Initial and Maintenance Antihypertensive Therapy under Uses: Hypertension in Adults.)

In children with hypertension with or without diabetes mellitus, blood pressure should be reduced to less than the corresponding age-adjusted 90th percentile value and to less than 130/80 mm Hg in adolescents at least 13 years of age. In children and adolescents with hypertension and CKD, the 24-hour mean arterial pressure (MAP) as determined by ambulatory blood pressure monitoring should be decreased to a value less than the 50th percentile.

Long-term Regimen Adjustments. A reduction in the dosage or number of antihypertensive drugs in the regimen may be possible in some patients after hypertension has been controlled effectively for an extended period. Such step-down therapy is more often successful in patients who are making lifestyle modifications. The reduction should be gradual and accompanied by frequent monitoring, since blood pressure often rises again to hypertensive levels.

Combination Therapy. When combination therapy is required in the management of hypertension, dosage of each agent can be adjusted first by administering each drug separately. If it is determined that the optimum maintenance dosage of both drugs corresponds to the ratio in a commercial combination preparation, a fixed combination may be used. Alternatively, therapy can be initiated with a fixed combination of 2 antihypertensive agents. Use of fixed-combination preparations may result in increased patient compliance. However, fixed-combination preparations containing 3 different antihypertensive agents may contain a thiazide diuretic dosage that is lower than recommended for the treatment of hypertension.

Whenever dosage adjustment is necessary, the drugs then can be administered separately again or increased with certain fixed combinations according to the manufacturer's recommendations. Initiating therapy and adjusting dosage with separate administration of each drug are particularly important with combination preparations containing antihypertensive agents that have wide ranges in their effective dosages and may require frequent dosage alterations (e.g., methyldopa, guanethidine).

For information on commercially available preparations containing hydrochlorothiazide in fixed combination with a potassium-sparing diuretic, see the individual monographs in 40:28.10.

■ **Dosage in Renal Impairment** For information on dosage of thiazide and thiazide-like diuretics in patient with renal impairment, see the individual monographs in 40:28.10.

Cautions

Adverse effects associated with some thiazides (e.g., hydrochlorothiazide) may be dose-related.

■ **Electrolyte, Fluid, and Renal Effects** One of the most common adverse effects of the thiazides is potassium depletion which occurs in most patients. Potassium depletion may cause cardiac arrhythmias and is particularly important in patients receiving cardiac glycosides because hypokalemia potentiates the cardiac toxicity (e.g., increased ventricular irritability) of these agents. Potassium concentrations may be especially low in patients with primary or secondary aldosteronism, in patients with a low potassium intake, in those receiving other potassium-depleting drugs, and in patients with other losses of potassium, as in vomiting and diarrhea. Intermittent rather than continuous administration of the thiazides and/or ingestion of potassium-rich foods may reduce or prevent potassium depletion; however, prophylactic administration of a potassium supplement such as potassium chloride solution or a potassium-sparing diuretic may be necessary in patients whose serum potassium concentration is less than about 3 mEq/L. Enteric-coated potassium-containing tablets should not be used because of the possibility of GI ulceration.

Rarely, sudden death from cardiac arrest has been associated with thiazide monotherapy, and this effect may be dose related. Since the risk of sudden cardiac death with thiazide therapy appears to be reduced by the addition of a potassium-sparing diuretic, it has been suggested that changes in serum concentrations of potassium or magnesium may contribute to the risk of sudden cardiac death; however, possible reductions in thiazide dosage that may have accompanied the addition of a potassium-sparing diuretic also may have contributed to the risk reduction with combined therapy.

Hypochloremic alkalosis may occur with hypokalemia, especially in patients with other losses of potassium and chloride such as those with vomiting, diarrhea, GI drainage, excessive sweating, paracentesis, or potassium-losing renal diseases. Patients with hepatic cirrhosis who are receiving thiazides are also very susceptible to hypokalemic hypochloremic alkalosis with the thiazides. Blood ammonia concentrations may be further increased in patients with previously elevated concentrations. The diuretic may induce hepatic encephalopathy secondary to electrolyte imbalances.

Dilutional hyponatremia may occasionally occur or be aggravated during thiazide therapy and can be life-threatening. Such hyponatremia usually develops insidiously during chronic therapy and is asymptomatic and of modest degree, and in such cases, serum sodium concentrations return rapidly to within the normal range following withdrawal of the diuretic, water restriction, and potassium and/or magnesium supplementation. However, severe hyponatremia (serum sodium concentration less than 120 mEq/L) can occur rarely. Dilutional hyponatremia most commonly occurs in hot weather in patients with chronic heart failure or hepatic disease, is usually present before diuretic therapy, and is manifested by signs of edema associated with hyponatremia. Geriatric patients, especially females who are underweight, have poor oral intake of fluid and electrolytes, and/or excessive intake of low-sodium nutritional supplements, may be at increased risk of dilutional hyponatremia induced by the drugs. Dilutional hyponatremia usually is treated by restriction of fluid intake to about 500 mL per day and withdrawal of the diuretic. Sodium chloride should not be administered unless the hyponatremia is life threatening. If sodium chloride is administered to correct severe, symptomatic hyponatremia, care should be taken to avoid early overcorrection to normonatremia or hypernatremia since resultant rapid osmolar changes may be associated with the development of central pontine myelinolysis. Therefore, although prognosis appears to depend on rapid correction of severe hyponatremia during the first 1 or 2 days, such correction initially should only be to a state of mild hyponatremia; it is recommended that serum sodium concentration be corrected by no more than 20 mEq/L during the first 24 hours. Avoidance of hypernatremia during subsequent days also is important. Patients with severe, symptomatic hyponatremia generally should be managed in an intensive care facility with frequent monitoring of fluid and electrolyte balance.

Hypercalcemia may also occur infrequently in patients receiving thiazides, especially in patients receiving vitamin D or having mild hyperparathyroidism. Hypomagnesemia may also occur.

Hyperuricemia occurs in many patients receiving a thiazide or related diuretic. Hyperuricemia is usually asymptomatic and rarely leads to clinical gout except in patients with a history of gout, familial predisposition to gout, or chronic renal failure. If therapy is required, hyperuricemia and gout may be treated with a uricosuric agent.

Impairment of renal function, interstitial nephritis (which may be allergic), and reversible renal failure have been reported mainly in patients with preexisting renal disease (proliferative glomerulonephritis or nephrotic syndrome) who were receiving thiazides; however, a direct causative relationship has not been demonstrated.

■ Metabolic and Endocrine Effects Pathologic changes in the parathyroid gland with hypercalcemia and hypophosphatemia have occurred occasionally during prolonged thiazide therapy. (See Cautions: Precautions and Contraindications.) Common complications of hyperparathyroidism such as nephrolithiasis, bone resorption, and peptic ulceration have not been reported.

Thiazides and related diuretics can produce hyperglycemia and glycosuria in diabetics. Insulin or oral antidiabetic agent requirements of diabetics may be altered by the thiazides and, in addition, diabetes mellitus has been precipitated in prediabetic patients receiving thiazides. However, results of a large, prospective, cohort study found that the increased risk of developing type 2 diabetes mellitus in patients receiving antihypertensive drug therapy (e.g., thiazide diuretics) appears to be related to the presence of hypertension. In this study, development of type 2 diabetes mellitus was shown to be almost 2.5 times more likely in hypertensive patients than in normotensive patients. In addition, once the study investigators accounted for the presence of hypertension, the risk of developing diabetes mellitus among hypertensive patients receiving thiazide diuretics was shown to be no greater than that among those receiving no drug therapy. Abnormal glucose tolerance usually does not develop in patients receiving thiazides who previously exhibited normal glucose tolerance. Hyperglycemia and impairment of glucose tolerance are almost always reversible by discontinuance of the drugs, and correction of hypokalemia may improve glucose tolerance.

Thiazides and related diuretics can slightly increase serum total cholesterol concentrations; increases in the low-density lipoprotein cholesterol and/or very low-density lipoprotein cholesterol subfractions appear to be principally responsible for these increases. The effect of these diuretics on high-density lipoprotein cholesterol concentrations has not been fully elucidated but appears to be variable. Increases in serum triglyceride concentrations also can occur in thiazide-treated patients. Whether changes in serum lipid and lipoprotein concentrations are dose-related and whether such changes persist during long-term diuretic therapy has not been established. In addition, the clinical importance of these effects is not known and further evaluation is needed. The diuretic-induced increase in serum cholesterol concentration can generally be counteracted by concomitant use of a diet low in saturated fat and cholesterol.

■ Uncommon Adverse Effects Adverse effects of thiazides other than electrolyte and metabolic disturbances are rare.

Dermatologic and Sensitivity Reactions Dermatologic reactions are uncommon with thiazides but purpura, photosensitivity, rash, alopecia, urticaria, erythema multiforme including Stevens-Johnson syndrome, exfoliative dermatitis including toxic epidermal necrolysis, and polyarteritis nodosa may occur. Cross-photosensitivity has been reported in a patient who received quinethazone after previously having photosensitivity reactions with 2 thiazides. Allergic reactions are most likely to occur in patients with a history of allergy or bronchial asthma, and the possibility of exacerbation or activation of systemic lupus erythematosus has been reported.

Most information reporting cross-reactivity among sulfonamide derivatives is based on case reports. The mechanism of sulfonamide sensitivity is poorly understood, and the contribution of allergens, haptens, and/or other immune mechanisms remains to be established. Although there is an association between hypersensitivity to sulfonamide anti-infectives and subsequent sensitivity reactions to non-anti-infective sulfonamides such as thiazides and thiazide manufacturers state that use of the diuretics is contraindicated in patients who are allergic to any sulfonamide derivative, this association appears to result from a predisposition to allergic reactions in general rather than to cross-reactivity to the sulfa moiety per se. In fact, a retrospective cohort study using the UK General Practice Research Database found that the risk of associated allergic reactions in sulfonamide anti-infective-sensitive patients was even greater following exposure to penicillins than following exposure to non-anti-infective sulfonamides such as thiazides. In addition, the risk of an allergic reaction following administration of a non-anti-infective sulfonamide (e.g., thiazides, sulfonylurea antidiabetic agents, furosemide, dapsone, probenecid) was lower in patients with a history of sensitivity to sulfonamide anti-infectives than in those with a history of penicillin sensitivity. There also is other evidence, including a pooled analysis of data from clinical trails with celecoxib (an arylsulfonamide) and a cohort study of the risk of cross-sensitivity between co-trimoxazole and dapsone (a sulfone), to support the apparent lack of chemical cross-reactivity among sulfa derivatives. Therefore, based on current evidence from cohort studies and pooled analyses, some researchers suggest that clinicians should understand that patients with a history of any allergic reaction to sulfonamides or penicillins may be at increased risk for reactions to other drugs in general, and a history of sensitivity to sulfonamide anti-infectives should not be considered an absolute contraindication to subsequent use of non-anti-infective sulfonamides.

Cardiovascular Effects Orthostatic hypotension may occur rarely, and hypotensive episodes have occurred during surgery in patients receiving thiazides. The hypotensive effect of the drugs may be enhanced in postsympathectomy patients. Transient cerebral ischemic attacks related to thiazide-induced hypotension have been reported.

GI Effects GI adverse effects reported with the thiazides include anorexia, gastric irritation, nausea, vomiting, sialadenitis, cramping, diarrhea, constipation, intrahepatic cholestatic jaundice, and pancreatitis.

CNS Effects CNS reactions associated with thiazides include dizziness, vertigo, paresthesia, headache, and xanthopsia.

Hematologic Effects Infrequently, hematologic reactions including leukopenia, hemolytic anemia, thrombocytopenic purpura, agranulocytosis, and aplastic anemia have been reported with some of the thiazides.

Other Adverse Effects Muscle spasms, impotence, renal failure, renal dysfunction, interstitial nephritis, weakness, restlessness, transient blurred vision, fever, respiratory distress, necrotizing angiitis (vasculitis and cutaneous vasculitis), and anaphylactic reactions have also been reported with thiazides.

Rarely, pulmonary edema and allergic pneumonitis have been reported with hydrochlorothiazide. Hematuria has been reported in at least one patient receiving IV chlorothiazide.

■ Precautions and Contraindications Electrolyte disturbances may occur during thiazide therapy, and patients should be observed for signs of electrolyte imbalance such as dryness of mouth, thirst, weakness, lethargy, drowsiness, restlessness, confusion, seizures, oliguria, or muscle pains or cramps, muscular fatigue, hypotension, tachycardia, or GI disturbances such as nausea and vomiting. Periodic determination of serum electrolyte concentrations (particularly potassium, sodium, chloride, and bicarbonate) should be performed and measures to maintain normal serum concentrations should be instituted if necessary. Serum and urinary electrolyte measurements are especially important in diabetic patients and in patients who are vomiting, have diarrhea, are receiving parenteral fluids, or are expected to undergo excessive diuresis. It has been recommended that electrolytes be measured weekly or more frequently early in the course of therapy. Once the electrolyte response has stabilized, it may be possible to extend the interval between electrolyte determinations to 3 months or longer.

Thiazides should be used with caution in patients with severe renal disease because the drugs decrease the glomerular filtration rate (GFR) and may precipitate azotemia. The effects of thiazides may be cumulative in patients with impaired renal function. If progressive renal impairment becomes evident as indicated by rising nonprotein nitrogen, BUN, or serum creatinine concentrations, careful reappraisal of therapy is necessary with consideration given to interrupting or discontinuing thiazide therapy. The drugs should also be used with caution in patients with impaired hepatic function or progressive liver disease, particularly when potassium deficiency exists, because they may precipitate hepatic coma as a result of alterations in electrolyte balance. Thiazides should be discontinued immediately if signs of impending hepatic coma appear.

Thiazides are contraindicated in patients with anuria and in those who are allergic to any of the thiazides. The manufacturers state that thiazides are contraindicated in patients who are allergic to other sulfonamide derivatives. However, there currently is limited evidence to support this latter contraindication, and some suggest that a history of sensitivity to sulfonamide anti-infectives ("sulfa sensitivity") should not be considered an absolute contraindication to non-anti-infective sulfonamides such as thiazides. (See Uncommon Adverse Effects: Dermatologic and Sensitivity Reactions, in Cautions.)

■ Pregnancy and Lactation The routine use of thiazides is contraindicated in pregnant women with mild edema who are otherwise healthy. Thiazides cross the placenta and appear in cord blood. Thrombocytopenia has been reported in newborn infants of women receiving thiazides; however, this appears to be an unpredictable idiosyncratic reaction. Amniotic fluid concentrations of uric acid and creatinine are elevated in women receiving thiazides near term. Jaundice may also occur in the fetus or neonate. These risks and the possibility that other effects of the thiazides may occur in the fetus or neonate must be weighed against the potential benefits of therapy.

Although some evidence suggests that thiazide use during pregnancy may be associated with an increased risk of fetal abnormalities, other data do not support such an association. Some experts have considered thiazide diuretics to be contraindicated during pregnancy, except in patients with heart disease or chronic hypertension, because of the theoretical fetal risk associated with plasma volume reduction. The American College of Obstetricians and Gynecologists (ACOG) states that thiazide diuretics may be used as second-line antihypertensive agents and may be particularly useful in women who are sodium sensitive. The goal of antihypertensive treatment in pregnant women with hypertension is to minimize the acute complications of maternal hypertension while avoiding therapy that could compromise fetal well-being. Antihypertensive therapy is recommended in pregnant women with chronic hypertension who have persistent, severely elevated blood pressure (e.g., systolic blood pressure [SBP] of 160 mm Hg or higher or diastolic blood pressure [DBP] of 105 mm Hg or higher); it is less clear whether antihypertensive therapy should be initiated in women with mild to moderate chronic hypertension. If initiation of antihypertensive therapy is necessary in a pregnant woman, use of labetalol, nifedipine, or methyldopa is recommended. Angiotensin-converting enzyme (ACE) inhibitors, angiotensin II receptor antagonists, and aldosterone antagonists should not be used in pregnant women. In women who are already receiving antihypertensive therapy prior to pregnancy, ACOG states there are insufficient data to make recommendations regarding the continuance or discontinuance of such therapy; treatment decisions should be individualized in these situations. Thiazide diuretics are not recommended for the prevention or management of gestational hypertension or preeclampsia.

Thiazides are distributed into the milk of nursing women in low concentrations; however, the drug is considered to be compatible with breastfeeding. The potential for idiosyncratic or allergic reactions in the infant should be considered, however, and some manufacturers state that women receiving thiazides should not nurse their infants.

Drug Interactions

■ Drugs Affected by or Causing Potassium Depletion In patients receiving digitalis glycosides, electrolyte disturbances produced by the thiazides (principally hypokalemia, but also hypomagnesemia and hypercalcemia) predispose the patient to digitalis toxicity. Periodic electrolyte determinations should be performed in patients receiving a thiazide and a digitalis glycoside, and correction of hypokalemia should be undertaken if warranted. (See Cautions: Electrolyte, Fluid, and Renal Effects.)

It has been stated that the thiazides and related diuretics may cause prolonged neuromuscular blockade in patients receiving nondepolarizing neuromuscular blocking agents, such as tubocurarine chloride or gallamine triethiodide (no longer commercially available in the US), presumably because of potassium depletion. Actual case reports are lacking, however.

Some drugs such as corticosteroids, corticotropin, and amphotericin B also cause potassium loss, and severe potassium depletion may occur when one of these drugs is administered during thiazide therapy.

■ Lithium Thiazides, sometimes used in combination with lithium to reduce lithium-induced polyuria, will reduce renal lithium clearance within several days. The reduced lithium clearance has resulted in increased serum lithium concentrations and several cases of lithium intoxication. When thiazide diuretics are used to treat lithium-induced polyuria, most clinicians recommend reducing lithium dosage by about 50% and carefully monitoring serum lithium concentrations. Thiazides and lithium should generally not be used concomitantly because of the increased risk of lithium toxicity.

■ Antidiabetic Agents The hyperglycemic effect of the thiazides may exacerbate diabetes mellitus, resulting in increased requirements of insulin or sulfonylurea antidiabetic agents, temporary loss of diabetic control, or secondary failure to the antidiabetic agent.

■ Hypotensive Agents The hypotensive effects of most other hypotensive agents are increased by the thiazide diuretics. This effect is usually used to therapeutic advantage in antihypertensive therapy, but severe postural hypotension may result if a thiazide is added to the regimen of a patient stabilized on a potent hypotensive agent such as guanethidine sulfate, methyldopa, or a ganglionic blocking agent. The hyperglycemic, hypotensive, and hyperuricemic effects of diazoxide may be potentiated by the thiazide diuretics. Caution should be used in administering the thiazides with diazoxide.

■ Probenecid Probenecid blocks thiazide-induced uric acid retention when administered concomitantly with the thiazides. It appears that probenecid enhances excretion of calcium, magnesium, and citrate during thiazide therapy, but urinary calcium concentrations remain below normal. The excretion of sodium, potassium, ammonia, chloride, bicarbonate, phosphate, and titratable acid during thiazide therapy do not seem to be affected by concomitant probenecid therapy. Probenecid also blocks the renal tubular secretion of the thiazides, but its effect on the duration of action of the thiazides has apparently not been studied.

■ Nonsteroidal Anti-inflammatory Agents Diuretics may increase the risk of nonsteroidal anti-inflammatory agent (NSAIA)-induced renal failure. Such NSAIA-induced renal failure appears to be secondary to decreased renal blood flow resulting from prostaglandin inhibition by the drugs. In addition, NSAIAs may interfere with the natriuretic, diuretic, and antihypertensive response to diuretics. Therefore, patients receiving the drugs concomitantly should be observed closely for possible adverse effects and/or attenuation of diuretic-induced therapeutic effects.

■ Other Drugs Since the pH of the urine becomes slightly more alkaline during thiazide therapy, the urinary excretion of some amines such as amphetamine and quinidine may be decreased somewhat when given concurrently with the thiazides; however, since the change in urine pH is not great during thiazide therapy, toxic blood concentrations of these drugs usually do not occur. Patients receiving amines (e.g., amphetamine, quinidine) should be monitored for signs of toxicity following initiation of thiazide therapy. Urinary alkalinization may decrease the effectiveness of methenamine compounds which require a urinary pH of 5.5 or less for optimal activity. The pH of the urine should be monitored during concurrent therapy with a thiazide and a methenamine compound.

Alcohol, barbiturates, and opiates are reported to increase the postural hypotensive effect of the thiazides.

It has been proposed that the thiazides may antagonize the effects of oral anticoagulants; however, studies which demonstrate this effect are lacking.

Cholestyramine or colestipol resin may bind thiazides and reduce their absorption from the GI tract, with cholestyramine reportedly producing greater binding in vitro. Thiazides should be administered at least 2 hours before cholestyramine or colestipol when these drugs are used concomitantly.

A decrease in arterial responsiveness to vasopressors has been reported during thiazide therapy; however, the clinical importance of this interaction has not been established.

Laboratory Test Interferences

In addition to alterations in laboratory test values resulting from the metabolic changes caused by the thiazides, the drugs may affect the results of a number of other tests. Thiazides may cause false-negative results in both the tyramine and phentolamine tests and probably the histamine test for pheochromocytoma. Protein-bound iodine values may be decreased during thiazide therapy, although usually not to subnormal levels. Triiodothyronine resin uptake may be decreased slightly, but the 24-hour I 131 uptake is not affected. Thyroid function is not affected by the thiazides.

Since thiazides may cause elevations in serum calcium in the absence of known disorders of calcium metabolism, the drugs should be discontinued prior to performing tests of parathyroid function.

It has been reported that hydrochlorothiazide causes falsely decreased values in the spectrophotometric assay of total urinary estrogen by interfering with formation of the Kober chromogen, and with the assay of estriol by degrading estriol at the acid hydrolytic stage of the assay. These interferences apparently do not occur with chlorothiazide.

Serum amylase values may be increased substantially in both asymptomatic patients and in patients developing acute pancreatitis who are receiving thiazides. Thiazides have been reported to decrease urinary corticosteroid values by interfering in vitro with the absorbance in the modified Glenn-Nelson technique for urinary 17-hydroxycorticosteroids. The drugs may also decrease urinary excretion of cortisol. The importance of the effect of thiazides on urinary corticosteroids is not clear.

Thiazides compete with phenolsulfonphthalein (PSP) for secretion by the proximal renal tubules, but the importance of this effect on PSP excretion is unknown.

Acute Toxicity

■ Manifestations In addition to diuresis and resultant dehydration, overdosage of thiazides may produce lethargy, nausea, weakness, and electrolyte imbalance; lethargy may progress to coma within a few hours with minimal depression of respiratory and cardiovascular function and without evidence of dehydration or serum electrolyte changes. The mechanism of thiazide-induced CNS depression is unknown. GI irritation and hypermotility may occur, and temporary elevation of the BUN has been reported. Serum electrolyte changes (e.g., hypokalemia, hypochloremia, hyponatremia) may occur, especially in patients with impaired renal function.

■ Treatment In the treatment of thiazide overdosage, gastric contents may be evacuated taking caution to avoid aspiration, especially in unconscious patients. If the patient is conscious, induction of vomiting with ipecac syrup is effective in removing the drug from the stomach. Cathartics should *not* be administered because they tend to promote loss of fluid and electrolytes. Treatment is generally supportive. Serum electrolytes and renal function should be monitored, and replacement of fluid and electrolytes may be indicated. Measures may be required to maintain respiratory, cardiovascular, and renal function. GI irritation is usually of short duration, but may be treated symptomatically.

Pharmacology

Thiazides and related diuretics enhance excretion of sodium, chloride, and water by interfering with the transport of sodium ions across the renal tubular epithelium. Their primary site of action appears to be the cortical diluting segment of the nephron. The exact mechanism of action of the thiazides is unclear; however, they may act by altering metabolism of the tubular cells.

Thiazides decrease the glomerular filtration rate (GFR), but whether this results from a direct effect on renal vasculature or is secondary to the decrease in intravascular fluid volume or an increase in tubular pressure caused by the inhibition of sodium and water reabsorption is unclear. The fall in GFR is not important in the mechanism of action of the drugs, but contributes to their decreased efficacy in patients with impaired renal function. Thiazides also exhibit a carbonic anhydrase inhibiting effect which varies considerably among the various agents.

In addition to increasing sodium and chloride excretion, thiazides affect excretion of other electrolytes. Potassium excretion is substantially increased because of the increased amount of sodium reaching the distal tubular site of sodium-potassium exchange. The ratio of potassium to sodium excreted may vary among the thiazides and related diuretics and at different dosages of the drugs; however, the differences in excretion are generally clinically insignificant. Long-term thiazide therapy can cause mild metabolic alkalosis associated with hypokalemia and hypochloremia.

Thiazides increase bicarbonate excretion (although to a lesser extent than chloride excretion) but change in urinary pH is usually minimal. The diuretic efficacy of the thiazides is not affected by the acid-base balance of the patient. Magnesium, phosphate, bromide, and iodide excretion are also increased. Excretion of ammonia may decrease slightly, and blood ammonia concentrations may be increased. Urinary calcium excretion may increase transiently when therapy is initiated; however, during long-term administration, it is substantially decreased. The hypocalciuric effect is thought to result from a decrease in extracellular fluid (ECF) volume, although calcium reabsorption in the nephron may be increased. Thiazides also have been reported to cause slight or intermittent elevations in serum calcium concentration. The rate of excretion of uric acid is decreased, probably because of competitive inhibition of uric acid secretion or a decrease in ECF volume and a secondary increase in uric acid reabsorption. Lithium excretion may also be decreased.

Thiazides have hypotensive activity in hypertensive patients, and they augment the action of other hypotensive agents. The precise mechanism of hypotensive action has not been determined, but it has been postulated that part of this effect is caused by direct arteriolar dilation. Initially, thiazides cause appreciable decreases in ECF volume, plasma volume, and cardiac output which may account for the decrease in blood pressure. After several weeks of therapy, however, plasma and ECF volumes approach, but remain slightly below, normal. Cardiac output returns to normal or slightly above, and peripheral vascular resistance remains decreased. Total body sodium also remains slightly below pretreatment values, which may be due to chronic depletion of sodium. Slight decreases in plasma and ECF volumes and total body sodium during prolonged thiazide therapy are not sufficient to explain the long-term decrease in blood pressure, but may explain the efficacy of thiazides in combination with most other hypotensive agents which tend to increase sodium retention and plasma volume.

Plasma renin activity is considerably elevated during thiazide therapy, probably because of plasma volume changes. The aldosterone secretion rate is slightly but substantially increased and contributes to the hypokalemia caused by thiazides.

Paradoxically, thiazides decrease urine volume in patients with diabetes insipidus. The urine becomes less hypotonic, but not hypertonic, and thirst and water consumption are decreased. This effect is thought to result mainly from the decrease in plasma volume and from sodium depletion with a resultant increase in renal water and sodium reabsorption, although other factors may play a role.

Thiazides can induce hyperglycemia, exacerbate preexisting diabetes mellitus, or precipitate diabetes in prediabetic patients. The mechanism of this action of the thiazides is not known, but there is evidence that the drugs act at both pancreatic and peripheral sites and that potassium depletion may decrease glucose tolerance.

Pharmacokinetics

■ **Absorption** Thiazides are absorbed from the GI tract in varying degrees. The onset of diuretic action of the thiazides following oral administration occurs within 2 hours, and the peak effect occurs 3–6 hours after administration. Following IV administration, chlorothiazide sodium has an onset of action within 15 minutes and a peak effect in 30 minutes. The duration of diuretic action of the individual agent is determined by the rate of its excretion. The approximate duration of diuretic action of a single dose of the thiazides and related diuretics is as follows:

Table 3. Duration of Diuretic Action

Drug	Duration of Diuretic Action (hours)
Chlorothiazide (IV)	2
Chlorothiazide (oral)	6–12
Hydrochlorothiazide	6–12
Metolazone	12–24
Hydroflumethiazide	12–24
Bendroflumethiazide	18–24
Methyclothiazide	24
Trichlormethiazide	24
Chlorthalidone	24–72

The onset of hypotensive action is generally 3 or 4 days, and the hypotensive action dissipates during the first week after discontinuing chronic therapy.

■ **Distribution** Thiazides are distributed in the extracellular space and cross the placenta. Thiazides also are distributed into milk.

■ **Elimination** Most thiazides are excreted in urine, principally unchanged. The drugs are excreted by glomerular filtration and active secretion in the proximal tubule. The renal clearance of the thiazides varies; those with the lowest renal clearance generally require the lowest dosage for therapeutic effect. In patients with uncompensated heart failure or impaired renal function, excretion of the drugs may be delayed.

Chemistry

Thiazide (benzothiadiazine) diuretics are derivatives of 1,2,4-benzothiadiazine-7-sulfonamide 1,1-dioxide. Substitution in the R^2 and R^3 positions of the thiazide nucleus increases the activity of the compound. In most thiazides, the 3-4 bond is saturated and all presently marketed compounds have a chloride or CF_3 substituent at the 6 position of the thiazide nucleus. Quinethazone and metolazone, which are pharmacologically similar to the thiazides, are quinazoline derivatives and differ from the thiazides in having a carbonyl group rather than a sulfoxide group at the 1 position. Chlorthalidone is also pharmacologically and structurally similar to the thiazides, but is a phthalimidine derivative of benzenesulfonamide. Diazoxide, a nondiuretic hypotensive agent, is structurally related to the thiazides, but lacks the 7-sulfamyl group common to the thiazide diuretics.

In general, thiazides occur as white or nearly white, crystalline powders and are very slightly soluble or practically insoluble in water.

For further information on chemistry and stability, pharmacology, pharmacokinetics, and dosage and administration of thiazides, see the individual monographs in 40:28.

†Use is not currently included in the labeling approved by the US Food and Drug Administration

hydroCHLOROthiazide HCTZ

■ Hydrochlorothiazide is a thiazide diuretic and antihypertensive agent.

Dosage and Administration

■ **Administration** Hydrochlorothiazide is administered orally.

■ **Dosage** Dosage of hydrochlorothiazide should be individualized according to the patient's requirements and response. The lowest dosage necessary to produce the desired clinical effect should be used. If hydrochlorothiazide is added to the regimen of a patient stabilized on a potent hypotensive agent, dosage of the hypotensive agent should initially be reduced to avoid the possibility of severe hypotension.

Edema For the management of edema, the usual adult dosage of hydrochlorothiazide is 25–100 mg daily in 1–3 divided doses. Many patients also may respond to intermittent therapy (e.g., on alternate days or on 3–5 days weekly). Excessive diuretic response and the resulting undesirable electrolyte imbalance are less likely to occur with such intermittent administration of the drug.

For the management of fluid retention (e.g., edema) associated with heart failure, some experts recommend initiating hydrochlorothiazide at a low dosage (e.g., 25 mg once or twice daily) and increasing the dosage (maximum of 200 mg daily) until urine output increases and weight decreases, generally by 0.5–1 kg daily. When hydrochlorothiazide is used for sequential nephron blockade in the management of fluid retention in heart failure, some experts recommend an initial dosage of 25–100 mg once or twice daily in combination with a loop diuretic. Experts state that diuretics should be administered at a dosage sufficient to achieve optimal volume status and relieve congestion without inducing an excessively rapid reduction in intravascular volume, which could result in hypotension, renal dysfunction, or both.

Hypertension **Usual Dosage.** For the management of hypertension in adults, the manufacturers recommend an initial hydrochlorothiazide dosage of 12.5–25 mg once daily and a usual maximum dosage of 50 mg daily (in 1 or 2 divided doses). Dosages of 25–100 mg daily (in 1 or 2 divided doses) have been used in randomized controlled studies; experts recommend a dosage of 25–50 mg daily for optimal balance between efficacy and safety in the management of hypertension in adults. Dosages exceeding 50 mg daily usually are associated with marked hypokalemia; some manufacturers state that such dosages are not recommended.

Fixed-combination Therapy. When combination therapy is required in the management of hypertension, dosage can first be adjusted by administering each drug separately. If it is determined that the optimum maintenance dosage corresponds to the ratio in the commercial combination preparation, the fixed combination may be used. Alternatively, therapy can be initiated with a fixed combination of 2 antihypertensive agents. Use of fixed-combination preparations may increase patient compliance.

For information on commercially available preparations containing hydrochlorothiazide in fixed combination with a potassium-sparing diuretic, see the individual monographs in 40:28.10.

Monitoring and Blood Pressure Treatment Goals. The patient's renal function and electrolytes should be assessed 2–4 weeks after initiation of diuretic therapy. Blood pressure should be monitored regularly (i.e., monthly) during therapy and dosage of the antihypertensive drug adjusted until blood pressure is controlled. If an adequate blood pressure response is not achieved with hydrochlorothiazide monotherapy, another antihypertensive agent with demonstrated benefit and preferably with a complementary mechanism of action (e.g., angiotensin-converting enzyme [ACE] inhibitor, angiotensin II receptor antagonist, calcium-channel blocker) may be added; if goal blood pressure is still not achieved, a third drug may be added. (See Uses: Hypertension in Adults, in the Thiazides General Statement 40:28.20.) In patients who develop unacceptable adverse effects with hydrochlorothiazide, the drug should be discontinued and another antihypertensive agent from a different pharmacologic class should be initiated.

The goal of hypertension management and prevention is to achieve and maintain optimal control of blood pressure. However, the optimum blood pressure threshold for initiating antihypertensive drug therapy and specific treatment goals remain controversial. A 2017 multidisciplinary hypertension guideline from the American College of Cardiology (ACC), American Heart Association (AHA), and a number of other professional organizations generally recommends a blood pressure goal of less than 130/80 mm Hg in all adults regardless of comorbidities or level of atherosclerotic cardiovascular disease (ASCVD) risk. Many patients will require at least 2 drugs from different pharmacologic classes to achieve this blood pressure goal; the potential benefits of hypertension management and drug cost, adverse effects, and risks associated with the use of multiple antihypertensive drugs also should be considered when deciding a patient's blood pressure treatment goal.

For additional information on target levels of blood pressure and on monitoring therapy in the management of hypertension, see Blood Pressure Monitoring and Treatment Goals under Dosage: Hypertension, in Dosage and Administration in the Thiazides General Statement 40:28.20.

Pediatric Dosage In children 6 months to 12 years of age, the usual dosage of hydrochlorothiazide for the management of hypertension or for diuresis is 1–2 mg/kg daily given as a single dose or in 2 divided doses. Infants younger than 6 months of age may require up to 3 mg/kg daily in 2 divided doses. The total daily dosage should not exceed 37.5 mg for children up to 2 years of age or 100 mg for children 2–12 years of age. Experts recommend initiation of the drug at the low end of the dosage range; the dosage may be increased every 2–4 weeks until blood pressure is controlled, the maximum dosage is reached, or adverse effects occur. For information on overall principles and expert recommendations for treatment of hypertension in pediatric patients, see Uses: Hypertension in Pediatric Patients, in the Thiazides General Statement 40:28.20.

Geriatric Dosage Because an increased incidence of adverse effects to hydrochlorothiazide and excessive reduction in blood pressure may occur in geriatric patients (older than 65 years of age), hydrochlorothiazide should be initiated at the lowest dosage (12.5 mg daily); dosage may be adjusted in increments of 12.5 mg if needed.

Cautions

Hydrochlorothiazide shares the pharmacologic actions, uses, and toxic potentials of the thiazides, and the usual precautions of thiazide administration should be observed. (See Cautions in the Thiazides General Statement 40:28.20)

When hydrochlorothiazide is used in fixed combination with other drugs, the cautions, precautions, contraindications, and interactions associated with the concomitant agent(s) should be considered in addition to those associated with hydrochlorothiazide.

Some commercially available formulations of hydrochlorothiazide contain sulfites that may cause allergic-type reactions, including anaphylaxis and life-threatening or less severe asthmatic episodes, in certain susceptible individuals. The overall prevalence of sulfite sensitivity in the general population is unknown but probably low; such sensitivity appears to occur more frequently in asthmatic than in nonasthmatic individuals.

Pharmacokinetics

Hydrochlorothiazide is well absorbed from the GI tract, with an oral bioavailability of approximately 65–75%. Although the rate and extent of absorption have been reported to vary depending on the formulation administered, no studies have been performed to determine the clinical importance (if any) of variations in absorption in patients receiving chronic hydrochlorothiazide therapy. Following oral administration of hydrochlorothiazide at doses of 12.5–100 mg, peak plasma concentrations of 70–490 ng/mL are observed within 1–5 hours of dosing. Food decreases the rate and extent of absorption of hydrochlorothiazide capsules (Microzide®). Bioavailability and peak plasma concentrations of the drug were decreased by about 10 and 20%, respectively, when hydrochlorothiazide capsules (Microzide®) were administered with food. Times to peak plasma concentration for such capsules were delayed by 1.3 hours (from 1.6 to 2.9 hours). Absorption of hydrochlorothiazide is reduced in patients with heart failure.

Approximately 40–68% of the drug is bound to plasma proteins.

Hydrochlorothiazide exhibits linear pharmacokinetics. Based on determination of plasma drug concentrations over a period of at least 24 hours, the plasma half-life of hydrochlorothiazide reportedly ranges from 5.6–15 hours. Hydrochlorothiazide apparently is not metabolized and is excreted unchanged in urine. At least 61% of the drug is reportedly eliminated from the body within 24 hours. Increased hydrochlorothiazide plasma concentrations and a prolonged elimination half-life have been reported in patients with renal impairment. The effect of hemodialysis on the elimination of the drug has not been determined.

Chemistry and Stability

■ **Chemistry** Hydrochlorothiazide is a thiazide diuretic. Hydrochlorothiazide occurs as a white or practically white, practically odorless, crystalline powder and has a slightly bitter taste. The drug is slightly soluble in water and soluble in alcohol and has pK_as of 7.9 and 9.2.

■ **Stability** Hydrochlorothiazide tablets and capsules should be stored in tightly closed containers at a controlled room temperature of 15–30°C and protected from light, moisture, and freezing. Hydrochlorothiazide oral solution should be stored in well-closed containers at a temperature less than 40°C, preferably at 15–30°C. Freezing of the oral solution should be avoided. Commercially available hydrochlorothiazide tablets have an expiration date of 3 or 5 years following the date of manufacture depending on the packaging.

For further information on chemistry and stability, pharmacology, pharmacokinetics, uses, cautions, acute toxicity, drug interactions, laboratory test interferences, and dosage and administration of hydrochlorothiazide, see the Thiazides General Statement 40:28.20.

Preparations

Excipients in commercially available drug preparations may have clinically important effects in some individuals; consult specific product labeling for details.

hydroCHLOROthiazide

Oral		
Capsules	12.5 mg*	**hydroCHLOROthiazide Capsules**
		Microzide®, Watson
Tablets	12.5 mg*	**hydroCHLOROthiazide Tablets**
	25 mg*	**hydroCHLOROthiazide Tablets**
	50 mg*	**hydroCHLOROthiazide Tablets**

*available from one or more manufacturer, distributor, and/or repackager by generic (nonproprietary) name

Amiloride Hydrochloride and hydroCHLOROthiazide

Oral		
Tablets	5 mg of Anhydrous Amiloride Hydrochloride and Hydrochlorothiazide 50 mg*	**Amiloride Hydrochloride and hydroCHLOROthiazide Tablets**

*available from one or more manufacturer, distributor, and/or repackager by generic (nonproprietary) name

Captopril and hydroCHLOROthiazide

Oral		
Tablets	25 mg Captopril and Hydrochlorothiazide 15 mg*	**Captopril and hydroCHLOROthiazide Tablets**
	25 mg Captopril and Hydrochlorothiazide 25 mg*	**Captopril and hydroCHLOROthiazide Tablets**
	50 mg Captopril and Hydrochlorothiazide 15 mg*	**Captopril and hydroCHLOROthiazide Tablets**
	50 mg Captopril and Hydrochlorothiazide 25 mg*	**Captopril and hydroCHLOROthiazide Tablets**

*available from one or more manufacturer, distributor, and/or repackager by generic (nonproprietary) name

Enalapril Maleate and hydroCHLOROthiazide

Oral		
Tablets	5 mg Enalapril Maleate and Hydrochlorothiazide 12.5 mg*	**Enalapril Maleate and hydroCHLOROthiazide Tablets**
	10 mg Enalapril Maleate and Hydrochlorothiazide 25 mg*	**Enalapril Maleate and hydroCHLOROthiazide Tablets**
		Vaseretic®, Valeant

*available from one or more manufacturer, distributor, and/or repackager by generic (nonproprietary) name

Methyldopa and hydroCHLOROthiazide

Oral		
Tablets, film-coated	250 mg Methyldopa and Hydrochlorothiazide 15 mg*	**Methyldopa and hydroCHLOROthiazide Tablets**
	250 mg Methyldopa and Hydrochlorothiazide 25 mg*	**Methyldopa and hydroCHLOROthiazide Tablets**

*available from one or more manufacturer, distributor, and/or repackager by generic (nonproprietary) name

Metoprolol Tartrate and hydroCHLOROthiazide

Oral		
Tablets	50 mg Metoprolol Tartrate and Hydrochlorothiazide 25 mg*	**Lopressor® HCT** (scored), Validus
		Metoprolol Tartrate and hydroCHLOROthiazide Tablets
	100 mg Metoprolol Tartrate and Hydrochlorothiazide 25 mg*	**Lopressor® HCT** (scored), Validus
		Metoprolol Tartrate and hydroCHLOROthiazide Tablets
	100 mg Metoprolol Tartrate and Hydrochlorothiazide 50 mg*	**Lopressor® HCT** (scored), Validus
		Metoprolol Tartrate and hydroCHLOROthiazide Tablets

*available from one or more manufacturer, distributor, and/or repackager by generic (nonproprietary) name

Propranolol Hydrochloride and hydroCHLOROthiazide

Oral		
Tablets	40 mg Propranolol Hydrochloride and Hydrochlorothiazide 25 mg*	**Propranolol Hydrochloride and hydroCHLOROthiazide Tablets**
	80 mg Propranolol Hydrochloride and Hydrochlorothiazide 25 mg*	**Propranolol Hydrochloride and hydroCHLOROthiazide Tablets**

*available from one or more manufacturer, distributor, and/or repackager by generic (nonproprietary) name

Spironolactone and hydroCHLOROthiazide

Oral		
Tablets, film-coated	25 mg Spironolactone and Hydrochlorothiazide 25 mg*	**Aldactazide®**, Pfizer
		Spironolactone and hydroCHLOROthiazide Tablets
	50 mg Spironolactone and Hydrochlorothiazide 50 mg	**Aldactazide®** (scored), Pfizer

*available from one or more manufacturer, distributor, and/or repackager by generic (nonproprietary) name

Triamterene and hydroCHLOROthiazide (Co-triamterzide)

Oral		
Capsules	37.5 mg Triamterene and Hydrochlorothiazide 25 mg*	**Dyazide®**, GlaxoSmithKline
		Triamterene and hydroCHLOROthiazide Capsules
Tablets	37.5 mg Triamterene and Hydrochlorothiazide 25 mg*	**Maxzide®** (scored), Mylan
		Triamterene and hydroCHLOROthiazide Tablets
	75 mg Triamterene and Hydrochlorothiazide 50 mg*	**Maxzide®** (scored), Mylan
		Triamterene and hydroCHLOROthiazide Tablets

*available from one or more manufacturer, distributor, and/or repackager by generic (nonproprietary) name

Other hydroCHLOROthiazide Combinations

Oral		
Tablets	12.5 mg with Candesartan 16 mg	**Atacand® HCT**, AstraZeneca
	12.5 mg with Candesartan 32 mg	**Atacand® HCT**, AstraZeneca
	12.5 mg with Fosinopril Sodium 10 mg*	**Fosinopril Sodium and hydroCHLOROthiazide Tablets**
	12.5 mg with Fosinopril Sodium 20 mg*	**Fosinopril Sodium and hydroCHLOROthiazide Tablets**
	12.5 mg with Irbesartan 150 mg	**Avalide®**, Bristol-Myers Squibb(also promoted by Sanofi-Synthelabo)
	12.5 mg with Irbesartan 300 mg	**Avalide®**, Bristol-Myers Squibb(also promoted by Sanofi-Synthelabo)
	12.5 mg with Lisinopril 10 mg*	**Lisinopril and hydroCHLOROthiazide Tablets**
		Prinzide®, Merck
		Zestoretic®, AstraZeneca
	12.5 mg with Lisinopril 20 mg*	**Lisinopril and hydroCHLOROthiazide Tablets**
		Prinzide®, Merck
		Zestoretic®, AstraZeneca
	12.5 mg with Telmisartan 40 mg*	**Micardis® HCT**, Boehringer Ingelheim
		Telmisartan and hydroCHLOROthiazide Tablets
	12.5 mg with Telmisartan 80 mg*	**Micardis® HCT**, Boehringer Ingelheim
		Telmisartan and hydroCHLOROthiazide Tablets
	25 mg with Irbesartan 300 mg	**Avalide®**, Bristol-Myers Squibb(also promoted by Sanofi-Synthelabo)
	25 mg with Lisinopril 20 mg*	**Lisinopril and hydroCHLOROthiazide Tablets**
		Prinzide®, Merck
		Zestoretic®, AstraZeneca
	25 mg with Telmisartan 80 mg*	**Micardis® HCT**, Boehringer Ingelheim
		Telmisartan and hydroCHLOROthiazide Tablets
Tablets, film-coated	6.25 mg with Benazepril Hydrochloride 5 mg*	**Benazepril Hydrochloride and hydroCHLOROthiazide Tablets**
		Lotensin® HCT (scored), Novartis
	6.25 mg with Bisoprolol Fumarate 2.5 mg*	**Bisoprolol Fumarate and hydroCHLOROthiazide Tablets**
		Ziac®, Duramed
	6.25 mg with Bisoprolol Fumarate 5 mg*	**Bisoprolol Fumarate and hydroCHLOROthiazide Tablets**
		Ziac®, Duramed
	6.25 mg with Bisoprolol Fumarate 10 mg*	**Bisoprolol Fumarate and hydroCHLOROthiazide Tablets**
		Ziac®, Duramed
	12.5 mg with Aliskiren Hemifumarate 150 mg (of aliskiren)	**Tekturna® HCT**, Noden
	12.5 mg with Aliskiren Hemifumarate 300 mg (of aliskiren)	**Tekturna® HCT**, Noden
	12.5 mg with Amlodipine Besylate 5 mg (of amlodipine) and Olmesartan Medoxomil 20 mg	**Tribenzor®**, Daiichi Sankyo
	12.5 mg with Amlodipine Besylate 5 mg (of amlodipine) and Olmesartan Medoxomil 40 mg	**Tribenzor®**, Daiichi Sankyo
	12.5 mg with Amlodipine Besylate 5 mg (of amlodipine) and Valsartan 160 mg*	**Amlodipine Besylate, Valsartan, and hydroCHLOROthiazide Tablets**
		Exforge HCT®, Novartis
	12.5 mg with Amlodipine Besylate 10 mg (of amlodipine) and Olmesartan Medoxomil 40 mg	**Tribenzor®**, Daiichi Sankyo
	12.5 mg with Amlodipine Besylate 10 mg (of amlodipine) and Valsartan 160 mg*	**Amlodipine Besylate, Valsartan, and hydroCHLOROthiazide Tablets**
		Exforge HCT®, Novartis
	12.5 mg with Benazepril Hydrochloride 10 mg*	**Benazepril Hydrochloride and hydroCHLOROthiazide Tablets**
		Lotensin® HCT (scored), Novartis
	12.5 mg with Benazepril Hydrochloride 20 mg*	**Benazepril Hydrochloride and Hydrochlorothiazide Tablets**
		Lotensin® HCT (scored), Novartis
	12.5 mg with Eprosartan Mesylate 600 mg (of eprosartan)	**Teveten® HCT**, Abbott
	12.5 mg with Losartan Potassium 50 mg	**Hyzaar®**, Merck
	12.5 mg with Losartan Potassium 100 mg	**Hyzaar®**, Merck
	12.5 mg with Moexipril Hydrochloride 7.5 mg*	**Moexipril Hydrochloride and hydroCHLOROthiazide Tablets**
		Uniretic® (scored), UCB
	12.5 mg with Moexipril 15 mg*	**Moexipril Hydrochloride and hydroCHLOROthiazide Tablets**
		Uniretic® (scored), UCB
	12.5 mg with Olmesartan Medoxomil 20 mg	**Benicar® HCT**, Daiichi-Sankyo
	12.5 mg with Olmesartan Medoxomil 40 mg	**Benicar® HCT**, Daiichi-Sankyo
	12.5 mg with Quinapril Hydrochloride 10 mg (of quinapril)*	**Accuretic®** (scored), Pfizer
		Quinapril Hydrochloride and hydroCHLOROthiazide Tablets
	12.5 mg with Quinapril Hydrochloride 20 mg (of quinapril)*	**Accuretic®** (scored), Pfizer
		Quinapril Hydrochloride and hydroCHLOROthiazide Tablets
	12.5 mg with Valsartan 80 mg*	**Diovan® HCT**, Novartis
		Valsartan and hydroCHLOROthiazide Tablets
	12.5 mg with Valsartan 160 mg*	**Diovan® HCT**, Novartis
		Valsartan and hydroCHLOROthiazide Tablets
	12.5 mg with Valsartan 320 mg*	**Diovan® HCT**, Novartis
		Valsartan and hydroCHLOROthiazide Tablets
	25 mg with Aliskiren Hemifumarate 150 mg (of aliskiren)	**Tekturna® HCT**, Noden

25 mg with Aliskiren Hemifumarate 300 mg (of aliskiren)	**Tekturna® HCT**, Noden
25 mg with Amlodipine Besylate 5 mg (of amlodipine) and Olmesartan Medoxomil 40 mg	**Tribenzor®**, Daiichi Sankyo
25 mg with Amlodipine Besylate 5 mg (of amlodipine) and Valsartan 160 mg*	**Amlodipine Besylate, Valsartan, and hydroCHLOROthiazide Tablets**
	Exforge HCT®, Novartis
25 mg with Amlodipine Besylate 10 mg (of amlodipine) and Olmesartan Medoxomil 40 mg	**Tribenzor®**, Daiichi Sankyo
25 mg with Amlodipine Besylate 10 mg (of amlodipine) and Valsartan 160 mg*	**Amlodipine Besylate, Valsartan, and hydroCHLOROthiazide Tablets**
	Exforge HCT®, Novartis
25 mg with Amlodipine Besylate 10 mg (of amlodipine) and Valsartan 320 mg*	**Amlodipine Besylate, Valsartan, and hydroCHLOROthiazide Tablets**
	Exforge HCT®, Novartis
25 mg with Benazepril Hydrochloride 20 mg*	**Benazepril Hydrochloride and hydroCHLOROthiazide Tablets**
	Lotensin® HCT (scored), Novartis
25 mg with Eprosartan Mesylate 600 mg (of eprosartan)	**Teveten® HCT**, Abbott
25 mg with Losartan Potassium 100 mg	**Hyzaar®**, Merck
25 mg with Moexipril Hydrochloride 15 mg*	**Moexipril Hydrochloride and hydroCHLOROthiazide Tablets**
	Uniretic® (scored), UCB
25 mg with Olmesartan Medoxomil 40 mg	**Benicar® HCT**, Daiichi-Sankyo
25 mg with Quinapril Hydrochloride 20 mg (of quinapril)*	**Accuretic®** (scored), Pfizer
	Quinapril Hydrochloride and hydroCHLOROthiazide Tablets
25 mg with Valsartan 160 mg*	**Diovan® HCT**, Novartis
	Valsartan and hydroCHLOROthiazide Tablets
25 mg with Valsartan 320 mg*	**Diovan® HCT**, Novartis
	Valsartan and hydroCHLOROthiazide Tablets

*available from one or more manufacturer, distributor, and/or repackager by generic (nonproprietary) name

Selected Revisions November 2019,

THIAZIDE-LIKE DIURETICS 40:28.24

Chlorthalidone

■ Chlorthalidone, which is structurally and pharmacologically similar to the thiazides, is a diuretic and antihypertensive agent.

Dosage and Administration

■ **Administration** Chlorthalidone is administered orally.

■ **Dosage** Dosage of chlorthalidone should be individualized according to the patient's requirements and response. If chlorthalidone is added to the regimen of a patient stabilized on a potent hypotensive agent, the dosage of the hypotensive agent should initially be reduced to avoid the possibility of severe hypotension.

Edema For the management of edema in adults, the usual initial dosage of chlorthalidone is 50–100 mg daily in a single dose after breakfast. Alternatively, therapy may be initiated at a dosage of 100 mg every other day or 3 times a week. Some patients require dosages of 150–200 mg daily or every other day. Dosages greater than 200 mg daily do not produce a greater response. In edematous patients, reduction of dosage to a lower maintenance level may be possible after several days or when nonedematous weight is attained.

For the management of fluid retention (e.g., edema) associated with heart failure, some experts recommend initiating chlorthalidone at a low dosage (e.g., 12.5–25 mg once daily) and increasing the dosage (maximum of 100 mg daily) until urine output increases and weight decreases, generally by 0.5–1 kg daily. Experts state that diuretics should be administered at a dosage sufficient to achieve optimal volume status and relieve congestion without inducing an excessively rapid reduction in intravascular volume, which could result in hypotension, renal dysfunction, or both.

Hypertension The usual manufacturer-recommended initial dosage of chlorthalidone for the management of hypertension in adults is 25 mg once daily. If blood pressure remains uncontrolled, the dosage may be increased to 50 mg once daily. Some experts recommend a chlorthalidone dosage of 12.5–25 mg once daily based on efficacy and tolerance demonstrated in clinical studies. Dosages of chlorthalidone exceeding 100 mg daily usually do not increase efficacy.

Fixed-combination Therapy. When combination therapy is required in the management of hypertension, dosage can be adjusted first by administering each drug separately. If it is determined that the optimum maintenance dosage corresponds to the ratio in a commercial combination preparation, the fixed combination may be used. The manufacturer states that commercially available preparations containing chlorthalidone in fixed combination with atenolol should not be used for initial antihypertensive therapy; however, some experts state that initiation of therapy with a fixed-combination preparation may increase patient compliance.

Monitoring and Blood Pressure Treatment Goals. The patient's renal function and electrolytes should be assessed 2–4 weeks after initiation of diuretic therapy. Blood pressure should be monitored regularly (i.e., monthly) during therapy and dosage of the antihypertensive drug adjusted until blood pressure is controlled. If an adequate blood pressure response is not achieved with chlorthalidone monotherapy, another antihypertensive agent with demonstrated benefit and preferably with a complementary mechanism of action (e.g., angiotensin-converting enzyme [ACE] inhibitor, angiotensin II receptor antagonist, calcium-channel blocker) may be added; if goal blood pressure is still not achieved, a third drug may be added. (See Uses: Hypertension in Adults, in the Thiazides General Statement 40:28.20.) In patients who develop unacceptable adverse effects with chlorthalidone, the drug should be discontinued and another antihypertensive agent from a different pharmacologic class should be initiated.

The goal of hypertension management and prevention is to achieve and maintain optimal control of blood pressure. However, the optimum blood pressure threshold for initiating antihypertensive drug therapy and specific treatment goals remain controversial. A 2017 multidisciplinary hypertension guideline from the American College of Cardiology (ACC), American Heart Association (AHA), and a number of other professional organizations generally recommends a blood pressure goal of less than 130/80 mm Hg in all adults, regardless of comorbidities or level of atherosclerotic cardiovascular disease (ASCVD) risk. Many patients will require at least 2 drugs from different pharmacologic classes to achieve this blood pressure goal; the potential benefits of hypertension management and drug cost, adverse effects, and risks associated with the use of multiple antihypertensive drugs also should be considered when deciding a patient's blood pressure treatment goal.

For additional information on target levels of blood pressure and on monitoring therapy in the management of hypertension, see Blood Pressure Monitoring and Treatment Goals under Dosage: Hypertension, in Dosage and Administration in the Thiazides General Statement 40:28.20.

Pediatric Dosage For the management of hypertension in children†, some experts recommend an initial dosage of 0.3 mg/kg once daily. Experts state that the dosage should be increased every 2–4 weeks until blood pressure is controlled, the maximum dosage is reached (2 mg/kg [up to 50 mg] daily), or adverse effects occur. For information on overall principles and expert recommendations for treatment of hypertension in pediatric patients, see Uses: Hypertension in Pediatric Patients, in the Thiazides General Statement 40:28.20.

Cautions

Chlorthalidone shares the pharmacologic actions, uses, and toxic potentials of the thiazides, and the usual precautions of thiazide administration should be observed. (See Cautions in the Thiazides General Statement 40:28.20.)

Pharmacokinetics

Chlorthalidone is absorbed from the GI tract. Little information is available on the extent of absorption of the drug.

About 90% of chlorthalidone is bound in the body, principally to or in red blood cells. The high degree of binding accounts for the long half-life of the drug which is reported to be 54 hours. During long-term oral administration, 30–60% of the daily dose is excreted unchanged in urine.

Chemistry and Stability

■ **Chemistry** Chlorthalidone is a phthalimidine derivative of benzenesulfonamide that is structurally and pharmacologically similar to the thiazide diuretics. The drug occurs as a white to yellowish-white, crystalline powder. The drug is practically insoluble in water and slightly soluble in alcohol and has a pK_a of 9.4.

■ **Stability** Chlorthalidone tablets should be stored in tight, light-resistant containers at 20–25°C.

For further information on chemistry, pharmacology, pharmacokinetics, cautions, acute toxicity, uses, drug interactions, laboratory test interferences, and dosage and administration of chlorthalidone, see the Thiazides General Statement 40:28.20.

Preparations

Excipients in commercially available drug preparations may have clinically important effects in some individuals; consult specific product labeling for details.

Chlorthalidone

Oral

Tablets	25 mg*	**Chlorthalidone Tablets**
	50 mg*	**Chlorthalidone Tablets**

*available from one or more manufacturer, distributor, and/or repackager by generic (nonproprietary) name

Atenolol and Chlorthalidone

Oral

Tablets	Atenolol 50 mg and Chlorthalidone 25 mg*	**Atenolol and Chlorthalidone Tablets**
		Tenoretic®, AstraZeneca
	Atenolol 100 mg and Chlorthalidone 25 mg*	**Atenolol and Chlorthalidone Tablets**
		Tenoretic®, AstraZeneca

*available from one or more manufacturer, distributor, and/or repackager by generic (nonproprietary) name

†Use is not currently included in the labeling approved by the US Food and Drug Administration

Selected Revisions January 2019,

ELECTROLYTIC, CALORIC, AND WATER BALANCE AGENTS, MISCELLANEOUS 40:92

Burosumab-twza

■ Burosumab is a recombinant fully human immunoglobulin G_1 (IgG_1) monoclonal antibody that binds to human fibroblast growth factor 23 (FGF23), a bone-derived hormone that regulates phosphate and vitamin D homeostasis.

Uses

■ **X-linked Hypophosphatemia** Burosumab-twza is used for the management of X-linked hypophosphatemia (previously known as familial vitamin D-resistant rickets). Burosumab-twza has been designated an orphan drug by FDA for use in this condition.

X-linked hypophosphatemia, a rare metabolic bone disease occurring in approximately 1 in 20,000 persons, is caused by loss-of-function mutations in the phosphate-regulating PHEX gene that result in elevated concentrations of fibroblast growth factor 23 (FGF23), a key regulator of phosphate homeostasis and vitamin D metabolism. Elevated FGF23 concentrations result in low serum phosphorus concentrations, low renal tubular reabsorption of phosphate, and impaired renal activation of vitamin D. Manifestations of rickets (e.g., impaired linear growth, progressive bowing of the femur and tibia) become apparent in early childhood; elevated serum alkaline phosphatase concentrations in children with X-linked hypophosphatemia are thought to correlate with severity of rickets. Osteomalacia and skeletal deformities in adults with X-linked hypophosphatemia may result in fractures or pseudofractures, bone and joint pain, osteoarthritis, and other debilitating musculoskeletal conditions. Severe dental disease (e.g., abscess) is common in patients with X-linked hypophosphatemia because of poorly mineralized dentin. Conventional therapy with oral phosphate supplements and activated vitamin D analogs (e.g., calcitriol) may improve bone mineralization but may be associated with development of hyperparathyroidism and nephrocalcinosis.

Osteomalacia in Adults Efficacy of burosumab for the management of X-linked hypophosphatemia in adults has been established in 2 phase 3 studies that demonstrated improvements in serum phosphorus concentrations and healing of osteomalacia-related bone lesions. The studies included a randomized, double-blind, placebo-controlled study in 134 adults with X-linked hypophosphatemia and a noncomparative, open-label study evaluating bone biopsy-derived histomorphometric parameters for 14 adults receiving the drug.

In the double-blind, placebo-controlled study, 134 adults (mean age 40 years, 35% male, 81% white, mean baseline serum phosphorus concentration 1.98 mg/dL) with skeletal pain associated with X-linked hypophosphatemia and osteomalacia were randomized in a 1:1 ratio to receive burosumab-twza 1 mg/kg (up to 90 mg) or placebo administered subcutaneously every 4 weeks for 24 weeks. Oral phosphate supplements and activated vitamin D analogs were discontinued at least 2 weeks prior to study enrollment. The primary efficacy end point was the proportion of patients achieving a mean serum phosphorus concentration (measured at the midpoint of each dosing interval) above the lower limit of normal (2.5 mg/dL); 94% of patients receiving burosumab achieved the primary efficacy end point compared with 8% of patients receiving placebo. In burosumab-treated patients, the mean phosphorus concentration was maintained above the lower limit of normal through the end of the 4-week dosing intervals. Similarly, the mean ratio of the maximum rate of renal tubular phosphate reabsorption (TmP) to the glomerular filtration rate (GFR) in burosumab-treated patients increased from 1.7 mg/dL at baseline to 2.7 and 2.2 mg/dL at the midpoint and end, respectively, of the final dosing interval of the double-blind treatment period (weeks 22 and 24, respectively); in placebo recipients, the ratio changed minimally, from 1.6 mg/dL at baseline to 1.7 mg/dL at both the midpoint and end of the final dosing interval. Burosumab also was associated with greater frequency of fracture healing than placebo. Active fractures, including both fractures and pseudofractures, were present at baseline in 47 or 58% of patients assigned to receive burosumab or placebo, respectively; a total of 65 active fractures (22% fractures, 78% pseudofractures) were identified at baseline in the burosumab group and 91 active fractures (14% fractures, 86% pseudofractures) were identified in the placebo group. At week 24, 43% of active fractures in burosumab-treated patients (including 50% of active fractures and 41% of active pseudofractures identified at baseline) were considered healed, and 8% of active fractures in placebo recipients (including none of the active fractures and 9% of the active pseudofractures identified at baseline) were considered healed, corresponding to a 16.8-fold greater odds of full healing at 24 weeks with burosumab treatment.

In the noncomparative, open-label study, 14 adults (mean age 40 years, 43% male) with X-linked hypophosphatemia received burosumab-twza 1 mg/kg every 4 weeks. After 48 weeks of treatment, histomorphometric evaluations of iliac crest bone biopsy specimens revealed healing of osteomalacia in 10 patients, as demonstrated by decreases of 57% in the ratio of osteoid volume to bone volume. Osteoid thickness was decreased in 11 patients by an average of 33%, and mineralization lag time was decreased in 6 patients by an average of 74%.

Rickets in Pediatric Patients Efficacy of burosumab for the management of X-linked hypophosphatemia has been established in 2 open-label phase 2 studies in pediatric patients that demonstrated improvements in serum phosphorus concentrations and radiographic measures of rickets severity.

In the first study, 52 children 5–12 years of age at Tanner stage 2 or less (mean age 8.5 years, 46% male, 88% white) with X-linked hypophosphatemia were randomized in a 1:1 ratio to receive burosumab-twza every 2 weeks or every 4 weeks for 64 weeks; 94% of the patients had radiographic evidence of rickets at baseline, and 96% of the patients had received prior therapy with oral phosphate supplements and activated vitamin D analogs (mean duration of therapy 7 years). The study design included a 16-week dosage titration period followed by a 48-week treatment period. Following an initial burosumab-twza dosage of 0.1–0.3 mg/kg every 2 weeks or 0.2–0.6 mg/kg every 4 weeks, dosage was adjusted every 4 weeks during the dosage titration period up to a maximum dose of 2 mg/kg (maximum of 90 mg) based on the fasting serum phosphorus concentration measured 2 weeks after administration of a dose to achieve a phosphorus concentration of 3.5–5 mg/dL. The primary efficacy end points were the change from baseline to week 40 and to week 64 in the Thacher Rickets Severity Score (RSS), which rates rachitic features observed on radiographic images of the wrist and knee on a scale of 0–10 with higher scores indicating greater disease severity. RSS scores in children with X-linked hypophosphatemia generally are in the range of 0–5. The 7-point Radiographic Global Impression of Change (RGI-C) scale was used to compare radiographic images of the wrist and knee taken at baseline and at weeks 40 and 64 to assess change in disease severity; RGI-C scores range from −3 (severe worsening) to 3 (complete healing).

In the first study in children receiving burosumab every 2 weeks, the mean RSS decreased from 1.9 at baseline to 0.8 and 0.9 at weeks 40 and 64, respectively; the RGI-C mean score was 1.7 at week 40 and 1.6 at week 64, with 69% of patients demonstrating substantial healing (defined as a score of 2 or greater) at week 40; mean serum phosphorus concentrations increased from 2.4 mg/dL at baseline to 3.3 and 3.4 mg/dL at weeks 40 and 64, respectively; and the mean TmP-to-GFR ratio increased from 2.2 mg/dL at baseline to 3.3 and 3.4 mg/dL at weeks 40 and 64, respectively. Decreases in alkaline phosphatase concentrations and increases in standing height-for-age Z-scores also were observed in children receiving burosumab every 2 weeks. Serum phosphorus concentrations exhibited less fluctuation when the drug was administered every 2 weeks rather than every 4 weeks, and responses generally appeared to be more favorable with administration every 2 weeks.

In the second study, 13 children 1–4 years of age (mean age 2.9 years, 69% male) with X-linked hypophosphatemia and radiographic evidence of rickets received burosumab-twza 0.8 mg/kg every 2 weeks for 64 weeks; the dose was increased to 1.2 mg/kg if 2 consecutive predose serum phosphorus concentrations were less than 3.2 mg/dL and the concentration had increased from baseline by less than 0.5 mg/dL. Mean serum phosphorus concentrations increased from 2.5 mg/dL at baseline to 3.5 mg/dL at week 40, the mean RSS decreased from 2.9 at baseline to 1.2 at week 40, and mean alkaline phosphatase concentrations decreased by 36% from baseline to week 40; the RGI-C mean score at week 40 was 2.3, with all patients demonstrating substantial healing (defined as a score of 2 of greater). Improvements in these outcome measures were maintained at week 64.

Dosage and Administration

■ **General** Oral phosphate supplements and activated vitamin D analogs (e.g., calcitriol) should be discontinued one week prior to initiation of treatment with burosumab. Fasting serum phosphorus concentration should be less than the reference range for age prior to the initiation of treatment with burosumab; the manufacturer states that initiation of the drug is contraindicated if the serum phosphorus concentration is within or exceeds the normal range for age.

Restricted Distribution Burosumab-twza is available only from a limited network of specialty pharmacies. The manufacturer should be contacted for additional information.

■ **Administration** Burosumab-twza is administered by subcutaneous injection. The drug should be administered by a clinician.

Burosumab-twza injection must be stored at 2–8°C and kept in the original carton for protection from light until time of use. Because burosumab-twza injection contains no preservatives, vials of the drug are intended for single dose only; unused portions remaining in the vial should be discarded.

Burosumab-twza injection should be inspected visually prior to administration. Burosumab-twza injection is a clear to slightly opalescent, colorless to pale brown-yellow solution. If the solution is discolored or cloudy or if any particles or foreign particulate matter is present, the drug must not be administered.

Subcutaneous injections should be made into the upper arms, upper thighs, buttocks, or any quadrant of the abdomen; injection sites should be rotated, with each injection administered at a different anatomic location than the previous injection. Injections should *not* be made into moles, scars, or areas where the skin is tender, bruised, erythematous, hard, or not intact.

No more than 1.5 mL of burosumab-twza solution should be injected subcutaneously at any one site; if the injection volume exceeds 1.5 mL, the total volume of the dose should be divided and administered at 2 separate injection sites.

If a dose of burosumab-twza is missed, the missed dose should be administered as soon as possible at the patient's usual dose.

■ **Dosage** ***Adult Dosage*** **Initial Dosage.** For the management of X-linked hypophosphatemia in adults, the recommended initial dosage of burosumab-twza is 1 mg/kg, rounded to the nearest 10 mg and not exceeding 90 mg, administered every 4 weeks.

Dosage Titration. Burosumab dosage in adults should be adjusted no more frequently than every 4 weeks based on fasting serum phosphorus concentrations.

Following initiation of burosumab therapy, fasting serum phosphorus concentrations should be measured monthly (with determinations made 2 weeks after a dose) for the first 3 months, then as clinically appropriate thereafter. Fasting serum phosphorus concentrations should be measured 2 weeks after dosage adjustments.

If the serum phosphorus concentration is within the normal range, burosumab should be continued at the same dosage.

If the serum phosphorus concentration exceeds the normal range, the next dose of burosumab should be withheld and the serum phosphorus concentration assessed again in 4 weeks. Once the serum phosphorus concentration is less than the normal range, therapy with burosumab may be reinitiated at a reduced dose of approximately one-half the initial dose (not exceeding 40 mg). (See Table 1.)

Table 1. Burosumab-twza Dose Reduction in Adults.

Previous Dose (mg)	Reduced Dose for Reinitiation (mg)
40	20
50	20
60	30
70	30
80 or greater	40

Pediatric Dosage **Initial Dosage.** For the management of X-linked hypophosphatemia in pediatric patients 1 year to less than 18 years of age, the recommended initial dosage of burosumab-twza is 0.8 mg/kg, rounded to the nearest 10 mg and not exceeding 90 mg, administered every 2 weeks. The minimum initial dose is 10 mg.

Dosage Titration. Burosumab dosage in pediatric patients should be adjusted no more frequently than every 4 weeks to maintain fasting serum phosphorus concentrations within the reference range for age.

Following initiation of burosumab therapy, fasting serum phosphorus concentrations should be measured every 4 weeks for the first 3 months, then as clinically appropriate thereafter. Fasting serum phosphorus concentrations should be measured 4 weeks after dosage adjustments.

If the serum phosphorus concentration exceeds the lower limit of the reference range for age but is below 5 mg/dL, burosumab should be continued at the same dosage.

If the serum phosphorus concentration is below the reference range for age, the dose may be increased in a stepwise manner, up to approximately 2 mg/kg (not exceeding 90 mg). (See Table 2.)

Table 2. Burosumab-twza Stepwise Dose Increases Based on Body Weight in Pediatric Patients 1 Year of Age or Older.

Body Weight (kg)	Initial Dose (mg)	Total Dose of First Stepwise Dose Increase (mg)	Total Dose of Second Stepwise Dose Increase (mg)
10–14	10	15	20
15–18	10	20	30
19–31	20	30	40
32–43	30	40	60
44–56	40	60	80
57–68	50	70	90
69–80	60	90	Not applicable
81–93	70	90	Not applicable
94–105	80	90	Not applicable
106 or greater	90	Not applicable	Not applicable

If the serum phosphorus concentration exceeds 5 mg/dL, the next dose of burosumab should be withheld and the serum phosphorus concentration assessed again in 4 weeks. Once the serum phosphorus concentration is less than the reference range for age, therapy with burosumab may be reinitiated at a reduced dose. (See Table 3.) The serum phosphorus concentration must be less than the reference range for age for reinitiation of the drug. If the concentration remains less than the reference range for age at 4 weeks after reinitiation at a reduced dose, the dosage can be increased. (See Table 2.)

Table 3. Burosumab-twza Dose Reduction in Pediatric Patients 1 Year of Age or Older.

Previous Dose (mg)	Reduced Dose for Reinitiation (mg)
10	5
15	10
20	10
30	10
40	20
50	20
60	30
70	30
80	40
90	40

■ **Special Populations** ***Hepatic Impairment*** The manufacturer makes no specific dosage recommendations for patients with hepatic impairment at this time.

Renal Impairment The manufacturer makes no specific dosage recommendations for patients with renal impairment at this time; however, the drug is contraindicated in patients with severe renal impairment or end-stage renal disease because of abnormal mineral metabolism in such patients.

Geriatric Patients The manufacturer makes no specific dosage recommendations for geriatric patients; in general, dosage selection should be cautious, usually initiating therapy at the low end of the usual range.

Cautions

■ **Contraindications** Use of burosumab is contraindicated in combination with oral phosphate supplements and activated vitamin D analogs (e.g., calcitriol) and in patients with severe renal impairment or end-stage renal disease. The drug should not be initiated if serum phosphorus concentration is within or exceeds the normal range for age.

■ **Warnings/Precautions** ***Sensitivity Reactions*** **Hypersensitivity Reactions.** Hypersensitivity reactions (e.g., rash, urticaria) have been reported in patients receiving burosumab. In noncomparative studies of burosumab-twza in pediatric patients, rash, injection site rash, and urticaria occurred in 22, 6, and 5%, respectively, of patients. In a comparative study in adults, hypersensitivity reactions were reported in approximately 6% of patients receiving either burosumab-twza or placebo; most events were mild or moderate and did not require drug discontinuance.

Burosumab should be discontinued if serious hypersensitivity reactions occur, and appropriate medical treatment should be initiated.

Hyperphosphatemia and Risk of Nephrocalcinosis Increases in serum phosphorus concentrations exceeding the upper limit of normal (ULN) may be associated with an increased risk of nephrocalcinosis. During clinical trials of burosumab-twza in pediatric patients with X-linked hypophosphatemia, no episodes of hyperphosphatemia were reported. In a comparative study in adults, 7% of patients receiving burosumab-twza experienced hyperphosphatemia at concentrations meeting the protocol-specified criteria for a 50% reduction in dosage (i.e., single serum phosphorus concentration exceeding 5 mg/dL or 2 sequential serum phosphorus concentrations exceeding the ULN [4.5 mg/dL]), and one patient required a second dosage reduction for continued hyperphosphatemia.

Treatment interruption and subsequent dosage reduction may be necessary if hyperphosphatemia occurs. (See Dosage and Administration: Dosage.)

Injection Site Reactions Injection site reactions (e.g., urticaria, erythema, rash, swelling, bruising, pain, pruritus, hematoma) have been reported in patients receiving burosumab. Injection site reactions were reported in approximately 58% of pediatric patients receiving burosumab-twza in noncomparative clinical studies and in approximately 12% of adults receiving either burosumab-twza or placebo in a comparative study. In general, the reactions were mild, occurred within one day of injection and persisted for 1–3 days, required no treatment, and resolved in nearly all cases.

Patients receiving burosumab should be monitored for injection site reactions. Burosumab should be discontinued if severe injection site reactions occur, and appropriate medical treatment should be administered.

Immunogenicity As with all therapeutic proteins, there is a potential for immunogenicity with burosumab therapy. Preexisting antiburosumab antibodies were detected in up to 10% of patients in clinical studies of the drug. Antiburosumab antibodies were not detected in patients who were antibody negative at initiation of therapy; however, the presence of burosumab-twza in the serum sample may interfere with the assay used to measure antibodies to the drug, potentially underestimating the true incidence of antibody formation. The clinical relevance of antiburosumab antibodies is unknown.

Specific Populations **Pregnancy.** Data regarding use of burosumab in pregnant women are lacking.

Burosumab crosses the placenta in monkeys. Reproduction studies in monkeys without X-linked hypophosphatemia have revealed no evidence of teratogenicity with IV burosumab-twza at exposure levels up to 64 times the exposure at the recommended adult dosage of 1 mg/kg every 4 weeks. Increases in late fetal loss and preterm births were observed but were not thought to indicate clinical risk since these effects were observed at the highest exposure and were accompanied by maternal hyperphosphatemia and placental mineralization. No adverse effects on prenatal and postnatal growth, including offspring survival, were observed.

If burosumab is used during pregnancy, serum phosphorus concentrations should be monitored throughout pregnancy. Pregnancies in patients receiving burosumab-twza should be reported to the Kyowa Kirin, Inc. Adverse Event reporting line at 888-756-8657.

Lactation. It is not known whether burosumab is distributed into human milk. Effects of the drug on the breast-fed infant (e.g., resulting from local GI exposure or limited systemic exposure) or milk production also are not known. The benefits of breast-feeding and the woman's clinical need for burosumab should be considered along with any potential adverse effects on the breast-fed infant from the drug or from the underlying maternal condition.

Pediatric Use. Safety and efficacy of burosumab have not been established in pediatric patients younger than 1 year of age.

Safety and efficacy of burosumab have been established in 2 open-label studies in 52 children 5–12 years of age and 13 children 1–4 years of age with X-linked hypophosphatemia. (See Rickets in Pediatric Patients under Uses: X-linked Hypophosphatemia.) Efficacy in adolescents with X-linked hypophosphatemia has been extrapolated from studies conducted in pediatric patients younger than 13 years of age, while dosage in adolescents was derived using modeling and simulation of both adult and pediatric pharmacokinetic and pharmacodynamic data.

No substantial age-related differences in the pharmacokinetics of burosumab have been observed.

Geriatric Use. Clinical trials of burosumab did not include sufficient numbers of patients 65 years of age or older to determine whether geriatric patients respond differently than younger patients. While other clinical experience has not revealed age-related differences in response, dosage of burosumab generally should be selected carefully in geriatric patients, usually initiating therapy at the low end of the dosage range, because of the greater frequency of decreased hepatic, renal, and/or cardiac function and of concomitant disease and drug therapy observed in the elderly.

No substantial age-related differences in the pharmacokinetics of burosumab have been observed.

Hepatic Impairment. The effect of hepatic impairment on the pharmacokinetics of burosumab is unknown.

Renal Impairment. The effect of renal impairment on the pharmacokinetics of burosumab is unknown. The manufacturer states that the drug is contraindicated in patients with severe renal impairment or end-stage renal disease because of abnormal mineral metabolism in such patients.

■ **Common Adverse Effects** Adverse effects reported in more than 10% of pediatric patients receiving burosumab-twza in clinical studies include headache, injection site reaction, vomiting, pyrexia, pain in extremity, decreased vitamin D concentration, rash, toothache, myalgia, tooth abscess, and dizziness.

Adverse effects reported in more than 5% of adults receiving burosumab-twza in a clinical study and in at least 2 more burosumab-treated patients than placebo recipients include back pain, headache, tooth infection, new or worsening restless legs syndrome, decreased vitamin D concentration, dizziness, constipation, and hyperphosphatemia.

In phase 2 and 3 studies of burosumab-twza in adults with X-linked hypophosphatemia, 3.4% of patients underwent spinal surgery. Spinal stenosis is prevalent in adults with X-linked hypophosphatemia, and spinal cord compression also has been reported. Most cases requiring spinal surgery during these studies appeared to involve progression of preexisting spinal stenosis, but it is unknown whether burosumab exacerbates spinal stenosis or spinal cord compression.

Drug Interactions

Formal drug interaction studies have not been conducted with burosumab to date.

■ **Phosphate Supplements** Use of burosumab in combination with oral phosphate supplements increases the risk of hyperphosphatemia. Concomitant use of oral phosphate supplements and burosumab is contraindicated. Oral phosphate supplements should be discontinued one week prior to initiation of treatment with burosumab.

■ **Vitamin D Analogs** Use of burosumab in combination with activated vitamin D analogs (e.g., calcitriol) increases the risk of hyperphosphatemia. Concomitant use of activated vitamin D analogs and burosumab is contraindicated. Activated vitamin D analogs should be discontinued one week prior to initiation of treatment with burosumab.

Description

Burosumab is a recombinant, fully human immunoglobulin G_1 (IgG_1) monoclonal antibody that binds to human fibroblast growth factor 23 (FGF23), a principally bone-derived hormone. FGF23 is the principal regulator of phosphate homeostasis, controlling reabsorption of phosphate in the kidney; FGF23 also regulates expression of 1α-hydroxylase, the rate-limiting enzyme in the renal activation of vitamin D. In X-linked hypophosphatemia, loss-of-function mutations in the phosphate-regulating endopeptidase homolog X-linked (*PHEX*) gene lead to excess FGF23 and resultant suppression of renal tubular phosphate reabsorption and renal synthesis of 1,25-dihydroxyvitamin D, renal phosphate wasting, and impaired bone mineralization. Burosumab binds at the *N*-terminal domain to both intact FGF23 and FGF23 polypeptide fragments and inhibits the biologic activity of the hormone, restoring renal phosphate reabsorption and increasing serum concentrations of 1,25-dihydroxyvitamin D.

The magnitude and duration of response to burosumab are dose related. Renal tubular phosphate reabsorption, serum phosphorus concentrations, and 1,25-dihydroxyvitamin D concentrations increase linearly with increasing burosumab exposure. Such treatment effects (e.g., increases in serum phosphorus concentrations) are reversible and return to baseline with elimination of the drug. Elevations in serum total FGF23 have been observed after initiation of burosumab-twza treatment; while the clinical implication of such increases is unknown, it has been suggested that this could indicate a need for higher doses with long-term therapy.

Following subcutaneous injection in patients with X-linked hypophosphatemia, bioavailability of burosumab-twza was nearly 100% and the drug exhibited linear pharmacokinetics within the dosage range of 0.1–1 mg/kg. Peak plasma concentrations of burosumab-twza were achieved in a mean of 8–11 days. The exact metabolic pathway of burosumab-twza has not been characterized; however, the drug is expected to be degraded into small peptides and amino acids via catabolic pathways. The half-life of burosumab-twza is approximately 13–19 days.

Advice to Patients

Risk of hypersensitivity reactions. Importance of patients contacting their clinician if such reactions (e.g., rash, injection site rash, urticaria) occur.

Risk of injection site reactions. Importance of patients contacting their clinician if such reactions (e.g., erythema, rash, swelling, bruising, pain, pruritus, urticaria, hematoma) occur.

Risk of new-onset or worsening restless legs syndrome. Importance of patients contacting their clinician if such a reaction occurs.

Importance of women informing clinicians if they are or plan to become pregnant or plan to breast-feed. Importance of reporting pregnancies to the manufacturer's adverse event reporting line at 888-756-8657. (See Pregnancy under Warnings/Precautions: Specific Populations, in Cautions.)

Importance of informing clinicians of existing or contemplated concomitant therapy, including prescription and OTC drugs and dietary or herbal supplements, as well as any concomitant illnesses.

Importance of informing patients of other important precautionary information. (See Cautions.)

Overview® (see Users Guide). For additional information on this drug until a more detailed monograph is developed and published, the manufacturer's labeling should be consulted. It is *essential* that the manufacturer's labeling be consulted for more detailed information on usual cautions, precautions, contraindications, potential drug interactions, laboratory test interferences, and acute toxicity.

Preparations

Distribution of burosumab-twza is restricted. (See Restricted Distribution under Dosage and Administration: General.)

Excipients in commercially available drug preparations may have clinically important effects in some individuals; consult specific product labeling for details.

Burosumab-twza

Parenteral

Injection, for subcutaneous use	10 mg/mL	**Crysvita**®, Ultragenyx
	20 mg/mL	**Crysvita**®, Ultragenyx
	30 mg/mL	**Crysvita**®, Ultragenyx

44:00 Enzymes

Agalsidase Beta§
Alglucosidase Alfa§
Asfotase Alfa§
Cerliponase Alfa§
Collagenase (Clostridium histolyticum)§
Elapegademase-lvlr§
Elosulfase Alfa§
Galsulfase§
Idursulfase§
Imiglucerase§
Laronidase§
Pegvaliase-pzpq§
Rasburicase§
Sacrosidase§
Sebelipase Alfa§
Taliglucerase Alfa§
Velaglucerase Alfa§
Vestronidase alfa-vjbk§

see also:
Alteplase 20:12.20
Asparaginase (Erwinia chrysanthemi) 10:00
Collagenase 84:92
Dornase Alfa 48:24
Pancrelipase 56:16
Pegaspargase 10:00
Reteplase 20:12.20
Tenecteplase 20:12.20

§ Omitted from the print version of *AHFS Drug Information*® because of space limitations. This monograph is available on the *AHFS Drug Information*® website, http://ahfsdruginformation.com. Username: ahfs2020; Password: ASHP94498.

48:00 Respiratory Tract Agents

48:48 Vasodilating Agents

48:92 Respiratory Agents, Miscellaneous

§ Omitted from the print version of *AHFS Drug Information*® because of space limitations. This monograph is available on the *AHFS Drug Information*® website, http://ahfsdruginformation.com. Username: ahfs2020; Password: ASHP94498.

* Please see the full *AHFS Pharmacologic-Therapeutic Classification*© on p. viii. Not all classes are used in the printed edition.

RESPIRATORY TRACT AGENTS 48:00

ANTIFIBROTIC AGENTS 48:02

Nintedanib Esylate

Intedanib

■ Nintedanib esylate, an inhibitor of multiple tyrosine kinases (including receptor tyrosine kinases [RTKs] and nonreceptor tyrosine kinases [nRTKs]), reduces fibroblast activity in idiopathic pulmonary fibrosis (IPF).

Uses

■ **Idiopathic Pulmonary Fibrosis** Nintedanib esylate is used for the treatment of idiopathic pulmonary fibrosis (IPF). Nintedanib is designated an orphan drug by FDA for this use.

Idiopathic pulmonary fibrosis is a specific form of chronic, progressive fibrosing interstitial pneumonia of unknown etiology characterized by worsening dyspnea, nonproductive cough, and progressive loss of lung function. IPF occurs mainly in older adults, is limited to the lungs, and is associated with the histopathologic and/or radiologic pattern of usual interstitial pneumonia. Although the pathogenesis is not well understood, IPF is characterized by abnormal alveolar epithelial cell signaling, which results in fibroblast proliferation and differentiation, leading to excessive collagen deposition in the lungs, lung fibrosis, and remodeling. The condition is more common in men than women, and the majority of patients have a history of cigarette smoking. The typical age of onset is 60–70 years; IPF rarely occurs in patients younger than 50 years of age. The clinical course of IPF is variable; most patients experience a gradual worsening of lung function over several years, but some may experience rapid declines or episodes of acute respiratory worsening. Acute exacerbation is estimated to affect 5–20% of patients with IPF and is defined as rapid worsening of dyspnea, hypoxemia, and new radiographic alveolar infiltrates in the absence of other causes; these events are associated with a mortality rate exceeding 60% during hospital admission, and over 90% within 6 months after hospital discharge. Median survival time has been reported to be 2.5–3.5 years after diagnosis; death usually occurs from respiratory failure.

Management of IPF has historically consisted of supportive treatment (i.e., supplemental oxygen, pulmonary rehabilitation) and lung transplantation in appropriate patients; pharmacologic therapies used for interstitial lung disease, such as corticosteroids or immunosuppressants, have not demonstrated a clinical benefit in IPF and generally are not recommended by most experts.

In clinical studies, nintedanib was more effective than placebo in reducing the annual rate of decline in forced vital capacity (FVC) in patients with IPF. Efficacy of nintedanib for the treatment of IPF was established in one phase 2 study (study 1) and two phase 3 studies (studies 2 and 3). All 3 studies were multicenter, randomized, double-blind, placebo-controlled studies that compared nintedanib 150 mg twice daily with placebo for 52 weeks in a total of 1231 patients with IPF. Patients in these studies were 40 years of age or older, had a diagnosis of IPF consistent with the American Thoracic Society (ATS) and European Respiratory Society (ERS) criteria for less than 5 years at the time of screening, had an FVC that was 50% or more of their predicted value, and a diffusing lung capacity for carbon monoxide (DLCO) 30–79% of their predicted value. All patients included in these studies had undergone high-resolution computed tomography (HRCT) of the chest within the previous year. The mean age of patients enrolled in the studies was 67 years and the mean FVC was 80% of their predicted values.

The primary end point for these studies was the annual rate of decline in FVC; secondary end points included time to first acute IPF exacerbation, change in FVC as a percent of predicted value from baseline, and survival. In all 3 studies, nintedanib was substantially more effective than placebo in reducing the annual rate of decline in FVC. Over 1 year, FVC declined by 60, 115, and 114 mL in nintedanib-treated patients compared with 191, 240, and 207 mL in those receiving placebo in studies 1, 2, and 3, respectively. Nintedanib therapy also improved several secondary measures of efficacy, including risk of first acute IPF exacerbation (in studies 1 and 3) and change from baseline in FVC as a percent of predicted value; there was no difference in all-cause mortality between the treatment groups.

While nintedanib dosages of 50 mg once or twice daily and 100 mg twice daily were evaluated in the phase 2 study, further information on the efficacy of these dosage regimens is not available. The FDA approved only the 150-mg twice daily dosage for the treatment of IPF. (See Dosage and Administration: Dosage.)

Dosage and Administration

■ **General** Liver function tests should be performed prior to initiation of nintedanib esylate therapy, monthly for the first 3 months, then every 3 months, and as clinically indicated.

Restricted Distribution Program Nintedanib esylate can only be obtained through a limited network of specialty pharmacies. Clinicians may consult the Ofev® website for specific ordering and availability information (http://www.hcp.ofev.com/).

■ **Administration** Nintedanib esylate is administered orally twice daily, approximately 12 hours apart, with food. The capsules should be swallowed whole with liquid and should not be chewed or crushed because of a bitter taste.

If a dose is missed, the missed dose should be skipped and the next dose should be taken at the regularly scheduled time; the recommended maximum daily dosage of 300 mg should not be exceeded.

■ **Dosage** Dosage of nintedanib esylate is expressed in terms of nintedanib.

Idiopathic Pulmonary Fibrosis The recommended dosage of nintedanib for the treatment of idiopathic pulmonary fibrosis (IPF) is 150 mg twice daily.

Dosage Modification for Toxicity **Hepatic Toxicity.** For serum transaminase (ALT or AST) elevations exceeding 3 times, but not more than 5 times, the upper limit of normal (ULN) *without* signs or symptoms of severe liver damage, nintedanib therapy should be interrupted or the dosage reduced to 100 mg twice daily until the liver function test results return to baseline values. Nintedanib therapy may be resumed at a reduced dosage of 100 mg twice daily and may subsequently be increased to the full dosage of 150 mg twice daily.

For ALT or AST elevations exceeding 5 times the ULN, or exceeding 3 times the ULN *with* signs or symptoms of severe liver damage, therapy with nintedanib should be discontinued. (See Hepatic Toxicity under Cautions: Warnings/Precautions.)

Other Adverse Effects. Interruption of nintedanib therapy or dosage reduction may be required in patients who develop intolerable adverse reactions (even with symptomatic treatment, if applicable) until the specific adverse reaction resolves to a level that allows continuation of therapy. (See Cautions: Warnings/Precautions.) Nintedanib may be resumed at the original dosage of 150 mg twice daily; alternatively, the drug may be resumed at a reduced dosage of 100 mg twice daily and may subsequently be increased to the full dosage of 150 mg twice daily. Nintedanib should be discontinued in patients who experience intolerable adverse reactions at a dosage of 100 mg twice daily.

■ **Special Populations** No initial dosage adjustment is necessary in patients with mild hepatic impairment (Child-Pugh class A); however, such patients should be closely monitored and interruption of therapy and/or dosage reduction should be considered in patients experiencing adverse reactions. (See Hepatic Toxicity under Dosage: Dosage Modification for Toxicity, in Dosage and Administration.) Nintedanib has not been studied in patients with moderate or severe hepatic impairment (Child-Pugh class B or C) and is not recommended for use in such patients.

No initial dosage adjustment is necessary in patients with mild to moderate renal impairment (creatinine clearance 30–90 mL/minute). Nintedanib has not been studied in patients with severe renal impairment (creatinine clearance less than 30 mL/minute) or end-stage renal disease.

The manufacturer makes no specific dosage recommendations for geriatric patients.

Cautions

■ **Contraindications** The manufacturer states there are no known contraindications to the use of nintedanib.

■ **Warnings/Precautions** ***Hepatic Toxicity*** Abnormal liver function test results, including elevated transaminase (ALT or AST), alkaline phosphatase, γ-glutamyltransferase, and bilirubin concentrations, have been reported in patients receiving nintedanib. Liver enzyme elevations were reported in 14% of patients receiving nintedanib compared with 3% of patients receiving placebo in clinical studies. Increases in liver enzymes were not associated with clinical signs or symptoms of liver injury and were reversible following dosage modification or interruption of therapy. In patients with ALT and/or AST elevations, most (94%) did not exceed 5 times the upper limit of normal (ULN) and in patients with bilirubin elevations, most (95%) did not exceed 2 times the ULN.

Liver function tests including serum ALT, AST, and total bilirubin concentrations should be performed prior to initiation of nintedanib therapy, monthly for the first 3 months, then every 3 months thereafter, and as clinically indicated. Interruption of therapy and/or dosage reduction may be necessary in patients who develop transaminase (ALT or AST) elevations during nintedanib therapy. (See Hepatic Toxicity under Dosage: Dosage Modification for Toxicity, in Dosage and Administration.)

GI Effects Nintedanib can cause adverse GI effects, including diarrhea, abdominal pain, nausea, and vomiting. Diarrhea occurred in 62% of patients receiving nintedanib compared with 18% of patients receiving placebo in clinical trials. Nausea and vomiting were reported in 24 and 12% of nintedanib-treated patients compared with 7 and 3% of patients receiving placebo, respectively. In most patients, these events were mild to moderate in severity; diarrhea generally occurred within the first 3 months of treatment. Diarrhea resulted in permanent dosage reduction in 11% of nintedanib-treated patients; diarrhea, nausea, and vomiting resulted in discontinuance of nintedanib in 5, 2, and 1% of patients, respectively.

Patients receiving nintedanib should be monitored for development of adverse GI effects and treated as necessary with appropriate therapy (e.g., antidiarrhea agents [e.g., loperamide], antiemetics, fluid replacement).

Interruption of therapy and/or dosage reduction may be necessary in patients experiencing diarrhea or if nausea or vomiting persists despite appropriate supportive care. Nintedanib should be discontinued if severe diarrhea persists despite symptomatic treatment or if severe nausea or vomiting does not resolve. (See Other Adverse Effects under Dosage: Dosage Modification for Toxicity, in Dosage and Administration.)

Fetal/Neonatal Morbidity and Mortality Based on animal findings, nintedanib may cause fetal harm if administered to pregnant women. Embryofetal toxicity and teratogenicity have been demonstrated in rats and rabbits given nintedanib dosages less than and approximately 5 times the maximum recommended human dose. Teratogenic effects included missing or additional major blood vessels, skeletal abnormalities, or missing urogenital organs. Women of childbearing potential should use effective contraception while receiving nintedanib and for at least 3 months after the drug is discontinued. If nintedanib is used during pregnancy or if the patient becomes pregnant while receiving the drug, the patient should be apprised of the potential fetal hazard. (See Advice to Patients.)

Arterial Thromboembolic Events Arterial thromboembolic events (e.g., myocardial infarction [MI]) have been reported in patients receiving nintedanib. In clinical studies, arterial thromboembolism was reported in 2.5% of nintedanib-treated patients compared with 0.8% of placebo recipients. MI occurred in 1.5% of patients receiving nintedanib.

Nintedanib should be used with caution in patients with cardiovascular risks, including coronary artery disease. The manufacturer states that treatment interruption should be considered in patients who develop signs or symptoms of acute myocardial ischemia.

Hemorrhage Because nintedanib inhibits vascular endothelial growth factor receptor [VEGFR], the risk of bleeding may be increased. Bleeding events were reported in 10% of patients receiving nintedanib compared with 7% of patients receiving placebo. Nintedanib should be used in patients with risk factors for bleeding only if the potential benefit outweighs the risk.

GI Perforation Nintedanib may increase the risk of GI perforation based on its mechanism of action. GI perforation was reported in 0.3% of nintedanib-treated patients in clinical studies.

Nintedanib should be used with caution in patients who have had recent abdominal surgery. In patients with risk factors for GI perforation, nintedanib should be used only if the potential benefit outweighs the risk. Nintedanib therapy should be discontinued in patients who develop GI perforation.

Specific Populations **Pregnancy.** Category D. (See Users Guide and see Fetal/Neonatal Morbidity and Mortality under Cautions: Warnings/Precautions.)

Lactation. Nintedanib and its metabolites are distributed into milk in rats; it is not known whether the drug is distributed into human milk. Because of the potential for serious adverse reactions to nintedanib in nursing infants, a decision should be made whether to discontinue nursing or the drug, taking into account the importance of the drug to the woman.

Pediatric Use. Safety and efficacy of nintedanib have not been established in pediatric patients.

Geriatric Use. In phase 2 and 3 clinical studies, 60.8% of patients were 65 years of age or older and 16.3% were 75 years of age or older. No overall differences in safety and efficacy were observed between geriatric patients and younger adults in phase 3 studies; however, the possibility of increased sensitivity to the drug in some geriatric patients cannot be ruled out.

Hepatic Impairment. Nintedanib is principally eliminated through biliary/fecal excretion. Formal pharmacokinetic studies of nintedanib have not been conducted in patients with hepatic impairment, and clinical studies excluded patients with AST, ALT, or bilirubin concentrations greater than 1.5 times the ULN. Patients with mild hepatic impairment (Child-Pugh class A) should be closely monitored and interruption of therapy and/or dosage reduction should be considered in patients experiencing adverse reactions. (See Hepatic Toxicity under Dosage: Dosage Modification for Toxicity, in Dosage and Administration.) Safety and efficacy of nintedanib have not been established in patients with moderate or severe hepatic impairment (Child-Pugh class B or C).

Renal Impairment. Less than 1% of nintedanib is excreted renally. Systemic exposure to nintedanib was not affected in individuals with mild or moderate (creatinine clearance 30–90 mL/minute) renal impairment. No initial dosage adjustment is recommended in patients with mild to moderate renal impairment; nintedanib has not been studied in patients with severe renal impairment (creatinine clearance less than 30 mL/minute) or end-stage renal disease.

■ **Common Adverse Effects** Adverse effects reported in 5% or more of patients receiving nintedanib and at an incidence greater than with placebo include diarrhea, nausea, abdominal pain, elevated concentrations of hepatic enzymes (e.g., ALT, AST, alkaline phosphatase), vomiting, decreased appetite, decreased weight, headache, and hypertension.

Drug Interactions

Nintedanib is a substrate of P-glycoprotein (P-gp) and, to a minor extent, cytochrome P-450 (CYP) 3A4.

In vitro studies indicate that nintedanib and its metabolites do not inhibit or induce CYP isoenzymes.

In vitro studies indicate that nintedanib does not inhibit organic anion-transporting polypeptide (OATP) 1B1, OATP1B3, OATP2B1, organic cation transporter (OCT) 2, or multidrug resistance protein (MRP) 2. In vitro, the drug has a weak inhibitory potential on OCT1, breast cancer resistance protein (BCRP), and P-gp; these findings are not expected to be clinically important.

■ **Drugs Affecting Hepatic Microsomal Enzymes and the P-glycoprotein Transport System** Concomitant use of nintedanib with inhibitors of P-gp and CYP3A4 (e.g., erythromycin, ketoconazole) may increase exposure to nintedanib. Patients should be monitored for adverse effects of nintedanib if an inhibitor of both P-gp and CYP3A4 is used concomitantly. Interruption of therapy and/or dosage reduction may be necessary in patients who experience adverse effects during such concomitant therapy. (See Dosage and Administration: Dosage Modification for Toxicity.)

Inducers of P-gp and CYP3A4 may decrease exposure to nintedanib. Concomitant use of nintedanib with P-gp and CYP3A4 inducers (e.g., carbamazepine, phenytoin, rifampin, St. John's wort [*Hypericum perforatum*]) should be avoided.

Ketoconazole Concomitant oral administration of nintedanib and ketoconazole (an inhibitor of P-gp and CYP3A4) increased peak plasma concentrations and systemic exposure of nintedanib by 1.8- and 1.6-fold, respectively.

Rifampin Concomitant oral administration of nintedanib and rifampin (an inducer of P-gp and CYP3A4) decreased peak plasma concentrations and systemic exposure of nintedanib by about 60 and 50%, respectively.

■ **Drugs Affecting Gastric Acidity** Because the aqueous solubility of nintedanib is pH dependent (i.e., increased solubility at pH less than 3), drugs that increase gastric pH may potentially affect the bioavailability of nintedanib. However, concomitant administration of proton-pump inhibitors or H_2-receptor antagonists in clinical studies did not affect trough concentrations of nintedanib.

■ **Drugs Affecting Hemostasis** Nintedanib may increase the risk of bleeding. (See Hemorrhage under Cautions: Warnings/Precautions.) The manufacturer states that patients receiving full-dose anticoagulation therapy should be monitored closely for bleeding; dosage adjustment of the anticoagulant may be necessary.

■ **Antineoplastic Agents** Concomitant use of nintedanib with pemetrexed or carboplatin in combination with paclitaxel in patients with non-small cell lung cancer (NSCLC) did not substantially alter the pharmacokinetics of these antineoplastic agents.

Concomitant use of nintedanib with docetaxel in patients with prostate cancer did not substantially alter the pharmacokinetics of docetaxel.

■ **Cigarette Smoking** Cigarette smoking reduces exposure to nintedanib by approximately 21%. Dosage adjustments are not required in smokers; however, the manufacturer recommends that patients be encouraged to stop smoking prior to initiation of nintedanib and to avoid smoking during therapy.

■ **Pirfenidone** In a multiple dose study in Japanese patients with idiopathic pulmonary fibrosis (IPF), addition of nintedanib to ongoing pirfenidone therapy resulted in a 41 and 32% decrease in nintedanib peak plasma concentrations and area under the concentration-time curve (AUC), respectively, compared with nintedanib alone. Concomitant use of nintedanib and pirfenidone did not have an effect on the pharmacokinetics of pirfenidone. In this study, nausea and vomiting were reported more frequently with concomitant nintedanib and pirfenidone therapy compared with nintedanib alone; all adverse effects reported in the study were mild or moderate in severity.

Description

Nintedanib esylate, an inhibitor of multiple tyrosine kinases (including receptor tyrosine kinases [RTKs] and nonreceptor tyrosine kinases [nRTKs]), reduces fibroblast activity in idiopathic pulmonary fibrosis (IPF); the drug also is an antineoplastic agent. Chemically, nintedanib is a substituted indolinone derivative. Nintedanib inhibits RTKs including vascular endothelial growth factor receptors (VEGFR)-1, VEGFR-2, and VEGFR-3; fibroblast growth factor receptors (FGFR)-1, FGFR-2, and FGFR-3; and platelet-derived growth factor receptors (PDGFR)-α and PDGFR-β. The VEGFR, FGFR, and PDGFR signaling pathways have been implicated in the pathogenesis of IPF; the binding of nintedanib to the ATP binding pocket of these receptors interrupts various signaling pathways that lead to the proliferation, migration, and differentiation of fibroblasts in the lungs. Nintedanib also inhibits the RTK Fms-like tyrosine kinase (FLT)-3, and the nRTKs Lck, Lyn, and Src; the effect of FLT-3 and nRTK inhibition in IPF is unknown.

Nintedanib exhibits dose-proportional pharmacokinetics following oral dosages ranging from 50–450 mg once daily and 150–300 mg twice daily. Following oral administration under fed conditions, peak plasma concentrations of nintedanib are achieved within 2–4 hours. Steady-state concentrations are achieved within 1 week. The absolute oral bioavailability of a 100-mg dose of nintedanib is 4.7%. Administration with food increases the systemic exposure of nintedanib by 20% and delays absorption by approximately 2 hours compared with administration in the fasting state. Nintedanib is 97.8% bound to plasma proteins in vitro (mainly albumin). Nintedanib is metabolized principally by hydrolytic cleavage via esterases to the carboxylate metabolite, BIBF 1202, which then undergoes glucuronidation by uridine diphosphate-glucuronosyltransferase (UGT) 1A1, 1A7, 1A8, and 1A10; cytochrome P-450 (CYP) isoenzymes, mainly CYP3A4, play a minor role in the drug's overall metabolism. Following oral administration of radiolabeled nintedanib, 93.4% of the dose is eliminated via fecal/biliary excretion, mainly as the metabolite BIBF 1202, and 0.65% is eliminated renally. The effective half-life of nintedanib in patients with IPF is 9.5 hours.

Advice to Patients

Importance of reading the manufacturer's patient information prior to beginning nintedanib therapy and each time the prescription is refilled.

Importance of taking nintedanib with food. Importance of swallowing capsules whole with liquid and not to chew or crush the capsules.

If a dose of nintedanib is missed, the missed dose should be skipped and the next dose taken at the regularly scheduled time; the dose should not be doubled to make up for a missed dose.

Risk of hepatotoxicity and importance of periodic liver function test monitoring. Importance of immediately reporting any manifestations of hepatotoxicity (e.g., jaundice, unusually dark or "tea-colored" urine, right upper quadrant pain, bleeding or bruising more easily than normal, lethargy) to clinician.

Importance of clinician informing patients that diarrhea, nausea, and vomiting are the most common adverse effects associated with nintedanib therapy, and that the clinician may recommend supportive treatment (e.g., hydration, antidiarrhea agents, and/or antiemetics). Importance of informing clinician at first sign of diarrhea or if severe or persistent diarrhea, nausea, or vomiting occurs.

Risk of arterial thromboembolic events. Importance of advising patients to seek emergency help and to contact clinician if any symptoms suggestive of acute myocardial ischemia or other thromboembolic event occur (e.g., chest pain or pressure; arm, back, neck, or jaw pain; shortness of breath; numbness or weakness on one side of the body; trouble talking; headache; or dizziness).

Risk of GI perforation; importance of immediately informing clinician of any manifestations of GI perforation (e.g., abdominal pain or swelling).

Increased risk of bleeding. Importance of promptly informing clinician of any unusual bleeding.

Risk of fetal harm. Necessity of women of childbearing potential to avoid pregnancy and to use effective methods of contraception while receiving nintedanib and for at least 3 months after the drug is discontinued. Importance of patients informing their clinicians if they are pregnant or think they may be pregnant.

Importance of advising women to avoid breast-feeding while receiving nintedanib therapy.

Importance of informing clinicians of existing or contemplated concomitant therapy, including prescription and OTC drugs and dietary or herbal supplements (e.g., anticoagulants, aspirin, laxatives, St. John's wort [*Hypericum perforatum*]), as well as any concomitant illnesses (e.g., hepatic impairment, cardiovascular disease).

Importance of informing patients of other important precautionary information. (See Cautions.)

Overview® (see Users Guide). For additional information on this drug until a more detailed monograph is developed and published, the manufacturer's labeling should be consulted. It is *essential* that the manufacturer's labeling be consulted for more detailed information on usual cautions, precautions, contraindications, potential drug interactions, laboratory test interferences, and acute toxicity.

Preparations

Distribution of nintedanib esylate is restricted. (See Restricted Distribution Program under Dosage and Administration: General.)

Excipients in commercially available drug preparations may have clinically important effects in some individuals; consult specific product labeling for details.

Nintedanib Esylate

Oral		
Capsules	100 mg (of nintedanib)	**Ofev®**, Boehringer Ingelheim
	150 mg (of nintedanib)	**Ofev®**, Boehringer Ingelheim

Pirfenidone

■ Pirfenidone, a synthetic pyridone, is an antifibrotic agent.

Uses

■ **Idiopathic Pulmonary Fibrosis** Pirfenidone is used for the treatment of idiopathic pulmonary fibrosis (IPF). Pirfenidone is designated an orphan drug by FDA for this use.

Idiopathic pulmonary fibrosis is a specific form of chronic, progressive fibrosing interstitial pneumonia of unknown etiology characterized by worsening dyspnea, nonproductive cough, and progressive loss of lung function. IPF occurs mainly in older adults, is limited to the lungs, and is associated with the histopathologic and/or radiologic pattern of usual interstitial pneumonia. Although the pathogenesis is not well understood, IPF is characterized by abnormal alveolar epithelial cell signaling, which results in fibroblast proliferation and differentiation, leading to excessive collagen deposition in the lungs, lung fibrosis, and remodeling. The condition is more common in men than women, and the majority of patients have a history of cigarette smoking. The typical age of onset is 60–70 years; IPF rarely occurs in patients younger than 50 years of age. The clinical course of IPF is variable; most patients experience a gradual worsening of lung function over several years, but some may experience rapid declines or episodes of acute respiratory worsening. Acute exacerbation is estimated to affect 5–20% of patients with IPF and is defined as rapid worsening of dyspnea, hypoxemia, and new radiographic alveolar infiltrates in the absence of other causes; these events are associated with a mortality rate exceeding 60% during hospital admission and over 90% within 6 months after hospital discharge. Median survival time has been reported to be 2.5–3.5 years after diagnosis; death usually occurs from respiratory failure.

Management of IPF has historically consisted of supportive treatment (i.e., supplemental oxygen, pulmonary rehabilitation) and lung transplantation in appropriate patients; pharmacologic therapies used for interstitial lung disease, such as corticosteroids or immunosuppressants, have not demonstrated a clinical benefit in IPF and generally are not recommended by most experts. The 2011 statement from the American Thoracic Society (ATS), European Respiratory Society (ERS), Japanese Respiratory Society (JRS), and the Latin American Thoracic Association (ALAT) on guidelines for diagnosis and management of IPF states that the majority of patients with IPF should not be treated with pirfenidone; however, the drug may be a reasonable choice in a small subset of patients, based on the potential risks and benefits of pirfenidone therapy.

In clinical studies, pirfenidone was more effective than placebo in reducing the mean rate of decline in percent of predicted forced vital capacity (FVC) in patients with IPF. Efficacy of pirfenidone for the treatment of IPF was established in 3 multicenter, randomized, double-blind, placebo-controlled phase 3 studies comparing pirfenidone 2403 mg daily with placebo in a total of 1247 patients with IPF (studies 1, 2, and 3). The primary end point in these studies was the change in percent of predicted FVC from baseline to study end; all-cause mortality was also evaluated as an exploratory end point. Patients in these studies were 40–80 years of age, had a diagnosis of IPF based on findings from high-resolution computed tomography (HRCT) with or without lung biopsy, had an FVC that was 50% or more of their predicted value and a diffusing lung capacity for carbon monoxide (DLCO) that was at least 30% (study 1) or 35% (studies 2 and 3) of their predicted value. The mean age of patients enrolled in the studies was 67 years; 74% were male, 65% were current or former smokers, and baseline mean FVC and DLCO were 72 and 46% of their predicted values, respectively.

In studies 1 and 2, pirfenidone was substantially more effective than placebo in reducing the mean rate of decline in percent of predicted FVC over 52 and 72 weeks, respectively. Study 3 did not show a substantial difference between the treatment groups over 72 weeks. In studies 1 and 2, patients who received pirfenidone 2403 mg daily experienced a mean FVC decline of 3.7 and 8% of their predicted value compared with 6.6 and 12.4% in those who received placebo, respectively, over each study duration. In study 1, FVC declined by a mean of 235 mL in pirfenidone-treated patients compared with 428 mL in placebo recipients over 52 weeks. In pooled analyses, there were no substantial differences between the treatment groups in all-cause mortality assessed over the study durations and follow-up periods.

Dosage and Administration

■ **General** Liver function tests should be performed prior to initiation of pirfenidone therapy, monthly for the first 6 months, and then every 3 months.

■ **Administration** Pirfenidone is administered orally 3 times daily with food, at the same time every day.

If a dose of pirfenidone is missed, the next dose should be administered as soon as it is remembered; a double dose should not be administered to make up for a missed dose. No more than 3 doses should be taken per day.

■ **Dosage** ***Idiopathic Pulmonary Fibrosis*** For the treatment of idiopathic pulmonary fibrosis (IPF), the recommended maintenance dosage is 801 mg (three 267-mg capsules) 3 times daily. The dosage should be titrated upward to the full dosage over a 2-week period beginning with 267 mg (1 capsule) 3 times daily for the first 7 days, followed by 534 mg (two 267-mg capsules) 3 times daily for an additional 7 days, and then 801 mg (three 267-mg capsules) 3 times daily thereafter. The maximum recommended daily dosage of pirfenidone is 2403 mg (801 mg 3 times daily).

Following treatment interruptions of 14 or more days, dosage of pirfenidone must be titrated upward using the initial 2-week dosage titration regimen. If treatment has been interrupted for less than 14 days, therapy can be resumed at the dosage received prior to the interruption.

Dosage Modification **Hepatic Toxicity.** For serum transaminase (ALT and/or AST) elevations exceeding 3 times, but not more than 5 times, the upper limit of normal (ULN) in patients *without* symptoms or hyperbilirubinemia, pirfenidone may be continued at the full dosage if clinically appropriate, therapy may be interrupted, or the dosage of the drug reduced until liver function test results return to normal. Pirfenidone therapy may be resumed and subsequently increased to the full dosage as tolerated. Patients should be monitored carefully; other drugs that could cause liver enzyme elevations should be discontinued and other causes of liver enzyme elevations should be excluded.

For ALT or AST elevations exceeding 3 times, but not more than 5 times, the ULN in patients *with* symptoms or hyperbilirubinemia, pirfenidone therapy should be permanently discontinued.

For ALT or AST elevations exceeding 5 times the ULN, pirfenidone should be permanently discontinued. (See Hepatic Toxicity under Cautions: Warnings/Precautions.)

Other Adverse Effects. Interruption of pirfenidone therapy or temporary dosage reduction should be considered in patients who develop clinically important adverse reactions (i.e., GI effects such as nausea, diarrhea, dyspepsia, vomiting or photosensitivity reaction or rash) to allow for resolution of symptoms. (See GI Effects and also see Photosensitivity under Cautions: Warnings/Precautions.)

Concomitant Use with Drugs Affecting Hepatic Microsomal Enzymes. If pirfenidone is used concomitantly with a potent inhibitor of cytochrome P-450 (CYP) isoenzyme 1A2 (e.g., fluvoxamine), pirfenidone dosage should be reduced to 267 mg (1 capsule) 3 times daily.

If pirfenidone is used concomitantly with the moderate CYP1A2 inhibitor ciprofloxacin (at a dosage of 750 mg twice daily), pirfenidone dosage should be reduced to 534 mg (two 267-mg capsules) 3 times daily. (See Drug Interactions: Drugs Affecting Hepatic Microsomal Enzymes.)

■ **Special Populations** No initial dosage adjustment is recommended in patients with mild or moderate hepatic impairment (Child-Pugh class A or B); patients should be closely monitored and interruption of therapy and/or dosage reduction should be considered in patients experiencing adverse reactions. (See Hepatic Toxicity under Dosage: Dosage Modification, in Dosage and Administration.) Pirfenidone has not been studied in patients with severe hepatic impairment (Child-Pugh class C) and is not recommended for use in such patients.

No initial dosage adjustment is recommended in patients with mild, moderate, or severe renal impairment; patients should be closely monitored and interruption of therapy and/or dosage reduction should be considered in patients experiencing adverse reactions. Pirfenidone has not been studied in patients with end-stage renal disease requiring dialysis and is not recommended for use in such patients.

No dosage adjustment is required for geriatric patients. (See Specific Populations under Cautions: Warnings/Precautions.)

Cautions

■ **Contraindications** The manufacturer states there are no known contraindications to the use of pirfenidone.

■ **Warnings/Precautions** ***Hepatic Toxicity*** Elevations in serum transaminase (ALT and/or AST) concentrations exceeding 3 times the upper limit of normal (ULN) have occurred in patients receiving pirfenidone; concomitant elevations in bilirubin concentrations have been reported rarely. ALT or AST elevations of at least 3 times the ULN were reported in 3.7% of patients receiving pirfenidone compared with 0.8% of patients receiving placebo in clinical studies; ALT or AST elevations of 10 times the ULN or greater occurred in 0.3% of pirfenidone-treated patients. Increases in liver enzymes were reversible following dosage modification or interruption of therapy. No cases of liver transplant or death due to liver failure related to pirfenidone use have been reported to date; however, the manufacturer states that the combination of transaminase elevations and hyperbilirubinemia without evidence of obstruction is generally recognized as an important predictor of severe liver injury possibly resulting in death or the need for liver transplant in some patients.

Liver function tests including ALT, AST, and bilirubin concentrations should be performed prior to initiation of pirfenidone therapy, monthly for the first 6 months, and then every 3 months thereafter. Interruption of therapy and/or dosage reduction may be necessary in patients experiencing liver enzyme elevations. (See Hepatic Toxicity under Dosage: Dosage Modification, in Dosage and Administration.)

Photosensitivity Photosensitivity manifested as rash or other reactions was reported in 9% of patients receiving pirfenidone in clinical studies. Most of the reactions occurred during the first 6 months following initiation of pirfenidone. Interruption of therapy and/or dosage reduction may be necessary in some patients experiencing photosensitivity reaction or rash. (See Adverse Reactions under Dosage: Dosage Modification, in Dosage and Administration and see Advice to Patients.)

GI Effects Nausea, diarrhea, dyspepsia, vomiting, gastroesophageal reflux disease (GERD), and abdominal pain were frequently reported in pirfenidone-treated patients in clinical studies. The incidence of adverse GI effects was highest during the first 3 months of pirfenidone therapy and decreased over time. Adverse GI effects (e.g., nausea, diarrhea, vomiting, dyspepsia) resulted in dosage interruption or modification in 18.5% of patients and discontinuance of therapy in 2.2% of patients receiving pirfenidone in clinical studies. Interruption of therapy and/or dosage reduction may be necessary in some patients experiencing adverse GI effects. (See Adverse Reactions under Dosage: Dosage Modification, in Dosage and Administration.)

Specific Populations **Pregnancy.** Category C. (See Users Guide.)

Lactation. Pirfenidone or its metabolites are distributed into milk in rats; it is not known whether the drug is distributed into human milk. Because of the potential for serious adverse reactions to pirfenidone in nursing infants, a decision should be made whether to discontinue nursing or the drug, taking into account the importance of the drug to the woman.

Pediatric Use. Safety and efficacy of pirfenidone have not been established in pediatric patients.

Geriatric Use. In clinical studies, 67% of patients were 65 years of age or older and 22% were 75 years of age or older. No overall differences in safety and efficacy were observed between geriatric patients and younger adults.

Hepatic Impairment. In individuals with moderate hepatic impairment (Child-Pugh class B), systemic exposure and peak plasma concentrations were increased approximately 1.6- and 1.4-fold, respectively, compared with individuals with normal hepatic function, but systemic exposure to 5-carboxy-pirfenidone (a metabolite expected to be pharmacologically inactive) was not substantially altered. Pirfenidone has not been studied in patients with severe hepatic impairment (Child-Pugh class C). (See Dosage and Administration: Special Populations.)

Renal Impairment. In individuals with mild (creatinine clearance 50–80 mL/minute), moderate (creatinine clearance 30–50 mL/minute), or severe renal impairment (creatinine clearance less than 30 mL/minute), systemic exposure was increased approximately 1.4-, 1.5-, or 1.2-fold, respectively, compared with individuals with normal renal function. Systemic exposure to 5-carboxy-pirfenidone (a metabolite expected to be pharmacologically inactive) was not substantially altered in individuals with mild renal impairment; however systemic exposure was increased 3.4- and 5.6-fold in individuals with moderate and severe renal impairment, respectively. Pirfenidone has not been studied in patients with end-stage renal disease requiring dialysis. (See Dosage and Administration: Special Populations.)

■ **Common Adverse Effects** Adverse effects reported in 10% or more of patients receiving pirfenidone and at an incidence greater than with placebo include nausea, rash, abdominal pain, upper respiratory tract infection, diarrhea, fatigue, headache, dyspepsia, dizziness, vomiting, anorexia, GERD, sinusitis, insomnia, decreased weight, and arthralgia.

Drug Interactions

Pirfenidone is metabolized principally (70–80%) by cytochrome P-450 (CYP) isoenzyme 1A2, and, to a lesser extent, by CYP isoenzymes 2C9, 2C19, 2D6, and 2E1.

In vitro studies indicate that pirfenidone has a weak inhibitory potential on P-glycoprotein (P-gp); effects of pirfenidone on P-gp substrates have not been studied to date.

Pirfenidone also demonstrated concentration-dependent inhibition of CYP2C9, 2C19, 1A2, 2D6, and 3A4 in vitro; effects of pirfenidone on drugs metabolized by these isoenzymes have not been studied to date.

■ **Drugs Affecting Hepatic Microsomal Enzymes** ***Inhibitors of CYP1A*** Concomitant use of pirfenidone with potent inhibitors of CYP1A2 (e.g., fluvoxamine) may result in substantially increased systemic exposure to pirfenidone and should be avoided. Fluvoxamine or other potent CYP1A2 inhibitors should be discontinued prior to initiation of pirfenidone therapy. If concomitant use of pirfenidone and fluvoxamine or other potent CYP1A2 inhibitors cannot be avoided, pirfenidone dosage should be reduced. (See Concomitant Use with Drugs Affecting Hepatic Microsomal Enzymes under Dosage: Dosage Modification, in Dosage and Administration.) Patients should be monitored closely for adverse effects; discontinuance of therapy should be considered as needed.

Concomitant use of pirfenidone with moderate inhibitors of CYP1A2 (e.g., ciprofloxacin) may result in moderately increased systemic exposure to pirfenidone.

Ciprofloxacin. Concomitant administration of pirfenidone (single 801-mg dose on day 6) with the moderate CYP1A2 inhibitor ciprofloxacin (750 mg twice daily on days 2–7) increased the systemic exposure to pirfenidone by 81%. Pirfenidone dosage should be reduced if used concomitantly with ciprofloxacin at a dosage of 750 mg twice daily. (See Concomitant Use with Drugs Affecting Hepatic Microsomal Enzymes under Dosage: Dosage Modification, in Dosage and Administration.) No initial dosage adjustment is recommended if pirfenidone is used concomitantly with ciprofloxacin at a dosage of 250 or 500 mg once daily; however, patients receiving such concomitant therapy should be monitored closely for adverse effects.

Fluvoxamine. Concomitant administration of a single dose of pirfenidone with the potent CYP1A2 inhibitor fluvoxamine (initially 50 mg daily, titrated upward to 150 mg daily for 10 days) in nonsmokers and smokers increased pirfenidone exposure approximately fourfold in nonsmokers and sevenfold in smokers.

Inhibitors of CYP1A2 and Other CYP Isoenzymes Concomitant use of pirfenidone with agents or a combination of agents that are potent or moderate inhibitors of both CYP1A2 and one or more other CYP isoenzymes involved with pirfenidone metabolism (i.e., CYP2C9, 2C19, 2D6, and 2E1) should be avoided.

Inducers of CYP1A2 Concomitant use of pirfenidone and CYP1A2 inducers may result in decreased exposure to and reduced efficacy of pirfenidone. (See Drug Interactions: Cigarette Smoking.) The manufacturer of pirfenidone recommends that potent CYP1A2 inducers be avoided during pirfenidone therapy.

■ **Cigarette Smoking** Cigarette smoking reduces peak plasma concentrations and systemic exposure to pirfenidone by 32 and 54%, respectively. The manufacturer recommends that patients be encouraged to stop smoking prior to initiation of pirfenidone and to avoid smoking during therapy.

■ **Nintedanib** In a multiple dose study in Japanese patients with idiopathic pulmonary fibrosis (IPF), addition of nintedanib to ongoing pirfenidone therapy resulted in a 41 and 32% decrease in nintedanib peak plasma concentrations and area under the concentration-time curve (AUC) compared with nintedanib alone, respectively. Concomitant use of nintedanib and pirfenidone did not have an effect on the pharmacokinetics of pirfenidone. In this study, nausea and vomiting were reported more frequently with combination nintedanib and pirfenidone therapy compared with nintedanib alone; all adverse effects reported in the study were mild or moderate in severity.

Description

Pirfenidone, a synthetic pyridone, is an antifibrotic agent. Although the precise mechanism of action of pirfenidone in the treatment of idiopathic pulmonary fibrosis (IPF) has not been fully elucidated, it is thought to be related to the drug's antifibrotic, anti-inflammatory, and antioxidant properties.

Pirfenidone has been shown to inhibit the activation of transforming growth factor-β (TGF-β), a profibrotic, proinflammatory cytokine. In vitro, pirfenidone suppressed TGF-β-mediated proliferation of human lung fibroblasts and differentiation into myofibroblasts, a process that may lead to excessive collagen deposition and fibrosis in the lungs. Pirfenidone also inhibited the release of proinflammatory cytokines (e.g., IL-1β, IL-6, tumor necrosis factor [TNF]-α, platelet derived growth factor [PDGF]) in animal models and in vitro. In addition, pirfenidone demonstrated antioxidant activity in vitro through its ability to scavenge reactive oxygen species (ROS), including hydroxyl radicals and superoxide anions.

Following oral administration, peak plasma concentrations of pirfenidone are achieved at a median of 0.5 hours (range 0.5–4 hours). Administration with food decreases the systemic exposure of pirfenidone by 16%, delays median time to peak plasma concentrations by 2.5 hours, and reduces the incidence of adverse effects compared with administration in the fasting state. Pirfenidone is 58% bound to plasma proteins (mainly albumin) at therapeutic concentrations. Pirfenidone is metabolized principally (70–80%) by cytochrome P-450 (CYP) isoenzyme 1A2; CYP2C9, 2C19, 2D6, and 2E1 also play a role in the drug's overall metabolism. Approximately 80% of a dose is excreted in urine within 24 hours, mainly as its major metabolite, 5-carboxy-pirfenidone, which is expected to be pharmacologically inactive. The mean terminal half-life of pirfenidone in healthy individuals is approximately 3 hours. Data from a population pharmacokinetic analysis indicate that age, gender, body mass index (BMI), and race do not have clinically important effects on the pharmacokinetics of pirfenidone.

Advice to Patients

Importance of reading the manufacturer's patient information prior to beginning pirfenidone therapy and each time the prescription is refilled.

Importance of taking pirfenidone with food to reduce the incidence of adverse effects (e.g., nausea and dizziness).

Importance of advising patients that if a dose of pirfenidone is missed, the dose should be taken as soon as it is remembered; 2 doses should not be taken at the same time to make up for a missed dose. No more than 3 doses should be taken per day.

Risk of hepatotoxicity and importance of periodic liver function test monitoring. Importance of immediately reporting any manifestations of hepatotoxicity (e.g., jaundice, unusually dark or "tea-colored" urine, right upper quadrant pain, bleeding or bruising more easily than normal, lethargy).

Risk of photosensitivity manifested as rash or other reactions. Importance of using sunscreen and protective clothing; limit exposure to sunlight, including sunlamps, during therapy. Importance of immediately reporting any symptoms of photosensitivity reaction or rash to a clinician.

Risk of adverse GI effects (e.g., nausea, diarrhea, dyspepsia, vomiting, gastroesophageal reflux disease [GERD], abdominal pain). Importance of contacting clinician if persistent adverse GI effects occur.

Importance of advising cigarette smokers to avoid smoking during pirfenidone therapy because plasma concentrations of the drug and efficacy may be reduced.

Importance of informing clinicians of existing or contemplated concomitant therapy, including prescription and OTC drugs and dietary or herbal supplements as well as any concomitant illnesses (e.g., hepatic impairment).

Importance of women informing clinicians if they are or plan to become pregnant or plan to breast-feed.

Importance of informing patients of other important precautionary information. (See Cautions.)

Overview® (see Users Guide). For additional information on this drug until a more detailed monograph is developed and published, the manufacturer's labeling should be consulted. It is *essential* that the manufacturer's labeling be consulted for more detailed information on usual cautions, precautions, contraindications, potential drug interactions, laboratory test interferences, and acute toxicity.

Preparations

Excipients in commercially available drug preparations may have clinically important effects in some individuals; consult specific product labeling for details.

Pirfenidone

Oral		
Capsules	267 mg	**Esbriet®**, InterMune

ANTITUSSIVES 48:08

Codeine Phosphate
Codeine Sulfate

■ Codeine is a phenanthrene-derivative opiate agonist antitussive agent.

Uses

■ **Cough** Codeine is used, alone or in combination with other antitussives or expectorants, in the symptomatic relief of nonproductive cough. Since the cough reflex may be a useful physiologic mechanism which clears the respiratory passages of foreign material and excess secretions and may aid in preventing or reversing atelectasis, cough suppressants should not be used indiscriminately.

Antitussives containing codeine should *not* be used in patients younger than 18 years of age. (See Cautions: Pediatric Precautions.)

■ **Pain** For use of codeine as an analgesic, see 28:08.08.

Dosage and Administration

■ **Administration** Codeine sulfate and codeine phosphate are administered orally as antitussives.

■ **Dosage** ***Cough*** Codeine preparations should be given in the smallest effective dose and as infrequently as possible to minimize the development of tolerance and physical dependence. Reduced dosage is indicated in poor-risk patients and in very old patients.

The usual oral antitussive dosage of codeine phosphate or codeine sulfate conventional (immediate-release) preparations in adults is 10–20 mg every 4–6 hours, not to exceed 120 mg daily.

Cautions

■ **Adverse Effects** Adverse reactions occur infrequently with usual oral antitussive doses of codeine. Nausea, vomiting, constipation with repeated doses, dizziness, sedation, palpitation, pruritus, and, rarely, excessive perspiration and agitation have been reported. Although equianalgesic doses of codeine and morphine produce similar degrees of respiratory depression, respiratory depression seldom occurs with oral antitussive doses of codeine.

■ **Precautions and Contraindications** Codeine is *contraindicated* in children younger than 12 years of age for the management of cough and cold. In addition, FDA states that use of antitussives containing codeine is *not* recommended in pediatric patients younger than 18 years of age. (See Cautions: Pediatric Precautions.)

Individuals who are ultrarapid metabolizers of cytochrome P-450 (CYP) 2D6 substrates are likely to have higher than expected serum concentrations of morphine, the active metabolite of codeine; therefore, FDA states that codeine should *not* be used in such patients. (See Pharmacokinetics: Pharmacogenomics.)

Because concomitant use of opiate agonists and benzodiazepines or other CNS depressants may result in profound sedation, respiratory depression, coma, and death, opiate antitussives should be *avoided* in patients receiving CNS depressants. (See Drug Interactions.) Patients receiving codeine and/or their caregivers should be apprised of the risks associated with concomitant therapeutic or illicit use of benzodiazepines, alcohol, or other CNS depressants.

When preparations containing codeine in fixed combination with other drugs are used, the cautions, precautions, and contraindications applicable to each ingredient must be considered.

In patients with asthma or pulmonary emphysema, the indiscriminate use of antitussives may precipitate respiratory insufficiency resulting from increased viscosity of bronchial secretions and suppression of the cough reflex.

Tolerance and physical dependence may occur following prolonged administration of codeine. Patients should be warned that codeine may impair their ability to perform activities requiring mental alertness or physical coordination (e.g., operating machinery, driving a motor vehicle). Codeine should be used with caution in debilitated patients. The drug should also be used with caution in patients who have undergone thoracotomies or laparotomies, since suppression of the cough reflex may lead to retention of secretions postoperatively in these patients.

FDA states that use of codeine is *not* recommended in nursing women, especially those who have evidence of ultrarapid metabolism of CYP2D6 substrates. Serious adverse events (i.e., excessive sedation, difficulty nursing, respiratory depression), including death, have been reported in nursing infants exposed to codeine. One case of opiate toxicity resulting in neonatal death has been reported in the nursing infant of a woman receiving codeine; genetic testing of the woman indicated that she was an ultrarapid metabolizer of codeine. (See Pharmacokinetics: Pharmacogenomics.) Higher than expected concentrations of morphine were found in breast milk and in the blood of the infant. Somnolence also has been reported more frequently in nursing infants whose mothers received codeine in combination with acetaminophen compared with those whose mothers received acetaminophen alone; evidence of ultrarapid metabolism of CYP2D6 substrates was identified in some of these women. Concentrations of morphine in breast milk are low and dose dependent in women who are normal metabolizers of codeine. Although not routinely used in clinical practice, FDA-approved tests (e.g., AmpliChip® CYP450 Test) are available to identify an individual's CYP2D6 genotype. However, testing alone may not adequately predict the risk of adverse reactions. Infants exposed to codeine through breast milk should be monitored closely for clinical manifestations of opiate toxicity (e.g., sedation, difficulty breast-feeding or breathing, hypotonia). If such manifestations occur, caregivers should seek immediate medical treatment for the infant.

Codeine is contraindicated in patients with known hypersensitivity to the drug.

For additional information on the usual precautions of opiate agonist therapy, see Cautions in the Opiate Agonists General Statement 28:08.08.

■ **Pediatric Precautions** Pediatric patients receiving codeine for the management of cough and cold, especially those who are obese, have obstructive sleep apnea or severe lung disease, or have evidence of ultrarapid metabolism of CYP2D6 substrates, are at increased risk of respiratory depression. Between January 1969 and May 2015, the FDA Adverse Event Reporting System (AERS) received 64 reports of respiratory depression, including 24 reports of death, worldwide that were associated with codeine use in pediatric patients younger than 18 years of age; in all 10 of the reports that provided information about CYP2D6 metabolizer status, the patients were ultrarapid or extensive metabolizers of CYP2D6 substrates. (See Pharmacokinetics: Pharmacogenomics.) Most of the cases of respiratory depression, including most of the deaths, occurred in children younger than 12 years of age. Respiratory depression may occur despite serum concentrations of codeine or morphine being within the therapeutic range; one patient who had concentrations within the therapeutic range died following use of codeine for management of pain after tonsillectomy and adenoidectomy. In addition, a review initiated by the European Medicines Agency (EMA) in 2014 identified 14 cases of morphine toxicity, including 4 deaths, in children 17 days to 6 years of age receiving codeine for relief of symptoms of upper respiratory tract infection (e.g., cough).

Because the risks of respiratory depression, misuse, abuse, addiction, overdosage, and death outweigh the potential benefit in pediatric patients, FDA states that antitussive agents containing opiates, including codeine, should *not* be used in pediatric patients younger than 18 years of age. In addition, use of codeine for the management of cough is *contraindicated* in children younger than 12 years of age. FDA is requiring inclusion of this warning against antitussive use of codeine in pediatric patients younger than 18 years of age and this contraindication to antitussive use of codeine in children younger than 12 years of age in the labeling of codeine-containing cough and cold preparations available by prescription; FDA also is considering additional regulatory action for fixed-combination codeine-containing cough and cold preparations available without a prescription in some states. FDA and EMA consider that cough and cold generally are self-limiting conditions and that evidence of codeine's efficacy in the management of these conditions in children is limited.

Serious adverse events, including deaths, also have been reported in children receiving codeine for management of pain. For additional information on precautions and contraindications associated with the use of codeine as an analgesic in pediatric patients, see Cautions: Pediatric Precautions in Codeine 28:08.08.

Drug Interactions

Concomitant use of opiate agonists and benzodiazepines or other CNS depressants (e.g., anxiolytics, sedatives, hypnotics, tranquilizers, muscle relaxants, general anesthetics, antipsychotics, other opiate agonists, alcohol) may result in profound sedation, respiratory depression, coma, and death. Opiate agonist antitussives should be avoided in patients taking benzodiazepines, other CNS depressants, or alcohol. Concomitant use of opiate agonists with serotonergic drugs can cause serotonin syndrome. (See Drug Interactions in the Opiate Agonists General Statement 28:08.08.)

Acute Toxicity

Toxic doses of codeine may produce exhilaration, excitement, seizures, delirium, hypotension, miosis, slow pulse, tachycardia, narcosis, flushed facies, tinnitus, lassitude, muscular weakness, and circulatory collapse or respiratory paralysis. Codeine should be discontinued if any of the aforementioned effects occur. Respiratory arrest, coma, and death have occurred in young children receiving oral codeine doses of 5–12 mg/kg. Severe respiratory depression resulting from acute toxicity may be reversed by administration of an opiate antagonist (i.e., naloxone hydrochloride).

Pharmacology

Codeine causes suppression of the cough reflex by a direct effect on the cough center in the medulla of the brain and appears to exert a drying effect on respiratory tract mucosa and to increase viscosity of bronchial secretions. On a weight basis, antitussive activity of codeine is less than that of morphine. Codeine also has mild analgesic and sedative effects.

Pharmacokinetics

Codeine is well absorbed from the GI tract. Following oral administration, peak antitussive effects usually occur within 1–2 hours and antitussive activity may persist for 4 hours. Codeine is distributed into milk.

Like other phenanthrene derivatives, codeine is metabolized in the liver. The drug undergoes *O*-demethylation (by cytochrome P-450 [CYP] isoenzyme 2D6), *N*-demethylation (by CYP3A4), and partial conjugation with glucuronic acid and is excreted in the urine as norcodeine and morphine in the free and conjugated forms. Negligible amounts of codeine and its metabolites are found in the feces.

Codeine is metabolized by the CYP microsomal enzyme system, principally by CYP3A4, and to a lesser extent by CYP2D6 (debrisoquine hydroxylase). Although the CYP2D6 isoenzyme accounts for only 10% of the metabolism of codeine, it plays an essential role in converting the drug to its active *O*-demethylated metabolite, morphine.

Pharmacogenomics: Metabolism of certain drugs, including codeine, is influenced by CYP2D6 polymorphism. Individuals who lack functional alleles of the CYP2D6 gene are described as poor metabolizers, those with one or two functional alleles are described as extensive metabolizers, and those who carry a duplicate or amplified gene are described as ultrarapid metabolizers. Genetically determined differences in drug metabolism can affect an individual's response to a drug or risk of having an adverse event. Individuals who are poor metabolizers experience no analgesic effects of codeine; individuals who are ultrarapid metabolizers are likely to have higher than expected serum concentrations of morphine.

Variations in CYP2D6 polymorphism occur at different frequencies among subpopulations of different ethnic or racial origin. Approximately 1–7% of Caucasians and 10–30% of Ethiopians and Saudi Arabians carry the genotype associated with ultra-rapid metabolism of CYP2D6 substrates.

Chemistry and Stability

■ **Chemistry** Codeine is a phenanthrene-derivative opiate agonist antitussive agent. Codeine occurs as colorless or white crystals or as a white, crystalline powder and is slightly soluble in water and freely soluble in alcohol. The phosphate and sulfate salts of codeine occur as white, needle-shaped crystals or white, crystalline powders. Codeine phosphate is freely soluble in water and slightly soluble in alcohol. Codeine sulfate is soluble in water and very slightly soluble in alcohol. Because of its greater water solubility, codeine phosphate is most frequently used for extemporaneous compounding.

■ **Stability** Codeine sulfate tablets should be stored in well-closed, light-resistant containers at a temperature less than 40°C, preferably between 15–30°C.

For further information on chemistry and stability, pharmacokinetics, uses, cautions, and dosage and administration of codeine, see 28:08.08. See also the Opiate Agonists General Statement 28:08.08.

Preparations

Codeine preparations are subject to control under the Federal Controlled Substances Act of 1970.

Excipients in commercially available drug preparations may have clinically important effects in some individuals; consult specific product labeling for details.

Codeine Phosphate

Crystals		
Powder		

Guaifenesin and Codeine Phosphate

Oral		
Solution	100 mg/5 mL Guaifenesin and Codeine Phosphate 6.3 mg/5 mL	**RelCof-C®** (C-V), Burel
		M-Clear® WC (C-V), R.A. McNeil
	100 mg/5 mL Guaifenesin and Codeine Phosphate 10 mg/5 mL*	**Cheratussin® AC** (C-V), Qualitest
		Guaiatussin® AC (C-V), Hi-Tech
		Guaifenesin AC Cough Syrup (C-V)
		Guaifenesin and Codeine Phosphate Oral Solution (C-V)
		Robafen® AC (C-V), Major
	200 mg/5 mL Guaifenesin and Codeine Phosphate 8 mg/5 mL	**Codar® GF** (C-V), Respa
	200 mg/5 mL Guaifenesin and Codeine Phosphate 10 mg/5 mL	**Coditussin® AC** (C-V), Glendale
	225 mg/5 mL Guaifenesin and Codeine Phosphate 7.5 mg/5 mL	**Mar-Cof® CG** (C-V), Marnel

Codeine phosphate is also commercially available in combination with other antihistamines, decongestants, and expectorants.

*available from one or more manufacturer, distributor, and/or repackager by generic (nonproprietary) name

Codeine Sulfate

Powder		
Oral		
Solution	30 mg/5 mL*	**Codeine Sulfate Oral Solution** (C-II)
Tablets	15 mg*	**Codeine Sulfate Tablets** (C-II)
	30 mg*	**Codeine Sulfate Tablets** (C-II)
	60 mg*	**Codeine Sulfate Tablets** (C-II)

*available from one or more manufacturer, distributor, and/or repackager by generic (nonproprietary) name

Dextromethorphan Dextromethorphan Hydrobromide

Dextromethorphan Hydrobromide, DM

■ Dextromethorphan, a derivative of levorphanol, is an antitussive agent.

Uses

Dextromethorphan is used for the temporary relief of coughs caused by minor throat and bronchial irritation such as may occur with common colds or with inhaled irritants. Dextromethorphan is most effective in the treatment of chronic, nonproductive cough. The drug is a common ingredient in commercial cough mixtures available without prescription.

Although cough and cold preparations that contain cough suppressants (including dextromethorphan), nasal decongestants, antihistamines, and/or expectorants commonly are used in pediatric patients younger than 2 years of age, systematic reviews of controlled trials have concluded that nonprescription (over-the-counter, OTC) cough and cold preparations are *not* more effective than placebo in reducing acute cough and other symptoms of upper respiratory tract infection in these patients. Furthermore, adverse events, including deaths, have been (and continue to be) reported in pediatric patients younger than 2 years of age receiving these preparations. (See Cautions: Pediatric Precautions and see Acute Toxicity: Manifestations.)

For information on abuse of dextromethorphan, see Cautions.

For use of dextromethorphan hydrobromide in fixed combination with quinidine sulfate in the treatment of pseudobulbar affect (PBA), see Dextromethorphan Hydrobromide and Quinidine Sulfate 28:92.

Dosage and Administration

■ **Administration** Dextromethorphan preparations are administered orally. Lozenges containing dextromethorphan hydrobromide should not be used in children younger than 6 years of age and liquid-filled capsules containing the drug should not be used in children younger than 12 years of age, unless otherwise directed by a clinician.

■ **Dosage** Dosages of dextromethorphan hydrobromide and dextromethorphan polistirex are expressed in terms of dextromethorphan hydrobromide.

The usual dosage of dextromethorphan hydrobromide for adults and children 12 years of age or older is 10–20 mg every 4 hours or 30 mg every 6–8 hours, not to exceed 120 mg daily, or as directed by a clinician. The usual dosage for children 6 to younger than 12 years of age is 5–10 mg every 4 hours or 15 mg every 6–8 hours, not to exceed 60 mg daily, or as directed by a clinician. Children 2 to younger than 6 years of age may receive 2.5–5 mg every 4 hours or 7.5 mg every 6–8 hours, not to exceed 30 mg daily, or as directed by a clinician. Dosage in children younger than 2 years of age must be individualized. Suggested dosages for children younger than 2 years of age† for some cough and cold preparations have been published in various references for prescribing and parenting. Using recommended dosages for adults and older children, some clinicians have extrapolated dosages for these preparations based on the weight or age of children younger than 2 years of age. However, these extrapolations were based on assumptions that pathology of the disease and pharmacology of the drugs are similar in adults and pediatric patients. There currently are *no* specific dosage recommendations (i.e., approved by the US Food and Drug Administration [FDA]) for cough and cold preparations for this patient population. (See Cautions: Pediatric Precautions.)

The usual dosage of dextromethorphan hydrobromide as the extended-release oral suspension containing the polistirex for adults and children 12 years of age or older is 60 mg twice daily. The usual dosage as the extended-release oral suspension for children 6 to younger than 12 years of age is 30 mg twice daily; children 2 to younger than 6 years of age may receive 15 mg twice daily.

Cautions

Adverse effects with dextromethorphan are rare, but nausea and/or other GI disturbances, slight drowsiness, and dizziness sometimes occur. The drug produces no analgesia or addiction and little or no CNS depression.

■ **Abuse** Abuse and recreational use of dextromethorphan have been reported with nonprescription (over-the-counter [OTC]) dextromethorphan-containing preparations and with dextromethorphan powder sold illicitly. Dextromethorphan is a safe and effective cough suppressant with minimal adverse effects when used at recommended dosages; however, the drug can have euphoric, stimulant, and dissociative effects at higher dosages. Abuse of the drug for its euphoric and dissociative effects occurs mainly in adolescents.

While dextromethorphan abuse is not a new phenomenon, a more recent trend involving illicit sale of pure dextromethorphan powder that has been encapsulated and sold as a street drug has caused concern. There also has been an increasing trend in abuse of dextromethorphan-containing OTC preparations. One study that analyzed the trend in dextromethorphan abuse in California identified Coricidin® HBP® Cough and Cold tablets as the most commonly abused OTC product. Abuse of dextromethorphan can result in serious adverse events, including death. (See Acute Toxicity.) Fatalities have been reported in adolescents that were possibly associated with consumption of powdered dextromethorphan sold illicitly in capsules.

■ **Precautions and Contraindications** Administration of dextromethorphan may be associated with histamine release, and the drug should be used with caution in atopic children. Dextromethorphan also should be used with caution in sedated or debilitated patients and in patients confined to the supine position. Dextromethorphan should not be taken for persistent or chronic cough (e.g., with smoking, emphysema, asthma) or when coughing is accompanied by excessive secretions, unless directed by a clinician. If cough persists for longer than 1 week, tends to recur, or is accompanied by high fever, rash, or persistent headache, a clinician should be consulted.

Individuals with phenylketonuria (i.e., homozygous deficiency of phenylalanine hydroxylase) and other individuals who must restrict their intake of phenylalanine should be warned that some commercially available preparations of dextromethorphan contain aspartame (NutraSweet®), which is metabolized in the GI tract to phenylalanine following oral administration.

Because cases of apparent serotonin syndrome, including 2 fatalities, have been reported in patients receiving dextromethorphan and monoamine oxidase (MAO) inhibitors concomitantly, dextromethorphan preparations should not be used in patients receiving these drugs or for 2 weeks after discontinuing them. For detailed information on serotonin syndrome, including its management, see Drug Interactions: Drugs Associated with Serotonin Syndrome, in the Monoamine Oxidase Inhibitors General Statement 28:16.04.12.

■ **Pediatric Precautions** Despite the lack of efficacy in children younger than 2 years of age, dextromethorphan use in such children has continued, in some cases with other prescription and/or nonprescription (over-the-counter, OTC) cough and cold preparations containing other agents (e.g., antihistamines, expectorants, nasal decongestants). In a report published by the US Centers for Disease Control and Prevention (CDC), cough and cold preparations containing dextromethorphan, acetaminophen, carbinoxamine, doxylamine, and/or pseudoephedrine were determined by medical examiners or coroners to be the underlying cause of death in 3 infants 6 months of age or younger during 2005. The actual cause of death might have been overdosage of one drug, interaction of different drugs, an underlying medical condition, or a combination of drugs and underlying medical conditions. In addition, an estimated 1519 children younger than 2 years of age were treated in emergency departments in the US during 2004–2005 for adverse events, including overdoses, associated with cold and cough preparations. (See Acute Toxicity: Manifestations; also see Cautions: Pediatric Precautions in Pseudoephedrine Hydrochloride 12:12.12.)

The dosages at which cough and cold preparations can cause illness or death in pediatric patients younger than 2 years of age are not known, and there are no specific dosage recommendations (i.e., approved by the US Food and Drug Administration [FDA]) for patients in this age group. (See Dosage and Administration: Dosage.) Because of the absence of dosage recommendations, limited published evidence of effectiveness, and risks for toxicity (including fatal overdosage), FDA stated that nonprescription cough and cold preparations should not be used in children younger than 2 years of age; the agency continues to assess safety and efficacy of these preparations in older children. Meanwhile, because children 2–3 years of age also are at increased risk of overdosage and toxicity, some manufacturers of oral nonprescription cough and cold preparations agreed to voluntarily revise the product labeling to state that such preparations should not be used in children younger than 4 years of age. FDA recommends that parents and caregivers adhere to the dosage instructions and warnings on the product labeling that accompanies the preparation if administering to children and consult with their clinician about any concerns. Clinicians should ask caregivers about use of nonprescription cough and cold preparations to avoid overdosage.

Acute Toxicity

■ **Pathogenesis** Dextromethorphan has a low order of toxicity, with the potential for toxic effects following acute overdosage being low. Although a few cases of toxicity and death have been reported, doses in excess of 100 times the usual adult dose have not been fatal.

■ **Manifestations** Manifestations following acute overdosage of dextromethorphan have included nausea, vomiting, drowsiness, dizziness, blurred vision, nystagmus, ataxia, shallow respiration, urinary retention, stupor, toxic psychosis, seizures, and coma. However, the presentation of dextromethorphan intoxication depends on the ingested dose. Manifestations of minimal intoxication include tachycardia, hypertension, vomiting, mydriasis, diaphoresis, nystagmus, euphoria, loss of motor coordination, and giggling/laughing. Manifestations of moderate intoxication include those associated with minimal intoxication, hallucinations, and a plodding ataxic gait ("zombie-like" walking). Severely intoxicated individuals may be agitated or somnolent.

From 1969–1981, the US Food and Drug Administration received 15 case reports of adverse reactions to dextromethorphan in children 1–10 years of age; these reactions included hallucinations, urticaria, nausea, insomnia, and hysteria, but no fatalities. Deaths that were possibly associated with consumption of powdered dextromethorphan (sold illicitly in capsules) have been reported in adolescents. Ataxia, facial edema, and urticaria occurred following acute ingestion of 225 mg of dextromethorphan in a 2-year-old child, and lateral nystagmus, ataxia, unstable gait, and excitability occurred in a 22-month-old child who ingested 360 mg of the drug. Lethargy, somnolence, ataxia, and nystagmus occurred in a 3-year-old who ingested 270 mg of the drug.

■ **Treatment** Treatment of dextromethorphan overdosage includes symptomatic and supportive measures. In one child, ataxia resolved rapidly following IV naloxone, and other neurologic manifestations resolved within 8 hours. In another child, manifestations of toxicity resolved following IV naloxone and oral administration of activated charcoal.

Pharmacology

Dextromethorphan retains only the antitussive activity of other morphinan derivatives. The drug is about equal to codeine in depressing the cough reflex and has no expectorant action. In therapeutic dosages, dextromethorphan does not inhibit ciliary activity.

Pharmacokinetics

Dextromethorphan is rapidly absorbed from the GI tract and exerts its antitussive effect in 15–30 minutes after oral administration. The duration of action is approximately 3–6 hours with conventional dosage forms.

Chemistry and Stability

■ **Chemistry** Dextromethorphan is an antitussive agent. Dextromethorphan is the methyl ether of the dextrorotatory form of levorphanol, an opiate analgesic. Dextromethorphan hydrobromide occurs as practically white crystals or crystalline powder and is sparingly soluble in water and freely soluble in alcohol.

■ **Stability** Dextromethorphan preparations should be stored in tight containers, and solutions and liquid-filled capsules containing dextromethorphan should be stored in tight, light-resistant containers.

Dextromethorphan is incompatible with penicillins, tetracyclines, salicylates, phenobarbital sodium, hydriodic acid, and high concentrations of sodium or potassium iodide.

Preparations

Excipients in commercially available drug preparations may have clinically important effects in some individuals; consult specific product labeling for details.

Dextromethorphan Hydrobromide

Oral		
Capsules, liquid-filled	15 mg	**Robitussin® Long-Acting CoughGels®**, Pfizer
Lozenges	5 mg	**Hold® DM**, Ascher
	10 mg	**Sucrets® DM Cough Formula**, Insight
Solution	7.5 mg/5 mL*	**Dextromethorphan Hydrobromide Solution**
	10 mg/5 mL*	**Dextromethorphan Hydrobromide Solution**
		Vicks® 44 Custom Care Dry Cough, Procter & Gamble
	15 mg/5 mL*	**Dextromethorphan Hydrobromide Solution**

*available from one or more manufacturer, distributor, and/or repackager by generic (nonproprietary) name

Dextromethorphan Hydrobromide Combinations

Oral		
Capsules, liquid-filled	10 mg with Acetaminophen 325 mg, Chlorpheniramine Maleate 2 mg, and Phenylephrine Hydrochloride 5 mg	**Alka-Seltzer Plus® Cold & Cough Formula Liquid Gels®**, Bayer
		Tylenol® Cold Multi-Symptom Nighttime Rapid Release Gels®, McNeil
	10 mg with Acetaminophen 325 mg, Doxylamine Succinate 6.25 mg, and Phenylephrine Hydrochloride 5 mg	**Alka-Seltzer Plus® Night Cold Formula Liquid Gels®**, Bayer
	10 mg with Acetaminophen 325 mg and Phenylephrine Hydrochloride 5 mg	**Alka-Seltzer® Plus Day Cold Formula Liquid Gels®**, Bayer
		Vicks® DayQuil® Cold & Flu Relief LiquiCaps®, Procter & Gamble
	15 mg with Acetaminophen 325 mg and Doxylamine Succinate 6.25 mg	**Vicks® NyQuil® Cold & Flu Relief LiquiCaps®**, Procter & Gamble
For solution	30 mg with Acetaminophen 1 g, Guaifenesin 400 mg, and Pseudoephedrine Hydrochloride 60 mg per packet	**Theraflu® Max-D Severe Cold & Flu**, Novartis
Kit	12 Tablets, film-coated, Acetaminophen 325 mg with Dextromethorphan Hydrobromide 10 mg and Phenylephrine Hydrochloride 5 mg (Comtrex® Daytime Caplets®)	**Comtrex® Cold & Cough Day-Night Maximum Strength Caplets®**, Novartis
	12 Tablets, film-coated, Acetaminophen 325 mg with Chlorpheniramine Maleate 2 mg, Dextromethorphan Hydrobromide 10 mg, and Phenylephrine Hydrochloride 5 mg (Comtrex® Nighttime Caplets®)	
Solution	3.3 mg/5 mL with Acetaminophen 108.3 mg/5 mL, Doxylamine Succinate 1.25 mg/5 mL, and Phenylephrine Hydrochloride 1.6 mg/5 mL	**Tylenol® Cold Multi-Symptom Nighttime**, McNeil
	3.3 mg/5 mL with Acetaminophen 108.3 mg/5 mL, Guaifenesin 66.6 mg/5 mL, and Phenylephrine Hydrochloride 1.6 mg/5 mL	**Tylenol® Cold Multi-Symptom Severe**, McNeil
		Tylenol® Cold & Flu Severe, McNeil
	3.3 mg/5 mL with Acetaminophen 108.3 mg/5 mL and Phenylephrine Hydrochloride 1.6 mg/5 mL	**Tylenol® Cold Multi-Symptom Daytime**, McNeil
		Vicks® DayQuil® Cold & Flu Relief, Procter & Gamble
	5 mg/5 mL with Acetaminophen 108.3 mg/5 mL and Doxylamine Succinate 2.08 mg/5 mL	**Vicks® NyQuil® Cold & Flu Relief**, Procter & Gamble

	5 mg/5 mL with Acetaminophen 160 mg/5 mL	**Children's Tylenol® Plus Cough & Sore Throat,** Prestige Brands
		Triaminic® Cough and Sore Throat, Novartis
	5 mg/5 mL with Acetaminophen 160 mg/5 mL and Chlorpheniramine Maleate 1 mg/5 mL	**Children's Tylenol® Plus Cough & Runny Nose,** McNeil
	5 mg/5 mL with Acetaminophen 160 mg/5 mL, Chlorpheniramine Maleate 1 mg/5 mL, and Phenylephrine Hydrochloride 2.5 mg/5 mL	**Children's Dimetapp® Multi-Symptom Cold & Flu,** Pfizer
		Children's Tylenol® Plus Flu, McNeil
	5 mg/5 mL with Acetaminophen 166.6 mg/5 mL	**Tylenol® Cold & Cough Daytime,** McNeil
	5 mg/5 mL with Acetaminophen 166.6 mg/5 mL and Doxylamine Succinate 2.08 mg/5 mL	**Tylenol® Cold & Cough Nighttime,** McNeil
	5 mg/5 mL with Brompheniramine Maleate 1 mg/5 mL and Phenylephrine Hydrochloride 2.5 mg/5 mL	**Children's Dimetapp® Cold & Cough,** Pfizer
	5 mg/5 mL with Chlorpheniramine Maleate 0.67 mg/5 mL	**Children's Vicks® NyQuil® Cold/Cough,** Procter & Gamble
	5 mg/5 mL with Chlorpheniramine Maleate 1 mg/5 mL and Pseudoephedrine Hydrochloride 15 mg/5 mL	**Kidkare® Cough & Cold Liquid,** Watson
	5 mg/5 mL with Doxylamine Succinate 2.08 mg/5 mL	**Vicks® NyQuil® Cough,** Procter & Gamble
	5 mg/5 mL with Guaifenesin 50 mg/5 mL and Phenylephrine Hydrochloride 2.5 mg/5 mL	**Robitussin® Children's Cough & Cold CF,** Pfizer
	5 mg/5 mL with Guaifenesin 100 mg/5 mL	**Pediacare® Cough & Congestion,** Prestige Brands
	5 mg/5 mL with Phenylephrine Hydrochloride 2.5 mg/5 mL	**Children's Sudafed PE® Cold & Cough,** McNeil
		Pediacare® Multi-Symptom Cold, Prestige Brands
		Triaminic® Daytime Cold & Cough, Novartis
	6.7 mg/5 mL with Guaifenesin 66.7 mg/5 mL	**Vicks® Formula 44® Custom Care Chesty Cough,** Procter & Gamble
	7.5 mg/5 mL with Acetaminophen 160 mg/5 mL and Chlorpheniramine Maleate 1 mg/5 mL	**Triaminic® Multi-Symptom Fever,** Novartis
	10 mg/5 mL with Acetaminophen 216.7 mg/5 mL and Chlorpheniramine Maleate 1.3 mg/5 mL	**Vicks® Formula 44® Custom Care Cough & Cold PM,** Procter & Gamble
	10 mg/5 mL with Guaifenesin 100 mg/5 mL*	**Cheracol D® Cough Formula,** Lee
		Dextromethorphan Hydrobromide with Guaifenesin Syrup
		Diabetic Tussin® DM, Health Care Products
		Guiatuss DM®, Goldline
		Robitussin® Peak Cold Cough + Chest Congestion DM, Pfizer
		Robitussin® Sugar-Free Cough + Chest Congestion DM, Pfizer
	10 mg/5 mL with Guaifenesin 100 mg/5 mL and Phenylephrine Hydrochloride 5 mg/5 mL*	**Robitussin® Peak Cold Multi-Symptom Cold®,** Pfizer
	10 mg/5 mL with Guaifenesin 200 mg/5 mL	**Diabetic Tussin® DM Maximum Strength,** Health Care Products
		Robitussin® Maximum Strength Cough + Chest Congestion, Pfizer
		Robitussin® Peak Cold Maximum Strength Cough + Chest Congestion, Pfizer
	15 mg/5 mL with Guaifenesin 100 mg/5 mL*	**Safe Tussin®,** Kramer
	15 mg/5 mL with Promethazine Hydrochloride 6.25 mg/5 mL*	**Promethazine Hydrochloride with Dextromethorphan Hydrobromide Cough Syrup**
	5 mg/mL with Guaifenesin 50 mg/mL and Phenylephrine Hydrochloride 2.5 mg/mL	**Suppress® DX Pediatric Drops,** Kramer Novis
Suspension	5 mg/5 mL with Acetaminophen 160 mg/5 mL	**Pediacare® Fever Reducer Plus Cough & Sore Throat,** Prestige Brands
	5 mg/5 mL with Acetaminophen 160 mg/5 mL and Chlorpheniramine Maleate 1 mg/5 mL	**Pediacare® Fever Reducer Plus Cough & Runny Nose,** Prestige Brands
	5 mg/5 mL with Acetaminophen 160 mg/5 mL, Chlorpheniramine Maleate 1 mg/5 mL, and Phenylephrine Hydrochloride 2.5 mg/5 mL	**Children's Tylenol® Plus Multi-Symptom Cold,** McNeil
		Pediacare® Fever Reducer Plus Multi-Symptom Cold, Prestige Brands
		Pediacare® Fever Reducer Plus Flu, Prestige Brands
	5 mg/5 mL with Acetaminophen 160 mg/5 mL and Phenylephrine Hydrochloride 2.5 mg/5 mL	**Pediacare® Fever Reducer Plus Cold & Cough,** Prestige Brands
Tablets	10 mg with Acetaminophen 325 mg, Guaifenesin 200 mg, and Phenylephrine Hydrochloride 5 mg	**Tylenol® Cold & Flu Severe,** McNeil
		Tylenol® Cold Head Congestion Severe, McNeil
	10 mg with Acetaminophen 325 mg and Phenylephrine Hydrochloride 5 mg	**Tylenol® Cold Multi-Symptom Daytime,** McNeil
	10 mg with Acetaminophen 325 mg and Phenylephrine Hydrochloride 15 mg	**Comtrex® Cold & Cough Multi-Symptom Relief Maximum Strength Tablets,** Novartis
	30 mg with Chlorpheniramine Maleate 4 mg	**Coricidin® HBP® Cough & Cold,** Schering-Plough
Tablets, chewable	10 mg with Chlorpheniramine Maleate 2 mg and Pseudoephedrine Hydrochloride 30 mg	**Dicel® DM,** Centrix
Tablets, extended-release	15 mg with Acetaminophen 500 mg and Chlorpheniramine Maleate 2 mg	**Coricidin® HBP® Flu Maximum Strength,** Schering-Plough
	30 mg with Guaifenesin 600 mg	**Mucinex® DM,** Reckitt Benckiser
	60 mg with Guaifenesin 1200 mg	**Maximum Strength Mucinex® DM,** Reckitt Benckiser
Tablets, film-coated	10 mg with Acetaminophen 325 mg, Chlorpheniramine Maleate 2 mg, and Phenylephrine Hydrochloride 5 mg	**Theraflu® Warming Relief Nighttime Multi-Symptom Cold,** Novartis
	10 mg with Acetaminophen 325 mg and Phenylephrine Hydrochloride 5 mg	**Comtrex® Non-Drowsy Maximum Strength Caplets®,** Novartis
		Theraflu® Warming Relief Daytime Multi-Symptom Cold, Novartis
		Tylenol® Cold Multi-Symptom Daytime, McNeil
	15 mg with Acetaminophen 325 mg, Guaifenesin 200 mg, and Phenylephrine Hydrochloride 5 mg	**Tylenol® Cold Head Congestion Severe,** McNeil

Dextromethorphan hydrobromide is also commercially available in combination with analgesic-antipyretics, antihistamines, and decongestants.

*available from one or more manufacturer, distributor, and/or repackager by generic (nonproprietary) name

Dextromethorphan Polistirex

Oral		
Suspension, extended-release	equivalent to Dextromethorphan Hydrobromide 30 mg/5 mL	**Delsym®,** Reckitt Benckiser

†Use is not currently included in the labeling approved by the US Food and Drug Administration

HYDROcodone Bitartrate

Dihydrocodeinone Bitartrate

■ Hydrocodone bitartrate is a phenanthrene-derivative opiate agonist antitussive and analgesic agent.

REMS

FDA approved a REMS for hydrocodone to ensure that the benefits outweigh the risks. The REMS may apply to one or more preparations of hydrocodone and consists of the following: medication guide and elements to assure safe use. See the FDA REMS page (http://www.accessdata.fda.gov/scripts/cder/rems/index.cfm) or the ASHP REMS Resource Center (http://www.ashp.org/REMS).

Uses

■ **Cough** Hydrocodone bitartrate and hydrocodone polistirex are used in combination with other antitussives or expectorants for the symptomatic relief of nonproductive cough. Since the cough reflex may be a useful physiologic mechanism that clears the respiratory passages of foreign material and excess secretions and may aid in preventing or reversing atelectasis, cough suppressants should not be used indiscriminately.

Antitussives containing hydrocodone should *not* be used in patients younger than 18 years of age. (See Cautions: Pediatric Precautions.)

■ **Pain** For use of hydrocodone as an analgesic agent, see 28:08.08.

Dosage and Administration

■ **Administration** Hydrocodone bitartrate and hydrocodone polistirex are administered orally.

When the extended-release oral suspension containing hydrocodone polistirex and chlorpheniramine polistirex (e.g., Tussionex® Pennkinetic®) is used, patients and caregivers should be strongly advised to use an accurate, calibrated dosing device to measure doses of the suspension. Use of a household teaspoon as a measuring device could result in overdosage. The extended-release oral suspension should not be diluted with other liquids or mixed with other drugs, since this may alter resin binding, thereby altering the rate of hydrocodone absorption and possibly resulting in toxicity. The extended-release oral suspension should not be given more frequently than every 12 hours; if cough is not controlled, the clinician should be contacted. The extended-release oral suspension should be shaken well before each use.

■ **Dosage** ***Cough*** Hydrocodone bitartrate and hydrocodone polistirex are currently commercially available only in combination products. Dosage of hydrocodone polistirex is expressed in terms of hydrocodone bitartrate.

Hydrocodone preparations should be given in the smallest effective dose and as infrequently as possible to minimize the development of tolerance and physical dependence. Reduced dosage is indicated in debilitated or poor-risk patients and in very old patients.

The recommended adult antitussive dosage of hydrocodone bitartrate conventional (immediate-release) preparations is 5 mg every 4–6 hours as needed, not to exceed 30 mg in a 24-hour period. However, recommended and maximum dosages of other drugs included in the combination preparations must be considered and may further limit the maximum hydrocodone bitartrate dosage given in a 24-hour period.

In adults, the usual antitussive dosage of hydrocodone bitartrate using the extended-release oral suspension containing hydrocodone polistirex and chlorpheniramine polistirex (e.g., Tussionex® Pennkinetic®) is 10 mg (5 mL) every 12 hours; the dosage should not exceed 20 mg (10 mL) daily.

Cautions

■ **Adverse Effects** Adverse reactions occur infrequently with usual oral antitussive doses of hydrocodone. The most common adverse effects of hydrocodone are lightheadedness, dizziness, sedation, nausea, and vomiting. These adverse effects appear to be more prominent in ambulatory patients than in nonambulatory patients, and some of these effects may be alleviated if the patient lies down. Other adverse effects include constipation, rash, pruritus, euphoria, and dysphoria.

■ **Precautions and Contraindications** Hydrocodone shares the toxic potentials of the opiate agonists, and the usual precautions of opiate agonist therapy should be observed. (See Cautions in the Opiate Agonists General Statement 28:08.08.)

Because concomitant use of opiate agonists and benzodiazepines or other CNS depressants may result in profound sedation, respiratory depression, coma, and death, opiate antitussives should be *avoided* in patients receiving CNS depressants. (See Drug Interactions.) Patients receiving hydrocodone should be apprised of the risks associated with concomitant therapeutic or illicit use of benzodiazepines, alcohol, or other CNS depressants.

In patients with asthma or pulmonary emphysema, indiscriminate use of antitussives may precipitate respiratory insufficiency resulting from increased viscosity of bronchial secretions and suppression of the cough reflex. Tolerance and physical dependence may occur following prolonged administration of hydrocodone preparations.

Patients should be warned that hydrocodone may impair their ability to perform activities requiring mental alertness or physical coordination (e.g., operating machinery, driving a motor vehicle).

As with other opiate agonist antitussives, hydrocodone may cause respiratory depression in large doses, when given more frequently than recommended, or in sensitive patients; this effect seldom occurs with usual oral doses. Overdosage and toxicity (including fatal respiratory depression) have been reported in adults and children receiving hydrocodone. (See Cautions: Pediatric Precautions.) Patients should be advised to immediately seek medical attention if they have trouble breathing, slow heartbeat, severe sleepiness, dizziness, confusion, or cold, clammy skin. Severe respiratory depression resulting from acute toxicity may be reversed by administration of an opiate antagonist (e.g., naloxone hydrochloride).

Hydrocodone should be used with caution in geriatric or debilitated patients and in those with hypothyroidism, Addison's disease, prostatic hypertrophy, urethral stricture, pulmonary disease, or severe renal or hepatic impairment. Hydrocodone also should be used with caution in patients with head injury, other intracranial lesions, or preexisting increased intracranial pressure, since opiate agonists may increase CSF pressure and markedly exaggerate these conditions; in addition, adverse CNS effects of the drug may obscure the clinical course of the underlying condition. The drug should also be used with caution in patients who have undergone thoracotomies or laparotomies, since suppression of the cough reflex may lead to retention of secretions postoperatively in these patients.

Hydrocodone may obscure the diagnosis or clinical course in patients with acute abdominal conditions.

Long-term use of hydrocodone may result in obstructive bowel disease, especially in patients with an underlying intestinal motility disorder.

Hydrocodone is contraindicated in patients who are hypersensitive to the drug or any ingredient in the formulation.

■ **Pediatric Precautions** Because the risks of respiratory depression, misuse, abuse, addiction, overdosage, and death outweigh the potential benefit in pediatric patients, FDA states that antitussive agents containing opiates, including hydrocodone, should *not* be used in pediatric patients younger than 18 years of age. In addition, use of hydrocodone for the management of cough and cold is *contraindicated* in children younger than 6 years of age.

■ **Geriatric Precautions** Clinical studies of hydrocodone polistirex and chlorpheniramine polistirex extended-release suspension did not include sufficient numbers of patients 65 years of age and older to determine whether they respond differently than younger adults. While other clinical experience generally has not revealed age-related differences in safety or response to the drug, care should be taken in dosage selection in geriatric patients. Because of the greater frequency of decreased hepatic, renal, and/or cardiac function and of concomitant disease and drug therapy in geriatric patients, the manufacturer suggests that patients in this age group receive initial dosages of this preparation in the lower end of the usual range.

Hydrocodone is substantially eliminated in urine and the risk of toxicity may be increased in patients with impaired renal function. Because geriatric patients are more likely to have decreased renal function, caution should be used when selecting dosages for such patients and monitoring of renal function should be considered.

■ **Pregnancy and Lactation** Safe use of hydrocodone during pregnancy has not been established; therefore, the drug should not be administered to pregnant women unless the possible benefits outweigh the potential risks.

It is not known whether hydrocodone is distributed into human milk. A decision should be made to discontinue nursing or the drug, taking into account the importance of the drug to the woman.

Drug Interactions

Concomitant use of opiate agonists and benzodiazepines or other CNS depressants (e.g., anxiolytics, sedatives, hypnotics, tranquilizers, muscle relaxants, general anesthetics, antipsychotics, other opiate agonists, alcohol) may result in profound sedation, respiratory depression, coma, and death. Opiate agonist antitussives should be avoided in patients taking benzodiazepines, other CNS depressants, or alcohol. Concurrent use of anticholinergic agents with hydrocodone may produce paralytic ileus. Concomitant use of opiate agonists with serotonergic drugs can cause serotonin syndrome. (See Drug Interactions in the Opiate Agonists General Statement 28:08.08.)

Pharmacology

Hydrocodone causes suppression of the cough reflex by a direct effect on the cough center in the medulla of the brain. The drug also appears to exert a drying effect on respiratory tract mucosa and to increase viscosity of bronchial secretions. On a weight basis, antitussive activity of hydrocodone is slightly greater than that of codeine. At equivalent therapeutic doses, hydrocodone is more sedating than codeine. The constipating effect of hydrocodone is less than that of morphine and not greater than that of codeine.

Pharmacokinetics

Hydrocodone is well absorbed from the GI tract. Following oral administration of a single 10-mg dose of hydrocodone to adult males in one study, a mean peak serum hydrocodone concentration of 23.6 ng/mL occurred after 1.3 hours. Following oral administration, antitussive action is maintained for 4–6 hours. Following multiple doses of the extended-release oral suspension containing hydrocodone polistirex and chlorpheniramine polistirex (Tussionex®

Pennkinetic®), a mean peak plasma hydrocodone concentration of 22.8 ng/mL occurred after 3.4 hours.

The elimination half-life of hydrocodone is reportedly about 3.8 hours in healthy adults. Like other phenanthrene derivatives, hydrocodone is probably metabolized in the liver and excreted mainly in urine. Metabolism of hydrocodone includes *O*-demethylation, *N*-demethylation, and 6-keto reduction.

Chemistry and Stability

■ **Chemistry** Hydrocodone bitartrate is a phenanthrene-derivative opiate agonist that is used as an antitussive and analgesic agent. Hydrocodone is a hydrogenated ketone derivative of codeine. Hydrocodone bitartrate occurs as fine, white crystals or crystalline powder and is soluble in water and slightly soluble in alcohol. Hydrocodone polistirex consists of hydrocodone with a cation-exchange resin copolymer complex of sulfonated styrene-divinylbenzene. Hydrocodone bitartrate and hydrocodone polistirex are currently commercially available only in combination products.

■ **Stability** Hydrocodone bitartrate is affected by light. Hydrocodone bitartrate preparations should be stored in tight, light-resistant containers at 15–30°C.

For further information on the chemistry, pharmacology, pharmacokinetics, uses, cautions, chronic toxicity, acute toxicity, and dosage and administration of hydrocodone bitartrate, see the Opiate Agonists General Statement 28:08.08 and Hydrocodone Bitartrate 28:08.08.

Preparations

Fixed-combination preparations containing hydrocodone in a concentration of 15 mg or less per dosage unit or 5 mL combined with a therapeutic amount of one or more nonopiate drugs or with a fourfold or greater quantity of isoquinolone opium alkaloid previously were subject to control under the Federal Controlled Substances Act of 1970 as schedule III (C-III) drugs. However, because of increasing concerns about misuse, abuse, and diversion, these preparations have been rescheduled and, effective October 6, 2014, are subject to control as schedule II (C-II) drugs. For additional information on the rescheduling of hydrocodone preparations, see Cautions: Misuse and Abuse, in Hydrocodone Bitartrate 28:08.08.

Excipients in commercially available drug preparations may have clinically important effects in some individuals; consult specific product labeling for details.

HYDROcodone Bitartrate Combinations

Oral		
Solution	5 mg/5 mL with Chlorpheniramine Maleate 4 mg/5 mL	**Vituz®** (C-II), Hawthorn
	5 mg/5 mL with Chlorpheniramine Maleate 4 mg/5 mL and Pseudoephedrine Hydrochloride 60 mg/5 mL*	**HYDROcodone Bitartrate, Chlorpheniramine Maleate, and Pseudoephedrine Hydrochloride Oral Solution** (C-II)
		Zutripro® (C-II), Hawthorn
	5 mg/5 mL with Homatropine Methylbromide 1.5 mg/5 mL*	**HYDROcodone Bitartrate and Homatropine Methylbromide Syrup** (C-II)
		Hydromet® Syrup (C-II), Actavis
	5 mg/5 mL with Pseudoephedrine Hydrochloride 60 mg/5 mL*	**HYDROcodone Bitartrate and Pseudoephedrine Hydrochloride Oral Solution** (C-II)
		Rezira® (C-II), Hawthorn
Tablets	5 mg with Homatropine Methylbromide 1.5 mg*	**HYDROcodone Bitartrate and Homatropine Methylbromide Tablets** (C-II)
		Tussigon® (C-II; scored), Pfizer

*available from one or more manufacturer, distributor, and/or repackager by generic (nonproprietary) name

HYDROcodone Polistirex Combinations

Oral		
Suspension, extended-release	equivalent to HYDROcodone Bitartrate 10 mg/5 mL with Chlorpheniramine Polistirex equivalent to Chlorpheniramine Maleate 8 mg/5 mL*	**HYDROcodone Polistirex and Chlorpheniramine Polistirex Extended-Release Suspension** (C-II)
		Tussionex® Pennkinetic® (C-II), UCB

*available from one or more manufacturer, distributor, and/or repackager by generic (nonproprietary) name

ANTI-INFLAMMATORY AGENTS 48:10

INTERLEUKIN ANTAGONISTS 48:10.20

Benralizumab

■ Benralizumab, a recombinant DNA-derived afucosylated humanized monoclonal antibody specific for the alpha chain of the interleukin-5 (IL-5) receptor (IL-5Rα), is an antiasthmatic agent. The drug is an IgG_1 kappa immunoglobulin.

Uses

■ **Asthma** Benralizumab is used as adjunctive maintenance therapy in patients with severe eosinophilic asthma (i.e., having an eosinophilic phenotype).

Benralizumab is *not* indicated for the treatment of other eosinophilic conditions or for the relief of acute bronchospasm or status asthmaticus.

The American Thoracic Society (ATS), European Respiratory Society (ERS), and the Global Initiative for Asthma (GINA) classify asthma as severe when it requires treatment with high-dose inhaled corticosteroids plus a second asthma controller therapy (e.g., long-acting β_2-agonist), and/or systemic corticosteroids to prevent asthma from becoming or remaining uncontrolled despite this therapy. Although there are no widely accepted definitions for specific asthma phenotypes, an eosinophilic phenotype (i.e., eosinophilic asthma) is generally characterized by blood and sputum eosinophilia and eosinophilic inflammation, recurrent exacerbations, and, frequently, responsiveness to corticosteroids. Sputum eosinophil counts are used as a reliable biomarker for eosinophilic lung inflammation; ATS and ERS currently recommend treatment of severe asthma guided by sputum eosinophil counts in addition to clinical criteria in adults, and treatment guided by clinical criteria alone in pediatric patients. However, sputum eosinophil counts are difficult to use in routine practice because testing must be performed in specialized centers experienced in using the technique. While some studies indicate that blood eosinophil count is not a reliable predictor of sputum eosinophil count in patients with asthma, other studies have shown that the values are moderately correlated and may potentially serve as a more accessible surrogate marker of eosinophilic lung inflammation.

In clinical studies, benralizumab was more effective than placebo in reducing the incidence of asthma exacerbations, decreasing oral corticosteroid dosage requirements, and improving forced expiratory volume in 1 second (FEV_1) from baseline. In a phase 2 double-blind, placebo-controlled, dose-ranging study, 609 adults stratified by eosinophilic status were randomized in a 1:1:1:1 ratio to receive benralizumab 2 mg, benralizumab 20 mg, benralizumab 100 mg, or placebo (eosinophilic population) or a 1:1 ratio to receive benralizumab 100 mg or placebo (non-eosinophilic population) subcutaneously every 4 weeks for 3 doses, followed by every 8 weeks thereafter for 52 weeks. Patients were receiving medium- to high-dose inhaled corticosteroids in combination with a long-acting β_2-agonist and had 2–6 asthma exacerbations requiring systemic corticosteroids in the previous 12 months, an Asthma Control Questionnaire (ACQ-6) score of 1.5 or higher at least twice during screening, and reduced morning lung function at screening (i.e., pre-bronchodilator FEV_1 of 40% to less than 90% of predicted). The primary end point was the annual asthma exacerbation rate. The annual asthma exacerbation rate increased by 12% in patients receiving benralizumab 2 mg and was reduced by 34 and 29% in patients receiving benralizumab 20 and 100 mg, respectively, compared with placebo.

Efficacy of benralizumab for the treatment of asthma was established in three phase 3 randomized, double-blind, placebo-controlled confirmatory studies. In the first and second studies, 2510 patients (mean age 49 years, 64% female, 79% white, mean baseline blood eosinophil count of 472 cells/mm^3) were randomized to receive benralizumab 30 mg every 4 weeks, benralizumab 30 mg every 4 weeks for 3 doses then every 8 weeks thereafter, or placebo for 48 weeks (study 1) or 56 weeks (study 2). Patients had at least 2 asthma exacerbations that required systemic corticosteroid therapy or a temporary increase in maintenance oral corticosteroid dosage in the previous 12 months, an ACQ-6 score of at least 1.5 at screening, and baseline reduced lung function (i.e., pre-bronchodilator FEV_1 of less than 80 or 90% in adults or adolescents, respectively) while receiving high- (Study 1) or medium- to high-dose (i.e., greater than 250 mcg of fluticasone propionate daily or equivalent) (Study 2) inhaled corticosteroids with a long-acting β_2-agonist with or without oral corticosteroids and another asthma controller drug. Benralizumab or placebo was administered as an adjunct to patients' existing asthma therapy. The primary end point was the frequency of asthma exacerbation (defined as a worsening of asthma that required treatment with systemic corticosteroids, a temporary increase in a stable dosage of systemic corticosteroids for at least 3 days, or a single long-acting [depot] corticosteroid injection and/or an emergency department visit that required systemic corticosteroids and/or hospitalization for urgent asthma treatment) among patients with baseline blood eosinophil counts of at least 300 cells/mm^3 over the treatment period. In both studies, benralizumab substantially decreased the rate of asthma exacerbation compared with placebo. In addition, benralizumab improved mean pre-bronchodilator FEV_1 and responder rate, as assessed by the ACQ-6 and the Standardized Asthma

Quality of Life Questionnaire for 12 Years and Older (AQLQ[S] +12), from baseline substantially more than placebo in both studies. Pre-specified subgroup analyses indicated that potential predictors of improved treatment response to benralizumab in terms of both asthma exacerbation rates and FEV_1 were prior exacerbation history (i.e., a history of 3 or more asthma exacerbations within the previous 12 months) and baseline blood eosinophil count (i.e., blood eosinophil count of at least 300 cells/mm^3).

The third study evaluated the effect of benralizumab on reducing the use of maintenance oral corticosteroids. In this study, 220 patients (mean age 51 years, 61% female, 93% white, mean baseline blood eosinophil count of 575 cells/mm^3) requiring daily oral corticosteroid therapy for at least 6 months in addition to regular use of high-dose inhaled corticosteroids and a long-acting β_2-agonist with or without additional controller therapy were randomized to receive benralizumab 30 mg every 4 weeks, benralizumab 30 mg every 4 weeks for 3 doses then every 8 weeks thereafter, or placebo for 28 weeks. Patients entered a corticosteroid reduction phase (weeks 4–24) during which the dosage of oral corticosteroid was reduced every 4 weeks according to a pre-specified schedule based on asthma control. The primary end point was the percent reduction of oral corticosteroid dosage during the maintenance phase (weeks 24–28) compared with baseline while maintaining asthma control. Patients receiving benralizumab achieved a substantially greater median percent reduction in daily maintenance oral corticosteroid dosage compared with those receiving placebo (75 versus 25%); a reduction in oral corticosteroid dosage of at least 50% was achieved in 66 or 37% of patients receiving benralizumab or placebo, respectively. Furthermore, a greater percentage of patients receiving benralizumab had a 90–100% reduction in oral corticosteroid dosage compared with placebo (35 versus 12%). In contrast, the percentage of patients having any increase or no change in oral corticosteroid dosage was 22% for those receiving benralizumab and 47% for those receiving placebo.

In a supportive phase 3 double-blind, placebo-controlled study, 211 adults (mean age 48–51 years, 61% female, 93% white, median baseline blood eosinophil count of 205–210 cells/mm^3) with mild to moderate, persistent asthma† were randomized to receive benralizumab 30 mg every 4 weeks for 3 doses or placebo for 12 weeks. The primary end point was the change from baseline in pre-bronchodilator FEV_1 at week 12. Patients receiving benralizumab achieved a greater improvement in mean pre-bronchodilator FEV_1 from baseline of 80 mL as compared with those receiving placebo.

Dosage and Administration

■ **General** Patients should be monitored for hypersensitivity reactions after administration of benralizumab. (See Hypersensitivity under Warnings/Precautions: Sensitivity Reactions, in Cautions.)

■ **Administration** Benralizumab is administered by subcutaneous injection by a clinician.

Subcutaneous injections should be made into the upper arm, thigh, or abdomen.

Benralizumab injection is commercially available in prefilled syringes. Benralizumab injection is a clear to opalescent, colorless to slightly yellow solution that may contain a few translucent or white to off-white particles. Prior to administration, benralizumab solution should be inspected visually for particulate matter or discoloration and should not be used if the solution is cloudy, discolored, or if large particles or foreign particulate matter are present. Benralizumab prefilled syringes are intended for single use only; the drug contains no preservatives. The entire amount of solution (1 mL) contained within the prefilled syringe, providing 30 mg of benralizumab, should be injected.

Prior to use, benralizumab injection should be stored at 2–8°C in the original carton, protected from light, and should not be frozen or shaken. Prior to administration, benralizumab prefilled syringes should be allowed to warm at room temperature for about 30 minutes and should be used within 24 hours. If not used within 24 hours when stored at room temperature, the prefilled syringe should be discarded.

■ **Dosage** For adjunctive maintenance therapy of severe eosinophilic asthma in adults and adolescents 12 years of age or older, the initial dosage of benralizumab is 30 mg every 4 weeks for 3 doses followed by 30 mg every 8 weeks.

■ **Special Populations** The manufacturer makes no specific dosage recommendations for geriatric patients or for patients with renal or hepatic impairment. (See Specific Populations under Cautions: Warnings/Precautions.)

Cautions

■ **Contraindications** Benralizumab is contraindicated in patients with a history of hypersensitivity to the drug or any ingredient in the formulation. (See Hypersensitivity under Warnings/Precautions: Sensitivity Reactions, in Cautions.)

■ **Warnings/Precautions** ***Sensitivity Reactions*** **Hypersensitivity.** Hypersensitivity reactions, including anaphylaxis, angioedema, urticaria, and rash, have been reported following administration of benralizumab. Such reactions generally occur within hours of administration of the drug, but may be delayed occurring days after administration in some cases.

Benralizumab should be administered by a clinician, and monitoring of patients for hypersensitivity reactions following administration of the drug is recommended. If a hypersensitivity reaction occurs, benralizumab should be discontinued. (See Cautions: Contraindications.)

Deterioration of Disease and Acute Episodes Benralizumab should *not* be used for the treatment of acute asthma symptoms or exacerbations, acute bronchospasm, or status asthmaticus. (See Advice to Patients.)

Reduction of Corticosteroid Dosage Systemic or inhaled corticosteroid therapy should *not* be discontinued abruptly upon initiation of benralizumab therapy. If appropriate, reduction in corticosteroid dosage should be performed gradually and directly supervised by a clinician. Reduction in corticosteroid dosage may be associated with systemic withdrawal symptoms and/or unmask conditions previously suppressed by corticosteroid therapy.

Parasitic Infection Because eosinophils may be involved in the immunologic response to some parasitic (specifically helminth) infections, benralizumab may potentially affect the response against such infections. The drug has not been studied in patients with known parasitic infections. Patients with preexisting parasitic (helminth) infections should be treated before initiating therapy with benralizumab. If a patient becomes infected while receiving treatment with benralizumab and does not respond to anthelmintic treatment, benralizumab therapy should be interrupted until the infection resolves.

Immunogenicity There is a potential for immunogenicity with benralizumab therapy. Development of anti-benralizumab antibodies was detected in 13% of patients receiving benralizumab in placebo-controlled clinical studies; development of neutralizing antibodies occurred in 12% of patients receiving the drug. Anti-benralizumab antibody titers of at least 400 resulted in an approximately 4.6-fold increase in drug clearance. While anti-benralizumab antibodies were associated with increased clearance of the drug and increased blood eosinophil concentrations, there was no observed effect on the efficacy or safety of the drug; however, the incidence and impact of anti-benralizumab antibodies on drug pharmacokinetics and pharmacodynamics require further evaluation.

Specific Populations **Pregnancy.** Monoclonal antibodies, such as benralizumab, are transported across the placenta during the third trimester, and potential effects on the fetus are more likely to occur during this time. However, there was no evidence of fetal harm in monkeys following IV administration of benralizumab on gestation day 20 or 22, gestation day 35, and every 14 days thereafter during gestation and for up to 1 month postpartum at dosages producing exposures up to approximately 310 times the exposure at the maximum recommended human dosage.

Lactation. It is not known whether benralizumab is distributed into human milk. The effects of benralizumab on nursing infants or on milk production also are unknown. Since IgG is distributed into milk in humans, it is expected that benralizumab will be present in human milk. The benefits of breast-feeding and the woman's clinical need for benralizumab should be considered along with any potential adverse effects on the breast-fed child from the drug or from the underlying maternal condition.

Pediatric Use. Safety and efficacy of benralizumab in pediatric patients younger than 12 years of age have not been established.

Phase 3 clinical studies included 62 adolescent patients 12–17 years of age with asthma who received benralizumab. The adverse effect profile in adolescents generally was similar to that seen in the overall population. Based on a population pharmacokinetic analysis, pharmacokinetics of benralizumab in adolescents were similar to those in adults; reduction in blood eosinophil concentrations also was similar.

Geriatric Use. In clinical trials of benralizumab, 13% of patients were 65 years of age or older and 0.4% were 75 years of age or older. Although no overall differences in safety or efficacy have been observed between geriatric patients and younger adults in controlled studies or in other clinical experience, the possibility of increased sensitivity to benralizumab in some geriatric patients cannot be ruled out.

Hepatic Impairment. Formal pharmacokinetic studies of benralizumab have not been conducted in patients with hepatic impairment. Population pharmacokinetic analyses indicate that baseline biomarkers of hepatic function (e.g., serum aminotransferases [ALT, AST] and bilirubin concentrations) did not have a clinically meaningful effect on the clearance of benralizumab.

Renal Impairment. Formal pharmacokinetic studies of benralizumab have not been conducted in patients with renal impairment. Population pharmacokinetic analyses indicate that benralizumab clearance is comparable in patients with a creatinine clearance between 30–80 mL/minute and those with normal renal function. Data are limited in those with a creatinine clearance less than 30 mL/minute.

■ **Common Adverse Effects** Adverse effects reported in at least 3% of patients receiving benralizumab and at an incidence equal to or higher than that reported with placebo include headache, pharyngitis, pyrexia, and hypersensitivity reactions.

Drug Interactions

Specific drug interaction studies have not been conducted to date with benralizumab.

■ **Drugs Metabolized by Hepatic Microsomal Enzymes** Benralizumab is not expected to affect cytochrome P-450 (CYP) isoenzymes; therefore, pharmacokinetic interactions are unlikely with drugs that are substrates of these isoenzymes.

■ **Drugs Affected by Efflux Transport Systems** Benralizumab is not expected to affect efflux transport systems; therefore, pharmacokinetic interactions are unlikely with drugs that are substrates of these transporters.

Description

Benralizumab, a recombinant DNA-derived afucosylated humanized monoclonal antibody specific for the alpha chain of the interleukin-5 (IL-5) receptor (IL-5Rα), is an antiasthmatic agent. The drug is an IgG_1 kappa immunoglobulin. Inflammation, an important factor in the pathogenesis of asthma, involves the activity of several endogenous inflammatory cells (e.g., eosinophils) and inflammatory mediators (e.g., cytokines). Although the precise mechanism of action of benralizumab in the treatment of asthma has not been fully elucidated, the drug has demonstrated binding with high affinity to the D1 domain of IL-5Rα expressed on the surface of eosinophils and basophils. IL-5 plays an important role in the growth, differentiation, recruitment, activation, and survival of eosinophils. Binding of benralizumab to IL-5Rα results in the inhibition of activation of IL-5R and subsequent signal transduction. Benralizumab induces direct, rapid, and nearly complete depletion of eosinophils and basophils in the circulation, bone marrow, and target tissues through antibody-dependent cell-mediated cytotoxicity (ADCC), an apoptotic process involving natural killer cells. The afucosylation of benralizumab is responsible for its 1000-fold enhancement of ADCC. In patients with asthma, subcutaneous administration of benralizumab resulted in dose-dependent decreases in blood eosinophil counts. Reductions in blood eosinophil counts have been observed 24 hours after an IV dose, with effects lasting at least 8–12 weeks. Treatment with benralizumab also was associated with reductions in blood basophil counts across all clinical studies; however, it is unknown if the effect of benralizumab on basophils in addition to eosinophils will provide additional clinical benefits.

Based on a population pharmacokinetic analysis, the estimated absolute bioavailability of benralizumab following subcutaneous administration is approximately 58%. Following subcutaneous injection, the drug is slowly absorbed with an absorption half-life of approximately 3.6 days. There were no clinically important differences in the relative bioavailability of the drug administered in the abdomen, thigh, or arm. The pharmacokinetics of benralizumab are approximately dose proportional when administered subcutaneously over a dosage range of 20–200 mg or IV over a dosage range of 0.03–3 mg/kg. Benralizumab is degraded by proteolytic enzymes that are widely distributed throughout the body and not restricted to hepatic tissue. In a population pharmacokinetic analysis, benralizumab exhibited linear pharmacokinetics, and there is no evidence that clearance of the drug occurs renally or through a target receptor-mediated pathway. The elimination half-life is approximately 15 days.

Advice to Patients

Risk of hypersensitivity reactions (e.g., anaphylaxis, angioedema, urticaria, rash). Instruct patients to immediately contact a clinician if they experience symptoms of an allergic reaction. (See Hypersensitivity under Warnings/Precautions: Sensitivity Reactions, in Cautions.)

Importance of informing patients that benralizumab does not relieve acute asthma symptoms or exacerbations. Patients should contact their clinician if asthma remains uncontrolled or worsens after initiation of treatment.

Importance of informing patients with asthma who are receiving inhaled or systemic corticosteroid therapy not to discontinue or reduce corticosteroid dosage, since corticosteroid withdrawal symptoms or worsening of asthma may occur; any change in corticosteroid dosage should be made under direct supervision of a clinician.

Importance of informing clinicians of existing or contemplated concomitant therapy, including prescription and OTC drugs, as well as any concomitant illnesses.

Importance of women informing clinicians if they are or plan to become pregnant or plan to breast-feed.

Importance of informing patients of other important precautionary information. (See Cautions.)

Overview® (see Users Guide). For additional information on this drug until a more detailed monograph is developed and published, the manufacturer's labeling should be consulted. It is *essential* that the manufacturer's labeling be consulted for more detailed information on usual cautions, precautions, contraindications, potential drug interactions, laboratory test interferences, and acute toxicity.

Preparations

Excipients in commercially available drug preparations may have clinically important effects in some individuals; consult specific product labeling for details.

Benralizumab

Parenteral

Injection, for subcutaneous use	30 mg/mL	**Fasenra®** (available as single-dose prefilled syringes), AstraZeneca

†Use is not currently included in the labeling approved by the US Food and Drug Administration

Mepolizumab

■ Mepolizumab, a recombinant DNA-derived humanized monoclonal antibody specific for interleukin-5 (IL-5), is an antiasthmatic agent. The drug is an IgG_1 kappa immunoglobulin.

Uses

■ **Asthma** Mepolizumab is used as adjunctive maintenance therapy in patients with severe eosinophilic asthma (i.e., having an eosinophilic phenotype).

Mepolizumab is *not* indicated for the treatment of other eosinophilic conditions or for the relief of acute bronchospasm or status asthmaticus.

The American Thoracic Society (ATS) and European Respiratory Society (ERS) classify asthma as severe when it requires treatment with high-dose inhaled corticosteroids plus a second asthma controller therapy (e.g., long-acting β-$_2$ agonist), and/or systemic corticosteroids to prevent asthma from becoming or remaining uncontrolled despite this therapy. Although there are no widely accepted definitions for specific asthma phenotypes, an eosinophilic phenotype (i.e., eosinophilic asthma) is generally characterized by blood and sputum eosinophilia and eosinophilic inflammation, recurrent exacerbations, and frequently, responsiveness to corticosteroids. Sputum eosinophil counts are used as a reliable biomarker for eosinophilic lung inflammation; ATS and ERS currently recommend treatment of severe asthma guided by sputum eosinophil counts in addition to clinical criteria in adults, and treatment guided by clinical criteria alone in pediatric patients. However, sputum eosinophil counts are difficult to use in routine practice because testing must be performed in specialized centers experienced in using the technique. While some studies indicate that blood eosinophil count is not a reliable predictor of sputum eosinophil count in patients with asthma, other studies have shown that the values are moderately correlated and may potentially serve as a more accessible surrogate marker of eosinophilic lung inflammation.

In clinical studies, mepolizumab was more effective than placebo in reducing the incidence of asthma exacerbations and substantially decreasing oral corticosteroid dosage requirements. Efficacy of mepolizumab for the treatment of asthma was established in 3 randomized, double-blind, placebo-controlled studies in patients with severe eosinophilic asthma. Patients were characterized as having severe eosinophilic asthma in the first study if they had, in the past 12 months, at least one of the following: a blood eosinophil count of at least 300/mm^3, sputum eosinophil count of 3% or more, exhaled nitric oxide concentration of at least 50 ppb, or deterioration of asthma control after a 25% or less reduction in regular maintenance use of inhaled or oral corticosteroid therapy. In the second and third studies, an eosinophilic phenotype was determined if patients had a blood eosinophil count of at least 150/mm^3 at screening or at least 300/mm^3 within the past 12 months. Mepolizumab or placebo was administered every 4 weeks as an adjunct to patients' existing asthma therapy.

Patients in the first and second studies had a history of 2 or more exacerbations in the previous year that required systemic corticosteroids despite regular use of high-dose inhaled corticosteroids (at least 880 mcg of fluticasone propionate daily or equivalent) and additional asthma controller therapy, with or without oral corticosteroids. The first study evaluated mepolizumab 75, 250, or 750 mg IV or placebo for 52 weeks; the second study evaluated mepolizumab 75 mg IV, 100 mg subcutaneously, or placebo for 32 weeks. The primary end point in these studies was the frequency of exacerbations (defined as a worsening of asthma that required treatment with systemic corticosteroids, an emergency department visit, or hospitalization). In both studies, all dosages of mepolizumab substantially decreased the rate of asthma exacerbations, including exacerbations requiring hospitalization and/or emergency department visits, compared with placebo.

The third study evaluated the effect of mepolizumab on reducing the use of maintenance oral corticosteroids. In this study, patients with severe eosinophilic asthma requiring daily oral corticosteroid therapy for at least 6 months in addition to regular use of high-dose inhaled corticosteroids and additional controller therapy were randomized to receive mepolizumab 100 mg subcutaneously or placebo for 24 weeks. Patients entered a corticosteroid reduction phase (weeks 4–20) during which the dosage of oral corticosteroid was reduced every 4 weeks according to a pre-specified schedule based on asthma control and symptoms of adrenal insufficiency. The primary end point was the percent reduction of oral corticosteroid dosage during the maintenance phase (weeks 20–24) compared with baseline while maintaining asthma control. Reductions in oral corticosteroid dosage were categorized as ranging from 90–100%, 75 to less than 90%, 50 to less than 75%, greater than 0 to less than 50%, and no improvement. Patients who had no reduction or an increase in oral corticosteroid dosage, loss of asthma control, or withdrawal from treatment were categorized as having no improvement. From baseline to the maintenance phase, substantially more patients receiving mepolizumab had a reduction in oral corticosteroid dosage required for asthma control compared with those receiving placebo; a 50% or greater reduction in oral corticosteroid dosage was achieved in 54 or 33% of patients receiving mepolizumab or placebo, respectively. Furthermore, a greater percentage of patients receiving mepolizumab had a 90–100% reduction in oral corticosteroid dosage compared with placebo (23 versus 11%). In contrast, the percentage of patients classified as having no improvement was 36 or 56% for the mepolizumab or placebo group, respectively.

Mepolizumab did not substantially improve lung function as measured by change in baseline forced expiratory volume in 1 second (FEV_1) compared with placebo in any of these studies.

Dosage and Administration

■ Administration Mepolizumab is administered by subcutaneous injection every 4 weeks by a clinician; the drug should *not* be administered IV.

Subcutaneous injections of mepolizumab should be made into the upper arm, thigh, or abdomen.

Reconstitution Mepolizumab lyophilized powder must be reconstituted prior to administration by a clinician. Mepolizumab lyophilized powder for injection is reconstituted by slowly adding 1.2 mL of sterile water for injection (preferably using a 2- or 3-mL syringe with a 21-gauge needle) to a vial labeled as containing 100 mg of mepolizumab to provide a solution containing 100 mg/mL; the stream of sterile water diluent should be directed onto the lyophilized powder. The vial should be gently swirled for 10 seconds at 15-second intervals until the powder is dissolved, typically within 5 minutes. The reconstituted solution should not be shaken. The manufacturer states that if a mechanical reconstitution device (swirler) is used, the vial may be swirled at 450 rpm for no longer than 10 minutes; alternatively, the vial may be swirled at 1000 rpm for no longer than 5 minutes. The reconstituted solution should be clear to opalescent, colorless to pale yellow or pale brown, and essentially free from particulates (small air bubbles are acceptable).

Reconstituted mepolizumab solution should be inspected visually for particulate matter and clarity; the drug should be discarded if the solution is cloudy or milky, or if particulate matter is present. Following reconstitution, the solution should be administered immediately or may be stored below 30°C for up to 8 hours; the solution should not be frozen. Prior to reconstitution, vials containing mepolizumab lyophilized powder should be stored below 25°C in the original package and protected from light; vials should not be frozen.

■ Dosage For adjunctive maintenance therapy of severe eosinophilic asthma in adults and adolescents 12 years of age and older, the recommended dosage of mepolizumab is 100 mg subcutaneously every 4 weeks.

The optimum duration of mepolizumab therapy has not been established. In an unblinded follow-up study in patients with severe eosinophilic asthma who completed 1 year of mepolizumab therapy, cessation of mepolizumab resulted in increased blood and sputum eosinophil counts within 3 months, blood eosinophil counts returning to baseline over 6 months, and a substantially increased rate of severe exacerbations over 3–6 months. After 12 months, the frequency of asthma exacerbations was no different between patients previously receiving mepolizumab or placebo.

■ Special Populations The manufacturer makes no specific dosage recommendations for geriatric patients or for patients with renal or hepatic impairment. (See Specific Populations under Cautions: Warnings/Precautions.)

Dosage adjustments are not needed based on gender or race.

Cautions

■ Contraindications Mepolizumab is contraindicated in patients with a history of hypersensitivity to the drug or any ingredient in the formulation.

■ Warnings/Precautions ***Sensitivity Reactions*** **Hypersensitivity.** Hypersensitivity reactions, including angioedema, bronchospasm, hypotension, urticaria, and rash have been reported in patients receiving mepolizumab. Such reactions generally occur within hours of administration, but may be delayed occurring days after administration in some cases. If hypersensitivity reaction occurs, mepolizumab should be discontinued. (See Cautions: Contraindications.)

Deterioration of Disease and Acute Episodes Mepolizumab should *not* be used for the treatment of acute asthma symptoms or exacerbations, acute bronchospasm, or status asthmaticus. (See Advice to Patients.)

Infectious Complications **Herpes Zoster Infection.** Herpes zoster infection, including some serious cases, have occurred in patients receiving mepolizumab. The manufacturer states that varicella (zoster) vaccination should be considered before starting mepolizumab if medically appropriate.

Parasitic Infection. Because eosinophils may be involved in the immunologic response to some parasitic (specifically helminth) infections, mepolizumab may potentially affect the response against such infections. The drug has not been studied in patients with known parasitic infections. Patients with preexisting parasitic (helminth) infections should be treated before initiating mepolizumab. If a patient becomes infected while receiving treatment with mepolizumab and does not respond to anthelmintic treatment, mepolizumab therapy should be interrupted until infection resolves.

Reduction of Corticosteroid Dosage Systemic or inhaled corticosteroid therapy should *not* be discontinued abruptly upon initiation of mepolizumab therapy. If appropriate, reduction in corticosteroid dosage should be performed gradually and under the direct supervision of a clinician. Reduction in corticosteroid dosage may be associated with systemic withdrawal symptoms and/or unmask conditions previously suppressed by corticosteroid therapy.

Immunogenicity Antibodies to mepolizumab were detected in 6% of patients receiving the drug in clinical studies; neutralizing antibodies were detected in one patient. Anti-mepolizumab antibodies were associated with an approximately 20% increased clearance of mepolizumab; however, there was no apparent correlation between anti-mepolizumab antibody titers and change in eosinophil counts. The clinical importance of such antibodies is not known.

Specific Populations **Pregnancy.** Monoclonal antibodies, such as mepolizumab are transported across the placenta in a linear fashion as pregnancy progresses with potential effects on the fetus being more likely during the second and third trimesters. However, there was no evidence of fetal harm in cynomolgus monkeys following IV administration of mepolizumab throughout pregnancy at dosages that produced exposures up to approximately 30 times the exposure at the maximum recommended human dosage.

To monitor pregnancy outcomes in women exposed to mepolizumab, the manufacturer maintains a pregnancy registry. Clinicians may enroll their patients or encourage their patients to enroll themselves in the registry by calling 877-311-8972 or visiting http://mothertobaby.org/asthma/.

Lactation. It is not known whether mepolizumab is distributed into human milk. However, the drug is distributed into the milk of cynomolgus monkeys. Since IgG is distributed into milk in humans, it is expected that mepolizumab will be present in human milk. The potential risks of infant exposure to mepolizumab should be weighed against the mother's clinical need for the drug as well as the known benefits of breast-feeding.

Pediatric Use. Safety and efficacy of mepolizumab in pediatric patients younger than 12 years of age have not been established.

Phase 3 clinical studies included 28 adolescent patients 12–17 years of age, 19 of whom received mepolizumab. The overall adverse effect profile in adolescents generally was similar to that seen in adults. In the 9 adolescents who received mepolizumab 100 mg subcutaneously, the mean apparent clearance of the drug was 35% less than that of adults.

Geriatric Use. Clinical studies of mepolizumab did not include sufficient numbers of patients 65 years of age or older to determine whether geriatric patients respond differently than younger adults. Other reported clinical experience has not identified differences in responses between geriatric and younger patients, but greater sensitivity in some older patients cannot be ruled out.

Hepatic Impairment. The pharmacokinetics of mepolizumab have not been formally studied in patients with hepatic impairment. However, hepatic impairment is unlikely to affect the elimination of the drug, because mepolizumab is degraded by widely distributed proteolytic enzymes that are not restricted to hepatic tissue.

Renal Impairment. The pharmacokinetics of mepolizumab have not been formally studied in patients with renal impairment. In a population pharmacokinetics analysis, clearance of mepolizumab was similar between patients with mild renal impairment (creatinine clearance 50–80 mL/minute) and those with normal renal function. Data in patients with moderate to severe renal impairment (creatinine clearance less than 50 mL/minute) are limited; however, mepolizumab is not eliminated renally.

■ Common Adverse Effects Adverse effects reported in at least 3% of patients receiving mepolizumab and at an incidence higher than that reported with placebo include headache, injection site reaction, back pain, fatigue, influenza, urinary tract infection, upper abdominal pain, pruritus, eczema, and muscle spasm.

Drug Interactions

Specific drug interaction studies have not been conducted to date with mepolizumab.

Description

Mepolizumab, a recombinant DNA-derived humanized monoclonal antibody specific for the cytokine interleukin-5 (IL-5), is an antiasthmatic agent. The drug is an IgG_1 kappa immunoglobulin. Inflammation is an important factor in the pathogenesis of asthma involving the activity of several endogenous inflammatory cells (e.g., eosinophils) and inflammatory mediators (e.g., cytokines). Although the precise mechanism of action of mepolizumab in the treatment of asthma has not been fully elucidated, the drug binds to IL-5, preventing its binding to the alpha chain of the IL-5 receptor complex expressed on the cell surface of eosinophils. IL-5 plays an important role in the growth, differentiation, recruitment, activation, and survival of eosinophils; blockade of IL-5 signaling reduces the production and survival of eosinophils and decreases eosinophil-mediated inflammation. In patients with asthma and blood eosinophil counts greater than 200/mm^3, subcutaneous and IV administration of mepolizumab resulted in dose-dependent decreases in blood eosinophil counts observable by day 3 in one study. In another study, multiple doses of mepolizumab 100 mg administered subcutaneously every 4 weeks resulted in a reduced mean eosinophil count of 40/mm^3 corresponding to an 84% mean geometric reduction in eosinophils compared with placebo. Such reductions were observed within 4 weeks and maintained throughout treatment.

Mepolizumab exhibits dose-proportional pharmacokinetics in patients with asthma over a subcutaneous dosage range of 12.5–250 mg. The absolute bioavailability of mepolizumab following subcutaneous injection is approximately 80%. Maximum plasma concentrations of the drug occurred from 4–8 days following subcutaneous administration in healthy individuals or patients with asthma. Following repeated subcutaneous administration of mepolizumab every 4 weeks, steady-state concentrations of mepolizumab were reached by approximately 16 weeks and twofold accumulation of the drug was observed at steady state. Mepolizumab is metabolized by proteolytic enzymes widely distributed throughout the body. The mean terminal half-life of mepolizumab is 16–22 days following subcutaneous administration.

Advice to Patients

Risk of hypersensitivity reactions. Importance of patients informing clinicians if hypersensitivity reactions (e.g., angioedema, bronchospasm, hypotension, urticaria, rash) occur. (See Sensitivity Reactions under Cautions: Warnings/Precautions.)

Importance of informing patients that mepolizumab does not relieve acute asthma symptoms or exacerbations. Patients should contact their clinician if asthma remains uncontrolled or worsens after initiation of treatment.

Possible increased risk of herpes zoster infections. Importance of patients informing clinicians if they do not have a history of varicella infection or vaccination.

Importance of informing patients with asthma who are receiving inhaled or systemic corticosteroid therapy not to discontinue or reduce corticosteroid dosage, since corticosteroid withdrawal symptoms or worsening of asthma may occur; any change in corticosteroid dosage should be made under direct supervision of a clinician.

Importance of informing clinicians of existing or contemplated concomitant therapy, including prescription and OTC drugs, as well as any concomitant illnesses.

Importance of women informing clinicians if they are or plan to become pregnant or plan to breast-feed. Importance of clinicians informing women about the manufacturer's pregnancy registry and encouraging patient enrollment. (See Pregnancy under Warnings/Precautions: Specific Populations, in Cautions.)

Importance of informing patients of other important precautionary information. (See Cautions.)

Overview® (see Users Guide). For additional information on this drug until a more detailed monograph is developed and published, the manufacturer's labeling should be consulted. It is *essential* that the manufacturer's labeling be consulted for more detailed information on usual cautions, precautions, contraindications, potential drug interactions, laboratory test interferences, and acute toxicity.

Preparations

Excipients in commercially available drug preparations may have clinically important effects in some individuals; consult specific product labeling for details.

Mepolizumab

Parenteral		
For injection, for subcutaneous use only	100 mg	Nucala®, GlaxoSmithKline

Reslizumab

■ Reslizumab, a recombinant DNA-derived humanized monoclonal antibody specific for interleukin-5 (IL-5), is an antiasthmatic agent. The drug is an IgG_4 kappa immunoglobulin.

Uses

■ **Asthma** Reslizumab is used as adjunctive maintenance therapy in adults with severe eosinophilic asthma (i.e., having an eosinophilic phenotype).

Reslizumab is *not* indicated for the treatment of other eosinophilic conditions, or for the relief of acute bronchospasm or status asthmaticus.

The American Thoracic Society (ATS) and European Respiratory Society (ERS) classify asthma as severe when it requires treatment with high-dose inhaled corticosteroids plus a second asthma controller therapy (e.g., long-acting β_2-agonist), and/or systemic corticosteroids to prevent asthma from becoming or remaining uncontrolled despite this therapy. Although there are no widely accepted definitions for specific asthma phenotypes, an eosinophilic phenotype (i.e., eosinophilic asthma) is generally characterized by blood and sputum eosinophilia and eosinophilic inflammation, recurrent exacerbations, and, frequently, responsiveness to corticosteroids. Sputum eosinophil counts are used as a reliable biomarker for eosinophilic lung inflammation; ATS and ERS currently recommend treatment of severe asthma guided by sputum eosinophil counts in addition to clinical criteria in adults, and treatment guided by clinical criteria alone in pediatric patients. However, sputum eosinophil counts are difficult to use in routine practice because testing must be performed in specialized centers experienced in using the technique. While some studies indicate that blood eosinophil count is not a reliable predictor of sputum eosinophil count in patients with asthma, other studies have shown that the values are moderately correlated and may potentially serve as a more accessible surrogate marker of eosinophilic lung inflammation.

In clinical studies, reslizumab was more effective than placebo in reducing the incidence of asthma exacerbations and improving forced expiratory volume in 1 second (FEV_1) from baseline. Efficacy of reslizumab for the treatment of asthma was established in 4 randomized, double-blind, placebo-controlled studies.

In the first and second studies, 953 patients (mean age 47 years, 63% female, 73% white, mean baseline blood eosinophil count 649–660 cells/mm³) were randomized in a 1:1 ratio to receive reslizumab 3 mg/kg IV or placebo once every 4 weeks for a total of 13 doses. Patients had a baseline blood eosinophil count of at least 400 cells/mm³, were receiving medium- to high-dose inhaled corticosteroids (at least 440 mcg of fluticasone propionate daily or equivalent) with or without another asthma controller drug (including oral corticosteroids at dosages up to 10 mg of prednisone daily or equivalent), and had at least 1 asthma exacerbation requiring systemic corticosteroids in the previous 12 months. The primary end point in these studies was the frequency of asthma exacerbations (defined as a worsening of asthma that required treatment with systemic corticosteroids, doubling of the inhaled or systemic corticosteroid dosage for at least 3 days, an emergency department visit, hospitalization, and/or unscheduled physician's office visit for urgent asthma treatment) over the 52-week treatment period. In both studies, reslizumab substantially decreased the rate of asthma exacerbations, including exacerbations requiring use of systemic corticosteroids and those requiring hospitalization and/or emergency department visits, compared with placebo. In addition, reslizumab increased FEV_1 from baseline substantially more than placebo in both studies.

In the third study, 315 patients (mean age 44 years, 58% female, 81% white, mean baseline blood eosinophil count 614 cells/mm³) were randomized in a 1:1:1 ratio to receive reslizumab 0.3 mg/kg IV, reslizumab 3 mg/kg IV, or placebo once every 4 weeks for a total of 4 doses. Patients had inadequately controlled asthma, were receiving a medium- to high-dose inhaled corticosteroid, and had a baseline blood eosinophil count of at least 400 cells/mm³. Although patients were not permitted to receive maintenance oral corticosteroids, other baseline asthma medications were continued during the study. The primary end point was the change in FEV_1 from baseline to 16 weeks. Both dosages of reslizumab resulted in substantially increased mean FEV_1 from baseline when compared with placebo. However, FEV_1 improvements were numerically greater in patients receiving reslizumab 3 mg/kg than in those receiving reslizumab 0.3 mg/kg (160 mL and 115 mL, respectively).

In the fourth study, 496 patients (mean age 45 years, 64% female, 67% white, mean baseline blood eosinophil count 280 cells/mm³, 80% with baseline blood eosinophil counts less than 400 cells/mm³) were randomized in a 4:1 ratio to receive reslizumab 3 mg/kg IV or placebo once every 4 weeks for a total of 4 doses. Patients had inadequately controlled asthma and were receiving a medium- to high-dose inhaled corticosteroid; patients were *not* selected based on blood eosinophil counts. Although patients were not permitted to receive maintenance oral corticosteroids, other baseline asthma medications were continued. The primary end point was the change in FEV_1 from baseline to 16 weeks. Reslizumab resulted in numerically increased mean FEV_1 from baseline when compared with placebo (255 mL and 187 mL, respectively). Study results failed to show an association between the treatment effect of reslizumab on FEV_1 and baseline eosinophil counts.

Dosage and Administration

■ **Administration** Reslizumab is administered by IV infusion. The drug must *not* be administered by rapid IV injection (e.g., IV push or bolus).

Reslizumab injection concentrate must be diluted prior to administration.

Diluted reslizumab solution should be administered in a healthcare setting by a clinician who is prepared to manage anaphylaxis. If the diluted solution is refrigerated, it should reach room temperature prior to administration. An infusion set with a compatible, low-protein-binding 0.2-μm inline filter should be used (e.g., polyethersulfone [PES], polyvinylidene fluoride [PVDF], nylon, cellulose acetate inline infusion filter).

Diluted reslizumab solution should be administered by IV infusion over 20–50 minutes; infusion time may vary depending on the total volume of the solution based upon the patient's weight. To ensure that the entire dose of reslizumab has been administered, the IV administration set should be flushed with 0.9% sodium chloride injection after IV infusion of the drug is complete. The patient should be observed during the infusion and for an appropriate period of time following the infusion.

Reslizumab infusion should be immediately discontinued if the patient experiences a severe systemic reaction, including anaphylaxis. (See Sensitivity Reactions under Cautions: Warnings/Precautions.)

Diluted reslizumab solution should *not* be administered in the same IV line with any other drug. To date, no physical or biochemical compatibility studies with other drugs have been conducted.

Unopened vials containing reslizumab injection concentrate should be stored at 2–8°C in the original package, protected from light, and should *not* be shaken or frozen.

Dilution Prior to dilution, reslizumab injection concentrate should be inspected visually for particulate matter and discoloration. Since reslizumab is a protein, translucent to white amorphous particles may be present in the solution. The solution should not be administered if it appears discolored or if other foreign particles are present.

Reslizumab injection concentrate in single-use vials should be removed from the refrigerator and should *not* be shaken to avoid foaming. The appropriate dose (3 mg/kg) of reslizumab injection concentrate should be withdrawn from the vial labeled as containing 10 mg/mL. Any unused portion of the injection concentrate should be discarded. Reslizumab injection concentrate should be added to 50 mL of 0.9% sodium chloride injection in a polyvinylchloride (PVC) or polyolefin infusion bag; the solution should be added slowly to minimize foaming. The diluted reslizumab solution for infusion should be mixed by gentle inversion and should *not* be shaken.

Diluted reslizumab solution should be administered immediately or may be stored at 2–8°C or at room temperature up to 25°C and protected from light for up to 16 hours. The time between dilution and administration should not exceed 16 hours.

Diluted reslizumab solution should not be mixed or diluted with any other drugs.

■ **Dosage** For adjunctive maintenance therapy of severe eosinophilic asthma in adults, the recommended dosage of reslizumab is 3 mg/kg IV every 4 weeks.

■ **Special Populations** The manufacturer makes no specific dosage recommendations for geriatric patients or for patients with renal or hepatic impairment. (See Specific Populations under Cautions: Warnings/Precautions.)

Cautions

■ **Contraindications** Reslizumab is contraindicated in patients with a history of hypersensitivity to the drug or any ingredient in the formulation.

■ **Warnings/Precautions** ***Sensitivity Reactions*** **Hypersensitivity.** Hypersensitivity reactions, including anaphylaxis, have been reported in patients receiving reslizumab. In clinical studies, anaphylaxis has been observed in 0.3% of patients receiving the drug. Manifestations included dyspnea, decreased oxygen saturation, wheezing, vomiting, and skin and mucosal involvement, including urticaria. Anaphylaxis was reported as early as the second dose of reslizumab and occurred during the infusion or within 20 minutes after completion of the infusion.

Anaphylaxis can be life-threatening. Reslizumab should be administered in a healthcare setting by a clinician prepared to manage anaphylaxis. Patients should be observed for an appropriate period of time after reslizumab administration. If severe systemic reactions (e.g., anaphylaxis) occur, the reslizumab infusion should be immediately stopped and medical treatment should be provided. If anaphylaxis occurs, reslizumab should be permanently discontinued. (See Advice to Patients.)

Deterioration of Disease and Acute Episodes Reslizumab should *not* be used for the treatment of acute asthma symptoms or exacerbations, acute bronchospasm, or status asthmaticus. (See Advice to Patients.)

Malignancy In clinical studies, 0.6% of patients receiving reslizumab had at least one malignant neoplasm reported compared with 0.3% of patients receiving placebo. The malignancies observed in those receiving reslizumab occurred in various tissue types. The majority of malignancies were diagnosed within less than 6 months of exposure to reslizumab.

Reduction of Corticosteroid Dosage Systemic or inhaled corticosteroid therapy should *not* be discontinued abruptly upon initiation of reslizumab therapy. If appropriate, reduction in corticosteroid dosage should be performed gradually and directly supervised by a clinician. Reduction in corticosteroid dosage may be associated with systemic withdrawal symptoms and/or unmask conditions previously suppressed by corticosteroid therapy.

Parasitic Infection Because eosinophils may be involved in the immunologic response to some parasitic (specifically helminth) infections, reslizumab may potentially affect the response against such infections. The drug has not been studied in patients with known parasitic infections. Patients with preexisting parasitic (helminth) infections should be treated before initiating therapy with reslizumab. If a patient becomes infected while receiving treatment with reslizumab and does not respond to anthelminthic treatment, reslizumab therapy should be interrupted until the infection resolves.

Immunogenicity There is a potential for immunogenicity with reslizumab therapy. Development of anti-reslizumab antibodies was detected in 5.4% of patients receiving reslizumab in placebo-controlled clinical studies. The presence of neutralizing antibodies to reslizumab was not evaluated. There was no observed effect of the anti-reslizumab antibodies on the clinical pharmacokinetics, pharmacodynamics, clinical efficacy, and safety of the drug.

Specific Populations **Pregnancy.** Monoclonal antibodies, such as reslizumab, are transported across the placenta in a linear fashion as pregnancy progresses with potential effects on the fetus being more likely during the second and third trimesters. However, there was no evidence of fetal harm in mice and rabbits following administration of reslizumab during organogenesis at dosages producing exposures up to 17 times the exposure at the maximum recommended human dosage.

Lactation. It is not known whether reslizumab is distributed into human milk. However, the drug is distributed into the milk of lactating mice. Since human IgG is distributed into milk in humans, reslizumab is expected to distribute into human milk. The potential risks of infant exposure to reslizumab should be weighed against the mother's clinical need for the drug as well as the known benefits of breast-feeding.

Pediatric Use. Safety and efficacy of reslizumab in pediatric patients younger than 18 years of age have not been established.

Geriatric Use. In clinical trials, no overall differences in efficacy or safety were observed in patients 65 years of age or older when compared with younger patients.

Hepatic Impairment. Formal pharmacokinetic studies of reslizumab have not been conducted in patients with hepatic impairment. Population pharmacokinetic analyses indicate that there are no substantial differences in reslizumab pharmacokinetics in patients with mild hepatic impairment (i.e., total bilirubin concentrations exceeding the upper limit of normal [ULN] but no more than 1.5 times the ULN or total bilirubin concentrations not exceeding the ULN with AST concentrations exceeding the ULN) compared with those having normal hepatic function.

Renal Impairment. Formal pharmacokinetic studies of reslizumab have not been conducted in patients with renal impairment. Population pharmacokinetic analyses indicate that there are no substantial differences in reslizumab pharmacokinetics in patients with mild (estimated glomerular filtration rate [GFR] of 60–89 mL/minute per 1.73 m^2) or moderate (estimated GFR of 30–59 mL/minute per 1.73 m^2) renal impairment compared with those having normal renal function.

■ **Common Adverse Effects** Adverse effects reported in at least 2% of patients receiving reslizumab and at an incidence higher than that reported with placebo include headache, upper respiratory tract infection, allergic rhinitis, back pain, sinusitis, urinary tract infection, dyspnea, dizziness, oropharyngeal pain, nausea, and vomiting.

Drug Interactions

Specific drug interaction studies have not been conducted to date with reslizumab.

■ **Drugs Metabolized by Hepatic Microsomal Enzymes** In vitro data indicate that reslizumab is unlikely to affect cytochrome P-450 (CYP) isoenzymes 1A2, 2B6, or 3A4.

■ **Corticosteroids** Population pharmacokinetic analyses indicate that concomitant use of reslizumab and corticosteroids does not affect reslizumab pharmacokinetics.

■ **Leukotriene-receptor Antagonists** Population pharmacokinetic analyses indicate that concomitant use of reslizumab and leukotriene-receptor antagonists does not affect reslizumab pharmacokinetics.

Description

Reslizumab, a recombinant DNA-derived humanized monoclonal antibody specific for the cytokine interleukin-5 (IL-5), is an antiasthmatic agent. The drug is an IgG_4 kappa immunoglobulin. Inflammation, an important factor in the pathogenesis of asthma, involves the activity of several endogenous inflammatory cells (e.g., eosinophils) and inflammatory mediators (e.g., cytokines). Although the precise mechanism of action of reslizumab in the treatment of asthma has not been fully elucidated, the drug binds to IL-5, preventing its binding to the alpha chain of the IL-5 receptor complex expressed on the cell surface of eosinophils. IL-5 plays an important role in the growth, differentiation, recruitment, activation, and survival of eosinophils; blockade of IL-5 signaling reduces the production and survival of eosinophils. In patients with asthma and blood eosinophil counts exceeding 400 cells/mm^3, IV administration of reslizumab 3 mg/kg resulted in decreased blood eosinophil counts observable after the first dose; these reductions were sustained for the duration of the 52-week study. Early eosinophil reduction was observed in a subset of patients with blood eosinophil counts assessed following 2–3 days of therapy.

Peak plasma concentrations of reslizumab typically occur at the end of the IV infusion. Following repeated IV administration of reslizumab, a 1.5- to 1.9-fold accumulation of the drug was observed. Reslizumab is metabolized by proteolytic enzymes into small peptides and amino acids. The half-life of reslizumab is approximately 24 days.

Advice to Patients

Risk of hypersensitivity reactions, including anaphylaxis. Advise patients of the signs and symptoms of hypersensitivity reactions and anaphylaxis (e.g., skin or mucosal involvement, airway compromise, reduced blood pressure). Instruct patients to immediately contact a clinician if they experience symptoms of an allergic reaction after receiving reslizumab infusion. (See Sensitivity Reactions under Cautions: Warnings/Precautions.)

Importance of informing patients that reslizumab does not relieve acute asthma symptoms or exacerbations. Patients should contact their clinician if asthma remains uncontrolled or worsens after initiation of treatment.

Advise patients of the possible increased risk of malignancy.

Importance of informing patients with asthma who are receiving inhaled or systemic corticosteroid therapy not to discontinue or reduce corticosteroid dosage, since corticosteroid withdrawal symptoms or worsening of asthma may occur; any change in corticosteroid dosage should be made under direct supervision of a clinician.

Importance of informing clinicians of existing or contemplated concomitant therapy, including prescription and OTC drugs, as well as any concomitant illnesses.

Importance of women informing clinicians if they are or plan to become pregnant or plan to breast-feed.

Importance of informing patients of other important precautionary information. (See Cautions.)

Overview® (see Users Guide). For additional information on this drug until a more detailed monograph is developed and published, the manufacturer's labeling should be consulted. It is *essential* that the manufacturer's labeling be consulted for more detailed information on usual cau-

tions, precautions, contraindications, potential drug interactions, laboratory test interferences, and acute toxicity.

Preparations

Excipients in commercially available drug preparations may have clinically important effects in some individuals; consult specific product labeling for details.

Reslizumab

Parenteral		
Concentrate for injection, for IV infusion only	10 mg/mL (100 mg)	**Cinqair**®, Teva

LEUKOTRIENE MODIFIERS 48:10.24

Montelukast Sodium

■ Montelukast sodium, a synthetic leukotriene-receptor antagonist, is an antiasthmatic agent.

Uses

Montelukast is used in the management of asthma and for the prevention of exercise-induced bronchospasm. Montelukast is also used for the symptomatic treatment of seasonal or perennial allergic rhinitis and has been evaluated for the management of urticaria†.

■ **Bronchospasm** ***Asthma*** Montelukast is used for the prevention and long-term symptomatic management of asthma.

Montelukast is not a bronchodilator and should *not* be used to relieve symptoms of acute asthma, including status asthmaticus; however, therapy with the drug can be continued during acute asthmatic attacks. All patients receiving montelukast should be provided with a short-acting, orally inhaled β_2-adrenergic agonist (e.g., albuterol) to use as supplemental therapy for acute symptoms that may occur despite montelukast therapy. Patients receiving montelukast should be cautioned not to decrease the dose of, or discontinue therapy with, other antiasthmatic agents unless instructed to do so by a clinician.

Mild Persistent Asthma. Drugs for asthma may be categorized as relievers (e.g., bronchodilators taken as needed for acute symptoms) or controllers (principally inhaled corticosteroids or other anti-inflammatory agents taken regularly to achieve long-term control of asthma). When control of symptoms deteriorates in patients with intermittent asthma and symptoms become persistent (e.g., daytime symptoms of asthma more than twice weekly but less than once daily, and nocturnal symptoms of asthma 3–4 times per month), current asthma management guidelines and most clinicians recommend initiation of an anti-inflammatory agent, preferably with a low-dose orally inhaled corticosteroid (e.g., 88–264, 88–176, or 176 mcg of fluticasone propionate [or its equivalent] daily via a metered-dose inhaler in adolescents and adults, children 5–11 years of age, or children 4 years of age or younger, respectively) as first-line therapy for persistent asthma, supplemented by as-needed use of a short-acting, inhaled β_2-agonist. Alternatives to low-dose inhaled corticosteroids for mild persistent asthma include certain leukotriene modifiers (i.e., montelukast, zafirlukast), extended-release theophylline (in adults and children 5 years of age or older), or mast-cell stabilizers (e.g., cromolyn, nedocromil [preparation for oral inhalation no longer commercially available in the US]), but these agents are less effective and generally not preferred as initial therapy. Limited evidence suggests that montelukast may be considered for maintenance therapy in young children with mild persistent asthma when inhaled corticosteroid delivery is suboptimal as a result of poor technique or adherence.

Moderate Persistent Asthma. According to current asthma medication guidelines, therapy with a long-acting inhaled β_2-agonist such as salmeterol or formoterol generally is recommended in adults and adolescents who have moderate persistent asthma and daily asthmatic symptoms that are inadequately controlled following addition of low-dose inhaled corticosteroids to as-needed inhaled β_2-agonist treatment. However, the National Asthma Education and Prevention Program recommends that the beneficial effects of long-acting inhaled β_2-agonists should be weighed carefully against the increased risk (although uncommon) of severe asthma exacerbations and asthma-related deaths associated with daily use of such agents. (See Asthma-related Death and Life-threatening Events under Cautions: Respiratory Effects, in Salmeterol 12:12.08.12.)

Current asthma management guidelines also state that an alternative, but equally preferred option for management of moderate persistent asthma that is not adequately controlled with a low dosage of inhaled corticosteroid is to increase the maintenance dosage to a medium dosage (e.g., exceeding 264 but not more than 440 mcg of fluticasone propionate [or its equivalent] daily via a metered-dose inhaler in adults and adolescents). Alternative less effective therapies that may be added to a low dosage of an inhaled corticosteroid include oral extended-release theophylline or certain leukotriene modifiers (i.e., montelukast, zafirlukast). Considerations favoring these leukotriene modifiers in combination with orally inhaled corticosteroids include intolerance to long-acting β_2-adrenergic agonists, marked preference for oral therapy, and demonstration of superior responsiveness to these leukotriene modifiers. Limited data are available in infants and children 11 years of age or younger with moderate persistent asthma, and recommendations of care are based on expert opinion and extrapolation from studies in adults. According to current asthma management guidelines, a long-acting inhaled β_2-agonist (e.g., salmeterol, formoterol), a leukotriene modifier (i.e., montelukast, zafirlukast), or extended-release theophylline (with appropriate monitoring) may be added to low-dose inhaled corticosteroid therapy in children 5–11 years of age. Because comparative data establishing relative efficacy of these agents in this age group are lacking, there is no clearly preferred agent for use as adjunctive therapy with a low-dose inhaled corticosteroid for treatment of asthma in these children.

Severe Persistent Asthma. Maintenance therapy with an inhaled corticosteroid at medium (e.g., exceeding 264 but not more than 440 mcg of fluticasone propionate in adults and adolescents or 176 but not more than 352 mcg of the drug [or its equivalent] in children 5–11 years of age daily via a metered-dose inhaler) or high dosages (e.g., exceeding 440 mcg of fluticasone propionate in adults and adolescents or 352 mcg of the drug [or its equivalent] in children 5–11 years of age daily via a metered-dose inhaler) and adjunctive therapy with a long-acting inhaled β_2-agonist is the preferred treatment according to current asthma management guidelines in adults and children 5 years of age or older with severe persistent asthma (i.e., continuous daytime asthma symptoms, nighttime symptoms 7 times per week). Such recommendations in children 5–11 years of age are based on expert opinion and extrapolation from studies in older children and adults. Alternatives to a long-acting inhaled β_2-agonist for severe persistent asthma in adults and children 5 years of age or older receiving medium-dose inhaled corticosteroids include certain leukotriene modifiers (i.e., montelukast, zafirlukast) or extended-release theophylline, but these therapies are generally not preferred. Omalizumab may be considered in adults and adolescents with severe persistent asthma with an allergic component who are inadequately controlled with high-dose inhaled corticosteroids and a long-acting β_2-agonist. In infants and children 4 years of age or younger with severe asthma, maintenance therapy with an inhaled corticosteroid at medium (e.g., exceeding 176 but not more than 352 mcg of fluticasone propionate [or its equivalent] daily via a metered-dose inhaler) or high dosages (e.g., exceeding 352 mcg of fluticasone propionate [or its equivalent] daily via a metered-dose inhaler) and adjunctive therapy with either a long-acting inhaled β_2-agonist or montelukast is the only preferred treatment according to current asthma management guidelines. Recommendations for care of infants and children with severe asthma are based on expert opinion and extrapolation from studies in adolescents and adults. For additional details on the stepped-care approach to drug therapy in asthma, see Asthma under Uses: Bronchospasm, in Albuterol 12:12.08.12 and see Asthma under Uses: Respiratory Diseases, in the Corticosteroids General Statement 68:04.

Clinical Experience with Leukotriene Modifiers. While efficacy of montelukast in the management of asthma has not been directly compared with that of zafirlukast or zileuton, improvements in forced expiratory volume in 1 second (FEV_1) and asthma symptoms reported with montelukast generally have been similar to those reported with zafirlukast or zileuton. For the management of mild persistent asthma, advantages of leukotriene modifiers relative to orally inhaled corticosteroids include ease of administration of an oral dosage form (and presumably improved compliance) and rapid onset of action (1 day versus a week or longer). The effects of montelukast appear to be additive with those of orally inhaled corticosteroids, and such combination therapy may improve asthma control in patients with moderate to severe asthma. In addition, montelukast therapy reduces the requirements for long-term inhaled corticosteroids in stable patients. Leukotriene modifiers may be especially useful in children and adults in whom disadvantages of using, continuing, or increasing the dose of orally inhaled corticosteroids have been identified. Additional clinical settings where therapy with a leukotriene modifier may be especially useful include patients with aspirin-induced asthma, exercise-induced bronchospasm (e.g., children who want to exercise at school without having to use an orally inhaled β_2-adrenergic agonist, those whose jobs require exercise under atmospheric conditions likely to induce an asthmatic episode), nocturnal asthma, acute allergen-induced asthma, or coexisting allergic rhinitis. Conversely, because leukotrienes do not play a major role in asthma pathology in patients with naturally occurring mutations in the 5-lipoxygenase gene, such patients are unlikely to respond to therapy with leukotriene modifiers.

Current data indicate that leukotriene modifiers such as montelukast generally produce modest improvements in lung function, diminish asthma symptoms, and decrease the need for supplemental, short-acting β_2-adrenergic agonist therapy in patients with mild to moderate persistent asthma. However, not all patients receiving leukotriene modifiers have substantial clinical improvement. While patients with aspirin-sensitive asthma generally respond to leukotriene modifiers, it currently is not possible to identify patients most likely to benefit from such therapy.

Clinical Efficacy of Montelukast. Efficacy of montelukast has been established in 2 clinical trials in adults and adolescents 15 years of age or older with mild to moderate intermittent or persistent asthma (i.e., a baseline FEV_1 averaging 66% of the predicted normal value and an inhaled, short-acting β_2-adrenergic agonist requirement averaging 5 puffs daily) who generally received montelukast for 12 weeks. Efficacy of montelukast also has been established in a clinical trial in children 6–14 years of age with mild to moderate intermittent or persistent asthma (i.e., a baseline FEV_1 averaging 72% of the predicted normal value and an inhaled, short-acting β_2-adrenergic agonist requirement averaging 3 or 4 puffs daily) who generally received montelukast for 8 weeks. Approximately 77–95% of children, adolescents, and adults enrolled in these studies had a history of exercise-induced bronchospasm, and 61–96% had a history of allergic rhinitis. In these clinical trials, adults and pediatric patients received montelukast once daily in the evening; evening administration was selected to provide high montelukast plasma concentrations in the early morning, the time of maximal airway narrowing. In these trials, montelukast was more effective than placebo in alleviating respiratory symptoms (i.e., daytime asthma symptoms, nighttime awakenings), improving pulmonary function (as measured by FEV_1 and peak expiratory flow rate [PEFR]), and reducing the need for supplemental therapy with an orally inhaled β_2-adrenergic agonist. The therapeutic effects of montelukast are evident after the first dose and persist for at least 24 hours.

Studies to date indicate that tolerance to montelukast does not occur and the therapeutic effect has been maintained for over 2.5 years in patients 15 years of age or older and at least 1.5 years in children 6–14 years of age. Discontinuance of long-term (i.e., 12 weeks) montelukast therapy is not associated with rebound deterioration in asthma symptoms. Efficacy of montelukast in the management of asthma in children 2–5 years of age is supported by evidence from studies in adults, adolescents, and children 6–14 years of age, the similar pathophysiology of asthma and the drug's effect in these populations, and data regarding the pharmacokinetics of montelukast in these patients.

Montelukast has been evaluated for the management of asthma in 2 randomized, controlled studies (the US study, the multinational study) that included 1576 patients 15 years of age or older with mild to moderate asthma who were allowed to receive an orally inhaled β_2-adrenergic agonist on an as-needed basis. Patients in the US study were randomized to receive montelukast 10 mg daily or placebo; about 23% of these patients also received an orally inhaled corticosteroid on a routine basis. Patients in the multinational study were randomized to receive montelukast 10 mg daily, placebo, or active control (i.e., orally inhaled beclomethasone dipropionate 200 mcg [dose expressed as amount of drug released during actuation from the valve stem] twice daily). In these studies, therapy with montelukast was associated with greater improvement than placebo in daytime asthma symptom scores, fewer nighttime awakenings per week, and improvement in other asthma-related outcomes. Compared with baseline values, reductions in asthma symptom scores (on a scale of 0–6) averaged 0.45 or 0.22 for montelukast or placebo, respectively; nighttime awakenings per week were reduced by 1.84 or 0.79, respectively. Montelukast produced modest improvements in pulmonary function compared with baseline values in this study, with increases in FEV_1, morning PEFR, and evening PEFR averaging 0.32 L, 24.5 L/minute, and 17.9 L/minute, respectively. In the US study, montelukast produced improvements in FEV_1 of 13.1% versus 4.2% with placebo. Montelukast therapy also enabled a reduction averaging about 1.56 puffs/day in the use of supplemental orally inhaled β_2-adrenergic agonist.

Therapy with montelukast in these studies was associated with a reduction in the number of patients experiencing an acute asthma episode (11.6% versus 18.4%), number of patients requiring oral corticosteroid rescue (10.7% versus 17.5%), fewer days with exacerbations (12.8% versus 20.5%), more days without symptoms (38.5% versus 27.2%), and greater improvement in physician and patient global evaluation scores than placebo. In the US study, the clinical effects of montelukast were not affected by gender, age, race, history of exercise-induced bronchoconstriction, history of allergic rhinitis, or concomitant use of orally inhaled corticosteroids. In patients 15 years of age and older, montelukast dosages exceeding 10 mg daily are not associated with additional clinical benefit.

In the multinational study, orally inhaled beclomethasone dipropionate 200 mcg (dose expressed as amount of drug released during actuation from the valve stem) twice daily was more effective in the management of asthma than montelukast. In patients 15 years of age or older, improvements in FEV_1 reported with inhaled beclomethasone (13.3% versus 7.49%) and decreases in asthma symptom scores (0.7 versus 0.49) generally have been greater than those reported with montelukast.

In a randomized, placebo-controlled study in 336 children 6–14 years of age or older with mild to moderate asthma who were allowed to receive an orally inhaled β_2-adrenergic agonist on an as-needed basis (36% also received an orally inhaled corticosteroid on a routine basis), therapy with montelukast 5 mg (chewable tablet) daily produced modest improvements in pulmonary function compared with baseline values, with increases in FEV_1 and morning PEFR (determined in clinic setting) averaging 0.16 L and 27.85 L/minute, respectively. Montelukast produced improvements in FEV_1 of 8.7% versus 8.2% with placebo. Montelukast therapy also enabled a reduction averaging about 0.56 puffs daily in the use of supplemental orally inhaled β_2-adrenergic agonists. Therapy with montelukast and intermittent use of an orally inhaled β_2-adrenergic agonist (with or without an orally inhaled corticosteroid) was associated with fewer days with asthma exacerbations (20.6% versus 25.7%) and greater improvement in clinician and parent global evaluation scores than intermittent use of a β_2-adrenergic agonist (with or without an orally inhaled corticosteroid). Subgroup analysis indicates that improvement in FEV_1 in children 6–11 years of age (7.7%) was essentially the same as in children 12–14 years of age (9.8%). In this study, the effects of montelukast on FEV_1 and as-needed inhaled β_2-adrenergic agonist use were not affected by gender, race, Tanner stage, history of allergic rhinitis, history of exercise-induced bronchospasm, or use of orally inhaled corticosteroids.

Montelukast has been evaluated for the management of asthma in children 2–5 years of age with mild persistent asthma. In a randomized, double-blind, placebo-controlled study, children received either montelukast 4 mg (as a chewable tablet) or placebo daily; about 27–29% of these patients also were receiving an orally inhaled corticosteroid on a routine basis. Patients were allowed to receive an orally inhaled β_2-adrenergic agonist on an as-needed basis. The primary end point was determination of the safety profile of montelukast, and secondary end points evaluated asthma control. In this study, therapy with montelukast was associated with improvement in daytime asthma symptom scores, days without symptoms, and days requiring β-adrenergic agonist use. Therapy with montelukast also was associated with a reduction in the number of patients requiring oral corticosteroid rescue.

Concomitant Corticosteroid Therapy. The role of montelukast as a corticosteroid-sparing agent in patients receiving orally inhaled corticosteroids has been evaluated in asthmatic adults. In one study in adults with stable asthma (a baseline FEV_1 averaging 84% of the predicted normal value), addition of montelukast to therapy with orally inhaled corticosteroids allowed a reduction in inhaled corticosteroid use while maintaining adequate asthma control. In this study, inhaled corticosteroids (i.e., metered-dose aerosol or dry powder for oral inhalation) used and their mean baseline requirement (dosage may not be expressed as dosage delivered from the mouthpiece) include beclomethasone dipropionate (1203 mcg/day), triamcinolone acetonide (2004 mcg/day), fluticasone propionate (1083 mcg/day), and budesonide (1192 mcg/day). Prior to study initiation, the dosage of orally inhaled corticosteroid was reduced to the lowest effective dosage, a reduction of 37%. An additional 47 or 30% reduction in corticosteroid dosage was reported in patients receiving montelukast or placebo for 12 weeks. In addition, about 40 or 29% of patients receiving montelukast or placebo reportedly were no longer receiving orally inhaled corticosteroids at study conclusion. Whether results of this study are applicable to patients who are maintained on higher doses of orally inhaled corticosteroids or systemic corticosteroid therapy remains to be determined.

Montelukast has been evaluated for use in combination with orally inhaled corticosteroids in asthmatic adults whose symptoms were not controlled by 336 mcg/day of beclomethasone dipropionate. Patients were randomized to receive combined therapy with beclomethasone and montelukast, beclomethasone alone, montelukast alone (beclomethasone withdrawn), or placebo (beclomethasone withdrawn). Treatment with beclomethasone and montelukast was more effective in improving pulmonary function (as measured by FEV_1) than therapy with beclomethasone alone, montelukast alone, or placebo. In addition, beclomethasone alone was more effective than montelukast alone in alleviating respiratory symptoms (i.e., daytime asthma symptoms, nighttime awakenings), improving pulmonary function (as measured by FEV_1 and PEFR), and reducing the need for supplemental therapy with an orally inhaled β_2-adrenergic agonist. While combined therapy with orally inhaled corticosteroids and montelukast may improve asthma control in patients not adequately controlled with orally inhaled corticosteroids alone, substitution of montelukast for orally inhaled corticosteroids is not likely to result in improved asthma control in these patients. The relative merits of adding montelukast to a regimen of orally inhaled corticosteroids in patients whose symptoms are inadequately controlled versus doubling the dose of the orally inhaled corticosteroid remain to be determined.

In adults with documented aspirin sensitivity who were receiving orally inhaled and/or systemic corticosteroids, addition of montelukast improved asthma control compared with placebo. The magnitude of the effect of montelukast in aspirin-sensitive patients was similar to that observed in the general population of asthma patients enrolled in clinical trials. Montelukast-treated patients with aspirin sensitivity should avoid aspirin or nonsteroidal anti-inflammatory agents (NSAIAs) since montelukast has not been shown to truncate the bronchoconstrictor response to aspirin or other NSAIAs in aspirin-sensitive patients.

Exercise-induced Bronchospasm Montelukast is used for the prevention of exercise-induced bronchospasm. In adults and adolescents 15 years of age or older with a FEV_1 averaging 83% of the predicted normal value and exercise-induced exacerbation of asthma, montelukast (10 mg daily 20–24 hours prior to exercise) reduced the mean maximal fall in FEV_1 and time to recovery compared with placebo. In this study, the response to montelukast was similar after 4, 8, and 12 weeks; however, not all patients responded to montelukast. Montelukast did not prevent clinically important deterioration in the maximal fall in FEV_1 after exercise (i.e., a 20% or greater decrease from baseline [before exercise]) in 52% of patients. While about 23% of patients experienced complete protection (i.e., a decrease in FEV_1 of less than 10% after exercise), 25% had little or no response (i.e., decrease in FEV_1 of more than 30% after exercise). Additional placebo-controlled, crossover studies in adults and in children 6–14 years of age with exercise-induced bronchospasm have reported similar results.

Results of 2 randomized, controlled studies in adults (15–46 years of age) with exercise-induced bronchospasm indicate that the bronchoprotective effect of montelukast is similar to that of salmeterol. Efficacy of montelukast in exercise-induced bronchoconstriction versus other therapies (e.g., orally inhaled albuterol, cromolyn sodium, or nedocromil [preparation for oral inhalation no longer commercially available in the US]) has not been established.

Advantages of montelukast for the management of exercise-induced bronchospasm compared with some other therapies (e.g., orally inhaled albuterol, cromolyn sodium, nedocromil [no longer commercially available in the US]) include oral administration and a protective effect that persists for 20–24 hours. While leukotriene modifiers are not included as first-line agents or as alternative agents to orally inhaled β_2-adrenergic agonists for the prevention or treatment of exercise-induced bronchoconstriction in current guidelines, current evidence supports their bronchoprotective efficacy, and the addition of montelukast may provide an additional measure of control in patients currently maintained on long-term controller therapy. The National Collegiate Athletic Association, the US Olympic Committee, and the International Olympic Committee allow competitors to use leukotriene modifiers without prior approval. The manufacturer states that patients who experience exacerbations of asthma after exercise should have a short-acting orally inhaled β_2-adrenergic agonist available for rescue. Daily administration of montelukast for the chronic treatment of asthma has not been established to prevent acute episodes of exercise-induced bronchospasm.

■ **Allergic Rhinitis** Montelukast is used for the symptomatic treatment of seasonal or perennial allergic rhinitis. Montelukast has been evaluated in a number of placebo-controlled or comparative trials with loratadine or cetirizine for the treatment of seasonal or perennial allergic rhinitis in patients 15–82 years of age. Therapy with montelukast generally has been associated with modest improvement in rhinitis end points (scores evaluating nasal congestion, nasal itching, rhinorrhea, nasal pruritus, sneezing) compared with placebo. Therapy with montelukast alone or in combination with loratadine has been associated with improved ocular manifestations, daytime nasal symptoms, nighttime symptoms, global evaluations, and quality of life compared with placebo.

■ **Urticaria** Montelukast (5–20 mg daily) has been used successfully in a limited number of patients with chronic idiopathic urticaria†; one retrospective analysis involving 18 patients indicated that many patients may benefit from the addition of a leukotriene modifier to existing therapy. Additional study is needed to elucidate further the role of leukotriene modifiers in the treatment of urticaria.

Dosage and Administration

■ **Administration** In patients with asthma with or without coexisting allergic rhinitis, montelukast is administered orally as a single daily dose in the evening. Safety and efficacy of montelukast in the management of asthma were established in clinical trials in which the drug was administered in the evening without regard to meals in adults, adolescents, and children 2–14 years of age. Evening dosing has been employed so that achievement of peak plasma concentrations of the drug might coincide with peak airway reactivity in the morning. In patients with allergic rhinitis, the time of administration may be individualized to suit patient needs. Efficacy was demonstrated in patients with seasonal allergic rhinitis when montelukast was administered in the morning or evening without regard to food intake.

Pharmacokinetic and clinical data support use of the 10-mg film-coated tablet of montelukast in adults and adolescents 15 years of age or older, use of the 5-mg chewable tablet in children 6–14 years of age, use of the 4-mg chewable tablet or 4-mg oral granules formulation in children 2–5 years of age, and use of the 4-mg oral granules formulation in infants and children 12–23 months of age for the treatment of asthma and in infants and children 6–23 months of age for the treatment of perennial allergic rhinitis.

Oral granules may be administered orally alone (directly in the mouth) or mixed with 1 teaspoonful (5 mL) of cold or room temperature baby formula or breast milk, or a spoonful of cold or room temperature soft food (applesauce, carrots, rice, or ice cream only); the stability of the drug when mixed with other foods has not been determined. Oral granules are not intended to be dissolved in any liquid other than baby formula or breast milk prior to administration. However, liquids may be taken subsequent to administration, and oral granules can be administered without regard to meals. The packet should not be opened until ready to use. After opening the packet of granules, patients should receive the full dose within 15 minutes; do not store the opened packet or mixtures of the drug with food, breast milk, or baby formula. Any unused portions should be discarded.

■ **Dosage** Dosage of montelukast sodium is expressed in terms of montelukast.

Asthma Patients should be advised that montelukast must be taken at regular intervals (i.e., daily) to be therapeutically effective. In addition, patients should be advised that the drug will *not* provide immediate symptomatic relief and should *not* be used for relief of acute bronchospasm; however, montelukast therapy can be continued during acute exacerbations of asthma. Patients should *not* discontinue or reduce the dosage of other antiasthmatic agents, even if they feel better as a result of initiation of montelukast therapy, unless instructed to do so by their clinician. No additional dosage is needed for the treatment of allergic rhinitis in patients already receiving chronic therapy for asthma.

Adult Dosage. For the prevention and long-term symptomatic control of asthma with or without allergic rhinitis, the usual dosage of montelukast for adults and adolescents 15 years of age or older is 10 mg once daily as film-coated tablets. The pharmacokinetic profile of montelukast in geriatric adults generally is similar to that in younger adults, and the manufacturer states that dosage of the drug in geriatric patients does not need to be modified based solely on age.

Pediatric Dosage. Adolescents 15 years of age or older may receive the usual adult dosage of montelukast of 10 mg once daily as film-coated tablets.

For the prevention and long-term symptomatic control of asthma with or without allergic rhinitis, the usual dosage of montelukast for children 6–14 years of age is 5 mg once daily as chewable tablets. The usual dosage of montelukast for the prevention and long-term symptomatic control of asthma with or without allergic rhinitis in children 2–5 years of age is 4 mg once daily as chewable tablets or oral granules. The usual dosage of montelukast for the prevention and long-term symptomatic control of asthma with or without allergic rhinitis in pediatric patients 12–23 months of age is 4 mg once daily as oral granules.

Exercise-induced Bronchospasm For the prevention of exercise-induced bronchospasm, montelukast should be administered at least 2 hours before exercise. Patients already taking montelukast for another indication, including chronic asthma, should not take an additional dose of the drug to prevent exercise-induced bronchospasm. All patients should have a short-acting β_2-adrenergic agonist available for exacerbations of asthma that may occur after exercise despite montelukast therapy.

Adult Dosage. For the prevention of exercise-induced bronchospasm, the usual dosage of montelukast for adults and adolescents 15 years of age or older is 10 mg as film-coated tablets administered at least 2 hours prior to exercise; an additional dose should not be taken within 24 hours of the previous dose. The pharmacokinetic profile of montelukast in geriatric adults generally is similar to that in younger adults, and the manufacturer states that dosage of the drug in geriatric patients does not need to be modified based solely on age.

Pediatric Dosage. For the prevention of exercise-induced bronchospasm†, a montelukast dosage of 5 mg daily in children 6–14 years of age has been used.

Allergic Rhinitis **Adult Dosage.** For symptomatic control of seasonal or perennial allergic rhinitis with or without asthma, the usual dosage of montelukast is 10 mg once daily as film-coated tablets.

Pediatric Dosage. Adolescents 15 years of age or older with allergic rhinitis with or without asthma may be given 10 mg once daily as film-coated tablets.

For the symptomatic control of seasonal or perennial allergic rhinitis with or without asthma, the usual dosage of montelukast for children 6–14 years of age is 5 mg once daily as chewable tablets. In children 2–5 years of age with seasonal or perennial allergic rhinitis with or without asthma, the usual dosage is 4 mg once daily as chewable tablets or oral granules. In infants and children 12–23 months of age or older with allergic rhinitis and asthma, the usual dosage of montelukast is 4 mg once daily as oral granules. The usual dosage of montelukast in pediatric patients 6–23 months of age with perennial allergic rhinitis is 4 mg once daily as oral granules.

■ **Dosage in Renal and Hepatic Impairment** Limited evidence in patients with mild to moderate hepatic impairment and clinical evidence of cirrhosis indicate that area under the plasma concentration-time curve (AUC) of montelukast is increased 41% and plasma montelukast elimination half-life is prolonged in these patients relative to patients with normal hepatic function. However, the manufacturer makes no specific recommendations for adjustment of montelukast dosage in patients with mild to moderate hepatic impairment. The pharmacokinetics of montelukast in patients with severe hepatic impairment or with hepatitis have not been evaluated.

The manufacturer makes no specific recommendations for dosage adjustment in patients with renal impairment. The drug is extensively metabolized and excreted principally in feces.

Cautions

Montelukast generally is well tolerated. Safety of montelukast has been evaluated in adults and adolescents 15 years of age or older with asthma or allergic rhinitis, in children 2–14 years of age with allergic rhinitis, in children 12 months of age or older with asthma, and in infants 6–23 months with perennial allergic rhinitis. While most adults and children 2 years of age or older with asthma received montelukast in clinical trials of 12 weeks' duration, safety data also have been collected from long-term studies lasting up to 2 years. The types of adverse effects reported in long-term studies were comparable to those reported in short-term, controlled studies.

A causal relationship between many adverse effects and montelukast has not been established. In clinical studies in adults and adolescents 15 years of age or older with asthma, adverse effects occurring in at least 1% of patients receiving montelukast and more frequently than with placebo included headache, influenza, abdominal pain, cough, increased serum ALT or AST concentration, dyspepsia, dizziness, asthenia/fatigue, dental pain, nasal congestion, rash, fever, infectious gastroenteritis, trauma, and pyuria, and the safety profile did not change substantially over time. In studies in asthmatic children 6–14 years of age, influenza, fever, dyspepsia, diarrhea, laryngitis, pharyngitis, nausea, otitis, sinusitis, and viral infection occurred in at least 2% of patients and more frequently in those receiving montelukast than in those receiving placebo; the safety profile in these children generally was similar to that in adults and did not change substantially over time. In clinical studies in asthmatic children 2–5 years of age, adverse effects occurring in at least 2% of patients receiving montelukast and more frequently than with placebo included fever, cough, abdominal pain, diarrhea, headache, rhinorrhea, sinusitis, otitis, influenza, rash, otic pain, gastroenteritis, eczema, urticaria, varicella, pneumonia, dermatitis, and conjunctivitis. In clinical studies in asthmatic children 6–23 months of age, upper respiratory tract infection, wheezing, otitis media, pharyngitis, tonsillitis, cough, and rhinitis occurred in at least 2% of patients receiving montelukast and more frequently than with placebo.

Discontinuance of montelukast therapy was required in about 2% of adolescents and adults and 4% of children 6–14 years of age in clinical studies, principally because of exacerbation of asthma.

■ **Nervous System Effects** Headache is the most frequently reported adverse effect with montelukast, occurring in 18–19% of children 6 years of age or older, adolescents, and adults. Headache has been reported in at least 2% of children 2–8 years of age with asthma receiving montelukast and in at least 1% (and more frequently than with placebo) of adults and adolescents 15 years of age or older with asthma. Sinus headache has been reported in at least 1% of adult and adolescent patients 15 years of age or older with perennial allergic rhinitis receiving montelukast and more frequently than in those receiving placebo. Dizziness or asthenia/fatigue has occurred in about 1.8–1.9% of patients 15 years of age or older receiving the drug in clinical studies. Dream abnormalities, hallucinations, agitation including aggressive behavior or hostility, anxiousness, paresthesia/hypoesthesia, seizures, drowsiness, insomnia, somnambulism, irritability, depression, suicidal thinking and behavior (including suicide), tremor, and restlessness also have been reported. (See Cautions: Precautions and Contraindications.)

■ **GI Effects** Abdominal pain has occurred in 2.9% of patients 15 years of age or older receiving montelukast. Dyspepsia, infectious gastroenteritis, and dental pain have been reported in 2.1, 1.5, and 1.7% of patients in this age group, respectively. Diarrhea or nausea has been reported in at least 2% of children 6–14 years of age receiving montelukast. Abdominal pain, diarrhea, and gastroenteritis have been reported in at least 2% of children 2–5 years of age with asthma and more frequently than in those receiving placebo. Gastroenteritis has been reported in at least 2% of children 6–8 years of age with asthma and more frequently than in those receiving placebo. Nausea, vomiting, dyspepsia, pancreatitis (rarely), and diarrhea also have been reported with montelukast therapy during postmarketing experience.

■ **Hepatic Effects** Elevations in the results of one or more liver function tests have occurred in patients receiving montelukast in clinical studies. Increases in serum ALT (SGPT) or AST (SGOT) concentrations occurred in 2.1 or 1.6%, respectively, of patients 15 years of age or older with asthma receiving montelukast in clinical studies. Increases in ALT occurred in at least 1% of adult and adolescent patients 15 years of age or older with perennial allergic rhinitis receiving montelukast in clinical studies and more frequently than in those receiving placebo. Changes in laboratory values returned to normal despite continuing montelukast therapy or were not directly attributable to drug therapy. Elevations in serum aminotransferase (transaminase) concentrations also have been reported in children 2–14 years of age receiving montelukast, but the incidence of these elevations was similar to that in children receiving placebo. Hepatic eosinophilic infiltration has been reported very rarely through postmarketing experience with montelukast. (See Dermatologic and Sensitivity Reactions.) Hepatocellular injury, cholestatic hepatitis, or mixed-pattern liver injury also has been reported rarely through postmarketing experience with montelukast. Confounding factors were present in most of these patients, such as the concomitant use of other drugs or alcohol or in the presence of coexisting conditions (e.g., other forms of hepatitis).

■ **Dermatologic and Sensitivity Reactions** Rash has occurred in 1.6% of adults and adolescents 15 years of age or older receiving montelukast. Rash, eczema, dermatitis, or urticaria has been reported in at least 2% of children 2–5 years of age receiving the drug. Atopic dermatitis, varicella, and skin infection have been reported in at least 2% of children 6–8 years of age with asthma receiving montelukast and more frequently than in those receiving placebo. Hypersensitivity reactions, including anaphylaxis, angioedema, pruritus, urticaria, and rarely hepatic eosinophilic infiltration, have been reported in patients receiving montelukast.

Eosinophilia and Churg-Strauss Syndrome Although montelukast therapy generally is associated with a decrease in peripheral blood eosinophil counts in asthmatic patients (see Pharmacology: Effects on Eosinophils), systemic eosinophilia, sometimes presenting with clinical features of vasculitis consistent with Churg-Strauss syndrome, has been reported rarely in patients receiving leukotriene modifiers (e.g., montelukast, pranlukast, zafirlukast); in almost all cases, these events were associated with a reduction (tapered dosage) or withdrawal of oral or high-dose inhaled corticosteroid therapy.

Churg-Strauss syndrome (allergic granulomatosis and angiitis) is an uncommon vasculitis of unknown etiology that is potentially fatal and characterized by at least 4 of the following 6 features: moderate to severe asthma, peripheral blood eosinophilia (greater than 10% on differential leukocyte count), mononeuropathy or polyneuropathy, nonfixed pulmonary infiltrates on radiograph, paranasal sinus abnormality, and blood vessel biopsy with extravascular eosinophils. The incidence of this syndrome in patients receiving leukotriene modifiers (e.g., zafirlukast) has been estimated to be approximately 60 cases/million patient-years of exposures; this is similar to the estimated incidence of this syndrome reported in patients receiving other antiasthmatic drugs (bambuterol, salmeterol, nedocromil [preparation for oral inhalation no longer commercially available in the US]). The onset of Churg-Strauss syndrome has been reported to range from 2 days to 10 months after initiation of leukotriene modifier therapy, and in most cases corticosteroid therapy had been withdrawn or dosage tapered within 3 months of the development of the syndrome.

Although the exact mechanism of Churg-Strauss syndrome has not been determined, it is unlikely that its development during therapy with leukotriene modifiers is directly attributable to these drugs. Instead, the occurrence of Churg-Strauss syndrome in patients receiving leukotriene modifiers is believed to result from unmasking of an underlying vasculitic syndrome that initially was diagnosed as moderate to severe asthma. In such patients, it has been postulated that corticosteroid therapy had suppressed or delayed the development of overt Churg-Strauss syndrome, and initiation of therapy with leukotriene modifiers resulted in decreased steroid requirements, with a subsequent unmasking of the syndrome as corticosteroid therapy was tapered or withdrawn. Remission of the syndrome usually can be induced with systemic corticosteroid therapy alone, although other immunodulating agents (e.g., cyclophosphamide, methotrexate) may be necessary in some patients.

■ **Respiratory Effects** Influenza, cough, and nasal congestion have been reported in 4.2, 2.7, and 1.6%, respectively, of montelukast-treated patients with asthma 15 years of age or older. Upper respiratory tract infection occurred in 1.9 or at least 2% of patients 15 years of age or older or 2–14 years of age, respectively, with seasonal allergic rhinitis. Upper respiratory tract infection, wheezing, pharyngitis, tonsillitis, cough, and rhinitis occurred in at least 2% of patients 12–23 months of age with asthma. Pharyngitis occurred in at least 2% of patients 2–14 years of age with seasonal allergic rhinitis. Laryngitis, pharyngitis, sinusitis, and viral infection have occurred in at least 2% of children 6–14 years of age with asthma receiving montelukast and more frequently than in those receiving placebo. Rhinorrhea, cough, sinusitis, influenza, and pneumonia have been reported in at least 2% of montelukast-treated children 2–5 years of age with asthma and more frequently than in those receiving placebo. Sinusitis, upper respiratory tract infection, or cough occurred in at least 1% of adult and adolescent patients 15 years of age or older with perennial allergic rhinitis receiving montelukast and more frequently than in those receiving placebo. Infective rhinitis and acute bronchitis occurred in at least 2% of montelukast-treated children 6–8 years of age with asthma and more frequently than in those receiving placebo.

■ **Other Adverse Effects** Fever or trauma occurred in 1.5 or 1% of patients 15 years of age or older receiving montelukast. Fever also has been reported in children 2–14 years of age. Fever, otic pain, or otitis occurred in at least 2% of children 2–5 years of age with asthma and more frequently than in those receiving placebo. Otitis has occurred in at least 2% of the children 6–14 years of age with asthma and more frequently than in those receiving placebo. Otitis media has occurred in at least 2% of montelukast-treated patients 12–23 months of age with asthma or 2–14 years of age with seasonal allergic rhinitis and more frequently than in those receiving placebo. Pyuria has occurred in 1% of patients 15 years of age or older and more frequently than with placebo. At least 2% of montelukast-treated children 2–5 years of age experienced conjunctivitis, varicella, leg pain, or thirst, each occurring more frequently than with placebo. Tooth infection and myopia have been reported in at least 2% of montelukast-treated children 6–8 years of age with asthma and more frequently than in those receiving placebo. Epistaxis occurred in at least 1% of adult and adolescent patients 15 years of age or older with perennial allergic rhinitis receiving montelukast and more frequently than in those receiving placebo. Edema has been reported through postmarketing experience with montelukast. Myalgia (including muscle cramps) arthralgia, palpitations, bruising, edema, and an increased tendency for bleeding also has occurred in montelukast-treated patients.

■ **Precautions and Contraindications** Patients should be advised that montelukast must be taken at regular intervals to be therapeutically effective. In addition, patients should be advised that the drug will not provide immediate symptomatic relief and should *not* be used for the relief of acute bronchospasm; however, montelukast therapy can be continued during acute exacerbations of asthma. Patients receiving montelukast should be provided with and instructed in the use of a short-acting, inhaled β_2-adrenergic bronchodilator as supplemental therapy for acute asthma symptoms. Patients should not discontinue or reduce the dosage of other antiasthmatic agents, even if they feel better as a result of initiation of montelukast therapy, unless instructed to do so by their clinician.

The manufacturer states that patients who experience exacerbations of asthma after exercise should have a short-acting orally inhaled β_2-adrenergic agonist available for rescue. (See Exercise-induced Bronchospasm under Uses: Bronchospasm.)

Patients in whom asthma is precipitated by aspirin or other nonsteroidal anti-inflammatory agents (NSAIAs) should continue to avoid aspirin and NSAIAs while receiving montelukast. While montelukast can improve airway function in asthmatic patients with documented aspirin sensitivity, the drug has *not* been shown to truncate the bronchoconstrictor response to aspirin or other NSAIAs in such patients.

Although orally inhaled corticosteroid requirements in patients with stable asthma may be reduced during montelukast therapy, only gradual (e.g., at 2-week intervals) reduction of the steroid dosage should be undertaken. Montelukast should not be abruptly substituted for oral or inhaled corticosteroids.

Because of postmarketing reports of neuropsychiatric events (e.g., depression, anxiety, agitation, aggressive behavior, irritability, suicidal ideation and behavior [suicidality]) in adults, adolescents, and pediatric patients, the US Food and Drug Administration (FDA) reviewed the safety of montelukast and other leukotriene modifiers to evaluate a possible link between the use of these agents and such behavior or mood changes. Data from placebo-controlled trials with montelukast, zafirlukast, and zileuton submitted to FDA indicate that suicidal ideation occurred in 0.01% of 9929 patients treated with montelukast and in none of the patients treated with other leukotriene modifiers. In these studies, no completed suicide occurred during therapy with any leukotriene modifier. Following review of the postmarketing reports and analysis of available clinical data, FDA has concluded that some of the neuropsychiatric events reported during postmarketing surveillance with montelukast (e.g., agitation, aggressive behavior or hostility, anxiousness, depression, dream abnormalities, hallucinations, insomnia, irritability, somnambulism, restlessness, tremor) appear consistent with a drug-induced effect. The manufacturer of montelukast states that patients receiving the drug and their clinicians should be alert to the potential for neuropsychiatric events. Patients should be instructed to contact their clinician if behavior or mood changes occur during therapy with montelukast. Clinicians should carefully evaluate the risks and benefits of continuing montelukast therapy in patients who develop neuropsychiatric symptoms.

Eosinophilia, vasculitic rash, worsening pulmonary symptoms, cardiac complications, and/or neuropathy consistent with Churg-Strauss syndrome, a systemic eosinophilic vasculitis, have been reported rarely in patients receiving leukotriene modifiers (e.g., montelukast, pranlukast, zafirlukast). While a causal relationship between this syndrome and leukotriene modifiers has not been established, clinicians should be alert to the development of such manifestations in patients receiving leukotriene modifiers. Patients should inform their clinician immediately if symptoms of Churg-Strauss syndrome (e.g., feeling of pins and needles or numbness of extremities, flu-like symptoms, rash, sinusitis) occur. (See Eosinophilia and Churg-Strauss Syndrome under Cautions: Dermatologic and Sensitivity Reactions.)

Patients should be advised that an increase in frequency of administration of short-acting inhaled bronchodilators or inadequate control of symptoms while receiving the maximum prescribed dosage of an inhaled bronchodilator may indicate substantial worsening of asthma that requires evaluation.

Montelukast is contraindicated in patients hypersensitive to the drug or any ingredient in the formulation. Individuals with phenylketonuria (i.e., homozygous genetic deficiency of phenylalanine hydroxylase) and other individuals who must restrict their intake of phenylalanine should be advised that montelukast chewable tablets contain aspartame (Nutrasweet®), which is metabolized in the GI tract to provide 0.674 mg of phenylalanine for each 4-mg chewable tablet or 0.842 mg of phenylalanine for each 5-mg chewable tablet of montelukast.

■ **Pediatric Precautions** Safety and efficacy of montelukast for the treatment of asthma in children younger than 12 months of age have not been established. Safety and efficacy of montelukast for the prevention of exercise-induced bronchospasm in children and adolescents younger than 15 years of age have not been established. Safety and efficacy of montelukast in infants younger than 6 months of age with perennial allergic rhinitis have not been established. Safety and efficacy of montelukast in pediatric patients younger than 2 years of age with seasonal allergic rhinitis have not been established. Safety of montelukast oral granules in pediatric patients 12–23 months with asthma has been demonstrated in a placebo-controlled trial and other clinical experience. Efficacy of montelukast in this age group was explored as a secondary end point in a safety study and is extrapolated from demonstrated efficacy in patients 6 years of age or older based on similar mean systemic exposure to montelukast and the substantial similarity of the disease course, pathophysiology, and effects of the drug among these populations.

Safety and efficacy of montelukast have been established in adequate and well-controlled studies in children 6–14 years of age with asthma and are similar to those reported in adults. Safety of the drug in children 2–5 years of age with asthma is extrapolated from demonstrated efficacy in asthmatic adults, adolescents, and children 6 years of age or older based on similar mean systemic exposure to montelukast and the substantial similarity of the disease course, pathophysiology, and effects of the drug among these populations. Efficacy of montelukast in children 2–5 years of age is supported by exploratory efficacy assessments from a large, well-controlled safety study.

Efficacy of montelukast in pediatric patients 2–14 years or 6 months to 14 years of age with seasonal or perennial allergic rhinitis, respectively, is supported by extrapolation from demonstrated efficacy in patients 15 years of age and older with allergic rhinitis and the assumption that the disease course, pathophysiology, and drug's effect are substantially similar among these populations. Safety of the montelukast in pediatric patients aged 2–14 years of age with allergic rhinitis is supported by data from studies in pediatric patients 2–14 years of age with asthma. Data from a safety study of montelukast therapy in pediatric patients 2–14 years of age with seasonal allergic rhinitis demonstrated a safety profile similar to that of placebo. Safety of montelukast in pediatric patients 6–23 months with perennial allergic rhinitis is supported by data from studies in pediatric patients 6–23 months of age with asthma and by pharmacokinetic data comparing systemic exposure in such pediatric patients with that in adults.

The effect of long-term therapy with montelukast on linear growth in pediatric patients has been assessed in a 56-week, multicenter, double-blind, randomized study with an active control (beclomethasone dipropionate) and placebo control in 360 children 6–8 years of age with mild asthma. Montelukast (5 mg once daily) did not affect growth rate in children compared with placebo; however, growth rate was slowed in children taking orally inhaled beclomethasone dipropionate (168 mcg twice daily) with chlorofluorocarbon propellants (no longer commercially available in the US) compared with placebo.

■ **Geriatric Precautions** When the total number of patients studied in clinical trials of montelukast is considered, 3.5% were 65 years of age or older, while 0.4% were 75 years of age or older. Although no overall differences in safety or efficacy were observed between geriatric and younger patients, and other clinical experience revealed no evidence of age-related differences, the possibility that some older patients may exhibit increased sensitivity to the drug cannot be ruled out.

Changes in the plasma elimination half-life of montelukast occur in geriatric individuals but do not affect the dosing regimen.

■ **Mutagenicity and Carcinogenicity** Montelukast was not mutagenic or clastogenic in the microbial mutagenesis assay, the V-79 mammalian cell mutagenesis assay, the alkaline elution assay in rat hepatocytes, the chromosomal aberration assay in Chinese hamster ovary cells, or the in vivo mouse bone marrow chromosomal aberration assay.

Montelukast was not tumorigenic in a 2-year carcinogenicity study in rats at oral (gavage) dosages up to 200 mg/kg daily (estimated exposure approximately 120 and 75 times the area under the plasma concentration-time curve [AUC] for adults and children, respectively, at the maximum recommended daily oral dose) or in a 92-week carcinogenicity study in mice at oral (gavage) dosages up to 100 mg/kg daily (estimated exposure approximately 45 and 25 times the AUC for adults and children, respectively, at the maximum recommended daily oral dose).

■ **Pregnancy, Fertility, and Lactation** Montelukast crosses the placenta following oral dosing in rats and rabbits. Reproduction studies in rats using oral dosages up to 400 mg/kg daily (estimated exposure approximately 100 times the AUC for adults at the maximum recommended daily oral dose) and in rabbits using oral dosages up to 300 mg/kg daily (estimated exposure approximately 110 times the AUC for adults at the maximum recommended daily oral dose) have not revealed evidence of harm to the fetus.

There are no adequate and well-controlled studies to date using montelukast in pregnant women, and the manufacturer states that montelukast should be used during pregnancy only when clearly needed. The American College of Obstetricians and Gynecologists (ACOG) generally recommends use of leukotriene modifiers as an alternative to a long-acting β_2-agonist in pregnant women with moderate persistent asthma who are inadequately controlled with low to medium dosages of an inhaled corticosteroid. (See Uses: Asthma.)

During postmarketing experience with montelukast, congenital limb defects have been reported rarely in the children of women treated with the drug; however, most of these women were receiving other antiasthmatic agents during their pregnancies. A causal relationship between montelukast use and the development of these congenital anomalies has not been established. The manufacturer maintains a registry to monitor pregnancy outcomes in women exposed to montelukast during pregnancy. Patients may be enrolled by calling 800-986-8999.

While reproduction studies in female rats using oral montelukast doses up to 100 mg/kg (estimated exposure approximately 20 times the AUC for adults at the maximum recommended daily oral dose) have not revealed evidence of impaired fertility, oral doses of 200 mg/kg (estimated exposure approximately 70 times the AUC for adults at the maximum recommended daily oral dose) have been associated with reduced fertility and fecundity indices. Reproduction studies in male rats using oral montelukast doses up to 800 mg/kg (estimated exposure approximately 160 times the AUC for adults at the maximum recommended daily oral dose) have not revealed evidence of impaired fertility.

Montelukast is distributed into milk in rats. Since it is not known whether montelukast is distributed in human milk, the drug should be used with caution in nursing women.

Drug Interactions

Montelukast has been used concomitantly in clinical studies with other drugs used routinely for the prevention and long-term symptomatic management of asthma without an apparent increase in adverse effects. In addition, montelukast has been used concomitantly with benzodiazepines, decongestants, nonsteroidal anti-inflammatory agents (NSAIAs), sedative-hypnotics, or thyroid hormones without evidence of an increase in adverse effects.

In drug-interaction studies, usual dosages of montelukast did not have clinically important effects on the pharmacokinetics of theophylline, warfarin, terfenadine (no longer commercially available in the US), digoxin, oral contraceptives (ethinyl estradiol with norethindrone), prednisone, or prednisolone.

■ **Nonsteroidal Anti-inflammatory Agents** Montelukast-treated patients with known aspirin sensitivity should continue to avoid aspirin and other NSAIAs. Although montelukast can improve airway function in asthmatics with aspirin sensitivity, the drug has *not* been shown to truncate the bronchoconstrictor response to aspirin or other NSAIAs in such patients, and an anaphylactic reaction has been reported following exposure to a NSAIA (e.g., diclofenac) in at least one aspirin-sensitive individual receiving montelukast.

■ **Drugs Affecting Hepatic Microsomal Enzymes** Metabolism of montelukast is mediated in part by the cytochrome P-450 (CYP) isoenzymes 3A4 and 2C9, and the possibility exists that drugs that induce or inhibit these isoenzymes may alter the plasma concentrations of montelukast. Montelukast does not appear to have any inhibitory effect on CYP3A4, CYP2C9, CYP1A2, CYP2A6, CYP2C19, or CYP2D6. Data from in vitro studies indicate that montelukast is a potent inhibitor of CYP2C8. However, data from several clinical drug interaction studies evaluating montelukast and rosiglitazone or repaglinide, substrates for the CYP2C8 isoenzyme, indicate that montelukast does not inhibit CYP2C8 in vivo. Therefore, clinical drug interactions involving montelukast and CYP2C8 substrates (e.g., paclitaxel, rosiglitazone, repaglinide) are not anticipated.

The effect of drugs that inhibit CYP3A4 (e.g., erythromycin, ketoconazole) or CYP2C9 (e.g., fluconazole) on the pharmacokinetics of montelukast remains to be determined.

Phenobarbital Administration of phenobarbital, which induces cytochrome P-450 isoenzymes, and a single 10-mg dose of montelukast resulted in a reduction of 40% in area under the plasma montelukast concentration-time curve (AUC). The manufacturer of montelukast states that the drug can be administered without dosage adjustment in patients also receiving phenobarbital. However, patients receiving montelukast with drugs that are potent inducers of cytochrome P-450 isoenzymes (e.g., phenobarbital) should be monitored for alterations in clinical response and/or adverse effects.

Theophylline Although theophylline may be metabolized to some extent via the CYP3A4 isoenzyme, drug interaction studies did not reveal evidence of a pharmacokinetic interaction with usual dosages of montelukast; however, the potential for an interaction exists with higher than recommended montelukast dosages. Following IV administration of a single theophylline dose (4.65 mg/kg of anhydrous drug) in healthy adults who had achieved steady-state plasma montelukast concentrations while receiving montelukast 10 mg daily, clinically important changes in the pharmacokinetics of theophylline were not observed.

At daily montelukast dosages that were 20-fold higher (200 mg once daily) than the currently recommended dosage, montelukast decreased the peak concentration achieved with a single oral (250 mg) or IV (5 mg/kg) theophylline dose by 12 or 10% respectively, the AUC by 43 or 44%, respectively, and the elimination half-life by 44 or 39%, respectively. At a montelukast dosage that was 60-fold higher (200 mg 3 times daily) than recommended, the drug decreased the peak concentration of a single 250-mg oral dose of theophylline by 25%, AUC by 66%, and elimination half-life by 63%.

Warfarin Although warfarin is eliminated principally via CYP-dependent hepatic metabolism (see Pharmacokinetics: Elimination, in Warfarin 20:12.04.08) and montelukast is highly (99%) protein bound, drug interaction studies did not identify clinically important pharmacokinetic interactions between the drugs. Concomitant administration of montelukast and warfarin does not appear to affect the pharmacokinetics of warfarin. The effect of a single 30-mg dose of warfarin on prothrombin time (PT) or international normalized ratio (INR) was not altered in healthy adults who had achieved steady-state plasma montelukast concentrations while receiving montelukast 10 mg daily. Montelukast did not exhibit a clinically important effect on AUCs or peak plasma concentrations of *R*- or *S*-warfarin, although slight but statistically significant decreases in the time to peak for both warfarin enantiomers and in elimination half-life of the less potent *R*-enantiomer were observed; the latter changes were not considered clinically important.

Rifampin Although specific drug interaction studies have not been performed to date, the manufacturer states that it is reasonable to employ appropriate clinical monitoring when a potent cytochrome P-450 enzyme inducer such as rifampin is used concomitantly with montelukast.

Antihistamines Administration of terfenadine (60 mg twice daily; no longer commercially available in the US) following achievement of steady-state plasma montelukast concentrations in adults receiving montelukast 10 mg daily did not alter the plasma concentration profile of terfenadine or fexofenadine, the active carboxylated metabolite, and did not affect ECG parameters (i.e., QT_c interval).

■ **Digoxin** Administration of digoxin in adults who had achieved steady-state plasma montelukast concentrations while receiving montelukast 10 mg daily did not alter the pharmacokinetic profile or urinary excretion of digoxin.

■ **Estrogen-Progestin Combinations** Administration of an oral contraceptive (a fixed combination of ethinyl estradiol 35 mcg with norethindrone 1 mg) following achievement of steady-state plasma montelukast concentrations in women receiving montelukast 100 mg or more daily did not alter the plasma concentrations of either the estrogen or the progestin.

■ **Corticosteroids** Administration of oral prednisone or IV prednisolone in patients who had achieved steady-state plasma montelukast concentrations while receiving montelukast 100 mg or more daily did not result in clinically important changes in the plasma profiles of the corticosteroids.

Acute Toxicity

■ **Pathogenesis** Limited information is available on the acute toxicity of montelukast. Single oral doses of up to 5 g/kg in mice (estimated exposure approximately 335 and 210 times the area under the plasma concentration-time curve [AUC] for adults and children, respectively, at the maximum recommended daily oral dose) and rats (estimated exposure approximately 230 and 145 times the AUC for adults and children, respectively, at the maximum recommended daily oral dose) were not lethal.

■ **Manifestations** Montelukast has been administered to adults with asthma in dosages up to 200 mg daily for 22 weeks, and in dosages up to 900 mg daily for approximately 1 week without clinically important adverse experiences.

There have been reports of acute overdosage with montelukast doses of up to 1 g in adults and children. While adverse effects were not reported in most incidents of overdosage, the most frequently reported adverse experiences that were reported included abdominal pain, somnolence, thirst, headache, vomiting, and psychomotor hyperactivity. Clinical and laboratory findings associated with these reports were consistent with the safety profile of the drug in adults and pediatric patients. In one 43-month-old child who ingested 65 mg of the drug and complained only of thirst, most of the ingested tablets were recovered via saline gastric lavage.

■ **Treatment** If acute overdosage of montelukast occurs, supportive and symptomatic treatment should be initiated and the patient closely observed. If indicated, unabsorbed material should be removed from the GI tract. Whether peritoneal dialysis or hemodialysis removes montelukast is unknown.

Pharmacology

■ **Anti-inflammatory Effects** ***Asthma and Allergic Rhinitis*** Montelukast sodium, a selective, competitive leukotriene-receptor antagonist, affects inflammatory processes involved in asthma and allergic rhinitis. Current evidence indicates that asthma is a chronic inflammatory disorder of the airways involving the production and activity of several endogenous inflammatory mediators, including leukotrienes. Montelukast exerts beneficial effects in patients with asthma by inhibiting the action of leukotrienes at specific receptor sites (i.e., the cysteinyl leukotrienes C_4 [LTC_4], D_4 [LTD_4], and E_4 [LTE_4]) on airway smooth muscle and nasal mucosa. Cysteinyl leukotrienes are released from the nasal mucosa after allergen exposure and are associated with manifestations of allergic rhinitis (e.g., increased nasal airway resistance, nasal obstruction). Leukotriene modifiers (e.g., montelukast, zafirlukast, zileuton) have actions consistent with those of anti-inflammatory agents in that an expert panel of the National Asthma Education and Prevention Program has defined anti-inflammatory agents as those that reduce the markers of airway inflammation (e.g., eosinophils, mast cells, activated lymphocytes, macrophages, cytokines) in airway tissue or airway secretions and thereby reduce the intensity of airway hyperresponsiveness. However, the precise anti-inflammatory actions responsible for the therapeutic effects of drugs in asthma (e.g., symptom reduction, improvement in expiratory flow, reduction in airway hyperresponsiveness, prevention of exacerbations, prevention of airway wall remodeling) remain to be fully elucidated.

Effects on Leukotrienes Leukotrienes are products of arachidonic acid metabolism via the 5-lipoxygenase pathway; the contribution of this pathway to the inflammatory process is complemented by the cyclooxygenase pathway, which converts arachidonic acid into other biologic mediators (e.g., prostaglandins, thromboxanes). Arachidonic acid is liberated by cell membranes in response to various factors, such as antigen-antibody interactions, IgE-receptor activation, microorganisms, and physical stimuli (e.g., cold, altered ionic conditions). The cysteinyl leukotrienes (LTC_4, LTD_4, LTE_4) and leukotriene B_4 (LTB_4, a potent chemotactic mediator) are derived from the initial unstable product of arachidonic acid metabolism, leukotriene A_4 (LTA_4). Cysteinyl leukotrienes are produced by a number of cell types, including eosinophils, basophils, mast cells, macrophages, and monocytes; however, the physiologic effects of these leukotrienes appear to be mediated through binding to a common receptor, CysLT. While several other mediators (e.g., histamine, prostaglandins) also act on target cells within airways to induce manifestations typical of asthma, the cysteinyl leukotrienes (formerly referred to as "slow-reacting substance of anaphylaxis" [SRSA]) are especially important in the pathogenesis of this disease, causing increased mucus secretion and vascular permeability, airway edema, bronchoconstriction, and altered cellular activity associated with the inflammatory process.

The involvement of leukotrienes in asthma is supported by evidence of increased concentrations of leukotrienes in biologic fluids (i.e., urine, bronchoalveolar lavage fluid, nasal fluid, plasma) of some patients with asthma compared with healthy individuals; increased urinary leukotriene concentrations also have been observed in patients following allergen challenge, episodes of asthma, and exercise or aspirin challenge. Compared with histamine or prostaglandins, cysteinyl leukotrienes are 100–1000 times more potent as bronchoconstrictors. In addition, patients with asthma are substantially more responsive to the effects of leukotrienes than are healthy individuals. In one study, patients with asthma were 25–100 times more sensitive to the bronchoconstrictor effects of inhaled LTD_4 than nonasthmatic individuals. However, there is substantial interindividual variability in airway sensitivity to the contractile effects of leukotrienes among both healthy individuals and patients with asthma.

Because of the role of leukotrienes in the pathogenesis of asthma, modification of leukotriene activity may be used to reduce airway symptoms, decrease bronchial smooth muscle tone, and improve asthma control. Inhibition of leukotriene-mediated effects may be achieved by drugs that interrupt 5-lipoxygenase activity and prevent formation of leukotrienes (e.g., zileuton) or by antagonism of leukotriene activity at specific receptor sites in the airway (e.g., montelukast, zafirlukast). The antagonist activity of montelukast is selective, competitive, and reversible. Montelukast competitively inhibits the action of LTD_4 at a subgroup of CysLT receptors ($CysLT_1$) in airway smooth muscle. In vitro, montelukast possesses affinity for the $CysLT_1$ receptor that is similar to that of LTD_4. In in vitro studies, montelukast antagonized contraction of isolated animal smooth muscle produced by LTD_4, but did not antagonize contraction produced by LTC_4. In animal studies, montelukast antagonized contraction of airway smooth muscle produced by LTD_4 or antigen.

Inhibition of Bronchoconstriction In patients with asthma, oral montelukast inhibits bronchoconstriction induced by exposure to known precipitating factors (e.g., allergens, cold and/or dry air, exercise); in addition, both the acute bronchoconstrictor response (immediate/early asthmatic response [IAR, EAR]) and the delayed inflammatory response (late asthmatic response [LAR]) to inhaled antigen are inhibited. Montelukast reduces sensitivity to inhaled LTD_4 in patients with asthma. In studies evaluating the in vivo potency of montelukast, oral administration of a single 5-mg dose of montelukast attenuated LTD_4-induced bronchoconstriction. The effect of montelukast on LTD_4-induced bronchoconstriction is evident within 4 hours of drug administration and persists for 24 hours or longer. Montelukast is associated with a longer duration of inhibition of LTD_4-induced bronchoconstriction than oral zafirlukast. In addition, montelukast inhibits both the acute bronchoconstrictor response and the delayed inflammatory response to inhaled antigen. In one crossover, placebo-controlled study, montelukast inhibited the acute bronchoconstrictor and delayed inflammatory response to antigen by 75 and 57%, respectively. Following IV administration of montelukast 7 mg (not commercially available in the US) in patients with asthma, forced expiratory volume in 1 second (FEV_1) increased 15% over baseline at 15 minutes and 18.43% at 60 minutes; following administration of a single oral dose of montelukast 10 mg in patients with asthma, FEV_1 increased 4.67% at 15 minutes and 12.9% at 60 minutes.

In a limited number of patients with asthma, single oral doses of montelukast 100 or 250 mg increased the FEV_1 regardless of concomitant use of inhaled corticosteroids. In addition, data from one clinical study indicate the bronchodilatory effects of inhaled corticosteroids and montelukast are additive.

■ **Effects on Eosinophils** Montelukast therapy decreased mean peripheral blood eosinophil count 9–15% from baseline in pediatric (at least 2 years of age) and adult patients with asthma. While a decrease in peripheral blood eosinophil count may indicate that montelukast has important effects on parameters of asthmatic inflammation, the clinical importance of changes in eosinophil counts in asthmatic patients remains to be determined.

Similarly, therapy with montelukast in patients with seasonal allergic rhinitis (15 years of age or older) either prevented the rise in mean peripheral blood eosinophil counts observed with placebo or actually decreased mean peripheral blood eosinophil counts compared with placebo.

■ **Other Effects** Montelukast has essentially no affinity for prostanoid, cholinergic, or β-adrenergic receptors.

Pharmacokinetics

While safety and efficacy of montelukast (10 or 5 mg daily) have been established in clinical studies in which the drug was administered in the evening without regard to meals, pharmacokinetics have been studied principally in healthy nonasthmatic adults and in asthmatic children who received the drug in the morning. Pharmacokinetic studies have not revealed diurnal or gender-related differences in the pharmacokinetics of the drug; further study is needed to determine if there are race-related differences.

The plasma concentration profile following oral administration of montelukast 10 mg in adolescents 15 years of age or older is similar to that in young adults. In addition, the plasma concentration profile following oral administration of montelukast 4 or 5 mg chewable tablets in children 2–5 or 6–14 years of age, respectively, is similar to the profile in adults receiving montelukast 10 mg (as the commercially available film-coated tablet). In children 6–11 months of age, systemic exposure to montelukast and variability in plasma drug concentrations are greater than those observed in adults. Based on population analyses, the mean area under the plasma concentration-time curve (AUC) and the mean peak plasma drug concentration were 60 and 89% higher, respectively, than those observed in adults. Systemic exposure following administration of 4-mg granules in infants 12–23 months of age is less variable than that with the same formulation in younger children, but the mean AUC and mean peak plasma concentration were 33 and 60% higher, respectively, than that following administration of 10-mg film-coated tablets in adults. Changes in disposition kinetics of montelukast occur in geriatric individuals but do not affect the dosing regimen. Pharmacokinetics of montelukast are linear for oral doses up to 50 mg.

Bioequivalence of the 10-mg film-coated tablet versus the 5-mg chewable tablet (2 tablets) has not been evaluated; however, limited data indicate that absorption of montelukast administered as a 10-mg chewable tablet (not commercially available) is more rapid and more complete than when the drug is administered as the commercially available film-coated tablet. The 4-mg oral granule formulation is bioequivalent to the 4-mg chewable tablet when administered to fasting adults, and the oral granules can be used as an alternative to the chewable tablets in patients 2–5 years of age.

■ **Absorption** Montelukast is rapidly absorbed from the GI tract, and peak plasma concentrations are attained within 3–4, 2–2.5, or 2 hours following oral administration in the fasted state of a single 10-mg film-coated (in adults), 5-mg chewable (in adults), or 4-mg chewable (in children 2–5 years of age) tablet, respectively. Oral bioavailability of montelukast administered as a 10-mg tablet in adults is 58–66%; presence of food in the GI tract does not affect bioavailability when the 10-mg film-coated tablet is administered with a standard meal in the morning. Oral bioavailability of the drug administered as a 5-mg chewable tablet in adults is 73% when the drug is administered in fasting individuals and 63% when the drug is administered with a standard meal in the morning. Ingestion of a high-fat meal in the morning with the 4-mg oral granules formulation had no effect on the AUC of montelukast; however, the time to peak plasma concentrations was prolonged from 2.3 hours to 6.4 hours and peak plasma concentrations were reduced by 35%. Administration of montelukast granules with applesauce does not appear to have a clinically important effect on the pharmacokinetics of montelukast.

Following oral administration of montelukast 10 mg daily for 7 days in fasting young adults, peak plasma concentrations averaged 541 ng/mL on day 1 and 602.8 ng/mL on day 7. Trough concentrations on days 3–7 were essentially constant and ranged from 18–24 ng/mL. In this study, values for area under the plasma concentration-time curve (AUC) at steady-state were about 14–15% higher than those achieved with a single dose, and were reached within 2 days.

The therapeutic effects of montelukast (e.g., as determined by improvements in asthma symptoms and/or lung function test results, decreased use of β-agonist bronchodilators) are evident after the first dose and persist for at least 24 hours.

In patients receiving montelukast 10 mg daily with mild to moderate hepatic impairment and clinical evidence of cirrhosis, the AUC of the drug was increased by 41% compared with the AUC in healthy individuals receiving montelukast.

■ **Distribution** Distribution of montelukast in body tissues and fluids has not been fully characterized. The steady-state volume of distribution of montelukast is 8–11 L.

Studies in rats indicate that only minimal amounts of radiolabeled material are detected in all tissues at 24 hours after administration of radiolabeled montelukast. Minimal amounts of radiolabeled montelukast cross the blood-brain barrier in rats.

Montelukast is more than 99% bound to plasma proteins.

It is not known whether montelukast crosses the placenta in humans; the drug crosses the placenta following oral administration in rats and rabbits. While it is not known whether montelukast is distributed in human milk, the drug is distributed into milk in rats.

■ **Elimination** The metabolic fate of montelukast has not been fully determined, but the drug is extensively metabolized in the GI tract and/or liver and excreted in bile. Several metabolic pathways have been identified including acyl glucuronidation, and oxidation catalyzed by several cytochrome P-450 (CYP) isoenzymes. In vitro studies indicate that the microsomal P-450 isoenzyme CYP3A4 is the major enzyme involved in formation of the 21-hydroxy metabolite (M5) and a sulfoxide metabolite (M2), and CYP2C9 is the major isoenzyme involved in the formation of the 36-hydroxy metabolite (M6). Other identified metabolites include an acyl glucuronide (M1) and a 25-hydroxy (a phenol, M3) analog.

Following oral administration of 54.8 mg of radiolabeled montelukast, metabolites of the drug represented less than 2% of circulating radioactivity. Montelukast metabolites that have been identified in plasma in radiolabeled studies include the 21-hydroxy (diastereomers of a benzylic acid, M5a and M5b) and the 36-hydroxy (diastereomers of a methyl alcohol, M6a and M6b) metabolites. Following oral administration of therapeutic doses of montelukast, plasma concentrations of metabolites at steady-state in adults and children were below the level of detection.

The mean plasma elimination half-life of montelukast in adults 19–48 years of age is 2.7–5.5 hours, and plasma clearance averages 45 mL/minute. A plasma elimination half-life of 3.4–4.2 hours has been reported in children 6–14 years of age. Limited data indicate that the plasma elimination half-life of montelukast is prolonged slightly in geriatric adults and in patients with mild to moderate hepatic impairment, although dosage adjustment is not required. A plasma elimination half-life of 6.6 or 7.4 hours has been reported in geriatric adults 65–73 years of age or patients with mild to moderate hepatic impairment, respectively.

Pharmacokinetics of montelukast have not been evaluated in patients with renal impairment. It is not known whether montelukast is removed from the body by hemodialysis or peritoneal dialysis.

Following oral administration, montelukast is excreted principally in bile as unchanged drug and metabolites. Following oral administration of radiolabeled montelukast, 86% of administered radioactivity was recovered in feces and less than 2% was recovered in urine over a 5-day collection period.

Chemistry and Stability

■ **Chemistry** Montelukast sodium, a synthetic leukotriene-receptor antagonist, is an antiasthmatic agent. Montelukast is a cysteinyl leukotriene analog that was developed based on a quinoline-containing compound that was modified with leukotriene structural elements. Structural modifications resulted in improved potency, oral bioavailability, clinical efficacy, and/or safety profile relative to early leukotriene antagonists (e.g., MK-571, verlukast). Montelukast consists of a 7-chloro-2-quinolinyl ethenylphenyl connected to a {[(1-hydroxy-1-methylethyl)phenyl]propyl}thiomethyl cyclopropaneacetic acid. Because montelukast contains polar and nonpolar groups at opposite ends of the molecule, the drug has amphophilic physicochemical properties.

Montelukast is pharmacologically but not structurally related to zafirlukast. Montelukast, like zafirlukast, differs chemically and pharmacologically from other currently available antiasthmatic agents (e.g., corticosteroids, mast-cell stabilizers, β-adrenergic agonist bronchodilators, theophylline, zileuton).

Montelukast sodium occurs as a hygroscopic, white to off-white powder. Montelukast sodium has solubilities of 0.2–0.5 mcg/mL in water at 25°C; the drug is freely soluble in alcohol. The apparent pK_as of the drug in water are 2.8 and 5.7.

Montelukast sodium chewable tablets contain aspartame (Nutrasweet®).

Following metabolism of aspartame in the GI tract, each 4- or 5-mg chewable tablet of montelukast provides 0.674 or 0.824 mg of phenylalanine, respectively.

■ **Stability** Commercially available montelukast sodium film-coated and chewable tablets and oral granules should be stored at 25°C and protected from light and moisture with exposure for short periods to temperatures of 15–30°C permitted. When stored as directed, montelukast sodium film-coated and chewable tablets have an expiration date of 2 years after the date of manufacture.

Preparations

Excipients in commercially available drug preparations may have clinically important effects in some individuals; consult specific product labeling for details.

Montelukast Sodium

Oral		
Granules	4 mg (of montelukast)	**Singulair**®, Merck
Tablets, chewable	4 mg (of montelukast)*	**Singulair**®, Merck
	5 mg (of montelukast)*	**Singulair**®, Merck
Tablets, film-coated	10 mg (of montelukast)*	**Singulair**®, Merck

†Use is not currently included in the labeling approved by the US Food and Drug Administration

Selected Revisions January 2013, © Copyright, July 2000, American Society of Health-System Pharmacists, Inc.

CYSTIC FIBROSIS TRANSMEMBRANE CONDUCTANCE REGULATOR MODULATORS 48:14

CYSTIC FIBROSIS TRANSMEMBRANE CONDUCTANCE REGULATOR CORRECTORS 48:14.04

Lumacaftor and Ivacaftor

■ The fixed combination of lumacaftor and ivacaftor contains 2 drugs that act directly on the cystic fibrosis transmembrane conductance regulator (CFTR) protein in bronchial epithelial cells and other cell lines harboring the F508del-CFTR mutation; lumacaftor is a CFTR corrector and ivacaftor is a CFTR potentiator.

Uses

■ **Cystic Fibrosis** Lumacaftor in fixed combination with ivacaftor is used for the treatment of cystic fibrosis in patients who are homozygous for the F508del mutation in the cystic fibrosis transmembrane conductance regulator (CFTR) gene. Lumacaftor and ivacaftor in fixed combination has been designated an orphan drug by the FDA for this use. If the genotype of the patient is unknown, an FDA-approved cystic fibrosis mutation test should be used to detect the presence of the F508del mutation on both alleles of the CFTR gene.

Safety and efficacy of lumacaftor and ivacaftor in fixed combination for the treatment of cystic fibrosis in patients who are homozygous for the F508del mutation in the CFTR gene were evaluated in one randomized, double-blind, placebo-controlled dose-ranging phase 2 study and 2 randomized, double-blind, placebo-controlled phase 3 studies (TRAFFIC and TRANSPORT) in 1108 clinically stable patients with cystic fibrosis. The phase 2 study included patients 18 years of age or older with a baseline forced expiratory volume in 1 second (FEV_1) at least 40% of predicted; 76 patients (homozygous for F508del mutation) were randomized to receive lumacaftor alone (200, 400, or 600 mg once daily or 400 mg every 12 hours) for 28 days followed by the addition of ivacaftor (250 mg every 12 hours) and 27 patients (homozygous or heterozygous for the F508del mutation) were randomized to placebo. During the initial 28-day period, patients receiving lumacaftor monotherapy demonstrated a dose-dependent decrease in percent predicted FEV_1 compared with placebo. Changes in percent predicted FEV_1 from baseline reported after 28 days of lumacaftor monotherapy compared with placebo were 0.24, −1.4, −2.7, or −4.6 for dosages of 200, 400, or 600 mg once daily or 400 mg every 12 hours, respectively. After 56 days of lumacaftor therapy (following the addition of ivacaftor 250 mg every 12 hours for 28 days), the percent predicted FEV_1 changes from baseline compared with placebo were 3.8, 2.7, 5.6, or 4.2, respectively. Sweat chloride concentrations were also assessed in this trial. After 28 days of lumacaftor monotherapy, the changes in sweat chloride concentrations compared with placebo were −4.9, −8.3, −6.1, or −8.2 mmol/L for dosages of 200, 400, or 600 mg once daily or 400 mg every 12 hours, respectively. After 56 days of lumacaftor therapy (following the addition of ivacaftor 250 mg every 12 hours for 28 days), the changes in sweat chloride concentrations from baseline compared with placebo were −5, −9.8, −9.5, or −11 mmol/L, respectively.

The TRAFFIC study evaluated 549 patients 12 years of age or older (mean age: 25 years) with a baseline FEV_1 that was 40–90% of predicted (mean FEV_1: 61% of predicted [range: 31–94%]). The TRANSPORT study evaluated 559 patients 12 years of age or older (mean age: 25 years) with FEV_1 that was 40–90% of predicted (mean FEV_1: 61% of predicted [range: 31–100%]). Patients in both studies were randomized in a 1:1:1 ratio to receive lumacaftor 400 mg every 12 hours combined with ivacaftor 250 mg every 12 hours, lumacaftor 600 mg once daily combined with ivacaftor 250 mg every 12 hours, or placebo with fat-containing food for 24 weeks in addition to existing cystic fibrosis therapies (e.g., bronchodilators, inhaled antibiotics, dornase alfa, hypertonic saline). The primary efficacy end point was the mean absolute change from baseline in the percent predicted FEV_1 at 24 weeks (calculated by the mean treatment effect at weeks 16 and 24). In both studies, treatment with lumacaftor combined with ivacaftor resulted in substantial improvement in FEV_1. The mean absolute change from baseline in the percent predicted FEV_1 at 24 weeks in patients receiving a regimen of lumacaftor 400 mg every 12 hours combined with ivacaftor 250 mg every 12 hours was greater (2.6 and 3 percentage points in the first and second studies, respectively) than in patients receiving placebo. These changes persisted throughout the 24-week treatment period.

Efficacy of lumacaftor in fixed combination with ivacaftor in patients 6–11 years of age is extrapolated from efficacy results in patients 12 years of age or older with support from population pharmacokinetic analyses demonstrating similar drug exposures in patients 6–11 years of age and those 12 years of age or older.

Efficacy and safety of lumacaftor in fixed combination with ivacaftor have *not* been established in patients with cystic fibrosis other than those homozygous for the F508del mutation.

Dosage and Administration

■ **Administration** Lumacaftor in fixed combination with ivacaftor should be administered orally every 12 hours with fat-containing food, such as eggs, avocados, nuts, butter, peanut butter, cheese pizza, or whole milk dairy products. The manufacturer states that systemic absorption of the drug is optimal when the drug is administered with fatty food and that a typical diet recommended for patients with cystic fibrosis will satisfy the requirement for fat-containing food.

■ **Dosage** Lumacaftor in fixed combination with ivacaftor is commercially available as tablets containing 100 mg of lumacaftor and 125 mg of ivacaftor or 200 mg of lumacaftor and 125 mg of ivacaftor.

Cystic Fibrosis For the treatment of cystic fibrosis in patients who are homozygous for the F508del mutation in the cystic fibrosis transmembrane conductance regulator (CFTR) gene, the recommended dosage of lumacaftor in fixed combination with ivacaftor in adults and children 12 years of age or older is lumacaftor 400 mg/ivacaftor 250 mg every 12 hours with fat-containing food. The recommended dosage of lumacaftor in fixed combination with ivacaftor in children 6–11 years of age with cystic fibrosis of this genotype is lumacaftor 200 mg/ivacaftor 250 mg every 12 hours with fat-containing food.

When initiating lumacaftor in fixed combination with ivacaftor in adults and children 12 years of age or older receiving a potent inhibitor of cytochrome P-450 (CYP) isoenzyme 3A (e.g., itraconazole), the recommended dosage of the fixed combination is lumacaftor 200 mg/ivacaftor 125 mg once daily for 1 week, followed by an increase in dosage to lumacaftor 400 mg/ivacaftor 250 mg every 12 hours. When initiating lumacaftor in fixed combination with ivacaftor in children 6–11 years of age receiving a potent inhibitor of CYP3A (e.g., itraconazole), the recommended dosage of the fixed combination is lumacaftor 100 mg/ivacaftor 125 mg once daily for 1 week, followed by an increase in dosage to lumacaftor 200 mg/ivacaftor 250 mg every 12 hours.

If lumacaftor in fixed combination with ivacaftor is interrupted for more than 1 week and then reinitiated in adults and children 12 years of age or older receiving a potent inhibitor of CYP3A, the dosage of the fixed combination should be reduced to lumacaftor 200 mg/ivacaftor 125 mg once daily for 1 week, then increased to the recommended daily dosage of lumacaftor 400 mg/ivacaftor 250 mg every 12 hours. If lumacaftor in fixed combination with ivacaftor is interrupted for more than 1 week and then reinitiated in children 6–11 years of age receiving a potent inhibitor of CYP3A, the dosage of the fixed combination should be reduced to lumacaftor 100 mg/ivacaftor 125 mg once daily for 1 week, then increased to the recommended daily dosage of lumacaftor 200 mg/ivacaftor 250 mg every 12 hours. Dosage adjustment is not needed if a CYP3A inhibitor is initiated in adult or pediatric patients already receiving lumacaftor in fixed combination with ivacaftor.

■ **Special Populations** ***Hepatic Impairment*** Adults and children 12 years of age or older: Dosage adjustment of lumacaftor in fixed combination with ivacaftor is not necessary in patients with mild hepatic impairment (Child-Pugh class A). Dosage of lumacaftor in fixed combination with ivacaftor should be reduced to lumacaftor 400 mg/ivacaftor 250 mg in the morning and lumacaftor 200 mg/ivacaftor 125 mg in the evening in patients with moderate hepatic impairment (Child-Pugh class B). After weighing the risks and benefits of treatment in patients with severe hepatic impairment (Child-Pugh class C), lumacaftor in fixed combination with ivacaftor should be used with caution at a dosage of lumacaftor 200 mg/ivacaftor 125 mg twice daily (in the morning and in the evening) or less.

Children 6–11 years of age: Dosage adjustment of lumacaftor in fixed combination with ivacaftor is not necessary in patients with mild hepatic impairment (Child-Pugh class A). Dosage of lumacaftor in fixed combination with ivacaftor should be reduced to lumacaftor 200 mg/ivacaftor 250 mg in the morning and lumacaftor 100 mg/ivacaftor 125 mg in the evening in patients with moderate hepatic impairment (Child-Pugh class B). After weighing the risks and benefits of treatment in patients with severe hepatic impairment (Child-Pugh class C), lumacaftor in fixed combination with ivacaftor should be used with caution at a dosage of lumacaftor 100 mg/ivacaftor 125 mg twice daily (in the morning and in the evening) or less.

Renal Impairment Dosage adjustment of lumacaftor in fixed combination with ivacaftor is not necessary in patients with mild to moderate renal impairment. Caution is advised if the fixed-combination therapy is used in patients with severe renal impairment or in those with end-stage renal disease (ESRD).

Geriatric Patients The manufacturer makes no specific dosage recommendations for geriatric patients at this time.

Cautions

■ **Contraindications** The manufacturer states that there are no known contraindications to the use of lumacaftor in fixed combination with ivacaftor.

■ **Warnings/Precautions** ***Hepatic Effects*** Worsening hepatic function, including hepatic encephalopathy, in patients with advanced liver disease has been reported in some patients with cystic fibrosis receiving lumacaftor in fixed combination with ivacaftor. Hepatic decompensation, including liver failure leading to death, has been reported in patients with cystic fibrosis and preexisting cirrhosis with portal hypertension who were receiving lumacaftor in fixed combination with ivacaftor. Lumacaftor in fixed combination with ivacaftor should be used with caution in patients with advanced liver disease and should be used only if the benefits are expected to outweigh the risks. If lumacaftor in fixed combination with ivacaftor is used in such patients, the patient should be closely monitored after the initiation of treatment and the dosage should be reduced. (See Hepatic Impairment under Dosage and Administration: Special Populations.)

Serious adverse effects related to elevated aminotransferase (ALT or AST) concentrations, sometimes associated with elevated total serum bilirubin concentrations, have been reported in patients with cystic fibrosis receiving lumacaftor in fixed combination with ivacaftor. In placebo-controlled clinical studies in patients 12 years of age or older, the incidence of maximum aminotransferase concentrations exceeding 8, 5, or 3 times the upper limit of normal (ULN) was similar between patients receiving lumacaftor/ivacaftor fixed-combination therapy and those receiving placebo. Serious adverse hepatic effects occurred in 3 patients receiving lumacaftor in fixed combination with ivacaftor (i.e., 2 patients with elevated aminotransferase concentrations and 1 patient with hepatic encephalopathy); serious adverse hepatic effects were not observed in patients receiving placebo. In an open-label study in patients 6–11 years of age, the incidence of peak aminotransferase concentrations exceeding 8, 5, or 3 times the ULN was 5, 9, or 19%, respectively; administration of lumacaftor in fixed combination with ivacaftor was maintained or resumed after interruption of therapy in all patients with aminotransferase elevations with the exception of one patient who permanently discontinued treatment.

Serum ALT, AST, and bilirubin concentrations should be assessed prior to initiation of therapy with lumacaftor in fixed combination with ivacaftor, every 3 months during the first year of therapy, and annually thereafter. In patients with a history of AST, ALT, or bilirubin elevations, more frequent monitoring should be considered. Patients who develop increased aminotransferase or bilirubin concentrations should be closely monitored until the abnormalities resolve. Lumacaftor/ivacaftor fixed-combination therapy should be interrupted in patients with ALT or AST elevations exceeding 5 times the ULN or in patients with ALT or AST elevations exceeding 3 times the ULN when associated with elevated bilirubin concentrations exceeding 2 times the ULN. Following resolution of aminotransferase elevations, the benefits and risks of resuming lumacaftor/ivacaftor fixed-combination therapy should be considered.

Respiratory Effects Respiratory effects have been reported frequently during therapy with lumacaftor in fixed combination with ivacaftor. In placebo-controlled clinical studies, adverse respiratory effects (e.g., chest discomfort, dyspnea, abnormal respiration) were observed more commonly in patients during initiation of therapy with lumacaftor/ivacaftor fixed-combination therapy compared with those receiving placebo (22 and 14%, respectively). These effects resulted in drug discontinuance and can be serious, especially in patients with advanced lung disease (i.e., those with forced expiratory volume in 1 second [FEV_1] less than 40% of predicted). Clinical experience in patients with FEV_1 less than 40% of predicted is limited. Additional monitoring of such patients is recommended during initiation of lumacaftor/ivacaftor fixed-combination therapy.

Hypertensive Effects Hypertensive effects have been reported during therapy with lumacaftor in fixed combination with ivacaftor. In placebo-controlled clinical studies, increased blood pressure was observed in approximately 1% of patients receiving lumacaftor/ivacaftor fixed-combination therapy compared with no patients receiving placebo. The manufacturer states that blood pressure should be monitored periodically in all patients receiving lumacaftor/ivacaftor fixed-combination therapy.

Interactions with Cytochrome P-450 (CYP) Isoenzyme 3A Substrates and Inducers Lumacaftor is a potent inducer of cytochrome P-450 (CYP) isoenzyme 3A. Concomitant use of lumacaftor in fixed combination with ivacaftor and CYP3A substrates may decrease systemic exposure of such substrate drugs and may decrease therapeutic effect. Therefore, concomitant use of lumacaftor/ivacaftor fixed-combination therapy with sensitive CYP3A substrates or such substrates with a narrow therapeutic index is not recommended.

Concomitant use of lumacaftor/ivacaftor fixed-combination therapy with hormonal contraceptives may substantially decrease systemic exposure of the hormonal contraceptive and result in reduced effectiveness. In placebo-controlled clinical studies, the incidence of menstrual abnormalities (e.g., amenorrhea, dysmenorrhea, menorrhagia, irregular menstrual cycles) was increased in patients receiving hormonal contraceptives concomitantly with lumacaftor/ivacaftor fixed-combination therapy when compared with those not receiving hormonal contraceptives (27 and 3%, respectively). Hormonal contraceptives, including oral, injectable, transdermal, and implantable forms, are not considered a reliable method of contraception when used concomitantly with lumacaftor/ivacaftor fixed-combination therapy. (See Drug Interactions: Estrogens and Progestins.)

Ivacaftor is a substrate of CYP3A4 and 3A5. Concomitant use of lumacaftor/ivacaftor fixed-combination therapy and potent CYP3A inducers (e.g., rifampin, St. John's wort *[Hypericum perforatum]*) substantially decreases systemic exposure of ivacaftor, which may reduce the therapeutic efficacy of lumacaftor/ivacaftor fixed-combination therapy. Therefore, concomitant use of lumacaftor/ivacaftor fixed-combination therapy with potent CYP3A inducers is not recommended. (See Drug Interactions: Drugs Affecting or Metabolized by Hepatic Microsomal Enzymes.)

Ocular Effects Ocular lens opacities (not congenital in nature) have been reported in pediatric patients receiving ivacaftor monotherapy. Although other risk factors were present in some cases (e.g., corticosteroid use, radiation exposure), possible risk attributable to ivacaftor cannot be excluded. Baseline and follow-up ophthalmologic examinations are recommended in pediatric patients receiving lumacaftor/ivacaftor fixed-combination therapy.

Specific Populations **Pregnancy.** Limited data are available regarding use of lumacaftor/ivacaftor fixed-combination therapy or its individual components in pregnant women. Animal reproduction studies using lumacaftor have not revealed evidence of teratogenicity or adverse effects on fetal development in rats and rabbits at exposures approximately 8 and 5 times the maximum recommended human dose, respectively. Similarly, animal reproduction studies using ivacaftor have not revealed evidence of teratogenicity or adverse effects on fetal development in rats and rabbits at exposures 7 and 45 times the maximum recommended human dose, respectively. There are no animal reproduction studies with concomitant use of lumacaftor and ivacaftor. Placental transfer of lumacaftor or ivacaftor has been observed in pregnant rats and rabbits. Lumacaftor in fixed combination with ivacaftor should be used during pregnancy only when clearly needed.

Lactation. Both lumacaftor and ivacaftor are distributed into milk in rats. However, it is not known whether lumacaftor or ivacaftor is distributed into human milk. The developmental and health benefits of breast-feeding and the clinical importance of the therapy to the woman should be considered when deciding whether to use caution or discontinue nursing. The effects of lumacaftor and ivacaftor in fixed combination on nursing infants or on milk production are unknown.

Pediatric Use. Safety and efficacy of lumacaftor/ivacaftor fixed-combination therapy have not been established in pediatric patients younger than 6 years of age.

The safety profile of lumacaftor/ivacaftor fixed-combination therapy in patients 6–11 years of age is similar to that observed in patients 12 years of age or older.

Following oral administration of lumacaftor 400 mg in fixed combination with ivacaftor 250 mg every 12 hours, the mean steady-state area under the concentration-time curves (AUCs) of lumacaftor and ivacaftor were similar in patients 12 to less than 18 years of age when compared with AUCs in adult patients.

Following oral administration of lumacaftor 200 mg in fixed combination with ivacaftor 250 mg every 12 hours in patients 6–11 years of age, the mean steady-state AUCs of lumacaftor and ivacaftor were similar to those observed in patients 12 years of age or older receiving lumacaftor 400 mg in fixed combination with ivacaftor 250 mg every 12 hours.

Geriatric Use. Clinical trials evaluating lumacaftor/ivacaftor fixed-combination therapy did not include sufficient numbers of patients 65 years of age or older to determine whether they respond differently than younger adults; cystic fibrosis is generally a disease of children and young adults.

Hepatic Impairment. Following oral administration of lumacaftor in fixed combination with ivacaftor for 10 days in patients with moderate hepatic impairment (Child-Pugh class B), AUCs and peak plasma concentrations of lumacaftor and ivacaftor were increased by 50 and 30%, respectively, for both drugs when compared with exposures in healthy individuals. The pharmacokinetics of lumacaftor/ivacaftor fixed-combination therapy have not been evaluated in patients with mild or severe hepatic impairment (Child-Pugh class A or C). Systemic exposures of lumacaftor and ivacaftor are expected to be higher in patients with severe hepatic impairment when compared with those in patients with moderate hepatic impairment.

Dosage adjustment of lumacaftor in fixed combination with ivacaftor is not necessary in patients with mild hepatic impairment. Dosage of lumacaftor/ivacaftor fixed-combination therapy should be reduced in patients with moderate hepatic impairment. The risks and benefits of treatment in patients with severe hepatic impairment should be weighed; if a decision is made to initiate lumacaftor/ivacaftor fixed-combination therapy, the therapy should be used with caution at a reduced dosage. (See Hepatic Impairment under Dosage and Administration: Special Populations.)

Renal Impairment. The pharmacokinetics of lumacaftor in fixed combination with ivacaftor have not been evaluated in patients with mild, moderate, or severe renal impairment or in patients with end-stage renal disease (ESRD). Although dosage adjustment of lumacaftor/ivacaftor fixed-combination therapy is not necessary in patients with mild to moderate renal impairment, caution is advised in those with severe renal impairment (i.e., creatinine clearances of 30 mL/minute or less) and those with ESRD.

■ **Common Adverse Effects** Adverse effects occurring in at least 5% of patients receiving lumacaftor/ivacaftor fixed-combination therapy and more frequently than that with placebo include dyspnea, nasopharyngitis, nausea, diarrhea, upper respiratory tract infection, fatigue, abnormal respiration, increased creatine kinase (CK, creatine phosphokinase, CPK) concentrations, rash, flatulence, rhinorrhea, and influenza.

Drug Interactions

■ **Drugs Affecting or Metabolized by Hepatic Microsomal Enzymes** Lumacaftor is a potent inducer of cytochrome P-450 (CYP) isoenzyme 3A; ivacaftor is a CYP3A4 and 3A5 substrate and a weak inhibitor of CYP3A when the single-entity preparation of ivacaftor is used. Concomitant use of lumacaftor and ivacaftor, a sensitive CYP3A substrate, decreased ivacaftor exposure by 80%. The net effect of lumacaftor in fixed combination with ivacaftor on hepatic microsomal enzymes is potent CYP3A induction.

CYP3A Inhibitors Concomitant use of itraconazole, a potent CYP3A inhibitor, and lumacaftor in fixed combination with ivacaftor results in a 4.3-fold increased ivacaftor exposure and does not affect lumacaftor exposure. However, as a result of the induction effect of lumacaftor on CYP3A, the steady-state net exposure of ivacaftor is not expected to exceed the exposure of ivacaftor when the single-entity preparation is used at the recommended dosage. Therefore, dosage adjustment is not necessary when CYP3A inhibitors (e.g., clarithromycin, itraconazole, ketoconazole, posaconazole, telithromycin, voriconazole) are initiated in patients currently receiving lumacaftor/ivacaftor fixed-combination therapy.

However, when initiating lumacaftor/ivacaftor fixed-combination therapy in adults and children 12 years of age or older already receiving potent CYP3A inhibitors, the dosage of lumacaftor/ivacaftor fixed-combination therapy should be reduced to lumacaftor 200 mg/ivacaftor 125 mg once daily for the first week of therapy to allow for the induction effect of lumacaftor to reach steady state. After the first week of therapy, the dosage of lumacaftor/ivacaftor fixed-combination therapy should be increased to the recommended dosage of lumacaftor 400 mg/ivacaftor 250 mg every 12 hours.

If lumacaftor/ivacaftor fixed-combination therapy is initiated in children 6–11 years of age already receiving clarithromycin or telithromycin, the dosage of lumacaftor/ivacaftor fixed-combination therapy should be reduced to lumacaftor 100 mg/ivacaftor 125 mg once daily for the first week of therapy to allow for the induction effect of lumacaftor to reach steady state. After the first week, the dosage of lumacaftor/ivacaftor fixed-combination therapy should be increased to the recommended daily dosage of lumacaftor 200 mg/ivacaftor 250 mg every 12 hours.

If lumacaftor/ivacaftor fixed-combination therapy is interrupted for more than 1 week in adults and children 12 years of age or older and then reinitiated in such a patient receiving a potent inhibitor of CYP3A, the dosage of lumacaftor/ivacaftor fixed-combination therapy should be reduced to lumacaftor 200 mg/ivacaftor 125 mg once daily for 1 week, then increased to the recommended daily dosage of lumacaftor 400 mg/ivacaftor 250 mg every 12 hours.

If lumacaftor/ivacaftor fixed-combination therapy is interrupted for more than 1 week in children 6–11 years of age and then reinitiated in such a patient receiving a potent inhibitor of CYP3A, the dosage of lumacaftor/ivacaftor fixed-combination therapy should be reduced to lumacaftor 100 mg/ivacaftor 125 mg once daily for 1 week, then increased to the recommended daily dosage of lumacaftor 200 mg/ivacaftor 250 mg every 12 hours.

Dosage adjustment is not recommended if lumacaftor/ivacaftor fixed-combination therapy is used concomitantly with moderate or weak CYP3A inhibitors.

CYP3A Inducers Concomitant use of rifampin, a potent CYP3A inducer, and lumacaftor in fixed combination with ivacaftor has minimal effect on lumacaftor exposure and decreases ivacaftor area under the concentration-time curve (AUC) by 57%, which may reduce the therapeutic effect of lumacaftor/ivacaftor fixed-combination therapy. Concomitant use of lumacaftor/ivacaftor fixed-combination therapy and potent CYP3A inducers (e.g., carbamazepine, phenobarbital, phenytoin, rifabutin, rifampin, St. John's wort [*Hypericum perforatum*]) is not recommended. Dosage adjustment is not recommended if lumacaftor/ivacaftor fixed-combination therapy is used concomitantly with moderate or weak CYP3A inducers.

CYP3A Substrates Concomitant use of lumacaftor in fixed combination with ivacaftor and substrates of CYP3A may result in decreased systemic exposure and reduced therapeutic effect of such substrate drugs. Therefore, concomitant use of lumacaftor/ivacaftor fixed-combination therapy with sensitive CYP3A substrates or CYP3A substrates having a narrow therapeutic index is not recommended. Such substrate drugs include certain benzodiazepines (e.g., midazolam, triazolam). If concomitant therapy with benzodiazepines and lumacaftor/ivacaftor in fixed combination is required, alternative therapy to such benzodiazepines should be considered. Immunosuppressive agents (e.g., cyclosporine, everolimus, sirolimus, tacrolimus) also are considered sensitive CYP3A substrates. Data are not available in patients with cystic fibrosis and organ transplants, but the potential for drug interactions exists. The manufacturer states that concomitant use of immunosuppressive drugs with lumacaftor in fixed combination with ivacaftor should be avoided in patients with cystic fibrosis and organ transplants.

Other CYP Substrates In vitro, lumacaftor has shown potential to induce CYP2B6, 2C8, 2C9, and 2C19 and has been shown to inhibit CYP2C8 and 2C9; in vitro, ivacaftor also may inhibit CYP2C9. Concomitant use of lumacaftor/ivacaftor fixed-combination therapy with substrates of CYP2B6, 2C8, 2C9, or 2C19 may alter the exposure of such substrate drugs.

■ **Drugs Affecting or Affected by P-glycoprotein Transport** In vitro, lumacaftor has shown potential to inhibit and induce P-glycoprotein (P-gp) transport. In a clinical study evaluating ivacaftor monotherapy, ivacaftor was shown to be a weak inhibitor of P-gp. Concomitant use of lumacaftor in fixed combination with ivacaftor and substrates of P-gp may alter the exposure of such substrate drugs. If digoxin is used concomitantly with lumacaftor/ivacaftor fixed-combination therapy, serum digoxin concentrations should be monitored and digoxin dosage should be titrated to obtain the desired clinical effect.

■ **Antacids** Dosage adjustment is not necessary if calcium carbonate and lumacaftor/ivacaftor fixed-combination therapy are used concomitantly.

■ **Antibacterial Agents** Dosage adjustment is not necessary if azithromycin, aztreonam, ceftazidime, ciprofloxacin, colistin (commercially available in the US as colistimethate sodium), co-trimoxazole, levofloxacin, or tobramycin is used concomitantly with lumacaftor/ivacaftor fixed-combination therapy.

Macrolide Antibiotics Concomitant use of certain macrolide antibiotics (e.g., clarithromycin, erythromycin, telithromycin) and lumacaftor in fixed combination with ivacaftor may reduce the systemic exposure and therapeutic effect of the macrolide antibiotic. An alternative antibiotic (e.g., azithromycin, ciprofloxacin, levofloxacin) should be considered.

If concomitant use with clarithromycin or telithromycin is required, dosage adjustment is not necessary if such therapy is initiated in patients currently receiving lumacaftor/ivacaftor fixed-combination therapy. However, if lumacaftor/ivacaftor fixed-combination therapy is initiated in adults and children 12 years of age or older already receiving clarithromycin or telithromycin, the dosage of lumacaftor/ivacaftor fixed-combination therapy should be reduced to lumacaftor 200 mg/ivacaftor 125 mg once daily for the first week of therapy to allow for the induction effect of lumacaftor to reach steady state. After the first week, the dosage of lumacaftor/ivacaftor fixed-combination therapy should be increased to the recommended daily dosage of lumacaftor 400 mg/ivacaftor 250 mg every 12 hours.

If lumacaftor/ivacaftor fixed-combination therapy is initiated in children 6–11 years of age already receiving clarithromycin or telithromycin, the dosage of lumacaftor/ivacaftor fixed-combination therapy should be reduced to lumacaftor 100 mg/ivacaftor 125 mg once daily for the first week of therapy to allow for the induction effect of lumacaftor to reach steady state. After the first week, the dosage of lumacaftor/ivacaftor fixed-combination therapy should be increased to the recommended daily dosage of lumacaftor 200 mg/ivacaftor 250 mg every 12 hours.

If lumacaftor/ivacaftor fixed-combination therapy is interrupted for more than 1 week in adults and children 12 years of age or older and then reinitiated in such a patient receiving a potent inhibitor of CYP3A, the dosage of lumacaftor/ivacaftor fixed-combination therapy should be reduced to lumacaftor 200 mg/ivacaftor 125 mg once daily for 1 week, then increased to the recommended daily dosage of lumacaftor 400 mg/ivacaftor 250 mg every 12 hours.

If lumacaftor/ivacaftor fixed-combination therapy is interrupted for more than 1 week in children 6–11 years of age and then reinitiated in such a patient receiving a potent inhibitor of CYP3A, the dosage of lumacaftor/ivacaftor fixed-combination therapy should be reduced to lumacaftor 100 mg/ivacaftor 125 mg once daily for 1 week, then increased to the recommended daily dosage of lumacaftor 200 mg/ivacaftor 250 mg every 12 hours.

■ **Antidiabetic Agents** Concomitant use of repaglinide and lumacaftor in fixed combination with ivacaftor may decrease the exposure of repaglinide. Dosage adjustment of repaglinide may be required to obtain the desired therapeutic effect.

Dosage adjustment is not necessary if metformin is used concomitantly with lumacaftor/ivacaftor fixed-combination therapy.

■ **Antifungal Agents** Concomitant use of certain antifungal agents (e.g., itraconazole, ketoconazole, posaconazole, voriconazole) and lumacaftor in fixed combination with ivacaftor may reduce the systemic exposure and therapeutic effect of the antifungal agent. Concomitant use of these antifungal agents and lumacaftor/ivacaftor fixed-combination therapy is not recommended. An alternative antifungal agent (e.g., fluconazole) should be considered.

If concomitant use of such antifungal agents is required, dosage adjustment is not necessary if such therapy is initiated in patients currently receiving the fixed combination of lumacaftor and ivacaftor.

However, if lumacaftor/ivacaftor fixed-combination therapy is initiated in adults and children 12 years of age or older already receiving certain antifungal agents (e.g., itraconazole, ketoconazole, posaconazole, voriconazole), the dosage of lumacaftor/ivacaftor fixed-combination therapy should be reduced to lumacaftor 200 mg/ivacaftor 125 mg once daily for the first week of therapy to allow for the induction effect of lumacaftor to reach steady state. After the first week, the dosage of lumacaftor/ivacaftor fixed-combination therapy should be increased to the recommended daily dosage of lumacaftor 400 mg/ivacaftor 250 mg every 12 hours.

If lumacaftor/ivacaftor fixed-combination therapy is initiated in children 6–11 years of age already receiving certain antifungal agents (e.g., itraconazole, ketoconazole, posaconazole, voriconazole), the dosage of lumacaftor/ivacaftor fixed-combination therapy should be reduced to lumacaftor 100 mg/ivacaftor 125 mg once daily for the first week of therapy to allow for the induction effect of lumacaftor to reach steady state. After the first week, the dosage of lumacaftor/ivacaftor fixed-combination therapy should be increased to the recommended daily dosage of lumacaftor 200 mg/ivacaftor 250 mg every 12 hours.

If lumacaftor/ivacaftor fixed-combination therapy is interrupted for more than 1 week in adults and children 12 years of age or older and then reinitiated in such a patient receiving a potent inhibitor of CYP3A, the dosage of lumacaftor/ivacaftor fixed-combination therapy should be reduced to lumacaftor 200 mg/ivacaftor 125 mg once daily for 1 week, then increased to the recommended daily dosage of lumacaftor 400 mg/ivacaftor 250 mg every 12 hours. Such patients should be monitored for breakthrough fungal infections.

If lumacaftor/ivacaftor fixed-combination therapy is interrupted for more than 1 week in children 6–11 years of age and then reinitiated in such a patient receiving a potent inhibitor of CYP3A, the dosage of lumacaftor/ivacaftor fixed-combination therapy should be reduced to lumacaftor 100 mg/ivacaftor 125 mg once daily for 1 week, then increased to the recommended daily dosage of lumacaftor 200 mg/ivacaftor 250 mg every 12 hours. Such patients should be monitored for breakthrough fungal infections.

■ **Antimuscarinic Agents** Dosage adjustment is not necessary if ipratropium or tiotropium is used concomitantly with lumacaftor/ivacaftor fixed-combination therapy.

■ **Cetirizine** Dosage adjustment is not necessary if cetirizine is used concomitantly with lumacaftor/ivacaftor fixed-combination therapy.

■ **Corticosteroids** Concomitant use of methylprednisolone or prednisone with lumacaftor in fixed combination with ivacaftor may reduce the systemic exposure and therapeutic effect of the corticosteroid. If used concomitantly with lumacaftor/ivacaftor fixed-combination therapy, an increased dosage of methylprednisolone or prednisone may be needed to obtain the desired clinical effect.

Dosage adjustment is not necessary if budesonide or fluticasone is used concomitantly with lumacaftor/ivacaftor fixed-combination therapy.

■ **Digestive Enzymes** Dosage adjustment is not necessary if pancreatin or pancrelipase is used concomitantly with lumacaftor/ivacaftor fixed-combination therapy.

■ **Dornase Alfa** Dosage adjustment is not necessary if dornase alfa and lumacaftor/ivacaftor fixed-combination therapy are used concomitantly.

■ **Estrogens and Progestins** Concomitant use of hormonal contraceptives and lumacaftor in fixed combination with ivacaftor may reduce the systemic exposure and therapeutic effect of the hormonal contraceptive. In clinical trials, menstrual abnormalities occurred more frequently in patients receiving hormonal contraceptives concomitantly with lumacaftor/ivacaftor fixed-combination therapy than in patients not receiving hormonal contraceptives.

Hormonal contraceptives, including oral, injectable, transdermal, or implantable forms, are not considered reliable methods of contraception when used concomitantly with lumacaftor/ivacaftor fixed-combination therapy; concomitant use should be avoided unless benefits outweigh the risks of concomitant use.

■ **Histamine H_2-receptor Antagonists** Concomitant use of ranitidine and lumacaftor/ivacaftor fixed-combination therapy may alter the exposure of ranitidine. Dosage adjustment of ranitidine may be required to obtain the desired therapeutic effect.

■ **Montelukast** Concomitant use of montelukast and lumacaftor in fixed combination with ivacaftor may reduce the systemic exposure and therapeutic effect of montelukast. Although dosage adjustment is not necessary, the patient should be clinically monitored as appropriate when montelukast is used concomitantly with lumacaftor/ivacaftor fixed-combination therapy.

■ **Nonsteroidal Anti-inflammatory Agents** Concomitant use of ibuprofen and lumacaftor/ivacaftor fixed-combination therapy may reduce the systemic exposure and therapeutic effect of ibuprofen. An increased dosage of ibuprofen may be required to obtain the desired therapeutic effect.

■ **Proton-pump Inhibitors** Concomitant use of proton-pump inhibitors (e.g., esomeprazole, lansoprazole, omeprazole) and lumacaftor/ivacaftor fixed-combination therapy may reduce the exposure and therapeutic effect of the proton-pump inhibitor. Dosage adjustment of the proton-pump inhibitor may be required to obtain the desired therapeutic effect.

■ **Selective β_2-Adrenergic Agonists** Dosage adjustment is not necessary if albuterol or salmeterol is used concomitantly with lumacaftor/ivacaftor fixed-combination therapy.

■ **Selective Serotonin-Reuptake Inhibitors** Concomitant use of certain selective serotonin-reuptake inhibitors (SSRIs), such as citalopram, escitalopram, and sertraline, and lumacaftor/ivacaftor fixed-combination therapy may reduce the systemic exposure and therapeutic effect of the SSRI. An increased dosage of the SSRI may be required to obtain the desired therapeutic effect.

■ **Warfarin** Concomitant use of warfarin and lumacaftor/ivacaftor fixed-combination therapy may alter the systemic exposure of warfarin. If used concomitantly, the international normalized ratio (INR) should be monitored.

Description

The fixed combination of lumacaftor and ivacaftor contains 2 drugs acting directly on the cystic fibrosis transmembrane conductance regulator (CFTR) protein; lumacaftor is a CFTR corrector and ivacaftor is a CFTR potentiator. The CFTR protein is a chloride channel present at the surface of epithelial cells in multiple organs that is involved in salt and fluid transport. Cystic fibrosis is caused by mutations in the gene encoding the CFTR protein that affect the quantity or function of this protein at the cell surface resulting in the clinical manifestations of cystic fibrosis (e.g., GI, hepatic, pulmonary, or reproductive dysfunction or symptoms).

The F508del mutation in the CFTR protein results in protein misfolding, causing a defect in cellular processing and trafficking that targets the protein for degradation and reduces the quantity of CFTR at the cell surface. The small amount of F508del-CFTR that reaches the cell surface is less stable and has low probability for channel opening (defective gating activity) when compared with wild-type CFTR protein. Lumacaftor improves the conformational stability of F508del-CFTR, resulting in increased processing and trafficking of mature protein to the cell surface. Ivacaftor facilitates increased chloride transport by potentiating the probability of channel opening (or gating) of the CFTR protein at the cell surface. In vitro, lumacaftor and ivacaftor demonstrate direct activity on the CFTR protein in primary human bronchial epithelial cultures and other cell lines harboring the F508del-CFTR mutation to increase quantity, stability, and function of F508del-CFTR at the cell surface, resulting in increased chloride ion transport. In vitro responses do not necessarily correspond to in vivo pharmacodynamic response or clinical benefit.

Steady-state concentrations of lumacaftor and ivacaftor are achieved in approximately 7 days after twice-daily administration. As lumacaftor reaches steady state, systemic exposure increases with an accumulation ratio of approximately 1.9; steady-state exposure of ivacaftor is lower than that observed on the first day of administration as a result of cytochrome P-450 (CYP) isoenzyme 3A induction by lumacaftor. Peak plasma concentrations of lumacaftor and ivacaftor are attained approximately 4 hours after a dose administered in the fed state. The area under the concentration-time curve (AUC) of lumacaftor is approximately twofold higher in healthy adults when compared with patients with cystic fibrosis; the AUC of ivacaftor is similar between healthy adults and patients with cystic fibrosis. Following administration of a single dose of the fixed combination of lumacaftor and ivacaftor with fat-containing foods, exposures of lumacaftor and ivacaftor are increased approximately twofold and threefold, respectively, when compared with administration in the fasting state. Both lumacaftor and ivacaftor are extensively bound to plasma proteins (approximately 99%); lumacaftor principally binds to albumin and ivacaftor principally binds to α_1-acid glycoprotein and albumin. Lumacaftor is not extensively metabolized in humans; in vitro and in vivo studies indicate that lumacaftor is principally metabolized by oxidation and glucuronidation. Ivacaftor is extensively metabolized in humans; in vitro and in vivo studies indicate that ivacaftor is principally metabolized by CYP3A. The M1 and M6 metabolites are the 2 major metabolites of ivacaftor in humans. Following oral administration, lumacaftor is mainly excreted unchanged in feces (51%); lumacaftor and its metabolites are minimally excreted in urine (8.6%). Following oral administration of the single-entity preparation of ivacaftor, 87.8% is excreted in feces after metabolic conversion; ivacaftor and its metabolites are minimally excreted in urine (6.6%). The half-life of lumacaftor is approximately 26 hours in patients with cystic fibrosis; the half-life of ivacaftor is approximately 9 hours in healthy individuals.

Advice to Patients

Importance of advising patients to read the manufacturer's patient information.

Importance of taking lumacaftor/ivacaftor in fixed combination with fat-containing food (e.g., butter, cheese pizza, eggs, peanut butter) to increase systemic absorption of the drug.

If a dose of lumacaftor/ivacaftor in fixed combination is missed by less than 6 hours, take the dose with fat-containing food as soon as it is remembered. If a dose is missed by more than 6 hours, omit the dose and take the next dose at the regularly scheduled time. Do *not* take a double dose to make up for a missed dose.

Risk of worsening hepatic function in patients with advanced liver disease. Importance of dosage reduction and close monitoring in such patients after initiation of lumacaftor/ivacaftor in fixed combination.

Importance of dosage reduction in patients with moderate hepatic impairment (Child-Pugh class B). Importance of considering risks and benefits of lumacaftor/ivacaftor in fixed combination in patients with severe hepatic impairment (Child-Pugh class C) prior to initiating therapy; importance of dosage reduction in such patients.

Risk of elevated liver function tests. Importance of monitoring liver function tests prior to initiation of lumacaftor/ivacaftor fixed-combination therapy, every 3 months during the first year of therapy, and annually thereafter.

Risk of respiratory effects (e.g., chest discomfort, dyspnea, abnormal respiration), especially in patients with advanced lung disease. Importance of additional monitoring during initiation of lumacaftor/ivacaftor fixed-combination therapy in patients with forced expiratory volume in 1 second (FEV_1) less than 40% of predicted.

Risk of increased blood pressure. Importance of informing patients that periodic monitoring of blood pressure during therapy is recommended.

Ocular lens opacities (cataracts) observed in some pediatric patients receiving ivacaftor monotherapy. Importance of baseline and follow-up ophthalmologic examination in pediatric patients receiving lumacaftor/ivacaftor fixed-combination therapy.

Importance of informing clinicians of existing or contemplated concomitant therapy, including prescription and OTC drugs, vitamins, and herbal supplements, as well as any concomitant illnesses (e.g., hepatic impairment). Concomitant use of lumacaftor/ivacaftor fixed-combination therapy with sensitive cytochrome P-450 (CYP) isoenzyme 3A substrates, inhibitors, and inducers requires particular attention. (See Drug Interactions.)

Risk of menstrual abnormalities; hormonal contraceptives should not be considered a reliable method of contraception when used concomitantly. Importance of advising patients to use alternative methods of effective contraception.

Importance of women informing clinicians if they are or plan to become pregnant or plan to breast-feed.

Importance of informing patients of other important precautionary information. (See Cautions.)

Overview® (see Users Guide). For additional information on this drug until a more detailed monograph is developed and published, the manufacturer's labeling should be consulted. It is *essential* that the manufacturer's labeling be consulted for more detailed information on usual cautions, precautions, contraindications, potential drug interactions, laboratory test interferences, and acute toxicity.

Preparations

Excipients in commercially available drug preparations may have clinically important effects in some individuals; consult specific product labeling for details.

Lumacaftor and Ivacaftor

Oral		
Tablets, film-coated	Lumacaftor 100 mg and Ivacaftor 125 mg	**Orkambi®**, Vertex
	Lumacaftor 200 mg and Ivacaftor 125 mg	**Orkambi®**, Vertex

Tezacaftor and Ivacaftor

■ The combination of tezacaftor and ivacaftor contains 2 drugs that act directly on the cystic fibrosis transmembrane conductance regulator (CFTR) protein in bronchial epithelial cells and other cell lines harboring certain CFTR mutations; tezacaftor is a CFTR corrector and ivacaftor is a CFTR potentiator.

Uses

■ **Cystic Fibrosis** Tezacaftor in combination with ivacaftor is used for the treatment of cystic fibrosis in patients who are homozygous for the F508del mutation in the cystic fibrosis transmembrane conductance regulator (CFTR) gene or who have at least 1 mutation in the CFTR gene that is responsive to the combination drug regimen based on in vitro data and/or clinical evidence (i.e., E56K, P67L, R74W, D110E, D110H, R117C, E193K, L206W, R347H, R352Q, A455E, D579G, 711+3A→G, E831X, S945L, S977F, F1052V, K1060T, A1067T, R1070W, F1074L, D1152H, D1270N, 2789+5G→A, 3272-26A→G, 3849+10kbC→T). Tezacaftor/ivacaftor combination therapy has been designated an orphan drug by the FDA for this use.

If the genotype of the patient is not known, an FDA-approved cystic fibrosis mutation test should be used to detect the presence of a CFTR mutation followed by verification with bidirectional sequencing when recommended by the mutation test instructions.

Safety and efficacy of tezacaftor/ivacaftor combination therapy were evaluated in 1 double-blind, placebo-controlled phase 2 dose-ranging study and 3 randomized, double-blind, placebo-controlled phase 3 studies (Trial 1 [EVOLVE], Trial 2 [EXPAND], and Trial 3). The phase 2 study included 176 patients 18 years of age or older who were homozygous for F508del mutation and had a baseline forced expiratory volume in 1 second (FEV_1) at least 40% of predicted; 34 patients were randomized to receive tezacaftor alone (10, 30, 100, or 150 mg once daily) and 106 patients were randomized to receive tezacaftor (10, 30, 100, or 150 mg once daily) in combination with ivacaftor 150 mg every 12 hours. During the 28-day treatment period, patients receiving tezacaftor/ivacaftor combination therapy demonstrated a dose-dependent increase in mean percent predicted FEV_1 change from baseline. Tezacaftor/ivacaftor combination therapy generally had a greater mean treatment effect when compared with tezacaftor alone. No additional benefit was observed with tezacaftor dosages exceeding 100 mg daily.

The EVOLVE study evaluated 504 patients with cystic fibrosis 12 years of age or older (mean age: 26.3 years) who were homozygous for F508del mutation. The baseline mean FEV_1 was 60% of predicted (range: 27.8–96.2%). Patients were randomized in a 1:1 ratio to receive tezacaftor 100 mg in fixed combination with ivacaftor 150 mg once daily in the morning and single-entity ivacaftor 150 mg once daily in the evening (approximately 12 hours apart) or placebo for 24 weeks. The primary efficacy end point was the mean absolute change from baseline in the percent predicted FEV_1 at 24 weeks. Results showed that the mean absolute change from baseline in the percent predicted FEV_1 at 24 weeks in patients receiving tezacaftor/ivacaftor combination therapy was 3.4% compared with −0.6% in those receiving placebo. In patients receiving tezacaftor/ivacaftor combination therapy, an increased percent predicted FEV_1 was observed at the first assessment on day 15 of the study and persisted throughout the 24-week treatment period.

The EXPAND study evaluated 244 patients with cystic fibrosis 12 years of age or older (mean age 34.8 years) who were heterozygous for F508del mutation and had a second mutation with a residual CFTR function predicted to be responsive to tezacaftor/ivacaftor combination therapy; 146 patients had a class V noncanonical splice mutation and 98 patients had a missense mutation (e.g., class II to IV residual function mutation) as the second allele. The baseline mean FEV_1 was 62.3% of predicted (range: 34.6–93.5%). Patients were randomized to receive tezacaftor/ivacaftor combination therapy (tezacaftor 100 mg once daily and ivacaftor 150 mg every 12 hours), ivacaftor alone (150 mg every 12 hours), or placebo. The primary efficacy end point was the mean absolute change in the percent predicted FEV_1 from baseline to the average of those measured at 4 and 8 weeks. Overall, the mean absolute change from baseline in the percent predicted FEV_1 (average of values at week 4 and week 8) in patients receiving tezacaftor/ivacaftor combination therapy was 6.8 or 2.1% higher than the mean absolute change in those receiving placebo or ivacaftor alone, respectively; mean absolute change from baseline in those receiving ivacaftor alone was 4.7% higher than the mean absolute change in those receiving placebo. In patients receiving tezacaftor/ivacaftor combination therapy, an increased percent predicted FEV_1 was observed as early as day 15 of therapy and persisted throughout the 8-week treatment period. Substantial improvements were observed in subgroups of patients with splice mutations or missense mutations.

Trial 3 evaluated 168 patients with cystic fibrosis 12 years of age or older (mean age 26.1 years) who were heterozygous for F508del mutation and had a second mutation predicted to be *unresponsive* to tezacaftor/ivacaftor combination therapy. The baseline mean FEV_1 was 57.5% of predicted (range: 31–96.7%). Patients were randomized to receive tezacaftor/ivacaftor combination therapy or placebo. The primary efficacy end point was the mean absolute change from baseline in the percent predicted FEV_1 through week 12. Overall, the mean absolute change from baseline in the percent predicted FEV_1 at 12 weeks in patients receiving tezacaftor/ivacaftor combination therapy was 1.2% higher than the mean absolute change in those receiving placebo. Based on the results at the planned interim analysis, Trial 3 was terminated because the prespecified futility criteria were met.

Dosage and Administration

■ **Administration** Tezacaftor and ivacaftor combination therapy (fixed-combination tablets containing tezacaftor and ivacaftor and single-entity tablets containing ivacaftor) should be administered orally with fat-containing food, such as eggs, cheese, nuts, whole milk, meats, or food prepared with butter or oils.

■ **Dosage** Tezacaftor/ivacaftor combination therapy is commercially available as a kit containing 4 weekly blister cards of 7 tablets containing 100 mg of tezacaftor in fixed combination with 150 mg of ivacaftor copackaged with 7 tablets containing 150 mg of single-entity ivacaftor.

Cystic Fibrosis For the treatment of cystic fibrosis in patients who are homozygous for the F508del mutation in the cystic fibrosis transmembrane conductance regulator (CFTR) gene or have at least 1 mutation in the CFTR that is responsive to tezacaftor/ivacaftor combination therapy, the recommended dosage of tezacaftor/ivacaftor combination therapy in adults and children 12 years of age or older is the fixed combination of tezacaftor 100 mg/ivacaftor 150 mg once daily in the morning and single-entity ivacaftor 150 mg once daily in the evening, approximately 12 hours apart with fat-containing food.

Adults and children 12 years of age or older receiving a moderate inhibitor of cytochrome P-450 (CYP) isoenzyme 3A (e.g., erythromycin, fluconazole) should receive the fixed combination of tezacaftor 100 mg/ivacaftor 150 mg administered once every other day and single-entity ivacaftor 150 mg administered once every other day, given on alternate days in the morning. The evening dose of single-entity ivacaftor 150 mg should not be administered in such patients.

Adults and children 12 years of age or older receiving a potent inhibitor of

CYP3A (e.g., clarithromycin, itraconazole, ketoconazole, posaconazole, telithromycin, voriconazole) should receive the fixed combination of tezacaftor 100 mg/ivacaftor 150 mg twice weekly, approximately 3–4 days apart. The evening dose of single-entity ivacaftor 150 mg should not be administered in such patients.

■ **Special Populations** ***Hepatic Impairment*** Dosage adjustment is not necessary in patients with mild hepatic impairment (Child-Pugh class A).

Patients with moderate hepatic impairment (Child-Pugh class B) should receive the fixed combination of tezacaftor 100 mg/ivacaftor 150 mg once daily in the morning. The evening dose of single-entity ivacaftor 150 mg should not be administered in such patients.

After weighing the risks and benefits of treatment in patients with severe hepatic impairment (Child-Pugh class C), tezacaftor/ivacaftor fixed-combination therapy should be used with caution at a dosage of tezacaftor 100 mg/ivacaftor 150 mg once daily in the morning or less frequently. The evening dose of single-entity ivacaftor 150 mg should not be administered in such patients.

Renal Impairment Dosage adjustment is not necessary in patients with mild or moderate renal impairment. Caution is advised if tezacaftor/ivacaftor combination therapy is used in patients with severe renal impairment or in those with end-stage renal disease (ESRD).

Geriatric Patients The manufacturer makes no specific dosage recommendations for geriatric patients at this time.

Cautions

■ **Contraindications** The manufacturer states that there are no known contraindications to the use of tezacaftor in combination with ivacaftor.

■ **Warnings/Precautions** ***Hepatic Effects*** Elevated aminotransferase (ALT or AST) concentrations have been reported in patients with cystic fibrosis receiving tezacaftor and ivacaftor combination therapy. In placebo-controlled clinical studies in patients 12 years of age or older, the incidence of maximum aminotransferase concentrations exceeding 8, 5, or 3 times the upper limit of normal (ULN) was similar between patients receiving tezacaftor/ivacaftor combination therapy and those receiving placebo. No patients receiving tezacaftor/ivacaftor combination therapy experienced aminotransferase concentrations exceeding 3 times the ULN associated with elevated total bilirubin concentrations exceeding 2 times the ULN.

Serum ALT and AST concentrations should be assessed prior to initiation of tezacaftor/ivacaftor combination therapy, every 3 months during the first year of therapy, and annually thereafter. In patients with a history of AST or ALT elevations, more frequent monitoring should be considered. Patients who develop increased aminotransferase or bilirubin concentrations should be closely monitored until the abnormalities resolve. Tezacaftor/ivacaftor combination therapy should be interrupted in patients with ALT or AST elevations exceeding 5 times the ULN or in those with ALT or AST elevations exceeding 3 times the ULN when associated with elevated bilirubin concentrations exceeding 2 times the ULN. Following resolution of aminotransferase elevations, the benefits and risks of resuming tezacaftor/ivacaftor combination therapy should be considered.

Interactions with Cytochrome P-450 (CYP) Isoenzyme 3A Inducers Tezacaftor and ivacaftor are substrates of cytochrome P-450 (CYP) isoenzymes 3A4 and 3A5. Concomitant use of tezacaftor/ivacaftor combination therapy and potent CYP3A inducers (e.g., rifampin, St. John's wort *[Hypericum perforatum]*) substantially decreases systemic exposure of ivacaftor and may decrease exposure of tezacaftor. Decreased exposures of ivacaftor and tezacaftor may reduce the therapeutic efficacy of the combination therapy. Therefore, concomitant use of tezacaftor/ivacaftor combination therapy with potent CYP3A inducers is not recommended. (See Drug Interactions: Drugs Affecting or Metabolized by Hepatic Microsomal Enzymes.)

Ocular Effects Ocular lens opacities (not congenital in nature) have been reported in pediatric patients receiving tezacaftor/ivacaftor combination therapy or ivacaftor monotherapy. Although other risk factors were present in some cases (e.g., corticosteroid use, radiation exposure), possible risk attributable to tezacaftor/ivacaftor combination therapy cannot be excluded. Baseline and follow-up ophthalmologic examinations are recommended in pediatric patients receiving tezacaftor/ivacaftor combination therapy.

Specific Populations **Pregnancy.** Limited data are available regarding use of tezacaftor/ivacaftor combination therapy or its individual components in pregnant women. Animal reproduction studies using tezacaftor have not revealed evidence of teratogenicity or adverse effects on fetal development in rats and rabbits at exposures approximately 3 and 0.2 times the maximum recommended human dose, respectively. Animal reproduction studies using ivacaftor have not revealed evidence of teratogenicity or adverse effects on fetal development in rats and rabbits at exposures 6 and 16 times the maximum recommended human dose, respectively. There are no animal reproduction studies with concomitant use of tezacaftor and ivacaftor. Placental transfer of tezacaftor has been observed in pregnant rats and placental transfer of ivacaftor has been observed in pregnant rats and rabbits.

Lactation. Both tezacaftor and ivacaftor are distributed into milk in rats. However, it is not known whether tezacaftor or ivacaftor is distributed into human milk. The developmental and health benefits of breast-feeding and the clinical importance of the therapy to the woman should be considered when deciding whether to use caution or discontinue nursing. The effects of tezacaftor and ivacaftor in fixed combination on nursing infants or on milk production are unknown.

Pediatric Use. Safety and efficacy of tezacaftor/ivacaftor combination therapy have not been established in pediatric patients younger than 12 years of age.

Based on population pharmacokinetic analyses, exposures of tezacaftor and ivacaftor in patients 12 to younger than 18 years of age are similar to those observed in adults.

Geriatric Use. Clinical trials evaluating tezacaftor/ivacaftor combination therapy did not include sufficient numbers of patients 65 years of age or older to determine whether they respond differently than younger adults.

Hepatic Impairment. Following oral administration of tezacaftor in combination with ivacaftor for 10 days in individuals with moderate hepatic impairment (Child-Pugh class B), area under the concentration-time curves (AUCs) and peak plasma concentrations of tezacaftor and ivacaftor were increased by 36 and 50%, respectively, when compared with exposures in healthy individuals. In a separate study, individuals with moderate hepatic impairment had a twofold increased AUC compared with that of healthy individuals, but the peak plasma concentrations were similar between the 2 groups. The pharmacokinetics of tezacaftor/ivacaftor combination therapy have not been evaluated in patients with mild or severe hepatic impairment (Child-Pugh class A or C). Systemic exposures of tezacaftor and ivacaftor are expected to be higher in patients with severe hepatic impairment when compared with those in patients with moderate hepatic impairment.

Dosage adjustment of tezacaftor/ivacaftor combination therapy is not necessary in patients with mild hepatic impairment. Dosage of tezacaftor/ivacaftor combination therapy should be reduced in patients with moderate hepatic impairment. The risks and benefits of treatment in patients with severe hepatic impairment should be weighed; if a decision is made to initiate tezacaftor/ivacaftor combination therapy, the therapy should be used with caution at a reduced dosage. (See Hepatic Impairment under Dosage and Administration: Special Populations.)

Renal Impairment. The pharmacokinetics of tezacaftor in combination with ivacaftor have not been evaluated in patients with moderate or severe renal impairment or in those with end-stage renal disease (ESRD). Population pharmacokinetic data indicate that mild or moderate renal impairment does not substantially affect the clearance of tezacaftor. Tezacaftor, ivacaftor, and their metabolites are minimally eliminated into urine.

Although dosage adjustment of tezacaftor/ivacaftor combination therapy is not necessary in patients with mild or moderate renal impairment, caution is advised in those with severe renal impairment (i.e., creatinine clearances of 30 mL/minute or less) and those with ESRD.

■ **Common Adverse Effects** Adverse effects occurring in at least 3% of patients receiving tezacaftor/ivacaftor combination therapy and more frequently than that with placebo include headache, nausea, nasopharyngitis, increased sputum production, sinus congestion, diarrhea, dizziness, and increased creatine kinase (CK, creatine phosphokinase, CPK) concentrations.

Drug Interactions

■ **Drugs Affecting or Metabolized by Hepatic Microsomal Enzymes** Tezacaftor is a substrate of cytochrome P-450 (CYP) 3A isoenzymes (e.g., CYP3A4, 3A5) and ivacaftor is a sensitive substrate of CYP3A isoenzymes.

Concomitant use of rifampin (600 mg once daily), a potent CYP3A inducer, and ivacaftor (single 150-mg dose) decreases ivacaftor area under the concentration-time curve (AUC) by 89%. Concomitant use of a potent CYP3A inducer is expected to substantially decrease tezacaftor exposure. Concomitant use of tezacaftor/ivacaftor combination therapy and potent CYP3A inducers (e.g., carbamazepine, phenobarbital, phenytoin, rifabutin, rifampin, St. John's wort *[Hypericum perforatum]*) may result in decreased tezacaftor and ivacaftor exposures resulting in reduced efficacy. Therefore, concomitant use is not recommended.

Concomitant use of itraconazole (200 mg twice daily on day 1, then 200 mg once daily), a potent CYP3A inhibitor, and tezacaftor in fixed combination with ivacaftor (tezacaftor 25 mg/ivacaftor 50 mg once daily) results in 4- and 15.6-fold increases in the AUCs of tezacaftor and ivacaftor, respectively. Concomitant use of fluconazole (400 mg on day 1, then 200 mg once daily), a moderate CYP3A inhibitor, and ivacaftor 150 mg twice daily results in a threefold increase in the AUC of ivacaftor; concomitant use of fluconazole and tezacaftor may increase tezacaftor exposure approximately twofold. If tezacaftor/ivacaftor combination therapy is used concomitantly with a potent CYP3A inhibitor (e.g., clarithromycin, itraconazole, ketoconazole, posaconazole, telithromycin, voriconazole), the dosage of tezacaftor/ivacaftor combination therapy should be reduced to tezacaftor 100 mg/ivacaftor 150 mg twice weekly, approximately 3–4 days apart. The evening dose of single-entity ivacaftor 150 mg should not be administered. If tezacaftor/ivacaftor combination therapy is used concomitantly with a moderate CYP3A inhibitor (e.g., erythromycin, fluconazole), the dosage should be reduced to tezacaftor 100 mg/ivacaftor 150 mg once every other day in combination with single-entity ivacaftor 150 mg once every other day, given on alternate days.

In vitro, tezacaftor has shown low potential to inhibit CYP3A4 and to induce CYP3A. In vitro, ivacaftor has shown potential to inhibit CYP3A. Concomitant use of oral midazolam, a sensitive CYP3A substrate, and tezacaftor/

ivacaftor combination therapy does not affect midazolam exposures. Dosage adjustment is not necessary if CYP3A substrates are used concomitantly with tezacaftor/ivacaftor combination therapy.

In vitro, tezacaftor has shown low potential to inhibit CYP1A2, 2B6, 2C8, 2C9, 2C19, and 2D6; the drug does not induce CYP1A2 or 2B6. In vitro, ivacaftor may inhibit CYP2C9; the drug does not induce CYP isoenzymes. Concomitant use of rosiglitazone, a CYP2C8 substrate, and ivacaftor alone does not affect the exposure of rosiglitazone. Concomitant use of desipramine, a CYP2D6 substrate, and ivacaftor does not affect the exposure of desipramine.

■ Drugs Affecting or Affected by P-glycoprotein Transport

Tezacaftor is a substrate for P-glycoprotein (P-gp) transport; ivacaftor is not a P-gp substrate. In vitro, ivacaftor has shown potential to inhibit P-gp; tezacaftor has shown low potential to inhibit P-gp.

Concomitant use of digoxin (single 0.5-mg dose), a sensitive P-gp substrate, and tezacaftor/ivacaftor combination therapy (tezacaftor 100 mg/ivacaftor 150 mg every morning and ivacaftor 150 mg every evening) results in a 1.3-fold increased digoxin AUC, which is consistent with weak inhibition of P-gp by ivacaftor. Concomitant use of tezacaftor/ivacaftor combination therapy and substrates of P-gp may increase the exposure, prolong therapeutic effect, or increase risk of adverse effects of such substrate drugs. P-gp substrates with a narrow therapeutic index (e.g., cyclosporine, digoxin, everolimus, sirolimus, tacrolimus) and tezacaftor/ivacaftor combination therapy should be used concomitantly with caution and patients should be appropriately monitored.

■ Drugs Affecting or Affected by Other Membrane Transporters

In vitro, tezacaftor is a substrate of breast cancer resistance protein (BCRP) and organic anion transporting polypeptide (OATP) 1B1. Tezacaftor is not a substrate of OATP1B3. Ivacaftor is not a substrate of OATP1B1 or 1B3.

In vitro, tezacaftor has shown low potential to inhibit BCRP, OATP1B1, OATP1B3, organic cation transporter (OCT) 2, organic anion transporter (OAT) 1, and OAT3. Ivacaftor does not inhibit OATP1B1, OATP1B3, OCT1, OCT2, OAT1, or OAT3.

■ Ciprofloxacin Concomitant use of ciprofloxacin and tezacaftor/ivacaftor combination therapy does not have a clinically important effect on tezacaftor or ivacaftor exposures. Therefore, dosage adjustment is not necessary if ciprofloxacin is used concomitantly with tezacaftor/ivacaftor combination therapy.

■ Estrogens and Progestins Concomitant use of ethinyl estradiol and norethindrone and tezacaftor/ivacaftor combination therapy does not substantially affect exposures of ethinyl estradiol, norethindrone, tezacaftor, or ivacaftor. Concomitant use of tezacaftor/ivacaftor combination therapy and hormonal contraceptives is not expected to affect the efficacy of the hormonal contraceptive.

■ Grapefruit and Seville Oranges Concomitant use of tezacaftor/ivacaftor combination therapy with grapefruit products or Seville oranges, which contain components that are moderate CYP3A inhibitors, may increase tezacaftor and ivacaftor exposures. Therefore, concomitant use with such therapy should be avoided.

Description

The combination of tezacaftor and ivacaftor contains 2 drugs acting directly on the cystic fibrosis transmembrane conductance regulator (CFTR) protein; tezacaftor is a CFTR corrector and ivacaftor is a CFTR potentiator.

The CFTR protein is a chloride channel present at the surface of epithelial cells in multiple organs that is involved in salt and fluid transport. Cystic fibrosis, an autosomal recessive disease, is caused by mutations in the CFTR gene resulting in the lack of a properly functioning CFTR protein. The most common CFTR gene mutation is F508del, which results in CFTR protein misfolding, causing a defect in cellular processing and trafficking that targets the protein for degradation and reduces the quantity of CFTR at the cell surface. Other types of CFTR gene mutations result in protein dysfunction by a variety of mechanisms including defective protein synthesis, gating functions, or channel conductance. Tezacaftor facilitates processing and trafficking of normal and select mutant forms of CFTR protein to the cell surface. Ivacaftor facilitates increased chloride transport by potentiating the probability of channel opening (or gating) of the CFTR protein at the cell surface. The combined effect of tezacaftor and ivacaftor increases the quantity and function of CFTR at the cell surface, resulting in increased chloride transport.

In vitro, tezacaftor/ivacaftor combination therapy increased chloride transport by at least 10% compared with baseline in Fisher rat thyroid (FRT) cells expressing certain CFTR mutations. In phase 2 and phase 3 clinical studies, tezacaftor/ivacaftor combination therapy improved lung function and decreased sweat chloride concentrations in patients who were homozygous or heterozygous for F508del mutation. Based on these results, patients are expected to be responsive to tezacaftor/ivacaftor combination therapy if they possess a homozygous CFTR genotype with the F508del mutation or if they have at least 1 copy of a responsive CFTR mutation (i.e., E56K, P67L, R74W, D110E, D110H, R117C, E193K, L206W, R347H, R352Q, A455E, D579G, 711+3A→G, E831X, S945L, S977F, F1052V, K1060T, A1067T, R1070W, F1074L, D1152H, D1270N, 2789+5G→A, 3272-26A→G, 3849+10kbC→T). With the exception of the homozygous F508del genotype, CFTR gene mutations not responsive to ivacaftor monotherapy are not expected to respond to tezacaftor/ivacaftor combination therapy.

The pharmacokinetics of tezacaftor and ivacaftor are similar between healthy adults and patients with cystic fibrosis. Steady-state concentrations of tezacaftor (once daily) and ivacaftor (twice daily) are achieved within 8 and 3–5 days, respectively. As tezacaftor and ivacaftor reach steady state, systemic exposure increases with an accumulation ratio of approximately 1.5 and 2.2, respectively. Following administration of tezacaftor 100 mg once daily and ivacaftor 150 mg twice daily in the fed state, peak plasma concentrations are attained at approximately 4 and 6 hours, respectively. Following administration of a single dose of the fixed combination of tezacaftor and ivacaftor with fat-containing foods, exposure of tezacaftor is similar to that observed with administration in the fasting state and exposure of ivacaftor is increased approximately threefold when compared with administration in the fasting state. Both tezacaftor and ivacaftor are extensively bound to plasma proteins (approximately 99%); tezacaftor principally binds to albumin and ivacaftor principally binds to α_1-acid glycoprotein and albumin. Tezacaftor and ivacaftor are extensively metabolized principally by CYP3A4 and 3A5. Tezacaftor has 3 major circulating metabolites, M1, M2, and M5; M1 has similar potency to the parent drug and is pharmacologically active, M2 has less pharmacologic activity than M1, and M5 is an inactive metabolite. M3 is a minor metabolite of tezacaftor resulting from direct glucuronidation of the parent drug. Ivacaftor has 2 major metabolites, M1 and M6; M1 has approximately one-sixth the potency of ivacaftor and M6 is an inactive metabolite. Following oral administration, tezacaftor is mainly excreted in feces (72% as unchanged drug or the M2 metabolite); 14% of a dose is excreted in urine (mainly as the M2 metabolite). Following oral administration of the single-entity preparation of ivacaftor, 87.8% is excreted in feces after metabolic conversion; ivacaftor and its metabolites are minimally excreted in urine (6.6%). The half-lives of tezacaftor and ivacaftor in patients with cystic fibrosis are 15 and 13.7 hours, respectively.

Advice to Patients

Importance of advising patients to read the manufacturer's patient information.

Importance of taking tezacaftor/ivacaftor combination therapy with fat-containing food (e.g., eggs, butter, peanut butter, cheese pizza, whole milk dairy products) to increase systemic absorption of the drug.

If a dose of tezacaftor/ivacaftor combination therapy is missed by 6 hours or less, take the dose with fat-containing food as soon as it is remembered. If a dose is missed by more than 6 hours, omit the dose and take the next dose at the regularly scheduled time. Do *not* take a double dose to make up for a missed dose.

Importance of dosage reduction in patients with moderate hepatic impairment (Child-Pugh class B). Importance of considering risks and benefits of tezacaftor/ivacaftor combination therapy in patients with severe hepatic impairment (Child-Pugh class C) prior to initiating therapy; importance of dosage reduction in such patients.

Risk of elevated liver function test results. Importance of monitoring liver function tests prior to initiation of tezacaftor/ivacaftor combination therapy, every 3 months during the first year of therapy, and annually thereafter.

Ocular lens opacities (cataracts) observed in some pediatric patients. Importance of baseline and follow-up ophthalmologic examinations in pediatric patients receiving tezacaftor/ivacaftor combination therapy.

Importance of informing clinicians of existing or contemplated concomitant therapy, including prescription and OTC drugs, vitamins, and herbal supplements, as well as any concomitant illnesses (e.g., hepatic impairment). Concomitant use of tezacaftor/ivacaftor combination therapy with sensitive cytochrome P-450 (CYP) isoenzyme 3A inhibitors and inducers requires particular attention. (See Drug Interactions.)

Importance of women informing clinicians if they are or plan to become pregnant or plan to breast-feed.

Importance of informing patients of other important precautionary information. (See Cautions.)

Overview® (see Users Guide). For additional information on this drug until a more detailed monograph is developed and published, the manufacturer's labeling should be consulted. It is *essential* that the manufacturer's labeling be consulted for more detailed information on usual cautions, precautions, contraindications, potential drug interactions, laboratory test interferences, and acute toxicity.

Preparations

Excipients in commercially available drug preparations may have clinically important effects in some individuals; consult specific product labeling for details.

Tezacaftor and Ivacaftor

Oral

Kit	Tezacaftor 100 mg and Ivacaftor 150 mg (28 film-coated tablets) Ivacaftor 150 mg (28 film-coated tablets)	**Symdeko®** (available as blister cards containing 7 fixed-combination tablets and 7 single-entity tablets), Vertex

CYSTIC FIBROSIS TRANSMEMBRANE CONDUCTANCE REGULATOR POTENTIATORS 48:14.12

Ivacaftor

■ Ivacaftor is a cystic fibrosis transmembrane conductance regulator (CFTR) potentiator.

Uses

■ **Cystic Fibrosis** Ivacaftor is used for the treatment of cystic fibrosis in patients with a G551D mutation in the cystic fibrosis transmembrane conductance regulator (CFTR) gene. Ivacaftor has been designated an orphan drug by the US Food and Drug Administration (FDA) for this use. If the genotype of the patient is unknown, an FDA-approved cystic fibrosis mutation test should be used to detect the presence of the G551D mutation.

Safety and efficacy of ivacaftor for the treatment of cystic fibrosis in patients with a G551D mutation in the CFTR gene were evaluated in 2 randomized, double-blind, placebo-controlled studies in 213 clinically stable patients with cystic fibrosis having at least one copy of the G551D mutation in the CFTR gene. The first study evaluated 161 patients 12 years of age or older (mean age: 26 years) with a baseline forced expiratory volume in 1 second (FEV_1) that was 40–90% of predicted (mean FEV_1: 64% of predicted [range: 32–98%]). The second study evaluated 52 pediatric patients 6–11 years of age (mean age: 9 years) with a baseline FEV_1 that was 40–105% of predicted (mean FEV_1: 84% of predicted [range: 44–134%]). Patients in both studies were randomized to receive ivacaftor (150 mg every 12 hours) or placebo with fat-containing food for 48 weeks in addition to existing cystic fibrosis therapies (e.g., dornase alfa, tobramycin); the use of inhaled hypertonic saline was not permitted. In both studies, treatment with ivacaftor resulted in substantial improvement in FEV_1. The mean absolute change from baseline in percent predicted FEV_1 at 24 weeks (primary efficacy endpoint) was greater with ivacaftor than placebo by 10.6 and 12.5 percentage points in the first and second studies, respectively; these changes persisted through 48 weeks. Patients receiving ivacaftor also demonstrated improvements in secondary endpoints (e.g., risk of pulmonary exacerbations, symptoms of cystic fibrosis, gain in body weight).

Ivacaftor is not effective in patients with cystic fibrosis who are homozygous for the F508del mutation in the CFTR gene. The F508del mutation in the CFTR gene is the most common mutation causing cystic fibrosis, and patients homozygous for this mutation account for about 50% of the population with this disease. In a 16-week, randomized, double-blind, placebo-controlled study in 140 patients 12 years of age or older with cystic fibrosis who were homozygous for the F508del mutation in the CFTR gene and had an FEV_1 at least 40% of predicted, ivacaftor (150 mg every 12 hours) did not improve lung function (as determined by the mean absolute change from baseline in percent predicted FEV_1 at 16 weeks [primary efficacy endpoint]) compared with placebo. In addition, there were no clinically important differences in secondary endpoints (e.g., sweat chloride concentration, symptoms of cystic fibrosis, weight change) in patients receiving ivacaftor compared with those receiving placebo.

Ivacaftor has not been studied in other patient populations with cystic fibrosis.

Dosage and Administration

■ **Administration** Ivacaftor is administered orally every 12 hours with fat-containing food, such as butter, cheese pizza, eggs, or peanut butter. The manufacturer states that systemic absorption of the drug is optimal when the drug is administered with fatty food and that a typical diet recommended for patients with cystic fibrosis will satisfy the requirement for fat-containing food.

■ **Dosage** For the treatment of cystic fibrosis in patients who have a G551D mutation in the cystic fibrosis transmembrane conductance regulator (CFTR) gene, the recommended dosage of orally inhaled ivacaftor in adults and children 6 years of age or older is 150 mg every 12 hours (total daily dosage of 300 mg) with fat-containing food.

When ivacaftor is used concomitantly with potent inhibitors of cytochrome P-450 (CYP) isoenzyme 3A (e.g., clarithromycin, itraconazole, ketoconazole, posaconazole, telithromycin, voriconazole), dosage of orally inhaled ivacaftor should be reduced to 150 mg twice weekly. When ivacaftor is used concomitantly with moderate CYP3A inhibitors (e.g., erythromycin, fluconazole), dosage of ivacaftor should be reduced to 150 mg once daily. Grapefruit juice and food containing grapefruit or Seville oranges (e.g., orange marmalade) should be avoided during ivacaftor therapy. Concomitant use of ivacaftor with potent CYP3A inducers (e.g., carbamazepine, phenobarbital, phenytoin, rifabutin, rifampin, St. John's wort [*Hypericum perforatum*]) is not recommended. (See Drug Interactions.)

■ **Special Populations** Dosage adjustment of ivacaftor is not necessary in patients with mild hepatic impairment (Child-Pugh class A). Dosage of orally inhaled ivacaftor should be reduced to 150 mg once daily in patients with moderate hepatic impairment (Child-Pugh class B, score 7–9). Ivacaftor should be used with caution and at a dosage of 150 mg once daily or less frequently in patients with severe hepatic impairment (Child-Pugh class C, score 10–15) after weighing the risks and benefits of treatment. (See Hepatic Impairment under Warnings/Precautions: Specific Populations, in Cautions.)

Dosage adjustment of ivacaftor is not necessary in patients with mild or moderate renal impairment. However, caution is recommended when using ivacaftor in patients with severe renal impairment (creatinine clearance of 30 mL/minute or less) or in those with end-stage renal disease (ESRD). (See Renal Impairment under Warnings/Precautions: Specific Populations, in Cautions.)

The manufacturer makes no specific dosage recommendations for geriatric patients. (See Geriatric Use under Warnings/Precautions: Specific Populations, in Cautions.)

Dosage adjustment of ivacaftor is not necessary based on gender.

Cautions

■ **Contraindications** The manufacturer states that there are no known contraindications to the use of ivacaftor.

■ **Warnings/Precautions** ***Hepatic Effects*** Elevated aminotransferase (ALT [SGPT] or AST [SGOT]) concentrations have been reported in patients with cystic fibrosis receiving ivacaftor. In placebo-controlled clinical studies of 48 weeks' duration, the incidence of maximum aminotransferase (ALT or AST) concentrations exceeding 8, 5, or 3 times the upper limit of normal (ULN) was 2, 3, and 6%, respectively, in patients receiving ivacaftor and 2, 2, and 8%, respectively, in those receiving placebo. Treatment was permanently discontinued as a result of elevated aminotransferase concentrations in 0.5 or 2% of patients receiving ivacaftor or placebo, respectively; aminotransferase concentrations exceeded 8 times the ULN in these patients. Serious adverse hepatic effects from elevated aminotransferase concentrations occurred in at least 2 patients receiving ivacaftor compared with none of those receiving placebo.

Serum ALT and AST concentrations should be assessed prior to initiation of ivacaftor therapy, every 3 months during the first year of therapy, and annually thereafter. Patients who develop increased aminotransferase concentrations should be closely monitored until the abnormalities resolve. Ivacaftor therapy should be interrupted in patients with ALT or AST elevations exceeding 5 times the ULN. Following resolution of aminotransferase elevations, the benefits and risks of resuming ivacaftor therapy should be considered.

Interactions with Cytochrome P-450 (CYP) Isoenzyme 3A Inducers Concomitant use of ivacaftor with potent CYP3A inducers, such as rifampin, substantially decreases systemic exposure of ivacaftor, which may reduce the therapeutic efficacy of ivacaftor. Therefore, concomitant use of ivacaftor with potent CYP3A inducers (e.g., carbamazepine, phenobarbital, phenytoin, rifabutin, rifampin, and St. John's wort [*Hypericum perforatum*]) is not recommended. (See Drug Interactions.)

Specific Populations **Pregnancy.** Category B. (See Users Guide.)

Lactation. Ivacaftor is distributed into milk in rats. Ivacaftor is likely distributed into human milk. Caution is advised if ivacaftor is administered in nursing women.

Pediatric Use. Safety and efficacy of ivacaftor in pediatric patients 6–17 years of age with cystic fibrosis having a G551D mutation in the cystic fibrosis transmembrane conductance regulator (CFTR) gene have been established in 2 placebo-controlled clinical studies; one study evaluated 161 patients 12 years of age or older and the other study evaluated 52 patients 6–11 years of age. (See Uses: Cystic Fibrosis.)

Safety and efficacy of ivacaftor have not been established in pediatric patients younger than 6 years of age.

Geriatric Use. Clinical studies of ivacaftor did not include sufficient numbers of patients 65 years of age or older to determine whether geriatric patients respond differently than younger patients; cystic fibrosis is generally a disease of children and young adults.

Hepatic Impairment. The effect of mild hepatic impairment (Child-Pugh class A) on the pharmacokinetics of ivacaftor has not been studied; however, the increase in the area under the serum concentration-time curve (AUC) of ivacaftor is expected to be less than twofold. Therefore, dosage adjustment of ivacaftor is not necessary in patients with mild hepatic impairment.

Patients with moderate hepatic impairment (Child-Pugh class B, score 7–9) had similar ivacaftor peak plasma concentrations, but had an approximately twofold increase in ivacaftor AUC, compared with healthy individuals matched for demographics. Therefore, dosage of ivacaftor should be reduced in patients with moderate hepatic impairment. (See Dosage and Administration: Special Populations.)

The effect of severe hepatic impairment (Child-Pugh class C, score 10–15) on the pharmacokinetics of ivacaftor has not been studied. The magnitude of increase in systemic exposure to the drug in patients with severe hepatic impairment is unknown, but is expected to be substantially higher than that observed in patients with moderate hepatic impairment. Therefore, ivacaftor should be used with caution and at a reduced dosage in patients with severe hepatic impairment after weighing the risks and benefits of treatment. (See Dosage and Administration: Special Populations.)

Renal Impairment. Ivacaftor has not been studied in patients with mild, moderate, or severe renal impairment or in patients with end-stage renal disease (ESRD). Dosage adjustment of ivacaftor is not necessary in patients with mild or moderate renal impairment because ivacaftor and its metabolites are minimally excreted in urine. (See Description.) However, caution is recommended when using ivacaftor in patients with severe renal impairment (i.e., creatinine clearance of 30 mL/minute or less) or in those with ESRD.

■ **Common Adverse Effects** Adverse effects reported in 8% or more of patients receiving ivacaftor and more frequently than placebo include headache, oropharyngeal pain, upper respiratory tract infection, nasal congestion, abdominal pain, nasopharyngitis, diarrhea, rash, nausea, and dizziness.

Drug Interactions

In vitro and clinical studies indicate that ivacaftor is principally metabolized by cytochrome P-450 (CYP) isoenzyme 3A. In vitro studies show that ivacaftor and its M1 metabolite are substrates of CYP3A (i.e., 3A4, 3A5). In vitro studies also show that ivacaftor is a weak inhibitor of CYP3A, has the potential to inhibit P-glycoprotein (P-gp) at therapeutic concentrations, and may also inhibit CYP2C8 and 2C9. The M1 metabolite, but not M6, also has the potential to inhibit CYP3A and P-gp. Ivacaftor and the M1 and M6 metabolites are not inducers of CYP isoenzymes. (See Description.)

■ **Drugs or Foods Affecting Hepatic Microsomal Enzymes** Concomitant administration of ivacaftor with ketoconazole, a potent CYP3A inhibitor, substantially increased systemic exposure (i.e., area under the serum concentration-time curve [AUC]) of ivacaftor by 8.5-fold. Therefore, dosage of ivacaftor should be reduced to 150 mg twice weekly when ivacaftor is used concomitantly with potent CYP3A inhibitors, such as clarithromycin, itraconazole, ketoconazole, posaconazole, telithromycin, and voriconazole.

Concomitant administration of ivacaftor with fluconazole, a moderate CYP3A inhibitor, increased systemic exposure (i.e., AUC) of ivacaftor by threefold. Therefore, dosage of ivacaftor should be reduced to 150 mg once daily when ivacaftor is used concomitantly with moderate CYP3A inhibitors, such as erythromycin and fluconazole.

Concomitant administration of ivacaftor with grapefruit juice may increase systemic exposure of ivacaftor. Grapefruit juice and Seville oranges contain one or more components that moderately inhibit CYP3A. Therefore, grapefruit juice or food containing grapefruit or Seville oranges (e.g., orange marmalade) should be avoided during ivacaftor therapy.

Concomitant administration of ivacaftor with rifampin, a potent CYP3A inducer, substantially decreased systemic exposure (i.e., AUC) of ivacaftor by ninefold, which may reduce the therapeutic efficacy of ivacaftor. Therefore, concomitant use of ivacaftor with potent CYP3A inducers, such as carbamazepine, phenobarbital, phenytoin, rifabutin, rifampin, and St. John's wort (*Hypericum perforatum*), is not recommended.

■ **Drugs Metabolized by Hepatic Microsomal Enzymes and/or P-glycoprotein (P-gp) Transport System** Concomitant administration of ivacaftor with midazolam, a sensitive CYP3A substrate, increased systemic exposure (i.e., AUC) of midazolam by 1.5-fold, consistent with weak inhibition of CYP3A by ivacaftor. Therefore, caution is advised and adequate monitoring for benzodiazepine-related adverse effects (e.g., prolonged or increased sedation or respiratory depression) is recommended when ivacaftor is used concomitantly with alprazolam, diazepam, midazolam, or triazolam.

Concomitant administration of ivacaftor may increase systemic exposure of drugs that are substrates of CYP3A and/or P-gp (e.g., cyclosporine, digoxin, tacrolimus) potentially increasing or prolonging the therapeutic and adverse effects of the substrate. Therefore, caution is advised and appropriate monitoring is recommended (e.g., serum concentrations for digoxin, prolonged or increased immunosuppression for cyclosporine and tacrolimus) when ivacaftor is used concomitantly with CYP3A and/or P-gp substrates.

Concomitant administration of ivacaftor with oral contraceptives containing ethinyl estradiol and norethindrone, which are less sensitive CYP3A substrates, did not affect systemic exposures of ivacaftor or its M1 or M6 metabolites, ethinyl estradiol, or norethindrone. Therefore, dosage adjustment of ivacaftor or the oral contraceptives is not recommended when used concomitantly.

Concomitant administration of ivacaftor with rosiglitazone, a CYP2C8 substrate, did not substantially affect systemic exposure of rosiglitazone. Therefore, dosage adjustment of rosiglitazone is not recommended when used concomitantly with ivacaftor.

Concomitant administration of ivacaftor with warfarin, a CYP2C9 substrate, may increase the systemic exposure of warfarin. Because ivacaftor has the potential to inhibit CYP2C9, monitoring is recommended (e.g., international normalized ratio [INR]) when concomitant administration of ivacaftor with warfarin is required.

Concomitant administration of ivacaftor with desipramine, a CYP2D6 substrate, did not affect systemic exposure of desipramine. Therefore, no dosage adjustment of desipramine is recommended when used concomitantly with ivacaftor.

Description

Ivacaftor is a potentiator of the cystic fibrosis transmembrane conductance regulator (CFTR) protein. The CFTR protein is a chloride channel present at the surface of epithelial cells in multiple organs that is involved in salt and fluid transport. Cystic fibrosis is caused by mutations in the gene encoding the CFTR protein that affect the quantity or function of this protein at the cell surface resulting in the clinical manifestations of cystic fibrosis (e.g., endocrine, GI, hepatic, pulmonary, or reproductive dysfunction or symptoms). In patients with the G551D mutation in the CFTR protein, the mutated protein reaches the cell surface, but does not activate normally resulting in a low probability of channel opening and defective chloride transport. Ivacaftor facilitates increased chloride transport by potentiating the probability of channel opening (or gating) of the G551D-CFTR protein.

The systemic exposure of ivacaftor is increased approximately twofold to fourfold when administered with food containing fat; therefore, ivacaftor should be administered with fat-containing food (e.g., butter, cheese pizza, eggs, peanut butter). Ivacaftor is extensively metabolized in humans. In vitro and clinical studies indicate that ivacaftor is principally metabolized by cytochrome P-450 (CYP) isoenzyme 3A. The M1 and M6 metabolites are the two major metabolites of ivacaftor in humans. The M1 metabolite has approximately one-sixth the potency of ivacaftor and is considered pharmacologically active. The M6 metabolite has less than one-fiftieth the potency of ivacaftor and is not considered pharmacologically active. In vitro, ivacaftor and the M1 metabolite are substrates of CYP3A (i.e., 3A4, 3A5). In addition, ivacaftor is a weak inhibitor of CYP3A, has the potential to inhibit P-glycoprotein (P-gp) at therapeutic concentrations, and may also inhibit CYP2C8 and 2C9. The M1 metabolite, but not M6, also has the potential to inhibit CYP3A and P-gp. Ivacaftor and the M1 and M6 metabolites are not inducers of CYP isoenzymes. Following oral administration, ivacaftor is mainly excreted in feces (87.8%) after metabolic conversion. Approximately 65% of the total dose was excreted as the M1 (22%) and M6 (43%) metabolites. Ivacaftor and its metabolites are minimally excreted in urine (6.6% of total radioactivity recovered); negligible amounts of unchanged drug are excreted in urine. Following a single dose, the apparent terminal half-life is approximately 12 hours.

Advice to Patients

Importance of advising patients to read the manufacturer's patient information before beginning treatment and each time the prescription is refilled.

Importance of taking ivacaftor with fat-containing food (e.g., butter, cheese pizza, eggs, peanut butter) to increase systemic absorption of the drug.

Importance of advising patients to avoid grapefruit juice or food containing grapefruit or Seville oranges (e.g., orange marmalade) during ivacaftor therapy.

Risk of elevated hepatic function tests. Importance of monitoring hepatic function tests prior to initiation of ivacaftor therapy, every 3 months during the first year of therapy, and annually thereafter.

Importance of informing clinicians of existing or contemplated concomitant therapy, including prescription and OTC drugs, vitamins, and herbal supplements, as well as any concomitant illnesses (e.g., hepatic impairment).

Importance of women informing clinicians if they are or plan to become pregnant or plan to breast-feed.

Importance of informing patients of other important precautionary information. (See Cautions.)

Overview® (see Users Guide). For additional information on this drug until a more detailed monograph is developed and published, the manufacturer's labeling should be consulted. It is *essential* that the manufacturer's labeling be consulted for more detailed information on usual cautions, precautions, contraindications, potential drug interactions, laboratory test interferences, and acute toxicity.

Preparations

Excipients in commercially available drug preparations may have clinically important effects in some individuals; consult specific product labeling for details.

Ivacaftor

Oral

Tablets, film-coated	150 mg	**Kalydeco®**, Vertex

EXPECTORANTS 48:16

guaiFENesin

Glyceryl Guaiacolate, α-Glyceryl Guaiacol Ether, Guaianesin

■ Guaifenesin is an expectorant.

Uses

■ **Cough** Guaifenesin is used as an expectorant in the symptomatic management of coughs associated with the common cold, bronchitis, laryngitis, pharyngitis, pertussis, influenza, and measles, and coughs provoked by chronic paranasal sinusitis. While there is clinical evidence that guaifenesin is an effective expectorant (i.e., increasing expectorated sputum volume over the first 4–6 days of a productive cough, decreasing sputum viscosity and difficulty in expectoration, and improving associated symptoms), there currently is insufficient evidence to support efficacy of the drug as an antitussive (cough suppressant). Therefore, guaifenesin's principal benefit in the symptomatic treatment of coughs results from the drug's ability to loosen and thin sputum and bronchial secretions and ease expectoration. Although such facilitation of evacuation of secretions may indirectly diminish the tendency to cough, the mechanism of this effect differs from that of antitussives, which inhibit or suppress cough. In addition to usefulness in the management of productive cough, guaifenesin's effects on sputum production and viscosity and on ease of expectoration suggest that the drug may prove useful in the management of irritative nonproductive cough and coughs productive of scanty amounts of thick, viscous secretions.

Although cough and cold preparations that contain cough suppressants, nasal decongestants, antihistamines, and/or expectorants commonly are used in pediatric patients younger than 2 years of age, systematic reviews of controlled trials have concluded that over-the-counter cough and cold preparations are *not* more effective than placebo in reducing acute cough and other symptoms of upper respiratory tract infection in these patients. Furthermore, adverse events, including deaths, have been (and continue to be) reported in pediatric patients younger than 2 years of age receiving these preparations. (See Cautions: Pediatric Precautions.)

Guaifenesin is combined with bronchodilators, decongestants, antihistamines, or opiate antitussives in numerous commercial liquid cough preparations.

Dosage and Administration

■ **Administration** Guaifenesin is administered orally.

Mucinex® 600-mg extended-release tablets should not be broken, crushed, or chewed and should not be used in children younger than 12 years of age; the tablets should be kept out of reach of young children to avoid accidental swallowing and choking.

■ **Dosage** ***Cough*** The usual dosage of guaifenesin as an expectorant in adults and children 12 years of age and older is 200–400 mg as conventional preparations every 4 hours, not to exceed 2.4 g daily. The usual dosage of guaifenesin 600-mg extended-release tablets as an expectorant in adults and children 12 years of age and older is 600 mg or 1.2 g every 12 hours, not to exceed 2.4 g daily. The usual dosage of guaifenesin as an expectorant for children 6 to younger than 12 years of age is 100–200 mg as conventional preparations every 4 hours, not to exceed 1.2 g daily. Alternatively, children 6–12 years of age may receive 600 mg as an appropriate extended-release preparation every 12 hours, not to exceed 1.2 g daily. Children 2 to younger than 6 years of age may receive 50–100 mg as conventional preparations every 4 hours, not to exceed 600 mg daily. Alternatively, children 2–6 years of age may receive 300 mg as an appropriate extended-release preparation every 12 hours, not to exceed 600 mg daily. Dosage of guaifenesin in children younger than 2 years of age must be individualized. Suggested dosages for children younger than 2 years of age† for some cough and cold preparations have been published in various references for prescribing and parenting. Using recommended dosages for adults and older children, some clinicians have extrapolated dosages for these preparations based on the weight or age of children younger than 2 years of age. However, these extrapolations were based on assumptions that pathology of the disease and pharmacology of the drugs are similar in adults and pediatric patients. There currently are *no* specific dosage recommendations (i.e., approved by the US Food and Drug Administration [FDA]) for cough and cold preparations for this patient population. (See Cautions: Pediatric Precautions.)

Cautions

Doses of guaifenesin larger than those required for expectorant action may produce emesis, but GI upset at ordinary dosage levels is rare.

For *self-medication*, unless directed by a physician, guaifenesin should not be used for persistent or chronic cough such as that occurring with smoking, asthma, chronic bronchitis, or emphysema, or for cough accompanied by excessive phlegm. A persistent cough may be indicative of a serious condition. If cough persists for more than one week, is recurrent, or is accompanied by fever, rash, or persistent headache, a physician should be consulted.

When preparations containing guaifenesin in fixed combination with other agents (e.g., acetaminophen, chlorpheniramine, codeine, dextromethorphan, ephedrine, phenylephrine, pseudoephedrine) are used, the cautions, precautions, and contraindications applicable to each ingredient should be considered.

■ **Pediatric Precautions** Overdosage and toxicity (including death) have been reported in children younger than 2 years of age receiving nonprescription (over-the-counter, OTC) preparations containing antihistamines, cough suppressants, expectorants, and nasal decongestants alone or in combination for relief of symptoms of upper respiratory tract infection. There is limited evidence of efficacy for these preparations in this age group, and appropriate dosages (i.e., approved by the US Food and Drug Administration [FDA]) for the symptomatic treatment of cold and cough have not been established. Therefore, FDA stated that nonprescription cough and cold preparations should not be used in children younger than 2 years of age; the agency continues to assess safety and efficacy of these preparations in older children. Meanwhile, because children 2–3 years of age also are at increased risk of overdosage and toxicity, some manufacturers of oral nonprescription cough and cold preparations agreed to voluntarily revise the product labeling to state that such preparations should not be used in children younger than 4 years of age. FDA recommends that parents and caregivers adhere to the dosage instructions and warnings on the product labeling that accompanies the preparation if administering to children and consult with their clinician about any concerns. Clinicians should ask caregivers about use of nonprescription cough and cold preparations to avoid overdosage. For additional information on precautions associated with the use of cough and cold preparations in pediatric patients, see Cautions: Pediatric Precautions in Dextromethorphan 48:08.

Pharmacology

By increasing respiratory tract fluid, guaifenesin reduces the viscosity of tenacious secretions and acts as an expectorant.

Chemistry and Stability

■ **Chemistry** Guaifenesin is an expectorant. Guaifenesin occurs as a white to slightly gray, crystalline powder, having a bitter taste. Guaifenesin may have a slight characteristic odor. Guaifenesin is soluble in alcohol and in water.

■ **Stability** Guaifenesin powder tends to become lumpy on storage. Guaifenesin preparations should be stored in tight containers.

Preparations

Excipients in commercially available drug preparations may have clinically important effects in some individuals; consult specific product labeling for details.

guaiFENesin

Oral		
Granules	50 mg per packet	**Mucinex® Mini Melts®**, Reckitt Benckiser
	100 mg per packet	**Mucinex® Mini Melts®**, Reckitt Benckiser
Solution	100 mg/5 mL*	**Children's Mucinex® Chest Congestion,** Reckitt Benckiser
		Diabetic Tussin® Expectorant, Health Care Products
		Guaifenesin Oral Solution
		Guiatuss® Syrup, Goldline
	200 mg/5 mL	**Diabetic Tussin® Mucus Relief,** Health Care Products
Tablets	200 mg*	**Guaifenesin Tablets**
Tablets, extended-release	600 mg	**Mucinex®**, Reckitt Benckiser
	1.2 g	**Mucinex® Maximum Strength,** Reckitt Benckiser

*available from one or more manufacturer, distributor, and/or repackager by generic (nonproprietary) name

guaiFENesin and Codeine Phosphate

Oral		
Solution	100 mg/5 mL Guaifenesin and Codeine Phosphate 10 mg/5 mL*	**Cheratussin® AC** (C-V), Qualitest
		Guaiatussin® AC (C-V), Hi-Tech
		Guaifenesin AC Cough Syrup (C-V)
		Guaifenesin and Codeine Phosphate Oral Solution (C-V)
		Robafen® AC (C-V), Major
	200 mg/5 mL Guaifenesin and Codeine Phosphate 8 mg/5 mL	**Codar® GF** (C-V), Respa

*available from one or more manufacturer, distributor, and/or repackager by generic (nonproprietary) name

Other guaiFENesin Combinations

Oral		
For Solution	400 mg/packet with Acetaminophen 1 g/packet	**Theraflu® Flu & Chest Congestion,** Novartis
	400 mg/packet with Acetaminophen 1 g/packet, Dextromethorphan Hydrobromide 30 mg/packet, and Pseudoephedrine Hydrochloride 60 mg/packet	**Theraflu® Max-D® Severe Cold & Flu,** Novartis
Granules	50 mg per packet with Dextromethorphan Hydrobromide 5 mg/packet	**Mucinex® Cough Mini Melts®**, Reckitt Benckiser
Solution	33.3 mg/5 mL with Dextromethorphan Hydrobromide 3.3 mg/5 mL	**Vicks® Nature Fusion® Cough and Chest Congestion,** Procter & Gamble
	50 mg/5 mL with Dextromethorphan Hydrobromide 5 mg/5 mL and Phenylephrine Hydrochloride 2.5 mg/5 mL	**Children's Robitussin® Cold & Cough CF,** Pfizer

	50 mg/5 mL with Phenylephrine Hydrochloride 2.5 mg/5 mL	**Triaminic® Chest and Nasal Congestion,** Novartis
	66.6 mg/5 mL with Acetaminophen 108.3 mg/5 mL, Dextromethorphan Hydrobromide 3.3 mg/5 mL, and Phenylephrine Hydrochloride 1.6 mg/5 mL	**Tylenol® Cold Multi-Symptom Severe,** McNeil **Tylenol® Cold & Flu Severe,** McNeil
	66.6 mg/5 mL with Acetaminophen 108.3 mg/5 mL, and Phenylephrine Hydrochloride 1.6 mg/5 mL	**Theraflu Warming Relief® Cold & Chest Congestion,** Novartis
	66.6 mg/5 mL with Dextromethorphan Hydrobromide 3.3 mg/5 mL	**Vicks® DayQuil® Mucus Control DM,** Procter & Gamble
	66.6 mg/5 mL with Dextromethorphan Hydrobromide 6.6 mg/5 mL	**Vicks® Formula 44® Custom Care Chesty Cough,** Procter & Gamble
	100 mg/5mL with Acetaminophen 162.5 mg/5 mL, Dextromethorphan Hydrobromide 5 mg/5 mL, and Phenylephrine Hydrochloride 2.5 mg/5 mL	**Children's Mucinex® Cold, Cough, and Sore Throat,** Reckitt Benckiser **Children's Mucinex® Multi-symptom Cold & Fever,** Reckitt Benckiser
	100 mg/5 mL with Dextromethorphan Hydrobromide 5 mg/5 mL	**Children's Mucinex® Cough,** Reckitt Benckiser **Pediacare® Children's Cough & Congestion,** Prestige Brands
	100 mg/5 mL with Dextromethorphan Hydrobromide 5 mg/5 mL and Phenylephrine Hydrochloride 2.5 mg/5 mL	**Children's Mucinex® Multi-symptom Cold,** Reckitt Benckiser
	100 mg/5 mL with Dextromethorphan Hydrobromide 10 mg/5 mL	**Robitussin® Peak Cold Cough + Chest Congestion DM,** Pfizer
	100 mg/5 mL with Dextromethorphan Hydrobromide 10 mg/5 mL and Phenylephrine Hydrochloride 5 mg/5 mL	**Robitussin® Peak Cold Multi-Symptom Cold®,** Pfizer
	100 mg/5 mL with Phenylephrine Hydrochloride 2.5 mg/5 mL	**Children's Mucinex® Stuffy Nose & Cold,** Reckitt Benckiser
	100 mg/5 mL with Phenylephrine Hydrochloride 5 mg/5 mL	**Rescon®-GG,** Capellon
	200 mg/5 mL with Dextromethorphan Hydrobromide 10 mg/5 mL	**Robitussin® Peak Cold Maximum Strength Cough + Chest Congestion DM,** Pfizer
	200 mg/5 mL with Dextromethorphan Hydrobromide 10 mg/5 mL and Phenylephrine Hydrochloride 5 mg/5 mL	**Robitussin® Peak Cold Maximum Strength Multi-Symptom Cold®,** Pfizer
Tablets	200 mg with Acetaminophen 325 mg, Dextromethorphan 10 mg, and Phenylephrine Hydrochloride 5 mg	**Tylenol® Cold Multi-symptom Severe,** McNeil **Tylenol® Cold & Flu Severe,** McNeil
	200 mg with Ephedrine Hydrochloride 12.5 mg	**Primatene®,** Pfizer
	400 mg with Ephedrine Sulfate 25 mg	**Bronkaid® Dual Action Caplets®,** Bayer
	400 mg with Pseudoephedrine Hydrochloride 60 mg	**Congestac® Caplets®,** Ascher
Tablets, extended-release	600 mg with Dextromethorphan Hydrobromide 30 mg	**Mucinex® DM,** Reckitt Benckiser
	600 mg with Pseudoephedrine Hydrochloride 60 mg	**Mucinex® D,** Reckitt Benckiser
	1.2 g with Dextromethorphan Hydrobromide 60 mg	**Mucinex® DM Maximum Strength,** Reckitt Benckiser
	1.2 g with Pseudoephedrine Hydrochloride 120 mg	**Mucinex® D Maximum Strength,** Reckitt Benckiser

Guaifenesin also is commercially available in combination with antihistamines, antitussives, bronchodilators, decongestants, and expectorants.

†Use is not currently included in the labeling approved by the US Food and Drug Administration

Selected Revisions February 2016,

PHOSPHODIESTERASE TYPE 4 INHIBITORS 48:32

Roflumilast

■ Roflumilast is a selective phosphodiesterase type 4 (PDE4) inhibitor.

Uses

■ **Bronchospasm** ***Chronic Obstructive Pulmonary Disease*** Roflumilast is used to reduce the risk of chronic obstructive pulmonary disease (COPD) exacerbations in patients with severe COPD associated with chronic bronchitis and a history of exacerbations. Roflumilast is *not* a bronchodilator and is *not* indicated for the relief of acute bronchospasm. The effects of roflumilast on COPD exacerbations when added to a fixed-combination preparation containing a long-acting β_2-adrenergic agonist and orally inhaled corticosteroid have not been established.

Safety and efficacy of roflumilast have been evaluated in 8 randomized, double-blind, placebo- and active-controlled studies in adults 40 years of age or older with COPD. Data from two 6-month, placebo-controlled, dose-selection studies in patients with COPD of varying severity (forced expiratory volume in 1 second [FEV_1] 30–80% of predicted) resulted in a roflumilast dosage of 500 mcg once daily being selected, based mainly based on improvements in lung function (e.g., FEV_1) observed with this dosage compared with roflumilast 250 mcg once daily.

The effect of roflumilast 500 mcg once daily on COPD exacerbations has been evaluated in four 1-year, placebo-controlled studies in patients with severe COPD (FEV_1 50% of predicted or less). In the first 2 studies, roflumilast did not substantially reduce the rate of moderate (defined as requiring systemic corticosteroids and/or antibiotics) or severe (defined as resulting in hospitalization and/or death) COPD exacerbations compared with placebo. However, based on results of exploratory analyses of these studies, some patients with severe COPD associated with chronic bronchitis and COPD exacerbations within the previous year appeared to have a greater reduction in the incidence of COPD exacerbations compared with the overall study population. In 2 subsequent studies in patients with severe COPD associated with chronic bronchitis who had at least one COPD exacerbation in the previous year and a history of smoking (20 pack-years or more), roflumilast reduced the incidence of moderate (defined as requiring systemic corticosteroids) or severe (defined as resulting in hospitalization and/or death) exacerbations compared with placebo. In addition, in patients receiving concomitant long-acting β_2-adrenergic agonists or short-acting antimuscarinics in these studies, the reduction in moderate or severe COPD exacerbations with roflumilast was similar to that observed in the overall study populations.

While roflumilast is not a bronchodilator, the previous four 1-year studies also evaluated the effect of roflumilast on lung function (as determined by change in pre- or post-bronchodilator FEV_1). In these studies, roflumilast 500 mcg once daily improved lung function compared with placebo. In addition, in two 6-month comparative studies in patients with moderate or severe COPD (FEV_1 40–70% of predicted) receiving either roflumilast (500 mcg once daily) or placebo as add-on therapy to treatment with salmeterol or tiotropium, roflumilast improved lung function (as determined by mean change in prebronchodilator FEV_1) compared with placebo.

For additional information on the treatment of COPD, see Uses: Chronic Obstructive Pulmonary Disease, in Ipratropium Bromide 12:08.08.

Dosage and Administration

■ **Administration** Roflumilast is administered orally once daily without regard to meals.

■ **Dosage** The recommended adult dosage of roflumilast to reduce the risk of chronic obstructive pulmonary disease (COPD) exacerbations in patients with severe COPD associated with chronic bronchitis and a history of exacerbations is 500 mcg once daily.

■ **Special Populations** Clinicians should consider the risks and benefits of using roflumilast in patients with mild hepatic impairment (Child-Pugh class A). Roflumilast is not recommended for use in patients with moderate or severe hepatic impairment (Child-Pugh class B or C). (See Cautions: Contraindications and also see Hepatic Impairment under Warnings/Precautions: Specific Populations, in Cautions.)

Dosage adjustment is not necessary in geriatric patients or patients with renal impairment. In addition, dosage adjustment is not necessary based on gender or race.

Cautions

■ **Contraindications** Moderate or severe hepatic impairment (Child-Pugh class B or C). (See Hepatic Impairment under Warnings/Precautions: Specific Populations, in Cautions.)

■ **Warnings/Precautions** ***Acute Bronchospasm*** Roflumilast is *not* a bronchodilator and should *not* be used for the relief of acute bronchospasm.

Psychiatric Events and Suicidality Roflumilast therapy is associated with an increase in adverse psychiatric effects. Adverse psychiatric effects were reported in 5.9% of patients receiving roflumilast (500 mcg once daily) compared with 3.3% of those receiving placebo in clinical studies. The most frequently reported adverse psychiatric effects were insomnia, anxiety, and depression, which were reported at an increased incidence in patients receiving roflumilast compared with placebo (2.4, 1.4, and 1.2% versus 1, 0.9, and 0.9%, respectively). Suicidal ideation or behavior, including completed suicide, has been observed in clinical studies. Three patients experienced suicide-related adverse effects while receiving roflumilast (one completed suicide and two suicide attempts) compared with one patient who received placebo (suicidal ideation).

Clinicians should carefully weigh the risks and benefits of roflumilast therapy before using the drug in patients with a history of depression and/or suicidal thoughts or behavior. In addition, clinicians should carefully evaluate the risks and benefits of continuing therapy with roflumilast if such effects occur. Some clinicians state that roflumilast should be avoided in patients with depression. (See Advice to Patients.)

Weight Loss Weight loss was reported in clinical studies in 7.5% of patients receiving roflumilast (500 mcg once daily) compared with 2.1% of those receiving placebo. In addition to being reported as an adverse effect, weight loss was prospectively evaluated in 2 placebo-controlled studies of 1 year's duration. In these studies, moderate (5–10% of body weight) or severe (greater than 10% of body weight) weight loss was reported in 20 or 7%, respectively, of patients receiving roflumilast compared with 7 or 2%, respectively, of those receiving placebo. Most patients with decreased body weight during roflumilast therapy regained some of the lost weight after treatment discontinuance.

Weight should be regularly monitored in patients receiving roflumilast. If unexplained or clinically important weight loss occurs, decreased body weight should be evaluated and discontinuance of roflumilast should be considered. Some clinicians advise that roflumilast therapy be avoided in underweight patients.

Interactions Concomitant use of roflumilast with potent cytochrome P-450 (CYP) isoenzyme 3A4 inducers (e.g., carbamazepine, phenobarbital, phenytoin, rifampin) is not recommended. (See Drug Interactions.)

Specific Populations **Pregnancy.** Category C. (See Users Guide.)

Roflumilast should not be used during labor and delivery. The effect of roflumilast on preterm labor or labor at term in humans is unknown; however, disruption of labor and delivery has occurred in animals receiving the drug.

Lactation. Roflumilast and/or its metabolites are distributed into milk in rats. Roflumilast and/or its metabolites are likely distributed into human milk. The effects of roflumilast on breast-fed infants have not been established. Roflumilast should not be used in nursing women.

Pediatric Use. Safety and efficacy of roflumilast have not been established in pediatric patients; chronic obstructive pulmonary disease (COPD) does not occur in children.

Geriatric Use. Approximately 46% of patients with COPD who received roflumilast in clinical studies have been older than 65 years of age and about 11% have been older than 75 years of age. Although no substantial differences in safety and efficacy relative to younger adults have been observed, and other clinical experience revealed no evidence of age-related differences, the possibility of increased sensitivity in some older patients cannot be ruled out. Dosage adjustment is not necessary in geriatric patients.

Hepatic Impairment. In a pharmacokinetic study evaluating a roflumilast dosage of 250 mcg once daily for 14 days, areas under the plasma concentration-time curve (AUCs) of roflumilast and roflumilast *N*-oxide were 51 and 24% higher, respectively, in individuals with mild hepatic impairment (Child-Pugh class A) and 92 and 41% higher, respectively, in individuals with moderate hepatic impairment (Child-Pugh class B) compared with values in healthy individuals matched for age, weight, and gender. Peak plasma concentrations of roflumilast and roflumilast *N*-oxide were 3 and 26% higher, respectively, in individuals with mild hepatic impairment and 26 and 40% higher, respectively, in individuals with moderate hepatic impairment compared with values for healthy individuals matched for age, weight, and gender. A roflumilast dosage of 500 mcg once daily has not been studied in patients with hepatic impairment.

Clinicians should consider the risks and benefits of using roflumilast in patients with mild hepatic impairment (Child-Pugh class A). Roflumilast is contraindicated in patients with moderate or severe hepatic impairment (Child-Pugh class B or C).

Renal Impairment. After administration of a single 500-mcg dose of roflumilast to individuals with severe renal impairment, AUCs of roflumilast and roflumilast *N*-oxide were reduced by 21 and 7%, respectively, and peak plasma concentrations were reduced by 16 and 12%, respectively. Dosage adjustment is not necessary in patients with renal impairment.

■ **Common Adverse Effects** Adverse effects reported in 2% or more of patients receiving roflumilast include diarrhea, weight loss, nausea, headache, back pain, influenza, insomnia, dizziness, and decreased appetite.

Drug Interactions

In vitro, roflumilast and roflumilast *N*-oxide do not inhibit the P-glycoprotein transport system.

■ **Drugs Affecting Hepatic Microsomal Enzymes** A major pathway for roflumilast metabolism is pyridine *N*-oxidation of roflumilast to roflumilast *N*-oxide by cytochrome P-450 (CYP) isoenzymes 3A4 and 1A2. Roflumilast *N*-oxide is *O*-dealkylated mainly by CYP3A4, and to a lesser extent by CYP2C19 and extrahepatic CYP1A, and glucuronidated.

Potent CYP3A4 inducers decrease systemic exposure to roflumilast and may reduce the therapeutic efficacy of the drug. Therefore, concomitant use of potent CYP3A4 inducers (e.g., carbamazepine, phenobarbital, phenytoin, rifampin) with roflumilast is not recommended.

Concomitant administration of agents that inhibit CYP3A4 or inhibit both CYP3A4 and CYP1A2 (e.g., cimetidine, enoxacin [no longer commercially available in the US], erythromycin, fluvoxamine, ketoconazole) may increase systemic exposure to roflumilast and may result in increased adverse effects. The risk of such concurrent use should be weighed carefully against the benefit.

■ **Drugs Metabolized by Hepatic Microsomal Enzymes** In vitro, therapeutic plasma concentrations of roflumilast and roflumilast *N*-oxide do not inhibit CYP isoenzymes 1A2, 2A6, 2B6, 2C8, 2C9, 2C19, 2D6, 2E1, 3A4/5, or 4A9/11; clinically important pharmacokinetic interactions with drugs metabolized by these isoenzymes are unlikely. In vitro, roflumilast does not induce CYP isoenzymes 1A2, 2A6, 2C9, 2C19, or 3A4/5 and is a weak inducer of CYP2B6.

■ **Albuterol** No clinically important pharmacokinetic interactions were observed when roflumilast was administered concomitantly with orally inhaled albuterol; no dosage adjustment is recommended.

■ **Antacids** No clinically important pharmacokinetic interactions were observed when roflumilast was administered concomitantly with an aluminum and magnesium hydroxides antacid; no dosage adjustment is recommended.

■ **Budesonide** No clinically important pharmacokinetic interactions were observed when roflumilast was administered concomitantly with orally inhaled budesonide; no dosage adjustment is recommended.

■ **Cimetidine** Concomitant administration of cimetidine (400 mg twice daily for 7 days), a dual CYP3A4 and CYP1A2 inhibitor, and roflumilast (single 500-mcg dose) increased peak plasma concentrations and area under the plasma concentration-time curve (AUC) of roflumilast by 46 and 85%, respectively, and decreased peak plasma concentrations and increased AUC of roflumilast *N*-oxide by 4 and 27%, respectively. Roflumilast and cimetidine should be used concomitantly with caution; the risk of such concurrent use should be weighed carefully against the benefit.

■ **Digoxin** No clinically important pharmacokinetic interactions were observed when roflumilast was administered concomitantly with oral digoxin; no dosage adjustment is recommended.

■ **Enoxacin** Concomitant administration of enoxacin (400 mg twice daily for 12 days; no longer commercially available in the US), a dual CYP3A4 and CYP1A2 inhibitor, and roflumilast (single 500-mcg dose) increased peak plasma concentrations and AUC of roflumilast by 20 and 56%, respectively, and decreased peak plasma concentrations and increased AUC of roflumilast *N*-oxide by 14 and 23%, respectively. Roflumilast and enoxacin should be used concomitantly with caution; the risk of such concurrent use should be weighed carefully against the benefit.

■ **Erythromycin** Concomitant administration of erythromycin (500 mg three times daily for 13 days), a CYP3A4 inhibitor, and roflumilast (single 500-mcg dose) increased peak plasma concentrations and AUC of roflumilast by 40 and 70%, respectively, and decreased peak plasma concentrations and increased AUC of roflumilast *N*-oxide by 34 and 4%, respectively. Roflumilast and erythromycin should be used concomitantly with caution; the risk of such concurrent use should be weighed carefully against the benefit.

■ **Fluvoxamine** Concomitant administration of fluvoxamine (50 mg daily for 14 days), a dual CYP3A4 and CYP1A2 inhibitor, and roflumilast (single 500-mcg dose) increased peak plasma concentrations and AUC of roflumilast by 12 and 156%, respectively, and decreased peak plasma concentrations and increased AUC of roflumilast *N*-oxide by 210 and 52%, respectively. Roflumilast and fluvoxamine should be used concomitantly with caution; the risk of such concurrent use should be weighed carefully against the benefit.

■ **Formoterol** No clinically important pharmacokinetic interactions were observed when roflumilast was administered concomitantly with orally inhaled formoterol; no dosage adjustment is recommended.

■ **Ketoconazole** Concomitant administration of ketoconazole (200 mg twice daily for 13 days), a potent CYP3A4 inhibitor, and roflumilast (single 500-mcg dose) increased peak plasma concentrations and AUC of roflumilast by 23 and 99%, respectively, and decreased peak plasma concentrations and increased AUC of roflumilast *N*-oxide by 38 and 3%, respectively. Roflumilast and ketoconazole should be used concomitantly with caution; the risk of such concurrent use should be weighed carefully against the benefit.

■ **Midazolam** No clinically important pharmacokinetic interactions were observed when roflumilast was administered concomitantly with oral midazolam; no dosage adjustment is recommended.

■ **Montelukast** No clinically important pharmacokinetic interactions were observed when roflumilast was administered concomitantly with oral montelukast; no dosage adjustment is recommended.

■ **Oral Contraceptives** Concomitant administration of roflumilast and oral contraceptives containing gestodene (not commercially available in the US) and ethinyl estradiol may increase systemic exposure to roflumilast and may increase the risk of adverse effects. Concomitant administration of the fixed-combination preparation containing 0.075 mg of gestodene and 0.03 mg of ethinyl estradiol daily and roflumilast (single 500-mcg dose) increased peak plasma concentrations and AUC of roflumilast by 38 and 51%, respectively, and decreased peak plasma concentrations and increased AUC of roflumilast *N*-oxide by 12 and 14%, respectively. Roflumilast and contraceptives containing gestodene and ethinyl estradiol should be used concomitantly with caution; the risk of such concurrent use should be weighed carefully against the benefit.

■ **Rifampin** Potent CYP inducers decrease systemic exposure to roflumilast and may reduce the therapeutic efficacy of roflumilast. Concomitant administration of rifampin (600 mg daily for 11 days), a potent CYP3A4 inducer, and roflumilast (single 500-mcg dose) decreased peak plasma concentrations and AUC of roflumilast by 68 and 79%, respectively, and increased peak plasma concentrations and decreased AUC of roflumilast *N*-oxide by 30 and 56%, respectively. Concomitant use is not recommended.

■ **Sildenafil** No clinically important pharmacokinetic interactions were observed when roflumilast was administered concomitantly with oral sildenafil; no dosage adjustment is recommended.

■ **Theophylline** No clinically important pharmacokinetic interactions were observed when roflumilast was administered concomitantly with oral theophylline; no dosage adjustment is recommended. However, some clinicians do not recommend concomitant administration of roflumilast with theophylline.

■ **Warfarin** No clinically important pharmacokinetic interactions were observed when roflumilast was administered concomitantly with oral warfarin; no dosage adjustment is recommended.

Description

Roflumilast and its active metabolite, roflumilast *N*-oxide, are selective inhibitors of phosphodiesterase type 4 (PDE4), a major enzyme involved in the metabolism of cyclic adenosine-3′,5′-monophosphate (cAMP) in lung tissue. Selective inhibition of PDE4 results in accumulation of intracellular cAMP. Although the exact mechanism(s) of therapeutic action of roflumilast in patients with chronic obstructive pulmonary disease (COPD) has not been fully elucidated, it is thought to be related to the effects of increased cAMP in lung cells. Increased cAMP concentrations can lead to activation of protein kinase A, resulting in phosphorylation and inactivation of target transcription factors, and subsequent reduction of cellular inflammatory activity. An anti-inflammatory effect may account for the clinical efficacy of roflumilast; however, few studies have evaluated the potential anti-inflammatory effects of roflumilast in humans and available data are limited and inconclusive. Roflumilast reduced the number of neutrophils and eosinophils in the sputum of patients with COPD and the number of total cells, neutrophils, and eosinophils in bronchoalveolar lavage fluid in healthy individuals; the clinical importance of these results is unknown. Roflumilast is *not* a bronchodilator.

Roflumilast is extensively metabolized via cytochrome P-450 (CYP) and conjugation reactions. A major pathway for roflumilast metabolism is pyridine *N*-oxidation of roflumilast to roflumilast *N*-oxide by CYP isoenzymes 3A4 and 1A2. Roflumilast *N*-oxide is *O*-dealkylated mainly by CYP3A4, and to a lesser extent by CYP2C19 and extrahepatic CYP1A, and glucuronidated. The *N*-oxide metabolite is the only major metabolite detected in human plasma and its pharmacokinetics are distinct from the parent compound. Roflumilast and roflumilast *N*-oxide together account for most (87.5%) of the administered dose present in plasma. While roflumilast is threefold more potent than roflumilast *N*-oxide with respect to PDE4 inhibition in vitro, the area under the plasma concentration-time curve (AUC) of roflumilast *N*-oxide is about tenfold greater than that of roflumilast. The *N*-oxide metabolite appears to account for about 90% of the biologic action of roflumilast. Roflumilast was not detected in urine, while a trace amount (less than 1%) of roflumilast *N*-oxide was detected; other conjugated metabolites were detected in urine. Following IV or oral administration of radiolabeled roflumilast, about 70% of radioactivity was recovered in urine. The median plasma effective half-lives of roflumilast and roflumilast *N*-oxide are approximately 17 and 30 hours, respectively.

Advice to Patients

Importance of patients reading the manufacturer's patient information (medication guide) prior to initiation of therapy and each time the prescription is refilled.

Importance of informing patients that roflumilast is not a bronchodilator and should not be used for the relief of acute bronchospasm.

Risk of adverse psychiatric effects (e.g., insomnia, anxiety, depression, suicidal ideation or behavior). Importance of advising patients, their families, and caregivers to be alert for the emergence or worsening of insomnia, anxiety, depression, suicidal thoughts, or other mood changes, and to contact a clinician if such changes occur.

Risk of weight loss. Importance of patients being regularly monitored for weight loss. Importance of patients informing a clinician if weight loss occurs.

Importance of informing clinicians of existing or contemplated concomitant therapy, including prescription and OTC drugs, vitamins, and herbal supplements, as well as any concomitant illnesses.

Importance of women informing clinicians if they are or plan to become pregnant or plan to breast-feed.

Importance of informing patients of other important precautionary information. (See Cautions.)

Overview® (see Users Guide). For additional information on this drug until a more detailed monograph is developed and published, the manufacturer's labeling should be consulted. It is *essential* that the manufacturer's labeling be consulted for more detailed information on usual cautions, precautions, contraindications, potential drug interactions, laboratory test interferences, and acute toxicity.

Preparations

Excipients in commercially available drug preparations may have clinically important effects in some individuals; consult specific product labeling for details.

Roflumilast

Oral		
Tablets	500 mcg	**Daliresp®**, Forest

VASODILATING AGENTS 48:48

Ambrisentan

■ Ambrisentan, a selective propionic-acid endothelin-1 (ET-1) type A receptor antagonist, is a vasodilator.

REMS

FDA approved a REMS for ambrisentan to ensure that the benefits outweigh the risks. The REMS may apply to one or more preparations of ambrisentan and consists of the following: elements to assure safe use and implementation system. See the FDA REMS page (https://www.accessdata.fda.gov/scripts/cder/rems/index.cfm). See also Restricted Distribution Program under Dosage and Administration: General.

Uses

■ **Pulmonary Arterial Hypertension** Ambrisentan is used in the management of pulmonary arterial hypertension (PAH; World Health Organization [WHO] group 1 pulmonary hypertension) to improve exercise capacity and to delay clinical worsening. Clinical studies establishing efficacy of ambrisentan for this use were conducted principally in patients with New York Heart Association (NYHA)/WHO functional class II or III PAH (idiopathic, heritable, or associated with connective tissue diseases). For more information about etiologies of PAH, see Uses: Pulmonary Arterial Hypertension, in Epoprostenol 48:48. Ambrisentan has been designated an orphan drug by the US Food and Drug Administration (FDA) for use in the treatment of PAH.

In addition to general treatment measures and supportive therapy (e.g., warfarin anticoagulation, diuretics, supplemental oxygen, digoxin), experts recommend an endothelin-receptor antagonist (e.g., ambrisentan, bosentan, macitentan) as one of several treatment options for the initial management of PAH in patients with NYHA/WHO functional class II, III, or IV symptoms who are not candidates for calcium-channel blocker therapy or in whom such therapy has failed; alternative therapies include phosphodiesterase (PDE) type 5 inhibitors (e.g., sildenafil, tadalafil), prostanoids (e.g., IV epoprostenol; inhaled iloprost; inhaled, IV, or subcutaneous treprostinil), soluble guanylate cyclase stimulators (e.g., riociguat). Current guidelines for the management of PAH state that an oral agent such as an endothelin-receptor antagonist generally is preferred for initial therapy in patients with NYHA/WHO functional class II symptoms, while those with more advanced NYHA/WHO functional class III disease may be treated with any currently approved PAH therapy; IV epoprostenol generally is recommended as the treatment of choice for patients with NYHA/WHO class IV PAH because of its demonstrated survival benefit. In general, choice of therapy should be individualized, taking into account factors such as disease severity, route of administration, potential adverse effects, costs of treatment, clinician experience, and patient preference.

Efficacy of ambrisentan for the management of PAH has been established in 2 randomized, double-blind, multicenter, placebo-controlled trials of 12 weeks' duration in a total of 393 adults with WHO group 1 PAH; 64% of the patients had idiopathic or familial PAH and 36% had PAH associated with other disorders (connective tissue diseases [32%], HIV infection [3%], use of anorexigenic agents [1%]). Most patients enrolled in these trials had WHO functional class II (38%) or III (55%) PAH at study entry. The trials were identically designed except for differences in the ambrisentan dosages studied. Patients in these 2 trials were randomized to receive ambrisentan (2.5, 5, or 10 mg once daily) or placebo in addition to standard therapy (e.g., anticoagulants, diuretics, calcium-channel blocking agents, and/or cardiac glycosides, but not prostacyclin analogs [e.g., epoprostenol, treprostinil, iloprost], other endothelin receptor antagonists [e.g., bosentan], or PDE type 5 inhibitors [e.g., sildenafil]). The primary end point, exercise capacity, was assessed using the 6-minute walking test. Treatment with ambrisentan resulted in significant improvements in walking distance (placebo-corrected mean increases of 31–59 meters in the 5-mg group and 51 meters in the 10-mg group at 12 weeks). Clinical worsening (defined as the time to first occurrence of death, lung transplantation, hospitalization for PAH, atrial septostomy, or early termination based on disease progression), evaluated as a secondary outcome measure in these studies, was substantially delayed in patients receiving ambrisentan compared with those receiving placebo. At 12 weeks, 94–97% of ambrisentan-treated patients remained free of a clinical worsening event versus 79–89% of placebo-treated patients. In an open-label extension of the 2 randomized controlled studies, improvements in exercise capacity were maintained in patients who continued to receive ambrisentan; estimated rates of survival for the overall study group were 93, 85, and 79% at 1, 2, and 3 years, respectively.

Current expert consensus guidelines recommend combination therapy with a prostanoid, PDE type 5 inhibitor, or soluble guanylate cyclase stimulator (added sequentially) in patients who have an inadequate response to initial monotherapy. Combination therapy with drugs that target the different pathophysiologic pathways in PAH may provide additive and/or synergistic benefits. Data from several small studies suggest that use of an endothelin-receptor antagonist in combination with a prostanoid or a PDE type 5 inhibitor may improve outcomes (e.g., reduce clinical worsening, increase 6-minute walking distance, improve hemodynamic parameters) in patients who remain symptomatic on monotherapy.

Unlike some endothelin receptor antagonists (e.g., bosentan, sitaxsentan [not commercially available in the US]) that have been associated with clinically important elevations in serum aminotransferases and serious hepatic injury, ambrisentan appears to have a low potential for hepatotoxicity. (See Hepatic Effects under Warnings/Precautions: Other Warnings and Precautions, in Cautions.) Limited data are available regarding the use of ambrisentan in patients with PAH who have discontinued therapy with other endothelin receptor antagonists because of aminotransferase elevations (ALT and/or AST exceeding 3 times the upper limit of normal). In an open-label, uncontrolled extension study, ambrisentan therapy was initiated in 36 such patients in whom aminotransferase concentrations had returned to normal prior to study entry. At a median follow-up of 13 months, after dosage had been increased to 10 mg daily in 50% of the patients, 34 patients continued to receive the drug; one case of transient aminotransferase elevation occurred, but no patients were withdrawn from the study as a result of elevated hepatic enzymes. Based on results of this study, the manufacturer states that ambrisentan may be considered in patients who experience asymptomatic aminotransferase elevations while receiving other endothelin-receptor antagonists, after aminotransferase levels have normalized.

■ **Pulmonary Fibrosis** Results of a randomized, placebo-controlled trial in patients with idiopathic pulmonary fibrosis†, with or without pulmonary hypertension (WHO group 3), demonstrated no clinical benefit with ambrisentan therapy, but a relatively greater risk of disease progression, reduced pulmonary function, hospitalization, and death; the study was terminated early for these safety findings and lack of efficacy. (See Cautions: Contraindications.)

Dosage and Administration

■ **General** ***Restricted Distribution Program*** Because of the risk of embryofetal toxicity, ambrisentan is available to female patients only through a restricted distribution program called the Letairis® Risk Evaluation and Mitigation Strategy (REMS). (See REMS and also see Fetal/Neonatal Morbidity and Mortality under Warnings/Precautions: Warnings, in Cautions.) *All* female patients regardless of childbearing potential must enroll in the program prior to initiating ambrisentan; in addition, females of childbearing potential must comply with all pregnancy testing and contraception requirements of the program. Male patients are exempt from these restrictions and do not need to enroll in the program. Clinicians and pharmacies must also be registered with the Letairis® REMS and comply with all terms of the program (including patient education and safety requirements) before they can prescribe or dispense ambrisentan. In addition, pharmacies must only dispense the drug to authorized patients. For additional information about the Letairis® REMS program, clinicians may call 866-664-5327 or visit www.letairisrems.com.

As a condition of the Letairis® REMS program, ambrisentan therapy should be initiated in females of childbearing potential *only* after a negative pregnancy test is obtained; pregnancy tests should be performed monthly during therapy and at 1 month following discontinuance of therapy. (See Advice to Patients.) Prepubertal female patients and/or their parent or guardian should be advised to immediately report any changes in the child's reproductive status (e.g., breast development, pubic hair) to her clinician. The prepubertal female's healthcare provider should decide when the child has reached puberty; children may reach puberty before having their first menstrual period.

No more than a 30-day supply of ambrisentan may be dispensed at one time. Dispensing to females of childbearing potential should occur only after obtaining confirmation from the patient that the required pregnancy testing was completed.

■ **Administration** ***Oral Administration*** Ambrisentan is administered orally without regard to meals. Ambrisentan tablets should not be split, chewed, or crushed.

If a dose of ambrisentan is missed, the dose should be taken as soon as it is remembered that day, and the next dose taken at the regularly scheduled time; 2 doses should not be taken at the same time to make up for a missed dose.

■ **Dosage** ***Pulmonary Arterial Hypertension*** The initial dosage of ambrisentan for the treatment of pulmonary arterial hypertension (PAH) in adults is 5 mg once daily; if tolerated, dosage may be increased to 10 mg once daily. Safety and efficacy of dosages exceeding 10 mg daily have not been established.

When administered concomitantly with cyclosporine, dosage of ambrisentan should be limited to 5 mg once daily. (See Drug Interactions: Cyclosporine.)

■ **Special Populations** Ambrisentan should be avoided in patients with preexisting moderate or severe hepatic impairment. (See Hepatic Impairment under Warnings/Precautions: Specific Populations, in Cautions.)

Dosage adjustment is not required in patients with mild or moderate renal impairment; the drug has not been studied in those with severe renal impairment. (See Renal Impairment under Warnings/Precautions: Specific Populations, in Cautions.)

Cautions

■ **Contraindications** Pregnancy.

Patients with idiopathic pulmonary fibrosis, with or without pulmonary hypertension (World Health Organization [WHO] group 3). (See Uses: Pulmonary Fibrosis.)

■ **Warnings/Precautions** ***Warnings*** **Fetal/Neonatal Morbidity and Mortality.** Ambrisentan may cause fetal harm if used during pregnancy; teratogenic (e.g., craniofacial defects, cardiovascular malformations, agenesis of the thymus and thyroid glands) and embryotoxic (e.g., decreased survival) effects have been demonstrated in animals. (See Cautions: Contraindications.)

Pregnancy must be excluded in females of childbearing potential prior to initiation of ambrisentan therapy and prevented thereafter by the use of acceptable methods of contraception during and for 1 month following cessation of therapy. (See Advice to Patients.) Monthly pregnancy tests are required in females of childbearing potential. If ambrisentan is used during pregnancy or if the patient becomes pregnant during therapy, the patient should be apprised of the potential hazard to the fetus.

Because of the risk of fetal harm, distribution of ambrisentan is restricted in female patients. (See Restricted Distribution Program under Dosage and Administration: General.)

Other Warnings and Precautions **Fluid Retention.** Peripheral edema, usually mild to moderate in severity, has been reported in patients receiving ambrisentan; peripheral edema has occurred with greater frequency and severity in geriatric patients. Peripheral edema is a known class effect of endothelin-receptor antagonists and also a clinical consequence of pulmonary arterial hypertension (PAH). Fluid retention, sometimes requiring intervention (e.g., diuretic therapy, fluid management, hospitalization), has been reported during postmarketing experience.

If clinically important fluid retention occurs (with or without weight gain), the patient should be further evaluated to determine the cause and to assess the need for specific treatment or discontinuance of ambrisentan therapy.

Fertility in Males. Reduced sperm counts have been observed in some men with PAH receiving several months of treatment with another endothelin receptor antagonist (bosentan); therefore, the possibility of adverse effects on spermatogenesis with ambrisentan cannot be excluded. Patients should be advised about the potential adverse effects of ambrisentan on fertility.

Hematologic Effects. Decreases in hemoglobin concentration and hematocrit have been reported within the first few weeks of ambrisentan therapy, followed by stabilization; decreases in hemoglobin concentration do not appear to be related to hemorrhage or hemolysis but have required transfusion in some cases. In the principal efficacy studies of ambrisentan in patients with PAH, a mean decrease in hemoglobin concentration of 0.8 g/dL was reported in patients receiving the drug; hemoglobin concentration decreased by more than 15% from baseline in 7% of patients receiving ambrisentan compared with 4% of those receiving placebo.

Hemoglobin concentrations should be monitored prior to initiation of ambrisentan therapy, at 1 month of treatment, and periodically thereafter during ambrisentan therapy. The manufacturer states that the drug is not recommended in patients with clinically important anemia. Discontinuance of therapy should be considered in those who experience clinically important, otherwise unexplained reductions in hemoglobin concentration during therapy.

Pulmonary Effects. If acute pulmonary edema occurs during ambrisentan therapy, the possibility of pulmonary veno-occlusive disease should be considered; if confirmed, the drug should be discontinued.

Hepatic Effects. Serious hepatotoxicity, including cirrhosis and liver failure, has been reported in patients receiving some endothelin-receptor antagonists (e.g., bosentan, sitaxsentan [not commercially available in the US]). Because hepatotoxicity was previously thought to be a class effect of these drugs, a boxed warning regarding a potential risk of liver injury was included in the original FDA-approved labeling for ambrisentan. However, further evaluation of the available clinical trial data and postmarketing information indicate that the risk of liver injury with ambrisentan is low. In the pivotal 12-week controlled clinical trials of ambrisentan, elevations in serum aminotransferase (AST/ALT) concentrations to at least 3 or more times the upper limit of normal (ULN) were not observed in any patient receiving the drug but occurred in 2.3% of those who received placebo. Approximately 2% of those who continued to receive ambrisentan for up to 2 years in the open-label extension of these studies experienced aminotransferase abnormalities exceeding 3 times the ULN; most events were mild and did not result in drug discontinuance. Elevations of serum aminotransferase concentrations have been reported in some patients receiving ambrisentan during postmarketing experience; however, alternative causes of liver dysfunction (e.g., heart failure, hepatic congestion, hepatitis, alcohol use, concomitant use of hepatotoxic drugs) could be identified in nearly all cases. Based on these findings, FDA has concluded that the incidence of hepatic effects with ambrisentan is similar to that observed in the general population of patients with PAH and has removed the liver injury warning from the drug's approved labeling.

Liver function tests should be monitored as clinically indicated in patients receiving ambrisentan. The drug should be discontinued if AST or ALT concentrations exceed 5 times the upper limit of normal (ULN) or if elevations in aminotransferase concentrations are accompanied by bilirubin concentrations exceeding 2 times the ULN or by manifestations of hepatic injury (e.g., anorexia, nausea, vomiting, fever, malaise, fatigue, abdominal pain, jaundice, dark urine, pruritus) for which alternative causes have been excluded.

Specific Populations **Pregnancy.** Category X. (See Fetal/Neonatal Morbidity and Mortality under Warnings/Precautions: Warnings, in Cautions.)

Lactation. It is not known whether ambrisentan is distributed into human milk. Because many drugs are distributed into human milk and because of the potential for serious adverse reactions to ambrisentan in nursing infants, a decision should be made whether to discontinue nursing or the drug.

Pediatric Use. Safety and efficacy have not been established in children and adolescents younger than 18 years of age.

Geriatric Use. A higher incidence of peripheral edema has been observed in patients 65 years of age or older relative to younger adults.

Hepatic Impairment. Because ambrisentan is substantially metabolized and eliminated by the liver and biliary system, the drug should not be used in patients with preexisting moderate or severe hepatic impairment. No information is available on the use of ambrisentan in patients with mild hepatic impairment; however, systemic exposure to the drug may be increased in such patients.

Renal Impairment. Ambrisentan has not been studied in patients with severe renal impairment or in those undergoing hemodialysis.

Mild or moderate renal impairment had no clinically important effect on ambrisentan disposition. (See Renal Impairment under Dosage and Administration: Special Populations.)

■ **Common Adverse Effects** Peripheral edema, nasal congestion, sinusitis, flushing, palpitations, nasopharyngitis, abdominal pain, constipation, dyspnea, headache.

Drug Interactions

In vitro studies indicate that ambrisentan is metabolized by cytochrome P-450 (CYP) isoenzymes 3A4 and 2C19 and by uridine 5′-diphosphate glucuronosyltransferases (UGTs; uridine diphosphoglucuronosyltransferase, UDP-glucuronate β-D-glucuronosyltransferase [acceptor-unspecific]) 1A9S, 2B7S, and 1A3S. The drug appears to be a substrate of the organic anion transport protein (OATP) and a substrate, but not inhibitor, of the P-glycoprotein transport system. At clinically relevant concentrations, ambrisentan does not inhibit or induce CYP enzymes.

■ **Drugs Affecting Hepatic Microsomal Enzymes** ***Inhibitors or Inducers of CYP2C19*** Pharmacokinetic interaction is possible, but experience with concomitant use of a potent CYP2C19 inhibitor (omeprazole) or a potent CYP2C19 inducer (rifampin) suggests that such interactions are not likely to be clinically important.

Inhibitors or Inducers of CYP3A4 Pharmacokinetic interaction is possible, but experience to date has demonstrated a clinically important interaction only with cyclosporine, a CYP3A4 inhibitor.

■ **Drugs Affecting the Organic Anion Transport Protein** Potential pharmacokinetic interaction (e.g., increased ambrisentan exposure) with drugs that inhibit OATP (e.g., cyclosporine).

■ **Drugs Affecting the P-glycoprotein Transport System** Pharmacokinetic interaction is possible with drugs that induce the P-glycoprotein transport system (e.g., rifampin), but such interactions are not likely to be clinically important. Pharmacokinetic interaction (e.g., increased ambrisentan exposure) is possible with drugs that inhibit P-glycoprotein (e.g., cyclosporine).

■ **Drugs Affecting Uridine 5′-Diphosphate Glucuronosyltransferase Enzymes** Pharmacokinetic interaction is possible with drugs that induce UGT (e.g., rifampin), but such interactions are not likely to be clinically important.

■ **Cyclosporine** In healthy individuals, concomitant administration of ambrisentan and cyclosporine increased area under the concentration-time curve (AUC) and peak plasma concentrations of ambrisentan by a factor of 2 and 1.5, respectively, but did not alter systemic exposure to cyclosporine. Dosage of ambrisentan should be reduced to 5 mg once daily if administered concomitantly with cyclosporine. No adjustment of cyclosporine dosage is required.

■ **Digoxin** In healthy men, concomitant administration of ambrisentan and digoxin resulted in a modest increase in systemic exposure (increased plasma concentrations and AUC) to digoxin; however, such changes are not likely to be clinically important. No dosage adjustments are necessary.

■ **Ketoconazole** In healthy men, concomitant administration of ambrisentan and ketoconazole (a potent CYP3A4 inhibitor) modestly increased systemic exposure to ambrisentan and slightly prolonged elimination half-life of the drug; however, such changes were not considered clinically important. No dosage adjustments are necessary.

■ **Mycophenolate Mofetil** Peak plasma concentrations and systemic exposure of ambrisentan were not altered with concomitant use of mycophenolate mofetil; pharmacokinetics of the active metabolite of mycophenolate mofetil, mycophenolic acid, also were unchanged. No dosage adjustments are necessary.

■ **Omeprazole** Concomitant administration of ambrisentan and omeprazole did not substantially alter peak plasma concentrations or systemic exposure of ambrisentan. No dosage adjustments are necessary.

■ **Hormonal Contraceptives** Concomitant use of ambrisentan with an oral contraceptive containing ethinyl estradiol and norethindrone did not result in any clinically important changes in systemic exposure to the hormonal contraceptive. No dosage adjustments are necessary.

■ **Phosphodiesterase Inhibitors** Clinically important pharmacokinetic interactions have not been observed with concomitant use of ambrisentan and the phosphodiesterase (PDE) type 5 inhibitors sildenafil or tadalafil in healthy individuals. No dosage adjustments are necessary.

■ **Rifampin** In healthy individuals, concomitant administration of ambrisentan and rifampin (potent inducer of CYP3A4 and inhibitor of OATP) increased systemic exposure to ambrisentan by twofold, but the effect was transient and not considered clinically important. No dosage adjustments are necessary.

■ **Ritonavir** Peak plasma concentrations and systemic exposure of ambrisentan were not altered with concomitant use of ritonavir; no dosage adjustments are necessary.

■ **Tacrolimus** Peak plasma concentrations and systemic exposure of ambrisentan were not altered with concomitant use of tacrolimus; no dosage adjustments are necessary.

■ **Warfarin** No clinically important interaction has been observed with concomitant use of ambrisentan and warfarin. In a study in healthy individuals, administration of a single dose of warfarin (25 mg) with ambrisentan (10 mg daily) did not substantially alter the pharmacokinetics of either drug and had no clinically important effect on prothrombin time (PT) or international normalized ratio (INR). No dosage adjustments are necessary.

Description

Ambrisentan, a selective endothelin-1 (ET-1) type A receptor antagonist, is a vasodilator. Although pharmacologically related to other ET-1 receptor antagonists, ambrisentan differs structurally and exhibits greater selectivity for ET-1 type A receptors than other currently available endothelin receptor antagonists. Increased concentrations of ET-1, a potent vasoconstrictor, have been detected in the plasma and lung tissue of patients with pulmonary arterial hypertension (PAH), suggesting a pathogenic role for ET-1 in this disorder. Two ET-1 receptor subtypes, type A and type B, have been identified; activation of ET-1 type A receptors primarily mediates vasoconstriction and smooth muscle cell proliferation, while activation of ET-1 type B receptors results in vasodilation and facilitates clearance of ET-1. Ambrisentan is approximately 4000-fold more selective for the type A receptor compared with the type B receptor; however, the clinical implications of this selectivity remain to be established.

In vitro evidence indicates that ambrisentan is metabolized by cytochrome P-450 (CYP) isoenzymes 3A4 and 2C19, and by uridine diphosphate-glucuronosyltransferases (UGT) 1A9, 2B7, and 1A3. In vitro studies suggest that ambrisentan also is a substrate of the transporters p-glycoprotein and organic anion transport protein (OATP).

Advice to Patients

Risk of fetal harm; importance of advising females of childbearing potential to avoid pregnancy and to use acceptable methods of contraception during and for 1 month following discontinuance of ambrisentan therapy. Acceptable methods of contraception include one highly effective form of contraception (intrauterine device [IUD], progesterone implant, or tubal sterilization) or a combination of methods (either one hormonal and one barrier method or 2 barrier methods where one form is the male condom). Acceptable hormonal methods of contraception include estrogen-progestin combination oral contraceptives or transdermal contraceptive systems, vaginal ring, and progesterone injections. Acceptable barrier methods include male condoms, diaphragms with spermicide, and cervical caps with spermicide. Even if the partner has had a vasectomy, an additional hormonal or barrier method must be used.

Importance of advising females to inform their clinician immediately if a menstrual period is missed or pregnancy is suspected; clinicians should perform a pregnancy test if pregnancy is suspected for any reason and provide counseling on the use of emergency contraception in the event of unprotected sexual intercourse or known or suspected contraceptive failure. Apprise patient of potential risk to fetus if pregnancy occurs.

Importance of all female patients (regardless of childbearing potential) enrolling in the Letairis® REMS program and complying with requirements of the program, including pregnancy testing and contraception requirements in females of childbearing potential. Importance of monitoring reproductive status of prepubertal females and immediately reporting changes to clinician.

Importance of periodic monitoring of red blood cell counts during treatment.

Importance of patients not taking ambrisentan if they have idiopathic pulmonary fibrosis.

Potential risk of liver toxicity. Importance of patients informing clinicians of any unexplained nausea, vomiting, right upper quadrant pain, fatigue, anorexia, jaundice, dark urine, fever, or itching.

Importance of taking ambrisentan as prescribed and of not interrupting or discontinuing therapy without consulting a clinician.

Importance of not taking a double dose to make up for a missed dose but instead taking the next scheduled dose.

Importance of advising patients to swallow tablets whole and not to split, chew, or crush tablets.

Importance of distributing the FDA-approved medication guide to every patient who receives ambrisentan and reviewing the information with female patients. (See REMS.) Importance of patients carefully reading the medication guide before initiating therapy and each time prescription is refilled.

Importance of females informing their clinician if they are or plan to become pregnant or plan to breast-feed.

Importance of informing clinicians of existing or contemplated concomitant therapy, including prescription (e.g., cyclosporine) and OTC drugs or herbal supplements, as well as any concomitant illnesses.

Importance of informing patients of other important precautionary information. (See Cautions.)

Overview® (see Users Guide). For additional information on this drug until a more detailed monograph is developed and published, the manufacturer's labeling should be consulted. It is *essential* that the manufacturer's labeling be consulted for more detailed information on usual cautions, precautions, contraindications, potential drug interactions, laboratory test interferences, and acute toxicity.

Preparations

Distribution of ambrisentan is restricted. (See Restricted Distribution Program under Dosage and Administration: General.)

Excipients in commercially available drug preparations may have clinically important effects in some individuals; consult specific product labeling for details.

Ambrisentan

Oral		
Tablets, film-coated	5 mg	Letairis®, Gilead
	10 mg	Letairis®, Gilead

†Use is not currently included in the labeling approved by the US Food and Drug Administration

Bosentan

■ Bosentan, an endothelin-receptor antagonist, is a vasodilator.

REMS

FDA approved a REMS for bosentan to ensure that the benefits outweigh the risks. The REMS may apply to one or more preparations of bosentan and consists of the following: elements to assure safe use and implementation system. See the FDA REMS page (https://www.accessdata.fda.gov/scripts/cder/rems/index.cfm). Also see Restricted Distribution Program under Dosage and Administration: General.

Uses

■ **Pulmonary Arterial Hypertension** Bosentan is used in the management of pulmonary arterial hypertension (PAH) (World Health Organization [WHO] group 1 pulmonary hypertension) to improve exercise capacity and to delay clinical worsening. Clinical studies establishing efficacy of bosentan for this use were conducted principally in patients with New York Heart Association (NYHA)/WHO functional class II–IV PAH (idiopathic, heritable, or associated with connective tissue diseases or congenital systemic-to-pulmonary shunts). For more information about etiologies of PAH, see Uses: Pulmonary Arterial Hypertension, in Epoprostenol 48:48. Bosentan has been designated an orphan drug by the US Food and Drug Administration (FDA) for use in the treatment of PAH.

In addition to general treatment measures and supportive therapy (e.g., warfarin anticoagulation, diuretics, supplemental oxygen, digoxin), experts recommend an endothelin-receptor antagonist (e.g., ambrisentan, bosentan, macitentan) as one of several treatment options for the initial management of PAH in patients with NYHA/WHO functional class II, III, or IV symptoms who are not candidates for calcium-channel blocker therapy or in whom such therapy has failed; alternative therapies include phosphodiesterase (PDE) type 5 inhibitors (e.g., sildenafil, tadalafil), prostanoids (IV epoprostenol; inhaled iloprost; inhaled, IV or subcutaneous treprostinil), or soluble guanylate cyclase stimulators (e.g., riociguat). Current guidelines for the management of PAH state that an oral agent such as an endothelin-receptor antagonist generally is preferred for initial therapy in patients with NYHA/WHO functional class II symptoms, while those with more advanced NYHA/WHO functional class III disease may be treated with any currently approved PAH therapy; IV epoprostenol generally is recommended as the treatment of choice for patients with NYHA/WHO class IV PAH because of its demonstrated survival benefit. In general, choice of PAH therapy should be individualized, taking into account factors such as disease severity, route of administration, potential adverse effects, costs of treatment, clinician experience, and patient preference.

Efficacy of bosentan for the management of severe (NYHA/WHO functional class III or IV) PAH has been established in 2 randomized, double-blind, multicenter, placebo-controlled clinical trials in a total of 245 patients with WHO functional class III or IV PAH; 72% of patients had idiopathic or familial PAH and the remainder had PAH associated with other disorders (connective tissue diseases [21%], autoimmune diseases [7%]). In these 2 clinical trials, addition of bosentan (62.5 mg orally twice daily for 4 weeks, followed by a maintenance dosage of 125 or 250 mg twice daily) to standard therapy (e.g., cardiac glycosides, anticoagulants, diuretics, and/or vasodilators [e.g., calcium-channel blocking agents, angiotensin-converting enzyme {ACE} inhibitors] but not other prostacyclin analogs [e.g., epoprostenol]) substantially increased exercise capacity, as indicated by a mean increase, relative to placebo, of 35–54 or 76 m, respectively, in the 6-minute walking distance. Improvement in walking distance was apparent after approximately 1 month of therapy with bosentan 62.5 mg twice daily, with full effect evident by about 2 months of therapy with higher dosages. Improvement was maintained for up to 7 months of therapy. In one study, walking distance tended to be greater with bosentan 250 mg twice daily than with bosentan 125 mg twice daily; however, the difference between groups was not significant, and administration of the higher dosage is not recommended because of an increased risk of hepatic injury. Bosentan therapy also resulted in substantial hemodynamic changes (e.g., increases in cardiac index associated with substantial reductions in pulmonary artery pressure, pulmonary vascular resistance, and mean right atrial pressure, without changes in heart rate) following 12 weeks of therapy and slowed the rate of clinical worsening (defined as the combined incidence of death, hospitalization for PAH, and worsening PAH requiring discontinuance of therapy or supplemental epoprostenol) over up to 28 weeks of therapy. In addition, there were substantial reductions in dyspnea during walking distance tests (based on Borg dyspnea score) and improvements in NYHA/WHO functional class in patients treated with bosentan. Because short-term vasodilator testing was not performed as part of the studies, it is not known whether the patients with the best response to bosentan would have had a similar response to other vasodilators. In long-term, open-label studies of patients with NYHA/WHO class III or IV PAH, 93 and 84% of patients were still alive after 1 and 2 years of bosentan therapy, respectively. Improvements in exercise capacity were maintained in patients who continued to receive bosentan for longer than 1 year.

Efficacy of bosentan in patients with milder PAH symptoms (NYHA/WHO functional class II) was evaluated in a randomized, double-blind, multicenter, placebo-controlled study in patients 12 years of age or older with NYHA/WHO class II PAH (principally idiopathic PAH or PAH associated with congenital heart disease or connective tissue disorders). Patients were randomized to receive bosentan (62.5 mg orally twice daily for 4 weeks, followed by 125 mg twice daily) or placebo for 6 months; with the exception of sildenafil, no other treatments for PAH (prostacyclin analogs, other endothelin-receptor antagonists) were allowed. Bosentan was more effective than placebo in improving hemodynamic parameters (e.g., pulmonary vascular resistance) and NYHA/WHO functional class, as well as in decreasing the rate of clinical worsening (defined as death from any cause, hospitalization for PAH, or symptomatic progression of PAH). Although the mean 6-minute walking distance increased in patients receiving bosentan compared with an overall decrease in the placebo group, the difference was not statistically significant. When considering use of bosentan in patients with mild (NYHA/WHO class II) PAH, clinicians should determine whether these benefits are sufficient to outweigh the risk of hepatotoxicity; liver injury could preclude future use of the drug.

Current expert consensus guidelines recommend combination therapy with a prostanoid, PDE type 5 inhibitor, or soluble guanylate cyclase stimulator (added sequentially) in patients who have an inadequate response to initial monotherapy. Combination therapy with drugs that target the different pathophysiologic pathways in PAH may provide additive and/or synergistic benefits. Data from several small studies suggest that use of an endothelin-receptor antagonist in combination with a prostanoid or a PDE type 5 inhibitor may improve outcomes (e.g., reduce clinical worsening, increase 6-minute walking distance, improve hemodynamic parameters) in patients who remain symptomatic on monotherapy.

■ **Congestive Heart Failure** Bosentan is not effective in the treatment of congestive heart failure (CHF) with left ventricular dysfunction†. Results of clinical studies in patients with NYHA class III or IV heart failure did not show a benefit of bosentan on patient global assessment or mortality. In addition, an increased incidence of hospitalization for CHF associated with weight gain and leg edema has been reported in patients with severe chronic CHF receiving bosentan.

Dosage and Administration

■ **General** ***Restricted Distribution Program*** Because bosentan can cause serious hepatic injury and is very likely to cause major birth defects if administered during pregnancy, commercially available bosentan must be obtained through a restricted distribution program, the Tracleer® Access Program (TAP). TAP is part of a required risk management plan (Risk Evaluation and Mitigation Strategy, REMS) that has been developed for bosentan to minimize the risk of fetal exposure and hepatotoxicity and to promote informed risk-versus-benefit decisions regarding use of the drug. (See REMS.) Clinicians and pharmacies must be registered with TAP and comply with all terms of the program (including patient education and safety requirements) before they can prescribe or dispense bosentan. In addition, the drug may be dispensed only to patients enrolled in, and who meet all conditions of, the program; patient enrollment must be done annually. Only designated pharmacies from a specialty pharmacy network will be authorized to dispense the drug. For additional information about TAP, clinicians may call 866-228-3546.

Prior to initiating bosentan therapy, serum aminotransferase (AST [SGOT] or ALT [SGPT]) concentrations must be measured, and in women of childbearing potential, clinicians must ascertain that the patient is not pregnant by obtaining negative results from a urine or serum pregnancy test performed during the first 5 days of a normal menstrual period and at least 11 days after the last unprotected act of sexual intercourse. Serum or urine pregnancy testing and monitoring of serum aminotransferases should be performed monthly during bosentan therapy.

No more than a 30-day supply of bosentan may be dispensed at one time, and dispensing should occur only after obtaining confirmation from the patient that the required liver function and pregnancy tests were completed. In addition, a medication guide explaining the risks and benefits of therapy must be distributed each time the drug is dispensed and must be reviewed with the patient.

■ **Administration** ***Oral Administration*** Bosentan is administered orally twice daily (in the morning and evening) without regard to meals.

■ **Dosage** The recommended initial dosage of bosentan for the treatment of pulmonary arterial hypertension (PAH) in adults and adolescents older than 12 years of age is 62.5 mg twice daily for 4 weeks, followed by 125 mg twice daily. In patients older than 12 years of age who weigh less than 40 kg, the recommended dosage of bosentan for both initial and maintenance therapy is 62.5 mg twice daily. Whenever bosentan therapy is discontinued, gradual reduction of the dosage (e.g., 62.5 mg twice daily for 3–7 days) should be considered to minimize the risk of clinical deterioration.

When bosentan therapy is initiated in patients who have been receiving an HIV protease inhibitor for at least 10 days, bosentan should be initiated at a dosage of 62.5 mg once daily or every other day based on individual patient tolerance. When therapy with an HIV protease inhibitor is initiated in patients receiving bosentan, bosentan should be discontinued at least 36 hours prior to initiating the HIV protease inhibitor; after at least 10 days of HIV protease inhibitor therapy, bosentan can be resumed at a dosage of 62.5 mg once daily or every other day based on patient tolerance. Concomitant use of bosentan and atazanavir (without ritonavir) should be avoided. (See Interactions: HIV Protease Inhibitors.)

■ **Special Populations** Dose reduction or discontinuance of bosentan therapy may be necessary in patients who develop elevated serum aminotransferase (AST [SGOT] or ALT [SGPT]) concentrations during therapy with the drug. Dose reduction or interruption of therapy should be instituted in patients with confirmed (i.e., upon a repeat test) aminotransferase concentrations exceeding 3 times, but not more than 5 times, the upper limit of normal (ULN); in those with confirmed aminotransferase concentrations exceeding 5 times the ULN, as well as in those with aminotransferase elevations accompanied by manifestations of hepatic disease (e.g., nausea, vomiting, fever, abdominal pain, jaundice, lethargy, fatigue) or increases in bilirubin concentrations of 2 times the ULN or greater, the drug should be discontinued by gradually reducing the dosage (e.g., 62.5 mg twice daily for 3–7 days). Serum aminotransferase concentrations should be monitored at least every 2 weeks following dose reduction or discontinuance of the drug.

Reinitiation of bosentan therapy at a starting dosage of 62.5 mg twice daily may be considered following the return of aminotransferase concentrations to pretreatment levels if the aminotransferase elevations did *not* exceed 8 times the ULN; serum aminotransferase concentrations should be checked within 3 days of reinitiating therapy and every 2 weeks thereafter. The manufacturer states that reinitiation of bosentan therapy should *not* be considered in patients whose aminotransferase concentrations exceeded 8 times the ULN. Clinical experience with reinitiation of bosentan therapy is lacking in such patients, as well as in those with aminotransferase elevations accompanied by manifestations of hepatic disease or by increases in bilirubin concentrations of 2 times the ULN or greater.

Bosentan generally should be avoided in patients with preexisting moderate or severe hepatic impairment (Child-Pugh class B or C). No dosage adjustment is required in patients with mild hepatic impairment (Child-Pugh class A). (See Hepatic Impairment under Warnings/Precautions: Specific Populations, in Cautions.)

No dosage adjustment is necessary in patients with renal impairment. (See Renal Impairment under Warnings/Precautions: Specific Populations, in Cautions.)

Cautions

■ **Contraindications** Known or suspected pregnancy, concomitant therapy with cyclosporine or glyburide, or known hypersensitivity to bosentan or to any ingredient in the formulation.

■ **Warnings/Precautions** ***Warnings*** **Hepatotoxicity.** Risk of developing serious hepatic injury. With close monitoring, unexplained hepatic cirrhosis and liver failure have been reported rarely after prolonged (exceeding 12 months) bosentan therapy during postmarketing surveillance.

In at least one patient, marked elevations in liver function test results developed (after more than 20 months of bosentan therapy) accompanied by nonspecific symptoms. Following drug discontinuance, AST/ALT concentrations remained elevated and bilirubin concentrations continued to increase; liver failure and biopsy-confirmed cirrhosis developed. Causality to bosentan could not be excluded. Liver failure later abated and liver function tests slowly resolved (7 months after discontinuance).

The manufacturer reinforces the importance of strict adherence to the monthly monitoring schedule for the duration of bosentan therapy (see Restricted Distribution Program under Dosage and Administration: General) and to the dosage adjustment and monitoring guidelines. (See Dosage and Administration: Special Populations.)

Dose-dependent elevations in aminotransferase (AST or ALT) concentrations of more than 3 times the upper limit of normal (ULN) have been observed in 11% of patients receiving bosentan at dosages up to 2 g daily in clinical trials and have been accompanied in a few cases by elevations in bilirubin concentrations. Because such changes are a marker for potential serious hepatic injury, serum aminotransferase concentrations must be measured prior to initiation of therapy and then monthly thereafter. Dose reduction or discontinuance of the drug may be necessary depending on the degree of hepatic impairment. (See Dosage and Administration: Special Populations.)

Fetal/Neonatal Morbidity and Mortality. Bosentan may cause fetal harm if used during pregnancy; teratogenic effects (e.g., malformations to craniofacial and cardiovascular structures) have been demonstrated in animals and appear to be a class effect of endothelin-receptor antagonists. No adequate and well-controlled studies have been conducted in pregnant women.

Bosentan is contraindicated during pregnancy; pregnancy must be excluded before treatment is initiated and prevented thereafter by means of 2 reliable contraceptive methods during and for one month following treatment, unless the patient has undergone tubal sterilization or chooses to use a Copper T380A or LNg 20 intrauterine device (IUD), in which case no additional contraceptive is needed. (See Restricted Distribution Program under Dosage and Administration: General.) Because the reliability of oral or other systemic (e.g., injectable, transdermal, implantable) hormonal contraceptives may be affected by bosentan, such contraceptives should *not* be used as the sole contraceptive method in patients receiving bosentan. (See Drug Interactions: Hormonal Contraceptives.) Pregnancy testing should be repeated monthly during therapy with the drug. If bosentan is used during pregnancy or if the patient becomes pregnant during therapy, the patient should be apprised of the potential hazard to the fetus. Consultation with a gynecology specialist regarding adequate contraception should be sought as needed.

Sensitivity Reactions Angioedema occurring 8 hours to 21 days after initiating bosentan therapy has been reported during postmarketing surveillance. In some patients, angioedema was treated with an antihistamine and manifestations of angioedema resolved without discontinuance of bosentan.

Other Warnings and Precautions **Fluid Retention.** Fluid retention requiring diuretics, fluid management, or hospitalization for decompensating heart failure within weeks of initiating bosentan has been reported in patients with pulmonary arterial hypertension (PAH) during postmarketing experience. Peripheral edema is a known class effect of endothelin-receptor antagonists and also a clinical consequence of PAH.

If clinically important fluid retention occurs (with or without weight gain), the patient should be further evaluated to determine the cause and to assess the need for specific treatment or discontinuance of bosentan therapy.

Fertility in Males. Decreases in sperm count of at least 50% have been observed in some men with PAH receiving usual dosages of bosentan for several months. Sperm counts generally remained within the normal range in patients who completed 6 months of therapy, and no changes in sperm morphology, sperm motility, or hormone levels were observed. At least one case of marked oligospermia, which resolved following discontinuance of bosentan, has been reported. The possibility that bosentan may cause adverse effects on spermatogenesis cannot be excluded.

Hematologic Effects. Dose-related decreases in hemoglobin concentration (mean decrease: 0.9 g/dL) and hematocrit have occurred in clinical trials, particularly during the first few weeks following initiation of bosentan therapy; hemoglobin concentrations generally have stabilized after 4–12 weeks of continued therapy. The manufacturer recommends that hemoglobin concentrations be monitored 1 and 3 months after initiation of bosentan therapy and every 3 months thereafter. The occurrence of a substantial decrease in hemoglobin concentration should prompt further evaluation to determine the cause and need for specific treatment.

Pulmonary Effects. If manifestations of pulmonary edema occur during therapy, the possibility of associated pulmonary veno-occlusive disease (PVOD) should be considered and bosentan should be discontinued.

Specific Populations **Pregnancy.** Category X. (See Warnings: Fetal/Neonatal Morbidity and Mortality and also see Contraindications, in Cautions.)

Lactation. It is not known whether bosentan is distributed into milk; because of the potential for serious adverse reactions to bosentan in nursing infants, a decision should be made whether to discontinue nursing or the drug, taking into account the importance of the drug to the woman.

Pediatric Use. The manufacturer states that safety and efficacy of bosentan have not been established in children younger than 12 years of age; however, the drug has been used in a limited number of patients in this age group. Results of an open-label study found that the efficacy, safety, and pharmacokinetics of bosentan in pediatric patients 3–15 years of age with NYHA/WHO class II or III PAH (idiopathic or associated with congenital heart disease) were similar to those parameters reported in adults; in this study, dosage of bosentan was determined by body weight and ranged from 31.25–125 mg twice daily.

Geriatric Use. Experience with bosentan in those 65 years of age and older is insufficient to determine whether they respond differently than younger adults.

Hepatic Impairment. Because bosentan is extensively metabolized by the liver, hepatic impairment is expected to increase systemic exposure to the drug. Increased exposure to bosentan and its active metabolite was observed in a pharmacokinetic study in 8 patients with PAH associated with portal hypertension who had moderate hepatic impairment (Child-Pugh class B). Limited data suggest that the pharmacokinetics of bosentan are not altered in patients with mild hepatic impairment (Child-Pugh class A). The pharmacokinetics of bosentan have not been evaluated in patients with severe hepatic impairment (Child-Pugh class C). Use of bosentan generally is not recommended in patients with preexisting moderate to severe hepatic impairment and/or in those with elevated serum aminotransferase concentrations exceeding 3 times the upper limit of normal. (See Dosage and Administration: Special Populations.)

Renal Impairment. The effect of renal impairment on the pharmacokinetics of bosentan is considered minimal; plasma bosentan concentrations are essentially unchanged in patients with severe renal impairment (creatinine clearance 15–30 mL/minute). (See Dosage and Administration: Special Populations.)

■ **Common Adverse Effects** Adverse effects occurring in 3% or more of patients receiving bosentan and more frequently than with placebo include headache, nasopharyngitis, flushing, abnormal hepatic function, lower limb edema, hypotension, palpitations, dyspepsia, edema, fatigue, pruritus, rash, and anemia.

Drug Interactions

■ **Drugs Affecting or Metabolized by Hepatic Microsomal Enzymes** Because bosentan induces cytochrome P-450 (CYP) isoenzymes 2C9 and 3A and possibly 2C19, plasma concentrations of drugs metabolized by these enzymes may be decreased when such drugs are used concomitantly with bosentan. In vitro studies indicate that bosentan does not inhibit CYP isoenzymes 1A2, 2C9, 2C19, 2D6, or 3A and, therefore, is not expected to increase plasma concentrations of drugs metabolized by these enzymes.

Because bosentan is metabolized by CYP isoenzymes 2C9 and 3A, concomitant use of drugs that inhibit these enzymes may result in increased plasma concentrations of bosentan. Concomitant administration of both an inhibitor of CYP2C9 (e.g., amiodarone, fluconazole) and a potent (e.g., ketoconazole, itraconazole) or moderate (e.g., amprenavir, erythromycin, fluconazole, diltiazem) inhibitor of CYP3A with bosentan is not recommended.

■ **Drugs Affecting the Organic Anion Transport Protein** In vitro data suggest that bosentan is a substrate of the organic anion transport protein (OATP); therefore, pharmacokinetic interactions are possible with drugs that inhibit OATP (e.g., rifampin, ritonavir).

■ **Cyclosporine** Concomitant use of bosentan with cyclosporine increased steady-state plasma bosentan concentrations by about threefold to fourfold and decreased plasma cyclosporine concentrations by approximately 50%. Following the first concomitant dose, a 30-fold increase in bosentan trough concentrations was observed, possibly due to an inhibitory effect of cyclosporine on hepatic protein transporters. Concomitant use is contraindicated.

■ **Digoxin** Clinically important effects on digoxin pharmacokinetics have not been observed with concomitant use.

■ **Glyburide** An increased risk of elevated serum aminotransferase concentrations has been noted in patients receiving bosentan and glyburide concomitantly. Concomitant use is contraindicated; alternative hypoglycemic agents should be considered.

Plasma concentrations of both bosentan and glyburide were decreased following concomitant use. Bosentan is expected to also reduce plasma concentrations of other hypoglycemic agents metabolized principally by CYP2C9 or CYP3A; the potential for loss of blood glucose control should be considered in patients receiving these drugs.

■ **HIV Protease Inhibitors** In healthy individuals, concomitant administration of bosentan and lopinavir/ritonavir increased trough concentrations of bosentan by approximately 48- and 5-fold on days 4 and 10, respectively; systemic exposure to lopinavir/ritonavir was not altered to a clinically important extent. Other HIV protease inhibitors also are expected to increase plasma concentrations of bosentan. Therefore, dosage adjustment of bosentan is necessary when antiretroviral regimens containing an HIV protease inhibitor are initiated in patients receiving bosentan or when bosentan is initiated in patients receiving an HIV protease inhibitor. (See Dosage and Administration: Special Populations.) Because plasma concentrations of atazanavir may be decreased when bosentan is administered with atazanavir (without ritonavir), concomitant use of bosentan and atazanavir (without ritonavir) should be avoided.

■ **HMG-CoA Reductase Inhibitors (Statins)** Concomitant administration of bosentan and simvastatin (a CYP3A substrate) reduced plasma concentrations of simvastatin and its active metabolite by approximately 50%. Bosentan is expected to also reduce plasma concentrations of other statins substantially metabolized by CYP3A (lovastatin, atorvastatin). Patients receiving these statins should have their serum cholesterol concentrations monitored when bosentan is initiated, and dosage of the statin should be adjusted if necessary.

■ **Hormonal Contraceptives** Concomitant use of bosentan with an oral contraceptive containing ethinyl estradiol and norethindrone resulted in substantially decreased systemic exposure to the oral contraceptive. An alternative or concomitant nonhormonal contraceptive method should be used during bosentan therapy; hormonal contraceptives (including oral, injectable, transdermal, implantable forms) should not be used as the sole contraceptive method.

■ **Iloprost** Limited data suggest that bosentan may be used to therapeutic advantage in combination with inhaled iloprost (up to 5 mcg 6–9 times daily during waking hours); such concomitant therapy appears to be well tolerated.

■ **Phosphodiesterase Inhibitors** In healthy men, concomitant administration of bosentan and the phosphodiesterase (PDE) type 5 inhibitor tadalafil decreased systemic exposure to tadalafil by 42% but did not substantially alter bosentan exposure. Such concomitant therapy was well tolerated.

In healthy men, concomitant administration of bosentan and sildenafil reduced plasma sildenafil concentrations by approximately 63% and increased plasma bosentan concentrations by approximately 50%. When administered concomitantly in patients with pulmonary arterial hypertension (PAH), bosentan substantially decreased plasma concentrations of sildenafil. However, the manufacturer states that dosage adjustments are not necessary.

■ **Ketoconazole** Concomitant administration of bosentan with ketoconazole, a potent CYP3A inhibitor, increased plasma bosentan concentrations by about twofold. Dosage adjustment of bosentan is not necessary; however, clinicians should consider the potential for increased effects of bosentan.

■ **Losartan** Pharmacokinetic interaction is unlikely.

■ **Nimodipine** Pharmacokinetic interaction is unlikely.

■ **Rifampin** In healthy individuals receiving bosentan and rifampin concomitantly, plasma bosentan concentrations increased initially by about sixfold after the first concurrent dose, but subsequently decreased with continued concomitant administration. The initial increase in bosentan concentration is likely a result of rifampin-induced inhibition of the OATP system. If concomitant therapy is necessary, liver function tests should be monitored weekly for the first 4 weeks followed by resumption of the usual monthly testing schedule.

■ **Tacrolimus** Markedly increased plasma bosentan concentrations have been observed in animals following concomitant administration of bosentan and tacrolimus. Caution should be exercised with concomitant administration.

■ **Treprostinil** Pharmacokinetic interaction has not been noted between bosentan and an oral formulation of treprostinil in healthy individuals.

■ **Warfarin** In a study in healthy individuals, bosentan reduced plasma concentrations of warfarin and substantially reduced its anticoagulant effects. The manufacturer states that clinically important changes in international normalized ratio (INR) or warfarin dosage were not observed in patients with PAH receiving bosentan and warfarin concomitantly in clinical trials. Some clinicians, however, recommend that INR be monitored closely in patients receiving warfarin when bosentan is initiated or discontinued.

Description

Bosentan, an endothelin receptor antagonist, improves exercise capacity and hemodynamics in patients with pulmonary arterial hypertension (PAH) by inhibiting the vasoconstricting effects of endothelin-1. Endothelin-1 (ET-1) concentrations have been shown to be elevated in plasma and lung tissue of patients with PAH, suggesting a pathogenic role for ET-1 in this disorder. Two ET-1 receptor subtypes, type A and type B, have been identified; activation of ET-1 type A receptors mediates vasoconstriction and smooth muscle cell proliferation, while activation of ET-1 type B receptors results in vasodilation and facilitates clearance of ET-1. Bosentan exhibits specific and competitive antagonism of both endothelin type A and type B receptors in the endothelium and vascular smooth muscle, with slightly greater affinity for ET-1 type A receptors. The clinical importance of selective versus nonselective endothelin receptor blockade is not known.

Bosentan is metabolized by cytochrome P-450 (CYP) isoenzymes 2C9 and 3A. The drug is eliminated principally by biliary excretion following metabolism in the liver; less than 3% of an orally administered dose is recovered in urine. Bosentan has been shown to induce cytochrome P-450 isoenzymes 2C9 and 3A and may possibly induce isoenzyme 2C19. Bosentan appears to induce its own metabolism following oral administration of multiple doses of the drug.

Advice to Patients

Risk of liver injury. Importance of patients promptly informing clinicians of any nausea, vomiting, fever, unusual tiredness, abdominal pain, or yellowing of the skin or white of the eyes.

Importance of women informing clinicians if they are or plan to become pregnant or plan to breast-feed.

Risk of fetal harm; importance of advising females of childbearing potential to avoid pregnancy and to use 2 reliable methods of contraception (either one hormonal and one barrier method or 2 barrier methods where one form is the male condom) simultaneously during and for 1 month following bosentan therapy unless the patient has undergone tubal sterilization or chooses to use a Copper T380A or LNg 20 intrauterine device (IUD), in which case no additional contraceptive is needed. (See Restricted Distribution Program under Dosage and Administration: General.) Acceptable hormonal contraceptive methods include progesterone injections, progesterone implants, estrogen-progestin combination oral contraceptives, transdermal contraceptive systems, and vaginal ring. Acceptable barrier methods include diaphragms with spermicide, cervical caps with spermicide, and male condoms. If the partner has had a vasectomy, an additional hormonal or barrier method must be used. Advise women to inform their clinician immediately if a menstrual period is missed or pregnancy is suspected. Apprise patient of potential risk to fetus if pregnancy occurs.

Importance of monthly monitoring of serum aminotransferases and monthly urine or serum pregnancy testing.

Importance of patients taking bosentan as prescribed and of not interrupting or discontinuing therapy without consulting a clinician.

Importance of not taking a double dose to make up for a missed dose but instead taking the next scheduled dose.

Importance of carefully reading the patient information (medication guide) provided by the manufacturer before initiating therapy and each time the prescription is refilled. (See REMS.)

Importance of informing clinicians of existing or contemplated concomitant therapy, including prescription and OTC drugs, as well as concomitant illnesses.

Importance of informing patients of other important precautionary information. (See Cautions.)

Overview® (see Users Guide). For additional information on this drug

until a more detailed monograph is developed and published, the manufacturer's labeling should be consulted. It is *essential* that the manufacturer's labeling be consulted for more detailed information on usual cautions, precautions, contraindications, potential drug interactions, laboratory test interferences, and acute toxicity.

Preparations

Distribution of bosentan is restricted. (See Restricted Distribution Program under Dosage and Administration: General.)

Excipients in commercially available drug preparations may have clinically important effects in some individuals; consult specific product labeling for details.

Bosentan

Oral		
Tablets, film-coated	62.5 mg (of anhydrous bosentan)	**Tracleer®**, Actelion
	125 mg (of anhydrous bosentan)	**Tracleer®**, Actelion

†Use is not currently included in the labeling approved by the US Food and Drug Administration

Selected Revisions May 2019, © Copyright, July 2002, American Society of Health-System Pharmacists, Inc.

Epoprostenol Sodium

■ Epoprostenol (PGI_2, PGX, prostacyclin), a naturally occurring prostaglandin, is a short-acting vasodilator and platelet-aggregation inhibitor.

Uses

■ **Pulmonary Arterial Hypertension** Epoprostenol sodium is used in the management of pulmonary arterial hypertension (PAH; World Health Organization [WHO] group 1 pulmonary hypertension) to improve exercise capacity. Clinical studies establishing efficacy of the drug were conducted principally in patients with New York Heart Association (NYHA)/WHO functional class III or IV PAH (idiopathic, heritable, or associated with connective tissue diseases). Epoprostenol has been designated an orphan drug by the US Food and Drug Administration (FDA) for use in the treatment of PAH.

Pulmonary hypertension is defined by the National Institutes of Health Registry as a mean pulmonary artery pressure exceeding 25 mm Hg at rest with a pulmonary capillary or left atrial pressure less than 15 mm Hg.

Pulmonary hypertension is currently classified into 5 categories (updated during the Fifth World Symposium on Pulmonary Arterial Hypertension in 2013): pulmonary arterial hypertension (PAH; Group 1), pulmonary hypertension associated with left heart diseases (Group 2), pulmonary hypertension associated with chronic lung diseases and/or hypoxia (Group 3), pulmonary hypertension due to chronic thrombotic and/or embolic disease (Group 4), and pulmonary hypertension due to unclear multifactorial mechanisms (Group 5). PAH is further subdivided into 4 subgroups: idiopathic, heritable, drug and toxin induced, and PAH related to risk factors or associated conditions (e.g., connective tissue diseases, HIV infection, portal hypertension, congenital heart diseases, schistosomiasis). The purpose of this classification is to group individual categories of pulmonary hypertension with similar pathophysiologic mechanisms, clinical presentations, and therapeutic options.

In addition to general treatment measures and supportive therapy (e.g., warfarin anticoagulation, diuretics, supplemental oxygen, digoxin), experts recommend IV epoprostenol as one of several treatment options for the initial management of PAH in patients with NYHA/WHO functional class III or IV symptoms who are not candidates for calcium-channel blocker therapy or in whom such therapy has failed; alternative therapies include endothelin-receptor antagonists (e.g., ambrisentan, bosentan, macitentan), phosphodiesterase (PDE) type 5 inhibitors (e.g., sildenafil, tadalafil), soluble guanylate cyclase stimulators (e.g., riociguat), or other prostanoids (e.g., inhaled iloprost; inhaled, IV, or subcutaneous treprostinil). While current guidelines for the management of PAH state that patients with NYHA/WHO functional class III disease may be treated with any currently approved PAH therapy, IV epoprostenol generally is recommended as the treatment of choice for patients with NYHA/WHO class IV PAH because of its demonstrated benefit on survival. In general, choice of PAH therapy should be individualized, taking into account factors such as disease severity, route of administration, potential adverse effects and costs of treatment, clinician experience, and patient preference.

Current expert consensus guidelines recommend combination therapy with an endothelin-receptor antagonist, PDE type 5 inhibitor, or soluble guanylate cyclase stimulator (added sequentially) in patients who have an inadequate response to initial monotherapy. Combination therapy with drugs that target the different pathophysiologic pathways in PAH may provide additive and/or synergistic benefits. Data from several studies suggest that use of a prostanoid in combination with an endothelin-receptor antagonist or a PDE type 5 inhibitor may improve outcomes (e.g., reduce clinical worsening, increase 6-minute walking distance, improve hemodynamic parameters) in patients who remain symptomatic on monotherapy.

Idiopathic or Heritable Pulmonary Arterial Hypertension Efficacy of epoprostenol in the treatment of idiopathic or heritable PAH has been established in 2 prospective, multicenter, randomized, open-label studies; these studies were of 8 or 12 weeks' duration and were conducted principally in adults with NYHA/WHO class III or IV PAH. In these studies, epoprostenol (infused IV at a mean dosage of 9.2 ng/kg per minute by the end of the studies) added to standard therapy (e.g., anticoagulants, oral vasodilators, diuretics, cardiac glycosides, supplemental oxygen) and titrated according to clinical response, was compared with standard therapy alone. Pooled data from these studies indicate that epoprostenol's effect on exercise capacity (i.e., a median increase of 47 m from baseline in the distance walked in 6 minutes) was statistically significant compared with a median decrease of 29 m in patients receiving standard therapy alone. Improvement in walking distance was apparent after 1 week of therapy with epoprostenol. Epoprostenol therapy was associated with improvements of indices of dyspnea and fatigue. Patients receiving epoprostenol also experienced improvements in hemodynamic parameters (e.g., increases in cardiac index, stroke volume, and arterial oxygen saturation, associated with reductions in mean pulmonary arterial pressure, total pulmonary resistance, pulmonary vascular resistance, mean right atrial pressure, mean systemic arterial pressure, and systemic vascular resistance) compared with baseline; hemodynamic effects generally were similar following acute and long-term administration of epoprostenol. Although a 20% decrease in mortality was reported at the end of the 12-week clinical study in patients receiving epoprostenol compared with those receiving standard therapy alone, some clinicians suggest that mortality data interpretation was confounded by baseline differences in exercise capacity between surviving and dying patients.

Pulmonary Arterial Hypertension Associated with Scleroderma Spectrum of Diseases Efficacy of epoprostenol in the treatment of PAH associated with the scleroderma spectrum of diseases has been established in a 12-week multicenter, randomized, open-label study principally in 111 adults with NYHA/WHO class III or IV symptoms. In this study, epoprostenol (infused IV at a mean dosage of 11.2 ng/kg per minute by week 12) added to standard therapy (e.g., anticoagulants, oral vasodilators, diuretics, cardiac glycosides, supplemental oxygen) and titrated according to clinical response, was compared with standard therapy alone. Results from this study indicate that epoprostenol's improvement on exercise capacity (i.e., a median increase of 46 m from baseline in the distance walked in 6 minutes) was statistically significant compared with a median decrease of 48 m in patients receiving standard therapy alone. Improvement in 6-minute walking distance (the primary end point) was apparent in some patients after 1 week of therapy with epoprostenol.

Patients receiving epoprostenol experienced a reduction in symptoms, as determined by substantial improvement in Borg dyspnea score and dyspnea fatigue index. While no change in NYHA/WHO functional class at 12 weeks of therapy was observed in 55 or 73% of patients receiving epoprostenol therapy or standard therapy alone, respectively, NYHA/WHO functional class improved in 41 or 0% of patients receiving epoprostenol therapy or standard therapy alone, respectively; worsening of functional status was reported in the remaining patients of both groups. In addition, epoprostenol therapy resulted in substantial hemodynamic changes (e.g., increases in cardiac index associated with reductions in mean pulmonary arterial pressure, mean right arterial pressure, pulmonary vascular resistance, and mean systemic arterial pressure) compared with baseline. Epoprostenol therapy was not associated with a survival benefit when compared with standard therapy alone. Safety and efficacy of epoprostenol have not been systematically evaluated in patients with pulmonary hypertension associated with other diseases.

Dosage and Administration

■ **General** ***Restricted Distribution*** Epoprostenol sodium and the portable controlled-infusion device used to administer the drug are available only through specialty pharmacies. For information about prescribing and obtaining epoprostenol sodium products, clinicians may contact the manufacturers.

■ **Administration** Epoprostenol sodium is administered by continuous IV infusion via a central venous catheter with a portable controlled-infusion device. A peripheral IV catheter may be used temporarily to administer the infusion until central venous access is established. The manufacturer's labeling should be consulted for ambulatory infusion-device specifications.

Delivery system malfunctions (e.g., infusion-device failure, occluded catheter) may result in inadvertent overdosage or underdosage. To avoid potential interruptions in drug delivery secondary to equipment malfunction, patients should have access to a back-up IV infusion device and infusion sets. A multi-lumen catheter should be considered for patients who routinely receive other IV drugs.

Reconstitution and Dilution Commercially available epoprostenol sodium for injection must be reconstituted with the appropriate diluent specified by the respective manufacturer (sterile diluent for Flolan® supplied by the manufacturer, sterile diluent for generic preparations of epoprostenol sodium for injection supplied by the specific manufacturer (e.g., Teva), and sterile water for injection or 0.9% sodium chloride injection [not supplied] for the Veletri® preparation); the drug is stable only when reconstituted as directed using the recommended diluent(s). The manufacturers' labeling should be consulted for details on reconstitution, preparation of solutions of epoprostenol, and selection of drug concentration in solutions.

Reconstituted solutions of epoprostenol sodium should *not* be admixed or administered with other parenteral solutions or medications.

Flolan® or Generic Epoprostenol Sodium for Injection (Teva). Epoprostenol sodium lyophilized powder for injection (Flolan® or Teva generic preparation) must be reconstituted *only* with the sterile diluent provided by the respective manufacturer. The reconstituted solution should be further diluted with a sufficient volume of the same diluent to provide a final concentration of epoprostenol sodium that is compatible with the infusion pump (with respect to minimum and maximum flow rates and other infusion pump criteria) and capacity of the drug delivery reservoir. Typical drug reservoirs used for long-term epoprostenol therapy contain a total reservoir volume of at least 100 mL.

Following reconstitution, epoprostenol sodium solutions (Flolan® or Teva generic preparation) may be administered immediately or stored under refrigeration at 2–8°C for up to 40 hours (if administration at room temperature is planned) or up to 24 hours (if administration with a cold pouch is planned); the solution should be protected from light. Reconstituted solutions should not be frozen; solutions that have been frozen or stored at 2–8°C for longer than 48 hours should be discarded.

When epoprostenol sodium (Flolan® or Teva generic preparation) is administered at room temperature (without a cold pouch), a single reservoir of reconstituted solution should be administered over a period not exceeding 8 hours. When a cold pouch is employed during the infusion, a single reservoir of reconstituted solution should be administered over a period not exceeding 24 hours. The gel packs in the cold pouch should be changed every 12 hours. The manufacturers' labeling should be consulted for cold pouch specifications and stability of epoprostenol sodium solutions (Flolan® or Teva generic preparation).

Veletri®. Epoprostenol sodium lyophilized powder for injection (Veletri®) should be reconstituted *only* with sterile water for injection or 0.9% sodium chloride injection. The reconstituted solution should be further diluted immediately with a sufficient volume of the same diluent to provide a final concentration of epoprostenol sodium that is compatible with the infusion pump being used (with respect to minimum and maximum flow rates and other specified infusion pump criteria) and the capacity of the drug delivery reservoir. Typical drug reservoirs used for long-term epoprostenol therapy contain a total reservoir volume of 100 mL. Reconstituted solutions of Veletri® should not be exposed to direct sunlight.

Following reconstitution and dilution, Veletri® solutions may be administered immediately or stored for up to 8 days under refrigeration (2–8°C). The stability of the solution is temperature and concentration dependent. When reconstituted and diluted as directed, Veletri® solutions are stable at room temperature for 24, 48, or 72 hours depending on the final concentration of the solution and timing of administration (immediately or after storage for up to 8 days at 2–8°C); use of cold pouches is not required during administration. Veletri® solutions with a final concentration of at least 3000 ng/mL but less than 15,000 ng/mL (prepared with the vial labeled as containing 0.5 mg of drug) may be infused at room temperature for a maximum of 48 hours if administered immediately or 24 hours if stored for up to 8 days at 2–8°C; short excursions to 40°C for up to 2 hours are permitted. Solutions with a final concentration of at least 15,000 ng/mL but less than 60,000 ng/mL (prepared with 1.5-mg vials of drug) may be infused at room temperature (either immediately or after refrigerator storage) for a maximum of 48 hours; short excursions to 40°C for up to 4 hours are permitted. For solutions with a concentration of 60,000 ng/mL or greater (prepared with 1.5-mg vials of drug), the maximum duration of infusion at room temperature is 72 hours if administered immediately or 48 hours if stored for up to 8 days at 2–8°C; short excursions to 40°C for up to 8 hours are permitted. Because the proportion of active ingredient to excipient is different for the different vial sizes of Veletri® (0.5 mg versus 1.5 mg), the manufacturer states that the stability of a solution at a given concentration may be different if prepared using vial sizes other than what is recommended.

Veletri® solutions also may be administered at higher temperatures (up to 40°C) according to the following guidelines. At temperatures of greater than 25°C and up to 30°C, Veletri® solutions with a concentration of at least 60,000 ng/mL may be infused (either immediately or after storage for up to 8 days at 2–8°C) for up to 48 hours; solutions with a concentration less than 60,000 ng/mL are less stable at these temperatures and should therefore be infused for no longer than 24 hours. At temperatures exceeding 30°C and up to 40°C, Veletri® solutions with a concentration of at least 60,000 ng/mL may be infused only if administered immediately after preparation and for a period of up to 24 hours.

Rate of Administration Abrupt discontinuance or sudden large reductions in dosage of epoprostenol may result in worsening of disease symptoms and should be avoided. (See Abrupt Withdrawal of Therapy under Warnings/Precautions: Warnings, in Cautions.) The infusion rate should be adjusted only under the direction of a physician, except in life-threatening situations (e.g., unconsciousness, collapse). Following changes in infusion rates, the patient should be observed; standing and supine blood pressure and heart rate should be monitored for several hours.

Infusion rates may be calculated using the following formula:

$$\text{Infusion rate (mL/hr)} = \frac{\text{dose (ng/kg per min)} \times \text{wt (in kg)} \times 60 \text{ min/hr}}{\text{final concentration of epoprostenol solution (ng/mL)}}$$

■ Dosage

Dosage of epoprostenol sodium is expressed in terms of epoprostenol. There is considerable interindividual variability in patient response to epoprostenol and dosage must be individualized. Dosage should be carefully titrated until therapeutic effect is achieved or adverse effects become intolerable.

Pulmonary Arterial Hypertension **Initiation and Titration of Therapy.** For the treatment of idiopathic/heritable pulmonary arterial hypertension (PAH) or PAH associated with the scleroderma spectrum of disease in adults, the recommended initial dosage of epoprostenol is 2 ng/kg per minute. If the initial dosage is *not* tolerated, a lower dosage should be used.

The initial tolerated epoprostenol dosage should be increased in increments of 2 ng/kg per minute at intervals of at least 15 minutes until dose-limiting pharmacologic effects are elicited or a tolerance limit to the drug is established and further increases in the infusion rate are not clinically warranted. Epoprostenol dosage should be maintained at a level where pharmacologic effects are tolerated.

In clinical studies in adults with PAH associated with the scleroderma spectrum of disease, the average initial dosage of 2.2 ng/kg per minute was increased during the first week of therapy to 4.1 ng/kg per minute on day 7, and the mean dosage was 11.2 ng/kg per minute by the end of week 12; incremental increases in dosage averaged 2–3 ng/kg per minute every 3 weeks.

Long-term Therapy. During long-term infusion, dosage increases generally are required based on persistence, recurrence, or worsening of disease symptoms; dosage reductions may be needed because of adverse effects. In addition, tolerance (tachyphylaxis) to therapeutic effects may occur in patients receiving long-term epoprostenol therapy and periodic dosage adjustment generally is required. (See Dosage Titration under Warnings/Precautions: General Precautions, in Cautions.)

Epoprostenol dosage should be adjusted in increments of 1–2 ng/kg per minute at intervals of at least 15 minutes. In clinical studies, incremental dosage adjustments were made in intervals of at least 24–48 hours. If dose-limiting adverse effects (nausea, vomiting, hypotension, sepsis, headache, abdominal pain, and/or respiratory disorder) occur, dosage should be decreased gradually in decrements of 2 ng/kg per minute at intervals of at least 15 minutes until dose-limiting effects resolve; abrupt withdrawal of epoprostenol or sudden large reductions in infusion rates should be avoided. (See Abrupt Withdrawal of Therapy under Warnings/Precautions: Warnings, in Cautions.) Adverse effects occasionally may resolve without dosage adjustment.

In clinical studies, epoprostenol therapy was tapered in patients receiving lung transplantation after initiation of cardiopulmonary bypass.

After 1 year of therapy, epoprostenol dosages in patients with PAH reportedly ranged from 20–35 ng/kg per minute.

Limited data from several open-label studies indicate that patients on a stable dosage of epoprostenol sodium (Flolan®) may be transitioned directly to the Veletri® preparation at the same dosage without any change in clinical efficacy or tolerability.

■ Special Populations

Initial dosage in geriatric patients should be selected with caution (usually at the low end of the dosage range) and titrated carefully because of age-related decreases in hepatic, renal, and/or cardiac function and concomitant disease and drug therapy.

Cautions

■ Contraindications

Long-term use in congestive heart failure (CHF) due to severe left ventricular systolic dysfunction.

Long-term use in patients who develop pulmonary edema during initial dosage titration.

Known hypersensitivity to epoprostenol or structurally related drugs.

■ Warnings/Precautions

Warnings **Solution and Drug Compatibility.** Epoprostenol sodium should be reconstituted and diluted using *only* the appropriate diluent specified by the manufacturer.

Epoprostenol sodium should *not* be admixed or infused in the same IV line with other solutions or drugs.

Abrupt Withdrawal of Therapy. Abrupt withdrawal (including interruptions in drug delivery) or sudden large reductions in dosage of epoprostenol may result in symptoms associated with rebound pulmonary hypertension (e.g., dyspnea, dizziness, asthenia) and should be avoided. Brief interruptions in therapy can lead to rapid clinical deterioration, including death, in patients with severe pulmonary hypertension who are dependent on the hemodynamic effects of epoprostenol. To avoid potential interruptions in drug delivery secondary to equipment malfunction, patients should have access to a back-up IV infusion device and infusion sets.

Sepsis. Aseptic technique must be used in routine catheter care and in the reconstitution and administration of drug solutions. In clinical studies of up to 12 weeks duration in patients with pulmonary arterial hypertension (PAH), local infection (reported in about 18% of patients) and sepsis (reported at a rate of 0.3 infections/patient per year) associated with the drug delivery system (long-term indwelling central venous catheter) have been reported.

General Precautions **Adequate Patient Evaluation and Monitoring.** Epoprostenol sodium should be used only under the supervision of a qualified clinician experienced in the diagnosis and management of pulmonary hypertension. The diagnosis of idiopathic or heritable PAH or PAH associated with connective tissue disorders should be carefully established.

Because epoprostenol is a potent pulmonary and systemic vasodilating agent, therapy with the drug should be initiated in a setting with adequate medical personnel and equipment for providing physiologic monitoring and emergency care.

The decision to initiate epoprostenol therapy must include careful consideration of the high likelihood that therapy will be needed for prolonged periods (possibly years), and the patient's ability to accept and care for a permanent IV catheter and infusion device.

Because of the complex nature of the disease and the potential for treatment-related complications, experts recommend referral of patients with pulmonary hypertension to specialized centers experienced in the management of pulmonary vascular diseases.

Increases in Pulmonary Arterial Pressure. Asymptomatic increases in pulmonary artery pressure coincident with increases in cardiac output have been reported rarely during initial dosage titration. Such increases in pulmonary arterial pressure do not necessarily preclude long-term epoprostenol therapy and may be controlled with dosage reduction.

Initial dosage titration has been performed with and without right heart catheterization during clinical studies.

Hematologic Effects. Because epoprostenol is a potent inhibitor of platelet aggregation, there is a potential risk of bleeding. Hemorrhagic events, including bleeding related to the delivery system (central venous catheter), have been reported with use of the drug. The risk of potential bleeding complications should be considered in patients receiving epoprostenol, particularly in those receiving concomitant antiplatelet or anticoagulant therapy and in those with clinical conditions associated with a higher risk of bleeding. (See Drug Interactions.)

Prophylaxis of Thromboembolism. Unless contraindicated, concomitant anticoagulant therapy should be administered to reduce the risk of pulmonary thromboembolism, systemic embolism (associated with the permanent indwelling central venous catheter), and other thromboembolic complications (secondary to decreased activity, slower blood flow, dilated right-sided heart chambers, and thrombosis commonly observed in the distal pulmonary arterial microvascular beds in patients with PAH). Experts generally recommend that patients with idiopathic or heritable PAH receive anticoagulant therapy with warfarin; there are fewer data to support use of anticoagulant therapy in patients with PAH associated with other conditions (e.g., scleroderma, congenital heart disease). In patients receiving epoprostenol, the benefits of concomitant anticoagulant therapy should be weighed against the risks of hemorrhage, particularly in those who may be predisposed to bleeding. (See Hematologic Effects under Warnings/Precautions: General Precautions, in Cautions.)

Dosage Titration. In clinical studies, the acute hemodynamic response to epoprostenol did not correlate well with improved exercise tolerance or survival during long-term use of the drug; therefore, adjustments in dosage during long-term use should be made immediately upon occurrence of dose-limiting adverse effects or worsening of symptoms associated with pulmonary hypertension. Following dosage adjustments, standing and supine blood pressure and heart rate should be monitored closely for several hours. (See Rate of Administration under Dosage and Administration: Administration.)

The practice of aggressively titrating epoprostenol to high dosages to overcome the effects of tachyphylaxis may lead to elevated cardiac output and/or high output heart failure. Dosage adjustments should be based on frequent assessments of PAH symptoms, exercise capacity, adverse effects, and hemodynamic function. Some experts recommend periodic cardiac catheterizations in patients receiving long-term treatment with epoprostenol to prevent underdosing or overdosing of the drug. The risks of cardiac catheterization should be weighed against potential benefits.

Specific Populations **Pregnancy.** Category B. (See Users Guide.) Safety and efficacy of epoprostenol during labor, vaginal delivery, or cesarean section have not been established.

Lactation. Not known whether epoprostenol is distributed into milk. Caution is advised if the drug is administered in nursing women.

Pediatric Use. The manufacturer states that safety and efficacy of epoprostenol have not been established in pediatric patients.

Treatment strategies in children† are generally similar to those used in adults.

Geriatric Use. Clinical studies of epoprostenol sodium did not include sufficient numbers of patients 65 years of age or older to determine whether geriatric patients respond differently than younger patients. Other reported clinical experience has not identified differences in responses between geriatric and younger patients. In general, dosage should be titrated carefully in geriatric patients. The greater frequency of decreased hepatic, renal, and/or cardiac function and of concomitant disease and drug therapy observed in the elderly should be considered.

■ **Common Adverse Effects** In long-term controlled clinical trials in patients with idiopathic or heritable PAH, adverse effects reported at least 10% more frequently with epoprostenol sodium than with standard therapy alone included dizziness, headache, nausea, vomiting, jaw pain, myalgia, flushing, diarrhea, tachycardia, nonspecific musculoskeletal pain, chills/fever/sepsis/flu-like symptoms, anxiety/nervousness/tremor, and hypoesthesia/hyperesthesia/paresthesia.

In long-term controlled clinical trials in patients with PAH associated with the scleroderma spectrum of diseases, adverse effects reported at least 10% more frequently with epoprostenol sodium than with standard therapy alone included pain/neck pain/arthralgia, jaw pain, anorexia, diarrhea, headache, nausea/vomiting, skin ulcer, eczema/rash/urticaria, flushing, and hypotension.

Drug Interactions

During clinical trials, epoprostenol sodium was used concomitantly with anticoagulants, cardiac glycosides, diuretics, oral vasodilators, and supplemental oxygen.

■ **Anticoagulants** Concomitant use of epoprostenol and anticoagulants may increase the risk of bleeding; however, patients in clinical trials of epoprostenol were maintained on anticoagulants without evidence of increased bleeding. (See Hematologic Effects under Warnings/Precautions: General Precautions, in Cautions.)

■ **Antihypertensive Agents** Concomitant use of epoprostenol and antihypertensive agents can result in additive hypotensive effects.

■ **Antiplatelet Agents** Concomitant use of epoprostenol and antiplatelet agents may increase the risk of bleeding. (See Hematologic Effects under Warnings/Precautions: General Precautions, in Cautions.)

■ **Digoxin** In patients with congestive heart failure receiving digoxin, oral clearance of digoxin was reduced by 15% during concurrent epoprostenol therapy, but returned to baseline values. Elevations in serum digoxin concentration that occur upon initiation of epoprostenol therapy may be clinically important in patients who are prone to digoxin toxicity.

■ **Diuretics** Concomitant use of epoprostenol and diuretics can result in additive hypotensive effects.

In patients with congestive heart failure receiving furosemide, oral clearance of furosemide was reduced by 13% during concurrent epoprostenol therapy, but returned to baseline values; this change is not considered clinically important.

■ **Vasodilating Agents** Concomitant use of epoprostenol and other vasodilating agents can result in additive hypotensive effects.

Description

Epoprostenol sodium (PGI_2, PGX, prostacyclin), the synthetic salt of a naturally occurring prostaglandin, possesses the pharmacologic actions (e.g., vasodilation of pulmonary and systemic arterial vascular beds, inhibition of platelet aggregation) of endogenous prostacyclin, a naturally occurring prostaglandin and arachidonic acid metabolite. Epoprostenol, a short-acting vasodilating agent and a platelet-aggregation inhibitor, produces dose-related increases in cardiac index and stroke volume and dose-related decreases in pulmonary vascular resistance, total pulmonary resistance, and mean systemic arterial pressure.

In animals, epoprostenol reduces right and left ventricular afterload and increases cardiac output and stroke volume as a result of the drug's vasodilatory effects. Studies have shown that cardiac effects of the drug are dose dependent; low doses of epoprostenol may cause a vagally mediated bradycardia while high doses of the drug cause a reflex tachycardia secondary to direct vasodilation and hypotension. Epoprostenol and synthetic prostacyclin analogs may have antiproliferative effects, including inhibition of fibromuscular proliferation of the intima of precapillary arteries which may be involved in the pathogenesis of pulmonary hypertension. Major effects on cardiac conduction have not been reported. Additional pharmacologic effects of epoprostenol observed in animals include bronchodilation, inhibition of gastric acid secretion, and decreased gastric emptying.

Since epoprostenol is unstable at pH values below 10.2–10.8 (for Flolan®), 11–11.8 (for the Teva generic preparation), and 11–13 (for the Veletri® preparation), oral administration is not possible and continuous IV administration is necessary, because of the drug's short half-life (about 6 minutes). Administration of the drug is complex, because of the requirements for continuous IV infusion (using permanent indwelling catheters), drug reconstitution by patients, operation of infusion pump, and maintenance of stability of the drug by constant refrigeration (using cold packs) and protection from light. The benefits of epoprostenol therapy in patients with pulmonary arterial hypertension (e.g., improvement in survival, exercise capacity, and quality of life assessments) and the logistical issues associated with drug's administration have led to the development of more stable synthetic prostacyclin analogs with similar pharmacologic actions and less complicated routes of administration (e.g., iloprost by oral inhalation, treprostinil by continuous subcutaneous infusion).

Several epoprostenol sodium formulations are commercially available in the US; these formulations differ principally with regard to their excipients, which result in products with slightly different pH values and stability. (See Dosage and Administration: Reconstitution and Dilution.) The epoprostenol sodium formulation containing sucrose and arginine excipients (Veletri®) has prolonged stability compared with formulations containing glycine and mannitol (e.g., Flolan®); however, the different formulations appear to be comparable in their pharmacokinetic and pharmacodynamic (e.g., cardiac output, heart rate, cardiac index) effects. Epoprostenol is rapidly hydrolyzed at neutral pH in plasma and also undergoes enzymatic degradation. Chemical assays with sufficient sensitivity and specificity to assess the in vivo pharmacokinetics of epoprostenol in humans are not currently available. Epoprostenol is metabolized to 2 major metabolites, 6-keto-$PGF_{1\alpha}$ (formed by spontaneous degradation) and 6,15-diketo-13,14-dihydro-$PGF_{1\alpha}$ (formed by enzymatic degradation), which appear to have minimal pharmacological activity based on laboratory animal data. In addition, 14 minor metabolites have been isolated from urine. Following IV administration of radiolabeled epoprostenol in adults, 82 and 4% of the total radioactivity was recovered in urine and feces, respectively, over 7 days.

Advice to Patients

Importance of advising patients that epoprostenol therapy is infused continuously through a permanent indwelling central venous catheter via a portable infusion device and requires sustained commitment to drug reconstitution and administration, and care of the permanent central venous catheter.

Importance of advising patients that epoprostenol therapy probably will be needed for prolonged periods, possibly years. Importance of access to a backup IV infusion device and infusion sets. Advise patients that even brief interruptions in the administration of epoprostenol may result in rapid symptomatic deterioration (e.g., dyspnea, dizziness, asthenia) and/or death.

Importance of careful consideration of patient's ability to accept and care for a permanent central venous catheter and infusion device.

Importance of advising patients that sterile technique must be adhered to in drug preparation and catheter care to prevent sepsis.

Advise patients that epoprostenol must be reconstituted only with the appropriate diluent specified by the manufacturer.

Importance of women informing their clinician if they are or plan to become pregnant or plan to breast-feed.

Importance of patient informing clinicians of existing or contemplated concomitant therapy, including prescription and OTC drugs, as well as any concomitant illnesses.

Importance of informing patients of other important precautionary information. (See Cautions.)

Overview® (see Users Guide). For additional information on this drug until a more detailed monograph is developed and published, the manufacturer's labeling should be consulted. It is *essential* that the manufacturer's labeling be consulted for more detailed information on usual cautions, precautions, contraindications, potential drug interactions, laboratory test interferences, and acute toxicity.

Preparations

Epoprostenol sodium for injection is available only through specialty pharmacies. (See Restricted Distribution under Dosage and Administration: General.)

Excipients in commercially available drug preparations may have clinically important effects in some individuals; consult specific product labeling for details.

Epoprostenol Sodium

Parenteral

For injection, for IV infusion	0.5 mg (of epoprostenol)*	**Epoprostenol Sodium for Injection** (available with diluent)
		Flolan® (available with diluent), GlaxoSmithKline
		Veletri®, Actelion
	1.5 mg (of epoprostenol)*	**Epoprostenol Sodium for Injection** (available with diluent)
		Flolan® (available with diluent), GlaxoSmithKline
		Veletri®, Actelion

*available from one or more manufacturer, distributor, and/or repackager by generic (nonproprietary) name

†Use is not currently included in the labeling approved by the US Food and Drug Administration

Macitentan

■ Macitentan, an endothelin-receptor antagonist, is a vasodilator.

REMS

FDA approved a REMS for macitentan to ensure that the benefits outweigh the risks. The REMS may apply to one or more preparations of macitentan and consists of the following: elements to assure safe use and implementation system. See the FDA REMS page (https://www.accessdata.fda.gov/scripts/cder/rems/index.cfm). See also Restricted Distribution Program under Dosage and Administration: General.

Uses

■ **Pulmonary Arterial Hypertension** Macitentan is used in the management of pulmonary arterial hypertension (PAH; World Health Organization [WHO] group 1 pulmonary hypertension) to delay disease progression (i.e., death, initiation of IV or subcutaneous prostanoids, clinical worsening). Clinical studies establishing efficacy of the drug for this use were conducted principally in patients with New York Heart Association (NYHA)/WHO functional class II or III PAH (idiopathic, heritable, associated with connective tissue diseases, or caused by congenital heart disease) who were receiving macitentan as monotherapy or in combination with a phosphodiesterase type 5 inhibitor or inhaled prostanoid for an average of 2 years. For more information about etiologies of PAH, see Uses: Pulmonary Arterial Hypertension, in Epoprostenol 48:48. Macitentan has been designated an orphan drug by the US Food and Drug Administration (FDA) for use in the treatment of PAH.

In addition to general treatment measures and supportive therapy (e.g., warfarin anticoagulation, diuretics, supplemental oxygen, digoxin), experts recommend the use of an endothelin-receptor antagonist (e.g., ambrisentan, bosentan, macitentan) as one of several treatment options for the initial management of PAH in patients with NYHA/WHO functional class II, III, or IV symptoms who are not candidates for calcium-channel blocker therapy or in whom such therapy has failed; alternative therapies include phosphodiesterase type 5 inhibitors (e.g., sildenafil, tadalafil), prostanoids (e.g., IV epoprostenol; inhaled iloprost; inhaled, IV, or subcutaneous treprostinil), or soluble guanylate cyclase stimulators (e.g., riociguat). Current guidelines for the management of PAH state that an oral agent such as an endothelin-receptor antagonist generally is preferred for initial therapy in patients with NYHA/WHO functional class II symptoms, while those with more advanced NYHA/WHO functional class III disease may be treated with any currently approved PAH therapy; IV epoprostenol generally is recommended as the treatment of choice for patients with NYHA/WHO functional class IV PAH because of its demonstrated survival benefit. In general, choice of therapy should be individualized, taking into account factors such as disease severity, route of administration, potential adverse effects and costs of treatment, clinician experience, and patient preference.

Efficacy of macitentan for the management of PAH has been established in a long-term (average treatment duration approximately 2 years), randomized, double-blind, placebo-controlled study (Study with an Endothelin Receptor Antagonist in Pulmonary Arterial Hypertension to Improve Clinical Outcome [SERAPHIN]) in 742 patients with WHO group 1 PAH (57% idiopathic or heritable, 31% associated with connective tissue disorders, and 12% caused by other etiologies [congenital heart disease, drugs/toxins, HIV]). Most patients had NYHA/WHO functional class II (52%) or III (46%) symptoms at study entry and 64% were receiving concomitant therapy with a phosphodiesterase type 5 inhibitor and/or an oral/inhaled prostanoid. Macitentan (10 mg once daily) was substantially more effective than placebo in reducing the progression of PAH; the primary composite end point of time to first occurrence of death, atrial septostomy, lung transplantation, initiation of IV/subcutaneous prostanoid therapy, or worsening of PAH (defined as a sustained decrease in 6-minute walking distance of at least 15% from baseline in addition to worsening of WHO functional class and need for additional PAH treatments) was reduced by 45% with macitentan therapy. The median duration of treatment with macitentan or placebo was 118 or 101 weeks, respectively. The beneficial effect of macitentan was driven largely by a reduction in clinical worsening events (deterioration in 6-minute walking distance, worsening of PAH symptoms, and need for additional PAH treatments). Macitentan therapy also improved several secondary measures of efficacy, including PAH-related death or hospitalization (50% risk reduction) and 6-minute walking distance (placebo-corrected mean increase of 22 meters at 6 months); there was no difference in all-cause mortality between the treatment groups.

In the SERAPHIN study, patients received macitentan either as monotherapy or in combination with another PAH-specific agent (a phosphodiesterase type 5 inhibitor and/or an oral/inhaled prostanoid); efficacy of macitentan was demonstrated with both regimens. In the treatment of PAH, combination therapy with drugs that target the different pathophysiologic pathways of the disease may provide additive and/or synergistic benefits. Current expert consensus guidelines recommend combination therapy with a prostanoid, phosphodiesterase type 5 inhibitor, or soluble guanylate cyclase stimulator (added sequentially) in patients who have an inadequate response to initial monotherapy. Data from several small studies suggest that use of an endothelin-receptor antagonist in combination with a prostanoid or a phosphodiesterase type 5 inhibitor may improve outcomes (e.g., reduce clinical worsening, increase 6-minute walking distance, improve hemodynamic parameters) in patients who remain symptomatic on monotherapy.

Dosage and Administration

■ **General** ***Restricted Distribution Program*** Because of the risk of embryofetal toxicity, macitentan is available to female patients only through a restricted distribution program called the Opsumit® Risk Evaluation and Mitigation Strategy (REMS). (See REMS and also see Fetal/Neonatal Morbidity and Mortality under Warnings/Precautions: Warnings, in Cautions.) *All* female patients regardless of childbearing potential must enroll in the program prior to initiating macitentan; in addition, females of childbearing potential must comply with all pregnancy testing and contraception requirements of the program. Male patients are exempt from these restrictions and do not need to enroll in the program. Clinicians and pharmacies must also be registered with the Opsumit® REMS and comply with all terms of the program (including patient education and safety requirements) before they can prescribe or dispense macitentan. In addition, pharmacies must only dispense the drug to authorized patients. For additional information about the Opsumit® REMS program, including certified pharmacies or wholesale distributors, clinicians may call 866-228-3546 or consult www.OPSUMITREMS.com.

As a condition of the Opsumit® REMS Program, macitentan therapy should be initiated in females of childbearing potential *only* after a negative pregnancy test is obtained; pregnancy tests must be performed monthly during therapy and at 1 month following discontinuance of therapy. (See Fetal/Neonatal Morbidity and Mortality under Warnings/Precautions: Warnings, in Cautions, and also see Advice to Patients.)

No more than a 30-day supply of macitentan may be dispensed at one time to prepubertal females and females of childbearing potential. Prepubertal female patients and/or their parent or guardian should be advised to immediately report any changes in the child's reproductive status (e.g., breast development, pubic hair) to her clinician. The prepubertal female's healthcare provider should decide when the child has reached puberty; such children may reach puberty before having their first menstrual period. Dispensing to females of childbearing potential should occur only after obtaining confirmation from the patient (or prescriber, if patient cannot be reached) that the required pregnancy tests were completed. In addition, a medication guide explaining the risks and benefits of macitentan therapy must be distributed to all patients with each prescription of the drug.

■ **Administration** *Oral Administration* Macitentan is administered orally without regard to meals. Macitentan tablets should not be split, chewed, or crushed.

If a dose of macitentan is missed, the dose should be taken as soon as it is remembered that day, and the next dose should be resumed at the regularly scheduled time; 2 doses should not be taken at the same time to make up for a missed dose.

■ **Dosage** *Pulmonary Arterial Hypertension* The recommended dosage of macitentan for the treatment of pulmonary arterial hypertension (PAH) in adults is 10 mg once daily. The manufacturer states that dosages exceeding 10 mg daily have not been evaluated in patients with PAH and are therefore not recommended.

■ **Special Populations** Dosage adjustment is not required in patients with renal or hepatic impairment. (See Specific Populations under Cautions: Warnings/Precautions.)

Cautions

■ **Contraindications** Pregnancy.

■ **Warnings/Precautions** *Warnings* **Fetal/Neonatal Morbidity and Mortality.** Macitentan may cause fetal harm if used during pregnancy; teratogenic (e.g., cardiovascular abnormalities, mandibular arch fusion abnormalities) and embryotoxic (e.g., reduced survival) effects have been demonstrated in animals. (See Cautions: Contraindications.)

Pregnancy must be excluded in females of childbearing potential prior to initiation of macitentan therapy and prevented thereafter by the use of acceptable methods of contraception during and for 1 month following cessation of therapy. (See Advice to Patients.) Monthly pregnancy tests are required in females of childbearing potential. If macitentan is used during pregnancy or if the patient becomes pregnant during therapy, the patient should be apprised of the potential hazard to the fetus.

Because of the risk of fetal harm, distribution of macitentan is restricted in female patients. (See Restricted Distribution Program under Dosage and Administration: General.)

Other Warnings and Precautions **Hepatic Effects.** Serious hepatotoxicity and liver failure have been reported in patients receiving other endothelin-receptor antagonists (e.g., bosentan, sitaxsentan [not commercially available in the US]). (See Description.) Elevations in serum aminotransferase (AST/ALT) concentrations to more than 3 times the upper limit of normal (ULN) were reported in 3.4% of patients receiving macitentan and 4.5% of those receiving placebo in the principal clinical study of the drug; AST/ALT elevations to more than 8 times the ULN occurred in 2.1 and 0.4% of patients in these respective treatment groups.

Although findings to date do not suggest a high potential for macitentan to cause hepatotoxicity, such a risk cannot be ruled out and patients should be monitored closely for adverse hepatic effects. (See Advice to Patients.) Liver function tests should be obtained prior to initiation of macitentan therapy and repeated thereafter as clinically indicated. The drug should be discontinued if clinically important elevations of aminotransferase concentrations occur or if aminotransferase elevations are accompanied by manifestations of hepatic disease (e.g., nausea, vomiting, fever, right upper quadrant pain, fatigue, anorexia, jaundice, dark urine, fever, itching) or an increase in bilirubin concentrations to more than 2 times the ULN. Reinitiation of macitentan therapy may be considered in patients who experience asymptomatic aminotransferase elevations after such concentrations normalize.

Hematologic Effects. As with other endothelin-receptor antagonists, reductions in hemoglobin concentration and hematocrit have been reported with macitentan; these decreases generally occur early during therapy and stabilize thereafter. In the principal efficacy study of macitentan in patients with PAH, a mean decrease in hemoglobin concentration of about 1 g/dL was reported in patients receiving the drug; hemoglobin concentrations decreased to less than 10 g/dL in 8.7% of patients receiving macitentan compared with 3.4% of those receiving placebo. Such decreases rarely have required transfusion.

Hemoglobin concentrations should be monitored prior to initiation of macitentan therapy and as clinically indicated thereafter. The drug should not be initiated in patients with severe anemia.

Pulmonary Effects. If manifestations of pulmonary edema occur during macitentan therapy, the possibility of pulmonary veno-occlusive disease should be considered; if confirmed, the drug should be discontinued.

Fertility in Males. Macitentan may cause adverse effects on spermatogenesis. Decreased sperm counts have been reported in some men who were receiving other endothelin-receptor antagonists. Although the effects of macitentan on spermatogenesis have not been established in humans, preclinical chronic toxicity studies have demonstrated some abnormal, but reversible testicular findings (e.g., tubular dilatation, tubular atrophy) in animals. Patients should be advised about the potential adverse effects of macitentan on fertility.

Specific Populations **Pregnancy.** Category X. (See Fetal/Neonatal Morbidity and Mortality under Warnings/Precautions: Warnings, in Cautions.)

Lactation. Macitentan and its metabolites are distributed into milk in rats; it is not known whether the drug is distributed into human milk. Because of the potential for serious adverse reactions to macitentan in nursing infants, a decision should be made whether to discontinue nursing or the drug.

Pediatric Use. Safety and efficacy of macitentan have not been established in pediatric patients.

Geriatric Use. In the principal clinical study of macitentan in patients with PAH, 14% of the patients were 65 years of age or older. No overall differences in safety or efficacy were observed between these geriatric patients and younger individuals.

Hepatic Impairment. Systemic exposure of macitentan is decreased by about 6–34% in patients with hepatic impairment, but this change is not considered to be clinically important. (See Dosage and Administration: Special Populations.)

Renal Impairment. Systemic exposure to macitentan and its active metabolite is increased by 30 and 60%, respectively, in patients with severe renal impairment (creatinine clearance of 15–29 mL/minute); these changes are not considered to be clinically important. (See Dosage and Administration: Special Populations.)

■ **Common Adverse Effects** The most common adverse effects reported with macitentan in clinical trials and occurring at least 3% more frequently with the drug than with placebo include anemia, nasopharyngitis/pharyngitis, bronchitis, headache, influenza, and urinary tract infection.

Drug Interactions

Macitentan is metabolized principally by cytochrome P-450 (CYP) isoenzyme 3A4, and to a lesser extent by CYP2C19. At clinically relevant concentrations, macitentan does not appear to inhibit or induce CYP enzymes. The drug also does not appear to be a substrate or inhibitor of the P-glycoprotein (P-gp) efflux transporter or the organic anion transport proteins (OATP) 1B1 and 1B3.

■ **Drugs Affecting Hepatic Microsomal Enzymes** Concomitant use of macitentan with potent inhibitors of CYP3A4 (e.g., ketoconazole, ritonavir) may increase exposure to macitentan and should be avoided.

Concomitant use of macitentan with potent inducers of CYP3A4 (e.g., rifampin) may decrease exposure to macitentan and should be avoided.

■ **Cyclosporine** In healthy individuals, concomitant administration of macitentan and cyclosporine (a CYP3A4 inhibitor) did not substantially alter systemic exposure to macitentan or its metabolites at steady state. No dosage adjustment is necessary when these drugs are administered concomitantly.

■ **HIV Protease Inhibitors** HIV protease inhibitors such as ritonavir are potent inhibitors of CYP3A4 and can therefore increase systemic exposure to macitentan if used concomitantly. Although the effects of ritonavir coadministration on macitentan pharmacokinetics have not been established, ritonavir is expected to increase macitentan exposure to a similar extent as that observed with ketoconazole. Concomitant use of macitentan and HIV protease inhibitors that are potent inhibitors of CYP3A4 is not recommended. In patients who require the use of a potent CYP3A4 inhibitor drug as part of their HIV treatment regimen, PAH therapies other than macitentan are recommended.

■ **Ketoconazole** In healthy individuals, concomitant administration of macitentan and ketoconazole (a potent CYP3A4 inhibitor) increased systemic exposure to macitentan by approximately twofold and reduced exposure to the active metabolite by about 26%. While some experts suggest that these changes are not clinically important, the manufacturer recommends that concomitant use of macitentan and ketoconazole be avoided.

■ **Rifampin** In healthy individuals, concomitant administration of macitentan and rifampin (a potent CYP3A4 inducer) substantially reduced systemic exposure and trough plasma concentrations of macitentan. Concomitant use of these drugs should be avoided.

■ **Sildenafil** In healthy individuals, concomitant administration of macitentan and sildenafil did not substantially alter systemic exposure or peak plasma concentrations of macitentan; exposure to sildenafil was increased by 15%, but this degree of change is not considered clinically important. No dosage adjustment is necessary when these drugs are administered concomitantly.

■ **Warfarin** Concomitant administration of warfarin and macitentan did not alter exposure to warfarin and had no effect on the international normalized ratio (INR).

Description

Macitentan, a nonselective (dual receptor) endothelin-1 (ET-1) receptor antagonist, is a vasodilator. ET-1 is a potent vasoconstrictor and mediator of a variety of deleterious effects (e.g., fibrosis, proliferation, hypertrophy, inflammation); increased concentrations of ET-1 have been detected in the plasma and lung tissue of patients with pulmonary arterial hypertension (PAH), suggesting a pathogenic role for ET-1 in this disorder. Macitentan binds with sustained and high affinity to both ET-1 type A and type B receptors in pulmonary arterial smooth muscle cells. Selectivity for these ET-1 receptors differs among the various endothelin-receptor antagonists; although dual blockade is thought to be advantageous in fully inhibiting the effects of ET-1-induced endothelial dysfunction, the clinical importance of selective versus nonselective endothelin receptor blockade is not known. Macitentan improves hemodynamics (e.g., pulmonary vascular resistance, cardiac output) in patients with

PAH and also has shown some beneficial effects on right ventricular hypertrophy in preclinical studies.

Macitentan exhibits dose-proportional pharmacokinetics following oral doses ranging from 1–30 mg. Peak concentrations of the drug are attained by about 8 hours after a dose. Macitentan is metabolized principally by cytochrome P-450 (CYP) isoenzyme 3A4, with minor contribution by CYP2C19. An oxidative depropyl metabolite has been identified as the main active metabolite, which represents about 40% of the pharmacologic activity of macitentan and has a systemic exposure approximately threefold higher than that of the parent drug. Following administration of radiolabeled macitentan in healthy individuals, approximately 50 and 24% of total radioactivity is recovered in urine and feces, respectively. Elimination half-lives of the drug and its active metabolite are approximately 16 and 48 hours, respectively. Neither macitentan nor its active metabolite interacts with proteins involved in hepatic bile transport (i.e., bile salt export pump [BSEP]) or with the organic anion-transporting polypeptides (i.e., OATP 1B1 and 1B3); such effects have been demonstrated with other endothelin-receptor antagonists and may be a contributing factor to the apparent differences observed in hepatotoxic potential between the agents.

Advice to Patients

Risk of fetal harm; importance of advising females of childbearing potential to avoid pregnancy and to use acceptable methods of contraception during and for 1 month following discontinuance of macitentan therapy. Acceptable methods of contraception include one highly effective form of contraception (intrauterine device [IUD], progesterone implant, or tubal sterilization) or a combination of methods (either one hormonal and one barrier method or 2 barrier methods where one form is the male condom). Acceptable hormonal methods of contraception include estrogen-progestin combination oral contraceptives or transdermal contraceptive systems, vaginal ring, and progesterone injections. Acceptable barrier methods include male condoms, diaphragms with spermicide, and cervical caps with spermicide. Even if the partner has had a vasectomy, an additional hormonal or barrier method must be used.

Importance of advising females to inform their clinician immediately if a menstrual period is missed or pregnancy is suspected; clinicians should perform a pregnancy test if pregnancy is suspected for any reason and provide counseling on the use of emergency contraception in the event of unprotected sexual intercourse or known or suspected contraceptive failure. Apprise patient of potential risk to fetus if pregnancy occurs.

Importance of all female patients (regardless of childbearing potential) enrolling in the Opsumit® REMS program and complying with all contraceptive and pregnancy testing requirements. Importance of monitoring reproductive status of prepubertal females and immediately reporting any changes to a clinician.

Importance of periodic monitoring of red blood cell counts during treatment.

Potential risk of liver toxicity. Importance of patients informing clinicians of any unexplained nausea, vomiting, right upper quadrant pain, fatigue, anorexia, jaundice, dark urine, fever, or itching.

Importance of taking macitentan as prescribed and of not interrupting or discontinuing therapy without consulting a clinician.

Importance of not taking a double dose to make up for a missed dose but instead taking the missed dose as soon as it is remembered, and then resuming the next dose at the regularly scheduled time.

Importance of advising patients to not split, chew, or crush tablets.

Importance of distributing the FDA-approved medication guide with every prescription and reviewing the information with female patients. (See REMS.) Importance of patients carefully reading the medication guide before initiating therapy and each time prescription is refilled.

Importance of females informing their clinician if they are or plan to become pregnant or plan to breast-feed.

Importance of informing clinicians of existing or contemplated concomitant therapy, including prescription (e.g., drugs for HIV) and OTC drugs or herbal supplements, as well as any concomitant illnesses.

Importance of informing patients of other important precautionary information. (See Cautions.)

Overview® (see Users Guide). For additional information on this drug until a more detailed monograph is developed and published, the manufacturer's labeling should be consulted. It is *essential* that the manufacturer's labeling be consulted for more detailed information on usual cautions, precautions, contraindications, potential drug interactions, laboratory test interferences, and acute toxicity.

Preparations

Distribution of macitentan is restricted. (See Restricted Distribution Program under Dosage and Administration: General.)

Excipients in commercially available drug preparations may have clinically important effects in some individuals; consult specific product labeling for details.

Macitentan

Oral		
Tablets, film-coated	10 mg	**Opsumit®**, Actelion

Selected Revisions November 2018, © Copyright, August 2014, American Society of Health-System Pharmacists, Inc.

Riociguat

■ Riociguat, a soluble guanylate cyclase (sGC) stimulator, is a vasodilator.

REMS

FDA approved a REMS for riociguat to ensure that the benefits outweigh the risks. The REMS may apply to one or more preparations of riociguat and consists of the following: elements to assure safe use and implementation system. See the FDA REMS page (https://www.accessdata.fda.gov/scripts/cder/rems/index.cfm). See also Restricted Distribution Program under Dosage and Administration: General.

Uses

■ **Pulmonary Hypertension** Riociguat is used for the management of persistent/recurrent chronic thromboembolic pulmonary hypertension (CTEPH; World Health Organization [WHO] group 4 pulmonary hypertension) and for pulmonary arterial hypertension (PAH; WHO group 1 pulmonary hypertension). CTEPH and PAH are characterized by pulmonary vascular obstruction but differ based on their underlying causes. Clinical studies establishing efficacy of riociguat for these uses were conducted principally in patients with New York Heart Association (NYHA)/WHO functional class II or III disease. For more information about etiologies of PAH, see Uses: Pulmonary Arterial Hypertension, in Epoprostenol 48:48. Riociguat has been designated an orphan drug by the US Food and Drug Administration (FDA) for the treatment of CTEPH and PAH.

Chronic Thromboembolic Pulmonary Hypertension Riociguat is used to improve exercise capacity and NYHA/WHO functional class in patients with CTEPH who have inoperable disease or persistent/recurrent pulmonary hypertension after surgery (i.e., pulmonary endarterectomy). In clinical studies, riociguat was more effective than placebo in improving the primary efficacy outcome of exercise capacity as well as other clinical outcome measures (e.g., hemodynamic parameters, NYHA/WHO functional class). The standard treatment for patients with CTEPH is pulmonary endarterectomy. Because such surgery is potentially curative, patients should always be assessed by an experienced clinician to determine if they are candidates for pulmonary endarterectomy before medical therapy is considered.

Efficacy and safety of riociguat for the management of CTEPH in adults were established in the Chronic Thromboembolic Pulmonary Hypertension Soluble Guanylate Cyclase-Stimulator Trial 1 (CHEST-1), a 16-week randomized, double-blind, multicenter, placebo-controlled study in 261 adults with CTEPH who were not considered to be candidates for pulmonary endarterectomy or had persistent or recurrent pulmonary hypertension after undergoing such surgery. Patients received riociguat (titrated up to a dosage of 2.5 mg 3 times daily) or placebo in addition to standard therapies including oral anticoagulants, diuretics, cardiac glycosides, calcium-channel blocking agents, and supplemental oxygen; concomitant use of nitric oxide donors, endothelin-receptor antagonists, prostacyclin analogs, phosphodiesterase (PDE) type 5 inhibitors (e.g., sildenafil, tadalafil, vardenafil), and nonspecific PDE inhibitors (e.g., dipyridamole, theophylline) was not permitted. Riociguat substantially improved exercise capacity as demonstrated by a mean increase of 46 m, relative to placebo, in 6-minute walking distance from baseline to 16 weeks; the improvement was apparent as early as the second week of therapy and continued throughout the study. The treatment effect of riociguat was consistent across various patient subgroups, including patients who were ineligible for surgery and those with persistent/recurrent disease after surgery. In addition, improvements in hemodynamics (e.g., pulmonary vascular resistance), N-terminal pro-brain natriuretic peptide concentrations, and NYHA/WHO functional class were observed in patients who received riociguat. There was no substantial difference in time to clinical worsening between the treatment groups. Preliminary results of an open-label extension study (CHEST-2) indicate that the benefits of riociguat with respect to exercise capacity (i.e., 6-minute walking distance) are sustained with continued therapy; estimated survival rates of 97 and 94% were reported at 1 and 2 years, respectively.

Pulmonary Arterial Hypertension Riociguat is used to improve exercise capacity and NYHA/WHO functional class and to delay clinical worsening in adults with PAH. Clinical studies establishing efficacy of the drug for this use were conducted principally in patients with NYHA/WHO functional class II or III PAH (idiopathic, heritable, or associated with connective tissue diseases) who were receiving riociguat as monotherapy or in combination with an endothelin-receptor antagonist or a prostanoid.

In addition to general treatment measures and supportive therapy (e.g., warfarin anticoagulation, diuretics, supplemental oxygen, digoxin), experts recommended riociguat as one of several drugs that can be used for the initial management of PAH in patients with NYHA/WHO functional class II, III, or IV symptoms who are not candidates for calcium-channel blocker therapy or in whom such therapy has failed; alternative therapies include endothelin-receptor antagonists (e.g., ambrisentan, bosentan, macitentan), PDE type 5 inhibitors (e.g., sildenafil, tadalafil), or prostanoids (e.g., IV epoprostenol; inhaled iloprost; inhaled, IV, or subcutaneous treprostinil). In general, choice of therapy should be individualized, taking into account factors such as disease severity, route of administration, potential adverse effects and costs of treatment, clinician experience, and patient preference.

Efficacy and safety of riociguat for the treatment of PAH were established in the Pulmonary Arterial Hypertension Soluble Guanylate Cyclase-Stimulator Trial 1 (PATENT-1), a 12-week randomized, double-blind, multicenter, placebo-controlled study in 443 patients with symptomatic PAH (61% idiopathic, 2% heritable, 25% associated with connective tissue diseases, 12% related to other etiologies [congenital heart disease, portal hypertension, anorexigen/amphetamine use]). The study included patients who were receiving no other PAH-specific therapies (50% of the study population) as well as patients who were receiving endothelin-receptor antagonists (44%) or oral/inhaled/subcutaneous prostacyclin analogs (6%). Riociguat was administered at individually titrated dosages up to 2.5 mg 3 times daily; concomitant use of oral anticoagulants, diuretics, cardiac glycosides, calcium-channel blocking agents, and supplemental oxygen, but not PDE type 5 inhibitors, was permitted. Riociguat substantially improved exercise capacity, as demonstrated by a mean increase of 36 m (placebo-corrected) in 6-minute walking distance from baseline to 12 weeks; the improvement was apparent as early as the second week of therapy and continued throughout the study. The treatment effect of riociguat was consistent in various patient subgroups, including those receiving no other PAH therapies and those receiving concomitant therapy with an endothelin-receptor antagonist or a prostacyclin analog. Riociguat therapy also was associated with substantial improvements in pulmonary vascular resistance, N-terminal pro-brain natriuretic peptide concentrations, NYHA/WHO functional class, rate of clinical worsening, and Borg dyspnea score. Preliminary results of an open-label extension study (PATENT-2) indicate that the benefits of riociguat with respect to exercise capacity (i.e., 6-minute walking distance) are sustained with continued therapy; estimated survival rates of 97 and 93% were reported at 1 and 2 years, respectively.

Current expert consensus guidelines recommend that patients who have an inadequate response to initial monotherapy with a PAH-specific agent may be treated with combination therapy. Combination therapy with drugs that target the different pathophysiologic pathways in PAH may provide additive and/or synergistic benefits. These experts state that combined use of riociguat with a prostanoid or an endothelin-receptor antagonist (added sequentially) may be considered; however, concomitant use of riociguat and PDE type 5 inhibitors is contraindicated because of the risk of hypotension. (See Cardiovascular Effects under Warnings/Precautions: Other Warnings and Precautions, in Cautions.)

Dosage and Administration

■ **General** ***Restricted Distribution Program*** Because of the risk of embryofetal toxicity, riociguat is available to female patients only through a restricted distribution program called the Adempas® Risk Evaluation and Mitigation Strategies (REMS) Program. (See Fetal/Neonatal Morbidity and Mortality under Warnings/Precautions: Warnings, in Cautions and also see REMS.) *All* female patients regardless of childbearing potential must enroll in the program prior to initiating riociguat therapy; in addition, females of childbearing potential must comply with all pregnancy testing and contraception requirements of the program. Male patients are exempt from these restrictions and do not need to enroll in the program. Clinicians and pharmacies (including both inpatient and outpatient) must be certified with the Adempas® REMS Program in order to prescribe and dispense the drug. In addition, pharmacies must only dispense to authorized patients. For additional information about the Adempas® REMS Program, clinicians may call 855-423-3672 or consult http://www.AdempasREMS.com.

As a condition of the Adempas® REMS Program, riociguat therapy should be initiated in females of childbearing potential *only* after a negative pregnancy test is obtained; pregnancy tests should be performed monthly during therapy and at 1 month following discontinuance of therapy. (See Advice to Patients.)

No more than a 30-day supply of riociguat may be dispensed at one time to females of childbearing potential. Prepubertal female patients and/or their parent or guardian should be advised to immediately report any changes in the child's reproductive status (e.g., breast development, pubic hair) to her clinician. The prepubertal female's healthcare provider should decide when the child has reached puberty; such children may reach puberty before having their first menstrual period. Dispensing to females of childbearing potential should occur only after obtaining confirmation from the patient that the required pregnancy tests were completed.

■ **Administration** ***Oral Administration*** Riociguat is administered orally. The drug may be given without regard to meals.

If a dose of riociguat is missed, the next dose should be taken at the regularly scheduled time; if treatment is interrupted for 3 or more days, retitration of the dosage is recommended.

■ **Dosage** ***Pulmonary Hypertension*** Dosage of riociguat should be individualized based on patient response and tolerance to the hypotensive effects of the drug. For the treatment of chronic thromboembolic pulmonary hypertension (CTEPH) or pulmonary arterial hypertension (PAH) in adults, the recommended initial dosage of riociguat is 1 mg 3 times daily (doses should be given approximately 6–8 hours apart). A reduced initial dosage of 0.5 mg 3 times daily should be considered in patients who may not tolerate the hypotensive effects of the drug. In patients without any manifestations of hypotension and in whom systolic blood pressure remains above 95 mm Hg, dosage may be titrated up to the maximum recommended dosage of 2.5 mg 3 times daily, if tolerated. Dosage increases should be made in increments of 0.5 mg 3 times daily at intervals of no less than every 2 weeks. If symptoms of hypotension occur at any time during therapy, dosage should be decreased by 0.5 mg 3 times daily.

Dosage Modification in Smokers Because smoking can decrease plasma concentrations of riociguat, consideration should be given to using a dosage higher than the usual recommended maximum dosage of 2.5 mg 3 times daily, if tolerated, in patients who smoke. (See Drug Interactions: Smoking.) This recommendation is based on pharmacokinetic modeling; safety and efficacy of such dosages have not been established. Conversely, a dosage reduction may be required in patients who stop smoking.

Concomitant Use with Drugs Affecting Hepatic Microsomal Enzymes and Transport Systems In patients receiving concomitant therapy with potent inhibitors of cytochrome P-450 (CYP) and P-glycoprotein (P-gp)/breast cancer resistance protein (BCRP), a reduced initial dosage of riociguat 0.5 mg 3 times daily should be considered. Patients should be monitored for hypotension upon initiation of and during such concomitant therapy. (See Drug Interactions.)

Cautions

■ **Contraindications** Pregnancy.

Concomitant therapy with nitrates or nitric oxide donors in any form (e.g., amyl nitrite, nitroglycerin).

Concomitant therapy with phosphodiesterase (PDE) inhibitors, including specific PDE type 5 inhibitors (e.g., sildenafil, tadalafil, vardenafil) and nonspecific PDE inhibitors (e.g., dipyridamole, theophylline).

■ **Warnings/Precautions** ***Warnings*** **Fetal/Neonatal Morbidity and Mortality.** Riociguat may cause fetal harm if used during pregnancy; teratogenic (e.g., cardiac ventricular-septal defect) and embryotoxic (e.g., spontaneous abortions, resorptions) effects have been demonstrated in animals. (See Cautions: Contraindications.)

Pregnancy must be excluded in females of childbearing potential prior to initiation of riociguat therapy and prevented thereafter by the use of acceptable methods of contraception during and for 1 month following cessation of therapy. (See Advice to Patients.) Monthly pregnancy tests are required during riociguat therapy in females of childbearing potential, with an additional test performed 1 month following discontinuance of therapy. If riociguat is used during pregnancy or if the patient becomes pregnant during therapy, the patient should be apprised of the potential hazard to the fetus.

Because of the risk of fetal harm, distribution of riociguat is restricted in female patients. (See Restricted Distribution Program under Dosage and Administration: General.)

Other Warnings and Precautions **Cardiovascular Effects.** Riociguat has general vasodilating properties and can therefore reduce systemic blood pressure. In the principal efficacy studies of the drug in patients with pulmonary hypertension, hypotension was reported in about 10% of patients who received riociguat compared with 4% of those who received placebo.

Nitrates, nitric oxide donors, or PDE inhibitors may potentiate the hypotensive effects of riociguat. (See Cautions: Contraindications.)

The potential for symptomatic hypotension or ischemia should be considered in patients who have predisposing risk factors (e.g., hypovolemia, severe left-ventricular outflow obstruction, resting hypotension, autonomic dysfunction, concomitant use of antihypertensive agents or drugs that can increase exposure to riociguat). (See Drug Interactions.) If manifestations of hypotension occur at any time during therapy, dosage of riociguat should be reduced. (See Dosage and Administration: Dosage.)

Bleeding. Bleeding has been reported in patients receiving riociguat. In the principal efficacy studies of the drug, serious hemorrhagic events, including hemoptysis, vaginal bleeding, catheter site bleeding, subdural hematoma, hematemesis, and intra-abdominal bleeding, occurred in 2.4% of patients receiving riociguat compared with none of the patients receiving placebo. At least 1 death has occurred as a result of a bleeding event.

Pulmonary Effects. Because of the possibility that riociguat may worsen the cardiovascular status of patients with pulmonary veno-occlusive disease, use of the drug in such patients is not recommended. If manifestations of pulmonary edema occur during riociguat therapy, the possibility of pulmonary veno-occlusive disease should be considered; if confirmed, the drug should be discontinued.

Specific Populations **Pregnancy.** Category X. (See Fetal/Neonatal Morbidity and Mortality under Warnings/Precautions: Warnings, in Cautions.)

Lactation. Riociguat and its metabolites are distributed into milk in rats; it is not known whether the drug is distributed into human milk. Because of the potential for serious adverse reactions to riociguat in nursing infants, a decision should be made whether to discontinue nursing or the drug.

Pediatric Use. Safety and efficacy of riociguat have not been established in pediatric patients.

Geriatric Use. In clinical studies of riociguat, approximately 23% of the patients were 65 years of age or older and 6% were 75 years of age or older. Although no overall differences in safety or efficacy were observed between geriatric and younger patients in these studies, the possibility that some older patients may exhibit increased sensitivity to the drug cannot be ruled out.

In geriatric patients, systemic exposure to riociguat may be increased.

Hepatic Impairment. In patients with mild to moderate hepatic impairment (Child-Pugh class A or B), systemic exposure to riociguat may be increased; however, peak plasma concentrations of the drug do not appear to be substantially altered. Safety and efficacy of riociguat in patients with severe hepatic impairment (Child-Pugh class C) have not been established.

Renal Impairment. Safety and efficacy of riociguat have not been established in patients with severe renal impairment (i.e., creatinine clearance less than 15 mL/minute) or in those undergoing dialysis; however, systemic exposure to the drug and its major active M-1 metabolite may be increased by about twofold in patients with severe renal impairment.

Systemic exposure to riociguat also may be increased in patients with mild or moderate renal impairment.

■ **Common Adverse Effects** The most common adverse effects of riociguat occurring more frequently than placebo by at least 3% include headache, dyspepsia/gastritis, dizziness, nausea, diarrhea, hypotension, vomiting, anemia, gastroesophageal reflux disease, and constipation.

Drug Interactions

■ **Drugs Affecting or Metabolized by Hepatic Microsomal Enzymes** Riociguat is metabolized principally by cytochrome P-450 (CYP) isoenzymes 1A1, 3A, 2C8, and 2J2. Concomitant use of drugs that inhibit or induce these isoenzymes may potentially alter plasma concentrations of riociguat.

CYP3A4 Inhibitors or Inducers CYP3A4 inhibitors (e.g., clarithromycin) can potentially increase plasma concentrations of riociguat.

Potent CYP3A4 inducers such as rifampin, phenytoin, carbamazepine, phenobarbital, or St. John's Wort (*Hypericum perforatum*) can potentially decrease concentrations of riociguat and should be used concomitantly with caution. Although no data are available to make specific dosing recommendations, the manufacturer states that titration to riociguat dosages higher than 2.5 mg 3 times daily may be considered in patients receiving potent CYP3A4 inducers.

CYP1A1 Inhibitors or Inducers Concomitant use of riociguat with potent inhibitors of CYP1A1 (e.g., erlotinib, gefitinib) can potentially increase exposure to riociguat and, thus, risk of hypotension. Caution is advised when these drugs are used concomitantly.

CYP1A1 inducers such as cigarette smoke can potentially decrease plasma concentrations of riociguat; adjustment of riociguat dosage may be required. (See Dosage Modification in Smokers under Dosage and Administration: Dosage.)

CYP1A1 Substrates In vitro studies indicate that riociguat and its main active metabolite are potent inhibitors of CYP1A1; therefore, clinically important interactions with drugs that are substantially metabolized by the CYP1A1 isoenzyme (e.g., erlotinib, granisetron) are possible.

■ **Drugs Affecting Efflux Transport Systems** Riociguat is a substrate of the efflux transporters P-glycoprotein (P-gp) and breast cancer resistance protein (BCRP); concomitant use of drugs that inhibit or induce these transport proteins may potentially alter plasma concentrations of riociguat.

Potent P-gp/BCRP Inhibitors Concomitant use of riociguat with potent inhibitors of P-gp/BCRP (e.g, cyclosporine) can potentially increase exposure to riociguat and, thus, risk of hypotension. Caution is advised when these drugs are used concomitantly.

■ **Drugs Affecting Hepatic Microsomal Enzymes and Efflux Transport Systems** ***Potent Inhibitors of Both CYP and P-gp/BCRP*** Concomitant use of riociguat with potent inhibitors of both CYP isoenzymes and P-gp/BCRP (e.g., azole antifungals, HIV protease inhibitors) is expected to substantially increase exposure to riociguat and, thus, risk of hypotension; dosage adjustments may be required. (See Concomitant Use with Drugs Affecting Hepatic Microsomal Enzymes and Transport Systems under Dosage and Administration: Dosage.)

■ **Drugs Affecting Gastric Acidity** Because the aqueous solubility of riociguat is dependent on pH, drugs that increase pH of the upper GI tract (e.g., antacids, histamine H_2-receptor antagonists, proton-pump inhibitors) may potentially decrease the bioavailability of riociguat.

Concomitant administration of an antacid containing aluminum hydroxide and magnesium hydroxide decreased peak plasma concentrations and systemic exposure of riociguat by approximately 56 and 34%, respectively. To reduce the possibility of decreased absorption of riociguat, antacids should not be administered within 1 hour of taking riociguat.

Concomitant administration of the proton-pump inhibitor omeprazole decreased peak plasma concentrations and systemic exposure of riociguat by approximately 35 and 26%, respectively; this interaction is considered to be modest, and no dosage adjustments are necessary when riociguat is administered with omeprazole.

Concomitant administration of the H_2-receptor antagonist ranitidine with riociguat resulted in slight reductions in peak plasma concentrations and systemic exposure of riociguat (by approximately 15 and 10%, respectively).

■ **Antihypertensive Agents** Additive blood pressure-lowering effects may occur if riociguat is administered in conjunction with antihypertensive agents.

■ **Aspirin** Concomitant administration of aspirin and riociguat did not substantially alter pharmacokinetics of riociguat or its active metabolite; in addition, no change in bleeding time or platelet aggregation was observed. No dosage adjustment is necessary when these drugs are used concomitantly.

■ **Azole Antifungals** The azole antifungals itraconazole and ketoconazole are potent multi-pathway CYP and P-gp/BCRP inhibitors and can substantially increase exposure to riociguat if administered concomitantly. Concomitant administration of ketoconazole increased mean peak plasma concentrations and area under the concentration-time curve (AUC) of riociguat by about 46 and 150%, respectively; in addition, half-life of riociguat was prolonged.

Concomitant use of riociguat with itraconazole or ketoconazole is not recommended; if such concomitant use is necessary, a reduced dosage of riociguat should be considered when initiating therapy and in patients who may not tolerate the hypotensive effect of riociguat. In addition, patients should be monitored for hypotension upon initiation of and during such concomitant therapy. (See Concomitant Use with Drugs Affecting Hepatic Microsomal Enzymes and Transport Systems under Dosage and Administration: Dosage.)

■ **Bosentan** Bosentan, a moderate inducer of CYP3A4, decreased steady-state plasma concentrations of riociguat by 27% but did not compromise efficacy of the drug combination. No dosage adjustments are necessary when these drugs are administered concomitantly.

■ **Clarithromycin** Clarithromycin, a CYP3A4 inhibitor, increased systemic exposure (geometric mean AUCs) to riociguat and its major active M-1 metabolite by 41 and 19%, respectively; peak plasma concentrations of riociguat were not altered. No dosage adjustments are necessary when these drugs are used concomitantly, but caution is advised.

■ **HIV Protease Inhibitors** HIV protease inhibitors such as ritonavir are potent multi-pathway CYP and P-gp/BCRP inhibitors and can substantially increase exposure to riociguat and, therefore, risk of hypotension, if administered concomitantly.

Concomitant use of riociguat with these HIV protease inhibitors is not recommended; however, if concomitant use is necessary, adjustment of riociguat dosage should be considered and patients should be monitored for hypotension upon initiation of and during such concomitant therapy. (See Concomitant Use with Drugs Affecting Hepatic Microsomal Enzymes and Transport Systems under Dosage and Administration: Dosage.)

■ **Midazolam** Riociguat does not appear to affect the pharmacokinetics of midazolam.

■ **Nitrates and Nitric Oxide Donors** Additive hypotensive effects can occur if riociguat is used concomitantly with nitrates (e.g., nitroglycerin) or nitric oxide donors (e.g., amyl nitrate). The blood pressure-lowering effects of sublingual nitroglycerin (0.4 mg) were potentiated by riociguat (2.5 mg) in a study in which patients were given nitroglycerin 4 and 8 hours after a dose of riociguat. In addition, syncope was reported in some of the patients.

Because of the risk of hypotension, concomitant administration of riociguat and nitrates or nitric oxide donors in any form is contraindicated. (See Cautions: Contraindications.)

■ **Phosphodiesterase Inhibitors** Additive hypotensive effects can occur if riociguat is used concomitantly with phosphodiesterase (PDE) inhibitors. In a study in patients with PAH who were receiving stable dosages of sildenafil (20 mg 3 times daily), administration of single doses of riociguat resulted in additive hemodynamic effects. In another study, concomitant use of sildenafil and riociguat resulted in no clinical benefit and a high rate of treatment discontinuance due to hypotension. At least one death, possibly related to the combined use of these drugs, also was reported. Riociguat does not appear to affect the pharmacokinetics of sildenafil.

Because of the risk of hypotension, concomitant use of riociguat with any phosphodiesterase inhibitor, including specific PDE type 5 (PDE5) inhibitors (e.g., sildenafil, tadalafil, vardenafil) or nonspecific PDE inhibitors (e.g., dipyridamole, theophylline), is contraindicated. (See Cautions: Contraindications.)

■ **Smoking** Cigarette smoking reduces plasma concentrations of riociguat by approximately 50–60%, presumably due to CYP1A1-inducing effects. Patients should be advised to stop smoking prior to the initiation of riociguat therapy. Dosage adjustments may be required in patients who smoke or stop smoking during riociguat therapy. (See Dosage Modification in Smokers under Dosage and Administration: Dosage.)

■ **Warfarin** Concomitant administration of warfarin and riociguat in healthy individuals did not affect pharmacodynamics (e.g., prothrombin time [PT]) or pharmacokinetics of warfarin. Although peak plasma riociguat concentrations were increased, the extent of increase (16%) was not considered to be clinically important. No dosage adjustment is necessary when warfarin and riociguat are used concomitantly.

Description

Riociguat, a soluble guanylate cyclase (sGC) stimulator, promotes vasodilation via its effects on the nitric oxide-sGC-cyclic guanosine monophosphate (cGMP) pathway. Binding of nitric oxide to sGC in smooth muscle cells increases the generation of intracellular cGMP, a signaling molecule involved in the regulation of vascular tone. Impairment of this nitric oxide signaling pathway, including decreased synthesis of nitric oxide and insufficient stimulation of sGC, has been demonstrated in patients with pulmonary hypertension. Riociguat has a dual mechanism of action in that it increases the sensitivity of sGC to endogenous nitric oxide and also directly stimulates sGC independent of nitric oxide to increase levels of cGMP. Riociguat improves hemodynamics (e.g., pulmonary vascular resistance, pulmonary artery pressure, cardiac output) in patients with pulmonary arterial hypertension (PAH) and also has been shown to reduce concentrations of N-terminal prohormone of brain (pro-brain) natriuretic peptide, a biomarker of heart function. In addition, preclinical studies have demonstrated some antiproliferative and antifibrotic effects of the drug.

Riociguat is rapidly absorbed with peak plasma concentrations attained approximately 0.5–1.5 hours following oral administration. Absolute bioavailability (oral versus IV) of the drug is about 94%. Riociguat is metabolized principally by hepatic cytochrome P-450 (CYP) isoenzymes 1A1, 3A, 2C8, and 2J2, with CYP1A1 responsible for conversion of the drug to its major active M-1 metabolite; the drug is further metabolized to the inactive *N*-glucuronide conjugate. Plasma concentrations of M-1 are about 50% of those of the parent drug in patients with PAH. Riociguat also is a substrate of the efflux transporters p-glycoprotein (P-gp) and breast cancer resistance protein (BCRP). Following oral administration of radiolabeled riociguat in healthy individuals, approximately 40 and 53% of the total radioactivity is recovered in urine and feces, respectively. Elimination half-life of the drug is about 7 hours in healthy individuals and 12 hours in patients with PAH.

Advice to Patients

Risk of fetal harm; importance of advising females of childbearing potential to avoid pregnancy and to use acceptable methods of contraception during and for 1 month following discontinuance of riociguat therapy. Acceptable methods of contraception include one highly effective form of contraception (intrauterine device [IUD], progesterone implant, or tubal sterilization) or a combination of methods (either one hormonal and one barrier method or 2 barrier methods where one form is the male condom). Acceptable hormonal methods of contraception include estrogen-progestin combination oral contraceptives or transdermal contraceptive systems, vaginal ring, and progesterone injections. Acceptable barrier methods include male condoms, diaphragms with spermicide, and cervical caps with spermicide. Even if the partner has had a vasectomy, an additional hormonal or barrier method must be used.

Importance of advising females to inform their clinician immediately if a menstrual period is missed or pregnancy is suspected; clinicians should provide counseling on the use of emergency contraception in the event of unprotected sexual intercourse or contraceptive failure. Apprise patient of potential risk to fetus if pregnancy occurs.

Importance of monthly pregnancy testing.

Importance of all female patients (regardless of childbearing potential) enrolling in the Adempas® REMS program and complying with contraceptive and pregnancy testing requirements. Importance of monitoring reproductive status of prepubertal females and immediately and reporting any changes to a clinician.

Risk of hemoptysis; importance of advising patients to report any potential manifestations of hemoptysis to their clinician.

Importance of advising patients that smoking during riociguat therapy may decrease concentrations of the drug and reduce efficacy; importance of informing clinician if smoking is started or stopped during riociguat therapy as riociguat dosage adjustment may be needed.

Importance of advising patients to not take antacids within 1 hour of riociguat administration and to avoid use of nitrates, nitric oxide donors, and phosphodiesterase (PDE) inhibitors while receiving riociguat therapy.

Risk of dizziness; importance of advising patients to avoid driving or operating machinery until effects of the drug on the individual are known and to consult their clinician, if necessary.

Importance of taking riociguat as prescribed and of not discontinuing therapy or altering dosage without consulting a clinician.

Importance of informing clinicians of existing or contemplated concomitant therapy, including prescription (e.g., azole antifungal agents, HIV protease inhibitors) and OTC drugs, as well as any concomitant illnesses.

Importance of women informing their clinician if they are or plan to become pregnant or plan to breast-feed.

Importance of informing patients of other important precautionary information. (See Cautions.)

Overview® (see Users Guide). For additional information on this drug until a more detailed monograph is developed and published, the manufacturer's labeling should be consulted. It is *essential* that the manufacturer's labeling be consulted for more detailed information on usual cautions, precautions, contraindications, potential drug interactions, laboratory test interferences, and acute toxicity.

Preparations

Distribution of riociguat is restricted. (See Restricted Distribution Program under Dosage and Administration: General.)

Excipients in commercially available drug preparations may have clinically important effects in some individuals; consult specific product labeling for details.

Riociguat

Oral		
Tablets, film-coated	0.5 mg	**Adempas®**, Bayer
	1 mg	**Adempas®**, Bayer
	1.5 mg	**Adempas®**, Bayer
	2 mg	**Adempas®**, Bayer
	2.5 mg	**Adempas®**, Bayer

Selexipag

■ Selexipag, a selective nonprostanoid prostacyclin receptor (IP receptor) agonist, is a vasodilator.

Uses

■ **Pulmonary Arterial Hypertension** Selexipag is used in the management of pulmonary arterial hypertension (PAH; World Health Organization [WHO] group 1 pulmonary hypertension) to delay disease progression and reduce the risk of hospitalization. Efficacy of the drug has been established principally in patients with WHO functional class II–III PAH (idiopathic, heritable, or associated with connective tissue disease or congenital heart disease with repaired shunts) who were receiving selexipag as monotherapy or in combination with an endothelin-receptor antagonist and/or a phosphodiesterase (PDE) type 5 inhibitor. For more information about etiologies of PAH, see Uses: Pulmonary Arterial Hypertension, in Epoprostenol 48:48. Selexipag has been designated an orphan drug by the US Food and Drug Administration (FDA) for use in the treatment of PAH.

In addition to general treatment measures and supportive therapy (e.g., oral anticoagulation, diuretics, supplemental oxygen, digoxin), experts recommend the use of a PAH-specific drug for initial management of PAH in patients who are not candidates for calcium-channel blocker therapy or in whom such therapy has failed; available treatment options include endothelin-receptor antagonists (e.g., ambrisentan, bosentan, macitentan), PDE type 5 inhibitors (e.g., sildenafil, tadalafil), soluble guanylate cyclase stimulators (e.g., riociguat), prostanoids (e.g., epoprostenol, iloprost, treprostinil), and selexipag. Combination therapy with drugs that target the different pathophysiologic pathways of PAH also may be considered since such therapy can provide additive and/or synergistic benefits. Treatment with selexipag alone or in combination with an endothelin receptor antagonist and/or a PDE type 5 inhibitor has been shown to reduce the risk of disease progression and hospitalization in patients with PAH, but has not been shown to reduce mortality. Data are lacking on the relative efficacy and tolerability of selexipag compared with prostacyclins or other oral agents used in the treatment of PAH. In general, choice of PAH therapy should be individualized, taking into account factors such as disease severity, route of administration, potential adverse effects and costs of treatment, clinician experience, and patient preference. For additional information on the treatment of PAH, see Uses: Pulmonary Arterial Hypertension, in Epoprostenol 48:48.

Efficacy of selexipag for the treatment of PAH has been established in a randomized, double-blind, placebo-controlled study (GRIPHON) in 1156 adults with WHO functional class I–IV PAH (58% idiopathic or heritable, 29% associated with connective tissue disease, and 13% caused by other etiologies [corrected congenital shunts, drugs/toxins, or human immunodeficiency virus {HIV}]). Most patients had WHO functional class II (46%) or III (53%) symptoms at study entry and 80% were receiving therapy with an endothelin-receptor antagonist and/or a PDE type 5 inhibitor at baseline; the remaining 20% of patients were treatment naive. Patients received placebo or selexipag (initial dosage of 200 mcg twice daily titrated to the highest tolerated dosage up to 1600 mcg twice daily); the median treatment duration at the time of the primary analysis was 63.7 weeks (with placebo) and 70.7 weeks (with selexipag). The primary end point was time to death from any cause or first occurrence of a complication related to PAH (disease progression [defined as a decrease of at least 15% in the distance walked in 6 minutes in addition to worsening functional class or need for additional therapy], hospitalization, initiation of parenteral prostanoid therapy or chronic oxygen, or need for lung transplantation or balloon atrial septostomy) up to the end of the treatment period. Because the study design allowed for patients in the placebo group to transition to open-label selexipag after any primary end point event, analysis of the primary end point was censored 7 days after the last dose of study drug (selexipag or placebo) was administered.

Selexipag substantially reduced the risk of the primary composite end point compared with placebo (event rate of 27 versus 41.6%; 40% risk reduction). The benefit of selexipag was attributed principally to a reduction in hospitalization and disease progression. In the analysis of primary end point events, there was an excess number of deaths in the selexipag treatment group compared with the placebo group; however, this was considered to be a chance finding because there were so few deaths and the imbalance was not observed until late into the study (after 18 months). When all-cause mortality was assessed through the end of the study (and included deaths that occurred after a complication of PAH), there was no substantial difference between the treatment groups. The treatment effect of selexipag with respect to the primary composite end point was consistent across various patient subgroups, including those who received the drug as monotherapy and those who received concomitant therapy with an endothelin-receptor antagonist, PDE type 5 inhibitor, or both. In addition, selexipag showed similar efficacy regardless of the dosage achieved after patients were titrated to their highest tolerated dosage. Treatment with selexipag modestly improved exercise capacity from baseline to 26 weeks, as indicated by an improvement in the distance walked in 6 minutes (placebo-corrected median treatment effect of 12 m); the subgroup of patients who were treatment-naive appeared to derive greater benefit.

Dosage and Administration

■ **General** ***Restricted Distribution*** Selexipag is available only through specialty pharmacies. For additional information, the manufacturer should be contacted at 866-228-3546.

■ **Administration** ***Oral Administration*** Selexipag is administered orally twice daily without regard to meals; however, tolerability of the drug may be improved when taken with food. Selexipag tablets should not be split, crushed, or chewed.

If a dose of selexipag is missed, the missed dose should be taken as soon as it is remembered. If the next scheduled dose is due within 6 hours, the missed dose should be skipped and the next dose should be taken at the regularly scheduled time. If treatment is missed for 3 or more days, the drug should be restarted at a lower dose and retitrated.

■ **Dosage** Dosage of selexipag should be individualized based on patient tolerability. The recommended initial dosage of selexipag for the treatment of pulmonary arterial hypertension (PAH) in adults is 200 mcg twice daily. Subsequent dosage should be increased in increments of 200 mcg twice daily (usually at weekly intervals) to the highest tolerated dosage up to 1600 mcg twice daily. Adverse effects tend to occur more frequently during the dose titration phase and may be managed with analgesics, antidiarrheals, and antiemetics.

■ **Special Populations** ***Hepatic Impairment*** No dosage adjustment is necessary in patients with mild hepatic impairment (Child-Pugh class A). A reduced initial dosage of selexipag 200 mcg *once* daily is recommended in patients with moderate hepatic impairment (Child-Pugh class B), and dosage should be increased in increments of 200 mcg *once* daily at weekly intervals as tolerated. Use of selexipag should be avoided in patients with severe hepatic impairment (Child-Pugh class C). (See Hepatic Impairment under Warnings/Precautions: Specific Populations, in Cautions.)

Renal Impairment No dosage adjustment is necessary in patients with an estimated glomerular filtration rate (eGFR) exceeding 15 mL/minute per 1.73 m^2. Selexipag has not been studied in patients with eGFR less than 15 mL/minute per 1.73 m^2 and those undergoing dialysis. (See Renal Impairment under Warnings/Precautions: Specific Populations, in Cautions.)

Cautions

■ **Contraindications** Concomitant use of potent inhibitors of cytochrome P-450 (CYP) isoenzyme 2C8 (e.g., gemfibrozil).

■ **Warnings/Precautions** ***Pulmonary Effects*** If manifestations of pulmonary edema occur during therapy, the possibility of associated pulmonary veno-occlusive disease (PVOD) should be considered and selexipag should be discontinued.

Specific Populations **Pregnancy.** There are no adequate and well-controlled studies of selexipag in pregnant women. Selexipag did not affect embryofetal development and survival in animal studies.

Lactation. It is not known whether selexipag is distributed into human milk. The drug and its metabolites are distributed into milk in rats. Because of the potential for serious adverse reactions to selexipag in nursing infants, a decision should be made whether to discontinue nursing or the drug, taking into account the importance of the drug to the woman.

Pediatric Use. Safety and efficacy of selexipag have not been established in pediatric patients.

Geriatric Use. Of the 1368 patients in clinical studies of selexipag, 18% were 65 years of age or older. No overall differences in safety and efficacy were observed between geriatric and younger patients; however, increased sensitivity in some older individuals cannot be ruled out.

Hepatic Impairment. In patients with mild hepatic impairment (Child-Pugh class A), exposure to selexipag was increased twofold compared with that observed in healthy individuals; exposure to the active metabolite was unchanged. In patients with moderate hepatic impairment (Child-Pugh class B), exposure to selexipag was increased fourfold compared with that observed in healthy individuals, and exposure to the active metabolite was doubled. Dosage adjustments are recommended for patients with moderate hepatic impairment. Use of selexipag should be avoided in patients with severe hepatic impairment (Child-Pugh class C). (See Hepatic Impairment under Dosage and Administration: Special Populations.)

Renal Impairment. In patients with severe renal impairment (estimated glomerular filtration rate [eGFR] of 15–29 mL/minute per 1.73 m^2), plasma concentrations and area under the plasma concentration-time curve (AUC) of selexipag and its active metabolite were increased by 40–70%. Selexipag has not been studied in patients undergoing dialysis or in those with eGFR less than 15 mL/minute per 1.73 m^2. (See Renal Impairment under Dosage and Administration: Special Populations.)

■ **Common Adverse Effects** The most common adverse effects reported with selexipag in clinical studies and occurring at least 3% more frequently with the drug than with placebo include headache, diarrhea, jaw pain, nausea, myalgia, vomiting, pain in extremity, flushing, arthralgia, anemia, decreased appetite, and rash.

Drug Interactions

Selexipag and its active metabolite are metabolized principally by cytochrome P-450 (CYP) isoenzyme 2C8 (CYP2C8) and to a lesser extent by CYP3A4. In vitro studies indicate that selexipag and its active metabolite do not inhibit or induce CYP enzymes at clinically relevant concentrations nor do they inhibit hepatic or renal transport proteins.

In vitro studies indicate that selexipag and its active metabolite are substrates of organic anion transport protein (OATP) 1B1 and 1B3. Selexipag is a substrate of P-glycoprotein (P-gp), and the active metabolite is a substrate of breast cancer resistance protein (BCRP).

■ **Drugs Affecting Hepatic Microsomal Enzymes** Potent CYP2C8 inhibitors: Concomitant use of selexipag with potent inhibitors of CYP2C8 (e.g., gemfibrozil) may substantially increase exposure to the active metabolite of selexipag, and is therefore contraindicated.

Moderate CYP2C8 inhibitors: Although not specifically evaluated, concomitant use of selexipag with moderate inhibitors of CYP2C8 (e.g., teriflunomide, deferasirox) also may increase exposure to selexipag and its active metabolite. A less frequent dosing regimen (e.g., once daily) should be considered when initiating selexipag in patients receiving a moderate CYP2C8 inhibitor, and dosage of selexipag should be reduced when initiating a moderate CYP2C8 inhibitor. Patients receiving such concomitant therapy should be monitored to ensure that the dosage of selexipag is tolerated.

CYP2C8 inducers: Concomitant use of selexipag with CYP2C8 inducers may decrease exposure to the active metabolite of selexipag.

CYP3A4 inhibitors: Concomitant administration of selexipag and the fixed combination of lopinavir and ritonavir (lopinavir/ritonavir; a potent CYP3A4 inhibitor) did not alter the pharmacokinetics of selexipag or its active metabolite to a clinically important extent; therefore, dosage adjustment of selexipag does not appear to be necessary when administered concomitantly with drugs that inhibit CYP3A4.

■ **Drugs Affecting Transport Proteins** Concomitant administration of selexipag and lopinavir/ritonavir (a known inhibitor of OATP1B1, OATP1B3, and P-gp) did not alter the pharmacokinetics of selexipag or its active metabolite to a clinically important extent; therefore, dosage adjustment of selexipag does not appear to be necessary when administered concomitantly with drugs that inhibit these transport proteins.

■ **Endothelin Receptor Antagonists** In the GRIPHON study, 16.4% of patients received concomitant therapy with an endothelin-receptor antagonist and selexipag without evidence of any clinically relevant drug interaction. No dosage adjustment is necessary with such concomitant therapy.

■ **Gemfibrozil** Concomitant administration of selexipag and gemfibrozil, a potent CYP2C8 inhibitor, increased exposure to selexipag by twofold and its active metabolite by 11-fold; such concomitant use is contraindicated.

■ **Lopinavir/Ritonavir** In healthy men, concomitant administration of selexipag with lopinavir/ritonavir increased exposure to selexipag by approximately twofold; however, systemic exposure to the active selexipag metabolite was increased by only 8%, which was not considered to be clinically important. No dosage adjustment is necessary when selexipag is administered concomitantly with lopinavir/ritonavir.

■ **Phosphodiesterase Type 5 Inhibitors** In the GRIPHON study, 32.9% of patients received concomitant therapy with a phosphodiesterase (PDE) type 5 inhibitor and selexipag without evidence of any clinically relevant drug interaction. No dosage adjustment is necessary with such concomitant therapy.

■ **Rifampin** Concomitant administration of selexipag and rifampin may decrease exposure to the active metabolite of selexipag. Dosage of selexipag should be increased (up to twofold) when used concomitantly with rifampin and decreased when rifampin is discontinued.

■ **Warfarin** Concomitant administration of warfarin and selexipag in healthy men did not alter the pharmacokinetics of warfarin or selexipag and had no effect on the international normalized ratio (INR). No dosage adjustment is necessary when these drugs are administered concomitantly.

Description

Selexipag is a selective nonprostanoid prostacyclin receptor (IP receptor) agonist that is structurally distinct from prostacyclin and its analogs. Selexipag is a prodrug that is rapidly hydrolyzed to its active metabolite (ACT-333679), which is approximately 37 times as potent as selexipag. Selexipag and its active metabolite have similar mechanisms of action to endogenous prostacyclin (i.e., IP receptor agonism). The binding affinity of the active metabolite for the IP receptor is more than 130 times greater than its affinity for other human prostanoid receptors. This high selectivity for the IP receptor may potentially minimize some of the known adverse effects of prostacyclins such as those affecting the GI system (e.g., nausea, vomiting). Activation of the IP receptor causes an increase in cyclic adenosine monophosphate (cAMP) production which leads to vascular smooth muscle relaxation. In a phase 2 clinical study, selexipag decreased pulmonary vascular resistance, increased cardiac index, and decreased systemic vascular resistance without causing systemic hypotension in patients with pulmonary arterial hypertension (PAH). Although selexipag and its active metabolite inhibit platelet aggregation in vitro, no effect on platelet aggregation was observed when the drug was administered to healthy individuals.

Selexipag exhibits dose-proportional pharmacokinetics with no accumulation following multiple doses. The absolute oral bioavailability of the drug is approximately 49%, most likely due to first-pass metabolism. Following oral administration, selexipag is rapidly absorbed and undergoes hydrolysis by hepatic and intestinal carboxylesterases to yield the active metabolite. Peak plasma concentrations of the drug and its active metabolite are obtained within 1–3 hours and 3–4 hours, respectively, following oral administration. Steady-state exposure of the active metabolite is approximately three- to fourfold that of the parent compound. In healthy individuals, administration with a high-fat meal prolonged absorption of selexipag, but did not substantially alter exposure to the drug or its active metabolite. Selexipag and its active metabolite are metabolized and predominantly eliminated in feces. Both the parent compound and active metabolite undergo oxidative metabolism, principally by cytochrome P-450 (CYP) isoenzyme 2C8 and to lesser extent by CYP3A4, to form less active metabolites (hydroxylated and dealkylated products). The active metabolite also is metabolized by uridine diphosphate-glucuronosyltransferases (UGT) 1A3 and 2B7. Following administration of radiolabeled selexipag in healthy individuals, approximately 93 and 12% of total radioactivity was recovered in feces and urine (only inactive metabolites present in urine), respectively. Terminal elimination half-lives of the drug and its active metabolite are approximately 0.8–2.5 and 6.2–13.5 hours, respectively. The effective half-life of the active metabolite is approximately 3–4 hours.

Advice to Patients

Importance of advising patients not to split, chew, or crush tablets.

Importance of taking a missed dose as soon as it is remembered but not within 6 hours of the next regularly scheduled dose.

Importance of women informing clinicians if they are or plan to become pregnant or plan to breast-feed.

Importance of informing clinicians of existing or contemplated concomitant therapy, including prescription and OTC drugs, as well as any concomitant illnesses.

Importance of informing patients of other important precautionary information. (See Cautions.)

Overview® (see Users Guide). For additional information until a more detailed monograph is developed and published, the manufacturer's labeling should be consulted. It is *essential* that the manufacturer's labeling be consulted for more detailed information on usual cautions, precautions, contraindications, potential drug interactions, laboratory test interferences, and acute toxicity.

Preparations

Selexipag is available only through specialty pharmacies. (See Restricted Distribution under Dosage and Administration: General.)

Excipients in commercially available drug preparations may have clinically important effects in some individuals; consult specific product labeling for details.

Selexipag

Oral		
Tablets, film-coated	200 mcg	Uptravi®, Actelion
	400 mcg	Uptravi®, Actelion
	600 mcg	Uptravi®, Actelion
	800 mcg	Uptravi®, Actelion
	1000 mcg	Uptravi®, Actelion
	1200 mcg	Uptravi®, Actelion
	1400 mcg	Uptravi®, Actelion
	1600 mcg	Uptravi®, Actelion
Titration Pack	140 Tablets, Selexipag 200 mcg (Uptravi®) 60 Tablets, Selexipag 800 mcg (Uptravi®)	Uptravi® Titration Pack, Actelion

Treprostinil
Treprostinil Diolamine

■ Treprostinil and treprostinil diolamine, synthetic analogs of prostacyclin, are vasodilators.

Uses

■ **Pulmonary Arterial Hypertension** Treprostinil is used parenterally (as a continuous subcutaneous or IV infusion) for the management of pulmonary arterial hypertension (PAH; World Health Organization [WHO] group 1 pulmonary hypertension) to reduce symptoms associated with exercise. Clinical studies establishing efficacy of the drug for this indication were conducted in patients with New York Heart Association (NYHA) functional class II–IV (predominantly class III) symptoms and a diagnosis of idiopathic or heritable PAH or PAH associated with connective tissue disease or congenital systemic-to-pulmonary shunts. For more information about etiologies of PAH, see Uses: Pulmonary Arterial Hypertension, in Epoprostenol 48:48. Parenteral treprostinil also is used to reduce the rate of clinical deterioration in PAH patients who require conversion from epoprostenol therapy; the risks and benefits of each drug should be carefully considered prior to transition.

Treprostinil is used by oral inhalation to improve exercise ability in patients with PAH; efficacy of the drug for this indication has been established principally in patients with NYHA/WHO functional class III PAH (idiopathic, heritable, or associated with connective tissue disease). Controlled clinical experience supporting the use of orally inhaled treprostinil is based principally on short-term trials in patients receiving the drug as add-on therapy to bosentan, an endothelin-receptor antagonist, or sildenafil, a phosphodiesterase (PDE) type 5 inhibitor.

Treprostinil diolamine is used orally (as extended-release tablets) to improve exercise ability in patients with PAH; efficacy of the drug for this indication has been established principally in patients with WHO functional class II–III PAH (idiopathic, heritable, or associated with connective tissue disease). Oral treprostinil may be more convenient than inhaled or parenteral formulations of the drug; however, studies have shown only modest benefits of the oral formulation on exercise capacity. The manufacturer states that when the drug is used as the sole vasodilator in patients with PAH, the effect on exercise capacity is approximately 10% of the deficit, and the effect, if any, in combination with other vasodilators is probably even less.

Treprostinil and treprostinil diolamine have been designated orphan drugs by the US Food and Drug Administration (FDA) for use in the treatment of PAH.

In addition to general treatment measures and supportive therapy (e.g., oral anticoagulation, diuretics, supplemental oxygen, digoxin), experts recommend treprostinil (parenteral or inhaled) as one of several treatment options for the initial management of PAH in patients with NYHA/WHO functional class III or IV symptoms who are not candidates for calcium-channel blocker therapy or in whom such therapy has failed; alternative therapies include endothelin-receptor antagonists (e.g., ambrisentan, bosentan, macitentan), PDE type 5 inhibitors (e.g., sildenafil, tadalafil), soluble guanylate cyclase stimulators (e.g., riociguat), or other prostanoids (IV epoprostenol, inhaled iloprost). While current guidelines for the management of PAH state that patients with NYHA/WHO functional class III symptoms may be treated with any currently approved PAH therapy, IV epoprostenol generally is recommended as the treatment of choice for patients with NYHA/WHO functional class IV because of its demonstrated survival benefit. Although oral treprostinil may be a potential initial treatment option for patients with less severe PAH, there are currently no guideline recommendations for the drug; additional studies are needed to establish the role of oral treprostinil in the treatment of PAH. In general, choice of PAH therapy should be individualized, taking into account factors such as disease severity, route of administration, potential adverse effects and costs of treatment, clinician experience, and patient preference.

Combination therapy with drugs that target the different pathophysiologic pathways in PAH may provide additive and/or synergistic benefits. Experts state that combination therapy should be considered in the management of PAH. Results of studies evaluating combination therapy with treprostinil have been variable with some studies (e.g., inhaled treprostinil in combination with an endothelin-receptor antagonist or a PDE type 5 inhibitor) demonstrating improvements in 6-minute walking distance, and other studies (e.g., oral treprostinil in combination with an endothelin-receptor antagonist and/or a PDE type 5 inhibitor) not demonstrating any benefit.

Clinical Experience with Parenteral Treprostinil Efficacy of subcutaneous treprostinil is based principally on the results of 2 multicenter, randomized, double-blind studies of 12 weeks' duration in a total of 470 patients with idiopathic/heritable PAH (58%) or PAH associated with either connective tissue disease (19%) or congenital systemic-to-pulmonary shunts (23%) who had NYHA class II–IV symptoms; most patients (81%) had NYHA class III symptoms. In these studies, treprostinil (infused subcutaneously at a mean dosage of 9.3 ng/kg per minute at week 12) or placebo was added to standard therapy (e.g., oral vasodilators, oral anticoagulants, diuretics, and/or cardiac glycosides). Pooled data from these studies indicate that treprostinil's effect on exercise capacity (i.e., a median increase of 10 m from baseline in the distance walked in 6 minutes) was small relative to the primary study end point (an increase in 6-minute walking distance of 55 m over baseline) and did not achieve conventional levels of statistical significance. The moderate clinical improvement has been attributed to suboptimal dosing of treprostinil. Because of infusion site pain, the average treprostinil dosage achieved in these studies was only 9.3 ng/kg per minute, which was considerably less than the target dosage of 22.5 ng/kg per minute; patients who were able to tolerate the highest dosages had greater improvements in 6-minute walk distance. Significant improvements in secondary end points were observed in these studies; patients receiving subcutaneous treprostinil experienced a reduction in symptoms, as determined by substantial improvement in Borg dyspnea score during the 6-minute walking test, and a substantial effect, compared with placebo, on an assessment that combined walking distance with Borg dyspnea score. Treprostinil therapy also was associated with improvements in indices of dyspnea, fatigue, and signs and symptoms of pulmonary hypertension, but interpretation of these results was confounded by incomplete blinding to treatment assignment that resulted from infusion site symptoms associated with administration of the drug. In addition, treprostinil therapy resulted in small but significant hemodynamic changes consistent with pulmonary and systemic vasodilation (e.g., increases in cardiac index associated with substantial reductions in mean pulmonary artery pressure, mean right atrial pressure, pulmonary or systemic vascular resistance index, and mixed venous oxygen saturation without substantial changes in heart rate) following 12 weeks of therapy. Subgroup analysis in these studies suggested a trend toward greater improvement in exercise capacity associated with treprostinil therapy in severely compromised patients compared with less compromised patients; however, further study is necessary to confirm this finding.

Although the principal efficacy studies of subcutaneous treprostinil failed to show substantial improvements in 6-minute walking distance and there was no trend toward decreased mortality or need for transplantation, the FDA Cardiovascular and Renal Drugs Advisory Committee recommended that the drug be approved based on improvements in perceived quality of life and dyspnea scores, decreases in other signs and symptoms of pulmonary hypertension (e.g., syncope, fatigue), a lack of safety concerns, and the absence in clinical studies of treprostinil of complications (e.g., infections, thrombosis) and logistical problems associated with administering epoprostenol.

The long-term effects of subcutaneous treprostinil were evaluated in a retrospective study of 860 PAH patients who received the drug subcutaneously for up to 4 years. Overall survival rates of 68–87% were reported; however, 59% of patients discontinued therapy by the end of the study period for various reasons (e.g., death, clinical deterioration, adverse effect). The majority of patients who discontinued therapy as a result of infusion site pain or reaction did so within the first year of therapy. For those who remained on subcutaneous treprostinil for more than 1 year, survival rates of 79–90% were reported.

Use of subcutaneous treprostinil is limited by infusion site pain, which can be intolerable in some patients and lead to discontinuance of therapy. The parenteral formulation of treprostinil may be administered as a continuous IV infusion in patients who are unable to tolerate the subcutaneous route. However, the risks associated with continuous IV infusion (e.g., catheter-related infections) should be considered in patients in whom continuous IV infusion is being considered. Efficacy of IV treprostinil for the treatment of PAH is supported primarily by data for subcutaneous treprostinil since bioequivalence between the 2 routes of administration has been demonstrated. In addition, an open-label study in 16 patients with PAH (primary/idiopathic PAH or PAH associated with connective tissue disease or congenital heart disease) demonstrated improvements in 6-minute walking distance, exercise capacity, dyspnea, and hemodynamics following 12 weeks of treatment with IV treprostinil.

Parenteral treprostinil also is used to reduce the rate of clinical deterioration in patients who require conversion from epoprostenol therapy. This indication is based on the results of a randomized, double-blind, placebo-controlled study in which PAH patients receiving stable dosages of IV epoprostenol were converted to subcutaneous treprostinil or placebo and monitored for clinical deterioration (defined as an increase in epoprostenol dosage, PAH-related hospitalization, or death). Seven out of 8 patients who transitioned to placebo had clinical deterioration by the end of the study period compared with only 1 out of 14 patients who transitioned to subcutaneous treprostinil. Although placebo-controlled conversion studies have not been conducted to date with IV treprostinil, several uncontrolled, open-label studies have demonstrated successful and safe conversions of patients from epoprostenol to IV treprostinil.

Clinical Experience with Orally Inhaled Treprostinil Efficacy of inhaled treprostinil is based principally on data from a 12-week randomized, double-blind, placebo-controlled study (TRIUMPH I) that evaluated the addition of inhaled treprostinil to an endothelin-receptor antagonist (bosentan) or a PDE type 5 inhibitor (sildenafil) in clinically stable patients with PAH; nearly all patients had NYHA/WHO class III symptoms. Patients were randomized to receive inhaled treprostinil (titrated to a target dose of 54 mcg per treatment session) or placebo 4 times daily while receiving stable dosages of bosentan (125 mg twice daily) or sildenafil (at least 20 mg 3 times daily). The addition of inhaled treprostinil to bosentan or sildenafil resulted in substantial improvements in exercise capacity, as measured by the change in 6-minute walking distance from baseline to 12 weeks. The median change in the placebo-corrected 6-minute walking distance was 20 m at peak treprostinil exposure (between 10–60 minutes after dosing) and 14 m at trough drug exposure (at least 4 hours after dosing). Improvement in walking distance was apparent as early as 6 weeks after initiation of therapy with inhaled treprostinil and was maintained throughout the duration of the trial. Long-term follow-up of patients who received inhaled treprostinil therapy during the principal efficacy study and open-label extension revealed survival rates of 97, 91, or 82% at 1, 2, or 3 years, respectively. However, these uncontrolled observations should be interpreted cautiously.

Clinical Experience with Oral Treprostinil Efficacy of oral treprostinil is based principally on data from a 12-week randomized, double-blind, placebo-controlled study (FREEDOM-M) in patients (predominantly WHO functional class II or III) who received the drug as monotherapy. Dosage of treprostinil was titrated based on clinical response and tolerability up to a maximum of 12 mg twice daily; the mean dosage achieved at 12 weeks was 3.4 mg twice daily. In the primary efficacy analysis that was conducted in 228 patients, oral treprostinil increased exercise capacity, as indicated by a median increase of approximately 23 m in 6-minute walking distance from baseline to 12 weeks relative to placebo. Although the treatment difference was statistically significant, the magnitude of effect was considered to be nominal. A complicating factor in the analysis of these results was the large number of patients who discontinued study drug prior to assessing 6-minute walking distance. Oral treprostinil also was evaluated as add-on therapy in 2 randomized, double-blind, placebo-controlled studies (FREEDOM-C and FREEDOM-C2) in patients (predominantly WHO functional class II or III) who were already receiving stable therapy with an endothelin-receptor antagonist and/or a PDE type 5 inhibitor. Approximately 40% of the patients were receiving both a PDE type 5 inhibitor and an endothelin-receptor antagonist. In both studies, the addition of oral treprostinil to existing vasodilator therapy did not result in an improvement in 6-minute walking distance from baseline to 16 weeks relative to placebo. It has been suggested that this lack of benefit may be due in part to the inability to titrate to an effective oral treprostinil dosage as a result of adverse effects. Additional studies of longer duration are needed to evaluate the clinical benefit of oral treprostinil in combination with other PAH therapies.

Following completion of the placebo-controlled studies of oral treprostinil, patients entered a long-term, uncontrolled open-label extension study. The average exposure to oral treprostinil was approximately 2 years (maximum of 6 years). Continued dosage increases were permitted up to a maximum of 21 mg twice daily. Patients who completed the 12-month efficacy assessment had an improvement from baseline of 24 m in mean 6-minute walking distance; the average treprostinil dosage achieved at 12 months was 4.2 mg twice daily. Among patients who remained in the study and continued to receive oral treprostinil therapy, overall survival rates were 92, 87, and 82% at the end of 1, 2, and 3 years, respectively; however, these uncontrolled observations should be interpreted cautiously.

Safety and tolerability of transitioning patients from parenteral treprostinil to oral treprostinil therapy were evaluated in a 24-week, uncontrolled, open-label study in low-risk patients with PAH (WHO functional class I or II) who were hemodynamically stable. All patients were transitioned successfully from parenteral to oral therapy, with most patients (94%) completing the transition over a 5-day period (range 2–29 days; median 3 days). After 24 weeks of oral treprostinil therapy, 6-minute walking distance and hemodynamic parameters remained stable. According to the transition protocol, patients were administered increasing doses of oral treprostinil 3 times daily while their dosage of parenteral treprostinil was simultaneously reduced; the mean total daily dose of oral treprostinil at the end of the transition was 27 mg compared with a mean parenteral treprostinil dosage prior to transition of 59 ng/kg per minute.

Dosage and Administration

■ **General** ***Restricted Distribution*** All commercially available preparations of treprostinil can be obtained only through specialty pharmacies. For additional information, the manufacturer should be contacted at 877-864-8437.

■ **Administration** Treprostinil is administered parenterally (by continuous subcutaneous or IV infusion) using a controlled-infusion device. Treprostinil also is available as an inhalation solution that is administered by oral inhalation using the Tyvaso® Inhalation System.

Treprostinil diolamine is administered orally as extended-release tablets (Orenitram®).

Parenteral Administration When treprostinil is administered parenterally, the subcutaneous route generally is preferred because of the potential for complications associated with long-term IV administration of the drug (e.g., bloodstream infections). The manufacturer states that the IV route should be reserved for patients who are not able to tolerate the subcutaneous route (e.g., due to infusion site pain or reaction) or in whom the risks of IV therapy are considered warranted. Continuous infusions of treprostinil are delivered using controlled-infusion devices (ambulatory infusion pumps) designed specifically for subcutaneous or IV drug delivery. The manufacturer's labeling should be consulted for ambulatory pump specifications. Delivery system malfunctions such as infusion-device failure or an occluded catheter may result in inadvertent overdosage or underdosage of treprostinil. To avoid potential interruptions in drug delivery, patients receiving subcutaneous or IV treprostinil therapy should have immediate access to a backup infusion pump and infusion sets.

Conversions from epoprostenol to subcutaneous or IV treprostinil therapy should be performed in a hospital setting where patients can be closely monitored.

Subcutaneous Administration. Treprostinil is administered as a continuous subcutaneous infusion through a self-inserted subcutaneous catheter. For subcutaneous administration, treprostinil injection should be given as supplied without further dilution. A single reservoir (syringe) of undiluted treprostinil can be administered for up to 72 hours at 37°C. Infusion rates for subcutaneous administration may be calculated using the following formula:

$$\text{subcutaneous infusion rate (mL/hr)} = \frac{\text{dose (ng/kg per minute)} \times \text{weight (in kg)} \times 0.00006}{\text{treprostinil vial strength (mg/mL)}}$$

IV Administration. Prior to IV infusion, commercially available treprostinil injection *must* be diluted with one of the following diluents: sterile water for injection, 0.9% sodium chloride injection, Remodulin® (treprostinil) sterile diluent for injection, Flolan® (epoprostenol sodium) sterile diluent for injection, or sterile diluent for generic epoprostenol sodium. Solutions of treprostinil prepared with a high-pH glycine diluent (Remodulin® [treprostinil] sterile diluent for injection, Flolan® [epoprostenol sodium] sterile diluent for injection, or sterile diluent for generic epoprostenol sodium) are stable (and may be stored) at room temperature for up to 14 days at concentrations as low as 0.004 mg/mL (4 mcg/mL); the diluted solution may be administered for up to 48 hours at 40°C. Solutions of treprostinil prepared with sterile water for injection or 0.9% sodium chloride for injection are stable (and may be stored) at room temperature for up to 4 hours or under refrigeration for up to 24 hours; the diluted solution may be administered for up to 48 hours at 40°C.

The diluted treprostinil solution should be prepared by adding the drug to a sufficient volume of diluent in an appropriate pump reservoir. Typical IV infusion system reservoirs have a total volume capacity of 50 or 100 mL. The concentration of the diluted treprostinil solution should be determined by first selecting an infusion rate that will allow for an infusion period of up to 48 hours. The following formulas can then be used to calculate the concentration and amount of treprostinil required to prepare the diluted solution:

$$\text{diluted IV treprostinil concentration (mg/mL)} = \frac{\text{dose (ng/kg per minute)} \times \text{weight (in kg)} \times 0.00006}{\text{IV infusion rate (mL/hr)}}$$

$$\text{amount of treprostinil injection (mL)} = \frac{\text{diluted IV treprostinil concentration (mg/mL)}}{\text{treprostinil vial strength (mg/mL)}} \times \text{total reservoir volume (mL)}$$

The diluted solution is administered as a continuous IV infusion through a surgically placed indwelling central venous catheter. If necessary, a peripheral IV catheter (preferably placed in a large vein) may be used temporarily to administer the drug until central venous access can be established.

The manufacturer's labeling should be consulted for additional information on the preparation and administration of IV treprostinil.

Oral Inhalation Treprostinil inhalation solution should be administered by oral inhalation only; the drug should *not* be ingested orally. The drug must be administered only with the Tyvaso® Inhalation System, which consists of an ultrasonic, pulsed delivery device and related accessories. To avoid potential interruptions in drug delivery secondary to equipment malfunction, patients should have access to a backup Tyvaso® Inhalation System device. Patients should be instructed on proper administration of orally inhaled treprostinil, including use and maintenance of the Tyvaso® Inhalation System device.

Prior to the first inhalation session, the entire contents of a single 2.9-mL ampul containing 1.74 mg of treprostinil inhalation solution should be transferred into the medicine cup supplied by the manufacturer. One ampul should contain enough drug for one day of treatment. Between daily treatment sessions, the inhalation device should be capped and stored upright with the remaining inhalation solution stored inside for up to 24 hours. At the end of the day, the medicine cup and any remaining drug solution should be discarded and the Tyvaso® Inhalation System device cleaned in accordance with the manufacturer's instructions.

Treprostinil for oral inhalation should *not* be mixed with other drugs in the Tyvaso® Inhalation System device. The solution should not be allowed to come in contact with the eyes or skin.

Oral Administration Treprostinil diolamine extended-release tablets are administered orally 2 or 3 times daily (approximately every 12 or 8 hours, respectively) with food. A thrice-daily regimen may produce less variation in drug concentrations and reduce the occurrence or severity of adverse events, which may improve tolerability. The tablets should be swallowed whole and not split, crushed, or chewed.

If a dose of treprostinil is missed, the missed dose should be taken as soon as it is remembered; if a patient misses 2 or more doses, the drug should be restarted at a lower dosage and retitrated.

Patients receiving treprostinil extended-release tablets should be advised that the tablet shell is designed to remain intact during passage through the GI tract and may be passed in the stool.

■ Dosage *Pulmonary Arterial Hypertension*

Parenteral Dosage. For the treatment of pulmonary arterial hypertension (PAH) in adults with New York Heart Association (NYHA) class II–IV symptoms, the recommended initial dosage of treprostinil is 1.25 ng/kg per minute given by continuous subcutaneous or IV infusion. If this initial dosage is not tolerated, the infusion rate should be decreased to 0.625 ng/kg per minute. Dosage should be titrated to achieve symptomatic improvement while minimizing adverse effects (e.g., infusion site reactions or pain, headache, nausea, vomiting, restlessness, anxiety). The infusion rate should be increased in increments of 1.25 ng/kg per minute at weekly intervals for the first 4 weeks and then 2.5 ng/kg per minute at weekly intervals for the remaining duration of infusion, depending on clinical response. More frequent dosage adjustments may be attempted if tolerated. Several months may be required to identify the optimal dosage in an individual patient.

Abrupt withdrawal or sudden large reductions in dosage of treprostinil may result in worsening of pulmonary hypertension symptoms and should be avoided. (See Withdrawal of Therapy under Cautions: Warnings/Precautions.) If therapy is interrupted for brief periods (e.g., a few hours), treprostinil may be restarted at the same dosage; longer periods of interruption may require retitration of therapy.

When converting patients from IV epoprostenol to parenteral treprostinil therapy, the manufacturer recommends that treprostinil be initiated at a dosage equal to 10% of the current epoprostenol dosage; dosage of treprostinil should then be gradually increased while simultaneously decreasing the dosage of epoprostenol. The following titration protocol is recommended by the manufacturer:

Step	Epoprostenol Dosage	Treprostinil Dosage
1	Unchanged	10% of starting epoprostenol dosage
2	80% of starting epoprostenol dosage	30% of starting epoprostenol dosage
3	60% of starting epoprostenol dosage	50% of starting epoprostenol dosage
4	40% of starting epoprostenol dosage	70% of starting epoprostenol dosage
5	20% of starting epoprostenol dosage	90% of starting epoprostenol dosage
6	5% of starting epoprostenol dosage	110% of starting epoprostenol dosage
7	0	110% of starting epoprostenol dosage + additional 5–10% increments as needed

Treprostinil dosage should be titrated according to individual requirements to a dosage that will allow for withdrawal of epoprostenol therapy while balancing symptoms of PAH and prostacyclin-related adverse effects. Any increase in PAH symptoms that occurs during the transition should be managed initially by increasing the dosage of treprostinil, and any adverse effects related to excess prostacyclin (e.g., facial flushing, headache, jaw pain) should be managed initially by decreasing the epoprostenol dosage. Other transition protocols have been used successfully to convert patients from epoprostenol to treprostinil therapy, including a rapid transition method in which the drug reservoir containing IV epoprostenol is switched directly with one containing IV treprostinil. Although data are limited, patients who transition from epoprostenol to IV treprostinil appear to require higher average dosages of treprostinil (in some cases, at least double) to maintain the same clinical benefits.

Oral Inhalation Dosage. The recommended initial dosage of orally inhaled treprostinil is 18 mcg (3 breaths) per treatment session. If this initial dosage is not tolerated, dosage should be reduced to 1 or 2 breaths per treatment session, then subsequently increased to 3 breaths as tolerated. A total of 4 treatment sessions should be administered daily, spaced equally apart at intervals of approximately 4 hours during waking hours. Dosage of orally inhaled treprostinil should be further increased by 3 breaths every 1–2 weeks until the target maintenance dosage of 54 mcg (9 breaths) per treatment session is achieved. Patients who are unable to reach the target dosage due to adverse effects should be maintained on the highest possible tolerated dosage that does not exceed the maximum recommended dosage of 9 breaths per treatment session. If a treatment session is missed or interrupted, therapy should be resumed as soon as possible at the usual dosage.

Oral Dosage. Dosage of treprostinil diolamine is expressed in terms of treprostinil.

The recommended initial oral dosage of treprostinil in adults is 0.25 mg twice daily (taken approximately every 12 hours) or 0.125 mg 3 times daily (taken approximately every 8 hours) as extended-release tablets. Dosage should be increased every 3–4 days in recommended increments of 0.25 or 0.5 mg twice daily or 0.125 mg 3 times daily until the highest tolerated dosage is achieved. A slower titration should be considered for patients not tolerating such increases. The appropriate maintenance dosage of oral treprostinil is determined by patient tolerability. If intolerable adverse effects occur, dosage should be decreased in decrements of 0.25 mg.

Abrupt discontinuance of treprostinil therapy should be avoided. When discontinuing oral treprostinil therapy, dosage should be reduced by 0.5–1 mg daily. (See Withdrawal of Therapy under Cautions: Warnings/Precautions.)

When used concomitantly with potent inhibitors of cytochrome P-450 (CYP) 2C8 (e.g., gemfibrozil), oral treprostinil should be initiated at a dosage of 0.125 mg twice daily and increased in increments of 0.125 mg twice daily every 3–4 days as tolerated.

When transitioning from parenteral to oral treprostinil therapy, the manufacturer recommends decreasing the dosage of subcutaneous or IV treprostinil while simultaneously increasing the dosage of oral treprostinil. Dosage of parenteral treprostinil may be reduced up to 30 ng/kg per minute per day and dosage of oral treprostinil may be simultaneously increased up to 6 mg per day (administered as 2 mg 3 times daily) if tolerated. The following equation can be used to estimate a comparable dose of oral treprostinil using the patient's current parenteral treprostinil dose:

$$\text{total daily dose of oral treprostinil (mg)} = 0.0072 \times \text{dose of parenteral treprostinil (ng/kg per minute)} \times \text{weight (kg)}$$

Temporary infusion of subcutaneous or IV treprostinil may be considered in the event of a planned, short-term interruption of oral treprostinil therapy in patients who are unable to take oral medications. The following formula can be used to calculate a comparable dose of parenteral treprostinil using the patient's current dose of oral treprostinil:

$$\text{dose of parenteral treprostinil (ng/kg per minute)} = \frac{139 \times \text{total daily dose of oral treprostinil (mg)}}{\text{weight (kg)}}$$

■ **Special Populations** ***Hepatic Impairment*** In patients with mild-to-moderate hepatic impairment, the initial dosage of subcutaneous or IV treprostinil should be decreased to 0.625 ng/kg per minute (based on ideal body weight), and dosage should be titrated slowly.

Orally inhaled treprostinil should be titrated slowly in patients with hepatic impairment because of the possibility of increased systemic exposure to the drug.

In patients with mild hepatic impairment (Child-Pugh class A), oral treprostinil should be initiated at a dosage of 0.125 mg twice daily and increased in increments of 0.125 mg twice daily every 3–4 days. (See Hepatic Impairment under Warnings/Precautions: Specific Populations, in Cautions.)

Renal Impairment The manufacturer makes no specific dosage recommendations for parenteral or orally inhaled treprostinil in patients with renal impairment; however, treprostinil should be titrated slowly in such patients because of the possibility of increased systemic exposure to the drug.

Dosage adjustments of oral treprostinil are not needed in patients with renal impairment. Oral treprostinil is not removed by dialysis.

Geriatric Patients Dosage of treprostinil should be selected with caution in geriatric patients because of the greater frequency of decreased hepatic, renal, or cardiac function and of concomitant disease or other drug therapy observed in such patients.

Cautions

■ **Contraindications** The manufacturer states that there are no known contraindications to the use of parenteral or orally inhaled treprostinil.

Oral treprostinil is contraindicated in patients with severe hepatic impairment (Child-Pugh class C).

■ **Warnings/Precautions** ***Risk of Infection with IV Administration*** Serious and potentially fatal bloodstream infections (BSI) and sepsis associated with the drug delivery system (long-term indwelling central venous catheter) have been reported in patients receiving continuous IV infusions of treprostinil. In an open-label study, 7 catheter-related infections were reported among 47 patients who received IV treprostinil (approximately 1 BSI event per 5 years of use). In a retrospective survey of 7 pulmonary hypertension treatment centers, a higher rate of overall and gram-negative bloodstream infections were identified among patients with pulmonary arterial hypertension (PAH) receiving IV treprostinil compared with IV epoprostenol. Approximately 1 BSI event (defined as any positive blood culture) was reported for every 3 years of use for patients receiving IV treprostinil. The reason for the reported difference in infection rate between IV treprostinil and IV epoprostenol is unknown, but may be related to differences in preparation and storage, infection-control practices, or anti-inflammatory activity of the agents.

To decrease the risk of infection, strict aseptic technique must be followed in routine catheter care and in the preparation and administration of IV treprostinil. Use of a high-pH glycine diluent (e.g., Remodulin® [treprostinil] sterile diluent for injection, Flolan® [epoprostenol sodium] sterile diluent for injection, sterile diluent for generic epoprostenol sodium for injection) with IV treprostinil has been associated with a lower incidence of blood stream infections compared with neutral diluents such as sterile water for injection and 0.9% sodium chloride injection. Because of the increased risk of infections associated with long-term IV administration of treprostinil, the manufacturer states that the subcutaneous route of administration is preferred over IV when the drug is administered parenterally.

Precautions Related to Orally Inhaled Treprostinil Safety and efficacy of orally inhaled treprostinil have not been established in patients with substantial lung disease such as asthma or chronic obstructive pulmonary disease. Patients who develop acute pulmonary infections while receiving inhaled treprostinil should be monitored for any worsening of lung disease and loss of drug effect.

Precautions Related to Oral Treprostinil The tablet shell of treprostinil extended-release tablets (Orenitram®) does not dissolve and may become lodged in a diverticulum in patients with diverticulosis. (See Oral Administration under Dosage and Administration: Administration.)

Adequate Patient Evaluation and Monitoring Because of the complex nature of the disease and the potential for treatment-related complications, the American College of Chest Physicians (ACCP) and other experts recommend referral of patients with PAH to specialized centers experienced in the management of pulmonary vascular diseases.

Withdrawal of Therapy Abrupt withdrawal or sudden large reductions in dosage of treprostinil may result in worsening of pulmonary hypertension symptoms and should be avoided.

Hematologic Effects Because treprostinil inhibits platelet aggregation, there is a potential increased risk of bleeding, particularly in patients receiving anticoagulant therapy. (See Drug Interactions: Anticoagulants.)

Hypotensive Effects Treprostinil is a potent vasodilator. There is a risk of symptomatic hypotension in patients with low systemic arterial pressure receiving orally inhaled treprostinil. Hypotension also has occurred in patients receiving subcutaneous treprostinil during clinical trials.

Specific Populations **Pregnancy.** Parenteral and orally inhaled treprostinil: Category B. (See Users Guide.) There are no adequate and well-controlled studies of parenteral or orally inhaled treprostinil in pregnant women. In an animal reproduction study in rats, subcutaneous infusion of treprostinil during organogenesis and late gestational development at dosages approximately 16 times higher than the average dosage used in clinical trials did not result in any fetal harm. In another study in rabbits, subcutaneous infusion of treprostinil during organogenesis at dosages approximately 5 times higher than the average dosage used in clinical trials resulted in an increased incidence of fetal skeletal variations associated with maternal toxicity. Animal reproduction studies have not been conducted with orally inhaled treprostinil.

Oral treprostinil: Category C. (See Users Guide.) There are no adequate and well-controlled studies of oral treprostinil in pregnant women. In animal studies, increased postimplantation loss, decreased fetal viability, and increased soft tissue and fetal skeletal malformations were observed in rats and rabbits treated with oral treprostinil at dosages corresponding to at least 5 times the expected human exposure.

Lactation. It is not known whether treprostinil is distributed into milk. Some manufacturers state that a decision should be made whether to discontinue nursing or the drug.

Pediatric Use. Safety and efficacy of parenteral treprostinil have not been established in children younger than 16 years of age. Clinical studies of parenteral treprostinil did not include sufficient numbers of patients 16 years of age and younger to determine whether pediatric patients respond differently than adults. In general, dosage should be titrated carefully in pediatric patients.

Safety and efficacy of oral or orally inhaled treprostinil have not been established in pediatric patients younger than 18 years of age.

Geriatric Use. Clinical studies of treprostinil did not include sufficient numbers of patients 65 years of age and older to determine whether geriatric patients respond differently than younger patients. In general, dosage should be selected carefully in geriatric patients. The greater frequency of decreased hepatic, renal, and/or cardiac function and of concomitant disease and drug therapy observed in the elderly should be considered.

Hepatic Impairment. In patients with portopulmonary hypertension and mild or moderate hepatic impairment, systemic exposure to subcutaneous treprostinil was increased by threefold or fivefold, respectively, compared with healthy individuals. Clearance of subcutaneous treprostinil was reduced by up to 80% in patients with hepatic impairment compared with that in healthy individuals. Dosage adjustment is recommended in patients with mild or moderate hepatic impairment receiving subcutaneous or IV treprostinil. (See Hepatic Impairment under Dosage and Administration: Special Populations.) Parenteral and orally inhaled treprostinil have not been studied in patients with severe hepatic impairment.

In patients with mild, moderate, or severe hepatic impairment, peak plasma concentrations and systemic exposure of oral treprostinil were increased by 1.6-, 4-, or 4.8-fold and 2.1-, 4.8-, or 7.6-fold, respectively, compared with healthy individuals. Use of oral treprostinil should be avoided in patients with moderate hepatic impairment and is contraindicated in patients with severe hepatic impairment.

Renal Impairment. Parenteral and orally inhaled treprostinil have not been studied in patients with renal impairment. Since treprostinil and its metabolites are eliminated principally by the kidneys, clearance of the drug may be reduced in patients with renal impairment.

Pharmacokinetics of oral treprostinil were not substantially altered in patients with severe or end-stage renal disease, including those undergoing dialysis.

■ **Common Adverse Effects** Infusion site pain and reactions (excluding bleeding/bruising but including reactions such as erythema, induration, and rash) are the most common adverse effects reported in patients receiving subcutaneous infusions of treprostinil; in some cases, these reactions may be severe or require discontinuance of the drug. Adverse effects attributed specifically to the IV route of administration of treprostinil include arm swelling, paresthesias, hematoma, and pain. Headache, diarrhea, nausea, rash, jaw pain, and vasodilation are other common adverse effects frequently reported in clinical trials of patients receiving either subcutaneous or IV treprostinil.

Common adverse effects associated with orally inhaled treprostinil include cough, throat irritation, headache, GI effects, muscle pain, jaw pain, bone pain, flushing, and syncope.

Common adverse effects associated with oral treprostinil include headache, diarrhea, nausea, flushing, jaw pain, extremity pain, hypokalemia, and abdominal discomfort.

Drug Interactions

■ **Drugs Affecting or Metabolized by Hepatic Microsomal Enzymes** Treprostinil is extensively metabolized in the liver, principally by cytochrome P-450 (CYP) isoenzyme 2C8 and to a lesser extent by CYP2C9. Based on pharmacokinetic studies with the oral formulation of treprostinil, concomitant administration of treprostinil with inhibitors (e.g., gemfibrozil) or inducers (e.g., rifampin) of CYP2C8 may increase or decrease exposure to treprostinil, respectively. When oral treprostinil is administered concomitantly with a potent CYP2C8 inhibitor, dosage reduction is recommended. (See Oral Dosage under Dosage: Pulmonary Arterial Hypertension, in Dosage and Administration.) Because treprostinil does not appear to inhibit or induce major CYP isoenzymes (see Description), pharmacokinetic interactions with drugs metabolized by CYP enzymes are considered unlikely.

■ **Acetaminophen** Results of drug interaction studies in healthy individuals indicate that acetaminophen (4 g daily) did not affect the pharmacokinetics of treprostinil administered subcutaneously or orally.

■ **Anticoagulants** Concomitant use of treprostinil and anticoagulants may increase the risk of bleeding. (See Hematologic Effects under Cautions: Warnings/Precautions.)

In healthy individuals receiving a single 25-mg dose of warfarin, treprostinil (as a subcutaneous infusion at a rate of 10 ng/kg per minute) did not affect the pharmacokinetics of *R*- and *S*-warfarin or the international normalized ratio (INR). No clinically important effects on the pharmacokinetics of treprostinil have been observed with concomitant administration of warfarin.

■ **Antihypertensive Agents** Additive hypotensive effects may occur if treprostinil is used concomitantly with antihypertensive agents.

■ **Bosentan** No pharmacokinetic interaction has been observed with bosentan (250 mg daily) and the oral formulation of treprostinil in healthy individuals. Dosage adjustments of oral treprostinil are not necessary when used concomitantly with bosentan.

■ **Diuretics** Additive hypotensive effects may occur if treprostinil is used concomitantly with diuretics.

■ **Esomeprazole** No pharmacokinetic interaction has been observed with concomitant use of esomeprazole (40 mg daily) and oral treprostinil (1 mg). Dosage adjustments of oral treprostinil are not necessary when used concomitantly with esomeprazole.

■ **Fluconazole** Results of drug interaction studies in healthy individuals indicate that fluconazole 200 mg daily did not affect the pharmacokinetics of treprostinil administered subcutaneously or orally. The manufacturer states that dosage adjustments of oral treprostinil are not necessary when used concomitantly with fluconazole.

■ **Gemfibrozil** Drug interaction studies with the oral formulation of treprostinil indicate that systemic exposure to treprostinil is increased with concomitant administration of gemfibrozil, a potent CYP2C8 inhibitor. Such increased exposure may be expected to increase the incidence of treprostinil-related adverse effects. When oral treprostinil is administered concomitantly with gemfibrozil, an initial treprostinil dosage of 0.125 mg twice daily is recommended, and the dosage should be increased in increments of 0.125 mg twice daily every 3–4 days as tolerated.

■ **Rifampin** Drug interaction studies with the oral formulation of treprostinil indicate that systemic exposure and peak plasma concentrations of treprostinil are decreased with concomitant administration of rifampin, a CYP2C8 and 2C9 inducer. Such decreased exposure may be expected to reduce the efficacy of treprostinil. The manufacturer states that dosage adjustments of oral treprostinil are not necessary when used concomitantly with rifampin.

■ **Sildenafil** No pharmacokinetic interaction has been observed between sildenafil (60 mg daily) and the oral formulation of treprostinil. The manufacturer states that dosage adjustments of oral treprostinil are not necessary when used concomitantly with sildenafil.

■ **Other Vasodilating Agents** Additive hypotensive effects may occur if treprostinil is used concomitantly with other vasodilating agents.

Description

Treprostinil, a synthetic analog of prostacyclin, has pharmacologic actions (e.g., vasodilation of pulmonary and systemic arterial vascular beds, inhibition of platelet aggregation) similar to those of epoprostenol. Treprostinil diolamine is a salt form of treprostinil that is commercially available as an osmotic extended-release tablet designed to release the drug at a controlled rate. In animals, the vasodilatory effects of treprostinil reduce right and left ventricular afterload and increase cardiac output and stroke volume. Studies have shown that treprostinil causes a dose-related negative inotropic and lusitropic effect. Orally inhaled treprostinil has been shown to exhibit high pulmonary selectivity and sustained pulmonary vasodilation without producing substantial systemic effects. Modest and temporary effects on the QT interval corrected for rate (QT_c) have been observed following single oral inhalation doses of treprostinil up to 84 mcg, but this may be an artifact of the rapidly changing heart rate produced by the drug. The effects of oral or parenteral treprostinil on the QT_c interval have not been established.

Unlike epoprostenol, treprostinil is chemically stable at neutral pH and room temperature and has a longer half-life (4 hours), which permits continuous subcutaneous infusion in addition to continuous IV infusion, which is currently the sole method of administration of epoprostenol. Treprostinil is substantially metabolized by the liver, principally by cytochrome P-450 (CYP) isoenzyme 2C8. Based on results of in vitro studies, treprostinil does not appear to inhibit CYP 1A2, 2A6, 2C8, 2C9, 2C19, 2D6, 2E1, or 3A isoenzymes, nor does it appear to induce 1A2, 2B6, 2C9, 2C19, or 3A isoenzymes.

Advice to Patients

Importance of informing patients that abrupt discontinuance of treprostinil therapy could result in worsening of pulmonary arterial hypertension (PAH) symptoms.

Importance of advising patients that parenteral treprostinil is infused continuously via an infusion pump through a subcutaneous or surgically placed indwelling central venous catheter, which will require a long-term commitment on the part of the patient to care for and operate. Importance of advising patients that subsequent management of the disease may require therapy with an alternate IV prostacyclin therapy (e.g., epoprostenol).

Importance of instructing patients regarding proper administration of extended-release tablets. Necessity of swallowing the tablets without splitting, chewing, crushing, or breaking. Importance of administering oral treprostinil with food.

Importance of advising patients to use sterile technique when preparing and administering parenteral treprostinil.

Importance of patients receiving adequate training in the proper administration of orally inhaled treprostinil, including dosing and setup, operation, and maintenance of the Tyvaso® Inhalation System device.

Importance of having immediate access to a backup pump and infusion sets (when administered parenterally) or a backup Tyvaso® Inhalation System device (when administered via oral inhalation) in order to avoid potential interruptions in drug therapy secondary to drug delivery device failure or equipment malfunction.

Importance of advising patients that if a scheduled treatment session of inhaled treprostinil is missed to resume treatment as soon as possible.

Importance of informing patients that the biologically inert components of the extended-release tablets remain intact during GI transit and are eliminated in the feces as an insoluble shell.

Importance of advising patients to avoid skin or eye contact with treprostinil oral inhalation solution. If skin or eye contact occurs, instruct patients to immediately rinse affected area with water.

Importance of understanding potential risks associated with therapy. Importance of women informing clinicians if they are or plan to become pregnant or plan to breast-feed. Importance of informing clinicians of existing or contemplated concomitant therapy, including prescription and OTC drugs, as well as concomitant illnesses.

Overview® (see Users Guide). For additional information until a more detailed monograph is developed and published, the manufacturer's labeling should be consulted. It is *essential* that the manufacturer's labeling be consulted for more detailed information on usual cautions, precautions, contraindications, potential drug interactions, laboratory test interferences, and acute toxicity.

Preparations

Treprostinil diolamine extended-release tablets (Orenitram®), treprostinil injection (Remodulin®), treprostinil inhalation solution (Tyvaso®), and the Tyvaso® Inhalation System are available only through specialty pharmacies. (See Restricted Distribution under Dosage and Administration: General.)

Excipients in commercially available drug preparations may have clinically important effects in some individuals; consult specific product labeling for details.

Treprostinil

Oral Inhalation		
Solution, for nebulization	0.6 mg/mL (1.74 mg)	**Tyvaso®** (available with Tyvaso® Inhalation System), United Therapeutics
Parenteral		
Injection, for continuous subcutaneous or IV infusion via controlled-infusion device only	1 mg/mL	**Remodulin®**, United Therapeutics
	2.5 mg/mL	**Remodulin®**, United Therapeutics
	5 mg/mL	**Remodulin®**, United Therapeutics
	10 mg/mL	**Remodulin®**, United Therapeutics

Treprostinil Diolamine

Oral		
Tablets, extended-release	0.125 mg (of treprostinil)	**Orenitram®**, United Therapeutics
	0.25 mg (of treprostinil)	**Orenitram®**, United Therapeutics
	1 mg (of treprostinil)	**Orenitram®**, United Therapeutics
	2.5 mg (of treprostinil)	**Orenitram®**, United Therapeutics
	5 mg (of treprostinil)	**Orenitram®**, United Therapeutics

52:00 Eye, Ear, Nose, and Throat Preparations*

52:02 Antiallergic Agents

Alcaftadine§
Azelastine§
Bepotastine§
Cetirizine§
Cromolyn§
Emedastine§
Epinastine§
Ketotifen§
Lodoxamide§
Nedocromil§
Olopatadine§
Pemirolast§
see also:
Cromolyn Sodium 48:10.32

52:04 Anti-infectives

52:04.04 Antibacterials

Bacitracin§
Besifloxacin§
Ciprofloxacin§
Doxycycline§
Erythromycin§
Gatifloxacin§
Gentamicin§
Levofloxacin§
Minocycline§
Moxifloxacin§
Neomycin§
Ofloxacin§
Polymyxin B§
Sulfacetamide§
Tobramycin§

52:04.16 Antifungals

Natamycin§

52:04.20 Antivirals

Ganciclovir§
Trifluridine§

52:04.92 EENT Anti-infectives, Miscellaneous

Carbamide Peroxide§
Chlorhexidine§
Zinc Sulfate§

52:08 Anti-inflammatory Agents

52:08.08 Corticosteroids

EENT Corticosteroids General Statement§
Beclomethasone§
Budesonide§
Ciclesonide§
Dexamethasone§
Difluprednate§
Flunisolide§
Fluocinolone§
Fluorometholone§
Fluticasone§
Hydrocortisone§
Loteprednol§
Mometasone§
Prednisolone§
Rimexolone§
Triamcinolone§

52:08.20 Nonsteroidal Anti-inflammatory Agents

Bromfenac§
Flurbiprofen§
Ketorolac§
Nepafenac§

52:08.92 Anti-inflammatory Agents, Miscellaneous

Cyclosporine§
Lifitegrast§

52:16 Local Anesthetics

Benzocaine§
Cocaine§
Dyclonine§
Proparacaine§
Tetracaine§

52:24 Mydriatics

Atropine§
Cyclopentolate§
Epinephrine§
Homatropine§
Phenylephrine§
Scopolamine§
Tropicamide§

52:28 Mouthwashes and Gargles

Hydrogen Peroxide§

52:32 Vasoconstrictors

Epinephrine§
Naphazoline§
Oxymetazoline§
Phenylephrine§
Propylhexedrine§
Tetrahydrozoline§

52:40 Antiglaucoma Agents

52:40.04 α-Adrenergic Agonists

Brimonidine§

52:40.08 β-Adrenergic Blocking Agents

Betaxolol§
Levobunolol§
Timolol§

52:40.12 Carbonic Anhydrase Inhibitors

Carbonic Anhydrase Inhibitors General Statement§
Acetazolamide§
Brinzolamide§
Dorzolamide§
Methazolamide§
see also:
Dichlorphenamide 92:26

52:40.20 Miotics

Miotics General Statement§
Acetylcholine§
Carbachol§
Pilocarpine§

52:40.28 Prostaglandin Analogs

Bimatoprost§
Latanoprost§
Latanoprostene Bunod§
Tafluprost§
Travoprost§

52:40.32 Rho Kinase Inhibitors

Netarsudil§

52:40.92 Antiglaucoma Agents, Miscellaneous

see also:
Epinephrine 52:24

52:92 EENT Drugs, Miscellaneous

Aflibercept§
Apraclonidine§
Cenegermin-bkbj§
Cysteamine§
Ocriplasmin§
Pegaptanib§
Ranibizumab§
Verteporfin§

§ Omitted from the print version of *AHFS Drug Information*® because of space limitations. This monograph is available on the *AHFS Drug Information*® website, http://ahfsdruginformation.com. Username: ahfs2020; Password: ASHP94498.

* Please see the full *AHFS Pharmacologic-Therapeutic Classification*© on p. viii. Not all classes are used in the printed edition.

56:00 Gastrointestinal Drugs

56:04 Antacids and Adsorbents

Aluminum Carbonate, see Antacids
Aluminum Hydroxide, see Antacids
Aluminum Phosphate, see Antacids
Antacids *p. 2993*
Calcium Carbonate, see Antacids
Charcoal, Activated *p. 2997*
Dihydroxyaluminum Aminoacetate, see Antacids
Dihydroxyaluminum Sodium Carbonate, see Antacids
Magaldrate, see Antacids
Magnesium Carbonate, see Antacids
Magnesium Hydroxide, see Antacids
Magnesium Oxide, see Antacids
Magnesium Trisilicate, see Antacids
Sodium Bicarbonate, see Antacids

56:08 Antidiarrhea Agents

Bismuth Salts *p. 3000*
Crofelemer§
Diphenoxylate§
Lactobacillus Acidophilus§
Loperamide *p. 3002*
Opium Preparations§
Paregoric, see Opium Preparations
Telotristat Etiprate§

56:10 Antiflatulents

Simethicone§

56:12 Cathartics and Laxatives

Cathartics and Laxatives General Statement *p. 3005*
Anthraquinone Laxatives *p. 3010*
Bisacodyl *p. 3011*
Bulk-Forming Laxatives *p. 3012*
Casanthranol, see Anthraquinone Laxatives
Cascara Sagrada, see Anthraquinone Laxatives
Castor Oil§
Docusate Calcium, see Stool Softeners
Docusate Sodium, see Stool Softeners
Glycerin, see Hyperosmotic Laxatives
Hyperosmotic Laxatives *p. 3013*
Magnesium Citrate, see Saline Laxatives
Magnesium Hydroxide, see Saline Laxatives
Magnesium Sulfate (Epsom Salt), see Saline Laxatives
Malt Soup Extract, see Bulk-Forming Laxatives
Methylcellulose, see Bulk-Forming Laxatives
Mineral Oil§
Polyethylene glycol, see Hyperosmotic Laxatives
Psyllium, see Bulk-Forming Laxatives
Saline Laxatives *p. 3015*
Senna, see Anthraquinone Laxatives
Sennosides, see Anthraquinone Laxatives
Sodium Phosphates, see Saline Laxatives
Sorbitol, see Hyperosmotic Laxatives
Stool Softeners§

56:14 Cholelitholytic Agents

Chenodiol§
Ursodiol§

56:16 Digestants

Pancrelipase§

56:22 Antiemetics

56:22.08 Antihistamines

Dimenhydrinate *p. 3018*
Meclizine *p. 3019*
Prochlorperazine *p. 3019*
Trimethobenzamide§
see also:
Antihistamines 4:00

56:22.20 5-HT_3 Receptor Antagonists

Dolasetron§
Granisetron *p. 3021*
Ondansetron *p. 3022*
Palonosetron *p. 3025*
see also:
Netupitant and Palonosetron 56:22.32

56:22.32 Neurokinin-1 Receptor Antagonists

Aprepitant/Fosaprepitant *p. 3027*
Netupitant and Palonosetron *p. 3030*
Rolapitant§

56:22.92 Antiemetics, Miscellaneous

Diphenidol§
Dronabinol§
Nabilone§
see also:
Olanzapine 28:16.08.04
Phenothiazines 28:16.08.24
Promethazine 28:24.92
Scopolamine 12:08.08

56:28 Antiulcer Agents and Acid Suppressants

see also:
Amoxicillin 8:12.16.08
Antacids 56:04
Clarithromycin 8:12.12.92
Metronidazole 8:30.92
Tetracycline 8:12.24

56:28.12 Histamine H_2-Antagonists

Cimetidine§
Famotidine *p. 3033*
Nizatidine§
Ranitidine *p. 3040*

56:28.28 Prostaglandins

Misoprostol§

56:28.32 Protectants

Sucralfate§

56:28.36 Proton-pump Inhibitors

Dexlansoprazole *p. 3047*
Esomeprazole *p. 3050*
Lansoprazole *p. 3054*
Omeprazole *p. 3060*
Pantoprazole *p. 3070*
Rabeprazole *p. 3074*

56:32 Prokinetic Agents

Cisapride§
Metoclopramide *p. 3077*
Prucalopride *p. 3084*
Tegaserod§

56:36 Anti-inflammatory Agents

Alosetron§
Balsalazide *p. 3086*
Mesalamine *p. 3087*
Olsalazine§
see also:
Sulfasalazine 8:12.20

56:92 GI Drugs, Miscellaneous

Alvimopan *p. 3096*
Cholic Acid§
Eluxadoline *p. 3098*
Linaclotide *p. 3100*
Lubiprostone *p. 3102*
Methylnaltrexone *p. 3104*
Naldemedine *p. 3107*
Naloxegol *p. 3108*
Obeticholic Acid§
Orlistat§
Plecanatide *p. 3111*
Teduglutide§
Tenapanor§
Vedolizumab *p. 3112*
see also:
Adalimumab 92:36
Certolizumab 92:36
Golimumab 92:36
Infliximab 92:36
Octreotide 68:29.04
Ustekinumab 84:92

§ Omitted from the print version of *AHFS Drug Information*® because of space limitations. This monograph is available on the *AHFS Drug Information*® website, http://ahfsdruginformation.com. Username: ahfs2020; Password: ASHP94498.
Please see the full AHFS Pharmacologic-Therapeutic Classification© on p. viii. Not all classes are used in the printed edition.

GASTROINTESTINAL DRUGS 56:00

ANTACIDS AND ADSORBENTS 56:04

Antacids

■ Antacids are inorganic salts that dissolve in acid gastric secretions releasing anions that partially neutralize gastric hydrochloric acid.

Uses

Antacids are used as an adjunct to other drugs for the relief of peptic ulcer pain and to promote the healing of peptic ulcers. Antacids also are used for the relief of esophageal reflux, acid indigestion, heartburn, dyspepsia, and sour stomach; for the prevention of stress ulceration and GI bleeding; to reduce the risk associated with gastric aspiration; and for the management of hyperphosphatemia.

■ **Considerations in Choosing an Antacid** The choice of a specific antacid preparation depends on palatability, cost, adverse effects, acid neutralizing capacity, the sodium content of the antacid, and the patient's renal and cardiovascular function. Because of its high sodium content, sodium bicarbonate generally is used only for occasional heartburn or indigestion and not for chronic high-dose management of peptic ulcer disease. The role of calcium carbonate in the management of peptic ulcers is controversial because this antacid may cause acid rebound, which is especially important when the drug is administered at bedtime. Most clinicians believe that calcium carbonate should not be used in the management of peptic ulcers. However, some clinicians postulate that frequent administration of calcium carbonate may ameliorate acid rebound and reduce the clinical importance of gastric hypersecretion and believe that calcium carbonate is useful because it has a rapid onset of action, high acid neutralizing capacity, and a prolonged effect and is relatively inexpensive. Magnesium and/or aluminum antacids are the most commonly used and are often administered concurrently or in commercially available combinations to control the frequency and consistency of bowel movements. In any antacid combination product, each active antacid ingredient must contribute at least 25% of the in vitro acid neutralizing capacity. With administration of fixed combinations, ideal regulation of bowel function is seldom achieved, and patients should be taught to supplement their antacid therapy with appropriate doses of magnesium, calcium, or aluminum antacids to regulate bowel function.

Fixed combinations of antacids and histamine H_2-receptor antagonists can be used for relief of *occasional* symptoms of heartburn (pyrosis) associated with acid indigestion (hyperchlorhydria) and sour stomach, with the antacid providing intital rapid relief and the histamine H_2-receptor antagonist providing more prolonged relief.

Fixed combinations of antacids with nonantacid laxatives are rational only if the laxative is used to counteract the constipating effect of the antacid. Antacid combinations containing analgesics or simethicone should be administered only when concurrent symptoms require the effects of both an antacid and the nonantacid drug. However, fixed combinations of antacids and analgesics are not indicated for the management of peptic ulcers. Antacid combinations containing an anticholinergic, sedative-hypnotic, antiemetic, antipepsin, or proteolytic agents, bile, or bile salts are irrational, unsafe, and ineffective. Optimal use of antacids and anticholinergics or sedative-hypnotics requires that the dosage of each drug be adjusted by administering each drug separately. Bismuth salts and milk have no appreciable acid neutralizing activity.

■ **Peptic Ulcers** Few well-designed clinical studies are available demonstrating the efficacy or inefficacy of antacids in the healing of peptic ulcers or for the relief of peptic ulcer pain. However, most clinicians believe that based upon the ability of antacids to increase gastric pH these drugs are useful in the management of peptic ulcers. In one well-controlled 4-week trial in outpatients, placebo was compared with 1- and 3-hour postprandial and bedtime administration of a suspension containing magnesium and aluminum hydroxides and simethicone (about 144 mEq of acid neutralizing capacity per dose); the antacid regimen was more effective than placebo in healing duodenal ulcer craters (endoscopically proven), but the antacid was no more effective than placebo in relieving ulcer pain.

In another study in outpatients with gastric or duodenal ulcers, calcium carbonate (about 8.2 mEq of acid neutralizing capacity) in tablet form administered every hour while the patient was awake and as necessary for abdominal discomfort produced a greater incidence of radiologically confirmed healing and pain relief in patients with gastric ulcers but not in those with duodenal ulcers after 30 days as compared with placebo. In a third well-controlled 3-week trial in hospitalized gastric ulcer patients, placebo was compared to administration of 30 mL of a suspension containing magnesium and aluminum hydroxides and simethicone (acid neutralizing capacity not specified) every 2 hours while the patient was awake; gastric ulcer healing and pain relief were not different in antacid-treated and placebo-treated patients. In a 5-day clinical study, 15 mL of an antacid (30 mEq of acid neutralizing capacity per dose) was alternately administered every 30 minutes with placebo as needed to relieve duodenal ulcer pain; antacid was not different from placebo. In the same study, a single 30-mL dose of the antacid was not more effective than placebo in relieving duodenal ulcer pain.

In one well-controlled study, 4 weeks of oral therapy with 1.2 g of cimetidine daily was compared to that with 1- and 3-hour postprandial and bedtime administration of magnesium and aluminum hydroxides antacid suspension (about 123 mEq of acid neutralizing capacity per dose); cimetidine and antacid did not differ significantly (64 *vs* 52%) in healing of duodenal ulcer craters and erosions or pain relief. Well-controlled clinical studies are not available comparing the efficacy of anticholinergic agents to antacids in the management of peptic ulcers.

Current epidemiologic and clinical evidence supports a strong association between gastric infection with *Helicobacter pylori* and the pathogenesis of duodenal and gastric ulcers; long-term *H. pylori* infection also has been implicated as a risk factor for gastric cancer. For additional information on the association of this infection with these and other GI conditions, see Helicobacter pylori infection, under Uses, in Clarithromycin 8:12.12.92.

Conventional antiulcer therapy with antacids, H_2-receptor antagonists, proton-pump inhibitors, and/or sucralfate heals ulcers but generally is ineffective in eradicating *H. pylori*, and such therapy is associated with a high rate of ulcer recurrence (e.g., 60–100% per year). The American College of Gastroenterology (ACG), the National Institutes of Health (NIH), and most clinicians currently recommend that *all* patients with initial or recurrent duodenal or gastric ulcer and documented *H. pylori* infection receive anti-infective therapy for treatment of the infection. Although 3-drug regimens consisting of a bismuth salt (e.g., bismuth subsalicylate) and 2 anti-infective agents (e.g., tetracycline or amoxicillin plus metronidazole) administered for 10–14 days have been effective in eradicating the infection, resolving associated gastritis, healing peptic ulcer, and preventing ulcer recurrence in many patients with *H. pylori*-associated peptic ulcer disease, current evidence principally from studies in Europe suggests that 1 week of such therapy provides comparable *H. pylori* eradication rates. Other regimens that combine one or more anti-infective agents (e.g., clarithromycin, amoxicillin) with a bismuth salt and/or an antisecretory agent (e.g., omeprazole, lansoprazole, H_2-receptor antagonist) also have been used successfully for *H. pylori* eradication, and the choice of a particular regimen should be based on the rapidly evolving data on optimal therapy, including consideration of the patient's prior exposure to anti-infective agents, the local prevalence of resistance, patient compliance, and cost of therapy.

Current evidence suggests that inclusion of a proton-pump inhibitor (e.g., omeprazole, lansoprazole) in anti-*H. pylori* regimens containing 2 anti-infectives enhances effectiveness, and limited data suggest that such regimens retain good efficacy despite imidazole (e.g., metronidazole) resistance. Therefore, the ACG and many clinicians currently recommend 1 week of therapy with a proton-pump inhibitor and 2 anti-infective agents (usually clarithromycin and amoxicillin or metronidazole), or a 3-drug, bismuth-based regimen (e.g., bismuth-metronidazole-tetracycline) concomitantly with a proton-pump inhibitor, for treatment of *H. pylori* infection. For a more complete discussion of *H. pylori* infection, including details about the efficacy of various regimens and rationale for drug selection, see Helicobacter pylori Infection, under Uses, in Clarithromycin 8:12.12.92.

■ **Acid Indigestion** Although the efficacy of antacids for the relief of acid indigestion, heartburn, sour stomach, and pressure and/or bloating (commonly referred as gas), generally has not been established systematically by well-designed studies, most experts believe that, since these symptoms may be caused by gastric acid, antacids are probably useful.

■ **Gastroesophageal Reflux** Antacids also may be useful to increase gastric pH and to increase lower esophageal sphincter pressure in the management of esophageal reflux. The ACG states that antacids and antirefluxants such as alginic acid are more effective than placebo in relieving symptoms of heartburn induced by a meal, and are useful for *self-medication* as initial therapy for milder forms of gastroesophageal reflux disease (GERD). However, suppression of gastric acid secretion with a proton-pump inhibitor or histamine H_2- receptor antagonist to control symptoms and prevent complications of the disease is considered by the ACG to be the principal therapeutic goal in the management of GERD. Other measures such as avoidance of constrictive clothing, treatment of obesity, reducing meal size and dietary fat intake, avoidance of foods that increase reflux, avoiding recumbency after meals, and elevating the head of the bed should be initiated and continued throughout the course of treatment. For further information on the treatment of GERD, see Uses: Gastroesophageal Reflux, in Omeprazole 56:28.36.

■ **Upper GI Bleeding** Antacids may be effective in the prevention of stress ulceration and GI bleeding. In one randomized controlled study in critically ill patients, antacids administered prophylactically to maintain gastric pH above 3.5 decreased the incidence of acute GI bleeding.

■ **Gastric Aspirations** Antacids have been administered prophylactically as an adjunct to reduce the risk of gastric acid aspiration in patients undergoing cesarean section or emergency surgery.

■ **Hyperphosphatemia** The hypophosphatemic effect of aluminum-containing antacids (except aluminum phosphate) has been used in conjunction with a low phosphate diet in the management of calcinosis universalis, in hyperparathyroidism secondary to chronic hemodialysis, and to prevent recurrent phosphatic renal calculi. Since aluminum carbonate reportedly binds phosphate more than does aluminum hydroxide, aluminum carbonate is generally preferred.

■ **Calcium Replacement** For the use of calcium carbonate as replacement therapy, see Calcium Salts 40:12. For the use of magnesium preparations as laxatives, see the Cathartics and Laxatives General Statement 56:12. For the use of sodium bicarbonate as an alkalinizing agent, see Sodium Bicarbonate 40:08.

Dosage and Administration

Antacids are administered orally. The dose of antacids should be expressed in terms of mEq of acid neutralizing capacity. Dose and frequency of administration depend on the acid secretory rate of the stomach, gastric emptying time, and the disorder being treated. The duration of action of antacids is determined principally by gastric emptying time. In fasting subjects, antacids have a duration of action of 20–60 minutes. However, if the drugs are administered 1 hour after meals, acid neutralizing effects may persist up to 3 hours. Sodium bicarbonate generally has a shorter duration of action than other antacids. Antacids should be used for longer than 2-week periods only under the management of a physician and as part of a carefully planned therapeutic regimen.

There is considerable variation in in vivo acid neutralizing capacity of equal volumes of different antacids and antacid products. Since suspensions are more rapidly and effectively solubilized than powders or tablets, antacid suspensions have a greater ability to react with and neutralize gastric acid. Antacid suspensions have a smaller particle size than do tablets and drying of antacid suspensions to prepare powders and tablets causes substantial loss of ability to neutralize acid. In general, an antacid suspension is preferable to a tablet or powder; tablets should be reserved for chronic use in patients who refuse suspensions because they are inconvenient or unpalatable. Tablets should be thoroughly chewed before swallowing.

The US Food and Drug Administration (FDA) requires that antacids have a minimum in vitro acid neutralizing capacity of 5 mEq per dose and that antacid labeling contain the in vitro acid neutralizing capacity; however, this FDA in vitro test does not correlate with in vivo acid neutralizing capacity.

For peptic ulcer disease, dosages of antacids are empirical and various antacid dosages have been used. In patients with uncomplicated duodenal ulcers or gastric ulcers, an antacid is administered 1 and 3 hours postprandially and at bedtime. In patients with duodenal ulcers, antacids are usually given for 4–6 weeks, and in patients with gastric ulcers, antacids are administered until healing is complete. If symptoms of duodenal ulcer recur, some clinicians recommend that antacids be administered 1 and 3 hours postprandially and at bedtime for 1 week and, if pain is relieved, less frequently for an additional 1–2 weeks; these patients should consult their physicians if pain worsens or is not relieved after the first week of therapy. Additional doses of antacids may be administered to relieve ulcer pain which occurs between regularly scheduled doses.

For the acute management of moderate or severe esophageal reflux, an antacid suspension is administered every hour; if symptoms persist, antacids may be given every 30 minutes. For long-term therapy of esophageal reflux, antacids are administered 1 and 3 hours postprandially and at bedtime and whenever symptoms recur.

In the management of GI bleeding and stress ulceration, antacids are usually administered every hour and, for GI bleeding, the antacid dosage should be titrated to maintain the nasogastric aspirate above pH 3.5. For severe symptoms, antacid suspensions may be diluted with water or milk and given by continuous intragastric infusion.

To reduce the risk of anesthesia-induced gastric acid aspiration, an antacid suspension has been given 30 minutes before anesthesia.

In conjunction with dietary phosphate restriction in the management of hyperphosphatemia, 30–40 mL of aluminum hydroxide or aluminum carbonate suspension is administered 3 or 4 times daily.

Cautions

■ **Precautions and Contraindications** Most antacids contain sodium as an impurity, and antacid products must be labeled with their sodium content if they contain more than 0.2 mEq of sodium per dose. Sodium bicarbonate is contraindicated and use of other sodium-containing antacids should be restricted in patients on low-sodium diets and in those with congestive heart failure, renal failure, edema, or cirrhosis. Antacid products containing more than 25 mEq of potassium in the recommended daily dosage should be used cautiously in patients with renal disease and only under the supervision of a physician.

Since antacids may alter the absorption of certain concomitantly administered oral drugs, patients taking oral drugs should be advised to consult their physician or other health professional before taking concomitant antacids. (See Drug Interactions.)

The most common adverse effects associated with prolonged administration of antacids are constipation and diarrhea. Although fixed-combination antacid products are frequently administered to balance the laxative and cathartic effects of each, bowel function must often be regulated by administering supplemental doses of an antacid with constipating (i.e., aluminum salt) or laxative (i.e., magnesium salt) action.

Some commercially available antacids contain the dye tartrazine (FD&C yellow No. 5), which may cause allergic reactions including bronchial asthma in susceptible individuals. Although the incidence of tartrazine sensitivity is low, it frequently occurs in patients who are sensitive to aspirin. Individuals with phenylketonuria (i.e., homozygous genetic deficiency of phenylalanine hydroxylase) and other individuals who must restrict their intake of phenylalanine should be warned that some antacids may contain aspartame, which is metabolized in the GI tract to phenylalanine following oral administration.

Serious medication errors have been reported to the US Food and Drug Administration (FDA) in which consumers used Maalox® Total Relief (bismuth subsalicylate) when they intended to use traditional Maalox® liquid antacid products containing aluminum hydroxide, magnesium hydroxide, and simethicone (e.g., Maalox® Advanced Regular Strength, Maalox® Advanced Maximum Strength). Because of the potential for serious adverse effects associated with accidental use of bismuth subsalicylate (which is chemically related to aspirin), the manufacturer of Maalox® Total Relief initially agreed to change the trade name of the product to one that did not include "Maalox"; however, the manufacturer instead discontinued the bismuth subsalicylate preparation in the summer of 2010.

Aluminum Antacids The most frequent adverse effect of aluminum antacids is constipation. Decreased bowel motility, dehydration, or fluid restriction may predispose patients to intestinal obstruction. Hemorrhoids and fissures or fecal impaction may occur.

Long-term administration of aluminum antacids in patients with renal failure or chronic renal failure may result in hyperaluminemia since small amounts of aluminum are absorbed from the GI tract and excretion of aluminum is decreased in patients with renal failure. Absorbed aluminum becomes bound to serum proteins (e.g., albumin, transferrin) and therefore is not easily dialyzed; aluminum may then accumulate in bones, lungs, and nerve tissue. Aluminum accumulation in the CNS may be the cause of dialysis encephalopathy, while aluminum accumulation in the bones may result in or worsen dialysis osteomalacia. Dialysis dementia also may occur in patients with renal failure receiving long-term aluminum antacid therapy for hyperphosphatemia. Several cases of dialysis encephalopathy have been associated with increased aluminum concentrations in the dialysate water. Aluminum intoxication with severe osteomalacia and extensive aluminum deposition at the junction between calcified and noncalcified bone has been reported in several young children who were receiving large dosages of aluminum hydroxide for the management of hyperphosphatemia associated with azotemia; the children were not undergoing hemodialysis during aluminum hydroxide therapy.

Aluminum salts may cause phosphorus depletion which is generally negligible. However, with prolonged administration or large doses, hypophosphatemia may occur, especially in patients with inadequate dietary intake of phosphorus; hypercalciuria secondary to bone resorption and increased intestinal absorption of calcium results. This phosphorus depletion syndrome is characterized by anorexia, malaise, and muscle weakness, and prolonged aluminum antacid therapy may cause urinary calculi, osteomalacia, and osteoporosis. A low-phosphorus diet, diarrhea, excessive phosphorus losses from malabsorption, and restoration of renal function after a kidney transplant increase the likelihood of the syndrome. Serum phosphate concentrations should be monitored at monthly or bimonthly intervals in patients on maintenance hemodialysis who are receiving chronic aluminum antacid therapy.

Calcium Carbonate The major limiting factor to the chronic use of calcium carbonate is gastric hypersecretion and acid rebound. Increased gastric acid secretion begins within 2 hours after administration of the drug and has occurred following a single 500-mg dose of calcium carbonate. In one study in peptic ulcer patients receiving large doses of calcium carbonate (500 mg/kg daily), hypercalcemia occurred in 14% of patients within 3 days of initiating therapy. Calcium carbonate may cause the milk-alkali syndrome which is characterized by hypercalcemia, metabolic alkalosis and, rarely, renal insufficiency; hypercalcemia may cause nausea, vomiting, anorexia, weakness, headache, dizziness, and change in mental status. Patients with renal impairment or dehydration and electrolyte imbalance are predisposed to developing the milk-alkali syndrome. Hypercalcemia has also been reported in chronic hemodialysis patients receiving calcium carbonate. Serum calcium concentrations should be monitored weekly and whenever symptoms of hypercalcemia occur in patients receiving large doses of calcium carbonate. Calcium carbonate reportedly causes constipation. Belching and flatulence may occur. When dietary phosphate is low, hypophosphatemia may occur.

Magnesium Antacids Magnesium-containing antacids commonly cause a laxative effect and frequent administration of these antacids alone often cannot be tolerated; repeated doses cause diarrhea which may cause fluid and electrolyte imbalances. Chronic administration of magnesium trisilicate infrequently produces silica renal stones.

In patients with severe renal impairment, hypermagnesemia characterized by hypotension, nausea, vomiting, ECG changes, respiratory or mental depression, and coma has occurred after administration of magnesium-containing antacids. Magnesium-containing antacids should not be administered in patients with renal failure, and antacid products containing more than 50 mEq of magnesium in the recommended daily dosage should be used cautiously and only under the supervision of a physician who should monitor electrolytes in patients with renal disease.

Sodium Bicarbonate Gastric distension and flatulence may occur with sodium bicarbonate preparations. Sodium bicarbonate, when given in large doses or in patients with renal insufficiency, may cause metabolic alkalosis. Chronic administration of bicarbonate with milk or calcium may cause the milk-alkali syndrome which is characterized by hypercalcemia, renal insufficiency, metabolic alkalosis, nausea, vomiting, headache, mental confusion, and anorexia. During the acute phase of the milk-alkali syndrome, the condition is reversible when the calcium and alkali are withdrawn. However, in patients with chronic milk-alkali syndrome, reduced renal function may persist even after calcium and alkali are discontinued. Patients with a salt-losing nephropathy have an increased risk of developing the milk-alkali syndrome.

The maximum daily dosage of sodium or bicarbonate is 200 mEq in patients younger than 60 years of age and 100 mEq in patients older than 60 years of age. Sodium bicarbonate is contraindicated for prolonged therapy because it may cause metabolic alkalosis or sodium overload.

Drug Interactions

All antacids potentially may increase or decrease the rate and/or extent of absorption of concomitantly administered oral drugs by changing GI transit time or by binding or chelating the drug. In vitro studies indicate that magnesium hydroxide or trisilicate has the greatest potential for drug binding and aluminum hydroxide and calcium carbonate are intermediate. Antacid-induced increases in GI pH may affect the disintegration, dissolution, solubility, or ionization of enteric-coated preparations and weakly acidic or basic drugs.

Simultaneous administration of aluminum-, calcium-, or magnesium-containing antacids with orally administered tetracyclines reduces the absorption of the tetracycline, probably because of chelation of these antacids by the tetracycline. Therefore, doses of tetracyclines should be spaced 1–2 hours from doses of antacids.

Concurrent administration of antacids and orally administered digoxin, indomethacin, or iron salts may decrease the absorption of these drugs. Doses of these drugs should be spaced as far apart as possible from doses of antacids. Concurrent administration of isoniazid and aluminum hydroxide gel may decrease the absorption of isoniazid; therefore, isoniazid should be administered at least 1 hour before aluminum-containing antacids. Absorption of buffered or enteric-coated aspirin is increased by simultaneous administration of antacids. Antacid-induced changes in urine pH increase urinary excretion and decrease blood concentrations of salicylates. Concurrent administration of dicumarol and an aluminum and magnesium hydroxides preparation reportedly increases the absorption of dicumarol; patients receiving antacids and oral anticoagulants should probably use warfarin rather than dicumarol. Concurrent administration of aluminum hydroxide and pseudoephedrine or diazepam increases the rate of absorption of the latter drugs. Administration of a magnesium and aluminum hydroxide preparation with chlordiazepoxide decreases the rate of chlordiazepoxide absorption. Administration of sodium bicarbonate with naproxen increases the rate of naproxen absorption, while concurrent administration of magnesium oxide or aluminum hydroxide with naproxen decreases the rate of naproxen absorption.

Antacid-induced increases in urine pH may decrease excretion of weakly basic drugs and increase excretion of weakly acidic drugs. Urinary excretion of amphetamines and quinidine are markedly decreased in patients whose urine is alkalinized with sodium bicarbonate and patients receiving these drugs concomitantly may have increased amphetamine or quinidine effects.

Pharmacology

The clinical use of antacids is based on their ability to increase the pH of gastric secretions. With usual doses, antacids generally do not increase and maintain gastric pH above 4–5. Although antacids do not neutralize all gastric acid, increasing gastric pH from 1.3 to 2.3 neutralizes 90% and increasing pH to 3.3 neutralizes 99% of gastric acid. Consequently, the amount of gastric acid back-diffusing through the gastric mucosa and the amount of acid reaching the duodenum is decreased. It is not known how much or for how long neutralization is required for optimal healing of peptic ulcers, but most clinicians believe that gastric pH should be maintained at about 3–3.5 for as many of the 24 hours as is possible. Antacids, in decreasing order of their ability to neutralize a given amount of acid, are calcium carbonate, sodium bicarbonate, magnesium salts, and aluminum salts. Magnesium hydroxide and aluminum hydroxide are the most potent magnesium and aluminum salts. Magnesium oxide has essentially the same acid neutralizing effect as magnesium hydroxide. Because magnesium trisilicate is slowly solubilized, it is a less effective buffer than magnesium hydroxide, carbonate, or phosphate.

Sodium bicarbonate rapidly reacts with hydrochloric acid to form sodium chloride, carbon dioxide, and water; excess bicarbonate that does not neutralize gastric acid rapidly empties into the small intestine and is absorbed. When sodium bicarbonate is given orally, gastric acid is neutralized by exogenous bicarbonate instead of intestinal bicarbonate. The net effect of administering sodium bicarbonate whether it reacts with gastric acid or reaches the small intestine is that all of a dose reaches the extracellular fluid. Mild metabolic alkalosis occurs; in patients with normal renal function, the kidneys excrete the excess sodium and bicarbonate ions and the urine becomes alkaline.

Antacids other than sodium bicarbonate neutralize gastric secretions but generally do not cause metabolic alkalosis, because the cation formed in the stomach is minimally absorbed and regains a basic anion in the small intestine. However, to the extent that the cation is absorbed and does not react with intestinal bicarbonate, the extracellular fluid receives a bicarbonate load; urinary pH is usually increased.

Calcium carbonate is slowly solubilized in the stomach and reacts with hydrochloric acid to form calcium chloride, carbon dioxide, and water. About 90% of the calcium chloride formed is converted to insoluble calcium salts (mainly calcium carbonate and to a lesser extent calcium phosphate) and calcium soaps in the small intestine and is not absorbed. When calcium carbonate is administered orally, a limited amount of calcium and intestinal bicarbonate are absorbed and hypercalcemia may occur. In some patients, metabolic alkalosis and the milk-alkali syndrome may occur. Calcium is excreted by the kidneys and hypercalciuria frequently occurs in patients receiving calcium carbonate.

Aluminum hydroxide or oxide is slowly solubilized in the stomach and reacts with hydrochloric acid to form aluminum chloride and water. In addition to forming aluminum chloride, dihydroxyaluminum sodium carbonate and aluminum carbonate form carbon dioxide, and aluminum phosphate forms phosphoric acid. About 17–30% of the aluminum chloride formed is absorbed and is rapidly excreted by the kidneys in patients with normal renal function. In the small intestine, aluminum chloride is rapidly converted to insoluble, poorly absorbed basic aluminum salts which are probably a mixture of hydrated aluminum oxide, oxyaluminum hydroxide, various basic aluminum carbonates, and aluminum soaps. Aluminum-containing antacids (except aluminum phosphate) also combine with dietary phosphate in the intestine forming insoluble, nonabsorbable aluminum phosphate which is excreted in the feces. If phosphate intake is limited in patients with normal renal function, aluminum antacids (except aluminum phosphate) decrease phosphate absorption and hypophosphatemia and hypophosphaturia occur; calcium absorption is increased. In vitro studies indicate that aluminum hydroxide binds bile salts with an affinity and capacity similar to that of cholestyramine; aluminum phosphate binds bile salts, but to a much lesser degree than does aluminum hydroxide.

Magnesium hydroxide rapidly reacts with hydrochloric acid to form magnesium chloride and water. In addition, magnesium carbonate forms carbon dioxide. Magnesium trisilicate is slowly solubilized and reacts with hydrochloric acid to form magnesium chloride, silicon dioxide, and water. About 15–30% of the magnesium chloride formed is absorbed and is rapidly excreted by the kidneys in patients with normal renal function. Any magnesium hydroxide that is not converted to magnesium chloride in the stomach is presumably subsequently changed in the small intestine to soluble but poorly absorbed salts. Magnesium hydroxide binds bile salts in vitro, but to a much lesser extent than does aluminum hydroxide. Magnesium-containing antacids have a laxative action. (See Saline Laxatives 56:12.)

Antacid-induced increases in gastric pH inhibit the proteolytic action of pepsin, an effect which is particularly important in patients with peptic ulcer disease. The optimum pH for pepsin activity is 1.5–2.5 and progressive inhibition occurs as gastric pH increases; above pH 4, the proteolytic activity of pepsin is minimal. Although some investigators have reported that aluminum- or calcium-containing antacids adsorb pepsin and thus have direct antipepsin effects, one study in which pH was controlled indicates that the antipepsin effects of antacids are due entirely to increased pH. Antacids do not coat the lining of peptic ulcers or the GI mucosa. Although some antacids, such as aluminum hydroxide, have astringent and demulcent actions, these effects are probably not important in the treatment of peptic ulcers.

In patients with peptic ulcers, antacids increase serum gastrin concentrations probably by increasing gastric pH. Single dose studies indicate that calcium carbonate causes gastric acid hypersecretion and acid rebound probably as a result of a local effect of calcium on gastrin-producing cells. Other antacids also increase secretion of gastric acid but do not cause acid rebound after the antacid has left the stomach. Aluminum-containing antacids delay gastric emptying time, an effect that is related to the concentration of aluminum in the stomach.

Chemistry and Stability

■ **Chemistry** Antacids are inorganic salts that dissolve in acid gastric secretions releasing anions that partially neutralize gastric hydrochloric acid.

Aluminum Antacids **Aluminum Carbonate.** Dried basic aluminum carbonate gel occurs as a white powder and is insoluble in water and in alcohol. Aluminum carbonate suspension is a white, creamy, thixotropic gel and contains the equivalent of 4.9–5.3% aluminum oxide and not less than 2.4% carbon dioxide.

Aluminum Hydroxide Dried aluminum hydroxide gel occurs as a white, odorless, tasteless, amorphous powder and is insoluble in water and in alcohol. The powder contains 50–57.5% aluminum oxide as the hydrated oxide and may contain varying amounts of aluminum carbonate and bicarbonate. Tablets of dried aluminum hydroxide gel contain 62–72% of the labeled amount of aluminum hydroxide as aluminum oxide. Aluminum hydroxide gel is a white, viscous suspension. The suspension contains the equivalent of 3.6–4.4% w/w aluminum oxide in the form of aluminum hydroxide and hydrated oxide. The suspension also may contain basic aluminum carbonate and bicarbonate, flavoring agents, sweeteners and antimicrobial agents. Aluminum hydroxide gel suspension should not be frozen.

Aluminum Phosphate Aluminum phosphate gel is a white, viscous suspension. The suspension contains 4–5% w/w aluminum phosphate and may contain preservatives.

Dihydroxyaluminum Aminoacetate Dihydroxyaluminum aminoacetate occurs as a white, odorless powder that has a faintly sweet taste and is insoluble in water. The powder contains 35.5–38.5% aluminum oxide calculated on a dried basis and may contain small amounts of aluminum oxide or aminoacetic acid.

Calcium Carbonate Precipitated calcium carbonate occurs as a fine, white, odorless, tasteless, microcrystalline powder and is practically insoluble in water and insoluble in alcohol.

Magnesium Antacids **Magnesium Carbonate.** Magnesium carbonate occurs as light, white, friable masses (heavy magnesium carbonate) or as a bulky, white powder (light magnesium carbonate). The drug is odorless and is practically insoluble in water and insoluble in alcohol. Magnesium carbonate contains the equivalent of 40–43.5% magnesium oxide.

Magnesium Hydroxide Magnesium hydroxide occurs as a bulky, white powder which is practically insoluble in water and in alcohol. Milk of Magnesia, Double-strength Milk of Magnesia, and Triple-strength Milk of Magnesia are suspensions containing 80, 160, and 240 mg of magnesium hydroxide per mL, respectively. Milk of Magnesia USP occurs as a white, opaque, more or less viscous suspension.

Magnesium Oxide Magnesium oxide occurs as a very bulky, white, powder (light magnesium oxide) or as a relatively dense, white powder (heavy magnesium oxide). Magnesium oxide is practically insoluble in water and insoluble in alcohol. Light magnesium oxide suspends more readily in liquids than does heavy magnesium oxide.

Magnesium Trisilicate Magnesium trisilicate, a compound of magnesium oxide and silicon dioxide, occurs as a fine, white, odorless, tasteless powder free from grittiness. The powder is insoluble in water and in alcohol. The powder contains not less than 20% magnesium oxide and not less than 45% silicon dioxide.

Miscellaneous Antacids **Dihydroxyaluminum Sodium Carbonate.** Dihydroxyaluminum sodium carbonate is a single molecule that reportedly combines the antacid properties of aluminum hydroxide and sodium bicarbonate. Dihydroxyaluminum sodium carbonate occurs as a fine, white, odorless powder that is slightly hygroscopic at room temperature. The powder is practically insoluble in water and contains the equivalent of 34.8–38.2% aluminum oxide.

Sodium Bicarbonate Sodium bicarbonate occurs as a white, crystalline powder with a saline and slightly alkaline taste. The drug is soluble in water and insoluble in alcohol. Aqueous solutions of sodium bicarbonate, when freshly prepared, are alkaline to litmus; alkalinity increases as the solutions stand, are agitated, or are heated.

Magaldrate Magaldrate, a chemical combination of aluminum and magnesium hydroxides and sulfate, occurs as a white, odorless, crystalline powder and is insoluble in water and in alcohol. The powder contains the equivalent of 34–46% magnesium oxide, the equivalent of 21–30% aluminum oxide, and 13.3–17.5% sulfur trioxide, calculated on the dried basis. Each gram of magaldrate in the oral suspension and tablets contains the equivalent of 340–460 mg of magnesium oxide and 210–300 mg of aluminum oxide.

■ **Stability** *Aluminum Antacids* **Aluminum Hydroxide.** Aluminum hydroxide gel suspension should not be frozen. On standing, small amounts of clear liquid may separate from aluminum hydroxide gel suspension.

Aluminum Phosphate On standing, small amounts of water may separate from aluminum phosphate gel suspension.

Magnesium Antacids **Magnesium Hydroxide.** Milk of Magnesia USP should preferably be stored at less than 35°C; however, freezing should be avoided. On standing, varying proportions of water usually separate from Milk of Magnesia USP suspension.

Magnesium Oxide Magnesium oxide readily absorbs water and carbon dioxide when exposed to air and, in the presence of a limited amount of water, forms a cement-like mass. In water, magnesium oxide is converted to magnesium hydroxide.

Preparations

Excipients in commercially available drug preparations may have clinically important effects in some individuals; consult specific product labeling for details.

Aluminum Carbonate, Basic

Oral		
Capsules	equivalent to dried aluminum hydroxide gel 608 mg or aluminum hydroxide 500 mg	**Basaljel®**, Wyeth
Tablets	equivalent to dried aluminum hydroxide gel 608 mg or aluminum hydroxide 500 mg	**Basaljel®** (scored), Wyeth

Aluminum Hydroxide

Oral		
Capsules	475 mg	**Alu-Cap®**, 3M
Suspension	320 mg/5 mL*	**Aluminum Hydroxide Suspension**
		Amphojel®, Wyeth
	600 mg/5 mL	**ALternaGEL®**, J&J-Merck
Tablets	300 mg	**Amphojel®**, Wyeth
Tablets, film-coated	600 mg	**Alu-Tab®**, 3M

*available from one or more manufacturer, distributor, and/or repackager by generic (nonproprietary) name

Calcium Carbonate, Precipitated (Precipitated Chalk)

Powder*		
Oral		
Pieces, chewing gum	500 mg	**Chooz®**, Insight
Suspension	400 mg/5 mL	**Mylanta® Children's Upset Stomach Relief**, J&J-Merck
	1.25 g/5 mL*	**Calcium Carbonate Suspension**
Tablets	1.25 g*	**Calcium Carbonate Tablets** (scored)
Tablets, chewable	400 mg	**Mylanta® Children's Upset Stomach Relief**, J&J-Merck
	420 mg	**Titralac® Regular**, 3M
	500 mg	**Tums® Antacid/Calcium Supplement**, GlaxoSmithKline
	650 mg*	**Calcium Carbonate Chewable Tablets**
	750 mg	**Titralac® Extra Strength**, 3M
		Tums® E-X Antacid/Calcium Supplement, GlaxoSmithKline
	850 mg	**Alka-Mints®**, Bayer
	1 g	**Tums® Ultra Antacid/Calcium Supplement**, GlaxoSmithKline
Tablets, chewable, rapidly disintegrating	600 mg	**Maalox® Quick Dissolve® Chewables**, Novartis
	1 g	**Maalox® Quick Dissolve® Chewables Maximum Strength**, Novartis

*available from one or more manufacturer, distributor, and/or repackager by generic (nonproprietary) name

Dihydroxyaluminum Sodium Carbonate

Powder*

*available from one or more manufacturer, distributor, and/or repackager by generic (nonproprietary) name

Magaldrate (Aluminum Magnesium Hydroxide)

Oral		
Suspension	540 mg/5 mL	**Lowsium®**, Rugby

Magaldrate Combinations

Oral		
Suspension	540 mg/5 mL with Simethicone 40 mg/5 mL	**Lowsium® Plus**, Rugby
		Riopan Plus®, Wyeth
	1080 mg/5 mL with Simethicone 40 mg/5mL	**Riopan Plus® Double Strength**, Wyeth

Magnesium Carbonate

Powder*

*available from one or more manufacturer, distributor, and/or repackager by generic (nonproprietary) name

Magnesium Hydroxide

Powder*		
Oral		
Suspension	400 mg/5 mL*	**Milk of Magnesia**
		Phillips'® Milk of Magnesia, Bayer
	800 mg/5 mL	**Phillips'® Milk of Magnesia Concentrate**, Bayer
	1.2 g/5 mL*	**Milk of Magnesia Concentrate**, Roxane
Tablets	300 mg*	**Phillips'® Milk of Magnesia**, Bayer

*available from one or more manufacturer, distributor, and/or repackager by generic (nonproprietary) name

Magnesium Oxide

Powder*		
Oral		
Capsules	140 mg	**Uro-Mag®**, Blaine
Tablets	400 mg*	**Magnesium Oxide Tablets**
		Mag-Ox® 400, Blaine
	420 mg*	**Magnesium Oxide Tablets**

*available from one or more manufacturer, distributor, and/or repackager by generic (nonproprietary) name

Magnesium Trisilicate

Powder*

*available from one or more manufacturer, distributor, and/or repackager by generic (nonproprietary) name

Sodium Bicarbonate (Baking Soda)

Powder*

Oral		
For solution	0.78 g/3.9 g	**Citrocarbonate® Granules,** Lee
Tablets	325 mg*	**Sodium Bicarbonate Tablets**
	650 mg*	**Sodium Bicarbonate Tablets**

*available from one or more manufacturer, distributor, and/or repackager by generic (nonproprietary) name

Aluminum Hydroxide and Magnesium Carbonate

Oral		
Suspension	Aluminum Hydroxide 31.7 mg/5 mL and Magnesium Carbonate 119.3 mg/5 mL	**Gaviscon® Liquid,** GlaxoSmithKline
		Genaton® Liquid, Teva
	Aluminum Hydroxide 254 mg/ 5 mL and Magnesium Carbonate 237.5 mg/5 mL	**Gaviscon® Extra Strength,** GlaxoSmithKline
Tablets, chewable	Aluminum Hydroxide 160 mg and Magnesium Carbonate 105 mg	**Gaviscon® Extra Strength,** GlaxoSmithKline

Aluminum Hydroxide and Magnesium Hydroxide

Oral		
Suspension	Aluminum Hydroxide 200 mg/ 5 mL and Magnesium Hydroxide 200 mg/5 mL	**Mag-Al®,** Pharmaceutical Associates
	Aluminum Hydroxide 225 mg/ 5 mL and Magnesium Hydroxide 200 mg/5 mL	**Alamag®,** Teva, URL
		Maalox®, Novartis
		Rulox®, Rugby
	Aluminum Hydroxide 600 mg/ 5 mL and Magnesium Hydroxide 300 mg/5 mL	**Maalox® TC,** Novartis
Tablets, chewable	Aluminum Hydroxide 200 mg and Magnesium Hydroxide 200 mg	**Rulox® #1,** Rugby

Aluminum Hydroxide and Magnesium Hydroxide Combinations

Oral		
Suspension	Aluminum Hydroxide 200 mg/ 5 mL, Magnesium Hydroxide 200 mg/5 mL, and Simethicone 20 mg/5 mL	**Almacone®,** Rugby
		Di-Gel®, Schering-Plough
		Maalox Advanced Regular Strength®, Novartis
		Mag-Al® Plus, Pharmaceutical Associates
		Mygel®, Sandoz
		Mylanta® Fast-Acting, J&J-Merck
	Aluminum Hydroxide 225 mg/ 5 mL, Magnesium Hydroxide 200 mg/5 mL, and Simethicone 25 mg/5 mL	**Alamag® Plus,** Teva
	Aluminum Hydroxide 400 mg/ 5 mL, Magnesium Hydroxide 400 mg/5 mL, and Simethicone 40 mg/5 mL	**Almacone® II Hi-Potency,** Rugby
		Antacid Double Strength®, Teva
		Maalox Advanced Maximum Strength®, Novartis
		Mag-Al® XS, Pharmaceutical Associates
		Mygel® II, Sandoz
		Mylanta® Fast-Acting Double Strength, J&J-Merck
	Aluminum Hydroxide 500 mg/ 5 mL, Magnesium Hydroxide 450 mg/5 mL, and Simethicone 40 mg/5 mL	**Kudrox®,** Schwarz
		Maalox® Antacid/Anti-Gas Maximum Strength, Novartis
Tablets, chewable	Aluminum Hydroxide 200 mg, Magnesium Hydroxide 200 mg, and Simethicone 20 mg	**Almacone®,** Rugby
	Aluminum Hydroxide 200 mg, Magnesium Hydroxide 200 mg, and Simethicone 25 mg	**Tempo®,** Blairex

Aluminum Hydroxide and Magnesium Trisilicate

Oral		
Tablets, chewable	Aluminum Hydroxide 80 mg and Magnesium Trisilicate 20 mg	**Gaviscon®,** GlaxoSmithKline
		Genaton®, Teva

Calcium Carbonate and Magnesium Carbonate

Oral		
Suspension	Calcium Carbonate 520 mg/5 mL and Magnesium Carbonate 400 mg/5 mL	**Marblen®,** Fleming

Calcium Carbonate and Magnesium Hydroxide

Oral		
Suspension	Calcium Carbonate 400 mg/5 mL and Magnesium Hydroxide 135 mg/5 mL	**Mylanta® Supreme Fast Acting,** J&J-Merck
Tablets	Calcium Carbonate 550 mg and Magnesium Hydroxide 125 mg	**Mylanta® Gelcaps®,** J&J-Merck
Tablets, chewable	Calcium Carbonate 350 mg and Magnesium Hydroxide 150 mg	**Mylanta® Fast-Acting,** J&J-Merck
	Calcium Carbonate 500 mg and Magnesium Hydroxide 110 mg	**Rolaids® Antacid,** Pfizer
	Calcium Carbonate 700 mg and Magnesium Hydroxide 300 mg	**Mylanta® Fast-Acting Maximum Strength,** J&J-Merck

Calcium Carbonate and Magnesium Hydroxide Combinations

Oral		
Tablets	Calcium Carbonate 280 mg, Magnesium Hydroxide 128 mg, and Simethicone 20 mg	**Di-Gel®,** Schering-Plough
Tablets, chewable	Calicum Carbonate 800 mg, Magnesium Hydroxide 165 mg, and Famotidine 10 mg	**Pepcid® Complete,** J&J-Merck

Other Calcium Carbonate Combinations

Oral		
Tablets	420 mg with Simethicone 21 mg	**Titralac® Plus,** 3M
Tablets, chewable, rapidly disintegrating	1 g with Simethicone 60 mg	**Maalox® Max® Quick Dissolve Chewables Antacid/Antigas Maximum Strength,** Novartis

Potassium Bicarbonate and Sodium Bicarbonate

Oral		
Tablets, for solution	Potassium Bicarbonate 312 mg and Sodium Bicarbonate 958 mg	**Alka-Seltzer® Gold Effervescent Antacid,** Bayer

Charcoal, Activated

Activated Carbon, Active Carbon, Adsorbent Charcoal, Decolorizing Carbon, Medicinal Charcoal

■ Activated charcoal, which is used clinically as an adsorbent and antidote based on its adsorptive property, is the residue from the destructive distillation of various organic materials that has been treated to increase its adsorptive power.

Uses

■ **Poisonings** Activated charcoal is an adsorbent used in the treatment (i.e., GI decontamination) of most oral poisonings except those caused by corrosive agents (e.g., strong acids or alkalis) or substances for which its absorptive capacity is too low to be clinically useful (e.g., iron salts, lithium, boric acid, arsenic, malathion, or organic solvents such as methanol, ethanol, or ethylene glycol). Randomized, controlled studies demonstrating the efficacy of GI decontamination measures, including activated charcoal, in reducing morbidity and mortality associated with most oral poisonings generally are lacking, and an expert panel of the American Academy of Clinical Toxicology and European Association of Poisons Centres and Clinical Toxicologists (AACT/EAPCCT) states that activated charcoal should not be administered *routinely* in the management of poisoned patients. However, since beneficial effects of activated charcoal have not been ruled out and the risks of a single dose of activated charcoal appear to be low, many clinicians currently consider single-dose activated charcoal the sole intervention needed for the immediate treatment of most oral poisonings. Activated charcoal is the most commonly used agent for GI decontamination in poisoned patients; however, use of activated charcoal has declined from 7.7% of all exposures reported to US poison control centers in 1995 to 5.6% of such exposures in 2004. Although the American Academy of Pediatrics (AAP) and other experts no longer recommend the routine use of ipecac syrup for out-of-hospital management of poisonings (see Uses: Acute Poisoning, in Ipecac Syrup 56:20), they state that current evidence does not support the routine administration of activated charcoal in the home as an alternative since safety and efficacy have not been established.

A few comparative studies in healthy individuals have shown that early GI decontamination with activated charcoal decreases absorption of ingested substances as well as or better than either induction of emesis or gastric lavage, and the combination of gastric emptying or ipecac plus activated charcoal generally does not appear to be more effective than activated charcoal alone. In addition, available data do not support the routine use of cathartics in combination with activated charcoal to remove the toxin/charcoal complex. Specialized references and experts should be consulted for additional information about the use of activated charcoal in the management of poisoning caused by specific agents.

Studies in healthy individuals suggest that activated charcoal may be beneficial if it is administered early (e.g., within 30–60 minutes of ingestion) in the management of acute poisoning and that the effectiveness of activated charcoal decreases over time. Therefore, the AACT/EAPCCT state that administration of activated charcoal may be considered up to 1 hour after ingestion of a potentially toxic amount of a poison known to be adsorbed by activated charcoal. AACT/EAPCCT also state that, although results of studies in healthy individuals suggest that the reduction in drug absorption achieved when activated charcoal is administered more than 1 hour after poison ingestion is of questionable clinical importance, the potential for benefit from use of activated charcoal more than 1 hour after ingestion cannot be excluded. Some clinicians suggest that administration of activated charcoal more than 1 hour following acute poisoning may be appropriate because of the difficulty in obtaining accurate histories regarding the time of ingestion of the toxic agent from pediatric or obtunded patients or suicidal individuals. Late administration of activated charcoal may be beneficial if the ingested substance undergoes enterohepatic circulation and reabsorption because of charcoal's ability to promote efflux of selected drugs (e.g., theophylline, phenobarbital, carbamazepine) from the blood into the bowel lumen. Some clinicians state that activated charcoal also may be of some benefit when given several hours after ingestion of extended-release drugs or drugs that slow gastric emptying, although others have suggested that charcoal may not be effective in reducing absorption of extended-release preparations because of their prolonged dissolution.

Although activated charcoal adsorbs some aliphatic hydrocarbons (e.g., gasoline, kerosene), its use is not recommended to treat ingestion of these substances (unless they also contain toxic additives) since they rarely produce toxicity other than that associated with aspiration. Activated charcoal is unlikely to enhance elimination of agents that are rapidly absorbed (e.g., strychnine, cyanides).Although a quantity of potassium cyanide (1.75–2.1 g) equivalent to several potentially lethal (e.g., 200 mg) doses may be adsorbed by a 50- to 60-g dose of activated charcoal, the adsorbent will not be useful in many ingestions of simple cyanide salts because of the rapid onset of life-threatening cyanide toxicity.

While multiple-dose administration of activated charcoal is unlikely to be an important measure for most intoxications, repeated doses of activated charcoal may enhance the elimination of some drugs even after systemic absorption (e.g., theophylline) by interrupting enterohepatic circulation or reducing reabsorption of drugs that diffuse or are excreted into the intestines. In animal studies, multiple doses of charcoal increased the total body clearance of acetaminophen, digoxin, phenobarbital, phenytoin, and theophylline. The use of multiple doses of activated charcoal may be considered for drugs that undergo enterohepatic or enteroenteric circulation, those with a small volume of distribution, those that are not extensively protein bound, and those with a low endogenous clearance. Multiple-dose activated charcoal also may be considered if a life-threatening amount of phenobarbital, carbamazepine, quinine, dapsone, theophylline, paraquat, or *Amanita phalloides* is ingested; such treatment may obviate the need for more invasive interventions (e.g., extracorporeal techniques). Multiple-dose activated charcoal does not enhance the elimination of cyclic antidepressants, and its efficacy in the treatment of intoxication with digoxin, digitoxin, phenytoin, sodium valproate, meprobamate, dapsone, carbamazepine, or cyclosporine has not been fully elucidated.

The "universal antidote" (2 parts activated charcoal, 1 part magnesium oxide, and 1 part tannic acid) is inferior to activated charcoal alone, and the tannic acid component is potentially hepatotoxic. Thus, there is no justification for the use of the "universal antidote."

■ **Hemoperfusion** Hemoperfusion through columns of activated charcoal is used to remove endogenous or exogenous toxins and has been performed in patients with uremia, hepatic failure, or acute toxicity caused by acetaminophen, barbiturates, glutethimide, methaqualone, methyprylon, or theophylline. Hemoperfusion through activated charcoal has been associated with substantial damage to formed blood elements including platelets, leukocytes, and erythrocytes (e.g., platelet aggregation, thrombocytopenia) and has been associated with the formation of free charcoal particle emboli. These hazards have been minimized by coating the activated charcoal with a biocompatible polymer such as poly (hydroxyethylmethacrylate).

■ **GI Disorders** Activated charcoal has been used to adsorb intestinal gases in the treatment of flatulence, intestinal distension, and dyspepsia; however, the US Food and Drug Administration (FDA) has classified activated charcoal as lacking substantial evidence of efficacy as an antiflatulent or digestive aid. Activated charcoal has been used alone or in combination with kaolin in the management of diarrhea but its value has not been established.

■ **Wounds and Ulcers** Activated charcoal also has been used topically in wound or ulcer dressings to decrease odor and promote healing.

■ **Other Uses** Activated charcoal has been used in the management of erythropoietic porphyria† (to interrupt the enterohepatic recycling of protoporphyrin and lower plasma porphyrin concentrations) and for symptomatic relief of pruritis in patients with renal failure†.

Dosage and Administration

■ **Administration** Activated charcoal is administered orally or via nasogastric or orogastric tube. Activated charcoal powder can be administered as an extemporaneously prepared aqueous slurry or suspension and is commercially available as a suspension.

Activated charcoal is most effective when administered early in the management of acute poisoning, preferably within 30–60 minutes of ingestion of the poison, although some benefit is possible with later administration in patients with gastric concretions or those who have ingested extended-release drugs or drugs that delay gastric emptying. Continuous instillation of activated charcoal slurry into the duodenum via a small nasogastric tube may improve the retention of activated charcoal when an ingested agent produces protracted vomiting (e.g., theophylline). Tablets or granules of activated charcoal are less effective than the powdered form of the drug and should not be used in the treatment of poisonings.

Many clinicians previously recommended that vomiting be induced with ipecac syrup before activated charcoal was administered. However, because administration of ipecac syrup may delay the administration of activated charcoal and there is little evidence to demonstrate improved outcome with its use, most clinicians no longer recommend routine use of ipecac syrup in the emergency department or hospital setting. However, under rare circumstances, use of ipecac syrup in the home setting may be appropriate if not contraindicated and if recommended by a poison control center or other qualified clinician. (See Uses: Acute Poisoning, in Ipecac Syrup 56:20.) Although activated charcoal does not appear to diminish the emetic effects of ipecac syrup when given 10 minutes following the ipecac dose, vomiting should be completed before administration of activated charcoal. (See Drug Interactions: Ipecac Syrup.)

For extemporaneous preparation, activated charcoal powder should be mixed with sufficient tap water (e.g., 20–30 g in at least 240 mL) to form a slurry. Some clinicians state that more concentrated slurries generally should be avoided to minimize the risk of airway obstruction if aspiration occurs, to aid in dispersion of the charcoal, and possibly to increase palatability. Sorbitol may reduce the gritty sensation and improve the palatability of activated charcoal, and acts as a hyperosmotic laxative that may help prevent constipation associated with the drug. Therefore, sorbitol has been used in the extemporaneous preparation of activated charcoal suspensions and is found in some commercial preparations. However, sorbitol should be administered only with single-dose activated charcoal or with the first dose of a multiple-dose regimen of the drug, and no more than 1 or 2 doses of sorbitol or another cathartic (if required) should be used in a 24-hour period because of the potential for dehydration, hypotension, and electrolyte disturbances (e.g., hypernatremia) associated with excessive catharsis. Sorbitol-containing preparations of activated charcoal should be used with caution in children and geriatric patients; hydration and electrolytes should be monitored with such use. Also, if sorbitol is used with an initial dose of activated charcoal, a second cathartic generally should not be administered. Sorbitol content may vary between commercially available preparations of activated charcoal, and the label should be consulted to determine the amount of sorbitol contained in such products.

The palatability of the activated charcoal slurry also can be improved by the addition of a thickening agent such as bentonite or carboxymethylcellulose. Some evidence suggests that a small amount of a flavoring agent such as concentrated fruit juice or chocolate syrup may be added without substantially interfering with the adsorptive capacity of activated charcoal. However, some clinicians state that flavoring agents have been shown to decrease the adsorptive capacity of activated charcoal and generally should not be used. If chocolate syrup is used for flavoring, it should be added just prior to administration since the sweetness and flavor reportedly disappear after a few minutes of contact with activated charcoal. Milk, ice cream, or sherbet should not be used as a vehicle for the administration of activated charcoal since the adsorptive capacity of activated charcoal was substantially decreased when ice cream (or sherbet) was mixed with activated charcoal in a 2.5:1 ratio by weight.

■ **Dosage** ***Poisonings*** If possible, individuals attempting to manage an acute poisoning in a medically unsupervised setting (e.g., at home) should attempt to contact a poison control center, emergency medical facility, or other qualified health professional. If such help cannot be obtained quickly, the directions on the container of activated charcoal should be followed. Because activated charcoal can adsorb ipecac syrup, individuals attempting to manage an acute poisoning in a medically unsupervised setting should not administer activated charcoal to a patient who has received ipecac syrup until after the patient has vomited unless otherwise directed by a health professional.

Adults and Adolescents. The optimum dose of activated charcoal for the treatment of poisoning in adults and adolescents has not been established. For *single-dose* treatment, a dose of 25–100 g (e.g., 50 g) of activated charcoal, given as a slurry in water, has been recommended in adults or adolescents 13 years of age or older. Some clinicians suggest a dose of 50–100 g in adults and state that a large dose (i.e., 1 g/kg) is required to promote adsorption and prevent desorption of the ingested substance, although others state that desorption of toxins from charcoal does not appear to be clinically important. Other clinicians state that a dose of 0.5–1 g /kg usually is appropriate, but that doses of 1.5–2 g/kg may be desirable for treatment of massive ingestions of highly toxic substances that are known to be well adsorbed by activated charcoal (e.g., aspirin, theophylline, extended-release verapamil) or when substantial clinical benefit may be provided by adsorption of a limited amount of a lethal substance (e.g., cyanide). Activated charcoal doses of up to 120 g reportedly have been well tolerated.

The usual dosage of activated charcoal for *multiple-dose* treatment in adults or adolescents 13 years of age or older is 50–100 g initially, followed by not less than 12.5 g every hour; alternatively, 25 g every 2 hours or 50 g every 4 hours may be given. Some clinicians recommend that 150–200 g of activated charcoal be administered in divided doses via a nasogastric tube over 4–8 hours in severely poisoned adults; the total dose administered may be more important than the frequency of administration. Other clinicians suggest a dosage of 0.5–1 g/kg administered every 4–6 hours for lower-risk ingestions and larger individual doses for more serious ingestions (e.g., administration of the highest dosage tolerated by the patient [e.g., 1–1.5 g/kg per hour] for life-threatening acute poisoning with extended-release theophylline). Higher dosages may be better tolerated by some patients when administered via continuous nasogastric infusion or when divided into smaller amounts and given more frequently. An antiemetic often is required to successfully administer high dosages of activated charcoal; however, because some antiemetics (e.g., phenothiazines) may decrease GI motility and lower the seizure threshold, use of a type 3 serotonin (5-HT_3) receptor antagonist (e.g., ondansetron) or metoclopramide may be preferred. Multiple-dose therapy with activated charcoal generally should be continued until the patient recovers or until major symptoms of toxicity resolve.

Pediatric Dosage. The optimum dose of activated charcoal in the treatment of poisoning in pediatric patients has not been established. Some clinicians state that optimal adsorption appears to occur at a charcoal-to-toxin ratio of 10 to 1 or higher but that a fixed dose of 1 g/kg generally is recommended in children. A dose of 25–50 g or 0.5–1 g/kg of body weight given as a slurry in water has been recommended for children 1–12 years of age. Infants up to 1 year of age may receive 10–25 g or 0.5–1 g/kg. Other clinicians suggest a dose of 15–30 g of activated charcoal in children with substantial overdoses of toxic substances when less than 1 hour has elapsed since ingestion. In children who have not swallowed the dose of activated charcoal within 20 minutes following ingestion of the toxic agent, some clinicians recommend that activated charcoal be administered through a nasogastric tube by personnel trained in the identification and treatment of complications of this procedure.

The usual dosage of activated charcoal used in *multiple-dose* therapy in children up to 13 years of age is 10–25 g initially, followed by 1–2 g/kg every 2–4 hours. An expert panel of the American Academy of Clinical Toxicology and European Association of Poisons Centres and Clinical Toxicologists (AACT/EAPCCT) states that doses of 10–25 g may be used in children younger than 5 years of age because of their smaller gut lumen capacity and the usually smaller overdoses in these individuals. Multiple-dose therapy with activated charcoal generally should be continued until the patient recovers or until major symptoms of toxicity resolve. An IV antiemetic may be necessary to minimize the risk of vomiting during administration of multiple doses of charcoal even when given by nasogastric tube.

GI Disorders In the management of GI disturbances such as flatulence or dyspepsia, activated charcoal has been administered in single doses of 0.6–5 g or in a dosage of 0.975–3.9 g 3 times daily after meals.

Cautions

Activated charcoal is generally well tolerated when given orally, particularly as a single-dose treatment. However, potential risks associated with administration of the drug include vomiting, pulmonary aspiration (fatalities have been reported), and intestinal obstruction (with multiple-dose administration).

■ **GI Effects** Adverse GI effects associated with the use of activated charcoal include vomiting, constipation, diarrhea, and GI obstruction or fecal impaction in dehydrated patients; constipation and intestinal obstruction have not been reported to occur with single-dose administration of activated charcoal. GI obstruction or pseudo-obstruction has been reported rarely with multiple-dose administration, generally when doses were administered at 3- to 6-hour intervals for 36–120 hours. At least one patient developed a rectal ulcer with massive hemorrhage following multiple-dose activated charcoal administration.

Vomiting reportedly occurs in about 7–20% of patients following administration of activated charcoal. Although some data suggest that vomiting occurs more frequently when activated charcoal is administered with sorbitol, other data suggest that sorbitol content does not substantially increase the risk for vomiting but rather that risk is increased in children with prior episodes of vomiting and in those receiving activated charcoal via nasogastric or orogastric tube administration.

Activated charcoal may produce black stools.

■ **Pulmonary Effects** Aspiration of activated charcoal has occurred rarely, and has resulted in granulomatous reactions, bronchiolitis obliterans, tissue reaction to suspension agents (sorbitol, povidone), and increased lung permeability. In one study of patients following acute overdosage, aspiration of activated charcoal occurred in about 2% of patients receiving activated charcoal alone and about 2% of those undergoing gastric emptying followed by activated charcoal. In rare cases, activated charcoal has been inadvertently introduced into the lung by a misplaced nasogastric tube. Death resulting from aspiration of activated charcoal has been reported rarely.

■ **Ocular Effects** Transient corneal abrasions have occurred when activated charcoal came in direct contact with the eye during administration.

■ **Precautions and Contraindications** Activated charcoal is not effective in adsorbing all drugs and toxic substances and its administration should not preclude other measures used in the emergency treatment of poisoning. In addition to a lack of evidence documenting the beneficial effects of activated charcoal following ingestion of corrosives or petroleum distillates, activated charcoal should not be used in the management of ingestion of these agents since vomiting may occur following its administration and charcoal may obscure endoscopic evaluation of gastroesophageal lesions. Activated charcoal only moderately adsorbs petroleum distillates (e.g., gasoline, kerosene), and the ingestion of these substances rarely result in toxicity other than that associated with aspiration (unless they also contain toxic additives). Although activated charcoal alone is not usually associated with an increased risk of aspiration, its administration may cause vomiting (e.g., because of concomitant water load and/or co-administration of sorbitol as a vehicle) and increase the potential for aspiration of gastric contents. Measures should be taken to reduce the risk of aspiration (e.g., placement of a cuffed endotracheal tube in patients with impaired laryngeal reflexes) since aspiration of activated charcoal may lead to more severe complications than aspiration of gastric contents alone. (See Cautions: Pulmonary Effects.) Sorbitol or other cathartics should not be administered with *each* dose of activated charcoal because of the potential for dehydration, hypotension and electrolyte disturbances (e.g., hypernatremia) associated with excessive catharsis.

Generally, activated charcoal should not be used when there is decreased peristalsis (i.e., reduced or absent bowel sounds); risk of GI obstruction, perforation or hemorrhage; recent surgery; electrolyte imbalance; or volume depletion. Activated charcoal is contraindicated prior to endoscopy, following ingestion of corrosive agents unless it is necessary to adsorb another ingested toxin. Administration of activated charcoal is contraindicated in patients with an unprotected airway, a GI tract that is not anatomically intact, and in poisonings in which the risk or severity of aspiration may be increased (e.g., hydrocarbon ingestions with a high aspiration potential). In addition, multiple-dose activated charcoal is contraindicated in the presence of ileus or bowel obstruction.

Drug Interactions

In general, activated charcoal can decrease the absorption of and therapeutic response to other orally administered drugs. Medications other than those used for GI decontamination or antidotes for ingested toxins should not be taken orally within 2 hours of administration of activated charcoal; if necessary, concomitant drug therapy can be given parenterally.

■ **Acetylcysteine** Acetylcysteine may be administered orally concomitantly with activated charcoal without impairment of its efficacy. Although acetylcysteine is adsorbed by activated charcoal in vitro, studies in humans indicate that efficacy of orally administered acetylcysteine is not substantially affected by the administration of activated charcoal. Alternatively, IV administration of acetylcysteine obviates concerns about interactions between activated charcoal and orally administered acetylcysteine.

■ **Ipecac Syrup** The adsorptive efficacy of activated charcoal may be decreased by the emesis induced by ipecac syrup; if both are to be used in the management of oral poisoning, activated charcoal should be administered after vomiting has ceased. The emetic properties of ipecac are apparently not substantially affected by the administration of activated charcoal. In some studies of healthy individuals, the emetic effects of ipecac syrup were not decreased when activated charcoal was administered within 10 minutes following administration of ipecac syrup, but prior to emesis. However, activated charcoal has been reported to adsorb ipecac alkaloids, and concurrent administration of activated charcoal and ipecac syrup is inconsistent with current practice. (See Dosage and Administration: Administration.)

■ **Polyethylene Glycol and Electrolyte Solutions** The adsorptive capacity of activated charcoal may be decreased by concurrent use of polyethylene glycol and iso-osmolar electrolyte solution (PEG-ELS) for whole-bowel irrigation.

Pharmacology

The clinical use of activated charcoal is based on its adsorptive property. Activated charcoal is an effective, nonspecific adsorbent of a wide variety of drugs and chemicals and thus inhibits GI absorption of these agents. Activated charcoal has a broader spectrum of adsorptive activity than other adsorbents, including attapulgite, Arizona montmorillonite, or evaporated milk. Results of animal and limited human studies indicate that some of the adsorbed chemicals may be released from the charcoal in the GI tract, but this effect is not usually of clinical importance. The effectiveness of activated charcoal in the lower GI tract is questionable, since passage through the upper GI tract generally saturates the adsorptive capacity of the drug.

Activated charcoal also adsorbs enzymes, vitamins, amino acids, minerals, and other nutrients from the GI tract; however, this effect is of no importance when the drug is used in the management of acute poisoning.

Activated charcoal does not adequately adsorb alcohols (e.g., ethanol, methanol), ethylene glycol, iron salts, lithium, strong acids and alkalis, corrosive agents, boric acid, arsenic, malathion, or organic solvents for clinical use in GI decontamination with these ingestants.Although potassium cyanide equivalent to several potentially lethal doses may be adsorbed by 50–60 g of activated charcoal, the rapid onset of life-threatening cyanide toxicity limits the usefulness of the adsorbent in many ingestions of simple cyanide salts. Burnt toast is not a form of activated charcoal and is not a useful antidote in the management of acute poisoning.

Pharmacokinetics

Activated charcoal is neither absorbed in the GI tract nor metabolized, and it is excreted in feces. Since it colors the feces black, activated charcoal can be used as a fecal marker.

Chemistry and Stability

■ **Chemistry** Activated charcoal is the residue from the destructive distillation of various organic materials which has been treated to increase its adsorptive power. Activated charcoal occurs as a fine, black, odorless, tasteless powder and is free from gritty matter. To be an effective adsorbent, the particle size of activated charcoal must be small (thus increasing the total surface area) and the mineral content should be low. For medicinal purposes, only the "activated" grade of charcoal should be used, since it is specifically treated to increase its total surface area and adsorptive capacity. Although commercial varieties of activated charcoal may vary in adsorptive capacity, 1 g of the drug must adsorb at least 100 mg of strychnine sulfate from 50 mL of water to meet the USP standard.

Activated charcoal is insoluble in water and in alcohol.

■ **Stability** Activated charcoal should be stored in well-closed glass or metal containers.

Preparations

Excipients in commercially available drug preparations may have clinically important effects in some individuals; consult specific product labeling for details.

Activated Charcoal

Powder*		
Extracorporeal		
Hemoperfusion System	150 g	**Adsorba® 150 C Pediatric,** Gambro
	300 g	**Adsorba® 300 C,** Gambro
Oral		
Capsules	260 mg*	**Charcoal Activated Capsules**
		CharcoCaps®, Requa
For suspension	15 g	**CharcoAid® G,** Little Remedies
Pellets	25 g	**EZ-Char®,** Paddock
Suspension	0.625 g/5 mL (15 or 25 g)	**Actidose-Aqua®,** Paddock
	1 g/5 mL (15, 25, or 50 g)	**Actidose-Aqua®,** Paddock
		Actidose® with Sorbitol, Paddock
		Insta-Char® Adult, Kerr
		Insta-Char® Pediatric, Kerr
		Liqui-Char®, Monarch
Tablets, delayed-release (enteric-coated core)	250 mg	**Charcoal Plus DS®,** Kramer

*available from one or more manufacturer, distributor, and/or repackager by generic (nonproprietary) name

Activated Charcoal Combinations

Oral		
Tablets, delayed-release (enteric-coated core)	250 mg with Simethicone 80 mg	**Flatulex®,** Dayton
	250 mg with Simethicone 125 mg	**Flatulex® Maximum Strength,** Dayton

†Use is not currently included in the labeling approved by the US Food and Drug Administration

ANTIDIARRHEA AGENTS 56:08

Bismuth Salts

Pink Bismuth

■ Bismuth subsalicylate is an antidiarrheal agent and antidyspepsia agent; bismuth subgallate is an internal deodorant.

Bismuth subcitrate potassium and bismuth subsalicylate are antiulcer agents (used as part of multiple-drug regimens for *Helicobacter pylori* infection).

Uses

■ **Diarrhea** Bismuth subsalicylate is used as *self-medication* in children and adults for symptomatic control of acute nonspecific diarrhea and travelers' diarrhea.

Bismuth subsalicylate has been used in adults for prevention of travelers' diarrhea†; however, the drug is less effective than anti-infective agents.

■ **Helicobacter pylori Infection and Duodenal Ulcer Disease** Bismuth subsalicylate or bismuth subcitrate potassium is used for treatment of *Helicobacter pylori* infection and duodenal ulcer disease (active disease or history of duodenal ulcer); eradication of *H. pylori* has been shown to reduce the risk of duodenal ulcer recurrence.

Bismuth subsalicylate or bismuth subcitrate potassium is used in multiple-drug regimens that also include metronidazole, tetracycline hydrochloride, and a histamine H_2-receptor antagonist or proton-pump inhibitor (quadruple therapy); such drug combinations are recommended by the American College of Gastroenterology (ACG) as a first-line treatment option for eradication of *H. pylori* infection. ACG recommends consideration of such quadruple-drug regimens in penicillin-allergic patients and those who have previously received a macrolide antibiotic. If the initial 14-day regimen does not eradicate *H. pylori*, retreat with a multiple-drug regimen that does not include metronidazole to avoid possible development of metronidazole resistance.

Multiple-drug regimens including bismuth subsalicylate, metronidazole, tetracycline hydrochloride, and a proton-pump inhibitor (instead of a histamine H_2-receptor antagonist) may be more effective against metronidazole-resistant strains of *H. pylori*; such regimens are recommended by ACG as an acceptable treatment option for persistent *H. pylori* infection ("salvage" treatment).

The fixed combination containing bismuth subcitrate potassium, metronidazole, and tetracycline hydrochloride (Pylera®) is used in conjunction with omeprazole for the treatment of *H. pylori* infection and duodenal ulcer disease (active ulcer or history of duodenal ulcer within past 5 years).

■ **Flatulence or Stool Odor** Bismuth subgallate is used as *self-medication* in children and adults for the reduction of flatulence or stool odor from a colostomy or ileostomy.

Bismuth subgallate has been used as *self-medication* for the reduction of odor from fecal incontinence†, irritable bowel syndrome†, or bariatric surgery†.

Bismuth subgallate is *not* expected to be effective for the reduction of odor from faulty personal hygiene†.

■ **Dyspepsia (Upset Stomach)** Bismuth subsalicylate is used as *self-medication* in children and adults for the symptomatic relief of dyspepsia (e.g., upset stomach, nausea, heartburn, fullness, belching, gas) secondary to over-indulgence in food and drink.

The effectiveness of bismuth salts in the treatment of nonulcer dyspepsia† is uncertain. The drugs are not recommended as first-line therapy because of the potential risk of neurotoxicity with long-term use; they may be useful as second-line agents.

Dosage and Administration

■ **Administration** ***Oral Administration*** **Capsules.** Bismuth subgallate: Administer orally up to 4 times daily with meals. Swallow the capsule whole.

Bismuth subcitrate potassium in fixed combination with metronidazole and tetracycline hydrochloride (Pylera®): Administer orally 4 times daily after meals and at bedtime; give omeprazole concomitantly as part of the regimen. (See Fixed Combination Containing Bismuth Subcitrate Potassium, Metronidazole, and Tetracycline Hydrochloride [Pylera®] under Dosage: Helicobacter pylori Infection and Duodenal Ulcer Disease, in Dosage and Administration.) Swallow the capsule whole. Administer with a full glass (240 mL) of water, particularly with bedtime doses, to reduce the risk of esophageal irritation and ulceration by the tetracycline hydrochloride component. If a dose of Pylera® is missed, take the next dose at the regularly scheduled time; do not double the dose. Contact a clinician if more than 4 doses are missed.

Suspension. Bismuth subsalicylate: Shake the suspension well prior to administration. Use the dose cup provided by the manufacturer for accurate dosing. For Diotame®, twist off the lid and dispense the appropriate dose by squeezing the tube.

Chewable Tablets. Bismuth subgallate: Administer orally up to 4 times daily with meals. Chew or swallow whole.

Bismuth subsalicylate: Chew or dissolve in the mouth and swallow.

Bismuth subsalicylate (with metronidazole and tetracycline hydrochloride in the Helidac® Therapy kit): Administer each component orally 4 times daily with meals and at bedtime. Chew and swallow the bismuth subsalicylate tablets. Administer the tetracycline hydrochloride and metronidazole components with a full glass (240 mL) of water, particularly with bedtime doses, to reduce the risk of esophageal irritation and ulceration by the tetracycline hydrochloride component. If a dose of Helidac® Therapy is missed, take the next dose at the regularly scheduled time; do not double the dose. If more than 4 doses are missed, contact a clinician.

Conventional Tablets. Bismuth subsalicylate (e.g., Pepto-Bismol® Easy-to-Swallow Caplets): Swallow with water; do not chew.

■ **Dosage** Bismuth salts are available as bismuth subgallate, bismuth subcitrate potassium, and bismuth subsalicylate; dosages are expressed in terms of the salts.

Bismuth subcitrate potassium is available in fixed combination with metronidazole and tetracycline hydrochloride (Pylera®); dosage of Pylera® is expressed as number of capsules.

Acute Nonspecific Diarrhea and Travelers' Diarrhea **Bismuth Subsalicylate.** Adults and children 12 years of age or older: 525 mg every 30–60 minutes or 1.05 g every hour as needed, not to exceed 4.2 g in a 24-hour period. Use until diarrhea stops, but not for more than 2 days. Alternatively, administer 1.05 g every 30 minutes† to every hour as needed, not to exceed 4.2 g in a 24-hour period. *Self-medication* should not exceed 2 days.

Prevention of Travelers' Diarrhea **Bismuth Subsalicylate.** Adults: For prevention of travelers' diarrhea†, 525 mg 4 times daily has been recommended.

Helicobacter pylori Infection and Duodenal Ulcer Disease **Bismuth Subsalicylate, Metronidazole, and Tetracycline Hydrochloride Regimen.** Adults: Administer 525 mg of bismuth subsalicylate in conjunction with metronidazole (250 mg) and tetracycline hydrochloride (500 mg) 4 times daily for 10–14 days; give concomitantly with ranitidine (150 mg) twice daily or the usual dosage of a proton-pump inhibitor once or twice daily.

Salvage therapy for persistent *H. pylori* infection: Administer for 7–14 days.

Bismuth Subsalicylate (with Metronidazole and Tetracycline Hydrochloride) in Helidac® Therapy Kit. Adults: Administer 525 mg of bismuth subsalicylate in conjunction with metronidazole (250 mg) and tetracycline hydrochloride (500 mg) 4 times daily (at meals and at bedtime) for 14 days; give concomitantly with usual dosage of H_2-receptor antagonist.

Fixed Combination Containing Bismuth Subcitrate Potassium, Metronidazole, and Tetracycline Hydrochloride (Pylera®). Adults: Administer 3 capsules 4 times daily (after meals and at bedtime) for 10 days; give concomitantly with omeprazole 20 mg twice daily (after morning and evening meal) for 10 days.

Flatulence or Stool Odor **Bismuth Subgallate.** Adults and children 12 years of age or older: Administer 200–400 mg up to 4 times daily.

Dyspepsia (Upset Stomach) **Bismuth Subsalicylate.** Adults and children 12 years of age or older: Administer 525 mg every 30–60 minutes as needed, not to exceed 4.2 g in a 24-hour period. Do not use for more than 2 days. Alternatively, administer 1.05 g every 30–60 minutes† as needed, not to exceed 4.2 g in a 24-hour period. *Self-medication* should not exceed 2 days.

■ **Special Populations** No special population dosage recommendations at this time. (See Cautions: Geriatric Use and also see Cautions: Renal Impairment.)

Cautions

■ **Contraindications** Helidac® Therapy (kit containing bismuth subsalicylate, metronidazole, tetracycline hydrochloride) is contraindicated in pregnant or nursing women, pediatric patients, patients with hepatic or renal impairment, patients with known allergy to aspirin or salicylates, and those with known hypersensitivity to any component of the kit.

Pylera® (fixed-combination capsule containing bismuth subcitrate potassium, metronidazole, tetracycline hydrochloride) is contraindicated in pregnant or nursing women, pediatric patients, patients with hepatic or renal impairment, and those with known hypersensitivity to any ingredient in the capsule.

■ **Warnings/Precautions** ***Warnings*** **GI Disorders.** Bismuth subsalicylate should not be used for *self-medication* in patients with an ulcer, bleeding disorder, or bloody or black stools.

Reye's Syndrome. A risk of Reye's syndrome exists with bismuth subsalicylate in children or adolescents who have or are recovering from varicella or influenza-like symptoms. (See Pediatric Use under Warnings/Precautions: Specific Populations, in Cautions.)

Neurotoxicity. Neurotoxicity associated with excessive doses of bismuth salts has been reported rarely; this effect is reversible following discontinuance of the drug.

Discoloration of Tongue and/or Stool. A transient and harmless darkening of the tongue and/or black stool is possible with bismuth treatment; do not confuse stool darkening with melena.

Lead Content. Bismuth mined from the ground, and commercially available Pepto-Bismol® preparations, may contain small amounts of naturally occurring lead. Amounts of lead in Pepto-Bismol® preparations are low compared with average daily lead exposure. Pepto-Bismol® preparations are *not* intended for chronic use.

Sensitivity Reactions **Hypersensitivity.** Bismuth subsalicylate contains salicylate; do not use in patients allergic to salicylates (including aspirin).

General Precautions **Selection and Use of Anti-infectives in H. pylori Regimens.** To reduce the development of drug-resistant bacteria and maintain effectiveness of Helidac® Therapy, Pylera®, and other anti-infective agents, use only for the treatment or prevention of infections proven or strongly suspected to be caused by susceptible bacteria.

When selecting or modifying anti-infective therapy, use results of culture and in vitro susceptibility testing. In the absence of such data, consider local epidemiology and susceptibility patterns when selecting anti-infectives for empiric therapy.

Phenylketonuria. Diotame® chewable tablets contain aspartame (Nutra-Sweet®), which is metabolized in the GI tract to phenylalanine following oral administration.

Medication Errors. Serious medication errors have been reported to the US Food and Drug Administration (FDA) in which consumers used Maalox® Total Relief (bismuth subsalicylate) when they intended to use traditional Maalox® liquid antacid products containing aluminum hydroxide, magnesium hydroxide, and simethicone (e.g., Maalox® Advanced Regular Strength, Maalox® Advanced Maximum Strength). Because of the potential for serious adverse effects associated with accidental use of bismuth subsalicylate (which is chemically related to aspirin), the manufacturer of Maalox® Total Relief initially agreed to change the trade name of the product to one that did not include "Maalox"; however, the manufacturer instead discontinued the bismuth subsalicylate preparation in the summer of 2010.

Use of Fixed Combinations or Multiple-Drug Kits. When the fixed-combination preparation containing bismuth subcitrate potassium, metronidazole, and tetracycline hydrochloride (Pylera®) or the kit containing bismuth subsalicylate, metronidazole, and tetracycline hydrochloride (Helidac® Therapy) is used for the treatment of *H. pylori* infection and duodenal ulcer disease, the cautions, precautions, and contraindications associated with metronidazole and tetracycline hydrochloride must be considered in addition to those associated with bismuth subcitrate potassium or bismuth subsalicylate.

Laboratory Test Interferences Bismuth absorbs x-rays; may interfere with radiographic diagnostic procedures of the GI tract.

Darkening of stool from bismuth salts does not interfere with any tests for occult blood.

Specific Populations **Pregnancy.** Bismuth subsalicylate: Category C (Category D in third trimester). (See Users Guide.)

Helidac® Therapy, Pylera®: Category D. (See Users Guide.)

Helidac® Therapy, Pylera®: Effect on labor and delivery unknown.

Lactation. Bismuth subsalicylate: Use with caution.

Helidac® Therapy, Pylera®: Discontinue nursing or the drug.

Pediatric Use. Do *not* use bismuth subsalicylate in children or adolescents who have or are recovering from varicella or influenza-like symptoms. Changes in behavior accompanied by nausea and vomiting in children or adolescents taking the drug may be an early sign of Reye's syndrome.

Safety and efficacy of the commercially available Helidac® Therapy kit or the fixed-combination preparation Pylera® in pediatric patients infected with *H. pylori* have not been established. Pylera® or the Helidac® Therapy kit should not be used in children younger than 8 years of age. (See Contraindications under Cautions.)

Geriatric Use. There is insufficient experience in patients 65 years of age or older to determine whether they respond differently than younger adults to the commercially available Helidac® Therapy kit or the fixed-combination preparation Pylera® for treatment of *H. pylori* infection and duodenal ulcer disease.

Consider age-related decreases in hepatic, renal, and/or cardiac function and concomitant disease and drug therapy.

Hepatic Impairment. Accumulation of bismuth salts may occur in patients with severe hepatic disease, presumably because of biliary excretion of bismuth from the body. The commercially available Helidac® Therapy kit and the fixed-combination preparation Pylera® are contraindicated in patients with hepatic impairment. (See Cautions: Contraindications.)

Renal Impairment. Use bismuth subsalicylate with caution, if at all, in patients with renal impairment. The commercially available Helidac® Therapy kit and the fixed-combination preparation Pylera® are contraindicated in patients with renal impairment. (See Contraindications under Cautions.)

■ **Common Adverse Effects** Bismuth: Transient and harmless darkening of the tongue and/or black stools, decreased peristalsis (with bismuth subgallate).

Helidac® Therapy: Nausea, diarrhea, abdominal pain, melena, upper respiratory infection.

Pylera®: Stool abnormality, diarrhea, dyspepsia, abdominal pain, nausea, headache, flu syndrome, taste perversion, asthenia, vaginitis, dizziness.

Drug Interactions

■ **Anticoagulants** Salicylate salts (e.g., bismuth subsalicylate) may increase the risk of bleeding with concomitant anticoagulant therapy. Monitor anticoagulant therapy and adjust anticoagulant dosage as needed.

■ **Antidiabetic Agents** Possibly enhanced hypoglycemic effects with concomitant salicylate salt therapy. Use with caution.

■ **Aspirin** Use with caution.

■ **Ciprofloxacin** Bismuth subsalicylate slightly decreases peak plasma concentrations and area under the concentration-time curve (AUC) of ciprofloxacin. This effect is not considered clinically important.

■ **Doxycycline** Bismuth subsalicylate may decrease absorption of doxycycline. Avoid using bismuth subsalicylate for *self-medication* in travelers taking doxycycline for malaria prophylaxis.

■ **Methotrexate** Avoid using bismuth subsalicylate for *self-medication* concomitantly with methotrexate.

■ **Omeprazole** Omeprazole increases the extent of absorption of bismuth from Pylera® capsules following concomitant administration.

■ **Probenecid** Use concomitantly with caution, if at all.

■ **Salicylates** Do not use bismuth subsalicylate for *self-medication* concomitantly with other salicylate drugs.

■ **Sulfinpyrazone** Use concomitantly with caution.

■ **Tetracycline** Bismuth and/or calcium carbonate (excipient of bismuth subsalicylate tablets) reduces systemic absorption of tetracycline; the clinical importance is unknown since relative contribution of systemic versus local antimicrobial activity against *H. pylori* has not been determined.

Description

Bismuth subsalicylate may protect gastric mucosa, bind to ulcer base and mucosa, bind bile acids, and decrease endogenous prostaglandin and bicarbonate secretion.

Bismuth subsalicylate reduces number of bowel movements, aids in firming stool, normalizes fluid movement via antisecretory mechanisms, binds bacterial toxins, and exhibits antimicrobial activity in patients with diarrhea.

Mechanism of antibacterial action of bismuth salts not fully elucidated.

Bismuth salts may exert bactericidal action by complexing in bacterial wall and periplasmic space, inhibiting urease, catalase and lipase/phospholipase, ATP synthesis, and *H. pylori* adherence.

Multiple-drug regimen of bismuth subsalicylate, metronidazole, and tetracycline hydrochloride and the fixed-combination preparation containing bismuth subcitrate potassium, metronidazole, and tetracycline hydrochloride (Pylera®) active against most strains of *H. pylori* in vitro and in clinical infections.

Bismuth subgallate may reduce number of odor-producing anaerobic intestinal microbes and/or directly interact with sulfur-containing compounds; reduces flatulence odor but not flatulence itself.

Each 262.4-mg tablet of bismuth subsalicylate contains an amount of salicylate comparable to that in approximately 130 mg of aspirin.

Advice to Patients

Importance of advising patients of the cautions, precautions, and contraindications associated with metronidazole and tetracycline hydrochloride when using Helidac® Therapy or Pylera®.

Importance of informing patient that temporary and harmless darkening of the tongue and/or black stool may occur with bismuth salts, and that stool darkening should not be confused with blood in the stool.

Do not use bismuth subsalicylate for *self-medication* in presence of peptic ulcers, bleeding disorders, bloody or black stool, known allergy to salicylates (including aspirin), or if taking other salicylates; consult clinician before use if diarrhea is accompanied by fever, mucus in stools, or if patient is on a sodium-restricted diet or currently taking drugs for anticoagulation, diabetes, gout, or arthritis.

Importance of instructing patients to discontinue bismuth subsalicylate for *self-medication* and inform clinician if symptoms worsen, ringing in the ears or loss of hearing occurs, or if diarrhea or other symptoms do not improve after 2 days of therapy.

Importance of advising patients *not* to use bismuth subsalicylate in children or adolescents who have or are recovering from chickenpox or flu-like symptoms. Importance of informing clinician if changes in behavior accompanied by nausea and vomiting occur while using bismuth subsalicylate, because these symptoms may be an early sign of Reye's syndrome.

Importance of adequate hydration (with clear fluids) to help prevent dehydration caused by diarrhea.

Importance of informing patients with phenylketonuria that Diotame® chewable tablets contain aspartame.

Importance of instructing patients about correct administration of Helidac® Therapy or Pylera® capsules, including administration of each dose after meals and at bedtime and with a full glass of water (particularly at bedtime to reduce risk of esophageal irritation and ulceration), swallowing Pylera® capsules whole, chewing and swallowing bismuth subsalicylate tablets, and about duration of therapy.

Importance of informing patients that Helidac® Therapy contains salicylates, and to contact a clinician if ringing in the ears occurs with concomitant aspirin therapy.

Importance of advising patient that if a dose of Helidac® Therapy or Pylera® is missed, the next dose should be taken at the regularly scheduled time; the dose should not be doubled. Importance of informing clinicians if more than 4 doses of Helidac® Therapy or Pylera® are missed.

Importance of advising patients that antibacterials (including Helidac® Therapy and Pylera®) should only be used to treat bacterial infections and not used to treat viral infections (e.g., the common cold).

Importance of completing full course of therapy, even if feeling better after a few days.

Advise patients that skipping doses or not completing the full course of therapy may decrease effectiveness and increase the likelihood that bacteria will develop resistance and will not be treatable with Helidac® Therapy or other anti-infective agents in the future.

Advise patients that Helidac® Therapy or the Pylera® fixed combination may reduce the effectiveness of oral contraceptives and that alternative nonhormonal contraceptive measures should be used.

Importance of informing clinician of existing or contemplated concomitant therapy, including prescription and OTC drugs and dietary or herbal products, as well as any concomitant illnesses.

Importance of women informing clinicians if they are or plan to become pregnant or plan to breast-feed.

Importance of advising patients of other important precautionary information. (See Cautions.)

Overview® (see Users Guide). For additional information on this drug until a more detailed monograph is developed and published, the manufacturer's labeling should be consulted. It is *essential* that the manufacturer's labeling be consulted for more detailed information on usual cautions, precautions, contraindications, potential drug interactions, laboratory test interferences, and acute toxicity.

Preparations

Excipients in commercially available drug preparations may have clinically important effects in some individuals; consult specific product labeling for details.

Bismuth Subcitrate Potassium Combinations

Oral		
Capsules	140 mg with Metronidazole 125 mg and Tetracycline Hydrochloride 125 mg	**Pylera®**, Axcan Pharma

Bismuth Subgallate

Oral		
Capsules	200 mg	**Devrom®**, Parthenon
Tablets, chewable	200 mg	**Devrom®**, Parthenon

Bismuth Subsalicylate

Oral		
Suspension	87.3 mg/5 mL*	**Bismatrol®**, Major
		Bismuth Subsalicylate Oral Suspension
		Diotame® Instydose, Medique
		Kaopectate®, Chattem
		Kao-Tin®, Major
		Peptic Relief®, Rugby
		Pepto-Bismol®, Procter & Gamble
		Pink Bismuth Suspension
	175 mg/5 mL*	**Bismatrol® Maximum Strength**, Major
		Bismuth Subsalicylate Oral Suspension
		Kaopectate® Extra Strength, Chattem
		Pepto-Bismol® Maximum Strength, Procter & Gamble
		Pink Bismuth Maximum Strength Suspension
Tablets	262 mg*	**Bismuth Subsalicylate Tablets**
		Pepto-Bismol® Easy-to-Swallow Caplets, Procter & Gamble
		Pink Bismuth Caplets
Tablets, chewable	262 mg*	**Bismatrol®**, Major
		Bismuth Subsalicylate Chewable Tablets
		Diotame®, Medique
		Peptic Relief®, Rugby
		Pepto-Bismol® Chewables, Procter & Gamble
		Pink Bismuth Chewable Tablets

*available from one or more manufacturer, distributor, and/or repackager by generic (nonproprietary) name

Bismuth Subsalicylate Combinations

Oral		
Kit	8 Tablets, chewable, Bismuth Subsalicylate 262.4 mg 4 Tablets, Metronidazole 250 mg 4 Capsules, Tetracycline Hydrochloride 500 mg	**Helidac® Therapy** (available as 14 blister cards), Prometheus

†Use is not currently included in the labeling approved by the US Food and Drug Administration

Loperamide Hydrochloride

■ Loperamide hydrochloride, a synthetic piperidine-derivative, is an antiperistaltic antidiarrhea agent.

Uses

■ **Diarrhea** Loperamide hydrochloride is used in the control and symptomatic relief of acute, nonspecific diarrhea and in the control and symptomatic relief of chronic diarrhea associated with inflammatory bowel disease. The drug has also been effective in controlling chronic functional (idiopathic) diarrhea† and chronic diarrhea caused by bowel resection or organic lesions†.

For *self-medication*, loperamide hydrochloride is used for symptomatic control of diarrhea, including travelers' diarrhea. The fixed combination containing loperamide hydrochloride and simethicone is used for *self-medication* for symptomatic control of diarrhea and symptomatic control of gas (gastric bloating, pressure, cramps).

Double-blind clinical studies have shown that loperamide is at least as effective as diphenoxylate for control of acute diarrhea and more effective than diphenoxylate in decreasing daily stool frequency, improving fecal consistency, and controlling chronic diarrhea.

Loperamide should not be used as primary therapy in patients with acute dysentery (characterized by blood in stools and high fever), acute ulcerative colitis, bacterial enterocolitis caused by invasive organisms (e.g., *Salmonella, Shigella, Campylobacter*), or pseudomembranous colitis associated with the use of anti-infectives. Fluid and electrolyte depletion may occur in patients who have diarrhea, and the use of loperamide does not preclude administration of appropriate fluid and electrolyte therapy.

Travelers' Diarrhea Antiperistaltic agents (e.g., loperamide, diphenoxylate) are used for symptomatic treatment of mild or uncomplicated travelers' diarrhea, including that occurring in adult travelers with human immunodeficiency virus (HIV) infection, and also have been used for adjunctive therapy when anti-infectives are indicated for the treatment of moderate to severe travelers' diarrhea.

The most common cause of travelers' diarrhea (80–90% of cases) is bacteria (e.g., enterotoxigenic *Escherichia coli, Campylobacter jejuni, Shigella, Salmonella, Aeromonas, Plesiomonas*). Travelers' diarrhea caused by bacteria often is self-limited and resolves within 3–7 days without treatment. In travelers with only mild diarrhea (without fever or bloody stools), use of loperamide may provide symptomatic relief in less that 24 hours. If diarrhea is moderate to severe, associated with fever or bloody stools, or extremely disruptive to travel plans, short-term (1–3 days) empiric treatment with an appropriate anti-infective (e.g., ciprofloxacin or levofloxacin, azithromycin, rifaximin) is recommended. Adjunctive therapy with an antiperistaltic agent during the first few days may shorten the duration of illness or reduce the frequency of bowel movements so that travelers can continue with travel plans while waiting for the beneficial effects of anti-infective treatment. However, loperamide and diphenoxylate are not usually recommended in travelers with high fever or bloody diarrhea or in young children. (See Cautions.)

For additional information on treatment of travelers' diarrhea, see Travelers' Diarrhea under Uses: GI Infections, in Ciprofloxacin 8:12.18.

■ **Ileostomy Discharge** Loperamide hydrochloride is used to reduce the volume of discharge from ileostomies. Although not statistically significant, in one study loperamide appeared to have a greater effect on ileostomy discharge than did diphenoxylate with atropine. The greater the initial ileostomy discharge, the more benefit obtained by the patient from loperamide therapy.

Dosage and Administration

■ **Administration** Loperamide hydrochloride is administered orally.

The oral solution or suspension should be administered using only the calibrated measuring cup provided by the manufacturer; the suspension should be shaken well prior to each dose.

Patients should receive appropriate fluid and electrolyte replacement as needed. Patients using the drug for *self-medication* should be advised to drink plenty of clear fluids to help prevent dehydration caused by diarrhea.

■ **Dosage** Dosage of loperamide hydrochloride is expressed in terms of the salt.

Adult Dosage **Acute Diarrhea.** For control and symptomatic relief of acute, nonspecific diarrhea in adults, the initial dosage of loperamide hydrochloride is 4 mg, followed by 2 mg after each unformed stool. The maximum recommended dosage of loperamide hydrochloride for adults is 16 mg daily.

For *self-medication* to control symptoms of diarrhea, including travelers' diarrhea, in adults, the initial dosage of loperamide hydrochloride (alone or in fixed combination with simethicone) is 4 mg, followed by 2 mg after each subsequent unformed stool. The maximum recommended dosage of loperamide hydrochloride for *self-medication* in adults is 8 mg in a 24-hour period; the duration of therapy should not exceed 2 days unless directed by a clinician.

Clinical improvement of acute diarrhea usually occurs within 48 hours after initiation of loperamide. The drug should be discontinued and a clinician consulted if there is no improvement after 48 hours of therapy.

Chronic Diarrhea. For control and symptomatic relief of chronic diarrhea associated with inflammatory bowel disease in adults, the initial dosage of loperamide hydrochloride is 4 mg, followed by 2 mg after each unformed stool until symptoms are controlled; dosage should then be reduced for maintenance as required. When the optimal dosage for maintenance therapy has been established, the daily dosage may then be administered as a single dose or in divided doses. In clinical trials, the average adult maintenance dosage was 4–8 mg daily and only rarely exceeded 16 mg daily. If improvement does not occur in patients with chronic diarrhea after treatment with loperamide hydrochloride given in a dosage of 16 mg daily for at least 10 days, symptoms are unlikely to be controlled by further administration of the drug. Loperamide therapy may be continued if diarrhea cannot be adequately controlled with diet or specific treatment.

Pediatric Dosage **Acute Diarrhea.** For control and symptomatic relief of acute, nonspecific diarrhea in children 2–12 years of age, dosage of loperamide hydrochloride is based on age and body weight. (See Table 1 for initial pediatric dosage for the *first day* of therapy.) On the second and subsequent days of therapy, children 2–12 years of age should receive a dosage of 0.1 mg/kg only after each unformed stool. Dosage on the second and subsequent days should not exceed the age-appropriate dosages recommended for the initial 24 hours of therapy.

Table 1. Initial Dosage of Loperamide Hydrochloride in Children 2–12 Years of Age

Age (weight)	Dosage (initial 24 hours)
2–5 years (13–20 kg)	1 mg 3 times daily
6–8 years (20–30 kg)	2 mg twice daily
8–12 years (>30 kg)	2 mg 3 times daily

For *self-medication* in children 12 years of age or older to control symptoms of diarrhea, including travelers' diarrhea, the initial dosage of loperamide hydrochloride (alone or in fixed combination with simethicone) is 4 mg, followed by 2 mg after each subsequent unformed stool. The maximum recommended dosage of loperamide hydrochloride for *self-medication* in children 12 years of age or older is 8 mg in a 24-hour period; the duration of therapy should not exceed 2 days unless directed by a clinician.

For *self-medication* in children 9–11 years of age (27.3–43.2 kg) to control symptoms of diarrhea, including travelers' diarrhea, the usual dosage of loperamide hydrochloride (alone or in fixed combination with simethicone) is 2 mg after the first unformed stool, followed by 1 mg after each subsequent unformed stool. The maximum recommended dosage of loperamide hydrochloride for *self-medication* in children 9–11 years of age is 6 mg daily in a 24-hour period; the duration of therapy should not exceed 2 days unless directed by a clinician.

For *self-medication* in children 6–8 years of age (21.8–26.8 kg) to control symptoms of diarrhea, including travelers' diarrhea, the usual dosage of loperamide hydrochloride (alone or in fixed combination with simethicone) is 2 mg after the first unformed stool, followed by 1 mg after each subsequent unformed stool. The maximum recommended dosage of loperamide hydrochloride for *self-medication* in children 6–8 years of age is 4 mg in a 24-hour period; the duration of therapy should not exceed 2 days unless directed by a clinician.

Loperamide hydrochloride (alone or in fixed combination with simethicone) should *not* be used for *self-medication* in children younger than 6 years of age unless directed by a clinician.

Clinical improvement of acute diarrhea usually occurs within 48 hours after initiation of loperamide. The drug should be discontinued and a clinician consulted if there is no improvement after 48 hours of therapy.

Chronic Diarrhea. A therapeutic dosage of loperamide hydrochloride for the treatment of chronic diarrhea in pediatric patients has not been established. A dosage of 0.08–0.24 mg/kg daily in 2 or 3 divided doses† has been used in a limited number of children for the management of chronic diarrhea and has been recommended by some clinicians.

■ **Dosage in Renal and Hepatic Impairment** Dosage adjustments are not necessary when loperamide hydrochloride is used in patients with renal impairment.

Loperamide hydrochloride should be used with caution in patients with hepatic impairment since first-pass metabolism may be decreased in such patients. (See Cautions: Precautions and Contraindications.)

Cautions

■ **Adverse Effects** In clinical trials evaluating loperamide hydrochloride for the treatment of diarrhea, adverse effects generally were minor and self-limiting and were reported more frequently in patients receiving the drug for treatment of chronic diarrhea than in those receiving the drug for treatment of acute diarrhea. Some adverse effects reported with loperamide during clinical trials and postmarketing experience are difficult to distinguish from symptoms of the underlying diarrheal syndrome.

The most frequently reported adverse effects in patients receiving recommended dosages of the drug are nausea, constipation, abdominal cramps, and dizziness. Dry mouth, abdominal pain, abdominal distention or discomfort, vomiting, flatulence, dyspepsia, drowsiness, fatigue, and urinary retention also have been reported. Children may be more sensitive to adverse CNS effects of the drug than adults.

Paralytic ileus and megacolon (including toxic megacolon) have been reported in patients receiving loperamide. There have been rare reports of toxic megacolon in patients with human immunodeficiency virus (HIV) infection who had infectious colitis associated with viral or bacterial pathogens and received loperamide. (See Cautions: Precautions and Contraindications.)

Hypersensitivity reactions, including rash, pruritus, urticaria, and angioedema, have been reported in patients receiving loperamide. There have been rare reports of severe hypersensitivity reactions (e.g., anaphylactic shock, anaphylactoid reactions) and bullous eruptions (e.g., erythema multiforme, Stevens-Johnson syndrome, toxic epidermal necrolysis).

Potentially fatal, serious cardiovascular effects (e.g., QT interval prolongation, torsades de pointes or other ventricular arrhythmias, syncope, cardiac arrest) have been reported in patients taking loperamide. Cardiovascular effects have been reported rarely in patients receiving recommended dosages of loperamide hydrochloride; the majority of reported cases involved higher than recommended dosages, usually in individuals misusing or abusing the drug. (See Misuse and Abuse Potential under Cautions: Precautions and Contraindications.)

■ **Precautions and Contraindications** Loperamide is contraindicated in patients with known hypersensitivity to the drug or any ingredient in the formulation.

Loperamide is contraindicated in patients with abdominal pain in the absence of diarrhea.

The drug is used only for control and symptomatic relief of diarrhea. Whenever an underlying etiology for the diarrhea can be determined, specific treatment should be given if indicated or appropriate.

Loperamide is contraindicated in patients with acute dysentery (characterized by blood in stools and high fever), acute ulcerative colitis, bacterial enterocolitis caused by invasive organisms (e.g., *Salmonella*, *Shigella*, *Campylobacter*), or pseudomembranous colitis associated with anti-infective therapy.

Because of the possible risk of serious sequelae, including ileus, megacolon, and toxic megacolon, loperamide should *not* be used when inhibition of peristalsis should be avoided. The drug *must* be discontinued promptly if constipation, abdominal distention, or ileus occurs. Based on rare reports of toxic megacolon in HIV-infected patients with infectious colitis associated with viral or bacterial pathogens, loperamide should be discontinued in HIV-infected patients at the earliest signs of abdominal distention.

Fluid and electrolyte depletion often occurs in patients with diarrhea, and administration of appropriate fluid and electrolytes is important in such cases. Loperamide therapy does not preclude administration of appropriate fluid and electrolyte therapy. When loperamide is used for *self-medication*, patients should be advised to drink plenty of clear fluids to help prevent dehydration caused by diarrhea.

Because tiredness, dizziness, or drowsiness may occur in the setting of diarrheal syndromes treated with loperamide, patients should be advised to use caution when driving a car or operating machinery.

Loperamide should be used with caution in patients with hepatic impairment. Such patients should be monitored closely for signs and symptoms of CNS toxicity during loperamide therapy, since first-pass metabolism of the drug may be decreased in patients with hepatic impairment.

Patients receiving loperamide should be advised to consult a clinician if diarrhea persists for longer than 2 days, if blood is present in stools, or if fever or abdominal distention develops.

Loperamide should be used with caution in patients predisposed to QT interval prolongation, torsades de pointes, or other serious arrhythmias. The drug also should be used with caution in patients who are receiving drugs that inhibit loperamide metabolism or transport (i.e., inhibitors of hepatic cytochrome P-450 [CYP] isoenzymes 3A4 and 2C8, inhibitors of P-glycoprotein [P-gp]) since increased plasma concentrations of loperamide may increase the risk of serious cardiovascular effects. (See Misuse and Abuse Potential under Cautions: Precautions and Contraindications and see Drug Interactions.)

Precautions Related to Self-medication For *self-medication*, loperamide should not be used for longer than 2 days unless directed by a clinician. Loperamide also should not be used for *self-medication* if diarrhea is accompanied by fever, if mucus or blood is present in the stool, or if rash or other allergic reaction to the drug has occurred previously.

If a patient is receiving an anti-infective or has a history of liver disease, a clinician should be consulted before the drug is used for *self-medication*.

When loperamide is used for *self-medication*, patients should be advised to discontinue the drug and contact a clinician if diarrhea symptoms worsen or last longer than 2 days or if abdominal swelling or bulging develops.

Precautions Related to Use of Fixed Combinations When the fixed combination containing loperamide and simethicone is used, the cautions, precautions, contraindications, and drug interactions associated with both drugs should be considered. Cautionary information applicable to specific populations (e.g., pregnant or nursing women, individuals with hepatic or renal impairment, geriatric patients) should be considered for both loperamide and simethicone.

Misuse and Abuse Potential FDA has warned clinicians to consider the potential for misuse and abuse of loperamide hydrochloride.

Serious cardiovascular effects, including fatalities, have occurred when loperamide hydrochloride was used at dosages higher than recommended. The majority of serious cardiovascular effects reported with loperamide have occurred in individuals who were intentionally misusing and abusing high dosages of the drug in an attempt to self-treat opioid withdrawal symptoms or to achieve a feeling of euphoria. The maximum recommended adult dosage of loperamide hydrochloride is 8 mg daily for *self-medication* or 16 mg daily for prescription use; in some cases of misuse and abuse, individuals ingested loperamide hydrochloride dosages of 70–1600 mg daily.

FDA recommends that clinicians consider loperamide as a possible cause of unexplained cardiac events (e.g., QT interval prolongation, torsades de pointes or other ventricular arrhythmias, syncope, cardiac arrest).

If loperamide-induced cardiotoxicity is suspected, loperamide should be promptly discontinued and appropriate therapy initiated to manage and prevent cardiac arrhythmias and severe outcomes. In some cases of torsades de pointes, drug treatment may be ineffective and electrical pacing or cardioversion may be required. Patients with opioid use disorders should be referred for treatment. When excessive loperamide ingestion is suspected, specific testing may be required to measure blood levels of the drug; standard drug screens for opioids may not include an assay for loperamide and may yield negative results even in the presence of loperamide.

Individuals abusing loperamide often take other drugs with the antidiarrheal agent in an attempt to increase loperamide absorption and penetration across the blood-brain barrier, inhibit loperamide metabolism, and enhance its euphoric effects. FDA warns that the risk of serious cardiac problems (e.g., abnormal heart rhythms) may be increased if high loperamide dosages are taken with drugs that interact with loperamide (e.g., cimetidine, clarithromycin, erythromycin, gemfibrozil, itraconazole, ketoconazole, quinidine, quinine, ranitidine, ritonavir). (See Drug Interactions.)

FDA states that patients and consumers should be advised to take loperamide *only* in the dosage prescribed by their clinician or stated on the label of the over-the-counter (OTC, nonprescription) product and should be warned that taking larger doses of loperamide (either intentionally or unintentionally) may lead to abnormal heart rhythms and serious cardiac events that can be fatal. In addition, patients and consumers should be warned that taking loperamide with some commonly used drugs also may increase the risk of serious cardiac adverse events. To help deter misuse and abuse of OTC loperamide products, FDA is working with manufacturers to limit the number of doses per package and to use single-dose (e.g., blister) packaging.

Patients and consumers should be advised to immediately seek medical attention if they or someone else taking loperamide experiences fainting, rapid heartbeat or irregular heart rhythm, or are unresponsive (i.e., can't be wakened or is not answering or reacting normally).

■ **Pediatric Precautions** Loperamide is contraindicated in children younger than 2 years of age because of the risks of respiratory depression and serious adverse cardiac reactions.

There have been rare reports of paralytic ileus associated with abdominal distention in patients receiving loperamide; most cases occurred in the setting of acute dysentery, overdosage, and with infants younger than 2 years of age.

Loperamide should not be used for *self-medication* in children younger than 6 years of age unless directed by a clinician.

Loperamide should be used with particular caution in young children because of the greater variability of response in this age group. The presence of dehydration, especially in younger children, may further influence the variability of response to the drug.

■ **Geriatric Precautions** Formal studies have not been conducted to evaluate loperamide in geriatric patients. There are no apparent differences in disposition of the drug in elderly patients with diarrhea relative to younger adults.

■ **Mutagenicity and Carcinogenicity** In a study in rats using loperamide hydrochloride dosages up to 40 mg/kg daily (21 times the maximum human dose of 16 mg daily based on body surface area comparison) for 18 months, there was no evidence of carcinogenicity.

Loperamide was not genotoxic in the Ames test, the SOS chromotest in *Escherichia coli*, the dominant lethal test in female mice, or the mouse embryo cell transformation assay.

■ **Pregnancy, Fertility, and Lactation** ***Pregnancy*** There are no adequate and well-controlled studies using loperamide in pregnant women, and the drug should be used during pregnancy only if potential benefits to the woman justify potential risks to the fetus.

Reproduction studies in rats and rabbits using loperamide hydrochloride dosages up to 40 mg/kg daily (43 times the human dosage based on body surface comparison) did not reveal evidence of teratogenicity; however, a dosage of 40 mg/kg daily in rats produced impaired growth and survival of offspring.

Fertility Although reproduction studies in female and male rats using loperamide hydrochloride dosages up to 10 mg/kg daily (5 times the human dosage based on body surface area comparison) did not reveal evidence of impaired fertility, a dosage of 20 or 40 mg/kg daily resulted in marked impairment of fertility in females and a dosage of 40 mg/kg daily resulted in impairment of fertility in males.

Lactation Because loperamide is distributed into milk in low concentrations, the drug is not recommended in nursing women.

Drug Interactions

■ **Drugs Affecting Hepatic Microsomal Enzymes** Loperamide hydrochloride is metabolized principally by hepatic cytochrome P-450 (CYP) isoenzymes 3A4 and 2C8.

Concomitant use of loperamide with drugs that are CYP3A4 inhibitors (e.g., clarithromycin, erythromycin, itraconazole, ketoconazole) or CYP2C8 inhibitors (e.g., gemfibrozil) may increase plasma loperamide concentrations and may increase the risk of serious cardiovascular effects. Caution is advised if loperamide is used in patients receiving a CYP3A4 or CYP2C8 inhibitor.

■ **Drugs Affecting P-glycoprotein Transport** Loperamide hydrochloride is a P-glycoprotein (P-gp) substrate.

Concomitant use of loperamide with drugs that are P-gp inhibitors (e.g., quinidine, quinine, ritonavir) may increase plasma loperamide concentrations and may increase the risk of enhanced central effects or serious cardiovascular effects. Caution is advised if loperamide is used in patients receiving a P-gp inhibitor.

■ **GI Drugs** Cimetidine or ranitidine can potentially interact with loperamide if the drugs are used concomitantly.

■ **Antiretroviral Agents** Concomitant use of loperamide hydrochloride (single 16-mg dose) and ritonavir (single 600-mg dose) resulted in up to a threefold increase in plasma loperamide concentrations. Loperamide should be used concomitantly with ritonavir with caution since increased plasma loperamide concentrations may result in enhanced central effects of the drug.

Concomitant use of loperamide hydrochloride (single 16-mg dose) and saquinavir (single 600-mg dose) resulted in a 54% decrease in saquinavir exposure, which may result in decreased efficacy of the antiretroviral agent. If loperamide and saquinavir are used concomitantly, therapeutic efficacy of saquinavir should be closely monitored.

■ **Quinidine** Concomitant use of loperamide hydrochloride (single 16-mg dose) and quinidine (single 600-mg dose) resulted in up to a threefold increase in plasma loperamide concentrations. Loperamide should be used concomitantly with quinidine with caution since increased plasma loperamide concentrations may result in enhanced central effects of the drug and may increase the risk of serious cardiovascular effects.

Acute Toxicity

■ **Manifestations** Overdosage of loperamide hydrochloride (including relative overdosage due to hepatic dysfunction) may be manifested by urinary retention, paralytic ileus, CNS depression, and GI effects (e.g., vomiting, abdominal pain or burning). Children may be more sensitive to CNS effects than adults. An adult who took three 20-mg doses of loperamide hydrochloride within 24 hours was nauseated after the second dose and vomited after the third dose. In studies designed to evaluate the potential for adverse effects, intentional ingestion of single doses of up to 60 mg did not result in any clinically important adverse effects.

Intentional or unintentional overdosage of loperamide (intentional misuse or abuse in an attempt to self-treat opioid withdrawal symptoms or to achieve a feeling of euphoria, suspected suicide attempt) or long-term use of high loperamide dosages has resulted in serious cardiovascular effects, including fatalities. Use of excessive loperamide dosage also has resulted in severe CNS effects (e.g., catatonia). In some cases of misuse and abuse, individuals ingested loperamide hydrochloride dosages of 70–1600 mg daily. (See Misuse and Abuse Potential under Cautions: Precautions and Contraindications.)

■ **Treatment** In the treatment of loperamide overdosage, gastric lavage is recommended, followed by administration of 100 g of activated charcoal slurry through the gastric tube. If vomiting has occurred spontaneously, 100 g of activated charcoal slurry should be administered orally as soon as fluids can be retained. Patients should be monitored for signs of CNS depression for at least 24 hours. Naloxone may be administered if CNS depression occurs. Because the duration of action of loperamide is greater than that of naloxone, the patient must be closely watched and additional doses of naloxone administered as necessary. Vital signs should be monitored for recurrence of symptoms of drug overdose for at least 24 hours after the last dose of naloxone. Forced diuresis would not be expected to be effective in loperamide overdosage, since relatively little drug is excreted in urine.

Pharmacology

Loperamide hydrochloride slows intestinal motility through a direct effect on the nerve endings and/or intramural ganglia of the intestinal wall. The drug is generally believed to act by interfering with the cholinergic and noncholinergic mechanisms involved in the peristaltic reflex, decreasing the activity of circular and longitudinal muscles in the intestinal wall. However, some data indicate that the drug may act, like diphenoxylate and morphine, by enhancing contractions of intestinal circular musculature, thus increasing segmentation and retarding forward motion through the intestine.

Loperamide prolongs the transit time of intestinal contents and therefore reduces fecal volume, increases fecal viscosity and bulk density, and diminishes loss of fluid and electrolytes. As an antidiarrhea agent, loperamide is reported to be more specific, longer acting, and 2–3 times more potent on a weight basis than diphenoxylate. Tolerance to the antidiarrheal effect of loperamide has not been reported.

In animals, loperamide has no analgesic activity even in extremely high doses. Although loperamide binds to opiate receptors in the brain and myenteric plexus, the drug has not produced opiate-like CNS effects in rats, even in large doses. Studies in monkeys, however, have demonstrated that high doses of loperamide can produce morphine-like symptoms of physical dependence and prevent signs of morphine withdrawal in morphine-dependent animals. In humans, the naloxone challenge pupil test, which when positive indicates opiate-like effects, was negative when performed after a single 16-mg dose of loperamide, and after more than 2 years of therapeutic use of the drug. Physical dependence on loperamide has not been reported in humans.

Pharmacokinetics

■ **Absorption** Peak plasma concentrations of loperamide occur about 5 or 2.5 hours following administration of loperamide hydrochloride capsules or oral solution, respectively. After a 2-mg oral dose of loperamide hydrochloride capsules, peak plasma concentrations of 2 ng/mL have been reported. The oral bioavailability of capsules and solution of the drug, as determined by area under the plasma concentration-time curve (AUC), is reportedly similar. Peak plasma concentrations of loperamide metabolites are reached 8 hours following oral administration of capsules of the drug.

■ **Distribution** It is not known whether loperamide crosses the placenta. The drug is distributed into milk in low concentrations.

■ **Elimination** Loperamide undergoes oxidative metabolism, principally by hepatic cytochrome P-450 (CYP) isoenzymes 2C8 and 3A4; CYP2B6 and CYP2D6 may also be involved.

The unchanged drug and metabolites are excreted principally in feces. A manufacturer reports that after oral administration of 4 mg of loperamide hydrochloride, less than 2% of the dose is excreted in urine and 30% of the dose is excreted in feces as intact drug. In animals, loperamide has been shown to undergo enterohepatic circulation.

The apparent elimination half-life of loperamide in healthy adults receiving recommended dosages of the drug is 10.8 hours (range 9.1–14.4 hours). Half-lives as high as 41 hours have been reported in individuals who ingested higher than recommended dosages of the drug.

Chemistry and Stability

■ **Chemistry** Loperamide hydrochloride is a synthetic piperidine-derivative antidiarrhea agent. The drug occurs as a white to slightly yellow powder and is slightly soluble in water and freely soluble in alcohol. Loperamide hydrochloride oral solution has a pH of about 5. The drug has a pK_a of 8.6.

■ **Stability** Loperamide hydrochloride capsules should be stored at 20–25°C in a well-closed container.

Loperamide hydrochloride solutions, suspensions, film-coated tablets, and chewable tablets commercially available for *self-administration* should be stored at 20–25°C.

Tablets containing a fixed combination of loperamide hydrochloride and simethicone commercially available for *self-administration* should be stored at 20–25°C and protected from light.

Preparations

Excipients in commercially available drug preparations may have clinically important effects in some individuals; consult specific product labeling for details.

Loperamide Hydrochloride

Oral		
Capsules	2 mg*	**Loperamide Hydrochloride Capsules**
Solution	1 mg/5 mL*	**Imodium® A-D,** McNeil
		Loperamide Hydrochloride Oral Solution
Suspension	1 mg/7.5 mL*	**Imodium® A-D,** McNeil
		Loperamide Hydrochloride Oral Suspension
Tablets, film-coated	2 mg*	**Imodium® A-D Caplets®,** McNeil
		Loperamide Hydrochloride Tablets
Tablets, chewable	2 mg	**Imodium® A-D EZ Chews,** McNeil

*available from one or more manufacturer, distributor, and/or repackager by generic (nonproprietary) name

Loperamide Hydrochloride Combinations

Oral		
Tablets	2 mg with Simethicone 125 mg*	**Imodium® Multi-Symptom Relief Caplets®,** McNeil
		Loperamide Hydrochloride and Simethicone Tablets
Tablets, chewable	2 mg with Simethicone 125 mg*	**Imodium® Multi-Symptom Relief Chewable Tablets,** McNeil
		Loperamide Hydrochloride and Simethicone Chewable Tablets

*available from one or more manufacturer, distributor, and/or repackager by generic (nonproprietary) name

†Use is not currently included in the labeling approved by the US Food and Drug Administration

CATHARTICS AND LAXATIVES 56:12

Cathartics and Laxatives General Statement

■ Cathartic, laxative, and purgative are terms describing drugs that promote evacuation of the intestine; the difference between the terms is largely one of degree.

General

Cathartic, laxative, and purgative are terms describing drugs that promote evacuation of the intestine; the difference between the terms is largely one of degree. Cathartic and purgative are interchangeable terms describing drugs that promote rapid evacuation of the intestine and noticeable alteration of stool consistency. The evacuant action of a laxative is less pronounced, but large doses of a laxative may produce catharsis or purgation. Cathartic, laxative, and purgative drugs will be referred to as laxatives.

Laxatives are usually subdivided into several categories, including the bulk-forming, hyperosmotic, lubricant, saline, and stimulant laxatives and the stool softeners. The bulk-forming laxatives include cellulose derivatives, karaya, malt soup extract, psyllium preparations, and dietary bran. Glycerin, sorbitol, and polyethylene glycol are commonly termed hyperosmotic laxatives. Mineral oil is a lubricant laxative. Laxatives containing magnesium cations or phosphate anions are commonly termed saline laxatives. Anthraquinone laxatives (aloe [preparations containing aloe are no longer commercially available in the US], cascara sagrada [preparations containing cascara sagrada are no longer commercially available in the US], senna), the diphenylmethane derivatives (bisacodyl, phenolphthalein [preparations containing phenolphthalein are no longer commercially available in the US]), castor oil, and dehydrocholic acid are stimulant laxatives. The stool softeners include the calcium, potassium, and sodium salts of docusate.

Pharmacology

The precise mechanisms of action of the laxatives are not known. Recent evidence indicates that the actions of the various laxatives may be pharmacologically similar but dose dependent and that most laxatives promote defecation by altering intestinal fluid and electrolyte transport. Active ion secretion stimulated by most laxatives may be the driving force for intestinal fluid accumulation and subsequent defecation.

■ **Bulk-forming Laxatives** Bulk-forming laxatives dissolve or swell in water to form an emollient gel or viscous solution. It is thought that the resulting bulk in the feces promotes peristalsis and reduces transit time. Reductions in fecal pH and in serum cholesterol, and altered composition of fecal bile acids have been observed following administration of some bulk-forming laxatives; some pharmacologists believe these actions may also contribute to the laxative effect of some of these drugs.

■ **Hyperosmotic Laxatives** When administered rectally, glycerin and sorbitol exert a hygroscopic and/or local irritant action, drawing water from the tissues into the feces and reflexly stimulating evacuation. The extent to which the simple physical distention of the rectum and the hygroscopic and/or local irritant actions are responsible for the laxative effects of some of these drugs is not known. Only extremely high oral doses of sorbitol (25 g daily) or glycerin exert laxative action.

Polyethylene glycol 3350 electrolyte solution is a nonabsorbable solution that passes through the bowel without net absorption or secretion; therefore, substantial fluid and electrolyte shifts are avoided. Polyethylene glycol 3350 electrolyte solution osmotically increases intraluminal fluids to induce diarrhea and rapidly cleanse the bowel.

■ **Mineral Oil** Oral mineral oil appears to lubricate fecal material and the intestinal mucosa by retarding reabsorption of water from the intestinal tract. Increased water retention may secondarily increase the bulk of the stool and hasten evacuation. Mineral oil emulsion reportedly has better wetting properties than does nonemulsified mineral oil and penetration of the feces thus may be enhanced. Rectal enemas of heavy or light mineral oil exert laxative action via a lubricant effect and/or simple physical distention of the rectum.

■ **Saline Laxatives** It is commonly believed that the action of the saline laxatives results from the hyperosmotic effect of poorly absorbed magnesium or phosphate ions within the small intestine and from the retention of water which indirectly stimulates stretch receptors and increases peristalsis. These mechanisms of action are unproven, and conversely, it has been noted that isosmolarity is present at the ligament of Treitz following ingestion of hyperosmolar meals. The laxative action of magnesium also may be the result of cholecystokinin release or decreased transit time. The effectiveness of phosphate enemas may simply reflect the volume of liquid introduced rectally.

Orally administered saline laxatives act mainly on the small intestine. Saline suppositories or enemas generally promote evacuation of the colon only.

The amount of sodium biphosphate in rectal suppositories containing sodium acid pyrophosphate, sodium bicarbonate, and sodium biphosphate is probably insufficient to exert an effect as a saline laxative, but it is included to facilitate the chemical reaction that produces carbon dioxide (CO_2). Rectal suppositories containing potassium bitartrate and sodium bicarbonate also produce CO_2. The expanding CO_2 promotes laxation by exerting pressure in the rectum.

■ **Stimulant Laxatives** It has commonly been thought that the stimulant laxatives induce defecation by stimulating propulsive peristaltic activity of the intestine through local irritation of the mucosa or through a more selective action on the intramural nerve plexus of intestinal smooth muscle, thus increasing motility. However, recent studies show that these drugs alter fluid and electrolyte absorption, producing net intestinal fluid accumulation and laxation. Some of these drugs may directly stimulate active intestinal ion secretion. Increased concentrations of cyclic 3′,5′-adenosine monophosphate (cAMP), occurring in colonic mucosal cells following administration of stimulant laxatives, may alter the permeability of these cells and mediate active ion secretion thereby producing net fluid accumulation and laxative action.

Stimulant laxatives mainly promote evacuation of the colon; however, castor oil and phenolphthalein (laxatives containing phenolphthalein are no longer commercially available in the US) also directly or reflexly increase activity of the small intestine. Rectal suppositories of some stimulant laxatives reportedly promote laxation by physical distention of the rectum.

With the exception of aloe (preparations containing aloe extract or aloe flower extract are no longer commercially available in the US) and aloin which are reportedly very irritating, the anthraquinone laxatives are considered to be the mild laxatives in the stimulant category. The laxative action of dehydrocholic acid also appears to be relatively mild. The diphenylmethanes have a more pronounced laxative effect. Castor oil produces violent purgation in therapeutic doses.

■ **Stool Softeners** In vitro studies suggest that the stool softeners soften fecal material and ease defecation by lowering surface tension at the oil-water interface of fecal material, permitting water and lipids to penetrate. Recent in vivo evidence suggests that the laxative properties of these drugs may result from stimulation of electrolyte and water secretion in the colon. Increased concentrations of cAMP, occurring in colonic mucosal cells following administration of these drugs, may alter the permeability of these cells and mediate active ion secretion thereby producing net fluid accumulation and laxative action.

Uses

■ **GI Conditions** Although there are few valid indications for laxatives, these drugs are self-prescribed and overused by a large portion of the population. Constipation usually is best avoided or relieved with proper diet (high fiber content such as bran), adequate fluid intake, prompt response to the defecation reflex, and exercise. The normal frequency of bowel movements varies from once daily to 1–2 times weekly. If constipation (i.e., decreased frequency of bowel movements with prolonged and difficult passage of stools) occurs, the cause should be identified carefully before initiating laxative use. Use of laxatives in infants and children should be avoided; childhood constipation is best treated by counseling the parents regarding acceptable variations in the frequency of bowel movements.

When laxatives are indicated, the *mildest* effective laxative should be used. Rectal suppositories or enemas are routinely used to empty the colon prior to surgery or radiologic or colonoscopic procedures but, except for these uses, should not be used when oral laxatives are effective. Single-ingredient laxative products facilitate necessary dosage adjustment and usually are as effective as and safer than combination products. Combinations of two different types of laxatives may be desirable in some patients such as those with both painful and infrequent bowel movements, but there is no rationale for combinations containing more than 2 laxatives. Most clinicians consider fixed combinations of laxatives with other drugs (e.g., belladonna alkaloids, other antimuscarinics, bismuth salts, vitamins, minerals, trace elements) unsafe and irrational.

Most clinicians consider bulk-forming laxatives to be the laxatives of choice for the initial treatment of most cases of simple constipation which is usually caused by a low-fiber and/or low-fluid diet; use of saline or stimulant laxatives for simple constipation is seldom necessary or desirable. If a stimulant laxative is used, most clinicians prefer senna or cascara (preparations containing cascara sagrada are no longer commercially available in the US) derivatives or dehydrocholic acid to the other stimulant laxatives. Aloin, aloe (preparations containing aloe extract or aloe flower extract are no longer commercially available in the US), and castor oil are avoided because they reportedly produce violent purgation, and phenolphthalein (laxatives containing phenolphthalein are no longer commercially available in the US) is avoided because it causes fixed skin eruptions.

Bulk-forming laxatives, stool softeners, or mineral oil are preferred to other laxatives in patients with conditions in which straining at defecation should be avoided (e.g., myocardial infarction, vascular diseases, diseases of the anus or rectum, hernias, recent rectal surgery). Oral stool softeners or mineral oil are preferred to bulk-forming laxatives to ease evacuation of feces in patients with constipation associated with hard, dry stools. Many clinicians consider the stool softeners to be the treatment of choice in childhood constipation associated with hard, dry stools and to be safer and more efficacious than mineral oil for conditions in which straining at defecation is to be avoided.

Bulk-forming and stimulant laxatives have been used to treat constipation that occurs following prolonged bed rest or hospitalization. These laxatives have also been used to treat constipation resulting from diminished colonic motor response in geriatric patients but, because this type of constipation is frequently due to psychological or physical laxative dependence, the bulk-forming laxatives are preferred.

Bulk-forming, hyperosmotic, stimulant, and mild saline laxatives (e.g., oral magnesium hydroxide or milk of magnesia) and stool softeners have been used to treat constipation occurring during pregnancy or the puerperium, but bulk-forming laxatives or stool softeners are usually preferred. Because the anthraquinone and diphenylmethane stimulant laxatives may be distributed into milk, other laxatives usually are used for postpartum constipation.

Mineral oil or stool softeners may be administered orally or rectally for the treatment of constipation associated with stricture of the colon or to soften fecal impactions. Some clinicians consider stool softeners to be safer and more efficacious than mineral oil for these purposes. After softening impacted feces with a stool softener or mineral oil, stimulant or saline laxatives may be administered rectally to evacuate the impacted colon. Alternatively, phosphate-containing saline enemas may be administered rectally to promote evacuation of fecal impactions after manual disimpaction.

Stimulant laxatives are used to treat constipation occurring secondary to idiopathic slowing of transit time, to constipating drugs, or to irritable bowel or spastic colon syndrome. They have also been used to treat constipation in patients with neurologic constipation.

Saline laxatives have been used to eliminate parasites and toxic anthelmintics prior to and/or after therapy with some anthelmintics (e.g., quinacrine hydrochloride). Because oral or rectal preparations of sodium phosphate and sodium biphosphate apparently do not destroy osmotically sensitive trophozoites of *Entamoeba histolytica* or *Giardia lamblia*, these preparations have been used to facilitate collection of stool samples for parasitic examination. However, most clinicians agree that with the newer anthelmintics use of laxatives to eliminate parasites or the anthelmintic is not necessary, may complicate identification of the parasite, and may be harmful to the patient.

Oral saline (usually magnesium citrate or sodium phosphates) and/or oral stimulant laxatives (usually castor oil, bisacodyl, or standardized senna fruit extract) are used to empty the bowel prior to surgery or radiologic, proctoscopic, or sigmoidoscopic procedures. These laxatives are usually supplemented with administration of rectal evacuants, such as saline, stimulant, or soapsuds enemas, immediately before radiologic procedures. Polyethylene glycol 3350 electrolyte solutions also are used to empty the bowel prior to colonoscopy and barium enema radiologic examinations. The American Society of Colon and Rectal Surgeons (ASCRS), American Society for Gastrointestinal Endoscopy (ASGE), and Society of American Gastrointestinal and Endoscopic Surgeons (SAGES) recommend the use of polyethylene glycol 3350 electrolyte solutions in patients with electrolyte or fluid imbalances (e.g., those with renal or liver insufficiency, congestive heart failure, liver failure, or advanced liver disease with ascites). These experts also recommend use of polyethylene glycol 3350 electrolyte solutions for colonic cleansing in infants and children. Glycerin and sorbitol also have been used before these procedures, but these laxatives do not always entirely empty the colon. Bisacodyl tannex has been added to barium sulfate enemas to aid in coating the intestinal mucosa and enhance colonic evacuation prior to radiologic examination of the colon. Bisacodyl and mineral oil enemas are used to cleanse the colon postoperatively. Bisacodyl suppositories may be used to cleanse the colon in pregnant women prior to delivery if they are given at least 2 hours before onset of the second stage of labor.

Sorbitol is used orally or rectally to facilitate the passage of sodium polystyrene sulfonate through the intestinal tract, to prevent constipation caused by the resin, and, by acting as a hyperosmotic laxative, to aid in potassium removal; sorbitol also improves the palatability of the resin.

Bisacodyl has been used to facilitate flushing of colostomies, but the value and safety of the drug as compared to irrigations have not been established.

Semisynthetic celluloses and psyllium bulk-forming laxatives have been used to increase the bulk of stools in patients with chronic, watery diarrhea; subjective improvement has been noted in these patients but the total water content of the stool has been unchanged. Bulk-forming laxatives and dietary bran have also been used, with some success, to reduce intraluminal and rectosigmoid pressure, and pain in patients with diverticular disease. One manufacturer suggests that stool softeners may be useful in the treatment of ulcerative colitis or diverticulitis.

Malt soup extract, in conjunction with other therapy such as proper diet and hygiene, has been used in the treatment of pruritus ani; however, evidence that the drug is effective for this condition is lacking. Bulk-forming laxatives have also been used in the management of obesity but their effectiveness in this condition is questionable.

■ **Other Uses** Saline laxatives are also used, after inducing emesis or performing gastric lavage, to hasten removal of some poisons from the GI tract, but should not be used after poisonings with ingested acids or alkalies. Magnesium laxatives should not be used to remove poisons producing CNS depression or renal function impairment.

Some manufacturers have suggested that oral phosphate saline laxatives may be useful for the symptomatic relief of gallbladder disorders, but their effectiveness in these conditions has not been proven.

When used as an adjunct to dietary therapy, oral psyllium hydrophilic mucilloid (3.4 g 3 times daily before meals as a sugar-free preparation) has produced modest reductions in serum total cholesterol, low-density lipoprotein (LDL)-cholesterol, and apolipoprotein B concentrations and the ratio of LDL cholesterol to high-density lipoprotein (HDL)-cholesterol in adults with mild to moderate hypercholesterolemia†.

Cautions

When used in appropriate dosages for a limited period of time (one week or less), most laxatives are relatively free from adverse effects such as diarrhea, GI irritation, and fluid and electrolyte depletion. Stimulant laxatives are the laxatives most likely to produce these adverse effects. Chronic use or overdosage of laxatives may produce persistent diarrhea, hypokalemia, loss of essential nutritional factors, and dehydration. Long-term use of laxatives, especially the stimulant laxatives, has been associated with laxative dependence, chronic constipation, and loss of normal bowel function.

Because magnesium, potassium, or sodium accumulation may occur in patients with renal disease, laxative products containing more than 50 mEq of magnesium, 25 mEq of potassium, or 1 mEq of sodium per dose should be used by these patients only under the supervision of a physician who should monitor electrolytes. Although no information is available on the amount of sodium absorbed following ingestion of carboxymethylcellulose sodium, this drug usually contains 2.7–4 mEq of sodium per gram. Congestive heart failure has occurred following indiscriminate use of saline laxatives containing sodium. Use of carboxymethylcellulose sodium and sodium-containing saline laxatives should be restricted in patients on low-sodium diets. Use of sodium-containing saline laxatives should also be restricted in those with congestive heart failure, edema, or cirrhosis.

Because standardized senna fruit extract and some psyllium preparations contain large amounts of sugar, the caloric value of these preparations should be considered in patients with diabetes mellitus.

All laxatives are contraindicated in patients with acute abdominal pain, nausea, vomiting, or other symptoms of appendicitis or undiagnosed abdominal pain. Stimulant laxatives are contraindicated in patients with intestinal obstruction. Bulk-forming laxatives are *not* useful when prompt or thorough bowel evacuation is necessary (e.g., poisonings, radiologic examination, bowel surgery) and are contraindicated in patients with partial obstruction of the bowel or dysphagia. Patients should consult their clinicians if sudden changes in bowel habits persist for longer than 2 weeks or if use of a laxative for one week has no effect. Polyethylene glycol 3350 electrolyte solutions are contraindicated in patients with GI obstruction, gastric retention, bowel perforation, toxic colitis, toxic megacolon, or ileus. Sodium phosphates are contraindicated in patients with biopsy-proven acute phosphate nephropathy, GI obstruction, gastric bypass or stapling surgery, bowel perforation, toxic colitis, toxic megacolon, congestive heart failure, history of kidney disease or clinically important renal function impairment, paralytic ileus, active inflammatory bowel disease, imperforate anus, decreased intravascular volume or dehydration, uncorrected electrolyte abnormalities, or known hypersensitivity to sodium phosphate salts or any ingredient in the formulation. (See Sodium Phosphates Preparations under Cautions: Saline Laxatives.)

■ **Bulk-forming Laxatives** Adverse effects occur rarely with the use of bulk-forming laxatives. Rare cases of allergic reactions and urticaria have been associated with the use of karaya. Bowel and/or esophageal obstruction, swelling or blockage of the throat, choking, or asphyxiation has occurred when insufficient liquid was administered with some of these laxatives; some of these effects probably result from formation of a viscous, semi-solid mass rather than the emollient gel or viscous solution that results when sufficient fluid is added to these laxatives. Therefore, at least one full glass (250 mL) of liquid should be administered with each dose of bulk-forming laxatives. Patients should be informed of the symptoms of esophageal obstruction and instructed to contact their physician if chest pain and/or pressure, regurgitation, vomiting, or difficulty in swallowing and/or breathing occur. Bulk-forming laxatives should not be used in individuals with esophageal obstruction, problems of the throat, or those who have difficulty in swallowing.

Potentially severe hypersensitivity reactions, including rhinoconjunctivitis, acute bronchospasm, and anaphylaxis, can occur in susceptible individuals (e.g., those with psyllium sensitivity or suffering from respiratory disorders) following inhalation of psyllium dust particles. Therefore, inhalation of psyllium hydrophilic mucilloid particles should be avoided. To minimize exposure and, therefore, sensitization to airborne particles of psyllium, one manufacturer suggests that health-care personnel dispense powdered psyllium preparations with a spoon rather than pouring them directly from the container into the glass for administration. In some cases, reassignment of health-care personnel to areas (e.g., nongeriatric units) where use of bulk powder formulations of psyllium was minimal has been necessary.

■ **Hyperosmotic Laxatives** Adverse effects occur rarely following rectal administration of glycerin or sorbitol. Glycerin may produce rectal discomfort, irritation, burning or griping, cramping pain and tenesmus. Hyperemia of the rectal mucosa with minimal amounts of hemorrhage and mucus discharge may also occur. These adverse effects occur less frequently following rectal administration of sorbitol. Diarrhea frequently occurs with the dosages of sorbitol used as adjuncts to sodium polystyrene sulfonate therapy.

Polyethylene glycol 3350 electrolyte solutions (oral or nasogastric) may produce malaise, nausea, abdominal distention, abdominal fullness and/or bloating, abdominal cramps, vomiting, anal irritation, and thirst. Generalized tonic-clonic seizures associated with electrolyte abnormalities (e.g., hyponatremia, hypokalemia) have been reported following use of polyethylene glycol 3350 electrolyte solutions for bowel cleansing in patients without a history of seizures. Such neurologic effects resolved with correction of fluid and electrolyte abnormalities. Polyethylene glycol 3350 electrolyte solutions (Golytely®, Colyte®, MoviPrep®) should be used with caution in patients with severe ulcerative colitis. In addition, polyethylene glycol 3350 electrolyte solutions should be used with caution in patients receiving drugs that increase the risk of electrolyte abnormalities (e.g., diuretics, angiotensin-converting enzyme [ACE] inhibitors). Consideration should be given to measuring electrolyte, BUN, and creatinine concentrations before and after colonoscopy in patients receiving such drugs and in those with known or suspected hyponatremia. Since MoviPrep® contains sodium ascorbate and ascorbic acid, the drug should be used with caution in patients with glucose-6-phosphate dehydrogenase (G-6-PD) deficiency, especially those with an active infection, with a history of hemolysis, or those taking concomitant drugs known to precipitate hemolytic reactions. If severe bloating, distention, or abdominal pain occurs in patients receiving therapy with polyethylene glycol 3350 electrolyte solutions, administration should be slowed or temporarily discontinued until symptoms subside. If GI obstruction or perforation is suspected, appropriate tests should be performed to rule out these conditions before administration of polyethylene glycol 3350 electrolyte solution.

If rectal bleeding, nausea, bloating, cramping, or abdominal pain worsens, or the patient experiences diarrhea or requires more than 7 days of use of polyethylene glycol 3350 solution (MiraLAX®) for the treatment of constipation, the drug should be discontinued and a clinician notified.

■ **Mineral Oil** Adverse effects associated with the proper use of mineral oil are few. Seepage of mineral oil from the rectum may occur following oral or rectal administration, particularly when high doses are given. Seepage may cause soiling of the skin and clothing, anal irritation, and pruritus ani; impair normal rectal reflex mechanisms; and increase infection of anorectal lesions and interfere with their healing. Seepage of mineral oil may be minimized by reducing dosage.

Infrequently, aspiration of orally administered mineral oil may occur, particularly in young children and geriatric or debilitated patients, causing lipid pneumonitis.

Rarely, and only with chronic, oral use of plain mineral oil, absorption of fat-soluble vitamins, including provitamin A and vitamins A, D, and K, may be impaired. Hypoprothrombinemia and hemorrhagic disease of the newborn has occurred when mineral oil was chronically administered orally to pregnant women. Clinically important malabsorption of fat-soluble vitamins can be minimized by administering mineral oil on an empty stomach and limiting use of the drug to periods of less than 1 week.

Systemic absorption of mineral oil has caused foreign-body granulomatous reactions or paraffinomas, particularly in mesenteric lymph nodes and in the liver and spleen. Tissue depositions of mineral oil have simulated neoplasms and, in rare instances, carcinomas have been associated with industrial exposure to unrefined mineral oils or injection of refined mineral oil in animals and humans.

Oral administration of mineral oil is contraindicated in children younger than 6 years of age; in bedridden, geriatric, debilitated, or pregnant patients; and in patients with esophageal or gastric retention, dysphagia, or hiatal hernia.

■ **Saline Laxatives** Saline laxatives generally do not produce serious adverse effects except when used for prolonged periods or when overdoses are administered. The bitter taste of magnesium sulfate, which may cause nausea, can be masked by mixing the drug with lemon juice. Common adverse effects associated with sodium phosphates preparations include dehydration, abdominal pain, bloating, nausea, vomiting, headache, and dizziness. Rectal discomfort and burning sensations have occurred occasionally in patients receiving carbon dioxide-releasing suppositories, because of inadequate moistening of the suppository prior to insertion and/or the sudden stretch reflex caused by expanding gas.

Dehydration may result from repeated administration of hypertonic solutions of saline laxatives but can be avoided by administering the laxatives with sufficient fluid. Serious, potentially life-threatening electrolyte disturbances may occur with long-term use or overdosage of saline laxatives.

Magnesium Sulfate Preparations Symptoms of hypermagnesemia, including muscle weakness, ECG changes, sedation, and confusion, may occur when plasma magnesium concentrations exceed 1.5–2.2 mEq/L. When plasma magnesium concentrations exceed 4 mEq/L, deep tendon reflexes become depressed and at 12–15 mEq/L, respiratory paralysis may occur. Complete heart block occasionally occurs when plasma magnesium concentrations are elevated. In patients with impaired renal function, oral or rectal administration of 30 g (243 mEq magnesium) or greater of magnesium sulfate has been fatal. If hypermagnesemia occurs, urinary excretion of magnesium may be increased by administration of diuretics (e.g., furosemide, ethacrynic acid, ammonium chloride).

Sodium Phosphates Preparations **Overdosage.** Overdosage has been reported in adults and pediatric patients receiving nonprescription (over-the-counter, OTC) sodium phosphates preparations (i.e., oral solution, enema) for *self-medication* of occasional constipation.

In 1998, following reports of inadvertent overdosage and death associated with the use of large-size containers of sodium phosphates oral solution, FDA limited the container size of the drugs to no more than 90 mL when used as a nonprescription laxative. In addition, FDA required that the product information of nonprescription oral and rectal sodium phosphates preparations contain warning and direction statements to inform patients that exceeding the recommended dosages in a 24-hour period can be harmful. According to a subsequent FDA review of the safety of oral sodium phosphates preparations, use of more than 45 mL (usually 90 mL or more) of sodium phosphates oral solution in a 24-hour period and/or use in patients at increased risk for electrolyte abnormalities has been associated with severe electrolyte abnormalities, dehydration, metabolic acidosis, renal failure, tetany, and death.

Between 1957 and August 2013, a total of 54 cases of serious adverse effects associated with oral or rectal sodium phosphate laxative preparations, including severe dehydration, electrolyte abnormalities (e.g., hypernatremia, hyperphosphatemia, hypocalcemia), acute kidney injury, cardiac arrhythmias, and/or death, have been identified in the FDA Adverse Event Reporting System (AERS) and the medical literature. Nearly half (12/25) of adult cases and 3% (1/29) of pediatric cases resulted in a fatal outcome. The remaining nonfatal cases were life-threatening in more than two-thirds of affected adults and in all of the affected children; these included acute deterioration in respiratory status, mental status, and heart function; dialysis; suspected bowel perforation requiring surgery; abdominal distention requiring surgery; and residual neurologic defects. The severity of reported adverse events was similar regardless of whether the drugs were administered orally or rectally.

In the 50 cases (27 pediatric, 23 adult) for which the administered dose was reported, the majority of adverse events occurred in patients who received higher than recommended dosages in a 24-hour period (i.e., a single dose that was larger than recommended or more than one dose in a day) or in patients at increased risk of developing sodium phosphate-induced toxicity (e.g., those with dehydration, kidney disease, acute colitis, or delayed bowel emptying or receiving concomitant therapy with drugs that affect renal function [e.g., diuretics, angiotensin converting-enzyme [ACE] inhibitors, angiotensin II receptor antagonists, nonsteroidal anti-inflammatory agents [NSAIAs]). Forty percent (11/27) of the pediatric cases for which the dose was reported occurred in young children for whom FDA has not proposed a safe and effective dose (9 cases in children younger than 2 years of age receiving a rectal preparation, and 2 cases in children younger than 5 years of age receiving an oral preparation); these children received doses comparable to those recommended on the label for use in adults or older children. The duration of sodium phosphates use in the majority of the overdose cases was 1–2 days.

In light of these findings, FDA issued a drug safety communication in 2014, warning patients of possible harm from exceeding the recommended dosages of nonprescription sodium phosphates preparations. The agency stated that the maximum recommended oral or rectal dosage of nonprescription sodium phosphates preparations should not be exceeded, and that additional doses are not recommended within 24 hours, even in patients who do not have a bowel movement after receiving a dose. FDA also stated that clinicians should be cautious in recommending use of nonprescription sodium phosphates preparations in patients older than 55 years of age; patients with hypovolemia, decreased intravascular volume, kidney disease, decreased bowel transit time, or active colitis; and patients receiving drugs that affect renal perfusion or function (e.g., diuretics, ACE inhibitors, angiotensin II receptor antagonists, NSAIAs). FDA recommended that serum electrolytes and renal function be assessed in patients who may be at increased risk of serious adverse effects, including those who have retained a rectal dose for more than 30 minutes, who are vomiting, or who may have signs of dehydration. Nonprescription sodium phosphates preparations should not be used concomitantly with other laxatives containing sodium phosphate. Patients should be advised to discontinue sodium phosphates therapy and to immediately seek medical attention if symptoms of kidney injury (e.g., drowsiness; sluggishness; decreased urine; swelling of the ankles, feet, or legs) occur.

Nonprescription sodium phosphates oral solution should not be used for *self-medication* of occasional constipation in children 5 years of age or younger, and nonprescription sodium phosphates enema should not be used for such *self-medication* in children 2 years of age or younger. Sodium phosphates preparations should not be used for *self-medication* of occasional constipation for longer than 3 days.

Serious Adverse Effects Associated with Oral Sodium Phosphates. Electrolyte abnormalities (e.g., hyperphosphatemia, hypernatremia, hypocalcemia, hypokalemia) resulting in prolongation of the QT interval, generalized tonic-clonic seizures, and/or loss of consciousness have been reported rarely with sodium phosphates preparations. Renal failure, acute phosphate nephropathy, and nephrocalcinosis, often resulting in *permanent* renal impairment and sometimes requiring long-term dialysis, also have been reported rarely in patients receiving oral sodium phosphates preparations (i.e., oral solution, OsmoPrep® tablets) for bowel cleansing prior to colonoscopy or other procedures. Onset of kidney injury occurred from several days to several months after use of the oral sodium phosphates preparation. Although certain patients (e.g., patients older than 55 years of age; patients with hypovolemia, increased bowel transit time, bowel obstruction, active colitis, or kidney disease; patients receiving drugs that affect renal perfusion or function, such as diuretics, ACE inhibitors, angiotensin II receptor antagonists, and possibly NSAIAs) appear to be at increased risk of developing acute phosphate nephropathy, this adverse effect has occurred in patients *without* identifiable risk factors; however, FDA states that the possibility that some of these patients were dehydrated prior to or did not drink sufficient fluids after ingestion of oral sodium phosphates preparations cannot be ruled out. Death secondary to substantial fluid shifts, severe electrolyte abnormalities, and cardiac arrhythmias also has occurred in patients with renal impairment, patients with bowel perforation, and patients who misused or administered overdosages of sodium phosphates preparations prior to colonoscopy. Prolonged use or overdosage of phosphate laxatives may result in inorganic phosphate poisoning, which reduces plasma calcium concentrations; acidosis also may occur.

Regulatory Actions in 2008 Involving Oral Sodium Phosphates. Because of continued reports of acute renal injury in patients receiving oral sodium phosphates preparations for bowel cleansing, in 2008 FDA required the manufacturer to add a boxed warning to the labeling of OsmoPrep®, an oral sodium phosphates preparation available by prescription only.

Because acute phosphate nephropathy also had been reported following use of nonprescription oral sodium phosphates preparations (i.e., oral solutions) as bowel cleansing regimens (i.e., at dosages higher than those used for relief of constipation), FDA stated that these preparations should be used for bowel cleansing *only* when a prescription for such use has been issued by a clinician. In response to FDA's announcement, at least one manufacturer (i.e., Fleet Laboratories) ceased distribution and initiated a voluntary recall of some of its nonprescription oral sodium phosphates preparations used for bowel cleansing (i.e., Fleet® Phospho-soda® Oral Saline Laxative, Fleet® Phospho-soda® EZ-PREP® Bowel Cleansing System) effective December 12, 2008. Health-care professionals were advised to cease recommending oral sodium phosphates preparations for bowel cleansing and to remove them from pharmacy shelves; patients requesting a nonprescription oral sodium phosphates preparation for bowel cleansing should be advised to consult their clinician for an alternative bowel cleansing preparation (i.e., one available by prescription only).

Because nonprescription oral sodium phosphates preparations had not been associated with acute kidney injury when used as laxatives (i.e., for relief of constipation), FDA concluded that these preparations should continue to be available over-the-counter for such use.

Subsequent Regulatory Actions Involving Oral Sodium Phosphates. Despite efforts to inform healthcare professionals and consumers about the risks associated with the use of sodium phosphates oral solution for bowel cleansing, FDA reported in 2011 that the agency continued to receive reports of acute kidney injury following administration of usual recommended dosages of the drugs for *self-medication* (i.e., approximately 60 g of sodium phosphates [dibasic sodium phosphate and monobasic sodium phosphate salts] administered as two 45-mL doses given 12 hours apart, or approximately 50 g of sodium phosphates administered as a 45-mL dose initially, followed by a 30-mL dose 12 hours later).

A review of reports received from 1969–2005 revealed 33 reports of acute kidney injury (i.e., chronic kidney failure requiring hospitalization or dialysis, end-stage kidney disease requiring transplantation) associated with the use of nonprescription sodium phosphates oral solution for bowel cleansing; in most cases, acute kidney injury occurred within the recommended dosages for *self-medication* for bowel cleansing, including the lower-dose regimen (i.e., approximately 50 g of sodium phosphates administered as a 45-mL dose initially, followed by a 30-mL dose 10–12 hours later). Seizures, serious cardiac events, and death also have been reported with nonprescription sodium phosphates oral solution, although most of these cases occurred following use of dosages higher than those recommended for *self-medication* for bowel cleansing.

As a result of these findings, FDA has tentatively concluded that the usual recommended dosage of nonprescription oral sodium phosphates *for self-medication* for bowel cleansing based on professional labeling in an OTC monograph poses an unacceptable risk of serious adverse events. Therefore, in February 2011, the agency issued a proposed rule amending the tentative final monograph on nonprescription laxative drug products to classify the individual sodium phosphate salts (i.e., dibasic sodium phosphate, monobasic sodium phosphate) as *not* generally recognized as safe (GRAS) for bowel cleansing. In the proposed rule, FDA also suggested that the professional labeling for sodium phosphates (which discusses use of the drugs as part of a bowel cleansing regimen) be removed from the 1985 tentative final monograph for over-the-counter laxative drug products. In response to FDA's proposed rule, some manufacturers have removed the indication for bowel cleansing from labeling of nonprescription sodium phosphates preparations.

Precautions and Contraindications Involving Use of Oral Sodium Phosphates for Bowel Cleansing. FDA states that use of prescription-only oral sodium phosphates preparations as bowel cleansing regimens should be *avoided* in patients younger than 18 years of age; these agents should be used with caution as bowel cleansing regimens in patients older than 55 years of age; patients with dehydration, kidney disease, delayed bowel emptying, or acute colitis; and patients receiving drugs that may affect renal perfusion or function (e.g., diuretics, ACE inhibitors, angiotensin II receptor antagonists, possibly NSAIAs).

Furthermore, the manufacturer of sodium phosphates tablets (OsmoPrep®) states that these preparations (which are intended for use in cleansing the bowel prior to colonoscopy) should be used with caution in patients with renal disease or renal impairment (creatinine clearance less than 30 mL/minute), congestive heart failure, ascites, unstable angina, gastric retention, ileus, pseudo-obstruction of the bowel, severe chronic constipation, severe active ulcerative colitis, acute exacerbation of chronic inflammatory bowel disease, or hypomotility syndrome. Sodium phosphates tablets also should be used with caution in patients with a history of acute phosphate nephropathy or inflammatory bowel disease, known or suspected electrolyte disturbances (e.g., dehydration), an increased risk of arrhythmias (i.e., history of cardiomyopathy or uncontrolled arrhythmias, recent history of myocardial infarction, evidence of prolonged QT interval), or a history or an increased risk of seizures (e.g., those receiving drugs that lower the seizure threshold [e.g., tricyclic antidepressants], those in alcohol or benzodiazepine withdrawal, those with known or suspected hyponatremia). Electrolyte abnormalities (e.g., hypernatremia, hyperphosphatemia, hypokalemia, hypocalcemia) should be corrected prior to initiation of oral sodium phosphates therapy for bowel cleansing.

Patients receiving oral sodium phosphates preparations for bowel cleansing should receive instructions on preparation for the procedure and be informed of symptoms of acute phosphate nephropathy (e.g., malaise; lethargy; drowsiness; decreased amount of urine; swelling of the ankles, feet, and legs). Patients should be advised not to exceed recommended dosages and to *avoid* use of additional laxatives, particularly sodium phosphate-based preparations. Patients also should be advised to drink sufficient quantities of clear fluids before, during, and after bowel cleansing.

IV hydration in a hospital setting may be used to support frail patients who are unable to drink an appropriate volume of fluid or who do not have adequate assistance at home. The fluid intake volume necessary to minimize electrolyte abnormalities and to lower the risk of acute phosphate nephropathy is not known; furthermore, it is not known whether fluid intake should be individualized based on weight, age, gender, concomitant drug therapy, or medical conditions. However, some data indicate that use of an electrolyte or carbohydrate-electrolyte replacement solution may help minimize electrolyte abnormalities and hypovolemia associated with bowel cleansing with oral sodium phosphates preparations.

The manufacturer states that sodium phosphates tablets are contraindicated in patients with biopsy-proven acute phosphate nephropathy, GI obstruction, gastric bypass or stapling surgery, bowel perforation, toxic colitis, toxic megacolon, or known hypersensitivity to sodium phosphate salts or any ingredient in the formulation.

FDA recommends that baseline and postprocedural (e.g., postcolonoscopy) laboratory measurements, including serum concentrations of electrolytes (e.g., potassium, sodium), phosphate, calcium, creatinine, and BUN, be obtained in patients who may be at increased risk of acute phosphate nephropathy, including those with vomiting and/or manifestations of dehydration. FDA also recommends monitoring of the glomerular filtration rate in smaller, frail patients. In addition, the manufacturers of sodium phosphates tablets recommend that baseline and postprocedural laboratory measurements also be considered in patients with a history of renal impairment, history of acute phosphate nephropathy, known or suspected electrolyte disorders, seizures, arrhythmias, cardiomyopathy, prolonged QT interval, recent history of myocardial infarction, or known or suspected hyperphosphatemia, hypocalcemia, hypokalemia, or hypernatremia. In addition, baseline and postprocedural ECGs should be considered in patients at high risk of serious cardiac arrhythmias.

Precautions and Contraindications Involving Use of Oral Sodium Phosphates for Occasional Constipation. When oral sodium phosphates solution is used for *self-medication* for the relief of occasional constipation, patients should be advised to drink sufficient quantities of fluids and should be advised not to exceed recommended dosages. The manufacturer states that use of oral sodium phosphates solution for *self-medication* of occasional constipation should be avoided in patients with a history of kidney disease or clinically important renal function impairment, congestive heart failure, decreased intravascular volume, dehydration, or uncorrected electrolyte abnormalities and in children younger than 5 years of age. Patients should be advised to consult their clinician before initiating *self-medication* with oral sodium phosphates solution if they are under a clinician's care for any medical condition, if their dietary sodium intake is restricted, or if they are receiving therapy with other prescription or nonprescription drugs.

Precautions and Contraindications Involving Sodium Phosphates Enemas. Because dehydration, hypocalcemia, hyperphosphatemia, hypernatremia, hypokalemia, and acidosis may occur following administration of sodium phosphates rectal solutions, these preparations should be used with caution in patients with cardiac disease, colostomy, or preexisting electrolyte disturbances (e.g., patients receiving diuretics) and in those receiving drugs that may affect serum electrolyte concentrations (e.g., diuretics). If fluid or electrolyte disturbances occur or if sodium phosphates rectal solutions are retained, fluid and electrolyte balance should be restored promptly as necessary; serum concentrations of calcium, phosphorus, chloride, and sodium should be monitored. Children with anatomic abnormalities of the colon or with abnormal colonic motility (e.g., megacolon) appear to be at particular risk of developing marked, potentially life-threatening fluid and electrolyte disturbances and altered acid-base balance during therapy with phosphate laxatives.

Sodium phosphates rectal solutions are contraindicated in patients with congestive heart failure, clinically important renal function impairment, known or suspected GI obstruction, congenital or acquired megacolon, paralytic ileus, perforation, active inflammatory bowel disease, imperforate anus, dehydration, or increased absorption capacity or decreased elimination capacity; sodium phosphates rectal solutions also are contraindicated in children younger than 2 years of age and patients with known hypersensitivity to sodium phosphate salts or any ingredient in the formulation.

The manufacturer states that patients should be advised to consult their clinician before initiating *self-medication* with sodium phosphates rectal solutions for the relief of occasional constipation if they have kidney disease or if their dietary sodium intake is restricted. Recommended dosages of sodium phosphates rectal solutions should not be exceeded.

■ Stimulant Laxatives

In therapeutic oral doses, all stimulant laxatives may produce some degree of abdominal discomfort, nausea, mild cramps, griping, and/or faintness. Rectal administration of bisacodyl suspensions or suppositories may cause irritation and a sensation of burning of the rectal mucosa and mild proctitis. Some clinicians state that stimulant laxative suppositories or enemas should not be used in patients with abdominal cramps, anal or rectal fissures, or ulcerated hemorrhoids. Aloe (preparations containing aloe extract or aloe flower extract are no longer commercially available in the US), aloin, and castor oil reportedly cause excessive irritation of the colon, and violent purgation usually accompanies administration of therapeutic doses. Castor oil may rarely cause pelvic congestion.

Stimulant laxatives are habit-forming and long-term use of these drugs may result in laxative dependence and loss of normal bowel function. With long-term use or overdosage of stimulant laxatives, electrolyte disturbances including hypokalemia, hypocalcemia, metabolic acidosis or alkalosis, abdominal pain, diarrhea, malabsorption, weight loss, and protein-losing enteropathy may occur. Electrolyte disturbances may produce vomiting and muscle weakness; rarely, osteomalacia, secondary aldosteronism, and tetany may occur. Pathologic changes including structural damage to the myenteric plexus, severe and permanent interference with colonic motility, and hypertrophy of the muscularis mucosae may occur with chronic use. "Cathartic colon" with atony and dilation of the colon, especially of the right side, has occurred with habitual use (often for several years) and often resembles ulcerative colitis.

Anthraquinone laxatives may discolor colonic mucosa (melanosis coli), but this adverse effect is usually innocuous and reversible. Anthraquinones also produce a pink to red or brown to black discoloration of the urine; phenolphthalein (laxatives containing phenolphthalein are no longer commercially available in the US) colors alkaline urine pink to red. The diphenylmethane and anthraquinone laxatives may be distributed into the milk of nursing women but usually in amounts insufficient to produce a laxative effect. Although specific evidence of carcinogenic potential in humans is not available, danthron-containing preparations were withdrawn from the US market in 1987 because mice and rats developed intestinal and hepatic tumors following chronic administration of high dosages of the laxative. In addition, danthron and other anthraquinone laxatives have been shown to be mutagenic in some in vitro studies.

Phenolphthalein and dehydrocholic acid rarely have produced hypersensitivity reactions. Phenolphthalein allergy often has been manifested by dermal reactions including polychromatic, fixed skin eruptions with macules and nonspecific rashes, itching, burning, and pigmentation that may last for several months. Phenolphthalein allergy also has produced renal irritation, encephalitis, cardiac arrest, respiratory disturbances, and, rarely, death.

Current evidence indicates that phenolphthalein is potentially genotoxic and carcinogenic in humans. FDA reached this conclusion after reviewing animal data demonstrating carcinogenic activity of the drug in rodents and subsequent data indicating that the mechanism of this activity probably was secondary to a genotoxic effect. Drug exposures used in the in vivo and in vitro studies showing the carcinogenic and genotoxic effects of phenolphthalein were in the range of those that could occur with human laxative use. These findings indicate that chronic use of the drug could result in damage to the human genome (including p53, which is known to be a tumor suppressor gene) and could increase the risk of malignancy; some human cancers have been associated with alterations of the p53 gene. As a result, all preparations containing phenolphthalein for *self-medication* (over-the-counter [OTC] use) are no longer generally recognized as safe and effective. Therefore, US manufacturers have reformulated phenolphthalein-containing preparations to include other laxatives.

As part of its ongoing review of OTC drug products, the FDA has determined that existing data are insufficient to establish safety and efficacy of aloe and cascara sagrada as stimulant laxatives. This determination was made after no comments or data were submitted in response to the FDA's request for mutagenicity, genotoxicity, and carcinogenicity data on these agents. Therefore, any OTC drug product containing laxative ingredients derived from aloe (i.e., aloe extract, aloe flower extract) or cascara sagrada (i.e., casanthranol, cascara fluidextract aromatic, or cascara sagrada bark, extract, or fluidextract) is considered by the FDA to be misbranded. Effective November 5, 2002, any such OTC drug product introduced or initially delivered for introduction into interstate commerce is considered to be misbranded, and manufacturers are required to reformulate preparations containing aloe or cascara sagrada to delete and/or replace these ingredients. In addition, previously marketed OTC products containing aloe or cascara sagrada may not be repackaged or relabeled after this date.

Hepatotoxicity may result if sufficient tannic acid is absorbed from bisacodyl tannex laxatives. Bisacodyl tannex should be used with caution, if at all, in patients receiving multiple enemas or in those with extensive ulceration of the colon since increased tannic acid absorption may occur.

In general, use of stimulant laxatives should be avoided in children younger than 6–10 years of age. Because the possibility of tannic acid absorption has not been studied adequately in children younger than 10 years of age, bisacodyl tannex is contraindicated in these patients. Castor oil is contraindicated in pregnant or menstruating women. Safe use of bisacodyl tannex during pregnancy has not been established.

■ **Stool Softeners** Adverse effects associated with the use of stool softeners are rare. Occasionally, mild, transitory GI cramping pains or rashes may occur. Irritation of the throat has occurred following oral administration of docusate sodium solutions. In one study, docusate sodium was found to be toxic to hepatic cells in vitro.

Drug Interactions

By increasing intestinal motility, all laxatives may potentially decrease transit time of concomitantly administered oral drugs and thereby decrease their absorption.

Mineral oil may impair absorption of many orally administered drugs including fat-soluble vitamins (i.e., vitamins A, D, E, and K), carotene, oral contraceptives, and coumarin and indandione derivative anticoagulants. By mixing with nonabsorbable sulfonamides (e.g., phthalylsulfathiazole) in the feces, mineral oil may interfere with antibacterial activity of these drugs. Patients receiving any of these drugs should be discouraged from ingesting more than therapeutic amounts of mineral oil and from taking these drugs concurrently with mineral oil.

Stool softeners (i.e., docusate salts) theoretically may enhance the absorption of many orally administered drugs. Docusate sodium increases the extent of mineral oil absorption and the rate of phenolphthalein (laxatives containing phenolphthalein are no longer commercially available in the US) absorption. Greater intestinal mucosal damage has reportedly occurred following concomitant administration of aspirin and docusate sodium than occurs with aspirin alone. Oral stool softeners should not be administered concurrently with oral mineral oil, and some clinicians recommend that stool softeners not be administered concurrently with any oral drugs having low therapeutic indices.

Magnesium hydroxide, in antacid preparations also containing aluminum hydroxide, has been shown to decrease the rate and extent of chlordiazepoxide, chlorpromazine, dicumarol, digoxin, and isoniazid absorption. The effect of magnesium hydroxide laxative preparations on drug bioavailability is not known.

Cellulose binds orally administered digitalis, nitrofurantoin, and salicylates in the GI tract. Although the clinical importance of these interactions has not been determined for other cellulose derivatives such as methylcellulose, patients taking bulk-forming laxatives concurrently with digitalis, nitrofurantoin, or salicylates should consult their physician or pharmacist before initiating or discontinuing use of these laxatives. Some clinicians recommend that bulk-forming laxatives be administered at least 3 hours after or before administration of these drugs.

Several manufacturers of polyethylene glycol 3350 electrolyte solution suggest that other oral drugs should be administered at least 1 hour before polyethylene glycol 3350 electrolyte solutions.

Laboratory Test Interferences

By discoloring the urine, anthraquinone laxatives and phenolphthalein (laxatives containing phenolphthalein are no longer commercially available in the US) may produce an apparent increase in the urinary excretion of phenolsulfonphthalein (PSP). These laxatives may also give false-positive test results for urinary urobilinogen and for estrogens when measured by the Kober procedure.

Dosage and Administration

■ **Administration** Laxatives are usually administered orally and in conjunction with adequate fluid intake. Rectal suppositories or enemas may be used when oral laxatives are not effective or to prepare for surgery, or radiologic or colonoscopic procedures.

Suppositories should be moistened with lukewarm water before being inserted high into the rectum and retained in the rectum for as long as possible. Before administering laxative enemas, the patient should lie on his left side with knees bent or should kneel on the bed with the head and chest lowered and forward until the left side of the face is resting on the surface of the bed. With steady pressure, the enema nozzle should be inserted into the rectum, with the nozzle toward the navel, and the container squeezed until the entire dose is expelled. Enema fluids, if properly introduced, usually provide adequate evacuation if retained until definite lower abdominal cramping is felt.

■ **Dosage** Laxatives should be used as infrequently as possible, at the lowest effective dosage level, and usually for periods not exceeding one week; laxatives should be used for longer periods only under the management of a physician and as part of a carefully planned therapeutic regimen.

For further information on chemistry, pharmacology, pharmacokinetics, uses, and dosage and administration of the Cathartics and Laxatives, see the individual monographs in 56:12.

†Use is not currently included in the labeling approved by the US Food and Drug Administration

Anthraquinone Laxatives

■ The anthraquinone group of stimulant laxatives includes the plant-derived compounds aloe (preparations containing aloe are no longer commercially available in the US), cascara sagrada (preparations containing cascara sagrada are no longer commercially available in the US), frangula, and senna.

Dosage and Administration

■ **Administration** Anthraquinone laxatives are administered orally, usually in a single dose at bedtime.

■ **Dosage** ***Senna*** Doses of the calcium sennosides, standardized senna concentrate, and standardized senna fruit extract are expressed in terms of sennosides.

The usual adult oral dose of senna is 0.5–2 g. The usual oral dosage of sennosides in adults and children 12 years of age and older is 12–50 mg once or twice daily. The usual laxative dosage of the senna preparations is 50% of the adult dosage for children 6–11 years of age, or 33% of the adult dosage for children 2–5 years of age.

When used to evacuate the bowel prior to colonic radiologic examinations, a dose of standardized senna fruit extract or standardized senna concentrate, to provide 105–157.5 mg of sennosides, should be administered orally 12–14 hours before the examination. To prepare for the examination, the patient should receive a residue-free diet one day before the examination; castor oil may be administered 16 hours before the examination, and a cleansing enema (e.g., tap water, soap suds, saline laxative, bisacodyl tannex enema) administered rectally on the day of the examination. Alternatively, magnesium citrate and magnesium sulfate (e.g., Citralax®) or commercially available tablets of standardized senna concentrate in fixed-combination with docusate sodium may be administered the day before the examination, and a suppository containing bisacodyl administered rectally on the day of the examination.

Pharmacokinetics

■ **Absorption** Following oral administration, the anthraquinone laxatives are absorbed only slightly from the small intestine. In the colon, most of the glycosides are hydrolyzed by the enzymes of colonic flora to the pharmacologically active, free anthraquinones.

Orally administered anthraquinone laxatives usually produce laxation within 6–12 hours but the effect may not occur for 24 hours. Rectally administered anthraquinone suppositories produce evacuation of the colon within 30 minutes to 2 hours.

■ **Distribution** Distribution of anthraquinones and their metabolites into body tissues and fluids has not been fully characterized. The drugs may be distributed into bile, saliva, and the colonic mucosa. Distribution of anthraquinones into milk remains controversial; however, if the drugs are distributed into milk, it is unlikely that they appear in sufficient amounts to affect nursing infants. Although an increase in bowel activity in infants nursed by women receiving aloe (preparations containing aloe are no longer commercially available in the US), cascara sagrada (preparations containing cascara sagrada are no longer commercially available in the US), or senna preparations has been suggested, there is insufficient supporting documentation. Some studies indicate that nursing infants are not affected by maternal ingestion of usual doses of senna and that senna is not detectable in milk with usual doses.

■ **Elimination** The absorbed anthraquinones are metabolized in the liver. Anthraquinones and their metabolites are excreted in feces via biliary elimination and/or in urine.

Chemistry and Stability

■ **Chemistry** The anthraquinone group of stimulant laxatives includes the plant-derived compounds aloe (preparations containing aloe are no longer commercially available in the US), cascara sagrada (preparations containing cascara sagrada are no longer commercially available in the US), and senna. The active laxative principles are hydroxymethylanthraquinone derivatives that occur naturally in plants as glycosides. The amount of active drug obtained from the plants may vary widely with seasonal and other conditions.

Aloe Aloe (no longer commercially available in the US) is the dried latex of the leaves of various species of *Aloe* found in the West Indies and Africa. Aloe differs in its texture and color depending on the species of *Aloe;* the drug has a nauseating, bitter taste and a characteristic, somewhat sour and disagreeable odor. Aloin is a microcrystalline powder consisting of a mixture of active ingredients (chiefly of barbaloin and isobarbaloin) extracted from aloe.

Cascara Sagrada Cascara sagrada (or cascara) (preparations containing cascara sagrada are no longer commercially available in the US) is the dried bark of the buckthorn tree, *Rhamnus purshiana,* and occurs as flattened or transversely curved pieces or as a coarse, moderate yellowish-brown to dusky, yellowish-orange powder. Cascara sagrada has a distinct odor and a bitter and slightly acrid taste. The main active principles of cascara sagrada are 4 primary anthraquinone glycosides, cascarosides A and B (glycosides of barbaloin) and cascarosides C and D (glycosides of chrysaloin). Cascara sagrada extract, fluidextract, and aromatic fluidextract are obtained by percolating and evaporating coarse cascara sagrada powder. Cascara sagrada extract occurs as a fine powder; *1 gram of cascara sagrada extract represents 3 grams of cascara sagrada.* The fluidextract and aromatic fluidextract are hydroalcoholic solutions of cascara sagrada; the fluidextract is bitter-tasting, but the aromatic fluidextract's palatability is improved by addition of magnesium oxide. *Cascara sagrada fluidextract and aromatic cascara fluidextract each represent in 1 mL the active principles from 1 gram of cascara sagrada.*

Casanthranol (preparations containing casanthranol are no longer commercially available in the US) is a purified, water-soluble mixture of the anthranol glycosides extracted from cascara sagrada. Casanthranol occurs as a light tan to brown, amorphous, hygroscopic powder and is freely soluble in water, with some residue. Each gram of casanthranol contains not less than 200 mg of total hydroxyanthracene derivatives, calculated on the dried basis as cascaroside A, of which not less than 80% of the derivatives consists of cascarosides (calculated as cascaroside A).

Senna Senna, which may be unground or powdered, consists of the dried leaflet of *Cassia acutifolia* or of *Cassia angustifolia*. The primary active cathartic principles of senna are the stereoisomeric glucosides, sennosides A and B. Sennosides (formerly known as sennosides A and B) is a partially purified natural complex of anthraquinone glucosides and is prepared from *Cassia angustifolia* or *C. acutifolia* as calcium salts. The calcium salts of sennosides occur as a brownish powder. Standardized senna concentrate is a dry powder prepared from whole deseeded senna pod. Standardized senna fruit extract is a liquid extract obtained from whole senna pod. Senna fluidextract is obtained by percolating and evaporating coarse senna (leaf) powder and senna syrup is prepared from the fluidextract and syrup.

■ **Stability** ***Senna*** Senna fluidextract should be stored in tight, light-resistant containers and exposure to temperatures above 40°C should be avoided.

For further information on pharmacology, uses, cautions, drug interactions, laboratory test interferences, and dosage and administration of anthraquinone laxatives, see the Cathartics and Laxatives General Statement 56:12.

Preparations

Excipients in commercially available drug preparations may have clinically important effects in some individuals; consult specific product labeling for details.

Senna Leaf

Oral		
Powder*		
Tablets	equivalent to Senna 600 mg	**Black Draught®**, Monticello

*available from one or more manufacturer, distributor, and/or repackager by generic (nonproprietary) name

Senna Concentrate, Standardized

Oral		
Pieces, chewable	15 mg Sennosides	**Ex-Lax® Chocolated,** Novartis
Powder	15 mg Sennosides per 3 g	**Senokot® Granules,** Purdue
Tablets	8.6 mg Sennosides*	**Nature's Remedy®**, Block
		Senexon®, Rugby
		Senna-Gen®, Teva
		Sennatural®, G&W
		Senokot®, Purdue Frederick
	15 mg Sennosides	**Ex-Lax® Regular Strength,** Novartis
	17 mg Sennosides	**SenokotXTRA®**, Purdue Frederick
	25 mg Sennosides	**Ex-Lax® Maximum Strength,** Novartis

*available from one or more manufacturer, distributor, and/or repackager by generic (nonproprietary) name

Senna Concentrate, Standardized Combinations

Oral		
Powder	123 mg/g Sennosides with Psyllium Hydrophilic Mucilloid 542 mg/g	**Perdiem® Overnight Relief,** Novartis
Tablets	8.6 mg Sennosides with Docusate Sodium 50 mg	**Gentlax® S,** Purdue Frederick
		Peri-Colace®, Purdue
		Senokot® S, Purdue Frederick

Senna Fluidextract

Oral		
Solution	3 mg Sennosides per mL	**Dr. Caldwell® Senna Laxative,** Denison
		Fletcher's® Castoria®, Mentholatum Company

Senna Fruit Extract, Standardized

Oral		
Solution	8.8 mg Sennosides per 5 mL	**Senna X-Prep® Liquid,** Purdue Frederick
		Senokot® Children's Syrup, Purdue Frederick
		Senokot® Syrup, Purdue Frederick

Sennosides Combinations

Oral		
Tablets	Sennosides 20 mg with Docusate Sodium 100 mg	**Correctol® 50 Plus,** Schering-Plough
Tablets, film-coated	Sennosides 10 mg with Docusate Sodium 65 mg	**Ex-Lax® Gentle Strength Caplets®**, Novartis

Bisacodyl

■ Diphenylmethane laxatives (e.g., bisacodyl) are stimulant laxatives.

Dosage and Administration

■ **Administration** Bisacodyl is administered orally. Bisacodyl also is administered rectally as a suppository or enema. Bisacodyl tannex is administered rectally as an enema. For occasional use as an oral laxative, bisacodyl should be administered the evening before a morning bowel movement is desired. Rectal bisacodyl suppositories and enemas may be administered at the time a bowel movement is desired. To avoid gastric irritation and the possibility of vomiting, enteric-coated bisacodyl tablets must be swallowed whole and not crushed, chewed, or taken within 1 hour of antacids or milk.

■ **Dosage** The recommended dosages of the diphenylmethane laxatives should not be exceeded.

Bisacodyl and Bisacodyl Tannex The usual oral laxative dosage of bisacodyl for adults and children 12 years of age and older is 5–15 mg daily given as a single dose. Children older than 3 years of age may be given bisacodyl in an oral dosage of 5–10 mg or 0.3 mg/kg daily given as a single dose. The usual rectal dosage of bisacodyl for adults and children 12 years of age and older is 10 mg daily given as a single dose, and for children 2–11 years of age the usual rectal dosage is 5–10 mg (one-half to one suppository) daily given as a single dose. For children younger than 2 years of age, the usual rectal dosage is 5 mg (one-half suppository) daily given as a single dose.

For surgical, radiologic, proctoscopic, or sigmoidoscopic preparation, the usual dose of bisacodyl may be given orally on the night preceding and rectally on the morning of surgery or examination. Up to 30 mg of the drug may be given orally to adults when complete evacuation of the colon is required for special procedures. In preparation for barium sulfate enemas, the patient should not eat following administration of the tablets and a bisacodyl suppository should be given 1–2 hours before the procedure. Preparatory regimens using magnesium citrate, which acts mainly on the small intestine, in addition to administration of the usual oral and rectal dose of bisacodyl have also been used. The usual dose of bisacodyl as a rectal suppository may be used to cleanse the colon prior to delivery if administered at least 2 hours before onset of the second stage of labor.

Alternatively, bisacodyl tannex may be used prior to radiologic examinations or sigmoidoscopic or proctoscopic procedures. Patients should receive a residue-free diet one day before, and 30–60 mL of castor oil should be administered 16 hours before the examination or procedure. A cleansing enema is prepared by dissolving bisacodyl tannex equivalent to 1.5 mg of bisacodyl and 2.5 g of tannic acid (one packet of the commercially available bisacodyl tannex product) in 1 liter of lukewarm water. When used as a radiopaque enema adjuvant, bisacodyl tannex equivalent to 1.5–3 mg of bisacodyl (1–2 packets of the commercially available product) is dissolved in 1 liter of barium sulfate suspension. The concentration of bisacodyl tannex should not exceed 0.5% (2 packets of the commercially available product per liter). The cleansing enema containing bisacodyl tannex may be administered on the day of the examination. If necessary, the cleansing enema may be repeated, but the total dosage for one entire colonic examination (including the cleansing enema) should not exceed 4.5 mg of bisacodyl and 7.5 g of tannic acid (3 packets of the commercially available preparation), and no more than 6 mg of bisacodyl and 10 g of tannic acid (4 packets of the commercially available product) should be administered during a 72-hour period.

Cautions

Diphenylmethane laxatives share the toxic potentials of other stimulant laxatives, and the usual precautions of such laxative therapy should be observed. (See Cautions in the Cathartics and Laxatives General Statement 56:12.)

Since current evidence indicates that phenolphthalein is potentially genotoxic and carcinogenic in humans (see Cautions: Stimulant Laxatives, in the Cathartics and Laxatives General Statement 56:12), all preparations containing phenolphthalein for *self-medication* (over-the-counter [OTC] use) are no longer generally recognized as safe and effective. Therefore, US manufacturers have reformulated phenolphthalein-containing preparations to include other laxatives.

Pharmacology

Bisacodyl shares the actions of the stimulant laxatives. The tannic acid present in the bisacodyl tannex complex precipitates protein and its astringent effect decreases mucus secretion in the large intestine. Tannic acid also reportedly facilitates adherence of contrast media to mucous membranes, but this is disputed by some clinicians. Although some reports state that tannic acid increases evacuation of the colon, others state that its astringent effect produces constipation.

Pharmacokinetics

Absorption of bisacodyl or bisacodyl tannex is minimal following oral or rectal administration. Any bisacodyl that is absorbed is metabolized in the liver and excreted in the urine and/or distributed into milk. Tannic acid may be absorbed following rectal administration; however, very little is known about the degree of absorption and circumstances under which absorption may occur with bisacodyl tannex.

Following oral administration of therapeutic dosages of diphenylmethane derivatives, evacuation is produced in 6–8 hours. Rectally administered bisacodyl or bisacodyl tannex produces evacuation of the colon within 15 minutes to 1 hour.

Chemistry and Stability

■ **Chemistry**

Bisacodyl and Bisacodyl Tannex Bisacodyl and bisacodyl tannex are diphenylmethane derivative stimulant laxatives.

Bisacodyl occurs as a white to off-white, crystalline powder and is practically insoluble in water and sparingly soluble in alcohol. Bisacodyl tannex is a complex of bisacodyl and tannic acid which occurs as a light tan, microcrystalline powder and is very soluble in water and in alcohol.

■ **Stability** ***Bisacodyl and Bisacodyl Tannex*** Bisacodyl rectal suppositories and enteric-coated tablets should be stored at less than 30°C. Reconstituted solutions of bisacodyl tannex should be used immediately following preparation.

For further information on pharmacology, uses, cautions, drug interactions, laboratory test interferences, and dosage and administration of the diphenylmethane laxatives, see the Cathartics and Laxatives General Statement 56:12.

Preparations

Excipients in commercially available drug preparations may have clinically important effects in some individuals; consult specific product labeling for details.

Bisacodyl

Oral		
Tablets, enteric-coated	5 mg*	**Alophen® Pills,** Numark
		Bisac-Evac®, G&W
		Bisacodyl Enteric-coated Tablets
		Carter's Little Pills®, Carter
		Correctol® Caplets®, Schering-Plough
		Correctol® Tablets, Schering-Plough
		Dulcolax®, Novartis
		Feen-A-Mint®, Schering-Plough
		Fleet® Bisacodyl, Fleet
Rectal		
Suppositories	10 mg*	**Bisac-Evac®,** G&W
		Bisacodyl Suppositories
		Bisacodyl Uniserts®, Upsher-Smith
		Dulcolax®, Novartis
		Fleet® Bisacodyl, Fleet
Suspension	10 mg/30 mL	**Fleet® Bisacodyl Enema,** Fleet

*available from one or more manufacturer, distributor, and/or repackager by generic (nonproprietary) name

Bisacodyl Combinations

4 Tablets, enteric-coated, Bisacodyl 5 mg (Dulcolax®) 1 Suppository, rectal, Bisacodyl 10 mg (Dulcolax®)	**Dulcolax® Bowel Prep Kit,** Novartis

Bulk-Forming Laxatives

■ Cellulose derivatives (methylcellulose), malt soup extract, and psyllium preparations are bulk-forming laxatives.

Dosage and Administration

■ **Administration** Bulk-forming laxatives are administered orally. Commercially available powders, flakes, granules, tablets, and liquids should be dissolved and/or diluted according to the instructions of the manufacturer. In the treatment of constipation, at least one full glass (250 mL) of liquid should be administered with each laxative dose. When used to increase the bulk of stools in patients with chronic, watery diarrhea, one manufacturer suggests that one-third of a glass (80 mL) of liquid be administered with each dose.

■ **Dosage** Bulk-forming laxatives are usually administered 1–3 times daily. To reduce the risk of esophageal obstruction in patients receiving large (e.g., the maximum daily dosage recommended by the manufacturer) dosages of bulk-forming laxatives, these laxatives should be administered in divided doses instead of a single daily dose. The usual dosages for the individual bulk-forming laxatives are below; for dosages in children younger than the ages listed, a physician should be consulted.

Methylcellulose **Adults and Children 12 and Older.** The usual dosage is up to 6 g daily given in divided doses of 0.45–3 g per dose.

Children 6–11 Years of Age. The usual dosage is up to 3 g daily given in divided doses of 0.45–1.5 g per dose.

Malt Soup Extract **Adults and Children 12 and Older.** The usual dosage is up to 64 g daily given in divided doses of 3–32 g per dose.

Children 6–11 Years of Age. The usual dosage is up to 32 g daily given in divided doses of 3–16 g per dose.

Children 2–5 Years of Age. The usual dosage is up to 16 g daily given in divided doses of 3–8 g per dose.

Psyllium Preparations **Adults and Children 12 and Older.** The usual dosage is up to 30 g daily given in divided doses of 2.5–7.5 g per dose.

Children 6–11 Years of Age. The usual dosage is up to 15 g daily given in divided doses of 2.5–3.75 g per dose.

Constipation and pain from diverticular disease appear to respond to daily doses of about 18 g of dietary bran.

Cautions

■ **Precautions and Contraindications** Potentially severe hypersensitivity reactions, including rhinoconjunctivitis, acute bronchospasm, and anaphylaxis, can occur in susceptible individuals (e.g., those with psyllium sensitivity or suffering from respiratory disorders) following inhalation of psyllium dust particles. Therefore, inhalation of psyllium hydrophilic mucilloid particles should be avoided. To minimize exposure and, therefore, sensitization to airborne particles of psyllium, one manufacturer suggests that health-care personnel dispense powdered psyllium preparations with a spoon rather than pouring them directly from the container into the glass for administration. In some cases, resassignment of health-care personnel to areas (e.g., non-geriatric units) where use of bulk powder formulations of psyllium was minimal has been necessary.

Individuals with phenylketonuria (i.e., homozygous genetic deficiency of phenylalanine hydroxylase) and other individuals who must restrict their intake of phenylalanine should be warned that each 3.4-g dose of psyllium hydrophilic mucilloid given as Metamucil® Smooth Texture Sugar Free Orange Flavor contains aspartame (NutraSweet®) which is metabolized in the GI tract to provide about 25 mg of phenylalanine following oral administration.

For a complete discussion of the precautions associated with bulk-forming laxatives, see Cautions in the Cathartics and Laxatives General Statement 56:12.

Pharmacokinetics

Bulk-forming laxatives generally are not absorbed from the GI tract. However, malt soup extract has been reported to be hydrolyzed in the colon, absorbed, and then metabolized by the liver. A laxative effect of the bulk-forming laxatives is usually apparent within 12–24 hours, but the full effect may not be apparent for 2–3 days.

Chemistry

Cellulose derivatives (methylcellulose), malt soup extract, and psyllium preparations are bulk-forming laxatives.

■ **Methylcellulose** Methylcellulose occurs as a white, fibrous powder or granules. When mixed with water, methylcellulose produces clear to opalescent viscous colloidal suspensions; the drug is insoluble in alcohol.

■ **Malt Soup Extract** Malt soup extract is obtained from the grain of one or more varieties of barley and contains 73% maltose, 12% other polymeric carbohydrates, 7% protein, and 1.5% potassium in addition to small amounts of calcium, phosphorus, magnesium, and vitamins. The drug swells in water.

■ **Psyllium Preparations** Psyllium preparations are obtained from the seeds of a variety of species of *Plantago*. Plantago or psyllium seed is the cleaned, dried, ripe seed of *Plantago psyllium* and related species. The coating of the dried, ripe *Plantago* seed has a high content of hemicellulose mucillages; psyllium hydrophilic mucilloid, obtained from the coating of *Plantago ovata,* contains about 50% hemicellulose.

For further information on pharmacology, uses, cautions, drug interactions, and dosage and administration of the bulk-forming laxatives, see the Cathartics and Laxatives General Statement 56:12.

Preparations

Excipients in commercially available drug preparations may have clinically important effects in some individuals; consult specific product labeling for details.

Malt Soup Extract

Oral		
Powder	1 g/g	**Maltsupex®**, Wallace
Solution	5.3 g/5 mL	**Maltsupex®**, Wallace
Tablets	750 mg	**Maltsupex®**, Wallace

Malt Soup Extract Combinations

Oral		
Powder	500 mg/g with Psyllium Hydrophilic Mucilloid 500 mg/g	**Syllamalt®**, Wallace

Methylcellulose

Powder*

Oral		
Powder	105 mg/g	**Citrucel®**, GlaxoSmithKline
	196 mg/g	**Citrucel®**, GlaxoSmithKline

*available from one or more manufacturer, distributor, and/or repackager by generic (nonproprietary) name

Psyllium Hydrophilic Mucilloid

Oral		
Pieces, chewable	3 g/piece	**Metamucil® Wafers,** Procter & Gamble
Powder	250 mg/g	**Metamucil® Smooth Texture,** Procter & Gamble
	273 mg/g	**Metamucil® Coarse Milled,** Procter & Gamble
	390 mg/g	**Serutan® Toasted Granules,** Numark
	429 mg/g	**Metamucil® Coarse Milled,** Procter & Gamble
	500 mg/g	**Genfiber®**, Teva
		Konsyl-D®, Konsyl Pharmaceuticals
		Modane® Bulk, Savage
		Natural Vegetable Laxative Powder, Major
		Reguloid®, Rugby
		Syllact®, Wallace
	517 mg/g	**Metamucil® Sugar Free Smooth Texture,** Procter & Gamble
	555 mg/g	**Metamucil® Sugar Free Smooth Texture,** Procter & Gamble
	672 mg/g	**Perdiem® Fiber,** Novartis
	946 mg/g	**Hydrocil® Instant,** Numark
	1 g/g	**Konsyl®**, Konsyl Pharmaceuticals

Psyllium Hydrophilic Mucilloid Combinations

Oral		
Powder	542 mg/g with Sennosides 123 mg/g	**Perdiem® Overnight Relief,** Novartis

Selected Revisions January 2009,

Hyperosmotic Laxatives

■ Glycerin (glycerol), polyethylene glycol (PEG), and sorbitol are hyperosmotic laxatives.

Dosage and Administration

Prior to bowel cleansing, a copy of the patient information (containing careful instructions on the proper methods of reconstitution and administration of the laxatives) provided by the manufacturer should be given to the patient.

■ **Reconstitution and Administration** Glycerin solutions and suppositories should be administered rectally. Polyethylene glycol 3350 electrolyte solutions are administered orally or through a nasogastric tube. Solutions of sorbitol (25–30%) usually are administered rectally.

Oral or Nasogastric Administration (Polyethylene glycol 3350, Polyethylene glycol 3350 with Electrolytes) **Reconstitution.** When polyethylene glycol is used for constipation, polyethylene glycol 3350 powder for oral solution (MiraLAX®) should be reconstituted with 120–240 mL of water (cold, room temperature, or hot).

When polyethylene glycol is used for bowel cleansing, polyethylene glycol 3350 powder (with electrolytes) for oral or nasogastric solution should be reconstituted with the appropriate amount of lukewarm water as directed by the manufacturer. The solution should be shaken vigorously until the ingredients are dissolved; additional ingredients (e.g., flavorings other than those provided by the manufacturers) are not recommended.

The reconstituted solutions should be refrigerated. Palatability of the oral solution may be increased if the reconstituted solution is chilled prior to administration; however, a chilled polyethylene glycol 3350 electrolyte solution is *not* recommended for infants.

Administration of Polyethylene Glycol 3350 Electrolyte Solutions for Bowel Cleansing. Patients should fast for approximately 3 or 4 hours before administration of polyethylene glycol 3350 electrolyte solution. In addition, patients should be advised not to eat solid foods for at least 2 hours prior to administration of the drug. Polyethylene glycol 3350 electrolyte solutions are administered orally, but may be given through a nasogastric tube if patients are unwilling or unable to drink the solution. Rapid drinking of each polyethylene glycol 3350 electrolyte solution portion is preferred to drinking small amounts continuously.

Polyethylene glycol 3350 electrolyte solutions may be given by single-dose regimens (usually on the evening prior to the colonoscopy [e.g., 6 p.m.]) or, if the procedure is scheduled for midmorning or later, patients should be allowed 3 hours for drinking the solution and 1 hour for complete bowel evacuation). Alternatively, a divided-dose regimen (usually consuming a portion on the evening prior to the colonoscopy and the remaining solution on the morning of the colonoscopy) may be used. Clinical studies suggest that the divided-dose polyethylene glycol 3350 electrolyte solution regimen (e.g., 2–3 L the evening before and 1 L the morning of the procedure) is superior to the standard single-dose regimen (e.g., 4 L administered on the evening prior to the procedure). In one study, polyethylene glycol 3350 electrolyte solution consumption less than 5 hours before colonoscopy was superior to a regimen administered 19 hours or more before the procedure. If a patient has an afternoon colonoscopy, a portion of the polyethylene glycol 3350 solution should be administered on the morning of the colonoscopy to improve bowel cleansing results.

Administration Precautions for Polyethylene glycol 3350 Electrolyte Solutions. Polyethylene glycol 3350 electrolyte solutions should be used with caution in patients with impaired gag reflex, unconscious or semiconscious patients, and those prone to regurgitation or aspiration; these patients should be observed during administration, especially if the solution is administered through a nasogastric tube.

If severe discomfort or distention occurs while consuming polyethylene glycol 3350 electrolyte solutions, administration of the drug should be slowed or temporarily discontinued until symptoms abate.

Rectal Administration (Glycerin) Regular glycerin suppositories should be moistened with lukewarm water before insertion high into the rectum. (See Dosage and Administration: Administration, in the Cathartics and Laxatives General Statement 56:12.) With steady pressure, the tip of the suppository should be inserted gently high into rectum. Patients should be instructed to retain the suppository for 15 minutes; melting of the suppository is not required to produce laxative action.

Before administering glycerin laxative enemas, the patient should initially lie on the left side with the right knee bent and arms resting comfortably or should kneel on the bed with the head and chest lowered and forward until the left side of the face is resting on the surface of the bed. With steady pressure, the enema nozzle should be inserted into the rectum with side-to-side movement with the tip pointing toward navel until the entire dose is expelled. While squeezing the container, the tip should be removed from rectum and the unit discarded. Use of glycerin laxative enemas should be discontinued if resistance is encountered. Enema fluids, if properly introduced, usually provide adequate evacuation if retained until definite lower abdominal cramping is felt. (See Dosage and Administration: Administration, in the Cathartics and Laxatives General Statement 56:12.)

■ **Dosage** ***Constipation*** For the treatment of constipation, hyperosmotic laxatives should be administered only at infrequent intervals in single doses at the lowest effective dosage level, and usually for periods not exceeding 1 week; laxatives should be used for longer periods only under the management of a clinician and as part of a carefully planned therapeutic regimen. (See Dosage and Administration: Dosage, in the Cathartics and Laxatives General Statement 56:12.)

Only extremely high oral doses of sorbitol (25 g daily) or glycerin exert laxative action. (See Pharmacology: Hyperosmotic Laxatives, in the Cathartics and Laxatives General Statement 56:12.)

Glycerine. For the treatment of constipation, the usual rectal dose of glycerin for adults is 2–3 g as a suppository or 5.6–15.3 g (5–15 mL) as an enema. Children 2 to younger than 6 years of age may receive 1–1.2 g as a suppository or 2.3 g (2.3 mL) as an enema; children 6 years of age and older may be given 2–2.1 g as a suppository or 5.6 g (5.5 mL) as an enema.

If a bowel movement does not occur after using the glycerin suppository or enema, the drug should be discontinued.

Sorbitol. For the treatment of constipation, the usual rectal dose of sorbitol as a 25–30% solution is (administered as enemas) 120 mL for adults and children 12 years of age and older or 30–60 mL for children 2–11 years of age.

When used as an adjunct to sodium polystyrene sulfonate resin, 15 mL of a 70% sorbitol solution may be administered orally until diarrhea occurs or 20–100 mL of the solution may be used as an oral vehicle for the resin. Alternatively, the resin may be given rectally as a 25% solution of sorbitol (see Sodium Polystyrene Sulfonate 40:18.18.)

Polyethylene Glycol 3350. For the treatment of constipation, the usual oral dosage in adults is 17 g (MiraLAX®) daily as needed for up to 7 days.

Bowel Cleansing **Polyethylene Glycol 3350 (with Electrolytes).** To empty the bowel prior to colonoscopy or barium radiologic examination, children 6 months of age or older may receive orally or by nasogastric tube 25 mL/kg (2.6 g/kg) per hour (NuLYTELY®or Trilyte®) until watery stool is clear and free of solid matter (NuLYTELY®or Trilyte®) or 4 L is consumed (Trilyte®).

To empty the bowel prior to colonoscopy or barium radiologic examination, the recommended dosage given by nasogastric tube in adults is 4 L administered at a rate of 20–30 mL (1.18–1.77 g [Golytely®]; 2.1–3.15 g [Nulytely®]; 1.2–1.8 g [Colyte®]) per minute (1.2–1.8 L/hour).

To empty the bowel prior to colonoscopy or barium radiologic examination, adults may receive 240 mL (about 14 g [GoLYTELY®], 25 g [NuLYTELY®], about 14 g [Colyte®], 25 g [Trilyte®]) orally every 10 minutes until rectal output is clear or 4 L is consumed. Alternatively, adults may receive a single-dose regimen of 240 mL (24 g [MoviPrep®]) orally every 15 minutes until 1 L is consumed followed by drinking of an additional 1 L (for a total of 2 L of MoviPrep®) 1.5 hours later. An additional 1 L of clear liquid shoudl be ingested during the evening prior the procedure.

When using a divided-dose regimen, adults may receive 240 mL (24 g [MoviPrep®]) every 15 minutes until 1 L is consumed followed by drinking an additional 0.5 L of clear liquid in the evening before the procedure, On the morning of the procedure, these adults should receive 240 mL (24 g [MoviPrep®]) every 15 minutes until 1 L is consumed followed by drinking an additional 0.5 L of clear liquid at least 1 hour prior to the procedure.

Alternatively, adults may receive a combination regimen of polyethylene glycol 3350 electrolyte solution and bisacodyl (HalfLytely®). In this regimen, patients initially should receive 20 mg of bisacodyl (four 5-mg bisacodyl delayed-release tablets) and wait for a bowel movement or a maximum of 6 hours, then drink 240 mL of polyethylene glycol 3350 electrolyte solution every 10 minutes until a total of 2 L has been consumed.

Pharmacokinetics

■ **Absorption** Following rectal administration, glycerin and sorbitol are poorly absorbed; colonic evacuation of glycerin rectal suppositories or enemas occurs within 15–60 minutes, while colonic evacuation of oral sorbitol occurs within 24–48 hours.

The manufacturers of polyethylene glycol 3350 preparations state that the osmotic effects of the drug result in virtually no net absorption or excretion of ions or water. Following oral administration of polyethylene glycol 3350 (MiraLAX®), colonic evacuation occurs in 1–3 days, while following oral administration of polyethylene glycol 3350 electrolyte solutions (GoLYTELY®, NuLYTELY®, Colyte®, MoviPrep®, Trilyte®), initial bowel movement usually occurs within 1 hour. In addition, following oral administration of polyethylene glycol 3350 electrolyte solutions (GoLYTELY®, NuLYTELY®, Trilyte®), complete bowel evacuation usually occurs within 4 hours. Following oral administration of polyethylene glycol 3350 electrolyte solution and bisacodyl (HalfLytely® bowel kit), initial bowel movement usually occurs within 1–6 hours after ingesting the bisacodyl tablets; a watery bowel movement usually occurs within 1 hour after ingesting the polyethylene glycol 3350 electrolyte solution portion of the kit.

■ **Distribution** It is not known whether polyethylene glycol 3350 (MiraLAX®) is distributed into human milk.

■ **Elimination** Sorbitol, a nonabsorbable disaccharide, is metabolized by colonic bacteria into acetic and other short chain fatty acids.

Chemistry and Stability

■ **Chemistry** Glycerin (glycerol) and sorbitol are hyperosmotic laxatives.

Glycerin Glycerin (glycerol), a trihydroxy alcohol, occurs as a clear, colorless, syrupy, hygroscopic liquid with a sweet taste and not more than a slight characteristic odor, which is neither harsh nor disagreeable. The drug is miscible with water and with alcohol and has a specific gravity of not less than 1.249.

Sorbitol Sorbitol (D-glucitol), a polyalcohol of sorbose, occurs as white, hygroscopic powder, granules, or flakes having a sweet taste and is very soluble in water and slightly soluble in alcohol. Sorbitol solutions occur as clear, sweet-tasting liquids.

■ **Stability** ***Glycerin*** Glycerin rectal suppositories should preferably be stored at less than 25°C.

Oral Polyethylene Glycol Powder for Solution Polyethylene glycol 3350 Powder for Solution (MiraLAX®) should be stored at 20–25°C.

Oral Polyethylene Glycol (with Electrolytes) Powder for Solution Colyte® should be stored at 20–25°C (may be exposed to 15–30°C). Following reconstitution, the solution should be refrigerated and used within 48 hours; unused portions should be discarded.

GoLYTELY® should be stored in tight containers at 15–30°C. Following reconstitution, the solution should be refrigerated and used within 48 hours; unused portions should be discarded.

MoviPrep®should be stored at 25°C (may be exposed to 15–30°C). Following reconstitution, the solution should be refrigerated and used within 48 hours; unused portions should be discarded.

NuLyTELY® should be stored in tight containers at 25°C. Following reconstitution the solution should be refrigerated and used within 48 hours; unused portions should be discarded.

Sorbitol Oral or rectal sorbitol 70% solution should be stored at 15–30°C.

For further information on the pharmacology, uses, cautions, drug interactions, and dosage and administration of the hyperosmotic laxatives, see the Cathartics and Laxatives General Statement 56:12.

Preparations

Excipients in commercially available drug preparations may have clinically important effects in some individuals; consult specific product labeling for details.

Glycerin (Glycerol)

Rectal		
Solution	2.3 g	**Fleet® Babylax®**, Fleet
	5.6 g	**Fleet® Liquid Glycerin Suppositories,** Fleet

Suppositories	1 g*	**Fleet® Child Glycerin Suppositories,** Fleet
	1.2 g*	**Colace® Glycerin Suppositories,** Purdue
	2 g*	**Fleet® Adult Glycerin Suppositories,** Fleet
	2.1 g*	**Colace® Glycerin Suppositories,** Purdue
	82.5%*	**Sani Supp® Adult Glycerin Suppositories,** G&W
		Sani Supp® Pediatric Glycerin Suppositories, G&W

*available from one or more manufacturer, distributor, and/or repackager by generic (nonproprietary) name

Polyethylene Glycol 3350

Oral		
For solution	17 g	**MiraLAX®,** Schering-Plough

Polyethylene Glycol 3350 and Electrolytes

Oral		
For solution	Polyethylene glycol 200 g, ascorbic acid 9.4 g/, potassium chloride 2.03 g, sodium ascorbate 11.8 g, sodium chloride 5.38 g, and sodium sulfate 15 g/2 L	**MoviPrep®,** Salix
	Polyethylene glycol 236 g, potassium chloride 2.97 g/L, sodium bicarbonate 6.74 g, sodium chloride 5.86 g, and sodium sulfate 22.74 g/4 L	**GoLYTELY®,** Braintree
	Polyethylene glycol 240 g, potassium chloride 2.98 g, sodium bicarbonate 6.72 g, sodium chloride 5.84 g, and sodium sulfate 22.72 g/4 L	**Colyte®,** Schwarz
	Polyethylene glycol 420 g, potassium chloride 1.48 g/4 L, sodium bicarbonate 5.72 g, and sodium chloride 11.2 g/4 L	**NuLYTELY®,** Braintree **Trilyte®,** Schwarz

Polyethylene Glycol 3350, Electrolytes and Bisacodyl Kit

Oral		
Kit	For solution, oral, Polyethylene glycol 210 g, sodium chloride 5.6 g, sodium bicarbonate 2.86 g, and potassium chloride 0.74 g/2 L	**HalfLytely®,** Braintree
	4 Tablets, enteric-coated, Bisacodyl 5 mg	

Sorbitol (D-Glucitol)

Powder*	
Oral or Rectal	
Solution	70%*

*available from one or more manufacturer, distributor, and/or repackager by generic (nonproprietary) name

Saline Laxatives

■ Laxatives containing magnesium cations or phosphate anions are commonly termed saline laxatives.

Dosage and Administration

For precautions that should be considered before administration of saline laxatives in patients susceptible to adverse effects, see Cautions: Saline Laxatives, in the Cathartics and Laxatives General Statement 56:12.

■ **Administration** ***Magnesium-containing Saline Laxatives*** Magnesium-containing saline laxatives are administered orally in the form of chewable tablets, suspensions, or solutions. A full (240 mL) glass of liquid should be ingested following administration of each dose.

Magnesium citrate oral solution may be chilled prior to administration.

Magnesium hydroxide suspension should be shaken well before each use. The fixed combination of magnesium hydroxide and mineral oil typically is administered at bedtime and should *not* be administered with meals.

Magnesium sulfate oral solution may be prepared by dissolving an appropriate dose of the crystals in at least 240 mL of water; lemon juice may be added to improve taste. Each level teaspoonful of magnesium sulfate crystals provides approximately 5 g of the drug and 495 mg (40.7 mEq) of magnesium.

Sodium Phosphates Phosphate-containing laxatives are administered orally as solutions or tablets and rectally as enemas in combinations containing dibasic sodium phosphate and monobasic sodium phosphate; commercially available phosphate-containing laxatives intended for rectal use (i.e., enema solutions) are *not* intended for oral administration.

When sodium phosphates are administered orally as solutions or tablets, a full (240 mL) glass of clear liquid (e.g., water) should be ingested following administration of each dose. Sodium phosphates tablets should be used with caution in patients with impaired gag reflex and those prone to regurgitation or aspiration; these patients should be observed during administration of sodium phosphates tablets.

When sodium phosphates are administered rectally as enemas, additional liquid should be ingested during therapy to ensure adequate hydration.

Enemas. Phosphate-containing enemas should be administered at room temperature. The protective shield (if present) should be removed from the tip of the enema. For administration of the enema, patients should be advised to lie on their left side with knees bent or to kneel on the bed with the head and chest lowered and forward until the left side of the face is resting on the surface of the bed. The enema nozzle should be inserted into the rectum with steady pressure and a slight side-to-side movement; the nozzle should be pointed toward the navel. To ease insertion, the patient should be advised to bear down as if having a bowel movement. The nozzle should not be forced into the rectum as this can cause injury. The container should be squeezed until nearly all of the liquid is expelled; it is not necessary to empty the container as it contains more liquid than needed. The nozzle should then be removed from the rectum, and the patient should be advised to maintain the position until the urge to evacuate is strong (usually within 1–5 minutes).

For children 2–4 years of age, an enema containing dibasic sodium phosphate 1.75 g and monobasic sodium phosphate 4.75 g in approximately 29 mL can be prepared for administration as follows. The cap of a pediatric-strength enema containing dibasic sodium phosphate 3.5 g and monobasic sodium phosphate 9.5 g in 59 mL (e.g., Fleet® Pedia-Lax® Enema) can be unscrewed and 30 mL of solution removed. The cap should then be replaced and the enema administered as directed.

Oral Solutions. When used as a laxative for *self-medication* of occasional constipation, oral solutions of dibasic sodium phosphate and monobasic sodium phosphate should be diluted before administration by adding the appropriate dose of the solution to 240 mL of cool water.

When used as a purgative in a bowel cleansing regimen prior to surgery or radiographic or endoscopic examination of the colon, oral solutions of dibasic sodium phosphate and monobasic sodium phosphate should be diluted before administration, as directed by a clinician. FDA states that nonprescription (over-the-counter, OTC) oral sodium phosphates preparations (e.g., oral solutions) should be used for bowel cleansing *only* when a prescription for such use has been issued by a clinician. (See Sodium Phosphates Oral Solution under Dosage: Bowel Cleansing, in Dosage and Administration.)

Carbon Dioxide-releasing Laxatives Carbon dioxide-releasing suppositories (e.g., CEO-TWO®) are administered rectally. Prior to insertion into the rectum, the wrapper should be removed, and the suppository should be moistened under a warm-water tap for 30 seconds or in a cup of water for at least 10 seconds. Mineral oil or petroleum jelly should *not* be used to lubricate these suppositories.

■ **Dosage** Saline laxatives should be administered only at infrequent intervals. Most studies suggest that the minimum effective oral laxative dose of magnesium is 80 mEq. The usual dosages of the various saline laxatives are below; for dosages in children younger than the ages listed, a physician should be consulted.

Constipation The manufacturers state that laxatives should not be used for *self-medication* of constipation for longer than 7 days without consulting a clinician. FDA states that sodium phosphates preparations should not be used for *self-medication* of occasional constipation for longer than 3 days.

Magnesium Citrate. The recommended oral dosage of magnesium citrate for *self-medication* of occasional constipation in adults and children 12 years of age and older is 8.75–25 g (usually 150–300 mL [8.75–17.5 g] of a 291-mg/5-mL oral solution) daily given as a single dose or in divided doses. The recommended oral dosage for *self-medication* in children 6–11 years of age is 5.5–12.5 g (usually 90–150 mL [5.25–8.75 g] of a 291-mg/5-mL oral solution) daily given as a single dose or in divided doses. The recommended oral dosage for *self-medication* in children 2–5 years of age is 2.7–6.25 g (usually 60–90 mL [3.5–5.25 g] of a 291-mg/5-mL oral solution) daily given as a single dose or in divided doses.

Magnesium Hydroxide. The usual oral dosage of magnesium hydroxide for *self-medication* of occasional constipation is 2.4–4.8 g daily in adults and children 12 years of age and older, 1.2–2.4 g daily in children 6–11 years of age, and 0.4–1.2 g daily in children 2–5 years of age. The usual dosage should be given as a single dose (preferably at bedtime), in divided doses, or as directed by a clinician.

Magnesium Sulfate. The usual oral dosage of magnesium sulfate for *self-medication* of occasional constipation is 10–30 g daily in adults and children 12 years of age and older, 5–10 g daily in children 6–11 years of age, and 2.5–5 g daily in children 2–5 years of age. The usual dosage may be given as a single dose or in divided doses.

Sodium Phosphates. When administered as an oral solution for *self-medication* of occasional constipation, the usual oral dosage in adults and children 12 years of age and older is dibasic sodium phosphate 2.7 g and monobasic sodium phosphate 7.2 g given as a single daily dose; the maximum dosage is dibasic sodium phosphate 8.1 g and monobasic sodium phosphate 21.6 g given as a single daily dose. The usual and maximum oral dosage for *self-medication* in children 10–11 years of age is dibasic sodium phosphate 2.7 g and monobasic sodium phosphate 7.2 g given as a single daily dose. The usual and maximum oral dosage for *self-medication* in children 5–9 years of age is dibasic sodium phosphate 1.35 g and monobasic sodium phosphate 3.6 g given as a single daily dose. The manufacturer states that nonprescription oral sodium phosphates preparations (e.g., oral solutions) should not be used for *self-medication* of occasional constipation in children 5 years of age or younger; FDA states that clinicians should be cautious in recommending use of these preparations in this patient population. FDA also states that nonprescription sodium phosphates preparations should not be used for *self-medication* of occasional constipation for longer than 3 days.

When administered as an enema for *self-medication* of occasional constipation, the usual rectal dosage in adults and children 12 years of age and older is dibasic sodium phosphate 7 g and monobasic sodium phosphate 19 g (one bottle of Fleet® Enema [approximately 118 mL] or Fleet® Enema Extra [approximately 197 mL]) daily given as a single dose. The usual rectal dosage for *self-medication* in children 5–11 years of age is dibasic sodium phosphate 3.5 g and monobasic sodium phosphate 9.5 g (one bottle [approximately 59 mL] of Fleet® Pedia-Lax® Enema) daily given as a single dose, or as directed by a clinician. The usual rectal dosage for *self-medication* in children 2–4 years of age is dibasic sodium phosphate 1.75 g and monobasic sodium phosphate 4.75 g (one-half of a bottle [approximately 29 mL] of Fleet® Pedia-Lax® Enema) daily given as a single dose. The manufacturer and FDA state that nonprescription rectal sodium phosphates preparations should not be used for *self-medication* of occasional constipation in children younger than 2 years of age. FDA also states that these preparations should not be used for *self-medication* of occasional constipation for longer than 3 days. Caution should be exercised when selecting phosphate-containing enemas since the commercially available enemas are available in various volumes (i.e., adult and pediatric); use of preparations with volumes appropriate for age should be ensured in order to minimize the risk of overdosage.

Severe dehydration, electrolyte abnormalities (e.g., hypernatremia, hyperphosphatemia, hypocalcemia), acute kidney injury, cardiac arrhythmias, and/or death have been reported rarely in adults and children receiving nonprescription sodium phosphates preparations (i.e., oral solution, enema) for *self-medication* of occasional constipation. The majority of reported adverse events occurred in patients who received higher than recommended dosages in a 24-hour period (i.e., a single dose that was larger than recommended or more than one dose in a day) or in patients at increased risk of developing sodium phosphate-induced toxicity. Therefore, FDA states that the maximum recommended oral or rectal dosage of nonprescription sodium phosphates preparations should not be exceeded, and that additional doses are not recommended within 24 hours, even in patients who do not have a bowel movement after receiving a dose. FDA also states that clinicians should be cautious in recommending use of nonprescription sodium phosphates preparations in patients older than 55 years of age; patients with hypovolemia, decreased intravascular volume, kidney disease, decreased bowel transit time, or active colitis; and patients receiving drugs that affect renal perfusion or function (e.g., diuretics, angiotensin converting-enzyme [ACE] inhibitors, angiotensin II receptor antagonists, nonsteroidal anti-inflammatory agents [NSAIAs]). FDA recommends that serum electrolytes and renal function be assessed in patients who may be at increased risk of serious adverse effects, including those who have retained a rectal dose for more than 30 minutes, who are vomiting, or who may have signs of dehydration. Patients should be advised to discontinue sodium phosphates therapy and to immediately seek medical attention if symptoms of kidney injury (e.g., drowsiness; sluggishness; decreased urine; swelling of the ankles, feet, or legs) occur. Nonprescription sodium phosphates preparations should not be used concomitantly with other laxatives containing sodium phosphate. For further information on adverse effects associated with sodium phosphates preparations, see Cautions: Saline Laxatives in the Cathartics and Laxatives General Statement 56:12.

Carbon Dioxide-releasing Laxatives. The usual rectal dosage for *self-medication* of occasional constipation in adults and children 12 years of age and older is 1 suppository (0.9 g of potassium bitartrate and 0.6 g of sodium bicarbonate) daily given as a single dose.

Bowel Cleansing **Sodium Phosphates Tablets.** When the fixed-combination oral tablets (OsmoPrep®) containing 0.398 g of dibasic sodium phosphate and 1.102 g of monobasic sodium phosphate are used to empty the bowel prior to colonoscopy, tablets should be taken in 2 regimens, one on the night before and one on the day of the procedure.

On the night before the procedure, 1.592 g of dibasic sodium phosphate and 4.408 g of monobasic sodium phosphate (4 tablets) should be taken with at least 240 mL of a clear liquid every 15 minutes until a total dose of 7.96 g of dibasic sodium phosphate and 22.04 g of monobasic sodium phosphate (total of 20 tablets) has been ingested. On the day of the procedure (starting 3–5 hours before the procedure), 1.592 g of dibasic sodium phosphate and 4.408 g of monobasic sodium phosphate (4 tablets) should be taken with at least 240 mL of a clear liquid every 15 minutes until a total dose of 4.776 g of dibasic sodium phosphate and 13.224 g of monobasic sodium phosphate (total of 12 tablets) has been ingested. Total dosage of the 2 regimens is 12.736 g of dibasic sodium phosphate and 35.264 g of monobasic sodium phosphate (32 tablets).

Sodium Phosphates Enemas. When sodium phosphates is administered rectally as an enema for bowel cleansing prior to rectal examinations, the usual dosage for *self-medication* in adults and children 12 years of age and older is dibasic sodium phosphate 7 g and monobasic sodium phosphate 19 g (one bottle of Fleet® Enema [approximately 118 mL] or Fleet® Enema Extra [approximately 197 mL]) daily given as a single dose. The usual rectal dosage for *self-medication* in children 5–11 years of age is dibasic sodium phosphate 3.5 g and monobasic sodium phosphate 9.5 g (one bottle [approximately 59 mL] of Fleet® Pedia-Lax® Enema) daily given as a single dose, or as directed by a clinician. The usual rectal dosage for *self-medication* in children 2–4 years of age is dibasic sodium phosphate 1.75 g and monobasic sodium phosphate 4.75 g (one-half bottle [approximately 29 mL] of Fleet® Pedia-Lax® Enema) daily given as a single dose.

Sodium Phosphates Oral Solution. When sodium phosphates oral solution is used as a purgative in a bowel cleansing regimen prior to surgery or radiographic or endoscopic examination of the colon, dosage of the oral solution should be prepared and administered as directed by a clinician.

Use of sodium phosphates oral solution for *self-medication* for bowel cleansing prior to surgery or radiographic or endoscopic rectal examinations rarely has resulted in fluid shifts, severe electrolyte abnormalities, cardiac arrhythmias, renal failure, acute phosphate nephropathy, generalized tonic-clonic seizures, loss of consciousness, and/or death. Therefore, in December 2008, FDA stated that oral sodium phosphates preparations should be used for bowel cleansing *only* when a prescription for such use has been issued by a clinician. FDA and some manufacturers of oral sodium phosphates preparations recommended that baseline and postprocedural (e.g., postcolonoscopy) laboratory measurements (i.e., serum concentrations of calcium, phosphate, potassium, sodium, creatinine, and BUN) be obtained in patients who may be at increased risk of serious adverse effects, including those with a history of renal impairment, history of acute phosphate nephropathy, known or suspected electrolyte disorders, seizures, arrhythmias, cardiomyopathy, prolonged QT interval, recent myocardial infarction, or known or suspected hyperphosphatemia, hypocalcemia, hypokalemia, or hypernatremia. In addition, postprocedural laboratory measurements should be obtained in patients with vomiting or signs of dehydration. FDA also recommended monitoring of the glomerular filtration rate in smaller, frail patients. Baseline and postprocedural ECGs should be considered in patients at high risk for serious cardiac arrhythmias.

Despite efforts to inform healthcare professionals and consumers about the risks associated with the use of sodium phosphates oral solution for bowel cleansing, FDA continued to receive reports of acute kidney injury (some resulting in kidney transplantation, dialysis, long-term renal failure, and, rarely, death) following administration of usual recommended dosages of the drugs for *self-medication* for bowel cleansing (approximately 60 g of sodium phosphates [dibasic sodium phosphate and monobasic sodium phosphate salts] administered as two 45-mL doses given 12 hours apart or approximately 50 g of sodium phosphates administered as a 45-mL dose initially, followed by a 30-mL dose 10–12 hours later). Therefore, as part of its ongoing review of over-the-counter drug products, FDA has tentatively concluded that the usual recommended dosage of nonprescription oral sodium phosphates *for self-medication* for bowel cleansing based on professional labeling in an OTC monograph poses an unacceptable risk of serious adverse events. In February 2011, the agency issued a proposed rule amending the tentative final monograph on nonprescription laxative drug products to classify the individual sodium phosphate salts (i.e., dibasic sodium phosphate, monobasic sodium phosphate) as *not* generally recognized as safe (GRAS) for bowel cleansing. In the proposed rule, FDA also suggested that the professional labeling for sodium phosphates (which discusses use of the drugs as part of a bowel cleansing regimen) be removed from the 1985 tentative final monograph for over-the-counter laxative drug products. In response to FDA's proposed rule, some manufacturers have removed the indication for bowel cleansing from labeling of nonprescription sodium phosphates preparations. For further information on adverse effects associated with sodium phosphates preparations, see Sodium Phosphates Preparations under Cautions: Saline Laxatives in the Cathartics and Laxatives General Statement 56:12.

Pharmacokinetics

Approximately 15–30% of orally administered magnesium-containing saline laxatives may be absorbed, probably from the small intestine by an active process. However, the exact extent of phosphate and sodium absorption from oral phosphate laxatives is unknown. The extent of phosphate absorption from rectally administered phosphate enemas is unknown, but about 1–20% of the sodium and phosphate in such preparations is reportedly absorbed. Magnesium and phosphate are excreted principally by the kidneys. Small amounts of magnesium are distributed into milk and saliva.

Therapeutic oral doses of saline laxatives produce a semifluid or watery stool in 0.5–6 hours. Purgative effects of sodium phosphates tablets (OsmoPrep®) persist for 1–3 hours. Carbon dioxide-releasing suppositories produce evacuation of the colon within 5–30 minutes. Rectal enemas containing phosphate salts produce evacuation within 1–5 minutes.

Chemistry and Stability

■ **Chemistry** Laxatives containing magnesium cations or phosphate anions are commonly termed saline laxatives. Saline laxatives containing magnesium include magnesium citrate, magnesium hydroxide (e.g., milk of magnesia), and magnesium sulfate. Phosphate-containing saline laxatives include dibasic sodium phosphate and monobasic sodium phosphate.

Magnesium Citrate Magnesium citrate is formed *in situ* when magnesium carbonate, anhydrous citric acid, and sodium or potassium bicarbonate are mixed in solution. Magnesium citrate solution occurs as a colorless to slightly yellow, clear, effervescent liquid having a sweet, acidulous taste and lemon flavor. The citric acid and sodium citrate in magnesium citrate solution act as sequestering agents, holding magnesium in solution in a complex anion form which is soluble but nonreactive. In addition, citric acid combined with sodium or potassium bicarbonate enables the solution to effervesce. Magnesium citrate solution contains an equivalent of 77.5–95 mg of magnesium oxide or 3.85–4.71 mEq of magnesium ion per 5 mL.

Magnesium Hydroxide Magnesium hydroxide occurs as a bulky, white powder and is practically insoluble in water and in alcohol. Milk of Magnesia, Double-strength Milk of Magnesia, and Triple-strength Milk of Magnesia are suspensions containing 80, 160, and 240 mg of magnesium hydroxide per mL, respectively. Milk of magnesia occurs as a white, opaque, more or less viscous suspension; on standing, varying proportions of water usually separate from the suspension. Magnesium hydroxide contains about 34.3 mEq of magnesium per gram and milk of magnesia contains about 2.4–2.9 mEq of magnesium per gram or approximately 13.66 mEq of magnesium per 5 mL.

Magnesium Sulfate Magnesium sulfate occurs as small, colorless, usually needle-like crystals having a cool, saline, bitter taste and is freely soluble in water and sparingly soluble in alcohol. One gram of the drug contains about 8.1 mEq of magnesium.

Sodium Phosphates Dibasic sodium phosphate (heptahydrate) occurs as a colorless or white, granular salt that is freely soluble in water and very slightly soluble in alcohol. Solutions of dibasic sodium phosphate are alkaline. Monobasic sodium phosphate occurs as monohydrate, colorless crystals or a white, crystalline powder. It is odorless and is freely soluble in water and practically insoluble in alcohol. Sodium phosphates rectal enemas and oral solutions contain 4–6% and 18% dibasic sodium phosphate, respectively, and 10–16% and 48% monobasic sodium phosphate, respectively, and have pHs of 5–5.8 and 4.4–5.2, respectively. Potency of dibasic sodium phosphate is calculated on the dried basis and that of monobasic sodium phosphate is calculated on the anhydrous basis; however, in sodium phosphates rectal enemas and oral solutions, potency of dibasic sodium phosphate is expressed in terms of the heptahydrate and that of monobasic sodium phosphate is expressed in terms of the monohydrate. In addition, in sodium phosphates oral tablets (OsmoPrep®), potency of dibasic sodium phosphate is calculated on the anhydrous basis and that of monobasic sodium phosphate is calculated in terms of the monohydrate.

Carbon Dioxide-releasing Laxatives Rectal suppositories containing potassium bitartrate and sodium bicarbonate, which release carbon dioxide, are commonly called carbon dioxide-releasing suppositories.

■ **Stability** ***Magnesium Citrate*** Magnesium citrate solution should be stored at 2–30°C to retard decomposition. The solution should be protected from excessive heat and freezing and should be discarded within 24 hours of opening.

Magnesium Hydroxide Milk of magnesia should preferably be stored at room temperature; freezing should be avoided. Magnesium hydroxide chewable tablets should be stored at room temperature.

Magnesium Sulfate Magnesium sulfate effervesces in warm, dry air and is incompatible with sodium and potassium tartrates, with soluble phosphates and arsenates, and with alkali carbonates and bicarbonates unless mixed in dilute proportions.

Sodium Phosphates Dibasic sodium phosphate (heptahydrate) effloresces in warm, dry air.

Monobasic sodium phosphate is slightly deliquescent.

Tablets of dibasic sodium phosphate and monobasic sodium phosphate should be stored at 25°C but may be exposed to temperatures ranging from 15–30°C. Oral solutions of dibasic sodium phosphate and monobasic sodium phosphate may be refrigerated but should not be frozen.

Carbon Dioxide-releasing Laxatives Rectal suppositories containing potassium bitartrate and sodium bicarbonate should be stored between 20–25°C, not to exceed 30°C. The suppositories should not be refrigerated.

For further information on pharmacology, uses, cautions, drug interactions, and dosage and administration of the saline laxatives, see the Cathartics and Laxatives General Statement 56:12. For use of magnesium preparations as antacids, see 56:04.

Preparations

Excipients in commercially available drug preparations may have clinically important effects in some individuals; consult specific product labeling for details.

Magnesium Citrate (Citrate of Magnesia)

Powder

Oral		
Solution*	291 mg/5 mL*	**Magnesium Citrate Oral Solution**

*available from one or more manufacturer, distributor, and/or repackager by generic (nonproprietary) name

Magnesium Hydroxide

Powder

Oral		
Suspension*	400 mg/5 mL*	**Milk of Magnesia**
		Phillips'® Milk of Magnesia, Bayer
	800 mg/5 mL	**Little Phillips'® Milk of Magnesia,** Bayer
		Phillips'® Concentrated Milk of Magnesia, Bayer
	1.2 g/5 mL*	**Milk of Magnesia Concentrate**
Tablets, chewable	311 mg	**Phillips'® Chewable Tablets,** Bayer
	400 mg	**Fleet® Pedia-Lax® Chewable Tablets,** Fleet

*available from one or more manufacturer, distributor, and/or repackager by generic (nonproprietary) name

Magnesium Hydroxide Combinations

Oral		
Suspension	300 mg (magnesium hydroxide)/5 mL with Mineral Oil 1.25 mL/5 mL*	**Magnesium Hydroxide and Mineral Oil Suspension**
		Phillips' M-O®, Bayer
	4 mL (milk of magnesia)/5 mL with Mineral Oil 1 mL/5 mL*	**Magnesium Hydroxide and Mineral Oil Suspension**

*available from one or more manufacturer, distributor, and/or repackager by generic (nonproprietary) name

Magnesium Sulfate (Epsom Salt)

Crystals*

Powder*

*available from one or more manufacturer, distributor, and/or repackager by generic (nonproprietary) name

Sodium Phosphate, Dibasic

Powder*

*available from one or more manufacturer, distributor, and/or repackager by generic (nonproprietary) name

Sodium Phosphate, Monobasic

Powder*

*available from one or more manufacturer, distributor, and/or repackager by generic (nonproprietary) name

Carbon Dioxide-releasing Suppositories

Rectal		
Suppository	Potassium Bitartrate 0.9 g and Sodium Bicarbonate 0.6 g	**Ceo-Two®,** Beutlich

Sodium Phosphates

Oral		
Solution	Dibasic Sodium Phosphate 900 mg/5 mL with Monobasic Sodium Phosphate 2.4 g/5 mL*	**Sodium Phosphate Oral Saline Laxative**
Tablet	Dibasic Sodium Phosphate (anhydrous) 0.398 g with Monobasic Sodium Phosphate (monohydrate) 1.102 g	**OsmoPrep®,** Salix
Rectal		
Solution	Dibasic Sodium Phosphate 36 mg/mL with Monobasic Sodium Phosphate 96 mg/mL	**Fleet® Enema Extra,** Fleet
	Dibasic Sodium Phosphate 59 mg/mL with Monobasic Sodium Phosphate 161 mg/mL	**Fleet® Enema,** Fleet **Fleet® Pedia-Lax® Enema,** Fleet

*available from one or more manufacturer, distributor, and/or repackager by generic (nonproprietary) name

ANTIEMETICS 56:22

ANTIHISTAMINES 56:22.08

dimenhyDRINATE

■ Dimenhydrinate, an ethanolamine-derivative antihistamine containing a diphenhydramine moiety, is an antiemetic.

Uses

■ **Motion Sickness** Dimenhydrinate is used principally in the prevention and treatment of nausea, vomiting, and/or vertigo associated with motion sickness, although scopolamine, promethazine, or meclizine may be more effective. Dimenhydrinate is most effective against motion sickness when given prophylactically, although susceptibility to motion sickness may vary with the patient's age, previous exposure to motion, and the type, severity, and duration of motion.

■ **Other Uses** Dimenhydrinate has been used for symptomatic treatment of Ménière's disease† and other vestibular disturbances†. Like other antihistamines, dimenhydrinate may be less effective than the phenothiazines in controlling nausea and vomiting not related to vestibular stimulation.

Although dimenhydrinate is a histamine antagonist, its use in allergic states has not been evaluated.

Dosage and Administration

■ **Administration** Dimenhydrinate may be administered orally or by IM or IV injection. For IV injection, each 50 mg of dimenhydrinate must be diluted with 10 mL of 0.9% sodium chloride injection and administered slowly over a period of 2 minutes.

■ **Dosage** For the prevention of motion sickness, dimenhydrinate should be taken orally 30 minutes before exposure to motion. For the prevention and treatment of nausea, vomiting, and/or vertigo associated with motion sickness, the usual oral dosage of dimenhydrinate for *self-medication* in adults and children 12 years of age or older is 50–100 mg every 4–6 hours, not to exceed 400 mg in 24 hours, or as directed by a clinician. The same dosage can be given parenterally in adults to treat motion sickness. Children 6 to younger than 12 years of age may receive 25–50 mg orally every 6–8 hours, not to exceed 150 mg in 24 hours, or as directed by a clinician. Children 2 to younger than 6 years of age may receive 12.5–25 mg orally every 6–8 hours, not to exceed 75 mg in 24 hours, or as directed by a clinician. Alternatively, children may be given 1.25 mg/kg or 37.5 mg/m^2, orally or IM 4 times daily, up to a maximum of 300 mg daily. Children younger than 2 years of age should receive oral dimenhydrinate only under the direction of a clinician. IV dosage has not been established for children.

For symptomatic relief of Ménière's disease, 25–50 mg of dimenhydrinate has been given orally 3 times daily for maintenance, or 50 mg has been given IM for acute attacks.

Cautions

■ **Adverse Effects** Drowsiness commonly occurs after administration of dimenhydrinate. Paradoxical CNS stimulation may occur in children and occasionally in adults.

Other adverse effects include headache, blurred vision, tinnitus, dryness of the mouth and respiratory passages, incoordination, palpitation, dizziness, and hypotension. Anorexia, constipation or diarrhea, urinary frequency, and dysuria are less common. Pain may occur at the site of IM injection. Because dimenhydrinate contains diphenhydramine, the possibility of other diphenhydramine-related adverse effects should also be considered. (See the Antihistamines General Statement 4:00 and Diphenhydramine Hydrochloride 4:04.)

■ **Precautions and Contraindications** Patients should be warned that dimenhydrinate may impair their ability to perform hazardous activities requiring mental alertness or physical coordination (e.g., operating machinery or driving a motor vehicle). Sedation may be enhanced by other CNS depressants. (See Drug Interactions: CNS Depressants.)

Dramamine® chewable tablets contain the dye tartrazine (FD&C yellow No. 5), which may cause allergic reactions including bronchial asthma in certain susceptible individuals. Although the incidence of tartrazine sensitivity is low, it frequently occurs in individuals who are sensitive to aspirin.

Dimenhydrinate should be used with caution in patients with seizure disorders. The anticholinergic effects of the drug should be considered when administering dimenhydrinate to patients with conditions that might be aggravated by anticholinergic therapy (e.g., angle-closure glaucoma, enlargement of the prostate gland). The drug may mask symptoms of ototoxicity and therefore should be administered with caution to patients receiving known ototoxic drugs. These patients should be closely monitored during therapy with dimenhydrinate.

■ **Pregnancy, Fertility, and Lactation** Reproduction studies in rats and rabbits using dimenhydrinate doses up to 20 and 25 times the human dose (on a mg/kg basis), respectively, have not revealed evidence of harm to the fetus. There are no adequate and well-controlled studies using dimenhydrinate in pregnant women. Clinical studies to date in pregnant women receiving the drug have not indicated an increased risk of abnormalities when administered during any trimester. Although the possibility of harm to the fetus appears remote, dimenhydrinate should be used during pregnancy only when clearly needed.

Reproduction studies in rats and rabbits using dimenhydrinate doses up to 20 and 25 times the human dose (on a mg/kg basis), respectively, have not revealed evidence of impaired fertility.

Small amounts of dimenhydrinate are distributed into milk. Because of the potential for adverse reactions to dimenhydrinate in nursing infants, a decision should be made whether to discontinue nursing or the drug, taking into account the importance of the drug to the woman.

Drug Interactions

■ **CNS Depressants** Dimenhydrinate may enhance the effects of other CNS depressants such as alcohol and barbiturates. If dimenhydrinate is used concomitantly with other CNS depressants, caution should be used to avoid overdosage.

■ **Drugs with Anticholinergic Effects** Because dimenhydrinate also has anticholinergic activity, it may potentiate the effects of other drugs with anticholinergic activity including tricyclic antidepressants.

■ **Ototoxic Drugs** When given concurrently with aminoglycoside antibiotics or other ototoxic drugs, dimenhydrinate may mask the early symptoms of ototoxicity. (See Cautions: Precautions and Contraindications.)

■ **Other Drugs** Although dimenhydrinate has been reported to induce hepatic microsomal enzymes in animals, there is no clinical evidence that dimenhydrinate influences the metabolism of other drugs in humans.

Acute Toxicity

■ **Manifestations** Accidental antihistamine overdose occurs frequently in infants and children. Symptoms of dimenhydrinate toxicity in children may resemble atropine overdosage and include dilated pupils, flushed face, excitation, hallucinations, confusion, ataxia, intermittent clonic convulsions, coma, cardiorespiratory collapse, and death. Symptoms may be delayed for up to 2 hours after ingestion; death may occur within 18 hours.

In adults, 500 mg or more of dimenhydrinate may cause extreme difficulty in speech and swallowing, and produces a psychosis indistinguishable from that of atropine poisoning. CNS excitation may be preceded by sedation, leading to a cycle of CNS excitation, seizures, and postictal depression.

■ **Treatment** Treatment of dimenhydrinate toxicity is symptomatic and supportive. Emetics are usually ineffective, but in the absence of seizures, early gastric lavage (with an endotracheal tube with cuff inflated in place to prevent aspiration of gastric contents) may be beneficial. Patients should be kept quiet to minimize CNS stimulation; seizures may be treated with diazepam in adults and phenobarbital in children. Mechanical respiratory assistance may be required.

Pharmacology

The pharmacologic effects of dimenhydrinate are believed to result principally from its diphenhydramine moiety. Like diphenhydramine, dimenhydrinate has CNS depressant, anticholinergic, antiemetic, antihistaminic, and local anesthetic effects. Although its exact mechanism of antiemetic action is unknown, dimenhydrinate has been shown to inhibit vestibular stimulation, acting first on the otolith system, and in larger doses on the semicircular canals. Dimenhydrinate inhibits acetylcholine; some investigators believe this is its primary mechanism of action, since cholinergic stimulation in the vestibular and reticular systems may be responsible for the nausea and vomiting of motion sickness. Tolerance to CNS depressant effects usually occurs after a few days of treatment, and some decrease in antiemetic effectiveness may be noted after prolonged use.

Pharmacokinetics

■ **Absorption** Dimenhydrinate is well absorbed after oral or parenteral administration. Antiemetic effects occur almost immediately after IV administration, within 15–30 minutes after oral administration, and 20–30 minutes after IM administration. The duration of action is 3–6 hours.

■ **Distribution and Elimination** Little information is available on the distribution and metabolic fate of dimenhydrinate. Like other antihistamines, the drug probably is widely distributed into body tissues, crosses the placenta, is metabolized by the liver, and is excreted in urine. Small amounts of dimenhydrinate are distributed into milk.

Chemistry and Stability

■ **Chemistry** Dimenhydrinate is an ethanolamine-derivative antihistamine that is used as an antiemetic. The drug contains 53–55.5% diphenhydramine and 44–47% 8-chlorotheophylline. Dimenhydrinate occurs as a white, odorless, crystalline powder with a bitter, numbing taste, and is slightly soluble in water and freely soluble in alcohol and in propylene glycol. Dimenhydrinate injection is a sterile solution of the drug in a mixture of propylene glycol and water and has a pH of 6.4–7.2.

■ **Stability** Dimenhydrinate preparations should be stored at room temperature; freezing of the oral solution and injection should be avoided. Dimenhydrinate tablets should be stored in well-closed containers and the oral solution in tight containers.

Dimenhydrinate injection has been reported to be incompatible with many drugs, but the compatibility depends on several factors (e.g., concentrations of the drugs, specific diluents used, resulting pH, temperature). Specialized references should be consulted for specific compatibility information.

Preparations

Excipients in commercially available drug preparations may have clinically important effects in some individuals; consult specific product labeling for details.

dimenhyDRINATE

Oral		
Solution	12.5 mg/5 mL*	**DMH® Syrup,** Alra
		Dramamine® Children's (with methylparaben), Pfizer
Tablets	50 mg*	**Dramamine®** (scored), Pfizer
Tablets, chewable	50 mg	**Dramamine® Children's** (with sorbitol and tartrazine; scored), Pfizer
Tablets, film-coated	50 mg	**TripTone® Caplets®** (scored), Del
Parenteral		
Injection	50 mg/mL*	**dimenhyDRINATE Injection** (with propylene glycol and benzyl alcohol), Abraxis

*available from one or more manufacturer, distributor, and/or repackager by generic (nonproprietary) name

†Use is not currently included in the labeling approved by the US Food and Drug Administration

Meclizine Hydrochloride

Meclozine Hydrochloride

■ Meclizine, a piperazine-derivative antihistamine, is an antiemetic.

Uses

■ **Motion Sickness** Meclizine hydrochloride is used in the prevention and treatment of nausea, vomiting, and/or vertigo associated with motion sickness. Meclizine is most effective against motion sickness when given prophylactically, although susceptibility to motion sickness may vary with the patient's age, previous exposure to motion, and the type, severity, and duration of motion. Although scopolamine generally is considered to be the most effective drug for the treatment of motion sickness, most clinicians prefer an antihistamine such as meclizine because it produces fewer adverse anticholinergic effects than does scopolamine. Meclizine and dimenhydrinate generally are considered to be equally effective in the treatment of motion sickness, but dimenhydrinate causes drowsiness more frequently. Meclizine has a longer duration of action than scopolamine and most other antihistamines. Promethazine may be more effective than other antihistamines in the treatment of motion sickness.

■ **Other Uses** Meclizine has been used in the symptomatic treatment of vertigo associated with diseases affecting the vestibular system (e.g., labyrinthitis, Ménière's disease), but the value of the drug in these conditions has not been established. Like other antihistamines, meclizine is less effective than the phenothiazines in controlling nausea and vomiting not related to vestibular stimulation.

Although meclizine is a histamine H_1-receptor antagonist, its use in allergic states has not been evaluated.

Dosage and Administration

■ **Administration** Meclizine hydrochloride is administered orally.

■ **Dosage** For the prevention and treatment of nausea, vomiting, and/or vertigo associated with motion sickness, the usual oral dosage of meclizine hydrochloride in adults and children 12 years of age or older is 25–50 mg once daily or as directed by a physician. For the prevention of motion sickness, 25–50 mg of the drug may be given 1 hour before exposure to motion.

For the control of vertigo associated with diseases affecting the vestibular system, the usual adult dosage is 25–100 mg daily, administered in divided doses.

For further information on pharmacology, cautions, and acute toxicity in therapy with meclizine, see the Antihistamines General Statement 4:00.

Cautions

■ **Adverse Effects** Drowsiness, fatigue, dry mouth, and, rarely, blurred vision have occurred after administration of meclizine.

■ **Precautions and Contraindications** Patients should be warned that meclizine may impair their ability to perform hazardous activities requiring mental alertness or physical coordination (e.g., operating machinery, driving a motor vehicle). In addition, additive CNS depression may occur when antihistamines, such as meclizine, are administered concomitantly with other CNS depressants including barbiturates, tranquilizers, and alcohol. If meclizine is used concomitantly with other depressant drugs, caution should be used to avoid overdosage. The anticholinergic effects of the drug should be considered when administering meclizine to patients with angle-closure glaucoma or prostatic hypertrophy.

Meclizine is contraindicated in patients who are hypersensitive to it.

■ **Pediatric Precautions** Safety and efficacy of meclizine in children younger than 12 years of age have not been established; therefore, the manufacturers state that use of the drug in this age group is not recommended. If the drug is used in this age group (e.g., for the prevention and treatment of nausea, vomiting, and/or vertigo associated with motion sickness), it should be only under the advice and supervision of a physician.

■ **Pregnancy** Meclizine is teratogenic in animals. Although retrospective studies in humans suggest that the use of meclizine during pregnancy is probably not associated with teratogenic effects, the manufacturers state that the drug is contraindicated in women who are or may become pregnant.

Pharmacology

Meclizine has CNS depressant, anticholinergic, antiemetic, antispasmodic, and local anesthetic effects in addition to antihistaminic activity. The drug depresses labyrinth excitability and conduction in vestibular-cerebellar pathways. The antiemetic and antimotion-sickness actions of meclizine result, at least in part, from its central anticholinergic and CNS depressant properties.

Pharmacokinetics

The onset of action of meclizine hydrochloride is about 1 hour and the drug has a prolonged duration of action, with effects persisting 8–24 hours following administration of a single oral dose. The drug has a plasma half-life of 6 hours. The metabolic fate of meclizine in humans is unknown. In rats, meclizine is metabolized (probably in the liver) to norchlorcyclizine. This metabolite is distributed throughout most body tissues and crosses the placenta. The drug is excreted in feces unchanged and in urine as norchlorcyclizine.

Chemistry and Stability

■ **Chemistry** Meclizine is a piperazine-derivative antihistamine that is used as an antiemetic. Meclizine hydrochloride occurs as a white or slightly yellowish, crystalline powder, has a slight odor and is tasteless, and is practically insoluble in water and slightly soluble in alcohol.

■ **Stability** Meclizine hydrochloride preparations should be stored at a temperature less than 40°C, preferably between 15–30°C; the conventional tablets should be stored in well-closed containers.

Preparations

Excipients in commercially available drug preparations may have clinically important effects in some individuals; consult specific product labeling for details.

Meclizine Hydrochloride

Oral		
Capsules	25 mg	**Meni-D®**, Seatrace
Tablets	12.5 mg*	**Antivert®**, Pfizer
	25 mg*	**Antivert®**, Pfizer
		Dramamine® Less Drowsy, Pfizer
	50 mg*	**Antivert®** (scored), Pfizer
Tablets, chewable	25 mg*	**Bonine®** (scored), Insight

*available from one or more manufacturer, distributor, and/or repackager by generic (nonproprietary) name

Prochlorperazine
Prochlorperazine Edisylate
Prochlorperazine Maleate

■ Prochlorperazine, a phenothiazine derivative, is an antiemetic.

Uses

Prochlorperazine is used for the control of severe nausea and vomiting of various etiologies. The drug is effective for the management of postoperative nausea and vomiting, and that caused by toxins, radiation, or cytotoxic drugs. Prochlorperazine also is effective for the relief of acute migraine attacks and associated nausea and vomiting. (For further information on management and classification of migraine headache, see Vascular Headaches: General Principles in Migraine Therapy, under Uses in Sumatriptan 28:32.28.) Prochlorperazine is not effective in preventing vertigo or motion sickness, or for the management of emesis caused by the action of drugs on the nodose ganglion or locally on the GI tract. Because safety of prochlorperazine for the prevention and treatment of nausea and vomiting associated with pregnancy has not been established, use of the drug is not recommended during pregnancy except in cases of severe nausea and vomiting so serious and intractable that, in the judgment of the clinician, pharmacologic intervention is required and the potential benefits justify the possible risks to the fetus. (See Cautions: Pregnancy, Fertility, and Lactation in the Phenothiazines General Statement 28:16.08.24.)

For the use of prochlorperazine as an antipsychotic agent, see 28:16.08.24.

Dosage and Administration

■ **Administration** Prochlorperazine edisylate is administered orally, by deep IM injection, or by direct IV injection or by IV infusion. When administered by direct IV injection, prochlorperazine is administered at a rate not exceeding 5 mg/minute; the drug should *not* be given as a bolus injection. Subcutaneous administration of the drug is *not* recommended because of local irritation. Prochlorperazine maleate is administered orally. Prochlorperazine is administered rectally.

For IV infusion, 20 mg (4 mL) of prochlorperazine injection should be diluted in 1 L of a compatible IV infusion solution (e.g., 0.9% sodium chloride).

■ **Dosage** Dosage of prochlorperazine and its salts is expressed in terms of prochlorperazine. Dosage must be carefully adjusted according to individual requirements and response, using the lowest possible effective dosage. Dosage should be increased more gradually in debilitated, emaciated, or geriatric patients. Since geriatric patients may be more susceptible to hypotension and neuromuscular reactions, these patients should be observed closely; in general, dosages in the lower end of the range are sufficient for most geriatric patients. Since children appear to be more prone to extrapyramidal reactions, even at moderate dosages, they should receive the lowest possible effective dosage and parents should be instructed not to exceed the prescribed dosage.

For the control of severe nausea and vomiting in patients who can tolerate oral administration of the drug, the usual adult oral dosage of prochlorperazine is 5 or 10 mg 3 or 4 times daily. Alternatively, a dosage of 15 mg (as the extended-release Spansule®) once daily upon arising or 10 mg (as the extended-release Spansule®) every 12 hours may be used; some patients subsequently may require a dosage of 30 mg (using the appropriate number of 10- or 15-mg extended-release Spansules®) once daily in the morning. Oral dosages exceeding 40 mg daily should be used only in resistant cases. The usual adult rectal dosage of prochlorperazine for the control of severe nausea and vomiting is 25 mg twice daily. The usual initial adult IM dose of prochlorperazine for the control of severe nausea and vomiting is 5–10 mg. If necessary, the initial IM dose may be repeated every 3 or 4 hours, but total IM dosage should not exceed 40 mg daily. For the control of severe nausea and vomiting, the usual adult IV dose of prochlorperazine is 2.5–10 mg; single IV doses of the drug should not exceed 10 mg and total IV dosage should not exceed 40 mg daily. For the control of severe nausea and vomiting in children older than 2 years of age and weighing more than 9 kg, the usual oral or rectal dosage of prochlorperazine is 0.4 mg/kg or 10 mg/m^2 daily given in 3 or 4 divided doses. Alternatively, the oral or rectal dosage of prochlorperazine for the control of severe nausea and vomiting in children older than 2 years of age and weighing 9.1–13.2 kg is 2.5 mg once or twice daily, but not exceeding 7.5 mg daily; children weighing 13.6–17.7 kg may receive 2.5 mg 2 or 3 times daily, but no more than 10 mg daily; and children weighing 18.2–38.6 kg may receive 2.5 mg 3 times daily or 5 mg twice daily, but no more than 15 mg daily. Generally, it is not necessary to continue oral or rectal therapy for longer than 24 hours in most pediatric patients. The usual IM dose of prochlorperazine for the control of severe nausea and vomiting in children 2 years of age or older and weighing more than 9 kg is 0.13 mg/kg. Generally, a single IM dose is sufficient to control nausea and vomiting in most pediatric patients.

For the control of severe nausea and vomiting during surgery, the usual initial adult IM dose of prochlorperazine is 5–10 mg given 1–2 hours before induction of anesthesia. If necessary, the initial IM dose may be repeated once, 30 minutes after the initial dose. To control acute symptoms during or after surgery, the usual adult IM dose is 5–10 mg, repeated once in 30 minutes, if necessary. For the control of severe nausea and vomiting during surgery, the usual adult IV dose of prochlorperazine is 5–10 mg given 15–30 minutes before induction of anesthesia. If necessary, the initial IV dose may be repeated once before surgery. To control acute symptoms during or after surgery, the usual adult IV dose is 5–10 mg, repeated once, if necessary; however, single IV doses of the drug should not exceed 10 mg. For the control of severe nausea and vomiting during surgery, prochlorperazine also may be given by IV infusion. For IV infusion, an infusion containing prochlorperazine 20 mg/L is begun 15–30 minutes before induction of anesthesia. Prochlorperazine is *not* recommended for the control of severe nausea and vomiting during surgery in children.

For further information on chemistry and stability, pharmacology, pharmacokinetics, uses, cautions, acute toxicity, drug interactions, laboratory test interferences, and dosage and administration of prochlorperazine, see the Phenothiazines General Statement 28:16.08.24. For information on the use of prochlorperazine in psychiatric disorders, see 28:16.08.24.

Cautions

■ **Precautions** Prochlorperazine shares the toxic potentials of other phenothiazines, and the usual precautions of phenothiazine therapy should be observed. (See Cautions in the Phenothiazines General Statement 28:16.08.24.) The incidence of extrapyramidal reactions associated with prochlorperazine therapy appears to be relatively high in hospitalized psychiatric patients and in children.

Care should be taken to avoid skin contact with prochlorperazine edisylate oral solution or injection, since contact dermatitis has occurred rarely.

■ **Pediatric Precautions** Safety and efficacy of prochlorperazine in children younger than 2 years of age or those weighing less than 9 kg have not been established.

Use of prochlorperazine should be avoided in children and adolescents with suspected Reye's syndrome, since the antiemetic and potential extrapyramidal effects produced by the drug may obscure the diagnosis of or be confused with the CNS signs of this condition; the drug also is hepatotoxic.

Prochlorperazine should not be used in children during surgery or in conditions for which pediatric dosage has not been established.

Pharmacology

The precise mechanism of antiemetic action of prochlorperazine is unclear, but the drug inhibits apomorphine-induced vomiting and has been shown to directly affect the medullary chemoreceptor trigger zone (CTZ), apparently by blocking dopamine receptors in the CTZ.

Pharmacokinetics

Following oral administration of prochlorperazine maleate in a tablet formulation, the drug has an onset of action of approximately 30–40 minutes and a duration of action of 3–4 hours. The onset of action following oral administration of prochlorperazine maleate in an extended-release formulation is approximately 30–40 minutes; the duration of action is 10–12 hours. Rectally administered prochlorperazine in a suppository has an onset of action of approximately 60 minutes and a duration of action of approximately 3–4 hours. Following IM administration of prochlorperazine edisylate, the drug has an onset of action within 10–20 minutes and a duration of action of 3–4 hours.

Chemistry and Stability

■ **Chemistry** Prochlorperazine is a phenothiazine antiemetic. The drug is a propylpiperazine derivative of phenothiazine. Prochlorperazine is commercially available as the base, edisylate salt, and maleate salt. Each 7.5 mg of prochlorperazine edisylate or 8 mg of prochlorperazine maleate is approximately equivalent to 5 mg of prochlorperazine.

Prochlorperazine occurs as a clear, pale yellow, viscous liquid and is very slightly soluble in water and freely soluble in alcohol. Prochlorperazine edisylate occurs as a white to very light yellow, odorless, crystalline powder and has approximate solubilities of 500 mg/mL in water and 0.67 mg/mL in alcohol at 25°C. Prochlorperazine maleate occurs as a white to pale yellow, practically odorless, crystalline powder and is practically insoluble in water and has a solubility of approximately 0.83 mg/mL in alcohol at 25°C. Prochlorperazine edisylate injection is a sterile solution of the drug in water for injection. The commercially available injection has a pH of 4.2–6.2 and may contain benzyl alcohol as a preservative and other excipients. The commercially available prochlorperazine edisylate oral solution has a pH of 4.5–5.

■ **Stability** Commercially available preparations of prochlorperazine should be stored in tight, light-resistant containers. Prochlorperazine edisylate oral solutions and injection, and prochlorperazine maleate tablets and extended-release capsules should be stored at a temperature less than 40°C, preferably between 15–30°C; freezing of the oral solutions and injection should be avoided. Prochlorperazine suppositories should be stored at a temperature less than 37°C. Slight yellowish discoloration of the oral solutions or injection will not affect potency or efficacy, but they should not be used if markedly discolored or if a precipitate is present. Prochlorperazine edisylate injection is physically and/or chemically incompatible with some drugs, but the compatibility depends on several factors (e.g., concentrations of the drugs, specific diluents used, resulting pH, temperature). Specialized references should be consulted for specific compatibility information.

Preparations

Excipients in commercially available drug preparations may have clinically important effects in some individuals; consult specific product labeling for details.

Prochlorperazine

Rectal

Suppositories	2.5 mg	**Compazine®**, GlaxoSmithKline
	5 mg	**Compazine®**, GlaxoSmithKline
	25 mg	**Compazine®**, GlaxoSmithKline
		Compro®, Paddock
		Prochlorperazine Suppositories

Prochlorperazine Edisylate

Oral		
Solution	5 mg (of prochlorperazine) per 5 mL	**Compazine® Syrup**, GlaxoSmithKline
Parenteral		
Injection	5 mg (of prochlorperazine) per mL*	**Compazine®**, GlaxoSmithKline

*available from one or more manufacturer, distributor, and/or repackager by generic (nonproprietary) name

Prochlorperazine Maleate

Oral		
Capsules, extended-release	10 mg (of prochlorperazine)	**Compazine® Spansule®**, GlaxoSmithKline
	15 mg (of prochlorperazine)	**Compazine® Spansule®**, GlaxoSmithKline
Tablets, film-coated	5 mg (of prochlorperazine)*	**Compazine®**, GlaxoSmithKline **Prochlorperazine Film-coated Tablets**
	10 mg (of prochlorperazine)*	**Compazine®**, GlaxoSmithKline **Prochlorperazine Film-coated Tablets**

*available from one or more manufacturer, distributor, and/or repackager by generic (nonproprietary) name

5-HT$_3$ Receptor Antagonists 56:22.20

Granisetron Hydrochloride

■ Granisetron hydrochloride, a selective, first-generation inhibitor of type 3 serotonergic (5-HT$_3$) receptors, is an antiemetic.

Uses

Granisetron hydrochloride is used orally or IV for the prevention of nausea and vomiting associated with initial and repeat courses of emetogenic cancer chemotherapy. The drug also is used orally for the prevention of radiation-induced nausea and vomiting. In addition, granisetron hydrochloride is used IV for the prevention and treatment of postoperative nausea and vomiting.

■ **Cancer Chemotherapy-induced Nausea and Vomiting** Granisetron is used IV for the prevention of nausea and vomiting associated with initial and repeat courses of emetogenic cancer chemotherapy, including high-dose cisplatin therapy, in adults and children 2–16 years of age. Granisetron is used orally in adults for the prevention of nausea and vomiting associated with initial and repeat courses of emetogenic cancer chemotherapy, including high-dose cisplatin therapy. The drug has been used effectively for the prevention of chemotherapy-induced emesis in patients receiving cisplatin alone or in combination with other antineoplastic agents.

To prevent chemotherapy-induced nausea and vomiting associated with *highly emetogenic* chemotherapy regimens (including an anthracycline plus cyclophosphamide), the American Society of Clinical Oncology (ASCO) currently recommends a 3-drug antiemetic regimen consisting of a neurokinin-1 (NK$_1$) receptor antagonist (e.g., either oral aprepitant or IV fosaprepitant dimeglumine), a type 3 serotonin (5-HT$_3$) receptor antagonist (e.g., dolasetron, granisetron, ondansetron, palonosetron, ramosetron [not commercially available in the US], tropisetron [not commercially available in the US]), and dexamethasone. ASCO states that the oral, fixed-combination of netupitant and palonosetron plus dexamethasone is an additional antiemetic treatment option in this setting.

For patients receiving *moderately emetogenic* chemotherapy regimens, ASCO recommends a 2-drug antiemetic regimen preferably consisting of palonosetron and dexamethasone. If palonosetron is not available, a first-generation 5-HT$_3$ receptor antagonist (preferably granisetron or ondansetron) may be substituted. Limited evidence suggests that aprepitant may be added to this regimen; in such cases, ASCO states that any of the 5-HT$_3$ receptor antagonists is appropriate.

For patients receiving chemotherapy regimens with a *low emetogenic risk*, ASCO recommends administration of a single dose of dexamethasone prior to chemotherapy.

In patients receiving chemotherapy regimens with a *minimal emetogenic risk*, antiemetics should not be routinely administered prior to or following chemotherapy.

■ **Radiation-induced Nausea and Vomiting** Granisetron is used orally for the prevention of radiation-induced nausea and vomiting in adults. The drug has been used effectively to prevent nausea and vomiting in patients receiving total body irradiation or daily fractionated radiation to the abdomen.

■ **Postoperative Nausea and Vomiting** Granisetron is used IV for the prevention and treatment of postoperative nausea and vomiting. The drug has been used effectively to prevent nausea and vomiting in surgical patients in whom nausea and vomiting must be avoided postoperatively and to treat patients who have developed postoperative nausea and/or vomiting. The manufacturer states that as with other antiemetics, routine prophylaxis with granisetron is not recommended in patients in whom there is little expectation that nausea and/or vomiting will occur postoperatively. However, use of the drug is recommended for patients in whom nausea and/or vomiting must be avoided postoperatively, even when the anticipated incidence of such nausea and/or vomiting is low.

Dosage and Administration

■ **Reconstitution and Administration** Granisetron hydrochloride is administered orally, by IV infusion, or by direct IV injection. For IV infusion, the drug should be diluted in 5% dextrose or 0.9% sodium chloride injection to a total volume of 20–50 mL and infused IV over 5 minutes. For direct IV injection, the drug is administered undiluted over 30 seconds.

■ **Dosage** The manufacturer states that safety and efficacy of IV granisetron for cancer chemotherapy-induced nausea and vomiting in children younger than 2 years of age have not been established. Safety and efficacy of IV granisetron for the prevention and treatment of postoperative nausea and vomiting, and safety and efficacy of oral granisetron have not been established in children of any age.

Dosage of granisetron, which is available for oral or IV use as the hydrochloride, is expressed in terms of granisetron.

The manufacturer states that a dose of granisetron oral solution is bioequivalent to the corresponding dose of the oral tablets, and the dosage forms may be used interchangeably.

The manufacturer states that dosage modification in geriatric patients is not necessary.

Cancer Chemotherapy-induced Nausea and Vomiting For the prevention of cancer chemotherapy-induced emesis in adults and children 2–16 years of age, 10 mcg/kg of granisetron is given as a 5-minute IV infusion or direct IV injection within 30 minutes before administration of an emetogenic drug. If the drug is administered orally, the usual adult dosage is 1 mg twice daily, or, alternatively, 2 mg once daily. When the twice-daily dosing regimen is used, the first dose (1 mg) is given up to 1 hour before chemotherapy and the second dose (1 mg) is given 12 hours after the first dose. When the once-daily dosing regimen is used, 2 mg is given up to 1 hour before chemotherapy. Oral or IV granisetron is administered only on the days when emetogenic chemotherapy is administered. The manufacturer states that continued granisetron therapy while patients are not receiving emetogenic chemotherapy has *not* been found to be useful.

Radiation-induced Nausea and Vomiting For the prevention of radiation-induced nausea and vomiting in adults undergoing total body irradiation or daily fractionated radiation to the abdomen, the usual oral dosage of granisetron is 2 mg once daily. Patients should receive oral granisetron within 1 hour of radiation. The manufacturer states that there is no experience with use of oral granisetron for the prevention of radiation-induced nausea and vomiting in children.

Postoperative Nausea and Vomiting For the prevention of postoperative nausea and vomiting in adults, a single granisetron IV dose of 1 mg is given undiluted over 30 seconds before induction of anesthesia or immediately before reversal of anesthesia. For the treatment of postoperative nausea and vomiting in adults, 1 mg of undiluted granisetron injection is administered IV over 30 seconds. The manufacturer states that clinical studies of granisetron for postoperative nausea and vomiting did not include sufficient numbers of patients 65 years of age and older to determine whether geriatric patients respond differently than younger patients; however, other clinical experience has not revealed age-related differences in response.

■ **Dosage in Renal and Hepatic Impairment** The manufacturer states that dosage modification is not necessary when granisetron is used in patients with renal or hepatic impairment.

Description

Granisetron hydrochloride, a selective inhibitor of type 3 serotonergic (5-HT$_3$) receptors, is an antiemetic. The drug is structurally and pharmacologically related to ondansetron. The antiemetic activity of granisetron appears to be mediated both centrally and peripherally via inhibition of 5-HT$_3$ receptors. Current evidence indicates that 5-HT$_3$ receptors play a major role in acute emesis, but only a minor role in delayed nausea and vomiting.

The role of serotonin as a mediator of acute chemotherapy (e.g., cisplatin)-induced emesis has been strongly suggested by the temporal relationship between the emetogenic action of such drugs and the release (e.g., from GI enterochromaffin cells) of serotonin (e.g., as reflected by increases in plasma and urine concentrations of the serotonin metabolite 5-hydroxyindoleacetic acid [5-HIAA]) as well as by the clinical efficacy of antiemetic agents that act as inhibitors of 5-HT$_3$ receptors (e.g., granisetron, metoclopramide, ondansetron). Studies in animals have shown that such chemotherapy-induced emesis can be prevented completely by ablation of the area postrema (the locus of the chemoreceptor trigger zone [CTZ]) or depletion of serotonin from this area; in addition, high levels of 5-HT$_3$ receptors have been demonstrated in this area, and direct injection of 5-HT$_3$ receptor antagonists into the area postrema also can prevent such chemotherapy-induced emesis. Therefore, current evidence suggests that the emetogenic action of such chemotherapy may be initiated by degenerative changes in the GI tract (e.g., small intestine) induced by these drugs and associated increases in endogenous serotonin release; serotonin then stimulates vagal and splanchnic nerve receptors that project to the medullary vomiting (emetic) center of the brain and also appears to stimulate 5-HT$_3$ receptors in the area postrema. Thus, 5-HT$_3$ receptor antagonists appear to prevent or ameliorate acute chemotherapy-induced emesis by inhibiting visceral (from the GI tract) afferent stimulation of the emetic center probably indirectly at the level of the area postrema and by directly inhibiting serotonin activity within the area postrema and CTZ.

Alternative mechanisms appear to be principally responsible for delayed nausea and vomiting induced by such chemotherapy (e.g., cisplatin), since similar temporal relationships between serotonin and emesis beyond the first day after a dose have not been established, and inhibitors of 5-HT$_3$ receptors do not appear to be effective alone in preventing or ameliorating delayed effects.

SumMon® (see Users Guide). For additional information on this drug until a more detailed monograph is developed and published, the manufacturer's labeling should be consulted. It is *essential* that the labeling be consulted for detailed information on the usual cautions, precautions, and contraindications.

Preparations

Excipients in commercially available drug preparations may have clinically important effects in some individuals; consult specific product labeling for details.

Granisetron Hydrochloride

Oral		
Solution	1 mg (of granisetron) per 5 mL	**Kytril®**, Roche
Tablets, film-coated	1 mg (of granisetron)	**Kytril®**, Roche
Parenteral		
Injection, for IV use	0.1 mg (of granisetron) per mL (0.1 mg)	**Kytril®**, Roche
	1 mg (of granisetron) per mL (1 and 4 mg)	**Kytril®**, Roche

Ondansetron Hydrochloride

■ Ondansetron hydrochloride, a selective, first-generation inhibitor of type 3 serotonin (5-HT$_3$) receptors, is an antiemetic.

Uses

■ **Cancer Chemotherapy-induced Nausea and Vomiting** Ondansetron is used orally or IV for the prevention of nausea and vomiting associated with emetogenic cancer chemotherapy. The drug is used IV with initial and repeat courses of emetogenic cancer chemotherapy, including high-dose cisplatin therapy. Ondansetron is used orally with highly emetogenic cancer chemotherapy (including cisplatin at a dosage of 50 mg/m^2 or greater). Ondansetron also is used orally with initial and repeat courses of moderately emetogenic cancer chemotherapy. The drug has been used effectively for the prevention of chemotherapy-induced emesis in patients receiving cisplatin alone or in combination with other antineoplastic agents and in those receiving other antineoplastic regimens (e.g., cyclophosphamide plus fluorouracil, doxorubicin, methotrexate, and/or vincristine) that did not include cisplatin.

To prevent chemotherapy-induced nausea and vomiting associated with *highly emetogenic* chemotherapy regimens (including an anthracycline plus cyclophosphamide), the American Society of Clinical Oncology (ASCO) currently recommends a 3-drug antiemetic regimen consisting of a neurokinin-1 (NK$_1$) receptor antagonist (e.g., either oral aprepitant or IV fosaprepitant dimeglumine), a type 3 serotonin (5-HT$_3$) receptor antagonist (e.g., dolasetron, granisetron, ondansetron, palonosetron, ramosetron [not commercially available in the US], tropisetron [not commercially available in the US]), and dexamethasone. ASCO states that the oral, fixed-combination of netupitant and palonosetron plus dexamethasone is an additional antiemetic treatment option in this setting.

For patients receiving *moderately emetogenic* chemotherapy regimens, ASCO recommends a 2-drug antiemetic regimen preferably consisting of palonosetron and dexamethasone. If palonosetron is not available, a first-generation 5-HT$_3$ receptor antagonist (preferably granisetron or ondansetron) may be substituted. Limited evidence suggests that aprepitant may be added to this regimen; in such cases, ASCO states that any of the 5-HT$_3$ receptor antagonists is appropriate.

For patients receiving chemotherapy regimens with a *low emetogenic risk*, ASCO recommends administration of a single dose of dexamethasone prior to chemotherapy.

In patients receiving chemotherapy regimens with a *minimal emetogenic risk*, antiemetics should not be routinely administered prior to or following chemotherapy.

■ **Postoperative Nausea and Vomiting** Ondansetron is used orally or IV for the prevention of postoperative nausea and vomiting. Oral or IV ondansetron has been used effectively to prevent nausea and vomiting in surgical patients where nausea and vomiting must be avoided postoperatively; IV ondansetron also has been used effectively to prevent further episodes of nausea and vomiting in patients who did not receive prophylactic antiemetic therapy and developed postoperative nausea and/or vomiting. Studies of oral ondansetron for the prevention of postoperative nausea and vomiting to date have included only women undergoing inpatient surgical procedures; no studies have been performed in males. Controlled studies comparing oral versus IV administration of ondansetron have not been performed to date. The manufacturer states that as with other antiemetics, routine prophylaxis with ondansetron is not recommended in patients in whom there is little expectation that nausea and/or vomiting will occur postoperatively. However, use of the drug is recommended for patients in whom nausea and/or vomiting must be avoided postoperatively, even when the anticipated incidence of such nausea and/or vomiting is low.

■ **Radiation-induced Nausea and Vomiting** Ondansetron is used orally for the prevention of radiation-induced nausea and vomiting. The drug has been used effectively to prevent nausea and vomiting in patients receiving total body irradiation or single high-dose fraction or daily fractionated radiation to the abdomen.

Dosage and Administration

■ **Reconstitution and Administration** Ondansetron hydrochloride generally is administered orally or IV; the manufacturer states that, alternatively, the drug may be administered *undiluted* by IM injection in adults for prevention of postoperative nausea and vomiting. (See Dosage: Postoperative Nausea and Vomiting.) For prevention of cancer chemotherapy-induced nausea and vomiting, ondansetron hydrochloride injection should be diluted in 50 mL of 5% dextrose injection or 0.9% sodium chloride injection and infused IV over 15 minutes.

For prevention of postoperative nausea and vomiting, ondansetron hydrochloride injection in single- or multiple-dose vials does *not* require dilution. The undiluted drug is administered by IV injection over a period of at least 30 seconds and, preferably, over a period of 2–5 minutes.

Ondansetron hydrochloride occasionally precipitates at the stopper/vial interface in vials that are stored upright; the manufacturer states that potency and safety of the drug are not affected. If a precipitate is found, the drug may be resolubilized by vigorous shaking of the vial.

Patients receiving ondansetron orally disintegrating tablets should be instructed not to remove a tablet from the blister until just prior to dosing. The tablet should not be pushed through the foil. With dry hands, the blister backing should be peeled completely off the blister. The tablet should then be gently removed and immediately placed on the tongue to dissolve and be swallowed with the saliva; administration with liquid is not necessary.

■ **Dosage** Dosage of ondansetron, which is available for oral or IV use as the hydrochloride dihydrate and also for oral use as ondansetron base (orally disintegrating tablets), is expressed in terms of ondansetron.

Cancer Chemotherapy-induced Nausea and Vomiting **Oral Dosage.** For the prevention of nausea and vomiting associated with moderately emetogenic cancer chemotherapy in adults and children 12 years of age and older, an initial ondansetron dose of 8 mg is given 30 minutes before administration of an emetogenic drug and the dose is repeated 8 hours after the initial dose. An 8-mg dose should be administered at 12-hour intervals for 1–2 days following completion of the emetogenic chemotherapy.

For children 4–11 years of age, an initial ondansetron dose of 4 mg is given 30 minutes before administration of a moderately emetogenic cancer chemotherapy drug, with subsequent doses 4 and 8 hours after the initial dose. A 4-mg dose should then be administered at 8-hour intervals for 1–2 days following completion of emetogenic cancer chemotherapy. Little information currently is available regarding dosages for children younger than 4 years of age.

For the prevention of nausea and vomiting associated with highly emetogenic cancer chemotherapy in adults, a single oral 24-mg dose of ondansetron is given 30 minutes before administration of single-day chemotherapy. The manufacturer states that multiple-day, single-daily-dose oral administration of ondansetron 24 mg has not been studied to date. In addition, safety and efficacy of single-daily-dose oral administration of the 24-mg dose have not been established in pediatric patients.

The manufacturer states that dosage modification is not necessary in geriatric patients.

IV Dosage. For the prevention of cancer chemotherapy-induced nausea and vomiting in adults and pediatric patients 6 months of age and older, an initial IV ondansetron dose of 0.15 mg/kg (up to a maximum of 16 mg per dose) is given as a 15-minute infusion beginning 30 minutes before administration of an emetogenic drug and is repeated twice at 4-hour intervals following the initial dose. Because of the risk of QT interval prolongation (see Cautions: Cardiovascular Effects), an antiemetic regimen consisting of a single IV ondansetron dose of 32 mg no longer is recommended for prevention of cancer chemotherapy-induced nausea and vomiting. Efficacy and safety of alternative single-dose IV ondansetron regimens for prevention of cancer chemotherapy-induced nausea and vomiting have not been established.

The manufacturer states that dosage modification is not necessary in geriatric patients. Little information currently is available regarding dosages for pediatric patients younger than 6 months of age.

Postoperative Nausea and Vomiting For the prevention of postoperative nausea and vomiting in adults, a single ondansetron IV dose of 4 mg is given immediately before induction of anesthesia or postoperatively if the patient experiences nausea and/or vomiting shortly after surgery. In pediatric patients 1 month to 12 years of age, the recommended dosage of ondansetron is a single IV dose of 4 mg in patients weighing more than 40 kg or a single IV dose of 0.1 mg/kg in patients weighing 40 kg or less; the dose should be given immediately before or after induction of anesthesia or postoperatively if the patient experiences nausea and/or vomiting shortly after surgery. Little information is available regarding dosages for patients weighing more than 80 kg. The manufacturer states that adults who do not achieve adequate control of postoperative nausea and vomiting with a single 4-mg IV dose of ondansetron given prior to induction of anesthesia will not obtain additional benefit from administration of a second 4-mg dose of the drug postoperatively. Efficacy of a second dose of ondansetron in pediatric patients who did not achieve adequate control of postoperative nausea and vomiting following a single prophylactic dose of the drug has not been evaluated.

If ondansetron is used orally for the prevention of postoperative nausea and vomiting in adults, a single 16-mg dose is given 1 hour before induction of anesthesia. The manufacturer states that oral or IV dosage modification is not necessary in geriatric patients and that there is no experience with the use of oral ondansetron for the prevention of postoperative nausea and vomiting in children.

As an alternative to IV administration for the prevention of postoperative nausea and vomiting in adults, an ondansetron dose of 4 mg may be given IM *undiluted* as a single injection.

Radiation-induced Nausea and Vomiting For prevention of radiation-induced nausea and vomiting in adults undergoing total body irradiation or single high-dose fraction or daily fractionated radiation to the abdomen, the usual oral dosage of ondansetron is 8 mg 3 times daily. Patients undergoing total body irradiation should receive one 8-mg dose 1–2 hours before each fraction of radiation therapy each day. Patients undergoing single high-dose fraction radiation therapy to the abdomen should receive one 8-mg dose 1–2 hours before radiation, with subsequent doses administered every 8 hours for 1–2 days after completion of radiation therapy. For patients undergoing daily fractionated radiation to the abdomen, one 8-mg dose should be given 1–2 hours before radiation therapy and then every 8 hours, with this regimen repeated for each day radiation therapy is given. The manufacturer states that dosage modification is not necessary in geriatric patients and that there is no experience with use of the drug for the prevention of radiation-induced nausea and vomiting in children.

■ **Dosage in Renal and Hepatic Impairment** The manufacturer states that patients with renal impairment do not require ondansetron dosage adjustment, but there is no experience with continuing ondansetron beyond the first day of therapy in such patients. Although only about 5% of the drug is eliminated by the kidneys and renal impairment was not expected to substantially alter elimination of ondansetron, mean plasma clearance has been decreased by about 41–50% in patients with severe renal impairment (creatinine clearances less than 30 mL/minute). However, the decrease in clearance was variable and not consistent with an increase in plasma half-life of the drug. In patients with severe hepatic impairment (Child-Pugh score of 10 or greater) clearance is decreased and apparent volume of distribution of ondansetron is increased with a resultant increase in plasma half-life; therefore, the manufacturer recommends that the total daily dose not exceed 8 mg in such patients.

Cautions

Ondansetron generally is well tolerated. Most adverse effects reported in clinical trials have been mild to moderate in severity. Adverse effects rarely have resulted in discontinuance of the drug. The most frequent adverse effects of ondansetron in patients receiving the drug for the prevention of chemotherapy-induced nausea and vomiting involve the nervous system (e.g., headache) and GI tract (e.g., diarrhea, constipation). Because most patients receiving ondansetron in clinical trials for chemotherapy-induced nausea and vomiting had serious underlying disease (e.g., cancer) and were receiving toxic drugs (e.g., cisplatin), diuretics, and IV fluids concomitantly, it may be difficult to attribute various adverse effects to ondansetron. In trials comparing ondansetron and metoclopramide, adverse effects occurring substantially more frequently for one drug compared with the other included headache and constipation for ondansetron and diarrhea and extrapyramidal/dystonic manifestations for metoclopramide; adverse effects resulting in drug discontinuance were less common with ondansetron.

The adverse effect profile of ondansetron in patients receiving the drug for the prevention of radiation-induced nausea and vomiting is similar to that in patients receiving the drug for the prevention of chemotherapy-induced nausea and vomiting, although specific incidences of effects may vary; the most common adverse effects of the drug in patients undergoing radiation were headache, constipation, and diarrhea.

In clinical trials in patients receiving ondansetron for the prevention of postoperative nausea and vomiting, the incidences of adverse effects associated with ondansetron, with the exception of headache, did not differ substantially from those associated with placebo. Most such patients were receiving concomitantly multiple preoperative and postoperative drugs. Studies of oral ondansetron for the prevention of postoperative nausea and vomiting to date have included only women undergoing inpatient surgical procedures; no studies have been performed in males.

■ **Nervous System Effects** Headache is the most common adverse nervous system effect of ondansetron, occurring in 11–24% of patients receiving the drug orally or IV in recommended dosages for prevention of chemotherapy-induced nausea and vomiting and in 9–17% of those receiving the drug for postoperative nausea and vomiting in controlled clinical trials; headache occurred in 5% of patients receiving ondansetron for radiation-induced nausea and vomiting. Preliminary observations in a small number of patients suggest that headache occurs more frequently when ondansetron orally disintegrating tablets are taken with water as compared to ingestion without water. Headache generally is mild to moderate in severity and generally responds to mild analgesics. While some evidence suggests that the incidence of headache may be dose related, other evidence failed to establish a clear relationship, particularly regarding severity. Migraine headache has been reported rarely with oral or IV ondansetron.

Dizziness has been reported in 7% of patients receiving ondansetron orally in recommended dosages for prevention of postoperative nausea and vomiting in controlled clinical trials. Dizziness has occurred occasionally in patients receiving the drug IV (mainly during or shortly after IV infusion) and in 4–5% of patients receiving ondansetron orally for prevention of chemotherapy-induced nausea and vomiting; however, a direct causal relationship to the drug has not been established. Although not directly attributed to the drug, other adverse nervous system effects reported include drowsiness or sedation, which occurred in 8%, and paresthesia, which occurred in 2%, of patients receiving the drug IV in the recommended dosage for prevention of postoperative nausea and vomiting; these effects also occurred occasionally in patients receiving the drug orally or IV for prevention of chemotherapy-induced nausea and vomiting. Drowsiness/sedation occurred in 20%, and anxiety/agitation in 6%, of patients receiving oral ondansetron for prevention of postoperative nausea and vomiting in clinical trials. Anxiety or agitation also has occurred in patients receiving the drug IV for prevention of postoperative nausea and vomiting.

Although extrapyramidal reactions were not reported with ondansetron in clinical trials comparing the drug with metoclopramide, manifestations consistent with, but not necessarily diagnostic of, such reactions have been reported rarely in patients receiving ondansetron. Oculogyric crisis, appearing alone, as well as other dystonic reactions, have been reported during postmarketing experience in patients receiving IV ondansetron.

Restlessness, akathisia, ataxia, lightheadedness, and insomnia have been reported rarely with IV ondansetron. Lightheadedness was reported mainly during IV infusion of ondansetron and resolved rapidly. Panic attacks also have been reported rarely.

Seizures (including tonic-clonic seizures) have been reported rarely in patients receiving ondansetron.

■ **GI Effects** Diarrhea is the most common adverse GI effect of ondansetron, occurring in 16% of patients receiving the drug IV in recommended dosages for prevention of chemotherapy-induced nausea and vomiting in controlled clinical trials and in 4–6% of patients receiving the drug orally in recommended dosages. Because most patients receiving ondansetron IV for chemotherapy-induced nausea and vomiting were receiving cisplatin concomitantly, which can cause diarrhea, a causal relationship to ondansetron has not been established. Constipation occurred in 3% of ondansetron-treated patients receiving single-day IV therapy, but is more common in patients receiving multiple-day therapy, occurring in 11% of patients receiving multiple-day IV therapy and in 6–9% of patients receiving multiple-day oral therapy in the recommended dosage for chemotherapy-induced nausea and vomiting. The incidence of constipation may be dose related. Dyspepsia or heartburn, thirst, flatulence, abdominal cramps, abdominal pain, abnormal taste, anorexia, xerostomia, and intestinal obstruction also have been reported with oral or IV ondansetron for prevention of chemotherapy-induced nausea and vomiting.

■ **Hepatic Effects** Increased serum concentrations of ALT (SGPT) and AST (SGOT) exceeding twice the upper limit of normal have been reported in approximately 1–2% of patients receiving ondansetron orally for prevention of chemotherapy-induced nausea and vomiting, in approximately 5% of patients receiving the drug IV for prevention of chemotherapy-induced nausea and vomiting, and in approximately 1% of patients receiving the drug IV for prevention of postoperative nausea and vomiting. The increases were transient and appeared to be unrelated to dose or duration of ondansetron therapy; however, similar transient increases recurred in some courses of therapy with repeat exposure to the drug, but symptomatic hepatic disease did not occur. In patients with cancer, the role of cancer chemotherapy in these increases cannot be clearly determined. Hepatosplenomegaly, jaundice, and increased serum concentrations of bilirubin and γ-glutamyltransferase (GGT, γ-glutamyltranspeptidase, GGTP) also have been reported rarely.

Liver failure and death have been reported rarely in patients with cancer receiving ondansetron concomitantly with other drugs, including potentially hepatotoxic cytotoxic chemotherapy and antibiotics; the etiology of the liver failure is unclear.

■ **Dermatologic and Sensitivity Reactions** Pruritus has been reported in 2% of patients receiving ondansetron IV and in 5% of those receiving the drug orally for prevention of postoperative nausea and vomiting in controlled clinical trials. Rash, which may be maculopapular and/or accompanied by pruritus, has occurred in approximately 1% of patients receiving the drug orally or IV for prevention of chemotherapy-induced nausea and vomiting in controlled clinical trials. Rarely, rash may be followed by desquamation and hyperpigmentation.

Serious hypersensitivity reactions have occurred in patients receiving ondansetron orally or IV. In patients with cancer, these reactions have been reported to occur mainly following the first dose during the second or third course of cancer chemotherapy. These reactions may include anaphylaxis/anaphylactoid reactions, angioedema, bronchospasm, cardiopulmonary arrest, hypotension, laryngeal edema, laryngospasm, shock, shortness of breath, stridor, wheezing, facial edema, and urticaria. Sensitivity reactions also have been reported in patients who have exhibited sensitivity to other selective 5-HT$_3$-receptor antagonists. If a hypersensitivity reaction occurs during ondansetron therapy, the drug should be discontinued, and severe acute hypersensitivity reactions should be treated with appropriate therapy (e.g., epinephrine, corticosteroids, maintenance of an adequate airway, oxygen, IV fluids, antihistamines, maintenance of blood pressure) as indicated.

■ **Cardiovascular Effects** Prolongation of the QT interval and cases of torsades de pointes have been reported in patients receiving ondansetron. Preliminary results of a randomized, double-blind, placebo- and active-controlled crossover study conducted in healthy adults to assess the drug's effects on the QT interval indicate that ondansetron prolongs the QT interval in a dose-dependent manner. Following IV infusion of ondansetron 8 or 32 mg over 15 minutes, the maximum mean baseline-corrected increase in the QT$_c$ interval (QT interval corrected for heart rate using Fridericia's formula) relative to placebo was 5.8 or 19.6 milliseconds, respectively. Other studies in postoperative patients or healthy individuals also suggest that ondansetron can prolong the QT interval. Based on these findings, an antiemetic regimen consisting of a single IV ondansetron dose of 32 mg given prior to emetogenic cancer chemotherapy no longer is recommended. Individual IV doses of the drug should *not* exceed 16 mg. (See Cautions: Precautions and Contraindications.)

Hypotension has occurred in 5% of patients receiving oral ondansetron for prevention of postoperative nausea and vomiting. Unspecified chest pain and hypotension have been reported in patients receiving ondansetron IV for prevention of postoperative nausea and vomiting in controlled clinical trials, but these effects have not been directly attributed to the drug.

Angina (chest pain), hypotension, flushing, tachycardia, ECG alterations (including arrhythmias and prolongation of PR, QRS, and QT intervals), and vascular occlusive events (e.g., myocardial infarction, cerebrovascular accident, pulmonary embolism, deep-vein thrombosis) have been reported rarely during clinical trials or postmarketing experience in patients receiving ondansetron orally or IV for prevention of chemotherapy-induced nausea and vomiting; a definite causal relationship to the drug has not been established. Arrhythmias (including ventricular and supraventricular tachycardia, premature ventricular complexes, and atrial fibrillation), bradycardia, ECG alterations (including second-degree heart block and ST-segment depression), hypertension, syncope, and palpitations have been reported in patients receiving IV ondansetron, although these effects have not been directly attributed to the drug. Transient ECG alterations including QT-interval prolongation have been reported rarely, mainly in patients receiving the drug IV; cases of torsades de pointes have been reported during postmarketing experience in patients receiving ondansetron. Bradycardia also was reported in 6% of patients receiving oral ondansetron in clinical trials for prevention of postoperative nausea and vomiting.

■ **Ocular Effects** Transient blurred vision, occasionally associated with abnormalities of accommodation, has been reported rarely in patients during or shortly after IV infusion of ondansetron. This adverse effect may be ameliorated with a slower infusion rate or following discontinuance of the infusion. Transient blindness, which resolved within a few minutes to 48 hours, also has been reported, generally during IV administration of the drug.

■ **Other Adverse Effects** Fever occurred in 8% of patients receiving ondansetron IV for prevention of chemotherapy-induced nausea and vomiting and in 2% of patients receiving the drug IV for prevention of postoperative nausea and vomiting in controlled clinical trials. Malaise or fatigue was reported in 9–13% and weakness was reported in up to 2% of patients receiving ondansetron orally for prevention of chemotherapy-induced nausea and vomiting. Pyrexia was reported in 8% of patients receiving oral ondansetron for prevention of postoperative nausea and vomiting in controlled trials. Shivers have been reported in 5% of patients receiving ondansetron orally for prevention of postoperative nausea and vomiting in controlled clinical trials, and occasionally in patients receiving the drug orally for prevention of chemotherapy-induced nausea and vomiting. However, these effects have not been directly attributed to the drug. Sweating also has been reported rarely with IV ondansetron.

Injection site reactions (including pain, erythema, swelling, and burning) occurred in 4% of patients receiving ondansetron IV for prevention of postoperative nausea and vomiting and occasionally in patients receiving the drug IV for prevention of chemotherapy-induced nausea and vomiting in controlled clinical trials. Wound problems were reported in 28% of patients receiving ondansetron orally for postoperative nausea and vomiting in controlled trials. Throat problems and hemorrhage also have been reported in patients receiving ondansetron orally or IV for prevention of postoperative nausea and vomiting.

Cold sensation occurred in 2% of patients receiving ondansetron IV for prevention of postoperative nausea and vomiting in controlled clinical trials, although a causal relationship has not been established. Urinary retention has occurred in 5%, and gynecologic disorder in 7%, of patients receiving oral ondansetron for prevention of postoperative nausea and vomiting. Sensation of cold has been reported in patients receiving ondansetron IV for prevention of chemotherapy-induced nausea and vomiting; sensation of warmth also has been reported rarely with IV ondansetron therapy. Musculoskeletal pain has been reported in patients receiving IV ondansetron. Hypoxia has been reported in 9% of those receiving the drug orally for postoperative nausea and vomiting. Dyspnea, hypoxia, and hiccups also have been reported with ondansetron.

Although a definite causal relationship to ondansetron has not been established, hypokalemia has been reported rarely in patients receiving the drug orally or IV for prevention of cancer chemotherapy-induced nausea and vomiting.

■ **Precautions and Contraindications** Because of the risk of QT-interval prolongation, ondansetron should be avoided in patients with congenital long QT syndrome. ECG monitoring is recommended in patients with electrolyte abnormalities such as hypokalemia or hypomagnesemia, congestive heart failure, or bradyarrhythmias and in those receiving other drugs known to prolong the QT interval. Electrolyte abnormalities should be corrected prior to IV administration of ondansetron. Because effects of ondansetron on the QT interval are dose related, use of single IV doses exceeding 16 mg should be avoided. Patients receiving ondansetron should be advised to seek immediate medical care if feelings of faintness, lightheadedness, irregular heartbeat, shortness of breath, or dizziness occur.

Like other antiemetics, ondansetron may mask a progressive ileus and/or gastric distention in patients undergoing abdominal surgery or in patients with chemotherapy-induced nausea and vomiting.

Because ondansetron does not stimulate gastric or intestinal peristalsis, it should not be used as a substitute for nasogastric suction.

Because clearance of ondansetron is decreased and apparent volume of distribution and plasma half-life are increased in patients with severe hepatic impairment, the drug should be used with caution and at reduced dosage in such patients. (See Dosage and Administration: Dosage in Renal and Hepatic Impairment.)

Ondansetron rarely may cause serious hypersensitivity reactions, and patients should be advised of this possibility and instructed to discontinue the drug and contact their clinician at the first sign of rash or any other sign of hypersensitivity. (See Cautions: Dermatologic and Sensitivity Reactions.) Ondansetron is contraindicated in patients with known hypersensitivity to the drug or any ingredient in the formulation.

Because profound hypotension and loss of consciousness have been reported when ondansetron was administered concomitantly with apomorphine, concomitant use of these drugs is contraindicated.

Individuals with phenylketonuria (i.e., homozygous genetic deficiency of phenylalanine hydroxylase) and other individuals who must restrict their intake of phenylalanine should be warned that each 4- and 8-mg Zofran® ODT® orally disintegrating tablet contains aspartame (NutraSweet®), which is metabolized in the GI tract to provide less than 0.03 mg of phenylalanine following oral administration.

■ **Pediatric Precautions** The manufacturer states that little information is available on IV use of ondansetron for the prevention of postoperative nausea and vomiting in pediatric patients younger than 1 month of age or for the prevention of cancer chemotherapy-induced nausea and vomiting in pediatric patients younger than 6 months of age. Little information is available on oral dosage of ondansetron in pediatric patients 4 years of age or younger. Efficacy of the single 24-mg oral dose of ondansetron for the prevention of nausea and vomiting induced by highly emetogenic cancer chemotherapy in pediatric patients younger than 18 years of age has not been established. Efficacy of oral ondansetron for prevention of radiation-induced and postoperative nausea and vomiting in pediatric patients younger than 18 years of age has not been established. In prevention of cancer chemotherapy-induced emesis, safety and efficacy of the drug orally and IV generally are comparable to that observed in older children and adults.

In placebo-controlled trials evaluating IV ondansetron for prevention of postoperative nausea and vomiting in pediatric patients, adverse effects occurred at similar frequencies in pediatric patients receiving recommended dosages of ondansetron and those receiving placebo; however, among pediatric patients 1–24 months of age, diarrhea occurred more frequently in those receiving ondansetron compared with those receiving placebo (2 versus less than 1%).

Pediatric cancer or surgical patients younger than 18 years of age generally tend to have higher clearances and shorter half-lives of ondansetron compared with adults. However, in infants 1–4 months of age, clearance of the drug is reduced and half-life is prolonged (by approximately 2.5-fold relative to values in infants older than 4 months up to 24 months of age); thus, the manufacturer recommends that infants younger than 4 months of age receiving ondansetron therapy be closely monitored.

■ **Geriatric Precautions** While safety and efficacy of ondansetron have not been established specifically in geriatric patients, a large proportion of patients treated with the drug for chemotherapy-induced nausea and vomiting and prevention of postoperative nausea and/or vomiting have been 65 years of age or older. Plasma clearance of ondansetron may be decreased and elimination half-life increased in patients older than 75 years of age. In clinical studies with ondansetron that included patients 65 years of age and older, no overall differences in efficacy or safety were observed between patients in this age group and younger patients. However, the possibility that some older patients may exhibit increased sensitivity to the drug cannot be ruled out.

■ **Mutagenicity and Carcinogenicity** Ondansetron was not mutagenic in standard tests performed for mutagenicity. In rats and mice receiving oral dosages up to 10 and 30 mg/kg daily, respectively (approximately 3.6 and 5.4 times, respectively, the recommended human IV dosage of 0.15 mg/kg given 3 times daily [calculated on the basis of body surface area]), ondansetron did not produce evidence of carcinogenicity.

■ **Pregnancy, Fertility, and Lactation** Reproduction studies in rats and rabbits receiving oral ondansetron dosages up to 15 and 30 mg/kg daily, respectively, and IV ondansetron dosages up to 4 mg/kg daily (approximately 1.4 and 2.9 times, respectively, the recommended human IV dosage of 0.15 mg/kg given 3 times daily [calculated on the basis of body surface area]) have not revealed evidence of harm to the fetus. There are no adequate and controlled studies to date using ondansetron in pregnant women, and the drug should be used during pregnancy only when clearly needed.

Reproduction studies in male and female rats using oral ondansetron dosages up to 15 mg/kg daily (approximately 3.8 times the recommended human IV dosage based on body surface area) have not revealed evidence of impaired fertility.

It is not known whether ondansetron is distributed into human milk; however, the drug is distributed into the milk of lactating rats. Because many drugs are distributed in human milk, ondansetron should be used with caution in nursing women.

Description

Ondansetron hydrochloride, a selective inhibitor of type 3 serotonin (5-HT$_3$) receptors, is an antiemetic. The antiemetic activity of ondansetron appears to be mediated both centrally and peripherally via inhibition of 5-HT$_3$ receptors. Current evidence indicates that 5-HT$_3$ receptors play a major role in acute emesis, but only a minor role in delayed nausea and vomiting.

The role of serotonin as a mediator of acute chemotherapy (e.g., cisplatin) induced emesis has been strongly suggested by the temporal relationship between the emetogenic action of such drugs and the release (e.g., from GI enterochromaffin cells) of serotonin (e.g., as reflected by increases in plasma and urine concentrations of the serotonin metabolite 5-hydroxyindoleacetic acid [5-HIAA]) as well as by the clinical efficacy of antiemetic agents that act as inhibitors of 5-HT$_3$ receptors (e.g., ondansetron, metoclopramide, granisetron). Studies in animals have shown that such chemotherapy-induced emesis can be prevented completely by ablation of the area postrema (the locus of the chemoreceptor trigger zone [CTZ]) or depletion of serotonin from this area; in addition, high levels of 5-HT$_3$ receptors have been demonstrated in this area, and direct injection of 5-HT$_3$ receptor antagonists into the area postrema also can prevent such chemotherapy-induced emesis. Therefore, current evidence suggests that the emetogenic action of such chemotherapy may be initiated by degenerative changes in the GI tract (e.g., small intestine) induced by these drugs and associated increases in endogenous serotonin release; serotonin then stimulates vagal and splanchnic nerve receptors that project to the medullary vomiting (emetic) center of the brain and also appears to stimulate 5-HT$_3$ receptors in the area postrema. Thus, 5-HT$_3$ receptor antagonists appear to prevent or ameliorate acute chemotherapy-induced emesis by inhibiting visceral (from the GI tract) afferent stimulation of the emetic center probably indirectly at the level of the area postrema and by directly inhibiting serotonin activity within the area postrema and CTZ.

Alternative mechanisms appear to be principally responsible for delayed nausea and vomiting induced by such chemotherapy (e.g., cisplatin), since similar temporal relationships between serotonin and emesis beyond the first day after a dose have not been established, and inhibitors of 5-HT$_3$ receptors do not appear to be effective alone in preventing or ameliorating delayed effects.

SumMon® (see Users Guide). For additional information on this drug until a more detailed monograph is developed and published, the manufacturer's labeling should be consulted. It is *essential* that the labeling be consulted for detailed information on the usual cautions, precautions, and contraindications concerning potential drug interactions and/or laboratory test interferences and for information on acute toxicity.

Preparations

Excipients in commercially available drug preparations may have clinically important effects in some individuals; consult specific product labeling for details.

Ondansetron

Oral		
Tablets, orally disintegrating	4 mg*	**Ondansetron Orally Disintegrating Tablets**
		Zofran® ODT®, GlaxoSmithKline
	8 mg*	**Ondansetron Orally Disintegrating Tablets**
		Zofran® ODT®, GlaxoSmithKline

*available from one or more manufacturer, distributor, and/or repackager by generic (nonproprietary) name

Ondansetron Hydrochloride

Oral		
Solution	4 mg (of ondansetron) per 5 mL*	**Ondansetron Hydrochloride Oral Solution**
		Zofran®, GlaxoSmithKline
Tablets, film-coated	4 mg (of ondansetron)*	**Ondansetron Hydrochloride Tablets**
		Zofran®, GlaxoSmithKline
	8 mg (of ondansetron)*	**Ondansetron Hydrochloride Tablets**
		Zofran®, GlaxoSmithKline
Parenteral		
Injection, for IV use	2 mg (of ondansetron) per mL*	**Ondansetron Hydrochloride Injection**
		Zofran®, GlaxoSmithKline

*available from one or more manufacturer, distributor, and/or repackager by generic (nonproprietary) name

Palonosetron Hydrochloride

■ Palonosetron hydrochloride, a selective, second-generation inhibitor of type 3 serotonergic (5-HT$_3$) receptors, is an antiemetic.

Uses

Palonosetron hydrochloride is used IV for the prevention of nausea and vomiting associated with initial and repeat courses of emetogenic cancer chemotherapy. Palonosetron hydrochloride also is used IV for the prevention and treatment of postoperative nausea and vomiting.

■ **Cancer Chemotherapy-induced Nausea and Vomiting** Palonosetron hydrochloride is used IV for the prevention of acute and delayed nausea and vomiting associated with initial and repeat courses of moderately emetogenic cancer chemotherapy. The drug also is used IV for the prevention of acute nausea and vomiting associated with initial and repeat courses of highly emetogenic cancer chemotherapy.

To prevent chemotherapy-induced nausea and vomiting associated with *highly emetogenic* chemotherapy regimens (including an anthracycline plus cyclophosphamide), the American Society of Clinical Oncology (ASCO) currently recommends a 3-drug antiemetic regimen consisting of a neurokinin-1 (NK$_1$) receptor antagonist (e.g., either oral aprepitant or IV fosaprepitant dimeglumine), a type 3 serotonin (5-HT$_3$) receptor antagonist (e.g., dolasetron, granisetron, ondansetron, palonosetron, ramosetron [not commercially available in the US], tropisetron [not commercially available in the US]), and dexamethasone. ASCO states that the oral, fixed-combination of netupitant and palonosetron plus dexamethasone is an additional antiemetic treatment option in this setting.

For patients receiving *moderately emetogenic* chemotherapy regimens, ASCO recommends a 2-drug antiemetic regimen preferably consisting of palonosetron and dexamethasone. If palonosetron is not available, a first-generation 5-HT$_3$ receptor antagonist (preferably granisetron or ondansetron) may be substituted. Limited evidence suggests that aprepitant may be added to this regimen; in such cases, ASCO states that any of the 5-HT$_3$ receptor antagonists is appropriate.

For patients receiving chemotherapy regimens with a *low emetogenic risk*, ASCO recommends administration of a single dose of dexamethasone prior to chemotherapy.

In patients receiving chemotherapy regimens with a *minimal emetogenic risk*, antiemetics should not be routinely administered prior to or following chemotherapy.

Clinical Experience Efficacy and safety of a single IV dose of palonosetron hydrochloride for the prevention of acute and delayed nausea and vomiting associated with moderately emetogenic cancer chemotherapy in adults were established in 2 comparative studies with single-dose ondansetron hydrochloride or dolasetron mesylate. In the first study, complete responses (i.e., no emetic episodes and no rescue antiemetic therapy) at 0–24 or 24–120 hours were achieved in 81 or 74%, respectively, of patients receiving palonosetron (0.25 mg IV) and 69 or 55%, respectively, of patients receiving ondansetron (32 mg IV). In the second study, complete responses at 0–24 or 24–120 hours were achieved in 63 or 54%, respectively, of patients receiving palonosetron (0.25 mg IV) and 53 or 39%, respectively, of patients receiving dolasetron mesylate (100 mg IV). Concomitant corticosteroids were not used prophylactically in the first study, and such use occurred in 4–6% of patients in the second study.

Efficacy and safety of a single IV dose of palonosetron hydrochloride for the prevention of acute nausea and vomiting associated with highly emetogenic cancer chemotherapy in adults were established in a dose-ranging study and a comparative study with ondansetron hydrochloride. In the comparative study, complete responses (i.e., no emetic episodes and no rescue antiemetic therapy) at 0–24 hours were achieved in 59 or 57% of patients receiving palonosetron (0.25 mg IV) or ondansetron (32 mg IV), respectively. Corticosteroids were administered prophylactically in 67% of patients.

Efficacy and safety of a single IV dose of palonosetron hydrochloride for the prevention of acute nausea and vomiting associated with emetogenic cancer chemotherapy in pediatric cancer patients were established in a comparative study with multiple-dose IV ondansetron hydrochloride in 327 pediatric cancer patients (mean age of 8.3 years; range: 2 months–16.9 years). In this study, complete responses (i.e., no vomiting or retching and no rescue antiemetic therapy) in the first 24 hours after starting chemotherapy were achieved in approximately 59% of pediatric patients receiving either palonosetron (single dose of 20 mcg/kg prior to chemotherapy; maximum of 1.5 mg IV) or ondansetron (0.15 mg/kg IV prior to chemotherapy and 4 and 8 hours after the first dose; maximum total dose of 32 mg). Concomitant corticosteroids were administered prophylactically in 55% of patients.

For oral use of palonosetron hydrochloride in fixed combination with netupitant as an antiemetic, see Netupitant and Palonosetron Hydrochloride 56:22.32.

■ **Postoperative Nausea and Vomiting** Palonosetron hydrochloride is used IV for the prevention of postoperative nausea and vomiting for up to 24 hours following surgery. Efficacy of the drug beyond 24 hours has not been demonstrated. The manufacturer states that, as with other antiemetics, routine prophylaxis with palonosetron is not recommended in patients in whom there is little expectation that nausea and/or vomiting will occur postoperatively. However, use of the drug is recommended for patients in whom nausea and/or vomiting must be avoided postoperatively, even when the anticipated incidence of such nausea and/or vomiting is low.

Efficacy of a single IV dose of palonosetron hydrochloride for the prevention of postoperative nausea for up to 24 hours following surgery was established in a randomized, double-blind clinical study. Outpatients (mean age of about 38 years; range: 21–74 years) undergoing elective gynecologic or abdominal laparoscopic surgery received either a single IV dose of palonosetron (0.025, 0.05, or 0.075 mg) or placebo immediately prior to induction of anesthesia. The primary efficacy measures were complete response (i.e., no emetic episode and no use of rescue drug in the 0–24 and in the 24–72 hour periods postoperatively). The complete response rate (0–24 hours) was higher in patients who received palonosetron 0.075 mg IV (42.8%) compared with those who received placebo (25.9%). Palonosetron 0.075 mg IV also reduced the severity of nausea compared with placebo.

In a randomized, double-blind, dose-ranging study, the efficacy of 5 IV palonosetron doses (0.1, 0.3, 1, 3, and 30 mcg/kg) for the prevention of postoperative nausea and vomiting following abdominal or vaginal hysterectomy was evaluated in 381 patients. The primary efficacy measure was proportion of patients with complete response in the first 24 hours following recovery from surgery. Palonosetron 1 mcg/kg (approximately 0.075 mg) was the lowest effective dose in this study and had a complete response rate of 44% compared with 19% for placebo. Palonosetron 1 mcg/kg also substantially reduced the severity of nausea compared with placebo.

Dosage and Administration

■ **Administration** Palonosetron hydrochloride is administered IV. The solution should be inspected visually for particulate matter and discoloration prior to administration. Palonosetron hydrochloride should not be mixed with other drugs, and the IV line should be flushed with 0.9% sodium chloride injection before and after administration of the drug.

■ **Dosage** Dosage of palonosetron hydrochloride is expressed in terms of palonosetron.

Cancer Chemotherapy-induced Nausea and Vomiting For the prevention of cancer chemotherapy-induced nausea and vomiting in adults, a single palonosetron dose of 0.25 mg (administered IV over 30 seconds) is given approximately 30 minutes before the start of chemotherapy.

For the prevention of cancer chemotherapy-induced nausea and vomiting in pediatric patients 1 month to less than 17 years of age, a single palonosetron dose of 20 mcg/kg (maximum dose of 1.5 mg) administered IV over 15 minutes is given approximately 30 minutes before the start of chemotherapy. The manufacturer states that a clinical study in pediatric patients 2 months to less than 17 years of age demonstrated that pediatric patients require a higher dose of palonosetron to prevent cancer chemotherapy-induced nausea and vomiting compared with adults.

Postoperative Nausea and Vomiting For the prevention of postoperative nausea and vomiting in adults, a single palonosetron dose of 0.075 mg (administered IV over 10 seconds) is given immediately before induction of anesthesia.

■ **Special Populations** No dosage adjustment is required in patients with any degree of hepatic impairment. (See Hepatic Impairment under Warnings/Precautions: Specific Populations, in Cautions.)

No dosage adjustment is required in patients with any degree of renal impairment. (See Renal Impairment under Warnings/Precautions: Specific Populations, in Cautions.)

No dosage adjustment is necessary in geriatric patients. (See Geriatric Patients under Warnings/Precautions: Specific Populations, in Cautions.)

Cautions

■ **Contraindications** Known hypersensitivity to palonosetron hydrochloride or any ingredient in the formulation. (See Sensitivity Reactions under Cautions: Warnings/Precautions.)

■ **Warnings/Precautions** ***Sensitivity Reactions*** Hypersensitivity reactions, including anaphylaxis, have been reported in patients receiving palonosetron; these reactions have occurred in patients with or without known hypersensitivity to other type 3 serotonergic (5-HT$_3$) receptor antagonists. (See Advice to Patients.)

Other Warnings and Precautions **Serotonin Syndrome.** Development of serotonin syndrome has been reported in patients receiving 5-HT$_3$ receptor antagonists. Most of the cases have been associated with concomitant use of other serotonergic drugs (e.g., selective serotonin-reuptake inhibitors [SSRIs], serotonin- and norepinephrine-reuptake inhibitors [SNRIs], monoamine oxidase [MAO] inhibitors, mirtazapine, fentanyl, lithium, tramadol, IV methylene blue). Some of the reported cases of serotonin syndrome were fatal. Serotonin syndrome occurring with overdosage of another 5-HT$_3$ receptor antagonist alone (ondansetron) also has been reported. The majority of reports of serotonin syndrome related to 5-HT$_3$ receptor antagonist use have occurred in a post-anesthesia care unit or an infusion center.

Manifestations associated with serotonin syndrome may include mental status changes (e.g., agitation, hallucinations, delirium, coma), autonomic instability (e.g., tachycardia, labile blood pressure, dizziness, diaphoresis, flushing, hyperthermia), neuromuscular symptoms (e.g., tremor, rigidity, myoclonus, hyperreflexia, incoordination), and seizures with or without GI symptoms (e.g., nausea, vomiting, diarrhea).

Patients receiving 5-HT$_3$ receptor antagonists, including palonosetron, should be monitored for the emergence of serotonin syndrome, particularly with concomitant use of other serotonergic drugs. If symptoms of serotonin syndrome occur, palonosetron should be discontinued, and supportive treatment should be initiated. (See Drug Interactions: Serotonergic Agents and also see Advice to Patients.)

For further information on serotonin syndrome, including manifestations and treatment, see Drug Interactions: Serotonergic Drugs, in Fluoxetine Hydrochloride 28:16.04.20.

Specific Populations **Pregnancy.** Category B. (See Users Guide.)

Lactation. Not known whether palonosetron is distributed into milk. Discontinue nursing or the drug, taking into account the importance of the drug to the woman.

Pediatric Use. Safety and efficacy of IV palonosetron have not been established in neonates younger than 1 month of age for prevention of chemotherapy-induced nausea and vomiting. (See Clinical Experience under Uses; Cancer Chemotherapy-induced Nausea and Vomiting.)

Safety and efficacy of IV palonosetron have not been established in pediatric patients for the prevention of postoperative nausea and vomiting.

Geriatric Use. In the clinical studies for palonosetron in chemotherapy-induced nausea and vomiting, 23% of adult cancer patients were 65 years of age or older and 5% were 75 years of age or older. No overall differences in safety and effectiveness were observed between these geriatric patients and younger adults in these studies, but increased sensitivity cannot be ruled out. A population pharmacokinetic analysis did not reveal any differences in palonosetron pharmacokinetics between cancer patients 65 years of age or older and younger cancer patients (18–64 years of age). The manufacturer states that no dosage adjustment or special monitoring is required for geriatric patients receiving palonosetron.

In the clinical studies for palonosetron in postoperative nausea and vomiting, 5% of adult patients were 65 years of age or older. No overall differences in safety were observed between these older individuals and younger individuals in these studies, although the possibility that some older patients may exhibit increased sensitivity to the drug cannot be ruled out.

No differences in efficacy were observed in geriatric patients for the chemotherapy-induced nausea and vomiting indication and none are expected for geriatric postoperative nausea and vomiting patients. However, efficacy of palonosetron in geriatric patients has not been adequately evaluated to date.

Hepatic Impairment. Hepatic impairment does not substantially affect total body clearance of palonosetron compared with values in healthy individuals. The manufacturer states that dosage adjustment is not necessary in patients with any degree of hepatic impairment.

Renal Impairment. Mild to moderate renal impairment does not substantially affect the pharmacokinetics of palonosetron. Total systemic exposure was approximately 28% higher in patients with severe renal impairment relative to healthy individuals. The manufacturer states that dosage adjustment is not necessary in patients with any degree of renal impairment.

■ **Common Adverse Effects** Adverse effects reported in 1% or more of adults receiving palonosetron for prevention of chemotherapy-induced nausea and vomiting include headache, constipation, diarrhea, dizziness, nonsustained tachycardia, bradycardia, hypotension, weakness, hyperkalemia, and anxiety.

Adverse effects reported in 2% or more of adults receiving palonosetron for postoperative nausea and vomiting include QT-interval prolongation, bradycardia, headache, and constipation.

Drug Interactions

■ **Drugs Affecting or Affected by Hepatic Microsomal Enzymes** Clinically important pharmacokinetic interactions unlikely. Metabolized principally by cytochrome P-450 (CYP) isoenzyme 2D6, but pharmacokinetics of palonosetron are not substantially different between poor and extensive metabolizers of isoenzyme 2D6 substrates. Metabolized to a lesser extent by isoenzymes 3A and 1A2. Does not inhibit activity of isoenzymes 1A2, 2A6, 2B6, 2C9, 2D6, 2E1, or 3A4/5; effect on isoenzyme 2C19 activity undetermined. Does not induce activity of isoenzymes 1A2, 2D6, or 3A4/5.

■ **Serotonergic Agents** Serotonin syndrome (including altered mental status, autonomic instability, and neuromuscular symptoms) has been reported following the concomitant use of type 3 serotonin (5-HT_3) receptor antagonists and other serotonergic drugs, including selective serotonin-reuptake inhibitors (SSRIs), serotonin- and norepinephrine-reuptake inhibitors (SNRIs), monoamine oxidase (MAO) inhibitors, mirtazapine, fentanyl, lithium, tramadol, and IV methylene blue. Patients should be monitored for the emergence of serotonin syndrome, especially with concomitant use of palonosetron and other serotonergic drugs. If symptoms of serotonin syndrome occur, palonosetron should be discontinued, and supportive treatment should be initiated. (See Serotonin Syndrome under Warnings/Precautions: Other Warnings and Precautions, in Cautions and also see Advice to Patients.)

■ **Antineoplastic Agents** Pharmacologic interaction unlikely. Palonosetron did not inhibit antineoplastic activity of cisplatin, cyclophosphamide, cytarabine, doxorubicin, or mitomycin in animal tumor models.

■ **Aprepitant** In healthy individuals, concomitant administration of a single dose of palonosetron (0.25 mg IV on day 1) and oral aprepitant given for 3 days (125 mg on day 1 and 80 mg on days 2 and 3) did not substantially alter the pharmacokinetics of palonosetron. The area under the concentration-time curve (AUC) of palonosetron was unchanged and peak plasma concentrations of the drug increased by 15%.

■ **Dexamethasone** Concomitant administration of a single dose of palonosetron (0.25 mg IV) and dexamethasone (20 mg IV) in healthy individuals revealed no pharmacokinetic interactions between the 2 drugs. (See Drug Interactions: Other Drugs.)

■ **Metoclopramide** In healthy individuals, concomitant administration of a single dose of palonosetron (0.75 mg IV on day 1) and steady-state oral metoclopramide (10 mg 4 times daily) revealed no clinically important pharmacokinetic interaction between the 2 drugs.

■ **Other Drugs** Palonosetron has been administered safely in controlled studies with corticosteroids (see Drug Interactions: Dexamethasone), analgesics, antiemetics, antispasmodics, and anticholinergic agents.

Description

Palonosetron hydrochloride, a selective inhibitor of type 3 serotonergic (5-HT_3) receptors, is an antiemetic. The drug is pharmacologically related to other 5-HT_3 receptor antagonists (e.g., dolasetron, granisetron, ondansetron), but the 5-HT_3 receptor antagonists differ structurally. Palonosetron has high binding affinity for 5-HT_3 receptors and little or no affinity for other receptors. The antiemetic activity of palonosetron appears to be mediated both centrally and peripherally via inhibition of 5-HT_3 receptors.

Current evidence suggests that chemotherapeutic agents produce acute nausea and vomiting by inducing degenerative changes in the GI tract (e.g., small intestine), thus increasing endogenous serotonin release from the enterochromaffin cells of the small intestine; serotonin then stimulates 5-HT_3 receptors on vagal and splanchnic nerves that project to the medullary vomiting (emetic) center of the brain and also appears to stimulate 5-HT_3 receptors in the area postrema. Thus, 5-HT_3 receptor antagonists appear to prevent or ameliorate acute chemotherapy-induced emesis by inhibiting visceral (from the GI tract) afferent stimulation of the emetic center probably indirectly at the level of the area postrema and by directly inhibiting serotonin activity within the area postrema and chemoreceptor trigger zone (CTZ).

Alternative mechanisms appear to be principally responsible for delayed nausea and vomiting induced by emetogenic chemotherapy, since similar temporal relationships between serotonin and emesis beyond the first day after a dose have not been established, and 5-HT_3 receptor antagonists generally have not appeared to be effective alone in preventing or ameliorating delayed effects. In addition, other antiemetic drugs (e.g., aprepitant) that have *no* activity at 5-HT_3 receptors effectively augment the activity of dexamethasone and ondansetron to inhibit both acute and delayed nausea and vomiting induced by highly emetogenic chemotherapy. Effective prevention of acute nausea and vomiting may decrease the risk of delayed nausea and vomiting in the same chemotherapy cycle. Although efficacy of a 5-HT_3 receptor antagonist appears to depend more on its interaction at the receptor than its plasma half-life, it has been hypothesized that palonosetron's potency and long plasma half-life (i.e., 4–5 times longer than those of other commercially available 5-HT_3 receptor antagonists) may contribute to its observed efficacy in preventing delayed nausea and vomiting caused by moderately emetogenic cancer chemotherapy.

Postoperative nausea and vomiting is influenced by a number of patient-, surgical-, and anesthesia-related factors and is triggered by a release of serotonin in a cascade of neuronal events involving both the CNS and the GI tract.

Approximately 80% of a single IV dose of palonosetron is recovered in urine within 144 hours following administration; about 40% of the dose is recovered in urine as unchanged drug. Following single-dose IV administration in healthy individuals, palonosetron appears to have a mean terminal elimination half-life of about 40 hours.

Advice to Patients

Importance of reading the palonosetron hydrochloride patient information provided by the manufacturer before beginning therapy and rereading it each time the preparation is given.

Importance of informing patients that hypersensitivity reactions, including anaphylaxis, have been reported in patients receiving palonosetron. Clinicians should advise patients to seek immediate medical attention if any signs or symptoms of a hypersensitivity reaction occur while receiving the drug.

Importance of informing patients of the possibility of serotonin syndrome, particularly with concomitant use of palonosetron and another serotonergic agent such as antidepressants and antimigraine agents. Clinicians should advise patients to seek immediate medical attention should they experience any of the following serotonin syndrome symptoms: changes in mental status, autonomic instability, neuromuscular symptoms, or seizures with or without GI symptoms.

Importance of informing clinicians of existing or contemplated concomitant therapy, including prescription and OTC drugs and dietary or herbal supplements, as well as any concomitant illnesses.

Importance of women informing clinicians if they are or plan to become pregnant or plan to breast-feed.

Importance of informing patients of other important precautionary information. (See Cautions.)

Overview® (see Users Guide). For additional information on this drug until a more detailed monograph is developed and published, the manufacturer's labeling should be consulted. It is *essential* that the manufacturer's labeling be consulted for more detailed information on usual cautions, precautions, contraindications, potential drug interactions, laboratory test interferences, and acute toxicity.

Preparations

Excipients in commercially available drug preparations may have clinically important effects in some individuals; consult specific product labeling for details.

Palonosetron Hydrochloride

Parenteral

Injection, for IV use	0.05 mg (of palonosetron) per mL	**Aloxi®** (available as 1.5- or 5-mL single-use vials), Helsinn

Selected Revisions March 2019, © Copyright, November 2003, American Society of Health-System Pharmacists, Inc.

NEUROKININ-1 RECEPTOR ANTAGONISTS 56:22.32

Aprepitant
Fosaprepitant Dimeglumine

■ Fosaprepitant dimeglumine, a prodrug of aprepitant, and aprepitant, a selective, high-affinity antagonist at substance P/neurokinin-1 (NK_1) receptors, are antiemetics.

Uses

■ **Cancer Chemotherapy-induced Nausea and Vomiting** Aprepitant and fosaprepitant dimeglumine are used in combination with other antiemetic agents for the prevention of acute and delayed nausea and vomiting associated with initial and repeat courses of moderately to highly emetogenic cancer chemotherapy, including high-dose cisplatin therapy in adults.

To prevent chemotherapy-induced nausea and vomiting associated with *highly emetogenic* chemotherapy regimens (including an anthracycline plus cyclophosphamide), the American Society of Clinical Oncology (ASCO) currently recommends a 3-drug antiemetic regimen consisting of a neurokinin-1 (NK_1) receptor antagonist (e.g., either oral aprepitant or IV fosaprepitant dimeglumine), a type 3 serotonin (5-HT_3) receptor antagonist (e.g., dolasetron, granisetron, ondansetron, palonosetron, ramosetron [not commercially available in the US], tropisetron [not commercially available in the US]), and dexamethasone. ASCO states that the oral, fixed-combination of netupitant and palonosetron plus dexamethasone is an additional antiemetic treatment option in this setting.

For patients receiving *moderately emetogenic* chemotherapy regimens, ASCO recommends a 2-drug antiemetic regimen preferably consisting of palonosetron and dexamethasone. If palonosetron is not available, a first-generation 5-HT_3 receptor antagonist (preferably granisetron or ondansetron) may be substituted. Limited evidence suggests that aprepitant may be added to this regimen; in such cases, ASCO states that any of the 5-HT_3 receptor antagonists is appropriate.

For patients receiving chemotherapy regimens with a *low emetogenic risk*, ASCO recommends administration of a single dose of dexamethasone prior to chemotherapy.

In patients receiving chemotherapy regimens with a *minimal emetogenic risk*, antiemetics should not be routinely administered prior to or following chemotherapy.

Safety and efficacy of aprepitant for chronic use or for treatment of established nausea and vomiting have not been established.

Clinical Experience Pivotal clinical efficacy studies for the prevention of acute and delayed nausea and vomiting associated with chemotherapy were conducted with oral aprepitant. Efficacy of aprepitant in patients receiving highly emetogenic chemotherapy was established in 2 controlled clinical studies comparing a regimen containing aprepitant in combination with a 5-HT_3 receptor antagonist (ondansetron) and a corticosteroid (dexamethasone) with a standard regimen containing ondansetron and dexamethasone alone. In these studies, 63–73% of those receiving the regimen with oral aprepitant or 43–52% of those receiving the standard regimen experienced a complete response (i.e., no emetic episodes and no use of rescue therapy) from 0–120 hours after treatment with cisplatin. In the acute phase (0–24 hours) after cisplatin treatment, 83–89% of patients receiving the aprepitant regimen or 68–78% of those receiving the standard regimen experienced a complete response. In the delayed phase (25–120 hours) after cisplatin treatment, 68–75% of patients receiving the aprepitant regimen or 47–56% of those receiving the standard regimen experienced complete response. In addition, antiemetic efficacy of the regimen containing aprepitant was maintained through up to 5 additional chemotherapy cycles in patients who continued into a multiple-cycle extension phase of these 2 studies.

Efficacy of aprepitant in patients receiving moderately emetogenic chemotherapy was established in a double-blind clinical study comparing a regimen containing aprepitant in combination with a 5-HT_3 receptor antagonist (ondansetron) and a corticosteroid (dexamethasone) with a standard regimen containing ondansetron and dexamethasone alone. In this study, a significantly higher proportion of patients with breast cancer receiving the aprepitant regimen (51%) had a complete response (i.e., no emetic episodes and no use of rescue therapy) compared with those receiving the standard regimen (42%) from 0–120 hours after treatment with cyclophosphamide and doxorubicin or epirubicin. In addition, more patients in the aprepitant group than in the standard regimen group reported minimal or no impact of chemotherapy-induced nausea and vomiting on daily living overall (64 versus 56%, respectively). Antiemetic efficacy of the regimen containing aprepitant was maintained through up to 3 additional chemotherapy cycles in patients who continued into a multiple-cycle extension phase of this study.

■ **Postoperative Nausea and Vomiting** Aprepitant is used for the prevention of postoperative nausea and vomiting in adults. Efficacy of aprepitant was established in 2 randomized, double-blind, active-comparator (ondansetron) clinical studies of similar design in 1658 patients. Patients were randomized to receive an oral aprepitant dose of 40 or 125 mg given 1–3 hours prior to anesthesia, or an IV ondansetron dose of 4 mg immediately before anesthesia induction. Aprepitant doses of 125 mg did not appear to provide additional benefit compared with 40-mg aprepitant doses. In the first study, significantly more patients receiving aprepitant 40-mg doses experienced no emesis (i.e., no emetic episodes regardless of use of rescue therapy) compared with patients receiving IV ondansetron (84 versus 71%, respectively) in the initial 24-hour period following surgery. Complete response (i.e., no emetic episodes and no use of rescue therapy) was reported in about 64 or 55% of those receiving aprepitant or ondansetron, respectively. Similar results were observed for up to 48 hours following surgery; no emesis was reported in about 82 or 66% of patients receiving aprepitant or ondansetron, respectively. Although aprepitant delayed the time to first emetic episode, it did not affect time to first use of rescue therapy compared with ondansetron.

The second study failed to support the primary hypothesis that a 40-mg oral aprepitant dose is superior to a 4-mg IV ondansetron dose in the prevention of postoperative nausea and vomiting as measured by the proportion of patients with complete response in the 24 hours following end of surgery. A similar percentage of patients who received 40 mg of aprepitant orally or 4 mg of IV ondansetron (45 versus 42%, respectively) achieved a complete response, and did not require rescue therapy for established emesis or nausea in the initial 24-hour period following surgery. A higher proportion of patients receiving aprepitant had a clinically meaningful effect compared with those receiving IV ondansetron (about 90 versus 74%, respectively) in the initial 24-hour period following surgery.

A combined analysis of the 2 pivotal studies showed that both aprepitant doses (40 and 125 mg) improved protection against nausea and vomiting and reduced the need for rescue therapy, compared with ondansetron. The 40-mg aprepitant dose also was found to be superior to ondansetron on the 3 measures of efficacy (accounting for any nausea, any vomiting, and any use of rescue therapy in the same patient).

Aprepitant capsules and fosaprepitant dimeglumine for injection have not been studied for chronic use or treatment of established nausea and vomiting.

Dosage and Administration

■ **Administration** ***Dispensing and Administration Precautions*** Because of similarities in spelling and/or pronunciation between Emend® (the trade name for aprepitant) and Amen® (a former trade name for medroxyprogesterone acetate; no longer commercially available under this trade name in the US) or Vfend® (the trade name for voriconazole), extra care should be exercised in ensuring the accuracy of prescriptions for these drugs. (See Dispensing and Administration Precautions under Warnings/Precautions: General Precautions, in Cautions.)

Oral Administration Aprepitant is administered orally without regard to meals.

IV Administration Fosaprepitant dimeglumine is administered by IV infusion over a period of 15 minutes. Fosaprepitant should not be mixed or reconstituted with solutions containing divalent cations (e.g., lactated Ringer's injection, Hartmann's solution).

For the prevention of cancer chemotherapy-induced nausea and vomiting, fosaprepitant dimeglumine injection should be reconstituted with 5 mL of 0.9% sodium chloride injection. The solution should be gently swirled; shaking and jetting saline into the vial should be avoided. The entire volume from the vial should be withdrawn aseptically and transferred into an infusion bag containing 110 mL of 0.9% sodium chloride injection, yielding a total volume of 115 mL and a final concentration of 1 mg/mL. The solution should be mixed by gentle inversion of the bag 2–3 times.

■ **Dosage** Dosage of fosaprepitant dimeglumine is expressed in terms of fosaprepitant.

■ **Cancer Chemotherapy-induced Nausea and Vomiting** Aprepitant is administered orally for 3 days as part of a regimen that includes a 5-HT_3 receptor antagonist and a corticosteroid.

The recommended oral adult dosage of aprepitant for moderately to highly emetogenic cancer chemotherapy is 125 mg administered 1 hour before chemotherapy on day 1, followed by 80 mg once daily in the morning on days 2 and 3 of the treatment regimen.

Alternatively, a 115-mg dose of fosaprepitant, infused over 15 minutes and administered 30 minutes prior to chemotherapy, may be substituted for aprepitant 125 mg on day 1 *only* of the 3-day regimen.

In clinical studies, the aprepitant regimen included 1 or 4 days of ondansetron and dexamethasone for moderately or highly emetogenic chemotherapy, respectively. For moderately emetogenic chemotherapy, ondansetron 8 mg was administered orally 30–60 minutes before chemotherapy and repeated 8 hours later on day 1 and dexamethasone 12 mg was administered orally 30 minutes prior to chemotherapy on day 1. For highly emetogenic chemotherapy, ondansetron 32 mg was administered IV 30 minutes before chemotherapy on day 1. Dexamethasone was given orally as 12 mg administered 30 minutes before chemotherapy on day 1, followed by 8 mg once daily in the morning on days 2–4. These are reduced dexamethasone dosages relative to the dosages often used to prevent cancer chemotherapy-induced nausea and vomiting to account for decreased dexamethasone metabolism when aprepitant is used concomitantly.

■ **Postoperative Nausea and Vomiting** The recommended oral adult dosage of aprepitant for the prevention of postoperative nausea and vomiting is 40 mg administered once within 3 hours before anesthesia induction.

■ **Special Populations** No special population dosage recommendations at this time.

Cautions

■ **Contraindications** Concomitant use of aprepitant or fosaprepitant dimeglumine with astemizole (no longer commercially available in the US), cisapride (currently commercially available in the US only under a limited-access protocol), pimozide, or terfenadine (no longer commercially available in the US). (See Drug Interactions: Drugs Metabolized by Hepatic Microsomal Enzymes.)

Known hypersensitivity to aprepitant, fosaprepitant dimeglumine, polysorbate 80, or any ingredient in the formulations.

■ **Warnings/Precautions** ***Sensitivity Reactions*** Stevens-Johnson syndrome has been reported in one patient receiving aprepitant with antineoplastic agents. Hypersensitivity reactions, including anaphylaxis, hives, rash, itching, and urticaria, which may be serious and can cause difficulty in breathing or swallowing, have been reported in patients receiving aprepitant or fosaprepitant. Angioedema was reported in one patient receiving aprepitant.

General Precautions **Dispensing and Administration Precautions.** A potential dispensing error exists because of the similarity in spelling and/or pronunciation of Emend® (the trade name for aprepitant and fosaprepitant dimeglumine) and Amen® (a former trade name for medroxyprogesterone acetate; no longer commercially available under this trade name in the US) or Vfend® (the trade name for voriconazole). The manufacturer advises precautionary measures, including removal of Amen® from the drug database, alerting pharmacy personnel about the potential for error, verifying verbal or telephone orders by spelling the drug name to the prescriber, and confirmation of the patient's understanding of the prescribed drug's purpose and use during patient counseling.

Specific Populations **Pregnancy.** Category B. (See Users Guide.)

Lactation. Aprepitant is distributed into milk in rats; it is not known whether the drug is distributed into milk in humans. Discontinue nursing or the drug, taking into account the importance of the drug to the woman.

Gender. In women, peak plasma concentrations of oral aprepitant are 16% higher, and plasma half-life is decreased compared with those reported in men. Not considered to be clinically important, and no dosage adjustment is necessary.

Pediatric Use. Safety and efficacy of fosaprepitant dimeglumine and aprepitant not established in children younger than 18 years of age.

Geriatric Use. No substantial differences in safety, efficacy, or pharmacokinetics of oral aprepitant relative to younger adults; no dosage adjustment necessary.

Hepatic Impairment. Oral aprepitant has not been adequately studied in patients with severe hepatic impairment (Child-Pugh score exceeding 9). No specific dosage adjustment is recommended by the manufacturer, but caution is advised in such patients. Area under the plasma concentration-time curve (AUC) decreased in patients with mild hepatic impairment, but increased in those with moderate hepatic impairment. However, these changes were not considered clinically important, and no dosage adjustment is necessary.

Fosaprepitant is metabolized by extrahepatic tissue; therefore hepatic insufficiency not expected to alter conversion of fosaprepitant to aprepitant.

Renal Impairment. Total (protein bound and unbound) aprepitant AUCs and peak plasma concentrations are decreased in patients with severe renal impairment or end-stage renal disease requiring hemodialysis, but AUC of active unbound drug is unaffected. No dosage adjustment necessary in such patients. Hemodialysis had no substantial effect on pharmacokinetics of aprepitant.

■ **Common Adverse Effects** Adverse effects occurring in 3% or more of patients receiving oral aprepitant capsules and more frequently than in those receiving standard therapy include asthenia and/or fatigue, dizziness, hypoesthesia, disorientation, nausea, anorexia, constipation, diarrhea, dyspepsia, heartburn, abdominal pain, epigastric discomfort, stomatitis, gastritis, hiccups, perforating duodenal ulcer, enterocolitis, neutropenia, alopecia, bradycardia, hypotension, hypertension, sinus tachycardia, hot flush, pharyngolaryngeal pain, neutropenic sepsis, pneumonia, pruritus, and dehydration.

Since fosaprepitant dimeglumine for injection is converted into aprepitant, adverse effects associated with aprepitant also may be expected to occur with the injection. Adverse effects occurring with IV fosaprepitant dimeglumine include infusion site reactions (e.g., pain, induration) and headache.

Drug Interactions

Because fosaprepitant is rapidly metabolized to aprepitant in vivo, interactions reported with aprepitant are expected to occur with fosaprepitant.

■ **Drugs Metabolized by Hepatic Microsomal Enzymes** Substrates of cytochrome P-450 (CYP) 3A4 (CYP3A4) isoenzyme: Potential pharmacokinetic interaction (altered metabolism of CYP3A4 substrates). Aprepitant is an inhibitor and inducer of CYP3A4 and an inducer of CYP2C9. There is evidence that aprepitant-induced CYP3A4 inhibition is dose dependent. A single 40-mg dose of aprepitant is a weak inhibitor of CYP3A4 and is not expected to have a clinically important effect on plasma concentrations of concomitantly administered drugs that are primarily metabolized by this enzyme. However, when given at higher dosages (i.e., in a regimen consisting of 125 mg on day 1 followed by 80 mg on days 2 and 3) or in repeated doses at any dose level, aprepitant is a moderate inhibitor of CYP3A4, and concomitant administration with drugs metabolized primarily by this enzyme may result in a clinically important effect. Aprepitant (at a dosage level of 125 mg on day 1 followed by 80 mg on days 2 and 3) may increase plasma concentrations of a CYP3A4 substrate to a lesser extent when the substrate is given IV rather than orally. Use with caution; dosage adjustment of concomitantly administered drugs (e.g., dexamethasone) may be necessary. (See Dosage and Administration: Cancer Chemotherapy-induced Nausea and Vomiting and see Drug Interactions: Corticosteroids.) Serious or life-threatening reactions may occur if aprepitant is used concomitantly with astemizole (no longer commercially available in the US), cisapride (currently commercially available in the US only under a limited-access protocol), pimozide, or terfenadine (no longer commercially available in the US).

Substrates of CYP2C9: Potential pharmacokinetic interaction (increased metabolism of CYP2C9 substrates [e.g., phenytoin, tolbutamide, *S*-warfarin] resulting in decreased plasma concentrations).

■ **Drugs Affecting Hepatic Microsomal Enzymes** Inhibitors of CYP3A4 (e.g., clarithromycin, diltiazem, itraconazole, ketoconazole, nefazodone, nelfinavir, ritonavir, troleandomycin): Potential pharmacokinetic interaction (decreased aprepitant metabolism, resulting in increased plasma aprepitant concentrations). Use with caution.

Inducers of CYP3A4 (e.g., carbamazepine, phenytoin, rifampin): Potential pharmacokinetic interaction (increased aprepitant metabolism). Decreased efficacy possible with strong CYP3A4 inducers (e.g., rifampin).

■ **Antineoplastic Agents** Potential pharmacokinetic interaction (increased plasma antineoplastic concentrations) with antineoplastic agents that are metabolized by CYP3A4. Use with caution and careful monitoring.

■ **5-HT$_3$ Receptor Antagonists** Pharmacokinetic interaction unlikely.

■ **Corticosteroids** Potential pharmacokinetic interaction (increased plasma corticosteroid concentrations) with corticosteroids that are metabolized by CYP3A4 (e.g., dexamethasone, methylprednisolone), particularly when given concomitantly with the 3-day aprepitant regimen (consisting of 125 mg on day 1 followed by 80 mg on days 2 and 3) or with fosaprepitant followed by aprepitant. Decreased dosage of oral and IV corticosteroids may be necessary. The manufacturer of fosaprepitant dimeglumine and aprepitant recommends that dosages of oral dexamethasone and methylprednisolone be reduced by 50% and IV dosage of methylprednisolone be reduced by 25% when these drugs are used concomitantly with fosaprepitant dimeglumine followed by aprepitant, or the 3-day oral aprepitant regimen. Because of weak inhibition of CYP3A4 associated with single 40-mg doses of aprepitant, dosage adjustments of corticosteroids are not required when used concomitantly with this aprepitant regimen.

■ **Digoxin** Pharmacokinetic interaction unlikely.

■ **Diltiazem** Potential pharmacokinetic interaction (increased plasma aprepitant and diltiazem concentrations), but no clinically important changes in ECG, heart rate, or blood pressure were observed in one study with oral aprepitant. The manufacturer recommends caution when aprepitant is used concomitantly with diltiazem.

In studies with fosaprepitant dimeglumine, a small but clinically meaningful decrease in diastolic blood pressure and a small but possibly clinically meaningful decrease in systolic blood pressure were reported. However, no clinically important changes in heart rate or PR interval beyond those induced by diltiazem were reported.

■ **Docetaxel** Pharmacokinetic interaction unlikely when administered with the 3-day aprepitant regimen (consisting of 125 mg on day 1 followed by 80 mg on days 2 and 3).

■ **Midazolam** Potential pharmacokinetic interaction (altered plasma midazolam concentrations). Dosage adjustment for IV midazolam may be necessary when administered concomitantly with the 3-day oral aprepitant regimen. Consider the potential effect of increased benzodiazepine plasma concentrations when midazolam is used concomitantly with the 3-day regimen of aprepitant or fosaprepitant followed by aprepitant.

Increase in plasma midazolam concentrations not considered clinically important when concomitantly administered with a single dose of fosaprepitant 100 mg or aprepitant 40 mg.

■ **Oral Contraceptives** Potential pharmacokinetic interaction (decreased plasma steroid concentrations). Use alternative or additional contraceptive methods during fosaprepitant and aprepitant treatment and for 1 month following the last dose.

■ **Paroxetine** Potential pharmacokinetic interaction (decreased plasma aprepitant and paroxetine concentrations.

■ **Vinorelbine** Pharmacokinetic interaction unlikely when administered with the 3-day aprepitant regimen (consisting of 125 mg on day 1 followed by 80 mg on days 2 and 3).

■ **Warfarin** Potential pharmacokinetic interaction (decreased plasma *S*-warfarin concentrations). Monitor prothrombin time closely for 2 weeks (particularly 7–10 days) after initiation of fosaprepitant followed by aprepitant, the 3-day oral aprepitant regimen, or aprepitant 40 mg as a single dose.

Description

Fosaprepitant dimeglumine, a prodrug of aprepitant, is rapidly (within 30 minutes of infusion completion) converted in hepatic and extrahepatic tissues to aprepitant, a selective, high-affinity antagonist at substance P/neurokinin 1 (NK_1) receptors. Aprepitant crosses the blood-brain barrier and occupies NK_1 receptors in the brain. The drug acts in the CNS to inhibit emesis induced by cytotoxic chemotherapy, including both the acute and delayed emesis induced by cisplatin therapy. Studies indicate that aprepitant augments the antiemetic activity of ondansetron and dexamethasone and inhibits both the acute and delayed phases of cisplatin-induced emesis.

Aprepitant is extensively metabolized to weakly active metabolites by the cytochrome P-450 (CYP) enzyme system, principally by CYP3A4, and to a lesser extent by CYP1A2 and CYP2C19. Aprepitant is both a moderate inhibitor and an inducer of CYP3A4; the drug also is an inducer of CYP2C9.

Advice to Patients

Importance of reading the fosaprepitant and aprepitant patient information provided by the manufacturer before beginning therapy and rereading each time the prescription is renewed.

Importance of using fosaprepitant and aprepitant only as directed by the clinician.

Advise patients that aprepitant may be taken with or without food.

Importance of taking first oral aprepitant (125-mg) dose 1 hour before initiation of antineoplastic chemotherapy.

Importance of taking aprepitant (40-mg) dose within 3 hours prior to induction of anesthesia for prevention of postoperative nausea and vomiting.

Importance of discontinuing aprepitant and promptly contacting a clinician if symptoms of an allergic reaction occur.

Importance of women informing clinicians if they are or plan to become pregnant or plan to breast-feed. Importance of women using alternative or additional contraceptive methods during fosaprepitant or aprepitant use (and for 1 month after last dose) if oral contraceptives are being taken.

Importance of informing clinician of existing or contemplated concomitant therapy, including prescription and OTC drugs and herbal products. Importance of closely monitoring prothrombin time in patients receiving chronic warfarin therapy during the 2 weeks (particularly 7–10 days) after initiation of the 3-day regimen of fosaprepitant followed by aprepitant or the 3-day oral aprepitant regimen for each antineoplastic chemotherapy cycle, or administration of aprepitant for prevention of postoperative emesis.

Importance of informing patients of other important precautionary information. (See Cautions.)

Overview® (see Users Guide). For additional information on this drug until a more detailed monograph is developed and published, the manufacturer's labeling should be consulted. It is *essential* that the manufacturer's labeling be consulted for more detailed information on usual cautions, precautions, contraindications, potential drug interactions, laboratory test interferences, and acute toxicity.

Preparations

Excipients in commercially available drug preparations may have clinically important effects in some individuals; consult specific product labeling for details.

Aprepitant

Oral		
Capsules	40 mg	Emend®, Merck
	80 mg	Emend®, Merck
	125 mg	Emend®, Merck

Fosaprepitant Dimeglumine

Parenteral		
For injection, for IV infusion only	115 mg (of fosaprepitant)	Emend®, Merck

Netupitant and Palonosetron Hydrochloride

NEPA, Palonosetron and Netupitant

■ Netupitant and palonosetron hydrochloride (netupitant/palonosetron) is a fixed combination of 2 antiemetic agents; netupitant is a selective antagonist at substance P/neurokinin-1 (NK_1) receptors and palonosetron is a selective, second-generation inhibitor of type 3 serotonergic (5-HT_3) receptors.

Uses

■ **Cancer Chemotherapy-induced Nausea and Vomiting** Netupitant and palonosetron hydrochloride are used orally in fixed combination (Akynzeo®) for the prevention of acute and delayed nausea and vomiting associated with initial and repeat courses of cancer chemotherapy, including, but not limited to, highly emetogenic chemotherapy. Palonosetron prevents nausea and vomiting during the acute phase and netupitant prevents nausea and vomiting during both the acute and delayed phase after cancer chemotherapy. Fixed-combination netupitant and palonosetron is used in an antiemetic regimen that also includes dexamethasone.

To prevent chemotherapy-induced nausea and vomiting associated with *highly emetogenic* chemotherapy regimens (including an anthracycline plus cyclophosphamide), the American Society of Clinical Oncology (ASCO) currently recommends a 3-drug antiemetic regimen consisting of a neurokinin-1 (NK_1) receptor antagonist (e.g., either oral aprepitant or IV fosaprepitant dimeglumine), a type 3 serotonin (5-HT_3) receptor antagonist (e.g., dolasetron, granisetron, ondansetron, palonosetron, ramosetron [not commercially available in the US], tropisetron [not commercially available in the US]), and dexamethasone. ASCO states that oral, fixed-combination netupitant and palonosetron plus dexamethasone is an additional antiemetic treatment option in this setting.

For patients receiving *moderately emetogenic* chemotherapy regimens, ASCO recommends a 2-drug antiemetic regimen preferably consisting of palonosetron and dexamethasone. If palonosetron is not available, a first-generation 5-HT_3 receptor antagonist (preferably granisetron or ondansetron) may be substituted. Limited evidence suggests that aprepitant may be added to this regimen; in such cases, ASCO states that any of the 5-HT_3 receptor antagonists is appropriate.

For patients receiving chemotherapy regimens with a *low emetogenic risk*, ASCO recommends administration of a single dose of dexamethasone prior to chemotherapy.

In patients receiving chemotherapy regimens with a minimal emetogenic risk, antiemetics should not be routinely administered prior to or following chemotherapy.

Clinical Experience Efficacy and safety of fixed-combination netupitant and palonosetron in combination with dexamethasone in the prevention of acute and delayed nausea and vomiting associated with initial and repeat courses of chemotherapy have been established in 2 randomized, double-blind, multicenter, controlled clinical studies. One of the trials was conducted in patients receiving highly emetogenic chemotherapy and the other trial was conducted in patients receiving moderately emetogenic chemotherapy. In both trials, complete response rates (i.e., no emetic episodes and no use of rescue therapy) were substantially higher with fixed-combination netupitant and palonosetron than with palonosetron alone.

In study 1, which was dose-finding in design, efficacy and safety of a single oral dose of netupitant (300 mg) in combination with oral palonosetron (0.5 mg), administered with oral dexamethasone (12 mg on day 1 and 8 mg once daily on days 2–4), were compared with a single oral dose of palonosetron (0.5 mg), administered with oral dexamethasone (20 mg on day 1 and 8 mg twice daily on days 2–4), in 694 chemotherapy-naive, adult cancer patients receiving a highly emetogenic, cisplatin-based chemotherapy regimen (median cisplatin dose was 75 mg/m^2). In this study, 86% of the patients who received netupitant in combination with palonosetron concomitantly received an antineoplastic agent in addition to protocol-mandated cisplatin. The most common antineoplastic agents and the percentage of patients exposed were cyclophosphamide (34%), fluorouracil (24%), etoposide (21%), and doxorubicin (16%). Primary efficacy endpoints were complete responses (i.e., no emetic episodes and no use of rescue therapy) in the delayed phase (25–120 hours), complete responses in the acute phase (0–24 hours), and complete responses in the overall phase (0–120 hours) after the initiation of treatment with cisplatin. A substantially greater proportion of patients in the netupitant and palonosetron treatment arm attained complete responses (90.4% [delayed phase], 98.5% [acute phase], and 89.6% [overall phase]) compared with those who received palonosetron alone (80.1% [delayed phase], 89.7% [acute phase], and 76.5% [overall phase]).

In study 2, efficacy and safety of a single oral dose of netupitant (300 mg) in combination with oral palonosetron (0.5 mg) were compared with a single dose of oral palonosetron (0.5 mg) in 1455 chemotherapy-naive, adult cancer patients scheduled to receive their first cycle of a moderately emetogenic chemotherapy regimen containing an anthracycline and cyclophosphamide for treatment of a solid malignant tumor. All patients also received a single oral dose of dexamethasone (12 or 20 mg on day 1 in patients who received netupitant in combination with palonosetron or palonosetron alone, respectively). After completion of cycle 1, patients had the option to enter a multiple-cycle extension phase and receive the same treatment assigned in cycle 1. Of the 1450 patients who received either netupitant in combination with palonosetron or palonosetron alone, 1438 patients (99%) completed cycle 1; 1286 patients (88%) continued treatment in the multiple-cycle extension phase, and 907 patients (62%) completed the multiple-cycle extension phase up to a maximum of 8 treatment cycles. The majority of patients who received netupitant in combination with palonosetron were treated with cyclophosphamide, and all patients also received either doxorubicin (68%) or epirubicin (32%). During the first cycle, 32% of patients treated with fixed-combination netupitant and palonosetron received a concomitant chemotherapeutic agent in addition to protocol-mandated regimens; the most common chemotherapeutic agents administered were fluorouracil (28%) and docetaxel (3%).

The primary efficacy endpoint in study 2 was the complete response rate in the delayed phase (25–120 hours) following initiation of the chemotherapy regimen; secondary endpoints included complete response in the acute phase (0–24 hours) and overall phase (0–120 hours). Patients continued into the multiple-cycle extension phase for up to 7 additional cycles of chemotherapy; however, only a limited number of patients received treatment beyond cycle 6. In cycle 1, a greater proportion of patients in the fixed-combination netupitant and palonosetron treatment arm attained a complete response (77% [delayed phase], 88% [acute phase], and 74% [overall phase]) compared with those who received palonosetron alone (70% [delayed phase], 85% [acute phase], and 67% [overall phase]). During all subsequent cycles, the complete response rate in the delayed phase was higher in patients who received netupitant in combination with palonosetron compared with those who received palonosetron alone. In addition, the antiemetic activity of netupitant in combination with palonosetron was maintained throughout repeat cycles in those patients who continued to receive the fixed combination in each of the multiple cycles.

Two additional clinical trials were conducted to support the efficacy of netupitant and palonosetron in fixed combination. In study 3, which was multinational, randomized, and double-blind in design, efficacy of a single oral dose of netupitant (300 mg) in fixed combination with palonosetron (0.5 mg) given on day 1 with oral dexamethasone was maintained throughout all cycles in 309 chemotherapy-naive, adult cancer patients undergoing initial and repeat cycles of moderately or highly emetogenic chemotherapy (including carboplatin, cisplatin, oxaliplatin, and doxorubicin-containing regimens). The fixed-dose combination of netupitant and palonosetron also was found to be well tolerated when given over multiple chemotherapy cycles in this study.

In a multinational, randomized, active-controlled, double-blind, clinical noninferiority study (study 4), efficacy and safety of a single oral dose of palonosetron (0.5 mg) were compared with IV palonosetron (0.25 mg) in 739 cancer patients scheduled to receive highly emetogenic cisplatin-based chemotherapy (70 mg/m^2 or more). The intent of this study was to demonstrate that oral palonosetron (0.5 mg) contributes to the efficacy of fixed-combination netupitant and palonosetron during the acute phase (i.e., the first 24 hours after cancer chemotherapy) in the setting of cisplatin-based chemotherapy. The primary efficacy endpoint was complete response (defined as no emetic episode and no use of rescue medication) within 24 hours (acute phase) following initiation of cisplatin-based chemotherapy. In patients who received oral palonosetron, 89.4% attained a complete response in the acute phase compared with 86.2% of those who received IV palonosetron; noninferiority of oral versus IV palonosetron was demonstrated in a statistical analysis of the complete response results.

For IV use of palonosetron hydrochloride as an antiemetic, see Palonosetron Hydrochloride 56:22.20.

Dosage and Administration

■ **Administration** The fixed-combination capsules containing netupitant and palonosetron hydrochloride (netupitant/palonosetron; Akynzeo®) are administered orally approximately one hour before the start of chemotherapy without regard to meals.

The manufacturer states that the antiemetic regimen also should include oral dexamethasone administered 30 minutes prior to chemotherapy on days 1–4 for highly emetogenic chemotherapy (including cisplatin-based chemotherapy), or on day 1 only for anthracycline- and cyclophosphamide-based chemotherapy and chemotherapy not considered highly emetogenic.

■ **Dosage** Netupitant and palonosetron hydrochloride is a fixed combination preparation containing 300 mg of netupitant and 0.5 mg of palonosetron.

The netupitant component is provided as netupitant; the palonosetron component is provided as palonosetron hydrochloride (dosage of this component is expressed in terms of palonosetron).

Cancer Chemotherapy-induced Nausea and Vomiting For the prevention of acute and delayed nausea and vomiting associated with initial and repeat courses of *highly emetogenic cancer chemotherapy, including cisplatin-based chemotherapy*, in adults, the recommended dosage of fixed-combination netupitant and palonosetron is 1 capsule (300 mg of netupitant and 0.5 mg of palonosetron) administered approximately 1 hour prior to the start of chemotherapy; dexamethasone 12 mg should be administered orally 30 minutes prior to chemotherapy on day 1, followed by 8 mg orally once daily on days 2–4 of the treatment regimen. (See Drug Interactions: Dexamethasone.)

For the prevention of acute and delayed nausea and vomiting associated with initial and repeat courses of *anthracycline- and cyclophosphamide-based chemotherapy and chemotherapy not considered highly emetogenic* in adults, the recommended dosage of fixed-combination netupitant and palonosetron is 1 capsule (300 mg of netupitant and 0.5 mg of palonosetron) administered approximately 1 hour prior to the start of chemotherapy; dexamethasone 12 mg should be administered orally 30 minutes prior to chemotherapy on day 1 of the treatment regimen. The manufacturer states that administration of dexamethasone on days 2–4 is not necessary. (See Drug Interactions: Dexamethasone.)

■ **Special Populations** Dosage adjustments are not necessary when fixed-combination netupitant and palonosetron is used in patients with mild or moderate hepatic impairment (Child-Pugh score of 5–8). However, fixed-combination netupitant and palonosetron should *not* be used in patients with severe hepatic impairment (Child-Pugh score exceeding 9) because the fixed combination has not been adequately studied in such patients.

Dosage adjustments are not necessary when fixed-combination netupitant and palonosetron is used in patients with mild to moderate renal impairment. However, fixed-combination netupitant and palonosetron should not be used in patients with severe renal impairment or end-stage renal disease.

Caution generally should be used when dosing fixed-combination netupitant and palonosetron in geriatric patients because of the greater frequency of decreased hepatic, renal, and/or cardiac function and concomitant diseases and other drug therapy in such patients.

Cautions

■ **Contraindications** The manufacturer states there are no known contraindications to the use of the fixed combination of netupitant and palonosetron hydrochloride.

■ **Warnings/Precautions** ***Sensitivity Reactions*** Hypersensitivity reactions, including anaphylaxis, have been reported in patients receiving palonosetron; the reactions have occurred in patients with or without known hypersensitivity to other type 3 serotonergic (5-HT_3) receptor antagonists. (See Advice to Patients.)

Other Warnings and Precautions **Serotonin Syndrome.** Development of serotonin syndrome has been reported in patients receiving 5-HT_3 receptor antagonists. Most of the cases have been associated with concomitant use of other serotonergic drugs (e.g., selective serotonin-reuptake inhibitors [SSRIs], serotonin- and norepinephrine-reuptake inhibitors [SNRIs], monoamine oxidase [MAO] inhibitors, mirtazapine, fentanyl, lithium, tramadol, IV methylene blue). Some of the reported cases of serotonin syndrome were fatal. Serotonin syndrome occurring with overdosage of another 5-HT_3 receptor antagonist alone (ondansetron) also has been reported. The majority of reports of serotonin syndrome related to 5-HT_3 receptor antagonist use have occurred in a post-anesthesia care unit or an infusion center.

Manifestations associated with serotonin syndrome may include mental status changes (e.g., agitation, hallucinations, delirium, coma), autonomic instability (e.g., tachycardia, labile blood pressure, dizziness, diaphoresis, flushing, hyperthermia), neuromuscular symptoms (e.g., tremor, rigidity, myoclonus, hyperreflexia, incoordination), and seizures with or without GI symptoms (e.g., nausea, vomiting, diarrhea).

Patients receiving 5-HT_3 receptor antagonists, including fixed-combination netupitant and palonosetron, should be monitored for the emergence of serotonin syndrome, particularly with concomitant use of other serotonergic drugs. If symptoms of serotonin syndrome occur, fixed-combination netupitant and palonosetron should be discontinued, and supportive treatment should be initiated. (See Drug Interactions: Serotonergic Agents and also see Advice to Patients.)

For further information on serotonin syndrome, including manifestations and treatment, see Drug Interactions: Serotonergic Drugs, in Fluoxetine Hydrochloride 28:16.04.20.

Specific Populations **Pregnancy.** Category C. (See Users Guide.)

Lactation. It is not known whether netupitant or palonosetron is distributed into human milk. Because many drugs are excreted in milk and because of the potential tumorigenicity palonosetron demonstrated in an animal carcinogenicity study, a decision should be made whether to discontinue nursing or the fixed combination of netupitant and palonosetron, taking into account the importance of the drugs to the woman.

Pediatric Use. The manufacturer states that the safety and efficacy of netupitant and palonosetron hydrochloride have not been established in pediatric patients younger than 18 years of age.

Geriatric Use. In the main clinical studies with the fixed combination of netupitant and palonosetron, 18% of adult cancer patients were 65 years of age or older and 2% were 75 years of age or older. No overall differences in safety were observed in these geriatric patients compared with younger adults in these studies. Exploratory analyses of the effect of age on efficacy were performed in 2 clinical studies comparing the fixed combination of netupitant and palonosetron with palonosetron. In study 1 in patients receiving cisplatin chemotherapy, the difference in complete response rates between fixed-combination netupitant and palonosetron and palonosetron alone was similar between patients 65 years of age or older and those younger than 65 years of age in both the acute and delayed phases. In study 2 in patients receiving anthracycline plus cyclophosphamide chemotherapy, the difference in complete response rates between fixed-combination netupitant and palonosetron and palonosetron alone also was similar between patients 65 years of age or older and those younger than 65 years of age in the acute phase. In the delayed phase, the difference in complete response rates between fixed-combination netupitant and palonosetron and palonosetron alone was higher in patients younger than 65 years of age; this difference may be explained, at least in part, by a higher complete response rate in the delayed phase with palonosetron alone in geriatric patients (81%) compared with younger patients treated with palonosetron alone (67%).

In a population pharmacokinetic analysis, age (within the range of 29–75 years of age) did not affect the pharmacokinetics of netupitant or palonosetron in cancer patients receiving the fixed combination of the 2 drugs. In healthy individuals older than 65 years of age, mean systemic exposure and peak plasma concentrations were 25 and 36% higher for netupitant, respectively, and 37 and 10% higher for palonosetron, respectively, compared with those in healthy younger adults (22–45 years of age).

Caution is advised when dosing fixed-combination netupitant and palonosetron in geriatric patients because of the greater frequency of decreased hepatic, renal, and/or cardiac function and of concomitant diseases and other drug therapy in such patients.

Hepatic Impairment. The effects of hepatic impairment on the pharmacokinetics of netupitant and palonosetron were studied following administration of a single oral dose of the fixed combination to patients with mild (Child-Pugh score of 5–6), moderate (Child-Pugh score of 7–9), or severe (Child-Pugh score exceeding 9) hepatic impairment. In patients with mild or moderate hepatic impairment, mean exposure of netupitant was 67 and 86% higher, respectively, than in healthy individuals and mean peak plasma concentration for netupitant was approximately 40 and 41% higher, respectively, than in healthy individuals. In patients with mild or moderate hepatic impairment, mean exposure of palonosetron was 33 and 62% higher, respectively, than in healthy individuals and mean peak plasma concentration for palonosetron was approximately 14% higher and unchanged, respectively, compared with healthy individuals. The manufacturer states that no dosage adjustment is necessary in patients with mild to moderate hepatic impairment.

The pharmacokinetics of netupitant and palonosetron were available from only 2 patients with severe hepatic impairment, and the manufacturer states that the data are too limited to draw a conclusion. Use of fixed-combination netupitant and palonosetron should therefore be avoided in patients with severe hepatic impairment.

Renal Impairment. In a population pharmacokinetic analysis, mild and moderate renal impairment did not substantially affect the pharmacokinetics of netupitant in cancer patients. The manufacturer states that no dosage adjustment of fixed-combination netupitant and palonosetron is necessary in patients with mild to moderate renal impairment.

The pharmacokinetics and safety of netupitant have not been studied in patients with severe renal impairment; however, severe renal impairment did not substantially affect the pharmacokinetics of palonosetron. In a study with IV palonosetron, total systemic exposure to palonosetron increased by approximately 28% in patients with severe renal impairment, compared with healthy individuals. The pharmacokinetics of netupitant and palonosetron have not been studied in patients with end-stage renal disease requiring hemodialysis. The manufacturer states that use of fixed-combination netupitant and palonosetron should be avoided in patients with severe renal impairment or end-stage renal disease.

■ **Common Adverse Effects** Adverse effects reported in 3% or more of patients receiving the oral fixed combination of netupitant and palonosetron concomitantly with highly emetogenic, cisplatin-based chemotherapy and that occurred more frequently than in those receiving palonosetron alone include dyspepsia, fatigue, constipation, and erythema.

Adverse effects reported in 3% or more of patients receiving fixed-combination netupitant with palonosetron concomitantly with anthracycline- and cyclophosphamide-based chemotherapy (cycle 1) and that occurred at a rate that exceeded palonosetron alone include headache, asthenia, and fatigue.

Drug Interactions

Metabolism of netupitant is primarily mediated by cytochrome P-450 (CYP) isoenzyme 3A4 and, to a lesser extent, by CYP2C9 and CYP2D6.

Based on in vitro studies and confirmed in an in vivo study, netupitant is a moderate inhibitor of CYP3A4; its M1 metabolite also is an inhibitor of

CYP3A4 based on in vitro studies. Based on in vitro studies, netupitant and its metabolites are unlikely to have clinically important pharmacokinetic drug interactions via inhibition of CYP isoenzymes 1A2, 2B6, 2C8, 2C9, 2C19, and 2D6 at the usual clinical dose of 300 mg.

Netupitant and its metabolites (M1, M2, and M3) do not induce CYP isoenzymes 1A2, 2B6, 2C9, 2C19, and 3A4.

Based on in vitro studies, netupitant inhibits P-glycoprotein (P-gp) and breast cancer resistance protein (BCRP) transporters. Netupitant is not a substrate for P-gp, but its M2 metabolite is a P-gp substrate.

In vitro studies indicate that netupitant and its 3 major metabolites are unlikely to have clinically important drug interactions with human efflux transporters bile salt export pump (BSEP), multidrug resistance protein (MRP) 2, and human uptake transporters organic anion transport protein (OATP) 1B1 or 1B3, organic anion transporter (OAT) 1 or 3, and organic cation transporter (OCT) 1 or 2 at the usual clinical dose of 300 mg.

In vitro studies suggest that CYP2D6 and, to a lesser extent, CYP3A4 and CYP1A2 are involved in the metabolism of palonosetron. Palonosetron does not inhibit CYP isoenzymes 1A2, 2A6, 2B6, 2C9, 2D6, 2E1, and 3A4/5 or induce CYP isoenzymes 1A2, 2D6, or 3A4/5 based on in vitro studies; CYP2C19 was not studied.

■ **Drugs Affecting or Metabolized by Hepatic Microsomal Enzymes** Concomitant use of fixed-combination netupitant and palonosetron with potent CYP3A4 inhibitors (e.g., ketoconazole) can substantially increase systemic exposure to the netupitant component of the fixed combination. (See Drug Interactions: Ketoconazole.) However, the manufacturer states that dosage adjustment is not necessary for single-dose administration of fixed-combination netupitant and palonosetron during concomitant use of potent CYP3A4 inhibitors.

Plasma concentrations of CYP3A4 substrates may increase when used concomitantly with fixed-combination netupitant and palonosetron. The inhibitory effect of netupitant on CYP3A4 can last for multiple days. Therefore, fixed-combination netupitant and palonosetron should be used with caution in patients concomitantly receiving drugs that are principally metabolized by CYP3A4.

Potent CYP3A inducers can decrease the efficacy of fixed-combination netupitant and palonosetron by substantially reducing plasma concentrations of the netupitant component. The manufacturer therefore states that concomitant use of fixed-combination netupitant and palonosetron should be avoided in patients who are receiving long-term therapy with a potent CYP3A4 inducer (e.g., rifampin). (See Drug Interactions: Rifampin.)

■ **Antineoplastic Agents** Systemic exposure to antineoplastic agents that are metabolized by CYP3A4 (e.g., docetaxel, paclitaxel, etoposide, irinotecan, cyclophosphamide, ifosfamide, imatinib, vinorelbine, vinblastine, vincristine) can increase when administered concomitantly with the fixed combination of netupitant and palonosetron. Systemic exposure to IV docetaxel, etoposide, and cyclophosphamide was increased when administered with fixed-combination netupitant with palonosetron. Systemic exposure to IV docetaxel, etoposide, and cyclophosphamide was increased when administered with fixed-combination netupitant with palonosetron compared with palonosetron administration alone in patients with cancer.

Concurrent administration of fixed-combination netupitant and palonosetron increased the mean peak plasma concentration and area under the concentration-time curve (AUC) of docetaxel by 49 and 35%, respectively, and increased the mean peak plasma concentration and AUC of etoposide by 10 and 28%, respectively, compared with palonosetron administration alone.

Following concomitant administration of fixed-combination netupitant and palonosetron, mean peak plasma concentration and AUC of cyclophosphamide were 27 and 20% higher, respectively, compared with concomitant administration of palonosetron alone.

The mean AUC of palonosetron was approximately 65% higher when fixed-combination netupitant and palonosetron was concomitantly administered with docetaxel than with etoposide or cyclophosphamide; the mean AUC of netupitant was similar among groups that received docetaxel, etoposide, or cyclophosphamide.

Caution and monitoring for chemotherapy-related adverse effects are advised in patients concomitantly receiving antineoplastic agents that are principally metabolized by CYP3A4.

■ **Serotonergic Agents** Serotonin syndrome (including altered mental status, autonomic instability, and neuromuscular symptoms) has been reported following the concomitant use of type 3 serotonin (5-HT_3) receptor antagonists and other serotonergic drugs, including selective serotonin-reuptake inhibitors (SSRIs), serotonin- and norepinephrine-reuptake inhibitors (SNRIs), monoamine oxidase (MAO) inhibitors, mirtazapine, fentanyl, lithium, tramadol, and IV methylene blue. Patients should be monitored for the emergence of serotonin syndrome, particularly during concomitant use of fixed-combination netupitant and palonosetron and other serotonergic drugs. If symptoms of serotonin syndrome occur, fixed-combination netupitant and palonosetron should be discontinued, and supportive treatment should be initiated. (See Serotonin Syndrome under Warnings/Precautions: Other Warnings and Precautions, in Cautions and also see Advice to Patients.)

■ **Netupitant and Palonosetron** The pharmacokinetics of netupitant and palonosetron were not substantially affected when oral netupitant (450 mg) and oral palonosetron (0.75 mg) were concurrently administered.

■ **Dexamethasone** Concomitant administration of a single dose of netupitant (300 mg on day 1) and a dexamethasone regimen (20 mg on day 1, followed by 8 mg twice daily on days 2–4) increased systemic exposure to dexamethasone approximately twofold. The mean AUC of dexamethasone increased by 1.7-fold on day 1 and up to 2.4-fold on days 2 and 4; the duration of this effect was not studied beyond 4 days. Therefore, the manufacturer states that a reduced dose of dexamethasone (i.e., 8 or 12 mg orally) should be administered when used with fixed-combination netupitant and palonosetron. (See Dosage and Administration: Dosage.)

■ **Digoxin** Concurrent administration of netupitant (450 mg) did not substantially affect systemic exposure and urinary excretion of digoxin, a P-gp substrate, at steady state. Therefore, concurrent administration of fixed-combination netupitant and palonosetron and digoxin is not expected to affect systemic exposure of digoxin.

■ **Erythromycin** Systemic exposure of erythromycin was highly variable and the mean peak concentration and AUC of erythromycin were increased by 92 and 56%, respectively, when erythromycin (500 mg) was concurrently administered with netupitant (300 mg). The pharmacokinetics of netupitant were not affected by concurrent administration of erythromycin.

■ **Ketoconazole** A single dose of fixed-combination netupitant and palonosetron was administered with ketoconazole (a potent CYP3A4 inhibitor) following once-daily administration of ketoconazole 400 mg for 12 days. Concurrent administration of ketoconazole increased the mean peak plasma concentrations and AUC of netupitant by 25 and 140%, respectively, and increased mean AUC and peak plasma concentrations of palonosetron by 10 and 15%, respectively, compared with administration of fixed-combination netupitant and palonosetron alone. Although ketoconazole can substantially increase systemic exposure to the netupitant component of the fixed combination, the manufacturer states that dosage adjustment is not necessary for single-dose administration of fixed-combination netupitant and palonosetron.

■ **Midazolam** Systemic exposure of midazolam was substantially higher when administered with netupitant. Following concomitant administration of netupitant (300 mg) and a single oral dose of midazolam (7.5 mg), the mean peak plasma concentration and AUC of midazolam were 36 and 126% higher, respectively. The pharmacokinetics of netupitant were unaffected by concomitant administration of midazolam. The manufacturer states that the potential effects of increased plasma concentrations of midazolam or other benzodiazepines metabolized by CYP3A4 (e.g., alprazolam, triazolam) should be considered when administering these drugs with fixed-combination netupitant and palonosetron.

■ **Oral Contraceptives** Single-dose netupitant in fixed combination with palonosetron, when given with a single oral dose of ethinyl estradiol 60 mcg and levonorgestrel 300 mcg, increased the AUC of levonorgestrel by 46%. However, fixed-combination netupitant and palonosetron did not substantially affect the AUC of ethinyl estradiol. A clinically important effect of fixed-combination netupitant and palonosetron on the efficacy of oral contraceptives containing levonorgestrel and ethinyl estradiol is therefore considered unlikely, and dosage adjustments are not necessary during concomitant use of these drugs.

■ **Rifampin** Single-dose, fixed-combination netupitant and palonosetron was administered with rifampin, a potent CYP3A4 inducer, following once-daily administration of rifampin (600 mg for 17 days). Concurrent administration of rifampin decreased the mean peak plasma concentration and exposure of netupitant by 62 and 82%, respectively, compared with those following administration of fixed-combination netupitant and palonosetron alone. Concurrent administration of rifampin decreased the mean peak plasma concentration and AUC of palonosetron by 15 and 19%, respectively.

Because potent CYP3A4 inducers can decrease the efficacy of fixed-combination netupitant and palonosetron by substantially reducing plasma concentrations of the netupitant component, use of fixed-combination netupitant and palonosetron should be avoided in patients receiving long-term therapy with potent CYP3A4 inducers such as rifampin.

Description

Netupitant and palonosetron hydrochloride is a fixed oral combination of 2 antiemetic agents: netupitant, a highly selective antagonist at substance P/neurokinin-1 (NK_1) receptors, and palonosetron, a selective, second-generation inhibitor of type 3 serotonergic (5-HT_3) receptors.

Palonosetron is pharmacologically related to first-generation 5-HT_3 receptor antagonists (e.g., dolasetron, granisetron, ondansetron). However, palonosetron has a higher potency, higher binding affinity for 5-HT_3 receptors, a longer elimination half-life, and a different molecular interaction with 5-HT_3 receptors than other commercially available 5-HT_3 receptor antagonists and exhibits little or no affinity for other receptors.

Current evidence suggests that chemotherapeutic agents produce acute nausea and vomiting by inducing degenerative changes in the GI tract (e.g., small intestine), thereby increasing endogenous serotonin release from the enterochromaffin cells of the small intestine. Serotonin then stimulates 5-HT_3 receptors on vagal and splanchnic nerves that project to the medullary vomiting (emetic) center of the brain and also appears to stimulate 5-HT_3 receptors in the area postrema. Thus, 5-HT_3 receptor antagonists appear to prevent or ameliorate acute chemotherapy-induced emesis by inhibiting visceral (from the GI tract) afferent stimulation of the emetic center probably indirectly at the level of the area postrema and by directly inhibiting serotonin activity within the area postrema and chemoreceptor trigger zone (CTZ).

Delayed emesis has been mainly associated with the activation of tachykinin family NK_1 receptors, which are widely distributed in the central and peripheral nervous systems, by substance P. Netupitant has been shown to inhibit substance P-mediated responses in in vitro and in vivo studies. Netupitant crosses the blood-brain barrier and occupies NK_1 receptors in the brain. In addition, the combination of palonosetron and netupitant may inhibit the action of substance P synergistically.

Following single-dose, oral administration of fixed-combination netupitant and palonosetron hydrochloride in healthy individuals, peak plasma concentrations of netupitant and palonosetron are achieved within approximately 5 hours.

In a pooled analysis, peak plasma concentration of netupitant was 35% higher in females than in males, while AUC was similar between males and females. In females, mean AUC and peak plasma concentration of palonosetron were 35 and 26% higher, respectively, compared with males.

Plasma protein binding of netupitant is greater than 99.5% at drug concentrations ranging from 10–1300 ng/mL and protein binding of its principal metabolites is greater than 97% at drug concentrations ranging from 100–2000 ng/mL. Approximately 62% of palonosetron is bound to plasma proteins. Netupitant is extensively metabolized to form 3 principal metabolites: a desmethyl derivative (M1), an *N*-oxide derivative (M2), and a OH-methyl derivative (M3). Following a single oral dose of netupitant, the apparent elimination half-life in cancer patients is 80 hours. The elimination half-life of palonosetron in cancer patients is 48 hours. Approximately 50% of a single, oral radiolabeled dose of netupitant was recovered in urine and feces within 120 hours following oral administration. A total of approximately 4 and 71% of a radiolabeled dose of netupitant was recovered in urine and feces collected over 336 hours, respectively; less than 1% of the dose was recovered in urine as unchanged drug. Following oral administration of a single dose of radiolabeled palonosetron in healthy individuals, 85–93% of the dose was excreted in urine and 5–8% was excreted in feces; approximately 40% of the dose was recovered in urine as unchanged drug.

Advice to Patients

Importance of reading patient information provided by the manufacturer before beginning therapy and rereading it each time the fixed-combination netupitant and palonosetron hydrochloride is taken.

Importance of informing patients to take fixed-combination netupitant and palonosetron hydrochloride with or without food approximately 1 hour before initiation of antineoplastic chemotherapy.

Importance of informing patients that hypersensitivity reactions, including anaphylaxis, have been reported in patients receiving palonosetron. Clinicians should advise patients to seek immediate medical attention if any signs or symptoms of a hypersensitivity reaction occur while receiving netupitant and palonosetron in fixed combination.

Importance of informing patients of the possibility of serotonin syndrome, particularly with concomitant use of fixed-combination netupitant and palonosetron and another serotonergic agent such as antidepressants and antimigraine agents. Clinicians should advise patients to seek immediate medical attention should they experience any of the following serotonin syndrome symptoms: changes in mental status, autonomic instability, or neuromuscular symptoms, either with or without GI symptoms.

Importance of women informing their clinician if they are or plan to become pregnant or plan to breast-feed.

Importance of informing clinicians of existing or contemplated concomitant therapy, including prescription and OTC drugs and dietary or herbal supplements, as well as any concomitant illnesses.

Importance of informing patients of other precautionary information. (See Cautions.)

Overview® (see Users Guide). For additional information on this drug until a more detailed monograph is developed and published, the manufacturer's labeling should be consulted. It is *essential* that the manufacturer's labeling be consulted for more detailed information on usual cautions, precautions, contraindications, potential drug interactions, laboratory test interferences, and acute toxicity.

Preparations

Excipients in commercially available drug preparations may have clinically important effects in some individuals; consult specific product labeling for details.

Netupitant and Palonosetron Hydrochloride

Oral

Capsules	Netupitant 300 mg and Palonosetron Hydrochloride 0.5 mg (of palonosetron)	**Akynzeo®**, Helsinn

ANTIULCER AGENTS AND ACID SUPPRESSANTS 56:28

HISTAMINE H_2-ANTAGONISTS 56:28.12

Famotidine

■ Famotidine is a histamine H_2-receptor antagonist.

Uses

Famotidine is used orally for the treatment of active duodenal or gastric ulcer, gastroesophageal reflux disease, endoscopically diagnosed erosive esophagitis, and as maintenance therapy for duodenal ulcer. Oral famotidine also is used for the management of pathological GI hypersecretory conditions. IV famotidine is used in hospitalized individuals with pathological GI hypersecretory conditions or intractable ulcers, or when oral therapy is not feasible.

■ **Duodenal Ulcer** ***Acute Therapy*** Famotidine is used for the short-term treatment of endoscopically or radiographically confirmed active duodenal ulcer. Antacids may be used concomitantly as needed for relief of pain. In controlled studies in patients with endoscopically confirmed duodenal ulcers, reported rates of ulcer healing for famotidine were substantially higher than those for placebo. In a multicenter, double-blind study in patients with endoscopically confirmed duodenal ulcer, reported rates of ulcer healing for oral famotidine dosages of 40 mg at bedtime daily, 20 mg twice daily, or 40 mg twice daily vs placebo were 32, 38, or 34%, respectively, vs 17%, at 2 weeks; 70, 67, or 75%, respectively, vs 31%, at 4 weeks; and 82–83% for these famotidine dosage regimens vs 45% for placebo, at 8 weeks. Famotidine also produced greater reductions in daytime and nocturnal pain and antacid consumption than did placebo, with complete relief of pain in most patients usually occurring within 2 weeks after initiation of famotidine therapy.

Famotidine appears to be at least as effective as cimetidine or ranitidine for the short-term treatment of active duodenal ulcer. An oral famotidine dosage of 40 mg at bedtime daily generally appears to be more effective than an oral cimetidine dosage of 800 mg daily and as effective as an oral ranitidine dosage of 300 mg daily (as a single or divided dose) in this condition. In a multicenter, double-blind study in patients with endoscopically confirmed duodenal ulcers, 68–81 or 76% of ulcers were healed following administration of famotidine (20 mg twice daily, 40 mg at bedtime daily, or 40 mg twice daily) or ranitidine (150 mg twice daily), respectively, for 4 weeks and 87–92 or 90%, respectively, were healed following therapy for 8 weeks. In geriatric patients, famotidine and ranitidine, in dosages of 40 mg at bedtime daily and 150 mg twice daily, respectively, were equally effective in healing active duodenal ulcers and providing symptomatic relief; 57 and 51% of ulcers were healed following administration of famotidine and ranitidine, respectively, for 8 weeks. In several studies, there appeared to be little difference between famotidine and ranitidine in reductions of daytime and nocturnal pain and antacid consumption.

Daily bedtime doses of famotidine generally appear to be as effective as a twice-daily regimen of the drug in healing active duodenal ulcer, although the bedtime regimen may be slightly less effective than twice-daily regimens at 4 but not 8 weeks. Ulcer healing rates averaged 32, 34, or 38% at 2 weeks; 68–70, 75–81, or 67–77% at 4 weeks; and 83–87, 82–92, or 82–92 at 8 weeks following oral famotidine dosages of 40 mg at bedtime daily, 40 mg twice daily, or 20 mg twice daily, respectively. Antacid consumption appeared to be similar with the various famotidine dosage regimens employed. Evidence from a multicenter, controlled study indicates that healing rates for duodenal ulcers in patients receiving famotidine may not be affected substantially by cigarette smoking or alcohol consumption, although healing rates were slightly higher in nonsmokers than in smokers.

Safety and efficacy of long-term famotidine therapy for active duodenal ulcer have not been determined. Studies to date have been limited to short-term treatment of active duodenal ulcer, and the safety and efficacy of treatment for active disease beyond 8 weeks have not been determined. Most patients with duodenal ulcer respond to famotidine therapy during the initial 4-week course of therapy; an additional 4 weeks of therapy may contribute to healing in some patients. However, short-term famotidine therapy (i.e., up to 8 weeks) for the treatment of active duodenal disease will not prevent recurrence following acute healing and discontinuance of the drug. Current epidemiologic and clinical evidence supports a strong association between gastric infection with *Helicobacter pylori* and the pathogenesis of duodenal and gastric ulcers; long-term *H. pylori* infection also has been implicated as a risk factor for gastric cancer. For additional information on the association of this infection with these and other GI conditions, see Helicobacter pylori Infection, under Uses, in Clarithromycin 8:12.12.92.

Conventional antiulcer therapy with H_2-receptor antagonists, proton-pump inhibitors, sucralfate, and/or antacids heals ulcers but generally is ineffective in eradicating *H. pylori*, and such therapy is associated with a high rate of ulcer recurrence (e.g., 60–100% per year). Duodenal ulcers have recurred within 6 months in 52–73% of patients following discontinuance of famotidine therapy. The American College of Gastroenterology (ACG), the National Institutes of Health (NIH), and most clinicians currently recommend that *all* patients with initial or recurrent duodenal or gastric ulcer and documented *H. pylori* infection receive anti-infective therapy for treatment of the infection. Although 3-drug regimens consisting of a bismuth salt (e.g., bismuth subsalicylate) and 2 anti-infective agents (e.g., tetracycline or amoxicillin plus metronidazole) administered for 10–14 days have been effective in eradicating the infection, resolving associated gastritis, healing peptic ulcer, and preventing ulcer recurrence in many patients with *H. pylori*-associated peptic ulcer disease, current evidence principally from studies in Europe suggests that 1 week of such therapy provides comparable *H. pylori* eradication rates. Other regimens that combine one or more anti-infective agents (e.g., clarithromycin, amoxicillin) with a bismuth salt and/or an antisecretory agent (e.g., omeprazole, lansoprazole, H_2-receptor antagonist) also have been used successfully for *H. pylori* eradication, and the choice of a particular regimen should be based on the rapidly evolving data on optimal therapy, including consideration of the patient's prior exposure to anti-infective agents, the local prevalence of resistance, patient compliance, and costs of therapy.

Current evidence suggests that inclusion of a proton-pump inhibitor (e.g., omeprazole, lansoprazole) in anti-*H. pylori* regimens containing 2 anti-infectives enhances effectiveness, and limited data suggest that such regimens retain good efficacy despite imidazole (e.g., metronidazole) resistance. Therefore, the ACG and many clinicians currently recommend 1 week of therapy with a proton-pump inhibitor and 2 anti-infective agents (usually clarithromycin and amoxicillin or metronidazole), or a 3-drug, bismuth-based regimen (e.g., bismuth-metronidazole-tetracycline) concomitantly with a proton-pump inhibitor, for treatment of *H. pylori* infection. For a more complete discussion of *H. pylori* infection, including details about the efficacy of various regimens and rationale for drug selection, see Helicobacter pylori Infection, under Uses, in Clarithromycin 8:12.12.92.

Maintenance Therapy Famotidine is used in reduced dosage as maintenance therapy following healing of active duodenal ulcer to reduce ulcer recurrence. In placebo-controlled studies, duodenal ulcer recurrence rates after 3, 6, and 12 months ranged from 9–14, 16–30, and 23–38%, respectively, for 20 or 40 mg of famotidine at bedtime daily vs 39, 52–73, and 57–77%, respectively, for placebo. Because the efficacy of H_2-receptor antagonists in preventing duodenal ulcer recurrence appears to be substantially reduced in patients who are cigarette smokers compared with nonsmokers, patients who are cigarette smokers should be advised of the importance of discontinuing smoking in the prevention of ulcer recurrence. Maintenance therapy with famotidine has not been studied for longer than 1 year in placebo-controlled studies, and the effect of maintenance therapy with the drug in patients with previously healed duodenal ulcers remains to be more fully evaluated.

■ Pathologic GI Hypersecretory Conditions Famotidine is used for the treatment of pathologic GI hypersecretory conditions (e.g., Zollinger-Ellison syndrome, multiple endocrine adenomas). Famotidine reduces gastric acid secretion and associated symptoms (including diarrhea, nausea, and epigastric burning and pain) in patients with these conditions. Antimuscarinics (e.g., isopropamide iodide) have been used concomitantly with famotidine to augment famotidine-induced inhibition of gastric acid secretion in some patients with GI hypersecretory conditions.

In a limited number of patients with GI hypersecretory conditions, famotidine has effectively inhibited gastric acid hypersecretion and produced inhibition of longer duration than cimetidine and somewhat longer than that of ranitidine. However, these drugs appear to be comparably effective for the treatment of hypersecretion when adequate, equipotent dosages are used and patient compliance is optimal. In one study, patients with GI hypersecretory conditions who were successfully treated with 1.2–9 or 0.6–5.4 g of cimetidine or ranitidine, respectively, alone daily subsequently were treated successfully with 50–800 mg of famotidine alone daily. Although famotidine, cimetidine, and ranitidine were equally effective in controlling gastric hypersecretion, substantially lower doses of famotidine were required and with less frequency than with cimetidine or ranitidine. Famotidine therapy alone or in combination with an antimuscarinic agent has been continued in a few patients for up to 34 months.

■ Gastric Ulcer Famotidine is used for short-term treatment of active, benign gastric ulcer. The efficacy of famotidine in the treatment of gastric ulcer appears to be similar to that of cimetidine or ranitidine, with 40–47, 36–71, or 40–76% of ulcers healed at 4 weeks; 65–68, 66–95, or 68–90% healed at 6 weeks; and 64–80, 67–86, or 79–91% healed at 8 weeks following therapy with famotidine, cimetidine, or ranitidine, respectively. In several other studies in patients with gastric ulcer, famotidine promoted healing of ulcers in about 42–65, 60–95, and 78 to greater than 91% of patients after 4, 6, and 8 weeks of treatment, respectively. Response of gastric ulcers to famotidine therapy does not appear to be affected by patient age or gender, cigarette smoking, alcohol consumption, or duration of disease. Patients with a history of chronic gastric ulcers (history of disease of 10 years or longer) appear to respond as well to famotidine therapy as patients with a brief history of disease. Famotidine also generally produced greater reductions in pain (fasting, postprandial, nocturnal) and other symptoms (including belching, nausea, anorexia) and in antacid consumption than did placebo. Safety and efficacy of famotidine in the treatment of gastric ulcer have not been established for periods exceeding 8 weeks; therefore, use of the drug for more prolonged treatment of active disease or for maintenance therapy of previously healed gastric ulcer remains to be more fully evaluated. If famotidine is used in the treatment of gastric ulcer, it should be kept in mind that symptomatic response does not preclude the presence of gastric malignancy.

Current epidemiologic and clinical evidence supports a strong association between gastric infection with *H. pylori* and the pathogenesis of gastric ulcers, and the ACG, NIH, and most clinicians currently recommend that *all* patients with initial or recurrent gastric ulcer and documented *H. pylori* infection receive anti-infective therapy for treatment of the infection. The choice of a particular regimen should be based on the rapidly evolving data on optimal therapy, including consideration of the patient's prior exposure to anti-infective agents, the local prevalence of resistance, patient compliance, and costs of therapy (See Duodenal Ulcer: Acute Therapy, in Uses.) For a more complete discussion of *H. pylori* infection, including details about the efficacy of various regimens and rationale for drug selection,see Helicobacter pylori Infection, under Uses, in Clarithromycin 8:12.12.92.

■ Gastroesophageal Reflux Disease Famotidine is used to provide short-term symptomatic relief of gastroesophageal reflux disease (GERD). Famotidine also is used for short-term treatment of esophagitis associated with gastroesophageal reflux, including endoscopically proven erosive or ulcerative disease. By increasing gastric pH, H_2-receptor antagonists have relieved heartburn and other symptoms of reflux and have been associated with somewhat higher healing rates of endoscopically proven esophagitis when compared with placebo and have reduced antacid consumption.

Suppression of gastric acid secretion is considered by the ACG to be the mainstay of treatment for GERD, and a proton-pump inhibitor or histamine H_2-receptor antagonist is used to achieve acid suppression, control symptoms, and prevent complications of the disease. The ACG states that a histamine H_2-receptor antagonist administered daily in divided doses is effective in many patients with less severe GERD, and over-the-counter (OTC) antacids and histamine H_2- receptor antagonists are appropriate for *self*-medication as initial therapy in such individuals. A histamine H_2-receptor antagonist is particularly useful when taken before certain activities (e.g., heavy meal, exercise) that may result in acid reflux symptoms in some patients. The ACG states that H_2-receptor antagonists generally may be used interchangeably, although the drugs may differ in potency and in their onset and duration of action. However, proton-pump inhibitors are more effective (i.e., provide more frequent and more rapid symptomatic relief and healing of esophagitis) than histamine H_2-receptor antagonists in the treatment of GERD. Although higher doses and more frequent administration of histamine H_2-receptor antagonists appear to increase their efficacy, such dosages are less effective and more expensive than proton-pump inhibitor therapy. Once-daily administration of a histamine H_2-receptor antagonist at full dosage is *not* considered to be appropriate therapy for GERD.

Based on data from a limited number of patients, famotidine 20 mg administered twice daily appears to be at least as effective as famotidine 40 mg administered at bedtime and more effective than placebo in improving symptoms of gastroesophageal reflux in patients who had no evidence of endoscopically proven erosive or ulcerative disease. Within 2 weeks of therapy, symptomatic relief was reported in a higher percentage of patients receiving famotidine compared with those receiving placebo; symptoms improved in 82, 69, and 62% of these patients at 6 weeks for famotidine 20 mg twice daily, famotidine 40 mg at bedtime, or placebo, respectively. In controlled studies in patients with endoscopically evaluated gastroesophageal reflux disease, reported rates of ulcer healing for famotidine were higher than those for placebo. Healing rates from controlled studies employing various dosage regimens were approximately 48, 32–34, 29, and 7–18% at 6 weeks and 69, 50–54, 43, and 26–29% at 12 weeks for famotidine 40 mg twice daily, 20 mg twice daily, 40 mg at bedtime, and placebo, respectively. Patients receiving famotidine reported faster relief of daytime and nocturnal heartburn and greater reduction in antacid consumption than those receiving placebo. Nocturnal heartburn relief was reported in a higher percentage of patients receiving famotidine than those receiving placebo; nocturnal heartburn relief occurred in about 58, 50, and 49% of patients receiving famotidine 20 mg twice daily, 40 mg at bedtime, and placebo, respectively, while daytime heartburn relief occurred in approximately 56, 42, and 46% of such patients, respectively. In a study in patients with gastroesophageal reflux who had endoscopically evaluated erosive or ulcerative disease, reported rates of ulcer or erosion healing at 6 weeks were 48 and 42% in patients receiving famotidine 40 mg twice daily or ranitidine 150 mg twice daily, respectively, while at 12 weeks rates of healing were 71 or 60% in patients receiving famotidine 40 mg twice daily or ranitidine 150 mg twice daily, respectively. However, ranitidine was as effective as famotidine in improving symptoms of gastroesophageal reflux.

H_2-receptor antagonists also have been used in combination with metoclopramide in a limited number of patients who failed to respond to an H_2-receptor antagonist alone, but the ACG states that frequent and potentially severe adverse CNS effects of metoclopramide have appropriately decreased regular use of the drug for GERD. Although some clinicians have suggested that a histamine H_2-receptor antagonist also may be used in combination with bethanechol† in patients who fail to respond to a histamine H_2-receptor antagonist alone, the ACG states that bethanechol has limited efficacy in the treatment of GERD.

Short-term therapy (i.e., up to 12 weeks) with H_2-receptor antagonists for the treatment of GERD will not prevent recurrence following ulcer healing and discontinuance of such therapy. Esophagitis has recurred within 6 months in up to 80% of patients following discontinuance of H_2-receptor antagonist therapy. Because GERD is considered a chronic disease, many patients with GERD require long-term, even lifelong, treatment. The ACG states that proton-pump inhibitors are effective and appropriate as maintenance therapy in many patients with the disease. Maintenance therapy† with an H_2-receptor antagonist also has been used to reduce recurrence of GERD. However, many patients initially responding to proton-pump inhibitors experience symptomatic relapse and failure of esophageal healing with subsequent use of a histamine H_2-receptor antagonist.

For further information on the treatment of GERD, see Uses: Gastroesophageal Reflux, in Omeprazole 56:28.36.

■ **Other Uses** Famotidine may be used for *self-medication* for relief of symptoms of *occasional* heartburn (pyrosis), acid indigestion (hyperchlorhydria), or sour stomach and for prevention of such symptoms caused by consumption of food or beverages. Famotidine also may be used in fixed combination with calcium carbonate and magnesium hydroxide (Pepcid® Complete) for *self-medication* for relief of symptoms of *occasional* heartburn (pyrosis) associated with acid indigestion (hyperchlorhydria) or sour stomach.

Famotidine also has been used in a limited number of patients to control intragastric pH and/or stress-induced GI bleeding in critically ill patients (e.g., traumatized or postoperative patients, patients in shock or with respiratory insufficiency)†. In patients with GI bleeding† secondary to duodenal or stress ulcers or gastritis, the drug may control GI bleeding and reduce the need for emergency surgery, but may not prevent bleeding recurrence. Additional study to further evaluate the effect of famotidine on morbidity and mortality in patients with these conditions is necessary.

Dosage and Administration

■ **Reconstitution and Administration** Famotidine is usually administered orally. The drug may also be given by slow IV injection or by slow IV infusion in hospitalized patients with pathologic hypersecretory conditions or intractable duodenal ulcers, or when oral therapy is not feasible. Antacids may be administered concomitantly as necessary for relief of pain. (See Drug Interactions: Food and Antacids.)

Parenteral solutions of famotidine should be inspected visually for particulate matter and discoloration prior to administration whenever solution and container permit.

Oral Suspension For oral administration, famotidine oral suspension may be substituted for famotidine tablets in patients who are unable to swallow tablets. The powder for suspension should be reconstituted at the time of dispensing by adding 46 mL of water to a bottle containing 400 mg of famotidine to provide a suspension containing 40 mg/5 mL. The suspension should be agitated well for 5–10 seconds after adding the water for reconstitution and again immediately prior to administration of each dose.

Orally Disintegrating Tablets Patients receiving famotidine orally disintegrating tablets should be instructed not to remove a tablet from the blister until just prior to dosing. The tablet should *not* be pushed through the foil. With dry hands, the blister package should be peeled completely off the blister. The tablet should then be gently removed and immediately placed on the tongue to dissolve and be swallowed with the saliva; administration with liquid is not necessary.

IV Injection. Famotidine concentrate for injection must be diluted prior to IV administration. For IV injection, 20 mg of famotidine is diluted to a total of 5 or 10 mL with 0.9% sodium chloride injection or another comparable IV solution (see Chemistry and Stability: Stability) to provide a solution containing approximately 4 or 2 mg/mL, respectively. The appropriate dose is injected IV at a rate no faster than 10 mg/minute.

IV Infusion. For intermittent IV infusion, 20 mg of famotidine as the concentrate is added to 100 mL of 5% dextrose injection or another compatible IV solution (see Chemistry and Stability: Stability) to provide a solution containing approximately 0.2 mg/mL. This solution is infused IV over 15–30 minutes.

Alternatively, famotidine that is commercially available as a diluted solution (0.4 mg of famotidine per mL) in 0.9% sodium chloride may be used for intermittent IV infusion. The commercially available diluted solution should only be administered by IV infusion over 15–30 minutes. The container should be checked for minute leaks by firmly squeezing the bag. The injection should be discarded if the seal is not intact or leaks are found or if the solution is cloudy or contains a precipitate. Additives should not be introduced into the injection container. The injection should not be used in series connections with other plastic containers, since such use could result in air embolism from residual air being drawn from the primary container before administration of fluid from the secondary container is complete.

■ **Dosage** ***Duodenal Ulcer*** For the treatment of active duodenal ulcer, the usual adult oral dosage of famotidine is 40 mg at bedtime daily. Alternatively, 20 mg twice daily may be administered orally in adults. The advantage of one oral regimen over another for particular patients with active duodenal ulcer has not been determined, although a once-daily bedtime dosage may be used for patients in whom dosing convenience is considered important for patient compliance. Healing may occur within 2 weeks in some patients and within 4 weeks in most patients. Some patients may benefit from an additional 4 weeks of therapy. It occasionally may be necessary to continue full-dose famotidine therapy for longer than 6–8 weeks; however, the safety and efficacy of continuing full-dose therapy beyond 8 weeks have not been determined. In hospitalized adults with intractable duodenal ulcers or when oral therapy is not feasible, the manufacturer states that famotidine may be administered IV in a dosage of 20 mg every 12 hours.

For maintenance therapy following healing of acute duodenal ulcer to reduce ulcer recurrence, the usual adult oral dosage of famotidine is 20 mg at bedtime daily.

For the treatment of duodenal ulcer in children 1–16 years of age, the manufacturer recommends an oral famotidine dosage of 0.5 mg/kg daily given at bedtime or in 2 divided doses, up to a total daily dosage of 40 mg. In hospitalized children 1–16 years of age with intractable ulcers or when oral therapy is not feasible, the manufacturer states that a famotidine dosage of 0.25 mg/kg may be administered IV (over not less than 2 minutes or as a 15-minute infusion) every 12 hours, up to a total daily dosage of 40 mg. Data from uncontrolled studies in pediatric patients suggest that famotidine is effective for gastric acid suppression when given in dosages of up to 1 mg/kg daily; however, data are insufficient to establish the percentage of these patients who respond to a given dose and duration of therapy. (See Cautions: Pediatric Precautions.) Therefore, treatment duration (initially based on recommendations in adults) and dosage in such patients should be individualized based on clinical response and/or gastric or esophageal pH determination and endoscopy.

Pathologic GI Hypersecretory Conditions For the treatment of pathologic GI hypersecretory conditions (e.g., Zollinger-Ellison syndrome, multiple endocrine adenomas), dosages of famotidine should be individualized according to patient response and tolerance. The usual initial adult dosage is 20 mg orally every 6 hours; however, higher initial dosages may be necessary in some patients. Subsequent famotidine dosage should be adjusted according to the patient's requirements and response, and therapy continued as long as clinically necessary. Periodic (e.g., once to several times yearly) increases in famotidine dosage may be necessary during long-term therapy. Oral dosages ranging from 20–160 mg every 6 hours generally have been necessary to maintain basal gastric acid secretion at less than 10 mEq/hour; determination of gastric acid secretion during the hour prior to a dose may be useful in establishing optimum dosage. Dosages up to 800 mg daily in divided doses have been administered to individuals with severe disease, although the manufacturer recommends dosages only up to 160 mg every 6 hours (640 mg daily). In hospitalized patients with pathologic GI hypersecretory conditions or when oral therapy is not feasible, the manufacturer states that famotidine may be administered IV in a dosage of 20 mg every 6 hours in adults; however, higher initial doses may be necessary in some patients. Subsequent IV dosage should be adjusted according to the patient's requirements and response.

The famotidine dosage necessary in patients who have previously received therapy with cimetidine or ranitidine is directly related to the severity of the GI hypersecretory condition and the dosage regimen of cimetidine or ranitidine. Patients who require low or high dosages of cimetidine or ranitidine will also require low or high dosages, respectively, of famotidine.

Gastric Ulcer For the short-term treatment of active, benign gastric ulcer, the usual adult oral dosage of famotidine is 40 mg daily at bedtime. Most patients demonstrate complete healing of gastric ulcers within 8 weeks; the safety and efficacy of continuing famotidine therapy beyond 8 weeks have not been determined.

For the treatment of gastric ulcer in children 1–16 years of age, the manufacturer recommends an oral famotidine dosage of 0.5 mg/kg daily given at bedtime or in 2 divided doses, up to a total daily dosage of 40 mg. In hospitalized children 1–16 years of age with intractable ulcers or when oral therapy is not feasible, the manufacturer states that a famotidine dosage of 0.25 mg/kg may be administered IV (over not less than 2 minutes or as a 15-minute infusion) every 12 hours, up to a total daily dosage of 40 mg. Data from uncontrolled studies in pediatric patients suggest that famotidine is effective for gastric acid suppression when given in dosages of up to 1 mg/kg daily; however, data are insufficient to establish the percentage of these patients who respond to a given dose and duration of therapy. (See Cautions: Pediatric Precautions.) Therefore, treatment duration (initially based on recommendations in adults) and dosage in such patients should be individualized based on clinical response and/or gastric or esophageal pH determination and endoscopy.

Gastroesophageal Reflux For the symptomatic relief of gastroesophageal reflux, the usual adult oral dosage of famotidine is 20 mg twice daily for up to 6 weeks. Famotidine dosages of 40 mg at bedtime also have been used for the symptomatic relief of gastroesophageal reflux; however, famotidine administered twice daily appears to be more effective in improving symptoms of gastroesophageal reflux than famotidine administered just at bedtime. In addition, the American College of Gastroenterology (ACG) states that once-daily administration of a histamine H_2-receptor antagonist at full dosage is *not* considered to be appropriate therapy for gastroesophageal reflux disease (GERD). For the symptomatic relief of esophagitis associated with gastroesophageal reflux, including endoscopically proven erosive or ulcerative disease, the usual adult oral dosage of famotidine is 20 or 40 mg twice daily for up to 12 weeks.

For the symptomatic relief of gastroesophageal reflux with or without esophagitis including erosions and ulcerations in children 1–16 years of age, the manufacturer recommends an initial oral famotidine dosage of 1 mg/kg daily in 2 divided doses, up to 40 mg twice daily. Data from uncontrolled studies in pediatric patients suggest that famotidine is effective in the management of gastroesophageal reflux with or without esophagitis including erosions and ulcerations when given in oral dosages of up to 2 mg/kg daily; however, data are insufficient to establish the percentage of these patients who respond to a given dose and duration of therapy. (See Cautions: Pediatric Precautions.) Therefore, treatment duration (initially based on recommendations in adults) and dosage in such patients should be individualized based on clinical response and/or gastric or esophageal pH determination and endoscopy.

The manufacturer states that dosages and dosage regimens for parenteral famotidine in patients with gastroesophageal reflux disease have not been established.

Self-medication For *self-medication* in relieving symptoms of occasional heartburn, acid indigestion, or sour stomach or in preventing such symptoms caused by consumption of food or beverages in patients 12 years of age or older, a famotidine dosage of 10 or 20 mg once or twice daily is recommended; when used prophylactically, the dose should be taken 10 minutes to 1 hour before eating or drinking. When the fixed combination of famotidine, calcium carbonate, and magnesium hydroxide (Pepcid® Complete) is used for *self-medication* for relief of occasional heartburn associated with acid indigestion or sour stomach, the usual dosage in adults and children 12 years of age or older is 1 tablet (10 mg of famotidine) once or twice daily. When famotidine chewable tablets are used for *self-medication*, the tablets should be chewed thoroughly before swallowing. When the 10-mg tablets are used for *self-medication*, the manufacturer recommends that the dosage of famotidine not exceed 20 mg in 24 hours. Alternatively, when the 20-mg tablets are used for *self-medication*, the manufacturer recommends that dosage of famotidine not exceed 40 mg in 24 hours. Famotidine for *self-medication* should not exceed 2 weeks of *continuous* therapy unless otherwise directed by a clinician. Persistent symptoms should be reported to a clinician.

■ **Dosage in Renal Impairment** In patients with renal impairment, doses and/or frequency of administration of famotidine can be modified in response to the degree of renal impairment. Adverse CNS effects have been reported in patients with moderate or severe renal insufficiency receiving famotidine, and modification of dosage and/or dosing interval may be used to avoid excess accumulation of the drug in such patients. In adults with moderate (creatinine clearances less than 50 mL/minute) or severe (creatinine clearances less than 10 mL/minute) renal impairment, the manufacturer states that dosage of famotidine may be reduced to half the usual dosage or the dosing interval may be prolonged to 36–48 hours as necessary according to the patient's clinical response. Some clinicians have recommended that one-half the usual adult dosage be administered in adults with creatinine clearances of 30–60 mL/minute per 1.48 m^2 and that one-fourth the usual adult dosage be administered in those with creatinine clearances less than 30 mL/minute per 1.48 m^2.

Based on the comparison of pharmacokinetic parameters of famotidine in adults and children, dosage adjustment also should be considered in children with moderate or severe renal impairment.

Cautions

Famotidine generally is well tolerated. A causal relationship between many adverse reactions and the drug has not been established but cannot be excluded. In some studies, the incidence of reported adverse effects was similar in patients receiving famotidine or placebo. The frequency of adverse effects of the drug does not appear to be affected by patient age in adults.

Overall, the frequency of adverse effects produced by famotidine is similar to that produced by ranitidine. Famotidine does not appear to exhibit substantial antiandrogenic activity nor to substantially affect serum prolactin concentrations, and the drug also does not appear to affect hepatic clearance of other drugs. Adverse nervous system effects (e.g., headache, dizziness) and GI effects (e.g., constipation, diarrhea) occur most frequently during famotidine therapy. Although adverse effects of the drug generally are not severe, discontinuance of famotidine therapy has been necessary in up to 14% of patients. Adverse effects generally are similar when famotidine is administered orally or IV.

■ **Nervous System Effects** Headache and dizziness occur in about 5 and 1% of patients, respectively, receiving famotidine. Weakness (asthenia), fatigue, paresthesia, tonic-clonic (grand mal) seizure, insomnia, drowsiness, and reversible psychic disturbances such as depression, disorientation, confusion, anxiety, agitation, decreased libido, and hallucinations have been reported in 1% or less of patients receiving famotidine but have not been directly attributed to the drug in many cases. The risk of adverse CNS effects of famotidine may be greater in patients with impaired renal function.

■ **GI Effects** Constipation and diarrhea occur in 1–2% of patients receiving famotidine. Nausea, vomiting, abdominal discomfort, flatulence, belching, anorexia, dry mouth, heartburn, and dysgeusia have been reported in 1% or less of patients receiving famotidine but have not been directly attributed to the drug in many cases.

■ **Dermatologic and Sensitivity Reactions** Adverse dermatologic effects occur in 1% or less of patients receiving famotidine, but a causal relationship to the drug has not been established. Dermatologic effects include acne, pruritus, urticaria, and dry skin. Rash also has been reported and occasionally has required discontinuance of the drug. Some of these adverse dermatologic effects appear to be hypersensitivity reactions. Anaphylaxis, angioedema, bronchospasm, orbital or facial edema, and conjunctival congestion also have been reported. Alopecia has occurred during famotidine therapy but was attributed to removal of the antiandrogenic effects of the previously administered high-dose cimetidine therapy. Toxic epidermal necrolysis has been reported very rarely with famotidine therapy. Transient irritation at the site of injection may occur following IV administration of famotidine.

■ **Renal Effects** Increases in BUN or serum creatinine concentrations and proteinuria have been reported occasionally during famotidine therapy. There is limited evidence that, unlike cimetidine, famotidine does not substantially inhibit renal tubular secretion of creatinine.

■ **Hepatic Effects** Increases in total serum bilirubin, and cholestatic jaundice have been reported rarely during famotidine therapy and have required discontinuance of the drug in some patients. Increases in serum aminotransferase (transaminase) (AST [SGOT] and ALT [SGPT]) and alkaline phosphatase concentrations also have occurred, occasionally requiring discontinuance of the drug. Hepatomegaly was reported in one patient during famotidine therapy.

■ **Respiratory Effects** ***Community-acquired Pneumonia*** Administration of gastric antisecretory agents (e.g., H_2-receptor antagonists, proton-pump inhibitors) has been associated with an increased risk for developing certain infections (e.g., community-acquired pneumonia). A possible association between chronic administration of gastric acid-suppressive drugs and occurrence of community-acquired pneumonia has been evaluated using a large Dutch database (Integrated Primary Care Information [IPCI]) containing information on approximately 500,000 patients, 364,683 of whom (average follow-up: 2.7 years) were selected for evaluating any such association. During the 8-year population-based, case-control study, gastric acid suppressants were first prescribed in 19,459 individuals (10,177 received H_2-receptor antagonists [mean duration of use: 2.8 months] and 12,337 received proton-pump inhibitors [mean duration of use: 5 months]; some individuals received both drugs). Most patients did not undergo endoscopy and were treated empirically for upper GI symptoms. In this study, first occurrence of pneumonia (confirmed by radiography or microbiologic testing in 18% of patients) was reported in 5551 individuals; development of pneumonia occurred in 185 individuals while receiving gastric acid suppressants and in 292 individuals who had discontinued such use.

The adjusted relative risk for development of pneumonia (or the incidence rate) was 0.6, 2.3 and 2.5 per 100 person-years for individuals not receiving acid-suppressive drugs, for those receiving H_2-receptor antagonists, and for those receiving proton-pump inhibitors, respectively. Patients using gastric acid suppressants developed community-acquired pneumonia 4.5 (95% confidence interval of 3.8–5.1) times more often than those who never used such drugs. When evaluating use of all gastric acid suppressants, current use of the drugs was associated with a small (27%) overall increase in the risk of pneumonia (adjusted odds ratio 1.27 and 95% confidence interval of 1.06–1.54). Higher risks were observed for current users of H_2-receptor antagonists and proton-pump inhibitors; the adjusted relative risk for developing community-acquired pneumonia was 1.63 (95% confidence interval of 1.07–2.48) or 1.89 (95% confidence interval of 1.36–2.62), respectively, for these classes of drugs compared with those who discontinued using these agents. Estimates for developing pneumonia were higher (1.7 [95% confidence interval of 0.8–2.9] for H_2-receptor antagonists) and 2.2 [95% confidence interval of 1.4–3.5] for proton-pump inhibitors) when only laboratory-confirmed cases of pneumonia were considered for analysis.

Although there was variation among individual H_2-receptor antagonists and individual proton-pump inhibitors, the numbers were small and the heterogeneity was not considered significant. For patients currrently receiving proton-pump inhibitors, a dose-response relationship for developing pneumonia was observed; individuals using more than one defined daily dose of these drugs had a 2.3-fold increased risk for developing pneumonia compared with those who discontinued gastric acid suppressants. Such a dose-response relationship for developing pneumonia was not observed in patients receiving H_2-receptor antagonists; however, dose variation of these drugs was limited. Among current users of H_2-receptor antagonists or proton-pump inhibitors, the risk for developing pneumonia was most pronounced among those who initiated such therapies within the past 30 days.

Although the exact mechanism for development of community-acquired pneumonia in patients receiving gastric acid suppressants has not been fully elucidated, it has been suggested that reduction of gastric acid secretion by acid suppressive therapy and consequent increases of gastric pH may result in a favorable environment for the development of infection. Intragastric acidity constitutes a major nonspecific defense mechanism of the stomach to ingested pathogens; when gastric pH is less than 4, most pathogens are killed, while at higher gastric pH, pathogens may survive. Since for the effective management of upper GI symptoms, intragastric pH should be maintained above 4 for several hours, acid suppressive therapy may lead to insufficient elimination or, even, increased colonization of ingested pathogens. Some evidence indicates that acid-supressive therapy may result in nosocomial infections.

It should be considered that certain patients (e.g., those with pleuritic chest pain, hypothermia, systolic hypotension, tachypnea, diabetes mellitus, neoplastic disease, neurologic disease, bacteremia, leukopenia, multilobar pulmonary infiltrate) are at increased risk for developing infections and in these individuals community-acquired pneumonia may be associated with increased mortality. Some clinicians state that gastric acid-suppressive drugs should be used in patients in whom community-acquired pneumonia may be severe (e.g., those with asthma or chronic obstructive lung disease, immunocompromised patients, pediatric or geriatric individuals) only when clearly needed and the lowest effective dose should be employed.

■ **Other Adverse Effects** Fever, hypertension, flushing, musculoskeletal pain (including muscle cramps), arthralgia, and tinnitus have been reported in 1% or less of patients receiving famotidine, but a causal relationship to the drug has not been established in many cases. An acute episode of gout occurred in one patient during therapy with the drug.

Leukocytosis, leukopenia, neutropenia, pancytopenia, agranulocytosis, eosinophilia, prolonged erythrocyte sedimentation rate (ESR), and thrombocytopenia have occurred rarely in patients receiving famotidine. Changes in serum protein or cholesterol concentrations also have occurred.

Unlike cimetidine, famotidine does not appear to exhibit substantial antiandrogenic activity. (See Pharmacology: Endocrine and Gonadal Effects.) Famotidine did not produce gynecomastia, impotence, or decreased libido in one study in males with GI hypersecretory conditions who were receiving dosages of 80–640 mg daily for periods longer than 12 months, but such effects occasionally have been associated with therapy with the drug. The manufacturer states that in controlled studies the incidence of impotence in patients receiving famotidine was not greater than that in patients receiving placebo. Impotence and gynecomastia, which developed in one male during cimetidine therapy, continued during subsequent therapy with ranitidine and then with famotidine, but did not resolve following discontinuance of famotidine. In at least one patient, androgenic activity that had been inhibited by cimetidine appeared to become disinhibited (as evidenced by worsening of preexisting alopecia) when famotidine was substituted. Menstrual abnormalities have occurred in at least one woman receiving famotidine.

Cardiac arrhythmias, palpitations, and AV block have been reported in 1% or less of patients receiving famotidine. There is limited evidence suggesting that famotidine may have a negative inotropic effect, but further study is necessary to confirm these preliminary findings.

■ **Precautions and Contraindications** Symptomatic response to famotidine should *not* be interpreted as precluding the presence of gastric malignancy.

The possibility that gastric acid-suppressive therapy may increase the risk of community-acquired pneumonia should be considered. (See Respiratory Effects: Community-acquired Pneumonia, in Cautions.)

Adverse CNS effects have been reported in patients with moderate (i.e., creatinine clearance less than 50 mL/minute) or severe (i.e., creatinine clearance less than 10 mL/minute) renal impairment receiving famotidine, and the drug should be used with caution and dosage and/or frequency of administration reduced in such patients, since the drug is excreted principally by the kidneys. (See Dosage and Administration: Dosage in Renal Impairment.)

Unless otherwise directed by a clinician, patients receiving famotidine for *self-medication* should be advised to discontinue the drug and consult a clinician if symptoms of heartburn (pyrosis), acid indigestion (hyperchlorhydria), or sour stomach persist after 2 weeks of continuous use of the drug.

Individuals with phenylketonuria (i.e., homozygous genetic deficiency of phenylalanine hydroxylase) and other individuals who must restrict their intake of phenylalnine should be warned that Pepcid AC® chewable tablets and Pepcid RPD® orally disintegrating tablets contain aspartame (NutraSweet®), which is metabolized in the GI tract to phenylalanine following oral administration.

Famotidine is contraindicated in patients with known hypersensitivity to the drug or any ingredient in the formulation. Since cross-sensitivity has been observed among H_2-receptor antagonists, famotidine should not be administered to patients with a history of hypersensitivity to other drugs in this class.

■ **Pediatric Precautions** Safety and efficacy of famotidine in children 1–16 years of age is supported by evidence from adequate and well-controlled studies in adults and by a limited number of studies in pediatric patients. In studies in a limited number of pediatric patients 1–15 years of age, clearance and area under the curve (AUC) were similar to those values reported in adults. Limited evidence also suggests that the relationship between serum concentration and acid suppression is similar in children 1–15 years of age as compared with adults. While uncontrolled studies suggest efficacy of famotidine in the treatment of gastroesophageal reflux disease and peptic ulcer, data in pediatric patients are insufficient to establish percent response with dose and duration of therapy. Therefore, treatment duration (initially based on adult duration recommendations) and dose should be individualized based on clinical response and/or pH determination (gastric or esophageal) and endoscopy. In uncontrolled clinical studies in pediatric patients, dosages of up to 1 mg/kg daily for peptic ulcer and 2 mg/kg daily for gastroesophageal reflux disease with or without esophagitis including erosions and ulcerations have been used. The manufacturer states that no pharmacokinetic or pharmacodynamic data for famotidine are available in children younger than 1 year of age. Famotidine should not be used for *self-medication* in children younger than 12 years of age unless directed by a clinician.

■ **Geriatric Precautions** Of almost 5000 patients in clinical studies of famotidine, 9.8% were 65 years of age or older, while 1.7% were older than 75 years of age. Although no overall differences in efficacy and safety were observed between geriatric and younger patients, the possibility that some older patients may exhibit increased sensitivity to the drug cannot be ruled out. Clinically important changes in the pharmacokinetics of famotidine have not been observed in geriatric individuals, and dosage of the drug does not need to be modified based on age alone. However, famotidine dosage should be selected carefully in geriatric patients because these individuals may have decreased renal function, and patients with renal impairment may be at increased risk of famotidine-induced toxicity. Monitoring of renal function may be useful for patients in this age group. Doses and/or frequency of administration of famotidine should be modified in geriatric patients with moderate (creatinine clearance less than 50 mL/minute) or severe (creatinine clearance less than 10 mL/minute) renal impairment. (See Dosage and Administration: Dosage in Renal Impairment)

■ **Mutagenicity and Carcinogenicity** No evidence of mutagenicity was observed in in vitro studies using famotidine concentrations up to 10 mg per plate in the Ames microbial mutagen test with or without metabolic activation and in in vivo studies in mice using a micronucleus test and a chromosomal aberration test.

No evidence of carcinogenicity was seen in long-term studies in mice or rats receiving oral famotidine dosages up to 2 g/kg daily (approximately 2500 times the usual human dosage). Although famotidine did not produce changes in gastric mucosal cells in animals, long-term effects of the drug on human gastric mucosal morphology are not known, and the risk, if any, of gastric neoplasms and long-term therapy with an H_2-receptor antagonist remains controversial.

■ **Pregnancy, Fertility, and Lactation** Reproduction studies in rats and rabbits using oral famotidine dosages up to 2 (approximately 2500 times the maximum human dosage) and 0.5 g/kg daily, respectively, or IV dosages up to 0.2 (approximately 250 times the maximum human dosage) and 0.1 g/kg daily, respectively, have not revealed evidence of harm to the fetus. Oral dosages of 2 g/kg daily inhibited weight gain in pregnant rats, and those of 0.5 and/or 2 g/kg daily on days 7–17 of gestation decreased fetal weight and delayed sternal ossification in the offspring. Decreased food intake and decreased weight gain also occurred in offspring of rats receiving these dosages from days 10–28 post partum. Death and locomotor dysfunction were observed in pregnant rats receiving IV famotidine dosages of 100 or 200 mg/kg daily. IV dosages of 100 or 200 mg/kg daily in rats have decreased pup body weight during the post-weaning period. Although no direct fetotoxic effects have been observed, sporadic abortions and decreases in fetal weight occurred secondary to substantial decreases in food intake in pregnant rabbits receiving oral dosages of 200 mg/kg (250 times the usual human dosage) or more daily. Decreased number of sacrocaudal vertebrae and delayed ossification have occurred in rabbits receiving oral famotidine dosages of 0.5 g/kg daily. There are no adequate and controlled studies to date using famotidine in pregnant women, and the drug should be used during pregnancy only when clearly needed. Women who are pregnant or nursing should seek the advice of a health professional before using famotidine for *self-medication*.

Reproduction studies in rats and rabbits using oral famotidine dosages up to 2 (approximately 2500 times the maximum human dosage) and 0.5 g/kg daily, respectively, or IV dosages up to 0.2 (approximately 250 times the maximum human dosage) and 0.1 g/kg daily, respectively, have not revealed evidence of impaired fertility.

Famotidine is distributed into milk in humans and in animals. The drug has produced transient growth depression in the offspring of lactating rats receiving dosages at least 600 times the usual human dosage. Because of the potential for serious adverse reactions to famotidine in nursing infants, a decision should be made whether to discontinue nursing or the drug, taking into account the importance of the drug to the woman.

Drug Interactions

■ **Food and Antacids** Food appears to slightly enhance, and antacids appear to slightly decrease, the bioavailability of famotidine, but these effects do not appear to be clinically important. Famotidine can be administered concomitantly with antacids.

In one study following concomitant administration of food and a single oral 40-mg dose of famotidine, mean peak plasma concentration, fraction of the dose excreted in urine, bioavailability, and renal clearance of famotidine increased slightly; however, area under the plasma concentration-time curve (AUC) and time to reach the peak were decreased slightly. In the same study following concomitant administration of 10 mL of an aluminum and magnesium hydroxides antacid (Mylanta-II®) and 40 mg of famotidine orally, the mean peak plasma concentration decreased from 81 to 60 ng/mL, and the mean AUC decreased from 443 to 355 mcg/hour per L. The time to reach the peak and the fraction of the dose excreted in urine also decreased slightly, and renal clearance increased slightly.

■ **Effects on Hepatic Clearance of Drugs** Unlike cimetidine or ranitidine, famotidine does not appear to inhibit the metabolism of drugs, including warfarin, theophylline, phenytoin, diazepam, or procainamide, by the hepatic cytochrome P-450 (microsomal) enzyme system. Metabolism of aminopyrine or antipyrine and clearance and/or half-life of the drugs also do not appear to be affected substantially by famotidine therapy. However, minimal effects of the drug on cytochrome P-450 enzymes have been suggested, and additional experience with long-term therapy and with relatively high dosages is necessary to determine the potential, if any, for clinically important effects. Famotidine does not appear to affect elimination of indocyanine green.

Acute Toxicity

There has been no experience to date with acute overdosage of famotidine.

■ **Pathogenesis** The oral and IV LD_{50}s of famotidine have been reported to be greater than 3000 and 254–563 mg/kg, respectively, in both mice and rats, and the intraperitoneal and subcutaneous LD_{50}s have been reported to be greater than 778 and greater than 800 mg/kg, respectively, in these animals. The minimum acute oral and IV lethal doses have been reported to be greater than 2000 and about 300 mg/kg, respectively, in dogs. In rabbits, oral famotidine dosages of 200 mg/kg or more daily produce substantial anorexia and growth retardation; however, no evidence of toxicity was observed following high oral dosages in dogs and rats. In dogs, IV dosages of 5–200 mg/kg daily produce vomiting; restlessness; pallor of the mucous membranes or redness of the mouth and ears; and cardiovascular effects, including hypotension, tachycardia, and collapse.

Oral dosages up to 800 mg of famotidine daily produced no evidence of serious toxicity when the drug was used in patients with pathologic GI hypersecretory conditions.

■ **Treatment** In acute famotidine overdose, usual measures to remove unabsorbed drug from the GI tract and clinical monitoring should be employed. Supportive and symptomatic treatment should be initiated.

Pharmacology

■ **GI Effects** Famotidine competitively inhibits the action of histamine on the H_2 receptors of parietal cells, reducing gastric acid secretion and concentration under daytime and nocturnal basal conditions and also when stimulated by food, histamine, or pentagastrin. The H_2-receptor antagonist activity of famotidine reportedly is slowly reversible, since the drug dissociates slowly from the H_2 receptor. Famotidine has been shown to be 20–150 or 3–20 times as potent on a molar basis as cimetidine or ranitidine, respectively, in inhibiting stimulated gastric acid secretion.

The degree of inhibition of gastric acid secretion by famotidine is similar to that observed following equipotent doses of cimetidine or ranitidine. A 5-mg dose of famotidine appears to produce inhibition of gastric acid secretion similar in degree to that produced by a 300-mg dose of cimetidine. The degree of inhibition of gastric acid secretion (especially nocturnal or food-stimulated) by famotidine is directly related to the dose and the time of administration of the drug. In one study in healthy individuals who were hypersecretors of gastric acid (basal gastric acid output of 5 or more mEq/hour), the total volume of gastric acid secretion was decreased 55–65% following single 20-mg oral or 10- or 20-mg IV doses of the drug, but the largest decrease was observed following the 20-mg IV dose. In another study in healthy individuals, a single 40-mg evening dose of famotidine inhibited 95 and 32% of nocturnal and daytime gastric acid secretion, respectively; 24-hour gastric acid secretion was inhibited about 70%.

Evening (bedtime) doses produce maximal inhibitory effects on nocturnal or breakfast-stimulated gastric acid secretion, but produce minimal inhibition of lunch- or dinner-stimulated secretion; administration of famotidine twice daily before meals produces substantial inhibition of meal-stimulated gastric acid secretion.

Basal and nocturnal gastric acid secretion appear to be inhibited to a greater extent than are food- or pentagastrin-stimulated gastric acid secretion following a given dose of famotidine in both healthy individuals and patients with duodenal ulcer or GI hypersecretory conditions. Following oral administration of a single 20- or 40-mg evening dose of famotidine, 86 or 94% of nocturnal gastric acid secretion, respectively, is inhibited for at least 10 hours. Following oral administration of a single 20- or 40-mg morning dose, 76 or 84% of food-stimulated gastric acid secretion, respectively, is inhibited for up to 3–5 hours and 25 or 30%, respectively, for up to 8–10 hours. However, inhibition of food-stimulated gastric acid secretion disappeared within 6–8 hours following administration of a 20-mg dose in some individuals. Following oral administration of a single 40-mg bedtime dose of the drug, basal or pentagastrin-stimulated gastric acid secretion is inhibited by 70 or 30%, respectively, for 12 hours and by 55 or 9%, respectively, for 20 hours.

The inhibitory effects of famotidine on gastric acid secretion do not appear to be cumulative following repeated administration of the drug, and tolerance to the drug's effects does not develop rapidly.

The increases in gastric pH that occur secondary to inhibition of gastric acid secretion by famotidine also are dose dependent. Nocturnal gastric pH increased to a mean of 5 or 6.4 following oral administration of a single 20- or 40-mg evening dose of famotidine, respectively, and basal gastric pH increased to about 5 for 3–8 hours after a single 20- or 40-mg morning (after breakfast) dose of the drug. Following administration of a single evening dose of 20 mg orally, 10 mg IV, 20 mg IV, or placebo, nocturnal gastric pH averaged 4.4, 5.5, 6.2, or 1.7, respectively, 2 hours after the dose; nocturnal gastric pH averaged 6, 5.4, and 4.4 at 7, 8, and 10 hours after the 20-mg IV dose or 4, 3.3, and 3 at 7, 8, and 10 hours after the 10-mg IV dose. Gastric pH for a 24-hour period (measured every 5 seconds) was greater than 6 about half the time during continuous IV infusion of famotidine dosages of 3.2 or 4 mg/hour in patients with duodenal ulcer; however, during postprandial periods of the day, pH exceeded 6 only 10% of the time.

Famotidine indirectly causes a dose-dependent reduction in pepsin secretion by decreasing the volume of gastric acid secretion. The drug appears to have minimal effects on fasting and postprandial serum gastrin concentrations. Serum gastrin concentrations have increased in some patients during famotidine therapy but remained within the normal range. Famotidine may protect the gastric mucosa from the irritant effects caused by certain drugs (e.g., aspirin, nonsteroidal anti-inflammatory agents).

Famotidine does not appear to affect gastric emptying, lower esophageal sphincter pressure, or biliary secretion.

Famotidine concentrations ranging from 128–1024 mcg/mL are necessary to inhibit growth of various strains of *Helicobacter pylori* (formerly *Campylobacter pylori* or *C. pyloridis*), an organism possibly contributing to the etiology of duodenal and gastric ulcers. The MIC_{50} and MIC_{90} of famotidine for susceptible strains of *H. pylori* are reportedly 512 and greater than 1024 mcg/mL, respectively.

■ **Endocrine and Gonadal Effects** Famotidine has been shown to have little, if any, effect on serum prolactin concentrations. Although changes in serum prolactin concentrations occurred following a 20-mg IV dose of the drug in some healthy individuals and patients with duodenal ulcer, these changes were considered within normal physiologic variations. Serum prolactin concentrations remained unchanged following single IV doses of 20 mg or following oral dosages of 80–640 mg daily for periods longer than 12 months.

Famotidine does not appear to have substantial antiandrogenic effects. Unlike cimetidine but like ranitidine, famotidine has been shown to have little, if any, effect on serum concentrations of testosterone, luteinizing hormone (LH), follicle-stimulating hormone (FSH), estradiol, parathyroid hormone (PTH), cortisol, insulin, glucagon, thyrotropin (TSH), thyroxine (T_4), triiodothyronine (T_3), or thyroxine-binding globulin (TBG).

■ **Other Effects** Famotidine has been shown to produce few, if any, CNS, cardiovascular, or respiratory effects. The drug does not appear to affect hepatic or portal blood flow in healthy individuals or patients with chronic liver disease. Unlike cimetidine, famotidine does not inhibit hepatic metabolism of antipyrine. Famotidine does not appear to affect the volume or bicarbonate or amylase content of exocrine pancreatic secretions.

In animals, famotidine did not inhibit immediate hypersensitivity reactions involving antigen-induced mediator release from mast cells or cellular and humoral immune responses.

Pharmacokinetics

■ **Absorption** Famotidine is incompletely absorbed from the GI tract following oral administration, and the drug reportedly undergoes minimal first-pass metabolism. The oral bioavailability of famotidine in adults is about 40–50%. Studies in a limited number of children 11–15 years of age indicate a similar oral bioavailability of famotidine (mean bioavailability: 50%). The film-coated tablets, oral suspension, and orally disintegrating tablets of famotidine reportedly are bioequivalent. Food may slightly enhance and antacids may slightly decrease the bioavailability of famotidine, but these alterations do not appear to be clinically important. (See Drug Interactions: Food and Antacids.)

Following IV injection of a single 20-mg dose of famotidine, peak plasma concentrations of 272 ng/mL occur within 20 minutes and decrease to 163, 98, 64, 25, and 11 ng/mL 1, 2, 4, 8, and 12 hours, respectively, after the dose. Following oral administration of a 5-, 10-, 20-, or 40-mg dose of famotidine, peak plasma concentrations of 17–22, 29–39, 40–71, or 78–132 ng/mL, respectively, occur within 1–4 hours.

Plasma famotidine concentrations necessary to inhibit 50% of tetragastrin-stimulated gastric acid secretion (IC_{50}) are estimated to be 13 ng/mL. Plasma famotidine concentrations greater than 50 ng/mL result in inhibition of more than 80% of gastric acid secretion; however, inhibition generally appears to diminish at lower concentrations. Data are conflicting regarding the relationship between plasma famotidine concentrations and a given therapeutic effect of acid inhibition. However, in one study, the decline in the degree of inhibition of gastric acid secretion appeared to be proportional to decreases in plasma famotidine concentrations.

Inhibition of gastric acid secretion is apparent within 1 hour following IV or oral administration of famotidine. Peak inhibition occurs within 0.5–3 or 1–4 hours following IV or oral administration, respectively. The duration of inhibition of gastric acid secretion and maximal inhibition produced by famotidine are dose dependent. The duration of inhibition of basal and nocturnal secretion following a single 20- or 40-mg oral dose of the drug reportedly is 10–12 hours. Inhibition of food-stimulated secretion generally persists for 8–10 hours when these doses are administered in the morning, but this inhibition may dissipate within 6–8 hours after a 20-mg oral dose in some patients. Following equipotent doses of famotidine (60 mg), cimetidine (1.9 g), or ranitidine (530 mg) in one study in patients with GI hypersecretory conditions, gastric acid secretion 12 hours after discontinuance of the drugs was reduced by 58, 27, or 38%, respectively, compared with basal secretion, and the time required for secretion to return to 20 mEq/hour averaged 12, 9, or 10 hours, respectively, following discontinuance of the drugs. The duration of inhibition of nocturnal gastric acid secretion is 10–15 hours following a single 10- or 20-mg IV famotidine dose. In one study in healthy individuals who were hypersecretors of gastric acid (basal gastric acid output of 5 or more mEq/hour), maximal inhibition of gastric acid secretion was 97.4, 99.7, or 99.4% 2–4 hours and 73.8, 77.2, or 83.3% 12 hours following a single famotidine dose of 10 or 20 mg IV or 20 mg orally, respectively.

■ **Distribution** Distribution of famotidine into human body tissues and fluids has not been fully characterized. The apparent volume of distribution of the drug is reported to be 1.1–1.4 L/kg in adults and does not appear to be altered substantially in patients with renal dysfunction. In children 1–15 years of age, a volume of distribution of 1.5–2.07 L/kg has been reported. Following oral or IV administration in rats, famotidine is widely distributed, appearing in highest concentrations in the kidney, liver, pancreas, and submandibular gland. The drug is 15–20% protein bound.

In rats, famotidine appears to distribute only minimally into the CNS, and does not cross the placenta. It is not known whether the drug crosses the placenta in humans. Famotidine is distributed into milk in rats; however, it is not known whether the drug is distributed into milk in humans.

■ **Elimination** The elimination half-life of famotidine averages 2.5–4 hours in adults with normal renal function. An elimination half-life of 2.3–3.38 hours has been reported in children 1–15 years of age. The elimination of famotidine does not appear to be affected substantially by age in adults, but is prolonged in patients with renal impairment; adjustment of dosage or dosing interval may be necessary to avoid excess accumulation of the drug in patients with moderate or severe renal impairment. (See Dosage and Administration: Dosage in Renal Impairment.) In adults with creatinine clearances of 10 mL or less per minute, the elimination half-life of the drug may exceed 20 hours, with an elimination half-life of about 24 hours in anuric patients. There is some evidence that plasma concentrations of famotidine decline in a biphasic manner. In adults with normal renal function and those with creatinine clearances of 60–90, 30–60, or less than 30 mL/minute per 1.48 m^2, the plasma half-life in the distribution phase ($t_{1/2\alpha}$) was not affected substantially by renal function, averaging 0.18, 0.23, 0.25, or 0.24 hours, respectively; the half-life in the terminal elimination phase ($t_{1/2\beta}$) averaged 2.6, 2.9, 4.7, or 12 hours, respectively.

Famotidine is metabolized in the liver to famotidine *S*-oxide (*S*-famotidine). The metabolite does not appear to inhibit gastric acid secretion. Orally administered famotidine undergoes minimal metabolism on first pass through the liver.

Famotidine is excreted principally in urine via glomerular filtration and tubular secretion. Approximately 25–30 or 65–80% of a dose is excreted unchanged in urine within 24 hours following oral or IV administration, respectively, and approximately 13–49 or 52–82% of a single 40-mg oral or IV dose, respectively, is excreted within 72 hours. The cumulative renal excretion of famotidine is decreased in patients with renal dysfunction, with 72, 69, 65, or 21% of an administered dose excreted in individuals with normal renal function or those with creatinine clearances of 60–90, 30–60, or less than 30 mL/minute per 1.48 m^2, respectively. A small fraction of an orally administered dose is excreted in urine as famotidine *S*-oxide. The remainder of an orally administered dose is eliminated in feces. Nonrenal excretion of famotidine did not show a compensatory increase in patients with severe renal impairment, but rather decreased by about 40% in these patients. Interindividual variation in the metabolism and excretion of famotidine has been reported. Following oral administration of a 20-mg dose, 24–56 or 28–79% of the administered dose reportedly was excreted in urine or feces, respectively.

Total body clearance of famotidine from plasma averages 381–483 mL/minute, and renal clearance of the drug averages 250–450 mL/minute. Total body and renal clearances are decreased in patients with renal dysfunction. In patients with creatinine clearances of 30–60 or less than 30 mL/minute per 1.48 m^2, total body clearance from plasma averaged 241 or 71–83 mL/minute, respectively, and renal clearance averaged 157 or 9.5–21 mL/minute, respectively.

Famotidine does not appear to be removed by hemodialysis.

Chemistry and Stability

■ **Chemistry** Famotidine is a histamine H_2-receptor antagonist. Unlike the earlier histamine H_2-receptor antagonists, burimamide and metiamide, which are not commercially available, and cimetidine and ranitidine, famotidine contains a guanidine-substituted thiazole ring rather than an imidazole or furan ring.

Famotidine occurs as a white to pale yellow, odorless, crystalline powder having a moderately bitter taste. Famotidine has solubilities of 740 mcg/mL in water and 360 mcg/mL in alcohol at 20°C. The drug has a pK_a of 7.1 in water at 25°C.

Famotidine is commercially available for oral administration as film-coated, chewable, gelatin-coated, or orally disintegrating tablets and as a powder for oral suspension. Some famotidine chewable tablet preparations (Pepcid® AC) and famotidine orally disintegrating tablets (Pepcid RPD®) contain aspartame (Nutrasweet®). (See Cautions: Precautions and Contraindications.) Following metabolism of aspartame in the GI tract, each 20- or 40-mg orally disintegrating tablet provides 1.05 or 2.1 mg, respectively, of phenylalanine.

Famotidine powder for suspension occurs as a white to off-white powder. When reconstituted as directed, oral suspensions of the drug occur as smooth, mobile, off-white homogenous suspensions and have a pH of 6.5–7.5.

Famotidine concentrate for injection is a clear, colorless, sterile solution of the drug in water for injection. The concentrate also contains mannitol; multiple-dose vials also contain benzyl alcohol as a preservative. Famotidine concentrate for injection has a pH of 5–5.6. The preservative-free injection has an osmolarity of 217 mOsm/L, and the injection preserved with benzyl alcohol has an osmolarity of 290 mOsm/L. Famotidine injection that is commercially available as a diluted solution in 0.9% sodium chloride is iso-osmotic and has a pH of 5.7–6.4. This injection contains approximately 7.8 mEq of sodium per 50 mL.

■ **Stability** Commercially available famotidine film-coated tablets (Pepcid®) should be stored in well-closed, light-resistant containers at 25°C, but may be exposed to temperatures ranging from 15–30°C. These tablets have an expiration date of 30 months following the date of manufacture when stored under these conditions. Famotidine orally disintegrating tablets (Pepcid RPD®) should be stored at 25°C, but may be exposed to temperatures ranging from 15–30°C. Famotidine tablets and chewable tablets for *self-medication* (Pepcid® AC, Pepcid® Complete) should be stored at a temperature between 25–30°C and protected from moisture.

Commercially available famotidine powder for oral suspension should be stored in tight containers at 25°C, but may be exposed to temperatures ranging from 15–30°C. The powder for oral suspension has an expiration date of 18 months following the date of manufacture when stored at a temperature less than 40°C. Following reconstitution, oral suspensions of the drug should be stored at a temperature less than 30°C and, although not necessary, may be refrigerated; freezing should be avoided. Any unused suspension should be discarded after 30 days.

Commercially available famotidine concentrate for injection should be refrigerated at 2–8°C and has an expiration date of 24 months following the date of manufacture when stored at this temperature. If freezing occurs, the injection should be thawed at room temperature or by warming it in a water bath or under running hot tap water, allowing sufficient time for dissolution of all ingredients. The injection should not be thawed by exposure to microwave radiation because of the potential hazard of rapidly increased temperature and vapor pressure in a closed system. When diluted with most commonly used IV solutions (e.g., 0.9% sodium chloride injection, 5 or 10% dextrose injection, lactated Ringer's, water for injection), famotidine solutions are stable for 7 days at room temperature. However, the manufacturer states that data on the maintenance of sterility of these solutions after dilution are unavailable. Therefore, the manufacturer recommends that solutions prepared by dilution of famotidine concentrate for injection, if not used immediately after dilution, should be refrigerated and used within 48 hours.

Famotidine injection that is commercially available as a diluted solution in 0.9% sodium chloride should be stored at room temperature (25°C) and is stable for 15 months when stored as recommended. Brief exposure to temperatures up to 35°C will not adversely affect the stability of the solution, but the solution should be protected from exposure to excessive heat. The commercially available injection of famotidine in 0.9% sodium chloride is provided in a plastic container fabricated from specially designed multilayered plastic PL 2501 (Galaxy® container). Solutions in contact with the plastic can leach out some of its chemical components in very small amounts within the expiration period of the injection; however, safety of the plastic has been confirmed in tests in animals according to USP biological tests for plastic containers as well as by tissue culture toxicity studies.

Preparations

Excipients in commercially available drug preparations may have clinically important effects in some individuals; consult specific product labeling for details.

Famotidine

Oral		
For suspension	40 mg/5 mL	**Pepcid®**, Merck
Tablets	10 mg	**Pepcid® AC Gelcaps,** J&J-Merck
Tablets, chewable	10 mg	**Pepcid® AC,** J&J-Merck
Tablets, film-coated	10 mg	**Pepcid® AC,** J&J-Merck
	20 mg*	**Pepcid®**, Merck
		Pepcid® AC Maximum Strength, J&J-Merck
	40 mg	**Pepcid®**, Merck
Tablets, orally disintegrating	20 mg	**Pepcid® RPD,** Merck
	40 mg	**Pepcid® RPD,** Merck
Parenteral		
For injection, concentrate	10 mg/mL (pharmacy bulk package)	**Famotidine for Injection**
For injection concentrate, for IV use	10 mg/mL	**Famotidine for Injection**
		Pepcid® I.V., Merck

*available from one or more manufacturer, distributor, and/or repackager by generic (nonproprietary) name

Famotidine in Sodium Chloride

Parenteral		
Injection, for IV use only	0.4 mg/mL (20 mg) in 0.9% Sodium Chloride	**Pepcid® Premixed in Iso-osmotic Sodium Chloride Injection** (Galaxy® [Baxter]), Merck

Famotidine Combinations

Oral		
Tablets, chewable	10 mg with calcium carbonate 800 mg and magnesium hydroxide 165 mg	**Pepcid® Complete,** J&J-Merck

†Use is not currently included in the labeling approved by the US Food and Drug Administration

raNITIdine Hydrochloride

■ Ranitidine is a histamine H_2-receptor antagonist.

Uses

Ranitidine is used orally for the treatment of active duodenal or gastric ulcer, gastroesophageal reflux disease, or endoscopically diagnosed erosive esophagitis, and as maintenance therapy for duodenal or gastric ulcer. Oral ranitidine also is used for the management of pathologic GI hypersecretory conditions and as maintenance therapy to prevent recurrence of erosive esophagitis. Ranitidine is used parenterally in hospitalized patients with pathologic GI hypersecretory conditions or intractable duodenal ulcer, or for short-term use when oral therapy is not feasible.

■ **Duodenal Ulcer** ***Acute Therapy*** Ranitidine is used orally for the short-term treatment of endoscopically or radiographically confirmed active duodenal ulcer. Ranitidine is used parenterally in hospitalized adults with intractable duodenal ulcer or for short-term use when oral therapy is not feasible. Ranitidine also is used IV in children 1 month to 16 years of age for the treatment of duodenal ulcer. Ranitidine bismuth citrate (no longer commercially available in the US) has been used in combination with clarithromycin for the treatment of *Helicobacter pylori* infection in adults with active duodenal ulcer. Antacids may be used concomitantly as needed for relief of pain.

In a multicenter, double-blind study in patients with endoscopically diagnosed duodenal ulcers who were receiving supplemental antacids, reported rates of ulcer healing for ranitidine (150 mg twice daily) versus placebo were 38 vs 19% at 2 weeks and 73 vs 45% at 4 weeks. Ranitidine also produced greater reductions in daytime and nocturnal pain and antacid consumption than did placebo. Similar rates of ulcer healing occur following oral ranitidine 150 mg twice daily or 300 mg at bedtime daily; ulcer healing rates of 85–86 or 83–87%, respectively, have been reported at 4 weeks and 92 or 87%, respectively, at 8 weeks. Although there was a trend favoring the twice-daily regimen in a large, multinational study, the differences in healing rates between the regimens were small and might be offset by the benefits derived from once-daily administration of the drug at bedtime.

Ranitidine appears to be as effective as cimetidine for the short-term treatment of active duodenal ulcer. In a multicenter, double-blind study in patients with active duodenal ulcers, 71 or 68% of ulcers were healed following administration of 150 mg of ranitidine twice daily or 300 mg of cimetidine 4 times daily, respectively, for 4 weeks. In another study in patients with endoscopically diagnosed duodenal ulcers, 77 or 84% of ulcers were healed following administration of 150 mg of ranitidine twice daily or 200 mg of cimetidine 3 times daily after meals and 400 mg at bedtime, respectively, for 4 weeks; there appeared to be no difference in healing rates in males or females, the number of episodes of pain was decreased by both drugs during the first 2 weeks of therapy, and fewer antacid tablets were consumed by all individuals as therapy continued. Ranitidine has been effective in some patients whose duodenal ulcers were refractory to cimetidine therapy.

Safety and efficacy of long-term ranitidine therapy for active duodenal ulcer have not been determined. Studies to date have been limited to short-term treatment of active duodenal ulcer, and the safety and efficacy of treatment for active disease beyond 8 weeks have not been determined. Most patients with duodenal ulcer respond to ranitidine therapy during the initial 4-week course of therapy; an additional 4 weeks of therapy may contribute to healing in some patients. However, short-term ranitidine therapy (i.e., up to 8 weeks) for the treatment of active duodenal disease will not prevent recurrence following acute healing and discontinuance of the drug. Current epidemiologic and clinical evidence supports a strong association between gastric infection with *H. pylori* and the pathogenesis of duodenal and gastric ulcers; long-term *H. pylori* infection also has been implicated as a risk factor for gastric cancer. For additional information on the association of this infection with these and other GI conditions, see Helicobacter pylori Infection, under Uses, in Clarithromycin 8:12.12.

Conventional antiulcer therapy with H_2-receptor antagonists, proton-pump inhibitors, sucralfate, and/or antacids heals ulcers but generally is ineffective in eradicating *H. pylori*, and such therapy is associated with a high rate of ulcer recurrence (e.g., 60–100% per year). Duodenal ulcers have recurred within 6 months in approximately 50–80% of individuals following discontinuance of ranitidine therapy. In one study in patients who agreed to retreatment, recurring duodenal ulcers rehealed within 8 weeks following an additional course of ranitidine therapy; however, the effect of continued, full-dose ranitidine treatment on the recurrence rate of duodenal ulcers remains to be more fully evaluated. The American College of Gastroenterology (ACG), the National Institutes of Health (NIH), and most clinicians currently recommend that *all* patients with initial or recurrent duodenal or gastric ulcer and documented *H. pylori* infection receive anti-infective therapy for treatment of the infection. Although 3-drug regimens consisting of a bismuth salt (e.g., bismuth subsalicylate) and 2 anti-infective agents (e.g., tetracycline or amoxicillin plus metronidazole) administered for 10–14 days have been effective in eradicating the infection, resolving associated gastritis, healing peptic ulcer, and preventing ulcer recurrence in many patients with *H. pylori*-associated peptic ulcer disease, current evidence principally from studies in Europe suggests that 1 week of such therapy provides comparable *H. pylori* eradication rates. Other regimens that combine one or more anti-infective agents (e.g., clarithromycin, amoxicillin) with a bismuth salt and/or an antisecretory agent (e.g., omeprazole, lansoprazole, H_2-receptor antagonist) also have been used successfully for *H. pylori* eradication, and the choice of a particular regimen should be based on the rapidly evolving data on optimal therapy, including consideration of the patient's prior exposure to anti-infective agents, the local prevalence of resistance, patient compliance, and costs of therapy.

Current evidence suggests that inclusion of a proton-pump inhibitor (e.g., omeprazole, lansoprazole) in anti-*H. pylori* regimens containing 2 anti-infectives enhances effectiveness, and limited data suggest that such regimens retain good efficacy despite imidazole (e.g., metronidazole) resistance. Therefore, the ACG and many clinicians currently recommend 1 week of therapy with a proton-pump inhibitor and 2 anti-infective agents (usually clarithromycin and amoxicillin or metronidazole), or a 3-drug, bismuth-based regimen (e.g., bismuth-metronidazole-tetracycline) concomitantly with a proton-pump inhibitor, for treatment of *H. pylori* infection.

Therapy with an antisecretory drug and a single anti-infective agent (i.e., "dual therapy") also has been used successfully for treatment of *H. pylori* infection. However, while some studies demonstrate that certain 2-drug anti-*H. pylori* regimens (e.g., clarithromycin-omeprazole, ranitidine bismuth citrate-omeprazole, amoxicillin-omeprazole) can successfully eradicate *H. pylori* infection and prevent recurrence of duodenal ulcer at least in the short term (e.g., at 6 months following completion of anti-*H. pylori* therapy), the ACG and some clinicians currently state that anti-*H. pylori* regimens consisting of at least 3 drugs (e.g., 2 anti-infective agents plus a proton-pump inhibitor) are recommended because of enhanced *H. pylori* eradication rates, decreased failures due to resistance, and shorter treatment periods compared with those apparently required with 2-drug regimens. Additional randomized, controlled studies comparing various anti-*H. pylori* regimens are needed to clarify optimum drug combinations, dosages, and durations of treatment for *H. pylori* infection. For a more complete discussion of *H. pylori* infection, including details about the efficacy of various regimens and rationale for drug selection, see Helicobacter pylori Infection, under Uses, in Clarithromycin 8:12.12.

Maintenance Therapy Ranitidine is used orally in reduced dosage as maintenance therapy following healing of active duodenal ulcer to reduce ulcer recurrence. In placebo-controlled studies, duodenal ulcer recurrence rates after 4 months, 8 months, and 1 year were 12–20, 21–24, and 28–35%, respectively, for 150 mg of ranitidine at bedtime daily vs 44–56, 54–64, and 59–68%, respectively, for placebo. In one placebo-controlled study, the 1-year reduction in recurrence persisted for almost 2 years of therapy. Because the efficacy of $_2$-receptor antagonists in preventing duodenal ulcer recurrence appears to be substantially reduced in patients who are cigarette smokers compared with nonsmokers, patients who are cigarette smokers should be advised of the importance of discontinuing smoking in the prevention of ulcer recurrence. Maintenance therapy with ranitidine has not been studied for longer than 2 years in placebo-controlled studies.

■ **Pathologic GI Hypersecretory Conditions** Ranitidine is used orally or parenterally for the treatment of pathologic GI hypersecretory conditions (e.g., Zollinger-Ellison syndrome, systemic mastocytosis, postoperative hypersecretion, "short-gut" syndrome). Ranitidine reduces gastric acid secretion and associated symptoms (e.g., diarrhea, anorexia, and pain) and promotes healing of intractable ulcers in patients with these conditions. Administration of ranitidine as a continuous IV infusion for up to 15 days in a limited number of patients with Zollinger-Ellison syndrome has resulted in control of gastric acid secretion to 10 mEq/hour or less; no patient developed acid-related disease complications (e.g., bleeding, perforation). Antacids may be used concomitantly as needed for relief of pain. Antimuscarinics (e.g., propantheline bromide, isopropamide iodide) have been used concomitantly with ranitidine to prolong and/or augment ranitidine-induced inhibition of gastric acid secretion in some patients with GI hypersecretory conditions.

The manufacturers state that, in a limited number of patients with GI hypersecretory conditions, ranitidine therapy has resulted in healing of ulcers in 42% of patients who had not responded to previous cimetidine therapy. In one study, patients with Zollinger-Ellison syndrome in whom cimetidine failed to control symptoms of the disease or who did not tolerate cimetidine therapy were successfully treated with 600–900 mg of ranitidine daily for up to 1–12 months. In another study, patients with GI hypersecretory conditions (e.g., Zollinger-Ellison syndrome, idiopathic gastric hypersecretion) who were successfully treated with 1.2–12.6 g of cimetidine daily alone or in combination with an antimuscarinic (i.e., propantheline bromide or isopropamide iodide) for up to 60 months were subsequently successfully treated with 450 mg to 6.3 g of ranitidine daily alone or in combination with an antimuscarinic for up to 25 months; both drugs appeared to be equally effective in controlling gastric hypersecretion but lower daily doses of ranitidine were required.

In one study, ranitidine was used successfully IV in the treatment of postoperative hypersecretion in patients whose condition was apparently resistant to cimetidine therapy or in whom adverse effects of cimetidine required discontinuance of the drug.

■ **Gastric Ulcer** ***Acute Therapy*** Ranitidine is used orally for short-term treatment of active, benign gastric ulcer. Antacids may be used concomitantly as needed for relief of pain. The efficacy of ranitidine in the treatment of gastric ulcer appears to be similar to that of cimetidine. Ranitidine promotes healing of ulcers in about 60–70% of patients after 4 weeks of treatment and about 70–80% of patients after 6 weeks of treatment. The usefulness of ranitidine therapy for longer than 6 weeks in the treatment of active, benign gastric ulcer remains to be clearly determined. When ranitidine is used in the treatment of gastric ulcer, it should be kept in mind that symptomatic response does not preclude the presence of a gastric malignancy.

Current epidemiologic and clinical evidence supports a strong association between gastric infection with *H. pylori* and the pathogenesis of gastric ulcers, and the ACG, NIH, and most clinicians currently recommend that *all* patients with initial or recurrent gastric ulcer and documented *H. pylori* infection receive anti-infective therapy for treatment of the infection. The choice of particular regimen should be based on the rapidly evolving data on optimal therapy, including consideration of the patient's exposure to anti-infective agents, the local prevalence of resistance, patient compliance, and costs of therapy. (See Duodenal Ulcer: Acute Therapy, in Uses.) For a more complete discussion of *H. pylori* infection, including details about the efficacy of various regimens and rationale for drug selection, see Helicobacter pylori Infection, under Uses, in Clarithromycin 8:12.12.

Maintenance Therapy Ranitidine is used orally in reduced dosage following healing of active, benign gastric ulcer to reduce ulcer recurrence. In 12-month controlled trials in patients with previously healed gastric ulcers, therapy with ranitidine 150 mg at bedtime each night was more effective than placebo in maintaining healing of gastric ulcers.

■ **Gastroesophageal Reflux** Ranitidine is used orally in the management of gastroesophageal reflux disease (GERD). Symptomatic relief generally occurs within 24 hours of initiating ranitidine therapy as conventional tablets or within 45 minutes as effervescent tablets. By increasing gastric pH, H_2-antagonists have relieved heartburn and other symptoms of reflux and have been associated with somewhat higher healing rates of endoscopically proven esophagitis when compared with placebo and have reduced antacid consumption.

Suppression of gastric acid secretion is considered by the ACG to be the mainstay of treatment for gastroesophageal reflux disease (GERD), and a proton-pump inhibitor or histamine H_2-receptor antagonist is used to achieve acid suppression, control symptoms, and prevent complications of the disease. Because GERD is considered to be a chronic disease, many patients with GERD require long-term, even lifelong, treatment. The ACG states that histamine H_2-receptor antagonists administered daily in divided doses are effective in many patients with less severe GERD, and over-the-counter (OTC) antacids and histamine H_2-receptor antagonists are appropriate for *self-medication* as initial therapy in such individuals. A histamine H_2-receptor antagonist is particularly useful when taken before certain activities (e.g., heavy meal, exercise) that may result in acid reflux symptoms in some patients. The ACG states that H_2-receptor antagonists generally may be used interchangeably, although the drugs may differ in potency and in their onset and duration of action. However, proton-pump inhibitors are more effective (i.e., provide more frequent and more rapid symptomatic relief and healing of esophagitis) than do histamine H_2-receptor antagonists in the treatment of GERD, and are effective and appropriate as maintenance therapy in many patients with the disease. Although higher doses and more frequent administration of histamine H_2-receptor antagonists appear to increase their efficacy, such dosages are less effective and more expensive than proton-pump inhibitor therapy. Once-daily administration of a histamine H_2-receptor antagonist at full dosage is *not* considered to be appropriate therapy for GERD.

H_2-antagonists have also been used in combination with metoclopramide in a limited number of patients who failed to respond to an H_2-antagonist alone†, but the ACG states that frequent and potentially severe adverse CNS effects of metoclopramide have appropriately decreased regular use of the drug for the treatment of GERD. Although some clinicians have suggested that a histamine H_2-receptor antagonist may also be used in combination with bethanechol† in patients who fail to respond to a histamine H_2-receptor antagonist alone, the ACG states that bethanechol has limited efficacy in the treatment of GERD.

Short-term therapy (i.e., up to 12 weeks) with H_2-receptor antagonists for the treatment of GERD will not prevent recurrence following ulcer healing and discontinuance of such therapy. Esophagitis has recurred within 6 months in up to 80% of patients following discontinuance of H_2-receptor antagonist therapy. Because GERD is considered to be a chronic disease, many patients with GERD require long-term, even lifelong, treatment. The ACG states that proton-pump inhibitors are effective and appropriate as maintenance therapy in many patients with the disease. Maintenance therapy† with an H_2-receptor antagonist also has been used to reduce recurrence of GERD. However, many patients initially responding to proton-pump inhibitors experience symptomatic relapse and failure of esophageal healing with subsequent use of a histamine H_2-receptor antagonist.

For further information on the treatment of GERD, see Uses: Gastroesophageal Reflux, in Omeprazole 56:40.

■ **Erosive Esophagitis** ***Acute Therapy*** Ranitidine is used orally for the treatment of endoscopically diagnosed erosive esophagitis. In two multicenter, double-blind, placebo-controlled trials of the drug, healing rates of 47, 71, and 84% were reported after 4, 8, and 12 weeks, respectively, of therapy with ranitidine at dosages of 150 mg 4 times daily; concomitant antacids were used as needed for relief of pain. Symptomatic improvement in heartburn generally occurred within 24 hours of initiation of drug therapy. No additional benefit in treatment of esophagitis or relief of heartburn symptoms was observed in patients receiving the drug at dosages of 300 mg 4 times daily.

Maintenance Therapy Ranitidine is used orally as maintenance therapy to prevent recurrence of erosive esophagitis in adults. In controlled trials of 48-weeks duration, ranitidine 150 mg twice daily was more effective than placebo in maintaining healing in patients with previously healed erosive esophagitis.

■ **Increasing Gastric pH in Neonates Undergoing Extracorporeal Membrane Oxygenation (ECMO)** Limited data suggest that ranitidine administered IV may be useful and safe for increasing gastric pH in neonates younger than 1 month of age receiving ECMO who are at risk of GI hemorrhage. Following a 2 mg/kg IV dose of ranitidine in 5 neonates receiving ECMO, gastric pH was increased from less than 4 to above 4 and remained above 4 for at least 15 hours after administration. (See Cautions: Pediatric Precautions)

■ **Other Uses** Ranitidine may be used for *self-medication* for relief or prevention of symptoms of occasional heartburn (pyrosis), acid indigestion (hyperchlorhydria), or sour stomach.

Ranitidine has been used for the treatment of recurrent postoperative ulcer† and upper GI bleeding† (e.g., secondary to gastric ulcer, duodenal ulcer, or hemorrhagic gastritis). Because ranitidine can increase gastric pH, the drug has also been used prophylactically to prevent acid-aspiration pneumonitis† during surgery.

Dosage and Administration

■ **Administration** Ranitidine hydrochloride usually is administered orally. The drug also may be given by IM or slow IV injection or by intermittent or continuous slow IV infusion in hospitalized patients with pathologic hypersecretory conditions or intractable duodenal ulcer, or when oral therapy is not feasible. In addition, ranitidine hydrochloride may be given by intermittent slow IV injection or intermittent infusion for the treatment of duodenal ulcer in children 1 month to 16 years of age, and by intermittent slow IV injection, intermittent infusion, or continuous slow IV infusion to decrease gastric pH in neonates younger than 1 month of age receiving extracorporeal membrane oxygenation (ECMO). Because of the risk of inducing bradycardia (see Cautions: Other Adverse Effects), the recommended rates of IV administration should not be exceeded. Antacids may be administered concomitantly as necessary for relief of pain. (See Drug Interactions: Food and Antacids.)

The 1-g pharmacy bulk package of ranitidine hydrochloride is *not* intended for direct IV infusion; doses of the drug from the bulk package must be further diluted in a compatible IV solution prior to administration.

Oral Administration Patients receiving 150-mg effervescent tablets of ranitidine hydrochloride should be advised that the preparation must be diluted in 180–240 mL (6–8 ounces) of water as directed prior to ingestion. For pediatric patients receiving the 25-mg effervescent tablets, 1 tablet should be dissolved in at least 5 mL (1 teaspoonful) of water in an appropriate measuring cup. The tablet should be dissolved completely before the solution is administered to the infant or child. For infants, the solution may be administered using a medicine dropper or oral syringe. Effervescent tablets should not be chewed, swallowed whole, or dissolved on the tongue.

IM Injection For IM administration, ranitidine hydrochloride injection may be given undiluted.

Intermittent Direct IV Injection Ranitidine hydrochloride injection must be diluted prior to IV administration. For slow IV injection, 50 mg of ranitidine is diluted to a concentration no greater than 2.5 mg/mL (i.e., a total of 20 mL) with 0.9% sodium chloride injection or another compatible IV solution (See Chemistry and Stability: Stability) and injected at a rate not exceeding 4 mL per minute (i.e., over a period of not less than 5 minutes).

Intermittent IV Infusion For intermittent slow IV infusion, 50 mg of ranitidine is diluted to a concentration no greater than 0.5 mg/mL (i.e., a total of 100 mL) of 5% dextrose injection or another compatible IV solution (See Chemistry and Stability: Stability) and infused at a rate not exceeding 5–7 mL per minute (i.e., over 15–20 minutes). Alternatively, the commercially available IV infusion solution of the drug in 0.45% sodium chloride can be infused IV over 15–20 minutes. The commercially available diluted solution should only be administered by IV infusion. The container should be checked for minute leaks by firmly squeezing the bag. The injection should be discarded if the seal is not intact or leaks are found or if the solution is cloudy or contains a precipitate. Additives should not be introduced into the injection container. The injection should not be used in series connections with other plastic containers, since such use could result in air embolism from residual air being drawn from the primary container before administration of fluid from the secondary container is complete.

Continuous IV Infusion For continuous IV infusion, 150 mg of ranitidine injection is diluted in 250 mL of 5% dextrose injection or another compatible IV solution (See Chemistry and Stability: Stability) and infused at a rate of 6.25 mg/hour over a 24-hour period. For use in patients with Zollinger-Ellison syndrome or other hypersecretory conditions, ranitidine injection should be diluted to a concentration no greater than 2.5 mg/mL with 5% dextrose or another compatible IV solution and the infusion initiated at a rate of 1 mg/kg per hour; the rate should be adjusted to individual patient requirements.

■ **Dosage** Although USP currently states that potency of ranitidine hydrochloride preparations should be expressed both in terms of the salt and the base ("active moiety"), dosage currently is expressed in terms of the base. (See Chemistry and Stability: Chemistry.)

Because geriatric patients are more likely to have decreased renal function, caution should be exercised in dosage selection, and it may be useful to monitor renal function. (See Cautions: Geriatric Precautions.)

Oral Dosage Oral dosages recommended for the treatment of duodenal and gastric ulcers and for maintenance therapy for duodenal and gastric ulcers in children 1 month to 16 years age are extrapolated from clinical adult studies and pharmacokinetic data in children. Dosages of oral ranitidine recommended for the treatment of gastroesophageal reflux disease or erosive esophagitis in children 1 month to 16 years of age or older are based on published medical literature; however, only limited data is available for these conditions in children.

Duodenal Ulcer. For the treatment of active duodenal ulcer, the usual adult oral dosage of ranitidine is 150 mg twice daily. Alternatively, 300 mg daily after the evening meal or at bedtime may be used for patients in whom dosing convenience is considered important for optimum compliance. The advantage of one regimen over another for particular patients with active duodenal ulcer has not been determined to date. Lower dosages have been effective in inhibiting gastric acid secretion in US studies to date; in several foreign studies, 100 mg twice daily was as effective as 150 mg twice daily in healing ulcers.

For the treatment of active duodenal ulcer in children 1 month to 16 years of age, the usual oral dosage of ranitidine is 2–4 mg/kg twice daily up to a maximum daily dosage of 300 mg.

Although the optimum duration of ranitidine therapy has not been established, healing may occur within the first 2 weeks in some patients and within 4 weeks in most patients; some patients may benefit from an additional 4 weeks of therapy. Safety and efficacy of continuing full-dose therapy beyond 8 weeks have not been determined.

Multiple-drug regimens currently recommended by the American College of Gastroenterology (ACG) and many clinicians for the treatment of *Helicobacter pylori* infection in patients with active duodenal ulcer consist of a proton-pump inhibitor (e.g., omeprazole) and 2 anti-infective agents (e.g., clarithromycin and amoxicillin or metronidazole) or a 3-drug, bismuth-based regimen (e.g., bismuth-metronidazole-tetracycline) concomitantly with a proton-pump inhibitor. (See Uses: Helicobacter pylori Infection, in Clarithromycin 8:12.12.92.)

For maintenance therapy following healing of acute duodenal ulcer to reduce ulcer recurrence, the usual adult oral dosage of ranitidine is 150 mg daily at bedtime. For maintenance therapy following healing of acute duodenal ulcer, the usual oral dosage of ranitidine in children 1 month to 16 years of age is 2–4 mg/kg once daily up to a maximum daily dosage of 150 mg.

Pathologic GI Hypersecretory Conditions. For the treatment of pathologic GI hypersecretory conditions (e.g., Zollinger-Ellison syndrome), the usual adult oral dosage of ranitidine is 150 mg twice daily. It may be necessary to administer 150-mg doses of ranitidine more frequently than twice daily in some patients; dosage should be adjusted according to individual response, and therapy continued as long as clinically necessary. Oral dosages up to 6 g daily have been administered to individuals with severe disease.

Gastric Ulcer. For the treatment of active, benign gastric ulcer, the usual adult oral dosage of ranitidine is 150 mg twice daily. For the treatment of active, benign gastric ulcer in children 1 month to 16 years of age, the usual oral dosage of ranitidine is 2–4 mg/kg twice daily up to a maximum daily dosage of 300 mg. Most patients demonstrate complete healing of gastric ulcers within 6 weeks, and the safety of ranitidine therapy for longer periods in the treatment of gastric ulcer have not been established.

For maintenance therapy following healing of active, benign gastric ulcer to reduce ulcer recurrence, the usual adult oral dosage of ranitidine is 150 mg daily at bedtime. For maintenance therapy following healing of active benign gastric ulcer in children 1 month to 16 years of age, the usual oral dosage of ranitidine is 2–4 mg/kg once daily up to a maximum daily dosage of 150 mg.

Gastroesophageal Reflux. For the management of gastroesophageal reflux disease (GERD), the usual adult oral dosage of ranitidine is 150 mg twice daily. An oral ranitidine dosage of 5–10 mg/kg daily, usually given as 2 equally divided doses, is recommended for the management of GERD in children 1 month to 16 years of age. Symptomatic relief often occurs within 24 hours after initiating therapy with the drug. The optimum duration of acute ranitidine therapy for reflux has not been established.

Erosive Esophagitis. For the treatment of endoscopically diagnosed erosive esophagitis, the usual adult oral dosage of ranitidine is 150 mg 4 times daily. An oral ranitidine dosage of 5–10 mg/kg daily, usually given as 2 equally divided doses, is recommended for the management of erosive esophagitis in children 1 month to 16 years of age.

For maintenance therapy following healing of endoscopically diagnosed erosive esophagitis, the usual adult oral dosage of ranitidine is 150 mg twice daily.

Self-medication. For *self-medication* for the relief or prevention of symptoms of occasional heartburn, acid indigestion, or sour stomach in patients 12 years of age and older, an oral ranitidine dosage of 75 or 150 mg once or twice daily is recommended; for the prevention of symptoms, the dose should be taken 30–60 minutes before consuming foods or beverages that cause heartburn. For *self-medication*, the manufacturers recommend that no more than 2 doses be administered in 24 hours and that such therapy not exceed 2 weeks of *continuous* use unless otherwise recommended by a clinician. Patients should be instructed to take the tablets with water. Use for *self-medication* should be discontinued and a clinician consulted if stomach pain is persistent, or if heartburn continues or worsens.

The manufacturers state that ranitidine should not be used for *self-medication* in children younger than 12 years of age unless otherwise directed by their clinician.

Parenteral Dosage **Adult Dosage.** The usual adult IM or intermittent IV dosage of ranitidine is 50 mg every 6–8 hours. If necessary, dosage may be increased by increasing the frequency of administration, but dosage should not exceed 400 mg daily.

When ranitidine is administered by continuous slow IV infusion, 150 mg of ranitidine is infused at a rate of 6.25 mg/hour over 24 hours. When the drug is administered by continuous slow IV infusion in adults with Zollinger-Ellison syndrome or other hypersecretory conditions, the infusion is usually started at a rate of 1 mg/kg per hour. If after 4 hours the patient is still symptomatic or if the measured gastric acid secretion is greater than 10 mEq/hour, the dose should be titrated upward in increments of 0.5 mg/kg per hour; the gastric acid secretion should then be redetermined. Doses up to 2.5 mg/kg per hour and infusion rates as high as 220 mg/hour have been used.

Pediatric Dosage. For the treatment of active duodenal ulcer in children 1 month to 16 years of age, the recommended IV dosage of ranitidine is 2–4 mg/kg daily in divided doses administered every 6–8 hours up to a maximum of 50 mg given every 6–8 hours.

Ranitidine IV dosages recommended for the treatment of duodenal ulcers in children 1 month to 16 years of age are extrapolated from clinical adult studies as well as limited pharmacokinetic data in children and published medical literature.

For neonatal patients (less than 1 month of age) receiving ECMO and at risk for GI hemorrhage, doses of 2 mg/kg given IV every 12–24 hours or as a continuous IV infusion should be considered; limited data indicate that a dose of 2 mg/kg usually is sufficient to increase gastric pH above 4 for at least 15 hours.

■ **Dosage in Renal Impairment** In patients with creatinine clearances less than 50 mL/minute, the manufacturer recommends an oral ranitidine dosage of 150 mg once every 24 hours and an IM or IV (intermittent slow infusion or direct injection) dosage of 50 mg every 18–24 hours; the administration of ranitidine as a continuous IV infusion has not been evaluated in patients with impaired renal function. Dosage intervals may be decreased cautiously from every 24 hours to every 12 hours or less, if necessary. Because hemodialysis reduces serum ranitidine concentrations, the dosage regimen should be adjusted so that a scheduled dose of ranitidine is administered at the end of dialysis.

Cautions

Adverse effects of ranitidine are generally infrequent and minor.

■ **Nervous System Effects** Headache (sometimes severe) occurs in approximately 3% of patients receiving ranitidine. Malaise, dizziness, somnolence,insomnia, and vertigo have been reported less frequently with ranitidine therapy. Reversible mental confusion, agitation, mental depression, and hallucinations have occurred, mainly in debilitated geriatric patients. Reversible involuntary motor disturbances have been reported rarely in patients receiving ranitidine. A child who was receiving prolonged, high-dose oral ranitidine therapy (8 mg/kg once daily for 10 months) developed altered consciousness, drowsiness, dysarthria, hyporeflexia, positive Babinski's sign, diaphoresis, and bradycardia, which resolved within 24 hours after discontinuance of the drug.

■ **GI Effects** Constipation, nausea, vomiting, and abdominal discomfort or pain have occurred in patients receiving ranitidine. Pancreatitis has been reported rarely.

■ **Dermatologic and Sensitivity Reactions** Rash, which may be urticarial, maculopapular, and/or pruritic, has been reported during ranitidine therapy. Rash, including rare cases of erythema multiforme, has occurred with ranitidine therapy. Urticaria at the site of injection has occurred following IV administration of ranitidine. Alopecia has occurred rarely.

Hypersensitivity reactions such as bronchospasm, fever, rash, and eosinophilia have occurred rarely in patients receiving ranitidine. Anaphylaxis, characterized by severe urticaria and a decrease in blood pressure in one patient following administration of a single dose of ranitidine, has occurred rarely; exacerbation of asthma and angioedema also has occurred. Mild erythema multiforme-like rash and alopecia also have occurred rarely.

■ **Hematologic Effects** Leukopenia, granulocytopenia, agranulocytosis, thrombocytopenia, aplastic anemia, acquired immune hemolytic anemia, and pancytopenia, which may be accompanied by bone marrow hypoplasia, have been reported rarely in patients receiving ranitidine. Alterations in blood cell counts (leukopenia, granulocytopenia, and thrombocytopenia) usually were reversible. At least one case of leukocytosis has been reported 6–8 days after initiating ranitidine therapy, which resolved following discontinuance of the drug. Although a causal relationship to the drug was not established, aplastic anemia has occurred in at least one patient receiving ranitidine.

■ **Renal and Genitourinary Effects** Small increases in serum creatinine, without concomitant increases in BUN, have been reported during ranitidine therapy; however, the manufacturers state that these increases have occurred less frequently than with cimetidine therapy and may result from competitive inhibition by ranitidine of creatinine secretion into the urine.

Loss of libido has been reported in male patients receiving ranitidine.

■ Hepatic Effects Increases in serum aminotransferase (transaminase) (AST [SGOT] and ALT [SGPT]), alkaline phosphatase, LDH, total bilirubin, and γ-glutamyl transferase (γ-glutamyltranspeptidase, GGT, GGTP) concentrations have been reported in patients receiving ranitidine. Hepatitis, which may be hepatocellular and/or hepatocanalicular, cholestatic, and may or may not be accompanied by jaundice, has occurred occasionally in individuals receiving ranitidine and usually was reversible; however, death has been reported rarely. Ranitidine should be discontinued immediately in patients with hepatitis. Hepatic failure has been reported rarely. In several multiple-dose studies in healthy individuals, increases in serum AST and ALT concentrations from pretreatment concentrations were greater in individuals receiving IV ranitidine dosages of 100 mg 4 times daily for 7 days than in those receiving 50 mg 4 times daily for 5 days.

■ Ocular Effects Reversible blurred vision suggestive of a change in accommodation has occurred rarely in patients receiving ranitidine. Exacerbation of ocular pain and blurred vision associated with increased intraocular pressure and chronic glaucoma have been reported in at least one patient during ranitidine therapy. Loss of color vision, which recurred following rechallenge, also has occurred in at least one patient.

■ Endocrine Effects The manufacturers state that ranitidine has not been associated with clinically important effects on endocrine or gonadal function. (See Pharmacology: Endocrine and Gonadal Effects.) Sexual impotence has occurred in at least one male during ranitidine therapy, but disappeared following discontinuance of the drug; impotence recurred upon rechallenge. Painful gynecomastia in men also has occurred during oral administration of ranitidine, but disappeared gradually following discontinuance of the drug; gynecomastia reappeared upon rechallenge.

■ Cardiovascular Effects As with other histamine H_2-receptor antagonists, cardiac arrhythmias have occurred rarely in patients receiving ranitidine. Bradycardia, sometimes associated with dyspnea, has occurred. Because bradycardia has been associated with rapid IV injection of the drug in some cases, usually in patients with underlying conditions predisposing to cardiac rhythm disturbances, recommended rates of IV administration should not be exceeded. Tachycardia, AV block, asystole, and ventricular premature complexes have also been reported rarely. Vasculitis has been reported rarely.

■ Respiratory Effects ***Community-acquired Pneumonia*** Administration of gastric antisecretory agents (e.g., H_2-receptor antagonists, proton-pump inhibitors) has been associated with an increased risk for developing certain infections (e.g., community-acquired pneumonia). A possible association between chronic administration of gastric acid-suppressive drugs and occurrence of community-acquired pneumonia has been evaluated using a large Dutch database (Integrated Primary Care Information [IPCI]) containing information on approximately 500,000 patients, 364,683 of whom (average follow-up: 2.7 years) were selected for evaluating any such association. During the 8-year population-based, case-control study, gastric acid suppressants were first prescribed in 19,459 individuals (10,177 received H_2-receptor antagonists [mean duration of use: 2.8 months] and 12,337 received proton-pump inhibitors [mean duration of use: 5 months]; some individuals received both drugs). Most patients did not undergo endoscopy and were treated empirically for upper GI symptoms. In this study, first occurrence of pneumonia (confirmed by radiography or microbiologic testing in 18% of patients) was reported in 5551 individuals; development of pneumonia occurred in 185 individuals while receiving gastric acid suppressants and in 292 individuals who had discontinued such use. The adjusted relative risk for development of pneumonia (or the incidence rate) was 0.6, 2.3 and 2.5 per 100 person-years for individuals not receiving acid-suppressive drugs, for those receiving H_2-receptor antagonists, and for those receiving proton-pump inhibitors, respectively. Patients using gastric acid suppressants developed community-acquired pneumonia 4.5 (95% confidence interval of 3.8–5.1) times more often than those who never used such drugs. When evaluating use of all gastric acid suppressants, current use of the drugs was associated with a small (27%) overall increase in the risk of pneumonia (adjusted odds ratio 1.27 and 95% confidence interval of 1.06–1.54). Higher risks were observed for current users of H_2-receptor antagonists and proton-pump inhibitors; the adjusted relative risk for developing community-acquired pneumonia was 1.63 (95% confidence interval of 1.07–2.48) or 1.89 (95% confidence interval of 1.36–2.62), respectively, for these classes of drugs compared with those who discontinued using these agents. Estimates for developing pneumonia were higher (1.7 [95% confidence interval of 0.8–2.9] for H_2-receptor antagonists and 2.2 [95% confidence interval of 1.4–3.5] for proton-pump inhibitors) when only laboratory-confirmed cases of pneumonia were considered for analysis. Although there was variation among individual H_2-receptor antagonists and individual proton-pump inhibitors, the numbers were small and the heterogeneity was not considered significant. For patients currently receiving proton-pump inhibitors, a dose-response relationship for developing pneumonia was observed; individuals using more than one defined daily dose of these drugs had a 2.3-fold increased risk for developing pneumonia compared with those who discontinued gastric acid suppressants. Such a dose-response relationship for developing pneumonia was not observed in patients receiving H_2-receptor antagonists; however, dose variation of these drugs was limited. Among current users of H_2-receptor antagonists or proton-pump inhibitors, the risk for developing pneumonia was most pronounced among those who initiated such therapies within the past 30 days.

Although the exact mechanism for development of community-acquired pneumonia in patients receiving gastric acid suppressants has not been fully elucidated, it has been suggested that reduction of gastric acid secretion by acid suppressive therapy and consequent increases of gastric pH may result in a favorable environment for the development of infection. Intragastric acidity constitutes a major nonspecific defense mechanism of the stomach to ingested pathogens; when gastric pH is less than 4, most pathogens are killed, while at higher gastric pH, pathogens may survive. Since for the effective management of upper GI symptoms, intragastric pH should be maintained above 4 for several hours, acid suppressive therapy may lead to insufficient elimination or, even, increased colonization of ingested pathogens. Some evidence indicates that acid-supressive therapy may result in nosocomial infections.

It should be considered that certain patients (e.g., those with pleuritic chest pain, hypothermia, systolic hypotension, tachypnea, diabetes mellitus, neoplastic disease, neurologic disease, bacteremia, leukopenia, multilobar pulmonary infiltrate) are at increased risk for developing infections and in these individuals community-acquired pneumonia may be associated with increased mortality. Some clinicians state that gastric acid-suppressive drugs should be used in patients in whom community-acquired pneumonia may be severe (e.g., those with asthma or chronic obstructive lung disease, immunocompromised patients, pediatric or geriatric individuals) only when clearly needed and the lowest effective dose should be employed.

■ Other Adverse Effects Arthralgias and myalgias have been reported rarely with ranitidine therapy. Rare reports suggest that ranitidine may precipitate acute attacks of porphyria in patients with acute porphyria; therefore, the drug should be avoided in patients with a history of acute porphyria.

■ Precautions and Contraindications Ranitidine should be used with caution and in reduced dosage in patients with impaired renal function, since ranitidine is excreted principally by the kidneys. Ranitidine should also be used with caution in patients with hepatic dysfunction since the drug is metabolized in the liver.

Limited evidence suggests that ranitidine may precipitate acute porphyria in patients with a history of this condition; therefore, therapy with ranitidine should be avoided in patients with a history of acute porphyria.

Since increases in serum ALT concentrations have occurred in healthy individuals receiving higher than recommended IV dosages of an H_2-receptor antagonist for 5 days or longer during clinical trials, the manufacturers suggest that it may be advisable to monitor serum ALT concentrations daily from the fifth day to the remainder of IV therapy in patients receiving IV ranitidine dosages of 400 mg or more daily for 5 days or longer. Hepatotoxicity has also been reported occasionally during oral therapy with the drug.

Individuals with phenylketonuria (i.e., homozygous genetic deficiency of phenylalanine hydroxylase) and other individuals who must restrict their intake of phenylalanine should be warned that each EFFERdose® effervescent tablet (containing 25 or 150 mg of ranitidine) contains aspartame (NutraSweet®), which is metabolized in the GI tract to provide about 2.81 or 16.84 mg, respectively, of phenylalanine following oral administration.

Symptomatic response to ranitidine should *not* be interpreted as precluding the presence of gastric malignancy.

Ranitidine should not be used for *self-medication* if the patient has difficulty swallowing and should not be used with other drugs that decrease gastric acid secretion. Patients with heartburn that has persisted for more than 3 months or heartburn in conjunction with lightheadedness, sweating, or dizziness should consult their clinician before using ranitidine for *self-medication*. Patients also should be advised to consult their clinician before using ranitidine for *self-medication* if they are experiencing chest or shoulder pain with lightheadedness, shortness of breath, sweating, or pain spreading to arms, neck, or shoulders. Those with frequent chest pain, unexplained weight loss, nausea and vomiting, stomach pain, or frequent wheezing (especially with heartburn) also should consult their clinician before using ranitidine for *self-medication*. Patients should discontinue ranitidine *self-medication* and consult their clinician if heartburn or stomach pain worsens or persists after 14 days of therapy. Patients with difficulty or pain with swallowing, vomiting with blood, or bloody or blackened stools should not use ranitidine for *self-medication*; such manifestations should be reported promptly to a clinician, since they may be indicative of a serious condition requiring alternative treatment. Women who are pregnant or breast feeding should consult their clinician before using ranitidine for *self-medication*.

Ranitidine is contraindicated in patients with known hypersensitivity to the drugs or any of the ingredients in the respective formulation.

■ Pediatric Precautions The manufacturer states that safety and efficacy of oral ranitidine for the treatment of active duodenal or gastric ulcer, gastroesophageal reflux disease, or endoscopically diagnosed erosive esophagitis, and as maintenance therapy for duodenal or gastric ulcer in pediatric patients 1 month to 16 years of age have been established. In addition, use of oral ranitidine in pediatric patients is supported by adequate and well-controlled studies in adults, pharmacokinetic data in children, and published reports in the medical literature.

Safety and efficacy of ranitidine administered IV for the treatment of active duodenal ulcer in pediatric patients 1 month to 16 years of age have been established and are supported by adequate and well-controlled studies in adults, pharmacokinetic data in children, and published reports in the medical literature. In a limited study of 20 critically ill pediatric patients receiving IV ranitidine 1 mg/kg every 6 hours, 10 patients with a baseline pH of 4 or higher maintained this baseline throughout the study, and 8 of the remaining patients with a baseline pH of 2 or lower achieved a pH of 4 or higher throughout variable periods after dosing. However, such data should be interpreted with caution when determining dosages for less seriously ill patients. Limited data suggest that ranitidine administered IV may be useful and safe for increasing gastric pH in neonates receiving extracorporeal membrane oxygenation (ECMO) who are at risk of GI hemorrhage.

Safety and efficacy of oral or parenteral ranitidine for the treatment of pathologic GI hypersecretory conditions have not been established in pediatric patients. Safety and efficacy of oral ranitidine as maintenance therapy to prevent recurrence of erosive esophagitis have not been established in pediatric patients. Safety and efficacy of oral ranitidine in neonates younger than 1 month of age have not been established.

■ **Geriatric Precautions** When the total number of patients studied in clinical trials of oral ranitidine is considered, 4197 were 65 years of age or older, while 899 were 75 years of age or older. Although no overall differences in efficacy or safety were observed between geriatric and younger patients, and other clinical experience revealed no evidence of age-related differences, the possibility that some older patients may exhibit increased sensitivity to the drug cannot be ruled out. Because geriatric patients may have decreased renal function and because patients with renal impairment may be at increased risk of ranitidine-induced toxicity, dosage should be selected carefully, and it may be useful to monitor renal function in these individuals.

■ **Mutagenicity and Carcinogenicity** It is not known if ranitidine is mutagenic or carcinogenic in humans. In vitro tests have generally not shown ranitidine or its *N*-oxide, *S*-oxide, and desmethyl metabolites to be mutagenic. No evidence of carcinogenicity was seen in long-term studies in dogs, mice, or rats receiving ranitidine dosages up to 2 g/kg daily; evidence of gastric neoplasm or premalignant gastric changes was not observed in these studies. Like cimetidine, ranitidine increases nitrate-reducing bacterial flora in the GI tract; however, the clinical importance of this effect is not known.

■ **Pregnancy, Fertility, and Lactation** Reproduction studies in rats and rabbits using oral ranitidine dosages up to 160 times the usual human oral dosage have not revealed evidence of harm to the fetus. There are no adequate and controlled studies to date using ranitidine in pregnant women, and the drug should be used during pregnancy only when clearly needed. Women who are pregnant or nursing should seek the advice of a health professional before using ranitidine for *self-medication.*

Reproduction studies in rats and rabbits using oral ranitidine dosages up to 160 times the usual human oral dosage have not revealed evidence of impaired fertility.

Since ranitidine is distributed into milk, the drug should be used with caution in nursing women.

Drug Interactions

■ **Food and Antacids** Concomitant administration of food or low-dose antacids (neutralizing capacity of 10–15 mEq of hydrochloric acid per 10 mL) does not appear to substantially decrease the absorption of ranitidine or the mean peak plasma concentration of the drug. However, in one study, concomitant administration of 30 mL of an aluminum and magnesium hydroxides antacid (Mylanta-II®; neutralizing capacity of 150 mEq of hydrochloric acid per 30 mL), 30 mL of water, and a single 150-mg dose of ranitidine resulted in a 33% decrease in the absorption of ranitidine; peak serum ranitidine concentration decreased from 613 to 432 ng/mL and the area under the serum concentration-time curve (AUC) decreased from 3613 to 2394 mcg·hour/L. The time to reach the peak and the rate of absorption of the drug were not substantially altered by concurrent administration of the antacid in this study; elimination half-life and renal clearance of ranitidine remained unchanged, but the fraction of the dose excreted in urine as unchanged drug and as the desmethyl metabolite was reduced by concomitant administration of antacid.

■ **Propantheline Bromide** Propantheline bromide appears to delay the absorption and increase the peak serum concentration of ranitidine, probably by delaying gastric emptying and prolonging transit time; the relative bioavailability of ranitidine reportedly is increased approximately 23% with concomitant administration of propantheline.

■ **Smoking** Cigarette smoking reportedly adversely affects the healing of duodenal ulcers and also appears to decrease the efficacy of ranitidine. In a controlled study, 62 and 100% of duodenal ulcers in smokers and nonsmokers, respectively, healed following oral administration of 150 mg of ranitidine twice daily; in the placebo group, 0 and 36% of duodenal ulcers in smokers and nonsmokers, respectively, healed. The number of cigarettes smoked per day did not appear to influence the ulcer healing rate.

■ **Effects on Hepatic Clearance of Drugs** Since ranitidine interacts with the hepatic cytochrome P-450 (microsomal) enzyme system differently than does cimetidine, ranitidine appears to only minimally inhibit hepatic metabolism of some drugs (e.g., coumarin anticoagulants, theophylline, diazepam, propranolol). Ranitidine forms a ligand complex with the cytochrome P-450 enzyme system; however, ranitidine appears to interact with different forms of cytochrome P-450 than does cimetidine. The affinity of ranitidine for cytochrome P-450 is about 10% that of cimetidine and the extent of inhibition of the enzyme system is about 2.4 times less than that with cimetidine. Inhibition of hepatic microsomal enzyme activity appears to be structurally determined rather than associated with H_2-receptor blockade, since ranitidine and cimetidine differ substantially in their effects on this enzyme system. Hepatic microsomal mixed-function oxidase activity appears to be unchanged following concomitant administration of ranitidine and aminopyrine or antipyrine, since demethylation of aminopyrine and clearance of antipyrine are essentially unaltered by ranitidine therapy.

Although cimetidine and ranitidine have been reported to reduce hepatic blood flow in some studies, other studies have not confirmed this finding. Ranitidine does not appear to affect elimination of indocyanine green.

Coumarin Anticoagulants The manufacturers state that increased or decreased prothrombin time (PT) has been reported during concomitant therapy with ranitidine and warfarin; however, pharmacokinetic studies of ranitidine at dosages of up to 400 mg daily and warfarin demonstrated no effect on warfarin clearance and/or PT. Ranitidine dosages exceeding 400 mg daily have not been studied for potential interaction with warfarin. In one study following concomitant administration of 200 mg of ranitidine twice daily for 14 days and daily warfarin doses (2.5–4.5 mg) designed to prolong the PT by 2–5 seconds, neither the PT nor plasma warfarin concentration was altered substantially. In another study, although the effect on PT was not determined, ranitidine (150 mg twice daily orally for 7 days prior to and 5 days after administration of warfarin) reportedly decreased total body clearance of warfarin (a single 10-mg oral dose) but did not substantially affect warfarin's plasma half-life; the mechanism of this apparent decrease in warfarin clearance was not determined.

Theophyllines In one controlled, crossover study in healthy adults who received 300 mg of ranitidine, 1.2 g of cimetidine, or 2.4 g of cimetidine orally for 4 days prior to and 1 day after an IV aminophylline dose of 6 mg/kg, cimetidine 1.2 or 2.4 g daily decreased plasma theophylline clearance by 22–49 or 11–52%, respectively, while ranitidine did not alter theophylline clearance. Similar results were reported in another controlled, crossover study in which healthy adults received ranitidine or cimetidine concomitantly with theophylline. Although decreased theophylline clearance has been reported in at least one patient receiving ranitidine and an extended-release theophylline preparation (Theo-Dur®) concomitantly, the change in theophylline clearance may have resulted from discontinuance of an aluminum and magnesium hydroxides antacid rather than from initiation of ranitidine therapy and documentation of a potential ranitidine/theophylline interaction in this case has been questioned.

Benzodiazepines In one study, concomitant administration of diazepam and 150 mg of ranitidine twice daily did not substantially affect the area under the plasma diazepam concentration-time curve (AUC) or the mean half-life of diazepam. In another study, concomitant administration of a single 2-mg dose of lorazepam and 150 mg of ranitidine every 12 hours did not affect the elimination half-life, volume of distribution, or clearance of lorazepam.

Administration of oral ranitidine appears to increase the systemic availability of oral triazolam. In healthy adults (18–60 years of age), concomitant administration of triazolam and ranitidine 75 or 150 mg twice daily resulted in a 10 or 28% increase in the AUC of triazolam, respectively, compared with administration of triazolam alone; in individuals older than 60 years of age, such concomitant administration resulted in a 30% increase in the AUC of triazolam compared with administration of triazolam alone. Elimination of triazolam and α-hydroxytriazolam (a major metabolite) were not altered in individuals receiving ranitidine. It has been suggested that increased ranitidine-induced gastric pH may increase bioavailability of triazolam. The clinical importance of this interaction is not known.

For information on the potential interaction between midazolam and ranitidine, see Drug Interactions in Midazolam Hydrochloride 28:24.08.

β-Adrenergic Blocking Agents Mean serum propranolol concentrations do not appear to differ substantially in individuals receiving ranitidine and propranolol concomitantly vs those receiving propranolol alone. In one study, combined therapy with 150 mg of ranitidine and 100 mg of atenolol daily for 7 days did not appear to alter the pharmacokinetics of atenolol; however, in the same study, the pharmacokinetics of 100 mg of metoprolol were altered by ranitidine. The AUC for metoprolol increased about 80% (1167 vs 2140 ng·hour/mL) and the mean peak serum concentration of metoprolol increased about 50% (177.2 vs 265 ng/mL) during concomitant ranitidine therapy. In the same study, the elimination half-life of metoprolol increased from 4.4 to 6.5 hours when ranitidine was used concomitantly.

Acetaminophen Although the clinical importance is not known, ranitidine reportedly produced dose-dependent inhibition of acetaminophen metabolism in one in vitro study; in another study in which rats were pretreated with 120 mg/kg of ranitidine and then administered 250 mg/kg of radiolabeled acetaminophen, ranitidine appeared to decrease the oxidation of acetaminophen as determined by liver concentrations of glutathione and a covalently bound toxic metabolite of acetaminophen.

Phenytoin Ranitidine does not appear to affect serum concentrations of phenytoin following administration of 150 mg of ranitidine twice daily for 14 days in individuals receiving chronic phenytoin therapy of 180 or 300 mg daily.

■ **Alcohol** Currently available data suggest that consumption of moderate amounts of alcohol (e.g., 0.3 g/kg of body weight) by individuals receiving H_2-receptor antagonists, including ranitidine, is unlikely to result in clinically important alterations in blood alcohol concentrations and/or alcohol metabolism, although the possibility of such alterations in predisposed individuals cannot be definitely excluded. Increases in blood alcohol concentrations have been noted in some studies in healthy individuals receiving ranitidine or some other H_2 antagonists concomitantly with alcohol; however, conflicting data exist, which may be related to the effects of various patient-specific factors (e.g., gender, ethnic group, hepatic function, chronic alcoholism) on alcohol metabolism and/or to differences in study design (e.g., alcohol dose and time of administration, fasting vs fed state). Although controversy exists regarding the potential for psychomotor impairment with increases in alcohol absorption and/or blood alcohol concentration induced by H_2-receptor antagonists, patients receiving these drugs should observe the usual precautions regarding alcohol intake and performance of hazardous tasks requiring mental alertness or physical coordination (e.g., driving, operating machinery).

■ **Other Drugs** The manufacturers state that ranitidine may affect the oral bioavailability of certain drugs by some yet unidentified mechanism (e.g., a pH-dependent effect on GI absorption or a change in volume of distribution).

Preliminary evidence indicates that concomitant administration of ranitidine may increase the AUC for nifedipine by about 30%.

Although ranitidine appears to only minimally affect the secretion of gastric intrinsic factor, malabsorption of, and resultant deficiency in, vitamin B_{12} may occur during long-term ranitidine therapy.

Ranitidine does not appear to alter peak serum concentration or AUC for ethanol following administration of 0.8 g/kg of ethanol 20% v/v in individuals pretreated for 7 days with 300 mg of ranitidine daily.

Laboratory Test Interferences

Ranitidine reportedly causes false-positive results in urine protein determinations using Multistix®; the manufacturers recommend that sulfosalicylic acid reagent be used for urinary protein determinations during ranitidine therapy.

Acute Toxicity

The manufacturers state that there has been limited experience to date with overdosage of ranitidine. Reported acute oral ingestions of up to 18 g of ranitidine have been associated with transient adverse effects similar to those encountered in usual clinical experience. In addition, gait abnormalities and hypotension have been reported with ranitidine overdosage.

Patients receiving ranitidine should be instructed to contact their physician or local poison control center immediately if they accidentally ingest an overdose of the drug.

For the treatment of ranitidine overdosage, usual measures to remove unabsorbed drug from the GI tract, clinical monitoring, and supportive treatment should be employed. Elimination of ranitidine may be enhanced by hemodialysis.

Pharmacology

■ **GI Effects** Ranitidine competitively inhibits the action of histamine on the H_2 receptors of parietal cells, reducing gastric acid secretion under daytime and nocturnal basal conditions and also when stimulated by food, insulin, amino acids, histamine, or pentagastrin. Ranitidine has been shown to be 3–13 times as potent on a molar basis as cimetidine in inhibiting stimulated gastric acid secretion.

Basal, nocturnal, and betazole-stimulated gastric acid secretion appear to be inhibited to a greater extent than are meal- and pentagastrin-stimulated gastric acid secretion following a given dose of ranitidine. Following oral administration of 150 mg of ranitidine, 95% of basal gastric acid secretion is inhibited for up to 4 hours, 92% of nocturnal gastric acid secretion is inhibited for up to 13 hours, and 99% of betazole-stimulated gastric acid secretion is inhibited for up to 3 hours. Following oral administration of 150 mg of ranitidine, 72% of pentagastrin-stimulated gastric acid secretion is inhibited for up to 5 hours and 79% of meal-stimulated gastric acid secretion is inhibited for up to 3 hours. In one study, hydrogen ion secretion was reduced by 29, 50, and 70% and volume of gastric secretion was reduced by 21, 37, and 47% following oral administration of 20, 40, and 80 mg of ranitidine, respectively. Following treatment with 80 mg of ranitidine in another study, 85% of the gastric acid samples obtained from individuals with duodenal ulcers had a pH greater than 3 and 71% of these samples had a pH greater than 5 for up to 12 hours after administration of the drug; 92% of pretreatment gastric acid samples had a pH less than 2.

Following IV administration of 20, 60, and 100 mg of ranitidine, 93, 99, and 99% of betazole-stimulated gastric acid secretion is inhibited, respectively, for up to 2 hours and 47, 66, and 77% of pentagastrin-stimulated gastric acid secretion is inhibited, respectively, for up to 3 hours.

Ranitidine indirectly causes a dose-dependent reduction in pepsin secretion by decreasing the volume of gastric acid secretion. The drug appears to have little, if any, effect on gastric secretion of mucus, gastric intrinsic factor secretion, or fasting and postprandial serum gastrin concentrations. Ranitidine may protect the gastric mucosa from bleeding and the irritant effects caused by certain drugs (e.g., aspirin, nonsteroidal anti-inflammatory agents).

The manufacturers state that ranitidine does not reduce serum calcium concentration in individuals with hypercalcemia and is not an anticholinergic agent. In one in vitro study, ranitidine appeared to inhibit human erythrocyte acetylcholinesterase and plasma pseudocholinesterase; however, in another study in vivo, ranitidine did not inhibit cholinesterases. Ranitidine inconsistently increases lower esophageal sphincter pressure; however, the drug may have some therapeutic value in the inhibition of acid gastroesophageal reflux. Although ranitidine has been shown to delay gastric emptying, the clinical importance of this effect is not known.

■ **Endocrine and Gonadal Effects** Ranitidine generally has been shown to have little, if any, effect on serum prolactin concentration in healthy individuals or in those with clinically diagnosed duodenal ulcers. In one study, IV administration of 50 or 100 mg of ranitidine did not substantially alter basal prolactin secretion; however, an increase in serum prolactin concentration occurred following IV administration of 200 or 300 mg. The increase in serum prolactin caused by IV administration of 300 mg of ranitidine was comparable to that observed following IV administration of 200 mg of cimetidine. (See Cautions: Endocrine Effects).

Ranitidine has been shown to have little, if any, effect on serum concentrations of testosterone, luteinizing hormone (LH), follicle-stimulating hormone (FSH), thyrotropin (TSH), cortisol, aldosterone, growth hormone (GH), progesterone, or estradiol. In one study, basal serum concentrations of thyroxine (T_4) and serum concentrations of T_4 40 minutes after protirelin stimulation were decreased slightly during ranitidine therapy, while basal and protirelin-stimulated serum concentrations of triiodothyronine (T_3) and reverse triiodothyronine (rT_3) were not altered by ranitidine therapy. Ranitidine therapy also has been shown to have little, if any, effect on sperm count, motility, or morphology, or on penile erection. Ranitidine may possibly inhibit vasopressin release; the clinical importance of this effect is not fully understood.

Ranitidine does not appear to alter mean fasting blood glucose concentration or mean daily insulin requirement in patients with type 1 (insulin-dependent) diabetes mellitus; sensitivity of the serum glucose concentration to IV infusion of insulin also does not appear to be affected by prolonged (4 weeks) ranitidine therapy.

■ **Other Effects** Although cimetidine and ranitidine have been reported to reduce hepatic blood flow in some studies, other studies have not confirmed this finding. Unlike cimetidine, ranitidine does not inhibit hepatic metabolism of antipyrine. Although ranitidine affects the cytochrome P-450 enzyme system in the liver, the drug appears to interact with the enzyme system differently than does cimetidine. (See Drug Interactions: Effects on Hepatic Clearance of Drugs.)

Secretin- and cholecystokinin-induced pancreatic secretion volume and bicarbonate and protein secretion do not appear to be altered by IV infusion of ranitidine. Ranitidine increases nitrate-reducing bacterial flora in the GI tract; however, the clinical importance of this effect is not known.

Pharmacokinetics

■ **Absorption** Ranitidine is rapidly absorbed from the GI tract following oral administration and from parenteral sites following IM injection; however, following oral administration, the drug undergoes extensive first-pass metabolism. (See Pharmacokinetics: Elimination.) The absolute bioavailability of orally administered ranitidine has been reported to be about 50%, and similar oral bioavailability of the drug has been reported in children 3.5–16 years of age. The manufacturer states that the average bioavailability of orally administered ranitidine is about 48% in pediatric patients. The oral solution and effervescent tablets of ranitidine hydrochloride have been shown to be bioequivalent to conventional tablets of the drug. Following oral administration, area under the plasma concentration-time curve may be substantially increased in geriatric individuals compared with younger adults. Following IM administration, the absolute bioavailability of ranitidine is 90–100%. Following oral administration of 150-mg doses of ranitidine hydrochloride, mean peak serum ranitidine concentrations of 372–545 ng/mL occur within 2–3 hours and may be positively correlated with age in adults. Following oral administration of ranitidine 150 mg twice daily in geriatric patients, average peak plasma concentrations of 526 ng/mL occur in about 3 hours. Following oral administration of single doses of the drug in one study, peak serum concentrations were biphasic in some individuals with an initial peak occurring at 0.5–1.5 hours after administration and a second peak occurring about 3 hours after administration. Following IM administration of a single 50-mg dose of ranitidine hydrochloride, mean peak serum ranitidine concentrations of 576 ng/mL occur within 15 minutes.

Absorption and mean peak plasma concentration of ranitidine are not substantially decreased by concomitant administration of food or low-potency antacids (neutralizing capacity of 10–15 mEq of hydrochloric acid per 10 mL); however, concomitant administration of higher potency antacids may decrease absorption of ranitidine. (See Drug Interactions: Food and Antacids.) Concomitant administration of propantheline appears to increase peak serum concentrations of ranitidine. (See Drug Interactions: Propantheline Bromide.)

The manufacturers state that serum ranitidine concentrations necessary to inhibit 50% of pentagastrin-stimulated gastric acid secretion (IC_{50}) are estimated to be 36–94 ng/mL. However, the manufacturers state that a consistent relationship between serum ranitidine concentrations and a given dose or given therapeutic effect of acid inhibition does not appear to exist. Following administration of a single 150-mg oral or 50-mg IM or IV dose, serum ranitidine concentrations remain in the IC_{50} range for up to 12 hours and 6–8 hours, respectively. Following chronic oral administration of 150 mg of ranitidine twice daily, trough serum concentrations range between 53–57 ng/mL. In one study following intraduodenal administration of ranitidine in individuals with duodenal ulcers, the IC_{50} of the drug was estimated to be 100 ng/mL. Substantial inhibition of gastric acid secretion reportedly continues for about 9.5 hours after ingestion of a single 150-mg dose of the drug.

Following oral administration of a single 1- to 2-mg/kg dose of ranitidine as tablets in children 3.5–16 years of age with gastric or duodenal ulcer, peak plasma ranitidine concentrations of 54–492 ng/mL were achieved in 2 hours.

Following administration of a single 2-mg/kg dose of ranitidine as the oral solution in otherwise healthy children 8 months to 14 years of age who required ranitidine therapy, peak plasma ranitidine concentrations of 244 ng/mL were achieved in 1.61 hours. Peak plasma concentrations of 320 ng/mL were achieved in 1.7 hours in these children following multiple dosing with 2 mg/kg. The manufacturer states that a serum ranitidine concentration of 40–60 ng/mL has been reported to be required for at least 90% suppression of basal acid secretion in pediatric patients with duodenal or gastric ulcers. In pediatric patients, oral ranitidine dosages of 6–10 mg/kg daily (given in 2 or 3 divided doses) maintain the gastric pH above 4 throughout most of the dosing interval.

■ **Distribution** Ranitidine is widely distributed throughout the body and is 10–19% protein bound. The apparent volume of distribution of ranitidine is reported to be 1.7 (1.2–1.9) L/kg. The apparent volume of distribution in children 3.5–16 years of age is reported to be 2.3–2.5 L/kg (range: 1.1–3.7 L/kg).

Following oral administration, ranitidine is distributed into CSF. In one study in patients undergoing diagnostic lumbar puncture, CSF concentrations of 0.01–0.04 mcg/mL were achieved 2–6 hours after a dose following 6 days of oral ranitidine 150 mg twice daily. In individuals with uninflamed meninges, CSF ranitidine concentrations are reported to be approximately 3–5% of concurrent peak serum concentrations.

Ranitidine is distributed into milk; concentrations in milk reportedly range from 25–100% of concurrent serum concentrations.

■ **Elimination** The elimination half-life of ranitidine in adults averages 1.7–3.2 hours and may be positively correlated with age in adults. The elimination half-life is prolonged in patients with renal impairment. In one study following oral administration of a single 150-mg dose of ranitidine in patients with creatinine clearances averaging 27.2 mL/minute, the terminal elimination half-life of ranitidine was 8.7 hours; a correlation between the degree of impairment and the elimination half-life of the drug was not apparent. However, in another study in patients with GFRs (as determined by inulin clearance) ranging from 3–69 mL/minute per 1.73 m^2, ranitidine clearance was shown to correlate with GFR and elimination half-life of ranitidine was correlated with degree of renal impairment. In a study in patients with creatinine clearances of 0.5–34 mL/minute, the elimination half-life ranged from 3–10 hours following IV administration of a single 50-mg dose. The manufacturers state that following oral administration of 150 mg of ranitidine twice daily for 4 weeks in patients with renal impairment, mean serum ranitidine concentrations were higher after 24 hours than the concentration observed 12 hours after the same dosage in patients with normal renal function.

There are no substantial differences in pharmacokinetics for ranitidine in pediatric patients 1 month to 16 years of age and healthy adults when correction is made for body weight; however, plasma clearance is decreased and elimination half-life prolonged in neonates younger than 1 month of age. In pharmacokinetic studies of pediatric patients with peptic ulcer disease receiving a 1.25- or 2.5-mg/kg IV dose of ranitidine, plasma clearance averaged 11.41, 8.96, or 9.89 mL/minute per kg, and the elimination half-life averaged 2.2, 2.1, or 1.7 hours in those younger than 6, 6–12, or older than 12 years of age, respectively; in adults receiving 2.5 mg/kg IV, plasma clearance averaged 8.77 mL/minute per kg and elimination half-life averaged 1.9 hours. Following a 0.13–0.8 mg/kg IV dose of ranitidine in pediatric patients 3.5–16 years of age with peptic ulcer disease, plasma clearance averaged 795 mL/minute per 1.73 m^2, and the elimination half-life averaged 1.8 hours. However, following a 2 mg/kg IV dose of ranitidine in neonatal patients less than 1 month of age receiving ECMO, plasma clearance averaged 4.3 mL/minute per kg and the elimination half-life averaged 6.6 hours. In pediatric patients in an intensive care setting who were 1 day to 12.6 years of age, ranitidine plasma clearance averaged 11.7 mL/minute per kg, and the ranitidine elimination half-life averaged 2.4 hours following a 1-mg/kg IV dose of ranitidine.

In geriatric patients, elimination half-life of ranitidine is prolonged and total clearance is reduced because of a decrease in renal function; although the manufacturer states that the half-life is 3–4 hours in geriatric patients following parenteral or oral administration, the half-life of ranitidine has been reported to be prolonged to about 6 hours in geriatric individuals following oral administration of a 100-mg dose of the drug.

Ranitidine is metabolized in the liver to ranitidine *N*-oxide, desmethyl ranitidine, and ranitidine *S*-oxide. Orally administered ranitidine undergoes extensive metabolism on first pass through the liver. Following oral administration of ranitidine to individuals with cirrhosis, the manufacturers state that there are minor but clinically unimportant alterations in the half-life, distribution, clearance, and bioavailability of ranitidine. Peak serum ranitidine concentrations in patients with cirrhosis appear to be higher than those in healthy individuals because of reduced first-pass metabolism of the drug and resultant increased bioavailability; bioavailability of ranitidine appears to average 70% following oral administration in patients with cirrhosis.

Ranitidine is excreted principally in urine via glomerular filtration and tubular secretion. The majority of urinary excretion of ranitidine occurs within the first 6 hours after administration. The portion of an orally administered dose that is excreted unchanged in urine is dose dependent; however, approximately 16–36% of an orally administered dose is excreted unchanged in urine within 24 hours. Approximately 4, 1–2, and 1% are excreted in urine as ranitidine *N*-oxide, desmethyl ranitidine, and ranitidine*S*-oxide, respectively, within 24 hours. The remainder of the administered dose is eliminated in feces, apparently via biliary excretion. Approximately 70% of an IV dose of ranitidine is excreted in urine as unchanged drug.

Renal clearance of ranitidine in healthy individuals is reported to average 410–530 mL/minute. In one study following oral administration of 100-mg doses of ranitidine in healthy adults, plasma, renal, and hepatic clearances of the drug were reported to be 20.8, 5.6, and 16.4 mL/minute per kg, respectively. Plasma clearance of ranitidine appears to be decreased in patients with renal dysfunction. In one study following IV administration of a single 50-mg dose of the drug in patients with creatinine clearances of 0.5–34 mL/minute, plasma clearance of the drug correlated with creatinine clearance and ranged from 1.7–10.9 mL/minute per kg. Plasma clearance appears to be reduced in geriatric patients and in patients with cirrhosis.

Ranitidine is removed by hemodialysis. The amount of ranitidine removed during hemodialysis depends on several factors (e.g., type of coil used, dialysis flow rate); however, preliminary evidence indicates that a single 6-hour period of hemodialysis removes about 10% of a 120-mg dose of ranitidine into the dialysate.

Chemistry and Stability

■ **Chemistry** Ranitidine is a histamine H_2-receptor antagonist. Unlike the earlier histamine H_2-receptor antagonists, burimamide and metiamide, which are not commercially available, and cimetidine, ranitidine contains an aminoalkyl-substituted furan ring rather than an imidazole ring.

Ranitidine hydrochloride has solubilities of 660 mg/mL in water and 190 mg/mL in alcohol. The drug has pK_as of 8.2 and 2.7. Ranitidine hydrochloride occurs as a white to pale yellow granular substance having a slightly bitter taste and sulfur-like odor.

Ranitidine hydrochloride is commercially available for oral administration as conventional and effervescent tablets, capsules, and solution. Each effervescent tabletcontaining 25 or 150 mg of ranitidine provides 1.33 or 7.96 mEq of sodium, respectively.

Ranitidine hydrochloride injection is a clear, colorless to yellow, sterile solution of the drug in water for injection. Ranitidine hydrochloride injection and the commercially available injection of the drug in 0.45% sodium chloride have a pH of 6.7–7.3. The latter preparation has a calculated osmolarity of approximately 180 mOsm/L. Each 50 mL of the commercially available IV infusion solution in 0.45% sodium chloride provides 5.1 mEq of sodium.

Potency of ranitidine hydrochloride preparations and dosage of the drug generally are expressed in terms of the base. Each 168 mg of ranitidine hydrochloride is approximately equivalent to 150 mg of ranitidine.

■ **Stability** Ranitidine hydrochloride 150 and 300 mg tablets should be stored at 15–30°C in tight, light-resistant containers in a dry place; the cap should be replaced securely each time the container is opened. Ranitidine hydrochloride tablets for *self-medication* should be stored at 20–25°C. The oral solution should be stored in a tight, light-resistant container at 4–25°C. USP states that the oral solution should be stored below 25°C and freezing should be avoided. The individually foil-packaged effervescent tablets should be stored at 2–30°C. Ranitidine hydrochloride injection should be stored at a temperature of 4–25°C and protected from light but may be exposed to temperatures up to 30°C. Commercially available ranitidine injection in 0.45% sodium chloride should be stored at 2–25°C and protected from light. Brief exposure to temperatures up to 40°C will not adversely affect stability of the injections, but freezing should be avoided; in addition, darkening of the undiluted injection will not affect potency.

Ranitidine hydrochloride injection is stable for up to 48 hours at room temperature when added to or diluted with most IV solutions (e.g., 0.9% sodium chloride, 5 or 10% dextrose, lactated Ringer's, 5% sodium bicarbonate). The commercially available IV infusion solution of the drug in 0.45% sodium chloride is provided in containers fabricated from a specially formulated, nonplasticized, thermoplastic copolyester (CR3). Water can permeate from inside the container into the overwrap in amounts insufficient to substantially affect the solution. Solutions in contact with the plastic can leach out some of its chemical components in very small amounts within the expiration period of the injection; however, safety of the plastic has been confirmed in tests in animals according to USP biological tests for plastic containers. Additives should not be introduced into the injection container of the commercially available diluted solution of the drug. The commercially available IV infusion solution of the drug in 0.45% sodium chloride is stable through the expiration date noted on the container when stored as recommended. When the pharmacy bulk package is used, infusion solutions of ranitidine hydrochloride should be prepared within 24 hours after the vial is first entered; any drug remaining in the bulk package after this period should be discarded.

Preparations

Excipients in commercially available drug preparations may have clinically important effects in some individuals; consult specific product labeling for details.

raNITIdine Hydrochloride

Oral		
Capsules, liquid-filled	150 mg (of ranitidine)	**raNITIdine Hydrochloride Capsules**
	300 mg (of ranitidine)	**raNITIdine Hydrochloride Capsules**
Solution	75 mg (of ranitidine) per 5 mL	**Zantac® Syrup,** GlaxoSmithKline

Tablets, film-coated	75 mg (of ranitidine)*	**raNITIdine Hydrochloride Tablets**
		Zantac® 75, Pfizer
	150 mg (of ranitidine)*	**raNITIdine Hydrochloride film-coated Tablets**
		Zantac®, GlaxoSmithKline
		Zantac® 150 Maximum Strength, GlaxoSmithKline
	300 mg (of ranitidine)*	**raNITIdine Hydrochloride film-coated Tablets**
		Zantac®, GlaxoSmithKline
Tablets, for solution	25 mg (of ranitidine)	**Zantac® EFFERdose® Tablets,** GlaxoSmithKline
	150 mg (of ranitidine)	**Zantac® EFFERdose® Tablets,** GlaxoSmithKline
Parenteral		
Injection	25 mg (of ranitidine) per mL	**raNITIdine Injection,** Bedford
		Zantac®, GlaxoSmithKline
Injection, for preparation of IV admixtures	25 mg (of ranitidine) per mL (1 g) pharmacy bulk package	**Zantac®,** GlaxoSmithKline

*available from one or more manufacturer, distributor, and/or repackager by generic (nonproprietary) name

raNITIdine Hydrochloride in Sodium Chloride

Parenteral		
Injection	1 mg (of ranitidine) per mL (50 mg) in 0.45% Sodium Chloride	**Zantac® Premixed** (in flexible plastic container), GlaxoSmithKline

†Use is not currently included in the labeling approved by the US Food and Drug Administration

Selected Revisions January 2009, © Copyright, April 1984, American Society of Health-System Pharmacists, Inc.

PROTON-PUMP INHIBITORS 56:28.36

Dexlansoprazole

■ Dexlansoprazole, commonly referred to as an acid- or proton-pump inhibitor, is a gastric antisecretory agent. Dexlansoprazole is the *R*-isomer of lansoprazole.

Uses

■ **Gastroesophageal Reflux** Dexlansoprazole is used for short-term (up to 8 weeks) treatment of all grades of erosive esophagitis, as maintenance therapy (for up to 6 months) following healing of erosive esophagitis to reduce recurrence of the disease, and for short-term (up to 4 weeks) management of symptoms (e.g., heartburn) of gastroesophageal reflux disease (GERD) in patients without erosive esophagitis.

Suppression of gastric acid secretion is considered by the American College of Gastroenterology (ACG) to be the mainstay of treatment for GERD, and a proton-pump inhibitor or histamine H_2-receptor antagonist is used to achieve acid suppression, control symptoms, and prevent complications of the disease. Because GERD is a chronic condition, the ACG states that continuous therapy to control symptoms and prevent complications is appropriate, and chronic, even lifelong, use of a proton-pump inhibitor is effective and appropriate as maintenance therapy in many patients with GERD. The ACG states that proton-pump inhibitors are more effective (i.e., provide more frequent and more rapid symptomatic relief and healing of esophagitis) than histamine H_2-receptor antagonists in the treatment of GERD. Proton-pump inhibitors also provide greater control of acid reflux than do prokinetic agents (e.g., cisapride [no longer commercially available in the US], metoclopramide) without the risk of severe adverse effects associated with these agents.

Efficacy of dexlansoprazole in the treatment of endoscopically diagnosed erosive esophagitis was established in 2 controlled studies in patients receiving dexlansoprazole 60 or 90 mg daily or lansoprazole 30 mg daily for 8 weeks. Healing rates at 4 weeks were similar for dexlansoprazole 60 mg daily and lansoprazole 30 mg daily (66–70 and 65%, respectively). Findings of one study showed higher rates of healing (85 versus 79%) for dexlansoprazole 60 mg daily versus lansoprazole 30 mg daily at 8 weeks; however, in the other study, healing rates at 8 weeks for these 2 regimens did not differ significantly (87 versus 85%, respectively). No additional benefit of the 90-mg dosage over the 60-mg dosage of dexlansoprazole was reported.

Efficacy of dexlansoprazole as maintenance therapy following healing of erosive esophagitis was established in a controlled study in patients with endoscopically confirmed healing of erosive esophagitis who received dexlansoprazole 30 or 60 mg daily or placebo for 6 months. Healing was maintained in 66% of patients receiving dexlansoprazole 30 mg daily compared with 14% of patients receiving placebo. In addition, patients receiving dexlansoprazole 30 mg daily reported a higher percentage of heartburn-free 24-hour periods over 6 months of maintenance therapy than did patients receiving placebo. Most patients receiving placebo discontinued such treatment between months 2 and 6 because of recurrent erosive esophagitis. No additional clinical benefit of the 60-mg dosage over the 30-mg dosage was reported.

Efficacy in patients with symptomatic nonerosive GERD was established in a controlled study in patients with a 6-month or longer history of heartburn episodes, no endoscopic evidence of erosive esophagitis, and heartburn for at least 4 of the 7 days immediately prior to randomization; patients received dexlansoprazole 30 or 60 mg daily or placebo for 4 weeks. The median percentage of days (24-hour periods) without heartburn was 55 or 19% during 4 weeks of therapy with dexlansoprazole or placebo, respectively; no additional benefit of the 60-mg dosage over the 30-mg dosage was reported.

For further information on the treatment of GERD, see Uses: Gastroesophageal Reflux, in Omeprazole 56:28.36.

■ **Crohn's Disease-associated Ulcers** Although evidence currently is limited, proton-pump inhibitors have been used for gastric acid-suppressive therapy as an adjunct in the symptomatic treatment of upper GI Crohn's disease†, including esophageal, gastroduodenal, and jejunoileal disease. Most evidence of efficacy to date has been from case studies in patients with Crohn's-associated peptic ulcer disease unresponsive to other therapies (e.g., histamine H_2-receptor antagonists, cytoprotective agents, antacids, and/or sucralfate). (See Uses: Crohn's Disease-associated Ulcers in Omeprazole 56:28.36.)

For further information on the management of Crohn's disease, see Uses: Crohn's Disease, in Mesalamine 56:36.

Dosage and Administration

■ **Administration** Dexlansoprazole is administered orally once daily. The drug may be taken without regard to food; however, because the effect on gastric pH during the initial 4 hours after a dose may be decreased slightly when dexlansoprazole is taken after a meal, patients with postprandial symptoms that do not respond adequately to postprandial administration may benefit from preprandial administration of the drug. Dexlansoprazole capsules should be swallowed whole; alternatively, the contents of a capsule may be sprinkled on a tablespoonful of applesauce and swallowed immediately without chewing.

Dispensing and Administration Precautions Dispensing errors have occurred because of similarity in spelling between Kapidex® (the former trade name for dexlansoprazole) and Casodex® (the trade name for bicalutamide, a nonsteroidal antiandrogenic antineoplastic agent) or Kadian® (a trade name for an extended-release capsule preparation of morphine sulfate, an opiate agonist analgesic). Therefore, in April 2010, the manufacturer of Kapidex® changed the trade name for dexlansoprazole from Kapidex® to Dexilant® to avoid future dispensing errors. (See Dispensing and Administration Precautions under Cautions: Warnings/Precautions.)

■ **Dosage** ***Gastroesophageal Reflux*** For short-term treatment of erosive esophagitis, the recommended adult dosage of dexlansoprazole is 60 mg once daily for up to 8 weeks. For maintenance therapy following healing of erosive esophagitis, the recommended adult dosage of dexlansoprazole is 30 mg once daily for up to 6 months. The manufacturer states that controlled studies of dexlansoprazole maintenance therapy beyond 6 months have not been performed. For short-term management of symptomatic gastroesophageal reflux disease (GERD) in patients without erosive esophagitis, the recommended adult dosage of dexlansoprazole is 30 mg once daily for 4 weeks. However, the American College of Gastroenterology (ACG) states that chronic, even lifelong, therapy with a proton-pump inhibitor is appropriate in many patients with GERD.

■ **Special Populations** No adjustment of dexlansoprazole dosage is necessary in geriatric patients, patients with renal impairment, or patients with mild hepatic impairment (Child-Pugh class A). The manufacturer states that a maximum dosage of 30 mg daily should be considered in patients with moderate hepatic impairment (Child-Pugh class B). The drug has not been studied in patients with severe hepatic impairment (Child-Pugh class C).

Cautions

■ **Contraindications** Known hypersensitivity to dexlansoprazole or any ingredient in the formulation.

■ **Warnings/Precautions** ***Sensitivity Reactions*** **Hypersensitivity Reactions.** Hypersensitivity reactions (e.g., anaphylaxis, toxic epidermal necrolysis, Stevens-Johnson syndrome) have been reported with dexlansoprazole.

Gastric Malignancy Symptomatic response to therapy with dexlansoprazole does not preclude the presence of gastric malignancy.

Clostridium difficile Infection Available data suggest a possible association between use of proton-pump inhibitors and risk of *Clostridium difficile* infection, including *C. difficile*-associated diarrhea and colitis (CDAD; also known as antibiotic-associated diarrhea and colitis or pseudomembranous colitis). In most observational studies to date, the risk of *C. difficile* infection in patients exposed to proton-pump inhibitors has ranged from 1.4–2.75 times that in patients not exposed to proton-pump inhibitors; however, some observational studies have found no increase in risk. Although many of the cases occurred in patients who had other risk factors for CDAD, including advanced age, comorbid conditions, and/or use of broad-spectrum anti-infectives, the US Food and Drug Administration (FDA) concluded that a contributory role for proton-pump inhibitors could not be definitively ruled out. The mechanism by which proton-pump inhibitors might increase the risk of CDAD has not been elucidated. Although it has been suggested that reduction of gastric acidity by gastric antisecretory agents might facilitate colonization with *C. difficile*, some studies have raised questions about this proposed mechanism or have suggested that the observed association is the result of confounding with other risk factors for CDAD. FDA also is reviewing the risk of CDAD in patients exposed to histamine H_2-receptor antagonists.

CDAD can be serious in patients who have one or more risk factors for *C. difficile* infection and are receiving concomitant therapy with a proton-pump inhibitor; colectomy and, rarely, death have been reported. FDA recommends that patients receive proton-pump inhibitors at the lowest effective dosage and for the shortest possible time appropriate for their clinical condition. Patients experiencing persistent diarrhea should be evaluated for CDAD and should be managed with appropriate supportive therapy (e.g., fluid and electrolyte management), anti-infective therapy directed against *C. difficile* (e.g., metronidazole, vancomycin), and surgical evaluation as clinically indicated.

Musculoskeletal Effects Findings from several observational studies suggest that therapy with proton-pump inhibitors, particularly in high dosages (i.e., multiple daily doses) and/or for prolonged periods of time (i.e., one year or longer), may be associated with an increased risk of osteoporosis-related fractures of the hip, wrist, or spine. The magnitude of risk is unclear; causality has not been established. (See Cautions: Musculoskeletal Effects, in Omeprazole 56:28.36.) FDA is continuing to evaluate this safety concern. Although controlled studies are required to confirm these findings, patients should receive proton-pump inhibitors at the lowest effective dosage and for the shortest possible time appropriate for their clinical condition. Individuals who are at risk for osteoporosis-related fractures should receive an adequate intake of calcium and vitamin D and should have their bone health assessed and managed according to current standards of care.

Hypomagnesemia Hypomagnesemia, symptomatic and asymptomatic, has been reported rarely in patients receiving long-term therapy (for at least 3 months or, in most cases, for longer than one year) with proton-pump inhibitors, including dexlansoprazole. Clinically serious adverse effects associated with hypomagnesemia, which are similar to manifestations of hypocalcemia, include tetany, seizures, tremors, carpopedal spasm, arrhythmias (e.g., atrial fibrillation, supraventricular tachycardia), and abnormal QT interval. Other reported adverse effects include paresthesia, muscle weakness, muscle cramps, lethargy, fatigue, and unsteadiness. In most patients, treatment of hypomagnesemia required magnesium replacement and discontinuance of the proton-pump inhibitor. Following discontinuance of the proton-pump inhibitor, hypomagnesemia resolved within a median of one week; upon rechallenge, hypomagnesemia recurred within a median of 2 weeks.

In patients expected to receive long-term therapy with a proton-pump inhibitor or in those receiving a proton-pump inhibitor concomitantly with digoxin or drugs that may cause hypomagnesemia (e.g., diuretics), clinicians should consider measurement of serum magnesium concentrations prior to initiation of prescription proton-pump inhibitor therapy and periodically thereafter. (See Cautions: Hypomagnesemia and also Cautions: Precautions and Contraindications, in Omeprazole 56:28.36.)

Respiratory Effects Administration of proton-pump inhibitors has been associated with an increased risk for developing certain infections (e.g., community-acquired pneumonia). For further precautionary information about this adverse effect, see Community-acquired Pneumonia under Cautions: Respiratory Effects, in Omeprazole 56:28.36.

Dispensing and Administration Precautions Because of similarity in spelling between Kapidex® (the former trade name for dexlansoprazole) and Casodex® (the trade name for bicalutamide, a nonsteroidal antiandrogenic antineoplastic agent) or Kadian® (a trade name for morphine sulfate, an opiate agonist), dispensing errors have been reported. Therefore, in April 2010, the manufacturer of Kapidex® changed the trade name for dexlansoprazole from Kapidex® to Dexilant® to avoid future dispensing errors. The potential exists for serious adverse effects to occur if patients receive the incorrect drug. Bicalutamide may cause fetal harm if used during pregnancy, and use of this drug is contraindicated in women. Kadian® is an extended-release morphine sulfate preparation intended for use in managing moderate to severe pain when a continuous around-the-clock opiate analgesic is needed for an extended period of time; ingestion of 100- or 200-mg Kadian® capsules by patients who are not opiate tolerant can cause fatal respiratory depression. In addition, there is a potential for the trade name Kapidex® to be confused with Capadex® (a trade name for a fixed-combination preparation containing propoxyphene and acetaminophen that is available via the Internet and marketed in certain other countries [e.g., Australia]). Some experts recommend that pharmacists assess measures of avoiding dispensing errors and implement them as appropriate (e.g., by using computerized name alerts, matching the prescribed drug with the patient's medical history, verifying orders for these drugs) and that clinicians consider including the intended use of the drug on the prescription.

Specific Populations **Pregnancy.** Category B. (See Users Guide.)

Lactation. It is unknown whether dexlansoprazole is distributed into milk. However, lansoprazole and its metabolites are distributed into milk in rats; the manufacturer states that a decision should be made whether to discontinue nursing or the drug, taking into account the importance of the drug to the woman.

Pediatric Use. Safety and efficacy have not been established in pediatric patients younger than 18 years of age.

Geriatric Use. No substantial differences in safety and efficacy relative to younger adults, but increased sensitivity of some older patients cannot be ruled out.

Hepatic Impairment. Systemic exposure to dexlansoprazole is increased approximately twofold in individuals with moderate hepatic impairment. The drug has not been studied in severe hepatic impairment. (See Dosage and Administration: Special Populations.)

Renal Impairment. Because dexlansoprazole is extensively metabolized in the liver to inactive metabolites, and unchanged drug is not recovered in urine following administration of an oral dose, renal impairment is not expected to affect the pharmacokinetics of the drug.

■ **Common Adverse Effects** Adverse effects reported in 2% or more of patients receiving dexlansoprazole and more frequently than with placebo include diarrhea, abdominal pain, nausea, upper respiratory infection, vomiting, and flatulence.

Drug Interactions

■ **Drugs Affecting or Metabolized by Hepatic Microsomal Enzymes** Dexlansoprazole is metabolized by cytochrome P-450 (CYP) isoenzymes 2C19 and 3A4. In vitro studies indicate that dexlansoprazole is unlikely to inhibit CYP isoenzymes 1A1, 1A2, 2A6, 2B6, 2C8, 2C9, 2C19, 2D6, 2E1, or 3A4; therefore, interactions with drugs metabolized by these isoenzymes are considered unlikely. Dexlansoprazole did not alter the pharmacokinetics of diazepam (a CYP2C19 substrate) in healthy individuals (mainly extensive or intermediate metabolizers of CYP2C19 substrates), nor did dexlansoprazole alter the pharmacokinetics of phenytoin (a CYP2C9 substrate) or theophylline (a CYP1A2 substrate) in healthy individuals; CYP1A2 genotypes were not determined.

■ **Drugs that Cause Hypomagnesemia** Potential pharmacologic interaction (possible increased risk of hypomagnesemia). In patients receiving diuretics (i.e., loop or thiazide diuretics) or other drugs that may cause hypomagnesemia, monitoring of magnesium concentrations should be considered prior to initiation of prescription proton-pump inhibitor therapy and periodically thereafter. (See Hypomagnesemia under Warnings/Precautions: General Precautions, in Cautions.)

■ **Gastric pH-dependent Drugs** Pharmacokinetic interaction is possible when dexlansoprazole is used concomitantly with gastric pH-dependent drugs (e.g., ketoconazole, iron salts, digoxin, ampicillin esters); altered absorption at increased gastric pH values.

■ **Antiretroviral Agents** ***Atazanavir*** Potential pharmacokinetic interaction with atazanavir (possible altered oral absorption of atazanavir at increased gastric pH, resulting in decreased plasma atazanavir concentrations). Concomitant use of omeprazole 40 mg once daily and atazanavir (with or without low-dose ritonavir) results in a substantial decrease in plasma concentrations of atazanavir and possible loss of the therapeutic effect of the antiretroviral agent. The manufacturer of dexlansoprazole states that concomitant administration with atazanavir is not recommended. If atazanavir is administered in a treatment-naive patient receiving a proton-pump inhibitor, a *ritonavir-boosted* regimen of 300 mg of atazanavir once daily with ritonavir 100 mg once daily with food is recommended. The dose of the proton-pump inhibitor should be administered approximately 12 hours before *ritonavir-boosted* atazanavir; the dose of the proton-pump inhibitor should not exceed omeprazole 20 mg daily (or equivalent). Concomitant use of proton-pump inhibitors with atazanavir is not recommended in treatment-experienced patients.

Fosamprenavir Concomitant use of esomeprazole with fosamprenavir (with or without ritonavir) did not substantially affect concentrations of amprenavir (active metabolite of fosamprenavir). No dosage adjustment is required when proton-pump inhibitors are used concomitantly with fosamprenavir (with or without ritonavir).

Lopinavir Concomitant use of omeprazole with the fixed combination of lopinavir and ritonavir (lopinavir/ritonavir) did not have a clinically important effect on plasma concentrations or area under the concentration-time curve (AUC) of lopinavir. No dosage adjustment is required when proton-pump inhibitors are used concomitantly with lopinavir/ritonavir.

Raltegravir Pharmacokinetic interaction with omeprazole (substantially increased peak plasma concentration and AUC of raltegravir); however, no dosage adjustment is recommended when proton-pump inhibitors are used concomitantly with raltegravir.

Rilpivirine Pharmacokinetic interaction with omeprazole (decreased plasma concentrations and AUC of rilpivirine). Concomitant use of other proton-pump inhibitors also may result in decreased plasma concentrations of rilpivirine. Concomitant use of rilpivirine and proton-pump inhibitors is contraindicated.

Saquinavir Potential pharmacokinetic interaction (increased peak plasma concentration and AUC of saquinavir). Concomitant use of omeprazole 40 mg once daily and *ritonavir-boosted* saquinavir (saquinavir 1 g twice daily and ritonavir 100 mg twice daily) increased the peak plasma concentration and AUC of saquinavir by 75 and 82%, respectively. Caution is advised if proton-pump inhibitors are used concomitantly with *ritonavir-boosted* saquinavir, and patients should be monitored for saquinavir toxicity.

■ **Clopidogrel** Potential pharmacokinetic interaction (decreased plasma concentration of the active metabolite of clopidogrel) and pharmacodynamic interaction (reduced antiplatelet effects) between proton-pump inhibitors and clopidogrel. Clopidogrel is metabolized to its active metabolite by CYP2C19. Concurrent use of omeprazole or esomeprazole, which inhibit CYP2C19, with clopidogrel reduces exposure to the active metabolite of clopidogrel and decreases platelet inhibitory effects. Although the clinical importance has not been fully elucidated, a reduction in the effectiveness of clopidogrel in preventing cardiovascular events is possible. Proton-pump inhibitors vary in their potency for inhibiting CYP2C19. The change in inhibition of adenosine diphosphate (ADP)-induced platelet aggregation associated with concomitant use of proton-pump inhibitors is related to the change in exposure to the active metabolite of clopidogrel. In pharmacokinetic and pharmacodynamic studies in healthy individuals, concomitant use of dexlansoprazole, lansoprazole, or pantoprazole had less effect on the antiplatelet activity of clopidogrel than did concomitant use of omeprazole or esomeprazole. In individuals who were extensive metabolizers of CYP2C19 substrates, use of dexlansoprazole (60 mg once daily) concomitantly with clopidogrel (75 mg once daily) for 9 days reduced exposure to the active metabolite of clopidogrel by about 9% compared with use of clopidogrel alone. The observed effects of dexlansoprazole on metabolite exposure and clopidogrel-induced platelet inhibition were not considered clinically important, and the manufacturer of dexlansoprazole states that no adjustment of clopidogrel dosage is necessary if clopidogrel is used concomitantly with recommended dosages of dexlansoprazole.

The decision to use a proton-pump inhibitor concomitantly with clopidogrel should be based on the assessed risks and benefits in individual patients. The American College of Cardiology Foundation/American College of Gastroenterology/American Heart Association (ACCF/ACG/AHA) states that the reduction in GI bleeding risk with proton-pump inhibitors is substantial in patients with risk factors for GI bleeding (e.g., advanced age; concomitant use of warfarin, corticosteroids, or nonsteroidal anti-inflammatory agents [NSAIAs]; *H. pylori* infection) and may outweigh any potential reduction in the cardiovascular efficacy of antiplatelet treatment associated with a drug-drug interaction. In contrast, ACCF/ACG/AHA states that patients without such risk factors receive little if any absolute risk reduction from proton-pump inhibitor therapy, and the risk/benefit balance may favor use of antiplatelet therapy without a proton-pump inhibitor in these patients.

If concomitant therapy with a proton-pump inhibitor and clopidogrel is considered necessary, use of an agent with little or no CYP2C19-inhibitory activity should be considered. Alternatively, treatment with a histamine H_2-receptor antagonist (ranitidine, famotidine, nizatidine) may be considered, although such agents may not be as effective as a proton-pump inhibitor in providing gastric protection; cimetidine should *not* be used since it also is a potent CYP2C19 inhibitor. There currently is no evidence that histamine H_2-receptor antagonists (other than cimetidine) or other drugs that reduce gastric acid (e.g., antacids) interfere with the antiplatelet effects of clopidogrel. For further information on interactions between proton-pump inhibitors and clopidogrel, see Drug Interactions: Proton-Pump Inhibitors, in Clopidogrel Bisulfate 20:12.18.

■ **Digoxin** Hypomagnesemia (e.g., resulting from long-term use of proton-pump inhibitors) sensitizes the myocardium to digoxin and, thus, may increase the risk of digoxin-induced cardiotoxic effects. In patients receiving digoxin, monitoring of magnesium concentrations should be considered prior to initiation of prescription proton-pump inhibitor therapy and periodically thereafter.

■ **Methotrexate** Potential pharmacokinetic interaction (increased serum methotrexate concentrations, possibly resulting in toxicity) when proton-pump inhibitors, including dexlansoprazole, are used concomitantly with methotrexate. Increased serum concentrations and delayed clearance of methotrexate and/or its metabolite hydroxymethotrexate, with or without symptoms of methotrexate toxicity, have been reported in patients receiving methotrexate (usually at doses of 300 mg/m^2 to 12 g/m^2) concomitantly with a proton-pump inhibitor. Although most of the reported cases occurred in patients receiving high doses of methotrexate, toxicity also has been reported in patients receiving low dosages of methotrexate (e.g., 15 mg per week) concomitantly with a proton-pump inhibitor. No formal studies of interactions between high-dose methotrexate and proton-pump inhibitors have been conducted to date.

The manufacturer of dexlansoprazole states that temporary discontinuance of proton-pump inhibitor therapy may be considered in some patients receiving high-dose methotrexate therapy. Some clinicians recommend either withholding proton-pump inhibitor therapy for several days before and after methotrexate administration or substituting a histamine H_2-receptor antagonist for the proton-pump inhibitor when acid suppressive therapy is indicated during methotrexate therapy. Pending further evaluation, some clinicians state that these recommendations should extend to patients receiving low-dose methotrexate.

■ **Tacrolimus** Potential pharmacokinetic interaction (increased whole blood concentrations of tacrolimus, particularly in transplant patients who are intermediate or poor metabolizers of CYP2C19 substrates).

■ **Warfarin** When warfarin 25 mg was administered orally on day 6 of an 11-day course of dexlansoprazole 90 mg once daily in healthy individuals, the pharmacokinetics of warfarin and the international normalized ratio (INR) were not altered; however, increased INR and prothrombin time have been reported in patients receiving warfarin concomitantly with proton-pump inhibitors. The INR and prothrombin time may need to be monitored when dexlansoprazole is used concomitantly with warfarin.

Description

Dexlansoprazole, a proton-pump inhibitor, is a gastric antisecretory agent that is structurally and pharmacologically related to esomeprazole, lansoprazole, omeprazole, pantoprazole, and rabeprazole. The drugs are substituted benzimidazoles and are chemically and pharmacologically unrelated to H_2-receptor antagonists or antimuscarinics. Dexlansoprazole is the *R*-isomer of lansoprazole, which is a racemic mixture of *R*- and *S*-isomers. Both isomers inhibit hydrogen-potassium ATPase, but plasma clearance of dexlansoprazole is slower than that of *S*-lansoprazole.

Dexlansoprazole binds to hydrogen-potassium ATPase in gastric parietal cells; inactivation of this enzyme system (also known as the proton, hydrogen, or acid pump) blocks the final step in the secretion of hydrochloric acid by these cells, resulting in potent, long-lasting inhibition of gastric acid secretion.

The commercially available delayed-release capsules of dexlansoprazole contain 2 types of enteric-coated granules of the drug that dissolve at different pH values. Following oral administration of this formulation, an initial (smaller) peak plasma concentration of the drug occurs at 1–2 hours followed by a second (larger) peak concentration at 4–5 hours. Following once-daily administration for 5 days, gastric pH exceeds 4 for 17 hours per day with dexlansoprazole 60 mg versus 14 hours per day with lansoprazole 30 mg. Dexlansoprazole is extensively metabolized in the liver by oxidation, reduction, and subsequent formation of inactive sulfate, glucuronide, and glutathione conjugates. Cytochrome P-450 (CYP) isoenzymes 2C19 and 3A4 are involved in the metabolism of dexlansoprazole. The drug is eliminated in urine (51%) and feces (48%); unchanged drug is not recovered in urine. Because the CYP2C19 isoenzyme is polymorphically expressed, systemic exposure to the drug generally is increased in individuals who are intermediate or poor metabolizers of CYP2C19 substrates. In one small study in Japanese men, systemic exposure (as measured by area under the serum concentration-time curve [AUC]) was increased twofold in intermediate metabolizers and up to 12-fold in poor metabolizers compared with extensive metabolizers.

Increased gastric pH during dexlansoprazole therapy stimulates gastrin secretion via a negative feedback mechanism. Enterochromaffin-like (ECL) cell hyperplasia has been reported during proton-pump inhibitor therapy. Gastric biopsy specimens obtained from 653 patients receiving dexlansoprazole 30–90 mg daily for up to one year revealed no instances of ECL cell hyperplasia. Although rats have demonstrated carcinoid lesions, no adenomatoid, dysplastic, or neoplastic changes have occurred to date in patients receiving long-term proton-pump inhibitor therapy.

Therapy with proton-pump inhibitors, particularly in high dosages and/or for prolonged periods of time, may be associated with an increased risk of osteoporosis-related fractures of the hip, wrist, or spine. (See Cautions: Musculoskeletal Effects.) The mechanism by which these drugs may increase risk of such fractures has not been elucidated but may involve decreased insoluble calcium absorption secondary to increased gastric pH.

Advice to Patients

Necessity of swallowing dexlansoprazole capsules whole or, alternatively, of sprinkling the capsule contents on a tablespoonful of applesauce and swallowing immediately without chewing.

Dexlansoprazole may be administered without regard to food.

Importance of continuing therapy for the entire treatment course, unless directed otherwise.

Importance of advising patients that use of multiple daily doses of the drug for an extended period of time may increase the risk of fractures of the hip, wrist, or spine.

Risk of hypomagnesemia; importance of advising patients to immediately report and seek care for any cardiovascular or neurologic manifestations (e.g., palpitations, dizziness, seizures, tetany).

Possible increased risk of *Clostridium difficile* infection; importance of contacting a clinician if persistent watery stools, abdominal pain, and fever occur.

Importance of informing clinicians of existing or contemplated concomitant therapy, including prescription and OTC drugs and herbal supplements, as well as any concomitant illnesses.

Importance of informing clinicians of any symptoms suggestive of an allergic reaction (e.g., facial swelling, rash).

Importance of women informing clinicians if they are or plan to become pregnant or plan to breast-feed.

Importance of informing patients of other important precautionary information. (See Cautions.)

Overview® (see Users Guide). For additional information on this drug until a more detailed monograph is developed and published, the manufacturer's labeling should be consulted. It is *essential* that the manufacturer's labeling be consulted for more detailed information on usual cautions, precautions, contraindications, potential drug interactions, laboratory test interferences, and acute toxicity.

Preparations

Excipients in commercially available drug preparations may have clinically important effects in some individuals; consult specific product labeling for details.

Dexlansoprazole

Oral		
Capsules, delayed-release (containing enteric-coated granules)	30 mg	**Dexilant®**, Takeda
	60 mg	**Dexilant®**, Takeda

†Use is not currently included in the labeling approved by the US Food and Drug Administration

Esomeprazole Magnesium
Esomeprazole Sodium

■ Esomeprazole, commonly referred to as an acid- or proton-pump inhibitor, is a gastric antisecretory agent. Esomeprazole is the *S*-isomer of omeprazole.

Uses

■ **Gastroesophageal Reflux** Esomeprazole magnesium is used for short-term (4–8 weeks) treatment of diagnostically confirmed erosive esophagitis in patients with gastroesophageal reflux disease (GERD). The drug also is used as maintenance therapy following healing of erosive esophagitis to reduce recurrence of the disease. In addition, esomeprazole is used for short-term (4–8 weeks) treatment of symptoms (e.g., heartburn) of GERD in patients without erosive esophagitis. In infants, esomeprazole is used for short-term (up to 6 weeks) treatment of erosive esophagitis due to acid-mediated GERD. Potential benefits of proton-pump inhibitors in gastroesophageal reflux and esophagitis are thought to result principally from reduced acidity of gastric contents induced by the drugs and resultant reduced irritation of esophageal mucosa; the drugs can effectively relieve symptoms of esophagitis (e.g., heartburn) and promote healing of ulcerative and erosive lesions. Because esomeprazole (*S*-omeprazole) is not eliminated as rapidly as *R*-omeprazole, more drug reaches and blocks the proton pump, providing greater control of intragastric pH than racemic omeprazole.

Suppression of gastric acid secretion is considered by the American College of Gastroenterology (ACG) to be the mainstay of treatment for GERD, and a proton-pump inhibitor or histamine H_2-receptor antagonist is used to achieve acid suppression, control symptoms, and prevent complications of the disease. Because GERD is considered to be a chronic disease, the ACG states that many patients with GERD will require long-term, even lifelong, treatment. The ACG states that proton-pump inhibitors are more effective (i.e., provide more frequent and more rapid symptomatic relief and healing of esophagitis) than histamine H_2-receptor antagonists for treatment of GERD, and are effective and appropriate as maintenance therapy in many patients with the disease. Proton-pump inhibitors also provide greater control of acid reflux than do prokinetic agents (e.g., cisapride [no longer commercially available in the US], metoclopramide) without the risk of severe adverse effects associated with these agents.

Efficacy of esomeprazole in the treatment of endoscopically diagnosed erosive esophagitis was established in 4 controlled studies in patients receiving esomeprazole 20 or 40 mg daily or omeprazole 20 mg daily for 8 weeks. Rates of healing and sustained resolution of heartburn achieved with esomeprazole were similar to or exceeded those achieved with omeprazole.

Efficacy in the long-term maintenance of healing was established in 2 controlled studies in patients with endoscopically confirmed healing of erosive esophagitis receiving esomeprazole 10, 20, or 40 mg daily or placebo for 6 months. Patients receiving esomeprazole remained in remission longer and experienced fewer recurrences than patients receiving placebo; although esomeprazole 10 mg daily provided less benefit than esomeprazole 20 or 40 mg daily, no additional benefit of the 40-mg daily dosage over the 20-mg daily dosage was reported.

Efficacy in patients with symptomatic GERD was established in 2 controlled studies in patients with a 6-month or longer history of heartburn episodes, no endoscopic evidence of erosive esophagitis, and heartburn for at least 4 of the 7 days immediately prior to randomization; patients received esomeprazole 20 or 40 mg daily or placebo for 4 weeks. The percentage of patients who were symptom-free was substantially higher in the group receiving esomeprazole than in the group receiving placebo; no additional benefit of the 40-mg dosage over the 20-mg dosage was reported.

In patients with erosive esophagitis who are unable to take esomeprazole orally, esomeprazole sodium may be used IV for short-term treatment of GERD. In several open-label crossover studies in patients with symptoms of GERD with or without erosive esophagitis, IV administration of esomeprazole 20 or 40 mg as either a 3-minute injection or a 15-minute infusion once daily for 10 days inhibited gastric acid secretion to a similar extent as the corresponding (20 or 40 mg) oral dosage of the drug.

For further information on the treatment of GERD, see Uses: Gastroesophageal Reflux, in Omeprazole 56:28.36.

■ **Duodenal Ulcer** Esomeprazole magnesium is used in combination with amoxicillin and clarithromycin (triple therapy) for short-term (10 days) treatment of patients with *H. pylori* infection and duodenal ulcer disease (active duodenal ulcer or a history of duodenal ulcer within the preceding 5 years).

Efficacy of esomeprazole-based triple therapy for *H. pylori* eradication was established in 2 controlled studies in patients with documented *H. pylori* infection and at least one endoscopically verified duodenal ulcer (or documented history of duodenal ulcer disease in the preceding 5 years). At 4 weeks after treatment, *H. pylori* eradication rates were substantially higher in patients receiving triple therapy (esomeprazole 40 mg once daily, amoxicillin 1 g twice daily, and clarithromycin 500 mg twice daily) for 10 days than in those receiving dual therapy (esomeprazole 40 mg daily and clarithromycin 500 mg twice daily) or monotherapy with esomeprazole 40 mg daily for 10 days.

■ **Prevention of Nonsteroidal Anti-inflammatory Agent-induced Ulcers** Esomeprazole magnesium is used for reducing the occurrence of gastric ulcers associated with chronic nonsteroidal anti-inflammatory agent (NSAIA) therapy in patients at risk for developing these ulcers, including individuals 60 years of age or older and/or those with a documented history of gastric ulcers. Efficacy for this indication was established in two 6-month randomized, controlled studies in patients receiving chronic therapy with either a prototypical NSAIA or a selective cyclooxygenase-2 (COX-2) inhibitor; individuals enrolled in these studies were considered to be at risk for developing NSAIA-associated ulcers because of their age (60 years or older) and/or a history of documented gastric or duodenal ulcer within the previous 5 years, but they had no evidence of gastric or duodenal ulcers on endoscopic examination at the start of the studies. Results of the studies indicated that esomeprazole 20 or 40 mg daily was more effective than placebo in preventing gastric ulcer occurrence during 6 months of treatment; however, no additional benefit was observed with the 40-mg daily dosage compared with the 20-mg daily dosage. In these studies, 94.7–95.4% of patients receiving esomeprazole 20 mg daily, 95.3–96.7% of those receiving esomeprazole 40 mg daily, and 83.3–88.2% of those receiving placebo remained free of gastric ulcers, as determined by serial endoscopic examinations, throughout the 6-month study. The occurrence rate of duodenal ulcers was too low to determine the effect of esomeprazole therapy on duodenal ulcer occurrence.

In 2 other randomized studies, combined therapy with esomeprazole and naproxen was associated with a lower cumulative incidence of gastric ulcer compared with naproxen therapy alone over 6 months of treatment (4.1–7.1 versus 23.1–24.3%). Patients in these studies were randomized to receive either esomeprazole in fixed combination with naproxen (as immediate-release esomeprazole 20 mg and delayed-release naproxen 500 mg twice daily) or delayed-release naproxen (500 mg twice daily) alone. In both studies, patients receiving combined therapy with esomeprazole and naproxen were less likely than patients receiving naproxen alone to discontinue therapy because of adverse upper GI effects, including duodenal ulcers (4 versus 12%). Most patients (83%) in these studies were 50–69 years of age; those younger than 50 years of age were required to have a history of documented gastric or duodenal ulcer within the previous 5 years. About one-fourth of patients also received low-dose aspirin. Efficacy in patients receiving concomitant aspirin therapy was similar to that in the overall study population.

■ **Pathologic GI Hypersecretory Conditions** Esomeprazole magnesium is used for the long-term treatment of pathologic GI hypersecretory conditions. Efficacy for this indication was established in an open-label study in a limited number of patients with previously diagnosed pathologic GI hypersecretory conditions (e.g., Zollinger-Ellison syndrome, idiopathic gastric acid hypersecretion); patients received total daily dosages of esomeprazole ranging from 80 mg–240 mg. The drug generally was well tolerated at these dosages for the duration of the study (12 months). At 12 months of therapy, 90% of patients treated with esomeprazole had controlled basal acid output (BAO) levels, defined as BAO of less than 5 or 10 mEq/hour in patients who had or had not previously undergone gastric acid-reducing surgery, respectively.

■ **Crohn's Disease-associated Ulcers** Although evidence currently is limited, proton-pump inhibitors have been used for gastric acid-suppressive therapy as an adjunct in the symptomatic treatment of upper GI Crohn's disease†, including esophageal, gastroduodenal, and jejunoileal disease. Most evidence of efficacy to date has been from case studies in patients with Crohn's-associated peptic ulcer disease unresponsive to other therapies (e.g., H_2-receptor antagonists, cytoprotective agents, antacids, and/or sucralfate). (See Uses: Crohn's Disease-associated Ulcers in Omeprazole 56:28.36.)

For further information on the management of Crohn's disease, see Uses: Crohn's Disease, in Mesalamine 56:36.

Dosage and Administration

■ **Administration** ***Oral Administration*** Esomeprazole magnesium is administered orally once or twice daily. Because the area under the plasma concentration-time curve (AUC) of a single 40-mg dose of esomeprazole administered after the intake of food is decreased by 43–53%, the manufacturer states that esomeprazole magnesium delayed-release capsules and delayed-release oral suspension should be taken at least 1 hour before a meal. The manufacturer states that tablets containing immediate-release esomeprazole magnesium in fixed combination with delayed-release naproxen should taken at least 30 minutes before a meal.

Esomeprazole Oral Capsules. Esomeprazole magnesium delayed-release capsules should be swallowed whole and the contents should not be crushed or chewed. Alternatively, for patients with difficulty swallowing, the contents of a capsule may be mixed with a tablespoon of applesauce and swallowed immediately. The applesauce should not be hot and should be soft enough to be swallowed without chewing. The applesauce and esomeprazole enteric-coated granule mixture should *not* be stored for future use.

For patients with a nasogastric tube, the contents of a capsule can be mixed with 50 mL of water in a 60-mL catheter-tipped syringe. The syringe should be shaken vigorously for 15 seconds and then held with the tip pointed up and inspected for dissolved or disintegrated granules and granules remaining in the tip. The mixture should not be used if dissolved or disintegrated granules are observed. The mixture should be administered immediately and the tube should be flushed with additional water.

Esomeprazole Oral Suspension. For reconstitution of esomeprazole magnesium for delayed-release oral suspension in single-dose packets, the contents of a 2.5- or 5-mg packet should be mixed thoroughly with 5 mL of water and the contents of a 10-, 20-, or 40-mg packet should be mixed thoroughly with 15 mL of water; the mixture should be allowed to thicken for 2–3 minutes. If a single dose requires 2 packets, the oral suspension may be reconstituted with twice the amount of water needed for 1 packet. Within 30 minutes of preparation, the mixture should be stirred and consumed. If any material remains after the mixture is ingested, additional water should be added, mixed, and ingested immediately.

For patients with a nasogastric or gastric tube, the contents of a 2.5- or 5-mg packet should be mixed with 5 mL of water and the contents of a 10-, 20-, or 40-mg packet should be mixed with 15 mL of water in a catheter-tipped syringe and then shaken immediately. The mixture should be allowed to thicken for 2–3 minutes. The mixture should be administered within 30 minutes of reconstitution; prior to administration, the syringe should be shaken again and the mixture injected into the stomach through the nasogastric or gastric tube (French size 6 or larger). The syringe should be refilled with additional water (5 or 15 mL, respectively), shaken, and used to flush any remaining drug mixture from the nasogastric or gastric tube into the stomach.

Esomeprazole and Naproxen Fixed-combination Tablets. Tablets containing immediate-release esomeprazole magnesium in fixed combination with delayed-release naproxen should be swallowed whole with liquid, and should not be split, chewed, crushed, or dissolved.

IV Administration Esomeprazole sodium is administered by IV injection over no less than 3 minutes or by IV infusion over 10–30 minutes.

For direct IV injection of a 20- or 40-mg dose in adults, esomeprazole sodium powder for injection is reconstituted by adding 5 mL of 0.9% sodium chloride injection to a vial labeled as containing 20 or 40 mg of esomeprazole. A volume of 5 mL of reconstituted solution (20 or 40 mg, respectively) should be withdrawn from the vial and injected over a period of no less than 3 minutes. Reconstituted solutions should be stored at room temperature (up to 30°C) and used within 12 hours of reconstitution. Each vial of esomeprazole sodium is intended for single use only.

For IV infusion of a 20- or 40-mg dose in adults, esomeprazole sodium powder for injection is reconstituted by adding 5 mL of 0.9% sodium chloride injection, lactated Ringer's injection, or 5% dextrose injection to a vial labeled as containing 20 or 40 mg of esomeprazole. The reconstituted solution should be further diluted with 0.9% sodium chloride injection, lactated Ringer's injection, or 5% dextrose injection to a final volume of 50 mL prior to IV infusion over 10–30 minutes. Esomeprazole sodium infusion solutions prepared using 0.9% sodium chloride injection or lactated Ringer's injection should be stored at room temperature (up to 30°C) and used within 12 hours of preparation; infusion solutions prepared using 5% dextrose injection should be stored at room temperature (up to 30°C) and used within 6 hours.

For IV infusion in pediatric patients 1 month to 17 years of age, esomeprazole sodium powder for injection is reconstituted by adding 5 mL of 0.9% sodium chloride injection to a vial labeled as containing 20 or 40 mg of esomeprazole to provide a solution containing 4 or 8 mg/mL, respectively. The reconstituted 4- or 8-mg/mL solution should be further diluted with 0.9% sodium chloride injection to a final volume of 50 mL to yield a final concentration of 0.4 or 0.8 mg/mL, respectively. The appropriate dose of esomeprazole should be withdrawn from the diluted solution and administered as an IV infusion over 10–30 minutes.

Parenteral esomeprazole sodium solutions should be inspected visually for particulate matter and discoloration prior to administration whenever solution and container permit.

The manufacturer states that esomeprazole sodium should not be administered simultaneously through the same IV line with other drugs. The IV line should be flushed with 0.9% sodium chloride injection, lactated Ringer's injection, or 5% dextrose injection before and after esomeprazole administration.

■ Dosage

Dosage of esomeprazole magnesium or esomeprazole sodium is expressed in terms of esomeprazole.

Duration of therapy with a proton-pump inhibitor should be based on safety and efficacy data associated with a specific indication, dosing frequency as described by the manufacturer, and the needs of individual patients. The potential benefits versus possible risks of initiating or continuing proton-pump inhibitor therapy should be weighed carefully.

Adult Dosage **Gastroesophageal Reflux.** The recommended oral dosage of esomeprazole for short-term treatment of erosive esophagitis in adults with GERD is 20 or 40 mg once daily for 4–8 weeks; an additional 4- to 8-week course of treatment may be considered if esophageal healing is incomplete after the first course of treatment. For maintenance therapy following healing of erosive esophagitis, the recommended adult oral dosage of esomeprazole is 20 mg once daily; the manufacturer states that controlled studies of esomeprazole maintenance therapy beyond 6 months have not been performed. The recommended oral dosage for the short-term treatment of symptomatic GERD in adults without erosive esophagitis is 20 mg once daily for 4 weeks; the manufacturer states that an additional 4-week course of therapy may be considered in patients whose symptoms have not completely resolved after the first course of treatment. However, the American College of Gastroenterology (ACG) states that chronic, even lifelong, therapy with a proton-pump inhibitor is appropriate in many patients with GERD.

In adults with erosive esophagitis who are unable to take esomeprazole orally, the usual dosage of IV esomeprazole for treatment of GERD is 20 or 40 mg administered by IV injection (over no less than 3 minutes) or by IV infusion (over 10–30 minutes) once daily; safety and efficacy of IV use beyond 10 days have not been established. Treatment with IV esomeprazole should be discontinued as soon as the patient is able to take the drug orally.

Duodenal Ulcer. When esomeprazole is used in combination with amoxicillin and clarithromycin (triple therapy) for eradication of *H. pylori* infection in patients with duodenal ulcer disease (active duodenal ulcer or a history of duodenal ulcer in the preceding 5 years), the recommended adult oral dosage is 40 mg once daily for 10 days.

Prevention of Nonsteroidal Anti-inflammatory Agent-induced Ulcers. For reducing the risk of nonsteroidal anti-inflammatory agent (NSAIA)-induced gastric ulcer, the usual adult oral dosage of esomeprazole is 20 or 40 mg once daily for up to 6 months; the manufacturer states that controlled studies of esomeprazole therapy in patients considered to be at risk for NSAIA-induced gastric ulcers did not extend beyond 6 months. When esomeprazole is administered in fixed combination with naproxen, the recommended adult dosage of esomeprazole is 20 mg (with naproxen 375 or 500 mg) twice daily. The fixed-combination preparation should not be used in patients requiring a total daily esomeprazole dosage of less than 40 mg.

Pathologic GI Hypersecretory Conditions. The recommended adult oral dosage of esomeprazole for the treatment of pathologic GI hypersecretory conditions (e.g., Zollinger-Ellison syndrome) is 40 mg twice daily. The manufacturer states that the dosage should be adjusted to individual patient needs; dosages up to 240 mg daily for up to 12 months have been administered.

Pediatric Dosage Oral dosage of esomeprazole for short-term (up to 6 weeks) treatment of erosive esophagitis due to acid-mediated GERD in infants 1 month to less than 1 year of age is based on weight. Infants weighing 3–5 kg may receive an oral esomeprazole dosage of 2.5 mg once daily, those weighing more than 5 kg but not more than 7.5 kg may receive 5 mg once daily, and those weighing more than 7.5 kg but not more than 12 kg may receive 10 mg once daily. The manufacturer states that dosages exceeding 1.33 mg/kg daily have not been studied in infants 1 month to less than 1 year of age.

The recommended oral dosage for the short-term treatment of symptomatic GERD in children 1–11 years of age without erosive esophagitis is 10 mg once daily for up to 8 weeks. The recommended oral dosage of esomeprazole for the short-term treatment of erosive esophagitis in children 1–11 years of age weighing less than 20 kg is 10 mg once daily for 8 weeks; 10 or 20 mg once daily for 8 weeks is recommended in children 1–11 years of age weighing 20 kg or more. The manufacturer states that dosages exceeding 1 mg/kg daily have not been studied in children 1–11 years of age.

The recommended oral dosage of esomeprazole for the short-term treatment of GERD in adolescents 12–17 years of age is 20 or 40 mg once daily for up to 8 weeks.

Pediatric patients who are unable to take esomeprazole orally for the treatment of GERD with erosive esophagitis may receive the drug IV. Infants 1 month to less than 1 year of age may receive an IV esomeprazole dosage of 0.5 mg/kg once daily; children and adolescents 1– 17 years of age may receive an IV dosage of 10 mg once daily if they weigh less than 55 kg or 20 mg once daily in they weigh 55 kg or more. Esomeprazole should be administered by IV infusion (over 10–30 minutes) in infants, children, and adolescents. Treatment with IV esomeprazole should be discontinued as soon as the patient is able to take the drug orally.

■ Special Populations

The oral or IV dosage of esomeprazole in patients with severe hepatic impairment (Child-Pugh class C) should *not* exceed 20 mg daily because AUCs of esomeprazole in such patients are 2–3 times greater than those in patients with normal hepatic function. Dosage adjustment is not necessary in patients with mild to moderate (Child-Pugh class A or B) hepatic impairment, patients with renal impairment, or geriatric patients. However, the commercially available tablets containing esomeprazole magnesium in fixed combination with naproxen are not recommended for use in patients with severe hepatic impairment or moderate to severe renal impairment (creatinine clearance less than 30 mL/minute).

Cautions

■ Contraindications

Known hypersensitivity to esomeprazole or other substituted benzimidazoles (e.g., lansoprazole, omeprazole, pantoprazole, rabeprazole) or any ingredient in the formulation.

■ Warnings/Precautions

Sensitivity Reactions **Hypersensitivity Reactions.** Hypersensitivity reactions (e.g., angioedema, anaphylactic shock) have been reported with esomeprazole.

Gastric Malignancy Symptomatic response to therapy with esomeprazole does not preclude the presence of gastric malignancy.

Atrophic Gastritis Atrophic gastritis has been noted occasionally in patients receiving long-term treatment with omeprazole.

Clostridium difficile Infection Available data suggest a possible association between use of proton-pump inhibitors and risk of *Clostridium difficile* infection, including *C. difficile*-associated diarrhea and colitis (CDAD; also known as antibiotic-associated diarrhea and colitis or pseudomembranous colitis). In most observational studies to date, the risk of *C. difficile* infection in patients exposed to proton-pump inhibitors has ranged from 1.4–2.75 times that in patients not exposed to proton-pump inhibitors; however, some observational studies have found no increase in risk. Although many of the cases occurred in patients who had other risk factors for CDAD, including advanced age, comorbid conditions, and/or use of broad-spectrum anti-infectives, the US

Food and Drug Administration (FDA) concluded that a contributory role for proton-pump inhibitors could not be definitively ruled out. The mechanism by which proton-pump inhibitors might increase the risk of CDAD has not been elucidated. Although it has been suggested that reduction of gastric acidity by gastric antisecretory agents might facilitate colonization with *C. difficile*, some studies have raised questions about this proposed mechanism or have suggested that the observed association is the result of confounding with other risk factors for CDAD. FDA also is reviewing the risk of CDAD in patients exposed to histamine H_2-receptor antagonists.

CDAD can be serious in patients who have one or more risk factors for *C. difficile* infection and are receiving concomitant therapy with a proton-pump inhibitor; colectomy and, rarely, death have been reported. FDA recommends that patients receive proton-pump inhibitors at the lowest effective dosage and for the shortest possible time appropriate for their clinical condition. Patients experiencing persistent diarrhea should be evaluated for CDAD and should be managed with appropriate supportive therapy (e.g., fluid and electrolyte management), anti-infective therapy directed against *C. difficile* (e.g., metronidazole, vancomycin), and surgical evaluation as clinically indicated.

Musculoskeletal Effects Findings from several observational studies suggest that therapy with proton-pump inhibitors, particularly in high dosages (i.e., multiple daily doses) and/or for prolonged periods of time (i.e., one year or longer), may be associated with an increased risk of osteoporosis-related fractures of the hip, wrist, or spine. The magnitude of risk is unclear; causality has not been established. (See Cautions: Musculoskeletal Effects, in Omeprazole 56:28.36.) FDA is continuing to evaluate this safety concern. Although controlled studies are required to confirm these findings, patients should receive proton-pump inhibitors at the lowest effective dosage and for the shortest possible time appropriate for their clinical condition. Individuals who are at risk for osteoporosis-related fractures should receive an adequate intake of calcium and vitamin D and should have their bone health assessed and managed according to current standards of care.

Hypomagnesemia Hypomagnesemia, symptomatic and asymptomatic, has been reported rarely in patients receiving long-term therapy (for at least 3 months or, in most cases, for longer than one year) with proton-pump inhibitors, including esomeprazole. Clinically serious adverse effects associated with hypomagnesemia, which are similar to manifestations of hypocalcemia, include tetany, seizures, tremors, carpopedal spasm, arrhythmias (e.g., atrial fibrillation, supraventricular tachycardia), and abnormal QT interval. Other reported adverse effects include paresthesia, muscle weakness, muscle cramps, lethargy, fatigue, and unsteadiness. In most patients, treatment of hypomagnesemia required magnesium replacement and discontinuance of the proton-pump inhibitor. Following discontinuance of the proton-pump inhibitor, hypomagnesemia resolved within a median of one week; upon rechallenge, hypomagnesemia recurred within a median of 2 weeks.

In patients expected to receive long-term therapy with a proton-pump inhibitor or in those receiving a proton-pump inhibitor concomitantly with digoxin or drugs that may cause hypomagnesemia (e.g., diuretics), clinicians should consider measurement of serum magnesium concentrations prior to initiation of prescription proton-pump inhibitor therapy and periodically thereafter. (See Cautions: Hypomagnesemia and also Cautions: Precautions and Contraindications, in Omeprazole 56:28.36.)

Interactions with Diagnostic Tests for Neuroendocrine Tumors Increases in intragastric pH may result in hypergastrinemia, enterochromaffin-like cell hyperplasia, and increased serum chromogranin A (CgA) concentrations. Increased CgA concentrations may produce false-positive results for diagnostic tests for neuroendocrine tumors. Clinicians should temporarily discontinue esomeprazole therapy before assessing CgA concentrations and consider repeating the test if initial CgA concentrations are high.

Cardiac Effects Although preliminary safety data from 2 long-term clinical trials comparing esomeprazole or omeprazole with antireflux surgery in patients with severe gastroesophageal reflux disease (GERD) raised concerns about a potential increased risk of cardiac events (myocardial infarction, heart failure, and sudden death) in patients receiving these drugs, the US Food and Drug Administration (FDA) has reviewed safety data from these and other studies of the drugs and has concluded that long-term use of esomeprazole or omeprazole is not likely to be associated with an increased risk of such cardiac events. FDA has concluded that the apparent increase in cardiac events observed in the early analyses is not a true effect of the drugs and recommends that clinicians continue to prescribe and patients continue to use these drugs in the manner described in the manufacturers' labelings. (See Cautions: Cardiovascular Effects, in Omeprazole 56:28.36.)

Respiratory Effects Administration of proton-pump inhibitors has been associated with an increased risk for developing certain infections (e.g., community-acquired pneumonia). (For further precautionary information about this adverse effect, see Community-acquired Pneumonia under Cautions: Respiratory Effects, in Omeprazole 56:28.36.)

Use of Fixed Combinations When esomeprazole is used in fixed combination with naproxen, the usual cautions, precautions, and contraindications associated with naproxen must be considered in addition to those associated with esomeprazole.

Specific Populations **Pregnancy.** Category B. (See Users Guide.)

Lactation. It is unknown whether esomeprazole is distributed into milk. However, omeprazole is distributed into human milk; discontinue nursing or drug because of potential risk in nursing infants.

Pediatric Use. Safety and efficacy of oral esomeprazole for short-term (4–8 weeks) treatment of GERD in pediatric patients 1–17 years of age are supported by evidence from controlled clinical trials in adults and by safety and pharmacokinetic studies in children and adolescents. Safety and tolerability of oral esomeprazole 5, 10, or 20 mg daily for up to 8 weeks were evaluated in children 1–11 years of age with endoscopically diagnosed GERD; the presence or absence of erosive esophagitis was confirmed endoscopically in this study. Safety and tolerability of oral esomeprazole 20 or 40 mg daily for up to 8 weeks were evaluated in adolescents 12–17 years of age with clinically diagnosed GERD; the presence or absence of erosive esophagitis was not confirmed endoscopically in this study. Adverse effects reported in children and adolescents were similar to those reported during clinical trials in adults; however, a higher incidence of somnolence was reported in children.

Safety and efficacy of oral esomeprazole for short-term (up to 6 weeks) treatment of erosive esophagitis due to acid-mediated GERD in infants 1 month to less than 1 year of age are supported by controlled clinical trials in adults and by safety, pharmacokinetic, and pharmacodynamic studies in pediatric patients. The most commonly reported adverse effects in infants 1–11 months of age receiving oral esomeprazole include irritability and vomiting.

Safety and efficacy of oral esomeprazole for other uses in pediatric patients have not been established. In a randomized, controlled, treatment-withdrawal study in infants 1–11 months of age with symptomatic GERD (diagnosed clinically in most patients), the proportion of patients discontinuing treatment because of worsening symptoms was similar in the esomeprazole and placebo groups.

Safety and efficacy of IV esomeprazole for short-term treatment of GERD with erosive esophagitis in pediatric patients 1 month to 17 years of age are supported by pharmacokinetic studies of IV esomeprazole in pediatric patients and adults and by pharmacodynamic studies of oral esomeprazole in pediatric patients and of IV esomeprazole in adults. Adverse effects of IV esomeprazole in pediatric patients 1 month to 17 years of age were consistent with the known safety profile of the drug.

Safety and efficacy of IV esomeprazole in neonates younger than 1 month of age have not been established.

Geriatric Use. No substantial differences in safety and efficacy relative to younger adults, but increased sensitivity of some older patients cannot be ruled out.

Severe Hepatic Impairment. Use with caution. (See Dosage and Administration: Special Populations.)

■ **Common Adverse Effects** Adverse effects occurring in 1% or more of patients receiving oral esomeprazole include headache, diarrhea, nausea, flatulence, abdominal pain, constipation, and dry mouth. Common adverse effects of IV esomeprazole generally are similar to those reported with oral esomeprazole, although injection site reaction, dizziness/vertigo, and pruritus also occur commonly with IV administration.

Drug Interactions

■ **Drugs Affecting or Metabolized by Hepatic Microsomal Enzymes** Esomeprazole is extensively metabolized by the cytochrome P-450 (CYP) 2C19 isoenzyme and to a lesser extent by CYP3A4. Esomeprazole also may interfere with CYP2C19 activity.

Potential pharmacokinetic interaction with drugs metabolized by CYP2C19 (esomeprazole-induced inhibition of metabolism). Concomitant administration of esomeprazole and diazepam (a CYP2C19 substrate) decreased diazepam clearance by 45%.

Concomitant use of esomeprazole and cilostazol, a substrate of CYP3A4 and CYP2C19, is expected to result in increased concentrations of cilostazol and its active metabolite; therefore, reduction of cilostazol dosage (from 100 mg twice daily to 50 mg twice daily) should be considered during such concomitant use.

Pharmacokinetic interaction with drugs metabolized by CYP isoenzymes 3A4, 1A2, 2A6, 2C9, 2D6, or 2E1 is considered unlikely.

Potential pharmacokinetic interaction (esomeprazole exposure may increase more than twofold) with combined inhibitors of CYP2C19 and CYP3A4 (e.g., voriconazole); dosage adjustment of esomeprazole usually is not required but may be considered in patients receiving high dosages (up to 240 mg daily), such as those with Zollinger-Ellison syndrome.

Potential pharmacokinetic interaction (decreased esomeprazole concentrations) with drugs that induce CYP2C19 and/or CYP3A4 (e.g., St. John's wort [*Hypericum perforatum*], rifampin). Concomitant use of omeprazole, of which esomeprazole is an enantiomer, and St. John's wort (300 mg 3 times daily for 14 days) in healthy men resulted in decreased systemic exposure to omeprazole; peak plasma concentrations and area under the plasma concentration-time curve (AUC) of omeprazole were decreased by 37.5 and 37.9%, respectively, in poor CYP2C19 metabolizers and by 49.6 and 43.9%, respectively, in extensive metabolizers. Concomitant use of esomeprazole with St. John's wort or rifampin should be avoided.

■ **Drugs that Cause Hypomagnesemia** Potential pharmacologic interaction (possible increased risk of hypomagnesemia). In patients receiving diuretics (i.e., loop or thiazide diuretics) or other drugs that may cause hypomagnesemia, monitoring of magnesium concentrations should be considered prior to initiation of prescription proton-pump inhibitor therapy and periodically thereafter. (See Hypomagnesemia under Cautions: Warnings/Precautions.)

■ **Gastric pH-dependent Drugs** Potential pharmacokinetic interaction (altered absorption at increased gastric pH) with gastric pH-dependent drugs (e.g., ketoconazole, iron salts, digoxin, atazanavir, erlotinib).

Concomitant use of omeprazole 20 mg once daily and digoxin in healthy individuals increased digoxin bioavailability by 10% (up to 30% in some individuals). Because esomeprazole is an enantiomer of omeprazole, concomitant use of esomeprazole with digoxin is expected to increase systemic exposure to digoxin; therefore, monitoring for manifestations of digoxin toxicity may be required during such concomitant use.

Absorption of ketoconazole, iron salts, atazanavir, or erlotinib may be decreased in patients receiving esomeprazole concomitantly.

■ **Antiretroviral Agents** ***Atazanavir*** Potential pharmacokinetic interaction (possible altered oral absorption of atazanavir at increased gastric pH, resulting in decreased plasma atazanavir concentrations). Concomitant use of omeprazole 40 mg once daily and atazanavir (with or without low-dose ritonavir) results in a substantial decrease in plasma concentrations of atazanavir and possible loss of the therapeutic effect of the antiretroviral agent or development of drug resistance. Concomitant use of omeprazole 40 mg once daily (administered 2 hours before atazanavir) and atazanavir 400 mg once daily decreased the AUC and peak plasma concentration of atazanavir by 94 and 96%, respectively. The manufacturer of esomeprazole states that concomitant administration with atazanavir is not recommended. If atazanavir is administered in an antiretroviral treatment-naive patient receiving a proton-pump inhibitor, a *ritonavir-boosted* regimen of 300 mg of atazanavir once daily with ritonavir 100 mg once daily with food is recommended. The dose of the proton-pump inhibitor should be administered approximately 12 hours before *ritonavir-boosted* atazanavir; the dose of the proton-pump inhibitor should not exceed omeprazole 20 mg daily (or equivalent). Concomitant use of proton-pump inhibitors with atazanavir is not recommended in antiretroviral treatment-experienced patients.

Fosamprenavir Concomitant use of esomeprazole and fosamprenavir increased the AUC of esomeprazole by about 55% but did not substantially alter plasma concentrations of amprenavir (active metabolite of fosamprenavir). Concomitant use of esomeprazole and *ritonavir-boosted* fosamprenavir did not substantially affect concentrations of either amprenavir or esomeprazole. No dosage adjustment is required when proton-pump inhibitors are used concomitantly with fosamprenavir (with or without ritonavir).

Lopinavir Concomitant use of omeprazole with the fixed combination of lopinavir and ritonavir (lopinavir/ritonavir) did not have a clinically important effect on plasma concentrations or AUC of lopinavir. No dosage adjustment is required when proton-pump inhibitors are used concomitantly with lopinavir/ritonavir.

Nelfinavir Potential pharmacokinetic interaction (decreased plasma nelfinavir concentrations). Concomitant use of omeprazole 40 mg once daily (given 30 minutes before a nelfinavir dose) and nelfinavir 1.25 g twice daily decreased peak plasma concentrations and AUCs of nelfinavir by 37 and 36%, respectively, and of its major active metabolite M8 by 89 and 92%, respectively. The manufacturer of esomeprazole states that concomitant administration with nelfinavir is not recommended.

Raltegravir Pharmacokinetic interaction with omeprazole (substantially increased peak plasma concentration and AUC of raltegravir); however, no dosage adjustment is recommended when proton-pump inhibitors are used concomitantly with raltegravir.

Rilpivirine Pharmacokinetic interaction with omeprazole (decreased plasma concentrations and AUC of rilpivirine). Concomitant use of other proton-pump inhibitors also may result in decreased plasma concentration of rilpivirine. Concomitant use of rilpivirine and proton-pump inhibitors is contraindicated.

Saquinavir Potential pharmacokinetic interaction (increased peak plasma concentration and AUC of saquinavir). Concomitant use of omeprazole 40 mg once daily and *ritonavir-boosted* saquinavir (saquinavir 1 g twice daily and ritonavir 100 mg twice daily) increased the peak plasma concentration and AUC of saquinavir by 75 and 82%, respectively. Caution is advised if proton-pump inhibitors are used concomitantly with *ritonavir-boosted* saquinavir, and patients should be monitored for saquinavir toxicity. The manufacturer of esomeprazole states that dosage reduction of saquinavir may be considered on an individual basis.

■ **Clopidogrel** Potential pharmacokinetic interaction (decreased plasma concentration of the active metabolite of clopidogrel) and pharmacodynamic interaction (reduced antiplatelet effects) between proton-pump inhibitors and clopidogrel. Clopidogrel is metabolized to its active metabolite by CYP2C19. Concurrent use of omeprazole or esomeprazole, which inhibit CYP2C19, with clopidogrel reduces exposure to the active metabolite of clopidogrel and decreases platelet inhibitory effects. Although the clinical importance has not been fully elucidated, a reduction in the effectiveness of clopidogrel in preventing cardiovascular events is possible. Proton-pump inhibitors vary in their potency for inhibiting CYP2C19. The change in inhibition of adenosine diphosphate (ADP)-induced platelet aggregation associated with concomitant use of proton-pump inhibitors is related to the change in exposure to the active metabolite of clopidogrel. In pharmacokinetic and pharmacodynamic studies in healthy individuals, concomitant use of dexlansoprazole, lansoprazole, or pantoprazole had less effect on the antiplatelet activity of clopidogrel than did concomitant use of omeprazole or esomeprazole. In individuals who were extensive metabolizers of CYP2C19 substrates, use of esomeprazole (40 mg once daily) concomitantly with clopidogrel (75 mg once daily) for 9 days reduced exposure to the active metabolite of clopidogrel by about 16% compared with use of clopidogrel alone. The manufacturer of clopidogrel states that concomitant use of esomeprazole and clopidogrel should be avoided.

The decision to use a proton-pump inhibitor concomitantly with clopidogrel should be based on the assessed risks and benefits in individual patients. The American College of Cardiology Foundation/American College of Gastroenterology/American Heart Association (ACCF/ACG/AHA) states that the reduction in GI bleeding risk with proton-pump inhibitors is substantial in patients with risk factors for GI bleeding (e.g., advanced age; concomitant use of warfarin, corticosteroids, or nonsteroidal anti-inflammatory agents [NSAIAs]; *H. pylori* infection) and may outweigh any potential reduction in the cardiovascular efficacy of antiplatelet treatment associated with a drug-drug interaction. In contrast, ACCF/ACG/AHA states that patients without such risk factors receive little if any absolute risk reduction from proton-pump inhibitor therapy, and the risk/benefit balance may favor use of antiplatelet therapy without a proton-pump inhibitor in these patients.

If concomitant therapy with a proton-pump inhibitor and clopidogrel is considered necessary, use of an agent with little or no CYP2C19-inhibitory activity should be considered. Alternatively, treatment with a histamine H_2-receptor antagonist (ranitidine, famotidine, nizatidine) may be considered, although such agents may not be as effective as a proton-pump inhibitor in providing gastric protection; cimetidine should *not* be used since it also is a potent CYP2C19 inhibitor. There currently is no evidence that histamine H_2-receptor antagonists (other than cimetidine) or other drugs that reduce gastric acid (e.g., antacids) interfere with the antiplatelet effects of clopidogrel. For further information on interactions between proton-pump inhibitors and clopidogrel, see Drug Interactions: Proton-Pump Inhibitors, in Clopidogrel Bisulfate 20:12.18.

■ **Digoxin** Hypomagnesemia (e.g., resulting from long-term use of proton-pump inhibitors) sensitizes the myocardium to digoxin and, thus, may increase the risk of digoxin-induced cardiotoxic effects. In patients receiving digoxin, monitoring of magnesium concentrations should be considered prior to initiation of prescription proton-pump inhibitor therapy and periodically thereafter.

■ **Methotrexate** Potential pharmacokinetic interaction (increased serum methotrexate concentrations, possibly resulting in toxicity) when proton-pump inhibitors, including esomeprazole, are used concomitantly with methotrexate. Increased serum concentrations and delayed clearance of methotrexate and/or its metabolite hydroxymethotrexate, with or without symptoms of methotrexate toxicity, have been reported in patients receiving methotrexate (usually at doses of 300 mg/m^2 to 12 g/m^2) concomitantly with a proton-pump inhibitor. Although most of the reported cases occurred in patients receiving high doses of methotrexate, toxicity also has been reported in patients receiving low dosages of methotrexate (e.g., 15 mg per week) concomitantly with a proton-pump inhibitor. No formal studies of interactions between high-dose methotrexate and proton-pump inhibitors have been conducted to date.

The manufacturer of esomeprazole states that temporary discontinuance of proton-pump inhibitor therapy may be considered in some patients receiving high-dose methotrexate therapy. Some clinicians recommend either withholding proton-pump inhibitor therapy for several days before and after methotrexate administration or substituting a histamine H_2-receptor antagonist for the proton-pump inhibitor when acid suppressive therapy is indicated during methotrexate therapy. Pending further evaluation, some clinicians state that these recommendations should extend to patients receiving low-dose methotrexate.

■ **Nonsteroidal Anti-inflammatory Agents** Pharmacokinetic interactions with naproxen or rofecoxib (no longer commercially available in the US) are unlikely.

■ **Sucralfate** In a single-dose study, concomitant administration of omeprazole 20 mg and sucralfate 1 g resulted in delayed absorption of omeprazole and decreased omeprazole bioavailability by 16%. Proton-pump inhibitors should be administered at least 30 minutes before sucralfate.

■ **Tacrolimus** Potential pharmacokinetic interaction (increased serum concentrations of tacrolimus).

■ **Warfarin** Potential increased international normalized ratio (INR) and prothrombin time when warfarin is used concomitantly with proton-pump inhibitors, including esomeprazole. Potential for abnormal bleeding and death; monitor for INR and prothrombin time increases when esomeprazole is used concomitantly with warfarin.

Description

Esomeprazole, a proton-pump inhibitor, is a gastric antisecretory agent that is structurally and pharmacologically related to lansoprazole, omeprazole, pantoprazole, and rabeprazole. The drugs are substituted benzimidazoles and are chemically and pharmacologically unrelated to H_2-receptor antagonists, antimuscarinics, or prostaglandin analogs. Esomeprazole is the *S*-isomer of omeprazole, which is a racemic mixture of *R*- and *S*-isomers.

Esomeprazole binds to hydrogen-potassium ATPase in gastric parietal cells; inactivation of this enzyme system (also known as the proton, hydrogen, or acid pump) blocks the final step in the secretion of hydrochloric acid by these cells, resulting in potent, long-lasting inhibition of gastric acid secretion.

Because the esomeprazole molecule is acid labile, the commercially available delayed-release capsules and packets for delayed-release oral suspension containing enteric-coated granules of the drug increase oral bioavailability. Esomeprazole is extensively metabolized, principally by the hepatic cytochrome P-450 (CYP) 2C19 isoenzyme and to a lesser extent by CYP3A4, to form metabolites lacking antisecretory activity. The CYP2C19 isoenzyme is polymorphically expressed; poor metabolizers (about 3% of Caucasians and 15–20% of Asians) lack the isoenzyme, and the metabolism of esomeprazole and omeprazole is decreased in such individuals compared with the rest of the population (i.e., extensive or rapid metabolizers). However, esomeprazole undergoes less metabolic transformation by CYP2C19 and may exhibit less variation in plasma concentrations between slow and rapid metabolizers than omeprazole. At steady state, the ratio of the area under the plasma concentration-time curve (AUC) of esomeprazole in poor metabolizers to the AUC of the drug in rapid metabolizers is about 2:1.

A proton-pump inhibitor (e.g., esomeprazole, omeprazole) can suppress but not eradicate gastric *Helicobacter pylori* in patients with duodenal ulcer and/or reflux esophagitis infected with the organism. Therapy with esomeprazole in combination with clarithromycin and amoxicillin can effectively eradicate *H. pylori* gastric infection.

Increased gastric pH during esomeprazole therapy stimulates gastrin secretion via a negative feedback mechanism and results in enterochromaffin-like cell (ECL) hyperplasia. Although rats have demonstrated carcinoid lesions, no adenomatoid, dysplastic, or neoplastic changes have occurred to date in patients receiving esomeprazole or other proton-pump inhibitors for up to 1 year.

Therapy with proton-pump inhibitors, particularly in high dosages and/or for prolonged periods of time, may be associated with an increased risk of osteoporosis-related fractures of the hip, wrist, or spine. (See Musculoskeletal Effects under Cautions: Warnings/Precautions.) The mechanism by which these drugs may increase risk of such fractures has not been elucidated but may involve decreased insoluble calcium absorption secondary to increased gastric pH.

Advice to Patients

Importance of taking oral esomeprazole at least 1 hour before a meal.

Necessity of swallowing capsules whole, without crushing or chewing the delayed-release granules. For patients with difficulty swallowing, necessity of mixing capsule contents with cool, soft applesauce and swallowing immediately without chewing. Importance of *not* storing mixture of applesauce and capsule contents for future use.

If using oral suspension, necessity of mixing packet contents with an appropriate amount of water, allowing suspension to thicken for 2–3 minutes, and stirring and drinking mixture within 30 minutes of preparation. Importance of swallowing suspension without crushing or chewing granules.

Antacid administration is permissible during esomeprazole therapy.

Importance of advising patients that use of multiple daily doses of the drug for an extended period of time may increase the risk of fractures of the hip, wrist, or spine.

Risk of hypomagnesemia; importance of advising patients to immediately report and seek care for any cardiovascular or neurologic manifestations (e.g., palpitations, dizziness, seizures, tetany).

Possible increased risk of *Clostridium difficile* infection; importance of contacting a clinician if persistent watery stools, abdominal pain, and fever occur.

Importance of informing clinicians of existing or contemplated concomitant therapy, including prescription and OTC drugs, as well as concomitant illnesses.

Importance of continuing therapy for the entire treatment course, unless directed otherwise.

Importance of women informing clinicians if they are or plan to become pregnant or plan to breast-feed.

Importance of informing patients of other important precautionary information. (See Cautions.)

Overview® (see Users Guide). For additional information until a more detailed monograph is developed and published, the manufacturer's labeling should be consulted. It is *essential* that the manufacturer's labeling be consulted for more detailed information on usual cautions, precautions, contraindications, potential drug interactions, laboratory test interferences, and acute toxicity.

Preparations

Excipients in commercially available drug preparations may have clinically important effects in some individuals; consult specific product labeling for details.

Esomeprazole Magnesium

Oral		
Capsules, delayed-release (containing enteric-coated granules)	20 mg (of esomeprazole)	**NexIUM®**, AstraZeneca
	40 mg (of esomeprazole)	**NexIUM®**, AstraZeneca
For Suspension, delayed-release (containing enteric-coated granules)	2.5 mg (of esomeprazole) per packet	**NexIUM®**, AstraZeneca
	5 mg (of esomeprazole) per packet	**NexIUM®**, AstraZeneca
	10 mg (of esomeprazole) per packet	**NexIUM®**, AstraZeneca
	20 mg (of esomeprazole) per packet	**NexIUM®**, AstraZeneca
	40 mg (of esomeprazole) per packet	**NexIUM®**, AstraZeneca

Esomeprazole Magnesium Combinations

Oral		
Tablets, delayed-release core (naproxen only)	20 mg (of esomeprazole) with Naproxen 375 mg	**Vimovo®**, AstraZeneca
	20 mg (of esomeprazole) with Naproxen 500 mg	**Vimovo®**, AstraZeneca

Esomeprazole Sodium

Parenteral		
For injection, for IV use	20 mg (of esomeprazole)	**NexIUM® IV**, AstraZeneca
	40 mg (of esomeprazole)	**NexIUM® IV**, AstraZeneca

†Use is not currently included in the labeling approved by the US Food and Drug Administration

Selected Revisions December 2012,

Lansoprazole

■ Lansoprazole, commonly referred to as an acid- or proton-pump inhibitor, is a gastric antisecretory agent.

Uses

Lansoprazole is used orally for the short-term treatment and symptomatic relief of active duodenal and benign gastric ulcer and as maintenance therapy following healing of duodenal ulcers. Lansoprazole also is used orally in combination with amoxicillin (dual therapy) or with clarithromycin and amoxicillin (triple therapy) for the treatment of *Helicobacter pylori* infection and duodenal ulcer disease. Lansoprazole also has been used in other multiple-drug regimens† for the treatment of *H. pylori* infection associated with peptic ulcer disease. Lansoprazole also is used orally for the treatment of nonsteroidal anti-inflammatory agent (NSAIA)-induced gastric ulcers in patients who continue NSAIA use, and for the prevention of NSAIA-induced gastric ulcers in patients with a documented history of gastric ulcer who require the use of an NSAIA. Oral lansoprazole also is used for short-term treatment and symptomatic relief of gastroesophageal reflux disease (e.g., erosive esophagitis), as maintenance therapy following healing of erosive esophagitis to reduce its recurrence and in the long-term treatment of pathologic GI hypersecretory conditions. Lansoprazole is used orally as *self-medication* for short-term treatment of frequent heartburn.

■ **Gastroesophageal Reflux** ***Acute Therapy*** Lansoprazole is used orally to provide short-term (up to 8 weeks) treatment and symptomatic relief of all grades of erosive esophagitis in patients with gastroesophageal reflux disease (GERD). Oral lansoprazole also is used for the short-term (up to 8 weeks) treatment of symptomatic GERD (e.g., heartburn). Potential benefits of lansoprazole in gastroesophageal reflux and esophagitis result principally from reduced acidity of gastric contents induced by the drug and resultant reduced irritation of esophageal mucosa; the drug can effectively relieve symptoms of esophagitis (e.g., heartburn) and promote healing of ulcerative and erosive lesions.

Suppression of gastric acid secretion is considered by the American College of Gastroenterology (ACG) to be the mainstay of treatment for GERD, and a proton-pump inhibitor or histamine H_2-receptor antagonist is used to achieve acid suppression, control symptoms, and prevent complications of the disease. The ACG states that proton-pump inhibitors are more effective (i.e., provide more frequent and more rapid symptomatic relief and healing of esophagitis) than histamine H_2-receptor antagonists in the treatment of GERD. Proton-pump inhibitors also provide greater control of acid reflux than do prokinetic agents (e.g., cisapride [no longer commercially available in the US], metoclopramide) without the risk of severe adverse effects associated with these agents.

In a controlled study in patients with manifestations of GERD (e.g., heartburn) and the absence of erosive esophageal lesions, symptomatic improvement (reduction in frequency and severity of heartburn) with lansoprazole was greater than that with placebo. In this study in patients with endoscopically confirmed GERD, the median percentage of days without heartburn was 84,

82, or 13% at week 8 of therapy with lansoprazole 15 mg daily, lansoprazole 30 mg daily, or placebo, respectively; the median percentage of nights without heartburn in these respective treatment groups was 92, 80, or 36% at week 8. Administration of 30 mg of lansoprazole daily did not provide improved relief compared with 15 mg daily in this study.

In controlled studies in patients with endoscopically evaluated GERD, reported rates of healing with lansoprazole were higher than those with placebo or an H_2-receptor antagonist and at least as high as those with omeprazole. Generally, antacids were used concomitantly for pain relief. In a controlled study in patients with esophagitis, reported rates of healing were 91, 95, 94, or 53% at 8 weeks in patients receiving lansoprazole 15 mg daily, 30 mg daily, 60 mg daily, or placebo, respectively. Healing rates from controlled studies were 80–84 or 39–52% at 4 weeks and 91–92 or 53–70% at 8 weeks for lansoprazole 30 mg daily or ranitidine 150 mg twice daily, respectively. Patients receiving lansoprazole reported faster relief of daytime and nocturnal heartburn and self-administered less antacid than those receiving placebo or an H_2-receptor antagonist; however, since the recommended dosage of ranitidine for esophagitis is 150 mg four times daily and patients treated with ranitidine received only 150 mg twice daily, further study is needed to evaluate relative efficacy. Lansoprazole also has been shown to be effective in promoting healing and providing symptomatic relief in a substantial proportion of patients failing to respond to usual or relatively high dosages of H_2-receptor antagonists.

Although lansoprazole has been used IV for short-term (up to 7 days) treatment of erosive esophagitis in patients who are unable to take the drug orally, a parenteral dosage form no longer is commercially available in the US. In one controlled study in patients with erosive esophagitis receiving oral lansoprazole, the degree of inhibition of gastric acid secretion following IV administration of lansoprazole 30 mg daily for 7 days was similar to that achieved following repeated oral administration of the drug.

Short-term lansoprazole therapy for the treatment of erosive esophagitis will not prevent recurrence of the disease following discontinuance of the drug. Most patients with erosive esophagitis respond to lansoprazole during an initial 8-week course of therapy; however, an additional 8 weeks of therapy may contribute to healing and symptomatic improvement in some patients (i.e., patients experiencing a recurrence of erosive esophagitis or patients who fail to heal after the initial course of therapy). If symptomatic GERD or severe esophagitis recur, the manufacturer states that additional 8-week courses of lansoprazole may be given. However, the ACG states that chronic, even lifelong, therapy with a proton-pump inhibitor is appropriate in many patients with GERD.

Maintenance Therapy Lansoprazole is used as maintenance therapy following healing of erosive esophagitis to reduce recurrence of the disease. In a multicenter, double-blind study, endoscopically documented remission of esophagitis was maintained at 6 months in 81, 93, or 27% of patients receiving lansoprazole 15 mg daily, 30 mg daily, or placebo, respectively, and such remission was maintained at 12 months in 79, 90, or 24% of patients, respectively. In another multicenter, double-blind study in patients with endoscopically confirmed healed esophagitis, remission of esophagitis was maintained at 6 months in 72, 72, or 13% of patients receiving lansoprazole 15 mg daily, 30 mg daily, or placebo, respectively, and at 12 months in 67, 55, or 13% of patients, respectively. Remission rates of esophagitis were independent of the patient's initial grade of erosive esophagitis and the daily dosage of lansoprazole (15 or 30 mg).

Because GERD is a chronic condition, the ACG states that continuous therapy to control symptoms and prevent complications is appropriate, and chronic, even lifelong, use of a proton-pump inhibitor is effective and appropriate as maintenance therapy in many patients with GERD. The frequent marked improvement in symptoms associated with full dosage of a proton-pump inhibitor generally is followed by rapid recurrence of symptoms once the drug is discontinued, and reduced-dosage regimens (e.g., every other day, "weekend" dosage) have not been shown to be consistently effective for maintenance therapy.

For further information on the treatment of GERD, see Uses: Gastroesophageal Reflux, in Omeprazole 56:28.36.

Self-medication Lansoprazole is used orally in adults 18 years of age or older as *self-medication* for short-term (14 days) treatment of frequent (2 or more days per week) heartburn. Because 1–4 days may be required for complete relief of symptoms, lansoprazole for *self-medication* is not intended for the immediate relief of heartburn. However, some individuals may experience complete relief of symptoms within 24 hours of taking the first dose of lansoprazole. In 2 controlled studies in adults with frequent (2 or more days per week) heartburn, the percentage of days (24-hour periods) without heartburn during 14 days of treatment was greater with lansoprazole 15 mg daily than with placebo (59.9–64.7 versus 45–45.7%). The percentage of heartburn-free nights during the 14-day treatment period was 79.5–81.6% with lansoprazole therapy compared with 76.3–77% with placebo. On day 1 of treatment, 50.4–50.7% of lansoprazole-treated patients experienced no heartburn compared with 33–37.9% of those receiving placebo. In a controlled study in adults with frequent nocturnal heartburn, the percentage of heartburn-free nights during 14 days of treatment was greater with lansoprazole 15 or 30 mg (61.3–61.7%) compared with placebo (47.8%). The percentage of days (24-hour periods) without heartburn and the percentage of patients without heartburn on day 1 of treatment also were greater with lansoprazole therapy than with placebo.

■ Gastric Ulcer

Acute Therapy Lansoprazole is used for the short-term treatment and symptomatic relief of active benign gastric ulcer. Antacids may be used concomitantly as needed for pain relief. In controlled studies in patients with endoscopically confirmed gastric ulcers, reported rates of ulcer healing for lansoprazole were substantially higher than those for placebo. In a multicenter, double-blind study in patients with endoscopically confirmed gastric ulcer, reported rates of ulcer healing in patients receiving lansoprazole 15 or 30 mg each morning or placebo were 65, 58, or 38%, respectively, at 4 weeks and 92, 97, or 77%, respectively, at 8 weeks. Lansoprazole also produced greater reductions in daytime and nocturnal pain and antacid consumption than did placebo.

Current epidemiologic and clinical evidence supports a strong association between gastric infection with *H. pylori* and the pathogenesis of gastric ulcers, and the ACG, NIH, and most clinicians currently recommend that *all* patients with initial or recurrent gastric ulcer and documented *H. pylori* infection receive anti-infective therapy for treatment of the infection. The choice of a particular regimen should be based on current data on optimal therapy, including consideration of the patient's prior exposure to anti-infective agents, the local prevalence of resistance, patient compliance, and costs of therapy. (See Duodenal Ulcer: Acute Therapy, in Uses.) For a more complete discussion of *H. pylori* infection, including details about the efficacy of various regimens and rationale for drug selection, see Uses: *Helicobacter pylori* Infection, in Clarithromycin 8:12.12.92.

■ NSAIA-induced Ulcers

Treatment Lansoprazole is used for the treatment of NSAIA-induced gastric ulcers in patients who continue NSAIA use. In 2 controlled studies in patients with endoscopically confirmed NSAIA-associated gastric ulcer who continued their NSAIA use, substantially more patients receiving lansoprazole 30 mg daily experienced ulcer healing at 8 weeks compared with those receiving an active control drug. In one study, healing of gastric ulcers occurred in 60 and 79% of patients receiving lansoprazole, compared with 28 and 55% of those receiving an active control drug at 4 and 8 weeks, respectively. In the second study, ulcer healing occurred in 77% of patients receiving lansoprazole or in 50% of those receiving an active control drug at 4 and 8 weeks. However, there was no substantial difference in the number of patients experiencing symptomatic (e.g., abdominal pain) relief between those receiving lansoprazole and those receiving the active control.

For treatment of NSAIA-induced ulcers, it is preferable to discontinue NSAIA therapy and initiate therapy with a drug (e.g., proton-pump inhibitor, histamine H_2-receptor antagonist) indicated for the treatment of ulcers. When NSAIA therapy must be continued, a proton-pump inhibitor is considered the drug of choice for treatment of ulcers since the efficacy of H_2-receptor antagonists is substantially decreased by continued use of NSAIAs. Treatment of *H. pylori* infection is recommended in patients receiving NSAIAs who have ulcers and are infected with this organism. For further information on *H. pylori* infection, including details about the efficacy of various regimens and rationale for drug selection, see Uses: *Helicobacter pylori* Infection, in Clarithromycin 8:12.12.92.

Prevention Lansoprazole is used for the prevention of NSAIA-induced gastric ulcers in patients with a documented history of gastric ulcer who require the use of an NSAIA. In a controlled study in patients with a history of gastric ulcer who required NSAIA therapy, lansoprazole 15 or 30 mg daily was more effective than placebo but less effective than misoprostol 200 mcg 4 times daily in preventing gastric ulcer recurrence at 4, 8, and 12 weeks of therapy. About one-half of the patients also had a history of duodenal ulcer. About 51, 93, 80, or 82% of those receiving placebo, misoprostol, or lansoprazole 15 or 30 mg, respectively, remained free of gastric ulcers at 12 weeks. In a subsequent subset analysis of patients receiving only naproxen or naproxen and aspirin (up to 325 mg daily), lansoprazole 15 or 30 mg daily was more effective than placebo and as effective as misoprostol in preventing gastric ulcer recurrence at 4, 8, and 12 weeks of therapy; about 33, 83, 89, or 83% of those receiving placebo, misoprostol, or lansoprazole 15 or 30 mg, respectively, remained free of gastric ulcers at 12 weeks. Serious NSAIA-related GI complications (e.g., bleeding, perforation, obstruction) were not reported during the study; however, the study was not designed to assess the effect of lansoprazole on the risk of such complications or on the risk of duodenal ulcers.

Serious adverse GI effects (e.g., bleeding, ulceration, perforation) can occur at any time in patients receiving chronic NSAIA therapy, and such effects may *not* be preceded by warning signs or symptoms. Results of studies to date are inconclusive concerning the relative risk of various NSAIAs in causing serious GI effects. In patients receiving prototypical NSAIAs and observed in clinical studies of several months' to 2-years' duration, symptomatic upper GI ulcers, gross bleeding, or perforation appeared to occur in approximately 1% of patients treated for 3–6 months and in about 2–4% of those treated for 1 year. These trends continue with long-term therapy and increase the likelihood of a serious GI event occurring at some time during the course of therapy. Studies have shown that patients with a history of peptic ulcer disease and/or GI bleeding who are receiving NSAIAs have a greater than tenfold higher risk for developing GI bleeding than patients without these risk factors. In addition to a history of ulcer disease, pharmacoepidemiologic studies have identified several comorbid conditions and concomitant therapies that may increase the risk for GI bleeding, including concomitant use of oral corticosteroids or anticoagulants, longer duration of NSAIA therapy, high NSAIA dosage, smoking, alcoholism, older age, and poor general health status. In addition, geriatric or debilitated patients appear to tolerate GI ulceration and bleeding less well than other individuals, and most spontaneous reports of fatal NSAIA-induced GI effects have been in such patients.

For patients at high risk for complications from NSAIA-induced GI ulceration (e.g., bleeding, perforation), concomitant use of misoprostol can be considered for preventive therapy. (See Misoprostol 56:28.28.) Alternatively, use of a proton-pump inhibitor (e.g., lansoprazole) may be used concomitantly to decrease the incidence of serious GI toxicity associated with NSAIA therapy. Another approach in high-risk patients who would benefit from NSAIA therapy is use of an NSAIA that is a selective inhibitor of cyclooxygenase-2 (COX-2), since these agents are associated with a lower incidence of serious GI bleeding than are prototypical NSAIAs. However, while celecoxib (200 mg twice daily) was comparably effective to diclofenac sodium (75 mg twice daily) plus omeprazole (20 mg daily) in preventing recurrent ulcer bleeding (recurrent ulcer bleeding probabilities of 4.9 versus 6.4%, respectively, during the 6-month study) in *H. pylori*-negative arthritis (principally osteoarthritis) patients with a recent history of ulcer bleeding, the protective efficacy was unexpectedly low for both regimens and it appeared that neither could completely protect patients at high risk. Additional study is necessary to elucidate optimal therapy for preventing GI complications associated with NSAIA therapy in high-risk patients.

■ **Duodenal Ulcer** ***Acute Therapy*** Lansoprazole is used for the short-term treatment of endoscopically or radiographically confirmed active duodenal ulcer. Antacids may be used concomitantly as needed for pain relief. In controlled studies in patients with endoscopically confirmed duodenal ulcers, reported rates of ulcer healing for lansoprazole were substantially higher than those for placebo. In a multicenter, double-blind study in patients with endoscopically confirmed duodenal ulcer, reported rates of ulcer healing for an oral lansoprazole dosage of 15 mg daily or placebo were 42 or 11%, respectively, at 2 weeks and 89 or 46%, respectively, at 4 weeks. A similar response was observed in patients receiving 30 or 60 mg of lansoprazole daily. Lansoprazole also produced greater reductions in daytime and nocturnal abdominal pain and antacid consumption than did placebo. Clinically important differences in the rates of ulcer healing between men and women receiving lansoprazole therapy do not appear to exist.

Lansoprazole appears to be at least as effective as H_2-receptor antagonists or other proton-pump inhibitors (e.g., omeprazole) for short-term treatment of active duodenal ulcer. In a multicenter, controlled study in patients with endoscopically confirmed duodenal ulcers, 35 or 31% of ulcers were healed following 2 weeks of oral therapy with lansoprazole 20 mg daily or ranitidine 300 mg twice daily, respectively, and 92 or 71%, respectively, were healed after 4 weeks of therapy. A lansoprazole dosage of 30 mg daily was similarly effective. In another multicenter, controlled study in patients with endoscopically confirmed duodenal ulcers, 88 or 82% of ulcers were healed following 2 weeks of oral therapy with lansoprazole 30 mg daily or omeprazole 20 mg daily, respectively, and 98 or 97%, respectively, were healed after 4 weeks of therapy.

Most patients with duodenal ulcer respond to lansoprazole therapy during the usual 4-week course of therapy. However, short-term lansoprazole therapy for the treatment of active duodenal disease will not prevent recurrence of the disease following acute healing and discontinuance of the drug.

Lansoprazole is used in combination with amoxicillin and clarithromycin for the treatment of *H. pylori* infection and duodenal ulcer disease. Lansoprazole also is used in combination with amoxicillin for the treatment of *H. pylori* infection and duodenal ulcer disease in patients who are either allergic to or intolerant of clarithromycin or in whom clarithromycin resistance is known or suspected. Lansoprazole also has been used in other multiple-drug regimens† for the treatment of *H. pylori* infection and peptic ulcer disease. Current epidemiologic and clinical evidence supports a strong association between gastric infection with *H. pylori* and the pathogenesis of duodenal and gastric ulcers; long-term *H. pylori* infection also has been implicated as a risk factor for gastric cancer. For additional information on the association of this infection with these and other GI conditions, see Helicobacter pylori Infection, under Uses, in Clarithromycin 8:12.12.92. Conventional antiulcer therapy with H_2-receptor antagonists, proton-pump inhibitors, sucralfate, and/or antacids heals ulcers but generally is ineffective in eradicating *H. pylori*, and such therapy is associated with a high rate of ulcer recurrence (e.g., 60–100% per year). The American College of Gastroenterology (ACG), the National Institutes of Health (NIH), and most clinicians currently recommend that *all* patients with initial or recurrent duodenal or gastric ulcer and documented *H. pylori* infection receive anti-infective therapy for treatment of the infection. Although 3-drug regimens consisting of a bismuth salt (e.g., bismuth subsalicylate) and 2 anti-infective agents (e.g., tetracycline or amoxicillin plus metronidazole) administered for 10–14 days have been effective in eradicating the infection, resolving associated gastritis, healing peptic ulcer, and preventing ulcer recurrence in many patients with *H. pylori*-associated peptic ulcer disease, current evidence principally from studies in Europe suggests that 1 week of such therapy provides comparable *H. pylori* eradication rates. Other regimens that combine one or more anti-infective agents (e.g., clarithromycin, amoxicillin) with a bismuth salt and/ or an antisecretory agent (e.g., omeprazole, lansoprazole, H_2-receptor antagonist) also have been used successfully for *H. pylori* eradication, and the choice of a particular regimen should be based on current data on optimal therapy, including consideration of the patient's prior exposure to anti-infective agents, the local prevalence of resistance, patient compliance, and costs of therapy.

Current evidence suggests that inclusion of a proton-pump inhibitor (e.g., lansoprazole, omeprazole) in anti-*H. pylori* regimens containing 2 anti-infectives enhances effectiveness, and limited data suggest that such regimens retain good efficacy despite imidazole (e.g., metronidazole) resistance. Therefore, the ACG and many clinicians currently recommend 1 week of therapy with a proton-pump inhibitor and 2 anti-infective agents (usually clarithromycin and amoxicillin or metronidazole), or a 3-drug, bismuth-based regimen (e.g., bismuth-metronidazole-tetracycline) concomitantly with a proton-pump inhibitor, for treatment of *H. pylori* infection.

Therapy with an antisecretory drug and a single anti-infective agent (i.e., "dual therapy") also has been used successfully for treatment of *H. pylori* infection. However, while some studies demonstrate that certain 2-drug anti-*H. pylori* regimens (e.g., clarithromycin-omeprazole, ranitidine bismuth citrate-omeprazole, amoxicillin-omeprazole) can successfully eradicate *H. pylori* infection and prevent recurrence of duodenal ulcer at least in the short term (e.g., at 6 months following completion of anti-*H. pylori* therapy), the ACG and some clinicians currently state that anti-*H. pylori* regimens consisting of at least 3 drugs (e.g., 2 anti-infective agents plus a proton-pump inhibitor) are recommended because of enhanced *H. pylori* eradication rates, decreased failures due to resistance, and shorter treatment periods compared with those apparently required with 2-drug regimens. Additional randomized, controlled studies comparing various anti-*H. pylori* regimens are needed to clarify optimum drug combinations, dosages, and durations of treatment for *H. pylori* infection. For a more complete discussion of *H. pylori* infection, including details about the efficacy of various regimens and rationale for drug selection,see Uses: Helicobacter pylori Infection, in Clarithromycin 8:12.12.92.

Maintenance Therapy Lansoprazole is used as maintenance therapy following healing of duodenal ulcers to reduce ulcer recurrence. In 2 controlled studies of patients with endoscopically documented healed duodenal ulcers, those receiving lansoprazole 15 or 30 mg daily remained healed substantially longer, and experienced substantially fewer recurrences than those receiving placebo over a 12 month period. In one study, 90, 87, and 84% of patients receiving lansoprazole 15 mg daily, and 49, 41, and 39% of patients receiving placebo, remained in endoscopically documented remission over 3, 6, and 12 months, respectively. In another study, 94, 94, and 85% of patients receiving lansoprazole 30 mg daily and 87, 79, and 70% of those receiving lansoprazole 15 mg daily were still in endoscopically documented remission at 3, 6, and 12 months, respectively. In comparison, only 33% of those receiving placebo remained in endoscopically documented remission over 3 months, and none were in remission at 6 or 12 months. There was no substantial difference between lansoprazole 15 or 30 mg daily in maintaining remission.

■ **Pathologic GI Hypersecretory Conditions** Lansoprazole is used for the long-term treatment of pathologic GI hypersecretory conditions (e.g., Zollinger-Ellison syndrome, multiple endocrine adenomas, systemic mastocytosis). The drug reduces gastric acid secretion and associated symptoms (including diarrhea, anorexia, and pain) in patients with these conditions. In dosages ranging from 15 mg every other day to 180 mg daily, lansoprazole can maintain basal acid secretion below 5 or 10 mEq/hour in patients who have or have not undergone gastric surgery, respectively. Lansoprazole therapy has been continued in some patients for longer than 4 years.

■ **Crohn's Disease-associated Ulcers** Although evidence currently is limited, proton-pump inhibitors have been used for gastric acid-suppressive therapy as an adjunct in the symptomatic treatment of upper GI Crohn's disease†, including esophageal, gastroduodenal, and jejunoileal disease. Most evidence of efficacy to date has been from case studies in patients with Crohn's-associated peptic ulcer disease unresponsive to other therapies (e.g., H_2-receptor antagonists, cytoprotective agents, antacids, and/or sucralfate). (See Uses: Crohn's Disease-associated Ulcers in Omeprazole 56:28.36.)

For further information on the management of Crohn's Disease, see Uses: Crohn's Disease, in Mesalamine 56:36.

Dosage and Administration

■ **Administration** Lansoprazole is administered orally. Lansoprazole also has been administered by IV infusion; however, a parenteral dosage form no longer is commercially available in the US.

If a dose of lansoprazole is missed, the dose should be taken as soon as possible. However, if the next scheduled dose is due, the missed dose should be omitted, and the next dose taken at the regularly scheduled time. A double dose should not be administered to make up for a missed dose.

Oral Administration Lansoprazole is administered orally as capsules or orally disintegrating tablets. To avoid decomposition of lansoprazole in the acidic pH of the stomach, the commercially available delayed-release capsules contain enteric-coated granules of the drug, and the orally disintegrating tablets contain enteric-coated microgranules of the drug. The contents of the capsules should *not* be chewed or crushed, nor should the orally disintegrating tablets be broken, cut, or chewed.

Lansoprazole usually is administered once daily, generally in the morning; however, the manufacturer states that administration of the drug in 2 equally divided doses in the morning and evening may improve efficacy in patients receiving more than 120 mg daily. When lansoprazole is used in combination with amoxicillin or with clarithromycin and amoxicillin for the treatment of *Helicobacter pylori* infection associated with duodenal ulcer, lansoprazole is given in 2 or 3 divided doses daily.

Following administration of lansoprazole with meals, the rate and extent of GI absorption are reduced. Therefore, lansoprazole should be taken before meals. Since an acidic environment in the parietal cell canaliculi is required for conversion of proton-pump inhibitors (e.g., lansoprazole) to their active sulfenamide metabolites, the American College of Gastroenterology suggests that proton-pump inhibitors are most effective when given about 30 minutes prior to meals and that effectiveness may be compromised if these drugs are administered during the basal state (e.g., to fasting patients at bedtime) or concomitantly with other antisecretory agents (e.g., anticholinergics, histamine H_2-receptor antagonists, somatostatin analogs, misoprostol). Lansoprazole may be administered concomitantly with antacids but should be administered at least 30 minutes before sucralfate (see Drug Interactions).

Oral Capsules. Lansoprazole capsules may be swallowed whole. Alternatively, the contents of a capsule may be sprinkled on a tablespoonful of a suitable soft food and swallowed without chewing; mixed with apple, orange, or tomato juice and consumed; or mixed with apple juice and given via a nasogastric tube.

In patients who have difficulty swallowing capsules, the contents of a capsule may be sprinkled on a tablespoonful of applesauce, liquid dietary supplement (e.g., Ensure®) pudding, cottage cheese, yogurt, or strained pears and ingested immediately without a clinically important effect on the drug's bioavailability. The granules should not be chewed or crushed. The manufacturer states that administration of lansoprazole mixed in other foods has not been evaluated clinically and is not recommended.

Alternatively, the contents of a capsule may be emptied into a small volume (i.e., 60 mL, about 2 ounces) of apple, orange, or tomato juice, mixed briefly, and swallowed immediately. To ensure complete consumption of the dose, the glass should be rinsed with 120 mL or more of juice, and the contents swallowed immediately. The manufacturer states that administration of lansoprazole mixed in other beverages has not been evaluated clinically and is not recommended.

For patients with a nasogastric tube, the contents of a capsule can be mixed with 40 mL of apple juice in a syringe and administered immediately (i.e., within 3–5 minutes) without any clinically important effect on the drug's bioavailability; the manufacturer states that other liquids should not be used. To facilitate delivery of the entire dose and to maintain patency of the nasogastric tube, the syringe and tube should be flushed with additional apple juice.

The manufacturer states that lansoprazole capsules for *self-medication* should be swallowed whole with a glass of water; the capsules should not be crushed or chewed.

Orally Disintegrating Tablets. Lansoprazole orally disintegrating tablets containing enteric-coated microgranules of the drug may be allowed to disintegrate on the tongue and then swallowed without chewing; alternatively, a tablet may be dispersed in a compatible liquid and administered orally using an oral syringe or given via a nasogastric tube. The orally disintegrating tablets should not be broken or cut.

For oral administration, the orally disintegrating tablet should be placed on the tongue and allowed to disintegrate (usually in less than 1 minute) with or without water, and the particles swallowed without chewing.

For administration using an oral syringe, a 15- or 30-mg orally disintegrating tablet should be placed in an oral syringe, about 4 or 10 mL, respectively, of water should be drawn into the syringe, and the syringe should be shaken gently to ensure rapid dispersal of the particles. The contents of the syringe should be administered within 15 minutes of preparation. An additional 2 mL (for a 15-mg dose) or 5 mL (for a 30-mg dose) of water should be drawn into the syringe, mixed gently, and the entire contents ingested to ensure complete consumption of the dose.

For administration via a nasogastric tube, a 15- or 30-mg orally disintegrating tablet should be placed in a syringe, about 4 or 10 mL, respectively, of water should be drawn into the syringe, and the syringe should be shaken gently to ensure rapid dispersal of the particles. The contents of the syringe should be administered through a nasogastric tube (8 French or larger) within 15 minutes of preparation. An additional 5 mL of water should be drawn into the syringe, mixed gently, and used to flush the nasogastric tube.

■ Dosage

Adult Dosage

Gastroesophageal Reflux. For the short-term treatment of symptomatic gastroesophageal reflux disease (GERD), the usual adult dosage of lansoprazole is 15 mg once daily for up to 8 weeks.

For the short-term symptomatic treatment of all grades of erosive esophagitis, the usual adult dosage of lansoprazole is 30 mg once daily. Therapy is continued until healing occurs, usually within 8 weeks; an additional 8 weeks of therapy (up to 16 weeks for a single course) may contribute to healing and symptomatic improvement in some patients. If the erosive esophagitis recurs, the manufacturer states that an additional 8-week course of lansoprazole may be given. However, the American College of Gastroenterology (ACG) states that chronic, even lifelong, therapy with a proton-pump inhibitor is appropriate in many patients with GERD.

For maintenance therapy following healing of erosive esophagitis to reduce recurrence, the usual adult dosage of lansoprazole is 15 mg daily. Safety and efficacy of lansoprazole maintenance therapy for longer than 1 year have not been established.

For *self-medication* to relieve symptoms of frequent heartburn in adults 18 years of age or older, a lansoprazole dosage of 15 mg once daily in the morning for 14 days is recommended. For *self-medication*, the manufacturer recommends that the dosage of lansoprazole not exceed 15 mg in 24 hours. In addition, the drug should not be used for *self-medication* for longer than 14 days of *continuous* use and individuals should not exceed one course of therapy every 4 months unless otherwise directed by a clinician.

Gastric Ulcer. For the short-term treatment of active benign gastric ulcer, the usual adult dosage of lansoprazole is 30 mg daily for up to 8 weeks.

Nonsteroidal Anti-inflammatory Agent (NSAIA)-induced Ulcers. For the treatment of nonsteroidal anti-inflammatory agent (NSAIA)-associated gastric ulcers in patients continuing NSAIA use, the usual adult dosage of lansoprazole is 30 mg once daily for 8 weeks.

For prevention of NSAIA-associated gastric ulcers in patients with a documented history of gastric ulcer who require the use of an NSAIA, the usual adult dosage of lansoprazole is 15 mg once daily for up to 12 weeks. Efficacy of lansoprazole for periods exceeding 12 weeks in preventing of NSAIA-induced gastric ulcers has not been studied.

Duodenal Ulcer. For the short-term treatment of active duodenal ulcer, the usual adult dosage of lansoprazole is 15 mg once daily. Although an oral dosage of 30 mg daily often was administered in clinical studies, the manufacturer states that dosages of 30 or even 60 mg daily were no more effective at healing active duodenal ulcers than 15 mg daily. Therapy should be continued up to 4 weeks or until healing occurs.

When lansoprazole is used in combination with amoxicillin and clarithromycin (triple therapy) for the treatment of *H. pylori* infection in patients with active duodenal ulcer, the usual adult dosage is 30 mg every 12 hours (morning and evening) for 10 or 14 days. When lansoprazole is used in combination with amoxicillin (dual therapy) for the treatment of *H. pylori* infection in patients with active duodenal ulcer, the usual adult dosage is 30 mg every 8 hours for 14 days.

For maintenance therapy following healing of duodenal ulcer to reduce recurrence, the usual adult dosage of lansoprazole is 15 mg daily. Safety and efficacy of lansoprazole maintenance therapy for longer than 1 year have not been established.

Pathologic GI Hypersecretory Conditions. For the long-term treatment of pathologic GI hypersecretory conditions (e.g., Zollinger-Ellison syndrome, multiple endocrine adenomas, systemic mastocytosis), dosages of lansoprazole should be individualized according to patient response and tolerance. The usual initial adult dosage is 60 mg once daily. Subsequent lansoprazole dosage should be adjusted as tolerated and necessary to adequately suppress gastric acid secretion, and therapy continued as long as clinically necessary.

Oral dosages ranging from 15 mg every other day to 180 mg daily have been necessary to maintain basal gastric acid secretion at less than 10 mEq/hour in patients without a history of gastric surgery and less than 5 mEq/hour in those who have undergone gastric surgery; generally, determination of gastric acid secretion during the hour prior to a dose is useful in establishing optimum dosage. The manufacturer recommends that daily dosages exceeding 120 mg be administered in 2 equally divided doses in the morning and evening. Lansoprazole has been given continuously for longer than 4 years in some patients with Zollinger-Ellison syndrome.

Pediatric Dosage

Gastroesophageal Reflux. For the short-term treatment of symptomatic GERD or erosive esophagitis in children 1–11 years of age, the usual oral dosage of lansoprazole for children weighing 30 kg or less is 15 mg once daily for up to 12 weeks; dosage for children weighing more than 30 kg is 30 mg once daily for up to 12 weeks. Dosage in children 1–11 years of age has been increased to up to 30 mg twice daily in patients remaining symptomatic after 2 or more weeks of treatment.

For children 12–17 years of age, the usual oral dosage of lansoprazole for treatment of nonerosive GERD is 15 mg daily for up to 8 weeks, and that for erosive esophagitis is 30 mg daily for up to 8 weeks.

■ Special Populations

The manufacturer states that lansoprazole dosage adjustment is not necessary in geriatric patients. Although pharmacokinetics of lansoprazole may be altered slightly in patients with renal impairment, dosage adjustment is not necessary. However, the commercially available daily administration pack containing lansoprazole, amoxicillin, and clarithromycin (Prevpac®)is not recommended for use in patients with creatinine clearance values less than 30 mL/minute. In patients with severe hepatic impairment, lansoprazole dosage reduction should be considered. (See Specific Populations under Cautions: Warnings/Precautions.)

Cautions

■ Contraindications

Known severe hypersensitivity to lansoprazole or any ingredient in the formulation.

■ Warnings/Precautions

Gastric Malignancy

Symptomatic response to therapy with lansoprazole does not preclude the presence of gastric malignancy.

Clostridium difficile Infection

Available data suggest a possible association between use of proton-pump inhibitors and risk of *Clostridium difficile* infection, including *C. difficile*-associated diarrhea and colitis (CDAD; also known as antibiotic-associated diarrhea and colitis or pseudomembranous colitis). In most observational studies to date, the risk of *C. difficile* infection in patients exposed to proton-pump inhibitors has ranged from 1.4–2.75 times that in patients not exposed to proton-pump inhibitors; however, some observational studies have found no increase in risk. Although many of the cases occurred in patients who had other risk factors for CDAD, including advanced age, comorbid conditions, and/or use of broad-spectrum anti-infectives, the US Food and Drug Administration (FDA) concluded that a contributory role for proton-pump inhibitors could not be definitively ruled out. The mechanism by which proton-pump inhibitors might increase the risk of CDAD has not been elucidated. Although it has been suggested that reduction of gastric acidity by gastric antisecretory agents might facilitate colonization with *C. difficile*, some studies have raised questions about this proposed mechanism or have suggested that the observed association is the result of confounding with other risk factors for CDAD. FDA also is reviewing the risk of CDAD in patients exposed to histamine H_2-receptor antagonists.

CDAD can be serious in patients who have one or more risk factors for *C. difficile* infection and are receiving concomitant therapy with a proton-pump inhibitor; colectomy and, rarely, death have been reported. FDA recommends that patients receive proton-pump inhibitors at the lowest effective dosage and for the shortest possible time appropriate for their clinical condition. Patients experiencing persistent diarrhea should be evaluated for CDAD and should be managed with appropriate supportive therapy (e.g., fluid and electrolyte management), anti-infective therapy directed against *C. difficile* (e.g., metronidazole, vancomycin), and surgical evaluation as clinically indicated.

Respiratory Effects Administration of proton-pump inhibitors has been associated with an increased risk for developing certain infections (e.g., community-acquired pneumonia). For further precautionary information about this adverse effect, see Community-acquired Pneumonia under Cautions: Respiratory Effects, in Omeprazole 56:28.36.

Musculoskeletal Effects Findings from several observational studies suggest that therapy with proton-pump inhibitors, particularly in high dosages (i.e., multiple daily doses) and/or for prolonged periods of time (i.e., one year or longer), may be associated with an increased risk of osteoporosis-related fractures of the hip, wrist, or spine. The magnitude of risk is unclear; causality has not been established. (See Cautions: Musculoskeletal Effects, in Omeprazole 56:28.36.) FDA is continuing to evaluate this safety concern. Although controlled studies are required to confirm these findings, patients should receive proton-pump inhibitors at the lowest effective dosage and for the shortest possible time appropriate for their clinical condition. Individuals who are at risk for osteoporosis-related fractures should receive an adequate intake of calcium and vitamin D and should have their bone health assessed and managed according to current standards of care.

Hypomagnesemia Hypomagnesemia, symptomatic and asymptomatic, has been reported rarely in patients receiving long-term therapy (for at least 3 months or, in most cases, for longer than one year) with proton-pump inhibitors, including lansoprazole. Clinically serious adverse effects associated with hypomagnesemia, which are similar to manifestations of hypocalcemia, include tetany, seizures, tremors, carpopedal spasm, arrhythmias (e.g., atrial fibrillation, supraventricular tachycardia), and abnormal QT interval. Other reported adverse effects include paresthesia, muscle weakness, muscle cramps, lethargy, fatigue, and unsteadiness. In most patients, treatment of hypomagnesemia required magnesium replacement and discontinuance of the proton-pump inhibitor. Following discontinuance of the proton-pump inhibitor, hypomagnesemia resolved within a median of one week; upon rechallenge, hypomagnesemia recurred within a median of 2 weeks.

In patients expected to receive long-term therapy with a proton-pump inhibitor or in those receiving a proton-pump inhibitor concomitantly with digoxin or drugs that may cause hypomagnesemia (e.g., diuretics), clinicians should consider measurement of serum magnesium concentrations prior to initiation of prescription proton-pump inhibitor therapy and periodically thereafter. (See Cautions: Hypomagnesemia and also Cautions: Precautions and Contraindications, in Omeprazole 56:28.36.)

Phenylketonuria Individuals with phenylketonuria (i.e., homozygous genetic deficiency of phenylalanine hydroxylase) and other individuals who must restrict their intake of phenylalanine should be warned that each 15- or 30-mg Prevacid® SoluTab® orally disintegrating tablet contains aspartame (NutraSweet®), which is metabolized in the GI tract to provide about 2.5 or 5.1 mg, respectively, of phenylalanine following oral administration.

Specific Populations **Pregnancy.** Category B. (See Users Guide.)

Lactation. Lansoprazole or its metabolites are distributed into milk in rats; it is not known whether lansoprazole is distributed into human milk. The manufacturer states that a decision should be made whether to discontinue nursing or the drug, taking into account the importance of the drug to the woman.

Pediatric Use. Safety and efficacy of oral lansoprazole in pediatric patients 1–17 years of age have been established for short-term treatment of symptomatic gastroesophageal reflux disease (GERD) and erosive esophagitis. In an open-label study in children 1–11 years of age, symptomatic improvement occurred following 8–12 weeks of lansoprazole therapy in 76% of children with symptomatic GERD; in a limited subset of children with endoscopically documented erosive esophagitis, rates of symptomatic improvement and healing were 81 and 100%, respectively. Lansoprazole was initiated at a dosage of 15 mg daily in children weighing 30 kg or less and a dosage of 30 mg daily in those weighing more than 30 kg; dosage could be increased up to 30 mg twice daily in children who continued to experience symptoms 2 or more weeks after initiating therapy with the drug. In an open-label study in adolescents 12–17 years of age with GERD, symptomatic improvement occurred following 8 weeks of therapy with lansoprazole 15 mg daily in 71% of those with nonerosive disease; in a smaller group of adolescents with erosive esophagitis, rates of symptomatic improvement and healing were 78 and 96%, respectively, following 8–12 weeks of therapy with lansoprazole 30 mg daily. The most commonly reported adverse effects in pediatric patients receiving lansoprazole include headache, abdominal pain, constipation, nausea, and dizziness.

Efficacy of oral lansoprazole has not been established in infants younger than 1 year of age. In a controlled study in infants 1 month to younger than 1 year of age with symptomatic GERD, lansoprazole was no more effective than placebo in reducing feeding-associated episodes of crying, fussing, or irritability; in both the placebo and lansoprazole groups, the response rate was 54%.

Safety and efficacy of lansoprazole for *self-medication* of frequent heartburn have not been established in children younger than 18 years of age.

Geriatric Use. The frequency of adverse effects in geriatric patients appears to be similar to that in younger patients. Clearance of lansoprazole may be decreased in geriatric patients, but accumulation of the drug does not occur with once-daily dosing and dosage adjustment is not necessary.

Hepatic Impairment. Systemic exposure to lansoprazole, as measured by area under the serum concentration-time curve (AUC), may be increased by up to 500% in patients with chronic hepatic impairment. Dosage reduction should be considered in patients with severe hepatic impairment.

Renal Impairment. Although the pharmacokinetics of lansoprazole may be altered slightly in patients with renal impairment, dosage adjustment is not necessary.

■ **Common Adverse Effects** Adverse effects occurring in 1% or more of patients receiving oral lansoprazole and more frequently than with placebo include abdominal pain, diarrhea, nausea, and constipation.

Drug Interactions

■ **Drugs Metabolized by Hepatic Microsomal Enzymes** Lansoprazole is metabolized by cytochrome P-450 (CYP) isoenzymes 2C19 and 3A. In studies in healthy individuals, clinically important interactions were not observed between lansoprazole and other drugs (e.g., antipyrine, clarithromycin, diazepam, ibuprofen, indomethacin, phenytoin, prednisone, propranolol, warfarin) metabolized by CYP isoenzymes, including the 1A2, 2C9, 2C19, 2D6, and 3A isoenzymes.

■ **Drugs that Cause Hypomagnesemia** Potential pharmacologic interaction (possible increased risk of hypomagnesemia). In patients receiving diuretics (i.e., loop or thiazide diuretics) or other drugs that may cause hypomagnesemia, monitoring of magnesium concentrations should be considered prior to initiation of prescription proton-pump inhibitor therapy and periodically thereafter. (See Hypomagnesemia under Cautions: Warnings/Precautions.)

■ **Gastric pH-dependent Drugs** Pharmacokinetic interaction is theoretically possible when lansoprazole is used concomitantly with gastric pH-dependent drugs (e.g., ampicillin esters, digoxin, iron salts, ketoconazole); altered drug absorption at increased gastric pH values.

■ **Amoxicillin** Clinically important interaction is unlikely.

■ **Antacids** Efficacy of lansoprazole is not altered by concomitant administration of antacids.

■ **Antiretroviral Agents** ***Atazanavir*** Potential pharmacokinetic interaction with atazanavir (possible altered oral absorption of atazanavir at increased gastric pH, resulting in decreased plasma atazanavir concentrations). Concomitant use of omeprazole 40 mg once daily and atazanavir (with or without low-dose ritonavir) results in a substantial decrease in plasma concentrations of atazanavir and possible loss of the therapeutic effect of the antiretroviral agent. The manufacturer of lansoprazole states that concomitant administration with atazanavir is not recommended. If atazanavir is administered in an antiretroviral treatment-naive patient receiving a proton-pump inhibitor, a *ritonavir-boosted* regimen of 300 mg of atazanavir once daily with ritonavir 100 mg once daily with food is recommended. The dose of the proton-pump inhibitor should be administered approximately 12 hours before *ritonavir-boosted* atazanavir; the dose of the proton-pump inhibitor should not exceed omeprazole 20 mg daily (or equivalent). Concomitant use of proton-pump inhibitors with atazanavir is not recommended in antiretroviral treatment-experienced patients.

Fosamprenavir Concomitant use of esomeprazole with fosamprenavir (with or without ritonavir) did not substantially affect concentrations of amprenavir (active metabolite of fosamprenavir). No dosage adjustment is required when proton-pump inhibitors are used concomitantly with fosamprenavir (with or without ritonavir).

Lopinavir Concomitant use of omeprazole with the fixed combination of lopinavir and ritonavir (lopinavir/ritonavir) did not have a clinically important effect on plasma concentrations or area under the concentration-time curve (AUC) of lopinavir. No dosage adjustment is required when proton-pump inhibitors are used concomitantly with lopinavir/ritonavir.

Raltegravir Pharmacokinetic interaction with omeprazole (substantially increased peak plasma concentration and AUC of raltegravir); however, no dosage adjustment is recommended when proton-pump inhibitors are used concomitantly with raltegravir.

Rilpivirine Pharmacokinetic interaction with omeprazole (decreased plasma concentrations and AUC of rilpivirine). Concomitant use of other proton-pump inhibitors also may result in decreased plasma concentrations of rilpivirine. Concomitant use of rilpivirine and proton-pump inhibitors is contraindicated.

Saquinavir Potential pharmacokinetic interaction (increased peak plasma concentration and AUC of saquinavir). Concomitant use of omeprazole 40 mg once daily and *ritonavir-boosted* saquinavir (saquinavir 1 g twice daily and ritonavir 100 mg twice daily) increased the peak plasma concentration and AUC of saquinavir by 75 and 82%, respectively. Caution is advised if proton-pump inhibitors are used concomitantly with *ritonavir-boosted* saquinavir, and patients should be monitored for saquinavir toxicity.

■ **Clopidogrel** Potential pharmacokinetic interaction (decreased plasma concentration of the active metabolite of clopidogrel) and pharmacodynamic interaction (reduced antiplatelet effects) between proton-pump inhibitors and clopidogrel. Clopidogrel is metabolized to its active metabolite by CYP2C19. Concurrent use of omeprazole or esomeprazole, which inhibit CYP2C19, with clopidogrel reduces exposure to the active metabolite of clopidogrel and decreases platelet inhibitory effects. Although the clinical importance has not been fully elucidated, a reduction in the effectiveness of clopidogrel in preventing cardiovascular events is possible. Proton-pump inhibitors vary in their potency for inhibiting CYP2C19. The change in inhibition of adenosine diphosphate (ADP)-induced platelet aggregation associated with concomitant use of proton-pump inhibitors is related to the change in exposure to the active metabolite of clopidogrel. In pharmacokinetic and pharmacodynamic studies in healthy individuals, concomitant use of dexlansoprazole, lansoprazole, or pantoprazole had less effect on the antiplatelet activity of clopidogrel than did concomitant use of omeprazole or esomeprazole. In individuals who were extensive metabolizers of CYP2C19 substrates, use of lansoprazole (30 mg once daily) concomitantly with clopidogrel (75 mg once daily) for 9 days reduced exposure to the active metabolite of clopidogrel by about 14% compared with use of clopidogrel alone. The observed effects of lansoprazole on metabolite exposure and clopidogrel-induced platelet inhibition were not considered clinically important, and the manufacturer of lansoprazole states that no adjustment of clopidogrel dosage is necessary if clopidogrel is used concomitantly with recommended dosages of lansoprazole.

The decision to use a proton-pump inhibitor concomitantly with clopidogrel should be based on the assessed risks and benefits in individual patients. The American College of Cardiology Foundation/American College of Gastroenterology/American Heart Association (ACCF/ACG/AHA) states that the reduction in GI bleeding risk with proton-pump inhibitors is substantial in patients with risk factors for GI bleeding (e.g., advanced age; concomitant use of warfarin, corticosteroids, or nonsteroidal anti-inflammatory agents [NSAIAs]; *H. pylori* infection) and may outweigh any potential reduction in the cardiovascular efficacy of antiplatelet treatment associated with a drug-drug interaction. In contrast, ACCF/ACG/AHA states that patients without such risk factors receive little if any absolute risk reduction from proton-pump inhibitor therapy, and the risk/benefit balance may favor use of antiplatelet therapy without a proton-pump inhibitor in these patients.

If concomitant therapy with a proton-pump inhibitor and clopidogrel is considered necessary, use of an agent with little or no CYP2C19-inhibitory activity should be considered. Alternatively, treatment with a histamine H_2-receptor antagonist (ranitidine, famotidine, nizatidine) may be considered, although such agents may not be as effective as a proton-pump inhibitor in providing gastric protection; cimetidine should *not* be used since it also is a potent CYP2C19 inhibitor. There currently is no evidence that histamine H_2-receptor antagonists (other than cimetidine) or other drugs that reduce gastric acid (e.g., antacids) interfere with the antiplatelet effects of clopidogrel. For further information on interactions between proton-pump inhibitors and clopidogrel, see Drug Interactions: Proton-Pump Inhibitors, in Clopidogrel Bisulfate 20:12.18.

■ **Digoxin** Hypomagnesemia (e.g., resulting from long-term use of proton-pump inhibitors) sensitizes the myocardium to digoxin and, thus, may increase the risk of digoxin-induced cardiotoxic effects. In patients receiving digoxin, monitoring of magnesium concentrations should be considered prior to initiation of prescription proton-pump inhibitor therapy and periodically thereafter.

■ **Methotrexate** Potential pharmacokinetic interaction (increased serum methotrexate concentrations, possibly resulting in toxicity) when proton-pump inhibitors, including lansoprazole, are used concomitantly with methotrexate. Increased serum concentrations and delayed clearance of methotrexate and/or its metabolite hydroxymethotrexate, with or without symptoms of methotrexate toxicity, have been reported in patients receiving methotrexate (usually at doses of 300 mg/m² to 12 g/m²) concomitantly with a proton-pump inhibitor. Although most of the reported cases occurred in patients receiving high doses of methotrexate, toxicity also has been reported in patients receiving low dosages of methotrexate (e.g., 15 mg per week) concomitantly with a proton-pump inhibitor. In patients with rheumatoid arthritis receiving low-dose methotrexate (7.5–15 mg weekly), concomitant use of lansoprazole (30 mg daily) and naproxen (500 mg twice daily) for 7 days had no effect on the pharmacokinetics of methotrexate or 7-hydroxymethotrexate. However, no formal studies of interactions between high-dose methotrexate and proton-pump inhibitors have been conducted to date.

The manufacturer of lansoprazole states that temporary discontinuance of proton-pump inhibitor therapy may be considered in some patients receiving high-dose methotrexate therapy. Some clinicians recommend either withholding proton-pump inhibitor therapy for several days before and after methotrexate administration or substituting a histamine H_2-receptor antagonist for the proton-pump inhibitor when acid suppressive therapy is indicated during methotrexate therapy. Pending further evaluation, some clinicians state that these recommendations should extend to patients receiving low-dose methotrexate.

■ **Sucralfate** Potential pharmacokinetic interaction. Concomitant administration of lansoprazole with sucralfate resulted in delayed absorption and decreased (by 17%) bioavailability of lansoprazole. Lansoprazole should be administered at least 30 minutes before sucralfate.

■ **Tacrolimus** Potential pharmacokinetic interaction (increased whole blood concentrations of tacrolimus), particularly in transplant patients who are intermediate or poor metabolizers of CYP2C19 substrates.

■ **Theophylline** Potential pharmacokinetic interaction. Concomitant administration of theophylline and lansoprazole may result in a slight (10%) increase in theophylline clearance. The interaction is unlikely to be clinically important, although some patients may require adjustment of theophylline dosage when lansoprazole therapy is initiated or discontinued.

■ **Warfarin** When warfarin was administered concomitantly with single or multiple doses of lansoprazole 60 mg in healthy individuals, the pharmacokinetics of warfarin and the prothrombin time were not altered; however, increased international normalized ratio (INR) and prothrombin time have been reported in patients receiving warfarin concomitantly with proton-pump inhibitors, including lansoprazole. The INR and prothrombin time may need to be monitored when lansoprazole is used concomitantly with warfarin.

Description

Lansoprazole is a substituted benzimidazole gastric antisecretory agent. Lansoprazole is structurally and pharmacologically related to dexlansoprazole, esomeprazole, omeprazole, pantoprazole, and rabeprazole; lansoprazole differs structurally from omeprazole by the presence of a trifluoroethoxy group in position 4 of the pyridine ring and the absence of methyl and methoxy groups on the pyridine and benzimidazole rings, respectively. The drugs are chemically and pharmacologically unrelated to H_2-receptor antagonists, antimuscarinics, or prostaglandin analogs. Lansoprazole is a racemic mixture of *R*- and *S*-isomers. Both isomers inhibit hydrogen/potassium adenosine triphosphatase (H^+K^+-exchanging ATPase), but plasma clearance of the *R*-isomer (dexlansoprazole) is slower than that of the *S*-isomer; following oral administration of racemic lansoprazole, plasma concentrations of the *R*-isomer are markedly higher than those of the *S*-isomer.

Lansoprazole binds to H^+K^+-exchanging ATPase in gastric parietal cells; inactivation of this enzyme system (also known as the proton, hydrogen, or acid pump) blocks the final step in the secretion of hydrochloric acid by these cells. Therefore, gastric antisecretory agents such as lansoprazole are commonly referred to as acid- or proton-pump inhibitors. Lansoprazole, a weak base, does not directly inhibit this enzyme system, but instead, it concentrates under the acid conditions of the parietal cell secretory canaliculi, where the drug undergoes rearrangement to active sulfenamide metabolites; these active metabolites then react with the sulfhydryl groups of H^+K^+-exchanging ATPase inactivating the proton pump. Because the sulfenamide metabolites form an irreversible covalent bond to H^+K^+-exchanging ATPase, acid secretion is inhibited until additional enzyme is synthesized, resulting in a prolonged duration of action.

Lansoprazole inhibits basal and stimulated gastric acid secretion; in addition, because the drug inhibits the final step in the secretory pathway, it inhibits such secretion regardless of the stimulus. The degree of inhibition of gastric acid secretion is related to the dose and duration of therapy, but lansoprazole is a more potent inhibitor of such secretion than are H_2-receptor antagonists. Following oral administration of 15 or 30 mg of lansoprazole, inhibition of gastric acid secretion is apparent within 2–3 or 1–2 hours, respectively. After multiple daily doses, increased gastric pH is apparent within 1 hour of administration of 30 mg of lansoprazole and within 1–2 hours after administration of 15 mg of the drug.

Although lansoprazole has a short terminal plasma half-life, the drug has a long duration of action (secondary to the prolonged presence of active lansoprazole metabolites within the parietal cell where they bind to H^+K^+-exchanging ATPase). Following continuous oral administration of 15 or 30 mg of lansoprazole, the percent of time during a 24-hour period that the gastric pH exceeds 4 is 49 or 66%, respectively. Inhibition of basal gastric secretion is 71% after an initial oral dose of 30 mg and 80% or greater after 7 days of oral administration of 30 mg of lansoprazole daily. Stimulated gastric secretion initially is reduced 81% after an oral dose of 30 mg of lansoprazole and gastric secretion is reduced 88% after 7 days of oral administration of 30 mg of lansoprazole daily. Oral administration of lansoprazole 60 mg produced almost complete inhibition of gastric acid secretion in some patients. Following discontinuance of lansoprazole therapy, gastric acid secretion returns to baseline over a 2- to 4-day period, without rebound gastric acidity.

The degree of inhibition of gastric acid secretion is similar following oral or IV administration (a parenteral formulation no longer is commercially available in the US) of lansoprazole 30 mg daily for 7 days in healthy individuals. Following oral or IV administration of the drug, the percent of time during a 24-hour period that the gastric pH exceeds 4 is about 67 or 71%, respectively, after an initial dose of 30 mg and about 78 or 80%, respectively, after 5 days of administration of lansoprazole 30 mg daily in healthy individuals.

Lansoprazole increases plasma gastrin concentrations; this increase occurs in response to a negative feedback mechanism resulting from decreased gastric acid secretion. Although a single oral dose of 30 mg of lansoprazole did not affect serum gastrin levels in healthy adults, patients with gastric ulcer receiving 30–60 mg of lansoprazole once daily for 2 months developed a 50–100% increase from baseline in median fasting serum gastrin concentration; however, median serum gastrin levels remained within the normal range. Serum gastrin concentrations reach a plateau within 2 months of lansoprazole therapy and return to pretreatment values within 1–12 weeks after discontinuing therapy with the drug. Although marked hypergastrinemia with subsequent enterochromaffin-like (ECL) cell proliferation and carcinoid lesions have been observed in animal studies, no evidence of similar ECL cell effects were observed in patients receiving the drug for periods of at least one year. Longer-term study and experience are needed to rule out the possibility of an increased risk of gastric tumors in patients receiving prolonged lansoprazole therapy.

Lansoprazole also decreases pepsin secretion and activity and increases serum pepsinogen; however, these effects are not as pronounced as the drug's inhibition of gastric acid secretion. Suppression of pepsin activity appears to be secondary to increased gastric pH, as conversion of the inactive precursor pepsinogen to pepsin requires an acidic gastric milieu. Pepsin output is inhibited in healthy adults receiving 30 mg of lansoprazole daily for 7 days in the morning or evening by 42–58 or 67–88%, respectively. When the dose is increased to 60 mg daily, no additional inhibition of pepsin secretion is observed. Pepsin activity also is inhibited by lansoprazole 30 mg daily administered in the morning or evening by 23 or 35%, respectively. Lansoprazole also substantially prolongs gastric emptying of digestible solids, but does not appear to affect lower esophageal sphincter pressure.

Lansoprazole can suppress *Helicobacter pylori* (formerly *Campylobacter pylori* or *C. pyloridis*) in patients with gastric or duodenal ulcers infected with the organism. Combined therapy with lansoprazole and one or more appropriate anti-infectives (e.g., amoxicillin, clarithromycin) can effectively eradicate *H. pylori* gastric infection. (See Duodenal Ulcer: Acute Therapy, in Uses.)

Lansoprazole is extensively metabolized in the liver. Cytochrome P-450 (CYP) isoenzymes 2C19 and 3A4 are involved in the metabolism of the drug. Following single-dose oral administration of lansoprazole, approximately one-third of the administered dose is eliminated in urine and two-thirds in feces; unchanged drug is not recovered in urine.

Therapy with proton-pump inhibitors, particularly in high dosages and/or for prolonged periods of time, may be associated with an increased risk of osteoporosis-related fractures of the hip, wrist, or spine. (See Musculoskeletal Effects under Cautions: Warnings/Precautions.) The mechanism by which these drugs may increase risk of such fractures has not been elucidated but may involve decreased insoluble calcium absorption secondary to increased gastric pH.

Advice to Patients

Importance of instructing patients regarding proper administration of delayed-release oral preparations (see Oral Administration under Dosage and Administration: Administration). Necessity of swallowing the preparation without crushing or chewing the delayed-release granules. Importance of administering lansoprazole delayed-release oral preparations before eating.

Importance of advising patients that use of multiple daily doses of the drug for an extended period of time may increase the risk of fractures of the hip, wrist, or spine.

Risk of hypomagnesemia; importance of advising patients to immediately report and seek care for any cardiovascular or neurologic manifestations (e.g., palpitations, dizziness, seizures, tetany).

Advise patients that *self-medication* with lansoprazole is not intended for immediate relief of heartburn; the drug may relieve symptoms within 24 hours, but 1–4 days may be required for complete relief.

Importance of not using lansoprazole for *self-medication* for longer than 14 days of *continuous* use and of not exceeding one course of therapy every 4 months unless otherwise directed by a clinician. Advise patients to discontinue use of lansoprazole as *self-medication* and to consult a clinician if their heartburn persists or worsens or if they need to use the drug for longer than 14 days or require more than one course of therapy every 4 months.

Advise patients to consult a clinician before using lansoprazole for *self-medication* if they have liver disease, have had heartburn for longer than 3 months, or are experiencing heartburn with lightheadedness, dizziness, or sweating; chest or shoulder pain with shortness of breath, sweating, lightheadedness, or pain spreading to the arms, neck, or shoulders; frequent chest pain; frequent wheezing (especially with heartburn); unexplained weight loss; nausea or vomiting; or stomach pain. Advise patients with difficulty or pain with swallowing, those vomiting blood, and those with bloody or blackened stools that they should not use lansoprazole for *self-medication* and should consult a clinician.

Possible increased risk of *Clostridium difficile* infection; importance of contacting a clinician if persistent watery stools, abdominal pain, and fever occur.

Importance of informing clinicians of existing or contemplated concomitant therapy, including prescription and OTC drugs, as well as any concomitant illnesses. Antacid administration is permissible with lansoprazole delayed-release preparations.

Importance of informing patients with phenylketonuria that lansoprazole delayed-release orally disintegrating tablets contain aspartame.

Importance of women informing clinicians if they are or plan to become pregnant or plan to breast-feed.

Importance of informing patients of other important precautionary information. (See Cautions.)

Overview® (see Users Guide). For additional information on this drug until a more detailed monograph is developed and published, the manufacturer's labeling should be consulted. It is *essential* that the manufacturer's labeling be consulted for more detailed information on usual cautions, precautions, contraindications, potential drug interactions, laboratory test interferences, and acute toxicity.

Preparations

Excipients in commercially available drug preparations may have clinically important effects in some individuals; consult specific product labeling for details.

Lansoprazole

Oral		
Capsules, delayed-release (containing enteric-coated granules)	15 mg*	**Lansoprazole Delayed-Release Capsules**
		Prevacid®, Takeda
		Prevacid® 24HR, Novartis
	30 mg*	**Lansoprazole Delayed-Release Capsules**
		Prevacid®, Takeda
Tablets, delayed-release (containing enteric-coated microgranules), orally disintegrating	15 mg	**Prevacid® SoluTab®**, Takeda
	30 mg	**Prevacid® SoluTab®**, Takeda

*available from one or more manufacturer, distributor, and/or repackager by generic (nonproprietary) name

Lansoprazole Combinations

Oral		
Kit	4 Capsules, Amoxicillin (trihydrate) 500 mg (of amoxicillin) 2 Capsules, delayed-release (containing enteric-coated granules), Lansoprazole, 30 mg (Prevacid®) 2 Tablets, film-coated, Clarithromycin, 500 mg (Biaxin® Filmtab®)	**Prevpac®**, Takeda

†Use is not currently included in the labeling approved by the US Food and Drug Administration

Omeprazole
Omeprazole Magnesium

■ Omeprazole, commonly referred to as an acid- or proton-pump inhibitor, is a gastric antisecretory agent.

Uses

Omeprazole is used in adults for the short-term treatment of active duodenal and benign gastric ulcer. Omeprazole also is used in combination with clarithromycin (dual therapy) or with amoxicillin and clarithromycin (triple therapy) for the treatment of *Helicobacter pylori* infection and duodenal ulcer disease in adults. Omeprazole also has been used in other multiple-drug regimens (with or without clarithromycin)† for the treatment of *H. pylori* infection associated with peptic ulcer disease. Omeprazole is used in adults and children 1 year of age and older for short-term treatment and symptomatic relief of gastroesophageal reflux disease (e.g., erosive esophagitis, heartburn) and as maintenance therapy following healing of erosive esophagitis to reduce its recurrence. The drug also is used as *self-medication* for short-term treatment and symptomatic relief of frequent heartburn in adults. Omeprazole is used for the long-term treatment of pathologic GI hypersecretory conditions in adults. Omeprazole also is used to decrease the risk of upper GI bleeding in critically ill adults.

■ **Duodenal Ulcer** ***Acute Therapy*** Omeprazole immediate- and delayed-release capsules, omeprazole immediate-release oral suspension, and omeprazole magnesium delayed-release oral suspension are used in adults for the short-term treatment of endoscopically or radiographically confirmed active duodenal ulcer. Antacids may be used concomitantly as needed for pain relief. In controlled studies in patients with endoscopically confirmed duodenal ulcers, reported rates of ulcer healing for omeprazole were substantially higher than those for placebo. In a multicenter, double-blind study in patients with endoscopically confirmed duodenal ulcer, reported rates of ulcer healing for an oral omeprazole dosage of 20 mg each morning or placebo were 41 or 13%, respectively, at 2 weeks and 75 or 27%, respectively, at 4 weeks. Omeprazole also produced greater reductions in daytime and nocturnal pain and antacid consumption than did placebo, with complete relief of pain in most patients usually occurring within 4 weeks after initiation of omeprazole therapy.

Omeprazole appears to be at least as effective as histamine H_2-receptor antagonists for short-term treatment of active duodenal ulcer. In a multicenter, controlled study in patients with endoscopically confirmed duodenal ulcers, 42 or 34% of ulcers were healed following oral administration of omeprazole 20 mg each morning or ranitidine 150 mg twice daily, respectively, for 2 weeks and 82 or 63%, respectively, were healed after 4 weeks of therapy. In another multicenter, controlled study in patients with endoscopically confirmed duodenal ulcers, ulcer healing occurred faster in patients given omeprazole 20 or 40 mg daily compared with patients given ranitidine 150 mg twice daily. Ulcer healing rates averaged 83 or 53% at 2 weeks, 97–100 or 82% at 4 weeks, and 100 or 94% at 8 weeks with the omeprazole regimens or ranitidine 150 mg twice daily, respectively. In several studies, ulcer healing was less likely in patients who were smokers and in those with large ulcers than in other patients.

Most patients with duodenal ulcer respond to omeprazole therapy during the initial 4-week course of therapy; an additional 4 weeks of therapy may contribute to healing in some patients.

Omeprazole delayed-release capsules and omeprazole magnesium delayed-release oral suspension are used in combination with clarithromycin and amoxicillin (triple therapy) for the treatment of *H. pylori* infection and duodenal ulcer disease in adults. Omeprazole delayed-release capsules and omeprazole magnesium delayed-release oral suspension also are used in combination with clarithromycin (dual therapy) in adults for the treatment of *H. pylori* infection and duodenal ulcer disease. Omeprazole also has been used in other multiple-drug regimens† for the treatment of *H. pylori* infection associated with peptic ulcer disease. Current epidemiologic and clinical evidence supports a strong association between gastric infection with *H. pylori* and the pathogenesis of duodenal and gastric ulcers; long-term *H. pylori* infection also has been implicated as a risk factor for gastric cancer. For additional information on the association of this infection with these and other GI conditions, see Helicobacter pylori Infection, under Uses, in Clarithromycin 8:12.12.92. Conventional antiulcer therapy with histamine H_2-receptor antagonists, proton-pump inhibitors, sucralfate, and/or antacids heals ulcers but generally is ineffective in eradicating *H. pylori*, and such therapy is associated with a high rate of ulcer recurrence (e.g., 60–100% per year). The American College of Gastroenterology (ACG), the National Institutes of Health (NIH), and most clinicians currently recommend that *all* patients with initial or recurrent duodenal or gastric ulcer and documented *H. pylori* infection receive anti-infective therapy for treatment of the infection. Although 3-drug regimens consisting of a bismuth salt (e.g., bismuth subsalicylate) and 2 anti-infective agents (e.g., tetracycline or amoxicillin plus metronidazole) administered for 10–14 days have been effective in eradicating the infection, resolving associated gastritis, healing peptic ulcer, and preventing ulcer recurrence in many patients with *H. pylori*-associated peptic ulcer disease, current evidence principally from studies in Europe suggests that 1 week of such therapy provides comparable *H. pylori* eradication rates. Other regimens that combine one or more anti-infective agents (e.g., clarithromycin, amoxicillin) with a bismuth salt and/or an antisecretory agent (e.g., omeprazole, lansoprazole, histamine H_2-receptor antagonist) also have been used successfully for *H. pylori* eradication, and the choice of a particular regimen should be based on the rapidly evolving data on optimal therapy, including consideration of the patient's prior exposure to anti-infective agents, the local prevalence of resistance, patient compliance, and costs of therapy.

Current evidence suggests that inclusion of a proton-pump inhibitor (e.g., omeprazole, lansoprazole) in anti-*H. pylori* regimens containing 2 anti-infectives enhances effectiveness, and limited data suggest that such regimens retain good efficacy despite imidazole (e.g., metronidazole) resistance. Therefore, the ACG and many clinicians currently recommend 1 week of therapy with a proton-pump inhibitor and 2 anti-infective agents (usually clarithromycin and amoxicillin or metronidazole), or a 3-drug, bismuth-based regimen (e.g., bismuth-metronidazole-tetracycline) concomitantly with a proton-pump inhibitor, for treatment of *H. pylori* infection.

Therapy with an antisecretory drug and a single anti-infective agent (i.e., "dual therapy") also has been used successfully for treatment of *H. pylori* infection. However, while some studies demonstrate that certain 2-drug anti-*H. pylori* regimens (e.g., clarithromycin-omeprazole, ranitidine bismuth citrate-omeprazole, amoxicillin-omeprazole) can successfully eradicate *H. pylori* infection and prevent recurrence of duodenal ulcer at least in the short term (e.g., at 6 months following completion of anti-*H. pylori* therapy), the ACG and some clinicians currently state that anti-*H. pylori* regimens consisting of at least 3 drugs (e.g., 2 anti-infective agents plus a proton-pump inhibitor) are recommended because of enhanced *H. pylori* eradication rates, decreased failures due to resistance, and shorter treatment periods compared with those apparently required with 2-drug regimens. Additional randomized, controlled studies comparing various anti-*H. pylori* regimens are needed to clarify optimum drug combinations, dosages, and durations of treatment for *H. pylori* infection. For a more complete discussion of *H. pylori* infection, including details about the efficacy of various regimens and rationale for drug selection, see Uses: Helicobacter pylori Infection, in Clarithromycin 8:12.12.92.

■ **Gastric Ulcer** ***Acute Therapy*** Omeprazole immediate- and delayed-release capsules, omeprazole immediate-release oral suspension, and omeprazole magnesium delayed-release oral suspension are used in adults for the short-term treatment and symptomatic relief of active benign gastric ulcer. In controlled studies in patients with endoscopically confirmed gastric ulcers, reported rates of ulcer healing with omeprazole therapy were substantially higher than those with placebo. In a multicenter, double-blind study in patients with endoscopically confirmed gastric ulcer, reported rates of ulcer healing with omeprazole 20 or 40 mg daily or placebo were 48, 56, or 31%, respectively, at 4 weeks and 75, 83, or 48%, respectively, at 8 weeks. In patients with an ulcer larger than 1 cm in size, the percentage of patients with healed ulcers at 8 weeks was greater with the 40-mg dosage than with the 20-mg dosage of omeprazole. Otherwise, for patients with smaller ulcers, no difference in ulcer healing rates between the 40- and 20-mg dosages was observed.

In a multicenter, comparative study in patients with endoscopically confirmed gastric ulcer, ulcer healing occurred at 4 weeks in 64 or 78% of patients receiving omeprazole 20 or 40 mg daily, respectively, compared with 56% of those receiving ranitidine 150 mg twice daily; at 8 weeks, 82, 91, or 78% of patients receiving omeprazole 20 mg daily, omeprazole 40 mg daily, or ranitidine 150 mg twice daily, respectively, had healed ulcers.

■ **Crohn's Disease-associated Ulcers** Although evidence currently is limited, proton-pump inhibitors have been used for gastric acid-suppressive therapy as an adjunct in the symptomatic treatment of upper GI Crohn's disease†, including esophageal, gastroduodenal, and jejunoileal disease. The drugs have been used for symptomatic relief of upper GI symptoms and to promote healing of Crohn's disease-associated peptic ulcer disease. Most evidence of efficacy to date has been from case studies in patients with Crohn's-associated peptic ulcer disease unresponsive to other therapies (e.g., histamine H_2-receptor antagonists, cytoprotective agents, antacids, and/or sucralfate). Omeprazole (20 or 40 mg daily) was associated with resolution of symptoms and ulcer healing within about 2 and 4 weeks, respectively, in some patients, while others required several months of acid-suppressive therapy. Subsequent symptomatic relief may be maintained with prolonged acid-suppressive therapy with a proton-pump inhibitor or H_2-receptor antagonist, with or without an immunosuppressive agent (e.g., azathioprine). Adjunctive inhibition of gastric acid secretion is likely to be more effective in promoting ulcer healing in Crohn's disease than corticosteroid therapy. Pending accumulation of more definitive evidence, some experts and clinicians state that therapy with a proton-pump inhibitor may be a useful adjunct to provide symptomatic relief and promote ulcer healing in patients with upper GI Crohn's disease.

For further information on the management of Crohn's Disease, see Uses: Crohn's Disease, in Mesalamine 56:36.

■ **Gastroesophageal Reflux** Omeprazole delayed-release capsules and omeprazole magnesium delayed-release oral suspension are used in adults and children 1 year of age and older, and omeprazole immediate-release capsules and immediate-release oral suspension are used in adults for the short-term treatment and symptomatic relief of gastroesophageal reflux disease (GERD) (e.g., erosive esophagitis, heartburn) and as maintenance therapy following healing of erosive esophagitis to prevent its recurrence. Safety and efficacy of omeprazole immediate-release capsules and immediate-release oral suspension have not been established in pediatric patients. Omeprazole magnesium delayed-release capsules are used in adults as *self-medication* for the short-term treatment and symptomatic relief of frequent heartburn.

GERD is considered to be a chronic disease, and many patients with GERD require long-term, even lifelong, treatment. Typical GERD symptoms include heartburn and/or regurgitation, often occurring after meals, especially large and/or fatty meals. The symptoms often are aggravated by recumbency or bending, and are relieved by antacids. GERD symptoms generally are controlled by appropriate medical therapy. Suppression of gastric acid secretion is considered by the ACG to be the mainstay of treatment for GERD, and a proton-pump inhibitor or histamine H_2-receptor antagonist is used to achieve acid suppression, control symptoms, and prevent complications of the disease. The ACG states that proton-pump inhibitors are more effective than histamine H_2-receptor antagonists for acute therapy of GERD and also are appropriate as maintenance therapy in many patients with the disease. Lifestyle modifications (e.g., elevation of the head of the bed, decreased dietary fat intake, smoking cessation, avoidance of recumbency for 3 hours after a meal, avoidance of foods that increase reflux, weight loss) should be initiated and continued throughout the course of treatment.

Acute Therapy Omeprazole delayed-release capsules and omeprazole magnesium delayed-release oral suspension are used in adults and children 1 year of age and older, and omeprazole immediate-release capsules and immediate-release oral suspension are used in adults for the short-term (4–8 weeks) treatment of endoscopically diagnosed erosive esophagitis in patients with GERD. Omeprazole delayed-release capsules and omeprazole magnesium delayed-release oral suspension are used in adults and children 1 year of age and older, and omeprazole immediate-release capsules and immediate-release oral suspension are used in adults for the short-term (4–8 weeks) treatment of symptomatic GERD (e.g., heartburn). Potential benefits of omeprazole in gastroesophageal reflux and esophagitis are thought to result principally from reduced acidity of gastric contents induced by the drug and resultant reduced irritation of esophageal mucosa; the drug can effectively relieve symptoms of esophagitis (e.g., heartburn) and promote healing of ulcerative and erosive lesions.

Drug Selection Considerations The ACG states that proton-pump inhibitors are more effective (i.e., provide more frequent and more rapid symptomatic relief and healing of esophagitis) than histamine H_2-receptor antagonists in the treatment of GERD. Although higher doses and more frequent administration of histamine H_2-receptor antagonists appear to increase their efficacy, such dosages are less effective than proton-pump inhibitor therapy. In addition, the ACG states that proton-pump inhibitors provide greater control of acid reflux than do prokinetic agents (e.g., cisapride [no longer commercially available in the US], metoclopramide) without the risk of severe adverse effects associated with these agents. Correction of esophageal and gastric motility defects that cause GERD might theoretically control the disease and make suppression of normal gastric acid secretion unnecessary, and prokinetic agents have been used in the treatment of GERD. However, cisapride was withdrawn from the US market because of its association with serious cardiac arrhythmias and death (see Cisapride 56:32), and metoclopramide frequently is associated with adverse CNS effects (e.g., restlessness, drowsiness, fatigue, lassitude). The ACG states that the frequent occurrence of adverse CNS effects has appropriately decreased regular use of metoclopramide for treatment of GERD. Cisapride or metoclopramide therapy appears to provide symptomatic relief and esophageal healing as effectively as a standard dosage of a histamine H_2-receptor antagonist, and improved efficacy has been reported when a prokinetic agent has been used in combination with a histamine H_2-receptor antagonist. Bethanechol, a cholinergic drug that increases GI motility, may increase lower esophageal sphincter pressure to a small degree, but the ACG states that the drug has limited efficacy in the treatment of GERD.

The ACG states that a histamine H_2-receptor antagonist administered daily in divided doses is effective in many patients with less severe GERD, and over-the-counter (OTC) antacids and histamine H_2-receptor antagonists are appropriate for *self-medication* as initial therapy in such individuals. A histamine H_2-receptor antagonist is particularly useful when taken before certain activities (e.g., heavy meal, exercise) that may result in acid reflux symptoms in some patients.

Other Considerations The ACG states that initial empiric therapy including suppression of gastric acid secretion and lifestyle modification is appropriate for patients with typical symptoms of uncomplicated GERD, and a diagnosis of GERD is reasonably assumed in those who respond to such therapy. Diagnostic testing (e.g., endoscopy, endoscopic biopsy, ambulatory pH testing, esophageal manometry) may be indicated when empiric drug therapy is unsuccessful, continuous medical therapy is required for symptomatic relief, chronic symptoms occur in patients at risk for esophageal metaplasia (e.g., Barrett's epithelium), or manifestations suggestive of complicated disease (e.g., dysphagia, bleeding, weight loss, choking [acid causing cough, shortness of breath, or hoarseness], chest pain) occur. In patients with symptoms refractory to empiric drug therapy, the diagnosis of GERD should be carefully confirmed with diagnostic testing before chronic, high-dose acid-suppression therapy or antireflux surgery is undertaken. Higher dosage and a longer therapeutic trial of a gastric antisecretory agent may be required in patients with atypical or extraesophageal symptoms (e.g., chronic chest pain, cough, hoarseness, asthma, dental erosions).

Clinical Trials In a controlled study in patients with manifestations of GERD (e.g., heartburn) and the absence of erosive esophageal lesions, symptomatic improvement with omeprazole was better than that with placebo. Complete resolution of heartburn was reported in 56, 36, or 14% of patients with endoscopically confirmed GERD and in 46, 31, or 13% of all enrolled patients after up to 4 weeks of therapy with omeprazole 20 mg daily, omeprazole 10 mg daily, or placebo, respectively.

In an uncontrolled, open-label study of 113 pediatric patients 2–16 years of age with a history of symptoms suggestive of nonerosive GERD, patients received an omeprazole dosage of 10 or 20 mg once daily (based on body weight) either as an intact capsule or as an open capsule in applesauce. The number and intensity of either pain-related symptoms or vomiting/regurgitation episodes was successfully reduced in 60 or 59% of those receiving omeprazole 10 or 20 mg, respectively. In another uncontrolled study in 12 children 1–2 years of age with a history of clinically diagnosed GERD, administration of omeprazole (0.5–1.5 mg/kg as an opened capsule in 8.4% sodium bicarbonate solution) for 8 weeks reduced episodes of vomiting/regurgitation from baseline by at least 50% in 9 patients (75%).

In controlled studies in patients with endoscopically diagnosed erosive esophagitis and symptoms of GERD, reported rates of healing with omeprazole were higher than those with placebo or an H_2-receptor antagonist. Healing rates from a controlled study were 39, 45, or 7% at 4 weeks and 74, 75, or 14% at 8 weeks for omeprazole 20 mg daily, 40 mg daily, or placebo, respectively. In controlled studies in patients with esophagitis, reported rates of healing were 57–74 or 27–43% at 4 weeks and 78–87 or 28–56% at 8 weeks in patients given omeprazole or ranitidine, respectively. Patients receiving omeprazole reported faster relief of daytime and nocturnal heartburn than those receiving placebo or an H_2-receptor antagonist. Omeprazole also has been shown to be effective in promoting healing and providing symptomatic relief in a substantial proportion of patients who failed to respond to an adequate course of relatively high dosages of an H_2-receptor antagonist.

In an uncontrolled, open-label dose-titration study in 57 pediatric patients aged 1–16 years of age with erosive esophagitis, omeprazole dosages of 0.7–3.5 mg/kg daily were required to promote healing. Dosages were initiated at 0.7 mg/kg daily and if therapeutic goals (intraesophageal pH below 4 for less than 6% of a 24-hour period) were not achieved after 5–14 days of treatment, the dosage was increased to 1.4 mg/kg daily. Based on additional measurements of intraesophageal pH and/or presence of pathologic acid reflux, the dosages were increased up to a maximum dosage of 3.5 mg/kg or 80 mg daily. After titration of omeprazole dosage, patients remained on treatment for 3 months (healing phase); patients with persistent erosive esophagitis after 3 months received a discretionary dosage increase and treatment for an additional 3 months. Erosive esophagitis was healed in 90% of children completing the first course of treatment in the healing phase of the study; 5% received a second treatment course. Healing occurred in 44% of the patients receiving omeprazole 0.7 mg/kg daily, and an additional 28% were healed with 1.4 mg/kg daily. After 3 months of treatment, 33% of the children had no overall symptoms, 57% had mild reflux symptoms, and 40% had less frequent regurgitation or vomiting.

Most patients with GERD respond to omeprazole therapy during an initial 8-week course of therapy; however, an additional 4 weeks of therapy may contribute to healing and symptomatic improvement in some patients. Short-term omeprazole therapy for the treatment of GERD will not prevent recurrence following discontinuance of the drug. If symptomatic GERD or erosive esophagitis recur, the manufacturers state that additional 4- to 8-week courses of omeprazole may be given. However, the ACG states that chronic therapy with a proton-pump inhibitor is appropriate in many patients with GERD.

Maintenance Therapy Omeprazole delayed-release capsules and omeprazole magnesium delayed-release oral suspension are used in adults and children 1 year of age and older, and omeprazole immediate-release capsules and immediate-release oral suspension are used in adults as maintenance therapy following healing of erosive esophagitis to reduce recurrence of the disease. In a multicenter, double-blind study, endoscopically documented remission of esophagitis was maintained at 6 months in 70, 34, or 11% of patients receiving omeprazole 20 mg daily, 20 mg on 3 consecutive days each week, or placebo, respectively. In another multicenter, double-blind study in patients with endoscopically confirmed healed esophagitis, endoscopic remission of esophagitis was maintained at 12 months in 77, 58, or 46% of patients receiving omeprazole 20 mg daily, 10 mg daily, or ranitidine 150 mg twice daily, respectively. However, patients with initial grade 3 or 4 erosive esophagitis required 20 mg of omeprazole daily for maintenance of healing.

In an uncontrolled, open-label study in 46 pediatric patients, maintenance dosages were half the dosages that were required for promotion of healing in 54% of the children studied. The remaining patients required a dosage increase (0.7 to a maximum of 2.8 mg/kg daily) for all or part of the maintenance period. There was no relapse of erosive esophagitis in 41% of the patients, and no symptoms occurred in 63% of the pediatric patients receiving omeprazole maintenance therapy.

Because GERD is a chronic condition, the ACG states that continuous therapy to control symptoms and prevent complications of the disease is appropriate, and chronic, even lifelong, use of a proton-pump inhibitor is effective and appropriate as maintenance therapy in many patients with GERD. Although neither medical nor surgical therapy of GERD appears to result in regression of Barrett's epithelium in the esophagus, chronic use of a proton-pump inhibitor at full dosage decreases the recurrence of esophageal strictures, increases the interval between symptomatic relapses, and may improve esophageal motility. In a double-blind, controlled study, antisecretory therapy had no clinically important effect on Barrett's mucosa in 106 patients receiving omeprazole (40 mg twice daily for 12 months, followed by 20 mg twice daily for 12 months) or ranitidine (300 mg twice daily for 24 months). Although neosquamous epithelium developed during antisecretory therapy, complete elimination of Barrett's mucosa was not achieved.

The frequent marked improvement in symptoms associated with full dosage of a proton-pump inhibitor generally is followed by rapid recurrence of symptoms once the drug is discontinued, and reduced-dosage regimens (e.g., every other day, "weekend" dosage) have not been shown to be consistently effective for maintenance therapy. In addition, many patients initially responding to proton-pump inhibitors experience symptomatic relapse and failure of esophageal healing when switched subsequently to a histamine H_2-receptor antagonist or prokinetic agent (e.g., cisapride, metoclopramide). Furthermore, prokinetic agents have been associated with severe adverse effects. Cisapride has been withdrawn from the US market because of its association with serious cardiac arrhythmias and death (see Cisapride 56:32), and metoclopramide frequently is associated with CNS adverse effects (e.g., restlessness, drowsiness, fatigue, lassitude) and may cause irreversible tardive dyskinesia with prolonged use. Once-daily administration of a histamine H_2-receptor antagonist at full dosage is *not* considered to be appropriate therapy for GERD. Although antacids and lifestyle modifications may provide long-term symptomatic control in up to 20% of patients with GERD, frequent symptomatic relapses may occur despite appropriate therapy in up to 50% of patients with chronic gastroesophageal reflux.

Self-Medication Omeprazole magnesium delayed-release capsules are used in adults 18 years of age or older as *self-medication* for short-term (14 days) treatment and symptomatic relief of frequent (e.g., 2 or more days a week) heartburn. Because 1–4 days may be required for complete relief of symptoms, omeprazole for *self-medication* is not intended for the immediate relief of heartburn, and other agents (e.g., antacids, histamine H_2-receptor antagonists) may be needed for initial relief. However, some individuals may experience complete relief of symptoms within 24 hours of taking the first dose of omeprazole. In 2 controlled studies, 50% of patients receiving omeprazole 20 mg daily experienced no heartburn during the first day of therapy, and the percentage of patients experiencing complete relief continued to increase in subsequent days; 30% of those receiving placebo experienced no heartburn during the first day of therapy. Omeprazole should not be used for *self-medication* of occasional heartburn (i.e., heartburn that occurs once weekly or less frequently) or for prevention of occasional meal- or beverage-induced heartburn.

■ **Pathologic GI Hypersecretory Conditions** Omeprazole delayed-release capsules and omeprazole magnesium delayed-release oral suspension are used in adults for the long-term treatment of pathologic GI hypersecretory conditions (e.g., Zollinger-Ellison syndrome, multiple endocrine adenomas, systemic mastocytosis). The drug reduces gastric acid secretion and associated symptoms (including diarrhea, anorexia, and pain) in patients with these conditions. In dosages ranging from 20 mg every other day to 360 mg daily, omeprazole can maintain basal acid secretion below 5 or 10 mEq/hour in patients who have or have not undergone gastric surgery, respectively. In addition, dosages ranging from 20–360 mg daily have been effective in resolving acid-related pathology in most patients with Zollinger-Ellison syndrome, including those whose symptoms were unresponsive to H_2-receptor antagonist therapy.

■ **Upper GI Bleeding** Omeprazole immediate-release oral suspension is used to decrease the risk of upper GI bleeding in critically ill adults. Efficacy of omeprazole was evaluated in a controlled, double-blind randomized clinical trial in critically ill patients who were randomized to receive either omeprazole immediate-release oral suspension (2 doses of 40 mg 6–8 hours apart on the first day, then 40 mg daily) via a gastric tube or IV cimetidine (300 mg loading dose, then 50–100 mg/hour continuously) for up to 14 days. The primary efficacy end point of the study was clinically important upper GI bleeding (defined as bright red blood that did not clear after tube adjustment and 5–10 minutes of lavage or positive test for occult blood in gastric aspirate ["coffee ground material"] for 8 consecutive hours on days 1 and 2, or for 2–4 hours on days 3–14 that did not clear with 100 mL of lavage). Omeprazole was at least as effective as IV cimetidine in preventing clinically important upper GI bleeding. In the intent-to-treat population, clinically important gastric bleeding occurred in 3.9% of patients receiving omeprazole and in 5.5% of those receiving IV cimetidine.

Dosage and Administration

■ **Administration** Omeprazole immediate-release and delayed-release capsules and omeprazole magnesium delayed-release tablets for *self-administration* are administered orally; oral suspensions of the drug are administered orally or through a gastric tube. To avoid decomposition of omeprazole in the acidic pH of the stomach, the commercially available delayed-release capsules and delayed-release oral suspension contain enteric-coated granules of the drug, and the immediate-release capsules and immediate-release oral suspension contain sodium bicarbonate.

Omeprazole immediate-release capsules (Zegerid®) are administered orally and must be swallowed intact with water; other liquids should not be used. The capsules should not be opened and mixed with food. Both the 20- and 40-mg capsules contain the same amount of sodium bicarbonate (1100 mg). Therefore, two 20-mg capsules are not equivalent to and should not be substituted for one 40-mg capsule.

Patients should be advised that the delayed-release capsules must be swallowed intact and *not* chewed or crushed. However, for adult and pediatric patients with difficulty swallowing, the delayed-release capsule may be opened, the contents carefully emptied on and mixed with a tablespoon of applesauce in a bowl, and the mixture swallowed immediately with a glass of cool water to ensure complete swallowing of the pellets. The applesauce should not be hot and should be soft enough to be swallowed without chewing. The applesauce and omeprazole enteric-coated pellet mixture should *not* be stored for future use. The manufacturer states that the 40-mg capsule, but not the 20-mg capsule, is bioequivalent when administered with or without applesauce. When the contents of a 20-mg capsule were administered with applesauce, the peak plasma omeprazole concentration decreased by 25%, but the area under the concentration-time curve (AUC) was not substantially changed. However, the clinical importance of this is unknown.

Tablets used for *self-medication* must be swallowed intact with a glass of water; the tablets should *not* be chewed or crushed and should *not* be crushed in food.

Omeprazole magnesium powder for delayed-release oral suspension (Prilosec®) should be reconstituted prior to administration by pouring the contents of a single-dose packet containing 2.5 or 10 mg of the drug into a small cup containing 5 or 15 mL, respectively, of water. The suspension should be stirred well and allowed to thicken for 2–3 minutes. Within 30 minutes of preparation, the mixture should be stirred and consumed. If any material remains in the cup after the mixture is ingested, additional water should be added, mixed, and ingested immediately. If the delayed-release oral suspension is to be administered through a nasogastric or gastric tube, the contents of a 2.5- or 10-mg packet should be mixed with 5 or 15 mL of water, respectively, in a catheter-tipped syringe and then shaken immediately. The mixture should be allowed to thicken for 2–3 minutes. The mixture should be administered within 30 minutes of reconstitution; prior to administration, the syringe should be shaken again and the mixture injected into the stomach through the nasogastric or gastric tube (French size 6 or larger). The syringe should be refilled with additional water (5 or 15 mL, respectively), shaken, and used to flush any remaining drug mixture from the nasogastric or gastric tube into the stomach.

Omeprazole powder for immediate-release oral suspension (Zegerid®) should be reconstituted prior to administration by pouring the contents of a single-dose packet containing 20 or 40 mg of the drug into a small cup containing 15–30 mL of water. The 20- and 40-mg powder for oral suspension packets contain the same amount of sodium bicarbonate (1680 mg). Therefore, two 20-mg packets are not equivalent to and should not be substituted for one 40-mg packet. The suspension should be stirred well and ingested immediately. The cup should be refilled with water and the contents ingested to ensure complete consumption of the dose. The manufacturer states that omeprazole powder for immediate-release oral suspension should not be mixed with any liquids (other than water) or foods. If the oral suspension is to be administered through a nasogastric or orogastric tube, the contents of each packet should be reconstituted with approximately 20 mL of water, stirred well and administered immediately. An appropriate-sized syringe should be used to instill the suspension into the tube. The suspension should then be flushed through the tube with 20 mL of water.

Following administration of delayed-release capsules of omeprazole with meals, the rate of GI absorption is reduced. Therefore, omeprazole should be taken before meals; administration up to 2 minutes prior to a meal reportedly has no adverse effect on oral bioavailability. However, since an acidic environment in the parietal cell canaliculi is required for conversion of proton-pump inhibitors (e.g., omeprazole) to their active sulfenamide metabolites, the American College of Gastroenterology suggests that proton-pump inhibitors are most effective when given about 30 minutes prior to meals; effectiveness may be compromised if these drugs are administered during the basal state (e.g., to fasting patients at bedtime) or concomitantly with other antisecretory agents (e.g., anticholinergics, histamine H_2-receptor antagonists, somatostatin analogs, misoprostol). The manufacturer states that delayed-release preparations of omeprazole should be administered at least 1 hour before a meal. Antacids may be administered concomitantly with the delayed-release preparations of omeprazole.

The manufacturer states that immediate-release preparations of omeprazole (Zegerid®) should be administered on an empty stomach at least 1 hour prior to a meal. For patients receiving continuous feedings via a nasogastric or orogastric tube, enteral feeding should be stopped temporarily for 3 hours before, and for 1 hour after administration of omeprazole immediate-release oral suspension. Also, the manufacturer states that antacids, antacid/alginic acid combinations, histamine H_2-receptor antagonists, or histamine H_2-receptor antagonist and antacid combinations may be used for "breakthrough" symptoms; however, efficacy of these agents for this use has not been established.

Omeprazole usually is administered once daily in the morning; however, administering the drug in divided doses (e.g., every 12 hours) has been reported to improve efficacy in patients receiving more than 80 mg daily.

■ **Dosage** The manufacturer states that omeprazole dosage adjustments based on age are not necessary in geriatric patients. However, since the bioavailability of omeprazole appears to be increased substantially in Asians, the manufacturer states that dosage adjustment should be considered in Asian patients, especially when such patients are receiving long-term omeprazole therapy for maintenance of healing of erosive esophagitis. There is no evidence from the omeprazole prescription safety database that Asians experience excess risk from omeprazole, or that accumulation of omeprazole in the blood is harmful when used over a short period of time (e.g., 14 days of *self-medication*) in Asian patients.

Dosage of omeprazole magnesium is expressed in terms of omeprazole.

Duodenal Ulcer For the short-term treatment of active duodenal ulcer, the usual adult dosage of omeprazole is 20 mg once daily. Therapy should be continued until healing occurs, usually within 2–4 weeks; some patients may benefit from an additional 4 weeks of therapy. Occasionally, dosages up to 40 mg daily may be necessary in patients who have been poorly responsive to therapy with H_2-receptor antagonists.

When omeprazole is used in combination with clarithromycin (dual therapy) for the treatment of *Helicobacter pylori* infection in patients with active duodenal ulcer, the usual adult dosage of omeprazole is 40 mg once daily (in the morning) for 14 days. In patients who have an active ulcer present at the time anti-*H. pylori* therapy is initiated, an additional 14 days of therapy with omeprazole 20 mg once daily is recommended for ulcer healing and symptom relief. When omeprazole is used in combination with clarithromycin and amoxicillin (triple therapy) for the treatment of *H. pylori* infection in patients with active duodenal ulcer, the usual adult dosage of omeprazole is 20 mg *twice* daily (morning and evening) for 10 days. In patients who have an active ulcer present at the time anti-*H. pylori* therapy is initiated, an additional 18 days of therapy with omeprazole 20 mg *once* daily is recommended for ulcer healing and symptom relief. Multiple-drug regimens currently recommended by the American College of Gastroenterology (ACG) and many clinicians for the treatment of *H. pylori* infection consist of a proton-pump inhibitor (e.g., omeprazole) and 2 anti-infective agents (e.g., clarithromycin and amoxicillin or metronidazole) or a 3-drug, bismuth-based regimen (e.g., bismuth-metronidazole-tetracycline) concomitantly with a proton-pump inhibitor; when omeprazole has been used in these regimens, dosages of 20 mg once daily to 80 mg twice daily (generally 20 mg twice daily) for 7–28 days have been used. While the minimum duration of therapy required to eradicate *H. pylori* infection with these 3- or 4-drug regimens has not been fully elucidated, the ACG and many clinicians state that treatment for longer than 1 week probably is not necessary. However, more prolonged therapy is recommended for patients with complicated, large, or refractory ulcers; therapy in such patients should be continued at least until successful eradication of *H. pylori* has been confirmed. (See Uses: Helicobacter pylori Infection, in Clarithromycin 8:12.12.92.)

Gastric Ulcer For the short-term treatment of active benign gastric ulcer, the usual adult dosage of omeprazole is 40 mg once daily for 4–8 weeks.

Gastroesophageal Reflux For the short-term, symptomatic treatment of gastroesophageal reflux disease (GERD) without erosive esophageal lesions, the usual adult dosage of omeprazole is 20 mg once daily for 4 weeks. For the short-term treatment of erosive esophagitis, the usual adult dosage of omeprazole is 20 mg once daily for 4–8 weeks. Occasionally, dosages up to 40 mg daily may be necessary in some patients. Therapy is continued until healing occurs, usually within 4–8 weeks; an additional 4 weeks of therapy (up to 12 weeks for a single course) may contribute to healing and symptomatic improvement in some patients. If erosive esophagitis or symptomatic GERD (heartburn) recurs, the manufacturer states that additional 4- to 8-week courses of omeprazole may be considered. However, the American College of Gastroenterology (ACG) states that chronic, even lifelong, therapy with a proton-pump inhibitor is appropriate in many patients with GERD.

For maintenance therapy following healing of erosive esophagitis to reduce recurrence, the usual adult dosage of omeprazole is 20 mg daily. Safety and efficacy of omeprazole maintenance therapy for longer than 1 year have not been established.

For the treatment of symptomatic GERD or erosive esophagitis and for maintenance of healing of erosive esophagitis in pediatric patients 1–16 years of age, a dosage of 5 mg of omeprazole daily is recommended for pediatric patients weighing at least 5 kg but less than 10 kg, 10 mg daily is recommended for those weighing at least 10 kg but less than 20 kg, and 20 mg daily is recommended for those weighing 20 kg or more. Omeprazole was administered as a single daily dose for 4 weeks in one study of children with symptomatic nonerosive GERD. On a mg/kg basis, the dosage of omeprazole required to heal erosive esophagitis in pediatric patients is greater than that required in adults. In an uncontrolled open-label study, dosages of 0.7–3.5 mg/kg daily (up to a maximum dosage of 80 mg daily) for 3–6 months were required for healing in children 1–16 years of age; a dosage of 0.7 mg/kg daily resulted in healing of erosive esophagitis in 44% of children, but a dosage of 1.4 mg/kg daily was required for healing to occur in an additional 28% of the children. In an uncontrolled open-label study of 46 pediatric patients, dosages of omeprazole for maintenance therapy following healing of erosive esophagitis were half those required for initial healing in 54% of children, but the remainder required an increased dosage (0.7 to a maximum of 2.8 mg/kg daily) for all or part of the maintenance period; maintenance therapy was continued for about 2 years.

Self-Medication For *self-medication* to relieve symptoms of frequent heartburn in adults 18 years of age or older, an omeprazole dosage of 20 mg once daily in the morning for 14 days is recommended. For *self-medication*, the manufacturer recommends that the dosage of omeprazole not exceed 20 mg in 24 hours. In addition, the drug should not be used for *self-medication* for longer than 14 days of *continuous* use and individuals should not exceed one course of therapy every 4 months unless otherwise directed by a clinician.

Pathologic GI Hypersecretory Conditions For the treatment of pathologic GI hypersecretory conditions (e.g., Zollinger-Ellison syndrome, multiple endocrine adenomas, systemic mastocytosis), dosages of omeprazole should be individualized according to patient response and tolerance. The usual initial adult dosage is 60 mg (as delayed-release capsules or delayed-release oral suspension) once daily. Subsequent omeprazole dosage should be adjusted as tolerated and necessary to adequately suppress gastric acid secretion, and therapy continued as long as clinically necessary. Daily dosages exceeding 80 mg should be administered in divided doses.

Oral dosages ranging from 20 mg every other day to 360 mg daily (given in 3 divided doses) have been necessary to maintain basal gastric acid secretion at less than 10 mEq/hour in patients without a history of gastric surgery and less than 5 mEq/hour in those who have undergone gastric surgery; determination of gastric acid secretion during the hour prior to a dose may be useful in establishing optimum dosage. Omeprazole has been given continuously for more than 5 years in some patients with Zollinger-Ellison syndrome.

Upper GI Bleeding For reduction of risk of upper GI bleeding in critically ill adults, the initial loading dose of omeprazole is 40 mg (as immediate-release oral suspension) followed by another 40-mg dose after 6–8 hours on the first day; thereafter, 40 mg (as immediate-release oral suspension) is administered once daily for up to 14 days. Safety and efficacy of omeprazole immediate-release oral suspension in critically ill patients for longer than 14 days have not been established.

■ **Dosage in Renal and Hepatic Impairment** Although pharmacokinetics may be altered in patients with renal impairment, dosage adjustment does not appear necessary in patients with such impairment. However, the manufacturers state that dosage adjustment should be considered in patients with hepatic impairment, particularly in such patients receiving long-term omeprazole therapy for maintenance of healing of erosive esophagitis. Some clinicians recommend that such patients with hepatic dysfunction receiving dosages exceeding 20 mg daily should be monitored closely for possible adverse effects.

Cautions

Omeprazole generally is well tolerated. The most frequent adverse effects associated with omeprazole therapy involve the GI tract (e.g., diarrhea, nausea, constipation, abdominal pain, vomiting, flatulence) and the CNS (e.g., headache, dizziness). In short-term studies, the incidence of reported adverse effects was similar in patients receiving omeprazole or placebo. In addition, while the most common effects have been reported in 1–7% of patients receiving omeprazole, they were considered by investigators as being possibly, probably, or definitely related to the drug in only 0.2–2.4% of patients. Overall, the frequency and type of adverse effects produced by omeprazole appear to be similar to those produced by ranitidine, and the frequency of omeprazole-induced effects does not appear to be affected by age in adults. In dose-ranging studies, a relationship between doses ranging from 10–60 mg and the frequency of adverse effects was not observed. Adverse effects were severe enough to result in discontinuance of omeprazole therapy in less than 2% of patients in clinical studies. The manufacturer states that the adverse event profile of omeprazole in pediatric patients is similar to that in adults. However, the most frequently reported adverse effects in pediatric patients were respiratory effects, which were reported in about 75 or 18% of those 1–2 or 2–16 years of age, respectively; fever was frequently reported (33%) in children 1–2 years of age, and accidental injuries were frequently reported (about 4%) in those 2–16 years of age.

In controlled clinical trials with combined omeprazole-clarithromycin or omeprazole-clarithromycin-amoxicillin therapy, no adverse drug experiences peculiar to these combinations were noted.

In a controlled clinical trial, the adverse event profile was similar for critically ill patients receiving either omeprazole immediate-release suspension or IV cimetidine for up to 14 days. The most frequent adverse effects reported in patients receiving omeprazole were pyrexia (20.2%), hypokalemia (12.4%), nosocomial pneumonia (11.2%), hyperglycemia (10.7%), thrombocytopenia (10.1%), hypomagnesemia (10.1%), and hypotension (9.6%).

■ **GI Effects** Diarrhea, abdominal pain, nausea, vomiting, constipation, flatulence, and acid regurgitation are the most frequent adverse GI effects reported with omeprazole therapy, occurring in about 1–5% of patients. Constipation, diarrhea, and gastric hypomotility occurred in 4.5, 3.9, and 1.7%, respectively, of critically ill patients receiving omeprazole immediate-release oral suspension or in 4.4, 8.3, and 3.3%, respectively, of those receiving IV cimetidine in a controlled clinical trial. Dysphagia, abdominal swelling, anorexia, irritable colon, fecal discoloration, pancreatitis (sometimes fatal), esophageal candidiasis, mucosal atrophy of the tongue, taste perversion, dry mouth, stomatitis, and microscopic colitis have been reported during postmarketing surveillance in patients receiving omeprazole; a causal relationship to the drug was not established in many cases. Benign gastric fundic polyps have been reported rarely and appear to resolve upon discontinuation of omeprazole therapy. Long-term administration of omeprazole has produced dose-related increases in gastric carcinoid tumors and enterochromaffin-like (ECL) cell hyperplasia in rats. Carcinoid tumors also have been observed in rats subjected to fundectomy or long-term treatment with other proton-pump inhibitors or high dosages of H_2-receptor antagonists. Gastric biopsy specimens obtained from patients in long-term studies with omeprazole have demonstrated an increased frequency of ECL cell hyperplasia. However, no cases of ECL cell carcinoid tumor, dysplasia, or neoplasia were found. (See Cautions: Mutagenicity and Carcinogenicity.)

Adverse GI effects observed in controlled trials with combined omeprazole and clarithromycin therapy that were not reported with omeprazole monotherapy include taste perversion in 15% of such patients and tongue discoloration in 2%.

As with other agents that elevate intragastric pH, administration of omeprazole for 14 days in healthy individuals increased the intragastric concentration of viable bacteria. The pattern of bacteria isolated was similar to that of saliva. Alterations in the intragastric bacterial flora were reversible following discontinuance of omeprazole. Treatment with proton-pump inhibitors may result in a slight increase in the risk of GI infections caused by such organisms as *Salmonella* and *Campylobacter* species.

Available data suggest a possible association between use of proton-pump inhibitors and risk of *Clostridium difficile* infection, including *C. difficile*-associated diarrhea and colitis (CDAD; also known as antibiotic-associated diarrhea and colitis or pseudomembranous colitis). In most observational studies to date, the risk of *C. difficile* infection in patients exposed to proton-pump inhibitors has ranged from 1.4–2.75 times that in patients not exposed to proton-pump inhibitors; however, some observational studies have found no increase in risk. Although many of the cases occurred in patients who had other risk factors for CDAD, including advanced age, comorbid conditions, and/or use of broad-spectrum anti-infectives, the US Food and Drug Administration (FDA) concluded that a contributory role for proton-pump inhibitors could not be definitively ruled out. The mechanism by which proton-pump inhibitors might increase the risk of CDAD has not been elucidated. Although it has been suggested that reduction of gastric acidity by gastric antisecretory agents might facilitate colonization with *C. difficile*, some studies have raised questions about this proposed mechanism or have suggested that the observed association is the result of confounding with other risk factors for CDAD. FDA also is reviewing the risk of CDAD in patients exposed to histamine H_2-receptor antagonists.

CDAD can be serious in patients who have one or more risk factors for *C. difficile* infection and are receiving concomitant therapy with a proton-pump inhibitor; colectomy and, rarely, death have been reported. FDA recommends that patients receive proton-pump inhibitors at the lowest effective dosage and for the shortest possible time appropriate for their clinical condition. Patients experiencing persistent diarrhea should be evaluated for CDAD and should be managed with appropriate supportive therapy (e.g., fluid and electrolyte management), anti-infective therapy directed against *C. difficile* (e.g., metronidazole, vancomycin), and surgical evaluation as clinically indicated.

■ **Nervous System Effects** Headache and dizziness are the most common adverse nervous system effects of omeprazole, occurring in 6.9 and 1.5%, respectively, of patients in US clinical studies. In a controlled clinical trial in critically ill patients, agitation occurred in 3.4 or 8.8% of patients receiving omeprazole immediate-release oral suspension or IV cimetidine, respectively. Asthenia has been reported in 1.1–1.3% of patients receiving omeprazole; in controlled studies, the incidence of this effect was similar in patients receiving omeprazole, ranitidine, or placebo. Psychic and sleep disturbances, including depression, agitation, aggression, hallucinations, confusion, insomnia, nervousness, tremors, apathy, somnolence, anxiety, and dream abnormalities, have been reported during postmarketing surveillance in patients receiving omeprazole; a causal relationship to the drug was not established in many cases. Other infrequent nervous system effects for which a causal relationship may not have been established include pain, fatigue, malaise, vertigo, paresthesia, and hemifacial dysesthesia.

■ **Respiratory Effects** Upper respiratory tract infections and cough have occurred in 1.9 and 1.1%, respectively, of patients receiving omeprazole; in controlled studies, the incidence of these effects was similar in patients receiving omeprazole, ranitidine, or placebo. Acute respiratory distress syndrome, respiratory failure, and pneumothorax occurred in 3.4, 1.7, and 0.6%, respectively, of critically ill patients receiving omeprazole immediate-release oral suspension or in 3.9, 3.3, and 4.4%, respectively, of those receiving IV cimetidine in a controlled clinical trial. Epistaxis and pharyngeal pain have been reported during postmarketing surveillance in patients receiving omeprazole; a causal relationship to the drug was not established. Adverse respiratory effects have been reported in about 75% of children 1–2 years of age and in about 18% of those 2–16 years of age.

Other adverse respiratory effects observed in controlled trials with combined omeprazole and clarithromycin therapy that were not reported with omeprazole monotherapy were rhinitis in 2% of patients, pharyngitis in 1%, and flu syndrome in 1%.

Community-acquired Pneumonia Administration of gastric antisecretory agents (e.g., proton-pump inhibitors, H_2-receptor antagonists) has been associated with an increased risk for developing certain infections (e.g., community-acquired pneumonia). A possible association between chronic administration of gastric acid-suppressive drugs and occurrence of community-acquired pneumonia has been evaluated using a large Dutch database (Integrated Primary Care Information [IPCI]) containing information on approximately 500,000 patients, 364,683 of whom (average follow-up: 2.7 years) were selected for evaluating any such association. During the 8-year population-based, case-control study, gastric acid suppressants were first prescribed in 19,459 individuals (12,337 received proton-pump inhibitors [mean duration of use: 5 months] and 10,177 received H_2-receptor antagonists [mean duration of use: 2.8 months]; some individuals received both drugs). Most patients did not undergo endoscopy and were treated empirically for upper GI symptoms. In this study, first occurrence of pneumonia (confirmed by radiography or microbiologic testing in 18% of patients) was reported in 5551 individuals; development of pneumonia occurred in 185 individuals while receiving gastric acid suppressants and in 292 individuals who had discontinued such use.

The adjusted relative risk for development of pneumonia (or the incidence rate) was 0.6, 2.3 and 2.5 per 100 person-years for individuals not receiving acid-suppressive drugs, for those receiving H_2-receptor antagonists, and for those receiving proton-pump inhibitors, respectively. Patients using gastric acid suppressants developed community-acquired pneumonia 4.5 (95% confidence interval of 3.8–5.1) times more often than those who never used such drugs. When evaluating use of all gastric acid suppressants, current use of the drugs was associated with a small (27%) overall increase in the risk of pneumonia (adjusted odds ratio 1.27 and 95% confidence interval of 1.06–1.54). Higher risks were observed for current users of proton-pump inhibitors and H_2-receptor antagonists; the adjusted relative risk for developing community-acquired pneumonia was 1.89 (95% confidence interval of 1.36–2.62) or 1.63 (95% confidence interval of 1.07–2.48), respectively, for these classes of drugs compared with those who discontinued using these agents. Estimates for developing pneumonia were higher (2.2 [95% confidence interval of 1.4–3.5] for proton-pump inhibitors and 1.7 [95% confidence interval of 0.8–2.9] for H_2-receptor antagonists) when only laboratory-confirmed cases of pneumonia were considered for analysis.

Although there was variation among individual proton-pump inhibitors and individual H_2-receptor antagonists, the numbers were small and the heterogeneity was not considered significant. For patients currently receiving proton-pump inhibitors, a dose-response relationship for developing pneumonia was observed; individuals using more than one defined daily dose of these drugs had a 2.3-fold increased risk for developing pneumonia compared with those who discontinued gastric acid suppressants. Such a dose-response relationship for developing pneumonia was not observed in patients receiving H_2-receptor antagonists; however, dose variation of these drugs was limited. Among current users of proton-pump inhibitors or H_2-receptor antagonists, the risk for developing pneumonia was most pronounced among those who initiated such therapies within the past 30 days.

Although the exact mechanism for development of community-acquired pneumonia in patients receiving gastric acid suppressants has not been fully elucidated, it has been suggested that reduction of gastric acid secretion by acid suppressive therapy and consequent increases of gastric pH may result in a favorable environment for the development of infection. Intragastric acidity constitutes a major nonspecific defense mechanism of the stomach to ingested pathogens; when gastric pH is less than 4, most pathogens are killed, while at higher gastric pH, pathogens may survive. Since intragastric pH should be maintained above 4 for several hours for the effective management of upper GI symptoms, acid suppressive therapy may lead to insufficient elimination or even increased colonization of ingested pathogens. Some evidence indicates that acid-suppressive therapy may result in nosocomial infections.

It should be considered that certain patients (e.g., those with pleuritic chest pain, hypothermia, systolic hypotension, tachypnea, diabetes mellitus, neoplastic disease, neurologic disease, bacteremia, leukopenia, multilobar pulmonary infiltrate) are at increased risk for developing infections and in these individuals community-acquired pneumonia may be associated with increased mortality. Some clinicians state that gastric acid-suppressive drugs should be used in patients in whom community-acquired pneumonia may be severe (e.g., those with asthma or chronic obstructive lung disease, immunocompromised patients, pediatric or geriatric individuals) only when clearly needed and the lowest effective dose should be employed.

■ **Musculoskeletal Effects** Back pain has been reported in about 1% of patients receiving omeprazole. Other musculoskeletal effects have been reported during postmarketing surveillance; a causal relationship to the drug was not established in many cases. Such effects include muscle cramps, myalgia, muscle weakness, joint pain, and leg pain. Bone fracture also has been reported during postmarketing surveillance in patients receiving omeprazole.

Findings from several observational studies suggest that therapy with proton-pump inhibitors, particularly in high dosages (i.e., multiple daily doses) and/or for prolonged periods of time (i.e., one year or longer), may be associated with an increased risk of osteoporosis-related fractures of the hip, wrist, or spine. The magnitude of the risk is not clear. To date, most of the observational studies assessing fracture risk in patients receiving proton-pump inhibitor therapy have limited the study population to individuals at least 50 years of age or older. Some of the studies found that the risk of hip fracture was increased with use of higher dosages of the drugs (e.g., average dosage of at least 1.5 "pills" daily) or with long-term use of the drugs, particularly long-term use of high dosages (e.g., dosages exceeding 1.75 times the average daily dosage for more than one year). Study results relating duration of proton-pump inhibitor use to emergence of increased fracture risk have been variable; one study found an increased risk of hip fracture after more than one year of use, whereas another study found an increased risk of hip fracture or osteoporosis-related fracture after 5 or 7 years of use, respectively. In yet another study, an increased risk of hip or spinal fracture was observed when the drugs were last used within the previous year but not when last use was more distant. One study that excluded patients with major risk factors for hip fracture found no relationship between proton-pump inhibitor use and hip fracture occurrence. Because these observational studies relied extensively on claims data from computerized administrative databases, the clinical relevance of reported findings is difficult to determine. FDA states that a causal relationship between proton-pump inhibitor use and fracture occurrence has not been established. To further evaluate this safety issue, FDA intends to analyze data obtained from several large, long-term, placebo-controlled trials of bisphosphonates in women at risk for osteoporosis-related fractures to assess risk of fractures based on use or nonuse of proton-pump inhibitors.

The mechanism by which proton-pump inhibitors may increase risk of fractures has not been elucidated, but it has been suggested that the mechanism may involve decreased insoluble calcium absorption secondary to increased gastric pH. Results of 3 observational studies showed no consistent relationship between proton-pump inhibitor use and bone mineral density. Additional studies evaluating effects of these drugs on bone homeostasis, including effects on biomarkers of bone formation and resorption, are ongoing.

■ **Hypomagnesemia** Hypomagnesemia, symptomatic and asymptomatic, has been reported rarely in patients receiving long-term therapy (for at least 3 months or, in most cases, for longer than one year) with proton-pump inhibitors, including omeprazole. (See Cautions: Precautions and Contraindications.) On March 2, 2011, after reviewing reports of hypomagnesemia in patients receiving proton-pump inhibitors (i.e., 38 cases from the Adverse Event Reporting System [AERS] database, 23 cases from the medical literature [at least 8 of which have been identified in AERS]), FDA confirmed that long-term use (in most cases, longer than one year) of proton-pump inhibitors may be associated with an increased risk of hypomagnesemia; the incidence of this adverse effect could not be quantified because hypomagnesemia is likely underrecognized and underreported. The mechanism responsible for hypomagnesemia associated with long-term use of proton-pump inhibitors is unknown; however, long-term use of these agents may be associated with changes in intestinal absorption of magnesium.

Clinically serious adverse effects associated with hypomagnesemia, which are similar to manifestations of hypocalcemia, include tetany, seizures, tremors, carpopedal spasm, arrhythmias (e.g., atrial fibrillation, supraventricular tachycardia), and abnormal QT interval. Other reported adverse effects include paresthesia, muscle weakness, muscle cramps, lethargy, fatigue, and unsteadiness. Manifestations of hypomagnesemia secondary to proton-pump inhibitor therapy may not be present in all patients. Hypomagnesemia also produces impaired parathyroid hormone secretion, which may lead to hypocalcemia. In most patients, treatment of hypomagnesemia required magnesium replacement and discontinuance of the proton-pump inhibitor. Following discontinuance of the proton-pump inhibitor, hypomagnesemia resolved within a median of one week; upon rechallenge, hypomagnesemia recurred within a median of 2 weeks. In a few patients in whom reinitiation of proton-pump inhibitor therapy was necessary, use of pantoprazole, the least potent proton-pump inhibitor, in combination with oral magnesium supplements resulted in acceptable control of GI discomfort (e.g., dyspepsia, reflux symptoms) without causing recurrent hypomagnesemia; further study is needed to establish the role, if any, of pantoprazole in patients with proton-pump inhibitor-induced hypomagnesemia.

Because nonprescription (over-the-counter, OTC) proton-pump inhibitors are marketed at low dosages and are only intended for a 14-day course of treatment up to 3 times per year, FDA states that there is very little risk of hypomagnesemia when these preparations are used in accordance with the directions on the labeling.

■ **Hepatic Effects** Mild and, rarely, marked increases in serum ALT (SGPT), AST (SGOT), γ-glutamyltransferase (GGT, γ-glutamyltranspeptidase, GGTP), alkaline phosphatase, and bilirubin concentrations have been reported during postmarketing surveillance in patients receiving omeprazole, but in many cases a causal relationship has not been established. In a controlled clinical trial in critically ill patients, abnormal liver function test results (not otherwise specified) occurred in 1.7 or 3.3% of patients receiving omeprazole immediate-release oral suspension or IV cimetidine, respectively. Rare occurrences of symptomatic liver disease have been reported, including hepatocellular, cholestatic, or mixed hepatitis, jaundice, liver necrosis, hepatic failure, and hepatic encephalopathy. Fatalities have been reported in some patients with hepatic failure or liver necrosis.

■ **Dermatologic and Sensitivity Reactions** In a controlled clinical trial in critically ill patients, rash and decubitus ulcer occurred in 5.6 and 3.4%, respectively, of patients receiving omeprazole immediate-release oral suspension or in 6.1 and 2.8%, respectively, of those receiving IV cimetidine.

Rash has been reported during postmarketing surveillance in patients receiving omeprazole; severe generalized reactions such as toxic epidermal necrolysis (some fatal), Stevens-Johnson syndrome, erythema multiforme, exfoliative dermatitis, and lichenoid eruptions have been reported. Other adverse dermatologic effects reported during postmarketing surveillance include skin inflammation, urticaria, purpura and/or petechiae (some cases with rechallenge) angioedema, pruritus, photosensitivity, alopecia, dry skin, and hyperhidrosis. Hypersensitivity reactions, including anaphylaxis, anaphylactic shock, angioedema, bronchospasm, interstitial nephritis, and urticaria, have been reported with omeprazole therapy. In many cases, a causal relationship to omeprazole has not been established.

■ **Hematologic Effects** Short-term use of omeprazole does not appear to be associated with substantial changes in hematologic parameters. However, in a controlled clinical trial of critically ill patients, thrombocytopenia, anemia, and aggravated anemia occurred in 10.1, 7.9 and 2.2%, respectively, of those receiving omeprazole immediate-release oral suspension, or in 6.1, 7.7, and 3.9%, respectively, of those receiving IV cimetidine. Agranulocytosis (occasionally fatal) has been reported rarely with omeprazole therapy, but a causal relationship to the drug is uncertain. Other adverse hematologic effects reported during postmarketing surveillance include pancytopenia, thrombocytopenia, neutropenia, leukopenia, anemia, and leukocytosis. Hemolytic anemia has been reported rarely in patients receiving omeprazole. In many cases, a causal relationship with omeprazole has not been established.

■ **Genitourinary Effects** Acute interstitial nephritis (some cases with positive rechallenge), urinary tract infection, microscopic pyuria, urinary frequency, elevated serum creatinine concentration, proteinuria, hematuria, glycosuria, testicular pain, and gynecomastia have been reported during postmarketing surveillance in patients receiving omeprazole; in many cases a causal relationship to the drug has not been established. Sexual disturbances (e.g., priapism) have been reported occasionally in patients receiving omeprazole.

■ **Cardiovascular Effects** In a controlled clinical trial of critically ill patients, hypotension and hypertension occurred in 9.6 and 7.9%, respectively, of patients receiving omeprazole immediate-release oral suspension, or in 6.6 and 3.3%, respectively, of those receiving IV cimetidine. Atrial fibrillation, ventricular tachycardia, bradycardia, supraventricular tachycardia and tachycardia (not otherwise specified) occurred in 6.2, 4.5, 3.9, 3.4, and 3.4%, respectively, of patients receiving omeprazole or in 3.9, 3.3, 2.8, 1.1, and 3.3%, respectively, of patients receiving IV cimetidine.

Chest pain, angina pectoris, tachycardia, bradycardia, palpitation, elevated blood pressure, and peripheral edema have been reported during postmarketing surveillance in patients receiving omeprazole; a causal relationship to the drug has not been established in many cases.

Although preliminary safety data from 2 long-term clinical trials comparing omeprazole or esomeprazole with antireflux surgery in patients with severe gastroesophageal reflux disease (GERD) raised concerns about a potential increased risk of cardiac events (myocardial infarction, heart failure, and sudden death) in patients receiving these drugs, FDA has reviewed safety data from these and other studies of the drugs and has concluded that long-term use of omeprazole or esomeprazole is not likely to be associated with an increased risk of such cardiac events. FDA has concluded that the apparent increase in cardiac events observed in the early analyses is not a true effect of the drugs.

In one study (a 14-year study comparing omeprazole with antireflux surgery in 298 patients), death from cardiac causes (heart failure, sudden death) or nonfatal myocardial infarction occurred in 8 or 9 patients, respectively, randomized to receive omeprazole and in 2 or 2 patients, respectively, randomized to undergo surgery. However, the findings may have been biased by baseline differences between the 2 groups, since patients in the surgery group tended to be younger and healthier and were less likely to have a history of myocardial infarction than those receiving omeprazole. In addition, some patients withdrew from the study prior to undergoing surgery, and several underwent surgery and also received drug therapy. Fewer than half of the patients remained in the study until its completion. Preliminary data from the second study (an ongoing study comparing esomeprazole with antireflux surgery in 554 patients) also suggested a difference in occurrence of cardiac events between treatment groups; however, after 5 years of follow-up, a similar number of patients in each treatment group had experienced cardiac-related events. FDA reviewed safety data from 14 additional comparative studies of omeprazole (including 4 placebo-controlled studies) and indicated that these studies do not suggest that omeprazole is associated with an increased risk of cardiac events. None of the studies were designed to assess cardiac risk, and patient follow-up in the studies was incomplete.

■ **Ocular Effects** Blurred vision, ocular irritation, dry eye syndrome, optic atrophy, anterior ischemic optic neuropathy, optic neuritis, and double vision have been reported during postmarketing surveillance in patients receiving omeprazole; in many cases a causal relationship to the drug has not been established.

■ **Other Adverse Effects** In a controlled clinical trial of critically ill patients, hypophosphatemia, hypocalcemia, fluid overload, and hyponatremia occurred in 6.2, 6.2, 5.1, and 3.9%, respectively, of patients receiving omeprazole immediate-release oral suspension or in 3.9, 5.5, 7.7, and 2.8%, respectively, of patients receiving IV cimetidine. Hypoglycemia, hyperkalemia, and hypernatremia occurred in 3.4, 2.2, and 1.7%, respectively, of those receiving omeprazole or in 4.4, 3.3, and 5%, respectively, of patients receiving IV cimetidine. Hyperpyrexia and edema occurred in 4.5 and 2.8%, respectively, of patients receiving omeprazole or in 1.7 and 6.1%, respectively, of patients receiving IV cimetidine. Sepsis (not otherwise specified), oral candidiasis, urinary tract infection, and candidal infection (not otherwise specified) occurred in 5.1, 3.9, 2.2, and 1.7%, respectively, of patients receiving omeprazole or in 5, 0.6, 3.3, and 3.9%, respectively, of patients receiving IV cimetidine.

Hyponatremia, hypoglycemia, weight gain, fever, and tinnitus have been reported during postmarketing surveillance in patients receiving omeprazole, but in many cases were not attributed to the drug. Acute gout also has been reported during omeprazole therapy.

Accidental injury occurred in about 4% of pediatric patients 2–16 years of age receiving omeprazole in clinical studies.

Limited evidence suggests that omeprazole therapy may cause a dose-dependent reduction in cyanocobalamin absorption, although conflicting data also exist. In one study, absorption of protein-bound cyanocobalamin decreased from a median value of 2.2 or 2.3% at baseline to 0.8 or 0.5% in healthy men receiving 20 or 40 mg, respectively, of omeprazole daily for 2 weeks. (See Cautions: Precautions and Contraindications.)

■ **Precautions and Contraindications** Symptomatic response to omeprazole should not be interpreted as precluding the presence of gastric malignancy.

While available endoscopic and histologic examinations of gastric biopsy specimens from humans exposed short-term to omeprazole have failed to reveal any associated risk, a dose-related increase in gastric carcinoid tumors has been observed during long-term exposure in animals, and further data from humans are needed to rule out the possibility of an increased risk of tumors during long-term exposure to the drug. (See Cautions: Mutagenicity and Carcinogenicity.)

Atrophic gastritis occasionally has been noted in gastric corpus biopsies from patients receiving long-term treatment with omeprazole.

The possibility that gastric acid-suppressive therapy may increase the risk of community-acquired pneumonia should be considered. (See Respiratory Effects: Community-acquired Pneumonia, in Cautions.)

Findings from several observational studies suggest that therapy with proton-pump inhibitors, particularly in high dosages and/or for prolonged periods of time, may be associated with an increased risk of osteoporosis-related fractures of the hip, wrist, or spine. (See Cautions: Musculoskeletal Effects.) Although controlled studies are required to confirm these findings, patients should receive proton-pump inhibitors at the lowest effective dosage and for the shortest possible time appropriate for their clinical condition. Individuals using omeprazole for *self-medication* should be advised that they should use the drug only as directed for no longer than 14 days of *continuous* use and that they should not exceed one course of therapy every 4 months. Patients who are at risk for osteoporosis-related fractures should receive an adequate intake of calcium and vitamin D and should have their bone health assessed and managed according to current standards of care.

Long-term use (in most cases, longer than one year) of proton-pump inhibitors may be associated with an increased risk of hypomagnesemia. In patients expected to receive long-term therapy with a proton-pump inhibitor or in those receiving a proton-pump inhibitor concomitantly with digoxin or drugs that may cause hypomagnesemia (e.g., diuretics), clinicians should consider measurement of serum magnesium concentrations prior to initiation of prescription proton-pump inhibitor therapy and periodically thereafter. Patients receiving proton-pump inhibitors should be advised to seek immediate care if manifestations of hypomagnesemia (e.g., arrhythmias, tetany, tremor, seizures) occur; in children, abnormal heart rates may cause fatigue, upset stomach, dizziness, and lightheadedness. Patients receiving nonprescription proton-pump inhibitors should be advised to follow the manufacturer's directions on the package carefully; if therapy with a nonprescription proton-pump inhibitor is continued for longer than the maximum recommended duration (an unlabeled [off-label] use), patients should be informed of the potential increased risk of hypomagnesemia.

Although preliminary safety data from 2 long-term clinical trials comparing omeprazole or esomeprazole with antireflux surgery in patients with severe gastroesophageal reflux disease (GERD) raised concerns about a potential increased risk of cardiac events (myocardial infarction, heart failure, and sudden death) in patients receiving these drugs, FDA has reviewed safety data from these and other studies of the drugs and has concluded that long-term use of omeprazole or esomeprazole is not likely to be associated with an increased risk of such cardiac events. FDA has concluded that the apparent increase in cardiac events observed in the early analyses is not a true effect of the drugs and recommends that clinicians continue to prescribe and patients continue to use these drugs in the manner described in the manufacturers' labelings. (See Cautions: Cardiovascular Effects.)

Because available data suggest a possible association between use of proton-pump inhibitors and risk of *Clostridium difficile* infection, patients should be advised to contact a clinician if persistent watery stools, abdominal pain, and fever occur.

Limited data suggest that omeprazole therapy may cause a dose-dependent reduction in cyanocobalamin absorption. (See Cautions: Other Adverse Effects.) Whether such a reduction in cyanocobalamin absorption can result in a deficiency of the vitamin has not been determined, although it has been suggested that pending further study, serum cyanocobalamin concentrations should be monitored in patients receiving long-term therapy with omeprazole.

Increases in intragastric pH may result in hypergastrinemia, enterochromaffin-like cell hyperplasia, and increased serum chromogranin A (CgA) concentrations. Increased CgA concentrations may produce false-positive results for diagnostic tests for neuroendocrine tumors. Clinicians should temporarily discontinue omeprazole therapy before assessing CgA concentrations and consider repeating the test if initial CgA concentrations are high.

Each 20- or 40-mg packet of omeprazole powder for immediate-release oral suspension (Zegerid®) contains 1680 mg of sodium bicarbonate (460 mg [20 mEq] of sodium). Each 20- or 40-mg immediate-release capsule of omeprazole (Zegerid®) contains 1100 mg of sodium bicarbonate (304 mg [13 mEq] of sodium). The sodium content of these preparations should be taken into consideration in patients whose sodium intake must be restricted; increased sodium intake may produce edema and weight increase. Sodium bicarbonate may cause metabolic alkalosis, seizures, and tetany, and chronic use with calcium or milk may cause milk-alkali syndrome. Acute toxicity associated with sodium bicarbonate overdose may include hypocalcemia, hypokalemia, hypernatremia, and seizures. Sodium bicarbonate should be used with caution in patients with Bartter's syndrome, hypokalemia, respiratory alkalosis, or acid-base abnormalities. Sodium bicarbonate is contraindicated in patients with metabolic alkalosis or hypocalcemia.

In clinical trials in patients who received combined clarithromycin-omeprazole therapy for *H. pylori* infection, some *H. pylori* isolates demonstrated an increase in clarithromycin MICs over time, indicating decreased susceptibility and increasing resistance to the drug. Susceptibility testing should be performed if possible in patients with *H. pylori* infection in whom therapy with combined clarithromycin-omeprazole fails (i.e., as determined in clinical trials by a positive result for *H. pylori* on culture or histologic testing 4 weeks following completion of therapy); if resistance to clarithromycin is demonstrated or susceptibility testing is not possible, alternative anti-infective therapy should be instituted. The American College of Gastroenterology (ACG) states that clarithromycin or metronidazole should not be used subsequently in patients with *H. pylori* infection who fail therapy that includes these drugs since resistance consistently emerges during such unsuccessful therapy. (See Uses: *Helicobacter pylori* Infection, in Clarithromycin 8:12.12.92.)

Patients should be advised to consult their clinician before using omeprazole for *self-medication* if they are taking warfarin, an antifungal agent (e.g., ketoconazole), diazepam, or digoxin. Patients with heartburn that has persisted for more than 3 months or heartburn in conjunction with lightheadedness, sweating, or dizziness should consult their clinician before using omeprazole for *self-medication*. Patients should be advised to consult their clinician before using omeprazole for *self-medication* if they are experiencing chest or shoulder pain with lightheadedness, shortness of breath, sweating, or pain spreading to arms, neck, or shoulders. Those with frequent chest pain, unexplained weight loss, nausea and vomiting, stomach pain, or frequent wheezing (especially with heartburn) also should consult their clinician before using omeprazole for *self-medication*. Patients should discontinue taking omeprazole for *self-medication* and consult their clinician if heartburn persists, or worsens after 14 days of therapy, or a course of treatment is needed more frequently than every 4 months. Patients with difficulty or pain with swallowing, vomiting with blood, or bloody or blackened stools should not use omeprazole for *self-medication*; such manifestations should be reported promptly to a clinician, since they may be indicative of a serious condition requiring alternative treatment. Women who are pregnant or breast feeding should consult their clinician before using omeprazole for *self-medication*.

Omeprazole is contraindicated in patients with known hypersensitivity to the drug, esomeprazole, or other substituted benzimidazoles (e.g., lansoprazole, pantoprazole, rabeprazole), or any ingredient in the formulation.

■ Pediatric Precautions Safety and efficacy of omeprazole (omeprazole delayed-release capsules and omeprazole magnesium delayed-release oral suspension) have been established for the treatment of symptomatic gastroesophageal reflux disease (GERD), erosive esophagitis, and maintenance of healing of erosive esophagitis in pediatric patients 1–16 years of age. Use in pediatric patients is supported by adequate and well-controlled studies in adults and additional pharmacokinetic data and clinical and safety studies in children. (See Gastroesophageal Reflux: Clinical Trials and see Gastroesophageal Reflux: Maintenance Therapy, in Uses.)

Safety and efficacy of omeprazole in pediatric patients younger than 1 year of age have not been established. Safety and efficacy of omeprazole for *self-medication* in those younger than 18 years of age have not been established. Safety and efficacy of omeprazole immediate-release capsules and oral suspension (Zegerid®) have not been established in pediatric patients younger than 18 years of age.

■ Geriatric Precautions In US and European clinical trials, more than 2000 patients treated with omeprazole were 65 years of age or older. Although no overall differences in efficacy or safety were observed between geriatric and younger patients, and other clinical experience revealed no evidence of age-related differences, the possibility that some older patients may exhibit increased sensitivity to the drug cannot be ruled out.

Although elimination of omeprazole may be somewhat delayed and oral bioavailability increased in the elderly, clinically important differences in the pharmacokinetic profile of omeprazole between geriatric individuals and younger adults generally do not appear to exist. Therefore, dosage adjustment solely on the basis of age generally is not required for geriatric patients.

The adverse effect profile of omeprazole is similar in geriatric patients and those 65 years of age and younger.

■ Mutagenicity and Carcinogenicity No evidence of mutagenicity was observed in vivo in the rat liver DNA damage assay or in some in vitro test systems, including the microbial (Ames test) and mammalian (mouse lymphoma) assays. Omeprazole was positive for clastogenic effects in an in vitro human lymphocyte chromosome aberration assay, in 1 of 2 in vivo mouse micronucleus tests, and in an in vivo bone marrow cell chromosomal aberration assay.

In animals, long-term administration of relatively high dosages of omeprazole results in morphologic changes in the gastric mucosa. Such changes observed in rats during long-term (24-month) administration of the drug include dose-related increases in gastric carcinoid tumors and enterochromaffin-like (ECL) cell hyperplasia, which are thought to represent exaggerated physiologic responses occurring secondary to profound inhibition of gastric acid secretion and subsequent hypergastrinemia and reversible hypertrophy of oxyntic mucosa. While such changes have not been observed following short-term administration of the drug in humans, additional long-term data are needed to rule out the possibility of an increased risk of gastric tumors in patients receiving long-term omeprazole therapy. In two 24-month studies in rats given omeprazole dosages of 1.7, 3.4, 13.8, 44, and 140.8 mg/kg daily (about 0.7–57 times the human dosage of 20 mg daily based on body surface area), the drug caused a dose-related increase in gastric ECL cell carcinoids in both male and female rats; the increase in carcinoids occurred more frequently in female rats. In addition, ECL cell hyperplasia was observed in both male and female rats receiving omeprazole. In female rats given omeprazole dosages of 13.8 mg/kg daily (about 6 times the human dosage of 20 mg daily based on body surface area) for 1 year and then observed for another year without the drug, carcinoids were not detected but ECL hyperplasia occurred in 94% of rats given omeprazole versus 10% of controls at the end of 1 year; at the end of the second year, hyperplasia was observed in 46% of rats given omeprazole versus 26% of controls. Gastric adenocarcinoma was reported in one rat; similar tumors were not seen in male or female rats treated for 2 years. For this strain of rat no similar tumor had been noted historically, but the finding of this tumor in only one rat is difficult to interpret. In a 1-year toxicity study in Sprague-Dawley rats, brain astrocytomas were found in a small number of males (but not in females) given omeprazole at dosage levels of 0.4, 2, and 16 mg/kg daily (about 0.2–6.5 times the human dosage of 20 mg daily based on body surface area). In a 2-year carcinogenicity study in Sprague-Dawley rats, no astrocytomas were found in males or females at 140.8 mg/kg daily (about 57 times the human dosage of 20 mg daily based on body surface area). Long-term carcinogenicity studies (78 weeks) in mice did not demonstrate increased tumor occurrence; however, the manufacturer states that the study was inconclusive. The drug was not carcinogenic in a 26-week p53± transgenic mouse study.

A number of patients with Zollinger-Ellison syndrome receiving long-term therapy with omeprazole have developed gastric carcinoids; however, Zollinger-Ellison syndrome is known to be associated with such tumors, and these findings are believed to be related to the underlying disease rather than to omeprazole therapy. Gastric corpus biopsy specimens obtained from more than 3000 patients in long-term studies with omeprazole have demonstrated an increased frequency of ECL cell hyperplasia (including micronodular hyperplasia of argyrophil cells) in association with increased plasma gastrin concentrations and progression to subatrophic or atrophic gastritis. However, no evidence of ECL cell carcinoids, dysplasia, or neoplasia has been observed in these patients, and it has been suggested that the development of mucosal cell hyperplasia may be related to the severity and natural progression of gastritis rather than to hypergastrinemia.

■ Pregnancy, Fertility, and Lactation ***Pregnancy*** Omeprazole crosses the placenta in animals and in humans. Reproductive studies in rats or rabbits using omeprazole dosages up to 138 or 69 mg/kg daily (about 56 times the human dosage of 20 mg daily based on body surface area), respectively, have not revealed evidence of teratogenicity. However, in rabbits given omeprazole dosages of 6.9–69.1 mg/kg daily (about 5.6–56 times the human dosage of 20 mg daily based on body surface area), dose-related increases in embryolethality, fetal resorptions, and pregnancy loss occurred. In rats, dose-related embryo/fetal toxicity and postnatal developmental toxicity were observed in offspring resulting from administration of omeprazole in dosages of 13.8–138 mg/kg daily (about 5.6–56 times the human dosage of 20 mg daily based on body surface area) to parents.

There are no adequate and controlled studies using omeprazole in pregnant women. Most reported experience with omeprazole during human pregnancy has been first trimester exposure; duration of use (i.e., intermittent, long-term) rarely has been specified. A review of published data (considered fair in quality and quantity) by the Teratogen Information System (TERIS) concluded that therapeutic dosages of omeprazole during pregnancy are unlikely to pose a substantial teratogenic risk. Data from cohort studies have not demonstrated that omeprazole exposure is associated with a statistically significant increase in the rate of major birth defects; however, the studies lacked the power to detect small increases in birth defects or in rare malformations. Therefore, additional study is needed.

A population-based retrospective cohort epidemiologic study using data from the Swedish Medical Birth Registry reported on outcomes in infants whose mothers used omeprazole during pregnancy; most (about 86%) were exposed to omeprazole during the first trimester, 4% during and beyond the first trimester, and about 10% were exposed only after the first trimester of pregnancy. Exposure to omeprazole was not associated with increased risk of any malformation (odds ratio 0.82 and 95% confidence interval of 0.50–1.34), low birth weight, or low Apgar score. The number of infants born with ventricular septal defects and the number of stillborn infants was slightly higher in the omeprazole-exposed infants than the expected number in the normal population, but both effects may be random. In an earlier study using data from the Swedish Medical Birth Registry, exposure to proton-pump inhibitors was not associated with increased risk of congenital malformation.

In a retrospective cohort study, the incidence of congenital malformations in women who received omeprazole or histamine H_2-antagonists (cimetidine or ranitidine) in the first trimester of pregnancy was compared with a control group of women who were not exposed to acid-suppressant drugs. The overall malformation rate was 4.4% (95% confidence interval of 3.6–5.3), the malformation rate for nonexposed women was 3.8% (95% confidence interval of 3–4.9), and the malformation rate associated with omeprazole exposure was 3.6% (95% confidence interval of 1.5–8.1). The relative risk of malformations associated with first-trimester exposure to omeprazole (compared with nonexposed women) was 0.9 (95% confidence interval of 0.3–2.2). The study could effectively rule out a relative risk greater than 2.5 for all malformations. Rates of preterm delivery or growth retardation did not differ between the groups.

A controlled prospective observational study followed women exposed to omeprazole, disease-paired controls exposed to histamine H_2-receptor antagonists, and controls exposed to nonteratogenic agents (e.g., acetaminophen, dental radiation) during pregnancy; major congenital malformations occurred in 4, 2.8, and 2%, respectively, of live births, or in 5.1%, 3.1%, and 3%, respectively, of live births when exposure occurred during the first trimester of pregnancy. Rates of spontaneous and elective abortions, preterm deliveries, gestational age at delivery, and mean birth weight did not differ between the groups. The study lacked statistical power to detect a small increase in major malformations; the sample size had 80% power to detect a fivefold increase in the major malformation rate.

The manufacturers state that several studies reported that adverse short-term effects were not observed in infants when a single oral or IV dose of omeprazole was administered to pregnant women as premedication for cesarean section under general anesthesia.

Omeprazole immediate-release capsules and oral suspension contain sodium bicarbonate; chronic use of sodium bicarbonate may lead to systemic alkalosis, and increased sodium intake may produce edema and weight increase.

Because there are no adequate and controlled studies using omeprazole in pregnant women, and because studies to date in animals and pregnant women cannot rule out the possibility of harm, the drug should be used during pregnancy only when clearly needed and only when the potential benefits justify the possible risk to the fetus.

Fertility Reproductive studies in rats using omeprazole dosages of up to 138 mg/kg daily (about 56 times the human dose of 20 mg daily based on body surface area) have not revealed evidence of impaired fertility.

Lactation Omeprazole is distributed into human milk; following oral administration of omeprazole 20 mg in one lactating woman, the peak concentration of the drug in breast milk was less than 7% of the peak serum concentration. Because of the potential for serious adverse reactions to omeprazole in nursing infants, and because of the potential for tumorigenicity shown in animal studies, a decision should be made whether to discontinue nursing or the drug, taking account the importance of the drug to the woman. In addition, omeprazole immediate-release capsules and oral suspension contain sodium bicarbonate, which should be used with caution in nursing mothers.

Drug Interactions

■ **Drugs Affecting or Metabolized by Hepatic Microsomal Enzymes** Omeprazole can prolong the elimination of diazepam, warfarin (the *R*-isomer), phenytoin, cyclosporine, disulfiram, and benzodiazepines, and the possibility that dosages of these and other drugs that are metabolized by cytochrome P-450 (CYP)-mediated oxidation in the liver may require adjustment should be considered when concomitant omeprazole therapy is initiated or discontinued.

Omeprazole is extensively metabolized by the CYP enzyme system. Drugs that induce CYP2C19 or CYP3A4 (e.g., rifampin, St. John's wort [*Hypericum perforatum*]) can substantially decrease omeprazole concentrations. In a crossover study, concomitant use of omeprazole and St. John's wort (300 mg 3 times daily for 14 days) in healthy men resulted in decreased exposure to omeprazole; peak plasma concentrations and area under the concentration-time curve (AUC) of omeprazole were decreased by 37.5 and 37.9%, respectively, in poor CYP2C19 metabolizers and by 49.6 and 43.9%, respectively, in extensive metabolizers. Concomitant use of omeprazole with St. John's wort or rifampin should be avoided.

■ **Drugs that Cause Hypomagnesemia** In patients receiving diuretics (i.e., loop or thiazide diuretics) or other drugs that may cause hypomagnesemia, monitoring of magnesium concentrations should be considered prior to initiation of prescription proton-pump inhibitor therapy and periodically thereafter. (See Cautions: Hypomagnesemia.)

■ **Gastric pH-dependent Drugs** The possibility that omeprazole-induced increases in gastric pH may affect the bioavailability of drugs such as ketoconazole, ampicillin esters, iron salts, erlotinib, or digoxin (where gastric acidity is an important determinant in oral absorption) should be considered. Concomitant use of omeprazole 20 mg once daily and digoxin in healthy individuals increased digoxin bioavailability by 10% (up to 30% in some individuals); monitoring for manifestations of digoxin toxicity may be required when omeprazole is used concomitantly.

■ **Antiretroviral Agents** ***Atazanavir*** Concomitant use of omeprazole 40 mg once daily and atazanavir (with or without low-dose ritonavir) results in a substantial decrease in plasma concentrations of atazanavir and possible loss of the therapeutic effect of the antiretroviral agent. The manufacturers of omeprazole state that concomitant use of omeprazole with atazanavir is not recommended. If atazanavir is administered in an antiretroviral treatment-naive patient receiving a proton-pump inhibitor, a *ritonavir-boosted* regimen of 300 mg of atazanavir once daily with ritonavir 100 mg once daily with food is recommended. The dose of the proton-pump inhibitor should be administered approximately 12 hours before *ritonavir-boosted* atazanavir; the dose of the proton-pump inhibitor should not exceed omeprazole 20 mg daily (or equivalent). Concomitant use of proton-pump inhibitors with atazanavir is not recommended in antiretroviral treatment-experienced patients.

Darunavir Concomitant use of omeprazole with *ritonavir-boosted* darunavir resulted in decreased plasma concentrations of omeprazole; plasma concentrations of darunavir were not affected. However, no dosage adjustment of either drug is required when omeprazole is used concomitantly with *ritonavir-boosted* darunavir.

Fosamprenavir Concomitant use of esomeprazole and fosamprenavir increased the AUC of esomeprazole by about 55% but did not substantially alter plasma concentrations of amprenavir (active metabolite of fosamprenavir). Concomitant use of esomeprazole and *ritonavir-boosted* fosamprenavir did not substantially affect concentrations of either amprenavir or esomeprazole. No dosage adjustment is required when proton-pump inhibitors are used concomitantly with fosamprenavir (with or without ritonavir).

Lopinavir Concomitant use of omeprazole with the fixed combination of lopinavir and ritonavir (lopinavir/ritonavir) did not have a clinically important effect on plasma concentrations or AUC of lopinavir. No dosage adjustment is required when proton-pump inhibitors are used concomitantly with lopinavir/ritonavir.

Nelfinavir Concomitant use of omeprazole 40 mg once daily (given 30 minutes before a nelfinavir dose) and nelfinavir 1.25 g twice daily decreased peak plasma concentrations and AUCs of nelfinavir by 37 and 36%, respectively, and of its major active metabolite M8 by 89 and 92%, respectively. The manufacturers of omeprazole state that concomitant use with nelfinavir is not recommended.

Raltegravir Concomitant use of omeprazole with raltegravir resulted in substantially increased peak plasma concentration and AUC of raltegravir; however, no dosage adjustment is recommended when proton-pump inhibitors are used concomitantly with raltegravir.

Rilpivirine Concomitant use of omeprazole with rilpivirine resulted in decreased plasma concentrations and AUC of rilpivirine. Concomitant use of rilpivirine and proton-pump inhibitors is contraindicated.

Saquinavir Concomitant use of omeprazole 40 mg once daily and saquinavir 1 g twice daily (with ritonavir 100 mg twice daily) increased peak serum concentrations and AUC of saquinavir by 75 and 82%, respectively. If omeprazole is used concomitantly with *ritonavir-boosted* saquinavir, clinical and laboratory monitoring for saquinavir toxicity is recommended, and reduction of saquinavir dosage should be considered.

Tipranavir Concomitant use of omeprazole with *ritonavir-boosted* tipranavir resulted in decreased plasma concentrations of omeprazole; plasma concentrations of tipranavir were not affected. An increase in omeprazole dosage may be required when omeprazole is used concomitantly with *ritonavir-boosted* tipranavir.

■ **Cilostazol** Concomitant use of omeprazole (40 mg daily for one week) and cilostazol in healthy individuals resulted in increased peak plasma concentrations and AUC of cilostazol (by 18 and 16%, respectively) and one of its active metabolites (by 29 and 69%, respectively). Therefore, reduction of cilostazol dosage (from 100 mg twice daily to 50 mg twice daily) should be considered during such concomitant use.

■ **Clarithromycin** Concomitant administration of clarithromycin (500 mg 3 times daily) and omeprazole (40 mg daily) in healthy men resulted in increases of 30, 89, and 34% in the peak plasma concentration, AUC, and elimination half-life, respectively, of omeprazole. Increases in omeprazole AUC and half-life had a modest effect on gastric pH; mean 24-hour gastric pH was 5.2 when omeprazole was administered alone versus 5.7 with concomitant administration of clarithromycin. Acid suppression resulting from omeprazole appears to enhance the activity of anti-infective therapy against *H. pylori*. Serum concentrations and AUCs of clarithromycin and 14-hydroxyclarithromycin also are increased by concomitant administration of omeprazole. (See Pharmacokinetics: Absorption, in Clarithromycin 8:12.12.92.)

■ **Clopidogrel** Because omeprazole inhibits CYP2C19, concurrent use of omeprazole with clopidogrel, which is metabolized to its active metabolite by CYP2C19, reduces plasma concentrations of clopidogrel's active metabolite and potentially may reduce clopidogrel's clinical efficacy.

In a crossover clinical trial in healthy individuals who received clopidogrel (a 300-mg loading dose, followed by 75 mg daily) alone or with omeprazole (80 mg administered at the same time as the clopidogrel dose) for 5 days, exposure to the active metabolite of clopidogrel was decreased by 46% and 42% on days 1 and 5, respectively, when the drugs were administered simultaneously. In addition, mean inhibition of platelet aggregation was reduced by 47% at 24 hours and by 30% on day 5. When administration of the 2 drugs (at the same dosages) was separated by 12 hours in another study, results were similar. Concomitant use of clopidogrel and omeprazole also has been associated with decreased antiplatelet effects as determined by vasodilator-stimulated phosphoprotein (VASP) phosphorylation.

The clinical importance of these effects has not yet been established but reduction in clopidogrel's effectiveness in preventing cardiovascular events is possible. Several observational studies involving large numbers of patients suggest that proton-pump inhibitors reduce the effectiveness of clopidogrel in preventing cardiovascular events (e.g., recurrent myocardial infarction, rehospitalization for acute coronary syndromes, urgent target vessel revascularization, death). However, data discounting the clinical importance of an interaction between clopidogrel and proton-pump inhibitors also have been reported. Some experts, including the American College of Cardiology (ACC) and the American Heart Association (AHA), state that additional data from large, prospective trials are needed to fully elucidate the clinical consequences, if any, of the observed interaction between clopidogrel and certain proton-pump inhibitors, including omeprazole.

Proton-pump inhibitors vary in their potency for inhibiting CYP2C19. The change in inhibition of adenosine diphosphate (ADP)-induced platelet aggregation associated with concomitant use of proton-pump inhibitors with clopidogrel is related to the change in exposure to the active metabolite of clopidogrel. In pharmacokinetic and pharmacodynamic studies in healthy individuals, concomitant use of dexlansoprazole, lansoprazole, or pantoprazole had less effect on the antiplatelet activity of clopidogrel than did concomitant use of omeprazole or esomeprazole. For further information on interactions between proton-pump inhibitors and clopidogrel, see Drug Interactions: Proton-Pump Inhibitors, in Clopidogrel Bisulfate 20:12.18. Concomitant use of clopidogrel and either omeprazole or esomeprazole should be avoided. Administration of the drugs at separate times will not prevent the interaction.

The decision to use a proton-pump inhibitor concomitantly with clopidogrel should be based on the assessed risks and benefits in individual patients. The American College of Cardiology Foundation/American College of Gastroenterology/American Heart Association (ACCF/ACG/AHA) states that the reduction in GI bleeding risk with proton-pump inhibitors is substantial in patients with risk factors for GI bleeding (e.g., advanced age; concomitant use of warfarin, corticosteroids, or nonsteroidal anti-inflammatory agents [NSAIAs]; *H. pylori* infection) and may outweigh any potential reduction in the cardiovascular efficacy of antiplatelet treatment associated with a drug-drug interaction. In contrast, ACCF/ACG/AHA states that patients without such risk factors receive little if any absolute risk reduction from proton-pump inhibitor therapy, and the risk/benefit balance may favor use of antiplatelet therapy without a proton-pump inhibitor in these patients. (See Drug Interactions: Proton Pump Inhibitors, in Clopidogrel Bisulfate 20:12.18.)

If concomitant proton-pump inhibitor use is considered necessary, use of an agent with little or no CYP2C19-inhibitory activity should be considered. Alternatively, treatment with a histamine H_2-receptor antagonist (ranitidine, famotidine, nizatidine) may be considered, although such agents may not be as effective as a proton-pump inhibitor in providing gastric protection; cimetidine should *not* be used since it also is a potent CYP2C19 inhibitor. There currently is no evidence that histamine H_2-receptor antagonists (other than cimetidine) or other drugs that reduce gastric acid (e.g., antacids) interfere with the antiplatelet effects of clopidogrel.

■ **Digoxin** Hypomagnesemia (e.g., resulting from long-term use of proton-pump inhibitors) sensitizes the myocardium to digoxin and, thus, may increase the risk of digoxin-induced cardiotoxic effects. In patients receiving digoxin, monitoring of magnesium concentrations should be considered prior to initiation of prescription proton-pump inhibitor therapy and periodically thereafter.

■ **Methotrexate** Data from case reports, population pharmacokinetic studies, and retrospective analyses suggest that concomitant use of proton-pump inhibitors, including omeprazole, with methotrexate may result in increased serum methotrexate concentrations and possibly result in toxicity. Increased serum concentrations and delayed clearance of methotrexate and/or its metabolite hydroxymethotrexate, with or without symptoms of methotrexate toxicity, have been reported in patients receiving methotrexate (usually at doses of 300 mg/m^2 to 12 g/m^2) concomitantly with a proton-pump inhibitor. Although most of the reported cases occurred in patients receiving high doses of methotrexate, toxicity also has been reported in patients receiving low dosages of methotrexate (e.g., 15 mg per week) concomitantly with a proton-pump inhibitor. No formal studies of interactions between high-dose methotrexate and proton-pump inhibitors have been conducted to date.

The manufacturer of omeprazole states that temporary discontinuance of proton-pump inhibitor therapy may be considered in some patients receiving high-dose methotrexate therapy. Some clinicians recommend either withholding proton-pump inhibitor therapy for several days before and after methotrexate administration or substituting a histamine H_2-receptor antagonist for the proton-pump inhibitor when acid suppressive therapy is indicated during methotrexate therapy. Pending further evaluation, some clinicians state that these recommendations should extend to patients receiving low-dose methotrexate.

■ **Tacrolimus** Concomitant use of omeprazole with tacrolimus may result in increased serum concentrations of tacrolimus.

■ **Voriconazole** Concomitant use of omeprazole (40 mg daily for 7 days) with voriconazole (a combined inhibitor of CYP2C19 and CYP3A4; 400 mg every 12 hours for one day, then 200 mg for 6 days) in healthy individuals increased peak plasma concentrations and AUC of omeprazole by an average of twofold and fourfold, respectively. Dosage adjustment of omeprazole usually is not required but may be considered in patients receiving high dosages (up to 240 mg daily), such as those with Zollinger-Ellison syndrome.

■ **Warfarin** Increases in international normalized ratio (INR) and prothrombin time have been reported in patients receiving warfarin concomitantly with a proton-pump inhibitor, including omeprazole. Because such increases may lead to abnormal bleeding and death, monitoring of INR and prothrombin time may be necessary in patients receiving warfarin and a proton-pump inhibitor concomitantly.

Description

Omeprazole is a substituted benzimidazole gastric antisecretory agent. Omeprazole is structurally and pharmacologically related to esomeprazole, lansoprazole, pantoprazole, and rabeprazole. Omeprazole is a racemic mixture of *R*- and *S*-isomers; esomeprazole is the *S*-isomer of omeprazole. The drugs are chemically and pharmacologically unrelated to H_2-receptor antagonists, antimuscarinics, or prostaglandin analogs.

Because the omeprazole molecule is acid labile, the drug is administered orally as a delayed-release capsule, tablet, or oral suspension or as a buffered immediate-release capsule or oral suspension. The commercially available omeprazole delayed-release capsules increase oral bioavailability by delaying absorption until after the capsule leaves the stomach; peak plasma concentrations of omeprazole occur 30 minutes to 3.5 hours after administration. Following administration of omeprazole magnesium delayed-release oral suspension, the peak plasma concentration and area under the concentration-time curve (AUC) of the drug are 88 and 87%, respectively, of the values achieved following oral administration of omeprazole delayed-release capsules. Omeprazole immediate-release capsules and oral suspension are rapidly absorbed immediate-release formulations that contain sodium bicarbonate to neutralize gastric acid; mean peak plasma concentrations of omeprazole occur at about 30 minutes (range 10–90 minutes) after oral administration of a single dose or repeated doses of the immediate-release capsule or oral suspension on an empty stomach (1 hour prior to a meal).

Omeprazole binds to hydrogen/potassium adenosine triphosphatase (H^+K^+-exchanging ATPase) in gastric parietal cells; inactivation of this enzyme system (also known as the proton, hydrogen, or acid pump) blocks the final step in the secretion of hydrochloric acid by these cells. Therefore, gastric antisecretory agents such as omeprazole and lansoprazole are commonly referred to as acid- or proton-pump inhibitors. Omeprazole, a weak base, does not directly inhibit this enzyme system, but instead, it concentrates under the acid conditions of the parietal cell secretory canaliculi, where the drug undergoes rearrangement to its active sulfenamide metabolite; this metabolite then reacts with sulfhydryl groups of H^+K^+-exchanging ATPase, inactivating the proton pump. Because the sulfenamide metabolite forms an irreversible covalent bond to H^+K^+-exchanging ATPase, acid secretion is inhibited until additional enzyme is synthesized, resulting in a prolonged duration of action. In an animal model, the pharmacologic effect of the drug at this enzyme was shown to correlate directly with sulfenamide formation.

Omeprazole inhibits basal and stimulated gastric acid secretion; in addition, because the drug inhibits the final step in the secretory pathway, it inhibits such secretion regardless of the stimulus. The degree of inhibition of gastric acid secretion is related to the dose and duration of therapy, but omeprazole is a more potent inhibitor of such secretion than are H_2-receptor antagonists. Following oral administration of omeprazole, inhibition of gastric acid secretion is apparent within 1 hour, peaks within 2 hours, and persists for up to 72 hours. Inhibition of gastric acid secretion increases with continuous drug administration and reaches a plateau after about 4 days of omeprazole therapy. Although omeprazole has a short terminal plasma half-life, the drug has a long duration of action (presumably secondary to prolonged binding of the drug to H^+K^+-exchanging ATPase). Following continuous oral administration of omeprazole, 78 and 58–80% of basal gastric acid secretion is inhibited 2–6 and 24 hours, respectively, after a 20-mg dose, and 94 and 80–93% of basal gastric acid secretion is inhibited, respectively, after a 40-mg dose. Following continuous oral administration, 79 and 50–59% of peak gastric acid output is inhibited 2–6 and 24 hours, respectively, after a 20-mg dose, and 88 and 62–68% of peak gastric acid output is inhibited, respectively, after a 40-mg dose. Oral administration of omeprazole 10–40 mg daily has reduced 24-hour intragastric acidity by 100% in some patients. Following discontinuance of omeprazole therapy, gastric acid secretion returns to baseline over a 3–5 day period.

Following oral administration of omeprazole 20 or 40 mg daily (as the immediate-release oral suspension) in healthy individuals, the median decrease in 24-hour integrated gastric acidity from baseline was 82 or 84%, respectively, the percent of time during a 24-hour period that the gastric pH exceeded 4 was 51 or 77%, respectively, and the median 24-hour gastric pH was 4.2 or 5.2, respectively. In critically ill patients receiving omeprazole 40 mg daily as the immediate-release oral suspension via nasogastric or orogastric tube, the median daily gastric pH was above 4 in at least 95% of patients over the course of a 14-day trial. Gastric pH was above 4 in 99% of patients 1–2.5 hours after the first dose, and in 92% of patients 6 hours after the first dose.

Omeprazole increases plasma gastrin concentrations; this increase occurs via a negative feedback mechanism resulting from decreased gastric acid secretion. Because of omeprazole's greater potency as an inhibitor of gastric acid secretion, the drug also causes secondary increases in plasma gastrin concentrations that exceed those produced by H_2-receptor antagonists. For example, administration of omeprazole 20 mg once daily for 1–2 weeks results in a 1.3- to 3.6-fold increase in plasma gastrin concentration, whereas administration of an H_2-receptor antagonist usually results in only a 1.1- to 1.8-fold increase. Plasma gastrin concentrations return to pretreatment values with 1–4 weeks after discontinuing omeprazole therapy. Despite omeprazole-induced reductions in gastric acid secretion, the drug does not contribute appreciably to increased plasma gastrin concentrations in most patients with Zollinger-Ellison syndrome, since gastrin is produced principally by the tumor rather than in response to achlorhydria in such patients. Omeprazole also indirectly causes a dose-dependent reduction in pepsin secretion by decreasing the volume of gastric acid secretion. A systematic dose-dependent effect on basal or stimulated pepsin secretion has not been observed in humans; basal pepsin output is low and pepsin activity is decreased when intragastric pH is maintained above 4. The drug does not appear to affect intrinsic factor secretion.

Omeprazole can suppress gastric *Helicobacter pylori* (formerly *Campylobacter pylori* or *C. pyloridis*) in patients with duodenal ulcer and/or reflux esophagitis infected with the organism. Combined therapy with omeprazole and one or more appropriate anti-infectives (e.g., clarithromycin, amoxicillin), can effectively eradicate *H. pylori* gastric infection. (See Duodenal Ulcer: Acute Therapy, in Uses.) Omeprazole does not appear to affect gastric emptying or lower esophageal sphincter pressure.

Short-term administration (2–4 weeks) of omeprazole dosages of 30–40 mg daily does not appear to affect thyroid function, carbohydrate metabolism, or plasma/serum concentrations of parathyroid hormone (parathormone), cortisol, estradiol, testosterone, prolactin, cholecystokinin, or secretin. However, the drug may decrease antral somatostatin concentrations.

Therapy with proton-pump inhibitors, particularly in high dosages and/or for prolonged periods of time, may be associated with an increased risk of osteoporosis-related fractures of the hip, wrist, or spine. (See Cautions: Musculoskeletal Effects.) The mechanism by which these drugs may increase risk of such fractures has not been elucidated but may involve decreased insoluble calcium absorption secondary to increased gastric pH.

SumMon® (see Users Guide). For additional information on this drug until a more detailed monograph is developed and published, the manufacturer's labeling should be consulted. It is *essential* that the labeling be consulted for detailed information on the usual cautions, precautions, and contraindications concerning potential drug interactions and/or laboratory test interferences and for information on acute toxicity.

Preparations

Excipients in commercially available drug preparations may have clinically important effects in some individuals; consult specific product labeling for details.

Omeprazole

Oral		
Capsules	20 mg	**Zegerid®**, Santarus
	40 mg	**Zegerid®**, Santarus
Capsules, delayed-release (containing enteric-coated granules)	10 mg*	**Omeprazole Delayed-release Capsules**
		PriLOSEC®, AstraZeneca
	20 mg*	**Omeprazole Delayed-release Capsules**
		PriLOSEC®, AstraZeneca
	40 mg*	**Omeprazole Delayed-release Capsules**
		PriLOSEC®, AstraZeneca
For suspension, powder	20 mg/packet	**Zegerid®**, Santarus
	40 mg/packet	**Zegerid®**, Santarus

*available from one or more manufacturer, distributor, and/or repackager by generic (nonproprietary) name

Omeprazole Magnesium

Oral		
For suspension, delayed-release (containing enteric-coated granules)	2.5 mg (of omeprazole) per packet	**PriLOSEC®**, AstraZeneca
	10 mg (of omeprazole) per packet	**PriLOSEC®**, AstraZeneca
Tablets, delayed-release	20 mg (of omeprazole)	**PriLOSEC® OTC**, Procter & Gamble

†Use is not currently included in the labeling approved by the US Food and Drug Administration

Pantoprazole Sodium

■ Pantoprazole sodium, commonly referred to as an acid- or proton-pump inhibitor, is a gastric antisecretory agent that can suppress gastric *Helicobacter pylori* in patients with duodenal ulcer and/or reflux esophagitis infected with the organism.

Uses

■ **Gastroesophageal Reflux** Pantoprazole sodium is used orally for the short-term (up to 8 weeks) treatment and symptomatic relief of erosive esophagitis in patients with gastroesophageal reflux disease (GERD). Pantoprazole sodium also is used orally as maintenance therapy following healing of erosive esophagitis to reduce recurrence of the disease. Pantoprazole sodium is used IV for up to 7–10 days in the treatment of GERD in patients with a history of erosive esophagitis. IV pantoprazole should be discontinued as soon as the patient is able to initiate or resume treatment with oral pantoprazole. Potential benefits in gastroesophageal reflux and esophagitis result principally from reduced acidity of gastric contents induced by the drug and resultant reduced irritation of esophageal mucosa; the drug can effectively relieve symptoms of esophagitis (e.g., heartburn, regurgitation) and promote healing of ulcerative and erosive lesions.

Suppression of gastric acid secretion is considered by the American College of Gastroenterology (ACG) to be the mainstay of treatment for GERD, and a proton-pump inhibitor or histamine H_2-receptor antagonist is used to achieve acid suppression, control symptoms, and prevent complications of the disease. Because GERD is considered to be a chronic disease, the ACG states that many patients with GERD require long-term, even lifelong, treatment. The ACG states that proton-pump inhibitors are more effective (i.e., provide more frequent and more rapid symptomatic relief and healing of esophagitis) than histamine H_2-receptor antagonists in the treatment of GERD, and are effective and appropriate as maintenance therapy in many patients with the disease. Proton-pump inhibitors also provide greater control of acid reflux than do prokinetic agents (e.g., cisapride [no longer commercially available in the US], metoclopramide) without the risk of severe adverse effects associated with these agents.

Safety and efficacy of oral pantoprazole for treating GERD and erosive esophagitis (grade 2 or greater on the Hetzel-Dent scale) were established in 2 short-term (up to 8 weeks), controlled studies in adults; pantoprazole was more effective than placebo or nizatidine in healing lesions and providing symptomatic relief. In other studies, pantoprazole was more effective than famotidine or ranitidine and at least as effective as omeprazole.

Safety and efficacy of oral pantoprazole as maintenance therapy following healing of erosive esophagitis were established in two 12-month controlled studies in adults. Pantoprazole (40 mg daily) was more effective than ranitidine (150 mg twice daily) in maintaining healing and decreasing the number of daytime and nocturnal heartburn episodes.

Safety and efficacy of IV pantoprazole for short-term (up to 7–10 days) use in the treatment of GERD in patients with a history of erosive esophagitis have been established in several studies. In a controlled study in adults receiving oral pantoprazole prior to study entry, the degree of inhibition of gastric acid secretion following substitution of IV pantoprazole (40 mg once daily for 7 days) was similar to that achieved following oral administration of the drug at the same daily dosage. In 2 controlled studies evaluating short-term (up to 7 days) use of IV pantoprazole as initial treatment for GERD in adults, the degree of inhibition of gastric acid secretion following IV administration of pantoprazole 40 mg once daily was similar to that achieved following oral administration of pantoprazole at the same daily dosage. In addition, relief of GERD symptoms and healing of esophageal lesions were comparable for IV and oral administration of pantoprazole.

Safety and efficacy of IV pantoprazole use for more than 10 days have not been established.

For further information on the treatment of GERD, see Uses: Gastroesophageal Reflux, in Omeprazole 56:28.36.

■ Pathologic GI Hypersecretory Conditions Pantoprazole sodium is used orally or IV for the treatment of pathologic GI hypersecretory conditions associated with Zollinger-Ellison syndrome or other neoplastic conditions. The drug reduces the volume of gastric acid output and hydrogen ion concentration of gastric secretions in patients with these conditions.

In an uncontrolled study in a limited number of patients with pathologic GI hypersecretory conditions (e.g., Zollinger-Ellison syndrome with or without multiple endocrine neoplasia type I), oral administration of pantoprazole at dosages of 80–240 mg daily maintained gastric acid secretion below 5 or 10 mEq/hour in patients who had or had not undergone gastric acid-reducing surgery, respectively. The drug was well tolerated at these dosages for more than 2 years in some patients.

Administration of IV pantoprazole in a limited number of patients with Zollinger-Ellison syndrome (with or without multiple endocrine neoplasia type I) resulted in control of gastric acid secretion to 10 mEq/hour or less with substantial reductions in hydrogen ion concentration and volume of gastric secretions within 45 minutes of drug administration. In another study, control of gastric acid secretion was maintained or improved in a limited number of patients switched from an oral proton-pump inhibitor to IV pantoprazole. In both studies, IV pantoprazole 160 or 240 mg daily in divided doses for up to 6 days maintained basal gastric acid secretion below target levels (10 mEq/hour in patients without or 5 mEq/hour in those with prior gastric acid-reducing surgery) for at least 24 hours in all patients and through the end of treatment (3–7 days) in nearly all patients. Dosage was individualized in both studies, but a regimen of 80 mg every 12 hours controlled gastric acid secretion in more than 80% of patients. There was no evidence of tolerance once acid secretion was controlled.

■ Crohn's Disease-associated Ulcers Although evidence currently is limited, proton-pump inhibitors have been used for gastric acid-suppressive therapy as an adjunct in the symptomatic treatment of upper GI Crohn's disease, including esophageal, gastroduodenal, and jejunoileal disease. Most evidence of efficacy to date has been from case studies in patients with Crohn's-associated peptic ulcer disease unresponsive to other therapies (e.g., H_2-receptor antagonists, cytoprotective agents, antacids, and/or sucralfate). (See Uses: Crohn's Disease-associated Ulcers in Omeprazole 56:28.36.)

For further information on the management of Crohn's Disease, see Uses: Crohn's Disease, in Mesalamine 56:36.

■ Other Uses Pantoprazole also has been used orally for treatment of gastric† or duodenal ulcers†. The recommended dosage of IV pantoprazole does *not* raise gastric pH sufficiently to contribute to the treatment of some conditions (e.g., life-threatening GI bleeding), and the drug's safety and efficacy in the treatment of conditions other than GERD or pathologic GI hypersecretory conditions associated with Zollinger-Ellison syndrome or other neoplastic conditions have not been established.

Dosage and Administration

■ Reconstitution and Administration Pantoprazole sodium is administered orally or IV; the drug is *not* intended for other parenteral routes of administration. Pantoprazole is administered once daily in the management of gastroesophageal reflux disease (GERD) and erosive esophagitis; in the management of pathologic GI hypersecretory conditions, pantoprazole generally is given twice daily, although the drug may be given IV every 8 hours if necessary.

For the treatment of GERD, one vial of pantoprazole sodium for injection should be reconstituted with 10 mL of 0.9% sodium chloride injection to provide a solution containing about 4 mg/mL of pantoprazole; the reconstituted solution may be stored for up to 24 hours at room temperature and does not need to be protected from light prior to IV injection over not less than 2 minutes. Alternatively, the reconstituted solution may be stored for up to 6 hours at room temperature prior to further dilution with 100 mL of 0.9% sodium chloride injection, 5% dextrose injection, or lactated Ringer's injection to provide a final concentration of about 0.4 mg/mL. The diluted solution may be stored at room temperature but must be used within 24 hours after initial reconstitution. Neither the reconstituted nor diluted solution needs to be protected from light. The diluted solution may be infused IV over a period of about 15 minutes (about 2.7 mg of the drug or 7 mL of solution per minute).

For the treatment of hypersecretory conditions, each of two 40-mg (of pantoprazole) vials of pantoprazole sodium for injection should be reconstituted with 10 mL of 0.9% sodium chloride injection; the total volume (approximately 20 mL) of reconstituted solution may be stored for up to 24 hours at room temperature and does not need to be protected from light prior to IV injection over not less than 2 minutes. Alternatively, the contents of both vials may be combined and stored for up to 6 hours at room temperature prior to further dilution with 80 mL of 0.9% sodium chloride injection, 5% dextrose injection, or lactated Ringer's injection to a final volume of about 100 mL, providing a final concentration of about 0.8 mg/mL. The diluted solution may be stored at room temperature but must be used within 24 hours after initial reconstitution. Neither the reconstituted nor diluted solution needs to be protected from light. The diluted solution may be infused IV over a period of about 15 minutes (about 5.3 mg of the drug or 7 mL of solution per minute).

Health-care personnel (e.g., pharmacists, nurses) preparing reconstituted solutions using spiked IV system adapters should use caution because of the potential for breakage of the glass vial. (See Glass Vial Breakage under Cautions: Warnings/Precautions.)

Pantoprazole sodium should be administered IV through a dedicated IV line or via a Y-site. Parenteral pantoprazole sodium solutions should be inspected visually for particulate matter and discoloration prior to and during administration whenever solution and container permit. Pantoprazole sodium for injection is incompatible by Y-site administration with midazolam hydrochloride injection and may be incompatible with solutions containing zinc. Y-site administration of IV pantoprazole should be discontinued immediately if precipitation or discoloration occurs.

Pantoprazole sodium delayed-release tablets should be swallowed intact and not split, crushed, or chewed. For patients unable to swallow the 40-mg tablets, a 40-mg dose may be administered using two 20-mg tablets. Food may delay the rate but does not affect the extent of GI absorption of the tablets; therefore, pantoprazole delayed-release tablets may be administered without regard to meals. Antacids do not affect the absorption of pantoprazole and may be administered concomitantly with the delayed-release tablets.

Pantoprazole delayed-release oral suspension should be administered 30 minutes before a meal. Pantoprazole sodium delayed-release granules for oral suspension should be mixed with applesauce or apple juice prior to administration; the granules should *not* be mixed with any other foods or liquids (including water). The delayed-release granules in the suspension should be swallowed intact and not crushed or chewed. The contents of a single-dose packet of pantoprazole sodium delayed-release granules for oral suspension should be sprinkled onto one teaspoonful of applesauce and administered within 10 minutes of preparation. After swallowing the pantoprazole and applesauce mixture, the patient should take sips of water, repeated as necessary, to ensure complete delivery of the dose. Alternatively, the contents of a single-dose packet may be sprinkled into 5 mL of apple juice; the resulting suspension should be stirred for 5 seconds and then swallowed immediately. The granules will not dissolve. The container should be rinsed once or twice with apple juice and the rinsings swallowed immediately to ensure complete delivery of the dose. The contents of a packet of delayed-release granules for oral suspension should not be divided to prepare a dose that is smaller than the full labeled dose (e.g., a 40-mg packet should not be used to prepare a 20-mg dose for a pediatric patient who is unable to swallow the delayed-release tablets).

Pantoprazole delayed-release oral suspension also can be administered via a nasogastric or gastrostomy tube (16 French or larger). The plunger should be removed from a 60-mL syringe and the catheter tip of the syringe attached to the nasogastric or gastrostomy tube; then, the contents of a single-dose packet of pantoprazole sodium delayed-release granules for oral suspension should be emptied into the barrel of the syringe while the syringe is held as high as possible to prevent bending of the tubing. A volume of 10 mL of apple juice should be added to the syringe and the syringe gently tapped or shaken to facilitate emptying; the syringe and tubing should be rinsed with 10 mL of apple juice at least 2 more times (until no granules remain).

For the treatment of pathologic hypersecretory conditions associated with Zollinger-Ellison syndrome or other neoplastic conditions, pantoprazole sodium for injection is administered IV every 8 or 12 hours. The frequency of administration may be individualized based on acid output measurements. Patients with Zollinger-Ellison syndrome may be vulnerable to serious complications of increased gastric acid secretion, even after a brief loss of gastric acid suppression. Therefore, transition from oral to IV and IV to oral formulations of gastric acid inhibitors should be performed in such a manner to ensure continuity of gastric acid suppression effects.

■ Dosage Dosage of pantoprazole sodium is expressed in terms of pantoprazole.

Gastroesophageal Reflux For the treatment of erosive esophagitis associated with GERD, the recommended adult oral dosage of pantoprazole is 40 mg daily. The duration of therapy is 8 weeks, and therapy may be extended for an additional 8 weeks if esophageal healing is incomplete. For maintenance therapy following healing of erosive esophagitis, the recommended adult oral dosage of pantoprazole is 40 mg once daily. Although the American College of Gastroenterology (ACG) states that chronic, even lifelong, therapy with a proton-pump inhibitor is appropriate in many patients with GERD, the manufacturer states that the safety and efficacy of continuing pantoprazole maintenance therapy for more than 1 year has not been established.

For the treatment of GERD associated with a history of erosive esophagitis, the recommended adult IV dosage of pantoprazole is 40 mg once daily. Treatment with IV pantoprazole should be discontinued as soon as the patient is able to initiate or resume treatment with the oral drug; safety and efficacy of IV pantoprazole use for more than 10 days have not been established.

For the treatment of erosive esophagitis associated with GERD in children 5 years of age or older, the recommended oral dosage of pantoprazole is 20 mg once daily in children weighing at least 15 kg but less than 40 kg and 40 mg once daily in children weighing 40 kg or more. Treatment may be continued for up to 8 weeks; safety beyond 8 weeks has not been established in pediatric patients.

Pathologic GI Hypersecretory Conditions For the treatment of pathologic GI hypersecretory conditions (e.g., Zollinger-Ellison syndrome, multiple endocrine neoplasia type I), the recommended adult oral dosage of pantoprazole is 40 mg twice daily. Dosages should be individualized and continued for as long as clinically necessary. Oral dosages up to 240 mg daily have been administered, and some patients have received the drug for more than 2 years.

The recommended adult IV dosage of pantoprazole for the treatment of pathologic GI hypersecretory conditions is 80 mg administered IV every 12 hours. In patients requiring a higher daily dosage, 80 mg administered IV every 8 hours is expected to maintain acid output below 10 mEq/hour. Safety and efficacy of dosages exceeding 240 mg daily, and use of IV pantoprazole for longer than 6 days have not been established.

■ **Special Populations** Dosage adjustment is not necessary in patients with renal impairment, patients undergoing hemodialysis, patients with hepatic impairment, or in geriatric patients. However, dosages exceeding 40 mg daily have not been studied in patients with hepatic impairment.

Reduction of pantoprazole dosage should be considered in pediatric patients who are poor metabolizers of cytochrome P-450 (CYP) 2C19 substrates, since exposure to the drug is increased by more than sixfold compared with that in extensive or moderate metabolizers. However, no dosage adjustment is required in adults who are poor metabolizers of CYP2C19 substrates, since minimal (23% or less) accumulation of the drug occurs with once-daily dosing.

Cautions

■ **Contraindications** Known hypersensitivity to pantoprazole, any other ingredient in the formulation, or other substituted benzimidazoles (e.g., esomeprazole, lansoprazole, omeprazole, rabeprazole).

■ **Warnings/Precautions** ***Sensitivity Reactions*** Anaphylaxis has been reported with the use of IV pantoprazole sodium. Immediate medical intervention and drug discontinuance are required if anaphylaxis or other severe hypersensitivity reaction occurs.

Gastric Malignancy Symptomatic response to therapy with pantoprazole does not preclude the presence of gastric neoplasm. Because of the chronic nature of the disease, there may be a potential for prolonged administration of pantoprazole in patients with gastroesophageal reflux disease (GERD); in long-term animal studies, pantoprazole caused rare types of GI tumors, although the relevance of these findings to humans is unknown.

Atrophic Gastritis Atrophic gastritis occasionally has been noted in gastric corpus biopsy specimens from patients receiving long-term treatment with pantoprazole, especially those infected with *Helicobacter pylori*.

Clostridium difficile Infection Available data suggest a possible association between use of proton-pump inhibitors and risk of *Clostridium difficile* infection, including *C. difficile*-associated diarrhea and colitis (CDAD; also known as antibiotic-associated diarrhea and colitis or pseudomembranous colitis). In most observational studies to date, the risk of *C. difficile* infection in patients exposed to proton-pump inhibitors has ranged from 1.4–2.75 times that in patients not exposed to proton-pump inhibitors; however, some observational studies have found no increase in risk. Although many of the cases occurred in patients who had other risk factors for CDAD, including advanced age, comorbid conditions, and/or use of broad-spectrum anti-infectives, the US Food and Drug Administration (FDA) concluded that a contributory role for proton-pump inhibitors could not be definitively ruled out. The mechanism by which proton-pump inhibitors might increase the risk of CDAD has not been elucidated. Although it has been suggested that reduction of gastric acidity by gastric antisecretory agents might facilitate colonization with *C. difficile*, some studies have raised questions about this proposed mechanism or have suggested that the observed association is the result of confounding with other risk factors for CDAD. FDA also is reviewing the risk of CDAD in patients exposed to histamine H_2-receptor antagonists.

CDAD can be serious in patients who have one or more risk factors for *C. difficile* infection and are receiving concomitant therapy with a proton-pump inhibitor; colectomy and, rarely, death have been reported. FDA recommends that patients receive proton-pump inhibitors at the lowest effective dosage and for the shortest possible time appropriate for their clinical condition. Patients experiencing persistent diarrhea should be evaluated for CDAD and should be managed with appropriate supportive therapy (e.g., fluid and electrolyte management), anti-infective therapy directed against *C. difficile* (e.g., metronidazole, vancomycin), and surgical evaluation as clinically indicated.

Musculoskeletal Effects Findings from several observational studies suggest that therapy with proton-pump inhibitors, particularly in high dosages (i.e., multiple daily doses) and/or for prolonged periods of time (i.e., one year or longer), may be associated with an increased risk of osteoporosis-related fractures of the hip, wrist, or spine. The magnitude of risk is unclear; causality has not been established. (See Cautions: Musculoskeletal Effects, in Omeprazole 56:28.36.) FDA is continuing to evaluate this safety concern. Although controlled studies are required to confirm these findings, patients should receive proton-pump inhibitors at the lowest effective dosage and for the shortest possible time appropriate for their clinical condition. Individuals who are at risk for osteoporosis-related fractures should receive an adequate intake of calcium and vitamin D and should have their bone health assessed and managed according to current standards of care.

Hypomagnesemia Hypomagnesemia, symptomatic and asymptomatic, has been reported rarely in patients receiving long-term therapy (for at least 3 months or, in most cases, for longer than one year) with proton-pump inhibitors, including pantoprazole. Clinically serious adverse effects associated with hypomagnesemia, which are similar to manifestations of hypocalcemia, include tetany, seizures, tremors, carpopedal spasm, arrhythmias (e.g., atrial fibrillation, supraventricular tachycardia), and abnormal QT interval. Other reported adverse effects include paresthesia, muscle weakness, muscle cramps, lethargy, fatigue, and unsteadiness. In most patients, treatment of hypomagnesemia required magnesium replacement and discontinuance of the proton-pump inhibitor. Following discontinuance of the proton-pump inhibitor, hypomagnesemia resolved within a median of one week; upon rechallenge, hypomagnesemia recurred within a median of 2 weeks.

In patients expected to receive long-term therapy with a proton-pump inhibitor or in those receiving a proton-pump inhibitor concomitantly with digoxin or drugs that may cause hypomagnesemia (e.g., diuretics), clinicians should consider measurement of serum magnesium concentrations prior to initiation of prescription proton-pump inhibitor therapy and periodically thereafter. (See Cautions: Hypomagnesemia and also Cautions: Precautions and Contraindications, in Omeprazole 56:28.36.)

Cyanocobalamin Malabsorption Hypochlorhydria or achlorhydria resulting from daily treatment with acid-suppressive drugs over a long period (e.g., longer than 3 years) may lead to malabsorption of cyanocobalamin. Cyanocobalamin deficiency has been reported rarely. The possibility of such malabsorption should be considered if manifestations of cyanocobalamin deficiency occur.

Injection Site Reactions Injection site reactions, including thrombophlebitis and abscess, have been associated with IV administration of pantoprazole.

Edetate Disodium Content Pantoprazole sodium for injection contains edetate disodium (disodium EDTA), which is a potent metal ion (e.g., zinc) chelator. Zinc supplementation should be considered during IV pantoprazole therapy in patients who are prone to zinc deficiency and caution should be exercised when IV pantoprazole is used concomitantly with other IV preparations that contain edetate disodium.

Laboratory Test Interferences **Cannabinoid Tests.** False-positive results for urine screening tests for tetrahydrocannabinol (THC) have been reported in patients receiving proton-pump inhibitors, including pantoprazole. An alternative confirmatory test should be considered to verify positive urine THC screening results in these patients.

Respiratory Effects Administration of proton-pump inhibitors has been associated with an increased risk for developing certain infections (e.g., community-acquired pneumonia). For further precautionary information about this adverse effect, see Community-acquired Pneumonia under Cautions: Respiratory Effects, in Omeprazole 56:28.36.

Glass Vial Breakage The manufacturer and the US Food and Drug Administration (FDA) have received reports of glass vial breakage during attempts to connect pantoprazole sodium vials to spiked IV system adapters. Such breakage may be a safety issue for health-care personnel (e.g., pharmacists, nurses) attempting to connect these system components either manually or with mechanical assistance, but is not considered by the manufacturer to be a quality issue for pantoprazole sodium for injection. Although the manufacturer is reviewing the use of pantoprazole sodium vials with such systems in order to understand the problem, the manufacturer has not performed studies with these systems to date and currently does not recommend use of spiked IV system adapters with pantoprazole sodium vials. The manufacturer of pantoprazole sodium states that if a decision is made to use spiked adapters, the manufacturer of the adapters should be contacted to provide assistance.

Specific Populations **Pregnancy.** Category B. (See Users Guide.)

Lactation. Pantoprazole is distributed into milk; discontinue nursing or the drug because of potential risk in nursing infants.

Pediatric Use. Efficacy and safety of oral pantoprazole for short-term treatment of erosive esophagitis associated with GERD in pediatric patients 1–16 years of age are supported by controlled clinical trials in adults and additional safety, efficacy, and pharmacokinetic studies in pediatric patients. However, because an appropriate dosage formulation is not available for children younger than 5 years of age, oral pantoprazole is labeled for use only in children 5 years of age or older. Safety and efficacy of oral pantoprazole for uses other than treatment of erosive esophagitis have not been established in pediatric patients.

Oral pantoprazole was evaluated in several clinical trials in pediatric patients 1–16 years of age with endoscopically diagnosed or symptomatic GERD, including a limited number of patients with endoscopically diagnosed erosive esophagitis. Because these clinical trials had no placebo or active comparator group and provided no evidence of a dose-related response to the pantoprazole dosages studied, the results were inconclusive regarding efficacy of pantoprazole for the treatment of symptomatic GERD in pediatric patients. Adverse effects reported in more than 4% of patients included upper respiratory tract infection, headache, fever, diarrhea, vomiting, rash, and abdominal pain. Following oral administration of a single 40-mg dose of pantoprazole, exposure to the drug was about 39% higher in children 6–11 years of age and about 10% higher in adolescents 12–16 years of age compared with adults.

Efficacy of oral pantoprazole in infants younger than 1 year of age has not been established. In a treatment-withdrawal study in infants 1–11 months of age with symptomatic GERD, pantoprazole was not more effective than placebo.

Safety and efficacy of IV pantoprazole in pediatric patients have not been established.

Geriatric Use. There are no substantial differences in safety and efficacy relative to younger adults. No dosage adjustment is necessary in geriatric patients.

■ **Common Adverse Effects** Adverse effects occurring in more than 2% of patients receiving oral pantoprazole and reported more frequently with pantoprazole than with placebo include headache, diarrhea, abdominal pain, vomiting, flatulence, dizziness, and arthralgia.

Adverse effects occurring in more than 1% of patients receiving IV pantoprazole and that generally had an unclear relationship to the drug include headache, injection site reaction (including thrombophlebitis and abscess), abdominal pain, constipation, dyspepsia, nausea, diarrhea, insomnia, dizziness, and rhinitis.

Drug Interactions

■ **Drugs Affecting Hepatic Microsomal Isoenzymes** Pharmacokinetic interaction unlikely. Pantoprazole is extensively metabolized, mainly via hepatic cytochrome P-450 (CYP) 2C19 isoenzyme; CYP3A4, CYP2D6, and CYP2C9 isoenzymes metabolize the drug to a much lesser extent. However, no clinically important drug interactions between pantoprazole and other drugs metabolized by the same isoenzymes were identified in clinical studies. Pantoprazole may have a lower potential for drug interactions than lansoprazole, omeprazole, and rabeprazole.

■ **Drugs that Cause Hypomagnesemia** Potential pharmacologic interaction (possible increased risk of hypomagnesemia). In patients receiving diuretics (i.e., loop or thiazide diuretics) or other drugs that may cause hypomagnesemia, monitoring of magnesium concentrations should be considered prior to initiation of prescription proton-pump inhibitor therapy and periodically thereafter. (See Hypomagnesemia under Cautions: Warnings/Precautions.)

■ **Gastric pH-Dependent Drugs** Pharmacokinetic interaction theoretically possible when pantoprazole is used concomitantly with gastric pH-dependent drugs (e.g., ampicillin esters, iron salts, ketoconazole); increased or decreased drug absorption at increased gastric pH values.

■ **Antiretroviral Agents** ***Atazanavir*** Potential pharmacokinetic interaction with atazanavir (possible altered oral absorption of atazanavir at increased gastric pH, resulting in decreased plasma atazanavir concentrations). Concomitant use of omeprazole 40 mg once daily and atazanavir (with or without low-dose ritonavir) results in a substantial decrease in plasma concentrations of atazanavir and possible loss of the therapeutic effect of the antiretroviral agent or development of drug resistance. The manufacturer of pantoprazole states that concomitant use with atazanavir is not recommended. If atazanavir is administered in a treatment-naive patient receiving a proton-pump inhibitor, a *ritonavir-boosted* regimen of 300 mg of atazanavir once daily with ritonavir 100 mg once daily with food is recommended. The dose of the proton-pump inhibitor should be administered approximately 12 hours before *ritonavir-boosted* atazanavir; the dose of the proton-pump inhibitor should not exceed omeprazole 20 mg daily (or equivalent). Concomitant use of proton-pump inhibitors with atazanavir is not recommended in treatment-experienced patients.

Fosamprenavir Concomitant use of esomeprazole with fosamprenavir (with or without ritonavir) did not substantially affect concentrations of amprenavir (active metabolite of fosamprenavir). No dosage adjustment is required when proton-pump inhibitors are used concomitantly with fosamprenavir (with or without ritonavir).

Lopinavir Concomitant use of omeprazole with the fixed combination of lopinavir and ritonavir (lopinavir/ritonavir) did not have a clinically important effect on plasma concentrations or area under the concentration-time curve (AUC) of lopinavir. No dosage adjustment is required when proton-pump inhibitors are used concomitantly with lopinavir/ritonavir.

Nelfinavir Potential pharmacokinetic interaction (decreased plasma nelfinavir concentrations). Concomitant use of omeprazole 40 mg once daily (given 30 minutes before a nelfinavir dose) and nelfinavir 1.25 g twice daily decreased peak plasma concentrations and AUCs of nelfinavir by 37 and 36%, respectively, and of its major active metabolite M8 by 89 and 92%, respectively. The manufacturer of pantoprazole states that concomitant use of proton-pump inhibitors with nelfinavir is not recommended.

Raltegravir Pharmacokinetic interaction with omeprazole (substantially increased peak plasma concentration and AUC of raltegravir); however, no dosage adjustment is recommended when proton-pump inhibitors are used concomitantly with raltegravir.

Rilpivirine Pharmacokinetic interaction with omeprazole (decreased plasma concentrations and AUC of rilpivirine). Concomitant use of other proton-pump inhibitors also may result in decreased plasma concentrations of rilpivirine. Concomitant use of rilpivirine and proton-pump inhibitors is contraindicated.

Saquinavir Potential pharmacokinetic interaction (increased peak plasma concentration and AUC of saquinavir). Concomitant use of omeprazole 40 mg once daily and *ritonavir-boosted* saquinavir (saquinavir 1 g twice daily and ritonavir 100 mg twice daily) increased the peak plasma concentration and AUC of saquinavir by 75 and 82%, respectively. Caution is advised if proton-pump inhibitors are used concomitantly with *ritonavir-boosted* saquinavir, and patients should be monitored for saquinavir toxicity.

■ **Clopidogrel** Potential pharmacokinetic interaction (decreased plasma concentration of the active metabolite of clopidogrel) and pharmacodynamic interaction (reduced antiplatelet effects) between proton-pump inhibitors and clopidogrel. Clopidogrel is metabolized to its active metabolite by cytochrome P-450 (CYP) isoenzyme 2C19 (CYP2C19). Concurrent use of omeprazole or esomeprazole, which inhibit CYP2C19, with clopidogrel reduces exposure to the active metabolite of clopidogrel and decreases platelet inhibitory effects. Although the clinical importance has not been fully elucidated, a reduction in the effectiveness of clopidogrel in preventing cardiovascular events is possible. Proton-pump inhibitors vary in their potency for inhibiting CYP2C19. The change in inhibition of adenosine diphosphate (ADP)-induced platelet aggregation associated with concomitant use of proton-pump inhibitors is related to the change in exposure to the active metabolite of clopidogrel. In pharmacokinetic and pharmacodynamic studies in healthy individuals, concomitant use of dexlansoprazole, lansoprazole, or pantoprazole had less effect on the antiplatelet activity of clopidogrel than did concomitant use of omeprazole or esomeprazole. Use of pantoprazole (80 mg daily, administered at the same time as clopidogrel) concomitantly with clopidogrel (300-mg loading dose followed by 75 mg daily) for 5 days reduced exposure to the active metabolite of clopidogrel by about 14% compared with use of clopidogrel alone. The observed effects of pantoprazole on metabolite exposure and clopidogrel-induced platelet inhibition were not considered clinically important, and the manufacturer of pantoprazole states that no adjustment of clopidogrel dosage is necessary if clopidogrel is used concomitantly with recommended dosages of pantoprazole.

The decision to use a proton-pump inhibitor concomitantly with clopidogrel should be based on the assessed risks and benefits in individual patients. The American College of Cardiology Foundation/American College of Gastroenterology/American Heart Association (ACCF/ACG/AHA) states that the reduction in GI bleeding risk with proton-pump inhibitors is substantial in patients with risk factors for GI bleeding (e.g., advanced age; concomitant use of warfarin, corticosteroids, or nonsteroidal anti-inflammatory agents [NSAIAs]; *H. pylori* infection) and may outweigh any potential reduction in the cardiovascular efficacy of antiplatelet treatment associated with a drug-drug interaction. In contrast, ACCF/ACG/AHA states that patients without such risk factors receive little if any absolute risk reduction from proton-pump inhibitor therapy, and the risk/benefit balance may favor use of antiplatelet therapy without a proton-pump inhibitor in these patients.

If concomitant therapy with a proton-pump inhibitor and clopidogrel is considered necessary, use of an agent with little or no CYP2C19-inhibitory activity should be considered. Alternatively, treatment with a histamine H_2-receptor antagonist (ranitidine, famotidine, nizatidine) may be considered, although such agents may not be as effective as a proton-pump inhibitor in providing gastric protection; cimetidine should *not* be used since it also is a potent CYP2C19 inhibitor. There currently is no evidence that histamine H_2-receptor antagonists (other than cimetidine) or other drugs that reduce gastric acid (e.g., antacids) interfere with the antiplatelet effects of clopidogrel. For further information on interactions between proton-pump inhibitors and clopidogrel, see Drug Interactions: Proton-Pump Inhibitors, in Clopidogrel Bisulfate 20:12.18.

■ **Digoxin** Hypomagnesemia (e.g., resulting from long-term use of proton-pump inhibitors) sensitizes the myocardium to digoxin and, thus, may increase the risk of digoxin-induced cardiotoxic effects. In patients receiving digoxin, monitoring of magnesium concentrations should be considered prior to initiation of prescription proton-pump inhibitor therapy and periodically thereafter.

■ **Methotrexate** Potential pharmacokinetic interaction (increased serum methotrexate concentrations, possibly resulting in toxicity) when proton-pump inhibitors, including pantoprazole, are used concomitantly with methotrexate. Increased serum concentrations and delayed clearance of methotrexate and/or its metabolite hydroxymethotrexate, with or without symptoms of methotrexate toxicity, have been reported in patients receiving methotrexate (usually at doses of 300 mg/m^2 to 12 g/m^2) concomitantly with a proton-pump inhibitor. Although most of the reported cases occurred in patients receiving high doses of methotrexate, toxicity also has been reported in patients receiving low dosages of methotrexate (e.g., 15 mg per week) concomitantly with a proton-pump inhibitor. No formal studies of interactions between high-dose methotrexate and proton-pump inhibitors have been conducted to date.

The manufacturer of pantoprazole states that temporary discontinuance of proton-pump inhibitor therapy may be considered in some patients receiving high-dose methotrexate therapy. Some clinicians recommend either withholding proton-pump inhibitor therapy for several days before and after methotrexate administration or substituting a histamine H_2-receptor antagonist for the proton-pump inhibitor when acid suppressive therapy is indicated during methotrexate therapy. Pending further evaluation, some clinicians state that these recommendations should extend to patients receiving low-dose methotrexate.

■ **Sucralfate** Potential delayed absorption and decreased bioavailability of proton-pump inhibitor (e.g., lansoprazole, omeprazole); administer proton-pump inhibitor at least 30 minutes before sucralfate.

■ **Warfarin** Potential increased international normalized ratio (INR) and prothrombin time when warfarin is used concomitantly with proton-pump inhibitors, including pantoprazole. Potential for abnormal bleeding and death; monitor for INR and prothrombin time increases when pantoprazole is used concomitantly with warfarin.

Description

Pantoprazole sodium, a proton-pump inhibitor, is a gastric antisecretory agent that is structurally and pharmacologically related to esomeprazole, lansoprazole, omeprazole, and rabeprazole. The drugs are substituted benzimidazoles and are chemically and pharmacologically unrelated to H_2-receptor antagonists, antimuscarinics, or prostaglandin analogs.

Pantoprazole, a weak base, concentrates under the acidic conditions of the parietal cell secretory canaliculi, where it is activated by rearrangement to a cationic cyclic sulfenamide. The activated form covalently binds to 2 sites of the hydrogen/potassium ATPase in the gastric parietal cells; inactivation of this enzyme system (also known as the proton, hydrogen, or acid pump) blocks the final step in the secretion of hydrochloric acid by these cells, resulting in potent, long-lasting inhibition of gastric acid secretion.

The duration of antisecretory effect of orally administered pantoprazole continues for more than 24 hours. Within 2.5 hours of administration of a 40-mg oral dose to healthy individuals, gastric acid secretion was inhibited by a mean of 51%, which increased to a mean of 85% following administration of 40 mg orally once daily for 7 days. Gastric acid secretion returned to normal within a week after pantoprazole discontinuance, and there was no evidence of rebound hypersecretion. Because the pantoprazole molecule is acid labile, the drug is commercially available for oral administration as delayed-release, enteric-coated formulations (tablets, granules for oral suspension) that increase oral bioavailability by delaying absorption until after the preparation leaves the stomach. The duration of antisecretory effect of IV pantoprazole was 24 hours. Following IV administration of a single 20- to 120-mg dose of pantoprazole to healthy individuals, onset of gastric acid suppression occurred within 15–30 minutes, and suppression of cumulative 24-hour acid output was dose dependent for doses of 20–80 mg. Within 2 hours of IV administration of pantoprazole 80 mg, complete suppression of acid output was achieved; no substantial additional suppression was observed following a 120-mg dose of the drug.

Pantoprazole is extensively metabolized, mainly via hepatic cytochrome P-450 (CYP) 2C19 isoenzyme; CYP3A4, CYP2D6, and CYP2C9 isoenzymes metabolize the drug to a much lesser extent. (See Dosage and Administration: Special Populations.)

Pantoprazole can suppress gastric *Helicobacter pylori* in patients with duodenal ulcer and/or reflux esophagitis infected with the organism. Combined therapy with pantoprazole and one or more anti-infectives (e.g., amoxicillin, clarithromycin) can effectively eradicate *H. pylori* gastric infection.

A moderate increase in enterochromaffin-like cell (ECL) density, which began after the first year of therapy and appeared to plateau after 4 years, occurred in patients receiving pantoprazole dosages of 40–240 mg daily for up to 5 years. Dose-related increases in ECL-cell proliferation and gastric neuroendocrine-cell tumors were observed in animal studies.

Therapy with proton-pump inhibitors, particularly in high dosages and/or for prolonged periods of time, may be associated with an increased risk of osteoporosis-related fractures of the hip, wrist, or spine. (See Musculoskeletal Effects under Cautions: Warnings/Precautions.) The mechanism by which these drugs may increase risk of such fractures has not been elucidated but may involve decreased insoluble calcium absorption secondary to increased gastric pH.

Advice to Patients

Importance of informing clinicians of existing or contemplated concomitant therapy, including prescription and OTC drugs, as well as concomitant illnesses. Antacid administration is permissible with pantoprazole delayed-release tablets.

Importance of women informing clinicians if they are or plan to become pregnant or plan to breast-feed.

Importance of instructing patients regarding proper administration of delayed-release oral preparations. Necessity of swallowing delayed-release tablets whole, without crushing or chewing. Importance of preparing the delayed-release suspension according to the manufacturer's directions and of administering the suspension 30 minutes before a meal. Importance of not dividing the contents of a packet of delayed-release granules for oral suspension to prepare a dose that is smaller than the full labeled dose.

Importance of advising patients that use of multiple daily doses of the drug for an extended period of time may increase the risk of fractures of the hip, wrist, or spine.

Risk of hypomagnesemia; importance of advising patients to immediately report and seek care for any cardiovascular or neurologic manifestations (e.g., palpitations, dizziness, seizures, tetany).

Possible increased risk of *Clostridium difficile* infection; importance of contacting a clinician if persistent watery stools, abdominal pain, and fever occur.

Importance of continuing therapy for the entire treatment course, unless directed otherwise.

Importance of informing patients of other important precautionary information. (See Cautions.)

Overview® (see Users Guide). For additional information until a more detailed monograph is developed and published, the manufacturer's labeling should be consulted. It is *essential* that the manufacturer's labeling be consulted for more detailed information on usual cautions, precautions, contraindications, potential drug interactions, laboratory test interferences, and acute toxicity.

Preparations

Excipients in commercially available drug preparations may have clinically important effects in some individuals; consult specific product labeling for details.

Pantoprazole Sodium

Oral		
For suspension, delayed-release (containing enteric-coated granules)	40 mg (of pantoprazole) per packet	**Protonix®**, Pfizer
Tablets, delayed-release (enteric-coated)	20 mg (of pantoprazole)*	**Pantoprazole Sodium Delayed-release Tablets**
		Protonix®, Pfizer
	40 mg (of pantoprazole)*	**Pantoprazole Sodium Delayed-release Tablets**
		Protonix®, Pfizer
Parenteral		
For injection, for IV infusion	40 mg (of pantoprazole)	**Protonix® I.V.**, Pfizer

*available from one or more manufacturer, distributor, and/or repackager by generic (nonproprietary) name

†Use is not currently included in the labeling approved by the US Food and Drug Administration

RABEprazole Sodium

■ Rabeprazole, commonly referred to as an acid or proton-pump inhibitor, is a gastric antisecretory agent.

Uses

■ **Gastroesophageal Reflux** Rabeprazole is used for the short-term (4–8 weeks) treatment of erosive or ulcerative esophagitis in patients with gastroesophageal reflux disease (GERD). The drug also is used as maintenance therapy following healing of erosive or ulcerative esophagitis to reduce recurrence of the disease. In addition, rabeprazole is used for the treatment of symptoms (e.g., heartburn) of GERD in patients without erosive or ulcerative esophagitis. Potential benefits in gastroesophageal reflux and esophagitis are thought to result principally from reduced acidity of gastric contents induced by the drug and resultant reduced irritation of esophageal mucosa; the drug can effectively relieve symptoms of esophagitis (e.g., heartburn) and promote healing of ulcerative and erosive lesions.

Suppression of gastric acid secretion is considered by the American College of Gastroenterology (ACG) to be the mainstay of treatment for GERD, and a proton-pump inhibitor or histamine H_2-receptor antagonist is used to achieve acid suppression, control symptoms, and prevent complications of the disease. Because GERD is considered to be a chronic disease, the ACG states that many patients with GERD require long-term, even lifelong, treatment. The ACG states that proton-pump inhibitors are more effective (i.e., provide more frequent and more rapid symptomatic relief and healing of esophagitis) than histamine H_2-receptor antagonists in the treatment of GERD, and are effective and appropriate as maintenance therapy in many patients with the disease. Proton-pump inhibitors also provide greater control of acid reflux than do prokinetic agents (e.g., cisapride [no longer commercially available in the US], metoclopramide) without the risk of severe adverse effects associated with these agents.

Efficacy of rabeprazole for treating acute GERD was established in 2 short-term (up to 8 weeks) controlled studies in adults; rabeprazole was more effective than placebo or ranitidine and at least as effective as omeprazole in healing lesions and providing symptomatic relief. Efficacy as maintenance therapy following healing of erosive or ulcerative esophagitis was established in two 52-week controlled studies in adults; maintenance of lesion healing and symptomatic relief were superior with rabeprazole versus placebo. Efficacy in patients with symptomatic GERD without erosive or ulcerative esophagitis was established in 2 short-term (4 weeks) controlled studies in patients with daytime and nocturnal heartburn, no endoscopic evidence of esophageal erosion, and 5 or more episodes of heartburn during the 7 days immediately prior to randomization. The percentage of daytime or nocturnal periods free of heartburn symptoms was greater, daily antacid consumption was substantially decreased, and other GERD-associated symptoms (regurgitation, belching, early satiety) were improved in patients receiving rabeprazole sodium 20 mg daily compared with those receiving placebo.

Antacids may be used concomitantly as needed for pain relief.

For further information on the treatment of GERD, see Uses: Gastroesophageal Reflux, in Omeprazole 56:28.36.

■ **Duodenal Ulcer** Rabeprazole is used for the short-term (up to 4 weeks) treatment of active duodenal ulcers. Efficacy for treating acute duodenal ulcers was established in two 4-week studies; rabeprazole was more effective than placebo and at least as effective as omeprazole in healing ulcers and providing symptomatic relief. Antacids may be used concomitantly as needed for pain relief.

Rabeprazole is used in combination with amoxicillin and clarithromycin (triple therapy) for the treatment of *Helicobacter pylori* infection and duodenal ulcer disease in individuals with active duodenal ulcer or a history of duodenal ulcer within the preceding 5 years. Efficacy of rabeprazole-based triple therapy for *H. pylori* eradication was established in a double-blind, parallel-group comparison study in patients with *H. pylori* infection; patients were stratified in a 1:1 ratio between those with peptic ulcer disease (active ulcer or a history of ulcer in the past 5 years) and symptomatic patients with no endoscopic evidence of peptic ulcer disease. Patients received 3, 7, or 10 days of therapy with rabeprazole (20 mg twice daily), amoxicillin (1 g twice daily), and clarithromycin (500 mg twice daily) or 10 days of therapy with omeprazole (20 mg twice daily), amoxicillin (1 g twice daily), and clarithromycin (500 mg twice daily). *H. pylori* eradication was defined as a negative ^{13}C urea breath test 6 weeks or more after completion of the assigned regimen. *H. pylori* eradication rates achieved with the 7- and 10-day rabeprazole regimens (77.3 and 78.1%, respectively, by intent-to-treat analysis) were similar to those achieved with the 10-day omeprazole regimen (73.3%); eradication rates achieved with the 3-day rabeprazole regimen (27.3%) were inferior to those achieved with the other regimens. For a more complete discussion of *H. pylori* infection, including details about the efficacy of various regimens and rationale for drug selection, see Uses: Helicobacter pylori Infection, in Clarithromycin 8:12.12.92.

■ **Pathologic GI Hypersecretory Conditions** Rabeprazole is used in the long-term treatment of pathologic GI hypersecretory conditions (e.g., Zollinger-Ellison syndrome). Experience in the treatment of these conditions is limited, but rabeprazole has been used effectively for up to 12 months; the optimum duration of treatment has not been clearly established.

■ **Crohn's Disease-associated Ulcers** Although evidence currently is limited, proton-pump inhibitors have been used for gastric acid-suppressive therapy as an adjunct in the symptomatic treatment of upper GI Crohn's disease†, including esophageal†, gastroduodenal†, and jejunoileal disease†. Most evidence of efficacy to date has been from case studies in patients with Crohn's-associated peptic ulcer disease unresponsive to other therapies (e.g., H_2-receptor antagonists, cytoprotective agents, antacids, and/or sucralfate). (See Uses: Crohn's Disease-associated Ulcers in Omeprazole 56:28.36.)

For further information on the management of Crohn's Disease, see Uses: Crohn's Disease, in Mesalamine 56:36.

Dosage and Administration

■ **Administration** Rabeprazole sodium is administered orally, generally once daily. Rabeprazole sodium tablets should *not* be chewed, crushed, or split. Food may delay the rate but does not affect the extent of GI absorption of the drug; therefore, rabeprazole generally may be given without regard to meals.

Although the manufacturer currently recommends dosing rabeprazole after the morning meal for duodenal ulcers because clinical studies establishing efficacy for this use employed such dosing, other evidence indicates that the drug may be given without regard to meals in the morning or at bedtime. The possibility that time of administration could facilitate treatment compliance should be considered.

When rabeprazole is used in combination with clarithromycin and amoxicillin (triple therapy) for the treatment of *H. pylori* infection, all 3 drugs should be taken twice daily with the morning and evening meals. Although concomitant administration of rabeprazole with clarithromycin and amoxicillin may result in increased peak plasma concentrations and areas under the plasma concentration-time curves (AUCs) of rabeprazole and 14-hydroxyclarithromycin (the active metabolite of clarithromycin), the increased exposure to these drugs is not expected to be clinically important.

■ **Dosage** ***Gastroesophageal Reflux*** The recommended adult dosage of rabeprazole sodium for the short-term treatment of erosive or ulcerative esophagitis in patients with gastroesophageal reflux disease (GERD), maintenance therapy following healing of erosive or ulcerative esophagitis, and short-term treatment of symptomatic GERD in patients without erosive or ulcerative esophagitis is 20 mg once daily. The duration of therapy for acute treatment of erosive or ulcerative esophagitis in patients with GERD is 4–8 weeks; an additional 8-week course of therapy may be considered in patients if esophageal healing is incomplete after the first course of treatment. Controlled studies for maintenance therapy following healing of erosive or ulcerative esophagitis did not extend beyond 12 months. The manufacturer states that the duration of therapy for symptomatic GERD in patients without erosive or ulcerative esophagitis is 4 weeks; an additional 4-week course of therapy may be considered in patients whose symptoms have not completely resolved after the first course of treatment. However, the American College of Gastroenterology (ACG) states that chronic, even lifelong, therapy with a proton-pump inhibitor is appropriate in many patients with GERD.

The recommended dosage of rabeprazole sodium for the short-term treatment of symptomatic GERD in adolescents 12 years of age and older is 20 mg once daily for up to 8 weeks.

Duodenal Ulcer Disease The recommended adult dosage of rabeprazole sodium for short-term treatment of duodenal ulcers is 20 mg daily, and the usual duration of therapy is 4 weeks; most patients heal within 4 weeks, but some may require additional therapy to achieve healing.

When rabeprazole sodium is used in combination with clarithromycin and amoxicillin (triple therapy) for the treatment of *H. pylori* infection in patients with active duodenal ulcer or a history of duodenal ulcer in the preceding 5 years, the usual adult dosage of rabeprazole sodium is 20 mg twice daily for 7 days.

Pathologic GI Hypersecretory Conditions The recommended initial adult dosage of rabeprazole sodium for the treatment of pathologic GI hypersecretory conditions (e.g., Zollinger-Ellison syndrome) is 60 mg once daily. Dosages up to 100 mg once daily or 60 mg twice daily have been used. Some patients may require divided doses. Dosage should be adjusted as necessary and continued for as long as clinically indicated. Some patients have been treated continuously with the drug for up to 1 year.

■ **Special Populations** Caution should be exercised in dosing patients with severe hepatic impairment, particularly because of the lack of clinical data in this patient population. However, accumulation of rabeprazole at the usual dosage of 20 mg daily is unlikely, and dosage adjustment is not necessary in those with mild to moderate hepatic impairment.

Dosage adjustment also is not necessary in geriatric patients nor in patients with renal impairment.

Cautions

■ **Contraindications** Known hypersensitivity to rabeprazole, other substituted benzimidazoles (e.g., esomeprazole, lansoprazole, omeprazole, pantoprazole), or any ingredient in the formulation.

■ **Warnings/Precautions** ***Gastric Malignancy*** Symptomatic response to therapy with rabeprazole does not preclude the occult presence of gastric neoplasm. Approximately 4% of patients had intestinal metaplasia during follow-up (up to 40 months), with no consistent changes noted.

Clostridium difficile Infection Available data suggest a possible association between use of proton-pump inhibitors and risk of *Clostridium difficile* infection, including *C. difficile*-associated diarrhea and colitis (CDAD; also known as antibiotic-associated diarrhea and colitis or pseudomembranous colitis). In most observational studies to date, the risk of *C. difficile* infection in patients exposed to proton-pump inhibitors has ranged from 1.4–2.75 times that in patients not exposed to proton-pump inhibitors; however, some observational studies have found no increase in risk. Although many of the cases occurred in patients who had other risk factors for CDAD, including advanced age, comorbid conditions, and/or use of broad-spectrum anti-infectives, the US Food and Drug Administration (FDA) concluded that a contributory role for proton-pump inhibitors could not be definitively ruled out. The mechanism by which proton-pump inhibitors might increase the risk of CDAD has not been elucidated. Although it has been suggested that reduction of gastric acidity by gastric antisecretory agents might facilitate colonization with *C. difficile*, some studies have raised questions about this proposed mechanism or have suggested that the observed association is the result of confounding with other risk factors for CDAD. FDA also is reviewing the risk of CDAD in patients exposed to histamine H_2-receptor antagonists.

CDAD can be serious in patients who have one or more risk factors for *C. difficile* infection and are receiving concomitant therapy with a proton-pump inhibitor; colectomy and, rarely, death have been reported. FDA recommends that patients receive proton-pump inhibitors at the lowest effective dosage and for the shortest possible time appropriate for their clinical condition. Patients experiencing persistent diarrhea should be evaluated for CDAD and should be managed with appropriate supportive therapy (e.g., fluid and electrolyte management), anti-infective therapy directed against *C. difficile* (e.g., metronidazole, vancomycin), and surgical evaluation as clinically indicated.

Respiratory Effects Administration of proton-pump inhibitors has been associated with an increased risk for developing certain infections (e.g., community-acquired pneumonia). (For further precautionary information about this adverse effect, see Community-acquired Pneumonia under Cautions: Respiratory Effects, in Omeprazole 56:28.36.)

Musculoskeletal Effects Findings from several observational studies suggest that therapy with proton-pump inhibitors, particularly in high dosages (i.e., multiple daily doses) and/or for prolonged periods of time (i.e., one year or longer), may be associated with an increased risk of osteoporosis-related fractures of the hip, wrist, or spine. The magnitude of risk is unclear; causality has not been established. (See Cautions: Musculoskeletal Effects, in Omeprazole 56:28.36.) FDA is continuing to evaluate this safety concern. Although controlled studies are required to confirm these findings, patients should receive proton-pump inhibitors at the lowest effective dosage and for the shortest possible time appropriate for their clinical condition. Individuals who are at risk for osteoporosis-related fractures should receive an adequate intake of calcium and vitamin D and should have their bone health assessed and managed according to current standards of care.

Hypomagnesemia Hypomagnesemia, symptomatic and asymptomatic, has been reported rarely in patients receiving long-term therapy (for at least 3 months or, in most cases, for longer than one year) with proton-pump inhibitors, including rabeprazole. Clinically serious adverse effects associated with hypomagnesemia, which are similar to manifestations of hypocalcemia, include tetany, seizures, tremors, carpopedal spasm, arrhythmias (e.g., atrial fibrillation, supraventricular tachycardia), and abnormal QT interval. Other reported adverse effects include paresthesia, muscle weakness, muscle cramps, lethargy, fatigue, and unsteadiness. In most patients, treatment of hypomagnesemia required magnesium replacement and discontinuance of the proton-pump inhibitor. Following discontinuance of the proton-pump inhibitor, hypomagnesemia resolved within a median of one week; upon rechallenge, hypomagnesemia recurred within a median of 2 weeks.

In patients expected to receive long-term therapy with a proton-pump inhibitor or in those receiving a proton-pump inhibitor concomitantly with digoxin or drugs that may cause hypomagnesemia (e.g., diuretics), clinicians should consider measurement of serum magnesium concentrations prior to initiation of prescription proton-pump inhibitor therapy and periodically thereafter. (See Cautions: Hypomagnesemia and also Cautions: Precautions and Contraindications, in Omeprazole 56:28.36.)

Specific Populations **Pregnancy.** Category B. (See Users Guide.)

Lactation. It is unknown whether rabeprazole is distributed into milk; discontinue nursing or drug because of potential risk in nursing infants.

Pediatric Use. Efficacy and safety of rabeprazole for short-term treatment of symptomatic GERD in adolescents 12–16 years of age are supported by controlled clinical trials in adults and additional safety and pharmacokinetic studies in adolescents. The pharmacokinetic and adverse effect profiles of rabeprazole in adolescents with symptomatic or endoscopically diagnosed GERD were similar to those in adults. Safety and efficacy of rabeprazole for uses other than short-term treatment of symptomatic GERD have not been established in pediatric patients.

Safety and efficacy of the drug in children younger than 12 years of age have not been established.

Geriatric Use. No substantial differences in safety and efficacy relative to younger adults, but increased sensitivity cannot be ruled out.

Severe Hepatic Impairment. Use with caution. (See Dosage and Administration: Special Populations.)

■ **Common Adverse Effects** Adverse effects occurring in 2% or more of patients receiving rabeprazole in controlled clinical trials and reported more frequently with rabeprazole than with placebo include pain, pharyngitis, flatulence, infection, and constipation.

Drug Interactions

Rabeprazole is extensively metabolized, mainly via hepatic cytochrome P-450 (CYP) 3A and 2C19 isoenzymes.

■ **Drugs that Cause Hypomagnesemia** Potential pharmacologic interaction (possible increased risk of hypomagnesemia). In patients receiving diuretics (i.e., loop or thiazide diuretics) or other drugs that may cause hypomagnesemia, monitoring of magnesium concentrations should be considered prior to initiation of prescription proton-pump inhibitor therapy and periodically thereafter. (See Hypomagnesemia under Cautions: Warnings/Precautions.)

■ **Gastric pH-Dependent Drugs** Potential pharmacokinetic interaction; increased or decreased drug absorption at increased gastric pH values (e.g., digoxin, ketoconazole). Increased monitoring during concomitant use with rabeprazole.

■ **Antiretroviral Agents** ***Atazanavir*** Potential pharmacokinetic interaction (possible altered oral absorption of atazanavir at increased gastric pH, resulting in decreased plasma atazanavir concentrations). Concomitant use of omeprazole 40 mg once daily and atazanavir (with or without low-dose ritonavir) results in a substantial decrease in plasma concentrations of atazanavir and possible loss of the therapeutic effect of the antiretroviral agent. The manufacturer of rabeprazole states that concomitant administration with atazanavir is not recommended. If atazanavir is administered in an antiretroviral treatment-naive patient receiving a proton-pump inhibitor, a *ritonavir-boosted* regimen of 300 mg of atazanavir once daily with ritonavir 100 mg once daily with food is recommended. The dose of the proton-pump inhibitor should be administered approximately 12 hours before *ritonavir-boosted* atazanavir; the dose of the proton-pump inhibitor should not exceed omeprazole 20 mg daily (or equivalent). Concomitant use of proton-pump inhibitors with atazanavir is not recommended in antiretroviral treatment-experienced patients.

Fosamprenavir Concomitant use of esomeprazole with fosamprenavir (with or without ritonavir) did not substantially affect concentrations of amprenavir (active metabolite of fosamprenavir). No dosage adjustment is required when proton-pump inhibitors are used concomitantly with fosamprenavir (with or without ritonavir).

Lopinavir Concomitant use of omeprazole with the fixed combination of lopinavir and ritonavir (lopinavir/ritonavir) did not have a clinically important effect on plasma concentrations or area under the concentration-time curve (AUC) of lopinavir. No dosage adjustment is required when proton-pump inhibitors are used concomitantly with lopinavir/ritonavir.

Raltegravir Pharmacokinetic interaction with omeprazole (substantially increased peak plasma concentration and AUC of raltegravir); however, no dosage adjustment is recommended when proton-pump inhibitors are used concomitantly with raltegravir.

Rilpivirine Pharmacokinetic interaction with omeprazole (decreased plasma concentrations and AUC of rilpivirine). Concomitant use of other proton-pump inhibitors also may result in decreased plasma concentrations of rilpivirine. Concomitant use of rilpivirine and proton-pump inhibitors is contraindicated.

Saquinavir Potential pharmacokinetic interaction (increased peak plasma concentration and AUC of saquinavir). Concomitant use of omeprazole 40 mg once daily and *ritonavir-boosted* saquinavir (saquinavir 1 g twice daily and ritonavir 100 mg twice daily) increased the peak plasma concentration and AUC of saquinavir by 75 and 82%, respectively. Caution is advised if proton-pump inhibitors are used concomitantly with *ritonavir-boosted* saquinavir, and patients should be monitored for saquinavir toxicity.

■ **Clopidogrel** Potential pharmacokinetic interaction (decreased plasma concentration of the active metabolite of clopidogrel) and pharmacodynamic interaction (reduced antiplatelet effects) between proton-pump inhibitors and clopidogrel. Clopidogrel is metabolized to its active metabolite by cytochrome P-450 (CYP) isoenzyme 2C19 (CYP2C19). Concurrent use of omeprazole or esomeprazole, which inhibit CYP2C19, with clopidogrel reduces exposure to the active metabolite of clopidogrel and decreases platelet inhibitory effects. Although the clinical importance has not been fully elucidated, a reduction in the effectiveness of clopidogrel in preventing cardiovascular events is possible. Proton-pump inhibitors vary in their potency for inhibiting CYP2C19. The change in inhibition of adenosine diphosphate (ADP)-induced platelet aggregation associated with concomitant use of proton-pump inhibitors is related to the change in exposure to the active metabolite of clopidogrel. In pharmacokinetic and pharmacodynamic studies in healthy individuals, dexlansoprazole, lansoprazole, and pantoprazole had less effect on the antiplatelet activity of clopidogrel than did omeprazole or esomeprazole.

The decision to use a proton-pump inhibitor concomitantly with clopidogrel should be based on the assessed risks and benefits in individual patients. The American College of Cardiology Foundation/American College of Gastroenterology/American Heart Association (ACCF/ACG/AHA) states that the reduction in GI bleeding risk with proton-pump inhibitors is substantial in patients with risk factors for GI bleeding (e.g., advanced age; concomitant use of warfarin, corticosteroids, or nonsteroidal anti-inflammatory agents [NSAIAs]; *H. pylori* infection) and may outweigh any potential reduction in the cardiovascular efficacy of antiplatelet treatment associated with a drug-drug interaction. In contrast, ACCF/ACG/AHA states that patients without such risk factors receive little if any absolute risk reduction from proton-pump inhibitor therapy, and the risk/benefit balance may favor use of antiplatelet therapy without a proton-pump inhibitor in these patients.

If concomitant therapy with a proton-pump inhibitor and clopidogrel is considered necessary, use of an agent with little or no CYP2C19-inhibitory activity should be considered. Alternatively, treatment with a histamine H_2-receptor antagonist (ranitidine, famotidine, nizatidine) may be considered, although such agents may not be as effective as a proton-pump inhibitor in providing gastric protection; cimetidine should *not* be used since it also is a potent CYP2C19 inhibitor. There currently is no evidence that histamine H_2-receptor antagonists (other than cimetidine) or other drugs that reduce gastric acid (e.g., antacids) interfere with the antiplatelet effects of clopidogrel. For further information on interactions between proton-pump inhibitors and clopidogrel, see Drug Interactions: Proton-Pump Inhibitors, in Clopidogrel Bisulfate 20:12.18.

■ **Cyclosporine** Potential pharmacokinetic interaction (inhibition of cyclosporine metabolism).

■ **Digoxin** Hypomagnesemia (e.g., resulting from long-term use of proton-pump inhibitors) sensitizes the myocardium to digoxin and, thus, may increase the risk of digoxin-induced cardiotoxic effects. In patients receiving digoxin, monitoring of magnesium concentrations should be considered prior to initiation of prescription proton-pump inhibitor therapy and periodically thereafter.

■ **Methotrexate** Potential pharmacokinetic interaction (increased serum methotrexate concentrations, possibly resulting in toxicity) when proton-pump inhibitors, including rabeprazole, are used concomitantly with methotrexate. Increased serum concentrations and delayed clearance of methotrexate and/or its metabolite hydroxymethotrexate, with or without symptoms of methotrexate toxicity, have been reported in patients receiving methotrexate (usually at doses of 300 mg/m^2 to 12 g/m^2) concomitantly with a proton-pump inhibitor. Although most of the reported cases occurred in patients receiving high doses of methotrexate, toxicity also has been reported in patients receiving low dosages of methotrexate (e.g., 15 mg per week) concomitantly with a proton-pump inhibitor. No formal studies of interactions between high-dose methotrexate and proton-pump inhibitors have been conducted to date.

The manufacturer of rabeprazole states that temporary discontinuance of proton-pump inhibitor therapy may be considered in some patients receiving high-dose methotrexate therapy. Some clinicians recommend either withholding proton-pump inhibitor therapy for several days before and after methotrexate administration or substituting a histamine H_2-receptor antagonist for the proton-pump inhibitor when acid suppressive therapy is indicated during methotrexate therapy. Pending further evaluation, some clinicians state that these recommendations should extend to patients receiving low-dose methotrexate.

■ **Sucralfate** Potential pharmacokinetic interaction. Concomitant administration of lansoprazole or omeprazole with sucralfate resulted in delayed absorption and decreased bioavailability of these proton-pump inhibitors. Administer proton-pump inhibitors at least 30 minutes before sucralfate.

■ **Warfarin** Increases in the international normalized ratio (INR) and prothrombin time have been reported in patients receiving warfarin concomitantly with a proton-pump inhibitor, including rabeprazole. Because such increases may lead to abnormal bleeding and death, monitoring of INR and prothrombin time may be necessary during concomitant use with rabeprazole.

Description

Rabeprazole, a proton-pump inhibitor, is a gastric antisecretory agent structurally and pharmacologically related to lansoprazole and omeprazole. The drugs are substituted benzimidazoles and are chemically and pharmacologically unrelated to H_2-receptor antagonists, antimuscarinics, or prostaglandin analogs.

Rabeprazole binds to hydrogen-potassium ATPase in gastric parietal cells; inactivation of this enzyme system (also known as the proton, hydrogen, or acid pump) blocks the final step in the secretion of hydrochloric acid by these cells, resulting in potent, long-lasting inhibition of gastric acid secretion. The antisecretory effect is apparent within 1 hour following oral administration, with the median inhibitory effect on 24-hour gastric acidity being 88% of maximal after the first dose.

Because the rabeprazole molecule is acid labile, the delayed-release, enteric-coated tablet formulation increases oral bioavailability. Rabeprazole is extensively metabolized, mainly via hepatic cytochrome P-450 (CYP) 3A and 2C19 isoenzymes.

Rabeprazole can suppress gastric *Helicobacter pylori* in patients with duodenal ulcer and/or reflux esophagitis infected with the organism, probably via binding to the bacteria and resultant inhibition of urease activity. Combined therapy with rabeprazole and one or more appropriate anti-infectives (e.g., clarithromycin, amoxicillin) can effectively eradicate *H. pylori* gastric infection.

Increased gastric pH during rabeprazole therapy stimulates gastrin secretion via a negative feedback mechanism and results in enterochromaffin-like cell (ECL) hyperplasia. Although rats have demonstrated carcinoid lesions, *no* clinical sequelae (e.g., no adenomatoid, dysplastic, or neoplastic changes) have occurred to date in patients receiving the drug for up to 1 year.

Therapy with proton-pump inhibitors, particularly in high dosages and/or for prolonged periods of time, may be associated with an increased risk of osteoporosis-related fractures of the hip, wrist, or spine. (See Musculoskeletal Effects under Cautions: Warnings/Precautions.) The mechanism by which these drugs may increase risk of such fractures has not been elucidated but may involve decreased insoluble calcium absorption secondary to increased gastric pH.

Advice to Patients

Importance of informing clinicians of existing or contemplated concomitant therapy, including prescription and OTC drugs, as well as concomitant illnesses.

Necessity of swallowing tablets whole, without crushing or chewing.

Importance of continuing rabeprazole therapy for the entire treatment course, unless directed otherwise.

Importance of advising patients that use of multiple daily doses of the drug for an extended period of time may increase the risk of fractures of the hip, wrist, or spine.

Risk of hypomagnesemia; importance of advising patients to immediately report and seek care for any cardiovascular or neurologic manifestations (e.g., palpitations, dizziness, seizures, tetany).

Possible increased risk of *Clostridium difficile* infection; importance of contacting a clinician if persistent watery stools, abdominal pain, and fever occur.

Importance of women informing their clinicians if they are or plan to become pregnant or plan to breast-feed.

Importance of informing patients of other important precautionary information. (See Cautions.)

Overview® (see Users Guide). For additional information until a more detailed monograph is developed and published, the manufacturer's labeling should be consulted. It is *essential* that the manufacturer's labeling be consulted for more detailed information on usual cautions, precautions, contraindications, potential drug interactions, laboratory test interferences, and acute toxicity.

Preparations

Excipients in commercially available drug preparations may have clinically important effects in some individuals; consult specific product labeling for details.

RABEprazole Sodium

Oral

Tablets, delayed-release (enteric-coated)	20 mg	**AcipHex®**, Eisai (also promoted by Janssen [formerly Ortho-McNeil-Janssen])

†Use is not currently included in the labeling approved by the US Food and Drug Administration

PROKINETIC AGENTS 56:32

Metoclopramide Hydrochloride

■ Metoclopramide hydrochloride is a dopamine-receptor antagonist, an antiemetic, and a stimulant of upper GI motility (prokinetic agent).

Uses

Metoclopramide is used in a variety of GI disorders, but principally for the management of GI motility disorders, especially gastric stasis, for the management of gastroesophageal reflux, for the prevention of cancer chemotherapy-induced nausea and vomiting, and for the prevention of postoperative nausea and vomiting when nasogastric suction is considered undesirable. The drug is also used to facilitate intubation of the small intestine and as an adjunct during radiographic examination of the upper GI tract.

Therapy with the drug should not exceed 12 weeks' duration. Metoclopramide oral solution and tablets are recommended for use in adults *only*.

■ **Diabetic Gastric Stasis** Metoclopramide is used for the symptomatic treatment of acute and recurrent diabetic gastric stasis (gastroparesis). Treatment of diabetic gastric stasis with metoclopramide is not curative. Since diabetic gastric stasis is a chronic, recurrent disease, successful therapy may often require long-term, intermittent use of metoclopramide.

The motility of the stomach is abnormal in patients with diabetic gastric stasis; fundic and antral contractility are markedly diminished and gastric emptying of liquids and solids is delayed. Although a correlation between gastric stasis and autonomic neuropathy has not been shown in diabetics, these patients may have signs of vagal nerve damage.

In patients with diabetic gastric stasis, metoclopramide increases the rate of gastric emptying and decreases usual symptoms of gastric stasis including nausea, vomiting, heartburn, anorexia, persistent postprandial fullness, abdominal pain and distention, and early satiety. Symptoms of delayed gastric emptying appear to respond to metoclopramide within different time intervals. Relief of nausea usually occurs soon after initiating metoclopramide therapy and continues to improve over a 3-week period. Subsequently, relief of vomiting and anorexia may precede relief of abdominal fullness by 1 week or longer.

In most patients with diabetic gastric stasis, metoclopramide-induced reduction of symptoms does not correlate well with improvement in gastric emptying. In some patients, complete relief of symptoms occurs despite minimal increases in the rate of gastric emptying, while in others, symptoms of gastric stasis persist despite a normalization in gastric emptying.

■ **Postsurgical Gastric Stasis** Metoclopramide has been used for the symptomatic treatment of acute and chronic postsurgical gastric stasis† following vagotomy and gastric resection or vagotomy and pyloroplasty. The drug has improved gastric emptying and decreased the usual symptoms of gastric stasis in patients with these conditions.

■ **Prevention of Cancer Chemotherapy-induced Emesis** Metoclopramide is used parenterally in high doses for the prevention of nausea and vomiting associated with emetogenic cancer chemotherapy. The drug also has been administered orally† for the prevention of chemotherapy-induced nausea and vomiting.

To prevent chemotherapy-induced nausea and vomiting associated with chemotherapy regimens with a high emetic risk (i.e., incidence of emesis exceeds 90% if no antiemetics are administered), the American Society of Clinical Oncology (ASCO) currently recommends a 3-drug antiemetic regimen consisting of a type 3 serotonin (5-HT_3) receptor antagonist (e.g., dolasetron, granisetron, ondansetron, palonosetron, tropisetron [not commercially available in the US]), dexamethasone, and aprepitant.

Antiemetic agents with a lower therapeutic index (i.e., less efficacious and generally associated with more frequent adverse effects), including metoclopramide, cannabinoids (e.g., dronabinol, nabilone), butyrophenones, and phenothiazines are *not* considered by ASCO to be appropriate first-line antiemetics for any group of patients receiving chemotherapy of high emetic risk; ASCO states that these drugs should be reserved for patients unable to tolerate or refractory to first-line agents.

The antiemetic combination of a 5-HT_3 receptor antagonist, dexamethasone, and aprepitant also is preferred in patients receiving combination chemotherapy with an anthracycline and cyclophosphamide.

For patients receiving other chemotherapy of moderate emetic risk (i.e., incidence of emesis without antiemetics exceeds 30% but does not exceed 90%), ASCO recommends a 2-drug antiemetic regimen consisting of a 5-HT_3 receptor antagonist and dexamethasone.

For patients receiving chemotherapy regimens with a low emetic risk (i.e., incidence of emesis without antiemetics exceeds 10% but does not exceed 30%), ASCO recommends dexamethasone alone on the first day of chemotherapy.

Antiemetics can be prescribed on an as-needed basis in patients receiving chemotherapy with a minimal emetic risk (incidence of emesis is less than 10% without antiemetics).

In patients experiencing vomiting and nausea despite recommended prophylaxis regimens, ASCO recommends that clinicians consider adding a benzodiazepine (e.g., alprazolam, lorazepam) to the regimen, substituting high-dose intravenous metoclopramide for the 5-HT_3 receptor antagonist in the regimen, or adding a butyrophenone or phenothiazine to the regimen.

For the prevention of *delayed* emesis in patients receiving cisplatin or other chemotherapy associated with a high emetic risk, these authorities currently recommend a 2-drug combination of dexamethasone and aprepitant.

Although antihistamines (e.g., diphenhydramine) and benzodiazepines (e.g., alprazolam, lorazepam) may be useful as adjunctive antiemetic agents, they currently are not recommended as monotherapy as antiemetic agents. However, many clinicians find benzodiazepines useful in the management of anticipatory emesis.

Cisplatin Metoclopramide is used parenterally for the prevention of cisplatin-induced nausea and vomiting. The drug has been used effectively for the prevention of chemotherapy-induced emesis in patients receiving cisplatin alone or in combination with other antineoplastic agents. In patients receiving cisplatin, high-dose metoclopramide (2 mg/kg) reduces the number and duration of vomiting episodes and the volume of emesis. In some patients, cisplatin-induced nausea and vomiting are completely prevented with metoclopramide therapy. Clinical evaluations of metoclopramide in the prevention of cisplatin-induced emesis have shown that the antiemetic effect of metoclopramide is greater than that of placebo, prochlorperazine, or tetrahydrocannabinol (THC). However, it appears that type 3 serotonergic (5-HT_3) receptor antagonists (e.g., dolasetron, granisetron, ondansetron, palonosetron, tropisetron [not commercially available in the US]) and aprepitant generally are more effective and better tolerated than metoclopramide, which reportedly is pharmacologically less selective, and therefore, these 5-HT_3 receptor antagonists given in combination with dexamethasone and aprepitant may be preferred for the initial prophylaxis of acute emetic effects in many patients; in some cases, these drugs may be effective in treating nausea and emesis that develop despite metoclopramide prophylaxis. Currently available 5-HT_3 receptor antagonists (i.e., dolasetron, granisetron, ondansetron, palonosetron, tropisetron [not commercially available in the US]) appear to be comparably effective in preventing acute cisplatin- and other chemotherapy-induced nausea and vomiting. The addition of dexamethasone to monotherapy with a 5-HT_3 receptor antagonist or metoclopramide increases the antiemetic efficacy of either drug alone, and such combined therapy may be useful in patients whose nausea and vomiting are refractory to monotherapy. Although addition of diphenhydramine to metoclopramide and dexamethasone therapy may increase the antiemetic efficacy further and decrease metoclopramide-induced adverse effects, combined therapy with a selective 5-HT_3 receptor antagonist and dexamethasone appears to be more effective than this triple-drug combination. In addition, some evidence suggests that such combined therapy may be more effective, albeit not optimally, than monotherapy for the prevention and treatment of delayed emesis. Various combinations of antiemetic agents have been used, and comparative efficacy is continually being evaluated.

Remaining most problematic is the management of *delayed* and *anticipatory* nausea and vomiting; pending further elucidation of optimal regimens, some clinicians suggest combined regimens of 2 or 3 drugs that include a 5-HT_3 receptor antagonist (e.g., dolasetron, granisetron, ondansetron, palonosetron, tropisetron [not commercially available in the US]), aprepitant, a corticosteroid (e.g., dexamethasone), metoclopramide, and/or benzodiazepine (e.g., lorazepam for anxiolytic, amnesic, and possibly antiemetic effects). In several clinical trials, oral† metoclopramide has been effective when given in combination with dexamethasone for the prevention of delayed emesis in patients receiving chemotherapy.

Based on limited published data, maximum efficacy of metoclopramide appears to depend greatly on the use of the appropriate dose, route, and schedule during administration of the drug. (See Prevention of Cancer Chemotherapy-induced Emesis, in Dosage and Administration: Dosage.) The efficacy of lower than currently recommended doses and/or alternate administration schedules for metoclopramide in the prevention of cisplatin-induced emesis remains to be clearly established. In one study in patients receiving cisplatin, optimum antiemetic effect was generally associated with serum metoclopramide concentrations greater than 850 ng/mL.

Metoclopramide is more likely to be effective in patients who were not previously exposed to cancer chemotherapy than in patients whose symptoms are refractory to conventional antiemetic agents. The antiemetic efficacy of metoclopramide appears to be maintained during subsequent doses of cisplatin.

Other Antineoplastic Agents Metoclopramide is used for prevention of nausea and vomiting associated with other antineoplastic agents (e.g., cyclophosphamide, dacarbazine, doxorubicin, methotrexate) and with cancer chemotherapy regimens that do not include cisplatin. Since various antineoplastic agents may induce emesis by different mechanisms, the efficacy of metoclopramide depends on their relative potential and specific pharmacologic pathways for inducing emesis. In patients receiving dacarbazine, high-dose metoclopramide (2 mg/kg) appears to be an effective antiemetic. When oral metoclopramide (10 mg 1–2 hours before chemotherapy and then every 8 hours for a week) was combined with IV dexamethasone (10 mg immediately before initiation of IV chemotherapy) in patients receiving cyclophosphamide, methotrexate, and fluorouracil for breast cancer (a moderately emetogenic regimen), this antiemetic combination appeared to be comparably effective overall to oral ondansetron (8 mg 1–2 hours before chemotherapy and then every 8 hours for a week) in preventing emesis during the 7-day treatment period but was more effective than ondansetron in reducing the frequency of nausea during the first day of chemotherapy. Additional study is needed to further evaluate the role of metoclopramide alone or combined with other antiemetics in the prevention of nausea and vomiting associated with the many different regimens used for cancer chemotherapy.

■ **Intubation of the Small Intestine** Metoclopramide is used parenterally to facilitate intubation of the small intestine in adults and children in whom the tube (e.g., endoscope, biopsy tube) does not pass through the pylorus with conventional maneuvers. The beneficial effect of metoclopramide on intubation of the small intestine is principally related to the pharmacologic action of the drug on GI motility and contractility. (See Pharmacology: GI Effects.) Metoclopramide has little influence on the time required for biopsy capsules to reach the pylorus, but substantially reduces the time required for the capsules to pass through the pylorus.

In several controlled trials in patients with or without GI disease (e.g., inflammatory bowel disease, chronic diarrhea, malabsorption, celiac disease, peptic ulcer) undergoing intubation of the small intestine, IV metoclopramide (10 mg) reduced the time required for intubation and facilitated performance of the procedure; however, administration of the drug generally did not influence patient tolerance of the procedure.

■ **Radiographic Examination of the Upper GI Tract** Metoclopramide is used parenterally to stimulate gastric emptying and intestinal transit of barium in patients in whom delayed emptying interferes with radiographic examination of the stomach and/or small intestine. In patients receiving oral barium, IV metoclopramide increases the rate of gastric emptying and reduces transit time of the barium in the small intestine. Metoclopramide markedly reduces the time required for radiographic examination of the small intestine and is effective in preventing nausea or regurgitation of barium that occurs in some patients with gastric atonia, pylorospasm, or spasm of the duodenal bulb.

■ **Gastroesophageal Reflux** Metoclopramide is used orally for the short-term (up to 12 weeks) relief of symptomatic, documented gastroesophageal reflux in adults who are unresponsive to conventional therapy alone, including changes in lifestyle, habits, and/or diet, which may be contributing or precipitating factors, and weight reduction in obese patients. However, agents that suppress gastric acid secretion (e.g., proton-pump inhibitors, histamine H_2-receptor antagonists) currently are considered to be the mainstay of treatment for gastroesophageal reflux disease (GERD).

Metoclopramide produces a dose-related increase in the resting tone of the lower esophageal sphincter in healthy adults and in patients with gastroesophageal reflux. There reportedly is substantial interindividual variation in the effect of metoclopramide on lower esophageal sphincter pressure. In patients with gastroesophageal reflux, metoclopramide increases gastric emptying rate both in those with normal or delayed gastric emptying, and reduces daytime and nocturnal heartburn and regurgitation; however, metoclopramide therapy produces greater reductions in severity and occurrence of daytime and postprandial heartburn and regurgitation than in nocturnal symptoms associated with gastroesophageal reflux. If symptoms are associated with particular situations of precipitating factors (e.g., following the evening meal), administration of a single dose of metoclopramide prior to the provocative situation rather than daily administration of multiple doses of the drug should be considered.

Based on data from a limited number of patients, metoclopramide appears to be more effective than an aluminum hydroxide antacid or placebo and about as effective as cimetidine in improving the symptoms of gastroesophageal reflux. Objective parameters (i.e., endoscopy, lower esophageal sphincter pressure, esophageal contraction amplitude) for response were not consistently improved in these patients following short-term (4–8 weeks) administration of metoclopramide; however, in one unpublished study, endoscopic evidence of healing was observed following administration of metoclopramide (15 mg 4 times daily) for 12 weeks. Since there is no documented correlation between symptoms and healing of esophageal lesions in patients with gastroesophageal reflux, therapy in patients with documented lesions should be accompanied by appropriate endoscopic evaluation. In a study comparing single oral doses of metoclopramide (15 mg) with an aluminum hydroxide antacid (30 mL) or placebo in patients with reflux esophagitis, metoclopramide was reportedly more effective than antacid in reducing the symptoms associated with reflux. Metoclopramide increased the resting tone of the lower esophageal sphincter in all patients for at least 1 hour and prevented gastroesophageal reflux following administration of an intragastric acid load. Although metoclopramide may be effective for the short-term relief of gastroesophageal reflux, safety and efficacy of metoclopramide therapy beyond 12 weeks have not been evaluated and such prolonged use is not recommended.

Although metoclopramide appears to provide symptomatic relief and esophageal healing as effectively as a standard dosage of a histamine H_2-receptor antagonist, and improved efficacy has been reported when metoclopramide has been used with a histamine H_2-receptor antagonist, the potential risks (e.g., severe and potentially irreversible adverse CNS effects) and benefits of metoclopramide relative to other effective therapies must be considered. The American College of Gastroenterology (ACG) states that the frequent occurrence of adverse CNS effects has appropriately decreased the regular use of metoclopramide for treatment of GERD. Furthermore, the American Gastroenterological Association (AGA) recommends against use of metoclopramide for treatment of GERD because of the drug's adverse effect profile and a lack of high-quality data supporting its use. The ACG and AGA state that proton-pump inhibitors provide greater control of acid reflux than do other currently available agents, including prokinetic agents (e.g., cisapride [no longer commercially available in the US], metoclopramide). Suppression of gastric acid secretion is considered by these experts to be the mainstay of treatment for

GERD, and a proton-pump inhibitor or histamine H_2-receptor antagonist is used to achieve acid suppression, control symptoms, and prevent complications of the disease. Because GERD is considered to be a chronic disease, many patients with GERD will require long-term, even lifelong, treatment. For further information on the treatment of GERD, see Uses: Gastroesophageal Reflux, in Omeprazole 56:28.36.

■ **Other Uses** Metoclopramide is used parenterally for the prevention of postoperative nausea and vomiting when nasogastric suction is considered undesirable.

Metoclopramide has been used for the management of migraine†. Some experts state that IM metoclopramide may be considered as adjunctive therapy for control of nausea in patients with acute migraine attacks and that the IV drug may be considered as monotherapy for relief of migraine pain. For further information on management and classification of migraine headache, see Vascular Headaches: General Principles in Migraine Therapy, under Uses in Sumatriptan 28:32.28.

Metoclopramide has been used in a limited number of patients for the treatment of peptic ulcer†. Metoclopramide has also been used as an antiemetic for the prevention of nausea and vomiting associated with drugs other than antineoplastic agents†, radiation therapy†, and other causes†. The drug has also been used for the management of anorexia nervosa†, vertigo†, and intractable hiccups†. Metoclopramide has been used to promote postpartum lactation†. Metoclopramide has also been used to empty the stomach of blood prior to endoscopy in patients with upper GI hemorrhage†. The safety and efficacy of metoclopramide in these conditions have not been established.

Dosage and Administration

■ **Administration** Metoclopramide is administered orally, by IM or direct IV injection, or by IV infusion.

Therapy with the drug should not exceed 12 weeks' duration. Metoclopramide oral solution and tablets are recommended for adults *only*.

For IM or direct IV injection, the commercially available metoclopramide injection is used without further dilution. For direct IV injection, each 10 mg of the drug should be administered slowly over 1–2 minutes, since a transient but intense feeling of anxiety and restlessness, followed by drowsiness, may occur with rapid IV injection.

For doses exceeding 10 mg, metoclopramide injection should be diluted in 50 mL of a compatible IV solution.

For IV infusion, metoclopramide hydrochloride injection should be diluted in 50 mL of one of the following IV solutions: 5% dextrose, 0.9% sodium chloride, 5% dextrose and 0.45% sodium chloride, Ringer's, or lactated Ringer's. Because the drug is most stable when diluted in 0.9% sodium chloride injection, the manufacturers state that this is the preferred solution for preparing IV infusions. IV infusions should be given slowly over at least 15 minutes. Other IV solutions flowing through a common administration tubing or site generally should be discontinued while metoclopramide is being infused unless the solutions are known to be compatible and the flow rate is adequately controlled.

Metoclopramide injection and diluted solutions of the drug should be inspected for particulate matter and discoloration prior to administration whenever solution and container permit; the solution should be discarded if particulate matter or discoloration is observed.

■ **Dosage** Although USP currently states that potency of metoclopramide hydrochloride preparations should be expressed both in terms of the salt and the base ("active moiety"), dosage currently is expressed in terms of the base. (See Chemistry and Stability: Chemistry.)

Diabetic Gastric Stasis For relief of symptoms associated with diabetic gastric stasis in patients who can tolerate oral administration of the drug, the usual adult oral dosage of metoclopramide is 10 mg 4 times daily, given 30 minutes before meals and at bedtime. In patients who have severe symptoms, or when oral administration of metoclopramide is not feasible, the drug should be given by IM or IV injection. The usual adult IM or IV dosage of metoclopramide for symptomatic relief of diabetic gastric stasis is 10 mg 4 times daily, given 30 minutes before meals and at bedtime; parenteral administration of metoclopramide for up 10 days may be required until symptoms subside sufficiently to allow oral administration of the drug.

Oral therapy with metoclopramide is usually continued for 2–8 weeks, depending on patient response and the likelihood of continued well-being if the drug is discontinued. Since diabetic gastric stasis is frequently recurrent, metoclopramide therapy should be reinstituted at the earliest recurrence of symptoms. However, a thorough assessment of the risks and benefits should be made prior to continuing further metoclopramide therapy.

Prevention of Cancer Chemotherapy-induced Emesis For the prevention of cancer chemotherapy-induced emesis, the manufacturer states that metoclopramide is usually given by IV infusion 30 minutes before administration of cancer chemotherapy, and repeated every 2 hours for 2 additional doses, then every 3 hours for 3 additional doses. For adults, the manufacturer states that the initial 2 doses of metoclopramide should be 2 mg/kg if highly emetogenic drugs (e.g., cisplatin, dacarbazine, dactinomycin) are used alone or in combination, while a metoclopramide dose of 1 mg/kg may be sufficient for less emetogenic drugs or chemotherapy regimens. However, combinations of other antiemetic agents generally are preferred as first-line antiemetic regimens in patients receiving chemotherapy of moderate or high emetic risk (see Uses: Prevention of Cancer Chemotherapy-induced Emesis). If extrapyramidal symptoms occur during these IV metoclopramide dosage regimens, diphenhydramine hydrochloride (e.g., 25–50 mg given IV or IM) may be administered.

Metoclopramide has been administered orally† for the prevention of chemotherapy-induced emesis. For prevention of emesis in patients receiving an IV chemotherapy regimen with low emetic risk, some experts state that 10–40 mg of metoclopramide may be administered orally† or IV before the chemotherapy dose and then repeated every 4 or 6 hours as needed; these experts state that patients receiving oral chemotherapy requiring only as-needed ("prn") antiemetic therapy may receive oral metoclopramide† (10–40 mg orally before the chemotherapy dose and then every 4 or 6 hours as needed). If dystonic reactions occur, patients may receive diphenhydramine hydrochloride (e.g., 25–50 mg orally or IV every 4 or 6 hours).

Metoclopramide also has been administered orally† for the prevention of delayed emesis in patients receiving chemotherapy (i.e., vomiting occurring 24 or more hours after chemotherapy). When given in combination with dexamethasone in clinical trials, oral metoclopramide dosages of 20–40 mg (or 0.5 mg/kg) given 2–4 times daily for 3 or 4 days have been used.

Prevention of Postoperative Nausea and Vomiting For the prevention of postoperative nausea and vomiting when nasogastric suction is considered undesirable, the manufacturer states that the usual adult IM dose of metoclopramide is 10 mg administered near the end of the surgical procedure, although a 20-mg dose also may be used.

Intubation of the Small Intestine For patients undergoing intubation of the small intestine in whom the tube has not passed through the pylorus during 10 minutes of conventional maneuvers, the usual dose of metoclopramide to facilitate intubation in adults and children older than 14 years of age is 10 mg, given as a single, direct IV injection. To facilitate intubation in children, the usual single IV dose of metoclopramide is 0.1 mg/kg in children younger than 6 years of age or 2.5–5 mg in children 6–14 years of age.

Radiographic Examination of the Upper GI Tract For patients in whom delayed gastric emptying interferes with radiographic examination of the stomach and/or small intestine, the usual adult dose of metoclopramide to stimulate gastric emptying and intestinal transit of barium is 10 mg, given as a single, direct IV injection.

Gastroesophageal Reflux For the symptomatic treatment of gastroesophageal reflux, the usual adult oral dosage of metoclopramide is 10–15 mg given up to 4 times daily 30 minutes before each meal and at bedtime, depending on the symptoms being treated and the patient's clinical response. (See Uses: Gastroesophageal Reflux.) If symptoms occur only intermittently or at specific times of the day, single oral doses up to 20 mg given prior to the provoking situation may be preferred to daily administration of multiple doses of the drug. Some patients (e.g., geriatric patients) who are sensitive to the therapeutic and/or adverse effects of the drug may require individual doses of only 5 mg. Although experience in patients with esophageal erosion and ulceration associated with gastroesophageal reflux is limited, a metoclopramide dosage of 15 mg 4 times daily has been suggested in such patients. Because of the poor correlation between symptoms and endoscopic appearance of the esophagus, therapy in patients with documented esophageal lesions is best guided by endoscopic evaluation. The safety and efficacy of continuing metoclopramide therapy beyond 12 weeks in patients with gastroesophageal reflux have not been established and such prolonged use is not recommended.

■ **Dosage in Renal and Hepatic Impairment** Because metoclopramide is eliminated principally via renal excretion, doses and/or frequency of administration of the drug should be modified in response to the degree of impairment in patients with impaired renal function. The manufacturers recommend that patients with creatinine clearances less than 40 mL/minute receive initial metoclopramide dosages that are approximately 50% of the usual recommended dosages. Dosage subsequently should be increased or decreased according to the patient's clinical response and tolerance.

Modification of metoclopramide dosage in patients with impaired hepatic function does not appear to be necessary.

Cautions

Adverse reactions to metoclopramide generally involve the CNS and GI tract and are usually mild, transient, and reversible following discontinuance of the drug. In general, the incidence of metoclopramide-induced adverse effects is related to dosage and duration of therapy.

■ **Nervous System Effects** The most frequent adverse effects of metoclopramide involve the CNS. Restlessness, drowsiness, fatigue, and lassitude have been reported in patients receiving the drug; these effects occur in about 10% of patients receiving a dosage of 10 mg 4 times daily. Insomnia, headache, confusion, dizziness, or depression with suicidal ideation occurs less frequently. The risk of drowsiness is increased at higher doses, occurring in about 70% of patients receiving doses of 1–2 mg/kg. Seizures have been reported rarely, although a causal relationship to metoclopramide has not been established. Hallucinations also have been reported rarely. Feelings of anxiety or agitation also may occur, especially following rapid IV injection of the drug.

Extrapyramidal reactions (e.g., acute dystonic reactions, akathisia) may occur in patients receiving metoclopramide and apparently are mediated via blockade of central dopaminergic receptors involved in motor function. Although extrapyramidal reactions may occur in all age groups and at any dose, they occur more frequently in pediatric patients and adults younger than 30 years of age and following IV administration of high doses of the drug (e.g., those used in prophylaxis of cancer chemotherapy-induced vomiting). Extrapyramidal reactions generally occur within 24–48 hours after starting therapy and usually subside within 24 hours following discontinuance of the drug. Most patients respond rapidly to treatment with diazepam or an agent with central anticholinergic activity such as diphenhydramine or benztropine.

Acute dystonic reactions, which resemble the acute dyskinesias produced by antipsychotic drugs (e.g., phenothiazines, butyrophenones), reportedly occur in less than 1% of adults receiving low dosages of metoclopramide (e.g., 30–40 mg daily) and are not necessarily related to dose. However, dystonic reactions occur in approximately 25% of young adults (i.e., 18–30 years of age) receiving high dosages of metoclopramide (e.g., 2 mg/kg per dose) during cancer chemotherapy; in adults older than 30 years of age who are receiving similar dosages of metoclopramide, the incidence of dystonic reactions is only about 1.8%. Dystonic reactions associated with metoclopramide therapy include involuntary movements of limbs, trismus, torticollis, facial spasms, rhythmic protrusions of the tongue, bulbar type of speech, opisthotonos, and oculogyric crisis. A dystonic reaction resembling tetanus has been reported in at least one patient, and dystonic reactions rarely may present as upper airway obstruction with stridor and dyspnea, possibly secondary to laryngospasm or supraglottic dystonia; cardiorespiratory arrest, which was fatal, also has occurred in at least one patient with an acute dystonic reaction. An acute dystonic reaction combined with myoclonus and asterixis also has been reported.

Akathisia combined with severe dysphoria and anxiety has been reported. Akathisia appears to be related to the peak plasma metoclopramide concentration and usually resolves following a reduction in dosage.

Treatment with metoclopramide may result in tardive dyskinesia, a potentially irreversible disorder manifested by involuntary movements of the tongue, face, mouth, or jaw, and sometimes by involuntary movements of the trunk and/or extremities; movements may be choreoathetotic in appearance. Although the risk of tardive dyskinesia with metoclopramide has not been extensively studied, the syndrome has been reported in about 20% of patients receiving the drug for at least 12 weeks. Treatment with metoclopramide for longer than 12 weeks should be avoided in all but rare cases where therapeutic benefit is thought to outweigh the risk of developing tardive dyskinesia. Although the risk of developing tardive dyskinesia in the general population may be increased in geriatric patients, women, and patients with diabetes mellitus, it is not possible to predict which patients will develop metoclopramide-induced tardive dyskinesia. The risk of developing tardive dyskinesia and the likelihood that it will become irreversible increase with increasing duration of therapy and total cumulative dose. Metoclopramide should be discontinued in patients who develop signs or symptoms of tardive dyskinesia. The syndrome may remit, either partially or completely, in some patients within several weeks to months after metoclopramide is discontinued. Metoclopramide itself may suppress or partially suppress the manifestations of tardive dyskinesia, thereby masking the underlying disease process. Whether this symptomatic suppression affects the long-term course of tardive dyskinesia is unknown. Therefore, metoclopramide should not be used for symptomatic control of tardive dyskinesia. Vesicular monoamine transporter 2 (VMAT2) inhibitors (e.g., deutetrabenazine, valbenazine tosylate) have been shown to be effective in reducing symptoms of tardive dyskinesia in controlled clinical studies. (See Deutetrabenazine 28:56 and Valbenazine Tosylate 28:56.) For additional information on tardive dyskinesia, including manifestations and treatment, see Tardive Dyskinesia under Cautions: Nervous System Effects, in the Phenothiazines General Statement 28:16.08.24.

Rarely, neuroleptic malignant syndrome (NMS) has occurred in patients receiving metoclopramide. NMS is a hypermetabolic reaction to dopamine antagonists, which may be characterized by hyperthermia, varying levels of consciousness, muscular rigidity, and autonomic dysfunction. In patients with clinical manifestations consistent with NMS, it is important to determine whether untreated or inadequately treated extrapyramidal reactions and serious medical illness (e.g., pneumonia, systemic infection) may coexist. Other important considerations in the differential diagnosis of NMS include the possibility of central anticholinergic toxicity, heat stroke, malignant hyperthermia, drug fever, and primary CNS pathology. Treatment of NMS includes immediate discontinuance of metoclopramide therapy and other drugs not considered essential to concurrent therapy, intensive symptomatic treatment and medical monitoring, and treatment of any concomitant serious medical condition for which specific therapies are available. Although drugs such as dantrolene and bromocriptine have been used in the treatment of NMS, their efficacy for this use has not been established and there currently is no specific drug therapy for NMS.

Parkinsonian symptoms, including tremor, rigidity, bradykinesia, and akinesia, rarely occur in patients receiving metoclopramide but may be associated with usual or excessive doses or with decreased renal function. Such symptoms develop more commonly during the first 6 months of metoclopramide therapy but occasionally after longer periods; following discontinuance of the drug, parkinsonian symptoms generally subside within 2–3 months.

Depression has been reported in patients receiving metoclopramide; in some of these patients, there was no history of an underlying depressive disorder. In some patients, depression has been severe and included unprovoked episodes of uncontrollable crying, suicidal ideation, and suicide. In most patients, signs of depression resolved following discontinuance of the drug and, in some, did not recur when metoclopramide was reinstituted at a lower dosage and gradually increased if necessary. Delirium, severe dysphoria, obsessive rumination, and mania have been reported occasionally.

■ GI Effects Nausea and bowel disturbances, principally diarrhea but also constipation, have occurred in some patients receiving metoclopramide. Xerostomia also has occurred.

■ Sensitivity Reactions Hypersensitivity reactions, including bronchospasm, urticaria, and rash (e.g., maculopapular), have been reported occasionally in patients receiving metoclopramide, especially in patients with a history of asthma. Angioedema, including laryngeal, glossal, or periorbital edema, has been reported rarely.

■ Hematologic Effects Agranulocytosis, neutropenia, and leukopenia have been reported rarely in patients receiving metoclopramide, but a causal relationship to the drug has not been established. Methemoglobinemia also has occurred in patients receiving the drug, particularly following overdosage in neonates, but also in adults receiving the drug. Sulfhemoglobinemia has been reported in adults receiving metoclopramide. (See Cautions: Precautions and Contraindications.) One child reportedly developed symptoms of acute intermittent porphyria immediately following IM administration of metoclopramide; the patient had a known history of acute intermittent porphyria exacerbated by various drugs.

■ Genitourinary Effects Metoclopramide is a potent stimulator of prolactin secretion in both genders; however, the clinical importance of the drug's effect on prolactin has not been fully determined. (See Cautions: Mutagenicity and Carcinogenicity.) Galactorrhea, gynecomastia, and menstrual disorders (e.g., amenorrhea) may occur in some patients during administration of metoclopramide. Impotence secondary to hyperprolactinemia can occur. Serum prolactin concentration usually returns to normal within 1 week following discontinuance of metoclopramide; adverse effects associated with increased serum prolactin concentration usually subside within a few weeks to months following discontinuance of the drug. Urinary frequency and incontinence also have been reported.

■ Cardiovascular Effects The risk of metoclopramide-induced, clinically important adverse cardiovascular effects appears to be low. AV block, hypotension, acute congestive heart failure, and hypertension have been reported. In addition, the drug may cause hypertensive crisis in patients with pheochromocytoma, apparently by causing release of catecholamines from the tumor. Metoclopramide-induced hypertensive crisis in patients with pheochromocytoma may be controlled with phentolamine. Supraventricular tachycardia has been reported rarely following parenteral administration of the drug. Transient flushing of the face and upper body have occurred with large IV doses of the drug. Severe bradycardia has reportedly occurred in one patient immediately following IV administration of 15–17 mg of metoclopramide.

■ Other Adverse Effects Visual disturbances have been reported in patients receiving metoclopramide. Fluid retention secondary to transient metoclopramide-induced elevations in serum aldosterone concentration also can occur. Rarely, hepatotoxicity, manifested as jaundice and alterations in liver function test results, has occurred in patients receiving metoclopramide concomitantly with other drugs with hepatotoxic potential.

■ Precautions and Contraindications The manufacturer's medication guide should be provided to the patient or caregiver each time metoclopramide is dispensed. The patient or caregiver should be instructed to read the medication guide before initiating therapy and each time the prescription is refilled. The clinician should assist the patient or caregiver in understanding the contents of the medication guide.

Patients should be warned that metoclopramide may impair their ability to perform activities requiring mental alertness or physical coordination (e.g., operating machinery, driving a motor vehicle). Patients also should be warned that metoclopramide may enhance their response to alcohol, barbiturates, or other CNS depressants. Patients should be informed that metoclopramide oral solution and tablets are recommended for use in adults *only*.

Extrapyramidal reactions may occur during metoclopramide therapy, especially in pediatric patients and adults younger than 30 years of age, or when high doses such as those used for prophylaxis of cancer chemotherapy-induced nausea and vomiting are administered. Because use of metoclopramide may result in tardive dyskinesia, a syndrome of potentially irreversible, involuntary, dyskinetic movements, therapy for longer than 12 weeks should be avoided in all but rare cases where therapeutic benefit is thought to outweigh the risk of developing tardive dyskinesia. Metoclopramide should be discontinued in patients who develop signs or symptoms of tardive dyskinesia. Because metoclopramide can exacerbate parkinsonian symptoms, the drug should be used with caution, if at all, in patients with parkinsonian syndrome. Neuroleptic malignant syndrome (NMS), a potentially fatal syndrome requiring immediate discontinuance of the drug and intensive symptomatic treatment, has been reported rarely in patients receiving metoclopramide. (See Cautions: Nervous System Effects.)

Metoclopramide should be used with extreme caution, and only when the anticipated benefits are expected to outweigh the possible risks, in patients with a history of mental depression, especially those with suicidal tendencies.

Because metoclopramide can stimulate GI motility, the drug theoretically could produce increased pressure on suture lines following GI anastomosis or closure. This possibility should be considered and weighed when deciding whether to use metoclopramide or nasogastric suction for the prevention of postoperative nausea and vomiting.

Metoclopramide should be used with caution and in reduced dosage during prolonged therapy in patients with impaired renal function. Because of the potential for transient increases in plasma aldosterone concentrations and sodium retention, the manufacturer and some clinicians state that certain patients (e.g., those with cirrhosis or congestive heart failure) may be at risk of developing fluid retention and volume overload or hypokalemia and should be closely monitored while receiving the drug. The manufacturer states that if fluid retention or volume overload occurs at any time during metoclopramide therapy, the drug should be discontinued. Metoclopramide should be used with caution in patients with hypertension since there is limited evidence that the drug may increase circulating catecholamines in such patients.

Adverse reactions, particularly those involving the CNS, may occur following discontinuance of metoclopramide therapy. A limited number of patients may experience withdrawal symptoms including dizziness, nervousness, and/or headaches following discontinuance.

Patients with cytochrome-b_5 reductase deficiency have an increased risk of methemoglobinemia and/or sulfhemoglobinemia when metoclopramide is administered. In patients with glucose-6-phosphate dehydrogenase (G-6-PD) deficiency who experience metoclopramide-induced methemoglobinemia, methylene blue treatment is not recommended. (See Acute Toxicity: Treatment.)

Metoclopramide is contraindicated in patients with a history of sensitivity or intolerance to the drug. Although there are no reports to date, patients allergic to procainamide theoretically may exhibit cross-sensitivity to metoclopramide, since the drugs are structurally similar.

Metoclopramide is contraindicated in patients in whom stimulation of GI motility might be dangerous (e.g., in the presence of mechanical obstruction or perforation). Although the manufacturers state that metoclopramide also is contraindicated in patients with GI hemorrhage, the drug has been used by some clinicians to empty the stomach of blood prior to endoscopy in patients with acute upper GI hemorrhage.

Metoclopramide is contraindicated in patients with pheochromocytoma, since the drug may cause hypertensive crisis in these patients.

Metoclopramide is contraindicated in patients with a history of seizure disorders since the frequency and severity of seizures may be increased by the drug. Metoclopramide is also contraindicated in patients receiving drugs that are likely to cause extrapyramidal reactions (e.g., phenothiazines, butyrophenones), since the frequency and severity of these reactions may be increased by metoclopramide.

■ **Pediatric Precautions** The safety profile of metoclopramide in adults cannot be extrapolated to pediatric patients.

Metoclopramide should be used with caution in pediatric patients, since the incidence of extrapyramidal reactions is increased in these patients.

Following oral or IV administration of metoclopramide in infants and children, pharmacodynamics of the drug are highly variable, and a relationship between drug plasma concentrations and pharmacodynamic effects has not been established. Data are insufficient to determine whether the pharmacokinetics of the drug in children is similar to those in adults.

Metoclopramide should be administered with caution to neonates because decreased clearance may result in increased serum concentrations of the drug. (See Pharmacokinetics: Elimination.) In addition, since neonates have reduced concentrations of cytochrome-b_5 reductase, they may be more susceptible to methemoglobinemia.

The manufacturers currently recommend that metoclopramide be used in children only to facilitate intubation of the small intestine. Metoclopramide has been effective for the management of gastric stasis† and gastroesophageal reflux† in infants and children. The drug has also been used in children for evacuation of the stomach prior to administration of anesthesia for emergency surgery†.

■ **Geriatric Precautions** Clinical studies of metoclopramide did not include sufficient numbers of patients 65 years of age and older to determine whether geriatric patients respond differently than younger patients.

The risk of developing parkinsonian symptoms increases with increasing dosage. Geriatric patients should receive the lowest effective dosage of metoclopramide. If parkinsonian symptoms develop in a geriatric patient receiving metoclopramide, metoclopramide generally should be discontinued before any specific antiparkinsonian therapy is considered. Geriatric patients also may be at increased risk for tardive dyskinesia. Sedation has been reported in patients receiving metoclopramide and may be manifested as confusion and oversedation in geriatric patients.

Metoclopramide is known to be substantially eliminated by the kidneys, and the risk of adverse reactions to the drug may be increased in patients with impaired renal function. In general, dosage should be selected carefully in geriatric patients, usually initiating therapy at the low end of the dosage range; the greater frequency of decreased renal function and of concomitant disease and drug therapy observed in geriatric patients also should be considered.

■ **Mutagenicity and Carcinogenicity** No evidence of metoclopramide-induced mutagenicity was observed in the Ames microbial mutagen test.

Although an increase in mammary neoplasms has been found in rodents following long-term administration of prolactin-stimulating antipsychotic agents (e.g., phenothiazines), no clinical or epidemiologic studies conducted to date have shown an association between long-term administration of prolactin-stimulating drugs and mammary tumorigenesis in humans. Current evidence is considered too limited to be conclusive, and further study is needed to determine the clinical importance in most patients of elevated serum prolactin concentrations associated with metoclopramide administration. Since in vitro tests indicate that approximately one-third of human breast cancers are prolactin-dependent, metoclopramide should be used with caution in patients with previously detected breast cancer.

■ **Pregnancy, Fertility, and Lactation** Reproduction studies in mice, rats, and rabbits using metoclopramide dosages up to 250 times the usual human dosage have not revealed evidence of harm to the fetus. There are no adequate and controlled studies to date using metoclopramide in pregnant women, and the drug should be used during pregnancy only when clearly needed.

It is not known whether metoclopramide affects fertility in humans. Menstrual disturbances have occurred in some individuals during metoclopramide therapy. (See Cautions: Other Adverse Effects.) Reproduction studies in male and female mice, rats, and rabbits using metoclopramide dosages 12–250 times the usual human dosage have not revealed evidence of impaired fertility.

Since metoclopramide is distributed into milk, the drug should be used with caution in nursing women.

Drug Interactions

■ **Effects on GI Absorption of Drugs** Because of its pharmacologic effects on transit time in the stomach and small intestine, metoclopramide may alter the absorption of certain drugs. The extent of absorption of drugs that disintegrate, dissolve, and/or are absorbed mainly in the stomach (e.g., digoxin) may be diminished by metoclopramide, whereas the rate and extent of absorption of drugs that are mainly absorbed in the small intestine (e.g., acetaminophen, aspirin, cyclosporine, diazepam, ethanol, levodopa, lithium, tetracycline) may be enhanced. The clinical importance of these effects has not been determined. Metoclopramide reportedly does not affect the absorption of Lanoxin® tablets, since these digoxin preparations have a small drug-particle size and are rapidly absorbed.

■ **CNS Depressants** Metoclopramide may be additive with, or may potentiate the action of, other CNS depressants such as opiates or other analgesics, barbiturates or other sedatives, anesthetics, or alcohol. When metoclopramide is used concomitantly with other CNS depressants, caution should be used to avoid excessive sedation.

■ **Insulin** Gastric stasis may be responsible for poor diabetic control in some patients; exogenously administered insulin may begin to act before food has left the stomach, potentially resulting in hypoglycemia. Since metoclopramide influences the delivery of food to the intestine and thus the rate of its absorption, adjustment in, or timing of, insulin dosage may be necessary in insulin-controlled diabetics.

■ **Other Drugs** Metoclopramide should not be used in patients receiving drugs that are likely to cause extrapyramidal reactions. (See Cautions: Precautions and Contraindications.)

The effects of metoclopramide on GI motility are antagonized by anticholinergic agents (e.g., atropine) and opiate analgesics.

Acute hypotension reportedly occurred in some patients receiving IV metoclopramide during neurosurgical procedures in which hypotensive anesthetic agents were used; various anesthetic agents, with or without concomitant administration of ganglionic blocking agents, were used. The mechanism and clinical importance of this adverse reaction are not known.

Metoclopramide should be used cautiously, if at all, in patients receiving concomitant therapy with monoamine oxidase (MAO) inhibitors because metoclopramide has been shown to cause release of catecholamines in patients with essential hypertension.

Acute Toxicity

Limited information is available on the acute toxicity of metoclopramide.

■ **Pathogenesis** The acute lethal dose of metoclopramide in humans is not known. In addition, there is no clearly defined relationship between plasma metoclopramide concentration and severity of intoxication. The oral LD_{50} of metoclopramide is 465 mg/kg in mice, 760 mg/kg in rats, and 870 mg/kg in rabbits. In animals, lethal doses produced dyspnea, excessive lacrimation, decreased activity, ataxia, miosis, tachycardia, tremors, and tonic seizures. Oral metoclopramide dosages up to 1 g daily have been used for several weeks in some patients receiving the drug for the management of psychiatric disorders.

■ **Manifestations** One patient who intentionally ingested 360 mg of metoclopramide experienced only drowsiness and disorientation. Although the patient was not lucid at the time of hospitalization, no focal neurologic abnormalities or cardiovascular symptoms were present, and gastric lavage was performed. Another patient had an uneventful recovery after ingesting 800 mg of metoclopramide; the patient had no abnormal neurologic, autonomic, or cardiovascular signs or symptoms. There have been numerous reports of overdosage in children; most of these children were younger than 1 year of age and were inadvertently given excessive amounts (1–11.6 mg/kg) orally over a 2- to 3-day period. One 5-month-old infant who weighed 7 kg was given a single 5-mg IM dose of metoclopramide; symptoms of overdose appeared within 30 minutes following administration and subsided within 12 hours. Manifestations of overdosage in these children included drowsiness, ataxia, agitation, hyperexcitability, dystonic extrapyramidal reactions, attacks of muscular contractions of the face or neck, oculogyric crisis, opisthotonos, and seizures. None of these patients lost consciousness, and all recovered spontaneously within 12–48 hours.

Methemoglobinemia, which responded to methylene blue therapy, and reduced oxyhemoglobin saturation occurred in a neonate who inadvertently received 1 mg/kg of metoclopramide orally every 6 hours for 36 hours. The neonate presented with manifestations of cyanosis, lethargy, poor feeding, diarrhea, and respiratory distress. Methemoglobinemia also has developed in several other infants following overdosage with the drug, and this age group may be predisposed to developing this toxicity.

In general, overdosage of metoclopramide may be expected to produce effects that are extensions of common adverse reactions; drowsiness, disorientation, and extrapyramidal reactions have been the principal effects reported. Other reported effects associated with metoclopramide overdosage have included feelings of anxiety or restlessness, headache, vertigo, nausea, vomiting, constipation, weakness, hypotension, and xerostomia; in addition, generalized seizures and methemoglobinemia have occurred in infants.

■ **Treatment** Treatment of metoclopramide overdosage generally involves symptomatic and supportive care. There is no specific antidote for metoclopramide intoxication; however, agents with central anticholinergic activity (e.g., diphenhydramine, benztropine) may be useful in controlling extrapyramidal reactions. Following acute ingestion of the drug, the stomach should be emptied immediately. If the patient is comatose, having seizures, or lacks the gag reflex, gastric lavage may be performed if an endotracheal tube with cuff inflated is in place to prevent aspiration of gastric contents. Symptoms of metoclopramide overdosage are generally self-limiting and usually subside within 24 hours. Appropriate therapy should be instituted if hypotension or excessive sedation occurs. Methemoglobinemia should be treated with methylene blue. However, in patients with glucose-6-phosphate dehydrogenase (G-6-PD) deficiency, methylene blue can induce hemolytic anemia, which may be fatal. Hemodialysis or peritoneal dialysis is unlikely to enhance the elimination of metoclopramide.

Pharmacology

The pharmacology of metoclopramide is complex and its mechanism(s) of action has not been fully elucidated. The principal pharmacologic effects of metoclopramide involve the GI tract and CNS.

■ **GI Effects** Metoclopramide has several effects on mechanical activity of GI smooth muscle. At low concentrations in vitro, metoclopramide increases the resting tone and phasic contractile activity of GI smooth muscle, while at high concentrations, the drug inhibits mechanical activity. Metoclopramide increases lower esophageal sphincter pressure in patients with hiatal hernia with or without associated gastroesophageal reflux and in healthy individuals. Following oral or IV administration of the drug, lower esophageal sphincter pressure generally increases to a greater extent in healthy individuals than in patients with reflux; there appears to be substantial interindividual variation in the effect of metoclopramide on lower esophageal sphincter pressure.

Metoclopramide accelerates gastric emptying and intestinal transit from the duodenum to the ileocecal valve by increasing the amplitude and duration of esophageal contractions, the resting tone of the lower esophageal sphincter, and the amplitude and tone of gastric (especially antral) contractions and by relaxing the pyloric sphincter and the duodenal bulb, while increasing peristalsis of the duodenum and jejunum. Unlike nonspecific cholinergic-like stimulation of upper GI smooth muscle, the stimulant effects of metoclopramide on GI smooth muscle coordinate gastric, pyloric, and duodenal motor activity. Metoclopramide is most effective in patients with reduced antral tone and duodenal activity. Metoclopramide lowers the pressure threshold for occurrence of the peristaltic reflex and enhances the frequency and amplitude of longitudinal muscle contractions. In addition to its ability to enhance motor activity of upper GI smooth muscle, metoclopramide may also increase gastric emptying by inhibiting receptive relaxation of the gastric fundus.

Although metoclopramide has been reported to have little, if any, effect on motility of the colon in several studies, there is some evidence that the drug may increase colonic motility. The effect of metoclopramide on motility of the gallbladder has been variable.

The pharmacologic actions of metoclopramide on the upper GI tract are similar to those of cholinergic drugs (e.g., bethanechol); however, unlike cholinergic drugs, metoclopramide does not stimulate gastric, biliary, or pancreatic secretions and does not affect serum gastrin concentration.

Although the exact mechanism of action of metoclopramide is unclear, the effects of metoclopramide on GI motility may be mediated via enhancement of cholinergic excitatory processes at the postganglionic neuromuscular junction; antagonism of nonadrenergic, noncholinergic inhibitory motor nerves (i.e., dopaminergic); and/or a direct effect on smooth muscle.

The effects of metoclopramide on GI motility do not depend on intact vagal innervation but are reduced or abolished by anticholinergic drugs (e.g., atropine) and potentiated by cholinergic drugs (e.g., carbachol, methacholine). These findings suggest that metoclopramide's effects on GI motility may depend in part on intramural cholinergic neurons of smooth muscle that are intact after vagal denervation. Unlike cholinergic drugs, metoclopramide requires intrinsic neuronal storage sites of acetylcholine to exert its pharmacologic effects. Postsynaptic activity results from metoclopramide's ability to enhance release of acetylcholine from postganglionic cholinergic neurons in the GI tract and to sensitize muscarinic receptors of GI smooth muscle to the actions of acetylcholine.

Metoclopramide does *not* exhibit anticholinesterase activity and its GI stimulant actions are not affected by ganglionic blocking drugs; however, the sensitization to acetylcholine may be prevented by ganglionic blocking drugs (e.g., hexamethonium).

Metoclopramide is a potent dopamine-receptor antagonist, and some of the actions of metoclopramide on GI smooth muscle may be mediated via antagonism of dopaminergic neurotransmission, Specific dopamine receptors in the esophagus and stomach have been identified; however, it is not known if there is a dopaminergic control system for smooth muscle function in the upper GI tract. In the GI tract, dopamine is principally an inhibitory neurotransmitter. Dopamine decreases the intensity of esophageal contractions, relaxes the proximal stomach, and reduces gastric secretion. Although metoclopramide blocks these inhibitory effects of dopamine, the actual role of dopamine in the peripheral control of GI motility has not been fully elucidated. Since cholinergic mechanisms are responsible for most excitatory motor activity in the GI tract, it appears that metoclopramide's therapeutic effects are principally caused by the drug's cholinergic-like activity; however, antagonism of GI dopaminergic activity may augment metoclopramide's cholinergic-like activity.

■ **Nervous System Effects** Metoclopramide is a potent central dopamine-receptor antagonist. The drug has antiemetic and sedative activity.

Antiemetic Effect The precise mechanism of antiemetic action of metoclopramide is unclear, but the drug has been shown to directly affect the medullary chemoreceptor trigger zone (CTZ) in the area postrema, apparently by blocking dopamine (e.g., D_2) receptors in the CTZ. Metoclopramide increases the CTZ threshold and decreases the sensitivity of visceral nerves that transmit afferent impulses from the GI tract to the vomiting center in the lateral reticular formation. The drug also enhances gastric emptying, which is believed to minimize stasis that precedes vomiting. It also has been suggested that inhibition of serotonin (i.e., 5-HT_3) receptors, at least when relatively high doses of metoclopramide are used, may contribute to the antiemetic action of the drug. Metoclopramide inhibits the central and peripheral emetic effects of apomorphine, hydergine, and levodopa.

Other Nervous System Effects In animals, metoclopramide exhibits neuroleptic effects similar to those of antipsychotic agents (e.g., phenothiazines); metoclopramide produces catalepsy and reverses behavioral effects mediated by amphetamine and apomorphine. Following administration of usual dosages (e.g., 40 mg daily), metoclopramide exhibits little, if any, antipsychotic or tranquilizing activity in psychiatric patients; however, antipsychotic effects have been observed in a limited number of patients with chronic schizophrenic disorder receiving oral metoclopramide dosages of 520–1000 mg daily for up to 24 days.

Metoclopramide produces varying degrees of sedation and lethargy in healthy adults. The drug may cause EEG changes, including increased slow-wave activity. Based on limited data in animals, usual IV doses of metoclopramide do not appear to lower the seizure threshold.

Like other dopamine-receptor antagonists (e.g., phenothiazines), metoclopramide may cause extrapyramidal reactions. (See Cautions: Nervous System Effects.) Metoclopramide may worsen symptoms in patients with parkinsonian syndrome.

■ **Cardiovascular and Renal Effects** Although metoclopramide does *not* appear to have clinically important antiarrhythmic activity, transient antiarrhythmic effects have been observed in animals and humans following administration of large IV doses. Following IV administration of a single 20-mg dose to patients with valvular heart disease (e.g., mitral stenosis) in one study, metoclopramide did *not* produce ECG changes nor did it exert a clinically important effect on hemodynamic parameters, including cardiac output, left ventricular end-diastolic pressure, or pulmonary artery pressure. At doses greater than 40 mg/kg in animals, metoclopramide produces only minimal ECG changes, including enhancement of R and T waves and a transient decrease in heart rate.

In healthy adults in one study, metoclopramide potentiated the vasopressor response to dopamine; however, in animals, metoclopramide reportedly blocks the hypertensive effect of dopamine. Potentiation of the vasopressor response to dopamine in humans may result from inhibition of a central homeostatic reflex by metoclopramide.

Limited data suggest that metoclopramide decreases renal plasma flow, at least at high doses given IV. The mechanism of this effect and its clinical importance remain to be established.

■ **Metabolic and Endocrine Effects** Metoclopramide indirectly stimulates secretion of prolactin from the anterior pituitary gland by inhibiting dopamine receptors in the pituitary and hypothalamus. The elevated prolactin concentrations persist during long-term administration and, like other prolactin-stimulating drugs, may be associated with galactorrhea, amenorrhea, gynecomastia, and impotence.

Metoclopramide does *not* appear to substantially alter the secretion of growth hormone, corticotropin, luteinizing hormone (LH), or follicle-stimulating hormone (FSH); however, following oral administration of a single 10-mg dose in one study in healthy adults, metoclopramide caused a small decrease in serum growth hormone, LH, and FSH concentrations. In another study in hypogonadal males, metoclopramide caused an increase in serum growth hormone concentration following IV administration of 10 mg of the drug. Serum thyrotropin concentrations may be increased by metoclopramide; however, serum thyrotropin concentrations usually remain within normal limits, and the clinical importance of this alteration has not been determined.

Metoclopramide produces a transient increase in plasma aldosterone concentrations. Although the exact mechanism has not been fully determined, metoclopramide appears to increase plasma aldosterone concentrations by stimulating the secretion of aldosterone via a direct effect on adrenal tissue; metoclopramide does not affect the metabolic clearance of aldosterone. There is no correlation between the changes in aldosterone and prolactin concentrations, suggesting that the effect on plasma aldosterone is not mediated via prolactin secretion. Metoclopramide does *not* alter plasma renin activity or plasma potassium or cortisol concentrations. Although the possibility of sodium retention and hypokalemia exists, especially in patients with edema (e.g., those with cirrhosis or congestive heart failure), plasma aldosterone concentrations reportedly return to pretreatment levels during prolonged administration of metoclopramide.

Pharmacokinetics

In all studies described in the Pharmacokinetics section, metoclopramide was administered as the monohydrochloride monohydrate salt; dosages and concentrations of the drug are expressed in terms of metoclopramide.

■ **Absorption** Metoclopramide is rapidly and almost completely absorbed from the GI tract following oral administration; however, absorption may be delayed or diminished in patients with gastric stasis. Considerable interindividual variations (up to fivefold) in peak plasma concentration have been reported with the same oral dose of metoclopramide. This variability apparently results from interindividual differences in first-pass metabolism of the drug. Bioavailability of metoclopramide appears to correlate with the ratio of free-:conjugated metoclopramide concentrations in urine. It appears that sulfate conjugation in the GI lumen and/or during first pass through the liver is the principal determinant of bioavailability of orally administered metoclopramide. The absolute bioavailability of orally administered metoclopramide has not been clearly established in humans, but limited data indicate that 30–100% of an oral dose of the drug reaches systemic circulation as unchanged metoclopramide. Following IM administration, the absolute bioavailability of metoclopramide is 74–96%.

Following oral administration of a single 10-mg dose of the drug in healthy, fasting adults in one study, peak plasma metoclopramide concentrations of 32–44 ng/mL occurred at 1–2 hours; following oral administration of a single 20-mg dose, peak plasma metoclopramide concentrations of 72–87 ng/mL occurred at an average of 2 hours. In a study in infants (3.5 weeks–5.4 months of age) with gastroesophageal reflux who received 0.15-mg/kg oral doses of metoclopramide every 6 hours for 10 doses as an oral solution, the mean peak plasma concentration (56.8 ng/mL) of the drug after the 10th dose was twofold higher compared with that after the first dose (29 ng/mL), suggesting that metoclopramide accumulates in plasma following multiple oral dosing in this age group. In these patients, time to reach mean peak plasma concentrations (2.2 hours) was similar after the 10th dose to that occurring after the first dose.

The onset of the principal pharmacologic actions of metoclopramide on the GI tract is 1–3 minutes following IV administration, 10–15 minutes following IM administration, and 30–60 minutes following oral administration. Pharmacologic effects persist for 1–2 hours following administration of a single dose.

The therapeutic range for plasma metoclopramide concentrations and the relationship of plasma concentration to clinical response and toxicity have not been clearly established. In one study, a maximum change in lower esophageal sphincter pressure correlated poorly with peak plasma metoclopramide concentration. Data from patients receiving large IV doses of metoclopramide (8 mg/kg in 4 divided doses) for the prevention of cisplatin-induced nausea and vomiting indicate that serum metoclopramide concentrations greater than 850 ng/mL may be required for optimum antiemetic effect in patients receiving cisplatin. Metoclopramide-induced akathisia is reportedly associated with peak plasma metoclopramide concentrations greater than 120 ng/mL.

■ **Distribution** Distribution of metoclopramide into human body tissues and fluids has not been fully characterized. The apparent volume of distribution of metoclopramide is reportedly 2.2–3.5 L/kg in adults and 1.93–4.4 L/kg in children. Following IM administration of metoclopramide in mice, the drug is rapidly distributed into most body tissues and fluids with high concentrations in the GI mucosa, liver, biliary tract, and salivary glands, and lower concentrations in brain, heart, thymus, adrenals, adipose tissue, and bone marrow. Metoclopramide crosses the blood-brain barrier and enters the CNS in animals, with high concentrations in the area postrema, which contains the chemoreceptor trigger zone (CTZ).

Metoclopramide is weakly bound to plasma proteins; in vitro, metoclopramide is 13–30% protein bound, principally to albumin.

Metoclopramide crosses the placenta and is distributed into milk; concentrations of the drug in milk are higher than those in plasma 2 hours after oral administration.

■ **Elimination** Plasma concentrations of metoclopramide decline in a biphasic manner.

Although limited data from single-dose studies have suggested that elimination of metoclopramide is dose dependent, other studies using oral doses up to 100 mg have *not* shown a dose-dependent pharmacokinetic profile. In addition, one pharmacokinetic study using high doses of metoclopramide did *not* demonstrate dose-dependent elimination. In adults, the half-life of metoclopramide in the initial phase ($t_{1/2\alpha}$) is about 5 minutes, and the half-life in the terminal phase ($t_{1/2\beta}$) ranges from 2.5–6 hours. In children receiving oral or IV metoclopramide, the elimination half-life of the drug reportedly is 4.1–4.5 hours. Following oral administration of 0.15-mg/kg doses of metoclopramide every 6 hours for 10 doses in an infant (3.5 weeks of age), elimination half-lives of 23.1 and 10.3 hours were observed after the first and 10th dose, respectively, which were substantially longer than those reported in older infants, suggesting a reduced clearance in the neonate possibly being associated with immature renal and hepatic functions present at birth. Total body clearance of metoclopramide is reportedly 10.9–11.7 mL/minute per kg in adults with normal renal function. Plasma metoclopramide concentrations may be higher and the half-life prolonged in patients with impaired renal function. In children receiving oral or IV metoclopramide, clearance of the drug reportedly is 6.16–11.1 mL/minute per kg.

Although the exact metabolic fate of metoclopramide is not clearly established, it appears that metoclopramide is only minimally metabolized. The major metabolite found in urine is 2-[(4-amino-5-chloro-2-methoxybenzoyl)amino]acetic acid; it is not known if this metabolite is pharmacologically active. Metoclopramide is conjugated with sulfuric and/or glucuronic acid.

Metoclopramide and its metabolites are excreted in urine and feces. In a limited number of adults with normal renal function, approximately 85% of an oral dose of radiolabeled metoclopramide was excreted in urine within 72 hours of administration, principally as unchanged drug and glucuronide or sulfate conjugates of metoclopramide. About 5–10% of an oral dose of metoclopramide is excreted in urine as 2-[(4-amino-5-chloro-2-methoxybenzoyl)amino]acetic acid and about 20% is excreted unchanged. Approximately 5% of an oral dose of the drug is excreted in feces via biliary elimination.

Limited evidence indicates that metoclopramide is only minimally removed by hemodialysis or peritoneal dialysis.

Chemistry and Stability

■ **Chemistry** Metoclopramide hydrochloride, a synthetic substituted benzamide, is a dopamine-receptor antagonist, an antiemetic, and a stimulant of upper GI motility. The drug is a derivative of *p*-aminobenzoic acid and is structurally related to procainamide, but lacks local anesthetic and antiarrhythmic properties. Metoclopramide differs structurally from procainamide by the presence of 5-chloro and 2-methoxy aryl substituents.

Metoclopramide hydrochloride occurs as a monohydrate, white, odorless, crystalline powder. The drug has solubilities of approximately 1.43 g/mL in water and 333 mg/mL in alcohol. Metoclopramide hydrochloride has pK_as of 0.6 and 9.3. Commercially available metoclopramide hydrochloride oral solution occurs as an orange-colored, palatable, aromatic, sugar-free liquid. The oral solution has a pH of 2–5.5 and contains parabens as preservatives. Metoclopramide hydrochloride injection is a clear, colorless, sterile, nonpyrogenic solution of the drug in water for injection. The injection also contains sodium chloride. The injection has a pH of 4.5–6.5.

USP currently states that potency of metoclopramide hydrochloride preparations should be expressed both in terms of the salt and the base ("active moiety"). Previously, potency was expressed only in terms of metoclopramide base. Dosage currently continues to be expressed in terms of the base. Therefore, care should be taken to avoid confusion between labeled potencies as the salt and base and dosage of metoclopramide hydrochloride.

■ **Stability** Metoclopramide hydrochloride is photosensitive and will degrade when exposed to light. Commercially available preparations of metoclopramide hydrochloride should be protected from light. Metoclopramide hydrochloride tablets, injection, and oral solution should be stored at controlled room temperature between 20–25°C. Metoclopramide hydrochloride tablets and metoclopramide hydrochloride oral solution should be stored in tight, light-resistant containers (i.e., amber glass bottles). The commercially available tablets are stable for 3 years and the oral solution and injection are stable for 5 years after manufacture.

Metoclopramide hydrochloride injection is reportedly stable at pH 2–9. Metoclopramide hydrochloride injection is physically and chemically compatible with the following IV solutions: 5% dextrose, 0.9% sodium chloride, 5% dextrose and 0.45% sodium chloride, Ringer's, and lactated Ringer's. Solutions of metoclopramide hydrochloride that have been prepared by dilution of the injection with 50 mL of one of these compatible IV solutions are stable for up to 48 hours when stored at 4–30°C and protected from light or for up to 24 hours when stored at these temperatures and exposed to normal light conditions. Solutions prepared by dilution of the injection with 0.9% sodium chloride injection may be frozen in PVC bags immediately after preparation and are stable for up to 4 weeks at −20°C. Solutions prepared by dilution of the injection with 5% dextrose injection should *not* be frozen in PVC bags since loss of potency of up to about 40% occurs within 4 weeks. Any unused portion remaining in the vial should be discarded and not stored for later use.

Admixtures containing metoclopramide hydrochloride have been reported to be physically compatible for at least 24 hours at 15–30°C with the following injections: ascorbic acid, benztropine mesylate, cimetidine hydrochloride (when admixed in 0.9% sodium chloride), clindamycin phosphate (when admixed in 0.9% sodium chloride), cyclophosphamide, cytarabine, dexamethasone sodium phosphate, diphenhydramine hydrochloride, doxorubicin hydrochloride, heparin sodium, hydrocortisone sodium phosphate, lidocaine hydrochloride, magnesium sulfate, mannitol, potassium acetate, potassium chloride, or monobasic and dibasic potassium phosphates. Metoclopramide hydrochloride is reportedly potentially incompatible with cisplatin when the drugs are admixed in 0.9% sodium chloride in a concentration of 0.1 and 0.5 mg/

mL, respectively, or 0.88 and 0.55 mg/mL, respectively, and therefore, the admixed solution should be used immediately after mixing. Metoclopramide hydrochloride also is reportedly potentially incompatible with methotrexate sodium (preserved with benzyl alcohol) when the drugs are admixed in a concentration of 2.5 and 12.5 mg/mL, respectively, or 4 and 5 mg/mL, respectively, and therefore, the admixed solution should be used immediately after mixing. Since the compatibility of these and other admixtures with metoclopramide hydrochloride depends on several factors (e.g., concentration of the drugs, resulting pH, temperature), specialized references should be consulted for specific conditions of compatibility. Cephalothin sodium (no longer commercially available in the US) and other cephalosporins, chloramphenicol sodium, and sodium bicarbonate are reported to be physically incompatible with metoclopramide hydrochloride.

Preparations

Excipients in commercially available drug preparations may have clinically important effects in some individuals; consult specific product labeling for details.

Metoclopramide Hydrochloride

Oral		
Solution	5 mg (of metoclopramide) per 5 mL*	**Metoclopramide Hydrochloride Syrup**
Tablets	5 mg (of metoclopramide)*	**Metoclopramide Hydrochloride Tablets**
		Reglan®, Alaven
	10 mg (of metoclopramide)*	**Metoclopramide Hydrochloride Tablets**
		Reglan® (scored), Alaven
Parenteral		
Injection	5 mg (of metoclopramide) per mL*	**Metoclopramide Hydrochloride Injection**
		Reglan®, Baxter

*available from one or more manufacturer, distributor, and/or repackager by generic (nonproprietary) name

†Use is not currently included in the labeling approved by the US Food and Drug Administration

Selected Revisions November 2017,

Prucalopride Succinate

■ Prucalopride succinate, a selective type 4 serotonin (5-HT_4) receptor agonist, is a GI prokinetic agent.

Uses

■ **Chronic Idiopathic Constipation** Prucalopride succinate is used for the symptomatic treatment of chronic idiopathic constipation.

Efficacy and safety of prucalopride for the symptomatic treatment of chronic idiopathic constipation have been evaluated in 6 similarly designed, phase 3 or 4, randomized, double-blind, placebo-controlled studies in a total of 2484 adults (mean age: 47 years, 76% female, 76% Caucasian, mean duration of constipation: 16 years) with chronic constipation not considered to be drug induced or caused by other medical conditions. An integrated analysis of data from the 6 studies indicated that prucalopride increases the frequency of complete spontaneous bowel movements (CSBMs) in patients with chronic idiopathic constipation.

Although there were minor variations among the studies in inclusion criteria, chronic constipation generally was defined as fewer than 3 CSBMs per week for at least 6 months *and* the presence of one of 3 symptoms (hard or very hard stools, a sensation of incomplete evacuation, straining during defecation) during at least 25% of bowel movements. Most of the patients randomized to receive prucalopride in these studies received a dosage of 2 mg daily. A prucalopride dosage of 4 mg daily also was evaluated in 3 studies. In 2 studies, geriatric patients received an initial dosage of 1 mg daily, with dosage increased to 2 mg daily if response was insufficient; dosage was increased in 81% of patients receiving the lower initial dosage. Treatment was continued for 12 weeks in 5 studies and for 24 weeks in one study. The prespecified primary end point in all 6 studies defined response as a mean of 3 or more CSBMs per week evaluated over 12 or 24 weeks of treatment. In a post hoc analysis, an alternative definition of response, based on FDA's efficacy standard for chronic idiopathic constipation, was utilized: 3 or more CSBMs per week *and* an increase of at least 1 CSBM per week compared with baseline for at least 9 weeks during a 12-week treatment period and for at least 3 of the last 4 weeks of the 12-week treatment period. On a daily basis, patients recorded information on bowel function and symptoms in an electronic diary.

In 5 of the 6 studies, both the prespecified primary end point and the alternative (post hoc) end point were achieved in greater proportions of patients receiving prucalopride 1 or 2 mg daily for 12 weeks compared with those receiving placebo (33, 38, 19, 29, and 24% versus 10, 18, 10, 13, and 12%, respectively, for the prespecified end point; 26, 32, 13, 19, and 16% versus 9, 14, 5, 8, and 5%, respectively, for the alternative end point). In the sixth study (24-week study), response rates for prucalopride-treated patients and placebo recipients did not differ significantly (25 versus 20%, respectively, for the prespecified end point; 17 versus 13%, respectively, for the alternative end point). In all studies, an increase in the frequency of CSBMs (i.e., number of CSBMs per week) was observed as early as the first week of therapy and was sustained through week 12. The median time to first spontaneous bowel movement or first CSBM following initiation of therapy was 0.1–0.4 or 1.4–4.7 days, respectively, for patients receiving prucalopride 1 or 2 mg daily compared with 1–1.6 or 9.1–20.6 days, respectively, for placebo recipients.

The 4-mg daily dosage of prucalopride was not found to provide any additional benefit over the 2-mg dosage.

Dosage and Administration

■ **Administration** Prucalopride succinate is administered orally once daily without regard to food.

■ **Dosage** Dosage of prucalopride succinate is expressed in terms of prucalopride.

For the symptomatic treatment of chronic idiopathic constipation, the recommended adult dosage of prucalopride is 2 mg once daily. In clinical trials, a dosage of 4 mg daily was not found to provide any additional benefit over the 2-mg dosage. In addition, most patients (81%) who received an initial dosage of 1 mg daily required an increase in dosage to 2 mg daily. (See Uses: Chronic Idiopathic Constipation.)

■ **Special Populations** No dosage adjustment is required in patients with hepatic impairment or those with mild or moderate renal impairment (creatinine clearance of 30 mL/minute or greater). For patients with severe renal impairment (creatinine clearance less than 30 mL/minute), dosage of prucalopride should be reduced to 1 mg once daily. Use of the drug should be avoided in patients with end-stage renal disease requiring dialysis. Dosage in geriatric patients should be based on renal function. (See Specific Populations under Cautions: Warnings/Precautions.)

Cautions

■ **Contraindications** Prucalopride is contraindicated in patients with intestinal perforation or obstruction due to a structural or functional disorder of the gut wall, obstructive ileus, or severe inflammatory conditions of the intestinal tract including Crohn's disease, ulcerative colitis, and toxic megacolon/megarectum. Prucalopride also is contraindicated in patients with known hypersensitivity to the drug.

■ **Warnings/Precautions** ***Sensitivity Reactions*** Hypersensitivity reactions including dyspnea, rash, pruritus, urticaria, and facial edema have been reported in patients receiving prucalopride.

Suicidal Ideation and Behavior In clinical trials, suicides, suicide attempts, and suicidal ideation have been reported in patients receiving prucalopride. However, a causal relationship to the drug has not been established. In double-blind trials, suicide attempt was reported in one patient 7 days after discontinuance of prucalopride therapy (2 mg daily) and by no patients receiving placebo. In open-label trials, suicide attempt was reported in 2 patients receiving the drug and suicidal ideation was reported in one additional patient. Completed suicide was reported in 2 patients who had discontinued prucalopride therapy (2 or 4 mg daily) at least one month prior to the event.

Patients receiving prucalopride should be monitored for persistent worsening of depression and for emergence of suicidal thoughts and behaviors. Families and caregivers of patients receiving the drug should be advised to monitor patients for unusual changes in mood or behavior and to report such changes to a clinician. Patients should be instructed to discontinue prucalopride therapy immediately and to contact their clinician if they experience persistent worsening of depression or emerging suicidal thoughts or behaviors.

Cardiovascular Safety Although certain nonselective type 4 serotonin (5-HT_4) receptor agonists (i.e., cisapride, tegaserod) have been associated with adverse cardiovascular events, results of a retrospective, observational, population-based cohort study revealed no increase in the risk of major adverse cardiovascular events (i.e., myocardial infarction, stroke, cardiovascular death) in patients receiving prucalopride, a selective 5-HT_4 receptor agonist. (See Description.) The observational study utilized data from European healthcare databases to estimate the risk of major adverse cardiovascular events with prucalopride versus polyethylene glycol 3350 therapy in patients with chronic constipation. The incidence estimates (6.57 or 10.24 per 1000 patient-years of exposure to prucalopride or polyethylene glycol 3350, respectively) excluded an increase in risk above the prespecified safety margin of a threefold increase in risk for prucalopride compared with polyethylene glycol use.

In double-blind clinical trials of prucalopride, the incidence of major adverse cardiovascular events was 3.5 per 1000 patient-years of prucalopride exposure compared with 5.2 per 1000 patient-years of placebo exposure; the incidence was 3.3 per 1000 patient-years of prucalopride exposure in double-blind and open-label trials combined. In healthy individuals, prucalopride did not cause clinically important prolongation of the QT interval at doses of 5 times the recommended dose.

Specific Populations **Pregnancy.** Available data from case reports of prucalopride use in pregnant women are insufficient to identify any drug-associated risks of spontaneous abortion, major birth defects, or adverse maternal or fetal outcomes. In animal reproduction studies in rats and rabbits, no adverse embryofetal developmental effects were observed at dosages up to approximately 390 and 780 times, respectively, the recommended human dosage. The highest dosage in rats was maternally toxic; a slight decrease in pup survival was observed at this dosage.

Lactation. Prucalopride is distributed into human milk. It is not known whether prucalopride affects the breast-fed child or affects milk production. The benefits of breast-feeding should be considered along with the importance of the drug to the woman and any potential adverse effects on the breast-fed child from the drug or underlying maternal condition.

During weaning, prucalopride was distributed into human breast milk with a milk-to-plasma ratio of 2.65:1 (based on area under the concentration-time curve [AUC]); mean infant exposure was estimated to be 1.74 mcg/kg daily (about 6% of the maternal dose) adjusted for body weight. However, the manufacturer states that the prucalopride concentration in breast milk during weaning may not reflect the concentration attained during full milk production.

Pediatric Use. Safety and efficacy of prucalopride have not been established in pediatric patients.

Geriatric Use. In controlled trials of at least 12-weeks' duration in patients with chronic idiopathic constipation, 15% of patients receiving prucalopride 1 or 2 mg daily were 65 years of age or older, while 5% were 75 years of age or older. No overall differences in safety and efficacy were observed in these studies between geriatric patients and younger adults, and no unanticipated safety concerns were identified in an additional 4-week double-blind, placebo-controlled, dose-escalation study in 89 geriatric nursing home patients with chronic idiopathic constipation. Geriatric patients had higher prucalopride exposure (26–28% higher AUC and peak plasma concentrations) compared with younger adults; however, the effect of age on the pharmacokinetics of prucalopride appears to be related to decreased renal function. Therefore, dosage of the drug in geriatric patients should be based on renal function.

Hepatic Impairment. Following oral administration of a single 2-mg dose of prucalopride, peak plasma concentration and AUC averaged 10–20% higher in patients with moderate or severe (Child-Pugh class B or C) hepatic impairment compared with individuals with normal hepatic function, but these increases in exposure were not considered to be clinically important.

Renal Impairment. Prucalopride is eliminated mainly by the kidneys, and the risk of adverse effects may be increased in patients with renal impairment. Following oral administration of a single 2-mg dose of prucalopride, AUC in patients with mild, moderate, or severe renal impairment (creatinine clearances of 60–89, 30–59, or 15–29 mL/minute, respectively) was increased by 1.23-, 1.4-, or 2.38-fold, respectively, compared with that in individuals with normal renal function. No dosage adjustment of prucalopride is necessary in patients with mild to moderate renal impairment; however, reduced dosage is recommended in patients with severe renal impairment. (See Dosage and Administration: Special Populations.) The pharmacokinetic profile of prucalopride in patients with end-stage renal disease or requiring dialysis has not been fully established, and the manufacturer states that use of the drug should be avoided in patients with end-stage renal disease requiring dialysis.

■ **Common Adverse Effects** Adverse effects reported in clinical trials in 2% or more of patients with chronic idiopathic constipation receiving prucalopride and at an incidence greater than that reported with placebo include headache, abdominal pain, nausea, diarrhea, abdominal distension, dizziness, vomiting, flatulence, and fatigue.

Drug Interactions

■ **Drugs Affecting or Metabolized by Hepatic Microsomal Enzymes** In vitro, prucalopride is a substrate of cytochrome P-450 (CYP) isoenzyme 3A4. In vitro studies indicate that prucalopride has limited potential to inhibit CYP isoenzymes 1A2, 2A6, 2B6, 2C8, 2C9, 2C19, 2D6, 2E1, and 3A4 or to induce CYP isoenzymes 1A2, 2B6, and 3A4 at clinically relevant concentrations.

■ **Drugs Affecting or Affected by Transport Systems** In vitro, prucalopride is a substrate of P-glycoprotein (P-gp) and breast cancer resistance protein (BCRP). In vitro studies indicate that prucalopride has limited potential to inhibit P-gp, BCRP, organic anion transport protein (OATP) 1B1 or 1B3, organic anion transporter (OAT) 1 or 3, organic cation transporter (OCT) 1 or 2, multidrug and toxin extrusion (MATE) 1 or 2-K transporters, bile salt export pump (BSEP), or multidrug resistance protein (MRP) 2 at clinically relevant concentrations.

■ **Cimetidine** No clinically important effect on the pharmacokinetics of prucalopride was observed when cimetidine, an inhibitor of multiple CYP isoenzymes and transport systems, was administered concomitantly with prucalopride.

■ **Digoxin** No clinically important effect on the pharmacokinetics of digoxin, a P-gp substrate, was observed when digoxin was administered concomitantly with prucalopride.

■ **Erythromycin** When prucalopride was administered with erythromycin (500 mg orally 4 times daily), a substrate and moderate inhibitor of CYP3A4 and an inhibitor of P-gp and OATP 1B1 and 1B3, the mean peak plasma concentration and area under the concentration-time curve (AUC) of erythromycin were increased by 40 and 28%, respectively. The mechanism for this interaction is not clear, but the increased exposure to erythromycin is unlikely to be clinically important. No clinically important effect on the pharmacokinetics of prucalopride was observed.

■ **Estrogens and Progestins** When a combination oral contraceptive containing ethinyl estradiol and norethisterone was administered concomitantly with prucalopride, no clinically important effect on the pharmacokinetics of either the estrogen or progestin was observed.

■ **Ketoconazole** When prucalopride was administered with ketoconazole (200 mg twice daily), a potent CYP3A4 inhibitor and an inhibitor of P-gp and BCRP, the peak plasma concentration and AUC of prucalopride were increased by approximately 40%. However, the manufacturer states that this effect is unlikely to be clinically important.

■ **Paroxetine** When paroxetine, a substrate and potent inhibitor of CYP2D6, was administered concomitantly with prucalopride, no clinically important effect on the pharmacokinetics of either drug was observed.

■ **Probenecid** No clinically important effect on the pharmacokinetics of prucalopride was observed when probenecid, an OAT1 and OAT3 inhibitor, was administered concomitantly with prucalopride.

■ **Warfarin** No clinically important effect on the pharmacokinetics of warfarin, a CYP2C9 substrate, was observed when warfarin was administered concomitantly with prucalopride.

Description

Prucalopride, a selective type 4 serotonin (5-HT_4) receptor agonist, is a GI prokinetic agent. The drug increases bowel motility by binding with high affinity to 5-HT_4 receptors, facilitating release of acetylcholine to enhance the amplitude of contractions and stimulate colonic peristalsis. In animal studies, prucalopride has been shown to induce contractions starting from the proximal colon to the anal sphincter. Following oral administration of a single 2-mg dose of prucalopride in patients with chronic idiopathic constipation, the number of high-amplitude propagating contractions was increased during the first 12 hours; with once-daily administration, mean colonic transit time was reduced by 12 hours from a baseline of 65 hours.

Prucalopride is devoid of effects mediated via type 2A, 2B, or 3 serotonin (5-HT_{2A}, 5-HT_{2B}, or 5-HT_3), motilin, or cholecystokinin A receptors in vitro at concentrations exceeding the 5-HT_4 receptor affinity by 150-fold or greater. In animal pharmacology studies, prucalopride had no clinically relevant effects on cardiovascular and cardiac electrophysiologic parameters at concentrations of at least 50 times the therapeutic peak plasma concentration in humans. Certain nonselective 5-HT_4 receptor agonists (i.e., cisapride, tegaserod) have been associated with adverse cardiovascular events; while cardiac arrhythmias associated with cisapride use have been attributed to the drug's lack of selectivity for the 5-HT_4 receptor (i.e., affinity for the human ether-a-go-go gene [hERG]-encoded cardiac potassium channel), the precise mechanism by which tegaserod use may be associated with ischemic cardiovascular events has not been fully established. (See Cardiovascular Safety under Cautions: Warnings/Precautions.)

Following oral administration, bioavailability of prucalopride exceeds 90% and peak plasma concentrations are achieved within 2–3 hours. Administration with a high-fat meal does not alter oral bioavailability. Pharmacokinetics of prucalopride are dose proportional and time independent during continued use. The elimination half-life is approximately 1 day. The parent drug accounts for 92–94% of plasma exposure. Prucalopride is eliminated mainly by the kidneys by passive filtration and active secretion and to a lesser extent (up to 35%) by nonrenal mechanisms. Approximately 84.2% of an orally administered dose is excreted in urine, with 60–65% of the dose excreted in urine as unchanged drug; 13.3% of an administered dose is excreted in feces, with 5% of the dose excreted in feces as unchanged drug. Prucalopride is a substrate of cytochrome P-450 (CYP) isoenzyme 3A4 in vitro. Seven minor metabolites have been identified; the most common metabolite (*O*-desmethylprucalopride acid) accounts for only 3.2 or 3.1% of the dose recovered in urine or feces, respectively. Age, sex, race, and body weight (after adjustment for renal function) do not appear to affect the pharmacokinetics of prucalopride.

Advice to Patients

Importance of advising patients to read the manufacturer's patient information.

Importance of advising patients and their caregivers and families that suicidal thoughts and behavior have been reported in patients receiving prucalopride. Importance of being alert for persistent worsening of symptoms of depression, unusual changes in mood or behavior, and emergence of suicidal thoughts or behavior. Importance of immediately discontinuing prucalopride and contacting a clinician if such symptoms occur.

Importance of women informing clinicians if they are or plan to become pregnant or plan to breast-feed.

Importance of patients informing clinicians of existing or contemplated concomitant therapy, including prescription and OTC drugs, as well as any concomitant illnesses.

Importance of informing patients of other important precautionary information. (See Cautions.)

Overview® (see Users Guide). For additional information on this drug until a more detailed monograph is developed and published, the manufacturer's labeling should be consulted. It is *essential* that the manufacturer's labeling be consulted for more detailed information on usual cautions, precautions, contraindications, potential drug interactions, laboratory test interferences, and acute toxicity.

Preparations

Excipients in commercially available drug preparations may have clinically important effects in some individuals; consult specific product labeling for details.

Prucalopride Succinate

Oral		
Tablets, film-coated	1 mg (of prucalopride)	Motegrity®, Shire
	2 mg (of prucalopride)	Motegrity®, Shire

Selected Revisions October 2019, © Copyright, January 2019, American Society of Health-System Pharmacists, Inc.

ANTI-INFLAMMATORY AGENTS 56:36

Balsalazide Disodium

■ Balsalazide is a GI anti-inflammatory agent.

Uses

■ Ulcerative Colitis Balsalazide is used in the management of mildly to moderately active ulcerative colitis. Safety and efficacy of balsalazide therapy have not been established beyond 12 weeks.

Safety and efficacy of balsalazide have been evaluated in 2 randomized, double-blind studies of 8 weeks' duration in patients with mildly to moderately active ulcerative colitis with sigmoidoscopic findings of friable or spontaneously bleeding mucosa. In these studies, improvements in rectal bleeding, stool frequency, or sigmoidoscopic findings were reported in 55–65, 49–59, or 74–79% of patients, respectively, who received balsalazide 6.75 g daily for 8 weeks. Balsalazide also reduced abdominal pain and improved functional assessment scores.

Results of clinical studies indicate that balsalazide 6.75 g daily appears to be at least as effective as sulfasalazine 3 g daily or mesalamine 2.4 g daily in improving symptoms in patients with ulcerative colitis who received the drugs orally for up to 12 weeks. In one randomized, double-blind study, symptomatic improvement or complete remission (defined as asymptomatic or with mild symptoms, sigmoidoscopy grade 0 or 1, and no rectal steroid use within 4 days) was achieved in 88 or 62%, respectively, of patients receiving balsalazide 6.75 mg daily and in 57 or 37%, respectively, of those who received mesalamine 2.4 g daily for 12 weeks. Treatment with balsalazide appears to be associated with more rapid symptomatic improvement (12–14 days earlier) compared to that with mesalamine. However, some clinicians state that a relative therapeutic advantage of balsalazide over mesalamine remains to be established.

■ Crohn's Disease Although controlled studies assessing the efficacy of balsalazide are lacking, limited data indicate that use of the drug may be beneficial in the management of Crohn's disease† involving the colon.

(For further information about the use of 5-aminosalicylic acid derivatives in the management of Crohn's Disease, see Uses: Crohn's Disease, in Mesalamine 56:36.)

Dosage and Administration

■ General Balsalazide disodium is administered orally 3 times daily.

■ Dosage ***Ulcerative Colitis*** Dosage of balsalazide disodium is expressed in terms of balsalazide. The recommended adult dosage of balsalazide is 6.75 g (equivalent to 2.4 g of mesalamine) daily administered as 3 equally divided doses of 2.25 g (three 750-mg capsules 3 times daily) for 8 weeks; some patients may require up to 12 weeks of therapy. The total daily dosage of balsalazide (6.75 g) is equivalent to approximately 2.4 g of mesalamine.

Crohn's Disease For the management of Crohn's disease† (involving the colon), a balsalazide dosage of 2–6 g daily may be used.

■ Special Populations No special population dosage recommendations at this time.

Cautions

■ Contraindications Known hypersensitivity to salicylates, balsalazide, or its metabolites, or any ingredient in the formulation.

■ Warnings/Precautions ***Major Toxicities*** **GI Effects.** Exacerbation of preexisting symptoms of ulcerative colitis has been reported rarely.

General Precautions **Gastric Retention.** Potential for prolonged gastric retention of the drug in patients with pyloric stenosis.

Specific Populations **Pregnancy.** Category B. (See Users Guide.)

Nursing Women. It is not known whether balsalazide is distributed in human milk. Because many drugs are excreted in human milk, caution is advised if the drug is administered in nursing women.

Pediatric Use. Safety and efficacy not established in children younger than 18 years of age.

Geriatric Use. Experience in those 65 years of age and older insufficient to determine whether they respond differently from younger adults.

Hepatic Impairment. Safety and efficacy not established in patients with hepatic impairment.

Renal Impairment. Safety and efficacy not established in patients with renal impairment. However, since renal toxicity has been reported in patients receiving other preparations of mesalamine, the manufacturer recommends that balsalazide be used with caution in patients with renal impairment or a history of renal disease.

■ Common Adverse Effects Adverse effects occurring in 4% or more of patients receiving balsalazide include headache, abdominal pain, diarrhea, nausea, vomiting, respiratory infection, arthralgia, flatulence, and fatigue.

Some adverse effects (e.g., abdominal pain, fatigue, nausea) appear to occur more frequently in women. The manufacturer states that certain adverse effects (e.g., abdominal pain, rectal bleeding, anemia) may be manifestations of ulcerative colitis.

Drug Interactions

No formal drug interaction studies have been performed.

■ Oral Anti-Infective Agents Potential pharmacologic interaction (e.g., interference with release of mesalamine in the colon).

■ Azathioprine and 6-Mercaptopurine Potential pharmacokinetic interaction (balsalazide may interfere with metabolism of these drugs by inhibition of thiopurine methyltransferase, an enzyme involved in the metabolism of the immunosuppressants).

Description

Balsalazide is a GI anti-inflammatory agent. Balsalazide is a prodrug of mesalamine (5-aminosalicylic acid) and has little or no pharmacologic activity until enzymatically cleaved in the colon to provide mesalamine and the inert 4-aminobenzoyl-β-alanine. Thus, the spectrum of pharmacologic activity of balsalazide generally is similar to that of mesalamine.

Mesalamine exhibits anti-inflammatory activity in the GI tract. Although the exact mechanism of action of mesalamine has not been fully elucidated, the drug appears to exert its anti-inflammatory effects locally, in the GI tract, rather than systemically. Limited data indicate that mesalamine may reduce inflammation in the colon by inhibiting cyclooxygenase, an enzyme that catalyzes the formation of prostaglandin precursors (endoperoxides) from arachidonic acid. Mesalamine also inhibits leukotriene synthesis, possibly by inhibiting lipoxygenase, an enzyme that catalyzes the formation of leukotrienes and hydroxyeicosatetraenoic acids (HETEs) from arachidonic acid and its metabolites. Although the role of arachidonic acid metabolites in the pathogenesis of inflammatory bowel disease remains to be determined, mucosal production of these metabolites, both through the cyclooxygenase and the lipoxygenase pathways, appears to be increased in patients with inflammatory bowel disease.

Following oral administration, balsalazide disodium passes intact into the colon where the azo-linkage is cleaved by intestinal flora to form mesalamine and 4-aminobenzoyl-β-alanine. A small portion of mesalamine is absorbed and undergoes N^4-acetylation. Balsalazide and/or its metabolites are excreted principally in feces. Approximately 65% of an administered dose is excreted in feces as mesalamine, 4-aminobenzoyl-β-alanine, or *N*-acetylated metabolites, and up to 25% is excreted in urine as *N*-acetylated metabolites; less than 1% of the dose is excreted in urine or feces as unchanged drug. (For further information on chemistry, pharmacology, and pharmacokinetics of mesalamine, see Mesalamine 56:36.)

Each g of balsalazide disodium (as commercially available 750-mg capsules) provides approximately 5 mEq (115 mg) of sodium.

Advice to Patients

Importance of women informing clinicians if they are or plan to become pregnant or to breast-feed.

Importance of informing clinicians of existing or contemplated concomitant therapy, including prescription and OTC drugs.

Overview (see Users Guide). For additional information until a more detailed monograph is developed and published, the manufacturer's labeling should be consulted. It is *essential* that the manufacturer's labeling be consulted for more detailed information on usual cautions, precautions, contraindications, potential drug interactions, laboratory test interferences, and acute toxicity.

Preparations

Excipients in commercially available drug preparations may have clinically important effects in some individuals; consult specific product labeling for details.

Balsalazide Disodium

Oral		
Capsules	750 mg	Colazal®, Salix

†Use is not currently included in the labeling approved by the US Food and Drug Administration

Selected Revisions January 2006, © Copyright, August 2001, American Society of Health-System Pharmacists, Inc.

Mesalamine

5-Aminosalicylic Acid, *m*-Aminosalicylic Acid, Fisalamine, Mesalazine, 5-ASA

■ Mesalamine, the 5-amino derivative of salicylic acid, is a GI anti-inflammatory agent.

Uses

■ **Ulcerative Colitis** Oral mesalamine (as delayed-release tablets or extended-release capsules) is used for the management of mildly to moderately active ulcerative colitis. In addition, mesalamine 400-mg delayed-release tablets (Asacol®) are used to maintain clinical remission in patients with ulcerative colitis, while mesalamine extended-release capsules (Pentasa®) and mesalamine 1.2-g delayed-release tablets (Lialda®) are used to induce clinical remission in patients with mildly to moderately active ulcerative colitis. Mesalamine rectal suspension is used in the management of mildly to moderately active distal ulcerative colitis, including ulcerative proctosigmoiditis and ulcerative proctitis. Mesalamine rectal suppositories are used in the management of active ulcerative proctitis. The drug is used in the management of these conditions in conjunction with usual supportive and dietary measures. Oral preparations of the drug may be preferable to rectal preparations in patients with extensive inflammatory bowel disease, since efficacy of rectal preparations may be limited to disease distal to the splenic flexure.

Mildly to Moderately Active Ulcerative Colitis Delayed- or extended-release oral preparations of mesalamine have been effective in patients with mildly to moderately active ulcerative colitis, including those with proctitis. When used in the management of mildly to moderately active ulcerative colitis, oral mesalamine has reduced disease activity, including improvement in sigmoidoscopic appearance of the bowel, rectal bleeding, abdominal/rectal pain, and stool consistency, frequency, and urgency.

Efficacy of mesalamine 400-mg delayed-release tablets (Asacol®) for the management of mildly to moderately active ulcerative colitis has been established in 2 placebo-controlled studies. In one randomized, double-blind, multicenter, dose-ranging (1.6 or 2.4 g daily) study, reduction of disease activity (measured by improvement in sigmoidoscopic appearance) was reported in 49 or 27% of patients receiving mesalamine (2.4 g daily) or placebo, respectively, while no consistent evidence of efficacy was observed with the 1.6-g daily dosage. In addition, substantially more patients receiving mesalamine (2.4 g daily) showed improvement in rectal bleeding and stool frequency than those receiving placebo.

In the other randomized, double-blind, 6-week study, sigmoidoscopic improvement occurred in 74 or 26% of patients receiving mesalamine delayed-release tablets (4.8 g daily) or placebo, respectively. More patients receiving mesalamine have shown improvement in overall symptoms than those receiving placebo.

Efficacy of mesalamine extended-release capsules for the management of mildly to moderately active ulcerative colitis has been established in 2 randomized, double-blind, placebo-controlled, dose-ranging studies. Primary efficacy parameters in these studies were measured by clinical improvement assessed by clinician global assessment (proportion of patients with complete or marked improvement), sigmoidoscopic index (objective measure of disease activity rated by mucosal vascular pattern, erythema, friability, granularity/ulcerations, improvement from baseline in mucopus), and treatment failure (proportion of patients developing severe or fulminant ulcerative colitis requiring corticosteroid therapy, hospitalization, or worsening of the disease within 7 days of therapy or lack of substantial improvement by 14 days of therapy). Secondary efficacy parameters were assessed by clinical symptoms (e.g., stool consistency/frequency/urgency, rectal bleeding, abdominal/rectal pain). Patients received 2 g (1 g twice daily) or 4 g (1 g 4 times daily) of mesalamine extended-release capsules daily. In one of these studies, clinician global index of treatment success was reported in 59, 57, or 36% of patients receiving a daily 4-g dosage of mesalamine, 2-g dosage of mesalamine, or placebo, respectively, while reductions in sigmoidoscopic index (rated by a standard 15-point scale) were 5, 4.3, or 2.5, respectively. Treatment failure was reported in 9, 18, or 22% of patients receiving a daily 4-g dosage of mesalamine, 2-g dosage of mesalamine, or placebo, respectively. Similar efficacy was observed in the other placebo-controlled study; clinician global index of treatment success was reported in 55, 41, or 31% of patients receiving a daily 4-g dosage of mesalamine, 2-g dosage of mesalamine, or placebo, respectively, while reductions in sigmoidoscopic index were 3.8, 2.6, or 1.6, respectively, and treatment failure was reported in 9, 17, or 31% of patients, respectively. While the 4-g daily dosages of mesalamine produced consistent improvement in primary parameters in these studies, the 2-g daily dosage was associated with inconsistent results. Consistent improvement in secondary parameters and induction of remission (assessed by endoscopic and symptomatic endpoints) also were observed with the 4-g daily dosages.

Induction of Remission of Ulcerative Colitis. Safety and efficacy of oral mesalamine 1.2-g delayed-release tablets (Lialda®) for induction of remission in patients with active, mild to moderate ulcerative colitis were evaluated in two 8-week randomized, double-blind, placebo-controlled trials that included 517 patients. Patients were randomized to receive a 2.4- or 4.8-g daily dosage of mesalamine or placebo. The primary efficacy end point at week 8 of treatment was the percentage of patients achieving remission (defined as an Ulcerative Colitis Disease Activity Index [UC-DAI] of 1 or less, with scores of zero for rectal bleeding and stool frequency, and a sigmoidoscopy score reduction of 1 point or more from baseline). The incidence of remission at 8 weeks was about 34–41, 29–41, or 13–22% in patients receiving mesalamine 2.4 g daily, mesalamine 4.8 g daily, or placebo, respectively. Patients receiving mesalamine 2.4 or 4.8 g daily also experienced greater benefit in secondary efficacy parameters (e.g., clinical improvement, treatment failure, clinical remission, sigmoidoscopic appearance) compared with patients receiving placebo.

Maintenance of Remission of Ulcerative Colitis. Safety and efficacy of oral mesalamine 400-mg delayed-release tablets (Asacol®) for maintenance therapy in patients with ulcerative colitis were evaluated in a 6-month randomized, double-blind, placebo-controlled study that included 264 patients. Patients were randomized to receive a daily 0.8-g dosage of mesalamine (90 patients), 1.6-g dosage of mesalamine (87 patients), or placebo (87 patients). Treatment success or failure was defined as maintenance of remission after 6 months or relapse during the study, respectively. Treatment success in patients receiving a daily 0.8-g mesalamine dosage was not statistically different from patients receiving placebo. Endoscopic remission of ulcerative colitis (based on intention-to-treat analysis) in all 174 patients receiving either 1.6 g of mesalamine daily or placebo, was reported in 61 out of 87 patients (70.1%) receiving mesalamine or 42 out of 87 patients (48.3%) in those receiving placebo. Pooled analysis of data from 4 comparator-drug (sulfasalazine) controlled maintenance trials indicate that treatment success occurred in 59 or 69% of patients receiving mesalamine extended-release capsules (0.8–2.8 g daily) or sulfasalazine (2–4 g daily), respectively; however, the difference in response was not statistically significant.

Mildly to Moderately Active Distal Ulcerative Colitis When used in the management of active distal ulcerative colitis, including proctosigmoiditis or proctitis, mesalamine rectal suspension has reduced stool frequency, rectal bleeding, mucosal inflammation, and abdominal pain. When used in the management of active ulcerative proctitis, mesalamine rectal suppositories have reduced stool frequency, rectal bleeding, and mucosal inflammation. Patients most likely to respond to rectal mesalamine are those with disease confined to the distal 20–40 cm of the colon. Clinical remission has occurred in 30–90% of patients with these conditions receiving rectal mesalamine; however, relapse usually has occurred following discontinuance and, rarely, during continued use of the drug. In responsive disease, improvement usually is evident within 1 week to 3 months of initiation of therapy, and some patients may need prolonged periods of rectal mesalamine therapy to achieve improvement. However, some clinicians have suggested that if clinical remission is not achieved within 2–4 months of initiation of rectal mesalamine therapy, it is unlikely that further improvement would be achieved with more prolonged therapy. There is limited evidence that the efficacy of rectal mesalamine can be sustained during chronic therapy, but additional study and experience are needed.

The optimum role of rectal mesalamine in the management of active ulcerative colitis remains to be elucidated, particularly relative to other therapies (e.g., oral sulfasalazine) and in patients with severe and/or refractory disease. Clinical studies have shown that rectal mesalamine is more effective than placebo and at least as effective as oral sulfasalazine in reducing signs and symptoms (e.g., stool frequency, rectal bleeding, mucosal inflammation) of these conditions. However, many patients who were already receiving oral sulfasalazine therapy continued to receive the drug when rectal mesalamine was initiated, and combined therapy may be necessary for optimal response in many such patients. In addition, some clinicians state that sulfasalazine therapy should be continued to minimize the risk of an exacerbated flare developing secondary to withdrawal of the drug and the delayed onset of mesalamine. Rectal mesalamine also was at least as effective as rectal hydrocortisone in patients with sigmoidoscopically or radiographically confirmed mild to moderate distal ulcerative colitis.

In patients with ulcerative colitis whose symptoms progress despite a recommended regimen of oral sulfasalazine and/or rectal or oral corticosteroids, therapy with rectal mesalamine may be beneficial. Combined therapy with rectal mesalamine and oral sulfasalazine and/or rectal or oral corticosteroids may produce additive effects in reducing signs and symptoms of refractory ulcerative colitis, although combined rectal mesalamine and oral corticosteroid therapy may be no more effective than an oral corticosteroid alone in severe disease. In addition, although efficacy of rectal mesalamine may be limited in patients with severe ulcerative colitis, the drug has been effective in some patients refractory to, or intolerant of, oral sulfasalazine and/or rectal or oral corticosteroids.

Clinical studies have shown that mesalamine rectal suppositories are more effective than placebo in reducing signs and symptoms (e.g., stool frequency, rectal bleeding, mucosal inflammation) of active ulcerative proctitis. Efficacy of mesalamine rectal suppositories appears to be independent of patients' gender, duration and extent of disease, or duration of current episode.

■ **Crohn's Disease** Mesalamine has been used for the management of active Crohn's disease†.

Overview Crohn's disease, a chronic inflammatory bowel disease, is characterized by focal, asymmetric, transmural, and occasionally, granulomatous inflammation affecting the GI tract (most frequently the ileum and colon) with a potential for systemic and extraintestinal complications and recurrent flare-ups.The etiology and pathogenesis of Crohn's disease have not been elucidated, but they appear to be multifactorial. Many clinicians have suggested that environmental (e.g., smoking, intestinal bacterial flora), immunologic (increased mucosal IgG), and genetic factors may contribute to the development of the disease. The disease can develop in any age group, although disease onset is more frequent in adolescents and young adults. Diagnosis of Crohn's disease is difficult because of the heterogenicity of manifestations, overlapping features with other inflammatory bowel diseases, and/or presentation without GI symptoms (i.e., extraintestinal symptoms). Symptoms of chronic or nocturnal diarrhea, abdominal pain, weight loss, fever, and rectal bleeding may be indicative of underlying inflammatory processes. Clinical manifestations of the disease include pallor, cachexia, abdominal mass or tenderness, and perianal fissures, fistulae, or abscesses. In children, growth arrest or loss of height may be one of the initial manifestations of Crohn's disease. Diagnosis and consequent treatment of Crohn's disease is based on clinical, laboratory, and diagnostic evaluations, including radiologic examinations and/or endoscopy.

Treatment Crohn's disease is not medically or surgically curable and generally is managed by reducing inflammation, improving quality of life, and minimizing short- and long-term toxicity (associated with treatment) and complications. Choice of treatment depends on several factors, including the severity, location (stomach/duodenum, jejunum, ileum, colon, rectum, anus), extent (localized, diffused), and pattern/behavior (principally inflammatory, fistulizing, or fibrostenotic) of the disease. In addition, previous history of the disease (e.g., intestinal surgery, response to previous treatment), extraintestinal complications, certain patient characteristics (e.g., age, gender, lifestyle, nutrition, compliance, social and emotional status, resources, education, functional ability), and other factors (e.g., growth in children) should be considered when initiating therapy. Most currently available drugs for Crohn's disease including amino derivatives of salicylic acid (e.g., mesalamine, balsalazide, olsalazine, sulfasalazine), conventional corticosteroids (hydrocortisone, methylprednisolone, prednisolone, prednisone), more recently available corticosteroids (e.g., budesonide, having substantial topical anti-inflammatory activity and lower systemic availability than conventional corticosteroids), corticotropin, biologic response modifiers (e.g., adalimumab, infliximab, natalizumab), and immunosuppressive or immunomodulating agents (e.g., azathioprine, cyclosporine, mercaptopurine, methotrexate, mycophenolate mofetil, tacrolimus, thalidomide,) are used to manage chronic inflammation of the intestinal mucosa. In addition, since the intestinal bacterial flora may be associated with intestinal inflammation, anti-infective agents (metronidazole and/or ciprofloxacin) may be used in the management of mildly to moderately and moderately to severely active disease. Many clinicians currently state that therapy for inflammatory bowel disease (e.g., Crohn's disease) should be disease modifying rather than merely symptomatic whenever possible.

According to criteria established by the American College of Gastroenterology, severity of Crohn's disease may be classified as mildly to moderately active, moderately to severely active, or severely active to fulminant disease. Patients generally considered to be in remission are those who are asymptomatic, those without inflammatory sequelae, or those who have responded to acute medical intervention or have undergone surgical resection and have no gross evidence of residual disease.

Mildly to Moderately Active Crohn's Disease. Patients are considered to have mildly to moderately active Crohn's disease if they are ambulatory and can tolerate oral alimentation without experiencing more than 10% of body weight loss or presenting manifestations of dehydration, toxicity (e.g., high fever, rigor, prostration), or abdominal tenderness/painful mass/obstruction. For the initial management of ileal, ileocolonic, or colonic mildly to moderately active Crohn's disease, many clinicians recommend preparations containing or being metabolized to 5-aminosalicylic acid (e.g., mesalamine, sulfasalazine) or possibly, budesonide (a relatively new corticosteroid). In general, the choice of 5-aminosalicylic acid derivatives should be based on the location of the disease.

Oral formulations of mesalamine that are in a slow- or pH-dependent matrix can deliver therapeutic concentrations of the drug to the stomach, small bowel, or distal ileum and therefore are used in patients with gastroduodenal and/or ileal Crohn's disease. Results of placebo-controlled studies on the efficacy of oral mesalamine preparations in the management of mildly to moderately active Crohn's disease have been equivocal, since administration of the drug was not consistently more effective than placebo. (See Active Crohn's Disease under Crohn's Disease: Use of Mesalamine in Crohn's Disease, in Uses.)

Sulfasalazine has not been consistently effective in patients with ileal disease and it is recommended that the drug be used in ileocolonic or colonic disease, preferably with left-sided condition, restricted to the colon. Budesonide, which appears to be more effective than mesalamine in the treatment of mildly to moderately active disease, generally is used in patients with Crohn's disease involving the ileum and/or ascending colon. (See Uses: Crohn's Disease, in Budesonide 68:04.) Therefore, some clinicians recommend that for initial management of Crohn's disease involving the ileum and/or ascending colon, patients should receive 8–16 weeks of therapy with budesonide delayed-release capsules and those with left-sided disease restricted to the colon should receive 16 weeks of therapy with sulfasalazine. Individuals who do not respond to therapy with sulfasalazine or budesonide or those who develop hypersensitivity to sulfasalazine should receive a conventional corticosteroid (e.g., prednisone, prednisolone). Therapy with metronidazole and/or ciprofloxacin also has been recommended in patients who do not respond to sulfasalazine. (See Uses: Crohn's Disease, in Metronidazole 8:30.92 and see Uses: Crohn's Disease, in Ciprofloxacin 8:12.18.)

Currently, there are inadequate data regarding the management of upper GI (e.g., esophageal, gastroduodenal, jejunoileal) Crohn's disease. Results of uncontrolled studies in a limited number of patients indicate that symptoms of upper GI Crohn's disease may respond to proton-pump inhibitors (e.g., omeprazole), frequently given in conjunction with corticosteroids or other immunosuppressant agents. Jejunoileitis, which is often accompanied by overgrowth of bacteria in the small intestine, may be treated with anti-infective therapy.

Response to initial therapy should be evaluated within several weeks. Treatment of active disease should be continued until remission of symptoms or, alternatively, treatment failure (lack of continued improvement) occurs. Patients who achieve remission should be considered for maintenance therapy (see Maintenance of Remission of Crohn's Disease under Crohn's Disease: Treatment, in Uses), while alternative therapy (according to clinical status and possible reassessment of disease severity) should be instituted in those whose disease continues to be symptomatic. (See Moderately to Severely Active Crohn's Disease under Crohn's Disease: Treatment, in Uses.)

Moderately to Severely Active Crohn's Disease. Patients are considered to have moderately to severely active Crohn's disease if they have failed to respond to therapy for mildly to moderately active disease or have developed more severe symptoms (e.g., fever, substantial weight loss, abdominal pain/tenderness, intermittent nausea or vomiting, significant anemia) than those with mildly to moderately active disease, but no evidence of obstruction. Conventional corticosteroids (e.g., prednisone, prednisolone) or possibly, budesonide may be used for the management of moderately to severely active disease until resolution of symptoms and appropriate weight gain occurs (usually within 7–28 days). Most patients (greater than 50%), however, become corticosteroid dependent or resistant. Addition of 5-aminosalicylic acid derivatives to corticosteroids has not been associated with short- or long-term benefit, while adjunctive use of azathioprine or mercaptopurine with corticosteroids has been found to be beneficial. It should be considered, however, that up to 3–4 months of adjunctive therapy with these immunosuppressants may be needed before substantial benefits (including remission) become apparent, and, therefore, these drugs mainly are used for maintenance therapy. Parenteral methotrexate also has been shown to be effective in allowing corticosteroids to be tapered in corticosteroid-dependent patients. In addition, limited data indicate that mycophenolate mofetil may be beneficial in the management of moderately to severely active Crohn's disease.

Infliximab or, possibly, thalidomide may be used in patients who have had an inadequate response to conventional therapies (e.g., corticosteroids, mesalamine sulfasalazine, azathioprine, mercaptopurine, methotrexate) or in whom conventional therapies are contraindicated. (For further information about the use of infliximab in moderately to severely active Crohn's disease, see Uses: Crohn's Disease, in Infliximab 92:36.)

Anti-infective therapy (e.g., metronidazole, ciprofloxacin, other broad spectrum antibiotics) or drainage (percutaneous or surgical) may be necessary when infection or abscess is present in patients with moderately to severely active Crohn's disease.

Severely Active to Fulminant Crohn's Disease. Patients with severely active to fulminant Crohn's disease usually include those who have persisting symptoms despite oral corticosteroid or infliximab therapy or those who develop severe manifestations (e.g., high fever, persistent vomiting, rebound tenderness, evidence of GI obstruction or abscess) of the disease. Individuals without an abscess or those who have been receiving oral corticosteroids should be treated with parenteral corticosteroids, given as a continuous IV infusion or, possibly, by intermittent IV injections in divided doses. In patients with severe disease, IV corticotropin (ACTH) has been used rarely. Patients with an inflammatory abdominal mass should receive broad-spectrum anti-infectives in conjunction with parenteral corticosteroids; these individuals usually have intestinal perforation and surgery would be needed after an appropriate waiting period. In those unable to tolerate nutritional requirements, elemental feeding or parenteral hyperalimentation is indicated after 5–7 days of parenteral corticosteroid therapy.

Limited data indicate that patients who do not respond to parenteral corticosteroids may respond to other immunosuppressive agents (e.g., IV cyclosporine, tacrolimus). Although definitive data are lacking concerning the use of infliximab in patients with severe Crohn's disease, some clinicians state that the drug may be used in patients with severe disease who do not respond to parenteral corticosteroids. Individuals who have responded to parenteral therapy (e.g., corticosteroids, cyclosporine, tacrolimus) may be switched gradually to the equivalent oral therapy, while surgery is indicated in those who do not respond or whose symptoms worsen.

Perianal and Fistulizing Crohn's Disease. Patients with acute suppurative disease, including perianal and/or perirectal abscesses, often require surgical intervention. Although controlled studies regarding the use of anti-infective agents in the management of perianal and fistulizing Crohn's disease are lacking, limited data suggest that use of metronidazole or ciprofloxacin alone or, alternatively, combination therapy with the 2 anti-infectives may provide benefit in nonsuppurative fistulizing disease.

Metronidazole and/or ciprofloxacin mainly are used for short-term therapy, although relapse usually occurs upon discontinuance; however, safety and efficacy of long-term anti-infective therapy have not been established and further study and experience are needed to elucidate fully the long-term benefits of such therapy. In addition, there are no controlled studies with fistula closure, as the primary end point, demonstrating that immunosuppressive therapy with azathioprine or mercaptopurine is effective in fistulizing disease. Current clinical practice concerning use of these agents is based on a pooled analysis of 5 controlled trials in which fistula closure was considered a secondary end point and in several uncontrolled case studies. Data from these studies indicate that long-term (several years) therapy with azathioprine or mercaptopurine may be effective in the management of fistulizing Crohn's disease. Use of cyclosporine for fistulizing disease is based on results of uncontrolled case studies; short-term administration of cyclosporine has been beneficial in several patients. Results of one controlled and several uncontrolled case studies have shown that tacrolimus also may be beneficial in the management of fistulizing Crohn's disease.

Infliximab has been effective in the management of fistulizing Crohn's disease; the drug is used to reduce the number of draining enterocutaneous and rectovaginal fistulas and to maintain fistula closure. Further study is needed to determine the relative safety and efficacy of infliximab and other therapies used for the management of fistulizing Crohn's disease (e.g., azathioprine, ciprofloxacin and/or metronidazole, mercaptopurine, surgical intervention). Some clinicians suggest that, although data are not available to date to support use of infliximab as first-line therapy for fistulizing Crohn's disease, use of the drug should be considered when fistulas have not responded to appropriate anti-infective regimens (e.g., ciprofloxacin and/or metronidazole) and/or immunosuppressive therapy (e.g., azathioprine, mercaptopurine).

For further information on the use of infliximab in Fistulizing Crohn's Disease, see Fistulizing Crohn's Disease under Uses: Crohn's Disease, in Infliximab 92:36.

Maintenance of Remission of Crohn's Disease. The goals of maintenance therapy are to prolong periods of remission and improve quality of life. Once remission has been achieved, choice of maintenance therapy should be evaluated individually, based on the condition (e.g., length of remission, type of remission [medical or surgical]) and characteristics of each patient. Maintenance of remission remains problematic because of the difficulty in identifying subgroups of patients who undergo early clinical or subclinical flare-ups and who would benefit from appropriate and timely treatment.

There are no drug treatments available to prevent relapse of Crohn's disease; however, clinical relapse may be delayed by using anti-inflammatory or anti-infective agents, or to a greater extent by using immunomodulating drugs. Most patients who have received corticosteroid therapy for active Crohn's disease (including conventional corticosteroids or budesonide) usually develop relapse within a year, unless they receive maintenance therapy. Neither sulfasalazine nor mesalamine appears to be effective in maintaining remission of Crohn's disease after medically induced clinical remission. Some clinicians state that mesalamine may be the optimal therapy for maintenance of remission in patients with ileal or jejunoileal disease, although the drug is associated with substantially lower efficacy in those with colonic disease. Mesalamine has been used with equivocal results for maintenance therapy of Crohn's disease. In some, but not other, placebo-controlled studies in patients with medically induced remission, relapse rates were lower with mesalamine relative to placebo. In several placebo-controlled studies, budesonide was effective for maintenance therapy in patients with medically-induced remission for up to about 6 months of therapy; however, no substantial difference was observed at 1 year of therapy.

Both azathioprine and mercaptopurine are effective for maintenance therapy in patients with medically-induced remission of Crohn's disease. Response generally is apparent after 3–6 months of therapy. Although clinical benefits beyond 4 years of therapy remain to be established, limited data indicate that such benefits may persist longer than 4 years. Methotrexate also has been used effectively for maintenance of Crohn's disease. Infliximab may be used to maintain clinical remission in patients with moderately to severely active disease who have had an inadequate response to conventional therapies (e.g., azathioprine, corticosteroids, mercaptopurine, mesalamine, sulfasalazine). (See Maintenance of Remission of Crohn's Disease under Crohn's Disease: Active Crohn's Disease, in Uses, in Infliximab 92:36.)

Drug therapy for prevention of disease relapse following surgically induced remission has not been firmly established. Limited data indicate that mesalamine or, possibly, sulfasalazine may reduce the risk of postoperative recurrence for up to 3 years. However, equivocal results were reported in patients with surgically induced remission receiving mesalamine. (See Maintenance of Remission of Crohn's Disease under Crohn's Disease: Use of Mesalamine in Crohn's Disease, in Uses.) In patients with surgically induced remission of Crohn's disease, mercaptopurine appears to be more effective than placebo and efficacy of azathioprine appears to be similar to that of mesalamine. Limited data also indicate that high-dose (20 mg/kg) metronidazole therapy may reduce postoperative recurrence for up to 1 year; however, long-term studies are needed to elucidate further the efficacy of such therapy. Ornidazole (another nitroimidazole-derivative anti-infective agent; currently not commercially available in the US) has been shown to prevent early postoperative endoscopic recurrence and postpone symptomatic relapse.

Surgery in Patients with Crohn's Disease. Surgical resection is not a cure for Crohn's disease. However, surgical intervention is needed in greater than 60% of patients to treat intractable hemorrhage, perforation, persistent or recurrent obstruction, abscess, or unresponsive fulminant disease. Some clinicians state that since therapy to reduce the risk of postoperative recurrence is available (see Maintenance of Remission of Crohn's Disease under Crohn's Disease: Treatment, in Uses), there is little justification to prolong ineffective drug therapy and delay surgery in patients with complications of Crohn's disease whose quality of life would be improved by surgical intervention.

Crohn's Disease in Pediatric Patients. Crohn's disease in pediatric patients generally is managed by controlling disease activity and symptoms, providing nutritional intervention (to ensure adequate food intake and reverse impaired weight and growth velocities) and psychologic support, and monitoring for extraintestinal manifestations (e.g., arthralgias, arthritis). Similar to adults, choice of therapy depends on severity and location of the disease.

Sulfasalazine (initial dosage of 25–40 mg/kg daily increased to 50–75 mg/kg daily [up to 4 g daily], given with 1 mg of folic acid daily) or mesalamine (initial oral dosage of 20–30 mg/kg daily increased up to 60 mg/kg daily) has been used in pediatric patients with mild ileal, ileocecal, ileocolonic, or colonic Crohn's disease; topical mesalamine or corticosteroid enemas may be used in left-sided colitis. Systemic corticosteroids (e.g., prednisone 1–2 mg/kg daily up to 60 mg daily) usually have been used in those with mild esophageal or gastroduodenal disease. Children with mild perianal disease or those intolerant to sulfasalazine or mesalamine may receive metronidazole (10–20 mg/kg daily, up to a maximum of 1 g daily). Budesonide (as pH-dependent-release preparations administered in a dosage of 0.45 mg/kg daily up to a maximum dosage of 9 mg daily) has been used for the management of mildly to moderately active Crohn's disease in a limited number of children 9.5–18 years of age. Budesonide is more effective than mesalamine, but less effective than conventional corticosteroids (e.g., prednisone).

For the management of moderately to severely active disease, systemic corticosteroids (e.g., prednisone or methylprednisolone 1–2 mg/kg daily up to 60 mg daily) may be used; some clinicians suggest that an immunosuppressive agent (e.g., mercaptopurine) be used conjunctively with corticosteroids, once initial diagnosis is made. IV metronidazole or another anti-infective should be used with corticosteroids if infection or abscess is present.

In pediatric patients who become corticosteroid dependent or resistant, mercaptopurine or azathioprine may be used, while methotrexate therapy (10–15 mg/m^2) should be considered in those who had an inadequate response to or did not tolerate mercaptopurine or azathioprine. Infliximab has been used in a limited number of pediatric patients for the management of the signs and symptoms of active Crohn's disease. For further information about the use of infliximab in children, see Crohn's Disease in Pediatric Patients under Uses: Crohn's Disease, in Infliximab 92:00. In children with refractory perianal fistulas, use of cyclosporine (4 mg/kg daily) may be considered.

Use of Mesalamine in Crohn's Disease **Active Crohn's Disease.** Extended-release oral mesalamine preparations have been used in the management of Crohn's disease†. It has been suggested that administration of extended-release oral mesalamine may be especially useful in the management of this condition since the drug is partially released from these preparations in the ileum, which may facilitate an anti-inflammatory effect in patients with ileitis.

Efficacy of oral mesalamine has been studied in several placebo-controlled studies in patients with mildly to moderately active Crohn's disease. In many of these studies, the Crohn's Disease Activity Index (CDAI) was used for clinical assessment. The CDAI score is based on subjective observations by the patient (e.g., the daily number of liquid or very soft stools, severity of abdominal pain, general well-being) and objective evidence (e.g., number of extraintestinal manifestations, presence of an abdominal mass, use or nonuse of antidiarrheal drugs, the hematocrit, body weight). Results of these studies have been equivocal.

In a 16-week multicenter, randomized, double-blind, dose-ranging, placebo-controlled study in 310 adults with mildly to moderately active ileal, ileocolonic, or colonic Crohn's disease†, patients were randomized to receive placebo or oral mesalamine extended-release capsules (Pentasa®) in a dosage of 1, 2, or 4 g daily. Remission (defined as a reduction from baseline CDAI of more than 50 points and a final CDAI score of less than 150 assessed at the final visit) was observed in 43 or 18% of patients receiving mesalamine 4 g daily or placebo, respectively, while a mean reduction of 72 or 21 points from baseline CDAI was observed, respectively. In addition, substantial improvements in time to remission and percentage of treatment failures (secondary parameters) also were observed in patients receiving the highest mesalamine dosage, when compared with placebo. CDAI reductions from baseline in patients receiving 1- or- 2 g daily dosages of mesalamine did not differ significantly from those receiving placebo. Location of the active disease was not associated with statistically different responses, although mean reductions of 93 points from baseline CDAI were observed in patients with ileitis receiving mesalamine 4 g daily compared with reductions of 2 points from baseline CDAI in those receiving placebo.

Investigators of this study conducted a second trial, very similar to the one described. In this 16-week randomized, double-blind, placebo-controlled study, patients with mildly to moderately active Crohn's disease were randomized to receive placebo or mesalamine (2 or 4 g daily) administered orally as extended-release capsules. Pooled analysis of the 2 trials in combination with data from another randomized, double-blind, placebo-controlled study in patients with mildly to moderately active Crohn's disease indicate that mesalamine, given in 4-g daily dosages, was associated with an 18-point greater reduction in CDAI than placebo, a difference that was not considered clinically important.

Results of several other placebo-controlled studies also failed to show an improved clinical response to oral mesalamine extended-release preparations when compared with placebo; however, in several of the studies, a lower dosage (e.g., 1 or 2 g daily) was used. Some clinicians state that high oral mesalamine dosages (exceeding 3 g daily) usually are needed for the treatment of Crohn's disease.

Substantial benefit of mesalamine versus placebo was observed in a small 16-week randomized, double-blind, placebo-controlled study in 38 adults with mildly to moderately active ileocolonic or colonic Crohn's disease (mean baseline CDAI of 231.7 or 204.8 in patients receiving mesalamine or placebo, respectively) who were randomized to receive oral mesalamine 400-mg delayed-release tablets (Asacol®; 20 patients) in a dosage of 800 mg 4 times daily or placebo (18 patients). Individuals were permitted to continue oral corticosteroids if they were receiving fixed dosages of the drugs (not exceeding 20 mg of prednisone daily or equivalent). Complete clinical response (defined as a reduction from baseline CDAI of 70 points or more and a final CDAI score of less than 150, assessed after 4, 8, and 16 weeks of treatment) was observed in 60 or 22% of patients receiving mesalamine or placebo, respectively. Partial clinical response (defined as a reduction from baseline CDAI of 70 points or more, and a final CDAI score of 150 or more, assessed after 4, 8, and 16 weeks of treatment) was observed in 15 or 0% of patients receiving mesalamine or placebo, respectively.

Conventional or more recently available corticosteroids appear to be more effective than mesalamine in the management of active Crohn's disease. Results of a comparator-drug (mesalamine versus budesonide) controlled study (patients having a median baseline CDAI score of 272) have shown that clinical improvement was substantially lower in adults receiving 2-g twice daily dosages of oral mesalamine delayed-release tablets than in those receiving 9-mg daily dosages of oral budesonide delayed-release capsules (45% for mesalamine versus 69% for budesonide). In addition to a higher clinical improvement rate, quality-of-life scores (e.g., anxiety, depressed mood, sense of well-being, self-control, general health, vitality) also were improved to a greater extent in patients receiving budesonide than in those receiving mesalamine.

Rectal administration of mesalamine has been effective in a limited number of patients for the management of active Crohn's disease, but the role of such therapy in this condition is not as well defined as in the management of ulcerative colitis. In addition, rectal mesalamine appears to be less effective in reducing signs and symptoms of Crohn's disease than those of ulcerative colitis. Efficacy in patients with ileitis alone has not been established, but many clinicians suggest that the limited delivery of rectally administered drug to the ileum makes it unlikely that substantial clinical benefit would be achieved in such patients.

Maintenance of Remission Crohn's Disease. The relative efficacy of mesalamine as maintenance therapy for Crohn's disease is controversial, since the drug has been used with equivocal results. Some clinicians state that oral mesalamine may be the optimal treatment in patients with ileal or jejunoileal disease; however, the drug is associated with substantially lower efficacy in those with colonic disease. Several controlled studies indicate that use of oral mesalamine in the management of inactive ileitis is associated with a substantially lower frequency of relapse than placebo. In one double-blind placebo-controlled trial, oral mesalamine extended-release capsules (2 g daily) reduced frequency of relapse only in those patients who were in remission for less than 3 months at initiation of therapy; average remission rates at 2 years of therapy were 45 or 29% in patients receiving oral mesalamine or placebo, respectively. In addition, results of a double-blind, placebo-controlled trial in 125 patients in remission (CDAI score of less than 150) indicate that oral mesalamine delayed-release tablets (2.4 g daily) did not substantially reduce the frequency of relapse at 3 or 6 months; relapse (defined as CDAI score of greater than 150) rates at 3 months of therapy were 12 or 22%, respectively, in patients receiving oral mesalamine or placebo, while such rates at 6 months of therapy were 28 or 41%, respectively. However, relapse rates in patients receiving mesalamine (34%) or placebo (55%) were significantly different at 12 months of therapy.

Efficacy of controlled- or delayed-release oral mesalamine has been evaluated in several placebo-controlled trials in patients achieving remission following medical or surgical therapy. While in some of these studies in patients with medically or surgically induced remission, fewer relapses were reported with mesalamine than with placebo, in others, no statistically significant differences were found when the drug was compared with placebo. Results of a pooled analysis in patients receiving mesalamine to reduce postoperative recurrence of Crohn's disease have indicated that in 4 out of 7 studies, administration of oral mesalamine (compared with no therapy) was beneficial in reducing endoscopic or clinical recurrence, while in 2 other studies, a statistically non-significant trend in favor of therapy was shown. Results of another pooled analysis using oral mesalamine indicate that following surgically induced remission, clinical recurrence may be substantially reduced in patients with ileal disease or in those with prolonged disease duration. However, the overall effect usually was modest and further study is needed to evaluate the role of the drug in maintenance therapy of Crohn's disease.

Dosage and Administration

■ **Administration** Mesalamine is administered orally as delayed-release tablets and as extended-release capsules. Mesalamine is administered rectally as a retention enema or suppositories.

Oral Administration Mesalamine delayed-release tablets should be swallowed whole without breaking the outer coating, since the coating is designed to maintain the integrity of the tablets prior to entering the colon, where the drug is released. In clinical trials using mesalamine 400-mg delayed-release tablets (Asacol®), about 2–3% of patients noticed intact or partially intact tablets in their stools; if this occurs repeatedly, patients should notify their clinician.

The manufacturer of mesalamine 1.2-g delayed-release tablets (Lialda®) states that the tablets should be taken with food.

Rectal Administration Mesalamine suppositories are administered rectally. A small amount of lubricating gel may be applied onto the tip of the suppository to assist insertion. The suppository should be inserted completely into the rectum with gentle pressure, pointed end first, and should be retained for 1–3 hours or longer, if possible, to achieve maximum benefit.

Mesalamine suspension is administered rectally as a retention enema, preferably at bedtime. Best results are achieved if the bowel is emptied just prior to enema administration. Mesalamine rectal suspension must be shaken well and the protective sheath removed from the applicator before administration. Lubrication of the applicator tip may facilitate insertion and minimize the risk of local trauma.

The patient should be given a copy of the mesalamine administration instructions provided by the manufacturer. To administer the enema, the patient should first lie on their left side with the lower leg extended and the upper right leg flexed forward for balance during and for 30 minutes after administration of the retention enema so that the drug will distribute throughout the sigmoid colon; the enema should be retained for approximately 8 hours, usually during sleeping. Alternatively, the patient may assume the "knee-chest" position, kneeling with their upper chest and one arm resting on a bed. The bottle should be held at its neck to avoid premature discharge of the suspension and the applicator tip inserted gently into the rectum, pointing the tip slightly toward the umbilicus. The bottle then should be grasped firmly and tilted slightly so that the nozzle is aimed toward the patient's back. A steady squeezing of the bottle will discharge most of the suspension. Following rectal instillation of the enema, the bottle should be withdrawn from the rectum and discarded. The rectal suspension and suppositories will cause staining of direct contact surfaces, including, but not limited to, fabrics, flooring, painted surfaces, marble, granite, vinyl, and enamel. Therefore, patients are advised to carefully choose a suitable location for administration of the rectal suspension.

■ **Dosage** ***Oral Dosage*** **Ulcerative Colitis.** For the management of mildly to moderately active ulcerative colitis, the usual adult oral dosage of mesalamine delayed-release tablets (Asacol®) is 2.4 g daily (given as two 400-mg tablets 3 times daily) for 6 weeks. Mesalamine delayed-release tablets also have been administered in dosages up to 4.8 g daily† (in divided doses). For the treatment and induction of remission of mildly to moderately active ulcerative colitis, the usual adult oral dosage of mesalamine extended-release capsules is 4 g daily, given in equally divided doses (as four 250-mg extended-release capsules or two 500-mg extended-release capsules) 4 times daily; treatment duration in controlled clinical trials was up to 8 weeks. Mesalamine extended-release capsules also have been administered in lower dosages (e.g., 2–4 g daily [in divided doses])†.

For induction of remission in patients with mildly to moderately active ulcerative colitis, the recommended adult oral dosage of mesalamine 1.2-g delayed-release tablets (Lialda®) is 2.4 or 4.8 g daily (given as two or four 1.2-g tablets once daily). Safety and efficacy beyond 8 weeks of treatment have not been established.

For maintenance of remission of ulcerative colitis, the recommended adult oral dosage of mesalamine delayed-release tablets (Asacol®) is 1.6 g daily (four 400-mg delayed-release tablets) given in divided doses; treatment duration in the prospective, well-controlled trial was 6 months. For maintenance of remission, mesalamine delayed-release tablets also have been given in dosages of 800 mg to 4.8 g (in divided doses). In addition, mesalamine extended-release capsules (1.5–3 g) have been used for maintenance of remission. Patients should be advised that ulcerative colitis rarely remits completely, and that continued use of maintenance dosages of mesalamine may substantially decrease the risk of relapse.

Crohn's Disease. For the treatment of mildly to moderately active Crohn's disease† in adults, oral mesalamine dosages of 3.2–4.8 g daily (as delayed-release tablets) or 4 g daily (as extended-release capsules) have been given, generally in divided doses. Lower dosages do not appear to be effective. For maintenance of remission of Crohn's disease† in adults, oral mesalamine dosages of 800 mg to 4.8 g daily (as delayed-release tablets) or 1.5– 3 g daily (as extended-release capsules) in divided doses have been given.

Rectal Dosage **Distal Ulcerative Colitis.** The usual adult rectal dosage of mesalamine as suppositories is 1 g once daily at bedtime (using 1-g suppositories) and as the enema suspension is 4 g once daily (preferably at bedtime). Although clinical response may be apparent within 3–21 days, therapy with the drug usually is continued for 3–6 weeks or until clinical and/or sigmoidoscopic remission is achieved. Efficacy of mesalamine therapy (in terms of modification of relapse rates) beyond 6 weeks has not been established, but the drug has been used rectally for prolonged periods (e.g., longer than 1 year) in some patients.

There is some evidence that lower dosages or less frequent administration of rectal mesalamine may be effective in some patients†, particularly after initial remission is achieved. In a limited number of adults with distal ulcerative colitis in whom clinical remission occurred following daily administration of 4 g of mesalamine rectal suspension, dosage of mesalamine was reduced to 4 g every 2 or 3 nights or, occasionally, less frequently. If clinical relapse occurred with this less frequent administration, dosage was increased to more frequent administration. In a limited number of adults with distal ulcerative colitis or ulcerative proctosigmoiditis, mesalamine rectal suspension also has been used effectively in dosages of 1–3 g daily. Further long-term studies are needed to evaluate the optimal maintenance dosage of mesalamine rectal suspension.

Cautions

Frequency of some adverse effects associated with oral or rectal mesalamine generally appears to be less than that associated with oral sulfasalazine (a prodrug of mesalamine). Some adverse effects (e.g., hematologic effects, nervous system effects, hypersensitivity reactions, fever, male infertility) associated with sulfasalazine have been attributed to sulfapyridine, another metabolite of sulfasalazine, rather than to mesalamine.

Oral and rectal mesalamine preparations usually are well tolerated. The most common adverse effects of oral or rectal mesalamine are GI effects and headache. In clinical studies, most adverse effects associated with oral or rectal preparations were mild in severity and were transient or reversible. However, adverse effects have been severe enough to require discontinuance of the drug in less than 1% or in up to about 4–5% of patients receiving rectal or oral mesalamine, respectively, although in some studies, the rate of discontinuance of the drug was similar to or less than in those receiving placebo. Most of the adverse effects reported with the use of oral mesalamine 400-mg delayed-release tablets (Asacol®) were similar in short- and long-term studies.

■ GI Effects In controlled clinical trials in patients receiving oral mesalamine 400-mg delayed-release tablets (Asacol®), abdominal pain, eructation, nausea, diarrhea, dyspepsia, vomiting, constipation, flatulence, exacerbation of colitis, abdominal enlargement, gastroenteritis, GI hemorrhage, rectal disorder (e.g., hemorrhage, tenesmus), and stool abnormalities, were the most common adverse GI effects, occurring in about 2–18% of patients; dry mouth, indigestion, stomatitis, and cramping were reported rarely. Frequency of these GI effects did not seem to increase with increased dosages, although in uncontrolled studies, the incidence of abdominal pain, flatulence, and GI bleeding were dose related. In patients receiving oral mesalamine 1.2-g delayed-release tablets (Lialda®), flatulence was reported in about 3–4% of patients. The most common adverse GI effects of oral mesalamine extended-released capsules were diarrhea (including melena), nausea, abdominal pain, dyspepsia, vomiting, anorexia, worsening of ulcerative colitis, and rectal urgency, occurring in greater than 0.4–3% of patients.

Exacerbation of colitis symptoms was reported in 3% of patients receiving oral mesalamine 400-mg delayed-release tablets (Asacol®). Exacerbation of colitis symptoms resulting in discontinuance of therapy was reported in 0.8% of patients receiving oral mesalamine 1.2-g delayed-release tablets (Lialda®). Other adverse GI effects associated with oral mesalamine 1.2-g delayed-release tablets and occurring in less than 1% of patients include abdominal distention, diarrhea, pancreatitis, rectal polyp, and vomiting. Other adverse GI effects associated with oral mesalamine extended-release capsules and occurring in less than 1% of patients include abdominal distention, constipation, duodenal ulcer, dysphagia, eructation, esophageal or mouth ulcer, fecal incontinence, GI bleeding (e.g., rectal bleeding), stool abnormalities (e.g., change in color or texture), oral moniliasis, and thirst, although a causal relationship to the drug of many of these adverse effects has not been established.

Abdominal pain, cramps, and/or discomfort are the most common adverse GI effects of rectal mesalamine, occurring in about 4–8% of patients, and occasionally have occurred as components of an acute intolerance syndrome. (See Cautions: Sensitivity Reactions.) Flatulence and nausea occur in about 1–6% of patients receiving the drug rectally, and worsening or development of diarrhea, colitis, constipation, hemorrhoids, and rectal pain, burning, and/or soreness occur in about 1–3% of patients. Difficulty in retaining the enema occurs occasionally in patients receiving mesalamine rectal suspension, but retention time may increase during continued use of the drug. Pain on insertion of the enema applicator tip and anal irritation occur in about 1% of patients receiving mesalamine rectal suspension. Anal irritation may be severe enough to require topical analgesic or anti-inflammatory therapy. Anal fissures or lacerations following insertion of the enema applicator tip also have been reported rarely. Lubrication of the applicator tip may minimize these effects. In some patients receiving rectal mesalamine, inflammation has extended to the entire colon (pancolitis); however, extension of inflammation occurs in about 5–10% of patients as part of the natural progression of the disease, and a causal relationship to the drug has not been established. In addition, extension and/or acute exacerbations of inflammation reportedly occurred less frequently in patients receiving rectal mesalamine than placebo. Worsening of colitis or symptoms of inflammatory bowel disease (e.g., melena, hematochezia) may occur after initiation of mesalamine therapy.

Although previously it was suggested that sulfasalazine-induced pancreatitis resulted from the sulfonamide (sulfapyridine) component of the drug, current evidence suggests that 5-aminosalicylic acid (mesalamine) also may be responsible, at least in part, for the development of this adverse effect. The possibility of acute pancreatitis should be considered in any patient who develops new abdominal complaints while receiving mesalamine therapy. Acute pancreatitis has occurred rarely in patients receiving mesalamine or one of its prodrugs (e.g., olsalazine, sulfasalazine). Evidence of pancreatitis included severe upper abdominal pain (radiating to the back) and elevated serum amylase concentrations. In several of these patients, pancreatitis recurred upon rechallenge with mesalamine or one of its prodrugs. Increased serum lipase or amylase concentrations have been reported in less than 1% of patients, receiving mesalamine extended-release capsules; however, a causal relationship to the drug has not been established.

Other adverse GI effects associated with preparations containing or being metabolized to mesalamine and reported in clinical studies, medical literature, or postmarketing reports include anorexia, taste perversion, gastritis, increased appetite, perforated peptic ulcer, and bloody diarrhea.

■ Nervous System Effects Headache is the most common adverse nervous system effect of oral and rectal mesalamine, occurring in about 2–18 and 7% of patients, respectively. In controlled clinical trials in patients receiving oral mesalamine 400-mg delayed-release tablets (Asacol®), dizziness, asthenia, malaise, insomnia, anxiety, migraine, nervousness, paresthesia, and hypertonia were the most common adverse nervous system effects, occurring in about 2–8% of patients; lethargy, mild disorientation, and stuffy head were reported rarely. Frequency of these nervous system effects did not seem to increase with increased dosages, although in uncontrolled studies, the incidence of asthenia and fever were dose related. Adverse nervous system effects associated with oral mesalamine 1.2-g delayed-release tablets (Lialda®) and occurring in less than 1% of patients include asthenia, fatigue, somnolence, and tremor. Adverse nervous system effects associated with oral mesalamine extended-release capsules and occurring in less than 1% of patients include depression, dizziness, insomnia, somnolence, malaise, asthenia, and paresthesia, although a causal relationship to the drug of many of these adverse effects has not been established.

Fatigue, asthenia, malaise, and weakness occur in about 3% and dizziness in about 2–3% of patients receiving mesalamine rectally. Mental depression and insomnia have been reported rarely in patients receiving rectal mesalamine.

Other adverse nervous system effects associated with preparations containing or being metabolized to mesalamine and reported in clinical studies, medical literature, or postmarketing reports include depression, somnolence, emotional lability, hyperesthesia, vertigo, confusion, tremor, peripheral neuropathy, transverse myelitis, and Guillain-Barré syndrome.

■ Sensitivity Reactions An acute intolerance syndrome (sensitivity reaction), characterized by cramping, abdominal pain, bloody diarrhea, and, occasionally, fever, headache, malaise, conjunctivitis, pruritus, and rash, has occurred in a few patients receiving mesalamine and required prompt discontinuance of the drug. In patients manifesting such intolerance, a history of sulfasalazine intolerance, if any, should be reevaluated. In at least one sulfasalazine-sensitive patient, administration of mesalamine produced headache, fever, intense abdominal colic, and profuse diarrhea within 8–24 hours after administration of the drug; oral corticosteroid and rectal cromolyn therapy was ineffective, and colectomy was required 2 weeks after rechallenge with mesalamine. Intolerance to mesalamine, which occasionally required corticosteroid therapy, also has occurred in several other sulfasalazine-sensitive patients, although most sulfasalazine-sensitive patients reportedly tolerated mesalamine well. Nonetheless, mesalamine therapy should be initiated cautiously in patients with a history of sulfasalazine sensitivity, and patients should be advised to discontinue mesalamine and contact their clinician if signs of sensitivity (e.g., fever, rash) develop or increased diarrhea or rectal bleeding occurs during mesalamine therapy. In addition, some clinicians recommend challenge with 1 or 2 test enemas before a complete course of rectal mesalamine therapy is initiated in patients with sulfasalazine sensitivity. In patients with mesalamine sensitivity, rechallenge with the drug should be undertaken only if mesalamine therapy is clearly needed and under close supervision. Reduced dosage should be considered for such rechallenge.

Photosensitivity has been reported in less than 1% of patients receiving oral mesalamine extended-release capsules; however, a causal relationship to the drug has not been definitely established. Stevens-Johnson syndrome, manifested by buccal ulceration and fever, has occurred rarely in patients receiving rectal mesalamine.

■ Dermatologic Effects Rash, pruritus, and acne have been reported in less than 1 to about 6% of patients receiving mesalamine. (See Cautions: Sensitivity Reactions.) Alopecia has been reported in up to about 1% of patients receiving oral mesalamine 1.2-g delayed-release tablets (Lialda®). Other dermatologic effects associated with oral mesalamine 1.2-g delayed-release tablets and occurring in less than 1% of patients include prurigo and urticaria. Other dermatologic effects associated with oral mesalamine extended-release capsules and occurring in less than 1% of patients include alopecia, dry skin, eczema, lichen planus, erythema nodosum, nail disorder, and urticaria, although a causal relationship to the drug of many of these adverse effects has not been established.

Alopecia has been reported in about 1% of patients receiving mesalamine rectal suspension. Alopecia usually is mild, being characterized as accelerated or excessive hair loss such as observably more hair in a comb, and usually is reversible following discontinuance of the drug. The manufacturer of rectal mesalamine preparations states that alopecia may not recur following reinstitution of mesalamine therapy and some clinicians have postulated that alopecia may result from flare-up of the disease rather than from the drug itself. Alopecia also has been reported in patients receiving sulfasalazine.

Other adverse dermatologic effects associated with preparations containing or being metabolized to mesalamine and reported in clinical studies, medical literature, or postmarketing reports include psoriasis and pyoderma gangrenosum.

■ Renal and Genitourinary Effects Mesalamine may adversely affect renal function.

In preclinical studies in animals, nephrotoxicity was the major adverse effect observed with oral or parenteral mesalamine and appeared to be dose related. Studies in rats, mice, and dogs receiving single oral mesalamine doses exceeding 900 mg/kg or single IV doses exceeding 214 mg/kg have revealed evidence of renal lesions (e.g., medullary and focal cortical lesions, papillary necrosis). In addition, renal lesions (e.g., granular and hyaline casts, tubular degeneration, tubular dilation, renal infarct, papillary necrosis, tubular necrosis, interstitial nephritis) have been reported in mice or rats receiving oral mesalamine dosages of 2400 or 1150 mg/kg daily, respectively. In cynomolgus monkeys receiving oral mesalamine dosages of 250 mg/kg daily, nephrosis, papillary edema, and interstitial fibrosis have been observed. It has been postulated that mesalamine-induced renal toxicity may be similar to analgesic nephropathy observed after chronic ingestion of large dosages of analgesics (e.g., aspirin), since these analgesics are structurally similar to mesalamine. Following single oral doses of 200 mg/kg in rats and dogs, no changes in urinary flow, specific gravity, or electrolyte excretion were observed; however, at higher doses (i.e., 600 mg/kg), increases in urinary sodium and protein excretion and in specific gravity were observed. Dose-related renal lesions were observed in male but not female rats and in dogs receiving oral mesalamine dosages of 160 mg/kg daily. Reversible, minimal tubular epithelial damage was observed in male rats receiving dosages of 40 mg/kg daily; however, no evidence of adverse renal effects was seen in dogs receiving such dosages for 6 months. Following oral mesalamine dosages of 640 mg/kg daily for 13 weeks in rats and dogs, death, probably secondary to renal failure, occurred; dose-related renal lesions (e.g., papillary necrosis and/or multifocal tubular injury) also were observed. In a combined 52-week toxicity and 127-week carcinogenicity study in rats receiving daily mesalamine dosages of 100-mg/kg and above, degeneration of kidneys was observed at 52 weeks, while at 127 weeks, increased incidence of kidney degeneration and hyalinization of basement membranes of Bowman's capsule was reported.

Renal impairment (e. g., minimal change nephropathy, acute and chronic interstitial nephritis, and, rarely, renal failure) and increases in blood urea nitrogen (BUN) and serum creatinine concentrations have been reported in patients receiving oral preparations containing or being metabolized to mesalamine. Nephrotoxicity also has occurred in patients receiving oral sulfasalazine. Adverse genitourinary effects associated with preparations containing or being metabolized to mesalamine and reported in clinical studies, medical literature, or postmarketing reports include dysuria, albuminuria, urinary urgency, hematuria, epididymitis, decreased libido, amenorrhea, dysmenorrhea, menorrhagia, and hypomenorrhea.

Rectal mesalamine has not been associated with overt adverse renal effects in humans to date. Although the limited systemic absorption of rectally administered mesalamine suggests that the potential for inducing nephrotoxicity by this route of administration is low, the possibility that adverse renal effects may occur in patients receiving rectal mesalamine must be considered. Urinary tract infection and/or urinary burning have been reported in less than 1% of patients receiving mesalamine rectal suspension.

■ Cardiovascular Effects In controlled clinical trials, chest pain and peripheral edema were reported in 3% of patients receiving oral mesalamine 400-mg delayed-release tablets (Asacol®). Tachycardia, hypertension, and hypotension were reported in less than 1% of patients receiving oral mesalamine 1.2-g delayed-release tablets (Lialda®). Palpitations and vasodilation were reported in less than 1% of patients receiving oral mesalamine extended-release capsules; however, a causal relationship to the drug of these adverse effects has not been established. Myocarditis, pericarditis, and facial edema have been reported in patients receiving preparations containing or being metabolized to mesalamine.

Peripheral or generalized edema has been reported in about 1% of patients receiving the drug rectally. Pericarditis, manifested as chest pain, fever, and/or dyspnea, has occurred rarely in patients receiving rectal mesalamine. Evidence of pericarditis occurred within several days to weeks after initiation of rectal mesalamine therapy and resolved following discontinuance of the drug. In most patients, pericarditis recurred with mesalamine or olsalazine rechallenge. However, the risk of cross-sensitivity with sulfasalazine or other 5-aminosalicylic acid (mesalamine) prodrugs (e.g., olsalazine) currently is not known. Other evidence of pericarditis included pericardial friction rub, radiographic evidence of pleural effusion and/or cardiac enlargement with possible tamponade, echocardiographic evidence of pericardial effusion, and/or ECG abnormalities (e.g., ST- and T-wave changes and inferior Q waves suggestive of myocardial infarction, ST-segment depression). Although there appears to be an association between mesalamine use and the development of pericarditis in these patients, the mechanism is unknown and pericarditis also has been reported in patients with inflammatory bowel disease who were not receiving mesalamine. In some of these latter patients, pericarditis developed during sulfasalazine therapy and therefore, may have been secondary to the drug rather than to the underlying condition. The possibility of pericarditis should be considered in any patient who develops chest pain or dyspnea during mesalamine therapy. Discontinuance of therapy with the drug may be warranted in some such patients, while mesalamine rechallenge may be performed under careful clinical observation if there is a continued therapeutic need for the drug.

Because mesalamine prodrugs have been used safely (i.e., without exacerbating preexisting pericarditis) and effectively in patients with inflammatory bowel disease and preexisting pericarditis, use of mesalamine or its prodrugs in such patients in whom the development of pericarditis was not previously associated with the drugs is *not* contraindicated.

■ Hepatic Effects Adverse hepatic effects associated with oral mesalamine extended-release capsules (and with other mesalamine-containing preparations) and occurring in less than 1% of patients include increased serum concentrations of AST (SGOT), ALT (SGPT), alkaline phosphatase, γ-glutamyltransferase (GGT, γ-glutamyltranspeptidase, GGTP), LDH, and amylase, although a causal relationship to the drug of many of these adverse effects has not been established. Increased serum bilirubin concentrations were reported in less than 1% of patients receiving oral mesalamine 1.2-g delayed-release tablets (Lialda®). Other adverse hepatic effects, some of them fatal, associated with preparations containing or being metabolized to mesalamine and reported in clinical studies, medical literature, or postmarketing reports include hepatotoxicity (e.g., jaundice [including cholestatic], hepatitis, cirrhosis, possible hepatocellular damage [liver necrosis, liver failure]), elevated serum bilirubin concentrations, cholecystitis, and (in at least one patient) Kawasaki-like disease (with changes in hepatic enzymes). Asymptomatic elevations of hepatic enzymes, which usually disappear with continued use or upon discontinuance of mesalamine, also have been reported.

■ Pulmonary and Respiratory Effects In controlled clinical trials in patients receiving oral mesalamine 400-mg delayed-release tablets (Asacol®), pharyngitis, rhinitis, increased cough, sinusitis, and bronchitis were reported in about 2–18% of patients. The frequency of these pulmonary and respiratory effects did not seem to increase with increasing dosages, although in uncontrolled studies, the incidence of rhinitis was dose related. Pharyngolaryngeal pain was reported in less than 1% of patients receiving oral mesalamine 1.2-g delayed-release tablets (Lialda®).

Upper respiratory infection has been reported in about 2% of patients receiving mesalamine rectally. Other adverse pulmonary and respiratory effects associated with preparations containing or being metabolized to mesalamine and reported in clinical studies, medical literature, or postmarketing reports include eosinophilic pneumonia, interstitial pneumonitis, fibrosing alveolitis, dyspnea, exacerbation of asthma, pulmonary infiltrates, and pleuritis.

■ Hematologic Effects Ecchymosis, thrombocythemia, and thrombocytopenia have been reported in less than 1% of patients receiving oral mesalamine extended-release capsules; however, a causal relationship to the drug of these adverse effects has not been established. Thrombocytopenia has been reported in less than 1% of patients receiving oral mesalamine 1.2-g delayed-release tablets (Lialda®). Adverse hematologic effects associated with preparations containing or being metabolized to mesalamine and reported in clinical studies, medical literature, or postmarketing reports include agranulocytosis, aplastic anemia, eosinophilia, leukopenia, anemia, and lymphadenopathy. In at least one patient receiving mesalamine rectal suppositories (500 mg every evening) for 7 months, leukopenia and thrombocytopenia occurred.

■ Musculoskeletal Effects In controlled clinical studies in patients receiving oral mesalamine 400-mg delayed-release tablets (Asacol®), back pain/lower back discomfort, arthralgia, myalgia, arthritis, and joint pain/disorder were reported in 2–5% of patients; muscle cramps occurred rarely. The frequency of these musculoskeletal effects did not seem to increase with increasing dosages, although in the uncontrolled studies the incidence of back pain and arthralgia were dose related. Arthralgia and back pain were reported in less than 1% of patients receiving oral mesalamine 1.2-g delayed-release tablets (Lialda®). Arthralgia, myalgia, and leg cramps were reported in less than 1% of patients receiving oral mesalamine extended-release capsules; however, a causal relationship to the drug of some of these adverse effects has not been established.

Leg or joint pain and/or stiffness has been reported in about 2% of patients receiving the drug rectally. Other musculoskeletal adverse effects associated with preparations containing or being metabolized to mesalamine and reported in clinical studies, medical literature, or postmarketing reports include neck pain and gout.

■ Ocular and Otic Effects In controlled clinical studies in patients receiving oral mesalamine 400-mg delayed-release tablets (Asacol®), otic disorder and otic pain were reported in 2% or more of patients; plugged ears were reported rarely. Otic pain was reported in less than 1% of patients receiving oral mesalamine 1.2-g delayed-release tablets (Lialda®). Conjunctivitis was reported in less than 1% of patients receiving oral mesalamine extended-release capsules; however, a causal relationship to the drug has not been established.

Adverse ocular and otic effects associated with preparations containing or being metabolized to mesalamine and reported in clinical studies, medical literature, or postmarketing reports include eye pain, blurred vision, and tinnitus. Keratoconjunctivitis sicca was reported in animals following oral administration of mesalamine; however, this ocular effect has not been reported in humans to date.

■ Other Adverse Effects In controlled clinical trials in patients receiving oral mesalamine 400-mg delayed-release tablets (Asacol®), pain/aching and fever were reported in 14 and 6% of patients, respectively; flu syndrome, chills, and sweating occurred in 3% of patients. The frequency of these adverse effects did not seem to increase with increasing dosages, although in uncontrolled studies, the incidence of flu syndrome, fever, and pain were dose related. Pyrexia was reported in less than 1% of patients receiving oral mesalamine 1.2-g delayed-release tablets (Lialda®).

Fever has been reported in about 1–3% of patients receiving rectal mesalamine. Fever also has been reported as a component of an acute mesalamine intolerance syndrome. (See Cautions: Sensitivity Reactions.) At least one patient died after receiving mesalamine rectal suspension, but a causal relationship to the drug has not been established.

■ **Precautions and Contraindications** Because mesalamine has been associated with adverse renal effects (see Cautions: Renal Effects),the drug should be used with caution in patients with renal impairment and only if the benefits outweigh the risks. Renal function should be evaluated in all patients prior to initiation of therapy with mesalamine and periodically thereafter. Although the potential for adverse mesalamine-induced renal effects appears to be low following rectal administration, the possibility of such effects occurring in patients receiving the drug should be considered, particularly when increased GI absorption or decreased renal elimination of the drug is possible or when a nonsteroidal anti-inflammatory agent or an oral preparation containing or metabolized to mesalamine is administered concomitantly. The manufacturers state that renal function should be monitored carefully during mesalamine therapy (especially during the initial phase of treatment, in patients with preexisting renal impairment, or in those receiving concomitant therapy with drugs that are a source of mesalamine [e.g., sulfasalazine]). Mesalamine-induced nephrotoxicity should be suspected in patients who develop renal dysfunction during treatment.

The possibility of extension and/or acute exacerbation of colitis occurring during mesalamine therapy should be considered. (See Cautions: GI Effects.)

Mesalamine therapy should be initiated with caution in patients with conditions predisposing them to the development of myocarditis or pericarditis. The possibility of pericarditis should be considered in any patient who develops chest pain or dyspnea during mesalamine therapy. (See Cautions: Cardiovascular Effects.)

Mesalamine therapy should be initiated with caution in patients with sulfasalazine sensitivity, although cross-sensitivity to mesalamine rectal suspension appears to be low. These patients should be instructed to discontinue mesalamine therapy and contact their clinician if signs of sensitivity (e.g., rash, fever) develop or increased diarrhea or rectal bleeding occur. The possibility that acute intolerance (sensitivity reaction) to mesalamine could occur in any patient receiving the drug should be considered. (See Cautions: Sensitivity Reactions.) Some clinicians also state that mesalamine, like other inhibitors of prostaglandin synthesis, should be used with caution in patients with aspirin sensitivity, although the risk of cross-sensitivity with mesalamine is not known.

Mesalamine should be used with caution in patients with hepatic impairment.

The possibility of acute pancreatitis should be considered in any patient who develops new abdominal complaints while receiving mesalamine therapy. (See Cautions: GI Effects.)

Patients with pyloric stenosis may experience prolonged gastric retention of oral mesalamine delayed-release tablets resulting in delayed release of the drug in the colon.

Mesalamine rectal suspension contains potassium metabisulfite, a sulfite that may cause allergic-type reactions, including anaphylaxis and life-threatening or less severe asthmatic episodes, in certain susceptible individuals. The overall prevalence of sulfite sensitivity in the general population is unknown but probably low; such sensitivity appears to occur more frequently in asthmatic than in nonasthmatic individuals. If a severe hypersensitivity reaction occurs during therapy with mesalamine rectal suspension, the drug should be discontinued and the patient given appropriate treatment (e.g., epinephrine). The presence of sulfites in the parenteral epinephrine preparation and the possibility of allergic-type reactions should *not* deter use of epinephrine when indicated for the treatment of serious allergic reactions or for other emergency situations. Epinephrine is the preferred treatment for such conditions, and currently available alternatives to epinephrine may not be optimally effective. Preparations containing mesalamine are contraindicated in patients with known hypersensitivity to the drug or any ingredient in the respective formulation. The manufacturers of oral mesalamine extended-release capsules (Pentasa®), oral mesalamine 1.2-g delayed-release tablets (Lialda®), and mesalamine rectal suppositories (Canasa®) state that the drug is contraindicated in patients with hypersensitivity to salicylates (including aspirin and mesalamine).

■ **Pediatric Precautions** Safety and efficacy of oral delayed-release tablets, oral extended-release capsules, rectal suspensions, and rectal suppositories of mesalamine in pediatric patients have not been established.

Mesalamine (oral delayed-release tablets given as an initial dosage of 20–30 mg/kg daily and increased up to 60 mg/kg daily) has been used in a limited number of pediatric patients† with inflammatory bowel disease (i.e., mild ileal, ileocecal, ileocolonic, or colonic disease) while rectal mesalamine suspension has been used in those with left-sided colitis. Limited data from a retrospective comparative study indicate that efficacy in maintaining remission of inflammatory bowel disease is similar in children receiving oral mesalamine delayed-release tablets compared with those receiving oral sulfasalazine. However, some patients may prefer mesalamine to sulfasalazine, because of ease and frequency of administration and better tolerance.

■ **Geriatric Precautions** Clinical studies of oral mesalamine delayed-release tablets and rectal suppositories of the drug did not include sufficient numbers of patients 65 years of age and older to determine whether geriatric patients respond differently than younger patients. While other clinical experience has not revealed differences in response, drug dosage should be selected cautiously in geriatric patients. The greater frequency of decreased hepatic, renal, and/or cardiac function and of concomitant disease and drug therapy observed in the elderly also should be considered. Reports from uncontrolled studies suggest that a higher incidence of blood dyscrasias (i.e., agranulocytosis, neutropenia, pancytopenia) may occur in patients 65 years of age or older receiving oral mesalamine delayed-release tablets; complete blood cell counts (CBCs) should be monitored closely in these patients during therapy with these oral preparations.

Mesalamine is substantially eliminated by the kidneys, and the risk of toxic reactions may be greater in patients with impaired renal function. Because of the greater frequency of decreased renal function observed in geriatric individuals, mesalamine should be used with caution in these patients and renal function monitored prior initiation of and during administration of oral mesalamine delayed-release tablets.

■ **Mutagenicity and Carcinogenicity** Mesalamine did not produce mutagenic activity in the Ames mutagen test using *Salmonella typhimurium*, in mouse lymphoma cells, or in in vitro chromosomal aberrations in Chinese hamster ovary cells. In addition, there was no evidence of mutagenicity of forward mutation test or reverse mutations in an in vitro test system using an *Escherichia coli* strain, and there was no evidence of adverse chromosomal effects in an in vivo micronucleus test in mice receiving single oral doses of mesalamine up to 600 mg/kg or in an in vivo sister chromatid exchange test in mice receiving single oral doses up to 610 mg/kg.

When compared with controls, an increased incidence of neoplastic lesions was not observed in a 2-year carcinogenicity study in rats receiving oral mesalamine dosages of up to 320 mg/kg daily. In addition, no carcinogenic or tumorigenic potential was seen in mice or rats receiving mesalamine in dosages up to 2500 or up to 800 mg/kg daily, respectively, for up to 2 years.

■ **Pregnancy, Fertility, and Lactation** Reproduction studies in rats and rabbits using oral mesalamine dosages of up to 1000 mg/kg daily and up to 800 mg/kg daily, respectively, have not revealed evidence of teratogenic effects or harm to the fetus. In addition, reproduction studies in rats and rabbits using oral mesalamine daily doses up to 5 and 8 times the maximum recommended human rectal dose, respectively, have not revealed evidence of fetal malformation. Sulfasalazine (a prodrug of mesalamine) has been used for the treatment of inflammatory bowel disease, including Crohn's disease and ulcerative colitis, during pregnancy. Although fetal abnormalities have been reported in infants born to women with inflammatory bowel disease who received sulfasalazine alone or combined with corticosteroids during pregnancy, most evidence indicates that sulfasalazine is not associated with a substantial risk of teratogenicity. The effect of sulfasalazine on subsequent growth, development, and functional maturation in children whose mothers received sulfasalazine during pregnancy has not been determined. Although the relevance to mesalamine of the experience with sulfasalazine in pregnant women currently is not known, placental transfer of mesalamine, but not sulfasalazine or sulfapyridine, has been reported to be negligible in pregnant women receiving oral sulfasalazine. Mesalamine crosses the placental barrier. Because there are no adequate and controlled studies to date using mesalamine or sulfasalazine in pregnant women, and animal studies are not always predictive of human response, the drugs should be used during pregnancy only when clearly needed.

Reproduction studies in rats receiving oral mesalamine dosages up to 320–480 mg/kg daily have not revealed evidence of impaired fertility and/or reproductive performance. Oligospermia, abnormal sperm forms, impaired sperm motility, and infertility have occurred in men receiving sulfasalazine; however, these effects on sperm maturation appear to be caused by effects of sulfapyridine rather than mesalamine and appear to be reversible following discontinuance of sulfasalazine. Evidence of infertility has been reported very rarely following administration of rectal mesalamine, and sulfasalazine-induced infertility has resolved and not recurred in some males in whom mesalamine replaced sulfasalazine. In addition, there is evidence from comparative studies in animals that sulfapyridine rather than mesalamine is responsible for sulfasalazine-induced effects on male fertility.

Following oral administration, low concentrations of mesalamine and higher concentrations of its *N*-acetyl metabolite have been detected in human breast milk. Although the clinical importance of this effect is not known, mesalamine should be used with caution and only if the benefits outweigh the risks in nursing women. The manufacturer of mesalamine extended-release capsules states that hypersensitivity reactions (e.g., diarrhea) in the infant of a breast-feeding woman receiving mesalamine cannot be excluded. The manufacturer of mesalamine rectal suspension recommends that the drug not be used in nursing women.

Drug Interactions

■ **Azathioprine** Use of mesalamine in patients receiving azathioprine may increase the risk of hematologic toxicity.

■ **Digoxin** Sulfasalazine and aminosalicylic acid (the 4-amino [para-amino] derivative of salicylic acid) may decrease GI absorption of digoxin, possibly by altering properties of the intestinal wall. In vitro, sulfasalazine did not appear to adsorb digoxin. After 2 weeks of concomitant oral administration of sulfasalazine or aminosalicylic acid with digoxin, absorption of digoxin was reduced 25 or 20%, respectively. It is not known whether concomitant administration of mesalamine (5-aminosalicylic acid) and digoxin results in similar alterations in absorption of the cardiac glycoside.

■ **Mercaptopurine** Use of mesalamine in patients receiving mercaptopurine may increase the risk of hematologic toxicity.

■ **Nephrotoxic Drugs** Use of mesalamine in patients receiving other nephrotoxic drugs (e.g., nonsteroidal anti-inflammatory agents [NSAIAs]) may increase the risk of nephrotoxicity.

Acute Toxicity

■ **Pathogenesis** The oral LD_{50} of mesalamine is 3.2 and 5.5 g/kg in male and female rats, respectively. In dogs, oral administration of single 6-g doses of mesalamine delayed-release tablets resulted in nonfatal renal papillary necrosis. A high incidence of lethality was reported in mice, rats, and cynomolgus monkeys receiving single oral 5000-, 4595-, and 3000-mg/kg doses of uncoated mesalamine, respectively.

■ **Manifestations** Two cases of overdosage of mesalamine 400-mg delayed-release tablets (Asacol®) have been reported in children. In one case, a 3-year old boy ingested 2 g of mesalamine as the 400-mg delayed-release tablets; the patient was treated with ipecac and activated charcoal and experienced no adverse effects. In a second case, a 3-year old boy (weighing approximately 16 kg) ingested up to 24 g of mesalamine as the 400-mg delayed-release tablets crushed in solution (resulting in uncoated drug); he was treated with orange juice and activated charcoal and no adverse effects were observed.

The manufacturers state that there have been no reported cases of overdosage with mesalamine controlled-release capsules or with mesalamine 1.2-g delayed-release tablets (Lialda®). Because mesalamine is an aminosalicylate, manifestations of overdosage likely would include symptoms of salicylate toxicity (e.g., tinnitus, vertigo, headache, confusion, drowsiness, sweating, hyperventilation, vomiting, diarrhea); severe intoxication may result in electrolyte imbalance, blood pH disorder, hyperthermia, and dehydration.

The manufacturers of mesalamine rectal suspension and suppositories state that there have been no documented cases of serious toxicity following acute overdosage of mesalamine. Because the drug is poorly absorbed following rectal administration, the likelihood of acute toxicity is low with this route of administration.

■ **Treatment** Since mesalamine is a derivative of salicylic acid, conventional therapy (e.g., induction of emesis and possible performance of gastric lavage to prevent further GI absorption of the drug, correction of fluid and electrolyte imbalance with appropriate IV therapy, maintenance of adequate renal function) for salicylate toxicity may be beneficial in case of overdosage of oral mesalamine preparations (e.g., extended-release capsules or delayed-release tablets). (See Acute Toxicity in the Salicylates General Statement 28:08.04.24.)

Pharmacology

■ **Anti-inflammatory Effect** Mesalamine exhibits anti-inflammatory activity in the GI tract. Due in part to the complexity of the inflammatory response, the exact mechanisms of the anti-inflammatory effect of mesalamine have not been fully elucidated, but it appears that several actions may contribute to the drug's activity in inflammatory bowel disease, and that they are local rather than systemic. Unlike salicylates, mesalamine is not metabolized to salicylic acid for pharmacologic activity.

Limited data have shown that the anti-inflammatory effect of mesalamine may be positively correlated with its ability to inhibit prostaglandin and leukotriene synthesis during inflammation; however, the relative contribution of these and other mechanisms of action remains to be determined. Although the role of arachidonic acid metabolites in the pathogenesis of inflammatory bowel disease has not been fully elucidated, mucosal production of these metabolites, both through the cyclooxygenase (e.g., prostaglandins) and the lipoxygenase pathways (e.g., leukotrienes, hydroxyeicosatetraenoic acids [HETEs]), appears to be increased in patients with inflammatory bowel disease. In patients with active ulcerative colitis, prostaglandin concentrations in feces, colorectal venous plasma, urine, and rectal biopsy specimens have been shown to be increased. Mesalamine may inhibit prostaglandin synthesis in the colon by inhibiting cyclooxygenase, an enzyme that catalyzes the formation of prostaglandin precursors (endoperoxides) from arachidonic acid. Since prostaglandins appear to mediate many inflammatory effects and have been shown to directly produce many signs and symptoms of inflammation, it has been suggested that the anti-inflammatory effect of mesalamine may be due in part to inhibition of prostaglandin synthesis and release during inflammation. However, because nonsteroidal anti-inflammatory agents (NSAIAs) such as flurbiprofen and indomethacin, which are more potent inhibitors of prostaglandin synthesis than is mesalamine, have not improved the clinical manifestations of inflammatory bowel disease despite decreasing prostaglandin concentrations, some clinicians have suggested that prostaglandins may not play an important role as mediators of inflammation in inflammatory bowel disease. Inhibition of prostaglandin synthesis also may reduce diarrhea and GI mucosal transport.

Mesalamine, unlike most NSAIAs, also inhibits leukotriene synthesis, possibly by inhibiting lipoxygenase, an enzyme that catalyzes the formation of leukotrienes and HETEs from arachidonic acid and its metabolites; however, steps in the pathway other than lipoxygenase activity may be affected by the drug. While it has been suggested that GI anti-inflammatory activity of mesalamine may depend principally on inhibition of the lipoxygenase pathway, the precise role of the leukotrienes remains to be more fully elucidated since benoxaprofen, a NSAIA that inhibits this pathway, has lacked substantial activity in the management of inflammatory bowel disease. Mesalamine also appears to inhibit colonic mucosal sulfidopeptide leukotriene synthesis, which may contribute to GI anti-inflammatory activity. Mesalamine also may inhibit conversion of 12-hydroperoxyeicosateraenoic acid (12-HPTE) to 12-HETE and 5,12-di-HETE, which appear to be chemotactic stimuli for polymorphonuclear leukocytes, and the drug has been shown to inhibit migration of leukocytes into inflamed tissue.

Mesalamine may inhibit production of soluble mediators of inflammation from arachidonic acid, which appear to be produced by colonic epithelial cells and mononuclear inflammatory cells. The drug also inhibits accumulation of thromboxane A in rectal mucosa, and has been shown to inhibit superoxide formation, which may contribute to its anti-inflammatory effect. Mesalamine has been shown to inhibit the migration and superoxide production of polymorphonuclear leukocytes.

It also has been suggested that low concentrations of mesalamine may enhance prostacyclin formation, a prostaglandin that is believed to exhibit cytoprotective effects on GI mucosa; however, at mesalamine concentrations achieved with usual dosages, the drug reduces prostaglandin concentrations in patients with ulcerative colitis, suggesting that this proposed mechanism may not be important in the drug's GI anti-inflammatory activity. Other actions of mesalamine may include alteration in the secretion and absorption of fluids and electrolytes by the colon, immunosuppression, and/or alteration of the GI bacterial flora. Mesalamine also may inhibit the activation of NFκB, a nuclear transcription factor that regulates the transcription of many genes for proinflammatory proteins.

There is limited evidence that mesalamine also may exhibit anti-inflammatory activity in patients with Crohn's disease, but additional study is necessary.

■ **Hematologic Effects** Mesalamine does not appear to inhibit adenosine diphosphate- or epinephrine-induced platelet aggregation, nor does the drug appear to have any fibrinolytic activity. The low potency of mesalamine as a cyclooxygenase inhibitor might explain the lack of appreciable effect on platelet aggregation.

■ **Other Effects** In animals, mesalamine does not appear to exhibit antipyretic, analgesic, negative or positive inotropic, anticonvulsant, antispasmodic, serotonergic agonist, or antitremor activity. The drug also does not appear to affect spontaneous motor activity or hexobarbital-induced sleeping time, and has no effect on blood pressure, heart rate, or breathing.

Pharmacokinetics

■ **Absorption** Following oral administration of conventional capsules or uncoated tablets of mesalamine, the drug is absorbed extensively from the proximal part of the GI tract. Therefore, to achieve a local effect in lower portions of the GI tract, oral mesalamine is administered as delayed-release tablets or extended-release capsules.

Following oral administration of the 400-mg delayed-release tablets (Asacol®), approximately 28% of mesalamine is absorbed and the remainder of the dose is available for topical activity and fecal excretion; absorption is similar in fed and fasting individuals. Peak plasma mesalamine concentrations usually occur within 4–12 hours following oral administration of the 400-mg delayed-release tablets; however, there is a relatively large interindividual variation in the plasma concentrations of mesalamine and *N*-acetyl-5-aminosalicylic acid following administration of these tablets. Following oral administration of a single 2.4-g dose of delayed-release mesalamine in healthy adults, average peak serum mesalamine and *N*-acetyl-5-aminosalicylic acid concentrations of 1.27 and 2.3 mcg/mL, respectively, occurred within about 6 hours.

Mesalamine appears to be more extensively absorbed from the 400-mg delayed-release tablets than when released from sulfasalazine (a prodrug of mesalamine). Following multiple-dose administration of the 400-mg delayed-release tablets, peak plasma concentrations of mesalamine and *N*-acetyl-5-aminosalicylic acid usually are achieved within 4–12 hours and are about 1.5–2 times higher than those following the equivalent mesalamine dose contained in sulfasalazine.

Following oral administration of 1.2-g delayed-release tablets (Lialda®) to healthy individuals at a dosage of 2.4 or 4.8 g once daily for 14 days, approximately 21–22% of the mesalamine dose is absorbed. Following oral administration of a single 1.2-, 2.4-, or 4.8-g (as the 1.2-g delayed-release tablets) dose of mesalamine in fasting healthy adults, the drug is detectable in plasma after 2 hours, and peak plasma mesalamine concentrations occur at approximately 9–12 hours. Following oral administration of 1.2-g mesalamine delayed-release tablets, pharmacokinetics of the drug are highly variable. Peak plasma mesalamine concentrations of 857, 1595, and 2154 ng/mL were reported following oral administration of a single mesalamine dose of 1.2-, 2.4-, or 4.8-g (as 1.2-g delayed-release tablets), respectively, in healthy fasting individuals. When administered as 1.2-g delayed-release tablets, mesalamine exhibits slightly nonlinear pharmacokinetics over the dosage range of 1.2–4.8 g daily. Dose-proportional increases in peak plasma mesalamine concentrations were observed with oral administration of a single dose between 1.2 and 2.4 g of mesalamine and less-than-proportional increases reported with a single dose between 2.4 and 4.8 g, with the dose-normalized value at 4.8 g representing an average of 74% that at 2.4 g based on geometric mean calculations.

Following administration of a single 4.8-g dose of mesalamine (as the 1.2-g delayed-release tablets) with a high-fat meal, there is a delay in absorption compared with fasting administration, with detectable plasma concentrations occurring about 4 hours after administration. Administration of mesalamine 1.2-g delayed release tablets with a high-fat meal also results in increased systemic mesalamine exposure, with increases of 91 and 16% in peak plasma concentration and area under the concentration-time curve (AUC), respectively. Following administration of mesalamine in single or multiple doses of 2.4 or 4.8 g (as the 1.2-g delayed-release tablets) once daily with a meal to healthy individuals, plasma concentrations of mesalamine were detectable 4 hours after a single dose and reached a peak 8 hours after a single dose. Steady-state plasma concentrations generally were achieved within 2 days of multiple-dose administration. Mean AUC values at steady state following multiple-dose administration were about 1.1–1.4 times those predicted based on single-dose pharmacokinetics.

Following oral administration of extended-release capsules (Pentasa®), about 20–30% of the drug is absorbed. Peak plasma mesalamine and *N*-acetyl-5-aminosalicylic acid concentrations of 1 and 1.8 mcg/mL, respectively, usually are attained in about 3 hours following oral administration of a 1-g dose of extended-release capsules. When administered as oral extended-release capsules, mesalamine exhibits nonlinear pharmacokinetics (unlike *N*-acetyl-5-aminosalicylic acid that exhibits linear kinetics) over the dosage range of 1–4 g daily, with plasma mesalamine concentrations at steady state being about 9 times higher (increasing from 0.14 to 1.21 mcg/mL) than those after a single oral dose of the drug, suggesting that mesalamine undergoes saturable first-pass elimination.

Rectal mesalamine suspension is poorly absorbed from the GI tract following rectal administration. Approximately 15% (range: 5–35%) of a rectally administered dose is absorbed. There is considerable interindividual variation in the extent of absorption of mesalamine rectal suspension. Absorption may depend on retention time of the enema, pH, and/or volume of mesalamine rectal suspension and also on the patient's underlying GI disease state. Rectal mesalamine suspension usually is retained for about 3.5–12 hours after administration as an enema; prolonged retention may increase absorption of the drug. Mesalamine is variably absorbed following rectal administration of the suppositories. Following rectal administration of a 500-mg suppository every 8 hours for 6 days in patients with ulcerative colitis, mean peak plasma mesalamine and *N*-acetyl-5-aminosalicylic acid plasma concentrations are about 353 and 467–1399 ng/mL, respectively, after the initial dose, while mean peak steady-state plasma concentrations of mesalamine and *N*-acetyl-5-aminosalicylic acid are about 361 and 193–1304 ng/mL, respectively; the mean minimum steady-state plasma concentrations are of mesalamine 89 ng/mL. Following rectal administration, mesalamine does not appear to accumulate in plasma. Mesalamine rectal suppositories usually are retained for 1–3 hours after administration.

Absorption of mesalamine appears to be decreased and delayed at acidic compared with higher (e.g., neutral) pH. Absorption of the drug appears to be decreased substantially in patients with active inflammatory bowel disease, probably secondary to local inflammatory changes, and increased with increasing volumes of the rectal suspension in patients whose disease is in remission. Following rectal administration of a single 4-g dose of mesalamine suspension in adults with ulcerative colitis in remission or with active disease, peak total plasma mesalamine concentrations occur within 3–6 hours and average about 4 or 3 mcg/mL, respectively. Following rectal administration of a single 2- or 4-g dose of mesalamine in patients with ulcerative colitis, average peak plasma *N*-acetyl-5-aminosalicylic acid (the principal metabolite of mesalamine) concentrations of 2 or 2.5 mcg/mL, respectively, occur within 4–7 hours. When mesalamine is administered directly into the small intestine, systemic absorption is increased. Following jejunal administration of a single 150-mg dose of mesalamine in healthy adults, peak plasma mesalamine concentrations of 5.8 mcg/mL (range: 4.6–9.1 mcg/mL) occur within about 1 hour.

Steady-state plasma mesalamine and *N*-acetyl-5-aminosalicylic acid concentrations averaged 0.29 and 0.7 mcg/mL, respectively, in patients receiving rectal mesalamine dosages of 1 g daily for 10 days; appreciable accumulation of mesalamine or the acetylated metabolite does not appear to occur.

■ **Distribution** Distribution of mesalamine into human body tissues and fluids has not been fully characterized. Following oral or IV administration of mesalamine in animals, the drug may be distributed into kidneys. Following rectal administration of mesalamine suspension in adults, the drug distributes from the rectum into the colon, generally reaching the splenic flexure and possibly the ascending colon. Following rectal administration of mesalamine suppositories, the drug distributes to some extent in rectal tissues. The apparent volume of distribution (V_d) of the drug in adults is approximately 0.2 L/kg.

In vitro, mesalamine and *N*-acetyl-5-aminosalicylic acid are approximately 44–55 and 80% bound, respectively, to plasma proteins. Mesalamine is approximately 43% bound to plasma proteins at a concentration of 2.5 mcg/mL. Protein binding of *N*-acetyl-5-aminosalicylic acid does not appear to be concentration dependent at concentrations ranging from 1–10 mcg/mL.

Mesalamine and *N*-acetyl-5-aminosalicylic acid cross the placenta following oral administration; however, serum concentrations of mesalamine in umbilical cord and amniotic fluid are very low. It is not known whether mesalamine crosses the placenta following rectal administration.

Following oral administration, low concentrations of mesalamine and higher concentrations of its metabolite, *N*-acetyl-5-aminosalicylic acid, have been detected in human breast milk. It is not known whether mesalamine or its metabolites are distributed into milk in humans following rectal administration.

■ **Elimination** Serum mesalamine concentrations appear to decline in a biphasic manner following IV administration of the drug. Following IV infusion of 0.5 g of the drug in healthy adults, the half-life of mesalamine averaged about 17 minutes in the distribution phase ($t_{1/2\alpha}$) and about 42 minutes in the terminal elimination phase ($t_{1/2\beta}$). Following oral administration of a single 1-g dose of mesalamine extended-release capsules (Pentasa®), the drug may undergo biphasic elimination; however, because of the continuous release and absorption of mesalamine throughout the GI tract, the correct elimination half-life of the drug cannot be determined. There is a relatively large interindividual variation in the elimination half-lives of mesalamine and *N*-acetyl-5-aminosalicylic acid following oral administration of mesalamine delayed-release tablets (Asacol®). Following oral administration of mesalamine 400-mg delayed-release tablets (Asacol®), the elimination half-lives of mesalamine and *N*-acetyl-5-aminosalicylic acid are about 12 hours (range: 2–15 hours). Following oral administration of a single 2.4- or 4.8-g dose as the 1.2-g delayed-release tablets (Lialda®) in healthy individuals, the elimination half-lives of mesalamine and *N*-acetyl-5-aminosalicylic acid are about 7–9 and 8–12 hours, respectively.

Following rectal administration of mesalamine suspension in healthy adults or those with inflammatory bowel disease, the elimination half-lives of mesalamine and *N*-acetyl-5-aminosalicylic acid are 0.5–1.5 hours and 5–10 hours, respectively. Following rectal administration of a 500-mg mesalamine suppository every 8 hours for 6 days in patients with ulcerative proctitis, the elimination half-lives of mesalamine and *N*-acetyl-5-aminosalicylic acid are 5 and 6 hours, respectively, after the initial dose, while the elimination half-lives of both the drug and its principal metabolite at steady-state are 7 hours.

The exact metabolic fate of mesalamine has not been clearly established. The drug undergoes rapid *N*-acetylation, probably in the liver and intestinal mucosa, to form *N*-acetyl-5-aminosalicylic acid; mesalamine and *N*-acetyl-5-aminosalicylic acid also may undergo conjugation with glucuronic acid. Several other, unidentified metabolites also may be formed. It has been suggested that *N*-acetylation also may occur (to a limited extent) in the intestinal wall and/or the lumen. The intestinal flora probably are involved in this acetylation, and extensive floral acetylation may adversely affect clinical efficacy of the drug. Correlation between acetylator phenotype of patients receiving mesalamine and the degree of *N*-acetylation does not appear to exist.

Although it has been suggested that *N*-acetyl-5-aminosalicylic acid may be pharmacologically active, therapeutic response has been poor in some patients treated rectally with this metabolite, and the relative contribution of this metabolite to the therapeutic effect of mesalamine remains questionable. *N*-acetyl-5-aminosalicylic acid did not inhibit lipoxygenase in vitro.

Following oral administration of mesalamine in healthy adults, approximately 20% of a dose is excreted in urine mainly as *N*-acetyl-5-aminosalicylic acid. Following oral administration of delayed- or extended-release mesalamine in patients with an ileorectal anastomosis or with colitis, amounts of mesalamine and *N*-acetyl-5-aminosalicylic acid excreted in urine appear to be similar to those excreted in healthy individuals; approximately 22% of a dose is excreted in urine (about 21% [i.e., about 4% of the dose] as *N*-acetyl-5-aminosalicylic acid). Of the approximately 21–22% of the dose absorbed following oral administration of mesalamine as the 1.2-g delayed-release tablets, less than 8% of the dose is excreted unchanged in the urine, compared with greater than 13% of the dose for *N*-acetyl-5-aminosalicylic acid. Following oral administration of delayed-release mesalamine, excretion of *N*-acetyl-5-aminosalicylic acid may be decreased in patients with Crohn's disease and in ileostomy patients. Following oral administration, mesalamine also is eliminated in feces. The amount of free mesalamine and salicylates excreted in feces in patients receiving mesalamine extended-release capsules, increase proportionally with the dose.

Following rectal administration of mesalamine suspension, unchanged drug and *N*-acetyl-5-aminosalicylic acid are excreted mainly in feces; small amounts of the drug and/or its metabolites are excreted in urine, mainly via tubular secretion. It is believed that the fraction of a rectal dose excreted in feces represents mainly unabsorbed drug. Biliary elimination of mesalamine appears to be negligible, although the drug may undergo some enterohepatic circulation. Following administration of a single rectal dose of mesalamine in patients with inflammatory bowel disease, about 50% of the dose is excreted in feces and about 10–35% (range: 6–79%) in urine within 24–48 hours. In patients with inflammatory bowel disease, about 44% of a single rectal dose is excreted in feces as unchanged drug, 3% as *N*-acetyl-5-aminosalicylic acid, and the remainder as unidentified metabolites. Following rectal administration, mesalamine is excreted in urine mainly as *N*-acetyl-5-aminosalicylic acid. It appears that urinary excretion characteristics may depend on the underlying disease state, dosage or volume of mesalamine suspension, and luminal pH. The presence of blood and mucus in the GI tract also may affect urinary excretion of the drug. The extent of urinary excretion of *N*-acetyl-5-aminosalicylic acid may be decreased at steady state, at low dosages, and in patients with active disease. Following rectal administration of mesalamine in patients with ulcerative colitis, approximately 10 (range: 2–18%) or 20% (range 10–37%) of the dose is excreted in urine of patients with active disease or those whose disease is in remission, respectively. Following rectal administration of a 4-g dose as a 100- or 200-mL suspension in patients with ulcerative colitis, approximately 16 or 25% of the dose was excreted in urine, respectively.

Following jejunal administration of mesalamine in healthy adults, approximately 54% (range: 47–70%) of the dose was excreted in urine and less than 2% in feces as *N*-acetyl-5-aminosalicylic acid within 24 hours.

Following oral administration of mesalamine in healthy individuals, the apparent renal clearance of *N*-acetyl-5-aminosalicylic acid is reported to average approximately 2.8–4.3 mL/minute per kg (range: 1–6.5 mL/minute per kg). The apparent renal clearance of this metabolite may be decreased in patients with ulcerative colitis or Crohn's disease.

Chemistry and Stability

■ **Chemistry** Mesalamine is an anti-inflammatory agent. Mesalamine is the 5-amino derivative of salicylic acid and therefore is related structurally to salicylates. Although there is limited in vitro evidence that metabolism of mesalamine to salicylate (ionized salicylic acid) can occur, formation of this metabolite appears to be minimal and is *not* necessary for the pharmacologic activity of the drug; therefore, mesalamine is not considered a true salicylate.

While the position of the amino group (5 [*meta*], as in mesalamine, versus 4 [*para*], as in aminosalicylic acid) may not be an important determinant of GI anti-inflammatory activity, presence of the group does appear to be important since salicylic acid (as the sodium salt), which lacks an amino group, does not appear to possess such activity in inflammatory bowel disease. Mesalamine appears to be the principal therapeutically active moiety of sulfasalazine. Mesalamine also is related structurally to aminobenzoic acid, differing from aminobenzoic acid by the presence of the amino group at position 5 rather than 4 and by the addition of a hydroxy group at position 2 (*ortho*). Mesalamine is commercially available for oral administration as delayed-release tablets or extended-release capsules. The drug is commercially available for rectal administration as an aqueous suspension or as suppositories.

Mesalamine occurs as white to slightly grey crystals or a light tan to pink crystalline powder and has a solubility of 1 mg/mL in water at 20°C and also is slightly soluble in alcohol. The drug has pK_as of 3, 6, and 13.9.

Mesalamine 400-mg delayed-release tablets (Asacol®) are coated with an acrylic-based resin that delays the release of the drug at least until the tablets reach the terminal ileum. Mesalamine 1.2-g delayed-release tablets (Lialda®) are coated with a pH-dependent polymer film that delays release of the drug from the tablet core (which contains mesalamine with hydrophilic and lipophilic excipients) until it reaches a pH of at least 7, usually in the terminal ileum. Mesalamine extended-release capsules are coated with ethylcellulose and are designed to release therapeutic amounts of the drug throughout the GI tract. Mesalamine rectal suspension contains sodium benzoate as a preservative, potassium metabisulfite as an antioxidant, carbomer 943P, xanthan gum, edetate disodium, and potassium acetate and has a pH of 4–5. Commercially available mesalamine suppositories contain the drug in a base of glycerides of saturated fatty acids (hard fat NF) base.

■ **Stability** Mesalamine is unstable in the presence of water and light, since oxidation and, to a lesser extent, light-catalyzed degradation of the drug occur. Therefore, the commercially available rectal suspension contains sodium metabisulfite as an antioxidant and is packaged in an airtight foil wrap in which air is replaced with nitrogen to minimize oxidation.

Commercially available mesalamine rectal suspension should be stored at controlled room temperature of 20–25°C but may be exposed to temperatures ranging from 15–30°C; the manufacturer states that mesalamine rectal suspension should be stored out of the reach of children. When stored at this temperature in the unopened foil-wrapped package, mesalamine rectal suspension has an expiration date of 2 years following the date of manufacture. Mesalamine rectal suspension may darken with time once the container has been removed from the foil wrap. While slight darkening of the off-white/tan suspension will not affect potency and some evidence indicates that even severely darkened suspensions remain potent, the manufacturer currently recommends that dark brown mesalamine suspensions be discarded. Based on experience to date, it appears that at least 1 year of exposure of mesalamine rectal suspensions to light (i.e., without foil protection) at room temperature is required for the drug to oxidize (darken) sufficiently to affect potency. No adverse effects have been attributed to oxidation products of the drug to date. Commercially available mesalamine suppositories should be stored below 25°C and out of the reach of children; freezing should be avoided.

Commercially available oral mesalamine 400-mg delayed-release tablets (Asacol®) should be stored at a controlled room temperature of 20–25°C, while the commercially available 1.2-g delayed-release tablets (Lialda®) should be stored at a controlled room temperature of 15–25°C but may be exposed to temperatures up to 30°C. The commercially available oral extended-release capsules should be stored at 25°C but may be exposed to temperatures ranging from 15–30°C.

Preparations

Excipients in commercially available drug preparations may have clinically important effects in some individuals; consult specific product labeling for details.

Mesalamine

Oral		
Capsules, extended-release	250 mg	**Pentasa®**, Shire
	500 mg	**Pentasa®**, Shire
Tablets, delayed-release	400 mg	**Asacol®**, Procter & Gamble
	1.2 g	**Lialda®**, Shire
Rectal		
Suppositories	1 g	**Canasa®**, Axcan
Suspension	4 g/60 mL	**Mesalamine Suspension Enema**
		Rowasa® Suspension Enema, Alaven

†Use is not currently included in the labeling approved by the US Food and Drug Administration

GI Drugs, Miscellaneous 56:92

Alvimopan

■ Alvimopan is a peripherally acting μ-opiate receptor antagonist.

REMS

FDA approved a REMS for alvimopan to ensure that the benefits outweigh the risks. The REMS may apply to one or more preparations of alvimopan and consists of the following: elements to assure safe use and implementation system. (See Dosage and Administration: Restricted Distribution Program.) See the FDA REMS page (https://www.accessdata.fda.gov/scripts/cder/rems/index.cfm).

Uses

■ **Postoperative Ileus** Alvimopan is used to accelerate upper and lower GI recovery following partial large or small bowel resection with primary anastomosis.

Efficacy of alvimopan in the management of postoperative ileus has been established in 5 multicenter, randomized, double-blind, parallel-group, placebo-controlled studies in over 1800 patients 18 years of age and older who underwent partial large or small bowel resection with primary anastomosis. Patients in these studies were randomized to receive alvimopan (6 or 12 mg) or placebo. The initial dose of the drug was administered 0.5–5 hours prior to the scheduled start of surgery with subsequent doses administered twice daily beginning on the first postoperative day and continuing until hospital discharge or for a maximum of 7 days. Opiates were provided for postoperative pain management and were administered as IV patient-controlled analgesia in 4 studies and as either IV patient-controlled analgesia or conventional IV or IM therapy in one study. Patients who received more than 3 doses of an opiate within 7 days prior to surgery, those with complete bowel obstruction, and those scheduled to undergo a total colectomy, colostomy, or ileostomy were excluded from study participation. Standard postoperative care included early removal of the nasogastric tube, ambulation the day following surgery, and early advancement of diet, as tolerated.

Results of the 5 studies indicated that alvimopan was superior to placebo in accelerating recovery of upper and lower GI function (i.e., tolerance of solid food and occurrence of first bowel movement). Recovery of GI function began approximately 48 hours following surgery, and recovery times were 10–26 hours shorter in alvimopan-treated patients compared with placebo-treated patients. The proportion of patients able to tolerate solid foods and pass a bowel movement was higher with alvimopan compared with placebo at all times throughout the study period. In addition, alvimopan reduced the time to hospital discharge compared with placebo. In these studies, no gender-, age-, or race-related differences in efficacy were noted. Alvimopan did not reverse opiate analgesia, as measured by opiate requirements and visual analog scale assessments of pain severity.

Although alvimopan has been studied for the management of postoperative ileus in women undergoing total abdominal hysterectomy† under general anesthesia, efficacy of the drug for this indication has not been established to date.

Dosage and Administration

■ **Restricted Distribution Program** Because of an increased risk of ischemic cardiovascular events (see Myocardial Infarction under Warnings/Precautions: Other Warnings and Precautions, in Cautions) associated with long-term alvimopan therapy, the drug is available only to hospitals for short-term inpatient use through a restricted distribution program (Entereg® Access Support and Education [EASE] program). (See REMS.)

In order to enroll in the EASE program, hospitals must perform bowel resection surgeries and confirm that staff who prescribe, dispense, or administer alvimopan have been provided with the EASE program enrollment kit (which contains the registration form, ordering information, hospital brochure, and the manufacturer's prescribing information for alvimopan). Hospitals enrolled in this program must have systems, order sets, protocols, or other measures in place to limit use of alvimopan to short-term (no more than 15 doses) therapy in inpatients. Hospitals must ensure that alvimopan will not be dispensed for outpatient use and that the drug will not be transferred to another hospital not registered with the EASE program. A database of registered hospitals is available on the program's website (http://www.entereg.com). Information about the EASE program is available at 866-423-6567 (866-4ADOLOR) or at http://www.entereg.com.

■ **Administration** ***Oral Administration*** Alvimopan is administered orally. In clinical studies, the preoperative dose was administered in the fasting state with subsequent doses administered without regard to meals.

■ **Dosage** Dosage of alvimopan, which is commercially available as the dihydrate, is calculated on the anhydrous basis.

To accelerate GI recovery in hospitalized patients following partial large or small bowel resection with primary anastomosis, the recommended adult dosage of alvimopan is 12 mg administered 30 minutes to 5 hours prior to surgery followed by 12 mg twice daily beginning the day after surgery and continuing for a maximum of 7 days or until discharge. Alvimopan is indicated for short-term (no more than 15 doses) use in hospitalized patients only. The drug should not be used for longer than 7 days following bowel resection.

■ **Special Populations** Dosage adjustments are not required in patients with mild to severe renal impairment; however, such patients should be monitored for possible adverse effects. Patients with severe renal impairment should be monitored closely for adverse effects (e.g., diarrhea, abdominal pain or cramping) that may indicate elevated concentrations of the drug or metabolite, and the drug should be discontinued if such events occur. Alvimopan is not recommended for use in patients with end-stage renal disease. (See Renal Impairment under Warnings/Precautions: Specific Populations, in Cautions.)

Dosage adjustments are not required in patients with mild to moderate hepatic impairment; such patients should be monitored for adverse effects (e.g., diarrhea, abdominal pain or cramping) that may indicate elevated concentrations of the drug or metabolite, and the drug should be discontinued if such events occur. Because clinical experience with alvimopan is limited in patients with severe hepatic impairment, the drug is not recommended for use in these patients. (See Hepatic Impairment under Warnings/Precautions: Specific Populations, in Cautions.)

Dosage adjustments based solely on age are not required in geriatric patients. (See Geriatric Use under Warnings/Precautions: Specific Populations, in Cautions.)

Cautions

■ **Contraindications** Patients who have taken opiates in therapeutic dosages for more than 7 consecutive days immediately prior to alvimopan administration.

■ **Warnings/Precautions** ***Warnings*** **Short-term, Inpatient Use.** Alvimopan is available only for short-term (no more than 15 doses) use in hospitalized patients. Alvimopan may be used only by hospitals enrolled in the Entereg® Access Support and Education (EASE) program. (See Dosage and Administration: Restricted Distribution Program.)

Other Warnings and Precautions **Myocardial Infarction.** A numerically higher incidence of myocardial infarction was reported in patients receiving alvimopan 0.5 mg twice daily compared with placebo in a 12-month clinical study evaluating long-term use of the drug for management of opiate-induced bowel dysfunction† in patients with chronic pain; a majority of events occurred 1–4 months after initiation of therapy.Similar results have not been observed in patients receiving short-term alvimopan therapy (12 mg twice daily for 7 days or less) following bowel resection. A causal relationship between myocardial infarction and alvimopan has not been established.

Because of an increased risk of ischemic cardiac events with long-term therapy, alvimopan is available only to hospitals through a restricted distribution program (EASE program). (See Dosage and Administration: Restricted Distribution Program.)

Recent Opiate Use. Patients recently exposed to opiates may exhibit increased sensitivity to alvimopan, which may be manifested principally as GI symptoms (e.g., abdominal pain, nausea, vomiting, diarrhea). Alvimopan should be used with caution in patients who have received more than 3 doses of an opiate within one week prior to surgery; such patients were excluded from clinical studies evaluating use of the drug for management of postoperative ileus. (See Cautions: Contraindications.)

Bowel Obstruction. Use of alvimopan in patients undergoing surgical correction of complete bowel obstruction is not recommended.

Crohn's Disease. Increased variability in alvimopan pharmacokinetics has been observed in patients with active or quiescent Crohn's disease; exposure to the drug generally was twofold higher in patients with quiescent disease compared with healthy individuals or patients with active disease. Concentrations of alvimopan's metabolite were lower in patients with Crohn's disease. However, the manufacturer states that dosage adjustments are not necessary.

Specific Populations **Pregnancy.** Category B. (See Users Guide.)

Lactation. Alvimopan and its metabolite are distributed into milk in rats; it is unknown whether the drug or its metabolite is distributed into human milk. Alvimopan should be used with caution in nursing women.

Pediatric Use. Safety and efficacy not established in children younger than 18 years of age.

Geriatric Use. Approximately 45% of patients enrolled in 5 clinical trials evaluating use of alvimopan for postoperative ileus were 65 years of age or older, and 18% were 75 years of age or older. Although no overall differences in efficacy or safety were observed between geriatric and younger patients and other clinical experience has not revealed any evidence of age-related differences, the possibility that some older patients may exhibit increased sensitivity to the drug cannot be ruled out.

Hepatic Impairment. Exposure to alvimopan may be slightly increased (1.5-fold to twofold) in patients with mild to moderate hepatic impairment (Child-Pugh class A or B); accumulation of alvimopan after multiple doses is possible in such patients. Patients with mild to moderate hepatic impairment should be monitored for possible adverse effects. (See Dosage and Administration: Special Populations.)

Exposure to alvimopan may be substantially increased (tenfold) in patients with severe hepatic impairment (Child-Pugh class C). Use in such patients is not recommended.

Renal Impairment. Because renal clearance accounts for only about 35% of the total clearance of alvimopan, renal impairment is thought to have a small effect on alvimopan clearance. The half-life of alvimopan in patients with mild to moderate renal impairment (creatinine clearance of 31–80 mL/minute) is similar to that in healthy individuals, but the half-life is prolonged in patients with severe renal impairment (creatinine clearance of 30 mL/minute or less).

Exposure to alvimopan's metabolite is increased twofold to fivefold in patients with moderate to severe renal impairment compared with patients with mild impairment and healthy individuals; accumulation of alvimopan and its metabolite after multiple doses is possible in patients with severe renal impairment.

Patients with renal impairment, particularly those with severe impairment, should be monitored for possible adverse effects. (See Dosage and Administration: Special Populations.)

Alvimopan has not been studied in patients with end-stage renal disease. Use in these patients is not recommended.

■ **Common Adverse Effects** Adverse effects reported in 3% or more of patients receiving alvimopan in clinical trials and more frequently (by a difference of at least one percentage point) with alvimopan than with placebo include constipation, hypokalemia, flatulence, dyspepsia, anemia, back pain, and urinary retention.

Drug Interactions

■ **Drugs Metabolized by Hepatic Microsomal Enzymes** Alvimopan and its metabolite do not inhibit cytochrome P-450 (CYP) isoenzyme 1A2, 2C9, 2C19, 3A4, 2D6, or 2E1 in vitro or induce isoenzyme 1A2, 2B6, 2C9, 2C19, or 3A4; therefore, pharmacokinetic interactions with substrates of these isoenzymes are unlikely.

■ **Drugs Affecting Hepatic Microsomal Enzymes** Pharmacokinetic interactions with inducers or inhibitors of the CYP isoenzyme system are unlikely.

■ **Drugs that are Substrates for or Inhibitors of P-glycoprotein Transport System** Alvimopan and its metabolite are substrates for the efflux transporter P-glycoprotein. Pharmacokinetic interactions are unlikely when alvimopan is administered with a mild to moderate inhibitor of this transport system. The effect, if any, of potent inhibitors (e.g., amiodarone, bepridil, cyclosporine, diltiazem, itraconazole, quinidine, quinine, spirinolactone, verapamil) of the P-glycoprotein transport system on the pharmacokinetics of alvimopan has not been established.

In vitro studies indicate that alvimopan is not an inhibitor of the P-glycoprotein transport system; therefore, pharmacokinetic interactions with substrates for this transport system are unlikely.

■ **Antibiotics** Plasma concentrations of alvimopan's metabolite were reduced (by 81%) in patients receiving preoperative oral antibiotics; however, the pharmacokinetics of alvimopan do not appear to be altered. Dosage adjustments are not necessary. (See Description.)

■ **Histamine H_2-receptor Antagonists and Proton-pump Inhibitors** Plasma concentrations of alvimopan's metabolite were reduced (by 49%) in patients receiving agents that block gastric acid secretion; however, the pharmacokinetics of alvimopan do not appear to be altered. Dosage adjustments are not necessary. (See Description.)

■ **Morphine** Concomitant administration of alvimopan with IV morphine sulfate did not result in clinically important alterations in the pharmacokinetics of morphine or morphine-6-glucuronide; dosage adjustments of IV morphine sulfate are not necessary.

Description

Alvimopan is a peripherally acting μ-opiate receptor antagonist.

Multiple factors (e.g., neurogenic, inflammatory, hormonal, pharmacologic) contribute to impaired GI motility following intra-abdominal surgery. The mechanism of action of alvimopan in the treatment of postoperative ileus stems from the drug's ability to block μ-opiate receptors in the GI tract, thereby antagonizing the peripheral inhibitory effects of opiates on GI motility and improving GI function. The drug does not readily cross the blood-brain barrier and therefore does not affect opiate analgesic activity or precipitate opiate withdrawal, as is observed with centrally active opiate antagonists (e.g., naloxone). Alvimopan exhibits greater affinity for μ-opiate receptors than for δ- and κ-opiate receptors and is a more potent μ-opiate receptor antagonist than is naloxone. Alvimopan does not appear to possess opiate agonist activity, nor does it possess affinity for nonopiate receptors, including α_1-, α_2-, and β-adrenergic; dopamine types 1 and 2 (D_1, D_2); serotonin type 2 (5-hydroxytryptamine [5-HT_{2A}]); histamine (H_1); γ-aminobutyric acid (GABA); benzodiazepine; and muscarinic receptors. In vitro studies have identified some differences in how alvimopan and methylnaltrexone (both peripheral μ-receptor antagonists) interact with opiate receptors (e.g., differences in binding affinity and functional activity) (see Description in Methylnaltrexone Bromide 56:92); however, it remains to be determined whether these differences are clinically important.

The absolute bioavailability of oral alvimopan averages 6% (range 1–19%). Orally administered alvimopan (unabsorbed drug and unmetabolized drug that reenters the intestine via biliary secretions) is metabolized by intestinal flora to an active, amide hydrolysis compound; however, the presence of this metabolite is not required for pharmacologic activity of alvimopan. Concentrations of alvimopan and its metabolite tend to be higher in patients with postoperative ileus than in healthy individuals; however, there is substantial intraindividual and interindividual variation in plasma concentrations of the metabolite. The drug and its metabolite are 80 and 94% bound to albumin, respectively. Alvimopan is not a substrate for, nor an inducer or inhibitor of, the cytochrome P-450 (CYP) isoenzyme system; hepatic metabolism is not an important route of elimination for alvimopan. The drug is eliminated mainly through biliary secretion (65%) and, to a lesser extent (35%), in the urine. The mean terminal-phase half-lives of alvimopan and its metabolite following multiple doses of the drug are 10–17 and 10–18 hours, respectively.

Advice to Patients

Importance of informing clinicians of long-term or intermittent opiate therapy, including any use of opiates in the week prior to receiving alvimopan. Potential for alvimopan to precipitate GI symptoms (e.g., abdominal pain, nausea, vomiting, diarrhea) in patients who have recently received opiate therapy; importance of informing clinician if such adverse events occur.

Importance of informing patients that alvimopan is indicated for hospital use only and for no more than 7 days following bowel resection.

Importance of women informing clinicians if they are or plan to become pregnant or plan to breast-feed. Importance of informing clinicians of existing or contemplated concomitant therapy, including prescription and OTC drugs, as well as any concomitant illnesses. Importance of informing patients of other important precautionary information. (See Cautions.)

Overview® (see Users Guide). For additional information on this drug until a more detailed monograph is developed and published, the manufacturer's labeling should be consulted. It is *essential* that the manufacturer's labeling be consulted for more detailed information on usual cautions, precautions, contraindications, potential drug interactions, laboratory test interferences, and acute toxicity.

Preparations

Distribution of alvimopan is restricted. (See Dosage and Administration: Restricted Distribution Program.)

Excipients in commercially available drug preparations may have clinically important effects in some individuals; consult specific product labeling for details.

Alvimopan

Oral		
Capsules	12 mg (of anhydrous alvimopan)	**Entereg®**, Adolor (comarketed by GlaxoSmithKline)

†Use is not currently included in the labeling approved by the US Food and Drug Administration

Selected Revisions December 2014.

Eluxadoline

■ Eluxadoline is a mixed μ-opiate receptor agonist and δ-opiate receptor antagonist; eluxadoline has poor oral bioavailability and is used for its local effects at opiate receptors in the GI tract.

Uses

■ **Irritable Bowel Syndrome** Eluxadoline is used for the management of irritable bowel syndrome (IBS) with diarrhea. The drug has been shown to reduce abdominal pain and improve stool consistency in such patients. Responses have been observed in both men and women with IBS with diarrhea.

Efficacy and safety of eluxadoline for the management of IBS with diarrhea were established in 2 randomized, double-blind, phase 3 studies in 2426 patients (age range 18–80 years, mean age 45 years; 66% female; 86% white, 27% Hispanic, and 11% black) who met Rome III criteria for IBS with diarrhea, defined as loose (mushy) or watery stools for at least 25% of bowel movements and hard or lumpy stools for less than 25% of bowel movements. Patients also were required to meet the following criteria over the week prior to randomization: the average of each day's worst abdominal pain score exceeded 3 (on a scale of 0–10), the average daily stool consistency score (assessed using the Bristol Stool Scale) was at least 5.5 (on a scale of 1–7), the Bristol Stool Scale score was 5 or greater on at least 5 days, and the average IBS with diarrhea global symptom score was 2 or greater (on a scale of 0–4). Patients with a history of pancreatitis, alcohol abuse, cholecystitis within the prior 6 months, sphincter of Oddi dysfunction, inflammatory bowel disease, celiac disease, intestinal obstruction, GI infection or diverticulitis within the prior 3 months, serum lipase concentrations exceeding 2 times the upper limit of normal (ULN), and serum aminotransferase (ALT or AST) concentrations exceeding 3 times the ULN were excluded from the study. Both studies included identical 26-week double-blind, placebo-controlled periods in which patients received oral eluxadoline 75 or 100 mg or placebo twice daily. Study 1 continued in a double-blind fashion for an additional 26 weeks, followed by a 2-week follow-up period, to evaluate long-term safety of eluxadoline; study 2 included a 4-week, single-blind, withdrawal phase following completion of the 26-week treatment period to assess the risk of rebound symptoms following drug discontinuance. Loperamide rescue therapy (maximum dosage of 8 mg daily, with no more than 14 mg over a 2-day period and no more than 22 mg over a 7-day period) for acute management of uncontrolled diarrhea and aspirin-containing drugs or nonsteroidal anti-inflammatory agents for abdominal pain were permitted during the double-blind treatment phase and single-blind withdrawal period. Other antidiarrheal agents, antispasmodic agents, or rifaximin for diarrhea and opiate-containing preparations for abdominal pain were not allowed.

In both studies, the primary measure of efficacy (composite response rate) was the proportion of patients simultaneously achieving both a daily abdominal pain response and a daily stool consistency response on at least 50% of days during weeks 1–12 of treatment. Daily abdominal pain response was achieved if the worst abdominal pain score in the previous 24 hours was improved by at least 30% compared with the average score for the week prior to randomization; daily stool consistency response was defined as Bristol Stool Scale score of less than 5 or as the absence of a bowel movement if accompanied by a daily pain response. Results for end points were based on electronic daily diary entries by patients. In both studies, the composite response rate at 12 weeks was higher for patients receiving eluxadoline 75 or 100 mg twice daily compared with those receiving placebo. Composite responses were achieved at 12 weeks by 25 or 24% (study 1) and 30 or 29% (study 2) of patients who received eluxadoline 100 or 75 mg, respectively, compared with 16–17% of patients who received placebo. At 26 weeks, composite response rates remained higher in both studies for patients receiving eluxadoline 100 mg compared with those receiving placebo and were higher in study 2 (but not in study 1) for patients receiving eluxadoline 75 mg compared with those receiving placebo. Similar proportions of male and female patients in both studies achieved a composite response. The proportion of patients achieving a composite response at each 4-week interval was numerically higher for eluxadoline 75 or 100 mg than for placebo as early as week 4 and continuing through week 24, demonstrating that efficacy was maintained throughout the treatment period. Among patients who reported receiving prior therapy with loperamide without adequate symptom control, the composite response rate was higher for those receiving eluxadoline 75 or 100 mg twice daily compared with those receiving placebo. Patients in all 3 treatment groups used loperamide infrequently during the study period (average of less than one 2-mg dose per week). No worsening of diarrhea or abdominal pain, compared with baseline, was reported following discontinuance of eluxadoline 75 or 100 mg during the 4-week, single-blind withdrawal period in study 2.

Dosage and Administration

■ **Administration** Eluxadoline is administered orally with food.

■ **Dosage** ***Irritable Bowel Syndrome with Diarrhea*** The recommended adult dosage of eluxadoline for the management of irritable bowel syndrome (IBS) with diarrhea is 100 mg twice daily. In patients who cannot tolerate the 100-mg dose of eluxadoline or are receiving concomitant therapy with an organic anion transporter protein (OATP) 1B1 inhibitor, the recommended adult dosage is 75 mg twice daily. (See Drug Interactions.) Eluxadoline should be discontinued if severe constipation lasting more than 4 days develops.

■ **Special Populations** In patients with mild or moderate (Child-Pugh class A or B) hepatic impairment, the recommended adult dosage of eluxadoline is 75 mg twice daily. The drug is contraindicated in patients with severe (Child-Pugh class C) hepatic impairment. The manufacturer makes no specific recommendations for geriatric patients or patients with renal impairment. (See Specific Populations under Cautions: Warnings/Precautions.)

Cautions

■ **Contraindications** Eluxadoline is contraindicated in patients who do not have a gallbladder because of the increased risk for pancreatitis and/or sphincter of Oddi spasm in such patients; the drug also is contraindicated in patients with known or suspected biliary duct obstruction or sphincter of Oddi disease or dysfunction because of the increased risk for sphincter of Oddi spasm. (See Pancreatitis and also see Sphincter of Oddi Spasm under Cautions: Warnings/Precautions.)

Because of the increased risk of acute pancreatitis, eluxadoline is contraindicated in patients with alcoholism, alcohol abuse or addiction, alcohol consumption in excess of 3 alcoholic beverages per day, or a history of pancreatitis or structural pancreatic diseases, including known or suspected pancreatic duct obstruction. (See Pancreatitis under Cautions: Warnings/Precautions.)

Eluxadoline is contraindicated in patients with severe hepatic impairment (Child-Pugh class C) because of the potential for substantially increased plasma concentrations of the drug. (See Hepatic Impairment under Warnings/Precautions: Specific Populations, in Cautions.)

Eluxadoline also is contraindicated in patients with a history of chronic or severe constipation or sequelae from constipation and those with known or suspected mechanical GI obstruction, since these patients may be at risk for severe complications of bowel obstruction.

■ **Warnings/Precautions** ***Pancreatitis*** Pancreatitis with or without sphincter of Oddi spasm, sometimes requiring hospitalization, has been reported in patients receiving eluxadoline, mainly in those without a gallbladder. Fatal cases of pancreatitis also have been reported in patients without a gallbladder. Cases of serious pancreatitis generally have occurred within the first week of therapy, with some patients experiencing the onset of symptoms following administration of 1 or 2 doses of the drug. Pancreatitis has been reported in some patients who did not consume alcohol and has developed in patients receiving eluxadoline dosages of either 75 or 100 mg twice daily. FDA states that alternative treatment options should be considered prior to initiating therapy with eluxadoline.

Pancreatitis not associated with sphincter of Oddi spasm was reported in less than 1% of patients receiving eluxadoline in clinical studies. Three of the 5 reported cases were associated with excessive alcohol consumption, one case was associated with biliary sludge, and one case occurred 2 weeks following discontinuance of the drug. All 5 cases resolved with normalization of lipase concentrations upon discontinuance of eluxadoline, with 4 of the cases resolving within 1 week of drug discontinuance. Patients did not experience organ failure or local or systemic complications.

From May 2015 through February 2017, FDA received 120 reports of serious cases of pancreatitis or death in patients receiving eluxadoline. Of the 68 patients with known gallbladder status, 56 did not have a gallbladder; most of these patients (44 patients) received the dosage of eluxadoline (75 mg twice daily) previously recommended for patients without a gallbladder. According to FDA, 76 patients were hospitalized and 2 patients died. The 2 fatalities occurred in patients without a gallbladder and were associated with pancreatitis or sphincter of Oddi spasm (one case each). In some cases of serious pancreatitis or death, sphincter of Oddi spasm (6 cases) or abdominal pain (16 cases) also was reported. Based on these postmarketing reports indicating increased risk of serious pancreatitis in patients without a gallbladder, use of eluxadoline in patients without a gallbladder is contraindicated.

Risk of developing pancreatitis also is increased in those who consume more than 3 alcoholic beverages per day. Patients' alcohol intake should be evaluated prior to initiation of eluxadoline, and chronic or acute excessive alcohol consumption should be avoided during eluxadoline therapy. Patients receiving the drug should be monitored for symptoms of pancreatitis (e.g., new or worsening abdominal pain that may radiate to the back or shoulder, with or without nausea and vomiting). Eluxadoline should be discontinued and medical attention should be sought immediately if symptoms suggestive of pancreatitis develop. (See Cautions: Contraindications and also see Advice to Patients.)

Sphincter of Oddi Spasm Because eluxadoline is a μ-opiate receptor agonist, patients receiving the drug are at risk for spasm of the sphincter of Oddi, which can result in pancreatitis or increases in hepatic enzyme concentrations associated with acute abdominal pain (e.g., biliary-type pain). Spasm generally has occurred within the first week of therapy, with some patients experiencing symptoms following administration of 1 or 2 doses of the drug. Sphincter of Oddi spasm occurred in less than 1% of patients receiving eluxadoline in clinical studies. All cases resolved upon discontinuance of therapy, with symptoms typically improved by the following day. In clinical studies, the one reported case of pancreatitis induced by sphincter of Oddi spasm occurred within minutes of the first dose of eluxadoline and resolved within 24 hours of drug discontinuance. Sphincter of Oddi spasm (with or without pancreatitis) resulting in hospitalization also has been reported during postmarketing experience, mainly in patients without a gallbladder. Use of eluxadoline in patients without a gallbladder is contraindicated. (See Cautions: Contraindications and also see Pancreatitis under Cautions: Warnings/Precautions.)

Eluxadoline should be discontinued and medical attention should be sought immediately if symptoms suggestive of sphincter of Oddi spasm (e.g., acute worsening of abdominal pain that may radiate to the back or shoulder, with or without nausea and vomiting) develop. Eluxadoline should not be reinitiated in patients who develop biliary duct obstruction or sphincter of Oddi spasm while receiving the drug.

Dependence and Abuse Eluxadoline is subject to control as a schedule IV (C-IV) drug. In clinical trials in patients with irritable bowel syndrome (IBS), the incidence of euphoria or feelings of drunkenness was 0–0.2% at dosages of 75 or 100 mg twice daily. In abuse-potential studies in recreational opiate-experienced individuals, supratherapeutic oral and intranasal doses of eluxadoline produced small but significant subjective responses (e.g., drug liking or disliking, high, dysphoria) and rates of euphoria (14–28%) that were intermediate to those produced by placebo (0–5%) or oxycodone (44–76%), suggesting the potential for psychological dependence. In animal studies, discontinuance of the drug following chronic administration did not produce behavioral signs of withdrawal, but responses in a self-administration study in animals suggested that the drug is sufficiently self-rewarding to produce reinforcement.

Specific Populations **Pregnancy.** There are no studies in pregnant women assessing eluxadoline-associated risks. Reproduction studies in rats and rabbits have not revealed evidence of teratogenicity, and a prenatal and postnatal development study in rats revealed no evidence of adverse effects in the offspring.

Lactation. It is not known whether eluxadoline is distributed into human milk; however, the drug is distributed into milk in rats. The benefits of breastfeeding and the importance of eluxadoline to the woman should be considered along with any potential adverse effects on the breast-fed child from the drug or from the underlying maternal condition.

Pediatric Use. Safety and efficacy of eluxadoline have not been established in pediatric patients.

Geriatric Use. In clinical studies evaluating eluxadoline in patients with IBS, 7.7% of those who received the study drug were 65 years of age or older, while 0.8% were 75 years of age or older. No overall differences in efficacy or types of adverse effects were observed between geriatric patients and younger adults. However, a higher proportion of geriatric patients, compared with younger adults, experienced adverse effects (66 versus 59%), serious adverse effects (9 versus 4%), and adverse GI effects (39 versus 28%).

Hepatic Impairment. In patients with mild, moderate, or severe (Child-Pugh class A, B, or C) hepatic impairment, plasma concentrations of eluxadoline were increased by 6-, 4-, and 16-fold, respectively, compared with individuals with normal hepatic function following a single oral 100-mg dose of the drug. Dosage of eluxadoline should be reduced in patients with mild or moderate hepatic impairment. (See Dosage and Administration: Special Populations.) Eluxadoline is contraindicated in patients with severe hepatic impairment; safety of the drug in this patient population has not been established. Patients with any degree of hepatic impairment who are receiving eluxadoline should be monitored for impairment of mental or physical abilities required for the performance of potentially hazardous activities (e.g., driving a car, operating machinery) and for other eluxadoline-related adverse effects.

■ **Common Adverse Effects** Adverse effects reported in more than 2% of patients receiving eluxadoline 75 or 100 mg twice daily for irritable bowel syndrome (IBS) with diarrhea (and with greater frequency than in patients receiving placebo) include constipation, nausea, abdominal pain, upper respiratory tract infection, vomiting, nasopharyngitis, abdominal distention, bronchitis, dizziness, flatulence, rash, increased ALT concentrations, fatigue, and viral gastroenteritis.

Drug Interactions

Metabolism of eluxadoline via the cytochrome P-450 (CYP) enzyme system has not been clearly established, and the potential for eluxadoline to inhibit CYP3A4 in the gut has not been established.

In vitro, eluxadoline is neither an inducer of CYP isoenzymes 1A2, 2C9, 2C19, or 3A4 nor an inhibitor of CYP isoenzymes 1A2, 2A6, 2B6, 2C9, 2C19, 2D6, or 3A4 at clinically relevant systemic concentrations. Although CYP2E1 was slightly inhibited by eluxadoline, clinically meaningful pharmacokinetic interactions are unlikely. However, in vitro studies were not adequate to establish the potential for eluxadoline to inhibit CYP3A4 in the gut.

In vitro studies suggest that eluxadoline is a substrate for organic anion transporter (OAT) 3, organic anion transport protein (OATP) 1B1, bile salt export pump (BSEP), and multidrug resistance protein (MRP) 2, but is not a substrate for organic cation transporter (OCT) 1 or 2, OAT1, OATP1B3, P-glycoprotein (P-gp), and breast cancer resistance protein (BCRP). Based on in vitro studies, clinically meaningful pharmacokinetic interactions via inhibition of OCT1, OCT2, OAT1, OAT3, OATP1B3, BSEP, and MRP2 by eluxadoline are unlikely. However, in vitro studies were not adequate to establish the potential for eluxadoline to inhibit P-gp in the gut.

■ **Drugs Affecting or Metabolized by Hepatic Microsomal Enzymes** ***Cytochrome P-450 Inhibitors*** Metabolic pathways of eluxadoline have not been fully elucidated, and the potential exists for concomitant use of potent CYP inhibitors (e.g., bupropion, ciprofloxacin, clarithromycin, fluconazole, gemfibrozil, paroxetine) to increase exposure to eluxadoline. As a precautionary measure, patients should be monitored for impairment of mental or physical abilities required for the performance of potentially hazardous tasks (e.g., driving a car, operating machinery) and for other eluxadoline-related adverse effects.

Cytochrome P-450 Isoenzyme 3A Substrates The potential for eluxadoline to inhibit CYP3A4 in the gut has not been established, and the potential exists for exposure to CYP3A substrates to be increased when eluxadoline is used concomitantly. If eluxadoline is initiated or discontinued in a patient receiving a CYP3A substrate that has a narrow therapeutic index (e.g., alfentanil, cyclosporine, dihydroergotamine, ergotamine, fentanyl, pimozide, quinidine, sirolimus, tacrolimus), plasma concentrations or pharmacodynamic effects of the CYP3A substrate should be monitored.

■ **Drugs Affecting or Affected by Organic Anion Transport Proteins** ***Organic Anion Transport Protein 1B1 Inhibitors*** Concomitant use of eluxadoline and OATP1B1 inhibitors (e.g., certain antiretrovirals [e.g., atazanavir, lopinavir, ritonavir, saquinavir, tipranavir], cyclosporine, eltrombopag, gemfibrozil, rifampin) may increase exposure to eluxadoline. (See Drug Interactions: Cyclosporine.) When eluxadoline is used concomitantly with an OATP1B1 inhibitor, dosage of eluxadoline should be reduced to 75 mg twice daily and the patient should be monitored for impairment of mental or physical abilities required for the performance of potentially hazardous tasks (e.g., driving a car, operating machinery) and for other eluxadoline-related adverse effects.

Organic Anion Transport Protein 1B1 Substrates Concomitant use of eluxadoline and OATP1B1 substrates may increase exposure to the OATP1B1 substrate. (See Drug Interactions: Rosuvastatin.)

■ **Drugs Affected by Breast Cancer Resistance Protein** Concomitant use of eluxadoline and BCRP substrates may increase exposure to the BCRP substrate. (See Drug Interactions: Rosuvastatin.)

■ **Constipating Drugs** Concomitant use of eluxadoline and drugs that cause constipation (e.g., alosetron, anticholinergics, opiates) increases the risk of constipation-related adverse effects, including serious constipation-related adverse effects. Use of eluxadoline with other drugs that may cause constipation should be avoided; loperamide may be used *occasionally* for acute management of severe diarrhea, but chronic use should be avoided. Loperamide should be discontinued immediately if constipation occurs.

■ **Cyclosporine** Concomitant administration of eluxadoline (single 100-mg dose) with cyclosporine (single 600-mg dose) (an inhibitor of OATP1B1 and MRP2) in healthy individuals increased the area under the concentration-time curve (AUC) and peak plasma concentration of eluxadoline by 4.4- and 6.2-fold, respectively, compared with administration of eluxadoline alone. When eluxadoline is used concomitantly with cyclosporine, dosage of eluxadoline should be reduced to 75 mg twice daily and the patient should be monitored for impairment of mental or physical abilities required for the performance of potentially hazardous tasks (e.g., driving a car, operating machinery) and for other eluxadoline-related adverse effects. Because cyclosporine also is a substrate of CYP3A4, the potential exists for increased cyclosporine exposure. (See Cytochrome P-450 Isoenzyme 3A Substrates under Drug Interactions: Drugs Affecting or Metabolized by Hepatic Microsomal Enzymes.)

■ **Oral Contraceptives** Concomitant administration of eluxadoline (100 mg twice daily) with an oral contraceptive containing 35 mcg of ethinyl estradiol and 0.5 mg of norethindrone in healthy individuals did not substantially alter steady-state exposure to the oral contraceptive components or to eluxadoline.

■ **Probenecid** Concomitant administration of eluxadoline (single 100-mg dose) with the dual OAT3 and MRP2 inhibitor probenecid (single 500-mg dose) in healthy individuals increased peak plasma concentration and AUC of eluxadoline by 31 and 35%, respectively, compared with administration of eluxadoline alone; however, these alterations in exposures are not expected to be clinically important.

■ **Rosuvastatin** Concomitant administration of eluxadoline (100 mg twice daily) with the dual OATP1B1 and BCRP substrate rosuvastatin (single 20-mg dose) in healthy individuals increased peak plasma concentration and AUC of rosuvastatin by 18 and 40%, respectively, compared with administration of rosuvastatin alone. Effects on the active major metabolite, *N*-desmethyl rosuvastatin, were similar. Because concomitant use of eluxadoline and rosuvastatin increases exposure to rosuvastatin and may increase risk of myopathy or rhabdomyolysis, the lowest effective dosage of rosuvastatin should be used.

Description

Eluxadoline is a mixed μ-opiate receptor agonist and δ-opiate receptor antagonist. Binding affinities of eluxadoline for the human μ- and δ-opiate receptors are 1.8 and 430 nM, respectively. The drug also exhibits agonist activity at the κ-opiate receptor, but binding affinity for this receptor in humans has not been determined. Eluxadoline has poor oral bioavailability and is used for its local effects at opiate receptors in the GI tract. In animals, eluxadoline interacts with opiate receptors in the gut, reduces contractility in intestinal tissue, and inhibits neurogenically mediated secretion in vitro; the drug has been shown to normalize GI transit and reduce fecal output in several animal models of altered GI function.

Eluxadoline is poorly absorbed after oral administration; some data suggest that the drug may undergo moderate hepatic first-pass extraction. Absolute oral bioavailability of eluxadoline has not been established. Eluxadoline exhibits approximately linear pharmacokinetics with no evidence of accumulation with twice-daily dosing. Substantial interpatient variability in pharmacokinetic parameters is observed. Following oral administration of a single 100-mg dose of eluxadoline in healthy individuals, the median time to peak plasma concentration is 1.5 (range: 1–8) or 2 (range: 0.5–6) hours under fed or fasting conditions, respectively. Administration of eluxadoline 100 mg with a high-fat meal decreases the peak plasma concentration and area under the concentration-time curve (AUC) by 50 and 60%, respectively. Eluxadoline is 81% bound to plasma proteins and has a mean plasma elimination half-life of 3.7–6 hours. Possible metabolic pathways of the drug have not been fully determined, although an acyl glucuronide metabolite has been detected in urine. Following administration of a single oral 300-mg dose of radiolabeled eluxadoline in healthy males, approximately 82% of the drug was recovered in feces within 14 days and less than 1% was recovered in urine within 8 days.

Advice to Patients

Importance of advising patients to read the manufacturer's medication guide before beginning treatment and each time the prescription is refilled.

Importance of patients informing their clinicians prior to initiating eluxadoline therapy if they do not have a gallbladder or have a history of pancreatic or gallbladder disease.

Importance of advising all patients to immediately discontinue eluxadoline and seek medical attention if symptoms of sphincter of Oddi spasm or pancreatitis (e.g., new or worsening abdominal, epigastric, or biliary pain that may radiate to the back or shoulder, with or without nausea and vomiting) develop.

Importance of advising patients to inform their clinician if they cannot tolerate eluxadoline.

Importance of advising patients to discontinue eluxadoline and inform their clinician if they experience constipation lasting more than 4 days.

Importance of advising patients that eluxadoline and alosetron should not be used concomitantly and that loperamide should not be used on a *chronic* basis with eluxadoline because of the potential for constipation; however, loperamide may be used *occasionally* with eluxadoline for acute management of severe diarrhea. Loperamide should be discontinued if constipation develops. Importance of advising patients receiving eluxadoline to avoid taking other drugs that may cause constipation (e.g., opiates, anticholinergics).

Importance of advising patients to avoid chronic or acute excessive alcohol consumption while taking eluxadoline since consumption of more than 3 alcoholic beverages per day increases the risk of pancreatitis.

Importance of informing patients that if a dose of eluxadoline is missed, therapy should be resumed with the next scheduled dose; the dose should *not* be doubled to make up for the missed dose.

Importance of advising patients with hepatic impairment that they should not drive, operate machinery, or perform other potentially hazardous activities until they know how eluxadoline affects them.

Importance of women informing clinicians if they are or plan to become pregnant or plan to breast-feed.

Importance of informing clinicians of existing or contemplated concomitant therapy, including prescription and OTC drugs, as well as any concomitant illnesses.

Importance of informing patients of other important precautionary information. (See Cautions.)

Overview® (see Users Guide). For additional information on this drug until a more detailed monograph is developed and published, the manufacturer's labeling should be consulted. It is *essential* that the manufacturer's labeling be consulted for more detailed information on usual cautions, precautions, contraindications, potential drug interactions, laboratory test interferences, and acute toxicity.

Preparations

Eluxadoline is subject to control under the Federal Controlled Substances Act of 1970 as a schedule IV (C-IV) drug.

Excipients in commercially available drug preparations may have clinically important effects in some individuals; consult specific product labeling for details.

Eluxadoline

Oral		
Tablets, film-coated	75 mg	Viberzi® (C-IV), Allergan
	100 mg	Viberzi® (C-IV), Allergan

Selected Revisions November 2017, © Copyright, March 2016, American Society of Health-System Pharmacists, Inc.

Linaclotide

■ Linaclotide, a guanylate cyclase-C (GC-C) agonist, stimulates secretion of chloride and bicarbonate into the intestinal lumen, which increases intestinal fluid and accelerates intestinal transit.

Uses

■ **Irritable Bowel Syndrome with Constipation** Linaclotide is used in adults for the symptomatic treatment of irritable bowel syndrome (IBS) with constipation.

Efficacy and safety of linaclotide for the symptomatic treatment of IBS with constipation have been evaluated in 2 randomized, double-blind, placebo-controlled studies (trial 31 and trial 302) in adults (mean age 44 years; 90% female; 77% white, 19% black, and 12% Hispanic) who met Rome II criteria for IBS. Eligible patients also were required to meet the following criteria during the 14-day baseline period: a mean abdominal pain score of at least 3 (on a scale of 0–10), fewer than 3 complete spontaneous bowel movements (CSBMs) per week, and 5 or fewer spontaneous bowel movements (SBMs) per week. In both studies, patients were randomized to receive linaclotide 290 mcg once daily or placebo. In trial 31, the assigned treatment was continued for 12 weeks; patients who completed 12 weeks of linaclotide therapy then were rerandomized to receive linaclotide 290 mcg once daily or placebo for 4 additional weeks, while those who had received placebo for 12 weeks were reassigned to receive linaclotide 290 mg once daily for 4 weeks. In trial 302, the originally assigned treatment was continued for 26 weeks. In both studies, the primary end point was efficacy over the first 12 weeks. Data on patients' symptoms were collected via daily patient reports.

In the first study (trial 31), 34% of patients receiving linaclotide and 21% of patients receiving placebo achieved the combined efficacy end point (defined as at least 30% improvement in mean abdominal pain score and an increase of one or more CSBMs per week compared with baseline) in the same week for at least 6 out of 12 weeks of treatment. The individual components of this end point were achieved by 50 and 49%, respectively, of patients receiving linaclotide and 37 and 30%, respectively, of those receiving placebo. In patients who switched to placebo after completing 12 weeks of linaclotide therapy, abdominal pain scores and CSBM frequency returned toward baseline values within 1 week following drug discontinuance; those who continued receiving linaclotide maintained their response over 4 additional weeks of treatment.

In the second study (trial 302), 34% of patients receiving linaclotide and 14% of those receiving placebo achieved the combined efficacy end point (at least 30% improvement in mean abdominal pain score and an increase of one or more CSBMs per week compared with baseline) in the same week for at least 6 out of the first 12 weeks of treatment. The individual components of this end point were achieved by 49 and 48%, respectively, of patients receiving linaclotide and 34 and 23%, respectively, of those receiving placebo. Results for the entire 26-week treatment period were consistent with those for the first 12 weeks, with 32% of linaclotide-treated patients and 13% of placebo recipients achieving the combined end point for at least 13 out of 26 weeks.

In both studies, assessments of changes in individual symptoms of IBS, measures of bowel function (frequency of SBMs, stool consistency, amount of straining with bowel movements), and patient ratings of the adequacy and degree of relief also favored linaclotide over placebo. Improvements in abdominal pain scores were apparent within the first week of linaclotide therapy and were maximal in 6–9 weeks; maximal effects on CSBM frequency were achieved within the first week of therapy.

A post-hoc analysis of data from trials 31 and 302 indicated that linaclotide improved abdominal symptoms in subsets of patients with severe symptoms at baseline (defined as any baseline abdominal pain, discomfort, bloating, fullness, or cramping rated 7 or greater on a scale of 0–10). At 12 weeks, the mean change in abdominal symptom scores from baseline in these subsets of patients was substantially greater in patients receiving linaclotide compared with those receiving placebo.

■ **Chronic Idiopathic Constipation** Linaclotide is used in adults for the symptomatic treatment of chronic idiopathic constipation.

Efficacy and safety of linaclotide (145 or 290 mcg daily) for the symptomatic treatment of chronic idiopathic constipation have been evaluated in 2 randomized, double-blind, placebo-controlled studies (trial 01 and trial 303) in adults who reported having had fewer than 3 SBMs per week and having experienced straining, lumpy or hard stools, and/or a sensation of incomplete evacuation during more than 25% of bowel movements for at least 12 weeks out of the previous 12 months. Patients were excluded if they met Rome II criteria for IBS. In the 2 studies combined, the mean age of patients was 48 years, and most patients were female (89%) and white (76%; 22% black, 10% Hispanic). In each study, patients were randomized to receive linaclotide 290 mcg, linaclotide 145 mcg, or placebo once daily for 12 weeks. In trial 303, patients who completed 12 weeks of linaclotide therapy were rerandomized to receive linaclotide (at the originally assigned dosage) or placebo for 4 additional weeks, while those who had received placebo for 12 weeks were reassigned to receive linaclotide 290 mcg daily for 4 weeks. Data on bowel function and patients' symptoms were collected via daily patient reports. The combined primary efficacy end point was defined as 3 or more CSBMs per week *and* an increase of at least 1 CSBM per week compared with baseline for at least 9 weeks during the 12-week treatment period.

Results from trial 303 showed that 19, 20, or 3% of patients receiving linaclotide 290 mcg, linaclotide 145 mcg, or placebo, respectively, achieved the combined efficacy end point. In patients who switched to placebo after receiving 12 weeks of linaclotide therapy, CSBM and SBM frequency returned toward baseline values within 1 week following drug discontinuance; those who continued receiving linaclotide maintained their response over 4 additional weeks of treatment.

Results from trial 01 showed that 20, 15, or 6% of patients receiving linaclotide 290 mcg, linaclotide 145 mcg, or placebo, respectively, achieved the combined efficacy end point.

Although both dosages of linaclotide were effective, the studies provided no consistent evidence indicating that the 290-mcg daily dosage confers additional clinical benefit beyond that produced by the 145-mcg daily dosage.

In both studies, assessments of changes in individual symptoms of constipation, measures of bowel function (frequency of SBMs, stool consistency, amount of straining with bowel movements), and overall severity of constipation also favored linaclotide over placebo. Maximal effects on CSBM frequency were achieved within the first week of therapy and were sustained throughout the treatment period.

Efficacy of linaclotide at a dosage of 72 mcg daily was established in a third randomized, double-blind, placebo-controlled study in adults who met modified Rome III criteria for functional constipation. The study design through week 12 was the same as that in trial 01 and trial 303. The mean age of patients was 46 years, and most patients were female (77%) and white (71%). The combined efficacy end point (3 or more CSBMs in a given week and an increase of at least 1 CSBM from baseline in the same week for a minimum of 9 weeks out of the 12-week treatment period) was achieved by 13% of patients receiving linaclotide 72 mcg daily compared with 5% of those receiving placebo. In a separate analysis using an alternate definition of response (3 or more CSBMs in a given week and an increase of at least 1 CSBM from baseline in the same week for a minimum of 9 weeks out of the 12-week treatment period and for at least 3 of the last 4 weeks of the treatment period), response rates were 12% for patients receiving linaclotide 72 mcg daily and 5% for those receiving placebo.

Dosage and Administration

■ **Administration** Linaclotide is administered orally on an empty stomach, at least 30 minutes prior to the first meal of the day. Administration immediately after a high-fat breakfast resulted in looser stools and increased frequency of stools when compared with administration in the fasted state. In clinical trials, linaclotide was administered at least 30 minutes before breakfast.

Linaclotide capsules should be swallowed whole. Alternatively, for patients who are unable to swallow whole capsules, linaclotide capsules may be opened and the contents (beads) may be sprinkled on applesauce and administered orally or dispersed in water and administered orally or via a nasogastric or gastrostomy tube. The manufacturer states that sprinkling the capsule contents of linaclotide capsules on soft foods other than applesauce or dispersing the contents in liquids other than water has not been studied. The capsules or capsule contents should not be crushed or chewed.

For administration in applesauce, the entire contents of one capsule of linaclotide should be sprinkled on one teaspoonful of room-temperature applesauce in a clean container. The entire mixture should be consumed (without chewing) immediately and should not be stored for later use.

For oral administration mixed in water, the entire contents of one capsule of linaclotide should be added to a clean cup containing approximately 30 mL of room-temperature bottled water, the mixture should be gently swirled for at least 20 seconds, and then the entire contents should be consumed immediately. Any beads remaining in the cup should be dispersed in an additional 30 mL of water, gently swirled again for at least 20 seconds, and then consumed immediately. The mixture should not be stored for later use. The manufacturer states that linaclotide is coated on the surface of the beads and will dissolve off the beads into the water. Thus, consumption of all the beads is not necessary to deliver a complete dose of the drug.

For administration via nasogastric or gastrostomy feeding tube, the entire contents of one linaclotide capsule should be added to a clean cup containing 30 mL of room-temperature bottled water, the mixture should be gently swirled for at least 20 seconds, and then the entire contents should be drawn up into an appropriately sized catheter-tipped syringe and administered into the nasogastric or gastrostomy tube rapidly (10 mL per 10 seconds) using steady pressure. Any beads remaining in the cup should be dispersed in an additional 30 mL of water and the process should be repeated. Following administration of the dose, the nasogastric or gastrostomy tube should be flushed with at least 10 mL of water. Because linaclotide is coated on the surface of the beads and will dissolve off the beads into the water, the manufacturer states that it is not necessary to administer all the beads to deliver a complete dose of the drug.

■ **Dosage** ***Adult Dosage*** **Irritable Bowel Syndrome with Constipation.** The recommended adult dosage of linaclotide for the symptomatic treatment of irritable bowel syndrome (IBS) with constipation is 290 mcg once daily.

Chronic Idiopathic Constipation. The recommended adult dosage of linaclotide for the symptomatic treatment of chronic idiopathic constipation is 145 mcg once daily. A dosage of 72 mcg once daily may be used based on individual presentation and tolerability.

■ **Special Populations** Dosage adjustments are not needed in patients with renal or hepatic impairment.

The manufacturer makes no specific dosage recommendations for geriatric patients.

Cautions

■ **Contraindications** Linaclotide is contraindicated in infants and children younger than 6 years of age. (See Pediatric Use under Warnings/Precautions: Specific Populations, in Cautions.) The drug also is contraindicated in any patient with known or suspected mechanical GI obstruction.

■ **Warnings/Precautions** ***Warnings*** **Pediatric Risk.** In toxicology studies, linaclotide caused deaths due to dehydration in neonatal mice when administered in single, clinically relevant, adult oral doses. Linaclotide is contraindicated in infants and children younger than 6 years of age and should be avoided in children and adolescents 6 years to younger than 18 years of age. (See Pediatric Use under Warnings/Precautions: Specific Populations, in Cautions.)

Other Warnings and Precautions **Diarrhea.** Diarrhea may occur, generally during the first 2 weeks of linaclotide therapy. The incidence of diarrhea is similar in patients with either irritable bowel syndrome (IBS) with constipation or chronic idiopathic constipation. In clinical trials in patients with these conditions, severe diarrhea was reported in 2% of patients receiving a linaclotide dosage of 145 or 290 mcg daily and in less than 1% of those receiving a dosage of 72 mcg daily. Cases of severe diarrhea that were associated with dizziness, syncope, hypotension, and electrolyte abnormalities (hypokalemia and hyponatremia) and that required hospitalization or administration of IV fluids have been reported during postmarketing experience with the drug. If severe diarrhea occurs, linaclotide therapy should be interrupted and the patient should be rehydrated.

Specific Populations **Pregnancy.** Since systemic absorption of linaclotide and its active metabolite is negligible following oral administration, the drug is not expected to result in fetal exposure if administered to pregnant women. However, available data on use of linaclotide in pregnant women are insufficient to inform fetal risk.

No adverse effects on embryofetal development were observed in rats or rabbits when linaclotide was administered orally during organogenesis at dosages of up to 100,000 or 40,000 mcg/kg daily, respectively. Severe maternal toxicity and associated effects on fetal morphology were observed in mice at dosages of at least 40,000 mcg/kg daily. No developmental abnormalities and no effects on growth, learning and memory, or fertility were observed in the offspring of rats that received linaclotide orally at dosages up to 100,000 mcg/kg daily during the period of organogenesis through lactation. Limited systemic exposure to linaclotide was achieved in rats, rabbits, and mice during the period of organogenesis. Animal and human doses should not be compared directly for evaluating relative exposure.

Lactation. It is not known whether linaclotide is distributed into human milk, affects milk production, or affects the breast-fed infant.

Systemic absorption of linaclotide and its active metabolite is negligible following oral administration. It is not known whether the negligible systemic absorption observed in adults will result in clinically important exposure in breast-fed infants. The benefits of breast-feeding and the importance of linaclotide to the woman should be considered along with potential adverse effects on the breast-fed infant from the drug or from the underlying maternal condition. Exposure of infants to linaclotide could result in serious adverse effects. (See Pediatric Use under Warnings/Precautions: Specific Populations, in Cautions.)

Pediatric Use. Linaclotide is contraindicated in infants and children younger than 6 years of age and should be avoided in children and adolescents 6 years to younger than 18 years of age.

Safety and efficacy of linaclotide in pediatric patients younger than 18 years of age have not been established, and the drug has caused deaths within 24 hours of administration in toxicology studies in neonatal mice (age approximately equivalent to a human age of 0–28 days). In neonatal mice, administration of linaclotide 10 mcg/kg daily caused deaths on postnatal day 7. Tolerability to linaclotide increased with age in juvenile mice. In 2-week-old mice, linaclotide was well tolerated at a dosage of 50 mcg/kg daily, but deaths occurred after a single oral dose of 100 mcg/kg. In 3-week-old mice, linaclotide was well tolerated at a dosage of 100 mcg/kg daily, but deaths occurred after a single oral dose of 600 mcg/kg. The deaths in neonatal mice were due to rapid and severe dehydration resulting from increased fluid secretion into the intestine as a consequence of guanylate cyclase-C (GC-C) stimulation. Because of increased intestinal expression of GC-C, infants and children younger than 6 years of age may be at greater risk of developing diarrhea and its potentially serious consequences compared with individuals 6 years of age and older. Although no deaths occurred in older juvenile mice, use of the drug in children and adolescents 6 years to younger than 18 years of age should be avoided because of the deaths reported in younger mice and the lack of safety and efficacy data in pediatric patients.

Geriatric Use. Clinical studies of linaclotide did not include sufficient numbers of patients 65 years of age and older to determine whether geriatric patients respond differently than younger adults. In clinical trials in patients with IBS with constipation, 5% of patients were 65 years of age or older, while 1% were 75 years of age and older; in clinical trials in patients with chronic idiopathic constipation, 11% were 65 years of age or older, while 2% were 75 years of age and older. In general, dosage should be selected with caution in geriatric patients because of the greater frequency of decreased hepatic, renal, and/or cardiac function and of concomitant disease and/or drug therapy.

Hepatic Impairment. Linaclotide has not been studied in patients with hepatic impairment. However, because linaclotide is metabolized within the GI tract and has negligible systemic bioavailability following oral administration, hepatic impairment is not expected to affect metabolism or clearance of the drug or its metabolite.

Renal Impairment. Linaclotide has not been studied in patients with renal impairment. However, because linaclotide is metabolized within the GI tract and has negligible systemic bioavailability following oral administration, renal impairment is not expected to affect clearance of the drug or its metabolite.

■ **Common Adverse Effects** Adverse effects reported in 2% or more of patients receiving linaclotide 290 mcg daily for the treatment of IBS with constipation, and more frequently with the drug than with placebo, include diarrhea, abdominal pain, flatulence, abdominal distension, viral gastroenteritis, and headache.

Adverse effects reported in 2% or more of patients receiving linaclotide 145 mcg daily for the treatment of chronic idiopathic constipation, and more frequently with the drug than with placebo, include diarrhea, abdominal pain, flatulence, abdominal distension, upper respiratory tract infection, and sinusitis.

Adverse effects reported in 2% or more of patients receiving linaclotide 72 mcg daily for the treatment of chronic idiopathic constipation, and more frequently with the drug than with placebo, include diarrhea and abdominal distension.

Drug Interactions

No formal drug interaction studies have been conducted with linaclotide to date. However, systemic exposure to linaclotide and its active metabolite is negligible following oral administration at recommended dosages, and in vitro studies indicate that linaclotide does not interact with cytochrome P-450 (CYP) isoenzymes or with common efflux and uptake transporters, including the P-glycoprotein (P-gp) efflux transporter. Thus, no interactions mediated by CYP enzymes or common transporters are anticipated.

Description

Linaclotide, a guanylate cyclase-C (GC-C) agonist, is a 14-amino acid peptide structurally related to endogenous guanylin peptide hormones that regulate fluid and electrolyte balance in the intestine. The parent drug and its active metabolite bind to GC-C receptors on the luminal surface of the intestinal epithelium, which increases intracellular and extracellular concentrations of cyclic guanosine monophosphate (cGMP). In turn, increased intracellular concentrations of cGMP trigger a signal-transduction cascade activating the cystic fibrosis transmembrane conductance regulator (CFTR) ion channel. This results in secretion of chloride and bicarbonate into the intestinal lumen causing increased intestinal fluid and accelerated intestinal transit. Linaclotide has been shown to change stool consistency and increase stool frequency.

In animal models, linaclotide also decreased visceral hyperalgesia and abdominal pain. This effect in animals is thought to be mediated by activation of GC-C leading to increased extracellular concentrations of cGMP, which inhibits colonic nociceptors. Further research is needed to determine the precise mechanism(s) by which linaclotide relieves abdominal pain in patients with irritable bowel syndrome (IBS) with constipation.

After oral administration, linaclotide is minimally absorbed with negligible systemic bioavailability. Linaclotide is metabolized by carboxypeptidase A within the GI tract to an active metabolite; both the parent drug and active metabolite are further degraded within the intestinal lumen to smaller peptides and amino acids. Following multiple-dose oral administration, about 3–5% of the drug is recovered in feces as active peptide, principally as active metabolite.

Advice to Patients

Importance of reading the manufacturer's patient information (medication guide) prior to initiation of therapy and each time the prescription is refilled.

Importance of advising patients that accidental ingestion of linaclotide by a child, especially a child younger than 6 years of age, may result in severe diarrhea and dehydration; importance of keeping linaclotide out of reach of children and of properly disposing of any unused drug. (See Pediatric Use under Warnings/Precautions: Specific Populations, in Cautions.)

Importance of advising patients that abdominal pain or diarrhea may occur and that they should discontinue linaclotide and contact their clinician if severe diarrhea or unusual or severe abdominal pain occurs, especially if associated with hematochezia or melena.

Importance of taking linaclotide once daily on an empty stomach; the capsule should be swallowed whole, and the capsule or capsule contents should not be crushed or chewed. Importance of advising patient of alternative forms of administration if patient is unable to swallow whole capsule.

Importance of storing linaclotide in the original container, with the lid tightly closed and the contents protected from moisture; importance of not removing the desiccant from the container and of not repackaging the capsules.

If a dose is missed, the missed dose should be omitted and the next dose taken at the regularly scheduled time. Two doses should not be taken at the same time to make up for a missed dose.

Importance of informing clinicians of existing or contemplated concomitant therapy, including prescription and OTC drugs, as well as any concomitant illnesses.

Importance of women informing clinicians if they are or plan to become pregnant or plan to breast-feed.

Importance of informing patients of other important precautionary information. (See Cautions.)

Overview® (see Users Guide). For additional information on this drug until a more detailed monograph is developed and published, the manufacturer's labeling should be consulted. It is *essential* that the manufacturer's labeling be consulted for more detailed information on usual cautions, precautions, contraindications, potential drug interactions, laboratory test interferences, and acute toxicity.

Preparations

Excipients in commercially available drug preparations may have clinically important effects in some individuals; consult specific product labeling for details.

Linaclotide

Oral		
Capsules	72 mcg	**Linzess®**, Allergan (comarketed by Ironwood)
	145 mcg	**Linzess®**, Allergan (comarketed by Ironwood)
	290 mcg	**Linzess®**, Allergan (comarketed by Ironwood)

Lubiprostone

■ Lubiprostone, a bicyclic fatty acid that selectively activates intestinal ClC-2 chloride channels, increases intestinal fluid secretion.

Uses

■ **Chronic Idiopathic Constipation** Lubiprostone is used for the management of chronic idiopathic constipation in adults.

Safety and efficacy of lubiprostone have been evaluated in 2 randomized, double-blind, placebo-controlled studies in a total of 479 adults (mean age: about 47 years, range: 20–81 years; 89% female; 80.8% white; 9.6% black; 7.3% Hispanic; 1.5% Asian) with chronic idiopathic constipation. In these studies, constipation was characterized by an average of less than 3 spontaneous bowel movements per week and the presence of one or more of 3 symptoms (very hard stools, sensation of incomplete evacuation, straining at defecation) occurring at least 25% of the time over a 6-month period prior to randomization. In these trials, patients receiving lubiprostone (24 mcg twice daily) had a higher frequency of spontaneous bowel movements, a decrease in signs and symptoms of constipation (including abdominal bloating, abdominal discomfort, stool consistency, and straining), and a decrease in constipation severity ratings compared with those receiving placebo. 57–63% of patients receiving lubiprostone (24 mcg twice daily) experienced spontaneous bowel movements within 24 hours after administration of treatment compared with 32–37% of those receiving placebo. In addition, the time to first spontaneous bowel movement was shorter in patients receiving the drug than in those receiving placebo. A rebound effect was not observed upon withdrawal of the drug following 4 weeks of treatment.

In 3 long-term, open-label safety trials in a total of 871 patients with chronic idiopathic constipation, lubiprostone (24 mcg twice daily for 6–12 months) was associated with decreases in abdominal bloating, abdominal discomfort, and severity of constipation throughout the treatment period.

■ **Irritable Bowel Syndrome with Constipation in Women** Lubiprostone is used for the treatment of irritable bowel syndrome (IBS) with constipation in women 18 years of age or older.

Safety and efficacy of lubiprostone have been evaluated in 2 double-blind, placebo-controlled studies in a total of 1154 adults (mean age: about 47 years, range: 18–85 years; 91.6% female; 77.4% white; 13.2% black; 8.5% Hispanic; 0.4% Asian) with IBS with constipation. In these studies, IBS was defined as abdominal pain or discomfort occurring over at least 6 months with 2 or more of 3 characteristics (relief with defecation, onset associated with change in stool frequency, or onset associated with change in stool form). The subtype of IBS with constipation was defined by the presence of 2 of 3 symptoms (less than 3 spontaneous bowel movements per week, more than 25% hard stools, more than 25% of spontaneous bowel movements associated with straining). Patients were randomized to receive lubiprostone 8 mcg twice daily (16 mcg daily) or placebo twice daily for 12 weeks. The primary end point was the number of "overall responders" as determined by patients' response (frequency of IBS) to a questionnaire. The percentage of patients qualifying as overall responders was 13.8 and 12.1% in study 1 and 2, respectively, while percentages of overall responders were 7.8 and 5.7% in those receiving placebo in study 1 and 2, respectively. In study 1, a rebound effect was not observed upon withdrawal of the drug following 12 weeks of treatment. Results of an open-label extension of these studies found that lubiprostone remained safe and effective for an additional 36 weeks.

Dosage and Administration

■ **General** Lubiprostone is administered orally twice daily with food and water. Food may decrease peak plasma concentrations of the drug by 55%; however, the clinical importance of this effect has not been elucidated and the manufacturer states that lubiprostone should be taken with food and water to reduce symptoms of nausea.

■ **Dosage** Clinicians and patients (with chronic idiopathic constipation or irritable bowel syndrome with constipation) should periodically assess the need for continued therapy.

Chronic Idiopathic Constipation The recommended adult dosage of lubiprostone for the treatment of chronic idiopathic constipation is 24 mcg twice daily.

Because dose-dependent nausea (sometimes severe) occurred frequently in patients receiving lubiprostone 24 mcg twice daily, dosage reduction to 24 mcg daily was allowed in such patients in the open-label, long-term studies.

Irritable Bowel Syndrome with Constipation in Women The recommended adult dosage of lubiprostone for the treatment of irritable bowel syndrome with constipation in women is 8 mcg twice daily.

■ **Special Populations** No special population recommendations at this time.

Cautions

■ **Contraindications** Known hypersensitivity to lubiprostone or any ingredient in the formulation. Known or suspected mechanical GI obstruction.

■ **Warnings/Precautions** ***Warnings*** **GI Obstruction.** Patients with symptoms suggestive of mechanical GI obstruction should be evaluated thoroughly to confirm absence of such obstruction prior to initiating lubiprostone therapy. (See Cautions: Contraindications.)

Fetal/Neonatal Morbidity and Mortality. Women of childbearing potential should have a negative pregnancy test prior to receiving lubiprostone and should use an effective method of contraception during therapy with the drug.

General Precautions **GI Effects.** Dose-dependent nausea may occur. Symptoms may be reduced by coadministration with food and water.

Possible diarrhea (may be severe). Lubiprostone should not be prescribed to patients experiencing severe diarrhea.

Respiratory Effects. Possible dyspnea (may result in discontinuance of drug). Acute onset of symptoms (e.g., sensation of chest tightness, difficulty in breathing) may occur, generally within 30–60 minutes after taking first dose. Symptoms usually resolve within a few hours; however, they frequently recur with subsequent doses.

Specific Populations **Pregnancy.** Category C. (See Users Guide.) (Also see Fetal/Neonatal Morbidity and Mortality under Warnings/Precautions: Warnings, in Cautions.)

Lactation. Not known whether lubiprostone is distributed into human milk; discontinue nursing or the drug, taking into account the importance of the drug to the woman.

Pediatric Use. Safety and efficacy not established in patients younger than 18 years of age.

Geriatric Use. Efficacy of lubiprostone in geriatric patients (65 years of age and older) with chronic idiopathic constipation was consistent with efficacy of the drug in the overall study population. Geriatric patients experienced a lower incidence (18 versus 29%) of associated nausea than the overall study population.

Experience in those 65 years of age or older with irritable bowel syndrome (IBS) with constipation was insufficient to determine whether they respond differently from younger adults. Safety profile of lubiprostone in these patients was consistent with the safety profile in the overall study population.

Hepatic or Renal Impairment. Lubiprostone has not been studied in patients with renal or hepatic impairment.

■ **Common Adverse Effects** Adverse effects reported in about 2% or more of patients receiving lubiprostone for the management of chronic idiopathic constipation include nausea, diarrhea, headache, abdominal distention, abdominal pain, flatulence, vomiting, dizziness, edema, loose stools, abdominal discomfort (abdominal tenderness, abdominal rigidity, GI discomfort), dyspepsia, chest discomfort/pain, dyspnea, and fatigue.

Adverse effects reported in about 3% or more of women receiving lubiprostone for the treatment of IBS with constipation include nausea, diarrhea, abdominal pain, and abdominal distention.

Drug Interactions

■ **Drugs Affecting or Metabolized by Hepatic Microsomal Enzymes** Pharmacokinetic interactions unlikely. In vitro, lubiprostone does not inhibit cytochrome P-450 (CYP) isoenzymes 1A2, 2A6, 2B6, 2C9, 2C19, 2D6, 2E1, or 3A4 or induce isoenzymes 1A2, 2B6, 2C9, or 3A4. Lubiprostone is not metabolized by CYP isoenzymes.

■ **Highly Protein-bound Drugs** Pharmacokinetic interaction unlikely.

Description

Lubiprostone, a bicyclic fatty acid that selectively activates intestinal ClC-2 chloride channels, increases intestinal chloride and fluid secretion without affecting serum sodium and potassium concentrations. Lubiprostone activates the ClC-2 chloride channel which is located on the apical (luminal) membrane of the human intestinal epithelium, independent of the actions of protein kinase A.

Decreased intestinal motility is a possible cause of chronic idiopathic constipation. Lubiprostone increases intestinal motility by increasing intestinal fluid secretion, consequently increasing the passage of stool and alleviating symptoms of chronic idiopathic constipation. Activation of ClC-2 by lubiprostone also may stimulate recovery of mucosal barrier function by restoring tight junction protein complexes in the intestine.

The drug also delays gastric emptying, which may cause nausea (the most common adverse effect associated with lubiprostone therapy).

Lubiprostone has low systemic bioavailability following oral administration, and plasma concentrations of the drug are below the limit of quantitation (10 pg/mL).

Lubiprostone is rapidly and extensively metabolized, probably in the stomach and jejunum, by processes mediated by carbonyl reductase; hepatic cytochrome P-450 enzymes are not involved in the metabolism of the drug. About 60% of an orally administered dose is excreted in the urine within 24 hours, while about 30% of such dose is excreted in feces within 168 hours.

Advice to Patients

Advise patients to take the drug twice daily (morning and evening) with food and water.

Importance of advising patients to swallow capsules whole without chewing or breaking apart.

Importance of advising patients that nausea may occur. Administration of the drug with food and water may reduce symptoms of nausea. Advise patients to contact a clinician if nausea becomes severe.

Clinicians and patients should periodically assess the need for continued treatment.

Importance of advising patients that diarrhea may occur. Advise patients to notify a clinician and not to take lubiprostone if they experience severe diarrhea.

Advise patients that dyspnea may occur; notify clinician if dyspnea becomes severe.

Importance of women informing clinicians if they are or plan to become pregnant or plan to breast-feed. Advise pregnant women of risk to the fetus. Importance of using effective method of contraception.

Importance of informing clinicians of existing or contemplated concomitant therapy, including prescription and OTC drugs, as well as any concomitant illnesses.

Importance of informing patients of other important precautionary information. (See Cautions.)

Overview® (see Users Guide). For additional information on this drug until a more detailed monograph is developed and published, the manufacturer's labeling should be consulted. It is *essential* that the manufacturer's labeling be consulted for more detailed information on usual cautions, precautions, contraindications, potential drug interactions, laboratory test interferences, and acute toxicity.

Preparations

Excipients in commercially available drug preparations may have clinically important effects in some individuals; consult specific product labeling for details.

Lubiprostone

Oral		
Capsules	8 mcg	Amitiza®, Sucampo
	24 mcg	Amitiza®, Sucampo

Methylnaltrexone Bromide

■ Methylnaltrexone bromide is a peripherally acting μ-opiate receptor antagonist.

Uses

■ **Opiate-induced Constipation** Methylnaltrexone bromide tablets or injection is used for the management of opiate-induced constipation in patients with chronic non-cancer-related pain, including those with chronic pain related to prior cancer or its treatment who do not require frequent (e.g., weekly) increases in opiate dosage. Methylnaltrexone bromide injection also is used for the management of opiate-induced constipation in patients with advanced illness or pain caused by active cancer who require opiate dosage escalation for palliative care.

Experience in Patients with Advanced Illness Efficacy of methylnaltrexone bromide injection for the management of opiate-induced constipation in patients with advanced illness has been established in 2 randomized, double-blind, placebo-controlled studies in 287 patients with advanced illness who were receiving palliative therapy and were suffering from opiate-induced constipation (defined as fewer than 3 bowel movements in the preceding week or no bowel movement for more than 2 days). Patients in these studies received a stable opiate regimen for at least 3 days prior to randomization and were maintained on their regular laxative therapy for at least 3 days prior to study entry and throughout the study.

In the first study, patients received a single subcutaneous dose of methylnaltrexone bromide (0.15 or 0.3 mg/kg) or placebo during the initial double-blind phase of the study, followed by 4 weeks of open-label treatment with methylnaltrexone bromide (0.075–0.3 mg/kg administered subcutaneously as needed, but no more frequently than one dose in a 24-hour period). During the single-dose, double-blind comparison, laxation occurred within 4 hours of the dose without the need for additional ("rescue") laxatives in a greater proportion of patients receiving methylnaltrexone bromide 0.15 or 0.3 mg/kg (62 or 58%, respectively) compared with those receiving placebo (14%).

In the second study, patients received subcutaneous doses of methylnaltrexone bromide (0.15 mg/kg) or placebo every other day for 2 weeks; if by day 8 patients experienced fewer than 3 rescue-free laxations, the dose of methylnaltrexone bromide could be increased to 0.3 mg/kg. A greater proportion of patients receiving methylnaltrexone, compared with those receiving placebo, experienced laxation without the need for additional ("rescue") laxatives within 4 hours of the first dose (48 versus 16%, respectively) and within 4 hours after at least 2 of the first 4 doses (52 versus 9%, respectively). The laxation response rate was consistent over all 7 doses during the 2-week double-blind period.

In both studies, approximately 30% of patients experienced laxation within 30 minutes of a dose of methylnaltrexone. There were no clinically important changes from baseline in pain scores or median daily opiate dosage in either the methylnaltrexone or placebo groups in either study. In these studies, no gender- or age-related differences in efficacy or safety were noted.

Following completion of both studies, 103 patients were enrolled in 2 open-label extension studies and received methylnaltrexone bromide for periods of up to 3 months. Response rates observed for methylnaltrexone during the double-blind phases of studies 1 and 2 were maintained during the 1-month open-label treatment period in study 1 and during the 2 open-label extension studies.

Experience in Patients with Chronic Non-cancer-related Pain Efficacy of methylnaltrexone bromide tablets or injection for the management of opiate-induced constipation in patients with chronic non-cancer-related pain has been established in 2 randomized, double-blind, placebo-controlled studies. In study 1, 803 patients received oral methylnaltrexone bromide (150, 300, or 450 mg once daily) or placebo for 4 weeks. In study 2, 460 patients received subcutaneous methylnaltrexone bromide (12 mg once daily or every other day) or placebo for 4 weeks. Patients (mean age 48–53 years, 60–63% female, 82–90% white) enrolled in these studies had received opiate analgesics for at least 1 month and had received a stable opiate regimen (equivalent to 50 mg or more of oral morphine sulfate daily) for at least 2 weeks prior to screening; the median baseline opiate dosage for each treatment group was equivalent to morphine sulfate 132–178 mg daily. Back pain was the most common indication for opiate analgesia in both studies; other commonly reported pain conditions were arthritis (including rheumatoid arthritis), neurologic or neuropathic pain, joint or extremity pain, and fibromyalgia. Opiate-induced constipation was defined as fewer than 3 spontaneous bowel movements per week during the 14-day screening period, with at least 25% of the bowel movements associated with a Bristol Stool Form Scale score of 1 or 2, straining, or a sensation of incomplete evacuation.

No laxatives other than a "rescue" laxative regimen given for an episode of no bowel movements for 3 days were permitted during the studies. The laxative regimen consisted of up to 3 or 4 bisacodyl tablets (in study 1 or study 2, respectively) taken orally once during a 24-hour period, 5 hours or longer and up to 8 hours following oral administration of the study drug in study 1 and at least 4 hours following injection of the study drug in study 2. In study 1, if bisacodyl did not result in a bowel movement within 24 hours, a second dose of bisacodyl or an enema was allowed; enema use was permitted after bisacodyl had failed at least once.

FDA labeling of oral methylnaltrexone for the management of opiate-induced constipation in patients with chronic non-cancer-related pain was based on response, a secondary end point in study 1 that was defined as 3 or more spontaneous bowel movements per week and an increase from baseline of 1 or more spontaneous bowel movements per week for at least 3 of the 4 study weeks, for the highest studied dosage. On this end point, methylnaltrexone bromide 450 mg daily was superior to placebo (response rate of 52 versus 38%).

FDA labeling of methylnaltrexone injection for the management of opiate-induced constipation in patients with chronic non-cancer-related pain also was based on response, which was defined as 3 or more spontaneous bowel movements per week for each of the 4 study weeks. On this end point, methylnaltrexone bromide 12 mg daily was superior to placebo; response rates for once-daily methylnaltrexone, alternate-day methylnaltrexone, and placebo were 59, 45, and 38%, respectively. In addition, 33% of patients who received the drug once daily experienced a spontaneous bowel movement within 4 hours following the first dose and approximately 50% experienced a spontaneous bowel movement prior to the second dose of the drug. Adverse effects, including nausea, diarrhea, vomiting, tremor, sensation of body temperature change, piloerection, and chills, were reported more frequently with alternate-day than with once-daily therapy.

Dosage and Administration

■ **General** In patients with chronic non-cancer-related pain and opiate-induced constipation, all maintenance laxative therapy should be discontinued prior to initiating methylnaltrexone; laxatives may be used as needed if the patient's response to methylnaltrexone is suboptimal after 3 days of therapy. Patients with chronic non-cancer-related pain who have been receiving opiates for less than 4 weeks may be less responsive to methylnaltrexone. If the opiate regimen is changed in patients with chronic non-cancer-related pain, the continued need for methylnaltrexone therapy should be reevaluated to avoid potential adverse effects (e.g., diarrhea).

Methylnaltrexone should be discontinued if therapy with opiate analgesics is discontinued.

■ **Administration** For the management of opiate-induced constipation, methylnaltrexone bromide is administered orally or by subcutaneous injection in patients with chronic non-cancer-related pain and by subcutaneous injection in those with advanced illness. Patients should be in close proximity to toilet facilities following administration of the drug.

Subcutaneous Administration Methylnaltrexone bromide is administered by subcutaneous injection into the upper arm, abdomen, or thigh; injection sites should be rotated. If the patient is self-administering the drug, injection sites in the abdomen and thigh are preferred; the upper arm should be used only if another person is administering the injection. Injections should not be made into areas where skin is bruised, tender, red, or hard, or where scars or stretch marks are present.

Methylnaltrexone bromide injection is commercially available in prefilled syringes and single-use vials. The prefilled syringes should be used only in patients who require an 8- or 12-mg dose of the drug; for administration of all other doses, the vials should be used. Once methylnaltrexone bromide is withdrawn from the vial into a syringe, the dose should be administered immediately or, if immediate administration is not possible, the syringe should be stored at room temperature and the dose administered within 24 hours. Any unused portion in the vial should be discarded. The prefilled syringes should not be removed from the tray until just prior to administration.

Methylnaltrexone bromide injection should be inspected visually for particulate matter and discoloration prior to administration. Methylnaltrexone bromide should not be administered if discoloration or particulates are observed.

Oral Administration Methylnaltrexone bromide tablets should be administered with water on an empty stomach at least 30 minutes before the first meal of the day.

■ **Dosage** ***Opiate-induced Constipation in Patients with Advanced Illness*** When methylnaltrexone bromide is used for the management of opiate-induced constipation in adults with advanced illness, dosage of the drug is based on the patient's weight. For patients weighing 38–61 kg, the recommended dosage is 8 mg (0.4 mL) given by subcutaneous injection as a single dose every other day as needed. For patients weighing 62–114 kg, the recommended dosage is 12 mg (0.6 mL) given as a single dose every other day as needed. For patients weighing less than 38 kg or more than 114 kg, the recommended dosage is 0.15 mg/kg given as a single dose every other day as needed. The injection volume for these patients is determined by multiplying the patient's weight in *kg* by 0.0075 and rounding up to the nearest 0.1 mL.

No more than one dose should be administered in any 24-hour period.

Opiate-induced Constipation in Patients with Chronic Non-cancer-related Pain For the management of opiate-induced constipation in adults with chronic non-cancer-related pain, the recommended dosage of methylnaltrexone bromide is 12 mg by subcutaneous injection once daily or 450 mg orally once daily. In patients with chronic non-cancer-related pain, subcutaneous therapy with methylnaltrexone bromide 12 mg every other day is not recommended, since adverse effects have been reported more frequently with alternate-day than with once-daily subcutaneous administration. (See Experience in Patients with Chronic Non-cancer-related Pain under Uses: Opiate-induced Constipation.)

■ **Special Populations** Dosage adjustments of methylnaltrexone bromide are not required in patients with mild renal or hepatic impairment. Reduced oral or subcutaneous dosage of the drug is recommended in patients with moderate or severe renal impairment. Patients with moderate hepatic impairment may receive the usual subcutaneous dosage of methylnaltrexone bromide but should receive a reduced oral dosage of the drug. In patients with severe hepatic impairment, reduced oral or subcutaneous dosage is recommended in those with chronic non-cancer-related pain. The manufacturer makes no specific dosage recommendations for patients with advanced illness and severe hepatic impairment. Dosage adjustments based solely on age are not required in geriatric patients. (See Specific Populations under Cautions: Warnings/Precautions.)

In patients with moderate or severe renal impairment (creatinine clearance less than 60 mL/minute) and chronic non-cancer-related pain, the recommended dosage of methylnaltrexone bromide for the management of opiate-induced constipation is 6 mg by subcutaneous injection once daily or 150 mg orally once daily.

Patients with moderate or severe renal impairment and advanced illness should receive one-half the usual recommended subcutaneous dosage. The recommended dosage in such patients is 4 mg (0.2 mL) every other day as needed in those weighing 38–61 kg, 6 mg (0.3 mL) every other day as needed in those weighing 62–114 kg, and 0.075 mg/kg every other day as needed in those weighing less than 38 kg or more than 114 kg. The injection volume for these patients is determined by multiplying the patient's weight in *kg* by 0.00375 and rounding up to the nearest 0.1 mL.

In patients with moderate or severe hepatic impairment (Child-Pugh class B or C) and chronic non-cancer-related pain, a reduced oral dosage of 150 mg once daily is recommended. In patients with severe hepatic impairment and chronic non-cancer-related pain, the recommended subcutaneous dosage is 4 mg (0.2 mL) once daily in those weighing 38–61 kg, 6 mg (0.3 mL) once daily in those weighing 62–114 kg, and 0.075 mg/kg once daily in those weighing less than 38 kg or more than 114 kg. The injection volume for these patients is determined by multiplying the patient's weight in *kg* by 0.00375 and rounding up to the nearest 0.1 mL.

Cautions

■ **Contraindications** Because of the potential for GI perforation, methylnaltrexone is contraindicated in patients with known or suspected GI obstruction and in patients at increased risk for recurrent GI obstruction (see GI Perforation under Cautions: Warnings/Precautions).

■ **Warnings/Precautions** ***GI Perforation*** GI perforation has been reported with use of methylnaltrexone in patients with advanced illness who have underlying conditions that may be associated with localized or diffuse reduction of structural integrity in the GI tract wall (e.g., peptic ulcer disease, Ogilvie's syndrome, diverticular disease, infiltrative GI tract malignancies or peritoneal metastases). Risks and benefits of methylnaltrexone therapy should be carefully considered in patients with these underlying conditions or with other conditions that might result in impaired integrity of the GI tract wall (e.g., Crohn's disease). Patients receiving methylnaltrexone should be monitored for the development of severe, persistent, or worsening abdominal pain. Methylnaltrexone should be discontinued if such symptoms occur.

Severe or Persistent Diarrhea If severe or persistent diarrhea occurs during methylnaltrexone therapy, discontinuance of the drug is recommended.

Opiate Withdrawal Symptoms consistent with opiate withdrawal (e.g., hyperhidrosis, chills, diarrhea, abdominal pain, anxiety, yawning) have occurred in patients receiving methylnaltrexone. Patients with disruptions in the blood-brain barrier may be at increased risk for opiate withdrawal or reduced analgesia; risks and benefits of methylnaltrexone therapy should be carefully considered in such patients, and these patients should be monitored for adequacy of analgesia and symptoms of opiate withdrawal.

Specific Populations **Pregnancy.** Because of the immature fetal blood-brain barrier, use of methylnaltrexone during pregnancy may precipitate opiate withdrawal in the fetus. Limited available data regarding use of the drug in pregnant women are insufficient to inform a drug-associated risk of major birth defects and spontaneous abortion. No adverse effects of the drug on embryofetal development have been observed in animal reproduction studies. Pregnant women should be advised of potential fetal risk.

Lactation. It is unknown whether methylnaltrexone is distributed into human milk, affects milk production, or affects nursing infants. Methylnaltrexone is distributed into milk in rats; the drug is detected in milk within 30 minutes after a single subcutaneous injection and is concentrated in milk (up to 24 times plasma concentrations) at 8 hours after administration. Because of the potential for serious adverse effects, including opiate withdrawal, in nursing infants, women should not breast-feed while receiving the drug.

Pediatric Use. Safety and efficacy of methylnaltrexone have not been established in children younger than 18 years of age.

Seizures, tremors, and labored breathing were observed in juvenile rats receiving IV methylnaltrexone for 13 weeks, and the juvenile animals exhibited greater sensitivity to adverse effects of the drug compared with adult animals. The toxicity profile in juvenile dogs was similar to that in adult dogs.

Geriatric Use. In clinical studies evaluating oral methylnaltrexone, 10% of patients were 65 years of age and older, while 2% were 75 years of age and older. In clinical studies evaluating methylnaltrexone injection, 28% of patients were 65 years of age and older, while 13% were 75 years of age and older. No overall differences in efficacy were observed in these studies between geriatric patients and younger adults. Although adverse effects were similar in geriatric patients and younger adults, a higher incidence of diarrhea was reported in geriatric patients receiving oral methylnaltrexone. Following IV administration of a single 24-mg dose of methylnaltrexone bromide in healthy individuals, clearance of the drug was decreased by approximately 20% and systemic exposure (area under the plasma concentration-time curve [AUC]) was increased by 26% in geriatric adults compared with younger adults. Based on these clinical and pharmacokinetic findings, geriatric patients should be monitored for adverse effects while receiving methylnaltrexone therapy, but dosage adjustments based on age are not necessary.

Hepatic Impairment. Following subcutaneous administration of a single 0.3-mg/kg dose of methylnaltrexone bromide, AUC and peak plasma concentrations of the drug were not altered substantially in patients with mild to moderate hepatic impairment compared with healthy individuals. Methylnaltrexone injection has not been evaluated in patients with severe hepatic impairment. Patients with severe hepatic impairment should be monitored for adverse effects.

Following oral administration of a single 450-mg dose of methylnaltrexone bromide, peak plasma concentrations of the drug were increased by 1.7-, 4.8-, or 3.8-fold in patients with mild, moderate, or severe hepatic impairment, respectively, compared with individuals with normal hepatic function; AUC was increased by approximately 2.1-fold in patients with moderate or severe hepatic impairment, but AUC in patients with mild hepatic impairment was similar to that in individuals with normal hepatic function.

Dosage adjustments are necessary based on the route of administration and degree of hepatic impairment. (See Dosage and Administration: Special Populations.)

Renal Impairment. Following subcutaneous administration of a single 0.3-mg/kg dose of methylnaltrexone bromide, AUC of the drug was increased by 1.3-, 1.7-, or 1.9-fold in patients with mild, moderate, or severe renal impairment, respectively, compared with individuals with normal renal function; renal impairment did not substantially alter peak plasma concentrations of the drug. Dosage reduction is recommended in patients with moderate or severe renal impairment. (See Dosage and Administration: Special Populations.) Methylnaltrexone has not been evaluated in patients with end-stage renal disease requiring dialysis.

■ **Common Adverse Effects** Adverse effects reported in 5% or more of patients with opiate-induced constipation and advanced illness receiving methylnaltrexone bromide injection, and at an incidence at least twice that reported with placebo, include transient abdominal pain, flatulence, nausea, dizziness, and diarrhea.

Adverse effects reported in 2% or more of patients with opiate-induced constipation and chronic non-cancer-related pain receiving oral methylnaltrexone, and at an incidence greater than that reported with placebo, include abdominal pain, diarrhea, headache, abdominal distention, vomiting, hyperhidrosis, anxiety, muscle spasms, rhinorrhea, and chills.

Adverse effects reported in 1% or more of patients with opiate-induced constipation and chronic non-cancer-related pain receiving methylnaltrexone injection, and at an incidence greater than that reported with placebo, include abdominal pain, nausea, diarrhea, hyperhidrosis, hot flush, tremor, and chills.

Drug Interactions

Methylnaltrexone does not substantially inhibit or induce cytochrome P-450 (CYP) isoenzymes 1A2, 2A6, 2B6, 2C9, 2C19, or 3A4 in vitro. In addition, methylnaltrexone does not induce CYP2E1 in vitro. Major metabolites of methylnaltrexone (i.e., methylnaltrexone sulfate, methyl-6α-naltrexol, methyl-6β-naltrexol) do not inhibit CYP isoenzymes 1A2, 2B6, 2C8, 2C9, 2C19, 2D6, or 3A4, nor do they induce CYP isoenzymes 1A2, 2B6, or 3A4 in vitro.

Results of in vitro studies indicate that methylnaltrexone and its major metabolites are not likely to cause clinically important interactions via inhibition of P-glycoprotein (P-gp), breast cancer resistance protein (BCRP), multidrug resistance protein 2 (MRP2), organic anion transport protein (OATP) 1B1 or 1B3, organic cation transporter (OCT) 1 or 2, organic anion transporter (OAT) 1 or 3, or multidrug and toxin extrusion transporter (MATE) 1 or 2K at methylnaltrexone bromide dosages of 450 mg orally or 12 mg subcutaneously once daily.

Methylnaltrexone, methyl-6α-naltrexol, and methyl-6β-naltrexol are substrates of OCT1, OCT2, MATE1, and MATE2K in vitro. Methyl-6α-naltrexol also is a substrate of BCRP, and methylnaltrexone sulfate is a substrate of MATE2K and a potential substrate of BCRP. Neither methylnaltrexone nor methyl-6β-naltrexol is a substrate of BCRP. In addition, methylnaltrexone sulfate is not a substrate of OCT1, OCT2, or MATE1. Neither methylnaltrexone nor its 3 major metabolites are substrates of P-gp, MRP2, OATP1B1, OATP1B3, OAT1, or OAT3.

■ **Cimetidine** In healthy individuals, concomitant administration of cimetidine (400 mg every 8 hours for 6 days) (an inhibitor of renal organic cation secretion) and methylnaltrexone bromide (single 24-mg IV dose) increased peak plasma concentration and area under the plasma concentration-time curve (AUC) of methylnaltrexone by 10% and decreased renal clearance of methylnaltrexone by approximately 40%; the change was not considered clinically important.

■ **Dextromethorphan** In healthy individuals, a single 0.3-mg/kg subcutaneous dose of methylnaltrexone bromide did not substantially affect the metabolism of dextromethorphan, a CYP2D6 substrate.

■ **Opiate Antagonists** Concomitant use of methylnaltrexone and other opiate antagonists should be avoided because of the potential for additive opiate receptor antagonism and an increased risk of opiate withdrawal.

Description

Methylnaltrexone bromide is a peripherally acting μ-opiate receptor antagonist. The drug is a quaternary amine derivative of the μ-receptor antagonist naltrexone.

Opiates slow intestinal motility and increase GI transit time. The mechanism of action of methylnaltrexone in the management of opiate-induced constipation stems from the drug's ability to block μ-opiate receptors in the GI tract, blocking the intestinal smooth muscle relaxation caused by opiates and thereby reversing opiate-induced slowing of GI transit time. The drug does not readily cross the blood-brain barrier and therefore does not affect opiate analgesic activity or precipitate opiate withdrawal, as is observed with centrally active opiate antagonists (e.g., naltrexone, naloxone). Methylnaltrexone exhibits greater affinity for μ-opiate receptors than for κ-opiate receptors; the drug does not interact with δ-opiate receptors nor does it substantially bind to non-opiate receptors. Methylnaltrexone has 2–4% of the opiate antagonist activity and potency of naloxone. Methylnaltrexone appears to possess some μ-receptor agonist activity. In vitro studies have identified some differences in how methylnaltrexone and alvimopan (both peripheral μ-receptor antagonists) interact with opiate receptors (e.g., differences in binding affinity and functional activity) (see Description in Alvimopan 56:92); however, it remains to be determined whether these differences are clinically important.

Following subcutaneous injection or oral administration of methylnaltrexone bromide, peak plasma concentrations and area under the concentration-time curve (AUC) of the drug increase in a dose-proportional manner over oral and subcutaneous dose ranges of 150–450 mg and 0.15–0.5 mg/kg, respectively. No substantial accumulation of the drug occurs following repeated subcutaneous (12 mg once daily) or oral (450 mg once daily) administration. Peak plasma concentrations are achieved within approximately 0.5 or 1.5 hours following subcutaneous or oral administration, respectively. The absolute bioavailability of methylnaltrexone bromide tablets has not been established. Administration of a single 450-mg oral dose of the drug with a high-fat meal (approximately 800–1000 calories, with 60% of calories from fat) decreased peak plasma concentration and AUC by 60 and 43%, respectively, and delayed the time to peak plasma concentration by 2 hours. The drug is 11–15% bound to plasma proteins. Following oral administration of a single 450-mg dose of methylnaltrexone bromide, concentrations of the drug decline in a multiphasic manner with a terminal half-life of approximately 15 hours.

The primary metabolic pathways of methylnaltrexone involve metabolism by aldo-keto reductase 1C enzymes to form methyl-6-naltrexol isomers and conjugation by sulfotransferase (SULT) 1E1 and 2A1 to form methylnaltrexone sulfate; the drug is not appreciably demethylated to form naltrexone. Methylnaltrexone does not undergo first-pass hepatic metabolism following subcutaneous administration, and systemic exposure to methylnaltrexone metabolites is greater following oral administration of a single 450-mg dose than following subcutaneous injection of a single 12-mg dose. The mean steady-state ratio of metabolite AUC to methylnaltrexone AUC was 30, 19, or 9% for methylnaltrexone sulfate, methyl-6α-naltrexol, or methyl-6β-naltrexol, respectively, following subcutaneous administration of 12 mg once daily and 79, 38, or 21%, respectively, following oral administration of 450 mg once daily. Methylnaltrexone sulfate is a weak μ-opiate receptor antagonist; methyl-6α-naltrexol and methyl-6β-naltrexol are active μ-opiate receptor antagonists.

Following IV administration of radiolabeled methylnaltrexone bromide, approximately 44% of the administered radioactivity was recovered in urine over 24 hours; several metabolites were detected, none of which was recovered in urine in amounts exceeding 6% of the administered radioactivity. After 7 days, 71% of administered radioactivity was recovered (54% in urine and 17% in feces). Following oral administration of methylnaltrexone bromide 450 mg once daily, approximately 1% of the administered dose was recovered in urine as unchanged drug on both day 1 and day 7. Methylnaltrexone appears to undergo active renal secretion.

Advice to Patients

Importance of patient and/or caregiver reading the manufacturer's patient information. Importance of discontinuing methylnaltrexone therapy following cessation of opiate analgesic therapy. Patients should be advised to inform their clinician if opiate therapy for chronic non-cancer-related pain is altered.

Importance of instructing patient and/or caregiver regarding proper dosage and administration of methylnaltrexone bromide injection, including the use of aseptic technique and proper disposal of needles and syringes, if it is determined that the patient and/or caregiver is competent to safely administer the drug.

Importance of advising patients with advanced illness or their caregivers to inject one dose of methylnaltrexone every other day as needed and to never administer more than one dose in a 24-hour period.

Importance of advising patients with chronic non-cancer-related pain to inject one dose of methylnaltrexone daily or to take methylnaltrexone tablets with water on an empty stomach at least 30 minutes prior to the first meal of the day.

Importance of informing patients that close proximity to a toilet is advised after drug administration.

Importance of advising patients with chronic non-cancer-related pain that they should discontinue all maintenance laxative therapy prior to initiation of methylnaltrexone and that laxatives may be used on an as-needed basis if response to methylnaltrexone is suboptimal following 3 days of therapy with the drug.

Possible risk of GI perforation. Importance of discontinuing methylnaltrexone and promptly seeking medical attention if unusually severe, persistent, or worsening abdominal pain occurs.

Importance of advising patients that symptoms consistent with opiate withdrawal (e.g., sweating, chills, diarrhea, abdominal pain, anxiety, yawning) may occur.

Importance of discontinuing methylnaltrexone and informing the clinician if severe or persistent diarrhea occurs.

Importance of women informing clinicians if they are or plan to become pregnant or plan to breast-feed. Women should be informed that methylnaltrexone use during pregnancy may precipitate opiate withdrawal in the fetus because the fetal blood-brain barrier is immature. Women also should be advised *not* to breast-feed while receiving methylnaltrexone because of the potential for opiate withdrawal in nursing infants.

Importance of informing clinicians of existing or contemplated concomitant therapy, including prescription and OTC drugs. Importance of informing patients of other important precautionary information. (See Cautions.)

Overview® (see Users Guide). For additional information on this drug until a more detailed monograph is developed and published, the manufacturer's labeling should be consulted. It is *essential* that the manufacturer's labeling be consulted for more detailed information on usual cautions, precautions, contraindications, potential drug interactions, laboratory test interferences, and acute toxicity.

Preparations

Excipients in commercially available drug preparations may have clinically important effects in some individuals; consult specific product labeling for details.

Methylnaltrexone Bromide

Oral		
Tablets, film-coated	150 mg	**Relistor®**, Salix
Parenteral		
Injection, for subcutaneous use	8 mg/0.4 mL	**Relistor®** (available as disposable prefilled syringes with needle-guard system), Salix
	12 mg/0.6 mL	**Relistor®** (available as single-dose vials and as disposable prefilled syringes with needle-guard system), Salix

Naldemedine Tosylate

■ Naldemedine tosylate is a peripherally acting μ-opiate receptor antagonist.

Uses

■ **Opiate-induced Constipation** Naldemedine tosylate is used for the management of opiate-induced constipation in patients with chronic non-cancer-related pain, including those with chronic pain related to prior cancer or its treatment who do not require frequent (e.g., weekly) increases in opiate dosage.

Safety and efficacy of naldemedine were established in 2 identical, randomized, double-blind, placebo-controlled studies (COMPOSE-1 and COMPOSE-2) in 1100 patients (mean age of 54 years, 59% women, 80% white) with chronic non-cancer-related pain and active opiate-induced constipation who had received a stable opiate dosage (equivalent to 30 mg or more of oral morphine sulfate daily) for at least 4 weeks prior to study enrollment. Opiate-induced constipation was defined as no more than 4 spontaneous bowel movements over 14 consecutive days and fewer than 3 spontaneous bowel movements per week with at least 25% of spontaneous bowel movements associated with straining, hard or lumpy stools, a sensation of incomplete evacuation, and/or a sensation of anorectal obstruction or blockage. Patients with evidence of substantial structural abnormalities of the GI tract, those with no bowel movements during a 3-week period (the 2-week qualifying period and the preceding 7 days), and patients who had never received laxatives for the management of opiate-induced constipation were excluded from these studies. Patients in these studies received naldemedine 0.2 mg once daily or placebo without regard to food for 12 weeks. No laxatives other than a "rescue" laxative regimen (bisacodyl for an episode of no bowel movements for 72 hours, followed by one-time use of an enema if no bowel movement occurred within 24 hours following bisacodyl administration) were permitted during the studies.

Patients enrolled in the studies had received their current opiate analgesic for an average of approximately 5 years; the mean baseline opiate dosage was equivalent to morphine sulfate 121–132 mg daily. Back or neck pain (61%) was the most common indication for opiate analgesia. The mean baseline number of spontaneous bowel movements was 1.2–1.3 per week.

The primary end point of the studies was response, defined as 3 or more spontaneous bowel movements per week and a change from baseline of 1 or more spontaneous bowel movements per week for at least 9 of the 12 study weeks and at least 3 of the final 4 weeks of the study. Response to naldemedine was superior to the placebo response in both studies; response rates for naldemedine and placebo were 48 and 35%, respectively, in COMPOSE-1 and 53 and 34%, respectively, in COMPOSE-2.

Secondary end points included the change in frequency of spontaneous bowel movements, spontaneous bowel movements without straining, and complete spontaneous bowel movements per week from baseline to the final 2 weeks of treatment, as well as the change in frequency of spontaneous bowel movements per week from baseline to week 1 of treatment. On each of these secondary end points, naldemedine was superior to placebo. From baseline to the final 2 weeks of treatment, spontaneous bowel movements, spontaneous bowel movements without straining, and complete spontaneous bowel movements in naldemedine-treated patients versus placebo recipients increased in frequency by a mean of 3.1 versus 2, 1.3 versus 0.7, and 2.3 versus 1.5 bowel movements per week, respectively, in COMPOSE-1 and by 3.3 versus 2.1, 1.8 versus 1.1, and 2.6 versus 1.6 bowel movements per week, respectively, in COMPOSE-2. From baseline to week 1 of treatment, spontaneous bowel movements in naldemedine-treated patients versus placebo recipients increased in frequency by a mean of 3.3 versus 1.3 and by 3.7 versus 1.6 bowel movements per week in these respective studies.

Dosage and Administration

■ **General** Changes in the analgesic dosing regimen are not required prior to initiation of naldemedine therapy. Patients receiving opiates for less than 4 weeks may be less responsive to naldemedine therapy. Naldemedine should be discontinued if therapy with opiate analgesics is discontinued.

■ **Administration** Naldemedine tosylate is administered orally without regard to food.

■ **Dosage** Dosage of naldemedine tosylate is expressed in terms of naldemedine.

The recommended adult dosage of naldemedine for the management of opiate-induced constipation in patients with chronic non-cancer-related pain is 0.2 mg once daily.

■ **Special Populations** No dosage adjustment of naldemedine is required in patients with mild or moderate hepatic impairment. Use of naldemedine should be avoided in patients with severe hepatic impairment. The manufacturer makes no specific dosage recommendations for geriatric patients or patients with renal impairment. (See Specific Populations under Cautions: Warnings/Precautions.)

Cautions

■ **Contraindications** Because of the potential for GI perforation, naldemedine is contraindicated in patients with known or suspected GI obstruction and in patients at increased risk for recurrent GI obstruction. (See GI Perforation under Cautions: Warnings/Precautions.)

Naldemedine also is contraindicated in patients with known hypersensitivity to the drug.

■ **Warnings/Precautions** ***GI Perforation*** GI perforation has been reported with use of methylnaltrexone, another peripherally acting opiate antagonist, in patients with underlying conditions that may be associated with localized or diffuse reduction of structural integrity in the GI tract wall (e.g., peptic ulcer disease, Ogilvie's syndrome, diverticular disease, infiltrative GI tract malignancies or peritoneal metastases). Risks and benefits of naldemedine therapy should be carefully considered in patients with these conditions or with other conditions that might result in impaired integrity of the GI tract wall (e.g., Crohn's disease). Patients receiving naldemedine should be monitored for the development of severe, persistent, or worsening abdominal pain. Naldemedine should be discontinued if such symptoms occur.

Opiate Withdrawal Manifestations consistent with opiate withdrawal, including hyperhidrosis, chills, increased lacrimation, hot flush/flushing, pyrexia, sneezing, feeling cold, abdominal pain, diarrhea, nausea, and vomiting, have been reported in patients receiving naldemedine.

Pooled data from the COMPOSE-1 and COMPOSE-2 studies indicated that the incidence of opiate-withdrawal manifestations (defined as same-day or consecutive-day occurrence of 3 or more adverse effects potentially related to opiate withdrawal) over 12 weeks of treatment was similar (1%) in patients receiving naldemedine and those receiving placebo. In a long-term (52-week) safety study, opiate-withdrawal manifestations occurred in 3 or 1% of patients receiving naldemedine or placebo, respectively. In most naldemedine-treated patients, the incidence of withdrawal manifestations confined solely to the GI tract was approximately equivalent to that of combined GI and non-GI manifestations.

Patients with disruptions in the blood-brain barrier may be at increased risk for opiate withdrawal or reduced analgesia; risks and benefits of naldemedine therapy should be carefully considered in such patients, and these patients should be monitored for symptoms of opiate withdrawal.

Sensitivity Reactions Hypersensitivity reactions, including bronchospasm and rash, have been reported in patients receiving naldemedine.

Specific Populations **Pregnancy.** Naldemedine should be used in pregnant women only if the potential benefits justify the potential risk to the fetus. There are no adequate and well-controlled studies of naldemedine in pregnant women. Naldemedine crosses the placenta; because of the immature fetal blood-brain barrier, use of naldemedine during pregnancy may precipitate opiate withdrawal in the fetus. No adverse effects of the drug on embryofetal development have been observed in animal reproduction studies.

Lactation. It is not known whether naldemedine is distributed into human milk, affects milk production, or affects the breast-fed infant. Naldemedine is distributed into milk in rats. Because of the potential for serious adverse effects, including opiate withdrawal, in nursing infants, a decision should be made whether to discontinue nursing or the drug, taking into account the importance of the drug to the woman. If naldemedine is discontinued, nursing may be resumed 3 days after the final dose of the drug.

Pediatric Use. Safety and efficacy of naldemedine have not been established in pediatric patients.

Geriatric Use. In clinical studies, 16% of patients who received naldemedine were 65 years of age and older, while 3% were 75 years of age and older. Although no overall differences in safety and efficacy were observed between geriatric patients and younger adults, the possibility that some older patients may exhibit increased sensitivity to the drug cannot be ruled out. A population pharmacokinetic analysis revealed no age-related differences in the pharmacokinetics of naldemedine.

Hepatic Impairment. The pharmacokinetic profile of naldemedine in patients with mild or moderate (Child-Pugh class A or B) hepatic impairment is similar to that in individuals with normal hepatic function. The effect of severe (Child-Pugh class C) hepatic impairment on the pharmacokinetics of naldemedine has not been established. Use of naldemedine should be avoided in patients with severe hepatic impairment.

Renal Impairment. The pharmacokinetic profile of naldemedine in patients with renal impairment (mild, moderate, or severe renal impairment or end-stage renal disease requiring hemodialysis) is similar to that in individuals with normal renal function. Naldemedine is not removed by hemodialysis.

■ **Common Adverse Effects** Adverse effects reported in 2% or more of patients receiving naldemedine and at a greater incidence than that observed with placebo include abdominal pain, diarrhea, nausea, vomiting, and gastroenteritis.

Drug Interactions

Naldemedine is metabolized principally by cytochrome P-450 (CYP) isoenzyme 3A4 (CYP3A4), with minimal contribution from uridine diphosphate-glucuronosyltransferase (UGT) 1A3; naldemedine also is a substrate of P-glycoprotein (P-gp). Naldemedine did not inhibit CYP isoenzyme 1A2, 2A6, 2B6, 2C8, 2C9, 2C19, 2D6, 2E1, 3A4/5, or 4A11 in vitro at clinically relevant concentrations. The drug also did not substantially induce CYP isoenzyme 1A2, 2B6, or 3A4 or UGT 1A2, 1A6, or 2B7.

Naldemedine does not inhibit organic anion transport protein (OATP) 1B1 or 1B3, organic cation transporter (OCT) 1 or 2, organic anion transporter (OAT) 1 or 3, breast cancer resistance protein (BCRP), or P-gp.

■ **Drugs Affecting Hepatic Microsomal Enzymes** Concomitant use of naldemedine with moderate (e.g., aprepitant, atazanavir, diltiazem, erythromycin, fluconazole) or potent (e.g., clarithromycin, itraconazole, ketoconazole, ritonavir, saquinavir) CYP3A inhibitors may result in increased plasma concentrations of naldemedine. Patients receiving naldemedine concomitantly with moderate or potent CYP3A inhibitors should be monitored for naldemedine-related adverse effects.

Potent CYP3A inducers (e.g., carbamazepine, phenytoin, rifampin, St. John's wort [*Hypericum perforatum*]) can substantially reduce plasma naldemedine concentrations and may decrease efficacy of the drug. Use of naldemedine with potent CYP3A inducers should be avoided.

■ **Drugs that Inhibit P-glycoprotein** Concomitant use of naldemedine and inhibitors of P-gp (e.g., amiodarone, captopril, cyclosporine, quercetin, quinidine, verapamil) may result in increased plasma concentrations of naldemedine. Patients receiving such concomitant therapy should be monitored for naldemedine-related adverse effects.

■ **Cyclosporine** Concomitant administration of naldemedine (single 0.4-mg dose) and the combined P-gp and weak CYP3A inhibitor cyclosporine (single 600-mg dose) increased the peak plasma concentration and area under the plasma concentration-time curve (AUC) of naldemedine by 45 and 78%, respectively. Patients receiving concomitant therapy with naldemedine and cyclosporine should be monitored for naldemedine-related adverse effects.

■ **Efavirenz** Pharmacokinetic simulations suggest that concomitant use of efavirenz, a moderate CYP3A inducer, decreases exposure to naldemedine by 43%. The clinical importance of this reduced exposure is unknown.

■ **Fluconazole** Concomitant administration of naldemedine (single 0.2-mg dose) and the combined P-gp and moderate CYP3A inhibitor fluconazole (400 mg on day 1, then 200 mg daily for 6 days) increased peak plasma concentration and AUC of naldemedine by 38 and 90%, respectively. Patients receiving concomitant therapy with naldemedine and fluconazole should be monitored for naldemedine-related adverse effects.

■ **Itraconazole** Concomitant administration of naldemedine (single 0.2-mg dose) and the combined P-gp and potent CYP3A inhibitor itraconazole (200 mg twice daily on day 1, then 200 mg once daily for 6 days) increased the peak plasma concentration and AUC of naldemedine by 12% and 2.91-fold, respectively. Patients receiving concomitant therapy with naldemedine and itraconazole should be monitored for naldemedine-related adverse effects.

■ **Opiate Antagonists** Concomitant use of naldemedine and other opiate antagonists should be avoided because of the potential for additive opiate receptor antagonism and an increased risk of opiate withdrawal.

■ **Rifampin** Concomitant administration of naldemedine (single 0.2-mg dose) and the combined P-gp and potent CYP3A inducer rifampin (600 mg once daily for 17 days) reduced the peak plasma concentration and AUC of naldemedine by approximately 38 and 83%, respectively. Concomitant use of rifampin and naldemedine may decrease the efficacy of naldemedine and should be avoided.

Description

Naldemedine tosylate, a derivative of naltrexone, is a peripherally acting μ-opiate receptor antagonist that also binds to and exhibits antagonistic activity at δ- and κ-opiate receptors. The mechanism of action of naldemedine in the management of opiate-induced constipation stems from the drug's ability to block μ-opiate receptors in the GI tract, thereby reversing opiate-induced constipating effects (e.g., slowing of GI transit). Naldemedine differs structurally from naltrexone by the addition of a large polar side chain that decreases the ability of the drug to cross the blood-brain barrier. In addition, naldemedine is a substrate of the P-glycoprotein (P-gp) efflux transporter. Because of these properties, CNS penetration of naldemedine is expected to be negligible at the recommended dosage, limiting the potential for interference with centrally mediated opiate analgesia.

Following oral administration in the fasted state, peak plasma concentrations of naldemedine are attained in approximately 45 minutes. Peak plasma concentration and area under the plasma concentration-time curve (AUC) increase in a dose-proportional or almost dose-proportional manner. Administration of naldemedine with a high-fat meal decreases the peak plasma concentration by approximately 35% and delays the time to peak plasma concentration by approximately 1.75 hours, but does not affect the extent of absorption. Naldemedine is 93–94% bound to plasma proteins and has a terminal elimination half-life of 11 hours. Naldemedine is metabolized principally by cytochrome P-450 isoenzyme 3A4 (CYP3A4), with minor contribution by uridine diphosphate-glucuronosyltransferase (UGT) isoenzyme 1A3 (UGT1A3), to form metabolites (nornaldemedine and naldemedine 3-glucuronide, respectively) that are less-potent opiate receptor antagonists. At usual clinical concentrations, these metabolites are not expected to contribute to the drug's pharmacologic effects. Naldemedine also is cleaved in the GI tract to form benzamidine and naldemedine carboxylic acid. Following oral administration of a radiolabeled dose of naldemedine, 57% of the dose was excreted in urine and 35% in feces, with 16–18% of the administered dose excreted as unchanged drug in urine. Benzamidine was the principal metabolite excreted in urine and feces, accounting for 32 and 20%, respectively, of the administered dose.

Advice to Patients

Importance of advising patients to read the manufacturer's medication guide.

Importance of discontinuing naldemedine following discontinuance of opiate analgesic therapy.

Possible risk of GI perforation. Importance of discontinuing naldemedine and promptly seeking medical attention if unusually severe, persistent, or worsening abdominal pain occurs.

Importance of advising patients that manifestations consistent with opiate withdrawal may occur and that they should inform their clinician if such manifestations occur.

Importance of women informing clinicians if they are or plan to become pregnant or plan to breast-feed. Women of child-bearing potential should be informed that naldemedine use during pregnancy may precipitate opiate withdrawal in the fetus because the fetal blood-brain barrier is immature. Women also should be advised *not* to breast-feed while receiving naldemedine and for 3 days following the final dose of the drug because of the potential for opiate withdrawal in nursing infants.

Importance of informing clinicians of existing or contemplated concomitant therapy, including prescription and OTC drugs and dietary supplements (especially those that alter activity of cytochrome P-450 isoenzyme 3A4 [CYP3A4]), as well as any concomitant illnesses.

Importance of informing patients of other important precautionary information. (See Cautions.)

Overview® (see Users Guide). For additional information on this drug until a more detailed monograph is developed and published, the manufacturer's labeling should be consulted. It is *essential* that the manufacturer's labeling be consulted for more detailed information on usual cautions, precautions, contraindications, potential drug interactions, laboratory test interferences, and acute toxicity.

Preparations

Excipients in commercially available drug preparations may have clinically important effects in some individuals; consult specific product labeling for details.

Naldemedine Tosylate

Oral

Tablets, film-coated	0.2 mg (of naldemedine)	**Symproic®**, Purdue

Naloxegol Oxalate

■ Naloxegol is a peripherally acting μ-opiate receptor antagonist.

Uses

■ **Opiate-induced Constipation** Naloxegol oxalate is used for the management of opiate-induced constipation in patients with chronic non-cancer-related pain, including those with chronic pain related to prior cancer or its treatment who do not require frequent (e.g., weekly) increases in opiate dosage.

Safety and efficacy of naloxegol were established in 2 identical randomized, double-blind, placebo-controlled, phase 3 studies (KODIAC-04 and KODIAC-05) in 1352 patients (mean age of 52 years) with non-cancer-related pain and active opiate-induced constipation who had received an oral opiate analgesic (at a stable dosage equivalent to 30 mg to 1 g of morphine sulfate daily) for at least 4 weeks prior to study enrollment. Opiate-induced constipation was defined as fewer than 3 spontaneous bowel movements per week during the 4 weeks prior to screening, with at least 25% of spontaneous bowel movements associated with straining, hard or lumpy stools, and/or a sensation of incomplete evacuation or anorectal obstruction. Patients with suspected clinically important disruptions of the blood-brain barrier were not enrolled in the studies. Patients in the studies were randomized to receive naloxegol 12.5 or 25 mg once daily or placebo for 12 weeks. No laxatives or bowel-therapy regimens other than a "rescue" laxative regimen (up to three 10- to 15-mg doses of bisacodyl followed, if necessary, by one-time use of an enema for an episode of no bowel movements for 72 hours) were permitted during the studies. Back pain (56–57%) and arthritis (10%) were the most common indications for opiate analgesia in the 2 studies. Patients enrolled in the studies had received their current opiate analgesic for an average of 3.6–3.7 years. The mean baseline opiate dosage was equivalent to 136–140 mg of morphine sulfate daily.

Laxative use on at least one occasion within 2 weeks prior to study enrollment was reported by 71% of patients. Approximately 53–55% of patients enrolled in the studies had an inadequate response to laxatives prior to study enrollment. Inadequate response to laxatives was defined as laxative use on at least 4 of the previous 14 days with at least 1 of the following symptoms of moderate, severe, or very severe intensity: incomplete bowel movements, hard stool, straining, or sensation of needing to pass a bowel movement but being unable to do so. In the subgroup of patients with inadequate response to laxatives, 42–50% of patients reported daily use of laxatives, most frequently stool softeners (18–24%), stimulants (16–18%), and polyethylene glycol (5–6%), prior to enrollment. Combined use of 2 laxative classes was reported by 27–31% of these patients at any time during the 14 days prior to enrollment; the most commonly reported combination was stimulants and stool softeners (8–10%).

The primary end point of the studies was response, defined as 3 or more spontaneous bowel movements per week and a change from baseline of 1 or more spontaneous bowel movements per week for at least 9 of the 12 study weeks and at least 3 of the final 4 study weeks. Response to naloxegol 25 mg daily was superior to the placebo response in both studies; however, response to naloxegol 12.5 mg daily was superior to the placebo response in only one of the studies. Response rates for naloxegol 25 mg, naloxegol 12.5 mg, and placebo were 44, 41, and 29%, respectively, in KODIAC-04 and 40, 35, and 29%, respectively, in KODIAC-05.

Key secondary end points of the studies included time to first postdose spontaneous bowel movement, change from baseline in the mean number of days per week with 1–3 spontaneous bowel movements, and response rate in patients with an inadequate response to laxatives prior to study enrollment. On each of these 3 key secondary end points, naloxegol 25 mg daily was superior to placebo in both studies and naloxegol 12.5 mg daily was superior to placebo in KODIAC-04; statistical significance for secondary end points could not be established for the 12.5-mg dosage in KODIAC-05 since this study failed to established efficacy of the 12.5-mg dosage for the primary efficacy end point. In the subgroup of patients with an inadequate response to laxatives, response rates were 49, 43, and 29% in KODIAC-04 for naloxegol 25 mg, naloxegol 12.5 mg, and placebo, respectively, and 47 and 31% in KODIAC-05 for naloxegol 25 mg and placebo, respectively. In KODIAC-04, median times to first postdose spontaneous bowel movement were 6, 20, and 36 hours with naloxegol 25 mg, naloxegol 12.5 mg, and placebo, respectively. In KODIAC-05, median times to first postdose spontaneous bowel movement were 12 and 37 hours with naloxegol 25 mg and placebo, respectively. A spontaneous bowel movement occurred within 24 hours of the first dose in 61–70 or 58% of patients receiving naloxegol 25 or 12.5 mg, respectively.

Mean daily opiate dosages remained stable during the studies, and mean changes from baseline in pain intensity (as measured on a scale of 0–10) were small and not clinically important.

Dosage and Administration

■ **General** All maintenance laxative therapy should be discontinued prior to initiating naloxegol; laxatives may be used as needed if the patient's response to naloxegol is suboptimal after 3 days of therapy.

Changes in the analgesic dosing regimen are not required prior to initiation of naloxegol therapy. Patients receiving opiates for less than 4 weeks may be less responsive to naloxegol therapy.

■ **Administration** Naloxegol oxalate is administered orally on an empty stomach at least 1 hour before or 2 hours after the first meal of the day. For patients who have cannot swallow naloxegol oxalate tablets whole, the tablet may be crushed to a powder and mixed with 120 mL of water in a glass; the resulting mixture should be stirred and then swallowed immediately. To ensure consumption of the entire dose, the glass should be rinsed with 120 mL of water; the resulting mixture should be stirred and then swallowed immediately.

For administration through a nasogastric tube, the nasogastric tube should first be flushed with 30 mL of water using a 60-mL syringe. The tablet should then be crushed to a powder and mixed with approximately 60 mL of water in a container. The resulting mixture should be drawn up into the 60-mL syringe and administered through the nasogastric tube. To facilitate delivery of the entire dose, the container should be rinsed with approximately 60 mL of water, the mixture should be drawn up into the same syringe, and the entire contents of the syringe should be used to flush the nasogastric tube.

Plasma concentrations of naloxegol attained when a crushed naloxegol oxalate tablet is mixed in water and administered either orally or through a nasogastric tube are comparable to those attained following oral administration of an intact tablet of the drug.

■ **Dosage** Dosage of naloxegol oxalate is expressed in terms of naloxegol.

The recommended adult dosage of naloxegol for the management of opiate-induced constipation in patients with chronic non-cancer-related pain is 25 mg once daily in the morning. If patients cannot tolerate the 25-mg daily dosage, dosage of naloxegol may be reduced to 12.5 mg once daily in the morning.

If concomitant use of moderate cytochrome P-450 (CYP) 3A4 inhibitors (e.g., diltiazem, erythromycin, verapamil) is unavoidable, dosage of naloxegol should be reduced to 12.5 mg once daily, and the patient should be monitored for adverse effects. (See Drug Interactions.)

■ **Special Populations** The recommended initial dosage of naloxegol in patients with moderate or severe renal impairment (i.e., creatinine clearance less than 60 mL/minute), including those with end-stage renal disease, is 12.5 mg once daily. If the initial naloxegol dosage is well tolerated but symptoms of opiate-induced constipation persist, dosage may be increased to 25 mg once daily, taking into consideration the potential for markedly increased systemic exposure to the drug in some patients with renal impairment and the associated increased risk of adverse effects. (See Renal Impairment under Warnings/Precautions: Specific Populations, in Cautions.)

No dosage adjustment is needed in patients with mild (Child-Pugh class A) or moderate (Child-Pugh class B) hepatic impairment. Use of naloxegol should be avoided in patients with severe (Child-Pugh class C) hepatic impairment; an appropriate dosage has not been established. (See Hepatic Impairment under Warnings/Precautions: Specific Populations, in Cautions.)

No dosage adjustment is required in geriatric patients based solely on age.

Cautions

■ **Contraindications** Because of the potential for GI perforation, naloxegol is contraindicated in patients with known or suspected GI obstruction and in patients at increased risk for recurrent GI obstruction (see GI Perforation under Cautions: Warnings/Precautions).

Naloxegol is contraindicated in patients receiving potent inhibitors of cytochrome P-450 (CYP) isoenzyme 3A4 (CYP3A4) (e.g., clarithromycin, ketoconazole) because of the potential for increased exposure to naloxegol and precipitation of opiate withdrawal (see Drug Interactions).

Naloxegol also is contraindicated in patients with known serious or severe hypersensitivity reactions to the drug or any ingredient in the formulation.

■ **Warnings/Precautions** ***Opiate Withdrawal*** In 2 controlled clinical trials of naloxegol in patients with opiate-induced constipation, possible opiate withdrawal (defined as the same-day occurrence of at least 3 adverse effects, not all related to the GI tract, that are potential manifestations of opiate withdrawal [e.g., hyperhidrosis, chills, diarrhea, abdominal pain, anxiety, irritability, yawning]) occurred in 1% of patients receiving naloxegol 12.5 mg daily, 3% of patients receiving naloxegol 25 mg daily, and less than 1% of those receiving placebo. In both trials, the incidence of adverse GI effects potentially related to opiate withdrawal was higher in patients receiving methadone compared with those receiving other opiate analgesics (39 versus 26% of those receiving naloxegol 12.5 mg daily and 75 versus 34% of those receiving naloxegol 25 mg daily).

Patients with disruptions in the blood-brain barrier may be at increased risk for opiate withdrawal or reduced analgesia; risks and benefits of naloxegol therapy should be carefully considered in such patients, and these patients should be monitored for symptoms of opiate withdrawal.

Severe Abdominal Pain and Diarrhea Severe abdominal pain and/or diarrhea, sometimes resulting in hospitalization, have been reported in patients receiving naloxegol. Most cases of severe abdominal pain have been reported in patients receiving a naloxegol dosage of 25 mg daily. Symptoms generally have occurred within a few days following initiation of therapy. Patients receiving naloxegol should be monitored for the development of abdominal pain and/or diarrhea. Naloxegol should be discontinued if severe symptoms occur. If appropriate, consideration can be given to reinitiating naloxegol therapy at a dosage of 12.5 mg once daily.

GI Perforation GI perforation has been reported with use of methylnaltrexone, another peripherally acting opiate antagonist, in patients with underlying conditions that may be associated with localized or diffuse reduction of structural integrity in the GI tract wall (e.g., peptic ulcer disease, Ogilvie's syndrome, diverticular disease, infiltrative GI tract malignancies or peritoneal metastases). Risks and benefits of naloxegol therapy should be carefully considered in patients with these conditions or with other conditions that might result in impaired integrity of the GI tract wall (e.g., Crohn's disease). Patients receiving naloxegol should be monitored for the development of severe, persistent, or worsening abdominal pain. Naloxegol should be discontinued if such symptoms occur.

Specific Populations **Pregnancy.** Category C. (See Users Guide.)

Naloxegol should be used in pregnant women only if the potential benefits justify the potential risk to the fetus. There are no adequate and well-controlled studies of naloxegol in pregnant women. Because of the immature fetal blood-brain barrier, use of naloxegol during pregnancy may precipitate opiate withdrawal in the fetus. No adverse effects of the drug on embryofetal development have been observed in animal reproduction studies.

Lactation. It is not known whether naloxegol is distributed into human milk; however, naloxegol is distributed into milk in rats and is absorbed in nursing rat pups. Because of the potential for serious adverse effects, including opiate withdrawal, in nursing infants, a decision should be made whether to discontinue nursing or the drug, taking into account the importance of the drug to the woman.

Pediatric Use. Safety and efficacy of naloxegol have not been established in pediatric patients.

Geriatric Use. In clinical studies of naloxegol, 11% of patients were 65 years of age and older, while 2% were 75 years of age and older. Although no overall differences in efficacy or safety were observed between geriatric patients and younger adults, and other clinical experience revealed no evidence of age-related differences in response, the possibility that some older patients may exhibit increased sensitivity to the drug cannot be ruled out.

Naloxegol exposure was higher in healthy geriatric Japanese individuals compared with younger individuals; however, no dosage adjustment is required in geriatric patients.

Hepatic Impairment. Following oral administration of a single 25-mg dose of naloxegol, slight decreases in area under the concentration-time curve (AUC) of the drug were observed in patients with mild (Child-Pugh class A) or moderate (Child-Pugh class B) hepatic impairment compared with those with normal hepatic function. No dosage adjustment is required in patients with mild or moderate hepatic impairment. The effect of severe hepatic impairment (Child-Pugh class C) on the pharmacokinetics of naloxegol has not been established. Use of naloxegol in patients with severe hepatic impairment should be avoided, as appropriate dosage in these patients has not been determined.

Renal Impairment. Following oral administration of a single 25-mg dose of naloxegol in patients with moderate or severe renal impairment or end-stage renal disease not yet requiring dialysis (i.e., creatinine clearance less than 60 mL/minute), the pharmacokinetic profile of naloxegol in most patients was similar to that observed in healthy individuals. However, some patients with renal impairment (including patients with moderate, severe, or end-stage renal disease) had markedly increased systemic exposure to the drug (e.g., up to tenfold higher than that observed in healthy individuals). Some patients with end-stage renal disease requiring dialysis also were included in the pharmacokinetic study. Plasma concentrations of naloxegol in these patients were similar to concentrations observed in healthy individuals whether the drug was administered before or after hemodialysis.

The reason for the high exposures observed in some patients with renal impairment is unknown; however, because the risk of adverse effects increases as systemic exposure increases, a reduced initial dosage of naloxegol is recommended in patients with creatinine clearances of less than 60 mL/minute. (See Dosage and Administration: Special Populations.) No dosage adjustment is required in patients with mild renal impairment.

■ **Common Adverse Effects** Adverse effects reported in 3% or more of patients receiving naloxegol 12.5 or 25 mg daily and at an incidence greater than that observed with placebo include abdominal pain, diarrhea, nausea, flatulence, vomiting, headache, and hyperhidrosis.

Drug Interactions

Naloxegol is metabolized principally by cytochrome P-450 (CYP) 3A isoenzymes and is a substrate, but not a clinically important inhibitor, of P-glycoprotein (P-gp). Naloxegol did not inhibit CYP 1A2, 2C9, 2C19, 2D6, or 3A4 nor substantially induce CYP 1A2, 2B6, or 3A4 in vitro at clinically relevant concentrations, and is not expected to alter metabolic clearance of drugs metabolized by these enzymes.

Naloxegol does not substantially inhibit breast cancer resistance protein (BCRP), organic anion transporter (OAT) 1 or 3, organic cation transporter (OCT) 2, or organic anion transport protein (OATP) 1B1 or 1B3.

■ **Drugs Affecting Hepatic Microsomal Enzymes** Concomitant use of naloxegol with potent CYP3A4 inhibitors (e.g., clarithromycin, itraconazole, ketoconazole) or moderate CYP3A4 inhibitors (e.g., diltiazem, erythromycin, verapamil) may result in increased plasma concentrations of naloxegol and increased risk of adverse effects. Use of naloxegol with potent CYP3A4 inhibitors is contraindicated. Use of naloxegol with moderate CYP3A4 inhibitors should be avoided; if concomitant use is unavoidable, dosage of naloxegol should be reduced to 12.5 mg once daily and the patient should be monitored for adverse effects. When naloxegol is used concomitantly with weak CYP3A4 inhibitors (e.g., cimetidine, quinidine), clinically important increases in naloxegol concentrations are not expected and dosage adjustments are not required.

Potent CYP3A4 inducers (e.g., carbamazepine, rifampin, St. John's wort [*Hypericum perforatum*]) can substantially decrease plasma naloxegol concentrations and may decrease the efficacy of naloxegol. Use of naloxegol with potent CYP3A4 inducers is not recommended.

■ **Diltiazem** Concomitant administration of naloxegol (single 25-mg dose) and the combined P-gp and moderate CYP3A4 inhibitor diltiazem (240 mg of extended-release diltiazem hydrochloride once daily) increased peak plasma concentration and area under the concentration-time curve (AUC) of naloxegol by 2.9- and 3.4-fold, respectively. Concomitant use of naloxegol with diltiazem should be avoided; if concomitant use cannot be avoided, dosage of naloxegol should be reduced to 12.5 mg once daily and the patient should be monitored for adverse effects.

■ **Efavirenz** Pharmacokinetic simulations suggested that concomitant administration of a single 25-mg dose of naloxegol with the moderate CYP3A inducer efavirenz (400 mg once daily) results in naloxegol exposures similar to those achieved with administration of naloxegol 12.5 mg alone (i.e., a 50% reduction in exposure).

■ **Grapefruit or Grapefruit Juice** When consumed concomitantly with naloxegol, grapefruit or grapefruit juice can increase plasma naloxegol concentrations. Consumption of grapefruit or grapefruit juice should be avoided by patients receiving naloxegol. The manufacturer states that the effect of grapefruit juice varies widely among brands and is dependent on the concentration, dose, and preparation. Studies have demonstrated that some preparations of grapefruit juice (e.g., high dose, double strength) are potent CYP3A inhibitors, while other preparations (e.g., low dose, single strength) are moderate CYP3A inhibitors.

■ **Ketoconazole** Concomitant administration of naloxegol (single 25-mg dose) and the combined P-gp and potent CYP3A4 inhibitor ketoconazole (400 mg once daily) increased peak plasma concentration and AUC of naloxegol by 9.6- and 12.9-fold, respectively. Concomitant use of naloxegol with ketoconazole is contraindicated.

■ **Morphine** In healthy individuals receiving IV morphine sulfate (5 mg per 70 kg), single doses of naloxegol (8 mg to 1 g) had no meaningful effect on systemic exposure to morphine or its major circulating metabolites. With increasing naloxegol dose, there was no trend toward increasing or decreasing morphine exposure compared with morphine administered alone.

■ **Opiate Antagonists** When naloxegol is used concomitantly with other opiate antagonists, the potential exists for additive opiate receptor antagonism and an increased risk of opiate withdrawal. Concomitant use of naloxegol with other opiate antagonists should be avoided.

■ **Quinidine** Because of its inhibitory effect on P-gp, the combined potent P-gp and weak CPY3A4 inhibitor quinidine sulfate (single 600-mg dose) increased peak plasma concentration and AUC of naloxegol (given as a single 25-mg dose) by 2.5- and 1.4-fold, respectively. However, no dosage adjustment is necessary.

■ **Rifampin** Concomitant administration of naloxegol (single 25-mg dose) and the combined P-gp and potent CYP3A4 inducer rifampin (600 mg once daily) decreased peak plasma concentration and AUC of naloxegol by 76 and 89%, respectively. Concomitant use of naloxegol with rifampin is not recommended.

Description

Naloxegol, a covalent conjugate of naloxone and polyethylene glycol (PEG), is a peripherally acting μ-opiate receptor antagonist. Naloxegol exhibits antagonist effects at the μ- and δ-opiate receptors and weak partial agonist activity at κ-opiate receptors, but has highest affinity for μ-opiate receptors; affinity of naloxegol for μ-opiate receptors is approximately 20-fold lower than that of naloxone. The mechanism of action of naloxegol in the management of opiate-induced constipation stems from the drug's ability to block μ-opiate receptors in the GI tract, thereby reversing opiate-induced constipating effects (e.g., slowing of GI motility and transit). Conjugation with PEG results in reduced passive permeability of the drug across the blood-brain barrier and renders naloxegol a substrate for P-glycoprotein, which results in increased efflux of the drug across the blood-brain barrier. CNS penetration of naloxegol is expected to be negligible at recommended dosages, limiting the potential for interference with centrally mediated opiate analgesia.

Naloxegol is rapidly absorbed from the GI tract, with peak plasma concentrations attained in less than 2 hours following oral administration. The presence of a secondary peak concentration has been observed approximately 0.4–3 hours after the first peak concentration in most individuals, suggesting that the drug undergoes enterohepatic circulation. Peak plasma concentration and area under the concentration time-curve (AUC) increase in a dose-proportional or almost dose-proportional manner. Administration with a high-fat meal increases the extent and rate of absorption of naloxegol; peak plasma concentration and AUC were increased by approximately 30 and 45%, respectively, when the drug was administered with a high-fat meal. Naloxegol is minimally bound to plasma proteins (approximately 4%) and has a half-life of 6–11 hours. Naloxegol is extensively metabolized, principally via cytochrome P-450 (CYP) 3A isoenzymes; the drug undergoes *N*-dealkylation, *O*-demethylation, oxidation, and shortening of the PEG chain. Approximately 68% of an oral dose is eliminated in feces (approximately 16% of which is unchanged drug) and 16% is eliminated in urine.

Advice to Patients

Importance of advising patients to read the manufacturer's medication guide before initiating therapy and each time the prescription is refilled.

Importance of discontinuing all maintenance laxative therapy prior to initiation of naloxegol therapy. Laxatives may be used as needed if the response to naloxegol is suboptimal after 3 days.

Importance of taking naloxegol on an empty stomach at least 1 hour before or 2 hours after the first meal of the day. If the patient cannot swallow the tablets intact or the drug must be administered through a nasogastric tube, the tablets may be crushed, mixed with water, and administered according to the manufacturer's instructions.

Importance of informing clinician if naloxegol therapy is not tolerated, as dosage adjustment may be appropriate.

Importance of informing clinician if opiate analgesics are discontinued, since naloxegol should be discontinued if opiate analgesics are discontinued.

Importance of advising patients that symptoms consistent with opiate withdrawal (e.g., sweating, chills, diarrhea, abdominal pain, anxiety, irritability, yawning) may occur. Importance of informing patients who are receiving methadone that they may be more likely than patients receiving other opiates to experience adverse GI effects that may be related to opiate withdrawal.

Importance of advising patients that severe abdominal pain and/or diarrhea may occur following initiation of naloxegol therapy; patients should be advised to discontinue therapy with the drug and contact their clinician if they experience such severe symptoms.

Possible risk of GI perforation. Importance of discontinuing naloxegol and promptly seeking medical attention if unusually severe, persistent, or worsening abdominal pain occurs.

Importance of women informing clinicians if they are or plan to become pregnant or plan to breast-feed. Women should be informed that naloxegol use during pregnancy may precipitate opiate withdrawal in the fetus because the fetal blood-brain barrier is immature. Women also should be advised *not* to breast-feed while receiving naloxegol because of the potential for opiate withdrawal in nursing infants.

Importance of informing clinicians of existing or contemplated concomitant therapy, including prescription and OTC drugs (especially those that alter activity of cytochrome P-450 isoenzyme 3A4 [CYP3A4]), as well as any concomitant illnesses. Patients receiving naloxegol should be advised to avoid consumption of grapefruit or grapefruit juice and to inform their clinician when they initiate or discontinue any concomitant drug therapy.

Importance of informing patients of other important precautionary information. (See Cautions.)

Overview® (see Users Guide). For additional information on this drug until a more detailed monograph is developed and published, the manufacturer's labeling should be consulted. It is *essential* that the manufacturer's labeling be consulted for more detailed information on usual cautions, precautions, contraindications, potential drug interactions, laboratory test interferences, and acute toxicity.

Preparations

Excipients in commercially available drug preparations may have clinically important effects in some individuals; consult specific product labeling for details.

Naloxegol Oxalate

Oral

Tablets, film-coated	12.5 mg (of naloxegol)	**Movantik®**, AstraZeneca
	25 mg (of naloxegol)	**Movantik®**, AstraZeneca

Plecanatide

■ Plecanatide, a guanylate cyclase-C (GC-C) agonist, stimulates secretion of chloride and bicarbonate into the intestinal lumen, which increases intestinal fluid and accelerates intestinal transit.

Uses

■ **Chronic Idiopathic Constipation** Plecanatide is used in adults for the symptomatic treatment of chronic idiopathic constipation.

Efficacy and safety of plecanatide for the symptomatic treatment of chronic idiopathic constipation have been evaluated in 2 randomized, double-blind, placebo-controlled studies in adults who met modified Rome III criteria for functional constipation for a minimum of 3 months prior to screening, with symptom onset at least 6 months prior to diagnosis. The modified Rome III criteria specified fewer than 3 defecations per week, rare occurrence of loose stool in the absence of laxative use, no use of manual maneuvers to facilitate defecation, failure to meet criteria for irritable bowel syndrome with constipation, and presence of 2 or more of the following symptoms for at least 25% of defecations: straining, lumpy or hard stool, sensation of incomplete evacuation, or sensation of anorectal obstruction/blockage. Patients also were required to meet the following 3 criteria during the last 2 weeks of the screening period: fewer than 3 complete spontaneous bowel movements (CSBMs) in each of the 2 weeks, a score of 6 or 7 on the Bristol Stool Form Scale for fewer than 25% of spontaneous bowel movements (SBMs), and one of the following criteria: a score of 1 or 2 on the Bristol Stool Form Scale for 25% or more of defecations, a straining value recorded on at least 25% of days when a bowel movement was reported, or a sense of incomplete evacuation following at least 25% of bowel movements. In the 2 studies combined, the mean age of patients was 45 years, and most patients were female (80%) and white (72%). Eligible patients were randomized to receive plecanatide 3 or 6 mg once daily or placebo for 12 weeks and then were followed for an additional 2 weeks. In the 2 studies combined, the intention-to-treat population included 2656 patients.

On a daily basis, patients recorded information on bowel function and symptoms in an electronic diary. The primary efficacy end point of both studies was the proportion of patients who achieved a response, defined as 3 or more CSBMs in a given week and an increase of 1 or more CSBMs from baseline in the same week for a minimum of 9 weeks out of the 12-week treatment period and for at least 3 of the last 4 weeks of the study. In both studies, a greater proportion of patients receiving plecanatide 3 mg daily compared with those receiving placebo (21 versus 10–13%, respectively) achieved a response. An increase in CSBM frequency (i.e., number of CSBMs per week) was observed within the first week of therapy and was sustained through week 12. The difference between patients receiving plecanatide 3 mg daily and those receiving placebo in the mean change in CSBM frequency from baseline to week 12 was approximately 1.1 CSBMs per week.

Over the 12-week treatment period, improvements were observed in stool frequency (number of CSBMs and SBMs per week), stool consistency (as measured by the Bristol Stool Form Scale), and/or amount of straining with bowel movements in patients receiving plecanatide 3 mg daily compared with those receiving placebo. During the 2-week period following discontinuance of treatment, patients' diary entries generally reverted to baseline status.

Plecanatide 6 mg once daily did not provide additional clinical benefit beyond that provided by the 3-mg daily dosage and was associated with an increased incidence of adverse effects. A response was achieved by 20% of patients receiving the 6-mg daily dosage.

Dosage and Administration

■ **Administration** Plecanatide is administered orally without regard to food. Although administration with a meal resulted in looser stools when compared with administration in the fasted state, plecanatide was administered with or without food in clinical trials.

Plecanatide tablets should be swallowed whole. Alternatively, for patients who are unable to swallow whole tablets, plecanatide tablets may be crushed and administered orally mixed in applesauce or dispersed in water and administered orally or via a nasogastric or gastric feeding tube. The manufacturer states that mixing crushed plecanatide tablets in soft foods other than applesauce or dispersing the tablets in liquids other than water has not been studied.

If a dose of plecanatide is missed, a double dose should not be administered to make up for the missed dose. The next dose should be taken at the regularly scheduled time.

For administration in applesauce, a plecanatide 3-mg tablet should be crushed to a powder and mixed with one teaspoonful of room-temperature applesauce in a clean container. The entire mixture should be consumed immediately and should not be stored for later use.

For oral administration as an aqueous dispersion, a plecanatide 3-mg tablet should be placed in a clean cup, approximately 30 mL of room-temperature water should then be added to the cup, and the mixture should be gently swirled for at least 10 seconds to disperse the disintegrating tablet. The entire mixture should be consumed immediately. Any residue remaining in the cup should be dispersed in an additional 30 mL of water, gently swirled again for at least 10 seconds, and then consumed immediately. The mixture should not be stored for later use.

For administration via nasogastric or gastric feeding tube, a plecanatide 3-mg tablet should be placed in a clean cup, approximately 30 mL of room-temperature water should be added to the cup, and the mixture should be gently swirled for at least 15 seconds to disperse the disintegrating tablet. The nasogastric or gastric feeding tube should be flushed with 30 mL of water and then the entire contents of the mixture should be drawn up into a syringe and administered immediately. Any residue remaining in the cup should be dispersed in an additional 30 mL of water, gently swirled again for at least 15 seconds, and then administered via the nasogastric or gastric feeding tube using the same syringe. Following administration of the dose, the nasogastric or gastric feeding tube should be flushed with at least 10 mL of water using either the same syringe or a new syringe. The mixture should not be stored for later use.

■ **Dosage** The recommended adult dosage of plecanatide for the symptomatic treatment of chronic idiopathic constipation is 3 mg once daily. A dosage of 6 mg daily is not recommended; in clinical trials, the 6-mg daily dosage did not provide additional clinical benefit beyond that provided by the 3-mg daily dosage and was associated with an increased incidence of adverse effects.

■ **Special Populations** The manufacturer makes no specific dosage recommendations for geriatric patients or for patients with renal or hepatic impairment. (See Specific Populations under Cautions: Warnings/Precautions.)

Cautions

■ **Contraindications** Plecanatide is contraindicated in infants and children younger than 6 years of age. (See Pediatric Use under Warnings/Precautions: Specific Populations, in Cautions.) The drug also is contraindicated in any patient with known or suspected mechanical GI obstruction.

■ **Warnings/Precautions** ***Warnings*** **Pediatric Risk.** In toxicology studies, plecanatide caused deaths due to dehydration in young juvenile mice within 24 hours following single-dose oral administration. Plecanatide is contraindicated in infants and children younger than 6 years of age and should be avoided in children and adolescents 6 years to younger than 18 years of age. (See Pediatric Use under Warnings/Precautions: Specific Populations, in Cautions.)

Other Warnings and Precautions **Diarrhea.** In clinical trials in patients with chronic idiopathic constipation, diarrhea resulting in drug discontinuance occurred in 2% of patients receiving plecanatide 3 mg daily compared with 0.5% of patients receiving placebo, while severe diarrhea was reported in 0.6 or 0.3% of patients receiving plecanatide 3 mg daily or placebo, respectively. Most reported cases of diarrhea occurred within 4 weeks of drug initiation, and severe diarrhea occurred within the first 3 days of treatment. Plecanatide therapy should be interrupted and the patient should be rehydrated if severe diarrhea develops.

Specific Populations **Pregnancy.** Since systemic absorption of plecanatide and its active metabolite is negligible following oral administration, the drug is not expected to result in fetal exposure if administered to pregnant women. However, available data on use of plecanatide in pregnant women are insufficient to inform fetal risk.

No adverse effects on embryofetal development were observed in mice or rabbits when plecanatide was administered orally during organogenesis at dosages up to 800 or 250 mg/kg daily, respectively. In addition, no developmental abnormalities and no effects on growth, learning and memory, or fertility were observed in the offspring of mice that received plecanatide orally at dosages up to 600 mg/kg daily during the period of organogenesis through lactation. Limited systemic exposure to plecanatide was achieved in rabbits during the period of organogenesis. Animal and human doses should not be compared directly for evaluating relative exposure.

Lactation. It is not known whether plecanatide is distributed into human milk, affects milk production, or affects the breast-fed infant.

Systemic absorption of plecanatide and its active metabolite is negligible following oral administration. It is not known whether the negligible systemic absorption observed in adults will result in clinically important exposure in breast-fed infants. The benefits of breast-feeding and the importance of plecanatide to the woman should be considered along with potential adverse effects on the breast-fed infant from the drug or from the underlying maternal condition. Exposure of infants to plecanatide could result in serious adverse effects. (See Pediatric Use under Warnings/Precautions: Specific Populations, in Cautions.)

Pediatric Use. Plecanatide is contraindicated in infants and children younger than 6 years of age and should be avoided in children and adolescents 6 years to younger than 18 years of age.

Safety and efficacy of plecanatide in pediatric patients younger than 18 years of age have not been established, and the drug has caused deaths within 24 hours of administration in toxicology studies in juvenile mice (age approximately equivalent to a human age of 1 month to younger than 2 years). The deaths in young juvenile mice occurred following single oral doses of plecanatide 0.5 and 10 mg/kg administered on postnatal days 7 and 14, respectively. The deaths apparently were due to dehydration resulting from increased fluid secretion into the intestine as a consequence of guanylate cyclase-C (GC-C) stimulation. Because of increased intestinal expression of GC-C, infants and children younger than 6 years of age may be at greater risk of developing diarrhea and its potentially serious consequences compared with individuals 6 years of age and older. Although no deaths were observed in older juvenile mice, use of plecanatide should be avoided in children and adolescents 6 years to younger than 18 years of age because of the deaths reported in younger mice and the lack of safety and efficacy data in pediatric patients. Although administration of the recommended plecanatide dosage (approximately 0.05 mg/kg daily in a 60-kg individual) in adults does not result in measurable plasma concentrations of the drug, systemic absorption was observed in juvenile animal toxicology studies; animal and human doses should not be compared directly for evaluating relative exposure.

Geriatric Use. Clinical trials of plecanatide did not include sufficient numbers of patients 65 years of age and older to determine whether geriatric patients respond differently than younger adults. In clinical trials in patients with chronic idiopathic constipation, 10% of patients were 65 years of age and older, while 2% were 75 years of age and older. Because of the greater frequency of decreased hepatic, renal, and/or cardiac function and of concomitant disease and drug therapy observed in the elderly, dosage selection for geriatric patients should be cautious.

Hepatic Impairment. The pharmacokinetics of plecanatide have not been formally studied in patients with hepatic impairment since the drug is not appreciably absorbed after oral administration.

Renal Impairment. The pharmacokinetics of plecanatide have not been formally studied in patients with renal impairment since the drug is not appreciably absorbed after oral administration.

■ **Common Adverse Effects** Diarrhea was reported in 5% of patients with chronic idiopathic constipation receiving plecanatide 3 mg daily and more frequently with the drug than with placebo.

Drug Interactions

Because plasma concentrations of plecanatide and its active metabolite are not measurable in adults following oral administration at the recommended dosage, only enzyme and transporter systems that are expressed in the GI tract have been evaluated for interaction potential. In vitro studies indicate that plecanatide and its active metabolite do not inhibit cytochrome P-450 (CYP) isoenzyme 2C9 or 3A4, do not induce CYP3A4, and are not substrates or inhibitors of P-glycoprotein (P-gp) or breast cancer resistance protein (BCRP).

Description

Plecanatide, a guanylate cyclase-C (GC-C) agonist, is a 16-amino acid peptide structurally related to endogenous uroguanylin peptide hormone. The parent drug and its active metabolite bind to GC-C receptors on the luminal surface of the intestinal epithelium, which increases intracellular and extracellular concentrations of cyclic guanosine monophosphate (cGMP). In turn, increased intracellular concentrations of cGMP trigger a signal-transduction cascade activating the cystic fibrosis transmembrane conductance regulator (CFTR) ion channel. This results in secretion of chloride and bicarbonate into the intestinal lumen causing increased intestinal fluid and accelerated intestinal transit.

In animal models, plecanatide has been shown to reduce abdominal muscle contractions (a measure of intestinal pain), increase fluid secretion into the GI tract, accelerate intestinal transit, and change stool consistency. Further research is needed to determine the precise mechanism(s) by which plecanatide relieves intestinal pain.

After oral administration, plecanatide is minimally absorbed with negligible systemic bioavailability. Administration of a single 9-mg dose of plecanatide with either a low-fat, low-calorie or a high-fat, high-calorie meal resulted in looser stools compared with administration in the fasting state. Plecanatide is metabolized in the GI tract to an active metabolite via lysis of the terminal leucine moiety. Plecanatide and its metabolite are proteolytically degraded within the intestinal lumen to smaller peptides and naturally occurring amino acids.

Advice to Patients

Importance of reading the manufacturer's patient information (medication guide) prior to initiation of therapy and each time the prescription is refilled.

Importance of advising patients that accidental ingestion of plecanatide by a child, especially a child younger than 6 years of age, may result in severe diarrhea and dehydration; importance of keeping plecanatide out of reach of children and of properly disposing of any unused drug. (See Pediatric Use under Warnings/Precautions: Specific Populations, in Cautions.)

Importance of advising patients that diarrhea may occur and that they should discontinue plecanatide and notify their clinician if diarrhea becomes severe.

Importance of advising patient of alternative forms of administration if patient is unable to swallow whole tablets.

Importance of storing plecanatide in the original container, with the lid tightly closed and the contents protected from moisture; importance of removing the polyester coil after opening the container, of not removing the desiccant from the container, and of not repackaging the tablets.

If a dose is missed, the missed dose should be omitted and the next dose taken at the regularly scheduled time. Two doses should not be taken at the same time to make up for a missed dose.

Importance of informing clinicians of existing or contemplated concomitant therapy, including prescription and OTC drugs, as well as any concomitant illnesses.

Importance of women informing clinicians if they are or plan to become pregnant or plan to breast-feed.

Importance of informing patients of other important precautionary information. (See Cautions.)

Overview® (see Users Guide). For additional information on this drug until a more detailed monograph is developed and published, the manufacturer's labeling should be consulted. It is *essential* that the manufacturer's labeling be consulted for more detailed information on usual cautions, precautions, contraindications, potential drug interactions, laboratory test interferences, and acute toxicity.

Preparations

Excipients in commercially available drug preparations may have clinically important effects in some individuals; consult specific product labeling for details.

Plecanatide

Oral

Tablets	3 mg	**Trulance®**, Synergy

Vedolizumab

■ Vedolizumab, a recombinant humanized anti-$\alpha 4\beta 7$-integrin monoclonal antibody, is an immunomodulatory agent that selectively inhibits lymphocyte recruitment to the GI tract.

Uses

■ **Ulcerative Colitis** Vedolizumab is used to induce and maintain clinical response and clinical remission, improve endoscopic appearance of mucosa, and achieve corticosteroid-free remission in adults with moderately to severely active ulcerative colitis who have had an inadequate response to, have lost response to, or were intolerant to a tumor necrosis factor (TNF; TNF-α) blocking agent or immunosuppressive agent (e.g., azathioprine, mercaptopurine), or who have had an inadequate response to, were intolerant to, or have demonstrated dependence on corticosteroids.

In clinical trials, vedolizumab has been shown to be more effective than placebo for induction of remission, clinical response, and endoscopic evidence of improved mucosal appearance and for prevention of relapse in patients with moderately to severely active ulcerative colitis.

Safety and efficacy of vedolizumab were evaluated in 2 randomized, double-blind, placebo-controlled, phase 3 studies (GEMINI 1) in adults with moderately to severely active ulcerative colitis (as defined by a Mayo score of 6–12 with an endoscopy subscore of 2 or 3). Mayo score ranges from 0–12 and includes 4 subscales (i.e., stool frequency, rectal bleeding, findings on endoscopy, and physician global assessment), each scored from 0–3 (normal to most severe, respectively). An endoscopy subscore of 2 is defined by marked erythema, lack of vascular pattern, friability, and erosions, whereas an endoscopy subscore of 3 is defined by spontaneous bleeding and ulceration. GEMINI 1 included separate induction and maintenance therapy studies, and these studies included patients who had been treated unsuccessfully with other therapies, including patients with an inadequate response or intolerance to azathioprine or mercaptopurine; patients with an inadequate response, loss of response, or intolerance to a TNF blocking agent; and, at centers outside of the US, patients who were corticosteroid dependent or had an inadequate response or intolerance to corticosteroid therapy. Patients who had received natalizumab, vedolizumab, efalizumab, or rituximab at any time in the past, TNF blocking agents within 60 days prior to enrollment, or cyclosporine, thalidomide, or investigational drugs within 30 days before enrollment were excluded from the study. Concomitant therapy with natalizumab or a TNF blocking agent was not permitted in GEMINI 1.

In study 1 of GEMINI 1, a total of 374 patients were randomized in a 3:2 ratio to receive induction therapy with vedolizumab (300 mg IV at weeks 0 and 2) or placebo. The proportion of patients with prior exposure to TNF blocking agents was limited to 50%. About 39% of patients had an inadequate response, loss of response, or intolerance to prior TNF blocking agent therapy; about 18% of patients had not received prior immunosuppressive or TNF blocking agent therapy but had an inadequate response to, inability to taper, or intolerance to corticosteroid therapy. Patients receiving stable dosages of aminosalicylates, corticosteroids (equivalent to 30 mg of prednisone daily or less), and immunosuppressive agents (i.e., azathioprine, mercaptopurine) were permitted to continue receiving these drugs throughout study 1 (i.e., through week 6). At baseline, 54% of patients were receiving corticosteroids, 30% were receiving azathioprine or mercaptopurine, and 74% were receiving aminosalicylates. The median baseline Mayo score was 9 or 8 in patients receiving vedolizumab or placebo, respectively. Clinical response (the primary end point), clinical remission, and mucosal appearance were evaluated at week 6. Clinical response was defined as a reduction in Mayo score of at least 3 points and at least 30% from baseline score, with a decrease in rectal bleeding subscore of at least 1 point or an absolute rectal bleeding subscore of 0 or 1. Clinical remission was defined as a Mayo score of 0–2 and no individual subscore exceeding 1. Improved mucosal appearance was defined as a Mayo endoscopy subscore of 0 (normal mucosa or inactive disease) or 1 (erythema, decreased vascular pattern, mild friability). At week 6, clinical response rates (47 versus 26%), clinical remission rates (17 versus 5%), and rates of improved mucosal appearance (41 versus 25%) were higher in patients receiving induction therapy with vedolizumab compared with those receiving placebo.

Study 2 of GEMINI 1 evaluated maintenance therapy with vedolizumab in patients who had achieved a clinical response to induction therapy with the drug. Patients in study 2 were enrolled from study 1 of GEMINI 1 or from an open-label group receiving the same vedolizumab induction regimen used in study 1; the open-label group was included in GEMINI 1 to provide an adequate number of patients for the maintenance therapy study. At week 6, a total of 373 patients with a clinical response to vedolizumab induction therapy were randomized to receive vedolizumab 300 mg IV every 8 weeks, vedolizumab 300 mg IV every 4 weeks, or placebo every 4 weeks. About 32% of the patients in study 2 had experienced an inadequate response, loss of response, or intolerance to prior TNF blocking agent therapy. Patients were allowed to receive concomitant aminosalicylates and corticosteroids through week 52. Concomitant therapy with azathioprine or mercaptopurine was allowed outside of the US but was not permitted past week 6 in the US. At week 6, 61% of patients were receiving corticosteroids, 32% were receiving azathioprine or mercaptopurine, and 75% were receiving aminosalicylates. A corticosteroid-tapering regimen was initiated at week 6 in patients who were receiving corticosteroids. The median Mayo score at week 6 was 8 in all 3 treatment groups. The primary end point was clinical remission at week 52. Secondary end points included durable clinical response (response at both weeks 6 and 52), durable clinical remission (remission at both weeks 6 and 52), improved mucosal appearance (defined as Mayo endoscopy subscore of 0 or 1) at week 52, and corticosteroid-free remission at week 52 (assessed in patients who were receiving corticosteroids at baseline). On each of these end points, vedolizumab was superior to placebo for maintenance therapy; however, administration of the drug every 4 weeks did not provide additional benefit beyond that achieved with administration every 8 weeks. Clinical remission was achieved at week 52 in 42, 45, or 16% of patients receiving vedolizumab every 8 weeks, vedolizumab every 4 weeks, or placebo, respectively. In these respective groups, durable clinical response was achieved in 57, 52, or 24% of patients; durable clinical remission was achieved in 21, 24, or 9% of patients; improved mucosal appearance was evident at week 52 in 52, 56, or 20% of patients; and corticosteroid-free remission was achieved at week 52 in 31, 45, or 14% of patients.

■ **Crohn's Disease** Vedolizumab is used to achieve clinical response, clinical remission, and corticosteroid-free remission in adults with moderately to severely active Crohn's disease who have had an inadequate response to, have lost response to, or were intolerant to a TNF blocking agent or immunosuppressive agent (e.g., azathioprine, mercaptopurine, methotrexate), or who had an inadequate response to, were intolerant to, or have demonstrated dependence on corticosteroids.

In several studies, efficacy of vedolizumab has been assessed at various time points in different populations of patients with moderately to severely active Crohn's disease; despite some inconsistencies in findings, modest effects have been observed and the overall findings suggest that vedolizumab provides clinical benefits in these patients. Additional studies are needed to fully characterize the time course of response and to identify which patients might derive greatest benefit from the drug.

Safety and efficacy of vedolizumab were evaluated in 3 randomized, double-blind, placebo-controlled, phase 3 clinical studies (GEMINI 2 and GEMINI 3) in adults with moderately to severely active Crohn's disease, defined as a Crohn's Disease Activity Index (CDAI) score of 220–450. GEMINI 2 included separate induction and maintenance therapy studies. The GEMINI 2 and GEMINI 3 studies included patients who had been treated unsuccessfully with other therapies, including patients with an inadequate response or intolerance to immunosuppressive therapy with azathioprine, mercaptopurine, or methotrexate; patients with an inadequate response, loss of response, or intolerance to 1 or more TNF blocking agents; and, at centers outside of the US, patients who were corticosteroid dependent or had an inadequate response or intolerance to corticosteroid therapy. Patients who had received natalizumab, vedolizumab, efalizumab, or rituximab at any time in the past or had received a TNF blocking agent within 30–60 days before enrollment were excluded from the studies. Concomitant therapy with natalizumab or a TNF blocking agent was not permitted.

In study 1 of GEMINI 2, a total of 368 patients were randomized in a 3:2 ratio to receive induction therapy with vedolizumab (300 mg IV at weeks 0 and 2) or placebo. The proportion of patients with prior exposure to TNF blocking agents was limited to 50%. About 48% of patients had an inadequate response, loss of response, or intolerance to TNF blocking agent therapy; about 17% of patients had not received prior immunosuppressive or TNF blocking agent therapy but had an inadequate response to, inability to taper, or intolerance to corticosteroid therapy. Patients receiving stable dosages of aminosalicylates, corticosteroids (equivalent to 30 mg of prednisone daily or less), antibiotics, and immunosuppressive agents (i.e., azathioprine, mercaptopurine, or methotrexate) were permitted to continue receiving these drugs throughout study 1 (i.e., through week 6). At baseline, 49% of patients were receiving corticosteroids; 35% were receiving azathioprine, mercaptopurine, or methotrexate; and 46% were receiving aminosalicylates. Median baseline CDAI scores for the 2 groups were similar (319–324). The 2 primary end points of the study were clinical remission (defined as a CDAI score of 150 or less) and CDAI-100 response (defined as a reduction in CDAI score from baseline of at least 100 points) at week 6. Patients receiving induction therapy with vedolizumab were more likely than those receiving placebo to achieve clinical remission (15 versus 7%) but not to achieve a CDAI-100 response (31 versus 26%).

Study 2 of GEMINI 2 evaluated maintenance therapy with vedolizumab in patients who had achieved a clinical response (defined as a decrease in CDAI score from baseline to week 6 of at least 70 points) to induction therapy with the drug. Patients in study 2 were enrolled from study 1 of GEMINI 2 or from an open-label group receiving the same vedolizumab induction regimen used in study 1; the open-label group was included in GEMINI 2 to provide an adequate number of patients for the maintenance therapy study. At week 6, a total of 461 patients with a clinical response to vedolizumab induction therapy were randomized to receive vedolizumab 300 mg IV every 8 weeks, vedolizumab 300 mg IV every 4 weeks, or placebo every 4 weeks. About 51% of the patients in study 2 had experienced an inadequate response, loss of response, or intolerance to prior TNF blocking agent therapy. Patients were allowed to receive concomitant therapy with aminosalicylates and corticosteroids through week 52. Concomitant therapy with azathioprine, mercaptopurine, or methotrexate was permitted outside of the US but was not allowed past week 6 in the US. At week 6, 59% of patients were receiving corticosteroids; 31% were receiving azathioprine, mercaptopurine, or methotrexate; and 41% were receiving aminosalicylates. A corticosteroid-tapering regimen was initiated at week 6 in patients who were receiving corticosteroids. The median CDAI score at week 6 was similar (315–322) in all 3 treatment groups. The primary end point was clinical remission at week 52. Secondary end points included CDAI-100 response at week 52, corticosteroid-free remission at week 52 (assessed in patients who were receiving corticosteroids at baseline), and durable clinical remission (clinical remission at 80% or more of study visits, including the final visit). Patients receiving maintenance therapy with vedolizumab were more likely than those receiving placebo to achieve clinical remission, CDAI-100 response, and corticosteroid-free remission at week 52, but not to achieve a durable clinical remission. Clinical remission was achieved at week 52 in 39, 36, or 22% of patients receiving vedolizumab every 8 weeks, vedolizumab every 4 weeks, or placebo, respectively. In these respective groups, CDAI-100 response was achieved at week 52 in 44, 46, or 30% of patients; corticosteroid-free remission was attained at week 52 in 32, 29, or 16% of patients; and durable clinical response was achieved in 21, 16, or 14% of patients.

Use of vedolizumab as induction therapy for Crohn's disease also was evaluated in GEMINI 3. Compared with GEMINI 2, this study included a greater proportion of patients (76%) who had experienced an inadequate response, loss of response, or intolerance to 1 or more TNF blocking agents. A total of 416 patients were randomized to receive either vedolizumab (300 mg IV at weeks 0, 2, and 6) or placebo. Concomitant treatment with aminosalicylates, corticosteroids, and immunosuppressive agents (i.e., azathioprine, mercaptopurine, or methotrexate) was allowed through week 10. At baseline, 54% of patients were receiving corticosteroids; 34% were receiving azathioprine, mercaptopurine, or methotrexate; and 31% were receiving aminosalicylates. Median baseline CDAI score was 317 in patients who received vedolizumab and 301 in patients who received placebo. The primary end point was clinical remission (CDAI score of 150 of less) at week 6 in patients who had experienced an inadequate response, loss of response, or intolerance to 1 or more TNF blocking agents. In this subset of 315 patients, clinical remission rates at week 6 did not differ significantly between those receiving induction therapy with vedolizumab and those receiving placebo (15 versus 12%, respectively); exploratory analysis indicated that clinical remission rates for vedolizumab-treated patients were higher at week 10 (27%, compared with 12% for placebo recipients), suggesting that assessment of remission at 6 weeks might not have been optimal in this patient population.

Dosage and Administration

■ **General** Because infusion-related or hypersensitivity reactions may occur, patients should be observed closely during infusions of vedolizumab. (See Hypersensitivity and Infusion-related Reactions under Cautions: Warnings/Precautions.)

Aminosalicylates, corticosteroids, and immunosuppressive agents (azathioprine, mercaptopurine) could be continued in clinical studies evaluating vedolizumab in patients with ulcerative colitis. Aminosalicylates, corticosteroids, antibiotics, and immunosuppressive agents (azathioprine, mercaptopurine, or methotrexate) could be continued in clinical studies evaluating vedolizumab in patients with Crohn's disease. (See Uses.)

■ **Administration** Vedolizumab is administered by IV infusion over 30 minutes. Vedolizumab should *not* be administered by rapid IV injection, such as IV push or bolus.

Commercially available vedolizumab lyophilized powder must be reconstituted and diluted prior to administration. The vials should be stored under refrigeration and brought to room temperature prior to reconstitution.

Vedolizumab powder for injection is reconstituted by adding 4.8 mL of sterile water for injection (using a syringe with a 21- to 25-gauge needle) to a vial labeled as containing 300 mg of the drug to provide a solution containing 60 mg/mL. The diluent should be directed toward the wall of the vial to avoid excessive foaming. The vial should then be swirled gently for at least 15 seconds to facilitate dissolution. The vial should *not* be shaken vigorously or inverted. The solution should be allowed to stand for up to 20 minutes at room temperature to allow for reconstitution and for any foam to settle. The vial can be swirled and inspected for dissolution during this time. If complete dissolution does not occur within 20 minutes, an additional 10 minutes should be allowed. The vial should *not* be used if dissolution does not occur within 30 minutes. Reconstituted vedolizumab solutions should be inspected visually for particulate matter and discoloration and should be discarded if either is present. Solutions of the drug should be clear or opalescent, colorless to light brownish yellow, and free of visible particulates.

Prior to preparation of the final diluted vedolizumab solution for infusion, the vial should be inverted gently 3 times. A total of 5 mL (300 mg) of reconstituted vedolizumab solution should then be withdrawn using a syringe with a 21- to 25-gauge needle and added to an infusion bag containing 250 mL of 0.9% sodium chloride injection; the solution should be gently mixed. The infusion solution should be used as soon as possible following preparation, but may be stored for up to 4 hours at 2–8°C. Any unused portions of reconstituted or diluted solutions of the drug should be discarded.

Vedolizumab should not be mixed with or administered through the same administration set as other drugs. The IV line should be flushed with 30 mL of 0.9% sodium chloride injection after each infusion of the drug.

■ **Dosage** ***Ulcerative Colitis*** The recommended dosage of vedolizumab in adults with moderately or severely active ulcerative colitis is 300 mg given by IV infusion over 30 minutes at 0, 2, and 6 weeks and then every 8 weeks thereafter. Therapy should be discontinued in patients who show no evidence of therapeutic benefit by week 14.

Crohn's Disease The recommended dosage of vedolizumab in adults with moderately or severely active Crohn's disease is 300 mg given by IV infusion over 30 minutes at 0, 2, and 6 weeks and then every 8 weeks thereafter. Therapy should be discontinued in patients who show no evidence of therapeutic benefit by week 14.

■ **Special Populations** The manufacturer makes no special population dosage recommendations at this time. (See Specific Populations under Cautions: Warnings/Precautions.)

Cautions

■ **Contraindications** Vedolizumab is contraindicated in patients with a known history of serious or severe hypersensitivity reaction (e.g., dyspnea, bronchospasm, urticaria, flushing, rash, increased heart rate) to the drug or any ingredient in the formulation.

■ **Warnings/Precautions** ***Hypersensitivity and Infusion-related Reactions*** Hypersensitivity and infusion-related reactions have been reported in patients receiving vedolizumab. Although such reactions generally are mild to moderate in severity, severe reactions, including anaphylaxis, have occurred. Infusion-related reactions may include nausea, headache, pruritus, dizziness, fatigue, pyrexia, urticaria, and vomiting. These reactions generally occur within the first 2 hours after an infusion and resolve without treatment or following administration of an antihistamine and/or IV hydrocortisone. Hypersensitivity reactions may include dyspnea, bronchospasm, urticaria, flushing, rash, and increased blood pressure and heart rate. Experience with other biologic agents suggests that hypersensitivity reactions, including anaphylaxis, to vedolizumab may vary in their time of onset, occurring during, immediately after, or several hours after an infusion.

Clinicians administering vedolizumab should be prepared to treat hypersensitivity and infusion-related reactions. Appropriate equipment and agents for the treatment of such reactions should be available for immediate use in patients receiving the drug. Patients receiving infusions of the drug should be observed until the infusion has been completed. If anaphylaxis or other serious allergic reactions occur, administration of vedolizumab should be discontinued immediately and appropriate treatment (e.g., epinephrine, antihistamines) should be initiated. In clinical trials, patients who had experienced a mild infusion-related or hypersensitivity reaction to vedolizumab could receive premedication (e.g., antihistamine, hydrocortisone, and/or acetaminophen) prior to subsequent infusions.

Infectious Complications Patients receiving vedolizumab are at increased risk of developing infections. The most commonly reported infections are nasopharyngeal and upper respiratory tract infections. However, serious infections, including anal abscess, sepsis (sometimes fatal), tuberculosis, *Salmonella* sepsis, *Listeria* meningitis, giardiasis, and cytomegaloviral colitis, have been reported and have occurred more commonly in patients with Crohn's disease than in those with ulcerative colitis. Anal abscess is the most frequently reported serious adverse effect in patients with Crohn's disease. In the GEMINI 1 and GEMINI 2 clinical trials, the rate of infection was 0.85 or 0.7 per patient-year in individuals receiving vedolizumab or placebo, respectively, and the rate of serious infection was 0.07 or 0.06 per patient-year, respectively. No increase in the rate of serious infections over 48 months was reported.

Patients with active severe infections should not begin vedolizumab therapy until the infection(s) has been controlled. If a patient develops a severe infection while receiving vedolizumab, interruption of therapy with the drug should be considered. Clinicians should exercise caution when considering use of vedolizumab in patients with a history of recurring severe infections. Screening for active or latent tuberculosis infection also should be considered.

Progressive Multifocal Leukoencephalopathy Progressive multifocal leukoencephalopathy (PML), an opportunistic infection of the brain caused by the JC virus, has been reported in patients receiving natalizumab, an anti-α4-integrin monoclonal antibody. PML generally occurs only in patients who are immunocompromised and usually progresses to death or severe disability. In clinical trials of vedolizumab, patients were actively monitored for PML. Although no cases of PML were reported among patients who were exposed to vedolizumab for at least 24 months, risk of this infection cannot be ruled out and safety of vedolizumab relative to other integrin receptor antagonists has not been fully established.

Patients receiving vedolizumab should be monitored for any new or worsening neurologic manifestations suggestive of PML (see Advice to Patients). If PML is suspected, the drug should be withheld and the patient should be referred to a neurologist for diagnostic evaluation. If PML is confirmed, vedolizumab should be permanently discontinued.

Hepatic Effects Increases in serum aminotransaminase (ALT and AST) and/or bilirubin concentrations, including several cases of hepatitis, have been reported in patients receiving vedolizumab. These adverse effects occurred following 2–5 doses of the drug; it is unclear whether the reactions were drug induced or autoimmune in etiology. All patients recovered following discontinuance of therapy, although some individuals also required corticosteroid treatment.

Vedolizumab should be discontinued in patients with jaundice or other evidence of clinically important hepatic injury.

Immunization Prior to initiation of vedolizumab therapy, patients should receive all appropriate vaccines as recommended by current immunization guidelines. Patients receiving vedolizumab may receive inactivated vaccines (e.g., parenteral influenza virus vaccine inactivated) and may receive live vaccines if the potential benefits justify the possible risks. (See Drug Interactions: Vaccines.)

Malignancies In GEMINI 1 and GEMINI 2 studies, malignancies (excluding dysplasia and basal cell carcinoma) were reported in 0.4% of patients who received vedolizumab and 0.3% of those who received placebo. Malignancies also have been reported during extension phases of the trials; however, data regarding effects of long-term exposure to the drug are limited.

Immunogenicity As with all therapeutic proteins, there is potential for immunogenicity in patients who receive vedolizumab. In GEMINI 1 and GEMINI 2 studies, antibodies to the drug were detected at any time during 52 weeks of continuous therapy in 56 patients (4%); however, antibodies were detected at 24 weeks after the last dose in 13% of patients who received the drug. Among the 56 patients who tested positive for antibody formation during treatment, 9 patients had persistently positive test results (positive at 2 or more time points) and 33 patients had evidence of neutralizing antibodies to the drug. None of the 9 patients with persistently positive anti-vedolizumab antibodies achieved clinical remission at week 6 or 52. Concentration data were available for 8 of the 9 patients and showed undetectable or reduced drug concentrations.

Specific Populations **Pregnancy.** Category B. (See Users Guide.) Monoclonal antibodies are transported across the placenta in a linear fashion as pregnancy progresses, with the largest amount transferred during the third trimester. Therefore, any adverse effect of vedolizumab on pregnancy outcomes would likely be greater during the second and third trimesters of pregnancy.

To monitor pregnancy outcomes in women who have been exposed to vedolizumab, a pregnancy registry has been established. Information about the registry can be obtained by calling 877-825-3327.

Lactation. Vedolizumab is distributed into milk in monkeys. It is not known whether the drug is distributed into human milk. Vedolizumab should be used with caution in nursing women.

Pediatric Use. Safety and efficacy of vedolizumab have not been established in pediatric patients.

Geriatric Use. Clinical studies of vedolizumab did not include sufficient numbers of patients 65 years of age and older to determine whether geriatric patients respond differently than younger adults. However, no overall differences in efficacy or safety were observed between geriatric and younger patients, and other clinical experience revealed no evidence of age-related differences.

Hepatic Impairment. Pharmacokinetic studies of vedolizumab have not been conducted in patients with hepatic impairment, and the manufacturer makes no specific dosage recommendations for such patients.

Renal Impairment. Pharmacokinetic studies of vedolizumab have not been conducted in patients with renal impairment, and the manufacturer makes no specific dosage recommendations for such patients.

■ **Common Adverse Effects** Adverse effects reported in 3% or more of patients with Crohn's disease or ulcerative colitis receiving vedolizumab in controlled clinical studies, and at an incidence that was at least 1% higher than that reported with placebo, include nasopharyngitis, headache, arthralgia, nausea, pyrexia, upper respiratory tract infection, fatigue, cough, bronchitis, influenza, back pain, rash, pruritus, sinusitis, oropharyngeal pain, and pain in extremities.

Drug Interactions

■ **Natalizumab** Concomitant use of vedolizumab with natalizumab, an anti-α4-integrin monoclonal antibody, should be avoided because of the potential for increased risk of progressive multifocal leukoencephalopathy (PML) and other infections. (See Progressive Multifocal Leukoencephalopathy under Cautions: Warnings/Precautions.)

■ **Tumor Necrosis Factor Blocking Agents** Concomitant use of vedolizumab with tumor necrosis factor (TNF) blocking agents should be avoided because of the potential for increased risk of infections.

■ **Vaccines** ***Inactivated Vaccines*** Following a 3-dose IM immunization series with a recombinant hepatitis B vaccine, seroconversion rates were similar in healthy individuals who received a single IV dose of vedolizumab (750 mg) and those who received placebo 4 days prior to initiation of the immunization series. The study participants also received a 2-dose immunization series with an oral inactivated cholera vaccine (not commercially available in the US), also beginning 4 days after vedolizumab or placebo administration; seroconversion rates and titers of antibody to cholera toxin were lower in individuals who received vedolizumab compared with those who received placebo. The effect of vedolizumab on immune responses to other oral or intranasal vaccines is not known. The manufacturer states that patients receiving vedolizumab may receive inactivated vaccines (e.g., parenteral influenza virus vaccine inactivated).

Live Vaccines Data are not available to date on the secondary transmission of infection by live vaccines in patients receiving vedolizumab. The manufacturer states that patients receiving vedolizumab may receive live vaccines if the potential benefits justify the possible risks.

Description

Vedolizumab, a recombinant humanized immunoglobulin G_1 (IgG_1) monoclonal antibody produced in Chinese hamster ovary cells, specifically binds to and inhibits the function of $\alpha4\beta7$ integrin. The $\alpha4\beta7$ integrin is involved principally in recruitment of lymphocytes into the GI tract and is present on the surface of a small subset of memory T-lymphocytes that preferentially migrate into the GI tract. Binding of vedolizumab to $\alpha4\beta7$ integrin blocks the interaction of $\alpha4\beta7$ integrin with mucosal addressin cell adhesion molecule-1 (MAdCAM-1), a major ligand for $\alpha4\beta7$ integrin that is expressed mainly on vascular endothelial cells in the GI tract, and inhibits migration of memory T-lymphocytes across the endothelium into inflamed GI parenchymal tissue. MAdCAM-1 plays a major role in the migration of T-lymphocytes into gut lymphoid tissue. Interaction of $\alpha4\beta7$ integrin with MAdCAM-1 has been implicated as an important contributor to the chronic inflammation that is characteristic of ulcerative colitis and Crohn's disease. Vedolizumab does not bind to or inhibit the function of $\alpha4\beta1$ and $\alpha E\beta7$ integrins and does not antagonize the interaction of $\alpha4$ integrins with vascular cell adhesion molecule-1 (VCAM-1). Vedolizumab appears to exert a more selective effect on the GI tract than does natalizumab, which binds to $\alpha4$ subunits of $\alpha4\beta1$ and $\alpha4\beta7$ integrins expressed on the surface of all leukocytes except neutrophils.

Saturation of $\alpha4\beta7$ receptors on subsets of circulating lymphocytes involved in gut immune surveillance was observed at vedolizumab doses of 0.2–10 mg/kg in clinical studies. In patients with ulcerative colitis, rectal biopsy specimens obtained following 4–6 weeks of vedolizumab therapy have revealed reductions in GI inflammation as compared with placebo controls. In healthy individuals and patients with ulcerative colitis or Crohn's disease, vedolizumab did not increase neutrophils, basophils, eosinophils, B-helper and cytotoxic T-lymphocytes, total memory helper T-lymphocytes, monocytes, or natural killer cells at doses of 0.2–10 mg/kg or 180–750 mg. In healthy individuals, vedolizumab did not alter $CD4^+$ or $CD8^+$ lymphocyte counts or $CD4^+/CD8^+$ lymphocyte ratio in CSF, and the drug was not detected in CSF at 5 weeks after IV administration of a single 450-mg dose.

Vedolizumab clearance is dependent on both linear and nonlinear pathways, and nonlinear clearance decreases with increasing concentrations of the drug. The serum half-life of vedolizumab is approximately 25 days in individuals receiving doses of 300 mg. Vedolizumab pharmacokinetics are similar in patients with ulcerative colitis and those with Crohn's disease. Population pharmacokinetic analyses indicate that pharmacokinetics of the drug are not substantially altered by disease severity, body weight, prior treatment with tumor necrosis factor (TNF) blocking agents, age (within the range of 18–78 years), serum albumin concentration, or concomitant therapy with azathioprine, mercaptopurine, methotrexate, or aminosalicylates. Plasma concentrations of the drug appear to be dose proportional over a dosage range of 2–10 mg/kg; however, the presence of persistent anti-vedolizumab antibodies reduces serum concentrations of the drug to undetectable or negligible levels.

Advice to Patients

Importance of providing patients with a copy of the manufacturer's patient information (medication guide).

Patients should be advised to immediately report symptoms consistent with a hypersensitivity reaction (e.g., rash, pruritus, shortness of breath or difficulty breathing, wheezing, dizziness, flushing, palpitations, swelling of the lips, tongue, throat, or face) that occur during or following an infusion of vedolizumab.

Importance of informing patients that they may be more likely to develop infections while receiving vedolizumab. Patients should be instructed to inform a clinician if they develop any signs or symptoms of infection (e.g., fever, chills, cough, dyspnea, fatigue, red or painful skin or sores, myalgia, rhinorrhea, sore throat, pain on urination) while receiving vedolizumab.

Importance of informing patients that progressive multifocal leukoencephalopathy (PML) has occurred in patients who received a different integrin receptor antagonist. Patients should be instructed to report any new or worsening neurologic manifestations (e.g., progressive weakness on one side of the body or clumsiness of limbs; changes in speech or walking; vision changes; changes in thinking, memory, and orientation leading to confusion and personality changes) immediately to their clinician.

Importance of informing patients that increased serum aminotransferase (ALT and AST) concentrations with or without elevated bilirubin concentrations have occurred in patients who received vedolizumab. Patients should be instructed to promptly report any symptoms suggestive of hepatic injury (e.g., fatigue, anorexia, right upper abdominal discomfort, dark urine, jaundice) while receiving vedolizumab.

Importance of reviewing vaccination status with clinician and receiving all appropriate vaccines prior to initiation of vedolizumab therapy.

Importance of informing clinician of existing or contemplated concomitant therapy, including prescription and OTC drugs and dietary or herbal supplements, as well as any concomitant illnesses (e.g., hepatic disease, tuberculosis or other infection) or any history of recurrent infections.

Importance of women informing their clinician if they are or plan to become pregnant or plan to breast-feed. (See Pregnancy under Warnings/Precautions: Specific Populations, in Cautions.)

Importance of informing patients of other important precautionary information. (See Cautions.)

Overview® (see Users Guide). For additional information on this drug until a more detailed monograph is developed and published, the manufacturer's labeling should be consulted. It is *essential* that the manufacturer's labeling be consulted for more detailed information on usual cautions, precautions, contraindications, potential drug interactions, laboratory test interferences, and acute toxicity.

Preparations

Excipients in commercially available drug preparations may have clinically important effects in some individuals; consult specific product labeling for details.

Vedolizumab

Parenteral

For injection, for IV infusion	300 mg	**Entyvio®**, Takeda

60:00 Gold Compounds

§ Omitted from the print version of *AHFS Drug Information*® because of space limitations. This monograph is available on the *AHFS Drug Information*® website, http://ahfsdruginformation.com. Username: ahfs2020; Password: ASHP94498.

64:00 Heavy Metal Antagonists

§ Omitted from the print version of *AHFS Drug Information*® because of space limitations. This monograph is available on the *AHFS Drug Information*® website, http://ahfsdruginformation.com. Username: ahfs2020; Password: ASHP94498.

68:00 Hormones and Synthetic Substitutes

68:04 Adrenals

68:08 Androgens

68:12 Contraceptives

68:16 Estrogens, Antiestrogens, and Estrogen Agonist-Antagonists

68:16.04 Estrogens

68:16.08 Antiestrogens

68:16.12 Estrogen Agonist-Antagonists

68:18 Gonadotropins

68:18.04 Antigonadotropins

68:18.08 Gonadotropins

68:20 Antidiabetic Agents

68:20.02 α-Glucosidase Inhibitors

* Please see the full AHFS Pharmacologic-Therapeutic Classification© on p. viii. Not all classes are used in the printed edition.

§ Omitted from the print version of *AHFS Drug Information®* because of space limitations. This monograph is available on the *AHFS Drug Information®* website, http://ahfsdruginformation.com. Username: ahfs2020; Password: ASHP94498.

HORMONES AND SYNTHETIC SUBSTITUTES 68:00

ADRENALS 68:04

Corticosteroids General Statement

■ Corticosteroids are hormones secreted by the adrenal cortex or synthetic analogs of these hormones. They exhibit glucocorticoid and/or mineralocorticoid activity and affect almost all body systems, but are used principally for their potent anti-inflammatory and immunosuppressant effects and for replacement.

Uses

In physiologic dosages, corticosteroids are used to replace deficient endogenous hormones. In pharmacologic dosages, the drugs have both therapeutic and diagnostic applications based on their ability to suppress secretion of normal adrenal hormones. Glucocorticoids are also used in pharmacologic dosages for their anti-inflammatory and immunosuppressant properties and their effects on blood and lymphatic systems in the palliative treatment of various diseases.

When glucocorticoids are used for their anti-inflammatory and immunosuppressant properties, synthetic glucocorticoids that have minimal mineralocorticoid activity are preferred to cortisone or hydrocortisone. *Glucocorticoid therapy is not curative and is rarely indicated as the primary method of treatment, but rather as supportive therapy to be used adjunctively with other indicated therapies.* If prolonged oral administration of glucocorticoids is required, alternate-day therapy should be used whenever possible to minimize adverse reactions, and continual attempts should be made to reduce the dosage or, preferably, to withdraw glucocorticoid therapy completely. (See General Dosage under Dosage and Administration: Dosage.)

■ **Adrenocortical Insufficiency** Corticosteroids are administered in physiologic dosages to replace deficient endogenous hormones in patients with adrenocortical insufficiency. Because production of both mineralocorticoids and glucocorticoids is deficient in these patients, hydrocortisone or cortisone (in conjunction with liberal salt intake) is usually the corticosteroid of choice for replacement therapy. Concomitant administration of a more potent mineralocorticoid (fludrocortisone) may be required in some patients, particularly in infants. If synthetic glucocorticoids are used instead of hydrocortisone or cortisone, a mineralocorticoid must also be given. In suspected or known adrenal insufficiency, parenteral therapy may be used preoperatively or during serious trauma, illness, or shock unresponsive to conventional therapy. In shock caused by acute adrenocortical insufficiency, IV administration of hydrocortisone (or a synthetic glucocorticoid) in conjunction with other therapy for shock is essential.

■ **Adrenogenital Syndrome** In salt-losing forms of congenital adrenogenital syndrome, cortisone or hydrocortisone is administered in conjunction with liberal salt intake. Because of the risk of growth retardation with excessive dosage (see Cautions: Pediatric Precautions), the minimum dosage of the corticosteroid required to suppress adrenocortical hyperfunction should be used. If sodium loss and hypotension are not adequately controlled by cortisone or hydrocortisone, an additional mineralocorticoid drug should be given. Mineralocorticoid replacement can usually be discontinued in children 5–7 years of age, but a glucocorticoid must be continued throughout life. Patients with the hypertensive form of congenital adrenogenital syndrome (who secrete excessive amounts of desoxycorticosterone) should be treated with a "short-acting" glucocorticoid with minimal mineralocorticoid activity (e.g., prednisone). Longer acting glucocorticoids (e.g., dexamethasone) should not be used in such patients because there is a tendency toward overdosage and growth may be retarded.

■ **Hypercalcemia** Glucocorticoids promote a reduction in serum calcium concentrations and are effective as hypocalcemic agents in patients with steroid-sensitive malignancies (e.g., multiple myeloma, lymphoma) and in patients with hypercalcemia due to sarcoidosis or vitamin D intoxication. Glucocorticoids are not effective in hypercalcemia caused by hyperparathyroidism.

■ **Thyroiditis** The anti-inflammatory action of glucocorticoids dramatically relieves symptoms such as fever and acute thyroid pain and swelling in granulomatous (subacute, nonsuppurative) thyroiditis. The drugs are indicated in moderate to high dosages for palliative therapy in severely ill patients unresponsive to salicylates and thyroid hormones. Glucocorticoids may also be effective in reducing orbital edema in endocrine exophthalmos (thyroid ophthalmopathy). Changes in thyroid status may necessitate adjustment of glucocorticoid dosage.

■ **Rheumatic Disorders and Collagen Diseases** In rheumatic disorders and collagen diseases, glucocorticoids relieve inflammation and suppress symptoms, but do not affect progression of the disease. The drugs are rarely indicated except for palliative, short-term treatment of acute exacerbations and systemic complications in patients refractory to more conservative therapy. Dosage in life-threatening situations is often high and is reduced rapidly after the crisis is past. Maintenance therapy with glucocorticoids is rarely indicated in rheumatoid arthritis, acute gouty arthritis, or systemic lupus erythematosus, but may be used as part of a total treatment program in selected patients when more conservative therapies have proven ineffective. Glucocorticoid withdrawal is extremely difficult in patients with these conditions, as relapses or rebounds usually occur upon discontinuance of the drugs.

In the symptomatic treatment of rheumatoid arthritis that involves only a few persistently inflamed joints or in the treatment of inflammation of tendons or bursae, local injections of slightly soluble glucocorticoids may be beneficial. Patients usually experience dramatic relief initially. Although inflammation tends to recur and sometimes it is more intense after cessation of therapy, the drugs can prevent invalidism by facilitating movement of joints that might otherwise become immobile.

Systemically administered glucocorticoids control acute manifestations of rheumatic carditis more rapidly than salicylates and may be life-saving in certain conditions, but glucocorticoids, like salicylates, cannot prevent valvular damage and are no better than salicylates for long-term treatment. Salicylates used concomitantly with glucocorticoids may decrease inflammatory rebound when the steroids are withdrawn. (See Drug Interactions: Nonsteroidal Anti-Inflammatory Agents.) Cytotoxic therapy is the treatment of choice in Wegener's granulomatosis, but glucocorticoids may be used adjunctively for severe systemic complications.

Glucocorticoids remain the primary treatment to control symptoms and prevent severe, often life-threatening complications in patients with dermatomyositis and polymyositis, polyarteritis nodosa, relapsing polychondritis, polymyalgia rheumatica and giant-cell (temporal) arteritis, or mixed connective tissue disease syndrome. High dosage may be required for acute situations; after a response has been obtained, glucocorticoids must often be continued for long periods at low dosage. Polymyositis associated with malignancy and childhood dermatomyositis may not respond well to glucocorticoids.

Systemic glucocorticoids are rarely indicated in psoriatic arthritis, diffuse scleroderma (progressive systemic sclerosis), acute and subacute bursitis, and osteoarthritis. Risks outweigh benefits received, and more conservative therapy should be used. In osteoarthritis, intra-articular injections of glucocorticoids may be beneficial but should be limited in number as joint damage may occur.

■ **Dermatologic Diseases** In dermatologic diseases such as pemphigus and pemphigoid, exfoliative dermatitis, bullous dermatitis herpetiformis, severe erythema multiforme (Stevens-Johnson syndrome), uncontrollable eczema, cutaneous sarcoidosis, mycosis fungoides, and lichen planus, systemic glucocorticoids should generally be reserved for acute exacerbations unresponsive to conservative therapy. In all these dermatologic diseases, high dosage of glucocorticoids may be required. Early initiation of systemic glucocorticoid therapy may be life-saving in pemphigus vulgaris and pemphigoid, and high or massive doses may be required. Dosage should be reduced gradually to the lowest effective level, but discontinuance may not be possible; alternate-day therapy may often be used beneficially.

Although chronic skin disorders are seldom an indication for systemic glucocorticoids, intralesional or sublesional injections may occasionally be indicated for localized chronic disorders (including keloids, psoriatic plaques, alopecia areata, discoid lupus erythematosus, and granuloma annulare) unresponsive to topical therapy. Systemic glucocorticoids are rarely indicated for psoriasis or alopecia (areata, totalis, or universalis). When systemic corticosteroids are used in the treatment of psoriasis, exacerbation of the disease may occur when the drugs are withdrawn or dosage is decreased. Although glucocorticoids may stimulate hair growth in patients with alopecia, hair loss returns when the drugs are discontinued.

■ **Allergic Conditions** Systemic glucocorticoids are used for control of severe or incapacitating allergic conditions that do not respond to adequate trials of conventional therapy in patients with bronchial asthma, seasonal or perennial allergic rhinitis, atopic dermatitis, urticaria associated with transfusion, or acute noninfectious laryngeal edema (although epinephrine is the drug of choice). Systemic glucocorticoids also may be used in acute manifestations of angioedema, serum sickness, contact dermatitis, drug hypersensitivity, and allergic symptoms of trichinosis. In acute conditions, the drugs may be used for short periods in high dosage with other therapy such as antihistamines and sympathomimetics.

In the symptomatic treatment of chronic allergic conditions, systemic glucocorticoids generally should be reserved for acute conditions and severe exacerbations. Prolonged treatment of chronic allergic conditions should be reserved for patients with disabling conditions unresponsive to more conservative therapy and for whom the risks of long-term glucocorticoid therapy are justified.

■ **Ocular Disorders** ***Optic Neuritis*** Systemic glucocorticoids have been used for the treatment of acute optic neuritis†. Interest in the use of IV methylprednisolone in the management of acute relapses of multiple sclerosis has been heightened as a result of the Optic Neuritis Treatment Trial. In this trial in which short-term glucocorticoid therapy (IV methylprednisolone 1 g daily for 3 days followed by oral prednisone 1 mg/kg daily for 11 days versus oral prednisone alone at this dosage for 14 days) was compared with placebo for the treatment of initial episodes of acute optic neuritis, the rate of vision recovery was faster with the methylprednisolone regimen, with the greatest benefit being observed in patients with visual acuity of 20/50 or worse at entry; however, there were no substantial differences in visual outcomes between the groups at 6 months. Use of oral prednisone alone did not improve the rate of vision recovery compared with placebo and was associated with an increased risk of new episodes of optic neuritis in either eye.

At 2-year follow-up, patients who had received the methylprednisolone regimen had a lower rate of progression to clinically definite multiple sclerosis than those who received placebo. This beneficial effect was most evident in patients at the highest risk for multiple sclerosis (i.e., those with multicentric brain lesions on magnetic resonance imaging [MRI] at study entry). However, after 3 years, differences between the treatment groups were no longer significant, suggesting that IV methylprednisolone delayed but did not arrest the development of multiple sclerosis after optic neuritis. At 5-year follow-up, most patients who had received the methylprednisolone regimen retained good to excellent vision, even if there had been single or multiple recurrences of optic neuritis during the 5-year period. The cumulative probability of having a new episode of optic neuritis over the 5-year follow-up period was 19% for affected eyes, 17% for fellow eyes, and 30% for either eye.

Patients who developed clinically diagnosed multiple sclerosis over the follow-up period were more likely to have recurrences of optic neuritis in the affected or fellow eye and also were more likely to have slight worsening of vision between the 6-month and 5-year follow-up examinations than patients without clinically diagnosed multiple sclerosis.

Other Ocular Disorders Systemic glucocorticoids may be used to suppress a variety of allergic and nonpyogenic ocular inflammations and to reduce scarring in ocular injuries. Glucocorticoids have been used for the treatment of severe acute and chronic allergic and inflammatory processes involving the eye that are intractable to adequate trials of conventional treatment (e.g., allergic conjunctivitis, keratitis, allergic corneal marginal ulcers, herpes zoster ophthalmicus, iritis and iridocyclitis, chorioretinitis, diffuse posterior uveitis and choroiditis, anterior segment inflammation, temporal arteritis, sympathetic ophthalmia). Moderate dosage is used initially and is quickly discontinued after the acute condition is controlled. Some disorders may relapse upon discontinuance of therapy and low-dose maintenance therapy may be required. Glucocorticoids are of no value in the treatment of degenerative ocular diseases such as cataracts.

Topically applied glucocorticoids appear to be as effective as systemic steroids for the treatment of most anterior ocular inflammations. Systemic glucocorticoid therapy may be required, however, in stubborn cases of anterior segment eye disease and is necessary when deeper ocular structures are involved.

■ **Respiratory Diseases** *Asthma* **Considerations in Initiating Antiasthma Therapy.** In the current stepped-care approach to antiasthmatic drug therapy, asthma is classified according to severity upon initial presentation (intermittent asthma or mild, moderate, or severe persistent asthma) and also by response to treatment (i.e., asthma control). While classification of asthma severity is useful for determining initial treatment, disease severity may vary over time and with treatment; therefore, after therapy is initiated, periodic assessment of asthma control is emphasized for guiding treatment decisions. Current asthma management guidelines state that initial therapy should correspond to disease severity, with subsequent monitoring and adjustments in therapy to achieve and maintain control of asthma according to the goals of treatment. Asthma therapy is aimed at achieving and maintaining control of asthma by reducing ongoing impairment (e.g., prevention of chronic and troublesome symptoms, reducing use of reliever drugs, maintaining normal or near-normal lung function and activity levels) and risk of future events (e.g., exacerbations requiring systemic glucocorticoids, treatment-related adverse effects). These 2 components of asthma control (i.e., current impairment and future risk) may respond differently to treatment.

The National Asthma Education and Prevention Program (NAEPP) classifies the levels of asthma control as well controlled, not well controlled, or very poorly controlled. In the stepped-care approach, the treatment step selected for asthma control in patients already receiving asthma therapy is based on the patient's current treatment and level of asthma control. Stepwise therapy is meant to assist, not replace, the clinical decision-making process in selecting therapy for individual patients. Once initiated, treatment is adjusted continuously according to changes in asthma control. Patients should be monitored every 2–6 weeks following initiation of therapy to ensure that asthma control is achieved. If asthma symptoms are not controlled with the current treatment regimen, treatment is stepped up until control is achieved. If an alternative treatment was used and produced an inadequate response, the preferred treatment should be used before stepping up to the next level of therapy. Regular monitoring at 1- to 6-month intervals, depending on the level of control, is recommended to ensure that control of asthma is maintained and that appropriate adjustments in therapy are made. When control has been maintained for at least 3 months, treatment intensity may be stepped down to find the lowest dosage and/or number of drugs required to maintain asthma control, with continued follow-up at 3-month intervals.

Mild Persistent Asthma. Drugs for asthma may be categorized as relievers (e.g., bronchodilators taken as needed for acute symptoms) or controllers (principally inhaled glucocorticoids or other anti-inflammatory agents taken regularly to achieve long-term control of asthma). In the stepped-care approach to antiasthmatic drug therapy, current asthma management guidelines and most clinicians recommend initiation of a controller drug such as an anti-inflammatory agent, preferably a low-dose orally inhaled glucocorticoid (e.g., 88–264, 88–176, or 176 mcg of fluticasone propionate [or its equivalent] daily via a metered-dose inhaler in adolescents and adults, children 5–11 years of age, or children 4 years of age or younger, respectively) as first-line therapy for persistent asthma (i.e., patients with daytime symptoms of asthma more than twice weekly but less than once daily, and nocturnal symptoms of asthma 3–4 times per month), supplemented by as-needed use of a short-acting, inhaled β_2-agonist. Alternatives to low-dose inhaled glucocorticoids as long-term control therapy for mild persistent asthma include certain leukotriene modifiers (i.e., montelukast, zafirlukast), extended-release theophylline, or mast-cell stabilizers (e.g., cromolyn sodium, nedocromil [preparation for oral inhalation no longer commercially available in the US]), but these therapies are less effective and generally not preferred as initial therapy. Some experts recommend that long-term control therapy be considered in infants and children 4 years of age or younger who have identifiable risk factors for asthma (e.g., parental history of asthma, clinician-diagnosed atopic dermatitis, sensitization to aeroallergens, or 2 of the following conditions: sensitization to foods, peripheral blood eosinophilia exceeding 4%, or wheezing unrelated to colds) and who in the previous year have had at least 4 episodes of wheezing that lasted more than 1 day and symptoms that affected sleep. Low-dose inhaled glucocorticoids also are recommended as the preferred initial therapy in such children. Cromolyn sodium is suggested (based on extrapolation of data from studies in older children) or montelukast is recommended by some experts as an alternative, but not preferred, therapy for children 4 years of age or younger with mild persistent asthma. Other experts do not consider mast cell stabilizers or extended-release theophylline to be acceptable alternatives to inhaled glucocorticoids for routine use as initial long-term therapy for such patients. Montelukast may be considered for maintenance therapy in young children with mild persistent asthma when inhaled glucocorticoid delivery is suboptimal as a result of poor technique or adherence.

Moderate Persistent Asthma. According to current asthma management guidelines, therapy with a long-acting inhaled β_2-agonist such as salmeterol or formoterol generally is recommended in adults and adolescents who have moderate persistent asthma and daily asthmatic symptoms that are inadequately controlled following addition of low-dose inhaled glucocorticoids to as-needed inhaled β_2-agonist treatment. However, the NAEPP recommends that the beneficial effects of long-acting inhaled β_2-agonists should be weighed carefully against the increased risk (although uncommon) of severe asthma exacerbations and asthma-related deaths associated with daily use of such agents. (See Asthma-related Death and Life-threatening Events under Cautions: Respiratory Effects, in Salmeterol 12:12.08.12.) Current asthma management guidelines also state that an alternative, but equally preferred option for management of moderate persistent asthma that is not adequately controlled with a low dosage of inhaled glucocorticoid is to increase the maintenance dosage to a medium dosage (e.g., exceeding 264 but not more than 440 mcg of fluticasone propionate [or its equivalent] daily via a metered-dose inhaler in adults and adolescents). Alternative less effective therapies that may be added to a low dosage of an inhaled glucocorticoid include oral extended-release theophylline or certain leukotriene modifiers (i.e., montelukast, zafirlukast).

Limited data are available in infants and children 11 years of age or younger with moderate persistent asthma, and recommendations of care are based on expert opinion and extrapolation from studies in adults. A long-acting inhaled β_2-agonist (e.g., salmeterol, formoterol), a leukotriene modifier (i.e., montelukast, zafirlukast), or extended-release theophylline (with appropriate monitoring) may be added to low-dose inhaled glucocorticoid therapy in children 5–11 years of age according to current asthma management guidelines. Because comparative data establishing relative efficacy of these agents are lacking in this age group, there is no clearly preferred agent as adjunctive therapy with a low-dose inhaled glucocorticoid for treatment of asthma in these children. In children 5–11 years of age with moderate persistent asthma that is not controlled with a low dosage of an inhaled glucocorticoid, another preferred option in current asthma management guidelines is to increase the maintenance dosage of the inhaled glucocorticoid to a medium dosage (e.g., exceeding 176 but not more than 352 mcg of fluticasone propionate [or its equivalent] daily via a metered-dose inhaler). In infants and children 4 years of age or younger with moderate persistent asthma that is not controlled by a low dosage of an inhaled glucocorticoid, the only preferred option is to increase the maintenance dosage of the inhaled glucocorticoid to a medium dosage (e.g., exceeding 176 but not more than 352 mcg of fluticasone propionate [or its equivalent] daily via a metered-dose inhaler).

Severe Persistent Asthma. Maintenance therapy with an inhaled glucocorticoid at medium dosages or high dosages (e.g., exceeding 440 mcg of fluticasone propionate [or its equivalent] in adults and adolescents or 352 mcg of the drug in children 5–11 years of age [or its equivalent] daily via a metered-dose inhaler) and adjunctive therapy with a long-acting inhaled β_2-agonist is the preferred treatment according to current asthma management guidelines in adults and children 5 years of age or older with severe persistent asthma (i.e., continuous daytime asthma symptoms, nighttime symptoms 7 times per week). Such therapy is appropriate in patients who have recurrent severe exacerbations requiring oral glucocorticoids, emergency department visits, or hospitalizations during therapy with low-dose inhaled corticosteroids. Treatment recommendations in children 5–11 years of age with severe persistent asthma are based on expert opinion and extrapolation from studies in older children and adults. Alternatives to a long-acting inhaled β_2-agonist for severe persistent asthma in adults and children 5 years of age or older receiving medium-dose inhaled glucocorticoids include extended-release theophylline or certain leukotriene modifiers (i.e., montelukast, zafirlukast), but these therapies are generally not preferred. Omalizumab may be considered in adults and adolescents with severe asthma with an allergic component who are inadequately controlled with high-dose inhaled glucocorticoids and a long-acting inhaled β_2-agonist. IM glucocorticoids have no advantage over a short oral course of oral glucocorticoids in preventing recurrent exacerbations. However, some glucocorticoids are recommended for IM use for control of severe or incapacitating allergic bronchial asthma in patients whose disease is intractable to adequate trials of conventional oral glucocorticoid treatment, those who are vomiting, or those who are noncompliant with oral glucocorticoid therapy. In infants and children 4 years of age or younger with severe asthma, maintenance therapy with an inhaled glucocorticoid at medium or high dosages (e.g., exceeding 352 mcg of fluticasone propionate [or its equivalent] daily via a metered-dose inhaler) and adjunctive therapy with either a long-acting inhaled β_2-agonist or montelukast is the only preferred treatment according to current asthma management guidelines. Recommendations for care of infants and children with severe asthma are based on expert opinion and extrapolation from studies in adolescents and adults. Patients with severe persistent asthma (including allergic asthma that may require immunotherapy or omalizumab) who have difficulty in achieving and maintaining control of asthma, or an exacerbation that requires hospitalization generally should be managed in consultation with an asthma specialist.

Poorly Controlled Asthma. If asthma symptoms in adults and children 5 years of age or older with moderate to severe asthma are very poorly controlled (i.e., at least 2 exacerbations per year requiring oral corticosteroids) with low to high maintenance dosages of an inhaled glucocorticoid and a long-acting inhaled β_2-agonist bronchodilator, a short course (3–10 days) of an oral glucocorticoid may be added to gain prompt control of asthma. In infants and children 4 years of age or younger with moderate-to-severe asthma who are very poorly controlled (i.e., more than 3 exacerbations per year requiring oral glucocorticoids) with medium-to-high maintenance dosages of an inhaled glucocorticoid with or without adjunctive therapy (i.e., a long-acting inhaled β_2-agonist, montelukast), a short course (3–10 days) of an oral glucocorticoid may be added to gain prompt control of asthma.

While clinical efficacy of oral glucocorticoids as add-on therapy in adults and children 5 years of age or older with severe asthma who are inadequately controlled with a high-dose inhaled glucocorticoid, intermittent oral glucocorticoid therapy, and a long-acting inhaled β_2-agonist bronchodilator has not been established in randomized controlled studies, some experts suggest regular use of oral glucocorticoids in such patients, based on consensus and clinical experience. A short course (2 weeks) of oral glucocorticoids may be considered to confirm clinical response prior to implementing long-term therapy with these agents. Once long-term oral glucocorticoid therapy is initiated, the lowest possible effective dosage (i.e., alternate-day or once-daily administration) should be used and the patient should be monitored carefully for adverse effects. Once asthma is well controlled, repeated attempts should be made to reduce the oral glucocorticoid dosage. Similarly, some experts, based on consensus and clinical experience, suggest regular use of oral glucocorticoid therapy in infants and children 4 years of age or younger with severe asthma who are not controlled with high-dose inhaled glucocorticoid and either a long-acting inhaled β_2-agonist or montelukast and intermittent oral glucocorticoid therapy. However, other experts do not consider regular use of oral glucocorticoid therapy to be appropriate therapy in children with severely uncontrolled asthma.

When asthma symptoms at any stage are not controlled with maintenance therapy plus supplemental, as-needed therapy with a short-acting inhaled β_2-agonist bronchodilator (e.g., if there is a need to increase the dose or frequency of administration of the short-acting sympathomimetic agent), prompt reevaluation is required to adjust dosage of the maintenance regimen or institute an alternative maintenance regimen.

Home Management of Acute Asthma Exacerbations. For acute exacerbations of asthma, initial home treatment consists of use of an inhaled short-acting β_2-agonist (no more than 2 doses via a metered-dose inhaler with 2–6 inhalations per dose or via nebulization every 20 minutes). Patients who have exacerbations of less severity may require a reduced dosage of a short-acting β_2-agonist. If response is good (peak expiratory flow [PEF] returns to at least 80% of predicted value or personal best and response is maintained for 3–4 hours), therapy with a short-acting β_2-agonist should be continued every 3–4 hours for 24–48 hours, and a short course of an oral glucocorticoid may be considered. If response is incomplete (PEF 50–79% of predicted value or personal best), therapy with an inhaled short-acting β_2-agonist should be continued, and an oral glucocorticoid should be added. If patients have a poor response to bronchodilator therapy (PEF less than 50% of predicted value or personal best), administration of an inhaled short-acting β_2-agonist should be repeated immediately, and an oral glucocorticoid should be added. Some clinicians recommend adding oral glucocorticoids (0.5–1 mg/kg prednisolone [or its equivalent] during a 24-hour period) to quickly resolve all but the mildest exacerbations of asthma, especially in patients whose response to a short-acting inhaled β_2-agonist is not prompt or sustained (e.g., PEF exceeding 80% of predicted value or personal best) after 1 hour or in those who have a history of exacerbations that required oral glucocorticoids. Oral glucocorticoids such as prednisone, prednisolone, or methylprednisolone are preferred over parenteral glucocorticoids because of their minimal mineralocorticoid effect, their relatively short half-life, and their limited effects on striated muscle. However, effects of glucocorticoids may not be evident for 4–6 hours; therefore, such drugs should not be the only treatment in an emergency.

For management of exacerbations due to viral respiratory infections, a short-acting inhaled β_2-agonist every 4–6 hours for 24 hours (longer therapy requires consultation with a clinician) in patients with mild symptoms may be sufficient to control symptoms and improve lung function. If viral infection-associated exacerbations occur more frequently than every 6 weeks, use of long-term control therapy should be considered. If a viral respiratory infection provokes moderate-to-severe exacerbations, a short course of an oral glucocorticoid should be considered. For those with a history of severe exacerbations associated with viral infections, initiation of oral glucocorticoids should be considered at the first sign of infection.

Prehospital Management of Acute Asthma Exacerbations. Should the response to home-initiated drug therapy be incomplete (PEF 50–79% of predicted value or personal best) or poor (PEF less than 50% of predicted value or personal best) after short-acting β_2-agonist therapy, the patient should seek medical attention urgently (same day if response is incomplete) or proceed immediately to the emergency department of a hospital (if response is poor). Other clinicians recommend seeking urgent medical attention in patients at a high risk of asthma-related death and those with continuing severe exacerbations (e.g., PEF remains less than 60% of predicted or personal best following use of a short-acting inhaled β_2-agonist, response to bronchodilator therapy has a duration of less than 2 hours). Orally inhaled, selective short-acting β_2-adrenergic agonists (i.e., albuterol, levalbuterol, pirbuterol) currently are recommended by an expert panel of NAEPP for prehospital management of asthma exacerbations (e.g., in emergency medicine facilities and/or ambulances). During prolonged emergency transport, NAEPP recommends that other asthma therapies such as ipratropium bromide and oral glucocorticoids should also be available for use.

Management of Acute Asthma Exacerbations in Acute-care Settings. In the emergency department, orally inhaled, selective β_2-adrenergic agonists via metered-dose inhaler or nebulization (not exceeding 3 doses every 20 minutes during the first hour) and supplemental oxygen currently also are recommended for asthma management in patients with mild-to-moderate acute exacerbations (forced expiratory volume in 1 second [FEV_1] or PEF at least 40% of predicted or personal best). If response to a β_2-adrenergic agonist in patients with mild-to-moderate asthma exacerbations is not immediate or if patients used oral glucocorticoids as self-medication prior to hospitalization, systemic oral glucocorticoids should be added to the regimen in the emergency department. Some clinicians suggest that *adjunctive* therapy with an inhaled anticholinergic bronchodilator (i.e., ipratropium) be considered in the emergency department in patients with moderate or severe exacerbations (PEF 60–80% or less than 60%, respectively, of predicted or personal best) of asthma who fail to respond adequately to β_2-adrenergic agonists and oral glucocorticoids. NAEPP recommends adjunctive therapy with ipratropium (via nebulization or a metered-dose inhaler) and oral glucocorticoids in patients with severe asthma exacerbations (FEV_1 or PEF less than 40% of predicted or personal best) in the emergency department who fail to respond adequately to short-acting, inhaled β_2-agonists. If the episode is severe, 1 dose of a short-acting β_2-agonist should be given, and the patient should be assessed for potential hospitalization. Adjunctive therapy such as IV magnesium sulfate or a nebulization gas mixture of helium and oxygen (heliox) may be considered to decrease the likelihood of intubation, but intubation should not be delayed if the procedure is deemed necessary. In patients with impending respiratory failure, intubation and mechanical ventilation with 100% oxygen, a short-acting β_2-adrenergic agonist in combination with ipratropium via nebulization given hourly or continuously, and an IV glucocorticoid should be administered in the emergency department. However, NAEPP recommends discontinuance of ipratropium upon hospitalization for severe asthma exacerbations for patients of all age groups. (See Asthma under Uses: Bronchospasm, in Albuterol 12:12.08.12.)

A repeat assessment of response should be made in all patients after the initial hour of intensive conventional treatment in the emergency department. In patients who have a moderate asthma exacerbation (FEV_1 or PEF of 40–69% of predicted or personal best) after the initial hour of intensive conventional treatment, an oral glucocorticoid and an inhaled short-acting β_2-agonist (once every hour) should be continued for 1–3 hours provided there is improvement; assessment of response and decision to hospitalize the patient should be made in less than 4 hours after admittance to the emergency department. For severe asthma exacerbations not responding to 1 hour of intensive conventional therapy, oxygen and oral glucocorticoids should be continued, and an inhaled short-acting β_2-agonist and ipratropium should be administered via nebulization either continuously or hourly in the emergency department. Assessment of response in patients with severe asthma exacerbations should be repeated at 2 hours, and discharge is appropriate in patients with a good response (FEV_1 or PEF at least 60–70% of predicted value or personal best that is sustained for 60 minutes after last treatment, normal physical examination). If response is incomplete (FEV_1 or PEF 40–69% of predicted or personal best and continuing mild-to-moderate symptoms), the decision to hospitalize the patient should be individualized.

Upon hospitalization, therapy with oxygen and an inhaled short-acting β_2-agonist should be continued, and therapy with oral glucocorticoids should be continued or intensified (switched from oral to IV). Adjunctive therapies (e.g., magnesium sulfate, heliox) could be considered in patients with an incomplete response to several hours of intensive therapy. Patients admitted to the hospital should be reassessed at regular intervals. Patients with a poor response to such hospitalization and interventions (FEV_1 or PEF less than 40% of predicted or personal best) and those with an incomplete response after 6–12 hours of hospitalization should be admitted to an intensive care unit (ICU). Patients with a poor response to several hours of intensive therapy and patients with impending respiratory failure also should be admitted to an ICU. Upon ICU admission, therapy with ipratropium should be discontinued, but therapy with a short-acting β_2-agonist, an IV glucocorticoid, and possible adjunctive therapy should be continued. Discharge is appropriate in hospitalized patients with a good response. Upon discharge, treatment with a short-acting β_2-agonist and an oral glucocorticoid (3–10 days) should be continued, and initiation of an inhaled glucocorticoid should be considered. Patients who were already taking an inhaled glucocorticoid prior to the acute exacerbation should continue therapy following discharge.

For more information on the stepped-care approach to drug therapy in asthma, see Asthma under Uses: Bronchospasm, in Albuterol 12:12.08.12.

Chronic Obstructive Pulmonary Disease The effects of oral and inhaled glucocorticoids in patients with stable chronic obstructive pulmonary disease† (COPD) are much less dramatic than in those with asthma, and the role of glucocorticoids in the management of stable COPD is limited to very specific indications. Because inhaled glucocorticoids do not affect the decline in lung function or reliably improve quality of life in patients with COPD, use of inhaled glucocorticoids is not considered first-line therapy for the treatment of COPD. However, in patients with severe to very severe COPD (e.g., FEV_1 less than 50% of predicted, history of exacerbations), the addition of an inhaled glucocorticoid to one or more long-acting bronchodilators may reduce the frequency of exacerbations and improve health status. Use of an inhaled glucocorticoid/long-acting bronchodilator combination should be reserved for patients with are symptomatic (repeated exacerbations) despite optimal or maximal dosages of long-acting bronchodilators. Beneficial effects of inhaled glucocorticoids in such patients have been seen with dosages equivalent to 800 mcg of budesonide daily. Short-acting bronchodilators may be used as needed for relief of acute symptoms that occur despite regular use of an inhaled glucocorticoid and long-acting bronchodilators. If symptoms are not adequately controlled with inhaled glucocorticoids and a long-acting bronchodilator, or if limiting adverse effects occur, oral extended-release theophylline may be added or substituted. Long-term treatment with oral glucocorticoids should be avoided in patients with COPD.

Management of acute exacerbations of COPD at home is based initially on the same drugs used for management of the stable patient. A short-acting β_2-adrenergic agonist is the preferred bronchodilator for treatment of acute exacerbations of COPD. For more severe exacerbations of COPD (e.g., FEV_1 less than 50% of predicted), a short (e.g., 10–14 days) course of oral glucocorticoids (e.g., equivalent to 30–40 mg of prednisone daily) can be added to bronchodilator therapy. Some clinicians consider inhaled glucocorticoids as an alternative to oral glucocorticoids for management of acute exacerbations of COPD. Oral glucocorticoids are especially helpful within the first 72 hours of an acute exacerbation and should be initiated early at the first signs of an exacerbation. If symptoms of COPD continue to deteriorate several hours after administration of oral glucocorticoids (e.g., sudden development of resting dyspnea, cyanosis, peripheral edema, changes in mental status, inability to eat or sleep because of symptoms), hospital assessment or admission should be considered. If patients cannot tolerate oral glucocorticoids, IV glucocorticoids should be used.

For additional information on the stepped-care approach to COPD, see Chronic Obstructive Pulmonary Disease under Uses: Bronchospasm, in Albuterol 12:12.08.12 and in Ipratropium 12:08.08.

Sarcoidosis In the management of sarcoidosis, systemic glucocorticoids are indicated for ocular, CNS, glandular, myocardial, or severe pulmonary involvement or for hypercalcemia or severe skin lesions unresponsive to intralesional or sublesional injections of glucocorticoids. Long-term therapy may be required.

Advanced Pulmonary and Extrapulmonary Tuberculosis Systemic glucocorticoids have been used as adjunctive therapy in some patients with severe pulmonary or extrapulmonary tuberculosis in an attempt to suppress manifestations related to the host's inflammatory response to the *Mycobacterium tuberculosis* bacillus and ameliorate complications of the disease. While evidence from studies of *M. tuberculosis* infection in both animals and humans indicates that glucocorticoids can have deleterious effects (e.g., increased virulence of the organism) in the absence of adequate antituberculosis therapy, such effects generally appear to be prevented by coadministration of effective antimycobacterial agents (e.g., streptomycin, isoniazid). Data from randomized, controlled trials are limited and principally consist of studies conducted before the use of current 4-drug, short-course antituberculosis regimens; however, an analysis of available evidence suggests that adjunctive glucocorticoid therapy may enhance short-term resolution of disease manifestations (e.g., clinical and radiographic abnormalities) in patients with advanced pulmonary tuberculosis and also may reduce mortality associated with certain forms of extrapulmonary disease (e.g., meningitis, pericarditis). Additional randomized, controlled studies in patients receiving current short-course antituberculosis regimens are needed to fully elucidate the potential benefits and risks of adjunctive glucocorticoid therapy in pulmonary or extrapulmonary tuberculosis. Dosage of adjunctive corticosteroids may need to be adjusted upward in patients receiving rifampin-containing antituberculosis regimens as a result of rifampin-induced increases in corticosteroid metabolism. (See Drug Interactions: Drugs Undergoing Hepatic Metabolism, in Rifampin 8:16.04.)

Advanced Pulmonary Tuberculosis. Adjunctive systemic glucocorticoid therapy has been used to treat severe systemic and respiratory manifestations in patients with advanced pulmonary tuberculosis. Although benefit to the patient is unclear, radiographically evident abnormalities (other than cavities) usually resolve more rapidly with glucocorticoid therapy. No improvement in long-term outcomes (chronic respiratory disease or death) has been observed. In patients receiving adequate antituberculosis therapy (2 or more effective agents), glucocorticoid use does not appear to delay the time to conversion of sputum culture to negative or affect long-term cure rates.

Tuberculous Meningitis. Use of systemic adjunctive glucocorticoids (e.g., dexamethasone, prednisone) in patients with moderate to severe tuberculous meningitis appears to reduce sequelae (e.g., intellectual impairment) and/or improve survival. In a randomized, controlled study in young children (mean age younger than 36 months) with tuberculous meningitis, therapy with prednisone (2–4 mg/kg daily) reduced mortality in patients with stage III disease from 17% to 4% but did not reduce the incidence of permanent motor deficits (hemiparesis and quadriparesis). Results from a prospective, randomized, placebo-controlled study in adults and adolescents older than 14 years of age with tuberculous meningitis (with or without HIV infection) also showed reduced mortality (relative risk of death of 0.69; 95% confidence interval of 0.52–0.92) in patients receiving dexamethasone (IV therapy tapered over 2–4 weeks, depending on disease severity, followed by oral therapy tapered over 4 weeks), but dexamethasone therapy was not associated with a substantial reduction in the proportion of severely disabled patients among survivors or in the proportion of patients who had either died or were severely disabled after 9 months. A faster resolution of abnormal CSF parameters (e.g., elevated intracranial pressure, basal exudate, CNS tuberculomas) occurs with glucocorticoids use, which may aid in patient management. Available data suggest that response is most favorable in patients with disease of intermediate severity (as opposed to early or late disease) and that continuation of glucocorticoid therapy for at least 4 weeks may be associated with better outcomes than with shorter regimens.

Tuberculous Pericarditis. Limited data suggest that adjunctive systemic glucocorticoid therapy is effective in the management of acute tuberculous pericarditis, rapidly reducing the size of pericardial effusions and the need for drainage procedures and decreasing mortality (probably through control of hemodynamically threatening effusion). However, glucocorticoid therapy does not appear to alter the incidence of progression to constrictive disease when used for treatment of either the acute or intermediate stage of pericarditis.

Tuberculous Pleurisy. While most studies of adjunctive systemic glucocorticoid therapy in patients with tuberculous pleurisy have not been randomized or controlled, limited evidence suggests that such therapy hastens the resolution of pain, dyspnea, and fever associated with this form of the disease. However, glucocorticoids appear to have little efficacy in preventing fibrotic changes and resultant constrictive lung disease, and some clinicians advise against their routine use.

Other Tuberculosis Complications. Limited data suggest that intrathoracic adenopathy associated with primary tuberculosis may resolve more rapidly with the use of adjunctive systemic glucocorticoids. While a few studies have reported a reduced frequency of complications (e.g., recurrent abdominal pain, intestinal obstruction) with adjunctive glucocorticoid therapy in patients with peritoneal tuberculosis, data from randomized trials are lacking, and rapid improvement in symptoms occurred in these patients with antituberculosis therapy alone. Although it has been suggested that atelectasis associated with endobronchial tuberculosis may benefit from glucocorticoid therapy, results of a randomized, controlled trial in a limited number of patients with this form of the disease suggested no important benefit of glucocorticoid therapy over antituberculosis therapy alone with regard to healing rates and changes in pulmonary function. Inadequate data are available regarding the safety and efficacy of adjunctive glucocorticoid therapy in patients with tuberculous lymphadenitis, miliary or laryngeal tuberculosis, or HIV-associated tuberculosis.

Lipid Pneumonitis In lipid pneumonitis, glucocorticoids appear to promote the breakdown or dissolution of pulmonary lesions and eliminate lipids in the sputum. Although high doses of glucocorticoids are commonly used in hydrocarbon pneumonitis to prevent pulmonary edema and fibrosis, there is no evidence that they prevent any complications or improve the recovery rate.

Pneumocystis carinii Pneumonia The use of systemic glucocorticoids as adjunctive therapy for *Pneumocystis carinii* pneumonia in patients with acquired immunodeficiency syndrome† (AIDS) can decrease the likelihood of deterioration of oxygenation, respiratory failure, and/or death in those with moderate to severe pneumonia. Based on the results of controlled, randomized studies, the National Institutes of Health-University of California (NIH-UC) Expert Panel currently recommends that adults and adolescents older than 13 years of age with documented or suspected human immunodeficiency virus (HIV) infection and documented or suspected pneumocystis pneumonia be given systemic glucocorticoid therapy in addition to anti-infective treatment if they have moderate to severe pulmonary dysfunction, defined as an arterial oxygen pressure of less than 70 mm Hg or an arterial-alveolar gradient exceeding 35 mm Hg on room air. It is not known whether patients with mild pneumocystis pneumonia (arterial oxygen pressure exceeding 70 mm Hg or arterial-alveolar gradient less than 35 mm Hg on room air) might have clinically important benefit with adjunctive glucocorticoid therapy, and such benefit may be difficult to demonstrate in clinical studies because of the generally good clinical outcome of this group.

Current data suggest that glucocorticoids prevent the early deterioration in oxygenation associated with antipneumocystis therapy, and it is recommended that adjunctive glucocorticoid therapy be initiated as early as possible in patients with pneumocystis pneumonia. Benefit in controlled studies has not been demonstrated with initiation of glucocorticoid therapy more than 72 hours after initiation of specific antipneumocystis therapy. Therefore, glucocorticoid therapy can be started in patients with presumed AIDS-associated pneumocystis pneumonia if these patients meet the oxygenation criteria recommended by the Expert Panel. The diagnosis of HIV infection and pneumocystis pneumonia should be confirmed promptly to minimize the likelihood of masking and/or exacerbating other treatable diseases (e.g., tuberculosis) and to avoid adverse effects of unnecessary drugs. Pending the availability of specific efficacy or safety data, it may be reasonable to consider adjunctive systemic glucocorticoid therapy for pneumocystis pneumonia in immunosuppressed patients *without* HIV infection or in pregnant women with HIV infection according to the same criteria as for nonpregnant adults with HIV infection.

Pending further accumulation of data, the NIH-UC Expert Panel recommends specific regimens of prednisone or, if parenteral therapy is required, methylprednisolone. (See Dosage and Administration, in Prednisone 68:04 and Methylprednisolone 68:04.) Higher dosages for patients whose condition is not improving on glucocorticoids, or newly initiated glucocorticoid therapy for those patients in whom standard treatment alone is failing, may or may not be beneficial; available evidence is inadequate to provide specific recommendations. Data also are needed to elucidate further the safety of adjunctive systemic glucocorticoid therapy in adolescents older than 13 years of age and adults with pneumocystis pneumonia and to establish the safety and efficacy of such therapy in pediatric AIDS patients with pneumocystis pneumonia. The regimen recommended by the Expert Panel was associated with a possible increased risk of reactivation of localized herpetic lesions and oral thrush lesions but no increase in the incidence of other opportunistic infections or malignancies (i.e., Kaposi's sarcoma).

Other Respiratory Diseases Systemic glucocorticoids may be used for symptomatic relief of acute manifestations of respiratory diseases including symptomatic idiopathic eosinophilic pneumonias (e.g., Löffler's syndrome) not manageable by other means, idiopathic pulmonary fibrosis, allergic bronchopulmonary aspergillosis, idiopathic bronchiolitis obliterans with organizing pneumonia, aspiration pneumonitis, hypersensitivity pneumonitis, and berylliosis. Glucocorticoids also are used in fulminating or disseminated tuberculosis (see Advanced Pulmonary and Extrapulmonary Tuberculosis under Uses: Respiratory Diseases) in conjunction with appropriate antituberculosis therapy. High dosage may be required for several days. Glucocorticoids are not indicated for uncomplicated chronic respiratory diseases.

■ Complications of Prematurity ***Antenatal Use in Preterm Labor*** Short-course IM therapy with glucocorticoids (e.g., dexamethasone, betamethasone) is used in selected women with preterm labor to hasten fetal maturation (e.g., lungs, cerebral blood vessels), including women with preterm premature rupture of membranes, preeclampsia, or third-trimester hemorrhage. Antenatal administration of glucocorticoids generally appears to reduce the incidence and/or severity of neonatal respiratory distress syndrome (RDS) as indicated by a reduction in requirements for neonatal ventilatory support or surfactant therapy, and the beneficial effects are additive with those of surfactant.

Antenatal glucocorticoid therapy also can improve neonatal circulatory stability and reduce the incidence or severity of intraventricular hemorrhage. The incidence of necrotizing enterocolitis also is reduced by the use of antenatal glucocorticoids. The combined effects on multiple organ maturation during glucocorticoid therapy reduces the incidence of neonatal mortality, and the beneficial effects extend to a broad range of gestational ages (i.e., 24–34 weeks) and are not limited by gender or race.

Data are conflicting concerning the effects of antenatal glucocorticoids on the incidence of bronchopulmonary dysplasia, and patent ductus arteriosus in neonates, and the efficacy and safety of antenatal therapy with the drugs before 24 weeks or after 34 weeks of gestation have not been established. Short-term adverse effects of antenatal glucocorticoid administration include transient neonatal and maternal adrenal suppression and increased risk of infection. No long-term sequelae were noted in children up to 12 years of age who had been exposed to short-term antenatal glucocorticoids.

Antenatal use of glucocorticoids to reduce infant morbidity and mortality in women with preterm premature rupture of membranes is somewhat controversial, since the magnitude of neonatal benefit on RDS appears to be less and the risk of neonatal infection is greater than those in women with intact membranes. However, even in the presence of preterm premature rupture of membranes, the incidence of neonatal mortality and intraventricular hemorrhage is reduced with antenatal glucocorticoid therapy. In addition, the magnitude of increased risk of neonatal infection associated with such therapy appears to be small. Therefore, because of the benefit on mortality and hemorrhage in fetuses younger than 30–32 weeks' gestation and the apparently small risk, antenatal maternal glucocorticoid therapy is considered appropriate in the absence of clinically important chorioamnionitis.

Antenatal therapy with IM dexamethasone phosphate (6 mg every 12 hours for 2 days) or IM betamethasone sodium phosphate in fixed combination with betamethasone acetate (12 mg once daily for 2 days) has been studied most extensively, and some experts state that these drugs generally have been preferred for use in preterm labor because of similarities in potency and efficacy and their ability to readily cross the placenta, as well as the relative absence of mineralocorticoid activity and relatively weak immunosuppressive effects. These glucocorticoids also have been preferred because of their longer duration of action compared with hydrocortisone or methylprednisone.

Beneficial effects of IM glucocorticoids on fetal maturation are greatest more than 24 hours after initiating therapy and extend up to at least 7 days; however, clinically important improvement in neonatal outcomes also has been observed in women receiving an incomplete course of glucocorticoid therapy (i.e., less than 24 hours), and antenatal administration of even a partial course of glucocorticoids should be attempted unless immediate delivery is anticipated. Some experts recommend a single course of treatment for all pregnant women between 24–34 weeks' gestation who are at risk of preterm delivery within 7 days and state that repeat courses of antenatal glucocorticoids should not be used routinely because data evaluating the risks and benefits of such therapy are insufficient. A recent clinical study evaluated the overall effect on neonatal morbidity of repeated weekly courses of antenatal glucocorticoid therapy compared with a single course of treatment in pregnant women at risk of preterm delivery. The incidence of neonatal morbidity (defined as the presence of severe RDS, bronchopulmonary dysplasia, severe intraventricular hemorrhage [IVH], periventricular leukomalacia, necrotizing enterocolitis, proven sepsis, or death between randomization and nursery discharge) observed with weekly treatment courses (22.5%) was similar to that observed with single courses of therapy (28%). Other clinical studies are in progress to determine if a specific number of exposures to antenatal corticosteroids or an increased interval between treatment courses will improve neonatal outcomes in women at risk of preterm delivery.

Maternal use of tocolytic agents in conjunction with glucocorticoids may delay delivery in patients with preterm labor long enough for the fetus to derive benefit from glucocorticoid-induced accelerated fetal maturation. Combined use of the drugs has been shown to reduce the risk of neonatal RDS, and women between 24–34 weeks' gestation at risk of preterm delivery are candidates for antenatal glucocorticoid therapy regardless of fetal race, gender, or availability of surfactant. Because β-adrenergic tocolytic monotherapy may be associated with an increased risk of intraventricular hemorrhage, the addition of antenatal glucocorticoid therapy could have a secondary benefit of reducing this risk.

Antenatal glucocorticoid therapy appears to have an additive effect with postnatal prophylactic lung surfactant therapy in reducing the incidence of RDS and neonatal mortality. In addition, antenatal glucocorticoids can reduce the incidence and/or severity of intraventricular hemorrhage, which surfactant therapy alone does not appear to benefit. However, data are limited concerning the prophylactic use of combination therapy for respiratory distress syndrome in women less than 28 weeks' gestation.

Postnatal Use for Bronchopulmonary Dysplasia Although some evidence indicates that postnatal IV glucocorticoids (e.g., dexamethasone) may be useful in preventing or treating bronchopulmonary dysplasia in preterm neonates with very low birth weight (i.e., less than 1.5 kg) who require mechanical ventilation, other evidence suggests that such therapy may be associated with an increased risk of serious adverse effects. Glucocorticoid therapy may provide short-term pulmonary benefits (e.g., reduced incidence of bronchopulmonary dysplasia, facilitation of weaning from mechanical ventilation) but does not reduce overall mortality and may be associated with both short-term adverse effects (e.g., hyperglycemia, hypertension, GI bleeding or intestinal perforation, hypertrophic obstructive cardiomyopathy, poor weight gain, poor growth of head circumference) and long-term sequelae. Long-term follow-up of preterm infants receiving IV glucocorticoids within 12 hours after birth indicates that postnatal glucocorticoid therapy is associated with an increased incidence of neurodevelopmental delay, cerebral palsy, impaired cognitive function, and stunted growth at or before school age. Therefore, the American Academy of Pediatrics (AAP) currently states that routine use of systemic glucocorticoids for prevention or treatment of bronchopulmonary dysplasia in very low birth weight infants is *not* recommended.

■ Hematologic Disorders Glucocorticoids are used in the management of acquired (autoimmune) hemolytic anemia, idiopathic thrombocytopenic purpura (ITP), secondary thrombocytopenia, erythroblastopenia, congenital (erythroid) hypoplastic anemia (Diamond-Blackfan syndrome), and pure red cell aplasia.

Although there is no evidence that glucocorticoids affect the course or duration of hematologic disorders, high or even massive dosage of the drugs is often used to decrease bleeding tendencies and normalize blood counts. When treatment is indicated in adults or children with moderate to severe idiopathic thrombocytopenic purpura (ITP), glucocorticoids, immune globulin IV (IGIV), or splenectomy are considered first-line therapies depending on the extent of bleeding involved. Other methods of treatment, such as splenectomy, should be considered if glucocorticoids must be continued for prolonged periods (exceeding several months), especially in patients with idiopathic or secondary thrombocytopenia, acquired (autoimmune) hemolytic anemia, erythroblastopenia (RBC anemia), or congenital (erythroid) hypoplastic anemia. Cytotoxic drugs produce better results in erythroblastopenia, but glucocorticoids may enhance response.

Glucocorticoids may not affect or prevent renal complications in Henoch-Schoenlein purpura. Glucocorticoids have been widely used in aplastic anemia in children, but there is no evidence to prove their effectiveness.

■ GI Diseases In ulcerative colitis, regional enteritis, and celiac disease, moderate to high dosage glucocorticoids may be useful as short-term palliative therapy for acute exacerbations and systemic complications of these chronic conditions. Glucocorticoids should not be used if there is a probability of impending perforation, abscess, or other pyogenic infection. Systemic and topical (rectal enema) glucocorticoids may be useful in acute ulcerative colitis. Sulfasalazine is the drug of choice for chronic ulcerative colitis, and a gluten-free diet is the primary method of therapy for celiac disease.

Glucocorticoids are rarely indicated for maintenance therapy in chronic GI diseases (ulcerative colitis, celiac disease) as they do not prevent relapses and may produce severe adverse reactions with long-term administration. Gastric hemorrhage and malignant hypertension are especially frequent. Occasionally, however, low dosages of glucocorticoids, in conjunction with other supportive therapy, may be useful for patients unresponsive to the usual therapy indicated for chronic conditions.

Crohn's Disease Conventional systemic glucocorticoids (e.g., prednisone, prednisolone, methylprednisolone) have been used for the management of mildly to moderately active and moderately to severely active Crohn's disease†, while budesonide (a more recently approved glucocorticoid) is used orally as delayed-release capsules for the management of mildly-to-moderately active Crohn's disease involving the ileum and/or ascending colon. Conventional glucocorticoids are at least as effective as sulfasalazine, mesalamine, budesonide, or azathioprine in patients with Crohn's disease; however, many clinicians and experts state that conventional glucocorticoids should not be used for the management of mildly to moderately active disease, because of their high incidence of adverse effects and, therefore, their use should be reserved for patients with moderately to severely active disease.

Although no appropriate dose-ranging studies have been performed to evaluate conventional glucocorticoid dosing or dosage schedules for Crohn's disease, comparable clinical effects have been reported in placebo-controlled and active comparator clinical trials in which 50–70% of patients received glucocorticoid dosages equivalent to prednisone (40 mg daily; tapered after clinical response). In these patients, resolution of certain symptoms and resumption of weight gain usually occurred after 1–4 weeks of therapy, while clinical remission was achieved over 8–12 weeks. Parenteral glucocorticoids (dosages equivalent to prednisone 40–60 mg, given as divided doses or as a continuous infusion) are recommended for patients with severe fulminant Crohn's disease†; individuals with inflammatory abdominal mass should receive broad-spectrum anti-infective agents in conjunction with glucocorticoids. Once patients respond to parenteral therapy, they should gradually be switched to an equivalent regimen of an oral glucocorticoid. About 50% of patients with active Crohn's disease, who are receiving systemic glucocorticoids, become glucocorticoid-dependent or glucocorticoid-resistant; such patients should receive drugs with steroid-sparing effects (e.g., azathioprine, mercaptopurine) or, alternatively, infliximab. Glucocorticoids should not be used for maintenance therapy of Crohn's disease, because both conventional glucocorticoids and budesonide usually do not prevent relapses and the drugs (especially conventional glucocorticoids) may produce severe adverse reactions with long-term administration.

Systemic conventional glucocorticoids (e.g., prednisone 1–2 mg/kg daily up to 60 mg daily) have been used in pediatric patients with mild esophageal or gastroduodenal Crohn's disease†. In addition, glucocorticoids (e.g., prednisone or methylprednisolone 1–2 mg/kg daily up to 60 mg daily) are recommended for the management of moderately to severely active Crohn's disease, in children. Results of a 12-week comparator-drug (prednisone versus budesonide) controlled study in pediatric patients 8–18 years of age (weighing more than 20 kg) with mildly to moderately active Crohn's disease (Pediatric Crohn's Disease Activity Index [PCDI] score of 12.5–40) indicate that remission rates in children receiving prednisone (40 mg daily for 2 weeks and then tapered until discontinuance) were similar (50% for prednisone versus 47% for budesonide) to those receiving budesonide (9 mg daily for 8 weeks, tapered until discontinuance). Incidence of adverse effects was substantially lower (about 32% for budesonide versus 71% for prednisone) and less severe in pediatric patients receiving budesonide than in those receiving prednisone.

For further information about the management of Crohn's disease, see Uses: Crohn's Disease, in Mesalamine 56:36.

Trichinosis Glucocorticoids are used in the treatment of trichinosis with neurologic or myocardial involvement.

■ **Neoplastic Diseases** Glucocorticoids in high dosage are used alone or as a component of various chemotherapeutic regimens in the palliative treatment of neoplastic diseases of the lymphatic system (e.g., leukemias and lymphomas in adults and acute leukemias in children). Massive dosage of glucocorticoids has occasionally been used in the treatment of neoplastic diseases but rarely offers any additional benefit and greatly increases adverse effects. Beneficial results are enhanced, however, when glucocorticoids are used as part of a total treatment regimen in combination with cytotoxic and immunosuppressive drugs; such a regimen should be administered only by an experienced oncologist.

In adults, acute lymphocytic (lymphoblastic) leukemia, chronic lymphocytic leukemia, and Hodgkin's disease respond well to combination regimens that include a glucocorticoid (usually prednisone or prednisolone). Acute myeloblastic leukemia, lymphosarcoma, and the blast crisis of chronic myelocytic leukemia may fail to respond or may relapse upon discontinuance of therapy.

In moderate dosage, glucocorticoids induce tumor remission in approximately 15% of patients with breast cancer. Because glucocorticoids used alone are not as effective as other agents (e.g., cytotoxic agents, hormones, antiestrogens) in the treatment of breast cancer, their use should be reserved for patients unresponsive to other therapy.

Glucocorticoids (e.g., prednisone) also have been used alone or as a component of various combination chemotherapeutic regimens in the treatment of advanced, symptomatic (i.e., painful) hormone-refractory prostate cancer. Use of glucocorticoids and/or chemotherapeutic agents in the treatment of advanced, hormone-resistant prostate cancer is palliative, with patients having median survival durations of less than 1 year; no therapy has been shown to improve survival to date, and therefore the principal goal of therapy in such cancer currently is improvement in quality of life, particularly pain. Randomized studies have shown that the addition of an antineoplastic agent (e.g., mitoxantrone) to glucocorticoid therapy results in a greater proportion of patients achieving a palliative response (i.e., pain reduction) and a longer duration of such response compared with glucocorticoid treatment alone. Improvement in certain quality-of-life measures, including indicators related to pain, physical activity or function, constipation, and mood, also may favor combination therapy.

Glucocorticoids (e.g., dexamethasone, prednisone) also have been used as a component of various combination chemotherapeutic regimens in the treatment of multiple myeloma. Dexamethasone has been used in combination chemotherapeutic regimens in various doses (20–40 mg) and schedules. Although high-dose dexamethasone has been associated with increased adverse effects (e.g., hyperglycemia, psychiatric effects, insomnia, hyperactivity, infectious complications), high-dose dexamethasone is an effective component of combination chemotherapeutic regimens for the treatment of multiple myeloma.

■ **Cancer Chemotherapy-induced Nausea and Vomiting** Glucocorticoid (e.g., dexamethasone, methylprednisolone) regimens have been used extensively for the prevention of nausea and vomiting associated with emetogenic cancer chemotherapy† including that associated with cisplatin. Most clinical experience to date has been with dexamethasone.

Clinical evaluations of dexamethasone in the prevention of chemotherapy-induced emesis have shown that the antiemetic effect of the glucocorticoid is greater than that of placebo or prochlorperazine. The addition of a glucocorticoid (e.g., dexamethasone) to therapy with a type 3 serotonin (5-HT_3) receptor antagonist (e.g., granisetron, ondansetron), aprepitant, and/or a substituted benzamide (e.g., metoclopramide appears to increase the antiemetic efficacy of either drug alone, and such combined therapy may be useful in preventing acute or delayed emesis in patients receiving emetogenic cancer chemotherapy.

To prevent chemotherapy-induced nausea and vomiting associated with chemotherapy regimens with a high emetic risk (i.e., incidence of emesis exceeds 90% if no antiemetics are administered), the American Society of Clinical Oncology (ASCO) currently recommends a 3-drug antiemetic regimen consisting of dexamethasone, aprepitant, and a 5-HT_3 receptor antagonist (e.g., dolasetron, granisetron, ondansetron, palonosetron, tropisetron [not commercially available in the US]). Antiemetic agents with a lower therapeutic index (i.e., less efficacious and generally associated with more frequent adverse effects), including cannabinoids (e.g., dronabinol, nabilone), metoclopramide, butyrophenones, and phenothiazines are *not* considered by ASCO to be appropriate first-line antiemetics for any group of patients receiving chemotherapy of high emetic risk; ASCO states that these drugs should be reserved for patients unable to tolerate or refractory to first-line agents.

The antiemetic combination of dexamethasone, aprepitant, and a 5-HT_3 receptor antagonist also is preferred in patients receiving combination chemotherapy with an anthracycline and cyclophosphamide.

For patients receiving other chemotherapy of moderate emetic risk (i.e., incidence of emesis without antiemetics exceeds 30% but does not exceed 90%), ASCO recommends a 2-drug antiemetic regimen consisting of dexamethasone and a 5-HT_3 receptor antagonist. For patients receiving chemotherapy regimens with a low emetic risk (i.e., incidence of emesis without antiemetics exceeds 10% but does not exceed 30%), ASCO recommends dexamethasone alone on the first day of chemotherapy.

Antiemetics can be prescribed on an as-needed basis in patients receiving chemotherapy with a minimal antiemetic risk (incidence of emesis is less than 10% without antiemetics).

For the prevention of *delayed* emesis in patients receiving cisplatin or other chemotherapy associated with a high emetic risk, these authorities currently recommend a 2-drug combination of dexamethasone and aprepitant.

Although antihistamines (e.g., diphenhydramine) and benzodiazepines (e.g., alprazolam, lorazepam) may be useful as adjunctive antiemetic agents, they currently are not recommended as monotherapy as antiemetic agents. However, many clinicians find benzodiazepines useful in the management of anticipatory emesis.

■ **Liver Diseases** Glucocorticoids may be beneficial or harmful in patients with liver disease. Although evidence is conflicting, the drugs probably are of no value in patients with acute hepatitis and massive necrosis. In patients with subacute hepatic necrosis and chronic active hepatitis, administration of glucocorticoids in high dosage can decrease serum bilirubin, ascites, and mortality rate. Prolonged low-dosage maintenance therapy may be necessary. In nonalcoholic cirrhosis in women, glucocorticoids increase survival rate in the absence of ascites, but not when ascites is present. The drugs are ineffective in men with nonalcoholic cirrhosis. Glucocorticoids may decrease mortality rate in patients with alcoholic cirrhosis with hepatic encephalopathy, but they should not be used in less seriously ill patients. Acute viral hepatitis is usually benign and self-limited, and glucocorticoids are rarely indicated.

■ **Cerebral Edema** Glucocorticoids administered parenterally, in high dosage, may be useful to decrease cerebral edema associated with brain tumors and neurosurgery. Some patients with cerebral edema associated with pseudotumor cerebri may also benefit from use of glucocorticoids, but the efficacy of the drugs is controversial and remains to be established. Edema resulting from brain abscesses is less responsive than that resulting from brain tumors.

The use of glucocorticoids in the management of cerebral edema is not a substitute for careful neurosurgical evaluation and definitive management such as neurosurgery or other specific therapy. Effects of glucocorticoids are not apparent for several hours and in acute situations the drugs should only be used adjunctively with other indicated therapy. Although any glucocorticoid may be effective, those having minimal mineralocorticoid activity are preferable. Glucocorticoids do not appear to be beneficial in cerebral edema associated with cerebral infarction.

Head Injury Pooled analyses of small controlled studies of glucocorticoids in patients with head injury have failed to clearly establish the efficacy of glucocorticoid therapy in this patient population. Because of a lack of evidence of efficacy, some experts have recommended against the use of glucocorticoids for improving outcomes or reducing intracranial pressure in patients with head injury. More recent evidence from a large, international, randomized, placebo-controlled study (Corticosteroid Randomization after Significant Head Injury [CRASH]) indicates that use of glucocorticoids in patients with head injuries may be detrimental. Results from this study in more than 10,000 patients with head injury and a Glasgow coma score not exceeding 14 within 8 hours of injury indicate that glucocorticoid therapy (e.g., methylprednisolone 2 g administered by IV infusion over 1 hour, followed by methylprednisolone 0.4 g/hour by IV infusion for 48 hours) is associated with a substantial increase in risk of death (21.1% with methylprednisolone versus 17.9% with placebo) within 2 weeks after head injury; the relative risk of death from all causes within 2 weeks in patients receiving methylprednisolone compared with placebo in this study was 1.18 (95% confidence interval of 1.09–1.27). The cause of the observed increase in mortality in patients receiving glucocorticoids is unclear because cause of death was not documented. Recruitment of patients for this study was halted after results from interim analyses were reported. Results regarding effects of glucocorticoid therapy on disability 6 months after head injury are pending.

Cerebral Malaria Glucocorticoids are not effective and can have detrimental effects in the management of cerebral malaria caused by *Plasmodium falciparum*; the drugs are no longer recommended for this condition.

■ **Acute Spinal Cord Injury** Some evidence indicates that therapy with large IV doses of glucocorticoids (i.e., methylprednisolone) can improve motor and sensory function in patients with acute spinal cord injury† when treatment is initiated promptly following injury. However, benefit in controlled studies in humans has been demonstrated to date only in patients receiving high-dose IV methylprednisolone within 8 hours after spinal cord injury, and whether improvement in neurologic function with such therapy will routinely lead to specific improvements in disability has not been established.

In a multicenter, comparative study, patients with acute spinal cord injuries† who received an initial 30-mg/kg dose of methylprednisolone (as the sodium succinate salt) by rapid IV injection (over 15 minutes) within 8 hours of injury, followed by infusion of the drug at 5.4 mg/kg per hour for an additional 23 hours, had substantial improvement in motor function and pinprick and touch sensation at 6 weeks and 6 months compared with those who received IV naloxone hydrochloride (5.4 mg/kg by rapid IV injection followed by 4 mg/kg per hour for an additional 23 hours) or placebo. The benefits of methylprednisolone therapy were observed in patients with complete as well as incomplete loss of motor and sensory function, and neurologic improvement observed at 6 weeks in methylprednisolone-treated patients was still evident at 6 months. Patients receiving naloxone or placebo and those in whom therapy with high-dose methylprednisolone was initiated later than 8 hours (but usually within 14 hours) after injury did not have substantial improvement in motor function or touch sensation. Mortality at 6 months was similar among treatment groups, and overall mortality was low (6%) compared with that of previous studies. Although the use of glucocorticoids in patients with spinal cord injuries has been associated with increased morbidity in some studies, clinically important differences in the incidence of wound infections, GI bleeding, and other complications among treatment groups in this study were not observed.

Limited evidence in animals suggests that the ameliorative effects of glucocorticoids in spinal cord injury† are related to dose and time of initiation of therapy; these effects appear to be characterized by a biphasic, bell-shaped response curve. In one study in animals with experimentally induced spinal cord injury, posttraumatic spinal cord ischemia was effectively minimized by a 30-mg/kg dose of methylprednisolone administered 30 minutes but not several hours after injury; at 30 minutes, a 15-mg/kg dose produced little benefit, while a dose of 60 mg/kg was ineffective or deleterious. Such studies suggest that the lack of appreciable benefit observed in an earlier controlled study of patients with acute spinal cord injury who were treated up to 48 hours after injury using a methylprednisolone dose of 100 mg or 1 g (approximately 15 mg/kg) daily for 10 days may have been related in part to delayed administration of the drug or administration of an insufficient dose. Additional studies are needed to determine the optimal timing, dosage, and duration of therapy with methylprednisolone or other glucocorticoids in patients with acute spinal cord injury and to elucidate further the potential benefits of glucocorticoid therapy on functional status in such patients.

■ **Low Back Pain** Glucocorticoids (alone or combined with a local anesthetic and/or an opiate analgesic) have been used epidurally† for symptomatic relief of low back pain†. Although this use remains controversial and convincing evidence of efficacy remains to be established, most experts state that this invasive form of therapy is an option for short-term relief of acute, subacute, or chronic radicular pain in patients with low back pain and radiculopathy associated with disk disease or herniation or spinal stenosis when more conservative therapies (e.g., rest, analgesics, physical therapy) fail and as a means of potentially avoiding surgery. The effect of epidural glucocorticoid injections on long-term outcomes of unremitting low back pain remains unclear. Epidural therapy for low back pain and radiculopathy involves injection of the drug(s) into the epidural space near the site where the nerve roots pass before entering the intervertebral foramen. Such therapy theoretically allows a concentrated amount of drug(s) to be deposited and retained locally, exposing nerves to the drug(s) for prolonged periods in an attempt to reduce inflammation, swelling, and pain. Epidural injections may be performed by caudal, interlaminar, or transforaminal approaches; the transforaminal approach requires the smallest injection volume and appears to be the most specific and possibly most effective route.

Because of the potential for complications related to improper needle placement or drug administration, many experts state that epidural injections should be performed by an experienced clinician using fluoroscopic guidance and contrast control to ensure that the needle is correctly positioned and that the injection is not performed intravascularly, intrathecally, or into tissues other than the epidural space. While some clinicians suggest that fluoroscopic guidance may not be necessary in patients who have not undergone previous surgery and whose spinal anatomy is normal, and for whom there are no other factors making the procedure technically difficult (e.g., obesity), serious adverse neurologic effects have been reported following epidural glucocorticoid injection both with and without fluoroscopic guidance. (See Cautions: Nervous System Effects.) Long-acting injectable suspension formulations of methylprednisolone, triamcinolone, and betamethasone are the most commonly used preparations for epidural injections. Optimal technique, dosage, timing of initial injection, and injection frequency, as well as maximum number of epidural glucocorticoid injections, remain to be established.

Water-soluble glucocorticoid preparations typically have not been used for epidural injection because they are cleared rapidly from the spinal canal and have been associated with adverse neurologic effects (e.g., seizures, segmental hyperalgesia) when injected intrathecally in animals. Limited evidence suggests that large particles (e.g., exceeding 50 μm) in glucocorticoid suspension preparations potentially may cause embolic vascular occlusion during inadvertent intra-arterial injection; it appears that some particulate suspensions (e.g., methylprednisolone acetate, triamcinolone hexacetonide) may contain substantial amounts of these large particles, and some clinicians have suggested that a glucocorticoid solution preparation (e.g., dexamethasone sodium phosphate) or a suspension with an overall smaller size of particulate matter (e.g., fixed combination of betamethasone sodium phosphate and betamethasone acetate) may be preferred for epidural injections. Long-acting injectable suspension preparations of glucocorticoids (e.g., Aristospan®, Celestone® Soluspan®, Depo-Medrol®, Kenalog®) also contain preservatives and/or suspending agents (e.g., benzalkonium chloride, benzyl alcohol, myristyl-γ-picolinium chloride, polyethylene glycol) that have been associated with neurotoxic effects in animals or humans. While most reports of neurotoxicity with intraspinal glucocorticoid therapy in humans have involved intrathecal administration, the safety of epidural injections using preserved glucocorticoid formulations is controversial, and epidural administration of these formulations is not recommended by the manufacturers. Currently there are no studies supporting the use of any one formulation over any other in terms of safety.

The principal risk of epidural injection therapy for low back pain and radiculopathy is rare epidural abscess. However, other serious adverse effects, including infectious complications (e.g., meningitis), neurologic effects (e.g., arachnoiditis, spinal cord trauma, increased intracranial pressure, nerve injury, seizures, bladder or bowel dysfunction, paraparesis or paralysis, brain damage), ocular effects, embolic vascular complications, and death may occur following attempted epidural injection (see Cautions). Systemic glucocorticoid effects (e.g., hypothalamic-pituitary-adrenal [HPA] axis suppression, hypercorticism, Cushing's syndrome, osteoporosis, fluid retention, hyperglycemia) also may occur after epidural glucocorticoid administration.

Data from the American Society of Anesthesiologists (ASA) Closed Claims Project database, which includes closed anesthesia malpractice claims arising from chronic pain management, suggest that serious injuries (e.g., brain damage, death) can occur when glucocorticoids are combined with local anesthetics and/or opiate analgesics for epidural injection and that patient safety may be improved by excluding typical epidural doses (volumes in excess of intrathecal test doses) of local anesthetics and/or opiate analgesics from epidural glucocorticoid injections.

Limited evidence suggests that therapeutic facet joint† and intradiscal glucocorticoid injections† are minimally effective or ineffective in the treatment of low back pain, although some clinicians report that facet joint injections may be useful in some patients with facet arthropathy. Inclusion of a glucocorticoid in trigger point injections also does not appear to be beneficial. Sacroiliac joint injections performed using fluoroscopic guidance may provide temporary pain relief in some patients when the principal source of spinal pain is the sacroiliac joint.

Although oral glucocorticoids have been used by some clinicians in the treatment of low back pain†, they do not appear to be effective and evidence supporting such use is lacking.

■ **Bacterial Meningitis** Although the use of glucocorticoids as adjunctive therapy in patients with bacterial meningitis† has been controversial, some evidence suggests that short-term adjunctive therapy (i.e., IV dexamethasone for the first 2–4 days of anti-infective therapy) may provide some benefit (e.g., on CSF abnormalities involving prostaglandin, lactate, glucose, and protein concentrations and on the development of hearing loss as a sequela) in patients with bacterial meningitis. Analysis of combined data from several placebo-controlled studies in which audiometric testing was performed suggests that the risk of moderate or more severe hearing loss in infants and children with *Haemophilus influenzae* meningitis treated with cefuroxime, ceftriaxone, or cefotaxime is reduced by adjunctive therapy with dexamethasone. In another placebo-controlled study, mortality and hearing loss were reduced in severely ill adults and children with *Streptococcus pneumoniae* meningitis who received IM dexamethasone phosphate therapy (8–12 mg every 12 hours) during the first 3 days of treatment with ampicillin and chloramphenicol.

The applicability of these results to all patients with bacterial meningitis has been questioned based on differences in patient characteristics (e.g., disease severity) between treatment groups or among studies, the use of different anti-infective and/or dexamethasone regimens, and the current lack of data on glucocorticoid therapy for bacterial meningitis in infants younger than 6 weeks of age or in geriatric patients. However, the frequency of neurologic sequelae has been decreased (but with varying degrees of statistical significance) in all studies to date when dexamethasone-treated patients with bacterial meningitis are compared with those who did not receive such adjunctive therapy, and some clinicians suggest that current evidence justifies the use of dexamethasone therapy in infants and children with bacterial meningitis and also in adults with associated severe CNS manifestations (e.g., high concentrations of bacteria in CSF, impaired mental status, intracranial hypertension). Other clinicians suggest that they would use dexamethasone therapy in all patients with bacterial meningitis.

AAP currently recommends that adjunctive therapy with IV dexamethasone for bacterial meningitis be considered on an individualized basis in infants and children 6 weeks of age and older after weighing the relative risks and benefits. AAP states that dexamethasone therapy should be used only when the diagnosis of bacterial meningitis has been proved or is strongly suspected based on CSF examination, Gram-stained smear, or antigen test results, and that such therapy should not be used in patients with suspected or proved aseptic or nonbacterial meningitis or partially treated meningitis with negative cultures. However, some clinicians suggest that rather than waiting for confirmation of the diagnosis, they would initiate therapy with dexamethasone in patients with suspected bacterial meningitis and discontinue the drug if the diagnosis proved incorrect. AAP recommends adjunctive dexamethasone therapy for infants and children with *H. influenzae* type b meningitis, and states that such therapy also should be considered for those with pneumococcal or meningococcal meningitis; however, because efficacy in these latter 2 infections has not been established by prospective studies (because the limited number of cases was insufficient to determine efficacy), some clinicians only recommend the use of adjunctive dexamethasone for *H. influenzae* type b infections.

Current data suggest that protective effects of dexamethasone therapy on hearing loss may be greater in patients with milder forms of the disease, and if the decision is made to use dexamethasone therapy for bacterial meningitis, such therapy should be given to patients with mild as well as severe illness; the decision to use dexamethasone should *not* be based on the severity of the prescribing illness. The efficacy and safety of adjunctive dexamethasone therapy in bacterial meningitis has not been established in infants younger than 6 weeks of age or in those with congenital or acquired abnormalities of the CNS with or without placement of a prosthetic device. If dexamethasone is used in patients with pneumococcal meningitis, a repeat lumbar puncture should be considered after 24–48 hours to assess the response to therapy since the drug may interfere with the ability to interpret clinical indicators of response to anti-infective therapy.

In almost all controlled studies to date of dexamethasone therapy for bacterial meningitis, a dosage of 0.15 mg/kg of dexamethasone phosphate has been given IV 4 times daily for the first 2–4 days of anti-infective treatment.

Limited data in animals suggest that dexamethasone may be superior to methylprednisolone in reversing certain CSF abnormalities (e.g., intracranial hypertension, elevated lactate concentrations) associated with bacterial meningitis, and experience is insufficient to allow recommendation of other dexamethasone dosage regimens or other glucocorticoids for use in bacterial meningitis.

Since current data indicate that dexamethasone's beneficial effects involve reduction of the inflammatory response to anti-infective-liberated bacterial endotoxins and cell-wall components, including reduction of the release of cytokines (e.g., interleukin-1 beta, tumor necrosis factor) in CSF, dexamethasone therapy should be initiated before or concurrently with the first dose of anti-infective therapy to achieve optimal effects.

Although serious adverse effects appear to be uncommon with IV dexamethasone therapy in patients with bacterial meningitis, GI bleeding, sometimes requiring transfusion, has been reported in a few patients receiving such therapy. Regular determinations of hemoglobin concentration and tests for occult blood in the stool are recommended in patients with bacterial meningitis receiving dexamethasone therapy; some clinicians also suggest the use of concomitant therapy with histamine H_2-receptor antagonists in these patients. If melena or obvious bleeding is observed, dexamethasone should be discontinued and appropriate therapeutic measures (e.g., blood transfusion) instituted as necessary.

Additional controlled studies are necessary to elucidate further the safety and efficacy of adjunctive glucocorticoid therapy in patients with bacterial meningitis of various etiologies, including in neonates and geriatric patients, and to determine the optimum timing and dosage of glucocorticoid therapy in these patients; some studies currently are ongoing.

For information on the use of glucocorticoids in tuberculous meningitis, see Tuberculous Meningitis under Respiratory Diseases: Advanced Pulmonary and Extrapulmonary Tuberculosis, in Uses.

■ **Multiple Sclerosis** Glucocorticoids currently are considered the drugs of choice for the management of acute relapses of multiple sclerosis. The anti-inflammatory and immunomodulating effects of the drugs can accelerate neurologic recovery by restoring the blood-brain barrier, reducing edema, and possibly improving axonal conduction. Glucocorticoids can shorten the duration of relapse and accelerate recovery; however, it remains to be established whether the drugs can improve the overall degree of recovery or alter the long-term course of the disease. Although corticotropin was considered the therapy of choice in the past, short-term, high-dose IV glucocorticoids (e.g., methylprednisolone) generally have replaced such therapy because of a more rapid onset of action, more consistent effects, and fewer adverse effects.

For moderate to severe relapses, methylprednisolone has been administered IV in a dosage of 1 g daily for 3–5 days, followed by 60 mg of oral prednisone daily, tapering the dosage over 12 days. Alternative regimens have included 1 g or 15 mg/kg of IV methylprednisolone tapered over 15 days to 1 mg/kg and followed by oral prednisone or prednisolone in gradually decreasing dosages over several weeks to months.

Interest in the use of IV methylprednisolone in the management of acute relapses of multiple sclerosis heightened as a result of the Optic Neuritis Treatment Trial in which the rate of recovery in vision was faster in those receiving the drug and the risk of development of clinically definite multiple sclerosis was reduced during the first 2 years of follow-up. (See Uses: Ocular Disorders.) The beneficial effect of the methylprednisolone regimen on disease progression was transient since results at 3- and 5-year follow-up indicate that there were not clinically important differences among treatment groups in the rate of development of clinically definite multiple sclerosis or the degree of neurologic disability among those who developed the disease during the 5-year follow-up period. Additional study is needed and under way to determine whether pulsed doses of glucocorticoids given every other month can slow progression of the disease in patients with moderate disability and secondary progressive multiple sclerosis.

■ **Myasthenia Gravis** Glucocorticoids (e.g., prednisone) are used in the management of myasthenia gravis, usually in patients who have had an inadequate response to anticholinesterase therapy. Glucocorticoids also have been administered parenterally in the treatment of myasthenic crisis.

■ **Organ Transplants** In massive dosage, glucocorticoids may be used concomitantly with other immunosuppressive drugs to prevent rejection of transplanted organs. Because the incidence of secondary infections is high in patients receiving these drugs, such therapy should be administered by physicians experienced in its use.

■ **Nephrotic Syndrome** Glucocorticoids can induce diuresis and remission of proteinuria in children and adults with nephrotic syndrome secondary to primary renal disease, especially when there is minimal renal histologic change. Lupus nephritis may also respond to glucocorticoids. High dosage may be required for prolonged periods, and alternate-day therapy should be used to decrease adverse effects. Nephrotic syndrome secondary to diabetes mellitus, renal amyloidosis, glomerulonephritis, or other diseases is generally refractory to glucocorticoids.

■ **Diagnostic Uses** Dexamethasone inhibits pituitary adrenocorticotropic hormone (ACTH) release and decreases output of endogenous corticosteroids when given in an amount which does not itself appreciably affect concentrations of urinary 17-hydroxycorticosteroids. This effect is utilized in the dexamethasone suppression test for the diagnosis of Cushing's syndrome and the differential diagnosis of adrenocortical tumors. (See Dexamethasone 68:04.)

The dexamethasone suppression test (DST) has been used for the detection, diagnosis, and management of mental depression; however, considerable controversy currently exists regarding the clinical utility of the test. The sensitivity of the DST in patients with major depression is relatively modest (about 40–50%), and a positive test result (nonsuppression) does not appear to reliably predict response to antidepressant therapy and a negative test result (suppression) is not an indication for withholding antidepressant therapy. Therefore, the American Psychiatric Association, American College of Physicians, and other experts currently state that, pending further studies and evaluation, the DST should not be used *routinely* for the diagnosis and management of depression, although judicious use of the DST may be a useful adjunct in clinical decision making in selected situations and as a research tool.

■ **Duchenne Muscular Dystrophy** The current standard of care for patients with Duchenne muscular dystrophy includes the use of corticosteroids (e.g., prednisone, deflazacort) for improving muscle function and strength. The American Academy of Neurology recommends the use of prednisone or deflazacort to improve muscle strength, pulmonary function, and possibly also slow the development of scoliosis and need for surgery in patients with Duchenne muscular dystrophy. Results of direct comparative studies suggest that prednisone and deflazacort are similarly effective in improving motor function, but differ in their adverse effect profiles (e.g., prednisone may be associated with more weight gain while deflazacort may be associated with a greater risk of cataracts).

■ **Cardiovascular Disorders** ***Shock*** Although IV glucocorticoids may be life-saving in shock secondary to adrenocortical insufficiency, the value of the drugs in the treatment of shock resulting from other causes is controversial. Management of shock should be based on specific treatment of the primary cause and secondary abnormalities, and glucocorticoids, if used, should be regarded only as adjunctive supportive treatment.

The value of glucocorticoids in the treatment of septic shock has been particularly controversial. Although some controlled studies have shown beneficial effects of high-dose regimens on morbidity and mortality in septic shock, many studies have not. Results of one prospective, controlled study suggest that glucocorticoids do not improve overall survival in patients with severe, late septic shock but may be beneficial early in the course of septic shock and in certain subgroups of patients. However, 2 subsequent, prospective, controlled studies failed to show a benefit of high-dose glucocorticoid therapy that was initiated *early* (i.e., within 2.8 hours of diagnosis) in patients with presumed sepsis or septic shock. In addition, there was some evidence that such therapy may be associated with an increased risk of mortality in certain patients (i.e., those with serum creatinine concentrations exceeding 2 mg/dL at diagnosis and those who developed secondary infection). Some clinicians state that, despite current evidence, additional, well-designed studies to evaluate the role of the drugs in septic shock are needed, particularly in patients with gram-negative sepsis.

Pericarditis Systemic glucocorticoids have been used to reduce the pain, fever, and inflammation of pericarditis†, including that associated with myocardial infarction.

The most common cardiac causes of recurrent chest pain following an acute myocardial infarction are acute pericarditis and ischemia, with the latter being the more common and potentially more serious. Recurrent pain occurring during the initial 12 hours after onset of infarction usually is considered related to the original infarction itself. Pericarditis probably is not responsible for clinically important chest pain during the initial 24 hours after infarction and may not become evident for up to several weeks after an acute myocardial infarction. Pericarditis in acute myocardial infarction occurs with extension of myocardial necrosis throughout the epicardial wall. The Multicenter Investigation of the Limitation of Infarct Size (MILIS) study found that pericarditis (defined as presence of pericardial friction rub) occurred in about 20% of patients following acute myocardial infarction. In patients not treated with thrombolytic therapy, pericarditis occurs in about 25% of patients as evidenced by either typical symptoms or pericardial friction rub, but the incidence averages only 14% when the presence of a friction rub is required for diagnosis. Patients with pericarditis have larger infarcts, lower ejection fractions, and a higher incidence of congestive heart failure. Although anterior chest discomfort mimicking ischemia can occur with pericarditis, pericardial pain usually exhibits distinguishing characteristics, including pleural or positional discomfort, radiation to the left shoulder, scapula, or trapezius muscle and a pericardial rub, electrocardiogram (ECG) J-point elevation with concave upward ST-segment elevation, and PR depression. It is important to distinguish between pain caused by pericarditis and that caused by ischemia since management will differ. In addition, the possibility that cardiac rupture, which occurs in about 1–4% of patients hospitalized for acute myocardial infarction, may account for recurrent pain should be considered since use of glucocorticoids may be a risk factor in its development.

While glucocorticoids can provide effective symptomatic relief, there is evidence that the drugs may cause thinning of developing scar and myocardial rupture. Glucocorticoids should be reserved for use only in patients with pericarditis refractory to therapy with aspirin or other nonsteroidal anti-inflammatory agents; aspirin is considered the treatment of choice for postmyocardial infarction pericarditis.

Glucocorticoids also have been used in the management of tuberculous pericarditis. (See Tuberculous Pericarditis under Respiratory Diseases: Advanced Pulmonary and Extrapulmonary Tuberculosis, in Uses.)

■ **Chronic Fatigue Syndrome** Because of evidence that chronic fatigue syndrome† is associated with subnormal cortisol secretion secondary to impaired activation of the hypothalamic-pituitary-adrenal (HPA) axis, glucocorticoid supplementation has been studied in patients with this condition. In a study in patients 18–55 years of age who met the US Centers for Disease Control and Prevention (CDC) case criteria for chronic fatigue syndrome, low-dose oral glucocorticoid therapy (approximately 13 mg/m^2 [20–30 mg] of hydrocortisone every morning and 3 mg/m^2 [5 mg] every afternoon for about 12 weeks) produced some symptomatic improvement as determined by a global self-rating wellness scale; however, there was no evidence of improvement in several other self-rating scales, including mood, depression, and activity scales. Because the modest symptomatic improvement with glucocorticoid therapy was associated with clinically important adrenal suppression, such therapy is not practical nor advisable for the chronic management of chronic fatigue syndrome.

■ **Anthrax** Glucocorticoid therapy has been used as an adjunct to anti-infective therapy in the treatment of anthrax† in an attempt to ameliorate toxin-mediated effects associated with *Bacillus anthracis* infections. Some experts suggest that glucocorticoids may be indicated in the treatment of cutaneous anthrax if there are signs of systemic involvement or extensive edema involving the neck and thoracic region. Glucocorticoid therapy also has been used as an adjunct in the treatment of anthrax meningitis. The US Centers for Disease Control and Prevention (CDC) suggest that adjunctive use of glucocorticoids be considered in the treatment of inhalational anthrax that occurs as the result of exposure to anthrax spores in the context of biologic warfare or bioterrorism if extensive edema, respiratory compromise, or meningitis is present. For information on treatment of anthrax and recommendations for prophylaxis following exposure to anthrax spores, see Uses: Anthrax, in Ciprofloxacin 8:12.18.

■ **Other Uses** In miscellaneous inflammatory reactions, such as those resulting from dental procedures, short-term glucocorticoid therapy can decrease edema and may alleviate pain associated with such inflammations.

Local injection of glucocorticoids (e.g., methylprednisolone, betamethasone) into the tissue near the carpal tunnel has been used in a limited number of patients to relieve symptoms (e.g., pain, edema, sensory deficit) of carpal tunnel syndrome. In clinical studies, short-term response was noted in most patients, but the improvement in symptoms waned during the following 11–24 months. Limited evidence suggests that injection technique may influence the duration of effect.

Glucocorticoids (e.g., betamethasone, dexamethasone, methylprednisolone) have been used by local injection for the management of cystic tumors of an aponeurosis or tendon (ganglia).

For EENT and topical uses of the corticosteroids, see 52:08.08 and 84:06.08.

Dosage and Administration

■ **Administration** Glucocorticoids, in appropriate forms, may be administered orally, by oral inhalation, and by IV, IM, subcutaneous, intra-articular, intrabursal, intradermal, intrasynovial, intralesional, or soft tissue injection. Long-acting injectable suspension formulations of some glucocorticoids (e.g., betamethasone, methylprednisolone, triamcinolone) have been administered by epidural injection, although the safety of epidural injections using preserved glucocorticoid formulations is controversial and epidural administration of these formulations is not recommended by the manufacturers. (See Uses: Low Back Pain and see Cautions: Nervous System Effects.) The manufacturer of Depo-Medrol® (sterile methylprednisolone acetate suspension) states that this formulation of methylprednisolone acetate contains benzyl alcohol, which is potentially toxic when administered locally to neural tissue, and that this formulation should *not* be administered intrathecally because of reports of severe adverse events with such use. (See Cautions: Nervous System Effects.) Whenever possible, topical corticosteroid therapy (see 52:08.08 and 84:06.08) is preferable to systemic therapy.

Because injections of slightly soluble glucocorticoids may produce atrophy at the site of injection, IM injections of these products should be made deeply into gluteal muscle; repeated IM injections at the same site should be avoided, and these products should not be administered subcutaneously. Knee, ankle, wrist, elbow, shoulder, phalangeal, and hip joints are suitable sites for intra-articular injections of glucocorticoids; spinal joints and joints without synovial spaces are not suitable for intra-articular injection. For intra-articular injections, a 20- to 24-gauge needle should be used; needle placement should be verified by aspirating a few drops of synovial fluid prior to drug administration with a second syringe. Joints should be injected where the synovial cavity is most superficial and free from large vessels and nerves. Joint fluid should be examined to exclude sepsis, and injection into an infected site should be avoided; if joint sepsis is evident, appropriate antibacterial therapy should be instituted. Symptoms of septic arthritis include local swelling, further restriction of joint motion, fever, or malaise. Glucocorticoids should not be injected into unstable joints and patients should be cautioned not to overuse joints in which the inflammatory process is still active despite symptomatic improvement.

For management of tenosynovitis and tendinitis, glucocorticoids should be injected into affected tendon sheaths rather than into tendons.

For disorders of the foot (bursitis, tenosynovitis, acute gouty arthritis), a tuberculin syringe with a 25-gauge, ¾-inch needle should be used for intra-articular or soft-tissue administration.

For dermatologic conditions, a tuberculin syringe with a 25-gauge, ½-inch needle should be used for intralesional administration.

In treatment of intercostal neuritis or neuralgia, local injections of glucocorticoids should be made cautiously to avoid penetration of the pleura, which may be indicated by appearance of sudden sharp pain during the injection.

■ **Dosage** ***General Dosage*** In the management of acute disorders, glucocorticoid dosage should be sufficient to ensure that symptoms are controlled quickly, and treatment should be discontinued as soon as possible. Acute disorders respond most rapidly to divided daily doses. In life-threatening situations where adrenal insufficiency may be the precipitating cause, glucocorticoids can be administered in any dosage required without serious complications, even before a definite diagnosis has been made.

Dosage ranges for glucocorticoids are extremely wide, and patient responses are quite variable. The amount of drug each patient receives should be individualized according to the diagnosis, severity, prognosis and probable duration of the disease, and patient response and tolerance. Occasionally, patients may respond better to one glucocorticoid than another but this is unpredictable.

Types of dosages generally used in various disease states are: *physiologic* or *replacement* (amount of glucocorticoid normally secreted by the adrenal cortex each day—approximately 20 mg of hydrocortisone), *pharmacologic* (any dosage greater than a physiologic dosage) which includes *maintenance* or *low* (dosage slightly in excess of physiologic amounts—e.g., 5–15 mg of prednisone daily), *moderate* (approximately 0.5 mg of prednisone/kg daily), *high* (approximately 1–3 mg of prednisone/kg daily), and *massive* (approximately 15–30 mg of prednisolone/kg daily). The *approximate* equivalent oral glucocorticoid dosages established by various laboratory assays are as follows:

Table 1. Equivalent Oral Dosages of Glucocorticoids

Drug	Equivalent Dosage
Cortisone	25 mg
Hydrocortisone	20 mg
Prednisolone	5 mg
Prednisone	5 mg
Methylprednisolone	4 mg
Triamcinolone	4 mg
Dexamethasone	0.75 mg
Betamethasone	0.6 mg

"Equivalent dosages" are general approximations and may not apply to all diseases or routes of administration (especially oral inhalation, IM or intrasynovial injections). In addition, duration of HPA-axis suppression and degree of mineralocorticoid activities must be considered separately. (See Pharmacology.)

Estimated equivalent daily dosages of inhaled glucocorticoids for the treatment of asthma for adults and adolescents 12 years of age or older are as follows:

Table 2. Equivalent Daily Dosages of Inhaled Glucocorticoids for Adults and Adolescents

Drug	Low Daily Dosage (mcg)	Medium Daily Dosage (mcg)	High Daily Dosage (mcg)
Beclomethasone with Fluoroethane Propellant	80–240	>240–480	>480
Budesonide Powder for Oral Inhalation	180–600	>600–1200	>1200
Flunisolide with Hydrofluoroalkane (HFA) Propellant	320	>320–640	>640
Fluticasone with Fluoroethane Propellant	88–264	>264–440	>440
Fluticasone Powder for Oral Inhalation	100–300	>300–500	>500
Mometasone Powder for Oral Inhalation	200	400	>400
Triamcinolone Acetonide with Dichlorodifluoromethane Propellant	300–750	>750–1500	>1500

Estimated equivalent daily dosages of inhaled glucocorticoids for the treatment of asthma for infants and children are as follows (Table 3):

Table 3. Equivalent Daily Dosages of Inhaled Glucocorticoids for Infants and Children

Drug	Low Daily Dosage		Medium Daily Dosage		High Daily Dosage	
	Infants and Children 0–4 years of age[a]	Children 5–11 years of age	Infants and Children 0–4 years of age[a]	Children 5–11 years of age	Infants and Children 0–4 years of age[a]	Children 5–11 years of age
Beclomethasone with Fluoroethane Propellant	NA[b]	80–160 mcg	NA	>160–320 mcg	NA	>320 mcg
Budesonide Powder for Oral Inhalation	NA	180–400 mcg	NA	>400–800 mcg	NA	>800 mcg
Budesonide Suspension for Nebulization	0.25–0.5 mg	0.5 mg	>0.5–1 mg	1 mg	>1 mg	2 mg
Flunisolide with Hydrofluoroalkane (HFA) Propellant	NA	160 mcg[c]	NA	320 mcg[c]	NA	≥640 mcg[c]
Fluticasone with Fluoroethane Propellant	176 mcg	88–176 mcg	>176–352 mcg	>176–352 mcg	>352 mcg	>352 mcg
Fluticasone Powder for Oral Inhalation	NA	100–200 mcg	NA	>200–400 mcg	NA	>400 mcg
Triamcinolone Acetonide with Dichlorodifluoromethane Propellant	NA	300–600 mcg	NA	>600–900 mcg	NA	>900 mcg

[a] Safety and efficacy of inhaled corticosteroids in children younger than 1 year of age have not been established.

[b] NA: not applicable.

[c] Safety and efficacy of flunisolide inhalation aerosol in children younger than 6 years of age have not been established.

Long-term glucocorticoid therapy should not be initiated without due consideration of its risks. Other less dangerous drugs should be used if possible. If glucocorticoids are clearly necessary, the drugs should be administered in the smallest dosage possible and should generally be used only as adjuncts to other treatments. Patients should be continually monitored for signs that indicate dosage adjustment is necessary, such as remission or exacerbations of the disease and stress (surgery, infection, trauma). Periodic attempts should be made to decrease dosage or, preferably, to withdraw the drugs completely. Prescription refills should always be limited so that periodic evaluations can be made of the patient's condition.

Alternate-Day Therapy Alternate-day therapy is the dosage regimen of choice for long-term oral glucocorticoid treatment of most conditions. In alternate-day therapy, a single dose is administered every other morning. The drug is administered in the morning to simulate the natural circadian rhythm of corticosteroid secretion which is high in the morning and low in the evening. This regimen provides relief of symptoms while minimizing adrenal suppression, protein catabolism, and other adverse effects. However, some patients, especially those with rheumatoid arthritis or ulcerative colitis, require daily glucocorticoid therapy because symptoms of the underlying disease cannot be controlled by alternate-day therapy. Only "short-acting" steroids (e.g., prednisone, prednisolone, methylprednisolone) that suppress the HPA axis for less than 1.5 days after a single oral dose should be used for alternate-day therapy.

Several methods of transferring patients from initial divided-dose oral therapy to alternate-day therapy have been described. Twice the total daily dose that has been found to be effective may be administered as a single dose every other morning; this dose may then be gradually decreased to maintenance levels. Alternatively, the daily dose may be decreased to maintenance levels prior to initiation of alternate-day therapy; then twice the daily dose is given every other day. A third method is to establish a maintenance dose that is administered every morning as a single dose; alternate-day therapy is then introduced by gradual increases of this dose on alternate mornings with corresponding decreases in the dose administered on intervening mornings until twice the daily dose is being taken on alternate mornings.

Because an intact HPA axis is necessary for alternate-day therapy to be effective, it may be difficult to transfer a patient who has been maintained on divided-dose therapy for prolonged periods to alternate-day therapy, but continual attempts should be made to do so. Symptomatic treatment with other drugs on the "off day" or a trial of more than double the daily dose every other day may be helpful. When alternate-day therapy is not possible, the entire daily dose of glucocorticoid can usually be administered as a single morning dose; however, some patients will require divided daily doses of glucocorticoids.

Discontinuance of Therapy Although high-dose glucocorticoid therapy used for only brief periods in emergency situations may be reduced and discontinued quite rapidly, withdrawal following long-term therapy with pharmacologic dosages of systemic glucocorticoids should be very gradual until recovery of HPA-axis function occurs. (See Cautions: Adrenocortical Insufficiency.) These precautions also apply when a patient is transferred from a systemic glucocorticoid to oral or nasal inhalation therapy with beclomethasone dipropionate, budesonide, fluticasone propionate, or flunisolide.

For certain acute allergic conditions (e.g., contact dermatitis such as poison ivy), glucocorticoids may be administered short term (e.g., for 6 days), giving an initially high dose (e.g., 30 mg of prednisone in divided doses) on the first day of therapy, and then withdrawing therapy by tapering the dose over several days (e.g., by 5 mg of prednisone daily). (See Dosage and Administration: Dosage, in Methylprednisolone 68:04 and also Prednisone 68:04.)

Many methods of slow withdrawal or "tapering" have been described. In one suggested regimen, glucocorticoid dosage is decreased by the equivalent of 2.5–5 mg of prednisone every 3–7 days until the physiologic dose (e.g., 5 mg of prednisone or prednisolone, 0.75 mg of dexamethasone, or 20 mg of hydrocortisone) is reached. Other recommendations state that decrements usually should not exceed 2.5 mg of prednisone (or its equivalent) every 1–2 weeks except in patients on alternate-day therapy in whom it may be possible to decrease dosage in decrements of 5 mg of prednisone (or its equivalent) at 1- to 2-week intervals. If the disease flares up during withdrawal, dosage may need to be increased and followed by a more gradual withdrawal. In addition, increased dosage will be required during periods of stress. When a physiologic dosage has been reached, it has been suggested that single 20-mg oral morning doses of hydrocortisone be substituted for whatever glucocorticoid the patient has been receiving. After 2–4 weeks, the dosage of hydrocortisone may be decreased by 2.5 mg every week until a single morning dosage of 10 mg daily is reached.

The time required for complete HPA function recovery following discontinuance of glucocorticoid therapy is variable. Tests of adrenal function may be used to measure recovery of adrenocortical function. Normal morning plasma cortisol concentrations (exceeding 10 mcg/dL) indicate that basal pituitary-adrenal function is adequate and that maintenance therapy can be discontinued. However, this does not assure that adrenal function has recovered sufficiently to adequately increase cortisol production in response to stress and, therefore, supplemental glucocorticoids may still be required during stress. Complete recovery of HPA function generally can be assumed and supplementary therapy during stress can usually be discontinued when response to a corticotropin or cosyntropin test is normal.

Cautions

Short-term administration of glucocorticoids, even in massive dosages, is unlikely to produce harmful effects. When the drugs are used for longer than brief periods, however, they can produce a variety of devastating effects, including adrenocortical atrophy and generalized protein depletion.

■ **Adrenocortical Insufficiency** When given in supraphysiologic doses for prolonged periods, glucocorticoids may cause decreased secretion of endogenous corticosteroids by suppressing pituitary release of corticotropin (secondary adrenocortical insufficiency). The degree and duration of adrenocortical insufficiency produced by the drugs is highly variable among patients and depends on the dose, frequency and time of administration, and duration of glucocorticoid therapy. This effect may be minimized by use of alternate-day therapy. (See Alternate-Day Therapy under Dosage and Administration: Dosage.)

As in patients with primary adrenocortical insufficiency maintained on corticosteroids, patients who develop secondary adrenocortical insufficiency require higher corticosteroid dosage when they are subjected to stress (e.g., infection, surgery, trauma). In addition, acute adrenal insufficiency (even death) may occur if the drugs are withdrawn abruptly or if patients are transferred from systemic glucocorticoid therapy to oral inhalation therapy. Therefore, the drugs should be withdrawn very gradually following long-term therapy with pharmacologic dosages. (See Discontinuance of Therapy under Dosage and Administration: Dosage.) Adrenal suppression may persist up to 12 months in patients who receive large dosages for prolonged periods. Until recovery occurs, patients may show signs and symptoms of adrenal insufficiency when they are subjected to stress and replacement therapy may be required. Since mineralocorticoid secretion may be impaired, sodium chloride and/or a mineralocorticoid should also be administered.

■ **Musculoskeletal Effects** Muscle wasting, muscle pain or weakness, delayed wound healing, and atrophy of the protein matrix of the bone resulting in osteoporosis, vertebral compression fractures, aseptic necrosis of femoral or humeral heads, or pathologic fractures of long bones are manifestations of protein catabolism which may occur during prolonged therapy with glucocorticoids. These adverse effects may be especially serious in geriatric or debilitated patients. Before initiating glucocorticoid therapy in postmenopausal women, the fact that they are especially prone to osteoporosis should be considered. Glucocorticoids should be withdrawn if osteoporosis develops, unless their use is life-saving. A high-protein diet may help to prevent adverse effects associated with protein catabolism.

An acute myopathy has been observed with the use of high doses of glucocorticoids, particularly in patients with disorders of neuromuscular transmission (e.g., myasthenia gravis) or in patients receiving concomitant therapy with neuromuscular blocking agents (e.g., pancuronium). This acute myopathy is generalized, may involve ocular and respiratory muscles, and may result in quadriparesis. Myopathy may be accompanied by elevated serum creatine kinase [CK, creatine phosphokinase, CPK] concentrations. Resolution or clinical improvement of the myopathy may occur weeks to years after discontinuance of glucocorticoid therapy.

Tendon rupture, particularly of the Achilles tendon, has occurred in patients receiving glucocorticoids.

Osteoporosis Osteoporosis and related fractures are some of the most serious adverse effects of long-term glucocorticoid therapy. More than 10% of patients are diagnosed with a fracture and 30–40% have radiographic evidence of vertebral fractures during long-term glucocorticoid use. Glucocorticoid-induced bone loss and osteoporosis result from increased osteoclast-mediated bone resorption and decreased osteoblast-mediated bone formation. Contributing mechanisms include: 1) effects on calcium homeostasis (e.g., decreased intestinal absorption of calcium and phosphate, increased urinary calcium excretion possibly secondary to a direct effect on tubular reabsorption, resultant secondary hyperparathyroidism leading to increased bone resorption if persistent), 2) effects on sex hormones (e.g., decreased sex hormone production both indirectly by reducing endogenous pituitary hormone concentrations and adrenal androgen production and directly through effects on gonadal hormone release, decreased pituitary secretion of luteinizing hormone with resultant decreased ovarian estrogen and testicular androgen production), 3) inhibition of bone formation (e.g., inhibition of osteoblast proliferation and attachment to matrix, inhibition of the synthesis of type I collagen and noncollagenous proteins by osteoblasts, and dose-related decreases in circulating osteocalcin, possibly mediated by effects on oncogene expression, prostaglandin E production, and the production of insulin-like growth factors and transforming growth factor), and 4) other effects (e.g., effects on the normal forces of muscle contraction on bone resulting from glucocorticoid-induced myopathy and muscle weakness, contribution of the underlying inflammatory condition being treated). Bone loss is most rapid during the first 3–6 months following initiation of glucocorticoid therapy and continues at a slower, steadier rate with prolonged use.

Patients with such bone loss are predisposed to fractures (particularly vertebral fractures because of greater effects of glucocorticoids on trabecular than cortical bone). The risk of fractures is both dose and duration dependent, with higher daily or cumulative doses of glucocorticoids and longer durations of use associated with greater risk. A high glucocorticoid dosage generally is considered a daily dosage equivalent to more than 7.5 mg of prednisone. However, some studies have reported an increased risk of fracture with daily dosages as low as 2.5–7.5 mg of prednisolone or equivalent, while others have found no appreciable decline in bone density with prednisone dosages averaging 8 mg daily or dosages of less than 5 mg daily. Alternate-day regimens have not been shown to be associated with less risk of bone loss than daily regimens. Bone loss has even been associated with oral inhalation of glucocorticoids. However, risk of osteoporosis is uncertain in patients receiving recommended doses of inhaled glucocorticoids.

Glucocorticoid-induced bone loss can be both prevented and treated; however, many patients receiving long-term glucocorticoid therapy do not receive appropriate therapies to prevent bone loss or are treated only after a fracture has occurred. The American College of Rheumatology (ACR) recommends that preventive therapy be considered for patients in whom the benefits of such therapy outweigh the potential harms. ACR recommendations are based on a risk-stratification approach in which an individual's risk level for developing a fracture (low, moderate, or high) is determined based on predisposing factors including the individual's preexisting or anticipated glucocorticoid dosage. An initial clinical fracture risk assessment is recommended as soon as possible, but at least within 6 months of initiating long-term glucocorticoid therapy and reassessments are recommended every 12 months during continued treatment. ACR states that the available data on fracture risk and risk reduction are more limited in children and adults younger than 40 years of age; nevertheless such patients also should be assessed for their fracture risk and managed accordingly.

To minimize the risk of glucocorticoid-induced bone loss, the smallest possible effective dosage and duration should be used. Topical and inhaled preparations should be used whenever possible. Lifestyle modifications to reduce the risk of osteoporosis (e.g., cigarette smoking cessation, limitation of alcohol consumption, participation in a weight-bearing exercise for 30–60 minutes daily) should be encouraged in all patients. In addition, patients should receive adequate calcium and vitamin D supplementation to preserve bone mass and limit the extent of glucocorticoid-induced bone loss. Patients who are considered to be at moderate-to-high risk of fracture generally should receive additional pharmacologic therapy. Bisphosphonates generally are preferred and have been shown to reduce the incidence of radiographic vertebral fractures in patients with glucocorticoid-induced osteoporosis.

The ACR guideline for the prevention and treatment of glucocorticoid-induced osteoporosis recommends calcium and vitamin D supplementation in addition to lifestyle modification in any patient receiving long-term (at least 3 months) glucocorticoid therapy at a daily dosage equivalent to at least 2.5 mg of prednisone. No further preventive measure is generally recommended in patients who are considered to be at low risk of fracture; however, such patients should be monitored closely during continued glucocorticoid therapy, with fracture risk assessments and bone mineral density (BMD) measurements performed at regular intervals. ACR recommends an additional pharmacologic agent in patients who are considered to be at moderate-to-high risk of fracture. Oral bisphosphonates generally are preferred in most situations because of their demonstrated benefits in reducing fracture risk as well as their safety and low cost; other suggested options include IV bisphosphonates, teriparatide, denosumab, and raloxifene (for postmenopausal women if no other therapy is appropriate). Because of some uncertainty regarding the relative benefits versus harms of these interventions, ACR states that most of their recommendations are conditional and that treatment decisions should be individualized based on patient preferences, values, and comorbidities.

■ **Increased Susceptibility to Infection** Glucocorticoids, especially in large doses, increase susceptibility to and mask symptoms of infection. Infections with any pathogen, including viral, bacterial, fungal, protozoan, or helminthic infections in any organ system, may be associated with glucocorticoids alone or in combination with other immunosuppressive agents. These infections may be mild, but they can be severe or fatal, and localized infections may disseminate.

Patients who become immunosuppressed while receiving glucocorticoids have increased susceptibility to infections compared with healthy individuals. Some infections such as varicella (chickenpox) and measles can have a more serious or even fatal outcome in such patients, particularly in children.

Immunosuppression is most likely to occur in patients receiving high-dose (e.g., equivalent to at least 1 mg/kg of prednisone daily), systemic glucocorticoid therapy for any period of time, particularly in conjunction with glucocorticoid-sparing drugs (e.g., troleandomycin) and/or concomitant immunosuppressant agents; however, patients receiving moderate dosages of systemic glucocorticoids for short periods or low dosages for prolonged periods also may be at risk.

FDA states that the possibility of orally inhaled glucocorticoid therapy causing sufficient immunosuppression to place a patient at risk of infection also should be considered. However, the risk of such therapy, including any possible contribution of local pulmonary immunosuppressant effects of inhaled drug to the development of serious pulmonary infections (e.g., varicella pneumonia), remains to be more fully elucidated.

Glucocorticoid-dependent children should undergo anti-varicella-zoster virus antibody testing. Vaccination should be considered for those who have absent or inadequate antibody concentrations. In addition, such children and any adult who are not likely to have been exposed to varicella or measles should avoid exposure to these infections while receiving glucocorticoids. If exposure to varicella or measles occurs in such individuals, administration of varicella zoster immune globulin (VZIG) or immune globulin, respectively, may be indicated. If varicella develops, treatment with an antiviral agent (e.g., acyclovir) may be considered, although fatal outcome (e.g., in those developing hemorrhagic varicella) may not always be avoided even if such therapy is initiated aggressively.

The immunosuppressive effects of glucocorticoids may result in activation of latent infection or exacerbation of intercurrent infections, including those caused by *Candida*, *Mycobacterium*, *Toxoplasma*, *Strongyloides*, *Pneumocystis*, *Cryptococcus*, *Nocardia*, or *Ameba*. Glucocorticoids should be used with great care in patients with known or suspected *Strongyloides* (threadworm) infection. In such patients, glucocorticoid-induced immunosuppression may lead to *Strongyloides* hyperinfection and dissemination with widespread larval migration, often accompanied by severe enterocolitis and potentially fatal gram-negative septicemia.

Some experts advise that the need to continue at least physiologic replacement dosages of glucocorticoids in glucocorticoid-dependent patients developing serious infection should be considered since discontinuance of the drugs before or after the development of varicella may have contributed to fatal outcome in some reported cases. Additional insight is needed regarding the dosages, routes, and types of glucocorticoids as well as immunologic characteristics likely to place patients at substantial risk of immunosuppression and serious infection.

The most common adverse effect of oral inhalation therapy with glucocorticoids is *Candida albicans* or *Aspergillus niger* infections of the mouth, pharynx, and occasionally the larynx. Oral candidiasis also is one of the most frequent adverse effects of therapy with long-term oral glucocorticoids. The occurrence of these fungal infections appears to be dose dependent; they also occur more frequently in women than in men. Some clinicians recommend that patients rinse their mouths with water and swallow after each oral inhalation dose to prevent *Candida* infection. Usually, *Candida* or *Aspergillus* infections are of little clinical importance, but occasionally they may require antifungal therapy or discontinuance of the oral inhalation.

The principal risk of epidural injection therapy for low back pain and radiculopathy is rare epidural abscess. Infectious complications (including bacterial meningitis) have been reported following epidural injection. Fungal and bacterial infections (including meningitis) have been reported in patients who received epidural or intra-articular therapy with contaminated glucocorticoid injections prepared by compounding pharmacies.

■ **Fluid and Electrolyte Disturbances** Sodium retention with resultant edema, potassium loss, hypokalemic alkalosis, and hypertension may occur in patients receiving glucocorticoids. Congestive heart failure may occur in susceptible patients. These mineralocorticoid effects are less frequent with synthetic glucocorticoids (except fludrocortisone) than with hydrocortisone or cortisone, but may occur, especially when synthetic glucocorticoids are given in high dosage for prolonged periods. Dietary salt restriction is advisable and potassium supplementation may be necessary in patients receiving glucocorticoids for anti-inflammatory or immunosuppressant effects. When glucocorticoids with substantial mineralocorticoid activity are administered, patients should be instructed to notify their physicians if edema develops. All glucocorticoids increase calcium excretion and may cause hypocalcemia.

■ **Ocular Effects** Prolonged use of glucocorticoids may result in posterior subcapsular and nuclear cataracts (particularly in children), exophthalmos, or increased intraocular pressure which may result in glaucoma or may occasionally damage the optic nerve. However, data from several studies indicate that the risk of subcapsular and nuclear cataracts associated with inhaled glucocorticoid use is negligible in young asthmatic patients, but the risk of such cataracts may be elevated in older patients. Data from a case-control study indicate that the risk of ocular hypertension or open-angle glaucoma was increased in patients receiving high dosages of orally inhaled glucocorticoids (at least 1600 mcg of beclomethasone dipropionate, budesonide, or triamcinolone acetonide) daily for at least 3 months. Patients receiving lower dosages of orally inhaled or intranasal glucocorticoids were not at increased risk for these adverse ocular effects. Results from a population-based study indicate that use of orally inhaled corticosteroids is associated with development of posterior subcapsular and nuclear cataracts. Establishment of secondary fungal and viral infections of the eye may also be enhanced in patients receiving glucocorticoids. Blindness has occurred rarely following intralesional injection of glucocorticoids around the face and head. Ocular effects (e.g., transient blindness, amblyopia, acute retinal necrosis syndrome, intraocular hemorrhage, cortical blindness) also have occurred following epidural injection. Eye irritation and eyelid edema have been reported in patients receiving glucocorticoids in clinical trials.

■ **Endocrine Effects** When glucocorticoids are administered over a prolonged period, they may produce various endocrine disorders including hypercorticism (cushingoid state) and amenorrhea or other menstrual difficulties. Corticosteroids may decrease glucose tolerance, produce hyperglycemia, and aggravate or precipitate diabetes mellitus especially in patients predisposed to diabetes mellitus. If steroid therapy is required in patients with diabetes mellitus, changes in insulin or oral antidiabetic agent dosage or diet may be necessary. Corticosteroids have also been reported to increase or decrease motility and number of sperm in some men.

■ **GI Effects** Adverse GI effects of corticosteroids include nausea, vomiting, anorexia which may result in weight loss, increased appetite which may result in weight gain, diarrhea or constipation, abdominal distention, pancreatitis, gastric irritation, and ulcerative esophagitis. Indigestion is one of the most frequently occurring adverse effects in patients receiving long-term therapy with oral corticosteroids. Blood in the stool has been reported in patients receiving prednisolone orally disintegrating tablets in clinical trials. Corticosteroids have been implicated in the development, reactivation, perforation, hemorrhage, and delayed healing of peptic ulcers. Although concomitant administration of antacids or other antiulcer agents (e.g., cimetidine) has been suggested to prevent peptic ulcer formation in patients receiving high dosages of corticosteroids, routine concomitant use of these agents does not appear to be warranted since corticosteroid-induced ulcers occur infrequently (in 2% or less of patients receiving corticosteroids) and the efficacy of antiulcer therapy in preventing these ulcers has not been established. However, selective use of preventive antiulcer therapy may be considered in patients receiving corticosteroids who are at increased risk of peptic ulcer formation (e.g., those receiving other ulcerogenic drugs). Gastric irritation may be reduced if oral corticosteroids are taken immediately before, during, or immediately after meals, or with food or milk.

■ **Nervous System Effects** Adverse neurologic effects of glucocorticoids have included headache, vertigo, insomnia, restlessness and increased motor activity, ischemic neuropathy, electroencephalogram (EEG) abnormalities, and seizures. Glucocorticoids may precipitate mental disturbances ranging from euphoria, mood swings, depression and anxiety, and personality changes to frank psychoses. Emotional instability or psychotic tendencies may be aggravated by the drugs. Increased intracranial pressure with papilledema (i.e., pseudotumor cerebri) has been reported, generally in association with withdrawal of glucocorticoid therapy.

Aseptic meningitis, arachnoiditis, exacerbation of pain, spinal cord trauma, subdural injection, intracranial air injection, increased intracranial pressure, nerve injury, seizures, bladder or bowel dysfunction, paraparesis or paralysis, sensory disturbances, and brain damage have been reported following epidural injection and/or intrathecal administration. It is unclear whether reports of neurologic effects associated with epidural glucocorticoid administration involved improper needle placement or were related to administration of the drug and/or preservatives.

Serious, potentially permanent, adverse neurologic events (e.g., spinal cord infarction, paraplegia, quadriplegia, cortical blindness, stroke, seizures, nerve injury, brain edema), including death, have been reported rarely following epidural glucocorticoid injection both with and without fluoroscopic guidance. In addition to potential direct needle trauma to the spinal cord, such adverse events also may be the result of inadvertent intra-arterial injection of the particulate glucocorticoid suspension with subsequent embolization. Many of the events occurred within minutes to 48 hours after epidural injection of the glucocorticoid. In some cases, diagnoses of adverse neurologic events were confirmed by magnetic resonance imaging or computed tomography. Patients should be advised to immediately seek emergency medical attention for unusual symptoms (e.g., loss of or changes in vision, tingling in extremities, sudden weakness or numbness affecting the face or occurring unilaterally or bilaterally in the arms or legs, dizziness, severe headache, seizures) occurring after epidural glucocorticoid injection.

■ **Dermatologic Effects** Various adverse dermatologic effects are associated with systemic glucocorticoid administration and include impaired wound healing, skin atrophy and thinning, acne, increased sweating, hirsutism, facial erythema, striae, petechiae, ecchymoses, and easy bruising. Long-term therapy with high dosages of inhaled corticosteroids is associated with skin thinning and easy bruising, particularly among women. Dermatologic manifestations of hypersensitivity to the corticosteroids include hives and/or allergic dermatitis, urticaria, and angioedema. Burning or tingling of the perineal area may occur after IV injection of the drugs. Parenteral corticosteroid therapy has also produced hypopigmentation or hyperpigmentation, scarring, induration, delayed pain or soreness, subcutaneous and cutaneous atrophy, and sterile abscesses. Kaposi's sarcoma has been reported to occur in patients receiving glucocorticoid therapy; discontinuance of such therapy may result in remission of the disease.

Dermal and/or subdermal changes forming depressions in the skin at the injection site have been reported with use of methylprednisolone acetate injectable suspension (Depo-Medrol®). Caution should be used to minimize the incidence of dermal and subdermal atrophy.

■ **Other Adverse Effects** A steroid withdrawal syndrome seemingly unrelated to adrenocortical insufficiency and consisting of anorexia, nausea and vomiting, lethargy, headache, fever, joint pain, desquamation, easy bruising, myalgia, weight loss, and/or hypotension has been reported following abrupt withdrawal of glucocorticoids. Symptoms often occurred while plasma glucocorticoid concentrations were still high but were falling rapidly; apparently the abrupt change in glucocorticoid concentration rather than a low concentration per se was responsible for the phenomenon. Bradycardia has occurred during or after IV administration of large doses of methylprednisolone sodium succinate but did not appear to be related to the rate or duration of infusion.

A few patients have experienced hoarseness, dry mouth, and sore throat during oral inhalation therapy with glucocorticoids; these adverse effects have also occurred in patients receiving only the aerosol vehicle and may be minimized by rinsing the mouth and swallowing after using the aerosol. Pharyngolaryngeal pain has been reported in patients receiving glucocorticoids in clinical trials. Dysphonia also has been reported following epidural glucocorticoid injection.

Injections of slightly soluble glucocorticoids may produce atrophy at the site of injection. (See Dosage and Administration: Administration.) Intra-articularly administered corticosteroids have caused postinjection flare and Charcot-like arthropathy. Epidural lipomatosis has been reported with repeated epidural glucocorticoid injections but appears to resolve following discontinuance of such therapy. Cerebral or pulmonary embolism, hematoma formation, pneumothorax, intravascular injection, and vascular injury also have been reported following epidural injection therapy.

Minor transient complications of epidural glucocorticoid therapy include headache, nausea, facial flushing, fever, and inadvertent spinal tap. Headache appears to occur commonly with epidural injection of glucocorticoids presumably secondary to pressure changes in the epidural space or accidental puncture of the dura.

Intranasal administration of these drugs has been associated with allergic reactions and rhinitis. Temporary or permanent visual impairment, including blindness, has been reported with glucocorticoid administration by intranasal, ophthalmic, and other routes of administration. Increased intraocular pressure, infection, residue or slough at the injection site, and ocular and periocular inflammation, including allergic reactions, have been reported with ophthalmic administration of glucocorticoids.

Hypercholesterolemia, atherosclerosis, thrombosis, thromboembolism, fat embolism, and thrombophlebitis have also been associated with corticosteroid therapy, particularly with cortisone. Hypertrophic cardiomyopathy has been reported in premature infants receiving glucocorticoids (e.g., prednisolone). Thrombocytopenia has been observed in a few patients following prolonged, high-dose glucocorticoid therapy. Palpitation, tachycardia, swelling of mouth and tongue, frequency and urgency of urination, and enuresis have been reported rarely. Anaphylactic reactions also have been reported rarely with parenteral glucocorticoid therapy. Glucocorticoids may decrease serum concentrations of ascorbic acid (vitamin C) and vitamin A; symptoms of vitamin A or C deficiency may occur rarely.

Transient, mild, asymptomatic elevations in ALT (SGPT), AST (SGOT), and alkaline phosphatase concentrations have been reported in patients receiving glucocorticoids; these effects are not associated with any clinical syndrome and generally resolve upon discontinuance of glucocorticoid therapy.

■ **Precautions and Contraindications** Prior to initiation of long-term glucocorticoid therapy, baseline ECGs, blood pressures, chest and spinal radiographs, glucose tolerance tests, and evaluations of HPA-axis function should be performed on all patients. Upper GI radiographs should be performed in patients predisposed to GI disorders, including those with known or suspected peptic ulcer disease. During long-term therapy, periodic height, weight, chest and spinal radiographs, hematopoietic, electrolyte, glucose tolerance, and ocular and blood pressure evaluations should be performed.

Patients receiving glucocorticoids should be instructed to notify their physicians of any infections, signs of infections (e.g., fever, sore throat, pain during urination, muscle aches), or injuries that develop during therapy or within 12 months after therapy is discontinued, so that adjustments in dosage can be made or glucocorticoid therapy reintroduced if necessary. In addition, when surgery is required, patients should be advised to inform the attending physician, dentist, or anesthesiologist that they are receiving or have recently (within 12 months) received glucocorticoids. Patients should carry identification cards listing the diseases for which they are being treated, the glucocorticoid they are receiving and its dosage, and the name and telephone number of their physician. Patients being transferred from systemic corticosteroid to oral inhalation therapy should carry special identification (e.g., card, bracelet) indicating the need for supplementary systemic corticosteroids during periods of stress. Patients receiving orally inhaled glucocorticoid therapy who are currently being withdrawn or who have been withdrawn from systemic corticosteroids should be advised to immediately resume full therapeutic dosages of systemic corticosteroids and to contact their clinician for further instructions during stressful periods (e.g., severe infection, severe asthmatic attack).

Because anaphylactoid reactions have occurred in patients receiving glucocorticoids parenterally, precautionary measures should be taken prior to parenteral administration of the drugs, particularly in patients with history of a drug allergy. Some patients who appear to be hypersensitive to parenteral glucocorticoids may actually be hypersensitive to the paraben preservatives present in some injectable formulations.

Because an apparent association has been suggested between use of corticosteroids and left ventricular free-wall rupture after a recent myocardial infarction, corticosteroids should be used with extreme caution in these patients.

Some commercially available oral preparations of prednisolone, and triamcinolone contain the dye tartrazine (FD&C yellow No. 5), which may cause allergic reactions including bronchial asthma in susceptible individuals. Although the incidence of tartrazine sensitivity is low, it frequently occurs in patients who are sensitive to aspirin.

Some commercially available formulations of dexamethasone, hydrocortisone, and prednisolone contain sulfites that may cause allergic-type reactions, including anaphylaxis and life-threatening or less severe asthmatic episodes, in certain susceptible individuals. The overall prevalence of sulfite sensitivity in the general population is unknown but probably low; such sensitivity appears to occur more frequently in asthmatic than in nonasthmatic individuals.

Glucocorticoids should be used with caution in patients with hypothyroidism or cirrhosis, because such patients often show exaggerated response to the drugs. Glucocorticoids should be used with caution in psychotic patients or patients with hypertension or congestive heart failure.

Corticosteroids should be used with caution in patients with active or latent peptic ulcer, diverticulitis, nonspecific ulcerative colitis (if there is a probability of impending perforation, abscess, or other pyogenic infection), and in those with recent intestinal anastomoses. Manifestations of peritoneal irritation following GI perforation may be minimal or absent in patients receiving glucocorticoids.

Glucocorticoids should be used cautiously in patients with myasthenia gravis, particularly in those receiving anticholinesterase therapy. If possible, anticholinesterase agents should be withdrawn at least 24 hours prior to initiating glucocorticoid therapy. Because cortisone has been reported rarely to increase blood coagulability and to precipitate intravascular thrombosis, thromboembolism, and thrombophlebitis, corticosteroids should be used with caution in patients with thromboembolic disorders. Glucocorticoids should be used with caution in patients with seizure disorders, renal insufficiency, osteoporosis, or herpes simplex infections of the eye; some manufacturers state that glucocorticoids should not be used in patients with active ocular herpes simplex infections. Corneal perforation may occur in patients with ocular herpes simplex infections who are receiving glucocorticoids. Glucocorticoids are not recommended for use in the treatment of optic neuritis as such use may increase the risk of new episodes.

Corticosteroids are contraindicated in patients with known hypersensitivity to any of the other corticosteroids. Specific corticosteroid preparations are contraindicated in patients with known hypersensitivity to any ingredient in the respective formulation. Fludrocortisone is contraindicated in all conditions except those which require a high degree of mineralocorticoid activity.

Because glucocorticoids increase susceptibility to and mask symptoms of infection, the drugs should not be used, except in life-threatening situations, in patients with viral infections or bacterial infections not controlled by anti-infectives. Manufacturers state that glucocorticoid oral inhalation therapy should be used with caution, if at all, in patients with untreated systemic fungal, bacterial, viral, or parasitic infections. Patients whose susceptibility to infection is high, such as those receiving glucocorticoids as immunosuppressive therapy, are especially likely to develop secondary infections. Patients receiving glucocorticoids who are potentially immunosuppressed should be warned of the risk of exposure to certain infections (e.g., chickenpox, measles) and of the importance of obtaining medical advice if such exposure occurs. (See Cautions: Increased Susceptibility to Infection.) Since glucocorticoid therapy can reactivate tuberculosis, treatment of latent tuberculosis infection should be included in the regimen of patients with a history of active tuberculosis undergoing prolonged glucocorticoid therapy. If glucocorticoids are indicated in patients with latent tuberculosis or tuberculin reactivity, close observation is necessary. Use of glucocorticoids in patients with active tuberculosis should be restricted to those with fulminating or disseminated tuberculosis in which glucocorticoids are used in conjunction with appropriate antimycobacterial chemotherapy. Manufacturers state that glucocorticoid oral inhalation therapy should be used with caution, if at all, in patients with clinical or asymptomatic *Mycobacterium tuberculosis* infections of the respiratory tract. Since glucocorticoids can reactivate latent amebiasis, any patient who has been in the tropics or who has unexplained diarrhea should be evaluated for amebiasis to exclude these patients prior to initiating therapy. In the treatment of acute or disseminated tuberculosis, glucocorticoids should only be used as part of a total antituberculosis regimen. Corticosteroids should not be used in patients with cerebral malaria. The manufacturers of methylprednisolone warn that the efficacy of glucocorticoids in the treatment of sepsis syndrome and septic shock has not been established (see Uses: Other Uses), and that at least one study suggested that such use in certain patients (e.g., those with serum creatinine concentrations exceeding 2 mg/dL at diagnosis and those who develop secondary infections) may be associated with an increased risk of mortality.

Some clinicians state that glucocorticoid oral inhalation therapy probably should be avoided when the risk of activating bronchopulmonary mycoses appears high, as in patients with bronchiectasis or inadequate immunologic responses. Although manufacturers state that glucocorticoids are contraindicated in patients with systemic fungal infections, most authorities believe that glucocorticoid therapy may be initiated in patients with known infections (including those from fungi) if effective specific chemotherapy is administered concomitantly. The manufacturers of methylprednisolone acetate state that although the drug is contraindicated in patients with systemic fungal infections, it may be used as an intra-articular injection for localized joint conditions. In patients with acute infection, methylprednisolone acetate should not be administered intra-articularly, bursally, or into a tendon for local effects.

FDA states that the efficacy and safety of epidural administration of glucocorticoids have not been established, and glucocorticoids are not FDA-labeled for such use. Prior to initiating such therapy, healthcare providers should discuss with patients the potential benefits and risks of epidural glucocorticoid injections and alternative treatments. Epidural administration of glucocorticoids is contraindicated in patients with local or systemic infection; individuals with bleeding disorders or receiving concurrent anticoagulant therapy (e.g., warfarin, heparin, antiplatelet agents); patients with known hypersensitivity to local anesthetic agents, contrast agents, or glucocorticoids; and patients who experienced complications with prior glucocorticoid injections. Epidural glucocorticoid therapy should be used with caution in patients with congestive heart failure or diabetes mellitus. Fluoroscopy (recommended for ensuring proper needle placement) is contraindicated in pregnant women.

IM administration of corticosteroids is contraindicated in patients with idiopathic thrombocytopenic purpura.

■ **Pediatric Precautions** The effects of glucocorticoids on the pathophysiology and course of diseases are considered to be similar in adults and children. Evidence of safety and efficacy for prednisolone in pediatric patients has been provided through studies using the drug in pediatric patients for the treatment of nephrotic syndrome (in patients older than 2 years of age) and aggressive leukemias and lymphomas (in patients older than 1 month of age). However, some of the conclusions of these studies, and evidence of safety and efficacy for other pediatric indications (e.g., severe asthma and wheezing), are based on controlled trials in adults.

The adverse effects of prednisolone in pediatric patients are similar to those in adults. As in adults, periodic evaluations of height, weight, ocular pressure, and blood pressure should be performed in children receiving glucocorticoids. Children, like adults, also should undergo clinical evaluation for the presence of infection, psychosocial disturbances, thromboembolism, peptic ulcers, cataracts, and osteoporosis.

Long-term administration of pharmacologic dosages of glucocorticoids to children should be avoided if possible, since the drugs may retard bone growth when administered by any route. If prolonged therapy is necessary, the growth and development of infants and children should be closely monitored, and the potential effects on growth should be weighed against clinical benefits and the availability of alternative therapy. Most children receiving recommended dosages of inhaled glucocorticoids achieved their predicted adult heights but at a later than normal age, and the potential but small risk of delayed growth is well balanced by the improved health outcomes associated with inhaled glucocorticoid therapy for mild or moderate persistent asthma in such children. Therapy with low-to-medium dose inhaled glucocorticoids is associated with a short-term (first year of treatment) decrease in growth rates (approximately 1 cm), but such effects appear to be temporary and do not predict final adult height. Effects on growth are not likely with inhaled glucocorticoid dosages of up to 200 mcg daily, and HPA-axis suppression is unlikely at dosages of less than 200 mcg daily of budesonide [or its equivalent] daily dosage. Results of controlled longitudinal studies and several cross-sectional studies in children with asthma receiving long-term inhaled glucocorticoid (2–5 years) therapy indicate that bone mineral density was not affected by use of inhaled glucocorticoids. High dosages of inhaled glucocorticoids for prolonged periods of time (e.g., exceeding 1 year), particularly in combination with frequent courses of systemic glucocorticoid therapy may be associated with adverse growth effects and/or reduced bone mineral density. Retardation of bone growth has been observed at low systemic doses of glucocorticoids and in the absence of hypothalamic-pituitary-adrenal (HPA) axis suppression (e.g., as determined by tests of HPA axis function such as cosyntropin stimulation and basal plasma cortisol concentrations). Growth velocity may therefore be a more sensitive indicator of systemic glucocorticoid exposure than some commonly used tests of HPA axis function. In order to minimize the potential effects of glucocorticoids on growth, dosage in children should be titrated to the lowest effective level. Alternate-day therapy minimizes growth suppression and should be instituted if growth suppression occurs.

Glucocorticoid-induced osteoporosis and associated fractures are common in children and adolescents receiving long-term systemic therapy with the drugs since bone turnover is high and the rates of bone formation required to maintain adequate mineralization of the rapidly growing skeleton also are high in this age group. In addition, glucocorticoids by inhibiting bone formation may prevent achievement of peak bone mass during adolescence. The underlying pediatric condition for which glucocorticoids are prescribed also may be associated independently with an increased risk of osteoporosis. Methods for monitoring bone mineralization (e.g., dual-energy x-ray absorptiometry [DXA]) in children and adolescents are similar to those in adults. However, the roles of various preventive or corrective therapies for glucocorticoid-induced bone loss in children currently are not well defined. At this time, the most prudent approach to minimizing the negative effects of glucocorticoids on BMD in children and adolescents is by ensuring that the patients consistently ingest either through diet or supplementation adequate calcium and vitamin D. (See Uses: Corticosteroid-induced Osteoporosis, in the Vitamin D Analogs General Statement 88:16.)

High dosages of glucocorticoids in children may cause acute pancreatitis leading to pancreatic destruction. Children have developed increases in intracranial pressure (pseudotumor cerebri), causing papilledema, oculomotor or abducens nerve paralysis, visual loss, and headache. Pseudotumor cerebri has occurred most frequently following reduction of dosage or a change in the steroid administered.

Some commercially available injections of dexamethasone, hydrocortisone, methylprednisolone, and triamcinolone contain benzyl alcohol as a preservative. Although a causal relationship has not been established, administration of injections preserved with benzyl alcohol has been associated with toxicity in neonates. Toxicity appears to have resulted from administration of large amounts (i.e., 100–400 mg/kg daily) of benzyl alcohol in these neonates. Although manufacturers of some benzyl alcohol-containing injectable glucocorticoids state that these drugs are contraindicated in premature infants and use of drugs preserved with benzyl alcohol should be avoided in neonates whenever possible, the American Academy of Pediatrics states that the presence of small amounts of the preservative in a commercially available injection should not proscribe its use when the medication is indicated in neonates and comparable benzyl alcohol-free preparations are not available.

■ **Pregnancy and Lactation** Glucocorticoids may cause fetal damage when administered to pregnant women. One retrospective study of 260 women who received pharmacologic dosages of glucocorticoids during pregnancy revealed 2 instances of cleft palate, 8 stillbirths, 1 spontaneous abortion, and 15 premature births. Another study reported 2 cases of cleft palate in 86 births. Occurrence of cleft palate in these studies is higher than in the general population but could have resulted from the underlying diseases as well as from the steroids. Other fetal abnormalities that have been reported following glucocorticoid administration in pregnant women include hydrocephalus and gastroschisis. Women should be instructed to inform their physicians if they become or wish to become pregnant while receiving glucocorticoids. If glucocorticoids must be used during pregnancy or if the patient becomes pregnant while taking one of these drugs, the potential risks should be carefully considered.

In a retrospective study of 260 women, administration of glucocorticoids throughout pregnancy has been reported to precipitate adrenal crisis in one neonate, but in other studies there was no evidence of this. Infants born to women who receive glucocorticoids during pregnancy should be carefully monitored for symptoms of adrenal insufficiency and appropriate therapy begun immediately if such symptoms appear.

Corticosteroids may be distributed into milk and could suppress growth, interfere with endogenous glucocorticoid production, or cause other adverse effects in nursing infants. Since adequate reproductive studies have not been performed in humans with glucocorticoids, these drugs should be administered to nursing mothers only if the benefits of therapy are judged to outweigh the potential risks to the infant.

Drug Interactions

■ **Drugs Affecting Hepatic Microsomal Enzymes** Metabolism of certain glucocorticoids is mediated by the cytochrome P-450 (CYP) isoenzyme 3A4, and the possibility exists that drugs that induce, inhibit, or compete for this isoenzyme may alter metabolism and clearance of glucocorticoids. Conversely, some glucocorticoids (e.g. betamethasone) inhibit the action of CYP3A4, and some glucocorticoids (e.g., dexamethasone) induce CYP3A4. These glucocorticoids may alter the metabolism of drugs metabolized by CYP3A4.

Cyclosporine Concomitant administration of prednisolone and cyclosporine may result in decreased plasma clearance of prednisolone, and plasma concentrations of cyclosporine may be increased during concomitant therapy with methylprednisolone. In addition, seizures reportedly have occurred in adult and pediatric patients receiving high-dose glucocorticoid therapy concurrently with cyclosporine. The mechanism of this interaction may involve competitive inhibition of hepatic microsomal enzymes. The potential drug interaction between cyclosporine and prednisolone or methylprednisolone and the possibility of exacerbated toxicity, as well as the need for appropriate dosage adjustment, should be considered when these drugs are administered concomitantly.

Other Drugs Drugs that induce cytochrome P-450 (CYP) isoenzyme 3A4 (e. g., barbiturates, phenytoin, rifampin, ephedrine, carbamazepine) may enhance metabolism of, and reduce, glucocorticoid concentrations. Dosage of glucocorticoids given in combination with such cytochrome P-450 inducers may need to be increased to achieve the desired response. Conversely, concomitant administration of certain glucocorticoids with drugs that inhibit CYP3A4 (e.g., macrolide antibiotics, ketoconazole) may decrease glucocorticoid clearance; dosage of glucocorticoids given in combination with cytochrome P-450 inhibitors may need to be decreased to avoid potential adverse effects.

■ **Antidiabetic Therapy** Because glucocorticoids may increase blood glucose concentrations, patients with diabetes mellitus receiving concurrent insulin and/or oral hypoglycemic agents may require adjustments in the dosage of such therapy.

■ **Estrogens** Estrogens may potentiate effects of hydrocortisone, possibly by increasing the concentration of transcortin and thus decreasing the amount of hydrocortisone available to be metabolized. Effects of other glucocorticoids that bind to transcortin could be similarly potentiated and dosage adjustments may be required if estrogens are added to or withdrawn from a stable dosage regimen.

■ **Nonsteroidal Anti-inflammatory Agents** Concomitant administration of ulcerogenic drugs such as indomethacin during corticosteroid therapy may increase the risk of GI ulceration. Aspirin should be used cautiously in conjunction with glucocorticoids in patients with hypoprothrombinemia. Although concomitant therapy with salicylates and corticosteroids does not appear to increase the incidence or severity of GI ulceration, the possibility of this effect should be considered.

Serum salicylate concentrations may decrease when corticosteroids are administered concomitantly. Likewise, when corticosteroids are discontinued in patients receiving salicylates, serum salicylate concentration may increase; salicylate intoxication has been precipitated rarely. Several mechanisms may be involved in this interaction. In one study in healthy individuals and in patients with polyarthritis who received both drugs concomitantly, corticosteroids increased the renal clearance of salicylate, possibly by increasing glomerular filtration rate. Corticosteroids may also induce the metabolism of salicylate. Salicylates and corticosteroids should be used concurrently with caution. Patients receiving both drugs should be observed closely for adverse effects of either drug. It may be necessary to increase salicylate dosage when corticosteroids are administered concurrently or decrease salicylate dosage when corticosteroids are discontinued in patients receiving salicylates.

In one study in patients with rheumatoid arthritis, concomitant administration of indomethacin and prednisolone resulted in increased plasma concentrations of free prednisolone; total plasma prednisolone concentrations were unchanged. It was suggested that indomethacin may have a steroid-sparing effect.

■ **Potassium-depleting Drugs** Potassium-depleting diuretics (e.g., thiazides, furosemide, ethacrynic acid) and other drugs that deplete potassium, such as amphotericin B, may enhance the potassium-wasting effect of glucocorticoids. Serum potassium should be closely monitored in patients receiving glucocorticoids and potassium-depleting drugs.

■ **Vaccines and Toxoids** Because corticosteroids inhibit antibody response, the drugs may cause a diminished response to toxoids and live or inactivated vaccines. In addition, corticosteroids may potentiate replication of some organisms contained in live, attenuated vaccines and supraphysiologic dosages of the drugs can aggravate neurologic reactions to some vaccines. Routine administration of vaccines or toxoids should generally be deferred until corticosteroid therapy is discontinued. Administration of live virus or live, attenuated vaccines, including smallpox vaccine, is contraindicated in patients receiving immunosuppressive dosages of glucocorticoids. In addition, if inactivated vaccines are administered to such patients, expected serum antibody response may not be obtained. The Advisory Committee on Immunization Practices (ACIP) states that administration of live virus vaccines usually is not contraindicated in patients receiving corticosteroid therapy as short-term (less than 2 weeks) treatment, in low to moderate dosages, as long-term alternate-day treatment with short-acting preparations, in maintenance physiologic dosages (replacement therapy), or if corticosteroids are administered topically, ophthalmically, intra-articularly, bursally, or into a tendon. If immunization is necessary in a patient receiving corticosteroid therapy, serologic testing may be needed to ensure adequate antibody response and additional doses of the vaccine or toxoid may be necessary. Immunization procedures may be undertaken in patients receiving nonimmunosuppressive doses of glucocorticoids or in patients receiving glucocorticoids as replacement therapy (e.g., Addison's disease). For specific information on administration of vaccines or toxoids in patients receiving corticosteroids, see the individual monographs in 80:00.

■ **Oral Anticoagulants** The effect of glucocorticoids on oral anticoagulant therapy is variable, and the efficacy of oral anticoagulants has been reported to be enhanced or diminished with concomitant glucocorticoid administration. Patients receiving glucocorticoids and oral anticoagulants concomitantly should be monitored (e.g., using coagulation indices) in order to maintain desired anticoagulant effect.

Laboratory Test Interferences

Glucocorticoids may decrease iodine 131 uptake and protein-bound iodine concentrations, making it difficult to monitor the therapeutic response of patients receiving the drugs for thyroiditis. Glucocorticoids may produce false-negative results in the nitroblue tetrazolium test for systemic bacterial infection.

Glucocorticoids may suppress reactions to skin tests. Phenytoin interferes with dexamethasone suppression tests.

Pharmacology

Pharmacology of the corticosteroids is complex and the drugs affect almost all body systems. Maximum pharmacologic activity lags behind peak blood concentrations, suggesting that most effects of the drugs result from modification of enzyme activity rather than from direct actions by the drugs.

Aldosterone is a naturally occurring mineralocorticoid, and it affects electrolyte and fluid balance by acting on the distal renal tubule to promote sodium reabsorption and potassium and hydrogen excretion. Although glomerular filtration rate is also increased which promotes sodium excretion, the net effect is almost always sodium retention with resultant edema and hypertension. The naturally occurring glucocorticoids, hydrocortisone (cortisol) and cortisone, have some mineralocorticoid activity in addition to their glucocorticoid activity. Synthetic glucocorticoids also exhibit some degree of mineralocorticoid activity, especially with prolonged, high-dose therapy. Fludrocortisone has extremely potent mineralocorticoid properties and is only used for this purpose; prednisone and prednisolone have approximately half the mineralocorticoid activity of hydrocortisone and cortisone; and betamethasone, dexamethasone, meprednisone (no longer commercially available in the US), methylprednisolone, and triamcinolone have relatively little mineralocorticoid activity.

In physiologic doses (see General Dosage under Dosage and Administration: Dosage), corticosteroids are administered to replace deficient endogenous hormones. In larger (pharmacologic) doses, glucocorticoids decrease inflammation by stabilizing leukocyte lysosomal membranes, preventing release of destructive acid hydrolases from leukocytes; inhibiting macrophage accumulation in inflamed areas; reducing leukocyte adhesion to capillary endothelium; reducing capillary wall permeability and edema formation; decreasing complement components; antagonizing histamine activity and release of kinin from substrates; reducing fibroblast proliferation, collagen deposition, and subsequent scar tissue formation; and possibly by other mechanisms as yet unknown. The drugs suppress the immune response by reducing activity and volume of the lymphatic system, producing lymphocytopenia, decreasing immunoglobulin and complement concentrations, decreasing passage of immune complexes through basement membranes, and possibly by depressing reactivity of tissue to antigen-antibody interactions. Glucocorticoids stimulate erythroid cells of bone marrow, prolong survival time of erythrocytes and platelets, and produce neutrophilia and eosinopenia. Glucocorticoids promote gluconeogenesis, redistribution of fat from peripheral to central areas of the body, and protein catabolism, which results in negative nitrogen balance. They reduce intestinal absorption and increase renal excretion of calcium.

In pharmacologic doses, systemically administered glucocorticoids suppress release of corticotropin (adrenocorticotropic hormone, ACTH) from the pituitary; thus the adrenal cortex ceases secretion of endogenous corticosteroids (secondary adrenocortical insufficiency). The degree and duration of hypothalamic-pituitary-adrenal (HPA) axis suppression produced by the drugs is highly variable among patients and depends on the dose, frequency and time of administration, and duration of glucocorticoid therapy. If suppressive doses of glucocorticoids are administered for prolonged periods, the adrenal cortex atrophies and patients develop cushingoid (hypercorticism) features and respond to stress like patients with primary adrenocortical insufficiency (Addison's disease, hypocorticism). (See Cautions: Adrenocortical Insufficiency.)

The duration of anti-inflammatory activity of glucocorticoids approximately equals the duration of HPA-axis suppression. In one study, the duration of HPA-axis suppression after a single oral dose of glucocorticoids was as follows:

Table 4. Duration of HPA-Axis Suppression After Single-Dose Oral Glucocorticoids

Drug	Duration of Suppression
Hydrocortisone 250 mg	1.25–1.5 days
Cortisone 250 mg	1.25–1.5 days
Methylprednisolone 40 mg	1.25–1.5 days
Prednisone 50 mg	1.25–1.5 days
Prednisolone 50 mg	1.25–1.5 days
Triamcinolone 40 mg	2.25 days
Dexamethasone 5 mg	2.75 days
Betamethasone 6 mg	3.25 days

Following IM administration of a single dose of 40–80 mg of triamcinolone acetonide, 50 mg of triamcinolone diacetate, 9 mg of betamethasone sodium phosphate and betamethasone acetate suspension, or 40–80 mg of methylprednisolone, the duration of HPA suppression is 2–4 weeks, 1 week, 1 week, and 4–8 days, respectively. Suppression of the HPA axis below the normal clinical range did not occur when beclomethasone dipropionate was administered by oral inhalation in dosages up to and including 640 mcg daily; however, a dose-dependent reduction of adrenal cortisol production was observed. Since inhaled beclomethasone dipropionate is absorbed into circulation and can be systemically active, HPA axis suppression could occur when recommended dosages are exceeded or in particularly sensitive individuals. With recommended dosages of triamcinolone acetonide administered by oral inhalation, suppression of the HPA axis has occurred within 6–12 weeks in some patients.

In a comparative pharmacodynamic study in healthy geriatric individuals (65–89 years of age) and in younger adults (23–34 years of age), geriatric individuals receiving a single dose of IV prednisolone (0.8 mg/kg, no longer commercially available in the US) or oral prednisone (0.8 mg/kg) exhibited a higher area under the concentration-time curve (AUC) for cortisol than that observed in younger adults. Increased cortisol concentrations in geriatric patients may be the result of attenuated suppression of endogenous cortisol or decreased hepatic clearance of cortisol compared with younger adults.

The mechanism of antiemetic action of corticosteroids remains to be established.

Pharmacokinetics

■ **Absorption** Most glucocorticoids appear to be readily absorbed when administered orally as free alcohols, ketones, cypionates, or acetates. Following IM administration, absorption of the water-soluble sodium phosphate and sodium succinate salts is rapid; the rate of absorption of the lipid-soluble acetate and acetonide esters is much slower. Following intra-articular administration of betamethasone sodium phosphate and betamethasone acetate injectable suspension, systemic absorption of the soluble portion (betamethasone sodium phosphate) is rapid. When the most rapid onset of action is desired, a water-soluble glucocorticoid ester should be administered IV. Systemic absorption occurs slowly following intra-articular, intrabursal, intrasynovial, intradermal, or soft tissue injection of most glucocorticoids.

Following oral inhalation, glucocorticoids are absorbed from the GI and respiratory tracts. After oral inhalation of beclomethasone dipropionate given via metered-dose aerosol with a tetrafluoroethane (non-CFC) propellant, most of the dose (e.g., 51–60% is deposited in the respiratory tract; approximately 27–33% of a dose is deposited in the oropharynx. Systemic bioavailability of fluticasone propionate is about 30 or 13.5% following oral inhalation of the aerosol (via metered spray) or of the powder (via the Diskhaler® device, no longer commercially available in the US), respectively. Systemic bioavailability of budesonide is about 39% in healthy individuals following oral inhalation of the powder (via the Turbuhaler® device) and about 6% in asthmatic children (4–6 years of age) following administration of the micronized suspension for nebulization (via jet nebulizer). Following oral inhalation of 320 mcg of flunisolide, the oral bioavailability is less than 7%. Absolute (compared with IV administration) bioavailability of orally inhaled mometasone furoate as a powder averaged less than 1%. Bioavailability following oral administration of fluticasone propionate is negligible (less than 1%), principally because of incomplete absorption and presystemic metabolism of the drug. Systemic bioavailability of a single orally ingested dose of budesonide is higher in patients with Crohn's disease (21%) than in healthy individuals (about 9%); however, bioavailabilities approach those of healthy individuals following multiple dosing.

Prednisolone sodium phosphate orally disintegrating tablets and solution are bioequivalent based on comparison of area under the plasma concentration-time curves (AUCs) and peak plasma concentrations of the 2 formulations.

Results of a pharmacokinetic study in healthy geriatric adults and younger adults (23–34 years of age) receiving a single IV dose of prednisolone (0.8 mg/kg, no longer commercially available in the US) or oral dose of prednisone (0.8 mg/kg) indicate that the plasma prednisolone concentrations and AUCs of total and unbound prednisolone in geriatric adults are higher than that reported in younger adults. (See Pharmacokinetics: Elimination.)

Normal endogenous plasma concentrations of cortisol and cortisone are 4–30 mcg/dL and 1–2 mcg/dL, respectively.

■ **Distribution** Animal studies indicate that most glucocorticoids are rapidly removed from the blood and distributed to muscles, liver, skin, intestines, and kidneys.

Glucocorticoids vary in the extent to which they are bound to plasma proteins. Cortisol (hydrocortisone) is extensively bound to corticosteroid-binding globulin (transcortin) and albumin, which are plasma proteins. With physiologic concentrations, cortisol is bound primarily to transcortin and only 5–10% of cortisol in plasma is unbound and is biologically active. Prednisolone (unlike other synthetic glucocorticoids such as betamethasone, dexamethasone, or triamcinolone) has a high affinity for transcortin and competes with cortisol for this binding protein. Results of a pharmacokinetic study in healthy geriatric adults and younger adults (23-34 years of age) receiving a single IV dose of prednisolone (0.8 mg/kg, no longer commercially available in the US) or oral dose of prednisone (0.8 mg/kg) indicate that the mean unbound fraction of prednisolone was higher, and the steady-state volume of distribution of unbound prednisolone was reduced in geriatric adults compared with younger adults. Because only unbound drug is pharmacologically active, patients with low serum albumin concentrations may be more susceptible to effects of glucocorticoids than patients with normal serum albumin concentrations.

Glucocorticoids cross the placenta and may be distributed into milk.

■ **Elimination** Glucocorticoids having a ketone group at C-11 (e.g., cortisone, prednisone, and meprednisone [no longer commercially available in the US]) must be reduced (primarily in the liver) to their corresponding 11-hydroxy analogs (hydrocortisone, prednisolone, and meprednisolone) in order to be pharmacologically active. Prednisone is rapidly converted to prednisolone, but much of cortisone is inactivated before it can be converted to hydrocortisone.

Pharmacologically active glucocorticoids are metabolized in most tissues, but primarily in the liver, to biologically inactive compounds. The metabolic clearance of hydrocortisone may be decreased in patients with hypothyroidism and increased in those with hyperthyroidism. Changes in thyroid status may necessitate adjustment of glucocorticoid dosage. The metabolic clearance of prednisolone is impaired in geriatric patients (as evidenced by a reduced fractional urinary clearance of 6β-hydroxyprednisolone) compared with younger adults. Inactive metabolites are excreted by the kidneys, primarily as glucuronides and sulfates, but also as unconjugated products. Small amounts of unmetabolized drugs are also excreted in urine. Negligible amounts of most of the drugs are excreted in bile; enterohepatic circulation does not occur.

Chemistry

Corticosteroids are hormones secreted by the adrenal cortex or synthetic analogs of these hormones. Traditionally, corticosteroids have been classified as mineralocorticoids or glucocorticoids based on their primary pharmacologic activity; however, separation of the drugs into these classes is not absolute. (See Pharmacology.) Of the corticosteroids that are used clinically, beclomethasone, betamethasone, budesonide, cortisone, dexamethasone, flunisolide, fluticasone, hydrocortisone, meprednisone (no longer commercially available in the US), methylprednisolone, paramethasone (no longer commercially available in the US), prednisolone, prednisone, and triamcinolone are classified as glucocorticoids. Although fludrocortisone is also a glucocorticoid, it has very potent mineralocorticoid properties and is used for its mineralocorticoid effects.

Glucocorticoids are 21-carbon steroids with the following general structure:

The glucocorticoids contain a hydroxyl group or an ester at position 17. In the glucocorticoids, position 11 also bears an oxygen atom as a hydroxyl or ketone group and substitutions may occur at positions 6, 9, and 16. Modifications of the glucocorticoid nucleus affect the pharmacologic activity, and multiple modifications may produce more pronounced effects than would be predicted on the basis of individual changes. The presence of a C-1 to C-2 double bond enhances glucocorticoid without enhancing mineralocorticoid activity. Although substitution of an α-methyl group on C-6 has no consistent effect on activity, a 6α-fluoro substituent enhances glucocorticoid without enhancing mineralocorticoid activity. Substitution of a fluorine atom in the 9α-position profoundly increases both mineralocorticoid and glucocorticoid activity. When the C-11 oxygen occurs as a ketone, the compound is inactive until it is converted to the 11β-hydroxy analog. Substitution at C-16 of an α-hydroxyl or an α- or β-methyl group profoundly decreases mineralocorticoid activity; an α-hydroxyl group lessens glucocorticoid activity, while an α- or β-methyl group has no consistent effect on glucocorticoid activity.

For further information on chemistry and stability, uses, cautions, and dosage and administration of corticosteroids, see the individual monographs in 68:04.

†Use is not currently included in the labeling approved by the US Food and Drug Administration

Selected Revisions February 2018,

Budesonide

■ Budesonide is a synthetic, nonhalogenated corticosteroid that has potent glucocorticoid and weak mineralocorticoid activity.

Uses

Budesonide is used orally for the management of mild to moderate Crohn's disease. Budesonide is used by oral inhalation for the management of bronchial asthma. Budesonide in fixed combination with formoterol fumarate is used by oral inhalation for the treatment of asthma and also for maintenance treatment of airflow obstruction in patients with chronic obstructive pulmonary disease (COPD), including chronic bronchitis and emphysema.

■ **Crohn's Disease** Budesonide is used orally as delayed-release capsules for the management of mildly to moderately active Crohn's disease involving the ileum and/or ascending colon and for maintenance of clinical remission for up to 3 months in this condition.

Safety and efficacy of delayed-release budesonide capsules in the management of active Crohn's disease were evaluated in 5 randomized, double-blind (2 placebo-controlled and 3 comparative) studies that included 994 adults (17–85 years of age [mean age: 35 years]; 40% male; 97% white) with mild to moderately active Crohn's disease involving the ileum and/or the ascending colon. For clinical assessment, the Crohn's Disease Activity Index (CDAI) was used. The CDAI score is based on subjective observations by the patient (e.g., the daily number of liquid or very soft stools, severity of abdominal pain, general well-being) and objective evidence (e.g., number of extraintestinal manifestations, presence of an abdominal mass, use or nonuse of antidiarrheal drugs, the hematocrit, body weight). Clinical improvement, defined as a CDAI score of 150 or less, assessed after 8 weeks of treatment, was the primary efficacy parameter in these studies. In the 2 placebo-controlled studies, patients were randomized to receive placebo or budesonide dosages of 3, 9, or 15 mg daily. In one of these studies (patients having a median CDAI score of 290), a statistically significant difference in clinical improvement was observed in patients receiving 9-mg (4.5 mg twice daily) daily dosages of budesonide (as the delayed-release capsules) when compared with those receiving placebo (51% for budesonide versus 20% for placebo). Improvements in the quality of life, as measured by the patients' responses to the inflammatory bowel disease questionnaire, highly correlated with CDAI scores. In this study, no additional benefit in the management of active Crohn's disease was observed when budesonide dosages were increased to 15 mg daily (7.5 mg twice daily). Clinical improvement was similar in patients receiving 3-mg (1.5 mg twice daily) daily dosages of budesonide to those receiving placebo. In the other placebo-controlled study (patients having a median CDAI score of 263), no statistically significant difference in clinical improvement was observed in patients receiving 9-mg (9 mg once daily or 4.5 mg twice daily) daily dosages of budesonide delayed-release capsules when compared with those receiving placebo (48–53% for budesonide versus 33% for placebo).

Results of a comparator-drug (budesonide versus mesalamine) controlled study (patients having a median CDAI score of 272) indicate that clinical improvement was substantially higher in adults receiving 9-mg daily dosages of budesonide delayed-release capsules than in those receiving 2-g twice daily dosages of mesalamine delayed-release tablets (69% for budesonide versus 45% for mesalamine). In addition to a higher clinical improvement rate, quality-of-life scores (e.g., anxiety, depressed mood, sense of well-being, self-control, general health, vitality) were improved to a greater extent in patients receiving budesonide than in those receiving mesalamine. Similar or lower clinical improvement rates were observed (although the difference was not statistically significant) in 2 comparative clinical trials (patients having a median CDAI score of 277) when oral budesonide delayed-release capsules were compared with oral prednisolone (40 mg daily initially and then tapered). In one 12-week study, clinical improvement was observed in 42–60% of patients receiving budesonide (42% in patients receiving 4.5 mg twice daily and 60% in those receiving 9 mg once daily for 8 weeks; dosage was tapered thereafter) compared with 60% of those receiving prednisolone (40 mg daily for 2 weeks and tapered thereafter). In the second trial (10 weeks' duration), clinical improvement was observed in 52 or 65% of patients receiving budesonide (9 mg daily for 8 weeks followed by 6 mg daily for 2 weeks) or prednisolone (40 mg daily for 2 weeks, 30 mg for 2 weeks, 25 mg for 2 weeks; daily dosage was then decreased by 5 mg each week for the last 4 weeks), respectively.

Results of a pooled analysis of randomized clinical trials have shown that adults with an active episode of mildly to moderately active Crohn's disease receiving budesonide are 82 or 73% more likely to achieve remission than those receiving placebo (relative risk of 1.82) or mesalamine (relative risk of 1.73), respectively. In addition, results of the pooled analysis indicate that budesonide (using preparations other than Entocort® EC) and conventional corticosteroids (e.g., prednisolone) were associated with similar remission rates in patients with mildly to moderately active Crohn's disease (CDAI scores of 200–300), although conventional corticosteroids were more likely to induce remission than oral budesonide when the patient population included individuals with severely active Crohn's disease.

Safety and efficacy of oral budesonide delayed-release capsules for maintenance therapy of Crohn's disease has been established in 4 randomized, double-blind, placebo-controlled studies of 12 months' duration in patients 18–73 (mean: 37) years of age, 60% of whom were female and 99% of whom were Caucasian. The mean CDAI score at study entry was 96 and approximately 75% had exclusively ileal disease. Budesonide has been effective in prolonging time to relapse defined as an increase in CDAI score of at least 60 units to a total score exceeding 150 or withdrawal secondary to disease deterioration. The median time to relapse in pooled analysis was 268 or 154 days for budesonide (6 mg daily) or placebo, respectively, and budesonide reduced the portion of patients with loss of symptom control relative to placebo at 3 months (28 versus 45%, respectively).

The potential benefits of corticosteroids for maintenance therapy of Crohn's disease should be considered carefully, because both conventional corticosteroids and budesonide do not prevent relapses and the drugs (especially conventional corticosteroids) may produce severe adverse reactions with long-term administration. (See Uses: GI Diseases, in Corticosteroids General Statement 68:04.)

Crohn's Disease in Pediatric Patients Although safety and efficacy of budesonide delayed-release capsules in pediatric patients have not been established, budesonide (using preparations other than Entocort® EC) has been used for the management of mildly to moderately active Crohn's disease† in a limited number of children 9.5–18 years of age. In one retrospective study in pediatric patients 9.5–18 years of age with mild to moderately active Crohn's disease (Pediatric Crohn's Disease Activity Index [PCDI] score of 12.5–40), budesonide pH-dependent-release preparations (0.45 mg/kg daily up to a maximum dosage of 9 mg daily) were compared with prednisone (2 mg/kg daily up to a maximum dosage of 40 mg daily). Remission was defined as the absence of clinical symptoms and a PCDI score of 10 or less, assessed after 8 weeks of treatment. Results of this study showed that 48 or 77% of pediatric patients achieved remission with budesonide or prednisone, respectively. In addition, 59% of pediatric patients who had shown no improvement with previous mesalamine therapy achieved remission with budesonide.

In addition, results of a 12-week comparator-drug (prednisone versus budesonide) controlled study in pediatric patients† 8–18 years of age (weighing more than 20 kg) with mildly to moderately active Crohn's disease (Pediatric Crohn's Disease Activity Index [PCDI] score of 12.5–40), indicate that remission rates in children receiving prednisone (40 mg daily for 2 weeks and then tapered to discontinuance) were similar (50% for prednisone versus 47% for budesonide) to those receiving budesonide pH- dependent-release preparations (9 mg daily for 8 weeks and then tapered to discontinuance). Total incidence of adverse effects was substantially lower (about 32% for budesonide versus 71% for prednisone) and less severe in pediatric patients receiving budesonide than those receiving prednisone.

For further information on the management of Crohn's disease, see Uses: Crohn's Disease, in Mesalamine 56:36.

■ **Asthma** Budesonide powder is used by oral inhalation, via the Flexhaler®, for the treatment of bronchial asthma in adults and pediatric patients 6 years of age or older who require chronic administration of corticosteroids to control symptoms. Budesonide inhalation suspension (administered via nebulization) is used by oral inhalation for the treatment of bronchial asthma in children 1–8 years of age. The inhalation aerosol containing budesonide in fixed combination with formoterol fumarate (Symbicort®) is used by oral inhalation for the treatment of asthma in adults and children 6 years of age or older. The fixed combination of budesonide and formoterol fumarate is used only in patients with asthma who have not responded adequately to long-term asthma controller therapy, such as inhaled corticosteroids, or whose disease severity clearly warrants initiation of treatment with both an inhaled corticosteroid and a long-acting β_2-adrenergic agonist. Once asthma control is achieved and maintained, the patient should be assessed at regular intervals and therapy should be stepped down (e.g., discontinuance of budesonide in fixed combination with formoterol fumarate), if possible without loss of asthma control, and the patient should be maintained on long-term asthma controller therapy, such as inhaled corticosteroids. Budesonide in fixed combination with formoterol fumarate should not be used in patients whose asthma is adequately controlled on low or medium dosage of inhaled corticosteroids. (See Serious Asthma-related Events under Warnings/Precautions: Warnings, in Cautions.) Orally inhaled budesonide, alone or in fixed combination with formoterol fumarate, should not be used in the management of acute bronchospasm.

Well-controlled clinical studies have shown that oral inhalation of budesonide improves pulmonary function and relieves symptoms of bronchial asthma. Following continuous use of the oral inhalation of budesonide powder (administered via a Flexhaler®) or the micronized suspension (administered via nebulization), improvement may occur within 1 or 2–8 days of therapy, respectively; however, maximum symptomatic relief may require at least 1–2 or 4–6 weeks, respectively. In corticosteroid-dependent patients, use of budesonide oral inhalation therapy may permit a reduction in the daily maintenance dosage of the systemic corticosteroid and gradual discontinuance of corticosteroid maintenance dosages. In 2 randomized, double-blind, placebo-controlled clinical studies in patients with mild to severe asthma, orally inhaled budesonide (160 or 320 mcg twice daily) in fixed combination with formoterol fumarate (9 mcg twice daily) produced greater improvement in most indices of pulmonary function (e.g., mean percent change from baseline in forced expiratory volume in 1 second [FEV_1] or morning and evening peak expiratory flow rate [PEFR]) than either drug alone and similar efficacy as concurrent therapy with both agents given separately. For information on the stepped-care approach to drug therapy in asthma, see Asthma under Uses: Respiratory Diseases, in the Corticosteroids General Statement 68:04.

■ **Chronic Obstructive Pulmonary Disease** The inhalation aerosol containing budesonide in fixed combination with formoterol fumarate is used by oral inhalation for maintenance treatment of airflow obstruction in patients with chronic obstructive pulmonary disease (COPD), including chronic bronchitis and emphysema. Orally inhaled budesonide in fixed combination with formoterol fumarate is *not* indicated for the relief of acute bronchospasm.

In 2 randomized, double-blind, placebo-controlled studies of 6 or 12 months' duration in patients with COPD, orally inhaled budesonide (320 mcg twice daily) in fixed combination with formoterol fumarate (9 mcg twice daily) produced greater improvements in the mean percent change from baseline in predose FEV_1 than formoterol alone or placebo and in 1-hour postdose FEV_1 than budesonide alone or placebo. The fixed combination containing 160 mcg of budesonide and 9 mcg of formoterol fumarate twice daily did not produce greater improvements from baseline in predose FEV_1 than formoterol alone or placebo. Therefore, the fixed combination containing 320 mcg of budesonide and 9 mcg of formoterol fumarate twice daily is the only recommended dosage for the treatment of airflow obstruction in COPD. For information on the stepped-care approach to drug therapy in COPD, see Chronic Obstructive Pulmonary Disease under Uses: Bronchospasm, in Ipratropium Bromide 12:08.08.

Dosage and Administration

■ **Administration** Budesonide is administered orally as delayed-release capsules. For oral inhalation, budesonide is available as an inhalation powder administered via an inhaler device (Flexhaler®), as a micronized suspension administered via nebulization, and as an inhalation aerosol containing budesonide in fixed combination with formoterol fumarate (Symbicort®) administered via an oral aerosol inhaler with hydrofluoroalkane (HFA) propellant. Patients receiving orally inhaled budesonide should rinse their mouth with water after each dose to remove residual drug in the oropharyngeal area and to minimize the development of fungal overgrowth and/or infection.

Oral Administration Budesonide is administered orally once daily as delayed-release capsules containing enteric-coated granules. The capsules should be swallowed intact; they should not be chewed or broken. However, limited data indicate that the release characteristics of the delayed-release capsules were not affected when the unencapsulated granules were added to applesauce for 30 minutes. Because grapefruit juice has been shown to inhibit cytochrome P-450 (CYP) isoenzyme 3A4, an enzyme involved in the metabolism of budesonide, concomitant use of budesonide capsules with grapefruit juice should be avoided. (See Drug Interactions: Drugs or Foods Affecting Hepatic Microsomal Enzymes.) Although administration with a high-fat meal delays time to reach peak plasma concentrations of budesonide by about 2.5 hours, the manufacturer makes no specific recommendation regarding administration of budesonide capsules with food.

Oral Inhalation via Powder Inhaler Budesonide oral inhalation powder (Pulmicort®) is administered by oral inhalation using an inhaler device (Flexhaler®). Budesonide inhalation powder should only be used with the inhaler supplied with the product. Before initial use, the inhaler must be primed; the priming procedure does not have to be repeated even if the inhaler is not used for a long period of time. The inhaler device should not be shaken. Before inhaling the dose, the patient should exhale fully, being careful not to blow into the mouthpiece. The patient should place the mouthpiece between the lips and inhale deeply and forcefully. The patient should not use another dose even if they did not sense the presence of the drug entering their lungs from the Flexhaler® device. Rinsing the mouth after inhalation of budesonide inhalation powder and spitting out the water are advised. The outside of the mouthpiece of the inhaler should be wiped clean with a dry tissue every 7 days. The inhaler should be discarded when the dose indicator reads zero. The canister should never be immersed in water to determine if the canister is empty.

Each actuation of the oral powder inhaler containing budesonide delivers 80 mcg of budesonide from the inhaler labeled as containing 90 mcg or 160 mcg of budesonide from the inhaler labeled as containing 180 mcg (based on testing at 60 L/minute for 2 seconds). Dose delivery for the oral powder inhaler is dependent on airflow through the device. The commercially available inhalation powder contains 60 actuations per 90-mcg inhaler device and 120 actuations per 180-mcg inhaler device.

Oral Inhalation via Nebulization Commercially available budesonide suspension for oral inhalation is administered via nebulization. *The oral inhalation suspension should not be administered parenterally or used with ultrasonic nebulizers.* Budesonide inhalation suspension should be administered using a jet nebulizer (with face mask or mouthpiece) connected to a compressor that has an adequate air flow. The face mask should be properly adjusted to optimize delivery and to avoid exposure of the eyes to nebulized drug. When a face mask is used for nebulization of budesonide suspension, the face should be washed after each use to avoid dermatologic corticosteroid effects (e.g., rash, contact dermatitis). In clinical trials, a Pari-LC-Jet Plus® Nebulizer was used to deliver budesonide inhalation suspension (Pulmicort® Respules®). The manufacturer states that safety and efficacy of budesonide inhalation suspension administered by a nebulizer other than the Pari-LC-Jet Plus® Nebulizer or a compressor other than the Pari Master compressor have not been established. Since stability and safety of budesonide suspension mixed with other drugs in a nebulizer have not been established, budesonide oral inhalation suspension for nebulization should not be mixed with other drugs. When the commercially available Pulmicort® Respules® are used, the amount of drug delivered to the lungs depends on the type of jet nebulizers used, performance of the compressor, and on factors such the patient's inspiratory flow. Using standardized in vitro testing at a flow rate of 5.5 L per minute, the mean delivered dose at the mouthpiece of the commercially available budesonide suspension (Pulmicort® Respules®) is 17% of the nominal dose.

Oral Inhalation via Aerosol Inhaler Budesonide in fixed combination with formoterol fumarate (Symbicort®) is administered by oral inhalation using an oral aerosol inhaler with hydrofluoroalkane (HFA) propellant. Budesonide/formoterol fumarate inhalation aerosol should only be used with the actuator supplied with the product. Before each inhalation, the inhaler must be shaken well for 5 seconds. The aerosol inhaler should be test sprayed twice into the air (away from the face) before initial use, and shaken well for 5 seconds before each spray. If the inhaler has not been used for more than 7 days or if the inhaler was dropped, the inhaler should be test sprayed twice into the air (away from the face) and shaken well for 5 seconds before each spray. Rinsing the mouth after inhalation of budesonide/formoterol fumarate inhalation aerosol and spitting out the water are advised. The mouthpiece of the inhaler should be wiped clean with a dry cloth every 7 days. The inhaler should be discarded when the labeled number of inhalations have been used or within 3 months after removal from the foil pouch. The canister should never be immersed in water to determine the amount of drug remaining in the canister ("float test").

Each actuation of the oral aerosol inhaler containing the fixed combination of budesonide and formoterol fumarate delivers 91 or 181 mcg of budesonide and 5.1 mcg of formoterol fumarate from the valve. Dosages of budesonide and formoterol fumarate in the fixed-combination inhalation aerosol are expressed in terms of drug delivered from the mouthpiece; each actuation of the inhaler delivers 80 or 160 mcg of budesonide and 4.5 mcg of formoterol fumarate from the actuator per metered spray. The amount of drug delivered to the lungs depends on factors such as the patient's coordination between the actuation of the inhaler and inspiration through the delivery system. The commercially available inhalation aerosol containing budesonide in fixed combination with formoterol fumarate delivers 60 metered sprays per 6- or 6.9-g canister and 120 metered sprays per 10.2-g canister.

■ **Dosage** ***Crohn's Disease*** For the management of mild to moderately active Crohn's disease involving the ileum and/or the ascending colon, the recommended adult oral dosage of delayed-release budesonide capsules is 9 mg administered daily in the morning for 8 weeks. Results of a double-blind, multicenter study indicate that in patients who have not experienced remission during the initial 8-week course of budesonide, a second 8-week (16 weeks of continuous therapy) course with the drug may be beneficial in some patients. The manufacturer states that for recurrent episodes of active Crohn's disease, a repeated 8-week course of oral budesonide may be given.

For maintenance of clinical remission following 8 weeks of active treatment once symptoms have been controlled (CDAI score of less than 150), the recommended adult oral dosage of delayed-release budesonide capsules is 6 mg once daily for up to 3 months. If symptom control is maintained at 3 months, an attempt to taper dosage to complete cessation is recommended. The manufacturer states that continued therapy beyond 3 months has not been shown to provide substantial clinical benefit.

Reduction of budesonide dosage should be considered in patients receiving a known inhibitor of the CYP3A4 isoenzyme concomitantly. (See Drugs and Foods that Inhibit CYP3A4 under Drug Interactions: Drugs or Foods Affecting Hepatic Microsomal Enzymes.)

No episodes of adrenal insufficiency have been reported in patients with mild to moderately active Crohn's disease (involving the ileum and/or the ascending colon) who have been switched from oral prednisolone to oral budesonide therapy. It should be considered, however, that abrupt discontinuance of prednisolone is not recommended and, therefore, dosage of prednisolone should be tapered when initiating budesonide therapy. (See Withdrawal of Systemic Corticosteroid Therapy under Warnings/Precautions: Warnings, in Cautions.)

Asthma The recommended initial and maximum dosages of budesonide suspension for oral inhalation are based on previous asthma therapy. The recommended initial dosage of the oral inhalation aerosol containing budesonide in fixed combination with formoterol fumarate is based on the patient's asthma severity. Safety and efficacy of dosages exceeding those recommended by the manufacturer have not been established. The manufacturer suggests that in patients who were receiving prior oral corticosteroid therapy, reduction of alternate-day or daily dosing should be initiated approximately 1 week after starting budesonide oral inhalation, followed by further reductions after an interval of 1 or 2 weeks; decrements usually should not exceed 2.5 mg or 25% of prednisone (or its equivalent) in patients receiving budesonide inhalation suspension administered via nebulization. The manufacturer of budesonide oral inhalation powder states that patients who were receiving prior oral corticosteroid therapy should be withdrawn slowly from systemic corticosteroid use after transferring to oral inhalation therapy by reducing the prednisone daily dosage by 2.5 mg (or its equivalent) on a weekly basis. The manufacturer of the oral inhalation aerosol containing budesonide in fixed combination with formoterol fumarate states that patients requiring oral corticosteroids should be withdrawn slowly from systemic corticosteroid use after transferring to budesonide in fixed combination with formoterol fumarate. The manufacturer also states that prednisone dosage reduction may be accomplished by reducing the daily dosage by 2.5 mg on a weekly basis during therapy with the oral inhalation aerosol containing budesonide in fixed combination with formoterol fumarate. Once oral corticosteroids are discontinued and symptoms of asthma have been controlled, the dosage of budesonide should be titrated to the lowest effective level. (See Withdrawal of Systemic Corticosteroid Therapy under Warnings/Precautions: Warnings, in Cautions and also see Advice to Patients.)

Oral Inhalation via Powder Inhaler. In asthmatic adults 18 years of age or older, the recommended initial dosage of budesonide oral inhalation powder is 320 mcg (labeled 360 mcg) twice daily. In some patients, an initial dosage of 160 mcg (labeled 180 mcg) twice daily may be adequate. If required, the dosage of budesonide may be increased to a maximum of 640 mcg (labeled 720 mcg) twice daily.

In asthmatic children and adolescents 6–17 years of age, the recommended initial dosage of budesonide oral inhalation powder is 160 mcg (labeled 180 mcg) twice daily. In some patients, an initial dosage of 320 mcg (labeled 360 mcg) twice daily may be appropriate. If required, the dosage may be increased to a maximum of 320 mcg (labeled 360 mcg) twice daily.

For all patients, the dosage of budesonide oral inhalation powder should be titrated to the lowest effective dosage after adequate asthma stability is achieved.

Oral Inhalation via Nebulization in Children (1–8 years of age). When budesonide suspension is administered via a nebulizer in children who previously were receiving bronchodilators alone, the recommended initial dosage of budesonide is 0.5 mg, given in 1 or 2 divided daily doses; the recommended maximum dosage is 0.5 mg daily. In children who were previously receiving inhaled corticosteroids, the recommended initial dosage of budesonide suspension, given via a nebulizer, is 0.5 mg, given in 1 or 2 divided daily doses; the recommended maximum dosage is 1 mg daily. In children who previously were receiving oral corticosteroids, the recommended initial dosage of budesonide inhalation suspension, given via a nebulizer, is 1 mg, given in 1 or 2 divided daily doses; the recommended maximum dosage is 1 mg daily. In children who are not receiving oral corticosteroids and who do not respond adequately to the initial once-daily administration of budesonide suspension, increasing the dosage or giving the drug in 2 divided doses daily should be considered.

In children with asthma symptoms who do not respond to nonsteroidal (e.g., bronchodilator, mast-cell stabilizer) therapy, an initial 0. 25-mg daily dosage of budesonide inhalation suspension, given via a nebulizer, may be considered. However, if the once-daily dosage does not provide adequate control of asthma symptoms, the total daily dosage should be increased and/or administered in divided doses.

Budesonide/Formoterol Fumarate Fixed-combination Therapy. In asthmatic adults and adolescents 12 years of age or older, the recommended initial dosage of the oral inhalation aerosol containing budesonide in fixed combination with formoterol fumarate is based on the patient's asthma severity, level of control of asthma symptoms, and/or risk of asthma exacerbations during current therapy with inhaled corticosteroids. The dosage of the inhalation aerosol fixed-combination preparation is 160 or 320 mcg of budesonide and 9 mcg of formoterol fumarate (2 inhalations) twice daily, given approximately 12 hours apart (morning and evening). The maximum recommended dosage of budesonide in fixed combination with formoterol fumarate is 320 mcg of budesonide with 9 mcg of formoterol fumarate (2 inhalations) twice daily. The manufacturer states that administration of the inhalation aerosol containing budesonide in fixed combination with formoterol fumarate more frequently than twice daily or in excess of 2 inhalations twice daily is not recommended. Patients receiving the fixed combination of budesonide and formoterol fumarate should not use additional long-acting β_2-agonists for any reason.

In asthmatic children 6 to less than 12 years of age, the recommended dosage of the oral inhalation aerosol containing budesonide in fixed combination with formoterol fumarate is 160 mcg of budesonide and 9 mcg of formoterol fumarate (2 inhalations) twice daily, given approximately 12 hours apart (morning and evening).

Improvement in asthma control following inhalation of budesonide in fixed combination with formoterol fumarate may occur within 15 minutes of initiating treatment, although maximum benefit may not be achieved for 2 weeks or longer after therapy initiation. Individual patients will experience a variable time to onset and degree of symptom relief. If control of asthma is inadequate after 1–2 weeks of therapy at the lower dosage, increasing the strength of the fixed combination (higher strengths contain higher dosages of budesonide only) may provide additional asthma control. If acute asthmatic symptoms arise despite therapy with budesonide in fixed combination with formoterol fumarate, a short-acting inhaled β_2-adrenergic agonist should be administered for immediate relief. Patients should be advised not to discontinue budesonide in fixed combination with formoterol fumarate without medical supervision, as symptoms may recur after treatment discontinuance. If a previously effective dosage of budesonide in fixed combination with formoterol fumarate fails to provide adequate asthma control, the therapeutic regimen should be reevaluated and additional therapeutic options should be considered (e.g., increasing the strength of the fixed combination [higher strengths contain higher dosages of budesonide only], adding additional inhaled corticosteroids, initiating systemic corticosteroids). The manufacturer warns that therapy with the fixed combination of budesonide and formoterol fumarate should *not* be initiated in patients during rapidly deteriorating or potentially life-threatening episodes of asthma.

Chronic Obstructive Pulmonary Disease **Budesonide/Formoterol Fumarate Fixed-combination Therapy.** For maintenance therapy of airflow obstruction in patients with chronic obstructive pulmonary disease (COPD), the recommended dosage of the oral inhalation aerosol containing budesonide in fixed combination with formoterol fumarate in adults is 320 mcg of budesonide and 9 mcg of formoterol fumarate (2 inhalations) twice daily (morning and evening). In clinical studies, the fixed combination containing 160 mcg of budesonide and 9 mcg of formoterol fumarate (2 inhalations) twice daily did not produce greater improvements from baseline in predose FEV_1 than formoterol alone or placebo; therefore, the fixed combination containing 320 mcg of budesonide and 9 mcg of formoterol fumarate (2 inhalations) twice daily is the only recommended dosage for the treatment of airflow obstruction in COPD. If shortness of breath occurs despite therapy with budesonide in fixed combination with formoterol fumarate, a short-acting inhaled β_2-adrenergic agonist should be taken for immediate relief. Patients should be advised not to discontinue budesonide in fixed combination with formoterol fumarate without medical supervision, as symptoms may recur after treatment discontinuance. The manufacturer warns that therapy with the fixed combination of budesonide and formoterol fumarate should *not* be initiated in patients during rapidly deteriorating or potentially life-threatening episodes of COPD. The manufacturer states that administration of the inhalation aerosol containing budesonide in fixed combination with formoterol fumarate more frequently than twice daily or in excess of 2 inhalations twice daily is not recommended. Patients receiving the fixed combination of budesonide and formoterol fumarate should not use additional long-acting β_2-agonists for any reason.

■ **Special Populations** Patients with Crohn's disease and moderate to severe hepatic impairment should be monitored for increased signs and symptoms of hypercorticism; reduction of budesonide oral dosage is recommended in these patients.

When budesonide is used in fixed combination with formoterol fumarate, dosage requirements for formoterol fumarate should be considered.

The manufacturer of budesonide in fixed combination with formoterol fumarate states that dosage adjustment is not required in geriatric patients. The manufacturer of budesonide in fixed combination with formoterol fumarate makes no specific dosage recommendations for patients with hepatic or renal impairment at this time. However, since budesonide and formoterol fumarate are cleared predominantly by the liver, impaired liver function theoretically may lead to accumulation of the drugs in plasma. Therefore, the manufacturer of budesonide in fixed combination with formoterol fumarate states that patients with hepatic disease should be closely monitored.

Cautions

■ **Contraindications** Known hypersensitivity to budesonide or any ingredient in the formulation.

Orally inhaled budesonide is contraindicated as primary treatment of acute asthmatic attacks or status asthmaticus when intensive measures (e.g., an orally inhaled $\beta_2$adrenergic agonist, an orally inhaled anticholinergic agent, subcutaneous epinephrine, IV aminophylline, and/or an oral/IV glucocorticoid) are required.

Orally inhaled budesonide powder (Pulmicort® Flexhaler®) is contraindicated in patients with severe hypersensitivity to milk proteins.

Budesonide in fixed combination with formoterol fumarate (Symbicort®) is contraindicated as primary treatment of status asthmaticus or other acute episodes of asthma or chronic obstructive pulmonary disease (COPD) when intensive measures are required.

When budesonide is used in fixed combination with formoterol fumarate, contraindications associated with formoterol fumarate should be considered.

■ Warnings/Precautions

Warnings **Use of Fixed Combinations.** When budesonide is used in fixed combination with formoterol fumarate, the usual cautions, precautions, contraindications, and interactions associated with formoterol fumarate should be considered. Cautionary information applicable to specific populations (e.g., pregnant or nursing women, individuals with hepatic or renal impairment, geriatric patients) should be considered for each drug in the fixed combination.

Serious Asthma-related Events. Monotherapy with long-acting β_2-adrenergic agonists, such as formoterol, a component of Symbicort®, increases the risk of asthma-related death. Data from a large (approximately 26,000 patients), placebo-controlled study (Salmeterol Multi-center Asthma Research Trial [SMART]) evaluating the safety of another long-acting β_2-adrenergic agonist, salmeterol, in patients with asthma showed an increase in asthma-related deaths in patients receiving salmeterol. (See Asthma-related Death and Life-threatening Events under Cautions: Respiratory Effects, in Salmeterol 12:12.08.12.) In addition, available data from controlled clinical trials suggest that monotherapy with long-acting β_2-adrenergic agonists increases the risk of asthma-related hospitalization in pediatric and adolescent patients.

However, FDA has concluded that there is no clinically important increased risk of serious asthma-related events, including hospitalization, intubation, or death, associated with concomitant use of long-acting β_2-adrenergic agonists (e.g., formoterol) and inhaled corticosteroids (e.g., budesonide) compared with inhaled corticosteroids alone based on the results of several large clinical studies. In addition, these studies showed that combination therapy with long-acting β_2-adrenergic agonists and inhaled corticosteroids was more effective in reducing the incidence of asthma exacerbations (i.e., events requiring use of systemic corticosteroids for at least 3 outpatient days or an asthma-related hospitalization or emergency department visit requiring use of systemic corticosteroids) compared with use of inhaled corticosteroids alone. (See Asthma-related Death and Serious Asthma-related Events under Warnings/Precautions: Warnings, in Cautions, in Formoterol 12:12.08.12.)

In the treatment of asthma, the fixed combination of budesonide and formoterol fumarate is used only in patients who have not responded adequately to long-term asthma controller therapy, such as inhaled corticosteroids, or whose disease severity warrants initiation of treatment with both an inhaled corticosteroid and a long-acting β_2-adrenergic agonist. (See Uses: Asthma.)

Withdrawal of Systemic Corticosteroid Therapy. In patients being switched from systemic corticosteroids to oral or orally inhaled budesonide, systemic corticosteroid therapy should be withdrawn gradually because life-threatening adrenal insufficiency may occur. Patients who have been maintained on 20 mg or more of prednisone (or its equivalent) daily may be most susceptible to such adverse events, particularly when their systemic corticosteroid therapy has been almost completely withdrawn. *In most patients, following withdrawal of systemic corticosteroid therapy, several months are required for total recovery of HPA function.* These patients should be carefully monitored during and for a number of months after withdrawal of systemic corticosteroids because of the risk of corticosteroid withdrawal symptoms (e.g., joint pain, muscular pain, lassitude, depression); acute adrenal insufficiency during exposure to trauma, surgery, or infection (particularly gastroenteritis) or other conditions associated with acute electrolyte loss; or symptomatic exacerbation of allergic conditions previously controlled by systemic corticosteroid therapy (e.g., rhinitis, conjunctivitis, eczema, arthritis, eosinophilic conditions). Clinicians should be alert for the potential for eosinophilia, vasculitic rash, worsening of pulmonary symptoms, cardiac complications, and/or neuropathy consistent with Churg-Strauss syndrome. In asthmatic patients, death, possibly resulting from acute adrenal insufficiency, has occurred rarely during and after transfer from a systemic corticosteroid to budesonide oral inhalation therapy. Systemic corticosteroid dosage should be carefully tapered and patients should be monitored during dosage reduction for objective signs of adrenal insufficiency and for benign intracranial hypertension. In general, the greater the dosage and duration of systemic corticosteroid therapy, the greater the time required for withdrawal of systemic corticosteroids and replacement by orally inhaled corticosteroids.

Immunosuppressed Patients. Patients who are taking immunosuppressant drugs have increased susceptibility to infections compared with healthy individuals, and certain infections (e.g., varicella [chickenpox], measles) can have a more serious or even fatal outcome in such patients, particularly in children. In patients who have not had these diseases or been properly vaccinated, particular care should be taken to avoid exposure. If exposure to varicella occurs in such individuals, administration of varicella zoster immune globulin (VZIG) or pooled IV immunoglobulin (IVIG) may be indicated; if exposure to measles occurs, pooled IM immune globulin (IG) may be indicated. If varicella (chickenpox) develops, treatment with an antiviral agent may be considered. It is not known how the dosage, route and duration of administration of a corticosteroid, or the contribution of the underlying disease and/or prior corticosteroid therapy affect the risk of developing a disseminated infection.For additional information, see Cautions: Increased Susceptibility to Infection and also see Precautions and Contraindications, in the Corticosteroids General Statement 68:04.

Hypothalamic-Pituitary-Adrenal (HPA) Axis Suppression. Since glucocorticoids can reduce HPA-axis response to stress (e.g., surgery), supplementation with a systemic corticosteroid in patients undergoing such stress is recommended.

Bronchospasm. As with other inhaled drugs for asthma, bronchospasm may occur, resulting in an immediate increase in wheezing following oral inhalation of budesonide. If bronchospasm occurs, appropriate treatment (e.g., use of a short-acting β-adrenergic agonist) should be initiated immediately, and budesonide therapy should be discontinued and alternate therapy instituted.

General Precautions **Infections.** Localized candidal infections of the mouth and/or pharynx have been reported in patients receiving orally inhaled budesonide therapy. When infection occurs, appropriate local or systemic antifungal treatment may be necessary while still continuing with inhaled budesonide therapy, although discontinuance of such therapy (under close medical supervision) may be required in some patients. Inhaled corticosteroid therapy should be used with extreme caution, if at all, in patients with clinical or asymptomatic *Mycobacterium tuberculosis* infections of the respiratory tract; untreated systemic fungal, bacterial, viral, or parasitic infections; or ocular herpes simplex. Clinicians should remain vigilant for the possible development of pneumonia in patients with COPD who are receiving budesonide in fixed combination with formoterol fumarate, since the clinical features of pneumonia and COPD exacerbations frequently overlap. Lower respiratory tract infections, including pneumonia, have been reported in patients with COPD following the administration of inhaled corticosteroids.

Ophthalmic Effects. Glaucoma, increased intraocular pressure (IOP), and cataracts have been reported rarely in patients receiving orally inhaled corticosteroids.

Concomitant Disease States. The manufacturer states that budesonide delayed-release capsules should be used with caution in patients with tuberculosis, hypertension, diabetes mellitus, osteoporosis, peptic ulcer, glaucoma or cataracts, a family history of diabetes or glaucoma, or any other condition in which glucocorticoids may be associated with adverse effects.

Systemic Corticosteroid Effects. Administration of higher than recommended dosages of orally inhaled budesonide or prolonged oral administration of budesonide capsules may result in manifestations of hypercorticism and suppression of HPA function.

Long-Term Administration. The long-term local and systemic effects of budesonide in humans, particularly local effects on developmental or immunologic processes in the mouth, pharynx, trachea, and lung, are unknown.

Musculoskeletal Effects. Long-term use of orally inhaled corticosteroids may affect normal bone metabolism, resulting in a loss of bone mineral density. (See Osteoporosis under Cautions: Musculoskeletal Effects, in the Corticosteroids General Statement 68:04.) The manufacturer of budesonide in fixed combination with formoterol states that patients with major risk factors for decreased bone mineral density, such as prolonged immobilization, family history of osteoporosis, postmenopausal status, tobacco use, advanced age, poor nutrition, or chronic use of drugs that can reduce bone mass (e.g., anticonvulsants, oral corticosteroids) should be monitored and treated using established standards of care. Since patients with COPD often have multiple risk factors for reduced bone mineral density, assessment of bone mineral density is recommended prior to initiation of therapy with budesonide in fixed combination with formoterol fumarate and periodically thereafter. If appreciable reductions in bone mineral density are seen and use of budesonide in fixed combination with formoterol fumarate is considered to be important for the patient's COPD therapy, use of agents to treat or prevent osteoporosis should be strongly considered.

Specific Populations **Pregnancy.** Category B (orally inhaled powder and inhalation suspension); category C (oral capsules and the fixed combination of budesonide and formoterol fumarate oral inhalation aerosol). (See Users Guide.) Hypoadrenalism may occur in infants of women receiving corticosteroid therapy during pregnancy. These infants should be carefully monitored.

Lactation. Like other corticosteroids, budesonide is distributed into milk; however, data are not available on the effects of the drug on the breast-fed child or on milk production. The benefits of breast-feeding and the importance of budesonide to the woman should be considered along with any potential adverse effects on the breast-fed infant from the drug or underlying maternal condition. The manufacturer of budesonide oral inhalation powder (Pulmicort® Flexhaler®) states that the drug should be used in nursing women only if clinically appropriate and that therapy should be titrated to the lowest effective dosage. In addition, budesonide powder inhaler should be used immediately after nursing to minimize infant exposure to the drug.

Pediatric Use. Safety and efficacy of oral budesonide delayed-release capsules have not been established in pediatric patients younger than 18 years of age with Crohn's disease. Oral budesonide (using preparations other than Entecort® EC) has been used for the management of mild to moderately active Crohn's disease in a limited number of pediatric patients without unusual adverse effects. Benign intracranial hypertension has been reported in at least one pediatric patient with Crohn's disease receiving the drug.

Safety and efficacy of budesonide inhalation powder have not been established in children younger than 6 years of age. Efficacy of budesonide inhalation suspension has not been established in children younger than 1 year of age, while safety of the suspension has not been established in children younger than 6 months of age. Safety and efficacy of budesonide in fixed combination with formoterol fumarate (Symbicort®) inhalation aerosol in patients 12 years of age or older with asthma have been established in studies of up to 12 months' duration; in addition, safety and efficacy of the fixed-combination preparation in children 6 to less than 12 years of age with asthma have been established in studies of up to 12 weeks' duration. The manufacturer states that safety and efficacy of the fixed-combination preparation in children younger than 6 years of age with asthma have not been established. Use of corticosteroids may lead to suppression of growth in children and adolescents. Therefore, children receiving prolonged therapy with orally inhaled budesonide should be monitored periodically for possible adverse effects on growth and development. (See Cautions: Pediatric Precautions, in the Corticosteroids General Statement 68:04.)

Geriatric Use. Clinical studies of oral budesonide delayed-release capsules or budesonide oral inhalation powder did not include sufficient numbers of patients 65 years of age or older to determine whether geriatric patients respond differently than younger patients. While other clinical experience with budesonide inhalation powder or inhalation suspension or with the inhalation aerosol containing budesonide in fixed combination with formoterol fumarate has not revealed age-related differences in response, oral drug dosage generally should be titrated carefully in geriatric patients, usually initiating therapy at the low end of the dosage range. Safety of budesonide inhalation powder in patients 65 years of age or older was similar to that observed in younger adults. No substantial differences in safety and efficacy of budesonide in fixed combination with formoterol fumarate were observed in geriatric patients relative to younger adults. The greater frequency of decreased hepatic, renal, and/or cardiac function and of concomitant disease and drug therapy observed in the elderly also should be considered. (See Dosage and Administration: Special Populations.)

Hepatic Impairment. May affect elimination of corticosteroids; increased systemic availability of oral budesonide capsules has been reported in patients with liver cirrhosis. Patients with mild hepatic impairment are minimally affected. Pharmacokinetics were not studied in patients with severe hepatic impairment. The manufacturer states that patients with hepatic disease receiving budesonide in fixed combination with formoterol fumarate should be closely monitored. (See Dosage and Administration: Special Populations.)

Renal Impairment. Pharmacokinetics of budesonide have not been studied in patients with renal impairment. However, since only the metabolites (having negligible glucocorticoid activity), and not the unchanged drug, are excreted by the kidneys, increased adverse effects are not expected in such patients receiving the drug.

■ **Common Adverse Effects** Adverse effects occurring in at least 5% of patients receiving budesonide oral capsules include headache, dizziness, nausea, vomiting, dyspepsia, diarrhea, abdominal pain, flatulence, sinusitis, respiratory infection, viral infection, pain (including back pain), arthralgia, and fatigue. Adverse effect profile in long-term treatment was similar to that of short-term treatment.

Adverse effects occurring in 1% or more of patients receiving budesonide by oral inhalation (as a powder using a Flexhaler® or a Turbuhaler® [no longer commercially available in the US] or as an inhalation suspension, administered via nebulization) include infections (e.g., respiratory infection, ocular infection), nasopharyngitis, pharyngitis, nasal congestion, allergic rhinitis, sinusitis, viral infection (e.g., herpes simplex), cough, voice alteration, stridor, earache, otitis (media or externa), viral infection, flu-like syndrome, moniliasis, oral candidiasis, flu syndrome, fever, headache, migraine, insomnia, dysphonia, hyperkinesia, asthenia, fatigue, emotional lability, pain (e.g., back pain), arthralgia, myalgia, hypertonia, fractures, dyspepsia, gastroenteritis, nausea, vomiting, diarrhea, abdominal pain, dry mouth, taste perversion, weight gain, anorexia, epistaxis, ecchymosis, purpura, cervical lymphadenopathy, conjunctivitis, rash (may be pustular), pruritus, allergic reaction, contact dermatitis, syncope, and chest pain.

Drug Interactions

The following information addresses potential interactions with budesonide. When budesonide is used in fixed combination with formoterol fumarate, interactions associated with formoterol fumarate should be considered. No formal drug interaction studies have been performed to date with the fixed-combination preparation containing budesonide and formoterol fumarate.

■ **Drugs or Foods Affecting Hepatic Microsomal Enzymes**

Drugs and Foods that Inhibit Isoenzyme CYP3A4 Since budesonide is metabolized in the liver by the cytochrome P-450 (CYP) 3A4 isoenzyme, concomitant use with drugs that are potent inhibitors of the CYP3A4 isoenzyme may result in increased plasma budesonide concentrations. Concomitant use of oral budesonide with oral ketoconazole resulted in an eightfold increase in budesonide systemic exposure. Patients in whom concomitant use of a known inhibitor of the CYP3A4 isoenzyme (e.g., erythromycin, itraconazole, clarithromycin, ketoconazole, indinavir, ritonavir, saquinavir) with oral budesonide capsules is indicated should be carefully monitored for increased signs and symptoms of hypercorticism and reduction of budesonide dosage should be considered.

Oral contraceptives containing ethinyl estradiol (also metabolized by CYP3A4 isoenzyme) do not appear to affect the pharmacokinetics of budesonide; in addition, budesonide does not appear to affect plasma concentrations of these oral contraceptives.

Concomitant use of oral budesonide delayed-release capsules with grapefruit juice resulted in a twofold increase in budesonide systemic exposure; therefore, such concomitant use should be avoided.

Drugs that Induce Isoenzyme CYP3A4 Concomitant administration of budesonide with drugs that induce CYP3A4 isoenzyme may result in decreased budesonide plasma concentrations.

■ **Drugs Affecting GI pH** Because budesonide delayed-release oral capsules containing enteric-coated granules are formulated to dissolve at a relatively nonacidic pH (exceeding 5.5) (see Description), concomitant use of drugs that affect GI pH may affect release properties and systemic uptake of oral budesonide delayed-release capsules. Although administration of gastric antisecretory agents (e.g., omeprazole, cimetidine) did not appear to affect the pharmacokinetic parameters (e.g., absorption) of the commercially available budesonide delayed-release capsules, slightly increased peak plasma concentrations and rate of absorption of budesonide have been reported following concomitant use of cimetidine (1 g daily) with a nonenteric-coated formulation of budesonide, resulting in substantial suppression of the hypothalamic-pituitary-adrenal (HPA) axis.

Description

Budesonide is a synthetic, nonhalogenated corticosteroid. Budesonide has potent glucocorticoid and weak mineralocorticoid activity. The exact mechanism of action of budesonide in the management of Crohn's disease is not known. The drug appears to have immunosuppressant and substantial topical anti-inflammatory activity and lower systemic availability than conventional corticosteroids. Budesonide oral delayed-release capsules have been formulated to release the drug at the site of inflammation (usually in the terminal ileum and ascending colon). For further information on the pharmacology of corticosteroids, see Pharmacology in the Corticosteroids General Statement 68:04.

Budesonide is commercially available as oral delayed-release capsules, oral inhalation powder, oral micronized suspension for nebulization, and an oral inhalation aerosol containing budesonide in fixed combination with formoterol fumarate.

Budesonide oral delayed-release capsules contain enteric-coated granules in an extended-release matrix. The enteric coating of the granules is formulated to dissolve at a relatively nonacidic pH (exceeding 5.5; i.e., in the small intestine); thereafter, budesonide is released slowly (in a time-dependent manner) from the matrix of ethylcellulose within the intestinal lumen. Budesonide powder for inhalation is administered by an inhaler (Flexhaler®), micronized sterile budesonide inhalation suspension for oral inhalation is administered by a jet nebulizer (with face mask or mouthpiece) connected to a compressor that has an adequate air flow, and budesonide in fixed combination with formoterol fumarate (Symbicort®) for oral inhalation is administered via an oral aerosol inhaler with hydrofluoroalkane (HFA) propellant. (See Dosage and Administration: Administration.)

In healthy individuals, following oral administration of 9 mg of budesonide as delayed-release capsules, the drug appears to be completely absorbed; peak plasma concentrations of 2.2 ng/mL are achieved within 0.5–10 hours. Systemic bioavailability of a single orally ingested dose of budesonide is higher (21%) in patients with Crohn's disease than in healthy individuals (about 9–15%); however, bioavailabilities approach those of healthy individuals following multiple dosing.

In healthy individuals, systemic bioavailability of budesonide inhalation powder (administered via a metered-dose inhaler [no longer commercially available in the US]), has been about 39%. The absolute bioavailability of budesonide inhalation suspension administered via a jet nebulizer in asthmatic children (4–6 years of age) has been reported to be 6%. Following oral inhalation of 1 mg of budesonide inhalation suspension for nebulization in asthmatic children (4–6 years of age), peak plasma concentrations of 1.1 ng/mL occurred about 20 minutes after nebulization. Following oral inhalation of budesonide powder, peak plasma concentrations in adults with asthma occur within about 10 minutes. The therapeutic effects of orally inhaled budesonide are thought to result from local actions of the deposited inhaled dose on the respiratory tract rather than from the systemic actions of the swallowed portion of the dose.

Budesonide undergoes extensive (about 80–95%) metabolism on first pass through the liver via the cytochrome P-450 enzyme system, mainly by the isoenzyme 3A4 (CYP3A4) to 2 metabolites with negligible (less than 1%) glucocorticoid activity when compared with the parent compound. Following oral or IV administration, the drug is excreted in urine (60%) and feces as metabolites; unchanged budesonide has not been detected in urine.

Race, gender, or advanced age does not appear to affect pharmacokinetics of budesonide.

Advice to Patients

When budesonide is used in fixed combination with formoterol fumarate, importance of informing patients of important cautionary information about formoterol fumarate.

Importance of informing patients receiving the fixed combination of budesonide and formoterol fumarate that monotherapy with long-acting β_2-adrenergic agonists, including formoterol, a component of Symbicort®, increases the risk of asthma-related death and may increase the risk of asthma-related hospitalization in pediatric and adolescent patients.

Necessity of swallowing budesonide capsules whole, without chewing or breaking. Patients should be advised that concomitant use of budesonide capsules with grapefruit juice should be avoided.

Advise that oral inhalation of budesonide must be used at regular intervals to be therapeutically effective. Importance of adherence to prescribed budesonide dosage, unless otherwise instructed by a clinician.

Advise that although improvement may occur within 1 or 2–8 days of therapy with budesonide oral inhalation powder or inhalation suspension, respectively; at least 1–2 or 4–6 weeks, respectively, of continuous therapy may be required for optimum effects to be achieved. Advise that although improvement in asthma control following administration of the oral inhalation aerosol containing budesonide in fixed combination with formoterol fumarate may occur within 15 minutes of initiating treatment, maximum benefit may not be achieved for 2 weeks or longer.

Patients should be carefully instructed in the use of the oral aerosol inhaler containing budesonide alone or in fixed combination with formoterol fumarate. Provide copy of manufacturer's patient information and medication guide.

Advise that orally inhaled budesonide alone or in fixed combination with formoterol fumarate should not be used as a bronchodilator and that the drug is not indicated for emergency use (e.g., relief of acute bronchospasm).

Importance of all patients being provided with a short-acting, inhaled β_2-adrenergic agonist as supplemental therapy for acute asthma symptoms. Importance of informing a clinician if a short-acting β_2-adrenergic agonist is not available for use.

Importance of discontinuing *regular* use of a short-acting, inhaled β_2-adrenergic agonist when initiating therapy with the fixed combination of budesonide and formoterol fumarate.

Advise patients being transferred from systemic corticosteroid to budesonide oral inhalation therapy to carry special identification (e.g., card) indicating the need for supplementary systemic corticosteroids during periods of stress or severe exacerbation of asthma. Such patients should immediately resume therapy with large doses of systemic corticosteroids and contact their clinician for further instructions during stressful periods (e.g., stress, severe asthmatic attack).

Importance of not exceeding the recommended dosage and of contacting a clinician immediately if asthma symptoms do not improve or worsen.

Importance of contacting a clinician if decreased effectiveness of a short-acting, inhaled β_2-adrenergic agonist (requiring more inhalations than usual) for acute symptoms occurs.

Importance of not using additional formoterol or other long-acting inhaled β_2-adrenergic agonists for any reason when the fixed combination of budesonide and formoterol fumarate is used.

In immunosuppressed patients, importance of avoiding exposure to chickenpox or measles, and, if exposed, of immediately consulting their clinician.

Importance of informing patients that corticosteroids may decrease bone mineral density.

Importance of informing patients that long-term use of inhaled corticosteroids may increase the risk for development of some ocular disorders (cataracts or glaucoma); regular eye examinations should be considered.

Importance of informing patients that orally inhaled corticosteroids may cause a reduction in growth velocity when administered to pediatric patients.

Importance of adequate understanding of proper storage and inhalation techniques, including use of the inhalation delivery systems.

Advise patients receiving orally inhaled budesonide to rinse their mouth with water after each dose to remove residual drug in the oropharyngeal area and to minimize the development of fungal overgrowth and/or infection.

Importance of informing patients with COPD receiving budesonide in fixed combination with formoterol fumarate that they have a higher risk of pneumonia and to contact their clinician if they develop symptoms of pneumonia.

Importance of women informing clinicians if they are or plan to become pregnant or plan to breast-feed.

Importance of informing clinicians of existing or contemplated concomitant therapy, including prescription and OTC drugs, as well as any concomitant illnesses.

Importance of informing patients of other important precautionary information. (See Cautions.)

Overview® (see Users Guide). For additional information on this drug until a more detailed monograph is developed and published, the manufacturer's labeling should be consulted. It is *essential* that the manufacturer's labeling be consulted for more detailed information on usual cautions, precautions, contraindications, potential drug interactions, laboratory test interferences, and acute toxicity.

Preparations

Excipients in commercially available drug preparations may have clinically important effects in some individuals; consult specific product labeling for details.

Budesonide

Oral		
Capsules, delayed-release (containing enteric-coated granules)	3 mg	**Entocort® EC**, AstraZeneca
Oral Inhalation		
Powder, for oral inhalation only	90 mcg (delivers 80 mcg per inhalation)	**Pulmicort® Flexhaler®**, AstraZeneca
	180 mcg (delivers 160 mcg per inhalation)	**Pulmicort® Flexhaler®**, AstraZeneca
Suspension, for nebulization	0.25 mg/2 mL	**Pulmicort® Respules®** (available in flexible ampuls), AstraZeneca
	0.5 mg/2 mL	**Pulmicort® Respules®** (available in flexible ampuls), AstraZeneca

Budesonide Combinations

Oral Inhalation		
Aerosol	80 mcg with Formoterol Fumarate Dihydrate 4.5 mcg per metered spray	**Symbicort®** (with hydrofluoroalkane propellant), AstraZeneca
	160 mcg with Formoterol Fumarate Dihydrate 4.5 mcg per metered spray	**Symbicort®** (with hydrofluoroalkane propellant), AstraZeneca

†Use is not currently included in the labeling approved by the US Food and Drug Administration

Dexamethasone

■ Dexamethasone is a synthetic glucocorticoid.

Uses

Dexamethasone is used principally as an anti-inflammatory or immunosuppressant agent. Because it has only minimal mineralocorticoid properties, the drug is inadequate alone for the management of adrenocortical insufficiency. If dexamethasone is used in the treatment of this condition, concomitant therapy with a mineralocorticoid is also required.

■ **Diagnostic Uses** Dexamethasone inhibits pituitary corticotropin (ACTH) release and decreases output of endogenous corticosteroids when given in an amount which does not itself appreciably affect levels of urinary 17-hydroxycorticosteroids. This effect is used in the dexamethasone suppression test for the diagnosis of Cushing's syndrome and the differential diagnosis of adrenal hyperplasia and adrenal adenoma.

■ **Cancer Chemotherapy-induced Nausea and Vomiting** Dexamethasone regimens are used extensively for the prevention of nausea and vomiting associated with emetogenic cancer chemotherapy†. To prevent chemotherapy-induced nausea and vomiting associated with chemotherapy regimens with a high emetic risk (i.e., incidence of emesis exceeds 90% if no antiemetics are administered), the American Society of Clinical Oncology (ASCO) currently recommends a 3-drug antiemetic regimen consisting of dexamethasone, aprepitant, and a type 3 serotonin (5-HT_3) receptor antagonist (e.g., dolasetron, granisetron, ondansetron, palonosetron, tropisetron [not commercially available in the US]). The antiemetic combination of dexamethasone, aprepitant, and a 5-HT_3 receptor antagonist also is preferred in patients receiving combination chemotherapy with an anthracycline and cyclophosphamide. For patients receiving other chemotherapy of moderate emetic risk (i.e., incidence of emesis without antiemetics exceeds 30% but does not exceed 90%), ASCO recommends a 2-drug antiemetic regimen consisting of dexamethasone and a 5-HT_3 receptor antagonist. For patients receiving chemotherapy regimens with a low emetic risk (i.e., incidence of emesis without antiemetics exceeds 10% but does not exceed 30%), ASCO recommends dexamethasone alone on the first day of chemotherapy. Antiemetics can be prescribed on an as needed basis in patients receiving chemotherapy with a minimal antiemetic risk (incidence of emesis is less than 10% without antiemetics). For the prevention of *delayed* emesis in patients receiving cisplatin or other chemotherapy associated with a high emetic risk, these authorities currently recommend a 2-drug combination of dexamethasone and aprepitant. (See Uses: Cancer Chemotherapy-induced Nausea and Vomiting, in the Corticosteroids General Statement 68:04.)

■ **Bacterial Meningitis** There is some evidence that short-term adjunctive therapy with IV dexamethasone may decrease the incidence of audiologic and/or neurologic sequelae in infants and children with *Haemophilus influenzae* meningitis and possibly may provide some benefit in patients with *Streptococcus pneumoniae* meningitis. The American Academy of Pediatrics (AAP) and other clinicians suggest that use of adjunctive dexamethasone therapy may be considered during the initial 2–4 days of anti-infective therapy in infants and children 6–8 weeks of age or older with known or suspected bacterial meningitis, especially in those with suspected or proven *H. influenzae* infection. If used, dexamethasone should be initiated before or concurrently with the first dose of anti-infective.

Dosage and Administration

The route of administration and dosage of dexamethasone and its derivatives depend on the condition being treated and the response of the patient. IM or IV therapy is generally reserved for patients who are not able to take the drugs orally or for use in an emergency situation. Dosage for infants and children should be based on the severity of the disease and the response of the patient rather than on strict adherence to dosage indicated by age, body weight, or body surface area. After a satisfactory response is obtained, dosage should be decreased in small decrements to the lowest level that maintains an adequate clinical response, and the drug should be discontinued as soon as possible. Patients should be continually monitored for signs that indicate dosage adjustment is necessary, such as remissions or exacerbations of the disease and stress (surgery, infection, trauma). Following long-term therapy, dexamethasone should be withdrawn gradually. (See the Corticosteroids General Statement 68:04.)

■ **Dexamethasone** Dexamethasone is administered orally as tablets, elixir, solution, or concentrate solution. The oral concentrate may be diluted in juice or other flavored liquid diluent or in semisolid food (e.g., applesauce) prior to administration.

The usual initial adult dosage of dexamethasone may range from 0.75–9 mg daily, depending on the disease being treated, and the drug usually is administered in 2–4 divided doses. In less severe diseases, dosages lower than 0.75 mg daily may be sufficient while severe diseases may require dosages higher than 9 mg daily. Children may be given a dosage of 0.02–0.3 mg/kg daily or 0.6–9 mg/m^2 daily, administered in 3 or 4 divided doses.

When dexamethasone is given for the prevention of chemotherapy-induced nausea and vomiting†, single doses or once-daily doses of the drug usually are given.

Diagnostic Uses When dexamethasone suppression is used as a screening test for Cushing's syndrome, 0.5 mg of dexamethasone is administered orally every 6 hours for 48 hours after baseline 24-hour urinary 17-hydroxycorticosteroid (17-OHCS) concentrations are determined. During the second 24 hours of dexamethasone administration, urine is collected and analyzed for 17-OHCS. Alternatively, after a baseline plasma cortisol determination, a 1-mg oral dose of dexamethasone may be administered at 11 p.m. and plasma cortisol determined at 8 a.m. the following morning. Plasma cortisol and urinary output of 17-OHCS are depressed following dexamethasone administration in normal individuals but remain at basal levels in patients with Cushing's syndrome. To distinguish adrenal tumor from adrenal hyperplasia, 2 mg of dexamethasone is administered orally every 6 hours for 48 hours. During the second 24 hours of dexamethasone administration, urine is collected and analyzed for 17-OHCS. Urinary 17-OHCS levels are decreased in patients with adrenal hyperplasia and remain at basal levels in patients with adrenocortical tumors.

Cancer Chemotherapy-induced Nausea and Vomiting When oral dexamethasone is used to prevent chemotherapy-induced nausea and vomiting† associated with cancer chemotherapy regimens with a high emetic risk in adults, the American Society of Clinical Oncology (ASCO) currently recommends that 12 mg of dexamethasone be administered with or without aprepitant prior to chemotherapy on the first day followed by 8 mg administered once daily on days 2–4. When oral dexamethasone is given in combination with aprepitant in patients receiving chemotherapy regimens of moderate emetic risk, ASCO currently recommends that a single 12-mg dose of the drug be given prior to chemotherapy on the first day. In patients receiving chemotherapy of low emetic risk, ASCO recommends dexamethasone be given alone as a single 8-mg dose prior to chemotherapy on the first day.

■ **Dexamethasone Sodium Phosphate** Dexamethasone sodium phosphate may be administered by intra-articular, intrasynovial, intralesional, soft-tissue, IM, or IV injection, or by IV infusion. IM or IV administration of dexamethasone sodium phosphate is indicated in emergency situations or when oral therapy is not feasible. Although dexamethasone sodium phosphate is rapidly absorbed from IM injection sites, the slower rate of absorption compared to IV administration should be kept in mind. When dexamethasone sodium phosphate is administered by IV infusion, the drug can be added to dextrose or sodium chloride injections.

Dosage of dexamethasone sodium phosphate is expressed in terms of dexamethasone phosphate. IM or IV dosage depends on the condition being treated and the patient's response, but usually ranges from 0.5–24 mg daily. Some clinicians state that children may be given 6–40 mcg/kg or 0.235–1.25 mg/m^2 IM or IV 1 or 2 times daily.

Shock In life-threatening shock, massive doses of dexamethasone phosphate (such as 1–6 mg/kg as a single IV injection or a 40-mg IV injection repeated every 2–6 hours if needed) have been recommended by some clinicians. Alternatively, 20 mg may be administered IV initially followed by continuous IV infusion of 3 mg/kg per 24 hours. High-Dose therapy should be continued only until the patient's condition has stabilized and usually should not be continued beyond 48–72 hours.

Cerebral Edema In the management of cerebral edema, 10 mg of dexamethasone phosphate is usually given IV followed by 4 mg IM every 6 hours until the symptoms of cerebral edema subside. Response usually is evident within 12–24 hours, and dosage may be reduced after 2–4 days and gradually discontinued over a period of 5–7 days. When possible, oral dexamethasone (1–3 mg 3 times daily) should replace IM administration of the drug. In patients with recurrent or inoperable brain tumors, dexamethasone phosphate in a maintenance dosage of 2 mg IM or IV 2 or 3 times daily may be effective in relieving symptoms of increased intracranial pressure.

Allergic Conditions In the management of acute self-limited allergic conditions or acute exacerbations of chronic allergic disorders, one manufacturer recommends administration of 4–8 mg of dexamethasone phosphate IM on the first day; 3 mg of dexamethasone orally in 2 divided doses on the second and third days; 1.5 mg orally in 2 divided doses on the fourth day; and a single oral daily dose of 0.75 mg on the fifth and sixth days; then the drug is discontinued.

Inflammatory Diseases For intra-articular, intrasynovial, intralesional, or soft-tissue injection, the dosage of dexamethasone phosphate varies with the degree of inflammation and the size and location of the affected area. For large joints such as the knee, 2–4 mg may be used. For smaller joints, 0.8–1 mg may be adequate. The dose for bursae is 2–3 mg and for ganglia, 1–2 mg. For soft-tissue injection, dosage varies from 0.4–1 mg in tendon sheath inflammation to as much as 2–6 mg for soft tissue infiltration. Injections may be repeated from once every 3–5 days (for bursae) to once every 2–3 weeks (for joints).

Cancer Chemotherapy-induced Nausea and Vomiting The optimum dosage of dexamethasone phosphate for the prevention of cancer chemotherapy-induced nausea and vomiting† has not been established, but the usual dose has been 8–20 mg IV before administration of the chemotherapy; in some cases, additional IV or oral doses were administered for 24–72 hours. ASCO currently recommends that dexamethasone phosphate be given in single 8-mg doses when used IV in patients receiving moderately emetogenic chemotherapy; this initial IV dose may be followed by single oral 8-mg doses on days 2 and 3.

Bacterial Meningitis When dexamethasone is used for adjunctive therapy in selected patients with bacterial meningitis†, a dosage of 0.15 mg/kg of dexamethasone phosphate given IV 4 times daily for the first 2–4 days of anti-infective therapy has been recommended for infants, children, and adults. Dexamethasone should be initiated 10–20 minutes before or concurrently with the first dose of anti-infective. Dexamethasone should not be given to patients who have already received anti-infective therapy; administration of dexamethasone in this circumstance is unlikely to improve patient outcome.

Tuberculous Meningitis For reducing the risk of sequelae and improving survival in patients with tuberculous meningitis, an IM dexamethasone phosphate dosage of 8–12 mg daily tapered over 6–8 weeks has been effective; higher dosages appear to provide no additional benefit and may be associated with more frequent adverse effects. It has been suggested that continuation of corticosteroid therapy for at least 4 weeks may be associated with better outcomes than shorter regimens. (See Respiratory Diseases: Advanced Pulmonary and Extrapulmonary Tuberculosis, in Uses in the Corticosteroids General Statement 68:04.)

Other Uses To prevent hyaline membrane disease (respiratory distress syndrome [RDS]) in premature infants†, 4 mg of dexamethasone phosphate has been given IM to the mother 3 times daily for 2 days before delivery.

Chemistry and Stability

■ **Chemistry** Dexamethasone is a synthetic glucocorticoid. Dexamethasone occurs as a white to practically white, odorless, crystalline powder and is practically insoluble in water and sparingly soluble in alcohol. Dexamethasone sodium phosphate occurs as a white or slightly yellow, crystalline powder that is odorless or has a slight odor of alcohol. Dexamethasone sodium phosphate is very hygroscopic and is freely soluble in water and slightly soluble in alcohol.

Commercially available dexamethasone sodium phosphate injection has a pH of 7.5–10.5. Dexamethasone oral solution is alcohol-free and the elixir and oral concentrate contain 3.8–5.7% and about 30% alcohol, respectively.

■ **Stability** Dexamethasone sodium phosphate injection is heat labile and must not be autoclaved. Dexamethasone preparations should generally be stored at a temperature less than 40°C, preferably between 15–30°C, unless otherwise specified by the manufacturer.

Dexamethasone sodium phosphate injection has been reported to be incompatible with various drugs, but the compatibility depends on several factors (e.g., concentrations of the drugs, resulting pH, temperatures). Specialized references should be consulted for more specific compatibility information.

For further information on chemistry, pharmacology, pharmacokinetics, uses, cautions, drug interactions, laboratory test interferences, and dosage and administration of dexamethasone, see the Corticosteroids General Statement 68:04. For EENT uses, see 52:08.08.

Preparations

Excipients in commercially available drug preparations may have clinically important effects in some individuals; consult specific product labeling for details.

Dexamethasone

Oral

Elixir	0.5 mg/5 mL*	**Dexamethasone Elixir**
Solution	0.5 mg/5 mL*	**Dexamethasone Oral Solution**
Solution, concentrate	0.5 mg/0.5 mL*	**Dexamethasone Intensol®**

Tablets	0.5 mg*	Dexamethasone Tablets
	0.75 mg*	Dexamethasone Tablets
	1 mg*	Dexamethasone Tablets
	1.5 mg*	Dexamethasone Tablets
		Dexpak® Taperpak® (scored; available as 6-, 10-, or 13-day mnemonic pack of 21, 35, or 51 tablets, respectively), ECR
	2 mg*	Dexamethasone Tablets
	4 mg*	Dexamethasone Tablets
	6 mg*	Dexamethasone Tablets

*available from one or more manufacturer, distributor, and/or repackager by generic (nonproprietary) name

Dexamethasone Sodium Phosphate

Parenteral		
Injection, for IM or IV use	4 mg (of dexamethasone phosphate) per mL*	Dexamethasone Sodium Phosphate Injection
	10 mg (of dexamethasone phosphate) per mL*	Dexamethasone Sodium Phosphate Injection

*available from one or more manufacturer, distributor, and/or repackager by generic (nonproprietary) name
†Use is not currently included in the labeling approved by the US Food and Drug Administration

Flunisolide

■ Flunisolide is a synthetic fluorinated glucocorticoid.

Uses

■ **Asthma** Flunisolide is used by oral inhalation for the long-term prevention of bronchospasm in patients with asthma. Orally inhaled flunisolide also may permit a reduction in dosage or discontinuance of systemic corticosteroids in patients who require prolonged administration of oral corticosteroids to control asthma symptoms.

Oral inhalation of flunisolide is contraindicated in the primary treatment of severe acute asthmatic attacks or status asthmaticus when intensive measures (e.g., oxygen, parenteral bronchodilators, IV corticosteroids) are required. Flunisolide oral inhalation is not a bronchodilator, and patients should be warned that the drug should not be used for rapid relief of bronchospasm.

Mild Persistent Asthma Drugs for asthma may be categorized as relievers (e.g., bronchodilators taken as needed for acute symptoms) or controllers (principally inhaled corticosteroids or other anti-inflammatory agents taken regularly to achieve long-term control of asthma). In the stepped-care approach to antiasthmatic drug therapy, current asthma management guidelines and most clinicians recommend initiation of a controller drug such as an anti-inflammatory agent, preferably a low-dose orally inhaled corticosteroid (e.g., 88–264, 88–176, or 176 mcg of fluticasone propionate [or its equivalent] daily via a metered-dose inhaler in adolescents and adults, children 5–11 years of age, or children 4 years of age or younger, respectively) as first-line therapy for persistent asthma (i.e., patients with daytime symptoms of asthma more than twice per week, but less than once daily, and nocturnal symptoms of asthma 3–4 times per month), supplemented by as-needed use of a short-acting, inhaled β_2-agonist. For equivalent orally inhaled dosages of corticosteroids, see General Dosage under Dosage and Administration: Dosage, in the Corticosteroids General Statement 68:04.

Moderate Persistent Asthma According to current asthma management guidelines, therapy with a long-acting β_2-agonist such as salmeterol or formoterol generally is recommended in adults and adolescents who have moderate persistent asthma and daily asthmatic symptoms that are inadequately controlled following addition of low-dose inhaled corticosteroids to as-needed inhaled β_2-agonist treatment. However, the National Asthma Education and Prevention Program (NAEPP) recommends that the beneficial effects of long-acting inhaled β_2-agonists should be weighed carefully against the increased risk (although uncommon) of severe asthma exacerbations and asthma-related deaths associated with daily use of such agents. (See Asthma-related Death and Life-threatening Events, under Cautions: Respiratory Effects, in Salmeterol 12:12.08.12.) Current asthma management guidelines also state that an alternative, but equally preferred option for management of moderate persistent asthma that is not adequately controlled with a low dosage of inhaled corticosteroid is to increase the maintenance dosage to a medium dosage (e.g., exceeding 264 but not more than 440 mcg of fluticasone propionate [or its equivalent] daily via a metered-dose inhaler in adults and adolescents).

In children 5–11 years of age with moderate persistent asthma that is not controlled with a low dosage of an inhaled corticosteroid, a long-acting inhaled β_2-agonist (e.g., salmeterol, formoterol), a leukotriene modifier (i.e., montelukast, zafirlukast), or extended-release theophylline (with appropriate monitoring) may be added to low-dose inhaled corticosteroid therapy according to current asthma management guidelines; another preferred option is to increase the maintenance dosage of the inhaled corticosteroid to a medium dosage (e.g., exceeding 176 but not more than 352 mcg of fluticasone propionate [or its equivalent] daily via a metered-dose inhaler). In infants and children 4 years of age or younger with moderate persistent asthma that is not controlled by a low dosage of an inhaled corticosteroid, the only preferred option is to increase the maintenance dosage of the inhaled corticosteroid to a medium dosage (e.g., exceeding 176 but not more than 352 mcg of fluticasone propionate [or its equivalent] daily via a metered-dose inhaler).

Severe Persistent Asthma Maintenance therapy with an inhaled corticosteroid at medium or high dosages (e.g., exceeding 440 mcg of fluticasone propionate in adults and adolescents or 352 mcg of the drug in children 5–11 years of age [or its equivalent] daily via a metered-dose inhaler) and adjunctive therapy with a long-acting inhaled β_2-agonist is the preferred treatment according to current asthma management guidelines for adults and children 5 years of age or older with severe persistent asthma (i.e., continuous daytime asthma symptoms, nighttime symptoms 7 times per week). In infants and children 4 years of age or younger with severe asthma, maintenance therapy with an inhaled corticosteroid at medium or high dosages (e.g., exceeding 352 mcg of fluticasone propionate [or its equivalent] daily via a metered-dose inhaler) and adjunctive therapy with either a long-acting inhaled β_2-agonist or montelukast is recommended in current asthma management guidelines as the only preferred treatment.

Poorly Controlled Asthma If asthma symptoms in patients with moderate to severe asthma are very poorly controlled (i.e., at least 2–3 exacerbations per year requiring oral corticosteroids), a short course of an oral corticosteroid (3–10 days) may be added to gain prompt control of asthma. Regular use of oral corticosteroids as add-on therapy in adults and children 5 years of age or older with severe asthma who are inadequately controlled with a high-dose inhaled corticosteroid, intermittent oral corticosteroid therapy, and a long-acting inhaled β_2-agonist bronchodilator is suggested, based on consensus and clinical experience. A short (2-week) course of oral corticosteroids may be considered to confirm clinical response prior to implementing long-term oral corticosteroid therapy. Once long-term oral corticosteroid therapy is initiated, the lowest possible effective dosage (i.e., alternate-day or once-daily administration) should be used, and the patient should be monitored carefully for adverse effects. Once asthma is well-controlled, repeated attempts should be made to reduce the oral corticosteroid dosage. Use of orally inhaled flunisolide as adjunctive therapy in patients who require prolonged administration of systemic corticosteroids to control asthma symptoms may permit a reduction in dosage or discontinuance of systemic corticosteroids. When used in recommended dosages in responsive patients, flunisolide oral inhalation may permit control of asthmatic symptoms with less suppression of hypothalamic-pituitary-adrenal (HPA) function compared with therapeutically equivalent oral doses of prednisone. For additional details on the stepped-care approach to drug therapy in asthma, see Asthma under Uses: Bronchospasm, in Albuterol 12:12.08.12 and see Asthma under Uses: Respiratory Diseases, in the Corticosteroids General Statement 68:04.

■ **Other Uses** **For EENT uses of flunisolide, see 52:08.08.**

Dosage and Administration

■ **Administration** Flunisolide is administered by oral inhalation using a metered-dose oral aerosol inhaler with an internal spacer device. This oral inhaler should not be used with external spacers or holding chambers. Patients should be carefully instructed in the use of the oral inhaler. To obtain optimum results, patients should also be given a copy of the patient instructions provided by the manufacturer. An adult should carefully supervise a child in the administration of flunisolide for oral inhalation. *The manufacturer states that the flunisolide oral inhaler should be used by oral inhalation only.*

The inhaler should be prepared for use by pulling the purple actuator out from the gray spacer and snapping it into place forming an "L" shape. The guide lines on the spacer should match up with the lines on the actuator. Before the first use, and any time the inhaler has not been used for more than 2 weeks, the inhaler should be primed with 2 test sprays by pressing down on the metal canister 2 times for 1 second each time with the mouthpiece pointed away from the face. The inhaler should be held between the thumb and index finger and shaken well immediately prior to use.

After inhaling then exhaling normally through the mouth, the mouthpiece of the inhaler should be placed into the mouth and the lips closed firmly around it. The patient should begin to inhale slowly through the mouth and then press the metal canister down with the index finger for at least 1 second; the patient should continue inhaling through the mouth for 3 more seconds. After inhalation is complete, the patient should remove the inhaler from the mouth, close the lips, and hold the breath for at least 10 seconds or as long as comfortable. The patient should then exhale and breathe normally. If additional inhalations are required, the patient should wait 20 seconds between inhalations, shake the inhaler again, and repeat the procedure. Following each treatment, the patient should rinse the mouth thoroughly with water and expectorate to remove drug deposited in the oropharyngeal area. The teeth also may be brushed if desired.

Appearance of a white residue at the opening of the mouthpiece and inside the spacer is normal with use and does not affect the performance of the inhaler. Cleaning the oral inhaler is not necessary.

■ **Dosage** Dosage of flunisolide hemihydrate is expressed in terms of flunisolide. Orally inhaled flunisolide with hydrofluoroalkane (HFA: tetrafluoroethane) propellants delivers 80 mcg of flunisolide per metered spray; the commercially available aerosol inhaler delivers 60 metered sprays per 5.1-g canister or 120 metered sprays per 8.9-g canister. Dosage must be carefully adjusted according to individual requirements and response. After a satisfactory response is obtained, dosage should be decreased gradually to the lowest possible dosage that maintains an adequate clinical response. The lowest effective dosage should be achieved, particularly in children, since inhaled corticosteroids have the potential to affect growth.

The usual initial dosage of flunisolide for adults and adolescents 12 years of age or older given as the inhalation aerosol is 160 mcg (2 sprays) twice daily (320 mcg total daily dosage). If required, the dosage may be increased to 320 mcg (4 sprays) twice daily. The manufacturer states that a dosage of 320 mcg twice daily (640 mcg total daily dosage) should not be exceeded in adults and adolescents, although higher dosages have been recommended for patients with severe persistent asthma. Patients should be monitored periodically for effects on the hypothalamic-pituitary-adrenal (HPA) axis.

In children 6–11 years of age, an initial dosage of 80 mcg (1 spray) twice daily (160 mcg total daily dosage) is recommended. If required, the dosage may be increased to 160 mcg (2 sprays) twice daily. When the drug is administered on a long-term basis to children, patients should be monitored for effects on growth as well as on the HPA axis. The manufacturer states that insufficient information is available to warrant use of the drug in children younger than 6 years of age.

When orally inhaled flunisolide is administered to patients receiving systemic corticosteroids, the aerosol initially is given concurrently with the maintenance dosage of the systemic corticosteroid. After at least 1 week, the systemic corticosteroid is gradually withdrawn. (See Dosage and Administration in the Corticosteroids General Statement 68:04.) *Gradual withdrawal of systemic corticosteroids following long-term therapy is strongly recommended, since death has occurred in some individuals in whom systemic corticosteroids were withdrawn too rapidly.* After systemic corticosteroids have been withdrawn, if exacerbations of asthma occur during flunisolide oral inhalation therapy, short courses of systemic corticosteroids should be given, then tapered as symptoms subside.

Patients who respond to the drug usually show improvement in pulmonary function within 2–4 weeks of continuous therapy.

Chemistry and Stability

■ **Chemistry** Flunisolide is a synthetic fluorinated corticosteroid.

Flunisolide occurs as a hemihydrate, white to creamy white, crystalline powder and is soluble in acetone and ethyl alcohol and practically insoluble in water.

For oral inhalation, flunisolide is commercially available as an aerosol containing a solution of the drug in a vehicle of ethanol and 1,1,1,2-tetrahydrofluoroethane (HFA 134a) propellant.

■ **Stability** Because the contents of flunisolide oral inhaler are under pressure, the aerosol container should *not* be punctured, used or stored near heat or an open flame, exposed to temperatures exceeding 49°C, or placed into a fire or incinerator for disposal. Freezing temperatures and prolonged exposure to sunlight also should be avoided.

For further information on chemistry, pharmacology, pharmacokinetics, cautions, and dosage and administration of flunisolide, see the Corticosteroids General Statement 68:04. For EENT uses, see 52:08.08.

Preparations

Excipients in commercially available drug preparations may have clinically important effects in some individuals; consult specific product labeling for details.

Flunisolide Hemihydrate

Oral Inhalation

Aerosol	80 mcg (of flunisolide) per metered spray	**Aerospan® Inhalation Aerosol** (with hydrofluoroalkane propellant), Acton

Fluticasone Propionate

■ Fluticasone propionate is a synthetic trifluorinated glucocorticoid.

Uses

■ **Bronchospasm** *Asthma* Fluticasone propionate is used for the long-term prevention of bronchospasm in patients with asthma. The fixed combination of fluticasone propionate and salmeterol xinafoate is used only in patients with asthma who have not responded adequately to long-term asthma controller therapy, such as inhaled corticosteroids, or whose disease severity clearly warrants initiation of treatment with both an inhaled corticosteroid and a long-acting β_2-adrenergic agonist. Once asthma control is achieved and maintained, the patient should be assessed at regular intervals and therapy should be stepped down (e.g., discontinuance of fluticasone propionate in fixed combination with salmeterol xinafoate), if possible without loss of asthma control, and the patient should be maintained on long-term asthma controller therapy, such as inhaled corticosteroids. Fluticasone propionate in fixed combination with salmeterol xinafoate should not be used in patients whose asthma is adequately controlled on low or medium dosage of inhaled corticosteroids. (See Serious Asthma-related Events under Warnings/Precautions: Warnings, in Cautions.)

Orally inhaled fluticasone propionate alone or combined with salmeterol xinafoate should not be used for the primary treatment of severe acute asthmatic attacks or status asthmaticus when intensive measures (e.g., oxygen, parenteral bronchodilators, IV corticosteroids) are required. Fluticasone propionate oral inhalation is not a bronchodilator, and patients should be warned that the drug alone or in fixed combination with salmeterol xinafoate should not be used for rapid relief of bronchospasm.

Mild Persistent Asthma. Drugs for asthma may be categorized as relievers (e.g., bronchodilators taken as needed for acute symptoms) or controllers (principally inhaled corticosteroids or other anti-inflammatory agents taken regularly to achieve long-term control of asthma). In the stepped-care approach to antiasthmatic drug therapy, current asthma management guidelines and most clinicians recommend initiation of a controller drug such as an anti-inflammatory agent, preferably a low-dose orally inhaled corticosteroid (e.g., 88–264, 88–176, or 176 mcg of fluticasone propionate [or its equivalent] daily via a metered-dose inhaler in adolescents and adults, children 5–11 years of age, or children 4 years of age or younger, respectively) as first-line therapy for persistent asthma (e.g., patients with daytime symptoms of asthma more than twice per week, but less than once daily, and nocturnal symptoms of asthma 3–4 times per month), supplemented by as-needed use of a short-acting, inhaled β_2-agonist.

Moderate Persistent Asthma. According to current asthma management guidelines, therapy with a long-acting β_2-agonist such as salmeterol or formoterol generally is recommended in adults and adolescents who have moderate persistent asthma and daily asthma symptoms that are inadequately controlled following addition of low-dose inhaled corticosteroids to as-needed inhaled β_2-agonist treatment. However, the National Asthma Education and Prevention Program (NAEPP) recommends that the beneficial effects of long-acting inhaled β_2-agonists should be weighed carefully against the increased risk (although uncommon) of severe asthma exacerbations and asthma-related deaths associated with daily use of such agents. (See Asthma-related Death and Life-threatening Events under Cautions: Respiratory Effects, in Salmeterol 12:12.08.12.) Current asthma management guidelines also state that an alternative, but equally preferred option for management of moderate persistent asthma that is not adequately controlled with a low dosage of inhaled corticosteroid is to increase the maintenance dosage to a medium dosage (e.g., exceeding 264 but not more than 440 mcg of fluticasone propionate [or its equivalent] daily via a metered-dose inhaler in adults and adolescents).

In children 5–11 years of age with moderate persistent asthma that is not controlled with a low dosage of an inhaled corticosteroid, a long-acting inhaled β_2-agonist (i.e., salmeterol, formoterol), a leukotriene modifier (i.e., montelukast, zafirlukast), or extended-release theophylline (with appropriate monitoring) may be added to low-dose inhaled corticosteroid therapy; another preferred option according to current asthma management guidelines is to increase the maintenance dosage of the inhaled corticosteroid to a medium dosage (e.g., exceeding 176 but not more than 352 mcg of fluticasone propionate [or its equivalent] daily via a metered-dose inhaler). In infants and children 4 years of age or younger with moderate persistent asthma that is not controlled by a low dosage of an inhaled corticosteroid, the only preferred option is to increase the maintenance dosage of the inhaled corticosteroid to a medium dosage (e.g., exceeding 176 but not more than 352 mcg of fluticasone propionate [or its equivalent] daily via a metered-dose inhaler).

Severe Persistent Asthma. Maintenance therapy with an inhaled corticosteroid at medium or high dosages (e.g., exceeding 440 mcg of fluticasone propionate [or its equivalent] daily in adults and adolescents or 352 mcg of the drug daily in children 5–11 years of age via a metered-dose inhaler) and adjunctive therapy with a long-acting inhaled β_2-agonist is the preferred treatment according to current asthma management guidelines for adults and children 5 years of age or older with severe persistent asthma (i.e., continuous daytime asthma symptoms, nighttime symptoms 7 times per week). In infants and children 4 years of age or younger with severe asthma, maintenance therapy with an inhaled corticosteroid at medium or high dosages (e.g., exceeding 352 mcg of fluticasone propionate or its equivalent daily via a metered-dose inhaler) and adjunctive therapy with either a long-acting inhaled β_2-agonist or montelukast is the only preferred treatment according to current asthma management guidelines.

Poorly Controlled Asthma. If asthma symptoms in patients with moderate to severe asthma are very poorly controlled (i.e., at least 2–3 exacerbations per year requiring oral corticosteroids), a short course of an oral corticosteroid (3–10 days) may be added to gain prompt control of asthma. Regular use of oral corticosteroids as add-on therapy in adults and children 5 years of age or older with severe asthma who are inadequately controlled with high-dose inhaled corticosteroid, intermittent oral corticosteroid therapy, and a long-acting inhaled β_2-agonist bronchodilator is suggested, based on consensus and clinical experience. A short (2-week) course of oral corticosteroids may be considered to confirm clinical response prior to implementing long-term therapy with these agents. Once long-term oral corticosteroid therapy is initiated, the lowest possible effective dosage (i.e., alternate-day or once-daily administration) should be used, and the patient should be monitored carefully for adverse effects. Once asthma is well-controlled, repeated attempts should be made to reduce the oral corticosteroid dosage. (See Asthma under Uses: Respiratory Diseases, in the Corticosteroids General Statement 68:04.) Use of orally inhaled fluticasone propionate as adjunctive therapy in patients who require chronic administration of systemic corticosteroids to control asthma symptoms may permit a reduction in dosage or discontinuance of systemic corticosteroids. When used in recommended dosages in responsive patients, fluticasone propionate oral inhalation may permit control of asthmatic symptoms with less suppression of hypothalamic-pituitary-adrenal (HPA) function than therapeutically equivalent oral dosages of prednisone. For additional details on the stepped-care approach to drug therapy in asthma, see Asthma under Uses: Bronchospasm, in Albuterol 12:12.08.12 and see Asthma under Uses: Respiratory Diseases, in the Corticosteroids General Statement 68:04.

Clinical Experience with Fluticasone Propionate. Well-controlled clinical studies have shown that oral inhalation of fluticasone propionate relieves symptoms of bronchial asthma (cough, dyspnea, wheezing) and improves pulmonary function. Although substantial improvement may occur within the first day of therapy, optimum symptomatic relief may require at least 1–2 weeks of continuous fluticasone propionate oral inhalation therapy. In corticosteroid-dependent patients, use of fluticasone propionate oral inhalation therapy may permit a substantial reduction in the daily maintenance dosage of the systemic corticosteroid and gradual discontinuance of corticosteroid maintenance dosages.

In several randomized, double-blind, placebo-controlled clinical trials in adults or children with mild to severe persistent asthma, fluticasone propionate (50, 100, 250, 500, or 1000 mcg twice daily) powder for oral inhalation produced greater improvement in pulmonary function (e.g., mean percent change from baseline in forced expiratory volume in 1 second [FEV_1] or morning or evening peak expiratory flow [PEF]) than placebo. Data from an open-label extension study in pediatric patients (4–11 years of age) with mild to moderate persistent asthma indicate that fluticasone propionate (100 mcg twice daily or 200 mcg once daily) maintained improvement in lung function for up to 1 year.

In several randomized, double-blind, placebo-controlled clinical trials in patients with mild to severe asthma, fluticasone propionate (100, 250, or 500 mcg) in fixed combination with salmeterol xinafoate (50 mcg as salmeterol) for oral inhalation produced greater improvement in most indices of pulmonary function (e.g., mean percent change from baseline in FEV_1, morning FEV_1, or PEF) than either drug alone and similar efficacy as concurrent therapy with both agents given separately. Additional randomized, double-blind, comparative trials in patients with mild to moderate persistent asthma who were not optimally controlled with their current antiasthma therapy, the fixed combination of fluticasone propionate 90, 230, or 460 mcg twice daily and salmeterol (42 mcg twice daily) with a hydrofluoroalkane propellant (HFA) for oral inhalation via a metered-dose inhaler (Advair® HFA) produced greater improvement in indices of pulmonary function (e.g., mean percent change from baseline in FEV_1 or morning and evening PEF) than either drug alone.

Chronic Obstructive Pulmonary Disease Fluticasone propionate in fixed combination with salmeterol xinafoate as the inhalation powder (Advair® Diskus®) is used for the maintenance treatment of airflow obstruction in patients with chronic obstructive pulmonary disease (COPD), including chronic bronchitis and/or emphysema. Fluticasone propionate in fixed combination with salmeterol xinafoate as the inhalation powder (Advair® Diskus®) also is used to reduce exacerbations of COPD in patients with a history of such exacerbations. Fluticasone propionate in fixed combination with salmeterol xinafoate is *not* indicated for the relief of acute bronchospasm.

In several randomized, double-blind, placebo-controlled studies of 6 or 12 months' duration in patients with COPD, orally inhaled fluticasone propionate (250 or 500 mcg twice daily) in fixed combination with salmeterol (50 mcg twice daily) as the inhalation powder produced greater improvement in lung function (defined as predose and postdose FEV_1) than either drug alone or placebo. The improvement in lung function with fluticasone propionate 500 mcg and salmeterol 50 mcg in fixed combination was similar to that observed with fluticasone propionate 250 mcg and salmeterol 50 mcg in fixed combination. In two randomized, double-blind studies of 12 months' duration in patients with COPD, orally inhaled fluticasone propionate (250 mcg twice daily) in fixed combination with salmeterol (50 mcg twice daily) as the inhalation powder produced a greater reduction in the annual incidence of moderate/severe COPD exacerbations and exacerbations requiring treatment with oral corticosteroids compared with salmeterol alone. No studies have been conducted to directly compare the efficacy of fluticasone propionate 250 mcg and salmeterol 50 mcg in fixed combination with fluticasone propionate 500 mcg and salmeterol 50 mcg in fixed combination in reducing exacerbations; however, in clinical studies, the reduction in exacerbations observed with fluticasone propionate 500 mcg and salmeterol 50 mcg in fixed combination was not greater than the reduction in exacerbations observed with fluticasone propionate 250 mcg and salmeterol 50 mcg in fixed combination. In a double-blind, placebo-controlled study of 3 years' duration in patients with COPD, orally inhaled fluticasone propionate (500 mcg) in fixed combination with salmeterol (50 mcg) as the inhalation powder did not improve all-cause mortality compared with either drug alone or placebo. Fluticasone propionate 250 mcg and salmeterol 50 mcg in fixed combination twice daily is the only recommended dosage for the treatment of COPD; an efficacy advantage of the higher dosage of the fixed combination (500 mcg of fluticasone propionate and 50 mcg of salmeterol) over the lower dosage (250 mcg of fluticasone propionate and 50 mcg of salmeterol) has not been established.

■ **Other Uses** Fluticasone also has been administered as oral tablets (formulation currently not commercially available in the US) in the management of ulcerative colitis†, Crohn's disease†, and celiac sprue†.

Dosage and Administration

■ **General** Dosage of fluticasone propionate alone or in fixed combination with salmeterol xinafoate should be adjusted carefully according to individual requirements and response. The recommended initial and maximum dosages of fluticasone propionate for oral inhalation are based on previous asthma therapy. The recommended initial dosage of the inhalation powder preparation containing fluticasone propionate in fixed combination with salmeterol (Advair® Diskus®) is based on the patient's asthma severity, and the recommended initial dosage of the inhalation aerosol containing fluticasone propionate in fixed combination with salmeterol (Advair® HFA) is based on the patient's current asthma therapy. The lowest effective dosage of fluticasone should be achieved, particularly in children, since inhaled corticosteroids have the potential to affect growth.

■ **Administration** Fluticasone propionate alone and in fixed combination with salmeterol is administered as a microcrystalline suspension by oral inhalation using an oral aerosol inhaler with hydrofluoroalkane (HFA; nonchlorofluorocarbon) propellant or as the inhalation powder using the Diskus® device that delivers the drug from foil-wrapped blisters. Fluticasone propionate in fixed combination with salmeterol xinafoate is also administered as an inhalation powder using the Diskus® device that delivers the drugs from foil-wrapped blisters.

Oral Inhalation via Aerosol Inhaler The fluticasone propionate HFA inhalation aerosol canister should be shaken well for 5 seconds immediately prior to use. The fluticasone propionate HFA aerosol canister should be used only with the supplied actuator (inhaler). The aerosol inhaler should be actuated 4 times prior to the initial use of fluticasone propionate. In addition, the inhaler should be shaken well for 5 seconds and actuated once prior to use if it has not been used for longer than 1 week or if the inhaler has been dropped. Patients should exhale slowly and completely and place the mouthpiece of the inhaler well into the mouth with lips closed around it. Patients should inhale slowly and deeply through the mouth while actuating the inhaler. Patients should hold their breath for up to 10 seconds, withdraw the mouthpiece from the mouth, and then exhale slowly. Subsequent actuations of the aerosol inhaler should be performed 30 seconds after the previous inhalation. Following each treatment, the patient should rinse the mouth thoroughly. The inhaler should be cleaned at least once a week after the evening dose by removing the mouthpiece cap from the inhaler and washing the mouthpiece with moistened cotton; the actuator should be allowed to air-dry overnight. When the dose counter on the inhaler reads "020", the patient should contact the pharmacy for a refill or consult their clinician to determine whether a refill is needed. The inhaler should be discarded when the dose counter reads "000". The canister should never be immersed in water to determine the amount of drug remaining in the canister ("float test").

Fluticasone propionate/salmeterol inhalation aerosol (Advair® HFA) should only be used with the actuator provided with the product. Before each inhalation, the inhaler must be shaken well for 5 seconds. The aerosol inhaler should be test sprayed 4 times into the air (away from the face) before initial use, and shaken well for 5 seconds before each spray. If the inhaler has not been used for more than 4 weeks or if the inhaler was dropped, the inhaler should be test sprayed twice into the air (away from the face) and shaken well for 5 seconds before each spray.

The cap covering the mouthpiece should be removed; the strap on the cap will stay attached to the actuator. The patient should look for foreign objects inside the inhaler prior to use and verify that the canister is fully inserted into the actuator. After exhaling as completely as possible, the patient should place the mouthpiece of the inhaler well into the mouth and close the lips firmly around it. Then the patient should inhale slowly and deeply through the mouth while actuating the inhaler. The patient should remove the mouthpiece from the mouth and hold the breath for as long as possible, up to 10 seconds, and then exhale normally. It is recommended that 30 seconds should elapse between inhalations. Rinsing the mouth thoroughly after inhalation of fluticasone propionate/salmeterol inhalation aerosol and spitting out the water are advised. The opening for the spray of the metal canister should be wiped dry with a dry cotton swab and the mouthpiece should be wiped clean with a dampened tissue at least once a week after the evening dose. The actuator should be allowed to air-dry overnight. When the dose counter on the inhaler reads "020," the patient should contact the pharmacy for a refill or consult their clinician to determine whether a refill is needed. The inhaler should be discarded when the dose counter reads "000." The counter should never be altered or removed from the canister.

Oral Inhalation via Dry Powder Inhaler The oral inhalation powder of fluticasone propionate alone or in fixed combination with salmeterol xinafoate is administered using a special preloaded oral inhaler (Diskus®). To obtain optimal benefit, the patient should be given a copy of the patient instructions or medication guide provided by the manufacturer with Flovent® Diskus® or Advair® Diskus®, respectively. Children should use Flovent® Diskus® or Advair® Diskus® under adult supervision as instructed by a clinician. The patient should hold the Diskus® device in one hand, put the thumb of the other hand on the thumbgrip, and push the thumbgrip until the mouthpiece appears and snaps into position. The lever on the Diskus® should then be depressed in a direction away from the patient while the inhaler is held in a level, horizontal position until a click is heard; the lever pierces the foil blister and releases the powdered drug into an exit port. To avoid releasing and wasting additional doses of the drug, the patient should not tilt or close the Diskus® device, play with the lever, or advance the lever more than once at this point. A dose counter will advance each time the lever is depressed.

Before inhaling the dose, the patient should exhale as completely as possible; the patient should *not* exhale into the Diskus® device because pressure from the exhalation will interfere with proper inhaler operation. The patient should then place the mouthpiece of the inhaler between the lips and inhale deeply and quickly through the inhaler with a steady, even breath; pressure from the inhalation will disperse drug from the exit port into the air stream created by the patient's inhalation. The patient should remove the inhaler from the mouth, hold his or her breath for a few seconds (i.e., 10 seconds), and then exhale slowly. While patients may or may not taste or feel a dose of drug delivered from the Diskus® device, they should be instructed not to use an extra dose even if they do not perceive that the dose has been delivered. Rinsing the mouth after inhalation of fluticasone propionate alone or in fixed combination with salmeterol is advised. The Diskus® device may be closed and reset for the next dose by sliding the thumbgrip towards the patient as far as it will go. The inhaler should not be washed but should be stored in a dry place away from direct heat or sunlight. The Flovent® Diskus® inhaler should be discarded when every blister has been used (when the dose indicator reads "0") or 6 weeks after removal from its foil overwrap pouch. The Advair® Diskus® inhaler should be discarded when every blister has been used or 1 month after removal from its foil overwrap pouch, whichever comes first. The inhaler should not be taken apart.

■ **Dosage** Unless otherwise stated, the dose of fluticasone propionate administered as an aerosol via metered-dose inhaler with a hydrofluoroalkane (HFA) propellant is expressed as the amount of drug delivered from the actuator of the inhaler per metered spray; the dose of fluticasone propionate (and of salmeterol in the combination preparation Advair®) administered as an oral inhalation powder is expressed as the nominal (labeled) dose contained in each foil-wrapped blister. The manufacturer states that spacer devices should not be used with Advair® or Flovent® Diskus®.

Each actuation of the commercially available fluticasone propionate HFA oral inhalation aerosol labeled as containing 44, 110, or 220 mcg of fluticasone propionate per metered spray delivers 50, 125, or 250 mcg from the valve, respectively, and 44, 110, or 220 mcg from the actuator, respectively. The 10.6-g (labeled as containing 44 mcg of fluticasone propionate) or 12-g canister (labeled as containing 110 or 220 mcg of fluticasone propionate) delivers 120 metered sprays of fluticasone propionate.

Each actuation of the oral aerosol inhaler containing the fixed combination of fluticasone propionate and salmeterol xinafoate delivers 50, 125, or 250 mcg of fluticasone propionate and 25 mcg of salmeterol from the valve. Dosages of fluticasone propionate and salmeterol in the fixed-combination inhalation aerosol are expressed in terms of drug delivered from the mouthpiece; each actuation of the inhaler delivers 45, 115, or 230 mcg of fluticasone propionate and 21 mcg of salmeterol from the mouthpiece. The commercially available inhalation aerosol of fluticasone propionate in fixed combination with salmeterol delivers 60 or 120 metered sprays per 8- or 12-g canister, respectively.

With commercially available fluticasone propionate inhalation powder (Flovent® Diskus®, Advair® Diskus®) delivered via the Diskus® device, the amount of drug delivered to the lungs depends on factors such as the patient's inspiratory flow. Using standardized in vitro testing at a flow rate of 60 L per minute for 2 seconds, the Flovent® Diskus® labeled as containing 50, 100, or 250 mcg of fluticasone propionate delivers 46, 94, or 235 mcg of fluticasone propionate, respectively. In adults with obstructive lung disease and severely compromised lung function (FEV_1 20–30% of predicted), mean peak inspiratory flow through the Diskus® device was 82.4 L/minute. In children 4 and 8 years of age with asthma, mean peak inspiratory flow through the Diskus® device was 70 and 104 L/minute, respectively. Using standardized in vitro testing at a flow rate of 60 L per minute for 2 seconds, the Advair® Diskus® device delivered 93, 233, and 465 mcg of fluticasone propionate and 45 mcg of salmeterol per activation from a Diskus® labeled as containing 100, 250, or 500 mcg of fluticasone propionate and 50 mcg of salmeterol, respectively. In adults with obstructive lung disease and severely compromised lung function (FEV_1 20–30% of predicted), mean peak inspiratory flow through the Diskus® device was 82.4 L/minute for Advair®. In adults and adolescents with asthma, mean peak inspiratory flow through the Diskus® device was 122.2 L/minute. In a group of children 4 years of age, mean peak inspiratory flow through the Advair® Diskus® device averaged 75.5 L/minute; in children 8 years of age, mean peak inspiratory flow averaged 107.3 L/minute.

Asthma **Fluticasone Propionate.** When the fluticasone propionate HFA oral inhalation aerosol is used, the initial, maintenance, and maximum dosage in children 4–11 years of age is 88 mcg twice daily. The recommended initial dosage of fluticasone propionate for adults and adolescents 12 years of age or older who previously were receiving bronchodilators alone is 88 mcg twice daily; the maximum recommended dosage is 440 mcg twice daily. In adults and adolescents 12 years of age or older who previously were receiving inhaled corticosteroids, the recommended initial dosages of fluticasone propionate, using the HFA oral inhalation aerosol, are 88–220 mcg twice daily; the maximum recommended dosage is 440 mcg twice daily. Initial dosages exceeding 88 mcg twice daily should be considered in patients with poorer asthma control or in those who were receiving inhaled corticosteroids at the higher end of the dosing range. In adults and adolescents 12 years of age or older who previously were receiving oral corticosteroids, the recommended initial and maximum dosage of fluticasone propionate, using the HFA oral inhalation aerosol, is 440 and 880 mcg twice daily, respectively. If control of asthma is inadequate after 2 weeks of therapy at the initial dosage, replacing the current strength with a higher strength may provide additional asthma control.

When fluticasone propionate inhalation powder is administered via the Diskus® device, the recommended initial dosage of fluticasone propionate in adults and adolescents 12 years of age or older who previously were receiving bronchodilators alone is 100 mcg twice daily; the maximum recommended dosage is 500 mcg twice daily. In adults and adolescents 12 years of age or older who previously were receiving inhaled corticosteroids, the recommended initial dosage of fluticasone propionate using the inhalation powder (administered via a Diskus®) is 100–250 mcg twice daily; the maximum recommended dosage is 500 mcg twice daily. Initial dosages exceeding 100 mcg twice daily should be considered in patients with poorer asthma control or in those who were receiving inhaled corticosteroids at the higher end of the dosing range. In adults and adolescents 12 years of age or older who previously were receiving oral corticosteroids, the recommended initial dosage of fluticasone propionate using the powdered drug is 500–1000 mcg twice daily (administered via the Diskus® device); the maximum recommended dosage for the Diskus® device is 1000 mcg twice daily.

When the fluticasone propionate inhalation powder is administered via the Diskus® device in children 4 to younger than 12 years of age who previously were receiving bronchodilators alone or with inhaled corticosteroids, the recommended initial dosage of fluticasone propionate is 50 mcg twice daily; the recommended maximum dosage is 100 mcg twice daily. Initial dosages exceeding 50 mcg twice daily should be considered in children with poorer asthma control or in those who were receiving inhaled corticosteroids at the higher end of the dosing range. Because patient responses may vary, pediatric patients previously maintained on fluticasone propionate inhalation powder administered via the Diskhaler® (50 or 100 mcg twice daily) may require dosage adjustments upon transfer to the drug administered via the Diskus® device.

Conversion to Orally Inhaled Therapy in Patients Receiving Systemic Corticosteroids. When orally inhaled corticosteroids are administered to patients receiving systemic corticosteroids, the patient's asthma should be reasonably stable before treatment with the oral inhalation begins. Initially, fluticasone propionate inhalation powder is given concurrently with the maintenance dosage of the systemic corticosteroid. The manufacturer suggests that in patients who were receiving prior oral corticosteroid therapy, reduction of oral corticosteroid dosage should be initiated at least 1 week after starting fluticasone propionate oral inhalation and decrements usually should not exceed 2.5–5 mg of prednisone (or its equivalent) each week. Once oral corticosteroids are discontinued and symptoms of asthma have been controlled, the dosage of fluticasone propionate should be titrated to the lowest effective level. The inability to decrease the dosage of oral corticosteroids during systemic corticosteroid withdrawal may indicate the need to increase the dosage of fluticasone propionate up to a maximum of 1000 mcg twice daily. The manufacturer of the oral inhalation powder containing fluticasone propionate in fixed combination with salmeterol (Advair® Diskus®) states that patients requiring oral corticosteroids should be withdrawn slowly from systemic corticosteroid use after transferring to fluticasone propionate in fixed combination with salmeterol inhalation powder. The manufacturer also states that prednisone dosage reduction may be accomplished by reducing the daily dosage of prednisone by 2.5 mg on a weekly basis during therapy with the oral inhalation powder containing fluticasone propionate in fixed combination with salmeterol. The oral inhalation aerosol containing fluticasone propionate in fixed combination with salmeterol (Advair® HFA) should *not* be used to transfer patients from systemic corticosteroid therapy. (See Dosage and Administration in the Corticosteroids General Statement 68:04.) *Particular care is needed in gradually withdrawing systemic corticosteroids following long-term therapy, since death has occurred in some individuals in whom systemic corticosteroids were withdrawn too rapidly.* (See Withdrawal of Systemic Corticosteroid Therapy under Warnings/Precautions: Warnings, in Cautions.)

Fluticasone Propionate/Salmeterol Fixed-combination Therapy. In asthmatic patients 4–11 years of age who are inadequately controlled on an inhaled corticosteroid, the recommended dosage of the commercially available inhalation powder preparation containing fluticasone propionate in fixed combination with salmeterol (Advair® Diskus®) is 100 mcg of fluticasone propionate and 50 mcg of salmeterol (1 inhalation) twice daily, given approximately 12 hours apart (morning and evening).

In asthmatic patients 12 years of age or older, the recommended initial dosage of the commercially available inhalation powder preparation containing fluticasone propionate in fixed combination with salmeterol (Advair® Diskus®) is based on the patient's asthma severity. The dosage of the inhalation powder fixed-combination preparation is 100, 250, or 500 mcg of fluticasone propionate and 50 mcg of salmeterol (1 inhalation) twice daily, given approximately 12 hours apart (morning and evening). The maximum recommended dosage of fluticasone propionate in fixed combination with salmeterol is 500 mcg of fluticasone propionate and 50 mcg of salmeterol twice daily. The manufacturer states that administration of the inhalation powder containing fluticasone propionate in fixed combination with salmeterol more frequently than twice daily or exceeding 1 inhalation twice daily is not recommended.

In asthmatic patients 12 years of age or older, the recommended initial dosage of the inhalation aerosol containing fluticasone propionate in fixed combination with salmeterol (Advair® HFA) is based on the patient's current asthma therapy. The dosage of the inhalation aerosol fixed-combination preparation is 90, 230, or 460 mcg of fluticasone propionate and 42 mcg of salmeterol (2 inhalations) twice daily, given approximately 12 hours apart (morning and evening). The maximum recommended dosage of fluticasone propionate is 460 mcg in fixed combination with 42 mcg of salmeterol (2 inhalations) twice daily. The manufacturer states that administration of the inhalation aerosol containing fluticasone propionate in fixed combination with salmeterol more frequently than twice daily or exceeding 2 inhalations twice daily is not recommended.

If control of asthma is inadequate after 2 weeks of therapy at the initial dosage, replacing the current strength of the fixed combination with a higher strength (higher strengths contain higher dosages of fluticasone propionate only) may provide additional asthma control. Patients receiving the fixed combination of fluticasone propionate and salmeterol twice daily should not use additional salmeterol or other long-acting β_2-adrenergic agonists (e.g., formoterol) for any reason, including the treatment of asthma or prevention of exercise-induced bronchospasm. Patients also should be advised not to discontinue fluticasone propionate in fixed combination with salmeterol without medical supervision, as symptoms may recur after treatment discontinuance. If a previously effective dosage of fluticasone propionate in fixed combination with salmeterol fails to provide adequate improvement in asthma control, the therapeutic regimen should be reevaluated and additional therapeutic options should be considered (e.g., increasing the strength of the fixed combination [higher strengths contain higher dosages of fluticasone propionate only], adding additional inhaled corticosteroids, initiating systemic corticosteroids). The manufacturer warns that therapy with the fixed combination of fluticasone propionate and salmeterol should *not* be initiated in patients during rapidly deteriorating or potentially life-threatening episodes of asthma. (See Respiratory Effects under Cautions: Warnings/Precautions and also see Cautions: Precautions and Contraindications, in Salmeterol 12:12.08.12.)

Chronic Obstructive Pulmonary Disease **Fluticasone Propionate/Salmeterol Fixed-combination Therapy.** For maintenance therapy of COPD, the recommended dosage of fluticasone propionate in fixed combination with salmeterol (Advair® Diskus®) in adults is 250 mcg of fluticasone propionate and 50 mcg of salmeterol (1 inhalation) twice daily, given approximately every 12 hours (morning and evening). If shortness of breath occurs between doses, an inhaled, short-acting β_2-agonist should be used for immediate relief. Higher dosages of salmeterol in fixed combination with fluticasone propionate (e.g., 500 mcg of fluticasone propionate and 50 mcg of salmeterol twice daily) do not result in additional benefit and are not recommended. Patients receiving fluticasone propionate in fixed combination with salmeterol should not use additional salmeterol or other long-acting β_2-agonists (e.g., arformoterol, formoterol) for any reason, including the treatment of COPD.

■ **Special Populations** The following information addresses dosage of fluticasone propionate in special populations. When fluticasone propionate is used in fixed combination with salmeterol, dosage requirements for salmeterol should be considered.

Dosage of fluticasone propionate HFA inhalation aerosol in geriatric patients should be selected with caution, reflecting the greater frequency of decreased hepatic function, presence of coexisting conditions, or other drug therapies in such patients. Dosage adjustments based solely on age are not recommended in geriatric patients receiving fluticasone propionate inhalation powder alone or fluticasone propionate inhalation powder or aerosol in fixed combination with salmeterol.

Cautions

■ **Contraindications** Primary treatment of severe acute asthmatic attacks or status asthmaticus when intensive measures (e.g., oxygen, parenteral bronchodilators, IV corticosteroids) are required.

Fluticasone propionate in fixed combination with salmeterol is contraindicated as primary treatment of status asthmaticus or other acute episodes of asthma or chronic obstructive pulmonary disease (COPD) when intensive measures are required.

Known hypersensitivity to fluticasone propionate or any ingredient (e.g., milk protein) in the formulation.

When fluticasone propionate is used in fixed combination with salmeterol, contraindications associated with salmeterol should be considered.

■ **Warnings/Precautions** ***Warnings*** **Use of Fixed Combinations.** When preparations containing fluticasone propionate in fixed combination with salmeterol are used, the usual cautions, precautions, and contraindications associated with salmeterol should be considered. Cautionary information applicable to specific populations (e.g., pregnant or nursing women, individuals with hepatic or renal impairment, geriatric patients) should be considered for each drug in the fixed combination.

Serious Asthma-related Events. Monotherapy with long-acting β_2-adrenergic agonists, such as salmeterol, a component of Advair® Diskus® and Advair® HFA, increases the risk of asthma-related death. Data from a large (approximately 26,000 patients), placebo-controlled study (Salmeterol Multi-center Asthma Research Trial [SMART]) evaluating the safety of salmeterol in patients with asthma showed an increase in asthma-related deaths in those receiving the drug. Results of a post hoc analysis revealed a statistically significant greater risk of asthma-related deaths or life-threatening experiences with salmeterol therapy in African-American patients and in patients not receiving concomitant inhaled corticosteroid therapy (53% of study patients) compared with placebo. In addition, available data from controlled clinical trials suggest that monotherapy with long-acting β_2-adrenergic agonists increases the risk of asthma-related hospitalization in pediatric and adolescent patients. (See Asthma-related Death and Life-threatening Events under Cautions: Respiratory Effects, in Salmeterol 12:12.08.12.)

However, FDA has concluded that there is no clinically important increased risk of serious asthma-related events, including hospitalization, intubation, or death, associated with concomitant use of long-acting β_2-adrenergic agonists (e.g., salmeterol) and inhaled corticosteroids (e.g., fluticasone) compared with inhaled corticosteroids alone based on the results of several large clinical studies. In addition, these studies showed that combination therapy with long-acting β_2-adrenergic agonists and inhaled corticosteroids was more effective in reducing the incidence of asthma exacerbations (i.e., events requiring use of systemic corticosteroids for at least 3 outpatient days or an asthma-related hospitalization or emergency department visit requiring use of systemic corticosteroids) compared with use of inhaled corticosteroids alone. (See Asthma-related Death and Life-Threatening Events under Cautions: Respiratory Effects, in Salmeterol 12:12.08.12.)

In the treatment of asthma, the fixed combination of fluticasone propionate and salmeterol xinafoate is used only in patients who have not responded adequately to long-term asthma controller therapy, such as inhaled corticosteroids, or whose disease severity clearly warrants initiation of treatment with both an inhaled corticosteroid and a long-acting β_2-adrenergic agonist. (See Asthma under Uses: Bronchospasm.)

Withdrawal of Systemic Corticosteroid Therapy. The fixed combination of fluticasone propionate and salmeterol xinafoate as the inhalation aerosol (Advair® HFA) should not be used for transferring patients from systemic corticosteroid therapy. In patients being switched from systemic corticosteroids to orally inhaled fluticasone propionate, systemic corticosteroid therapy should be withdrawn gradually and patients should be monitored during dosage reduction for objective signs of adrenal insufficiency (e.g., hypotension, fatigue, lassitude, weakness, nausea, vomiting) since a life-threatening exacerbation of asthma or adrenal insufficiency could occur. Lung function (FEV_1 or morning PEF), adjunctive β_2-adrenergic agonist use, and asthma symptoms should be carefully monitored during withdrawal of systemic corticosteroid therapy. *In most patients, several months are required for total recovery of HPA function following withdrawal of systemic corticosteroid therapy.* Patients who have been previously maintained on a corticosteroid dosage equivalent to 20 mg or more of prednisone daily may be most susceptible to adrenal insufficiency, particularly when systemic corticosteroids have been almost completely withdrawn. Corticosteroid withdrawal symptoms (e.g., joint pain, muscular pain, fatigue, lassitude, depression) may occur. Acute adrenal insufficiency may occur during exposure to trauma, surgery, or infection (particularly gastroenteritis or other conditions associated with acute electrolyte loss). Clinicians should be alert for the potential for eosinophilia, vasculitic rash, worsening of pulmonary symptoms, cardiac complications, and/or neuropathy consistent with Churg-Strauss syndrome; or unmasking of conditions previously controlled by systemic corticosteroid therapy (e.g., rhinitis, conjunctivitis, eczema, arthritis, eosinophilic conditions).

Immunosuppressed Patients. Patients who become immunosuppressed while receiving corticosteroids have increased susceptibility to infections compared with healthy individuals, and certain infections (e.g., varicella [chickenpox], measles) can have a more serious or even fatal outcome in such patients, particularly in children. Patients receiving corticosteroids who are potentially immunosuppressed should be warned of the risk of exposure to certain infections (e.g., chickenpox, measles) and of the importance of obtaining medical advice if such exposure occurs. Such patients should take particular care to avoid exposure to these infections. If exposure to varicella (chickenpox) or measles occurs in susceptible patients, administration of varicella zoster immune globulin (VZIG) or pooled immune globulin (IG), respectively, should be considered. If chickenpox develops, treatment with an antiviral agent should be considered. For additional information, see Cautions: Increased Susceptibility to Infection and also see Cautions: Precautions and Contraindications, in the Corticosteroids General Statement 68:04.

Bronchospasm. As with other inhaled drugs for asthma, bronchospasm may occur, resulting in an immediate increase in wheezing following oral inhalation of fluticasone propionate. If bronchospasm occurs, appropriate treatment (e.g., use of a short-acting β_2-adrenergic agonist) should be instituted immediately and fluticasone propionate therapy should be discontinued.

Acute Exacerbations of Asthma or Chronic Obstructive Pulmonary Disease. Therapy with the fixed combination of fluticasone propionate and salmeterol xinafoate should not be initiated in patients with substantially worsening or acutely deteriorating asthma or acute symptoms of chronic obstructive pulmonary disease (COPD). Failure to respond to a previously effective dosage of fluticasone propionate in fixed combination with salmeterol xinafoate may indicate substantially worsening asthma or COPD that requires reevaluation. If inadequate control of symptoms persists with supplemental β_2-agonist bronchodilator therapy (i.e., if there is a need to increase the dose or frequency of administration of the short-acting bronchodilator) or an appreciable decrease in lung function (e.g., peak expiratory flow [PEF]) occurs, prompt reevaluation of asthma therapy is required; however, extra/increased doses of salmeterol or other long-acting inhaled β_2-agonists (e.g., formoterol) should not be used in such situations or for any indication. Such reevaluation may include increasing the strength of the fixed combination (higher strengths contain higher dosages of fluticasone propionate only), adding additional inhaled corticosteroid, or initiating systemic corticosteroids. Patients should not increase the frequency of administration of the fixed combination. (See Cautions: Precautions and Contraindications, in Salmeterol 12:12.08.12.)

Sensitivity Reactions Immediate hypersensitivity reactions, including urticaria, angioedema, rash, bronchospasm, hypotension, and anaphylaxis, may occur following oral inhalation of fluticasone in fixed combination with salmeterol.

Anaphylactic reactions, including reactions in patients with severe milk protein allergy, have been reported following oral inhalation of powder products containing lactose, such as fluticasone in fixed combination with salmeterol (Advair® Diskus®). (See Cautions: Contraindications.)

General Precautions **Infections.** Localized candidal infections of the pharynx have been reported in patients receiving orally inhaled fluticasone propionate therapy. When infection occurs, appropriate local or systemic treatment of the infection may be necessary and/or discontinuance of orally inhaled fluticasone propionate therapy may be required. Inhaled corticosteroid therapy should be used with extreme caution, if at all, in patients with clinical or asymptomatic *Mycobacterium tuberculosis* infections of the respiratory tract; untreated fungal, bacterial, or parasitic infections; or ocular herpes simplex or untreated systemic viral infections. Clinicians should remain vigilant for the possible development of pneumonia in patients with COPD who are receiving the inhalation powder preparation containing fluticasone propionate in fixed combination with salmeterol (Advair® Diskus®), since the clinical features of pneumonia and COPD exacerbations frequently overlap. Lower respiratory tract infections, including pneumonia, have been reported in patients with COPD following the administration of inhaled corticosteroids, including fluticasone propionate and the inhalation powder preparation containing fluticasone propionate in fixed combination with salmeterol (Advair® Diskus®).

Ophthalmic Effects. Glaucoma, increased intraocular pressure, and cataracts rarely have been reported in patients receiving orally inhaled corticosteroids, including fluticasone propionate; regular eye examinations should be considered.

Systemic Corticosteroid Effects. Administration of higher than recommended dosages of orally inhaled fluticasone propionate may result in manifestations of hypercorticism and suppression of HPA function. If such changes occur, the dosage of fluticasone propionate should be reduced slowly, consistent with accepted procedures for reducing corticosteroid dosage and management of asthma symptoms. Particular care should be taken in monitoring patients postoperatively or during periods of stress for evidence of inadequate adrenal response.

Musculoskeletal Effects. Long-term use of orally inhaled corticosteroids may affect normal bone metabolism, resulting in a loss of bone mineral density. (See Osteoporosis under Cautions: Musculoskeletal Effects, in the Corticosteroids General Statement 68:04.) In a 2-year study in adults with asthma, orally inhaled fluticasone propionate was not associated with appreciable changes in lumbar spine bone mineral density. The manufacturer of fluticasone propionate in fixed combination with salmeterol states that use of this preparation can pose additional risks in patients with major risk factors for decreased bone mineral density, such as tobacco use, advanced age, sedentary lifestyle, poor nutrition, family history of osteoporosis, or chronic use of drugs that can reduce bone mass (e.g., anticonvulsants, corticosteroids). Since patients with chronic obstructive pulmonary disease (COPD) often have multiple risk factors for reduced bone mineral density, assessment of bone mineral density is recommended prior to initiation of therapy and periodically thereafter. If appreciable reductions in bone mineral density are seen and use of fluticasone propionate and salmeterol in fixed combination is considered to be important for the patient's COPD therapy, use of agents to treat or prevent osteoporosis should be strongly considered.

Specific Populations **Pregnancy.** Category C. (See Users Guide.)

Lactation. While it is not known whether fluticasone propionate is distributed into milk in humans, the drug is distributed into milk in rats. In addition, other corticosteroids are distributed into milk. Data also are not available on the effects of the drug on the breast-fed child or on milk production. Since data are not available on the use of fluticasone propionate oral inhalation aerosol in nursing women, caution is advised if the drug is administered in nursing women. The benefits of breast-feeding should be considered along with the woman's clinical need for fluticasone propionate oral inhalation and any potential adverse effects on the breast-fed child from the drug or underlying maternal condition.

Pediatric Use. Safety and efficacy of fluticasone propionate inhalation aerosol or powder alone in children younger than 4 years of age have not been established. Safety and efficacy of the inhalation powder containing fluticasone propionate in fixed combination with salmeterol (Advair® Diskus®) in children younger than 4 years of age have not been established. Safety and efficacy of the inhalation aerosol containing fluticasone propionate in fixed combination with salmeterol (Advair® HFA) in children younger than 12 years of age have not been established. Use of the inhalation powder containing fluticasone propionate in children 4–11 years of age is supported by data from several clinical trials. Use of fluticasone propionate inhalation aerosol or the inhalation powder containing fluticasone propionate in fixed combination with salmeterol (Advair® Diskus®) in children 4–11 years of age is supported by data from several clinical trials and by extrapolation of efficacy data from older patients. The adverse effect profile of Flovent® HFA in pediatric patients (4–11 years of age) generally is similar to that observed in adolescents and adults.

Use of corticosteroids or inadequate control of chronic diseases (e.g., asthma) may lead to suppression of growth in children and adolescents. Therefore, children receiving prolonged therapy with orally inhaled fluticasone propionate should be monitored periodically (e.g., via stadiometry) for possible adverse effects on growth and development. The benefits of corticosteroid therapy should be weighed against the possibility of growth suppression and the risks associated with alternative therapies. Children should be maintained on the lowest possible dosage of fluticasone propionate that controls asthma symptoms. (See Cautions: Pediatric Precautions, in the Corticosteroids General Statement 68:04.)

Geriatric Use. Although no overall differences in safety and efficacy of orally inhaled fluticasone propionate alone or fluticasone propionate in fixed combination with salmeterol as the inhalation aerosol (Advair® HFA) were observed relative to younger adults, the possibility that some older patients may exhibit increased sensitivity to the drug cannot be ruled out. Experience with the inhalation powder containing fluticasone propionate in fixed combination with salmeterol (Advair® Diskus®) in those 65 years of age or older with asthma is insufficient to determine whether geriatric patients respond differently than younger patients. In clinical studies evaluating the inhalation powder containing fluticasone propionate in fixed combination with salmeterol for COPD, patients 65 years of age or older experienced a higher incidence of serious adverse effects compared with those younger than 65 years of age, although the distribution of adverse effects was similar in the two groups. Dosage of fluticasone propionate HFA inhalation aerosol in geriatric patients should be selected with caution, reflecting the greater frequency of decreased hepatic function, presence of coexisting conditions, or other drug therapies in such patients. Dosage adjustments based solely on age are not recommended in geriatric patients receiving fluticasone propionate inhalation powder alone or fluticasone propionate inhalation powder or aerosol in fixed combination with salmeterol.

■ **Common Adverse Effects** Adverse effects occurring in more than 3% of patients older than 12 years of age receiving fluticasone propionate HFA oral inhalation aerosol in controlled clinical trials include upper respiratory tract infection, headache, throat irritation, upper respiratory inflammation, sinusitis/sinus infection, candidiasis (including oral candidiasis), cough, hoarseness/dysphonia, and bronchitis. Adverse effects reported in clinical trials with fluticasone propionate HFA inhalation aerosol in pediatric patients (4–11 years of age) generally were similar to those observed in adolescents and adults.

Adverse effects occurring in more than 3% of patients receiving fluticasone propionate oral inhalation powder in controlled clinical trials include upper respiratory tract infection, throat irritation, sinusitis/sinus infection, upper respiratory inflammation, rhinitis, viral respiratory infection, cough, bronchitis, oral candidiasis, nausea and vomiting, GI discomfort and pain, viral GI infection, musculoskeletal pain, muscle injury, headache, fever, and viral infection.

Drug Interactions

The following information addresses potential interactions with fluticasone propionate. When fluticasone propionate is used in fixed combination with salmeterol, interactions associated with salmeterol should be considered. No formal drug interaction studies have been performed to date with the fixed-combination preparations containing fluticasone propionate and salmeterol.

■ **Drugs Affecting Hepatic Microsomal Enzymes** Since fluticasone propionate is metabolized in the liver by the cytochrome P-450 (CYP) 3A4 isoenzyme, concomitant use of drugs that affect cytochrome P-450 hepatic microsomal enzymes could alter the metabolism of fluticasone.

Cushing's syndrome and adrenal suppression have been reported during postmarketing experience in patients receiving concomitant therapy with fluticasone propionate and ritonavir, a highly potent CYP3A4 inhibitor. Concomitant use of ritonavir and fluticasone propionate is not recommended unless the potential benefit is considered to outweigh the risk of systemic corticosteroid adverse effects.

Administration of a single 1-mg dose of orally inhaled fluticasone propionate in healthy individuals receiving ketoconazole (200 mg once daily to steady state) increased mean plasma fluticasone concentrations, resulting in a depression of certain indices of HPA-axis function (as determined by a reduction in area under the plasma cortisol concentration-time curve [AUC]). Care should be exercised when fluticasone propionate is used concomitantly with long-term ketoconazole or other potent isoenzyme CYP3A4 inhibitors.

Concomitant use of fluticasone propionate (500 mcg twice daily) and erythromycin (333 mg 3 times daily) did not affect fluticasone propionate pharmacokinetics.

Description

Fluticasone propionate is a synthetic trifluorinated glucocorticoid. For a discussion of the pharmacology of fluticasone propionate, see Pharmacology in the Corticosteroids General Statement 68:04 and in Fluticasone Propionate 52:08.08.

Bioavailability following oral administration of fluticasone propionate is negligible (less than 1%), principally because of incomplete absorption and presystemic metabolism of the drug. Following oral inhalation, fluticasone propionate is absorbed into systemic circulation from the surface of the lungs; in healthy adults, the systemic bioavailability of the drug was about 18% following oral inhalation of the powder for inhalation (via the Diskus® device). However, results of comparative studies using fluticasone propionate administered orally or by inhalation indicate that the clinical efficacy of the orally inhaled drug appears to result from local action rather than from systemic absorption.

Fluticasone propionate is metabolized in the liver by the cytochrome P-450 (CYP) isoenzyme 3A4; the only identified metabolite is the inactive 17 β-carboxylic acid derivative. Fluticasone propionate is excreted principally in the feces, both as unchanged drug and metabolites. Following oral administration of radiolabeled fluticasone propionate, less than 5% of the administered dose was excreted in urine as metabolites.

Advice to Patients

When fluticasone propionate is used in fixed combination with salmeterol xinafoate, importance of informing patients of important cautionary information about salmeterol xinafoate.

A copy of the manufacturer's patient information (medication guide) for fluticasone propionate in fixed combination with salmeterol (Advair® Diskus® and Advair® HFA) must be provided to all patients with each prescription of the drug. Importance of instructing patients to read the medication guide prior to initiation of therapy and each time the prescription is refilled.

Importance of informing patients receiving the fixed combination of fluticasone propionate and salmeterol xinafoate that monotherapy with long-acting β_2-adrenergic agonists, including salmeterol, a component of Advair® Diskus® and Advair® HFA, increases the risk of asthma-related death and may increase the risk of asthma-related hospitalization in pediatric and adolescent patients.

Importance of instructing patients in the use of oral inhaler and Diskus® devices and providing a copy of the manufacturer's instructions for patients.

Importance of pediatric patients receiving therapy under adult supervision.

Importance of adequate understanding of proper storage, preparation, and inhalation techniques, including use of the inhalation delivery systems.

Importance of rinsing the mouth after oral inhalation.

Importance of advising patients that fluticasone propionate oral inhalation must be used at regular intervals to be therapeutically effective.

Importance of not exceeding the recommended dosage and of contacting a clinician immediately if symptoms of asthma or chronic obstructive pulmonary disease (COPD) occur that are not responsive to bronchodilators.

Importance of advising patients that if a dose of fluticasone propionate alone or in fixed combination with salmeterol is missed, the next dose should be taken at the regularly scheduled time; the dose should not be doubled.

Importance of not discontinuing therapy with fluticasone propionate, alone or in fixed combination with salmeterol, without clinician guidance, as symptoms may recur.

Importance of discontinuing *regular* use of oral or inhaled, short-acting β_2-adrenergic agonists and using inhaled, short-acting β_2-adrenergic agonists only for relief of acute symptoms (e.g., shortness of breath) after initiation of therapy with the fixed combination of fluticasone propionate and salmeterol.

Importance of availability of a short-acting, inhaled β_2-adrenergic agonist for acute asthma symptoms. Importance of informing a clinician if a short-acting, inhaled β_2-adrenergic agonist is not available for use.

Importance of contacting a clinician if decreased effectiveness of a short-acting β_2-adrenergic agonist (exceeding 4 inhalations for greater than 2 consecutive days or 1 canister in an 8-week period) for acute symptoms occurs.

Importance of advising patients that although substantial improvement may occur within the first day of therapy with fluticasone propionate, at least 1–2 weeks or more of continuous therapy may be required for optimum effects.

Importance of advising patients using fluticasone in fixed combination with salmeterol that at least 1 week of therapy may be required for optimum effects to be achieved. Importance of contacting a clinician if asthma symptoms do not improve after 1 week of therapy with the fixed-combination preparation.

Importance of informing patients receiving therapy with the fixed combination of fluticasone propionate and salmeterol regarding common adverse effects associated with β_2-adrenergic agonists such as palpitations, chest pain, rapid heart rate, tremor, or nervousness.

Importance of informing patients that corticosteroids may decrease bone mineral density.

Importance of informing patients that long-term use of inhaled corticosteroids may increase the risk for development of some eye problems (cataracts or glaucoma).

Importance of informing a clinician of heart problems, high blood pressure, seizures, thyroid disorders, diabetes mellitus, liver disorders, osteoporosis, or immune disorders prior to initiation of therapy.

Importance of advising patients that orally inhaled fluticasone propionate should not be used as a bronchodilator and that the drug is not indicated for emergency use (e.g., relief of acute bronchospasm).

Importance of advising patients that additional salmeterol or other long-acting inhaled β_2-adrenergic agonists should not be used for prevention of exercise-induced bronchospasm, treatment of asthma or COPD, or any other reason when the fixed combination of fluticasone propionate and salmeterol xinafoate is used.

Importance of advising patients being transferred from systemic corticosteroid to fluticasone propionate oral inhalation therapy to carry special identification (e.g., card, bracelet) indicating the need for supplementary systemic corticosteroids during periods of stress. Importance of advising such patients that they should immediately resume full therapeutic dosages of systemic corticosteroids and contact their clinician for further instructions during stressful periods (e.g., severe infection, severe asthmatic attack).

Importance of patients avoiding exposure to chickenpox or measles, and, if exposed, of immediately consulting their clinician.

Importance of informing patients with COPD receiving the inhalation powder preparation containing fluticasone propionate in fixed combination with salmeterol (Advair® Diskus®) that they have a higher risk of pneumonia and to contact their clinician if they develop symptoms of pneumonia.

Importance of informing clinicians of existing or contemplated concomitant therapy, including therapy with prescription drugs, particularly ritonavir, other orally inhaled bronchodilators or corticosteroids, OTC drugs, vitamins, or herbal supplements.

Importance of informing clinicians of allergies to fluticasone, salmeterol (in fixed combination), other drugs, or foods.

Importance of women informing clinicians if they are or plan to become pregnant or plan to breast-feed.

Importance of informing patients of other important precautionary information. (See Cautions.)

Overview® (see Users Guide). For additional information on this drug until a more detailed monograph is developed and published, the manufacturer's labeling should be consulted. It is *essential* that the manufacturer's labeling be consulted for more detailed information on usual cautions, precautions, contraindications, potential drug interactions, laboratory test interferences, and acute toxicity.

Preparations

Excipients in commercially available drug preparations may have clinically important effects in some individuals; consult specific product labeling for details.

Fluticasone Propionate

Oral Inhalation		
Aerosol	44 mcg/metered spray	**Flovent® HFA** (with tetrafluoroethane propellant), GlaxoSmithKline
	110 mcg/metered spray	**Flovent® HFA** (with tetrafluoroethane propellant), GlaxoSmithKline
	220 mcg/metered spray	**Flovent® HFA** (with tetrafluoroethane propellant), GlaxoSmithKline
Powder for inhalation	50 mcg/inhalation	**Flovent® Diskus®**, GlaxoSmithKline
	100 mcg/inhalation	**Flovent® Diskus®**, GlaxoSmithKline
	250 mcg/inhalation	**Flovent® Diskus®**, GlaxoSmithKline

Fluticasone Propionate Combinations

Oral Inhalation		
Aerosol	45 mcg with salmeterol xinafoate 21 mcg (of salmeterol) per metered spray (from the actuator)	**Advair® HFA** (with hydrofluoroalkane propellant), GlaxoSmithKline
	115 mcg with salmeterol xinafoate 21 mcg (of salmeterol) per metered spray (from the actuator)	**Advair® HFA** (with hydrofluoroalkane propellant), GlaxoSmithKline
	230 mcg with salmeterol xinafoate 21 mcg (of salmeterol) per metered spray (from the actuator)	**Advair® HFA** (with hydrofluoroalkane propellant), GlaxoSmithKline
Powder for inhalation	100 mcg with salmeterol xinafoate 50 mcg (of salmeterol) per inhalation	**Advair® Diskus®**, GlaxoSmithKline
	250 mcg with salmeterol xinafoate 50 mcg (of salmeterol) per inhalation	**Advair® Diskus®**, GlaxoSmithKline
	500 mcg with salmeterol xinafoate 50 mcg (of salmeterol) per inhalation	**Advair® Diskus®**, GlaxoSmithKline

†Use is not currently included in the labeling approved by the US Food and Drug Administration

Hydrocortisone

Compound F, Cortisol

■ Hydrocortisone (cortisol) is a glucocorticoid secreted by the adrenal cortex.

Uses

Hydrocortisone or cortisone is usually the corticosteroid of choice for replacement therapy in patients with adrenocortical insufficiency, because these drugs have both glucocorticoid and mineralocorticoid properties. Concomitant administration of a more potent mineralocorticoid (fludrocortisone) may be required in some patients. For anti-inflammatory or immunosuppressive uses, synthetic glucocorticoids which have minimal mineralocorticoid activity are preferred.

Dosage and Administration

■ **Administration** The route of administration and dosage of hydrocortisone and its derivatives depend on the condition being treated and the response of the patient.

Hydrocortisone Hydrocortisone is administered orally; the drug also was previously administered by IM injection, but absorption of the drug from the injection site is slow (4–8 hours) and a parenteral dosage form currently is not commercially available in the US.

Hydrocortisone Sodium Succinate Hydrocortisone sodium succinate may be administered by IM or IV injection or by IV infusion. Hydrocortisone sodium succinate is reconstituted for IM or IV injection with bacteriostatic water for injection or bacteriostatic 0.9% sodium chloride injection according to the manufacturer's instructions. When the drug is administered by direct IV injection, it should be administered over a period of at least 30 seconds. For IV infusion, the reconstituted hydrocortisone sodium succinate should be further diluted with 5% dextrose, 0.9% sodium chloride, or 5% dextrose in 0.9% sodium chloride injection to a concentration of 0.1–1 mg/mL.

■ **Dosage** Dosage of hydrocortisone sodium succinate is expressed in terms of hydrocortisone. IM or IV therapy is generally reserved for patients who are unable to take the drug orally or for use in emergency situations. Hydrocortisone sodium succinate is absorbed rapidly, and peak plasma concentrations are attained within 1 hour following IM administration. Parenteral injection of hydrocortisone sodium succinate must be given at 4- to 6-hour intervals if constant high blood concentrations of hydrocortisone are required. After the initial emergency period, a longer-acting injectable corticosteroid preparation or oral administration of a corticosteroid should be considered. Dosage for infants and children should be based on the severity of the disease and the response of the patient rather than on strict adherence to dosage indicated by age, body weight, or body surface area. After a satisfactory response is obtained, dosage should be decreased in small decrements to the lowest level that maintains an adequate clinical response. Patients should be continually monitored for signs that indicate dosage adjustment is necessary, such as remissions or exacerbations of the disease and stress (surgery, infection, trauma). If hydrocortisone is used orally for prolonged anti-inflammatory therapy, an alternate-day dosage regimen should be considered. Following long-term therapy, hydrocortisone should be withdrawn gradually. (See the Corticosteroids General Statement 68:04.)

Hydrocortisone The initial adult oral dosage of hydrocortisone as the free alcohol may range from 10–320 mg daily, depending on the disease being treated, and is usually administered in 3 or 4 divided doses. Some clinicians state that children may be given an oral dosage of 0.56–8 mg/kg daily or 16–240 mg/m² daily, administered in 3 or 4 divided doses.

Hydrocortisone Sodium Succinate The IM or IV dosage of hydrocortisone as the sodium succinate may range from 100 mg to 8 g daily. The usual dosage is 100–500 mg IM or IV initially and every 2–10 hours as needed. Some clinicians state that the usual IM or IV dosage for children is 0.16–1 mg/kg or 6–30 mg/m² administered 1 or 2 times daily.

In life-threatening shock, massive IV doses of hydrocortisone as the sodium succinate (such as 50 mg/kg initially and repeated in 4 hours and/or every 24 hours if needed, or 0.5–2 g IV initially and repeated at 2- to 6-hour intervals as required) have been recommended by some clinicians. In such cases, the drug is administered by direct IV injection over a period of one to several minutes. High-dose therapy should be continued only until the patient's condition has stabilized and usually should not be continued beyond 48–72 hours. If massive corticosteroid therapy is needed beyond 72 hours, a corticosteroid which causes less sodium retention (such as methylprednisolone sodium succinate or dexamethasone sodium phosphate) should be used to minimize the risk of hypernatremia.

Chemistry and Stability

■ **Chemistry** Hydrocortisone (cortisol) is a corticosteroid secreted by the adrenal cortex. The corticosteroid is commercially available as hydrocortisone and hydrocortisone sodium succinate. Hydrocortisone occurs as an odorless, white to practically white, crystalline powder. Hydrocortisone is very slightly soluble in water and sparingly soluble in alcohol. Hydrocortisone sodium succinate occurs as a white or nearly white, odorless, amorphous solid and is very soluble in water and in alcohol. The sodium succinate ester of hydrocortisone is hygroscopic.

Following reconstitution with bacteriostatic water for injection, hydrocortisone sodium succinate injection has a pH of 7–8.

■ **Stability** Commercially available preparations of hydrocortisone should be stored at a temperature less than 40°C, preferably between 15–30°C. Hydrocortisone tablets should be stored in well-closed containers. Reconstituted solutions of hydrocortisone sodium succinate should be stored at 25°C or below. Reconstituted solutions of the drug should not be used unless they are clear, and unused solutions should be discarded after 3 days. Solutions of hydrocortisone and its derivatives are heat labile and must not be autoclaved.

Injections of hydrocortisone and its esters have been reported to be incompatible with various drugs, but the compatibility depends on several factors (e.g., concentration of the drugs, resulting pH, temperatures). Specialized references should be consulted for more specific compatibility information.

For further information on chemistry, pharmacology, pharmacokinetics, uses, cautions, drug interactions, laboratory test interferences, and dosage and administration of hydrocortisone, see the Corticosteroids General Statement 68:04. For EENT and topical uses, see 52:08.08 and 84:06.08, respectively.

Preparations

Excipients in commercially available drug preparations may have clinically important effects in some individuals; consult specific product labeling for details.

Hydrocortisone

Powder

Oral

Tablets	5 mg*	**Cortef®** (scored), Pfizer **Hydrocortisone Tablets**
	10 mg*	**Cortef®** (scored), Pfizer **Hydrocortisone Tablets**
	20 mg*	**Cortef®** (scored), Pfizer **Hydrocortisone Tablets**

*available from one or more manufacturer, distributor, and/or repackager by generic (nonproprietary) name

Hydrocortisone Sodium Succinate

Parenteral

For injection	100 mg (of hydrocortisone)	**A-hydroCort®**, Hospira **Solu-CORTEF®**, Pfizer
	250 mg (of hydrocortisone)	**Solu-CORTEF®**, Pfizer
	500 mg (of hydrocortisone)	**Solu-CORTEF®**, Pfizer
	1 g (of hydrocortisone)	**Solu-CORTEF®**, Pfizer

methylPREDNISolone

6-α-Methylprednisolone

■ Methylprednisolone is a synthetic glucocorticoid.

Uses

Methylprednisolone and its derivatives are used principally as anti-inflammatory or immunosuppressant agents. Because methylprednisolone has only minimal mineralocorticoid properties, the drug is inadequate alone for the management of adrenocortical insufficiency. If methylprednisolone is used in the treatment of this condition, concomitant therapy with a mineralocorticoid also is required.

Dosage and Administration

■ **Administration** The route of administration and dosage of methylprednisolone and its derivatives depend on the condition being treated and the response of the patient. IM or IV therapy is generally reserved for patients who are unable to take the drug orally or for use in emergency situations. After the initial emergency period, a longer-acting injectable corticosteroid preparation or oral administration of a corticosteroid should be considered.

■ **Dosage** Dosage for infants and children should be based on the severity of the disease and the response of the patient rather than on strict adherence to dosage indicated by age, body weight, or body surface area. After a satisfactory response is obtained, dosage should be decreased in small decrements to the lowest level that maintains an adequate clinical response. Patients should be continually monitored for signs that indicate dosage adjustment is necessary, such as remissions or exacerbations of the disease and stress (surgery, infection, trauma). When long-term oral methylprednisolone therapy is necessary, an alternate-day dosage regimen should be considered. Following long-term therapy, methylprednisolone should be withdrawn gradually. (See the Corticosteroids General Statement 68:04.)

Methylprednisolone Methylprednisolone is administered orally. The initial adult dosage may range from 2–60 mg daily, depending on the disease being treated, and is usually administered in 4 divided doses. Some clinicians state that children may be given a dosage of 0.117–1.66 mg/kg daily or 3.3–50 mg/m² daily, administered in 3 or 4 divided doses.

For certain allergic conditions (e.g., contact dermatitis including poison ivy), methylprednisolone may be administered for short-term use (e.g., 6 days) using 4-mg tablets; the recommended initial dosage is 24 mg (6 tablets) for the first day, which is then tapered by 4 mg daily until 21 tablets have been administered. On the first day, 8 mg (2 tablets) is administered twice daily (before breakfast and at bedtime) and 4 mg (1 tablet) is administered twice daily (after lunch and dinner). On the second day, 4 mg (1 tablet) is administered 3 times daily (before breakfast, after lunch, and after dinner) and 8 mg (2 tablets) is administered at bedtime. On the third day, 4 mg (1 tablet) is administered 4 times daily (before breakfast, after lunch, after dinner, and at bedtime). On the fourth day, 4 mg (1 tablet) is administered 3 times daily (before breakfast, after lunch, and at bedtime). On the fifth day, 4 mg (1 tablet) is administered twice daily (before breakfast and at bedtime). On the sixth day, 4 mg (1 tablet) is administered before breakfast. Some clinicians state that tapering the dosage of the drug over a longer period (e.g., 12 days instead of 6 days) may be associated with a lower incidence of flare-up of the dermatitis than that associated with 6-day therapy.

To gain prompt control of asthma in infants and children 4 years of age or younger with very poorly controlled, moderate-to-severe asthma (i.e., more than 3 exacerbations per year requiring oral corticosteroids) and in children 5–11 years of age with asthma of comparable control and severity (i.e., at least 2 exacerbations per year requiring oral corticosteroids), methylprednisolone 1–2 mg/kg daily (maximum 60 mg daily) may be added to existing asthma therapy. (See Asthma under Uses: Respiratory Diseases, in the Corticosteroids General Statement 68:04.) In adults and adolescents with very poorly controlled, moderate-to-severe asthma (i.e., at least 2 exacerbations per year requiring oral corticosteroids), methylprednisolone 40–60 mg daily as a single dose or in 2 divided doses may be added to low-to-high maintenance dosages of the inhaled corticosteroid and a long-acting inhaled β_2-agonist bronchodilator. A short course (usually 3–10 days) of oral corticosteroid therapy should be continued until the patient achieves a peak expiratory flow (PEF) of 80% of his or her personal best and until symptoms resolve. However, a longer duration of treatment may be needed in some patients. There is no evidence that tapering the dosage after improvement will prevent a relapse.

Methylprednisolone 7.5–60 mg daily in the morning or every other day is suggested in adults and adolescents with severe asthma who are inadequately controlled with a high-dose inhaled corticosteroid, intermittent oral corticosteroid therapy, and a long-acting inhaled β_2-agonist bronchodilator, based on consensus and clinical experience. A short course (2 weeks) of oral corticosteroids may be considered to confirm clinical response prior to implementing long-term therapy with these agents. Once long-term oral corticosteroid therapy is initiated, the lowest possible effective dosage (i.e., alternate-day or once-daily administration) should be used and the patient should be monitored carefully for adverse effects. Once asthma is well controlled, repeated attempts should be made to reduce the oral corticosteroid dosage.

For emergency department treatment of moderate-to-severe acute asthma exacerbations not controlled with an inhaled β_2-adrenergic agonist in children 11 years of age or younger, methylprednisolone 1–2 mg/kg daily in 2 divided doses (maximum 60 mg daily) can be added. For treatment of such exacerbations in adults and adolescents, methylprednisolone 40–80 mg daily as a single dose or in 2 divided doses can be added to an inhaled β_2-adrenergic agonist. Treatment should be continued until the patient achieves a PEF of 70% of predicted or personal best. For additional information on the stepped-care approach to drug therapy in asthma, see Asthma under Uses: Respiratory Diseases, in the Corticosteroids General Statement 68:04.

Methylprednisolone Acetate Methylprednisolone acetate may be administered by IM, intra-articular, intralesional, intrasynovial, or soft tissue injection. The manufacturer of Depo-Medrol® states that this formulation of methylprednisolone acetate should *not* be administered intrathecally because of reports of severe adverse events with such use. (See Cautions: Other Adverse Effects, in the Corticosteroids General Statement 68:04.) Because it is slowly absorbed, IM administration of methylprednisolone acetate suspension is not indicated when an immediate effect of short duration is required. The usual adult IM dose of methylprednisolone acetate is 10–80 mg. When methylprednisolone acetate suspension is given as a temporary substitute for oral therapy, the dose of the suspension should be equal to the total daily oral dose of methylprednisolone and should be administered IM once daily. If a prolonged effect is desired, a dose of methylprednisolone acetate equal to 7 times the daily oral dose of methylprednisolone may be administered IM once weekly. For maintenance therapy in patients with rheumatoid arthritis, 40–120 mg may be administered IM weekly. In patients with congenital adrenogenital syndrome, 40 mg of methylprednisolone acetate administered IM every 2 weeks may be adequate.

For intra-articular, intralesional, or soft tissue injection, the dosage of methylprednisolone acetate varies with the degree of inflammation and the size and location of the affected area. A local anesthetic such as 1% procaine hydrochloride may be infiltrated into the tissue surrounding the joint before administration of methylprednisolone acetate. For large joints such as the knee, 20–80 mg of methylprednisolone acetate may be used. For smaller joints, 4–40 mg may be adequate. The dose for bursae, ganglia, and soft tissue infiltration is 4–30 mg. Methylprednisolone acetate in a dosage of 20–60 mg may be administered intralesionally. Absorption of methylprednisolone acetate from intra-articular injection sites is usually very slow and continues for about 7 days. Intra-articular, intralesional, intrasynovial, and soft tissue injections may be repeated every 1–5 weeks depending on the response of the patient.

For control of severe or incapacitating allergic conditions (e.g., bronchial asthma, seasonal or perennial allergic rhinitis) intractable to adequate trials of conventional therapy, the usual IM dose of methylprednisolone acetate is 80–120 mg in adults. For pediatric patients with such conditions, the American Academy of Pediatrics (AAP) recommends an initial IM methylprednisolone acetate dose of 1–2 mg/kg. A single methylprednisolone acetate IM injection of 7.5 mg/kg or 240 mg is recommended by the National Asthma Education and Prevention Program (NAEPP) in infants and children 4 years of age or younger or adults and children 5 years of age or older, respectively, with very poorly-controlled, moderate-to-severe asthma as an alternative to a short course of an oral corticosteroid to gain prompt control of asthma in those who are vomiting or noncompliant with oral corticosteroid therapy. Relief of asthma symptoms should occur within 6–48 hours and persist for several days to 2 weeks. Relief of coryzal symptoms of allergic rhinitis should occur within 6 hours and persist for several days to 3 weeks.

Methylprednisolone Sodium Succinate Methylprednisolone sodium succinate may be administered by IM or IV injection or by IV infusion; absorption from IM injection sites is rapid. Methylprednisolone sodium succinate is reconstituted for IM or IV injection with bacteriostatic water for injection containing 0.9% benzyl alcohol according to the manufacturer's instructions. When the drug is administered by direct IV injection it should be administered over a period of at least 1 minute. For IV infusion, the reconstituted methylprednisolone sodium succinate should be further diluted with 5% dextrose, 0.9% sodium chloride, 5% dextrose in 0.9% sodium chloride injection, or other compatible IV solution.

Dosage of methylprednisolone sodium succinate is expressed in terms of methylprednisolone. IM or IV dosage of methylprednisolone as the sodium succinate may range from 10 mg to 1.5 g daily; however, much higher IV dosages have been used in the management of life-threatening shock. The usual adult dosage is 10–250 mg IM or IV and may be repeated up to 6 times daily. Some clinicians state that children may be given 0.03–0.2 mg/kg or 1–6.25 mg/m² IM 1–2 times daily.

For control of severe or incapacitating allergic conditions intractable to adequate trials of conventional treatment, such as bronchial asthma in pediatric patients, the AAP recommends an initial IV methylprednisolone dose of 1–2 mg/kg.

In adults and adolescents older than 13 years of age with acquired immunodeficiency syndrome† (AIDS) who require parenteral glucocorticoid therapy as an adjunct to anti-infective treatment of moderate to severe *Pneumocystis carinii* pneumonia, an IV methylprednisolone regimen of 30 mg twice daily for 5 days, followed by 30 mg once daily for 5 days, and then 15 mg once daily for 11 days (or until completion of the anti-infective regimen) currently is recommended. Such adjunctive glucocorticoid therapy preferably should be initiated within 24–72 hours of initial antipneumocystis therapy. However, it should be recognized that this recommendation is based on limited data and may not represent the optimum dosage and schedule. Therefore, clinicians should consult published protocols and the most current clinical guidelines. Shorter courses of glucocorticoid therapy would be desirable, but rebound deterioration in pulmonary function has occurred in some patients following discontinuance of glucocorticoid therapy, and some clinicians discourage the use of shorter treatment courses.

In life-threatening shock, massive IV doses of methylprednisolone as the sodium succinate (such as 30 mg/kg initially and repeated every 4–6 hours if needed or 100–250 mg initially and repeated at 2- to 6-hour intervals as required) have been recommended. In such cases, the drug is administered by direct IV injection over a period of 3–15 minutes. Alternatively, following the initial dose by direct IV injection, additional doses of 30 mg/kg may be administered by slow continuous IV infusion every 12 hours for 24–48 hours. High-dose therapy should be continued only until the patient's condition has stabilized and usually should not be continued beyond 48–72 hours.

When used to treat motor and/or sensory deficits and potentially minimize disability in patients with acute spinal cord injury†, an initial dose of 30 mg/kg of methylprednisolone given by rapid IV injection over 15 minutes, followed in 45 minutes by IV infusion of 5.4 mg/kg per hour for 23 hours (total dose administered over 24 hours), has been recommended. Other glucocorticoids and other methylprednisolone dosage regimens have not been shown to be effective in humans to date, and glucocorticoid therapy should be initiated as early as possible after spinal cord injury since appreciable benefit has been observed only when methylprednisolone therapy was initiated within 8 hours of injury.

In the successful management of severe lupus nephritis†, methylprednisolone as the sodium succinate has been administered by so-called "pulse" therapy. In adults, a daily dose of 1 g has been given IV over a 1-hour period for 3 consecutive days; children have been given 30 mg/kg IV every other day for 6 doses. "Pulse" therapy with methylprednisolone sodium succinate has been followed by long-term oral prednisone or prednisolone therapy (0.5–1 mg/kg daily).

For the management of croup† in pediatric patients, AAP recommends an initial IV methylprednisolone dose of 1–2 mg/kg.

Chemistry and Stability

■ **Chemistry** Methylprednisolone is a synthetic glucocorticoid. The free alcohol and the acetate ester of methylprednisolone occur as white or practically white, odorless, crystalline powders and are practically insoluble in water and sparingly soluble in alcohol. The sodium succinate ester of methylprednisolone occurs as a white or nearly white, odorless, hygroscopic, amorphous solid and is very soluble in water and in alcohol.

Hydrochloric acid and/or sodium hydroxide may be added during manufacture of methylprednisolone acetate sterile suspensions to adjust pH to 3.5–7. Following reconstitution with the diluent supplied by the manufacturers, methylprednisolone sodium succinate injection has a pH of 7–8.

■ **Stability** Commercially available preparations of methylprednisolone should be stored at a temperature less than 40°C, preferably between 15–30°C; freezing of methylprednisolone acetate sterile suspension should be avoided. Unreconstituted methylprednisolone sodium succinate sterile powder and reconstituted solutions of the drug, and methylprednisolone sodium acetate solution for injection should be stored at a controlled room temperature of 20–25°C. Reconstituted solutions of methylprednisolone sodium succinate should not be used unless they are clear, and unused solutions should be discarded after 48 hours.

Injections of methylprednisolone acetate and methylprednisolone sodium succinate have been reported to be incompatible with various drugs, but the compatibility depends on several factors (e.g., concentrations of the drugs, resulting pH, temperatures). Specialized references should be consulted for specific compatibility information. Methylprednisolone acetate sterile suspension should not be diluted or mixed with any other solution.

For further information on chemistry, pharmacology, pharmacokinetics, uses, cautions, drug interactions, laboratory test interferences, and dosage and administration of methylprednisolone, see the Corticosteroids General Statement 68:04. For EENT and topical uses, see 84:06.08.

Preparations

Excipients in commercially available drug preparations may have clinically important effects in some individuals; consult specific product labeling for details.

methylPREDNISolone

Oral		
Tablets	2 mg	**Medrol®** (scored), Pfizer
	4 mg*	**Medrol®** (scored), Pfizer
		Medrol® Dosepak® (scored; available as 6-day mnemonic pack of 21 tablets), Pfizer
		Methylprednisolone Tablets
	8 mg*	**Medrol®** (scored), Pfizer
		Methylprednisolone Tablets
	16 mg*	**Medrol®** (scored), Pfizer
		Methylprednisolone Tablets
	32 mg*	**Medrol®** (scored), Pfizer
		Methylprednisolone Tablets

*available from one or more manufacturer, distributor, and/or repackager by generic (nonproprietary) name

methylPREDNISolone Acetate

Parenteral		
Injectable suspension	20 mg/mL	**DEPO-Medrol®**, Pfizer
	40 mg/mL*	**DEPO-Medrol®**, Pfizer
		Methylprednisolone Acetate Injectable Suspension
	80 mg/mL*	**DEPO-Medrol®**, Pfizer
		Methylprednisolone Acetate Injectable Suspension

*available from one or more manufacturer, distributor, and/or repackager by generic (nonproprietary) name

methylPREDNISolone Sodium Succinate

Parenteral		
For injection	40 mg (of methylprednisolone)*	**A-methaPred®**, Hospira
		Methylprednisolone Sodium Succinate Injection
		SOLU-Medrol®, Pfizer
	125 mg (of methylprednisolone)*	**A-methaPred®**, Hospira
		Methylprednisolone Sodium Succinate Injection
		SOLU-Medrol®, Pfizer
	500 mg (of methylprednisolone)	**SOLU-Medrol®**, Pfizer
	1 g (of methylprednisolone)*	**Methylprednisolone Sodium Succinate Injection**
		SOLU-Medrol®, Pfizer
	2 g (of methylprednisolone)	**SOLU-Medrol®**, Pfizer

*available from one or more manufacturer, distributor, and/or repackager by generic (nonproprietary) name

†Use is not currently included in the labeling approved by the US Food and Drug Administration

Mometasone Furoate

■ Mometasone furoate is a synthetic glucocorticoid.

Uses

■ **Bronchospasm** ***Asthma*** Mometasone furoate is used for the maintenance treatment of asthma as prophylactic therapy.

The fixed combination of mometasone furoate and formoterol fumarate (mometasone/formoterol) is used for the treatment of asthma in patients not responding adequately to long-term asthma controller therapy (e.g., inhaled corticosteroids) or whose asthma severity warrants initiation of treatment with both an inhaled corticosteroid and a long-acting β_2-adrenergic agonist.

Orally inhaled mometasone furoate alone or in fixed combination with formoterol fumarate should *not* be used for the primary treatment of severe acute asthmatic attacks or status asthmaticus when intensive measures (e.g., oxygen, parenteral bronchodilators, IV corticosteroids) are required. Mometasone furoate alone or in fixed combination with formoterol fumarate should *not* be used as a bronchodilator or for the rapid relief of bronchospasm.

National Asthma Education and Prevention Program (NAEPP) guidelines include recommendations for assessing asthma severity and asthma control as principal components for effective management of asthma. Assessment of asthma severity is used principally to determine initial therapy; once therapy is initiated, asthma control is assessed to guide decisions about adjusting or maintaining therapy using a stepped-care approach.

In the stepped-care approach to antiasthmatic drug therapy, asthma management guidelines and most clinicians recommend initiation of a controller drug such as an anti-inflammatory agent, preferably a low-dose orally inhaled corticosteroid (e.g., 88–264, 88–176, or 176 mcg of fluticasone propionate [or its equivalent] daily via a metered-dose inhaler in adolescents and adults, children 5–11 years of age, or children 4 years of age or younger, respectively) as first-line therapy for persistent asthma (i.e., patients with daytime symptoms of asthma more than twice per week, but less than once daily, and nocturnal symptoms of asthma 3 or 4 times per month), supplemented by as-needed use of a short-acting, inhaled β_2-agonist. For equivalent orally inhaled dosages of corticosteroids, see General Dosage under Dosage and Administration: Dosage, in the Corticosteroids General Statement 68:04.

According to asthma management guidelines, therapy with a long-acting β_2-agonist (e.g., formoterol, salmeterol) generally is recommended in adults and adolescents who have moderate persistent asthma and daily asthmatic symptoms that are inadequately controlled following addition of low-dose inhaled corticosteroids to as-needed short-acting inhaled β_2-agonist treatment. However, NAEPP recommends that the beneficial effects of long-acting β_2-agonists should be weighed carefully against the increased risk (although uncommon) of severe asthma exacerbations and asthma-related deaths associated with daily use of such agents. (See Asthma-Related Death and Life-Threatening Events under Cautions: Respiratory Effects, in Salmeterol 12:12.08.12.) Asthma management guidelines also state that an alternative, but equally preferred option for management of moderate persistent asthma that is not adequately controlled with a low dosage of inhaled corticosteroid is to increase the maintenance dosage to a medium dosage (e.g., exceeding 264 but not more than 440 mcg of fluticasone propionate [or its equivalent] daily via a metered-dose inhaler in adults and adolescents).

Maintenance therapy with an inhaled corticosteroid at medium or high dosages (e.g., exceeding 440 mcg of fluticasone propionate in adults and adolescents or 352 mcg of the drug in children 5–11 years of age [or its equivalent] daily via a metered-dose inhaler) and adjunctive therapy with a long-acting inhaled β_2-agonist is the preferred treatment according to current asthma management guidelines for adults and children 5 years of age or older with severe persistent asthma (i.e., continuous daytime asthma symptoms, nighttime symptoms 7 times per week).

If asthma symptoms in patients with moderate to severe asthma are very poorly controlled (i.e., at least 2–3 exacerbations per year requiring oral corticosteroids), a short course of an oral corticosteroid (3–10 days) may be added to gain prompt control of asthma. Regular use of oral corticosteroids as add-on therapy in adults and children 5 years of age or older with severe asthma who are inadequately controlled with a high-dose inhaled corticosteroid, intermittent oral corticosteroid therapy, and a long-acting inhaled β_2-agonist bronchodilator is suggested, based on consensus and clinical experience. A short (2-week) course of oral corticosteroids may be considered to confirm clinical response prior to implementing long-term oral corticosteroid therapy. Once long-term oral corticosteroid therapy is initiated, the lowest possible effective dosage (i.e., alternate-day or once-daily administration) should be used, and the patient should be monitored carefully for adverse effects. Once asthma is well controlled, repeated attempts should be made to reduce the oral corticosteroid dosage. (See Dosage: Discontinuance of Therapy, under Dosage and Administration in the Corticosteroids General Statement 68:04.)

Well-controlled clinical studies have shown that oral inhalation of mometasone relieves symptoms of bronchial asthma and improves pulmonary function. Optimum symptomatic relief may require at least 1–2 weeks of continuous mometasone oral inhalation therapy. In corticosteroid-dependent patients, use of mometasone oral inhalation therapy may permit a substantial reduction in the daily maintenance dosage, or discontinuance, of the systemic corticosteroid.

Clinical Experience with Mometasone Furoate. In several studies in patients with mild to moderate asthma who were receiving short-acting β_2-adrenergic agonists alone, orally inhaled mometasone furoate (220 mcg once or twice daily or 440 mcg once daily) produced greater improvements in pulmonary function (e.g., morning predose forced expiratory volume in 1 second [FEV_1], morning or evening peak expiratory flow rate [PEFR]) than placebo. In adolescents and adults with mild to moderate asthma who were receiving inhaled corticosteroids, substitution of mometasone furoate (220 or 440 mcg once daily; 110, 220, or 440 mcg twice daily) for the previous inhaled corticosteroid (at existing or reduced dosage) maintained or improved pulmonary function (e.g., as assessed by morning predose FEV_1). In pediatric patients 4–11 years of age with mild to moderate asthma who were receiving inhaled corticosteroids, substitution of mometasone furoate (110 mcg once or twice daily) for the previous inhaled corticosteroid improved pulmonary function (e.g., change in percentage of predicted FEV_1 from baseline to end point).

In a 12-week, double-blind, placebo-controlled study in patients with severe persistent asthma who were receiving chronic oral therapy with prednisone (approximately 12 mg daily) usually in conjunction with inhaled corticosteroids, discontinuance of oral prednisone therapy was achieved in 40 or 0% of patients receiving orally inhaled mometasone furoate 440 mcg twice daily or placebo, respectively, following discontinuance of any previous inhaled corticosteroid therapy. At the study end point, oral prednisone dosage was decreased by 46% in patients receiving orally inhaled mometasone furoate 440 mcg twice daily and increased by 164% in those receiving placebo.

Clinical Experience with Fixed Combination of Mometasone Furoate and Formoterol Fumarate. In one randomized, double-blind, placebo-controlled, 26-week study in patients with asthma 12 years of age or older, orally inhaled mometasone/formoterol (2 inhalations of a preparation containing mometasone furoate 100 mcg/formoterol fumarate dihydrate 5 mcg administered twice daily) was compared with either orally inhaled mometasone furoate 100 mcg, formoterol fumarate dihydrate 5 mcg, or placebo (2 inhalations administered twice daily). A co-primary efficacy end point in this study was the change from baseline in FEV_1 AUC from 0–12 hours. In this study, patients receiving the mometasone/formoterol fixed combination had substantially greater increases in FEV_1 AUC 0–12 hours at 12 weeks compared with those receiving single-entity mometasone furoate or placebo; such improvements were maintained over the 26-week study period. Another primary end point in this study was deterioration in asthma or reduction in lung function. Patients who received the mometasone/formoterol fixed combination had fewer reports of asthma deterioration compared with patients receiving single-entity formoterol fumarate.

In a randomized, double-blind, 12-week study in patients with asthma 12 years of age or older, orally inhaled mometasone/formoterol (2 inhalations of a preparation containing mometasone furoate 100 or 200 mcg/formoterol fumarate dihydrate 5 mcg administered twice daily) was compared with orally inhaled mometasone furoate 200 mcg (2 inhalations administered twice daily). Patients with asthma who received either dosage of the mometasone/formoterol fixed combination had substantially greater increases in FEV_1 from baseline and over 12 weeks compared with those receiving single-entity mometasone furoate.

For EENT and topical uses of mometasone furoate, see 52:08.08 and 84:06.08, respectively.

Dosage and Administration

■ **Administration** ***Oral Inhalation*** Mometasone furoate (Asmanex® Twisthaler®) is administered by oral inhalation as an oral inhalation powder using the Twisthaler® breath-actuated dry powder inhalation device.

Mometasone furoate (Asmanex® HFA) is administered by oral inhalation as an oral inhalation suspension using a metered-dose aerosol inhaler with a hydrofluoroalkane (HFA; non-chlorofluorocarbon) propellant.

Mometasone furoate in fixed combination with formoterol fumarate (mometasone/formoterol; Dulera®) is administered by oral inhalation as an oral inhalation suspension using a metered-dose aerosol inhaler with an HFA propellant.

Following each mometasone furoate or mometasone/formoterol oral inhalation treatment, the mouth should be rinsed thoroughly with water without swallowing.

Children should only use the oral inhalation devices under adult supervision as instructed by a clinician.

Oral Inhalation via Dry-Powder Inhaler. Mometasone furoate (Asmanex® Twisthaler®) is administered by oral inhalation as an oral inhalation powder. This preparation should be administered as a single inhalation once or twice daily. When administered once daily, it should be used at the same time each day, preferably in the evening for optimal efficacy.

Removal of the cap from the Twisthaler® device (by twisting in a counter-clockwise direction) loads a single dose of drug from the drug storage unit into the inhalation channel, making the dose available for administration via oral inhalation through the mouthpiece. The dose counter will decrease by 1 each time the cap is removed. Before inhaling the dose, the patient should exhale as completely as possible; the patient should *not* exhale into the Twisthaler® device. The patient should then place the mouthpiece of the inhaler between the lips and inhale quickly and deeply through the inhaler. Patients should not cover the ventilation holes on either side of the inhaler while inhaling the dose. The patient should remove the inhaler from the mouth, hold the breath for about 10 seconds, then exhale slowly.

The Twisthaler® device should be closed and reloaded for the next dose by twisting the cap in a clockwise direction until a click is heard. Patients should wipe the mouthpiece dry with a dry cloth or tissue and store the device in a dry place. The inhaler should not be washed. The inhaler should be discarded when every inhalation has been used (when the dose indicator reads "00") or 45 days after removal from its foil pouch, whichever comes first.

Oral Inhalation via Aerosol. Mometasone furoate (Asmanex® HFA) is administered by oral inhalation using an oral aerosol inhaler with HFA propellant. This preparation should be administered as 2 inhalations twice daily (morning and evening). The aerosol inhaler should be primed by releasing 4 test sprays into the air (away from the face) before initial use and shaken well before each spray. If the inhaler has not been used for more than 5 days, the inhaler should be primed again by releasing 4 test sprays into the air (away from the face) and shaken well before each spray. The cap from the mouthpiece of the actuator should be removed before use. The mouthpiece should be cleaned using a dry wipe after every 7 days of use; water should not be used to clean the inhaler. Mometasone oral inhalation aerosol should only be used with the actuator supplied with the product.

Mometasone/formoterol fixed combination (Dulera®) is administered by oral inhalation using an aerosol inhaler with HFA propellant. The fixed combination should be administered as 2 inhalations twice daily (morning and evening). Mometasone/formoterol should only be used with the actuator supplied with the product. The aerosol inhaler should be primed by releasing 4 test sprays into the air (away from the face) before initial use and shaken well before each spray. If the inhaler has not been used for more than 5 days, it should be primed again by releasing 4 test sprays into the air (away from the face) and shaken well before each spray. Before each inhalation, the inhaler must be shaken well. The mouthpiece of the inhaler should be wiped clean with a dry cloth every 7 days; water should not be used to clean the inhaler.

■ **Dosage** Dosage of mometasone furoate is expressed in terms of the salt.

Mometasone/formoterol is a fixed combination of mometasone furoate and formoterol fumarate dihydrate; dosage of the mometasone component is expressed in terms of the salt and dosage of the formoterol component is expressed in terms of the hydrated salt.

The strength and dosage of mometasone furoate administered as an oral inhalation powder (Asmanex® Twisthaler®) is expressed as the nominal (labeled) dose contained in the Twisthaler® device. The actual amount of drug delivered to the lungs depends on factors such as the patient's inspiratory flow. Based on standardized in vitro testing at a flow rate of 30 and 60 L/minute at a constant volume of 2 L, each actuation of the Twisthaler® inhaler labeled as containing 220 or 110 mcg of mometasone furoate delivers 200 or 100 mcg of mometasone furoate, respectively, from the mouthpiece. In adults and adolescents 12 years of age or older with asthma of varying severity, mean peak inspiratory flow through the Twisthaler® device was 69 L/minute. Mean peak inspiratory flow through the Twisthaler® device in pediatric patients 5–8 or 9–12 years of age exceeded 50 or 60 L/minute, respectively.

Each actuation of the mometasone furoate oral aerosol metered-dose inhaler (Asmanex® HFA) delivers 115 or 225 mcg of mometasone furoate from the valve and 100 or 200 mcg of mometasone furoate from the actuator, depending on the preparation used. The strength and dosage of these mometasone preparations are expressed in terms of drug delivered from the mouthpiece of the actuator. The actual amount of drug delivered to the lungs may depend on factors such as the patient's coordination between actuation of the device and inspiration through the delivery system. Commercially available Asmanex® HFA aerosol inhaler delivers 120 actuations per 13-g canister.

Each actuation of the oral aerosol inhaler containing the fixed combination of mometasone furoate and formoterol fumarate (Dulera®) delivers 115 or 225 mcg of mometasone furoate and 5.5 mcg of formoterol fumarate dihydrate from the valve and delivers 100 or 200 mcg of mometasone furoate and 5 mcg of formoterol fumarate dihydrate from the actuator per metered spray, depending on the preparation used. The strength and dosage of mometasone/formoterol preparations are expressed in terms of drug delivered from the mouthpiece of the actuator. The actual amount of drug delivered to the lungs may depend on factors such as the patient's coordination between actuation of the device and inspiration through the delivery system. Commercially available mometasone/formoterol aerosol inhaler delivers 60 or 120 metered sprays per 8.8- or 13-g canister, respectively.

Asthma Dosage of mometasone furoate alone or in fixed combination with formoterol fumarate should be adjusted carefully according to individual requirements and response. The recommended initial and maximum dosages of mometasone furoate are based on previous asthma therapy. The lowest effective dosage of mometasone furoate should be used, particularly in children and adolescents, since inhaled corticosteroids have the potential to affect growth. (See Pediatric Use under Warnings/Precautions: Specific Populations, in Cautions.) Safety and efficacy of mometasone furoate dosages exceeding those recommended by the manufacturer have not been established.

Mometasone Furoate. When mometasone furoate oral inhalation powder (Asmanex® Twisthaler®) is used, the initial and maximum dosage in children 4–11 years of age is 110 mcg once daily in the evening, regardless of previous therapy. The recommended initial dosage of mometasone furoate for adults and adolescents 12 years of age or older who were previously receiving bronchodilators alone or inhaled corticosteroids is 220 mcg once daily in the evening. If control of asthma is inadequate in patients 12 years of age or older after 2 weeks of mometasone furoate therapy at the initial dosage, a higher dosage of the drug may provide additional asthma control. If required, the dosage may be increased to a maximum of 440 mcg daily (given as 440 mcg once daily or 220 mcg twice daily). The recommended initial and maximum dosage of mometasone furoate in adults and adolescents 12 years of age or older who were previously receiving oral corticosteroids is 440 mcg twice daily.

When mometasone furoate oral inhalation aerosol (Asmanex® HFA) is used, the initial dosage is based on previous asthma therapy. The initial dosage in adults and adolescents 12 years of age or older previously receiving inhaled medium-dose corticosteroids is 200 mcg (2 inhalations of preparation containing 100 mcg) twice daily. The initial dosage in adolescents 12 years of age or older previously receiving inhaled high-dose corticosteroids or oral corticosteroids is 400 mcg (2 inhalations of preparation containing 200 mcg) twice daily. If control of asthma is inadequate after 2 weeks of mometasone furoate therapy at the lower dosage, switching to a higher strength preparation of the drug, initiating therapy with an oral corticosteroid, or initiating oral inhalation therapy with a fixed-combination preparation containing a corticosteroid and a long-acting β_2-agonist should be considered.

Fixed Combination of Mometasone Furoate and Formoterol Fumarate. When the mometasone/formoterol fixed-combination oral inhalation aerosol (Dulera®) is used in patients with asthma, the recommended initial dosage is based on the patient's asthma severity, previous asthma therapy (including previous inhaled corticosteroid dosage), current control of asthma symptoms, and risk of future asthma exacerbations.

In adults and adolescents 12 years of age or older, the dosage of orally inhaled mometasone/formoterol fixed combination is 200 or 400 mcg of mometasone furoate and 10 mcg of formoterol fumarate dihydrate (2 inhalations of preparation containing 100 or 200 mcg of mometasone furoate and 5 mcg of formoterol fumarate dihydrate) twice daily. If control of asthma is inadequate after 2 weeks of mometasone/formoterol therapy at the lower dosage, switching to a higher strength preparation of the fixed combination (higher strengths contain higher dosages of mometasone only) may provide additional asthma control. The maximum recommended daily dosage of the mometasone/formoterol fixed combination in asthmatic adults and adolescents 12 years of age or older is 800 mcg of mometasone and 20 mcg of formoterol fumarate dihydrate (maximum of 2 inhalations of preparation containing mometasone furoate 200 mcg and formoterol fumarate 5 mcg dihydrate twice daily).

Conversion to Orally Inhaled Therapy in Patients Receiving Systemic Corticosteroids. When switching to an orally inhaled corticosteroid in patients receiving systemic corticosteroids, the patient's asthma should be reasonably stable before oral inhalation therapy begins. Initially, mometasone furoate inhalation powder is given concurrently with the maintenance dosage of the systemic corticosteroid. Reduction of the systemic corticosteroid dosage should be initiated at least 1 week after starting mometasone furoate oral inhalation, and dosage reductions should not exceed 2.5 mg daily of prednisone (or its equivalent) each week. *Particular care is needed in gradually withdrawing systemic corticosteroids following long-term therapy with these drugs, since death due to adrenal insufficiency has occurred in some individuals in whom systemic corticosteroids were withdrawn too rapidly.* (See Withdrawal of Systemic Corticosteroids under Cautions: Warnings/Precautions.)

■ **Special Populations** Patients with hepatic impairment should be closely monitored for signs of increased drug exposure during mometasone therapy.

In patients with renal impairment, there are no specific dosage recommendations for mometasone at this time.

When the mometasone/formoterol fixed combination is used, dosage requirements for formoterol fumarate should be considered.

Cautions

■ **Contraindications** Mometasone furoate and the fixed combination containing mometasone furoate and formoterol fumarate (mometasone/formoterol) are contraindicated for primary treatment of severe acute asthmatic attacks or status asthmaticus when intensive measures (e.g., oxygen, parenteral bronchodilators, IV corticosteroids) are required.

Mometasone furoate is contraindicated in patients hypersensitive to the drug or any ingredient (e.g., milk proteins) in the formulation. Mometasone oral inhalation powder contains small amounts of lactose, which has trace amounts of milk proteins. Anaphylactic reactions in patients with milk protein allergy have been reported; therefore, patients with known milk protein allergy should not receive mometasone oral inhalation powder.

Mometasone/formoterol fixed combination is contraindicated in patients hypersensitive to mometasone, formoterol, or any ingredient in the formulation.

■ **Warnings/Precautions** ***Use of Fixed Combinations*** When mometasone furoate is used in fixed combination with formoterol fumarate, cautions, precautions, contraindications, and interactions associated with formoterol fumarate should be considered. (See Risk of Serious Asthma-related Events under Cautions: Warnings/Precautions.)

Cautionary information applicable to specific populations (e.g., pregnant or nursing women, individuals with hepatic or renal impairment, geriatric patients) should be considered for each drug in the fixed combination.

Acute Exacerbations of Asthma Orally inhaled mometasone furoate alone or in fixed combination with formoterol fumarate should *not* be used as a bronchodilator and is not indicated for emergency use (e.g., status asthmaticus) or relief of acute bronchospasm. Acute asthma symptoms should be treated with a short-acting β_2-agonist bronchodilator. If inadequate control of symptoms persists with supplemental β_2-agonist bronchodilator therapy, prompt reevaluation of asthma therapy is required. Such reevaluation may include dosage adjustment of inhaled corticosteroids or initiation of systemic corticosteroids.

Localized Candidal Infections Candidal infections of the mouth and pharynx have been reported in patients receiving orally inhaled mometasone therapy. If such infections occur, appropriate local or systemic antifungal treatment of the infection may be necessary while still continuing orally inhaled mometasone therapy, although interruption of mometasone therapy may be required in some patients. Patients receiving mometasone or mometasone/formoterol should be instructed to rinse their mouths with water (without swallowing) after each dose to help reduce the risk of oropharyngeal candidiasis.

Immunosuppressed Patients Patients who are taking immunosuppressant drugs have increased susceptibility to infections compared with healthy individuals, and certain infections (e.g., varicella [chickenpox], measles) can have a more serious or even fatal outcome in such patients. Patients receiving corticosteroids who are potentially immunosuppressed and who have not had these diseases or have not been properly vaccinated against these diseases should be warned of the risk of exposure to certain infections (e.g., chickenpox, measles) and take particular care to avoid exposure. If exposure to chickenpox or measles occurs in susceptible individuals, administration of varicella zoster immune globulin (VZIG) or immune globulin IM (IGIM), respectively, may be indicated. If chickenpox develops, treatment with an antiviral agent may be considered.

It is not known how the dosage, route, and duration of administration of a corticosteroid, or the contribution of the underlying disease and/or prior corticosteroid therapy, affect the risk of developing a disseminated infection. Inhaled corticosteroid therapy should be used with caution, if at all, in patients with clinical or asymptomatic *Mycobacterium tuberculosis* infections of the respiratory tract; untreated systemic fungal, bacterial, parasitic, or viral infections; or ocular herpes simplex. For additional information, see Cautions: Increased Susceptibility to Infection and also see Precautions and Contraindications, in the Corticosteroids General Statement 68:04.

Withdrawal of Systemic Corticosteroids Systemic corticosteroid therapy should be withdrawn gradually in patients being switched from systemic corticosteroids to less systemically available orally inhaled corticosteroids. Patients should be monitored during dosage reduction for objective signs and symptoms of adrenal insufficiency (e.g., fatigue, lassitude, weakness, nausea, vomiting, hypotension) since life-threatening adrenal insufficiency could occur. Lung function (forced expiratory volume in 1 second [FEV_1] or peak expiratory flow rate [PEFR]), adjunctive β_2-adrenergic agonist use, and asthma symptoms should be carefully monitored during withdrawal of systemic corticosteroid therapy. *In most patients, several months are required for total recovery of hypothalamic-pituitary-adrenal (HPA) function following withdrawal of systemic corticosteroid therapy.* Patients who have been maintained on a systemic corticosteroid dosage equivalent to 20 mg or more of prednisone daily may be most susceptible to adrenal insufficiency, particularly when systemic corticosteroids have been almost completely withdrawn. These patients should be carefully monitored during and for a number of months after withdrawal of systemic corticosteroids for corticosteroid withdrawal symptoms (e.g., joint pain, muscular pain, lassitude, depression); acute adrenal insufficiency during exposure to trauma, surgery, or infection (particularly gastroenteritis) or other conditions associated with acute electrolyte loss; or symptomatic exacerbation of allergic conditions previously controlled by systemic corticosteroid therapy (e.g., rhinitis, conjunctivitis, eczema, arthritis, eosinophilic conditions).

In patients who have been withdrawn from systemic corticosteroids, reinitiation of systemic corticosteroid therapy will likely be necessary during periods of stress or severe asthmatic attack. Since glucocorticoids can reduce HPA-axis response to stress, supplementation with a systemic corticosteroid in patients undergoing such stress is recommended.

Systemic Corticosteroid Effects Although minimal absorption of mometasone furoate into systemic circulation occurs following oral inhalation of the drug at recommended dosages, manifestations of hypercorticism and HPA-axis suppression could occur if recommended dosages are exceeded over prolonged periods of time or in particularly sensitive individuals. If such changes occur, the dosage of mometasone furoate should be reduced slowly, consistent with accepted procedures for reducing systemic corticosteroid dosage and management of asthma symptoms. Particular care should be taken in monitoring patients postoperatively or during periods of stress for evidence of inadequate adrenal response.

Musculoskeletal Effects Long-term use of orally inhaled corticosteroids, including mometasone furoate, may affect normal bone metabolism, resulting in a loss of bone mineral density. (See Osteoporosis under Cautions: Musculoskeletal Effects, in the Corticosteroids General Statement 68:04.) Although appreciable reduction in lumbar spine bone mineral density was noted in a 2-year study in adults receiving 220 mcg of mometasone furoate twice daily, this adverse effect was not confirmed in another 2-year study in adults receiving 440 mcg of the drug twice daily.

Patients with major risk factors for decreased bone mineral density, such as family history of osteoporosis, prolonged immobilization, or chronic use of drugs that can reduce bone mass (e.g., anticonvulsants, corticosteroids), should be monitored and treated using established standards of care.

Ophthalmic Effects Glaucoma, increased intraocular pressure (IOP), and cataracts have been reported in patients receiving long-term therapy with orally inhaled corticosteroids. Referral to an ophthalmologist should be considered in patients who develop ophthalmic symptoms or in those receiving long-term therapy with mometasone furoate.

Bronchospasm As with other inhaled drugs for asthma, paradoxical bronchospasm may occur, resulting in an immediate increase in wheezing following oral inhalation of mometasone furoate.

If paradoxical bronchospasm occurs, appropriate treatment (e.g., use of a short-acting inhaled β_2-adrenergic agonist) should be instituted immediately, and mometasone therapy should be discontinued.

Sensitivity Reactions Cases of anaphylaxis, rash, pruritus, angioedema, urticaria, flushing, allergic dermatitis, and bronchospasm have been reported with mometasone furoate oral inhalation therapy in clinical trials and during postmarketing experience. Orally inhaled mometasone furoate should be discontinued if such reactions occur.

Mometasone furoate oral inhalation powder contains small amounts of lactose with trace amounts of milk proteins. Anaphylactic reactions in patients with milk protein allergy have been reported; therefore, patients with known milk protein allergy should not receive this preparation of mometasone furoate. (See Cautions: Contraindications.)

Risk of Serious Asthma-related Events Monotherapy with long-acting β_2-adrenergic agonists, such as formoterol, a component of the mometasone/formoterol fixed combination, increases the risk of asthma-related death. Data from a large placebo-controlled safety study (Salmeterol Multi-center Asthma Research Trial [SMART]) evaluating the safety of another long-acting β_2-adrenergic agonist, salmeterol, in patients with asthma showed an increase in asthma-related deaths in patients receiving salmeterol. (See Asthma-related Death and Life-threatening Events under Cautions: Respiratory Effects, in Salmeterol 12:12.08.12.) In addition, available data from controlled clinical trials suggest that monotherapy with long-acting β_2-adrenergic agonists increases the risk of asthma-related hospitalization in pediatric and adolescent patients.

However, FDA has concluded that there is no clinically important increased risk of serious asthma-related events, including hospitalization, intubation, or death, associated with concomitant use of long-acting β_2-adrenergic agonists (e.g., formoterol) and inhaled corticosteroids (e.g., mometasone) compared with inhaled corticosteroids alone based on the results of several large clinical studies. In addition, these studies showed that combination therapy with long-acting β_2-adrenergic agonists and inhaled corticosteroids was more effective in reducing the incidence of asthma exacerbations (i.e., events requiring use of systemic corticosteroids for at least 3 outpatient days or an asthma-related hospitalization or emergency department visit requiring use of systemic corticosteroids) compared with use of inhaled corticosteroids alone. (See Asthma-related Death and Serious Asthma-related Events under Warnings/Precautions: Warnings, in Cautions, in Formoterol Fumarate 12:12.08.12.)

In the treatment of asthma, the mometasone/formoterol fixed combination should be used only in patients who have not responded adequately to long-term asthma controller therapy, such as inhaled corticosteroids, or whose disease severity warrants initiation of treatment with both an inhaled corticosteroid and a long-acting β_2-adrenergic agonist.

Specific Populations **Pregnancy.** Category C. (See Users Guide.)

There are no adequate and well-controlled studies with mometasone furoate in pregnant women. The drug should be used during pregnancy only if potential benefits justify potential risks to the fetus.

There is an increased risk of adverse perinatal outcomes (e.g., preeclampsia, premature birth, low birth weight, neonates small for gestational age) in women with poorly or moderately controlled asthma. Pregnant women with asthma should be closely monitored and therapy adjusted as necessary to maintain optimal asthma control.

The effects of mometasone furoate in fixed combination with formoterol fumarate during labor and delivery are not known. Because of the potential for β-agonist interference with uterine contractility, use of the mometasone/formoterol fixed combination during labor should be restricted to those patients in whom the benefits clearly outweigh the risks.

Hypoadrenalism may occur in infants of women who have received substantial oral corticosteroid dosages during pregnancy. These infants should be carefully monitored.

Lactation. It is not known whether mometasone furoate is distributed into milk; however, other corticosteroids are distributed into milk. Data are not available on the effects of the drug on the breast-fed child or milk production. The benefits of breast-feeding and the importance of mometasone to the woman should be considered along with any potential adverse effects on the breast-fed infant from the drug or underlying maternal condition. The manufacturer of mometasone oral inhalation powder (Asmanex® Twisthaler®) states that caution is advised if mometasone furoate is administered in nursing women.

The manufacturer of the mometasone/formoterol fixed combination states that a decision should be made whether to discontinue nursing or the drug, taking into account the importance of the drug to the woman.

Pediatric Use. Safety and efficacy of mometasone furoate oral inhalation powder have not been established in children younger than 4 years of age.

Safety and efficacy of mometasone furoate oral inhalation aerosol have not been established in children younger than 12 years of age.

Safety and efficacy of the mometasone/formoterol fixed combination have not been established in children younger than 12 years of age.

Use of corticosteroids may lead to suppression of growth in children and adolescents. Therefore, pediatric patients receiving prolonged therapy with orally inhaled mometasone should be monitored periodically (e.g., via stadiometry) for possible adverse effects on growth and development. The benefits of corticosteroid therapy should be weighed against the possibility of growth suppression and the availability of safe and effective alternative therapies. Pediatric patients should be maintained on the lowest possible dosage of mometasone that controls asthma symptoms. (See Cautions: Pediatric Precautions, in the Corticosteroids General Statement 68:04.)

Geriatric Use. Although no overall differences in safety and efficacy of orally inhaled mometasone furoate were observed in geriatric patients relative to younger adults, the possibility that some older patients may exhibit increased sensitivity to the drug cannot be ruled out.

■ **Common Adverse Effects** Adverse effects occurring in 5% or more of patients receiving mometasone furoate oral inhalation powder for the treatment of asthma include headache, allergic rhinitis, pharyngitis, upper respiratory tract infection, sinusitis, oral candidiasis, dysmenorrhea, musculoskeletal pain, back pain, and dyspepsia.

Adverse effects occurring in 3% or more of patients receiving mometasone furoate oral inhalation aerosol for the treatment of asthma include nasopharyngitis, headache, sinusitis, bronchitis, and influenza.

Adverse effects occurring in 3% or more of patients receiving the mometasone/formoterol fixed combination for the treatment of asthma and more frequently than in those receiving placebo include nasopharyngitis, sinusitis, and headache.

Drug Interactions

The following information addresses potential interactions with mometasone furoate. When mometasone furoate is used in fixed combination with formoterol fumarate (mometasone/formoterol), interactions associated with formoterol also should be considered. No formal drug interaction studies have been performed to date with the mometasone/formoterol fixed combination.

■ **Drugs Affecting Hepatic Microsomal Enzymes** ***Drugs that Inhibit Isoenzyme CYP3A4*** Since mometasone furoate is principally metabolized in the liver by the cytochrome P-450 (CYP) 3A4 isoenzyme, concomitant use with drugs that are potent inhibitors of the CYP3A4 isoenzyme (e.g., atazanavir, clarithromycin, cobicistat-containing preparations, indinavir, itraconazole, ketoconazole, nefazodone, nelfinavir, ritonavir, saquinavir) may result in increased plasma mometasone concentrations.

Caution should be exercised when considering concomitant use of mometasone furoate with ketoconazole and other known inhibitors of the CYP3A4 isoenzyme. The benefits of such concomitant use should be weighed against the risk of systemic corticosteroid effects. If concomitant use is necessary, patients should be monitored for adverse systemic corticosteroid effects related to increased systemic exposure to mometasone furoate.

Description

Mometasone furoate is a synthetic nonfluorinated glucocorticoid. For a discussion of the pharmacology of mometasone, see Pharmacology in the Corticosteroids General Statement 68:04.

Systemic bioavailability of mometasone furoate following oral inhalation of a single 400-mcg dose is reported to be less than 1%. Most of an orally inhaled dose of the drug is swallowed and excreted unchanged in feces. Any systemically absorbed drug is extensively metabolized in the liver, principally by the cytochrome P-450 (CYP) 3A4 isoenzyme, and is excreted principally in feces and to a lesser extent in urine.

Advice to Patients

When mometasone furoate is used in fixed combination with formoterol fumarate, importance of informing patients of important cautionary information about formoterol fumarate.

Importance of instructing patients to read manufacturer's patient instructions prior to initiation of therapy.

Importance of pediatric patients receiving therapy under adult supervision.

Importance of adequate understanding of proper storage, preparation, and inhalation techniques, including use of the oral inhalation delivery systems.

Importance of informing clinician of any history of hypersensitivity reactions to mometasone or other ingredients in the formulations or of known allergy to milk proteins.

Importance of rinsing the mouth with water without swallowing after oral inhalation.

Importance of advising patients that mometasone furoate oral inhalation must be used at regular intervals to be therapeutically effective. Importance of adherence to prescribed dosage regimen; do not increase the frequency of administration without consulting a clinician.

Importance of advising patients that if a dose of mometasone furoate alone or in fixed combination with formoterol fumarate is missed, the next dose should be taken at the regularly scheduled time; the dose should not be doubled.

Importance of advising patients that at least 1–2 weeks of continuous therapy may be required for optimum effects to be achieved. Importance of contacting a clinician if asthma symptoms do not improve in such a time frame.

Importance of advising patients that orally inhaled mometasone furoate should not be used as a bronchodilator and that the drug is not indicated for emergency use (e.g., relief of acute bronchospasm).

Importance of availability and use of a short-acting β_2-adrenergic agonist for relief of acute asthma symptoms.

Importance of contacting a clinician immediately when asthmatic attacks are not controlled by current bronchodilator therapy.

Importance of gradual withdrawal from systemic corticosteroids during transfer to orally inhaled mometasone furoate and of monitoring by a clinician during such transfer of therapy. (See Conversion to Orally Inhaled Therapy in Patients Receiving Systemic Corticosteroids under Dosage: Asthma, in Dosage and Administration.)

Importance of advising patients being transferred from systemic corticosteroid to mometasone furoate oral inhalation therapy to carry special identification (e.g., card) indicating the need for supplementary systemic corticosteroids during periods of stress or severe exacerbation of asthma. Importance of advising patients to immediately resume therapy with large doses of systemic corticosteroids and contact their clinician for further instructions during stressful periods (e.g., stress, severe asthmatic attack, surgery, trauma, infection).

Importance of informing patients that corticosteroids may decrease bone mineral density. (See Musculoskeletal Effects under Cautions: Warnings/Precautions.)

Risk of localized candidal infections of mouth and pharynx. (See Localized Candidal Infections under Cautions: Warnings/Precautions.)

Risk for development of cataracts or glaucoma associated with long-term use of inhaled corticosteroids (e.g., mometasone). Importance of reporting any vision changes to a clinician. (See Ophthalmic Effects under Cautions: Warnings/Precautions.)

Risk of systemic corticosteroid effects (e.g., hypercorticism, potentially life-threatening adrenal suppression). Importance of informing a clinician of fatigue, weakness, nausea, vomiting, dizziness, or fainting. (See Systemic Corticosteroid Effects under Cautions: Warnings/Precautions.)

Risk of reduction in growth velocity in children and adolescents with orally inhaled corticosteroids. (See Pediatric Use under Warnings/Precautions: Specific Populations, in Cautions.)

Importance of immunosuppressed patients avoiding exposure to chickenpox or measles, and, if exposed, of immediately consulting a clinician. (See Immunosuppressed Patients under Cautions: Warnings/Precautions.)

Importance of advising immunosuppressed patients of potential worsening of existing tuberculosis; fungal, bacterial, parasitic, or viral infections; or ocular herpes simplex. Importance of immunosuppressed patients informing clinician of a history of infections.

Importance of women informing clinicians if they are or plan to become pregnant or plan to breast-feed.

Importance of informing clinicians of existing or contemplated concomitant therapy, including prescription (e.g., anticonvulsants, systemic corticosteroids) and OTC drugs, as well as any concomitant illnesses (e.g., infections).

Importance of informing patients of other important precautionary information. (See Cautions.)

Overview® (see Users Guide). For additional information on this drug until a more detailed monograph is developed and published, the manufacturer's labeling should be consulted. It is *essential* that the manufacturer's labeling be consulted for more detailed information on usual cautions, precautions, contraindications, potential drug interactions, laboratory test interferences, and acute toxicity.

Preparations

Excipients in commercially available drug preparations may have clinically important effects in some individuals; consult specific product labeling for details.

Mometasone Furoate

Oral Inhalation		
Aerosol	100 mcg per metered spray	**Asmanex® HFA** (with hydrofluoroalkane propellant), Merck
	200 mcg per metered spray	**Asmanex® HFA** (with hydrofluoroalkane propellant), Merck
Powder, for oral inhalation	110 mcg (delivers 100 mcg per inhalation)	**Asmanex® Twisthaler®**, Teva
	220 mcg (delivers 200 mcg per inhalation)	**Asmanex® Twisthaler®**, Teva

Mometasone Furoate Combinations

Oral Inhalation		
Aerosol	100 mcg with Formoterol Fumarate Dihydrate 5 mcg per metered spray	**Dulera®** (with hydrofluoroalkane propellant), Merck
	200 mcg with Formoterol Fumarate Dihydrate 5 mcg per metered spray	**Dulera®** (with hydrofluoroalkane propellant), Merck

Prasterone

Dehydroepiandrosterone, DHEA

■ Prasterone is an inactive endogenous steroid that is converted intracellularly into active androgens and/or estrogens.

Uses

■ **Dyspareunia** Prasterone is used for the treatment of moderate to severe dyspareunia, a symptom of vulvar and vaginal atrophy, associated with menopause.

The safety and efficacy of prasterone vaginal inserts were evaluated in 2 randomized, double-blind, placebo-controlled trials of 12 weeks' duration and 1 open-label trial of 52 weeks' duration in healthy postmenopausal women with signs of vulvar and vaginal atrophy (defined as having 5% or fewer superficial cells on a vaginal smear and a vaginal pH of greater than 5) who identified moderate to severe dyspareunia as their most bothersome symptom.

The primary efficacy outcomes in both 12-week studies were the change in percentage of vaginal parabasal cells, percentage of vaginal superficial cells, change in vaginal pH, and mean change from baseline in severity of the most bothersome moderate to severe symptom of dyspareunia; symptoms were rated by the patients using a 4-point scale [0, none; 1, mild; 2, moderate; 3, severe]). The first study evaluated 255 postmenopausal women with vulvar and vaginal atrophy who reported moderate to severe dyspareunia as their most bothersome symptom. Patients were randomized in a 1:1:1 ratio to receive intravaginal administration of prasterone 3.25 or 6.5 mg or placebo once daily for 12 weeks. Baseline characteristics were similar among groups (mean age 58.6 years, mean time since last menstrual period 14.5 years, 92% white). Reduction of the mean severity score from baseline to 12 weeks was substantially greater in patients receiving prasterone 6.5 mg compared with those receiving placebo (−1.27 versus −0.87, respectively). The percentage of parabasal cells on vaginal smear between baseline and 12 weeks decreased by 37.3 or 47.4% in patients receiving prasterone 3.25 or 6.5 mg daily, respectively, compared with a decrease of 1.6% in those receiving placebo. Patients receiving prasterone 3.25 or 6.5 mg daily showed an increased percentage of superficial cells on the vaginal smear (increase of 4.8 or 5.6%, respectively) compared with those receiving placebo (increase of 0.9%). Over the same time period, vaginal pH decreased by 0.78 or 1.04 in patients receiving prasterone 3.25 or 6.5 mg daily, respectively, compared with a decrease of 0.2 in those receiving placebo.

The second study evaluated 558 postmenopausal women with vulvar and vaginal atrophy who reported moderate to severe dyspareunia as the most bothersome symptom at baseline. Patients were randomized in a 2:1 ratio to receive intravaginal administration of prasterone 6.5 mg or placebo once daily for 12 weeks. At 12 weeks, reduction of the mean severity score for dyspareunia (compared with baseline values) was substantially greater in patients receiving prasterone compared with those receiving placebo (−1.42 versus −1.06, respectively). The mean decrease from baseline to 12 weeks in the percentage of parabasal cells on the vaginal smear was 41.5% in patients receiving prasterone compared with 12% in those receiving placebo; the mean percentage of superficial cells on the vaginal smear increased by 10.2 or 1.75% in patients receiving prasterone or placebo, respectively. During the same time period, the mean decrease in vaginal pH was 0.94 in patients receiving prasterone and 0.27 in those receiving placebo.

In an open-label, 52-week study, 521 postmenopausal women (mean age 57.9 years, mean time since last menstrual period 8.4 years, 92% white) received prasterone 6.5 mg intravaginally once daily. Reduction of the mean severity score from baseline to 12 weeks was −1.37 and the severity score continued to decrease at weeks 26 and 52 (−1.6 and −1.7, respectively, from baseline). At week 52, the percentage of parabasal cells decreased by 42.68%, the percentage of superficial cells increased by 7.4%, and vaginal pH decreased by 1.14 compared with baseline values. Most of the changes in the percentage of parabasal and superficial cells and vaginal pH were observed by week 12 of treatment, but continued improvement was demonstrated after 26 and 52 weeks of treatment.

Dosage and Administration

■ **Administration** Prasterone vaginal inserts are administered intravaginally using the disposable applicator provided by the manufacturer.

■ **Dosage** *Dyspareunia* For the treatment of moderate to severe dyspareunia associated with menopause, the recommended dosage of prasterone is 6.5 mg (1 vaginal insert) once daily at bedtime.

■ **Special Populations** *Hepatic Impairment* The manufacturer makes no specific recommendations for prasterone dosage adjustments in patients with hepatic impairment. The drug has not been studied in such patients.

Renal Impairment The manufacturer makes no specific recommendations for prasterone dosage adjustments in patients with renal impairment. The drug has not been studied in such patients.

Cautions

■ **Contraindications** Prasterone is contraindicated in postmenopausal women with undiagnosed abnormal genital bleeding. The cause of undiagnosed, persistent, or recurrent genital bleeding should be determined prior to considering therapy with the drug.

■ **Warnings/Precautions** *Breast Cancer* Estrogen is a metabolite of prasterone. Use of exogenous estrogen is contraindicated in women with a known or suspected history of breast cancer. Prasterone has not been studied in women with a history of breast cancer.

Specific Populations **Pregnancy.** Prasterone has not been studied in pregnant women and animal reproduction studies have not been conducted. The manufacturer states that the drug is labeled for use only in postmenopausal women.

Lactation. It is not known whether prasterone is distributed into human milk. Effects of the drug on the breast-fed infant or milk production also are unknown.

Pediatric Use. Safety and efficacy of prasterone have not been established in pediatric patients; the drug is not indicated in pediatric patients.

Geriatric Use. Of the prasterone-treated postmenopausal women enrolled in the placebo-controlled 12-week clinical trials and the open-label 52-week study, 19 and 11% of patients, respectively, were 65 years of age or older.

Hepatic Impairment. The effect of hepatic impairment on the pharmacokinetics of prasterone has not been studied.

Renal Impairment. The effect of renal impairment on the pharmacokinetics of prasterone has not been studied.

■ **Common Adverse Effects** In the 12-week, placebo-controlled trials, vaginal discharge occurred in at least 2% of patients receiving prasterone and more frequently than in those receiving placebo. Adverse effects occurring in at least 2% of patients receiving prasterone for up to 52 weeks included vaginal discharge and abnormal Papanicolaou test (Pap smear).

Drug Interactions

Drug interaction studies have not been performed using prasterone vaginal inserts.

Description

Prasterone (i.e., dehydroepiandrosterone [DHEA]) is an inactive endogenous steroid that is converted intracellularly into active androgens and/or estrogens. Although the exact mechanism of action of prasterone in the treatment of vulvar and vaginal atrophy in postmenopausal women is not fully established, clinical studies demonstrate that intravaginal application of the drug exhibits both androgenic and estrogenic activity. (See Uses: Dyspareunia.) Intravaginal administration of prasterone for up to 52 weeks does not have a stimulatory effect on the endometrium, but an increased incidence of abnormal Papanicolaou test (Pap smear) results was observed.

Following administration of prasterone 6.5 mg intravaginally for 7 days, the mean peak plasma concentrations and AUC of prasterone were substantially higher than those in patients who received placebo. At 12 weeks, serum trough prasterone concentrations increased 47% from baseline. Exogenous and endogenous prasterone are metabolized by human steroidogenic enzymes (e.g., hydroxysteroid dehydrogenases, 5α-reductases, aromatases) to form androgen and estrogen metabolites. Peak plasma concentrations of testosterone and estradiol, metabolites of prasterone, were slightly higher in patients receiving prasterone than in those who received placebo; after intravaginal administration of prasterone for 12 weeks, testosterone and estradiol serum trough concentrations increased 21 and 19%, respectively, from baseline. However, systemic concentrations of estrogens and androgens remained within the expected range for postmenopausal women.

Advice to Patients

Importance of instructing patients to read the manufacturer's patient information and instructions for use prior to initiation of therapy.

Importance of instructing patients to empty their bladder and wash their hands before handling the vaginal insert and applicator.

Importance of informing patients that vaginal discharge or abnormal Papanicolaou test (Pap smear) results may occur.

Importance of informing clinicians of existing or contemplated concomitant therapy, including prescription and OTC drugs, as well as any concomitant illnesses.

Importance of women informing clinicians if they are or plan to become pregnant or plan to breast-feed.

Importance of informing patients of other important precautionary information. (See Cautions.)

Overview® (see Users Guide). For additional information on this drug until a more detailed monograph is developed and published, the manufacturer's labeling should be consulted. It is *essential* that the manufacturer's labeling be consulted for more detailed information on usual cautions, precautions, contraindications, potential drug interactions, laboratory test interferences, and acute toxicity.

Preparations

Excipients in commercially available drug preparations may have clinically important effects in some individuals; consult specific product labeling for details.

Prasterone

Vaginal

Insert	6.5 mg	**Intrarosa® (with disposable applicators),** AMAG Pharmaceuticals Inc.

prednisoLONE

Deltahydrocortisone, Metacortandralone

■ Prednisolone is a synthetic glucocorticoid.

Uses

Prednisolone is used principally as an anti-inflammatory or immunosuppressant agent. Because prednisolone has only minimal mineralocorticoid properties, the drug is inadequate alone for the management of adrenocortical insufficiency. If prednisolone is used in the treatment of this condition, concomitant therapy with a mineralocorticoid is also required.

Dosage and Administration

■ **Dosage** The dosage of prednisolone and its derivatives depends on the condition being treated and the response of the patient. Dosage for infants and children should be based on the severity of the disease and the response of the patient rather than on strict adherence to dosage indicated by age, body weight, or body surface area. After a satisfactory response is obtained, dosage should be decreased in small decrements to the lowest level that maintains an adequate clinical response. Patients should be continually monitored for signs that indicate dosage adjustment is necessary, such as remissions or exacerbations of the disease and stress (surgery, infection, trauma). When long-term oral prednisolone therapy is necessary, an alternate-day dosage regimen should be considered. Following long-term therapy, prednisolone should be withdrawn gradually. (See the Corticosteroids General Statement 68:04.)

Prednisolone Prednisolone is administered orally. The initial adult dosage of prednisolone may range from 5–60 mg daily, depending on the disease being treated, and is usually administered in 2–4 divided doses. Some clinicians state that children may be given a prednisolone dosage of 0.14–2 mg/kg daily or 4–60 mg/m² daily, administered in 4 divided doses.

Prednisolone Sodium Phosphate Prednisolone sodium phosphate is administered orally as a solution or orally disintegrating tablets; the drug also has been given by IM, IV, intra-articular, intralesional, or soft tissue injection or by IV infusion (a parenteral preparation of prednisolone sodium phosphate no longer is commercially available in the US). Patients should be instructed not to remove the orally disintegrating tablet from the blister card until just prior to dosing. Prednisolone sodium phosphate orally disintegrating tablets should be allowed to dissolve on the tongue or should be swallowed whole with or without water; the tablets should not be broken. If the dosage of prednisolone required does not correspond to the strength of the commercially available prednisolone sodium phosphate orally disintegrating tablets, another formulation of prednisolone should be used.

Dosage of prednisolone sodium phosphate is expressed in terms of prednisolone. The amount of drug each patient receives should be individualized according to diagnosis, severity, and patient response. The initial dosage of prednisolone ranges from 5–60 mg daily depending on the disease being treated. In less severe diseases, a lower dosage may be sufficient, while in selected patients with severe disease, dosages greater than the initial dosage may be required. In pediatric patients, the initial dosage of prednisolone may range from 0.14–2 mg/kg daily in 3 or 4 divided doses or 4–60 mg/m² daily. The initial dosage should be maintained or adjusted until a satisfactory response is obtained. Patients should be continually monitored for signs that indicate dosage adjustment is necessary, such as remission or exacerbations of disease and stress. Patients may require higher dosages of prednisolone when they are subjected to stress. Following long-term therapy, prednisolone should be withdrawn gradually. (See Discontinuance of Therapy under Dosage and Administration: Dosage, in the Corticosteroids General Statement 68:04.)

Multiple Sclerosis. For the treatment of acute exacerbations of multiple sclerosis, the usual oral dosage of prednisolone is 200 mg daily for one week, followed by 80 mg every other day for a month.

Nephrotic Syndrome. In the treatment of nephrotic syndrome in children, the usual oral dosage of prednisolone solution is 60 mg/m² daily given in 3 divided doses for 4 weeks, followed by 4 weeks of alternate-day therapy at single doses of 40 mg/m².

Asthma. To gain prompt control of asthma in infants and children 4 years of age or younger with very poorly controlled, moderate-to-severe asthma (i.e., more than 3 exacerbations per year requiring oral corticosteroids) and in children 5–11 years of age with asthma of comparable control and severity (i.e., at least 2 exacerbations per year requiring oral corticosteroids), prednisolone 1–2 mg/kg daily (maximum 60 mg daily) may be added to existing asthma therapy. In adults and adolescents with very poorly controlled, moderate-to-severe asthma (i.e. at least 2 exacerbations per year requiring oral corticosteroids), prednisolone 40–60 mg daily as a single dose or in 2 divided doses may be added to low-to-high maintenance dosages of the inhaled corticosteroid and a long-acting inhaled β_2-agonist bronchodilator. A short course of oral corticosteroid therapy (usually 3–10 days) should be continued until the patient achieves a peak expiratory flow (PEF) of at least 80% of his or her personal best and until symptoms resolve. However, a longer duration of treatment may be needed in some patients. There is no evidence that tapering the dosage after improvement will prevent a relapse.

For the treatment of moderate-to-severe exacerbations of asthma associated with a viral respiratory infection in infants and children 4 years of age or younger with intermittent asthma, prednisolone 1 mg/kg daily for 3–10 days or equivalent daily dosage should be considered. For those with a history of viral-associated severe asthma exacerbations, initiation of oral corticosteroids should be considered at the first sign of infection.

For the treatment of acute asthma exacerbations in the community setting, 0.5–1 mg/kg of prednisolone or equivalent during a 24-hour period is recommended to quickly resolve all but the mildest exacerbations of asthma, especially in patients whose response to a short-acting inhaled β_2-agonist is not prompt or sustained. For emergency department treatment of moderate-to-severe acute asthma exacerbations not controlled with an inhaled β_2-adrenergic agonist in children 11 years of age or younger, prednisolone 1–2 mg/kg daily in 2 divided doses (maximum 60 mg daily) can be added. For treatment of such exacerbations in adults and adolescents, prednisolone 40–80 mg daily as a single dose or in 2 divided doses can be added to an inhaled β_2-agonist. Treatment should be continued until the patient achieves a PEF of 70% of predicted or personal best. For additional information on the stepped-care approach to drug therapy in asthma, see Asthma under Uses: Respiratory Diseases, in the Corticosteroids General Statement 68:04.

Chemistry and Stability

■ Chemistry Prednisolone is a synthetic glucocorticoid. Prednisolone occurs as white to practically white, odorless, crystalline powder. Prednisolone, which may be anhydrous or contain 1.5 molecules of water of hydration, is very slightly soluble in water and sparingly soluble in alcohol. The sodium phosphate ester of prednisolone occurs as white or slightly yellow, friable granules or powder which is odorless or has a slight odor and is freely soluble in water, soluble in methanol, slightly soluble in alcohol and chloroform, and very slightly soluble in acetone and dioxane. The sodium phosphate ester of prednisolone is hygroscopic. Each 6.7 mg of prednisolone sodium phosphate is equivalent to 5 mg of prednisolone.

■ Stability Commercially available preparations of prednisolone should be stored at a temperature less than 40°C, preferably between 15–30°C; freezing of the oral solutions should be avoided. Prednisolone oral solution should be stored at 15–30°C; such solutions should not be refrigerated. Prednisolone sodium phosphate oral solution (Pediapred®) should be stored at 4–25°C and may be refrigerated. Prednisolone sodium phosphate oral solutions (Orapred® and some generic preparations) should be stored at 2–8°C. Prednisolone sodium phosphate orally disintegrating tablets (Orapred ODT®) should be stored at 20–25°C and protected from moisture. Prednisolone and prednisolone sodium phosphate oral solutions should be protected from light. Solutions of prednisolone and its derivatives are heat labile and must not be autoclaved.

For further information on chemistry, pharmacology, pharmacokinetics, uses, cautions, drug interactions, laboratory test interferences, and dosage and administration of prednisolone, see the Corticosteroids General Statement 68:04. For EENT uses, see 52:08.08.

Preparations

Excipients in commercially available drug preparations may have clinically important effects in some individuals; consult specific product labeling for details.

prednisoLONE

Oral		
Solution	5 mg/5 mL*	**Prednisolone Syrup**
	15 mg/5 mL*	**Prednisolone Syrup**
		Prelone® Syrup, Aero
Tablets	5 mg*	**Prednisolone Tablets**

*available from one or more manufacturer, distributor, and/or repackager by generic (nonproprietary) name

prednisoLONE Sodium Phosphate

Oral		
Solution	5 mg (of prednisolone) per 5 mL*	**Pediapred®**, Celltech
		Prednisolone Sodium Phosphate Oral Solution
	15 mg (of prednisolone) per 5 mL	**Orapred®**, BioMarin
		Prednisolone Sodium Phosphate Oral Solution
Tablets, orally disintegrating	10 mg (of prednisolone)	**Orapred ODT®**, Alliant
	15 mg (of prednisolone)	**Orapred ODT®**, Alliant
	30 mg (of prednisolone)	**Orapred ODT®**, Alliant

*available from one or more manufacturer, distributor, and/or repackager by generic (nonproprietary) name

predniSONE

Deltacortisone, Deltadehydrocortisone

■ Prednisone is a synthetic glucocorticoid.

Uses

Prednisone is usually considered the oral glucocorticoid of choice for anti-inflammatory or immunosuppressant effects. Because it has only minimal mineralocorticoid properties, the drug is inadequate alone for the management of adrenocortical insufficiency. If prednisone is used in the treatment of this condition, concomitant therapy with a mineralocorticoid is also required.

Dosage and Administration

■ Administration Prednisone is administered orally. For patients unable to swallow tablets, prednisone may be administered orally as a commercially available solution, concentrate solution, or an extemporaneously prepared suspension. The oral concentrate may be diluted in juice or other flavored diluent or in semisolid food (e.g., applesauce) prior to administration.

An extemporaneous prednisone suspension containing 10 mg/mL can be prepared in the following manner. First, 5 g of prednisone as tablets is mixed with 200 mL of 0.1% sodium benzoate solution; 100 mL of an aqueous suspension containing 3% tragacanth, 3% acacia, and 0.1% sodium benzoate is then added, and the mixture is stirred until homogeneous. When the prednisone suspension is diluted to 500 mL with a mixture of 67% simple syrup and 33% cherry syrup, it contains prednisone 10 mg/mL and is apparently stable for 2 months at 2–8°C. (4 L of the tragacanth-acacia suspension may be prepared in a container that can be closed for vigorous agitation. Initially, 4 g of sodium benzoate is dissolved in 2 L of purified water. Then 120 g of powdered tragacanth and 120 g of acacia are added in that order and the container shaken vigorously. Additional water is added gradually over 24–48 hours with agitation at regular intervals until a volume of 4 L and a smooth suspension results. To mask the odor, 1 mL of anise oil may be added.)

■ Dosage Dosage of prednisone depends on the condition being treated and the response of the patient. Dosage for infants and children should be based on the severity of the disease and the response of the patient rather than on strict adherence to dosage indicated by age, body weight, or body surface area. After a satisfactory response is obtained, dosage should be decreased in small decrements to the lowest level that maintains an adequate clinical response. The drug should be discontinued as soon as possible. Patients should be continually monitored for signs that indicate dosage adjustment is necessary, such as remissions or exacerbations of the disease and stress (surgery, infection, trauma). When long-term prednisone therapy is necessary, an alternate-day dosage regimen should be considered. Following long-term therapy, prednisone should be withdrawn gradually. (See the Corticosteroids General Statement 68:04.)

The initial adult dosage of prednisone may range from 5–60 mg daily, depending on the disease being treated, and is usually administered in 2–4 divided doses. Some clinicians state that children may be given a dosage of 0.14–2 mg/kg daily or 4–60 mg/m² daily, administered in 4 divided doses.

Pneumocystis carinii Pneumonia For use as an adjunct to anti-infective therapy in the treatment of moderate to severe *Pneumocystis carinii* pneumonia in adults and adolescents older than 13 years of age with acquired immunodeficiency syndrome† (AIDS), an oral prednisone regimen of 40 mg twice daily for 5 days, followed by 40 mg once daily for 5 days, and then 20 mg once daily for 11 days (or until completion of the anti-infective regimen) currently is recommended. Such adjunctive glucocorticoid therapy preferably should be initiated within 24–72 hours of initial antipneumocystis therapy. However, it should be recognized that this recommendation is based on limited data and may not represent the optimum dosage and schedule. Therefore, clinicians should consult published protocols and the most current clinical guidelines. Shorter courses of therapy would be desirable, but rebound deterioration in pulmonary function has occurred in some patients following discontinuance of glucocortical therapy, and some clinicians discourage the use of shorter treatment courses.

Allergic Conditions For certain allergic conditions (e.g., contact dermatitis including poison ivy), prednisone may be administered for short-term use (e.g., 6 days) using 5-mg tablets; the recommended initial dosage is 30 mg (6 tablets) for the first day, which is then tapered by 5 mg daily until 21 tablets have been administered. On the first day, 10 mg (2 tablets) is administered twice daily (before breakfast and at bedtime) and 5 mg (1 tablet) is administered twice daily (after lunch and dinner). On the second day, 5 mg (1 tablet) is administered 3 times daily (before breakfast, after lunch, and after dinner) and 10 mg (2 tablets) is administered at bedtime. On the third day, 5 mg (1 tablet) is administered 4 times daily (before breakfast, after lunch, after dinner, and at bedtime). On the fourth day, 5 mg (1 tablet) is administered 3 times daily (before breakfast, after lunch, and at bedtime). On the fifth day, 5 mg (1 tablet) is administered twice daily (before breakfast and at bedtime). On the sixth day, 5 mg (1 tablet) is administered before breakfast.

Asthma To gain prompt control of asthma in infants and children 4 years of age or younger with very poorly controlled, moderate-to-severe asthma (i.e., more than 3 exacerbations per year requiring oral corticosteroids) and in children 5–11 years of age with asthma of comparable control and severity (i.e., at least 2 exacerbations per year requiring oral corticosteroids), prednisone 1–2 mg/kg daily (maximum 60 mg daily) may be added to existing asthma therapy. In adults and adolescents with very poorly controlled, moderate-to-severe asthma (i.e., at least 2 exacerbations per year requiring oral corticosteroids), prednisone 40–60 mg daily as a single dose or in 2 divided doses may be added to low-to-high maintenance dosages of the inhaled corticosteroid and a long-acting inhaled β_2-agonist bronchodilator. A short course of oral corticosteroid therapy (usually 3–10 days) should be continued until the patient achieves a peak expiratory flow (PEF) of at least 80% of his or her personal best and until symptoms resolve. However, a longer duration of treatment may be needed in some patients. There is no evidence that tapering the dosage after improvement will prevent a relapse.

For the treatment of moderate-to-severe exacerbations of asthma associated with a viral respiratory infection in infants and children 4 years of age or younger with intermittent asthma, prednisone 1 mg/kg daily for 3–10 days or equivalent daily dosage should be considered. For those with a history of viral-associated severe asthma exacerbations, initiation of oral corticosteroids should be considered at the first sign of infection.

For the treatment of acute asthma exacerbations in the community setting, 0.5–1 mg/kg of prednisone or equivalent during a 24-hour period is recommended to quickly resolve all but the mildest exacerbations of asthma, especially in patients whose response to a short-acting inhaled β_2-agonist is not prompt or sustained. For emergency department treatment of moderate-to-severe acute asthma exacerbations not controlled with an inhaled β_2-adrenergic agonist in children 11 years of age or younger, prednisone 1–2 mg/kg daily in

2 divided doses (maximum 60 mg daily) can be added. For treatment of such exacerbations in adults and adolescents, prednisone 40–80 mg daily as a single dose or in 2 divided doses can be added to an inhaled β_2-adrenergic agonist. Treatment should be continued until the patient achieves a PEF of 70% of predicted or personal best. For additional information on the stepped-care approach to drug therapy in asthma, see Asthma under Uses: Respiratory Diseases, in the Corticosteroids General Statement 68:04.

Advanced Pulmonary or Extrapulmonary Tuberculosis For enhancing resolution of severe systemic and respiratory complications of advanced pulmonary tuberculosis, corticosteroid dosages equivalent to 40–60 mg daily of prednisone, tapered over 4–8 weeks, have been used. (See Advanced Pulmonary and Extrapulmonary Tuberculosis under Uses: Respiratory Diseases, in the Corticosteroids General Statement 68:04.) A prednisone dosage of 1 mg/kg daily for 30 days, followed by gradual tapering of the dosage over a period of weeks, has been suggested in patients with tuberculous meningitis. Tuberculous pericarditis has been treated with prednisone (or prednisolone) dosages of 60 mg daily tapered over 6–12 weeks. For the treatment of pain, dyspnea, and fever associated with tuberculous pleurisy, corticosteroid dosages equivalent to 20–40 mg daily of prednisone tapered over 4–8 weeks have been suggested. Prednisone 2–5 mg/kg per day (or equivalent), with dosage reduction to 1 mg/kg per day over the first week and tapered over the next 5 weeks, has been used to hasten resolution of mediastinal lymphadenopathy associated with primary intrathoracic tuberculosis.

Chemistry and Stability

■ **Chemistry** Prednisone is a synthetic glucocorticoid. Prednisone occurs as a white to practically white, odorless, crystalline powder and is very slightly soluble in water and slightly soluble in alcohol. Prednisone oral solution has a pH of 2.6–3.6 and contains 4–6% alcohol, and the oral concentrate solution has a pH of 3–4 and contains about 30% alcohol.

■ **Stability** Prednisone tablets should be stored in well-closed containers at a temperature less than 40°C, preferably between 15–30°C. Prednisone oral solution and oral concentrate solution should be stored in tight containers at 15–30°C.

For further information on chemistry, pharmacology, uses, pharmacokinetics, cautions, drug interactions, laboratory test interferences, and dosage and administration of prednisone, see the Corticosteroids General Statement 68:04.

Preparations

Excipients in commercially available drug preparations may have clinically important effects in some individuals; consult specific product labeling for details.

predniSONE

Powder		
Oral		
Solution	5 mg/5 mL	**predniSONE Oral Solution,** Roxane
Solution, concentrate	5 mg/mL	**predniSONE Intensol®**, Roxane
Tablets	1 mg*	**predniSONE Tablets**
	2.5 mg*	**predniSONE Tablets**
	5 mg*	**Sterapred® 5 mg Unipak®**, Merz
		Sterapred® 5 mg 12 Day Unipak®, Merz
	10 mg*	**Sterapred® DS Unipak®**, Merz
		Sterapred® DS 12 Day Unipak®, Merz
	20 mg*	**predniSONE Tablets**
	50 mg*	**predniSONE Tablets**

*available from one or more manufacturer, distributor, and/or repackager by generic (nonproprietary) name

†Use is not currently included in the labeling approved by the US Food and Drug Administration

Selected Revisions March 2010,

Triamcinolone

■ Triamcinolone is a synthetic glucocorticoid.

Uses

Triamcinolone is used principally as an anti-inflammatory or immunosuppressant agent. Because it has virtually no mineralocorticoid properties, the drug is inadequate alone for the management of adrenocortical insufficiency. If triamcinolone is used in the treatment of this condition, concomitant therapy with a mineralocorticoid is also required.

■ **Asthma** Triamcinolone acetonide is used by oral inhalation for the long-term prevention of bronchospasm in patients with asthma.

Orally inhaled triamcinolone acetonide should not be used for the primary treatment of severe acute asthmatic attacks or status asthmaticus when intensive measures (e.g., oxygen, parenteral bronchodilators, IV corticosteroids) are required. Triamcinolone acetonide oral inhaler is not a bronchodilator, and patients should be warned that the drug should not be used for rapid relief of bronchospasm.

Mild Persistent Asthma Drugs for asthma may be categorized as relievers (e.g., bronchodilators taken as needed for acute symptoms) or controllers (principally inhaled corticosteroids or other anti-inflammatory agents taken regularly to achieve long-term control of asthma). In the stepped-care approach to antiasthmatic drug therapy, current asthma management guidelines and most clinicians recommend initiation of a controller drug such as an anti-inflammatory agent, preferably a low-dose orally inhaled corticosteroid (e.g., 88–264, 88–176, or 176 mcg of fluticasone propionate [or its equivalent] daily via a metered-dose inhaler in adolescents and adults, children 5–11 years of age, or children 4 years of age or younger, respectively) as first-line therapy for persistent asthma (i.e., patients with daytime symptoms of asthma more than twice per week, but less than once daily, and nocturnal symptoms of asthma 3–4 times per month), supplemented by as-needed use of a short-acting, inhaled β_2-agonist. For equivalent orally inhaled dosages of corticosteroids, see General Dosage under Dosage and Administration: Dosage, in the Corticosteroids General Statement 68:04.

Moderate Persistent Asthma According to current asthma management guidelines, therapy with a long-acting β_2-agonist such as salmeterol or formoterol generally is recommended in adults and adolescents who have moderate persistent asthma and daily asthmatic symptoms that are inadequately controlled following addition of low-dose inhaled corticosteroids to as-needed inhaled β_2-agonist treatment. However, the National Asthma Education and Prevention Program (NAEPP) recommends that the beneficial effects of long-acting inhaled β_2-agonists should be weighed carefully against the increased risk (although uncommon) of severe asthma exacerbations and asthma-related deaths associated with daily use of such agents. (See Asthma-related Death and Life-threatening Events under Cautions: Respiratory Effects, in Salmeterol 12:12.08.12.) Current asthma management guidelines also state that an alternative, but equally preferred option for management of moderate persistent asthma that is not adequately controlled with a low dosage of inhaled corticosteroid is to increase the maintenance dosage to a medium dosage (e.g., exceeding 264 but not more than 440 mcg of fluticasone propionate [or its equivalent] daily via a metered-dose inhaler in adults and adolescents).

In children 5–11 years of age with moderate persistent asthma that is not controlled with a low dosage of an inhaled corticosteroid, a long-acting inhaled β_2-agonist (e.g., salmeterol, formoterol), a leukotriene modifier (i.e., montelukast, zafirlukast), or extended-release theophylline (with appropriate monitoring) may be added to low-dose inhaled corticosteroid therapy according to current asthma management guidelines; another preferred option is to increase the maintenance dosage of the inhaled corticosteroid to a medium dosage (e.g., exceeding 176 but not more than 352 mcg of fluticasone propionate [or its equivalent] daily via a metered-dose inhaler). In infants and children 4 years of age or younger with moderate persistent asthma that is not controlled by a low dosage of an inhaled corticosteroid, the only preferred option is to increase the maintenance dosage of the inhaled corticosteroid to a medium dosage (e.g., exceeding 176 but not more than 352 mcg of fluticasone propionate [or its equivalent] daily via a metered-dose inhaler).

Severe Persistent Asthma Maintenance therapy with an inhaled corticosteroid at medium or high dosages (e.g., exceeding 440 mcg of fluticasone propionate or its equivalent daily in adults and adolescents or 352 mcg of the drug in children 5–11 years of age or its equivalent via a metered-dose inhaler) and adjunctive therapy with a long-acting inhaled β_2-agonist is the preferred treatment according to current asthma management guidelines for adults and children 5 years of age or older with severe persistent asthma (i.e., continuous daytime asthma symptoms, nighttime symptoms 7 times per week). In infants and children 4 years of age or younger with severe asthma, maintenance therapy with an inhaled corticosteroid at medium or high dosages (e.g., exceeding 352 mcg of fluticasone propionate daily or its equivalent via a metered-dose inhaler) and adjunctive therapy with either a long-acting inhaled β_2-agonist or montelukast is recommended in current asthma management guidelines as the only preferred treatment.

Poorly Controlled Asthma If asthma symptoms in patients with moderate to severe asthma are very poorly controlled (i.e., at least 2–3 exacerbations per year requiring oral corticosteroids), a short course of an oral corticosteroid (3–10 days) may be added to gain prompt control of asthma. Regular use of oral corticosteroids as add-on therapy in adults and children 5 years of age or older with severe asthma who are inadequately controlled with high-dose inhaled corticosteroid, intermittent oral corticosteroid therapy, and a long-acting inhaled β_2-agonist bronchodilator is suggested, based on consensus and clinical experience. A short (2-week) course of oral corticosteroids may be considered to confirm clinical response prior to implementing long-term therapy with these agents. Once long-term oral corticosteroid therapy is initiated, the lowest possible effective dosage (i.e., alternate-day or once-daily administration) should be used, and the patient should be monitored carefully for adverse effects. Once asthma is well-controlled, repeated attempts should be made to reduce the oral corticosteroid dosage. Use of orally inhaled triamcinolone acetonide as adjunctive therapy in patients who require chronic administration of systemic corticosteroids to control asthma symptoms may permit a reduction in dosage or discontinuance of systemic corticosteroids. When used in recommended dosages in responsive patients, triamcinolone acetonide oral inhalation may permit control of asthmatic symptoms with less suppression of hypothalamic-pituitary-adrenal (HPA) function than therapeutically equivalent oral dosages of prednisone. For additional details on the stepped-care approach to drug therapy in asthma, see Asthma under Uses: Bronchospasm, in Albuterol 12:12.08.12 and see Asthma under Uses: Respiratory Diseases, in the Corticosteroids General Statement 68:04.

Dosage and Administration

The route of administration and dosage of triamcinolone and its derivatives depend on the condition being treated and the response of the patient. IM therapy is generally reserved for patients who are not able to take the drug orally. Dosage for infants and children should be based on the severity of the disease and the response of the patient rather than on strict adherence to dosage indicated by age, body weight, or body surface area. After a satisfactory response is obtained, dosage should be decreased in small decrements to the lowest level that maintains an adequate clinical response, and the drug should be discontinued as soon as possible. Patients should be continually monitored for signs that indicate dosage adjustment is necessary, such as remissions or exacerbations of the disease and stress (surgery, infection, trauma). One manufacturer recommends that an alternate-day dosage regimen be considered when long-term oral triamcinolone therapy is necessary. However, most authorities state that only methylprednisolone, prednisolone, and prednisone have been proven to be suitable for alternate-day glucocorticoid therapy. Following long-term therapy, triamcinolone should be withdrawn gradually. (See Discontinuance of Therapy under Dosage and Administration: Dosage, in the Corticosteroids General Statement 68:04.)

■ **Triamcinolone** Triamcinolone is administered orally. The initial adult dosage of triamcinolone may range from 4–48 mg daily depending on the disease being treated and is usually administered in 1–4 doses. Some clinicians state that children may be given a dosage of 0.117–1.66 mg/kg daily or 3.3–50 mg/m^2 daily, administered in 4 divided doses.

■ **Triamcinolone Acetonide** Triamcinolone acetonide may be administered by IM, intra-articular, intrasynovial, intralesional (intradermal) or sublesional, and soft-tissue injection or by oral inhalation. Because it is slowly absorbed and its effects may persist for several weeks, IM administration of triamcinolone acetonide is not indicated when an immediate effect of short duration is required.

The usual IM dose for adults and children older than 12 years of age is 60 mg (using the 40-mg/mL sterile suspension). Additional IM doses of 20–100 mg (usually 40–80 mg) may be given when signs and symptoms recur. Some clinicians recommend that triamcinolone acetonide be administered IM at 6-week intervals, if possible, to minimize HPA suppression. Some clinicians state that children 6–12 years of age may receive 0.03–0.2 mg/kg or 1–6.25 mg/m^2 IM at 1- to 7-day intervals. IM dosage for children younger than 6 years of age has not been established, and triamcinolone acetonide should not be administered IM to children in this age group.

For intralesional (or sublesional) injections, the 10-mg/mL sterile suspension of triamcinolone acetonide is used. The usual intralesional or sublesional dose of triamcinolone acetonide is 1 mg per injection site and may be repeated 1 or more times a week depending on the response of the patient. A tuberculin syringe should be used to facilitate intralesional or sublesional dosage measurement. Multiple sites may be injected if they are at least 1 cm apart, but the total amount of triamcinolone acetonide administered intralesionally at any one time should not exceed 30 mg.

For intra-articular, intrasynovial, and soft-tissue injection, the usual dose of triamcinolone acetonide (using either the 10-mg/mL or 40-mg/mL sterile suspension) is 2.5–40 mg depending on the location of the affected area and the degree of inflammation; the dose may be repeated when signs and symptoms recur. Anti-inflammatory effects may be maintained for several weeks following intra-articular administration of the drug. A local anesthetic, such as procaine hydrochloride, may be infiltrated into the soft tissue surrounding the joint and/or injected into the joint before administration of triamcinolone acetonide. For large joints such as the knee, 15–40 mg of triamcinolone acetonide may be used. For smaller joints, 2.5–10 mg may be adequate. For soft-tissue injection in the treatment of tendon sheath inflammation, the usual dose is 2.5–10 mg.

For oral inhalation use, the triamcinolone acetonide oral aerosol inhaler delivers about 200 mcg of drug from the valve and 75 mcg from the spacer mouthpiece per metered spray under defined in vitro test conditions. The commercially available aerosol delivers at least 240 metered sprays; however, since reliable dosage delivery cannot be assured after 240 metered sprays, the aerosol inhaler should not be used after 240 actuations and patients should be cautioned against longer use of an individual inhaler. Patients should be carefully instructed in the use of the oral inhaler. To obtain optimum results, patients should also be given a copy of the patient instructions provided by the manufacturer. The inhaler should be shaken well immediately prior to use and inverted prior to actuation. After exhaling as completely as possible, the mouthpiece of the inhaler should be placed well into the mouth and the lips closed firmly around it. The patient should then inhale slowly and deeply through the mouth while pressing the metal canister down with the forefinger. After holding the breath for as long as possible (about 5–10 seconds), the mouthpiece should be removed and the patient should exhale slowly. If additional inhalations are required, the patient should wait 1 minute between inhalations, shake the inhaler again, and repeat the procedure. Following each treatment, the patient should rinse the mouth thoroughly with water or mouthwash to remove drug deposited in the oropharyngeal area.

Dosage of triamcinolone acetonide oral inhalation must be carefully adjusted according to individual requirements and response. The usual initial adult dosage by oral inhalation is 150 mcg (2 sprays) 3 or 4 times daily or 300 mcg (4 sprays) twice daily (450 or 600 mcg total). In adults with severe asthma, it may be advisable to start with 12–16 sprays daily (900–1200 mcg total), and then reduce the dosage to the lowest effective level. While the manufacturer states that a triamcinolone acetonide dosage of 1200 mcg (16 sprays) daily in adults should not be exceeded, some experts state that higher dosages may be used in adults with severe persistent asthma.

In children 6–12 years of age, the usual initial dosage is 75 or 150 mcg (1 or 2 sprays) 3 or 4 times daily (225–600 mcg total) or 150 or 300 mcg (2–4 sprays) twice daily (300–600 mcg total); dosage is adjusted according to patient response. While the manufacturer states that dosage for children 6–12 years of age should not exceed 900 mcg (12 sprays) daily, some experts state that higher dosages may be used in children with severe persistent asthma. The manufacturer states that the drug is not recommended for use in children younger than 6 years of age. When orally inhaled triamcinolone acetonide is administered to patients receiving systemic corticosteroids, the patient's asthma should be reasonably stable before treatment with the oral inhalation begins. Initially, the aerosol is given concurrently with the maintenance dosage of the systemic corticosteroid. After about 1 week, the systemic corticosteroid is gradually withdrawn. (See Discontinuance of Therapy under Dosage and Administration: Dosage, in the Corticosteroids General Statement 68:04.) *Gradual withdrawal of systemic corticosteroids following long-term therapy is strongly recommended, since death has occurred in some individuals in whom systemic corticosteroids were withdrawn too rapidly.* After systemic corticosteroids have been withdrawn, if exacerbations of asthma occur during triamcinolone acetonide oral inhalation therapy, short courses of systemic corticosteroids should be given, then tapered as symptoms subside.

■ **Triamcinolone Hexacetonide** Triamcinolone hexacetonide may be administered by intra-articular, intralesional, or sublesional injection. Sterile suspensions of triamcinolone hexacetonide may be diluted with a local anesthetic such as 1% or 2% lidocaine hydrochloride prior to intra-articular or intralesional injection or with sterile water for injection, 0.9% sodium chloride injection, or 5% or 10% dextrose in 0.9% sodium chloride injection prior to intralesional administration. Diluents containing preservatives such as parabens or phenols should be avoided. (See Chemistry and Stability: Stability.) For intralesional (or sublesional) injection, the 5-mg/mL sterile suspension of triamcinolone hexacetonide is used.

The usual dosage for intralesional (or sublesional) injection is up to 0.5 mg per square inch of affected skin. Additional injections should be administered according to the response of the patient. For intra-articular injections, the usual dosage of triamcinolone hexacetonide (using the 20-mg/mL sterile suspension) is 2–20 mg depending on the size of the joint, degree of inflammation and amount of fluid present; doses may be repeated at intervals of 3–4 weeks. For large joints such as the knee, 10–20 mg may be used. For smaller joints such as in the fingers, 2–6 mg may be adequate.

Chemistry and Stability

■ **Chemistry** Triamcinolone is a synthetic glucocorticoid. The free alcohol occurs as a white or practically white, odorless, crystalline powder and is very slightly soluble in water and slightly soluble in alcohol. Triamcinolone acetonide occurs as a white to cream-colored, crystalline powder having not more than a slight odor and is practically insoluble in water and very soluble in dehydrated alcohol. The diacetate ester of triamcinolone occurs as a white to off-white, fine crystalline powder with not more than a slight odor and is practically insoluble in water and sparingly soluble in alcohol. Triamcinolone hexacetonide occurs as a white to cream-colored powder and is practically insoluble in water and very slightly soluble in alcohol.

Commercially available sterile suspensions of triamcinolone acetonide and triamcinolone hexacetonide have a pH of 5–7.5 and 4–8, respectively.

For oral inhalation, triamcinolone acetonide is commercially available as an aerosol containing a microcrystalline suspension of the drug in a vehicle of a fluorocarbon propellant (dichlorodifluoromethane) and dehydrated alcohol. Although triamcinolone acetonide is administered by an oral inhaler that produces metered sprays containing 200 mcg of triamcinolone acetonide per spray, each actuation of the inhaler delivers a dose equivalent to 100 mcg of triamcinolone acetonide, since a portion of each spray is retained within the delivery device.

■ **Stability** Commercially available oral and parenteral preparations of triamcinolone should be stored at a temperature less than 40 °C, preferably between 15–30 °C; freezing of the sterile suspensions should be avoided. Exposure of sterile suspensions of the drug to freezing temperatures can result in irreversible clumping or agglomeration (granular appearance); such suspensions should *not* be used. Triamcinolone tablets should be stored in well-closed containers. Triamcinolone acetonide sterile suspension should be protected from light. Triamcinolone acetonide oral inhaler should be stored at controlled room temperature (20–25 °C). Because the contents of the oral inhaler are under pressure, the aerosol container should *not* be punctured, used or stored near heat or an open flame, exposed to temperatures exceeding 49 °C, or placed into a fire or incinerator for disposal.

Sterile suspensions of triamcinolone hexacetonide should not be mixed with diluents or local anesthetics containing preservatives (such as parabens or phenols) because flocculation of the suspension may result. Unused diluted suspensions of the hexacetonide esters of triamcinolone should be discarded after 7 days.

For further information on chemistry, pharmacology, pharmacokinetics, uses, cautions, drug interactions, laboratory test interferences, and dosage and administration of triamcinolone, see the Corticosteroids General Statement 68:04. For EENT and topical uses, see 52:08.08 and 84:06.08, respectively.

Preparations

Abbott discontinued the manufacture of triamcinolone acetonide oral inhalation aerosol (Azmacort®) effective December 31, 2009. The US Food and Drug Administration (FDA) states that triamcinolone acetonide oral inhalation aerosol with chlorofluorocarbon (CFC) propellants will not be manufactured, sold, or dispensed in the US after December 31, 2010.

Excipients in commercially available drug preparations may have clinically important effects in some individuals; consult specific product labeling for details.

Triamcinolone

Oral		
Tablets	4 mg	**Aristocort®** (scored), Astellas

Triamcinolone Acetonide

Parenteral		
Injectable suspension	10 mg/mL	**Kenalog®**, Bristol-Myers Squibb
	40 mg/mL	**Kenalog®**, Bristol-Myers Squibb

Triamcinolone Acetonide (Microcrystalline)

Oral Inhalation		
Aerosol	75 mcg/metered spray	**Azmacort® Oral Inhaler**, Abbott

Triamcinolone Hexacetonide (Microcrystalline)

Parenteral		
Injectable suspension	5 mg/mL	**Aristospan® Intralesional**, Sandoz
	20 mg/mL	**Aristospan® Intra-articular**, Sandoz

Selected Revisions January 2018,

ANDROGENS 68:08

Danazol

■ Danazol is a synthetic derivative of ethisterone (ethinyl testosterone) with weak androgenic and anabolic properties and no estrogenic or progestogenic activity.

Uses

■ **Endometriosis** Danazol is used for the palliative treatment of endometriosis in patients in whom alternative hormonal therapy is ineffective, intolerable, or contraindicated. Observation of the patient and analgesic therapy are usually adequate for patients with minimal symptoms or pelvic findings of endometriosis. Moderate endometriosis generally is treated conservatively with hormones, including estrogen and progestin (alone or in combination) or testosterone, while severe endometriosis generally requires surgery. When endometriosis is extensive, hormonal therapy may be administered prior to surgery, but danazol is not indicated when surgery alone is considered the treatment of choice. Uncontrolled clinical studies report symptomatic improvement, including relief of pain, in about 37–87% of patients with endometriosis who received danazol. Best results have occurred in patients with mild to moderate endometriosis. Resolution of endometrial lesions, as indicated by laparoscopy or laparotomy, has been reported to occur in 36–72% of patients receiving danazol. In most patients, endometriosis recurred within 8–12 months following discontinuance of the drug. Reports indicate that about 30–50% of previously infertile women with endometriosis are able to conceive within 6–8 months after danazol therapy, but this percentage is no greater than that expected following treatment with other hormones or surgery.

■ **Hereditary Angioedema** Danazol is used for the prophylactic treatment of all types (i.e., abdominal, cutaneous, laryngeal) of hereditary angioedema in males and females. In one well-controlled study in patients with hereditary angioedema, the number of attacks was substantially decreased during danazol therapy. However, long-term (i.e., exceeding 10 years) prophylaxis with danazol, even at low dosages, has been associated with adverse hepatic effects (e.g., hepatic adenomas). (See Cautions: Hepatic Effects.) Because the adverse androgenic effects of the drug may be hazardous to children and pregnant women, some clinicians believe fibrinolytic inhibitors (e.g., aminocaproic acid) may be preferable to danazol when treating angioedema in these patients.

■ **Fibrocystic Breast Disease** Danazol is used for the palliative treatment of fibrocystic breast disease in patients who are unresponsive to simple measures including the use of padded brassieres and/or analgesics. Danazol is usually effective in decreasing pain, tenderness, and nodularity; in most patients, breast pain and tenderness are substantially relieved during the first month of therapy and eliminated in 2–3 months, but elimination of nodularity usually requires 4–6 months of uninterrupted therapy. The patient should be warned that danazol therapy produces considerable alterations in hormone concentrations, and symptoms often recur following discontinuance of the drug; approximately 50% of patients may show evidence of recurrence of symptoms within 1 year after discontinuance of the drug.

■ **Other Uses** In precocious puberty, danazol has been used to produce regression of secondary sexual characteristics† but the drug does not halt the progression of bone age and, therefore, it should not be used for this purpose.

Danazol has been used for the management of patients with idiopathic thrombocytopenic purpura (ITP)†. In patients with ITP, danazol produced a marked increase in platelet counts in most patients and can produce prolonged remissions; response did not appear to be affected by duration of disease or by previous failure of splenectomy or other therapies (e.g., colchicine, vinca alkaloids, corticosteroids). About 50% of patients with ITP who had unsatisfactory responses to colchicine or vinca alkaloids responded to danazol and about 30% of those who had an unsatisfactory response to corticosteroids responded to danazol. There is some evidence that efficacy of danazol in ITP may be reduced in young, unsplenectomized patients, particularly those who are female. Further study is needed to determine the role of danazol in the treatment of these conditions.

■ **Misuse, Abuse, and Dependence** Because of their anabolic and androgenic effects on performance (ergogenic potential) and physique, androgens have been misused and abused by athletes, bodybuilders, weightlifters, and others, including high school- and college-aged individuals engaged in sports. Following review of data from published literature and case reports in October 2016, the FDA concluded that misuse and abuse of androgens are associated with serious adverse cardiovascular, hepatic, endocrine, and mental health effects. (See Cautions; see also Uses: Misuse, Abuse, and Dependence, in Testosterone 68:08.)

Serum testosterone concentrations should be evaluated in patients who may be misusing or abusing androgens (e.g., patients experiencing serious adverse cardiovascular or psychiatric effects); however, serum testosterone concentrations may be below or within the normal range in patients abusing synthetic derivatives of testosterone.

Dosage and Administration

Danazol is administered orally. For the treatment of endometriosis and fibrocystic breast disease, administration of the drug should be initiated during menstruation; otherwise, appropriate laboratory tests should be performed to ensure that the patient is not pregnant. (See Cautions: Pregnancy, Fertility, and Lactation.) Attempts should be made to determine the lowest possible effective dosage of the drug.

■ **Endometriosis** For the palliative treatment of endometriosis in patients with moderate to severe disease or in patients who are infertile because of endometriosis, the usual initial dosage of danazol is 800 mg daily given in 2 divided doses. Amenorrhea and a rapid improvement in painful symptoms are best achieved at this dosage. Subsequent dosage may be gradually reduced, depending on the patient's therapeutic response, to a level sufficient to maintain amenorrhea.

For the treatment of endometriosis in patients with mild disease, the usual initial dosage is 200–400 mg daily given in 2 divided doses. Subsequent dosage should be adjusted according to the patient's tolerance and therapeutic response.

Danazol therapy for the treatment of endometriosis should continue *uninterrupted* for 3–6 months; however, therapy may be extended to 9 months, if necessary. If symptoms recur following discontinuance of therapy, treatment with danazol may be reinstituted.

■ **Fibrocystic Breast Disease** For the symptomatic management of fibrocystic breast disease, the usual dosage of danazol is 100–400 mg daily given in 2 divided doses. Dosage should be individualized according to severity of the disease and the patient's response to treatment. Since ovulation may not be suppressed when danazol is administered at this dosage, an effective nonhormonal method of contraception is recommended during therapy with the drug. Regular menstrual patterns, irregular menstrual patterns, and amenorrhea each occur in approximately one-third of patients receiving danazol at a dosage of 100 mg daily. Irregular menstrual patterns and amenorrhea occur more frequently when higher dosages are used. In most patients, breast pain and tenderness are substantially relieved during the first month of therapy, and eliminated in 2–3 months, but elimination of nodularity usually requires 4–6 months of uninterrupted therapy. If symptoms recur following discontinuance of therapy, treatment with danazol may be reinstituted.

■ **Hereditary Angioedema** For the prophylactic treatment of hereditary angioedema, the usual initial dosage of danazol is 200 mg 2 or 3 times daily. After an initial response is obtained, as evidenced by prevention of episodes of edematous attacks, subsequent maintenance dosage should be determined by decreasing the dosage by 50% or less at intervals of 1–3 months or longer, depending on the frequency of attacks prior to initiation of danazol therapy. If an attack occurs during treatment with the drug, dosage may be increased by up to 200 mg daily. Dosage requirements for continuous prophylaxis should be individualized according to the patient's response to treatment. During the dosage adjustment phase, patients should be closely monitored, particularly if they have a history of airway involvement. If danazol therapy was initiated during exacerbation of angioedema resulting from trauma, stress, or other cause, periodic attempts to reduce dosage or withdraw therapy should be considered.

Cautions

■ Adverse Effects ***Endocrine Effects*** The most frequent adverse effects of danazol are androgenic effects, and include mild hirsutism, decreased breast size, voice changes (e.g., deepening, hoarseness, instability), sore throat, acne, increased oiliness of skin or hair, hair loss, weight gain, edema, and, rarely, clitoral hypertrophy or testicular atrophy. Adverse hypoestrogenic effects of the drug include flushing, sweating, nervousness, emotional lability, and vaginitis with itching, dryness, burning, and/or bleeding. Although these adverse effects usually subside following discontinuance of the drug, patients should be observed for signs of virilization because some adverse androgenic effects may not be reversible.

Glucose intolerance, increased insulin requirements in patients with diabetes mellitus and abnormalities in laboratory tests (e.g., serum creatine kinase [CK; creatine phosphokinase, CPK], oral glucose tolerance, glucagon, thyroxine-binding globulin, sex steroid binding globulin [sex hormone binding globulin, SHBG; testosterone-estradiol-binding globulin, TEBG], other plasma proteins, lipids and lipoproteins) also have been reported in patients receiving danazol; however, these effects have not been directly attributed to the drug.

Genitourinary Effects Menstrual irregularities (e.g., spotting, alteration of menstrual cycle, amenorrhea) occur in most females receiving the drug. Amenorrhea occurs during danazol therapy in most females but menstruation usually resumes within 2–3 months following discontinuance of the drug; however, persistent amenorrhea has been reported rarely.

Hematuria also has been reported; however, this effect has not been directly attributed to the drug.

Hepatic Effects Like other 17-alkylated steroids, danazol may cause cholestatic jaundice, peliosis of the liver, and benign or (rarely) malignant hepatic adenoma following long-term administration of the drug. Hepatic dysfunction, as evidenced by elevated concentrations of hepatic enzymes (e.g., alkaline phosphatase, AST [SGOT], ALT [SGPT]) and/or by jaundice, has been reported in patients receiving danazol dosages of 400 mg or more daily.

Nervous System Effects Benign intracranial hypertension (pseudotumor cerebri), manifested as headache, papilledema, nausea and vomiting, and/or visual disturbances (e.g., diplopia), may occur in patients receiving danazol. In addition, anxiety, depression, dizziness, fainting, emotional lability, fatigue, Guillain-Barré syndrome, headache, nervousness, seizures, sleep disorders, syncope, paresthesias, tremor, and weakness have occurred during danazol therapy; however, these effects have not been directly attributed to the drug.

Cardiovascular Effects Increased blood pressure, thromboembolism, and thrombotic or thrombophlebitic events (e.g., sagittal sinus thrombosis, life-threatening or fatal stroke) have been reported in patients receiving danazol.

Dermatologic and Sensitivity Reactions Allergic reactions, such as urticaria, pruritus, petechiae, rashes (e.g., maculopapular, vesicular, papular, purpuric), and erythema multiforme (including Stevens-Johnson syndrome), have occurred during danazol therapy. Photosensitivity also has been reported.

GI Effects Gastroenteritis, changes in appetite, nausea, vomiting, constipation, and bleeding gums have been reported with danazol therapy; however, these effects have not been directly attributed to the drug.

Musculoskeletal Effects Muscle cramps or spasms; joint pain or swelling; locked joints; pain in the back, neck, legs, or rarely, pelvis; and carpal tunnel syndrome (which may be secondary to fluid retention) have been reported in patients receiving danazol, although these effects have not been directly attributed to the drug.

Hematologic Effects Reversible erythrocytosis, leukocytosis, polycythemia, eosinophilia, leukopenia, thrombocytopenia, and increased erythrocyte and platelet counts have been reported with danazol therapy; however, these effects have not been directly attributed to the drug.

Ocular Effects Visual disturbances, conjunctival edema, and rarely, cataracts have been reported with danazol therapy; however, these effects have not been directly attributed to the drug.

Misuse, Abuse, and Dependence Serious adverse effects (e.g., increased aggression, antisocial behavior, manic episode, hostility, depression, changes in libido, increased risk of cardiovascular events, hepatotoxicity, testicular atrophy, sperm abnormalities) are associated with misuse and abuse of androgens (see Uses: Misuse, Abuse, and Dependence).

Manifestations of withdrawal (e.g., depressed mood, major depression, fatigue, cravings, restlessness, irritability, anorexia, insomnia, decreased libido, hypogonadotropic hypogonadism) may occur if androgens are discontinued abruptly or dosage is substantially reduced in physically dependent patients or in those taking supratherapeutic dosages of such drugs; withdrawal symptoms may persist for weeks or months.

Other Adverse Effects Fever, chills, and rarely, nasal congestion and pancreatitis also have been reported with danazol therapy; however, these effects have not been directly attributed to the drug.

■ Precautions and Contraindications Because danazol may cause fluid retention, the drug should be used with caution in patients who may be adversely affected by this condition such as those with seizure disorders, migraine, or cardiac or renal dysfunction.

Periodic evaluations of liver function should be performed in all patients receiving danazol, since the drug may cause hepatic dysfunction.

Semen should be evaluated for volume, viscosity, and sperm count and motility every 3–4 months during danazol therapy, especially in adolescents.

Patients should be carefully monitored for signs of virilization, since some adverse androgenic effects may not subside after discontinuance of the drug.

Danazol has been associated with peliosis of the liver and benign or malignant hepatic adenoma, and such hepatic effects may not be apparent until complicated by acute, potentially life-threatening intra-abdominal hemorrhage; clinicians should be aware that such hepatotoxicity may develop during long-term administration of danazol. (See Cautions: Hepatic Effects.)

Patients receiving danazol who develop signs and/or symptoms of pseudotumor cerebri (e.g., headache, nausea and vomiting, visual disturbances) should be examined for the presence of papilledema and informed to discontinue the drug immediately if any such manifestation is present; such patients should be referred to a neurologist for further evaluation and care.

Since substantial alterations in lipoprotein profiles (e.g., decreases in serum high-density lipoproteins, increases in serum low-density lipoproteins) have been reported in patients receiving danazol therapy, clinicians should consider the potential increased risk of cardiovascular disease (e.g., coronary artery disease, atherosclerosis) versus the possible benefits of therapy.

The possibility of carcinoma of the breast should be excluded before initiating danazol therapy in patients with fibrocystic breast disease. Nodularity, pain, and tenderness caused by fibrocystic breast disease may prevent recognition of underlying carcinoma before initiation of therapy. If any nodule persists or enlarges during danazol therapy, carcinoma should be considered and ruled out. Patients should be informed of the serious adverse effects associated with misuse and abuse of androgens. (See Uses: Misuse, Abuse, and Dependence, in Testosterone 68:08.)

Danazol is contraindicated in pregnant or nursing women and in patients with abnormal genital bleeding of unknown etiology. The drug is also contraindicated in patients with markedly impaired hepatic, renal, or cardiac function and in those with porphyria.

■ Pregnancy, Fertility, and Lactation Although there are no adequate and controlled studies to date in humans, danazol may cause fetal harm when administered to pregnant women. Androgenic effects including clitoral hypertrophy, labial fusion of the external genital fold to form a scrotal-like structure, ambiguous genitalia, abnormal vaginal development, and persistence of a urogenital sinus have occurred in the female offspring of women who were given danazol during pregnancy. Spontaneous abortions have also occurred in pregnant women who received the drug. Since the risks clearly outweigh the possible benefits in women who are or may become pregnant, danazol is contraindicated in such women. Women of childbearing age should be instructed to use an effective, nonhormonal method of contraception during danazol therapy and be informed of the potential hazard to the fetus should they become pregnant during therapy. In addition, a reliable pregnancy test (e.g., beta-subunit radioimmunoassay [RIA]) must be performed immediately prior to beginning danazol therapy. If the drug is inadvertently administered during pregnancy or if the patient becomes pregnant while receiving the drug, administration of danazol should be discontinued, and the woman should be apprised of the potential risk to the fetus.

Although the effect of danazol on fertility in humans has not been conclusively determined, the drug suppresses ovulation at high dosages and decreases libido in women and produces a reversible oligospermia or azoospermia with no apparent change in libido in men; abnormalities in the volume and viscosity of semen and in sperm motility also may occur. Studies to further evaluate the effect of danazol on fertility are under way.

Because of the potential for serious adverse reactions to danazol in nursing infants, a decision should be made whether to discontinue nursing or not use the drug, taking into account the importance of the drug to the woman.

Pharmacology

Danazol reportedly suppresses the pituitary-ovarian axis by inhibiting output of pituitary and hypothalamic gonadotropins. There is evidence that danazol directly inhibits the synthesis of sex steroids and binds to gonadal (sex) steroid receptors in the cytoplasm of target tissues and may thereby exhibit antiestrogen, anabolic, and weakly androgenic effects. The drug possesses weak androgenic and anabolic properties but exerts no estrogenic or progestogenic activity; androgenic activity is dose related. In addition, danazol has been shown to substantially decrease IgG, IgM, and IgA concentrations as well as phospholipid and IgG isotope autoantibodies in patients with endometriosis and associated elevations of autoantibodies, suggesting that this could be another mechanism by which the drug facilitates regression of this disorder. Danazol does not suppress normal pituitary release of corticotropin or adrenocortical release of cortisol.

When administered to women in some clinical studies, danazol suppressed the midcycle surge of follicle-stimulating hormone (FSH) and luteinizing hormone (LH) and decreased plasma estradiol and progesterone concentrations. However, other studies in women found little or no change in plasma concentrations of FSH, LH, estradiol, progesterone, and prolactin following administration of danazol. Regressive hypoestrogenic changes in the vaginal smear or in the pyknotic index of vaginal cytology, and reduced midcycle basal body temperatures have also been reported. Studies in men treated with danazol showed decreased plasma concentrations of FSH, LH, testosterone, and dihydroepiandrosterone. Investigators base claims of the antigonadotropic activity of danazol on these findings and on reports of decreased mean gonadal weight in animals treated with the drug.

In the treatment of endometriosis, suppression of ovarian steroidogenesis produces atrophy and involution of normal and ectopic endometrial tissue. Anovulation and resultant amenorrhea occur in most women after 6–8 weeks of danazol therapy. One study reported decreased sperm counts in males during danazol therapy, but another reported inconsistent changes in sperm production.

In one well-controlled study in patients with hereditary angioedema receiving danazol, serum levels of complement 1 (C1) esterase inhibitor were 4.5 times greater and C4 levels were 15 times greater than those prior to administration of the drug. In one study in several patients with factor VIII deficiency (hemophilia A) and in one patient with factor IX deficiency (hemophilia B), danazol produced substantial increases in plasma levels of factor VIII and IX, respectively. Danazol has also been shown to increase levels of alpha$_1$-antitrypsin in deficient individuals. In a study in patients with idiopathic thrombocytopenic purpura, danazol caused a marked decrease in platelet-reactive IgG.

Pharmacokinetics

■ **Absorption** In one study in healthy women, oral administration of 400 mg of danazol twice daily for 2 days produced plasma danazol concentrations ranging from 140–460 ng/mL, with an average plasma concentration of 260 ng/mL 2 hours after the last dose. Bioavailability studies indicate that plasma danazol concentrations do not increase proportionally with increases in dose; doubling the dose results in a 35–40% increase in plasma concentrations. However, bioavailability and peak plasma concentrations of danazol increased by 3- to 4-fold, respectively, in healthy women who received 100- and 200-mg of danazol as single doses with a high-fat meal (more than 30 g of fat) compared with those who received the drug under fasting conditions. In addition, administration with food delayed mean time to reach peak plasma danazol concentrations by about 30 minutes.

■ **Distribution and Elimination** Information regarding distribution and elimination of danazol is minimal. Danazol is metabolized to 2-hydroxymethylethisterone, which appears in the plasma in a concentration 5–10 times greater than that of the unchanged drug.

Chemistry and Stability

■ **Chemistry** Danazol is a synthetic derivative of ethisterone (ethinyl testosterone). The drug occurs as a white to pale yellow, crystalline powder and is practically insoluble in water and sparingly soluble in alcohol.

■ **Stability** Commercially available danazol capsules should be stored in well-closed containers at a temperature less than 40°C, preferably between 15–30°C.

Preparations

Excipients in commercially available drug preparations may have clinically important effects in some individuals; consult specific product labeling for details.

Danazol

Oral

Capsules	50 mg*	**Danazol Capsules**
	100 mg*	**Danazol Capsules**
	200 mg*	**Danazol Capsules**

*available from one or more manufacturer, distributor, and/or repackager by generic (nonproprietary) name

†Use is not currently included in the labeling approved by the US Food and Drug Administration

Selected Revisions November 2017, © Copyright, July 1977, American Society of Health-System Pharmacists, Inc.

methylTESTOSTERone

■ Methyltestosterone is a synthetic androgenic anabolic steroid hormone.

Uses

Methyltestosterone is used mainly for replacement or substitution of diminished or absent endogenous testicular hormone.

■ **Uses in Males** In males, methyltestosterone is used for the management of congenital or acquired primary hypogonadism such as that resulting from orchiectomy or from testicular failure caused by cryptorchidism, bilateral torsion, orchitis, or vanishing testis syndrome. Methyltestosterone also is used in males for the management of congenital or acquired hypogonadotropic hypogonadism such as that resulting from idiopathic gonadotropin or gonadotropin releasing hormone (luteinizing hormone releasing hormone) deficiency or from pituitary-hypothalamic injury caused by tumors, trauma, or radiation. If any of these conditions occur before puberty, androgen replacement therapy will be necessary during adolescence for the development of secondary sexual characteristics and prolonged therapy will be required to maintain these characteristics. Prolonged androgen therapy also is required to maintain sexual characteristics in other males who develop testosterone deficiency after puberty.

When the diagnosis is well established, methyltestosterone may be used to stimulate puberty in carefully selected males with delayed puberty. These males usually have a family history of delayed puberty that is not caused by a pathologic disorder. Brief treatment with conservative doses of an androgen may occasionally be justified in these males if they do not respond to psychologic support. Because androgens may adversely affect bone maturation in these prepubertal males, this potential risk should be fully discussed with the patient and his parents prior to initiation of androgen therapy. (See Cautions: Pediatric Precautions.) If androgen therapy is initiated in these prepubertal males, radiographs of the hand and wrist should be obtained at 6-month intervals to determine the effect of therapy on the epiphyseal centers.

The safety and efficacy of methyltestosterone in patients with low testosterone concentrations related to aging (i.e., late-onset hypogonadism) have not been established. Although endogenous testosterone concentrations decline with aging and manifestations of hypogonadism such as decreased libido, impotence, decreased body hair growth, decreased muscle mass, increased risk of cardiovascular disease, and decreased bone mass and resultant osteoporosis may occur, it is unclear whether these symptoms are related to such decreased concentrations or to normal aging; therefore, the need to replace testosterone in aging men is unclear. For further information on management of low testosterone concentrations related to aging, see Late-onset Hypogonadism under Uses: Uses in Males, in Testosterone 68:08.

For additional information on the management of male hypogonadism, see Uses: Uses in Males in Testosterone 68:08.

■ **Other Uses** In females, methyltestosterone is used for the palliative treatment of androgen-responsive, advanced, inoperable, metastatic (skeletal) carcinoma of the breast in women who are 1–5 years postmenopausal. Primary goals of therapy in these women include ablation of the ovaries. Other methods of counteracting estrogen activity include adrenalectomy, hypophysectomy, and/or antiestrogen therapy (e.g., tamoxifen). Androgen therapy also has been used in premenopausal women with carcinoma of the breast who have benefited from oophorectomy and are considered to have a hormone-responsive tumor. The decision to use androgen therapy in women with carcinoma of the breast should be made by an oncologist with expertise in the treatment of this carcinoma.

Methyltestosterone also has been used for the prevention of postpartum breast pain and engorgement; however, the drug does not appear to prevent or suppress lactation.

In females, methyltestosterone is used in combination with estrogens for the management of moderate to severe vasomotor symptoms† associated with menopause in patients who do not respond adequately to estrogens alone. While estrogen/androgen combinations were found to be effective for the management of vasomotor symptoms associated with menopause under a determination made by the FDA in 1976, formal administrative proceedings were initiated by the FDA in April 2003 to examine the effectiveness of estrogen/androgen combinations for this indication. FDA is undertaking this action because the agency does not believe there is substantial evidence available to establish the contribution of androgens to the effectiveness of estrogen/androgen combinations for the management of vasomotor symptoms in menopausal women who do not respond to estrogens alone. The FDA will allow continued marketing of combination estrogen/androgen products while the matter is under study.

Although methyltestosterone has been used in other conditions (e.g., fractures, surgery, convalescence, functional uterine bleeding), there is a lack of substantial evidence that androgens are effective in these conditions. In addition, the FDA states that there currently is no evidence to support the safety and efficacy of methyltestosterone as an aphrodisiac (i.e., to arouse or increase sexual desire or to improve sexual performance).

■ **Misuse, Abuse, and Dependence** Because of their anabolic and androgenic effects on performance (ergogenic potential) and physique, androgens have been misused and abused by athletes, bodybuilders, weight lifters, and others, including high school- and college-aged individuals engaged in sports. Following review of data from published literature and case reports in October 2016, the FDA concluded that misuse and abuse of androgens are associated with serious adverse cardiovascular, hepatic, endocrine, and mental health effects. (See Cautions; also see Uses: Misuse, Abuse, and Dependence, in Testosterone 68:08.)

Serum testosterone concentrations should be evaluated in patients who may be misusing or abusing androgens (e.g., patients experiencing serious adverse cardiovascular or psychiatric effects); however, serum testosterone concentrations may be below or within the normal range in patients abusing synthetic derivatives of testosterone.

Dosage and Administration

Diagnosis of male hypogonadism must be confirmed by laboratory testing prior to initiation of methyltestosterone therapy. To confirm this diagnosis, serum testosterone concentrations should be measured in the morning on at least 2 separate days and must be consistently below the normal range. Serum testosterone concentrations may be low later in the day in men with or without hypogonadism; therefore, measuring testosterone concentrations later in the day should be avoided.

■ **Administration** Methyltestosterone is administered orally; the drug usually is given in divided daily doses. Methyltestosterone also has been administered intrabuccally.

■ **Dosage** Dosage of methyltestosterone is variable and should be individualized according to the condition being treated, the severity of symptoms, and the patient's age, gender, and history of prior androgenic therapy.

Male Hypogonadism For replacement of endogenous testicular hormone in androgen-deficient males, the usual oral dosage of methyltestosterone is 10–50 mg daily as capsules. Alternatively, buccal tablets have been administered in a dosage of 5–25 mg daily. For the management of postpubertal cryptorchidism in patients with evidence of hypogonadism, several manufacturers recommend an oral methyltestosterone dosage of 30 mg daily as capsules. Alternatively, buccal tablets have been administered in a dosage of 15 mg daily.

Various dosage regimens have been used to induce pubertal changes in hypogonadal males. Some clinicians recommend that lower dosages be used initially, followed by gradual increases in dosage as puberty progresses; subsequently, the dosage may be decreased to maintenance levels. Other clinicians state that higher dosages are required initially to induce pubertal changes and lower dosages can then be used for maintenance therapy after puberty. The chronologic and skeletal ages of the patient must be considered when determining the initial dosage and subsequent dosage adjustment. In general, short-term administration (e.g., 4–6 months) of methyltestosterone and dosages in the lower end of the usual range for replacement (i.e., 10 mg daily) are used for the treatment of delayed puberty in males.

Inoperable Carcinoma of the Breast For the palliative treatment of advanced, inoperable, metastatic carcinoma of the breast in women, the usual oral dosage of methyltestosterone is 50–200 mg daily as capsules. Alternatively, buccal tablets have been administered in a dosage of 25–100 mg daily.

Postpartum Breast Pain and Engorgement For the prevention of postpartum breast pain and engorgement, the usual oral dosage of methyltestosterone is 80 mg daily as capsules for 3–5 days after parturition. Alternatively, buccal tablets have been administered in a dosage of 40 mg daily for 3–5 days after parturition.

Vasomotor Symptoms Associated with Menopause When methyltestosterone is used in combination with an estrogen (i.e., conjugated estrogens or esterified estrogens) for the short-term management of moderate to severe vasomotor symptoms† associated with menopause, the lowest possible effective dosage should be used and therapy should be discontinued as soon as possible. Attempts to reduce dosage or discontinue the drugs should be made at 3- to 6-month intervals. The combined drugs are administered for 21 consecutive days, followed by 7 days without the drugs, and then this regimen is repeated as necessary. The manufacturers' labeling for the respective drugs or drug combinations should be consulted for usual recommended dosages for combination therapy. Women with an intact uterus receiving combination therapy should be closely monitored for signs of endometrial carcinoma, and appropriate diagnostic measures should be employed if persistent or recurring abnormal vaginal bleeding occurs during therapy with the drugs.

Cautions

■ **Adverse Effects** Cardiovascular events (e.g., myocardial infarction [MI], stroke) have been reported with methyltestosterone therapy. Long-term clinical safety studies have not been conducted to date to determine the cardiovascular effects of testosterone replacement therapy in men. Epidemiologic data and results from randomized, controlled clinical trials have been inconclusive for determining the risk of serious adverse cardiovascular events (i.e., nonfatal MI, nonfatal stroke, death) with testosterone use compared with nonuse.

Because the current evidence regarding the cardiovascular risk associated with testosterone replacement therapy is weak because of the limited scope, quality, design, and size of the clinical trials, the FDA has requested additional evidence from well-designed studies to further elucidate the cardiovascular risk associated with testosterone use. Following review of data from several observational studies and meta-analyses in March 2015, the FDA concluded that use of testosterone is associated with a possible increased risk of serious adverse cardiovascular events. Clinicians should inform patients of this potential increased risk when deciding whether to use or continue to use testosterone replacement therapy. For further precautionary information about adverse cardiovascular effects, see Cautions: Cardiovascular Effects, in Testosterone 68:08.

Venous thromboembolic events, including deep-vein thrombosis (DVT) and pulmonary embolism (PE), have been reported during postmarketing experience with testosterone preparations, including methyltestosterone. Patients reporting symptoms of pain, edema, warmth, and erythema in a lower extremity or presenting with acute shortness of breath should be evaluated for possible DVT or PE, respectively. If venous thromboembolism is suspected, methyltestosterone therapy should be discontinued and appropriate evaluation and management should be initiated.

Adverse effects associated with methyltestosterone are similar to those of other synthetic or natural androgens and include acne, gynecomastia, and edema. If edema is present before or develops during therapy, administration of diuretics may be required. Gynecomastia frequently develops and occasionally persists in patients being treated for hypogonadism.

Oligospermia and decreased ejaculatory volume may occur in males receiving excessive dosage or prolonged administration of the drug. Priapism or excessive sexual stimulation in males, especially geriatric patients, also may occur. If priapism or excessive sexual stimulation develops during methyltestosterone therapy, the drug should be discontinued temporarily, since these are signs of excessive dosage; if therapy with methyltestosterone is reinstituted, a lower dosage should be used. Male pattern of baldness also may occur.

Amenorrhea and other menstrual irregularities and inhibition of gonadotropin secretion occur commonly in females. Virilization, including deepening of the voice, hirsutism, and clitoral enlargement, also occur commonly in females; these changes may not be reversible following discontinuance of the drug.

Hypersensitivity reactions, including skin manifestations and anaphylactoid reactions, have occurred rarely with methyltestosterone.

Hypercalcemia resulting from osteolysis, especially in immobile patients and those with metastatic carcinoma of the breast, has been reported in patients receiving methyltestosterone. The drug should be discontinued if hypercalcemia occurs in patients with cancer since this may indicate progression of metastases to the bone. Retention of water, sodium, chloride, potassium, and inorganic phosphates also has occurred in patients receiving the drug.

Cholestatic hepatitis and jaundice and abnormal liver function test results may occur in patients receiving 17-α-alkylandrogens such as methyltestosterone. These adverse hepatic effects may occur at relatively low doses of the drug. Drug-induced jaundice usually is reversible following discontinuance of the drug. Methyltestosterone should be discontinued if cholestatic jaundice or hepatitis occurs, or if liver function test results become abnormal during therapy with the drug, and the etiology of these disorders should be determined. Peliosis of the liver and hepatic neoplasms, including hepatocellular carcinoma, have been reported rarely in patients receiving long-term administration of androgenic anabolic steroids. Peliosis of the liver can be a life-threatening or fatal complication of androgen therapy.

Serious adverse effects (e.g., increased aggression, antisocial behavior, manic episode, hostility, depression, changes in libido, increased risk of cardiovascular events, hepatotoxicity, testicular atrophy, sperm abnormalities) are associated with misuse and abuse of androgens (see Uses: Misuse, Abuse, and Dependence). Methyltestosterone preparations currently are subject to control under the Federal Controlled Substances Act of 1970, as amended by the Anabolic Steroids Control Act of 1990 and 2004, as schedule III (C-III) drugs.

Manifestations of withdrawal (e.g., depressed mood, major depression, fatigue, cravings, restlessness, irritability, anorexia, insomnia, decreased libido, hypogonadotropic hypogonadism) may occur if androgens are discontinued abruptly or dosage is substantially reduced in physically dependent patients or in those taking supratherapeutic dosages of such drugs; withdrawal symptoms may persist for weeks or months.

Other adverse effects associated with methyltestosterone therapy include nausea, polycythemia, headache, anxiety, mental depression, generalized paresthesia, and suppression of clotting factors II, V, VII, and X. Serum cholesterol concentration may increase during androgen therapy.

■ **Precautions and Contraindications** Methyltestosterone shares the toxic potentials of other androgens, and the usual precautions of androgen therapy should be observed. When methyltestosterone is used in combination with estrogens, the usual precautions associated with estrogen therapy also should be observed. (See Cautions in Conjugated Estrogens 68:16.04.) Clinicians prescribing estrogens should be aware of the risks associated with these drugs, and the manufacturers' labeling should be consulted for further discussion of these risks and associated precautions.

Methyltestosterone should be used with caution in patients with cardiac, renal, or hepatic dysfunction since edema, with or without congestive heart failure, may occur as a result of sodium and water retention. If edema occurs during methyltestosterone therapy and it is considered a serious complication, the drug should be discontinued; diuretic therapy also may be necessary. Liver function should be evaluated periodically during use of methyltestosterone.

Some experts recommend that methyltestosterone be used with caution in patients at high risk for cardiovascular disease, such as older men or those with diabetes mellitus or obesity, since serious adverse cardiovascular events (i.e., MI, stroke, death) may occur. (See Cautions: Adverse Effects.)

Females should be carefully monitored for signs of virilization (e.g., deepening of the voice, hirsutism, clitoromegaly, menstrual irregularities) during methyltestosterone therapy. The drug should generally be discontinued when mild virilization is evident, since some adverse androgenic effects (e.g., voice changes) may not subside following discontinuance of the drug. The woman and physician may decide that some virilization is acceptable during treatment for carcinoma of the breast.

Males should be carefully monitored for the development of priapism or excessive sexual stimulation since these are signs of excessive dosage. Males, especially geriatric patients, may become overly stimulated. Stimulation to the point of increasing the nervous, mental, and physical activities beyond the patient's cardiovascular capacity should be avoided when methyltestosterone is used to treat climacteric in males. (See also Cautions: Adverse Effects.) Geriatric males may be at increased risk of developing prostatic hypertrophy and carcinoma during androgen therapy.

Adult or adolescent males should be advised to report too frequent or persistent penile erections to their physician. Females should be advised to report hoarseness, acne, menstrual changes, or the growth of facial hair to their physician. All patients should be advised to report nausea, vomiting, changes in skin color, or ankle swelling to their physician.

Patients receiving high dosages of methyltestosterone should have periodic hemoglobin and hematocrit determinations, since polycythemia may occur.

Methyltestosterone is contraindicated in males with carcinoma of the breast or known or suspected carcinoma of the prostate. Some manufacturers state that the drug also is contraindicated in patients with cardiac, renal, or hepatic decompensation; hypercalcemia; impaired liver function; and in patients who are easily sexually stimulated. Because of the potential risk of serious adverse health effects, methyltestosterone should not be used for enhancement of athletic performance or physique. (See Uses: Misuse, Abuse and Dependence, in Testosterone 68:08.) Patients should be informed of the serious adverse effects associated with misuse and abuse of androgens.

■ **Pediatric Precautions** Androgens should be used with extreme caution in children and only by specialists who are aware of the adverse effects of these drugs on bone maturation. Methyltestosterone should be used cautiously to stimulate puberty, and only in carefully selected males with delayed puberty. (See Uses: Uses in Males.) In children, methyltestosterone may accelerate bone maturation without producing compensatory gain in linear growth. This adverse effect may result in compromised adult stature. The younger the child, the greater the risk of methyltestosterone compromising final mature stature. If methyltestosterone is administered to prepubertal children (e.g., to stimulate puberty in males), the drug should be used with extreme caution, and radiographic examination of the hand and wrist should be performed every 6 months to determine the rate of bone maturation and to assess the effect of treatment on the epiphyseal centers. If methyltestosterone is to be used to stimulate puberty in a male with delayed puberty, the potential risk of therapy should be fully discussed with the patient and his parents prior to initiation of the drug.

■ **Mutagenicity and Carcinogenicity** Hepatocellular carcinoma reportedly has occurred in patients receiving long-term therapy with high dosages of androgens. Regression of the tumor does not always occur following discontinuance of androgen therapy. Geriatric patients may be at increased risk of developing prostatic hypertrophy and carcinoma during androgen therapy.

Following implantation of testosterone in mice, cervical-uterine tumors developed and occasionally metastasized. There is some evidence to suggest that injection of testosterone into some strains of female mice increases their susceptibility to hepatomas. Testosterone also has been shown to increase the number of tumors and decrease the degree of differentiation of chemically induced tumors in rats. It is not known whether androgens, including methyltestosterone, are mutagenic.

■ **Pregnancy, Fertility, and Lactation** Methyltestosterone may cause fetal harm when administered to pregnant women. Androgenic effects including clitoral hypertrophy, labial fusion of the external genital fold to form a scrotal-like structure, abnormal vaginal development, and persistence of a urogenital sinus have occurred in the female offspring of women who were given androgens during pregnancy. The degree of masculinization is related to the amount of drug given to the woman and the age of the fetus; masculinization is most likely to occur in a female fetus when exposure to androgens occurs during the first trimester. Since the risks clearly outweigh the possible benefits in women who are or may become pregnant, methyltestosterone is contraindicated in such women. Women who become pregnant while receiving the drug should be informed of the potential hazard to the fetus.

Although the effect of methyltestosterone on fertility in humans has not been conclusively determined, the drug produces oligospermia and decreased ejaculatory volume in males. Priapism and excessive sexual stimulation also have occurred in males receiving the drug. (See Cautions: Adverse Effects and Precautions and Contraindications.) Increased or decreased libido also has been reported.

It is not known whether methyltestosterone is distributed into milk. Because of the potential for serious adverse reactions to androgens in nursing infants, a decision should be made whether to discontinue nursing or to not use methyltestosterone, taking into account the importance of the drug to the woman.

Drug Interactions

Methyltestosterone may potentiate the action of oral anticoagulants, causing bleeding in some patients. When methyltestosterone therapy is initiated in patients receiving oral anticoagulants, dosage reduction of the anticoagulant may be required to prevent an excessive hypoprothrombinemic response. Patients receiving oral anticoagulants also should be closely monitored when androgen therapy is discontinued.

The metabolic effects of androgens may decrease blood glucose concentrations and insulin requirements in patients with diabetes.

Laboratory Test Interferences

Protein bound iodine (PBI) concentrations may be decreased in some patients during methyltestosterone therapy; however, this does not appear to be clinically important. Androgens may decrease thyroxine-binding globulin concentrations, resulting in decreased total serum thyroxine (T_4) concentrations and increased resin uptake of triiodothyronine (T_3) and T_4. Free thyroid hormone concentrations remain unchanged, and there is no clinical evidence of thyroid dysfunction.

Pharmacology

Endogenous androgens are essential hormones that are responsible for the normal growth and development of the male sex organs and for maintenance of secondary sex characteristics, including the growth and maturation of the prostate, seminal vesicles, penis, and scrotum; development of male hair distribution, such as beard, pubic, chest, and axillary hair; laryngeal enlargement and thickening of the vocal cords; and alterations in body musculature and fat distribution.

Like testosterone and other androgenic anabolic hormones, methyltestosterone also produces retention of nitrogen, potassium, sodium, and phosphorus; increases protein anabolism; and decreases amino acid catabolism and urinary calcium concentrations. Nitrogen balance is improved only when there is sufficient intake of calories and protein.

Androgens are responsible for the growth spurt that occurs during adolescence and for the eventual termination of linear growth that results from fusion of the epiphyseal growth centers. Although exogenous androgens accelerate linear growth rates in children, the drugs may cause a disproportionate advancement in bone maturation, and long-term administration of the drugs in prepubertal children may result in fusion of the epiphyseal growth centers and premature termination of the growth process.

Exogenous administration of androgens inhibits the release of endogenous testosterone via feedback inhibition of pituitary luteinizing hormone (LH). Following administration of large doses of exogenous androgens, spermatogenesis also may be suppressed as a result of feedback inhibition of pituitary follicle-stimulating hormone (FSH).

Androgens reportedly stimulate the production of erythrocytes, apparently by enhancing the production of erythropoietic stimulating factor.

Chemistry and Stability

■ **Chemistry** Methyltestosterone is a synthetic androgenic anabolic steroid hormone. The drug is structurally similar to testosterone, but is methylated at the 17 position of the steroid nucleus. Methylation at the 17 position is associated with less hepatic metabolism and enhanced pharmacologic activity following oral administration compared with testosterone.

Methyltestosterone occurs as white or creamy white, odorless, slightly hygroscopic crystals or a crystalline powder and is practically insoluble in water and soluble in alcohol.

■ **Stability** Commercially available preparations of methyltestosterone should be protected from light and stored in well-closed containers at a temperature less than 40°C, preferably between 2–30°C, unless otherwise specified by the manufacturer.

Preparations

Most methyltestosterone-containing preparations are subject to control under the Federal Controlled Substances Act of 1970, as amended by the Anabolic Steroids Control Act of 1990 and 2004, as schedule III (C-III) drugs. However, manufacturers of certain preparations containing androgenic anabolic steroids (principally combinations that also include estrogens) have applied for and obtained for their product(s) an exemption from the record-keeping and other regulatory requirements of the Federal Controlled Substances Act. (See the introductory paragraph under Preparations, in Testosterone 68:08.) Because regulatory requirements for a given preparation containing an androgenic anabolic steroid may be subject to change under the provisions of the Act, the manufacturer should be contacted when specific clarification about a preparation's status is required.

Excipients in commercially available drug preparations may have clinically important effects in some individuals; consult specific product labeling for details.

methylTESTOSTERone

Oral

Capsules	10 mg*	**Android®** (C-III), Valeant
		methylTESTOSTERone Capsules (C-III)
		Testred® (C-III), Valeant
Tablets	10 mg*	**Methitest®** (C-III; scored), Global
		methylTESTOSTERone Tablets (C-III)

*available from one or more manufacturer, distributor, and/or repackager by generic (nonproprietary) name

†Use is not currently included in the labeling approved by the US Food and Drug Administration

Testosterone

■ Testosterone, the principal endogenous androgen, is a naturally occurring androgenic anabolic steroid hormone.

REMS

FDA approved a REMS for testosterone to ensure that the benefits outweigh the risks. The REMS may apply to one or more preparations of testosterone and consists of the following: medication guide or elements to assure safe use and implementation system. See the FDA REMS page (https://www.accessdata.fda.gov/scripts/cder/rems/index.cfm).

Uses

Testosterone is used for replacement or substitution of diminished or absent endogenous testicular hormone caused by certain medical conditions.

Diagnosis of hypogonadism must be confirmed by laboratory testing prior to initiation of testosterone therapy. (See Dosage and Administration.)

The safety and efficacy of testosterone replacement therapy in men with low testosterone concentrations related to aging have not been established. (See Late-onset Hypogonadism under Uses: Uses in Males.)

■ **Uses in Males** ***Hypogonadism*** In males, testosterone is used for the management of congenital or acquired primary hypogonadism such as that resulting from orchiectomy or from testicular failure caused by cryptorchidism, bilateral torsion, orchitis, or vanishing testis syndrome. Testosterone also is used in males for the management of congenital or acquired hypogonadotropic hypogonadism such as that resulting from idiopathic gonadotropin or gonadotropin-releasing hormone (luteinizing hormone releasing hormone) deficiency or from pituitary-hypothalamic injury caused by tumors, trauma, or radiation. If any of these conditions occur before puberty, androgen replacement therapy will be necessary during adolescence for the development of secondary sexual characteristics and prolonged therapy will be required to maintain these characteristics. Prolonged androgen therapy also is required to maintain sexual characteristics in other males who develop testosterone deficiency after puberty.

Manifestations. Hypogonadism in males may manifest with signs and symptoms of testosterone deficiency and/or infertility, with manifestations depending principally on the age of the patient at the time of development. Hypogonadism seldom is recognized before the age of puberty unless it is associated with growth retardation or other anatomic and/or endocrine abnormalities. When hypogonadism develops before puberty onset, manifestations include small testes, phallus, and prostate; minimal pubic and axillary hair; disproportionately long arms and legs (secondary to delayed epiphyseal closure); reduced male musculature; gynecomastia; and a persistently high-pitched voice. Postpubertal loss of testicular function results in slowly evolving subtle clinical manifestations, which may be difficult to appreciate in aging men because they often are attributed to growing old. Growth of body hair usually slows, while the voice and size of the phallus and prostate remain unchanged. Patients with postpubertal hypogonadism may manifest a progressive decrease in muscle mass, libido loss, impotence, oligospermia or azoospermia, and/or occasionally menopause-type hot flushes (with acute onset of hypogonadism). Hypogonadism also is associated with a risk of osteoporosis and resultant fractures. Many cases of postpubertal hypogonadism are initially detected during fertility evaluations.

Hypogonadism Associated with HIV Infection. Hypogonadism occurs commonly in human immunodeficiency virus (HIV)-infected men, particularly as their disease progresses to acquired immunodeficiency syndrome (AIDS). Hypogonadism has been reported in up to 50% of HIV-infected men, being most likely in those with AIDS; however, the incidence may now be lower as a result of highly active antiretroviral therapy (HAART) and resultant improved overall health in HIV-infected patients. Such patients generally exhibit low serum testosterone concentrations and usually low (indicating hypothalamic-pituitary involvement) or occasionally high (indicating testicular involvement) gonadotropin concentrations. In addition to typical manifestations of hypogonadism (e.g., impaired sexual mood and functioning, loss of body hair, gynecomastia, bone loss, impaired sense of well-being), hypogonadal HIV-infected men may exhibit a disproportionate loss of lean body mass and muscle wasting. The etiology of hypotestosteronism in HIV-infected men likely is multifactorial and may show interindividual variation and may include primary testicular problems, changes in the hypothalamic-pituitary-gonadal axis, and/or changes caused by chronic illness, poor nutrition, or medications; approximately 25% of hypogonadism cases in HIV-infected men are primary. Testosterone replacement therapy is considered the androgen of choice for the treatment of androgen deficiency (e.g., hypogonadism) and AIDS wasting in HIV-infected men.

Late-onset Hypogonadism. The safety and efficacy of testosterone replacement therapy for men with late-onset hypogonadism (i.e., low testosterone concentrations related to aging) have not been established. Although endogenous testosterone concentrations decline with aging and manifestations of hypogonadism such as decreased libido, impotence, decreased body hair growth, decreased muscle mass, increased risk of cardiovascular disease, and decreased bone mass and resultant osteoporosis may occur, it is unclear whether these symptoms are related to such decreased concentrations or to normal aging; therefore, the need to replace testosterone in aging men is unclear.

There currently is a paucity of information from well-designed studies on the use of testosterone in middle-aged or older men who do not meet the clinical diagnostic criteria for established hypogonadism but who may have testosterone levels in the low range for young adults and/or who show one or more manifestations common to both aging and hypogonadism. In addition, studies that have been conducted generally have been of short duration, involved small numbers of patients, and often lacked adequate controls. Therefore, assessments of risks and benefits have been limited to date, and uncertainties remain about the value of testosterone therapy in older men without a clinical diagnosis of hypogonadism. In most studies to date, it appears that older men were given testosterone dosages that increased testosterone levels to the normal physiologic range for young adult males. Because of the potential risks of testosterone therapy and the availability of other safe and effective intervention options for some of the diseases and conditions it is intended to prevent or treat (e.g., bisphosphonates for osteoporosis), testosterone should be considered a therapeutic rather than a preventative measure in aging men. Although endogenous testosterone levels clearly decline with aging, it currently is unclear whether such decreased levels affect health outcomes in older men. Much remains unknown about how physiologic pathways are affected by changes in endogenous testosterone concentrations or by the administration of exogenous testosterone in aging men.

Current limited evidence suggests that testosterone therapy in aging men may produce beneficial effects on body composition, strength, bone density, frailty, cognitive function, mood, sexual function, and quality of life. However, additional evidence from well-designed studies is needed to further elucidate the role of testosterone therapy in men with low testosterone concentrations related to aging.

Testosterone Replacement Therapy for Hypogonadism. Men with symptomatic hypogonadism and clearly low testosterone concentrations (free or total, considering SHBG) are potential candidates for testosterone replacement therapy; however, the potential prostatic risk must be considered. Serum total (bound and free) testosterone concentrations less than 300 ng/dL generally are considered indicative of hypogonadism in men, and the biochemical goal of hormone replacement therapy with testosterone generally is to increase serum total testosterone concentrations to within the normal physiologic range of 300–1200 ng/mL. The principal goals of testosterone replacement are to restore sexual function, libido, well-being, and behavior; to stimulate and maintain virilization (e.g., secondary sex characteristics such as muscle mass, body hair, phallus growth); to optimize bone density and prevent osteoporosis; to possibly normalize somatotropin (growth hormone) concentrations in geriatric men; to potentially improve cardiovascular risk; and to restore fertility in cases of hypogonadotropic hypogonadism. In HIV-infected men, additional goals include improvement in mood (e.g., depression), energy level (fatigue), quality of life, and lean body mass (wasting syndrome); however, clinical response to testosterone therapy in HIV-infected men is not necessarily correlated to baseline serum testosterone concentrations, and eugonadal HIV-infected men may benefit from such therapy.

Delayed Puberty When the diagnosis is well established, testosterone may be used to stimulate puberty in carefully selected males with delayed puberty. These males usually have a family history of delayed puberty that is not caused by a pathologic disorder. Brief treatment with conservative doses of an androgen may occasionally be justified in these males if they do not respond to psychologic support. Because androgens may adversely affect bone maturation in these prepubertal males, this potential risk should be fully discussed with the patient and his parents prior to initiation of androgen therapy. (See Cautions: Pediatric Precautions.) If androgen therapy is initiated in these prepubertal males, radiographs of the hand and wrist should be obtained at 6-month intervals to determine the effect of therapy on the epiphyseal centers. Testosterone is designated an orphan drug by the FDA for use in this condition.

Corticosteroid-induced Hypogonadism and Osteoporosis Patients receiving long-term corticosteroid therapy may develop hypogonadism secondary to inhibition of secretion of luteinizing hormone (LH) and follicle-stimulating hormone (FSH) from the pituitary as well as secondary to direct effects on the testes and ovaries, and such hypogonadism may be associated with bone loss. Therefore, all patients receiving prolonged corticosteroid therapy should be assessed for possible hypogonadism, which should be corrected if present. Unlike experience with hormone replacement therapy (HRT, combined estrogen and progestin therapy) in postmenopausal women receiving chronic prednisone therapy, there currently is only limited information on the effect of androgen (e.g., testosterone) replacement therapy in men with hypogonadism secondary to long-term corticosteroid therapy. In a small study in men with corticosteroid-treated asthma and low serum testosterone concentrations, lumbar spine bone mass density (BMD) was increased nearly 4% after 12 months of monthly testosterone injections; lean body mass also was increased and fat mass was reduced. Therefore, men who develop low serum testosterone concentrations while receiving long-term corticosteroid therapy should be offered testosterone replacement therapy in an attempt to treat hypogonadism and possibly reduce the risk of corticosteroid-induced osteoporosis† when contraindications to androgen therapy are not present. Some experts (e.g., the American College of Rheumatology) recommend that such men with serum testosterone concentrations below the physiologic range (i.e., less than 300 ng/mL) receive replacement therapy. The goal of testosterone replacement therapy in men receiving long-term corticosteroid therapy is to provide serum testosterone concentrations within the therapeutic range. It is important that the possibility of prostate cancer be ruled out in any man being considered for such replacement therapy. For additional information on the management of corticosteroid-induced osteoporosis, see Cautions: Musculoskeletal Effects in the Corticosteroids General Statement 68:04.

Erectile Dysfunction Although testosterone replacement therapy may restore sexual function in hypogonadal men (see Uses in Males: Hypogonadism, in Uses), the American Urological Association (AUA) states that the drug is not indicated for the treatment of erectile dysfunction in men with normal serum testosterone concentrations†. Outcome measures in studies to date are inadequate to evaluate testosterone's efficacy in eugonadal men. In men with borderline testosterone concentrations, a clinical trial of replacement therapy may be warranted in the management of erectile dysfunction; however, the risks of hormone replacement must be weighed carefully.

■ **Uses in Females** ***Inoperable Carcinoma of the Breast*** In females, testosterone has been used for the palliative treatment of androgen-responsive, advanced, inoperable, metastatic (skeletal) carcinoma of the breast in women who are 1–5 years postmenopausal. Primary goals of therapy in these women include ablation of the ovaries. Other methods of counteracting estrogen activity include adrenalectomy, hypophysectomy, and/or antiestrogen therapy (e.g., tamoxifen). Androgen therapy also has been used in premenopausal women with carcinoma of the breast who have benefited from oophorectomy and are considered to have a hormone-responsive tumor. The decision to use androgen therapy in women with carcinoma of the breast should be made by an oncologist with expertise in the treatment of this carcinoma.

Postpartum Breast Pain and Engorgement Testosterone formerly was used for the prevention of postpartum breast pain and engorgement†; however, the drug does not appear to prevent or suppress lactation. Testosterone esters also have been used in combination with estrogens for the prevention of postpartum breast pain and engorgement; however, the FDA has withdrawn approval of estrogen-containing drugs for this indication. Data from controlled studies indicate that the incidence of substantial painful engorgement is low in untreated women, and the condition usually responds to analgesic or other supportive therapy.

Menopause In females, testosterone esters also are used in combination with estrogens for the management of moderate to severe vasomotor symptoms† associated with menopause in patients who do not respond adequately to estrogens alone. While estrogen/androgen combinations were found to be effective for the management of vasomotor symptoms associated with menopause under a determination made by the FDA in 1976, formal administrative proceedings were initiated by the FDA in April 2003 to examine the effectiveness of estrogen/androgen combinations for this indication. FDA is undertaking this action because the agency does not believe there is substantial evidence available to establish the contribution of androgens to the effectiveness of estrogen/androgen combinations for the management of vasomotor symptoms in menopausal women who do not respond to estrogens alone. The FDA will allow continued marketing of combination estrogen/androgen products while the matter is under study.

■ **Misuse, Abuse, and Dependence** Because of their anabolic and androgenic effects on performance (ergogenic potential) and physique, androgens have been misused and abused by athletes, bodybuilders, weight lifters, and others, including high school- and college-aged individuals engaged in sports. The drugs also have been misused and abused for cosmetic purposes by noncompetitors attempting to achieve bodies with lean muscle mass. Although historically the drugs have been regarded as ineffective for anabolic and androgenic uses in athletes, limited evidence suggests that androgens may increase skeletal muscle mass and strength when used in conjunction with proper (e.g., high-protein, high calorie) diet and training but that their use is not associated with increased power or capacity for aerobic work. There continues to be a lack of evidence of long-term beneficial effects, and the drugs have been associated with substantial adverse health effects and toxicity. When used to improve athletic performance and physique, dosages employed often substantially (e.g., 10- to 1000-fold) exceed usual therapeutic dosages of the drugs. In addition, several androgens often are taken concomitantly ("stacking") for extended periods. The extent of misuse and abuse of androgens has not been fully determined, but nonmedical use is believed to be widespread. Estimates for the rate of misuse and abuse by weight lifters and body builders have ranged up to 50–80%. However, in terms of actual numbers, it has been suggested that most misuse and abuse of androgens are by individuals who never compete in sports. Evidence from one study indicates that about 7% of male high school seniors use or have used the drugs. Although the likelihood of use was increased in males intending to participate in school-sponsored sports (particularly football and wrestling), 35% of users had no intention of participating in school-sponsored sports. About 40% of these high school students admitted initiating use of the drugs at 15 years of age or younger. In studies of college students, androgen use among athletes ranged up to about 20%.

Following review of data from published literature and case reports in October 2016, the FDA concluded that misuse and abuse of androgens are associated with serious adverse effects. Serious adverse effects including increased aggression, hostility, and antisocial behavior ("roid rage"); psychotic manifestations and affective disorders (e.g., manic episode, depression, paranoia, psychosis, delusions, hallucinations); changes in libido; cardiovascular events (e.g., cardiac arrest, myocardial infarction [MI], hypertrophic cardiomyopathy, congestive heart failure [CHF], cerebrovascular accident); and hepatotoxicity (e.g., abnormal liver function test results, liver tumors [hepatic adenomas, hepatocellular carcinoma], peliosis hepatis, jaundice) have been reported in individuals who misuse and abuse androgens. Other potential adverse effects of androgens in adolescents or younger children include premature bone maturation and epiphyseal closure with resultant irreversible short stature, precocious puberty, possible increased risk of ruptured tendons and ligaments and of tendinitis, and acne. Other potential adverse effects of androgens in males include transient ischemic attacks, convulsions, hypomania, irritability, dyslipidemias, gynecomastia, hair loss, testicular atrophy and sperm abnormalities (oligospermia, decreased motility, abnormal morphology, azoospermia), impotence, subfertility, infertility, and prostatic enlargement with resultant difficulty in urinating. Other potential adverse effects in females include clitoral enlargement (which may be irreversible), menstrual irregularities, hirsutism, androgenetic alopecia, deepened voice, breast atrophy, and virilization. Manifestations of withdrawal (e.g., depressed mood, major depression, fatigue, cravings, restlessness, irritability, anorexia, insomnia, decreased libido, hypogonadotropic hypogonadism) may occur if androgens, such as testosterone, are discontinued abruptly or the dosage is substantially reduced in patients who are physically dependent or receiving supratherapeutic doses of the drug; withdrawal symptoms may persist for weeks or months.

Serum testosterone concentrations should be evaluated in patients who may be misusing or abusing androgens (e.g., patients experiencing serious adverse cardiovascular or psychiatric effects); however, serum testosterone concentrations may be below or within the normal range in patients abusing synthetic derivatives of testosterone. Because of the potential for serious adverse effects associated with misuse and abuse of androgens, preventive measures have been initiated, including educational programs, interdiction of black market supplies, drug screening of athletes with associated penalties for use, and other control measures. The prescription, dispensing, distribution, and use of most androgens currently are restricted as controlled substances. In addition, medical and sports experts, including the American College of Sports Medicine, American Medical Association, American Academy of Pediatrics, American College Health Association, National Strength and Conditioning Association, National Collegiate Athletic Association, National Football League, US Olympic Committee, and the International Olympic Committee, consider the use of androgens to enhance athletic performance or physique inappropriate and unacceptable because of known adverse effects, lack of data regarding long-term gains in size and strength, and potential long-term adverse sequelae and because their use by athletes is contrary to the rules and ethical principles of athletic competition.

Dosage and Administration

Diagnosis of hypogonadism must be confirmed by laboratory testing prior to initiation of testosterone therapy. To confirm this diagnosis, serum testosterone concentrations should be measured in the morning on at least 2 separate days and must be consistently below the normal range. Serum testosterone concentrations may be low later in the day in men with or without hypogonadism; therefore, measuring testosterone concentrations later in the day should be avoided.

■ **Administration** Testosterone is administered by IM injection; percutaneously by topical application of a transdermal system, solution, or gel to the skin; intranasally; subcutaneously as a biodegradable implant; and intrabuccally (transmucosally) as a buccal tablet.

IM Injection Testosterone cypionate (Depo®-testosterone), testosterone enanthate (Delatestryl®), and testosterone undecanoate (Aveed®) are administered by deep IM injection into the gluteal muscle; the usual precautions for IM administration should be followed.

Because of the risk of serious pulmonary oil microembolism reactions and anaphylaxis following IM administration of testosterone undecanoate, patients should be observed for 30 minutes in a healthcare setting following each IM injection of the drug.

Restricted Distribution Program. Because of the potential for serious pulmonary oil microembolism reactions and anaphylaxis in patients receiving IM testosterone undecanoate (Aveed®) (see Cautions: Sensitivity Reactions and also Other Adverse Effects), testosterone undecanoate must be obtained through a restricted distribution program, the Aveed® Risk Evaluation and Mitigation Strategy (REMS) Program, designed to minimize the risk of pulmonary oil microembolism reactions and anaphylaxis. Clinicians and institutions that prescribe and/or dispense testosterone undecanoate must enroll in and comply with all requirements of the Aveed® REMS Program. Institutions are required to have appropriate equipment for the treatment of serious pulmonary oil microembolism and anaphylactic reactions for immediate use in patients receiving the drug. For additional information or to enroll in the Aveed® REMS program, clinicians may contact 855-755-0494 or visit www.AveedREMS.com.

Subcutaneous Administration Testosterone pellets are administered as a biodegradable implant subcutaneously into the hip or other fatty area by a clinician; the usual precautions for subcutaneous implantation should be followed.

Transdermal Administration Patients receiving transdermal testosterone therapy (Androderm®) should be carefully instructed in the proper use and disposal of the transdermal system. To obtain optimum results, patients should be given a copy of the patient instructions provided by the manufacturer. To expose the adhesive surface of the system, the protective liner should be peeled and discarded prior to administration.

The transdermal system should then be applied topically to a clean, dry area of skin on the back, abdomen, upper arm, or thigh by firmly pressing the system with the adhesive side touching the skin; the system should *not* be applied to the scrotum. The system should be applied immediately after removal from its protective pouch and removal of the protective liner. The system should be pressed firmly in place, ensuring good contact, particularly around the edges. The application site should not be oily, damaged, or irritated. Application of transdermal systems over bony prominences or on a part of the body that may be subject to prolonged pressure during sleep or sitting (e.g., the deltoid region of the upper arm, the greater trochanter of the femur, the ischial tuberosity) should be avoided, because burn-like blisters may occur. If the transdermal system becomes loose, the system should be smoothed down by firmly rubbing around the edges. If the system should inadvertently come off before noon following application the previous evening, a new system may be applied until the next scheduled application that evening. If the transdermal system comes off later in the day, the system should not be replaced until the next scheduled application that evening. If a system comes off, it should not be reapplied with tape.

To minimize and/or prevent potential skin irritation, each testosterone transdermal system should be applied at a different site, with an interval of at least 1 week allowed between applications to a particular site. Mild skin irritation may be ameliorated by application of over-the-counter topical hydrocortisone *cream* after system removal; alternatively, a small amount of triamcinolone acetonide *cream* 0.1% may be applied to the skin under the drug reservoir to minimize irritation (ointment formulations should *not* be used because they may reduce testosterone absorption).

Testosterone transdermal systems are applied once daily; to produce serum testosterone concentrations that mimic endogenous profiles, the system should be applied at night (e.g., 10 p.m.). The system should be left in place for approximately 24 hours; after this period, the system should be removed and discarded and a new system applied.

The transdermal system does not need to be removed during sexual intercourse nor while showering or bathing; however, patients should avoid swimming, showering, or washing the administration site for at least 3 hours following application.

Topical Administration Patients receiving testosterone topical gel (AndroGel®, Fortesta®, Testim®, Vogelxo®) or solution (Axiron®) should be instructed on use of the gel or solution and given a copy of the patient instructions provided by the manufacturer.

AndroGel® is commercially available as unit-dose packets or as a metered-dose pump. AndroGel® should be applied topically once daily, preferably in the morning, to clean, dry, intact skin only; testosterone topical gel 1% (AndroGel® 1%) should be applied on the shoulders, upper arms, and/or abdomen and testosterone topical gel 1.62% (AndroGel® 1.62%) should be applied only on the shoulders and upper arms. The gel should *not* be applied to other parts of the body (e.g., genitals, chest, axillae, knees, back). To apply a dose from the unit-dose packet, the entire contents of the packet should be squeezed into the palm of the hand and immediately applied to the application site; alternatively, a portion of the contents should be squeezed into the palm of the hand and applied to the application site and the procedure repeated until the entire contents of the packet has been applied. Alternatively, the gel can be applied directly to the application site. Patients using the metered-dose pump should be instructed to prime the pump prior to initial use by depressing the pump 3 times; this gel should be discarded by rinsing down the sink or placing in household trash in a manner that avoids accidental exposure or ingestion by household members or pets. To apply a dose from the metered-dose pump, the gel may be collected in the palm of the hand by pressing the pump firmly and fully; the gel is applied to the application site. Patients should immediately wash their hands with soap and water following application of the gel. Before dressing, the patient should allow the application site to dry; after the gel has dried, the application site should be covered with clothing (e.g., a shirt) to prevent transfer of testosterone to another individual. Following application of AndroGel® 1 or 1.62%, patients should avoid swimming, showering, or washing the application site for at least 5 or 2 hours, respectively.

Testim® is commercially available as unit-dose tubes. Testim® should be applied topically once daily, preferably in the morning, to clean, dry, intact skin only on the shoulders and/or upper arms; the gel should *not* be applied to the abdomen or genitals. Upon opening the tube, the entire contents should be squeezed into the palm of the hand and immediately applied to the application site. Patients should immediately wash their hands with soap and water following application of the gel. Before dressing, the patient should allow the application site to dry; after the gel has dried, the application site should be covered with clothing (e.g., a shirt) to prevent transfer of testosterone to another individual. Patients should avoid swimming, showering, or washing the administration site for at least 2 hours following application.

Vogelxo® is commercially available as unit-dose tubes or packets and as a metered-dose pump. Vogelxo® should be applied topically once daily to clean, dry, intact skin only on the shoulders and/or upper arms; the gel should *not* be applied to the abdomen or genitals. To apply a dose from the unit-dose tube or packet, the entire contents of the tube or packet should be squeezed into the palm of the hand and immediately applied to the application site. Patients using the metered-dose pump should be instructed to prime the pump prior to initial use by pressing the pump 3 times; this gel should be discarded by rinsing down the sink to avoid accidental exposure or ingestion by others. To apply a dose from the metered-dose pump, the gel may be collected in the palm of the hand by pressing the pump firmly and fully; the gel is applied to the application site. Patients should immediately wash their hands with soap and water following application of the gel. Before dressing, the patient should allow the application site to dry; after the gel has dried, the application site should be covered with clothing (e.g., a shirt) to prevent transfer of testosterone to another individual. Patients should avoid swimming, showering, or washing the application site for at least 2 hours following administration.

Fortesta® is commercially available as a metered-dose pump. Fortesta® should be applied topically once daily, in the morning, to clean, dry, intact skin only on the front and inner thighs; the gel should *not* be applied to the genitals or other parts of the body. Patients should be instructed to prime the pump prior to initial use by pressing the pump 8 times; this gel should be discarded by rinsing down the sink or placing in household trash in a manner that avoids accidental exposure or ingestion by others. To apply a dose from the metered-dose pump, the gel should be applied directly to the application site; the area of the thigh adjacent to the scrotum should be avoided. Patients should use one finger to gently and evenly rub the gel into the application site. Patients should immediately wash their hands with soap and water following application of the gel. Before dressing, the patient should allow the application site to dry; after the gel has dried, the application site should be covered with clothing (e.g., pants, shorts) to prevent transfer of testosterone to another individual. Patients should avoid swimming, showering, or washing the application site for at least 2 hours following administration.

Axiron® is commercially available as a metered-dose pump. Axiron® should be applied topically once daily to clean, dry, intact skin only on the axilla; the solution should *not* be applied to the genitals or other parts of the body (i.e., abdomen, shoulders, upper arms). Patients should be instructed to prime the pump prior to initial use by pressing the pump 3 times; this solution should be discarded by rinsing down a basin, sink, or toilet. To dispense a dose from the metered-dose pump, the solution should be dispensed into the applicator cup. To apply a dose from the applicator cup, the applicator cup should be held upright and placed onto the application site and then wiped steadily up and down. If the solution drips or runs, excess solution should be collected using the applicator cup; the solution should *not* be rubbed in with fingers or hands. Application sites should be allowed to dry completely prior to another application. Deodorants and antiperspirants should not affect the efficacy of Axiron®; however, application of a deodorant or antiperspirant (stick or roll-on) should occur prior to application of Axiron® to avoid contamination of the deodorant or antiperspirant product. Patients should immediately wash their hands with soap and water following application of the solution. Before dressing, the patient should allow the application site to dry; after the solution has dried, the application site should be covered with clothing (e.g., shirt) to prevent transfer of testosterone to another individual. Patients should avoid swimming, showering, or washing the application site for at least 2 hours following administration.

Prior to any situation in which skin-to-skin contact with other individuals at the site of testosterone gel or solution application is anticipated, patients should wash the application site(s) thoroughly with soap and water to remove any testosterone residue. If unwashed or unclothed skin at the site of testosterone gel or solution application comes in contact with the skin of another individual, the general area of contact should be washed with soap and water as soon as possible. Studies show that residual testosterone is removed from the skin surface by washing with soap and water. Signs of virilization in children (e.g., changes in genital size, libido, or development of pubic hair) and women (e.g., changes in body hair distribution, substantial increases in acne) and the possibility of secondary exposure to topical testosterone products (AndroGel®, Axiron®, Fortesta®, Testim®, Vogelxo®) should be brought to the attention of a clinician. (See Cautions: Precautions and Contraindications.)

Buccal Administration Patients receiving testosterone extended-release buccal (transmucosal) tablets (Striant®) should be instructed on use of the buccal system and given a copy of the patient instructions provided by the manufacturer. Testosterone extended-release buccal (transmucosal) tablets are applied to the gum region twice daily, morning and evening (approximately 12 hours apart). Upon opening the packet, the rounded-side surface of the buccal tablet should be placed against the gum and held in place with a finger over the lip and against the buccal tablet for 30 seconds. The buccal tablet should be placed just above the incisor tooth; the application site should be alternated between the left and right upper incisors. The buccal tablet is designed to stay in place until removed. Care should be taken not to dislodge the buccal tablet; placement of the tablet should be verified after tooth brushing, use of mouthwash, and eating or drinking liquids. The buccal tablet should not be chewed or swallowed. If the buccal tablet fails to properly adhere to the gum or falls off, the buccal tablet should be removed and a new tablet applied. If the buccal tablet must be replaced within 8 hours after application, the new tablet can remain in place until the next regularly scheduled dose (i.e., the application schedule employed should be continued). If the tablet must be replaced more than 8 hours after application, the replacement tablet can remain in place for the remainder of the current dosing interval as well as the next full dosing interval. To remove the buccal tablet, the tablet should be slid downward from the gum toward the tooth.

Intranasal Administration Testosterone nasal gel (Natesto®) is administered intranasally using a metered-dose nasal pump. Patients should be instructed carefully in the use of the nasal pump. To obtain optimum results, patients also should be given a copy of the patient instructions provided by the manufacturer. Testosterone nasal gel should be administered intranasally 3 times daily; the nasal gel should *not* be applied to other parts of the body. Patients should be instructed to prime the pump prior to initial use by depressing the pump 10 times; this gel should be discarded by rinsing down a sink with warm water. Prior to administration of testosterone nasal gel, patients should clear their nasal passages. Patients should place their right index finger on the pump of the actuator and slowly insert the actuator into the left nostril until the finger reaches the base of the nose. To ensure adequate application of the gel, the tip of the actuator should be in contact with the lateral wall of the nostril. To dispense a dose from the metered-dose pump, the pump should be slowly pressed until it stops and the tip of the actuator should be wiped along the inside of the lateral nostril wall upon removal from the nose. This procedure is then repeated using the patient's left index finger for administration to the right nostril. Patients should lightly massage the application site by pressing on the nostrils just below the nasal bridge. Patients should avoid blowing their nose or sniffing for 1 hour following application. If testosterone nasal gel gets on the hands, patients should wash their hands with soap and warm water.

■ **Dosage** Dosage of testosterone is variable and should be individualized according to the condition being treated; the severity of symptoms; the patient's age, gender, and history of prior androgenic therapy; and the specific testosterone preparation being used.

Various dosage regimens have been used to induce pubertal changes in hypogonadal males. Some clinicians recommend that lower dosages be used initially, followed by gradual increases in dosage as puberty progresses; subsequently, the dosage may be decreased to maintenance levels. Other clinicians state that higher dosages are required initially to induce pubertal changes and lower dosages can then be used for maintenance therapy after puberty. The chronologic and skeletal ages of the patient must be considered when determining the initial dosage and subsequent dosage adjustment.

IM Dosage **Male Hypogonadism.** For replacement of endogenous testicular hormone in androgen-deficient males, the usual IM dosage of testosterone cypionate or testosterone enanthate is 50–400 mg every 2–4 weeks. The recommended initial dosage of testosterone undecanoate is 750 mg every 4 weeks for the first 2 doses, then 750 mg every 10 weeks thereafter. In general, testosterone therapy is initiated with full therapeutic doses; subsequent dosage adjustment should be made according to the patient's tolerance and therapeutic response.

Alternatively, some clinicians state that complete androgen replacement in hypogonadal men generally can be achieved with 50–100 mg of testosterone cypionate or testosterone enanthate administered IM every 7–10 days. This regimen generally will achieve relatively physiologic testosterone concentrations throughout the time interval between doses. Longer time intervals between IM doses are more convenient but are associated with greater fluctuations in testosterone concentrations. Higher dosages produce longer-term effects but higher peak concentrations and wider swings between peak and nadir testosterone concentrations and resultant symptom fluctuation in many patients. If less frequent injection is desired, 100–150 mg IM every 2 weeks may be considered. While 300 mg IM every 3 weeks also may be considered for convenience, such dosing is associated with wider testosterone fluctuations and generally is inadequate to ensure a consistent clinical response. For men who develop pronounced symptoms in the week prior to the next dose with such prolonged dosing intervals, a smaller dose at a shorter dosing interval should be tried; in general, serum total testosterone concentrations should exceed 250–300 ng/dL just before the next dose.

If full androgen replacement is not required, lower testosterone dosages are used. For example, in adult males with prepubertal onset of hypogonadism who are going through puberty for the first time with IM testosterone replacement, testosterone therapy may be initiated at 50 mg every 3–4 weeks, gradually increasing the dose in subsequent months as tolerated up to full replacement within 1 year.

Attainment of full virilization in men with hypogonadism may require up to 3–4 years of IM testosterone replacement. Patients generally should be monitored at 4–6 months to assess clinical progress, review compliance, and determine whether any complications or psychologic adjustment problems are present.

For delayed puberty, the usual IM dosage of testosterone enanthate is 50–200 mg every 2–4 weeks for a limited period of time (e.g., 4–6 months).

Inoperable Carcinoma of the Breast. For the palliative treatment of advanced, inoperable, metastatic carcinoma of the breast in women, the usual IM dosage of testosterone enanthate is 200–400 mg every 2–4 weeks.

Subcutaneous Dosage For replacement of endogenous testicular hormone in androgen-deficient males, the usual dosage of testosterone pellets is 150–450 mg implanted subcutaneously every 3–6 months. Dosage adjustment should be made according to the patient's tolerance and therapeutic response.

For delayed puberty, the dosage of testosterone pellets is generally less than the dosage used for male hypogonadism and for a limited period of time (e.g., 4–6 months).

Transdermal Dosage Transdermal testosterone (Androderm®) is commercially available as a system delivering 2 mg/24 hours or 4 mg/24 hours. Dosage should be adjusted according to determinations of serum testosterone concentrations.

When Androderm® is used for the treatment of male hypogonadism, the usual initial transdermal dosage is 4 mg once daily administered nightly as one system delivering 4 mg/24 hours. Dosage should be adjusted according to morning serum testosterone concentrations approximately 2 weeks following initiation of therapy. Depending on requirements, dosage can be increased to 6 mg once daily administered nightly as one system delivering 4 mg/24 hours plus one delivering 2 mg/24 hours or can be decreased to 2 mg once daily administered nightly as one system delivering 2 mg/24 hours.

Patients currently maintained on a transdermal dosage of 2.5 mg once daily may be switched to one system delivering 2 mg/24 hours at the next scheduled dose. Patients currently maintained on a transdermal dosage of 5 mg once daily may be switched to one system delivering 4 mg/24 hours at the next scheduled dose. Patients currently maintained on a transdermal dosage of 7.5 mg once daily may be switched to 6 mg once daily with one system delivering 4 mg/24 hours plus one delivering 2 mg/24 hours.

Approximately 2 weeks after switching therapy, the early morning serum testosterone concentrations should be measured in patients following system application the previous evening to ensure proper dosing.

Topical Gel Dosage Topical testosterone is commercially available as a 1% gel in unit-dose packets containing a 25-mg dose of testosterone (2.5 g of gel) (AndroGel®) or a 50-mg dose of testosterone (5 g of gel) (AndroGel®, Vogelxo®); as a 1.62% gel in unit-dose packets (AndroGel®) containing a 20.25- or 40.5-mg dose of testosterone (1.25 or 2.5 g of gel, respectively); as a nonaerosol metered-dose pump (AndroGel® [each actuation of the pump delivers 1.25 g of gel containing 20.25 mg of testosterone after priming], Fortesta® [each actuation of the pump delivers 0.5 g of gel containing 10 mg of testosterone after priming], Vogelxo® [each actuation of the pump delivers 1.25 g of gel containing 12.5 mg of testosterone after priming]); or in unit-dose tubes (Testim®, Vogelxo®) containing a 50-mg dose (5 g of gel).

For the treatment of male hypogonadism, the usual initial dosage of testosterone gel 1% (AndroGel® 1%, Testim®, Vogelxo®) is the entire contents of a packet or tube containing 50 mg of testosterone, the entire contents of 2 packets containing 25 mg of testosterone, or 4 actuations of the pump (5 g of gel) applied topically once daily, preferably in the morning; this dose delivers about 5 mg of testosterone systemically. The usual initial dosage of testosterone gel 1.62% (AndroGel® 1.62%) is the entire contents of a packet containing 40.5 mg of testosterone or 2 actuations of the pump (2.5 g of gel) applied topically once daily in the morning. The usual initial dosage of Fortesta® is 40 mg of testosterone or 4 actuations of the pump (2 g of gel) applied topically once daily in the morning. Dosage should be adjusted according to serum testosterone concentrations obtained at regular intervals following initiation of AndroGel® 1% therapy, approximately 14 days after initiating daily application of Testim® or Vogelxo®, approximately 14 and 28 days after initiating daily application or dosage adjustment of AndroGel 1.62%, and approximately 14 and 35 days after initiating daily application or dosage adjustment of Fortesta®.

If serum testosterone concentrations are below the normal range in a patient receiving AndroGel® 1%, the dosage can be increased initially to 75 mg of testosterone (7.5 g of gel) and, if necessary, subsequently to 100 mg of testosterone (10 g of gel). If serum testosterone concentrations exceed the normal range in a patient receiving AndroGel® 1% therapy, the daily dosage may be decreased. AndroGel® 1% should be discontinued if the serum testosterone concentrations consistently exceed the normal range at a daily dosage of 50 mg of testosterone (5 g of gel).

If serum testosterone concentrations are below the normal range in a patient receiving Testim® or Vogelxo®, the dosage can be increased to 100 mg of testosterone (10 g of gel, 8 actuations of the pump).

If serum testosterone concentrations exceed 750 ng/dL in a patient receiving AndroGel® 1.62%, the dosage should be decreased to 20.25 mg of testosterone (1.25 g of gel, 1 actuation of the pump). If serum testosterone concentrations are below 350 ng/dL in a patient receiving AndroGel® 1.62%, the dosage should be increased initially to 60.75 mg of testosterone (3.75 g of gel, 3 actuations of the pump) and, if necessary, subsequently to 81 mg of testosterone (5 g of gel, 4 actuations of the pump).

In patients receiving Fortesta®, the dosage should be decreased by 20 mg of testosterone (2 actuations of the pump) if serum testosterone concentrations reach or exceed 2500 ng/dL or by 10 mg of testosterone (1 actuation of the pump) if serum testosterone concentrations are 1250 ng/dL or greater, but less than 2500 ng/dL; however, if a 10-mg dosage of testosterone requires further reduction, Fortesta® should be discontinued. If serum testosterone concentrations are below 500 ng/dL in a patient receiving Fortesta®, the dosage of testosterone can be adjusted in 10-mg increments (1 actuation of the pump); however, the daily dosage should not exceed 70 mg of testosterone (7 actuations of the pump).

Topical Solution Dosage Topical testosterone is commercially available as a solution in a metered-dose pump (Axiron®; each actuation of the pump delivers 1.5 mL of solution containing 30 mg of testosterone after priming). For the treatment of male hypogonadism, the recommended initial dosage of testosterone solution is 60 mg (2 actuations of the pump) applied topically once daily. Dosage should be adjusted according to serum testosterone concentrations obtained following initiation of therapy and at least 14 days after initiating daily application or dosage adjustment of testosterone solution. If serum testosterone concentrations exceed 1050 ng/dL in a patient receiving testosterone topical solution, the dosage should be decreased from 60 mg (2 actuations of the pump) to 30 mg (1 actuation of the pump); however, if a 30-mg dosage of testosterone requires further reduction, testosterone topical solution should be discontinued. If serum testosterone concentrations are below 300 ng/dL in a patient receiving testosterone topical solution, the dosage of testosterone can be adjusted in 30-mg increments (1 actuation of the pump); however, the daily dosage should *not* exceed 120 mg of testosterone (4 actuations of the pump).

Buccal (Transmucosal) Dosage When testosterone buccal (transmucosal) tablets (Striant®) are used for the treatment of male hypogonadism, the usual dosage is 30 mg (one extended-release tablet) twice daily, morning and evening (about 12 hours apart). Serum testosterone concentrations should be obtained just prior to the morning dose 4–12 weeks after initiation of therapy with testosterone buccal tablets. If total serum testosterone concentrations are consistently outside of the normal range, testosterone buccal tablets should be discontinued.

Intranasal Dosage Intranasal testosterone is commercially available as a gel in a metered-dose nasal pump (Natesto®; each actuation of the pump delivers 0.122 g of gel containing 5.5 mg of testosterone after priming). For the treatment of male hypogonadism, the recommended initial dosage of testosterone nasal gel is 1 actuation of the pump per nostril for a total dosage of 11 mg 3 times daily. Dosage should be adjusted according to serum testosterone concentrations obtained at least 1 month after initiating therapy and periodically thereafter. If serum testosterone concentrations consistently exceed 1050 ng/dL, testosterone nasal gel should be discontinued. If serum testosterone concentrations are consistently below 300 ng/dL, testosterone nasal gel should be discontinued and alternative therapy considered. If severe rhinitis occurs, testosterone nasal gel should be temporarily interrupted until resolution of symptoms; however, if severe rhinitis persists, testosterone nasal gel should be discontinued and alternative therapy considered.

■ **Dosage in Renal and Hepatic Impairment** The manufacturers of testosterone enanthate injection, testosterone undecanoate injection, and testosterone transdermal system, topical gel, topical solution, nasal gel, and buccal tablets state that clinical studies involving patients with renal or hepatic impairment have not been conducted. Therefore, there are no special population dosage recommendations at this time.

Cautions

Adverse effects associated with testosterone are similar to those of other synthetic or natural androgens and include acne, flushing of the skin, gynecomastia, increased or decreased libido, habituation, and edema. In addition, gynecomastia frequently develops and occasionally persists in patients being treated for hypogonadism.

■ **Cardiovascular Effects** Long-term clinical safety studies have not been conducted to date to determine the cardiovascular effects of testosterone replacement therapy in men. Epidemiologic data and results from randomized, controlled clinical trials have been inconclusive for determining the risk of serious adverse cardiovascular events (i.e., nonfatal myocardial infarction [MI], nonfatal stroke, death) with testosterone use compared with nonuse.

In 2 observational studies, the risk of serious adverse cardiovascular events was increased in patients receiving testosterone replacement therapy compared with those not receiving such therapy; however, 2 other observational studies found a mortality benefit with use of testosterone replacement therapy and one observational study was inconclusive. In addition, findings from 2 meta-analyses of data from published, randomized, controlled clinical trials show conflicting results. Because the current evidence regarding the cardiovascular risk associated with testosterone replacement therapy is weak because of the limited scope, quality, design, and size of the clinical trials, the FDA has requested additional evidence from well-designed studies to further elucidate the cardiovascular risk associated with testosterone use.

Following review of the data from several observational studies and meta-analyses in March 2015, the FDA concluded that use of testosterone is associated with a possible increased risk of serious adverse cardiovascular events. Clinicians should inform patients of this potential increased risk when deciding whether to use or continue to use testosterone replacement therapy. Although the FDA Bone, Reproductive and Urologic Drugs Advisory Committee (BRUDAC) and the Drug Safety and Risk Management Advisory Committee (DSaRM) concluded that there was insufficient evidence to suggest that the potential cardiovascular risk was confined to a certain subset of patients, some experts state that testosterone replacement therapy should be used with caution in patients at high risk for cardiovascular disease, such as older men or those with diabetes mellitus or obesity.

■ **Local Effects** IM administration of anabolic steroids has been associated with urticaria and inflammation at the injection site, postinjection induration, and furunculosis.

Pellet extrusion at or near the implantation site, generally during the first month following subcutaneous implantation of testosterone pellets (Testopel®), has been reported in postmarketing surveillance; infection also may occur at the implantation site. Infection and/or extrusion at the implantation site may be manifested with induration, inflammation, fibrosis, bleeding, contusions, wound drainage, pain, and pruritus.

The most common adverse effect associated with transdermal testosterone is local irritation at the site of application. In clinical studies with Androderm® transdermal systems, most patients developed mild to moderate erythema at the site of application at some time during therapy; 37% of patients receiving this preparation experienced pruritus at the application site, 12% experienced burn-like blisters (manifesting with bullae, epidermal necrosis, or ulceration) on the skin immediately under the system, and 6, 3, and 3% developed vesicles, burning, and induration, respectively, at the application site. In patients who developed burn-like blisters, most such lesions were associated with application of the system over bony prominences or on body parts that may have been subject to prolonged pressure during sleep or sitting (e.g., over the deltoid region of the upper arm, the greater trochanter of the femur, or the ischial tuberosity), and such administration should be avoided; the more severe lesions healed over several weeks with occasional scarring, and such lesions should be treated as burns. Application site reactions occurring in less than 3% of patients receiving Androderm® include bullae, mechanical irritation, and contamination.

In one comparative study, the incidence of application site reactions was substantially less with Testoderm® TTS (no longer commercially available in the US) than with Androderm®, possibly because of the lower amount of delivered alcohol (a permeation-enhancer excipient in the transdermal systems) per unit area of skin with Testoderm® TTS. The possibility exists that excipients other than alcohol also may play a role in application site reactions. Mild skin irritation may be ameliorated with topical application of over-the-counter hydrocortisone *cream;* alternatively, application of triamcinolone acetonide 0.1% *cream* under the central drug reservoir of the transdermal system may decrease the incidence and severity of application site reactions.

Application site reactions were reported in 5, 3, or 4% of patients who received 50, 75, or 100 mg, respectively, of testosterone gel 1% (as AndroGel® 1%) topically for up to 6 months in a clinical trial, but none of these patients required treatment or discontinued the drug because of these reactions. Application site reactions were reported in 2.14% of patients who received testosterone gel 1.62% (as AndroGel® 1.62%), but none of these patients discontinued the drug because of these reactions. In a long-term (up to 3 years) follow-up study, application site reactions were reported in 5.6% of patients. Application site reactions were reported in 2 or 4% of patients receiving 50- or 100-mg doses, respectively, of another testosterone gel formulation (Testim®, Vogelxo®) compared with placebo (3%). Application site reactions were reported in 16.1% of patients receiving another testosterone gel formulation (Fortesta®). AndroGel® 1% appears to have minimal potential for inducing phototoxic reactions. Other application site reactions reported with AndroGel® 1% during postmarketing surveillance include pruritus, dry skin, erythema, rash, discolored hair, and paresthesia. The possibility that testosterone transfer to another individual (including women and children) could occur when skin-to-skin contact is made with the application site should be considered. (See Cautions: Precautions and Contraindications.) In vitro studies have shown that 96% of residual testosterone is removed from the skin by washing with soap and water.

In clinical studies with a testosterone topical solution (Axiron®), irritation (5–7% of patients) or erythema (7–8% of patients) developed at the application site following 120 or 180 days of therapy, respectively.

The most common adverse effects associated with testosterone nasal gel are nasal discomfort, nasal scabbing, rhinorrhea, epistaxis, nasopharyngitis, bronchitis, upper respiratory tract infection, and sinusitis. In a clinical study with Natesto® nasal gel, most patients developed mild to moderate adverse effects; however, long-term effects of testosterone nasal gel are unknown because of limited data.

Gum or mouth irritation, bitter taste, and gum pain or tenderness have been reported in 9.2, 4.1, and 3.1%, respectively, of patients receiving testosterone buccal tablets (Striant®) in one controlled study. Gum edema or taste perversion occurred in 2% of patients receiving the drug in this study. Most gum-related adverse effects were transient; gum irritation generally resolved in 1–8 days and tenderness resolved in 1–14 days.

■ **Genitourinary Effects** Oligospermia and decreased ejaculatory volume may occur in males receiving excessive dosage or prolonged administration of testosterone. Priapism or excessive sexual stimulation in males, especially geriatric patients, may also occur. If priapism or excessive sexual stimulation develops during testosterone therapy, the drug should be discontinued temporarily, since these are signs of excessive dosage; if therapy with testosterone is reinstituted, a lower dosage should be used. Male pattern of baldness may also occur.

Amenorrhea and other menstrual irregularities and inhibition of gonadotropin secretion occur commonly in females.

Gynecomastia can occur in males receiving testosterone replacement therapy as a result of aromatization of testosterone to estradiol and changes in sex hormone binding globulin (SHBG). Surgery can be considered for such patients.

Testosterone, especially its active metabolite dihydrotestosterone (DHT), stimulates growth of the prostate and seminal vesicles. In hypogonadal men receiving testosterone replacement, such growth did not exceed the volumes expected in normal men. Testosterone therapy was associated with an overall mean increase in serum prostate-specific antigen (PSA) concentrations of 0.11–0.14, 0.13, 0.1–0.2, or 0.5 ng/mL in studies evaluating the effect of topical testosterone gel (AndroGel®), topical testosterone solution (Axiron®), testosterone nasal gel (Natesto®), or testosterone undecanoate injection (Aveed®), respectively, on serum PSA concentrations in men with hypogonadism. In one study, PSA was reduced in 21%, unchanged in 22%, and increased in 57% of patients receiving testosterone replacement therapy for 1 year. Increased serum PSA concentrations also were observed in 18% of hypogonadal men receiving AndroGel® 1% for up to 42 months; most of these increases occurred within the first year of therapy. No clear relationship between testosterone replacement therapy and prostate cancer has been established to date, although anecdotal reports have been published; additional long-term studies are needed to clarify the potential risk. (See Cautions: Mutagenicity and Carcinogenicity.)

Other adverse genitourinary effects of testosterone include epididymitis and bladder irritability. Impaired urination, prostatic enlargement, prostate cancer, testicular atrophy, oligospermia, priapism, gynecomastia, and mastodynia have been reported during postmarketing experience with topical testosterone gel (AndroGel® 1%).

■ **Endocrine and Metabolic Effects** Virilization, including deepening of the voice, hirsutism, and clitoral enlargement, occur commonly in females; these changes may not be reversible following discontinuance of the drug.

Secondary exposure to testosterone resulting in virilization of children has been reported with use of topical testosterone gel during postmarketing surveillance. (See Cautions: Precautions and Contraindications.) The FDA has fully reviewed 8 reports of secondary exposure to testosterone from testosterone gel products in children 9 months to 5 years of age. Additional cases in children have been reported and currently are under FDA review. Signs and symptoms have included enlargement of the penis or clitoris, development of pubic hair, increased erections and libido, aggressive behavior, and advanced bone age. In most cases, these signs and symptoms resolved with removal of the testosterone exposure. However, in a few cases, enlarged genitalia did not fully return to age-appropriate normal size, and bone age remained modestly greater than chronologic age. In some of these children, invasive diagnostic procedures were performed as a result of the delay in recognizing the underlying cause of the signs and symptoms. Direct contact of the child with application sites on the skin of men using testosterone gel was reported in most of the cases. The possibility of secondary exposure from contact with items such as shirts and bed linens of men receiving testosterone gel also may be considered.

Because of the aromatization of testosterone to estradiol, lipid abnormalities usually do not develop secondary to testosterone replacement, and the ratio of HDL to total cholesterol generally remains constant. However, the possibility that lipid abnormalities may develop should be considered. (See Cautions: Precautions and Contraindications.) Anabolic steroids that do not undergo aromatization increase LDL-cholesterol and lower HDL-cholesterol, which could increase cardiovascular risk.

Hypercalcemia resulting from osteolysis, especially in immobile patients and those with metastatic carcinoma of the breast, has been reported in patients receiving testosterone. (See Cautions: Precautions and Contraindications.) The drug should be discontinued if hypercalcemia occurs in patients with cancer, since this may indicate progression of metastases to the bone. Retention of water, sodium, chloride, potassium, and inorganic phosphates has also occurred in patients receiving the drug. If edema is present before or develops during therapy, administration of diuretics may be required.

■ **Nervous System Effects** Sleep apnea has occurred occasionally in men receiving testosterone replacement. Although the mechanism of testosterone-induced apnea remains to be elucidated, a relationship between sex hormones and sleep apnea has been suggested since untreated males are more likely than females to develop this disorder and disordered breathing during sleep is more common among healthy males than among premenopausal women. In addition, loud snoring is more common in untreated men than in women, and physiologic mechanisms for snoring and obstructive sleep apnea are similar. Therefore, it has been postulated that abnormal relaxation of pharyngeal muscles seen in both snoring and obstructive sleep apnea is affected by circulating concentrations of hormones, including testosterone. If manifestations of sleep apnea occur or worsen in testosterone-treated patients, sleep studies should be performed and testosterone replacement dosage should be decreased or the drug discontinued if sleep apnea is confirmed. In addition, patients receiving testosterone replacement should be advised to report any sleep-associated changes such as snoring, daytime somnolence, and emotional disturbances.

Sleeplessness, headache, anxiety, mental depression, and generalized paresthesia also have occurred in patients receiving testosterone. Headache, dizziness, sleep apnea, insomnia, depression, emotional lability, nervousness, hostility, amnesia, and anxiety have been reported during postmarketing experience with topical testosterone (AndroGel® 1%).

■ **Sensitivity Reactions** Hypersensitivity reactions, including skin manifestations and anaphylactoid reactions, have occurred rarely with testosterone. Allergic contact dermatitis has been reported with topical administration (e.g., as transdermal systems) of testosterone. (See Cautions: Local Effects.)

■ **Hematologic Effects** Supraphysiologic concentrations of testosterone can stimulate erythropoiesis. Increased hemoglobin and hematocrit and possibly adverse effects secondary to hyperviscosity may result. In addition, leukopenia, polycythemia, and suppression of clotting factors II, V, VII, and X also have occurred in patients receiving testosterone.

■ **Hepatic Effects** Cholestatic hepatitis, peliosis hepatis, hepatic neoplasms, jaundice and abnormal liver function test results have occurred in patients receiving androgens, principally 17-α-alkylandrogens such as fluoxymesterone or methyltestosterone. (See Cautions in Fluoxymesterone 68:08 and in Methyltestosterone 68:08.) Multiple hepatic adenomas have been reported with long-term use of testosterone enanthate injection. Abnormal liver function tests (e.g., ALT, AST, gamma-glutamyltranspeptidase [GGTP], bilirubin) also have been reported during postmarketing surveillance with topical testosterone (AndroGel® 1%).

■ **Other Adverse Effects** Other adverse effects associated with testosterone therapy include nausea, chills, and excitation. Nausea, asthenia, edema, malaise, dyspnea, acne, alopecia, sweating, weight gain, hypertension, and vasodilation (hot flushes) have been reported during postmarketing experience with topical testosterone (AndroGel® 1%).

Serious pulmonary oil microembolism reactions, including cough, urge to cough, dyspnea, hyperhidrosis, throat tightness, angina, dizziness, and syncope, have occurred rarely with IM testosterone undecanoate. In clinical trials, pulmonary oil microembolism reactions have occurred during or immediately following IM administration of 750 mg or 1 g of testosterone undecanoate; these reactions have been reported following administration of the third and tenth injection of the drug. Although these reactions generally lasted a few minutes and resolved following initiation of supportive measures, some reactions persisted for several hours and required emergency care and/or hospitalization. (See Dosage and Administration: Administration.)

■ **Precautions and Contraindications** Testosterone shares the toxic potentials of other androgens, and the usual precautions of androgen therapy should be observed. When testosterone esters are used in combination with estrogens, the usual precautions associated with estrogen therapy should also be observed. (See Cautions in Conjugated Estrogens 68:16.04.) Clinicians prescribing estrogens should be aware of the risks associated with use of these drugs and the manufacturers' labeling should be consulted for further discussion of these risks and associated precautions.

Patients receiving testosterone replacement therapy should be monitored periodically for response and tolerance. Some clinicians recommend that patients be monitored every 3–4 months during the first year of testosterone replacement, and periodically thereafter. Patients with benign prostatic hyperplasia (BPH) receiving androgen therapy are at increased risk for worsening of signs and symptoms of BPH. Patients treated with androgens also may be at increased risk for development of BPH and/or prostate cancer. (See Cautions: Mutagenicity and Carcinogenicity.) The manufacturers of testosterone transdermal system, nasal gel, and topical solution state that evaluation of patients for prostate cancer is appropriate prior to initiation of therapy, 3–6 months after initiation of therapy, and then in accordance with current standards of care. The manufacturers of testosterone topical gel, testosterone buccal tablets, and testosterone undecanoate injection state that evaluation of patients for prostate cancer is appropriate prior to initiating and during androgen therapy. Some clinicians recommend that rectal prostate examination be performed routinely along with assessment of prostate-related symptoms every 6–12 months. Additionally, determination of PSA should be performed annually in older men.

Increases in hematocrit may occur during testosterone therapy as a manifestation of increased red blood cell (RBC) mass, and may require dosage reduction or discontinuance of testosterone. Increased RBC mass also may increase the risk for a thromboembolic event. Annual determination of hematocrit is recommended by some clinicians during testosterone replacement therapy because of the hormone's erythropoietic potential. Determination of hematocrit should occur prior to initiation of therapy, and is appropriate 3–6 months after initiation of therapy, and then annually thereafter. Patients receiving high dosages of testosterone should have periodic hemoglobin and hematocrit determinations, since polycythemia may occur. Some clinicians state that hyperviscosity states are relative contraindications to testosterone therapy.

Changes in serum lipid profiles may require dosage adjustment or discontinuance of testosterone therapy. Some clinicians recommend that patients receiving testosterone replacement have a lipid profile performed at baseline, 6–12 months after initiation of therapy, and then annually thereafter. Androgen therapy should be used with caution in cancer patients at risk of hypercalcemia (and associated hypercalciuria). Regular monitoring of serum calcium concentrations is recommended in these patients.

Cardiovascular events, including MI or stroke, have been reported during postmarketing experience with testosterone preparations. Testosterone should be used with caution in patients at high risk for cardiovascular disease (e.g., older men, those with diabetes mellitus or obesity). Patients should be advised to immediately report symptoms suggestive of MI or stroke (e.g., chest pain, shortness of breath, unilateral weakness, difficulty talking) to their clinician.

Venous thromboembolic events, including deep-vein thrombosis (DVT) and pulmonary embolism (PE), have been reported during postmarketing experience with testosterone preparations. Patients reporting symptoms of pain, edema, warmth, and erythema in a lower extremity or presenting with acute shortness of breath should be evaluated for possible DVT or PE, respectively. If venous thromboembolism is suspected, testosterone therapy should be discontinued and appropriate evaluation and management should be initiated.

Testosterone should be used with caution in patients with cardiac, renal, and/or hepatic dysfunction since edema may occur as a result of sodium and water retention. Edema, with or without congestive heart failure, may be a serious complication in patients with preexisting cardiac, renal, and/or hepatic disease. If edema occurs during testosterone therapy and it is considered a serious complication, the drug should be discontinued; diuretic therapy may also be necessary. Testosterone cypionate (Depo®-testosterone) is contraindicated in patients with serious cardiac, hepatic, or renal disease.

Females should be carefully monitored for signs of virilization (e.g., deepening of the voice, hirsutism, clitoromegaly, menstrual irregularities) during testosterone therapy. The drug should generally be discontinued when mild virilization is evident, since some adverse androgenic effects (e.g., voice changes) may not subside following discontinuance of the drug. The woman and physician may decide that some virilization is acceptable during treatment for carcinoma of the breast.

Males should be carefully monitored for the development of priapism or excessive sexual stimulation since these are signs of excessive dosage. Males, especially geriatric patients, may become overly stimulated. Stimulation to the point of increasing the nervous, mental, and physical activities beyond the patient's cardiovascular capacity should be avoided when testosterone is used to treat decreased testosterone concentrations related to aging. Geriatric males may be at increased risk of developing prostatic hypertrophy and carcinoma during androgen therapy.

Adult or adolescent males should be advised to report too frequent or persistent penile erections to their physician. Females should be advised to report hoarseness, acne, menstrual changes, or the growth of facial hair to their physician. All patients should be advised to report nausea, vomiting, changes in skin color, or ankle swelling to their physician.

Treatment of hypogonadal men with testosterone products may potentiate sleep apnea in some patients, especially those with risk factors such as obesity or chronic lung diseases. Some clinicians also state that a history of sleep apnea is a relative contraindication to testosterone therapy. (See Cautions: Systemic Effects.)

Testosterone topical gels and topical solution contain a flammable vehicle (alcohol), and should not be exposed to an open flame or ignited materials (e.g., a lighted cigarette). The topical gel or topical solution is no longer flammable once the gel or solution has dried.

Virilization in children and women can occur following secondary exposure to testosterone in topical testosterone preparations, including gels or solution. Cases of secondary exposure resulting in virilization of children have been reported during postmarketing surveillance of topical testosterone preparations. (See Cautions: Endocrine and Metabolic Effects.) Signs and symptoms of virilization in children have included enlargement of the penis or clitoris, development of pubic hair, increased erections and libido, aggressive behavior, and advanced bone age. In most cases, these signs and symptoms regressed with removal of the testosterone exposure. However, in a few cases, enlarged genitalia did not fully return to age-appropriate normal size, and bone age remained modestly greater than chronologic age.

The risk of testosterone transfer in some of these reported cases was increased by lack of adherence to precautions for the appropriate use of the topical testosterone preparations. Men using topical testosterone gel or solution should strictly adhere to the recommended instructions for use and appropriate precautions from the manufacturers to minimize the potential for secondary exposure to testosterone in other individuals. (See Dosage and Administration: Administration.) Children and women should avoid contact with application sites on the skin of men using topical testosterone products.

Inappropriate changes in genital size or development of pubic hair or libido in children, changes in body hair distribution, substantial increase in acne, or other signs of virilization in adult women, and the possibility of secondary exposure to testosterone topical gel should be brought to the attention of a clinician. Testosterone topical gel should be promptly discontinued at least until the cause of virilization in such children and women has been identified.

Testosterone transdermal system (Androderm®) should be removed before undergoing magnetic resonance imaging (MRI), since the transdermal system contains aluminum and may cause skin burns at the application site.

Serious pulmonary oil microembolism reactions and anaphylaxis have been reported following IM administration of testosterone undecanoate. Patients should be monitored for 30 minutes following each dose of IM testosterone undecanoate.

Adverse nasal reactions have been reported with testosterone nasal gel. Because of limited data in patients with a history of nasal disorders (e.g., nasal or sinus surgery, nasal fracture within the previous 6 months, nasal fracture resulting in a deviated anterior nasal septum), mucosal inflammatory disorders (e.g., Sjogren's syndrome), and/or sinus disease, testosterone nasal gel is not recommended in such patients. Patients should be advised to report nasal symptoms to their clinician to determine if further evaluation by an ear, nose, and throat (ENT) specialist or discontinuance of testosterone nasal gel is necessary.

Testosterone topical gel, topical solution, nasal gel, transdermal system, and buccal tablets and testosterone undecanoate injection (Aveed®) are not indicated for use in women, have not been evaluated in women, and should not be used in women.

Testosterone is contraindicated in males with carcinoma of the breast or known or suspected carcinoma of the prostate. Testosterone also is contraindicated in women who are or may become pregnant or who are breastfeeding. (See Cautions: Pregnancy, Fertility, and Lactation.) Testosterone cypionate injection, testosterone enanthate injection, and testosterone undecanoate injection are contraindicated in patients with known hypersensitivity to the drug or any ingredient in the respective formulation. Because of the potential risk of serious adverse health effects, testosterone should not be used for enhancement of athletic performance or physique. (See Uses: Misuse, Abuse, and Dependence.) Patients should be informed of the serious adverse effects associated with misuse and abuse of androgens.

■ **Pediatric Precautions** Androgens should be used with extreme caution in children and only by specialists who are aware of the adverse effects of these drugs on bone maturation. Testosterone should be used cautiously to stimulate puberty, and only in carefully selected males with delayed puberty. (See Uses: Uses in Males.) In children, testosterone may accelerate bone maturation without producing compensatory gain in linear growth. This adverse effect may result in compromised adult stature. The younger the child, the greater the risk of testosterone compromising final mature stature. If testosterone is administered to prepubertal children (e.g., to stimulate puberty in males), the drug should be used with extreme caution, and radiographic examination of the hand and wrist should be performed every 6 months to determine the rate of bone maturation and to assess the effect of treatment on the epiphyseal centers. If testosterone is to be used to stimulate puberty in a male with delayed puberty, the potential risk of therapy should be fully discussed with the patient and his parents prior to initiation of the drug.

Safety and efficacy of testosterone topical gel, topical solution, nasal gel, transdermal system, and buccal tablets and testosterone undecanoate injection (Aveed®) in pediatric patients younger than 18 years of age have not been established. Safety and efficacy of testosterone cypionate injection (Depo®-testosterone) in pediatric patients younger than 12 years of age have not been established. Secondary exposure to testosterone in children can occur with the use of topical testosterone preparations, including gels or solution, in other individuals. (See Cautions: Precautions and Contraindications.)

■ **Geriatric Precautions** Clinical studies evaluating testosterone enanthate injection (Delatestryl®), testosterone undecanoate injection (Aveed®), and testosterone topical gel (AndroGel®, Fortesta®), topical solution, nasal gel, and transdermal system have not included sufficient numbers of adults 65 years of age or older to determine whether geriatric patients respond differently than younger adults. There also are insufficient long-term safety data with testosterone enanthate injection, testosterone undecanoate injection, and testosterone topical gel (AndroGel®, Fortesta®, Testim®, Vogelxo®). topical solution, nasal gel, and transdermal system to determine the potential risks of cardiovascular disease, prostate cancer, and prostatic hyperplasia in geriatric adults. The manufacturer of testosterone buccal tablets (Striant®) states that no substantial differences in safety and efficacy were observed in clinical studies in patients 65 years of age or older relative to younger adults. Differences in pharmacokinetics were observed between geriatric and younger adults in studies with Striant®, but it is not known whether these differences are clinically important.

■ **Mutagenicity and Carcinogenicity** Hepatocellular carcinoma has reportedly occurred in patients receiving long-term therapy with high dosages of androgens. Regression of the tumor does not always occur following discontinuance of androgen therapy. Geriatric patients may be at increased risk of developing prostatic hypertrophy and carcinoma during androgen therapy, although the manufacturers state that conclusive evidence to support this risk is lacking. Testosterone replacement is contraindicated in men with known or suspected prostate cancer or male breast cancer since the drug can stimulate tumor growth in androgen-dependent neoplasms. The prostate and breasts should be examined carefully prior to initiating testosterone therapy in men and at follow-up visits. Baseline and follow-up determinations of PSA also should be performed in older men (e.g., older than 50 years of age) at increased risk for prostate cancer.

Following implantation of testosterone in mice, cervical-uterine tumors developed which occasionally metastasized. There is some evidence to suggest that injection of testosterone into some strains of female mice increases their susceptibility to hepatomas. Testosterone has also been shown to increase the number of tumors and decrease the degree of differentiation of chemically induced tumors in rats. It is not known whether androgens, including testosterone, are mutagenic.

■ **Pregnancy, Fertility, and Lactation** Testosterone may cause fetal harm when administered to pregnant women due to the potential for virilization of a female fetus. Androgenic effects including clitoral hypertrophy, labial fusion of the external genital fold to form a scrotal-like structure, abnormal vaginal development, and persistence of a urogenital sinus have occurred in the female offspring of women who were given androgens during pregnancy. The degree of masculinization is related to the amount of drug given to the woman and the age of the fetus; masculinization is most likely to occur in a female fetus when exposure to androgens occurs during the first trimester. Since the risks clearly outweigh the possible benefits in women who are or may become pregnant, testosterone is contraindicated in such women. Women who become pregnant while receiving the drug should be informed of the potential hazard to the fetus.

Pregnant women or those who may become pregnant should be aware of the possibility that testosterone could be transferred from patients treated with topical preparations of the drug such as their sexual partners or other individuals in close physical contact. (See Cautions: Precautions and Contraindications.) Testosterone transdermal system (Androderm®) has an occlusive backing that prevents the partner from coming in contact with active ingredient in the system. Transdermal systems that inadvertently are transferred to a sexual partner should be removed immediately and the contacted skin washed. Pregnant women should avoid skin contact with testosterone topical gel application sites in men. (See Cautions: Precautions and Contraindications.) If unwashed or unclothed skin to which testosterone topical gel has been applied comes in direct contact with the skin of a pregnant woman, the general area of contact by the woman should be washed with soap and water immediately. In vitro studies show that residual testosterone is removed by such washing.

Although the effect of testosterone on fertility in humans has not been conclusively determined, the drug produces oligospermia and decreased ejaculatory volume in males. With high dosages of androgen therapy, spermatogenesis may be suppressed through feedback inhibition of pituitary follicle-stimulating hormone possibly leading to adverse effects on semen parameters including sperm count. Priapism and excessive sexual stimulation also have occurred in males receiving the drug. (See Cautions: Precautions and Contraindications.) Increased or decreased libido also has been reported.

It is not known whether testosterone is distributed into milk. The manufacturers of testosterone enanthate injection (Delatestryl®) and testosterone pellets (Testopel®) state that because of the potential for serious adverse reactions to androgens in nursing infants, a decision should be made whether to discontinue nursing or the drug, taking into account the importance of the drug to the woman. The manufacturer of testosterone cypionate injection (Depo®-testosterone) states that use in nursing women is not recommended. Testosterone topical gel, topical solution, nasal gel, transdermal system, and buccal tablets and testosterone undecanoate injection (Aveed®) are not indicated for use in women. Testosterone topical gel, topical solution, nasal gel, and buccal tablets and testosterone undecanoate injection also are contraindicated in nursing women because of the potential for serious adverse reactions in nursing infants. Exposure of a female nursing infant to androgens may result in varying degrees of virilization. Testosterone and other androgens also may adversely affect lactation.

Drug Interactions

Testosterone may potentiate the action of oral anticoagulants, causing bleeding in some patients. When testosterone therapy is initiated in patients receiving oral anticoagulants, dosage reduction of the anticoagulant may be required to prevent an excessive hypoprothrombinemic response. In patients receiving concomitant therapy with testosterone and anticoagulants, more frequent monitoring of INR and prothrombin time is recommended, especially during initiation or discontinuance of therapy.

Increased serum oxyphenbutazone concentrations have reportedly occurred in patients receiving androgens concurrently with oxyphenbutazone.

Changes in insulin sensitivity or glycemic control may occur in patients receiving androgen therapy. The metabolic effects of androgens may decrease blood glucose concentrations and insulin requirements in patients with diabetes.

Concomitant administration of testosterone with ACTH or corticosteroids may result in increased fluid retention and edema formation. Therefore, testosterone should be administered with caution in patients with cardiac, renal, and/or hepatic disease. Patients should be monitored for fluid retention and edema formation.

Administration of IM testosterone cypionate resulted in increased clearance of propranolol in one study. It is not known whether there is a potential for this interaction with topically administered testosterone gel.

Topical administration of 0.1% triamcinolone cream prior to application of a testosterone transdermal system did not alter absorption of testosterone; however, pretreatment with topical administration of triamcinolone ointment substantially reduced absorption of testosterone.

Administration of intranasal oxymetazoline, a sympathomimetic nasal decongestant, prior to administration of testosterone nasal gel (Natesto®) did not alter absorption of testosterone. Concomitant administration of testosterone nasal gel with other drugs administered intranasally has not been studied. The manufacturer does not recommend concomitant use with such drugs.

Laboratory Test Interferences

Protein bound iodine (PBI) concentrations may be decreased in some patients during testosterone therapy; however, this does not appear to be clinically important. Androgens may decrease thyroxine-binding globulin concentrations, resulting in decreased total serum thyroxine (T_4) concentrations and increased resin uptake of triiodothyronine (T_3) and T_4. Free thyroid hormone concentrations remain unchanged, and there is no clinical evidence of thyroid dysfunction.

Testosterone may cause a decrease in creatinine and creatine excretion and increase the excretion of 17-ketosteroids.

Electrolyte changes (e.g., nitrogen, calcium, potassium, phosphorus, sodium), changes in serum lipids (e.g., hyperlipidemia, elevated triglycerides, decreased high-density lipoprotein [HDL]-cholesterol), impaired glucose tolerance, and fluctuating testosterone concentrations have been reported during postmarketing surveillance with a topical testosterone gel (AndroGel®).

Pharmacology

Testosterone is the principal endogenous androgen. Endogenous androgens are essential hormones that are responsible for the normal growth and development of the male sex organs and for maintenance of secondary sex characteristics, including the growth and maturation of the prostate, seminal vesicles, penis, and scrotum; development of male hair distribution, such as beard, pubic, chest, and axillary hair; laryngeal enlargement and thickening of the vocal cords; and alterations in body musculature and fat distribution.

Testosterone, like other androgenic anabolic hormones, also produces retention of nitrogen, potassium, sodium, and phosphorus; increases protein anabolism; and decreases amino acid catabolism and urinary calcium concentrations. Nitrogen balance is improved only when there is sufficient intake of calories and protein.

Androgens are responsible for the growth spurt that occurs during adolescence and for the eventual termination of linear growth that results from fusion of the epiphyseal growth centers. Although endogenous androgens accelerate linear growth rates in children, the drugs may cause a disproportionate advancement in bone maturation, and long-term administration of the drugs in prepubertal children may result in fusion of the epiphyseal growth centers and premature termination of the growth process.

Exogenous administration of androgens inhibits the release of endogenous testosterone via feedback inhibition of pituitary luteinizing hormone (LH). Following administration of large doses of exogenous androgens, spermatogenesis may also be suppressed as a result of feedback inhibition of pituitary follicle-stimulating hormone (FSH).

Androgens reportedly stimulate the production of erythrocytes, apparently by enhancing the production of erythropoietic-stimulating factor.

Endogenous serum testosterone concentrations vary from hour to hour, and periodic declines below the normal range can occur occasionally in otherwise healthy men. Serum concentrations of the hormone exhibit diurnal variation, with highest concentrations of circulating testosterone occurring in the early morning hours. For a reliable testosterone determination, use of 3 pooled morning serum testosterone samples can minimize errors attributable to variation in concentrations of the hormone. Testosterone circulates principally in bound form, mainly to sex hormone binding globulin (SHBG; testosterone-estradiol binding globulin, TEBG) and albumin. Testosterone is tightly bound to SHBG and is not biologically active, whereas the fraction associated with albumin is only weakly bound and can dissociate to unbound, active hormone. Only about 2% of endogenous testosterone circulates unbound while 30–40% circulates bound to SHBG and the rest is bound to albumin and other proteins.

Pharmacokinetics

For information on the pharmacokinetics of endogenous testosterone, see Pharmacology.

■ **Absorption** Following oral administration of testosterone, only small amounts of the drug reach systemic circulation unchanged. The low bioavailability of orally administered testosterone results from metabolism of the drug in the GI mucosa during absorption and on first pass through the liver. The synthetic androgens (i.e., fluoxymesterone, methyltestosterone) are less extensively metabolized following oral administration.

Esterification of testosterone generally results in less polar compounds. The enanthate ester of testosterone is absorbed slowly from the lipid tissue phase at the IM injection site, achieving peak serum concentrations about 72 hours after IM injection; thus, this preparation has a prolonged duration of action (i.e., up to 2–4 weeks) following IM administration. Because IM injection of testosterone esters causes local irritation, the rate of absorption may be erratic.

Testosterone is absorbed systemically through the skin following topical application as a gel, solution, or transdermal system. Following topical application of a hydroalcoholic gel formulation of testosterone (AndroGel®, Testim®, Vogelxo®) to the skin, the gel quickly dries on the skin surface, which serves as a reservoir for sustained release of the hormone into systemic circulation. Approximately 10% of a testosterone dose applied topically to the skin as a 1% gel is absorbed percutaneously into systemic circulation.

The manufacturer of AndroGel® states that increases in serum testosterone concentrations were apparent within 30 minutes of topical application of a 100-mg testosterone dose of the 1% gel, with physiologic concentrations being achieved in most patients within 4 hours (pretreatment concentrations were not described); percutaneous absorption continues for the entire 24-hour dosing interval. Serum testosterone concentrations approximate steady-state levels by the end of the initial 24 hours and are at steady state by the second or third day of dosing of the 1% gel. With daily topical application of the 1% gel (AndroGel®), serum testosterone concentrations 30, 90, and 180 days after initiating treatment generally are maintained in the eugonadal range. Administration of 10 or 5 g of the 1% gel (AndroGel®) daily results in average daily serum testosterone concentrations of 792 or 566 ng/dL, respectively, at day 30. Following discontinuance of such topical therapy, serum testosterone concentrations remain within the normal range for 24–48 hours but return to pretreatment levels by the fifth day after the last application. The manufacturer states that mean concentrations of the active metabolite dihydrotestosterone (DHT) were within or about 7% above the normal range 180 days after initiating daily topical application of 50 or 100 mg, respectively, of testosterone as the gel. Increases in DHT concentrations appeared to parallel those of testosterone, and the mean steady-state ratio of DHT to testosterone was maintained in the normal range during the 180-day treatment period.

Following administration of testosterone gel (Testim®), physiologic concentrations of testosterone are achieved within 24 hours; percutaneous absorption continues for the entire 24-hour dosing interval. Administration of 10 or 5 g of Testim® daily results in average daily serum testosterone concentrations of 612 or 365 ng/dL, respectively, at day 30. DHT concentrations increase in parallel with testosterone concentrations; DHT concentrations have remained within the normal range during a 90-day treatment period.

Following topical application of testosterone solution (Axiron®) to the skin, ethanol and isopropyl alcohol evaporate leaving testosterone on the skin surface, which serves as a reservoir for sustained release of the hormone into systemic circulation. Following topical application of testosterone solution daily, serum testosterone concentrations reach steady-state levels by approximately 14 days. Following discontinuance of such topical therapy, serum testosterone concentrations return to pretreatment levels by 7–10 days after the last application. DHT concentrations increase in parallel with testosterone concentrations; mean steady-state ratios of testosterone to DHT have remained within the normal range during a 120-day treatment period.

Following topical application of transdermal systems of testosterone, the hormone is absorbed percutaneously into systemic circulation. Although interindividual variation in percutaneous testosterone absorption occurs, serum testosterone concentrations achieved with recommended dosages of transdermal systems of the drug generally reach the normal range during the first day of dosing and are maintained during continuous dosing without accumulation. Average daily serum testosterone concentrations in patients receiving Androderm® reportedly are 498 ng/dL at steady state. Mean ratios of testosterone to DHT are within the normal range.

With topical application of a transdermal preparation, the extent of percutaneous testosterone absorption varies according to the site of application, possibly secondary to regional differences in skin permeability, cutaneous blood flow, and/or degree of adhesion between the transdermal system and skin. In one study in which transdermal systems were applied to the abdomen, back, chest, shin, thigh, or upper arm, serum hormone profiles were qualitatively similar with each site, but steady-state serum concentrations showed significant differences, decreasing in order with the back, thigh, upper arm, abdomen, chest, and shin. Application of Androderm® transdermal systems to the abdomen, back, thighs, or upper arms results in achievement of similar serum testosterone concentration profiles, and these sites are recommended as optimal for rotation of application sites during chronic therapy. Daily nighttime (at approximately 10 p.m.) application of Androderm® transdermal system results in a serum testosterone concentration profile that mimics the endogenous diurnal pattern in healthy young men. In one study, showering 3 hours after application of Androderm® decreased peak plasma concentrations of testosterone by 0.4% compared with not showering 3 hours after application of the transdermal system. In addition, showering 3 hours after transdermal system application did not substantially alter the systemic exposure of testosterone.

Following intranasal administration of testosterone nasal gel (Natesto®), peak plasma concentrations occur approximately 40 minutes after administration. Average daily serum testosterone concentration in patients receiving 11 mg of the nasal gel 3 times daily is 421 ng/dL. DHT concentrations increase in parallel with testosterone concentrations; mean steady-state ratios of testosterone to DHT have remained within the normal range during a 90-day treatment period.

Following buccal (transmucosal) administration of testosterone (Striant®), the drug is absorbed transmucosally from the buccal mucosa; testosterone that is absorbed systemically via the oral mucosa bypasses first-pass metabolism. Following administration of testosterone buccal tablets every 12 hours, steady-state concentrations of testosterone are achieved after the second dose. Testosterone concentrations decrease to concentrations below the normal range about 2–4 hours after removal of the buccal tablet. Average daily serum testosterone concentrations in patients receiving the buccal tablet are 520–550 ng/dL at steady state. Increases in DHT concentrations appear to parallel those of testosterone, and mean steady-state ratios of testosterone to DHT are within the normal range.

Following IM administration of testosterone undecanoate (Aveed®), the drug is slowly absorbed from the lipid phase and hydrolyzed to testosterone. Following IM administration of testosterone undecanoate 750 mg, peak plasma concentrations of testosterone occur after a median of 7 days and steady-state concentrations are achieved after the third injection (14 weeks). Increases in DHT concentrations appear to parallel those of testosterone, and mean ratios of testosterone to DHT are within the normal range.

■ **Distribution** Circulating testosterone is chiefly bound in the serum to sex steroid binding globulin (sex hormone binding globulin, SHBG; testosterone-estradiol-binding globulin, TEBG) and albumin. Because testosterone easily dissociates from albumin, the albumin-bound drug is presumed to be pharmacologically active. The SHBG-bound portion is not considered to be pharmacologically active.

In serum, testosterone is bound with high affinity to SHBG and with low affinity to albumin. The amount of SHBG in serum and the total testosterone concentration determine the distribution of pharmacologically active and nonactive forms of the androgen. SHBG-binding capacity is high in prepubertal children, declines during puberty and adulthood, and increases again during the later decades of life. Approximately 30–40% of testosterone in plasma is bound to SHBG, 2% remains unbound (free), and the rest is bound to albumin and other proteins.

■ **Elimination** The plasma half-life of testosterone reportedly ranges from 10–100 minutes. The plasma half-life of testosterone cypionate after IM injection is approximately 8 days. Following removal of an Androderm® transdermal system, plasma testosterone concentrations decline with an apparent half-life of approximately 70 minutes and hypogonadal concentrations are reached within 24 hours.

Testosterone is metabolized principally in the liver to various 17-ketosteroids via 2 different pathways. The major active metabolites of testosterone are estradiol and DHT. In many tissues, the activity of testosterone appears to depend on reduction to DHT, which binds to SHBG with greater affinity than does testosterone. Testosterone and its metabolites are excreted in urine and feces. Approximately 90% of an IM dose of testosterone is excreted in urine as glucuronic and sulfuric acid conjugates of the drug and its metabolites; approximately 6% of a dose is excreted in feces, principally as unconjugated drug.

Chemistry and Stability

■ **Chemistry** Testosterone is a naturally occurring androgenic anabolic steroid hormone. The drug may be obtained from animal testes but is usually prepared synthetically from cholesterol. Dehydroepiandrosterone is an intermediate in the synthesis of the drug that can be treated by chemical or microbiologic processes to form testosterone. Testosterone is commercially available as the base, and as the cypionate, enanthate, and propionate esters.

Testosterone occurs as white or slightly creamy white, odorless crystals or as a crystalline powder and is practically insoluble in water, freely soluble in dehydrated alcohol, and soluble in vegetable oils. Testosterone cypionate occurs as a white or creamy white, crystalline powder that is odorless or has a slight odor and is insoluble in water, freely soluble in alcohol, and soluble in vegetable oils. Testosterone enanthate occurs as a white or creamy white, crystalline powder that is odorless or has a faint odor characteristic of heptanoic acid and is insoluble in water and soluble in vegetable oils. Testosterone undecanoate occurs as a white to off-white, crystalline powder.

Parenteral Preparations Testosterone cypionate injection is a sterile solution of the drug in a suitable vegetable oil (e.g., cottonseed oil), which may also contain benzyl alcohol as a preservative.

Testosterone enanthate injection is a sterile solution of the drug in a suitable vegetable oil (e.g., sesame oil), which may also contain chlorobutanol as a preservative.

Testosterone undecanoate injection is a sterile solution of the drug in a suitable vegetable oil (e.g., castor oil).

Transdermal Systems Transdermal testosterone (Androderm®) is commercially available as a system that consists of an outer layer of metallized polyester, ethylene-methacrylic acid copolymer (Surlyn®), and ethylene vinyl acetate; a drug reservoir of testosterone, alcohol, glycerin, glycerol monooleate, methyl laurate, and purified water, gelled with an acrylic acid copolymer; a permeable polyethylene microporous membrane; and a peripheral layer of acrylic adhesive surrounding the central, active drug delivery area of the system. The central delivery surface of the system is sealed with a peelable laminate disk composed of a 5-layer laminate containing polyester, polyesterurethane adhesive, aluminum foil, polyesterurethane adhesive, and polyethylene; the disk is attached to and removed with the release liner, a silicone-coated polyester film that should be removed prior to application.

Topical Gel Testosterone topical gel is a clear to translucent, colorless, hydroalcoholic gel containing testosterone. AndroGel® also contains alcohol, purified water, sodium hydroxide, carbomer 980, and isopropyl myristate; Testim® also contains alcohol 74%, purified water, pentadecactone, carbopol, acrylates, propylene glycol, glycerin, polyethylene glycol, and tromethamine; Fortesta® also contains alcohol, purified water, propylene glycol, 2-propanol, oleic acid, carbomer 1382, triethanolamine, and butylated hydroxytoluene; Vogelxo® also contains alcohol, oleyl alcohol, purified water, glycerin, carbomer copolymer Type B, carbomer homopolymer Type C, diisopropyl adipate, methyl laurate, polyethylene glycol, propylene glycol, and tromethamine. Each g of testosterone gel 1% contains 10 mg of testosterone. Each g of testosterone gel 1.62% contains 16.2 mg of testosterone. Each g of testosterone gel 2% contains 20 mg of testosterone.

Topical Solution Testosterone topical solution is a clear to colorless solution containing testosterone. Axiron® also contains alcohol, isopropyl alcohol, octisalate, and povidone. Each mL of testosterone solution contains 20 mg of testosterone.

Nasal Gel Testosterone nasal gel is a slightly yellow gel containing testosterone. Natesto® also contains castor oil, oleoyl polyoxylglycerides, and colloidal silicon dioxide. Each g of testosterone nasal gel contains approximately 45 mg of testosterone.

Buccal Tablets Testosterone buccal (transmucosal) preparations (Striant®) contain the drug in a system that provides controlled and extended release of testosterone as the buccal system gradually hydrates. In addition to testosterone, the system also contains lactose (anhydrous and monohydrate), carbomer 934P, hypromellose, magnesium stearate, polycarbophil, colloidal silicon dioxide, starch, and talc.

■ **Stability** Testosterone enanthate injection (Delatestryl®) should be stored at room temperature. A precipitate may form if the injection is stored at a low temperature; however, this will dissolve after warming and rolling the syringe or vial containing the drug between the palms of the hands. Testosterone undecanoate injection (Aveed®) should be stored at 25°C, but may be exposed to temperatures of 15–30°C. Testosterone cypionate injection (Depo®-testosterone) should be stored at 20–25°C.

Testosterone pellets (Testopel®) should be stored at 25°C, but may be exposed to temperatures of 15–30°C.

Testosterone topical gels (AndroGel®, Fortesta,® Testim®, Vogelxo®) should be stored at 20–25°C, but may be exposed to temperatures of 15–30°C. Testosterone topical solution (Axiron®) should be stored at 25°C, but may be exposed to temperatures of 15–30°C. Testosterone transdermal system (Androderm®) should be stored at 20–25°C and protected from excessive heat. Testosterone nasal gel (Natesto®) should be stored at 20–25°C, but may be exposed to temperatures of 15–30°C. Testosterone buccal (transmucosal) tablets (Striant®) should be stored at 20–25°C and should be protected from heat and moisture.

Testosterone transdermal systems, topical gels, topical solutions, nasal gels, and buccal tablets should be disposed of in household trash in a manner that prevents accidental application or ingestion by children or pets.

Preparations

Distribution of testosterone undecanoate injection (Aveed®) is restricted. (See REMS and also see Restricted Distribution Program under Administration: IM Injection, in Dosage and Administration.)

Most preparations containing testosterone or its salts, esters, or ethers are subject to control under the Federal Controlled Substances Act of 1970, as amended by the Anabolic Steroids Control Act of 1990 and 2004, as schedule III (C-III) drugs. (See Uses: Misuse and Abuse.) However, manufacturers of certain preparations containing androgenic anabolic steroid hormones (principally combinations that also include estrogens) have applied for and obtained for their products(s) an exemption from the record-keeping and other regulatory requirements of the Federal Controlled Substances Act. Under provisions of the Act, specific products can be exempted from such control by the Attorney General, in consultation with the Secretary of Health and Human Services, if the product is determined *not* to possess any significant potential for abuse because of concentration, preparation, combination, and/or delivery system. Because regulatory requirements for a given preparation containing an androgenic anabolic steroid may be subject to change based on these provisions, the manufacturer should be contacted when specific clarification about a preparation's status is required.

Excipients in commercially available drug preparations may have clinically important effects in some individuals; consult specific product labeling for details.

Testosterone

Buccal (Transmucosal)		
Tablets, extended-release	30 mg	**Striant®** (C-III), Columbia
Nasal		
Gel	5.5 mg	**Natesto®** (C-III), Aytu Bioscience
Parenteral		
Implant, pellets for subcutaneous use	75 mg	**Testopel®** (C-III), Endo
Topical		
Gel	1% (12.5 and 50 mg)*	**Testosterone Gel** (C-III)
		Vogelxo® (C-III), Upsher-Smith
	1% (25 and 50 mg)*	**AndroGel®** (C-III), AbbVie
		Testosterone Gel (C-III)
	1% (50 mg)*	**Testim®** (C-III), Endo
		Testosterone Gel (C-III)
	1.62% (20.25 and 40.5 mg)*	**AndroGel®** (C-III), AbbVie
	2% (10 mg)*	**Fortesta®** (C-III), Endo
Solution	30 mg/1.5 mL*	**Axiron®** (C-III), Lilly
		Testosterone Topical Solution (C-III)
Transdermal System	2 mg/24 hours (9.7 mg/32 cm²)	**Androderm®** (C-III), Allergan
	4 mg/24 hours (19.5 mg/39 cm²)	**Androderm®** (C-III), Allergan

*available from one or more manufacturer, distributor, and/or repackager by generic (nonproprietary) name

Testosterone Cypionate

Parenteral		
Injection (in oil)	200 mg/mL*	**Depo®-Testosterone** (C-III), Pfizer
		Testosterone Cypionate Injection (C-III)

*available from one or more manufacturer, distributor, and/or repackager by generic (nonproprietary) name

Testosterone Enanthate

Parenteral		
Injection (in oil)	200 mg/mL*	**Delatestryl®** (C-III), Endo
		Testosterone Enanthate Injection (C-III)

*available from one or more manufacturer, distributor, and/or repackager by generic (nonproprietary) name

Testosterone Undecanoate

Parenteral		
Injection (in oil)	250 mg/mL	**Aveed®** (C-III), Endo

†Use is not currently included in the labeling approved by the US Food and Drug Administration

CONTRACEPTIVES 68:12

Estrogen-Progestin Combinations BCs, OCs

■ Estrogen-progestin combinations are contraceptive combinations containing estrogenic and progestinic steroids.

Uses

■ **Contraception** Oral, intravaginal, and transdermal estrogen-progestin combinations are used for prevention of conception in women who elect to use one of these preparations as a method of contraception. When taken according to the prescribed regimen, these contraceptives provide almost completely effective contraception.

The pregnancy rate in women using conventional-dosage oral contraceptives (containing 35 mcg or more of ethinyl estradiol or 50 mcg or more of mestranol) is generally reported as less than one pregnancy per 100 woman-years of use. Slightly higher rates (somewhat more than one pregnancy per 100 woman-years) reportedly occur with some oral preparations containing 35 mcg or less of ethinyl estradiol, and rates of about 3 pregnancies per 100 woman-years reportedly occur with oral contraceptives containing progestins only. The pregnancy rate in women using the vaginal contraceptive ring containing ethinyl estradiol and etonogestrel (NuvaRing®) is reported as 1–2 pregnancies per 100 women-years of use. The pregnancy rate in women using the transdermal contraceptive system containing ethinyl estradiol and norelgestromin (Ortho Evra®) is reported as approximately one pregnancy per 100 women-years of use. Five out of the 15 pregnancies reported in large clinical trials in women using the transdermal contraceptive system Ortho Evra® occurred in women with a baseline weight of 90 kg or more; these data suggest that Ortho Evra® may be less effective in such women than in those with a lower body weight. Pregnancy rates for other methods of contraception reportedly range from about less than 1–6 pregnancies per 100 woman-years for intrauterine devices (IUDs) to about 14–47 pregnancies per 100 woman-years for the calendar method of periodic abstinence (rhythm). The pregnancy rate when no method of contraception is used is about 60–80 pregnancies per 100 woman-years. Pregnancy rates are derived from various studies conducted by different investigators in different population groups and, therefore, cannot be compared precisely.

Because a positive association between the dose of estrogens in oral contraceptives and the risk of thromboembolism has been shown in at least 2 studies, it is prudent and therapeutically desirable to minimize exposure to estrogens; therefore, the oral contraceptive used in a given patient should be that preparation which contains the least amount of estrogen and is compatible with an acceptable pregnancy rate and patient acceptance. Following a recommendation by the US Food and Drug Administration's (FDA) Fertility and Maternal Health Drugs Advisory Committee, oral contraceptive preparations containing more than 50 mcg of estrogen were discontinued in 1988 since these formulations were considered no more effective than those containing lower dosages of estrogen.

Because the pharmacokinetic profile for the transdermal contraceptive system containing ethinyl estradiol and norelgestromin (Ortho Evra®) differs from the profile for oral contraceptive preparations (see Pharmacokinetics: Absorption), the clinician and patient must weigh the possible risks of higher estrogen exposure with Ortho Evra® against the possibility of pregnancy if the oral contraceptive is not taken according to the prescribed regimen. Increased exposure to estrogen may increase the risk of certain adverse effects (e.g., venous thromboembolism). (See Thromboembolic Disorders in Cautions: Cardiovascular Effects.)

The clinician and patient must weigh the possible risks of estrogen-progestin contraception against those of other methods of contraception or no contraception. In addition, potential noncontraceptive benefits associated with use of oral contraceptives can be considered. (See Pharmacology: Other Effects.)

For information on parenteral use of fixed combinations of medroxyprogesterone acetate and estradiol cypionate (e.g., Lunelle®), see Uses: Contraception in Females, in Medroxyprogesterone Acetate 68:32.

Postcoital Contraception A short-course, high-dose regimen of an oral estrogen-progestin combination is used in women for the prevention of conception after unprotected intercourse (postcoital contraception, morning-after pills) as an emergency contraceptive (EC)†. If taken soon enough after intercourse (i.e., within 72–120 hours), the combination regimen can *prevent* not *terminate* pregnancy; therefore, the regimen is contraceptive not abortifacient.

Several regimens employing high-dose combinations of ethinyl estradiol and norgestrel or levonorgestrel have been used safely and effectively for postcoital contraception†. One widely studied and used regimen (the Yuzpe regimen) consists of administering 2 tablets containing 50 mcg of ethinyl estradiol and 0.5 mg of norgestrel each (i.e., a dose of 100 mcg and 1 mg, respectively) within 72 hours after unprotected intercourse, repeating this dose 12 hours later. Alternative combination regimens consisting of 100–120 mcg of ethinyl estradiol and 1.2 mg of norgestrel or 0.5–0.6 mg of levonorgestrel administered within 72 hours of intercourse and repeated 12 hours later also have been used. Raw pregnancy (failure) rates in trials employing such regimens have ranged from 0.2–7.4%. However, not all women given emergency postcoital contraception are at genuine risk for pregnancy, since unprotected intercourse that occurs in the early follicular or in the luteal phase is unlikely to result in conception. Therefore, a more accurate indication of efficacy would be based on the timing of unprotected intercourse and the probability that pregnancy would occur without treatment. When efficacy of postcoital contraception with such estrogen-progestin combination regimens is based on the likelihood of pregnancy (computed by matching the cycle day of unprotected intercourse with known conception rates for that cycle day), estimates from various studies of the proportionate reduction in pregnancy risk have ranged from about 55–94%, and pooled analysis of data from studies employing the Yuzpe regimen reveal that such therapy is approximately 74% (confidence interval: 68.2–79.3%) effective in preventing a single pregnancy. Because of study limitations of this pooled analysis, it is likely that true efficacy rates are higher than this estimate, perhaps exceeding 80%. However, postcoital (emergency) contraceptive regimens are not as effective as most other forms of long-term contraception. The efficacy of postcoital regimens employing lower estrogen/progestin doses currently is not known.

An emergency contraceptive regimen employing a progestin alone (levonorgestrel) appears to be more effective and better tolerated than the estrogen-progestin emergency contraceptive ("Yuzpe") regimen when the regimens are initiated within 72 hours of unprotected intercourse, and therefore, the progestin-alone regimen generally is preferred when readily available.

To prevent pregnancy, oral estrogen-progestin combination therapy ideally should begin within 72 hours following coitus. Studies show that emergency contraception is moderately effective when the first dose is administered up to 120 hours after unprotected intercourse. Postcoital contraceptive efficacy diminishes as the time period between intercourse and administration of the combination increases, with the regimen becoming completely ineffective by day 6 or 7, when implantation usually occurs.

Because of the short time frame for effective postcoital use, women should be informed of the availability of postcoital contraception before such use is warranted and offered advanced provision (e.g., provided a prescription for emergency contraception at the time of a routine gynecology visit), advised of the availability of an over-the-counter (OTC) emergency contraceptive preparation, or advised to contact a clinician immediately if the need arises. By informing women of this emergency option and advising them of steps to take to readily obtain the combinations before or when needed, effective postcoital contraception ultimately could reduce substantially the number of unintended pregnancies and induced abortions. Because of the high incidence of adverse effects (e.g., nausea and vomiting with estrogen-progestin combinations) decreased contraceptive efficacy compared with conventional long-term contraceptive methods, including cyclic use of estrogen-progestin combinations, postcoital contraception with the combinations generally should be limited to emergency situations following unprotected intercourse (e.g., rape, contraceptive failure, missed doses of oral or parenteral contraceptives, lack of planning). Postcoital contraceptive regimens should not be used as a routine method of contraception. Women should be informed that postcoital contraceptives do not protect against human immunodeficiency virus (HIV) infection or other sexually transmitted diseases. Women should be advised about various available routine methods of contraception when given emergency contraception and instructed as to when to begin an effective method of such contraception; the potential value of condoms as a supplement to other methods (e.g., to reduce the risk of sexually transmitted diseases) also should be discussed. Women who request emergency contraceptives repeatedly should be informed about other contraceptive options.

The American College of Obstetricians and Gynecologists (ACOG), other experts, and some states (e.g., Alaska, California, Hawaii, Maine, New Mexico, Washington) have advocated increased access to emergency postcoital contraception (e.g., nonprescription access via pharmacies, advance provision by clinicians) as a means of decreasing unintended pregnancy and abortion rates. There is some evidence that increased access to emergency postcoital contraception may not compromise conventional contraceptive use or sexual behavior, potentially allaying some concerns that have prompted others to advocate for restricted access. The US Food and Drug Administration (FDA) has approved one postcoital contraceptive (Plan B® One-Step; levonorgestrel) for nonprescription (OTC) status for women 17 years of age or older; the contraceptive will remain a prescription-only preparation for women younger than 17 years of age. For information on this preparation, see Progestins 68:12.

Use of high-dose oral estrogen-progestin combinations as emergency postcoital contraception may cause menstrual cycle disruption; if menstruation is delayed by a week or more, a sensitive pregnancy test should be performed. If pregnancy has already occurred, there is little, if any, evidence that postcoital regimens will adversely affect the fetus or pregnancy. (See Cautions: Pregnancy, Fertility, and Lactation.) Because postcoital regimens may not prevent ectopic (tubal or abdominal) pregnancies, women receiving such regimens should be informed that ectopic pregnancy is a medical emergency and to consult their clinician immediately if spotting or cramping occurs (usually beginning shortly after the first missed period with such pregnancy). Women should consult their clinician regarding when they can start or resume cyclic oral contraceptive regimens with a combination; they also should be instructed carefully regarding differences in administration schedule and any differences in formulation (e.g., potency, active versus inert tablets) of the preparations.

For the use of progestin-only therapy as a postcoital contraceptive, see Progestins 68:12.

■ **Contraception and Folate Supplementation** Certain estrogen-progestin combinations (Beyaz® [ethinyl estradiol 20 mcg in fixed combination with drospirenone 3 mg and levomefolate calcium 0.451 mg], Safyral®[ethinyl estradiol 30 mcg in fixed combination with drospirenone 3 mg and levomefolate calcium 0.451 mg]) are used in women choosing oral contraceptives as their method of contraception, for the additional purpose of increasing folate concentrations to reduce the risk of fetal neural tube defects when conception occurs while the woman is receiving the contraceptive or shortly after the contraceptive is discontinued. The US Preventive Services Task Force recommends that women of childbearing age receive supplemental folic acid at a dosage of at least 0.4 mg daily. Other folate supplementation that a woman may be taking should be considered before prescribing ethinyl estradiol in combination with drospirenone and levomefolate calcium (Beyaz®, Safyral®). Folate supplementation should be maintained if a woman discontinues this contraceptive because of pregnancy.

■ **Acne Vulgaris** Certain triphasic or estrophasic oral estrogen-progestin combinations (specifically, Ortho Tri-Cyclen® [ethinyl estradiol 35 mcg in fixed combination with norgestimate 0.18, 0.215, or 0.25 mg], or Estrostep® [ethinyl estradiol 20, 30, or 35 mcg in fixed combination with norethindrone acetate 1 mg]) can be used for the treatment of moderate acne vulgaris in females 15 years of age or older who have no known contraindications to oral contraceptive therapy, desire contraception, have achieved menarche, and are unresponsive to topical anti-acne medication. The manufacturer of Estrostep® states that the drug should be used for the treatment of acne vulgaris only in women who desire oral contraception and plan to take the drug for at least 6 months. Acne is a skin condition with a multifactorial etiology and the combination of ethinyl estradiol and norgestimate may increase sex hormone-binding globulin (SHBG) and decrease free testosterone serum concentrations. This may result in a decrease in the severity of facial acne in otherwise healthy women. In two double-blind, placebo-controlled, 6-month multicenter trials, therapy with the ethinyl estradiol/norgestimate combination resulted in clinically important decreases in inflammatory lesion count and total lesion count as compared with placebo (56.6% versus 36.6% and 49.6% versus 30.3%, respectively). In two 6-month, randomized, double-blind, placebo-controlled, multicenter studies in young women (mean age: 24 years) with acne vulgaris, therapy with the ethinyl estradiol/norethindrone combination or placebo resulted in a 52 or 41% reduction in inflammatory lesion count, respectively, and a 43 or 32% reduction in total lesion count, respectively.

The estrogen-progestin combinations (specifically, Yaz® [ethinyl estradiol 20 mcg in fixed combination with drospirenone 3 mg], Beyaz® [ethinyl estradiol 20 mcg in fixed combination with drospirenone 3 mg and levomefolate calcium 0.451 mg]) also are used for the treatment of moderate acne vulgaris in females at least 14 years of age who have no known contraindications to oral contraceptive therapy and who desire oral contraception and have achieved menarche.

■ **Premenstrual Dysphoric Disorder** The estrogen-progestin combinations (Yaz® [ethinyl estradiol 20 mcg in fixed combination with drospirenone 3 mg], Beyaz® [ethinyl estradiol 20 mcg in fixed combination with drospirenone 3 mg and levomefolate calcium 0.451 mg]) are used for the treatment of premenstrual dysphoric disorder (formerly known as late luteal phase dysphoric disorder) in women who desire oral contraception. Efficacy of ethinyl estradiol in combination with drospirenone (Yaz®) has been evaluated in 2 randomized, placebo-controlled, double-blind studies of 3 months' duration in adult women who met DSM-IV criteria for premenstrual dysphoric disorder. In these studies, ethinyl estradiol in combination with drospirenone was found to be superior to placebo in improving symptoms associated with this disorder. Efficacy of ethinyl estradiol 20 mcg in fixed combination with drospirenone 3 mg (Yaz®) or ethinyl estradiol 20 mcg in fixed combination with drospirenone 3 mg and levomefolate calcium 0.451 mg (Beyaz®) when used for more than 3 menstrual cycles has not been evaluated.

■ **Other Uses** Estrogen-progestin preparations have been used for the treatment of endometriosis† or dysfunctional uterine bleeding†.

Dosage and Administration

■ **Administration** Estrogen-progestin combination contraceptives are administered orally, intravaginally, and percutaneously by topical application of a transdermal system to the skin.

Contraception **Oral Administration.** To ensure maximum contraceptive efficacy, oral contraceptives should be taken as near as possible to the same time each day (i.e., at regular 24-hour intervals). Most oral contraceptives are commercially available in a mnemonic dispensing package that is designed to aid the user in complying with the prescribed dosage schedule; these containers should be used whenever possible.

To minimize nausea, oral contraceptives should be taken with or after the evening meal or at bedtime. As vomiting or diarrhea may decrease absorption of oral contraceptives and potentially result in treatment failures, a back-up method of contraception (e.g., condoms, foam, sponge) should be used until the next clinician contact.

Chewable tablets may be swallowed whole or chewed and consumed with 240 mL of liquid.

Intravaginal Administration. Patients receiving the vaginal contraceptive ring containing ethinyl estradiol and etonogestrel (NuvaRing®) should be carefully instructed in the use of the vaginal ring. To obtain optimum results, patients also should be given a copy of the patient information provided by the manufacturer. The ring should be inserted into the vagina by the patient; the manufacturer states that the exact position of the ring inside the vagina is not critical for its proper functioning. If the ring is accidentally expelled, it can be rinsed with cool or lukewarm water and reinserted or, if necessary, a new ring should be inserted as soon as possible; in either case, the administration schedule employed should be continued. If the contraceptive ring has been out of the vagina for longer than 3 hours, a back-up method of contraception (e.g., condoms, spermicides) must be used until the ring has been used continuously for 7 days.

Transdermal Administration. Women receiving the transdermal contraceptive containing ethinyl estradiol and norelgestromin (Ortho Evra®) should be instructed in the use of the transdermal system. To obtain optimum results, women also should be given a copy of the patient information provided by the manufacturer. The transdermal system is applied topically to a clean and dry area of intact skin on the buttock, abdomen, upper outer arm, or upper torso, by firmly pressing the system with the adhesive side touching the skin. The system should be pressed firmly in place with the palm of the hand for about 10 seconds, ensuring good contact, particularly around the edges. The application site should not be oily, damaged, or irritated. The transdermal system should *not* be applied to the breasts or to areas where tight clothing may cause the system to be rubbed off. If the system inadvertently gets detached during the period of use, and is off for less than one day, the system may be reapplied or, if necessary, a new system (if the system is no longer sticky) may be applied; in either case, the application schedule employed should be continued. If the system is off for longer than one day or for an unknown duration, a new system should be applied immediately and a new 4-week cycle should be started; a back-up method of contraception (e.g., condoms, spermicides, diaphragm) must be used for the first week of the new cycle. Patients should be instructed to handle the used transdermal system carefully (e.g., fold the system in half with the sticky sides together) and then discard the system.

Postcoital Contraception **Oral Administration.** Postcoital contraceptive regimens usually consist of 2–5 tablets per dose† administered 12 hours apart. The first dose should be administered *as soon as possible but preferably within 72 hours* following unprotected intercourse; the second dose is administered 12 hours later. Women should be advised of the importance of taking the second dose 12 hours after the initial dose, and to schedule the first dose as conveniently as possible so that the likelihood of missing the second dose 12 hours later is minimized (e.g., if the first dose were taken at 3 p.m., the second dose would need to be taken at 3 a.m., which might present a problem of compliance for heavy sleepers). The first dose can be taken up to 120 hours after unprotected intercourse if necessary, but efficacy decreases as initiation of contraception becomes more remote from unprotected intercourse.

Because the high dosage in the combination regimens may cause severe nausea and vomiting in a substantial proportion of women, which could limit compliance with postcoital contraception, use of an antiemetic 1 hour prior to administration of the first dose of the combination should be considered. Administering the dose with food is not effective in reducing adverse GI effects (i.e., nausea). If vomiting does occur within 2 hours after administration of a dose of the estrogen-progestin combination, consideration should be given to repeating the dose.

Because of the short time frame of effective postcoital use (i.e., therapy must commence within 72–120 hours of unprotected intercourse), clinicians ideally should inform women of the availability of postcoital contraception before such use is warranted, advising them to contact a clinician immediately if the need for such contraception arises. Alternatively, women can be given an appropriate estrogen-progestin combination in advance, with careful instructions on how to safely and effectively use the combination for emergency postcoital contraception; if a supply of the drugs is given to a woman in advance, she also should be advised that postcoital contraceptives are for emergency situations (e.g., unprotected intercourse, missed doses of oral contraceptives, missed parenteral contraceptive dose, contraceptive failure) only and should not be employed as the primary method of contraception.

If the menstrual period is delayed by a week or more, or if persistent irregular bleeding or lower abdominal pain occurs, professional medical follow-up care should be obtained.

■ **Dosage** ***Contraception*** Before initiating therapy, women receiving estrogen-progestin contraceptives should be given a copy of the patient labeling for the drugs.

Oral Dosage. Estrogen-progestin oral contraceptives are usually classified according to their formulation:

- those monophasic preparations containing 50 mcg of estrogen,
- those monophasic preparations containing less than 50 mcg of estrogen (usually 20–35 mcg),
- those containing less than 50 mcg of estrogen with 2 sequences of progestin doses (biphasic),
- those containing less than 50 mcg of estrogen with 3 sequences of progestin doses (triphasic), and
- those containing 3 sequences of estrogen (e.g., 20, 30, 35 mcg) with a fixed dose of progestin (estrophasic).

Although the progestin content of the formulations also varies, oral contraceptives usually are described in terms of their estrogen content. The estrogenic and progestinic dominance of oral contraceptives depends mainly on the amount of estrogen and the amount and specific progestin contained in the formulation. The estrogenic or progestinic dominance of an oral contraceptive may contribute to hormone-related adverse effects and may be useful in selecting an alternate formulation when unacceptable adverse effects occur with a given formulation.

Whenever possible, the smallest dosage of estrogen and progestin should be used. The amount of both hormones should be considered in the choice of an oral contraceptive preparation. It is prudent and in keeping with good principles of therapeutics to minimize exposure to estrogen and progestin. The combination used should be one which contains the least amount of estrogen and progestin that is compatible with a low failure rate and with the individual needs of the woman. Common adverse effects are usually most pronounced during the first oral contraceptive cycle and generally disappear or diminish after 3 or 4 cycles; there does not appear to be any advantage in changing preparations during this period. If minor adverse effects persist after the fourth cycle, a different combination of drugs or a different dosage may be tried.

Most fixed combinations are available as 21- or 28-day dosage preparations (conventional-cycle oral contraceptives). Some 28-day preparations contain 21 hormonally active tablets and 7 inert or ferrous fumarate-containing tablets; other 28-day preparations contain 24 hormonally active tablets and 4 inert or ferrous fumarate-containing tablets. In establishing an oral contraceptive dosage cycle, the menstrual cycle is usually considered to be 28 days. The first day of bleeding is counted as the first day of the cycle.

One fixed-combination extended-cycle oral contraceptive (e.g., Seasonale®) is available as a 91-day dosage preparation containing 84 hormonally active tablets and 7 inert tablets. Other extended-cycle oral contraceptive preparations (e.g., LoSeasonique®, Seasonique®,) are available as 91-day preparations with 84 hormonally active tablets containing estrogen/progestin and 7 tablets containing low-dose estrogen.

One fixed-combination continuous-regimen (noncyclic) oral contraceptive (i.e., Lybrel®) is available as a 28-day dosage preparation containing 28 hormonally active tablets.

Conventional-cycle Oral Contraceptives. Administration of **monophasic** fixed-combination conventional-cycle oral contraceptives usually begins on the first day of the menstrual cycle or on the first Sunday after menstrual bleeding has started. A back-up method of contraception (e.g., condoms, foam, sponge) should be employed for 7 days following initiation of oral contraceptive therapy if the first dose of the oral contraceptive is begun on the first Sunday after menstrual bleeding starts. A back-up method of contraception is not needed if the first dosage cycle is initiated on the first day of the menstrual cycle. When the 21-day conventional-cycle preparations are used, tablets containing estrogen/progestin are administered once daily for 21 consecutive days, followed by up to 7 days without drugs. When the 28-day dosage preparations containing 21 hormonally active tablets are used, tablets containing estrogen/progestin are administered once daily for 21 consecutive days, followed by inert tablets or tablets containing ferrous fumarate for 7 days. When the 28-day dosage preparations containing 24 hormonally active tablets are used, tablets containing estrogen/progestin are administered once daily for 24 consecutive days, followed by inert tablets or tablets containing ferrous fumarate for 4 days. Withdrawal bleeding usually occurs within 2 or 3 days after the last hormonally active tablet has been taken. Repeat dosage cycles begin on the same day of the week as the initial cycle. Repeat cycles should generally begin regardless of whether menstruation has stopped; after several cycles of fixed-combination preparations, menstrual flow may be considerably reduced. If a repeat 21-day cycle is started later than the eighth day after taking the last hormonally active tablet (or later than the next day after taking the last inactive tablet with 28-day dosage preparations), a back-up method of contraception should be employed until the patient has taken a hormonally active tablet daily for 7 consecutive days.

When a **biphasic** oral contraceptive (e.g., Ortho-Novum® 10/11) is used, each dosage cycle consists of 2 sequentially administered fixed combinations; the first sequence consists of 10 tablets containing a fixed combination of low-dose estrogen and low-dose progestin and the second sequence consists of 11 tablets containing a fixed combination of low-dose estrogen and higher-dose progestin. Although biphasic oral contraceptives consist of 2 sequentially administered fixed combinations, they are *not* the same as previously available "sequential" oral contraceptives which consisted of an estrogen alone for the first sequence. Administration of a biphasic oral contraceptive usually begins on the first Sunday after or on which bleeding has started. Tablets from the first sequence are administered once daily for 10 consecutive days, followed by once-daily administration of tablets from the second sequence for 11 consecutive days and then a period of 7 days without drug; when a 28-day dosage preparation is used, inert tablets are administered during this latter 7-day period. A back-up method of contraception (e.g., condoms, foam, sponge) should be employed for 7 days following initiation of oral contraceptive therapy if the first dose of the oral contraceptive is begun on the first Sunday on or after menstrual bleeding starts; a back-up method of contraception is not necessary if the first dosage cycle is initiated on the first day of the menstrual cycle. Repeat dosage cycles begin on the eighth day after taking the last hormonally active tablet.

Triphasic oral contraceptives contain graduated sequences of progestin or estrogen. With most commercially available triphasic oral contraceptives (e.g., Ortho-Novum® 7/7/7, Ortho-Tri-Cyclen®, Ortho-Tri-Cyclen® Lo, Tri-Levlen®, Tri-Norinyl®, Triphasil®), each dosage cycle consists of 3 sequentially administered fixed combinations of the hormones in which the ratio of progestin to estrogen progressively increases with each sequence. The first sequence consists of tablets containing a fixed combination of low-dose estrogen and low-dose progestin, the second sequence consists of tablets containing a fixed combination of low-dose (i.e., Ortho-Novum 7/7/7, Ortho-Tri-Cyclen®, Ortho-Tri-Cyclen® Lo, Tri-Norinyl®) or low but slightly higher-dose estrogen (i.e., Tri-Levlen®, Triphasil®) and higher-dose progestin, and the third sequence consists of tablets containing low-dose estrogen and either an even higher-dose progestin (i.e., Ortho-Novum® 7/7/7, Ortho-Tri-Cyclen®, Ortho-Tri-Cyclen® Lo, Tri-Levlen®, Triphasil®) or low-dose progestin (i.e., Tri-Norinyl®).

Triphasic oral contraceptives in which the estrogen component progressively increases with each sequence also are available; such contraceptives have been referred to as "**estrophasic**". With the currently commercially available estrophasic oral contraceptive (e.g., Estrostep®), the first sequence consists of tablets containing a fixed combination of a progestin and low-dose estrogen, the second sequence consists of tablets containing a fixed combination of a progestin and a slightly higher dosage of an estrogen, and the third sequence consists of tablets containing a progestin and an even higher dosage of an estrogen.

Administration of a triphasic oral contraceptive usually begins on the first Sunday after or on which bleeding has started or on the first day of the menstrual cycle. Tablets from the first sequence of Ortho-Novum® 7/7/7, Ortho-Tri-Cyclen®, or Ortho-Tri-Cyclen® Lo are administered once daily for 7 consecutive days, followed by once-daily administration of tablets from the second sequence for 7 consecutive days and then once-daily administration of tablets from the third sequence for 7 consecutive days. Tablets from the first sequence of Tri-Norinyl® are administered once daily for 7 consecutive days, followed by once-daily administration of tablets from the second sequence for 9 consecutive days and then once-daily administration of tablets from the third sequence for 5 consecutive days. Tablets from the first sequence of Tri-Levlen® or Triphasil® are administered once daily for 6 consecutive days, followed by once-daily administration of tablets from the second sequence for 5 consecutive days and then once-daily administration of tablets from the third sequence for 10 consecutive days. Tablets from the first sequence of Estrostep® are administered once daily for 5 consecutive days, followed by once-daily administration of tablets from the second sequence for 7 consecutive days and then once-daily administration of tablets from the third sequence for 9 consecutive days. The 3 sequences are then followed by a period of 7 days without drug; when a 28-day dosage preparation is used, inert tablets are administered during this latter 7-day period. Repeat dosage cycles begin on the eighth day after taking the last hormonally active tablet. If a repeat 21-day cycle is started later than the eighth day after taking the last hormonally active tablet (or later than the next day after taking the last inactive tablet with 28-day dosage preparations), a back-up method of contraception should be employed until the patient has taken a hormonally active tablet daily for 7 consecutive days.

If oral contraceptives are first taken postpartum or later than the fifth day of the menstrual cycle, the contraceptive effect should not be relied on until after 7 consecutive days of drug administration, since there is a possibility that ovulation and conception may have occurred. In all patients, additional contraceptive measures may be advisable through the first week of the *initial* regimen. In determining whether to initiate oral contraceptive therapy in the postpartum period, the increased risk of thromboembolism during this period must be considered since use of oral contraceptives is also associated with an increased risk of thromboembolic and thrombotic disorders. (See Thromboembolic Disorders in Cautions: Cardiovascular Effects.)

If spotting or breakthrough bleeding occurs during oral contraceptive use, the dosage cycle should generally be continued. Spotting or breakthrough bleeding usually stops within one week. If bleeding persists or is prolonged, nonfunctional causes should be considered. (See Cautions: Genitourinary Effects.) For information on the use of oral contraceptives when a menstrual period has been missed, see Cautions: Pregnancy, Fertility, and Lactation.

When a woman misses one estrogen/progestin tablet of a conventional cycle oral contraceptive, the missed dose should be taken as soon as it is remembered, followed by resumption of the regular schedule. Additional contraceptive methods are not necessary if only one tablet is missed. When 2 doses are missed during the first one or 2 weeks of the cycle, the 2 missed doses should both be taken as soon as they are remembered, then 2 tablets the next day, followed by resumption of the regular schedule. If 2 consecutive estrogen/progestin tablets are missed during the third or fourth week of a dosage cycle that was initiated on the first day of the menstrual cycle, the remainder of the tablets in the pack for that cycle should be discarded and a new dosage cycle started the same day. If 2 consecutive estrogen/progestin tablets are missed during the third or fourth week of a dosage cycle that was initiated on the first Sunday on or after menstruation started, the patient should continue to take one tablet daily until Sunday, then discard the remainder of the tablets for that cycle and start a new dosage cycle that same day. If 3 or more consecutive estrogen/progestin tablets are missed during a dosage cycle that was initiated on the first day of the menstrual cycle, the remainder of the tablets in that cycle should be discarded and a new dosage cycle started the same day. If 3 or more consecutive estrogen/progestin tablets are missed during a dosage cycle that was initiated on the first Sunday on or after menstruation started, the patient should continue to take one tablet daily until Sunday, then discard the remainder of the tablets for that cycle and start a new dosage cycle that same day. During the 28-day dosage cycle, any inactive tablets that are missed should be discarded and the patient should continue taking the remaining inactive tablets until the cycle is finished. A back-up contraceptive method is not required during the fourth week as a result of missed inactive tablets. With 28-day contraceptive cycles, a new cycle of tablets should be started the day after taking the last tablet of the previous 28-day dosage cycle (i.e., no days without tablets). If the patient is unsure of what drug regimen to take as a result of missed tablets, a back-up method of contraception should be used for each sexual encounter, and one active tablet should be taken each day until the next clinician contact.

Missed doses may cause light bleeding or spotting or amenorrhea, and ingestion of multiple tablets to make up for those missed (i.e., 2 doses at a time) may be associated with nausea. If breakthrough bleeding occurs following missed doses, it will usually be transient and of no consequence. If breakthrough bleeding resembling menstruation occurs during use of monophasic (conventional cycle) fixed-combination oral contraceptives, therapy should be discontinued, the remainder of the tablets in that cycle should be discarded, and the next cycle should be started on the next Sunday. There is little likelihood of ovulation when one dose is missed; however, the possibility of ovulation and spotting or breakthrough bleeding increases with each missed dose. Whenever 2 or more doses are missed, additional contraceptive methods should be used for the next 7 days.

In nonlactating postpartum women, oral contraceptives may be initiated no earlier than 28 days after delivery. In women who choose to breast-feed, oral contraceptives should not be given in the immediate postpartum period. Whenever possible, the use of oral contraceptives should be deferred until the infant has been weaned. (See Cautions: Pregnancy, Fertility, and Lactation.)

Extended-cycle Oral Contraceptives. When a fixed-combination extended-cycle oral contraceptive (e.g., LoSeasonique®, Seasonale®, Seasonique®) is used, the oral contraceptive is administered in a cyclic regimen using a 91-day cycle. Because extended-cycle oral contraceptives are administered using a 91-day cycle, women using these preparations should expect to have 4 menstrual periods per year. When an extended-cycle preparation is used, tablets containing estrogen/progestin are administered once daily for 84 days followed by administration of inert tablets or tablets containing 10 mcg of estrogen for 7 days. Administration of the extended-cycle preparation usually begins on the first Sunday after or on which bleeding begins. A back-up method of contraception (e.g., condom, spermicide) should be employed for 7 days following initiation of therapy. Withdrawal bleeding usually occurs during the 7 days after the last estrogen/progestin tablet. Repeat dosage cycles begin on the same day of the week (Sunday) as the initial cycle. If a repeat cycle is started later than the scheduled day, a back-up method of contraception should be employed until the patient has taken a hormonally active tablet daily for 7 consecutive days.

When a woman misses one estrogen/progestin tablet of an extended-cycle oral contraceptive (i.e., LoSeasonique®, Seasonale®, Seasonique®), the missed dose should be taken as soon as it is remembered, followed by resumption of the regular schedule. Additional contraceptive measures are not necessary if only one tablet is missed. When 2 estrogen/progestin tablets are missed, the 2 missed tablets should be taken as soon as they are remembered, then 2 tablets the next day, followed by resumption of the regular cycle. A back-up method of contraception (e.g., condom, spermicide) should be employed until the patient has taken an estrogen/progestin tablet daily for 7 consecutive days. When 3 or more consecutive estrogen/progestin tablets are missed, the patient should continue to take one tablet daily; the missed tablets should be discarded. A back-up method of contraception (e.g., condom, spermicide) should be employed when the patient misses a dose and until the patient has taken an estrogen/progestin tablet daily for 7 consecutive days. Inert tablets or estrogen-containing tablets that are missed should be discarded and the patient should continue taking the remaining tablets until the cycle is finished. A back-up contraceptive method is not required if the patient missed inert or estrogen-containing tablets. If the patient is unsure of what drug regimen to take as a result of missed tablets, a back-up method of contraception should be used for each sexual encounter, and one tablet taken each day until the next clinician contact. Missed doses may cause light bleeding or spotting, and ingestion of multiple tablets to make up for those missed doses may be associated with nausea.

In nonlactating postpartum women, fixed-combination extended-cycle oral contraceptives may be started no earlier than 28 days after delivery. Women may start taking fixed-combination extended-cycle oral contraceptives immediately following a complete first-trimester abortion; a back-up method of contraception is not needed.

Continuous-Regimen (Noncyclic) Oral Contraceptive. When a fixed-combination continuous-regimen oral contraceptive (i.e., Lybrel®) is used, the oral contraceptive is administered each day and continued daily without interruption (i.e., without a drug-free interval). Therefore, women using this preparation should expect no withdrawal menstruation-like bleeding; uterine bleeding and/or spotting does occur in some women. Administration of the continuous-regimen oral contraceptive usually begins on the first day of the menstrual cycle in women who did not use hormonal contraception in the preceding month. A back-up method of contraception is not needed if the oral contraceptive is started on the first day of the menstrual cycle. The manufacturer states that women switching from a cyclic estrogen-progestin oral contraceptive should start the continuous-regimen oral contraceptive on the first day of withdrawal bleeding, within 7 days of the last hormonally active tablet; a back-up method of contraception is not needed. Women switching from progestin-only oral contraceptives should start the continuous-regimen oral contraceptive on the day after the last dose of the progestin-only oral contraceptive. Women switching from a progestin-only implant should start the continuous-regimen oral contraceptive on the same day that the implant is removed. Women switching from a progestin-only contraceptive injection should start the continuous-regimen oral contraceptive on the day that the next contraceptive injection would have been due. A back-up method of contraception (e.g., condom, spermicide) is recommended in all women switching from progestin-only contraceptives until the fixed-combination continuous-regimen oral contraceptive has been used for 7 days.

When a woman misses one tablet of the fixed-combination continuous-regimen oral contraceptive (i.e., Lybrel®), the missed dose should be taken as soon as it is remembered, followed by resumption of the regular schedule (this may involve taking 2 tablets on one day). When 2 tablets are missed and the missed doses are remembered on the day of the second missed dose, the 2 missed tablets should be taken as soon as they are remembered, followed by resumption of the regular schedule. When 2 tablets are missed and the missed doses are remembered on the day after the second missed dose, the 2 missed tablets should be taken as soon as they are remembered, then 2 tablets the next day, followed by resumption of the regular schedule. When 3 or more tablets are missed, the patient should contact her clinician for advice and continue to take one tablet daily until the clinician is contacted. When one or more tablets are missed, a back-up method of contraception (e.g., condom, spermicide) should be used until the patient has taken the oral contraceptive for 7 days. If the patient is unsure of what drug regimen to take as a result of missed tablets, a back-up method of contraception should be used for each sexual encounter.

In nonlactating postpartum women, the fixed-combination continuous-regimen oral contraceptive may be started no earlier than 28 days after delivery. In addition, the continuous regimen oral contraceptive may be started no earlier than 28 days after a second-trimester abortion. A back-up method of contraception should be used until the patient has taken the oral contraceptive for 7 days. Women may start the continuous-regimen oral contraceptive immediately following a complete first-trimester abortion; a back-up method of contraception is not needed.

Intravaginal Dosage. Each vaginal contraceptive ring containing ethinyl estradiol and etonogestrel (NuvaRing®) is intended to be used for one cycle which consists of a 3-week period of continuous use of the ring followed by a 1-week ring-free period. When the vaginal ring is used for contraception, one ring (delivering ethinyl estradiol 0.015 mg/24 hours and etonogestrel 0.12 mg/24 hours) is inserted into the vagina at the beginning of the cycle. After 3 weeks, the vaginal ring is removed on the same day of the week as it was inserted and at about the same time of day. After a 1-week ring-free period, a new ring is inserted on the same day of the week as in the previous cycle. Withdrawal bleeding usually occurs within 2–3 days after removal of the ring. For contraceptive effectiveness, a new ring must be inserted 1 week after the previous ring was removed even if menstrual bleeding is not finished.

To initiate therapy, the vaginal ring (containing ethinyl estradiol and etonogestrel) usually is inserted on or before day 5 of the cycle (the first day of bleeding is counted as the first day of the menstrual cycle) in women who did not use hormonal contraception in the preceding month. During the first cycle, a back-up method of contraception (e.g., condom, spermicide) is recommended until the contraceptive ring has been used continuously for 7 days. The manufacturer states that women switching from estrogen-progestin oral contraceptives to the vaginal ring should insert the ring within 7 days of the last hormonally active tablet and no later than the day that a new oral contraceptive cycle would have been started; a back-up method of contraception is not needed. Women switching from progestin-only contraceptives to the vaginal ring should insert the ring on any day of the month if they are switching from a progestin-only oral contraceptive (without skipping any day between receiving the last progestin oral contraceptive and the initial administration of the vaginal ring). In addition, women switching from a progestin-only contraceptive injection should insert the vaginal ring on the same day as the next contraceptive injection would have been due. Women who are switching from a progestin-only implant or a progestin-containing intrauterine device should insert the vaginal ring on the same day as the implant or the intrauterine device is removed. A back-up method of contraception is recommended in all women switching from progestin-only contraceptives until the vaginal ring has been used continuously for 7 days.

When the woman forgets to insert a new vaginal ring at the start of any cycle, the ring should be inserted as soon as she remembers and back-up contraception must be employed until the ring has been used continuously for 7 days. If the vaginal ring is left in place for up to 1 extra week (up to 4 weeks total), the ring should be removed and a new ring can be inserted after a 1-week drug-free interval. If the ring is left in place for longer than 4 weeks, pregnancy should be ruled out and a back-up method of contraception must be used until a new ring has been used continuously for 7 days.

Women may start using the vaginal contraceptive ring in the first 5 days following a complete first-trimester abortion; a back-up method of contraception is not needed in these women. If the contraceptive preparation is not used within the mentioned 5 days, the woman should follow the general instructions for women who did not use hormonal contraception in the preceding month.

If a nonlactating woman chooses to initiate contraception postpartum with the contraceptive vaginal ring (NuvaRing®) before menstruation has started, the possibility that ovulation and conception may have occurred prior to initiation of contraceptive therapy should be considered, and back-up contraception must be employed for the first 7 days.

Transdermal Dosage. When the transdermal system containing ethinyl estradiol and norelgestromin (Ortho Evra®) is used for contraception, it is applied topically in a cyclic regimen using a 28-day cycle. One transdermal system (containing ethinyl estradiol 0.75 mg and norelgestromin 6 mg) is applied once weekly (same day each week) for 3 weeks, followed by a 1-week drug-free interval (drug-free interval should *not* exceed 7 days); then the regimen is repeated. Systemic exposure to estrogen is greater with the transdermal system (Ortho Evra®) than with oral contraceptive preparations because of differences in the pharmacokinetic profiles of the preparations. (See Pharmacokinetics: Absorption and see the introductory discussion under Cautions.)

Administration of the transdermal contraceptive system usually begins on the first day of the menstrual cycle or on the first Sunday after menstrual bleeding has started. A back-up method of contraception (condom, spermicide, diaphragm) should be employed for the first 7 days after application of the first system if therapy is started after day 1 of the menstrual cycle. A back-up method of contraception is not needed if the first system is applied on the first day of the menstrual cycle. The manufacturer states that women switching from estrogen-progestin oral contraceptives to the estrogen-progestin transdermal system should apply the transdermal system on the first day of withdrawal bleeding. If there is no withdrawal bleeding within 5 days of the last hormonally active tablet, pregnancy must be ruled out. If therapy with the transdermal system is initiated after the first day of bleeding, a back-up method of contraception should be used for 7 days. If more than 7 days elapse after receiving the last hormonally active tablet, the possibility of ovulation and conception should be considered.

When a woman has not adhered to the prescribed transdermal contraceptive regimen by not applying the estrogen and progestin-containing system at the initiation of any cycle (i.e., day 1/first week), the system should be applied as soon as it is remembered and a new dosage cycle started the same day; back-up contraception must be employed for the first 7 days of the new cycle. In addition, if the transdermal system has not been changed in the middle of the cycle (i.e., on day 8/week 2 or day 15/week 3) for 1–2 days (up to 48 hours), a new system should be applied as soon as it is remembered and the application schedule employed should be continued; back-up contraception is not needed. However, if the transdermal system has not been changed for more than 2 days (48 hours or more) in the middle of the cycle, a new dosage cycle should be started; back-up contraception must be employed for the first 7 days of the new cycle. When the transdermal system is not removed at the end of the application schedule (i.e., on day 22/week 4), the system should be removed as soon as it is remembered and the application schedule employed should be continued (i.e., system applied on day 28); back-up contraception is not needed.

Women may start using the transdermal contraceptive system immediately after a first-trimester abortion; a back-up method of contraception is not needed. If the contraceptive preparation is not used within 5 days of a first-trimester abortion, the woman should follow instructions as if initiating transdermal contraception for the first time.

Postcoital Contraception **Oral Dosage.** Several regimens employing short-course, high-dose oral combinations of ethinyl estradiol and norgestrel or levonorgestrel have been used safely and effectively for postcoital contraception†. One widely studied and used regimen (the "Yuzpe" regimen) consists of an oral dose of 100 mcg of ethinyl estradiol and 1 mg of norgestrel (administered as 2 tablets each containing 50 mcg and 0.5 mg of the drugs, respectively) within 72 hours after unprotected intercourse, initiating the first dose at a time when it would make convenient administering the subsequent repeat dose 12 hours later. Alternative combination regimens that have been used consist of a dose of 120 mcg of ethinyl estradiol and 1.2 mg of norgestrel or 0.5–0.6 mg of levonorgestrel (e.g., administered as 4 tablets each containing 30 mcg of ethinyl estradiol and 0.3 mg of norgestrel or 0.125–0.15 mg of levonorgestrel) within 72 hours after intercourse, repeating the dose 12 hours later. Another combination regimen that has been used consists of a dose of 100 mcg of ethinyl estradiol and 0.5 mg of levonorgestrel (e.g., administered as 5 tablets each containing 20 mcg of ethinyl estradiol and 0.1 mg of levonorgestrel) within 72 hours after intercourse, repeating the dose 12 hours later. Because postcoital efficacy diminishes as the time between intercourse and initiation of estrogen-progestin combination therapy increases, such therapy should be initiated *as soon as possible but preferably within 72 hours* following unprotected intercourse. If necessary, the first dose can be given up to 120 hours after unprotected intercourse. Women should be advised that taking more than the prescribed dose probably will not further decrease the risk of pregnancy, but will increase the risk of severe adverse GI effects.

If women are given a conventional mnemonic package of an oral estrogen-progestin combination for use in taking a postcoital contraceptive regimen, they should be instructed carefully regarding the number and color of the tablets to be taken with each dose and that only a portion of the contents of the package actually will be used.

Table 1. Dosage of estrogen-progestin combinations for postcoital contraception

Estrogen-progestin combination formulation [brand name]	Number and color of tablets per dose[a]
Ethinyl estradiol (50 mcg) with norgestrel (0.5 mg) [Ovral®]	2 white tablets (any of 21 tablets)
Ethinyl estradiol (50 mcg) with norgestrel (0.5 mg) [Ovral®-28]	2 white tablets (any of *first* 21 tablets)
Ethinyl estradiol (30 mcg) with norgestrel (0.3 mg) [Lo-Ovral®]	4 white tablets (any of 21 tablets)
Ethinyl estradiol (30 mcg) with norgestrel (0.3 mg) [Lo-Ovral®-28]	4 white tablets (any of *first* 21 tablets)
Ethinyl estradiol (30 mcg) with levonorgestrel (0.15 mg) [Nordette®]	4 light-orange tablets (any of 21 tablets)
Ethinyl estradiol (30 mcg) with levonorgestrel (0.15 mg) [Nordette®-28]	4 light-orange tablets (any of *first* 21 tablets)
Ethinyl estradiol (30 mcg) with levonorgestrel (0.15 mg) [Levlen® 21]	4 light-orange tablets (any of 21 tablets)
Ethinyl estradiol (30 mcg) with levonorgestrel (0.15 mg) [Levlen® 28]	4 light-orange tablets (any of *first* 21 tablets)
Ethinyl estradiol (30 mcg) with levonorgestrel (0.125 mg) [Tri-Levlen® 21]	4 yellow tablets (any of *last* 10 tablets)
Ethinyl estradiol (30 mcg) with levonorgestrel (0.125 mg) [Tri-Levlen® 28]	4 yellow tablets (any of tablets 12–21)
Ethinyl estradiol (30 mcg) with levonorgestrel (0.125 mg) [Tri-Phasil® 21]	4 yellow tablets (any of *last* 10 tablets)
Ethinyl estradiol (30 mcg) with levonorgestrel (0.125 mg) [Tri-Levlen® 28]	4 yellow tablets (any of tablets 12–21)
Ethinyl estradiol (20 mcg) with levonorgestrel (0.1 mg) [Lessina® 28]	5 pink tablets (any of *first* 21 tablets)

[a] Dose is administered initially and then repeated 12 hours later

Contraception and Folate Supplementation **Oral Dosage.** For increasing folate concentrations in women using oral contraceptives, the combination of ethinyl estradiol 20 mcg in fixed combination with drospirenone 3 mg and levomefolate calcium 0.451 mg (Beyaz®) or ethinyl estradiol 30 mcg in fixed combination with drospirenone 3 mg and levomefolate calcium 0.451 mg (Safyral®) is used in the same dosage and administration (i.e., timing of initiation of therapy) as used in contraception.

Acne Vulgaris **Oral Dosage.** For the treatment of acne vulgaris, the triphasic oral estrogen-progestin combination of ethinyl estradiol 35 mcg in fixed combination with norgestimate 0.18, 0.215, or 0.25 mg (Ortho-Tri-Cyclen®) or norethindrone 1 mg in fixed combination with ethinyl estradiol 20, 30, or 35 mcg (Estrostep®) is used in the same dosage and administration (i.e., timing of initiation of therapy) as used in contraception.

For the treatment of acne vulgaris, the estrogen-progestin combination of ethinyl estradiol 20 mcg in fixed combination with drospirenone 3 mg (Yaz®) or ethinyl estradiol 20 mcg in fixed combination with drospirenone 3 mg and levomefolate calcium 0.451 mg (Beyaz®) is used in the same dosage and administration (i.e., timing of initiation of therapy) as used in contraception.

Premenstrual Dysphoric Disorder **Oral Dosage.** For the treatment of premenstrual dysphoric disorder, the combination of ethinyl estradiol 20 mcg in fixed combination with drospirenone 3 mg (Yaz®) or ethinyl estradiol 20 mcg in fixed combination with drospirenone 3 mg and levomefolate calcium 0.451 mg (Beyaz®) is used in the same dosage and administration (i.e., timing of initiation of therapy) as used in contraception. (See Conventional-cycle Oral Contraceptives under Dosage: Contraception, in Dosage and Administration.)

Cautions

The potential risks of estrogen-progestin contraceptive use have been established in women of reproductive age. The risks should be identical for postpubertal adolescents under 16 years of age and users 16 years of age or older. Estrogen-progestin combination contraceptives including short-term, high-dose postcoital contraceptives are not indicated before menarche.

Exposure to ethinyl estradiol and norelgestromin is higher in women receiving the Ortho-Evra® transdermal system than in women receiving an oral contraceptive preparation containing ethinyl estradiol 35 mcg and norgestimate 0.25 mg per tablet. Increased exposure to estrogen may increase the risk for adverse effects.

Exposure to ethinyl estradiol and levonorgestrel is higher in women receiving Lybrel® (a fixed-combination continuous-regimen oral contraceptive) than in women receiving a conventional-cycle oral contraceptive containing the same ethinyl estradiol dose and a similar dose of the progestin component; use of Lybrel® results in 13 additional weeks of hormone intake per year.

Epidemiologic data are not available to determine whether safety and efficacy associated with the vaginal route of administration of estrogen-progestin contraceptives differ from the oral route. Adverse effects similar to those with oral estrogen-progestin contraceptives generally are expected with vaginal estrogen-progestin contraceptives.

Information on the potential risks of estrogen-progestin contraceptive use (and associated cautions, precautions, and contraindications) is based principally on studies and experience with preparations that contained higher estrogen and/or progestin doses than those in currently available preparations. The relative risks associated with use of currently available lower-dose preparations remains to be determined. For example, while previous experience indicated that the risk of adverse cardiovascular effects associated with oral contraceptives was increased in *nonsmoking* women older than 40 years of age, this risk may have resulted in part from the high estrogen content of previously available preparations. It currently is not known whether such increased cardiovascular risk also is associated with use of currently available, low-dose preparations, but some experts consider the possible benefits of low-dose (containing no more than 35 mcg of estrogen) oral contraceptives to outweigh the potential risks of pregnancy in healthy *nonsmoking* women older than 40 years of age who have no other risk factors. The risk of serious morbidity or mortality is very small in healthy women without underlying risk factors. The risk of morbidity and mortality increases significantly in the presence of other risk factors (e.g., hypertension, hyperlipidemias, obesity, diabetes).

Common adverse effects of oral estrogen-progestin contraceptives appear to be mainly caused by the estrogen, are usually most pronounced during the first oral contraceptive cycle, and disappear or diminish after 3 or 4 cycles; there does not appear to be any advantage in changing preparations during this period of time. If minor adverse effects persist after the fourth cycle, a different combination of drugs or a different dosage may be tried. Although conventional-dosage preparations (containing 35 mcg or more of ethinyl estradiol or 50 mcg or more of mestranol) are generally associated with slightly lower pregnancy rates than reduced-dosage preparations, conventional-dosage preparations are generally more frequently associated with adverse effects (e.g., edema, nausea and vomiting, thromboembolic disorders) than reduced-dosage preparations; however, reduced-dosage preparations are more frequently associated with bleeding irregularities, including breakthrough bleeding, spotting, and menstrual irregularities, than conventional-dosage preparations. Because of the increased risk of thromboembolic disorders associated with conventional-dosage preparations, reduced-dosage preparations are recommended for initial use in patients who have not previously received oral contraceptives. Although numerous adverse effects have been reported in women receiving oral contraceptives, many of the reported effects are conditions that could occur spontaneously in women of childbearing age and a causal relationship has, in many instances, been difficult to establish.

It is not known if oral contraceptive combinations containing desogestrel or norgestimate cause fewer androgenic effects (e.g., acne, hirsutism, weight gain) than estrogen-progestin combinations containing conventional progestins (e.g., levonorgestrel, norethindrone). There is some evidence that oral contraceptives containing desogestrel may be associated with an increased risk of nonfatal venous thrombosis. (See Thromboembolic Disorders in Cautions: Cardiovascular Effects.)

Limited data are available concerning the risk of using short-course, high-dose estrogen-progestin combinations for emergency contraception. No serious or long-term complications have been associated with such postcoital regimens in Europe, where experience is extensive. In addition, some evidence indicates that emergency postcoital contraception may not compromise conventional contraception use or sexual behavior (e.g., promiscuity, sexually transmitted disease [STD] risk).

■ GI Effects

The most frequent adverse effect of oral contraceptives is nausea. In addition, nausea has been reported in women using vaginal or transdermal estrogen-progestin contraceptives.

The principal risk associated with currently recommended high-dose, postcoital estrogen-progestin combination regimens appears to be moderate to severe adverse GI effects including severe vomiting and nausea, which occur in 12–22 and 30–66%, respectively, of women receiving the short-course regimens and may limit compliance with, and effectiveness of, the regimens. In 2 prospective, randomized studies, nausea and vomiting were less common with a high-dose postcoital progestin-only regimen (0.75 mg levonorgestrel every 12 hours for 2 doses) than with a high-dose estrogen-progestin regimen (100 mcg ethinyl estradiol and 0.5 mg levonorgestrel every 12 hours for 2 doses).

Other adverse GI effects include vomiting, abdominal cramps, abdominal pain, bloating, diarrhea, constipation, and inflammatory bowel disease. Gingivitis and dry socket also have been reported. Changes in appetite and changes in weight also may occur.

■ Dermatologic Effects

The most frequent dermatologic reaction to oral contraceptives is chloasma or melasma. Women who have had melasma during pregnancy appear to be most susceptible. Irregular brown macules may develop slowly on the face within 1 month to 2 years following initiation of oral contraceptive therapy. The macules fade more slowly than in melasma gravidarum and may be permanent.

Acne may improve during oral contraceptive therapy because of decreased sebum production and depression of sebaceous gland activity; however, it may increase in severity during initial therapy and may develop in some women who have not previously had acne.

Other dermatologic reactions include allergic rash, urticaria, erythema multiforme, erythema nodosum, hemorrhagic eruption, pruritus, and angioedema. Hirsutism and alopecia also have occurred. Herpes gestationis and porphyria cutanea have reportedly been adversely affected in women receiving oral contraceptives.

Application site reaction has occurred in women using the transdermal contraceptive system containing ethinyl estradiol and norelgestromin. The manufacturer states that if such skin irritation occurs, the transdermal system may be removed and a new patch applied to a different location until the next new application day.

■ Cardiovascular Effects

A positive association between the amount of estrogen and progestin in oral contraceptives and the risk of adverse cardiovascular effects has been observed. Adverse effects similar to those with oral combination estrogen-progestin contraceptives generally are expected with vaginal or transdermal estrogen-progestin contraceptives.

Elevated Blood Pressure Increases in blood pressure may occur in women receiving estrogen-progestin contraceptives. Blood pressure elevations are usually minor, but clinically important hypertension may occur in some women. Some women develop hypertension within 1–3 weeks after initiation of oral contraceptive therapy and become normotensive during the part of the oral contraceptive cycle when they do not receive the drugs. In others, blood pressure increases slowly and may not reach abnormal levels for several months. Elevated blood pressure may gradually decrease or persist after the oral contraceptive is discontinued.

The risk of hypertension increases with increasing duration of oral contraceptive use and is about 2.5–3 times greater in the fifth year of continual use than in the first year. Age also is positively correlated with the risk of hypertension in oral contraceptive users, becoming substantial in women about 35 years of age and older. Women with a history of hypertension, preexisting renal disease, a history of toxemia or elevated blood pressure during pregnancy, a familial tendency toward hypertension or its consequences, or a history of excessive weight gain or fluid retention during the menstrual cycle may be at increased risk of developing elevated blood pressure during estrogen-progestin contraceptive therapy and, therefore, should be monitored closely. Even though elevated blood pressure may remain within the normal range, the clinical implications of elevations should be considered in all patients. All women, but particularly those with other risk factors for cardiovascular disease or stroke, should have blood pressure measurements before an oral contraceptive is prescribed and at regular intervals during therapy.

Thromboembolic Disorders Oral contraceptive use is associated with an increased risk of thromboembolic and thrombotic disorders. One study has shown an increased relative risk of fatal venous thromboembolism (VTE) and several other studies have shown an increased relative risk of nonfatal VTE in oral contraceptive users. Case-controlled studies estimated that the relative risk for developing fatal or nonfatal thromboembolism (ranging in severity from superficial thrombosis to pulmonary embolism) was 3–11 times greater in oral contraceptive users than in nonusers and 1.5–6 times greater in women predisposed to venous thromboembolic disorders. However, cohort studies suggest that the overall relative risk is somewhat lower, ranging from 3 times greater for new cases to 4.5 times greater for new cases requiring hospitalization in oral contraceptive users when compared with nonusers. A prospective review failed to show increased mortality rates from cardiovascular disorders in oral contraceptive users; however, when a selected subset of this study was analyzed in a retrospective, case-controlled fashion, an increased risk of VTE was associated with oral contraceptive use. Hereditary coagulation disorders, such as factor V Leiden mutation, increase the risk of thromboembolic disease. The risk of thromboembolic disease from oral contraceptive use is not related to the duration of use and disappears when oral contraceptive use is discontinued.

The pharmacokinetic profile for the transdermal contraceptive system containing ethinyl estradiol and norelgestromin (Ortho Evra®) differs from the profile for oral contraceptive preparations. Overall exposure to ethinyl estradiol and norelgestromin is higher in women receiving Ortho Evra® than in women receiving an oral contraceptive preparation containing ethinyl estradiol 35 mcg and norgestimate 0.25 mg per tablet. (See Pharmacokinetics: Absorption.) Increased exposure to estrogen may increase the risk of certain adverse effects (e.g., VTE). The risk of VTE in women using Ortho Evra® relative to the risk in women using an oral contraceptive containing norgestimate or levonorgestrel and ethinyl estradiol 30–35 mcg has been investigated in several epidemiologic, case-controlled studies. In one study that used data from health care claims, current use of Ortho Evra® was not associated with an increased risk of nonfatal VTE compared with use of an oral contraceptive (odds ratio [OR] 0.9; 95% confidence interval: 0.5–1.6). In a subsequent analysis that included an additional 17 months of data from this study, current use of Ortho Evra® was not associated with an increased risk of nonfatal VTE compared with use of an oral contraceptive (OR 1.1; 95% confidence interval: 0.6–2.1). In another study that used claims data and chart review, current use of Ortho Evra® was associated with an increased risk of VTE compared with use of an oral contraceptive (OR 2.4; 95% confidence interval: 1.1–5.5). Findings from another study that used claims data indicated current use of Ortho Evra® might be associated with an increased risk of idiopathic VTE compared with use of an oral contraceptive (OR 2; 95% confidence interval: 0.9–4.1).

Because the fixed-combination continuous-regimen oral contraceptive (Lybrel®) is administered daily (not cyclically), overall exposure to estrogen and progestin is higher in women receiving this preparation than in women receiving a conventional-cycle oral contraceptive containing the same dose of ethinyl estradiol and a similar dose of the progestin component.

A review conducted by the US Food and Drug Administration (FDA) indicates that the use of oral contraceptive combinations that contain the progestins desogestrel (Desogen®, Ortho-Cept®) or gestodene (not commercially available in the US) may be associated with an increased risk of nonfatal venous thrombosis compared with oral contraceptives containing conventional progestins (e.g., levonorgestrel, norethindrone). This conclusion was based on interim results of 3 unpublished comparative studies (i.e., by the World Health Organization [WHO], by the Boston Drug Surveillance Program, by the European Transnational study coordinated by McGill University of Canada). Interim results of these unpublished studies indicate that, while the overall risk of nonfatal venous thrombosis is lower than that reported in previous studies, estrogen-progestin combinations containing desogestrel or gestodene appear to be associated with a twofold increased risk of venous thrombosis compared with oral contraceptives containing conventional progestins. Some experts have recommended that estrogen-progestin combinations containing desogestrel or gestodene not be prescribed routinely for prevention of conception in women; however, other clinicians state that further analysis of data is needed for such a recommendation. Although the FDA does not recommend that women currently using oral contraceptives containing desogestrel discontinue such use or switch to another estrogen-progestin combination contraceptive, the FDA states that women using an oral contraceptive containing desogestrel should be advised to discuss such use with their clinician, taking into consideration the relative risks and benefits associated with these oral contraceptives. It should be considered that the contraceptive vaginal ring (NuvaRing®) contains etonogestrel, the active metabolite of desogestrel; however, it is not known whether NuvaRing® is associated with an increased risk of venous thrombosis.

Another safety review conducted by the FDA indicates that use of combination oral contraceptives containing the progestin drospirenone may be associated with an increased risk of VTE compared with that of oral contraceptives containing levonorgestrel or other progestins. This conclusion was based on results of several epidemiologic studies (i.e., the US postapproval safety study by Ingenix, the European Active Surveillance Study [EURAS], the Long-Term Active Surveillance Study [LASS], 2 Danish cohort studies, the Dutch multiple environmental and genetic assessment of risk factors for venous thrombosis [MEGA] study, the UK General Practice Research Database [GPRD] study, the PharMetrics study, and the FDA-supported study) evaluating the risk of VTE in women using oral contraceptives containing drospirenone. These studies reported that the risk of VTE in such women ranged from no increase to a threefold increase in risk. The FDA's safety review was prompted by results of 2 recent case-control studies that showed a twofold to threefold increased risk of VTE (including deep-vein thrombosis and pulmonary embolism) in patients receiving oral contraceptives containing drospirenone compared with those receiving oral contraceptives containing the progestin levonorgestrel. These 2 studies evaluated cases of idiopathic VTE occurring in women 15–44 years of age who were current users of oral contraceptives containing 30 mcg of estrogen with either drospirenone or levonorgestrel; women with risk factors for VTE were excluded from the studies. The FDA has also reviewed data from a large US retrospective cohort study in more than 800,000 women evaluating thrombotic and thromboembolic risks (including VTE) associated with hormonal contraceptives. Final results from this study suggest an increased risk of VTE (hazard ratio greater than 1) in women using oral contraceptives containing drospirenone compared with women using other hormonal contraceptives. (See Cautions: Precautions and Contraindications.)

Given the conflicting results of the previous epidemiologic studies and the recent findings, the FDA held a joint meeting of the Reproductive Health Drugs Advisory Committee and the Drug Safety and Risk Management Advisory Committee on December 8, 2011, to review the risks and benefits of such therapy and specifically discuss the risk of VTE associated with drospirenone-containing hormonal contraceptives. The studies reviewed by the FDA did not provide consistent data for the comparative risk of thromboembolic events between oral contraceptives that contain drospirenone and those that do not. In addition, the studies did not account for important known and unknown patient characteristics that may influence prescribing patterns and may affect risk of VTE. For these reasons, the FDA states that it is unclear whether the increased risk of thromboembolic events observed in these epidemiologic studies actually resulted from use of drospirenone-containing oral contraceptives. At this time, the FDA has concluded that the risk of VTE may be higher for such oral contraceptives. The FDA will continue to communicate any new safety information as it becomes available.

An increased risk of cerebrovascular disorders, including thrombotic and hemorrhagic stroke, also is associated with oral contraceptive use, although the risk generally is greatest in older (i.e., older than 35 years of age), hypertensive women who also smoke. The use of estrogen-progestin contraceptives also is associated with an increased risk of stroke in women with other underlying risk factors. Hypertension is a risk factor in both users and nonusers of oral contraceptives for both thrombotic and hemorrhagic stroke, while smoking appears to increase the risk for hemorrhagic stroke. Although cigarette smoking alone has been associated with an increased risk of cerebrovascular disorders, concomitant cigarette smoking and oral contraceptive use is associated with a greater risk of these disorders than either alone. The relative risk of thrombotic stroke has been shown to range from 3 for normotensive users of oral contraceptives to 14 for users with hypertension. The relative risk of hemorrhagic stroke is reported to be 1.2 in nonsmoking women who use oral contraceptives, 2.6 in nonusers who do not smoke, 7.6 in users who smoke, 1.8 in normotensive users, and 25.7 in users with severe hypertension. The risk also appears to be greater in older women.

An increased relative risk of myocardial infarction has been associated with oral contraceptive use. In one study, oral contraceptive use was one of several risk factors for coronary artery disease which included cigarette smoking, hypertension, hypercholesterolemia, obesity, diabetes, and preeclamptic toxemia; the risk of myocardial infarction increased as the number of risk factors for coronary artery disease increased. The relative risk of developing fatal myocardial infarction has been estimated as twice as great in oral contraceptive users who do not smoke compared with nonusers who do not smoke, as 5 times greater in oral contraceptive users who smoke compared with users who do not smoke, and about 10–12 times greater in users who smoke compared with nonusers who do not smoke; women who smoke 15 or more cigarettes daily are especially at risk. However, other data suggest that the likelihood of myocardial infarction is not increased in young women who use oral contraceptives and do not smoke or have hypertension or diabetes.

A positive association between thromboembolic disorders and estrogen dosage of oral contraceptives also exists. The progestin content of oral contraceptives also appears to contribute to the risk of thromboembolic disorders. Use of oral contraceptive combinations that contain the progestins desogestrel or gestodene (not commercially available in the US) may be associated with an increased risk of nonfatal venous thrombosis compared with use of oral contraceptives containing conventional progestins (e.g., levonorgestrel, norethindrone). However, desogestrel has minimal androgenic activity and there is some evidence that the risk of myocardial infarction associated with oral contraceptives is lower when the progestin has minimal androgenic activity than when the activity is greater. A relationship between the estrogen and/or progestin dosage of oral contraceptives and the risk of myocardial infarction has not been established. However, a decrease in serum high-density lipoprotein (HDL) concentration has been reported with increasing progestational activity of oral contraceptives and decreased HDL has been associated with an increased risk of ischemic heart disease. (See Effects on Lipids and Lipoproteins, in Cautions: Endocrine and Metabolic Effects.)

The clinician and the woman using estrogen-progestin contraceptives should be alert to the earliest signs and symptoms of thromboembolic and thrombotic disorders (e.g., thrombophlebitis, pulmonary embolism, cerebrovascular insufficiency, coronary occlusion, retinal thrombosis, mesenteric thrombosis). Estrogen-progestin contraceptives should be discontinued immediately when any of these disorders occurs or is suspected. A two- to four-fold increased risk of postsurgery thromboembolic complications has been reported in oral contraceptive users; the risk in women predisposed to venous thromboembolic disorders is twice that in women who have no such predisposition. (See Cautions: Precautions and Contraindications.)

Other Cardiovascular Effects Oral contraceptives may cause some degree of fluid retention and edema. Oral contraceptives should be used with caution in patients with conditions that might be aggravated by fluid retention. (See Cautions: Precautions and Contraindications.) Premature ventricular and supraventricular complexes and other ECG abnormalities have been reported in women receiving oral contraceptives; however, a causal relationship has not been established.

■ Endocrine and Metabolic Effects Endocrine function test results may be altered in patients receiving oral contraceptives. If results of endocrine function tests are abnormal, the tests should be repeated 2 months after the drug has been discontinued.

Effects on Glucose Decreased glucose tolerance has been observed in a significant percentage of patients receiving oral contraceptives. Fasting blood glucose concentrations are not altered in most patients; however, increased plasma insulin and blood pyruvate concentrations may occur. Although decreased glucose tolerance appears to be directly related to the estrogen of oral contraceptives, estrogen alone does not appear to decrease glucose tolerance and therefore this effect appears to involve both estrogenic and progestinic components. Progestins increase insulin secretion and insulin resistance, and these effects vary among different progestin agents. Prediabetic and diabetic patients should be carefully monitored during estrogen-progestin contraceptive therapy.

Effects on Lipids and Lipoproteins Increased concentrations of plasma triglyceride, low-density lipoproteins, and total phospholipids may occur during therapy with estrogen-progestin contraceptives. The clinical importance of these alterations in lipid and lipoprotein concentrations has not been established; however, it may be advisable to avoid use of oral contraceptives in women with elevated serum lipids. Generally, the progestin component of oral contraceptives has been shown to decrease high-density lipoprotein cholesterol (HDL-cholesterol), whereas the estrogen component has been shown to increase it; however, some newer progestins (e.g., desogestrel, norgestimate) also may increase HDL-cholesterol. Therefore, it has been suggested that the net effect of estrogen-progestin contraceptives on high-density lipoprotein cholesterol depends on the specific formulation.

Effects on Thyroid The estrogenic component of estrogen-progestin contraceptives may produce elevations in thyroxine-binding globulin (TBG) resulting in elevated total circulating thyroid hormone, as measured by protein-bound iodine (PBI), thyroxine (T_4) (by column and radioimmunoassay), and butanol extractable iodine. Decreased triiodothyronine (T_3) resin uptake, reflecting elevated TBG, also occurs, while free T_4 concentrations are unaltered. Basal metabolic rate, cholesterol concentrations, iodine-131 uptake, and the free thyroxine index remain unchanged, suggesting that thyroid function is not affected. Abnormal thyroid function test results usually return to pretreatment levels within 2–4 months after estrogen therapy is discontinued.

Other Endocrine and Metabolic Effects Estrogen-progestin contraceptives also affect other serum proteins. Serum albumin may be increased or decreased and variable effects on immunoglobulins have been reported. Serum cholinesterase, haptoglobulins, and orosomucoid decrease; transferrin, plasminogen, α_2-macroglobulin, and testosterone- and estradiol-binding globulins are increased. Estrogen-progestin contraceptive therapy causes decreased pregnanediol excretion. Ceruloplasmin elevations may give plasma a green color. Cryofibrinogenemia has also been reported. The renin substrate (angiotensinogen) concentration is increased and the aldosterone excretion rate is moderately elevated. Some patients may have hyporesponsive plasma renin activity with normal aldosterone excretion for a few weeks after oral contraceptives are discontinued. Estrogen-progestin contraceptives may cause increased serum magnesium, copper, zinc, and iron concentrations as well as total iron-binding capacity; however, the clinical importance of these increased mineral concentrations has not been determined.

Oral contraceptives may also decrease the response to the metyrapone test. (See Laboratory Test Interferences.)

Because drospirenone has antimineralocorticoid activity, the potential exists for hyperkalemia to occur in high-risk patients (e.g., those with renal or hepatic impairment, adrenal insufficiency) receiving oral contraceptives containing this progestin.

■ Hepatic Effects Liver function test results may be altered in patients receiving oral contraceptives and if results of these tests are abnormal, they should be repeated 2 months after the drugs have been discontinued. Increased sulfobromophthalein retention occurs frequently, as a result of interference with the transfer of dye conjugates from liver cells into bile; uptake, conjugation, and storage do not appear to be affected. Less frequently, increased serum aminotransferase and alkaline phosphatase concentrations may occur. Liver function test results usually return to normal within several weeks after oral contraceptives are discontinued; occasionally, however, abnormal test results may persist for longer periods.

Cholestatic jaundice has been reported during oral contraceptive use. Cholestasis is manifested by the development of malaise, anorexia, and pruritus about 2 weeks to 2 months after the start of therapy. Occasionally, arthralgia, fever, and rash may occur. Serum bilirubin concentration may range from 3–10 mg/dL and is mostly conjugated. Women with a history of jaundice during pregnancy have an increased risk of jaundice recurrence while receiving oral contraceptives. If jaundice occurs during oral contraceptive therapy, the drugs should be discontinued. Oral contraceptives may precipitate hepatic forms of porphyria and these drugs probably should not be used by women who have a familial history of hepatic porphyrias, since the occurrence of these conditions appears to be genetically determined. Budd-Chiari syndrome has also occurred in oral contraceptive users. Many patients who develop oral contraceptive- or pregnancy-associated Budd-Chiari syndrome also may have inherited or acquired thrombophilia. Steroid hormones (including oral contraceptives) may be poorly metabolized in patients with hepatic dysfunction; therefore, the drugs should be administered with caution to these individuals.

Liver tumors have been associated with oral contraceptive use. Liver tumors have been benign or malignant and have occurred during short-term and long-term use of oral contraceptives. Most commonly, liver tumors are benign hepatocellular adenomas. Long-term oral contraceptive users have an estimated annual incidence of hepatocellular adenoma of 3–4 per 100,000; risk appears to increase after 4 or more years of use. In several women who developed benign hepatocellular adenomas during oral contraceptive use, these tumors regressed following discontinuance of the drugs. Although benign hepatocellular adenomas are apparently uncommon findings in oral contraceptive users, they may result in death because of their vascularity which predisposes them to rupture and massive hemorrhage. Therefore, the presence of a liver tumor should be considered in women who develop sudden severe abdominal pain or shock. Patients with liver tumors have shown variable clinical features which may make preoperative diagnosis difficult; some of these patients have had right upper quadrant masses, while most have had signs and symptoms of acute intraperitoneal hemorrhage. Routine radiologic and laboratory test evaluations may not be helpful. Liver scans may show a focal defect, and hepatic arteriography may be useful in diagnosing primary liver neoplasm. Hepatocellular carcinoma has also been reported rarely in women receiving oral contraceptives, although a causal relationship to the drugs has not been clearly established. For women using oral contraceptives for 8 or more years, several epidemiologic studies have suggested a relative risk that is up to 7–20 times that of nonusers, although the occurrence of this tumor is rare. It also has not been clearly established whether hepatic adenoma induced by oral contraceptives can differentiate into hepatic carcinoma.

■ Genitourinary Effects Breakthrough bleeding and/or spotting (especially within the first 3 months of use), changes in menstrual flow, missed menses (during use), or amenorrhea (after use) may occur in women receiving hormonal contraceptives. Bleeding irregularities are more frequently associated with reduced-dosage preparations than with conventional-dosage preparations. Breakthrough bleeding that occurs early in the cycle generally is caused by a lack of adequate estrogenic stimulation, whereas bleeding after midcycle generally indicates progestin deficiency. Changes in the estrogen and/or progestin dose, ratio, and/or sequence may control or alleviate breakthrough bleeding. In women who develop breakthrough bleeding while receiving a biphasic oral contraceptive, switching to a triphasic oral contraceptive may control or alleviate bleeding since the progestin dose is increased after day 7 with the triphasic regimen. Once the possibility of pregnancy has been ruled out in women with missed menses (absence of withdrawal bleeding) (see Pregnancy, in Cautions: Pregnancy, Fertility, and Lactation), switching to a preparation with higher estrogenic activity or dose or to a triphasic preparation (since it allows endometrial proliferation during the initial 7-day, low-dose progestin period) may be beneficial. However, the risks (e.g., adverse cardiovascular effects) associated with increased estrogen and progestin doses must be considered, and increasing the dose to minimize bleeding irregularities should only be done if necessary.

While use of an extended-cycle oral contraceptive (e.g., LoSeasonique®, Seasonale®, Seasonique®) results in fewer planned menses (4 per year) than conventional-cycle oral contraceptives (13 per year), bleeding irregularities occur more frequently in women using the extended-cycle preparation than in women using the conventional-cycle preparation. Irregular bleeding occurs most often during the first few 91-day cycles. In one study in women who had used oral contraceptives, administration of Seasonale® resulted in 7 or more and 20 or more days of intramenstrual bleeding and/or spotting in 65 and 35% of women, respectively, during cycle 1 and in 42 and 15% of women, respectively, during cycle 4. In another study, administration of Seasonique® resulted in 7 or more and 20 or more days of intramenstrual bleeding and/or spotting in 64 and 29% of women, respectively, during cycle 1 and in 39 and 11% of women, respectively, during cycle 4. In women receiving a conventional-cycle oral contraceptive, intramenstrual bleeding and/or spotting for 7 or more and 20 or more days occurred in 38 and 6% of women, respectively, during cycles 1–4 and in 39 and 4% of women, respectively, during cycles 10–13.

Use of extended-cycle oral contraceptive preparations is associated with fewer menstrual symptoms than use of conventional-cycle oral contraceptive preparations. Whether adding 10 mcg of estradiol to the final 7 tablets in the cycle (LoSeasonique®, Seasonique®) will further reduce withdrawal symptoms (e.g., migraine headache) remains to be determined.

While use of a continuous-regimen (noncyclic) estrogen-progestin oral contraceptive (Lybrel®) eliminates withdrawal bleeding, irregular bleeding and/or spotting occurs in some women. In one study, administration of Lybrel® resulted in 4 or more and 7 or more days of bleeding and/or spotting in 67 and 54% of women, respectively, during the second 28-day dosing period and in 31 and 20% of women, respectively, during the thirteenth 28-day dosing period.

Adequate diagnostic procedures should be performed in patients with undiagnosed persistent or recurrent vaginal bleeding. When pathology has been excluded, time or change to another preparation may resolve the problem. Women with a history of oligomenorrhea or secondary amenorrhea or young women with irregular cycles may tend to remain anovulatory or to become amenorrheic after discontinuance of oral contraceptives; women with these preexisting problems should be advised of this possibility and encouraged to use other contraceptive methods.

Dysmenorrhea also may occur. Post-use anovulation, occasionally accompanied by galactorrhea, and a premenstrual-like syndrome has been reported. Post-use anovulation may be prolonged and may occur in women who had no previous irregularities. Galactorrhea and pituitary tumors (e.g., adenomas) have been associated with amenorrhea in former oral contraceptive users. One study showed a 16-fold increased prevalence of prolactin-secreting pituitary tumors (prolactinomas) among former users of oral contraceptives who had amenorrhea with galactorrhea compared with those without galactorrhea. In another study, the relative risk of prolactinoma was 1.3 when oral contraceptives were used for contraception and 7.7 when the drugs were used for menstrual regulation. In patients with breakthrough bleeding or irregular vaginal bleeding, nonfunctional causes should be considered.

Changes in cervical erosion and secretions and endocervical hyperplasia may occur during oral contraceptive therapy. In addition, preexisting uterine leiomyoma may increase in size in women receiving oral contraceptives. Vaginitis, impaired renal function, and backache and a cystitis-like syndrome have been reported but have not been definitely attributed to the drugs.

An increased incidence of *Candida* vaginitis has been associated with oral contraceptive therapy. Decreased motility and tonus of the upper urinary tract may occur in some patients leading to overdistention of the ureters, thus promoting bacteriuria and its complications and making treatment of the infection more difficult. Because oral contraceptives change the vaginal pH from acidic to alkaline, it has been suggested that there may be an increased risk of gonorrhea infection upon exposure; however, there is some evidence that progestins may inhibit growth of *Neisseria gonorrhoeae* in vitro and that oral contraceptives may have some protective effect against gonococcal pelvic inflammatory disease (PID). Although some clinicians have suggested that the risk of PID may be decreased in oral contraceptive users, there is some evidence that the frequency of cervical chlamydial infections may be increased several-fold in women receiving oral contraceptives compared with nonusers or women using barrier contraceptives, possibly secondary to cervical ectopy induced by the drugs; therefore, it should *not* be assumed that oral contraceptives provide protection against PID (i.e., that caused by *Chlamydia trachomatis*).

Although it has been suggested (based on very limited data) that use of multiphasic estrogen-progestin oral contraceptives may be associated with an increased risk of functional ovarian cysts, there currently is insufficient evidence to determine whether such increased risk exists. Epidemiologic evidence with monophasic estrogen-progestin oral contraceptives, principally high-dose estrogen preparations, indicates that monophasic contraceptives are associated with a reduced risk of developing functional ovarian risks when compared with nonusers of oral contraceptives. Epidemiologic studies and postmarketing surveillance currently are under way to determine the incidences of ovarian cysts in users of various types of oral contraceptives and in similar women not using the drugs.

Coital problems, device expulsion, and vaginal symptoms (discomfort, vaginitis, leukorrhea, foreign body sensation) have occurred in women using the contraceptive vaginal ring containing ethinyl estradiol and etonogestrel.

■ Nervous System Effects Mental depression may occur in women receiving oral contraceptives. In a few cases, mental depression has been severe and has led to suicidal behavior. Mental depression appears to occur most frequently in patients with a history of depression, including premenstrual depression; however, relief of premenstrual tension occurs in some women. Patients with a history of mental depression should be observed carefully and the estrogen-progestin contraceptive discontinued if severe depression recurs during use.

Fatigue, dizziness, nervousness, aggressiveness, anxiety, emotional lability, and irritability have been reported in women receiving estrogen-progestin contraceptives; changes in libido may also occur. Psychotic behavior, chorea, and cerebrovascular disease (with associated mitral valve prolapse) have also been reported; however, a causal relationship has not been established.

Headache, especially migraine headache, may occur during estrogen-progestin contraceptive therapy. Estrogen-progestin contraceptives should be discontinued and the cause evaluated when migraine occurs or is exacerbated, or when a new headache pattern develops which is recurrent, persistent, or severe.

■ Ocular Effects Oral contraceptives have been reported to produce harmful ocular effects in myopic women. In women who developed myopia at or near puberty and in whom myopia became stable in adulthood, the drugs have reportedly increased the refractive error 2- to 3-fold, usually after 6 months of use. In women who are myopic and have considerable astigmatism, oral contraceptives may produce marked changes in the astigmatic error, possibly leading to frank keratoconus. In addition, oral contraceptives may produce a rapid advancement of the ocular disorder in patients with a family history of marked myopic astigmatism or keratoconus. Contact lens wearers receiving estrogen-progestin contraceptives may have more difficulties with their contact lenses than do nonusers who wear contact lenses. Contact lens wearers who develop visual disturbances or changes in lens tolerance during estrogen-progestin contraceptive use should be assessed by an ophthalmologist; temporary or permanent cessation of contact lens wear should be considered.

Neuro-ocular lesions such as optic neuritis or retinal thrombosis have been associated with estrogen-progestin contraceptive use. If unexplained, sudden or gradual, partial or complete loss of vision; proptosis or diplopia; papilledema; or retinal vascular lesions occur during therapy with estrogen-progestin contraceptives, the drugs should be discontinued and evaluation for retinal vein thrombosis should be instituted immediately along with other appropriate diagnostic and therapeutic measures. Cataracts have also occurred during oral contraceptive use but have not been directly attributed to the drugs.

■ Hematologic Effects Changes in various blood factors and blood components have been observed in patients receiving oral contraceptives; however, further studies are required before the clinical importance of these changes can be established. Increases in fibrinogen and blood coagulation factors II, VII, VIII, IX, X, and XII levels and decreases in antithrombin III activity may occur in women receiving hormonal contraceptives. Blood coagulation factor levels may return to normal one to several weeks after the oral contraceptive is discontinued. Hematocrit may be slightly increased and an increased rate of blood coagulation may occur. The estrogen component of the contraceptive appears to enhance norepinephrine-induced platelet aggregation, whereas the progestin causes increased fibrinolytic activity. Anemia and sickle cell disease have also been reported during oral contraceptive use.

■ Other Adverse Effects Breast changes, including tenderness, enlargement, and secretion, may occur during estrogen-progestin contraceptive use.

Oral contraceptive use and estrogen use have appeared to be associated with an increased risk of gallbladder disease, especially in young women. In one study, an increased risk of gallbladder disease occurred after 2 years of use of the drugs and doubled after 4 or 5 years of use. In another study, an increased risk was apparent between 6–12 months of use. However, recent evidence suggests that the risk of gallbladder disease may be minimal in patients using formulations of oral contraceptives containing relatively low dosages of estrogens and/or progestins.

The relationship between oral contraceptive use and systemic lupus erythematosus (SLE) is not well-defined. Positive lupus erythematosus (LE) cell test results and antinuclear antibodies have been associated with oral contraceptive use in some women. Precipitation of SLE and exacerbation of preexisting disease have also been associated with oral contraceptive use in some women, and some clinicians recommend that other methods of contraception be used in women with a history of SLE. Rheumatic symptoms and synovitis have been associated with oral contraceptive use. Although several epidemiologic studies have suggested that oral contraceptive use appears to be associated with a decreased incidence of rheumatoid arthritis compared with nonuse, one epidemiologic study found no such association and the relationship, if any, between oral contraceptive use and rheumatoid arthritis remains to be determined.

Other reported adverse effects of estrogen-progestin contraceptives include Raynaud's phenomenon, auditory disturbances, hemolytic uremic syndrome, colitis, pancreatitis, upper respiratory tract infection, sinusitis, and rhinitis.

■ Precautions and Contraindications Use of estrogen-progestin oral contraceptives is associated with an increased risk of several serious conditions including thromboembolism, arterial thrombosis (e.g., stroke, myocardial infarction), liver tumor, gallbladder disease, visual disturbances, fetal abnormalities, and hypertension. The risk of thrombotic events is even higher in women with other risk factors for these events. Cigarette smoking increases the risk of serious adverse cardiovascular effects during oral contraceptive use. This risk increases with age and with heavy smoking (15 or more cigarettes daily) and is markedly greater in women older than 35 years of age. Women who are receiving estrogen-progestin contraceptives should be *strongly* advised not to smoke. Women older than 35 years of age who smoke, and women with ischemic heart disease or a history of this disease, should not use estrogen-progestin contraceptives. Estrogen-progestin contraceptives should be used with caution in women with cardiovascular disease risk factors. Clinicians prescribing estrogen-progestin contraceptives should be aware of the risks associated with such use; the sections in Cautions and the manufacturers' labeling should be consulted for further discussion of these risks and associated precautions. In addition, potential noncontraceptive benefits associated with use of estrogen-progestin contraceptives can be considered. (See Pharmacology: Other Effects.)

Because of dose-related risks of vascular disease from oral contraceptives, the dosage regimen prescribed should contain the least amount of estrogen and progestin that is compatible with a low failure rate and the needs of the patient.

Adverse effects similar to those with oral combination estrogen-progestin contraceptives generally are expected with vaginal or transdermal estrogen-progestin contraceptives.

No data are available concerning the risk of using short-course, high-dose estrogen-progestin combinations for emergency contraception among women with contraindications to routine use of cyclic estrogen-progestin combinations for contraception. Since such postcoital contraceptive regimens do not appear to adversely affect clotting factors, vascular complications (e.g., abnormal blood clotting, stroke, myocardial infarction) are unlikely to occur. No serious or long-term complications have been associated with such postcoital contraceptive regimens in Europe, where experience is extensive. Most experts state that there currently is no real contraindication to postcoital (emergency) contraception with the recommended regimens and that the benefits generally outweigh any theoretical or proven risk.

Patients should be advised that emergency contraceptive regimens are not as effective as most other forms of long-term contraception and should not be used as a woman's routine form of contraception. Patients should be informed that as with all estrogen-progestin contraceptives and other nonbarrier contraceptive methods, emergency contraceptive regimens do not protect against human immunodeficiency virus (HIV) infection or other sexually transmitted diseases.

Women receiving estrogen-progestin contraceptives should be under supervision of a physician who should inform them of the possible risks involved. Women receiving these contraceptives also should be given a copy of the patient labeling for the drugs.

It is good medical practice that all women, including those receiving estrogen-progestin contraceptives, have a medical history and physical examination performed annually. The physical examination may be deferred until after initiation of these contraceptives if requested by the woman and judged appropriate by the clinician. Physical examination should include special attention to blood pressure, breasts, abdomen, and pelvic organs and should include a Papanicolaou test (Pap smear) and relevant laboratory tests.

Women receiving estrogen-progestin contraceptives (including drospirenone-containing oral contraceptives) should be advised to notify their clinician if signs or symptoms of thromboembolic or thrombotic disorders (e.g., thrombophlebitis, pulmonary embolism, cerebrovascular insufficiency, coronary occlusion, retinal thrombosis, mesenteric thrombosis) occur, including sudden severe headache or vomiting, disturbance of vision or speech, sudden partial or complete loss of vision, dizziness or faintness, weakness or numbness in an extremity, sharp or crushing chest pain, unexplained cough, hemoptysis, sudden shortness of breath, calf pain, or heaviness in the chest. Oral contraceptive combinations containing drospirenone should be discontinued if an arterial or venous thrombotic event occurs during therapy. Women currently receiving an oral contraceptive combination containing drospirenone should be informed of the potential risk of thromboembolic events. Patients also should be advised about the current information available regarding the risk of VTE with oral contraceptives containing drospirenone compared with those containing levonorgestrel. Known risk factors for development of VTE include smoking, obesity, family history, and other factors that contraindicate the use of oral contraceptive combinations. Patients should discuss their risk of VTE with their clinician before deciding which contraceptive method to use. The risk of thromboembolic disease associated with oral contraceptive use gradually disappears after such therapy is discontinued. However, the FDA states that patients should not discontinue oral contraceptives containing drospirenone without consulting a clinician.

Although the risk of VTE is higher in women using any oral contraceptives compared with nonusers, the risk remains lower than that associated with pregnancy and the postpartum period. The risk of VTE in women receiving estrogen-progestin oral contraceptives is estimated to be 3–9 per 10,000 woman-years. In comparison, if 10,000 women who are not pregnant and not users of oral contraceptives are followed for one year, 1–5 of these women will develop a VTE. The risk of VTE is highest during the first year of oral contraceptive use. Results from a large, prospective cohort safety study of various estrogen-progestin oral contraceptives suggest that this increased risk is highest during the first 6 months of use compared with that in nonusers. Data from this safety study indicate that the highest risk of VTE occurs after initiation of estrogen-progestin oral contraceptive therapy or resumption of therapy (following a 4-week or longer drug-free interval) with the same or a different oral contraceptive combination. Before initiating use of an estrogen-progestin combination containing drospirenone in a new user or in a woman who is switching from an oral contraceptive not containing drospirenone, clinicians should consider the risks and benefits of drospirenone-containing oral contraceptives, including risk for developing VTE, specific to that woman.

Women receiving estrogen-progestin contraceptives should also be advised to inform their physician if severe abdominal pain or mass (indicating a possible liver tumor), jaundice, severe mental depression, edema, or unusual bleeding occurs. Because severe nausea and vomiting have occurred following postcoital use of high-dose estrogen-progestin combinations as emergency contraception, women taking such therapy should be instructed carefully regarding what to do if vomiting occurs after administering a dose, and concomitant use of an antiemetic should be considered. (See Dosage and Administration: Administration.) Women receiving estrogen-progestin contraceptives should be instructed in self-examination of their breasts and should report nodules or fibrocystic disease in the breast or abnormal breast radiographic or mammographic findings to their physician.

Estrogen-progestin contraceptives should be used with caution, and only with careful monitoring, in patients with conditions that might be aggravated by fluid retention (e.g., asthma, seizure disorders, migraine, or cardiac, renal, or hepatic insufficiency) and in patients being treated for hyperlipidemia, since control of the condition may become difficult. Women with a history of hypertension, hypertension-related diseases, or renal disease should be encouraged to use another method of contraception. Women with hypertension who elect to use estrogen-progestin contraceptives should be monitored closely, and if a clinically important elevation of blood pressure occurs, use of the drugs should be discontinued.

Because a twofold to fourfold increased risk of postsurgery thromboembolic complications has been reported in oral contraceptive users, estrogen-progestin contraceptives should be discontinued whenever feasible, at least 4 weeks before surgery that is associated with an increased risk of thromboembolism or prolonged immobilization; it is also recommended that patients wait 2 weeks after elective surgery associated with an increased risk of thromboembolism or after immobilization before resuming the use of these contraceptives.

Although the absolute rates for developing VTE are increased for users of hormonal contraceptives compared with nonusers, the rates for VTE development are even greater during pregnancy, especially during the postpartum period. Since the immediate postpartum period is associated with an increased risk of thromboembolism, estrogen-progestin contraceptive use should be started no earlier than 4 weeks after delivery in women who elect not to breast-feed their infants or in women who have had a midtrimester pregnancy termination. The risk of thromboembolism decreases while the risk of ovulation increases after the first 3 weeks postpartum.

Oral contraceptives containing the progestin drospirenone should not be used in patients who are predisposed to developing hyperkalemia (e.g., those with renal or hepatic impairment or adrenal insufficiency). If a drospirenone-containing oral contraceptive is used in women receiving daily, long-term therapy with agents that may increase serum potassium concentrations (e.g., angiotensin-converting enzyme (ACE) inhibitors, angiotensin II type 1 (AT_1) receptor antagonists, potassium-sparing diuretics, heparin, aldosterone antagonists [spironolactone], nonsteroidal anti-inflammatory agents [NSAIAs]), the serum potassium concentration should be determined during the first oral contraceptive cycle.

Five out of the 15 pregnancies reported in large clinical trials in women using the transdermal contraceptive system containing ethinyl estradiol and norelgestromin (Ortho Evra®) occurred in women with a baseline weight of 90 kg or more; these results suggest that the contraceptive preparation may be less effective in such women than in those with a lower body weight. The clinician and the woman with high body weight should discuss the individual needs of such a patient when choosing an appropriate contraceptive option.

The contraceptive vaginal ring containing ethinyl estradiol and etonogestrel (NuvaRing®) may not be suitable for women with conditions that make the vagina susceptible to vaginal irritation or ulceration.

Estrogen-progestin contraceptives are contraindicated in women who are hypersensitive to the drug or any ingredient in the formulation and in those with known or suspected pregnancy, undiagnosed abnormal genital bleeding, diplopia or any ocular lesion arising from ophthalmic vascular disease, classical migraine, active liver disease, or history of cholestatic jaundice with pregnancy or with prior use of oral contraceptives. The drugs also are contraindicated during breast-feeding and in women who have or have had thrombophlebitis or thromboembolic disorders, cerebrovascular or coronary artery disease (including myocardial infarction), severe hypertension, diabetes with vascular involvement, known or suspected carcinoma of the breast, known or suspected estrogen-dependent neoplasia (e.g., carcinoma of the endometrium), or benign or malignant liver tumor that developed during oral contraceptive or other estrogen use. Oral contraceptives containing the progestin drospirenone are contraindicated in women with renal impairment, hepatic tumors (benign or malignant) or hepatic disease, adrenal insufficiency, high risk of arterial or venous thrombotic diseases, undiagnosed abnormal uterine bleeding, history of breast cancer or other estrogen- or progestin-sensitive cancer, and in pregnancy.

■ **Pediatric Precautions** Safety and efficacy of estrogen-progestin contraceptives have been established in women of reproductive age. Safety and efficacy are expected to be identical for postpubertal adolescents under 16 years of age and users 16 years of age or older. The manufacturers of estrogen-progestin contraceptives containing drospirenone state that safety and efficacy are expected to be the same for postpubertal adolescents under 18 years of age and users 18 years of age or older. Estrogen-progestin contraceptives are not indicated before menarche.

■ **Geriatric Precautions** Oral contraceptives have not been evaluated in women 65 years of age and older and are not indicated in this population.

■ **Mutagenicity and Carcinogenicity** Chromosomal abnormalities determined in peripheral lymphocytes have been increased in women receiving oral contraceptives compared with nonusers.

Prolonged continuous administration of natural or synthetic estrogen in certain animal species increases the frequency of certain benign or malignant tumors including those of the breast, cervix, uterus, vagina, ovary, pituitary, and liver. Certain synthetic progestins (none currently contained in oral contraceptives) have increased the frequency of benign and malignant mammary nodules in dogs. Drospirenone has increased the frequency of benign and total (benign plus malignant) adrenal gland pheochromocytomas in rats and the frequency of carcinomas of the harderian gland in mice.

The manufacturers state that there is at present no consistent evidence from human studies of an increased risk of cancer associated with oral contraceptive use; whether this statement also applies to vaginal or transdermal estrogen-progestin contraceptives is not known. Close clinical surveillance of all women using estrogen-progestin contraceptives is, nevertheless, essential. Appropriate diagnostic measures should be undertaken to rule out malignancy in all women with undiagnosed persistent or recurrent abnormal vaginal bleeding. Women with a strong family history of breast cancer or who have breast nodules, fibrocystic disease, or abnormal mammographic findings should be closely monitored if they elect to use estrogen-progestin contraceptives.

Cervical Cancer There is some evidence from epidemiologic studies that use of oral contraceptives may be associated with an increased risk of cervical carcinoma. In one study, the incidence of biopsy-proven cervical neoplasia (i.e., dysplasia, carcinoma *in situ*, or invasive carcinoma) was increased in long-term oral contraceptive users compared with women who used an intrauterine contraceptive device (IUD); it was recommended that particular attention to the importance of regular Papanicolaou tests be given in women who have used oral contraceptives for longer than 48 months. Although a causal relationship to the drugs could not be excluded, data from a population-based (Costa Rican women), case-control study suggest that the increased risk of carcinoma in situ associated with oral contraceptive use may have resulted from a detection bias secondary to more frequent use of Papanicolaou tests in oral contraceptive users. These data revealed no evidence of increased risk of invasive cervical cancer in users compared with nonusers. The FDA recommends that all estrogen-progestin contraceptive users be monitored carefully with physical examinations and Papanicolaou tests, at least yearly. (See Cautions: Precautions and Contraindications.)

Endometrial Cancer Several retrospective case-controlled studies have shown an increased relative risk of endometrial carcinoma in postmenopausal women who received prolonged estrogen replacement therapy for relief of menopausal symptoms. Although an increased risk of adenocarcinoma of the endometrium has been associated with sequential oral contraceptive use (sequential oral contraceptives are no longer available in the US), no association between increased risk of endometrial cancer and use of currently available estrogen-progestin combination preparations or progestin-only preparations has been shown, although individual cases have been reported. The Cancer and Steroid Hormone Study of the US Centers for Disease Control and Prevention (CDC) and the National Institute of Child Health and Human Development (NICHD) showed that women who used estrogen-progestin oral contraceptives had *decreased* relative risk of epithelial endometrial cancer (i.e., adenocarcinoma, adenoacanthoma, and adenosquamous cancers) compared with nonusers; the protective effect occurred in women who had used combination oral contraceptives for at least 12 months, and it persisted for at least 15 years after discontinuance of oral contraceptives. This decreased risk of endometrial cancer was not evident in women who had used oral contraceptives for less than 12 months.

Ovarian Cancer Several studies have shown a decreased risk of epithelial ovarian cancer in oral contraceptive users compared with nonusers. The Cancer and Steroid Hormone Study showed that women who used oral contraceptives had a *decreased* relative risk of epithelial ovarian cancer compared with nonusers; the protective effect occurred in women who had used oral contraceptives for as little as 3–6 months, and it persisted for at least 15 years after discontinuance of oral contraceptive use. The risk of ovarian cancer decreased with increasing duration of oral contraceptive use and did not appear to be affected by the age at the time of first use of oral contraceptives or the oral contraceptive type (i.e., combination or sequential) or specific formulation. Because of inadequate data, the association between use of oral contraceptives and nonepithelial (i.e., germ-cell, sex cord-stromal) ovarian cancers could not be fully assessed.

Breast Cancer Many studies have shown *no* increased risk of breast cancer in women receiving oral contraceptives or estrogens. Some studies, however, have suggested an overall increased risk of breast cancer in women receiving oral contraceptives and some studies have suggested that certain subgroups of women who use oral contraceptives may be at increased risk (e.g., women younger than 45 years of age who have used oral contraceptives, women who begin oral contraceptive use early in their childbearing years, women who use oral contraceptives for extended periods of time, women who use oral contraceptives before a first full-term pregnancy); however, these findings have occurred in only some studies and other large studies have shown no such possible associations. Because of several studies suggesting an increased risk of breast cancer with oral contraceptive use, the FDA Fertility and Maternal Health Drugs Advisory Committee reviewed these data in early 1989. The Committee concluded at that time that existing data suggested no *overall* increased risk of breast cancer associated with oral contraceptive use and that a change in prescribing practices by clinicians or in the use of oral contraceptives by women was not justified.

The Cancer and Steroid Hormone (CASH) study showed no association between oral contraceptive use and the risk of breast cancer; the duration of oral contraceptive use, time since first use, or menopause status did not alter the user's risk of breast cancer. In addition, in the CASH study, oral contraceptive use before a woman's first full-term pregnancy did not increase her risk of breast cancer compared with other methods of delaying first pregnancy. In a population based, case-controlled (Women's CARE) study in women 35–64 years of age, current or former use of oral contraceptives was not associated with an increased risk of breast cancer. Findings from the Women's CARE study generally are in agreement with results from the Cancer and Steroid Hormone Study. In the Women's CARE study, the relative risk of breast cancer did not increase consistently with longer periods of use or higher dosages of estrogen, nor was the risk increased with initiation of oral contraceptives at young age or in those with history of breast cancer in a first-degree relative. There was no consistent difference in risk between white and black women. The age at last use, use in relation to the first term pregnancy, duration of use before the first term pregnancy, or type of progestin did not change the oral contraceptive user's risk of breast cancer. A case-control study by the University of Southern California Cancer Surveillance Program indicated that use of "high-progestin" combination oral contraceptives (relative progestin potency determined by delay in menses test) before 25 years of age was associated with an increased risk of breast cancer; however, the validity of this study has been questioned and the CASH study found *no* such association. In this latter study, neither the type of estrogen nor the type of progestin contained in oral contraceptives was associated with increased risk of breast cancer; the type of progestin also was not associated with an increased risk of breast cancer in the Women's CARE study. In these studies, the type of oral contraceptive used (i.e., combination, sequential, progestin only, or more than one type) did not increase the risk.Another case-control study indicated that in women younger than 45 years of age use of oral contraceptives before their first full-term pregnancy was associated with an increased risk of breast cancer; the CASH study and the Women's CARE study found *no* such association. In a meta-analysis of numerous clinical trials, a small increase in the frequency of breast cancer localized to the breast was diagnosed in women within 10 years of current or past use of combined estrogen-progestin oral contraceptives. The Women's CARE study found no such association. No increase in the frequency of breast cancer was diagnosed in women who had not received estrogen-progestin combination oral contraception for at least 10 years.

While the relationship between breast cancer risk and use of oral contraceptives in women with a familial predisposition to breast cancer has not been precisely established, results from a multigenerational study suggest that women who used earlier formulations of oral contraceptives (i.e., high-dose formulations commercially available prior to 1975) and who also have a first-degree relative with breast cancer may be at increased risk of breast cancer. This multigenerational, historical cohort study included the relatives (i.e., daughters, sisters, granddaughters, nieces, women who married into the families) of over 400 women diagnosed with breast cancer between 1944 and 1952 (probands). In the entire cohort (i.e., daughters, sisters, granddaughters, nieces, women who married into the families), the relative risk (RR) of breast cancer was 1.4 in those who reported ever having used oral contraceptives. Risk was not influenced by duration of contraceptive use. After accounting for age and birth cohort, use of oral contraceptives was associated with an increased risk of breast cancer (RR of 3.3) among sisters and daughters of the probands but not among their nieces or granddaughters (RR of 1.2) or in women who married into the family (RR of 1.2). The risk to first-degree relatives increased with the number of relatives in the family with breast or ovarian cancer; the relative risk was 4.6 for families with at least 3 members who had breast or ovarian cancer and 11.4 for families with at least 5 members who had breast or ovarian cancer. The risk of breast cancer was not increased in first-degree relatives who reported use of oral contraceptives after 1975, although the small number of reported cases of cancer in this study (2 of 60 women who took oral contraceptives) limits the statistical reliability of this finding. While the increased risk of breast cancer among high-risk women in this study appeared to be limited to those who used earlier formulations containing higher dosages of estrogen and progestin than current oral contraceptives, the mean age for first-degree relatives who reported use of oral contraceptives after 1975 was 43 years, and breast cancer may not yet have occurred in many women in this group. The Women's CARE study found no association between use of oral combination contraceptives with high dose estrogen (50 mcg or more of ethinyl estradiol or 75 mcg or more of mestranol) and an increased risk of breast cancer in women with a family history of breast cancer. The relative risk of breast cancer in women with a family history of breast cancer who received high dose estrogen combinations for up to 15 years or longer was essentially the same as the relative risk in women with a family history of breast cancer who received lower-dose estrogen combinations for similar periods of time.

Other Cancers Although an increased occurrence of malignant melanoma, urinary tract cancers, and thyroid cancers has been reportedly associated with oral contraceptive use, these findings have not been established. Although liver tumors (mainly hepatocellular adenomas) have been associated with oral contraceptive use, these liver tumors have usually been benign. (See Cautions: Hepatic Effects.)

■ **Pregnancy, Fertility, and Lactation** ***Pregnancy*** Although preliminary evidence suggested that oral contraceptives could cause serious fetal toxicity when administered to pregnant women, current evidence does not suggest an association between inadvertent use of oral contraceptives in early pregnancy and teratogenic effects (including cardiovascular and limb defects, which have been reported following use of sex hormones). In addition, extensive epidemiologic studies have revealed no increased risk of birth defects in neonates born to women who used estrogen-progestin contraceptives prior to pregnancy. However, since the risks of estrogen-progestin contraceptive use clearly outweigh any possible benefit in women who are pregnant, these agents are contraindicated in such women. Although estrogens and/or progestins were previously used to treat threatened or habitual abortion, there is considerable evidence that estrogens are ineffective and no evidence from well-controlled studies that progestins are effective for these uses. Progestin-only or estrogen-progestin contraceptives should *not* be used to induce withdrawal bleeding as a test of pregnancy.

Data concerning pregnancy outcomes following unsuccessful emergency postcoital contraception with estrogen-progestin combinations are limited, in part because such women may choose abortion following failure of postcoital contraception. Pooled data from several controlled trials that followed pregnancies that occurred despite postcoital estrogen-progestin combinations indicate delivery of 45 healthy neonates, 1 neonate with absent left kidney, and 2 neonates with minor anomalies. In addition, numerous studies evaluating teratologic risk of conception during cyclic (routine) oral contraceptive regimens (for both currently available low-dose oral contraceptive regimens and older, high-dose preparations [e.g., 150 mcg of ethinyl estradiol daily] that are no longer available) indicate no increased fetal risks. Exposure to the amount of estrogen-progestin in postcoital contraceptive regimens is not large when compared with the total amount of the estrogen-progestin cyclic (routine) oral contraceptive regimens, and there currently is no evidence of substantial risk to the fetus with such short-term exposure. Estrogen-progestin postcoital contraceptive regimens are contraindicated in pregnancy because of lack of efficacy, not because of adverse effects on the fetus.

In women who have missed 2 consecutive menstrual periods during estrogen-progestin conventional-cycle contraceptive use, the drug should be withheld until pregnancy has been ruled out. In women using a fixed-combination extended-cycle oral contraceptive (e.g., LoSeasonique®, Seasonale®, Seasonique®), the possibility of pregnancy should be considered after one missed menstrual period. When the woman has not adhered to the prescribed oral contraceptive regimen, the possibility of pregnancy should be considered after one missed menstrual period and the drug should be withheld until pregnancy has been ruled out. A back-up method of contraception should be instituted until the possibility of pregnancy has been eliminated. If pregnancy is confirmed, the woman should be informed of the potential hazard to the fetus and the advisability of continuing the pregnancy should be weighed against the risks of exposure of the fetus to the drugs.

Fertility Studies have found a slight delay in return to fertility but no absolute impairment of fertility following discontinuance of fixed-combination conventional-cycle oral contraceptives. A survey of pregnant women attending antenatal clinics in England reported that the time to conception following discontinuance of long-term (i.e., longer than 2 years) use of fixed-combination oral contraceptives (8.2 months) was twofold longer than time to conception following condom use (4.2 months).

Lactation Estrogen-progestin contraceptives may decrease the quantity and quality of milk if given in the immediate postpartum period. Small amounts of the hormonal agents in estrogen-progestin contraceptives are distributed into milk and adverse effects such as jaundice and breast enlargement have been reported in nursing infants of women receiving cyclic regimens; therefore, because of the theoretical risk, some clinicians recommend that lactating women receiving high-dose postcoital contraceptive regimens use alternative milk sources for their infants for at least 24 hours after completion of the regimen. When possible, the use of cyclic estrogen-progestin contraceptives should be deferred until the infant has been weaned. Long-term follow-up after oral contraceptive use showed no apparent clinical effect on breast-feeding mothers or children whose mothers were breast-feeding and using oral contraceptives.

Drug Interactions

■ **Drugs Affecting Hepatic Microsomal Enzymes** Clinically important drug interactions may occur when estrogen-progestin oral contraceptives are administered with other drugs metabolized by the hepatic microsomal cytochrome P-450 (CYP) enzyme system. Metabolism of estrogens is mediated by the CYP3A4 isoenzyme, and the possibility exists that drugs that induce this isoenzyme may reduce ethinyl estradiol concentrations.

Rifampin reportedly decreases contraceptive efficacy and increases breakthrough bleeding during concomitant use with oral contraceptives. These effects have been attributed to enhanced metabolism of both the estrogenic and progestinic components of oral contraceptives, presumably by induction of hepatic microsomal enzymes. It has been suggested that similar effects may occur during concomitant therapy with other known inducers of hepatic microsomal enzymes, including barbiturates, bosentan, carbamazepine, dexamethasone, griseofulvin, phenylbutazone (no longer commercially available in the US), phenytoin, felbamate, oxcarbazepine, rifabutin, modafinil, topiramate, and primidone. Because herbal supplements containing St. John's wort (*Hypericum perforatum*) may induce hepatic cytochrome P-450 isoenzymes and the *p*-glycoprotein transport system, St. John's wort may decrease contraceptive efficacy of estrogen-progestin contraceptives, including that of high-dose estrogen-progestin postcoital contraceptive regimens, and increase breakthrough bleeding during concomitant use with estrogen-progestin contraceptives. Because of the risk of contraceptive failure during concomitant use of estrogen-progestin contraceptives with known inducers of hepatic microsomal enzymes, it has been suggested that alternate methods of contraception be considered in patients receiving these drugs or that oral contraceptive preparations with increased dosage be considered; however, the possibility that adverse effects may be increased with increased-dosage preparations should also be considered.

Data currently are not available concerning the effect of drugs that induce hepatic microsomal enzymes on the contraceptive efficacy of high-dose estrogen-progestin postcoital contraceptive regimens. However, because contraceptive failure has occurred during concomitant use of cyclic oral contraceptive regimens and known inducers of hepatic microsomal enzymes, some clinicians suggest that the dosage of postcoital estrogen-progestin contraceptive regimens may need to be increased, possibly doubled, in women receiving such inducers concomitantly.

Estrogens are inhibitors of the CYP enzyme and may alter the pharmacokinetics of drugs metabolized by this isoenzyme.

■ **Anti-infective Agents** ***Antiretroviral Agents*** Concomitant use of oral contraceptives and some HIV-protease inhibitors or nonnucleoside reverse transcriptase inhibitors may result in substantial changes in the area under the plasma concentration-time curve (AUC) of the estrogen and/or progestin. Concomitant use of oral contraceptives and some HIV-protease inhibitors or nonnucleoside reverse transcriptase inhibitors may reduce the efficacy of the oral contraceptive; whether this precaution applies to vaginal or transdermal estrogen-progestin contraceptives is not known. For additional information, see the individual monographs in 8:18:08 Antiretroviral Agents.

Other Anti-infective Agents It has been suggested that anti-infective agents which alter the GI bacterial flora may decrease the contraceptive efficacy of oral contraceptives and increase breakthrough bleeding. GI bacteria produce enzymes which hydrolyze conjugates of estrogens (e.g., ethinyl estradiol) that have been excreted into the GI tract via bile; hydrolysis of these conjugates allows enterohepatic circulation of the pharmacologically active drug. By disrupting the GI flora, anti-infective agents may decrease or eliminate enterohepatic circulation of oral contraceptives. The clinical importance of this potential interaction has not been determined; however, the manufacturers caution that concomitant use of anti-infective agents (e.g., ampicillin, chloramphenicol, neomycin, nitrofurantoin, penicillin V, sulfonamides, tetracyclines) with oral contraceptives may result in decreased efficacy of the contraceptive.

In one study in healthy women using the vaginal contraceptive ring containing ethinyl estradiol and etonogestrel (NuvaRing®), vaginal administration of a single oil-based suppository containing 1200 mg of miconazole nitrate on day 8 of the cycle increased the serum concentration of ethinyl estradiol or etonogestrel by 16 or 17%, respectively. While the clinical importance of these findings is unknown, the efficacy of the contraceptive vaginal ring is not expected to be affected. The effects of long-term administration of miconazole nitrate vaginal suppositories in women using the contraceptive vaginal ring are not known.

Fluconazole, itraconazole and ketoconazole also may increase plasma concentrations of contraceptive steroids.

Concurrent use of oral contraceptives and troleandomycin may increase the risk of cholestatic jaundice; therefore, the drugs should be used together cautiously.

■ **Benzodiazepines** Oral contraceptives appear to decrease oxidative metabolism by the liver of some benzodiazepines (e.g., diazepam, chlordiazepoxide), while they may increase metabolism of other benzodiazepines (e.g., lorazepam, oxazepam, temazepam) that undergo glucuronide conjugation in the liver. Although the clinical importance of these potential interactions between oral contraceptives and benzodiazepines has not been determined, alterations in benzodiazepine dosage may be necessary in some patients. Although interactions have not yet been documented, other benzodiazepines that undergo oxidative metabolism in the liver include alprazolam, clorazepate, flurazepam, halazepam (no longer commercially available in the US), and prazepam.

■ **β-Adrenergic Blocking Agents** Oral contraceptives have substantially increased the area under the plasma concentration-time curve (AUC) of orally administered metoprolol when the drugs were used concomitantly. It has been suggested that oral contraceptives decrease the first-pass metabolism of metoprolol. Although the clinical importance of this interaction has not been determined, women receiving oral contraceptives and metoprolol (and possibly other β-adrenergic blockers that undergo first-pass metabolism in the liver) concomitantly may require a decrease in the dosage of the β-adrenergic blocker.

■ **Corticosteroids** Estrogens have been reported to enhance the anti-inflammatory effect of hydrocortisone in patients with chronic inflammatory skin diseases. In addition, there is limited evidence that oral contraceptives decrease the metabolic clearance of prednisolone. Increased plasma concentrations of prednisolone and other corticosteroids have been observed when these drugs were used concomitantly with oral contraceptives. It has been suggested that estrogens and oral contraceptives may decrease the hepatic metabolism of corticosteroids and/or alter serum corticosteroid protein binding. Patients receiving concomitant oral contraceptive-corticosteroid therapy should be observed for signs of excessive corticosteroid effects, and alterations in corticosteroid dosage may be necessary when oral contraceptives are started or discontinued.

■ **Other Drugs** There is limited evidence that oral contraceptives may decrease the metabolism of tricyclic antidepressants; however, the clinical importance of this effect has not been determined. Although one report indicated that oral contraceptives may inhibit the metabolism of meperidine, a subsequent study was unable to confirm this finding.

The manufacturers caution that analgesics, isoniazid, antimigraine drugs, and tranquilizers may decrease the efficacy of oral contraceptives. Oral contraceptives may alter the effects of other drugs by impairing their metabolism, altering their protein binding, or by other mechanisms. Although the clinical importance of many of these interactions has not been determined, the manufacturers caution that concomitant use of oral contraceptives with oral anticoagulants, anticonvulsants, hypotensive agents (e.g., guanethidine), vitamins, or oral antidiabetic agents may result in decreased or increased effects of these drugs. Concomitant administration of atorvastatin with an oral contraceptive increased the area under the plasma concentration-time curve (AUC) of norethindrone and ethinyl estradiol by about 30 and 20%, respectively.

Increased plasma concentrations of cyclosporine and theophylline have been observed when these drugs were used concomitantly with oral contraceptives. Ascorbic acid or acetaminophen may increase plasma concentrations of some synthetic estrogens. Decreased plasma concentrations of acetaminophen and lamotrigine, and increased clearance of temazepam, salicylic acid, morphine, or clofibric acid have been observed when these drugs were administered concomitantly with oral contraceptives. The effects of oral contraceptives on plasma concentrations of lamotrigine may reduce seizure control in patients receiving concomitant therapy and dosage adjustment of lamotrigine may be necessary.

There is a potential for increased serum potassium concentrations in women receiving a drospirenone-containing oral contraceptive concomitantly with other drugs that increase serum potassium concentrations. In one study in mildly hypertensive postmenopausal women receiving enalapril maleate (10 mg twice daily) and drospirenone in fixed combination with ethinyl estradiol (Yasmin®) or placebo, mean serum potassium concentrations (evaluated every other day for 2 weeks) relative to baseline were 0.22 mEq/L higher in those receiving drospirenone in fixed combination with ethinyl estradiol than in those receiving placebo. If a drospirenone-containing oral contraceptive is used in women receiving daily, long-term therapy with agents that may increase serum potassium concentrations (e.g., angiotensin-converting enzyme (ACE) inhibitors, angiotensin II type 1 (AT_1) receptor antagonists, potassium-sparing diuretics, heparin, aldosterone antagonists [spironolactone], nonsteroidal anti-inflammatory agents [NSAIAs]), the serum potassium concentration should be determined during the first oral contraceptive cycle.

In one study in healthy women using the vaginal contraceptive ring containing ethinyl estradiol and etonogestrel (NuvaRing®), vaginal administration of a single dose of 100 mg of water-based nonoxynol 9 spermicide gel did not affect the serum concentrations of ethinyl estradiol or etonogestrel. The effects of long-term vaginal administration of nonoxynol 9 spermicide gel in women using the contraceptive vaginal ring are not known.

Laboratory Test Interferences

A decreased response to the metyrapone test may occur in women receiving oral contraceptives; however, the drugs do not interfere with the pituitary-adrenal reaction to stress. Because the adrenal responds to corticotropin, it appears that the estrogen acts on the adrenal gland to interfere with the metyrapone test. The estrogen component of oral contraceptives increases the level of circulating corticosteroid-binding globulin (transcortin) resulting in an increase in total plasma cortisol, a decrease in cortisol secretion rate, and a decrease in urinary excretion of 17-ketogenic steroids, 17-hydroxycorticosteroids, and 17-ketosteroids. Because plasma cortisol concentrations may be similar to those of patients with Cushing's syndrome and urinary steroids may suggest hypofunction, oral contraceptives should be discontinued for a few weeks before performing adrenal function tests. The dexamethasone suppression test, however, can exclude Cushing's syndrome and corticotropin tests can rule out primary adrenocortical insufficiency, even in patients receiving oral contraceptives.

Elevation in sex-hormone binding globulin (SHBG) concentration by combination estrogen-progestin contraceptives results in increased total circulating sex steroids and corticoids; however, free (unbound) concentrations of these steroids remain unchanged. Certain other endocrine and liver function tests may also be affected by oral contraceptives. (See Cautions: Endocrine and Metabolic Effects; Hepatic Effects.)

False-positive results in the nitro blue tetrazolium (NBT) test for the diagnosis of bacterial infection have occurred in women receiving oral contraceptives.

The manufacturers state that the pathologist should be advised of oral contraceptive use when relevant specimens from an oral contraceptive user are submitted.

Acute Toxicity

Acute overdosage of large doses of oral contraceptives in children reportedly produces almost no toxicity except nausea and vomiting. Withdrawal bleeding may occur in females.

Because drospirenone has antimineralocorticoid properties, serum potassium and sodium concentrations and indicators of metabolic acidosis should be monitored in the event of overdosage with a drospirenone-containing oral contraceptive.

Pharmacology

The pharmacologic effects of estrogen-progestin contraceptives are complex and appear to depend on many variables including the specific drugs used, the amount and proportion of each drug, the age of the user, and the duration of administration. In general, estrogen-progestin combinations elicit, to varying degrees, many of the pharmacologic responses usually produced by endogenous estrogens and progesterone and produce numerous effects on many organs.

■ **Contraceptive Effect** Estrogen-progestin combinations produce a contraceptive effect mainly by suppressing the hypothalamic-pituitary system resulting in prevention of ovulation. The estrogen acts mainly by suppressing secretion of follicle-stimulating hormone (FSH), resulting in prevention of follicular development and the rise of plasma estradiol concentration which is thought to be the stimulus for release of luteinizing hormone (LH). In combination products, the progestin appears to act mainly by inhibiting the preovulatory rise of LH. Long-term administration of these combination products results in inhibition of both FSH and LH secretion. It has been suggested that oral contraceptives may also produce a direct effect on ovarian steroidogenesis or the response of the ovary to gonadotropins. In addition, changes in the cervical mucus may prevent sperm penetration; however, further studies are required to determine the precise effects of estrogen-progestin combinations on sperm activity.

Endometrial changes depend on the type of oral contraceptive administered. Conventional-cycle combination products are usually associated with a shortened period of endometrial proliferation followed by an early but brief and limited secretory activity in the epithelium of endometrial glands. After several oral contraceptive cycles, thinning or regression of the endometrium may occur, resulting in reduced menstrual flow or possible amenorrhea.

The precise mechanism of contraceptive activity of estrogen-progestin combinations administered *after* intercourse (postcoital) is not known. However, the effect is contraceptive, not abortifacient, in nature; therefore, timing is critical to efficacy. High-dosage estrogen-progestin combinations are only effective before pregnancy is established. Once implantation occurs (i.e., usually within 6–7 days after ovulation), the combinations would be ineffective in preventing pregnancy. Estrogen-progestin combinations in high dosage provide a short, potent burst of hormonal exposure that may effectively prevent conception by delaying or inhibiting ovulation, and/or producing changes in endometrial development that are hostile to uterine implantation of the fertilized ovum, depending on when the drugs are administered relative to the menstrual cycle and the time period since intercourse. Postcoital contraceptives taken before midcycle may inhibit ovulation by suppressing the midcycle surge in luteinizing hormone that is necessary for final follicular growth and ovulation. Endometrial biopsies in women receiving high-dose estrogen-progestin combination contraceptives at midcycle indicate that coordinated timing of the maturation of glandular epithelium and stroma of the endometrial lining is disrupted. Possible alterations in transport of the ovum through the fallopian tube, fertilization, and corpus luteum development and function have been reported with postcoital use of estrogen-progestin combinations,but these effects are inconsistent and are thought to be of secondary importance as mechanisms in preventing pregnancy.

Ovulation usually resumes within 3 menstrual cycles after oral contraceptives have been discontinued; however, anovulation and amenorrhea may persist for 6 months or longer in some women. After the drug is discontinued, pituitary function recovers first, followed by ovarian function; the endometrium may require up to 3 months to regain its normal histology and enzymatic activity.

■ **Other Effects** Oral contraceptives may produce a wide variety of metabolic changes, possibly as a result of a direct action on the liver. The drugs may produce alterations in carbohydrate and lipid metabolism, increased serum hormone concentrations, and alterations in serum metals and plasma proteins. The estrogen appears to cause most of these metabolic effects. In one study, oral contraceptives containing mestranol and ethynodiol diacetate were shown to produce an increase in cardiac index and stroke volume, a small rise in plasma volume, and an elevation in blood pressure. Urinary tract dilatation may also occur in women receiving oral contraceptives. In nursing women, oral contraceptives may decrease the quantity and quality of milk when given immediately postpartum.

Potential noncontraceptive benefits of oral contraceptives, as evidenced from epidemiologic studies, include effects on menses, effects related to inhibition of ovulation, and effects from long-term use. Use of the drugs has been associated with improved menstrual cycle regularity and decreased incidences of blood loss, iron deficiency anemia, and dysmenorrhea. A decreased incidence of functional ovarian cysts and of ectopic pregnancies also has been associated with use of the drugs. Long-term use of oral contraceptives has been associated with a decreased incidence of formation of fibroadenomas and fibrocystic disease of the breast, a decreased incidence of some (e.g., gonococcal) pelvic inflammatory disease (see Cautions: Genitourinary Effects), and a decreased incidence of some cancers (e.g., endometrial or ovarian cancer) (see Cautions: Mutagenicity and Carcinogenicity).

Pharmacokinetics

■ **Absorption** ***Oral Administration*** Oral contraceptive steroids are generally well absorbed from the GI tract. Following oral administration, levonorgestrel is completely absorbed. Some oral contraceptive steroids are metabolized in the GI mucosa during absorption and on first pass through the liver. Desogestrel is metabolized in the intestinal mucosa and on first pass through the liver to 3-keto-desogestrel, a metabolite believed to be responsible for the pharmacologic activity of desogestrel. Following oral administration, the absolute bioavailability appears to be about 40% for ethinyl estradiol, 65% for norethindrone, and about 76% for desogestrel or drospirenone. Following oral administration, the relative bioavailability of desogestrel, as measured by serum concentrations of 3-keto-desogestrel (the active metabolite of desogestrel), reportedly is about 84%. Although the absolute bioavailabilities have not been determined, about 60% of norgestimate and 60% of ethynodiol diacetate are reportedly absorbed following oral administration.

Considerable interindividual variation in peak plasma concentrations attained and extent of absorption have been reported for oral contraceptive steroids. Peak plasma concentrations of 100–200 pg/mL are reached 1–2 hours after a 50-mcg dose of ethinyl estradiol; although higher plasma concentrations have been reported, these probably represent methodologic problems. Following single-dose oral administration of ethinyl estradiol 20 mcg (in a fixed combination with levonorgestrel 0.1 mg), mean peak serum concentration was reported to be 50–62 pg/mL at approximately 1.5 hours; at steady state, mean peak ethinyl estradiol concentration of 66–77 pg/mL was reported at approximately 1.3–1.4 hours after administration.

Peak plasma norethindrone concentrations of 1.7–5 ng/mL or 5–10 ng/mL have been reported following a 0.5- or a 1-mg oral dose, respectively. The time to peak plasma norethindrone concentrations varies between 0.5–4 hours, apparently being more delayed as the dose increases.

Following oral administration of a single 0.15-mg dose of desogestrel (given in fixed combination with 30 mcg of ethinyl estradiol), average peak plasma 3-keto-desogestrel concentrations of 2.8 ng/mL are reached within 1.4 hours; at steady state (attained after 19 days or more), average peak plasma 3-keto-desogestrel concentrations of 5.8 ng/mL are reached within 1.4 hours after a dose.

Peak plasma norgestimate and 17-deacetyl norgestimate (an active metabolite of norgestimate) concentrations of 0.1 and 3.6 ng/mL are reached within 1 and 1.5 hours, respectively, following oral administration of a single 0.36-mg dose of norgestimate (given in fixed combination with 70 mcg of ethinyl estradiol); at steady state, mean plasma 17-deacetyl norgestimate concentrations of 4.4 ng/mL are reached in about 1.4 hours after a dose. Following single-dose oral administration of levonorgestrel 0.1 mg (in a fixed combination with ethinyl estradiol 20 mcg), mean peak serum concentration was reported to be 2.4–2.8 ng/mL at approximately 1.3–1.6 hours; at steady state, mean peak levonorgestrel concentration of 4–6 ng/mL was reported at approximately 1–1.5 hours after administration.

Plasma concentrations of desogestrel, norethindrone, and levonorgestrel at steady state are higher than predicted from single-dose kinetics because of enhanced binding of these progestins following the induction of sex hormone binding globulin (SHBG) by ethinyl estradiol.

Following single-dose oral administration of drospirenone 3 mg (in fixed combination with ethinyl estradiol 30 mcg) in women, mean peak serum concentration was reported to be 36.9 ng/mL at about 1.7 hours; at steady state, mean peak drospirenone concentrations of 78.7–87.5 ng/mL are reached in about 1.6–1.8 hours after a dose. Although steady-state serum concentrations of drospirenone in women with mild renal impairment (creatinine clearance 50–80 mL/minute) generally are similar to those in women with normal renal function (creatinine clearance greater than or equal to 80 mL/minute), drug concentrations in women with moderate renal impairment (creatinine clearance 30–49 mL/minute) are about 37% higher than concentrations in women with normal renal function.

Vaginal Administration Ethinyl estradiol and etonogestrel are absorbed systemically through the mucous membrane. Following administration of one vaginal ring delivering ethinyl estradiol 0.015 mg/24 hours and etonogestrel 0.12 mg/24 hours (NuvaRing®), peak serum concentrations of ethinyl estradiol are reached on day 2–3 and peak serum concentrations of etonogestrel are reached by day 7. Mean serum concentrations of ethinyl estradiol 1, 2, or 3 weeks after insertion of the ring are 19.1, 18.3, or 17.6 pg/mL, respectively and mean serum concentration of etonogestrel at these time points are 1578, 1476, or 1374 pg/mL, respectively. Following vaginal administration of the ring, bioavailability appears to be about 56% for ethinyl estradiol and 100% for etonogestrel.

Transdermal Administration Ethinyl estradiol and norelgestromin are also absorbed systemically through the skin. Following topical application of one system containing ethinyl estradiol 0.75 mg and norelgestromin 6 mg (Ortho Evra®), peak serum concentrations of ethinyl estradiol and norelgestromin are reached within 48 hours and are maintained at approximately steady state throughout the application period (7 days). In clinical studies, steady state serum concentrations of ethinyl estradiol and norelgestromin were reached during the second week of patch wear; mean steady-state serum concentrations of ethinyl estradiol ranged from 11.2–137 pg/mL and steady-state concentrations of norelgestromin ranged from 0.305–1.53 pg/mL. Serum concentrations generally are consistent from all studies and application sites (i.e., abdomen, buttock, upper outer arm, upper torso). Results of multi-dose studies indicate that steady-state area under the plasma-concentration time curve (AUC) of ethinyl estradiol and norelgestromin may increase slightly over time compared with values from week 1 of cycle 1. Following 3 consecutive cycles of patch wear, mean steady-state serum concentrations of ethinyl estradiol were 49.6 pg/mL (coefficient of variation of 54.4%) and steady-state concentrations of norelgestromin were 0.7 ng/mL (coefficient of variation of 45.3%) at week 3. Health club activities (i.e., sauna, whirlpool, treadmill) or a cold water bath do not result in clinically important changes in the absorption of ethinyl estradiol or norelgestromin compared with normal wear.

The pharmacokinetic profile for the transdermal contraceptive system containing ethinyl estradiol and norelgestromin (Ortho Evra®) differs from the profile for oral contraceptive preparations. Overall exposure to ethinyl estradiol and norelgestromin is higher in women receiving Ortho Evra® than in women receiving an oral contraceptive preparation containing ethinyl estradiol 35 mcg and norgestimate 0.25 mg. The average plasma concentration and AUC (from 0–168 hours) of ethinyl estradiol at steady-state in women receiving Ortho Evra® are 55–60% higher and peak plasma concentrations are 25% lower than values in women receiving an oral contraceptive preparation containing ethinyl estradiol 35 mcg (average weekly exposure [AUC_{0-168}] to the oral contraceptive calculated as 7 times the AUC from 0–24 hours).

■ **Distribution** Contraceptive steroids are widely distributed into body tissues and fluids. The apparent volume of distribution for contraceptive steroids reportedly ranges from 1.5–4.3 L/kg.

Contraceptive steroids are extensively bound to plasma proteins. Ethinyl estradiol is about 98% protein bound, mainly to albumin. Norethindrone is highly (greater than 95%) protein bound to albumin and sex hormone binding globulin (SHBG). Levonorgestrel and 3-keto-desogestrel (the active metabolite of desogestrel) are 93–98 and 96% protein bound, respectively; levonorgestrel is about 34–50 or 48–65% bound to albumin or SHBG, respectively, while 3-keto-desogestrel is about 64 or 32% bound to albumin or SHBG, respectively. Drospirenone is about 97% protein bound, presumably to albumin. Etonogestrel is about 32% bound to SHBG and 66% bound to albumin. Norelgestromin is reportedly more than 97% bound to serum proteins (mainly albumin). Norgestimate, norelgestromin, drospirenone, and ethinyl estradiol do not appear to bind to SHBG. The binding capacity of SHBG for progestins is enhanced by ethinyl estradiol and by other enzyme-inducing drugs such as carbamazepine, phenobarbital, or rifampin. The binding of progestins to albumin and SHBG is low affinity, high capacity and high affinity, low capacity, respectively. Only the unbound fraction of contraceptive steroids is biologically active.

Contraceptive steroids may be distributed into bile. Small amounts of oral contraceptive steroids are also distributed into milk. The plasma-to-milk ratios of levonorgestrel and norethindrone concentrations are reportedly 100:15–100:25 and 100:10, respectively. It has been estimated that about 0.02% of a 50-mcg dose of ethinyl estradiol is distributed into milk.

■ **Elimination** The elimination half-life has been reported to be 11–45 hours for levonorgestrel, about 28 hours for norelgestromin, about 30 hours for drospirenone or etonogestrel, 5–14 hours for norethindrone, 6–45 hours for ethinyl estradiol, and 12–58 hours for 3-keto-desogestrel (the active metabolite of desogestrel). Serum concentrations of norethindrone return to near baseline levels 24 hours after a single 0.35-mg dose, making rigid adherence to once-daily administration necessary for efficacy. Plasma clearance of norethindrone and ethinyl estradiol each is about 0.4 L/hour per kg. Serum concentrations of norgestimate generally are below the lower detection limits of assay within 5 hours of single or multiple oral dosing, and determination of half-life of the drug may not be accurate. An elimination half-life of 12–30 hours has been reported for 17-acetyl norgestimate (an active metabolite of norgestimate). Following removal of the transdermal preparation containing ethinyl estradiol 0.75 mg and norelgestromin 6 mg (Ortho Evra®), serum concentrations of ethinyl estradiol and norelgestromin decline to low or undetectable concentrations within 3 days.

Oral contraceptive steroids are metabolized mainly in the liver and/or GI mucosa during absorption. Ethinyl estradiol and norethindrone appear to undergo extensive first-pass metabolism. Levonorgestrel does not appear to undergo first-pass metabolism.

Ethinyl estradiol is mainly metabolized via aromatic hydroxylation by hepatic microsomal isoenzyme cytochrome P-450 (CYP) 3A4. The major hydroxylated metabolite of ethinyl estradiol is 2-hydroxy-ethinylestradiol, which is thought to contribute to some of the adverse cardiovascular effects of the drug. The hydroxylated metabolite is further metabolized by methylation and glucuronidation prior to urinary and fecal excretion. Ethinyl estradiol and its metabolites undergo glucuronide and sulfate conjugation. The major first-pass metabolite of ethinyl estradiol is its sulfate conjugate. Ethinyl estradiol undergoes extensive enterohepatic circulation as glucuronide and sulfate conjugates. Bacteria in the GI tract hydrolyze these conjugates (excreted into the GI tract via bile), allowing reabsorption of ethinyl estradiol. Mestranol is rapidly metabolized mainly to ethinyl estradiol by demethylation; ethinyl estradiol is thought to be principally responsible for the estrogenic effects of mestranol. Following oral administration of a single 50- or 100-mcg dose of mestranol, the ratio of plasma mestranol to ethinyl estradiol concentrations is reportedly 0.24:1; in the usual oral dosages, mestranol and ethinyl estradiol are considered approximately equipotent.

Levonorgestrel and norethindrone are metabolized mainly by reduction, hydroxylation or oxidation, and glucuronide and sulfate conjugation. Unlike ethinyl estradiol, levonorgestrel and norethindrone do not undergo appreciable enterohepatic circulation; norethindrone is partially excreted, mainly as metabolites, in the feces via biliary elimination. Levonorgestrel and its metabolites are principally (40–68%) excreted in the urine. Desogestrel is rapidly and completely metabolized by hydroxylation in the intestinal mucosa and on first pass through the liver to 3-keto-desogestrel, a metabolite believed to be responsible for the pharmacologic actions of desogestrel; metabolites with no pharmacologic actions also have been identified and these metabolites may undergo glucuronide and sulfate conjugation. Norgestimate is metabolized extensively, mainly by hydrolysis, reduction, and hydroxylation to 17-deacetyl norgestimate, 3-keto-norgestimate, and levonorgestrel, metabolites that subsequently may undergo glucuronide and sulfate conjugation; however, it is believed that only 17-deactyl norgestimate contributes to the pharmacologic activity of norgestimate. Limited information is available on the pharmacokinetics of norethindrone acetate and ethynodiol diacetate; however, the drugs reportedly are rapidly metabolized to norethindrone. Drospirenone is metabolized to 2 major inactive metabolites, which according to one study are formed independently of the cytochrome P-450 enzyme system. The manufacturers state that drospirenone is metabolized only to a minor extent in vitro, mainly by CYP3A4. At least 20 metabolites have been detected in urine or feces.

Contraceptive steroids are excreted in urine and feces, principally as glucuronide and sulfate conjugates of the drugs and metabolites. Unchanged drug and unconjugated metabolites may also be excreted to some extent in urine and feces; although this may be particularly true for ethinyl estradiol, the metabolism and excretion of this and other oral contraceptive steroids is complex and variable, and specialized references should be consulted for more detailed information.

Chemistry and Stability

■ **Chemistry** Estrogen-progestin combination contraceptives contain estrogenic and progestinic steroids and are commercially available as oral tablets, an intravaginal ring, and a transdermal system.

The estrogenic component of commercially available oral contraceptive combinations is ethinyl estradiol or mestranol; the estrogenic component of vaginal and transdermal contraceptive combinations is ethinyl estradiol.

Ethinyl estradiol is a semisynthetic steroidal estrogen; the compound is the most orally active estrogenic drug currently available. The estrogenic potency of ethinyl estradiol is about 20 times that of diethylstilbestrol (no longer commercially available in the US). Mestranol, the 3-methyl ester of ethinyl estradiol, is slightly less active than ethinyl estradiol.

The progestinic component of commercially available oral contraceptive combinations is desogestrel, drospirenone, ethynodiol diacetate, levonorgestrel, norethindrone, norethindrone acetate, norgestimate, or norgestrel. These progestins are mainly derivatives of 19-nortestosterone; ethynodiol diacetate is a 17α-hydroxyprogesterone derivative, and drospirenone is structurally related to spironolactone. Norgestrel is a racemic mixture; levonorgestrel is the pharmacologically active isomer. In terms of oral progestational activity, desogestrel, levonorgestrel, and norgestrel are the most potent of these progestins and norethindrone is the least potent. Levonorgestrel and norgestrel have the greatest androgenic activity while norgestimate and norethindrone have the weakest androgenic activity. Desogestrel, etonogestrel, and norgestimate appear to have a substantially higher selectivity index (ratio of affinity for progesterone receptors versus affinity for androgen receptors) than conventional progestins (e.g., levonorgestrel, norethindrone). Drospirenone has progestational, antimineralocorticoid, and antiandrogenic activity.

The progestinic component of the commercially available transdermal system (Ortho Evra®) or contraceptive vaginal ring (NuvaRing®) is norelgestromin (the active metabolite of orally administered norgestimate) or etonogestrel (the active metabolite of desogestrel), respectively.

Intravaginal ethinyl estradiol in fixed combination with etonogestrel (NuvaRing®) is commercially available as a non-biodegradable, flexible ring that also contains magnesium stearate and ethylene vinyl acetate copolymers.

Transdermal ethinyl estradiol in fixed combination with norelgestromin (Ortho Evra®) is commercially available as a system that consists of an outer layer of polyethylene/polyester film and a drug reservoir consisting of ethinyl estradiol and norelgestromin in a polyisobutylene/polybutene adhesive matrix; a polyethylene terephthalate film is attached to the adhesive surface and should be removed prior to application.

■ **Stability** Estrogen-progestin combinations generally should be stored at room temperature in a well-closed container, unless otherwise specified by the manufacturer. Commercially available oral contraceptives are provided in mnemonic (memory-aid) dispensing packages which are exempted from the child-safety packaging requirements of the US Poison Prevention Packaging Act of 1970. Vaginal ethinyl estradiol in fixed combination with etonogestrel (Nuva Ring®) should be refrigerated at 2–8°C until dispensed. Once dispensed, the vaginal ring can be stored for up to 4 months at 25°C, but may be exposed to temperatures ranging from 15–30°C. Transdermal ethinyl estradiol in fixed combination with norelgestromin (Ortho Evra®) should be stored at 25°C, but may be exposed to temperatures ranging from 15–30°C. After removal from the protective pouch, the transdermal system should be applied immediately.

Preparations

Excipients in commercially available drug preparations may have clinically important effects in some individuals; consult specific product labeling for details.

Ethinyl Estradiol Combinations

Oral

Tablets, monophasic regimen	20 mcg with Drospirenone 3 mg*	**Beyaz®** (24 tablets with levomefolate calcium 0.451 mg plus 4 tablets containing only levomefolate calcium 0.451 mg), Bayer HealthCare
		Yaz® (24 tablets plus 4 inert tablets), Bayer HealthCare
	20 mcg with Levonorgestrel 0.09 mg	**Lybrel®** (28 tablets), Wyeth
	20 mcg with Levonorgestrel 0.1 mg	**Alesse®-21** (21 tablets), Wyeth
		Alesse®-28 (21 tablets plus 7 inert tablets), Wyeth
		Aviane® 28 (21 tablets plus 7 inert tablets), Barr
		Lessina® 28 (21 tablets plus 7 inert tablets), Barr
		Levlite® 28 (21 tablets plus 7 inert tablets), Berlex
		LoSeasonique® (84 tablets plus 7 tablets containing ethinyl estradiol 10 mcg), Duramed
	20 mcg with Norethindrone Acetate 1 mg	**Loestrin® 21 1/20** (21 tablets), Pfizer
		Loestrin® Fe 1/20 (21 tablets plus 7 tablets containing only ferrous fumarate 75 mg), Pfizer
		Loestrin® 24 Fe (24 tablets plus 4 tablets containing only ferrous fumarate 75 mg), Warner Chilcott
		Microgestin® Fe 1/20 (21 tablets plus 7 tablets containing only ferrous fumarate 75 mg), Watson
	30 mcg with Desogestrel 0.15 mg	**Apri® 28** (21 tablets plus 7 inert tablets), Barr
		Desogen® (21 tablets plus 7 inert tablets), Organon
		Ortho-Cept® 28 (21 tablets plus 7 inert tablets), Janssen (formerly Ortho-McNeil)
	30 mcg with Drospirenone 3 mg*	**Safyral®** (21 tablets with levomefolate calcium 0.451 mg plus 7 tablets containing only levomefolate calcium 0.451 mg), Bayer HealthCare
		Yasmin® (21 tablets plus 7 inert tablets), Bayer HealthCare
	30 mcg with Levonorgestrel 0.15 mg	**Levlen® 21** (21 tablets), Berlex
		Levlen® 28 (21 tablets plus 7 inert tablets), Berlex
		Levora® 0.15/30-28 (21 tablets plus 7 inert tablets), Watson
		Nordette®-28 (21 tablets plus 7 inert tablets), Monarch
		Portia® 28 (21 tablets plus 7 inert tablets), Barr
		Seasonale® (84 tablets plus 7 inert tablets), Duramed
		Seasonique® (84 tablets plus 7 tablets containing ethinyl estradiol 10 mcg), Duramed
	30 mcg with Norethindrone Acetate 1.5 mg	**Loestrin® 21 1.5/30** (21 tablets), Pfizer
		Loestrin® Fe 1.5/30 (21 tablets plus 7 tablets containing only ferrous fumarate 75 mg), Pfizer
		Microgestin® Fe 1.5/30 (21 tablets plus 7 tablets containing only ferrous fumarate 75 mg), Watson
	30 mcg with Norgestrel 0.3 mg	**Cryselle®** (21 tablets plus 7 inert tablets), Barr
		Lo/Ovral® (21 tablets), Wyeth
		Lo/Ovral®-28 (21 tablets plus 7 inert tablets), Wyeth
		Low-Ogestrel® 28 (21 tablets plus 7 inert tablets), Watson
	35 mcg with Ethynodiol Diacetate 1 mg	**Demulen 1/35®-21** (21 tablets), Pfizer
		Demulen 1/35®-28 (21 tablets plus 7 inert tablets), Pfizer
		Zovia® 1/35E-28 (21 tablets plus 7 inert tablets), Watson
	35 mcg with Norethindrone 0.4 mg	**Ovcon®/35. 21-Day** (21 tablets), Warner Chilcott
		Ovcon®/35 28-Day (21 tablets plus 7 inert tablets), Warner Chilcott
	35 mcg with Norethindrone 0.5 mg	**Brevicon® 28-Day** (21 tablets plus 7 inert tablets), Watson
		Modicon® 28 (21 tablets plus 7 inert tablets), Janssen (formerly Ortho-McNeil)
		Necon®-0.5/35-21 (21 tablets), Watson
		Necon®-0.5/35-28 (21 tablets plus 7 inert tablets), Watson
		Nelova® 0.5/35E 28 (21 tablets plus 7 inert tablets), Warner Chilcott
		Nortrel® 0.5/35 28 (21 tablets plus 7 inert tablets), Barr

Dosage Form	Strength	Brand Names
	35 mcg with Norethindrone 1 mg	**Necon®-1/35 28** (21 tablets plus 7 inert tablets), Watson
		Norinyl® 1+35 28-Day (21 tablets plus 7 inert tablets), Watson
		Nortrel® 1/35 21 (21 tablets), Barr
		Nortrel® 1/35 28 (21 tablets plus 7 inert tablets), Barr
		Ortho-Novum® 1/35 28 (21 tablets plus 7 inert tablets), Janssen (formerly Ortho-McNeil)
	35 mcg with Norgestimate 0.25 mg	**MonoNessa®** (21 tablets plus 7 inert tablets), Watson
		Ortho-Cyclen® 28 (21 tablets plus 7 inert tablets), Janssen (formerly Ortho-McNeil)
		Sprintec® (21 tablets plus 7 inert tablets), Barr
	50 mcg with Ethynodiol Diacetate 1 mg	**Demulen 1/50®-21** (21 tablets), Pfizer
		Demulen 1/50®-28 (21 tablets plus 7 inert tablets), Pfizer
		Zovia® 1/50E-28 (21 tablets plus 7 inert tablets), Watson
	50 mcg with Norethindrone 1 mg	**Ovcon®/50 28-Day** (21 tablets plus 7 inert tablets), Warner Chilcott
	50 mcg with Norgestrel 0.5 mg	**Ogestrel® 0.5/50-28** (21 tablets plus 7 inert tablets), Watson
		Ovral® (21 tablets), Wyeth
		Ovral®-28 (21 tablets plus 7 inert tablets), Wyeth
	20 mcg with Desogestrel 0.15 mg (21 tablets), and 10 mcg (5 tablets),	**Kariva®** (26 tablets plus 2 inert tablets), Barr
		Mircette® (26 tablets plus 2 inert tablets), Organon
Tablets, chewable	35 mcg with Norethindrone 0.4 mg	**Ovcon® 35 Fe** (21 tablets plus 7 tablets containing only ferrous fumarate 75 mg), Warner Chilcott
		Femcon® Fe (21 tablets plus 7 tablets containing only ferrous fumarate 75 mg), Warner Chilcott
Tablets, biphasic regimen	35 mcg with Norethindrone 0.5 mg (10 tablets) and 35 mcg with Norethindrone 1 mg (11 tablets)	**Necon® 10/11-21** (21 tablets), Watson
		Necon® 10/11-28 (21 tablets plus 7 inert tablets), Watson
Tablets, triphasic regimen	20 mcg with Norethindrone Acetate 1 mg (5 tablets), 30 mcg with Norethindrone Acetate 1 mg (7 tablets), and 35 mcg with Norethindrone Acetate 1 mg (9 tablets)	**Estrostep® 21** (21 tablets), Pfizer
		Estrostep® Fe (21 tablets plus 7 tablets containing only ferrous fumarate 75 mg), Pfizer
	25 mcg with Desogestrel 0.1 mg (7 tablets), 25 mcg with Desogestrel 0.125 mg (7 tablets), and 25 mcg with Desogestrel 0.150 mg (7 tablets)	**Cyclessa®** (21 tablets plus 7 inert tablets), Organon
	25 mcg with Norgestimate 0.18 mg (7 tablets), 25 mcg with Norgestimate 0.215 mg (7 tablets), and 25 mcg with Norgestimate 0.25 mg (7 tablets)	**Ortho Tri-Cyclen® Lo** (21 tablets plus 7 inert tablets), Janssen (formerly Ortho-McNeil)
	30 mcg with Levonorgestrel 0.05 mg (6 tablets), 40 mcg with Levonorgestrel 0.075 mg (5 tablets), and 30 mcg with Levonorgestrel 0.125 mg (10 tablets)	**Enpresse® 28** (21 tablets plus 7 inert tablets), Barr
		Tri-Levlen® 21 (21 tablets), Berlex
		Tri-Levlen® 28 (21 tablets plus 7 inert tablets), Berlex
		Triphasil®-21 (21 tablets), Wyeth
		Triphasil®-28 (21 tablets plus 7 inert tablets), Wyeth
		Trivora®-28 (21 tablets plus 7 inert tablets), Watson
	35 mcg with Norethindrone 0.5 mg (7 tablets), 35 mcg with Norethindrone 0.75 mg (7 tablets), and 35 mcg with Norethindrone 1 mg (7 tablets)	**Necon® 7/7/7** (21 tablets plus 7 inert tablets), Watson
		Ortho-Novum® 7/7/7 28 (21 tablets plus 7 inert tablets), Janssen (formerly Ortho-McNeil)
	35 mcg with Norethindrone 0.5 mg (7 tablets), 35 mcg with Norethindrone 1 mg (9 tablets), and 35 mcg with Norethindrone 0.5 mg (5 tablets)	**Tri-Norinyl®-28** (21 tablets plus 7 inert tablets), Watson
	35 mcg with Norgestimate 0.18 mg (7 tablets), 35 mcg with Norgestimate 0.215 mg (7 tablets), and 35 mcg with Norgestimate 0.25 mg (7 tablets)	**Ortho Tri-Cyclen® 28** (21 tablets plus 7 inert tablets), Janssen (formerly Ortho-McNeil)
		Tri-Sprintec® (21 tablets plus 7 inert tablets), Barr
Topical		
Transdermal System	0.75 mg with 6 mg Norelgestromin/20 cm²	**Ortho Evra®**, Janssen (formerly Ortho-McNeil)
Vaginal		
Ring	0.015 mg with 0.12 mg Etonogestrel/24 hours (2.7 mg with 11.7 mg Etonogestrel/ring	**NuvaRing®**, Organon

Mestranol Combinations

Dosage Form	Strength	Brand Names
Oral		
Tablets, monophasic regimen	50 mcg with Norethindrone 1 mg	**Necon® 1/50-21** (21 tablets), Watson
		Necon® 1/50-28 (21 tablets plus 7 inert tablets), Watson
		Norinyl® 1+50 28-Day (21 tablets plus 7 inert tablets), Watson
		Ortho-Novum® 1/50 28 (21 tablets plus 7 inert tablets), Janssen (formerly Ortho-McNeil)

†Use is not currently included in the labeling approved by the US Food and Drug Administration

Progestins

■ Etonogestrel, levonorgestrel, and norethindrone are synthetic progestin contraceptives.

Uses

■ **Contraception** ***Oral Contraceptives*** Norethindrone, in small doses (minipills), is used for the prevention of conception in women who elect to use oral contraceptives as a method of contraception. Progestin-only oral contraceptives are generally reserved for women who do not tolerate estrogens or in whom estrogens are contraindicated, since progestin-only oral contraceptives are less effective than estrogen-progestin combinations and require a high level of patient compliance. When taken according to the prescribed regimen, progestin-only oral contraceptives provide almost completely effective contraception. The efficacy of oral contraceptives mainly depends on compliance with the prescribed regimen. Progestin-only oral contraceptives must be taken daily, without interruption, to be effective.

Progestin-only oral contraceptives are reported to be somewhat less effective than estrogen-progestin combinations. The pregnancy rate in women using progestin-only oral contraceptives is generally reported to be about 3 pregnancies per 100 woman-years of use. For information on the pregnancy rates reported with other methods of contraception, including estrogen-progestin combinations, see Uses in Estrogen-Progestin Combinations 68:12. Pregnancy rates are derived from various studies conducted by different investigators in different population groups and, therefore, cannot be compared precisely.

In women receiving norethindrone, the pregnancy rate, especially during the first 6 months of use, is reportedly greater in women who had not previously received oral contraceptives than in those who had been immediately switched from an estrogen-progestin combination. The reported difference in pregnancy rates probably resulted from failure to comply with the prescribed regimen. Therefore, it is especially important that women who are prescribed progestin-only oral contraceptives as initial oral contraception be advised to strictly adhere to the prescribed regimen.

For the use of norethindrone or norethindrone acetate in combination with estrogens as an oral contraceptive, see Estrogen-Progestin Combinations 68:12. For the use of the drugs in the treatment of secondary amenorrhea, endometriosis, or abnormal uterine bleeding, see Norethindrone 68:32.

Intrauterine System Levonorgestrel-releasing intrauterine system is used for prevention of conception in women who elect to use this method of contraception. The manufacturer states that the system is recommended for use in women who have had one or more children; are in a stable, mutually monogamous relationship; have no history of pelvic inflammatory disease (PID); and have no history of ectopic pregnancy or any condition that would predispose to ectopic pregnancy. Each system may be used for up to 5 years; thereafter, the system should be removed and may be replaced with a new system if continued contraception is desired. The pregnancy rate in women using the levonorgestrel-releasing intrauterine system is reported as up to 0.2 pregnancies per 100 women during the first year of use; the cumulative 5-year pregnancy rate is reported to be approximately 0.7 pregnancies per 100 women.

Subcutaneous Implants Etonogestrel for subcutaneous implantation (Implanon®) is used for prevention of conception in women who elect to use this method of contraception. The system consists of a single rod containing etonogestrel that is implanted subcutaneously in the upper arm to provide contraception for up to 3 years.

Postcoital (Emergency) Contraception Levonorgestrel is used as an emergency contraceptive (EC) to prevent pregnancy following unprotected intercourse or known or suspected contraceptive failure. To achieve optimal efficacy, the postcoital contraceptive regimen should be initiated as soon as possible within 72 hours of unprotected intercourse. Studies show that emergency contraception is moderately effective when the regimen is administered up to 120 hours after unprotected intercourse. Postcoital contraceptive efficacy diminishes as the time period between intercourse and initiation of contraception increases.

An emergency contraceptive regimen employing a progestin alone (levonorgestrel) appears to be more effective and better tolerated than a common estrogen-progestin emergency contraceptive ("Yuzpe") regimen when the regimens are initiated within 72 hours of unprotected intercourse; therefore, the progestin-only regimen generally is preferred when readily available. In a double-blind, randomized multicenter study in women who reported unprotected intercourse within 72 hours of receiving emergency contraception, a single-dose of levonorgestrel 1.5 mg was as effective in preventing pregnancy as levonorgestrel 0.75 mg every 12 hours for 2 doses. In a double-blind, randomized, multicenter study in women who reported only one act of unprotected intercourse within 72 hours of receiving emergency contraception, the expected pregnancy (failure) rate of 8% (with no contraception) was reduced to approximately 1% with a progestin-only regimen (levonorgestrel 0.75 mg every 12 hours for 2 doses). In another prospective, randomized study in women who reported a single act of intercourse within 48 hours of receiving emergency contraception, failure rates with the 2-dose levonorgestrel regimen and Yuzpe regimens (levonorgestrel 0.5 mg and 0.1 mg ethinyl estradiol every 12 hours for 2 doses) were similar (2.6 versus 2.4%, respectively). The efficacy of treatment in both studies was greatest when the contraceptive was given during the first 24 hours after unprotected intercourse; efficacy declined during subsequent 24-hour periods. The 2-dose levonorgestrel regimen was better tolerated than the Yuzpe regimen. In these 2 studies, nausea occurred in 23.1 versus 50.5% and in 16.1 versus 46.5% of women receiving the 2-dose levonorgestrel regimen versus the Yuzpe regimen, respectively, while vomiting occurred in 5.6 versus 18.8% and in 2.7 versus 22.4% of women with the 2-dose levonorgestrel regimen or Yuzpe regimen, respectively.

Since unprotected intercourse that occurs outside the fertile period is unlikely to result in conception, not all women given emergency postcoital contraception are at genuine risk for pregnancy. Therefore, a more accurate indication of the efficacy of postcoital contraceptive regimens would be based on the timing of unprotected intercourse and the probability that pregnancy would occur without treatment. Analysis of data from the multicenter, progestin-only (levonorgestrel) study involving approximately 2000 women suggest that when efficacy of postcoital contraception is based on the observed versus expected number of pregnancies, the levonorgestrel-only regimen would prevent 85% of pregnancies; pooled analysis of observed-versus-expected pregnancy data from other studies employing the Yuzpe regimen suggest that such therapy is approximately 74% effective in preventing pregnancy. However, postcoital (emergency) contraceptive regimens are not as effective as most other forms of long-term contraception.

Since postcoital contraceptive efficacy diminishes as the time period between intercourse and administration of the regimen increases, available data suggest that as with combination estrogen-progestin regimens, progestin-only postcoital contraception should ideally begin within 72 hours of unprotected intercourse. Emergency contraception is moderately effective when the regimen is administered up to 120 hours after unprotected intercourse. The effectiveness of postcoital contraception administered after more than 120 hours has not been established.

The American College of Obstetricians and Gynecologists (ACOG), other experts, and some states (e.g., Alaska, California, Hawaii, Maine, New Mexico, Washington) have advocated increased access to emergency postcoital contraception (e.g., nonprescription access via pharmacies, advance provision by clinicians) as a means of decreasing unintended pregnancy and abortion rates. There is some evidence that increased access to emergency postcoital contraception may not compromise conventional contraceptive use or sexual behavior, potentially allaying some concerns that have prompted others to advocate for restricted access. The FDA has approved the single-dose levonorgestrel regimen (Plan B One-Step®) for nonprescription (over-the-counter [OTC]) status for women of childbearing potential regardless of age. Another FDA-approved product (Next Choice One Dose®) is commercially available as a single-dose levonorgestrel regimen for OTC status in women 17 years of age or older or as a prescription-only preparation in women younger than 17 years of age. A 2-dose levonorgestrel preparation is also commercially available as a prescription-only preparation for women younger than 17 years of age.

For information on the use of combination estrogen-progestin contraceptives for postcoital contraception, see Contraception: Postcoital Contraception under Uses, in Estrogen-Progestin Combinations 68:12.

Dosage and Administration

■ **Administration** Norethindrone is administered orally once daily. The tablets should be taken at the same time each day and continued daily without interruption, including throughout all bleeding episodes. Women should be advised to inform a clinician if prolonged bleeding, amenorrhea, or severe abdominal pain occurs.

Levonorgestrel is administered orally or as a levonorgestrel-releasing intrauterine device.

If vomiting occurs within 2 hours following administration of levonorgestrel (e.g., Plan B One-Step®, Next Choice One Dose®) for postcoital contraception, a clinician should be contacted to discuss the need for repeating the dose. If vomiting occurs within 2 hours following administration of the first or second dose of the levonorgestrel 2-dose regimen for emergency contraception, a clinician should be contacted to discuss the need for taking another dose.

Levonorgestrel-releasing intrauterine system should be inserted into the uterine cavity under strict aseptic conditions following a complete review of the patient's medical and social histories, exclusion of pregnancy, and physical examination (including pelvic examination, Papanicolaou test [Pap smear], and appropriate laboratory tests for other genital diseases [e.g., gonorrhea, chlamydia] as indicated). Special attention should be given to determining whether the woman is at risk for ectopic pregnancy or pelvic inflammatory disease (PID). Patients should be reexamined shortly after the first menstrual period following insertion of the device to verify that the device is properly positioned. The manufacturer's labeling should be consulted for proper methods of inserting and removing the levonorgestrel-releasing intrauterine system and for associated precautions.

Etonogestrel is administered as a nonbiodegradable implant that is inserted subcutaneously in the inner aspect of the upper arm. The manufacturer's labeling should be consulted for the proper method of administration and associated precautions.

■ **Dosage** ***Contraception*** **Oral Dosage.** The daily dose of progestin-only oral contraceptives is 0.35 mg of norethindrone. Therapy should begin on the first day of menstruation and should be continued each day of the year without interruption. If therapy begins on another day, the woman should be advised to use a back-up method of contraception (e.g., condom, spermicide) for each sexual encounter during the first 48 hours. Women who have had a miscarriage or an abortion may begin progestin-only oral contraceptives the next day.Women who are exclusively breast-feeding their infants may begin therapy 6 weeks after delivery; women whose infants are only partially breast-fed may begin therapy with the drug 3 weeks after delivery.

If a norethindrone dose is taken more than 3 hours late or if one or more consecutive doses are missed, the last missed dose should be taken as soon as it is remembered, followed by resumption of the regular schedule; a back-up method of contraception (e.g., condom, spermicide) should be used for each sexual encounter during the next 48 hours. If the woman is unsure of what drug regimen to take as a result of missed doses, a back-up method of contraception should be used for each sexual encounter, and one tablet should be taken each day until the clinician can be contacted.

If vomiting occurs soon after a dose, a back-up method of contraception (e.g., condom, spermicide) should be used for each sexual encounter during the next 48 hours.

If a menstrual period is delayed and norethindrone has not been taken exactly as directed, or if 45 days have elapsed since the beginning of the last menstrual period, the possibility of pregnancy should be excluded. If pregnancy is confirmed, the woman should be advised to discontinue the progestin-only oral contraceptive.

Intrauterine Dosage. Each levonorgestrel-releasing intrauterine system contains 52 mg of the drug and is intended to be used for periods of up to 5 years. When the levonorgestrel-releasing intrauterine system is used for contraception, the system is inserted into the uterine cavity within 7 days of the onset of menses. In postpartum women, the levonorgestrel-releasing intrauterine system should not be inserted until at least 6 weeks postpartum or until involution of the uterus is complete. The system may be inserted immediately after a first-trimester abortion, but insertion following a second-trimester abortion should be delayed until involution of the uterus is complete.

The levonorgestrel-releasing intrauterine system should be removed after 5 years of use, since contraceptive efficacy beyond 5 years has not been established. In women who wish to continue contraception with the levonorgestrel-releasing intrauterine system, a new system may be inserted immediately following removal of the existing system. The system can be removed and replaced with a new system at any time during the menstrual cycle. For women with regular menstrual cycles who wish to initiate an alternative contraceptive method, the intrauterine system should be removed during the first 7 days of a menstrual cycle and the new method started. For those with irregular cycles or amenorrhea or for those in whom the system is removed after the seventh day of the menstrual cycle, the new contraceptive method should be initiated at least 7 days before removal of the intrauterine system.

Subcutaneous Dosage. Etonogestrel implant contains 68 mg of the drug and is intended to be used for periods of up to 3 years.

When an etonogestrel implant is used for contraception, timing of insertion depends on the patient's history. To initiate therapy in women who did not use hormonal contraception in the preceding month, the etonogestrel implant usually is inserted on or before day 5 of the cycle (the first day of bleeding is counted as the first day of the menstrual cycle). When switching from other contraceptive methods, therapy with etonogestrel should be initiated in a manner that ensures continuous contraceptive coverage based on the mechanism of action of both methods (e.g., etonogestrel implant should be inserted within 7 days of the last hormonally active tablet, or removal of a transdermal patch or vaginal ring in women switching from combined estrogen-progestin contraceptives; etonogestrel implant may be inserted on any day of the month in women switching from a progestin-only oral contraceptive [without skipping any day between receiving the last progestin oral contraceptive and the initial administration of the implant]; etonogestrel implant should be inserted within the dosing period recommended for the parenteral contraceptive preparation in women switching from a progestin-only contraceptive injection; etonogestrel implant should be inserted on the same day as a progestin-containing intrauterine device is removed in women switching from this device). The implant may be inserted immediately after a first-trimester abortion or 21–28 days following a second-trimester abortion. Etonogestrel implant may be inserted 21–28 days postpartum in women who are only partially breast-feeding their infant or after the fourth postpartum week in women who are exclusively breast-feeding their infant. The manufacturer states that a back-up method of contraception is not needed when etonogestrel therapy is initiated according to one of these schedules. The implant is removed 3 years after insertion. In women who wish to continue contraception with etonogestrel implant, a new implant should be inserted on the same day as the existing implant is removed.

Postcoital (Emergency) Contraception When levonorgestrel is used alone as a short-course, progestin-only emergency postcoital contraceptive, a single 1.5-mg dose of levonorgestrel is administered as soon as possible within 72 hours of unprotected intercourse. Alternatively, a levonorgestrel dose of 0.75 mg is administered as soon as possible within 72 hours of unprotected intercourse, followed by a repeat dose of 0.75 mg 12 hours after the first dose. Regardless of regimen, the first dose can be taken up to 120 hours after unprotected intercourse if necessary, but efficacy decreases as initiation of contraception becomes more remote from unprotected intercourse. Commercial preparations containing one levonorgestrel 1.5-mg tablet (e.g., Plan B® One-Step, Next Choice One Dose®) are available for this purpose. The FDA has approved Plan B® One-Step for nonprescription (over-the-counter [OTC]) status for women of childbearing potential regardless of age. A commercial preparation containing 2 levonorgestrel 0.75-mg tablets also is available for postcoital contraception. The levonorgestrel postcoital contraceptive regimens may be used at any time during the menstrual cycle. Since postcoital contraceptive efficacy diminishes as the time period between intercourse and administration of the regimen increases, postcoital contraception with levonorgestrel should begin as soon as possible but within 72–120 hours of unprotected intercourse. The effectiveness of postcoital contraception administered after more than 120 hours has not been established.

Repeated postcoital (emergency) contraception use indicates the need for counseling about other contraceptive options. Safety of recurrent use has not been established but the risk appears to be low, even within the same menstrual cycle. The possibility that risk of adverse effects (e.g., menstrual irregularities) may be increased with frequently repeated postcoital contraception should be considered.

Cautions

■ Adverse Effects

Although common adverse effects of estrogen-progestin oral contraceptives appear to be mainly caused by the estrogen, it has not been determined whether the adverse effects associated with low-dose oral progestin regimens differ from those resulting from administration of estrogen-progestin combinations. There is some evidence that the progestin component plays a major role in the development of some adverse effects of oral contraceptives when combined with estrogens. The potency and type of progestin in estrogen-progestin combinations appear to have important effects on lipoprotein lipids (high-density and low-density lipoproteins) and may contribute to the increased risk of arteriosclerotic disease in oral contraceptive users. Pending further accumulation of data on progestin-only oral contraceptives, the same precautions associated with estrogen-progestin combination therapy should be observed with progestin-only preparations. For a complete discussion of the cautions, precautions, and contraindications of oral contraceptives, see Cautions in Estrogen-Progestin Combinations 68:12.

The most frequent adverse effects of continuous oral low-dose progestin administration are menstrual irregularity, changes in menstrual flow, and/or amenorrhea, which may be difficult to differentiate from pregnancy. In clinical trials, these adverse effects caused a higher drop-out rate than that observed with estrogen-progestin oral contraceptives. Like the estrogen-progestin combination oral contraceptives, progestins can cause breakthrough bleeding, spotting, edema, weight gain, nausea, breast tenderness, headache, and mental depression; however, the incidence and severity of these adverse effects are much less with progestins than with estrogen-progestin combinations. Progestin-only oral contraceptives occasionally may alter lipid metabolism, resulting in decreased concentrations of high-density lipoprotein [HDL]-cholesterol, HDL_2, apolipoprotein A-I (apo A-I), and apolipoprotein A-II (apo A-II), and increased concentrations of hepatic lipase. There usually is no effect on concentrations of total cholesterol, HDL_3, low-density lipoprotein (LDL)-cholesterol, or very low-density lipoprotein (VLDL)-cholesterol.

Adverse effects reported in 5% or more of women using the levonorgestrel-releasing intrauterine system include abdominal pain, leukorrhea, headache, vaginitis, back pain, breast pain, acne, depression, hypertension, upper respiratory infection, nausea, nervousness, dysmenorrhea, weight increase, skin disorder, decreased libido, abnormal Papanicolaou test (Pap smear), and sinusitis.

Adverse effects reported in 5% or more of women using the etonogestrel implant include headache, vaginitis, weight increase, acne, breast pain, upper respiratory infection, abdominal pain, pharyngitis, leukorrhea, influenza-like symptoms, dizziness, dysmenorrhea, back pain, emotional lability, nausea, pain, nervousness, sinusitis, depression, and insertion site pain.

Limited data from 2 comparative studies in which women receiving emergency postcoital contraception with either an estrogen-progestin regimen (levonorgestrel 0.5 mg and 100 mcg ethinyl estradiol every 12 hours for 2 doses) or a progestin-only regimen (levonorgestrel 0.75 mg every 12 hours for 2 doses) indicate a lower incidence of nausea or vomiting with the progestin-only (levonorgestrel) regimen. In these 2 studies, nausea occurred in 23.1 versus 50.5% and in 16.1 versus 46.5% of women receiving the 2-dose levonorgestrel regimen versus the estrogen-progestin regimen, respectively, while vomiting occurred in 5.6 versus 18.8% and in 2.7 versus 22.4% of women with the levonorgestrel- or estrogen-progestin regimen, respectively. Other adverse effects occurring in one of these studies with the 2-dose levonorgestrel regimen included nausea (23% of patients), abdominal pain (17.6% of patients), fatigue (16.9% of patients), headache (16.8% of patients), heavier or lighter menstrual bleeding (13.8 or 12.5% of patients, respectively), dizziness (11.2% of patients), breast tenderness (10.7% of patients), vomiting (5.6% of patients), or diarrhea (5% of patients). Adverse effects reported with the single-dose levonorgestrel regimen include heavier menstrual bleeding (30.9% of patients), nausea (13.7% of patients), lower abdominal pain (13.3% of patients), fatigue (13.3% of patients), headache (10.3% of patients), dizziness (9.6% of patients), breast tenderness (8.2% of patients), or more than a 7-day delay in menses (4.5% of patients). In addition, some evidence indicates that emergency postcoital contraception may not compromise conventional contraception use or sexual behavior (e.g., promiscuity, sexually transmitted disease [STD] risk).

Other adverse reactions which have been reported in women receiving progestins are weight gain or loss, changes in cervical erosion and secretions, cholestatic jaundice, allergic rash with or without pruritus, melasma or chloasma, breast changes (tenderness, enlargement, and secretion), and hirsutism.

■ Precautions and Contraindications

It is good medical practice that all women, including those receiving progestin-only oral contraceptives, have a complete medical history and physical examination performed periodically (e.g., annually); the physical examination may be deferred until after initiation of therapy if requested by the woman and judged appropriate by the clinician. Physical examination is not required prior to initiating therapy with oral levonorgestrel for postcoital (emergency) contraception. In women receiving the levonorgestrel-releasing intrauterine system, complete medical and social histories (including those of the partner) and physical examination (including pelvic examination, Papanicolaou test [Pap smear], and appropriate laboratory tests for other genital diseases [e.g., gonorrhea, chlamydia] as indicated) should be performed, and pregnancy should be excluded prior to insertion of the intrauterine system; special attention should be given to determining whether the woman is at risk for ectopic pregnancy or pelvic inflammatory disease (PID).

Safety and efficacy of progestin contraceptives have been established in women of reproductive age. Safety and efficacy of long-term progestin contraceptives are expected to be identical for postpubertal adolescents younger than 16 years of age and women 16 years of age or older. Safety and efficacy of progestin emergency contraceptives are expected to be identical for postpubertal adolescents younger than 17 years of age and women 17 years of age or older. Progestin contraceptives are not indicated before menarche.

Progestin contraceptives have not been evaluated in women older than 65 years of age and these drugs are not indicated for use in postmenopausal women.

Slight deterioration in glucose tolerance, coupled with increases in plasma insulin concentrations, may occur in some patients receiving progestin-only contraceptives. However, in women with diabetes mellitus receiving progestin-only contraceptives, insulin requirements generally are unchanged. Nevertheless, prediabetic or diabetic women should be carefully monitored while receiving these contraceptives.

Headache, including migraine headache, has been reported during progestin-only contraceptive therapy. Progestin-only oral contraceptives should be discontinued and the cause evaluated when migraine occurs or is exacerbated, or when severe, persistent, or recurrent headache develops.

Because the presence of organisms capable of causing PID cannot be determined by appearance, and because insertion of an intrauterine system may be associated with introduction of vaginal bacteria into the uterus, the levonorgestrel-releasing intrauterine system should be inserted under strict aseptic conditions. Administration of anti-infectives may be considered; however, the benefit of such prophylactic measure is unknown. Syncope, bradycardia, or other neurovascular episodes may occur during insertion or removal of the intrauterine system, particularly in women predisposed to these conditions or in those with cervical stenosis. If decreased pulse, perspiration, or pallor is observed, the woman should remain supine until these signs have disappeared. Women receiving the levonorgestrel-releasing intrauterine system who have certain types of valvular or congenital heart disease and surgically constructed systemic-pulmonary shunts are at increased risk of infective endocarditis and, possibly, septic embolism. Women with known congenital heart disease who may be at increased risk should receive appropriate anti-infectives at the time of insertion and removal of the intrauterine system. Women requiring chronic corticosteroid therapy or insulin for diabetes mellitus should be carefully monitored for development of infection. The levonorgestrel-releasing intrauterine system should be used with caution in women who have a coagulopathy or are receiving anticoagulants. Use of the intrauterine system in women with vaginitis or cervicitis should be postponed until appropriate treatment has eradicated the infection and until it has been determined that the cervicitis is not caused by *Neisseria gonorrhoeae* or *Chlamydia*.

Because the levonorgestrel-releasing intrauterine system may be displaced following insertion, women should be reexamined and evaluated shortly after the first postinsertion menses, but definitely within 3 months after insertion. During examination, the removal threads of the intrauterine system should be located; if the threads are not visible, location of the system should be verified (e.g., by radiograph or ultrasound, by gentle exploration of the uterine cavity with a probe). If the intrauterine system is in place with no evidence of perforation, no intervention is indicated. If the system is verified as displaced, it should be removed, and a new system may be inserted at that time or during the next menses if it is certain that conception has not occurred. If expulsion has occurred, the system may be replaced within 7 days of a menstrual period after pregnancy has been excluded. Partial or complete expulsion of any intrauterine system may result in bleeding or pain; however, expulsion may occur without the woman's knowledge.

Concomitant use of progestin-only contraceptives with drugs that induce hepatic microsomal enzymes (e.g., barbiturates, carbamazepine, phenytoin, HIV protease inhibitors, rifampin, St. John's wort [*Hypericum perforatum*]) reduces contraceptive efficacy, possibly resulting in unintended pregnancy or breakthrough bleeding. Effects of hepatic enzyme inducers on the contraceptive efficacy of the levonorgestrel-releasing intrauterine system have not been evaluated. No significant interaction has been found when progestin-only oral contraceptives are used concomitantly with broad-spectrum anti-infectives.

Women should be informed that progestin-only contraceptives do not protect against human immunodeficiency virus (HIV) infection or other sexually transmitted diseases.

Levonorgestrel 0.75 or 1.5 mg used for postcoital (emergency) contraception is not effective in terminating an existing pregnancy. Rapid return of fertility is likely following use of levonorgestrel for postcoital contraception. Routine methods of contraception should be continued or initiated as soon as possible following use of levonorgestrel to ensure ongoing pregnancy prevention.

Women receiving progestin-only oral contraceptives should be advised to take the tablets exactly as directed and at the same time every day, including throughout all bleeding episodes. (See Dosage and Administration.) Women should be advised to inform a clinician if prolonged bleeding, amenorrhea, or severe abdominal pain occurs. Although progestin-only oral contraceptives do not affect the quality or quantity of breast milk in lactating women, isolated cases of decreased milk production have been reported, and lactating women are advised to contact a clinician if they are not producing enough milk. The World Health Organization states that nursing women can continue to breastfeed without restriction during postcoital (emergency) contraceptive regimens.

Women considering use of the levonorgestrel-releasing intrauterine system should be encouraged to review the manufacturer's patient information and to discuss with a clinician the risks and benefits associated with the use of an intrauterine contraceptive system. Following insertion of the intrauterine system, women should be instructed on how to check after their menstrual period to ensure that the removal threads still protrude from the cervix and should be cautioned not to pull on the threads and displace the system.

Irregular menstrual patterns are common in women receiving progestin-only contraceptives. If genital bleeding patterns are suggestive of infection, malignancy, or other pathologic causes, such causes should be ruled out. If prolonged amenorrhea develops in women receiving progestin-only oral contraceptives, the possibility of pregnancy should be evaluated. In women using the levonorgestrel-releasing intrauterine system, the number of days of bleeding and spotting may be increased and bleeding patterns may be irregular during the first 3–6 months of use; thereafter, bleeding may remain irregular but the number of days with bleeding or spotting is decreased. If bleeding irregularities develop during prolonged use of the levonorgestrel-releasing intrauterine system, pathologic causes should be ruled out. Amenorrhea develops within 1 year in about 20% of women using the levonorgestrel-releasing intrauterine system. The possibility of pregnancy should be considered in women using this contraceptive method if menstruation does not occur within 6 weeks of the onset of the previous menstrual period. Once pregnancy has been excluded, repeated pregnancy tests are not required in women using the levonorgestrel-releasing intrauterine system in the absence of other evidence of pregnancy or unless pelvic pain is present.

Delayed atresia of ovarian follicles, with resulting follicular enlargement, may occur in patients receiving progestins. Follicular enlargement generally is asymptomatic or associated with mild abdominal pain and resolves spontaneously; in rare cases, surgery may be required.

The rate of ectopic pregnancy in women receiving progestin-only oral contraceptives has been reported as 5 ectopic pregnancies per 1000 woman-years of use. Up to 10% of pregnancies reported in clinical trials in women receiving progestin-only oral contraceptives have been ectopic. The possibility of ectopic pregnancy should be considered whenever a patient receiving a low-dose progestin oral contraceptive becomes pregnant or experiences severe lower abdominal pain. A follow-up physical or pelvic examination is recommended by the manufacturers if there is any question regarding the general health or pregnancy status of a woman following administration of levonorgestrel 0.75 or 1.5 mg for postcoital (emergency) contraception. The manufacturers state that a history of ectopic pregnancy does not need to be considered a contraindication to progestin-only oral contraceptives.

The rate of ectopic pregnancy in clinical trials in women using the levonorgestrel-releasing intrauterine system has been reported to be 1 ectopic pregnancy per 1000 woman-years of use, a rate not substantially different from that in sexually active women not using any contraceptive method. About one-half of the pregnancies reported during these clinical trials were ectopic. Patients with a history of ectopic pregnancy were excluded from clinical trials of the levonorgestrel-releasing intrauterine system, and use of this contraceptive method is not recommended in women with a history of ectopic pregnancy or conditions that may predispose to ectopic pregnancy. Women using the levonorgestrel-releasing intrauterine system should be taught to recognize and report symptoms of ectopic pregnancy.

In women who have intrauterine pregnancies while using an intrauterine contraceptive device, septic abortion (resulting in septicemia, septic shock, and death) can occur. If pregnancy occurs in a woman using the levonorgestrel-releasing intrauterine system, the intrauterine system should be removed. Removal or manipulation of the system may result in pregnancy loss. If the system cannot be removed or if the woman chooses not to have the system removed, she should be advised that failure to remove the system increases the risk of miscarriage, sepsis, and premature labor and delivery, and she should be followed closely and advised to report immediately any flu-like symptoms, fever, chills, cramping, pain, bleeding, vaginal discharge, or leakage of fluid. The long-term effects on the fetus of leaving the levonorgestrel-releasing system in place as the pregnancy progresses are unknown. Clinical experience with pregnancy outcomes in such cases is limited, and the possibility of teratogenic effects cannot be completely excluded. Congenital anomalies have been reported infrequently when the levonorgestrel-releasing system was not removed; however, the role of the levonorgestrel-releasing system in the development of these anomalies has not been established.

Group A streptococcal sepsis has been reported rarely following insertion of the levonorgestrel-releasing intrauterine system. Severe pain has occurred within hours of insertion, followed by onset of sepsis within several days. Use of strict aseptic technique during insertion of the device is essential.

Use of intrauterine contraceptive devices is associated with an increased risk of PID, with the highest risk occurring shortly (generally within 20 days) after insertion of the device. The decision to use the levonorgestrel-releasing intrauterine system should include consideration of the risk of PID. If the woman or her partner has multiple sexual partners, risk of PID is increased and the levonorgestrel-releasing intrauterine system should not be used. Risk also is increased in women with a history of PID, and use of the device is contraindicated in such women unless there has been a subsequent intrauterine pregnancy. All women who are considering use of the levonorgestrel-releasing intrauterine system should be informed of the possibility of PID and long-term sequelae (tubal damage resulting in ectopic pregnancy or infertility or, less often, hysterectomy or death) and should be taught to recognize signs and symptoms of PID (e.g., prolonged or heavy bleeding, unusual vaginal discharge, abdominal or pelvic pain or tenderness, dyspareunia, chills, fever). PID may be asymptomatic but still result in tubal damage and long-term sequelae. If PID is suspected or confirmed, the patient should be promptly evaluated and appropriate treatment initiated.

Actinomycosis also has been reported in association with intrauterine contraceptive devices. If symptomatic actinomycosis occurs, the intrauterine system should be removed and appropriate anti-infective treatment initiated. Management of asymptomatic patients is controversial.

Partial penetration or embedment of the levonorgestrel-releasing intrauterine system in the myometrium may decrease contraceptive efficacy and make removal of the device difficult. If perforation of the uterus or cervix occurs, the device must be removed and surgery may be required. Potential complications include adhesions, peritonitis, intestinal perforation or obstruction, abscesses, and erosion of adjacent viscera. The risk of perforation is increased in lactating women. To decrease the risk of perforation in postpartum women and in women who have undergone a second-trimester abortion, insertion of the device should be delayed until uterine involution is complete.

The levonorgestrel-releasing intrauterine system should be removed if any of the following occur: menorrhagia and/or metrorrhagia producing anemia, HIV infection, sexually transmitted disease, pelvic infection, endometritis, symptomatic genital actinomycosis, intractable pelvic pain, severe dyspareunia, pregnancy, endometrial or cervical malignancy, or uterine or cervical perforation. Removal of the intrauterine system also should be considered if any of the following conditions arise for the first time: migraine, focal migraine with asymmetrical visual loss or other manifestations indicating transient cerebral ischemia, exceptionally severe headache, jaundice, marked increase of blood pressure, or severe arterial disease (e.g., stroke, myocardial infarction).

The manufacturers state that progestin-only oral contraceptives are contraindicated in women who are hypersensitive to the drug or any ingredient in the formulation and in those with known or suspected pregnancy, undiagnosed abnormal genital bleeding, active liver disease, benign or malignant liver tumor, or known or suspected carcinoma of the breast. In addition to the usual contraindications associated with oral progestin therapy, the levonorgestrel-releasing intrauterine system is contraindicated in patients with congenital or acquired uterine anomalies (including fibroids) if they distort the uterine cavity, acute PID or a history of PID unless there has been a subsequent intrauterine pregnancy, postpartum endometritis or infected abortion in the previous 3 months, known or suspected uterine or cervical neoplasia or an unresolved abnormal Papanicolaou test (Pap smear) result, untreated acute cervicitis or vaginitis (including bacterial vaginosis or other lower genital tract infection until the infection is controlled), conditions associated with increased susceptibility to infection (e.g., leukemia, acquired immunodeficiency syndrome [AIDS], IV drug abuse), genital actinomycosis, or a history of ectopic pregnancy or any condition that would predispose to ectopic pregnancy. The levonorgestrel-releasing intrauterine system also is contraindicated if a previously inserted intrauterine contraceptive device has not been removed or if the woman or her partner has multiple sexual partners.

Most experts state that there currently is no real contraindication to postcoital (emergency) contraception with the recommended regimens and that the benefits generally outweigh any theoretical or proven risk. Levonorgestrel for emergency contraception should not be used as a woman's routine form of contraception. In addition, use of levonorgestrel for emergency contraception is not recommended in women who are hypersensitive to the drug or any ingredient in the formulation or in those with known or suspected pregnancy.

Drug Interactions

For information on drug interactions associated with oral contraceptives, see Drug Interactions in Estrogen-Progestin Combinations 68:12.

Laboratory Test Interferences

For information on laboratory test interferences associated with oral contraceptives, see Laboratory Test Interferences in Estrogen-Progestin Combinations 68:12.

Pharmacology

Norethindrone shares the actions of progestins. Although the exact mechanism of action of progestin-only oral contraceptives is not known, norethindrone, when administered in usual contraceptive doses, appears to act principally by altering cervical mucus so that sperm migration into the uterus is inhibited. Progestational changes in the endometrium also occur which may inhibit implantation of the fertilized ovum in the uterus. In addition, continuous administration of low doses of norethindrone alters the rate of ovum transport by changing motility and secretion in fallopian tubes. Norethindrone prevents pregnancy even in the presence of ovulation. Norethindrone suppresses ovulation and causes ovarian and endometrial atrophy at high doses; the drug does not consistently suppress ovulation when administered in a continuous low-dose regimen. In low doses, norethindrone causes variable suppression of follicle-stimulating hormone (FSH) and luteinizing hormone (LH). Norethindrone has mild androgenic activity. At low doses, norethindrone also has some estrogenic activity.

The precise mechanism of contraceptive activity of levonorgestrel administered *after* intercourse (postcoital) is not known. Levonorgestrel has been shown to inhibit or delay ovulation or fertilization; other mechanisms of action for preventing pregnancy presumably are involved. Levonorgestrel is only effective before pregnancy is established. Once implantation occurs, levonorgestrel is ineffective in preventing pregnancy.

Pharmacokinetics

For a discussion on the absorption, distribution, and elimination of oral contraceptive steroids, including norethindrone, see Pharmacokinetics in Estrogen-Progestin Combinations 68:12.

Following insertion of an intrauterine system containing 52 mg of levonorgestrel (Mirena®), the drug is initially released into the uterine cavity at a rate of 20 mcg per day. The rate of drug release decreases progressively to about one-half of the initial rate after 5 years of use. Plasma levonorgestrel concentrations stabilize at 150–200 pg/mL a few weeks following insertion of the system; concentrations at 12, 24, and 60 months following insertion of the device reportedly average 180, 192, and 159 pg/mL, respectively.

Following subcutaneous insertion of etonogestrel implant, the drug is released at a rate of 60–70 mcg per day at week 5–6; the rate decreases to 35–45 mcg per day at the end of the first year, to 30–40 mcg per day at the end of the second year, and then to 25–30 mcg per day at the end of the third year. Plasma etonogestrel concentrations of 781–894 pg/mL are achieved within a few weeks following insertion of the implant; concentrations at 12, 24, and 36 months following insertion of the device reportedly average 192–261, 154–194, and 156–177 pg/mL, respectively.

Following oral administration of a single 0.75- or 1.5-mg dose of levonorgestrel, the drug is rapidly and completely absorbed with peak plasma concentrations of 14 or 19 ng/mL achieved in 1.6 or 1.7 hours, respectively.

Chemistry and Stability

■ **Chemistry** Etonogestrel, levonorgestrel, and norethindrone are synthetic progestins which are used as contraceptives. Norethindrone occurs as a white to creamy white, crystalline powder and is practically insoluble in water and sparingly soluble in alcohol.

The commercially available levonorgestrel-releasing intrauterine system consists of a T-shaped polyethylene frame with a cylindrical drug reservoir around the vertical stem. The drug reservoir, a mixture of levonorgestrel and silicone, contains 52 mg of levonorgestrel and is covered by a silicone membrane. The polyethylene frame contains barium sulfate and is radiopaque. A monofilament polyethylene removal thread is attached to a loop at the end of the vertical stem of the frame.

Etonogestrel is commercially available as a nonbiodegradable implant. The implant is 4 cm long and has a diameter of 2 mm. The implant does not contain latex and is not radiopaque.

■ **Stability** Norethindrone tablets should be stored at a temperature of 25°C but may be exposed to temperatures ranging from 15–30°C. Commercially available oral contraceptives are provided in mnemonic dispensing packages which are exempted from the child safety packaging requirements of the US Poison Prevention Packaging Act. Levonorgestrel tablets should be stored at 20–25°C.

The levonorgestrel-releasing intrauterine system should be stored at a temperature of 25°C but may be exposed to temperatures ranging from 15–30°C. The system is supplied as a sterile device and should not be resterilized. The device should not be used if the inner package is damaged or has been opened.

Etonogestrel implant should be stored at a temperature of 25°C but may be exposed to temperatures ranging from 15–30°C.

Preparations

FDA has approved Next Choice One Dose® for nonprescription (over-the-counter [OTC]) status for women 17 years of age or older; the contraceptive will remain a prescription-only preparation for women younger than 17 years of age.

Excipients in commercially available drug preparations may have clinically important effects in some individuals; consult specific product labeling for details.

Etonogestrel

Parenteral		
Implant	68 mg	**Implanon®**, Organon

Levonorgestrel

Intrauterine		
Intrauterine System	52 mg	**Mirena®**, Berlex
Oral		
Tablets	0.75 mg*	**Levonorgestrel Tablets** (available in pack of 2 tablets), Perrigo
	1.5 mg*	**Fallback Solo®**, Lupin
		Levonorgestrel Tablets
		Next Choice One Dose®, Actavis
		Opcicon® One-Step, Sun
		Plan B One-Step®, Teva

*available from one or more manufacturer, distributor, and/or repackager by generic (nonproprietary) name

Norethindrone (Norethisterone)

Oral		
Tablets	0.35 mg	**Micronor®**, Ortho-McNeil
		Nor-Q.D.®, Watson

Selected Revisions April 2016,

Ulipristal Acetate

■ Ulipristal acetate, a synthetic selective progesterone receptor modulator, is a postcoital contraceptive.

Uses

■ **Postcoital Contraception** Ulipristal acetate is used as an emergency contraceptive (EC) to prevent unintended pregnancy following unprotected intercourse or known or suspected contraceptive failure. Postcoital (emergency) contraceptive regimens are not as effective as most other methods of long-term contraception and should not be used routinely for contraception.To achieve optimal efficacy, the first dose of ulipristal acetate should be taken as soon as possible within 120 hours of unprotected intercourse.

Efficacy and safety of ulipristal for use as an emergency contraceptive have been established in 2 phase 3 clinical studies. In an open-label, multicenter study in women 18 years of age or older who reported unprotected intercourse within 48–120 hours of emergency contraception with ulipristal acetate, the expected pregnancy rate of 5.5% (with no contraception) was reduced to an observed rate of approximately 2.2% following administration of a single 30-mg dose of the drug. In a randomized, single-blind, multinational comparative study, women 16 years of age or older who reported unprotected intercourse within 72 hours of emergency contraception were randomly assigned to receive single doses of either ulipristal acetate 30 mg or levonorgestrel 1.5 mg. In this study, the primary endpoint was the pregnancy rate in women who received emergency contraception within 72 hours of unprotected intercourse. Following administration within 72 hours of unprotected intercourse, ulipristal reduced the incidence of pregnancy from an expected rate of 5.6% to an observed rate of 1.9% compared with a reduction in pregnancy from an expected rate of 5.4% to an observed rate of 2.6% for levonorgestrel. These results indicate that ulipristal was noninferior to levonorgestrel as an emergency contraceptive. A secondary endpoint was the pregnancy rate in women who received emergency contraception within 120 hours of unprotected intercourse. The data from this study were combined with results from another direct comparison study of ulipristal and levonorgestrel to determine the efficacy of ulipristal for postcoital contraception within 120 hours of unprotected intercourse. Meta-analysis of the pooled data demonstrated that the rate of pregnancy in the ulipristal group was lower than that in the levonorgestrel group from 0–24 hours (0.9 vs 2.5%, respectively), 0–72 hours (1.4 vs 2.2%, respectively), and 0–120 hours (1.3 vs 2.2%, respectively); however, the differences in pregnancy rates between the two treatment groups were not statistically significant.

Levonorgestrel currently is the preferred postcoital contraceptive; however, efficacy of levonorgestrel diminishes as time between unprotected intercourse and initiation of contraception increases. Available data suggest that postcoital contraception with levonorgestrel should ideally begin within 72 hours of unprotected intercourse. Studies of ulipristal for emergency contraception have demonstrated sustained efficacy for up to 120 hours after unprotected intercourse; however, efficacy has not been established when the drug is administered more than 120 hours after unprotected intercourse.

Dosage and Administration

■ **Administration** Ulipristal acetate is administered orally without regard to meals. The drug may be used at any time during the menstrual cycle.

If vomiting occurs within 3 hours after administration, a repeat dose should be considered.

■ **Dosage** The recommended adult dosage of ulipristal acetate for the prevention of unintended pregnancy following unprotected intercourse is a single 30-mg dose administered as soon as possible within 120 hours of unprotected intercourse or known or suspected contraceptive failure.

■ **Special Populations** No special population dosage recommendations at this time.

Cautions

■ **Contraindications** Known or suspected pregnancy.

■ **Warnings/Precautions** ***Warnings*** **Fetal/Neonatal Morbidity and Mortality.** May cause fetal harm; embryofetal death reported in animals. No adequate and well-controlled studies to date in pregnant women. If the drug is inadvertently used during pregnancy, the woman should be apprised of the potential hazard to the fetus.

Existing Pregnancy. Ulipristal is *not* indicated for termination of an existing pregnancy. The possibility of pregnancy should be excluded prior to administration of the drug. If pregnancy cannot be excluded on the basis of history and/or physical examination, pregnancy testing should be performed. If there is any concern regarding the general health or pregnancy status of a woman after receiving ulipristal, a follow-up physical and/or pelvic examination is recommended.

Ectopic Pregnancy. Clinicians should consider the possibility of ectopic pregnancy in women who become pregnant or complain of severe lower abdominal pain after receiving ulipristal. The manufacturer states that a history of ectopic pregnancy is not a contraindication to use of ulipristal.

Repeated Use. Ulipristal is intended for occasional use as an emergency contraceptive. Postcoital (emergency) contraceptive regimens are not as effective as most other methods of long-term contraception and should not be used routinely for contraception. Repeated use of ulipristal within the same menstrual cycle is not recommended; safety and efficacy of such repeated use have not been evaluated.

Fertility Following Use. Rapid return of fertility is likely following treatment with ulipristal for emergency contraception. Therefore, routine methods of contraception should be continued or initiated as soon as possible to ensure ongoing prevention of pregnancy. Use of ulipristal may reduce the contraceptive action of other hormonal contraceptive agents. (See Drug Interactions.) Therefore, a reliable barrier method of contraception should be used by women after receiving ulipristal for subsequent acts of intercourse occurring within the same menstrual cycle.

Effect on Menstrual Cycle. Use of ulipristal may cause menstrual cycle disruption by a few days (onset of menstruation either earlier or later than expected). If onset of menstruation is delayed by a week or more, a sensitive pregnancy test should be performed to rule out pregnancy. Intermenstrual bleeding also has been reported in women after receiving ulipristal.

Risk of HIV Infection and Other STDs. Ulipristal does *not* protect against human immunodeficiency virus (HIV) infection or other sexually transmitted diseases (STDs).

Specific Populations **Pregnancy.** Category X. (See Fetal/Neonatal Morbidity and Mortality under Warnings/Precautions: Warnings and also see Contraindications, in Cautions.)

Lactation. Distributed into milk in rats; not known whether distributed into human milk. Not recommended for use in nursing women.

Pediatric Use. Safety and efficacy of ulipristal have been established in women of reproductive age. Safety and efficacy are expected to be identical for postpubertal adolescents younger than 18 years of age and women 18 years of age or older. Ulipristal is not intended for use before menarche.

Geriatric Use. Ulipristal has not been evaluated in women 65 years of age or older and is not intended for use for postmenopausal women.

Hepatic Impairment. No studies have been conducted to evaluate the effect of hepatic impairment on the pharmacokinetic disposition of ulipristal.

Renal Impairment. No studies have been conducted to evaluate the effect of renal impairment on the pharmacokinetic disposition of ulipristal.

■ **Common Adverse Effects** The most common adverse effects reported in clinical trials of ulipristal are headache, abdominal pain, nausea, dysmenorrhea, fatigue, and dizziness.

Drug Interactions

No formal drug interaction studies have been performed to date.

■ **Drugs Affecting or Metabolized by Hepatic Microsomal Enzymes** In vitro data indicate that the metabolism of ulipristal acetate is mediated predominantly by cytochrome P-450 (CYP) isoenzyme 3A4, and the possibility exists that drugs that induce or inhibit this isoenzyme may affect plasma ulipristal concentrations. Concomitant use of ulipristal with drugs that induce CYP3A4 (e.g., bosentan, carbamazepine, felbamate, griseofulvin, oxcarbazepine, phenobarbital and other barbiturates, phenytoin, rifampin, St. John's wort [Hypericum perforatum], topiramate) may result in decreased plasma concentrations and reduced efficacy of ulipristal. Concomitant use of ulipristal with drugs that inhibit CYP3A4 (e.g., itraconazole, ketoconazole) may result in increased plasma concentrations of ulipristal.

In vitro studies show that ulipristal does not induce or inhibit the activity of CYP isoenzymes.

■ **Hormonal Contraceptives** No data are available to date regarding concomitant use of ulipristal with other hormonal contraceptive agents. However, use of ulipristal may reduce the contraceptive action of other hormonal contraceptives as a result of the drug's high-affinity binding to progesterone receptors. The manufacturer states that a reliable barrier method of contraception should be used after a woman receives ulipristal for subsequent acts of intercourse occurring within the same menstrual cycle.

Description

Ulipristal acetate is a synthetic selective progesterone receptor modulator and a derivative of 19-norprogesterone. The drug is structurally and pharmacologically related to mifepristone. Ulipristal, like mifepristone, exhibits antagonist activity at progesterone receptors and inhibits progesterone from binding to its receptors; however, the drug also possesses partial agonist activity at the progesterone receptor. Animal studies indicate that the antiglucocorticoid activity of ulipristal is lower than its antiprogestin activity. The exact mechanism of action of ulipristal is unknown, but may involve inhibition or delay of ovulation or inhibition of follicular growth or rupture; alterations to the endometrium that may affect implantation also may contribute to efficacy. However, in doses used for postcoital contraception (30 mg), ulipristal acetate has no clinically important effect on the endometrium.

Peak plasma concentrations of ulipristal acetate and its active metabolite, monodemethyl ulipristal acetate, are reached 60–90 minutes following a single oral dose under fasting conditions. Administration of ulipristal with a high-fat meal reduced mean peak plasma concentrations by 40–45% and delayed the time to peak plasma concentration from a median of 0.75 to 3 hours. However, the differences resulting from administration of the drug with food are not expected to result in clinically important effects on efficacy or safety. Ulipristal acetate is more than 94% bound to plasma proteins, mainly high density lipoprotein (HDL)-cholesterol, alpha-1-acid glycoprotein, and albumin. In vitro data show that ulipristal is metabolized mainly by the cytochrome P-450 (CYP) 3A4 isoenzyme to mono-demethylated and di-demethylated metabolites. The terminal half-life of ulipristal acetate is approximately 32 hours following oral administration.

Advice to Patients

Importance of reading the patient information (medication guide) provided by the manufacturer before initiating therapy.

Importance of taking ulipristal acetate as soon as possible and not more than 120 hours after unprotected intercourse or a known or suspected contraceptive failure.

Importance of women informing clinicians if they know or suspect that they are pregnant. Ulipristal should *not* be used for termination of an existing pregnancy.

Importance of women informing clinicians if vomiting occurs within 3 hours of taking ulipristal to evaluate the need for a repeat dose.

Importance of advising patients to seek medical attention if they experience severe lower abdominal pain 3–5 weeks after taking ulipristal to rule out the possibility of ectopic pregnancy.

Importance of advising patients to contact their clinician after receiving ulipristal if menstruation is delayed by more than 1 week beyond the expected date to rule out the possibility of pregnancy.

Importance of advising patients not to use ulipristal for routine contraception or for repeated use within the same menstrual cycle.

Importance of advising patients that ulipristal may reduce the contraceptive action of other hormonal contraceptives and to use a reliable barrier method of contraception (e.g., condom with spermicide) after receiving ulipristal for any subsequent acts of intercourse occurring within the same menstrual cycle.

Importance of advising women that ulipristal should not be used if they are breast-feeding.

Importance of advising women that ulipristal is not effective in all cases and that the drug may be less effective in women with a body mass index exceeding 30 kg/m^2.

Importance of informing women that ulipristal does not provide protection against human immunodeficiency virus (HIV)-infection or other sexually transmitted diseases.

Importance of informing clinicians of existing or contemplated concomitant therapy, including prescription and OTC drugs, as well as any concomitant illnesses.

Importance of informing patients of other important precautionary information. (See Cautions.)

Overview® (see Users Guide). For additional information on this drug until a more detailed monograph is developed and published, the manufacturer's labeling should be consulted. It is *essential* that the manufacturer's labeling be consulted for more detailed information on usual cautions, precautions, contraindications, potential drug interactions, laboratory test interferences, and acute toxicity.

Preparations

Excipients in commercially available drug preparations may have clinically important effects in some individuals; consult specific product labeling for details.

Ulipristal Acetate

Oral

Tablets	30 mg	**ella®**, Watson

ESTROGENS, ANTIESTROGENS, AND ESTROGEN AGONIST-ANTAGONISTS 68:16

ESTROGENS 68:16.04

Estrogens General Statement

■ Estrogens are naturally occurring hormones or synthetic steroidal and nonsteroidal compounds with estrogenic activity.

Uses

■ **Estrogen Replacement Therapy** Estrogens are used for the treatment of moderate to severe vasomotor symptoms and other symptoms, including vulvar and vaginal atrophy, associated with menopause and for the prevention and treatment of osteoporosis. When estrogens are used alone, such therapy is referred to as estrogen replacement therapy (ERT); when estrogens are used in combination with progestins, such therapy usually is referred to as hormone replacement therapy (HRT) or postmenopausal hormone therapy. Another therapeutic option for postmenopausal women involves use of estrogens in combination with an estrogen agonist-antagonist (e.g., bazedoxifene); this combination is referred to as a tissue-selective estrogen complex (TSEC). Long-term therapy with estrogens is associated with an increased risk of endometrial hyperplasia and/or carcinoma in postmenopausal women; however, use of progestins in conjunction with estrogen therapy (HRT) substantially reduces the risk. Women with an intact uterus must receive progestin in addition to estrogen to avoid the increased risk of endometrial carcinoma; long-term use of estrogen alone in women with an intact uterus is not recommended. As an alternative to progestin therapy, the use of bazedoxifene (an estrogen agonist-antagonist) in fixed combination with conjugated estrogens reduces the risk of endometrial hyperplasia. HRT is associated with increased risks of myocardial infarction (MI), stroke, invasive breast cancer, pulmonary emboli, and deep-vein thrombosis. ERT is associated with increased risks of stroke and deep-vein thrombosis. Because of the potential risks associated with HRT and ERT, the benefit to risk should be assessed for each patient, considering alternative therapies as part of this assessment. If ERT or HRT is used, it should be prescribed at the lowest effective dosage and for the shortest duration consistent with treatment goals and risks for the individual woman.

In the past, estrogens were used for prevention of cardiovascular disease in postmenopausal women; however, recent data indicate that use of ERT or HRT does not decrease the incidence of cardiovascular disease, and estrogen replacement therapy alone (ERT) or combined with progestins (HRT) should *no longer* be used for the prevention of cardiovascular disease.

While estrogen or estrogen/progestin therapy is effective for the management of certain menopausal symptoms and for the prevention and treatment of osteoporosis, results of a recent controlled study (Women's Health Initiative [WHI] study of estrogen plus progestin) indicate that HRT, specifically conjugated estrogens 0.625 mg in conjunction with medroxyprogesterone acetate 2.5 mg daily, is associated with a small increase in the risk of breast cancer, cardiovascular disease, stroke, and venous thromboembolism. Results of the WHI study of estrogen alone indicate that ERT (specifically conjugated estrogens 0.625 mg daily) is associated with a small increase in the risk of stroke and deep-vein thrombosis. Results of the WHI also showed that HRT had no clinically important effect on measures of depression, insomnia, sexual function, or cognition (i.e., health-related quality-of-life measures) in women without menopausal symptoms. Based on the WHI findings, recommendations on the appropriate use of hormone therapy have been revised. Because the risks of hormone therapy exceed the benefits for the prevention of chronic diseases in postmenopausal women, experts state that ERT or HRT should not be used for the prevention of chronic conditions in postmenopausal women. The American Heart Association (AHA), the American College of Obstetricians and Gynecologists (ACOG), FDA, and manufacturers recommend that hormone therapy not be used to prevent heart disease in healthy women (primary prevention) or to protect women with preexisting heart disease (secondary prevention). ACOG, FDA, and the manufacturers also recommend that women receiving hormone therapy solely for the prevention of postmenopausal osteoporosis consider alternative therapy (e.g., alendronate, raloxifene, risedronate). Although these recommendations are based on results of the WHI study that evaluated one specific estrogen (conjugated estrogens 0.625 mg) and one estrogen/progestin preparation (conjugated estrogens 0.625 mg in conjunction with medroxyprogesterone acetate 2.5 mg), the risks should be assumed to be similar with other hormonal regimens, including different dosages of these drugs as well as other estrogen/progestin combinations not studied in WHI, in the absence of comparable data to the contrary.

While the risks of HRT are likely to exceed the benefits in most women receiving these agents for prevention of chronic diseases (e.g., cardiovascular disease, osteoporosis), the long-term safety of short-term use of HRT for the management of menopausal symptoms remains to be precisely established. Estrogen or estrogen/progestin therapy is the most effective therapy for the relief of vasomotor symptoms such as hot flushes (flashes) and sleep disturbances. The fixed combination of conjugated estrogens with bazedoxifene acetate also is used for the management of moderate to severe vasomotor symptoms associated with menopause. (See Uses: Vasomotor Symptoms, in Bazedoxifene Acetate 68:16.12.) Estrogen or estrogen/progestin therapy also is effective in the treatment of genitourinary symptoms such as vaginal dryness; however, the use of topical vaginal preparations should be considered when only vulvar and vaginal symptoms are being treated. The decision to use estrogen or estrogen/progestin therapy for management of menopausal symptoms should be individualized taking into account the woman's preference, her risk for specific chronic diseases, and the presence and severity of menopausal symptoms. ACOG, FDA, and the manufacturers recommend that women who choose hormone therapy for the relief of menopausal symptoms receive such therapy for the shortest possible time and in the lowest effective dosage; women also should regularly consult their clinician and undergo regular breast cancer screenings. ACOG recommends against routine discontinuance of systemic estrogen therapy when a women reaches 65 years of age, since some women 65 years of age or older may continue to need systemic hormone therapy for management of vasomotor symptoms. Continuation of hormone therapy for management of vasomotor symptoms should be individualized taking into account the woman's symptoms and the risks and benefits of hormone therapy, regardless of age.

Regardless of a woman's age or duration of hormone therapy, discontinuance may be associated with recurrent vasomotor symptoms in approximately 50% of women. There is insufficient evidence to recommend one method of stopping hormone therapy (e.g., abrupt discontinuance, dosage tapering) over another to prevent recurrent symptoms.

Lifestyle modifications that may help reduce menopausal symptoms such as hot flushes include smoking cessation, dietary manipulation (avoid/limit spicy foods, caffeine, and alcohol), stress reduction, and loose or layered clothing. There is increasing evidence that drugs other than hormone preparations may alleviate certain menopausal symptoms. For women experiencing vasomotor symptoms, selective serotonin-reuptake inhibitors (SSRIs), selective serotonin- and norepinephrine-reuptake inhibitors (SNRIs), gabapentin, or clonidine has been used for treatment. SSRIs, SNRIs, and gabapentin have been shown to be effective for treatment of vasomotor symptoms in randomized, controlled trials, while evidence supporting the efficacy of clonidine is limited. For symptoms such as vaginal dryness, topical administration of estrogen alone usually is effective. Although only limited amounts of estrogen are systemically absorbed from vaginal tablets and rings, limited data are available regarding long-term safety of vaginally administered estrogen.

Estrogens also are used in the treatment of a variety of other conditions associated with a deficiency of estrogenic hormones, including female hypogonadism and castration and primary ovarian failure. In addition, estrogens also may be used in the treatment of abnormal uterine bleeding caused by hormonal imbalance not associated with organic pathology; however, progestins are usually preferred.

Osteoporosis **Prevention in Postmenopausal Women.** Estrogen replacement therapy (ERT) is effective for the prevention of osteoporosis in women and has been shown to reduce bone resorption and retard or halt bone loss associated with estrogen deficiency in postmenopausal women. Oral estrogens (e.g., estradiol, estropipate, conjugated estrogens) and transdermal estrogens (e.g., estradiol) are used adjunctively with other therapeutic measures (e.g., diet, calcium, vitamin D, weight-bearing exercise, physical therapy) to retard further bone loss and the progression of osteoporosis in postmenopausal women. The fixed combination of conjugated estrogens with bazedoxifene acetate also is used for the prevention of osteoporosis. (See Prevention in Postmenopausal Women under Uses: Osteoporosis, in Bazedoxifene Acetate 68:16.12.)

In a placebo-controlled study in postmenopausal women, administration of estrogen replacement therapy (conjugated estrogens) with (HRT) or without (ERT) a progestin for 36 months was associated with a 1.7% increase in hip bone mineral density (BMD) and 3.5–5% increase in lumbar spine BMD compared with baseline, while placebo recipients lost an average of 1.7% in hip BMD and 1.8% in spinal BMD. Increases in BMD observed in women receiving estrogen replacement therapy without a progestin (ERT) generally have been essentially the same as those observed in women receiving combined estrogen/progestin therapy (HRT).

In case-controlled studies in Caucasian women, estrogen replacement therapy has been associated with a substantial (about 60%) reduction in the incidence of hip and wrist fractures in those in whom estrogen therapy was initiated within a few years of menopause; some studies suggest that estrogens may also reduce the incidence of vertebral fracture. In the WHI study, there was a 24% reduction in total fractures in postmenopausal women receiving HRT compared with those receiving placebo and a 30–39% reduction in total fractures in women receiving ERT compared with women receiving placebo. The number of cases of hip fracture per 10,000 patient-years of exposure was 10 or 15 in women receiving HRT or placebo, respectively. The number of cases of hip fracture per 10,000 patient-years of exposure was 11 or 17 in women receiving ERT or placebo, respectively. Estrogen replacement therapy reportedly prevents further estrogen deficiency-induced bone loss in postmenopausal women when started up to 6 years after menopause, but such therapy does not appear to restore bone mass to premenopausal levels. In addition, when estrogen therapy is discontinued, bone mass declines at a rate similar to that occurring in the immediate postmenopausal period. It has been suggested that optimum estrogen replacement therapy for the prevention of osteoporosis should be initiated within 5 years of menopause and be continued for long-term (exceeding 10 years); however, risks associated with such long-term use should be considered. (See Carcinogenicity.)

Caucasian or Asian women are at a higher risk for osteoporosis than black women. Other risk factors include premature ovarian failure; a family history of osteoporosis; a small, slim body frame; endocrine disorders such as thyrotoxicosis, hyperparathyroidism, Cushing's syndrome, hyperprolactinemia, insulin-dependent diabetes mellitus (type 1, IDDM); cigarette smoking; drinking excessive amounts of alcohol; a sedentary lifestyle and/or lack of physical exercise; low body weight; and low dietary calcium intake. Premature ovarian failure (surgical or nonsurgical) hastens the onset of osteoporosis, and estrogen deficiency in premenopausal women (e.g., secondary to anorexia nervosa- or exercise-induced amenorrhea or to hyperprolactinemia) induces bone loss and may reduce peak bone mass.

While estrogen or estrogen/progestin therapy is effective for the prevention of osteoporosis in postmenopausal women, results of a recent controlled study (WHI study) indicate that HRT, specifically conjugated estrogens 0.625 mg in conjunction with medroxyprogesterone acetate 2.5 mg daily, is associated with a small increase in the risk of breast cancer, cardiovascular disease, stroke, and venous thromboembolism. Results of the WHI estrogen-alone study indicate that ERT (specifically conjugated estrogens 0.625 mg daily) is associated with a small increase in the risk of stroke and deep-vein thrombosis. Because the risks of hormone therapy exceed the benefits for the prevention of chronic diseases in postmenopausal women, experts state that ERT or HRT should not be used for the prevention of chronic conditions (e.g., osteoporosis) in postmenopausal women. ACOG, FDA, and the manufacturers recommend that women receiving hormone therapy solely for the prevention of postmenopausal osteoporosis consider alternative therapy. Alternative agents that can be used for the prevention of osteoporosis include alendronate, raloxifene, or risedronate. However, experience with these agents is not as extensive as with HRT. (See Osteoporosis: Prevention in Postmenopausal Women, under Uses, in Alendronate 92:24, Raloxifene 68:16.12, and Risedronate 92:24.) In addition, alendronate and risedronate are associated with substantial adverse GI effects (e.g., esophagitis). (See Dosage and Administration: Administration, in Alendronate 92:24 and Risedronate 92:24.)

Women being considered for estrogen replacement therapy should have no contraindications to estrogen therapy and should fully understand the risks associated with estrogen use and agree to regular medical examinations. The choice of estrogen replacement therapy, alendronate, raloxifene, or risedronate for the prevention of postmenopausal osteoporosis should be individualized, taking into account differences in tolerability and safety and individual preference. For all women, lifestyle modifications for healthy bones include a diet high in calcium (postmenopausal women should receive 1.2–1.5 g of calcium daily), adequate intake of vitamin D (as supplied by a multivitamin), and regular weight-bearing exercise such as walking or jogging. Whether additional preventive therapy generally should be offered to all women or just recommended for selected women at highest risk of developing osteoporosis remains to be established.

Although there is no biologic reason to suspect that the effects of estrogens would differ in nonwhite women, the efficacy of estrogen replacement therapy in preventing osteoporosis in nonwhite women has not been established to date.

Treatment in Postmenopausal Women. Estrogen replacement therapy has been effective in the treatment of osteoporosis in postmenopausal women and has been recommended as first-line therapy for women with osteoporosis. However, results of a recent controlled study (WHI study) indicate that HRT, specifically conjugated estrogens 0.625 mg in conjunction with medroxyprogesterone acetate 2.5 mg daily, is associated with a small increase in the risk of breast cancer, cardiovascular disease, stroke, and venous thromboembolism. Results of the WHI estrogen-alone study indicate that ERT (specifically conjugated estrogens 0.625 mg daily) is associated with a small increase in the risk of stroke and deep-vein thrombosis. Based on these findings, recommendations on the appropriate use of hormone therapy are being revised. The risks and benefits of long-term use of hormone therapy in the management of osteoporosis should be evaluated taking into account the increased risk of breast cancer and cardiovascular disease, availability of other pharmacologic modalities (e.g., alendronate, calcitonin, calcium, raloxifene, risedronate, vitamin D), and life-style factors that can be modified.

Estrogen replacement therapy produces the most marked benefits when begun soon (e.g., within 5 years) following menopause; such therapy also appears to be effective even when initiated many years after menopause in older women. Some clinicians suggest that prolonged therapy (e.g., at least 5 years) with estrogens is necessary since the beneficial effects of estrogen replacement therapy do not appear to persist after discontinuance of treatment.

Various estrogen-containing therapies (e.g., conjugated estrogens, estrogen/progestin combinations) have been used concomitantly with bisphosphonates (e.g., alendronate, etidronate) and calcium in the treatment of osteoporosis in postmenopausal women. In several clinical trials in postmenopausal women with osteoporosis, the combination of estrogen-containing therapy and alendronate resulted in a greater degree of suppression of bone turnover than either therapy given alone. In a placebo-controlled, 2-year clinical trial comparing monotherapy with alendronate (10 mg daily) or conjugated estrogens (0.625 mg daily) with the combination of these drugs at the same monotherapy dosages in postmenopausal women with osteoporosis not currently receiving antiresorptive therapy, combination therapy increased bone mineral density (BMD) (as determined by dual-energy radiographic absorption measurements) in the lumbar spine and femoral neck compared with either agent given alone or placebo (calcium 500 mg daily). A bone histology study in these patients indicated that the bone formed during therapy was of normal quality. Compared with calcium supplementation alone, bone turnover after 18 months was suppressed by 98% with combined alendronate-estrogen replacement therapy, 94% with alendronate therapy alone, and 78% with estrogen replacement therapy alone. In another comparative study in postmenopausal women who had osteoporosis despite hormone replacement therapy with estrogen (conjugated estrogens) or estrogen plus progestin (medroxyprogesterone) for at least 1 year (mean duration about 10 years), the addition of alendronate (10 mg daily) increased BMD (as determined by dual-energy radiographic absorption measurements) in the lumbar spine and hip trochanter compared with hormone replacement therapy alone at 12 months; all patients also received calcium and vitamin D supplementation. In both trials, the incidence of new fractures was similar across treatment groups. In these trials, sample size and study duration may have been inadequate to detect differences in fracture incidence with combination therapy, monotherapy with alendronate or estrogen, or placebo, and further studies are needed. The safety of combination therapy was similar to that with each antiresorptive agent alone.

Prevention in Women with Anorexia Nervosa Estrogens have been used in a limited number of anorexic women with chronic amenorrhea to reduce calcium loss† and, thereby, reduce the risks of osteoporosis. However, results of various controlled and uncontrolled studies indicate that estrogens appear to benefit only a subset of low-weight (initial body weight less than 70% of ideal body weight) women with anorexia nervosa. Because data supporting use of estrogen therapy for the treatment or prevention of osteoporosis in female children, adolescents, or adults with anorexia nervosa are limited or lacking, the American Psychiatric Association (APA) concludes that therapy with estrogens alone does not appear to reverse osteoporosis or osteopenia, and unless there is weight gain, such therapy does not prevent further bone loss.Furthermore, many clinicians state that the decision to initiate estrogen therapy in these patients should be deferred until weight gain and normal menses have been restored, since artificially inducing menses carries the risk of supporting or reinforcing a patient's denial that she does not need to gain weight. For a complete discussion of diagnosis and treatment of anorexia nervosa and other eating disorders, see Uses: Eating Disorders, in Fluoxetine 28:16.04.20.

Cardiovascular Risk Reduction While results from earlier observational studies indicated that estrogen replacement therapy or combined estrogen/progestin therapy was associated with cardiovascular benefit in postmenopausal women, results of the Heart and Estrogen/Progestin Replacement Study (HERS) and the Women's Health Initiative (WHI) study indicate that use of estrogen replacement therapy (ERT) or combined estrogen/progestin replacement therapy (hormone replacement therapy, HRT) does *not* decrease the incidence of cardiovascular disease.

Substantial epidemiologic evidence has indicated that postmenopausal women receiving ERT may have a reduction of up to 50% in the risk of ischemic heart disease and a similar reduction in total mortality compared with women who have never received such therapy. In observational studies, the increase in life expectancy based on a reduced risk of coronary heart disease (CHD) in postmenopausal women receiving ERT has been estimated to be 2–3 years. While these studies generally enrolled healthy women, observational studies in women with preexisting coronary disease also suggest that ERT reduces the risk of reinfarction and CHD-related death. However, the conclusions of these studies have been criticized for methodological reasons.

Although some observational studies have shown a cardioprotective effect with estrogen alone or in combination with progestin, conflicting data have been reported in large prospective, randomized studies. In one of these studies (HERS), no overall cardiovascular benefit was reported with HRT in postmenopausal women with established coronary disease. In addition, results of the WHI study indicate that HRT, specifically conjugated estrogens 0.625 mg in conjunction with medroxyprogesterone acetate 2.5 mg daily, is associated with a small increase in the risk of cardiovascular disease and stroke in predominantly healthy postmenopausal women. Results from the WHI estrogen-alone study indicate that ERT (specifically conjugated estrogens 0.625 mg daily) does not affect the risk of CHD but is associated with a small increase in the risk of stroke in healthy postmenopausal women who have undergone a hysterectomy. In another randomized study, ERT (conjugated estrogens 0.625 mg daily) or HRT (conjugated estrogens 0.625 mg daily and medroxyprogesterone acetate 2.5 mg daily) was associated with reductions in LDL-cholesterol and increases in HDL-cholesterol concentrations but had no effect on progression of coronary atherosclerosis in women with established CHD.

In HERS, 2763 postmenopausal women with established CHD were randomized to receive HRT (conjugated estrogens 0.625 mg daily in conjunction with medroxyprogesterone acetate 2.5 mg daily) or placebo. After a follow-up averaging 6.8 years, HRT was not associated with an overall reduction in the rate of CHD events (e.g., nonfatal MI, CHD-related death). Based on year of randomization, women who received HRT experienced an increased incidence of CHD events during the first year and a lower incidence in the fourth year compared with women who received placebo. However, based on the entire 6.8 years of follow-up, a trend toward a lower or higher incidence of CHD over time was not evident. Analysis of data from 2 observational studies in postmenopausal women with cardiovascular disease (i.e., the Nurses' Health Study and a Group Health Cooperative study) indicate that the risk for a recurrent major coronary event in women with established coronary heart disease is increased early (up to 1 year) after initiation of HRT and decreases with long-term use. Women with CHD often have risk factors such as diabetes mellitus and obesity that influence the tendency to develop thrombosis, and any procoagulant effects of hormone therapy would be greatest in such women. Whether estrogen/progestin therapy (HRT) is associated in susceptible subgroups with immediate prothrombotic, proarrhythmic, or proischemic effects that are gradually outweighed by a beneficial effect on the underlying progression of atherosclerosis (perhaps as a result of favorable effects on lipoproteins) requires further study.

The WHI was a long-term study sponsored by the National Institutes of Health (NIH) that focused on strategies that can potentially reduce the incidence of heart disease, breast and colorectal cancer, and fractures in postmenopausal women. One part of this initiative followed 16,608 predominantly healthy women (with an intact uterus) who were 50–79 years of age who received HRT (i.e., conjugated estrogens 0.625 mg in conjunction with medroxyprogesterone acetate 2.5 mg daily) or placebo. The goal of this 8.5-year study was to evaluate the relationship between HRT and CHD, stroke, pulmonary embolism, breast cancer, endometrial carcinoma, colorectal cancer, hip fracture, and death from other causes. The study was stopped early because health risks exceeded benefits over an average follow-up of 5.2 years. At the time the study was stopped, the increased number of cases of invasive breast cancer, CHD, stroke, and pulmonary embolism in the estrogen/progestin group relative to the placebo group was not counterbalanced by reductions in the number of cases of hip fracture and colorectal cancer. Estrogen/progestin therapy did not affect all-cause mortality.

In the WHI estrogen plus progestin study, there was a 29% increase in the incidence of heart disease in postmenopausal women receiving HRT compared with those receiving placebo. The number of CHD events (e.g., MI) per 10,000 patient-years of exposure was 37 or 30 in women receiving HRT or placebo, respectively. In addition, there was a 41% increase in the incidence of stroke in postmenopausal women receiving HRT compared with those receiving placebo. The number of cases of stroke per 10,000 patient-years of exposure was 29 or 20 in women receiving HRT or placebo, respectively.

Another part of the WHI initiative followed 10,739 predominately healthy women who were 50–79 years of age and had undergone a prior hysterectomy, and received ERT (conjugated estrogens 0.625 mg daily) or placebo. The goal of this study was to evaluate the relationship between ERT and CHD, stroke, pulmonary embolism, breast cancer, colorectal cancer, hip fracture, and death from other causes. At the time the study was stopped (after nearly 7 years), results indicated that ERT did not affect the incidence of CHD or overall mortality but did increase the risk of stroke. There was a 39% increase in the incidence of stroke in women receiving ERT compared with those receiving placebo. Approximately 80% of all strokes were ischemic. The number of cases of stroke per 10,000 patient-years of exposure was 44 or 32 in women receiving ERT or placebo, respectively.

An ancillary substudy of the WHI examined the effect of ERT (conjugated estrogens 0.625 mg daily) or placebo on coronary-artery calcification in women 50–59 years of age at the time of randomization. Imaging of the coronary arteries 8.7 years after study start (7.4 years of treatment and 1.3 years after study completion) indicated that women who received estrogen had a lower prevalence and quantity of coronary-artery calcium than placebo-treated women. Intent-to-treat analysis showed that administration of estrogen reduced coronary calcification by 42%; in women with at least 80% adherence to study medication for 5 years, administration of estrogen reduced coronary calcification by 61%.

Based on the finding of no overall cardiovascular benefit observed in HERS and the WHI study and the lack of effect of ERT or HRT on angiographic progression of coronary artery disease, the AHA, ACOG, FDA, and manufacturers recommend that hormone therapy not be used to prevent heart disease in healthy women (primary prevention) or to protect women with preexisting heart disease (secondary prevention).

If a woman with cardiovascular disease receiving long-term HRT experiences an acute cardiovascular event (e.g., MI) or is immobilized, discontinuance of HRT or administration of venous thrombosis prophylaxis during hospitalization should be considered to reduce the risk of thromboembolism. Decisions to resume HRT should be based on established noncoronary risks and benefits and patient preference.

■ **Corticosteroid-induced Hypogonadism and Osteoporosis** Patients receiving long-term corticosteroid therapy may develop hypogonadism secondary to inhibition of secretion of luteinizing hormone (LH) and follicle-stimulating hormone (FSH) from the pituitary as well as secondary to direct effects on the ovaries and testes, and such hypogonadism may be associated with bone loss. Therefore, all patients receiving prolonged corticosteroid therapy should be assessed for possible hypogonadism, which should be corrected if present.

Hormone replacement therapy (HRT, combined estrogen and progestin therapy) has been effective in increasing lumbar spine but not femoral neck bone mass density (BMD) in postmenopausal women with asthma or rheumatoid arthritis who were receiving chronic corticosteroid therapy. HRT in a control group of women receiving long-term low-dose corticosteroid therapy in one study appeared to prevent BMD loss at the lumbar spine, hip, and distal radius over the course of 1 year. While there currently are no well-designed studies establishing the *preventive* efficacy of HRT on corticosteroid-induced bone loss and radiographic vertebral fractures, data from existing studies suggest that HRT is adequate to prevent bone loss in postmenopausal women receiving low-to-moderate-dose corticosteroid therapy†, and postmenopausal women receiving long-term corticosteroid therapy should be offered HRT if no contraindications exist. The protective efficacy of HRT in such women who are receiving moderate-to-high doses of corticosteroids remains to be established. Corticosteroid-treated women who develop fractures while receiving HRT or in whom HRT is not well tolerated should receive calcium and vitamin D supplementation along with bisphosphonate therapy (e.g., alendronate, risedronate) in an attempt to prevent bone loss and/or increase BMD as well as to prevent apoptosis of osteocytes and osteoblasts and reduce the risk of radiographic vertebral fractures.

There also currently are no controlled studies of HRT in premenopausal women receiving chronic corticosteroid therapy. However, observational studies in premenopausal female athletes with menstrual irregularities suggest that estrogen-progestin combination (e.g., oral contraceptive) use is associated with a higher adjusted bone mineral content and BMD relative to women who do not take estrogen-progestin combinations. Therefore, premenopausal women who develop menstrual irregularities (e.g., oligomenorrhea, amenorrhea) while receiving long-term corticosteroid therapy should be offered combined cyclic estrogen and progestin therapy (e.g., estrogen-progestin combination oral contraceptives) in an attempt to treat hypogonadism and possibly reduce the risk ofcorticosteroid-induced osteoporosis† when contraindications to estrogen-progestin therapy are not present. For additional information on the management of corticosteroid-induced osteoporosis, see Cautions: Musculoskeletal Effects in the Corticosteroids General Statement 68:04.

■ **Alzheimer's Disease** Some data from observational studies indicate that prior use of hormone replacement therapy (HRT), but not current HRT unless such use exceeds 10 years, is associated with reduced risk of Alzheimer's disease†. Estrogens have not been shown to prevent progression of Alzheimer's disease, and the American Academy of Neurology (AAN) recommends that estrogens not be used for the treatment of Alzheimer's disease.

Findings from the Women' Health Initiative Memory study (WHIMS; an ancillary study of the Women's Health Initiative [WHI] study in women 65 years of age or older without dementia at study entry) indicate that use of ERT (conjugated estrogens 0.625 mg daily) or HRT (conjugated estrogens 0.625 mg in conjunction with medroxyprogesterone acetate 2.5 mg daily) does not improve cognitive function relative to placebo in these women and may adversely affect cognition. In the WHIMS study, more women receiving ERT or HRT had substantial and clinically important declines in the Modified Mini-Mental State Examination total score compared with women receiving placebo, suggesting that some women receiving these hormonal therapies experience detrimental effects. In addition, the rate of probable dementia in women receiving ERT or HRT was higher than that in women receiving placebo. Women with relatively low baseline cognitive function were at particularly high risk for adverse cognitive effects. Use of hormone therapy to prevent dementia or cognitive decline in women 65 years of age or older is not recommended.

■ **Metastatic Breast Carcinoma** Estrogens are used in the palliative treatment of advanced, inoperable, metastatic carcinoma of the breast in postmenopausal women and in men. Estrogens are one of several second-line agents that can be used in certain postmenopausal women with metastatic breast cancer.

■ **Prostate Carcinoma** In males, estrogens are used for the palliative treatment of advanced carcinoma of the prostate; however, the risk of adverse cardiovascular effects of the drugs must be considered.

■ **Other Uses** Estrogens also are used in combination with progestins for ovulation control in the prevention of conception and for the treatment of moderate acne vulgaris; estrogen-progestin combinations also are used in short-course, high-dose regimens in women for the prevention of contraception after unprotected intercourse (postcoital contraception, "morning-after pills") as emergency contraceptives. (See Uses: Postcoital Contraception, in Estrogen-Progestin Combinations 68:12.)

Although in the past estrogens have been used for the prevention of postpartum breast engorgement†, FDA has withdrawn approval of estrogen-containing drugs for this indication since estrogens have not been shown to be safe for use in women with postpartum breast engorgement. Data from controlled studies indicate that the incidence of substantial painful engorgement is low in untreated women, and the condition usually responds to appropriate analgesic or other supportive therapy.

Estrogens have *not* been shown to be effective for any purpose during pregnancy.

For information on the uses of specific estrogens, see the individual monographs in 68:16.04.

Dosage and Administration

■ **Administration** Estrogens may be administered orally, parenterally, intravaginally, or topically.

■ **Dosage** Dosage equivalencies for estrogens have not been clearly established, and reported comparative values vary greatly. The dosage range of estrogens is generally wide, and dosage should be individualized according to the condition being treated and the response and tolerance of the patient. To minimize the risk of adverse effects, the lowest possible effective dosage and the shortest duration of therapy consistent with treatment goals and risks for the individual woman should be used. When estrogen therapy is used in the management of vasomotor symptoms or vulvar and vaginal atrophy associated with menopause, the lowest dosage that will control such symptoms should be used. When short-term estrogen therapy is indicated (e.g., for the management of vasomotor symptoms associated with menopause vulvar and vaginal atrophy), therapy should be discontinued as soon as possible; attempts to reduce dosage or discontinue the drug should be made at 3- to 6-month intervals.

Estrogen therapy is administered in a continuous daily regimen or, alternatively, estrogens are administered cyclically. When estrogens are administered cyclically, the drugs are usually given once daily for 3 weeks, followed by 1 week without the drugs, and then this regimen is repeated as necessary. While estrogen therapy alone may be appropriate in women who have undergone a hysterectomy, a progestin generally is added to estrogen therapy in women with an intact uterus. Addition of a progestin for 10 or more days of a cycle of estrogen administration or daily with estrogen in a continuous regimen reduces the incidence of endometrial hyperplasia and the attendant risk of endometrial carcinoma in women with an intact uterus. Morphologic and biochemical studies of the endometrium suggest that 10–13 days of progestin are needed to provide maximum maturation of the endometrium and to eliminate any hyperplastic changes. When a progestin is used in conjunction with estrogen therapy, the usual precautions associated with progestin therapy should be observed. Clinicians prescribing progestins should be aware of the risks associated with these drugs and the manufacturers' labeling should be consulted. The choice and dosage of a progestin may be important factors in minimizing potential adverse effects.

As an alternative to progestins, the use of bazedoxifene (an estrogen agonist-antagonist) in fixed combination with conjugated estrogens reduces the risk of endometrial hyperplasia. When bazedoxifene is used in fixed combination with estrogen therapy, the usual precautions associated with bazedoxifene therapy should be observed.

Cautions

Numerous adverse effects have been reported in patients receiving estrogens and these may be similar to the adverse effects associated with estrogen-progestin oral contraceptives. Most of the serious adverse effects of estrogen-progestin oral contraceptives (e.g., thromboembolic disorders, hepatocellular adenoma) generally have not been associated with postmenopausal estrogen therapy, which may reflect the comparatively low dosages of estrogens used in postmenopausal women. When larger dosages of estrogen are used (e.g., for the palliative treatment of carcinoma of the breast or prostate), an increased risk of the serious adverse effects may occur. For additional information on the adverse effects, precautions, and contraindications associated with estrogens, see Cautions in Estrogen-Progestin Combinations 68:12.

■ **GI Effects** Nausea has been frequently associated with estrogen therapy. Other adverse GI effects include vomiting, abdominal cramps, bloating, and diarrhea. Changes in appetite and changes in weight may also occur.

In patients with hypertriglyceridemia, estrogen therapy may be associated with further increases in plasma triglycerides resulting in pancreatitis and other complications. If acute pancreatitis occurs, estrogens should be discontinued. The risk of gallbladder disease appears to be increased 2- to 4-fold in postmenopausal women receiving estrogen replacement therapy. In one study, an increased risk of gallbladder disease occurred after 2 years of use of the drugs and doubled after 4 or 5 years of use. In another study, an increased risk of gallbladder disease was apparent between 6–12 months of use.

■ **Dermatologic Effects** The most frequent adverse dermatologic reaction associated with estrogen therapy is chloasma or melasma. Women who have had melasma during pregnancy appear to be most susceptible. Irregular brown macules may develop slowly on the face within 1 month to 2 years following initiation of estrogen therapy. The macules fade more slowly than in melasma gravidarum and may be permanent.

Other dermatologic reactions include erythema multiforme, erythema nodosum, and hemorrhagic eruption. Hirsutism and alopecia have also occurred. Porphyria cutanea has reportedly been adversely affected in some women receiving estrogen therapy.

■ **Cardiovascular Effects** In the absence of comparable data, the cardiovascular risks identified in the Women's Health Initiative (WHI) study with conjugated estrogens 0.625 mg daily alone or in conjunction with medroxyprogesterone acetate 2.5 mg daily should be assumed to be similar for other dosages of these drugs as well as for other combinations of estrogens and progestins.

Elevated Blood Pressure There is no evidence that estrogen replacement therapy in postmenopausal women is associated with elevated blood pressure; in fact, unopposed estrogen therapy in postmenopausal women has been associated with blood pressure reductions in some studies. However, increases in blood pressure may occur in some women receiving estrogens, particularly if high dosages are used. Blood pressure elevations are usually minor, but clinically important hypertension may occur in some women. Elevated blood pressure may gradually decrease or persist after discontinuance of estrogen therapy. The precise cause of increased blood pressure is not known, but it may result from a stimulatory effect of estrogen on the renin-angiotensin system.

Women receiving high dosages of estrogens or those with a history of hypertension, preexisting renal disease, a history of toxemia or elevated blood pressure during pregnancy, a familial tendency toward hypertension or its consequences, or a history of excessive weight gain or fluid retention during the menstrual cycle may be at increased risk of developing elevated blood pressure during estrogen therapy and, therefore, should be monitored closely. Even though elevated blood pressure may remain within the normal range, the clinical implications of elevations should be considered in all patients. All women, but particularly those with other risk factors for cardiovascular disease or stroke and those receiving high dosages of estrogens, should have blood pressure measurements before an estrogen is prescribed and at regular intervals during therapy. Estrogens should be discontinued if the patient becomes hypertensive during therapy.

Results of a recent controlled study (WHI study) indicate that hormone replacement therapy, specifically conjugated estrogens 0.625 mg in conjunction with medroxyprogesterone acetate 2.5 mg daily, is associated with a small increase in the risk of cardiovascular disease. In the WHI estrogen plus progestin study, there was a 29% increase in the incidence of heart disease in postmenopausal women receiving hormone replacement therapy compared with those receiving placebo. The number of coronary heart disease (CHD) events (e.g., myocardial infarction [MI]) per 10,000 patient-years of exposure was 37 or 30 in women receiving hormone replacement therapy or placebo, respectively. In the WHI estrogen-alone study, ERT did not affect the incidence of CHD.

Thromboembolic Disorders Oral contraceptive use is associated with an increased risk of thromboembolic and thrombotic disorders including thrombophlebitis, pulmonary embolism, stroke, subarachnoid hemorrhage, and MI. Retinal thrombosis and mesenteric thrombosis also have been reported in women receiving oral contraceptives. An increased risk of postsurgery thromboembolic complications has also been reported in patients receiving oral contraceptives.

Estrogen replacement therapy and hormone (estrogen/progestin) replacement therapy are associated with an increased risk of venous thromboembolic events. Results of some studies indicate that the risk of venous thromboembolic events with estrogen or hormone replacement therapy is about 2–3 times greater than that in women not receiving such therapy. In the WHI estrogen plus progestin study, the rate of venous thromboembolism, deep-vein thrombosis, or pulmonary embolism in women receiving hormone replacement therapy was twice the rate of these events in women receiving placebo. The number of cases of venous thromboembolism per 10,000 patient-years of exposure was 34 or 16 in women receiving hormone replacement therapy or placebo, respectively. In the WHI estrogen-alone study, the incidence of deep-vein thrombosis was increased in women receiving estrogen compared with women receiving placebo. Venous thrombosis is more likely to occur during the first year of therapy; patients with risk factors for thrombosis are at increased risk of venous thrombosis.

Data are conflicting on whether estrogen therapy alone or in combination with progestins is associated with an increased risk of stroke. While some studies suggest that estrogen replacement therapy may be associated with both an increased and a decreased risk of stroke in postmenopausal women, results from a large prospective study (the Nurses' Health Study) indicate no association between risk of stroke and use of estrogen replacement therapy either alone or in combination with progestins. In the WHI estrogen plus progestin study, there was a 41% increase in the incidence of stroke in postmenopausal women receiving hormone replacement therapy compared with those receiving placebo. The number of cases of stroke per 10,000 patient-years of exposure was 29 or 21 in women receiving hormone replacement therapy or placebo, respectively. In the WHI estrogen-alone study, there was a 39% increase in the incidence of stroke in women receiving estrogen compared with those receiving placebo. Approximately 80% of all strokes in the WHI estrogen-alone study were ischemic strokes. The number of cases of stroke per 10,000 patient-years of exposure was 44 or 32 in women receiving ERT or placebo, respectively; this represents an absolute excess risk of 12 additional strokes per 10,000 patient-years. The American Heart Association (AHA) states that hormone therapy should not be used to prevent stroke in postmenopausal women.

In a study in men, large dosages (i.e., 5 mg daily) of conjugated estrogens have been shown to increase the risk of nonfatal MI, pulmonary embolism, and thrombophlebitis.

The clinician and the patient using estrogens should be alert to the earliest signs and symptoms of thromboembolic and thrombotic disorders (e.g., thrombophlebitis, pulmonary embolism, cerebrovascular insufficiency, coronary occlusion, retinal thrombosis, mesenteric thrombosis). Estrogen therapy should be discontinued immediately when any of these disorders occurs or is suspected. (See Cautions: Precautions and Contraindications.)

Other Cardiovascular Effects Estrogens may cause some degree of fluid retention. Estrogen therapy should therefore be used with caution in patients with conditions that might be aggravated by fluid retention. (See Cautions: Precautions and Contraindications.)

■ Endocrine and Metabolic Effects Endocrine function test results (e.g., glucose tolerance, thyroid function) may be altered in patients receiving large dosages of estrogens. (See Laboratory Test Interferences.)

Decreased glucose tolerance has occurred in women receiving estrogen-containing oral contraceptives and may occur in patients receiving large dosages of estrogens. Prediabetic and diabetic patients should be carefully monitored during estrogen therapy.

Increased serum triglyceride concentrations have occurred in some women receiving estrogen-containing oral contraceptives and may occur during therapy with estrogens. The clinical importance of these alterations in lipid and lipoprotein concentrations has not been established; however, women with elevated serum lipid concentrations who have decided to use estrogens in combination with progestins should be monitored closely.

Estrogens have reportedly caused severe hypercalcemia in patients with breast cancer and bone metastases. If severe hypercalcemia occurs, estrogen therapy should be discontinued and appropriate therapy to decrease serum calcium concentration should be instituted.

Estrogen therapy should be used with caution in women with hypoparathyroidism because estrogen-induced hypocalcemia may occur.

■ Hepatic Effects Liver function test results may be altered in patients receiving estrogen therapy; if results of these tests are abnormal, they should be repeated 2 months after discontinuance of the drug. Increased sulfobromophthalein retention has reportedly occurred in women receiving estrogen-containing oral contraceptives, as a result of interference with the transfer of dye conjugates from liver cells into bile; uptake, conjugation, and storage do not appear to be affected. Less frequently, increased serum aminotransferase and alkaline phosphatase concentrations have occurred. Liver function test results usually return to normal within several weeks after estrogen-containing oral contraceptives are discontinued; occasionally, however, abnormal test results may persist for longer periods. The possibility that these alterations in liver function test results may occur in patients receiving estrogens should be considered.

Cholestatic jaundice has been reported in women receiving estrogen-containing oral contraceptives, and the possibility that this effect may occur during estrogen therapy should be considered. Cholestasis is manifested by the development of malaise, anorexia, and pruritus about 2 weeks to 2 months after the start of therapy. Occasionally, arthralgia, fever, and rash may occur. Serum bilirubin may range from 3–10 mg/dL and is mostly conjugated. Women with a history of jaundice during pregnancy have an increased risk of jaundice recurrence while receiving estrogen-containing oral contraceptives. If jaundice occurs during estrogen therapy, the drug should be discontinued. Estrogens may precipitate hepatic forms of porphyria, and the drugs probably should not be used by women who have a familial history of hepatic porphyrias, since the occurrence of these conditions appears to be genetically determined. Steroid hormones (including estrogens) may be poorly metabolized in patients with hepatic dysfunction; therefore, estrogens should be administered with caution to these individuals.

Liver tumors have been associated with use of estrogen-containing oral contraceptives. Liver tumors have been benign or malignant and have occurred during short-term and long-term use of oral contraceptives. Most commonly, liver tumors are benign hepatocellular adenomas and occur only rarely in oral contraceptive users; however, they may result in death because their vascularity predisposes them to rupture and cause massive hemorrhage. Although benign hepatocellular adenomas have not been reported to date with estrogens, the possibility of a liver tumor should be considered in any patient receiving an estrogen who develops sudden severe abdominal pain or shock.

■ Genitourinary Effects Breakthrough bleeding, spotting, changes in menstrual flow, missed menses (during use), or amenorrhea (after use) may occur in women receiving estrogen therapy. Dysmenorrhea and a premenstrual-like syndrome also have been reported. In patients with breakthrough bleeding or irregular vaginal bleeding, nonfunctional causes should be considered. Appropriate diagnostic procedures should be performed in patients with undiagnosed persistent or recurrent vaginal bleeding.

Changes in cervical erosion and secretions may occur during estrogen therapy. In addition, preexisting uterine leiomyoma may increase in size in women receiving estrogens. A cystitis-like syndrome has been reported but has not been definitely attributed to estrogens. An increased incidence of *Candida* vaginitis has been associated with estrogen therapy.

The possibility that estrogen replacement therapy in postmenopausal women, particularly prolonged use, may be associated with an increased risk of endometrial or ovarian cancer should be considered. (See Cautions: Mutagenicity and Carcinogenicity.)

■ Nervous System Effects Mental depression may occur in patients receiving estrogens. In a few women receiving estrogen-containing oral contraceptives, mental depression was severe and led to suicidal behavior. Patients with a history of mental depression should be observed carefully and estrogens discontinued if severe depression recurs during use.

Dizziness, changes in libido, and chorea have been reported in patients receiving estrogens.

Headache, especially migraine headache, may occur during estrogen therapy. Estrogens should be discontinued and the cause evaluated when migraine occurs or is exacerbated, or when a new headache pattern develops that is recurrent, persistent, and/or severe.

■ Ocular Effects Estrogens have been reported to produce keratoconus (steepening or corneal curvature) and intolerance to contact lenses. Contact lens wearers who develop visual disturbances or changes in lens tolerance during estrogen therapy should be assessed by an ophthalmologist; temporary or permanent cessation of contact lens wear should be considered.

Retinal vascular thrombosis has been reported in patients receiving estrogens. If unexplained, sudden or gradual, partial or complete loss of vision; proptosis or diplopia; papilledema; or retinal vascular lesions occur during therapy with an estrogen, the drug should be discontinued and appropriate diagnostic and therapeutic measures instituted.

■ Hematologic Effects Changes in various blood factors and blood components have been observed in women receiving estrogen-containing oral contraceptives and may occur in patients receiving estrogens; however, further studies are required before the clinical importance of these changes can be established. Estrogen (ERT) and hormone replacement therapy (estrogen/progestin, HRT) are associated with an increased risk of venous thromboembolic events in postmenopausal women. Increases in prothrombin and blood coagulation factors VII, VIII, IX, and X levels may occur in patients receiving estrogens; decreases in antithrombin III activity and decreased fibrinolysis also have been reported. In a clinical study in patients receiving conjugated estrogens in conjunction with medroxyprogesterone acetate, factors VII and X concentrations and plasminogen activity were increased and antithrombin III activity usually was decreased following 1 year of therapy. Estrogens may also enhance norepinephrine-induced platelet aggregation.

■ Other Adverse Effects Breast changes, including tenderness, enlargement, and secretion, may occur during estrogen therapy. The incidence of breast pain may be increased in patients receiving estrogens in conjunction with progestins compared with those receiving estrogens alone; breast pain was reported in about 33% of women receiving conjugated estrogens concomitantly with medroxyprogesterone acetate compared to 12% of women receiving unopposed conjugated estrogen therapy.

■ Precautions and Contraindications Use of estrogens may be associated with an increased risk of several serious conditions including deep-vein thrombosis, stroke, MI, pulmonary embolism, liver tumor, gallbladder disease, visual disturbances, and malignancy. Clinicians prescribing estrogens should be aware of the risks associated with the use of estrogens; the manufacturers' labeling also should be consulted for further discussion of these risks and associated precautions. When estrogens are used in combination with other drugs (e.g., androgens, progestins, bazedoxifene), the usual precautions associated with the other drugs should also be observed. If a progestin is administered concomitantly with estrogen therapy, potential risks may include adverse effects on lipid metabolism, glucose tolerance, or possible enhancement of mitotic activity in breast epithelial tissue.

Because of the potential increased risk of cardiovascular events, breast cancer, and venous thromboembolic events, estrogen and estrogen/progestin therapy should be limited to the lowest effective doses and shortest duration of therapy consistent with treatment goals and risks for the individual woman. Therapy with estrogen, estrogen/progestin, or conjugated estrogens in fixed combination with bazedoxifene should be periodically reevaluated.

Patients receiving estrogens should be under the supervision of a physician who should inform them of the possible risks involved. Patients receiving estrogens should also be given a copy of the patient labeling for the drugs.

A complete medical and family history should be taken prior to initiation of estrogen therapy and periodically thereafter. Estrogens should generally not be prescribed for longer than 1 year without a repeat physical examination being performed. Physical examination should include special attention to blood pressure, breasts, abdomen, and pelvic organs and should include a Papanicolaou test (Pap smear) and relevant laboratory tests.

Patients receiving estrogens should be informed to notify their physician if signs or symptoms of thromboembolic or thrombotic disorders (e.g., thrombophlebitis, pulmonary embolism, cerebrovascular insufficiency, coronary occlusion, retinal thrombosis, mesenteric thrombosis) occur, including sudden severe headache or vomiting, disturbance of vision or speech, sudden partial or complete loss of vision, dizziness or faintness, weakness or numbness in an extremity, sharp or crushing chest pain, unexplained cough, hemoptysis, sudden shortness of breath, calf pain, or heaviness in the chest. If signs or symptoms consistent with a thromboembolic or thrombotic disorder occur, hormone replacement therapy (HRT) should be discontinued immediately. Use of ERT or HRT is not advised in women with a history of stroke or transient ischemic attacks. If hormone therapy is initiated or discontinued in a woman receiving oral anticoagulant therapy, effectiveness of the anticoagulant may be altered and dosage adjustment needed. Patients receiving estrogens should also be advised to inform their physician if abdominal pain, swelling, or tenderness (indicating possible gallbladder disease), or an abdominal mass (indicating a possible liver tumor), jaundice, severe mental depression, or unusual bleeding occurs. Since endometrial hyperplasia and endometrial carcinoma have been reported in women receiving estrogen therapy, adequate diagnostic tests should be performed in women with undiagnosed, persistent, or recurring abnormal vaginal bleeding. (See Carcinogenicity.) Women receiving estrogens should be instructed in self-examination of their breasts and should report lumps in the breast to their physician.

Estrogens should be used with caution, and only with careful monitoring, in patients with conditions that might be aggravated by fluid retention (e.g., cardiac or renal insufficiency); in patients with cerebrovascular or coronary artery disease (including MI); and in women with a strong family history of breast cancer or who have breast nodules, fibrocystic disease, or abnormal mammographic findings (see Cautions: Carcinogenicity).

Women undergoing surgery and those with fracture or who are immobilized have a relatively high risk of venous thromboembolic events. Therefore, estrogens should be discontinued, whenever feasible, at least 4–6 weeks prior to surgery that is associated with an increased risk of thromboembolism or prolonged immobilization. The decision as to when to resume estrogen therapy following major surgery or immobilization should be based on the risks of postsurgery thromboembolic complications and the need for such therapy. In addition, some clinicians recommend that women discontinue estrogen replacement therapy during immobilization due to fracture, stroke, or other severe illness; estrogen replacement therapy can be restarted when normal activity is resumed. Since acute pancreatitis, associated with increased triglyceride concentrations, has been reported in a few women receiving estrogens alone or in conjunction with a progestin, it is recommended that serum lipid concentrations be monitored prior to and during estrogen therapy. (See Cautions: GI Effects.)

Because estrogens influence the metabolism of calcium and phosphorus, the drugs should be used with caution in patients with renal insufficiency and in patients with metabolic bone diseases that are associated with hypercalcemia.

Metabolism of estrogens may be decreased in patients with impaired hepatic function. Caution is advised in patients with a history of cholestatic jaundice associated with estrogen use or pregnancy; if cholestatic jaundice recurs, estrogen therapy should be discontinued.

Estrogens may exacerbate asthma, diabetes mellitus, epilepsy, migraine, porphyria, systemic lupus erythematosus, and hepatic hemangiomas and should be used with caution in women with these conditions. Estrogens also may exacerbate symptoms of angioedema in women with hereditary angioedema.

Estrogens are contraindicated in patients with known or suspected pregnancy, undiagnosed abnormal genital bleeding, known or suspected breast cancer or a history of breast cancer (except when used for the palliative treatment of metastatic disease in appropriately selected individuals), or known or suspected estrogen-dependent neoplasia. Estrogens also are contraindicated in patients with active deep-vein thrombosis or pulmonary embolism; a history of deep-vein thrombosis or pulmonary embolism; active or recent (within the past year) arterial thromboembolic disease (e.g., stroke, MI); liver disease or impairment; known protein C, protein S, or antithrombin deficiency, or other known thrombophilic disorders; or known hypersensitivity to estrogen or any ingredient in the formulation.

■ **Pediatric Precautions** Estrogen therapy has been used for the induction of puberty in adolescents with some forms of pubertal delay. Safety and efficacy of estrogens in children have not otherwise been established. Estrogen therapy should be used with caution in young individuals in whom bone growth is not yet complete, since estrogens may cause premature closure of the epiphyses.

■ **Geriatric Precautions** When the total number of patients studied in the Women's Health Initiative (WHI) study is considered, 44–46% were 65 years of age or older, while 6.6–7.1% were 75 years of age or older. In the estrogen plus progestin WHI study, there was a higher relative risk of nonfatal stoke or breast cancer in women 75 years of age or older compared with women younger than 75 years of age.

■ **Carcinogenicity** Prolonged continuous administration of natural or synthetic estrogen in certain animal species increases the frequency of certain benign or malignant tumors including those of the breast, cervix, uterus, vagina, ovary, pituitary, and liver.

Endometrial Cancer Several studies have shown an increased relative risk of endometrial carcinoma in postmenopausal women who received prolonged estrogen replacement therapy for relief of menopausal symptoms. This risk was independent of other known risk factors for endometrial carcinoma and appeared to depend on duration and dosage of estrogen therapy. While there appears to be no increased risk of endometrial carcinoma in postmenopausal women receiving estrogen therapy for less than 1 year, prolonged estrogen therapy may be associated with an increased risk of such carcinoma. The risk of endometrial carcinoma reportedly is increased 2- to 12-fold in postmenopausal women receiving unopposed estrogen therapy compared with those not receiving estrogens; such increased risk may depend on dosage and duration of therapy and may be 15- to 24-fold higher in women receiving long-term (5 years or more) estrogen therapy. Limited data indicate that a substantial increased risk of endometrial carcinoma may persist for up to 15 years following discontinuance of estrogen therapy. Because of the increased risk of endometrial carcinoma associated with prolonged estrogen therapy, patients receiving prolonged treatment with the drugs should be evaluated at least twice yearly to reassess the need for continued therapy. Results of several studies indicate that when progestins are used concomitantly with estrogen replacement therapy, the incidence of endometrial hyperplasia and endometrial carcinoma is reduced substantially. In a randomized, controlled, multicenter study in postmenopausal women, endometrial hyperplasia occurred in 20 or 1% or less of women receiving estrogen therapy alone or in conjunction with progestins, respectively. In the WHI study, the incidence of endometrial carcinoma in women receiving hormone replacement therapy (conjugated estrogens 0.625 mg in conjunction with medroxyprogesterone acetate 2.5 mg daily) was similar to the incidence in women receiving placebo. As an alternative to progestins, the use of bazedoxifene (an estrogen agonist-antagonist) in fixed combination with conjugated estrogens reduces the risk of endometrial hyperplasia, which may be a precursor to endometrial carcinoma.

Although estrogen-associated risk of endometrial carcinoma is substantially reduced when estrogens are administered concomitantly with progestins or bazedoxifene, a risk still exists. Therefore, clinical surveillance and evaluation of all menopausal women receiving estrogen therapy is essential. Diagnostic tests, including endometrial sampling when indicated, should be performed to rule out malignancy in all women who have undiagnosed, persistent, or abnormal vaginal bleeding.

Currently, there is no evidence that estrogens derived from natural sources are more or less hazardous than synthetic estrogens at equiestrogenic dosages.

Breast Cancer All women receiving estrogens should perform monthly self-examinations of their breasts and be monitored at least annually by a health-care provider for breast abnormalities and more frequently if there are any signs and symptoms. Periodic mammography should be scheduled based on patient age, risk factors, and prior mammogram results. Women with a strong family history of breast cancer or who have breast nodules, fibrocystic disease, or abnormal mammographic findings should be monitored particularly closely if they elect to use estrogens. Although the clinical importance remains to be established, therapy with estrogen/progestin increases mammographic breast density relative to therapy with estrogen alone or placebo.

Because breast tissue is sensitive to reproductive hormones, there has been long-standing concern about the risk of breast cancer in women receiving hormone replacement therapy (HRT). The estrogen/progestin arm of the WHI study recently was terminated prematurely because of an increased incidence of breast cancer in women receiving HRT. In the WHI study, the risk of invasive breast cancer was 26% higher in women receiving HRT (conjugated estrogens 0.625 mg in conjunction with medroxyprogesterone acetate 2.5 mg daily) compared with those receiving placebo; the estimated hazard ratio for breast cancer was 1.26. While there have been several observational studies evaluating the risk of breast cancer in women receiving HRT, conclusions are limited by healthy-user bias; variations in specific preparations, dosage, and duration of therapy; and differences in the methods used to determine breast cancer end points. In aggregate, breast cancer incidence is slightly increased among current (relative risk: 1.21–1.4) or long-term (longer than 5 years) recipients (relative risk: 1.23–1.35) compared with nonusers. Based on these findings, recommendations on the appropriate use of hormone therapy have been revised. Because the risks of hormone therapy exceed the benefits for the prevention of chronic diseases in postmenopausal women, experts state that ERT or HRT should not be used for the prevention of chronic conditions in postmenopausal women. The American Heart Association (AHA), the American College of Obstetricians and Gynecologists (ACOG), FDA, and manufacturers recommend that hormone therapy not be used to prevent heart disease in healthy women (primary prevention) or to protect women with preexisting heart disease (secondary prevention). ACOG, FDA, and the manufacturers also recommend that women receiving hormone therapy solely for the prevention of postmenopausal osteoporosis consider alternative therapy (e.g., alendronate, raloxifene, risedronate).

The decision to use estrogen or estrogen/progestin for management of menopausal symptoms should be individualized taking into account the women's preference, her risk for specific chronic diseases, and the presence and severity of menopausal symptoms.

Results of a large (involving more than 100,000 women) prospective cohort study (the Nurses' Health Study) in postmenopausal women who received conjugated estrogens indicated an increased risk of breast cancer in such women; in addition, an increased risk of breast cancer also was observed in individuals who received estrogen therapy in conjunction with progestins. The relative risk of breast cancer increased with age and duration of therapy, with the greatest risk being observed in women 60–64 years of age and in women who received estrogen replacement therapy for more than 10 years. In women receiving estrogens alone or in conjunction with progestins, the relative risk of developing breast cancer was 1.32 or 1.41, respectively. The relative risk of breast cancer was similar in women who had never received estrogen replacement therapy, women who received prior estrogen therapy, and women who received estrogen therapy for less than 5 years; however, the relative risk of developing breast cancer increased to 1.63 in women 60–64 years who received estrogens for at least 5 years. Results of this study also indicated that the relative risk of developing breast cancer was similar in women with and without a family history of the disease; consumption of alcohol did not affect results.

Data from the Nurses' Health Study, the Breast Cancer Detection Demonstration Project, and other studies indicate that estrogen/progestin regimens are associated with an increased risk of breast cancer beyond that associated with estrogen alone. In the Breast Cancer Detection Demonstration Project (a study that included 46,000 women), the relative risk of breast cancer in women who received estrogen or estrogen/progestin within the previous 4 years was 1.2 or 1.4, respectively. Similar to results from other studies, the increased risk was generally limited to current or recent recipients and was related to duration of use. The relative risk (adjusted for mammographic screening, age at menopause, body mass index [BMI], education, age) increased by 0.01 with each year of estrogen use and by 0.08 with each year of estrogen/progestin use in recent recipients. Among recent recipients of progestin for fewer than 15 days per month, the relative risk of breast cancer associated with therapy for less than 4 years was 1.1 while the relative risk associated with therapy for longer than 4 years was 1.5; estimates for risk were not available for recipients of progestins for 15 or more days per month due to insufficient data. The relative risk of breast cancer in recent recipients of estrogen or estrogen/progestin increased 0.03 or 0.12, respectively, each year in women with a BMI of 24.4 kg/m^2 or less; an increase in risk associated with duration of use was not observed in heavier women.

The WHI, a long-term study sponsored by the National Institutes of Health (NIH), followed 16,608 predominantly healthy women with an intact uterus who were 50–79 years of age and who received HRT (i.e., conjugated estrogens 0.625 mg in conjunction with medroxyprogesterone acetate 2.5 mg daily) or placebo with the goal of evaluating the relationship between HRT and coronary heart disease (CHD), stroke, pulmonary embolism, breast cancer, endometrial carcinoma, colorectal cancer, hip fracture, and death from other causes. The study was stopped early because health risks exceeded benefits over an average follow-up of 5.2 years. At the time the study was stopped, the increased number of cases of invasive breast cancer, CHD, stroke, and pulmonary embolism in the estrogen/ progestin group relative to the placebo group was not counterbalanced by reductions in the number of cases of hip fracture and colorectal cancer. The WHI study is the first randomized, controlled study to confirm that estrogen/progestin therapy increases the risk of breast cancer in postmenopausal women and to quantify the risk. In the WHI estrogen plus progestin study, the risk of invasive breast cancer was 26% higher in women receiving HRT (conjugated estrogens 0.625 mg in conjunction with medroxyprogesterone acetate 2.5 mg daily) compared with those receiving placebo; the estimated hazard ratio for breast cancer was 1.26. The number of cases of breast cancer per 10,000 patient-years of exposure was 38 or 30 in women receiving HRT or placebo, respectively. The increase in breast cancer risk was apparent after 4 years of estrogen/progestin therapy, and the risk appeared to be cumulative. In addition, the risk associated with HRT appeared to increase at a higher rate than would be expected based on advancing age. The hazard ratio for HRT was not higher in women with a family history or other risk factors for breast cancer, except for prior postmenopausal hormone therapy. In the WHI estrogen-alone study, use of estrogen was not associated with an increased risk of breast cancer.

Whether the effect of hormone replacement therapy on breast cancer incidence varies among histologic types of invasive carcinomas remains to be established. Findings from the Breast Cancer Detection Demonstration Project and the WHI estrogen plus progestin study indicate that such therapy is associated with an increase in risk for the majority of invasive tumors classified as lobular and/or ductal carcinomas. Findings from other studies indicate that estrogen/progestin therapy is associated with an increased risk of invasive lobular carcinoma. While data from some studies (e.g., the Iowa Women's Health Study) suggest that estrogen/progestin therapy is associated with an increased risk of invasive breast cancer with a favorable prognosis, findings from the WHI indicate that such therapy is associated with cancers that are at least as invasive as those in women not receiving estrogen/progestin therapy. Analysis of breast cancer characteristics in women enrolled in the WHI indicate that the invasive breast cancers diagnosed in women receiving estrogen/progestin were similar in histology and grade but were larger (1.7 versus 1.5 cm, respectively) and were at a more advanced grade (regional/metastatic disease in 25.4 versus 16%, respectively) than those diagnosed in women receiving placebo.

The US Department of Health and Human Services 1985 DES Task Force concluded that the weight of evidence to date indicates that women who used diethylstilbestrol (DES) during pregnancy may subsequently experience an increased risk of breast cancer; however, because of limitations of current data and study methodologies, a causal relationship to the drug has not been established. Data from studies to date suggest an overall relative risk of breast cancer for DES-treated women ranging from 1.2–1.5 times that for untreated women, an excess risk that is similar to that associated with a number of other breast cancer risk factors; however, in epidemiologic analyses, these levels of excess risk are difficult to evaluate since various sources of bias that could be responsible for such excesses cannot be easily ruled out. It should be noted that conclusions regarding the likelihood of causality for this association between DES use and breast cancer could be substantially influenced by further follow-up of exposed women who have already been identified and studied and by initiation of studies of other exposed women which pay particular attention to matching DES-exposed and unexposed groups based on indications for DES use, to evaluating dose-latency relationships, and to the possibility of bias toward early diagnosis of breast cancer among exposed women. Initiation of studies that investigate interactions with other risk factors, considering possible additive and cumulative risks, and endocrinologic and immunologic considerations may also influence conclusions about the likelihood of causality.

Ovarian Cancer While findings from epidemiologic (e.g., case-control) studies on the association between postmenopausal hormone replacement therapy and the risk of ovarian cancer have been inconsistent, results from 2 large, prospective cohort studies with average follow-up of 13–14 years indicate that postmenopausal estrogen use is associated with an increased risk of ovarian cancer.

In the American Cancer Society's Cancer Prevention Study II, which included over 200,000 postmenopausal women, women receiving oral estrogen replacement therapy at study entry (baseline) had higher death rates from ovarian cancer (adjusted rate ratio: 1.51) than women who had never received estrogen replacement therapy. Duration of estrogen use also was associated with increased risk; women who received estrogen replacement therapy for 10 or more years and who were receiving such therapy at baseline were more than twice as likely to have died from ovarian cancer as never users (adjusted rate ratio: 2.2). Estrogen use for less than 10 years was not associated with an increased risk of ovarian cancer mortality. Among women who discontinued estrogen after 10 or more years of use, the risk decreased with time; the adjusted rate ratio was 2.05 in those who received estrogen within the previous 15 years and 1.31 in those who had not received estrogen within the previous 15 years. Whether women receiving oral estrogen also received progestin was not evaluated in this study; however, most hormone replacement regimens for postmenopausal women contained only estrogenic compounds until the late 1970's and most women receiving hormone replacement therapy in 1982 (baseline) presumably were receiving unopposed estrogen therapy.

Data from the Breast Cancer Detection Demonstration Project also indicate that estrogen replacement therapy is associated with an increased risk of developing ovarian cancer and that the risk associated with estrogen-only hormone replacement therapy is greater than that associated with estrogen-progestin replacement therapy. In a study in over 40,000 postmenopausal women, those who received estrogen-only hormone replacement therapy were twice as likely to develop ovarian cancer as never users (adjusted relative risk: 2) with a lower risk (adjusted relative risk: 1.3) in women who received estrogen-progestin replacement therapy. Although the lifetime risk of ovarian cancer is low (1.7%), any increase in risk of ovarian cancer related to long-term estrogen therapy should be considered in the risk/benefit assessment of such therapy.

GI Cancers Data from observational studies, the Heart and Estrogen/progestin Replacement Study (HERS), and the WHI estrogen plus progestin study indicate that hormone replacement therapy reduces the incidence of colorectal cancer. In the WHI estrogen plus progestin study, the risk of colorectal cancer was reduced by 37% in women receiving hormone replacement therapy (conjugated estrogens 0.625 mg in conjunction with medroxyprogesterone acetate 2.5 mg daily) compared with those receiving placebo. The number of cases of colorectal cancer per 10,000 patient-years of exposure was 10 or 16 in women receiving hormone replacement therapy or placebo, respectively. Results from the WHI estrogen-alone study indicate that ERT (conjugated estrogens 0.625 mg daily) does not affect the incidence of colorectal cancer.

■ Pregnancy and Lactation

Estrogens can cause fetal harm when administered to pregnant women. *In utero* exposure of females to diethylstilbestrol (DES [no longer commercially available in the US]), a nonsteroidal estrogen, is associated with an increased risk of developing a rare form of vaginal or cervical cancer (clear-cell adenocarcinoma) in later life. In addition, such exposure to DES causes epithelial changes in the vagina and cervix in 30–90% of these exposed female offspring.

In utero exposure of females to DES is also associated with an increased risk of developing a rare form of vaginal or cervical cancer (clear-cell adenocarcinoma) in later life. In addition, such exposure to DES causes epithelial changes (adenosis) in the vagina and cervix in 30–90% of these exposed female offspring. Experience from the National Collaborative Diethylstilbestrol Adenosis (DESAD) Project indicates that women exposed to DES *in utero* appear to have an increased risk of dysplasia and carcinoma *in situ* of the cervix and vagina; the rate of these changes was 15.7 versus 7.9 cases per 1000 person-years of follow-up for exposed and unexposed women, respectively, and was even higher in exposed women with squamous metaplasia extending to the outer half of the cervix or onto the vagina. The 1985 DES Task Force concluded that, based on the results of the DESAD Project, women exposed to DES *in utero* may be at increased risk of cervical and vaginal dysplasia, particularly if they have extensive metaplasia; however, further documentation and evaluation of this association are necessary, and the relationship between DES exposure *in utero* and subsequent risk of squamous cell carcinoma of the cervix remains unclear.

In utero exposure to DES in females has not been associated with an increased risk of developing cancer other than an increased risk of developing vaginal or cervical clear-cell adenocarcinoma. *In utero* exposure of males to DES has been associated with an increased incidence of genital tract abnormalities including epididymal cysts, maldescended testes, hypoplastic testes, varicoceles, low sperm counts, and spermatozoal defects (e.g., decreased motility, possibly abnormal forms). Similar data are not available for other estrogens, but it cannot be presumed that they would not induce similar changes.

Although estrogens were previously used to treat threatened or habitual abortion, there is no evidence that estrogens are effective for these uses; in addition, the potential for adverse effects of the drugs on the fetus exists. Estrogens should not be used during pregnancy.

Administration of estrogens to nursing women has been associated with decreased amounts and lower quality of milk. In addition, detectable amounts of estrogens and progestins have been identified in milk of women receiving these drugs. Although estrogens were previously used for the prevention of postpartum breast engorgement, such use is no longer recommended. Caution is advised when estrogens are administered to nursing women. Conjugated estrogens in fixed combination with bazedoxifene should not be used in nursing women.

Drug Interactions

■ **Drugs Affecting Hepatic Microsomal Enzymes** Metabolism of estrogen is mediated in part by cytochrome P-450 (CYP) isoenzyme 3A4, and the possibility exists that drugs that induce or inhibit this isoenzyme may affect plasma estrogen concentrations. Concomitant use of estrogens with drugs that induce CYP3A4 (e.g., carbamazepine, phenobarbital, rifampin, St. John's wort [*Hypericum perforatum*]) may result in decreased plasma concentrations of estrogen, resulting in decreased therapeutic effects and/or changes in uterine bleeding profile. Concomitant use of estrogen with drugs or foods that inhibit CYP3A4 (e.g., clarithromycin, erythromycin, grapefruit juice, itraconazole, ketoconazole) may result in increased plasma concentrations of estrogens and an increase in the incidence of adverse effects.

Rifampin reportedly decreases estrogenic activity during concomitant use with estrogens. This effect has been attributed to enhanced metabolism of estrogen, presumably by induction of hepatic microsomal enzymes.

■ **Corticosteroids** Estrogens have been reported to enhance the anti-inflammatory effect of hydrocortisone in patients with chronic inflammatory skin diseases. It has been suggested that estrogens may decrease the hepatic metabolism of corticosteroids and/or alter serum corticosteroid protein binding. Patients receiving concomitant estrogen and corticosteroid therapy should be observed for signs of excessive corticosteroid effects, and alterations in corticosteroid dosage may be necessary when estrogens are started or discontinued.

■ **Oral Anticoagulants** Estrogens may decrease the action of oral anticoagulants. When estrogen therapy is initiated in patients receiving anticoagulants, an increase in anticoagulant dosage may be required.

Laboratory Test Interferences

Estrogen-containing oral contraceptives have caused abnormal thyroid function test results. (See Effects on Thyroid in Cautions: Endocrine and Metabolic Effects, in Estrogen-Progestin Combinations 68:12.) Estrogen-containing oral contraceptives have altered response to the metyrapone test (see Laboratory Test Interferences in Estrogen-Progestin Combinations 68:12) and liver function test results (see Cautions: Hepatic Effects, in Estrogen-Progestin Combinations 68:12). Estrogen-containing oral contraceptives have also caused decreased pregnanediol excretion.

The manufacturers state that the pathologist should be advised of estrogen use when relevant specimens from a patient exposed to estrogens are submitted.

Acute Toxicity

Acute overdosage of large doses of oral contraceptives in children reportedly produces almost no toxicity except nausea and vomiting. Acute overdosage of estrogens may cause nausea, and withdrawal bleeding may occur in females.

Pharmacology

Estrogens are hormones secreted principally by the ovarian follicles and also by the adrenals, corpus luteum, placenta, and testes, or are synthetic steroidal and nonsteroidal compounds. Estrogenic hormones are secreted at varying rates during the menstrual cycle throughout the period of activity of the ovaries. During pregnancy, the placenta becomes the main source of estrogens. At the menopause, ovarian secretion of estrogens declines at varying rates. The gonadotropins of the anterior pituitary regulate secretion of the ovarian hormones, estradiol and progesterone; hypothalamic control of pituitary gonadotropin production is in turn regulated by plasma concentrations of the estrogens and progesterone. This complex feedback system results in the cyclic phenomenon of ovulation and menstruation.

■ **Estrogen Receptors** Estrogens have an important role in the reproductive, skeletal, cardiovascular, and central nervous systems in women, and act principally by regulating gene expression. Biologic response is initiated when estrogen binds to a ligand-binding domain of the estrogen receptor resulting in a conformational change that leads to gene transcription through specific estrogen response elements (ERE) of target gene promoters; subsequent activation or repression of the target gene is mediated through 2 distinct transactivation domains (i.e., AF-1 and AF-2) of the receptor. The estrogen receptor also mediates gene transcription using different response elements (i.e., AP-1) and other signal pathways. Recent advances in the molecular pharmacology of estrogen and estrogen receptors have resulted in the development of selective estrogen receptor modulators (e.g., clomiphene, raloxifene, tamoxifen, toremifene), agents that bind and activate the estrogen receptor but that exhibit tissue-specific effects distinct from estrogen. Tissue-specific estrogen-agonist or -antagonist activity of these drugs appears to be related to structural differences in their estrogen receptor complex (e.g., specifically the surface topography of AF-2 for raloxifene) compared with the estrogen (estradiol)-estrogen receptor complex. A second estrogen receptor also has been identified, and existence of at least 2 estrogen receptors (ER_α, ER_β) may contribute to the tissue-specific activity of selective modulators. While the role of the estrogen receptor in bone, cardiovascular tissue, and the CNS continues to be studied, emerging evidence indicates that the mechanism of action of estrogen receptors in these tissues differs from the manner in which estrogen receptors function in reproductive tissue.

Intracellular cytosol-binding proteins for estrogens have been identified in estrogen-responsive tissues including the female genital organs, breasts, pituitary, and hypothalamus. The estrogen-binding protein complex (i.e., cytosol-binding protein and estrogen) distributes into the cell nucleus where it stimulates DNA, RNA, and protein synthesis. The presence of these receptor proteins is responsible for the palliative response to estrogen therapy in women with metastatic carcinoma of the breast.

■ **Estrogenic Effects** Exogenous estrogens elicit, to varying degrees, all the pharmacologic responses usually produced by endogenous estrogens. Endogenous estrogens are essential hormones that are responsible for the normal growth and development of the female sex organs and for maintenance of secondary sex characteristics, including the growth and maturation of the vagina, uterus, and fallopian tubes; enlargement of the breasts; maintenance of tone and elasticity of urogenital structures; growth of axillary and pubic hair; and pigmentation of the nipples and genitals.

Although the mechanism(s) has not been elucidated, estrogens contribute to the shaping of body contours and the skeleton, to the growth spurt that occurs during adolescence, and to the eventual termination of linear growth that results from fusion of the epiphyseal centers. Estrogens cause an increase in cell height and secretions of the cervical mucosa, thickening and cornification of the vaginal mucosa, proliferation of the endometrium, and an increase in uterine tone. The estrogen-stimulated endometrium may bleed within 48–72 hours after discontinuance of estrogen therapy. Paradoxically, prolonged estrogen therapy may cause shrinkage of the endometrium and an increase in size of the myometrium.

Menstrual Effects During the preovulatory or nonovulatory phase of the menstrual cycle, estrogen is the principal determinant in the onset of menstruation. A decline of estrogenic activity at the end of the menstrual cycle also may induce menstruation; however, the cessation of progesterone secretion is the most important factor during the mature ovulatory phase of the menstrual cycle.

Gonadotropic Effects Although the precise actions of estrogens on secretory activity of the pituitary have not been fully characterized, estrogens affect the release of gonadotropins (e.g., follicle-stimulating hormone [FSH]) from the pituitary, apparently as a result of feedback inhibition; the effect of estrogens on luteinizing hormone (LH) is complex and biphasic. The effects of estrogens on pituitary secretion of gonadotropins result in inhibition of lactation, inhibition of ovulation, development of a proliferative endometrium and, by inhibiting androgen secretion, a reduction of sebaceous secretions.

■ **Anabolic and Metabolic Effects** Estrogens have a weak anabolic effect and may cause sodium retention with associated fluid retention and edema. Estrogens also affect bone by increasing calcium deposition and accelerating epiphyseal closure, following initial growth stimulation.

■ **Cardiovascular Effects** Estrogens have generally favorable effects on blood cholesterol and phospholipid concentrations. Estrogens reduce LDL-cholesterol and increase HDL-cholesterol concentrations in a dose-related manner. The decrease in LDL-cholesterol concentrations associated with estrogen therapy appears to result from increased LDL catabolism, while the increase in triglyceride concentrations is caused by increased production of large, triglyceride-rich, very-low-density lipoproteins (VLDLs); changes in serum HDL-cholesterol concentrations appear to result principally from an increase in the cholesterol and apolipoprotein A-1 content of HDL_2- and a slight increase in HDL_3-cholesterol.

Results of several clinical studies in postmenopausal women indicate that replacement therapy with unopposed conjugated estrogens (estrogen replacement therapy, ERT) may reduce LDL-cholesterol and increase HDL-cholesterol by about 8–15%; however, use of progestins in conjunction with estrogen (hormone replacement therapy, HRT) may blunt these favorable effects on the lipid profile. In a 1-year prospective, randomized, double-blind study in healthy, postmenopausal, predominately white women at low risk for cardiovascular disease, HDL-cholesterol concentrations increased 14.1 or 4.4% in women receiving conjugated estrogens (0.625 mg daily) alone (ERT) or conjugated estrogens (0.625 mg daily) in conjunction with cyclic medroxyprogesterone acetate (5 mg daily on days 15–28 of the cycle) (HRT), respectively; decreases in LDL-cholesterol concentrations were similar in women receiving estrogens alone (ERT) or in conjunction with the progestin (HRT). In this study, serum triglyceride concentrations increased by 39.4 or 27.5% in women receiving estrogens alone (ERT) or in conjunction with the progestin (HRT), respectively. In addition, in a 3-year, placebo-controlled, multicenter study in postmenopausal women, HDL-cholesterol concentrations were higher in patients receiving conjugated estrogens alone (ERT) than in those receiving conjugated estrogens in conjunction with progestins (HRT); HDL-cholesterol concentrations were lower in patients receiving placebo than in those receiving estrogen replacement therapy. Concomitant progestin therapy blunts some of the favorable effects of estrogens on the lipid profile of postmenopausal women.

Although most experience to date on the lipid-lowering effect of estrogens included administration of conjugated estrogens, limited evidence indicates that postmenopausal women who received oral micronized estradiol (2 mg daily for 6 weeks) had changes in LDL- and HDL-cholesterol and triglyceride concentrations that were similar to those produced by low-dose conjugated estrogen therapy, but transdermal estradiol (0.1 mg twice weekly) did not substantially affect serum lipoprotein concentrations.

Other effects of estrogens that may contribute to effects on cardiovascular risk indicators include reduction of insulin and blood glucose concentrations and direct effects on blood vessels. Estrogen receptors have been identified in the heart and coronary arteries, suggesting that estrogens may have specific effects on these tissues.

The Women's Health Initiative (WHI) study provided evidence of increased cardiovascular risk associated with combined estrogen and progestin therapy (HRT). (See Cautions: Cardiovascular Effects.)

Pharmacokinetics

■ **Absorption** Following oral administration, the natural, unconjugated estrogens are inactivated in the GI tract and liver. Conjugated estrogens and some synthetic derivatives of the natural estrogens may be administered orally. Absorption and metabolism following oral administration of these drugs is rapid and daily doses are usually required. Chlorotrianisene (no longer commercially available in the US), however, has a prolonged duration of action which may result from the storage in and slow release of estrogenically active substance from adipose tissue. Similarly, quinestrol (no longer commercially available in the US) has a prolonged duration of action as a result of its extensive storage in and slow release from adipose tissue.

Following IM administration of estrogen oil solutions, absorption begins promptly and continues for several days. When estrogen is conjugated with aryl and alkyl groups, the rate of absorption of estrogen is slowed.

Estrogens are readily absorbed through the skin and mucous membranes. Depending on the amount of estrogen applied, systemic as well as local effects may occur following topical application.

■ **Distribution** Estrogens are distributed throughout most body tissues. Studies utilizing radioisotopes have indicated that the greatest concentrations of estrogens may occur in the fat deposits of the body; obese patients have demonstrated slower and more prolonged estrogen excretion. Estrogens are 50–80% bound to plasma proteins. Estriol is bound less to plasma proteins than is estrone or estradiol but all 3 estrogens are bound to approximately the same extent by erythrocytes. Studies using radioisotopes have demonstrated a rapid transfer of free estrone and estradiol between mother and fetus. Fetal estrogens appear to originate principally from the placenta and mother.

■ **Elimination** The steroidal estrogens are metabolized principally in the liver, although the kidneys, gonads, and muscle tissues may be involved to some extent. The steroids and their metabolites are conjugated at the hydroxyl group of the C 3 position with sulfuric or glucuronic acid; these conjugates may undergo further metabolic change. Conjugation increases water solubility and facilitates excretion in urine. Large amounts of free estrogens are also distributed into the bile, reabsorbed from the GI tract, and recirculated through the liver where further degradation occurs. Estrogens and their metabolites are excreted mainly in urine; however, small amounts are also present in feces.

The metabolic fate of the synthetic estrogens has not been fully elucidated. Diethylstilbestrol (no longer commercially available in the US) metabolism, however, appears to be similar to that of the natural estrogens with the drug being excreted mainly as the glucuronide in urine.

Chemistry

Estrogens are naturally occurring hormones or synthetic steroidal and nonsteroidal compounds with estrogenic activity. The estrogens can be divided into 2 groups based on their chemical structures: steroidal and nonsteroidal compounds. All naturally occurring estrogens are steroids that contain a cyclopentanoperhydrophenanthrene ring structure with an unsaturated A ring, a methyl group at the C 13 position, a phenolic hydroxyl group at the C 3 position, and a ketone or hydroxyl group at the C 17 position. Only a limited number of changes can be made in this basic steroid structure without losing estrogenic activity. These changes are limited to an interconversion of the hydroxyl and ketone groups or the addition of various side chains at the C 3 and C 17 positions.

The natural steroidal estrogens (estradiol, estrone, estriol, equilin, and equilenin) and their conjugates are usually obtained from pregnant mares' urine or prepared synthetically. The natural steroidal estrogens, both those obtained exclusively from natural sources and those prepared synthetically, are insoluble in water but when conjugated as the sulfates or glucuronides, these hormones become water soluble. Synthetic derivatives of the natural steroidal estrogens were previously available. The nonsteroidal estrogens include diethylstilbestrol (DES) (no longer commercially available in the US) and dienestrol (no longer commercially available in the US).

For further information on chemistry and stability, pharmacology, pharmacokinetics, uses, cautions, and dosage and administration of estrogens, see the individual monographs in 68:16.04. See also Estrogen-Progestin Combinations 68:12.

†Use is not currently included in the labeling approved by the US Food and Drug Administration

Estradiol

■ Estradiol (a principal endogenous estrogen) is a steroidal estrogen.

Uses

■ **Estradiol** Oral, transdermal, or topical estradiol is used for the management of moderate to severe vasomotor symptoms associated with menopause and for the management of vulvar and vaginal atrophy (atrophic vaginitis, kraurosis vulvae). Oral or transdermal estradiol is used for the treatment of female hypoestrogenism due to hypogonadism, castration, or primary ovarian failure. If estrogens are used solely for the management of vulvar and vaginal atrophy, use of topical vaginal preparations should be considered. Estradiol also may be administered intravaginally as a cream or tablet for the management of vulvar and vaginal atrophy. Estradiol vaginal ring is used for the management of urogenital symptoms associated with postmenopausal atrophy of the vagina (i.e., dryness, burning, pruritus, dyspareunia) and/or lower urinary tract (i.e., urinary urgency, dysuria).

Oral or transdermal estradiol (Alora®, Climara®, Climara Pro®, Estraderm®, Menostar®, Vivelle®, Vivelle-Dot®) is used adjunctively with other therapeutic measures (e.g., diet, calcium, weight-bearing exercise [including walking, running], physical therapy) to retard further bone loss and the progression of osteoporosis associated with estrogen deficiency in postmenopausal women. While estrogen replacement therapy is effective for the prevention of osteoporosis in women and has been shown to reduce bone resorption and retard or halt bone loss in postmenopausal women, such therapy is associated with a number of adverse effects. (See Uses: Estrogen Replacement Therapy, in the Estrogens General Statement 68:16.04.) If prevention of postmenopausal osteoporosis is the sole indication for estrogen therapy, alternative therapy (e.g., alendronate, raloxifene, risedronate) also should be considered.

While results from earlier observational studies indicated that estrogen replacement therapy (ERT) or combined estrogen/progestin therapy (HRT) was associated with cardiovascular benefit in postmenopausal women, results from recent controlled studies indicate that hormone therapy does not decrease the incidence of cardiovascular disease. The American Heart Association (AHA), American College of Obstetricians and Gynecologists (ACOG), US Food and Drug Administration (FDA) and manufacturers recommend that hormone therapy not be used to prevent heart disease in healthy women (primary prevention) or to protect women with preexisting heart disease (secondary prevention). (See Cardiovascular Risk Reduction under Uses: Estrogen Replacement Therapy, in the Estrogens General Statement 68:16.04.)

Oral estradiol is used for the palliative treatment of advanced, inoperable, metastatic carcinoma of the breast in postmenopausal women and in men. Estrogens are one of several second-line agents that can be used in certain postmenopausal women with metastatic breast cancer.

Oral estradiol is used for the palliative treatment of advanced carcinoma of the prostate in men; however, the risk of adverse cardiovascular effects of estrogens must be considered.

■ **Estradiol Acetate** Oral estradiol acetate and estradiol acetate vaginal ring are used for management of moderate to severe vasomotor symptoms associated with menopause. Estradiol acetate vaginal ring also is used for the management of moderate to severe symptoms of vulvar and vaginal atrophy associated with menopause. If estradiol acetate vaginal ring is used solely for the management of vulvar and vaginal atrophy, use of an alternative topical vaginal preparation should be considered.

■ **Estradiol Cypionate** Estradiol cypionate is used for the management of moderate to severe vasomotor symptoms associated with menopause. Estradiol cypionate also is used for the management of female hypogonadism.

Estradiol cypionate in fixed combination with testosterone cypionate is used for the management of moderate to severe vasomotor symptoms associated with menopause. While estrogen/androgen combinations were found to be effective for this indication under a determination made by the US Food and Drug Administration (FDA) in 1976, formal administrative proceedings were initiated by the FDA in April 2003 to examine the effectiveness of estrogen/androgen combinations for the management of vasomotor symptoms associated with menopause. FDA is undertaking this action because the agency does not believe there is substantial evidence available to establish the contribution of androgens to the effectiveness of estrogen/androgen combinations for the management of vasomotor symptoms in menopausal women who do not respond adequately to estrogen alone. The FDA will allow continued marketing of combination estrogen/androgen products while the matter is under study.

Estradiol cypionate in fixed combination with medroxyprogesterone acetate is used parenterally as a long-active contraceptive in women. For additional information on contraceptive use of estradiol cypionate in fixed combination with medroxyprogesterone acetate, see Uses: Contraception in Females in Medroxyprogesterone Acetate 68:32.

■ **Estradiol Valerate** In women, estradiol valerate is used for the management of moderate to severe vasomotor symptoms associated with menopause. Estradiol valerate also is used for the management of vulvar and vaginal atrophy, female hypogonadism and castration, and primary ovarian failure. If estrogens are used solely for the management of vulvar and vaginal atrophy, use of topical vaginal preparations should be considered.

Estradiol valerate is used for the palliative treatment of advanced carcinoma of the prostate in men; however, the risk of adverse cardiovascular effects of estrogens must be considered.

Although in the past estradiol valerate was used for the prevention of postpartum breast engorgement†, the FDA has withdrawn approval of estrogen-containing drugs for this indication since estrogens have not been shown to be safe for use in women with postpartum breast engorgement. Data from controlled studies indicate that the incidence of substantial painful engorgement is low in untreated women, and the condition usually responds to appropriate analgesic or other supportive therapy.

■ **Ethinyl Estradiol** Ethinyl estradiol in fixed combination with norethindrone acetate is used for the management of moderate to severe vasomotor symptoms associated with menopause. Ethinyl estradiol in fixed combination with norethindrone acetate also is used adjunctively with other therapeutic measures (e.g., diet, calcium, weight-bearing exercise [including walking, running], physical therapy) to retard further bone loss and the progression of osteoporosis associated with estrogen deficiency in postmenopausal women. While estrogen replacement therapy is effective for the prevention of osteoporosis in women and has been shown to reduce bone resorption and retard or halt bone loss in postmenopausal women, such therapy is associated with a number of adverse effects. (See Uses: Estrogen Replacement Therapy, in the Estrogens General Statement 68:16.04.) If prevention of postmenopausal osteoporosis is the sole indication for estrogen therapy, alternative therapy (e.g., alendronate, raloxifene, risedronate) also should be considered.

Dosage and Administration

■ **Reconstitution and Administration** Estradiol is administered orally, intravaginally, percutaneously by topical application of a transdermal system, and by topical application of a gel, emulsion, or transdermal spray to the skin. Estradiol acetate is administered orally and intravaginally. Ethinyl estradiol is administered orally. Estradiol cypionate and estradiol valerate are administered IM.

Patients receiving a transdermal estradiol system should be carefully instructed in the use of the transdermal system. To obtain optimum results, patients should also be given a copy of the patient instructions provided by the manufacturer. To expose the adhesive surface of the system, the protective strip should be peeled and discarded prior to administration. The transdermal system is applied topically to a clean, dry, and not excessively hairy area of intact skin on the trunk of the body, preferably the abdomen or buttocks, by firmly pressing the system with the adhesive side touching the skin. The system should be applied immediately after removal from its protective pouch and removal of the protective liner. The system should be pressed firmly in place with the palm of the hand for about 10 seconds, ensuring good contact, particularly around the edges. The application site should not be oily, damaged, or irritated. The transdermal system should *not* be applied to the breasts, and application at the waistline should be avoided, since tight clothing may cause the system to be rubbed off. If the system should inadvertently come off during the period of use, it may be reapplied or, if necessary, a new system may be applied; in either case, the application schedule employed should be continued. To minimize and/or prevent potential skin irritation, each transdermal system should be applied at a different site, with an interval of at least 1 week allowed between applications to a particular site. Estradiol transdermal systems are applied once (Climara®, Climara Pro®, Estradiol Transdermal System [Mylan], Menostar®) or twice (Alora®, Combipatch®, Estraderm®, Vivelle®, Vivelle-Dot®) weekly; the system in use is removed and discarded and a new system is applied. The transdermal systems for application twice weekly are commercially available in a dispensing package that is designed to aid the user in complying with the prescribed dosage regimen (the same 2 days each week). If a system is not changed on a designated day, it should be replaced as soon as possible.

Patients receiving estradiol topical gel (Elestrin®, EstroGel®) should be instructed in use of the gel and given a copy of the patient instructions provided by the manufacturer. Estradiol topical gel should be applied topically once daily at the same time each day to clean, dry, intact skin. To apply a dose of Elestrin®, the pump should be held with the tip facing the arm and the pump should be firmly and fully depressed. Elestrin® gel is applied to the upper arm and shoulder using 2 fingers.To apply a dose of EstroGel®, the gel should be collected in the palm of the hand by pressing the pump firmly and fully. EstroGel® gel is applied to one arm from shoulder to wrist using the hand. The topical gel should not be applied to the breasts or in or around the vagina. The application site should be allowed to dry for up for 5 minutes before dressing. Hands should be washed with soap and water after application of the gel. It is not known how long bathing and swimming should be delayed after application of the gel. Therefore, estradiol topical gel should be applied after bathing; the time allowed between application of the gel and swimming should be as long as possible (at least 2 hours). Application of sunscreen 10 minutes prior to application of Elestrin® increases exposure to estradiol by 55%, and application of sunscreen 25 minutes after application of Elestrin® does not alter exposure to estradiol. Application of sunscreen for 7 days to the site of application of Elestrin® increased estradiol exposure twofold; this effect was noted when sunscreen was applied before and after application of Elestrin®. Concomitant application of EstroGel® and sunscreen preparations has not been evaluated.

Patients receiving estradiol topical emulsion (Estrasorb®) should be instructed in use of the emulsion and given a copy of the patient instructions provided by the manufacturer. Estradiol topical emulsion should be applied topically once daily every morning to clean, dry, intact skin. To apply a dose, the contents of one pouch should be placed on the left thigh. The emulsion should be rubbed into the entire left thigh and calf for 3 minutes using one or both hands. Any excess emulsion remaining on the hands can be rubbed onto the buttocks. The contents of another pouch should be placed on the right thigh. The emulsion should be rubbed into the entire right thigh and calf for 3 minutes using one or both hands. Any excess emulsion remaining on the hands can be rubbed onto the buttocks. The emulsion should be applied immediately after opening the pouch. The application site should be allowed to dry before dressing. Hands should be washed with soap and water after application of the emulsion. Estradiol topical emulsion should not be applied in close proximity to application of sunscreen. Application of sunscreen 10 minutes prior to application of estradiol topical emulsion increases exposure to estradiol by 35%, and application of sunscreen 25 minutes after application of estradiol topical emulsion increases exposure to estradiol by 15%.

Patients receiving estradiol transdermal spray (Evamist®) should be instructed in use of the spray and given a copy of the patient instructions provided by the manufacturer. Estradiol transdermal spray should be applied topically once daily at the same time each day to clean, dry, intact skin on the inside of the forearm between the elbow and the wrist. Prior to initial use, estradiol transdermal spray pump must be primed; it is not necessary to prime the pump before each daily dose. To prime the pump, the applicator is held upright with the cover on and the pump depressed three times. To apply a dose of estradiol transdermal spray, the cover should be removed, the applicator held upright and the cone section of the applicator placed flat against the skin; the pump should then be depressed. One, two, or three sprays may be applied to non-overlapping areas of the inner forearm, starting near the elbow. Estradiol transdermal spray should not be applied to any area other than the inner forearm; the spray should not be applied to the breasts or around the vagina. The application site should be allowed to dry for up for 2 minutes before dressing and 30 minutes before washing the area. The application site should not be massaged or rubbed. Other individuals should not be allowed to have direct contact with the skin at the site of spray application for at least 30 minutes following administration. Patients receiving estradiol transdermal spray should ensure that children and pets avoid contact with the skin at the application site to prevent inadvertent exposure to the drug. (See Cautions.) If a child comes in direct contact with the patient's forearm where Evamist® was applied, the general area of contact should be washed with soap and water as soon as possible. Patients who cannot avoid such contact with children should wear clothing with long sleeves to cover the application site. Application of sunscreen 1 hour after application of estradiol transdermal spray decreases exposure to estradiol by 11%; application of sunscreen 1 hour prior to application of estradiol transdermal spray does not alter exposure to estradiol.

■ **Dosage** Dosage of estradiol, estradiol acetate, estradiol cypionate, estradiol valerate, and ethinyl estradiol must be individualized according to the condition being treated and the tolerance and therapeutic response of the patient. To minimize the risk of adverse effects, the lowest possible effective dosage should be used. When short-term estrogen therapy is indicated (e.g., for the management of vasomotor symptoms associated with menopause; vulvar and vaginal atrophy), therapy should be discontinued as soon as possible; attempts to reduce dosage or discontinue the drug should be made at 3- to 6-month intervals. Because of the potential increased risk of cardiovascular events, breast cancer, and venous thromboembolic events, estrogen and estrogen/progestin therapy should be limited to the lowest effective doses and shortest duration of therapy consistent with treatment goals and risks for the individual woman. Estrogen and estrogen/progestin therapy should be periodically reevaluated.

Estrogen therapy is administered continuously or cyclically. While estrogen therapy alone may be appropriate in women who have undergone a hysterectomy, many clinicians currently recommend that a progestin be added to estrogen therapy in women with an intact uterus. Addition of progestin therapy for 10 or more days of a cycle of estrogen administration or daily with estrogen in a continuous regimen reduces the incidence of endometrial hyperplasia and the attendant risk of endometrial carcinoma in women with an intact uterus. Morphologic and biochemical studies of the endometrium suggest that 10–13 days of progestin are needed to provide maximum maturation of the endometrium and to eliminate any hyperplastic changes. The manufacturer of Menostar® recommends that women with an intact uterus receive a progestin for 14 days every 6–12 months. When a progestin is used in conjunction with an estrogen, the usual precautions associated with progestin therapy should be observed. Clinicians prescribing progestins should be aware of the risks associated with these drugs and the manufacturers' labeling should be consulted. The choice and dosage of a progestin may be important factors in minimizing adverse effects.

When long-acting parenteral preparations are used in the management of conditions associated with estrogen deficiency, the drugs are usually administered once every 3–4 weeks.

Estradiol **Oral Dosage.** For the management of moderate to severe vasomotor symptoms associated with menopause or for the management of vulvar and vaginal atrophy, the usual initial oral dosage of estradiol is 1 or 2 mg daily in a cyclic regimen. For replacement therapy in female hypogonadism, female castration, or primary ovarian failure, the usual initial oral dosage of estradiol is 1 or 2 mg daily. Subsequent dosage should be adjusted according to the patient's therapeutic response, using the lowest possible effective maintenance dosage.

For the prevention of osteoporosis, an oral dosage of estradiol 0.5 mg daily in a cyclic regimen has been used. The lowest effective dosage of estradiol for this indication has not been determined.

When estradiol is used in fixed combination with norethindrone acetate (Activella®) for the management of moderate to severe vasomotor symptoms associated with menopause, the management of vulvar and vaginal atrophy associated with menopause, or prevention of postmenopausal osteoporosis, the usual dosage is 1 mg of estradiol combined with 0.5 mg of norethindrone acetate daily.

When estradiol is used in fixed combination with drospirenone (Angeliq®) for the management of moderate to severe vasomotor symptoms associated with menopause or for the management of vulvar and vaginal atrophy associated with menopause, the usual dosage is 1 mg of estradiol combined with 0.5 mg of drospirenone daily.

When estradiol is used with norgestimate (Prefest®) for the management of moderate to severe vasomotor symptoms associated with menopause, the management of vulvar and vaginal atrophy associated with menopause, or prevention of postmenopausal osteoporosis, the usual dosage is 1 mg of estradiol daily for 3 days followed by 1 mg of estradiol with 0.09 mg of norgestimate daily for 3 days; the regimen is continued without interruption.

For the palliative treatment of advanced, metastatic carcinoma of the breast in appropriately selected men and postmenopausal women, the usual oral dosage of estradiol is 10 mg 3 times daily. Estrogen therapy is usually continued in these patients for at least 3 months.

For the palliative treatment of advanced carcinoma of the prostate, the usual oral dosage of estradiol is 1–2 mg 3 times daily.

Transdermal System Dosage. Transdermal estradiol is commercially available as systems that are applied once or twice weekly. Estradiol transdermal systems that are applied twice weekly include Alora® (available as a system delivering 0.025 mg/24 hours, 0.05 mg/24 hours, 0.075 mg/24 hours, or 0.1 mg/24 hours), Estraderm® (available as a system delivering 0.05 mg/24 hours or 0.1 mg/24 hours), and Vivelle® and Vivelle-Dot® (available as a system delivering 0.025 mg/24 hours, 0.0375 mg/24 hours, 0.05 mg/24 hours, 0.075 mg/24 hours, or 0.1 mg/24 hours). Estradiol transdermal systems that are applied once weekly include Climara® (available as a system delivering 0.025 mg/24 hours, 0.0375 mg/24 hours, 0.05 mg/24 hours, 0.06 mg/24 hours, 0.075 mg/24 hours, or 0.1 mg/24 hours) and Menostar® (available as a system delivering 0.014 mg/24 hours). In addition, transdermal estradiol/norethindrone (CombiPatch®) is commercially available as a system delivering 0.05 mg/24 hours of estradiol and 0.14 mg/24 hours of norethindrone acetate and as a system delivering 0.05 mg/24 hours of estradiol and 0.25 mg/24 hours of norethindrone acetate. Transdermal estradiol/levonorgestrel (Climara Pro®) is commercially available as a system delivering 0.045 mg/24 hours of estradiol and 0.015 mg/24 hours of levonorgestrel.

When Alora® or Estraderm® is used for the management of moderate to severe vasomotor symptoms associated with menopause or for the management of vulvar and vaginal atrophy, the usual initial dosage of transdermal estradiol is one system delivering 0.05 mg/24 hours applied twice weekly in a continuous regimen in women who have undergone a hysterectomy or a cyclic regimen (3 weeks on drug followed by 1 week without the drug, and then the regimen is repeated as necessary) in women with an intact uterus.

When Climara® is used for the management of moderate to severe vasomotor symptoms associated with menopause, the usual initial dosage of transdermal estradiol is one system delivering 0.025 mg/24 hours applied once weekly in a continuous regimen. Subsequent dosage should be adjusted according to the severity of the symptoms and the patient's therapeutic response, using the lowest possible effective maintenance dosage.

When Vivelle® or Vivelle-Dot® is used for the management of moderate to severe vasomotor symptoms associated with menopause or for the management of vulvar and vaginal atrophy, the usual initial dosage of transdermal estradiol is one system delivering 0.0375 mg/24 hours applied twice weekly in a cyclic or continuous regimen. Subsequent dosage should be adjusted according to the patient's therapeutic response, using the lowest possible effective maintenance dosage. In women who have undergone hysterectomy, transdermal estradiol Vivelle-Dot® may be applied twice a week in a continuous regimen.

When estradiol/levonorgestrel (Climara Pro®) is used for the management of moderate to severe vasomotor symptoms associated with menopause in women with an intact uterus, one system delivering 0.045 mg/24 hours of estradiol and 0.015 mg/24 hours of levonorgestrel is applied once weekly in a continuous regimen.

When estradiol/norethindrone acetate (CombiPatch®) is used for the management of moderate to severe vasomotor systems associated with menopause, for the management of vulvar and vaginal atrophy, or for the treatment of hypoestrogenism secondary to hypogonadism, castration, or primary ovarian failure, CombiPatch® may be administered as a continuous combined regimen or as a continuous sequential regimen. In the continuous combined regimen, one CombiPatch® system delivering 0.05 mg/24 hours of estradiol and 0.14 mg/24 hours of norethindrone acetate is applied twice weekly in a continuous regimen. If necessary, the dosage of norethindrone acetate may be increased by using the dosage system that delivers 0.25 mg/24 hours of norethindrone acetate. In the continuous sequential regimen, one system of transdermal estradiol delivering 0.05 mg/24 hours (i.e., Vivelle®) is applied twice weekly for the first 14 days of a 28-day cycle then one estradiol/norethindrone acetate (CombiPatch®) system delivering 0.05 mg/24 hours of estradiol and 0.14 mg/24 hours of norethindrone acetate is applied twice weekly for the remaining 14 days of the cycle. If necessary, the dosage of norethindrone acetate may be increased by using the dosage system that delivers 0.25 mg/24 hours of norethindrone acetate.

When Alora® is used for the prevention of postmenopausal osteoporosis, the minimum dose that has been shown to be effective is one system delivering 0.025 mg/24 hours applied twice weekly in a continuous regimen.

When Climara® is used for the prevention of postmenopausal osteoporosis, the minimum dose that has been shown to be effective is one system delivering 0.025 mg/24 hours applied once weekly in a continuous regimen.

For the prevention of osteoporosis, the usual initial dosage of transdermal estradiol (Estraderm®) is one system delivering 0.05 mg/24 hours applied twice weekly in a cyclic regimen in women with an intact uterus. In women who have undergone hysterectomy, one Estraderm® system is applied twice weekly in a continuous regimen. Subsequent dosage can be adjusted according to the patient's response.

For the prevention of osteoporosis, the usual dosage of transdermal estradiol (Menostar®) is one system delivering 0.014 mg/24 hours applied once weekly in a continuous regimen.

When Vivelle® or Vivelle-Dot® is used for the prevention of postmenopausal osteoporosis, the usual dosage is one system delivering 0.025 mg/24 hours applied twice weekly.

When estradiol/levonorgestrel (Climara Pro®) is used for the prevention of postmenopausal osteoporosis in women with an intact uterus, one system delivering 0.045 mg/24 hours of estradiol and 0.015 mg/24 hours of levonorgestrel is applied once weekly in a continuous regimen.

In women who are currently not receiving an oral estrogen, transdermal estradiol therapy can be initiated immediately. In women who are currently receiving an oral estrogen, transdermal estradiol therapy can be initiated 1 week after discontinuance of oral therapy or sooner if symptoms reappear before the week has passed.

Topical Gel Dosage. Commercially available estradiol 0.06% topical gel (Elestrin®) is supplied in a non-aerosol metered-dose pump. Each depression of the pump delivers 0.87 g of gel containing 0.52 mg of estradiol. When estradiol gel (Elestrin®) is used for the management of moderate to severe vasomotor symptoms associated with menopause, the usual initial dosage is 0.87 g of gel (0.52 mg of estradiol) applied topically once daily. Prior to using the pump for the first time, the pump must be primed by fully depressing the pump 10 times; this gel should be discarded in a manner that avoids accidental exposure or ingestion by household members or pets.

Commercially available estradiol 0.06% topical gel (EstroGel®) is supplied in a non-aerosol metered-dose pump. Each depression of the pump delivers 1.25 g of gel containing 0.75 mg of estradiol. When estradiol gel (EstroGel®) is used for the management of moderate to severe vasomotor symptoms associated with menopause or the treatment of moderate to severe symptoms of vulvar and vaginal atrophy associated with menopause, 1.25 g of gel (0.75 mg of estradiol) is applied topically once daily. Prior to using the pump for the first time, the pump must be primed by fully depressing the 93-g pump twice or depressing the 25-g pump 3 times; this gel should be discarded in a manner that avoids accidental exposure or ingestion by household members or pets.

Topical Emulsion Dosage. Commercially available estradiol hemihydrate 0.25% topical emulsion (Estrasorb®) is supplied in foil-laminated pouches. Each pouch contains 1.74 g of emulsion. When estradiol topical emulsion (Estrasorb®) is used for the management of moderate to severe vasomotor symptoms associated with menopause, the contents of 2 pouches (delivering a total of 0.05 mg of estradiol/24 hours) are applied topically once daily.

Transdermal Spray Dosage. Commercially available estradiol transdermal spray (Evamist®) is supplied in a metered-dose pump. The metered pump delivers a metered 90-mcL spray that contains 1.53 mg of estradiol per actuation. When estradiol transdermal spray is used for the management of moderate to severe vasomotor symptoms associated with menopause, the recommended initial dose is one spray to the inner forearm once daily. Subsequent dosage is based on clinical response. One, two, or three sprays may be administered each morning to adjacent, non-overlapping areas of the inner forearm.

Vaginal Dosage. For the management of symptoms of vulvar and vaginal atrophy associated with menopause, 2–4 g of estradiol vaginal cream may be administered intravaginally once daily for 1–2 weeks, then gradually reduced to one-half the initial dosage for a similar period. Maintenance dosages of 1 g of estradiol vaginal cream administered intravaginally 1–3 times weekly may be used after restoration of the vaginal mucosa has occurred.

When estradiol vaginal ring (Estring®) is used for the management of postmenopausal urogenital symptoms, one ring (delivering estradiol 0.0075 mg/24 hours) is inserted into the upper third of the vaginal vault; the ring is to remain in place for 3 months. After 3 months, the ring should be removed and, if appropriate, replaced with a new ring. If the ring is expelled, the ring should be rinsed in lukewarm water and reinserted.

For the management of atrophic vaginitis, one vaginal tablet containing 25 mcg of estradiol (Vagifem®) is inserted intravaginally once daily (preferably at the same time each day) for 2 weeks (initial dosage). For maintenance therapy for this condition, one vaginal tablet containing 25 mcg of the drug is inserted intravaginally twice weekly.

Estradiol Acetate Estradiol acetate (Femtrace®) is commercially available for oral administration as tablets containing 0.45, 0.9, or 1.8 mg of estradiol acetate; the tablets are administered once daily. When estradiol acetate tablets are used for the management of moderate to severe vasomotor symptoms associated with menopause, therapy should be initiated with the lowest dose.

Estradiol acetate vaginal ring (Femring®) is commercially available as a ring delivering estradiol 0.05 mg/24 hours or 0.1 mg/24 hours. When estradiol acetate vaginal ring (Femring®) is used for the management of moderate to severe vasomotor symptoms or symptoms of vulvar and vaginal atrophy associated with menopause, therapy should be initiated with the lowest dose. To initiate therapy, one ring delivering estradiol 0.05 mg/24 hours is inserted into the vaginal vault; the ring remains in place for 3 months. After 3 months, the ring should be removed and, if appropriate, replaced with a new ring.

Estradiol Cypionate For the management of moderate to severe vasomotor symptoms associated with menopause, the usual dosage of estradiol cypionate is 1–5 mg administered IM once every 3–4 weeks.

For replacement therapy in female hypogonadism, the usual dosage of estradiol cypionate is 1.5–2 mg once every month.

When estradiol cypionate in fixed combination with testosterone cypionate is used for the management of moderate to severe vasomotor symptoms associated with menopause, the usual dosage of estradiol cypionate is 2 mg in combination with testosterone 50 mg administered IM every 4 weeks.

Estradiol Valerate For the management of moderate to severe vasomotor symptoms or for the management of vulvar and vaginal atrophy associated with menopause, and for replacement therapy in female hypogonadism, female castration, or primary ovarian failure, the usual dosage of estradiol valerate is 10–20 mg once every 4 weeks as necessary.

For the palliative treatment of advanced carcinoma of the prostate, the usual dosage of estradiol valerate is 30 mg or more once every 1 or 2 weeks.

Ethinyl Estradiol **Estrogen-Progestin Combination Therapy.** Ethinyl estradiol in fixed combination with norethindrone acetate (Femhrt®) is commercially available for oral administration as tablets containing 2.5 mcg of ethinyl estradiol with 0.5 mg of norethindrone acetate and as tablets containing 5 mcg of ethinyl estradiol with 1 mg of norethindrone acetate; the tablets are administered once daily. When ethinyl estradiol is used in combination with norethindrone acetate for the management of moderate to severe vasomotor symptoms associated with menopause or the prevention of postmenopausal osteoporosis, therapy should be initiated with the lowest dose.

Cautions

Estradiol, estradiol acetate, estradiol cypionate, estradiol valerate, and ethinyl estradiol share the toxic potentials of other estrogens, and the usual cautions, precautions, and contraindications associated with estrogen therapy should be observed. (See Cautions in the Estrogens General Statement 68:16.04.) In addition, when estradiol or ethinyl estradiol is used in conjunction with progestins, the cautions, precautions, and contraindications associated with progestins must be considered in addition to those associated with estrogens. For additional information, see Cautions in Estrogen-Progestin Combinations 68:12.

In clinical studies, the most common adverse effect reported with transdermal estradiol therapy was erythema and irritation at the application site. Dermatologic reactions have been reported in up to 97% of patients using transdermal systems. The irritation generally resolves completely within a day or so. Rash has been reported rarely in patients receiving transdermal estradiol therapy. Rotation of application sites minimizes and/or prevents potential skin irritation. If erythema persists or severe irritation or rash occurs, patients should contact their physician.

Estrace® 2-mg tablets contain the dye tartrazine (FD&C yellow No. 5), which may cause allergic reactions including bronchial asthma in susceptible individuals. Although the incidence of tartrazine sensitivity is low, it frequently occurs in patients who are sensitive to aspirin.

The US Food and Drug Administration (FDA) is reviewing reports of adverse effects associated with estradiol transdermal spray (Evamist®) in children and pets who may have been inadvertently exposed to the drug through skin contact with women receiving the drug. Children exposed to the drug may experience signs of premature puberty including nipple swelling and breast development in females and breast enlargement in males. If such a child shows signs of premature puberty (e.g., nipple or breast swelling, breast tenderness or enlargement), the parents should be advised to contact the child's clinician and to inform the clinician of the child's possible exposure to the drug.

Some estradiol topical preparations (e.g., gel, solution) contain alcohol. Preparations containing alcohol are flammable; exposure to open flame or lighted cigarettes should be avoided until the applied product has dried.

Pharmacology

Estradiol is the principal and most active endogenous estrogen. Ethinyl estradiol is one of the most potent synthetic estrogens, and unlike estradiol, ethinyl estradiol has similar activity following oral or parenteral administration. Following subcutaneous administration, ethinyl estradiol is equal in potency to estradiol, but following oral administration, ethinyl estradiol is 15–20 times more active than estradiol. The principal pharmacologic effects of estradiol, estradiol cypionate or valerate, and ethinyl estradiol are similar to those of other natural and synthetic estrogens. (See Pharmacology in the Estrogens General Statement 68:16.04.)

Estradiol valerate has a duration of action of 14–21 days, and estradiol cypionate has a duration of action of 14–28 days.

Chemistry and Stability

■ Chemistry

Estradiol Estradiol is a naturally occurring steroidal estrogen. The drug may be obtained from natural sources or prepared synthetically. Estradiol is structurally similar to estrone but differs from estrone in the substitution of a secondary alcohol group for the keto group at the 17 position on ring D of the steroid nucleus.

Estradiol occurs as white or creamy white, small crystals or as a crystalline powder, is odorless and hygroscopic, and is practically insoluble in water and has a solubility of approximately 35.7 mg/mL in alcohol at 25°C.

Transdermal estradiol (Alora®) is commercially available as a system that consists of an outer layer of polyethylene backing film and a drug reservoir consisting of estradiol and sorbitan monooleate dissolved in an acrylic adhesive matrix. A polyester overlapped release liner protects the adhesive matrix during storage and should be removed prior to application.

Transdermal estradiol (Climara®) is commercially available as a system that consists of an outer layer of translucent polyethylene film and an acrylate adhesive matrix that contains estradiol; a siliconized or fluoropolymer-coated polyester film is attached to the adhesive surface and should be removed prior to application.

Transdermal estradiol (Estraderm®) is commercially available as a system that consists of an outer layer of transparent polyester film; a drug reservoir of estradiol and alcohol gelled with hydroxypropyl cellulose; an ethylene-vinyl acetate copolymer membrane that controls the rate of diffusion of the drug; and a final adhesive layer consisting of light mineral oil and polyisobutylene. The adhesive layer is covered by a protective strip of siliconized polyester film which is removed prior to application.

Transdermal estradiol (Menostar®) is commercially available as a system that consists of an outer layer of translucent polyethylene film and an acrylate adhesive matrix that contains estradiol; a siliconized or fluoropolymer-coated polyester film is attached to the adhesive surface and should be removed prior to application.

Transdermal estradiol (Vivelle®, Vivelle-Dot®) is commercially available as a system that consists of an outer layer of translucent film and an adhesive formulation that contains estradiol; a polyester release liner is attached to the adhesive surface and should be removed prior to application.

Transdermal estradiol in fixed combination with levonorgestrel (Climara Pro®) is commercially available as a system that consists of an outer layer of translucent polyethylene film and an acrylate adhesive matrix that contains estradiol and levonorgestrel; a siliconized or fluoropolymer-coated polyester film is attached to the adhesive surface and should be removed prior to application.

Transdermal estradiol in fixed combination with norethindrone acetate (CombiPatch®) is commercially available as a system that consists of an outer layer of polyolefin film and a silicone and acrylic-based multipolymeric adhesive matrix that contains estradiol and norethindrone acetate; a protective liner is attached to the adhesive surface and should be removed prior to application.

Estradiol topical gel (Elestrin®) is commercially available as a hydroalcoholic gel containing estradiol 0.06%; the gel also contains purified water, alcohol, propylene glycol, diethylene glycol monoethyl ether, triethanolamine, carbomer 940, and edetate disodium. Elestrin® is supplied in a non-aerosol metered-dose pump. The pump contains 144 g of gel and delivers 100 metered doses of 0.87 g of gel.

Estradiol topical gel (EstroGel®) is commercially available as a clear, colorless, hydroalcoholic gel containing estradiol 0.06%; the gel also contains purified water, alcohol, triethanolamine, and carbomer 934P and is formulated to provide controlled release of estradiol. EstroGel® is supplied in a non-aerosol metered-dose pump. The pump containing 93 g of gel delivers 64 metered doses of 1.25 g of gel, and the pump containing 25 g of gel delivers 14 metered doses of 1.25 g of gel.

Estradiol topical emulsion (Estrasorb®) is commercially available as an emulsion containing estradiol hemihydrate 0.25%; estradiol is encapsulated using a micellar nanoparticle technology. The emulsion also contains soybean oil, water, polysorbate 80, and alcohol. Estradiol topical emulsion is supplied in foil-laminated pouches. Each pouch contains 1.74 g of emulsion and 4.35 mg of estradiol hemihydrate.

Estradiol transdermal spray (Evamist®) delivers a metered 90-mcL spray that contains 1.53 mg of estradiol per actuation. The commercially available pump contains 8.1 mL of solution and delivers 75 metered doses. The solution is packaged in a glass vial fitted with a metered-dose pump; this unit is encased in a plastic housing with a conical bell opening that controls the distance, angle, and area of application of the spray.

Estradiol also is commercially available as a vaginal tablet and as a vaginal ring that consists of estradiol, silicone polymers, and barium sulfate.

Estradiol Acetate Estradiol acetate is commercially available as an oral tablet and as a vaginal ring that consists of estradiol acetate, silicone polymers, and barium sulfate.

Estradiol Cypionate Estradiol cypionate is formed by esterification of estradiol with cyclopentanepropionic acid at C 17 on ring D of the steroid nucleus. Estradiol cypionate occurs as a white to practically white, crystalline powder, is odorless or may have a slight odor, and has solubilities of less than 0.1 mg/mL in water and approximately 25 mg/mL in alcohol at 25°C. The drug is also sparingly soluble in vegetable oils. Estradiol cypionate is commercially available alone and in fixed combination with testosterone cypionate for parenteral use. Commercially available estradiol cypionate injection is a sterile solution of the drug in a suitable oil (e.g., cottonseed oil); the injection may also contain chlorobutanol as a preservative.

Estradiol Valerate Estradiol valerate is formed by esterification of estradiol with valeric acid at C 17 on ring D of the steroid nucleus. Estradiol valerate occurs as a white, crystalline powder and is usually odorless but may have a faint, fatty odor. The drug is practically insoluble in water and sparingly soluble in sesame oil and in peanut oil. Estradiol valerate injection is a sterile solution of the drug in a suitable vegetable oil (e.g., sesame oil, castor oil); commercially available injections may also contain chlorobutanol or benzyl benzoate and benzyl alcohol as preservatives.

Ethinyl Estradiol Ethinyl estradiol is a semisynthetic estrogen. The presence of the ethinyl group at C 17 on ring D of the steroid nucleus prevents enzymatic degradation of the estradiol molecule and results in an orally active compound.

Ethinyl estradiol occurs as a white to creamy white, odorless, crystalline powder and is insoluble in water and soluble in alcohol and vegetable oils.

■ **Stability** Estradiol tablets should be stored in tight, light-resistant containers at a temperature of 20–25°C. The commercially available transdermal systems of estradiol should be stored at a temperature of 30°C or lower; after removal from the protective pouch, a transdermal system should be applied immediately and should not be stored. The commercially available transdermal systems of estradiol/norethindrone acetate should be refrigerated at 2–8°C until dispensed. Once dispensed, the transdermal systems may be stored at a temperature lower than 25°C for up to 6 months. The commercially available transdermal systems of estradiol/levonorgestrel should be stored at 20–25°C but may be exposed to temperatures ranging from 15–30°C. After removal from the protective pouch, the transdermal systems should be applied immediately and should not be stored. Estradiol vaginal ring should be stored at controlled room temperature (15–30°C). Estradiol topical gel, estradiol topical emulsion, estradiol transdermal spray, estradiol vaginal tablets, and estradiol acetate vaginal ring should be stored at a controlled room temperature of 25°C, but may be exposed to temperatures ranging from 15–30°C. Estradiol cypionate and estradiol valerate injections should be stored at room temperature. Estradiol acetate tablets should be stored at 25°C but may be exposed to temperatures ranging from 15–30°C.

For further information on chemistry, pharmacology, pharmacokinetics, cautions, acute toxicity, drug interactions, laboratory test interferences, and dosage and administration of estradiol and estradiol esters, see the Estrogens General Statement 68:16.04.

Preparations

Most preparations containing androgenic anabolic steroid hormones are subject to control under the Federal Controlled Substances Act of 1970, as amended by the Anabolic Steroids Control Act of 1990 and 2004, as schedule III (C-III) drugs. (See Uses: Misuse and Abuse, in Testosterone 68:08.) However, manufacturers of certain preparations containing androgenic anabolic steroids (principally combinations that also include estrogens) have applied for and obtained for their product(s) an exemption from the record-keeping and other regulatory requirements of the Federal Controlled Substances Act. (See the introductory paragraph under Preparations, in Testosterone 68:08.) Because regulatory requirements for a given preparation containing an androgenic anabolic steroid may be subject to change under the provisions of the Act, the manufacturer should be contacted when specific clarification about a preparation's status is required.

Excipients in commercially available drug preparations may have clinically important effects in some individuals; consult specific product labeling for details.

Estradiol

Topical		
Gel	0.06%	**Elestrin®**, Kenwood Therapeutics
		EstroGel®, Ascend Therapeutics
Solution	1.53 mg/meter spray	**Evamist®**, Ther-Rx
Transdermal System	0.014 mg/24 hours (1 mg/3.25 cm²)	**Menostar®**, Berlex
	0.025 mg/24 hours (0.77 mg/9 cm²)	**Alora®**, Watson
	0.025 mg/24 hours (2 mg/6.5 cm²)	**Climara®**, Berlex
	0.025 mg/24 hours (0.97 mg/7.75 cm²)*	**Estradiol Transdermal System** (once weekly)
	0.025 mg/24 hours (2.17 mg/7.25 cm²)	**Vivelle®**, Novartis
	0.025 mg/24 hours (0.39 mg/2.5 cm²)	**Vivelle-Dot®**, Novartis
	0.0375 mg/24 hours (2.85 mg/9.375 cm²)	**Climara®**, Berlex
	0.0375 mg/24 hours (1.46 mg/11.625 cm²)*	**Estradiol Transdermal System** (once weekly)
	0.0375 mg/24 hours (3.28 mg/11 cm²)	**Vivelle®**, Novartis
	0.0375 mg/24 hours (0.585 mg/3.75 cm²)	**Vivelle-Dot®**, Novartis
	0.05 mg/24 hours (1.5 mg/18 cm²)	**Alora®**, Watson
	0.05 mg/24 hours (3.8 mg/12.5 cm²)	**Climara®**, Berlex
	0.05 mg/24 hours (4 mg/10 cm²)	**Estraderm®**, Novartis
	0.05 mg/24 hours (1.94 mg/15.5 cm²)*	**Estradiol Transdermal System** (once weekly)
	0.05 mg/24 hours (4.33 mg/14.5 cm²)	**Vivelle®**, Novartis
	0.05 mg/24 hours (0.78 mg/5 cm²)	**Vivelle-Dot®**, Novartis
	0.06 mg/24 hours (4.55 mg/15 cm²)	**Climara®**, Berlex
	0.06 mg/24 hours (2.33 mg/18.6 cm²)*	**Estradiol Transdermal System** (once weekly)
	0.075 mg/24 hours (2.3 mg/27 cm²)	**Alora®**, Watson
	0.075 mg/24 hours (5.7 mg/18.75 cm²)	**Climara®**, Berlex
	0.075 mg/24 hours (2.91mg/23.25 cm²)*	**Estradiol Transdermal System** (once weekly)
	0.075 mg/24 hours (6.57 mg/22 cm²)	**Vivelle®**, Novartis
	0.075 mg/24 hours (1.17 mg/7.5 cm²)	**Vivelle-Dot®**, Novartis
	0.1 mg/24 hours (3 mg/36 cm²)	**Alora®**, Watson
	0.1 mg/24 hours (7.6 mg/25 cm²)	**Climara®**, Berlex
	0.1 mg/24 hours (8 mg/20 cm²)	**Estraderm®**, Novartis
	0.1 mg/24 hours (3.88 mg/31 cm²)*	**Estradiol Transdermal System** (once weekly)
	0.1 mg/24 hours (8.66 mg/29 cm²)	**Vivelle®**, Novartis
	0.1 mg/24 hours (1.56 mg/10 cm²)	**Vivelle-Dot®**, Novartis
Vaginal		
Cream	0.01%	**Estrace®**, Warner Chilcott
Ring	2 mg/ring (0.0075 mg/24 hours)	**Estring®**, Pfizer

*available from one or more manufacturer, distributor, and/or repackager by generic (nonproprietary) name

Estradiol Combinations

Oral		
Tablets, biphasic regimen	1 mg (15 tablets) and 1 mg with Norgestimate 0.09 mg (15 tablets)	**Prefest®**, Barr
Tablets, film-coated	1 mg with Norethindrone Acetate 0.5 mg	**Activella®** (28 tablets), Novo Nordisk
	1 mg with Drospirenone 0.5 mg	**Angeliq®** (28 tablets), Berlex
Topical		
Transdermal System	0.045 mg and 0.015 mg Levonorgestrel/24 hours (4.4 mg and 1.39 mg Levonorgestrel/22 cm²)	**Climara Pro®**, Berlex

	0.05 mg and 0.14 mg Norethindrone Acetate/24 hours (0.62 mg and 2.7 mg Norethindrone Acetate/9 cm²)	**CombiPatch®**, Novartis
	0.05 mg and 0.25 mg Norethindrone Acetate/24 hours (0.51 mg and 4.8 mg Norethindrone Acetate/16 cm²)	**CombiPatch®**, Novartis

Estradiol (Hemihydrate)

Topical		
Emulsion	0.25%	**Estrasorb®**, Espirit
Vaginal		
Tablets, film-coated	25 mcg (of estradiol)	**Vagifem®** (available as disposable applicators), NovoNordisk

Estradiol (Micronized)

Oral		
Tablets	0.5 mg*	**Estrace®** (scored), Warner Chilcott
	1 mg*	**Estrace®** (scored), Warner Chilcott
	2 mg*	**Estrace®** (scored), Warner Chilcott

*available from one or more manufacturer, distributor, and/or repackager by generic (nonproprietary) name

Estradiol Acetate

Oral		
Tablets	0.45 mg	**Femtrace®**, Warner Chillcott
	0.9 mg	**Femtrace®**, Warner Chillcott
	1.8 mg	**Femtrace®**, Warner Chilcott
Vaginal		
Ring	12.4 mg/ring (0.05 mg estradiol/24 hours)	**Femring®**, Warner Chilcott
	24.8 mg/ring (0.1 mg estradiol/24 hours)	**Femring®**, Warner Chilcott

Estradiol Cypionate

Parenteral		
Injection (in oil)	5 mg/mL	**Depo®-Estradiol**, Pfizer

Estradiol Cypionate Combinations

Parenteral		
Injection (in oil)	2 mg/mL with Testosterone Cypionate 50 mg/mL	**Depo-Testadiol®**, Pfizer

Estradiol Valerate

Parenteral		
Injection (in oil)	10 mg/mL	**Delestrogen®**, Monarch
	20 mg/mL	**Delestrogen®**, Monarch
	40 mg/mL	**Delestrogen®**, Monarch

Ethinyl Estradiol Combinations

Oral		
Tablets	2.5 mcg with Norethindrone Acetate 0.5 mg	**FemHRT®**, Warner Chillcott
	5 mcg with Norethindrone Acetate 1 mg	**FemHRT®**, Warner Chillcott

†Use is not currently included in the labeling approved by the US Food and Drug Administration

Estrogens, Conjugated

Estrogenic Substances, Conjugated

■ Conjugated estrogens is a mixture of estrogens that is available either as preparations that meet current official USP standards (i.e., conjugated estrogens USP) or as nonofficial preparations (i.e., synthetic conjugated estrogens A and synthetic conjugated estrogens B, which are prepared synthetically from plant sources).

Uses

In women, oral conjugated estrogens USP and synthetic conjugated estrogens A are used for the management of moderate to severe vasomotor symptoms associated with menopause and for the management of vulvar and vaginal atrophy (atrophic vaginitis). If estrogens are used solely for the management of vulvar and vaginal atrophy, use of topical vaginal preparations should be considered. Synthetic conjugated estrogens B is used for the management of moderate to severe vasomotor symptoms and for the management of severe vaginal dryness, pain with sexual intercourse, and symptoms of vulvar and vaginal atrophy associated with menopause. Oral conjugated estrogens USP also is used for the management of female hypoestrogenism secondary to hypogonadism, castration, or primary ovarian failure.

Oral conjugated estrogens USP is used adjunctively with other therapeutic measures (e.g., diet, calcium, weight-bearing exercise [including walking, running], physical therapy) to retard further bone loss and the progression of osteoporosis associated with estrogen deficiency in postmenopausal women. While estrogen replacement therapy is effective for the prevention of osteoporosis in women and has been shown to reduce bone resorption and retard or halt bone loss in postmenopausal women, such therapy is associated with a number of adverse effects. (See Uses: Estrogen Replacement Therapy, in the Estrogens General Statement 68:16.04.) If prevention of postmenopausal osteoporosis is the sole indication for therapy with oral conjugated estrogens, alternative therapy (e.g., alendronate, raloxifene, risedronate) should be considered.

Another therapeutic option involves use of conjugated estrogens in combination with an estrogen agonist-antagonist (bazedoxifene) for the management of moderate to severe vasomotor symptoms associated with menopause and for prevention of osteoporosis. The combination of conjugated estrogens with bazedoxifene is referred to as a tissue-selective estrogen complex (TSEC).

While results from earlier observational studies indicated that estrogen replacement therapy (ERT) or combined estrogen/progestin therapy (hormone replacement therapy, HRT) was associated with cardiovascular benefit in postmenopausal women, results of the Heart and Estrogen/progestin Replacement Study (HERS) evaluating estrogen/progestin and the Women's Health Initiative (WHI) study evaluating estrogen alone and estrogen/progestin therapy indicate that hormone therapy does not decrease the incidence of cardiovascular disease. The American Heart Association (AHA), American College of Obstetricians and Gynecologists (ACOG), FDA, and manufacturers recommend that hormone therapy not be used to prevent heart disease in healthy women (primary prevention) or to protect women with preexisting heart disease (secondary prevention). (See Cardiovascular Risk Reduction under Uses: Estrogen Replacement Therapy, in the Estrogens General Statement 68:16.04.)

Oral conjugated estrogens USP is used for the palliative treatment of advanced, inoperable, metastatic carcinoma of the breast in postmenopausal women and in men. Estrogens are one of several second-line agents that can be used in certain postmenopausal women with metastatic breast cancer.

Oral conjugated estrogens USP is used for the palliative treatment of advanced carcinoma of the prostate in men; however, the risk of adverse cardiovascular effects of estrogens must be considered.

Conjugated estrogens USP may be administered IM or IV for the treatment of abnormal uterine bleeding caused by hormonal imbalance not associated with organic pathology.

Conjugated estrogens USP may be administered intravaginally for the management of atrophic vaginitis or kraurosis vulvae.

Although in the past oral conjugated estrogens has been used for the prevention of postpartum breast engorgement†, the FDA has withdrawn approval of estrogen-containing drugs for this indication since estrogens have not been shown to be safe for use in women with postpartum breast engorgement. Data from controlled studies indicate that the incidence of substantial painful engorgement is low in untreated women, and the condition usually responds to appropriate analgesic or other supportive therapy.

Dosage and Administration

■ **Reconstitution and Administration** Conjugated estrogens USP is usually administered orally, but may also be administered intravaginally or by deep IM or slow IV injection. Synthetic conjugated estrogens A and synthetic conjugated estrogens B are administered orally.

When parenteral administration of conjugated estrogens USP is required, IV injection is preferred because of the more rapid response obtained following this route of administration compared to IM injection. For direct IV injection, the drug should be administered slowly to avoid the occurrence of a flushing reaction.

For parenteral administration, conjugated estrogens USP powder for injection is reconstituted with 5 mL of sterile water for injection. Using aseptic technique, the diluent should then be slowly added, directing the flow against the inner wall of the vial (Secule®), while gently agitating the container to facilitate dissolution of the contents; vigorous shaking of the container should be avoided. Premarin® solutions should be used immediately after reconstitution.

Oral dosage preparations containing medroxyprogesterone acetate in combination with conjugated estrogens USP as monophasic or biphasic regimens are commercially available in a mnemonic dispensing package that is designed to aid the user in complying with the prescribed dosage schedule. The monophasic combination (Prempro®) is available in a 28-day dosage preparation that contains 28 tablets of conjugated estrogens USP (0.625 mg) in fixed combination with medroxyprogesterone acetate (2.5 or 5 mg). The monophasic combination (Prempro®) also is available in a 28-day dosage preparation that contains 28 tablets of conjugated estrogens USP (0.3 or 0.45 mg) in fixed combination with medroxyprogesterone acetate (1.5 mg). The biphasic combination (Premphase®) is available in a 28-day dosage preparation that contains 14 tablets of conjugated estrogens USP (0.625 mg) and 14 tablets of conjugated estrogens USP (0.625 mg) in fixed combination with medroxyprogesterone acetate (5 mg).

The oral dosage preparation containing conjugated estrogens in fixed combination with bazedoxifene acetate is commercially available in a 30-day package that includes 2 blister packs of 15 tablets each containing conjugated estrogens 0.45 mg in fixed combination with bazedoxifene acetate 22.6 mg (equivalent to 20 mg of bazedoxifene).

■ Dosage

Dosage of conjugated estrogens USP, synthetic conjugated estrogens A, and synthetic conjugated estrogens B must be individualized according to the condition being treated and the tolerance and therapeutic response of the patient. To minimize the risk of adverse effects, the lowest possible effective dosage should be used. Because of the potential increased risk of cardiovascular events, breast cancer, and venous thromboembolic events, therapy with estrogen, estrogen/progestin, or conjugated estrogens in fixed combination with bazedoxifene should be limited to the lowest effective doses and shortest duration of therapy consistent with treatment goals and risks for the individual woman. Therapy with estrogen, estrogen/progestin, or conjugated estrogens in fixed combination with bazedoxifene should be periodically reevaluated.

Estrogen therapy is administered in a continuous daily dosage regimen or, alternatively, in a cyclic regimen. When estrogens are administered cyclically, the drugs usually are given once daily for 3 weeks followed by 1 week without the drugs or once daily for 25 days followed by 5 days off, and then the respective regimen is repeated as necessary.

While estrogen therapy alone (estrogen replacement therapy, ERT) may be appropriate in women who have undergone a hysterectomy, a progestin generally is added to estrogen therapy (hormone replacement therapy, HRT) in women with an intact uterus. Addition of a progestin for 10 or more days of a cycle of estrogen or daily with estrogen in a continuous regimen reduces the incidence of endometrial hyperplasia and the attendant risk of endometrial carcinoma in women with an intact uterus. Morphologic and biochemical studies of the endometrium suggest that 10–13 days of progestin are needed to provide maximum maturation of the endometrium and to eliminate any hyperplastic changes. As an alternative to progestins, the use of bazedoxifene (an estrogen agonist-antagonist) in fixed combination with conjugated estrogens reduces the risk of endometrial hyperplasia.

When estrogen therapy is used in conjunction with a progestin or in fixed combination with bazedoxifene, the usual precautions associated with progestins or bazedoxifene should be observed. Clinicians prescribing estrogens in conjunction with progestins or conjugated estrogens in fixed combination with bazedoxifene should be aware of the risks associated with these drugs and the manufacturers' labeling should be consulted. Clinical studies indicate that addition of a progestin to estrogen replacement therapy does not interfere with the efficacy of estrogen therapy in the management of vasomotor symptoms associated with menopause, treatment of vulvar and vaginal atrophy, or prevention of osteoporosis. The choice and dosage of a progestin may be important factors in minimizing potential adverse effects.

Exposure to conjugated estrogens USP vaginal cream has been reported to weaken latex condoms. The potential for conjugated estrogens USP vaginal cream to weaken and contribute to the protective failure of latex or rubber condoms, diaphragms, or cervical caps should be considered.

Menopausal Symptoms

Conjugated Estrogens USP. For the management of moderate to severe vasomotor symptoms and/or for the management of vulvar and vaginal atrophy associated with menopause, the usual initial oral dosage of conjugated estrogens USP is 0.3 mg daily. Subsequent dosage adjustment should be based on the patient's response. The drug may be administered in a continuous daily regimen or in a cyclic regimen (25 days on drug followed by 5 days off drug, then this regimen is repeated as necessary). Alternatively, for the management of vulvar and vaginal atrophy, 0.5–2 g of conjugated estrogens USP vaginal cream may be administered intravaginally once daily in the usual cyclic regimen.

When conjugated estrogens USP is used in conjunction with medroxyprogesterone for the management of moderate to severe vasomotor symptoms associated with menopause or for the management of vulvar and vaginal atrophy, conjugated estrogens USP is administered in a continuous daily dosage regimen while medroxyprogesterone may be administered in a continuous daily dosage regimen (Prempro®) or cyclically (Premphase®). When both drugs are administered in a continuous daily dosage regimen, conjugated estrogens is administered in a daily dosage of 0.3 mg in conjunction with oral medroxyprogesterone acetate in a daily dosage of 1.5 mg. Alternatively, conjugated estrogens is administered in a daily dosage of 0.45 mg in conjunction with medroxyprogesterone acetate in a daily dosage of 1.5 mg, or conjugated estrogens is administered in a daily dosage of 0.625 mg in conjunction with medroxyprogesterone acetate in a daily dosage of 2.5 or 5 mg. When conjugated estrogens USP is administered in a continuous daily dosage regimen and medroxyprogesterone is administered cyclically (Premphase®), conjugated estrogens USP is administered in a daily dosage of 0.625 mg, while oral medroxyprogesterone acetate is administered in a daily dosage of 5 mg on days 15–28 of the cycle. Therapy with conjugated estrogens in conjunction with medroxyprogesterone generally should be initiated with the lowest dosage (i.e., conjugated estrogens 0.3 mg in conjunction with medroxyprogesterone acetate 1.5 mg). Subsequent dosage should be adjusted based on the patient's therapeutic response and should be reevaluated periodically. If spotting or bleeding is problematic and has been appropriately evaluated, dosage can be adjusted.

When conjugated estrogens is used in conjunction with bazedoxifene for the treatment of moderate to severe vasomotor symptoms associated with menopause, conjugated estrogens is administered in a daily dosage of 0.45 mg in fixed combination with bazedoxifene 20 mg.

Synthetic Conjugated Estrogens A. For the management of moderate to severe vasomotor symptoms associated with menopause, the usual oral dosage of synthetic conjugated estrogens A is 0.45–1.25 mg daily. The usual initial oral dosage of synthetic conjugated estrogens A is 0.45 mg daily; subsequent dosage adjustment should be based on the patient's response. For the management of vulvar and vaginal atrophy, the usual oral dosage of synthetic conjugated estrogens A is 0.3 mg daily.

Synthetic Conjugated Estrogens B. For the management of moderate to severe vasomotor symptoms associated with menopause, the usual oral dosage of synthetic conjugated estrogens B is 0.3–1.25 mg daily. The usual initial oral dosage of synthetic conjugated estrogens B for this condition is 0.3 mg daily. Subsequent dosage adjustment should be based on the patient's response.

For the management of severe vaginal dryness, pain with sexual intercourse, and vulvar and vaginal atrophy associated with menopause, the usual oral dosage of synthetic conjugated estrogens B is 0.3 mg daily.

Osteoporosis

For the prevention of osteoporosis, the usual initial oral dosage of conjugated estrogens USP is 0.3 mg once daily. Subsequent dosage should be adjusted based on the patient's clinical and bone mineral density responses. The drug may be administered in a continuous daily regimen or in a cyclic regimen (25 days on drug followed by 5 days off drug, then this regimen is repeated as necessary).

When conjugated estrogens USP is used in conjunction with medroxyprogesterone, conjugated estrogens USP is administered in a continuous daily dosage regimen while medroxyprogesterone may be administered in a continuous daily dosage regimen (Prempro®) or cyclically (Premphase®). When both drugs are administered in a continuous daily dosage regimen, conjugated estrogens USP is administered in a daily dosage of 0.3 mg in conjunction with oral medroxyprogesterone acetate in a daily dosage of 1.5 mg. Alternatively, conjugated estrogens is administered in a daily dosage of 0.45 mg in conjunction with medroxyprogesterone acetate in a daily dosage of 1.5 mg, or conjugated estrogens is administered in a daily dosage of 0.625 mg in conjunction with medroxyprogesterone acetate in a daily dosage of 2.5 or 5 mg. When conjugated estrogens USP is administered in a continuous daily dosage regimen and medroxyprogesterone is administered cyclically, conjugated estrogens USP is administered in a daily dosage of 0.625 mg, while oral medroxyprogesterone acetate is administered in a daily dosage of 5 mg on days 15–28 of the cycle. Therapy with conjugated estrogens in conjunction with medroxyprogesterone generally should be initiated with the lowest dosage (i.e., conjugated estrogens 0.3 mg in conjunction with medroxyprogesterone acetate 1.5 mg). Subsequent dosage should be adjusted based on the patient's clinical and bone mineral density responses. If spotting or bleeding is problematic and has been appropriately evaluated, dosage can be adjusted.

When conjugated estrogens is used in conjunction with bazedoxifene for the prevention of osteoporosis, conjugated estrogens is administered once daily at a dosage of 0.45 mg in fixed combination with bazedoxifene 20 mg.

Female Hypoestrogenism

For replacement therapy in female hypoestrogenism, the usual oral dosage of conjugated estrogens USP is 0.3–0.625 mg daily in a cyclic regimen (3 weeks on drug, 1 week off). Dosage may be adjusted based on symptom severity and responsiveness of the endometrium.

For the management of female castration or primary ovarian failure, the usual initial oral dosage of conjugated estrogens USP is 1.25 mg daily in a cyclic regimen. Subsequent dosage should be adjusted according to the severity of the symptoms and the patient's therapeutic response, using the lowest possible effective maintenance dosage.

Inoperable Carcinoma of the Breast

For the palliative treatment of inoperable, advanced, metastatic carcinoma of the breast in appropriately selected men and postmenopausal women, the usual oral dosage of conjugated estrogens USP is 10 mg 3 times daily. Estrogen therapy is usually continued in these patients for at least 3 months.

Prostate Carcinoma

For the palliative treatment of advanced carcinoma of the prostate, the usual oral dosage of conjugated estrogens USP is 1.25–2.5 mg 3 times daily.

Abnormal Uterine Bleeding

For the emergency treatment of abnormal uterine bleeding caused by hormonal imbalance, the usual IV or IM dose of conjugated estrogens USP is 25 mg. If necessary, the dose may be repeated in 6–12 hours. The use of conjugated estrogens USP for this condition does not preclude the use of other appropriate measures.

Cautions

Conjugated estrogens USP, synthetic conjugated estrogens A, and synthetic conjugated estrogens B share the toxic potentials of other estrogens, and the usual cautions, precautions, and contraindications associated with estrogen therapy should be observed. (See Cautions in the Estrogens General Statement 68:16.04.)

Conjugated estrogens is contraindicated in patients who are hypersensitive to the drug or any ingredient in the respective formulation.

Pharmacology

The principal pharmacologic effects of conjugated estrogens are similar to those of other natural and synthetic estrogens. (See Pharmacology in the Estrogens General Statement 68:16.04.)

Chemistry and Stability

■ **Chemistry** Conjugated estrogens is a mixture of estrogens that is available either as preparations that meet current official USP standards (i.e., conjugated estrogens USP) or as nonofficial preparations (i.e., synthetic conjugated estrogens A, synthetic conjugated estrogens B).

Conjugated estrogens obtained from natural sources occurs as a buff-colored, amorphous powder and is odorless or has a slight, characteristic odor. Conjugated estrogens that is prepared synthetically occurs as a white to light buff, crystalline or amorphous powder and is odorless or has a slight odor. Conjugated estrogens is soluble in water.

Conjugated Estrogens USP Conjugated estrogens USP is a mixture containing the sodium salts of the water-soluble sulfate esters of estrone and equilin derived wholly or in part from equine urine or may be prepared synthetically from estrone and equilin. Conjugated estrogens USP also contains conjugated estrogenic substances of the type excreted by pregnant mares including 17α-dihydroequilin, 17α-estradiol, 17β-dihydroequilin, equilenin, 17α-dihydroequilenin, 17β-dihydroequilenin, $\delta^{8,9}$-dehydroestrone, and 17β-estradiol. Conjugated estrogens USP contains 52.5–61.5% sodium estrone sulfate and 22.5–30.5% sodium equilin sulfate. Conjugated estrogens contains, as sodium sulfate conjugates, 13.5–19.5% 17α-dihydroequilin, 2.5–9.5% 17α-estradiol, and 0.5–4% 17β-dihydroequilin.

Conjugated estrogens USP currently is commercially available as preparations (Premarin®, Premphase®, Prempro®) containing mixtures of estrogens obtained exclusively from natural sources and which are present in the formulations as the sodium salts of water-soluble estrogen sulfates blended to represent the average composition of material derived from pregnant mare urine; according to USP standards, the formulations include a mixture of sodium estrone sulfate and sodium equilin sulfate as well as the concomitant components 17α-dihydroequilin, 17α-estradiol, and 17β-dihydroequilin as sodium sulfate conjugates.

Conjugated estrogens USP injection is commercially available as a sterile, lyophilized cake. The lyophilized cake also contains lactose, sodium citrate, and simethicone; in addition, sodium hydroxide and/or hydrochloric acid may be added during manufacture of the powder for injection to adjust the pH. A sterile diluent containing water for injection and benzyl alcohol as a preservative is provided for reconstitution.

Synthetic Conjugated Estrogens A Synthetic conjugated estrogens A is a mixture of conjugated estrogens prepared synthetically from plant sources (i.e., soy and yams). Synthetic conjugated estrogens A is commercially available as preparations (Cenestin®) containing a mixture of 9 of the 10 known conjugated estrogenic substances present in currently available commercial preparations of conjugated estrogens USP. However, unlike currently available preparations of conjugated estrogens USP, the conjugated estrogenic substances present in synthetic conjugated estrogens A are prepared entirely synthetically.

Synthetic conjugated estrogens A is commercially available as preparations containing mixtures of estrogens prepared exclusively synthetically as the sodium salts of water-soluble estrogen sulfates blended into a 9-component mixture of estrone sulfate and sodium equilin sulfate as well as the concomitant components 17α-dihydroequilin, 17α-estradiol, 17β-dihydroequilin, 17α-dihydroequilenin, 17β-dihydroequilenin, equilenin, and 17β-estradiol as sodium sulfate conjugates.

Synthetic Conjugated Estrogens B Synthetic conjugated estrogens B is a mixture of conjugated estrogens prepared synthetically from plant sources. Synthetic conjugated estrogens B is commercially available as preparations (Enjuvia®) containing a mixture of the 10 conjugated estrogenic substances present in currently available commercial preparations of conjugated estrogens USP. Unlike currently available preparations of conjugated estrogens USP, the conjugated estrogenic substances present in synthetic conjugated estrogens B are prepared entirely synthetically.

Synthetic conjugated estrogens B is commercially available as preparations containing mixtures of estrogens prepared exclusively synthetically as the sodium salts of water-soluble estrogen sulfates blended into a 10-component mixture of estrone sulfate and sodium equilin sulfate as well as the concomitant components 17α-dihydroequilin, 17α-estradiol, 17β-dihydroequilin, 17α-dihydroequilenin, 17β-dihydroequilenin, equilenin, 17β-estradiol, and $\delta^{8,9}$-dehydroestrone as sodium sulfate conjugates.

■ **Stability** Commercially available conjugated estrogens USP tablets, synthetic conjugated estrogens A tablets, synthetic conjugated estrogens B tablets, and conjugated estrogens USP vaginal cream should be stored at controlled room temperature (20–25°C). Conjugated estrogens USP powder for injection should be stored at a temperature of 2–8°C prior to reconstitution. Following reconstitution, solutions of the drug should be used immediately.

Conjugated estrogens USP injection is physically and chemically compatible with the following IV solutions: 5% dextrose, 0.9% sodium chloride, and invert sugar solutions; the injection is physically and/or chemically incompatible with protein hydrolysate, ascorbic acid, or any solution with an acid pH. Specialized references should be consulted for specific compatibility information.

For further information on chemistry, pharmacology, pharmacokinetics, cautions, acute toxicity, drug interactions, laboratory test interferences, and dosage and administration of conjugated estrogens, see the Estrogens General Statement 68:16.04.

Preparations

Excipients in commercially available drug preparations may have clinically important effects in some individuals; consult specific product labeling for details.

Conjugated Estrogens USP

Oral		
Tablets	0.3 mg	**Premarin®**, Pfizer
	0.45 mg	**Premarin®**, Pfizer
	0.625 mg	**Premarin®**, Pfizer
	0.9 mg	**Premarin®**, Pfizer
	1.25 mg	**Premarin®**, Pfizer
Parenteral		
For injection	25 mg	**Premarin® Intravenous**, Pfizer
Vaginal		
Cream	0.0625%	**Premarin®**, Pfizer

Conjugated Estrogens Combinations

Oral		
Tablets	0.45 mg with Bazedoxifene Acetate 20 mg (of bazedoxifene)	**Duavee®**, Pfizer
Tablets, monophasic regimen	0.3 mg with Medroxyprogesterone Acetate 1.5 mg (28 tablets)	**Prempro®**, Pfizer
	0.45 mg with Medroxyprogersterone Acetate 1.5 mg (28 tablets)	**Prempro®**, Pfizer
	0.625 mg with Medroxyprogesterone Acetate 2.5 mg (28 tablets)	**Prempro®**, Pfizer
	0.625 mg with Medroxyprogesterone Acetate 5 mg (28 tablets)	**Prempro®**, Pfizer
Tablets, biphasic regimen	0.625 mg (14 tablets Premarin®) and 0.625 mg with Medroxyprogesterone Acetate 5 mg (14 tablets)	**Premphase®**, Pfizer

Conjugated Estrogens A, Synthetic

Oral		
Tablets, film-coated	0.3 mg	**Cenestin®**, Teva
	0.45 mg	**Cenestin®**, Teva
	0.625 mg	**Cenestin®**, Teva
	0.9 mg	**Cenestin®**, Teva
	1.25 mg	**Cenestin®**, Teva

Conjugated Estrogens B, Synthetic

Oral		
Tablets, film-coated	0.3 mg	**Enjuvia®**, Teva
	0.45 mg	**Enjuvia®**, Teva
	0.625 mg	**Enjuvia®**, Teva
	0.9 mg	**Enjuvia®**, Teva
	1.25 mg	**Enjuvia®**, Teva

†Use is not currently included in the labeling approved by the US Food and Drug Administration

ANTIESTROGENS 68:16.08

Anastrozole

■ Anastrozole, an aromatase inhibitor, is an antineoplastic agent.

Uses

■ **Breast Cancer** ***Reduction in the Incidence of Breast Cancer in Women at High Risk*** Randomized trials are under way to investigate the use of aromatase inhibitors, such as anastrozole, for reduction in the incidence of breast cancer† among women who are at high risk for developing the disease.

Initial or Sequential Adjuvant Therapy for Early-stage Breast Cancer Anastrozole is used alone as initial (primary) adjuvant therapy in postmenopausal women with early-stage hormone receptor-positive breast cancer. Anastrozole also is used as sequential adjuvant therapy following 2–3 years of adjuvant tamoxifen for early-stage hormone receptor-positive breast cancer† in postmenopausal women. Aromatase inhibitors, including anastrozole, currently are considered a treatment of choice for adjuvant hormonal therapy to lower the risk of breast cancer recurrence in postmenopausal women with early-stage hormone receptor-positive breast cancer. Although tamoxifen historically has been the drug of choice for adjuvant hormonal therapy in such patients, results of large, randomized clinical studies indicate that an aromatase inhibitor-containing regimen is modestly more effective than tamoxifen alone. Longer-term follow-up of these studies is needed to further clarify lasting clinical efficacy, effects on survival, and late adverse effects of aromatase inhibitor therapy.

Clinical Trials of Anastrozole as Initial Adjuvant Therapy. In a double-blind, multicenter trial (the Arimidex, Tamoxifen, Alone or in Combination [ATAC] trial), 9366 postmenopausal women with operable breast cancer were randomized to receive anastrozole 1 mg daily, tamoxifen 20 mg daily, or a combination of anastrozole 1 mg daily and tamoxifen 20 mg daily, as adjuvant therapy for 5 years or until recurrence of disease. About 84% of the patients in each group had hormone receptor-positive (i.e., estrogen receptor-positive, progesterone receptor-positive, or both) breast tumors. The primary end point of the trial was disease-free survival, which was defined as time to occurrence of any of the following events: distant or local recurrence, a contralateral primary breast tumor, or death from any cause.

Analysis of the data at a median follow-up of 68 months when patients had received treatment for a median of 60 months showed that disease-free survival was prolonged in patients receiving anastrozole compared with those receiving tamoxifen (hazard ratio of 0.87 with a 95% confidence interval of 0.78–0.97). The frequency of events observed in patients receiving anastrozole versus tamoxifen was locoregional recurrence in 3.8 versus 4.8%, contralateral breast cancer in 1.1 versus 1.9%, and distant recurrence in 10.4 versus 12% of patients. No difference was observed between the groups for the secondary endpoints of distant disease-free survival and overall survival. Subgroup analysis confirmed that disease-free survival was prolonged with anastrozole versus tamoxifen therapy for patients with hormone receptor-positive tumors, but benefit was less clear in patients who had received previous adjuvant therapy or patients who were 65 years of age or older.

Analysis of the data (both overall and for the subset of patients with hormone receptor-positive tumors) at a median follow-up of 10 years (120 months) showed that the benefit of prolonged disease-free survival was maintained in patients receiving anastrozole, but there was no difference in overall survival between the groups; time to recurrence, time to distant recurrence, and incidence of contralateral breast cancer also were improved in patients receiving anastrozole compared with those receiving tamoxifen. The greatest differences between anastrozole and tamoxifen in time to recurrence, rate of contralateral breast cancer, and disease-free survival were observed during the first 2 years of treatment; between-treatment differences in distant recurrence rates remained similar over 10 years of follow-up. Although recurrence rates for the anastrozole and tamoxifen treatment groups remained different throughout 10 years of follow-up, analyses conducted using data for patients with hormone receptor-positive tumors suggested that the difference between treatments might diminish after 8 years of follow-up. Assessment of quality of life during 5 years of treatment did not show any difference between the anastrozole and tamoxifen groups.

At a median follow-up of 33 months, combination therapy with anastrozole and tamoxifen was not associated with an improvement in disease-free survival compared with tamoxifen alone, and this treatment arm was discontinued.

In the ATAC trial, anastrozole was associated with a higher incidence of joint disorders (including arthritis, arthrosis, and arthralgia), fractures (including fractures of the spine, hip, and wrist), and elevations in serum cholesterol compared with tamoxifen. Postmenopausal women receiving aromatase inhibitors, such as anastrozole, as adjuvant therapy are at high risk for osteoporosis. (See Precautions and Contraindications and Musculoskeletal Effects sections in Cautions for further information on screening and treatment guidelines for osteoporosis in such patients.) Anastrozole was associated with a lower incidence of endometrial cancer, ischemic cerebrovascular events, venous thromboembolic events (including deep venous thrombosis), vaginal discharge, vaginal bleeding, and hot flushes compared with tamoxifen.

Clinical Trials of Anastrozole as Sequential Adjuvant Therapy. In a randomized trial involving 448 postmenopausal women with node-positive, estrogen receptor-positive breast cancer (Italian Tamoxifen Anastrozole [ITA] trial), patients who had received 2–3 years of adjuvant tamoxifen therapy were randomized to receive anastrozole or to continue receiving tamoxifen to complete a total of 5 years of adjuvant therapy. At a median follow-up of 36 months following randomization, those receiving tamoxifen followed by anastrozole had longer event-free survival and disease-free survival but similar overall survival as those receiving 5 years of tamoxifen therapy. Improvements in recurrence-free survival and event-free survival associated with anastrozole therapy were maintained at a median follow-up of 64 months; overall survival was not significantly different between treatment groups.

Analysis of combined data from 2 randomized trials involving a total of 3224 postmenopausal women with hormone-sensitive early-stage breast cancer who had received 2 years of adjuvant therapy with tamoxifen (Austrian Breast and Colorectal Cancer Study Group trial 8 [ABCSG-8] and Arimidex-Nolvadex [ARNO] 95 trial) showed that those receiving anastrozole for the remaining 3 years of adjuvant therapy had a higher rate of event-free survival (96%) compared with those receiving tamoxifen for the entire 5-year period (93%); at the completion of 5 years of endocrine therapy, overall survival did not differ between the groups. Analysis of data from ABCSG-8 alone showed a low overall rate of breast cancer recurrence and a high overall survival rate among patients enrolled in this study (reflecting inclusion in the study of women at low to moderate risk of recurrence) and no significant difference in recurrence-free survival between the 2 adjuvant regimens at a median follow-up of 5 years after initiation of adjuvant endocrine therapy. Analysis of data from the ARNO 95 trial at a median follow-up of 30 months, when patients who previously had received tamoxifen for 2 years had received randomized treatment with anastrozole or tamoxifen for a median of about 27 months, indicated that patients who were switched to anastrozole had prolonged disease-free and overall survival compared with those who continued receiving tamoxifen.

Analysis of pooled data for individual patients from these 3 randomized trials, conducted at a median follow-up of 30 months, suggested that disease-free survival, event-free survival, distant recurrence-free survival, and overall survival are longer in patients who switch to anastrozole following 2–3 years of tamoxifen than in those who remain on tamoxifen for the 5-year duration of adjuvant therapy for hormone receptor-positive early-stage breast cancer.

Clinical Role. Based on data from randomized controlled trials demonstrating prolonged disease-free survival in patients receiving anastrozole- or other aromatase inhibitor-based adjuvant regimens, the American Society of Clinical Oncology (ASCO) states that most postmenopausal women with early-stage hormone receptor-positive breast cancer should consider receiving an aromatase inhibitor (e.g., anastrozole) during the course of adjuvant therapy, either as primary (initial) therapy or following 2–3 years of tamoxifen therapy (sequential therapy), to complete a total of 5 years of adjuvant endocrine therapy. Clinically meaningful differences among the currently available aromatase inhibitors (i.e., anastrozole, exemestane, letrozole) have not been demonstrated to date. Data also support switching to an aromatase inhibitor following 5 years of adjuvant tamoxifen therapy (extended therapy) (see Extended Adjuvant Therapy for Early-stage Breast Cancer under Uses: Breast Cancer). The optimal time for switching from tamoxifen to an aromatase inhibitor is not known. The duration of aromatase inhibitor therapy should not exceed 5 years, since toxicity of long-term (e.g., beyond 5 years) use of aromatase inhibitors, including anastrozole, has not been determined. The optimal duration of adjuvant anastrozole therapy is not known. ASCO states that clinicians should consider adverse effects, patient preference, and preexisting conditions when selecting an adjuvant regimen; during the course of adjuvant therapy, patients who are intolerant of one aromatase inhibitor may be switched to a different aromatase inhibitor or to tamoxifen.

The use of a luteinizing hormone-releasing hormone (LHRH) agonist (e.g., goserelin) in combination with an aromatase inhibitor, such as anastrozole, as adjuvant therapy in *premenopausal* women with hormone receptor-positive breast cancer† is being investigated in large randomized trials. The use of an aromatase inhibitor as a single agent for adjuvant therapy is *not* appropriate in premenopausal women with breast cancer because these agents alone are not likely to provide sufficient suppression of ovarian function to be of clinical benefit. Similarly, the use of an aromatase inhibitor as monotherapy for adjuvant therapy for hormone receptor-positive breast cancer in premenopausal women experiencing a chemotherapy-induced disruption in ovarian function is not advised; a substantial number of such patients can expect resumption of ovarian function, and this would likely render therapy with an aromatase inhibitor ineffective.

Extended Adjuvant Therapy for Early-stage Breast Cancer Based on data from randomized controlled trials demonstrating prolonged disease-free survival in patients receiving aromatase inhibitors, including anastrozole, as extended adjuvant therapy following 5 years of adjuvant tamoxifen therapy, ASCO recommends extended therapy with an aromatase inhibitor (e.g., anastrozole) in postmenopausal women with early-stage hormone receptor-positive breast cancer who complete 5 years of adjuvant tamoxifen therapy. (See Extended Adjuvant Therapy for Early-stage Breast Cancer in Uses: Breast Cancer, in Letrozole 68:16.08.) Clinically meaningful differences among the currently available aromatase inhibitors (i.e., anastrozole, exemestane, letrozole) have not been demonstrated to date. Clinicians should consider adverse effects, patient preference, and preexisting conditions when selecting an adjuvant regimen. ASCO states that women who receive extended adjuvant therapy should receive a total of 8–10 years of adjuvant endocrine therapy, including 5 years of tamoxifen therapy followed by 3–5 years of aromatase inhibitor therapy. The optimal duration of extended adjuvant therapy is not known, and the toxicity of long-term (e.g., beyond 5 years) use of aromatase inhibitors in this setting has not been determined. Ongoing clinical trials are evaluating whether longer durations of aromatase inhibitor therapy are more effective.

Anastrozole is used as extended adjuvant therapy following adjuvant tamoxifen for hormone receptor-positive early-stage breast cancer† in postmenopausal women. In a randomized trial involving 856 postmenopausal women with hormone receptor-positive early-stage breast cancer who remained free of disease after completing 5 years of adjuvant therapy with tamoxifen (47% of whom had also received the aromatase inhibitor aminoglutethimide for the first 2 years of therapy), those receiving 3 years of extended adjuvant therapy with anastrozole had reduced risk of disease recurrence and similar overall survival compared with those who received no further treatment.

First-line Therapy for Advanced Breast Cancer Anastrozole is used for the first-line treatment of hormone receptor-positive or hormone receptor-unknown locally advanced or metastatic breast cancer in postmenopausal women. Data from 2 double-blind, randomized clinical trials indicate that anastrozole is at least as effective as tamoxifen for producing objective tumor response and delaying tumor progression in such patients. In the 2 studies, a total of 1021 patients (age range: 30–92 years) were randomized to receive anastrozole 1 mg once daily or tamoxifen 20 mg once daily for hormone receptor-positive (i.e., estrogen receptor-positive, progesterone receptor-positive, or both) breast tumors or hormone receptor-unknown breast tumors.

Results from trial 0030, a North American study involving 353 patients (about 90% with hormone receptor-positive breast tumors and 10% with hormone receptor-unknown breast tumors), showed a similar objective response rate (about 21 and 17%, respectively) and an increased median time to progression (11.1 versus 5.6 months, respectively) for patients receiving anastrozole compared with those receiving tamoxifen at a median follow-up of about 18 months. In trial 0027, a predominately European study involving 668 patients (about 45% with hormone receptor-positive breast tumors and 55% with hormone receptor-unknown breast tumors), a similar objective response rate (about 33% in both groups) and median time to progression (about 8 months in both groups) were reported at a median follow-up of 19 months in patients receiving anastrozole or tamoxifen.

Conclusions concerning differences in overall survival between the 2 treatments could not be made because of the low number of deaths occurring across treatment groups in either study at the time of data analysis. A later analysis of combined patient data for the 2 studies at a median of 43.7 months of follow-up showed no difference in survival between the treatment groups (death rate: 56%); analysis of pooled data from published studies for first-line, second-line, or subsequent therapy of advanced breast cancer that included these 2 studies suggests that treatment with third-generation aromatase inhibitors, such as anastrozole, as first-line therapy for advanced breast cancer offers a small survival advantage (about 11%) compared with standard hormonal therapy, such as tamoxifen. Analysis of combined data for the 2 studies shows that adverse effects occurred at a similar frequency in patients receiving anastrozole or tamoxifen.

Second-line Therapy for Advanced Breast Cancer Anastrozole is used for the treatment of advanced breast cancer in postmenopausal women with disease progression following tamoxifen therapy. The principal goal of therapy in patients with metastatic breast cancer generally has been palliative with an emphasis on extension of survival and improvement in the quality of life. Data from 2 comparative clinical trials suggest that anastrozole is at least as effective as megestrol acetate in postmenopausal women with advanced breast cancer who have had disease progression following tamoxifen therapy for either advanced or early breast cancer. Patients who have estrogen receptor-negative breast cancer and those who fail to respond to tamoxifen therapy rarely have responded to anastrozole.

In 2 well-controlled clinical trials, a total of 764 postmenopausal women with advanced breast cancer which progressed following tamoxifen therapy (for either advanced or early breast cancer) were randomized to receive anastrozole 1 mg or 10 mg daily, or megestrol acetate 40 mg 4 times daily. Most of the patients enrolled had ER-positive tumors; patients with ER-negative disease were eligible only if they previously had responded to tamoxifen (about 5% of the patients in each trial). Some patients also had received previous cytotoxic therapy. The primary efficacy variables were time to progression and objective response rate, and similar results were observed among treatment groups and between the 2 trials.

In trial 0004, a North American study involving 386 patients (about 80% with hormone receptor-positive breast tumors), a median time to progression of 5.7, 5.3, and 5.1 months, respectively, and an objective response rate of 12.5, 10, and 10.2%, respectively, were reported in patients receiving anastrozole 1 mg daily, anastrozole 10 mg daily, and megestrol acetate 40 mg 4 times daily. In trial 0005, a predominately European study involving 378 patients (about 60% with hormone receptor-positive breast tumors), a median time to progression of 4.4, 5.3, and 3.9 months, respectively, and an objective response rate of 12.6, 15.3, and 14.4%, respectively, were reported in patients receiving anastrozole 1 mg daily, anastrozole 10 mg daily, and megestrol acetate 40 mg 4 times daily.

Pooled analysis of data from the 2 trials showed a median time to progression of 4.8, 5.3, and 4.6 months, respectively, and an objective response rate of 12.5, 12.5, and 12.3%, respectively, in patients receiving anastrozole 1 mg daily, anastrozole 10 mg daily, and megestrol acetate 40 mg 4 times daily. Similar efficacy was observed for patients receiving anastrozole 1 mg and megestrol acetate, and there was no evidence of superior efficacy of the 10-mg daily dose of anastrozole compared with the 1-mg daily dose. Analysis of pooled data from published studies for first-line, second-line, or subsequent therapy of advanced breast cancer that included these 2 studies suggests that treatment with third-generation aromatase inhibitors, such as anastrozole, as second-line or subsequent therapy for advanced breast cancer offers a small survival advantage (about 14%) compared with standard hormonal therapy, such as megestrol acetate. Weight gain was reported less frequently with anastrozole (1 mg daily) than with megestrol acetate (40 mg 4 times daily) in these clinical trials.

Anastrozole is used as second-line hormonal therapy in postmenopausal women with estrogen receptor-positive or estrogen receptor-unknown advanced breast cancer. In premenopausal women with hormone receptor-positive advanced breast cancer†, ovarian ablation by surgery or external-beam radiation, or suppression of ovarian function with an LHRH agonist, is advised; the use of an LHRH agonist (e.g., goserelin) in combination with an aromatase inhibitor, such as anastrozole, is being investigated. The use of an aromatase inhibitor as single-agent therapy is *not* appropriate in premenopausal women with breast cancer because these agents alone are not likely to provide sufficient suppression of ovarian function to be of clinical benefit.

Dosage and Administration

■ Administration

Anastrozole is administered orally.

Food does not affect the absorption of anastrozole, and the drug may be administered without regard to meals.

■ Dosage

Unlike aminoglutethimide, a less selective aromatase inhibitor, anastrozole is highly selective for suppression of estrogen synthesis, and concomitant corticosteroid replacement therapy is not required.

Because no evidence of altered pharmacokinetics has been observed in women older than 80 years of age compared with women younger than 50 years of age, the manufacturer states that adjustment of anastrozole dosage is not necessary in geriatric patients.

Breast Cancer **Adjuvant Therapy for Early-stage Breast Cancer.** For adjuvant therapy in the treatment of early-stage, hormone receptor-positive breast cancer in postmenopausal women, the recommended dosage of anastrozole is 1 mg daily. The optimal duration of therapy is unknown. In a large, randomized clinical trial (the ATAC trial), the duration of anastrozole therapy was 5 years. Because adherence to adjuvant anastrozole therapy may decrease during the first year of therapy and further diminish over time, communication with the patient and interventions to improve compliance should be considered.

The American Society of Clinical Oncology (ASCO) states that an aromatase inhibitor (e.g., anastrozole) may be administered to postmenopausal women with early-stage, hormone receptor-positive breast cancer as initial adjuvant therapy and continued for a total of 5 years or may be administered following initial tamoxifen therapy as part of a sequential adjuvant regimen. The optimal time to switch from tamoxifen to aromatase inhibitor therapy is not known; however, based on clinical trials conducted to date, ASCO recommends that patients who are disease-free may be switched to an aromatase inhibitor after 2–3 years of tamoxifen therapy to complete a 5-year sequential adjuvant regimen. In patients who initially receive an aromatase inhibitor but discontinue therapy prior to 5 years, ASCO states that consideration should be given to administering tamoxifen to complete the 5-year adjuvant regimen. ASCO recommends that patients who receive an extended adjuvant regimen receive an aromatase inhibitor (e.g., anastrozole) for 3–5 years beyond the initial 5 years of tamoxifen therapy, to complete a total of 8–10 years of adjuvant endocrine therapy.

First-line Therapy for Advanced Breast Cancer. For the first-line treatment of hormone receptor-positive or hormone receptor-unknown locally advanced or metastatic breast cancer in postmenopausal women, the recommended dosage of anastrozole is 1 mg daily. Anastrozole therapy should be continued until tumor progression is evident.

Second-line Therapy for Advanced Breast Cancer. For the second-line treatment of advanced breast cancer in postmenopausal women with disease progression following tamoxifen therapy, the recommended dosage of anastrozole is 1 mg daily. Anastrozole therapy should be continued until tumor progression is evident.

■ Dosage in Renal and Hepatic Impairment

Reduction in renal clearance does not affect total body clearance of anastrozole since only about 10% of the drug is excreted unchanged in urine. Therefore, adjustment of anastrozole dosage is not required in patients with renal impairment.

The manufacturer states that no dosage adjustment is required in patients with mild to moderate hepatic impairment or stable hepatic cirrhosis. Anastrozole has not been studied in patients with severe hepatic impairment.

Cautions

The incidence of adverse effects is based on data from randomized trials of postmenopausal women receiving anastrozole 1 mg daily for breast cancer as initial adjuvant therapy (3092 patients, median duration of treatment: 60 months), as first-line therapy (506 patients), or as second-line therapy (262 patients). Unless the type of therapy (based on stage of breast cancer) is specified, incidence rates reflect the experience of all these patients receiving the drug. Unless otherwise noted, these adverse effects occurred at a similar rate in patients receiving treatments being compared with anastrozole (i.e., tamoxifen as adjuvant therapy for early breast cancer or as initial treatment for advanced breast cancer, and megestrol acetate as second-line therapy for advanced breast cancer).

In the ATAC trial in patients with early-stage breast cancer, the most frequent adverse effects of anastrozole were hot flushes (flashes), asthenia, arthritis, pain, arthralgia, pharyngitis, hypertension, depression, nausea and vomiting, rash, osteoporosis, fractures, back pain, insomnia, headache, peripheral edema, and lymphedema. The most common adverse effect resulting in discontinuance of either anastrozole or tamoxifen in this trial was hot flushes, although fewer patients discontinued therapy because of hot flushes in the anastrozole group. Serious treatment-related adverse events were reported less frequently during treatment in patients receiving anastrozole compared with those receiving tamoxifen, but occurred at similar rates during posttreatment follow-up. At a median follow-up of 10 years, safety results for the ATAC trial were similar to results reported during earlier analyses. The total number of deaths occurring during or following treatment was similar in the 2 treatment groups, although more deaths were related to breast cancer in the tamoxifen group than in the anastrozole group.

In patients with advanced breast cancer, the most frequent adverse effects of anastrozole are hot flushes, nausea, asthenia, pain, headache, back pain, bone pain, increased cough, dyspnea, pharyngitis, and peripheral edema. Anastrozole generally was well tolerated in patients with advanced breast cancer receiving the drug as second-line therapy in clinical trials; less than 3.3% of patients (compared with 4% for patients receiving megestrol acetate) withdrew from the clinical trials because of adverse effects. Less common adverse effects (i.e., those reported in 2–5% of patients) that occurred in patients receiving anastrozole as second-line therapy were similar to those observed in patients receiving the drug as first-line therapy in clinical trials.

■ **Cardiovascular Effects** ***Thromboembolic Events and Ischemic Disease*** Among patients receiving adjuvant therapy, venous thromboembolic events occurred less frequently in patients receiving anastrozole than in those receiving tamoxifen (3 versus 5%); this included deep venous thrombosis (2% of patients in each treatment group). Ischemic cerebrovascular events also occurred less frequently in patients receiving anastrozole compared with those receiving tamoxifen (2 versus 3%). Ischemic cardiovascular events were reported in similar proportions of patients receiving anastrozole or tamoxifen (4 versus 3%). Angina pectoris or myocardial infarction was reported in 2.3 or 1.2%, respectively, of those receiving adjuvant therapy with anastrozole compared with 1.6 or 1.1%, respectively, of those receiving tamoxifen. In the subset of patients with preexisting ischemic heart disease, ischemic cardiovascular events were reported in 17% of patients receiving anastrozole compared with 10% of those receiving tamoxifen; angina pectoris or myocardial infarction was reported in 11.6 or 0.9%, respectively of those receiving anastrozole compared with 5.2 or 3.2%, respectively, of those receiving tamoxifen. At a median follow-up of 10 years (median adjuvant treatment duration of 5 years), cardiovascular events in patients receiving adjuvant anastrozole or tamoxifen therapy were consistent with the known safety profiles of the drugs.

Among patients receiving anastrozole as first-line therapy, thromboembolic disease was reported in 18 patients (4%), with 5 patients experiencing venous thrombosis (including pulmonary embolus, thrombophlebitis, and retinal vein thrombosis) and 13 patients experiencing coronary and/or cerebral thrombosis (including myocardial infarction, myocardial ischemia, angina pectoris, cerebrovascular accident, cerebral ischemia, and cerebral infarct).

Among patients receiving anastrozole as second-line therapy, thromboembolic disease was reported in 3%, and thrombophlebitis occurred in 2–5%.

Vasomotor Symptoms Among patients receiving adjuvant therapy, hot flushes (flashes) occurred less frequently in patients receiving anastrozole than in those receiving tamoxifen (36 versus 41%). Among patients receiving anastrozole as first-line or second-line therapy, hot flushes occurred in 26 or 13%, respectively.

Effects on Lipoproteins Among patients receiving adjuvant therapy in the ATAC trial, increased serum cholesterol concentrations were reported more frequently in patients receiving anastrozole compared with those receiving tamoxifen (9 versus 3.5%). However, in another clinical trial, no clinically important changes in concentrations of total, high-density lipoprotein (HDL)-, or low-density lipoprotein (LDL)-cholesterol or concentrations of triglycerides were observed from baseline to 12 months in patients receiving anastrozole alone or in conjunction with risedronate.

Among patients receiving anastrozole as second-line therapy, mean total serum cholesterol concentrations increased by 19 mg/dL (0.5 mmol/L); increases in LDL cholesterol have been shown to contribute to these elevations.

Other Cardiovascular Effects Vasodilation was reported in 36 or 25% of patients receiving anastrozole as adjuvant or first-line therapy, respectively. Hypertension occurred in 13% and lymphedema and peripheral edema each occurred in 10% of patients receiving anastrozole as adjuvant therapy. Among patients receiving anastrozole as first-line or second-line therapy, peripheral edema was reported in 10 or 5%, respectively, and hypertension was reported in about 5%. Edema occurred in 7% of patients receiving anastrozole as second-line therapy.

■ **Genitourinary Effects** Among patients receiving adjuvant therapy, vaginal bleeding and vaginal discharge occurred less frequently in patients receiving anastrozole than in those receiving tamoxifen (5 versus 10% and 4 versus 13%, respectively). Endometrial cancer also was reported less frequently in patients receiving anastrozole than in those receiving tamoxifen (0.2 versus 0.6%). (Also see Cautions: Mutagenicity and Carcinogenicity.) Vulvovaginitis was reported in 6% of patients and vaginal hemorrhage (without further diagnosis) and vaginitis each were reported in 4% of patients receiving anastrozole as adjuvant therapy. In a subprotocol assessing quality of life during 5 years of treatment in the ATAC trial, analysis of gynecologic symptoms and sexual function showed that anastrozole was associated with less vaginal discharge but more vaginal dryness, pain on intercourse, and loss of sexual interest than tamoxifen; no difference in overall quality of life was detected between the groups. In another subprotocol assessing occurrence of endometrial disorders in a small subset of patients enrolled in the ATAC trial, endometrial abnormalities (mainly polyps) were reported after 6 years of follow-up in 12 or 20% of patients receiving anastrozole or tamoxifen, respectively; fewer patients receiving anastrozole appeared to require medical intervention for endometrial abnormalities (1.4 versus 9.8%). Most abnormalities occurred within the first year of treatment.

Among patients receiving anastrozole as first-line or second-line therapy, pelvic pain occurred in 5%, vaginal bleeding or hemorrhage occurred in 1 or 2%, respectively, and vaginal dryness was reported in 2%.

Breast pain and urinary tract infection each occurred in up to 8% of patients receiving anastrozole. Leukorrhea was reported in 3% of patients receiving anastrozole as adjuvant therapy and 2% of patients receiving the drug as first-line therapy.

■ **Musculoskeletal Effects** Among patients receiving adjuvant therapy, adverse musculoskeletal effects (e.g., joint symptoms including joint disorder, arthritis, arthrosis, and arthralgia) and fractures occurred more frequently in patients receiving anastrozole than in those receiving tamoxifen (36 versus 29% and 10 versus 7%, respectively); this included fractures of the spine, hip, and wrist (4 versus 3%). Arthritis, arthralgia, and arthrosis occurred in 17, 15, and 7%, respectively, of patients receiving anastrozole as adjuvant therapy; osteoporosis, bone pain, and joint disorder were reported in 11, 7, and 6%, respectively. Myalgia occurred in 6% of patients receiving anastrozole as adjuvant therapy. In clinical trials, carpal tunnel syndrome occurred more frequently in patients receiving anastrozole than in those receiving tamoxifen (2.5 versus 0.7%).

A syndrome consisting of arthralgia and other symmetrical bone and joint symptoms (e.g., pain, stiffness, achiness) that are not associated with other manifestations of rheumatologic disorders has been reported in patients receiving aromatase inhibitors. Symptoms generally resolve within 8–10 weeks following discontinuance of therapy.

Because anastrozole lowers circulating estrogen concentrations, it may cause a reduction in bone mineral density (BMD). Analysis of data at 12 and 24 months from a substudy of the ATAC trial showed that whereas mean values for lumbar spine and total hip BMD (compared with baseline) decreased in patients receiving anastrozole, these values increased in those receiving tamoxifen. For patients receiving adjuvant therapy with anastrozole, the rate of bone loss at the lumbar spine slowed at 2–5 years compared with the change measured from baseline to 2 years, but the rate of bone loss at the hip did not slow over the 5-year period. Analysis of the data at 5 years indicated accelerated bone loss at the lumbar spine and the hip in patients receiving anastrozole, compared with a slight increase in BMD in the lumbar spine but not in the hip in patients receiving tamoxifen. Among women who had normal BMD at baseline, none developed osteoporosis after 5 years of anastrozole therapy, but osteopenia was more frequent in these patients than in those receiving tamoxifen (17 versus 3%).

Analysis of data from the ATAC study at a median follow-up of 10 years (median adjuvant treatment duration of 5 years) showed that the cumulative incidence of all first fractures (both serious and nonserious, occurring either during or after treatment) was higher in the anastrozole group compared with the tamoxifen group (15 versus 11%). Fractures were reported more frequently during treatment in patients receiving anastrozole compared with those receiving tamoxifen; however, after completion of treatment, the incidence of fractures was similar between groups.

Postmenopausal women receiving anastrozole as adjuvant therapy are at high risk for osteoporosis. All postmenopausal women initiating adjuvant therapy with an aromatase inhibitor should be evaluated for risk of osteoporotic fractures. Screening with dual energy radiographic absorptiometry (DXA) to determine the BMD of the hip and spine should be performed in conjunction with assessment of other risk factors for fracture (e.g., age, low body mass index, family history of hip fracture, prior fragility fracture, history of cigarette smoking, excessive alcohol consumption, current or prior corticosteroid use). Patients should be monitored closely for changes in risk status during therapy, and BMD should be assessed at regular intervals (e.g., every 1–2 years in those with osteopenia or osteoporosis). Other potential causes of osteoporosis (e.g., vitamin D deficiency, hyperthyroidism, hyperparathyroidism, hypercalciuria) should be considered. Appropriate therapy to prevent further bone loss should be initiated as clinically indicated. The decision to initiate therapy with an antiresorptive agent (e.g., a bisphosphonate, denosumab) should be based on overall risk of fracture and rate of bone loss. (See Uses: Prevention of Aromatase Inhibitor-associated Bone Loss, in Zoledronic Acid 92:24.) All women receiving adjuvant therapy with anastrozole should be advised to adopt lifestyle changes (e.g., weight-bearing exercise, abstinence from smoking, moderation in alcohol consumption) and dietary supplementation with calcium and vitamin D to reduce the risk of osteoporosis.

Among patients receiving first-line therapy, there was no evidence of an increased incidence of fracture in patients receiving anastrozole compared with those receiving tamoxifen. Tumor flare was reported in 3% of such patients.

Among patients receiving anastrozole as first-line or second-line therapy, bone pain was reported in 11 or 6%, respectively. Myalgia, arthralgia, pathologic fracture, and neck pain each were reported in 2–5% of patients receiving anastrozole as second-line therapy, which was similar to experience in those receiving the drug as first-line therapy.

Back pain occurred in 10–12% of patients receiving anastrozole. Joint pain and stiffness also have been reported in patients receiving anastrozole. Joint pain (commonly affecting the hands, knees, hips, lower back, or shoulders) and stiffness, particularly early morning stiffness, have been reported within 2 months of initiation of therapy in patients receiving anastrozole as second-line therapy; none of these patients had a history of arthritis or arthralgia associated with menopause, prior chemotherapy, or hormone therapy. In a small number of patients experiencing severe arthralgia, symptoms resolved with discontinuance of the drug. Trigger finger has been reported in less than 1% of patients receiving anastrozole.

■ **GI Effects** Among patients receiving anastrozole as adjuvant therapy, nausea and vomiting were reported in 13%. Dyspepsia and unspecified GI disorder each occurred in 7% of such patients.

Among patients receiving anastrozole as first-line or second-line therapy, GI disturbance was reported in 34 or 29%, nausea in 19 or 16%, vomiting in 8 or 9%, and anorexia in 5 or 7%, respectively.

Among patients receiving second-line therapy, diarrhea occurred more frequently in patients receiving anastrozole than in those receiving megestrol acetate (8 versus 3%). Dry mouth was reported in 6% of such patients.

Diarrhea occurred in 8–9%, and abdominal pain and constipation each occurred in 7–9% of patients receiving anastrozole.

■ **Respiratory Effects** Pharyngitis occurred in 14, 10, and 6% of patients receiving anastrozole as adjuvant, first-line, or second-line therapy, respectively. Increased cough was reported in 8–11%, and dyspnea was reported in 8–10% of patients receiving anastrozole. Sinusitis occurred in 6% and bronchitis in 5% of patients receiving anastrozole as adjuvant therapy. Sinusitis, bronchitis, and rhinitis each were reported in 2–5% of patients receiving anastrozole as second-line therapy, which was similar to experience in those receiving the drug as first-line therapy.

■ **Nervous System Effects** Among patients receiving anastrozole as adjuvant therapy, mood disturbance was reported in 19%, depression in 13%, insomnia in 10%, and anxiety in 6%. Among patients receiving anastrozole as first-line or second-line therapy, depression occurred in 5% and insomnia occurred in about 5–6%. Headache occurred in 9–13% and dizziness in 6–8% of patients receiving anastrozole. Paresthesia occurred in 7 or 5% of patients receiving anastrozole as adjuvant or second-line therapy, respectively.

Somnolence, confusion, anxiety, and nervousness each were reported in 2–5% of patients receiving anastrozole as second-line therapy, which was similar to experience in those receiving the drug as first-line therapy. Hypertonia occurred in 3% of patients receiving anastrozole as first-line therapy.

■ **Dermatologic Effects** Rash occurred in 11, 8, or 6% of patients receiving anastrozole as adjuvant, first-line, or second-line therapy, respectively. Sweating occurred in 5 or 2% of patients receiving anastrozole as adjuvant or second-line therapy, respectively. Hair thinning, alopecia, and pruritus each were reported in 2–5% of patients receiving anastrozole as second-line therapy, which was similar to experience in those receiving the drug as first-line therapy.

Mucocutaneous disorders, including erythema multiforme and Stevens-Johnson syndrome, have been reported in patients receiving anastrozole.

■ **Metabolic Effects** Weight gain occurred in 9% of patients receiving anastrozole as adjuvant therapy and in 2% of those receiving anastrozole as first-line or second-line therapy. Among patients receiving second-line therapy, weight gain occurred less frequently in patients receiving anastrozole than in those receiving megestrol acetate (2 versus 12%). Weight loss was reported in 2–5% of patients receiving anastrozole as second-line therapy, which was similar to experience in those receiving the drug as first-line therapy.

■ **Hepatic Effects** Increased serum concentrations of γ-glutamyltransferase (GGT), AST, ALT, and alkaline phosphatase were reported in 2–5% of patients receiving anastrozole as second-line therapy, which was similar to experience in those receiving the drug as first-line therapy. During postmarketing surveillance, increased serum concentrations of AST, ALT, or alkaline phosphatase have been reported in up to 10% of patients receiving anastrozole; hepatitis and increased serum concentrations of GGT and bilirubin have been reported in less than 1% of patients.

■ **Hematologic Effects** Anemia occurred in 4% of patients receiving anastrozole as adjuvant therapy. Anemia and leukopenia each were reported in 2–5% of patients receiving anastrozole as second-line therapy, which was similar to experience in those receiving the drug as first-line therapy.

■ **Infectious Complications** Among patients receiving anastrozole as adjuvant therapy, infection was reported in 9%. Infection was reported in 2–5% of patients receiving anastrozole as second-line therapy, which was similar to experience in those receiving the drug as first-line therapy.

■ **Ocular Effects** Cataracts were reported in 6% of patients receiving anastrozole as adjuvant therapy. Retinal hemorrhage has been reported in patients receiving anastrozole as adjuvant therapy.

■ **Sensitivity Reactions** Systemic allergic reactions, including angioedema, urticaria, and anaphylaxis, have been reported in patients receiving anastrozole.

■ **Other Adverse Effects** Fatigue/asthenia occurred in 16–19%, pain (nonspecific) in 11–17%, and chest pain (nonspecific) in 5–7% of patients receiving anastrozole. Accidental injury was reported in 10% of patients receiving anastrozole as adjuvant therapy and in 2–5% of patients receiving anastrozole as first-line or second-line therapy. Flu syndrome was reported in up to 7% of patients receiving anastrozole. Cyst occurred in 5% of patients receiving anastrozole as adjuvant therapy. Lethargy was reported in 1% of patients receiving anastrozole as first-line therapy. Fever and malaise each were reported in 2–5% of patients receiving anastrozole as second-line therapy, which was similar to experience in those receiving the drug as first-line therapy.

■ **Precautions and Contraindications** Anastrozole currently is indicated for use in the treatment of breast cancer in postmenopausal women only. Anastrozole is *not* recommended for use in premenopausal women because safety and efficacy have not been established in this patient population.

Postmenopausal women with breast cancer receiving adjuvant therapy with an aromatase inhibitor, such as anastrozole, are at high risk for osteoporosis. Postmenopausal women initiating such therapy should undergo screening to determine BMD and be evaluated for other risk factors for osteoporotic fractures. Patients should be monitored closely for changes in risk status during therapy, and BMD should be assessed at regular intervals. Appropriate therapy to prevent further bone loss should be initiated as clinically indicated. All women receiving adjuvant therapy with anastrozole should be advised to adopt lifestyle changes (e.g., weight-bearing exercise) and dietary supplementation with calcium and vitamin D to reduce the risk of osteoporosis. (Also see Cautions: Musculoskeletal Effects.)

The effect of anastrozole on lipid metabolism has not been fully established, and serum lipoprotein concentrations should be monitored in patients receiving long-term therapy with the drug.

Because an increased incidence of ischemic cardiovascular events has been observed in women with preexisting ischemic heart disease who received anastrozole as adjuvant therapy, risks and benefits of the drug should be considered in patients with ischemic heart disease.

Anastrozole is contraindicated in patients with known hypersensitivity to the drug or any component of the commercially available formulation.

■ **Pediatric Precautions** Efficacy of anastrozole for the treatment of pubertal gynecomastia† in adolescent males and for the treatment of progressive precocious puberty associated with McCune-Albright syndrome† in girls has not been established.

Results of a randomized, double-blind, placebo-controlled trial in 80 adolescent males 11–18 years of age with pubertal gynecomastia failed to establish efficacy of anastrozole (1 mg daily for 6 months) in reducing gynecomastia or relieving breast pain. Serum estradiol concentrations were reduced by 15.4 or 4.5% in patients receiving anastrozole or placebo, respectively. Patients receiving anastrozole were more likely to experience treatment-related adverse effects (16.3 versus 8.1%), and the difference was related mainly to higher rates of acne and headache in those receiving anastrozole. One patient discontinued anastrozole therapy because of testicular enlargement.

Results of a noncomparative open-label trial of anastrozole (1 mg daily for 12 months) in 28 girls (2 to less than 10 years of age) with McCune-Albright syndrome and progressive precocious puberty showed no reduction from baseline in the frequency of vaginal bleeding days or in the rate of increase in bone age and no clinically important changes in Tanner staging, mean ovarian or uterine volume, or mean predicted adult height. A small reduction in growth rate was observed; however, because the study was uncontrolled, it is unclear whether this effect was related to anastrozole or to other confounding factors (e.g., variations in endogenous estrogen levels commonly observed in patients with McCune-Albright syndrome). Adverse effects (i.e., nausea, acne, extremity pain, increased aminotransferase concentrations, allergic dermatitis) were reported in 18% of patients.

Pharmacokinetics of anastrozole were similar in adolescent males with pubertal gynecomastia and in girls with McCune-Albright syndrome, and the elimination half-life in these pediatric populations (about 47 hours) was similar to that observed in postmenopausal women with breast cancer.

■ **Geriatric Precautions** Among patients receiving anastrozole as adjuvant therapy for early-stage breast cancer in the ATAC trial, 45% were 65 years of age or older. Subgroup analysis showed that anastrozole did not provide the same benefit for disease-free survival in women 65 years of age or older (hazard ratio of 0.93 with a 95% confidence interval of 0.8–1.08) that it provided in postmenopausal women younger than 65 years of age (hazard ratio of 0.79 with a 95% confidence interval of 0.67–0.94).

Among patients receiving anastrozole as first-line or second-line therapy in clinical trials, about 50% were 65 years of age or older. No difference in efficacy was observed for geriatric patients (65 years or older) compared with younger patients receiving anastrozole as second-line therapy for advanced breast cancer; moderately greater efficacy was observed for geriatric patients (65 years or older) receiving either anastrozole or tamoxifen as first-line therapy for advanced breast cancer.

■ **Mutagenicity and Carcinogenicity** ***Mutagenicity*** In vitro tests, including the Ames and *E. coli* bacterial tests and the CHO-K1 gene mutation assay, have not shown anastrozole to be mutagenic. In addition, the drug was not shown to be clastogenic in the in vitro chromosome aberration test in human lymphocytes or in the in vivo micronucleus test in rats.

Carcinogenicity At a median duration of treatment of 60 months, a lower incidence of endometrial cancer (0.2 versus 0.6%) was observed in patients receiving anastrozole versus tamoxifen as adjuvant therapy in a large, randomized trial; neoplasm and breast neoplasm each were reported as an adverse event in 5% of patients in each treatment group. At a median follow-up of 10 years, the incidence of endometrial cancer remained lower in patients who had received anastrozole compared with those who had received tamoxifen for a median of 60 months (0.2 versus 0.8%); the cumulative incidence of new primary cancers was similar (14%) in each treatment group.

Anastrozole has shown carcinogenic activity in animal models. In rats administered anastrozole 1–25 mg/kg daily (about 10–243 times the daily maximum recommended human dose on a mg/m² basis) by oral gavage for up to 2 years, an increase in the incidence of hepatocellular adenoma and carcinoma and uterine stromal polyps was observed in females and an increased incidence of thyroid adenoma was observed in males receiving the high dose. In female rats, a dose-related increase in the incidence of ovarian and uterine hyperplasia was observed. Area under the plasma concentration-time curve from 0 to 24 hours (AUC_{0-24h}) values in rats receiving anastrozole 25 mg/kg daily were 110–125 times higher than AUC_{0-24h} values in postmenopausal individuals receiving the recommended dose of the drug.

In mice, oral doses of anastrozole 5–50 mg/kg daily (about 24–243 times the daily maximum recommended human dose on a mg/m² basis) for up to 2 years resulted in an increased incidence of benign ovarian stromal, epithelial, and granulosa cell tumors in female mice at all dosage levels and an increased incidence of lymphosarcoma in male and female mice at the high dose. In female mice, a dose-related increase in the incidence of ovarian hyperplasia also was observed; the ovarian changes observed are considered to be rodent-specific effects of aromatase inhibition, and the clinical importance of these effects to humans is unknown. AUC values in mice receiving anastrozole 50 mg/kg daily were 35–40 times higher than AUC values in postmenopausal individuals receiving the recommended dosage of the drug.

■ **Pregnancy, Fertility, and Lactation** Anastrozole is contraindicated in women who are or may become pregnant (i.e., premenopausal women) since the drug can cause fetal toxicity when administered to pregnant women and clinical benefits of anastrozole therapy in premenopausal women with breast cancer have not been established. If the drug is administered during pregnancy or if the patient becomes pregnant while receiving the drug, the patient should be informed of the potential hazard to the fetus and the potential risk for loss of the pregnancy.

Adequate, well-controlled studies of anastrozole in pregnant women have not been conducted. Anastrozole has been shown to cross the placenta in rats and rabbits receiving oral doses of 0.1 mg/kg (approximately 1 and 1.9 times the recommended human dose, respectively, on a mg/m² basis). Increased pregnancy loss (increased preimplantation and/or postimplantation loss, increased resorption, and decreased numbers of live fetuses) was demonstrated in rats and rabbits receiving anastrozole dosages equal to or exceeding 0.1 and 0.02 mg/kg daily, respectively (about one and one-third times the recommended human dosage, respectively, on a mg/m² basis), during the period of organogenesis; in rats, this effect was dose-related. In rats receiving dosages equal to or exceeding 0.1 mg/kg daily, placental weights were increased.

In rats, anastrozole dosages of 1 mg/kg daily (which produced steady-state peak plasma anastrozole concentrations and AUC_{0-24h} values that were 19 and 9 times higher, respectively, than those observed in healthy postmenopausal women receiving the recommended dose) resulted in fetotoxicity, including delayed fetal development (i.e., incomplete ossification and depressed fetal body weights). In rats, no evidence of teratogenicity was observed at dosages of up to 1 mg/kg daily. In rabbits, anastrozole dosages equal to or exceeding 1 mg/kg daily (about 16 times the recommended human dosage on a mg/m² basis) caused pregnancy failure. No evidence of teratogenicity was observed in rabbits receiving anastrozole 0.2 mg/kg daily (about 3 times the recommended human dosage on a mg/m² basis).

Impairment of fertility and effects on the reproductive organs associated with anastrozole have been demonstrated in animal studies. In female rats, oral administration of anastrozole at a dosage of 1 mg/kg daily (about 10 times the recommended human dosage on a mg/m² basis and resulting in an AUC_{0-24h} about 9 times higher than that observed in postmenopausal women receiving the recommended dose) from 2 weeks before mating to pregnancy day 7 caused a high incidence of infertility and reduced numbers of viable pregnancies. Preimplantation loss of ova or fetus was increased at dosages equal to or exceeding 0.02 mg/kg daily (about one-fifth the recommended human dosage on a mg/m² basis). Recovery of fertility was observed following a 5-week nondosing period that followed 3 weeks of dosing. Whether the effects observed in rats are indicative of impaired fertility in humans receiving anastrozole is not known.

In multiple-dose studies in rats, anastrozole dosages equal to or exceeding 1 mg/kg daily for 6 months (which resulted in steady-state peak plasma anastrozole concentrations and AUC_{0-24h} values that were 19 and 9 times higher, respectively, than those observed in healthy postmenopausal humans receiving the recommended dosage) resulted in hypertrophy of the ovaries and development of follicular cysts. In multiple-dose studies in dogs receiving anastrozole dosages equal to or exceeding 1 mg/kg daily for 6 months (which produced steady-state peak plasma anastrozole concentrations and AUC_{0-24h} values that were 22 and 16 times higher, respectively, than those observed in postmenopausal women receiving the recommended dosage), hyperplastic uteri were observed. The relationship between the reproductive effects observed in animals and possible effects of the drug on fertility in humans is not known.

It is not known whether anastrozole is distributed into milk. Because many drugs are distributed into milk and because tumorigenic effects of anastrozole have been observed in animals and anastrozole has the potential to cause serious adverse reactions in nursing infants, a decision should be made whether to discontinue nursing or the drug, taking into account the importance of the drug to the woman.

Drug Interactions

■ **Selective Estrogen Receptor Modulators** The concomitant use of selective estrogen receptor modulators (e.g., tamoxifen, raloxifene) and aromatase inhibitors, such as anastrozole, is not recommended.

Data from a subprotocol of the ATAC trial indicate that concomitant use of anastrozole and tamoxifen does not affect the pharmacokinetics of tamoxifen or *N*-desmethyltamoxifen, its principal active metabolite. The mean plasma anastrozole concentration was reduced by an average of 27% in patients receiving tamoxifen and anastrozole versus anastrozole alone, but analysis of blood samples from a different subprotocol of the ATAC trial demonstrates similar degrees of suppression of plasma estradiol concentrations for anastrozole alone and in combination with tamoxifen. Although the clinical importance of this pharmacokinetic interaction is uncertain, combination therapy did not demonstrate greater efficacy than use of tamoxifen alone, and the concomitant use of anastrozole and tamoxifen is *not* recommended.

Because this pharmacokinetic interaction may occur with similar agents and reduce plasma concentrations of anastrozole, the concomitant use of other selective estrogen receptor modulators (e.g., raloxifene) is not recommended. Among women receiving anastrozole who require drug therapy for osteoporosis, the use of an oral bisphosphonate, rather than raloxifene, is advised.

■ **Estrogens** Because estrogens may diminish the pharmacologic action of anastrozole, the drugs should not be used concomitantly.

■ **Drugs Metabolized by Hepatic Microsomal Enzymes** Anastrozole has been shown to inhibit in vitro metabolic reactions catalyzed by cytochrome P-450 (CYP) isoenzymes 1A2, 2C8/9, and 3A4, but only at relatively high concentrations. Anastrozole did not inhibit CYP isoenzyme 2A6 or 2D6 in human liver microsomes, and the drug did not alter the pharmacokinetics of antipyrine. In addition, anastrozole did not alter systemic exposure (as measured by peak plasma concentrations and area under the concentration-time curve [AUC]) or anticoagulant effects of either *R*- or *S*-warfarin. It is considered unlikely that anastrozole, when administered at the recommended dosage, will result in clinically important interactions with drugs metabolized by CYP enzymes.

Acute Toxicity

■ **Pathogenesis** Limited information is available on the acute toxicity of anastrozole. In clinical trials, single doses of up to 60 mg (administered to healthy males) and multiple doses of up to 10 mg daily (administered to postmenopausal women with advanced breast cancer) have been well tolerated. A single dose of anastrozole that results in life-threatening manifestations has not been identified. Lethality occurred in rats receiving single doses exceeding 100 mg/kg (about 800 times the recommended human dose on a mg/m² basis); lethal doses of the drug were associated with severe irritation to the stomach, including necrosis, gastritis, ulceration, and hemorrhage. In dogs, a median lethal oral dosage exceeding 45 mg/kg daily was reported.

■ **Treatment** There is no known specific antidote for anastrozole overdosage. Management of overdosage should consist of symptomatic treatment and general supportive care, including frequent monitoring of vital signs and close observation of the patient. The possibility that multiple agents may have been taken should be considered. If the patient is alert, emesis may be induced. Because anastrozole is not highly bound to plasma proteins, dialysis may be helpful.

Pharmacology

Anastrozole, a benzyltriazole derivative, is a selective, nonsteroidal aromatase inhibitor. Anastrozole differs structurally from aminoglutethimide but shares the pharmacologic activity of competitive aromatase inhibition; although both drugs are selective nonsteroidal inhibitors, anastrozole is more potent and selective on a molar basis.

■ **Antineoplastic Effects** Because estrogen acts as a growth factor for hormone-dependent breast cancer cells, anastrozole-induced reduction of serum and tumor concentrations of estrogen (see Pharmacology: Hormonal Effects) inhibits tumor growth and delays disease progression.

Many breast cancers also contain aromatase; however, the importance of tumor-generated estrogens has not been determined.

■ **Hormonal Effects** Anastrozole selectively inhibits the conversion of androgens to estrogens. In postmenopausal women, ovarian secretion of estrogen declines and conversion of adrenal androgens (mainly androstenedione and testosterone) to estrone and estradiol in peripheral tissues (adipose, muscle, and liver), catalyzed by the aromatase enzyme, is the principal source of estrogens. Anastrozole inhibits the aromatase enzyme by competitively binding to the heme of the cytochrome P-450 unit of the enzyme; suppression of estrogen biosynthesis in all tissues reduces serum concentrations of circulating estrogens, including estrone, estradiol, and estrone sulfate.

Anastrozole selectively inhibits synthesis of estrogens and does not affect synthesis of adrenal corticosteroid, aldosterone, or thyroid hormone. In animals, anastrozole has not been shown to possess direct progestogenic, androgenic, or estrogenic activity, but alterations in the circulating concentrations of progesterone, androgens, and estrogens have been observed.

Clinically important suppression of serum estradiol concentrations has been observed in postmenopausal women with advanced breast cancer receiving multiple daily anastrozole doses of 0.5, 1, 3, 5, and 10 mg. Anastrozole doses equal to or exceeding 1 mg resulted in suppression of mean serum estradiol concentrations to the lower limit of detection (3.7 pmol/L). Administration of anastrozole at the recommended daily oral dose of 1 mg reduced serum estradiol concentrations by about 70% within 24 hours and by about 80% after 14 days of daily dosing. Suppression of serum estradiol concentrations was maintained for up to 6 days after discontinuance of anastrozole 1 mg daily. No effect on cortisol or aldosterone secretion at baseline or in response to corticotropin (adrenocorticotropic hormone, ACTH) was observed in multiple daily dosing trials with anastrozole 3, 5, or 10 mg. No increase in thyrotropin (thyroid-stimulating hormone, TSH) was observed in patients receiving multiple daily doses of anastrozole 5 or 10 mg.

The effect of anastrozole on serum estradiol concentrations in premenopausal women has not been studied. Ovarian secretion is the principal source of estrogen in premenopausal women; because it acts by suppressing other sources of estrogens, anastrozole would not be expected to lower serum estradiol concentrations in women with functioning ovaries.

Pharmacokinetics

The pharmacokinetics of anastrozole are linear over the dose range of 1–20 mg and are not altered with repeated dosing. The pharmacokinetic disposition of anastrozole is similar in female patients with breast cancer and in healthy postmenopausal women.

■ **Absorption** Anastrozole is rapidly and well absorbed into systemic circulation following oral administration; peak plasma concentrations generally are attained within 2 hours when the drug is administered in the fasted state. Plasma concentrations approach steady state after about 7 days of once-daily dosing, and steady-state concentrations are approximately 3–4 times higher than concentrations achieved after a single dose of the drug.

Food reduces the rate but does not affect the extent of oral absorption of anastrozole. When anastrozole was administered 30 minutes after food, the mean peak plasma concentration of the drug was decreased by 16% and the median time to peak plasma concentration was delayed by 3 hours.

■ **Distribution** Within the therapeutic plasma concentration range, anastrozole is 40% bound to plasma proteins.

It is not known whether anastrozole crosses the placenta in humans; however, the drug has been shown to cross the placenta in rats and rabbits. (See Cautions: Pregnancy, Fertility, and Lactation.)

It is not known whether anastrozole is distributed into milk in humans.

■ **Elimination** A mean terminal elimination half-life of approximately 50 hours has been reported.

Anastrozole is extensively metabolized in the liver. Hepatic metabolism accounts for about 85% of the elimination of anastrozole, with renal excretion accounting for only about 10% of total clearance. Studies with radiolabeled drug have shown that about 85% of an orally administered dose is recovered in urine and feces.

Metabolism of anastrozole occurs via *N*-dealkylation, hydroxylation, and glucuronidation. Three metabolites of anastrozole have been identified in human plasma and urine: triazole, a glucuronide conjugate of anastrozole, and a glucuronide conjugate of hydroxyanastrozole. Triazole, the major circulating metabolite of anastrozole, lacks pharmacologic activity, and the aromatase-inhibiting activity of anastrozole results principally from the parent drug.

Among healthy postmenopausal women and female patients with breast cancer, no age-related differences in pharmacokinetics of anastrozole have been observed in women older than 80 years of age compared with women younger than 50 years of age.

The apparent oral clearance of anastrozole was reduced by approximately 30% in individuals with stable hepatic cirrhosis related to alcohol abuse compared with controls with normal hepatic function. However, plasma anastrozole concentrations observed in individuals with hepatic cirrhosis were within the range of concentrations observed in normal individuals across all clinical trials.

Although the renal clearance of anastrozole decreases proportionally with creatinine clearance and is reduced by about 50% in individuals with severe renal impairment (creatinine clearance less than 30 mL/minute per 1.73 m^2) compared with controls, total body clearance of anastrozole is reduced by only 10% in patients with severe renal impairment.

Steady-state minimum plasma concentrations averaged 25.7 and 30.4 ng/mL, respectively, in white and Japanese postmenopausal women receiving anastrozole 1 mg daily for 16 days; serum estradiol and estrone sulfate concentrations were similar between the groups.

Chemistry and Stability

■ **Chemistry** Anastrozole, a benzyltriazole derivative, is a selective, nonsteroidal aromatase inhibitor. Competitive aromatase inhibitors, such as anastrozole, also have been referred to as type II inhibitors of the enzyme. Anastrozole differs structurally from aminoglutethimide but shares the pharmacologic activity of competitive aromatase inhibition. Anastrozole is a triazole derivative; the *N*-4 nitrogen of the triazole ring, which coordinates with the heme iron atom of the aromatase enzyme complex, is thought to be responsible for the high affinity of the drug for the estrogen synthetase enzyme.

Anastrozole occurs as an off-white powder. Anastrozole is very slightly soluble in water (0.5 mg/mL at 25°C), and solubility of the drug is independent of pH within the physiologic range. Anastrozole is freely soluble in methanol, acetone, alcohol, and tetrahydrofuran, and very soluble in acetonitrile.

■ **Stability** Commercially available anastrozole tablets should be stored at a controlled room temperature of 20–25°C.

For further information on the handling of antineoplastic agents, see the ASHP Guidelines on Handling Hazardous Drugs at http://www.ahfsdruginformation.com.

Preparations

Excipients in commercially available drug preparations may have clinically important effects in some individuals; consult specific product labeling for details.

Anastrozole

Oral

Tablets, film-coated	1 mg*	**Anastrozole Film-coated Tablets**
		Arimidex®, AstraZeneca

*available from one or more manufacturer, distributor, and/or repackager by generic (nonproprietary) name

†Use is not currently included in the labeling approved by the US Food and Drug Administration

Exemestane

■ Exemestane, an aromatase inhibitor, is an antineoplastic agent.

Uses

■ **Breast Cancer** ***Initial or Sequential Adjuvant Therapy for Early-stage Breast Cancer*** Exemestane is used as sequential adjuvant therapy in postmenopausal women with early-stage estrogen receptor-positive breast cancer who have received 2–3 years of adjuvant tamoxifen therapy and are switched to exemestane to complete a total of 5 consecutive years of adjuvant hormonal therapy. Exemestane also has been used alone as initial adjuvant therapy† in postmenopausal women with early-stage hormone receptor-positive breast cancer. Aromatase inhibitors, including exemestane, currently are considered a treatment of choice for adjuvant hormonal therapy to lower the risk of breast cancer recurrence in postmenopausal women with early-stage hormone receptor-positive breast cancer. Although tamoxifen historically has been the drug of choice for adjuvant hormonal therapy in such patients, results of large, randomized clinical studies indicate that an aromatase inhibitor-containing regimen is modestly more effective than tamoxifen alone. Longer-term follow-up of these studies is needed to further clarify lasting clinical efficacy, effects on survival, and late adverse effects of aromatase inhibitor therapy.

Clinical Trials of Exemestane as Sequential Adjuvant Therapy. In Intergroup Exemestane Study 031, a randomized double-blind trial, 4724 postmenopausal women who previously had been diagnosed with early-stage breast cancer and who remained free of disease after 2–3 years of adjuvant tamoxifen therapy were randomized to switch to exemestane therapy or to continue receiving tamoxifen to complete a total of 5 years of adjuvant hormonal therapy. The median duration of tamoxifen therapy prior to randomization was approximately 28 months. Exemestane was administered at a dosage of 25 mg daily, and tamoxifen was administered at a dosage of 20 or 30 mg daily (about 3% of patients received the 30-mg dosage). About 86% of patients enrolled in the study had estrogen receptor-positive disease. The primary end point of the trial was disease-free survival.

Analysis of the data at a median follow-up of 34.5 months, when patients had received study treatment for a median of 27 months, showed that disease-free survival was prolonged in patients who were switched from tamoxifen to exemestane compared with those who continued receiving tamoxifen (hazard ratio of 0.69). Distant recurrence-free survival and time to contralateral breast cancer also were prolonged in patients receiving exemestane. Breast cancer-related events in patients receiving exemestane versus tamoxifen included locoregional recurrence (1.4 versus 1.9%), distant recurrence (5.4 versus 7.7%), primary cancer in the contralateral breast (0.3 versus 1%), breast cancer-related death (0.04 versus 0.25%), and ipsilateral breast cancer (0.04 versus 0%). No difference in overall survival was observed between the 2 treatment groups overall or within the subset of patients with hormone receptor-positive disease.

Subsequent analyses showed that the disease-free survival benefit associated with switching to exemestane was maintained at a median follow-up of about 4.6 years (hazard ratio of 0.76, which corresponded to an absolute improvement in disease-free survival of 3.3 or 3.4% at 2.5 or 5 years, respectively, after randomization) and at a median follow-up of about 7.6 years (hazard ratio of 0.84, which corresponded to an absolute difference in disease-free survival of 2.8 or 4.1% at 5 or 8 years, respectively, after randomization). No difference in overall survival was observed between the 2 treatment groups. However, among patients with estrogen receptor-positive or estrogen receptor-unknown disease, use of exemestane as sequential adjuvant therapy was associated with a modest overall survival benefit at 7.6 years of follow-up (hazard ratio of 0.86, which corresponded to an absolute difference in disease-free survival of 1.4 or 2.4% at 5 or 8 years, respectively, after randomization).

Hypertension, other cardiovascular events (e.g., cardiac ischemia), musculoskeletal pain, arthralgia, arthritis, osteoporosis, fracture, carpal tunnel syndrome, paresthesia, diarrhea, and gastric ulcer occurred more frequently during treatment or posttreatment follow-up in patients receiving exemestane, whereas venous thromboembolism, muscle cramp, serious gynecologic event (e.g., vaginal bleeding, uterine dilatation and curettage), endometrial hyperplasia, and uterine polyp/fibroid occurred more frequently in patients receiving tamoxifen.

Clinical Trials of Exemestane as Initial Adjuvant Therapy. Data from two phase 3 randomized open-label clinical trials indicate that initial therapy† with exemestane is at least as effective as initial therapy with anastrozole or sequential therapy with tamoxifen followed by exemestane in postmenopausal women with early-stage hormone receptor-positive breast cancer.

In the first study (Tamoxifen Exemestane Adjuvant Multinational [TEAM]), 9779 postmenopausal women with early-stage hormone receptor-positive breast cancer were randomized to receive exemestane 25 mg daily for 5 years or sequential therapy with tamoxifen 20 mg daily for 2–3 years followed by exemestane 25 mg daily for a total treatment duration of 5 years. Most (98%) of the patients enrolled in the study had estrogen receptor-positive tumors. The primary end point of the study was disease-free survival. At a median follow-up of 5.1 years, no significant difference in estimated 5-year disease-free survival was observed between patients receiving sequential therapy and those receiving initial exemestane therapy (85 and 86%, respectively; hazard ratio of 0.97 with a 95% confidence interval of 0.88–1.08); in addition, no difference in 5-year overall survival was observed between the groups. Disease relapse or breast cancer-related death occurred in similar proportions of patients receiving sequential therapy (11%) or initial exemestane therapy (10%). In this study, fractures, osteoporosis, hyperlipidemia, hypertension, and cardiac failure occurred more frequently in patients receiving initial exemestane therapy, whereas venous thrombosis, vaginal bleeding, and endometrial disorders occurred more frequently in those receiving sequential therapy.

In the second study (MA.27), 7576 postmenopausal women with hormone receptor-positive primary invasive breast cancer were randomized to receive exemestane 25 mg daily or anastrozole 1 mg daily for 5 years, with or without celecoxib; however, random assignment to celecoxib was halted when data from another study suggested that celecoxib may increase cardiovascular risk. Patients were stratified according to lymph node status, receipt of prior adjuvant chemotherapy, use of concomitant trastuzumab therapy, and previous random assignment to celecoxib and concomitant prophylactic aspirin therapy. Most (99%) of the patients enrolled in the study had estrogen receptor-positive tumors. The primary end point of the study was event-free survival. At a median follow-up of 4.1 years, no significant difference in estimated 4-year event-free survival was observed between patients receiving exemestane and those receiving anastrozole (91 and 91.2%, respectively; hazard ratio of 1.02 with a 95% confidence interval of 0.87–1.18). In addition, no difference in overall survival was observed between the groups. Elevations in aminotransferase (ALT or AST) concentrations (3 versus 1%), elevations in serum bilirubin concentrations (2 versus 1%), and atrial fibrillation (2 versus 1%) occurred more frequently in patients receiving exemestane, whereas hyperlipidemia (18 versus 15%), hypertriglyceridemia (3 versus 2%), and osteoporosis (35 versus 31%) occurred more frequently in patients receiving anastrozole.

Clinical Role. Based on data from randomized controlled trials demonstrating prolonged disease-free survival in patients receiving aromatase inhibitor-based adjuvant regimens, use of exemestane may be considered a reasonable choice (accepted, with possible conditions) for initial adjuvant therapy in postmenopausal women with early-stage hormone receptor-positive breast cancer; factors that should be considered when selecting an appropriate aromatase inhibitor include tolerability, patient preference, and preexisting conditions.

The American Society of Clinical Oncology (ASCO) states that most postmenopausal women with early-stage hormone receptor-positive breast cancer should consider receiving an aromatase inhibitor (e.g., exemestane) during the course of adjuvant therapy, either as primary (initial) therapy or following 2–3 years of tamoxifen therapy (sequential therapy), to complete a total of 5 years of adjuvant endocrine therapy. Clinically meaningful differences among the currently available aromatase inhibitors (i.e., anastrozole, exemestane, letrozole) have not been demonstrated to date. Data also support switching to an aromatase inhibitor following 5 years of adjuvant tamoxifen therapy (extended therapy) (see Extended Adjuvant Therapy for Early-stage Breast Cancer under Uses: Breast Cancer). The optimal time for switching from tamoxifen to an aromatase inhibitor is not known. The duration of aromatase inhibitor therapy should not exceed 5 years, since toxicity of long-term (e.g., beyond 5 years) use of aromatase inhibitors, including exemestane, has not been determined. The optimal duration of adjuvant exemestane therapy is not known. ASCO states that clinicians should consider adverse effects, patient preference, and preexisting conditions when selecting an adjuvant regimen; during the course of adjuvant therapy, patients who are intolerant of one aromatase inhibitor may be switched to a different aromatase inhibitor or to tamoxifen.

The use of a luteinizing hormone-releasing hormone (LHRH) agonist (e.g., triptorelin) in combination with exemestane as adjuvant therapy in *premenopausal* women with hormone receptor-positive breast cancer† is being investigated in a large randomized trial. The use of an aromatase inhibitor as a single agent for adjuvant therapy is *not* appropriate in premenopausal women with breast cancer because these agents alone are not likely to provide sufficient suppression of ovarian function to be of clinical benefit. Similarly, the use of an aromatase inhibitor as monotherapy for adjuvant therapy for hormone receptor-positive breast cancer in premenopausal women experiencing a chemotherapy-induced disruption in ovarian function is not advised; a substantial number of such patients can expect resumption of ovarian function, and this would likely render therapy with an aromatase inhibitor ineffective.

Extended Adjuvant Therapy for Early-stage Breast Cancer

Exemestane has been used as extended adjuvant therapy† in postmenopausal women with early-stage breast cancer who have received 5 years of adjuvant tamoxifen therapy.

Clinical Trials. Efficacy of exemestane as extended adjuvant therapy in postmenopausal women with early-stage breast cancer who have received 5 years of adjuvant tamoxifen therapy has been evaluated in a double-blind, placebo-controlled, randomized phase 3 trial (National Surgical Adjuvant Breast and Bowel Project [NSABP] B-33) in postmenopausal women mostly with hormone receptor-positive breast cancer (97% hormone receptor-positive, 3% hormone receptor-unknown). In this trial, 1598 patients who had received adjuvant therapy with tamoxifen for approximately 5 years (range: approximately 4.75–5.6 years) were randomized to receive exemestane 25 mg daily or placebo for 5 years. Based on interim results from a similarly designed trial demonstrating benefit from extended adjuvant therapy with letrozole, recruitment of patients for the NSABP B-33 trial was halted early, the study was unblinded, and exemestane therapy was offered to all women who had been receiving placebo. After the study was unblinded, 44% of patients randomized to receive placebo crossed over to receive exemestane therapy and 72% of patients randomized to receive exemestane continued their assigned therapy.

At a median follow-up of 30 months, the estimated 4-year disease-free survival did not differ significantly between patients receiving exemestane and those receiving placebo (91 versus 89%, respectively, based on intent-to-treat analysis); in addition, no difference in overall survival was observed between the groups. A significant difference in estimated 4-year relapse-free survival was observed between patients randomized to receive exemestane and those randomized to receive placebo (96 versus 94%, respectively). Exemestane treatment was associated with numerically, but not significantly, fewer local or metastatic recurrences and with a significant reduction in the incidence of new contralateral breast cancer, as compared with placebo. An exploratory subset analysis suggested that the effect of exemestane on disease-free survival was greater in patients with tumors larger than 2 cm or with node-positive disease. Although grade 3 adverse effects occurred more commonly in patients receiving exemestane, the incidence of grade 4 adverse effects was similar for patients receiving exemestane or placebo.

Clinical Role. Based on data from randomized controlled trials demonstrating prolonged disease-free survival in patients receiving aromatase inhibitors as extended adjuvant therapy, use of exemestane may be considered a reasonable choice (accepted, with possible conditions) for extended adjuvant therapy in postmenopausal women with early-stage hormone receptor-positive breast cancer who have received 5 years of adjuvant tamoxifen therapy; factors that should be considered when selecting an appropriate aromatase inhibitor include tolerability, patient preference, and preexisting conditions.

ASCO recommends extended therapy with an aromatase inhibitor (e.g., exemestane) in postmenopausal women with early-stage hormone receptor-positive breast cancer who complete 5 years of adjuvant tamoxifen therapy. (See Extended Adjuvant Therapy for Early-stage Breast Cancer in Uses: Breast Cancer, in Letrozole 68:16.08.) Clinically meaningful differences among the currently available aromatase inhibitors (i.e., anastrozole, exemestane, letrozole) have not been demonstrated to date. Clinicians should consider adverse effects, patient preference, and preexisting conditions when selecting an adjuvant regimen. ASCO states that women who receive extended adjuvant therapy should receive a total of 8–10 years of adjuvant endocrine therapy, including 5 years of tamoxifen therapy followed by 3–5 years of aromatase inhibitor therapy. The optimal duration of exemestane as extended adjuvant therapy is not known, and the toxicity of long-term (e.g., beyond 5 years) use of aromatase inhibitors, including exemestane, in this setting has not been determined. Ongoing clinical trials are evaluating whether longer durations of aromatase inhibitor therapy are more effective.

Second-line Therapy for Advanced Breast Cancer Exemestane is used in the treatment of advanced breast cancer in postmenopausal women whose disease has progressed following tamoxifen therapy. Efficacy was evaluated in one comparative study (versus megestrol acetate) and 2 single-arm studies in postmenopausal women with advanced breast cancer that progressed after tamoxifen therapy for metastatic disease or as adjuvant therapy; some patients also received prior chemotherapy either for metastasis or as adjuvant therapy. The studies evaluated objective response rates (complete and partial response); time to tumor progression (TTP) and overall survival also were assessed in the comparative study. In the comparative study, objective response rates for exemestane and megestrol were comparable at 15 and 12.4%, respectively. Response rates for exemestane in the 2 single-arm studies were 23.4 and 28.1%. In the comparative study, the median duration of response was 76.1 and 71 weeks for exemestane and megestrol, respectively, and the median TTP was 20.3 and 16.6 weeks, respectively. No conclusions could be drawn related to overall survival differences with the limited study data available.

Dosage and Administration

■ **General** Exemestane is administered orally after a meal (to enhance GI absorption).

Breast Cancer Dosage adjustments are recommended when exemestane is used in conjunction with potent inducers of cytochrome P-450 (CYP) isoenzyme 3A4. (See Cytochrome P-450 Isoenzyme 3A4 Inducers under Drug Interactions: Drugs Affecting or Metabolized by Hepatic Microsomal Enzymes.)

Initial or Sequential Adjuvant Therapy for Early-stage Breast Cancer. For sequential adjuvant treatment in postmenopausal women with early-stage estrogen receptor-positive breast cancer, the recommended dosage of exemestane is 25 mg once daily. Exemestane is used in patients who have received 2–3 years of adjuvant tamoxifen therapy and are being switched to exemestane to complete a total of 5 consecutive years of adjuvant hormonal therapy.

When used for initial adjuvant treatment† in postmenopausal women with early-stage hormone receptor-positive breast cancer, exemestane has been administered at a dosage of 25 mg once daily for 5 years.

The American Society of Clinical Oncology (ASCO) states that an aromatase inhibitor (e.g., exemestane) may be administered to postmenopausal women with early-stage hormone receptor-positive breast cancer as initial adjuvant therapy and continued for a total of 5 years or may be administered following initial tamoxifen therapy as part of a sequential adjuvant regimen. The optimal time to switch from tamoxifen to aromatase inhibitor therapy is not known; however, based on clinical trials conducted to date, ASCO recommends that patients who are disease-free may be switched to an aromatase inhibitor after 2–3 years of tamoxifen therapy to complete a 5-year sequential adjuvant regimen. In patients who initially receive an aromatase inhibitor but discontinue therapy prior to 5 years, ASCO states that consideration should be given to administering tamoxifen to complete the 5-year adjuvant regimen.

Extended Adjuvant Therapy for Early-stage Breast Cancer. When used for extended adjuvant treatment† in postmenopausal women with early-stage breast cancer who have received 5 years of adjuvant tamoxifen therapy, exemestane has been administered at a dosage of 25 mg once daily. ASCO recommends that patients who receive an extended adjuvant regimen receive an aromatase inhibitor (e.g., exemestane) for 3–5 years beyond the initial 5 years of tamoxifen therapy, to complete a total of 8–10 years of adjuvant endocrine therapy.

Second-line Therapy for Advanced Breast Cancer. For the second-line treatment of advanced breast cancer in postmenopausal women whose disease has progressed following tamoxifen therapy, the recommended dosage of exemestane is 25 mg once daily. Higher dosages have not been shown to provide substantially greater suppression of plasma estrogens but may be associated with increased adverse effects. In clinical trials, treatment generally was continued until tumor progression or unacceptable toxicity occurred.

■ Special Populations

The safety of chronic dosing in patients with moderate to severe renal or hepatic impairment has not been studied. Although exemestane AUCs are increased (e.g., threefold) in patients with renal or hepatic insufficiency, the manufacturer states that experience with exemestane at repeated doses up to 200 mg daily in patients without such insufficiency (which demonstrated a moderate increase in non-life-threatening adverse effects) indicates that dosage adjustment does not appear to be necessary.

Cautions

■ Contraindications

Known hypersensitivity to exemestane or any ingredient in the formulation.

Pregnancy and premenopausal women. (See Fetal/Neonatal Morbidity and Mortality and also Premenopausal Women under Cautions: Warnings/Precautions.)

■ Warnings/Precautions

Fetal/Neonatal Morbidity and Mortality Exemestane may cause fetal harm; the drug has been shown to be embryotoxic, fetotoxic, and abortifacient in animals. There are no adequate and well-controlled studies in pregnant women. Exemestane is contraindicated in women who are or may become pregnant (i.e., premenopausal women). If exemestane is used during pregnancy or if the patient becomes pregnant while receiving the drug, the patient should be apprised of the potential hazard to the fetus and the potential risk for pregnancy loss.

Estrogenic Agents Estrogenic agents should not be administered concomitantly with exemestane. (See Drug Interactions: Estrogenic Agents.)

Effects on Bone Exemestane may cause a reduction in bone mineral density (BMD). Postmenopausal women receiving an aromatase inhibitor as adjuvant therapy are at high risk for osteoporosis. Following 2 years of adjuvant treatment with exemestane or tamoxifen, the reductions from baseline in lumbar spine and femoral neck BMD were 3.1 and 4.2%, respectively, in patients receiving exemestane and 0.2 and 0.3%, respectively, in those receiving tamoxifen. In a placebo-controlled trial, lumbar spine and femoral neck BMD were decreased by 3.5 and 4.6%, respectively, in patients receiving exemestane for 2 years, compared with 2.4 and 2.6%, respectively, in those receiving placebo. Concomitant bisphosphonate therapy and supplementation of vitamin D and calcium were not allowed in these clinical trials. In Intergroup Exemestane Study 031 (which was initiated after patients had completed 2–3 years of adjuvant tamoxifen therapy), patients switched to exemestane to complete 5 years of adjuvant therapy had a higher incidence of fracture during study treatment or posttreatment follow-up than did those who continued receiving tamoxifen (11 versus 8%).

All postmenopausal women initiating adjuvant therapy with an aromatase inhibitor should be evaluated for risk of osteoporotic fractures. Screening with dual energy radiographic absorptiometry (DXA) to determine the BMD of the hip and spine should be performed in conjunction with assessment of other risk factors for fracture (e.g., age, low body mass index, family history of hip fracture, prior fragility fracture, history of cigarette smoking, excess alcohol consumption, current or prior corticosteroid use). Patients should be monitored closely for changes in risk status during therapy, and BMD should be assessed at regular intervals (e.g., every 1–2 years in those with osteopenia or osteoporosis). Other potential causes of osteoporosis (e.g., vitamin D deficiency, hyperthyroidism, hyperparathyroidism, hypercalciuria) should be considered. The manufacturer states that concentrations of 25-hydroxyvitamin D should be measured routinely prior to initiation of exemestane therapy, and women with vitamin D deficiency should receive supplemental vitamin D. Appropriate therapy to prevent further bone loss should be initiated as clinically indicated. The decision to initiate therapy with an antiresorptive agent (e.g., a bisphosphonate, denosumab) should be based on overall risk of fracture and rate of bone loss. (See Uses: Prevention of Aromatase Inhibitor-associated Bone Loss, in Zoledronic Acid 92:24.) All women receiving adjuvant therapy with an aromatase inhibitor should be advised to adopt lifestyle changes (e.g., weight-bearing exercise, abstinence from smoking, moderation in alcohol consumption) and dietary supplementation with calcium and vitamin D to reduce the risk of osteoporosis.

Hematologic Effects Grade 3 or 4 lymphocytopenia was reported in 20% of patients with advanced breast cancer receiving exemestane therapy; however, 89% of these patients had preexisting lower-grade lymphocytopenia, and 40% either recovered or improved to a lesser severity lymphopenia during exemestane therapy. Patients did not experience a substantial increase in viral infections, and no opportunistic infections were observed.

In patients with early-stage breast cancer, hematologic abnormalities were reported less frequently in those receiving exemestane compared with those receiving tamoxifen; grade 3 or 4 abnormalities occurred rarely (about 0.1% of patients).

Hepatic Effects Serum aminotransferase (AST, ALT), alkaline phosphatase, and γ-glutamyltransferase (γ-glutamyltranspeptidase, GGT, GGTP) concentrations exceeding 5 times the upper limit of normal (i.e., grade 3 or worse) have been rarely reported in patients receiving exemestane for treatment of advanced breast cancer, but generally appear to be attributable to bone or liver metastasis. In one study, grade 3 or 4 elevations in GGT concentrations occurred in patients without evidence of liver metastasis in 3 or 2% of those receiving exemestane or megestrol acetate, respectively.

In patients with early-stage breast cancer, elevated serum concentrations of bilirubin and alkaline phosphatase were reported more frequently in patients receiving exemestane (5–7 and 14–15%, respectively) compared with those receiving tamoxifen (0.8 and 3%, respectively) or placebo (0 and 7%, respectively). Grade 3–4 elevations in bilirubin concentrations occurred rarely in patients receiving exemestane (0.9%) or tamoxifen (0.1%).

Renal Effects In clinical studies in patients with early-stage breast cancer, elevated serum creatinine concentrations were reported in 6% of patients receiving exemestane compared with 4% of those receiving tamoxifen and 0% of those receiving placebo.

Specific Populations **Pregnancy.** Category X. (See Fetal/Neonatal Morbidity and Mortality under Cautions: Warnings/Precautions.) (See Users Guide.)

Lactation. Exemestane is distributed into milk in rats; because of the potential for serious adverse effects in nursing infants, a decision should be made whether to discontinue the drug, taking into account the importance of the drug to the woman.

Pediatric Use. Exemestane is not indicated in pediatric patients; safety and efficacy have not been established.

Geriatric Use. Use of exemestane in geriatric patients requires no special precautions.

Premenopausal Women. Because of the lack of safety and efficacy data and because of concerns about possible incomplete estrogen suppression and reflex increases in gonadotrophin levels (ovarian hyperstimulation syndrome) in this population, the manufacturer states that exemestane is contraindicated in premenopausal women.

Hepatic or Renal Impairment. Although safety of chronic dosing in patients with moderate or severe hepatic or renal impairment has not been established, dosage adjustment does not appear to be necessary. (See Dosage and Administration: Special Populations.)

■ Common Adverse Effects

Adverse events reported in 10% or more of patients with early-stage breast cancer receiving exemestane include hot flushes (flashes), fatigue, arthralgia, headache, insomnia, increased sweating, alopecia, hypertension, nausea, and abdominal pain. Adverse events resulting in drug discontinuance occurred in similar proportions of exemestane- and tamoxifen-treated patients.

Adverse events reported in 10% or more of patients with advanced breast cancer receiving exemestane include fatigue, nausea, hot flushes, pain, depression, insomnia, anxiety, and dyspnea.

Drug Interactions

■ Drugs Affecting or Metabolized by Hepatic Microsomal Enzymes

Exemestane is metabolized by cytochrome P-450 isoenzyme 3A4 (CYP3A4). Exemestane does not inhibit CYP isoenzymes 1A2, 2C9, 2D6, 2E1, or 3A4.

Cytochrome P-450 Isoenzyme 3A4 Inhibitors Concomitant administration of ketoconazole, a potent CYP3A4 inhibitor, and exemestane did not substantially alter the pharmacokinetics of exemestane. Therefore, clinically important pharmacokinetic interactions between exemestane and CYP3A4 inhibitors appear to be unlikely.

Cytochrome P-450 Isoenzyme 3A4 Inducers Administration of the potent CYP3A4 inducer rifampin (600 mg daily for 14 days) followed by exemestane (single 25-mg dose) resulted in a 41% decrease in peak plasma concentrations and a 54% decrease in systemic exposure of exemestane. Concomitant use of other CYP3A4 inducers (e.g., carbamazepine, phenobarbital, phenytoin, St. John's wort [*Hypericum perforatum*]) also may result in decreased exposure to exemestane. An increase in exemestane dosage to 50 mg once daily is recommended in patients receiving concomitant therapy with a potent CYP3A4 inducer.

■ **Estrogenic Agents** Because estrogens may diminish the pharmacologic action of exemestane, the drugs should not be used concomitantly.

Pharmacokinetics

■ **Absorption** ***Bioavailability*** Rapidly absorbed following oral administration, with peak concentrations in women with breast cancer or healthy women attained within about 1.2 or 2.9 hours, respectively.

Steady-state plasma concentrations achieved in approximately 7 days.

Food High-fat meal increases plasma exemestane concentrations by approximately 40%.

■ **Distribution** ***Extent*** Extensively distributed into tissues.

Crosses placenta.

Distributed into milk in animals; not studied in pregnant or nursing women.

Plasma Protein Binding 90% (mainly α_1-acid glycoprotein and albumin).

■ **Elimination** ***Metabolism*** Extensively metabolized via CYP3A4 and aldoketoreductases; metabolites are inactive or inhibit aromatase with decreased potency compared with parent drug. One metabolite, 17-hydroexemestane, may have androgenic activity.

Elimination Route Excreted similarly (42%) in both urine and feces; <1% excreted as unchanged drug in urine.

Half-life Approximately 24 hours.

Special Populations In patients with moderate or severe hepatic or renal impairment, AUC is approximately 3 times higher than in healthy individuals.

Description

Exemestane is an irreversible, selective steroidal aromatase inhibitor structurally related to the natural substrate androstenedione. Unlike nonsteroidal (type II) aromatase inhibitors (e.g., aminoglutethimide, letrozole), steroidal inhibitors such as exemestane (type I aromatase inhibitors) act as false substrates and are converted by aromatase to reactive alkylating intermediates that bind covalently to the substrate binding site of the enzyme; this binding to the active site of aromatase is irreversible, resulting in its inactivation (i.e., "suicide" inhibition). As a result of these differences, there appears to be a lack of cross-resistance in susceptible cancers between type I and II inhibitors.

Exemestane selectively inhibits the conversion of androgens to estrogens. Because estrogen acts as a growth factor for hormone-dependent breast cancer cells, reduction of serum and tumor concentrations of estrogen inhibits tumor growth and delays disease progression. In postmenopausal women, ovarian secretion of estrogen declines and conversion of adrenal androgens (mainly androstenedione and testosterone) to estrone and estradiol in peripheral tissues (adipose, muscle, and liver), catalyzed by the aromatase enzyme, is the principal source of estrogens. Exemestane selectively inhibits the synthesis of estrogens and does not affect synthesis of adrenal corticosteroid, aldosterone, or thyroid hormone. In dose-ranging (0.5–800 mg) studies, 25 mg was the minimum dose to exhibit maximum suppression of plasma estrogens. A single 25-mg exemestane dose reduces plasma estrogen (estradiol, estrone, and estrone sulfate) concentrations in postmenopausal women by as much as 85–95% within 2–3 days, with maximal suppression persisting up to at least 4–5 days after dosing. After 4–12 weeks of exemestane therapy (25 mg daily) in postmenopausal women, plasma estrogen concentrations were suppressed by an average of 91–95%, and whole body aromatization was suppressed by 98%. Although an apparently lower suppression (e.g., by 60–70%) of plasma estrogens has been reported in some studies, these studies used a less-specific assay method (i.e., RIA) than the method (i.e., HPLC) used in studies reporting higher levels of suppression.

A dose-dependent decrease in sex hormone binding globulin (SHBG) has been observed with exemestane dosages of 2.5 mg or more daily. Slight, dose-independent increases in serum luteinizing hormone (LH) and follicle-stimulating hormone (FSH) concentrations have been observed even at low dosages as a result of negative feedback on the pituitary gland. At dosages up to 25 mg daily, no clinically important effect on circulating concentrations of androstenedione, dehydroepiandrostenedione sulfate, or 17-hydroxyprogesterone and only small decreases in circulating concentrations of testosterone are observed; however, at dosages of 200 mg or more daily, testosterone and androstenedione concentrations are increased. 17-Hydroexemestane, a metabolite, exhibits substantial intrinsic androgenic activity, which may become clinically important at high (e.g., 200 mg daily) exemestane dosages.

Exemestane is principally metabolized via oxidation by the cytochrome P-450 (CYP) 3A4 isoenzyme. Serum exemestane concentrations increased by approximately 40% after a high-fat breakfast. Unlike aminoglutethimide, exemestane does not adversely affect plasma total homocysteine concentrations.

Advice to Patients

Importance of informing clinicians of existing or contemplated concomitant therapy, including prescription and OTC drugs and herbal supplements, as well as any concomitant illnesses. Importance of not taking estrogenic agents concomitantly with exemestane.

Patients should be warned of the potential hazard to the fetus in cases of inadvertent exposure of pregnant women to exemestane. Patients also should be advised that exemestane is indicated for use only in postmenopausal women.

Risk of osteoporosis. Life-style changes (e.g., weight-bearing exercise, abstinence from smoking, moderation of alcohol consumption) and dietary supplementation with calcium and vitamin D are advised. Importance of bone mineral density (BMD) monitoring.

Importance of informing patients of other important precautionary information. (See Cautions.)

Overview (see Users Guide). For additional information until a more detailed monograph is developed and published, the manufacturer's labeling should be consulted. It is *essential* that the manufacturer's labeling be consulted for more detailed information on usual cautions, precautions, contraindications, potential drug interactions, laboratory test interferences, and acute toxicity.

Preparations

Excipients in commercially available drug preparations may have clinically important effects in some individuals; consult specific product labeling for details.

Exemestane

Oral		
Tablets	25 mg*	**Aromasin®**, Pfizer **Exemestane Tablets**

*available from one or more manufacturer, distributor, and/or repackager by generic (nonproprietary) name

†Use is not currently included in the labeling approved by the US Food and Drug Administration

Letrozole

■ Letrozole, an aromatase inhibitor, is an antineoplastic agent.

Uses

■ **Breast Cancer** ***Initial or Sequential Adjuvant Therapy for Early-stage Breast Cancer*** Letrozole is used as adjuvant therapy in postmenopausal women with early-stage hormone receptor-positive breast cancer. Aromatase inhibitors, including letrozole, currently are considered a treatment of choice for adjuvant hormonal therapy to lower the risk of breast cancer recurrence in postmenopausal women with early-stage hormone receptor-positive breast cancer. Although tamoxifen historically has been the drug of choice for adjuvant hormonal therapy in such patients, results of large, randomized clinical studies indicate that an aromatase inhibitor-containing regimen is modestly more effective than tamoxifen alone. Longer-term follow-up of these studies is needed to further clarify lasting clinical efficacy, effects on survival, and late adverse effects of aromatase inhibitor therapy.

Clinical Trials. Efficacy of letrozole as initial or sequential adjuvant therapy in postmenopausal women with early-stage breast cancer is based principally on results of a randomized double-blind trial (Breast International Group [BIG] 1-98) in approximately 8000 postmenopausal women with early-stage hormone receptor-positive breast cancer. The study was initially designed to compare 5 years of adjuvant letrozole therapy with 5 years of adjuvant tamoxifen therapy; however, the randomization scheme subsequently was modified to include 4 regimens (2 sequential regimens in addition to the 2 single-drug regimens) to evaluate whether, in women who are disease-free approximately 2 years after initiating adjuvant therapy, switching endocrine treatments (i.e., administering tamoxifen for 2 years followed by letrozole for 3 years, or vice versa) is superior to continuing the initial agent for a total of 5 years. Letrozole was administered at a dosage of 2.5 mg daily, and tamoxifen was administered at a dosage of 20 mg daily.

At a median follow-up of 26 months, when patients had received either letrozole or tamoxifen for a median of 24 months, analysis of the data showed that patients receiving letrozole had prolonged disease-free and systemic disease-free survival and a reduced risk of distant recurrence compared with patients receiving tamoxifen. Overall survival and risk of new contralateral breast cancer did not differ significantly between letrozole- and tamoxifen-treated patients. Estimated 5-year disease-free survival was 84 or 81.4% for patients receiving letrozole or tamoxifen, respectively. Based on recommendations of an independent data monitoring board, the tamoxifen-only treatment groups were unblinded and disease-free patients in these groups were allowed to complete initial adjuvant therapy with letrozole if they had received tamoxifen for at least 2 years or to initiate extended adjuvant therapy with letrozole if they had received tamoxifen for at least 4.5 years. Approximately 25% of patients originally randomized to receive tamoxifen only for 5 years crossed over to receive letrozole, generally at 3–5 years following initiation of tamoxifen therapy. Despite the confounding effect of selective patient crossover from tamoxifen to letrozole, subsequent analysis of data for patients originally randomized to receive either letrozole only or tamoxifen only for 5 years showed that a difference in disease-free survival persisted at a median follow-up of 6.1 years. At the time of this analysis, estimated 5-year disease-free survival rates for the letrozole and tamoxifen groups were 87.4 and 84.7%, respectively; overall survival did not differ significantly between treatment groups. At a median follow-up of 8.7 years, patients originally randomized to receive letrozole only had longer overall and disease-free survival and longer breast cancer-free and distant recurrence-free intervals compared with those originally randomized to receive tamoxifen.

In the primary analysis of sequential therapy, each sequential regimen was compared with the single-drug regimen for the first drug in that sequence (e.g., letrozole followed by tamoxifen was compared with letrozole alone) from the time of the switch; no significant differences in overall survival, disease-free survival, or systemic or distant disease-free survival were observed. However, because of emerging clinical trial data and changing medical practice, additional comparisons, including comparison of each sequential regimen with letrozole alone, also were conducted. At a median follow-up of 5.9 years following randomization, neither letrozole followed by tamoxifen nor tamoxifen followed by letrozole improved disease-free survival compared with letrozole alone; estimated 5-year disease-free survival for patients receiving one of these 3 regimens was 86–88%. Similar results were observed at a median follow-up of 8 years, when disease-free and overall survival rates were 77–79 and 86–88%, respectively, for patients who received either of the sequential regimens or letrozole alone; 88–90% of these patients had no evidence of distant recurrence, and 84–86% had no evidence of breast cancer recurrence.

In this study, fracture, myocardial infarction, hypercholesterolemia, and arthralgia occurred more frequently in patients receiving letrozole, whereas thromboembolic events, vaginal bleeding, and endometrial disorders (hyperplasia, cancer, proliferation) occurred more frequently in those receiving tamoxifen.

Clinical Role. Based on data from randomized controlled trials (including BIG 1-98) demonstrating prolonged disease-free survival in patients receiving letrozole- or other aromatase inhibitor-based adjuvant regimens, the American Society of Clinical Oncology (ASCO) states that most postmenopausal women with early-stage hormone receptor-positive breast cancer should consider receiving an aromatase inhibitor (e.g., letrozole) during the course of adjuvant therapy, either as primary (initial) therapy or following 2–3 years of tamoxifen therapy (sequential therapy), to complete a total of 5 years of adjuvant endocrine therapy. Clinically meaningful differences among the currently available aromatase inhibitors (i.e., anastrozole, exemestane, letrozole) have not been demonstrated to date. Data also support switching to an aromatase inhibitor following 5 years of adjuvant tamoxifen therapy (extended therapy) (see Extended Adjuvant Therapy for Early-stage Breast Cancer under Uses: Breast Cancer). The optimal time for switching from tamoxifen to an aromatase inhibitor is not known. The duration of aromatase inhibitor therapy should not exceed 5 years, since toxicity of long-term (e.g., beyond 5 years) use of aromatase inhibitors, including letrozole, has not been determined. The optimal duration of adjuvant letrozole therapy is not known. ASCO states that clinicians should consider adverse effects, patient preference, and preexisting conditions when selecting an adjuvant regimen; during the course of adjuvant therapy, patients who are intolerant of one aromatase inhibitor may be switched to a different aromatase inhibitor or to tamoxifen.

The use of an LHRH agonist (e.g., goserelin) in combination with an aromatase inhibitor, such as letrozole, as adjuvant therapy in *premenopausal* women with hormone receptor-positive breast cancer† is being investigated. The use of an aromatase inhibitor as a single agent for adjuvant therapy is *not* appropriate in premenopausal women with breast cancer because these agents alone are not likely to provide sufficient suppression of ovarian function to be of clinical benefit. Similarly, the use of monotherapy with aromatase inhibitors as adjuvant therapy for hormone receptor-positive breast cancer in premenopausal women experiencing a chemotherapy-induced disruption in ovarian function is not advised; a substantial number of such patients can expect resumption of ovarian function, and this would likely render therapy with an aromatase inhibitor ineffective.

Extended Adjuvant Therapy for Early-stage Breast Cancer

Letrozole is used as extended adjuvant therapy in postmenopausal women with early-stage breast cancer who have received 5 years of adjuvant tamoxifen therapy. Efficacy of letrozole as extended adjuvant therapy is based on analysis of disease-free survival in patients receiving the drug for a median of 5 years.

Clinical Trials. Efficacy of letrozole as extended adjuvant therapy in postmenopausal women with early-stage breast cancer who have received 5 years of adjuvant tamoxifen therapy is based principally on results of a double-blind, placebo-controlled randomized trial (National Cancer Institute of Canada Clinical Trials Group [NCIC CTC] MA.17) in postmenopausal women with mostly hormone receptor-positive breast cancer (98% hormone receptor-positive, 2% hormone receptor-unknown). In this trial, 5187 patients who had received adjuvant therapy with tamoxifen for approximately 5 years (range: 4.5–6 years) were randomized to receive letrozole 2.5 mg or placebo daily for 5 years; treatment was initiated within 3 months of discontinuance of tamoxifen therapy.

At a median follow-up of 2.4 years (based on 40% of the number of events required for the final analysis), an estimated 4-year disease-free survival rate of 93% in patients receiving letrozole and 87% in patients receiving placebo was reported. In addition, letrozole treatment was associated with reduction in the incidence of local or metastatic recurrence or new contralateral breast cancer (hazard ratio 0.57). The estimated 4-year overall survival rate was similar for patients receiving letrozole versus placebo (96 versus 94%). Based on the prolonged disease-free survival and a trend toward reduced overall mortality in patients receiving letrozole, the data and safety monitoring committee recommended early termination of the trial. The study was unblinded, all participants were informed of the findings, and letrozole therapy was offered to all women who had been receiving placebo.

After the study was unblinded, approximately 60% of patients randomized to receive placebo crossed over to receive letrozole therapy. Updated results at a median follow-up of 5.2 years (median treatment duration of 5 years) demonstrated a reduction in the incidence of breast cancer recurrence or new contralateral breast cancer in patients originally randomized to receive letrozole compared with that in patients originally randomized to receive placebo (hazard ratio 0.75). The effect of patients crossing over from placebo to letrozole therapy confounded the analysis of survival, as patients switching from placebo to letrozole accounted for 64% of the total patient-years of follow-up for the placebo group. The analysis of disease-free survival indicated that breast cancer recurrence, new contralateral breast cancer, or death from any cause occurred in 13.3% of patients originally randomized to receive letrozole compared with 15.5% of those originally randomized to receive placebo; the observed results were not statistically significant, but the treatment difference was diluted by patients crossing over from placebo to letrozole. Overall survival and distant disease-free survival of patients originally randomized to receive letrozole did not differ significantly from that of patients originally randomized to receive placebo.

An increased incidence of hot flushes (flashes), arthritis, arthralgia, and myalgia was observed in patients receiving letrozole. Patients receiving letrozole also experienced higher rates of bone fracture, newly diagnosed osteoporosis, and cardiovascular events. Because of the early stoppage of the study, long-term adverse effects associated with letrozole therapy may have been underestimated. Postmenopausal women receiving aromatase inhibitors, such as letrozole, as adjuvant therapy are at high risk for osteoporosis. (See Precautions and Contraindications and Musculoskeletal Effects sections in Cautions for further information on screening and treatment guidelines for osteoporosis in such patients.) Vaginal bleeding occurred less frequently in patients receiving letrozole than in those receiving placebo.

Clinical Role. Based on data from randomized controlled trials (including NCIC CTC MA.17) demonstrating prolonged disease-free survival in patients receiving letrozole or other aromatase inhibitors as extended adjuvant therapy following 5 years of adjuvant tamoxifen therapy, ASCO recommends extended therapy with an aromatase inhibitor (e.g., letrozole) in postmenopausal women with early-stage hormone receptor-positive breast cancer who complete 5 years of adjuvant tamoxifen therapy. Clinically meaningful differences among the currently available aromatase inhibitors (i.e., anastrozole, exemestane, letrozole) have not been demonstrated to date. Clinicians should consider adverse effects, patient preference, and preexisting conditions when selecting an adjuvant regimen. ASCO states that women who receive extended adjuvant therapy should receive a total of 8–10 years of adjuvant endocrine therapy, including 5 years of tamoxifen therapy followed by 3–5 years of aromatase inhibitor therapy. The optimal duration of letrozole as extended adjuvant therapy is not known, and the toxicity of long-term (e.g., beyond 5 years) use of aromatase inhibitors, including letrozole, in this setting has not been determined. Ongoing clinical trials are evaluating whether longer durations of aromatase inhibitor therapy are more effective. In one such trial, patients from the MA.17 trial and other patients who are disease-free after approximately 5 years of aromatase inhibitor therapy are randomized to receive 5 years of placebo or another 5 years of aromatase inhibitor therapy (i.e., letrozole).

First-Line Therapy for Advanced Breast Cancer Letrozole is used for the first-line treatment of hormone receptor-positive or hormone receptor-unknown locally advanced or metastatic breast cancer in postmenopausal women. Data from a double-blind, randomized clinical trial indicate that letrozole is superior to tamoxifen for delaying tumor progression and producing objective tumor response in such patients. In this trial, a total of 916 postmenopausal patients (about 65% with hormone receptor-positive breast tumors and 35% with hormone receptor-unknown breast tumors) were randomized to receive letrozole 2.5 mg daily or tamoxifen 20 mg daily.

At a median follow-up of about 32 months, patients receiving letrozole had a longer median time to progression (9.4 versus 6 months), a higher overall objective response rate (32 versus 21%), and a higher complete response rate (9 versus 3%) compared with patients receiving tamoxifen. Median duration of response was 18 months in patients receiving letrozole and 16 months in those receiving tamoxifen. Among the subset of patients who had received prior antiestrogen adjuvant therapy, letrozole was associated with a higher objective response rate (26 versus 8%) and a longer median time to progression (8.9 versus 5.9 months) compared with tamoxifen. Median overall survival (35 versus 32 months) was similar in patients randomized to receive letrozole or tamoxifen, respectively. The incidence of adverse effects was similar for patients receiving letrozole or tamoxifen; common adverse effects included bone pain, hot flushes (flashes), back pain, dyspnea, nausea, and arthralgia.

The design of the study allowed patients to cross over to the opposite treatment arm upon disease progression. Approximately 50% of the patients in the study crossed over to the opposite treatment arm, with crossover occurring by 36 months in almost all cases. The median time to crossover was 17 months in patients crossing over from letrozole to tamoxifen and 13 months in patients crossing over from tamoxifen to letrozole. Among the patients who did not cross over to the opposite treatment arm, median survival was 35 months in patients receiving letrozole and 20 months in patients receiving tamoxifen.

Letrozole also is used in combination with lapatinib ditosylate for the treatment of hormone receptor-positive metastatic breast cancer that overexpresses human epidermal growth factor receptor type 2 (HER2) in postmenopausal women who are candidates for hormonal therapy. (See Combination Therapy with Lapatinib and Letrozole under Breast Cancer: Advanced or Metastatic Breast Cancer in Uses in Lapatinib Ditosylate 10:00.)

Letrozole also is used in combination with ribociclib for the initial treatment of hormone receptor-positive, HER2-negative advanced or metastatic breast cancer in postmenopausal women. (See Initial Therapy for Advanced Breast Cancer under Uses: Breast Cancer, in Ribociclib Succinate 10:00.)

Second-Line Therapy for Advanced Breast Cancer Letrozole is used for the palliative treatment of advanced breast cancer in postmenopausal women with disease progression following antiestrogen therapy (e.g., tamoxifen). The principal goal of therapy in patients with metastatic breast cancer generally has been palliative with an emphasis on extension of survival and improvement in the quality of life.

Clinical Trials. The current labeled indication for letrozole in previously treated breast cancer is based on 2 randomized multicenter phase II trials involving postmenopausal women with locally advanced or metastatic breast cancer who had hormone receptor-positive or hormone receptor-unknown tumors; all patients had measurable or evaluable disease that had progressed following prior antiestrogen therapy. In both studies, the safety and efficacy of 2 dosages of letrozole were evaluated and the distribution of hormone receptor status was similar among the patients (about 55% with hormone receptor-positive breast tumors and 45% with hormone receptor-unknown breast tumors). In both studies, at least 60% of the patients had received therapeutic antiestrogens, and an objective response to this therapy had occurred in about one-fifth of these patients.

In a double-blind, randomized trial involving 552 postmenopausal women, patients receiving letrozole (2.5 mg daily) had a similar rate of objective response (24 versus 16%) and similar median survival (730 versus 659 days) compared with those receiving megestrol acetate (160 mg daily) at a minimum follow-up of 15 months. Responses to letrozole were observed in patients with advanced breast cancer that did not respond to first-line antiestrogen therapy. Similar objective response rate (12 versus 16%) also was observed in patients receiving the lower dosage of letrozole (0.5 mg daily) versus megestrol acetate. Adverse cardiovascular effects, principally thromboembolic events, and vaginal bleeding occurred less frequently in patients receiving either dose level of letrozole than in those receiving megestrol acetate.

In an open-label randomized trial involving 557 postmenopausal women, letrozole 2.5 mg daily was at least as effective as aminoglutethimide (250 mg twice daily) with a similar rate of objective response (about 18 versus 12%, respectively) and similar median survival (792 versus 592 days, respectively) at a minimum follow-up of 9 months; a similar rate of objective response (about 18 versus 12%, respectively) and similar median survival (636 days versus 592 days, respectively) also was observed in patients receiving the lower dosage of letrozole (0.5 mg daily) versus aminoglutethimide.

In a double-blind, randomized phase III trial comparing 2 doses of letrozole (2.5 mg or 0.5 mg) with megestrol acetate (40 mg 4 times daily) in women with advanced or metastatic breast cancer (hormone receptor-positive or hormone receptor-unknown tumors), similar rate of objective response was observed among the groups. No statistical difference in efficacy has been demonstrated between either dose level of letrozole (2.5 mg or 0.5 mg daily) and the comparison treatment (megestrol acetate or aminoglutethimide), and no statistical difference in the incidence of adverse effects has been noted for the 2 dose levels. Some clinicians question whether there is any clinically meaningful difference in efficacy and safety between these letrozole dosages; commercially available letrozole tablets are available for the 2. 5-mg dose only.

In a double-blind, randomized, crossover trial exploring the biochemical efficacy of letrozole versus anastrozole, another aromatase inhibitor, in 12 postmenopausal women with estrogen receptor-positive metastatic breast cancer, letrozole caused greater inhibition of in vivo aromatization and greater suppression of plasma concentrations of estrone and estrone sulfate than anastrozole. The clinical importance of differences in the degree of estrogen suppression between various aromatase inhibitors has not been established. In an open-label, randomized, multicenter trial involving 713 postmenopausal women with advanced or metastatic breast cancer (hormone receptor-positive tumors and hormone receptor-unknown tumors each in about half of the patients), no difference in time to progression of disease or incidence of adverse effects was observed among patients receiving letrozole or anastrozole.

Clinical Role. Letrozole is used as second-line hormonal therapy in postmenopausal women with hormone receptor-positive advanced breast cancer. In premenopausal women with hormone receptor-positive advanced breast cancer†, ovarian ablation by surgery or external-beam radiation, or suppression of ovarian function with a luteinizing hormone-releasing hormone (LHRH) agonist, is advised; the use of an LHRH agonist (e.g., goserelin) in combination with an aromatase inhibitor, such as letrozole, is being investigated. The use of an aromatase inhibitor as single-agent therapy is *not* appropriate in premenopausal women with breast cancer because these agents alone are not likely to provide sufficient suppression of ovarian function to be of clinical benefit.

Dosage and Administration

■ **Administration** Letrozole is administered orally. Food does not affect the absorption of letrozole, and the drug may be administered without regard to meals.

■ **Dosage** ***Breast Cancer*** **Initial or Sequential Adjuvant Therapy for Early-stage Breast Cancer.** For adjuvant treatment of early-stage hormone receptor-positive breast cancer in postmenopausal women, the recommended dosage of letrozole is 2.5 mg once daily. The optimal duration of adjuvant therapy is unknown. The planned duration of therapy in the study establishing use of letrozole as initial adjuvant therapy was 5 years; 73% of patients in this study completed adjuvant therapy. Treatment should be discontinued if relapse occurs.

The American Society of Clinical Oncology (ASCO) states that an aromatase inhibitor (e.g., letrozole) may be administered to postmenopausal women with early-stage hormone receptor-positive breast cancer as initial adjuvant therapy and continued for a total of 5 years or may be administered following initial tamoxifen therapy as part of a sequential adjuvant regimen. The optimal time to switch from tamoxifen to aromatase inhibitor therapy is not known; however, based on clinical trials conducted to date, ASCO recommends that patients who are disease-free may be switched to an aromatase inhibitor after 2–3 years of tamoxifen therapy to complete a 5-year sequential adjuvant regimen. In patients who initially receive an aromatase inhibitor but discontinue therapy prior to 5 years, ASCO states that consideration should be given to administering tamoxifen to complete the 5-year adjuvant regimen.

Extended Adjuvant Therapy for Early-stage Breast Cancer. For the extended adjuvant treatment of early-stage breast cancer in postmenopausal women who have completed 5 years of adjuvant therapy with tamoxifen, the recommended dosage of letrozole is 2.5 mg once daily. The optimal duration of therapy is unknown. The planned duration of therapy in the study establishing use of letrozole as extended adjuvant therapy was 5 years. In the final updated analysis of this study, the median treatment duration was 5 years (60 months); 71% of patients completed at least 3 years of extended adjuvant treatment, and 58% completed at least 4.5 years of such treatment. ASCO recommends that patients who receive an extended adjuvant regimen receive an aromatase inhibitor (e.g., letrozole) for 3–5 years beyond the initial 5 years of tamoxifen therapy, to complete a total of 8–10 years of adjuvant endocrine therapy. Treatment should be discontinued if relapse occurs.

First-line Therapy for Advanced Breast Cancer. For the first-line treatment of hormone receptor-positive or hormone receptor-unknown locally advanced or metastatic breast cancer in postmenopausal women, the recommended dosage of letrozole is 2.5 mg once daily. Treatment should be continued until disease progression occurs.

Second-line Therapy for Advanced Breast Cancer. For the second-line treatment of advanced or metastatic breast cancer in postmenopausal women with disease progression following antiestrogen therapy, the recommended dosage of letrozole is 2.5 mg once daily. Treatment should be continued until disease progression occurs.

■ **Dosage in Renal and Hepatic Impairment** Although letrozole is metabolized to an inactive metabolite whose glucuronide conjugate undergoes mainly renal excretion, the manufacturer states that no dosage adjustment is necessary in patients with a creatinine clearance of at least 10 mL/minute.

Letrozole is metabolized slowly in the liver, and modest increases in serum letrozole concentrations have been observed in patients with moderate hepatic impairment secondary to cirrhosis. The manufacturer states that no dosage adjustment is required in patients with mild to moderate hepatic impairment. A 50% reduction in letrozole dosage (to 2.5 mg every other day) is recommended in patients with cirrhosis and severe hepatic impairment. The effect of hepatic impairment on letrozole pharmacokinetics in patients with cancer and elevated bilirubin concentrations who do not have cirrhosis has not been determined.

Cautions

The incidence of reported adverse effects is based on data from randomized trials of postmenopausal women receiving letrozole 2.5 mg daily for breast cancer as initial adjuvant therapy for early-stage disease (2448 patients; median duration of treatment: 5 years; median follow-up: 6.1 years), extended adjuvant therapy for early-stage disease (2563 patients; median duration of treatment: 24 months; median follow-up: 28 months), first-line therapy for advanced disease (455 patients, median duration of treatment: 11 months), or second-line therapy for advanced disease (359 patients). Rates of adverse reactions were similar among women receiving letrozole as first-line or second-line therapy for advanced disease, and unless the type of therapy is specified, incidence rates reflect the experience of all these patients receiving the drug. For an additional 380 patients receiving a lower dosage of letrozole (0.5 mg daily) as second-line therapy, the incidences of adverse effects were similar to those in the patients receiving the higher dose. The most frequent adverse effects of letrozole are hypercholesterolemia, hot flushes (flashes), and arthralgia/arthritis in patients receiving the drug as initial adjuvant therapy; flushing, asthenia, arthralgia, headache, and increased sweating in those receiving the drug as extended adjuvant therapy; and bone pain in those receiving treatment for advanced disease.

In patients receiving initial adjuvant therapy for early-stage breast cancer, fracture, myocardial infarction, hypercholesterolemia, and arthralgia occurred more frequently in those receiving letrozole, whereas thromboembolic events, vaginal bleeding, endometrial hyperplasia or cancer, and endometrial proliferation disorders occurred more frequently in those receiving tamoxifen. In patients receiving letrozole as extended adjuvant therapy following 5 years of tamoxifen therapy, hot flushes (flashes), arthralgia/arthritis, and myalgia occurred more frequently in letrozole-treated patients than in placebo recipients.

The described adverse effects occurred at a similar rate in patients receiving letrozole or tamoxifen as first-line therapy for advanced breast cancer. Discontinuance of therapy because of adverse effects other than progression of tumor was required in 2% of patients receiving letrozole and 3% of patients receiving tamoxifen.

Unless otherwise noted, the adverse effects described occurred at a similar rate in patients receiving treatments being compared with letrozole (i.e., megestrol acetate or aminoglutethimide) as second-line therapy for advanced breast cancer. Adverse effects typically were mild to moderate in severity among patients in all treatment groups; in general, it was not possible to distinguish adverse reactions secondary to treatment from the consequences of metastatic breast cancer, the effects of estrogen deprivation, or intercurrent illness. In the 2 studies comparing letrozole with either megestrol acetate or aminoglutethimide, discontinuance of therapy because of adverse effects other than progression of tumor was required as follows: megestrol acetate (7.9%), letrozole 2.5 mg (2.3%), and letrozole 0.5 mg (2.7%); aminoglutethimide (3.9%), letrozole 2.5 mg (3.8%), and letrozole 0.5 mg (3.1%).

■ **Musculoskeletal Effects** In patients receiving letrozole as initial adjuvant therapy, arthralgia/arthritis was reported in 25% of patients and fracture was reported during treatment in 10% of patients; arthralgia/arthritis and fracture were reported less frequently in patients receiving tamoxifen (20 and 7%, respectively). The overall incidence of fractures, including those that occurred during posttreatment follow-up, was 14% in patients receiving letrozole and 10% in those receiving tamoxifen. Myalgia occurred in 9% and back pain, osteoporosis, osteopenia, bone pain, and pain in extremity each occurred in 4–5% of patients receiving letrozole as initial adjuvant therapy.

In patients receiving letrozole as extended adjuvant therapy following 5 years of adjuvant tamoxifen therapy, arthralgia was reported in 22% and arthritis, myalgia, and back pain each were reported in 5–7% of patients. At a median follow-up of 28 months, fracture was reported in 5.9% of patients receiving letrozole and 5.5% of those receiving placebo, and the incidence of self-reported osteoporosis was higher among patients receiving letrozole (6.9 versus 5.5%); about 19–21% of patients received bisphosphonate therapy. At a median follow-up of 62 months, fracture and newly diagnosed osteoporosis each were reported in 13–14% of patients receiving letrozole compared with 8% of those receiving placebo.

In patients receiving letrozole as first-line therapy for advanced disease, bone pain, back pain, and limb pain occurred in 22, 18, and 10% of patients, respectively. In patients receiving letrozole as second-line therapy for advanced disease, adverse musculoskeletal effects (including musculoskeletal, skeletal, back, arm, and leg pain) were reported in 21% and fracture was reported in less than 5% of patients. Arthralgia was reported in 16% of patients receiving letrozole as first-line therapy and in 8% of patients receiving the drug as second-line therapy. Hypercalcemia occurred in less than 5% of patients receiving letrozole as second-line therapy.

A syndrome consisting of arthralgia and other symmetrical bone and joint symptoms (e.g., pain, stiffness, achiness) that are not associated with other manifestations of rheumatologic disorders has been reported in patients receiving aromatase inhibitors. Symptoms generally resolve within 8–10 weeks following discontinuance of therapy.

Because letrozole lowers circulating estrogen concentrations, it may cause a reduction in bone mineral density (BMD). In a substudy of the controlled trial evaluating letrozole as initial adjuvant therapy, the change in lumbar spine BMD following 2 years of treatment was a median decrease of 4.1% in patients receiving letrozole compared with a median increase of 0.3% in those receiving tamoxifen (a difference of 4.4%). Results for total hip BMD were similar, although the difference between treatment groups was less pronounced. During the 2-year treatment period, osteoporosis developed in one patient with baseline osteopenia and fracture was reported in 4 or 6% of patients receiving letrozole or tamoxifen, respectively. In a substudy of the trial evaluating letrozole as extended adjuvant therapy in patients who had received 5 years of adjuvant tamoxifen therapy, the median decrease from baseline in hip BMD following 2 years of treatment was about 4% in patients receiving letrozole compared with 2% in those receiving placebo; letrozole- and placebo-treated patients had similar changes from baseline in lumbar spine BMD.

Postmenopausal women receiving an aromatase inhibitor, such as letrozole, as adjuvant therapy are at high risk for osteoporosis. All postmenopausal women initiating adjuvant therapy with an aromatase inhibitor should be evaluated for risk of osteoporotic fractures. Screening with dual energy radiographic absorptiometry (DXA) to determine the BMD of the hip and spine should be performed in conjunction with assessment of other risk factors for fracture (e.g., age, low body mass index, family history of hip fracture, prior fragility fracture, history of cigarette smoking, excessive alcohol consumption, current or prior corticosteroid use). Patients should be monitored closely for changes in risk status during therapy, and BMD should be assessed at regular intervals (e.g., every 1–2 years in those with osteopenia or osteoporosis). Other potential causes of osteoporosis (e.g., vitamin D deficiency, hyperthyroidism, hyperparathyroidism, hypercalciuria) should be considered. Appropriate therapy to prevent further bone loss should be initiated as clinically indicated. The decision to initiate therapy with an antiresorptive agent (e.g., a bisphosphonate, denosumab) should be based on overall risk of fracture and rate of bone loss. (See Uses: Prevention of Aromatase Inhibitor-associated Bone Loss, in Zoledronic Acid 92:24.) All women receiving adjuvant therapy with letrozole should be advised to adopt lifestyle changes (e.g., weight-bearing exercise, abstinence from smoking, moderation in alcohol consumption) and dietary supplementation with calcium and vitamin D to reduce the risk of osteoporosis.

■ **GI Effects** In patients receiving letrozole as initial adjuvant therapy, nausea occurred in 12% and vomiting, constipation, and anorexia each occurred in 3% or less of patients. In patients receiving letrozole as extended adjuvant therapy, constipation, nausea, or diarrhea occurred in 11, 9, or 5%, respectively, of patients.

In patients receiving letrozole as first-line or second-line therapy for advanced disease, nausea, vomiting, and diarrhea were reported in 13–17, 7, and 6–8% of patients, respectively. Constipation and anorexia were reported in 6–10 and 4–5% of patients, respectively. Abdominal pain and dyspepsia were reported in 6 and 3%, respectively, of patients receiving the drug as second-line therapy. Stomatitis, increased appetite, dry mouth, and disturbances of taste and thirst also have been reported in patients receiving letrozole as first-line or second-line therapy.

■ **Respiratory Effects** Dyspnea was reported in 6% of patients receiving letrozole as extended adjuvant therapy. Dyspnea also was reported in 18 or 7%, and coughing was reported in 13 or 6%, of patients receiving letrozole as first-line or second-line therapy for advanced disease, respectively. Chest wall pain was reported in 6% of patients receiving letrozole as first-line therapy. Pleural effusion occurred in less than 5% of patients receiving letrozole as second-line therapy.

■ **Nervous System Effects** In patients receiving letrozole as initial adjuvant therapy, depression, headache, and dizziness/lightheadedness each were reported in 3–5% of patients.

In patients receiving letrozole as extended adjuvant therapy, headache, dizziness, or insomnia was reported in 20, 14, or 6% of patients.

Headache was reported in 8–9% of patients receiving letrozole as first-line or second-line therapy for advanced disease. Insomnia occurred in 7% of patients receiving letrozole as first-line therapy. In patients receiving letrozole as second-line therapy, somnolence and dizziness each occurred in 3% of patients. Depression, anxiety, and vertigo each were reported in less than 5% of patients receiving letrozole as second-line therapy. Memory impairment, irritability, nervousness, and dysesthesia (including hypoesthesia and paresthesia) also have been reported in patients receiving letrozole as first-line or second-line therapy.

■ **Cardiovascular Effects** ***Thromboembolic Events and Ischemic Disease*** In patients receiving letrozole as initial adjuvant therapy, myocardial infarction or ischemia, angina, cerebrovascular accident, and thromboembolic events each were reported in 3% or less of patients during treatment or posttreatment follow-up. When compared with patients receiving tamoxifen as initial adjuvant therapy, myocardial infarction occurred more frequently in patients receiving letrozole (1 versus 0.5% during treatment), whereas thromboembolic events occurred more frequently in patients receiving tamoxifen (3 versus 4.5%). Cardiovascular ischemic events were reported in 7% of patients receiving letrozole as extended adjuvant therapy following 5 years of adjuvant tamoxifen therapy.

Peripheral thromboembolic events (including venous thrombosis, thrombophlebitis, portal vein thrombosis, and pulmonary embolism), cardiovascular events (including angina, myocardial infarction, myocardial ischemia, and coronary heart disease), and cerebrovascular events (including transient ischemic attacks, thrombotic or hemorrhagic strokes, and development of hemiparesis) occurred in 2% or less of patients receiving letrozole as first-line therapy for advanced disease. Among patients receiving second-line therapy for advanced disease, thromboembolic events occurred less frequently in patients receiving letrozole than in those receiving megestrol acetate (0.6 versus 4.7%). Chest pain was reported in 6–8% of patients receiving letrozole. Arterial thrombosis also has been reported in patients receiving letrozole as first-line or second-line therapy.

Vasomotor Symptoms Hot flushes (flashes) were reported in 34% of patients receiving letrozole as initial adjuvant therapy, 19% of patients receiving letrozole as first-line therapy, and 6% of patients receiving the drug as second-line therapy for advanced disease. Flushing occurred in 50% of patients receiving letrozole as extended adjuvant therapy following 5 years of adjuvant tamoxifen therapy.

Effects on Lipoproteins Hypercholesterolemia was reported in 52% of patients receiving letrozole as initial adjuvant therapy, 16% of patients receiving the drug as extended adjuvant therapy, and 3% of patients receiving the drug as second-line therapy for advanced disease.

In the trial evaluating letrozole as initial adjuvant therapy, hypercholesterolemia was reported more frequently in patients receiving letrozole than in those receiving tamoxifen (52 versus 29%), and a greater proportion of letrozole-treated patients received antilipemic agents (25 versus 16%). Grade 3 or 4 hypercholesterolemia was reported in 0.4 or 0.1% of patients receiving letrozole or tamoxifen, respectively. Among patients with normal baseline serum cholesterol concentrations, elevated total cholesterol concentrations were reported in 8 or 3% of those receiving letrozole or tamoxifen, respectively. In a phase 3 safety trial, 12 or 4% of postmenopausal women receiving letrozole or tamoxifen, respectively, as adjuvant therapy for breast cancer had at least one total cholesterol concentration during 2 years of treatment that was of higher adverse-event grade than the baseline concentration.

In the placebo-controlled trial evaluating letrozole as extended adjuvant therapy in patients who had received 5 years of adjuvant tamoxifen therapy, concentrations of total cholesterol and lipoprotein fractions in letrozole-treated patients were similar to those in placebo recipients throughout the 5 years of letrozole or placebo treatment. Similar proportions of letrozole- and placebo-treated patients received antilipemic agents.

Other Cardiovascular Effects In patients receiving letrozole as initial or extended adjuvant therapy, edema occurred in 7 or 18%, respectively, of patients. In patients receiving letrozole as initial adjuvant therapy, cardiovascular events (other than myocardial infarction or ischemia, angina, cerebrovascular accident, and thromboembolic event) occurred in 13% of patients during treatment or posttreatment follow-up. Cardiovascular events were reported in 10% of patients receiving letrozole as extended adjuvant therapy.

Hypertension occurred in 5–8% and peripheral edema occurred in 5% of patients receiving letrozole as first-line or second-line therapy for advanced disease. Postmastectomy lymphedema was reported in 7% of patients receiving letrozole as first-line therapy. Palpitation, cardiac failure, and tachycardia also have been reported in patients receiving letrozole as first-line or second-line therapy.

■ Hematologic Effects Moderate decreases in lymphocyte counts were observed in some patients receiving letrozole 2.5 mg daily. The decreased lymphocyte counts were transient in about half of the affected patients, and the clinical importance of this finding is uncertain. Thrombocytopenia was reported in at least 2 patients receiving letrozole. In one patient, pancytopenia occurred after approximately 5 months of letrozole therapy; transfusion with packed red blood cells was administered to increase the hemoglobin level, and leukocyte and platelet counts returned to normal levels within 2 weeks following discontinuance of the drug. Leukopenia has been reported in patients receiving letrozole as first-line or second-line therapy for advanced disease.

■ Infectious Complications Infection or infestation occurred in 6% of patients receiving letrozole as extended adjuvant therapy. Influenza and urinary tract infection each were reported in 6% of patients receiving letrozole as first-line therapy for advanced disease. Viral infection was reported in 6% of patients receiving letrozole as second-line therapy for advanced disease.

■ Dermatologic and Sensitivity Reactions Night sweats were reported in 15% and alopecia was reported in 3% of patients receiving letrozole as initial adjuvant therapy. Increased sweating was reported in 24% of patients receiving letrozole as extended adjuvant therapy.

In patients receiving letrozole as second-line therapy for advanced disease, rash (including rash, erythematous rash, maculopapular rash, psoriasiform rash, and vesicular rash) and pruritus were reported in 5 and 1%, respectively. Alopecia and increased sweating were reported in less than 5% of patients receiving letrozole as second-line therapy. Hair thinning also has been reported in patients receiving letrozole as first-line therapy for advanced disease. Urticaria and dryness of the skin and mucosa also have been reported in patients receiving letrozole as first-line or second-line therapy.

During postmarketing experience, angioedema, anaphylactic reaction, toxic epidermal necrolysis, and erythema multiforme have been reported in patients receiving letrozole.

■ Hepatic Effects During postmarketing experience, increased hepatic enzymes and hepatitis have been reported in patients receiving letrozole.

■ Genitourinary Effects Vaginal bleeding, vaginal irritation, and breast pain each were reported in 2–5% of patients receiving letrozole as initial adjuvant therapy. In patients receiving initial adjuvant therapy, endometrial hyperplasia or cancer and endometrial proliferation disorders occurred during treatment or posttreatment follow-up less frequently in patients receiving letrozole than in those receiving tamoxifen (less than 1 versus 2–4%). In patients receiving letrozole as extended adjuvant therapy, vaginal bleeding and vulvovaginal dryness each occurred in 5% of patients.

Breast pain was reported in 7% of patients receiving letrozole as first-line therapy for advanced disease. Among patients receiving second-line therapy for advanced disease, vaginal bleeding occurred less frequently in patients receiving letrozole than in those receiving megestrol acetate (0.3 versus 3.2%). Increased urinary frequency and vaginal discharge also have been reported in patients receiving letrozole as first-line or second-line therapy.

■ Metabolic Effects Weight loss or gain was reported in 6 or 13%, respectively, of patients receiving letrozole as initial adjuvant therapy. In patients with advanced disease, weight loss occurred in 7% of patients receiving letrozole as first-line therapy, and weight gain occurred in 2% of patients receiving letrozole as second-line therapy.

■ Other Adverse Effects Fatigue (including lethargy, malaise, and asthenia) was reported in 10% of patients receiving letrozole as initial adjuvant therapy, and asthenia was reported in 34% of patients receiving the drug as extended adjuvant therapy. Fatigue also was reported in 8–13% of patients receiving letrozole as first-line or second-line therapy for advanced disease. Weakness and pain (unspecified) were reported in 6 and 5%, respectively, of patients receiving letrozole as first-line therapy. Asthenia was reported in 4% of patients receiving letrozole as second-line therapy. Renal disorders were reported in 5% of patients receiving letrozole as extended adjuvant therapy. Cataract was reported in 2% of patients receiving letrozole as initial adjuvant therapy. Cataract, eye irritation, cancer pain, and pyrexia also have been reported in patients receiving letrozole as first-line or second-line therapy. Second malignancies occurred during treatment or posttreatment follow-up in 4% of patients receiving letrozole as initial adjuvant therapy. During postmarketing experience, blurred vision, carpal tunnel syndrome, and trigger finger also have been reported in patients receiving letrozole.

■ Precautions and Contraindications Letrozole currently is indicated for use in the treatment of breast cancer in postmenopausal women only. Letrozole is *not* recommended for use in premenopausal women because safety and efficacy have not been established in this patient population.

Because fatigue, dizziness, and, uncommonly somnolence have been reported during letrozole therapy, patients should be advised to use caution while driving or operating machinery.

Postmenopausal women with breast cancer receiving adjuvant therapy with an aromatase inhibitor, such as letrozole, are at high risk for osteoporosis. Postmenopausal women initiating such therapy should undergo screening to determine BMD and be evaluated for other risk factors for osteoporotic fractures. Patients should be monitored closely for changes in risk status during therapy, and BMD should be assessed at regular intervals. Appropriate therapy to prevent further bone loss should be initiated as clinically indicated. All women receiving adjuvant therapy with letrozole should be advised to adopt lifestyle changes (e.g., weight-bearing exercise) and dietary supplementation with calcium and vitamin D to reduce the risk of osteoporosis. (Also see Cautions: Musculoskeletal Effects.)

The effect of letrozole on lipid metabolism has not been fully established, and serum lipid concentrations should be monitored in patients receiving long-term therapy with the drug.

■ Pediatric Precautions The manufacturer states that safety and efficacy of letrozole in children have not been established.

Adverse effects on bone (bone maturation, bone mineral density) and neuroendocrine and reproductive development disorders of the hypothalamic-pituitary axis were reported following administration of letrozole 0.003–0.3 mg/kg daily in young rats (exposures less than that expected at the recommended human adult dosage) for 12 weeks beginning on postnatal day 7.

■ Geriatric Precautions In the clinical trial evaluating letrozole as initial adjuvant therapy for early-stage breast cancer, 36% of patients were 65 years of age or older at enrollment, while 12% were 75 years of age or older. Adverse effects generally occurred more frequently in geriatric patients regardless of their assigned study treatment; however, no overall differences in safety and efficacy of letrozole versus tamoxifen were observed between geriatric patients and younger adults.

In the clinical trial evaluating letrozole as extended adjuvant therapy for early-stage breast cancer, 41% of patients were 65 years of age or older at enrollment, while 12% were 75 years of age or older. Although no overall differences in safety or efficacy were observed between geriatric patients and younger adults, and other clinical experience revealed no evidence of age-related differences, the possibility that some older patients may exhibit increased sensitivity to the drug cannot be ruled out.

In clinical trials evaluating letrozole as first-line or second-line therapy for advanced or metastatic breast cancer, about one-third of patients were 70 years of age or older (median age: 64–65 years). Among patients receiving letrozole as first-line therapy in a clinical trial, higher response rate and longer time to tumor progression were observed in geriatric patients (70 years or older) compared with younger patients.

■ Mutagenicity and Carcinogenicity ***Mutagenicity*** In vitro tests, including the Ames and *E. coli* bacterial tests, have not shown letrozole to be mutagenic. Potential clastogenicity was demonstrated by the results of 2 in vitro assays (CHO K1 and CCL 61 Chinese hamster ovary cells), but the drug was not shown to be clastogenic in the in vivo micronucleus test in rats.

Carcinogenicity Letrozole has shown carcinogenic activity in animal models. In mice administered letrozole 0.6–60 mg/kg daily (about 1–100 times the daily maximum recommended human dosage on a mg/m^2 basis) by oral gavage for up to 2 years, a dose-related increase in the incidence of benign ovarian stromal tumors was observed. When the high-dose group was excluded (because of low survival), an increased incidence of combined hepatocellular adenoma and carcinoma was observed in female mice. In a separate study, plasma AUC_{0-12h} values in mice administered letrozole 60 mg/kg daily were 55 times higher than the AUC_{0-24h} values in patients with breast cancer receiving the recommended dose of the drug.

Oral administration of letrozole 0.1–10 mg/kg daily (about 0.4–40 times the daily maximum recommended human dosage on a mg/m^2 basis) for up to 2 years in rats resulted in an increase in the incidence of benign ovarian stromal tumors at the 10 mg/kg daily dose. Ovarian hyperplasia was observed in female rats receiving doses equal to or exceeding 0.1 mg/kg daily. Plasma AUC_{0-24h} values in rats at 10 mg/kg daily were 80 times higher than the AUC_{0-24h} values in breast cancer patients receiving the recommended dosage of the drug.

■ Pregnancy, Fertility, and Lactation Letrozole is contraindicated in women who are or may become pregnant (i.e., premenopausal women) since the drug can cause fetal toxicity when administered to pregnant women and clinical benefits of letrozole therapy in premenopausal women with breast cancer have not been established. Perimenopausal women and women who recently have become postmenopausal should be advised of the need to use adequate methods of contraception until the postmenopausal state is clinically well established. If letrozole is administered during pregnancy or if the patient becomes pregnant while receiving the drug, the patient should be informed of the potential hazard to the fetus.

Adequate, well-controlled studies of letrozole in pregnant women have not been conducted. In rats receiving doses equal to or exceeding 0.003 mg/kg (about 1/100 the daily maximum recommended human dose on a mg/m² basis) during the period of organogenesis, letrozole was embryotoxic and fetotoxic, causing intrauterine mortality, increased resorption, increased postimplantation loss, decreased numbers of live fetuses, and fetal anomalies (including absence and shortening of renal papilla, dilation of ureter, edema, and incomplete ossification of frontal skull and metatarsals). Letrozole was shown to be teratogenic in rats; administration of 0.03 mg/kg letrozole (about 1/10 the daily maximum recommended human dose on a mg/m² basis) resulted in fetal domed head and cervical/centrum vertebral fusion. In rabbits, letrozole was embryotoxic at doses equal to or exceeding 0.002 mg/kg (about 1/100,000 the daily maximum recommended human dose on a mg/m² basis) and fetotoxic at a dose of 0.02 mg/kg (about 1/10,000 the daily maximum recommended human dose on a mg/m² basis); fetal anomalies included incomplete ossification of the skull, sternebrae, forelegs, and hindlegs.

Studies have not been conducted to date to determine whether letrozole affects fertility in males or females. However, repeated administration of letrozole 0.6, 0.1, and 0.03 mg/kg in mice, rats, and dogs, respectively (about 1, 0.4, and 0.4 times the daily maximum recommended human dose on a mg/m² basis, respectively) caused sexual inactivity in females and atrophy of the reproductive tract in males and females. In young rats receiving doses of 0.003–0.3 mg/kg daily (exposures less than that expected at the recommended human dosage) for 12 weeks beginning on postnatal day 7, letrozole resulted in neuroendocrine and reproductive developmental disturbances of the hypothalamic-pituitary axis; decreased fertility was accompanied by pituitary gland hypertrophy, testicular changes including degeneration of the seminiferous tubular epithelium in males, and atrophy of the reproductive tract in females.

It is not known whether letrozole is distributed into milk. Because many drugs are distributed into milk and because of the potential for serious adverse reactions to letrozole in nursing infants, a decision should be made whether to discontinue nursing or the drug, taking into account the importance of the drug to the woman.

Drug Interactions

■ **Selective Estrogen Receptor Modulators** The concomitant use of selective estrogen receptor modulators (e.g., tamoxifen, raloxifene) and aromatase inhibitors, such as letrozole, is not recommended.

Concomitant use of tamoxifen 20 mg daily and letrozole 2.5 mg daily reduced letrozole plasma concentrations by an average of 38%. In a separate study, no effect of letrozole on the pharmacokinetics of tamoxifen, its principal active metabolite, *N*-desmethyltamoxifen, or 4-hydroxytamoxifen was observed. Analysis of blood samples from both of these studies demonstrates similar degrees of estrogen suppression for letrozole alone and in combination with tamoxifen. Although the clinical importance of this pharmacokinetic interaction is uncertain, the concomitant use of letrozole and tamoxifen is *not* recommended. Clinical experience in patients with previously treated advanced breast cancer indicates that administration of letrozole immediately after tamoxifen does not reduce the therapeutic effect of letrozole.

Because this pharmacokinetic interaction may occur with similar agents and reduce plasma concentrations of letrozole, the concomitant use of other selective estrogen receptor modulators (e.g., raloxifene) is not recommended. Among women receiving letrozole who require drug therapy for osteoporosis, the use of an oral bisphosphonate agent, rather than raloxifene, is advised.

■ **Estrogens** Because estrogens may diminish the pharmacologic action of aromatase inhibitors, such as letrozole, these agents should not be used concomitantly.

■ **Drugs Affecting or Metabolized by Hepatic Microsomal Enzymes** Because metabolism of letrozole is mediated by cytochrome P-450 (CYP) isoenzymes 3A4 and 2A6, agents that induce or inhibit these isoenzymes may alter the metabolism of the drug. Cimetidine, which inhibits hepatic microsomal enzymes, did not alter the pharmacokinetics of letrozole.

In human liver microsomes, letrozole has been shown to strongly inhibit in vitro metabolic reactions catalyzed by CYP2A6 and to moderately inhibit reactions catalyzed by CYP2C19; thus, concomitant use of letrozole may result in decreased metabolism and increased plasma concentrations of agents metabolized by these hepatic microsomal enzymes. An interaction study did not show a clinically important effect of letrozole on the pharmacokinetics of warfarin.

Acute Toxicity

■ **Pathogenesis** Limited information is available on the acute toxicity of letrozole. Isolated cases of letrozole overdose have been reported; among these cases, the highest single dose ingested was 62.5 mg (25 tablets), and no serious adverse events were reported. In clinical trials, single doses of up to 30 mg and multiple doses of up to 10 mg daily were well tolerated. A lethal single oral dose of 2 g/kg in mice and rats (about 4000–8000 times the daily maximum recommended human dose on a mg/m² basis) has been reported; lethal doses were associated with reduced motor activity, ataxia, and dyspnea. Decreased blood pressure and arrhythmias leading to death were observed in cats receiving single IV doses equal to or exceeding 10 mg/kg (about 50 times the daily maximum recommended human dose on a mg/m² basis).

■ **Treatment** Because of the limited data available, no firm recommendations for treatment of letrozole overdosage can be made. Management of overdosage should consist of symptomatic treatment and general supportive care, including frequent monitoring of vital signs. If the patient is alert, emesis may be induced.

Pharmacology

Letrozole, a benzyltriazole derivative, is a selective, nonsteroidal aromatase inhibitor. Letrozole differs structurally from aminoglutethimide but shares the pharmacologic activity of competitive aromatase inhibition; although both drugs are selective nonsteroidal inhibitors, letrozole is more potent and selective on a molar basis.

■ **Antineoplastic Effects** Suppression of plasma concentrations of estradiol, estrone, and estrone sulfate by 75–95% from baseline, with maximal suppression achieved within 2–3 days, has been observed in postmenopausal women with advanced breast cancer receiving daily letrozole doses of 0.1–5 mg. Suppression was dose-related, and letrozole doses equal to or exceeding 0.5 mg resulted in suppression to estrone and estrone sulfate concentrations below the lower limit of detection in many cases. Suppression of serum estrogen concentrations was maintained throughout treatment in all patients receiving daily letrozole doses equal to or exceeding 0.5 mg.

■ **Hormonal Effects** Letrozole selectively inhibits synthesis of estrogens and does not affect synthesis of adrenal corticosteroid, aldosterone, or thyroid hormone.

No clinically relevant effect on plasma concentrations of cortisol, aldosterone, 11-deoxycortisol, 17-hydroxyprogesterone, and adrenocorticotropic hormone, corticotropin (ACTH) or in plasma renin activity was observed in postmenopausal patients receiving letrozole 0.1–5 mg daily. No effect on cortisol or aldosterone secretion in response to ACTH stimulation was observed after 6–12 weeks in patients receiving letrozole 0.1, 0.25, 0.5, 1, 2.5, or 5 mg daily.

The blockade of estrogen synthesis does not result in the accumulation of androgenic precursors. Plasma concentrations of androgens (androstenedione and testosterone) in healthy postmenopausal women receiving single doses of letrozole 0.1, 0.5, or 2.5 mg were not altered. In addition, no effect on plasma androstenedione concentrations was observed in postmenopausal patients receiving daily letrozole doses of 0.1–5 mg. Plasma concentrations of luteinizing hormone (LH) and follicle-stimulating hormone (FSH) were not affected, and no effect on thyroid function, as measured by thyrotropin (thyroid-stimulating hormone, TSH) serum concentrations, triiodothyronine (T_3) uptake, and thyroxine (T_4) serum concentrations, was observed in patients receiving letrozole.

Pharmacokinetics

■ **Absorption** Letrozole is rapidly and completely absorbed from the GI tract following oral administration. Steady-state plasma concentrations of the drug are reached in 2–6 weeks in patients receiving letrozole 2.5 mg daily. Letrozole exhibits slightly nonlinear pharmacokinetics with repeated administration of 2.5 mg daily, with steady-state plasma concentrations 1.5–2 times higher than predicted based on plasma concentrations measured after a single dose. However, continuous accumulation of letrozole does not occur, and steady-state concentrations are maintained over extended periods of daily drug administration. Food does not affect the oral absorption of the drug.

■ **Distribution** Letrozole has a large volume of distribution of approximately 1.9 L/kg. Letrozole is weakly bound to plasma proteins.

It is not known whether letrozole is distributed into milk in humans.

■ **Elimination** Letrozole has a terminal elimination half-life of about 2 days.

The primary elimination pathway of letrozole consists of slow metabolism in the liver to a pharmacologically inactive carbinol metabolite (4,4′-methanol-bisbenzonitrile) followed by renal excretion of the glucuronide conjugate of this metabolite. Formation of the carbinol metabolite is mediated by cytochrome P-450 (CYP) isoenzymes 3A4 and 2A6, and formation of the ketone analog of the carbinol metabolite is mediated by isoenzyme 2A6.

Following oral administration of radiolabeled letrozole, 90% of the administered dose was excreted in the urine. Of the radiolabeled drug recovered in urine, at least 75% was the glucuronide of the carbinol metabolite, about 9% consisted of 2 unidentified metabolites, and 6% was unchanged drug.

Age-related differences in pharmacokinetics over the range of 35 years of age to greater than 80 years of age have not been observed in patients receiving letrozole in clinical trials. Age-related differences between adults and children or race-related differences in the pharmacokinetics of letrozole have not been evaluated.

Liver function influences serum concentrations of letrozole, and the need for dosage adjustment is determined by the extent of hepatic dysfunction. In individuals with liver cirrhosis and severe hepatic impairment (Child-Pugh classification C, which included serum bilirubin concentrations of about 2–11 times the upper limit of normal with minimal to severe ascites), a twofold increase in mean area under the plasma concentration-time curve (AUC) and a 47% reduction in systemic clearance of letrozole have been reported. Patients with severe hepatic impairment are exposed to higher concentrations of letrozole, and dosage reduction is necessary. (See Dosage and Administration: Dosage in Renal and Hepatic Impairment.) In individuals with moderate hepatic impairment unrelated to liver metastases (e.g., cirrhosis, Child-Pugh classification A and B), the mean AUC values for letrozole were increased by 37% but were still within the range observed for control subjects with normal hepatic function. The effect of hepatic impairment on letrozole pharmacokinetics in patients with cancer and elevated bilirubin concentrations who do not have cirrhosis has not been determined.

Letrozole pharmacokinetics were not altered in individuals with varying renal function (24-hour creatinine clearance 9–116 mL/minute) receiving single doses of 2.5 mg or in patients with advanced breast cancer and renal impairment (calculated creatinine clearance 20–50 mL/minute) receiving multiple doses of 0.5 or 2.5 mg daily.

Chemistry and Stability

■ **Chemistry** Letrozole, a benzhydryltriazole derivative, is a selective, nonsteroidal aromatase inhibitor. Letrozole, a nonsteroidal aromatase inhibitor, differs structurally from aminoglutethimide but shares the pharmacologic activity of competitive aromatase inhibition. Competitive aromatase inhibitors also have been referred to as type II inhibitors of the enzyme. Like anastrozole, letrozole is a triazole derivative. The *N*-4 nitrogen of the triazole ring, which coordinates with the heme iron atom of the aromatase enzyme complex, is thought to be responsible for the high affinity of the drug for the estrogen synthetase enzyme.

Letrozole occurs as a white to yellowish, practically odorless crystalline powder. Letrozole is freely soluble in dichloromethane, slightly soluble in alcohol, and practically insoluble in water and has a melting range of 184–185°C.

■ **Stability** Commercially available letrozole tablets should be stored at a controlled room temperature of 25°C but may be exposed to temperatures ranging from 15–30°C.

For further information on the handling of antineoplastic agents, see the ASHP Guidelines on Handling Hazardous Drugs at http://www.ahfsdruginformation.com.

Preparations

Excipients in commercially available drug preparations may have clinically important effects in some individuals; consult specific product labeling for details.

Letrozole

Oral

Tablets, film-coated	2.5 mg	**Femara®**, Novartis

Letrozole Combinations

Oral

Kit	Letrozole 2.5 mg (28 film-coated tablets)	**Kisqali® Femara® Co-Pack,** Novartis
	Ribociclib succinate 200 mg (of ribociclib) (21, 42, or 63 film-coated tablets)	

†Use is not currently included in the labeling approved by the US Food and Drug Administration

ESTROGEN AGONIST-ANTAGONISTS 68:16.12

Bazedoxifene Acetate

■ Bazedoxifene acetate is a tissue-selective, estrogen agonist-antagonist.

Uses

■ **Osteoporosis** ***Prevention in Postmenopausal Women*** Bazedoxifene acetate in fixed combination with conjugated estrogens is used for the prevention of osteoporosis in postmenopausal women with an intact uterus. Safety and efficacy of bazedoxifene/conjugated estrogens in fixed combination for prevention of osteoporosis in premenopausal women† have not been established; use in such patients is *not* recommended.

Safety and efficacy of bazedoxifene in fixed combination with conjugated estrogens have been evaluated for the prevention of osteoporosis in postmenopausal women in 2 double-blind, randomized, placebo- and active-controlled studies (SMART-1 and SMART-5). In the SMART-1 study, postmenopausal women with an intact uterus were randomized to 1 of 8 treatment groups; 6 treatment groups received various dosage combinations of bazedoxifene/conjugated estrogens fixed-combination therapy once daily, while the other 2 groups received raloxifene 60 mg once daily or placebo. Women also received supplemental calcium (600–1200 mg) and vitamin D (200–400 units) daily. The SMART-1 study consisted of 2 substudies. In Substudy I, women were more than 5 years postmenopausal, had a lumbar spine or total hip bone mineral density (BMD) T-score of −1 to −2.5, and had at least 1 additional risk factor for osteoporosis. Of the 1454 women in this substudy (mean age 58 years), 182 received bazedoxifene 20 mg in fixed combination with conjugated estrogens 0.45 mg once daily (mean baseline BMD T-score of −1.43) and 184 women received placebo (mean baseline BMD T-score of −1.52). Women in Substudy II were 1–5 years postmenopausal and had at least 1 additional risk factor for osteoporosis. Of the 861 women in this substudy (mean age 52 years), 111 received bazedoxifene 20 mg in fixed combination with conjugated estrogens 0.45 mg once daily (mean baseline BMD T-score of −0.81) and 108 women received placebo (mean baseline BMD T-score of −0.94). The primary end point of both substudies was change in BMD at the lumbar spine; change in BMD of the hip was evaluated as a secondary end point. At 24 months, women receiving bazedoxifene 20 mg in fixed combination with conjugated estrogens 0.45 mg experienced substantially increased lumbar spine BMD compared with women receiving placebo in Substudy I (treatment difference 3.11%) and Substudy II (treatment difference 3.62%). These women also had substantially increased total hip BMD compared with those receiving placebo in Substudy I (treatment difference 1.73%) and Substudy II (treatment difference 1.96%).

In the SMART-5 study, bazedoxifene in fixed combination with conjugated estrogens was evaluated for the prevention of osteoporosis in a substudy of 590 women less than 5 years postmenopausal with an intact uterus. Women were randomized to receive once daily therapy with bazedoxifene 20 mg in fixed combination with conjugated estrogens 0.45 mg, bazedoxifene 20 mg in fixed combination with conjugated estrogens 0.625 mg, bazedoxifene 20 mg alone, medroxyprogesterone acetate 1.5 mg in fixed combination with conjugated estrogens 0.45 mg, or placebo. All women also received supplemental calcium 600 mg daily and vitamin D 400 units daily. The primary end point of the osteoporosis substudy was percent change from baseline in lumber spine BMD; change in BMD of the hip was evaluated as a secondary end point. At 12 months, all active treatment groups showed an increased lumbar spine BMD and total hip BMD while women in the placebo group experienced decreased BMD. Women receiving bazedoxifene 20 mg in fixed combination with conjugated estrogens 0.45 mg experienced substantially increased mean lumbar spine and total hip BMD (treatment difference of 1.51 and 1.21%, respectively, compared with placebo).

Treatment in Postmenopausal Women Bazedoxifene 20 mg is commercially available in other countries for the treatment† of postmenopausal osteoporosis. However, the drug currently is *not* FDA-labeled for the treatment of osteoporosis in the US. Efficacy and safety of bazedoxifene were evaluated in a randomized, double-blind, placebo- and active-controlled, phase 3 clinical study in postmenopausal women with osteoporosis. Patients receiving bazedoxifene 20 or 40 mg once daily for up to 5 years experienced a substantially decreased incidence of new vertebral fractures, increased lumbar spine BMD, and decreased bone turnover markers (e.g., serum osteocalcin and C-telopeptide) compared with those receiving placebo.

■ **Vasomotor Symptoms** Bazedoxifene/conjugated estrogens fixed-combination therapy is used for the management of moderate to severe vasomotor symptoms associated with menopause in women with an intact uterus.

Safety and efficacy of bazedoxifene/conjugated estrogens fixed-combination therapy have been evaluated for the treatment of moderate to severe vasomotor symptoms associated with menopause in a randomized, double-blind, placebo-controlled study (SMART-2). Over 300 women (mean age 53 years, mean time since menopause 4.5 years) with a baseline of at least 7 moderate to severe hot flushes per day or at least 50 per week were randomized to receive once daily therapy with bazedoxifene 20 mg in fixed combination with conjugated estrogens 0.45 mg, bazedoxifene 20 mg in fixed combination with conjugated estrogens 0.625 mg, or placebo. The primary efficacy outcomes were change from baseline in the average daily number of hot flushes (moderate and severe) and severity rating of hot flushes. At 12 weeks, women receiving bazedoxifene 20 mg in fixed combination with conjugated estrogens 0.45 mg experienced a 74% reduction in number of hot flushes from baseline compared with a 47% reduction in women receiving placebo. The severity rating of hot flushes also was substantially decreased in women receiving bazedoxifene/conjugated estrogens fixed-combination therapy when compared with placebo. Reduction in severity of hot flushes was observed as early as 3 weeks following initiation of therapy with bazedoxifene 20 mg in fixed combination with conjugated estrogens 0.45 mg. In a secondary analysis of data from the SMART-2 study, women receiving bazedoxifene 20 mg in fixed combination with conjugated estrogens 0.45 mg showed a mean increase from baseline of 2.8 days per week *without* moderate to severe hot flushes compared with an increase of 1 day per week in women receiving placebo.

In a double-blind, randomized, placebo- and active-controlled study (SMART-1), the number and severity of hot flushes were evaluated in a subset of 216 women reporting at least 7 hot flushes per day or more than 50 per week at baseline. At 12 weeks, women receiving bazedoxifene 20 mg in fixed combination with conjugated estrogens 0.45 mg experienced a greater mean reduction from baseline in the average daily number of hot flushes and also experienced a decreased severity of hot flushes compared with those receiving placebo. These effects were sustained through 2 years of treatment with the fixed-combination therapy.

Dosage and Administration

■ **General** Bazedoxifene acetate in fixed combination with conjugated estrogens should be prescribed at the lowest effective dosage for the shortest duration consistent with treatment goals and risks for the individual woman. Postmenopausal women receiving the fixed-combination therapy should be re-evaluated periodically as clinically appropriate to determine if continued treatment is necessary.

Patients receiving bazedoxifene/conjugated estrogens fixed-combination therapy for prevention of osteoporosis should receive supplemental calcium and/or vitamin D if daily dietary intake is inadequate.

■ **Administration** Bazedoxifene/conjugated estrogens fixed-combination tablets are administered orally without regard to meals. Tablets should be swallowed whole.

■ **Dosage** Dosage of bazedoxifene acetate is expressed in terms of bazedoxifene.

Each tablet of bazedoxifene acetate in fixed combination with conjugated estrogens contains bazedoxifene 20 mg and conjugated estrogens 0.45 mg.

Osteoporosis For the prevention of osteoporosis in postmenopausal women, the recommended dosage of bazedoxifene/conjugated estrogens fixed-combination therapy is bazedoxifene 20 mg with conjugated estrogens 0.45 mg once daily.

Vasomotor Symptoms For the management of moderate to severe vasomotor symptoms associated with menopause, the recommended dosage of bazedoxifene/conjugated estrogens fixed-combination therapy is bazedoxifene 20 mg with conjugated estrogens 0.45 mg once daily.

■ **Special Populations** When bazedoxifene acetate is used in fixed combination with conjugated estrogens, dosage requirements for conjugated estrogens should be considered.

Hepatic Impairment Bazedoxifene/conjugated estrogens fixed-combination therapy is contraindicated in patients with hepatic impairment. (See Cautions: Contraindications.)

Renal Impairment Use of bazedoxifene/conjugated estrogens fixed-combination therapy is not recommended in patients with renal impairment.

Cautions

■ **Contraindications** Bazedoxifene acetate in fixed combination with conjugated estrogens is contraindicated in women with undiagnosed abnormal uterine bleeding, women with known or suspected estrogen-dependent neoplasia, and women with known or suspected breast cancer or a history of breast cancer. (See Genitourinary Effects under Warnings/Precautions: Warnings, in Cautions and also see Carcinogenicity under Warnings/Precautions: Other Warnings/Precautions, in Cautions.)

The fixed-combination therapy is contraindicated in women with active deep-vein thrombosis (DVT), pulmonary embolism (PE), active arterial thromboembolic disease (e.g., stroke, myocardial infarction [MI]), or history of these conditions. (See Cardiovascular Effects under Warnings/Precautions: Warnings, in Cautions.)

The fixed-combination therapy also is contraindicated in women with known hepatic impairment or disease; known protein C, protein S, or antithrombin deficiency; other known thrombophilic disorders; or hypersensitivity (e.g., anaphylaxis, angioedema) to any ingredient in the formulation.

Bazedoxifene/conjugated estrogens fixed-combination therapy is contraindicated in women who are or may become pregnant. (See Fetal/Neonatal Morbidity and Mortality under Warnings/ Precautions: Other Warnings/Precautions, in Cautions and also see Pregnancy under Warnings/Precautions: Specific Populations, in Cautions.) The drug also is contraindicated in women who are breast-feeding. (See Lactation under Warnings/Precautions: Specific Populations, in Cautions.)

■ **Warnings/Precautions** ***Warnings*** **Use of Fixed Combinations.**

Cardiovascular Effects. Risk factors for cardiovascular disorders, arterial vascular disease (e.g., hypertension, diabetes mellitus, tobacco use, hypercholesterolemia, obesity), and/or venous thromboembolism (VTE) including personal or family history of VTE, obesity, or systemic lupus erythematosus should be managed appropriately during bazedoxifene/conjugated estrogens fixed-combination therapy. Estrogen therapy should *not* be used for the prevention of cardiovascular disease.

When used individually, estrogen agonists-antagonists, including bazedoxifene, and conjugated estrogens are known to increase the risk of VTE. In the Women's Health Initiative (WHI) study of estrogen alone, an increased risk of stroke and VTE (including DVT and PE) was reported in postmenopausal women (50–79 years of age) receiving oral conjugated estrogens alone at a dosage of 0.625 mg daily over 7.1 years compared with women receiving placebo. Increased risk of stroke was demonstrated during the first year of the study and persisted; for VTE, increased risk was evident during the first 2 years of the study. In the WHI study, no overall effect on coronary heart disease (CHD) events (i.e., nonfatal or silent MI, CHD death) was reported in women receiving estrogen therapy alone versus placebo. In clinical studies of bazedoxifene/conjugated estrogens fixed-combination therapy, VTE was reported in 0% of women receiving the fixed combination and 0.1% of women receiving placebo. As a result of the low rate of VTE in both groups, it is not possible to conclude that the risk of VTE with bazedoxifene/conjugated estrogens fixed-combination therapy is different from that observed with other estrogen preparations.

Bazedoxifene/conjugated estrogens fixed-combination therapy should be discontinued immediately if VTE (including PE or DVT) or stroke occurs or is suspected. If possible, the drug should be discontinued at least 4–6 weeks prior to surgery associated with an increased risk of thromboembolism or during periods of prolonged immobilization and should not be resumed until the patient is fully ambulatory. Women receiving bazedoxifene/conjugated estrogens fixed-combination therapy should be advised to ambulate periodically during travel involving prolonged immobilization.

There have been reports of substantial increases in blood pressure attributed to idiosyncratic reactions to estrogens. A generalized effect of estrogens on blood pressure was not observed in a large, randomized, placebo-controlled study.

Bazedoxifene/conjugated estrogens fixed-combination therapy may cause increased plasma high-density lipoprotein [HDL]-cholesterol and HDL2-cholesterol subfraction concentrations, decreased low-density lipoprotein [LDL]-cholesterol concentrations, and increased triglyceride concentrations.

Estrogens may cause some degree of fluid retention. Therefore, women with conditions that might be aggravated by fluid retention (e.g., cardiac dysfunction, renal impairment) should be carefully observed when receiving estrogens.

Dementia. Results from the WHI Memory Study (WHIMS; an ancillary study of the WHI study in women 65–79 years of age without an intact uterus) indicate that use of conjugated estrogens 0.625 mg daily increases the risk of probable dementia in women receiving conjugated estrogens compared with women receiving placebo (absolute risk: 37 versus 25 cases per 10,000 women-years; relative risk: 1.49 [0.83–2.66]) after an average follow-up of 5.2 years. It is unknown whether this finding is applicable to younger postmenopausal women.

Estrogen therapy should *not* be used for the prevention of dementia.

Genitourinary Effects. Bazedoxifene is an estrogen agonist-antagonist, which reduces the risk of endometrial hyperplasia that can occur when conjugated estrogens are used alone. Postmenopausal women with an intact uterus receiving estrogen therapy alone are at increased risk of endometrial cancer. Such risk is dependent on duration of therapy and estrogen dosage and has been shown to persist for at least 8–15 years after estrogen therapy is discontinued. The use of bazedoxifene with conjugated estrogens reduces the risk of endometrial hyperplasia, which may be a precursor to endometrial cancer. In clinical studies of bazedoxifene/conjugated estrogens fixed-combination therapy, the incidence of endometrial hyperplasia or malignancy was less than 1% in women receiving the fixed combination for up to 24 months.

Clinical surveillance is important for all women receiving bazedoxifene/ conjugated estrogens fixed-combination therapy. Adequate diagnostic measures, including directed and random endometrial sampling when indicated, should be undertaken to rule out malignancy in postmenopausal women with undiagnosed persistent or recurrent abnormal genital bleeding. In addition, women receiving the fixed-combination therapy should *not* use additional estrogens as this may increase the risk of endometrial hyperplasia.

Other Warnings/Precautions **Fetal/Neonatal Morbidity and Mortality.** Bazedoxifene may cause fetal harm. No animal studies were performed to evaluate the effect of bazedoxifene in fixed combination with conjugated estrogens. Reduced numbers of live fetuses and/or reduction in fetal body weight have been observed in rats at bazedoxifene exposures of 0.3 or more times the human exposure with the 20-mg dose; abortions and an increased incidence of heart and skeletal system anomalies also occurred in rabbits at 2 times the human exposure associated with the 20-mg dose.

If the fixed combination of bazedoxifene and conjugated estrogens is used during pregnancy or if a woman becomes pregnant while receiving the drug, the patient should be informed of the potential hazard to the fetus.

Body Mass Index. Results from a population pharmacokinetic model of bazedoxifene/conjugated estrogens fixed-combination therapy show that systemic exposure of bazedoxifene is predicted to be reduced by 17% in women with a body mass index (BMI) greater than 27 kg/m^2 compared with women having a BMI of 27 kg/m^2 or less. Reduced bazedoxifene exposure may be associated with an increased risk of endometrial hyperplasia.

Regardless of BMI, adequate diagnostic measures, including directed and random endometrial sampling when indicated, should be undertaken to rule out malignancy in postmenopausal women with undiagnosed persistent or recurrent abnormal genital bleeding.

Carcinogenicity. In the WHI estrogen-alone study, postmenopausal women who received conjugated estrogens 0.625 mg once daily did not have an increased risk of invasive breast cancer when compared with those receiving placebo (average follow-up of 7.1 years). However, an increased incidence of abnormal mammograms requiring further evaluation has been reported with use of estrogen therapy alone. The effect of bazedoxifene/conjugated estrogens fixed-combination therapy on the risk of breast cancer is unknown. In a clinical study of women receiving bazedoxifene 20 mg in fixed combination with conjugated estrogens 0.45 mg, there was no observed increase in breast density after 12 months when compared with placebo. In a clinical study of up to 2 years' duration, there was no observed increased risk of breast cancer in women receiving the fixed-combination therapy. All women receiving bazedoxifene/ conjugated estrogens fixed-combination therapy should receive annual breast examinations by a clinician and perform monthly breast self-examinations. In addition, mammography examinations should be scheduled based on patient age, risk factors, and prior mammogram results.

Some epidemiologic studies suggest that use of estrogen-only preparations for 5 or more years is associated with an increased risk of ovarian cancer. However, data regarding the duration of exposure associated with this risk have been inconsistent. The effect of bazedoxifene/conjugated estrogens fixed-combination therapy on the risk of ovarian cancer is unknown.

Endocrine and Metabolic Effects. Estrogen administration leads to increased thyroxine-binding globulin (TBG) concentrations. Bazedoxifene/conjugated estrogens fixed-combination therapy also may increase TBG concentrations leading to increased circulating total thyroid hormone (as measured by protein-bound iodine [PBI]), thyroxine (T_4) concentrations (by column or radioimmunoassay [RIA]), or triiodothyronine (T_3) concentrations (by RIA). Women with normal thyroid function are able to compensate for increased TBG concentrations by synthesizing more thyroid hormone and, thereby, maintaining T_4 and T_3 concentrations in the normal range. Women receiving thyroid hormone replacement therapy and estrogens concomitantly may require an increased dosage of thyroid hormone. Thyroid function should be monitored in such patients to maintain free thyroid hormone concentrations in an acceptable range.

In women with preexisting hypertriglyceridemia, use of estrogens may be associated with increased plasma triglyceride concentrations leading to pancreatitis. Discontinuance of bazedoxifene/conjugated estrogens fixed-combination therapy should be considered if pancreatitis occurs.

Bazedoxifene/conjugated estrogens fixed-combination therapy may cause impaired glucose tolerance.

Bazedoxifene/conjugated estrogens fixed-combination therapy may decrease free hormone concentrations (e.g., testosterone, estradiol). Concentrations of certain binding proteins may be elevated (e.g., corticosteroid-binding globulin [CBG], sex hormone binding globulin [SHBG]) leading to increased total circulating corticosteroids and sex steroids, respectively. The fixed-combination therapy also may increase concentrations of certain plasma proteins (e.g., angiotensinogen/renin substrate, α_1-antitrypsin, ceruloplasmin).

Exacerbation of Other Conditions. Estrogens may exacerbate asthma, diabetes mellitus, epilepsy, migraine, porphyria, systemic lupus erythematosus, and hepatic hemangiomas and should be used with caution in women with these conditions.

GI Effects. A twofold to fourfold increased risk of gallbladder disease requiring surgery has been reported in postmenopausal women receiving estrogens.

Hematologic Effects. Bazedoxifene/conjugated estrogens fixed-combination therapy may cause accelerated prothrombin time (PT), partial thromboplastin time (PTT), or platelet aggregation time. The fixed-combination therapy also may increase platelet count and increase factors II, VII antigen, VIII antigen, VIII coagulant activity, IX, X, XII, VII-X complex, II-VII-X complex, and β-thromboglobulin.

Hepatic Effects. Bazedoxifene/conjugated estrogens fixed-combination therapy has not been studied in women with hepatic impairment or in those with a history of cholestatic jaundice. Women with hepatic impairment receiving bazedoxifene alone had a 4.3-fold increased overall exposure when compared with controls; estrogens also may be poorly metabolized in women with hepatic impairment.

Bazedoxifene/conjugated estrogens fixed-combination therapy is contraindicated in patients with hepatic impairment. (See Cautions: Contraindications.) The fixed-combination therapy should be used with caution in women with a history of cholestatic jaundice associated with previous estrogen use or with pregnancy. If such conditions recur, bazedoxifene/conjugated estrogens fixed-combination therapy should be discontinued.

Hereditary Angioedema. Use of estrogens may exacerbate symptoms of angioedema in women with hereditary angioedema.

Hypocalcemia. Estrogens should be used with caution in women with hypoparathyroidism; estrogen therapy may induce hypocalcemia in such patients.

Laboratory Monitoring. Monitoring of serum follicle-stimulating hormone (FSH) and estradiol concentrations has *not* been shown to be useful in the management of moderate to severe vasomotor symptoms.

Ocular Effects. Retinal vascular thrombosis has been reported in patients receiving estrogens. Bazedoxifene/conjugated estrogens fixed-combination therapy should be discontinued pending diagnostic evaluation if there is a sudden partial or complete loss of vision or a sudden onset of proptosis, diplopia, or migraine. The fixed combination should be permanently discontinued if ophthalmologic examination reveals papilledema or retinal vascular lesions.

Use in Premenopausal Women. Safety and efficacy of bazedoxifene in fixed combination with conjugated estrogens in premenopausal women† have not been established; use in such patients is *not* recommended.

Use with Progestins, Estrogens, or Estrogen Agonists-Antagonists. Postmenopausal women receiving bazedoxifene/conjugated estrogens fixed-combination therapy should *not* receive concomitant therapy with progestins, additional estrogens, or additional estrogen agonists-antagonists.

Specific Populations **Pregnancy.** Category X. (See Cautions: Contraindications and also see Fetal/Neonatal Morbidity and Mortality under Warnings/Precautions: Other Warnings/Precautions, in Cautions.)

Lactation. It is not known whether the fixed combination of bazedoxifene and conjugated estrogens is distributed into human milk. Estrogen administration to nursing women has been shown to decrease the quantity and quality of milk. The fixed-combination therapy should *not* be used in nursing women.

Pediatric Use. Bazedoxifene/conjugated estrogens fixed-combination therapy is *not* indicated for use in pediatric patients.

Geriatric Use. Bazedoxifene/conjugated estrogens fixed-combination therapy is *not* recommended in women older than 75 years of age. Women older than 75 years of age were not included in clinical studies of the fixed-combination therapy. Following a single 20-mg dose of bazedoxifene alone, area under the concentration-time curve (AUC) was 1.5-fold higher in women 65–74 years of age and 2.6-fold higher in women 75 years of age or older compared with women 51–64 years of age.

No overall differences in safety or efficacy were observed in women 65–74 years of age compared with younger women. However, greater sensitivity in some older women cannot be ruled out.

Hepatic Impairment. Bazedoxifene/conjugated estrogens fixed-combination therapy is contraindicated in patients with hepatic impairment. (See Cautions: Contraindications.)

Women with mild, moderate, or severe hepatic impairment (Child-Pugh class A, B, or C) receiving a single 20-mg dose of bazedoxifene had increased peak plasma concentrations (67, 32, or 20%, respectively) and increased AUC (143, 109, or 268%, respectively) compared with healthy women. The half-life of the drug was prolonged to 50 hours in women with severe hepatic impairment compared with 32 hours in healthy women. The pharmacokinetics, safety, and efficacy of bazedoxifene/conjugated estrogens fixed-combination therapy have not been studied in women with hepatic impairment.

Renal Impairment. Bazedoxifene/conjugated estrogens fixed-combination therapy is not recommended in women with renal impairment. Pharmacokinetics, safety, and efficacy of the fixed-combination therapy have not been studied in such patients.

When bazedoxifene 20 mg once daily was studied alone in postmenopausal women with mild, moderate, or severe renal impairment, results showed no increase in the incidence or severity of adverse effects compared with placebo.

■ **Common Adverse Effects** Adverse effects occurring in at least 5% of patients receiving bazedoxifene/conjugated estrogens fixed-combination therapy and more frequently than that with placebo include nausea, diarrhea, dyspepsia, upper abdominal pain, muscle spasms, neck pain, dizziness, nasopharyngitis, and oropharyngeal pain.

Drug Interactions

Formal drug interaction studies have not been performed to date with bazedoxifene acetate in fixed combination with conjugated estrogens.

■ **Drugs Affecting or Metabolized by Hepatic Microsomal Enzymes** Bazedoxifene undergoes little or no metabolism by cytochrome P-450 (CYP) isoenzymes. The drug does not induce or inhibit the activity of CYP isoenzymes; in vitro data suggest that bazedoxifene is unlikely to interact with drugs metabolized by these isoenzymes.

Estrogens are metabolized partially by CYP3A4. Inducers of CYP3A4 (e.g., carbamazepine, phenobarbital, rifampin, St. John's wort [*Hypericum perforatum*]) may decrease estrogen plasma concentrations and result in decreased therapeutic effect and/or changes in uterine bleeding. Inhibitors of CYP3A4 (e.g., clarithromycin, erythromycin, grapefruit juice, itraconazole, ketoconazole, ritonavir) may increase conjugated estrogen exposures resulting in increased risk of endometrial hyperplasia. If a patient receives a CYP3A4 inhibitor concomitantly with bazedoxifene/conjugated estrogens fixed-combination therapy for more than 30 days, adequate diagnostic measures, including directed and random endometrial sampling when indicated, should be undertaken to rule out malignancy in postmenopausal women with undiagnosed persistent or recurrent abnormal genital bleeding.

■ **Drugs Affecting or Metabolized by Uridine Diphosphate-glucuronosyltransferase** Bazedoxifene is metabolized by uridine diphosphate-glucuronosyltransferase (UGT) enzymes in the intestinal tract and liver. The metabolism of bazedoxifene may be increased if used concomitantly with drugs known to induce UGT enzymes (e.g., rifampin, phenobarbital, carbamazepine, phenytoin). Decreased bazedoxifene exposures may be associated with an increased risk of endometrial hyperplasia. Adequate diagnostic measures, including directed and random endometrial sampling when indicated, should be undertaken to rule out malignancy in postmenopausal women with undiagnosed persistent or recurrent abnormal genital bleeding.

■ **Antacids** Concomitant use of a single 40-mg dose of bazedoxifene with a single dose of antacid containing aluminum hydroxide 460 mg and magnesium hydroxide 400 mg increased bazedoxifene area under the concentration-time curve (AUC) by 7% and decreased peak plasma concentrations by 8%.

■ **Estrogens and Estrogen Agonists-Antagonists** There are no clinically important pharmacokinetic interactions between conjugated estrogens and bazedoxifene.

Concomitant use of conjugated estrogens 0.625 mg daily for 8 days and a single dose of bazedoxifene 20 mg in fixed combination with conjugated estrogens 0.625 mg decreased bazedoxifene AUC by 6% and increased peak plasma concentrations by 3%. Concomitant use of bazedoxifene 20 mg daily for 10 days and a single dose of bazedoxifene 20 mg in fixed combination with conjugated estrogens 0.625 mg increased AUC and peak concentrations of unconjugated estrone by 3 and 11%, respectively; the AUC and peak plasma concentrations of equilin increased by 14 and 17%, respectively.

Bazedoxifene/conjugated estrogens fixed-combination therapy should *not* be used concomitantly with additional estrogens as this may increase the risk of endometrial hyperplasia.

Bazedoxifene/conjugated estrogens fixed-combination therapy should *not* be used concomitantly with additional estrogen agonists-antagonists.

■ **HMG-CoA Reductase Inhibitors** Concomitant use of bazedoxifene 40 mg and atorvastatin 20 mg in healthy postmenopausal women did not substantially affect the pharmacokinetics of either drug.

■ **Macrolides** Concomitant use of azithromycin 500 mg daily for 9 days followed by azithromycin 250 mg daily for 4 days and a single 40-mg dose of bazedoxifene did not substantially affect the pharmacokinetics of bazedoxifene.

■ **Nonsteroidal Anti-inflammatory Agents** Concomitant use of bazedoxifene 20 mg and ibuprofen 600 mg did not substantially affect the pharmacokinetics of either drug.

■ **Progestins** Bazedoxifene/conjugated estrogens fixed-combination therapy should *not* be used concomitantly with progestins.

Description

Bazedoxifene acetate is a tissue-selective, estrogen agonist-antagonist; the drug also is referred to as a selective estrogen receptor modulator (SERM). Bazedoxifene has mixed estrogen agonist and antagonist activities resulting in activation of estrogenic pathways in some tissues and blockade of estrogenic pathways in other tissues. The drug binds to estrogen receptor (ER) α and ERβ, with slightly stronger binding occurring at the ERα receptor.

In animal studies, bazedoxifene exhibits estrogen antagonistic effects on the endometrium when given alone and when given concomitantly with conjugated estrogens; these effects also were demonstrated in clinical trials (e.g., no difference from placebo in the effect on endometrial thickness or endometrial hyperplasia). In vitro, bazedoxifene has been shown to have limited estrogen agonistic effects on human breast cancer cells and blocks stimulatory actions of estradiol and conjugated estrogens on breast cells, which reverses negative effects of estrogen in breast cancer cells. Bazedoxifene also has been shown to increase bone mass in animal models and in clinical studies.

The combination of a SERM (e.g., bazedoxifene) and estrogens is also referred to as a tissue-selective estrogen complex (TSEC). Bazedoxifene in fixed combination with conjugated estrogens produces a composite effect specific to each target tissue. The bazedoxifene component of the fixed-combination therapy reduces the risk of endometrial hyperplasia associated with use of conjugated estrogens alone.

Following oral administration of multiple doses of bazedoxifene 20 mg in fixed combination with conjugated estrogens 0.45 mg to healthy, postmenopausal women, peak bazedoxifene plasma concentrations are attained at approximately 2.5 hours after the dose. The absolute bioavailability of bazedoxifene is approximately 6%. Area under the concentration-time curve (AUC) of bazedoxifene is increased by 25% when the fixed combination is taken with a high-fat, high-calorie meal; peak plasma concentrations of bazedoxifene are not affected by food. In vitro, bazedoxifene is highly bound to plasma proteins (98–99%); the drug does not bind to sex hormone binding globulin (SHBG). Following oral administration of bazedoxifene 20 mg alone, the drug undergoes extensive metabolism principally by glucuronidation; little or no metabolism is mediated by cytochrome P-450 (CYP) isoenzymes. The major metabolite is bazedoxifene-5-glucuronide; plasma concentrations of the metabolite are approximately tenfold higher than those of unchanged drug. The drug is expected to undergo enterohepatic recycling from the gut to systemic circulation. Bazedoxifene undergoes biliary excretion followed by elimination in feces (85%); less than 1% of a dose is eliminated in urine. After oral administration of bazedoxifene/conjugated estrogens in fixed combination, the half-life of bazedoxifene is approximately 30 hours.

Advice to Patients

Importance of instructing patients to read the manufacturer's patient information prior to initiation of therapy and each time the prescription is refilled.

Importance of instructing patients to open only 1 foil pouch containing bazedoxifene/conjugated estrogens fixed-combination tablets at a time (if more than 1 blister package is dispensed) and to record the date the blister package is opened on the package label. The tablets should not be used if the package is opened for more than 60 days. Only 1 tablet should be removed from the blister package at the time of use. The tablets should be kept in the original package and should *not* be placed in pill boxes or pill organizers.

If a dose is missed, importance of advising patients to take it as soon as they remember. Patients should not take the missed dose if it is almost time for the next scheduled dose. Patients should be informed not to take 2 doses at the same time to make up for a missed dose.

Importance of advising patients to add supplemental calcium and/or vitamin D to the diet if daily intake is inadequate.

Importance of patients immediately reporting any signs or symptoms related to venous thrombosis and thromboembolic events to a clinician.

Importance of women reporting any unusual vaginal bleeding to a clinician as soon as possible.

Importance of informing women of possible serious adverse effects of estrogen therapy (e.g., cardiovascular disorders, malignant neoplasms, probable dementia).

Importance of informing women of possible less serious, but common adverse effects of bazedoxifene in fixed combination with conjugated estrogens (e.g., muscle spasms, nausea, diarrhea, dyspepsia, upper abdominal pain, throat pain, dizziness, neck pain).

Importance of informing clinicians of existing or contemplated concomitant therapy, including prescription and OTC drugs, as well as any concomitant illnesses.

Importance of women informing clinicians if they are or plan to become pregnant or plan to breast-feed. (See Cautions: Contraindications.)

Importance of informing patients of other important precautionary information. (See Cautions.)

Overview® (see Users Guide). For additional information on this drug until a more detailed monograph is developed and published, the manufacturer's labeling should be consulted. It is *essential* that the manufacturer's labeling be consulted for more detailed information on usual cautions, precautions, contraindications, potential drug interactions, laboratory test interferences, and acute toxicity.

Preparations

Excipients in commercially available drug preparations may have clinically important effects in some individuals; consult specific product labeling for details.

Bazedoxifene Acetate Combinations

Oral		
Tablets	20 mg (of bazedoxifene) with Conjugated Estrogens 0.45 mg	**Duavee®**, Pfizer

†Use is not currently included in the labeling approved by the US Food and Drug Administration

clomiPHENE Citrate

■ Clomiphene citrate is a nonsteroidal compound with both estrogenic and anti-estrogenic properties that is used to induce ovulation in anovulatory women.

Uses

■ **Female Infertility** Clomiphene citrate is used to induce ovulation in appropriately selected anovulatory women desiring pregnancy. Clomiphene citrate is ineffective in patients with primary pituitary or ovarian failure and is indicated only for patients in whom ovulatory dysfunction has been demonstrated. The drug is not a substitute for appropriate therapy of other conditions which may cause ovulatory dysfunction (e.g., thyroid or adrenal disease). Optimum results with clomiphene therapy are obtained in patients with adequately functioning anterior pituitary gland, adrenals, ovaries, and thyroid. Although better results are usually obtained in patients with adequate serum estrogen concentrations, reduced serum estrogen concentrations do not always preclude successful therapy.

Candidates for clomiphene therapy must be given a complete pelvic examination and endometrial biopsy before each course of treatment and neoplastic lesions must be ruled out. All impediments to achieving ovulation and conception must be excluded or treated before beginning clomiphene citrate therapy. The therapeutic effects of clomiphene citrate are temporary, and the anovulatory pattern usually resumes following discontinuance of therapy or when pregnancy is completed.

■ **Other Uses** Clomiphene citrate has been used in a limited number of patients for the treatment of a variety of menstrual abnormalities†, gynecomastia†, fibrocystic disease of the breast†, oligospermia†, persistent lactation†, endometrial hyperplasia†, endometrial anaplasia†, and regulation of cycles in patients using the rhythm method of contraception†. The drug also has been used in combination with estrogens or menotropins† in patients who are refractory to either drug alone. Efficacy of clomiphene citrate in these conditions has not been established.

Dosage and Administration

■ **Administration** Clomiphene citrate is administered orally.

■ **Dosage** The usual initial dosage of clomiphene citrate used to induce ovulation is 50 mg daily for 5 days. It is important to carefully time the dosage schedule. Therapy may be started at any time in patients who have had no recent uterine bleeding. If progestin-induced bleeding is planned, or if spontaneous uterine bleeding occurs prior to therapy, the regimen should be started on the fifth day of the cycle. Once ovulation has been established, each subsequent course of therapy should be started on the fifth day of the cycle. Although ovulation is slightly more likely to occur with a dosage of 100 mg daily for 5 days, the adverse effects and incidence of multiple ovulations with resulting plural gestations may be expected to increase at this higher dosage.

The majority of the patients who are going to respond to clomiphene citrate will ovulate after the first course of therapy, generally within 5–14 days. If ovulation has not occurred at this time, 100 mg of clomiphene citrate may be administered daily for 5 days, starting as early as 30 days after previous therapy. Dosage should be increased only in those patients who do not respond to the first course of therapy, and dosage should never be increased or extended beyond 100 mg daily for 5 days. Prolonged amenorrhea may be less responsive to clomiphene and may require 2 or more cycles of therapy. Three courses of clomiphene should constitute an adequate therapeutic trial; if ovulatory menses or pregnancy has not occurred at this time, the diagnosis should be reevaluated. The likelihood of conception decreases with each succeeding course of therapy.

Since the relative safety of long-term cyclic therapy with clomiphene has not been conclusively demonstrated, and since the majority of patients will ovulate after 3 courses of therapy, long-term cyclic therapy is not recommended.

Cautions

■ Adverse Effects The frequency and severity of adverse reactions to clomiphene citrate appear to be dose related and occur most frequently in patients receiving high doses (100 mg or more daily) and/or prolonged therapy.

The most common adverse effects of clomiphene citrate are ovarian enlargement or cyst formation and vasomotor symptoms such as hot flashes. When clomiphene is administered in recommended dosages, abnormal ovarian enlargement is infrequent; however, the usual cyclic variation in ovarian size may be exaggerated and mid-cycle ovarian pain (mittelschmerz) may be accentuated. Ovarian enlargement and cyst formation (usually luteal) may occur more frequently and the luteal phase of the menstrual cycle may be prolonged in patients receiving higher dosages or prolonged administration of the drug. Some patients with polycystic ovary syndrome are unusually sensitive to gonadotropin and may have an exaggerated response to usual doses of clomiphene citrate. Massive ovarian enlargement has been reported rarely. If abnormal enlargement of the ovary occurs during clomiphene therapy, the drug should be discontinued. (See Cautions: Precautions and Contraindications.) Maximal enlargement of the ovary does not occur until several days following discontinuance of clomiphene therapy; however, ovarian enlargement and cyst formation usually regress spontaneously a few days or weeks following discontinuance of the drug. Unless a strong indication for laparotomy exists, most patients with ovarian enlargement or cyst formation should be managed conservatively.

Vasomotor symptoms reported with clomiphene resemble menopausal hot flashes. These effects are usually mild and disappear after clomiphene therapy is discontinued.

Abdominal symptoms or pelvic discomfort including distention, bloating, or pain may occur with clomiphene therapy and may resemble mittelschmerz, premenstrual phenomena, or ovarian enlargement.

Adverse visual symptoms including transient blurring of vision, diplopia, scotomata, phosphenes, or photophobia have occurred in patients receiving clomiphene. These adverse ocular effects appear to be dose related and usually disappear within a few days or weeks following discontinuance of the drug. Visual symptoms seem to result from intensification and prolongation of afterimages and often first appear or are accentuated when the patient is exposed to a more brightly-lit environment. Rarely, decreased visual acuity may occur. One patient reportedly developed posterior cortical senile cataracts following clomiphene therapy, but the causal relationship between cataracts and the drug has not been determined. Ophthalmologically definable scotomata and electroretinographic changes in retinal function have also been reported.

Other adverse effects of clomiphene citrate include nausea or vomiting, increased urinary frequency or volume, heavier menses, increased appetite and weight gain, and various dermatologic conditions including urticaria, rash, or allergic dermatitis. Breast discomfort, increased nervous tension, headache, restlessness, insomnia, dizziness, lightheadedness, depression, fatigue, and reversible hair loss may also occur.

Clomiphene citrate has not been reported to produce any clinically important abnormalities in hematologic or renal systems, in protein-bound iodine, or in serum cholesterol when given for short periods; however, following prolonged, continuous administration, elevated concentrations of desmosterol have been reported, indicating a possible interference with cholesterol synthesis.

Increased retention of sulfobromophthalein has occurred during therapy with clomiphene while results of other liver function tests usually have been normal. One case of jaundice due to bile stasis has been reported.

■ Precautions and Contraindications Because of possible visual disturbances, dizziness, or lightheadedness, patients receiving clomiphene citrate should be cautioned against performing hazardous tasks requiring mental alertness or physical coordination (e.g., operating machinery, driving a motor vehicle), particularly under conditions of variable lighting. Clomiphene citrate should be used with caution in patients who are unusually sensitive to pituitary gonadotropins (e.g., patients with polycystic ovary syndrome).

Because further enlargement of the ovary may occur, clomiphene citrate should not be given in the presence of an ovarian cyst. Patients should be carefully monitored for signs and symptoms of excessive ovarian stimulation (e.g., pelvic pain) during clomiphene therapy. If ovarian enlargement or cyst development occurs, therapy should be interrupted until the ovaries have returned to pretreatment size, and the dosage or duration of the next course of therapy should be decreased.

If any adverse visual symptoms occur during clomiphene treatment, the drug should be discontinued and a complete ophthalmologic evaluation performed.

Clomiphene citrate is contraindicated in patients with liver disease or in those with a history of liver dysfunction, and clinical evaluation of liver function should always precede therapy. Clomiphene citrate is contraindicated in patients with abnormal uterine bleeding of undetermined origin.

■ Pregnancy The incidence of multiple ovulations with resulting plural gestations (mostly twins) is increased when conception occurs during a cycle in which clomiphene citrate is administered. Prior to clomiphene citrate therapy, the patient and her male sexual partner should be informed of the possibility and potential risks associated with plural gestation. Simultaneous bilateral tubal pregnancy, an extremely rare form of twin pregnancy, has been reported following combined therapy with clomiphene citrate and chorionic gonadotropin.

Clomiphene citrate is contraindicated during pregnancy. The drug has been shown to be teratogenic in rats and rabbits. Congenital abnormalities (e.g., Down's syndrome, exstrophy, club foot, tibial torsion, blocked tear duct, hemangioma, neural tube defects) have been reported in infants conceived following clomiphene citrate therapy. These effects have not been directly attributed to the drug and the manufacturers state that the cumulative rate of congenital abnormalities does not exceed that reported in the general population. To avoid inadvertent clomiphene citrate administration during early pregnancy, the patient should be carefully observed to determine if ovulation occurs. The basal body temperature should be recorded throughout all treatment cycles, and clomiphene therapy should be discontinued if pregnancy is suspected. If the basal body temperature is biphasic and not followed by menses, the possibility of an ovarian cyst and/or pregnancy should be excluded and subsequent clomiphene therapy should be delayed until a correct diagnosis has been made.

Pharmacology

Clomiphene citrate has both estrogenic and anti-estrogenic properties, but its precise mechanism of action in inducing ovulation in anovulatory females has not been determined. The drug appears to stimulate the release of the pituitary gonadotropins, follicle-stimulating hormone (FSH), and luteinizing hormone (LH), which results in development and maturation of the ovarian follicle, ovulation, and subsequent development and function of the corpus luteum. Gonadotropin release may result from direct stimulation of the hypothalamic-pituitary axis or from a decreased inhibitory influence of estrogens on the hypothalamic-pituitary axis by competing with the endogenous estrogens of the uterus, pituitary, or hypothalamus. Clomiphene citrate may also directly affect the biosynthesis of ovarian hormones.

Clomiphene citrate has no progestational, androgenic, or anti-androgenic effects and does not appear to interfere with pituitary-adrenal or pituitary-thyroid functions.

Pharmacokinetics

Clomiphene citrate is readily absorbed from the GI tract following oral administration. In studies using radiolabeled clomiphene citrate, blood concentrations of the drug were low and exhibited interpatient variation.

Clomiphene citrate appears to have a half-life of about 5 days; however, following oral administration of radiolabeled drug, radioactivity was present in feces for up to 6 weeks. Although the exact metabolic fate of clomiphene citrate is not clearly established, the drug appears to be metabolized in the liver. The drug and/or its metabolites are excreted principally in feces via biliary elimination. Limited studies suggest that the drug is excreted slowly from a sequestered enterohepatic recirculation pool or may be stored in body fat and subsequently released slowly.

Chemistry and Stability

■ Chemistry Clomiphene citrate is a nonsteroidal triarylethylene compound that is used to induce ovulation in anovulatory women. Clomiphene citrate is structurally related to chlorotrianisene (no longer commercially available in the US). Clomiphene citrate occurs as a white to pale yellow, crystalline powder and is sparingly soluble in water and in alcohol.

■ Stability Clomiphene citrate tablets should be protected from light and stored in well-closed containers at a temperature less than 40°C, preferably between 15–30°C.

Preparations

Excipients in commercially available drug preparations may have clinically important effects in some individuals; consult specific product labeling for details.

clomiPHENE Citrate

Oral

Tablets	50 mg*	**Clomid®** (scored), Sanofi-Aventis
		Serophene® (scored), Serono

*available from one or more manufacturer, distributor, and/or repackager by generic (nonproprietary) name

†Use is not currently included in the labeling approved by the US Food and Drug Administration

Ospemifene

■ Ospemifene, a triphenylethylene derivative, is a tissue-selective, estrogen agonist-antagonist.

Uses

■ **Dyspareunia** Ospemifene is used for the treatment of moderate to severe dyspareunia, a symptom of vulvar and vaginal atrophy, associated with menopause.

The safety and efficacy of ospemifene were evaluated in 3 randomized, double-blind, placebo-controlled trials of 12 or 52 weeks' duration in healthy postmenopausal women with signs and symptoms of vulvar and vaginal atrophy (defined as having 5% or fewer superficial cells on a vaginal smear, a vaginal pH of greater than 5, and the presence of at least one moderate to severe vaginal symptom). An additional long-term extension study of 1 year's duration evaluated the safety of ospemifene.

The primary efficacy outcomes in the first 2 studies were improvement in the maturation index (i.e., decreased percentage of parabasal cells and increased percentage of superficial cells in the vaginal epithelium), change in vaginal pH, and the mean change from baseline in severity of the most bothersome moderate to severe symptom reported (e.g., dyspareunia, vaginal dryness); vaginal symptoms were rated by the patients using a 4-point scale (0, none; 1, mild; 2, moderate; 3, severe). The first study evaluated 826 postmenopausal women with vulvar and vaginal atrophy who reported at least one moderate to severe vaginal symptom considered most bothersome (e.g., vaginal dryness, dyspareunia, or vaginal irritation/itching). Patients were randomized to receive ospemifene 30 or 60 mg or placebo once daily for 12 weeks. Baseline characteristics were similar among groups (mean age 58–59 years, mean time from last menstrual period 14–15 years, 90% white). For patients who reported the most bothersome symptom of dyspareunia, reduction of the mean severity score from baseline to 12 weeks was substantially greater in patients receiving ospemifene 60 mg daily compared with those receiving placebo (−1.39 versus −0.89, respectively). The percentage of parabasal cells on vaginal smear between baseline and 12 weeks decreased by 21.9 or 30.1% in patients receiving ospemifene 30 or 60 mg daily, respectively, compared with an increase of approximately 4% in those receiving placebo. Patients receiving ospemifene 30 or 60 mg daily showed an increased percentage of superficial cells on the vaginal smear (increase of 7.8 or 10.8%, respectively) compared with those receiving placebo (increase of 2.2%). Over the same time period, vaginal pH decreased by 0.67 or 1.01 in patients receiving ospemifene 30 or 60 mg daily, respectively, compared with a decrease of 0.1 in those receiving placebo.

The second study evaluated 605 postmenopausal women with vulvar and vaginal atrophy who reported the most bothersome symptom of dyspareunia as moderate to severe at baseline. Patients were randomized to receive ospemifene 60 mg or placebo once daily for 12 weeks. Baseline characteristics were similar between groups (mean age 58 years, 91% white, mean body mass index 26 kg/m²). At 12 weeks, reduction of the mean severity score for dyspareunia (compared with baseline values) was substantially greater in patients receiving ospemifene 60 mg daily compared with those receiving placebo (−1.55 versus −1.29, respectively). The mean decrease from baseline to 12 weeks in parabasal cells on the vaginal smear was 40.2% in patients receiving ospemifene compared with no reduction in those receiving placebo; the mean percentage of superficial cells on the vaginal smear increased by 12.3 or 1.7% in patients receiving ospemifene or placebo, respectively. During the same time period, the mean decrease in vaginal pH was 0.94 in patients receiving ospemifene and 0.07 in those receiving placebo.

A 52-week safety and efficacy study evaluated 426 postmenopausal women with an intact uterus who met criteria for diagnosis of vulvar and vaginal atrophy. Patients were randomized in a 6:1 ratio to receive ospemifene 60 mg or placebo once daily (mean age 62 years, 99.5% white, mean body mass index 24 kg/m²). Efficacy was evaluated after 12 weeks of treatment; all end points were compared with baseline values. Patients receiving ospemifene had a median decrease in parabasal cells of 40%, median increase in superficial cells of 5%, and mean decrease in vaginal pH of 1.21; symptoms of vulvar and vaginal atrophy were not evaluated in this study.

Dosage and Administration

■ **General** When a drug like ospemifene with estrogen agonistic effects on the endometrium is prescribed, concomitant use of progestin therapy should be considered in postmenopausal women with an intact uterus to reduce the risk of endometrial cancer. Progestin therapy is not necessary in postmenopausal women without an intact uterus. (See Genitourinary Effects under Warnings/Precautions: Warnings, in Cautions.)

Ospemifene therapy should be used for the shortest duration consistent with treatment goals and risks for the individual woman. Postmenopausal women receiving ospemifene should be reevaluated periodically as clinically appropriate to determine if continued treatment is necessary.

■ **Administration** Ospemifene is administered orally with food.

■ **Dosage** ***Dyspareunia*** For the treatment of moderate to severe dyspareunia associated with menopause, the recommended dosage of ospemifene is 60 mg once daily.

■ **Special Populations** ***Hepatic Impairment*** No dosage adjustments are needed in patients with mild or moderate hepatic impairment (Child-Pugh class A or B). The drug has not been studied and should not be used in patients with severe hepatic impairment (Child-Pugh class C). (See Hepatic Impairment under Warnings/Precautions: Specific Populations, in Cautions.)

Renal Impairment No dosage adjustments are needed in patients with renal impairment.

Cautions

■ **Contraindications** Ospemifene is contraindicated in women with undiagnosed abnormal genital bleeding and in women with known or suspected estrogen-dependent neoplasia. (See Genitourinary Effects under Warnings/Precautions: Warnings, in Cautions.)

The drug also is contraindicated in women with active deep-vein thrombosis (DVT), pulmonary embolism (PE), active arterial thromboembolic disease (e.g., stroke, myocardial infarction [MI]), or history of these conditions. (See Cardiovascular Effects under Warnings/Precautions: Warnings, in Cautions.)

Ospemifene is contraindicated in women who are or may become pregnant. (See Fetal/Neonatal Morbidity and Mortality under Warnings/Precautions: Other Warnings/Precautions, in Cautions and also see Pregnancy under Warnings/Precautions: Specific Populations, in Cautions.)

■ **Warnings/Precautions** ***Warnings*** **Cardiovascular Effects.** Risk factors for cardiovascular disorders, arterial vascular disease (e.g., hypertension, diabetes mellitus, tobacco use, hypercholesterolemia, obesity), and/or venous thromboembolism (VTE) including personal or family history of VTE, obesity, or systemic lupus erythematosus should be managed appropriately during ospemifene therapy.

In the Women's Health Initiative (WHI) estrogen-alone study, an increased risk of stroke and VTE (including DVT and PE) was reported in postmenopausal women (50–79 years of age) who received oral conjugated estrogen alone at a dosage of 0.625 mg daily over 7.1 years compared with women who received placebo. The increased risk of stroke was demonstrated during the first year of the study and persisted; for VTE, the increased risk was evident during the first 2 years of the study. In the WHI study, no overall effect on coronary heart disease (CHD) events (i.e., nonfatal or silent MI, CHD death) was reported in women receiving estrogen therapy alone versus placebo.

In studies with ospemifene, the incidence of DVT was 1.45 per 1000 women in patients receiving ospemifene 60 mg daily versus 1.04 per 1000 women in those receiving placebo. In studies with ospemifene (up to 15 months' duration), the incidence rates of thromboembolic and hemorrhagic stroke were 0.72 and 1.45 per 1000 women, respectively, in patients receiving ospemifene 60 mg daily versus 1.04 and 0 per 1000 women in those receiving placebo. In clinical studies, one MI was reported in a woman receiving ospemifene 60 mg daily.

Ospemifene should be discontinued immediately if VTE (including PE or DVT) or thromboembolic or hemorrhagic stroke occurs or is suspected. If possible, ospemifene should be discontinued at least 4–6 weeks prior to surgery associated with an increased risk of thromboembolism or during periods of prolonged immobilization.

Genitourinary Effects. Ospemifene is an estrogen agonist-antagonist with tissue-selective effects, including estrogen agonistic effects on the endometrium. Postmenopausal women with an intact uterus who use estrogen therapy alone are at increased risk of endometrial cancer. Such risk is dependent on duration of therapy and estrogen dosage and has been shown to persist for at least 8–15 years after estrogen therapy is discontinued. Adding a progestin to postmenopausal estrogen therapy reduces the risk of endometrial hyperplasia, which may be a precursor to endometrial cancer. There are possible risks that may be associated with the combined use of progestin and estrogen compared with estrogen therapy alone (e.g., increased risk of breast cancer). The concomitant use of progestin therapy with ospemifene was not evaluated in clinical trials.

In clinical trials, no cases of endometrial cancer were reported in patients receiving ospemifene 60 mg daily for periods of up to 52 weeks' duration; there was 1 report of simple hyperplasia without atypia. Endometrial thickening of 5 mm or greater was observed in patients receiving ospemifene at a rate of 60.1 per 1000 women versus 21.1 per 1000 women receiving placebo. Proliferative endometrium of any type occurred in 86.1 per 1000 women receiving ospemifene versus 13.3 per 1000 women receiving placebo. Uterine polyps occurred in 5.9 per 1000 women receiving ospemifene versus 1.8 per 1000 women receiving placebo.

Clinical surveillance is important for all women receiving ospemifene. Adequate diagnostic measures, including directed and random endometrial sampling when indicated, should be undertaken to rule out malignancy in postmenopausal women with undiagnosed persistent or recurrent abnormal genital bleeding.

Other Warnings/Precautions **Breast Cancer.** Ospemifene has not been adequately studied in women with breast cancer. Therefore, it should not be used in women with known or suspected breast cancer or with a history of breast cancer.

Fetal/Neonatal Morbidity and Mortality. Ospemifene may cause fetal harm. Embryofetal deaths and an increased rate of pup deaths at birth have been demonstrated in rats at dosages below human clinical exposures; embryofetal deaths also occurred in rabbits at 10 times the human clinical exposure based on mg/m^2 dosing. These reproductive effects are consistent with and considered to be related to the estrogen-receptor activity of ospemifene.

If ospemifene is used during pregnancy or if a woman becomes pregnant while receiving the drug, the patient should be informed of the potential hazard to the fetus.

Specific Populations **Pregnancy.** Category X. (See Users Guide.) (See Cautions: Contraindications and also see Fetal/Neonatal Morbidity and Mortality under Warnings/Precautions: Other Warnings/Precautions, in Cautions.)

Lactation. It is not known whether ospemifene is distributed into human milk. Ospemifene is distributed into milk in rats and detected at higher concentrations than in maternal plasma.

Pediatric Use. Ospemifene is not indicated in pediatric patients and has not been studied in this age group.

Geriatric Use. No substantial differences in safety and efficacy have been observed in women 65 years of age or older compared with younger women.

Hepatic Impairment. Ospemifene has not been studied in patients with severe hepatic impairment. Therefore, the manufacturer states that the drug should not be used in such patients. No dosage adjustments are needed in women with mild or moderate hepatic impairment.

Renal Impairment. Dosage adjustment is not required in patients with renal impairment.

■ **Common Adverse Effects** Adverse effects occurring in at least 1% of patients receiving ospemifene and more frequently with the drug than with placebo include hot flush, vaginal discharge, genital discharge, muscle spasms, and hyperhidrosis.

Drug Interactions

In vitro studies indicate that ospemifene is principally metabolized by cytochrome P-450 (CYP) isoenzymes 3A4 and 2C9; other isoenzymes (specifically CYP2C19 and 2B6) also are involved in the drug's metabolism. Ospemifene is a weak inhibitor of CYP2B6, 2C9, 2C19, 2C8, 2D6, and 3A4 in vitro. Ospemifene is not a clinically important substrate of the P-glycoprotein (P-gp) transport system in vitro.

■ **Drugs Affecting or Metabolized by Hepatic Microsomal Enzymes** Because ospemifene is principally metabolized by CYP isoenzymes 3A4 and 2C9, potent inhibitors or inducers of these isoenzymes are expected to alter the drug's pharmacokinetics. Concomitant use of ospemifene with a drug known to inhibit both CYP3A4 and 2C9 may increase the risk of ospemifene-related adverse reactions. Clinically important pharmacokinetic interactions between ospemifene and substrates of CYP2B6, 2C9, 2C19, 2C8, 2D6, and 3A4 are unlikely.

Concomitant administration of a single 60-mg dose of ospemifene with 400 mg on day 1 followed by 200 mg daily of fluconazole (a potent inhibitor of CYP2C9 and a moderate inhibitor of CYP3A4 and 2C19) resulted in increased ospemifene systemic exposure; peak concentrations and area under the concentration-time curve [AUC] of ospemifene increased by 1.7- and 2.7-fold, respectively. This pharmacokinetic interaction may increase the risk of ospemifene-related adverse effects. Fluconazole should not be used concomitantly with ospemifene.

Concomitant administration of a single 60-mg dose of ospemifene with 400 mg daily of ketoconazole (a potent CYP3A4 inhibitor) resulted in increased ospemifene systemic exposure; peak concentrations and AUC of ospemifene increased by 1.5- and 1.4-fold, respectively. This pharmacokinetic interaction may increase the risk of ospemifene-related adverse effects. Ospemifene and ketoconazole should be used concomitantly with caution.

Concomitant administration of a single 60-mg dose of ospemifene with 40 mg daily of omeprazole (a moderate CYP2C19 inhibitor) resulted in increased ospemifene systemic exposure; peak concentrations and AUC of ospemifene both increased by approximately 1.2-fold. Concomitant administration of a single 20-mg dose of omeprazole with 60 mg daily of ospemifene did not affect omeprazole pharmacokinetics. Clinically important pharmacokinetic interactions with concomitant administration of ospemifene and omeprazole are unlikely.

Concomitant administration of a single 60-mg dose of ospemifene with 600 mg daily of rifampin (a potent CYP3A4 inducer and a moderate CYP2C9 and 2C19 inducer) resulted in decreased ospemifene systemic exposure; peak concentrations and AUC of ospemifene decreased by 51 and 58%, respectively. Concomitant use of ospemifene with drugs that induce CYP3A4, 2C9, and/or 2C19 (e.g., rifampin) would be expected to decrease ospemifene systemic exposure and may decrease the drug's efficacy.

Concomitant administration of a single 10-mg dose of warfarin (a CYP2C9 substrate) with 60 mg daily of ospemifene had no effect on warfarin pharmacokinetics; studies were not conducted with multiple daily doses of warfarin. The effects of ospemifene on international normalized ratio (INR) or prothrombin time (PT) were not studied in patients receiving concomitant ospemifene and warfarin.

■ **Protein-bound Drugs** Ospemifene is more than 99% bound to serum proteins. The concomitant use of ospemifene with other highly protein-bound drugs may result in clinically important interactions through competition for protein-binding sites and may lead to increased exposure of either ospemifene or the other drug.

■ **Antiarrhythmic Agents** ***Quinidine*** Quinidine did not inhibit ospemifene metabolism in vitro.

■ **Bupropion** Concomitant administration of a single 150-mg dose of extended-release bupropion with 60 mg of ospemifene daily did not affect bupropion pharmacokinetics.

■ **Estrogen and Estrogen Agonists-Antagonists** The safety of ospemifene when used with estrogen or estrogen agonists-antagonists has not been studied. Therefore, ospemifene should not be used concomitantly with estrogen or estrogen agonists-antagonists.

Description

Ospemifene is a tissue-selective, estrogen agonist-antagonist; the drug also is referred to as a selective estrogen receptor modulator (SERM). Ospemifene has mixed estrogen agonist and antagonist activities, which result in activation of estrogenic pathways in some tissues and blockade of estrogenic pathways in other tissues. The drug binds to estrogen receptor (ER)α and ERβ, with stronger binding occurring at the ERα receptor. In animal studies, the drug exhibited strong estrogenic effects on vaginal epithelium; these effects were also demonstrated in clinical trials (e.g., improvement in the maturation index, decreased vaginal pH, decreased symptoms such as dyspareunia and vaginal dryness).

Ospemifene has been shown to have estrogenic effects on bone in rats; in healthy postmenopausal women, ospemifene reduced biochemical markers of bone turnover. However, further studies assessing bone mineral density (BMD) and fracture risk are needed to evaluate ospemifene's clinical effects on bone.

In postmenopausal women, ospemifene at a dosage of 60 mg daily did not have a substantial effect on serum lipoprotein concentrations (i.e., total, low-density lipoprotein [LDL]-, or high-density lipoprotein [HDL]-cholesterol, or triglyceride concentrations).

In clinical trials, ospemifene had weak estrogenic effects on the endometrium. Postmenopausal women receiving ospemifene for up to 1 year demonstrated slight dose-related mean increases in endometrial thickness compared with patients receiving placebo, but no cases of endometrial cancer were observed. (See Genitourinary Effects under Warnings/Precautions: Warnings, in Cautions.)

Preclinical in vitro and in vivo data suggest ospemifene may have breast antiestrogenic activity in several breast cancer models, but these effects have not been assessed in clinical trials. (See Breast Cancer under Other Warnings/Precautions: Warnings/Precautions, in Cautions.)

Following oral administration of a single 60-mg dose of ospemifene with a high-fat, high-calorie meal, the drug is rapidly absorbed with peak serum concentrations attained at approximately 2.5 hours after the dose. Peak serum concentration and area under the serum concentration-time curve (AUC) of ospemifene are increased when the drug is taken with food. Ospemifene is highly bound to serum proteins and has a half-life of approximately 26 hours. The drug undergoes metabolism mainly via cytochrome P-450 (CYP) isoenzymes 3A4 and 2C9; other isoenzymes (CYP2C19 and 2B6) also play a role in the metabolism of the drug. The major metabolite is 4-hydroxyospemifene. After oral administration of ospemifene, 75% of the dose is excreted in feces and 7% is excreted in urine.

Advice to Patients

Importance of instructing patients to read the manufacturer's patient information prior to initiation of therapy and each time the prescription is refilled.

Importance of advising patients that ospemifene may initiate or increase the occurrence of hot flushes in some women.

Importance of postmenopausal women reporting any unusual vaginal bleeding to a clinician as soon as possible.

Importance of informing clinicians of any current or previous occurrence of cancer, venous thromboembolism (VTE), stroke, or myocardial infarction (MI).

Importance of informing a clinician of any impending surgery or prolonged bed rest.

Importance of informing clinicians of existing or contemplated concomitant therapy, including prescription and OTC drugs, as well as any concomitant illnesses.

Importance of women informing clinicians if they are or plan to become pregnant or plan to breast-feed. Advise pregnant women of risk to the fetus.

Importance of informing patients of other important precautionary information. (See Cautions.)

Overview® (see Users Guide). For additional information on this drug until a more detailed monograph is developed and published, the manufacturer's labeling should be consulted. It is *essential* that the manufacturer's labeling be consulted for more detailed information on usual cautions, precautions, contraindications, potential drug interactions, laboratory test interferences, and acute toxicity.

Preparations

Excipients in commercially available drug preparations may have clinically important effects in some individuals; consult specific product labeling for details.

Ospemifene

Oral

Tablets, film-coated	60 mg	**Osphena®**, Shionogi

Raloxifene Hydrochloride

Keoxifene Hydrochloride

■ Raloxifene hydrochloride, a nonsteroidal benzothiophene derivative, is an estrogen agonist-antagonist.

Uses

■ **Osteoporosis** Raloxifene is used for the prevention and treatment of osteoporosis in postmenopausal women.

Osteoporosis, a systemic skeletal disease characterized by low bone mass and microarchitectural deterioration of bone tissue with consequent increased bone fragility and susceptibility to fracture, is observed in a large proportion of postmenopausal women. Adult women have less bone mass than men at all ages, and decreased production of estrogen at menopause is associated with accelerated bone loss, particularly from the lumbar spine, for about 5 years, during which time skeletal mass loss averages 3% per year. While the risk of postmenopausal osteoporosis cannot be quantified by a single clinical finding or test result, many risk factors have been identified, with the probability of developing osteoporosis increasing with multiple risk factors. Risk factors for postmenopausal osteoporosis and related fractures include early menopause, decreased bone mineral density (BMD), low body mass index (BMI), previous fracture or family history of fracture/osteoporosis, excessive alcohol intake, smoking, inadequate physical activity, low calcium and vitamin D intake, certain drugs (e.g., glucocorticoids), and medical conditions or diseases (e.g., rheumatoid arthritis, diabetes mellitus, Cushing syndrome, hyperparathyroidism).

In addition to adequate intake of calcium/vitamin D and other lifestyle modifications (e.g., exercise, avoidance of excessive alcohol and tobacco use), experts recommend that pharmacologic therapy for osteoporosis be considered in postmenopausal women who are at high risk of fractures (generally those who have experienced a previous hip or vertebral fracture or who have low BMD); pharmacologic therapy also may be considered in postmenopausal women who have low bone mass, although there is less evidence supporting overall fracture risk reduction in such patients. When selecting an appropriate pharmacologic agent, use of a drug with proven antifracture efficacy is recommended. Experts generally recommend raloxifene as a second- or third-line agent after other therapies (e.g., bisphosphonates) have been attempted. Choice of therapy should be individualized based on the potential benefits (with respect to fracture risk reduction) and adverse effects of therapy as well as patient preferences, comorbidities, and risk factors. For additional information on the prevention and treatment of osteoporosis, see Uses: Osteoporosis, in Alendronate 92:24.

Prevention in Postmenopausal Women Raloxifene is used for the *prevention* of osteoporosis in postmenopausal women; supplemental calcium and/or vitamin D should be used concomitantly if daily dietary intake is considered inadequate. The goal of preventive therapy is preservation of bone mass and a resultant decrease in fracture risk. Unlike estrogens, raloxifene is *not* effective in relieving vasomotor symptoms (hot flushes [flashes]) associated with estrogen deficiency. (See Cautions: Cardiovascular Effects.) The efficacy of raloxifene in preventing other forms of osteoporosis (e.g., drug [such as corticosteroid]-induced) remains to be established.

Raloxifene has been evaluated for the prevention of osteoporosis in postmenopausal women in 3 multinational (North American trial, European trial, International trial), randomized, placebo-controlled, double-blind studies that included 1764 women (median age: 54 years; median time since menopause: 5 years; 93.5% white; all women in the International trial had undergone hysterectomy; 12 or 19% of women in the European or North American trials, respectively, had undergone hysterectomy) with normal or low (osteopenia) BMD values (mean lumbar spine BMD value 0.74–1 standard deviations below the premenopausal mean). All women received 400–600 mg of elemental calcium daily in addition to their usual dietary calcium intake. In these studies, therapy with raloxifene hydrochloride 60 mg daily increased BMD, as determined by dual-energy radiographic absorption (DXA) measurements, in the lumbar spine, hip, and total body. While women receiving placebo (i.e., calcium) lost approximately 1% of BMD at 24 months, substantial increases in BMD were apparent at 12 months following initiation of raloxifene therapy and were maintained at 24 months. Increases in total body BMD of 1.3–2% compared with placebo (i.e., calcium) have been reported in raloxifene-treated women. In North American or European postmenopausal women receiving raloxifene hydrochloride 60 mg daily for 24 months, the increase in BMD (expressed as mean % increase versus placebo) was 2–2.4% for total hip, 2.1–2.5% for femoral neck, 2.2–2.7% for trochanter, 2.3–2.4% for intertrochanter, and 2–2.4% for lumbar spine. In women receiving raloxifene hydrochloride 60 mg daily who had undergone hysterectomy (the International trial), the increase in BMD (expressed as mean % increase versus placebo) was 1.3% for total hip, trochanter, and intertrochanter; 1.6% for femoral neck; and 1.8% for lumbar spine. The effect of raloxifene therapy for longer than 2 years is being investigated in ongoing studies. Whether increases in BMD are maintained following withdrawal of raloxifene has not been established. The effect of raloxifene therapy on forearm BMD remains to be determined. While raloxifene prevented bone loss at the ultradistal radius in one study (European trial), a protective effect at this site was not documented in another study (North American trial).

The effect of raloxifene on BMD versus estrogens or alendronate has been evaluated in several clinical studies. In one comparative study, therapy with conjugated estrogens 0.625 mg daily for 6 months was associated with substantially greater increases in BMD than therapy with raloxifene. Based on historical comparisons, the effect of raloxifene on hip BMD appears to be slightly less than that of estrogen/progestin or alendronate, and the effect of raloxifene on lumbar spine BMD appears to be about half that of estrogen/progestin or alendronate. In osteoporosis prevention studies that evaluated raloxifene (European trial), various estrogen/progestin combinations (HRT) (Early Postmenopausal Intervention Cohort Study), or alendronate therapy (Early Postmenopausal Intervention Cohort Study) for 24 months, raloxifene hydrochloride therapy (60 mg daily) was associated with 1.6% increases in hip BMD compared with baseline, HRT was associated with 1.8–3.2% increases, and alendronate (5 mg daily) therapy was associated with 1.3–1.9% increases. In these studies, raloxifene, HRT, or alendronate was associated with increases in BMD of lumbar spine of 1.6%, 4–5.1%, or 2.9–3.5%, respectively, compared with baseline. In a limited number of healthy postmenopausal women, administration of tamoxifen 20 mg daily for 24 months was associated with an increase in lumbar spine BMD compared with baseline of 1.4%.

While the exact role of raloxifene in the prevention of osteoporosis relative to other available agents (e.g., estrogens, alendronate, risedronate) remains to be clearly determined, advantages of raloxifene include a better adverse effect profile than that of estrogens (with or without progestin). In addition, raloxifene may be especially useful in patients who are unable or unwilling to comply with the recommended regimen for oral administration of alendronate. While estrogen replacement therapy is effective for the prevention of osteoporosis in women, such therapy is associated with a number of adverse effects and the proportion of postmenopausal women who take estrogens for prolonged periods of time is low. Because raloxifene appears to have a more favorable adverse effect profile than estrogen or estrogen/progestin therapy, long-term compliance with raloxifene may be better than that with estrogens. However, clinical experience with raloxifene is limited compared with estrogen replacement therapy, and the effect of raloxifene on fracture rates has not been established. The role of raloxifene versus alendronate also has not been established. The choice of alendronate, estrogen, raloxifene, or risedronate for the prevention of postmenopausal osteoporosis should be individualized, taking into account differences in tolerability and safety, and individual preference.

The optimal timing for initiation of preventive therapy for osteoporosis, including that with raloxifene, and the optimal duration of such therapy remain to be established. Although raloxifene preventive therapy was initiated at a median of 5 years postmenopause in clinical trials, experience with estrogen replacement therapy suggests that the protective effect may be greatest if the drug is initiated soon after menopause and continued into late life or indefinitely. If preventive therapy is not initiated soon after menopause, some benefit also may be likely with delayed initiation. In general, exercise and adequate calcium and vitamin D intake should be encouraged for all women. Whether additional preventive therapy generally should be offered to all women or just recommended for selected women at highest risk of developing osteoporosis remains to be established.

Treatment in Postmenopausal Women Raloxifene is used for the treatment of osteoporosis in postmenopausal women. While recent evidence indicates that raloxifene reduces the risk of vertebral fracture in women with osteoporosis, experience with the drug is limited and efficacy of raloxifene in the treatment of osteoporosis compared with that of estrogens or alendronate remains to be determined. The role of raloxifene in the treatment of osteoporosis may be determined by the effect of the drug on breast cancer. (See Breast Cancer: Reduction in the Incidence of Breast Cancer in Women with Osteoporosis, in Uses.)

The effects of raloxifene on BMD and fracture incidence have been evaluated in a 3-year, multinational, randomized, double-blind study that included 7705 postmenopausal women (median age: 67 years; median time since menopause: 19 years) with osteoporosis (vertebral or hip BMD values at least 2.5 standard deviations below premenopausal mean values without baseline vertebral fractures or one or more vertebral fractures). All women received 500 mg of elemental calcium daily and 10–15 mcg (400–600 units) of cholecalciferol daily in addition to their usual calcium and vitamin D intake. In this study, therapy with raloxifene increased BMD (as determined by dual-energy radiographic absorption [DXA] measurements) of the spine, hip, and total body, and reduced the risk of vertebral fracture (as determined radiographically).

In women receiving raloxifene 60 mg daily for 24 months, the increase in BMD (expressed as a mean percent increase versus placebo) was 2.2% for ultradistal radius, 0.9% for distal radius, and 1.1% for total body. In women receiving raloxifene 60 mg daily for 36 months, the increase in BMD was 2.6% for lumbar spine and 2.1% for femoral neck. In this study, women receiving raloxifene had fewer new vertebral fractures regardless of vertebral fracture status at the beginning of the study. In women without baseline vertebral fractures, radiographic evaluation at study completion revealed one or more new vertebral fractures in 4.3% of placebo-treated women and in 1.9% of raloxifene-treated women (relative risk reduction 55%). In women with one or more baseline fractures, radiographic evaluation at study completion revealed one or more new fractures in 20.2% of placebo-treated women and in 14.1% of women receiving raloxifene hydrochloride 60 mg daily (relative risk reduction 30%). In women with one or more baseline fractures, the incidence of new fractures was 10.7% in women receiving raloxifene hydrochloride 120 mg daily. Fewer raloxifene-treated women (1.8%) experienced one or more new symptomatic vertebral fractures than placebo-treated women (3.1%). Differences in the reduction in vertebral fracture risk associated with raloxifene therapy based on age, baseline femoral neck or lumbar spine BMD, prior hormone replacement therapy, or prior hysterectomy have not been observed in this study. A reduction in nonspinal fractures was not observed in raloxifene-treated women at month 36.

Use in Premenopausal Women Safety and efficacy of raloxifene in premenopausal women have not been established, and the role, if any, of the drug in the prevention or treatment of osteoporosis in such women remains to be determined.

■ **Glucocorticoid-induced Osteoporosis** Raloxifene has been used for the treatment and prevention of glucocorticoid-induced osteoporosis†.

The American College of Rheumatology (ACR) recommends optimizing calcium and vitamin D intake and lifestyle modifications (e.g., diet, smoking cessation, weight-bearing or resistance-training exercise) in all patients receiving long-term glucocorticoid therapy; in addition, pharmacologic therapy with an oral bisphosphonate is recommended in patients who are considered to be at moderate-to-high risk of fracture. Oral bisphosphonates generally are preferred because of their demonstrated antifracture benefits, safety, and cost; experts state that raloxifene may be used in postmenopausal women if no other therapy is available. For additional information on the management of glucocorticoid-induced osteoporosis, see Cautions: Musculoskeletal Effects in the Corticosteroids General Statement 68:04.

■ **Breast Cancer** Raloxifene is used to reduce the incidence of invasive breast cancer in postmenopausal women with osteoporosis and in postmenopausal women at high risk for developing invasive breast cancer. Raloxifene should *not* be used to reduce the risk of breast cancer in *premenopausal women*†.

Raloxifene is not indicated for the treatment of breast cancer or to reduce the risk of recurrence of breast cancer. Raloxifene is not indicated for reduction in the risk of noninvasive breast cancer.

Reduction in the Incidence of Breast Cancer in Women with Osteoporosis Raloxifene is used to reduce the incidence of invasive breast cancer in postmenopausal women with osteoporosis. Findings from the Multiple Outcomes of Raloxifene Evaluation (MORE) study, a double-blind study that evaluated effects of raloxifene on fracture incidence (primary end point) and incidence of breast cancer (secondary end point) in postmenopausal women with osteoporosis, provided the first evidence of possible breast cancer risk reduction effects of raloxifene. Results from the 4-year MORE study showed a 72 and 84% reduction in the incidence of newly diagnosed invasive breast cancer and estrogen receptor (ER)-positive breast cancer, respectively, in women receiving raloxifene compared with those receiving placebo. The Continuing Outcomes Relevant to Evista (CORE) study investigated the effect of 4 additional years of raloxifene therapy on the incidence of invasive breast cancer in a subset of the MORE cohort who agreed to continue therapy. During the 8 years of the MORE and CORE study, the incidence of invasive breast cancer and ER-positive breast cancer was reduced by 66 and 76%, respectively, in those receiving raloxifene compared with those receiving placebo. The incidence of noninvasive breast cancer in women receiving raloxifene was similar to that in women receiving placebo.

Reduction in the Incidence of Breast Cancer in Women at High Risk Raloxifene is used to reduce the incidence of invasive breast cancer in postmenopausal women at high risk for developing the disease.

Experts consider use of raloxifene an option in postmenopausal women 35 years of age or older who are considered at high risk for developing breast cancer (i.e., a 5-year projected risk of 1.67% or greater based on the calculated score derived from the Gail risk model) to reduce the risk of invasive breast cancer. Additionally, experts consider use of raloxifene an option to reduce the risk of invasive breast cancer in postmenopausal women 35 years of age or older with a history of lobular carcinoma in situ (LCIS), since these women are at increased risk for developing invasive breast cancer in both the affected and contralateral breast.

The effects of raloxifene versus tamoxifen on reducing the incidence of breast cancer were evaluated in a double-blind, randomized, phase 3 study (Study of Tamoxifen and Raloxifene [STAR]; also known as the National Surgical Adjuvant Breast and Bowel Project [NSABP] P-2 study). This study enrolled postmenopausal women at least 35 years of age who were at high risk for developing breast cancer. Breast cancer risk was determined using the National Cancer Institute (NCI) Breast Cancer Risk Assessment Tool based on a statistical model (the Gail model). High risk was defined as a 5-year projected breast cancer risk score of 1.67% or greater, calculated using the NCI (or Gail) assessment tool. Additionally, postmenopausal women 35 years of age or older with a history of LCIS, whose only prior treatment included local excision, were eligible to participate in the study. Patients enrolled in the STAR study were randomized to receive either tamoxifen (20 mg daily) or raloxifene (60 mg daily) for a maximum of 5 years.

Analysis of data from the STAR study at an average follow-up of approximately 4 years (47 months) showed that raloxifene and tamoxifen were equivalent in efficacy in lowering the risk of invasive breast cancer (4.3 cases per 1000 women in the tamoxifen group versus 4.41 cases per 1000 women in the raloxifene group; risk ratio of 1.02). Although the comparison did not reach statistical significance, there were fewer cases of noninvasive breast cancer in women receiving tamoxifen than in those receiving raloxifene (1.51 per 1000 in the tamoxifen group versus 2.11 per 1000 in the raloxifene group; risk ratio of 1.4). In contrast to these findings, longer-term follow-up (approximately 7 years) showed that tamoxifen had a greater effect than raloxifene in lowering the risk of invasive breast cancer, while the between-treatment difference in risk of noninvasive breast cancer was smaller than that observed at the time of the initial analysis. The updated analysis showed a 24% reduction in raloxifene efficacy in lowering the risk of invasive breast cancer compared with tamoxifen. Although raloxifene remained as effective as tamoxifen in lowering the risk of invasive breast cancer in women with LCIS (risk ratio of 1.13), the drug was less effective than tamoxifen in women with atypical hyperplasia (risk ratio of 1.48). Noninvasive breast cancer was reported slightly (risk ratio of 1.22), but not significantly, more frequently in those receiving raloxifene compared with those receiving tamoxifen at approximately 7 years' follow-up.

In the STAR study, use of raloxifene was associated with a lower risk of thromboembolic events than use of tamoxifen, but rates of myocardial infarction, severe angina, or acute ischemic syndrome did not differ between the raloxifene and tamoxifen groups. Rates of fracture were essentially identical in the raloxifene and tamoxifen groups. Fewer cataracts were reported in the raloxifene group than in the tamoxifen group. Between-treatment differences in adverse effects mostly remained similar over approximately 7 years' follow-up. Based on patient-reported symptoms and quality of life assessments performed during the STAR study, there were no differences in overall physical, mental health, or depressive symptoms among women receiving either raloxifene or tamoxifen. However, women receiving raloxifene reported more musculoskeletal problems, dyspareunia (painful intercourse), and weight gain; women receiving tamoxifen reported more bladder-control (e.g., urinary incontinence) problems, gynecologic problems, and leg cramps. At the time of the initial analysis, fewer cases of endometrial cancer were reported in women receiving raloxifene compared with tamoxifen, but the difference was not statistically significant; however, an increase in the risk of endometrial cancer and endometrial hyperplasia was reported in patients receiving tamoxifen compared with those receiving raloxifene at approximately 7 years. (See Cautions: Genitourinary Effects.)

The effect of raloxifene on the reduction in breast cancer incidence in women with BRCA1 or BRCA2 genetic mutations has not been established. Additionally, the effect of raloxifene (or tamoxifen) has not been studied in women with a history of exposure to thoracic radiation, which is considered a possible risk factor for breast cancer.

Reduction in the Incidence of Breast Cancer in Women at Increased Risk of Coronary Events The effect of raloxifene on the incidence of coronary events and invasive breast cancer was evaluated in postmenopausal women with coronary heart disease or increased risk for coronary heart disease (Raloxifene Use for the Heart; RUTH). Results from the 5-year RUTH study showed a 44 and 55% reduction in the incidence of newly diagnosed invasive breast cancer and estrogen receptor (ER)-positive breast cancer, respectively, in women receiving raloxifene compared with those receiving placebo. Treatment with raloxifene did not affect the risk of coronary events; an increased risk of venous thromboembolic events and fatal stroke was observed in women receiving raloxifene. (See Cautions: Cardiovascular Effects and Cautions: Precautions and Contraindications.)

Dosage and Administration

■ **Administration** Raloxifene is administered orally as a single daily dose. The manufacturer states that the drug may be taken without regard to meals or time of day. Raloxifene may be administered concomitantly with calcium carbonate or aluminum and magnesium hydroxide-containing antacids.

■ **Dosage** Dosage of raloxifene hydrochloride is expressed in terms of the hydrochloride. Raloxifene hydrochloride 60 mg contains 55.71 mg of raloxifene.

Patients receiving raloxifene for prevention or treatment of osteoporosis should receive supplemental calcium and/or vitamin D if their daily dietary intake is inadequate.

Osteoporosis **Prevention in Postmenopausal Women.** For the prevention of osteoporosis in postmenopausal women, the recommended dosage of raloxifene hydrochloride is 60 mg once daily.

Treatment in Postmenopausal Women. For the treatment of osteoporosis in postmenopausal women, the recommended dosage of raloxifene hydrochloride is 60 mg once daily.

Breast Cancer **Reduction in the Incidence of Breast Cancer.** To reduce the incidence of invasive breast cancer in postmenopausal women with osteoporosis and in postmenopausal women at high risk for developing invasive breast cancer, the recommended dosage of raloxifene hydrochloride is 60 mg once daily. The American Society of Clinical Oncology (ASCO) recommends a treatment duration of 5 years. If a patient is receiving raloxifene as treatment for osteoporosis, for which breast cancer reduction is a secondary goal, ASCO suggests that the treatment duration may be extended beyond 5 years.

■ **Dosage in Renal and Hepatic Impairment** Plasma concentrations are higher in individuals with moderate to severe renal impairment compared with individuals with normal renal function. The manufacturer makes no specific recommendations for raloxifene dosage adjustment in patients with renal impairment.

Limited evidence from patients with cirrhosis (Child-Pugh class A) and total serum bilirubin concentrations of 0.6–2 mg/dL indicate that plasma concentrations of raloxifene are 150% higher in such patients relative to plasma concentrations in patients with normal hepatic function. Raloxifene has not been evaluated in patients with hepatic impairment other than Child-Pugh class A. The manufacturer currently makes no specific recommendation for adjustment of raloxifene dosage in patients with hepatic impairment. However, the drug is extensively metabolized in the liver and excreted principally in feces.

Cautions

Information on the safety of raloxifene has been obtained from phase II and III clinical studies in postmenopausal women who received varying dosages of the drug for the prevention of osteoporosis for 2–30 months. Of the more than 2000 women who received raloxifene hydrochloride in these studies, about 40% received 60 mg daily, 40% received 120–600 mg daily, and 20% received 10–50 mg daily. Information has been obtained from clinical studies in women with osteoporosis who received raloxifene hydrochloride 60 or 120 mg daily for 36 months. Information on safety of raloxifene also has been obtained from the Multiple Outcomes of Raloxifene Evaluation (MORE) study, the Continuing Outcomes Relevant to Evista (CORE) study, the Raloxifene Use for the Heart (RUTH) trial, and the Study of Tamoxifen and Raloxifene (STAR) study. Safety of raloxifene in men or in premenopausal women has not been established.

Raloxifene generally is well tolerated. The incidence of reported adverse effects in clinical studies generally was similar in patients receiving raloxifene or placebo; however, the incidences of venous thromboembolic events, vasomotor symptoms (i.e., hot flushes [flashes]), and musculoskeletal pain (i.e., leg cramps) were higher in patients receiving raloxifene. In clinical studies that evaluated raloxifene for the prevention or treatment of osteoporosis, about 10.9–11.4% of patients receiving raloxifene hydrochloride discontinued therapy because of adverse effects; this was similar to the 8.8–12.2% discontinuance rate reported with placebo. The adverse effect profile suggests that long-term compliance with raloxifene therapy may be more likely than with estrogens.

■ **Cardiovascular Effects** Use of raloxifene did not affect the risk of coronary events in a study in postmenopausal women with coronary heart disease (CHD) or risk factors for CHD (RUTH study). In the STAR study, the incidence of ischemic heart disease (i.e., myocardial infarction, severe angina, acute ischemic syndrome) in those receiving raloxifene was similar to the incidence in those receiving tamoxifen.

Limited evidence suggests that women who experienced substantial hypertriglyceridemia (exceeding 5.6 mmol/L or 500 mg/dL) while receiving oral estrogen, alone or in combination with a progestin, may develop increased serum triglyceride concentrations during raloxifene therapy.

Thromboembolic Events Raloxifene therapy is associated with an increased risk of venous thromboembolic events such as deep-vein thrombosis and pulmonary embolism. The greatest risk for thromboembolic events occurs during the first 4 months of raloxifene therapy. In placebo-controlled osteoporosis prevention studies, the risk of deep-vein thrombosis or pulmonary embolism with raloxifene was about 3 times greater than that with placebo, a rate that appears similar to that reported in postmenopausal women receiving estrogen replacement therapy. Retinal vein occlusion and superficial thrombophlebitis have occurred in women receiving raloxifene. Such thromboembolic complications have been associated with raloxifene therapy despite favorable effects on certain clotting factors (e.g., fibrinogen) observed in women receiving the drug, and the relationship, if any, of raloxifene-induced clotting factor changes to thromboembolic phenomena is unclear.

In the CORE study and the MORE study, the incidence of thromboembolic events was higher in women receiving raloxifene than in those receiving placebo but the differences were not statistically significant. Use of raloxifene was associated with an increased risk of venous thromboembolic events in a study that evaluated safety of raloxifene in postmenopausal women with CHD or risk factors for CHD (RUTH study). The incidence of total stroke in those receiving raloxifene was similar to the incidence in those receiving placebo in this study; however, use of raloxifene was associated with an increased risk of fatal stroke. In the STAR study, the incidence of thromboembolic events (e.g., pulmonary embolism or deep vein thrombosis) was lower with raloxifene compared with tamoxifen. The incidence of stroke and transient ischemic attacks was similar for both the raloxifene and tamoxifen groups during the STAR study.

Vasomotor Symptoms In clinical studies in postmenopausal women receiving raloxifene for the prevention of osteoporosis, vasomotor symptoms (i.e., hot flushes [flashes]) occurred more frequently in women receiving raloxifene than in those receiving placebo or continuous combined or cyclic estrogen/progestin therapy. Vasomotor symptoms occurred in 24.6% of patients receiving raloxifene hydrochloride 60 mg daily and required discontinuance of therapy in 1.7% of patients receiving this dosage in clinical trials for the prevention of osteoporosis; the incidence of raloxifene-induced vasomotor symptoms appears to be dose related. The first episode of vasomotor symptoms generally occurs during the first 6 months of therapy. Whether clonidine ameliorates raloxifene-induced hot flushes has not been evaluated. In clinical studies in women with osteoporosis, vasomotor symptoms occurred in about 9.7% of women receiving raloxifene hydrochloride 60 mg daily. In the STAR study, women receiving tamoxifen reported more vasomotor symptoms than those receiving raloxifene.

Other Cardiovascular Effects Syncope or development of a varicose vein condition has occurred in up to 2.3% of patients receiving raloxifene in clinical studies. In clinical trials, peripheral edema occurred in up to 14.1% of raloxifene-treated women.

■ **Genitourinary Effects** Breast tenderness/pain or vaginal bleeding has been reported in 4.4 or 6.2%, respectively, of postmenopausal women receiving raloxifene in clinical trials for the prevention of osteoporosis. Breast pain and vaginal bleeding occur substantially (e.g., 10 times) less frequently in postmenopausal women receiving raloxifene compared with those receiving continuous combined or cyclic estrogen/progestin therapy. In addition, the incidence of these effects actually appeared to decrease with increasing raloxifene dosage in one study. Vaginitis, urinary tract infection, cystitis, leukorrhea, uterine disorder, urinary tract disorder, or endometrial disorder occurred in up to 4.3, 4, 4.6, 3.3, 3.3, 2.5, or 3.1%, respectively, of postmenopausal women receiving raloxifene in clinical trials. In the STAR study, bladder and gynecologic problems, endometrial cancer, and endometrial hyperplasia were reported more frequently in those receiving tamoxifen than in those receiving raloxifene; however, dyspareunia (painful intercourse) was reported more frequently in women receiving raloxifene.

The percentage of sexually active women was lower with raloxifene compared with tamoxifen at nearly every assessment point over the 5-year study duration; among sexually active women, there were increased reports of difficulty with sexual arousal, interest and enjoyment in women receiving raloxifene.

Clinically and histologically benign endometrial polyps have occurred in women receiving raloxifene. In osteoporosis studies in postmenopausal women, there was no evidence of endometrial changes (e.g., hyperplasia) associated with raloxifene therapy. (See Cautions: Mutagenicity and Carcinogenicity.)

■ **GI Effects** In clinical trials in postmenopausal women receiving raloxifene hydrochloride 60 mg daily, nausea, diarrhea, dyspepsia, or vomiting occurred in up to 8.8, 7.2, 5.9, or 4.8% of women, respectively. Adverse GI effects reported in 2.6–3.3% of patients include flatulence, GI disorder, and gastroenteritis.

■ **Musculoskeletal Effects** Musculoskeletal pain (i.e., leg cramps) has occurred more frequently in postmenopausal women receiving raloxifene compared with placebo. In controlled clinical trials, leg cramps/muscle spasms were reported in 7-12% of women receiving raloxifene. Arthralgia, myalgia, arthritis, or tendon disorder has been reported in up to 15.5, 7.7, 4, or 3.6% of patients receiving raloxifene.

■ **Sensitivity and Dermatologic Effects** In clinical trials in women receiving raloxifene hydrochloride 60 mg daily, rash occurred in 5.5% and sweating occurred in 3.1% of patients.

■ **Nervous System Effects** Depression or insomnia occurred in up to 6.4 or 5.5% of women receiving raloxifene in clinical trials. Vertigo, neuralgia, or hypoesthesia have been reported in up to 4.1, 2.4, or 2.1% of women receiving raloxifene.

Headache or migraine has been reported in 9.2 or 2.4% of women receiving raloxifene hydrochloride 60 mg daily in controlled studies.

■ **Respiratory Effects** Adverse respiratory effects such as sinusitis, rhinitis, bronchitis, pharyngitis, cough, pneumonia, or laryngitis occurred in up to 10.3, 10.2, 9.5, 7.6, 9.3, 2.6, or 2.2%, respectively, of women receiving raloxifene in clinical trials.

■ **Other Adverse Effects** Infection, flu-like syndrome, chest pain, or fever has been reported in up to 15.1, 14.6, 4, or 3.9%, respectively, of women receiving raloxifene in clinical trials. Weight gain occurred in 8.8% of raloxifene-treated women. Hepatitis has been reported rarely in women receiving raloxifene.Platelet counts have been decreased minimally in women receiving raloxifene.

Use of tamoxifen has been associated with increased rates of cataracts and cataract surgery. In the STAR study, fewer cataracts (RR 0.79; 95% confidence interval: 0.68–0.92) and cataract surgeries (RR 0.82; 95% confidence interval: 0.68–0.99) occurred in those receiving raloxifene than in those receiving tamoxifen.

■ **Precautions and Contraindications** Raloxifene is contraindicated in women with active or past episodes of venous thrombosis, including deep-vein thrombosis, pulmonary embolism, or retinal vein thrombosis. Potential therapeutic benefit versus risk should be assessed in women at risk of thromboembolic disease secondary to congestive heart failure, superficial thrombophlebitis, or active malignancy.

Patients receiving raloxifene should be informed to notify their clinician if signs or symptoms of a thromboembolic disorder (i.e., thrombophlebitis, pulmonary embolism, retinal thrombosis) occur. Because an increased risk of thromboembolic complications associated with prolonged immobilization may occur during raloxifene therapy, the drug should be discontinued at least 72 hours before and withheld during prolonged immobilization (e.g., postsurgery recovery, prolonged bed rest). Raloxifene therapy may be resumed once the patient is fully ambulatory. Patients receiving raloxifene should be advised to avoid prolonged restrictions in movement while traveling because of the increased risk of venous thromboembolic events.

Use of raloxifene has been associated with an increased risk of fatal stroke in women with coronary heart disease (CHD) or increased risk for CHD (in the RUTH study). Therefore, potential therapeutic benefit versus risk should be assessed in women at risk for stroke secondary to a history of stroke or transient ischemic attack [TIA], atrial fibrillation, hypertension, or smoking cigarettes.

Raloxifene should not be used for the primary or secondary prevention of cardiovascular disease. Therapy with raloxifene for 5 years was not associated with cardiovascular benefit in women with CHD or increased risk for CHD (in the RUTH study).

In women with a history of elevated triglyceride concentrations during therapy with oral estrogen (alone or in combination with a progestin), serum triglyceride concentrations should be monitored carefully during raloxifene therapy.

Postmenopausal women receiving raloxifene for the treatment or prevention of osteoporosis should be advised that the drug should be used in conjunction with other therapeutic measures (diet, adequate vitamin D and calcium intake, weight-bearing exercise) and lifestyle modifications (discontinuance of cigarette smoking, moderation of alcohol consumption).

Although raloxifene therapy has not been associated with endometrial proliferation, unexplained uterine bleeding should be investigated as clinically indicated. Some experts recommend an annual gynecologic examination in women with an intact uterus who are receiving raloxifene for breast cancer risk reduction. While raloxifene therapy has not been associated with breast enlargement, pain, or an increased risk of cancer, any unexplained breast abnormality occurring during raloxifene therapy should be investigated. Raloxifene has not been adequately studied to date in women with a history of breast cancer.

In women experiencing vision problems or who develop cataracts while receiving raloxifene, some experts recommend that an ophthalmology examination be performed.

Safety and efficacy of raloxifene have not been evaluated in men. Safety of raloxifene in premenopausal women has not been established. Because of the potential hazard to the fetus if raloxifene is inadvertently administered during pregnancy, use of the drug in premenopausal women is not recommended by the manufacturer.

Safety and efficacy of raloxifene have not been established in patients with hepatic impairment, and the drug should be used with caution in such patients.

Raloxifene should be used with caution in patients with moderate to severe renal impairment. Safety and efficacy of the drug have not been established in these patients.

Because of the embryotoxic and teratogenic effects of the drug, raloxifene is contraindicated in women who are pregnant. (See Cautions: Pregnancy, Fertility, and Lactation.)

■ **Pediatric Precautions** The manufacturer states that raloxifene should not be used in pediatric patients.

■ **Geriatric Precautions** Safety and efficacy of raloxifene in geriatric patients have not been studied specifically to date; however, prevention of osteoporosis, for which safety and efficacy have been established, occurs principally in patients older than 50 years of age. When the total number of patients studied in placebo-controlled clinical trials of raloxifene is considered, 61% were 65 years of age or older, while 15.5% were 75 years of age and older. No overall differences in efficacy or safety were observed between geriatric and younger patients. Pharmacokinetic studies have not revealed age-related differences in pharmacokinetic parameters of the drug in women 42–84 years of age. Based on clinical studies with raloxifene, special precautions based on age generally do not appear necessary.

■ **Mutagenicity and Carcinogenicity** The incidence of estrogen-dependent breast cancer or endometrial cancer is being evaluated in completed and ongoing clinical studies that involve over 17,000 women who received at least one dose of raloxifene. Analysis at up to 8 years indicates that raloxifene is *not* associated with an increased risk of endometrial cancer or ovarian cancer compared with placebo. Fewer cases of endometrial cancer were reported in women receiving raloxifene compared with tamoxifen in the STAR study; however, the difference between the treatment groups was not statistically significant. The annual incidence rates of endometrial cancer (per 1000 women) were 1.25 (raloxifene) and 2 (tamoxifen); the cumulative incidence over 7 years was 8.1 and 14.7 (per 1000 women) for raloxifene and tamoxifen, respectively. Although there was no difference in the incidence of endometrial cancer between treatment groups, a statistically significant decrease in uterine hyperplasia with atypia (a risk factor for endometrial cancer) was reported in at-risk women (i.e., those with an intact uterus) receiving raloxifene compared with tamoxifen during the STAR study.

Raloxifene has a protective effect against the development of hormone-sensitive breast cancer. (See Uses: Breast Cancer).

Raloxifene was not mutagenic in in vitro or in vivo studies, including the Ames microbial test with and without metabolic activation, the unscheduled DNA synthesis assay in rat hepatocytes, the mouse lymphoma assay for mammalian cell mutation, the chromosomal aberration assay in Chinese hamster ovary cells, the sister chromatid exchange assay in Chinese hamsters, and the micronucleus test in mice.

In a 21-month carcinogenicity study in mice, there was an increased incidence of ovarian tumors (i.e., benign and malignant tumors of granulosa/theca cell origin, benign tumors of epithelial cell origin) in female mice given oral raloxifene hydrochloride 9–242 mg/kg daily (equivalent to systemic exposure of about 0.3–34 times the area under the plasma concentration-time curve [AUC] in women receiving the recommended raloxifene hydrochloride dosage) and an increased incidence of testicular interstitial cell tumors, prostatic adenomas, and adenocarcinomas in male mice given raloxifene hydrochloride 41 or 210 mg/kg daily (4.7 or 24 times the AUC in women). In a 2-year carcinogenicity study in rats treated during their reproductive lives when ovaries were functional and responsive to hormonal therapy, there was an increased incidence in ovarian tumors (i.e., benign tumors of granulosa/theca cell origin) in female animals given raloxifene hydrochloride 270 mg/kg daily (about 400 times the AUC for women).

■ **Pregnancy, Fertility, and Lactation** Raloxifene may cause fetal toxicity when administered to pregnant women. Effects on reproductive function are expected because raloxifene is an estrogen agonist-antagonist. Since the risks clearly outweigh any possible benefits in women who are pregnant, raloxifene is contraindicated in such women; the drug also is not indicated for use in women of childbearing potential. If raloxifene is inadvertently administered during pregnancy or if the patient becomes pregnant while receiving the drug, raloxifene should be discontinued and the patient informed of the potential hazard to the fetus.

In reproductive studies in rabbits using raloxifene hydrochloride doses of 0.1 mg/kg or more (at least 0.04 times the recommended dose in humans on a mg/m^2 basis), abortion and a low rate of fetal heart anomalies (i.e., ventricular septal defects) were observed, and in rabbits using raloxifene doses of 10 mg/kg or more (at least 4 times the recommended dose in humans on a mg/m^2 basis), hydrocephaly was observed in the fetuses. In reproductive studies in rats using raloxifene hydrochloride doses of 1 mg/kg or more (at least 0.2 times the recommended dose in humans on a mg/m^2 basis), retardation of fetal development and developmental abnormalities (i.e., wavy ribs, kidney cavitation) were observed.

In studies in rats using raloxifene hydrochloride doses of 0.1–10 mg/kg (0.02–1.6 times the recommended dose in humans on a mg/m^2 basis) during gestation and lactation, delayed and disrupted parturition, decreased neonatal survival and altered physical development, sex- and age-specific reductions in growth and changes in pituitary hormone content, and decreased lymphoid compartment size in offspring were observed. Disruption of parturition, which resulted in maternal and progeny morbidity and/or death, was observed in rats given raloxifene hydrochloride 10 mg/kg. While ovarian or vaginal pathology was not observed in adult offspring (4 months of age), uterine hypoplasia and reduced fertility were noted.

In male and female rats given raloxifene hydrochloride doses of 5 mg/kg or more (at least 0.8 times the recommended human dose on a mg/m^2 basis) prior to and during mating, no pregnancies occurred. Estrous cycle disruption and inhibition of ovulation were observed in female rats given raloxifene hydrochloride doses of 0.1–10 mg/kg (0.02–1.6 times the recommended human dose on a mg/m^2 basis); these effects were reversible. In rats given raloxifene hydrochloride doses of 0.1 mg/kg or more (at least 0.02 times the recommended human dose on a mg/m^2 basis) during the preimplantation period, delayed and disrupted embryo implantation resulting in prolonged gestation and reduced litter size were observed. Changes in sperm production or quality or reproductive performance were not observed in male rats given raloxifene hydrochloride 100 mg/kg daily (16 times the recommended human dosage on a mg/m^2 basis) for 2 weeks. The reproductive and developmental effects observed in raloxifene-treated animals are consistent with the estrogen-receptor activity of the drug.

It is not known whether raloxifene distributes into human milk or if the drug affects milk production or the nursing infant; however, because raloxifene is an estrogen agonist-antagonist, estrogenic effects on mammary tissue during lactation may be affected.

Drug Interactions

■ **Protein-bound Drugs** Raloxifene is more than 95% bound to plasma proteins. The manufacturer states that concomitant administration of raloxifene with other highly protein-bound drugs is not expected to affect the plasma concentrations of raloxifene. In raloxifene-treated women with osteoporosis, concomitant administration of other highly protein-bound drugs (e.g., gemfibrozil) did not affect the plasma concentrations of raloxifene. Raloxifene reportedly does not affect the protein binding of phenytoin, tamoxifen, or warfarin (see Drug Interactions: Oral Anticoagulants) in vitro. The manufacturer states that caution is advised if raloxifene is used concomitantly with other highly protein-bound drugs such as diazepam, diazoxide, or lidocaine.

■ **Estrogens** The manufacturer states that concomitant use of systemic estrogens with raloxifene currently is not recommended because of the lack of experience from prospective clinical trials with such use.

■ **Antilipemic Agents** Administration of cholestyramine and raloxifene results in a 60% decrease in the absorption and enterohepatic cycling of raloxifene. The manufacturer states that raloxifene should not be administered with cholestyramine. Although not studied specifically, other anion-exchange resins would also be expected to decrease the absorption and enterohepatic cycling of raloxifene.

In raloxifene-treated women with osteoporosis, concomitant administration of gemfibrozil did not affect the plasma concentrations of raloxifene.

Concomitant use of raloxifene and other antilipemic agents has not been specifically studied.

■ **Cardiac Glycosides** Raloxifene reportedly does not affect the pharmacokinetics of digoxin.

■ **Oral Anticoagulants** While the effect of long-term administration of raloxifene in conjunction with warfarin has not been studied and the drug reportedly does not affect the protein binding of the anticoagulant, concomitant administration of single doses of raloxifene and warfarin has resulted in a 10% decrease in prothrombin time compared with administration of warfarin alone. In raloxifene-treated women with osteoporosis, concomitant administration of warfarin did not affect the plasma concentrations of raloxifene. If the drugs are used concomitantly, the patient and prothrombin time should be monitored closely and the dosage of the anticoagulant adjusted accordingly.

■ **Aminopenicillins** Concomitant administration of raloxifene and ampicillin results in a 28% decrease in peak plasma concentration and a 14% decrease in the extent of absorption of raloxifene. These changes in raloxifene absorption are consistent with decreased enterohepatic cycling associated with a reduction of enteric bacteria. Because systemic exposure and the elimination rate of raloxifene are not affected, raloxifene may be given concomitantly with ampicillin.

In raloxifene-treated women with osteoporosis, concomitant administration of amoxicillin did not affect the plasma concentrations of raloxifene. Raloxifene may be given concomitantly with amoxicillin.

■ **Antacids** Concomitant administration of raloxifene and calcium carbonate or aluminum and magnesium hydroxide-containing antacids does not affect the systemic exposure to raloxifene. Raloxifene may be given concomitantly with antacids.

■ **Corticosteroids** Pharmacokinetics of methylprednisolone following administration of a single oral dose were not altered in women receiving long-term therapy with raloxifene. Raloxifene may be given concomitantly with corticosteroids.

■ **Other Drugs** Use of raloxifene with cyclosporine has not been evaluated.

Acute Toxicity

■ **Manifestations** Limited information is available on the acute toxicity of raloxifene. Administration of raloxifene hydrochloride 600 mg daily for 8 weeks in a limited number of postmenopausal women was not associated with any unusual adverse effects.

Mortality was not observed in rats or mice following single oral doses of raloxifene hydrochloride 5000 mg/kg (810 or 405 times, respectively, the recommended human dose on a mg/m^2 basis). Mortality was not observed in monkeys following single oral doses of raloxifene hydrochloride 1000 mg/kg (80 times the recommended human dose on a mg/m^2 basis).

■ **Treatment** There is no known antidote for raloxifene overdosage. If acute overdosage of raloxifene occurs, supportive and symptomatic treatment should be initiated and the patient observed closely.

Pharmacology

Raloxifene is a selective estrogen receptor modulator (SERM) with mixed estrogen agonist or antagonist (antiestrogen) activity in specific tissues. Raloxifene exhibits estrogen agonist activity on bone and circulating lipoproteins, but estrogen antagonist activity on breast and uterine tissue.

Estrogens have an important role in the reproductive, skeletal, cardiovascular, and central nervous systems in women, and act principally by regulating gene expression. Biologic response is initiated when estrogen binds to a ligand-binding domain of the estrogen receptor resulting in a conformational change that leads to gene transcription through specific estrogen response elements (ERE) of target gene promoters; subsequent activation or repression of the target gene is mediated through 2 distinct transactivation domains (i.e., AF-1 and AF-2) of the receptor. The estrogen receptor also mediates gene transcription using different response elements (i.e., AP-1) and other signal pathways.

Recent advances in the molecular pharmacology of estrogen and estrogen receptors have resulted in the development of selective estrogen receptor modulators, agents that bind and activate the estrogen receptor but that exhibit tissue-specific effects distinct from estrogen. In addition to raloxifene, agents that have been described as antiestrogens (i.e., clomiphene, tamoxifen, toremifene) are selective estrogen receptor modulators. Although the precise mechanism of action of raloxifene has not been fully elucidated, tissue-specific estrogen-agonist or -antagonist activity of the drug appears to be related to structural differences in the raloxifene-estrogen receptor complex (specifically the surface topography of AF-2) compared with the estrogen (estradiol)-estrogen receptor complex. A second estrogen receptor also has been identified, and existence of at least 2 estrogen receptors (ERα, ERβ) may contribute to the tissue-specific activity of raloxifene. Tissue-selective conversion of metabolite to parent drug does not appear to play a role in the tissue-specific activity of raloxifene.

Raloxifene has estrogen agonist activity in bone and cardiovascular tissue. While the role of the estrogen receptor in bone, cardiovascular tissue, and the CNS continues to be studied, emerging evidence indicates that the mechanism of action of estrogen receptors in these tissues differs from the manner in which estrogen receptors function in reproductive tissue. In tissues where raloxifene exerts estrogen agonist activity, the raloxifene-estrogen receptor complex binds to DNA sequences distinct from the estrogen receptor element in reproductive tissues.

■ **Effects on Bone** The role of estrogen as a regulator of adult bone mass is well established. The progressive loss of bone mass observed in a large proportion of postmenopausal women is related to decreased ovarian function and to a reduction in the level of circulating estrogens. The loss of bone mineral density in these women is largely attributed to bone remodeling imbalances favoring osteoclastic cell-mediated bone resorption; impairment of osteoblasts (or their precursors) and bone formation also may be involved. Bone remodeling imbalances resulting from inadequate estrogen concentrations lead to bone formation that is inadequate to offset resorptive losses.

In postmenopausal women or women who have undergone oophorectomy, the principal pharmacologic action of raloxifene in bone, like that of estrogen replacement therapy, is to decrease the rate of bone resorption, thus slowing the rate of bone loss. Estrogens and raloxifene maintain bone mass, in part, through regulation of the gene-encoding transforming growth factor-β3 (TGF-β3). TGF-β3 is a bone matrix protein with antiosteoclastic properties. In in vitro cell-based assays, raloxifene activates TGF-β3 through pathways that are estrogen receptor-mediated but involve DNA sequences distinct from the estrogen response element. In addition, raloxifene binds to the estrogen receptor and acts as an estrogen agonist in human preosteoclastic cells resulting in inhibition of their proliferative capacity. Inhibition of the proliferative capacity of osteoclastic cells presumably contributes to raloxifene's effects on bone resorption. Other mechanisms involved in maintaining bone balance include estrogen-dependent down-regulation of the bone-resorbing cytokine interleukin-6. Raloxifene, like estrogens, suppresses cytokine interleukin-6 promoter activity. Results of in vitro studies indicate that the monoglucuronide conjugates of raloxifene are substantially less effective than raloxifene at inhibiting the resorbing activity of osteoclasts or producing TGF-β3.

Raloxifene reduces bone resorption and decreases bone turnover as manifested by reductions in serum and urine concentrations of bone turnover markers and increases in bone mineral density (BMD). In osteoporosis treatment and prevention studies, reductions in serum and urine markers of bone turnover (i.e., bone-specific alkaline phosphatase, osteocalcin, collagen breakdown products) generally occurred within 3 months following initiation of raloxifene therapy, peaked within 9–12 months, and persisted throughout the 36- and 24-month observation period.

The effect of raloxifene versus cyclic estrogen/progestin (conjugated estrogens 0.625 mg in conjunction with medroxyprogesterone acetate 2.5 mg daily, on days 15–28 of the cycle) on bone remodeling has been evaluated in a limited number of postmenopausal women using radiotracer techniques. Results of this study suggest that the effects of raloxifene on bone remodeling are similar to those of estrogen/progestin; at 31 weeks, remodeling suppression was greater with estrogen than raloxifene (i.e., positive shift in calcium balance of 91 versus 60 mg calcium daily, reduction in bone resorption of 162 versus 82 mg calcium daily) but remodeling balance was the same for both agents since bone formation was reduced by estrogen but not by raloxifene. Results from 56 paired bone biopsies obtained at baseline and at year 2 in patients receiving raloxifene for the treatment of osteoporosis indicate that raloxifene therapy is associated with substantial decreases in the bone formation rate per tissue volume; such an effect is consistent with a reduction in bone turnover. In addition, normal bone quality was maintained; no evidence of osteomalacia, marrow fibrosis, cellular toxicity, or woven bone was observed at year 2 in raloxifene-treated women.

The skeletal effects of raloxifene have been assessed in several animal models. In oophorectomized rats, raloxifene prevented increased bone resorption and bone loss; raloxifene was associated with positive effects on bone strength, but these effects varied with time. In cynomolgus monkeys, administration of raloxifene or conjugated estrogens for 2 years (equivalent to 6 years in humans) suppressed bone turnover and increased the BMD in the lumbar spine and in the central cancellous bone of the proximal tibia. In raloxifene- or estrogen-treated cynomolgus monkeys, bone strength (i.e., vertebral compression breaking force) was positively correlated with BMD of the lumbar spine. Histologic examination of bone from rats or monkeys given raloxifene did not reveal evidence of woven bone, marrow fibrosis, or mineralization defects.

The effects of raloxifene on bone in premenopausal women with normal menstrual cycles have not been evaluated. Although evidence from a pilot trial employing tamoxifen for the prevention of breast cancer suggested that the effects of estrogen agonist-antagonists on bone mineral density (BMD) may depend on menopausal status, with postmenopausal women experiencing positive effects on bone health and premenopausal women experiencing negative effects, evidence from animal studies indicates that raloxifene, unlike tamoxifen, does *not* antagonize the effects of estrogen on bone. Therefore, raloxifene, unlike tamoxifen, may not decrease BMD in premenopausal women with normal menstrual cycles.

■ **Effects on Lipoproteins** Raloxifene, like estrogens, has favorable effects on blood cholesterol. In a study in postmenopausal women with coronary heart disease or increased risk for coronary heart disease (RUTH study), use of raloxifene was associated with moderate effects on low-density lipoprotein (LDL)-cholesterol and high-density lipoprotein (HDL)-cholesterol concentrations. The magnitude of these effects were of lesser magnitude than changes achieved with other agents known to be cardioprotective.

■ **Effects on the Uterus and Breast** In contrast to raloxifene's estrogen-agonist effects on bone and on lipoproteins and the cardiovascular system, the drug has estrogen-antagonist activity in the uterus and breast. By comparison, tamoxifen exhibits estrogen antagonist activity in breast tissue but agonist activity in uterine tissue.

Raloxifene competitively inhibits the binding of estrogen to estrogen receptors in reproductive tissue. Because raloxifene competes with estrogens for binding to estrogen receptors, raloxifene prevents transcriptional activation of genes containing the estrogen response element. While the raloxifene-estrogen receptor complex activates genes through pathways that involve DNA sequences distinct from the estrogen response element in bone tissues, the raloxifene-estrogen receptor complex does not appear to have intrinsic activity in transcriptional activation of genes in reproductive tissues. Direct inhibition of estrogen binding to its receptor contributes to the estrogen-antagonist activity of raloxifene, but other mechanisms also are involved.

Raloxifene does not exhibit uterotropic activity. Studies in rats indicate that raloxifene, in contrast to estrogens and tamoxifen, produces marginal increases in uterine weight without endometrial proliferation. While estrogens (e.g., estradiol) and tamoxifen presumably mediate uterine activity through an AP-1 response element, raloxifene is not active at this site, and lack of affinity for the AP-1 site in uterine tissue may account for raloxifene's lack of uterine stimulatory activity.

In postmenopausal women, raloxifene does not appear to stimulate endometrial development and may inhibit endometrial proliferation that occurs in the presence of low concentrations of endogenous estrogen. Endometrial thickness has been evaluated in women enrolled in the osteoporosis treatment and prevention studies. In the osteoporosis treatment study, evaluation at 36 months indicated that raloxifene-treated women had a mean 0.06-mm increase in endometrial thickness over baseline and placebo-treated women had a mean 0.27-mm decrease. In the osteoporosis prevention study, endometrial thickness measurements in postmenopausal women receiving raloxifene were similar to measurements reported in women receiving placebo; evaluation at 24 months (using transvaginal ultrasonography) indicated that raloxifene-treated women had a mean 0.09-mm increase in endometrial thickness over baseline and placebo-treated women had a mean 0.04-mm increase. During the STAR study, women receiving both raloxifene and tamoxifen were required to undergo an annual gynecologic examination. Endometrial or uterine hyperplasia (with or without atypia) was reported in a small number of women receiving raloxifene as chemoprevention for breast cancer in this study; the number of cases of endometrial hyperplasia was considerably lower with raloxifene compared with tamoxifen (14 versus 84 cases).

The endometrial effect of raloxifene in premenopausal women with normal concentrations of endogenous estrogens differs from the effect in postmenopausal women. In a limited number of premenopausal women with normal menstrual cycles receiving raloxifene hydrochloride 100 or 200 mg daily for 28 days, subtle morphologic changes that could result from estrogen antagonist activity of the drug were noted in follicular and luteal phase biopsies; however, definite antagonist activity was not established.

Raloxifene inhibits estradiol-dependent proliferation of MCF-7 human mammary tumor cells in vitro. On a molar basis, raloxifene is about 60–1000 times more potent than tamoxifen as an inhibitor of estrogen-stimulated proliferation of the MCF-7 human mammary tumor cell line; however, potency of the 4-hydroxy metabolite of tamoxifen in inhibiting such proliferation is comparable to that of raloxifene. In vitro, raloxifene also has been shown to inhibit the invasiveness of these cells, whereas tamoxifen enhanced their invasiveness. In MCF-7 breast cancer cell-related assays, the monoglucuronide conjugates of raloxifene are substantially less potent than raloxifene at inhibiting cell proliferation. While raloxifene has antitumor activity in vivo, tamoxifen produced greater levels of efficacy against mammary tumors in most in vivo tumor prevention studies. The pharmacologic disparity between in vitro and in vivo results for tamoxifen and raloxifene has been attributed to activity of tamoxifen's 4-hydroxy metabolite in vivo. Raloxifene does not exhibit antiproliferative effects on nonestrogen-dependent (i.e., androgen-sensitive) mammary tumor cell lines.

■ **Other Effects** The activity of raloxifene on estrogen receptors in the CNS remains to be determined; however, the drug does not appear to ameliorate the vasomotor or psychologic manifestations associated with estrogen deficiency.

Pharmacokinetics

The pharmacokinetics of raloxifene have been studied principally in postmenopausal women. Pharmacokinetic parameters of raloxifene show considerable interindividual variation; however, studies in a limited number of individuals have not revealed gender- or race-related differences. In addition, there has been no evidence of age-related differences in the pharmacokinetics of the drug in women 42–84 years of age; the pharmacokinetics in children have not been determined. Limited information is available on the pharmacokinetics of raloxifene in individuals with hepatic and/or renal impairment.

■ **Absorption** Raloxifene is rapidly absorbed from the GI tract. Because raloxifene undergoes extensive first-pass glucuronidation, oral bioavailability of unchanged drug is low. While approximately 60% of an oral dose is absorbed, absolute bioavailability as unchanged raloxifene is only 2%. However, systemic availability of raloxifene may be greater than that indicated in bioavailability studies because circulating glucuronide conjugates are converted back to parent drug in various tissues.

Raloxifene undergoes extensive first-pass glucuronidation and enterohepatic circulation, and peak plasma concentrations of the glucuronide conjugates of raloxifene are achieved more rapidly than peak plasma concentrations of the parent drug. Following oral administration of a single 120- or 150-mg dose of raloxifene hydrochloride, peak plasma concentrations of raloxifene and its glucuronide conjugates are achieved at 6 and 1 hour, respectively. Plasma concentrations of raloxifene's glucuronide conjugates exceed those of the parent drug, and the time to achieve maximum concentrations of the drug and glucuronide metabolites depends on the extent and rate of systemic interconversion and enterohepatic circulation. Following oral administration of radiolabeled raloxifene, less than 1% of total circulating radiolabeled material in plasma represented parent drug.

Using data normalized for a single 60-mg dose and a 60-kg body weight, oral administration of raloxifene hydrochloride in postmenopausal women would be expected to result in mean peak plasma raloxifene concentrations of 0.5 ng/mL and oral administration of multiple 60-mg doses in mean peak plasma raloxifene concentrations of 1.36 ng/mL. Area under the plasma concentration-time curve (AUC) of raloxifene following a single dose is essentially the same as the AUC following multiple doses of the drug. Increasing the dose of raloxifene hydrochloride over a range of 30–150 mg results in a slightly less than proportional increase in the AUC of raloxifene. Administration of raloxifene with a standardized high-fat meal increases the peak plasma concentration and AUC of raloxifene 28 and 16%, respectively, compared with administration on an empty stomach but does not result in clinically important changes in systemic exposure.

Results of a single-dose study in patients with cirrhosis of the liver (Child-Pugh class A) and total serum bilirubin concentrations of 0.6–2 mg/dL indicate that plasma raloxifene concentrations correlate with serum bilirubin concentrations and are 150% higher in such individuals compared with individuals with normal hepatic function.

In postmenopausal women receiving raloxifene in clinical trials, plasma concentrations of raloxifene in those with mild renal impairment were similar to values in women with normal renal function.Results of a single-dose study in individuals with moderate renal impairment (creatinine clearance of 31–50 mL/minute) or severe renal impairment (creatinine clearance of 30 mL/minute or less) indicate that plasma raloxifene concentrations (area under the plasma concentration-time curve) are 122% higher in such individuals compared with individuals with normal renal function.

■ **Distribution** Distribution of raloxifene into body tissues and fluids has not been fully characterized. Raloxifene and raloxifene 4′-glucuronide have been detected in saliva following oral administration of radiolabeled drug. In studies in rats given radiolabeled raloxifene 6-glucuronide, the liver contained the highest concentration of radioactivity, followed by serum, lung, and kidney. While bone and the uterus contained relatively low concentrations of radiolabeled metabolite, 24% of the radioactivity in bone, 14% in the uterus, and 23% in the liver represented raloxifene. Results of this study indicate that the conversion of metabolite to parent drug occurs readily in a variety of tissues including the liver, lung, spleen, kidney, bone, and uterus.

The apparent volume of distribution following oral administration of single doses of raloxifene hydrochloride 30–150 mg is 2348 L/kg, suggesting extensive tissue distribution. The volume of distribution reportedly is not dose dependent over a dosage range of 30–150 mg daily.

Raloxifene and its monoglucuronide conjugates are more than 95% bound to plasma proteins. Raloxifene binds to albumin and α_1-acid glycoprotein (α_1-AGP), but not to testosterone-estradiol binding globulin (sex hormone binding globulin).

It is not known if raloxifene is distributed into milk.

■ **Elimination** Raloxifene undergoes extensive first-pass metabolism to the glucuronide conjugates raloxifene 4′-glucuronide, 6-glucuronide, and 6,4′-diglucuronide. Metabolism of raloxifene does not appear to be mediated by cytochrome P-450 enzymes, since metabolites other than glucuronide conjugates have not been identified.

The plasma elimination half-life of raloxifene at steady-state averages 32.5 hours (range: 15.8–86.6 hours). The terminal log-linear portions of the plasma clearance curves for raloxifene and its glucuronide conjugates generally are parallel. Following IV administration, raloxifene is cleared from systemic circulation at a rate approximating hepatic blood flow. Following oral administration of a single dose, apparent oral clearance of the drug is 44.1 L/hour per kg.

Raloxifene is excreted principally in feces as unabsorbed drug and via biliary elimination as glucuronide conjugates, which subsequently are metabolized by bacteria in the GI tract to the parent drug. Following oral administration, less than 6 or 0.2% of a raloxifene dose is excreted as glucuronide conjugates or parent drug, respectively, in urine.

Chemistry and Stability

■ **Chemistry** Raloxifene hydrochloride, a nonsteroidal benzothiophene derivative, is an estrogen agonist-antagonist. The drug also has been referred to as a selective estrogen receptor modulator (SERM). Raloxifene differs chemically and pharmacologically from naturally occurring estrogens, synthetic steroidal and nonsteroidal compounds with estrogenic activity, and agents that have been described as antiestrogens (e.g., clomiphene, tamoxifen, toremifene). However, like clomiphene, tamoxifen, and toremifene, raloxifene exhibits both estrogen agonist and antagonist (antiestrogen) activity, although the overall pharmacologic profiles of the drugs differ. Differences in the pharmacologic activity of raloxifene versus estradiol, tamoxifen, or toremifene are thought to depend on the 3-dimensional configuration of each drug.

Raloxifene consists of a 2-arylbenzothiophene core and a piperidine-containing basic side chain. Presence of hydroxy groups at positions 6 and 4′ of the 2-arylbenzothiophene core are important for estrogen receptor binding and correspond to the 3- and 17β-hydroxy substituents of estradiol. While raloxifene binds at the same site as estradiol within the ligand-binding domain of the estrogen receptor, the binding mode of the 4′ hydroxyl group and presence of the piperidine-containing basic side chain of raloxifene results in a drug-estrogen receptor complex that differs structurally and biologically from the estradiol-estrogen receptor complex. The orientation of the basic side chain is important in determining the uterine activity profile of selective estrogen-receptor modulators; the planar orientation and presence of the piperidine ring on the basic side chain of raloxifene result in a compound that lacks uterine estrogen agonist activity.

Raloxifene hydrochloride occurs as an off-white to pale yellow or greenish-yellow powder. The drug has solubilities of 0.3 mg/mL in water at 25°C and 1.6 mg/mL in alcohol at 25°C.

■ **Stability** Commercially available raloxifene hydrochloride tablets should be stored at controlled room temperature (20–25°C). When stored as directed, the tablets have an expiration date of 2 years following the date of manufacture.

Preparations

Excipients in commercially available drug preparations may have clinically important effects in some individuals; consult specific product labeling for details.

Raloxifene Hydrochloride

Oral		
Tablets, film-coated	60 mg*	**Evista®**, Lilly
		Raloxifene Hydrochloride Tablets

*available from one or more manufacturer, distributor, and/or repackager by generic (nonproprietary) name

†Use is not currently included in the labeling approved by the US Food and Drug Administration

Selected Revisions November 2019,

Tamoxifen Citrate

■ Tamoxifen, a triphenylethylene-derivative, nonsteroidal estrogen agonist-antagonist, is an antineoplastic agent.

Uses

■ **Breast Cancer** ***Adjuvant Therapy*** Tamoxifen is used as an adjunct to surgery and radiation therapy for the treatment of breast cancer in women with positive or negative axillary lymph nodes. Adjuvant tamoxifen therapy reduces the occurrence of contralateral breast cancer in premenopausal or postmenopausal women with breast cancer.

Systematic overviews of randomized clinical studies evaluating the effects of adjuvant tamoxifen therapy for early breast cancer have been conducted at regular intervals and have shown increases in 10-year survival and disease-free survival rates in patients receiving tamoxifen 20–40 mg daily for 1–5 years or longer (median 2 years). Among women with estrogen receptor-positive or estrogen receptor-unknown breast cancer and positive nodes who received about 5 years of tamoxifen therapy, overall survival at 10 years was 61.4% compared with 50.5% for patients who did not receive tamoxifen. Among women with estrogen receptor-positive or estrogen receptor-unknown breast cancer and negative nodes who received about 5 years of tamoxifen therapy, overall survival at 10 years was 78.9% compared with 73.3% for patients who did not receive tamoxifen. Both the absolute risk of relapse and the absolute benefit of treatment with tamoxifen were greater in women with positive nodes than in women with negative nodes. Greater reductions in disease recurrence and mortality were observed in patients with estrogen receptor-positive or estrogen receptor-unknown tumors than those with estrogen receptor-negative tumors. The reduction in disease recurrence and mortality was greater in those studies that used tamoxifen for about 5 years rather than shorter periods. There was no indication that dosages exceeding 20 mg daily were more effective. About 5 years of tamoxifen therapy generally reduced the rate of recurrence by one-third to one-half throughout the initial 10 years and reduced disease mortality by approximately one-third throughout the initial 15 years in women with estrogen receptor-positive breast cancer. Absolute risk reductions were independent of progesterone receptor status, patient age, axillary lymph node status, or use of chemotherapy.

Data from 2 large randomized phase 3 clinical studies (Adjuvant Tamoxifen: Longer Against Shorter [ATLAS] and Adjuvant Tamoxifen—To Offer More? [aTTom]) indicate that extended adjuvant tamoxifen therapy for 10 years further reduces the risk of breast cancer mortality and recurrence. In these studies, women who received adjuvant therapy with tamoxifen for 5 years were randomized to discontinue tamoxifen or to continue the drug for an additional 5 years (for a total of 10 years of adjuvant tamoxifen therapy). In the ATLAS study, extended adjuvant tamoxifen therapy reduced the risk of breast cancer mortality or recurrence by 3 or 10%, respectively, during years 5–9 and by 29 or 25%, respectively, beyond 10 years in women with estrogen receptor-positive breast cancer. In the aTTom trial, similar reductions in breast cancer mortality and recurrence were observed in women with estrogen receptor-positive or estrogen receptor-unknown breast cancer who received extended adjuvant tamoxifen therapy. Endometrial cancer occurred more frequently in patients who received extended adjuvant tamoxifen therapy compared with those who received 5 years of therapy in the ATLAS (3.1 versus 1.6% cumulative risk) and aTTom (2.9 versus 1.3% incidence) studies; an increased risk of pulmonary embolism also was observed in those receiving extended therapy.

Because the risk for breast cancer recurrence following 5 years of therapy is low in patients with small tumors and/or node-negative disease compared with those with large tumors and/or node-positive disease, the magnitude of benefit derived from extended therapy is expected to be lower in patients with lower-stage disease. Experts previously recommended an optimum duration of adjuvant tamoxifen therapy of 5 years in premenopausal women with hormone receptor-positive breast cancer, and a minimum of 5 years of adjuvant endocrine therapy (i.e., aromatase inhibitor or tamoxifen followed by an aromatase inhibitor for a total of at least 5 years) in those who are postmenopausal. Based on current evidence, the American Society of Clinical Oncology (ASCO) and other experts recommend continuation of initial adjuvant tamoxifen therapy for an additional 5 years (for a total of 10 years) in premenopausal or perimenopausal women and, in postmenopausal women who received 5 years of initial adjuvant tamoxifen therapy, an option of continuing tamoxifen or switching to an aromatase inhibitor for an additional 5 years (for a total of 10 years). The potential benefits of extended adjuvant endocrine therapy and drug cost, adverse effects, and risks associated with an extended duration of therapy also should be considered.

Tamoxifen is used as an adjunct to surgery and radiation therapy in the treatment of breast cancer in women with negative axillary lymph nodes. Several controlled studies have demonstrated an improvement in disease-free survival for women with node-negative breast cancer who received adjuvant therapy with tamoxifen or combination chemotherapy compared with no therapy until relapse. Adjuvant therapy with tamoxifen has been associated with reductions in tumor recurrence at both local and distant sites, including reductions in new primary tumors in the contralateral breast, with a relatively low incidence of clinically important adverse effects. Data indicate that adjuvant therapy with tamoxifen or combination chemotherapy generally reduces the rate of recurrence by one-fourth to one-third, although the reduction in absolute risk of recurrence appears to be relatively modest (e.g., 4–15%). Although all patients with node-negative breast cancer are at some risk for recurrence, patients with tumors smaller than 0.5 cm in diameter have a favorable prognosis, and the clinical benefit of adjuvant systemic therapy in these patients is minimal; adjuvant systemic therapy generally is not recommended in such patients, but some experts state that use of adjuvant endocrine therapy with or without sequential combination chemotherapy in patients with node-negative disease should be individualized based on consideration of the risk of recurrent disease without such adjuvant therapy, the expected reduction in risk and improvement in quality of life with such adjuvant therapy, and the potential adverse effects of such therapy. For patients with large tumors (exceeding 0.5 cm in diameter) and node-negative, hormone receptor-positive disease, ASCO and other experts state that the decision regarding use of adjuvant endocrine therapy with or without sequential combination chemotherapy may be guided by prognostic tools, such as the recurrence score based on 21-gene assay results, to predict the absolute benefits of combination chemotherapy in addition to adjuvant endocrine therapy.

Tamoxifen also is used as an adjunct to surgery and radiation therapy in the treatment of breast cancer in women with positive axillary lymph nodes. Numerous studies have shown that adjuvant therapy with tamoxifen alone increases disease-free survival in postmenopausal women whose tumors contain hormone receptors and who have positive axillary lymph nodes. The therapeutic benefit of tamoxifen alone may correlate with increasing quantity of hormone receptors in the tumor and may be greatest in patients with 4 or more positive nodes. Tamoxifen also has been used in conjunction with combination chemotherapy as adjuvant therapy following surgery in patients with positive nodes. Several studies indicate that disease-free survival in postmenopausal women with hormone receptor-containing tumors and positive nodes is greater following adjuvant therapy consisting of sequential tamoxifen and combination chemotherapy than following adjuvant therapy consisting of combination chemotherapy alone, but some data suggest that the benefit may be limited to the subgroup of patients with 4 or more positive nodes. Although the addition of combination chemotherapy to standard endocrine therapy is recommended in most patients with hormone receptor-positive tumors and positive nodes, some experts state that prognostic tools, such as the recurrence score based on

21-gene assay results, may be used to guide the decision to add adjuvant chemotherapy to endocrine therapy in certain patients with early-stage hormone receptor-positive breast cancer with 1–3 positive ipsilateral nodes.

Metastatic Breast Cancer Tamoxifen is used in the palliative treatment of metastatic breast cancer in women.

Selective estrogen receptor modulators (i.e., tamoxifen, toremifene) have been used for many years and are still considered an appropriate treatment option for postmenopausal women with hormone receptor-positive metastatic breast cancer; however, results of randomized clinical studies indicate that aromatase inhibitors are modestly more effective than tamoxifen in such patients. A randomized, open-label phase 3 study comparing tamoxifen with exemestane in postmenopausal women with hormone receptor-positive metastatic breast cancer demonstrated similar progression-free survival and overall survival outcomes in both treatment groups; however, findings from a meta-analysis of randomized controlled studies suggested a modest, but significant, survival benefit favoring aromatase inhibitors over other endocrine therapies (hazard ratio of 0.9; 95% confidence interval: 0.84–0.97). Tamoxifen and aromatase inhibitors were both well tolerated in clinical trials; however, thromboembolic events and vaginal bleeding occurred more frequently in patients receiving tamoxifen. Based on current evidence and because of the favorable toxicity profile, ASCO recommends aromatase inhibitors as initial endocrine therapy in postmenopausal women with metastatic hormone receptor-positive breast cancer.

Tamoxifen also is used in the palliative treatment of metastatic breast cancer in premenopausal women as an alternative to ovarian ablative therapy (oophorectomy or radiation). Patients with tumors containing estrogen receptors are more likely to respond to tamoxifen therapy than those with estrogen receptor-negative tumors. While objective response rate, time to treatment failure (relapse or progression), and overall survival appear to be similar in premenopausal women receiving tamoxifen or ovarian ablative therapy, current data and experience are inadequate to establish therapeutic equivalence. Some premenopausal women with disease progression during tamoxifen therapy subsequently respond to ovarian ablation. While some evidence suggests that an initial response to tamoxifen may be associated with a greater likelihood of subsequent response to ablative therapy following disease progression, failure to respond initially to tamoxifen does not preclude the possibility of subsequent response to ovarian ablation (i.e., some premenopausal women not responding initially to tamoxifen subsequently have responded to ablation).

Reduction in the Incidence of Invasive Breast Cancer in Women with Ductal Carcinoma in Situ Tamoxifen is used to reduce the risk of invasive breast cancer following surgery and radiation therapy in women with ductal carcinoma in situ (DCIS). The decision regarding use of tamoxifen to reduce the risk of invasive breast cancer in women with DCIS should be based on an individualized assessment of the benefits versus risks of such therapy. Current evidence suggests a duration of 5 years of tamoxifen therapy.

The current indication for tamoxifen is based principally on the results of a randomized, double-blind, placebo-controlled clinical trial (National Surgical Adjuvant Breast and Bowel Project [NSABP] B-24) in women undergoing surgery and radiation therapy for the treatment of DCIS. The primary measure of efficacy was reduced incidence of invasive breast cancer in the ipsilateral or contralateral breast. More than 80% of tumors were 1 cm or less in diameter, not palpable, and detected by mammography alone. Most patients (over 60%) were postmenopausal, 16% had positive surgical margins, and approximately 50% of tumors contained comedo necrosis. In this trial, 1804 women were randomized to receive tamoxifen (10 mg twice daily) or placebo for 5 years. Data available as of December 31, 1998, for 1798 women at a median follow-up of 74 months showed a 43% reduction in the incidence of invasive breast cancer in women receiving tamoxifen compared with those receiving placebo (44 versus 74 cases, respectively). At 5 years following study enrollment, survival was 97% in both treatment groups.

Reduction in the Incidence of Breast Cancer in Women at High Risk Tamoxifen is used to reduce the incidence of breast cancer in women at high risk for developing the disease.

ASCO considers use of tamoxifen an option for reducing the risk of invasive breast cancer in premenopausal or postmenopausal women 35 years of age or older who are considered at high risk for developing breast cancer (i.e., 5-year projected risk of 1.67% or greater based on the calculated score derived from the Gail risk model). In addition, ASCO considers use of tamoxifen an option for reducing the risk of invasive breast cancer in premenopausal or postmenopausal women 35 years of age or older with a history of lobular carcinoma in situ (LCIS), since these women are at increased risk for developing invasive breast cancer in both the affected and contralateral breast. (See Risk Assessment under Breast Cancer: Reduction in the Incidence of Breast Cancer in Women at High Risk, in Uses.)

Clinical Trials. The current indication for use of tamoxifen in reduction of the incidence of breast cancer is based principally on the results of the Breast Cancer Prevention Trial (BCPT; also known as the NSABP P-1 trial), a double-blind, randomized, placebo-controlled clinical trial conducted in the US, which was stopped early because of the clear evidence of a reduction in the incidence of invasive breast cancer among women at high risk for the disease who received tamoxifen therapy.

Tamoxifen has been shown to decrease the incidence of breast cancer among women at high risk for developing the disease and is considered an alternative to prophylactic bilateral mastectomy (typically total mastectomy accompanied by breast reconstruction), which generally is reserved for women with exceptionally high risk of developing breast cancer. The reduction in the incidence of a second primary cancer in the contralateral breast in women with early breast cancer who received adjuvant therapy with tamoxifen provided the rationale for the study of the drug in the primary prevention of breast cancer. No effect of tamoxifen on overall or breast cancer-related mortality was observed in this study.

In the BCPT, 13,388 women 35 years of age and older who were at high risk for developing breast cancer were randomized to receive either tamoxifen 10 mg twice daily or placebo twice daily for 5 years. Data available as of January 31, 1998, for 13,114 women at a median follow-up of 4.2 years showed a 44% reduction in the incidence of invasive breast cancer in women receiving tamoxifen versus placebo (86 versus 156 cases, respectively); data available as of March 31, 1998, for 13,175 women at a median follow-up of 4.6 years showed a 49% reduction in the incidence of invasive breast cancer among women receiving tamoxifen (89 cases) compared with those receiving placebo (175 cases); and data available as of March 31, 2005, for 13,207 women at a mean follow-up of 6 years showed a 43% reduction in the incidence of invasive breast cancer among women who received tamoxifen compared with those who received placebo. Reductions in the incidence of invasive breast cancer were observed in all age groups (35–49, 50–59, and 60 years of age and older), in women with or without LCIS, and in women at each risk level specified in the study; however, the reduction in the incidence of invasive breast cancer was substantial (75%) in those with a history of atypical hyperplasia. According to characteristics of the breast tumors that developed in women during the study, use of tamoxifen decreased the incidence of small, estrogen receptor-positive tumors but did not affect the incidence of estrogen receptor-negative or larger (exceeding 2 cm in diameter at the time of diagnosis) tumors. According to data available as of March 31, 2005, 23 participants in the study had died of breast cancer (12 in the tamoxifen group, 11 in the placebo group). A 37% reduction in the incidence of noninvasive breast cancer (DCIS and LCIS) also was observed among women who received tamoxifen compared with those who received placebo according to data available as of March 31, 2005.

Tamoxifen therapy is associated with an increased risk of serious adverse effects, including uterine malignancies (see Cautions: Mutagenicity and Carcinogenicity), pulmonary embolism, deep-vein thrombosis, and stroke (see Cautions: Cardiovascular Effects). In the BCPT, the risk of these adverse effects was increased particularly among tamoxifen-treated women who were 50 years of age or older.

Secondary objectives of the BCPT included study of the effects of tamoxifen on the incidence of ischemic heart disease (see Pharmacology: Effects on Lipoproteins) and bone fractures (see Pharmacology: Effects on Bone). No difference in the incidence of ischemic events was observed among women receiving tamoxifen or placebo. Data available as of March 31, 2005, showed a 29% reduction in the incidence of osteoporotic fractures in women 50 years of age or older at study entry who received tamoxifen compared with those who received placebo.

About 39% of the participants in the BCPT were women 35–49 years of age, 31% were 50–59 years of age, and 30% were 60 years of age or older. Despite efforts to enroll members of minority groups in the trial, only about 4% of participants represented minority groups (e.g., African American, Asian American, Hispanic), and the generalizability of the study results, including the size of the treatment effect as well as the risk of adverse effects, to these populations is uncertain.

Additional clinical trials investigating the use of 5 or 8 years of tamoxifen therapy for the prevention of breast cancer were conducted in other countries, including the UK and Italy. Following completion of a pilot study in the UK involving 2494 women (Royal Marsden Hospital study), 7154 women at high risk of breast cancer were enrolled in a tamoxifen chemoprevention study (International Breast Cancer Intervention Study [IBIS-I]). In 1992, recruitment of women 35 years of age or older who had undergone a hysterectomy was begun for a tamoxifen chemoprevention trial in Milan, Italy (Italian Tamoxifen Prevention study); following enrollment and randomization of 5408 women, recruitment was terminated earlier than planned because of the large number of women dropping out of the study and concerns regarding the adverse effects of tamoxifen.

In contrast to the findings of the BCPT, a reduction in the incidence of breast cancer among women who received tamoxifen compared with those who received placebo was not observed in the Royal Marsden Hospital and Italian Tamoxifen Prevention studies at a median follow-up of approximately 13 and 9 years, respectively; however, tamoxifen reduced the incidence of invasive estrogen receptor-positive tumors by 39% in the Royal Marsden Hospital study, particularly during the posttreatment period (reduction of 52%). In the Royal Marsden Hospital study, the posttreatment reduction in the incidence of invasive estrogen receptor-positive tumors did not differ according to menopausal status or concomitant use of hormone replacement therapy. The interaction of several factors may have contributed to the differing outcomes of the European studies of tamoxifen for the prevention of breast cancer compared with the results of the BCPT, including smaller sample size, differing study populations (e.g., fewer older women in the UK and Italian studies than in the BCPT), and differences in the degree of risk of developing breast cancer among study populations (e.g., lower risk of developing breast cancer among participants in the Italian study compared with those in the BCPT). Consistent with findings from the BCPT, an increased incidence of deep-vein thrombosis, pulmonary embolism, stroke, and endometrial cancer has been observed in patients receiving tamoxifen versus placebo in these trials.

Analysis of data from the IBIS-I study at a median follow-up of 16 years showed a 28% reduction in the incidence of breast cancer in patients who received tamoxifen compared with those who received placebo in the 10 years following initiation of therapy; a slightly greater reduction (31%) was observed in subsequent years. Consistent with findings from the BCPT, use of tamoxifen reduced the incidence of DCIS or invasive estrogen receptor-positive breast cancer by 35 or 34%, respectively, compared with placebo but did not affect the incidence of invasive estrogen receptor-negative tumors. The preventive effects of tamoxifen did not differ according to age, but reduced benefit was observed in women who used concomitant hormone replacement therapy during the 5-year treatment period. Increased incidences of deep-vein thrombosis during the initial 10 years and nonmelanoma skin cancers were observed in patients who received tamoxifen compared with those who received placebo.

Tamoxifen also has been compared with raloxifene in a double-blind, randomized, phase 3 study (Study of Tamoxifen and Raloxifene [STAR]; also known as the NSABP P-2 study). Patients enrolled in this study were randomized to receive either tamoxifen (20 mg daily) or raloxifene (60 mg daily) for a maximum of 5 years. Analysis of the data at an average follow-up of approximately 4 years (47 months) showed that tamoxifen and raloxifene were equivalent in efficacy in lowering the risk of invasive breast cancer. Although the comparison did not reach statistical significance, there were fewer cases of noninvasive breast cancer in women receiving tamoxifen than in those receiving raloxifene (1.51 per 1000 in the tamoxifen group versus 2.11 per 1000 in the raloxifene group; risk ratio of 1.4). In contrast to these findings, longer-term follow-up (approximately 7 years) showed that tamoxifen had a greater effect than raloxifene in lowering the risk of invasive breast cancer, while the between-treatment difference in risk of noninvasive breast cancer was smaller than that observed at the time of the initial analysis. The updated analysis showed a 24% reduction in raloxifene efficacy in lowering the risk of invasive breast cancer compared with tamoxifen. Although raloxifene remained as effective as tamoxifen in lowering the risk of invasive breast cancer in women with LCIS (risk ratio of 1.13), the drug was less effective than tamoxifen in women with atypical hyperplasia (risk ratio of 1.48). Noninvasive breast cancer was reported slightly (risk ratio of 1.22), but not significantly, more frequently in those receiving raloxifene compared with those receiving tamoxifen at approximately 7 years' follow-up.

In the STAR study, use of tamoxifen was associated with a higher risk of thromboembolic events than use of raloxifene, but rates of myocardial infarction, severe angina, or acute ischemic syndrome did not differ between the tamoxifen and raloxifene groups. Rates of fracture were essentially identical in the tamoxifen and raloxifene groups. Fewer cataracts were reported in the raloxifene group than in the tamoxifen group. Between-treatment differences in adverse effects mostly remained similar over approximately 7 years' follow-up. No differences in overall physical, mental health, or depressive symptoms were observed among women receiving either tamoxifen or raloxifene. However, women receiving tamoxifen reported more bladder-control (e.g., urinary incontinence) problems, gynecologic problems, and leg cramps. At the time of the initial analysis, endometrial cancer was reported more frequently in women receiving tamoxifen compared with those receiving raloxifene, but the difference was not statistically significant; however, an increase in the risk of endometrial cancer and endometrial hyperplasia was observed in patients receiving tamoxifen compared with those receiving raloxifene at approximately 7 years.

Risk Assessment. Benefit of tamoxifen for the primary prevention of breast cancer currently has been demonstrated only for women at high risk of developing breast cancer. Women are advised to consult with a health-care professional to determine their risk of developing breast cancer, and formal risk assessment by an oncology expert should be considered before the initiation of tamoxifen therapy. The National Cancer Institute (NCI) and NSABP have developed a computer-based tool that will help women consult with health-care providers regarding their personal risk and benefit for tamoxifen therapy. Examples of profiles that define a woman as being at high risk for developing breast cancer are included in the prescribing information for tamoxifen.

In the BCPT, women 60 years of age and older were eligible for enrollment based on age alone because the risk of breast cancer increases with increasing age. Women 35 years of age or older who had been diagnosed with LCIS were eligible for the study based on that diagnosis alone. Other women 35–59 years of age were eligible to participate in the study if they had a 5-year predicted risk of breast cancer scored as 1.67% or greater according to calculations with a statistical model known as the Gail model, which considers a combination of risk factors including number of first-degree relatives (i.e., mother, sister, daughter) diagnosed with breast cancer, number of breast biopsies, presence or absence of atypical hyperplasia on breast biopsy, age at menarche (i.e., first menstrual period), and either nulliparity or age at first live birth.

The following profiles are *examples* predicting a 5-year risk of 1.67% or greater according to the Gail model; although these examples are arranged in ascending order by age, *they do not necessarily represent ascending order of risk*:

- Age 35 years or older, one first-degree relative with a history of breast cancer, a personal history of 2 or more benign breast biopsies, and a personal history of a breast biopsy showing atypical hyperplasia
- Age 35 years or older, at least 2 first-degree relatives with a history of breast cancer, and a personal history of at least one breast biopsy
- Age 35 years or older and LCIS
- Age 40 years or older, one first-degree relative with a history of breast cancer, a personal history of 2 or more benign breast biopsies, age at first live birth 25 years or older, and age at menarche 11 years or younger
- Age 40 years or older, at least 2 first-degree relatives with a history of breast cancer, and age at first live birth 19 years or younger
- Age 40 years or older, one first-degree relative with a history of breast cancer, and a personal history of a breast biopsy showing atypical hyperplasia
- Age 45 years or older, at least 2 first-degree relatives with a history of breast cancer, and age at first live birth 24 years or younger
- Age 45 years or older, one first-degree relative with a history of breast cancer, a personal history of a benign breast biopsy, age at menarche 11 years or younger, and age at first live birth 20 years or older
- Age 50 years or older, at least 2 first-degree relatives with a history of breast cancer
- Age 50 years or older, history of one breast biopsy showing atypical hyperplasia, age at first live birth 30 years or older, and age at menarche 11 years or younger
- Age 50 years or older, history of at least 2 breast biopsies with a history of atypical hyperplasia, and age at first live birth 30 years or older
- Age 55 years or older, one first-degree relative with a history of breast cancer, a personal history of a benign breast biopsy, and age at menarche 11 years or younger
- Age 55 years or older, history of at least 2 breast biopsies with a history of atypical hyperplasia, and age at first live birth 20 years or older
- Age 60 years or older, 5-year predicted breast cancer risk of at least 1.67% according to the Gail model

Although each of the above profiles represents a 5-year predicted breast cancer risk of *at least* 1.67%, the absolute risk for these profiles varies (including both low and high risk scores) and must be calculated using the Gail model. Because the degree of risk differs according to the specific values applied to each variable in the Gail model and the combination of these individual risk factors, calculation of the 5-year predicted absolute risk for breast cancer provides the best estimate of risk to be used in judging possible benefit of tamoxifen therapy. In the BCPT, 25% of the women had a 5-year predicted breast cancer risk of 2% or less, 57.6% had a risk of 2.01–5%, and 17.4% had a risk of 5% or greater. Health-care professionals can request a Gail Model Risk Assessment Tool from the manufacturer or access a calculator based on the Gail model on the National Cancer Institute's website (https://bcrisktool.cancer.gov/).

For women 60 years of age or older, no additional risk factors were required for participation in the BCPT. However, a woman 50 years of age or older must consider other factors before choosing to take tamoxifen (e.g., whether she has had a hysterectomy). For women in the BCPT, particularly those 50 years of age or older, tamoxifen increased the risk of uterine malignancies (see Uterine Cancer in Cautions: Mutagenicity and Carcinogenicity), pulmonary embolism, deep-vein thrombosis, and stroke (see Cautions: Cardiovascular Effects). Following assessment of the risk of developing breast cancer, the decision regarding use of tamoxifen for reduction in the incidence of breast cancer should be based on an individual assessment of the benefits versus risks of tamoxifen therapy. (See Benefit Versus Risk under Breast Cancer: Reduction in the Incidence of Breast Cancer in Women at High Risk, in Uses.)

Although other criteria may identify women at high risk for the development of breast cancer, the benefit of tamoxifen therapy in these groups is unknown. Women with BRCA1 or BRCA2 genetic mutations are known to be at high risk for developing breast cancer, but data regarding the effect of tamoxifen on breast cancer incidence in women with inherited mutations are insufficient to support recommendations regarding tamoxifen use. Some evidence suggests that plasma insulin-like growth factor I (IGF-I) concentrations may be useful in identifying premenopausal women who are at high risk of breast cancer, but additional studies are needed to confirm this correlation and establish the benefit of tamoxifen therapy in such women.

Benefit Versus Risk. The benefit of tamoxifen as preventive therapy must be weighed against the risks associated with its use, and such treatment may not be appropriate in some women despite a high risk of breast cancer. The decision to initiate tamoxifen therapy for the prevention of breast cancer is complex and must be individualized.

Some experts state that for women with a life expectancy of less than 10 years, the benefit of tamoxifen as preventive therapy is likely minimal.

Women with risk factors for thrombosis, including hypertension, diabetes mellitus, smoking, and/or obesity, must consider that tamoxifen increases the risk of serious thrombosis.

Women with BRCA1 or BRCA2 genetic mutations, which place them at high risk for developing breast cancer, have been proposed as candidates for tamoxifen preventive therapy, but data regarding the effect of tamoxifen on breast cancer incidence in women with inherited mutations are insufficient to support recommendations regarding tamoxifen use. One small study showed that breast tumors arising in women with the BRCA1 mutation were less likely to be estrogen receptor-positive and thus may be less likely to respond to tamoxifen preventive therapy. Anonymous blood samples taken from 288 participants in the BCPT who developed invasive breast cancer were analyzed retrospectively to determine the incidence of breast cancer in women with BRCA1 or BRCA2 mutations who received tamoxifen compared with those who received placebo. The analysis indicated that tamoxifen use was associated with a reduction in breast cancer incidence in those with BRCA2 mutation but not in those with BRCA1 mutation. However, interpretation of the data are limited because only 19 of the samples (6.6%) were from patients with BRCA1 or BRCA2 mutations and because this question was not included in the initial design of the study. Further evidence is needed to establish the effect of tamoxifen therapy on the prevention of breast cancer in this population.

Because of the small number (about 4%) of minority participants (e.g., African American, Asian American, Hispanic) in the BCPT, the generalizability of the study results, including the size of the treatment effect as well as the risk of adverse effects, to these populations is uncertain.

Although tamoxifen therapy may reduce the incidence of breast cancer in women at high risk, it does not replace the need for clinical surveillance, and regular breast examination and screening with mammography are advised in such patients.

Duration of Therapy. The optimum duration of therapy with tamoxifen for the prevention of breast cancer has not been established; however, experts recommend a duration of 5 years.

Male Breast Cancer Tamoxifen is used in the palliative treatment of metastatic breast cancer in men. Breast cancer is a relatively rare disease in men and accounts only for about 0.5–1% of all breast cancers in the US. Cancer of the male breast appears to be biologically similar to the disease in women; however, centrally located lesions predominate in men, and tumors in males usually contain a higher frequency of hormone receptors than in females. Since the therapeutic benefit of tamoxifen may correlate with increasing quantity of hormone receptors in the tumor, the high frequency of hormone receptors in men may explain the high response rate of male breast carcinoma to endocrine therapy. Treatment to date has been similar to that for women with breast cancer; however, experience in men is very limited.

Combined results of several studies and published case reports showed an objective response (complete and partial) rate of about 50% in males with advanced (metastatic) breast cancer treated with tamoxifen. In addition to that in the breast, tumor regression is apparent in affected bone, soft tissue, liver, and lungs. Some experts consider tamoxifen the first-line hormonal therapy in males with estrogen receptor-containing tumors and positive nodes. Since limited evidence suggests that objective response rates may be similar in males receiving tamoxifen or testicular ablative therapy and drug therapy may be accepted better, tamoxifen is rapidly replacing orchiectomy in the palliative treatment of advanced breast cancer when estrogen receptors are present. Male breast cancer that progresses during tamoxifen therapy subsequently may respond to testicular ablation. Tamoxifen alone or in conjunction with combination chemotherapy also is used as an adjunct to surgery in the treatment of breast cancer in men with positive axillary lymph nodes†. Limited data indicate that disease-free 5-year survival is greater in males receiving adjuvant tamoxifen therapy compared with those not receiving the drug. Although randomized, controlled trials would be needed to evaluate systematically the role of tamoxifen in systemic adjuvant therapy in men with breast cancer, it is unlikely that such studies can be performed because of the rarity of this condition.

Pharmacogenomic Considerations for Tamoxifen Therapy **Cytochrome P-450 Isoenzyme 2D6 Polymorphism.** Studies indicate that exposure to endoxifen, the major active metabolite of tamoxifen, is strongly associated with cytochrome P-450 isoenzyme 2D6 (CYP2D6) metabolizer phenotype, and low endoxifen concentrations have been associated with an increased risk for disease recurrence in women receiving adjuvant tamoxifen therapy for breast cancer; however, the validity of CYP2D6 metabolizer phenotype as a predictor of the outcome of tamoxifen therapy is controversial.

Although tamoxifen is metabolized by multiple CYP isoenzymes, CYP2D6 is the principal isoenzyme responsible for formation of the active metabolites endoxifen (4-hydroxy-*N*-desmethyltamoxifen) and 4-hydroxytamoxifen. (See Pharmacokinetics: Elimination.) Activity of the CYP2D6 isoenzyme is under genetic control and is subject to individual variation; the CYP2D6 gene is highly polymorphic. Interindividual variability in systemic exposure to endoxifen is partially (approximately 30–53%) explained by CYP2D6 polymorphism.

The Clinical Pharmacogenetics Implementation Consortium (CPIC) guideline for CYP2D6 and tamoxifen therapy assigns the following metabolizer phenotypes and activity scores based on genotype; the activity score is the sum of activity score values assigned to each CYP2D6 allele, where 0 = no function and 1 = normal function. Individuals who lack functional alleles of the CYP2D6 gene have an activity score of 0 and are described as poor metabolizers; those with one decreased-function allele and one inactive allele have an activity score of 0.5 and are intermediate metabolizers; those with 2 decreased-function alleles or one normal-function allele and one inactive allele have an activity score of 1 and may be variably described as normal or intermediate metabolizers; those with 2 normal-function alleles or one normal-function allele and one decreased-function allele have an activity score of 2 or 1.5, respectively, and are normal metabolizers; and those who carry a duplicate or amplified gene have an activity score exceeding 2 and are ultrarapid metabolizers. The CYP2D6*4 allele (null activity) and CYP2D6*10 allele (reduced activity) are the most common variations reported in Caucasians and individuals of Asian ancestry, respectively, although variation exists in prevalence among various Asian populations. The ultrarapid metabolizer phenotype is more common in patients from Arabic and North African countries than in individuals of European ancestry.

Results from several studies demonstrated an approximately twofold to threefold higher risk of breast cancer recurrence in women with the CYP2D6 poor-metabolizer phenotype who received adjuvant tamoxifen therapy compared to those with the normal-metabolizer phenotype.

In a secondary analysis of the Austrian Breast and Colorectal Cancer Study Group 8 (ABCSG-8) study, postmenopausal women with the poor-metabolizer phenotype (2 inactive alleles) who received adjuvant tamoxifen therapy for 5 years had a substantially higher risk of disease recurrence or death compared with extensive metabolizers (those who lacked inactive or decreased-function alleles) (odds ratio of 2.45; 95% confidence interval of 1.05–5.73); a trend toward higher risk of disease recurrence or death was observed in women with one inactive allele (i.e., poor/intermediate metabolizer, poor/extensive metabolizer) compared with extensive metabolizers (odds ratio of 1.67; 95% confidence interval of 0.95–2.93). However, among patients who received sequential therapy with tamoxifen for 2 years followed by anastrozole for 3 years, CYP2D6 metabolizer phenotypes were not associated with increased risk of disease recurrence or death, suggesting that the risk of these events in patients with reduced CYP2D6 metabolic activity was negated by sequential use with another active drug that is not metabolized by CYP2D6.

In contrast to these findings, an association between CYP2D6 metabolizer phenotype and disease recurrence in postmenopausal women who received adjuvant tamoxifen therapy for 5 years was not demonstrated in secondary analyses of the Arimidex, Tamoxifen, Alone or in Combination (ATAC) and Breast International Group 1-98 (BIG 1-98) studies; however, limitations of these studies include potential genotype errors (e.g., genotyping from somatic rather than germline tissue) and analysis of DNA samples for only a small proportion of study participants.

A nested case-control study from the BCPT and STAR studies also failed to demonstrate an association between CYP2D6 metabolizer phenotype and breast cancer incidence in women 50 years of age or older who received tamoxifen therapy for the primary prevention of breast cancer for a duration of up to 5 years.

A meta-analysis conducted by the International Tamoxifen Pharmacogenomics Consortium (ITPC), which combined data from 12 clinical trials in 4973 tamoxifen-treated patients worldwide, found an increased risk of disease recurrence in CYP2D6 poor metabolizers; however, this risk was observed only when strict inclusion criteria were used (i.e., postmenopausal women with estrogen receptor-positive breast cancer receiving adjuvant tamoxifen therapy at a dosage of 20 mg daily for 5 years). In addition, a systematic review of 38 studies investigating associations between CYP2D6 genetic variation and survival outcomes after tamoxifen treatment found that 53% of the studies reported at least one statistically significant association between CYP2D6 genetic variation and survival; studies that used comprehensive genotyping panels were more likely to report such an association. Numerical, but not statistically significant, associations were observed based on the source of DNA for genotyping. Other study limitations (e.g., retrospective design, inadequate statistical power, use of convenience samples, differences in outcome definitions and phenotype classification, noncompliance with therapy, use of CYP2D6 inhibitors or chemotherapy, duration of follow-up) might have contributed to the discrepant findings reported to date.

In a clinical study evaluating CYP2D6 genotype-guided dosing, an increase in tamoxifen dosage from 20 mg daily to 40 mg daily in patients with poor or intermediate metabolizer phenotype increased endoxifen concentrations. Following 4 months of therapy at the 40-mg daily dosage, endoxifen concentrations in intermediate metabolizers were similar to those in extensive metabolizers receiving a standard tamoxifen dosage (20 mg daily); although endoxifen concentrations also increased in poor metabolizers following dosage escalation, the concentrations remained significantly lower than those achieved in extensive metabolizers receiving the standard dosage or in intermediate metabolizers receiving the genotype-guided dosage. Clinically meaningful increases in adverse effects or decreases in quality of life were not observed in those receiving genotype-guided dosing.

Although some experts do not recommend use of CYP2D6 genotyping to guide treatment decisions in patients with hormone receptor-positive breast cancer based on current levels of evidence, CPIC and other experts recommend that postmenopausal women with CYP2D6 poor-, intermediate-, or normal/intermediate-metabolizer phenotypes (activity scores of 0–1) receive adjuvant endocrine therapy with an alternative agent such as an aromatase inhibitor and that premenopausal women with these phenotypes receive an aromatase inhibitor plus ovarian ablation. If use of an aromatase inhibitor is contraindicated, CPIC and these experts state that an increased tamoxifen dosage of 40 mg daily may be considered; however, suboptimal concentrations of endoxifen may be achieved in patients with a CYP2D6 poor-metabolizer phenotype despite dosage adjustment. The safety of tamoxifen dosages exceeding 40 mg daily in patients with the poor-metabolizer phenotype has not been established.

Application of CYP2D6 genotyping as a tool to aid in treatment decisions has important limitations and should not substitute for appropriate clinical judgment and patient management. The potential for other patient characteristics, such as menopausal status, to influence the utility of CYP2D6 genotyping for optimizing tamoxifen therapy has not been adequately studied to date.

Other Polymorphic Cytochrome P-450 Isoenzymes. Although some data suggest a direct relationship between CYP2C19 polymorphism and endoxifen plasma concentrations and survival, analysis of data from the ITPC data set failed to confirm a clinically meaningful association between CYP2C19 genomic variants and disease recurrence in women who received adjuvant tamoxifen therapy for breast cancer. Therefore, CPIC and some other experts state that a clinical role for CYP2C19 polymorphisms in guiding tamoxifen treatment decisions has not been established. Pharmacogenetic variation in other CYP isoenzymes (e.g., 2C9, 3A4, and 3A5) appears to have only a small effect on endoxifen exposure.

■ **Other Uses** Tamoxifen has been used to stimulate ovulation† in appropriately selected anovulatory women desiring pregnancy, especially in those with oligomenorrhea or amenorrhea who were previously receiving oral contraceptives. Limited data suggest that tamoxifen therapy may be useful for the management of some types of mastalgia† (e.g., cyclical), but additional studies are needed to evaluate the efficacy, safety, and dosage of the drug for this condition. Tamoxifen also has been used to reduce the frequency of vaginal bleeding episodes and to reduce the rate of increase in bone age in girls with Albright syndrome† (also known as McCune-Albright syndrome) and precocious puberty; however, the effects of tamoxifen beyond one year of treatment in these patients have not been established. (See Cautions: Pediatric Precautions.)

Dosage and Administration

■ **Administration** Tamoxifen citrate is administered orally. Dosages exceeding 20 mg daily should be given in divided doses (morning and evening).

■ **Dosage** Dosage of tamoxifen citrate is expressed in terms of tamoxifen.

Breast Cancer **Adjuvant Therapy.** When tamoxifen is used as an adjunct to surgery and radiation therapy in the treatment of breast cancer, the usual dosage of the drug is 20–40 mg daily. In several clinical studies of adjuvant tamoxifen therapy, there was no evidence that dosages exceeding 20 mg daily are necessary. However, if tamoxifen is used as adjuvant therapy in patients with cytochrome P-450 isoenzyme 2D6 (CYP2D6) poor-, intermediate-, or normal/intermediate-metabolizer phenotypes (activity scores of 0–1), some experts state that a dosage of 40 mg daily may be considered, since a dosage of 20 mg daily may result in suboptimal concentrations of the active metabolite endoxifen. Although endoxifen concentrations may remain suboptimal in patients with the poor-metabolizer phenotype despite such dosage adjustment, the safety of tamoxifen dosages exceeding 40 mg daily in these patients has not been established. (See Cytochrome P-450 Isoenzyme 2D6 Polymorphism under Breast Cancer: Pharmacogenomic Considerations for Tamoxifen Therapy, in Uses.) The optimum duration of adjuvant tamoxifen therapy is 5 years in most patients; however, continuation of adjuvant therapy for an additional 5 years (for a total of 10 years) may be considered in women with early-stage hormone receptor-positive breast cancer based on their menopausal status. (See Adjuvant Therapy under Uses: Breast Cancer.) The magnitude of benefit of extended therapy (i.e., beyond 5 years) with tamoxifen is expected to be lower in women with small tumors and/or node-negative disease.

Metastatic Breast Cancer. For the treatment of metastatic breast cancer in women, the usual dosage of tamoxifen is 20–40 mg daily. Because there does not appear to be any significant difference in response rates with the two dosages, most clinicians believe that 20 mg daily usually should be used initially. If an objective response to the drug occurs, it usually is evident within 4–10 weeks; however, several months of therapy may be required before an objective response occurs in patients with bone metastases.

Reduction in the Incidence of Invasive Breast Cancer in Women with Ductal Carcinoma in Situ. For reduction in the incidence of invasive breast cancer in women with ductal carcinoma in situ (DCIS), the recommended dosage of tamoxifen is 20 mg daily for 5 years.

Reduction in the Incidence of Breast Cancer in Women at High Risk. For reduction in the incidence of breast cancer in women at high risk, the recommended dosage of tamoxifen is 20 mg daily. Experts recommend a 5-year duration of tamoxifen therapy for the prevention of breast cancer in women at high risk of the disease.

Male Breast Cancer. For the treatment of metastatic breast cancer in men, the usual dosage of tamoxifen is 20–40 mg daily. When tamoxifen alone or in combination with radiation therapy was used as an adjunct to surgery† in the treatment of breast cancer in men, a tamoxifen dosage of 20 mg daily was used. The optimum duration of adjuvant tamoxifen therapy has not been established; however, some clinicians suggest a similar duration of therapy in men as in women (i.e., 5–10 years). Decisions about the duration of adjuvant tamoxifen therapy may be individualized, as they are for women, based on risk of disease recurrence and adverse effects.

Other Uses To stimulate ovulation†, 5–40 mg of tamoxifen has been administered twice daily for 4 days.

Cautions

The manufacturer states that the adverse effect profile of tamoxifen in breast cancer patients generally appears to be similar for men and women. Adverse effects of tamoxifen citrate usually are relatively mild and rarely severe enough to necessitate discontinuance of the drug in patients with breast cancer. Tamoxifen usually is well tolerated in male patients with breast cancer. In the Breast Cancer Prevention Trial (BCPT), 15% of women receiving tamoxifen withdrew from the trial for medical reasons (e.g., hot flushes, vaginal discharge) compared with 9.7% of women receiving placebo.

Tamoxifen therapy is associated with increased risk of serious adverse effects, including uterine cancer, pulmonary embolism, deep-vein thrombosis, and stroke in women receiving the drug for reduction in the incidence of breast cancer (i.e., women at high risk for breast cancer or women with ductal carcinoma in situ). In the BCPT, the risk of these adverse effects was increased particularly among tamoxifen-treated women who were 50 years of age or older.

■ **Cardiovascular Effects** Adverse cardiovascular effects of tamoxifen include thrombotic and venous thromboembolic events such as stroke, pulmonary embolism, and deep-vein thrombosis.

Thromboembolic Events In the BCPT, women without a history of pulmonary emboli receiving tamoxifen had an approximately threefold increase in the risk of developing a pulmonary embolism (18 versus 6 cases; incidence rate of 0.75 versus 0.25 per 1000 women-years) compared with those receiving placebo. Three women in the study, all of whom were receiving tamoxifen, died of pulmonary embolism. Of the cases of pulmonary embolism, 87% occurred in women at least 50 years of age at the time of randomization; among women receiving tamoxifen in the BCPT, episodes of pulmonary embolism occurred on average at 27 months (range: 2–60 months) following initiation of therapy with the drug.

Although the difference was not significant, the risk of deep-vein thrombosis was increased (relative risk of 1.6) among women receiving tamoxifen versus placebo in the BCPT (35 versus 22 cases according to data available as of March 31, 1998). A similar increase in relative risk of deep-vein thrombosis was observed in women 49 years of age and younger as in women 50 years of age or older, although fewer events occurred in younger women. Women who had thromboembolic events were at risk for a second related event (7 of 25 women receiving placebo and 5 of 48 women receiving tamoxifen according to data available as of January 31, 1998). Among women receiving tamoxifen in the BCPT, episodes of deep-vein thrombosis occurred on average at 19 months (range: 2–57 months) following initiation of therapy with the drug. Thrombotic events, including deep-vein thrombosis, pulmonary embolism, and superficial phlebitis, also have been reported in 1.7% of women receiving tamoxifen as adjuvant therapy for the treatment of breast cancer; at least 2 deaths have occurred in patients with breast cancer who had thrombotic events during tamoxifen therapy. Clotting factor abnormalities have been observed with prolonged tamoxifen therapy at usual dosages, and antithrombin III, fibrinogen, and platelet counts have been decreased minimally; the relationship, if any, of such changes to thromboembolic phenomena is unclear. Results of a small substudy of the BCPT suggested that screening patients for factor V Leiden and prothrombin G20210A mutations would not be beneficial in identifying patients who should not receive tamoxifen.

Although the difference was not significant, an increase in the incidence of stroke was observed in women receiving tamoxifen (38 events) versus placebo (24 events) in the BCPT (relative risk of 1.59 and 95% confidence interval of 0.93–2.77 according to data available as of March 31, 1998). Hemorrhagic strokes accounted for 10 of 38 (26%) or 6 of 24 (25%) strokes in women receiving tamoxifen or placebo, respectively. Occlusive strokes accounted for 21 of 38 (55%) or 14 of 24 (58%) strokes in women receiving tamoxifen or placebo, respectively. Among women receiving tamoxifen or placebo, 7 of 38 (18%) or 4 of 24 (17%) strokes, respectively, were of unknown etiology. Fatal stroke occurred in 4 women receiving tamoxifen and in 3 women receiving placebo. Among women experiencing stroke, 88% occurred in women 50 years of age or older at the time of randomization. Among women receiving tamoxifen in the BCPT, episodes of stroke occurred on average at 30 months (range: 1–63 months) following initiation of therapy with the drug.

In the Arimidex, Tamoxifen, Alone or in Combination (ATAC) trial, venous thromboembolic events and ischemic cerebrovascular events were reported more frequently in women receiving adjuvant therapy with tamoxifen compared with those receiving anastrozole (5 versus 3% and 3 versus 2%, respectively).

Vasomotor Symptoms In clinical studies, vasomotor symptoms (i.e., hot flushes [flashes]) occur more frequently in patients receiving tamoxifen than in those receiving placebo. Hot flushes are one of the most common adverse effects reported in women receiving tamoxifen for the treatment or prevention of breast cancer. In the BCPT, hot flushes occurred in 80% of women receiving tamoxifen compared with 68% of those receiving placebo. In addition, more women who were receiving tamoxifen versus placebo reported severe hot flushes (45 versus 28%). Withdrawal from the trial because of hot flushes occurred more frequently among women receiving tamoxifen versus placebo (3.1 versus 1.5%). In the ATAC trial, hot flushes were reported more frequently in women receiving adjuvant therapy with tamoxifen compared with those receiving anastrozole (41 versus 36%). In some patients, clonidine may ameliorate tamoxifen-induced hot flushes.

Effects on Lipoproteins Hyperlipidemias have been reported in patients receiving tamoxifen. Hypertriglyceridemia has been reported in patients with breast cancer receiving tamoxifen and may be severe, particularly in patients with a known history of elevated triglyceride levels, such as those associated with familial hypertriglyceridemia. Although tamoxifen-induced hypertriglyceridemia may respond to withdrawal of the drug or treatment with lipid-lowering agents, at least one patient developed fulminant pancreatitis and subsequently died. Periodic monitoring of plasma triglyceride concentrations is advised in patients with preexisting hyperlipidemias during the entire duration of tamoxifen therapy since onset of hypertriglyceridemia may be delayed.

Potentially beneficial estrogenic effects, including decreased total and low-density lipoprotein concentrations and decreased cardiovascular morbidity and mortality (particularly in postmenopausal women), also have been observed in women receiving prolonged tamoxifen therapy. (See Pharmacology: Effects on Lipoproteins.)

Other Cardiovascular Effects Fluid retention has been reported in women receiving tamoxifen as adjuvant therapy for breast cancer. Edema has also been reported in women with metastatic breast cancer receiving tamoxifen.

■ **Genitourinary and Renal Effects** Vaginal discharge and menstrual irregularities occur more frequently in patients receiving tamoxifen than in those receiving placebo. Vaginal discharge, occurring in 55%, was one of the most common adverse effects reported among women receiving tamoxifen for the primary prevention of breast cancer in the BCPT. In addition, more women who were receiving tamoxifen versus placebo reported vaginal discharge that was moderately, quite a bit, or extremely bothersome (29 versus 13%). Withdrawal from the trial because of vaginal discharge occurred more frequently among women receiving tamoxifen versus placebo (0.5 versus 0.1%). Vaginal bleeding may occur with tamoxifen therapy. In the ATAC trial, vaginal bleeding and vaginal discharge were reported more frequently in women receiving tamoxifen compared with those receiving anastrozole (10 versus 5% and 13 versus 4%, respectively). Vaginal dryness and pruritus vulvae have been reported infrequently in women receiving tamoxifen for metastatic breast cancer. Amenorrhea also has been reported in women receiving tamoxifen.

An increased incidence of endometrial changes, including hyperplasia and polyps, has been associated with tamoxifen therapy. The underlying mechanism of these changes appears to be related to the estrogenic properties of tamoxifen. Endometriosis and uterine fibroids, possibly resulting from tamoxifen's partial estrogenic activity, have been reported rarely in women receiving tamoxifen. In addition, ovarian cysts have been observed in a small number of premenopausal patients with advanced breast cancer who have been treated with tamoxifen. An increased incidence of uterine fibroids (in premenopausal and postmenopausal women) and benign ovarian cysts (in premenopausal women) also was noted in women receiving tamoxifen in a study for the prevention of breast cancer.

Loss of libido and impotence have been reported in some male patients and resulted in discontinuance of tamoxifen therapy. In oligospermic men who were receiving tamoxifen therapy, increased lutropin (luteinizing hormone, LH), follitropin (follicle-stimulating hormone, FSH), testosterone, and estrogen concentrations were reported. Priapism has been reported in at least one patient receiving tamoxifen.

Increased serum BUN and/or creatinine also has been reported in patients receiving tamoxifen as adjuvant therapy for breast cancer.

■ **Musculoskeletal Effects** Musculoskeletal pain and bone pain have been reported in patients with breast cancer receiving tamoxifen. Increased bone and tumor pain or flare have occurred with tamoxifen therapy for metastatic breast cancer and are sometimes associated with a good tumor response. Patients with increased bone pain may require additional analgesics. Patients with soft tissue disease may demonstrate sudden increases in the size of preexisting lesions, sometimes associated with marked erythema within and surrounding the lesions, and/or development of new lesions. If bone pain and disease flare occur, they are usually apparent shortly after initiation of tamoxifen therapy and generally subside rapidly. Management of tamoxifen-related flare includes supportive care and possibly interruption of treatment with the drug, with subsequent reinstitution of therapy at a reduced dosage (i.e., 5–10 mg daily) and gradual increases to the usual dosage; in some cases, prednisone may be added concomitantly for 1–2 weeks.

Hypercalcemia, in some cases life-threatening, may occur during initial tamoxifen therapy in patients with metastatic breast cancer who have bone metastases. Periodic determination of serum calcium concentrations should be performed during initial therapy in these patients (e.g., once or twice weekly during the first 2–3 weeks of therapy) and appropriate treatment initiated if hypercalcemia occurs. If hypercalcemia is severe, the drug should be discontinued. Following appropriate management of hypercalcemia, tamoxifen therapy may be reinstituted with caution and careful monitoring, at a reduced dosage or concomitantly with a low dosage of prednisone.

A potentially beneficial estrogenic effect of prolonged tamoxifen therapy is preservation of bone mineral density (BMD) of the lumbar spine in postmenopausal women. (See Pharmacology: Effects on Bone.) Results of a substudy of the ATAC trial indicated that at 12 and 24 months postmenopausal women receiving adjuvant therapy with tamoxifen had a mean increase from baseline in both lumbar spine and total hip BMD, whereas those receiving anastrozole had a mean decrease from baseline in both lumbar spine and total hip bone BMD. In the ATAC trial, fractures of the spine, hip, or wrist were reported in 4% of patients receiving anastrozole compared with 3% of those receiving tamoxifen.

Joint symptoms also were reported more frequently in patients receiving anastrozole compared with those receiving tamoxifen (36 versus 29%) in the ATAC trial.

■ **Ocular Effects** Tamoxifen rarely has been associated with ocular toxicity. Retinopathy, corneal opacities, and decreased visual acuity have occurred in patients receiving extremely high dosages (e.g., 180–320 mg daily) of tamoxifen for longer than 1 year. Ocular effects such as visual disturbances, decrement in color vision perception, corneal changes, cataracts, need for cataract surgery, optic neuritis, retinal vein thrombosis, intraretinal crystals, posterior subcapsular opacities, and/or retinopathy have also been reported in patients receiving recommended dosages of the drug. A slightly increased rate of developing cataracts and a greater risk of developing cataracts and undergoing cataract surgery were observed in women receiving tamoxifen in the BCPT.

■ **Hepatic Effects** Changes in hepatic enzyme concentrations (e.g., increased serum AST [SGOT] or ALT [SGPT] concentrations) and increased bilirubin and/or alkaline phosphatase concentrations have been reported in patients receiving tamoxifen therapy. Rarely, more severe hepatic abnormalities, including fatty changes in the liver, cholestasis, hepatitis, hepatic necrosis, and death, have occurred. A causal relationship of these adverse hepatic effects to tamoxifen has not been established; however, following rechallenge with tamoxifen, adverse hepatic effects occurred in some patients.

■ **GI Effects** Adverse GI effects of tamoxifen, including nausea, anorexia, distaste for food, and abdominal cramps, have been reported in patients with breast cancer.

■ **Nervous System Effects** Adverse nervous system effects reported in patients receiving tamoxifen for metastatic breast cancer include dizziness, lightheadedness, headache, fatigue, and mental depression.

■ **Hematologic Effects** Thrombocytopenia (platelet counts of 50,000–100,000/mm^3 and, infrequently, lower) occasionally has occurred in patients receiving tamoxifen for the treatment of breast cancer; however, platelet counts returned to normal even though tamoxifen therapy was continued. Hemorrhagic episodes have occurred rarely in patients with severe thrombocytopenia. Neutropenia, pancytopenia, and leukopenia (sometimes associated with anemia and/or thrombocytopenia) also have been reported and may be severe. A causal relationship of the drug to some of these hematologic reactions has not been established.

Purpuric vasculitis, which was unresponsive to prednisone 25 mg daily but resolved completely following drug withdrawal, has been reported in at least one patient receiving tamoxifen.

■ **Dermatologic Effects** Thinning and/or partial loss of hair occurs infrequently in patients receiving tamoxifen for metastatic breast cancer. Erythema multiforme, Stevens-Johnson syndrome, and bullous pemphigoid have been reported rarely in patients receiving tamoxifen. Skin changes have occurred in patients receiving tamoxifen as adjuvant therapy for breast cancer.

■ **Other Adverse Effects** Other adverse effects reported in patients receiving tamoxifen as adjuvant therapy for breast cancer or for metastatic breast cancer include weight loss, fatigue, and cough. Hypersensitivity reactions, including angioedema, have been reported rarely in patients receiving tamoxifen, sometimes more than one year following initiation of therapy. Interstitial pneumonitis also has been reported rarely in patients receiving the drug.

■ **Precautions and Contraindications** Serious, life-threatening or fatal events associated with tamoxifen used for reduction in the incidence of breast cancer (i.e., women at high risk for breast cancer and women with ductal carcinoma in situ [DCIS]) include endometrial cancer, uterine sarcoma, stroke, and pulmonary embolism. Healthcare providers should discuss the potential benefits versus risks of tamoxifen therapy with women considering use of the drug to potentially reduce their risk of developing breast cancer.

Because of the increased risk of thromboembolic events associated with tamoxifen therapy in the BCPT, tamoxifen for reduction in the incidence of breast cancer is contraindicated in women with a history of deep-vein thrombosis or pulmonary embolism. Use of tamoxifen to reduce the incidence of breast cancer also is contraindicated in women who require anticoagulant therapy with a coumarin derivative. Women receiving or who have received tamoxifen should promptly seek medical attention for symptoms of unexplained shortness of breath or leg swelling/tenderness.

Use of tamoxifen is associated with an increased incidence of uterine malignancies. (See Cautions: Mutagenicity and Carcinogenicity.) Women receiving tamoxifen or women with a history of having received tamoxifen who report abnormal vaginal bleeding should be evaluated promptly. Women receiving or who have received tamoxifen should receive routine gynecologic care and should be advised to report promptly any abnormal gynecologic symptoms, such as menstrual irregularities, abnormal vaginal bleeding, change in vaginal discharge, or pelvic pain/pressure, to their physician.

Women receiving or who have received tamoxifen also should seek prompt medical attention for new breast lumps. Women should inform all care providers, regardless of the reason for evaluation, that they are receiving tamoxifen therapy.

Women receiving tamoxifen to reduce the incidence of breast cancer should receive clinical evaluation including a breast examination, a mammogram, and a gynecologic examination prior to the initiation of therapy with the drug. Such clinical evaluation should be repeated at regular intervals during tamoxifen therapy. The same type of clinical evaluation should be followed for women receiving tamoxifen as adjuvant therapy for breast cancer. Women receiving tamoxifen for the treatment of metastatic breast cancer should review this clinical monitoring plan with their care provider and select the appropriate modalities and schedule of evaluation.

The manufacturer states that tamoxifen should be used with caution in patients with leukopenia and thrombocytopenia, and periodic complete blood counts, including platelet counts, should be performed in patients receiving the drug. The manufacturer also states that periodic liver function tests should be obtained.

Because of infrequent reports of lipoprotein abnormalities in patients receiving tamoxifen, including cases of hypertriglyceridemia and marked hyperlipoproteinemia, periodic monitoring of serum triglycerides and cholesterol is recommended during tamoxifen therapy in patients with a preexisting hyperlipoproteinemia. However, potentially beneficial estrogenic effects on lipoproteins (e.g., decreased total and low-density lipoproteins concentrations) also may occur.

Patients complaining of visual changes or abnormalities during tamoxifen therapy should be assessed carefully for possible ocular toxicity. Women receiving or who have received tamoxifen should seek prompt medical attention for changes in vision.

Women who are at high risk of developing breast cancer may consider tamoxifen therapy to reduce the incidence of breast cancer. Women who are considering use of tamoxifen for reduction in the incidence of breast cancer should consult a health-care professional to assess their risk of breast cancer and weigh the potential benefits and risks of therapy. Women should be informed and understand that while tamoxifen therapy may reduce the incidence of breast cancer, it may not eliminate risk of the disease. Those electing to receive tamoxifen therapy should be advised to read the medication guide for tamoxifen prior to initiating therapy with the drug and each time the prescription is renewed. In the BCPT, tamoxifen decreased the incidence of small, estrogen receptor-positive tumors, but did not alter the incidence of larger (exceeding 2 cm in diameter) or estrogen receptor-negative breast tumors. In other clinical trials that were smaller than the BCPT and enrolled women at a lower risk for breast cancer, no difference in the number of cases of breast cancer was observed in women receiving tamoxifen or placebo. In women with breast cancer who are at high risk of developing a second breast cancer, treatment with about 5 years of tamoxifen reduced the annual incidence rate of a second breast cancer by approximately 50%.

Women who are pregnant or who plan to become pregnant should not use tamoxifen to reduce the risk of breast cancer. (See Cautions: Pregnancy, Fertility, and Lactation.)

Women with DCIS who are considering use of tamoxifen to reduce the risk of invasive breast cancer following surgery and radiation therapy should consult a health-care professional to assess the potential benefits and risks of therapy, since tamoxifen has been shown to reduce the incidence of invasive breast cancer but has not been shown to improve survival. Those electing to receive tamoxifen therapy should be advised to read the medication guide for tamoxifen prior to initiating therapy with the drug and each time the prescription is renewed.

Tamoxifen is contraindicated in patients with known hypersensitivity to the drug or other ingredients in the formulation.

■ **Pediatric Precautions** Tamoxifen has been used for the treatment of Albright syndrome† (also known as McCune-Albright syndrome) and precocious puberty in girls 2–10 years of age; however, the effects of tamoxifen beyond one year of treatment in these patients have not been established. In a noncomparative study, 28 girls 2–10 years of age with Albright syndrome and precocious puberty (manifested by physical signs of pubertal development, episodes of vaginal bleeding, and/or advanced bone age) received tamoxifen 20 mg once daily for up to 12 months. Tamoxifen therapy was associated with a 50% reduction in frequency of vaginal bleeding episodes and reductions in bone age maturation and linear growth velocity. An increase in mean uterine volume was observed following 6 months of therapy, with doubling of uterine volume observed after one year of therapy; however, a casual relationship to the drug has not been established. Because tamoxifen has been associated with an increased incidence of endometrial and uterine malignancies in adults, the manufacturer recommends continued monitoring for long-term uterine effects in pediatric patients receiving tamoxifen for the treatment of Albright syndrome.

■ **Geriatric Precautions** In the BCPT, 16% of the study participants were 65 years of age or older and 6% were at least 70 years of age. Reductions in the incidence of breast cancer were observed in women receiving tamoxifen across all age groups. Across all other outcomes, the results in the subset of women 65 years of age or older reflect the results observed in the subset of women at least 50 years of age. In this trial, the risk of serious adverse effects (e.g., endometrial cancer, pulmonary embolism, deep-vein thrombosis, stroke) was greatest in women 50 years of age and older.

In the National Surgical Adjuvant Breast and Bowel Project (NSABP) B-24 study evaluating tamoxifen in patients with DCIS, 23% of the study participants were 65 years of age or older and 10% were at least 70 years of age. Because invasive breast cancer occurred in relatively few tamoxifen- or placebo-treated women 65 years of age or older, the results were insufficient to determine whether geriatric patients respond differently than younger adults for this outcome. Across all other outcomes, no overall differences were observed between geriatric patients and younger adults. In this study, no overall differences in safety were observed between geriatric patients and younger adults.

■ **Mutagenicity and Carcinogenicity** ***Mutagenicity*** No evidence of tamoxifen-induced mutagenicity was observed in various in vivo and in vitro tests with prokaryotic and eukaryotic test systems in the presence of drug metabolizing systems. However, increased levels of DNA adducts have been found in cultured human lymphocytes and the livers of rats exposed to tamoxifen. Tamoxifen also has been found to increase levels of micronucleus formation in vitro in human lymphoblastoid cell lines (MCL-5). Thus, tamoxifen is potentially genotoxic in animals and in humans.

Carcinogenicity Tamoxifen is carcinogenic in animals and humans.

Uterine Cancer. In athymic mice, tamoxifen has stimulated the growth of certain endometrial tumors. An increased incidence of uterine sarcoma, endometrial cancer, and endometrial changes including hyperplasia and polyps has been reported in women receiving tamoxifen. The incidence and pattern of this increase is related to the estrogenic activity of tamoxifen. Some evidence suggests that prior exposure to hormone replacement therapy may contribute to the development of endometrial cancer and may be a confounding factor in determining the effect of tamoxifen therapy on the uterus.

An increased incidence of uterine cancer, sometimes fatal, has been reported in women receiving tamoxifen. Most uterine malignancies associated with tamoxifen therapy are classified as adenocarcinoma of the endometrium; however, rare uterine sarcomas, including malignant mixed mullerian tumors, also have been reported.

Uterine sarcoma has been reported more frequently among women receiving long-term therapy (i.e., exceeding 2 years) with tamoxifen than among women not receiving the drug. Among women enrolled in the BCPT, uterine sarcomas were reported in 4 women receiving tamoxifen versus one of the women receiving placebo (an incidence of 0.17 and 0.04 per 1000 women-years, respectively). Uterine sarcoma generally is associated with more advanced disease at the time of diagnosis, poorer prognosis, and shorter survival.

Long-term (i.e., exceeding 2 years) tamoxifen therapy has been associated with an increased risk (3.1–7.5 times that in untreated women) of developing endometrial cancer. In a large controlled study of adjuvant tamoxifen therapy (40 mg daily for 2–5 years) in women with early breast carcinoma, the relative risk of developing endometrial cancers associated with tamoxifen therapy was 5.6 times that of the control group (23 of 1372 tamoxifen-treated women and 4 of 1357 women in the control group developed cancers of the uterus). After approximately 6.8 years of follow-up in the National Surgical Adjuvant Breast and Bowel Project (NSABP) B-14 study, 15 of 1419 women randomized to receive tamoxifen 20 mg daily for 5 years developed uterine cancer; 2 of 1424 women who were receiving placebo initially, but who subsequently received tamoxifen for recurrent breast carcinoma, also developed uterine cancer. The relative risk of endometrial cancer in the tamoxifen-treated women was 7.5; most of the uterine cancers in tamoxifen-treated patients with breast cancer were diagnosed at an early stage, but deaths resulting from uterine cancer associated with tamoxifen therapy for the treatment of breast cancer have been reported.

Women receiving tamoxifen for the prevention of breast cancer in the Breast Cancer Prevention Trial (BCPT) had an approximately 3.1 times greater risk of developing an endometrial adenocarcinoma than women receiving placebo (53 versus 17 cases or an incidence of 2.2 versus 0.71 per 1000 women-years at a median follow-up of 6.9 years). The increased risk of developing endometrial cancer in women receiving tamoxifen for the prevention of breast cancer occurred predominantly in women 50 years of age or older at the time of randomization (relative risk of 4.5 according to data available as of January 31, 1998; relative risk of 4.01 according to data available as of March 31, 1998). According to age at the time of diagnosis of endometrial cancer, increase in risk of endometrial cancer was similar for women 49 years of age or younger (relative risk of 2.21) and women 50 years of age or older (relative risk of 2.5), although fewer cases of endometrial cancer occurred in younger women. Among women receiving tamoxifen in the BCPT, endometrial cancer was diagnosed on average at 32 months (range: 1–61 months) following initiation of therapy with the drug.

All but one of the women in the BCPT who developed endometrial cancer (a study participant receiving placebo who subsequently died of endometrial cancer) had early-stage disease that could be treated effectively with surgery (i.e., hysterectomy) with or without postoperative radiation therapy. The distribution according to stage of endometrial cancer (according to FIGO) was similar among women receiving tamoxifen or placebo.

Approximately 37% of the participants receiving tamoxifen or placebo in the BCPT had undergone a hysterectomy prior to enrollment in the study and therefore were not at risk for the development of endometrial cancer. For women in the BCPT who had an intact uterus, endometrial sampling (i.e., examination of cells from the lining of the uterus) did not alter the rate of detection of endometrial cancer; currently, no data suggest that routine endometrial sampling in asymptomatic women receiving tamoxifen to reduce the incidence of breast cancer would be beneficial. Endometrial cancer often is associated with clinical manifestations, such as abnormal vaginal bleeding or pelvic pain. About 88% of cases of endometrial cancer diagnosed in tamoxifen-treated women in the BCPT were associated with symptoms.

Endometrial hyperplasia can be a premalignant change. In one study of postmenopausal women receiving tamoxifen for the prevention of breast cancer, 16% developed atypical hyperplasia while no cases occurred in those receiving placebo; 8% of women receiving tamoxifen had an endometrial polyp compared with 2% of those receiving placebo. These findings were based on screening of a randomized cohort of women from the study who had not been screened before the initiation of therapy, and some of the women also were receiving hormone replacement therapy as permitted by the study protocol. Optimal management of women who develop endometrial changes during tamoxifen therapy remains to be elucidated; the value of progestins in reversing such hyperplasia is not established nor are their effects on breast cancer in tamoxifen-treated women adequately studied. Screening and management of women who develop endometrial hyperplasia during tamoxifen therapy should be individualized, weighing the risks and benefits of continued therapy with the drug.

Endometriosis also has been reported. In addition, variations in the karyopyknotic index on vaginal smears and varying degrees of estrogenic effects on the Papanicolaou test also have been reported in postmenopausal women receiving the drug. Patients receiving or having previously received tamoxifen should undergo routine gynecologic examinations, and they should be advised to report promptly any menstrual irregularities, abnormal vaginal bleeding, change in vaginal discharge, or pelvic pain/pressure to their clinician; the cause of such effects should be evaluated promptly.

Liver Cancer. In rats given 5, 20, or 35 mg/kg of tamoxifen daily (approximately 1, 3, or 7 times, respectively, the maximum recommended human dosage on a mg/m^2 basis) for up to 2 years, hepatocellular carcinoma occurred at all dosages. The incidence of this carcinoma in rats receiving 20 or 35 mg/kg daily (69%) was substantially greater than that in those given 5 mg/kg daily (14%), and the incidence in rats given 5 mg/kg daily was substantially greater than that in controls. In rats given 45 mg/kg of tamoxifen daily (approximately 9 times the maximum recommended human dosage on a mg/m^2 basis), hepatocellular neoplasms were evident at 3–6 months.

In a study of women with breast cancer receiving tamoxifen (40 mg daily) or no adjuvant endocrine therapy for 2–5 years, 3 cases of liver cancer were reported in women receiving tamoxifen versus 1 case in the control group. One case of liver cancer was reported among women receiving tamoxifen in the BCPT.

Other Cancers. Granulosa cell ovarian tumors and interstitial cell testicular tumors were observed in mice receiving trans and racemic formulations of the drug for 13–15 months at dosages of 5, 20, or 50 mg/kg daily (approximately 0.5, 2, or 5 times, respectively, the maximum recommended human dosage on a mg/m^2 basis); however, the relevance of these findings to humans is not known.

Data from the NSABP B-14 study did not reveal an increased incidence of carcinomas other than uterine carcinomas. However, several second primary tumors occurring at sites other than the endometrium have been reported in clinical studies; it currently is not known whether an increased risk of these carcinomas is associated with tamoxifen therapy, and additional studies are needed to evaluate the risk of this carcinogenicity. Tamoxifen therapy has been associated with a reduced incidence of second primary breast carcinomas.

■ **Pregnancy, Fertility, and Lactation** Tamoxifen may cause fetal harm when administered to pregnant women. Effects on reproductive function are expected from the antiestrogenic properties of the drug. In reproduction studies in rats using tamoxifen dosages equal to or less than the human dosage, nonteratogenic developmental skeletal changes were observed and were found to be reversible. In fertility studies in rats and teratology studies in rabbits using dosages at or below those used in humans, a lower incidence of egg implantation and a higher incidence of fetal death or retarded in utero growth were observed, reportedly with slower learning behavior in some rat offspring compared with historical controls, although this latter effect is not clearly established. No teratogenic effects were observed in monkeys receiving tamoxifen during the period of organogenesis or the last half of pregnancy; although the dosage employed was high enough to terminate pregnancy in some of the animals, those that maintained pregnancy delivered offspring without evidence of teratogenicity. In reproduction studies in rats using tamoxifen dosages 0.002–2.4 times the maximum recommended dosages in humans on a mg/m^2 basis, changes in both male and female similar to those caused by estradiol, ethynylestradiol, and diethylstilbestrol (DES) (no longer commercially available in the US) were observed. Although the clinical importance of these changes is unknown, some of these changes, especially vaginal adenosis, are similar to those observed in young women who were exposed to DES in utero; such women have a greater risk (1 in 1000) of developing clear-cell adenocarcinoma of the vagina or cervix. To date, in utero exposure to tamoxifen has not been shown to cause vaginal adenosis or clear-cell adenocarcinoma of the vagina or cervix in young women. However, only a small number of young women have been exposed to tamoxifen in utero; of these, a smaller number have been followed long enough (15–20 years) to determine whether vaginal or cervical neoplasia could occur as a result of exposure to tamoxifen.

There are no adequate and well-controlled studies using tamoxifen in pregnant women. There have been reports of spontaneous abortions, birth defects, fetal deaths, and vaginal bleeding. Women should not become pregnant while receiving tamoxifen or within 2 months after discontinuance of therapy with the drug, and those of childbearing potential should use an effective barrier or other nonhormonal method of contraception during tamoxifen therapy and for approximately 2 months after the drug has been discontinued. When tamoxifen is administered during pregnancy or if the patient becomes pregnant while receiving the drug or within approximately 2 months after discontinuance of therapy with tamoxifen, the patient should be informed of the potential hazard to the fetus, including the possible long-term risk of a DES-like syndrome.

For sexually active women of childbearing potential who are receiving tamoxifen for reduction in the incidence of breast cancer, therapy with the drug should be initiated during menstruation. In women with menstrual irregularity, pregnancy testing with a negative β-human chorionic gonadotropin (β-HCG) test result should be confirmed immediately prior to the initiation of tamoxifen therapy.

Marked reductions in fertility and reproductive indices, as well as death of all fetuses, were observed in reproduction studies in rats receiving tamoxifen. Tamoxifen has not been shown to cause infertility in women, including in the presence of menstrual irregularity.

It is not known if tamoxifen is distributed into milk. Direct exposure (not via breast milk) of neonatal mice and rat pups to tamoxifen has resulted in adverse reproductive tract effects (i.e., lesions in female pups that are similar to those observed in humans after intrauterine DES exposure; functional defects, including testicular atrophy and arrested spermatogenesis, in male pups). Because of the potential for serious adverse reactions to tamoxifen in nursing infants, a decision should be made whether to discontinue nursing or the drug, taking into account the importance of the drug to the woman. In 2 placebo-controlled trials, inhibition of early postpartum milk production was observed in women who received tamoxifen within 24 hours of delivery for a duration of 5–18 days. The effect of tamoxifen on established milk production is not known.

Drug Interactions

■ **Drugs Affecting Hepatic Microsomal Enzymes** Concomitant use of tamoxifen with inhibitors of cytochrome P-450 (CYP) isoenzyme 2D6 (e.g., bupropion, fluoxetine, paroxetine, quinidine) may result in decreased plasma concentrations of the active metabolite 4-hydroxy-*N*-desmethyltamoxifen (also known as endoxifen). (See Drug Interactions: Selective Serotonin-Reuptake Inhibitors.) However, studies investigating the effect of CYP2D6 inhibitors on tamoxifen efficacy have had substantial limitations and are inconclusive, as they have resulted in contradictory findings. Some experts recommend avoiding concomitant use of tamoxifen and weak, moderate, or potent CYP2D6 inhibitors in patients with a CYP2D6 intermediate- or normal/intermediate-metabolizer phenotype; these experts recommend that moderate or potent CYP2D6 inhibitors also be avoided in patients with CYP2D6 normal- or ultrarapid-metabolizer phenotype and that alternative adjuvant endocrine therapies (rather than tamoxifen) be used in patients with poor-metabolizer phenotype. (See Cytochrome P-450 Isoenzyme 2D6 Polymorphism under Breast Cancer: Pharmacogenomic Considerations for Tamoxifen Therapy, in Uses.) However, the role of CYP2D6 genotype testing in patients receiving tamoxifen remains controversial, and other experts make recommendations that are not dependent on genotyping results. Because the effect of CYP2D6-mediated interactions on long-term clinical outcomes of tamoxifen therapy is uncertain, these experts state that it is reasonable to avoid concomitant use of CYP2D6 inhibitors, particularly those with moderate or potent inhibitory activity, when possible in patients receiving tamoxifen.

Concomitant use of tamoxifen and drugs that induce CYP isoenzymes (e.g., phenobarbital, phenytoin, aminoglutethimide [no longer commercially available in the US]) may reduce plasma concentrations of tamoxifen and endoxifen. (See Drug Interactions: Other Drugs.) However, the clinical importance of this interaction has not been established. Nonetheless, some clinicians suggest that use of agents with the potential to induce multiple isoenzymes and transporters (e.g., carbamazepine, phenobarbital, phenytoin, rifabutin, rifampin, rifapentine, St. John's wort [*Hypericum perforatum*]) should be avoided in patients receiving tamoxifen.

■ **Anticoagulants** Tamoxifen has been reported to potentiate the hypoprothrombinemic effect of warfarin. In patients stabilized on warfarin therapy, substantial prolongations in prothrombin time have occurred within several days to weeks after initiation of tamoxifen therapy; overt signs of bleeding (e.g., hematemesis, hematuria, subdural hematoma, intraocular hemorrhage) also have occurred during concomitant therapy with the drugs. While the mechanism for this interaction currently is not known, tamoxifen and coumarin-derivative anticoagulants should be used concomitantly with caution. If the drugs are used concomitantly, the patient and prothrombin time should be monitored closely and dosage of the anticoagulant adjusted accordingly.

■ **Aromatase Inhibitors** Concomitant use of selective estrogen receptor modulators (e.g., tamoxifen) and aromatase inhibitors (e.g., anastrozole, exemestane, letrozole) is not recommended based on pharmacokinetic and clinical considerations. Data from a subprotocol of the Arimidex, Tamoxifen, Alone or in Combination (ATAC) trial indicate that concomitant use of tamoxifen and anastrozole does not affect the pharmacokinetics of tamoxifen or *N*-desmethyltamoxifen. The mean plasma anastrozole concentration was reduced by an average of 27% in patients receiving tamoxifen and anastrozole versus anastrozole alone, but analysis of blood samples from a different subprotocol of the ATAC trial demonstrated similar degrees of suppression of plasma estradiol concentrations for anastrozole alone and in combination with tamoxifen. Although the clinical importance of this pharmacokinetic interaction is uncertain, combination therapy did not demonstrate greater efficacy as adjuvant therapy for breast cancer than use of tamoxifen alone. When tamoxifen was used concomitantly with letrozole, the plasma letrozole concentration was reduced by 37%.

■ **Selective Serotonin-Reuptake Inhibitors** Substantial decreases in plasma concentrations of endoxifen have been observed in patients receiving concomitant therapy with tamoxifen and a selective serotonin-reuptake inhibitor (SSRI) with potent CYP2D6 inhibitory activity (i.e., paroxetine, fluoxetine). However, studies investigating the effect of SSRIs on tamoxifen efficacy have been inconclusive. SSRIs with moderate or potent CYP2D6 inhibitory activity should be avoided in patients receiving tamoxifen; if therapy with an antidepressant is required, use of an SSRI or selective serotonin- and norepinephrine-reuptake inhibitor (SNRI) with little or no inhibitory effect on CYP2D6 (e.g., citalopram, escitalopram, venlafaxine, desvenlafaxine) would be preferred. (See Drug Interactions: Drugs Affecting Hepatic Microsomal Enzymes.)

■ **Other Drugs** Concomitant use of rifampin and tamoxifen reportedly has decreased systemic exposure to tamoxifen and endoxifen by 84–86 and 70%, respectively. Following administration of aminoglutethimide (no longer commercially available in the US) in patients receiving tamoxifen therapy, systemic exposure to tamoxifen and endoxifen were decreased by 73 and 93%, respectively, while concentrations of other metabolites generally were reduced by about 50%; endoxifen concentrations were undetectable in 3 of 6 patients. Endoxifen concentrations also were markedly lower than predicted following initiation of tamoxifen therapy in a patient with CYP2D6 extensive-metabolizer phenotype who was receiving phenytoin. In at least one patient receiving tamoxifen and phenobarbital concomitantly, serum tamoxifen concentrations were decreased by about 80%. (See Drug Interactions: Drugs Affecting Hepatic Microsomal Enzymes.)

The effect of tamoxifen on the metabolism and excretion of other antineoplastic drugs, such as cyclophosphamide, and other drugs that require mixed function oxidases for activation, is unknown.

In vitro, erythromycin, cyclosporine, nifedipine, and diltiazem competitively inhibited formation of *N*-desmethyltamoxifen; however, the clinical importance of these interactions is unknown. Serum tamoxifen and *N*-desmethyltamoxifen concentrations reportedly were increased in patients receiving bromocriptine and tamoxifen concomitantly. Serum concentrations of *N*-desmethyltamoxifen, but not those of tamoxifen, are decreased in patients receiving medroxyprogesterone and tamoxifen concomitantly.

An increased risk of thromboembolic events has been observed in patients receiving tamoxifen concomitantly with cytotoxic drugs.

Laboratory Test Interferences

■ **Estrogen-Receptor Determinations** Because the elimination of tamoxifen and its principal metabolites is prolonged, false-negative estrogen-receptor determinations might result if the determination is performed too soon after discontinuance of tamoxifen therapy. To avoid this possibility it is recommended that estrogen-receptor determinations be delayed for 4–6 weeks after discontinuance of the drug.

■ **Thyroid Function Tests** Increased serum thyroxine concentrations, which were not accompanied by signs and symptoms of clinical hyperthyroidism and may be explained by increases in thyroxine-binding globulin, have occurred in a few postmenopausal women receiving tamoxifen.

Acute Toxicity

■ **Manifestations** In studies to determine the acute lethal dose of tamoxifen, respiratory difficulties and seizures were reported in animals receiving very high doses of tamoxifen. There currently is no information available on overdosage of tamoxifen in humans.

In one study to determine the maximum tolerated dose of tamoxifen, acute neurotoxicity, manifested by tremor, hyperreflexia, unsteady gait, and dizziness, occurred in patients with advanced (metastatic) carcinoma who were receiving very high dosages of tamoxifen (i.e., loading doses exceeding 400 mg/m^2 followed by maintenance dosages of 150 mg/m^2 given twice daily) to reverse multiple-drug resistance. These adverse effects occurred within 3–5 days of initiating tamoxifen therapy and disappeared 2–5 days after discontinuance of the drug. No permanent neurologic sequelae were reported in these patients. Although a causal relationship to tamoxifen has not been established, seizures were reported in at least one of these patients several days after discontinuance of the drug and disappearance of adverse nervous system effects. In patients receiving loading doses exceeding 250 mg/m^2 followed by maintenance doses of 80 mg/m^2 administered twice daily, prolongation of the QT interval was reported. In one female patient who had a body surface area of 1.5 m^2, the minimal loading and maintenance doses of the drug at which neurological symptoms and prolongation of the QT interval occurred were at least sixfold higher than the maximum recommended dose.

■ **Treatment** The manufacturer recommends no specific treatment for tamoxifen overdosage and states that treatment should be symptomatic.

Pharmacology

Tamoxifen citrate, a nonsteroidal antiestrogen, is a triphenylethylene derivative with both estrogen antagonist (antiestrogen) and agonist (estrogen-like) activity. Tamoxifen acts as an estrogen antagonist on breast tissue and in the CNS and as an estrogen agonist on endometrium, bone, and lipids. The precise mechanism(s) of action of the drug is not known. Tamoxifen and at least several of its metabolites compete with estradiol for binding to cytoplasmic estrogen receptors in tissues such as breast, uterus, vagina, anterior pituitary, and tumors containing high concentrations of estrogen receptors.

■ **Effects on the Breast** The competition of tamoxifen and at least several of its metabolites with estradiol for binding to cytoplasmic estrogen receptors in breast tissue is thought to contribute to its protective effect against the development of breast cancer. Although the tamoxifen-receptor and metabolite-receptor complexes are translocated to the nucleus, binding to nuclear chromatin appears to occur in an atypical manner and persists for longer periods of time than the estrogen-receptor complexes. DNA synthesis and estrogen responses are thus markedly reduced. Contrary to a previous hypothesis, a study in rats demonstrated that tamoxifen does not interfere with replenishment of cytoplasmic estrogen receptors. The in vivo antiestrogenic and antitumor effects of tamoxifen appear to result from the combined actions of unchanged drug and several of the identified metabolites, but their relative contribution remains to be fully elucidated.

Tamoxifen also appears to oppose the proliferative effects of estrogen on breast epithelium by increasing production of inhibitory factors (e.g., transforming growth factor [TGF]-β) and decreasing production of stimulatory factors (e.g., TGF-α, insulin-like growth factor-1) that influence breast cell growth.

■ **Effects on Bone** In vitro and animal studies show that tamoxifen acts as an estrogen agonist on bone. Results of an in vitro study show that tamoxifen inhibits the resorbing activity of osteoclasts. In oophorectomized rats, tamoxifen prevented increased bone resorption and bone loss. In humans, tamoxifen reduces bone resorption and decreases bone turnover as manifested by reductions in serum and urine concentrations of bone turnover markers (e.g., alkaline phosphatase, osteocalcin) and increases in bone mineral density. Tamoxifen appears to act mainly on sites of trabecular bone, such as the lumbar spine, and seems to have little effect on cortical bone (e.g., radial bone).

Healthy postmenopausal women receiving tamoxifen 20 mg daily for 2 years experienced a small increase in mean bone mineral density of the lumbar spine compared with those receiving placebo; no effect of tamoxifen was observed on bone mineral density of the proximal femur. In studies of postmenopausal women receiving long-term treatment (i.e., at least 2 years) with tamoxifen as adjuvant therapy for early-stage breast cancer, tamoxifen preserved bone mass in the lumbar spine. In the Breast Cancer Prevention Trial (BCPT), women receiving tamoxifen had fewer fractures of the hip than those receiving placebo (12 versus 22 cases, respectively), but the difference was not significant, and the total number of fractures identified as most likely to be associated with osteoporosis (hip, wrist, and spine) was similar (111 versus 137 cases, respectively); because of the small number of fracture events overall, no definitive conclusions could be drawn from this study regarding the effect of tamoxifen on the rate of fractures.

Some evidence suggests that the effects of tamoxifen on bone mineral density depend on menopausal status. In a pilot trial conducted in the UK for the prevention of breast cancer, postmenopausal women receiving tamoxifen had an increase in bone mineral density of the lumbar spine and hip compared with those receiving placebo; in contrast, premenopausal women receiving tamoxifen had loss of bone mineral density in the lumbar spine and hip, which may increase the risk of osteoporosis and fracture, compared with those receiving placebo. Similarly, subgroup analysis of data from the BCPT showed no evidence of bone loss at the lumbar spine and hip in tamoxifen-treated postmenopausal women, but tamoxifen was associated with substantial bone loss at the lumbar spine and hip in premenopausal women. Additional studies and long-term follow-up are needed to confirm the effects of tamoxifen on bone loss in premenopausal women. Although clinicians generally recommend evaluation and treatment of osteoporosis in postmenopausal women only, some experts propose investigation of preventive measures for osteoporosis (e.g., bisphosphonates, hormone replacement therapy) in premenopausal women receiving tamoxifen for the prevention and treatment of breast cancer. Further study is needed to evaluate the long-term effects of tamoxifen on bone mineral density and risk of osteoporosis and fracture in healthy women.

Further study is needed to establish the potentially beneficial effects of tamoxifen on bone density and risk of osteoporosis; although it may be considered in the risk-benefit analysis of tamoxifen for the prevention and/or treatment of breast cancer, this effect alone is *not* an indication for tamoxifen therapy.

■ **Effects on Lipoproteins** Tamoxifen, like estrogens, favorably affects serum cholesterol by decreasing total and low-density lipoprotein (LDL)-cholesterol concentrations. Less favorably, tamoxifen appears to moderately decrease high-density lipoprotein (HDL)-cholesterol concentrations and increase triglyceride concentrations.

Results of studies to determine whether favorable alterations in serum lipoproteins induced by tamoxifen result in reduced risk of cardiovascular events have been inconsistent. In a large randomized trial conducted in Scotland, postmenopausal women who received adjuvant therapy with tamoxifen for a 5-year period immediately following mastectomy for operable breast cancer had fewer fatal myocardial infarctions than patients who received tamoxifen for a minimum of 6 weeks upon first recurrence of breast cancer. In the Stockholm study, retrospective analysis showed that postmenopausal women with early-stage breast cancer who received adjuvant therapy with tamoxifen had less cardiac morbidity than those who received placebo; the reduction in cardiac morbidity was greater for women receiving tamoxifen for a longer duration (i.e., 5 versus 2 years). Findings from the NSABP protocol B-14 suggested a trend toward reduced mortality from coronary heart disease among women with node-negative, estrogen receptor-positive breast cancer receiving 5 years of therapy with tamoxifen versus placebo, but the difference between the groups was not significant. Although a 20% reduction in mortality from cardiovascular events was projected for women receiving tamoxifen in the BCPT, the incidence of fatal and nonfatal myocardial infarctions was similar among women receiving tamoxifen or placebo; the number of events of severe angina or acute ischemic syndrome also did not differ between the groups. Because of the age distribution of women in the BCPT (about 30% were 60 years of age or older), some experts have questioned whether the sample size of women at risk for myocardial infarction would be sufficient to detect a positive effect of tamoxifen on cardiovascular disease.

Further study and longer follow-up are needed to establish the effect of tamoxifen on serum lipoprotein concentrations and cardiovascular morbidity/mortality; although it may be considered in the risk-benefit analysis of tamoxifen for the prevention and/or treatment of breast cancer, this effect alone is *not* an indication for tamoxifen therapy.

■ **Effects on the Uterus** Tamoxifen acts as an estrogen agonist on the uterus and exhibits proliferative and tumor-promoting effects on the endometrium. (See Cautions: Mutagenicity and Carcinogenicity.)

■ **Other Effects** Following short-term administration in anovulatory women, tamoxifen may induce ovulation by stimulating the release of the hypothalamic gonadotropin-releasing factor with a resulting increase in secretion of pituitary gonadotropin.

Pharmacokinetics

■ **Absorption** Tamoxifen appears to be absorbed slowly following oral administration, with peak serum concentrations generally occurring about 3–6 hours after a single dose. The extent of absorption in humans has not been adequately determined, but limited data from animal studies suggest that the drug is well absorbed. Data from animal studies also suggest that tamoxifen and/or its metabolites undergo extensive enterohepatic circulation.

Following oral administration, peak serum tamoxifen concentrations average about 17 ng/mL after a single 10-mg dose, about 40 ng/mL after a single 20-mg dose, and 65–70 ng/mL after a single 40-mg dose; however, there is considerable interindividual variation in serum tamoxifen concentrations attained after single doses and at steady state with continuous dosing. Following a single oral dose of tamoxifen, peak serum concentrations of *N*-desmethyltamoxifen, the major metabolite of the drug, generally range from about 15–50% those of unchanged tamoxifen; however, with continuous dosing, steady-state serum concentrations of *N*-desmethyltamoxifen generally range from about 1–2 times those of unchanged tamoxifen. Following continuous administration in patients receiving oral tamoxifen 10 mg twice daily for 3 months, steady-state plasma concentrations of tamoxifen and *N*-desmethyltamoxifen average about 120 ng/mL (range: 67–183 ng/mL) and 336 ng/mL (range: 148–654 ng/mL), respectively. Steady-state serum concentrations of tamoxifen are generally attained after 3–4 weeks of continuous dosing, while those of *N*-desmethyltamoxifen are generally attained after 3–8 weeks of continuous dosing. Steady-state serum concentrations can be attained more rapidly with a loading-dose regimen, but there is no therapeutic advantage with such a regimen. In a 3-month crossover study, the steady-state oral bioavailability of 20-mg tamoxifen tablets (administered once daily) was similar to that of 10-mg tablets (administered twice daily).

In 27 girls 2–10 years of age receiving tamoxifen (20 mg once daily) for the treatment of Albright syndrome, the average steady-state peak plasma concentration of tamoxifen was achieved approximately 8 hours following administration. Systemic exposure to *N*-desmethyltamoxifen was comparable between pediatric patients and adults.

■ **Distribution** Distribution of tamoxifen and its metabolites into human body tissues and fluids has not been fully characterized. In a study in a limited number of women given radiolabeled tamoxifen prior to hysterectomy, concentrations of radioactivity in uterine tissues were greater than those in serum 4–96 hours after the drug was given; highest uterine concentrations of radioactivity were present in the endometrium. Tamoxifen metabolites are distributed into bile in animals. Distribution of tamoxifen and its principal metabolites in the cytosol of human breast tumor tissue generally appears to parallel the relative concentrations present in serum, although cytosol concentrations may exhibit even greater interindividual variation than serum concentrations.

It is not known if tamoxifen is distributed into milk.

■ **Elimination** Limited data suggest that tamoxifen has a distribution half-life of 7–14 hours and an elimination half-life of about 5–7 days (range: 3–21 days). The elimination half-life of *N*-desmethyltamoxifen, the major metabolite, is estimated to be approximately 14 days.

Tamoxifen is rapidly and extensively metabolized in the liver, principally by demethylation and hydroxylation. Although multiple cytochrome P-450 (CYP) isoenzymes, including 1A2, 2B6, 2C9, 2C19, 2D6, and 3A4/5, are involved in the metabolism of tamoxifen, the principal metabolic pathway involves demethylation of the parent drug, mediated mainly by CYP3A4/5, to form *N*-desmethyltamoxifen, followed by CYP2D6-mediated hydroxylation to form 4-hydroxy-*N*-desmethyltamoxifen (also known as endoxifen). *N*-Desmethyltamoxifen also undergoes CYP3A4/5-mediated demethylation to form *N,N*-didesmethyltamoxifen. Formation of *N*-desmethyltamoxifen accounts for approximately 92% of the metabolism of the parent drug. Tamoxifen also is metabolized to a lesser extent (approximately 7%) by CYP isoenzymes, mainly CYP2D6, to form 4-hydroxytamoxifen, which undergoes further metabolism to form endoxifen and polar conjugates. Other metabolites, including metabolite E, 4-hydroxy-*N,N*-didesmethyltamoxifen (norendoxifen), and tamoxifen bisphenol, also have been identified. Tamoxifen and its metabolites also are metabolized by multiple uridine diphosphate-glucuronosyltransferase (UGT) isoenzymes and to a lesser extent by sulfotransferases (mainly SULT1A1) to form glucuronide and sulfate conjugates, respectively.

Tamoxifen and its metabolites exhibit a range of affinities and effects (antagonistic or agonistic) at estrogen receptors. Whereas unchanged tamoxifen is a weak antiestrogen, both endoxifen and 4-hydroxytamoxifen are potent antiestrogens, exhibiting 100-fold greater affinity for estrogen receptors and 30- to 100-fold greater suppression of estrogen-dependent cell proliferation compared with tamoxifen; because plasma concentrations of endoxifen are up to tenfold higher than those of 4-hydroxytamoxifen, endoxifen is considered the major active metabolite of tamoxifen. The biologic activity of the metabolite *N*-desmethyltamoxifen appears to be similar to that of tamoxifen. Both interindividual and intraindividual variation in concentrations of tamoxifen and its metabolites have been observed. With continuous administration of tamoxifen, serum concentrations of *N*-desmethyltamoxifen are generally about 1–2 times those of unchanged tamoxifen, while those of *N,N*-desdimethyltamoxifen are about 20–40% of those of unchanged tamoxifen; concentrations of the hydroxylated metabolites and metabolite E appear to be less than 5% of those of unchanged tamoxifen.

Studies indicate that endoxifen exposure is strongly associated with CYP2D6 metabolizer phenotype, but genetic polymorphism of CYP2D6 explains only part (approximately 30–53%) of the observed variability in endoxifen concentrations. Individuals with low CYP2D6 activity (from CYP2D6 polymorphism or concomitant use with a potent CYP2D6 inhibitor) exhibit substantially lower serum concentrations of endoxifen; however, studies evaluating the effect of these pharmacogenomic factors and drug interactions on breast cancer recurrence have been inconclusive. (See Cytochrome P-450 Isoenzyme 2D6 Polymorphism under Breast Cancer: Pharmacogenomic Considerations for Tamoxifen Therapy, in Uses.)

The excretory fate of tamoxifen and its metabolites has not been well characterized. Following oral administration of a 20-mg dose of radiolabeled tamoxifen in women, approximately 65% of the administered dose was excreted in feces over a 2-week period, mainly as polar conjugates; unchanged tamoxifen and unconjugated metabolites accounted for less than 30% of the fecal radioactivity. Unchanged tamoxifen and *N*-desmethyltamoxifen have been detected in urine in small amounts. In animals, tamoxifen and/or its metabolites appear to undergo extensive enterohepatic circulation and are excreted in feces and urine as glucuronides, other conjugates, and unidentified polar metabolites.

In 27 girls 2–10 years of age receiving tamoxifen (20 mg once daily) for the treatment of Albright syndrome, clearance of the drug adjusted for body weight was approximately 2.3-fold higher than clearance in women with breast cancer; among those 2–6 or 7–10 years of age, clearance was increased by 2.6- or 1.9-fold, respectively.

The effects of age, gender, race, and hepatic impairment on the pharmacokinetics of tamoxifen have not been established.

Chemistry and Stability

■ **Chemistry** Tamoxifen is a triphenylethylene-derivative, nonsteroidal estrogen agonist-antagonist that is structurally related to clomiphene. Like clomiphene and toremifene, tamoxifen previously was referred to as an antiestrogen because it was thought to be devoid of clinically important estrogen agonist activity. However, like these drugs and raloxifene, tamoxifen exhibits both estrogen agonist and antagonist activity, although the overall pharmacologic profiles of the drugs differ.

Tamoxifen citrate occurs as a fine, white crystalline powder and has a solubility of 0.5 mg/mL in water at 37°C and is very slightly soluble in alcohol. The drug has a pK_a of 8.85.

■ **Stability** Commercially available tamoxifen tablets should be protected from light and stored in well-closed containers at controlled room temperature (20–25°C).

For further information on the handling of antineoplastic agents, see the ASHP Guidelines on Handling Hazardous Drugs at http://www.ahfsdruginformation.com.

Preparations

Excipients in commercially available drug preparations may have clinically important effects in some individuals; consult specific product labeling for details.

Tamoxifen Citrate

Oral		
Tablets	10 mg (of tamoxifen)*	**Tamoxifen Citrate Tablets**
	20 mg (of tamoxifen)*	**Tamoxifen Citrate Tablets**
Tablets, film-coated	10 mg (of tamoxifen)*	**Tamoxifen Citrate Tablets**
	20 mg (of tamoxifen)*	**Tamoxifen Citrate Tablets**

*available from one or more manufacturer, distributor, and/or repackager by generic (nonproprietary) name

†Use is not currently included in the labeling approved by the US Food and Drug Administration

Biguanides 68:20.04

metFORMIN Hydrochloride

Dimethylbiguanide Hydrochloride

■ Metformin hydrochloride is a biguanide antidiabetic agent.

Uses

■ **Diabetes Mellitus** Metformin is used as monotherapy as an adjunct to diet and exercise to improve glycemic control in patients with type 2 diabetes mellitus. Metformin may also be used in combination with a sulfonylurea or a thiazolidinedione antidiabetic agent as an adjunct to diet and exercise in patients with type 2 diabetes mellitus who do not achieve adequate glycemic control with metformin, sulfonylurea, or thiazolidinedione monotherapy.

Metformin may be used with repaglinide in patients with type 2 diabetes mellitus who have inadequate glycemic control with metformin or repaglinide monotherapy. Metformin is commercially available in fixed combination with repaglinide for use in patients with type 2 diabetes mellitus who are already receiving repaglinide and metformin concurrently as separate components or in those who have inadequate glycemic control with repaglinide or metformin monotherapy. Metformin also may be used concomitantly with nateglinide for the management of type 2 diabetes mellitus in treatment-naive patients (those not previously treated with antidiabetic agents) as well as in those who have previously received antidiabetic therapy.

Metformin is commercially available in fixed combination with glyburide or glipizide for use as an adjunct to diet and exercise to improve glycemic control in adults with diabetes mellitus; such fixed-combination preparations may be used as initial therapy in patients whose hyperglycemia cannot be controlled by diet and exercise alone, or as second-line therapy in patients who do not achieve adequate control of hyperglycemia with metformin or sulfonylurea monotherapy. A thiazolidinedione may be added to metformin in fixed combination with glyburide in patients who have inadequate glycemic control with fixed-combination therapy.

Metformin is commercially available in fixed combination with rosiglitazone for use in the management of type 2 diabetes mellitus when treatment with both rosiglitazone and metformin is appropriate. Metformin is commercially available in fixed combination with pioglitazone (as immediate- or extended-release tablets) for use as an adjunct to diet and exercise in patients with type 2 diabetes mellitus who have inadequate glycemic control with pioglitazone or metformin monotherapy or in those who are already receiving pioglitazone and metformin concurrently as separate components.

Metformin is commercially available in fixed combination with a dipeptidyl peptidase-4 [DPP-4] inhibitor (e.g., alogliptin, linagliptin, saxagliptin, sitagliptin) for use when treatment with both drug components is appropriate.

Metformin is commercially available in fixed combinations with the sodium-glucose cotransporter-2 (SGLT2) inhibitors canagliflozin, dapagliflozin, empagliflozin, or ertugliflozin for use when treatment with both drug components is appropriate.

Metformin also may be used as adjunctive therapy in patients with type 2 diabetes mellitus receiving insulin therapy to improve glycemic control and/or decrease the dosage of insulin needed to obtain optimal glycemic control.

The American Diabetes Association (ADA) currently classifies diabetes mellitus as type 1 (due to autoimmune β-cell destruction, usually leading to absolute insulin deficiency); type 2 (due to a progressive loss of β-cell insulin secretion, frequently on the background of insulin resistance); gestational diabetes mellitus (diabetes diagnosed in the second or third trimester of pregnancy that was not clearly overt diabetes prior to gestation); or specific types of diabetes due to other causes, such as monogenic diabetes syndromes (e.g., neonatal diabetes or maturity-onset diabetes of the young [MODY]), diseases of the exocrine pancreas (e.g., cystic fibrosis, pancreatitis), or drug- or chemical-induced diabetes (e.g., that associated with glucocorticoid use, the treatment of HIV/AIDS, organ transplantation). According to ADA and other experts, a diagnosis of diabetes mellitus currently is established by a fasting plasma glucose of 126 mg/dL or greater, a 2-hour plasma glucose of 200 mg/dL or greater during an oral glucose tolerance test, or a glycosylated hemoglobin (hemoglobin A_{1c}; HbA_{1c}) concentration of 6.5% or greater; results should be confirmed by repeat testing in the absence of unequivocal hyperglycemia. Alternatively, a random plasma glucose of 200 mg/dL or greater in a patient with classic symptoms of hyperglycemia or hyperglycemic crisis is considered confirmation of the diagnosis of diabetes mellitus.

Type 1 diabetes mellitus was previously described as juvenile-onset diabetes mellitus, since it usually occurs during youth. Type 2 diabetes mellitus previously was described as adult-onset diabetes mellitus. However, type 1 or type 2 diabetes mellitus can occur at any age, and the current classification is based on pathogenesis (e.g., autoimmune destruction of pancreatic β cells, insulin resistance) and clinical presentation rather than on age of onset. In both type 1 and type 2 diabetes mellitus, various genetic and environmental factors can result in the progressive loss of β-cell mass and/or function that manifests clinically as hyperglycemia. Epidemiologic data indicate that the incidence of type 2 diabetes mellitus is increasing in children and adolescents.

Patients with type 2 diabetes mellitus have insulin resistance and usually have relative (rather than absolute) insulin deficiency. Most patients with type 2 diabetes mellitus (about 80–90%) are overweight or obese; obesity itself also contributes to the insulin resistance and glucose intolerance observed in these patients. Patients with type 2 diabetes mellitus who are not obese may have an increased percentage of abdominal fat, which is an indicator of increased cardiometabolic risk. While children with immune-mediated type 1 diabetes mellitus generally are not overweight, the incidence of obesity in children with this form of diabetes is increasing with the increasing incidence of obesity in the US population. Distinguishing between type 1 and type 2 diabetes mellitus in children may be difficult since obesity may occur with either type of diabetes mellitus, and autoantigens and ketosis may be present in a substantial number of children with features of type 2 diabetes mellitus (e.g., obesity, acanthosis nigricans).

Metformin is *not* effective as sole therapy in patients with type 1 diabetes mellitus†; insulin is necessary in these patients.

Patients with type 2 diabetes mellitus are *not* dependent initially on insulin (although many patients eventually require insulin for glycemic control) nor are they prone to ketosis; however, insulin occasionally may be required for correction of symptomatic or persistent hyperglycemia that is not controlled by dietary regulation or oral antidiabetic agents (e.g., sulfonylureas), and ketosis occasionally may develop during periods of severe stress (e.g., acute infection, trauma, surgery, use of certain drugs [e.g., corticosteroids, atypical antipsychotics, SGLT2 inhibitors]). Type 2 diabetes mellitus is a heterogeneous subclass of the disease; hyperglycemia in these patients often is accompanied by other metabolic abnormalities such as obesity, hypertension, hyperlipidemia, and impaired fibrinolysis. Endogenous insulin is present in type 2 diabetic patients, although plasma insulin concentrations may be decreased, increased, or normal. In patients with type 2 diabetes mellitus, glucose-stimulated secretion of endogenous insulin is frequently, but not always, reduced and decreased peripheral sensitivity to insulin is almost always associated with glucose intolerance.

Glycemic Control and Microvascular Complications Current evidence from epidemiologic and clinical studies supports an association between chronic hyperglycemia and the pathogenesis of microvascular complications in patients with diabetes mellitus, and results of randomized, controlled studies in patients with type 1 diabetes mellitus indicate that intensive management of hyperglycemia with near-normalization of blood glucose and glycosylated hemoglobin (hemoglobin A_{1c} [HbA_{1c}]) concentrations provides substantial benefits in terms of reducing chronic microvascular (e.g., neuropathy, retinopathy, nephropathy) complications associated with the disease. HbA_{1c} concentration reflects the glycosylation of other proteins throughout the body as a result of recent hyperglycemia and is used as a predictor of risk for the development of diabetic microvascular complications (e.g., neuropathy, retinopathy, nephropathy). Microvascular complications of diabetes are the principal causes of blindness and renal failure in developed countries and are more closely associated with hyperglycemia than are macrovascular complications.

In the Diabetes Control and Complications Trial (DCCT), a reduction of approximately 50–75% in the risk of development or progression of retinopathy, nephropathy, and neuropathy was demonstrated during an average 6.5 years of follow-up in patients with type 1 diabetes mellitus receiving intensive insulin treatment (3 or more insulin injections daily with dosage adjusted according to results of at least 4 daily blood glucose determinations, dietary intake, and anticipated exercise) compared with that in patients receiving conventional insulin treatment (1 or 2 insulin injections daily, self-monitoring of blood or urine glucose values, education about diet and exercise). However, the incidence of severe hypoglycemia, including multiple episodes in some patients, was 3 times higher in the intensive-treatment group than in the conventional-treatment group. The reduction in risk of microvascular complications in the DCCT study correlated continuously with the reduction in HbA_{1c} concentration (hemoglobin A_{1c}) produced by intensive insulin treatment (e.g., a 40% reduction in risk of microvascular disease for each 10% reduction in hemoglobin A_{1c}). These data imply that any decrease in HbA_{1c} levels is beneficial and that complete normalization of blood glucose concentrations may prevent diabetic microvascular complications.

The DCCT was terminated prematurely because of the pronounced benefits of intensive insulin regimens, and all treatment groups were encouraged to institute or continue such intensive insulin therapy. In the Epidemiology of Diabetes Interventions and Complications (EDIC) study, the long-term, open-label continuation phase of the DCCT, the reduction in the risk of microvascular complications (e.g., retinopathy, nephropathy, neuropathy) associated with intensive insulin therapy has been maintained throughout 7 years of follow-up. In addition, the prevalence of hypertension (an important consequence of diabetic nephropathy) in those receiving conventional therapy has exceeded that of those receiving intensive therapy. Patients receiving conventional insulin therapy in the DCCT were able to achieve a lower HbA_{1c} when switched to intensive therapy in the continuation study, although the average HbA_{1c} values achieved during the continuation study were higher (i.e., worse) than those achieved during the DCCT with intensive insulin therapy. Patients who remained on intensive insulin therapy during the EDIC continuation study were not able to maintain the degree of glycemic control achieved during the DCCT; by 5 years of follow-up in the EDIC study, HbA_{1c} values were similar in both intensive and conventional therapy groups. The EDIC study demonstrated that the greater the duration of chronically elevated plasma glucose concentrations (as determined by HbA_{1c} values), the greater the risk of microvascular complications. Conversely, the longer patients can maintain a target HbA_{1c} of 7% of less, the greater the delay in the onset of these complications.

In another randomized, controlled study (Stockholm Diabetes Intervention Study) in patients with type 1 diabetes mellitus who were evaluated for up to 7.5 years, blood glucose control (as determined by HbA_{1c} concentrations) was improved, and the incidence of microvascular complications (e.g., decreased visual acuity, retinopathy, nephropathy, decreased nerve conduction velocity) reduced, with intensive insulin treatment (e.g., at least 3 insulin injections daily accompanied by intensive educational efforts) compared with that in patients receiving standard treatment (e.g., generally 2 insulin injections daily without intensive educational efforts).

Data from the United Kingdom Prospective Diabetes Study (UKPDS) and the Action in Diabetes and VAscular disease: preterax and diamicroN modified release Controlled Evaluation (ADVANCE) study in patients with type 2 diabetes mellitus generally are consistent with the same benefits of oral hypoglycemic agents on microvascular complications as those observed in type 1 diabetics receiving insulin therapy in the DCCT.

The UKPDS evaluated middle-aged, newly diagnosed, overweight (exceeding 120% of ideal body weight) or non-overweight patients with type 2 diabetes mellitus who received conventional or intensive treatment regimens with an oral sulfonylurea agent and/or insulin; overweight patients also could be allocated to metformin therapy in the same proportions as those allocated to sulfonylureas and insulin. Initial therapy consisted of an oral antidiabetic agent (sulfonylurea or metformin) or insulin, with stepwise addition of metformin (or glyburide in those initially allocated to metformin) in those poorly controlled on initial therapy or conversion to insulin alone in patients not adequately controlled with 2 oral agents. Intensive treatment consisted of antidiabetic therapy targeted to a fasting plasma glucose concentration of less than 108 mg/dL or, in patients receiving insulin, preprandial glucose concentrations of 72–126 mg/dL. Conventional treatment consisted of antidiabetic therapy targeted to a fasting plasma glucose concentration of less than 270 mg/dL without symptoms of hyperglycemia. Results of UKPDS indicate greater beneficial effects on retinopathy, nephropathy, and possibly neuropathy with intensive glucose-lowering therapy (median achieved HbA_{1c} concentration: 7%) in type 2 diabetics compared with that in the conventional treatment group (median achieved HbA_{1c} concentration: 7.9%). The overall incidence of microvascular complications was reduced by 25% with intensive therapy. Epidemiologic analysis of UKPDS results indicates a continuous relationship between the risks of microvascular complications and glycemia, with a 35% reduction in risk for each 1% reduction in HbA_{1c}, and no evidence of a glycemic threshold.

The ADVANCE study also evaluated the relatively short-term effects (median follow-up: 5 years) of conventional or intensive therapy on the development of major vascular complications. The primary end point was the composite of major macrovascular (death from cardiovascular events, nonfatal myocardial infarction, or nonfatal stroke) and major microvascular (new or worsening nephropathy or retinopathy) events. While the incidence of the primary composite end point was reduced by approximately 10% in the ADVANCE study, the beneficial effect was due principally to a 21% reduction in microvascular events (nephropathy); there was no appreciable reduction in macrovascular outcomes. Intensive antidiabetic therapy (mean achieved HbA_{1c} concentration: 6.5%) was associated with a reduction in new or worsening nephropathy compared with conventional treatment (mean achieved HbA_{1c} concentration of 7.3%), but there was no effect on the development of new or worsening retinopathy. Results of the Veterans Affairs Diabetes Trial (VADT), another study similar in design to the ADVANCE study, also indicated that intensive therapy in patients with poorly controlled type 2 diabetes mellitus (median baseline HbA_{1c} concentration of 9.4%) did not lessen the rate of microvascular complications compared with standard antidiabetic therapy.

In UKPDS, fasting plasma glucose concentrations and HbA_{1c} values steadily increased over 10 years in the patients receiving conventional therapy, and more than 80% of these patients eventually required antidiabetic therapy in addition to diet to maintain fasting plasma glucose concentrations within the desired goal of less than 270 mg/dL. In patients receiving intensive therapy initiated with chlorpropamide, glyburide, or insulin, fasting plasma glucose concentrations and HbA_{1c} values decreased during the first year of the study. Subsequent increases in these indices of glycemic control after the first year paralleled that in the conventional therapy group for the remainder of the study, indicating slow decline of pancreatic β-cell function and loss of glycemic control regardless of intensity of therapy. In contrast to UKPDS, no diminution in the effect on HbA_{1c} or fasting blood glucose concentrations with either intensive or conventional therapy was observed in ADVANCE or VADT over a median follow-up of 5 or 5.6 years, respectively.

Data from long-term follow-up (over 10 years) of middle-aged, newly diagnosed UKPDS patients with type 2 diabetes mellitus indicate that strict glycemic control (i.e., maintenance of fasting blood glucose concentrations below 108 mg/dL) was not achieved with initial intensive oral antidiabetic therapy (stepwise introduction of a sulfonylurea [i.e., chlorpropamide, glyburide], then insulin, or an oral sulfonylurea and insulin, or insulin alone to achieve fasting plasma glucose concentrations of 108 mg/dL) in most patients; at 3 and 9 years, 50 and 75%, respectively, of patients required combination therapy with sulfonylureas or initiation of insulin to maintain adequate glycemic control. While strict guidelines for insulin dosage adjustments were used in the DCCT study, adjustments of antidiabetic therapy dosage in UKPDS were not as frequent (dosage adjustments allowed every 3 months); in addition, the definition of secondary treatment failure with sulfonylureas and the time of institution of supplementary antidiabetic therapy changed as the study progressed. Because of the benefits of strict glycemic control, the goal of therapy for type 2 diabetes mellitus is to lower blood glucose to as close to normal as possible, which generally requires aggressive management efforts (e.g., mixing therapy with various antidiabetic agents including sulfonylureas, metformin, insulin, and/or possibly others) over time. For additional information on clinical studies demonstrating the benefits of strict glycemic control on microvascular complications in patients with type 1 or type 2 diabetes mellitus, see Glycemic Control and Microvascular Complications under Uses: Diabetes Mellitus, in the Insulins General Statement 68:20.08.

Macrovascular Outcomes and Cardiovascular Risk Reduction Current evidence indicates that appropriate management of dyslipidemia, blood pressure, and vascular thrombosis provides substantial benefits in terms of reducing macrovascular complications associated with diabetes mellitus; intensive glycemic control generally has not been associated with appreciable reductions in macrovascular outcomes in controlled trials. Reduction in blood pressure to a mean of 144/82 mm Hg ("tight blood pressure control") in patients with diabetes mellitus and uncomplicated mild to moderate hypertension in UKPDS substantially reduced the incidence of virtually all macrovascular (e.g., stroke, heart failure) and microvascular (e.g., retinopathy, vitreous hemorrhage, renal failure) outcomes and diabetes-related mortality; blood pressure and glycemic control were additive in their beneficial effects on these end points. While intensive antidiabetic therapy titrated with the goal of reducing HbA_{1c} to near-normal concentrations (6–6.5% or less) has not been associated with appreciable reductions in cardiovascular events during the randomized portion of controlled trials examining such outcomes, results of long-term follow-up (10–11 years) from DCCT and UKPDS indicate a delayed cardiovascular benefit in patients treated with intensive antidiabetic therapy early in the course of type 1 or type 2 diabetes mellitus. Recent evidence suggests that therapy with certain SGLT2 inhibitors or GLP-1 agonists can reduce the risk of major cardiovascular events (e.g., MI, stroke, cardiovascular death) or the risk of hospitalization for heart failure in patients with type 2 diabetes mellitus and established cardiovascular disease. For additional details regarding the effects of antidiabetic therapy on macrovascular outcomes, see Macrovascular Outcomes and Cardiovascular Risk Reduction under Uses: Type 2 Diabetes Mellitus, in Canagliflozin 68:20.18, Dapagliflozin Propanediol 68:20.18, and Liraglutide 68:20.06.

Treatment Goals The ADA generally states that it is reasonable to attempt to achieve in patients with type 2 diabetes mellitus the same blood glucose and HbA_{1c} goals recommended for patients with type 1 diabetes mellitus. Based on target values for blood glucose and HbA_{1c} used in clinical trials (e.g., DCCT) for type 1 diabetic patients, modified somewhat to reduce the risk of severe hypoglycemia, ADA currently recommends target preprandial (fasting) and peak postprandial (1–2 hours after the *beginning* of a meal) *plasma* glucose concentrations of 80–130 and less than 180 mg/dL, respectively, and HbA_{1c} concentrations of less than 7% (based on a nondiabetic range of 4–6%) *in general* in adults with type 1 or type 2 diabetes mellitus who are not pregnant. HbA_{1c} concentrations of 7% or greater should prompt clinicians to initiate or adjust antidiabetic therapy in nonpregnant patients with the goal of achieving HbA_{1c} concentrations of less than 7%. Patients with diabetes mellitus who have elevated HbA_{1c} concentrations despite having adequate preprandial glucose concentrations should monitor glucose concentrations 1–2 hours after the start of a meal.

More stringent treatment goals (i.e., an HbA_{1c} less than 6%) can be considered in selected patients. An *individualized* HbA_{1c} concentration goal that is closer to normal without risking substantial hypoglycemia is reasonable in patients with a short duration of diabetes mellitus, no appreciable cardiovascular disease, and a long life expectancy. Less stringent treatment goals may be appropriate in patients with long-standing diabetes mellitus in whom the general HbA_{1c} concentration goal of less than 7% is difficult to obtain despite adequate education on self-management of the disease, appropriate glucose monitoring, and effective dosages of multiple antidiabetic agents, including insulin. Achievement of HbA_{1c} values of less than 7% is not appropriate or practical for some patients, and clinical judgment should be used in designing a treatment regimen based on the potential benefits and risks (e.g., hypoglycemia) of more intensified therapy. For additional details on individualizing treatment in patients with diabetes mellitus, see Treatment Goals under Uses: Diabetes Mellitus, in the Insulins General Statement 68:20.08.

Considerations in Initiating and Maintaining Antidiabetic Therapy Recognizing that lifestyle interventions often fail to achieve or maintain the target glycemic goal within the first year of initiation of such interventions, ADA currently suggests initiation of metformin concurrently with lifestyle interventions at the time of diagnosis of type 2 diabetes mellitus. ADA and other clinicians state that lifestyle interventions should remain a principal consideration in the management of diabetes even after pharmacologic therapy is initiated. The importance of regular physical activity also should be emphasized, and cardiovascular risk factors should be identified and corrective measures employed when feasible.

Metformin Monotherapy Clinical studies indicate that metformin is as effective (approximately 1.5% decrease in HbA_{1c} values) as a sulfonylurea antidiabetic agent (e.g., chlorpropamide, glyburide, glipizide, tolbutamide) for the management of type 2 diabetes mellitus. Most clinicians currently recommend metformin as initial monotherapy in patients with type 2 diabetes mellitus whose hyperglycemia is not controlled despite dietary modification and exercise. Potential advantages of metformin compared with sulfonylurea antidiabetic agents or insulin include a minimal risk of hypoglycemia, more favorable effects on serum lipids, reduction of hyperinsulinemia, and weight loss or lack of weight gain. Type 2 diabetic patients who are very obese or who have baseline fasting blood glucose concentrations exceeding 200 mg/dL may be less likely to respond to therapy with sulfonylurea antidiabetic agents. Since metformin may stabilize or decrease body weight, the drug is particularly useful as initial monotherapy in obese individuals who might gain weight while receiving a sulfonylurea. Metformin is equally effective in lean or obese patients with type 2 diabetes mellitus. Metformin may be effective as replacement monotherapy in some patients with primary or secondary failure to sulfonylureas. (See Diabetes Mellitus: Combination Therapy, in Uses.)

In controlled studies of up to 8 months' duration in adults with type 2 diabetes mellitus, therapy with metformin hydrochloride (0.5–3 g daily) reduced fasting and postprandial glucose concentrations and HbA_{1c} substantially more than did placebo. The antihyperglycemic effect of metformin does not appear to correlate with duration of diabetes, age, obesity, race, fasting insulin concentrations, or baseline plasma lipid concentrations. In a placebo-controlled study in pediatric (10–16 years of age), treatment-naive (i.e., those receiving diet therapy only), obese patients with type 2 diabetes mellitus, the net difference in fasting plasma glucose concentrations in patients receiving metformin hydrochloride (up to 2 g daily) or placebo for up to 16 weeks was 64.3 mg/dL, reflecting an increase in fasting plasma glucose concentrations in the placebo group and an improvement in glycemic control with metformin therapy. The improvement in glycemic control with metformin in these pediatric patients was similar to that observed in clinical studies with the drug in adults. A small, similar weight loss occurred in patients receiving either metformin or placebo in this study. In a multicenter, randomized, controlled study in newly diagnosed, asymptomatic patients with type 2 diabetes mellitus, the efficacy of metformin therapy in reducing fasting plasma glucose (target value: less than 108 mg/dL) and HbA_{1c} concentrations in a subgroup of obese patients was similar to that of therapy with a sulfonylurea (chlorpropamide, glyburide, or glipizide) or insulin in nonobese patients; all drug regimens improved glycemic control compared with conventional (diet only) therapy. However, unlike sulfonylurea or insulin therapy, metformin therapy generally decreased plasma insulin concentrations and was not associated with weight gain or an increased incidence of hypoglycemia. In this long-term study, gradual deterioration in glycemic control occurred with all therapies over the study period despite increases in drug dosage or combined drug therapy; HbA_{1c} concentrations generally had increased to baseline levels after 4–5 years of therapy with any of the drug regimens. Such deterioration in glycemic control has been attributed to a progressive decline in pancreatic β-cell function rather than a reduction in insulin sensitivity.

Oral antidiabetic agents, including metformin, are *not* effective as sole therapy in patients with diabetes mellitus complicated by acidosis, ketosis, or coma; insulin is required in these conditions.

Combination Therapy Metformin may be used concomitantly with one or more oral antidiabetic agents (e.g., a sulfonylurea, a thiazolidinedione, a meglitinide, a DPP-4 inhibitor, an SGLT2 inhibitor, and/or an α-glucosidase inhibitor), a glucagon-like peptide-1 (GLP-1) agonist, or insulin to improve glycemic control in patients with type 2 diabetes.

In patients receiving initial monotherapy with metformin, the incidence of primary and secondary failures appears to be less than or similar to that in patients receiving sulfonylurea monotherapy. Secondary failure to metformin is characterized by progressively decreasing diabetic control following 1 month to several years of good control. Combined therapy with metformin and another oral antidiabetic agent generally is used in patients with longstanding type 2 diabetes mellitus who have poor glycemic control with monotherapy. ADA and most clinicians currently recommend initiating therapy with metformin and adding another antidiabetic agent if patients fail to achieve or maintain target HbA_{1c} goals. Optimum benefit generally is obtained by addition of a second antidiabetic agent as soon as monotherapy with metformin no longer provides adequate glycemic control (i.e., when the target glycemic goal is not achieved within 2–3 months of initiation of metformin therapy or at any other time when the HbA_{1c} goal is not achieved).

Combination Therapy with Oral Antidiabetic Agents. Combined therapy with metformin and other oral antidiabetic agents in patients not adequately controlled with monotherapy may reduce symptoms or allow reduced insulin dosages; some clinicians consider use of combination oral antidiabetic therapy as a means to delay or avoid institution of insulin. ADA considers the choice of additional second-line therapy to depend on the degree of glycemic control achieved during metformin monotherapy. Initiating antidiabetic therapy with 2 agents (metformin plus another agent) may be appropriate in patients whose HbA_{1c} is 7.5% or higher or is at least 1.5% above the target level. Insulin therapy should be considered when hyperglycemia is severe (e.g., blood glucose of at least 300 mg/dL, HbA_{1c} of at least 10%), especially in the presence of catabolic manifestations (e.g., weight loss, hypertriglyceridemia, ketosis), or if symptoms of hyperglycemia are present. (See Combination Therapy with Insulin under Uses: Diabetes Mellitus.)

When glycemic control is closer to the target HbA_{1c} goal with metformin monotherapy (e.g., HbA_{1c} less than 7.5%), an agent with a lesser potential to lower glycemia and/or slower onset of action may be considered (e.g., sulfonylurea, thiazolidinedione) as additional therapy to metformin. ADA states that other antidiabetic agents such as α-glucosidase inhibitors, meglitinides, exenatide, or pramlintide generally are less effective, less well studied, and/or more expensive than recommended therapies (i.e., metformin, a sulfonylurea, a thiazolidinedione, insulin). However, these agents may be appropriate for treatment of type 2 diabetes mellitus in selected patients.

Metformin is commercially available in fixed combination with glyburide or glipizide for use as initial therapy in the management of patients with type 2 diabetes mellitus whose hyperglycemia cannot be controlled by diet and exercise alone. In several comparative trials in such patients, therapy with metformin in fixed combination with glyburide or glipizide was more effective in improving glycemic control (as determined by HbA_{1c} values, fasting plasma glucose concentrations) than monotherapy with either component. A greater percentage of patients receiving metformin in fixed combination with glipizide or glipizide achieved strict glycemic control (e.g., HbA_{1c} values less than 7%) than patients receiving monotherapy with metformin, glyburide, or glipizide.

Metformin in fixed combination with glyburide or glipizide also is used to improve glycemic control in patients with type 2 diabetes mellitus who are inadequately controlled with either sulfonylurea or metformin monotherapy. In several comparative studies in such patients, greater glycemic control (as determined by HbA_{1c} values, fasting plasma glucose concentrations) was achieved with the fixed combination of metformin and glyburide or glipizide than with metformin, glyburide, or glipizide monotherapy. Strict glycemic control (e.g., HbA_{1c} values less than 7%) was achieved in a greater percentage of patients receiving fixed combinations of metformin with a sulfonylurea (glyburide or glipizide) than with sulfonylurea or metformin monotherapy. In a comparative clinical trial in pediatric patients (9–16 years of age) with type 2 diabetes mellitus, therapy with metformin in fixed combination with glyburide (titrated to a final mean daily dosage of 3.1 mg of glyburide and 623 mg of metformin hydrochloride) was no more effective in improving glycemic control (as determined by reductions in HbA_{1c} values) than monotherapy with either component (titrated to final mean daily dosages of 6.5 mg of glyburide or 1.5 g of metformin hydrochloride).

Metformin (immediate- or extended-release) is used in fixed combination with pioglitazone in patients with type 2 diabetes mellitus who have inadequate glycemic control with pioglitazone or metformin monotherapy or in those who are already receiving pioglitazone and metformin concurrently as separate components. No clinical trials have evaluated the fixed combination of metformin and pioglitazone; efficacy and safety of the fixed combination has been established based on concurrent administration of the 2 agents given separately. Safety and efficacy of the fixed combination of metformin and pioglitazone in patients with type 2 diabetes mellitus are extrapolated from clinical trials evaluating pioglitazone as add-on therapy to metformin.

Metformin also is used in combination with rosiglitazone (either as a fixed-combination preparation or as individual drugs given concurrently) in patients with type 2 diabetes mellitus when treatment with both metformin and rosiglitazone is appropriate. (See Combination Therapy under Uses: Diabetes Mellitus, in Rosiglitazone 68:20.28.)

The fixed-combination preparation containing metformin and rosiglitazone has not been specifically studied in patients previously receiving metformin monotherapy; however, clinical trials have evaluated rosiglitazone (4 or 8 mg once daily) as add-on therapy in patients who had inadequate glycemic control with metformin (2.5 g once daily). In these studies, substantial improvements in fasting plasma glucose and HbA_{1c} concentrations were observed with the combination of rosiglitazone and metformin compared with metformin alone. In a dose-ranging trial evaluating rosiglitazone 4 or 8 mg as add-on therapy to the maximum daily dosage of metformin hydrochloride, 28.1% of patients receiving the higher dosage of rosiglitazone concurrently with metformin achieved HbA_{1c} values of 7% or less.

A thiazolidinedione may be added to metformin in fixed combination with glyburide in patients with type 2 diabetes mellitus who have inadequate glycemic control with the fixed combination. In such patients, the addition of rosiglitazone to combined therapy with metformin and glyburide has reduced fasting glucose concentrations and HbA_{1c} values. Strict glycemic control (e.g., HbA_{1c} values less than 7%) was achieved in 42.4% of patients of receiving the triple combination of metformin, glyburide, and rosiglitazone compared with 13.5% of those receiving metformin and glyburide.

Metformin in fixed combination with repaglinide is used in patients with type 2 diabetes mellitus who have inadequate glycemic control with repaglinide or metformin monotherapy or in those who are already receiving repaglinide and metformin concurrently as separate components. In a double-blind, controlled trial in patients with type 2 diabetes mellitus who had inadequate glycemic control with metformin monotherapy, add-on therapy with repaglinide resulted in greater glycemic control (as determined by HbA_{1c} values, fasting plasma glucose concentrations) than metformin or repaglinide monotherapy. Combined therapy with metformin and repaglinide resulted in a greater reduction in HbA_{1c} and fasting plasma glucose concentrations at a lower repaglinide dosage than with repaglinide monotherapy. However, the incidence of hypoglycemia with combined metformin and repaglinide therapy was higher than with repaglinide monotherapy. In addition, body weight increased in patients receiving repaglinide alone or combined with metformin but remained stable in those receiving metformin monotherapy.

In a clinical trial in patients who had inadequate glycemic control (HbA_{1c} exceeding 7.1%) with metformin monotherapy, addition of repaglinide to metformin therapy produced reductions in fasting plasma glucose concentrations and HbA_{1c} averaging 39.6 mg/dL and 1.4%, respectively, compared with reductions averaging 4.5 mg/dL and 0.33%, respectively, with metformin alone; patients receiving repaglinide therapy alone had an increase in fasting plasma glucose concentrations of 8.8 mg/dL and a reduction of 0.38% in HbA_{1c}. In a clinical trial in treatment-naive patients or patients who had previously received antidiabetic therapy (followed by a washout period of at least 2 months), combined therapy with metformin hydrochloride and nateglinide resulted in greater reductions in HbA_{1c} and fasting plasma glucose concentrations than metformin or nateglinide monotherapy.

In another clinical trial in patients with type 2 diabetes mellitus who had inadequate glycemic control with metformin, a sulfonylurea, or insulin, the combination of pioglitazone (30 mg daily) and metformin (and withdrawal of other antidiabetic therapy) reduced fasting plasma glucose concentrations and HbA_{1c} values compared with metformin therapy alone, regardless of whether patients were receiving lower (less than 2 g daily) or higher (2 g daily or more) dosages of metformin hydrochloride.

In a multicenter, controlled study in patients whose hyperglycemia was inadequately controlled by diet and metformin therapy, the addition of acarbose produced appreciable improvement in postprandial plasma glucose concentrations and modest improvement in HbA_{1c}. Fasting plasma glucose concentrations generally are not reduced by addition of acarbose to therapy with metformin since acarbose acts principally during a meal to delay carbohydrate absorption. Limited data suggest that combined therapy with metformin and a sulfonylurea is as effective or more effective in reducing fasting blood glucose and HbA_{1c} concentrations than combined therapy with acarbose and a sulfonylurea; however, acarbose may provide better control of postprandial blood glucose concentrations.

Metformin (immediate-release) is used in fixed combination with alogliptin in patients with type 2 diabetes mellitus when treatment with both drugs is appropriate. Efficacy and safety of this fixed combination have been established based on concurrent administration of the 2 agents given separately. (See Combination Therapy under Uses: Diabetes Mellitus, in Alogliptin 68:20.05.)

Metformin (immediate- or extended-release) is used in fixed combination with linagliptin in patients with type 2 diabetes mellitus when treatment with both drugs is appropriate. Efficacy and safety of these fixed combinations have been established based on concurrent administration of the 2 agents given separately. (See Combination Therapy under Uses: Diabetes Mellitus, in Linagliptin 68:20.05.)

Extended-release metformin is used in fixed combination with saxagliptin in patients with type 2 diabetes mellitus when treatment with both drugs is appropriate. Efficacy and safety of this fixed combination have been established based on concurrent administration of metformin and saxagliptin given as separate tablets. (See Combination Therapy under Uses: Diabetes Mellitus, in Saxagliptin 68:20.05.)

Metformin (immediate- or extended-release) is used in fixed combination with sitagliptin in patients with type 2 diabetes mellitus when treatment with both drugs is appropriate. Efficacy and safety of these fixed combinations have been established based on concurrent administration of the 2 agents given separately and extrapolations from clinical trials evaluating sitagliptin as add-on therapy to metformin. (See Combination Therapy under Uses: Diabetes Mellitus, in Sitagliptin 68:20.05.)

Metformin is used in fixed combinations with the SGLT2 inhibitors canagliflozin, dapagliflozin, empagliflozin, or ertugliflozin. These fixed-combination preparations are used in patients with type 2 diabetes mellitus when treatment with both drugs is appropriate. Efficacy and safety of these fixed combinations have been established based on concurrent administration of the 2 drugs given separately. In clinical trials evaluating the efficacy of the combination of an SGLT2 inhibitor and metformin, patients who received both drugs had substantially greater improvements in HbA_{1c} than when either drug component was administered alone. (See Combination Therapy under Uses: Diabetes Mellitus, in the individual monographs on Canagliflozin 68:20.18, Dapagliflozin 68:20.18, Empagliflozin 68:20.18, and Ertugliflozin 68:20.18.)

Conflicting data regarding the long-term benefit of metformin as part of an intensive antidiabetic regimen have been reported in UKPDS, which consisted of middle-aged, newly diagnosed, overweight (exceeding 120% of ideal body weight) or non-overweight patients with type 2 diabetes mellitus who received long-term therapy (over 10 years) with intensive or conventional treatment. (See Glycemic Control and Microvascular Complications, under Uses: Diabetes Mellitus.) In a UKPDS substudy, overweight patients receiving metformin as initial therapy in a stepwise intensive regimen had a 32% lower risk of developing any diabetes-related endpoint (including macrovascular and microvascular complications) compared with those managed by dietary modification alone; the reduction in any diabetes-related end point was greater in those receiving metformin than in those receiving initial intensive therapy with a sulfonylurea or insulin. The risk for diabetes-related death or myocardial infarction (39% lower) was also lower with intensive therapy with metformin or sulfonylureas or insulin compared with conventional therapy; no differences between the effects of intensive therapies were noted. In contrast, a second UKPDS substudy in which metformin was added to sulfonylurea therapy to improve glycemic control resulted in an increase in the risk of diabetes-related death or death from any cause compared with continuing therapy with a sulfonylurea alone. A pooled analysis of both trials and epidemiologic analysis of other data from UKPDS in patients who received stepwise therapy with metformin and sulfonylurea therapy because of progressive hyperglycemia showed a small reduction in diabetes-related death, all-cause mortality, myocardial infarction, and stroke. Reasons for disparate results of these trials are unclear but may be related to trial design, the relatively smaller number of patients receiving metformin, analytical methods, or differences in response between overweight and non-overweight patients. Pending the results of additional studies, the ADA and other clinicians do not recommend changing current guidelines regarding the use of metformin as monotherapy or in combination with sulfonylureas.

When lifestyle interventions, metformin, and a second oral antidiabetic agent are not effective in maintaining the target glycemic goal in patients with type 2 diabetes mellitus, ADA and other clinicians generally recommend the addition of insulin therapy. In patients whose HbA_{1c} is close to the target level (less than 8%) on metformin and a second oral antidiabetic agent, addition of a third oral antidiabetic agent instead of insulin may be considered. However, ADA states that triple combination oral antidiabetic therapy is more costly and potentially not as effective as adding insulin therapy to dual combination oral antidiabetic therapy.

Combination Therapy with Insulin ADA and other clinicians state that combined therapy with insulin and metformin with or without other oral antidiabetic agents is one of several options for the management of hyperglycemia in patients not responding adequately to oral monotherapy with metformin, the preferred agent for initiation of oral antidiabetic therapy. In patients with a HbA_{1c} exceeding 8.5% or symptoms secondary to hyperglycemia) despite metformin monotherapy, consideration should be given to adding insulin. When glycemia is not controlled with metformin with or without other oral antidiabetic agents and basal insulin (e.g., given as intermediate- or long-acting insulin at bedtime or in the morning), therapy with insulin should be intensified by adding additional short-acting or rapid-acting insulin injections at mealtimes. Therapy with insulin secretagogues (i.e., sulfonylureas, meglitinides) should be tapered and discontinued when intensive insulin therapy is initiated, as insulin secretagogues do not appear to be synergistic with such insulin therapy.

Combined therapy with insulin and one or more oral antidiabetic agents appears to increase glycemic control with lower doses of insulin than would be required with insulin alone and with a decreased potential for body weight gain associated with insulin therapy. Data from a small, placebo-controlled, 24-week trial indicate that addition of metformin improved glycemic control (as measured by a reduction in HbA_{1c}) in patients who failed to achieve adequate glycemic control with insulin therapy; insulin dosage in patients receiving adjunctive metformin therapy was decreased by 16%. In another small, placebo-controlled study in patients adequately controlled with insulin therapy, insulin dosage requirements were reduced by 19% after addition of metformin.

Metformin has been used as an adjunct to insulin to reduce insulin requirements in a limited number of patients with type 1 diabetes mellitus†, but the potential benefits and risks require further evaluation before such combined therapy can be recommended.

■ **Polycystic Ovary Syndrome** Metformin has been used in the management of metabolic and reproductive abnormalities associated with polycystic ovary syndrome†. However, adequate and well-controlled clinical trials evaluating metformin therapy for polycystic ovary syndrome remain limited, particularly regarding long-term efficacy, and available data are conflicting regarding the benefits of the drug in ameliorating various manifestations of the condition.

While metformin has beneficial effects on cardiovascular risk factors such as insulin resistance and obesity, evidence from pooled analyses of data suggest that the drug has limited overall benefits on reproductive outcomes (e.g., live birth rates) in women with polycystic ovary syndrome. As with diabetes mellitus, lifestyle changes (e.g., diet, exercise, weight loss in obese patients) are strongly recommended for the initial management of polycystic ovary syndrome; however, long-term success with such measures alone is difficult to achieve and drug therapy, including metformin, often is used for symptomatic management of this condition.

Polycystic ovary syndrome is characterized by chronic anovulation (generally manifested as oligomenorrhea or amenorrhea) and hyperandrogenism (excessive production of male hormones in women) with clinical manifestations of irregular menstrual cycles, infertility, hirsutism, acne, and dyslipidemia. While the principal etiology is unknown, insulin resistance with compensatory hyperinsulinemia is a prominent manifestation of polycystic ovary syndrome. Hyperinsulinemia stimulates ovarian and adrenal androgen secretion, leading to hyperandrogenism and its associated clinical manifestations. In addition, cardiovascular risk factors such as obesity and impaired glucose tolerance, including metabolic syndrome and type 2 diabetes mellitus, are present in a substantial proportion of women with polycystic ovary syndrome, making the use of insulin-sensitizing drugs such as metformin reasonable in the treatment of this condition.

Metformin and other insulin-sensitizing agents (e.g., thiazolidinedione antidiabetic agents) improve insulin resistance, which leads to a reduction in androgen production in ovarian theca cells and potential beneficial effects on metabolic and hormonal abnormalities associated with polycystic ovary syndrome. Although metformin therapy has not been shown specifically to reduce cardiovascular events in women with polycystic ovary syndrome, the drug's pharmacologic and clinical effects support its use as maintenance therapy to ameliorate insulin resistance and hyperinsulinemia in such women.

Estrogen-progestin oral contraceptives with or without an antiandrogen (e.g., spironolactone) traditionally have been used in the long-term management of polycystic ovary syndrome; however, such therapy may worsen preexisting insulin resistance and glucose tolerance and potentially increase cardiovascular risk. In a meta-analysis based on a small number of randomized, controlled trials in patients with polycystic ovary syndrome, oral contraceptive therapy (ethinyl estradiol with cyproterone acetate [not commercially available in the US] or norgestimate) for up to 12 months was associated with improvement in menstrual pattern and serum androgen concentrations compared with metformin, while metformin was more effective than oral contraceptives in reducing fasting insulin and triglyceride concentrations. However, a preference for either drug as maintenance therapy for polycystic ovary syndrome could not be determined because of a lack of adequate trial data. Another meta-analysis was unable to determine clinically important effects of metformin or thiazolidinedione therapy on metabolic or hyperandrogenism parameters such as fasting insulin or glucose concentrations, hirsutism, or hormone levels. Because of a lack of adequate long-term clinical trials, the effects of therapy with oral contraceptives or metformin on long-term outcomes such as diabetes, cardiovascular disease, or endometrial cancer in women with polycystic ovary syndrome have not been established.

Variable effects have been reported with metformin therapy used alone or in combination with fertility-enhancing drugs (e.g., clomiphene) for the treatment of infertility in women with polycystic ovary syndrome. Currently available evidence suggests that metformin hydrochloride dosages of 1.5–2.5 g daily in women with polycystic ovary syndrome increase the frequency of spontaneous ovulation, menstrual cyclicity, and ovulatory response after ovarian stimulation (e.g., with clomiphene, recombinant follicle-stimulating hormone). However, improvement in the rate of live births with metformin therapy generally has not been comparable to that associated with clomiphene therapy in such women. Results of a meta-analysis also indicated improvement in ovulation and clinical pregnancy rates with combined metformin and clomiphene treatment compared with clomiphene alone in women with polycystic ovary syndrome. However, another meta-analysis found only minimal improvement in ovulation rate and no improvement in pregnancy rate with metformin therapy. Some clinicians suggest that metformin therapy may be useful for inducing ovulation in women with polycystic ovary syndrome who desire pregnancy at a more distant time (e.g., more than 6 months away), and that clomiphene therapy may be preferable in those who desire to become pregnant much sooner. A potential advantage of metformin therapy over clomiphene for infertility is a reduced chance of twin or triplet pregnancy with metformin. Additional large, randomized, well-controlled studies are needed to establish the effectiveness of metformin alone or in combination with other therapies for treatment of infertility associated with polycystic ovary syndrome.

Dosage and Administration

■ **Administration** Metformin hydrochloride is administered orally. In patients receiving metformin hydrochloride immediate-release tablets at a dosage of 2 g or less daily, the drug usually can be given as 2 divided doses daily; however, in patients who require more than 2 g daily, the drug usually should be administered as 3 divided doses daily. Immediate-release metformin hydrochloride in fixed combination with canagliflozin, dapagliflozin, empagliflozin, ertugliflozin, pioglitazone, rosiglitazone, repaglinide, alogliptin, linagliptin, or sitagliptin is administered in divided doses daily with meals to reduce the GI effects of the metformin hydrochloride component. Although food decreases the extent and slightly delays absorption of metformin immediate-release tablets, the manufacturer recommends that the drug be taken with meals to decrease adverse GI effects.

The fixed combination of metformin hydrochloride and repaglinide should be administered within approximately 15 minutes prior to meals; timing may vary from immediately before meals to 30 minutes before meals. Patients who skip a meal should omit the dose of the fixed combination of metformin hydrochloride and repaglinide for that meal.

Metformin hydrochloride extended-release tablets should be taken with the evening meal. The manufacturer of Fortamet® (metformin hydrochloride extended-release tablets) states that each dose of the drug should be taken with a full glass of water. The matrix core of some extended-release tablet preparations (e.g., Glucophage® XR, Glumetza®) usually is broken up in the GI tract, but patients should be advised that occasionally the biologically inert components of the tablet may remain intact and be passed in the stool as a soft, hydrated mass. Occasionally, Glumetza® may be eliminated in the feces as a soft, hydrated mass or an insoluble shell. The membrane coating surrounding the core of another extended-release tablet (Fortamet®) remains intact through the GI tract and is excreted in feces as a soft mass that may resemble the original tablet. (See Chemistry and Stability: Stability.)

Extended-release metformin hydrochloride in fixed combination with canagliflozin, dapagliflozin, or empagliflozin is administered once daily with the morning meal.

The fixed combination of extended-release metformin hydrochloride and linagliptin should be administered once daily with a meal. The fixed combination of extended-release metformin hydrochloride and sitagliptin should be administered once daily with a meal, preferably with the evening meal. Extended-release metformin hydrochloride in fixed combination with saxagliptin should be administered once daily with the evening meal.

Extended-release metformin hydrochloride tablets and fixed-combination preparations containing the extended-release form of the drug must be swallowed whole and not chewed, cut, or crushed; inactive ingredients occasionally may be eliminated in feces as a soft mass that may resemble the original tablet.

■ **Dosage** ***Diabetes Mellitus*** Dosage of metformin hydrochloride must be individualized carefully based on patient response and tolerance. The goal of therapy should be to reduce both fasting glucose and glycosylated hemoglobin (hemoglobin A_{1c} [HbA_{1c}]) values to normal or near normal using the lowest effective dosage of metformin hydrochloride, either when used as monotherapy or combined with another antidiabetic agent. Patients should be monitored with regular laboratory evaluations, including fasting blood (or plasma) glucose determinations, to assess therapeutic response and the minimum effective dosage of metformin hydrochloride. (*Glucose concentrations in plasma generally are 10–15% higher than those in whole blood; glucose concentrations also may vary according to the method and laboratory used for these determinations.*)

Following initiation of metformin therapy and dosage titration, determination of HbA_{1c} concentrations at intervals of approximately 3 months is useful for assessing the patient's continued response to therapy. HbA_{1c} is a better indicator of long-term glycemic control than fasting plasma glucose concentrations alone.

Since adverse GI effects with metformin appear to be dose related, it is recommended that dosage of the drug be increased gradually and that the drug be taken with meals. (See Cautions: GI Effects.)

Initial Dosage. For the management of type 2 diabetes mellitus in adults, the manufacturer states that the usual initial dosage of metformin hydrochloride as immediate-release tablets is 500 mg twice daily or 850 mg once daily with meals. Alternatively, an initial metformin hydrochloride dosage of 500 mg once daily has been suggested by some experts. When metformin hydrochloride oral solution is used, the usual initial dosage is 500 mg twice daily or 850 mg once daily with meals. The manufacturers state that in general, clinically important responses are not observed at metformin hydrochloride dosages of less than 1.5 g daily.

When metformin hydrochloride is administered as certain extended-release tablet preparations (e.g., Glucophage® XR), the usual initial dosage in adults is 500 mg once daily with the evening meal. With another extended-release tablet preparation (Fortamet®), the usual initial dosage is 1 g once daily with the evening meal, although the manufacturer states that 500 mg once daily may be used when clinically appropriate. The recommended initial dosage of another extended-release preparation of metformin hydrochloride (Glumetza®) is 1 g once daily with the evening meal. Subsequent dosage of metformin hydrochloride should be adjusted according to the patient's therapeutic response, using the lowest possible effective dosage. (See Dosage: Maintenance Dosage, under Dosage and Administration.)

Although satisfactory control of blood glucose concentrations may be achieved within a few days after dosage adjustment, the full effects of the drug may not be observed for up to 2 weeks.

Metformin should be used with caution in geriatric patients since aging is associated with reduced renal function, and accumulation of the drug resulting in lactic acidosis may occur in patients with renal impairment. In addition, renal function should be monitored regularly in geriatric patients to determine the appropriate dosage of metformin hydrochloride. Metformin should not be initiated in geriatric patients 80 years of age or older unless determinations of creatinine clearance indicate normal renal function. Initial dosages of metformin hydrochloride in geriatric patients should be conservative (initiated at the low end of the dosage range) and should be titrated carefully. It has been suggested, based on limited data, that initial dosages of metformin hydrochloride in geriatric patients be reduced by approximately 33% compared with such dosages in other patients with type 2 diabetes mellitus.

For the management of type 2 diabetes mellitus in children or adolescents 10–16 years of age, the usual initial dosage of metformin hydrochloride as immediate-release tablets or the oral solution is 500 mg twice daily given in the morning and evening with meals. Safety and efficacy of certain extended-release tablet preparations of metformin hydrochloride (Glucophage® XR, Fortamet®) have not been established in children or adolescents younger than 17 years of age. Safety and efficacy of another extended-release tablet preparation (Glumetza®) have not been established in children and adolescents younger than 18 years of age.

Transferring from Therapy with Other Antidiabetic Agents. When transferring from most sulfonylurea antidiabetic agents to metformin, a transition period generally is not required, and administration of the sulfonylurea antidiabetic agent may be abruptly discontinued. Because an exaggerated hypoglycemic response may occur in some patients during the transition from a sulfonylurea antidiabetic agent with a prolonged half-life (e.g., chlorpropamide) to metformin, patients being transferred from such agents should be monitored closely for the occurrence of hypoglycemia during the initial 2 weeks of the transition period.

Dosage Titration. In adults receiving an initial metformin hydrochloride dosage of 500 mg twice daily as immediate-release tablets or the oral solution, daily dosage may be increased by 500 mg at weekly intervals until the desired fasting blood glucose concentration (e.g., less than 140 mg/dL) is achieved or a dosage of 2 g daily is reached. Alternatively, in adults receiving 500 mg of metformin hydrochloride twice daily as immediate-release tablets or the oral solution, dosage may be increased to 850 mg twice daily after 2 weeks. In adults receiving an initial dosage of 500 mg of metformin hydrochloride once or twice daily (with breakfast and/or dinner), some experts recommend increasing the dosage to 850 mg or 1 g twice daily after 5–7 days if additional glycemic control is needed and the drug is well tolerated (e.g., no adverse GI effects). If adverse GI effects appear during dosage titration of metformin hydrochloride, dosage should be decreased to the previous lower dosage, and further dosage increments attempted at a later time. In adults receiving an initial metformin hydrochloride dosage of 850 mg daily as immediate-release tablets or the oral solution, daily dosage may be increased by 850 mg every *other* week (i.e., every 2 weeks) until the desired fasting blood glucose concentration (e.g., less than 140 mg/dL) is achieved or a total dosage of 2 g daily is reached. For patients requiring additional glycemic control with metformin hydrochloride, a maximum daily dosage of 2.55 g as immediate-release tablets or the oral solution may be used.

In adults (17–18 years of age or older) receiving certain metformin hydrochloride extended-release tablets (e.g., Glucophage® XR, Glumetza®), daily dosage may be increased by 500 mg at weekly intervals until the desired glycemic response is achieved or a maximum dosage of 2 g daily is reached. If glycemic control is not achieved with metformin hydrochloride extended-release tablets (e.g., Glucophage® XR, Glumetza®) at a dosage of 2 g once daily, a dosage of 1 g twice daily should be considered. If a dosage exceeding 2 g daily is needed in patients receiving certain metformin hydrochloride extended-release tablet preparations (e.g., Glucophage® XR), the manufacturers suggest that therapy be switched to immediate-release metformin hydrochloride tablets and dosage titrated up to a maximum dosage of 2.55 g daily in divided doses. Conversely, therapy with extended-release tablets may be substituted for immediate-release tablets at the same total daily dosage of immediate-release tablets; dosage subsequently should be adjusted according to glycemic response.

With another extended-release metformin hydrochloride tablet preparation (Fortamet®), daily dosage may be increased by 500 mg at weekly intervals up to a maximum of 2.5 g once daily with the evening meal. In patients transferring from immediate-release tablets to an extended-release tablet preparation, glycemic control should be closely monitored and dosage adjustments made accordingly.

Dosage in adults generally should not exceed 2.55 g daily when given as metformin hydrochloride immediate-release tablets or oral solution, 2.5 g daily when given as certain extended-release tablets (e.g., Fortamet®), or 2 g daily when given as certain other extended-release tablet preparations (e.g., Glucophage® XR). Metformin hydrochloride dosages of up to 3 g daily have been associated with modestly greater effectiveness than 1.7 g daily. However, adverse GI effects may limit the maximum dosage that can be tolerated. (Consult the manufacturer's labeling for product-specific details.) Dosages exceeding 2 g of metformin hydrochloride daily as immediate-release tablets or the oral solution may be better tolerated if given in 3 divided doses daily with meals. Maintenance dosage of metformin hydrochloride should be conservative in debilitated, malnourished, or geriatric patients because of an increased risk of hypoglycemia in these patients. Dosage of metformin hydrochloride in fixed combination with pioglitazone in such patients should not be titrated to the maximum recommended dosage. (See Cautions: Precautions and Contraindications.)

Metformin should be used with caution in geriatric patients since aging is associated with reduced renal function, and accumulation of the drug resulting in lactic acidosis may occur in patients with renal impairment. In addition, renal function should be monitored periodically in geriatric patients to determine the appropriate dosage of metformin hydrochloride. Any dosage adjustment in geriatric patients should be based on a careful assessment of renal function. It has been suggested, based on limited data, that maximum dosages in geriatric patients be reduced by approximately 33% compared with such dosages in other patients with type 2 diabetes mellitus.

In children or adolescents 10–16 years of age receiving metformin hydrochloride 500 mg twice daily as immediate-release tablets or the oral solution, daily dosage may be increased by 500 mg at weekly intervals until the desired glycemic response is achieved or up to a maximum dosage of 2 g daily given in divided doses.

Concomitant Therapy with Metformin and Sulfonylurea Antidiabetic Agents. The manufacturer of glipizide states that other oral antidiabetic agents may be added to glipizide therapy if glycemic control is inadequate with glipizide. The manufacturers of glimepiride or glyburide state that combination therapy with metformin may be used in patients who no longer respond adequately to either antidiabetic agent alone, despite appropriate antidiabetic monotherapy, diet, and exercise. ADA states that a second antidiabetic agent may be added as soon as monotherapy with metformin at the maximum tolerated dosage no longer provides adequate glycemic control (i.e., when the target glycemic goal is not achieved within 2–3 months of initiation of therapy with metformin or at any other time when the HbA_{1c} goal is not achieved).

The commercially available preparation containing metformin hydrochloride in fixed combination with glyburide (e.g., Glucovance®) may be used as initial therapy in patients with type 2 diabetes mellitus whose blood glucose is not adequately controlled with diet and exercise alone, or as second-line therapy in those in whom glycemic control with glyburide or metformin monotherapy is not adequate. If the fixed combination of metformin and glyburide is used as initial therapy, the recommended initial dosage is 250 mg of metformin hydrochloride and 1.25 mg of glyburide daily with a meal. Patients with more severe hyperglycemia (as determined by HbA_{1c} exceeding 9% or fasting plasma glucose concentrations exceeding 200 mg/dL) may receive an initial dosage of 250 mg of metformin hydrochloride and 1.25 mg of glyburide twice daily with the morning and evening meals. Daily dosage may be increased in increments of 1.25 mg of glyburide and 250 mg of metformin hydrochloride at 2-week intervals until the minimum effective dosage required to achieve adequate blood glucose control is reached. A total daily dosage exceeding 10 mg of glyburide and 2 g of metformin hydrochloride has not been evaluated in clinical trials in patients receiving the fixed-combination preparation as initial therapy. The manufacturer states that the fixed-combination preparation containing 5 mg of glyburide and 500 mg of metformin hydrochloride should not be used as initial therapy in treatment-naive patients because of the increased risk for hypoglycemia.

If the fixed combination of metformin hydrochloride and glipizide (e.g., Metaglip®) is used as initial therapy in patients who have inadequate glycemic control with diet and exercise alone, the recommended initial dosage is 250 mg of metformin hydrochloride and 2.5 mg of glipizide once daily with a meal. Patients with more severe hyperglycemia (as determined by fasting plasma glucose concentrations of 280–320 mg/dL) may receive an initial dosage of 500 mg of metformin hydrochloride and 2.5 mg of glipizide twice daily. The efficacy of metformin in fixed combination with glipizide has not been established in patients whose fasting plasma glucose concentrations exceed 320 mg/dL. Daily dosage may be increased in increments of one tablet (using the tablet strength at which therapy was initiated, either 2.5 mg of glipizide and 250 mg of metformin hydrochloride or 2.5 mg of glipizide and 500 mg of metformin in hydrochloride) at 2-week intervals until the minimum effective dosage required to achieve adequate blood glucose control is reached; there is no experience with total daily dosages exceeding 2 g of metformin hydrochloride and 10 mg of glipizide in clinical trials in patients receiving the fixed combination for initial therapy. A total daily dosage exceeding 2 g of metformin hydrochloride and 10 mg of glipizide has not been evaluated in clinical trials in patients receiving the fixed-combination preparation as initial therapy.

The commercially available preparations containing metformin hydrochloride in fixed combination with glyburide or glipizide also may be used as second-line therapy in patients with type 2 diabetes mellitus whose blood glucose is not adequately controlled with either glyburide or glipizide (or another sulfonylurea antidiabetic agent) or metformin alone. Dosage of the fixed combinations is based on the patient's current dosages of metformin hydrochloride and glyburide or glipizide, effectiveness, and tolerability. The recommended initial dosage of the commercially available fixed-combination tablets in previously treated patients is 500 mg of metformin hydrochloride and 2.5 or 5 mg of glyburide or glipizide twice daily with the morning and evening meals. In order to minimize the risk of hypoglycemia, the initial dosage of glyburide and metformin hydrochloride in fixed combination should not exceed the daily dosage of metformin hydrochloride, glyburide, or glipizide (or the equivalent dosage of another sulfonylurea) previously received. The daily dosage of the fixed combination of metformin hydrochloride and glyburide or glipizide should be titrated upward in increments not exceeding 500 mg of metformin hydrochloride and 5 mg of glyburide or glipizide until adequate control of blood glucose is achieved or a maximum daily dosage of 2 g of metformin hydrochloride and 20 mg of glyburide or glipizide is reached.

For patients being switched from combined therapy with separate preparations, the initial dosage of the fixed-combination preparation of metformin hydrochloride and glyburide or glipizide should not exceed the daily dosage of glyburide, glipizide (or equivalent dosage of another sulfonylurea antidiabetic agent), *and* metformin hydrochloride currently being taken. Such patients should be monitored for signs and symptoms of hypoglycemia following the switch. In the transfer from previous antidiabetic therapy to the fixed combination, the decision to switch to the nearest equivalent dosage or to titrate dosage should be based on clinical judgment. Hypoglycemia and hyperglycemia are possible in such patients, and any change in the therapy of type 2 diabetic patients should be undertaken with caution and appropriate monitoring. If blood glucose concentrations are not adequately controlled following initial administration of the fixed-combination preparations, the daily dosage may be titrated in increments of no more than 5 mg of glyburide and 500 mg of metformin hydrochloride daily until adequate glycemic control is achieved or a maximum daily dosage of 20 mg of glyburide or glipizide and 2 g of metformin hydrochloride is reached. The safety and efficacy of switching from another combined therapy with separate preparations of glyburide (or another sulfonylurea antidiabetic agent) and metformin in the fixed-combination preparation have not been established in clinical studies.

Therapy with metformin in fixed combination with glyburide should be used with caution in geriatric patients, since aging is associated with reduced renal function. The initial and maintenance dosages of metformin hydrochloride in fixed combination with glyburide should be conservative and should be titrated carefully in such patients. Renal function should be assessed with initial dosage selection and with each dosage adjustment, particularly in geriatric patients, to aid in prevention of lactic acidosis. To minimize the risk of hypoglycemia, maintenance dosage of the fixed combination of metformin hydrochloride and glyburide in geriatric, debilitated, or malnourished patients should *not* be titrated to the maximum dosage recommended for other patients.

For patients whose hyperglycemia is not adequately controlled on therapy with metformin in fixed combination with glyburide, a thiazolidinedione (e.g., pioglitazone, rosiglitazone) may be added at its recommended initial dosage and the dosage of the fixed combination may be continued unchanged. In patients requiring further glycemic control, the dosage of the thiazolidinedione may be titrated upward, based on the dosage regimen recommended by the manufacturer. Such triple therapy with glyburide, metformin, and a thiazolidinedione may increase the potential for hypoglycemia at any time of day. If hypoglycemia develops during such triple therapy, consideration should be given to reducing the dosage of the glyburide component; adjustment of the dosage of the other components of the antidiabetic regimen also should be considered as clinically indicated.

Combination Therapy with Metformin and a Thiazolidinedione. The commercially available fixed-combination preparation containing metformin hydrochloride and rosiglitazone (Avandamet®) may be used in patients with type 2 diabetes mellitus when treatment with both metformin and rosiglitazone is appropriate.

The commercially available fixed-combination preparations containing metformin hydrochloride (immediate- or extended-release) and pioglitazone (Actoplus Met®, Actoplus Met® XR) are used as second-line therapy in patients with type 2 diabetes mellitus who have inadequate glycemic control with pioglitazone or metformin monotherapy or in those who are already receiving each drug component separately.

When the commercially available fixed-combination preparations containing metformin hydrochloride and pioglitazone are used as second-line therapy in patients inadequately controlled on monotherapy with the individual drugs or to replace concurrent therapy with the drugs given as separate tablets, dosage of the fixed combinations should be based on the patient's current dosages of metformin hydrochloride and/or pioglitazone, effectiveness, and tolerability. If the fixed combination containing metformin hydrochloride and pioglitazone (Actoplus Met®) is used, the usual initial dosage is metformin hydrochloride 500 or 850 mg and pioglitazone 15 mg given once or twice daily. If the fixed combination containing extended-release metformin hydrochloride and immediate-release pioglitazone (Actoplus Met® XR) is used, the usual initial dosage is metformin hydrochloride 1 g and pioglitazone 15 or 30 mg given once daily with the evening meal. Dosage should be titrated gradually, based on assessment of therapeutic response, to a maximum daily dosage of 2.55 g of metformin hydrochloride and 45 mg of pioglitazone (as Actoplus Met®) or 2 g of extended-release metformin hydrochloride and 45 mg of immediate-release pioglitazone (as Actoplus Met® XR).

The safety and efficacy of transferring from therapy with other oral antidiabetic agents to the fixed combination of pioglitazone and metformin hydrochloride have not been specifically established in clinical studies. Any change in the therapy of patients with type 2 diabetes mellitus should be undertaken with caution and appropriate monitoring, as changes in glycemic control can occur. Ideally, long-term glycemic control should be evaluated using HbA_{1c} at 8–12 weeks following transfer of therapy unless there is evidence of deterioration of glycemic control as measured by fasting plasma glucose concentrations.

When the commercially available preparation containing metformin hydrochloride in fixed combination with rosiglitazone (Avandamet®) is used in patients with type 2 diabetes mellitus, selection of the fixed-combination dosage should be based on the patient's current dosages of the individual drugs. In patients currently receiving rosiglitazone monotherapy, the usual initial dosage of metformin hydrochloride (in fixed combination with rosiglitazone) is 1 g daily plus the patient's existing dosage of rosiglitazone, given in 2 divided doses. In patients currently receiving metformin hydrochloride monotherapy, the usual initial dosage of rosiglitazone (in fixed combination with metformin hydrochloride) is 4 mg daily plus the patient's existing dosage of metformin hydrochloride, given in 2 divided doses. (See Table 1.)

Table 1. Initial Dosage of the Fixed Combination of Rosiglitazone and Metformin Hydrochloride (Avandamet®) as Second-Line Therapy

Prior Therapy	Usual Initial Dosage of Avandamet®	
Total Daily Dosage	**Tablet Strength**	**Number of Tablets**
Metformin Hydrochloride		
1 g	2 mg/500 mg	1 tablet twice daily
2 g	2 mg/1 g	1 tablet twice daily
Rosiglitazone		
4 mg	2 mg/500 mg	1 tablet twice daily
8 mg	4 mg/500 mg	1 tablet twice daily

Therapy should be individualized in patients already receiving metformin hydrochloride at dosages not available in the fixed combination (i.e., dosages other than 1 or 2 g).

For patients switching from combined therapy with separate preparations of metformin hydrochloride and rosiglitazone, the initial dosage of the fixed-combination preparation of metformin hydrochloride and rosiglitazone should be the same as the daily dosage of metformin hydrochloride and rosiglitazone currently being taken.

If additional glycemic control is needed following initial therapy or transfer, the dosage of the fixed combination of metformin hydrochloride and rosiglitazone may be titrated upward in increments not exceeding 500 mg of metformin hydrochloride and/or 4 mg of rosiglitazone until adequate glycemic control is achieved or a maximum daily dosage of 2 g of metformin hydrochloride and 8 mg of rosiglitazone is reached.

Therapy with metformin in fixed combination with rosiglitazone should be used with caution in geriatric patients, since aging is associated with reduced renal function. The initial and maintenance dosages of metformin hydrochloride in fixed combination with rosiglitazone should be conservative and should be titrated carefully in such patients. Renal function should be assessed with initial dosage selection and with each dosage adjustment, particularly in geriatric patients, to aid in prevention of lactic acidosis. To minimize the risk of hypoglycemia, maintenance dosage of the fixed combination of metformin hydrochloride and glyburide in geriatric, debilitated, or malnourished patients should *not* be titrated to the maximum dosage recommended for other patients.

Combination Therapy with Metformin and Repaglinide. When the fixed combination of metformin hydrochloride and repaglinide (PrandiMet®) is used as second-line therapy in patients inadequately controlled on monotherapy with one of the drugs or to replace concurrent therapy with the drugs given as separate tablets, dosage of the fixed combination should be individualized based on the patient's current dosage regimen, effectiveness, and tolerability. In patients inadequately controlled on metformin hydrochloride monotherapy, the usual initial dosage of the fixed combination is metformin hydrochloride 500 mg and repaglinide 1 mg twice daily with meals, with gradual dosage escalation as needed to reduce the risk of hypoglycemia with repaglinide. In patients inadequately controlled on repaglinide monotherapy, the usual initial dosage of the metformin hydrochloride component (in fixed combination with repaglinide) is 500 mg twice daily with meals, with gradual dosage escalation as needed to reduce GI adverse effects with metformin.

For patients being switched from concurrent therapy with metformin hydrochloride and repaglinide given as separate tablets, the initial dosage of the fixed combination should be the one that most closely provides (but does not exceed) the patient's existing dosage of these drugs.

Dosage of the fixed combination should be titrated gradually, based on assessment of therapeutic response, to a maximum daily dosage of 2.5 g of metformin hydrochloride and 10 mg of repaglinide given in 2 or 3 divided doses. Dosages of metformin and repaglinide given in fixed combination should not exceed 1 g or 4 mg, respectively, per meal. Safety and efficacy of transferring from therapy with other oral antidiabetic agents to the fixed combination of repaglinide and metformin hydrochloride have not been specifically established in clinical studies. Any change in the therapy of patients with type 2 diabetes mellitus should be undertaken with caution and appropriate monitoring, as changes in glycemic control can occur.

Dosage of metformin hydrochloride in fixed combination with repaglinide should be titrated with caution in patients of advanced age, since aging is associated with reduced renal function. In geriatric patients, particularly those 80 years of age or older, dosage adjustment should be based on careful assessment of renal function.

Metformin Hydrochloride/Alogliptin Fixed-combination Therapy. Dosage of the fixed combination of metformin hydrochloride and alogliptin should be individualized based on the patient's current antidiabetic regimen, effectiveness, and tolerability. Dosage should be increased gradually to minimize the adverse GI effects of metformin. The maximum recommended dosage of the fixed combination of metformin hydrochloride and alogliptin is 2 g of metformin hydrochloride and 25 mg of alogliptin daily.

Metformin Hydrochloride/Linagliptin Fixed-combination Therapy. Dosage of the fixed combination of metformin hydrochloride and linagliptin should be individualized based on its effectiveness and patient tolerability. The dosage may be increased up to a maximum of 2 g of metformin hydrochloride and 5 mg of linagliptin daily.

In patients *not* currently receiving metformin hydrochloride, the recommended initial total daily dosage of the fixed combination is 1 g of metformin hydrochloride and 5 mg of linagliptin administered in 2 divided doses (when given as the fixed-combination preparation containing immediate-release metformin hydrochloride) or once daily (when given as the fixed-combination preparation containing extended-release metformin hydrochloride).

In patients currently receiving metformin hydrochloride, the recommended initial total daily dosage of the fixed combination is a total daily metformin hydrochloride dosage similar to what the patient is receiving and 5 mg of linagliptin, administered in 2 divided doses (when given as the fixed-combination preparation containing immediate-release metformin hydrochloride) or once daily (when given as the fixed-combination preparation containing extended-release metformin hydrochloride).

In patients currently receiving metformin hydrochloride and linagliptin, the recommended initial dosage of the fixed combination of immediate-release metformin hydrochloride and linagliptin is the same as the existing total daily dosage of each component administered in 2 divided doses daily. In patients already receiving linagliptin and metformin or the fixed combination of linagliptin and immediate-release metformin, the recommended initial dosage of the fixed combination of extended-release metformin hydrochloride and linagliptin is a total daily metformin hydrochloride dosage similar to the patient's existing dosage and 5 mg of linagliptin administered once daily.

Metformin Hydrochloride/Saxagliptin Fixed-combination Therapy. Dosage of extended-release metformin hydrochloride in fixed combination with saxagliptin hydrochloride should be individualized based on the patient's current antidiabetic regimen, clinical response, and tolerability. Any change in therapy should be undertaken with care and appropriate monitoring because changes in glycemic control can occur.

When the fixed-combination preparation containing extended-release metformin hydrochloride and saxagliptin is used in patients inadequately controlled on monotherapy with saxagliptin 5 mg daily, the recommended initial dosage of the fixed combination is 500 mg of extended-release metformin hydrochloride and 5 mg of saxagliptin once daily; dosage should be increased gradually to reduce adverse GI effects of metformin.

When the fixed-combination preparation containing extended-release metformin hydrochloride and saxagliptin is used in patients inadequately controlled on monotherapy with extended-release metformin hydrochloride, dosage of the fixed combination should provide metformin hydrochloride at the patient's current dosage or at the nearest therapeutically appropriate dosage. Following a switch from immediate-release to extended-release metformin, glycemic control should be closely monitored and dosage adjustments made accordingly.

In patients inadequately controlled on monotherapy with saxagliptin 2.5 mg daily, the recommended initial dosage of the fixed combination is 1 g of extended-release metformin hydrochloride and 2.5 mg of saxagliptin daily. Patients who require 2.5 mg of saxagliptin *and* who are either metformin naive or require a dose of metformin hydrochloride exceeding 1 g should use the individual components.

The maximum recommended dosages of extended-release metformin hydrochloride and saxagliptin in fixed combination are 2 g of extended-release metformin hydrochloride and 5 mg of saxagliptin daily.

When the fixed-combination preparation containing extended-release metformin hydrochloride and saxagliptin is used concomitantly with a potent cytochrome P-450 isoenzyme 3A4/5 (CYP3A4/5) inhibitor (e.g., atazanavir, clarithromycin, indinavir, itraconazole, ketoconazole, nefazodone, nelfinavir, ritonavir, saquinavir, telithromycin), dosage of saxagliptin should be limited to 2.5 mg once daily.

Metformin Hydrochloride/Sitagliptin Fixed-combination Therapy. Dosage of the fixed-combination preparation containing immediate- or extended-release metformin hydrochloride and sitagliptin (Janumet® or Janumet® XR) should be individualized based on the patient's current antidiabetic regimen, effectiveness, and tolerability. When the fixed combination containing immediate-release metformin hydrochloride and sitagliptin is used in patients *not* currently receiving metformin hydrochloride, the recommended initial dosage is 500 mg of immediate-release metformin hydrochloride and 50 mg of sitagliptin twice daily. When the fixed combination containing extended-release metformin hydrochloride and sitagliptin is used in patients *not* currently receiving metformin hydrochloride, the recommended initial dosage is 1 g of extended-release metformin hydrochloride and 100 mg of sitagliptin once daily. The dosage should be increased gradually to reduce adverse GI effects associated with the metformin hydrochloride component.

When the fixed combination of immediate-release metformin hydrochloride and sitagliptin is used in patients currently receiving metformin hydrochloride, the recommended initial dosage is 500 mg of metformin hydrochloride and 50 mg of sitagliptin or 1 g of metformin hydrochloride and 50 mg of sitagliptin twice daily, depending on the patient's existing dosage of metformin hydrochloride.

When the fixed combination of immediate-release metformin hydrochloride and sitagliptin is used in patients currently receiving immediate-release metformin hydrochloride 850 mg twice daily, the recommended initial dosage of the fixed combination is 1 g of immediate-release metformin hydrochloride and 50 mg of sitagliptin twice daily.

When the fixed combination of extended-release metformin hydrochloride and sitagliptin is used in patients currently receiving metformin hydrochloride, the recommended initial dosage of the fixed combination is 1 g of extended-release metformin hydrochloride and 100 mg of sitagliptin or 2 g of extended-release metformin hydrochloride and 100 mg of sitagliptin once daily, depending on the patient's existing dosage of metformin hydrochloride.

In patients currently receiving immediate-release metformin hydrochloride 850 or 1000 mg twice daily, the recommend initial dosage of the fixed combination containing extended-release metformin hydrochloride and sitagliptin is 2 g of extended-release metformin hydrochloride and 100 mg of sitagliptin once daily.

The same total daily dosage of sitagliptin and metformin hydrochloride should be maintained when transitioning between the fixed combination of immediate-release metformin hydrochloride and sitagliptin and the fixed combination of extended-release metformin hydrochloride and sitagliptin.

The safety and efficacy of transferring from therapy with other oral antidiabetic agents to the fixed combination of sitagliptin and immediate- or extended-release metformin hydrochloride have not been specifically established in clinical studies. Any change in the therapy of patients with type 2 diabetes mellitus should be undertaken with caution and appropriate monitoring, as changes in glycemic control can occur.

Concomitant administration of the fixed combination of immediate- or extended-release metformin hydrochloride and sitagliptin with a sulfonylurea or insulin may require reduced dosages of the sulfonylurea or insulin to reduce the risk of hypoglycemia.

Dosage of metformin hydrochloride in fixed combination with sitagliptin should be selected carefully in patients of advanced age, since aging is associated with reduced renal function. In geriatric patients, dosage adjustment should be based on careful and regular assessment of renal function.

Metformin Hydrochloride/Canagliflozin Fixed-combination Therapy. When the commercially available fixed combination of immediate-release metformin hydrochloride and canagliflozin (Invokamet®) is used in patients with type 2 diabetes mellitus in whom treatment with both drugs is appropriate, the initial dosage should be based on the patient's current regimen with canagliflozin and/or metformin hydrochloride. In patients with an estimated glomerular filtration rate (eGFR) of at least 60 mL/minute per 1.73 m^2, the dosage of the fixed-combination preparation may be gradually increased based on effectiveness and tolerability up to a maximum of 2 g of metformin hydrochloride and 300 mg of canagliflozin daily.

In patients *not* currently treated with either metformin hydrochloride or canagliflozin, the recommended initial total daily dosage of these drugs is 1 g of metformin hydrochloride and 100 mg of canagliflozin, administered in 2 divided doses (when given as the fixed-combination preparation containing immediate-release metformin hydrochloride) or once daily (when given as the fixed-combination preparation containing extended-release metformin hydrochloride).

In patients currently receiving metformin hydrochloride, the recommended initial total daily dosage of the fixed combination with canagliflozin is a metformin hydrochloride dosage similar to the patient's existing total daily dosage and 100 mg of canagliflozin, administered in 2 divided doses (when given as the fixed-combination preparation containing immediate-release metformin hydrochloride) or once daily (when given as the fixed-combination preparation containing extended-release metformin hydrochloride). Patients who are currently receiving an evening dose of extended-release metformin hydrochloride should skip their last dose prior to initiating therapy with the fixed combination of canagliflozin and metformin hydrochloride the following morning.

In patients currently receiving canagliflozin, the recommended initial total daily dosage of the fixed combination is 1 g of metformin hydrochloride and the same daily dosage of canagliflozin, administered in 2 divided doses (when given as the fixed-combination preparation containing immediate-release metformin hydrochloride) or once daily (when given as the fixed-combination preparation containing extended-release metformin hydrochloride).

In patients currently receiving metformin hydrochloride and canagliflozin as separate components, the recommended initial dosage of the fixed combination is a total daily metformin hydrochloride dosage similar to the patient's existing dosage and the same daily dosage of canagliflozin, administered in 2 divided doses (when given as the fixed-combination preparation containing immediate-release metformin hydrochloride) or once daily (when given as the fixed-combination preparation containing extended-release metformin hydrochloride).

Metformin Hydrochloride/Dapagliflozin Fixed-combination Therapy. When the commercially available fixed combination of extended-release metformin hydrochloride and dapagliflozin (Xigduo® XR) is used in patients with type 2 diabetes mellitus, the recommended initial dosage is based on the patient's current regimen of metformin hydrochloride and/or dapagliflozin. For patients *not* currently receiving dapagliflozin, the recommended initial dosage of the dapagliflozin component is 5 mg once daily. Dosage should be titrated gradually based on effectiveness and tolerability up to a maximum daily dosage of 2 g of extended-release metformin hydrochloride and 10 mg of dapagliflozin. Patients who are already receiving extended-release metformin hydrochloride in the evening who are switching to the fixed combination of dapagliflozin and metformin hydrochloride should skip their last dose of metformin hydrochloride before initiating therapy with the fixed combination the following morning.

Metformin Hydrochloride/Empagliflozin Fixed-combination Therapy. Dosage of metformin hydrochloride in fixed combination with empagliflozin should be individualized based on the patient's current antidiabetic regimen. The dosage of the fixed-combination preparation may be gradually increased based on effectiveness and tolerability up to a maximum of 2 g of metformin hydrochloride and 25 mg of empagliflozin daily.

In patients currently receiving metformin hydrochloride, the recommended initial total daily dosage of the fixed combination is a metformin hydrochloride dosage similar to the patient's existing total daily dosage and 10 mg of empagliflozin, administered in 2 divided doses (when given as the fixed-combination preparation containing immediate-release metformin hydrochloride) or once daily (when given as the fixed-combination preparation containing extended-release metformin hydrochloride).

In patients currently receiving empagliflozin, the recommended initial total daily dosage of the fixed combination is 1 g of metformin hydrochloride and the same daily dosage of empagliflozin administered in 2 divided doses (when given as the fixed-combination preparation containing immediate-release metformin hydrochloride) or once daily (when given as the fixed-combination preparation containing extended-release metformin hydrochloride).

In patients currently receiving metformin hydrochloride and empagliflozin as separate components, the recommended initial total daily dosage of the fixed combination is a metformin hydrochloride dosage similar to the patient's existing total daily dosage and the same daily dosage of empagliflozin, administered in 2 divided doses (when given as the fixed-combination preparation containing immediate-release metformin hydrochloride) or once daily (when given as the fixed-combination preparation containing extended-release metformin hydrochloride).

Metformin Hydrochloride/Ertugliflozin Fixed-combination Therapy. When the commercially available fixed-combination preparation containing immediate-release metformin hydrochloride and ertugliflozin (Segluromet®) is used in patients with type 2 diabetes mellitus, the recommended initial dosage is based on the patient's current regimen of metformin hydrochloride and/or ertugliflozin. The dosage of the fixed combination may be increased gradually based on effectiveness and tolerability up to a maximum of 2 g of metformin hydrochloride and 15 mg of ertugliflozin daily.

In patients currently receiving metformin hydrochloride, the recommended initial total daily dosage of the fixed combination is a metformin hydrochloride dosage similar to the patient's existing total daily dosage and 5 mg of ertugliflozin, administered in 2 divided doses.

In patients currently receiving ertugliflozin, the recommended initial total daily dosage of the fixed combination is 1 g of metformin hydrochloride and an ertugliflozin dosage similar to the patient's existing total daily dosage, administered in 2 divided doses.

For patients currently receiving metformin hydrochloride and ertugliflozin as separate components, the recommended initial total daily dosage of the fixed combination is a dosage of metformin hydrochloride similar to the patient's existing total daily dosage and the same daily dosage of ertugliflozin, administered in 2 divided doses.

Concomitant Therapy with Metformin and Insulin. Combination therapy with metformin and insulin may be used in patients who no longer respond adequately to therapy with oral antidiabetic agents. In such patients, an initial metformin hydrochloride dosage of 500 mg once daily is recommended. The daily dosage may be increased by 500 mg at weekly intervals up to a maximum of 2.5 g daily with immediate-release tablets, the oral solution, or an extended-release tablet preparation (Fortamet®); a maximum of 2 g daily with other extended-release tablet preparations (e.g., Glucophage® XR, Glumetza®); or until the desired fasting blood glucose concentration is achieved. Dosages up to 2 g may be given in 2 divided doses daily (e.g., 2 g daily given as 1 g with the morning and evening meals); dosages exceeding 2 g of metformin hydrochloride daily may be better tolerated if given in 3 divided doses daily with meals. Concurrent insulin dosage should initially remain unchanged. Patients should be monitored closely (e.g., with determination of fasting glucose concentrations) during the dosage titration. When fasting plasma glucose concentrations decrease to less than 120 mg/dL in patients receiving combined metformin and insulin therapy, the insulin dosage may be decreased by 10–25%. Further dosage adjustments should be individualized based on glycemic response. Periodic adjustments in dosage may be necessary during continued combination therapy, as guided by monitoring of fasting glucose and/or HbA_{1c} concentrations.

Polycystic Ovary Syndrome In women with polycystic ovary syndrome†, metformin hydrochloride dosages of 1.5–2.25 g daily in divided doses generally have been used to ameliorate symptoms of insulin resistance and hyperinsulinemia and to increase the frequency of spontaneous ovulation, menstrual cyclicity, and ovulatory response after ovarian stimulation.

■ **Dosage in Renal and Hepatic Impairment** Because of the risk of lactic acidosis, which occurs rarely but may be fatal, metformin should not be used in patients with severe renal disease or dysfunction and should be avoided in those with clinical or laboratory evidence of hepatic disease. In patients with moderate renal disease, the benefits and risks of continuing metformin therapy should be assessed. (See Cautions: Lactic Acidosis.)

While metformin has been contraindicated in patients with renal impairment (e.g., men or women with serum creatinine concentrations equal to or exceeding 1.5 or 1.4 mg/dL, respectively), an FDA review of clinical studies evaluating the safety of metformin in patients with reduced kidney function suggests that metformin can be used safely in patients with mild impairment in kidney function and in some patients with moderate impairment in kidney function.

The manufacturers and FDA state that renal function (estimated glomerular filtration rate [eGFR]) should be assessed prior to initiation of metformin and at least annually; more frequent monitoring has been recommended in patients with an increased risk of developing renal impairment (e.g., geriatric patients). The manufacturers and FDA state that metformin therapy should not be initiated in patients with an eGFR between 30–45 mL/minute per 1.73 m² and that the benefits and risks of continuing the drug should be assessed in those already receiving metformin whose eGFR falls below 45 mL/minute per 1.73 m². The manufacturers and FDA state that metformin should not be used in patients with an eGFR of less than 30 mL/minute per 1.73 m². The National Kidney Foundation Kidney Disease Outcomes Quality Initiative (NKF-KDOQI) states that the exact GFR cutoff for metformin use to avoid lactic acidosis is controversial. The NKF-KDOQI and other clinicians suggest that metformin therapy be avoided in patients with a GFR less than 30 mL/minute per 1.73 m² but that the risk-benefit of such therapy should be considered if GFR is stable. In addition, the NKF-KDOQI states that metformin therapy is probably safe when GFR is at least 45 mL/minute per 1.73 m² but that use of the drug should be reviewed when GFR falls below 45 mL/minute per 1.73 m². (See Cautions: Precautions and Contraindications.)

Cautions

Adverse effects, principally GI effects, reportedly occur in about 5–50% of patients receiving metformin therapy as immediate-release tablets in clinical trials and generally required discontinuance of the drug in 6% or less of patients.

■ **Lactic Acidosis** Accumulation of metformin may occur in patients with renal impairment, and such accumulation rarely can result in lactic acidosis, a serious, potentially fatal metabolic disease. The reported overall incidence of lactic acidosis in patients receiving metformin therapy is approximately 0.04 cases per 1000 patient-years of metformin therapy. (See Cautions: Precautions and Contraindications and also see Chemistry and Stability: Chemistry.) However, lactic acidosis constitutes a medical emergency requiring immediate hospitalization and treatment; in such cases, metformin should be discontinued and general supportive therapy (e.g., volume expansion, diuresis) should be initiated immediately. Prompt hemodialysis also is recommended. (See Acute Toxicity.)

Metformin-associated lactic acidosis has been characterized by elevated blood lactate concentrations (exceeding 45 mg/dL), anion gap acidosis (without evidence of ketonuria or ketonemia), and an increased lactate/pyruvate ratio. Lactic acidosis also may occur in association with a variety of pathophysiologic conditions, including diabetes mellitus, and generally whenever substantial tissue hypoperfusion and hypoxemia exist. Approximately 50% of cases of metformin-associated lactic acidosis have been reported to be fatal. However, it has been suggested that in such cases of lactic acidosis not accompanied by conditions predisposing to tissue anoxia (e.g., heart failure, renal or pulmonary disease), techniques for the elimination of metformin from the body may allow recovery rates exceeding 80%.

The manufacturer states that when metformin has been implicated as the cause of lactic acidosis, plasma metformin concentrations exceeding 5 mcg/mL generally have been observed. However, plasma metformin concentrations may not be an accurate indication of tissue accumulation of the drug in patients with metformin-induced lactic acidosis, and increased plasma concentrations of lactic acid or lactic acidosis have been demonstrated during metformin therapy despite normal plasma concentrations of the drug. Patients with lactic acidosis and normal plasma metformin concentrations also may have other conditions contributing to the development of lactic acidosis (e.g., hypoxia, dehydration). Some observational data suggest that neither plasma metformin concentrations nor plasma lactate concentrations are related to mortality in patients with lactic acidosis receiving metformin.

Lactic acidosis often has a subtle onset and may be accompanied only by nonspecific symptoms such as malaise, myalgias, respiratory distress, increasing somnolence, and nonspecific abdominal distress. Associated hypothermia, hypotension, and resistant bradyarrhythmias with more marked acidosis also may occur. Patients and clinicians should be aware of the possible importance of such symptoms, and patients should be instructed to notify their clinician immediately if these symptoms occur; metformin should be discontinued until the patient is hospitalized and a clinician has evaluated the patient's condition. Once a patient is stabilized at any dosage of metformin hydrochloride, GI symptoms, which are common during initiation of therapy, are unlikely to be drug related; later occurrence of GI symptoms could be manifestations of lactic acidosis or other serious disease.

Lactic acidosis associated with metformin therapy generally has occurred in diabetic patients with severe renal insufficiency; most cases of lactic acidosis have been reported in patients with concomitant medical and/or surgical problems who were receiving multiple drugs.

Some observational studies and meta-analyses suggest that the incidence of lactic acidosis in patients with type 2 diabetes mellitus who are receiving metformin therapy is similar to that in patients not receiving the drug. Analyses of pooled data that included all known prospective comparative trials and observational cohort studies of metformin therapy of at least 1 month's duration (up to 70,490 patient-years of metformin treatment) revealed no cases of fatal or nonfatal metformin-induced lactic acidosis; therefore, an incidence rate for metformin-associated lactic acidosis could not be calculated. While these analyses allowed for the inclusion of patients with at least one contraindication to metformin (e.g., renal insufficiency), information on the safety of metformin in the presence of such contraindications could not be evaluated because of the lack of information on the number of included patients with such conditions. In these analyses, all cases of lactic acidosis reportedly occurred in patients with comorbidities predisposing to lactic acidosis, suggesting that association of the condition with metformin use may be coincidental rather than causal.

The risk of lactic acidosis appears to increase with the degree of renal impairment and the patient's age; therefore, the risk of this condition can be minimized by periodic monitoring of renal function and cautious dosage selection (i.e., initiating drug therapy at the low end of the dosage range). Metformin therapy should be withheld promptly in patients with any condition associated with hypoxemia, sepsis, or dehydration, or in any patient who becomes acutely unwell. Therapy with the drug alone or in fixed combinations also should be avoided in patients with clinical or laboratory evidence of hepatic impairment since elimination of lactate may be reduced substantially in such patients. Patients should be advised not to consume excessive amounts of alcohol, either acutely or chronically, since alcohol may potentiate the effects of metformin on lactate metabolism by decreasing hepatic gluconeogenesis.

The manufacturers, FDA, and other clinicians state that metformin-containing therapy should be discontinued before or at the time of an intravascular (e.g., IV, intra-arterial) iodinated contrast imaging procedure in patients with an estimated glomerular filtration rate (eGFR) of 30–60 mL/minute per 1.73 m² and in patients with a history of liver disease, alcoholism, or heart failure. Therapy with metformin-containing preparations also should be withheld temporarily in patients undergoing surgery or receiving intra-arterial iodinated contrast agents. Renal function should be evaluated 48 hours after the imaging procedure and metformin therapy may be reinstituted if renal function is stable. (See Cautions: Precautions and Contraindications.)

■ **GI Effects** Adverse GI effects such as diarrhea, nausea, vomiting, flatulence, indigestion, and abdominal discomfort (e.g., bloating, abdominal cramping or pain) are the most common adverse effects associated with metformin-containing therapy as immediate-release tablets; diarrhea and nausea/vomiting are among the most common drug-related adverse effects reported in clinical trials with the extended-release tablets. Because substantial diarrhea and/or vomiting may cause dehydration and prerenal azotemia, metformin should be discontinued in patients who develop such potentially serious GI effects; persistent diarrhea resolves promptly upon discontinuance of the drug. Unpleasant or metallic taste (taste disorder/disturbance), which usually resolves spontaneously, has been reported in approximately 1–5% of patients receiving metformin immediate-release or extended-release tablets. Other adverse GI effects reported in 1–5% of patients receiving immediate-release or an extended-release metformin tablet preparation (Glucophage® XR) include abnormal stools, distended abdomen, constipation, or dyspepsia/heartburn. Other adverse GI effects reported in 1–5% of patients receiving another metformin extended-release tablet (Fortamet®) include dyspepsia, flatulence, and abdominal pain. Anorexia also has been reported with metformin therapy.

Metformin-induced adverse GI effects appear to be dose related, generally occur at initiation of therapy, and usually subside spontaneously during continued metformin therapy; in some cases, a reduction in metformin hydrochloride dosage may be useful in hastening resolution of these effects. Diarrhea severe enough to require discontinuance of metformin occurred in about 6% of patients receiving the immediate-release tablets and in about 0.6% of those receiving the extended-release tablets in controlled clinical trials. Since adverse GI effects occurring during initiation of metformin therapy appear to be dose related, they may be reduced by gradual dosage escalation and administration of the drug with meals.

Diarrhea was reported in up to 7.5% of patients receiving combined therapy with metformin hydrochloride and sitagliptin in clinical trials.

■ **Hypoglycemia** Hypoglycemia is uncommon in patients receiving metformin as monotherapy; however, it may occur when metformin is used concomitantly with an oral sulfonylurea antidiabetic agent, a thiazolidinedione, or insulin, when caloric intake is deficient, or when strenuous exercise is not accompanied by food intake. Symptoms of hypoglycemia (such as dizziness, shakiness, sweating, hunger) have occurred in 21.3, 11.4, or 37.7% of patients receiving glyburide (5.3 mg), glyburide in fixed combination with metformin hydrochloride (2.78 mg of glyburide, 557 mg of metformin hydrochloride), or glyburide in fixed combination with metformin hydrochloride at a final mean titrated dosage of 824 mg of metformin hydrochloride and 4.1 mg of glyburide in controlled clinical trials. In a controlled initial therapy trial of metformin hydrochloride in fixed combination with glipizide, symptomatic hypoglycemia and blood glucose concentrations 50 mg/dL or less occurred in 2.9, 0, 7.6, or 9.3% of patients receiving glipizide monotherapy (final mean dosage of 16.7 mg), metformin hydrochloride monotherapy (final mean dosage of 1.749 g of metformin hydrochloride), the fixed combination with glipizide (final mean dosage of 791 mg of metformin hydrochloride and 7.9 mg of glipizide), and the fixed combination with a higher dosage of the metformin hydrochloride component (final mean dosage of 1.477 g of metformin hydrochloride and 7.4 mg of glipizide). In a controlled trial in patients inadequately controlled by monotherapy with metformin hydrochloride or a sulfonylurea agent, documented hypoglycemia (as determined by blood glucose concentrations of 50 mg/dL or less) occurred in 0, 1.3, or 12.6% of patients receiving glipizide monotherapy (mean final dosage of 30 mg), metformin hydrochloride monotherapy (mean final dosage of 1.927 g), or metformin hydrochloride in fixed combination with glipizide at a final mean dosage of 1.747 g of metformin hydrochloride and 5 mg of glipizide. When rosiglitazone was added to fixed combination therapy of glyburide and metformin hydrochloride, documented hypoglycemia occurred in 22% of such patients compared to 3.3% of patients receiving glyburide in fixed combination with metformin hydrochloride. (See Cautions: Precautions and Contraindications.)

Hypoglycemia was reported in 16.4% of patients when sitagliptin was added to combined metformin hydrochloride and glimepiride therapy, compared with 0.9% of those receiving placebo in conjunction with metformin hydrochloride and glimepiride therapy.

■ **Hematologic Effects** Asymptomatic decreases in serum vitamin B_{12} concentration were reported in about 7–9% of patients receiving metformin alone, and in about 6% of those receiving metformin concomitantly with a sulfonylurea antidiabetic agent, during 29-week controlled clinical trials. Such decreases may be related to interference with absorption of vitamin B_{12} from B_{12}-intrinsic factor complex; however, they rarely are associated with anemia and are rapidly reversible following discontinuation of metformin or supplementation with vitamin B_{12}. Serum folic acid concentrations do not appear to decrease substantially in patients receiving metformin therapy. Megaloblastic anemia has been reported rarely in patients receiving metformin. No increased incidence of neuropathy has been observed in patients receiving the drug. Hematologic parameters (e.g., hemoglobin) should be monitored annually and serum vitamin B_{12} concentrations should be monitored every 2–3 years in patients receiving metformin; any apparent abnormalities should be appropriately investigated and managed (e.g., administration of supplemental vitamin B_{12} to those who develop neuropathy). Some individuals such as those who have inadequate vitamin B_{12} or calcium intake or absorption appear to be at an increased risk for developing subnormal vitamin B_{12} concentrations. Some clinicians have suggested that periodic supplementation with parenteral vitamin B_{12} be considered in such patients and in alcoholics. (See Cautions: Precautions and Contraindications.)

■ **Dermatologic Reactions** The manufacturer states that incidence of rash or dermatitis in patients receiving metformin monotherapy is similar to that with placebo, and that the incidence of these dermatologic effects in patients receiving metformin concomitantly with a sulfonylurea antidiabetic agent is similar to that in individuals receiving a sulfonylurea antidiabetic agent alone.

■ **Nervous System Effects** Headache, agitation, dizziness, and tiredness were reported in a small comparative study in geriatric diabetic patients receiving metformin. Headache was reported in 4.7 or 5.1% of patients receiving metformin as an extended-release tablet preparation (Fortamet®) or as immediate-release tablets, respectively. Headache has been reported in 9.3 or 8.9% of patients receiving metformin or metformin in fixed combination with glyburide, respectively. Headache has been reported in 5.3 or 12.6% of patients receiving metformin or metformin in fixed combination with glipizide, respectively. Headache has been reported in 5.9% of patients receiving combined therapy with metformin and sitagliptin and 6.9% of patients receiving combined therapy with metformin, sitagliptin, and glimepiride in clinical trials. Dizziness has been reported in 3.8 or 5.5% of patients receiving metformin or metformin in fixed combination with glyburide, respectively. Dizziness has been reported in 3.8 or 5.5% of patients receiving metformin or metformin in fixed combination with glyburide, respectively.

■ **Respiratory Effects** Pneumonitis with vasculitis has been reported rarely with concomitant metformin and oral sulfonylurea (e.g., glyburide) therapy. Upper respiratory tract infection was reported in 16.3 or 17.3% of patients receiving metformin or metformin in fixed combination with glyburide, respectively. Upper respiratory tract infection was reported in 8.5 or 8.1–9.9% of patients receiving metformin or metformin in fixed combination with glipizide, respectively, as initial therapy for type 2 diabetes mellitus. Upper respiratory tract infection was reported in 10.7 or 10.3% of patients receiving metformin or metformin in fixed combination with glipizide, respectively, as second-line therapy for type 2 diabetes mellitus. Upper respiratory tract infection was reported in 5.2 or 6.2% of patients receiving metformin or metformin combined with sitagliptin, respectively, in clinical trials. Rhinitis was reported in 4.2 or 5.6% of patients receiving metformin as an extended-release tablet preparation (Fortamet®) or as immediate-release tablets, respectively. Infection was reported in 20.5 or 20.9% of patients receiving an extended-release tablet preparation (Fortamet®) or immediate-release tablets, respectively.

■ **Other Adverse Effects** Urinary tract infection has been reported in 8 or 1.1% of patients receiving metformin alone or in fixed combination with glipizide, respectively. Hypertension has been reported in 5.6 or 2.9–3.5% of patients receiving metformin alone or in fixed combination with glipizide, respectively. Musculoskeletal pain has been reported in 6.7 or 8% of patients receiving metformin alone or in fixed combination with glipizide, respectively. Severe acute hepatitis associated with marked elevations in serum hepatic aminotransferase values and cholestasis has been reported following initiation of metformin therapy in a patient receiving glipizide and enalapril. Accidental injury was reported in 7.3 or 5.6% of patients receiving metformin as an extended-release tablet preparation (Fortamet®) or as immediate-release tablets, respectively.

■ **Precautions and Contraindications** When metformin hydrochloride is used in fixed combination with other drugs (e.g., sulfonylureas, thiazolidinediones, dipeptidyl peptidase-4 [DPP-4] inhibitors, meglitinides, sodium-glucose cotransporter 2 [SGLT2] inhibitors), the cautions, precautions, contraindications, and drug interactions associated with these concomitant agents must be considered in addition to those associated with metformin.

The diagnostic and therapeutic measures for managing diabetes mellitus that are necessary to ensure optimum control of the disease with insulin are generally necessary with metformin. Clinicians who prescribe metformin should be familiar with the indications, limitations, and patient-selection criteria for therapy with oral antidiabetic agents to ensure appropriate patient management. Patients receiving metformin should be monitored with regular laboratory evaluations, including blood glucose determinations, to determine the minimum effective dosage of metformin hydrochloride when used either as monotherapy or in combination with a sulfonylurea or thiazolidinedione antidiabetic agent. Glycosylated hemoglobin (hemoglobin A_{1c} [HbA_{1c}]) measurements also are useful, particularly for monitoring long-term control of blood glucose concentration.

Patients should be informed of the risks of lactic acidosis and conditions that predispose to its development. (See Cautions: Lactic Acidosis.) Since metformin is excreted substantially by the kidneys, accumulation of the drug resulting in lactic acidosis may occur in patients with renal impairment; the risk of lactic acidosis increases with degree of renal impairment. Hemodialysis has been used in patients with lactic acidosis to accelerate the clearance of metformin.(See Acute Toxicity.) The manufacturer states that renal function should be evaluated prior to initiation of therapy with metformin preparations and at least annually thereafter.

Metformin therapy is contraindicated in patients with an eGFR of less than 30 mL/minute per 1.73 m^2. In patients in whom development of impaired renal function is anticipated (e.g., those with blood glucose concentrations exceeding 300 mg/dL, who may develop renal dysfunction as a result of polyuria and volume depletion; geriatric patients), renal function should be monitored more frequently. In addition, drugs that may affect renal function, produce substantial hemodynamic changes, or interfere with metformin elimination (e.g., cimetidine) should be used with caution in patients receiving metformin. The National Kidney Foundation (NKF) Kidney Disease Outcomes Quality Initiative (KDOQI) recommends temporary discontinuance of potentially nephrotoxic and renally excreted drugs (e.g., angiotensin-converting enzyme [ACE] inhibitors, angiotensin II receptor antagonists, aldosterone inhibitors, direct renin inhibitors, diuretics, nonsteroidal anti-inflammatory agents [NSAIAs], metformin, lithium, digoxin) in patients with a GFR less than 60 mL/minute per 1.73 m^2.

Extended-release metformin hydrochloride tablets or fixed-combination preparations containing the extended-release form of the drug should not be chewed, cut, or crushed; these dosage forms must be swallowed whole. Patients should be aware that the biologically inert components of the tablet may occasionally be eliminated in the feces as a soft, hydrated mass.

Some clinicians state that metformin should not be used in patients with heart failure requiring drug therapy (e.g., digoxin, furosemide), such as those with unstable or acute heart failure. These patients are at risk for hypoperfusion and hypoxemia, which may lead to lactic acidosis. It has been suggested that metformin may be reinstituted once acute heart failure has resolved and renal function is normal (as measured by creatinine clearance); the decision to continue metformin therapy in such patients should be individualized.

Iodinated contrast agents are a potential concern for furthering renal damage in patients with acute kidney injury, and in patients with severe chronic kidney disease (stage IV or stage V). Since administration of iodinated contrast media may lead to acute alteration of renal function and has been associated with lactic acidosis in patients receiving metformin, metformin-containing preparations should be discontinued before or at the time of the procedure in patients with an eGFR between 30–60 mL/minute per 1.73 m^2; in patients with a history of liver disease, alcoholism, or heart failure; and in those receiving intra-arterial iodinated contrast agents. Renal function should be evaluated 48 hours after the imaging procedure and metformin therapy may be reinstituted if renal function is stable. However, the American College of Radiology states that in patients with no evidence of acute kidney injury and an eGFR of at least 30 mL/minute per 1.73 m^2, there is no need to discontinue metformin either prior to or following the administration of iodinated contrast media, nor is there a need to reassess the patient's renal function following the test or procedure.

The manufacturers state that metformin also should be discontinued temporarily in patients undergoing surgery, except minor surgery that is not associated with restricted food or fluid intake; the drug should be reinitiated only when the patient's oral intake has resumed and renal function has been shown to be normal. In addition, any diabetic patient previously well controlled with metformin therapy who develops a clinical illness (especially one that is vague and poorly defined) or whose laboratory test results deviate from normal should be evaluated promptly for evidence of ketoacidosis or lactic acidosis. (See Cautions: Lactic Acidosis.) Such evaluation should include determinations of serum electrolytes and ketones, blood glucose, and if indicated, blood pH, lactate, pyruvate, and metformin concentrations. Since cardiovascular collapse (shock), heart failure, ischemic heart disease (e.g., acute myocardial infarction), peripheral vascular disease (e.g., claudication), obstructive airways disease, or other conditions that are likely to cause central hypoxemia or reduced peripheral perfusion have been associated with lactic acidosis and prerenal azotemia, metformin should be discontinued in patients developing such conditions.

The cardiovascular risks associated with use of oral antidiabetic agents have not been fully determined. In 1970, the University Group Diabetes Program (UGDP) reported that administration of oral antidiabetic agents (i.e., tolbutamide or phenformin) was associated with increased cardiovascular mortality compared with treatment with dietary regulation alone or with dietary regulation and insulin. The UGDP reported that type 2 diabetic patients who were treated for 5–8 years with dietary regulation and a fixed dose (1.5 g daily) of tolbutamide or dietary regulation and a fixed dose (100 mg daily) of phenformin (currently not commercially available in the US) had a cardiovascular mortality rate approximately 2.5 times that of patients treated with dietary regulation alone. Although a substantial increase in total mortality was observed only with phenformin, both tolbutamide and phenformin were discontinued because of the increases in cardiovascular mortality. The results of the UGDP study have been analyzed exhaustively, and there has been general disagreement in the scientific and medical communities regarding the study's validity and clinical importance. The management of patients with type 2 diabetes mellitus has changed substantially since the UGDP was initiated in 1961. Dietary management, weight reduction, better control of blood glucose concentration, and regular physical activity have received greater emphasis in the management of diabetes in these patients. In addition, reduction of existing cardiovascular risk factors (e.g., management of hypertension, discontinuance of smoking) has been emphasized. The American Diabetes Association (ADA) currently recommends that clinician judgment in the management of type 2 diabetes mellitus be based on assessment of all available therapeutic information, including data on cardiovascular risk factors, the positive effect of metabolic control of diabetes on cardiovascular disease, the importance of dietary management and weight reduction in obese diabetic patients, the importance of regular physical activity, and objective reports in the scientific literature that pertain to the UGDP study and to the long-term use of sulfonylureas.

Results of several long-term studies by the UKPDS group indicate that effects of metformin on mortality and macrovascular outcomes vary considerably depending on the patient population evaluated. In one study, intensive therapy (target fasting plasma glucose of less than 108 mg/dL) initiated with metformin or other antidiabetic agents (chlorpropamide, glyburide, or insulin) was compared with conventional therapy (target fasting plasma glucose of less than 270 mg/dL) consisting of diet and supplemental therapy with the same antidiabetic agents for marked hyperglycemia in overweight (exceeding 120% of ideal body weight) patients. In this study, cardiovascular disease accounted for 62% of the total mortality observed in patients receiving conventional therapy. Intensive therapy initiated with metformin in these overweight patients was associated with a 36% reduction in all-cause mortality and a 30% lower risk of developing macrovascular disease (myocardial infarction, sudden death, angina, stroke, peripheral vascular disease) compared with conventional therapy; the reduction in macrovascular disease was similar among intensive therapies employing other antidiabetic agents.

In another study, metformin was given as supplemental therapy in overweight and non-overweight patients who were poorly controlled on existing sulfonylurea therapy, or sulfonylurea therapy alone was continued. In this study, intensive metformin and sulfonylurea therapy was associated with an *increase* in the risk of diabetes-related death or death from any cause compared with that in patients continuing to receive sulfonylurea therapy alone. Similarly, another study by the UKPDS group found no decrease in mortality when metformin was added to sulfonylurea therapy (i.e., chlorpropamide or glyburide) or insulin alone in an intensive regimen (target fasting plasma glucose concentration of 108 mg/dL) in obese and non-obese patients. A pooled analysis of both UKPDS trials and epidemiologic analysis of other non-overweight and overweight patients from UKPDS who received metformin and sulfonylurea therapy because of progressive hyperglycemia showed a small reduction in diabetes-related death, all-cause mortality, myocardial infarction, and stroke.

Patients should be advised fully and completely about the nature of diabetes mellitus, what they must do to prevent and detect complications, and how to control their condition. *Patients should be informed of the potential risks and advantages of metformin therapy and of alternative forms of treatment.* Patients should be instructed about the importance of adherence to dietary instructions, of a regular exercise program, and of regular assessment of blood glucose, HbA_{1c}, renal function, and hematologic parameters. The possibility of primary and secondary failure to metformin therapy also should be explained to patients.

Patients and responsible family members should be informed of the risks of hypoglycemia, symptoms and treatment of hypoglycemic reactions, and conditions that predispose to the development of such reactions, since these reactions occasionally may occur during therapy with metformin. Hypoglycemia occurs infrequently in patients receiving metformin therapy under usual conditions of use; the incidence of hypoglycemia with metformin is much lower than that in patients receiving sulfonylureas, meglitinides (e.g., repaglinide), or insulin. However, hypoglycemia may occur when the drug is used concomitantly with a sulfonylurea antidiabetic agent and/or insulin. In addition, certain other factors (e.g., deficient caloric intake, strenuous exercise not compensated by caloric supplementation, alcohol ingestion, adrenal or pituitary insufficiency) may predispose patients to the development of hypoglycemia. Debilitated, malnourished, or geriatric patients also may be particularly susceptible to hypoglycemia; this condition may be difficult to recognize in geriatric patients or in those receiving β-adrenergic blocking agents or other sympatholytic agents. (See Drug Interactions: β-Adrenergic Blocking Agents.)

To maintain control of diabetes during periods of stress (e.g., fever of any cause, trauma, infection, surgery), temporary discontinuance of metformin and administration of insulin may be required. Metformin therapy may be reinstituted after the acute episode is resolved. Patients should contact a clinician promptly concerning changes in dosage requirements during periods of stress.

Since decreases in serum vitamin B_{12} concentrations have been reported in some patients receiving metformin, hematologic parameters (e.g., hemoglobin, hematocrit, erythrocyte indices) should be evaluated prior to initiation of metformin therapy and at least annually during treatment and any abnormality properly investigated. Vitamin B_{12} concentrations should be monitored every 2–3 years in patients receiving metformin therapy and any abnormalities managed. Some patients (i.e., those with an inadequate absorption or intake of vitamin B_{12} or calcium) appear to be predisposed to developing decreased vitamin B_{12} concentrations.

Metformin alone or in fixed combination with other drugs is contraindicated in patients with severe renal impairment (eGFR less than 30 mL/minute per 1.73 m^2) , which may result from conditions such as cardiovascular collapse (shock), acute myocardial infarction, or septicemia. Initiation of therapy with metformin in fixed combination with pioglitazone or rosiglitazone is contraindicated in patients with New York Heart Association (NYHA) class III or IV heart failure. Patients with NYHA class III or IV heart failure were not studied in clinical trials of metformin in fixed combination with pioglitazone or rosiglitazone, and these fixed combinations are not recommended in these patients or in patients with symptomatic heart failure. Metformin-containing therapy also is contraindicated as *sole* therapy in patients with type 1 diabetes mellitus and in patients with diabetes complicated by acute or chronic metabolic acidosis, including diabetic ketoacidosis with or without coma. Insulin is required for the treatment of diabetic ketoacidosis. Metformin-containing therapy also is contraindicated in patients with known hypersensitivity to any ingredient in the respective formulations.

No studies have been performed evaluating the safety or efficacy of metformin and rosiglitazone in combination with insulin, and the manufacturer of Avandamet® states that use of such combination therapy is not indicated. An increased incidence of adverse cardiovascular events (e.g., edema, CHF) has occurred with rosiglitazone in combination with insulin. (See Congestive Heart Failure under Warnings/Precautions: Warnings, in Cautions in Rosiglitazone 68:20.28.) If metformin is used concomitantly with rosiglitazone and insulin, patients treated with this combination should be monitored for adverse cardiovascular events. Combination therapy with rosiglitazone, metformin, and insulin should be discontinued in patients who do not respond to such therapy (as determined by a reduction in HbA_{1c} values or insulin dosage within 4–5 months) or in those who develop clinically important adverse effects.

■ **Pediatric Precautions** Safety and efficacy of metformin immediate-release or certain extended-release tablets (Glucophage® XR, Fortamet®) in pediatric patients younger than 10 or younger than 17 years of age, respectively, have not been established. Safety and efficacy of another extended-release preparation (Glumetza®) have not been established in pediatric patients younger than 18 years of age. Safety and efficacy of metformin oral solution in children younger than 10 years of age have not been established. Data from a placebo-controlled clinical trial indicated a similar glycemic response and adverse effect profile for metformin in pediatric patients (10–16 years of age) as in adults. (See Diabetes Mellitus: Metformin Monotherapy, in Uses.) The safety and efficacy of metformin in fixed combination with glipizide, pioglitazone, rosiglitazone, repaglinide, or sitagliptin in pediatric patients have not been established. Data from a comparative trial evaluating the safety and efficacy of metformin in fixed combination with glyburide compared with monotherapy with each agent in pediatric patients (9–16 years of age) with type 2 diabetes mellitus indicate no unexpected safety concerns with such combination therapy. The American Diabetes Association (ADA) states that most pediatric diabetologists use oral antidiabetic agents in children with type 2 diabetes mellitus because of greater patient compliance and convenience for the patient's family and a lack of evidence demonstrating better efficacy of insulin as initial therapy for type 2 diabetes mellitus.

■ **Geriatric Precautions** Controlled clinical trials evaluating metformin hydrochloride immediate-release and extended-release tablets (Glucophage® XR, Glumetza®) did not include sufficient numbers of geriatric patients to determine whether geriatric patients respond differently to metformin than younger patients, although other reported clinical experience has not identified any differences in response between geriatric and younger patients. Data from controlled clinical trials evaluating another metformin hydrochloride extended-release preparation (Fortamet®) indicate no overall differences in safety or efficacy in geriatric patients compared with younger adults. Data from controlled clinical trials with metformin in fixed combination with glyburide or glipizide have not revealed age-related differences in safety and efficacy of the combination, but greater sensitivity of geriatric patients to these fixed combinations cannot be ruled out. Since metformin is excreted principally by the kidneys and renal function declines with age, the drug should be used with caution in geriatric patients. As geriatric patients are at risk for the development of lactic acidosis, metformin therapy should not be initiated in geriatric patients 80 years of age and older without confirmation of adequate renal function as measured by creatinine clearance. In addition, renal function should be monitored periodically and care should be taken in dosage selection for geriatric patients; such patients generally should not receive the maximum recommended dosage of metformin hydrochloride. (See Dosage: Maintenance Dosage in Dosage and Administration.)

■ **Mutagenicity and Carcinogenicity** No evidence of mutagenicity or chromosomal damage was observed in vivo in a micronucleus test in mice or in in vitro test systems, including microbial (Ames test) and mammalian (mouse lymphoma and human lymphocytes) assays.

No evidence of carcinogenic potential was seen in a 104-week study in male and female rats receiving metformin hydrochloride dosages up to and including 900 mg/kg daily or in a 91-week study in male and female mice receiving metformin hydrochloride at dosages up to and including 1500 mg/kg daily; these dosages are about 3 times the maximum recommended human daily dosage based on body surface area. However, an increased incidence of benign stromal uterine polyps was observed in female rats treated with 900 mg/kg of metformin hydrochloride daily.

■ **Pregnancy, Fertility, and Lactation** Reproduction studies in rats and rabbits given metformin hydrochloride dosages of 600 mg/kg daily (about twice the maximum recommended human daily dosage based on body surface area or about 2 and 6 times the maximum recommended human daily dosage of extended-release tablets [2 g] based on body surface area comparisons with rats and rabbits, respectively) have not revealed evidence of harm (e.g., teratogenicity) to the fetus. Determination of fetal concentrations of metformin suggest that a partial placental barrier to the drug exists. Since abnormal maternal blood glucose concentrations during pregnancy may be associated with a higher incidence of congenital abnormalities, most experts recommend that insulin be used during pregnancy to maintain optimum control of blood glucose concentration.

There are no adequate and controlled studies to date using metformin in pregnant women. Limited data from uncontrolled or retrospective studies are conflicting with regard to the effects of long-term maternal therapy with metformin hydrochloride (1.5–3 g daily) on neonatal morbidity (e.g., congenital malformations) and mortality. Metformin should be used during pregnancy only when clearly needed. Metformin in fixed combination with pioglitazone should not be used in pregnancy unless the potential benefit justifies the potential risk to the fetus. Metformin in fixed combination with rosiglitazone is not recommended for use in pregnant women.

No evidence of impaired fertility was observed in rats following administration of metformin hydrochloride dosages of 600 mg/kg daily (about twice the maximum recommended human dosage based on body surface area).

Metformin is distributed into milk in lactating rats and reaches concentrations comparable to those in plasma. Limited data indicate that small amounts of metformin also are distributed into breast milk in humans. In a study in 7 nursing women who received metformin hydrochloride (median dosage 1500 mg daily), the mean milk-to-plasma ratio for metformin was 0.35 and the overall average concentration in milk over the dosing interval was 0.27 mg/L. Metformin was present in low or undetectable amounts in the plasma of 4 breast-fed infants, and no adverse effects were noted in 6 infants that were evaluated. In another study, mean peak and trough metformin concentrations in 4 nursing women receiving metformin hydrochloride 500 mg twice daily were 1.06 and 0.42 mcg/mL, respectively, in serum and 0.42 and 0.39 mcg/mL, respectively, in breast milk. The mean milk-to-serum ratio was 0.63 and the mean estimated infant dose as a percentage of the mother's weight-adjusted dose was 0.65%. Blood glucose concentrations obtained in 3 infants 4 hours after breastfeeding were within normal limits (47-77 mg/dL). However, the manufacturer states that because of the potential for hypoglycemia in infants, a decision should be made whether to discontinue nursing or the drug, taking into account the importance of the drug to the woman. If metformin alone or in fixed combination with pioglitazone is discontinued in a nursing mother and dietary therapy is inadequate for glycemic control, insulin therapy should be considered.

Drug Interactions

■ **Antidiabetic Agents** Although hypoglycemia occurs infrequently in patients receiving metformin therapy alone, hypoglycemia may occur when the drug is used concomitantly with a sulfonylurea antidiabetic agent (e.g., glyburide), a meglitinide (e.g., repaglinide), and/or insulin. (See Cautions: Precautions and Contraindications.)

In a single-dose study in patients with type 2 diabetes mellitus, concomitant administration of glyburide with metformin did not alter the pharmacokinetics or pharmacodynamics of metformin. Although variable decreases in the area under the blood concentration-time curve (AUC) and peak blood concentration of glyburide were observed, the single-dose nature of this study and the lack of a relationship between glyburide blood concentrations and pharmacodynamic effects preclude evaluation of the clinical importance of these effects.

In a single-dose study, administration of metformin concomitantly with an α-glucosidase inhibitor (acarbose) resulted in an acute decrease in the bioavailability of metformin. Coadministration of guar gum (10 g) and metformin hydrochloride (1.7 g) with a standard meal in healthy individuals reduced and delayed the absorption of metformin from the GI tract.

■ **Diuretics** Thiazide diuretics can exacerbate diabetes mellitus, resulting in increased requirements of oral antidiabetic agents, temporary loss of diabetic control, or secondary failure to the antidiabetic agent. If control of diabetes is impaired by a thiazide diuretic, clinicians may consider substituting a less diabetogenic diuretic (e.g., potassium-sparing diuretic), reducing the dosage of or discontinuing the diuretic, or increasing the dosage of the oral antidiabetic agent.

In a single-dose study in healthy individuals, administration of furosemide concomitantly with metformin increased peak plasma and blood concentrations of metformin by approximately 22% and AUC of metformin by approximately 15%. Administration of metformin concomitantly with furosemide decreased peak plasma furosemide concentrations by approximately 31% and AUC by approximately 12%. The renal clearance of both drugs remained unchanged during such concomitant use, but the half-life of furosemide was decreased by 32%. The manufacturer states that no information is available on potential interactions between metformin and furosemide during long-term administration.

■ **Nifedipine** Concomitant administration of single doses of metformin and nifedipine in healthy individuals resulted in enhanced absorption of metformin, as indicated by increases of 20 and 9% in the peak plasma concentration and AUC, respectively, of metformin. Nifedipine also increased the urinary excretion of metformin; half-life and time to peak plasma concentration of metformin remained unchanged. Metformin appears to have minimal effects on the pharmacokinetics of nifedipine.

■ **Cationic Agents** Cimetidine may reduce the urinary excretion of metformin by competing for renal tubular organic cationic transport systems. In single- and multiple-dose studies in healthy individuals, concomitant administration of cimetidine and metformin increased the peak plasma and whole blood concentrations of metformin by approximately 60–81% and the area under the plasma or whole blood concentration-time curve (AUC) of metformin by approximately 40–50%. Metformin has negligible effects on cimetidine pharmacokinetics, possibly because cimetidine has a higher affinity for renal tubular transport sites. The manufacturer states that the possibility of other cationic drugs that undergo substantial tubular secretion (e.g., amiloride, digoxin, morphine, procainamide, quinidine, quinine, ranitidine, triamterene, trimethoprim, vancomycin) decreasing the urinary excretion of metformin should be considered. Patients receiving metformin concomitantly with a cationic drug that is excreted by the proximal renal tubules should be monitored carefully and the need for possible dosage adjustment of either agent considered.

■ ***β*-Adrenergic Blocking Agents** In single-dose studies in healthy individuals, concomitant administration of metformin and propranolol did not alter the pharmacokinetics of either drug. However, several potential interactions between β-adrenergic blocking agents and oral antidiabetic agents (e.g., sulfonylureas, metformin) exist. β-Adrenergic blocking agents may impair glucose tolerance; increase the frequency or severity of hypoglycemia; block hypoglycemia-induced tachycardia but not hypoglycemic sweating, which may actually be increased; delay the rate of recovery of blood glucose concentration following drug-induced hypoglycemia; alter the hemodynamic response to hypoglycemia, possibly resulting in an exaggerated hypertensive response; and possibly impair peripheral circulation. Nonselective β- adrenergic blocking agents (e.g., propranolol, nadolol) without intrinsic sympathomimetic activity are more likely to affect glucose metabolism than more selective β-adrenergic blocking agents (e.g., metoprolol, atenolol) or those with intrinsic sympathomimetic activity (e.g., acebutolol, pindolol). Signs of hypoglycemia (e.g., tachycardia, blood pressure changes, tremor, feelings of anxiety) mediated by catecholamines may be masked by either nonselective or selective β-adrenergic blocking agents. These drugs should be used with caution in patients with type 2 diabetes mellitus who are receiving antidiabetic agents, especially in those with labile disease or in those prone to hypoglycemia. Use of low-dose, selective β_1-adrenergic blockers (e.g., metoprolol) or β-adrenergic blocking agents with intrinsic sympathomimetic activity in patients receiving oral antidiabetic agents may theoretically decrease the risk of affecting glycemic control. When an oral antidiabetic agent and a β-adrenergic blocking agent are used concomitantly, the patient should be advised about and monitored closely for altered antidiabetic response.

■ **Alcohol** Combined use of alcohol and metformin can increase the risk of hypoglycemia and lactic acidosis, since alcohol decreases lactate clearance and hepatic gluconeogenesis and may increase insulin secretion. (See Cautions: Lactic Acidosis.) Excessive alcohol intake, on an acute or chronic basis, should be avoided in patients receiving metformin therapy.

■ **Protein-Bound Drugs** Binding of metformin to plasma proteins is negligible; therefore, metformin is less likely to interact with drugs that are highly protein bound compared with sulfonylurea antidiabetic agents, which are extensively bound to plasma proteins.

■ **Angiotensin-Converting Enzyme Inhibitors** Angiotensin-converting enzyme (ACE) inhibitors (e.g., captopril, enalapril) may reduce fasting blood glucose concentrations in nondiabetic individuals and have been associated with unexplained hypoglycemia in patients whose diabetes had been controlled with insulin or oral antidiabetic agents, including combined therapy with glyburide and metformin. Testing in some of these patients indicated that the ACE inhibitor (e.g., captopril) apparently increased insulin sensitivity; the mechanism of this effect is not known. Other investigators have reported no alterations in glycemic control with concomitant use of an ACE inhibitor and oral antidiabetic agents or insulin in diabetic patients. The potential risk of precipitating hypoglycemia or hyperglycemia appears to be low but should be considered when therapy with an ACE inhibitor is initiated or withdrawn in diabetic patients; blood glucose concentrations should be monitored during dosage adjustments with either agent.

■ **Clomiphene** In premenopausal patients with polycystic ovary syndrome, therapy with certain oral antidiabetic agents, including metformin, may result in the resumption of ovulation in a modest number of women. Ovulatory response is further increased in patients pretreated with metformin hydrochloride (500 mg 3 times daily for 35 days) receiving additional low-dose clomiphene (50 mg daily for 5 days); ovulation was associated with decreased insulin secretion and increased serum progesterone concentrations.

■ **Other Drugs** Drugs that cause hyperglycemia and may exacerbate loss of glycemic control in patients with diabetes mellitus include corticosteroids, oral contraceptives, thiazide diuretics, sympathomimetics, phenothiazines, niacin, calcium-channel blocking agents, and isoniazid. When such drugs are added to or withdrawn from therapy in patients receiving oral antidiabetic agents, patients should be observed closely for evidence of altered glycemic control.

Acute Toxicity

Limited information is available on the acute toxicity of metformin. Hypoglycemia has been reported in approximately 10% of cases after acute oral ingestion of amounts exceeding 50 g of metformin hydrochloride; lactic acidosis has been reported in approximately 32% of metformin overdose cases. (See Cautions: Lactic Acidosis.) Since metformin is eliminated by dialysis (with a clearance of up to 170 mL per minute under good hemodynamic conditions), prompt hemodialysis is recommended to correct acidosis and remove accumulated drug; such management often results in rapid reversal of symptoms and recovery.

Pharmacology

■ **Antidiabetic Effects** Metformin hydrochloride, a biguanide antidiabetic agent, is chemically and pharmacologically unrelated to sulfonylurea antidiabetic agents. Unlike sulfonylureas, biguanides such as metformin lower blood glucose concentrations in patients with type 2 diabetes mellitus without increasing insulin secretion from pancreatic β cells; however, metformin is ineffective in the absence of some endogenous or exogenous insulin. Biguanides usually do not produce hypoglycemia in diabetic patients and do not affect normal blood glucose concentrations in nondiabetic individuals; metformin, even in excessive dosage, normally does not lower glucose concentrations below euglycemia, although hypoglycemia occasionally may occur with overdosage. (See Acute Toxicity.) Therefore, while biguanides as well as sulfonylureas historically have been referred to as oral hypoglycemic agents, biguanides such as metformin are more appropriately referred to as antihyperglycemic agents.

Type 2 diabetes mellitus is characterized by insulin resistance (impaired uptake and disposal of glucose by peripheral tissues and excessive glucose production by the liver), and abnormal insulin secretion, which may result in insulin deficiency (impaired secretion of insulin from pancreatic β cells) during the late stage of the disease. (See Uses.) Although the underlying pathophysiology of type 2 diabetes mellitus may be similar in obese and nonobese patients with the disease, severe peripheral and hepatic insulin resistance appears to predominate in obese patients, while nonobese patients tend to have milder degrees of insulin resistance but more marked insulin deficiency; however, both abnormalities eventually occur in the course of the disease. Obesity itself often is associated with insulin resistance and an elevated rate of fatty acid oxidation, which may contribute to the glucose intolerance observed in obese patients with type 2 diabetes mellitus.

Metformin lowers both basal (fasting) and postprandial glucose concentrations in patients with type 2 diabetes mellitus. Although the precise mechanism(s) by which metformin exerts its antihyperglycemic effect has not been fully established, current evidence suggests that the drug improves both peripheral and hepatic sensitivity to insulin. Improved insulin sensitivity occurs principally as a result of decreased hepatic glucose production and enhanced insulin-stimulated uptake and utilization of glucose by peripheral tissues (e.g., skeletal muscle, adipocytes); the relative contribution of these mechanisms to the antihyperglycemic effect of metformin has not been fully elucidated. Increases of 18–29% in the rate of insulin-stimulated glucose uptake (principally by skeletal muscle) have been reported in patients with type 2 diabetes mellitus with metformin hydrochloride and in normoglycemic insulin-resistant individuals in whom glucose utilization during therapy (0.5–3 g daily) generally was evaluated using a euglycemic, hyperinsulinemic clamp technique (a high-dose, continuous IV infusion of insulin administered concurrently with a glucose infusion titrated to maintain euglycemia). However, some studies in which insulin and/or glucose concentrations were not regulated during metformin therapy have reported no increases and/or even decreases in glucose uptake, possibly because of the nonphysiologic conditions inherent in the euglycemic, hyperinsulinemic clamp technique.

The apparent improvement in peripheral glucose disposal with metformin therapy has been attributed principally to improved metabolism of glucose via nonoxidative (anaerobic) pathways (e.g., glycogen formation in skeletal muscle, postprandial lactate production in splanchnic tissues, lipogenesis in adipose tissue). Studies in animals and humans indicate that metformin, unlike phenformin, enhances glucose oxidation and does not affect fasting lactate production in peripheral tissues. While increases in postprandial plasma lactate concentrations have been demonstrated in type 2 diabetic patients receiving metformin alone or in combination with a sulfonylurea (e.g., glyburide), plasma lactate concentrations generally remain within the normal range during metformin therapy. Postprandial increases in serum lactate concentration observed with metformin therapy may occur as a result of increased conversion of glucose to lactate and glycogen in the splanchnic bed by metformin. While most of the lactate from the portal circulation serves as a substrate for gluconeogenesis and is thus cleared, some may escape into the systemic circulation as increased amounts are presented to the liver after a meal. Metformin does not increase lactate production or alter lactate uptake or release from skeletal muscle.

Metformin reduces basal hepatic glucose production by decreasing gluconeogenesis and possibly glycogenolysis, thereby lowering fasting plasma glucose concentrations. Although some investigators have suggested that reduction of hepatic glucose production may be the drug's principal antihyperglycemic mechanism, this effect has not been demonstrated in all studies. In vitro studies in hepatocytes indicate that metformin, at concentrations similar to or higher than those observed with therapeutic dosages, enhances insulin-induced suppression of gluconeogenesis and decreases glucagon-stimulated gluconeogenesis. Insulin secretion usually remains unchanged during metformin therapy; fasting insulin concentrations and day-long plasma insulin response remain the same or may even decrease. The magnitude of the decrease in fasting blood glucose concentrations generally is proportional to the level of fasting baseline hyperglycemia. Metformin also may decrease plasma glucose concentrations by enhancing basal glucose disposal through insulin-independent mechanisms (e.g., a decrease in free fatty acid oxidation), but such effects appear to be modest.

Receptor binding of insulin is decreased in patients with type 2 diabetes mellitus, and some studies using radiolabeled insulin in rat and human cell cultures have demonstrated improved insulin binding with metformin. However, conflicting data also have been reported, and a direct correlation between increases in insulin binding and decreases in blood glucose concentration has not been observed. In in vitro studies in animal and human skeletal muscle cells or adipocytes, metformin has increased glucose uptake through enhancement of insulin-stimulated recruitment of specific glucose transporters (e.g., GLUT-1, GLUT-4) to the plasma membrane of insulin target cells (e.g., adipose tissue, skeletal muscle) and through increases in the activity of these glucose transporters. In in vitro studies using metformin concentrations within the therapeutic range, metformin has not consistently enhanced basal glucose uptake, which is noninsulin-mediated; however, in vitro data may not accurately reflect in vivo actions of the drug, and further study is needed to determine whether metformin acts through insulin-dependent or -independent pathways, or both, to affect basal glucose uptake.

Metformin accumulates in the walls of the intestine but does not appear to have clinically important effects on glucose absorption.

■ **Antilipemic Effects** Metformin has demonstrated modest favorable effects on serum lipids, which are often abnormal in patients with type 2 diabetes mellitus. In clinical studies, particularly in patients with elevated baseline serum lipid concentrations (e.g., patients with type II, type III, or type IV hyperlipoproteinemia), metformin alone or combined with a sulfonylurea antidiabetic agent lowered fasting serum triglyceride concentrations and total and LDL-cholesterol concentrations without adversely affecting other serum lipids.

Modest reductions (e.g., 10–20%) in serum triglyceride concentrations noted with metformin therapy generally have been attributed to decreased hepatic synthesis of VLDL-cholesterol, particularly in patients with elevated baseline triglyceride concentrations. Characteristics of patients who are likely to exhibit a decrease in serum triglycerides with metformin therapy have not been determined, and correlation of potential antilipemic effect with the degree of glycemic control has been inconsistent. Small reductions (e.g., 5–10%) in serum total cholesterol also have been reported in some studies; these effects may be attributed to decreased LDL- or VLDL-cholesterol concentrations. Increases in HDL-cholesterol also have been reported with metformin therapy in nondiabetic patients and in those with type 2 diabetes mellitus. Consistent changes in plasma glycerol and free fatty acid concentrations have not been reported during metformin therapy in patients with type 2 diabetes mellitus or in nondiabetic individuals. A reduction in free fatty oxidation has been suggested as a possible mechanism for the decrease in plasma free fatty acids observed in some studies with metformin therapy.

■ Hematologic Effects Metformin may exert potentially beneficial effects on the fibrinolytic system by increasing the activity of tissue-type plasminogen activator (t-PA) and/or reducing concentrations of plasminogen activator inhibitor-1 (PAI-1) in nondiabetic, hypertensive patients and in patients with type 2 diabetes mellitus; serum fibrinogen concentrations do not appear to be affected by metformin therapy. Patients with type 2 diabetes mellitus, hypertension, and obesity often have hyperinsulinemia and a high incidence of vascular disease. PAI-1 concentrations, which are regulated by insulin, may be substantially increased in patients with type 2 diabetes mellitus and in obese individuals, and it has been suggested that the reduced fibrinolytic activity associated with elevated PAI-1 concentrations may be important in the pathogenesis of vascular disease in these individuals. Metformin has been shown to increase fibrinolytic activity (as measured by blood clot lysis time, euglobulin fibrinolytic activity, and by increases in t-PA activity) in patients with coronary artery disease, obese individuals, and in patients with mild hypertension; increases in fibrinolytic activity with metformin therapy generally occur in patients who have low fibrinolytic activity at baseline. Reduced platelet density, activation, and/or aggregation; decreased blood pressure; and decreased peripheral arterial resistance also have been reported in some normotensive patients with type 2 diabetes mellitus and in nondiabetic, mildly hypertensive patients receiving metformin; however, whether these effects are associated with the drug or are secondary to improvement in glycemic control or a reduction in body weight has not been determined.

■ Other Effects Therapy with metformin may be associated with weight stabilization or loss. Although the exact mechanism associated with such alterations in weight has not been established, suggested mechanisms include the absence of a hyperinsulinemic effect (which if present may increase appetite and/or lipogenesis) and decreased dietary intake associated with adverse GI effects of metformin. The antihyperglycemic effect of the drug does not appear to be related to weight loss in patients with type 2 diabetes mellitus receiving metformin, nor does weight loss appear to be dose related. Limited data from studies comparing metformin therapy with oral sulfonylurea (e.g., glyburide, chlorpropamide, tolbutamide) therapy indicate that patients with type 2 diabetes mellitus receiving oral sulfonylureas gained weight or lost less weight than patients receiving metformin.

Metformin has little or no effect on fasting plasma glucagon, somatostatin, serum growth hormone, or serum cortisol concentration in patients with normal renal function; glucagon, growth hormone, and cortisol concentrations are elevated in patients with lactic acidosis and renal failure who have been receiving metformin.

Pharmacokinetics

The pharmacokinetics of metformin in patients with normal renal function do not appear to be affected by gender, race, or the presence of diabetes mellitus. Following administration of a single 500-mg dose of metformin hydrochloride as immediate-release tablets with food in pediatric patients (12–16 years of age) with type 2 diabetes mellitus, mean peak plasma concentrations and area under the concentration-time curve (AUC) differed less than 5% compared with those values in healthy adults; all patients had normal renal function. In pediatric patients 11–16 years of age receiving a single dose of metformin in fixed combination with glyburide, mean dose-normalized glyburide peak plasma concentration and AUC differed less than 6% from historical values in healthy adults.

Bioequivalence has been demonstrated between the fixed combination of rosiglitazone and metformin and each agent given concurrently and also between the fixed combination of sitagliptin and metformin and each agent given concurrently. Bioequivalence also has been demonstrated between the fixed combination of pioglitazone and metformin and each agent (pioglitazone and extended-release metformin [Fortamet®]) given concurrently. Results of a bioequivalence study indicate that the fixed-combination tablets of canagliflozin and immediate-release metformin hydrochloride are bioequivalent to the corresponding doses of canagliflozin and metformin hydrochloride given as individual tablets under fed conditions. Bioequivalence between the fixed combination of dapagliflozin and extended-release metformin hydrochloride (Xigduo® XR) and each agent (dapagliflozin and extended-release metformin hydrochloride) given concurrently as separate tablets has been demonstrated; however, the relative bioavailability of the fixed combination of dapagliflozin and extended-release metformin hydrochloride (Xigduo® XR) and concomitantly administered dapagliflozin and immediate-release metformin hydrochloride has not been established. Bioequivalence between the fixed-combination tablets of empagliflozin and immediate-release metformin hydrochloride and the corresponding doses of empagliflozin and metformin hydrochloride as individual tablets also has been established. In healthy individuals who received the extended-release metformin hydrochloride preparation (Glumetza®) in a single-dose crossover study, a 1-g tablet has been shown to be bioequivalent to two 500-mg tablets based on peak plasma concentrations and AUC.

■ Absorption Metformin is slowly and incompletely absorbed from the GI tract, mainly from the small intestine; absorption is complete within 6 hours. The absolute oral bioavailability of the drug under fasting conditions is reported to be approximately 50–60% with metformin hydrochloride doses of 0.5–1.5 g; binding of the drug to the intestinal wall may explain the difference between the amount of drug absorbed (as determined by the urinary and fecal excretion of unchanged drug) and the amount bioavailable in some studies. In single-dose studies with metformin hydrochloride immediate-release tablets at doses of 0.5–1.5 g or 0.85–2.55 g, plasma metformin concentrations did not increase in proportion to increasing doses, suggesting an active saturable absorption process. Similarly, in single-dose studies with an extended-release tablet preparation (Glumetza®) at doses of 0.5–2.5 g, plasma metformin concentrations did not increase in proportion to increasing doses. At steady state after administration of a metformin hydrochloride extended-release tablet preparation (Glucophage® XR), the AUC and peak plasma concentrations were not dose proportional within the range of 0.5–2 g. However, limited data from studies in animals and in human intestinal cell cultures suggest that transepithelial transfer of metformin in the intestine may occur through a passive, nonsaturable mechanism, possibly involving a paracellular route. In several studies with another metformin hydrochloride extended-release tablet preparation (Fortamet®) using doses of 1–2.5 g, metformin exposure was dose-related.

Food decreases and slightly delays the absorption of metformin immediate-release tablets; the clinical importance of these effects is unknown. (See Dosage and Administration: Administration.) Administration of metformin hydrochloride immediate-release tablets with food reportedly has decreased peak plasma concentrations of the drug by 35–40%, reduced area under the plasma concentration-time curve (AUC) by 20–25%, and delayed time to peak plasma drug concentration by 35–40 minutes compared with these parameters in fasting individuals receiving this metformin preparation. However, in one study, concomitant administration of the drug as immediate-release tablets with food had a less pronounced effect (average reduction in bioavailability of 10%) on absorption.

Following oral administration of metformin hydrochloride as an extended-release tablet preparation (Glucophage® XR) with food, the extent of absorption (as measured by AUC) increased by approximately 50%, but peak plasma concentrations and time to achieve peak plasma concentrations were not altered. Following administration of another metformin hydrochloride extended-release tablet formulation (Fortamet®) with food, the extent of absorption (as measured by AUC) increased by approximately 60%, peak plasma concentrations were increased by approximately 30%, and time to achieve peak plasma concentrations was prolonged (6.1 hours versus 4 hours) compared with those in the fasting state. The pharmacokinetics of a certain metformin extended-release tablet preparation (Glucophage® XR) were not affected by the fat content of meals. However, following administration of another metformin hydrochloride extended-release preparation (Glumetza®) with low-fat and high-fat meals, the AUCs increased by 38 and 73%, respectively, compared with those in the fasting state. Following administration of the fixed combination of extended-release metformin hydrochloride 1 g and immediate-release pioglitazone 30 mg (Actoplus Met® XR) with food, there was no change in the extent of absorption (as measured by AUC) of pioglitazone but there was a decrease of approximately 18% in peak concentration. Peak concentrations of the extended-release metformin hydrochloride component were increased by approximately 98% and AUC exposure by approximately 85% when Actoplus Met® XR was given with food. Time to peak concentration was prolonged by approximately 3 hours for pioglitazone and 2 hours for extended-release metformin hydrochloride under fed conditions.

Following oral administration of metformin hydrochloride as an oral solution with food, the extent of absorption (as measured by AUC) increased by approximately 17–21% compared with administration in the fasted state. Food delayed the time to achieve peak plasma concentrations by 1.4 hours compared with administration in the fasted state. The pharmacokinetics of metformin oral solution were not appreciably affected by the fat content of meals.

Following oral administration of 0.5–1.5 g of metformin hydrochloride as immediate-release tablets in healthy individuals or in patients with type 2 diabetes mellitus, peak plasma drug concentrations of approximately 0.4–3 mcg/mL usually are attained within 2–4 hours. Following oral administration of a single dose (0.5–2 g) of metformin hydrochloride as extended-release tablets (Glucophage® XR), peak plasma drug concentrations of 0.6–1.8 mcg/mL usually are attained within a median of 7 hours (range: 4–8 hours). Following administration of a single dose (0.5–2.5 g) of another extended-release preparation (Glumetza®), peak plasma drug concentrations of 0.47–1.6 mcg/mL usually are attained within 7–8 hours. Peak plasma drug concentrations following administration of metformin extended-release tablets (Glucophage® XR) are approximately 20% lower than those following administration of the same dose as immediate-release tablets. The extent of absorption of metformin hydrochloride 2 g once daily as extended-release tablets is similar to that following administration of 1 g of the drug twice daily as immediate-release tablets.

Steady-state plasma concentrations with usual dosages of metformin hydrochloride as immediate-release tablets (e.g., 1.5–2.55 g daily in 1 to 3 divided doses) are attained within 24–48 hours and generally average about 1 mcg/mL or less.

A precise correlation between plasma metformin concentrations and the drug's antihyperglycemic effect has not been established. In addition, plasma metformin concentrations generally have shown no correlation with plasma lactate concentrations during metformin therapy in patients with type 2 diabetes mellitus. Although metformin-associated lactic acidosis generally has been associated with plasma metformin concentrations exceeding 5 mcg/mL (see Cautions: Lactic Acidosis), such high concentrations reportedly were not observed during controlled clinical trials with the drug, even at maximum dosage (2.5–2.55 g daily).

Satisfactory control of blood or plasma glucose concentration may occur within a few days to 1 week following initiation of metformin therapy in patients with type 2 diabetes mellitus, but the maximum antihyperglycemic effect may be delayed for up to 2 weeks. Following discontinuance of metformin therapy, blood glucose concentration increases within 2 weeks.

■ **Distribution** Metformin is distributed rapidly in animals and humans into peripheral body tissues and fluids, particularly the GI tract; the drug also appears to distribute slowly into erythrocytes and into a deep tissue compartment (probably GI tissues). The highest tissue concentrations of metformin (at least 10 times the plasma concentration) occur in the GI tract (e.g., esophagus, stomach, duodenum, jejunum, ileum), with lower concentrations (twice the plasma concentration) occurring in kidney, liver, and salivary gland tissue. The drug distributes into salivary glands with a half-life of about 9 hours. Metformin concentrations in saliva are tenfold lower than those in plasma and may be responsible for the metallic taste reported in some patients receiving the drug. Any local effect of metformin on glucose absorption in the GI tract may be associated with the relatively high GI concentrations of the drug compared with those in other tissues. It is not known whether metformin crosses the blood-brain barrier or the placenta in humans or if the drug is distributed into human milk; however, in lactating rats, metformin is distributed into breast milk at levels comparable to those in plasma.

Following oral administration of single 850-mg doses of metformin hydrochloride as immediate-release tablets, the apparent volume of distribution has been reported to average 654 L. Volume of distribution reported after IV administration of the drug generally has been smaller (e.g., 63–276 L) than that with oral administration, perhaps because of less drug binding in the GI tract and/or different methods of determining volume of distribution in various studies. Unlike oral sulfonylurea antidiabetic agents, which are more than 90% bound to plasma proteins, metformin is negligibly bound to plasma proteins. Metformin equilibrates freely between erythrocytes and plasma, most likely as a function of time; drug bound to erythrocytes is approximately 5% of total blood concentration.

■ **Elimination** Following oral administration of metformin hydrochloride (0.5–1.5 g) as immediate-release tablets in healthy individuals or in patients with type 2 diabetes mellitus, plasma concentrations decline in a triphasic manner. Following multiple-dose administration of metformin hydrochloride (500 mg twice daily for 7–14 days) as immediate-release tablets in a limited number of patients with type 2 diabetes mellitus, peak plasma concentrations remained unchanged, but trough drug concentrations were higher than with single-dose administration, suggesting some drug accumulation in a peripheral tissue compartment. (See Pharmacokinetics: Distribution.) No accumulation of metformin appears to occur following repeated oral doses of the drug as extended-release tablets. The principal plasma elimination half-life of metformin averages approximately 6.2 hours; 90% of the drug is cleared within 24 hours in patients with normal renal function. The decline in plasma metformin concentrations is slower after oral than after IV administration of the drug, indicating that elimination is absorption rate-limited. Urinary excretion data and data from whole blood indicate a slower terminal-elimination phase half-life of 8–20 hours (e.g., 17.6 hours) suggesting that the erythrocyte mass may be a compartment of distribution.

Metformin is not metabolized in the liver or GI tract and is not excreted in bile; no metabolites of the drug have been identified in humans. Renal elimination of metformin involves glomerular filtration and secretion by the proximal convoluted tubules as unchanged drug. Following single-dose oral administration of metformin hydrochloride (0.5–1.5 g) as immediate-release tablets, urinary recovery ranges from 35–52% of the total dose. Following administration of a single dose of metformin hydrochloride as an extended-release tablet (Fortamet®) in healthy individuals, urinary recovery was 40.9% over 24 hours. Approximately 20–33% of the total oral dose as immediate-release tablets is excreted in feces within 4–7 days. Total plasma clearance of metformin hydrochloride following single-dose oral administration (0.5–1.5 g) has ranged from 718–1552 mL/minute. Metformin is removed by hemodialysis with a clearance of up to 170 mL/minute under good hemodynamic conditions.

Renal clearance is approximately 3.5 times greater than creatinine clearance, indicating that tubular secretion is the principal route of metformin elimination. Following a single 850-mg oral dose of metformin hydrochloride, renal clearance averaged 552, 491, or 412 mL/minute in nondiabetic adults, diabetic adults, or healthy geriatric individuals, respectively. Renal impairment results in increased peak plasma concentrations of metformin, a prolonged time to peak plasma concentration, and a decreased volume of distribution. Renal clearance is decreased in patients with renal impairment (as measured by decreases in creatinine clearance) and, apparently because of reduced renal function with age, in geriatric individuals. In geriatric individuals, decreased renal and plasma clearance of metformin also results in increased plasma concentrations of the drug; volume of distribution remains unaffected. (See Cautions: Precautions and Contraindications.)

Chemistry and Stability

■ **Chemistry** Metformin hydrochloride, a dimethylbiguanide, is an orally active antidiabetic agent derived from guanidine. Guanidine occurs naturally in *Galega officinalis*, a medieval European remedy for diabetes mellitus.

Metformin is structurally and pharmacologically related to phenformin, a phenethylbiguanide (no longer commercially available in the US). However, the guanidinium group of metformin has 2 methyl substituents rather than a single hydrophobic phenethyl substituent as in phenformin, giving metformin improved water solubility and decreased binding affinity for biologic membranes (e.g., mitochondrial, plasma membranes) compared with phenformin. Consequently, metformin causes less disturbance to mitochondrial-mediated glucose oxidative pathways, resulting in a decrease in the formation of lactate from glucose via anaerobic metabolism and a reduced potential for the development of lactic acidosis compared with phenformin.

Metformin hydrochloride is commercially available as immediate-release or extended-release tablets alone or in fixed combination with dipeptidyl peptidase-4 [DPP-4] inhibitors, meglitinides, sodium-glucose cotransporter 2 [SGLT2] inhibitors, sulfonylureas, or thiazolidinediones.

Certain extended-release tablet formulations (Glucophage® XR, Glumetza®) contain hydrophilic polymer(s) that form a swellable gel matrix when in contact with gastric or intestinal fluids and release the drug by diffusion slowly over time. Another commercially available metformin hydrochloride extended-release tablet formulation (Fortamet®) contains the drug in an oral osmotic delivery system. This delivery system consists of an osmotically active core (comprised of a layer containing the drug and a coating that delays release of the drug from the core) surrounded by a semipermeable membrane with laser-drilled delivery orifices; the semipermeable membrane allows the passage of water but not higher molecular weight components of biological fluids. When exposed to water in the GI tract, the drug dissolves and is pushed out of the delivery orifices of the membrane into the GI tract at a constant rate. The rate of metformin hydrochloride delivery in the GI tract depends on the maintenance of a constant osmotic gradient across the membrane. The inert components of the drug delivery system (membrane coating) remain intact and are eliminated in feces.

The fixed combination of extended-release metformin hydrochloride and immediate-release pioglitazone (Actoplus Met® XR) consists of a core tablet of extended-release metformin hydrochloride with an immediate-release layer of pioglitazone. The metformin core tablet is an extended-release formulation using single composition osmotic technology (SCOT®) for once-daily oral administration. The extended-release tablet consists of an osmotically active core formulation of metformin hydrochloride surrounded by a semipermeable membrane and coated with a pioglitazone drug layer. The core formulation contains small amounts of excipients. The semipermeable membrane is permeable to water but not to higher molecular weight components of biologic fluids. Upon ingestion, the pioglitazone layer is dissolved and water is taken up through the membrane, which in turn dissolves the metformin and excipients in the core formulation. The dissolved metformin and excipients exit through laser-drilled ports in the membrane. The rate of drug delivery is constant and depends upon maintenance of a constant osmotic gradient across the membrane, which exists as long as there is undissolved metformin in the core tablet. Following dissolution of the core materials, the rate of drug delivery slowly decreases until the osmotic gradient across the membrane falls to zero and drug delivery ceases. The membrane coating remains intact during transit of the dosage form through the GI tract and is excreted in feces.

Metformin is a weak base; the pH of a 1% aqueous solution of metformin hydrochloride is 6.68. The pK_a of metformin base is 12.4. Metformin hydrochloride is freely soluble in water and practically insoluble in acetone, ether, and chloroform.

■ **Stability** Commercially available metformin hydrochloride immediate-release (including fixed-combination preparations with glipizide or rosiglitazone) and extended-release tablets should be stored at a controlled room temperature of 20–25°C and protected from light but may be exposed to temperatures ranging from 15–30°C . Metformin hydrochloride oral solution should be stored at 15–30°C. Fixed-combination preparations containing metformin hydrochloride and glyburide should be stored at a controlled room temperature up to 25°C and be protected from light. Metformin hydrochloride in fixed combination with pioglitazone should be stored at 25°C and protected from moisture and humidity, but may be exposed to temperatures ranging from 15–30°C. Fixed-combination preparations containing metformin hydrochloride and repaglinide should be stored at a controlled room temperature not exceeding 25°C and be protected from moisture. Preparations containing metformin hydrochloride and canagliflozin, dapagliflozin, ertugliflozin, saxagliptin, or sitagliptin in fixed combination should be stored at 20–25°C but may be exposed to temperatures ranging from 15–30°C. The fixed combination of metformin hydrochloride and ertugliflozin should be protected from moisture and stored in a dry place. Preparations containing metformin hydrochloride and empagliflozin, alogliptin, or linagliptin in fixed combination should be stored at 25°C but may be exposed to temperatures ranging from 15–30°C. The fixed combination of metformin hydrochloride and linagliptin should be protected from exposure to high humidity.

Preparations

Excipients in commercially available drug preparations may have clinically important effects in some individuals; consult specific product labeling for details.

metFORMIN Hydrochloride

Oral		
Solution	500 mg/5 mL*	**metFORMIN Hydrochloride Solution**
		Riomet®, Ranbaxy
Tablets, extended-release	500 mg*	**Fortamet®**, Shionogi Pharma
		Glucophage® XR®, Bristol-Myers Squibb
		Glumetza®, Depomed
		metFORMIN Hydrochloride Extended-Release Tablets
	750 mg*	**Glucophage® XR®**, Bristol-Myers Squibb
		metFORMIN Hydrochloride Extended-Release Tablets
	1 g*	**Fortamet®**, Shionogi Pharma
		Glumetza®, Depomed
Tablets, film-coated	500 mg*	**Glucophage®**, Bristol-Myers Squibb
		metFORMIN Hydrochloride Tablets
	625 mg*	**metFORMIN Hydrochloride Tablets**
	750 mg*	**metFORMIN Hydrochloride Tablets**
	850 mg*	**Glucophage®**, Bristol-Myers Squibb
		metFORMIN Hydrochloride Tablets
	1 g*	**Glucophage®**, Bristol-Myers Squibb
		metFORMIN Hydrochloride Tablets

*available from one or more manufacturer, distributor, and/or repackager by generic (nonproprietary) name

metFORMIN Hydrochloride Combinations

Oral		
Tablets, extended-release	500 mg with Immediate-release Canagliflozin (anhydrous) 50 mg	**Invokamet® XR**, Janssen
	500 mg with Immediate-release Canagliflozin (anhydrous) 150 mg	**Invokamet® XR**, Janssen
	500 mg with Immediate-release Dapagliflozin Propanediol 5 mg (of dapagliflozin)	**Xigduo® XR**, AstraZeneca
	500 mg with Immediate-release Dapagliflozin Propanediol 10 mg (of dapagliflozin)	**Xigduo® XR**, AstraZeneca
	500 mg with Immediate-release Saxagliptin 5 mg	**Kombiglyze® XR**, AstraZeneca
	500 mg with Immediate-release Sitagliptin 50 mg	**Janumet® XR**, Merck
	1 g with Immediate-release Canagliflozin (anhydrous) 50 mg	**Invokamet® XR**, Janssen
	1 g with Immediate-release Canagliflozin (anhydrous) 150 mg	**Invokamet® XR**, Janssen
	1 g with Immediate-release Dapagliflozin Propanediol 2.5 mg (of dapagliflozin)	**Xigduo® XR**, AstraZeneca
	1 g with Immediate-release Dapagliflozin Propanediol 5 mg (of dapagliflozin)	**Xigduo® XR**, AstraZeneca
	1 g with Immediate-release Dapagliflozin Propanediol 10 mg (of dapagliflozin)	**Xigduo® XR**, AstraZeneca
	1 g with Immediate-release Empagliflozin 5 mg	**Synjardy® XR**, Boehniger Ingelheim
	1 g with Immediate-release Empagliflozin 10 mg	**Synjardy® XR**, Boehniger Ingelheim
	1 g with Immediate-release Empagliflozin 12.5 mg	**Synjardy® XR**, Boehniger Ingelheim
	1 g with Immediate-release Empagliflozin 25 mg	**Synjardy® XR**, Boehniger Ingelheim
	1 g with Immediate-release Linagliptin 2.5 mg	**Jentadueto® XR**, Boehringer Ingelheim
	1 g with Immediate-release Linagliptin 5 mg	**Jentadueto® XR**, Boehringer Ingelheim
	1 g with Immediate-release Pioglitazone Hydrochloride 15 mg (of pioglitazone)	**Actoplus Met® XR**, Takeda
	1 g with Immediate-release Pioglitazone Hydrochloride 30 mg (of pioglitazone)	**Actoplus Met® XR**, Takeda
	1 g with Immediate-release Saxagliptin 2.5 mg	**Kombiglyze® XR**, AstraZeneca
	1 g with Immediate-release Saxagliptin 5 mg	**Kombiglyze® XR**, AstraZeneca
	1 g with Immediate-release Sitagliptin 50 mg	**Janumet® XR**, Merck
	1 g with Immediate-release Sitagliptin 100 mg	**Janumet® XR**, Merck
Tablets, film-coated	250 mg with Glipizide 2.5 mg*	**Metaglip®**, Bristol-Myers Squibb
		metFORMIN Hydrochloride and Glipizide Tablets
	250 mg with Glyburide 1.25 mg*	**Glucovance®**, Bristol-Myers Squibb
		metFORMIN Hydrochloride and Glyburide Tablets
	500 mg with Alogliptin Benzoate 12.5 mg (of alogliptin)	**Kazano®**, Takeda
	500 mg with Canagliflozin (anhydrous) 50 mg	**Invokamet®**, Janssen
	500 mg with Canagliflozin (anhydrous) 150 mg	**Invokamet®**, Janssen
	500 mg with Empagliflozin 5 mg	**Synjardy®**, Boehringer Ingelheim
	500 mg with Empagliflozin 12.5 mg	**Synjardy®**, Boehringer Ingelheim
	500 mg with Ertugliflozin L-pyroglutamic Acid 2.5 mg (of ertugliflozin)	**Segluromet®**, Merck
	500 mg with Ertugliflozin L-pyroglutamic Acid 7.5 mg (of ertugliflozin)	**Segluromet®**, Merck
	500 mg with Glipizide 2.5 mg*	**Metaglip®**, Bristol-Myers Squibb
		metFORMIN Hydrochloride and Glipizide Tablets
	500 mg with Glipizide 5 mg*	**Metaglip®**, Bristol-Myers Squibb
		metFORMIN Hydrochloride and Glipizide Tablets
	500 mg with Glyburide 2.5 mg*	**Glucovance®**, Bristol-Myers Squibb
		metFORMIN Hydrochloride and Glyburide Tablets
	500 mg with Glyburide 5 mg*	**Glucovance®**, Bristol-Myers Squibb
		MetFORMIN Hydrochloride and Glyburide Tablets
	500 mg with Linagliptin 2.5 mg	**Jentadueto®**, Boehringer Ingelheim
	500 mg with Pioglitazone Hydrochloride 15 mg (of pioglitazone)	**Actoplus Met®**, Takeda
	500 mg with Repaglinide 1 mg	**Prandimet®**, Novo Nordisk
	500 mg with Repaglinide 2 mg	**Prandimet®**, Novo Nordisk
	500 mg with Rosiglitazone Maleate 2 mg (of rosiglitazone)	**Avandamet®**, GlaxoSmithKline
	500 mg with Rosiglitazone Maleate 4 mg (of rosiglitazone)	**Avandamet®**, GlaxoSmithKline
	500 mg with Sitagliptin Phosphate 50 mg (of sitagliptin)	**Janumet®**, Merck
	850 mg with Linagliptin 2.5 mg	**Jentadueto®**, Boehringer Ingelheim

850 mg with Pioglitazone Hydrochloride 15 mg (of pioglitazone)	**Actoplus Met®**, Takeda
1 g with Alogliptin Benzoate 12.5 mg (of alogliptin)	**Kazano®**, Takeda
1 g with Canagliflozin (anhydrous) 50 mg	**Invokamet®**, Janssen
1 g with Canagliflozin (anhydrous) 150 mg	**Invokamet®**, Janssen
1 g with Empagliflozin 5 mg	**Synjardy®**, Boehringer Ingelheim
1 g with Empagliflozin 12.5 mg	**Synjardy®**, Boehringer Ingelheim
1 g with Ertugliflozin L-pyroglutamic Acid 2.5 mg (of ertugliflozin)	**Segluromet®**, Merck
1 g with Ertugliflozin L-pyroglutamic Acid 7.5 mg (of ertugliflozin)	**Segluromet®**, Merck
1 g with Linagliptin 2.5 mg	**Jentadueto®**, Boehringer Ingelheim
1 g with Rosiglitazone Maleate 2 mg (of rosiglitazone)	**Avandamet®**, GlaxoSmithKline
1 g with Rosiglitazone Maleate 4 mg (of rosiglitazone)	**Avandamet®**, GlaxoSmithKline
1 g with Sitagliptin Phosphate 50 mg (of sitagliptin)	**Janumet®**, Merck

*available from one or more manufacturer, distributor, and/or repackager by generic (nonproprietary) name

†Use is not currently included in the labeling approved by the US Food and Drug Administration

Dipeptidyl Peptidase IV (DPP-4) Inhibitors 68:20.05

Alogliptin Benzoate

■ Alogliptin benzoate, a dipeptidyl peptidase-4 (DPP-4) inhibitor, is an antidiabetic agent.

Uses

■ **Diabetes Mellitus** Alogliptin benzoate is used as monotherapy as an adjunct to diet and exercise to improve glycemic control in patients with type 2 diabetes mellitus. Alogliptin is used as initial therapy in combination with metformin hydrochloride or pioglitazone as an adjunct to diet and exercise to improve glycemic control in patients with type 2 diabetes mellitus when treatment with both alogliptin and metformin or pioglitazone is appropriate. Alogliptin also is used in combination with other oral antidiabetic agents (e.g., metformin, a sulfonylurea, a peroxisome proliferator-activated $receptor_{\gamma}$ [$PPAR_{\gamma}$] agonist [thiazolidinedione]) or insulin as an adjunct to diet and exercise in patients with type 2 diabetes mellitus who have not achieved adequate glycemic control.

While metformin generally is the preferred antidiabetic agent for initial therapy in patients with type 2 diabetes mellitus, the American Association of Clinical Endocrinologists/American College of Endocrinology (AACE/ACE) suggests a dipeptidyl peptidase-4 (DPP-4) inhibitor as one of several alternative antidiabetic agents for initial monotherapy in patients with a contraindication to metformin (e.g., renal disease, hepatic disease, GI intolerance, risk of lactic acidosis). DPP-4 inhibitors also are recommended by AACE/ACE as part of combination therapy, particularly when both postprandial and fasting plasma glucose concentrations are elevated.

Alogliptin should not be used in patients with type 1 diabetes mellitus or for the treatment of diabetic ketoacidosis.

Alogliptin Monotherapy Efficacy of alogliptin as monotherapy for the management of type 2 diabetes mellitus has been established in a double-blind, placebo-controlled study of 26 weeks' duration in a total of 329 patients. Alogliptin (12.5 or 25 mg once daily) improved glycemic control as evidenced by a reduction in glycosylated hemoglobin (HbA_{1c}) as well as in fasting plasma glucose concentrations compared with placebo. HbA_{1c} was reduced by approximately 0.6% (from a mean baseline HbA_{1c} concentration of about 8%) in patients receiving alogliptin 25 mg, compared with no change in HbA_{1c} in those receiving placebo.

In a double-blind, active-controlled study of 52 weeks' duration in 441 patients 65–87 years of age, alogliptin (25 mg once daily) was noninferior to glipizide (5–10 mg daily) in reducing HbA_{1c}. Mean reductions in HbA_{1c} from baseline (mean HbA_{1c} of 7.5%) were 0.14% with alogliptin and 0.09% with glipizide. Patients receiving alogliptin also experienced lower risk of hypoglycemia and lost weight (loss of 0.62 kg) compared with patients receiving glipizide, who experienced weight gain (0.6 kg).

Combination Therapy Efficacy of the combination of alogliptin and pioglitazone as *initial* therapy in patients with type 2 diabetes mellitus inadequately controlled with diet and exercise is supported by results of a 26-week randomized, active-controlled study. Patients receiving initial therapy with alogliptin (25 mg daily) in combination with pioglitazone (30 mg daily) had greater improvements in HbA_{1c} and fasting plasma glucose than those receiving alogliptin monotherapy or pioglitazone monotherapy. Mean reductions in HbA_{1c} from baseline (mean HbA_{1c} of 8.8%) were 1% with alogliptin 25 mg once daily, 1.2% with pioglitazone 30 mg once daily, and 1.7% with alogliptin 25 mg once daily in combination with pioglitazone 30 mg once daily. The proportion of patients who achieved an HbA_{1c} of 7% or less was greater with alogliptin and pioglitazone combination therapy (63%) than with alogliptin (24%) or pioglitazone (34%) monotherapy.

In another 26-week, randomized trial in patients who had inadequate glycemic control with diet and exercise, patients receiving *initial* therapy with the combination of alogliptin (12.5 mg twice daily) and metformin hydrochloride (500 mg or 1 g twice daily) had greater improvements in HbA_{1c} and fasting plasma glucose than those receiving placebo, metformin monotherapy, or alogliptin monotherapy. Mean reductions in HbA_{1c} from baseline (mean HbA_{1c} of 8.4%) were 0.6% with alogliptin 12.5 mg twice daily, 0.7% with metformin hydrochloride 500 mg twice daily, 1.1% with metformin hydrochloride 1 g twice daily, 1.2% with alogliptin 12.5 mg and metformin hydrochloride 500 mg twice daily, and 1.6% with alogliptin 12.5 mg and metformin hydrochloride 1 g twice daily, while HbA_{1c} increased by 0.1% with placebo. In this trial, 47% of patients receiving alogliptin 12.5 mg and metformin hydrochloride 500 mg twice daily and 59% of those receiving alogliptin 12.5 mg and metformin hydrochloride 1 g twice daily achieved a mean HbA_{1c} of less than 7%, compared with 20% of those receiving alogliptin 12.5 mg twice daily as monotherapy and 27 or 34% of those receiving metformin hydrochloride 500 mg or 1 g twice daily as monotherapy.

Efficacy of alogliptin in combination with metformin, a sulfonylurea, or a thiazolidinedione in the management of type 2 diabetes (in patients inadequately controlled with metformin monotherapy, metformin and a thiazolidinedione, or a sulfonylurea) has been established in several randomized, placebo- or active-controlled, double-blind studies. In these studies, addition of alogliptin (25 mg daily) to existing therapy improved glycemic control as evidenced by reductions in HbA_{1c} as well as in fasting plasma glucose concentrations, compared with placebo or existing therapy. In a 26-week study in patients receiving metformin hydrochloride (dosage of at least 1.5 g daily or maximum tolerated dosage), the addition of alogliptin resulted in a reduction of 0.6% in HbA_{1c} compared with a reduction of 0.1% in HbA_{1c} with placebo. In a 26-week study in patients receiving metformin hydrochloride (at least 1.5 g daily), the addition of alogliptin and pioglitazone (15, 30, or 45 mg daily) resulted in reductions of 1.3–1.6% in HbA_{1c}; addition of pioglitazone alone, alogliptin alone, or placebo resulted in HbA_{1c} reductions of 0.8–1, 0.9, or 0.1%, respectively.

In a 26-week study in patients receiving a thiazolidinedione alone or in combination with metformin or a sulfonylurea, addition of alogliptin (25 mg once daily) or placebo resulted in reductions of 0.8 or 0.2%, respectively, in HbA_{1c}. Patients receiving metformin or a sulfonylurea at baseline continued these agents at the same dosage throughout the study.

In a 52-week study in patients receiving metformin hydrochloride (at least 1.5 g daily or maximum tolerated dosage) and pioglitazone (30 mg daily), add-on therapy with alogliptin (25 mg daily) or increased dosage of pioglitazone (45 mg daily) resulted in a reduction of 0.7 or 0.3%, respectively, from a baseline HbA_{1c} of approximately 8.2%.

In a 26-week study in patients receiving glyburide, addition of alogliptin (25 mg daily) resulted in a reduction of 0.5% in HbA_{1c} compared with addition of placebo.

Efficacy of alogliptin in combination with insulin (with or without metformin) in the management of type 2 diabetes mellitus in patients who have inadequate glycemic control with insulin is supported by results of a 26-week, randomized, double-blind, placebo-controlled study. In this study, addition of alogliptin (25 mg once daily) to existing stable insulin (premixed insulin, or short-, intermediate- or long-acting [basal] insulin) therapy with or without metformin hydrochloride resulted in improvements in HbA_{1c} and fasting plasma glucose concentrations compared with the addition of placebo. Among patients also receiving metformin, addition of alogliptin reduced HbA_{1c} by 0.8% compared with 0.2% in those receiving add-on placebo; among patients receiving insulin monotherapy, addition of alogliptin reduced HbA_{1c} by 0.7% compared with 0.1% in those receiving add-on placebo.

Dosage and Administration

■ **Administration** When administered as monotherapy, alogliptin may be administered orally once daily without regard to meals.

When alogliptin is administered in fixed combination with metformin hydrochloride, the combination should be administered twice daily with food; dosage should be titrated gradually to minimize adverse GI effects of the metformin component. Fixed-combination tablets should be swallowed whole and should not be split before swallowing.

When alogliptin is administered in fixed combination with pioglitazone, the combination should be administered once daily without regard to meals. Fixed-combination tablets should be swallowed whole and should not be split before swallowing.

If a dose is missed, the missed dose should be taken as soon as it is remembered followed by resumption of the regular schedule. If the missed dose is not remembered until the time of the next dose, the missed dose should be skipped and the regular schedule resumed; the dose should not be doubled to replace a missed dose.

■ **Dosage** Dosage of alogliptin benzoate is expressed in terms of alogliptin.

Alogliptin Monotherapy The recommended dosage of alogliptin for the management of type 2 diabetes mellitus is 25 mg once daily.

Combination Therapy with Metformin Hydrochloride Dosage of alogliptin in fixed combination with metformin hydrochloride should be individualized based on the patient's current antidiabetic regimen, effectiveness, and tolerability. Dosage should be increased gradually to reduce adverse GI effects of metformin.

The maximum recommended dosage of alogliptin in fixed combination with metformin hydrochloride is 25 mg of alogliptin and 2 g of metformin hydrochloride daily.

Combination Therapy with Pioglitazone When the fixed-combination preparation containing alogliptin and pioglitazone is used in patients inadequately controlled with diet and exercise, the recommended initial dosage is 25 mg of alogliptin and 15 mg of pioglitazone once daily or 25 mg of alogliptin and 30 mg of pioglitazone once daily.

When the fixed-combination preparation containing alogliptin and pioglitazone is used in patients inadequately controlled on alogliptin monotherapy, the recommended initial dosage is 25 mg of alogliptin and 15 mg of pioglitazone once daily or 25 mg of alogliptin and 30 mg of pioglitazone once daily.

When the fixed-combination preparation containing alogliptin and pioglitazone is used in patients inadequately controlled on pioglitazone monotherapy, the recommended initial dosage is 25 mg of alogliptin and 15 mg of pioglitazone once daily, 25 mg of alogliptin and 30 mg of pioglitazone once daily, or 25 mg of alogliptin and 45 mg of pioglitazone once daily based on the patient's current antidiabetic therapy.

When the fixed-combination preparation containing alogliptin and pioglitazone is used in patients inadequately controlled on metformin monotherapy, the recommended initial dosage is 25 mg of alogliptin and 15 mg of pioglitazone once daily or 25 mg of alogliptin and 30 mg of pioglitazone once daily.

The maximum recommended dosage of alogliptin in fixed combination with pioglitazone is 25 mg of alogliptin and 45 mg of pioglitazone daily.

■ **Special Populations** No adjustment of alogliptin dosage is necessary in patients with mild renal impairment (creatinine clearance of 60 mL/minute or greater). In patients with moderate renal impairment (creatinine clearance of 30 to less than 60 mL/minute), the recommended dosage of alogliptin is 12.5 mg once daily. In patients with severe renal impairment (creatinine clearance of 15 to less than 30 mL/minute) or end-stage renal disease (creatinine clearance of 15 mL/minute or less or requiring hemodialysis), the recommended daily dosage is 6.25 mg once daily. Alogliptin may be administered without regard to the timing of hemodialysis.

The fixed combination of alogliptin and metformin hydrochloride is contraindicated in patients with renal impairment. Assessment of renal function is recommended prior to initiation of alogliptin therapy and periodically thereafter.

The fixed combination of alogliptin and pioglitazone is not recommended in patients with severe renal impairment or end-stage renal disease.

No adjustment of alogliptin dosage is recommended in patients with mild to moderate hepatic impairment; data are lacking in patients with severe hepatic impairment.

The fixed combination of alogliptin and metformin is not recommended in patients with hepatic impairment.

No dosage adjustment is necessary based on age, gender, or race.

The recommended initial dosage of the fixed combination of alogliptin and pioglitazone in patients with congestive heart failure (CHF) (New York Heart Association [NYHA] class I or II) is 25 mg of alogliptin and 15 mg of pioglitazone once daily.

Cautions

■ **Contraindications** Alogliptin is contraindicated in patients with known serious hypersensitivity (e.g., anaphylaxis, angioedema, severe adverse cutaneous reactions) to alogliptin.

■ **Warnings/Precautions** ***Pancreatitis and Pancreatic Precancerous Changes*** Acute pancreatitis has been reported during postmarketing experience in patients receiving alogliptin. In clinical studies in patients with type 2 diabetes mellitus, acute pancreatitis was reported in 0.2% of patients receiving alogliptin 25 mg compared with less than 0.1% of patients receiving active comparators or placebo. In a randomized, double-blind study (EXAMINE) in 5380 patients with type 2 diabetes mellitus and recent acute coronary syndrome, acute pancreatitis was reported in 0.4 or 0.3% of patients receiving alogliptin or placebo, respectively. FDA has been evaluating unpublished findings suggesting an increased risk of pancreatitis and precancerous pancreatic cell changes (pancreatic duct metaplasia) in patients with type 2 diabetes mellitus receiving incretin mimetics (exenatide, liraglutide, sitagliptin, saxagliptin, alogliptin, or linagliptin). These findings are based on examination of a small number of pancreatic tissue specimens taken from patients who died from unspecified causes while receiving an incretin mimetic. FDA will notify healthcare professionals of its conclusions and recommendations when the review is complete, or when the agency has additional information to report.

FDA has recommended that clinicians continue to follow the recommendations in the prescribing information for incretin mimetics. The manufacturer states that patients receiving alogliptin should be observed carefully for signs and symptoms of pancreatitis. If pancreatitis is suspected, alogliptin should be promptly discontinued and appropriate management instituted. It is not known whether patients with a history of pancreatitis are at increased risk for pancreatitis with alogliptin therapy.

Severe Arthralgia Severe, disabling joint pain has been reported during postmarketing experience in patients receiving DPP-4 inhibitors (e.g., alogliptin, linagliptin, saxagliptin, sitagliptin). Onset of such symptoms has ranged from 1 day to years following initiation of therapy. Fever, chills, rash, and swelling accompanied joint pain in some patients, suggesting an immunologic reaction; some patients have required hospitalization. Symptoms resolved upon discontinuance of the DPP-4 inhibitor, usually in less than a month. In some patients, symptoms recurred when the same or another DPP-4 inhibitor was restarted. DPP-4 inhibitors should be considered as a possible cause of severe joint pain and should be discontinued if appropriate. (See Advice to Patients.)

Sensitivity Reactions Hypersensitivity reactions (e.g., anaphylaxis, angioedema, severe adverse cutaneous reactions including Stevens-Johnson syndrome) have been reported in patients receiving alogliptin.

If a serious hypersensitivity reaction is suspected, alogliptin should be promptly discontinued, other potential causes of the event should be investigated, and alternative antidiabetic therapy should be instituted. (See Advice to Patients.) Alogliptin should be used with caution in patients with a history of angioedema to other dipeptidyl peptidase-4 inhibitors because it is unknown whether such patients will be predisposed to angioedema with alogliptin.

Hepatic Effects Fatal and nonfatal hepatic failure have been reported during postmarketing experience in patients receiving alogliptin. In randomized controlled trials, serum alanine aminotransferase (ALT) elevations exceeding 3 times the upper limit of normal were observed in 1.3% of patients receiving alogliptin and 1.5% of all comparator-treated patients.

Patients with type 2 diabetes mellitus may have fatty liver disease, which may cause liver function test abnormalities; such patients may also have other forms of liver function disease, many of which can be treated or managed. Therefore, hepatic function should be assessed prior to initiation of alogliptin, and the drug should be initiated with caution in patients with abnormal liver function test results.

Liver function should be assessed promptly in patients who report signs or symptoms that may indicate liver injury (e.g., fatigue, anorexia, right upper abdominal discomfort, dark urine, jaundice). If the patient has clinically important liver enzyme elevations and if liver function test abnormalities persist or worsen, alogliptin therapy should be interrupted. Alogliptin should not be restarted in these patients without another explanation for the liver function test abnormalities.

Concomitant Therapy with Hypoglycemic Agents When alogliptin is used in combination with an insulin secretagogue (e.g., a sulfonylurea) or insulin, the incidence of hypoglycemia is increased compared with sulfonylurea or insulin monotherapy. Therefore, patients receiving alogliptin may require a reduced dosage of the concomitant insulin secretagogue or insulin to reduce the risk of hypoglycemia.

Cardiovascular Effects **Macrovascular Outcomes.** The manufacturer states that evidence of macrovascular risk reduction with alogliptin or any other antidiabetic agent has not been conclusively demonstrated in clinical trials.

Heart Failure Risk. Alogliptin may increase the risk of heart failure, particularly in patients who have a history of heart failure or renal impairment. In a randomized, double-blind study (EXAMINE) in which alogliptin or placebo was added to standard care in 5380 patients with type 2 diabetes mellitus and recent acute coronary syndrome, 3.9% of patients receiving alogliptin experienced at least one hospitalization for heart failure compared with 3.3% of patients receiving placebo. The average duration of follow-up in this study was 1.5 years.

The potential risks and benefits of alogliptin therapy should be considered prior to use in patients at higher risk for heart failure. Patients receiving alogliptin-containing therapy should be monitored for manifestations of heart failure. (See Advice to Patients.) If heart failure develops, appropriate evaluation and management should be instituted and consideration given to discontinuing alogliptin.

Use of Fixed Combinations When alogliptin is used in fixed combination with metformin hydrochloride or pioglitazone, the cautions, precautions, and contraindications associated with metformin hydrochloride or pioglitazone should be considered.

Specific Populations **Pregnancy.** Category B. (See Users Guide.)

Lactation. Alogliptin is distributed into milk in lactating rats at a milk-to-plasma ratio of 2:1; it is not known whether the drug is distributed into human milk. Caution is advised if alogliptin is administered in nursing women.

Pediatric Use. Safety and efficacy of alogliptin alone, in fixed combination with metformin, or in fixed combination with pioglitazone have not been established in pediatric patients younger than 18 years of age.

Geriatric Use. Of 8507 patients in clinical trials of alogliptin, 24.3% were 65 years of age and older; 4% were 75 years of age and older. No substantial differences in safety and efficacy relative to younger adults were observed, but increased sensitivity cannot be ruled out.

Hepatic Impairment. In patients with moderate hepatic impairment (Child-Pugh class B), alogliptin total exposure was approximately 10% lower than values in healthy individuals. Alogliptin has not been studied in patients with severe hepatic impairment (Child-Pugh class C). Caution should be exercised in patients with liver disease.

Renal Impairment. In patients with mild renal impairment (creatinine clearance of 60 to less than 90 mL/minute), area under the plasma concentration-time curve (AUC) of alogliptin increased approximately 1.2-fold; the manufacturer does not recommend dosage adjustment of alogliptin in patients with mild renal impairment.

However, dosage adjustment is recommended when the drug is used in patients with moderate or severe renal impairment or end-stage renal disease. (See Special Populations under Dosage and Administration: Dosage.) Plasma AUC of alogliptin was increased approximately twofold in patients with moderate renal impairment (creatinine clearance of 30 to less than 60 mL/minute), threefold in those with severe renal impairment (creatinine clearance of 15 to less than 30 mL/minute), and fourfold in those with end-stage renal disease (creatinine clearance of 15 mL/minute or less or requiring hemodialysis).

■ **Common Adverse Effects** Adverse effects reported in at least 4% of patients receiving alogliptin monotherapy and more commonly than with placebo include nasopharyngitis, headache, and upper respiratory tract infection.

Adverse effects reported in at least 4% of patients receiving alogliptin in combination with metformin and more commonly than with placebo include upper respiratory tract infection, nasopharyngitis, diarrhea, hypertension, headache, back pain, and urinary tract infection.

Adverse effects reported in at least 4% of patients receiving alogliptin in combination with pioglitazone and more commonly than with placebo include nasopharyngitis, back pain, and upper respiratory tract infection.

Drug Interactions

Alogliptin is principally renally excreted; cytochrome P-450 (CYP)-related metabolism is negligible.

■ **Drugs Affecting or Metabolized by Hepatic Microsomal Enzymes** Alogliptin does not induce CYP1A2, 2B6, 2C9, 2C19, or 3A4 and does not inhibit CYP1A2, 2C8, 2C9, 2C19, 3A4, or 2D6.

Concurrent administration of alogliptin (100 mg once daily for 7 days) with a single dose of a CYP1A2 substrate (caffeine 200 mg), a CYP2C9 substrate (tolbutamide 500 mg), a CYP2D6 substrate (dextromethorphan 30 mg), or a CYP3A4 substrate (midazolam 4 mg) did not meaningfully increase the peak plasma concentrations or area under the concentration-time curve (AUC) of caffeine, tolbutamide, dextromethorphan, or midazolam. The manufacturer states that no dosage adjustment is necessary with such concomitant therapy.

■ **Drugs that are Substrates of P-glycoprotein Transport Systems** Concurrent administration of alogliptin (100 mg once daily for 7 days) with a single dose of a P-glycoprotein substrate (fexofenadine 80 mg) did not meaningfully increase the peak plasma concentration or AUC of fexofenadine. The manufacturer states that no dosage adjustment is necessary with such concomitant therapy.

■ **Atorvastatin** Concurrent administration of alogliptin (25 mg once daily for 7 days) and atorvastatin (80 mg once daily for 7 days) did not meaningfully alter the peak plasma concentrations or AUC of alogliptin or atorvastatin. The manufacturer states that no dosage adjustment is necessary.

■ **Cimetidine** Concurrent administration of alogliptin (100 mg once daily for 6 days) and cimetidine (400 mg once daily for 6 days) did not meaningfully alter the peak plasma concentrations or AUC of alogliptin or cimetidine. The manufacturer states that no dosage adjustment is necessary.

■ **Contraceptives, Hormonal** Concurrent administration of alogliptin (25 mg once daily for 21 days) and an estrogen-progestin contraceptive (ethinyl estradiol 35 mcg and norethindrone 1 mg once daily for 21 days) did not meaningfully alter the peak plasma concentrations or AUC of ethinyl estradiol or norethindrone; no dosage adjustment is necessary.

■ **Cyclosporine** Concurrent administration of a single dose of alogliptin (25 mg) and a single dose of cyclosporine (600 mg) did not meaningfully alter the peak plasma concentrations or AUC of alogliptin. The manufacturer states that no dosage adjustment is necessary.

■ **Digoxin** Concurrent administration of alogliptin (25 mg once daily for 10 days) and digoxin (0.2 mg once daily for 10 days) did not meaningfully alter the peak plasma concentrations or AUC of alogliptin or digoxin. The manufacturer states that no dosage adjustment is necessary.

■ **Fluconazole** Concurrent administration of a single dose of alogliptin (25 mg) and fluconazole (200 mg once daily for 7 days) did not meaningfully alter the peak plasma concentrations or AUC of alogliptin. The manufacturer states that no dosage adjustment is necessary.

■ **Gemfibrozil** Concurrent administration of a single dose of alogliptin (25 mg) and gemfibrozil (600 mg twice daily for 7 days) did not meaningfully alter the peak plasma concentrations or AUC of alogliptin. The manufacturer states that no dosage adjustment is necessary.

■ **Glyburide** Concurrent administration of alogliptin (25 mg once daily for 8 days) and a single dose of glyburide (5 mg) did not meaningfully alter the peak plasma concentrations or AUC of glyburide. No dosage adjustment is necessary.

■ **Ketoconazole** Concurrent administration of a single dose of alogliptin (25 mg) and ketoconazole (400 mg once daily for 7 days) did not meaningfully alter the peak plasma concentrations or AUC of alogliptin. The manufacturer states that no dosage adjustment is necessary.

■ **Metformin** Concurrent administration of alogliptin (100 mg once daily for 6 days) and metformin hydrochloride (1 g twice daily for 6 days) did not meaningfully alter the peak plasma concentrations or AUC of alogliptin or metformin. The manufacturer states that no dosage adjustment is necessary.

■ **Pioglitazone** Concurrent administration of alogliptin (25 mg once daily for 12 days) and pioglitazone (45 mg once daily for 12 days) did not meaningfully alter the peak plasma concentrations or AUC of alogliptin or pioglitazone. No dosage adjustment is necessary.

■ **Warfarin** Concurrent administration of alogliptin (25 mg once daily for 7 days) and warfarin sodium (stable dosage of 1–10 mg once daily for 7 days) did not alter the peak plasma concentrations or AUC of *R*- or *S*-warfarin; prothrombin time (PT) or international normalized ratio (INR) was not altered. The manufacturer states that no dosage adjustment is necessary.

Description

Alogliptin inhibits dipeptidyl peptidase-4 (DPP-4), an enzyme that inactivates the incretin hormones glucagon-like peptide-1 (GLP-1) and glucose-dependent insulinotropic polypeptide (GIP). Alogliptin selectively inhibits DPP-4 with no effect on DPP-8 or DPP-9 in vitro at concentrations approximating those from therapeutic exposures. Alogliptin increases circulating concentrations of GLP-1 and GIP in a glucose-dependent manner.

GLP-1 and GIP stimulate insulin secretion from pancreatic β-cells in a glucose-dependent manner (i.e., when glucose concentrations are elevated). GLP-1 also decreases glucagon secretion from pancreatic α-cells, leading to reduced hepatic glucose production.

Alogliptin did not increase the QT interval corrected for rate (QT_c) at daily dosages of 50 or 400 mg daily for 7 days in a randomized, placebo-controlled, active-comparator (moxifloxacin) study; the 400-mg dose produced plasma concentrations 19-fold higher than the maximum recommended clinical dose of 25 mg.

Following oral administration of a single dose of alogliptin (up to 800 mg) in healthy individuals, median time to peak plasma concentration was 1–2 hours; the drug has an absolute oral bioavailability of approximately 100%. Administration of alogliptin with food did not substantially alter total and peak exposure to the drug. Alogliptin does not undergo extensive metabolism; 60–80% of the dose is excreted unchanged. Following administration of a radiolabeled dose of alogliptin, approximately 89% of administered radioactivity was excreted in urine (76%) and feces (13%). Terminal elimination half-life of alogliptin is approximately 21 hours following a single dose of 25 mg.

Advice to Patients

Importance of patient reading medication guide before initiating therapy and each time the drug is dispensed.

Importance of informing patients of the potential risks and benefits of alogliptin. Importance of not using alogliptin in patients with type 1 diabetes mellitus or diabetic ketoacidosis.

Importance of informing patient about possibility of acute pancreatitis, which may be severe or fatal, with alogliptin therapy. Importance of patient informing clinicians about a history of pancreatitis, gallstones, alcoholism, or kidney or liver problems. Importance of informing patients about signs and symptoms of pancreatitis, including persistent severe abdominal pain sometimes radiating to the back that may or may not be accompanied by vomiting; importance of patient discontinuing alogliptin and promptly notifying clinician if such signs or symptoms are present.

Importance of informing patients about possibility of heart failure with alogliptin therapy. Importance of patients informing clinicians about a history of heart failure or renal impairment. Importance of informing patients about signs and symptoms of heart failure (e.g., shortness of breath, weight gain, edema); importance of patients immediately contacting a clinician if manifestations of heart failure occur.

Importance of informing patients of the possibility of severe and disabling joint pain with DPP-4 inhibitors (e.g., alogliptin, linagliptin, saxagliptin, sitagliptin). Advise patients to contact a clinician promptly if severe and persistent joint pain occurs; patients should not discontinue the DPP-4 inhibitor without consulting their clinician.

Importance of informing patient of risk of hypoglycemia, particularly if concomitant therapy with a sulfonylurea antidiabetic agent (i.e., insulin secretagogue) or insulin is used.

Risk of serious allergic (hypersensitivity) reaction. If signs or symptoms of such reactions occur (e.g., rash, hives, swelling of the face, lips, tongue, and throat that may cause difficulty in breathing or swallowing), importance of discontinuing alogliptin therapy and informing clinician promptly.

Importance of informing patients about possibility of liver injury, sometimes fatal, with alogliptin. If signs or symptoms of liver injury (e.g., nausea, vomiting, abdominal pain, unusual/unexplained fatigue, anorexia, dark urine, jaundice) occur, importance of discontinuing alogliptin therapy and informing clinician promptly.

Importance of taking alogliptin exactly as directed by clinician. (See Dosage and Administration: Administration.)

Importance of women informing their clinicians if they are or plan to become pregnant or plan to breast-feed.

Importance of informing clinicians of existing or contemplated concomitant therapy, including prescription and OTC drugs and dietary or herbal supplements, as well as any concomitant illnesses.

Importance of informing patients of other important precautionary information. (See Cautions.)

Overview® (see Users Guide). For additional information on this drug until a more detailed monograph is developed and published, the manufacturer's labeling should be consulted. It is *essential* that the manufacturer's labeling be consulted for more detailed information on usual cautions, precautions, contraindications, potential drug interactions, laboratory test interferences, and acute toxicity.

Preparations

Excipients in commercially available drug preparations may have clinically important effects in some individuals; consult specific product labeling for details.

Alogliptin Benzoate

Oral		
Tablets, film-coated	6.25 mg (of alogliptin)	**Nesina®**, Takeda
	12.5 mg (of alogliptin)	**Nesina®**, Takeda
	25 mg (of alogliptin)	**Nesina®**, Takeda

Alogliptin Benzoate Combinations

Oral		
Tablets, film-coated	12.5 mg (of alogliptin) with Metformin Hydrochloride 500 mg	**Kazano®**, Takeda
	12.5 mg (of alogliptin) with Metformin Hydrochloride 1 g	**Kazano®**, Takeda
	12.5 mg (of alogliptin) with Pioglitazone Hydrochloride 15 mg (of pioglitazone)	**Oseni®**, Takeda
	12.5 mg (of alogliptin) with Pioglitazone Hydrochloride 30 mg (of pioglitazone)	**Oseni®**, Takeda
	12.5 mg (of alogliptin) with Pioglitazone Hydrochloride 45 mg (of pioglitazone)	**Oseni®**, Takeda
	25 mg (of alogliptin) with Pioglitazone Hydrochloride 15 mg (of pioglitazone)	**Oseni®**, Takeda
	25 mg (of alogliptin) with Pioglitazone Hydrochloride 30 mg (of pioglitazone)	**Oseni®**, Takeda
	25 mg (of alogliptin) with Pioglitazone Hydrochloride 45 mg (of pioglitazone)	**Oseni®**, Takeda

Linagliptin

■ Linagliptin, a dipeptidyl peptidase-4 (DPP-4) inhibitor, is an antidiabetic agent.

Uses

■ **Type 2 Diabetes Mellitus** Linagliptin is used as monotherapy as an adjunct to diet and exercise to improve glycemic control in patients with type 2 diabetes mellitus. Linagliptin also is used as initial therapy in combination with metformin hydrochloride as an adjunct to diet and exercise to improve glycemic control in patients with type 2 diabetes mellitus. Linagliptin also is used in combination with other oral antidiabetic agents (e.g., metformin, a sulfonylurea, a peroxisome proliferator-activated receptor$_\gamma$ [PPAR$_\gamma$] agonist [thiazolidinedione]) or insulin as an adjunct to diet and exercise in patients with type 2 diabetes mellitus who have not achieved adequate glycemic control with oral antidiabetic agent monotherapy. Linagliptin is commercially available in fixed combination with the sodium-glucose cotransporter 2 (SGLT2) inhibitor, empagliflozin (Glyxambi®) or immediate- or extended-release metformin hydrochloride (Jentadueto®, Jentadueto® XR, respectively); these fixed-combination preparations are used as adjuncts to diet and exercise to improve glycemic control in patients with type 2 diabetes mellitus when treatment with both drugs in the fixed combination is appropriate.

While metformin generally is the preferred antidiabetic agent for initial therapy in patients with type 2 diabetes mellitus, the American Association of Clinical Endocrinologists/American College of Endocrinology (AACE/ACE) suggests a dipeptidyl peptidase-4 (DPP-4) inhibitor as one of several alternative antidiabetic agents for initial monotherapy in patients with a contraindication to metformin (e.g., renal disease, hepatic disease, GI intolerance, risk of lactic acidosis). DPP-4 inhibitors are also recommended by AACE/ACE as part of combination therapy, particularly when both postprandial and fasting plasma glucose concentrations are elevated.

Linagliptin should not be used in patients with type 1 diabetes mellitus or for the treatment of diabetic ketoacidosis.

Linagliptin Monotherapy Efficacy of linagliptin as monotherapy for the management of type 2 diabetes mellitus has been established in 2 double-blind, placebo-controlled studies of 18 or 24 weeks' duration. Linagliptin (5 mg once daily) improved glycemic control as evidenced by reductions in glycosylated hemoglobin (HbA$_{1c}$) as well as in fasting and 2-hour postprandial plasma glucose concentrations. HbA$_{1c}$ was reduced by a mean of 0.4% (from a mean baseline concentration of about 8%) in patients receiving linagliptin 5 mg daily, compared with an increase in HbA$_{1c}$ of 0.1–0.3% in those receiving placebo.

Combination Therapy Efficacy of linagliptin in combination with metformin, an SGLT2 inhibitor, a sulfonylurea, or a thiazolidinedione in the management of type 2 diabetes mellitus has been established in several randomized, placebo- or active-controlled, double-blind studies. In these studies, the addition of linagliptin (5 mg once daily) to current therapy (metformin and/or a sulfonylurea; pioglitazone; metformin and empagliflozin) improved glycemic control as evidenced by reductions in HbA$_{1c}$ as well as in fasting and/or 2-hour postprandial plasma glucose concentrations.

Efficacy of the combination of linagliptin and metformin as *initial* therapy in patients with type 2 diabetes mellitus inadequately controlled with diet and exercise is supported by results of a 24-week, randomized, double-blind trial. In this trial, concurrent therapy with linagliptin and metformin hydrochloride improved glycemic control (as evidenced by reductions in HbA$_{1c}$ and fasting plasma glucose) compared with linagliptin or metformin hydrochloride monotherapy or placebo. Reductions in HbA$_{1c}$ were 1.2 or 1.6% with linagliptin 2.5 mg plus metformin hydrochloride 0.5 or 1 g twice daily, respectively; 0.5% with linagliptin 5 mg once daily; 0.6 or 1.1% with metformin hydrochloride 0.5 or 1 g twice daily, respectively; and 0.1% with placebo.

In a 24-week study in patients receiving metformin hydrochloride monotherapy (at least 1.5 g daily), add-on therapy with linagliptin resulted in a reduction of 0.5% in HbA$_{1c}$ compared with an increase of 0.15% in patients receiving metformin hydrochloride and add-on placebo. In a 104-week, active-controlled, noninferiority study in patients receiving metformin hydrochloride monotherapy (at least 1.5 g daily), add-on therapy with linagliptin was noninferior at 52 weeks and resulted in a reduction of 0.4% in HbA$_{1c}$ from baseline, compared with a reduction of 0.6% from baseline in patients receiving add-on therapy with glimepiride (initiated at 1 mg daily and titrated over 12 weeks to a maximum dosage of 4 mg daily [mean dosage: 3 mg daily]). At 104 weeks, add-on therapy with linagliptin resulted in a reduction of 0.2% in HbA$_{1c}$ from baseline, compared with a reduction of 0.4% from baseline in those receiving add-on glimepiride therapy. Patients receiving add-on linagliptin therapy had a mean decrease in body weight (loss of 1.1 kg), while those receiving add-on glimepiride had a mean increase in body weight (gain of 1.4 kg). In a 24-week study in treatment-naive patients with type 2 diabetes mellitus, initial therapy with linagliptin and metformin hydrochloride produced substantially greater reductions in HbA$_{1c}$ compared with linagliptin therapy alone (reduction of 2.9 versus 2%, respectively).

In a 24-week study in patients receiving pioglitazone monotherapy (30 mg daily), add-on linagliptin or placebo resulted in a reduction of 1.1 or 0.6%, respectively, in HbA$_{1c}$.

In an 18-week study in patients receiving a sulfonylurea antidiabetic agent (sulfonylurea not specified), add-on therapy with linagliptin resulted in a reduction of 0.5% in HbA$_{1c}$ compared with a reduction of 0.1% in patients receiving add-on placebo.

In a 24-week study in patients receiving metformin and a sulfonylurea (generally glimepiride, glyburide [glibenclamide], or gliclazide [not commercially available in the US]), add-on therapy with linagliptin or placebo resulted in a reduction of 0.7 or 0.1%, respectively, in HbA$_{1c}$.

In an international, phase 3, randomized, double-blind trial, add-on therapy with linagliptin and empagliflozin in fixed combination was more effective in reducing HbA$_{1c}$ and fasting plasma glucose concentrations than add-on linagliptin or empagliflozin monotherapy in 686 adults with type 2 diabetes mellitus inadequately controlled with metformin hydrochloride (dosage of at least 1.5 g daily, or maximum tolerated dosage, or maximum labeled dosage). At 24 weeks, reduction in mean HbA$_{1c}$ from baseline was 1.19% with linagliptin 5 mg/empagliflozin 25 mg, 1.08% with linagliptin 5 mg/empagliflozin 10 mg, 0.62% with empagliflozin 25 mg, 0.66% with empagliflozin 10 mg, and 0.7% with linagliptin 5 mg. Glycemic efficacy (HbA$_{1c}$ reductions) with the fixed combinations of linagliptin and empagliflozin was maintained at week 52. The fixed combinations of linagliptin and empagliflozin also were associated with reductions from baseline in systolic blood pressure compared with linagliptin monotherapy. Body weight was reduced in patients receiving the fixed combinations of empagliflozin/linagliptin compared with linagliptin but not empagliflozin monotherapy.

Efficacy of linagliptin in combination with insulin in patients with type 2 diabetes mellitus inadequately controlled with insulin (with or without oral antidiabetic agents) is supported by the results of a 24-week randomized, placebo-controlled trial. In this trial, addition of linagliptin (5 mg once daily) to existing stable therapy with insulin resulted in improvements in HbA_{1c} and fasting plasma glucose concentrations at week 24 compared with addition of placebo. Mean reductions in HbA_{1c} were 0.6% in patients receiving linagliptin and 0.1% in those receiving placebo.

Dosage and Administration

■ **Administration** When administered as monotherapy, linagliptin is administered orally once daily without regard to meals.

The fixed combination of linagliptin and empagliflozin is administered orally once daily in the morning with or without food.

The fixed combination of linagliptin and *immediate-release* metformin hydrochloride is administered orally twice daily with meals.

The fixed combination of linagliptin and *extended-release* metformin hydrochloride is administered orally once daily with a meal.

If a dose of linagliptin alone or in fixed combination with empagliflozin or immediate- or extended-release metformin hydrochloride is missed, the missed dose should be taken as soon as it is remembered followed by resumption of the regular schedule. If the missed dose is not remembered until the time of the next dose, the missed dose should be skipped and the regular schedule resumed. The dose should not be doubled to replace a missed dose.

■ **Dosage** ***Linagliptin Monotherapy*** When used as monotherapy for the management of type 2 diabetes mellitus, the recommended dosage of linagliptin is 5 mg once daily.

Combination Therapy with a Sulfonylurea When used concomitantly with a sulfonylurea for the management of type 2 diabetes mellitus, the recommended dosage of linagliptin is 5 mg once daily; dosage of the sulfonylurea may need to be reduced to decrease risk of hypoglycemia.

Linagliptin/Empagliflozin Fixed-combination Therapy The recommended initial dosage of the fixed combination of linagliptin and empagliflozin is 5 mg of linagliptin and 10 mg of empagliflozin once daily in the morning. If this dosage is well tolerated, the dosage may be increased to 5 mg of linagliptin and 25 mg of empagliflozin once daily.

Linagliptin/Immediate- or Extended-release Metformin Hydrochloride Fixed-combination Therapy Dosage of the fixed combinations of linagliptin and immediate- or extended-release metformin hydrochloride should be individualized based on effectiveness and patient tolerability. Dosage of these fixed combinations may be increased up to a daily maximum of 5 mg of linagliptin and 2 g of metformin hydrochloride.

In patients *not* currently receiving metformin hydrochloride, the recommended initial total daily dosage of the fixed combination is 5 mg of linagliptin and 1 g of metformin hydrochloride administered in 2 divided doses (when given as the fixed combination containing *immediate-release* metformin hydrochloride) or once daily (when given as the fixed combination containing *extended-release* metformin hydrochloride).

In patients currently receiving metformin hydrochloride, the recommended initial total daily dosage of the fixed combination is 5 mg of linagliptin and a total daily metformin hydrochloride dosage similar to the patient's existing dosage, administered in 2 divided doses (when given as the fixed combination containing *immediate-release* metformin hydrochloride) or once daily (when given as the fixed combination containing *extended-release* metformin hydrochloride).

In patients currently receiving linagliptin *and* metformin hydrochloride, the recommended initial dosage of the fixed combination of linagliptin and *immediate-release* metformin hydrochloride is the same total daily dosage of each component administered in 2 divided doses daily.

In patients currently receiving linagliptin *and* metformin hydrochloride *or* the fixed combination of linagliptin and *immediate-release* metformin, the recommended initial dosage of the fixed combination of linagliptin and *extended-release* metformin is 5 mg of linagliptin and a total daily dosage of metformin hydrochloride similar to the patient's existing dosage, administered once daily.

■ **Special Populations** ***Hepatic Impairment*** **Linagliptin Monotherapy.** Dosage adjustment is not routinely required based on hepatic impairment.

Linagliptin/Empagliflozin Fixed-combination Therapy. The fixed combination of linagliptin and empagliflozin may be used in patients with hepatic impairment.

Linagliptin/Immediate- or Extended-release Metformin Hydrochloride Fixed-combination Therapy. The fixed combinations of linagliptin and immediate- or extended-release metformin hydrochloride are not recommended in patients with hepatic impairment.

Renal Impairment **Linagliptin Monotherapy.** Dosage adjustment is not routinely required based on renal impairment.

Linagliptin/Empagliflozin Fixed-combination Therapy. Dosage adjustment of the fixed combination of linagliptin and empagliflozin is not necessary in patients with an estimated glomerular filtration rate (eGFR) of at least 45 mL/minute per 1.73 m².

The fixed combination of linagliptin and empagliflozin should not be initiated in patients with an eGFR less than 45 mL/minute per 1.73 m². The fixed combination should be discontinued if the eGFR is persistently less than 45 mL/minute per 1.73 m².

Linagliptin/Immediate- or Extended-release Metformin Hydrochloride Fixed-combination Therapy. Initiation of the fixed combinations of linagliptin and immediate- or extended-release metformin hydrochloride is not recommended in patients with an eGFR of 30–45 mL/minute per 1.73 m².

If the eGFR decreases to 30–45 mL/minute per 1.73 m² during therapy with a fixed combination of linagliptin and metformin hydrochloride, the risks and benefits of continuing therapy with the fixed combination should be assessed.

The fixed combinations of linagliptin and immediate- or extended-release metformin hydrochloride are contraindicated in patients with an eGFR less than 30 mL/minute per 1.73 m².

If a fixed combination of linagliptin and metformin is discontinued due to evidence of renal impairment, linagliptin may be continued as a single-entity tablet at the same total daily dosage of 5 mg.

Geriatric Patients **Linagliptin Monotherapy.** Dosage adjustment of linagliptin is not recommended in geriatric patients based solely on age.

Cautions

■ **Contraindications** Linagliptin is contraindicated in patients with a history of hypersensitivity reaction (e.g., anaphylaxis, urticaria, angioedema, bronchial hyperreactivity) to linagliptin.

■ **Warnings/Precautions** ***Pancreatitis and Pancreatic Precancerous Changes*** Acute pancreatitis, including fatal pancreatitis, has been reported in patients receiving linagliptin therapy. In a multicenter, randomized, placebo-controlled trial evaluating linagliptin, acute pancreatitis was reported in 9 patients receiving linagliptin (0.3%) versus 5 patients receiving placebo (0.1%); 2 patients who developed acute pancreatitis while receiving linagliptin died.

FDA has been evaluating unpublished findings suggesting an increased risk of pancreatitis and precancerous pancreatic cell changes (pancreatic duct metaplasia) in patients with type 2 diabetes mellitus receiving incretin mimetics (alogliptin, exenatide, linagliptin, liraglutide, saxagliptin, and sitagliptin). These findings are based on examination of a small number of pancreatic tissue specimens taken from patients who died from unspecified causes while receiving an incretin mimetic. FDA will notify healthcare professionals of its conclusions and recommendations when the review is complete, or when the agency has additional information to report.

FDA has recommended that clinicians continue to follow the recommendations in the prescribing information for incretin mimetics. The manufacturer states that patients receiving linagliptin therapy should be monitored for signs and symptoms of pancreatitis. (See Advice to Patients.) If pancreatitis is suspected, linagliptin should be promptly discontinued and appropriate management instituted. Safety and efficacy of linagliptin have not been established in patients with a history of pancreatitis and it is not known whether such patients are at increased risk for pancreatitis with linagliptin therapy.

Severe Arthralgia Severe, disabling joint pain has been reported during postmarketing experience in patients receiving dipeptidyl peptidase-4 (DPP-4) inhibitors (e.g., alogliptin, linagliptin, saxagliptin, sitagliptin). Onset of such symptoms has ranged from 1 day to years following initiation of therapy. Fever, chills, rash, and swelling accompanied joint pain in some patients, suggesting an immunologic reaction; some patients required hospitalization. Symptoms resolved upon discontinuance of the DPP-4 inhibitor, usually in less than a month. In some patients, symptoms recurred when the same or another DPP-4 inhibitor was restarted. DPP-4 inhibitors should be considered as a possible cause of severe joint pain and should be discontinued if appropriate. (See Advice to Patients.)

Heart Failure Risk In cardiovascular outcomes studies conducted with other dipeptidyl peptidase-4 (DPP-4) inhibitors (alogliptin, saxagliptin) in patients with type 2 diabetes mellitus and atherosclerotic cardiovascular disease (ASCVD), an association between DPP-4 inhibitor treatment and heart failure was observed.

The potential risks and benefits of linagliptin therapy should be considered prior to use in patients at risk for heart failure (e.g., history of heart failure or renal impairment). Patients receiving linagliptin-containing therapy should be monitored for manifestations of heart failure. (See Advice to Patients.) If heart failure develops, appropriate evaluation and management should be instituted and consideration given to discontinuing linagliptin.

Concomitant Therapy with Hypoglycemic Agents Use of linagliptin in combination with an insulin secretagogue (e.g., a sulfonylurea) was associated with a higher rate of hypoglycemia compared with placebo in a clinical trial. Use of linagliptin in combination with insulin in patients with severe renal impairment also was associated with a higher rate of hypoglycemia compared with placebo in another clinical trial. A reduced dosage of an insulin secretagogue or insulin may be required to decrease the risk of hypoglycemia when used in combination with linagliptin.

Dermatologic and Sensitivity Reactions There have been postmarketing reports of serious allergic and hypersensitivity reactions (e.g., anaphylaxis, angioedema, exfoliative skin conditions) with linagliptin; rash also has been reported. The onset of such reactions usually was within the first 3 months following treatment initiation, but such reactions may occur after the first dose. (See Cautions: Contraindications.)

If a serious hypersensitivity reaction is suspected, promptly discontinue linagliptin, assess for other potential causes of the event, and initiate alternative antidiabetic therapy. (See Advice to Patients.) Linagliptin should be used with caution in patients with a history of angioedema with other DPP-4 inhibitors because it is unknown whether such patients will be predisposed to angioedema with linagliptin.

In a multicenter, randomized, placebo-controlled trial evaluating linagliptin, bullous pemphigoid was reported in 7 patients receiving linagliptin (0.2%) versus none of the patients receiving placebo. Postmarketing cases of bullous pemphigoid requiring hospitalization have been reported with DPP-4 inhibitor use. These cases usually resolved after discontinuation of the DPP-4 inhibitor and treatment with topical or systemic immunosuppressive therapy. Patients should be advised to report the development of blisters or erosions while receiving linagliptin. If bullous pemphigoid is suspected, the drug should be discontinued and referral to a dermatologist should be considered for diagnosis and appropriate treatment.

Use of Fixed Combinations When linagliptin is used in fixed combination with empagliflozin, metformin hydrochloride, or other drugs, the cautions, precautions, contraindications, and interactions associated with the concomitant agent(s) should be considered in addition to those associated with linagliptin.

Specific Populations **Pregnancy.** Data on use of linagliptin in pregnant women are insufficient to inform a drug-associated risk for major birth defects or miscarriage.

In animal reproduction studies, no adverse developmental effects were observed when linagliptin was administered to pregnant rats during the period of organogenesis.

Lactation. Linagliptin is distributed into milk in animals at a milk-to-plasma ratio of 4:1; it is not known whether the drug is distributed into human milk. The benefits of breast-feeding and the importance of linagliptin to the woman should be considered along with any potential adverse effects on the breast-fed infant from the drug or from the underlying maternal condition.

Pediatric Use. Safety and efficacy of linagliptin alone or in fixed combination with empagliflozin or fixed combination with immediate- or extended-release metformin hydrochloride have not been established in patients younger than 18 years of age.

Geriatric Use. Of 4040 patients in clinical studies of linagliptin, 27% were 65 years of age and older and 3% were 75 years of age and older. No substantial differences in safety and efficacy relative to younger adults were observed, but increased sensitivity cannot be ruled out.

Hepatic Impairment. In patients with mild hepatic impairment (Child-Pugh class A), linagliptin area under the concentration-time curve (AUC) and peak plasma concentration were reduced by 25 and 36%, respectively, compared with values in healthy individuals. In patients with moderate hepatic impairment (Child-Pugh class B), linagliptin AUC and peak plasma concentration were reduced by 14 and 8%, respectively, compared with values in healthy individuals. In patients with severe hepatic impairment (Child-Pugh class C), linagliptin AUC was comparable to that in healthy individuals, and peak plasma concentration was reduced by 23% relative to that in healthy individuals.

The fixed combination of linagliptin and empagliflozin may be used in patients with hepatic impairment.

Use of the fixed combinations of linagliptin and immediate- or extended-release metformin hydrochloride is not recommended in patients with hepatic impairment.

Renal Impairment. In patients with mild renal impairment (creatinine clearance 50 to less than 80 mL/minute), linagliptin exposure was comparable to that in healthy individuals. In patients with moderate renal impairment (creatinine clearance 30 to less than 50 mL/minute), linagliptin AUC and peak plasma concentration were increased by 71 and 46%, respectively, compared with values in healthy individuals. In patients with severe renal impairment (creatinine clearance less than 30 mL/minute) and type 2 diabetes mellitus, linagliptin AUC and peak plasma concentration were increased by 42 and 35%, respectively, compared with those values in patients with type 2 diabetes mellitus and normal renal function.

The fixed combination of linagliptin and empagliflozin should not be initiated in patients with an estimated glomerular filtration rate (eGFR) less than 45 mL/minute per 1.73 m^2. (See Renal Impairment under Dosage and Administration: Special Populations.)

Initiation of the fixed combinations of linagliptin and immediate- or extended-release metformin hydrochloride is not recommended in patients with an eGFR between 30–45 mL/minute per 1.73 m^2 and is contraindicated in patients with an eGFR less than 30 mL/minute per 1.73 m^2. (See Renal Impairment under Dosage and Administration: Special Populations.)

■ **Common Adverse Effects** Adverse effects reported in at least 5% of patients receiving linagliptin monotherapy include nasopharyngitis.

Adverse effects reported in at least 2% of patients receiving linagliptin concomitantly with pioglitazone, a sulfonylurea, metformin, or basal insulin include nasopharyngitis, hyperlipidemia, cough, hypertriglyceridemia, weight gain, urinary tract infection, constipation, back pain, arthralgia, upper respiratory tract infection, headache, and pain in extremity.

Adverse effects reported in at least 5% of patients receiving linagliptin and empagliflozin in clinical trials include urinary tract infection, nasopharyngitis, and upper respiratory tract infection.

Adverse effects reported in at least 5% of patients receiving linagliptin and metformin hydrochloride in clinical trials include nasopharyngitis and diarrhea.

Drug Interactions

■ **Drugs Affecting or Metabolized by Hepatic Microsomal Enzymes** Linagliptin is a weak to moderate inhibitor of cytochrome P-450 (CYP) isoenzyme 3A4; however, it does not inhibit or induce CYP isoenzymes 1A2, 2A6, 2B6, 2C8, 2C9, 2C19, 2D6, 2E1, or 4A11 in vitro.

In vivo studies indicate that drug interactions are unlikely with substrates of CYP isoenzymes 3A4, 2C9, or 2C8. No adjustment of linagliptin dosage is recommended based on results of pharmacokinetic studies.

Inducers of CYP3A4 (e.g., rifampin) decrease exposure to linagliptin, resulting in subtherapeutic and likely ineffective concentrations. The manufacturer states that alternatives to linagliptin are strongly recommended in patients who require therapy with potent CYP3A4 inducers.

■ **Drugs Affecting or Affected by P-glycoprotein Transport** Linagliptin is a P-glycoprotein substrate and inhibits P-glycoprotein-mediated transport of digoxin at high concentrations. At therapeutic concentrations, linagliptin is considered unlikely to cause interactions with other P-glycoprotein substrates; no adjustment of linagliptin dosage is recommended based on results of pharmacokinetic studies.

Inducers of P-glycoprotein (e.g., rifampin) decrease exposure to linagliptin, resulting in subtherapeutic and likely ineffective concentrations. The manufacturer states that alternatives to linagliptin are strongly recommended in patients who require therapy with potent P-glycoprotein inducers.

■ **Drugs Affected by Organic Cation Transporter** In vivo studies indicate that drug interactions are unlikely with substrates of organic cation transporter (OCT). No adjustment of linagliptin dosage is recommended based on results of pharmacokinetic studies.

■ **Digoxin** Concomitant use of linagliptin (5 mg once daily) and digoxin (0.25 mg once daily) in healthy individuals did not appreciably alter the pharmacokinetics of digoxin (e.g., a 2% increase in area under the concentration-time curve [AUC] and a 6% decrease in peak plasma concentration with concomitant use); no digoxin dosage adjustment is necessary.

■ **Estrogens or Progestins** Concomitant use of linagliptin (5 mg once daily) and an estrogen-progestin contraceptive (ethinyl estradiol 30 mcg with levonorgestrel 0.15 mg once daily) increased AUC and peak plasma concentration by 1 and 8%, respectively, for ethinyl estradiol and by 9 and 13%, respectively, for levonorgestrel. No dosage adjustments are necessary for ethinyl estradiol or levonorgestrel when given concomitantly with linagliptin.

■ **Metformin** Concomitant use of linagliptin (10 mg once daily) and metformin hydrochloride (850 mg 3 times daily) in healthy individuals increased linagliptin AUC and peak plasma concentration by 20 and 3%, respectively. Such concomitant use did not affect metformin AUC but reduced metformin peak plasma concentration by 11%. These alterations in pharmacokinetic parameters were not associated with clinically relevant effects (e.g., hypoglycemia), and no dosage adjustments are necessary for either drug.

■ **Pioglitazone** Concomitant use of linagliptin (10 mg once daily) and pioglitazone (45 mg once daily) in healthy individuals increased linagliptin AUC and peak plasma concentration by 13 and 7%, respectively. Pioglitazone AUC and peak plasma concentration were reduced by 6 and 14%, respectively, during concomitant linagliptin therapy; small changes (5% or less) in AUC and peak plasma concentrations of 2 pioglitazone active metabolites also occurred with such concomitant therapy. No dosage adjustments are necessary for either drug when given concomitantly.

■ **Rifampin** Concomitant use of linagliptin (5 mg once daily) and rifampin (600 mg once daily) reduced linagliptin AUC and peak plasma concentration by 40 and 44%, respectively; such concomitant therapy is not recommended. (See Drugs Affecting or Metabolized by Hepatic Microsomal Enzymes and see Drugs Affecting or Affected by P-glycoprotein Transport under Drug Interactions.)

■ **Ritonavir** Administration of a single dose of linagliptin (5 mg) to patients receiving ritonavir (200 mg twice daily) resulted in approximately a twofold increase in linagliptin AUC and approximately a threefold increase in linagliptin peak plasma concentration. The increase in exposure was not associated with an increase in linagliptin accumulation. No adjustment of linagliptin dosage is necessary when linagliptin is administered concurrently with ritonavir.

■ **Simvastatin** Concomitant use of linagliptin (10 mg once daily) and simvastatin (40 mg once daily) in healthy individuals increased simvastatin AUC and peak plasma concentration by 34 and 10%, respectively; these changes were not considered clinically important. No simvastatin dosage adjustment is necessary when given concomitantly with linagliptin.

■ **Sulfonylureas** When a sulfonylurea is administered concomitantly with linagliptin, reduction in the dosage of the sulfonylurea may be required to reduce the risk of hypoglycemia.

A single dose of glyburide (1.75 mg) given on day 6 to healthy individuals receiving linagliptin therapy (5 mg once daily for 6 days) decreased glyburide exposure (AUC and peak plasma concentration) by about 14%; these changes were not considered clinically important. No dosage adjustments are necessary for either drug when given concomitantly.

■ **Warfarin** Administration of a single dose of warfarin sodium (10 mg) to healthy individuals receiving linagliptin (5 mg once daily) had no apparent effect (i.e., change of 3% or less) on *R*- or *S*-warfarin AUC and peak plasma concentration and no clinically relevant effect on international normalized ratio (INR) or prothrombin time (PT); no warfarin dosage adjustment is necessary.

Description

Linagliptin is a xanthine-derived inhibitor of dipeptidyl peptidase-4 (DPP-4), an enzyme that inactivates incretin hormones glucagon-like peptide-1 (GLP-1) and glucose-dependent insulinotropic polypeptide (GIP). The drug selectively inhibits DPP-4 with no effect on DPP-8 or DDP-9 in vitro at concentrations approximating those achieved with therapeutic dosages. Linagliptin increases the concentrations of active incretin hormones (e.g., GLP-1, GIP), stimulating the release of insulin in a glucose-dependent manner and decreasing circulating levels of glucagon. GLP-1 and GIP are secreted at low basal levels throughout the day, and levels increase immediately after a meal. Both incretin hormones increase insulin biosynthesis and secretion from pancreatic β-cells in the presence of normal and elevated blood glucose concentrations. GLP-1 also reduces glucagon secretion from pancreatic α-cells, resulting in a reduction in hepatic glucose output.

Linagliptin monotherapy usually is not associated with hypoglycemia or substantial changes in body weight.

Peak plasma linagliptin concentrations usually are attained within 1.5 hours after a 5-mg oral dose, and the drug has an absolute oral bioavailability of approximately 30%. Administration of linagliptin with a high-fat meal reduced peak plasma concentration by 15% and increased area under the concentration-time curve (AUC) by 4%; these changes are not considered clinically important. Metabolism represents a minor elimination pathway for linagliptin; approximately 90% of a dose is excreted unchanged. Following administration of a radiolabeled dose of linagliptin, approximately 85% of administered radioactivity was eliminated via the enterohepatic system (80%) or in urine (5%). Terminal half-life of linagliptin exceeds 100 hours; plasma concentrations decline in at least a biphasic manner. The effective half-life for accumulation of linagliptin based on 5-mg multiple oral dosing is approximately 12 hours.

Results of bioequivalence studies indicate that the fixed-combination tablets containing linagliptin and empagliflozin or linagliptin and immediate-release metformin hydrochloride are bioequivalent to single-entity tablets of linagliptin given concomitantly with single-entity tablets of empagliflozin or single-entity tablets of immediate-release metformin hydrochloride, respectively, in corresponding doses.

Advice to Patients

When linagliptin is used in fixed combination with other drugs, importance of informing patients of important cautionary information about the concomitant agent(s).

Importance of patient reading medication guide before initiating therapy and each time the drug is dispensed.

Importance of informing patients of the potential risks and benefits of linagliptin and of alternative therapies. Importance of not using linagliptin in patients with type 1 diabetes mellitus or diabetic ketoacidosis.

Importance of informing patient about possibility of acute pancreatitis, which may be severe or fatal, with linagliptin therapy. Importance of patient informing clinicians about a history of pancreatitis, gallstones, alcoholism, or high triglyceride levels. Importance of informing patients about signs and symptoms of pancreatitis, including persistent severe abdominal pain sometimes radiating to the back that may or may not be accompanied by vomiting; importance of patient discontinuing linagliptin and promptly notifying clinician if such signs or symptoms are present.

Importance of informing patients about possibility of heart failure with linagliptin therapy. Importance of patients informing clinicians about a history of heart failure or renal impairment. Importance of informing patients about signs and symptoms of heart failure (e.g., shortness of breath, weight gain, edema); importance of patients immediately contacting a clinician if manifestations of heart failure occur.

Importance of informing patients of the possibility of severe and disabling joint pain with dipeptidyl peptidase-4 (DPP-4) inhibitors (e.g., alogliptin, linagliptin, saxagliptin, sitagliptin). Advise patients to contact a clinician promptly if severe and persistent joint pain occurs; patients should not discontinue the DPP-4 inhibitor without consulting their clinician.

Importance of informing patients that bullous pemphigoid may occur with the use of a DPP-4 inhibitor. Advise patients to contact a clinician if blisters or erosions occur.

Increased risk of hypoglycemia when linagliptin is used in combination with a sulfonylurea or insulin. Importance of informing patients that a lower dosage of the sulfonylurea or insulin may be required to reduce the risk of hypoglycemia if used concomitantly with linagliptin.

Risk of serious allergic (hypersensitivity) reactions, such as angioedema, anaphylaxis, and exfoliative skin conditions. If signs or symptoms of such reactions occur (e.g., rash, skin flaking or peeling, hives, swelling of the skin, swelling of the face, lips, tongue, and throat that may cause difficulty in breathing or swallowing), importance of discontinuing linagliptin-containing therapy and informing clinician promptly.

Importance of informing patients about the importance of adherence to dietary instructions, regular physical activity, periodic blood glucose monitoring and HbA_{1C} testing, recognition and management of hypoglycemia and hyperglycemia, and assessment of complications of diabetes mellitus.

Importance of seeking medical advice promptly during periods of stress such as fever, trauma, infection, or surgery as medication requirements may change.

Importance of informing patients that response to all antidiabetic therapies should be monitored by periodic measurements of blood glucose and HbA_{1C}, with a goal of decreasing these levels toward the normal range.

Importance of informing clinicians if any unusual symptom develops or if any existing symptom persists or worsens.

Importance of women informing their clinicians if they are or plan to become pregnant or plan to breast-feed.

Importance of informing clinicians of existing or contemplated concomitant therapy, including prescription and OTC drugs and dietary or herbal supplements, as well as any concomitant illnesses.

Importance of informing patients of other important precautionary information. (See Cautions.)

Overview® (see Users Guide). For additional information on this drug until a more detailed monograph is developed and published, the manufacturer's labeling should be consulted. It is *essential* that the manufacturer's labeling be consulted for more detailed information on usual cautions, precautions, contraindications, potential drug interactions, laboratory test interferences, and acute toxicity.

Preparations

Excipients in commercially available drug preparations may have clinically important effects in some individuals; consult specific product labeling for details.

Linagliptin

Oral		
Tablet, film-coated	5 mg	**Tradjenta®**, Boehringer Ingelheim

Linagliptin Combinations

Oral		
Tablets, extended-release	2.5 mg with Extended-release Metformin Hydrochloride 1 g	**Jentadueto® XR**, Boehringer Ingelheim
	5 mg with Extended-release Metformin Hydrochloride 1 g	**Jentadueto® XR**, Boehringer Ingelheim
Tablets, film-coated	2.5 mg with Metformin Hydrochloride 500 mg	**Jentadueto®**, Boehringer Ingelheim
	2.5 mg with Metformin Hydrochloride 850 mg	**Jentadueto®**, Boehringer Ingelheim
	2.5 mg with Metformin Hydrochloride 1 g	**Jentadueto®**, Boehringer Ingelheim
	5 mg with Empagliflozin 10 mg	**Glyxambi®**, Boehringer Ingelheim
	5 mg with Empagliflozin 25 mg	**Glyxambi®**, Boehringer Ingelheim

sAXagliptin Hydrochloride

■ Saxagliptin hydrochloride, a dipeptidyl peptidase-4 (DPP-4) inhibitor, is an antidiabetic agent.

Uses

■ **Type 2 Diabetes Mellitus** Saxagliptin is used as monotherapy as an adjunct to diet and exercise to improve glycemic control in patients with type 2 diabetes mellitus. Saxagliptin also is used as initial therapy in combination with metformin hydrochloride (given separately or as the fixed combination of saxagliptin and *extended-release* metformin hydrochloride) as an adjunct to diet and exercise to improve glycemic control in patients with type 2 diabetes mellitus when treatment with both saxagliptin and metformin is appropriate. Saxagliptin also is used in combination with other oral antidiabetic agents (e.g., metformin, a sulfonylurea, a thiazolidinedione [peroxisome proliferator-activated receptor-γ] agonist) or insulin as an adjunct to diet and exercise in patients with type 2 diabetes mellitus who have not achieved adequate glycemic control with one or more oral antidiabetic agents and/or insulin. Additionally, the fixed combination of saxagliptin and dapagliflozin is used as an adjunct to diet and exercise to improve glycemic control in patients with type 2 diabetes mellitus.

While metformin generally is the preferred antidiabetic agent for initial therapy in patients with type 2 diabetes mellitus, the American Association of Clinical Endocrinologists/American College of Endocrinology (AACE/ACE) suggests a dipeptidyl peptidase-4 (DPP-4) inhibitor as one of several alternative antidiabetic agents for initial monotherapy in patients with a contraindication to metformin (e.g., renal disease, hepatic disease, GI intolerance, risk of lactic acidosis). DPP-4 inhibitors also are recommended by AACE/ACE as part of combination therapy, particularly when both postprandial and fasting plasma glucose concentrations are elevated.

In pivotal clinical trials, glycemic efficacy and safety of saxagliptin in patients with type 2 diabetes mellitus was evaluated at dosages of 2.5, 5, and 10 mg once daily as monotherapy or in combination with other antidiabetic agents. In these trials, the 10-mg daily dosage (currently not an FDA-labeled dosage) of saxagliptin did not demonstrate greater efficacy than the 5-mg daily dosage.

Saxagliptin should not be used in patients with type 1 diabetes mellitus or for the treatment of diabetic ketoacidosis.

Saxagliptin Monotherapy Efficacy of saxagliptin as monotherapy in treatment-naive patients with type 2 diabetes mellitus is supported by results of 2 double-blind, placebo-controlled trials of 24 weeks' duration. In these trials, saxagliptin (2.5 or 5 mg once daily) improved glycemic control as evidenced by mean reductions in glycosylated hemoglobin (hemoglobin A_{1c}; HbA_{1c}) of about 0.4–0.7% (from a mean baseline HbA_{1c} of 7.9%) compared with a mean increase in HbA_{1c} of about 0.2–0.3% with placebo.

Combination Therapy Clinical trials evaluating the efficacy and safety of the *fixed combination* of saxagliptin and *extended-release* metformin hydrochloride (Kombiglyze® XR) in reducing HbA_{1c} have not been conducted; unless otherwise specified, clinical trials of saxagliptin in combination with metformin discussed in this monograph were conducted using concomitantly administered saxagliptin and *immediate-release* metformin. Bioequivalence between the fixed combination of saxagliptin and extended-release metformin hydrochloride (Kombiglyze® XR) and each agent (saxagliptin and extended-release metformin hydrochloride) given concurrently as separate tablets has been demonstrated. (See Description.) Safety and efficacy of the fixed combination of saxagliptin and dapagliflozin (Qtern®) have been established by clinical trials evaluating saxagliptin as add-on therapy to treatment with dapagliflozin and metformin hydrochloride or evaluating saxagliptin and dapagliflozin as add-on therapy to metformin hydrochloride treatment.

Efficacy of the combination of saxagliptin and metformin as *initial* therapy in patients with type 2 diabetes mellitus inadequately controlled with diet and exercise is supported by results of a 24-week randomized, active-controlled trial. In this trial, concurrent therapy with saxagliptin (5 or 10 mg once daily) and metformin hydrochloride (500 mg daily initially, titrated up to a maximum of 2 g daily given in 2 divided doses with meals) improved HbA_{1c}, fasting plasma glucose, and 2-hour postprandial glucose values compared with saxagliptin or metformin monotherapy. Mean reductions in HbA_{1c} from baseline were 2.5% in patients receiving saxagliptin 5 mg daily plus metformin, 2.5% in patients receiving saxagliptin 10 mg daily plus metformin, 2% with metformin plus placebo, and 1.7% with saxagliptin 10 mg daily plus placebo. The proportion of patients achieving an HbA_{1c} less than 7% at week 24 was approximately 60% in patients receiving saxagliptin 5 or 10 mg daily plus metformin, 32% in patients receiving saxagliptin 10 mg daily plus placebo, and 41% in patients receiving metformin plus placebo.

Efficacy of saxagliptin in combination with metformin, a sulfonylurea (glyburide), or a thiazolidinedione (pioglitazone or rosiglitazone) in patients with type 2 diabetes mellitus inadequately controlled on monotherapy with these drugs is supported by results of several long-term (24–52 weeks' duration), randomized, placebo- or active-controlled trials demonstrating improvements in HbA_{1c} and fasting and/or 2-hour postprandial plasma glucose concentrations. In a trial in patients already receiving metformin hydrochloride (1.5–2.55 g daily), add-on therapy with saxagliptin (2.5 or 5 mg daily) resulted in a mean HbA_{1c} decrease of about 0.6 or 0.7%, respectively, (from a mean baseline HbA_{1c} of 8.1%) compared with a mean HbA_{1c} increase of about 0.1% with add-on placebo. In patients receiving either pioglitazone (30–45 mg daily) or rosiglitazone (4–8 mg daily) therapy, addition of saxagliptin (2.5 or 5 mg daily) resulted in a mean HbA_{1c} reduction of 0.7 or 0.9%, respectively, (from a mean baseline HbA_{1c} of 8.3 or 8.4%, respectively) compared with a mean reduction of 0.3% (from a mean baseline HbA_{1c} of 8.2%) with add-on placebo. In patients receiving a submaximal dosage of glyburide (7.5 mg daily as a fixed dosage), addition of saxagliptin (2.5 or 5 mg daily) resulted in a mean HbA_{1c} reduction of 0.5 or 0.6%, respectively, (from a mean baseline HbA_{1c} of 8.4 or 8.5%, respectively) compared with a mean increase of 0.1% with placebo added to glyburide 10 mg daily and titrated up to a maximum dosage of 15 mg daily (about 92% of patients had glyburide dosage titrated up to 15 mg daily within the initial 4 weeks of the trial).

In a 24-week trial in patients already receiving metformin and a sulfonylurea, addition of saxagliptin (5 mg once daily) resulted in a mean HbA_{1c} reduction of 0.7% (from a mean baseline HbA_{1c} of 8.4%) compared with a mean reduction of 0.1% with placebo (from a mean baseline HbA_{1c} of 8.2%).

In another trial comparing add-on therapy with saxagliptin versus add-on therapy with glipizide in patients already receiving metformin hydrochloride (1.5–3 g daily), addition of saxagliptin (5 mg daily) resulted in a mean HbA_{1c} reduction of 0.6% (from a mean baseline HbA_{1c} of 7.7%) versus a reduction of 0.7% (from a mean baseline HbA_{1c} of 7.6%) with add-on glipizide therapy (initial glipizide dosage of 5 mg daily, titrated up to a mean final dosage of 15 mg daily).

Efficacy of saxagliptin in combination with insulin in patients with type 2 diabetes mellitus inadequately controlled with insulin (with or without metformin) is supported by results of a 24-week, randomized, placebo-controlled trial. In this trial, addition of saxagliptin (5 mg once daily) to existing stable therapy with premixed insulin or intermediate- or long-acting insulin (insulin given in combination with metformin in some patients) resulted in improvements in HbA_{1c} and 2-hour postprandial glucose concentrations at week 24 compared with addition of placebo. Mean reductions in HbA_{1c} were similar for patients receiving saxagliptin as add-on therapy with insulin alone or insulin with metformin (0.4% in both groups). The mean reduction from baseline in 2-hour postprandial glucose at week 24 was 27 mg/dL with add-on saxagliptin and 4 mg/dL with add-on placebo. The mean change from baseline in daily insulin dosage at the end of the study was 2 or 5 units with saxagliptin or placebo, respectively.

Efficacy of the combination of dapagliflozin and saxagliptin with metformin hydrochloride for the management of type 2 diabetes mellitus is supported by several randomized, double-blind, controlled clinical studies. In a 24-week study in patients with inadequate glycemic control (HbA_{1c} concentration of 7.5–10%) despite treatment with metformin hydrochloride, the addition of dapagliflozin and saxagliptin to existing therapy with metformin hydrochloride substantially improved glycemic control. Patients who received triple therapy with dapagliflozin, saxagliptin and metformin hydrochloride had a HbA_{1c} reduction of 1.02% compared with a reduction of 0.62 or 0.69% in those who received dual therapy with dapagliflozin and metformin hydrochloride or saxagliptin and metformin hydrochloride therapy, respectively. Additionally, a larger proportion who received triple therapy achieved HbA_{1c} below 7% compared with those who received dual therapy.

In another clinical study of 24 weeks' duration, adults with type 2 diabetes mellitus who had inadequate glycemic control on metformin alone (HbA_{1c} 8–12%) received add-on therapy with 10 mg of dapagliflozin and 5 mg of saxagliptin, 10 mg of dapagliflozin, or 5 mg of saxagliptin. After 24 weeks, concomitant therapy with dapagliflozin and saxagliptin resulted in substantial decreases in HbA_{1c}, and a greater proportion of patients receiving this therapy achieved a HbA_{1c} below 7%, compared with those receiving add-on therapy with only dapagliflozin or saxagliptin.

In a clinical study evaluating the efficacy of add-on therapy with saxagliptin in adults (mean age: 54.6 years, 52.7% female, 87.9% Caucasian) with type 2 diabetes mellitus (mean HbA_{1c}: 7.9%) already receiving concomitant dapagliflozin and metformin therapy, the addition of saxagliptin resulted in substantial reductions in HbA_{1c}. The combination of the 3 agents was well tolerated and patients receiving therapy with all 3 agents had a reduction in HbA_{1c} of 0.5% compared with a reduction of 0.2% in patients receiving only dapagliflozin and metformin therapy.

Dosage and Administration

■ Administration When saxagliptin is administered as monotherapy, the drug should be administered orally once daily without regard to meals. If a dose is missed, the missed dose should be taken as soon as it is remembered followed by resumption of the regular schedule. If the missed dose is not remembered until the time of the next dose, the missed dose should be skipped and the regular schedule resumed; the dose should not be doubled to replace a missed dose.

When saxagliptin is administered in fixed combination with dapagliflozin, the combination should be administered orally once daily in the morning with or without food. The fixed-combination tablets containing saxagliptin and dapagliflozin should be swallowed whole and should not be cut, chewed, or crushed. If a dose of the fixed combination is missed, the missed dose should be taken as soon as it is remembered followed by resumption of the regular schedule. If the missed dose is not remembered until it is almost time for the next dose, the missed dose should be skipped and the regular schedule resumed; the dose should not be doubled to replace a missed dose.

When saxagliptin is administered in fixed combination with *extended-release* metformin hydrochloride, the combination should be administered orally once daily with the evening meal; dosage should be titrated gradually to minimize adverse GI effects of the metformin component. The fixed-combination tablets of saxagliptin and *extended-release* metformin hydrochloride should be swallowed whole and should not be cut, chewed, or crushed. If a dose of the fixed combination of saxagliptin and *extended-release* metformin hydrochloride is missed, the next dose should be taken as prescribed unless a healthcare provider instructs otherwise; an extra dose should not be taken the next day.

■ Dosage Dosage of saxagliptin hydrochloride (anhydrous) is expressed in terms of saxagliptin.

Saxagliptin Monotherapy The recommended dosage of saxagliptin for the management of type 2 diabetes mellitus in adults is 2.5 or 5 mg once daily. In clinical trials, higher dosages (e.g., 10 mg once daily) did not provide additional benefit and are not recommended by the manufacturer.

When saxagliptin is used concomitantly with a potent inhibitor of cytochrome P-450 (CYP) isoenzymes 3A4/5 (e.g., atazanavir, clarithromycin, indinavir, itraconazole, ketoconazole, nefazodone, nelfinavir, ritonavir, saquinavir), dosage of saxagliptin should be limited to 2.5 mg once daily.

Saxagliptin/Dapagliflozin Fixed-combination Therapy In patients *not* already receiving dapagliflozin therapy, the recommended initial dosage of the fixed combination of saxagliptin and dapagliflozin is 5 mg of saxagliptin and 5 mg of dapagliflozin once daily in the morning. In patients who tolerate the initial dosage and require additional glycemic control, the dosage of the fixed combination may be increased to 5 mg of saxagliptin and 10 mg of dapagliflozin once daily in the morning.

The fixed combination of saxagliptin and dapagliflozin should *not* be used in patients receiving concomitant therapy with a potent cytochrome P-450 3A4/5 inhibitor (e.g., atazanavir, clarithromycin, indinavir, itraconazole, ketoconazole, nefazodone, nelfinavir, ritonavir, saquinavir). (See Drug Interactions: Drugs Affecting or Metabolized by Hepatic Microsomal Enzymes.)

Saxagliptin/Extended-release Metformin Hydrochloride Fixed-combination Therapy Dosage of saxagliptin hydrochloride in fixed combination with *extended-release* metformin hydrochloride should be individualized based on the patient's current antidiabetic regimen, clinical response, and tolerability. Any change in therapy should be undertaken with care and appropriate monitoring because changes in glycemic control can occur.

When the fixed-combination preparation containing saxagliptin and *extended-release* metformin hydrochloride is used in patients inadequately controlled on monotherapy with saxagliptin 5 mg daily, the recommended initial dosage is 5 mg of saxagliptin and 500 mg of extended-release metformin hydrochloride once daily; dosage should be increased gradually to reduce adverse GI effects of metformin.

In patients inadequately controlled on monotherapy with saxagliptin 2.5 mg daily, the recommended initial dosage of saxagliptin in fixed combination with *extended-release* metformin hydrochloride is 2.5 mg of saxagliptin and 1 g of extended-release metformin hydrochloride daily. Patients who require 2.5 mg of saxagliptin and who are either metformin naive or require a dose of metformin hydrochloride exceeding 1 g should use the individual components.

When the fixed-combination preparation containing saxagliptin and *extended-release* metformin hydrochloride is used in patients inadequately controlled on monotherapy with *extended-release* metformin hydrochloride, dosage of the fixed combination should provide metformin hydrochloride at the patient's current dosage, or the nearest therapeutically appropriate dosage.

Following a switch from *immediate-release* to *extended-release* metformin, glycemic control should be closely monitored and dosage adjustments made accordingly.

The maximum recommended dosage of saxagliptin in fixed combination with *extended-release* metformin hydrochloride is 5 mg of saxagliptin and 2 g of extended-release metformin hydrochloride daily. When the fixed combination preparation is used concomitantly with a potent CYP3A4/5 inhibitor (e.g., atazanavir, clarithromycin, indinavir, itraconazole, ketoconazole, nefazodone, nelfinavir, ritonavir, saquinavir), dosage of saxagliptin should be limited to 2.5 mg once daily.

■ **Special Populations** ***Hepatic Impairment*** **Saxagliptin Monotherapy.** The manufacturer makes no dosage recommendations for patients with hepatic impairment.

Saxagliptin/Dapagliflozin Fixed-combination Therapy. The manufacturer makes no dosage recommendations for patients with hepatic impairment.

Saxagliptin/Extended-release Metformin Hydrochloride Fixed-combination Therapy. The fixed-combination preparation containing saxagliptin and *extended-release* metformin hydrochloride is *not* recommended in patients with hepatic impairment.

Renal Impairment **Saxagliptin Monotherapy.** Dosage adjustment of saxagliptin is not recommended in patients with an estimated glomerular filtration rate (eGFR) of at least 45 mL/minute per 1.73 m^2.

In patients with an eGFR less than 45 mL/minute per 1.73 m^2 or end-stage renal disease requiring hemodialysis, the recommended dosage of saxagliptin is 2.5 mg once daily. In patients undergoing hemodialysis, saxagliptin should be administered *after* the dialysis procedure. Saxagliptin has not been studied in patients undergoing peritoneal dialysis.

Saxagliptin/Dapagliflozin Fixed-combination Therapy. Dosage adjustment of the fixed combination of saxagliptin and dapagliflozin is not needed in patients with an eGFR of at least 45 mL/minute per 1.73 m^2.

The fixed combination of saxagliptin and dapagliflozin is contraindicated in patients with an eGFR less than 45 mL/minute per 1.73 m^2 or end-stage renal disease and in those receiving hemodialysis.

Saxagliptin/Extended-release Metformin Hydrochloride Fixed-combination Therapy. Initiation of the fixed combination of saxagliptin and *extended-release* metformin hydrochloride is not recommended in patients with an eGFR between 30–45 mL/minute per 1.73 m^2. In patients receiving the fixed combination of saxagliptin and *extended-release* metformin hydrochloride whose eGFR decreases to 30 to less than 45 mL/minute per 1.73 m^2, the risks and benefits of continuing therapy should be assessed and the dosage of the saxagliptin component should be limited to 2.5 mg once daily.

The fixed combination of saxagliptin and *extended-release* metformin hydrochloride is contraindicated in patients with an eGFR less than 30 mL/minute per 1.73 m^2.

Geriatric Patients **Saxagliptin Monotherapy.** Dosage adjustment of saxagliptin is not recommended in geriatric patients based solely on age; however, because of the greater frequency of decreased renal function in geriatric patients, dosage in geriatric patients should be selected with caution.

Cautions

■ **Contraindications** Saxagliptin is contraindicated in patients with known serious hypersensitivity (e.g., anaphylaxis, angioedema, exfoliative skin reaction) to saxagliptin or any ingredient in the formulation.

■ **Warnings/Precautions** ***Pancreatitis and Pancreatic Precancerous Changes*** Acute pancreatitis has been reported during postmarketing experience in patients receiving saxagliptin therapy. In a randomized, double-blind study (SAVOR) in 16,492 patients with type 2 diabetes mellitus and established atherosclerotic cardiovascular disease or at high risk for the disease, acute pancreatitis was confirmed in 0.2 or 0.1% of patients receiving saxagliptin or placebo, respectively, in addition to standard care. Preexisting risk factors for pancreatitis were present in 88% of patients who developed pancreatitis while receiving saxagliptin and in 100% of those who developed pancreatitis while receiving placebo. FDA has been evaluating unpublished findings suggesting an increased risk of pancreatitis and precancerous pancreatic cell changes (pancreatic duct metaplasia) in patients with type 2 diabetes mellitus receiving incretin mimetics (exenatide, liraglutide, sitagliptin, saxagliptin, alogliptin, or linagliptin). These findings are based on examination of a small number of pancreatic tissue specimens taken from patients who died from unspecified causes while receiving an incretin mimetic.

FDA has recommended that clinicians continue to follow the recommendations in the prescribing information for incretin mimetics. The manufacturer states that patients receiving saxagliptin-containing therapy should be monitored for manifestations of pancreatitis. (See Advice to Patients.) If pancreatitis is suspected, saxagliptin should be promptly discontinued and appropriate management instituted. Safety and efficacy of saxagliptin have not been established in patients with a history of pancreatitis and it is not known whether such patients are at increased risk for pancreatitis with saxagliptin therapy.

Severe Arthralgia Severe, disabling joint pain has been reported during postmarketing experience in patients receiving dipeptidyl peptidase-4 (DPP-4) inhibitors (e.g., alogliptin, linagliptin, saxagliptin, sitagliptin). Onset of such symptoms has ranged from 1 day to years following initiation of therapy. Fever, chills, rash, and swelling accompanied joint pain in some patients, suggesting an immunologic reaction; some patients have required hospitalization. Symptoms resolved upon discontinuance of the DPP-4 inhibitor, usually in less than a month. In some patients, symptoms recurred when the same or another DPP-4 inhibitor was restarted. DPP-4 inhibitors should be considered as a possible cause of severe joint pain and should be discontinued if appropriate. (See Advice to Patients.)

Concomitant Therapy with Hypoglycemic Agents When saxagliptin is added to therapy with an insulin secretagogue (e.g., a sulfonylurea) or insulin, the incidence of hypoglycemia is increased compared with sulfonylurea or insulin monotherapy. Therefore, patients receiving saxagliptin may require a reduced dosage of a concomitant insulin secretagogue (e.g., a sulfonylurea) or insulin to reduce the risk of hypoglycemia.

Reduction in Lymphocyte Count Dose-related mean decreases in absolute lymphocyte count have been reported with saxagliptin dosages of 5 and 10 mg daily in clinical trials; clinical importance is not known. In most patients, recurrence of this effect was not observed with repeated exposure; however, some patients had reductions in lymphocyte count upon rechallenge that led to discontinuance of saxagliptin. Reductions in lymphocyte count were not associated with clinically relevant adverse effects. When clinically indicated (i.e., settings of unusual or prolonged infection), lymphocyte count should be measured.

Dermatologic and Sensitivity Reactions In a pooled analysis of data from 5 studies, hypersensitivity reactions (e.g., urticaria, facial edema) were reported in 1.5% of patients receiving saxagliptin 2.5 or 5 mg daily. In addition, there have been postmarketing reports of serious allergic and hypersensitivity reactions (e.g., anaphylaxis, angioedema, exfoliative skin conditions). The onset of such reactions usually was within the first 3 months following treatment initiation; some reactions occurred after the first dose. (See Cautions: Contraindications.)

If a serious hypersensitivity reaction is suspected, saxagliptin should be promptly discontinued, other potential causes of the event should be investigated, appropriate treatment for the reaction should be provided, and alternative antidiabetic therapy should be instituted. (See Advice to Patients.) Saxagliptin should be used with caution in patients with a history of angioedema to other DPP-4 inhibitors because it is unknown whether such patients will be predisposed to angioedema with saxagliptin.

Postmarketing cases of bullous pemphigoid requiring hospitalization have been reported with DPP-4 inhibitor use. These cases usually resolved after discontinuation of the DPP-4 inhibitor and treatment with topical or systemic immunosuppressive therapy. Patients should be advised to report the development of blisters or erosions while receiving saxagliptin. If bullous pemphigoid is suspected, the drug should be discontinued and referral to a dermatologist should be considered for diagnosis and appropriate treatment.

Cardiovascular Effects **Macrovascular Outcomes.** In a pooled analysis of 8 randomized, phase 2 or 3 clinical trials (total of 4607 patients) designed to evaluate the relative risk of cardiovascular events (cardiovascular death, myocardial infarction, stroke) in patients receiving saxagliptin versus other antidiabetic agents (metformin, glyburide) or placebo, no increased cardiovascular risk was noted with saxagliptin therapy. The manufacturer states that evidence of macrovascular risk reduction with saxagliptin, the fixed combination of saxagliptin and dapagliflozin, or the fixed combination of saxagliptin and extended-release metformin hydrochloride has not been conclusively demonstrated in clinical trials.

Heart Failure Risk. Saxagliptin may increase the risk of heart failure, particularly in patients who have a history of heart failure or renal impairment. In a randomized, double-blind study (SAVOR) in which saxagliptin or placebo was added to standard care in 16,492 patients with type 2 diabetes mellitus and established atherosclerotic cardiovascular disease or at high risk for the disease, more patients receiving saxagliptin were hospitalized for heart failure than patients receiving placebo (3.5 or 2.8%, respectively). After a median of 2 years of follow-up, treatment with saxagliptin was associated with a 27% increased risk of hospitalization for heart failure; however, therapy with the drug was not associated with increased or decreased rates of cardiovascular death or other ischemic events. Patients with a history of heart failure or renal impairment had a higher risk of hospitalization for heart failure in this study regardless of treatment (saxagliptin or placebo).

The potential risks and benefits of saxagliptin therapy should be considered prior to use in patients at higher risk for heart failure. Patients receiving saxagliptin-containing therapy should be monitored for manifestations of heart failure. (See Advice to Patients.) If heart failure develops, appropriate evaluation and management should be instituted and consideration given to discontinuing saxagliptin.

Use of Fixed Combinations When saxagliptin is used in fixed combination with metformin hydrochloride, dapagliflozin, or other drugs, the cautions, precautions, and contraindications associated with the concomitant agent(s) should be considered.

Specific Populations **Pregnancy.** Data on use of saxagliptin in pregnant women are not sufficient to determine a drug-associated risk for major birth defects or miscarriage.

In animal studies, no adverse developmental effects were observed when saxagliptin was administered to pregnant rats and rabbits during organogenesis (at exposures 1503 and 152 times the human 5-mg dose, respectively) or in pregnant or lactating rats (at exposures up to 470 times the human 5-mg dose) during the prenatal and postnatal period.

Lactation. Saxagliptin is distributed into milk in rats at a milk-to-plasma ratio of approximately 1:1; it is not known whether saxagliptin is distributed into human milk. The benefits of breast-feeding and the importance of saxagliptin to the woman should be considered along with any potential adverse effects on the breast-fed infant from the drug or from the underlying maternal condition.

Pediatric Use. Safety and efficacy of saxagliptin alone or in fixed combination with dapagliflozin or *extended-release* metformin hydrochloride have not been established in patients younger than 18 years of age.

Geriatric Use. No substantial differences in safety and efficacy of saxagliptin relative to younger adults have been observed, but increased sensitivity cannot be ruled out.

Saxagliptin and its active metabolite are eliminated in part by the kidneys; renal function should be assessed periodically since geriatric patients are more likely to have decreased renal function.

Hepatic Impairment. In patients with hepatic impairment (Child-Pugh class A, B, and C), mean peak concentrations and area under the plasma concentration-time curve (AUC) of saxagliptin were increased by up to 8 and 77%, respectively, compared with healthy individuals following a single 10-mg dose of the drug; peak concentrations and AUC of the active metabolite were increased by up to 59 and 33%, respectively. These differences were not considered clinically important.

The fixed combination of saxagliptin and dapagliflozin may be used in patients with hepatic impairment. However, safety and efficacy have not been studied in patients with severe hepatic impairment and the benefits and risks of the fixed combination in such patients should be considered.

Use of the fixed combination of saxagliptin and *extended-release* metformin hydrochloride is not recommended in patients with hepatic impairment.

Renal Impairment. In patients with mild, moderate, or severe renal impairment (including those with end-stage renal disease on hemodialysis), peak concentrations of saxagliptin and its active metabolite were not affected following a single 10-mg dose of the drug. In patients with moderate or severe renal impairment (including those with end-stage renal disease on hemodialysis), the AUC of saxagliptin and its active metabolite were increased by more than twofold, respectively, compared with individuals with normal renal function. No dosage adjustment of saxagliptin is recommended in patients with an estimated glomerular filtration rate (eGFR) of at least 45 mL/minute per 1.73 m^2. However, dosage adjustment of saxagliptin is recommended when the drug is used in patients with an eGFR less than 45 mL/minute per 1.73 m^2 or end-stage renal disease requiring hemodialysis. (See Renal Impairment under Dosage and Administration: Special Populations.) Renal function should be assessed prior to initiation of therapy and periodically thereafter. Saxagliptin is removed by hemodialysis.

The fixed combination of saxagliptin and dapagliflozin is contraindicated in patients with an eGFR less than 45 mL/minute per 1.73 m^2.

Initiation of the fixed combination of saxagliptin and *extended-release* metformin hydrochloride is not recommended in patients with an eGFR between 30–45 mL/minute per 1.73 m^2 and is contraindicated in patients with an eGFR less than 30 mL/minute per 1.73 m^2. A reduced dosage of the saxagliptin component is recommended for patients taking the fixed combination of saxagliptin and extended-release metformin hydrochloride whose eGFR later decreases below 45 mL/minute per 1.73 m^2 during therapy. (See Renal Impairment under Dosage and Administration: Special Populations.)

■ **Common Adverse Effects** In clinical trials, the incidence of hypoglycemic adverse reactions in patients receiving saxagliptin was based on all reports of hypoglycemia, although a concurrent glucose measurement was not required or was normal in some patients with reported hypoglycemic reactions; therefore, it is not possible to determine conclusively whether all these reports represent true hypoglycemic events. In the clinical trial in which saxagliptin or placebo was added to insulin therapy (with or without metformin), (see Uses: Diabetes Mellitus) the incidence of adverse effects (except for confirmed hypoglycemia) was similar with add-on saxagliptin and add-on placebo. However, the incidence of confirmed hypoglycemia (as determined by fingerstick blood glucose of 50 mg/dL or less) in this trial was higher with saxagliptin 5 mg daily (5.3%) than with placebo (3.3%).

Adverse effects reported in at least 5% of patients in clinical trials receiving saxagliptin 5 mg daily as monotherapy or in combination with metformin, a thiazolidinedione (pioglitazone or rosiglitazone), or glyburide and more frequently than with placebo include upper respiratory tract infection, urinary tract infection, and headache.

Adverse effects reported in at least 2% of patients receiving saxagliptin in combination with dapagliflozin and metformin hydrochloride include upper respiratory tract infection, urinary tract infection, dyslipidemia, headache, diarrhea, back pain, genital infection, and arthralgia.

Adverse effects reported in at least 5% of patients in clinical trials receiving saxagliptin in combination with immediate-release metformin and more frequently than with metformin alone include headache and nasopharyngitis.

Drug Interactions

■ **Drugs Affecting or Metabolized by Hepatic Microsomal Enzymes** Saxagliptin and its active metabolite do not inhibit cytochrome P-450 (CYP) isoenzymes 1A2, 2A6, 2B6, 2C9, 2C19, 2D6, 2E1, or 3A4 and do not induce CYP1A2, 2B6, 2C9, or 3A4 in vitro. Pharmacokinetic interactions with drugs metabolized by these isoenzymes are unlikely.

Saxagliptin is metabolized principally via CYP3A4 and CYP3A5. Administration of a single dose of saxagliptin (100 mg) to healthy individuals receiving ketoconazole (200 mg every 12 hours for 9 days) decreased the peak steady-state plasma concentration and area under the plasma concentration-time curve (AUC) of ketoconazole by 16 and 13%, respectively, and increased the peak plasma concentration and AUC of saxagliptin by 62 and 145% (2.5-fold), respectively. Similar increases in saxagliptin plasma concentrations and AUC are anticipated with concomitant use of saxagliptin and other potent CYP3A4/5 inhibitors (e.g. atazanavir, clarithromycin, indinavir, itraconazole, nefazodone, nelfinavir, ritonavir, saquinavir). Saxagliptin dosage should be limited to 2.5 mg daily when the drug is used concomitantly with a potent CYP3A4/5 inhibitor. The fixed combination of saxagliptin and dapagliflozin should not be used in patients receiving a potent CYP3A4/5 inhibitor.

■ **Inhibitors of P-glycoprotein Transport System** Saxagliptin is a substrate of the P-glycoprotein transport system but does not appreciably induce or inhibit P-glycoprotein.

■ **Antacids** Concurrent administration of a single dose of saxagliptin (10 mg) and a single dose of liquid antacid containing aluminum hydroxide (2.4 g), magnesium hydroxide (2.4 g), and simethicone (240 mg) decreased peak plasma concentrations of saxagliptin by 26% and AUC by 3%. The manufacturer states that no dosage adjustments are required with concurrent use.

■ **Dapagliflozin** Concurrent administration of saxagliptin (5-mg single dose) and dapagliflozin (10-mg single dose) decreased the peak plasma concentration of saxagliptin by 7% and the AUC by 1%. The manufacturer states that no dosage adjustments are required with concurrent use.

■ **Digoxin** Concurrent administration of saxagliptin (10 mg once daily for 7 days) and digoxin (0.25 mg every 6 hours the first day, then 0.25 mg every 12 hours the second day, then 0.25 mg once daily for 5 days), a P-glycoprotein substrate, increased the AUC and peak plasma concentration of digoxin by 6 and 9%, respectively; the AUC of saxagliptin was increased by 5% and peak plasma saxagliptin concentrations decreased by 1%. The manufacturer states that no dosage adjustments are required with concurrent use.

■ **Diltiazem** Concurrent administration of saxagliptin (10-mg single dose) and a long-acting formulation of diltiazem (360 mg daily for 9 days) increased the peak steady-state plasma concentration of diltiazem by 16% and the AUC by 10%; in addition, peak plasma saxagliptin concentrations increased by 63% and saxagliptin AUC was increased by 2.1-fold. The manufacturer states that no dosage adjustments are required with concurrent use.

■ **Famotidine** Administration of a single dose of saxagliptin (10 mg) concurrently with a single dose of famotidine (40 mg) increased the peak plasma concentration of saxagliptin by 14% and AUC by 3%. The manufacturer states that no dosage adjustments are required with concurrent use.

■ **Hormonal Contraceptives** Concurrent administration of saxagliptin (5 mg once daily for 21 days) and an estrogen-progestin combination contraceptive (ethinyl estradiol 35 mcg in fixed combination with norgestimate 0.25 mg once daily for 21 days) did not appreciably alter the steady-state pharmacokinetics of ethinyl estradiol or the primary active progestin component, norelgestromin. The mean AUC and peak plasma concentration of norgestrel, an active metabolite of norelgestromin, were increased by 13 and 17%, respectively, which is not considered clinically important. The manufacturer states that no dosage adjustments are required with concurrent use.

■ **Metformin** Concomitant administration of a single dose of saxagliptin (100 mg) and metformin hydrochloride (1 g) decreased the peak plasma concentration of saxagliptin by 21% and the AUC by 2%; metformin AUC and peak plasma concentration were increased by 20 and 9%, respectively. The manufacturer states that no dosage adjustments are required with concurrent use.

■ **Omeprazole** Concurrent administration of saxagliptin (10 mg daily) and omeprazole (40 mg daily for 5 days) increased saxagliptin AUC by 13%

and decreased peak plasma concentrations of the drug by 2%. The manufacturer states that no dosage adjustments are required with concurrent use.

■ **Pioglitazone** Concurrent administration of saxagliptin (10 mg once daily for 5 days) and pioglitazone (45 mg daily for 10 days) increased the peak plasma concentration of pioglitazone by 14% and the AUC by 8%. In addition, the AUC and peak plasma concentration of saxagliptin were each increased by 11%. The manufacturer states that no dosage adjustments are required with concurrent use.

■ **Rifampin** Concomitant administration of a single dose of saxagliptin (5 mg) with rifampin (600 mg daily for 6 days) decreased peak steady-state plasma concentrations and AUC of saxagliptin by 53 and 76%, respectively, while peak plasma concentration of the active metabolite was increased by 39%; there was no appreciable change in the AUC of the active metabolite of saxagliptin. The manufacturer states that no dosage adjustments are required with concurrent use.

■ **Simvastatin** Concomitant administration of saxagliptin (10 mg once daily for 4 days) and simvastatin (40 mg once daily for 8 days) increased the peak plasma concentration and AUC of saxagliptin by 21 and 12%, respectively, while simvastatin peak plasma concentrations were reduced by 12% and AUC was increased by 4%. The manufacturer states that no dosage adjustments are required with concurrent use.

■ **Sulfonylureas** Concomitant administration of single doses of saxagliptin (10 mg) and glyburide (5 mg) increased peak plasma concentrations of glyburide and saxagliptin by 16 and 8%, respectively; the AUC of glyburide was increased by 6% and that of saxagliptin was decreased by 2%. The manufacturer states that no dosage adjustments are required because of changes in systemic exposures when saxagliptin and glyburide are given concomitantly. However, in patients receiving saxagliptin concomitantly with a sulfonylurea antidiabetic agent, a reduced dosage of the sulfonylurea may be required to reduce the risk of hypoglycemia.

Description

Saxagliptin inhibits dipeptidyl peptidase-4 (DPP-4), an enzyme that inactivates incretin hormones glucagon-like peptide-1 (GLP-1) and glucose-dependent insulinotropic polypeptide (GIP). Both saxagliptin and its active metabolite (5-hydroxy saxagliptin) are more selective for inhibition of DPP-4 than for DPP-8 or DPP-9. Saxagliptin increases circulating levels of GLP-1 and GIP in a glucose-dependent manner.

GLP-1 and GIP stimulate insulin secretion from pancreatic β-cells in a glucose-dependent manner (i.e., when glucose concentrations are normal or elevated). GLP-1 also decreases glucagon secretion from pancreatic α-cells, leading to reduced hepatic glucose production.

Saxagliptin lowers fasting plasma glucose concentrations and reduces glucose excursions following a glucose load or meal in patients with type 2 diabetes mellitus.

Saxagliptin monotherapy usually is not associated with substantial changes in body weight.

Saxagliptin did not produce a clinically meaningful prolongation of the QT interval corrected for rate (QT_c) or heart rate at daily dosages up to 40 mg (8 times the maximum recommended human dose) in a randomized, double-blind, placebo-controlled, crossover active-comparator study using moxifloxacin in healthy individuals.

Following oral administration of a single dose of saxagliptin under fasted conditions, the median time to peak plasma concentration was 2 hours for saxagliptin and 4 hours for 5-hydroxy saxagliptin. Administration of saxagliptin with a high-fat meal increased the area under the plasma concentration-time curve (AUC) by 27% and delayed the time to peak plasma concentration by approximately 20 minutes. In vitro binding of saxagliptin and 5-hydroxy saxagliptin to serum proteins is negligible.

Metabolism of saxagliptin is principally mediated by cytochrome P-450 (CYP) 3A4 and 3A5 isoenzymes. Mean plasma half-life of saxagliptin or 5-hydroxy saxagliptin is 2.5 or 3.1 hours, respectively. Saxagliptin is eliminated by both renal and hepatic pathways; following administration of a single radiolabeled dose, 75% of the dose was excreted in urine (including 24% as unchanged drug and 36% as 5-hydroxy saxagliptin). A total of 22% of administered radioactivity was recovered in feces, representing the fraction of the saxagliptin dose excreted in bile and/or unabsorbed drug from the GI tract.

Bioequivalence between the fixed combination of saxagliptin and extended-release metformin hydrochloride (Kombiglyze® XR) and each agent (saxagliptin and *extended-release* metformin hydrochloride) given concurrently as separate tablets has been demonstrated; however, the relative bioavailability of the fixed combination of saxagliptin and extended-release metformin hydrochloride (Kombiglyze® XR) and concomitantly administered saxagliptin and *immediate-release* metformin hydrochloride has not been established. Metformin hydrochloride immediate-release and extended-release tablets have a similar extent of absorption (AUC), but peak plasma concentrations of metformin following administration of the drug as extended-release tablets are approximately 20% lower than peak concentrations following administration of the same dose as immediate-release tablets.

Advice to Patients

When saxagliptin is used in fixed combination with other drugs, importance of informing patients of important cautionary information about the concomitant agent(s).

Importance of patients reading medication guide before initiating therapy and each time the drug is dispensed.

Importance of informing patients of the potential risks and benefits of saxagliptin and of alternative therapies. Importance of not using saxagliptin in patients with type 1 diabetes mellitus or diabetic ketoacidosis.

Importance of informing patients about possibility of acute pancreatitis, which may be severe or fatal, with saxagliptin therapy. Importance of patients informing clinicians about a history of pancreatitis, gallstones, alcoholism, or high triglyceride levels. Importance of informing patients about signs and symptoms of pancreatitis, including persistent severe abdominal pain sometimes radiating to the back that may or may not be accompanied by vomiting; importance of patient discontinuing saxagliptin and promptly notifying clinician if such signs or symptoms are present.

Importance of informing patients of the possibility of severe and disabling joint pain with dipeptidyl peptidase-4 (DPP-4) inhibitors (e.g., alogliptin, linagliptin, saxagliptin, sitagliptin). Advise patients to contact a clinician promptly if severe and persistent joint pain occurs; patients should not discontinue the drug without consulting their clinician.

Importance of informing patients about possibility of heart failure with saxagliptin therapy. Importance of patients informing clinicians about a history of heart failure or renal impairment. Importance of informing patients about signs and symptoms of heart failure (e.g., shortness of breath, weight gain, edema); importance of patients immediately contacting a clinician if manifestations of heart failure occur.

Importance of informing clinician if hypoglycemia occurs, particularly if concomitant therapy with a sulfonylurea antidiabetic agent (i.e., insulin secretagogue) or insulin is used; a lower dosage of the sulfonylurea or insulin may be required in such cases.

Importance of informing patients about the importance of adherence to dietary instructions, regular physical activity, periodic blood glucose monitoring and glycosylated hemoglobin (hemoglobin A_{1c}; HbA_{1c}) testing, recognition and management of hypoglycemia and hyperglycemia, and assessment of diabetes complications.

Importance of seeking medical advice promptly during periods of stress such as fever, trauma, infection, or surgery as medication requirements may change.

Importance of informing patients that response to all diabetic therapies should be monitored by periodic measurements of blood glucose and HbA_{1c}, with a goal of decreasing these levels toward the normal range.

Importance of informing patients of the potential need to adjust their dosage based on changes in renal function over time.

Importance of informing their clinician if any unusual symptom develops or if any existing symptom persists or worsens.

Risk of serious allergic (hypersensitivity) reactions, such as angioedema, anaphylaxis, and exfoliative skin conditions. If signs or symptoms of such reactions occur (e.g., rash, skin flaking or peeling, hives, swelling of the skin, swelling of the face, lips, tongue, and throat that may cause difficulty in breathing or swallowing), importance of discontinuing saxagliptin-containing therapy and informing clinician promptly.

Importance of informing patients that bullous pemphigoid may occur with the use of a DPP-4 inhibitor. Advise patients to contact a clinician if blisters or erosions occur.

Importance of advising patient not to split, chew, or crush tablets of saxagliptin or the fixed combination of saxagliptin and dapagliflozin. Importance of swallowing tablets of the fixed-combination preparation of saxagliptin and extended-release metformin hydrochloride whole and not cutting, crushing, or chewing them. Importance of advising patients receiving the fixed-combination preparation of saxagliptin and extended-release metformin hydrochloride that occasionally the inactive components of the tablet may remain intact and be passed in the stool as a soft, hydrated mass resembling the original tablet.

Importance of taking saxagliptin exactly as directed by clinician. Importance of informing patients that if they miss a dose of saxagliptin or the fixed combination of saxagliptin and dapagliflozin, they should take the dose as soon as it is remembered unless it is almost time for the next dose. In that case, the missed dose should be skipped and the next dose taken at the regular time; patients should not take 2 doses at the same time unless instructed to do so by their clinician. Importance of informing patients that if they miss a dose of the fixed combination of saxagliptin and extended-release metformin hydrochloride, they should take the next dose as prescribed unless otherwise instructed by their clinician; patients should be instructed not to take an extra dose the next day.

Importance of women informing their clinicians if they are or plan to become pregnant or plan to breast-feed.

Importance of informing clinicians of existing or contemplated concomitant therapy, including prescription (e.g., antibiotics, antifungals, antiretrovirals) and OTC drugs and dietary or herbal supplements, as well as any concomitant illnesses (e.g., allergies, kidney disease).

Importance of informing patients of other important precautionary information. (See Cautions.)

Overview® (see Users Guide). For additional information on this drug until a more detailed monograph is developed and published, the manufacturer's labeling should be consulted. It is *essential* that the manufacturer's labeling be consulted for more detailed information on usual cautions, precautions, contraindications, potential drug interactions, laboratory test interferences, and acute toxicity.

Preparations

Excipients in commercially available drug preparations may have clinically important effects in some individuals; consult specific product labeling for details.

sAXagliptin Hydrochloride

Oral		
Tablets, film-coated	2.5 mg (of saxagliptin)	**Onglyza®**, AstraZeneca
	5 mg (of saxagliptin)	**Onglyza®**, AstraZeneca

sAXagliptin Hydrochloride Combinations

Oral		
Tablets, extended-release	2.5 mg (of saxagliptin) with Extended-release Metformin Hydrochloride 1 g	**Kombiglyze XR®**, AstraZeneca
	5 mg (of saxagliptin) with Extended-release Metformin Hydrochloride 500 mg	**Kombiglyze XR®**, AstraZeneca
	5 mg (of saxagliptin) with Extended-release Metformin Hydrochloride 1 g	**Kombiglyze XR®**, AstraZeneca
Tablets, film-coated	5 mg (of saxagliptin) with Dapagliflozin Propranediol 5 mg (of dapagliflozin)	**Qtern®**, AstraZeneca
	5 mg (of saxagliptin) with Dapagliflozin Propranediol 10 mg (of dapagliflozin)	**Qtern®**, AstraZeneca

SITagliptin Phosphate

■ Sitagliptin phosphate, a dipeptidyl peptidase-4 (DPP-4) inhibitor, is an antidiabetic agent.

Uses

■ **Type 2 Diabetes Mellitus** Sitagliptin is used as monotherapy as an adjunct to diet and exercise to improve glycemic control in patients with type 2 diabetes mellitus. Sitagliptin is used in combination with immediate- or extended release metformin hydrochloride given separately or as a fixed combination (Janumet® or Janumet® XR, respectively) as an adjunct to diet and exercise to improve glycemic control in patients with type 2 diabetes mellitus when treatment with both sitagliptin and metformin is appropriate. Sitagliptin also is commercially available in fixed combination with the sodium-glucose cotransporter 2 (SGLT2) inhibitor, ertugliflozin (Steglujan®); the fixed combination is used as an adjunct to diet and exercise to improve glycemic control in patients with type 2 diabetes mellitus when treatment with both drugs is appropriate. Sitagliptin also is used in combination with other oral antidiabetic agents (e.g., metformin, a sulfonylurea, a thiazolidinedione [peroxisome proliferator-activated receptor$_\gamma$ agonist]) or insulin as an adjunct to diet and exercise in patients with type 2 diabetes mellitus who have not achieved adequate glycemic control with one or more oral antidiabetic agents and/or insulin.

While metformin generally is the preferred antidiabetic agent for initial therapy in patients with type 2 diabetes mellitus, the American Association of Clinical Endocrinologists/American College of Endocrinology (AACE/ACE) suggests a dipeptidyl peptidase-4 (DPP-4) inhibitor as one of several alternative antidiabetic agents for initial monotherapy in patients with a contraindication to metformin (e.g., renal disease, hepatic disease, GI intolerance, risk of lactic acidosis). DPP-4 inhibitors also are recommended by AACE/ACE as part of combination therapy, particularly when both postprandial and fasting plasma glucose concentrations are elevated.

Sitagliptin should not be used in patients with type 1 diabetes mellitus or for the treatment of diabetic ketoacidosis.

Sitagliptin Monotherapy Efficacy of sitagliptin as monotherapy for the management of type 2 diabetes mellitus is supported by results of 2 controlled trials of 18 or 24 weeks' duration. Sitagliptin (100 or 200 mg once daily) improved glycemic control, as evidenced by reductions in glycosylated hemoglobin (hemoglobin A_{1c} [HbA_{1c}]) as well as fasting and 2-hour postprandial plasma glucose concentrations, compared with placebo. HbA_{1c} was reduced by 0.5–0.6% (from an average baseline value of about 8%) in patients receiving sitagliptin 100 mg daily, compared with an increase of 0.1–0.2% in those receiving placebo. Overall, use of a higher than recommended dosage of sitagliptin (200 mg daily) did not provide greater glycemic control than did the recommended dosage of 100 mg daily.

Combination Therapy Efficacy of the combination of sitagliptin and metformin as *initial* therapy in patients with type 2 diabetes mellitus inadequately controlled with diet and exercise is supported by results of a 24-week randomized, placebo-controlled trial. In this trial, patients receiving initial therapy with sitagliptin (50 mg twice daily) in combination with metformin hydrochloride (500 mg or 1 g twice daily) had greater improvements in HbA_{1c}, fasting plasma glucose, and 2-hour postprandial glucose concentrations than those receiving placebo, metformin monotherapy, or sitagliptin monotherapy. Mean reductions in HbA_{1c} from baseline in patients not receiving an antihyperglycemic agent at trial entry were 1.1% with sitagliptin 100 mg once daily, 1.1% with metformin hydrochloride 500 mg twice daily, 1.2% with metformin hydrochloride 1 g twice daily, 1.6% with sitagliptin 50 mg twice daily in combination with metformin hydrochloride 500 mg twice daily, 1.9% with sitagliptin 50 mg twice daily in combination with metformin hydrochloride 1 g twice daily, and 0.2% with placebo.

In another 24-week, randomized trial in patients who had inadequate glycemic control with diet and exercise, *initial* therapy with the combination of sitagliptin (100 mg once daily) and pioglitazone (30 mg once daily) produced greater improvements in HbA_{1c}, fasting plasma glucose, and 2-hour postprandial glucose concentrations than pioglitazone monotherapy (30 mg once daily). In this trial, patients receiving the sitagliptin/pioglitazone combination achieved a 0.9% mean reduction in HbA_{1c} compared with those receiving pioglitazone monotherapy, and 60% of patients receiving sitagliptin/pioglitazone achieved a mean HbA_{1c} less than 7%, compared with 28% of those receiving pioglitazone monotherapy.

Efficacy of sitagliptin in combination with metformin, a sulfonylurea, and/or a thiazolidinedione in the management of type 2 diabetes mellitus (in patients inadequately controlled with metformin or thiazolidinedione monotherapy) is supported by results from several long-term (24 weeks' duration), randomized, placebo-controlled trials. In these trials, the addition of sitagliptin (100 mg once daily) to existing metformin and/or glimepiride therapy or to pioglitazone or rosiglitazone/metformin therapy improved glycemic control, as evidenced by reductions in HbA_{1c} as well as fasting and/or 2-hour postprandial plasma glucose concentrations, compared with placebo or existing therapy.

In patients receiving metformin hydrochloride therapy (dosage of at least 1.5 g daily), the addition of sitagliptin resulted in a reduction of 0.7% in HbA_{1c}, while the addition of placebo resulted in no appreciable change in HbA_{1c}. In patients receiving glimepiride therapy (dosage of at least 4 mg daily), the addition of sitagliptin resulted in a reduction of 0.6% in HbA_{1c} compared with addition of placebo. In patients receiving glimepiride (dosage of at least 4 mg daily) in combination with metformin hydrochloride (dosage of at least 1.5 g daily), the addition of sitagliptin resulted in a reduction of 0.9% in HbA_{1c} compared with addition of placebo. In patients receiving pioglitazone therapy (30–45 mg daily), the addition of sitagliptin or placebo resulted in reductions of 0.9 or 0.2%, respectively, in HbA_{1c}.

In patients receiving metformin and rosiglitazone therapy in a 54-week trial, addition of sitagliptin 100 mg once daily or placebo resulted in mean reductions in HbA_{1c} of 1 or 0.3%, respectively; sulfonylurea (e.g., glipizide) rescue therapy was used in 18 or 40% of patients receiving sitagliptin or placebo, respectively. In a 52-week noninferiority trial in patients receiving metformin hydrochloride (dosage of at least 1.5 g daily), add-on therapy with sitagliptin (100 mg once daily) or glipizide (5–20 mg once daily; mean 10 mg once daily) was associated with similar mean reductions from baseline in HbA_{1c} (intent-to-treat analysis); results may be applicable principally to patients with baseline HbA_{1c} values less than 8–9%, comparable to those of this study population.

Efficacy of sitagliptin in combination with insulin (with or without metformin) in the management of type 2 diabetes mellitus in patients who have inadequate glycemic control with insulin is supported by results of a 24-week, randomized, placebo-controlled trial. In this trial, addition of sitagliptin (100 mg once daily) to existing stable insulin (premixed insulin or intermediate- or long-acting insulin) therapy with or without metformin hydrochloride (dosage of at least 1.5 g daily) resulted in improvements in HbA_{1c}, fasting plasma glucose, and 2-hour postprandial glucose concentrations compared with addition of placebo. In patients who received sitagliptin as add-on therapy to metformin and insulin, 14% had HbA_{1c} reductions to less than 7% compared with 5% of those receiving add-on placebo with metformin and insulin. Among patients also receiving metformin, the median daily dosage of insulin at baseline for patients treated with sitagliptin or placebo was 40 or 42 units, respectively; the median daily insulin dosage for both groups at the end of the study was unchanged. Hypoglycemia was more common in patients receiving add-on sitagliptin therapy.

Efficacy and safety of the fixed combinations of sitagliptin and immediate- or extended-release metformin hydrochloride have been established based on concurrent administration of the 2 agents given separately and extrapolations from clinical trials evaluating sitagliptin as add-on therapy to metformin. Bioequivalence has been demonstrated between the fixed combination of sitagliptin and metformin hydrochloride and the drugs administered concurrently as separate tablets.

Efficacy and safety of the combination of sitagliptin and ertugliflozin (as initial therapy or as add-on therapy) for the management of type 2 diabetes mellitus has been established in 3 randomized, placebo- and active comparator trials. In a trial in adults with type 2 diabetes mellitus inadequately controlled with metformin hydrochloride monotherapy (dosage of at least 1.5 g daily for at least 8 weeks), the addition of ertugliflozin and sitagliptin combination therapy substantially improved glycemic control compared with the addition of either ertugliflozin or sitagliptin alone. In this trial, patients received ertugliflozin 5 mg, ertugliflozin 15 mg, sitagliptin 100 mg, ertugliflozin 5 mg and sitagliptin 100 mg, or ertugliflozin 15 mg and sitagliptin 100 mg, once daily. At week 26, patients who received concomitant therapy with ertugliflozin 5 or 15 mg and sitagliptin 100 mg had greater reductions in HbA_{1c} (reduction of 1.4%), compared with ertugliflozin or sitagliptin alone (reduction of 1%). Additionally, a higher proportion of patients who received concomitant therapy with ertugliflozin 5 or 15 mg and sitagliptin 100 mg as an add-on to existing metformin therapy achieved an HbA_{1c} of less than 7% (53 or 51%, respectively) than those who received ertugliflozin 5 or 15 mg or sitagliptin 100 mg alone (29, 34, or 39%, respectively).

In a 26-week trial in patients receiving metformin hydrochloride (dosage of at least 1.5 g daily for at least 8 weeks) and sitagliptin (100 mg once daily), the addition of ertugliflozin 5 or 15 mg once daily resulted in a reduction in HbA_{1c} of 0.7 or 0.8%, respectively, compared with a 0.2% reduction in HbA_{1c} with placebo. In patients who received ertugliflozin 5 or 15 mg, approximately 35 or 42%, respectively, had HbA_{1c} reductions to less than 7%, compared with approximately 20% of patients receiving placebo. Patients receiving ertugliflozin 5 or 15 mg once daily also had greater reductions in fasting plasma glucose, body weight, and systolic blood pressure than those receiving placebo.

In another trial, concomitant therapy with ertugliflozin (5 or 15 mg once daily) and sitagliptin (100 mg daily) as initial therapy in patients with type 2 diabetes mellitus inadequately controlled with diet and exercise substantially improved glycemic control (as evidenced by reductions in HbA_{1c}) compared with placebo. Reductions in HbA_{1c} were 1.6 or 1.5% with ertugliflozin 5 or 15 mg once daily, respectively, plus sitagliptin and 0.6% with placebo. Additionally, a greater percentage of patients achieved an HbA_{1c} of less than 7% and greater reductions in fasting plasma glucose with ertugliflozin and sitagliptin combination therapy compared with placebo.

Dosage and Administration

■ **Administration** When sitagliptin is administered as monotherapy, the drug should be administered orally once daily with or without food. If a dose is missed, the missed dose should be taken as soon as it is remembered followed by resumption of the regular schedule. If the missed dose is remembered at the time of the next dose, the missed dose should be skipped and the regular schedule resumed. The dose should not be doubled to replace a missed dose.

The fixed combination of sitagliptin and ertugliflozin should be administered orally once daily in the morning, with or without food. If a dose is missed, the missed dose should be taken as soon as it is remembered followed by resumption of the regular schedule. If the missed dose is not remembered until it is almost time for the next dose, the missed dose should be skipped and the regular schedule resumed; the dose should not be doubled to replace a missed dose.

The fixed combination of sitagliptin and immediate-release metformin hydrochloride should be administered orally twice daily with meals. The fixed combination of sitagliptin and extended-release metformin hydrochloride should be administered orally once daily with a meal, preferably with the evening meal. The dosage of the fixed combination should be increased gradually to minimize the adverse GI effects of the metformin component. If a dose is missed, the missed dose should be taken with a meal as soon as it is remembered followed by resumption of the regular schedule. If a missed dose is remembered at the time of the next dose, the missed dose should be skipped and the regular schedule resumed. The dose should not be doubled to replace a missed dose.

■ **Dosage** Sitagliptin phosphate is commercially available as the monohydrate; dosage is expressed in terms of sitagliptin.

Sitagliptin Monotherapy The recommended dosage of sitagliptin for the management of type 2 diabetes mellitus in adults is 100 mg once daily. In clinical trials, higher dosages (200 mg daily) did not provide additional glycemic benefit.

Sitagliptin/Ertugliflozin Fixed-combination Therapy The recommended initial dosage of the fixed combination of sitagliptin and ertugliflozin is 100 mg of sitagliptin and 5 mg of ertugliflozin once daily in the morning without regard to meals. If tolerated, the dosage may be increased to a maximum dosage of 100 mg of sitagliptin and 15 mg of ertugliflozin in patients who require additional glycemic control. In patients currently receiving ertugliflozin and switching to the fixed combination of sitagliptin and ertugliflozin, the current dosage of ertugliflozin can be maintained. Volume depletion should be corrected before initiating therapy with the fixed combination of sitagliptin and ertugliflozin.

Sitagliptin/Immediate-release Metformin Hydrochloride Fixed-combination Therapy Dosage of the fixed combinations of sitagliptin and *immediate-release* metformin hydrochloride (Janumet®) should be individualized based on the patient's current antidiabetic regimen, effectiveness, and tolerability.

In patients *not* currently receiving metformin hydrochloride, the recommended initial dosage of the fixed combination of sitagliptin and *immediate-release* metformin hydrochloride is 50 mg of sitagliptin and 500 mg of immediate-release metformin hydrochloride twice daily. Dosage should be increased gradually to reduce adverse GI effects associated with the metformin hydrochloride component.

In patients currently receiving metformin hydrochloride, the recommended initial dosage of the fixed combination of sitagliptin and *immediate-release* metformin hydrochloride is 50 mg of sitagliptin and 500 mg of immediate-release metformin hydrochloride twice daily or 50 mg of sitagliptin and 1 g of immediate-release metformin hydrochloride twice daily, depending on the patient's existing dosage of metformin hydrochloride.

In patients currently receiving *immediate-release* metformin hydrochloride 850 mg twice daily, the recommended initial dosage of the fixed combination of sitagliptin and *immediate-release* metformin hydrochloride is 50 mg of sitagliptin and 1 g of immediate-release metformin hydrochloride twice daily.

The maximum recommended daily dosage of the fixed combinations containing sitagliptin and *immediate-release* metformin hydrochloride is 100 mg of sitagliptin and 2 g of metformin hydrochloride.

The same total daily dosage of sitagliptin and metformin hydrochloride should be maintained when transitioning between the fixed combination of sitagliptin and *immediate-release* metformin hydrochloride and the fixed combination of sitagliptin and *extended-release* metformin hydrochloride.

Efficacy and safety of switching therapy from oral antidiabetic agents other than sitagliptin or metformin hydrochloride specifically to the fixed combination of sitagliptin and immediate-release metformin hydrochloride have not been established.

Sitagliptin/Extended-release Metformin Hydrochloride Fixed-combination Therapy Dosage of the fixed combinations of sitagliptin and *extended-release* metformin hydrochloride (Janumet® XR) should be individualized based on the patient's current antidiabetic regimen, effectiveness, and tolerability.

In patients *not* currently receiving metformin hydrochloride, the recommended initial dosage of the fixed combination of sitagliptin and *extended-release* metformin hydrochloride is 100 mg of sitagliptin and 1 g of extended-release metformin hydrochloride once daily. Dosage should be increased gradually to reduce adverse GI effects associated with the metformin hydrochloride component.

In patients currently receiving metformin hydrochloride, the recommended initial dosage of the fixed combination of sitagliptin and *extended release* metformin hydrochloride is 100 mg of sitagliptin and 1 g of extended-release metformin hydrochloride once daily or 100 mg of sitagliptin and 2 g of extended-release metformin hydrochloride once daily, depending on the patient's existing dosage of metformin hydrochloride.

In patients currently receiving *immediate-release* metformin hydrochloride 850 mg or 1 g twice daily, the recommended initial dosage of the fixed combination of sitagliptin and *extended-release* metformin hydrochloride is 100 mg of sitagliptin and 2 g of extended-release metformin hydrochloride.

The same total daily dosage of sitagliptin and metformin hydrochloride should be maintained when transitioning between the fixed combination of sitagliptin and *immediate-release* metformin hydrochloride and the fixed combination of sitagliptin and *extended-release* metformin hydrochloride.

The maximum recommended daily dosage of the fixed combinations containing sitagliptin and *extended-release* metformin hydrochloride is 100 mg of sitagliptin and 2 g of metformin hydrochloride.

Efficacy and safety of switching therapy from oral antidiabetic agents other than sitagliptin or metformin hydrochloride specifically to the fixed combination of sitagliptin and extended-release metformin hydrochloride have not been established.

Combination Therapy with Sitagliptin and Other Oral Antidiabetic Agents or Insulin Given as Separate Components When given in combination with metformin hydrochloride as separate tablets, a sitagliptin dosage of 100 mg once daily has been used.

When given as separate tablets in combination with a sulfonylurea with or without metformin hydrochloride, a sitagliptin dosage of 100 mg once daily has been used. Dosage of the concomitant sulfonylurea may need to be reduced to decrease risk of hypoglycemia. For additional details, see Uses: Diabetes Mellitus.

When given as separate tablets in combination with a thiazolidinedione antidiabetic agent (e.g., pioglitazone, rosiglitazone) with or without metformin hydrochloride, a sitagliptin dosage of 100 mg once daily has been used. For additional details, see Uses: Diabetes Mellitus.

When given in combination with insulin with or without metformin hydrochloride, a sitagliptin dosage of 100 mg once daily has been used. Dosage of concomitant insulin may need to be reduced to decrease risk of hypoglycemia.

■ **Special Populations** ***Hepatic Impairment*** **Sitagliptin Monotherapy.** Dosage adjustment of sitagliptin is not necessary in patients with mild to moderate hepatic impairment (Child-Pugh score 9 or less). Efficacy and safety of sitagliptin have not been established in patients with severe hepatic impairment (Child-Pugh score greater than 9).

Sitagliptin/Ertugliflozin Fixed-combination Therapy. Dosage adjustment of the fixed combination of sitagliptin and ertugliflozin is not necessary in patients with mild to moderate hepatic impairment (Child-Pugh score 9 or less). Efficacy and safety of the fixed combination have not been established in patients with severe hepatic impairment (Child-Pugh score greater than 9).

Sitagliptin/Immediate- or Extended-release Metformin Hydrochloride Fixed-combination Therapy. The fixed combinations of sitagliptin and immediate- or extended-release metformin hydrochloride are not recommended in patients with hepatic impairment.

Renal Impairment **Sitagliptin Monotherapy.** Dosage adjustment of sitagliptin is not necessary in patients with an estimated glomerular filtration rate (eGFR) of at least 45 mL/minute per 1.73 m².

Dosage adjustment of sitagliptin is recommended in patients with an eGFR of less than 45 mL/minute per 1.73 m² or end-stage renal disease requiring hemodialysis or peritoneal dialysis. Caution should be used to ensure that the correct dosage of sitagliptin is prescribed for patients with moderate or severe renal impairment. (See Worsening of Renal Function under Cautions: Warnings/Precautions.)

In patients with an eGFR of 30 to less than 45 mL/minute per 1.73 m^2, the recommended dosage of sitagliptin is 50 mg once daily.

In patients with an eGFR less than 30 mL/minute per 1.73 m^2), the recommended dosage is 25 mg once daily.

Patients with end-stage renal disease requiring hemodialysis or peritoneal dialysis should receive a dosage of 25 mg once daily. Sitagliptin may be administered without regard to the timing of dialysis.

Sitagliptin/Ertugliflozin Fixed-combination Therapy. Dosage adjustment of the fixed combination of sitagliptin and ertugliflozin is not necessary in patients with mild renal impairment (eGFR 60–89 mL/minute per 1.73 m^2).

Initiation of the fixed combination of sitagliptin and ertugliflozin is not recommended in patients with moderate renal impairment (eGFR of 30 to less than 60 mL/minute per 1.73 m^2). Continued use of the fixed combination is not recommended in patients with an eGFR persistently between 30 and less than 60 mL/minute per 1.73 m^2.

The fixed combination of sitagliptin and ertugliflozin is contraindicated in patients with severe renal impairment (eGFR less than 30 mL/minute per 1.73 m^2) or end-stage renal disease and in those receiving dialysis. (See Renal Impairment under Warnings/Precautions: Specific Populations, in Cautions.)

Sitagliptin/Immediate- or Extended-release Metformin Hydrochloride Fixed-combination Therapy. Initiation of the fixed combinations of sitagliptin and immediate- or extended-release metformin hydrochloride is not recommended in patients with an eGFR of 30–45 mL/minute per 1.73 m^2.

In patients already receiving the fixed combination of sitagliptin and *extended-release* metformin hydrochloride whose eGFR decreases to 30–45 mL/minute per 1.73 m^2 during therapy, the benefits and risks of continuing the fixed combination should be assessed and the dosage of the sitagliptin component should be limited to 50 mg once daily.

The fixed combinations of sitagliptin and immediate- or extended-release metformin hydrochloride are contraindicated in patients with an eGFR less than 30 mL/minute per 1.73 m^2.

Geriatric Patients Dosage in geriatric patients should be selected with caution because of age-related decreases in renal function. (See Geriatric Use under Warnings/Precautions: Specific Populations, in Cautions.)

Cautions

■ Contraindications Sitagliptin is contraindicated in patients with known serious hypersensitivity (e.g., anaphylaxis, angioedema) to sitagliptin or to any ingredient in the formulation.

■ Warnings/Precautions ***Pancreatitis and Pancreatic Precancerous Changes*** Acute pancreatitis, including fatal and nonfatal hemorrhagic or necrotizing pancreatitis, has been reported during postmarketing experience in patients receiving sitagliptin with or without metformin hydrochloride. The most common manifestations associated with pancreatitis were abdominal pain, nausea, and vomiting. Hospitalization was required in 66% of 88 reported cases, including 2 cases of hemorrhagic or necrotizing pancreatitis that necessitated prolonged hospitalization and intensive-care unit (ICU) care. Pancreatitis occurred within 30 days of initiation of sitagliptin or sitagliptin/metformin therapy in 21% of cases; discontinuance of the drug led to resolution of pancreatitis in 53% of patients. At least one other risk factor (e.g., obesity, high cholesterol and/or triglyceride concentrations) was noted in 51% of cases.

FDA has been evaluating unpublished findings suggesting an increased risk of pancreatitis and precancerous pancreatic cell changes (pancreatic duct metaplasia) in patients with type 2 diabetes mellitus receiving incretin mimetics (exenatide, liraglutide, sitagliptin, saxagliptin, alogliptin, or linagliptin). These findings are based on examination of a small number of pancreatic tissue specimens taken from patients who died from unspecified causes while receiving an incretin mimetic.

FDA has recommended that clinicians continue to follow the recommendations in the prescribing information for incretin mimetics. The manufacturer states that patients receiving sitagliptin-containing therapy should be monitored for manifestations of pancreatitis, such as nausea, vomiting, anorexia, and persistent severe abdominal pain, sometimes radiating to the back; persistent severe abdominal pain, sometimes radiating to the back, which may or may not be accompanied by vomiting, is the hallmark symptom of acute pancreatitis. If pancreatitis is suspected, sitagliptin should be promptly discontinued and appropriate management instituted (e.g., including laboratory studies such as serum and urine amylase, amylase/creatinine clearance ratio, electrolytes, and serum calcium, glucose, and lipase). Safety and efficacy of sitagliptin have not been established in patients with a history of pancreatitis and it is not known whether such patients are at increased risk for pancreatitis with sitagliptin therapy.

Heart Failure Risk In cardiovascular outcomes studies conducted with other dipeptidyl peptidase-4 (DPP-4) inhibitors (alogliptin, saxagliptin) in patients with type 2 diabetes mellitus and atherosclerotic cardiovascular disease (ASCVD), an association between DPP-4 inhibitor treatment and heart failure was observed.

The potential risks and benefits of sitagliptin therapy should be considered prior to use in patients at risk for heart failure (e.g., history of heart failure or renal impairment). Patients receiving sitagliptin-containing therapy should be monitored for manifestations of heart failure. (See Advice to Patients.) If heart failure develops, appropriate evaluation and management should be instituted and consideration given to discontinuing sitagliptin.

Worsening of Renal Function Renal function should be assessed prior to initiation of sitagliptin and periodically thereafter. Worsening of renal function, including acute renal failure that sometimes required dialysis, has been reported in some patients during postmarketing experience. A subset of these patients had renal insufficiency, some of whom were prescribed inappropriate dosages of sitagliptin. A return to baseline levels of renal insufficiency has been observed with supportive treatment and discontinuance of potentially causative agents. Cautious reinitiation of sitagliptin can be considered if another etiology is deemed likely to have precipitated the acute worsening of renal function. The manufacturer states that sitagliptin has not been found to be nephrotoxic in clinical trials or in preclinical studies at clinically relevant dosages.

Severe Arthralgia Severe, disabling joint pain has been reported during postmarketing experience in patients receiving DPP-4 inhibitors (e.g., alogliptin, linagliptin, saxagliptin, sitagliptin). Onset of such symptoms has ranged from 1 day to years following initiation of therapy. Fever, chills, rash, and swelling accompanied joint pain in some patients, suggesting an immunologic reaction; some patients have required hospitalization. Symptoms resolved upon discontinuance of the DPP-4 inhibitor, usually in less than a month. In some patients, symptoms recurred when the same or another DPP-4 inhibitor was restarted. DPP-4 inhibitors should be considered as a possible cause of severe joint pain and should be discontinued if appropriate. (See Advice to Patients.)

Concomitant Therapy with Hypoglycemic Agents When sitagliptin was used in combination with a sulfonylurea or insulin, the incidence of hypoglycemia was greater than that in patients receiving placebo with a sulfonylurea or insulin. In a long-term (52-week) clinical noninferiority study, rates of hypoglycemia with sitagliptin/metformin combination therapy were lower than those observed with glipizide/metformin combination therapy. However, in a 24-week clinical study, rates of hypoglycemia in patients receiving sitagliptin and glimepiride with or without metformin were greater than those in patients receiving glimepiride and metformin. Patients receiving sitagliptin may require a lower dosage of a concomitant insulin secretagogue (e.g., sulfonylurea) or insulin to reduce the risk of hypoglycemia.

Dermatologic and Sensitivity Reactions There have been postmarketing reports of serious allergic and hypersensitivity reactions (e.g., anaphylaxis, angioedema, exfoliative skin conditions such as Stevens-Johnson syndrome); rash, urticaria, and cutaneous vasculitis also have been reported. The onset of such reactions usually was within the first 3 months following treatment initiation, but such reactions may occur after the first dose. (See Cautions: Contraindications.)

If hypersensitivity reactions occur, promptly discontinue the drug, assess for other potential causes of the event, institute appropriate monitoring and treatment, and initiate alternative antidiabetic therapy. (See Advice to Patients.) Sitagliptin should be used with caution in patients with a history of angioedema with other DPP-4 inhibitors because it is unknown whether such patients will be predisposed to angioedema with sitagliptin.

Postmarketing cases of bullous pemphigoid requiring hospitalization have been reported with DPP-4 inhibitor use. These cases usually resolved after discontinuation of the DPP-4 inhibitor and treatment with topical or systemic immunosuppressive therapy. Patients should be advised to report the development of blisters or erosions while receiving sitagliptin. If bullous pemphigoid is suspected, the drug should be discontinued and referral to a dermatologist should be considered for diagnosis and appropriate treatment.

Loss of Glycemic Control Loss of glycemic control may occur during periods of stress (e.g., fever, trauma, infection, surgery). (See Advice to Patients.)

Temporary discontinuance of sitagliptin and administration of insulin may be required. Sitagliptin therapy may be reinstituted after the acute episode of hyperglycemia has resolved.

Macrovascular Outcomes Evidence of macrovascular risk reduction with sitagliptin has not been conclusively demonstrated in controlled clinical trials.

Use of Fixed Combinations When sitagliptin is used in fixed combination with metformin hydrochloride or ertugliflozin, the cautions, precautions, and contraindications associated with metformin hydrochloride or ertugliflozin should be considered.

Specific Populations **Pregnancy.** Data are lacking on the use of sitagliptin in pregnant women. In animal studies, no adverse developmental effects were observed when sitagliptin was administered to pregnant rats and rabbits during organogenesis at doses up to 30 times the human 100-mg dose (based on area under the concentration-time curve [AUC]). Pregnancy registry may be contacted at 800-986-8999.

Lactation. Sitagliptin is distributed into milk in rats. It is not known whether the drug is distributed into human milk, affects the breastfed infant, or affects milk production. The benefits of breast-feeding and the importance of sitagliptin to the woman should be considered along with any potential adverse effects on the breast-fed infant from the drug or from the underlying maternal condition

Pediatric Use. Safety and efficacy of sitagliptin alone or in fixed combination with ertugliflozin or in fixed combination with immediate- or extended-release metformin hydrochloride have not been established in children younger than 18 years of age.

Geriatric Use. No substantial differences in safety and efficacy of sitagliptin relative to younger adults, but increased sensitivity cannot be ruled out. Renal function should be assessed more frequently in geriatric patients. (See Renal Impairment under Warnings/Precautions: Specific Populations, in Cautions.)

Renal Impairment. Sitagliptin is substantially eliminated by the kidneys; renal function should be assessed prior to initiation of therapy and periodically thereafter. (See Worsening of Renal Function under Cautions: Warnings/Precautions and also see Renal Impairment under Dosage and Administration: Special Populations.)

■ **Common Adverse Effects** Adverse effects reported in at least 5% of patients receiving sitagliptin as monotherapy or add-on therapy with metformin and/or a thiazolidinedione or glimepiride and more commonly than with placebo include nasopharyngitis, upper respiratory tract infection, peripheral edema, and headache.

Adverse effects reported in patients receiving sitagliptin concomitantly with ertugliflozin are similar to those reported with use of ertugliflozin alone.

Adverse effects reported in at least 5% of patients receiving sitagliptin and immediate-release metformin hydrochloride concomitantly and occurring more commonly than with placebo include diarrhea, upper respiratory infection, and headache.

Adverse effects reported in at least 5% of patients receiving sitagliptin in combination with immediate-release metformin and a sulfonylurea (glimepiride) and occurring more commonly than with placebo include hypoglycemia and headache.

Adverse effects reported in at least 5% of patients receiving sitagliptin in combination with insulin and occurring more commonly than with placebo include hypoglycemia.

Drug Interactions

■ **Drugs Metabolized by Hepatic Microsomal Enzymes** Sitagliptin is metabolized to a limited extent by cytochrome P-450 (CYP) isoenzymes 3A4 and 2C8 to inactive metabolites. Sitagliptin does not inhibit CYP isoenzymes 1A2, 2B6, 2C8, 2C9, 2C19, 2D6, or 3A4 in vitro or induce CYP3A4. Pharmacokinetic interactions with drugs metabolized by these isoenzymes are unlikely.

■ **Drugs Secreted by Renal Tubular Cationic Transport** Sitagliptin is a substrate of the organic anion transport system; pharmacokinetic interactions are unlikely with substrates of the organic cationic transport system.

■ **Drugs Affecting or Affected by P-glycoprotein Transport System** Sitagliptin is a substrate of the P-glycoprotein transport system (P-gp). There is a potential pharmacokinetic interaction (increased absorption and renal clearance of sitagliptin) with P-gp inhibitors.

Clinically important pharmacokinetic interactions with P-gp inhibitors appear to be unlikely. Sitagliptin does not appear to inhibit the P-gp transport system. Pharmacokinetic interactions are unlikely with substrates of P-gp.

■ **Protein-bound Drugs** Pharmacokinetic interactions between sitagliptin and protein-bound drugs are unlikely.

■ **Cyclosporine** Concomitant administration of cyclosporine and sitagliptin may increase absorption and plasma concentrations of sitagliptin. However, this interaction is not considered clinically important.

■ **Digoxin** Concomitant administration of sitagliptin (100 mg daily for 10 days) with digoxin resulted in a slight increase in plasma concentrations and area under the concentration-time curve (AUC) of digoxin (18 and 11%, respectively). While these increases are not considered clinically important, patients receiving digoxin should be monitored appropriately; however, no digoxin or sitagliptin dosage adjustment is needed.

■ **Ertugliflozin** Administration of a single dose of sitagliptin (100 mg) with a single dose of ertugliflozin (15 mg) did not have a clinically important effect on the pharmacokinetics of ertugliflozin or sitagliptin.

■ **Hormonal Contraceptives, Oral** Sitagliptin has no clinically important effect on the pharmacokinetics of norethindrone or ethinyl estradiol.

■ **Metformin** Sitagliptin and metformin have a potential additive effect on active glucagon-like peptide (GLP-1) concentrations. Pharmacokinetic interactions are unlikely.

The relevance of these effects to glycemic control in patients with type 2 diabetes mellitus is unclear.

■ **Simvastatin** Pharmacokinetic interactions between sitagliptin and simvastatin are unlikely.

■ **Sulfonylureas or Insulin** The incidence of hypoglycemia was increased compared with placebo when sitagliptin was added to therapy with an insulin secretagogue (e.g., sulfonylurea) or insulin. (See Concomitant Therapy with Hypoglycemic Agents under Cautions: Warnings/Precautions.) Clinically important pharmacokinetic interactions between sitagliptin and sulfonylureas (e.g., glimepiride, glipizide, glyburide, tolbutamide) are unlikely.

■ **Thiazolidinediones** Pharmacokinetic interactions between sitagliptin and thiazolidinediones are unlikely.

■ **Warfarin** Pharmacokinetic interactions between sitagliptin and warfarin are unlikely.

Description

Sitagliptin inhibits dipeptidyl peptidase-4 (DPP-4), an enzyme that inactivates glucagon-like peptide (GLP-1) and glucose-dependent insulinotropic polypeptide (GIP), which are incretin hormones. The drug inhibits DPP-4 selectively with no effect on DPP-8 or DDP-9 in vitro at concentrations approximating those from therapeutic dosage. Sitagliptin increases circulating concentrations of GIP and GLP-1 in a glucose-dependent manner. Coadministration of sitagliptin and metformin has an additive effect on active GLP-1 concentrations.

GIP and GLP-1 stimulate insulin synthesis and release from pancreatic β-cells in a glucose-dependent manner (i.e., when glucose concentrations are normal or elevated) by intracellular signaling pathways involving cyclic 3′,5′-adenosine monophosphate (cAMP). GLP-1 also decreases glucagon secretion from pancreatic α-cells in a glucose-dependent manner, leading to reduced hepatic glucose production.

Sitagliptin lowers fasting plasma glucose concentrations and reduces glucose excursions following glucose load or meal in patients with type 2 diabetes mellitus.

Sitagliptin monotherapy usually is not associated with hypoglycemia or substantial changes in body weight.

Peak plasma sitagliptin concentration is achieved within 3 hours following oral administration. Absolute bioavailability is approximately 87%. Administration of sitagliptin with a high-fat meal had no effect on the pharmacokinetics of the drug Sitagliptin is metabolized to a limited extent by CYP isoenzymes 3A4 and 2C8 to inactive metabolites. Terminal half-of sitagliptin is 12.4 hours following oral administration of a 100 mg oral dose. Following administration of a single radiolabeled dose, 87% of the dose was excreted in the urine (mainly as unchanged drug) and 13% was excreted in the feces.

Advice to Patients

When sitagliptin is used in fixed combination with other drugs, importance of informing patients of important cautionary information about the concomitant agent(s).

Importance of patient reading medication guide before initiating therapy and each time the drug is dispensed.

Inform patients of potential risks and advantages of sitagliptin-containing therapy and of alternative therapies. Importance of not using sitagliptin in patients with type 1 diabetes mellitus or diabetic ketoacidosis.

Importance of patient informing clinician if hypoglycemia occurs, particularly if concomitant therapy with a sulfonylurea antidiabetic agent (i.e., insulin secretagogue) or insulin is used; a lower dosage of the sulfonylurea or insulin may be required in such cases.

Importance of informing patient about possibility of acute pancreatitis, which may be severe or fatal, with sitagliptin-containing therapy. Importance of patients advising clinicians about a history of pancreatitis, gallstones, alcoholism, high triglyceride levels, or kidney problems. Importance of advising patients about signs and symptoms of pancreatitis, including nausea, vomiting, anorexia, and persistent severe abdominal pain sometimes radiating to the back; importance of patient discontinuing sitagliptin and promptly notifying clinician if such signs or symptoms are present.

Importance of informing patients of the possibility of severe and disabling joint pain with dipeptidyl peptidase-4 (DPP-4) inhibitors (e.g., alogliptin, linagliptin, saxagliptin, sitagliptin). Advise patients to contact a clinician promptly if severe and persistent joint pain occurs; patients should not discontinue the DPP-4 inhibitor without consulting their clinician.

Importance of informing patients about possibility of heart failure with sitagliptin therapy. Importance of patients informing clinicians about a history of heart failure or renal impairment. Importance of informing patients about signs and symptoms of heart failure (e.g., shortness of breath, weight gain, edema); importance of patients immediately contacting a clinician if manifestations of heart failure occur.

Importance of instructing patients regarding self-monitoring of blood glucose, periodic HbA_{1c} monitoring, adherence to meal planning, regular physical exercise, and management of hypoglycemia and hyperglycemia.

Discuss potential for alterations in dosage requirements in special situations (e.g., fever, trauma, infection, surgery, changes in renal function); importance of informing clinician promptly if such situations occur. (See Loss of Glycemic Control under Cautions: Warnings/Precautions.)

Risk of allergic reactions (e.g., rash; hives; swelling of face, lips, tongue, throat that may cause difficulty in breathing or swallowing). If such reactions occur, importance of discontinuing sitagliptin and informing clinicians promptly. (See Sensitivity Reactions under Cautions: Warnings/Precautions.)

Importance of informing patients that bullous pemphigoid may occur with the use of a DPP-4 inhibitor. Advise patients to contact a clinician if blisters or erosions occur.

Importance of swallowing tablets of the fixed combination of sitagliptin and immediate- or extended-release metformin hydrochloride whole and not cutting, crushing, or chewing them.

Importance of women informing their clinicians if they are or plan to become pregnant or plan to breast-feed.

Importance of informing clinicians of existing or contemplated concomitant therapy, including prescription and OTC drugs and dietary or herbal supplements, as well as any concomitant illnesses (e.g., allergies, kidney problems, history of pancreatitis).

Importance of informing patients of other important precautionary information. (See Cautions.)

Overview® (see Users Guide). For additional information on this drug until a more detailed monograph is developed and published, the manufacturer's labeling should be consulted. It is *essential* that the manufacturer's labeling be consulted for more detailed information on usual cautions, precautions, contraindications, potential drug interactions, laboratory test interferences, and acute toxicity.

Preparations

Excipients in commercially available drug preparations may have clinically important effects in some individuals; consult specific product labeling for details.

SITagliptin Phosphate

Oral

Tablets, film-coated	25 mg (of sitagliptin)	**Januvia®**, Merck
	50 mg (of sitagliptin)	**Januvia®**, Merck
	100 mg (of sitagliptin)	**Januvia®**, Merck

SITagliptin Phosphate Combinations

Oral

Tablets, extended-release	50 mg (of sitagliptin) with Extended-release Metformin Hydrochloride 500 mg	**Janumet® XR**, Merck
	50 mg (of sitagliptin) with Extended-release Metformin Hydrochloride 1 g	**Janumet® XR**, Merck
	100 mg (of sitagliptin) with Extended-release Metformin Hydrochloride 1 g	**Janumet® XR**, Merck
Tablets, film-coated	50 mg (of sitagliptin) with Metformin Hydrochloride 500 mg	**Janumet®**, Merck
	50 mg (of sitagliptin) with Metformin Hydrochloride 1 g	**Janumet®**, Merck
	100 mg (of sitagliptin) with Ertugliflozin L-pyroglutamic Acid 5 mg (of ertugliflozin)	**Steglujan®**, Merck
	100 mg (of sitagliptin) with Ertugliflozin L-pyroglutamic Acid 15 mg (of ertugliflozin)	**Steglujan®**, Merck

INCRETIN MIMETICS 68:20.06

Dulaglutide

■ Dulaglutide, a long-acting glucagon-like peptide-1 (GLP-1) receptor agonist (incretin mimetic), is an antidiabetic agent.

Uses

■ Type 2 Diabetes Mellitus Dulaglutide is used as an adjunct to diet and exercise to improve glycemic control in patients with type 2 diabetes mellitus. Dulaglutide has been used alone or as add-on therapy with metformin, the combination of metformin and a sulfonylurea, the combination of metformin and a thiazolidinedione, and prandial insulin with or without metformin. However, because of the uncertain relevance to humans of thyroid C-cell tumors found in rodents given dulaglutide, the drug is not recommended as first-line therapy for patients inadequately controlled on diet and exercise alone. (See Risk of Thyroid C-Cell Tumors under Warnings/Precautions: Warnings, in Cautions.)

Current guidelines for the treatment of type 2 diabetes mellitus generally recommend metformin as first-line therapy in addition to lifestyle modifications because of its well-established safety and efficacy (e.g., beneficial effects on glycosylated hemoglobin [hemoglobin A_{1c}; HbA_{1c}], weight, and cardiovascular mortality) in patients with recent-onset or newly diagnosed type 2 diabetes mellitus or mild hyperglycemia. Because of the progressive nature of the disease, patients initially receiving an oral antidiabetic agent will eventually require multiple oral and/or injectable antidiabetic agents of different therapeutic classes and/or insulin for adequate glycemic control. Patients with inadequate glycemic control with metformin monotherapy should receive treatment with additional antidiabetic agents; data suggest that the addition of each noninsulin agent to initial therapy lowers HbA_{1c} by approximately 0.7–1%. Some experts recommend initiating antidiabetic therapy with 2 agents (metformin plus another agent) in patients whose HbA_{1c} is 7.5% or higher, while other experts recommend initiating such dual therapy in patients whose HbA_{1c} is at least 1.5% above the target level. When the greater glucose-lowering effect of an injectable drug is needed, some experts suggest that glucagon-like peptide-1 (GLP-1) receptor agonists are preferred over insulin. Early introduction of insulin therapy should be considered when hyperglycemia is severe (e.g., blood glucose of at least 300 mg/dL, HbA_{1c} of at least 10%), especially in the presence of catabolic manifestations (e.g., weight loss, hypertriglyceridemia, ketosis), or if symptoms of hyperglycemia are present. For additional information regarding the initiation of insulin therapy, see Uses: Diabetes Mellitus, in the Insulins General Statement 68:20.08.

Experts state that a patient's comorbidities should be considered when selecting additional (in addition to metformin) antidiabetic agents. Patients with type 2 diabetes mellitus who have established atherosclerotic cardiovascular disease (ASCVD) should receive a drug with demonstrated cardiovascular disease benefit (e.g., GLP-1 receptor agonist [e.g., liraglutide], sodium-glucose cotransporter 2 [SGLT2] inhibitor [e.g., canagliflozin, empagliflozin]). In patients with ASCVD and heart failure or with an increased risk of heart failure, an SGLT2 inhibitor with demonstrated cardiovascular benefit may be preferred. An SGLT2 inhibitor or GLP-1 receptor agonist shown to reduce the risk of chronic kidney disease (CKD) progression, cardiovascular events, or both (e.g., canagliflozin, empagliflozin, liraglutide) should be considered in patients with type 2 diabetes mellitus and CKD. Experts state that SGLT2 inhibitors may be a good choice for patients at high risk of CKD progression (i.e., patients with albuminuria or a history of estimated glomerular filtration rate [eGFR] decline) because they may have a beneficial effect on the incidence of CKD; however, adequate renal function is required for their use. Some GLP-1 receptor agonists may be used in patients with lower eGFR and may provide greater benefits for reduction of ASCVD than for CKD progression or heart failure. In patients without ASCVD, heart failure, or CKD, the decision regarding the addition of other antidiabetic agents (e.g., sulfonylurea, thiazolidinedione, dipeptidyl peptidase-4 [DPP-4] inhibitor, SGLT2 inhibitor, GLP-1 receptor agonist, basal insulin) should be based on drug-specific effects and individual patient factors.

Dulaglutide has not been studied in patients with a history of pancreatitis; other antidiabetic agents should be considered in such patients. (See Pancreatitis and Pancreatic Precancerous Changes under Warnings/Precautions: Other Warnings and Precautions, in Cautions.)

Dulaglutide has not been studied in patients with severe GI disease, including severe gastroparesis, and the drug is not recommended for use in patients with preexisting severe GI disease. (See GI Effects under Warnings/Precautions: Other Warnings and Precautions, in Cautions.)

Dulaglutide is not a substitute for insulin in insulin-requiring patients; the drug should not be used in patients with type 1 diabetes mellitus or for the treatment of diabetic ketoacidosis.

Dulaglutide Monotherapy When given as monotherapy for the management of type 2 diabetes mellitus, dulaglutide improves glycemic control as evidenced by reductions from baseline in glycosylated hemoglobin (hemoglobin A_{1c}; HbA_{1c}). Efficacy and safety of dulaglutide as monotherapy have been established in a 52-week, randomized, double-blind, noninferiority study comparing dulaglutide (0.75 mg or 1.5 mg once weekly throughout the study) with metformin (median initial dosage of 1 g daily with upward titration to 1.5–2 g daily) in patients with type 2 diabetes mellitus. The primary study end point was the change in HbA_{1c} from baseline to week 26.

At week 26, HbA_{1c} was reduced in all treatment groups; both dosages of dulaglutide were noninferior to metformin at 26 and 52 weeks. Mean HbA_{1c} was reduced by 0.7 and 0.8% in patients receiving dulaglutide 0.75 and 1.5 mg, respectively, and by 0.6% in those receiving metformin. Patients in all 3 treatment groups also had decreased fasting plasma glucose and body weight at 26 and 52 weeks. Patients included in this trial had type 2 diabetes mellitus inadequately controlled by diet and exercise or one oral antidiabetic agent, and had a mean baseline HbA_{1c} of 7.6%. Approximately 75% of patients were taking an oral antidiabetic agent before the study; approximately 90% of these patients were receiving metformin and approximately 10% were receiving a sulfonylurea.

Combination Therapy When given as add-on therapy in combination with one or more oral antidiabetic agents (e.g., metformin, a sulfonylurea, a thiazolidinedione), dulaglutide improved glycemic control more than sitagliptin or exenatide. Dulaglutide was noninferior to insulin glargine in reducing HbA_{1c} when added to prandial insulin with or without metformin or to other oral antidiabetic agents, and was noninferior to liraglutide when added to metformin. Safety and efficacy of dulaglutide as add-on therapy to other antidiabetic agents in the management of type 2 diabetes mellitus have been established in several randomized, active-controlled, double-blind or open-label studies lasting 26–104 weeks in over 4000 patients. In these studies, patients randomized to dulaglutide received either 0.75 or 1.5 mg once weekly with no dosage adjustments.

In a 104-week, randomized, double-blind study, patients who received dulaglutide in addition to existing metformin therapy (at least 1.5 g daily) experienced a substantially greater reduction in HbA_{1c} at the 52-week primary end point than those who received sitagliptin (100 mg once daily) as add-on therapy to metformin. Both 0.75- and 1.5-mg dosages of dulaglutide were superior to placebo and sitagliptin in reducing HbA_{1c}, with greater reduction in HbA_{1c} with the higher dulaglutide dosage. More patients achieved HbA_{1c} less than 7% in the dulaglutide groups than in the sitagliptin group; patients who received dulaglutide also had substantially lowered fasting plasma glucose and greater weight loss compared with those who received sitagliptin.

In a 52-week study in patients inadequately controlled on pioglitazone (30–45 mg daily) and metformin (at least 1.5 g daily) therapy, add-on therapy with dulaglutide (0.75 or 1.5 mg once weekly) was superior to placebo and add-on exenatide (5 mcg twice daily for 4 weeks, then 10 mcg twice daily) in reducing HbA_{1c} at the 26-week primary end point. Superiority of dulaglutide over exenatide was maintained at 52 weeks. At 26 weeks, an HbA_{1c} less than 7% was achieved in 66 or 78% of patients receiving dulaglutide 0.75 or 1.5 mg, respectively, compared with 52% of those receiving exenatide.

In a 78-week, randomized, open-label noninferiority study, dulaglutide (0.75 or 1.5 mg once weekly) was compared with insulin glargine (10 units daily initially, titrated to a fasting plasma glucose goal of less than 100 mg/dL) as add-on therapy to maximally tolerated dosages of metformin and glimepiride. At the 52-week primary end point, dulaglutide 1.5 mg was superior, and 0.75 mg noninferior to insulin glargine (mean daily dosage 29.4 units) as add-on therapy with regard to HbA_{1c} reduction. Dulaglutide was associated with mean body weight losses of 1.3 and 1.9 kg for the 0.75- and 1.5-mg dosages, respectively, while insulin glargine treatment resulted in a mean body weight gain of 1.4 kg.

In a 52-week, randomized, open-label noninferiority trial, dulaglutide (0.75 or 1.5 mg once weekly) was compared with insulin glargine (initiated at 50% of the prerandomization total daily insulin dosage and titrated to a fasting plasma glucose of less than 100 mg/dL) as add-on therapy to prandial (3 times daily) insulin lispro with or without metformin. At the 26-week primary end point, HbA_{1c} was reduced in all treatment groups; both dosages of dulaglutide were noninferior to insulin glargine.

In a 26-week, open-label noninferiority study, dulaglutide (1.5 mg once weekly) was compared with liraglutide (titrated from 0.6 mg daily to 1.8 mg daily by week 3) as add-on therapy in patients with type 2 diabetes not adequately controlled with metformin (at least 1.5 g daily). At the 26-week primary end point, HbA_{1c} was reduced in both groups; the dulaglutide 1.5-mg dosage was noninferior to liraglutide.

Safety and efficacy of dulaglutide *in combination* with basal insulin have not been established.

Macrovascular Outcomes and Cardiovascular Risk Reduction Some GLP-1 receptor agonists (e.g., liraglutide) have demonstrated the ability to reduce the risk of cardiovascular events in those patients with type 2 diabetes mellitus and established cardiovascular disease. In addition to lowering blood glucose, GLP-1 receptor agonists appear to modify several nonglycemic cardiovascular risk factors such as blood pressure, body weight, and lipid profile. GLP-1 receptor agonists also may have beneficial endothelial effects. The manufacturer states there have been no clinical studies establishing conclusive evidence of macrovascular risk reduction with dulaglutide. For further discussion on the use of GLP-1 receptor agonists for cardiovascular risk reduction, see Macrovascular Outcomes and Cardiovascular Risk Reduction under Uses: Type 2 Diabetes Mellitus, in Liraglutide 68:20.06.

Beneficial Effects on Renal Function In several cardiovascular outcomes trials involving the use of GLP-1 receptor agonists (e.g., liraglutide) in patients with type 2 diabetes mellitus at increased risk for cardiovascular disease or with existing cardiovascular disease, beneficial effects on renal function have been observed as a secondary outcome. GLP-1 receptor agonists may be used in patients with lower eGFR compared with SGLT2 inhibitors; however, these drugs may have greater benefits for reduction of ASCVD than for CKD progression. For further discussion of the beneficial effects on renal function of GLP-1 receptor agonists, see Beneficial Effects on Renal Function, under Uses: Type 2 Diabetes Mellitus, in Liraglutide 68:20.06.

Dosage and Administration

■ **Administration** Dulaglutide is administered by subcutaneous injection; the drug should *not* be administered IV or IM. Dulaglutide is administered once weekly, on the same day each week, at any time of day without regard to meals. The day of weekly administration may be changed if necessary; however, at least 3 days should elapse between doses.

If a dose is missed, the missed dose should be administered as soon as possible if there are at least 3 days (72 hours) remaining before the next scheduled dose; the regular weekly schedule should then be resumed. If less than 3 days remain before the next scheduled dose, the missed dose should be skipped and the next dose should be administered on the usual weekly day, followed by resumption of the regular weekly schedule.

Dulaglutide is administered by subcutaneous injection into the abdomen, thigh, or upper arm using a single-dose, prefilled injection pen (the drug is not currently available in prefilled syringes in the US). The same area of the body may be used for weekly injections; however, injection sites should be rotated with each dose.

When using dulaglutide in combination with insulin, the drugs should be administered as separate injections; insulin and dulaglutide injections should never be mixed. Dulaglutide and insulin may be injected into the same body regions; however, the injections should not be adjacent to each other.

■ **Dosage** ***Type 2 Diabetes Mellitus*** The recommended initial dosage of dulaglutide for the management of type 2 diabetes mellitus in adults is 0.75 mg subcutaneously once weekly. If glycemic response is inadequate, the dosage may be increased to a maximum of 1.5 mg once weekly.

■ **Special Populations** No dosage adjustment is necessary in patients with renal or hepatic impairment, including end-stage renal disease. However, clinicians should use caution when initiating dulaglutide or escalating dosage in patients with renal impairment. (See Renal Effects under Warnings/Precautions: Other Warnings and Precautions, in Cautions.)

No dosage adjustment is necessary based on age, gender, race, ethnicity, or body weight.

Cautions

■ **Contraindications** Dulaglutide is contraindicated in patients with a personal or family history of medullary thyroid carcinoma (MTC) and in patients with multiple endocrine neoplasia syndrome type 2 (MEN 2).

Dulaglutide is also contraindicated in patients with a prior serious hypersensitivity reaction to dulaglutide or to any of the product components.

■ **Warnings/Precautions** ***Warnings*** **Risk of Thyroid C-Cell Tumors.** Glucagon-like peptide-1 (GLP-1) receptor agonists such as dulaglutide cause dose- and treatment duration-dependent thyroid C-cell tumors in rats and mice. It is unknown whether dulaglutide causes thyroid C-cell tumors, including MTC, in humans.

At least 1 case of MTC has been reported in a patient treated with dulaglutide. This patient had serum calcitonin concentrations approximately 8 times the upper limit of normal (ULN) prior to treatment. Very elevated serum calcitonin values may be indicative of MTC; patients with MTC usually have serum calcitonin values exceeding 50 ng/mL. Although routine monitoring of serum calcitonin is of uncertain value in patients treated with dulaglutide, patients should also be referred to an endocrinologist for further evaluation if serum calcitonin is found to be elevated. Patients with thyroid nodules noted on physical examination or neck imaging also should be referred to an endocrinologist. The role of monitoring serum calcitonin concentrations or thyroid ultrasounds for the purpose of early detection of MTC in patients receiving dulaglutide is unknown.

Sensitivity Reactions Serious hypersensitivity reactions (severe urticaria, systemic rash, facial edema, lip swelling) have been reported in patients receiving dulaglutide. If a hypersensitivity reaction occurs, the patient should discontinue dulaglutide and seek medical advice promptly.

Other Warnings and Precautions **Pancreatitis and Pancreatic Precancerous Changes.** Acute pancreatitis has been reported in association with dulaglutide in clinical trials. FDA is evaluating unpublished findings suggesting an increased risk of pancreatitis and precancerous pancreatic cellular changes (pancreatic duct metaplasia) in patients with type 2 diabetes mellitus receiving incretin mimetics (exenatide, liraglutide, sitagliptin, saxagliptin, alogliptin, or linagliptin). These findings are based on examination of a small number of pancreatic tissue specimens taken from patients treated with incretin mimetics who died from unspecified causes. FDA will notify healthcare professionals of its conclusions and recommendations when the review is complete or when the agency has additional information to report.

In clinical trials, 5 cases of confirmed pancreatitis occurred among dulaglutide-treated patients compared with 1 case in patients treated with a non-incretin comparator drug (1.4 versus 0.88 cases per 1000 patient years, respectively).

FDA states that at this time clinicians should continue to follow the recommendations in the prescribing information for incretin mimetics. The manufacturer states that if pancreatitis is suspected, dulaglutide should be discontinued promptly. If pancreatitis is confirmed, dulaglutide should not be restarted.

Efficacy and safety of dulaglutide have not been established in patients with a history of pancreatitis. Alternative antidiabetic therapy should be considered in patients with a history of pancreatitis.

Use with Drugs Known to Cause Hypoglycemia. Patients receiving dulaglutide in combination with an insulin secretagogue (e.g., sulfonylurea) or insulin have an increased risk of hypoglycemia. A lower dosage of the concomitant insulin secretagogue or insulin may be required to reduce the risk of hypoglycemia.

Renal Effects. During postmarketing experience, acute renal failure and worsening of chronic renal failure (which sometimes required hemodialysis) have been reported with GLP-1 receptor agonists. Some of these events have occurred in patients without known underlying renal disease. Most of these events have occurred in patients experiencing nausea, vomiting, diarrhea, or dehydration. Because these GI effects may worsen renal function, clinicians should use caution when initiating dulaglutide or escalating dosage in patients with renal impairment.

GI Effects. Use of dulaglutide may be associated with adverse GI effects, sometimes severe. In clinical trials, more patients receiving dulaglutide (1.3–3.5%) discontinued treatment because of adverse GI effects than patients receiving placebo (0.2%). Dulaglutide has not been studied in patients with severe GI disease, including severe gastroparesis; use of the drug is not recommended in such patients.

Specific Populations **Pregnancy.** Category C. (See Users Guide.)

Lactation. It is not known whether dulaglutide is distributed into milk in humans; a decision should be made whether to discontinue nursing or the drug, taking into account the importance of the drug to the woman.

Pediatric Use. Safety and efficacy of dulaglutide have not been established in children or adolescents younger than 18 years of age.

Geriatric Use. In a pool of 3342 patients in placebo- and active-controlled clinical trials, 18.6% of dulaglutide-treated patients were 65 years of age and older and 1.9% were 75 years of age and older. No substantial differences in safety and efficacy relative to younger adults were observed in these patients, but increased sensitivity in some geriatric individuals cannot be ruled out.

Hepatic Impairment. Because of the limited clinical experience of dulaglutide in patients with hepatic impairment, the drug should be used with caution in such patients. In a single-dose pharmacokinetic study, systemic exposure of dulaglutide decreased by 23, 33, and 21% in patients with mild, moderate, and severe hepatic impairment, respectively, compared with that in patients with normal hepatic function. These findings were not considered clinically important, and no dosage adjustment is considered necessary in patients with hepatic impairment.

Renal Impairment. In clinical trials, 1.2, 4.3, or 0% of dulaglutide-treated patients had mild, moderate, or severe renal impairment, respectively. No substantial differences in safety or efficacy relative to patients with normal renal function were observed. Because of the limited clinical experience of dulaglutide in patients with severe renal impairment or end-stage renal disease, the drug should be used with caution in such patients; the manufacturer recommends monitoring renal function in such patients with severe adverse GI reactions. (See Renal Effects under Warnings/Precautions: Other Warnings and Precautions, in Cautions.)

In a single-dose pharmacokinetic study in individuals with renal impairment, systemic exposure to dulaglutide was increased by 20, 28, 14, and 12% in patients with mild, moderate, and severe renal impairment, and end-stage renal disease, respectively, compared with patients with normal renal function. These findings were not considered clinically important, and no dosage adjustment is considered necessary in patients with renal impairment.

■ **Common Adverse Effects** Adverse effects other than hypoglycemia reported in at least 5% of patients receiving dulaglutide in placebo-controlled clinical trials and more frequently than with placebo include nausea, diarrhea, vomiting, abdominal pain/discomfort, decreased appetite, dyspepsia, and fatigue.

Drug Interactions

■ **Effects on GI Absorption of Other Drugs** Potential pharmacokinetic interaction (altered extent and rate of absorption because of dulaglutide-induced slowing of gastric emptying). In clinical pharmacology studies, dulaglutide did not affect the absorption of concomitantly administered oral drugs to any clinically relevant degree. However, caution should be exercised when dulaglutide is used concomitantly with oral drugs. In addition, concentrations of orally administered drugs with a narrow therapeutic index should be monitored adequately when such drugs are administered concomitantly with dulaglutide.

■ **Acetaminophen** Concomitant administration of dulaglutide and acetaminophen did not meaningfully alter the peak plasma concentration or area under the concentration-time curve (AUC) of acetaminophen. The manufacturer states that no adjustment of concomitant acetaminophen dosage is necessary.

■ **Atorvastatin** Concomitant administration of dulaglutide 1.5 mg and atorvastatin 40 mg decreased the AUC of atorvastatin by 21%, which is not considered clinically important. Peak plasma concentration of atorvastatin was reduced by 70%; the clinical importance of this is not known. The manufacturer states that no adjustment of concomitant atorvastatin dosage is necessary.

■ **Digoxin** Concomitant administration of dulaglutide and digoxin did not meaningfully alter the peak plasma concentration or AUC of digoxin. The manufacturer states that no adjustment of concomitant digoxin dosage is necessary.

■ **Lisinopril** Concomitant administration of dulaglutide and lisinopril did not meaningfully alter the peak plasma concentration or AUC of lisinopril. The manufacturer states that no adjustment of concomitant lisinopril dosage is necessary.

■ **Metformin** Concomitant administration of dulaglutide and metformin did not meaningfully alter the peak plasma concentration or AUC of metformin. The manufacturer states that no adjustment of concomitant metformin dosage is necessary.

■ **Metoprolol** Concomitant administration of dulaglutide and metoprolol did not meaningfully alter the peak plasma concentration or AUC of metoprolol. The manufacturer states that no adjustment of concomitant metoprolol dosage is necessary.

■ **Oral Contraceptives** Concomitant administration of dulaglutide and an oral contraceptive containing ethinyl estradiol and norgestimate did not substantially alter the AUC or peak plasma concentration of ethinyl estradiol or norelgestromin (a major metabolite of norgestimate); no adjustment of the concomitant oral contraceptive containing ethinyl estradiol and norgestimate dosage is necessary.

■ **Sitagliptin** Administration of single doses of dulaglutide 1.5 mg with sitagliptin 100 mg at steady state resulted in increases of approximately 38 and 27% in dulaglutide AUC and peak plasma concentration, respectively, which was not considered clinically important; no dosage adjustment of either drug is necessary.

■ **Warfarin** Concomitant administration of dulaglutide 1.5 mg and single 10-mg doses of warfarin sodium did not meaningfully alter the AUC of *R*- or *S*-warfarin; the manufacturer states that no adjustment of concomitant warfarin dosage is necessary.

Description

Dulaglutide is a long-acting glucagon-like peptide-1 (GLP-1) receptor agonist prepared from mammalian cell culture. The drug is a recombinant fusion protein that consists of 2 identical disulfide-linked chains, each containing an N-terminal GLP-1 analog covalently linked to the Fc portion of a modified human immunoglobulin G_4 (IgG_4) heavy chain by a small peptide linker. Each GLP-1 analog is 90% homologous to human GLP-1 (7–37) with structural modifications conferring resistance to degradation by dipeptidyl peptidase-4 (DPP-4). Both resistance to DPP-4 degradation and large molecule size (approximately 63 kilodaltons) extend the half-life of dulaglutide, allowing for weekly dosing.

Activation of GLP-1 receptors by dulaglutide stimulates insulin release in the presence of elevated glucose concentrations, suppresses glucagon release, and slows gastric emptying, resulting in lower fasting and postprandial blood glucose concentrations in patients with type 2 diabetes mellitus. The delay in gastric emptying produced by dulaglutide is largest after the first dose and diminishes with subsequent dosing.

Peak plasma dulaglutide concentrations are achieved 24–72 hours following subcutaneous administration. Steady-state concentrations are achieved 2–4 weeks following weekly administration. Absolute bioavailability following subcutaneous administration of single doses of 0.75 and 1.5 mg are 65 and 47%, respectively. Dulaglutide is thought to be degraded into its component amino acids by general protein catabolism pathways. The elimination half-life of dulaglutide is approximately 5 days.

Advice to Patients

Importance of patients reading the medication guide and instructions for use prior to initiating therapy and each time the prescription is refilled.

Importance of informing patients that dulaglutide causes benign and malignant thyroid C-cell tumors in rats and that relevance of this finding to humans is unknown. Patients should report symptoms of thyroid tumors (e.g., a lump in the neck, persistent hoarseness, dysphagia, dyspnea) to their clinician.

Importance of informing patients of the possibility of acute pancreatitis with dulaglutide therapy. Importance of patients informing clinicians if they have a history of pancreatitis. Importance of informing patients about signs and symptoms of pancreatitis, including persistent severe abdominal pain sometimes radiating to the back that may or may not be accompanied by vomiting; importance of patient discontinuing dulaglutide and promptly notifying clinician if such signs or symptoms occur.

Importance of informing patients of risk of hypoglycemia, particularly if concomitant therapy with an insulin secretagogue (e.g., sulfonylurea) or insulin is used. Importance of reviewing signs, symptoms, and management of hypoglycemia.

Importance of informing patients of possibility of hypersensitivity reactions. Patients should be instructed to discontinue dulaglutide and promptly seek medical advice if symptoms of hypersensitivity occur.

Importance of informing patients of potential risk of adverse GI effects and possibility of dehydration due to such adverse effects; patients should be advised to take precautions to avoid fluid depletion. Importance of informing patients of potential risk of worsening renal function, which may require dialysis in some cases.

Importance of patients reading the manufacturer's instructions for use before starting dulaglutide therapy. Importance of instructing patients regarding proper use, storage, and disposal of injection pen. After dispensing, pens should be stored in the refrigerator or may be stored at room temperature for up to 14 days; injection pens should be protected from light and not frozen.

Importance of informing patients not to take an extra dose of dulaglutide to make up for a missed dose. If a dose is missed, patients should take the dose as soon as possible if there are at least 3 days (72 hours) until the next dose; the next dose can be taken on their usual weekly day. If there are less than 3 days until the next dose, the missed dose should be skipped and patient should take the next dose on their usual weekly day.

Importance of women informing clinicians if they are or plan to become pregnant or plan to breast-feed.

Importance of informing clinicians of existing or contemplated concomitant therapy, including prescription and OTC drugs, as well as any concomitant illnesses (e.g., pancreatitis).

Importance of informing patients of other important precautionary information. (See Cautions.)

Overview® (see Users Guide). For additional information on this drug until a more detailed monograph is developed and published, the manufacturer's labeling should be consulted. It is *essential* that the manufacturer's labeling be consulted for more detailed information on usual cautions, precautions, contraindications, potential drug interactions, laboratory test interferences, and acute toxicity.

Preparations

Excipients in commercially available drug preparations may have clinically important effects in some individuals; consult specific product labeling for details.

Dulaglutide

Parenteral

Injection, for subcutaneous use only	0.75 mg/0.5 mL	**Trulicity®** (available as prefilled single-use injection pen), Lilly
	1.5 mg/0.5 mL	**Trulicity®** (available as prefilled single-use injection pen), Lilly

Selected Revisions November 2019,

Exenatide

■ Exenatide, a synthetic, human glucagon-like peptide-1 (GLP-1) receptor agonist (incretin mimetic), is an antidiabetic agent.

Uses

■ **Type 2 Diabetes Mellitus** Exenatide is used as an adjunct to diet and exercise to improve glycemic control in patients with type 2 diabetes mellitus. The drug is available as an injection for twice-daily administration (Byetta®) and as an extended-release for injectable suspension formulation for once-weekly administration (Bydureon®).

Current guidelines for the treatment of type 2 diabetes mellitus generally recommend metformin as first-line therapy in addition to lifestyle modifications because of its well-established safety and efficacy (i.e., beneficial effects on glycosylated hemoglobin [hemoglobin A_{1c}; HbA_{1c}], weight, and cardiovascular mortality) in patients with recent-onset type 2 diabetes mellitus or mild hyperglycemia. With declining β-cell function, patients initially receiving an oral antidiabetic agent will eventually require multiple oral and/or injectable antidiabetic agents of different therapeutic classes and/or insulin for adequate glycemic control. Patients with inadequate glycemic control with metformin monotherapy should receive treatment with additional antidiabetic agents; data suggest that the addition of each noninsulin agent added to initial therapy lowers HbA_{1c} by approximately 0.7–1%. Initiating antidiabetic therapy with 2 agents (metformin plus another agent) may be appropriate in patients with moderate hyperglycemia or when the HbA_{1c} is at least 1.5% above the target level. When the greater glucose-lowering effect of an injectable drug is needed, some experts suggest that GLP-1 receptor agonists are preferred over insulin. Insulin therapy should be considered when hyperglycemia is severe (e.g., blood glucose of at least 300 mg/dL, HbA_{1c} of at least 10%), especially in the presence of catabolic manifestations (e.g., weight loss, hypertriglyceridemia, ketosis). For additional information regarding the initiation of insulin therapy, see Uses: Diabetes Mellitus, in the Insulins General Statement 68:20.08.

Experts state that a patient's comorbidities should be considered when selecting additional (in addition to metformin) antidiabetic agents. Patients with type 2 diabetes mellitus who have established atherosclerotic cardiovascular disease (ASCVD) should receive a drug with demonstrated cardiovascular disease benefit (e.g., GLP-1 receptor agonist [e.g., liraglutide], sodium-glucose cotransporter 2 [SGLT2] inhibitor [e.g., canagliflozin, empagliflozin]). In patients with ASCVD and heart failure or with an increased risk of heart failure, an SGLT2 inhibitor with demonstrated cardiovascular benefit may be preferred. An SGLT2 inhibitor or GLP-1 receptor agonist with demonstrated ability to reduce the risk of chronic kidney disease (CKD) progression, cardiovascular events, or both (e.g., canagliflozin, empagliflozin, liraglutide) should be considered in patients with type 2 diabetes mellitus and CKD. Experts state that SGLT2 inhibitors may be a good choice for patients at high risk of CKD progression (i.e., patients with albuminuria or a history of estimated glomerular filtration rate [eGFR] decline) because they may have a beneficial effect on the incidence of CKD; however, adequate renal function is required for their use. Some GLP-1 receptor agonists may be used in patients with lower eGFR and may provide greater benefits for reduction of ASCVD than for CKD progression or heart failure. In patients without ASCVD, heart failure, or CKD, the decision regarding the addition of other antidiabetic agents (e.g., sulfonylurea, thiazolidinedione, dipeptidyl peptidase-4 [DPP-4] inhibitor, SGLT2 inhibitor, GLP-1 receptor agonist, basal insulin) should be based on drug-specific effects and individual patient factors.

Exenatide has been used as monotherapy or in combination with metformin, a sulfonylurea, or a thiazolidinedione; in combination with metformin and a sulfonylurea or a thiazolidinedione; or in combination with insulin glargine with or without metformin and/or a thiazolidinedione. The extended-release formulation of exenatide has been used as monotherapy or in combination with metformin, a sulfonylurea, or a thiazolidinedione; in combination with metformin and a sulfonylurea or a thiazolidinedione; in combination with an SGLT2 inhibitor and metformin; or in combination with basal insulinBecause of the uncertain relevance to humans of thyroid C-cell tumors found in rodents given extended-release exenatide, this formulation of the drug is not recommended as *first-line* therapy for patients with inadequate glycemic control on diet and exercise alone. (See Risk of Thyroid C-cell Tumors with Extended-release Exenatide under Warnings/Precautions: Warnings, in Cautions.)

Safety and efficacy of exenatide or extended-release exenatide have not been established in patients with a history of pancreatitis; other antidiabetic agents should be considered in such patients. (See Pancreatitis and Pancreatic Precancerous Changes under Warnings/Precautions: Other Warnings and Precautions, in Cautions.)

Exenatide or extended-release exenatide is not a substitute for insulin. The manufacturer states that exenatide or extended-release exenatide should not be used in patients with type 1 diabetes mellitus or for the treatment of diabetic ketoacidosis because the drug is not effective for these conditions. The safety and efficacy of exenatide or extended-release exenatide in combination with *prandial* insulin have not been established, and the manufacturer of exenatide states that such concomitant use is not recommended. (See Use with Drugs Known to Cause Hypoglycemia under Cautions: Warnings/Precautions: Other Warnings and Precautions, in Cautions.)

Exenatide and extended-release exenatide contain the same active ingredient and should not be used concomitantly.

Exenatide When given as monotherapy or add-on therapy, twice-daily exenatide improves glycemic control (e.g., as determined by changes in glycosylated hemoglobin [hemoglobin A_{1c}, HbA_{1c}]) more than placebo and similar to that of titrated insulin lispro or insulin aspart 70/30 therapy. In addition, therapy with GLP-1 receptor agonists such as exenatide generally is associated with weight loss compared with that observed with placebo and most other antidiabetic agents (e.g., sulfonylureas, thiazolidinediones, insulin).

Safety and efficacy of exenatide as monotherapy in patients with type 2 diabetes mellitus have been established in a 24-week, randomized, double-blind, placebo-controlled study. In this study, patients with baseline HbA_{1c} concentrations of 6.5–10% (mean: 7.8–7.9%) received exenatide 5 or 10 mcg or placebo subcutaneously twice daily before the morning and evening meals. Patients assigned to receive exenatide 10 mcg twice daily received 5 mcg twice daily for 4 weeks, then 10 mcg twice daily. The primary study end point was the change in HbA_{1c} concentration from baseline to week 24 (or the last value at time of early discontinuance of therapy). At week 24, therapy with exenatide 5 or 10 mcg twice daily resulted in mean reductions of 0.7 or 0.9%, respectively, in HbA_{1c} compared with baseline. HbA_{1c} concentrations below 7% were achieved in 48, 53, or 38% of patients receiving exenatide 5 mcg, exenatide 10 mcg, or placebo, respectively. Patients receiving exenatide also experienced greater weight reduction than those receiving placebo (−2.8, −3.1, or −1.4 kg with twice-daily dosages of exenatide 5 mcg, 10 mcg, or placebo, respectively).

In several studies of 30 weeks' duration in which exenatide (5 or 10 mcg twice daily) was given in combination with maximally effective dosages of metformin hydrochloride, a sulfonylurea (e.g., glipizide, glyburide, glimepiride, tolazamide, chlorpropamide), or metformin hydrochloride in combination with a sulfonylurea, combined therapy with subcutaneous exenatide and these oral antidiabetic agents or regimens resulted in a reduction from baseline in HbA_{1c} and progressive weight loss compared with that achieved with existing oral antidiabetic therapy.

Safety and efficacy of exenatide as add-on therapy to other antidiabetic agents also have been established in other studies. In a 16-week, placebo-controlled study in patients who had not achieved adequate glycemic control with a thiazolidinedione with or without metformin, the addition of subcutaneous exenatide (5 or 10 mcg twice daily) to existing oral antidiabetic therapy resulted in a reduction from baseline in HbA_{1c} at week 16 compared with that achieved with existing oral antidiabetic therapy. In a 30-week, placebo-controlled study in patients with type 2 diabetes mellitus who had inadequate glycemic control on titrated insulin glargine with or without metformin and/or a thiazolidinedione (i.e., pioglitazone), addition of exenatide (5 or 10 mcg twice daily) to existing antidiabetic therapy reduced HbA_{1c} from baseline at week 30 compared with that achieved with existing antidiabetic therapy. In a 26-week randomized, open-label study in patients with type 2 diabetes mellitus receiving metformin therapy (baseline HbA_{1c} 6.5–10%), addition of exenatide (5 mcg twice daily for 4 weeks, then 10 mcg twice daily) was noninferior to addition of titrated, premixed insulin aspart (70% long-acting insulin aspart protamine, 30% rapid-acting insulin aspart) in improving HbA_{1c} (least-squares mean HbA_{1c} reduction of 1 or 1.14% with exenatide or insulin aspart 70/30, respectively). In addition, exenatide therapy was associated with less hypoglycemia than insulin aspart and resulted in weight reduction while insulin aspart 70/30 caused weight gain.

Extended-release Exenatide Clinical studies indicate that the once-weekly extended-release formulation of exenatide generally is as effective as conventional regimens of metformin or pioglitazone and more effective than sitagliptin, titrated insulin glargine, insulin detemir, or twice-daily exenatide in improving glycemic control. Improvements in glycemic control have been maintained during long-term therapy (e.g., up to 6 years) with extended-release exenatide. In addition, compared with twice-daily exenatide, once-weekly extended-release exenatide generally has been associated with a similar degree of weight loss and GI adverse effects.

Safety and efficacy of once-weekly subcutaneous extended-release exenatide as monotherapy or in combination with other antidiabetic agents have been established in several randomized, open-label or double-blind clinical studies generally of 24–30 weeks' duration (e.g., DURATION studies) in adults with type 2 diabetes mellitus. In the 6 DURATION studies, once-weekly therapy with subcutaneous extended-release exenatide was compared with subcutaneous insulin glargine, liraglutide, or twice-daily exenatide or with oral antidiabetic agents (metformin, sitagliptin, pioglitazone) in patients who had inadequate glycemic control (mean baseline HbA_{1c} concentrations of 8.3–8.6%) with or without preexisting oral antidiabetic therapy. The primary efficacy end point in these studies was the mean change in HbA_{1c} from baseline to the end of the study; extended-release exenatide reduced HbA_{1c} by 1.3–1.9% compared with reductions of 0.9–1.5% for twice-daily exenatide, 1.2–1.6% for pioglitazone, 0.9–1.2% for sitagliptin, 1.5% for metformin, 1.3% for insulin glargine, and 1.5% for liraglutide. In general, extended-release exenatide was more effective than twice-daily exenatide overall in reducing HbA_{1c} and fasting plasma glucose, while twice-daily exenatide had a greater effect on postprandial hyperglycemia. In addition, the proportion of patients achieving an HbA_{1c} of less than 7% with extended-release exenatide in the DURATION studies generally was similar to that with pioglitazone and greater than that with sitagliptin or insulin glargine.

In the long-term therapy (up to 6 years) portions of the DURATION-1 study, improvements in glycemic control and weight generally were sustained in patients who continued once-weekly therapy with extended-release exenatide and sustained or enhanced in those whose therapy was switched from the twice-daily to the once-weekly formulation. Compared with insulin and most oral antidiabetic agents, therapy with subcutaneous extended-release exenatide resulted in slow but progressive weight loss, which was similar to that associated with twice-daily exenatide and sustained during long-term therapy. Extended-release exenatide therapy was well tolerated in these studies, with no major hypoglycemic episodes reported and a low risk of hypoglycemia compared with insulin and most other oral antidiabetic agent comparators; when hypoglycemic episodes occurred, patients generally were receiving concomitant sulfonylurea therapy.

Efficacy of extended-release exenatide in conjunction with basal insulin with or without metformin hydrochloride in the management of type 2 diabetes mellitus in patients with inadequate glycemic control despite treatment with titrated insulin glargine (dosage of at least 20 units daily) with or without metformin hydrochloride is supported by results of a 28-week, randomized, active-controlled study (DURATION-7). In this study, the addition of extended-release exenatide to existing therapy with insulin glargine with or without metformin hydrochloride resulted in substantially greater improvements in HbA_{1c} compared with insulin glargine therapy with or without metformin (reduction of 0.88 versus 0.24%, respectively). Greater reductions in fasting plasma glucose concentrations and body weight also were observed among patients who received therapy with extended-release exenatide therapy.

Efficacy of extended-release exenatide in conjunction with dapagliflozin as add-on therapy to metformin hydrochloride in the management of type 2 diabetes mellitus in patients who have inadequate glycemic control (HbA_{1c} concentration of 8 to less than 12%) with metformin hydrochloride is supported by results of a 28-week, randomized, active-controlled study (DURATION-8). In this study, the addition of dapagliflozin (10 mg daily) and extended-release exenatide (2 mg once weekly) to existing stable therapy with metformin hydrochloride (at least 1.5 g daily) resulted in substantially greater improvements in HbA_{1c} and fasting plasma glucose compared with dapagliflozin or extended-release exenatide therapy alone. In patients who received dapagliflozin 10 mg once daily and extended-release exenatide 2 mg once weekly as add-on therapy to metformin hydrochloride, addition of dapagliflozin and extended-release exenatide reduced HbA_{1c} by 1.77%, versus a 1.3 or 1.42% reduction in those receiving add-on therapy with dapagliflozin or extended-release exenatide alone, respectively. More weight loss and greater reductions in systolic blood pressure also were observed among those who received add-on therapy with dapagliflozin and extended-release exenatide compared with add-on therapy with either drug alone.

Macrovascular Outcomes and Cardiovascular Risk Reduction Some GLP-1 receptor agonists (e.g., liraglutide) have demonstrated the ability to reduce the risk of cardiovascular events in those patients with type 2 diabetes mellitus and established cardiovascular disease. In addition to lowering blood glucose, GLP-1 receptor agonists appear to modify several nonglycemic cardiovascular risk factors, such as blood pressure, body weight, and lipid profile. GLP-1 receptor agonists also may have beneficial endothelial effects. The Exenatide Study of Cardiovascular Event Lowering (EXSCEL) was designed to assess the cardiovascular safety and efficacy of extended-release exenatide in patients with type 2 diabetes mellitus with or without cardiovascular disease. This study included adults (mean age: 62 years) with type 2 diabetes mellitus; approximately 73% of patients had established cardiovascular disease (e.g., history of major clinical manifestation of coronary artery disease, ischemic cerebrovascular disease, atherosclerotic peripheral arterial disease). In this study, patients received 2 mg of extended-release exenatide or placebo subcutaneously once weekly. During the study, other antidiabetic agents also were used to achieve clinically appropriate HbA_{1c} concentrations. Other oral antidiabetic drugs used in the study included metformin hydrochloride (76.6%), sulfonylurea (36.6%), DPP-4 inhibitors (14.9%), thiazolidinediones (3.9%), and SGLT2 inhibitors (0.9%). Approximately 46.3% of patients also received insulin therapy (13.8% with insulin alone and 32.6% with insulin and one or more oral antidiabetic agents). The use of concomitant cardiovascular medications (e.g., angiotensin-converting enzyme [ACE] inhibitors, angiotensin II receptor antagonists, diuretics, β-adrenergic blocking agents, calcium-channel blocking agents, antithrombotics and anticoagulants, and lipid-lowering agents) was similar between the extended-release exenatide treatment group and the placebo group. The primary outcome was the composite of time to first occurrence of cardiovascular death, nonfatal myocardial infarction (MI), and nonfatal stroke. In this study, treatment with extended-release exenatide did not increase the risk of a major cardiovascular adverse event; additionally, there was no substantial difference in the incidence of major cardiovascular adverse events between those who received extended-release exenatide and those who received placebo (event rate 11.4 versus 12.2%, respectively).

Beneficial Effects on Renal Function In several cardiovascular outcomes trials involving the use of GLP-1 receptor agonists (e.g., liraglutide) in patients with type 2 diabetes mellitus at increased risk for cardiovascular disease or with existing cardiovascular disease, beneficial effects on renal function have been observed as a secondary outcome. GLP-1 receptor agonists may be used in patients with lower eGFR compared with SGLT2 inhibitors; however, these drugs may have greater benefits for reduction of ASCVD than for CKD progression. For further discussion of the beneficial renal effects of GLP-1 receptor agonists, see Beneficial Effects on Renal Function under Uses: Type 2 Diabetes Mellitus, in Liraglutide 68:20.06.

Dosage and Administration

■ **General** Patients should be monitored regularly (e.g., blood glucose determinations, HbA_{1c}) to determine therapeutic response.

■ **Administration** Exenatide and extended-release exenatide are intended for *self-administration* by the patient. Patients should be instructed by a healthcare professional in the preparation and use of exenatide or extended-release exenatide before first use.

Exenatide Exenatide is administered by subcutaneous injection into the abdomen, thigh, or upper arm; safety and efficacy of IV or IM administration have not been established.

Exenatide is administered within 60 minutes *before* the morning and evening meals (or before the 2 main meals of the day, approximately 6 hours or more apart); it should *not* be administered after a meal.

If a dose of exenatide is missed, that dose should be omitted and the next dose taken at the regularly scheduled time.

Exenatide should not be transferred from the injection pen to a syringe or vial. Exenatide should not be mixed with insulin in the same injection pen or vial even if they are taken at the same time. Exenatide should be used only if the solution is clear, colorless, and contains no particles.

Exenatide injection pens should be stored in the original carton and protected from light at 2–8°C before first use and at room temperature not exceeding 25°C after first use. Exenatide pens should not be frozen; the pen should be discarded if it has been frozen. Injection pens should be discarded 30 days after first use, even if some drug remains in the pen.

The manufacturer's instructions for use should be consulted for additional details about preparation and administration of exenatide.

Extended-release Exenatide Extended-release exenatide is administered by subcutaneous injection into the abdomen, thigh, or back of upper arm region; the drug must not be administered IV or IM. Patients should use a different injection site each week when administering extended-release exenatide in the same region.

Extended-release exenatide may be administered at any time during the dosing day, with or without a meal. The day of weekly administration of extended-release exenatide may be changed if necessary, provided the last dose was administered at least 3 days previously.

When extended-release exenatide is administered in conjunction with basal insulin, the drugs should be administered as separate injections; they should *not* be mixed together into a single injection. Extended-release exenatide and insulin may be injected into the same body region, but the injections should not be adjacent to each other.

If a dose of extended-release exenatide is missed, the missed dose should be administered as soon as noticed provided there are at least 3 days until the next scheduled dose; the usual regimen of extended-release exenatide (once weekly) may then be resumed. If a dose is missed and the next regularly scheduled dose is due in 1 or 2 days, the missed dose should *not* be administered; instead, the next dose should be taken on the regularly scheduled day.

Extended-release exenatide should be stored at 2–8°C up to the expiration date or until preparation for use. If needed, the drug can be stored for up to 4 weeks at room temperature *not* to exceed 25°C. Extended-release exenatide should be protected from light and should not be frozen; the drug should be discarded if it has been frozen.

The manufacturer's instructions for use should be consulted for additional details about preparation and administration of extended-release exenatide.

Reconstitution. Extended-release exenatide is supplied as a sterile, white to off-white powder in prefilled single-use injection pens and in single-dose vials; the powder must be reconstituted before administration. If the injection pen has been stored in the refrigerator, the patient should allow the pen to stand at room temperature for at least 15 minutes before starting the reconstitution procedure.

The diluent is contained in one compartment of the injection pen with the extended-release exenatide powder in another compartment; the diluent for the vial is supplied in a prefilled syringe within each single-dose tray. The diluent should only be used if it is clear and free of visible particulate matter when viewed through the prefilled syringe or the injection window of the pen.

The needle provided by the manufacturer should be attached to the injection pen and twisted clockwise until tight; the needle cover should *not* be removed at this point. Needles other than those provided by the manufacturer should not be used with the extended-release exenatide injection pen.

The injection pen is reconstituted by holding the pen upright and *slowly* turning the white knob at the bottom of the pen until a click is heard and the green label disappears; this allows the diluent and the drug powder to mix. The pen should then be tapped firmly against the palm of the hand (refer to manufacturer's instructions for use for detailed illustration) until the suspension is uniformly cloudy with no clumps when viewed through the mixing window; if particles are visible in the suspension, it should not be used. The suspension should not be injected until it is well mixed or the full dose of extended-release exenatide will not be delivered.

The vial is reconstituted by tapping it several times against a hard surface to loosen the drug powder and attaching the orange vial connector to the vial. After removing the white cap on the syringe, the orange connector is twisted onto the syringe until it is snug. While pressing down on the plunger of the syringe with the thumb, the vial and attached syringe should be shaken hard until the diluent and drug powder are mixed well and the suspension is cloudy and without clumps. The vial and syringe are then inverted and the vial is tapped gently to drain the drug suspension into the syringe. The connector is then removed from the syringe and the needle is attached to the syringe. The manufacturer's instructions for use should be consulted for additional details about reconstitution and administration of extended-release exenatide.

The reconstituted suspension in the injection pen or vial contains 2 mg of extended-release exenatide in 0.65 mL of diluent. Extended-release exenatide must be administered immediately after reconstitution; it cannot be stored for later use.

■ Dosage *Type 2 Diabetes Mellitus*

Exenatide. The recommended initial dosage of exenatide for the management of type 2 diabetes mellitus is 5 mcg subcutaneously twice daily. Based on clinical response, the dosage of exenatide may be increased to 10 mcg subcutaneously twice daily 1 month after treatment initiation.

Patients receiving exenatide in combination with a sulfonylurea may require a reduction in the dosage of the sulfonylurea to reduce the risk of hypoglycemia. (See Use with Drugs Known to Cause Hypoglycemia under Cautions: Warnings/Precautions.)

When exenatide is used in combination with insulin, the dosage of insulin should be evaluated. In patients at increased risk of hypoglycemia, a reduction in the dosage of insulin should be considered. (See Use with Drugs Known to Cause Hypoglycemia under Cautions: Warnings/Precautions.)

Extended-release Exenatide. The recommended dosage of extended-release exenatide for the management of type 2 diabetes mellitus is 2 mg subcutaneously once every 7 days (once weekly).

Patients receiving extended-release exenatide in combination with a sulfonylurea may require a reduction in the dosage of the sulfonylurea to reduce the risk of hypoglycemia.

Prior treatment with exenatide is not required when initiating extended-release exenatide therapy. If extended-release exenatide is initiated in an individual already receiving exenatide, exenatide should be discontinued. Patients changing from therapy with exenatide to extended-release exenatide may experience transient elevations (lasting approximately 2–4 weeks) in blood glucose concentrations.

■ Special Populations

No dosage adjustment of exenatide is required in patients with mild renal impairment (creatinine clearance 50–80 mL/minute). Caution should be used when initiating exenatide or increasing dosage from 5 mcg twice daily to 10 mcg twice daily in patients with moderate renal impairment (creatinine clearance 30–50 mL/minute). In a study of exenatide in patients with end-stage renal disease receiving dialysis, mean exenatide exposure increased by 3.4-fold compared with that in patients with normal renal function. Extended-release exenatide has not been studied in patients with severe renal impairment (creatinine clearance less than 30 mL/min) or in patients with end-stage renal disease receiving dialysis. However, population pharmacokinetic analysis of patients with renal impairment who received extended-release exenatide 2 mg indicates that exposure to the drug is increased by 62 or 33% in those with moderate or mild renal impairment, respectively. Exenatide and extended-release exenatide should not be used in patients with end-stage renal disease or severe renal impairment (creatinine clearance less than 30 mL/minute for exenatide or estimated glomerular filtration rate [eGFR] less than 45 mL/minute per 1.73 m^2 for extended-release exenatide) and should be used with caution in patients with moderate renal impairment or in those who have undergone renal transplantation. (See Renal Impairment under Warnings/Precautions: Specific Populations, in Cautions.)

The pharmacokinetics of exenatide have not been studied in patients with acute or chronic hepatic impairment. However, since exenatide is eliminated principally by the kidney, dosage adjustments are not expected to be necessary in patients with hepatic impairment.

Careful dosage selection is recommended in geriatric patients due to possible age-related decrease in renal function and concomitant disease and drug therapy; however, dosage requirements generally are similar in geriatric patients and younger adults. Caution should be used when initiating extended-release exenatide in geriatric patients.

Population pharmacokinetic analysis suggests that body mass index has no clinically important effect on the pharmacokinetics of exenatide, and gender and race do not affect steady-state concentrations of exenatide following administration of extended-release exenatide.

Cautions

■ Contraindications

Known hypersensitivity to exenatide or any ingredient in the formulation.

Extended-release exenatide is contraindicated in patients with a personal or family history of medullary thyroid carcinoma (MTC) and in patients with multiple endocrine neoplasia syndrome type 2 (MEN 2).

■ Warnings/Precautions

Warnings

Risk of Thyroid C-cell Tumors with Extended-release Exenatide. Extended-release exenatide causes a dose-dependent and treatment-duration-dependent increase in the incidence of thyroid C-cell tumors (adenomas and/or carcinomas) at clinically relevant exposures in male and female rats compared with controls. The manufacturer states the potential of extended-release exenatide to induce C-cell tumors in mice has not been established. Other glucagon-like peptide-1 (GLP-1) receptor agonists also have induced thyroid C-cell adenomas and carcinomas in male and female mice and rats at clinically relevant exposures. It is unknown whether extended-release exenatide causes thyroid C-cell tumors, including MTC, in humans. Serum calcitonin, a biologic marker of MTC, was not assessed in clinical trials evaluating the use of extended-release exenatide. Patients with MTC typically have serum calcitonin concentrations exceeding 50 ng/L. Patients receiving extended-release exenatide who have thyroid nodules noted on physical examination or neck imaging should be referred to an endocrinologist for further evaluation. Although routine monitoring of serum calcitonin or using thyroid ultrasound for early detection of MTC in patients receiving extended-release exenatide is of uncertain value, patients should also be referred to an endocrinologist for further evaluation if serum calcitonin is measured and found to be elevated.

Sensitivity Reactions

Generalized pruritus and/or urticaria and macular or papular rash have been reported during postmarketing experience with exenatide. Serious hypersensitivity reactions (e.g., angioedema, anaphylaxis) also have been reported. If a hypersensitivity reaction occurs, exenatide or extended-release exenatide and other suspect agents should be discontinued, and the patient should seek medical advice promptly. Patients with a history of anaphylaxis or angioedema with another GLP-1 receptor agonist should be monitored closely for allergic reactions; it is unknown whether such patients will be predisposed to anaphylaxis with extended-release exenatide.

Other Warnings and Precautions

Pancreatitis and Pancreatic Precancerous Changes. Acute pancreatitis, including fatal and nonfatal hemorrhagic or necrotizing pancreatitis requiring hospitalization, has been reported during postmarketing experience with exenatide. Persistent, severe abdominal pain, which may be accompanied by vomiting, is the hallmark symptom of acute pancreatitis. Most patients who have developed pancreatitis during exenatide therapy had at least one other risk factor for acute pancreatitis (e.g., gallstones, severe hypertriglyceridemia, alcohol use) and have required hospitalization. Some patients have developed serious complications including dehydration and renal failure, suspected ileus, phlegmon, and ascites. Acute or worsening pancreatitis has been associated temporally with an increase in exenatide dosage from 5 to 10 mcg twice daily, the maximum recommended dosage, in some patients. Symptoms of acute pancreatitis (e.g., nausea, vomiting, abdominal pain) recurred upon rechallenge with the drug in several patients; abdominal pain abated after permanent discontinuance of the drug in one patient. Most patients have improved upon discontinuance of exenatide.

FDA has been evaluating unpublished findings suggesting an increased risk of pancreatitis and precancerous pancreatic cellular changes (pancreatic duct metaplasia) in patients with type 2 diabetes mellitus receiving incretin mimetics (exenatide, liraglutide, sitagliptin, saxagliptin, alogliptin, or linagliptin). These findings are based on examination of a small number of pancreatic tissue specimens taken from patients who died from unspecified causes while receiving an incretin mimetic. FDA will notify healthcare professionals of its conclusions and recommendations when the review is complete, or when the agency has additional information to report.

FDA has recommended that clinicians continue to follow the recommendations in the prescribing information for incretin mimetics. The manufacturer states that after initiation of exenatide or extended-release exenatide and after increases in dosage, patients should be observed carefully for signs and symptoms of acute pancreatitis (e.g., unexplained, persistent severe abdominal pain that may radiate to the back; nausea; vomiting; elevated serum amylase or lipase concentrations). If pancreatitis is suspected, therapy with exenatide or extended-release exenatide and other potentially suspect drugs should be promptly discontinued, confirmatory tests performed (e.g., serum amylase or lipase concentrations, radiologic imaging), and appropriate therapy initiated. Exenatide or extended-release exenatide should *not* be resumed if pancreatitis is confirmed.

Safety and efficacy of exenatide or extended-release exenatide have not been established in patients with a history of pancreatitis; other antidiabetic therapies should be considered in such patients.

Use with Drugs Known to Cause Hypoglycemia. The risk of hypoglycemia is increased when exenatide or extended-release exenatide is used in combination with a sulfonylurea. Therefore, patients receiving exenatide or extended-release exenatide in combination with a sulfonylurea may require a reduction in the dosage of the sulfonylurea to reduce the risk of hypoglycemia.

When exenatide is used in combination with insulin, the dosage of insulin should be evaluated. In a clinical trial in which exenatide was added to insulin glargine therapy, the dosage of insulin glargine was reduced by 20% in patients with HbA_{1c} concentrations of 8% or less; however, some clinicians suggest that the relative safety and efficacy of this approach to dosage adjustment of basal insulin may not apply to patients with baseline HbA_{1c} concentrations of less than 7%, those with a recent history of major hypoglycemia, or those receiving long-acting GLP-1 receptor agonists. In patients at increased risk of hypoglycemia, a reduction in the dosage of insulin should be considered. (See Dosage and Administration: Dosage.) The safety and efficacy of exenatide or extended-release exenatide in combination with *prandial* insulin have not been established, and the manufacturer of exenatide states that such concomitant use is not recommended.

The use of exenatide or extended-release exenatide in combination with other glucose-independent insulin secretagogues (e.g., meglitinides) also may increase the risk of hypoglycemia.

Renal Effects. Deterioration of renal function (e.g., increased serum creatinine concentrations, renal impairment/insufficiency, worsened chronic renal failure, acute renal failure sometimes requiring hemodialysis or kidney transplantation) has been reported rarely with exenatide. Some of these events occurred in patients experiencing nausea, vomiting, and/or diarrhea with or without dehydration; these adverse effects may have contributed to development of altered renal function in these patients. Some of these events also occurred in patients receiving exenatide in combination with other agents known to affect renal function or hydration status (e.g., angiotensin-converting enzyme inhibitors, nonsteroidal anti-inflammatory agents, diuretics).

Exenatide has not been found to be directly nephrotoxic in preclinical or clinical studies. Renal effects usually have been reversible with supportive treatment and discontinuance of potentially causative agents, including exenatide. Altered renal function may be a consequence of diabetes mellitus, independent of any risk associated with exenatide therapy. Because exenatide or extended-release exenatide may induce nausea and vomiting with transient hypovolemia, treatment with this drug may worsen renal function.

Clinicians should closely monitor patients receiving exenatide for signs and symptoms of renal dysfunction and consider discontinuance of the drug if renal dysfunction is suspected and cannot be explained by other causes. (See Renal Impairment under Warnings/Precautions: Specific Populations, in Cautions.)

GI Effects. Data are lacking on the use of exenatide in patients with severe GI disease, including gastroparesis. Use of exenatide is commonly associated with adverse GI effects, including nausea, vomiting, and diarrhea. Nausea, vomiting, and/or diarrhea resulting in dehydration, abdominal distention, abdominal pain, eructation, constipation, flatulence, acute pancreatitis, and hemorrhagic and necrotizing pancreatitis sometimes resulting in death have been reported during postmarketing experience with exenatide. Use of exenatide or extended-release exenatide is not recommended in patients with severe GI disease.

Immunogenicity. Antibodies to exenatide have developed in patients receiving exenatide or extended-release exenatide therapy. Antibodies to exenatide were assessed in 90% of patients in the 30-, 16-, and 24-week clinical trials of exenatide with or without other antidiabetic therapy. Patients in these trials who had low-titer (e.g., less than 625) antibodies to exenatide (38, 31, or 28% of patients assessed for antibodies in the 3 clinical trials at 30, 16, or 24 weeks, respectively) generally had glycemic control (based on glycosylated hemoglobin [HbA_{1c}]) comparable to that of patients without antibodies. Of patients who had higher (e.g., 625 or higher) antibody titers (6, 9, or 2% of patients assessed for antibodies in the 3 clinical trials, respectively), 3, 4, or 1% of patients, respectively, appeared to have an attenuated glycemic response.

Anti-exenatide antibodies were measured in all patients who received extended-release exenatide in 5 comparator-controlled studies that ranged from 24–30 weeks in duration. In patients with low-titer antibodies (49% of patients at any time during the study and 45% of patients at study end point), the level of glycemic control was comparable to that observed in the 43% of patients without antibody titers. In addition, of patients with higher antibody titers at study end point (12% of patients), approximately half (6% of overall patients) treated with extended-release exenatide had an attenuated glycemic response. The remaining patients had a glycemic response comparable to that of patients without antibodies. If worsening glycemic control or failure to achieve targeted glycemic control occurs in patients receiving exenatide or extended-release exenatide therapy, alternative antidiabetic therapy should be considered.

Approximately 210 patients with anti-exenatide antibodies in clinical trials were evaluated for cross-reactive antibodies to GLP-1 and/or glucagon, and treatment-emergent cross-reactive antibodies were not observed across the range of titers.

Injection-site Reactions. Serious injection-site reactions (e.g., abscess, cellulitis, necrosis) with or without subcutaneous nodules have been reported during postmarketing experience in patients receiving extended-release exenatide; in isolated cases, surgical intervention was required. Injection-site reactions also have been reported with exenatide during postmarketing experience.

The incidence of injection-site reactions for patients treated with extended-release exenatide was similar for patients with antibodies to the drug and those without evidence of such antibody development (5.8 and 7%, respectively). In the 5 comparator-controlled clinical studies, injection-site reactions were observed more frequently in patients treated with extended-release exenatide (17.1%) than in patients treated with exenatide (12.7%), titrated insulin glargine (1.8%), or in those patients who received placebo injections (sitagliptin [10.6%], pioglitazone [6.4%], and metformin [13%] treatment arms). For patients treated with extended-release exenatide, injection-site reactions were more commonly observed in antibody-positive patients (14.2%) versus antibody-negative patients (3.1%), with a greater incidence in those with higher titer antibodies.

Risk Associated with Sharing of Injection Pens. Exenatide and extended-release exenatide injection pens must never be shared among patients, even if the needle has been changed. Sharing of injection pens poses a risk for transmission of blood-borne pathogens.

Acute Gallbladder Disease. Acute events of gallbladder disease have been reported with GLP-1 receptor agonist use, including extended-release exenatide, during clinical studies. In the EXSCEL study, 1.9% of patients who received extended-release exenatide and 1.4% of those who received placebo reported an acute event of gallbladder disease (e.g., cholelithiasis, cholecystitis). If cholelithiasis is suspected, the manufacturer states that gallbladder studies and appropriate clinical follow-up are indicated.

Specific Populations

Pregnancy. Data are lacking on the use of exenatide or extended-release exenatide in pregnant women. In animal reproduction studies in rats, exenatide or extended-release exenatide use during pregnancy was associated with reduced fetal growth and skeletal ossification deficits. In animal reproduction studies in mice, exenatide use was associated with an increased number of neonatal deaths. Exenatide or extended-release exenatide should be used during pregnancy only if the potential benefit justifies the potential risk to the fetus.

Lactation. Exenatide is distributed into milk in mice. It is not known whether exenatide is distributed into human milk. The benefits of breast-feeding and the importance of exenatide or extended-release exenatide to the woman should be considered along with any potential adverse effects on the breast-fed infant from the drug or from the underlying maternal condition.

Pediatric Use. Safety and efficacy of exenatide have not been established in patients younger than 17 years of age. Safety and efficacy of extended-release exenatide have not been established in pediatric patients, and the manufacturer states that use of the drug in this patient population is not recommended.

Geriatric Use. No substantial differences in safety and efficacy nor in pharmacokinetics have been observed in geriatric patients relative to younger adults. Because geriatric patients are more likely to have decreased renal function, caution should be used when initiating therapy with the drug in such patients.

Hepatic Impairment. Exenatide has not been studied in patients with a diagnosis of acute or chronic hepatic impairment. Because exenatide is cleared principally by the kidney, hepatic dysfunction is not expected to affect blood concentrations of the drug, and the manufacturer makes no specific dosage recommendations for patients with hepatic impairment.

Renal Impairment. Use of exenatide or extended-release exenatide is not recommended in patients with end-stage renal disease or severe renal impairment (creatinine clearance less than 30 mL/minute for exenatide or estimated glomerular filtration rate [eGFR] less than 45 mL/minute per 1.73 m^2 for extended-release exenatide); the drug should be used with caution in patients who have undergone renal transplantation. In patients with end-stage renal disease receiving dialysis, mean exenatide clearance was reduced to 0.9 L/hour compared with 9.1 L/hour in patients without renal disease, and single 5-mcg doses of exenatide were not well tolerated in patients with end-stage renal disease because of adverse GI effects. Because exenatide or extended-release exenatide may induce nausea and vomiting with transient hypovolemia, treatment with this drug may worsen renal function. (See Renal Effects under Cautions: Warnings/Precautions.) Safety and efficacy of extended-release exenatide have not been established in patients with end-stage renal disease or severe renal impairment.

In patients with mild renal impairment (creatinine clearance 50–80 mL/minute), no adjustment of exenatide dosage is required. Caution should be used when initiating exenatide or increasing exenatide dosage from 5 mcg twice daily to 10 mcg twice daily in patients with moderate renal impairment (creatinine clearance 30–50 mL/minute). Patients receiving extended-release exenatide who have mild renal impairment should be monitored for adverse effects (e.g., nausea and vomiting) that may lead to hypovolemia. In patients with mild to moderate renal impairment (creatinine clearance 30–80 mL/minute), systemic exposure to exenatide was similar to that in individuals with normal renal function. (See Renal Effects under Cautions: Warnings/Precautions.)

Extended-release exenatide should be used with caution in patients with moderate renal impairment (creatinine clearance 30–50 mL/minute).

■ Common Adverse Effects

Hypoglycemia occurred in at least 5% of patients receiving exenatide in overall clinical trials and more frequently than with placebo. In individual clinical trials, hypoglycemia was reported in 5.2 or 3.8% of patients receiving exenatide 5 or 10 mcg twice daily, respectively, as monotherapy; in 4.5 or 5.3% of patients receiving exenatide 5 or 10 mcg twice daily, respectively, in combination with metformin; in 14.4 or 35.7% of patients receiving exenatide 5 or 10 mcg twice daily, respectively, in combination with a sulfonylurea; in 19.2 or 27.8% of patients receiving exenatide 5 or 10 mcg twice daily, respectively, in combination with metformin and a sulfonylurea; in 10.7% of patients receiving exenatide 10 mcg twice daily in combination with a thiazolidinedione; and in 24.8% of patients receiving exenatide 10 mcg twice daily in combination with insulin glargine.

Adverse effects other than hypoglycemia reported in at least 2% of patients receiving exenatide in combination with other oral antidiabetic agents in clinical trials and more frequently than with placebo include nausea, vomiting, diarrhea, jittery feeling, dizziness, headache, dyspepsia, asthenia, gastroesophageal reflux disease, hyperhidrosis, constipation, abdominal distention, decreased appetite, and flatulence.

There were no reported cases of major hypoglycemia in 5 comparator-controlled, 24- to 30-week clinical studies in patients receiving 2 mg of extended-release exenatide once weekly. In these studies, major hypoglycemia was defined as a glucose concentration of less than 54 mg/dL accompanied by loss of consciousness, seizure, or coma (or other mental status change consistent with neuroglycopenia in the judgment of the investigator or clinician) that resolved after the administration of glucagon or glucose or required third-party assistance to resolve because of severe impairment in consciousness or behavior. Minor hypoglycemia (defined as symptoms of hypoglycemia with a concomitant glucose concentration of less than 54 mg/dL and ability of the patient to self-treat) in these studies was reported in 2% of patients receiving extended-release exenatide as monotherapy; 1.3 or 3.7% of patients receiving extended-release exenatide in combination with metformin; and in 20% of patients receiving extended-release exenatide in combination with metformin and a sulfonylurea. Minor hypoglycemia occurred in 12.5 or 14.5% of patients receiving extended-release exenatide with metformin, a sulfonylurea, a thiazolidinedione, or a combination of these agents but was *not* reported in patients who received one of these same regimens without concomitant sulfonylurea therapy.

Adverse effects other than hypoglycemia reported in at least 5% of patients receiving extended-release exenatide as monotherapy or in combination with other oral antidiabetic agents (metformin, a sulfonylurea, a thiazolidinedione, or a combination of these drugs) include nausea, diarrhea, injection-site pruritus, vomiting, injection-site nodule, constipation, headache, viral gastroenteritis, gastroesophageal reflux disease, dyspepsia, injection-site erythema, fatigue, injection-site hematoma, and decreased appetite.

Drug Interactions

■ **Effects on GI Absorption of Other Drugs** The effect of exenatide-induced slowing of gastric emptying may reduce the rate and extent of absorption of concomitantly administered oral drugs. Exenatide should be used with caution in patients receiving oral drugs that have a narrow therapeutic index or require rapid GI absorption. In patients receiving oral drugs for which efficacy depends on threshold concentrations, such as oral contraceptives and anti-infective agents, those drugs should be taken at least 1 hour before exenatide administration. If such drugs need to be administered with food, patients should take them with a meal or snack (e.g., lunch) at a time when exenatide is not administered.

Because of the potential for similar effects of extended-release exenatide on concomitant oral drug absorption, caution should be used with such concomitant use.

■ **Acetaminophen** When acetaminophen (1 g) was administered simultaneously with subcutaneous exenatide (10 mcg) or 1, 2, or 4 hours following exenatide injection, acetaminophen area under the concentration-time curve (AUC) decreased by 21, 23, 24, or 14%, respectively; peak plasma concentrations decreased by 37, 56, 54, or 41%, respectively; and time to peak plasma concentrations increased from 0.6 hours to 0.9, 4.2, 3.3, or 1.6 hours, respectively; however, acetaminophen AUC, peak plasma concentration, and time to peak plasma concentration were not appreciably changed when acetaminophen was given 1 hour prior to exenatide.

When acetaminophen (1 g) was administered either with or without a meal following 14 weeks of therapy with subcutaneous extended-release exenatide (2 mg once weekly), no substantial changes in acetaminophen AUC were observed compared with control. Acetaminophen peak plasma concentration was reduced by 16% (fasting) and 5% (fed), and time to peak plasma concentration was increased from approximately 1 hour in the control period to 1.4 and 1.3 hours in the fasting and fed states, respectively.

■ **Antidiabetic Agents** The risk of hypoglycemia is increased when exenatide or extended-release exenatide is used in combination with a sulfonylurea; patients receiving these exenatide formulations concomitantly with a sulfonylurea may require a reduction in the dosage of the sulfonylurea.

When exenatide is used in combination with insulin, the dosage of insulin should be evaluated; in patients at increased risk of hypoglycemia, a reduction in the dosage of insulin should be considered. (See Dosage and Administration: Dosage.) The safety and efficacy of exenatide or extended-release exenatide in combination with *prandial* insulin have not been established, and the manufacturer of exenatide states that such concomitant use is not recommended.

The use of exenatide or extended-release exenatide in combination with other glucose-independent insulin secretagogues (e.g., meglitinides) may increase the risk of hypoglycemia.

■ **Anti-infective Agents** The effect of exenatide-induced slowing of gastric emptying may reduce the rate and extent of absorption of concomitantly administered oral anti-infective agents. Oral anti-infective agents should be taken at least 1 hour before exenatide administration. (See Drug Interactions: Effects on GI Absorption of Other Drugs.)

■ **Digoxin** Administration of exenatide (10 mcg subcutaneously twice daily) 30 minutes before digoxin (0.25 mg orally once daily) decreased the peak plasma concentration of digoxin by 17% and delayed the time to peak plasma concentration of digoxin by approximately 2.5 hours; however, there was no change in the overall steady-state AUC and renal clearance of digoxin.

■ **Lisinopril** In patients with mild to moderate hypertension receiving stable dosages of lisinopril (5–20 mg daily), exenatide (10 mcg subcutaneously twice daily) did not alter the steady-state AUC or peak plasma concentration of lisinopril or the 24-hour mean systolic and diastolic blood pressure. However, the steady-state time to peak plasma concentration of lisinopril was delayed by 2 hours.

■ **Lovastatin** Administration of exenatide (10 mcg subcutaneously twice daily) 30 minutes before lovastatin (single 40-mg oral dose) decreased the lovastatin AUC and peak plasma concentration by approximately 40 and 28%, respectively, and delayed the time to peak plasma concentration of lovastatin by 4 hours. In clinical trials, the use of exenatide in patients already receiving HMG-CoA reductase inhibitors (statins) was not associated with consistent changes in lipid profiles compared to baseline.

■ **Oral Contraceptives** In healthy women, repeated daily administration of a fixed-combination oral contraceptive (30 mcg of ethinyl estradiol and 150 mcg of levonorgestrel) 30 minutes after subcutaneous injection of exenatide (10 mcg twice daily) decreased the peak plasma concentrations of ethinyl estradiol and levonorgestrel by 45 and 27%, respectively, and delayed the time to peak plasma concentrations of ethinyl estradiol and levonorgestrel by 3 and 3.5 hours, respectively. Repeated daily administration of the fixed-combination oral contraceptive 1 hour prior to administration of exenatide decreased the mean peak plasma concentration of ethinyl estradiol by 15%; however, the mean peak plasma concentration of levonorgestrel was not substantially changed. Exenatide did not alter the mean trough concentrations of levonorgestrel following repeated daily administration of the fixed-combination oral contraceptive for both regimens; however, the mean trough concentration of ethinyl estradiol increased by 20% when the fixed-combination oral contraceptive was administered 30 minutes after exenatide injection. In this study, the effect of exenatide on the pharmacokinetics of oral contraceptives was confounded by the possible effect of food on oral contraceptives. Therefore, oral contraceptives should be administered at least 1 hour prior to exenatide administration. (See Drug Interactions: Effects on GI Absorption of Other Drugs.)

■ **Warfarin** Increases in international normalized ratio [INR], sometimes associated with bleeding, have been reported during postmarketing experience with concomitant use of exenatide and warfarin. In a drug interaction study, no clinically important changes in warfarin (*S*- or *R*-enantiomer) AUC, peak plasma concentrations, or therapeutic response (as indicated by INR) were observed when warfarin sodium (single 25-mg dose) was administered 35 minutes after exenatide (5 mcg subcutaneously twice daily for 2 days, then 10 mcg twice daily for 7 days); however, the time to peak warfarin concentration was delayed by approximately 2 hours. In patients receiving warfarin, prothrombin time should be monitored more frequently after initiating or altering exenatide therapy; once a stable prothrombin time has been achieved, prothrombin times may be monitored at intervals usually recommended for patients receiving warfarin therapy.

Data are lacking on the effects of concomitant therapy with warfarin and extended-release exenatide. After initiation of extended-release exenatide in patients receiving warfarin concomitantly, the INR should be monitored more frequently. Once a stable INR has been documented, the INR can be monitored at intervals generally recommended for patients receiving warfarin therapy.

Description

Exenatide, a synthetic analog of a naturally occurring peptide isolated from the saliva of *Heloderma suspectum* (Gila monster), is a glucagon-like peptide-1 (GLP-1) mimetic (incretin mimetic). Exenatide has 53% amino acid similarity to human GLP-1 and is structurally and pharmacologically unrelated to insulin, sulfonylureas, meglitinides, biguanides, thiazolidinediones, and α-glucosidase inhibitors. Several antihyperglycemic actions of exenatide similar to the effects of human GLP-1 are involved in the lowering of fasting and postprandial glucose concentrations in patients with type 2 diabetes mellitus. The drug improves pancreatic β-cell function by increasing glucose-dependent insulin synthesis, secretion, and acute β-cell responsiveness (i.e., first phase insulin response). In contrast to sulfonylureas, stimulation of insulin secretion by exenatide subsides as blood glucose concentrations following a meal decrease and approach euglycemia. Exenatide inhibits inappropriately high glucagon secretion during episodes of hyperglycemia (e.g., after a meal) in patients with type 2 diabetes mellitus but does not impair the normal glucagon response to hypoglycemia. In addition, exenatide slows gastric emptying, which reduces the rate of glucose absorption from a meal, reduces food intake, and is associated with weight loss; the drug also may reduce appetite and promote early satiety. Exenatide does not appear to be associated with clinically important prolongation of the QT interval (corrected for rate using Bazett's formula [QT_c]).

Extended-release exenatide consists of exenatide incorporated in an extended-release microsphere formulation containing the 50:50 poly(D,L-lactide-co-glycolide) polymer along with sucrose. Each dose of extended-release exenatide contains 37.2 mg of the polymer and 0.8 mg of sucrose. Following a single dose of exenatide given as the extended-release formulation, the drug is released from the microspheres over approximately 10 weeks. Exenatide plasma concentration peaks around week 2 and week 6–7 after administration of the extended-release formulation, representing an initial surface-bound release and then a more gradual release of the drug from microspheres. Steady-state plasma concentrations of the drug are reached at approximately 6–7 weeks with once-weekly (every 7 days) administration. Plasma exenatide concentrations generally fall to undetectable levels approximately 10 weeks after discontinuance of dosing.

Advice to Patients

Importance of instructing patients on proper use and storage of the exenatide or extended-release exenatide injection pen, including proper reconstitution and injection technique to ensure delivery of a full dose, proper disposal of injection pens and needles using puncture-resistant containers, how and when to set up a new injection pen, and that only one setup step is necessary at initial use of exenatide. Importance of reading manufacturer's patient information (e.g., medication guide) and the injection pen user manual before starting therapy with exenatide or extended-release exenatide and of reviewing this information each time the prescription is refilled. Importance of patients not *self-administering* exenatide or extended-release exenatide if they are blind or unable to see well.

Importance of providing information regarding the potential risks and advantages of exenatide or extended-release exenatide therapy and of alternative modes of treatment. Importance of not using exenatide or extended-release exenatide in patients with type 1 diabetes mellitus or diabetic ketoacidosis.

Importance of providing instruction regarding diabetes self-management practices, such as regular physical activity, adhering to meal planning, periodic blood glucose monitoring, glycosylated hemoglobin (hemoglobin A_{1c} [HbA_{1c}]) testing, recognition and management of hypoglycemia and hyperglycemia, and assessment of other diabetic complications.

Importance of informing patients that extended-release exenatide causes benign and malignant thyroid C-cell tumors in rats and that the relevance of this finding in humans is unknown. Importance of not using extended-release exenatide in patients with a personal or family history of medullary thyroid cancer (MTC) or diagnosis of multiple endocrine neoplasia syndrome type 2 (MEN 2). Importance of advising patients receiving extended-release exenatide to report symptoms such as a lump or swelling in the neck, hoarseness, dysphagia, or dyspnea, which may be suggestive of thyroid cancer.

Importance of patients discontinuing exenatide or extended-release exenatide and other suspect drugs and seeking medical assistance immediately if signs and symptoms of a serious hypersensitivity reaction (e.g., anaphylaxis, angioedema) occur. Importance of patients informing their clinician if they have experienced a sensitivity reaction to exenatide or any ingredient in the formulations.

Importance of informing patients of the potential risk of acute pancreatitis, which may be severe and lead to death. Importance of patient informing clinicians about a history of pancreatitis, gallstones, alcoholism, or high triglyceride concentrations. Importance of patients discontinuing exenatide or extended-release exenatide and promptly informing clinician if unexplained, persistent, severe abdominal pain that may radiate to the back and may or may not be accompanied by nausea and vomiting occurs; these symptoms may be associated with acute pancreatitis. If pancreatitis is suspected, exenatide or extended-release exenatide should be promptly discontinued and not restarted if pancreatitis is confirmed.

Importance of informing patients of the potential risk for worsening renal function and about signs and symptoms of altered renal function (e.g., increased serum creatinine; changes in color, frequency, or amount of urination; unexplained swelling in extremities; increases in blood pressure; lethargy; changes in appetite or digestion; dull ache in the middle to lower back). Importance of patient informing clinician about development of nausea, vomiting, or diarrhea because of potential contribution of these effects to dehydration and consequent altered renal function. Importance of informing patients that chronic conditions such as hypertension or pancreatitis and concomitant therapy with nonsteroidal anti-inflammatory agents (NSAIAs), diuretics, or antihypertensive agents can increase the risk of developing altered renal function with exenatide therapy.

Importance of informing patients receiving exenatide that the dosage of concomitant insulin may need to be reduced in those at increased risk of hypoglycemia. Increased risk of hypoglycemia when exenatide or extended-release exenatide is used in combination with an agent that induces hypoglycemia, such as a sulfonylurea or other glucose-independent insulin secretagogue (e.g., meglitinide). Importance of informing patients that a lower dosage of sulfonylurea or other insulin secretagogue may be required to reduce the risk of hypoglycemia if used concomitantly with exenatide. Importance of reviewing with patients the symptoms, treatment, and conditions that predispose to development of hypoglycemia when initiating exenatide or extended-release exenatide treatment, especially when exenatide is administered concomitantly with a sulfonylurea or insulin; importance of clinician reinforcing instructions for management of hypoglycemia. (See Use with Drugs Known to Cause Hypoglycemia under Cautions: Warnings/Precautions.)

Importance of advising patients to seek medical advice if symptomatic subcutaneous injection-site nodules or any signs or symptoms of abscess, cellulitis, or necrosis occur.

Importance of informing patients of the potential risk for cholelithiasis or cholecystitis. Importance of instructing patients to contact a clinician for appropriate clinical follow-up if cholelithiasis or cholecystitis is suspected.

Importance of informing patients that reduced appetite, food intake, and/or body weight may occur with exenatide or extended-release exenatide therapy but do not require modification of dosage regimen. Importance of informing patient about occurrence of nausea, particularly upon initiation of exenatide or extended-release exenatide therapy, and that nausea decreases over time as the drug is continued.

Importance of informing patients that exenatide or extended-release exenatide injection pens should *not* be shared with another person, even if the needle has been changed. Sharing of the injection pen among patients may pose a risk of transmitting or acquiring infection.

Importance of informing patients regarding the timing of exenatide or extended-release exenatide administration with concomitant oral drugs, such as oral contraceptives and anti-infective agents, because of slowing of gastric emptying with these exenatide formulations. (See Drug Interactions: Effects on GI Absorption of Other Drugs.)

Importance of not mixing exenatide with insulin.

Importance of advising patients what to do if a dose of exenatide or extended-release exenatide is missed. (See Dosage and Administration: Administration.)

Importance of injecting extended-release exenatide immediately after reconstitution. Importance of *not* injecting exenatide or extended-release exenatide IV or IM. Importance of informing patient that extended-release exenatide should be administered as a subcutaneous injection at any time on the dosing day, with or without meals. Importance of informing patients that the day of once-weekly administration (once every 7 days) can be changed if necessary, provided the last dose was administered 3 or more days previously.

Importance of informing patients to discontinue exenatide once extended-release exenatide is initiated. Importance of informing patients that transient elevations in blood glucose concentrations may occur but generally improve within the first 2 weeks after initiation of extended-release exenatide therapy.

Importance of women informing clinicians if they are or plan to become pregnant or plan to breast-feed. Importance of informing women about enrolling in the pregnancy registry for exenatide or extended-release exenatide if they use the drugs at any time during pregnancy.

Importance of informing clinicians of existing or contemplated concomitant therapy, including prescription and OTC drugs, vitamins, and herbal supplements, as well as any concomitant illnesses (e.g., hypertension, history of liver disease, gastroparesis or serious digestive problems, severe kidney disease or kidney transplant).

Importance of informing patients of other important precautionary information. (See Cautions.)

Overview® (see Users Guide). For additional information on this drug until a more detailed monograph is developed and published, the manufacturer's labeling should be consulted. It is *essential* that the manufacturer's labeling be consulted for more detailed information on usual cautions, precautions, contraindications, potential drug interactions, laboratory test interferences, and acute toxicity.

Preparations

Excipients in commercially available drug preparations may have clinically important effects in some individuals; consult specific product labeling for details.

Exenatide

Parenteral		
Injection, for subcutaneous use	250 mcg/mL	Byetta® (available as prefilled cartridge pen), AstraZeneca
For injection, extended-release, for subcutaneous use	2 mg	Bydureon® (available as single-dose, prefilled, dual-chambered injection pen with diluent and as single-dose vial with vial connector and prefilled syringe containing diluent), AstraZeneca

Liraglutide

Insulin Degludec and Liraglutide

■ Liraglutide, a synthetic, long-acting human glucagon-like peptide-1 (GLP-1) receptor agonist (incretin mimetic), is an antidiabetic agent and antiobesity drug.

Uses

Liraglutide is used as an adjunct to diet and exercise to improve glycemic control in patients with type 2 diabetes mellitus and as an adjunct to caloric restriction and increased physical activity for the long-term management of obesity. Liraglutide also is used to reduce the risk of major adverse cardiovascular events (i.e., cardiovascular death, nonfatal myocardial infarction [MI], nonfatal stroke) in patients with type 2 diabetes mellitus and established cardiovascular disease. Liraglutide in fixed combination with insulin degludec (Xultophy®) is used as an adjunct to diet and exercise to improve glycemic control in adults with type 2 diabetes mellitus.

The fixed combination of insulin degludec and liraglutide should not be used for the treatment of diabetic ketoacidosis or for the treatment of type 1 diabetes mellitus. Insulin degludec and liraglutide in fixed combination should not be used in combination with any other preparation containing liraglutide or another glucagon-like peptide-1 (GLP-1) receptor agonist.

Saxenda® and Victoza® both contain liraglutide and therefore should not be used together.

■ **Type 2 Diabetes Mellitus** Liraglutide is used as an adjunct to diet and exercise to improve glycemic control in patients with type 2 diabetes mellitus. Liraglutide has been used alone or as add-on therapy with metformin, a sulfonylurea, insulin, or the combination of metformin and a sulfonylurea or thiazolidinedione.

Current guidelines for the treatment of type 2 diabetes mellitus generally recommend metformin as first-line therapy in addition to lifestyle modifications because of its well-established safety and efficacy (e.g., beneficial effects on glycosylated hemoglobin [hemoglobin A_{1c}; HbA_{1c}], weight, and cardiovascular mortality) in patients with recent-onset or newly diagnosed type 2 diabetes mellitus or mild hyperglycemia. Because of the progressive nature of the disease, patients initially receiving an oral antidiabetic agent will eventually require multiple oral and/or injectable antidiabetic agents of different therapeutic classes and/or insulin for adequate glycemic control. Patients with inadequate glycemic control with metformin monotherapy should receive treatment with additional antidiabetic agents; data suggest that the addition of each noninsulin agent to initial therapy lowers HbA_{1c} by approximately 0.7–1%. Some experts recommend initiating antidiabetic therapy with 2 agents (metformin plus another agent) in patients whose HbA_{1c} is 7.5% or higher, while other experts recommend initiating such dual therapy in patients whose HbA_{1c} is at least 1.5% above the target level. When the greater glucose-lowering effect of an injectable drug is needed, some experts suggest that glucagon-like peptide-1 (GLP-1) receptor agonists are preferred over insulin. Early introduction of insulin therapy should be considered when hyperglycemia is severe (e.g., blood glucose of at least 300 mg/dL, HbA_{1c} of at least 10%), especially in the presence of catabolic manifestations (e.g., weight loss, hypertriglyceridemia, ketosis), or if symptoms of hyperglycemia are present. For additional information regarding the initiation of insulin therapy, see Uses: Diabetes Mellitus, in the Insulins General Statement 68:20.08.

Experts state that a patient's comorbidities should be considered when selecting additional (in addition to metformin) antidiabetic agents. Patients with type 2 diabetes mellitus who have established atherosclerotic cardiovascular disease (ASCVD) should receive a drug with demonstrated cardiovascular disease benefit (e.g., GLP-1 receptor agonist [e.g., liraglutide], sodium-glucose cotransporter 2 [SGLT2] inhibitor [e.g., canagliflozin, empagliflozin]). In patients with ASCVD and heart failure or with an increased risk of heart failure, an SGLT2 inhibitor with demonstrated cardiovascular benefit may be preferred. An SGLT2 inhibitor or GLP-1 receptor agonist shown to reduce the risk of chronic kidney disease (CKD) progression, cardiovascular events, or both (e.g., canagliflozin, empagliflozin, liraglutide) should be considered in patients with type 2 diabetes mellitus and CKD. Experts state that SGLT2 inhibitors may be a good choice for patients at high risk of CKD progression (i.e., patients with albuminuria or a history of estimated glomerular filtration rate [eGFR] decline) because they may have a beneficial effect on the incidence of CKD; however, adequate renal function is required for their use. Some GLP-1 receptor agonists may be used in patients with lower eGFR and may provide greater benefits for reduction of ASCVD than for CKD progression or heart failure. In patients without ASCVD, heart failure, or CKD, the decision regarding the addition of other antidiabetic agents (e.g., sulfonylurea, thiazolidinedione, dipeptidyl peptidase-4 [DPP-4] inhibitor, SGLT2 inhibitor, GLP-1 receptor agonist, basal insulin) should be based on drug-specific effects and individual patient factors.

Liraglutide is not a substitute for insulin in insulin-requiring patients. The manufacturer states that liraglutide should not be used in patients with type 1 diabetes mellitus or for the treatment of diabetic ketoacidosis as it would not be effective in these settings.

Liraglutide Monotherapy When given as monotherapy for the management of type 2 diabetes mellitus, liraglutide improves glycemic control compared with glimepiride as evidenced by reductions from baseline in glycosylated hemoglobin (hemoglobin A_{1c}; HbA_{1c}) and fasting plasma glucose concentrations; liraglutide therapy also was associated with a reduction in body weight compared with an increase in body weight with glimepiride.

Efficacy and safety of liraglutide as monotherapy in adults with type 2 diabetes mellitus have been established in a 52-week randomized, double-blind, double-dummy trial. In this trial, 746 patients with a mean baseline HbA_{1c} concentration of 8.2% received liraglutide 1.2 or 1.8 mg subcutaneously once daily or glimepiride 8 mg orally once daily as well as corresponding placebo. All patients randomized to liraglutide received an initial dosage of 0.6 mg once daily for 1 week; dosage subsequently was titrated in increments of 0.6 mg weekly to a dosage of either 1.2 or 1.8 mg once daily. All patients randomized to glimepiride received an initial dosage of 2 mg once daily for 2 weeks, followed by 4 mg once daily for 2 weeks, and then 8 mg once daily. The primary study end point was the change in HbA_{1c} concentration from baseline to week 52 (or the last value at time of early discontinuance of therapy). At week 52, HbA_{1c} was reduced from baseline by about 0.8, 1.1, or 0.5% with once-daily liraglutide 1.2 mg, liraglutide 1.8 mg, or glimepiride 8 mg, respectively. HbA_{1c} concentrations below 7% were achieved in 43, 51, or 28% of patients receiving once-daily liraglutide 1.2 mg, liraglutide 1.8 mg, or glimepiride 8 mg, respectively. Body weight was reduced by 2.1 or 2.5 kg with liraglutide 1.2 or 1.8 mg once daily, respectively, but was increased by 1.1 kg in patients receiving glimepiride 8 mg once daily.

Combination Therapy When given as add-on therapy to metformin and/or a sulfonylurea, metformin and a thiazolidinedione, or metformin and insulin detemir in clinical trials, liraglutide was more effective than placebo and at least as effective as add-on therapy with sitagliptin, glimepiride, or exenatide in improving glycemic control (as evidenced by reduction in HbA_{1c} concentrations).

Efficacy and safety of liraglutide (1.2 or 1.8 mg subcutaneously once daily) as add-on therapy with maximally effective dosages of metformin, a sulfonylurea (e.g., glimepiride), or metformin in combination with a sulfonylurea or a thiazolidinedione were established in several studies of 26 weeks' duration. Combined therapy with subcutaneous liraglutide and these oral antidiabetic agents or regimens resulted in improved glycemic control (as indicated by a reduction in HbA_{1c} from baseline values) compared with that achieved with existing oral antidiabetic therapy.

In a multicenter, randomized, open-label comparative study, adults with type 2 diabetes mellitus who received liraglutide 1.8 mg once daily in addition to their current therapy (metformin, a sulfonylurea, or both) experienced a greater reduction in HbA_{1c} than those who received exenatide 10 mcg twice daily in addition to current therapy (1.12 or 0.79% with liraglutide or exenatide, respectively). Mean reductions in weight were similar with liraglutide (3.24 kg) or exenatide (2.87 kg).

In a 26-week, randomized, open-label comparative study, adults with type 2 diabetes mellitus who received liraglutide 1.2 or 1.8 mg once daily in addition to their current therapy (metformin hydrochloride at least 1.5 g daily) experienced a greater reduction in HbA_{1c} than those who received sitagliptin 100 mg once daily in addition to current therapy (HbA_{1c} reduction of 1.2, 1.5, or 0.9% with liraglutide 1.2 mg, liraglutide 1.8 mg, or sitagliptin 100 mg once daily, respectively).

Safety and efficacy of liraglutide in combination with insulin (i.e., insulin detemir) were established in a study of 26 weeks' duration in adult patients receiving metformin hydrochloride (at least 1.5 g daily). Treatment with liraglutide 1.8 mg in addition to insulin detemir and metformin resulted in greater reduction in HbA_{1c} than treatment with liraglutide 1.8 mg in addition to metformin (HbA_{1c} reduction of 0.5% or 0, respectively).

In another study, pediatric patients at least 10 years of age (mean age: 14.6 years) with type 2 diabetes mellitus and a HbA_{1c} of 7–11% (if previously treated with diet and exercise alone) or a HbA_{1c} of 6.5–11% (if previously treated with metformin with or without insulin) were randomized to receive liraglutide or placebo once daily; all patients received metformin with or without basal insulin therapy. Liraglutide was initiated at a dosage of 0.6 mg subcutaneously once daily and increased by increments of 0.6 mg every week over the course of 2–3 weeks based on tolerability and fasting plasma glucose concentrations (goal fasting plasma glucose concentration: 110 mg/dL or less). Most patients did not receive the maximum dosage of liraglutide because fasting plasma glucose concentrations of 110 mg/dL or less were achieved with lower dosages. After 26 weeks of therapy, treatment with liraglutide was superior to placebo in reducing HbA_{1c} from baseline (reduction of 0.64% or increase of 0.42%, respectively). Additionally, a larger proportion of patients who received liraglutide therapy obtained a HbA_{1c} of less than 7% compared with those who received placebo (63.7 versus 36.5%, respectively).

In a 26-week, randomized, double-blind, placebo-controlled study, adults with type 2 diabetes mellitus and moderate renal impairment (eGFR 30–59 mL/minute per 1.73 m^2) who received liraglutide 1.8 mg once daily in addition to their current therapy (basal or premixed insulin and/or metformin, pioglitazone, or sulfonylurea) experienced a greater reduction in HbA_{1c} than those who received placebo in addition to their current therapy (reduction of 0.9 versus 0.4%, respectively). There was no worsening of renal function in those who received liraglutide therapy.

If inadequate glycemic control or failure to achieve target glycemic control occurs with liraglutide, alternative antidiabetic therapy should be considered.

Safety and efficacy of liraglutide in combination with *prandial* insulin have not been established. (See Use with Drugs Known to Cause Hypoglycemia under Warnings/Precautions: Other Warnings and Precautions, in Cautions.)

Insulin Degludec/Liraglutide Fixed-combination Therapy Current data indicate that the fixed combination of insulin degludec and liraglutide is more effective than either drug (as add-on therapy to one or more oral antidiabetic agents) in improving glycemic control (as determined by reductions in HbA_{1c}) in adults with type 2 diabetes mellitus. Safety and efficacy of the fixed combination of insulin degludec and liraglutide for the treatment of type 2 diabetes mellitus have been established in 5 parallel, randomized, active- or placebo-controlled phase 3 clinical trials of 26 weeks' duration in adults with type 2 diabetes mellitus.

In 2 clinical studies, the use of the fixed combination of insulin degludec and liraglutide substantially improved glycemic control in adults with type 2 diabetes mellitus who had inadequate glycemic control with oral antidiabetic agents and who were naive to basal insulin or GLP-1 receptor agonists. In the first study, all patients continued on prestudy treatment with metformin with or without pioglitazone. In addition to the prestudy treatment, patients also received the fixed combination of liraglutide and insulin degludec (initial dosage: 10 units of insulin degludec and 0.36 mg liraglutide), liraglutide (initial dosage: 0.6 mg), or insulin degludec (initial dosage: 10 units) subcutaneously once daily. Patients in the fixed-combination group or the insulin degludec treatment group had their dosages titrated twice weekly towards a target fasting plasma glucose concentration of 72–90 mg/dL. Patients in the liraglutide treatment group followed a fixed-escalation scheme with weekly dosage increases of 0.6 mg until the liraglutide maintenance dosage of 1.8 mg was achieved. After 26 weeks, the reduction in HbA_{1c} from baseline was 1.81, 1.35, or 1.21% in patients treated with the fixed combination of insulin degludec and liraglutide, insulin degludec, or liraglutide, respectively. In the second study, all patients continued on prestudy treatment with a sulfonylurea with or without metformin. In addition to the prestudy treatment, patients also received the fixed combination of liraglutide and insulin degludec (initial dosage: 10 units of insulin degludec and 0.36 mg liraglutide) or placebo. Patients in the fixed-combination group had their dosage titrated twice weekly towards a target fasting plasma glucose concentration of 72–108 mg/dL. After 26 weeks, the reduction in HbA_{1c} from baseline was 1.42 or 0.62% in patients treated with the fixed combination of insulin degludec and liraglutide or placebo, respectively.

In another clinical trial, insulin-naive adults with type 2 diabetes mellitus who were inadequately controlled on metformin alone or in combination with pioglitazone and/or a sulfonylurea plus maximum-dose (or maximally tolerated) liraglutide (mean daily dose at baseline: 1.7 mg) continued to receive their pretrial therapy or had their therapy changed from liraglutide to the fixed combination of insulin degludec and liraglutide. Oral antidiabetic agents were continued at pretrial dosages throughout the trial in both treatment groups. The starting dosage of the fixed combination was insulin degludec 16 units and liraglutide 0.58 mg once daily; dosage adjustments were performed twice weekly based on fasting blood glucose concentrations (end-of-trial dosage of the fixed combination: insulin degludec 44 units and liraglutide 1.58 mg daily). After 26 weeks, the reduction in HbA_{1c} from baseline was 1.31 or 0.36% with the fixed combination of insulin degludec and liraglutide versus liraglutide, respectively. A mean weight gain from baseline of 2 kg was observed in patients receiving the fixed combination of insulin degludec and liraglutide compared with a weight loss of 0.8 kg in those receiving liraglutide. A higher rate of hypoglycemia was observed in the fixed-combination treatment group.

In another trial comparing the fixed combination of insulin degludec and liraglutide with insulin degludec therapy in adults with type 2 diabetes mellitus who were inadequately controlled with basal insulin and metformin with or without a sulfonylurea or a meglitinide, patients who received the fixed combination at equivalent insulin dosages achieved superior glycemic control. In this trial, all basal insulins and oral antidiabetic drugs except for metformin hydrochloride (mean daily dose: 1984 mg) were discontinued at randomization; patients received a starting insulin degludec dosage of 16 units (given separately or in the fixed combination with liraglutide 0.58 mg) once daily, which was titrated biweekly based on fasting plasma glucose concentrations. After 26 weeks, the mean daily dosage of insulin degludec was 46 units (with liraglutide 1.66 mg in the fixed combination) in both treatment groups. The reductions in HbA_{1c} from baseline were superior with the fixed combination of insulin degludec and liraglutide compared with insulin degludec treatment (reduction of 1.94 versus 1.05 %, respectively). There was no substantial difference between the 2 treatment groups with regard to hypoglycemia.

In another trial comparing the fixed combination of insulin degludec and liraglutide with insulin glargine therapy in adults with type 2 diabetes mellitus inadequately controlled on insulin glargine and metformin, patients who received the fixed combination of insulin degludec and liraglutide achieved substantially greater reductions in HbA_{1c} compared with those who received insulin glargine therapy. Patients in this trial either continued treatment with insulin glargine or were switched to the fixed combination of insulin degludec and liraglutide, both in conjunction with metformin. The starting insulin degludec dosage was 16 units daily (with liraglutide 0.58 mg in the fixed combination), irrespective of the patient's previous daily dosage of insulin glargine (mean insulin glargine pretrial dosage: 31 units daily). Patients whose therapy was switched from insulin glargine to the fixed combination of insulin degludec and liraglutide showed no worsening of blood glucose control immediately following the switch, despite the initial reduction in insulin dosage for patients who received the fixed combination. Each treatment was titrated biweekly based on fasting blood glucose concentrations with no upper dosing limit in the insulin glargine group and a maximum daily dosage of 50 units of insulin degludec in the fixed-combination treatment group. The mean dosage of the fixed combination was insulin degludec 41 units and liraglutide 1.48 mg daily; mean dosage of insulin glargine was 66 units daily. The reductions in HbA_{1c} from baseline were substantially greater with the fixed combination of insulin degludec and liraglutide compared with insulin glargine (reduction of 1.67 versus 1.16%, respectively).

Macrovascular Outcomes and Cardiovascular Risk Reduction Some GLP-1 receptor agonists (e.g., liraglutide) have demonstrated the ability to reduce the risk of cardiovascular events in those patients with type 2 diabetes mellitus and established cardiovascular disease. In addition to lowering blood glucose, GLP-1 receptor agonists appear to modify several nonglycemic cardiovascular risk factors, such as blood pressure, body weight, and lipid profile. GLP-1 receptor agonists also may have beneficial endothelial effects. When liraglutide is used for the management of type 2 diabetes mellitus in patients with established cardiovascular disease, liraglutide reduces the risk of adverse cardiovascular and renal outcomes. The Liraglutide Effect and Action in Diabetes: Evaluation of Cardiovascular Outcome Results (LEADER) study was designed to assess the cardiovascular safety and efficacy of liraglutide in patients with type 2 diabetes mellitus at high risk for or with cardiovascular disease. This study included adults with type 2 diabetes mellitus who were at least 50 years of age (mean age: 64 years) with at least one coexisting cardiovascular condition (e.g., coronary heart disease, cerebrovascular disease, peripheral vascular disease, CKD of stage 3 or greater, chronic heart failure New York Heart Association [NYHA] class II or III) or at least 60 years of age with at least one cardiovascular risk factor (e.g., microalbuminuria or proteinuria, hypertension and left ventricular hypertrophy, left ventricular systolic or diastolic dysfunction, an ankle-branchial index of less than 0.9). In this study, patients were randomized to receive liraglutide (1.8 mg [or maximally tolerated dose]) or placebo subcutaneously once daily for a median duration of 3.5 years. During the study, antidiabetic and cardiovascular therapies were modified to achieve standard of care treatment targets with respect to blood glucose, lipids, and blood pressure. Concomitant use of other standard of care treatments for diabetes mellitus (excluding DPP-4 inhibitors or other GLP-1 receptor agonists) and ASCVD (nondiuretic antihypertensives [92.4%], diuretics [41.8%], statins [72.1%], antiplatelet agents [66.8%]) was permitted. The primary outcome was the composite of time to first occurrence of cardiovascular death, nonfatal MI, and nonfatal stroke. In these studies, patients who received treatment with liraglutide had substantially lower rates of the primary cardiovascular outcome compared with those who received placebo (event rate 13 versus 14.9%). Deaths from cardiovascular causes were substantially reduced in the liraglutide group compared with placebo (event rate 4.7 versus 6%).

Beneficial Effects on Renal Function In several cardiovascular outcomes trials involving the use of GLP-1 receptor agonists (e.g., liraglutide) in patients with type 2 diabetes at increased risk for cardiovascular disease or with existing cardiovascular disease, beneficial effects on renal function have been observed as a secondary outcome. GLP-1 receptor agonists may be used in patients with lower eGFR compared with SGLT2 inhibitors; however, these drugs may have greater benefits for reduction of ASCVD than for CKD progression. In the LEADER study (see Macrovascular Outcomes and Cardiovascular Risk Reduction under Uses: Type 2 Diabetes Mellitus), liraglutide reduced the risk of new or worsening nephropathy (a composite of persistent macroalbuminuria, doubling of serum creatinine, end-stage renal disease, or death from end-stage renal disease) by 22%.

■ **Obesity** Liraglutide is used as an adjunct to caloric restriction and increased physical activity for the long-term management of body weight in patients who are obese (pretreatment body mass index [BMI] of 30 kg/m^2 or greater) or, in the presence of an underlying weight-related comorbid condition (e.g., hypertension, type 2 diabetes mellitus, dyslipidemia), those who are overweight (pretreatment BMI of 27 kg/m^2 or greater).

The manufacturer states that the Saxenda® preparation of liraglutide is not intended for use in the treatment of type 2 diabetes mellitus. When used for the management of body weight, liraglutide has not been studied in patients taking insulin; the manufacturer states that Saxenda® should not be used with insulin.

Safety and efficacy of liraglutide in combination with other products used to promote weight loss, including prescription and nonprescription (OTC) drugs and dietary or herbal supplements, have not been established.

When used in conjunction with a reduced-calorie diet and increased exercise, liraglutide substantially decreases body weight compared with placebo in obese and overweight diabetic and nondiabetic patients. In clinical trials, weight loss with liraglutide therapy has been maintained over 56 weeks. Efficacy and safety of liraglutide for the management of body weight were evaluated in 3 randomized, double-blind, placebo-controlled studies of 56 weeks' duration (studies 1, 2, and 3) in a total of 4788 patients who were obese (defined as a BMI of 30 kg/m^2 or greater) or overweight (defined as a BMI of 27–29.9 kg/m^2) with at least one weight-related comorbid condition such as hypertension or dyslipidemia. All patients received instruction regarding a reduced-calorie diet (approximately 500 kcal/day deficit) and exercise counseling (recommended increased physical activity for at least 150 minutes per week) initially and throughout the study. In all 3 studies, liraglutide was initiated at 0.6 mg subcutaneously once daily and titrated over 4 weeks to a dosage of 3 mg once daily. Across all 3 studies, 27% of patients in the liraglutide group and 35% of patients in the placebo group discontinued treatment. Approximately 10 or 4% of patients treated with liraglutide or placebo, respectively, discontinued treatment due to an adverse reaction; most such discontinuances occurred during the first few months of treatment.

Study 1 compared liraglutide with placebo in addition to caloric restriction and increased physical activity in 3731 obese or overweight nondiabetic patients. The mean baseline body weight for both treatment groups was 106.2 kg and mean BMI was 38.3 kg/m^2. Other baseline characteristics were similar between groups; mean age was 45 years, 79% were female, 85% Caucasian, 10% African American, and 11% Hispanic or Latino. Principal measures of efficacy were mean percent change in body weight from baseline, the proportion of patients who lost at least 5% of their baseline body weight, and the proportion who lost at least 10% of their baseline body weight. At 56 weeks, liraglutide 3 mg daily reduced body weight by a greater percentage from baseline than placebo (a mean reduction of 7.4% versus 3%, respectively). A substantially greater proportion of patients receiving liraglutide lost 5% or more of their baseline body weight compared with patients receiving placebo (62.3 versus 34.4%, respectively). Similarly, more patients receiving liraglutide lost 10% or more of their baseline body weight compared with patients receiving placebo (33.9 versus 15.4%, respectively). In a subset of patients who had abnormal blood glucose concentrations at randomization (prediabetes), a substantially greater proportion of patients receiving liraglutide lost 5% or more of their baseline body weight at week 56, 160, or both 56 and 160 weeks compared with patients receiving placebo (56, 28, or 26 versus 25, 14, or 10%, respectively). More patients in the liraglutide treatment group regressed from prediabetes to normoglycemia by week 160 than those patients who received placebo. In addition, liraglutide was superior to placebo on several secondary measures of efficacy: deceased BMI, waist circumference, systolic and diastolic blood pressure, total cholesterol and triglyceride concentrations, and measures of glycemic control (glycosylated hemoglobin [HbA_{1c}], fasting glucose, fasting insulin).

Study 2 compared liraglutide with placebo in addition to caloric restriction and increased physical activity in 635 obese or overweight patients with type 2 diabetes mellitus. Patients had baseline HbA_{1c} 7–10% and were treated with 1-3 oral antidiabetic agents (metformin, a sulfonylurea, a thiazolidinedione) or with diet and exercise alone. The mean baseline body weight was 105.9 kg and mean BMI was 37.1 kg/m²; mean age was 55 years, 50% were female, 83% Caucasian, 12% African American, and 10% Hispanic or Latino. Principal measures of efficacy were identical to those in study 1. At 56 weeks, liraglutide 3 mg daily reduced body weight by a greater percentage from baseline than placebo (a mean reduction of 5.4% versus 1.7%, respectively). More patients receiving liraglutide lost 5% or more (49%) or 10% or more (22.4%) of their baseline body weight compared with patients receiving placebo (16.4 or 5.5%, respectively). Liraglutide also improved several secondary measures of efficacy: waist circumference, systolic and diastolic blood pressure, total cholesterol and triglyceride concentrations, and measures of glycemic control (HbA_{1c}, fasting glucose).

Study 3 evaluated the effect of liraglutide or placebo in 422 obese or overweight nondiabetic patients who had lost at least 5% of their baseline body weight with diet and exercise. In this study, patients were initially treated with a low-calorie diet (total daily energy intake 1200–1400 kcal) and recommended physical activity of at least 150 minutes per week for up to 12 weeks. Patients who lost at least 5% of their baseline body weight received liraglutide 3 mg daily or placebo for 56 weeks in addition to a continued reduced-calorie diet (approximately 500 kcal/day deficit) and exercise counseling. The mean baseline body weight was 99.6 kg and mean BMI was 35.6 kg/m²; mean age was 46 years, 81% were female, 84% Caucasian, 13% African American, and 7% Hispanic or Latino. Principal measures of efficacy in this study were mean percent change in body weight from time of randomization, the proportion of patients that maintained their original weight loss (i.e., not gaining more than 0.5% body weight from time of randomization), and the proportion of patients who lost 5% or more of body weight after randomization. Liraglutide was superior to placebo on all primary efficacy end points at 56 weeks; liraglutide-treated patients experienced a weight loss of 4.9% of body weight at randomization compared with a weight gain of 0.3% in placebo recipients. A greater proportion of liraglutide-treated patients did not gain back more than 0.5% of their weight at randomization compared with placebo recipients, and more liraglutide-treated patients lost an additional 5% or more of their body weight at randomization compared with those who received placebo (44.2 versus 21.7%, respectively). Furthermore, a substantially greater proportion of patients receiving liraglutide lost 10% or more of their body weight at randomization compared with patients receiving placebo (25.4 versus 6.9%, respectively).

Dosage and Administration

■ **General** Dosage of the fixed combination of insulin degludec and liraglutide is expressed in terms of units of insulin degludec on the dose counter display of the Xultophy® injection pen; each dosage unit delivers 1 unit of insulin degludec and 0.036 mg of liraglutide.

Patients receiving liraglutide for the management of type 2 diabetes mellitus should be monitored regularly (e.g., blood glucose determinations, HbA_{1c}) to determine therapeutic response. The dosage of the fixed combination of insulin degludec and liraglutide is based on the results of blood glucose determinations and should be carefully individualized to obtain optimum therapeutic effect. Dosage adjustments of insulin degludec and the fixed combination of insulin degludec and liraglutide may be needed during acute illness or when used with other drugs or with changes in physical activity, meal patterns (i.e., macronutrient content or timing of food intake), or renal or hepatic function.

■ **Administration** Liraglutide or the fixed combination of insulin degludec and liraglutide is administered by subcutaneous injection into the abdomen, thigh, or upper arm using a prefilled injection pen; the drug must *not* be administered IV or IM.

Liraglutide is administered once daily at any time of day, without regard to meals. The injection site and timing can be changed without dosage adjustment. The fixed combination of insulin degludec and liraglutide is administered by subcutaneous injection once daily at the same time each day without regard to meals.

If a dose of liraglutide or the fixed combination of insulin degludec and liraglutide is missed, the regular schedule should be resumed with the next scheduled dose; an extra dose or increase in dose should not be taken to replace a missed dose. If more than 3 days have elapsed since the last dose of liraglutide or the fixed combination of insulin degludec and liraglutide, the initial dosage should be restarted and retitrated. (See Dosage and Administration: Dosage.)

When using liraglutide in combination with insulin for the management of type 2 diabetes mellitus, the drugs should be administered as separate injections; insulin and liraglutide should never be mixed. Liraglutide and insulin may be injected in the same body regions; however, the injections should not be adjacent to each other. Liraglutide in fixed combination with insulin degludec is commercially available as Xultophy®. The fixed combination of insulin degludec and liraglutide should not be mixed with any other insulin preparations or solutions.

■ **Dosage** ***Type 2 Diabetes Mellitus*** The recommended initial dosage of liraglutide for the management of type 2 diabetes mellitus in adults is 0.6 mg subcutaneously once daily. The 0.6-mg daily dosage of liraglutide is *not* effective for glycemic control and is intended only as a starting dosage to reduce GI intolerance. After one week, the dosage of liraglutide should be increased to 1.2 mg daily. If clinical response is inadequate, dosage may be increased to 1.8 mg daily after at least one week of treatment with the 1.2-mg daily dose.

The recommended initial dosage of liraglutide for the management of type 2 diabetes mellitus in children and adolescents at least 10 years of age is 0.6 mg subcutaneously once daily. After at least one week, the dosage may be increased to 1.2 mg daily if additional glycemic control is required. If clinical response is inadequate, dosage may be increased to 1.8 mg daily after at least one week of treatment with the 1.2-mg daily dose.

If more than 3 days have elapsed since the last dose of liraglutide, patients should be advised to reinitiate liraglutide at 0.6 mg subcutaneously once daily to minimize any adverse GI effects. Upon reinitiation, liraglutide should be titrated at the discretion of the clinician.

In adults with type 2 diabetes mellitus who are naive to basal insulin or a glucagon-like peptide-1 (GLP-1) receptor agonist, the recommended initial dosage of the fixed combination of insulin degludec and liraglutide (Xultophy®) is 10 units (10 units of insulin degludec and 0.36 mg of liraglutide) once daily.

In adults with type 2 diabetes mellitus who are currently receiving basal insulin or a GLP-1 receptor agonist (e.g., liraglutide), such therapy must be discontinued prior to initiation of the fixed combination of insulin degludec and liraglutide. The recommended initial dosage of the fixed combination in these patients is 16 units (16 units of insulin degludec and 0.58 mg of liraglutide) once daily.

The dosage of insulin degludec in the fixed combination with liraglutide may be increased or decreased by 2 units (2 units of insulin degludec and 0.072 mg of liraglutide) every 3–4 days as needed. The fixed combination of insulin degludec and liraglutide should not be administered more than once daily. Adjustments in concomitant oral antidiabetic therapy may be needed. The maximum daily dosage of insulin degludec in the fixed combination with liraglutide is 50 units (50 units of insulin degludec and 1.8 mg of liraglutide).

Obesity The recommended dosage of liraglutide for the management of body weight in obese or overweight adults is 3 mg subcutaneously once daily. To minimize adverse GI effects, dosage should be initiated at 0.6 mg daily and increased by 0.6 mg at weekly intervals until the maintenance dosage is reached. (See Table 1.)

Table 1. Dosage Escalation Schedule for the Treatment of Obesity

Week	Daily Dose
1	0.6 mg
2	1.2 mg
3	1.8 mg
4	2.4 mg
5 and onward	3 mg

If an increase in dosage is not tolerated (e.g., adverse GI effects), dosage escalation may be delayed for approximately 1 week. However, if a dosage of 3 mg daily is not tolerated, liraglutide should be discontinued, as efficacy has not been established at dosages lower than 3 mg daily.

If more than 3 days have elapsed since the last dose of liraglutide, the drug should be reinitiated at a dosage of 0.6 mg subcutaneously once daily to minimize any adverse GI effects; the dosage should then be retitrated to a maintenance dosage of 3 mg once daily.

Body weight should be evaluated 16 weeks after initiating liraglutide. Treatment should be discontinued in patients who do not experience a meaningful reduction in weight (at least 4% of baseline body weight) after 16 weeks since such patients are unlikely to achieve and sustain meaningful weight loss with continued liraglutide therapy.

■ **Special Populations** No dosage adjustment is recommended in patients with renal or hepatic impairment or based solely on age. However, clinicians should use caution when initiating liraglutide or escalating dosage in patients with renal impairment. (See Renal Effects under Warnings and Precautions: Other Warnings and Precautions, in Cautions.) Data are lacking on the use of the fixed combination of insulin degludec and liraglutide in patients with hepatic impairment. Safety and efficacy of the fixed combination of insulin degludec and liraglutide have not been established in patients with renal impairment; glucose monitoring should be intensified and the dosage of insulin degludec and liraglutide in the fixed combination adjusted on an individual basis.

Cautions

■ **Contraindications** Liraglutide alone or in fixed combination with insulin degludec (Xultophy®) is contraindicated in patients with a personal or family history of medullary thyroid carcinoma (MTC) and in patients with multiple endocrine neoplasia syndrome type 2 (MEN 2).

Liraglutide alone or in fixed combination with insulin degludec also is contraindicated in patients with a history of serious hypersensitivity to liraglutide or to any of the product components.

The fixed combination of insulin degludec and liraglutide is contraindicated during episodes of hypoglycemia.

Liraglutide is contraindicated for the management of obesity in women who are pregnant. (See Pregnancy under Warnings/Precautions: Specific Populations, in Cautions.)

■ **Warnings/Precautions** ***Warnings*** **Risk of Thyroid C-Cell Tumors.** Liraglutide causes dose-dependent and treatment duration-dependent thyroid C-cell tumors at clinically relevant exposures in both genders of rats and mice. Cases of MTC have been reported in patients receiving liraglutide during postmarketing experience; data from these reports are insufficient to establish or exclude a causal relationship between MTC and liraglutide use in humans. It is also unknown whether liraglutide causes thyroid C-cell tumors in humans, as relevance to humans of such tumors in rodents has not been determined. For this reason, liraglutide or the fixed combination of insulin degludec and liraglutide is contraindicated in patients with a history of MTC and in patients with MEN 2. (See Cautions: Contraindications.) In addition, liraglutide should not be used as first-line treatment for diabetes mellitus until additional studies are completed that support expanded use.

In clinical trials of diabetes mellitus treatment, adjusted mean serum calcitonin concentrations were higher in liraglutide-treated patients than in placebo-treated patients but not higher than in patients receiving an active comparator drug. Adjusted mean serum calcitonin concentrations were also higher in liraglutide-treated patients than in placebo-treated patients in clinical trials of obesity management. Very elevated serum calcitonin values may be indicative of MTC; patients with MTC usually have serum calcitonin values exceeding 50 ng/L. Although routine monitoring of serum calcitonin concentrations or thyroid ultrasounds for the purpose of early detection of MTC in patients receiving liraglutide is of uncertain value and may increase the risk of unnecessary procedures, patients should be further evaluated if serum calcitonin is measured and found to be elevated or thyroid nodules are noted on physical examination or neck imaging.

To specifically evaluate the risk of MTC, the FDA has required the manufacturer to establish a cancer registry to monitor the rate of this type of cancer in the US over a period of 15 years.

Sensitivity Reactions Serious hypersensitivity reactions (anaphylaxis, angioedema) have been reported in patients receiving liraglutide. If a hypersensitivity reaction occurs, patients should discontinue liraglutide or the fixed combination of insulin degludec and liraglutide and other suspect drugs and promptly seek medical advice.

Liraglutide should be used with caution in patients with a history of anaphylaxis or angioedema with another glucagon-like peptide-1 (GLP-1) receptor agonist, as it is unknown whether such patients will be predisposed to angioedema with liraglutide.

Other Warnings and Precautions **Use of Fixed Combinations.** When liraglutide is used in fixed combination with other drugs (e.g., insulin degludec), cautions, precautions, contraindications, and interactions associated with the concomitant agent(s) should be considered in addition to those associated with insulin degludec.

Pancreatitis and Pancreatic Precancerous Changes. Acute pancreatitis, including fatal and nonfatal hemorrhagic or necrotizing pancreatitis, has been reported during postmarketing experience with liraglutide. FDA has been evaluating unpublished findings suggesting an increased risk of pancreatitis and precancerous pancreatic cell changes (pancreatic duct metaplasia) in patients with type 2 diabetes mellitus receiving incretin mimetics (exenatide, liraglutide, sitagliptin, saxagliptin, alogliptin, or linagliptin). These findings are based on examination of a small number of pancreatic tissue specimens taken from patients who died from unspecified causes while receiving an incretin mimetic. FDA will notify healthcare professionals of its conclusions and recommendations when the review is complete or when the agency has additional information to report.

In clinical trials with liraglutide in type 2 diabetes mellitus, there were 13 cases of pancreatitis (9 acute, 4 chronic) among liraglutide-treated patients compared with 1 case in a glimepiride-treated patient (2.7 versus 0.5 cases per 1000 patient-years, respectively). One case of pancreatitis with necrosis was fatal, though clinical causality could not be established. Some patients had other risk factors for pancreatitis, including a history of cholelithiasis or alcohol abuse. In clinical trials with liraglutide in the treatment of obesity, acute pancreatitis was confirmed in 0.3% of liraglutide-treated patients (9 of 3291 patients) compared with 0.1% of patients who received placebo (1 of 1843 patients). In addition, there were 2 cases of acute pancreatitis in liraglutide-treated patients who withdrew prematurely from the clinical trials; these cases occurred 74 and 124 days after the last dose of liraglutide. Two additional cases of acute pancreatitis were reported during a follow-up period; one case occurred within 2 weeks of discontinuing liraglutide and the other occurred 106 days after completing treatment with liraglutide.

FDA has recommended that clinicians continue to follow the recommendations in the prescribing information for incretin mimetics. The manufacturer states patients receiving liraglutide should be observed carefully for manifestations of pancreatitis after initiation of the drug and after dosage increases. Patients should contact their clinician promptly if they experience symptoms of pancreatitis, including persistent severe abdominal pain that sometimes radiates to the back and that may or may not be accompanied by vomiting. If pancreatitis is suspected, liraglutide or the fixed combination of insulin degludec and liraglutide should be discontinued promptly and appropriate management initiated. If pancreatitis is confirmed, liraglutide or the fixed combination of insulin degludec and liraglutide should not be restarted.

Efficacy and safety of liraglutide or the fixed combination of insulin degludec and liraglutide have not been established in patients with a history of pancreatitis, and it is not known whether such patients would have an increased risk of pancreatitis while taking liraglutide; patients with a history of pancreatitis were excluded from clinical trials of liraglutide (Saxenda®) for the management of obesity.

Acute Gallbladder Disease. Liraglutide may increase the risk of acute gallbladder disease (e.g., cholelithiasis, cholecystitis). In clinical trials for obesity management, cholelithiasis was reported in 2.2% of patients receiving liraglutide and in 0.8% of placebo recipients, and cholecystitis occurred in 0.8% of liraglutide-treated patients compared with 0.4% of placebo recipients. Cholecystectomy was required in most liraglutide-treated patients experiencing cholelithiasis and cholecystitis. In the LEADER study, gallbladder disease (e.g., cholelithiasis or cholecystitis) occurred in 3.1% of liraglutide-treated patients compared with 1.9% of placebo recipients. Cholecystectomy or hospitalization was required in most liraglutide-treated patients experiencing gallbladder disease.

Although substantial or rapid weight loss can increase the risk of cholelithiasis, the incidence of acute gallbladder disease was greater in liraglutide-treated patients than in those who received placebo in clinical trials of obesity management, even after accounting for the degree of weight loss. If cholelithiasis is suspected, gallbladder studies and appropriate clinical follow-up are recommended.

Sharing of Injection Pens. Liraglutide (Victoza®, Saxenda®) or the fixed combination of insulin degludec and liraglutide (Xultophy®) injection pens must never be shared among patients, even if the needle has been changed. Sharing of injection pens poses a risk for transmission of blood-borne pathogens.

Use with Drugs Known to Cause Hypoglycemia. Patients receiving liraglutide in combination with an insulin secretagogue (e.g., a sulfonylurea) or insulin may have an increased risk of hypoglycemia. In 5 clinical trials of liraglutide for the treatment of diabetes mellitus, hypoglycemia requiring the assistance of another person for treatment occurred in 8 patients receiving liraglutide, and 7 of these patients were concomitantly receiving a sulfonylurea antidiabetic agent.

In a clinical study in pediatric patients (mean age: 14.6 years) with type 2 diabetes mellitus, 21.2% of liraglutide-treated patients experienced hypoglycemia (blood glucose concentration less than 54 mg/dL) with or without symptoms. None of the patients experienced severe hypoglycemia (i.e., a hypoglycemic episode requiring assistance of another person).

In clinical trials of obesity management in patients *without* type 2 diabetes mellitus, spontaneously reported symptomatic episodes of unconfirmed hypoglycemia were reported by 1.6 or 1.1% of patients receiving liraglutide or placebo, respectively.

When initiating liraglutide in patients taking insulin secretagogues (e.g., a sulfonylurea) or insulin, the risk of hypoglycemia may be reduced by decreasing the dosage of the concomitant insulin secretagogue or insulin. The manufacturer states that insulin should not be used concomitantly in patients receiving liraglutide for the management of obesity. Patients with type 2 diabetes mellitus should be monitored for an increase in blood glucose when liraglutide is discontinued.

Elevated Heart Rate. Liraglutide has been associated with increases in heart rate in patients receiving the drug for the management of obesity. In clinical trials in such patients, liraglutide was associated with a mean increase in resting heart rate of 2–3 beats per minute compared with placebo; in a clinical pharmacology study, liraglutide therapy was associated with an increase in heart rate of 4–9 beats per minute compared with placebo. Heart rate increases of more than 10 or 20 beats per minute at 2 consecutive study visits were reported in 34 or 5% of patients receiving liraglutide, respectively, compared with 19 or 2% of patients receiving placebo, respectively, in clinical studies of obesity management. At least one occurrence of resting heart rate exceeding 100 beats per minute was reported in 6% of liraglutide-treated patients compared with 4% of placebo recipients, and such heart rate increases occurred at 2 consecutive visits in 0.9 or 0.3% of liraglutide- or placebo-treated patients, respectively. The clinical importance of elevated heart rate is unclear, especially in patients with cardiovascular or cerebrovascular disease who had limited exposure to the drug in clinical trials of obesity management. Heart rate should be monitored regularly in patients receiving liraglutide; the drug should be discontinued in patients who experience a sustained increase in resting heart rate.

Renal Effects. Acute renal failure and worsening of chronic renal failure, sometimes requiring hemodialysis, have been reported with GLP-1 receptor agonists, including liraglutide. Some of these events occurred in patients without known underlying renal disease. Most of these events occurred in patients experiencing nausea, vomiting, diarrhea, or dehydration. Some of these events occurred in patients receiving liraglutide in combination with one or more agents known to affect renal function or hydration status.

Liraglutide has not been found to be directly nephrotoxic in preclinical or clinical studies. Renal effects usually have been reversible with supportive treatment and discontinuance of potentially causative agents, including liraglutide. (See Dosage and Administration: Special Populations.)

Suicidality. Suicidal ideation was observed in 9 patients (0.3%) receiving liraglutide in clinical trials for the management of obesity and in 2 patients (0.1%) receiving placebo; suicide attempt was reported in 1 of these patients. Patients receiving liraglutide should be monitored for the emergence or worsening of depression, suicidal thoughts or behavior (suicidality), and/or any unusual changes in mood or behavior. If a patient experiences suicidal thoughts or behaviors while receiving liraglutide, the drug should be discontinued. Liraglutide should be avoided in patients with a history of suicidal attempts or active suicidal ideation.

Immunogenicity. As with all therapeutic proteins, there is a potential for immunogenicity with liraglutide or the fixed combination of insulin degludec and liraglutide. In 5 double-blind clinical studies, antibodies to liraglutide were assessed in 50–70% of liraglutide-treated patients at the end of treatment (week 26 or greater). Low titers of anti-liraglutide antibodies were detected in 8.6% of these liraglutide-treated patients. The development of cross-reacting anti-liraglutide antibodies to native GLP-1 peptide also has occurred; however, the potential for clinically important neutralization of native GLP-1 has not been assessed. Antibody formation has not been associated with reduced efficacy of liraglutide or an increase in adverse events potentially related to immunogenicity (e.g., urticaria, angioedema). In a clinical study in pediatric patients 10–17 years of age, anti-liraglutide antibodies were detected in 1.5% of liraglutide-treated patients after 26 weeks of treatment and 8.5% of liraglutide-treated patients after 53 weeks of treatment. None of these patients developed cross-reactive antibodies to native GLP-1 or had neutralizing antibodies.

Specific Populations **Pregnancy.** Data are lacking on the use of liraglutide (Victoza®) in pregnant women. Reproduction studies in rats using liraglutide at dosages resulting in systemic exposures 0.8 times the exposure from the maximum recommended human dosage (1.8 mg daily) have shown teratogenic effects. Studies in rabbits have shown reduced growth and major abnormalities at systemic exposures below the maximum recommended human dosage. Liraglutide for the management of diabetes mellitus should be used during pregnancy only when the potential benefits justify the possible risks to the fetus.

The manufacturer states that liraglutide (Saxenda®) is contraindicated for the management of obesity in women who are pregnant because weight loss offers no potential benefit to pregnant women and may result in fetal harm. If a woman taking liraglutide for the management of obesity becomes pregnant or plans to become pregnant, the drug should be discontinued.

Lactation. Liraglutide is distributed into milk in rats. It is not known whether liraglutide is distributed into milk in humans; a decision should be made whether to discontinue nursing or the drug, taking into account the importance of the drug to the woman.

Pediatric Use. Safety and efficacy of liraglutide for the management of type 2 diabetes mellitus have not been established in children or adolescents younger than 10 years of age. Safety and efficacy of liraglutide for chronic weight management have not been established in children or adolescents younger than 18 years of age.

Safety and efficacy of the fixed combination of insulin degludec and liraglutide have not been established in pediatric patients.

Geriatric Use. No substantial differences in safety and efficacy relative to younger adults have been observed with liraglutide or the fixed combination of insulin degludec and liraglutide, but increased sensitivity of some older patients cannot be ruled out. Hypoglycemia may be difficult to recognize in geriatric patients.

Hepatic Impairment. Experience in patients with mild, moderate, or severe hepatic impairment is limited; liraglutide or the fixed combination of insulin degludec and liraglutide should be used with caution in such patients.

Renal Impairment. In a clinical study of 26 weeks' duration, patients with moderate renal impairment (estimated glomerular filtration rate [eGFR] 30–59 mL/minute per 1.73m^2) who received liraglutide 1.8 mg once daily had no worsening of renal function. Data regarding the use of liraglutide in patients with severe renal impairment are lacking. Caution should be used when initiating or escalating doses of liraglutide in patients with renal impairment. Experience with the fixed combination of insulin degludec and liraglutide in patients with mild, moderate, or severe renal impairment is limited; the combination should be used with caution in such patients. (See Renal Effects under Warnings/Precautions: Other Warnings and Precautions, in Cautions.)

Patients with Gastroparesis. Liraglutide slows gastric emptying and potentially may affect absorption of concomitantly administered oral drugs. (See Drug Interactions: Effects on GI Absorption of Other Drugs.) Liraglutide has not been studied in patients with preexisting gastroparesis.

■ **Common Adverse Effects** Adverse effects reported in at least 5% of patients receiving liraglutide monotherapy for the management of type 2 diabetes mellitus in clinical trials include nausea, diarrhea, vomiting, constipation, and headache.

Adverse effects reported in at least 2% of patients receiving liraglutide for the management of obesity and more frequently than with placebo include nausea, hypoglycemia (in patients with obesity and type 2 diabetes mellitus), diarrhea, constipation, vomiting, headache, decreased appetite, dyspepsia, fatigue, dizziness, abdominal pain, increased lipase concentrations, gastroesophageal reflux disease, gastroenteritis, abdominal distention, eructation, urinary tract infection, flatulence, viral gastroenteritis, injection site erythema, injection site reaction, insomnia, dry mouth, asthenia, and anxiety.

Adverse effects occurring in at least 5% of patients with type 2 diabetes mellitus who received the fixed combination of insulin degludec and liraglutide include nasopharyngitis, headache, nausea, diarrhea, increased lipase concentrations, and upper respiratory tract infection.

Drug Interactions

■ **Effects on GI Absorption of Other Drugs** Potential pharmacokinetic interaction (altered absorption because of liraglutide-induced slowing of gastric emptying). In clinical trials, liraglutide did not affect the absorption of concomitantly administered oral drugs to any clinically relevant degree. However, caution should be exercised when liraglutide is administered concomitantly with oral drugs.

■ **Acetaminophen** Potential pharmacokinetic interaction (decreased acetaminophen peak plasma concentration and rate of absorption following a single dose of acetaminophen); no change in overall acetaminophen exposure (area under the serum concentration-time curve [AUC]).

■ **Antidiabetic Agents** The risk of serious hypoglycemia is increased when liraglutide is used in conjunction with an insulin secretagogue (e.g., sulfonylurea) or basal insulin; patients receiving liraglutide concomitantly with such agents may require a reduction in the dosage of the insulin secretagogue or insulin. The safety and efficacy of liraglutide in conjunction with short-acting (e.g., prandial) insulin have not been established.

No pharmacokinetic interaction has been observed following administration of separate subcutaneous injections of insulin detemir (single dose of 0.5 units/kg) and liraglutide (1.8 mg at steady state) in patients with type 2 diabetes mellitus.

■ **Atorvastatin** Potential pharmacokinetic interaction (decreased atorvastatin peak plasma concentration and rate of absorption following a single dose of atorvastatin); no change in overall atorvastatin exposure (AUC).

■ **Digoxin** Potential pharmacokinetic interaction (decreased digoxin peak plasma concentration, AUC, and rate of absorption following a single dose of digoxin).

■ **Griseofulvin** Potential pharmacokinetic interaction (increased griseofulvin peak plasma concentration following a single dose of griseofulvin); no change in overall griseofulvin exposure (AUC).

■ **Lisinopril** Potential pharmacokinetic interaction (decreased lisinopril peak plasma concentration, AUC, and rate of absorption following a single dose of lisinopril).

■ **Oral Contraceptives** Potential pharmacokinetic interaction (decreased peak plasma concentrations and rates of absorption of ethinyl estradiol and levonorgestrel; increased AUC of levonorgestrel but no effect on AUC of ethinyl estradiol).

Description

Liraglutide is an acylated, long-acting, human glucagon-like peptide-1 (GLP-1) receptor agonist; the synthetic (recombinant DNA origin) peptide precursor of liraglutide has 97% amino acid sequence homology to endogenous human GLP-1-(7-37). Liraglutide is prepared by substituting arginine for lysine at position 34 and attaching palmitic acid with a glutamic acid spacer on the remaining lysine residue at position 26 of the peptide precursor. GLP-1-(7-37) represents less than 20% of total circulating endogenous GLP-1. Like GLP-1-(7-37), liraglutide activates the GLP-1 receptor in pancreatic β cells. Liraglutide also increases intracellular cyclic 3′,5′-adenosine monophosphate (cAMP) leading to insulin release in the presence of elevated glucose concentrations. This insulin secretion subsides as blood glucose concentrations decrease and approach euglycemia. In addition, liraglutide suppresses glucagon secretion in a glucose-dependent manner but does not impair normal glucagon response to hypoglycemia. Liraglutide delays gastric emptying, reducing the rate at which postprandial glucose appears in the circulation. As a result of these actions resulting in increased insulin secretion, suppression of glucagon secretion, and delays in gastric emptying, liraglutide effectively reduces fasting and postprandial plasma glucose concentrations in patients with type 2 diabetes mellitus.

GLP-1 is a physiological regulator of appetite. The GLP-1 receptor is located in several areas of the brain involved in appetite regulation. Weight loss effects of liraglutide are mediated by decreased calorie intake; the drug does not increase 24-hour energy expenditure.

Peak plasma liraglutide concentration is achieved an average of 11 hours (range: 8–12 hours) following subcutaneous administration. Glucose-lowering activity is sustained for 24 hours after a dose of liraglutide at steady state. Liraglutide exposure increases proportionally in the dosage range of 0.6–3 mg. Absolute bioavailability following subcutaneous administration is approximately 55%. Liraglutide is extensively (greater than 98%) bound to plasma proteins. Liraglutide is endogenously metabolized in a similar manner to large proteins without a specific organ as a major route of elimination. The endogenous enzymes dipeptidyl peptidase-4 (DPP-4) and neutral endopeptidase (NEP) are likely to be involved in degradation of the drug. The average terminal half-life of liraglutide is 13 hours following subcutaneous administration, making the drug suitable for once-daily administration. Following a dose of radiolabeled liraglutide, intact liraglutide was not detected in urine or feces, and only a minor amount of administered radioactivity was excreted as liraglutide-related metabolites in urine or feces (6 or 5%, respectively).

Advice to Patients

When liraglutide is used in fixed combination with other drugs, importance of informing patients of important cautionary information about the concomitant agents.

Importance of reading manufacturer's medication guide and the injection pen's patient instructions for use before starting therapy with liraglutide or the fixed combination of insulin degludec and liraglutide and of reviewing this information each time the prescription is renewed.

Importance of informing patients that liraglutide causes benign and malignant thyroid C-cell tumors in mice and rats and that relevance of this finding to humans is unknown. Importance of counseling patients to report symptoms of thyroid tumors (e.g., a lump in the neck, hoarseness, dysphagia, dyspnea) or a personal or family history of thyroid cancer, including medullary thyroid cancer (MTC) or multiple endocrine neoplasia type 2 (MEN 2), to their clinician.

Importance of informing patients of the potential risk of acute pancreatitis, which may be severe or fatal, with liraglutide therapy. Importance of patient informing clinicians about a history of pancreatitis. Importance of informing patients about signs and symptoms of pancreatitis, including persistent severe abdominal pain sometimes radiating to the back that may or may not be accompanied by vomiting. Importance of instructing patients to discontinue liraglutide or the fixed combination of insulin degludec and liraglutide promptly and contact their clinician if persistent, severe abdominal pain occurs.

Importance of informing patients of the risk of gallbladder disease, which can require cholecystectomy. Substantial or rapid weight loss increases the risk of cholelithiasis; however, cholelithiasis can occur in the absence of weight loss. Patients should be instructed to contact their clinician if they experience symptoms of gallbladder disease (e.g., abdominal pain, fever, jaundice, clay-colored stools).

Importance of informing patient of risk of hypoglycemia, particularly if concomitant therapy with an insulin secretagogue (e.g., a sulfonylurea) or insulin is used. Importance of reviewing signs, symptoms, and management of hypoglycemia.

Risk of increased resting heart rate; importance of advising patients that their heart rate should be measured periodically during therapy. Patients should be instructed to contact their clinician if they experience sustained palpitations or tachycardia at rest.

Importance of informing patients of possibility of risk of dehydration due to adverse GI reactions; patients should be advised to take precautions to avoid fluid depletion. Importance of informing patients of potential risk of worsening renal function, including renal failure that may require dialysis in some cases.

Importance of informing patients of possibility of serious hypersensitivity reactions. Patients should be instructed to discontinue liraglutide or the fixed combination of insulin degludec and liraglutide and promptly seek medical advice if symptoms of hypersensitivity occur.

Potential risk of suicidality; importance of patients being alert to and immediately reporting emergence of suicidality, worsening depression, or unusual changes in mood or behavior.

Importance of informing patients that they should never share an injection pen containing liraglutide or the fixed combination of insulin degludec and liraglutide with another person, even if the needle is changed; sharing of the pen may pose a risk of transmission of infection.

Importance of instructing patients with diabetes mellitus regarding self-monitoring of blood glucose, periodic glycosylated hemoglobin (hemoglobin A_{1c}, HbA_{1c}) monitoring, adherence to meal planning, and regular physical exercise.

Importance of informing patients of the most common adverse effects, including headache, nausea, and diarrhea. Nausea is most common when first starting liraglutide, but decreases over time in most patients and does not typically require discontinuance of the drug.

Importance of cautioning patients not to take an extra dose of liraglutide or the fixed combination of insulin degludec and liraglutide to make up for a missed dose. If a dose is missed, patients should resume the once-daily regimen with the next scheduled dose.

Importance of informing patients that if more than 3 days have passed since the last dose of liraglutide, the drug should be reinitiated at a dosage of 0.6 mg once daily to mitigate GI symptoms associated with reinitiation of treatment, then retitrated. (See Dosage and Administration: Dosage.)

Importance of informing patients that if more than 3 days have passed since the last dose of the fixed combination of insulin degludec and liraglutide, the drug should be reinitiated at the starting dose to mitigate GI symptoms due to the liraglutide component. (See Dosage and Administration: Dosage.)

Importance of instructing patients to discontinue use of liraglutide for the management of obesity if they have not achieved 4% weight loss after 16 weeks of therapy.

Response to all diabetic therapies should be monitored by periodic measurements of blood glucose and HbA_{1c} levels, with a goal of decreasing these levels towards the normal range.

Importance of women informing clinicians if they are or plan to become pregnant or plan to breast-feed.

Importance of informing clinicians of existing or contemplated concomitant therapy, including prescription and OTC drugs, as well as any concomitant illnesses (e.g., gallstones, hypertension, pancreatitis, history of alcoholism, high triglyceride concentrations, digestion problems, severe kidney disease, kidney transplant).

Importance of informing patients of other important precautionary information. (See Cautions.)

Overview® (see Users Guide). For additional information on this drug until a more detailed monograph is developed and published, the manufacturer's labeling should be consulted. It is *essential* that the manufacturer's labeling be consulted for more detailed information on usual cautions, precautions, contraindications, potential drug interactions, laboratory test interferences, and acute toxicity.

Preparations

Excipients in commercially available drug preparations may have clinically important effects in some individuals; consult specific product labeling for details.

Liraglutide

Parenteral		
Injection, for subcutaneous use	6 mg/mL	**Victoza®** (available as prefilled cartridge pen), Novo Nordisk
	6 mg/mL	**Saxenda®** (available as prefilled cartridge pen), Novo Nordisk

Liraglutide Combinations

Parenteral		
Injection, for subcutaneous use	3.6 mg/mL with Insulin Degludec 100 units/mL	**Xultophy®** (available as prefilled injection pens), Novo Nordisk

Selected Revisions November 2019, © Copyright, December 2011, American Society of Health-System Pharmacists, Inc.

Lixisenatide

■ Lixisenatide, a synthetic, short-acting glucagon-like peptide-1 (GLP-1) receptor agonist (incretin mimetic), is an antidiabetic agent.

Uses

■ **Type 2 Diabetes Mellitus** Lixisenatide is used as an adjunct to diet and exercise to improve glycemic control in patients with type 2 diabetes mellitus. Lixisenatide also is commercially available in fixed combination with insulin glargine; the fixed combination (insulin glargine/lixisenatide) is used as an adjunct to diet and exercise to improve glycemic control in patients with type 2 diabetes mellitus inadequately controlled on lixisenatide or on less than 60 units daily of basal insulin. Lixisenatide has been used alone or as add-on therapy in conjunction with other antidiabetic agents, including metformin with or without a sulfonylurea; a sulfonylurea or thiazolidinedione with or without metformin; basal insulin (insulin glargine, insulin detemir, or isophane [NPH] insulin) with or without metformin or a sulfonylurea; or insulin glargine with or without metformin with or without a thiazolidinedione.

Current guidelines for the treatment of type 2 diabetes mellitus generally recommend metformin as first-line therapy in addition to lifestyle modifications because of its well-established safety and efficacy (e.g., beneficial effects on glycosylated hemoglobin [hemoglobin A_{1c}; HbA_{1c}], weight, and cardiovascular mortality) in patients with recent-onset or newly diagnosed type 2 diabetes mellitus or mild hyperglycemia. Because of the progressive nature of the disease, patients initially receiving an oral antidiabetic agent will eventually require multiple oral and/or injectable antidiabetic agents of different therapeutic classes and/or insulin for adequate glycemic control. Patients with inadequate glycemic control with metformin monotherapy should receive treatment with additional antidiabetic agents; data suggest that the addition of each noninsulin agent to initial therapy lowers HbA_{1c} by approximately 0.7–1%. Some experts recommend initiating antidiabetic therapy with 2 agents (metformin plus another agent) in patients whose HbA_{1c} is 7.5% or higher, while other experts recommend initiating such dual therapy in patients whose HbA_{1c} is at least 1.5% above the target level. When the greater glucose-lowering effect of an injectable drug is needed, some experts suggest that glucagon-like peptide-1 (GLP-1) receptor agonists are preferred over insulin. Early initiation of insulin therapy should be considered when hyperglycemia is severe (e.g., blood glucose of at least 300 mg/dL, HbA_{1c} of at least 10%), especially in the presence of catabolic manifestations (e.g., weight loss, hypertriglyceridemia, ketosis), or if symptoms of hyperglycemia are present. For additional information regarding the initiation of insulin therapy, see Uses: Diabetes Mellitus, in the Insulins General Statement 68:20.08.

Experts state that a patient's comorbidities should be considered when selecting additional (in addition to metformin) antidiabetic agents. Patients with type 2 diabetes mellitus who have established atherosclerotic cardiovascular disease (ASCVD) should receive a drug with demonstrated cardiovascular disease benefit (e.g., GLP-1 receptor agonist [e.g., liraglutide], sodium-glucose cotransporter 2 [SGLT2] inhibitor [e.g., canagliflozin, empagliflozin]). In patients with ASCVD and heart failure or with an increased risk of heart failure, an SGLT2 inhibitor with demonstrated cardiovascular benefit may be preferred. An SGLT2 inhibitor or GLP-1 receptor agonist with demonstrated ability to reduce the risk of chronic kidney disease (CKD) progression, cardiovascular events, or both (e.g., canagliflozin, empagliflozin, liraglutide) should be considered in patients with type 2 diabetes mellitus and CKD. Experts state that SGLT2 inhibitors may be a good choice for patients at high risk of CKD progression (i.e., patients with albuminuria or a history of estimated glomerular filtration rate [eGFR] decline) because they may have a beneficial effect on the incidence of CKD; however, adequate renal function is required for their use. Some GLP-1 receptor agonists may be used in patients with lower eGFR and may provide greater benefits for reduction of ASCVD than for CKD progression or heart failure. In patients without ASCVD, heart failure, or CKD, the decision regarding the addition of other antidiabetic agents (e.g., sulfonylurea, thiazolidinedione, dipeptidyl peptidase-4 [DPP-4] inhibitor, SGLT2 inhibitor, GLP-1 receptor agonist, basal insulin) should be based on drug-specific effects and individual patient factors.

Data indicate that lixisenatide 20 mcg daily is capable of reducing glycosylated hemoglobin (hemoglobin A_{1c}; HbA_{1c}) by approximately 0.5–0.6% from a baseline of 8% after 6 months of therapy and is especially effective in reducing postprandial plasma glucose concentrations. Available data suggest that lixisenatide therapy may be useful for patients who need to lower their postprandial plasma glucose concentrations in order to achieve their goal HbA_{1c} despite having fasting plasma glucose concentrations that are within goal.

Safety and efficacy of lixisenatide alone or in combination with insulin glargine have *not* been established in patients with chronic pancreatitis or a history of unexplained pancreatitis. (See Pancreatitis under Cautions: Warnings/Precautions.) The manufacturer states that other antidiabetic therapies should be considered in patients with a history of pancreatitis.

Lixisenatide is not a substitute for insulin; the manufacturer states that lixisenatide alone or in combination with insulin glargine is not indicated in patients with type 1 diabetes mellitus or for the treatment of diabetic ketoacidosis. The safety and efficacy of lixisenatide or insulin glargine/lixisenatide in conjunction with *short-acting* (e.g., prandial) insulin have not been established, and such concomitant use is not recommended. (See Use with Drugs Known to Cause Hypoglycemia under Cautions: Warnings/Precautions.) Lixisenatide alone or in combination with insulin glargine is not recommended for use in patients with gastroparesis. (See Patients with Gastroparesis, under Warnings/Precautions: Specific Populations, in Cautions.)

Lixisenatide Monotherapy When given as monotherapy for the management of type 2 diabetes mellitus, lixisenatide improves glycemic control as evidenced by reductions from baseline in HbA_{1c}. Safety and efficacy of lixisenatide as monotherapy have been established in a 12-week, randomized, double-blind, placebo-controlled trial comparing lixisenatide (20 mcg once daily) with placebo in patients with a mean baseline HbA_{1c} concentration of 8.07%. At week 12, therapy with lixisenatide 20 mcg once daily was associated with a mean HbA_{1c} reduction of 0.83%. HbA_{1c} concentrations below 7% were achieved in 44 or 24% of patients receiving lixisenatide or placebo, respectively. There was no substantial difference in weight loss between lixisenatide and placebo treatment groups.

Combination Therapy When given as add-on therapy in conjunction with one or more oral antidiabetic agents (e.g., metformin, a sulfonylurea, a thiazolidinedione) with or without basal insulin, lixisenatide improved glycemic control and had a beneficial effect on body weight (i.e., no weight gain or weight loss). In trials comparing add-on therapy with lixisenatide versus add-on exenatide or insulin glulisine, lixisenatide was noninferior to exenatide, and lixisenatide in conjunction with insulin glargine was noninferior to insulin glulisine (administered once or 3 times daily) in conjunction with insulin glargine with regard to HbA_{1c} reduction from baseline; however, lixisenatide add-on therapy was associated with smaller mean reductions in HbA_{1c} compared with exenatide or insulin glulisine (3 times daily) add-on therapy.

In several trials of 24 weeks' duration in which lixisenatide (20 mcg once daily) was added to therapy with metformin hydrochloride alone or with a sulfonylurea, combined therapy with lixisenatide and these oral antidiabetic agents resulted in greater reductions from baseline in HbA_{1c} compared with those achieved with existing oral antidiabetic therapy. In a trial comparing lixisenatide 20 mcg once daily and exenatide 10 mcg twice daily (both in conjunction with metformin), lixisenatide was noninferior to exenatide; however, lixisenatide therapy was associated with less HbA_{1c} reduction than exenatide therapy (reduction of 0.73 versus 0.9%, respectively). Additionally, weight loss was greater with exenatide compared with lixisenatide therapy.

Safety and efficacy of lixisenatide as add-on therapy also have been established in clinical trials with other antidiabetic agents. In a 24-week, placebo-controlled trial in patients who had not achieved adequate glycemic control with a sulfonylurea with or without metformin, the addition of lixisenatide (20 mcg once daily) resulted in a greater reduction from baseline in HbA_{1c} at week 24 than that achieved with existing oral antidiabetic therapy (HbA_{1c} reduction of 0.77 versus 0.18%, respectively). Lixisenatide therapy also was associated with a substantially greater reduction in mean body weight (reduction of 1.63 versus 0.83 kg, respectively). In a 24-week, placebo-controlled trial in patients with type 2 diabetes mellitus who had inadequate glycemic control on pioglitazone with or without metformin, addition of lixisenatide (20 mcg once daily) resulted in improved glycemic control (as indicated by a reduction in HbA_{1c} from baseline) at week 24. There was no substantial difference in weight loss between the 2 treatment groups.

Safety and efficacy of lixisenatide in conjunction with basal insulin have been established in several trials of 24 or 26 weeks' duration in patients receiving insulin with or without oral antidiabetic agents (e.g., metformin, a sulfonylurea, a thiazolidinedione). In 2 trials of 24 weeks' duration, patients with type 2 diabetes mellitus who had inadequate glycemic control on basal insulin (e.g., insulin glargine, insulin detemir, NPH insulin) with or without metformin or a sulfonylurea demonstrated a reduction in HbA_{1c} from baseline at week 24 with the addition of lixisenatide (20 mcg once daily) to existing antidiabetic therapy. In another trial of 24 weeks' duration, patients with type 2 diabetes mellitus who had inadequate glycemic control with insulin glargine and metformin with or without a thiazolidinedione had substantial reductions in HbA_{1c} from baseline at week 24 with add-on lixisenatide (20 mcg once daily) compared with that achieved with existing antidiabetic therapy. In a 26-week, open-label trial, patients with type 2 diabetes mellitus who had inadequate glycemic control with insulin glargine with or without 1–3 oral antidiabetic agents (e.g., metformin, a dipeptidyl peptidase-4 [DPP-4] inhibitor, a sulfonylurea, a meglitinide) received lixisenatide 20 mcg once daily or insulin glulisine 1 or 3 times daily, all in conjunction with insulin glargine with or without metformin. Lixisenatide was noninferior to insulin glulisine (1 or 3 times daily) with regard to HbA_{1c} reduction from baseline; however, the HbA_{1c} reductions observed with lixisenatide were substantially less than those associated with insulin glulisine therapy administered 3 times daily (reduction of 0.6 versus 0.8%, respectively).

Insulin Glargine/Lixisenatide Fixed-combination Therapy Current data indicate that the fixed combination of insulin glargine and lixisenatide (insulin glargine/lixisenatide) is more effective than monotherapy with either drug in improving glycemic control (as determined by reductions in HbA_{1c}) in patients with type 2 diabetes mellitus. Additionally, therapy with insulin glargine/lixisenatide was associated with weight loss while weight gain was observed with insulin glargine monotherapy. Safety and efficacy of insulin glargine/lixisenatide have been established in an open-label trial in approximately 740 patients with type 2 diabetes mellitus inadequately controlled on basal insulin (e.g., insulin detemir, insulin glargine, NPH insulin) alone or in conjunction with 1 or 2 oral antidiabetic agents (e.g., metformin, a sulfonylurea, a meglitinide, a sodium-glucose cotransporter 2 [SGLT2] inhibitor, a DPP-4 inhibitor). Patients underwent a 6-week run-in period in which all oral antidiabetic drugs (except metformin) were discontinued and therapy with insulin glargine was initiated and titrated prior to randomization. Patients then received treatment with insulin glargine/lixisenatide or continued insulin glargine therapy. The dosages of insulin glargine or insulin glargine/lixisenatide were titrated once weekly based on fasting plasma glucose concentrations (mean final dosages of insulin glargine alone or in combination with lixisenatide were equivalent at week 30 [46.7 units]). At week 30, there was a substantially greater reduction in HbA_{1c} with insulin glargine/lixisenatide than with insulin glargine alone (reduction of 1.1 versus 0.6%, respectively). Patients receiving therapy with insulin glargine/lixisenatide had an average weight loss of 0.7 kg while those receiving insulin glargine monotherapy gained an average of 0.7 kg.

In another open-label trial of 30 weeks' duration, approximately 1170 patients with type 2 diabetes mellitus inadequately controlled on metformin with or without another antidiabetic agent (e.g., a sulfonylurea, a meglitinide, an SGLT2 inhibitor, a DPP-4 inhibitor) received therapy with insulin glargine/lixisenatide, insulin glargine, or lixisenatide, all in conjunction with metformin. Greater reductions in HbA_{1c} were observed with insulin glargine/lixisenatide than with either component alone (reduction of 1.6, 1.3, or 0.9% for insulin glargine/lixisenatide, insulin glargine, or lixisenatide therapy, respectively). Mean body weight was reduced by 0.3 or 2.3 kg in patients receiving insulin glargine/lixisenatide or lixisenatide, respectively. Mean body weight was increased by 1.1 kg in patients receiving insulin glargine monotherapy.

Insulin glargine/lixisenatide is not recommended for use with any other drug preparation containing lixisenatide or another GLP-1 receptor agonist.

Macrovascular Outcomes and Cardiovascular Risk Reduction Some GLP-1 receptor agonists (e.g., liraglutide) have demonstrated the ability to reduce the risk of cardiovascular events in those patients with type 2 diabetes mellitus and established cardiovascular disease. In addition to lowering blood glucose, GLP-1 receptor agonists appear to modify several nonglycemic cardiovascular risk factors, such as blood pressure, body weight, and lipid profile. GLP-1 receptor agonists also may have beneficial endothelial effects. The manufacturer states that there have been no clinical studies establishing conclusive evidence of macrovascular risk reduction with lixisenatide. For further discussion on the use of GLP-1 receptor agonists for cardiovascular risk reduction, see Macrovascular Outcomes and Cardiovascular Risk Reduction under Uses: Type 2 Diabetes Mellitus, in Liraglutide 68:20.06.

Safety and efficacy of lixisenatide in patients with type 2 diabetes mellitus who had a recent acute coronary event (myocardial infarction [MI], hospitalization for unstable angina) were evaluated in a double-blind, placebo-controlled, multinational trial (The Evaluation of Lixisenatide in Acute Coronary Syndrome [ELIXA]). No substantial difference in the rate of cardiovascular events was demonstrated in patients receiving lixisenatide in addition to conventional antidiabetic therapy (e.g., oral antidiabetic agents, insulin) compared with conventional therapy without lixisenatide. In this trial, patients received lixisenatide 20 mcg or placebo subcutaneously once daily for a median of 22.4–23.3 months. Approximately 93.9% of patients were receiving one antidiabetic drug (e.g., metformin, a sulfonylurea, insulin) prior to starting the trial; additionally, most patients also were receiving cardiovascular drugs at baseline (platelet aggregation inhibitors [97.5%], statins [92.7%], angiotensin-converting enzyme [ACE] inhibitors and/or angiotensin II receptor antagonists [86.8%], β-adrenergic blocking agents [84.4%]). The primary end point was the composite of the first occurrence of death from cardiovascular causes, nonfatal MI, nonfatal stroke, or hospitalization for unstable angina, which occurred in 13.4 versus 13.2% of patients treated with or without lixisenatide, respectively.

Beneficial Effects on Renal Function In several cardiovascular outcomes trials involving the use of GLP-1 receptor agonists (e.g., liraglutide) in patients with type 2 diabetes mellitus at increased risk for cardiovascular disease or with existing cardiovascular disease, beneficial effects on renal function have been observed as a secondary outcome. GLP-1 receptor agonists may be used in patients with lower eGFR compared with SGLT2 inhibitors; however, these drugs may have greater benefits for reduction of ASCVD than for CKD progression. For further discussion of the beneficial effects on renal function of GLP-1 receptor agonists, see Beneficial Effects on Renal Function under Uses: Type 2 Diabetes Mellitus, in Liraglutide 68:20.06.

Dosage and Administration

■ General The dosage of the fixed combination of insulin glargine and lixisenatide (insulin glargine/lixisenatide) has been expressed in terms of the insulin glargine component; however, each mL of insulin glargine/lixisenatide contains 100 units of insulin glargine *and* 33 mcg of lixisenatide.

Therapy with lixisenatide or basal insulin should be discontinued prior to initiating therapy with the fixed combination of insulin glargine and lixisenatide.

■ Administration Lixisenatide or insulin glargine/lixisenatide is administered by subcutaneous injection into the abdomen, thigh, or upper arm using a prefilled injection pen; the injection must *not* be administered IV, IM, or via an insulin pump. A planned rotation of injection sites within an area should be followed to reduce the risk of lipodystrophy.

Lixisenatide is administered once daily within 1 hour *before* the first meal of the day, preferably the same meal each day and the same time each day. If a dose of lixisenatide is missed, the dose should be administered within 1 hour before the next meal. Insulin glargine/lixisenatide is administered once daily within 1 hour *before* the first meal of the day. If a dose of insulin glargine/lixisenatide is missed, the patient should resume the once-daily regimen with the next scheduled dose.

Lixisenatide or insulin glargine/lixisenatide should be used only if the solution is clear, colorless (or almost colorless for insulin glargine/lixisenatide), and contains no particles. Insulin glargine/lixisenatide should not be mixed with any other insulin or solution.

Injections pens containing lixisenatide or insulin glargine/lixisenatide should be stored at 2–8°C in the original carton and protected from light before first use. After first use, injection pens containing lixisenatide or insulin glargine/lixisenatide should be stored at room temperature not exceeding 30 or 25°C, respectively. The injection pens should not be frozen; the pen should be discarded if it has been frozen. Injection pens containing lixisenatide or insulin glargine/lixisenatide should be discarded 14 or 28 days after first use, respectively, even if some drug remains in the pen.

The manufacturer's instructions for use should be consulted for additional details about the administration of lixisenatide or insulin glargine/lixisenatide.

■ Dosage ***Lixisenatide Monotherapy*** The recommended initial dosage of lixisenatide for the management of type 2 diabetes mellitus is 10 mcg subcutaneously once daily for 14 days. On day 15, the dosage should be increased to 20 mcg subcutaneously once daily.

Lixisenatide Combination Therapy Patients receiving lixisenatide in conjunction with a sulfonylurea or basal insulin may require a reduction in the dosage of the sulfonylurea or basal insulin to reduce the risk of hypoglycemia. (See Use with Drugs Known to Cause Hypoglycemia, under Cautions: Warnings/Precautions.)

Insulin Glargine/Lixisenatide Fixed-combination Therapy The recommended initial dosage of insulin glargine/lixisenatide for patients inadequately controlled on less than 30 units of basal insulin daily or on lixisenatide is 15 units (15 units insulin glargine/5 mcg lixisenatide) subcutaneously once daily. For patients inadequately controlled on 30–60 units of basal insulin daily, the recommended initial dosage of insulin glargine/lixisenatide is 30 units (30 units insulin glargine/10 mcg lixisenatide) subcutaneously once daily. The dosage should be titrated by 2–4 units every week based on the patient's metabolic needs, blood glucose concentrations, and glycemic control goal. The recommended dosage of insulin glargine/lixisenatide is 15–60 units (15–60 units insulin glargine/5–20 mcg lixisenatide) once daily. Alternative antidiabetic therapy should be used if the patient requires a dosage of insulin glargine/lixisenatide of less than 15 units (15 units insulin glargine/5 mcg lixisenatide) or exceeding 60 units (60 units insulin glargine/20 mcg lixisenatide) daily.

■ Special Populations ***Hepatic Impairment*** Dosage adjustments are not likely required in patients with hepatic impairment since hepatic impairment is not expected to affect lixisenatide pharmacokinetics. Frequent glucose monitoring and adjustments may be required for patients with hepatic impairment receiving insulin glargine/lixisenatide.

Renal Impairment No adjustment of lixisenatide dosage is required in patients with mild or moderate renal impairment (estimated glomerular filtration rate [eGFR] 30–89 mL/minute per 1.73 m^2). However, close monitoring for changes in renal function and for adverse effects (e.g., hypoglycemia, nausea, vomiting) is recommended in such patients when initiating lixisenatide or escalating dosage; such changes and adverse effects may lead to dehydration and acute renal failure or worsening of chronic renal failure in patients with moderate renal impairment. There is limited experience with the use of lixisenatide in patients with severe renal impairment (eGFR 15 to less than 30 mL/minute per 1.73 m^2), and these patients should be closely monitored for the occurrence of adverse GI effects and changes in renal function with lixisenatide use. Data and experience are lacking on the use of lixisenatide in patients with end-stage renal disease (eGFR less than 15 mL/minute per 1.73 m^2) and lixisenatide use is not recommended in such patients. Frequent glucose monitoring and dosage adjustments may be required for patients with renal impairment receiving insulin glargine/lixisenatide. Data and experience are lacking on the use of insulin glargine/lixisenatide in patients with end-stage renal disease; the fixed combination is not recommended in such patients. (See Renal Impairment under Warnings/Precautions: Specific Populations, in Cautions.)

Cautions

■ Contraindications Lixisenatide and the fixed combination of insulin glargine and lixisenatide (insulin glargine/lixisenatide) are contraindicated in patients with known hypersensitivity to lixisenatide or any ingredient in the formulation. Insulin glargine/lixisenatide also is contraindicated during episodes of hypoglycemia.

■ Warnings/Precautions ***Pancreatitis*** Acute pancreatitis, including fatal and nonfatal hemorrhagic or necrotizing pancreatitis, has been reported during postmarketing experience in patients treated with glucagon-like peptide-1 (GLP-1) receptor agonists. The US Food and Drug Administration (FDA) has been evaluating unpublished findings suggesting an increased risk of pancreatitis and precancerous pancreatic cell changes (pancreatic duct metaplasia) in patients with type 2 diabetes mellitus receiving incretin mimetics (exenatide, liraglutide, sitagliptin, saxagliptin, alogliptin, or linagliptin). These findings are based on examination of a small number of pancreatic tissue specimens taken from patients who died from unspecified causes while receiving an incretin mimetic.

In clinical trials, the incidence of pancreatitis in lixisenatide-treated patients versus patients who received other antidiabetic therapy was 21 versus 17 per 10,000 patient-years; some patients in these trials had risk factors for pancreatitis (e.g., history of cholelithiasis or alcohol abuse).

FDA has recommended that clinicians continue to follow the recommendations in the prescribing information for incretin mimetics. The manufacturer states that patients receiving lixisenatide or insulin glargine/lixisenatide should be observed carefully for manifestations of pancreatitis after initiation of the drug. Patients should contact their clinician promptly if they experience symptoms of pancreatitis, including persistent severe abdominal pain that sometimes radiates to the back and that may or may not be accompanied by vomiting. If pancreatitis is suspected, lixisenatide or insulin glargine/lixisenatide should be discontinued promptly and appropriate management initiated. If pancreatitis is confirmed, therapy with lixisenatide or insulin glargine/lixisenatide should not be restarted.

Data are lacking on use of lixisenatide in patients with chronic pancreatitis or a history of unexplained pancreatitis; other antidiabetic therapies should be considered in patients with a history of pancreatitis.

Sharing of Injection Pens Injection pens containing lixisenatide or insulin glargine/lixisenatide must never be shared among patients, even if the needle has been changed. Sharing of injection pens poses a risk for transmission of blood-borne pathogens.

Use with Drugs Known to Cause Hypoglycemia The risk of hypoglycemia is increased when lixisenatide is used in conjunction with a sulfonylurea or basal insulin. Therefore, patients receiving lixisenatide in conjunction with a sulfonylurea or basal insulin may require a reduction in the dosage of the sulfonylurea or insulin to reduce the risk of hypoglycemia. (See Dosage and Administration: Dosage.)

The safety and efficacy of lixisenatide in conjunction with *short-acting* (e.g., prandial) insulin have not been established, and such concomitant use is not recommended by the manufacturer.

Medication Errors Administration of insulin glargine/lixisenatide in a dose exceeding 60 units (of the insulin glargine component) may result in an overdose of the lixisenatide component. The maximum dosage of lixisenatide (20 mcg daily) should not be exceeded, and insulin glargine/lixisenatide should not be used in conjunction with another GLP-1 receptor agonist.

Renal Effects Deterioration of renal function (e.g., acute kidney injury and worsened chronic renal failure, sometimes requiring hemodialysis) has been reported in patients receiving GLP-1 receptor agonists. Some of these events occurred in patients without known underlying renal disease. Most of these events occurred in patients experiencing nausea, vomiting, diarrhea, or dehydration.

Clinicians should monitor renal function when initiating or escalating dosage of lixisenatide or insulin glargine/lixisenatide in patients with renal impairment and in those reporting severe adverse GI effects. (See Renal Impairment under Warnings/Precautions: Specific Populations, in Cautions.)

Immunogenicity As with all therapeutic proteins, there is a potential for immunogenicity with lixisenatide or insulin glargine/lixisenatide. Antibodies to lixisenatide have developed in patients receiving lixisenatide therapy. In a pooled analysis of 9 placebo-controlled studies, antibodies to lixisenatide were assessed in 70% of lixisenatide-treated patients at week 24. Patients in these studies who had higher antibody concentrations (exceeding 100 nmol/L) had an attenuated glycemic response. Additionally, a higher incidence of allergic reactions and injection-site reactions occurred in antibody-positive patients. After 30 weeks of treatment with insulin glargine/lixisenatide in clinical trials, the incidence of anti-insulin glargine or anti-lixisenatide antibodies was 21–26.2 or 43%, respectively. Alternative antidiabetic therapy should be considered if there is worsening glycemic control, failure to achieve targeted glycemic control, or clinically important injection-site reactions or allergic reactions with the use of lixisenatide or insulin glargine/lixisenatide.

Macrovascular Outcomes The manufacturer states that evidence of macrovascular risk reduction with lixisenatide or insulin glargine/lixisenatide has not been conclusively demonstrated in controlled clinical trials.

Use of Fixed Combinations When lixisenatide is used in fixed combination with insulin glargine or other drugs, the cautions, precautions, contraindications, and interactions associated with the concomitant agent(s) should be considered in addition to those associated with lixisenatide.

Sensitivity Reactions Serious hypersensitivity reactions (e.g., anaphylaxis, angioedema) have been reported with lixisenatide. In clinical trials, 0.1% of patients experienced an anaphylactic reaction. Patients with a history of anaphylaxis or angioedema with another GLP-1 receptor agonist should be monitored closely for allergic reactions when receiving lixisenatide because it is unknown whether such patients will be predisposed to anaphylaxis with lixisenatide. If a hypersensitivity reaction occurs, lixisenatide or insulin glargine/lixisenatide should be discontinued and the patient should seek medical attention promptly.

Specific Populations **Pregnancy.** Data are lacking on the use of lixisenatide or insulin glargine/lixisenatide in pregnant women. Lixisenatide has been associated with visceral closure and skeletal defects in rats and rabbits receiving the drug during organogenesis at dosages producing systemic exposures (based on plasma area under the concentration-time curve [AUC]) that were equal to or sixfold greater than, respectively, those achieved in humans at the highest recommended dosage (20 mcg daily). Lixisenatide or insulin glargine/lixisenatide should be used during pregnancy only if the potential benefit justifies the potential risk to the fetus.

Lactation. Lixisenatide is distributed into milk in rats. It is not known whether lixisenatide is distributed into milk in humans. The benefits of breastfeeding and the importance of lixisenatide to the woman should be considered along with any potential adverse effects on the breast-fed infant from the drug or from the underlying maternal condition.

Pediatric Use. Safety and efficacy of lixisenatide or insulin glargine/lixisenatide have not been established in patients younger than 18 years of age.

Geriatric Use. No substantial differences in safety and efficacy of lixisenatide or insulin glargine/lixisenatide have been observed in geriatric patients relative to younger adults, but increased sensitivity cannot be ruled out. Caution should be used when insulin glargine/lixisenatide is administered to geriatric patients; hypoglycemia may be difficult to recognize in such patients, and the initial dosing, dose increments, and maintenance dosage of insulin glargine/lixisenatide should be conservative to prevent hypoglycemia.

Hepatic Impairment. Data are lacking on use of lixisenatide in patients with acute or chronic hepatic impairment. Because lixisenatide is presumed to be cleared principally by the kidney, hepatic dysfunction is not expected to affect the pharmacokinetics of the drug, and the manufacturer makes no specific dosage recommendations for patients with hepatic impairment.

Renal Impairment. Use of lixisenatide is not recommended in patients with end-stage renal disease (estimated glomerular filtration rate [eGFR] less than 15 mL/minute per 1.73 m^2). In patients with mild, moderate, or severe renal impairment, lixisenatide plasma concentrations and systemic exposure were increased by 60, 42, or 83% and 34, 69, or 124%, respectively. The manufacturer recommends no dosage adjustments for patients with mild, moderate, or severe renal impairment receiving lixisenatide; however, the renal function of such patients should be closely monitored when initiating or escalating doses of lixisenatide and patients should be observed for adverse effects. (See Renal Impairment under Dosage and Administration: Special Populations.)

Patients with Gastroparesis. Lixisenatide slows gastric emptying and may affect absorption of concomitantly administered oral drugs. (See Drug Interactions: Effects on GI Absorption of Other Drugs.) Safety and efficacy of lixisenatide or insulin glargine/lixisenatide have not been established in patients with preexisting gastroparesis, and the manufacturer states that lixisenatide therapy is not recommended in patients with severe gastroparesis.

■ **Common Adverse Effects** Adverse effects reported in at least 5% of patients receiving lixisenatide include nausea, vomiting, headache, diarrhea, dizziness, and hypoglycemia.

Adverse effects reported in at least 5% of patients receiving insulin glargine in fixed combination with lixisenatide (insulin glargine/lixisenatide) include hypoglycemia, nausea, nasopharyngitis, diarrhea, upper respiratory tract infection, and headache.

Drug Interactions

In vitro, lixisenatide is neither an inducer nor an inhibitor of cytochrome P-450 (CYP) isoenzymes; lixisenatide is not metabolized by CYP isoenzymes.

■ **Effects on GI Absorption of Other Drugs** The effect of lixisenatide-induced slowing of gastric emptying may reduce the rate and extent of absorption of concomitantly administered oral drugs. Lixisenatide should be used with caution in patients receiving oral drugs that have a narrow therapeutic index or require careful clinical monitoring. In patients receiving oral drugs for which efficacy depends on threshold concentrations (e.g., anti-infective agents) or drugs for which a delay in effect would be undesirable (e.g., acetaminophen), those drugs should be taken at least 1 hour before the administration of lixisenatide or the fixed combination of insulin glargine and lixisenatide (insulin glargine/lixisenatide). If such drugs need to be administered with food, patients should take them with a meal or snack at a time when lixisenatide is not administered.

■ **Acetaminophen** Lixisenatide appears to reduce the rate but not the extent of acetaminophen absorption when the drugs are administered concurrently. With administration of a single 1-g oral dose of acetaminophen, acetaminophen area under the concentration-time curve (AUC) was not changed whether the dose of acetaminophen was administered before or after subcutaneous lixisenatide (10 mcg). In addition, peak plasma concentration and time to peak plasma concentration of acetaminophen were not affected when acetaminophen was administered 1 hour *before* lixisenatide. However, when acetaminophen was administered 1 or 4 hours *after* lixisenatide (10 mcg), the peak plasma concentration of acetaminophen was decreased by 29 or 31%, respectively, and the median time to acetaminophen peak plasma concentration was delayed by 2 or 1.75 hours, respectively. To facilitate a rapid onset of effect, acetaminophen should be administered at least 1 hour prior to injection of lixisenatide; no adjustment of acetaminophen dosage is necessary with concomitant lixisenatide.

■ **Antidiabetic Agents** The risk of hypoglycemia is increased when lixisenatide is used in conjunction with a sulfonylurea or basal insulin; patients receiving lixisenatide concomitantly with such agents may require a reduction in the dosage of the sulfonylurea or insulin. The safety and efficacy of lixisenatide in conjunction with *short-acting* (e.g., prandial) insulin have not been established, and the manufacturer states that such concomitant use is not recommended.

■ **Anti-infective Agents** The effect of lixisenatide-induced slowing of gastric emptying may reduce the rate and extent of absorption of concomitantly administered oral anti-infective agents. Oral anti-infective agents should be taken at least 1 hour prior to subcutaneous injection of lixisenatide.

■ **Atorvastatin** Concurrent administration of subcutaneous lixisenatide (20 mcg) and oral atorvastatin (40 mg) once daily in the morning for 6 days did not alter atorvastatin AUC; however, the peak plasma concentration and the time to peak plasma concentration of atorvastatin were decreased by 31% and delayed by 3.25 hours, respectively. When atorvastatin was administered in the evening and lixisenatide was administered in the morning, no change in the time to peak plasma concentration of atorvastatin was observed; however, the AUC and peak plasma concentration of atorvastatin were increased by 27 and 66%, respectively. Atorvastatin should be administered at least 1 hour prior to lixisenatide.

■ **Digoxin** Subcutaneous injection of lixisenatide (20 mcg) 30 minutes before oral digoxin (0.25 mg) decreased the steady-state peak plasma digoxin concentration by 26% and delayed the time to peak plasma digoxin concentration by approximately 1.5 hours. However, there was no change in the overall steady-state AUC of digoxin. No change in digoxin dosage or timing of administration is necessary. Patients receiving such concomitant therapy should be monitored appropriately.

■ **Oral Contraceptives** Administration of a single dose of a fixed-combination oral contraceptive (30 mcg of ethinyl estradiol and 150 mcg of levonorgestrel) 1 hour *before* or 11 hours *after* subcutaneous injection of lixisenatide (10 mcg) did not affect the peak plasma concentrations, AUCs, or time to peak plasma concentrations of the oral contraceptive components. Administration of the same oral contraceptive 1 or 4 hours *after* subcutaneous injection of lixisenatide (10 mcg) did not affect AUCs or terminal half-lives of the oral contraceptive components; however, the peak plasma concentration of ethinyl estradiol was decreased by 52 or 39%, respectively, and the peak plasma concentration of levonorgestrel was decreased by 46 or 20%, respectively. Therefore, oral contraceptives should be administered at least 1 hour *before* or 11 hours *after* lixisenatide.

■ **Ramipril** Concomitant administration of subcutaneous lixisenatide (20 mcg) and oral ramipril (5 mg) for 6 days did not affect the AUC and peak plasma concentration of ramiprilat (the active metabolite of ramipril); however, such concomitant administration increased the ramipril AUC by 21% and decreased its peak plasma concentration by 63%. The time to peak plasma concentration of ramipril and ramiprilat was delayed by approximately 2.5 hours. No change in ramipril dosage or timing of administration is necessary.

■ **Warfarin** Concomitant administration of warfarin 25 mg during repeated dosing with lixisenatide 20 mcg had no affect on warfarin AUC or on international normalized ratio (INR); however, the peak plasma concentration of warfarin was decreased by 19% and the time to peak plasma concentration was delayed by 7 hours. No change in warfarin dosage or timing of administration is necessary. INR should be monitored frequently in patients receiving warfarin and lixisenatide concomitantly. (See Drug Interactions: Effects on GI Absorption of Other Drugs.)

Description

Lixisenatide, a synthetic analog of endogenous exendin-4 (a naturally occurring peptide isolated from the saliva of *Heloderma suspectum* [Gila monster]), is a short-acting, glucagon-like peptide-1 (GLP-1) receptor agonist. Lixisenatide is a 44-amino acid amidated peptide that is similar in structure to exendin-4 with the exception of the addition of 6 lysine residues at the C-terminal amino acid and the deletion of a proline at position 36. These structural changes increase lixisenatide's binding affinity to the GLP-1 receptor, prevent the degradation of the peptide by dipeptidyl peptidase-4 (DPP-4), and increase its circulating half-life. Lixisenatide has a fourfold higher affinity for the GLP-1 receptor than endogenous human GLP-1.

Activation of GLP-1 receptors stimulates insulin release in the presence of elevated glucose concentrations, suppresses glucose-dependent glucagon release, and slows gastric emptying, resulting in lower fasting and postprandial blood glucose concentrations and, potentially, weight loss in patients with type 2 diabetes mellitus. Long-acting GLP-1 agonists (e.g., albiglutide, dulaglutide, exenatide extended-release, liraglutide) induce marked reductions in fasting plasma glucose concentrations (by stimulating insulin secretion) and modest reductions in postprandial glucose concentrations, while short-acting GLP-1 agonists (e.g., exenatide, lixisenatide) have less of an effect on fasting plasma glucose concentrations and more of an effect on reducing postprandial glucose concentrations (by slowing gastric emptying and inhibiting glucagon secretion). Lixisenatide does not appear to be associated with clinically important prolongation of the corrected QT interval (QT_c, Bazett's formula) or increases in heart rate.

Peak plasma lixisenatide concentrations are achieved 1–3.5 hours following subcutaneous administration. Lixisenatide is thought to be eliminated through glomerular filtration and proteolytic degradation. The elimination half-life of lixisenatide is approximately 3 hours.

Advice to Patients

Importance of patients reading the medication guide and instructions for use prior to initiating therapy and each time drug is dispensed.

Importance of instructing patient and caregivers on preparation and use of the injection pen prior to first use; training should include a practice injection.

Importance of *not* mixing or diluting the fixed combination of insulin glargine and lixisenatide (insulin glargine/lixisenatide) with any other insulin or solution.

Importance of informing patients of possibility of hypersensitivity reactions (e.g., anaphylaxis). Patients should be instructed to discontinue lixisenatide or insulin glargine/lixisenatide and promptly seek medical advice if symptoms of hypersensitivity occur.

Importance of informing patients of the possibility of acute pancreatitis with lixisenatide therapy. Importance of patients informing clinicians about a history of pancreatitis, gallstones, or alcoholism. Importance of informing patients about signs and symptoms of pancreatitis, including persistent severe abdominal pain sometimes radiating to the back that may or may not be accompanied by vomiting; importance of patient discontinuing lixisenatide or insulin glargine/lixisenatide and promptly notifying clinician if such signs or symptoms occur.

Importance of informing patients that they should never share injection pens containing lixisenatide or insulin glargine/lixisenatide with another person, even if the needle is changed; sharing of the pen may pose a risk of transmitting or acquiring infection.

Importance of informing patients of the risk of hypoglycemia, particularly if concomitant therapy with an insulin secretagogue (e.g., sulfonylurea) or insulin is used.

Importance of informing patients of the potential risk of dehydration due to adverse GI effects; importance of advising patients to take precautions to avoid fluid depletion. Importance of informing patients of the potential risk for worsening renal function, which in some cases may require dialysis.

Importance of women informing clinicians if they are or plan to become pregnant or plan to breast-feed.

Importance of informing clinicians of existing or contemplated concomitant therapy, including prescription and OTC drugs, as well as any concomitant illnesses.

Importance of informing patients of other important precautionary information. (See Cautions.)

Overview® (see Users Guide). For additional information on this drug until a more detailed monograph is developed and published, the manufacturer's labeling should be consulted. It is *essential* that the manufacturer's labeling be consulted for more detailed information on usual cautions, precautions, contraindications, potential drug interactions, laboratory test interferences, and acute toxicity.

Preparations

Excipients in commercially available drug preparations may have clinically important effects in some individuals; consult specific product labeling for details.

Lixisenatide

Parenteral		
Kit, injection, for subcutaneous use	2 injection pens, 100 mcg/mL	**Adlyxin® Pen Maintenance Pack** (available as prefilled injection pens), Sanofi-Aventis
Kit, injection, for subcutaneous use	1 injection pen, 50 mcg/mL 1 injection pen, 100 mcg/mL	**Adlyxin® Pen Starter Pack** (available as prefilled injection pens), Sanofi-Aventis

Lixisenatide Combinations

Parenteral		
Injection, for subcutaneous use	33 mcg/mL with Insulin Glargine 100 units/mL	**Soliqua® 100/33** (available as prefilled injection pens), Sanofi-Aventis

INSULINS 68:20.08

Insulins General Statement

■ Insulin is a hormone secreted by the beta cells of the pancreatic islets of Langerhans. Commercially available insulin preparations are classified as rapid-acting (insulin aspart, insulin glulisine, insulin lispro), short-acting (insulin human), intermediate-acting (insulin human isophane), or long-acting (insulin degludec, insulin detemir, insulin glargine).

Uses

■ **Diabetes Mellitus** ***Overview*** The American Diabetes Association (ADA) generally classifies diabetes mellitus as type 1 (due to autoimmune β-cell destruction, usually leading to absolute insulin deficiency); type 2 (due to a progressive loss of β-cell insulin secretion frequently on the background of insulin resistance); gestational diabetes mellitus (diabetes diagnosed in the second or third trimester of pregnancy that was not clearly overt diabetes prior to gestation); or specific types of diabetes due to other causes, such as monogenic diabetes syndromes (e.g., neonatal diabetes or maturity-onset diabetes of the young [MODY], diseases of the exocrine pancreas (e.g., cystic fibrosis, pancreatitis), or drug- or chemical-induced diabetes (e.g., that associated with glucocorticoid use, treatment of human immunodeficiency virus [HIV] /acquired immunodeficiency syndrome [AIDS], organ transplantation).

According to ADA and other experts, a diagnosis of diabetes mellitus currently is established by a fasting plasma glucose concentration of 126 mg/dL or greater, a 2-hour plasma glucose concentration of 200 mg/dL or greater during an oral glucose tolerance test, or a glycosylated hemoglobin (hemoglobin A_{1c}; HbA_{1c}) concentration of 6.5% or greater; results should be confirmed by repeat testing in the absence of unequivocal hyperglycemia. Alternatively, a random plasma glucose concentration of 200 mg/dL or greater in a patient with classic symptoms of hyperglycemia or hyperglycemic crisis is considered confirmation of the diagnosis of diabetes mellitus.

Type 1 diabetes mellitus was previously described as juvenile-onset diabetes mellitus, since it usually occurs during youth. Type 2 diabetes mellitus was previously described as adult-onset diabetes mellitus. However, type 1 or type 2 diabetes mellitus can occur at any age, and the current classification is based on pathogenesis (e.g., autoimmune destruction of pancreatic β cells, insulin resistance) and clinical presentation rather than on the age of onset. In both type 1 and type 2 diabetes mellitus, various genetic and environmental factors can result in the progressive loss of β-cell mass and/or function that manifests clinically as hyperglycemia. Many patients' diabetes mellitus does not easily fit into a single classification. Epidemiologic data indicate that the incidence of type 2 diabetes mellitus is increasing in children and adolescents.

Patients with type 2 diabetes mellitus (approximately 90–95% of all patients with diabetes mellitus) have insulin resistance and usually have relative (rather than absolute) insulin deficiency. Most patients with type 2 diabetes mellitus are overweight or obese; obesity itself also contributes to the insulin resistance and glucose intolerance observed in these patients. Patients with type 2 diabetes mellitus who are not obese may have an increased percentage of abdominal fat, which is an indicator of increased cardiometabolic risk. Distinguishing between type 1 and type 2 diabetes in children may be difficult since obesity may occur with either type of diabetes mellitus, and autoantigens and ketosis may be present in a substantial number of children with features of type 2 diabetes mellitus (e.g., obesity, acanthosis nigricans).

Considerations in Initiating Antidiabetic Therapy Lifestyle modifications (e.g., self-management of diabetes mellitus, medical nutrition therapy [promoting healthy eating to achieve and maintain body weight goals], increased physical activity, smoking cessation, psychosocial care) are an important aspect of diabetes mellitus care in patients of all ages. Such lifestyle/behavioral modifications decrease cardiovascular risk and microvascular complications, improve glycemic control, and remain an indispensable part of the management of diabetes mellitus. Lipid management aimed at lowering low-density lipoprotein (LDL)-cholesterol, raising high-density lipoprotein (HDL)-cholesterol, and lowering triglycerides in patients with type 2 diabetes mellitus has been shown to reduce macrovascular disease and mortality. Although data on risk reduction are not as definitive in patients with type 1 diabetes mellitus, lipid-lowering therapy also should be considered in patients with type 1 diabetes. Efforts also should be aimed at blood pressure control in both adults and children, as reduction in blood pressure in uncomplicated mild to moderately hypertensive patients with diabetes mellitus has reduced the incidence of virtually all macrovascular (stroke, heart failure) and microvascular (retinopathy, vitreous hemorrhage, renal failure) outcomes and diabetes-related mortality. For information on the treatment of hypertension in patients with diabetes mellitus, see Uses: Hypertension, in Captopril 24:24.

Treatment with insulin is essential in all patients with type 1 diabetes mellitus. (See Insulin Monotherapy under Uses: Diabetes Mellitus.) Current guidelines for the treatment of type 2 diabetes mellitus generally recommend metformin as first-line therapy in addition to lifestyle modifications because of its well-established safety and efficacy (e.g., beneficial effects on HbA_{1c}, weight, and cardiovascular mortality) in patients with recent-onset or newly diagnosed type 2 diabetes mellitus or mild hyperglycemia. However, insulin therapy should be considered in patients with type 2 diabetes mellitus when hyperglycemia is severe (e.g., blood glucose concentration of 300 mg/dL or higher, HbA_{1c} of at least 10%), especially in the presence of catabolic manifestations (e.g., weight loss, hypertriglyceridemia, ketosis), or if symptoms of hyperglycemia are present. When the greater glucose-lowering effect of an injectable drug is needed, some experts currently suggest that glucagon-like peptide-1 (GLP-1) receptor agonists may be preferred over insulin because of a lower risk of hypoglycemia and beneficial effects on body weight, although they are associated with a greater risk of adverse GI effects. Because of the progressive nature of the disease, patients initially receiving an oral antidiabetic agent will eventually require multiple oral and/or injectable antidiabetic agents of different therapeutic classes and/or insulin for adequate glycemic control. (See Combination Therapy with Other Antidiabetic Agents under Uses: Diabetes Mellitus.)

Insulin Monotherapy Insulin is used as replacement therapy in the management of diabetes mellitus. It supplements deficient concentrations of endogenous insulin and temporarily restores the ability of the body to properly utilize carbohydrates, fats, and proteins.

Insulin therapy is indicated in all cases of type 1 diabetes mellitus and is mandatory in the treatment of diabetic ketoacidosis and hyperosmolar hyperglycemic states. For additional information, see Diabetic Ketoacidosis and Hyperosmolar Hyperglycemic States under Dosage and Administration: Dosage, in Insulin Human 68:20.08.08. Insulin also is indicated in patients with type 2 diabetes mellitus when weight reduction, proper dietary regulation, and/or oral antidiabetic agents have failed to maintain satisfactory concentrations of blood glucose in both the fasting and postprandial state. In addition, insulin is indicated in otherwise stable, type 2 diabetic patients in the presence of major surgery, fever, severe trauma, infections, serious renal or hepatic dysfunction, hyperthyroidism or other endocrine dysfunction, gangrene, Raynaud's disease, or pregnancy.

In general, goals of insulin therapy in all patients should include maintenance of blood glucose as close as possible to euglycemia without an undue risk of hypoglycemia; avoidance of symptoms attributable to hyperglycemia, glycosuria, or ketonuria; and maintenance of ideal body weight and of normal growth and development in children.

Both conventional and intensive insulin treatment regimens have been used in patients with type 1 or severe type 2 diabetes mellitus. Conventional insulin therapy generally has consisted of 1 or 2 subcutaneous injections of insulin per day (e.g., before breakfast and/or dinner) using a mixture of an intermediate-acting insulin such as isophane (neutral protamine Hagedorn [NPH]) insulin and a short-acting (e.g., insulin human) or rapid-acting insulin (e.g., insulin lispro, insulin glulisine, insulin aspart). However, in most patients with type 1 diabetes mellitus who are able to understand and carry out the treatment regimen, who are not at increased risk for hypoglycemic episodes, and who do not have other characteristics that increase risk or decrease benefit, ADA and many clinicians currently recommend the use of physiologically based, intensive insulin regimens (i.e., 3 or more insulin injections daily of basal [intermediate- or long-acting] and prandial [short- or rapid-acting] insulin or continuous subcutaneous insulin infusion with dosage adjusted according to the results of multiple daily blood glucose determinations [e.g., 3 or 4 times daily], dietary intake, and anticipated exercise). (See Cautions: Precautions and Contraindications.)

The goal of intensive insulin therapy is to achieve near-normal glycemic control (some experts currently recommend a HbA_{1c} target of less than 7% as a reasonable goal for nonpregnant adults); however, some clinicians recommend more stringent goals (i.e., HbA_{1c} target of 6.5% or less), especially if this can be achieved without substantial hypoglycemia or other adverse effects. Because HbA_{1c} is slightly lower in normal pregnancy than in normal nonpregnant women due to increased red blood cell turnover, ADA states that the ideal HbA_{1c} in pregnant women is less than 6% but that target HbA_{1c} may be relaxed to less than 7% to prevent hypoglycemia. ADA recommends a HbA_{1c} target of less than 7.5% for older adults and even less stringent glycemic goals (i.e., HbA_{1c} target of less than 8–8.5%) in older adults with multiple comorbidities, cognitive impairment, or functional dependence. In children and adolescents, ADA recommends an HbA_{1c} target of less than 7.5% in those with type 1 diabetes mellitus (with individualization according to the needs of the patient and family), although a target less than 7% is reasonable if it can be achieved without excessive hypoglycemia. In children and adolescents with type 2 diabetes mellitus, ADA recommends an HbA_{1c} target of less than 7% (or less than 6.5% if it can be achieved without substantial hypoglycemia or other adverse effects). (See Glycemic Control and Microvascular Complications under Uses: Diabetes Mellitus.)

Insulin regimens should be tailored to the specific clinical circumstances in individual patients. In patients without acute illness who are eating discrete meals, physiologic insulin requirements are composed of basal insulin (the amount of exogenous insulin per unit of time required to prevent unchecked gluconeogenesis and ketogenesis), meal-related (prandial or "bolus") insulin, and supplemental (correction-dose) insulin to cover premeal or between-meal hyperglycemia. Correction-dose insulin should not be confused with "sliding-scale" insulin regimens, which generally consist of set amounts of short-acting insulin given several times daily based on capillary blood glucose measurements without regard to timing of food, presence or absence of other insulin requirements, or consideration of individual patient sensitivity to insulin; such regimens have been ineffective in hospitalized diabetic patients and are not recommended. Use of such sliding-scale regimens treats existing hyperglycemia rather than preventing its occurrence and may lead to rapid changes in blood glucose concentrations, which exacerbates both hyperglycemia and hypoglycemia. In addition, studies have found that sliding-scale insulin regimens prescribed upon hospital admission are likely to be used throughout the hospital stay without modifications for risk factors for hypoglycemia or hyperglycemia, prehospital insulin treatment regimens, or patient's sensitivity to insulin.

In hospitalized patients, nutritional intake may not be provided principally as discrete meals, and insulin requirements should be considered to comprise basal and nutritional needs (e.g., IV dextrose, parenteral nutrition, enteral feedings, nutritional supplements, discrete meals). Determination of insulin requirements in hospitalized patients also must take into account counterregulatory responses to stress and/or illness and use of diabetogenic drugs (e.g., corticosteroids, vasopressors).

Subcutaneous insulin may be used to achieve glucose control in most noncritically ill hospitalized patients with diabetes mellitus, and various types of insulin may be used to achieve the daily insulin dose requirements. Subcutaneous insulin regimens in hospitalized patients generally consist of regularly scheduled injections of intermediate- or long-acting insulin to fulfill basal insulin requirements, with supplemental injections of rapid- or short-acting insulin as prandial and correction-dose insulin.

IV administration of regular insulin provides the greatest flexibility in dosing and is used in preference to subcutaneous administration in hospitalized patients with established diabetes mellitus or hyperglycemia (e.g., unrecognized diabetes mellitus, hospital-related hyperglycemia) for diabetic ketoacidosis, nonketotic hyperosmolar states, poorly controlled diabetes mellitus and widely fluctuating blood glucose concentrations, or severe insulin resistance. In critically ill patients, continuous IV insulin infusion has been demonstrated to be the most effective method for achieving glycemic control. Other situations that may require IV infusion of regular insulin include diabetic or hyperglycemic hospitalized patients who are not eating, have cardiogenic shock, or are experiencing exacerbated hyperglycemia during high-dose corticosteroid therapy. IV infusion of regular insulin also is used in general preoperative, intraoperative, and postoperative care, including heart or solid organ transplantation or surgery, or surgical patients requiring mechanical ventilation. IV regular insulin is also used as a dose-finding strategy in anticipation of initiation or reinitiation of subcutaneous insulin therapy in diabetic patients.

Combination Therapy with Other Antidiabetic Agents Combined therapy with insulin and oral antidiabetic agents may be useful in some patients with type 2 diabetes mellitus whose blood glucose concentrations are not adequately controlled with maximal dosages of oral agent(s) and/or as a means of providing increased flexibility with respect to timing of meals and amount of food ingested. Some experts currently state that GLP-1 receptor agonists may be preferred over insulin in most patients who require the addition of a more potent glucose-lowering drug to achieve glycemic control. In clinical studies in patients receiving oral antidiabetic agents who required further blood glucose lowering, the efficacy of add-on therapy with a GLP-1 receptor agonist or insulin was similar. Additionally, use of GLP-1 receptor agonists was associated with beneficial effects on body weight and a lower risk of hypoglycemia compared with insulin, at the cost of a greater incidence of adverse GI effects.

Concomitant therapy with insulin (e.g., given as intermediate- or long-acting insulin at bedtime or rapid-acting insulin prior to meals) and one or more oral antidiabetic agents appears to improve glycemic control with lower dosages of insulin than would be required with insulin alone and may decrease the potential for body weight gain associated with insulin therapy. In addition, oral antidiabetic therapy combined with insulin therapy may delay progression to either more intensive insulin monotherapy or to a second daytime injection of insulin with oral antidiabetic agents. However, combined therapy may increase the risk of hypoglycemic reactions.

Patients who have inadequate glycemic control with basal insulin (with or without metformin) may benefit from the addition of a GLP-1 receptor agonist, a sodium glucose cotransporter-2 (SGLT2) inhibitor, or a dipeptidyl peptidase-4 (DPP-4) inhibitor (if not already receiving one of these agents). The combination of insulin and a DPP-4 inhibitor, GLP-1 receptor agonist, or SGLT2 inhibitor enhances blood glucose reductions and may minimize weight gain without increasing the risk of hypoglycemia. DPP-4 inhibitors and GLP-1 receptor agonists also increase endogenous insulin secretion in response to food, which may reduce postprandial hyperglycemia. Patients whose blood glucose concentrations remain uncontrolled despite treatment with basal insulin (e.g., given as intermediate-acting or long-acting insulin at bedtime or in the morning) in combination with oral antidiabetic agents or a GLP-1 receptor may require intensification of their insulin regimens through the addition of short-acting or rapid-acting insulin injections at mealtimes to control postprandial hyperglycemia.

Glycemic Control and Microvascular Complications Current evidence from epidemiologic and clinical studies supports an association between chronic hyperglycemia and the pathogenesis of microvascular complications in patients with diabetes mellitus, and results of randomized, controlled studies in patients with type 1 diabetes mellitus indicate that intensive management of hyperglycemia with near-normalization of blood glucose and glycosylated hemoglobin (hemoglobin A_{1c} [HbA_{1c}]) concentrations provides substantial benefits in terms of reducing chronic microvascular (e.g., neuropathy, retinopathy, nephropathy) complications associated with the disease. HbA_{1c} concentration reflects the nonenzymatic glycosylation of other proteins throughout the body as a result of hyperglycemia over the previous 6–8 weeks and is used as a predictor of risk for the development of diabetic microvascular complications (e.g., neuropathy, retinopathy, nephropathy). Microvascular complications of diabetes are the principal causes of blindness and renal failure in developed countries and are more closely associated with hyperglycemia than are macrovascular complications.

In the Diabetes Control and Complications Trial (DCCT), a reduction of approximately 50–75% in the risk of development or progression of retinopathy, nephropathy, and neuropathy was demonstrated during an average 6.5 years of follow-up in patients with type 1 diabetes mellitus receiving intensive insulin treatment (3 or more insulin injections daily with dosage adjusted according to results of at least 4 daily blood glucose determinations, dietary intake, and anticipated exercise) compared with that in patients receiving conventional insulin treatment (1 or 2 insulin injections daily, self-monitoring of blood or urine glucose values, education about diet and exercise). However, the incidence of severe hypoglycemia, including multiple episodes in some patients, was 3 times higher in the intensive-treatment group than in the conventional-treatment group. The reduction in risk of microvascular complications in the DCCT correlated continuously with the reduction in HbA_{1c} concentration produced by intensive insulin treatment (e.g., a 40% reduction in risk of microvascular disease for each 10% reduction in hemoglobin A_{1c} concentration). These data imply that any reduction in HbA_{1c} concentrations is beneficial and that complete normalization of blood glucose concentrations may prevent diabetic microvascular complications.

The DCCT was terminated prematurely because of the pronounced benefits of intensive insulin regimens, and all treatment groups were encouraged to institute or continue such intensive insulin therapy. In the Epidemiology of Diabetes Interventions and Complications (EDIC) study, the long-term, open-label continuation phase of the DCCT, the reduction in the risk of microvascular complications (e.g., retinopathy, nephropathy, neuropathy) associated with intensive insulin therapy has been maintained throughout 7 years of follow-up. In addition, the prevalence of hypertension (an important consequence of diabetic nephropathy) in those receiving conventional therapy has exceeded that of those receiving intensive therapy. Patients receiving conventional insulin therapy in the DCCT were able to achieve a lower HbA_{1c} concentration when switched to intensive therapy in the continuation study, although the average HbA_{1c} concentrations achieved during the continuation study were higher (i.e., worse) than those achieved during the DCCT with intensive insulin therapy. Patients who remained on intensive insulin therapy during the EDIC continuation study were not able to maintain the degree of glycemic control achieved during the DCCT; by 5 years of follow-up in the EDIC study, HbA_{1c} concentrations were similar in both intensive and conventional therapy groups. The EDIC study demonstrated that the greater the duration of chronically elevated plasma glucose concentrations (as determined by HbA_{1c} concentrations), the greater the risk of microvascular complications. Conversely, the longer patients can maintain a target HbA_{1c} concentration of 7% or less, the greater the delay in the onset of these complications.

In another randomized, controlled study (Stockholm Diabetes Intervention Study) in patients with type 1 diabetes mellitus who were evaluated for up to 7.5 years, blood glucose control (as determined by HbA_{1c} concentrations) was improved, and the incidence of microvascular complications (e.g., decreased visual acuity, retinopathy, nephropathy, decreased nerve conduction velocity) was reduced, with intensive insulin treatment (e.g., at least 3 insulin injections daily accompanied by intensive educational efforts) compared with that in patients receiving standard treatment (e.g., generally 2 insulin injections daily without intensive educational efforts).

Evidence from the United Kingdom Prospective Diabetes Study (UKPDS) and the Action in Diabetes and VAscular disease: preterax and diamicroN modified release Controlled Evaluation (ADVANCE) study in patients with type 2 diabetes mellitus generally is consistent with the same benefits of therapy with insulin and/or oral hypoglycemic agents on microvascular complications as those observed in type 1 diabetics receiving insulin therapy in the DCCT.

The UKPDS evaluated middle-aged, newly diagnosed, overweight (exceeding 120% of ideal body weight) or non-overweight patients with type 2 diabetes mellitus who received conventional or intensive treatment regimens with an oral antidiabetic agent and/or insulin. Intensive insulin (i.e., long-acting [UltraLente®, no longer commercially available in the US] or insulin human isophane [NPH] given once daily) therapy was initiated with a stepwise approach, in which the dosage of insulin is gradually increased, followed by addition of short-acting regular insulin at meals, and substitution of mixtures of short-acting and isophane (NPH) insulins given several times daily if preprandial or bedtime plasma glucose concentrations were above 126 mg/dL. Conventional treatment consisted of antidiabetic therapy targeted to a fasting plasma glucose concentration of less than 270 mg/dL without symptoms of hyperglycemia. Results of the UKPDS indicate greater beneficial effects on retinopathy, nephropathy, and possibly neuropathy with intensive glucose-lowering therapy (median achieved HbA_{1c} concentration: 7%) in type 2 diabetics compared with that in the conventional treatment group (median achieved HbA_{1c} concentration: 7.9%). The overall incidence of microvascular complications was reduced by 25% with intensive therapy. Epidemiologic analysis of the UKPDS results indicates a continuous relationship between the risks of microvascular complications and glycemia, with a 35% reduction in risk for each 1% reduction in HbA_{1c} concentrations, and no evidence of a glycemic threshold.

The ADVANCE study also evaluated the relatively short-term effects (median follow-up: 5 years) of conventional or intensive therapy on the development of major vascular complications. The primary end point was the composite of major macrovascular (death from cardiovascular events, nonfatal myocardial infarction, or nonfatal stroke) and major microvascular (new or worsening nephropathy or retinopathy) events. While the incidence of the primary composite end point was reduced by approximately 10% in the ADVANCE study, the beneficial effect was due principally to a 21% reduction in microvascular events (nephropathy); there was no appreciable reduction in macrovascular outcomes. Intensive antidiabetic therapy (mean achieved HbA_{1c} concentration: 6.5%) was associated with a reduction in new or worsening nephropathy compared with conventional treatment (mean achieved HbA_{1c} concentration of 7.3%), but there was no effect on the development of new or worsening retinopathy. Results of the Veterans Affairs Diabetes Trial (VADT), another study similar in design to the ADVANCE study, also indicated that intensive therapy in patients with poorly controlled type 2 diabetes mellitus (median baseline HbA_{1c} concentration of 9.4%) did not lessen the rate of microvascular complications compared with standard antidiabetic therapy.

In the UKPDS, fasting plasma glucose and HbA_{1c} concentrations steadily increased over 10 years in the patients receiving conventional therapy, and more than 80% of these patients eventually required antidiabetic therapy in addition to diet to maintain fasting plasma glucose concentrations within the desired goal of less than 270 mg/dL. In patients receiving intensive therapy initiated with insulin, chlorpropamide, or glyburide, fasting plasma glucose concentrations and HbA_{1c} concentrations decreased during the first year of the study. Subsequent increases in these indices of glycemic control after the first year paralleled that in the conventional therapy group for the remainder of the study, indicating slow decline of pancreatic β-cell function and loss of glycemic control regardless of intensity of therapy. In contrast to UKPDS, no diminution in the effect on HbA_{1c} or fasting blood glucose concentrations with either intensive or conventional therapy was observed in ADVANCE or VADT over a median follow-up of 5 or 5.6 years, respectively.

Macrovascular Outcomes and Cardiovascular Risk Reduction

Current evidence indicates that appropriate management of dyslipidemia, blood pressure, and vascular thrombosis provides substantial benefits in terms of reducing macrovascular complications associated with diabetes mellitus. In contrast to the demonstrated benefits of intensive glycemic control on microvascular complications, antidiabetic therapy titrated with the goal of reducing HbA_{1c} to near-normal concentrations (6–6.5% or less) has not been associated with appreciable reductions in cardiovascular events during the randomized portion of controlled trials examining such outcomes. Data from recent, relatively short-term (median duration: 3.5–5.6 years) clinical trials (ADVANCE, VADT, Action to Control Cardiovascular Risk in Diabetes [ACCORD]) in patients with type 2 diabetes mellitus who were at high risk for cardiovascular disease (e.g., mean age 60–66 years, 8–12 years older than patients in UKPDS, disease duration of 8–11.5 years, known cardiovascular disease or multiple risk factors suggestive of atherosclerosis present in approximately one-third of patients) and were receiving intensive antidiabetic therapy (median achieved HbA_{1c} concentrations of 6.3, 6.4, and 6.9% in ADVANCE, ACCORD, and VADT studies, respectively) have not demonstrated substantial reductions in the incidence of cardiovascular events beyond that associated with aggressive management of known cardiovascular risk factors (e.g., blood pressure control, dyslipidemia, smoking cessation).

However, results of long-term follow-up (10–11 years) from DCCT and UKPDS indicate a delayed cardiovascular benefit in patients treated with intensive antidiabetic therapy early in the course of type 1 or type 2 diabetes mellitus. Data from the DCCT-EDIC study, which reported the results of 11 years of follow-up from DCCT, have shown that patients with type 1 diabetes mellitus and without cardiovascular disease who were randomized to intensive insulin therapy at a relatively young age (13–40 years of age at time of randomization) had a 42% reduction in the risk of any cardiovascular event (i.e., myocardial infarction, stroke, angina, need for revascularization, cardiovascular death) and a 57% reduction in the risk of first nonfatal myocardial infarction, stroke, or cardiovascular death compared with those outcomes in patients randomized at baseline to conventional insulin therapy. Similarly, 10-year follow-up data from the UKPDS indicate that intensive therapy with sulfonylurea/insulin or metformin reduced the risk of myocardial infarction by 15 or 33%, respectively.

In middle-aged patients with well-established type 2 diabetes mellitus, some evidence of a cardiovascular benefit with intensive antidiabetic therapy also has been observed in certain subsets of patients with characteristics similar to those in the DCCT and UKPDS, such as those with a shorter duration of diabetes, lower baseline HbA_{1c} concentrations, and/or absence of known cardiovascular disease. In the ACCORD study, prespecified subgroup analyses suggested that patients with no cardiovascular events at study entry and those with a baseline HbA_{1c} concentration of 8% or less had a reduction in primary cardiovascular outcome (myocardial infarction, stroke, cardiovascular death). Posthoc subgroup analyses of the VADT suggested that patients with a duration of diabetes of less than 12 years appeared to have a cardiovascular benefit with intensive antidiabetic therapy while such therapy had a neutral or adverse effect on the development of cardiovascular disease in those with a longer duration of diabetes.

A relationship between glycemia (as determined by fasting glucose or HbA_{1c} concentration) and vascular intima-media thickness, a surrogate marker for coronary and cerebrovascular disease, has been demonstrated in patients with and without diabetes mellitus. The delayed benefits of intensive antidiabetic therapy on risk of cardiovascular events in patients with diabetes mellitus in whom such therapy was initiated relatively early in the course of the disease may relate to reduction in the accumulation of advanced glycosylation end products that lead to the development of atherosclerosis over a period of years. Clinical data from long-term follow-up studies and subgroup analyses of relatively short-term studies suggest that intensive therapy may delay or prevent the progression of cardiovascular disease optimally in those without substantial atherosclerosis while providing minimal protection from cardiovascular events when the disease is well established. Subset analyses from EDIC and VADT examining carotid intima-media thickness and vascular calcification also suggest that intensive therapy reduces the progression of atherosclerosis in those with minimal or less advanced atherosclerosis. Data from the EDIC follow-up study to DCCT suggest that patients receiving intensive insulin therapy during DCCT had less progression of carotid intima-media thickness 6 years after completion of the DCCT than patients receiving conventional therapy. The lower HbA_{1c} concentration attained in the intensive therapy group during DCCT was associated with a decrease in the progression of carotid-intima media thickness at the end of the EDIC follow-up study. Limited data from VADT suggest that middle-aged patients with less coronary arterial calcification at baseline (coronary artery calcification Agatson scores of less than 100) had a reduction in cardiovascular events with intensive treatment. In contrast, patients in VADT with higher coronary arterial calcification at baseline (coronary artery calcification Agatson scores exceeding 100) did not have a reduction in cardiovascular events with intensive treatment.

Current strategies for intensive treatment of hyperglycemia and the associated increased risk of severe hypoglycemia in patients with advanced type 2 diabetes mellitus may have counterbalancing consequences for cardiovascular disease (e.g., myocardial ischemia/infarction, increased cardiovascular morbidity and mortality, weight gain, other metabolic changes). Potential risks of very intensive therapy may outweigh benefits in patients with a very long duration of diabetes; known history of severe hypoglycemia; advanced atherosclerosis or other cardiovascular disease; positive risk factors for cardiovascular disease; or advanced age or frailty. In the ACCORD study, patients with type 2 diabetes mellitus who were at high risk for cardiovascular disease and received intensive antidiabetic therapy had a 22 or 35% increase in the relative risk of all-cause or cardiovascular death, respectively, compared with that in patients receiving conventional antidiabetic therapy. Differences in mortality in patients receiving intensive therapy became apparent after 1 year and continued throughout follow-up until premature discontinuance of the intensive-therapy regimen after a mean of 3.5 years of follow-up. Exploratory analyses of episodes of severe hypoglycemia, differences in the use of ancillary drug therapy between those receiving conventional and intensive therapy, weight changes, achieved HbA_{1c} concentrations and rate of achievement of target HbA_{1c} concentrations, drug interactions, and other factors did not provide an explanation for the increased mortality observed in the ACCORD study. However, intensive therapy was not associated with an increase in mortality in the ADVANCE trial, another trial of similar design, despite achievement of a target HbA_{1c} concentration (median of 6.3%) that was similar to that achieved in the ACCORD trial (median of 6.4%). Differences in patient characteristics and study design between the ADVANCE and ACCORD trials may provide additional hypotheses regarding discrepancies between the effects of intensive therapy on mortality in these trials. Patients in the ADVANCE trial had less-advanced diabetes (disease duration 2–3 years shorter than in ACCORD) and had lower baseline HbA_{1c} despite use of insulin in only a small proportion of patients (1.5% of patients in the ADVANCE study were receiving insulin at baseline versus 35% of those in the ACCORD study). HbA_{1c} concentration was lowered more gradually to the target goal in the ADVANCE trial (several years versus 1 year to achieve maximum separation between HbA_{1c} in the ADVANCE or ACCORD trial, respectively); the target goal was achieved in the ADVANCE trial without appreciable weight gain and with fewer episodes of severe hypoglycemia than in ACCORD or VADT. Severe hypoglycemia occurred in less than 3%, approximately 16%, or 21% of patients receiving intensive therapy in ADVANCE, ACCORD, or VADT, respectively. Future combined analyses of the ADVANCE, ACCORD, and other trials should provide further insight into the effects of intensive antidiabetic therapy on the development of macrovascular events.

Data from clinical trials also support the use of certain oral antidiabetic agents (e.g., some SGLT2 inhibitors [canagliflozin, empagliflozin] or GLP-1 receptor agonists [liraglutide, semaglutide]) to reduce the risk of cardiovascular events in patients with type 2 diabetes mellitus and established cardiovascular disease. For further discussion on the use of certain SGLT2 inhibitors or GLP-1 receptor agonists for cardiovascular risk reduction, see the individual drug monographs in 68:20.

Treatment Goals ADA generally recommends the same blood glucose and HbA_{1c} concentration goals for all nonpregnant adults with type 1 or type 2 diabetes mellitus but states that less stringent treatment goals may be appropriate for certain patients. ADA currently recommends target preprandial and peak postprandial (1–2 hours after the *beginning* of a meal) *plasma* glucose concentrations of 80–130 and less than 180 mg/dL, respectively, and HbA_{1c} concentrations of less than 7% (based on a nondiabetic range of 4–6%) *in general* in adults with type 1 or 2 diabetes mellitus who are not pregnant. HbA_{1c} concentrations of 7% or greater should prompt clinicians to initiate or adjust antidiabetic therapy in nonpregnant patients with the goal of achieving HbA_{1c} concentrations of less than 7%. Patients with diabetes mellitus who have elevated HbA_{1c} concentrations despite having adequate preprandial glucose concentrations should monitor glucose concentrations 1–2 hours after the start of a meal.

More stringent treatment goals (i.e., HbA_{1c} concentrations even lower than the general goal of less than 7 or less than 6% in nonpregnant or pregnant patients, respectively, can be considered in selected patients. An *individualized* HbA_{1c} concentration goal that is closer to normal without risking severe hypoglycemia is reasonable in patients with a short duration of diabetes mellitus, no appreciable cardiovascular disease, and a long life expectancy. ADA recommends target preprandial and 2-hour postprandial blood glucose concentrations less than 95 and 120 mg/dL, respectively, in women with gestational diabetes mellitus. (See Cautions: Pregnancy and see Uses: Gestational Diabetes Mellitus.)

In hospitalized patients, ADA recommends a target blood glucose concentration of 140–180 mg/dL for the majority of critically ill and noncritically ill patients. Higher target glucose concentrations may be appropriate in terminally ill patients, those with severe comorbidities, and in patient care settings where frequent glucose monitoring is not feasible. An HbA_{1c} concentration should be obtained in all hospitalized diabetic patients if a current (previous 3 months) test is not available. Hospitalized patients who have hyperglycemia (random blood glucose concentration exceeding 140 mg/dL) should have a follow-up appointment with a clinician within 1 month of hospital discharge.

Treatment goals should be individualized, and specific target values for blood glucose and HbA_{1c} concentration appropriately adjusted, based on the patient's capacity to understand and adhere to the treatment regimen, the risk of severe hypoglycemia, and other patient factors that may increase risk or decrease benefit (e.g., young children [less than 6 years of age]; advanced age or frailty; cognitive or functional impairment; advanced microvascular or macrovascular complications or extensive comorbid conditions; other diseases that materially shorten life expectancy). Less stringent treatment goals may be appropriate in patients with long-standing diabetes mellitus in whom the general HbA_{1c} concentration goal of less than 7% is difficult to obtain despite adequate education on self-management of the disease, appropriate glucose monitoring, and effective dosages of multiple antidiabetic agents, including insulin. Achievement of HbA_{1c} concentrations less than 7% is not appropriate or practical for some patients, and clinical judgment should be used in designing a treatment regimen based on the potential benefits and risks (e.g., hypoglycemia) of more intensified therapy. Higher target blood glucose concentrations are advisable in patients with a history of recurrent, severe hypoglycemia and in patients with hypoglycemic unawareness, after they have been advised of the risks of intensive insulin therapy. Some clinicians consider it inappropriate to institute intensive therapy in these patients because they may have defective glucose counterregulatory responses. Severe or frequent hypoglycemia is an absolute indication for modification of treatment regimens, including setting higher glycemic goals. Clinicians should be vigilant in the prevention of severe hypoglycemia in patients with advanced diabetes mellitus and should not aggressively attempt to achieve near-normal HbA_{1c} concentrations in patients in whom such a target cannot be achieved with reasonable ease and safety.

Data from a decision model based on extrapolated benefits of intensive glycemic control in type 1 diabetic patients (i.e., as demonstrated in the Diabetes Control and Complications Trial [DCCT]) suggest substantial benefits (i.e., in terms of reduction in years of blindness or end-stage renal disease) of reducing HbA_{1c} to near-normal concentrations (e.g., from 9 to 7%) in patients with early-onset (i.e., at 40–50 years of age) type 2 diabetes mellitus. Geriatric patients with a life expectancy long enough to reap the benefits of long-term intensive diabetes management who are active, cognitively intact, and willing to self-manage diabetes mellitus should be treated using the same goals for younger adults with diabetes mellitus. For frail geriatric patients, patients with an intermediate remaining life expectancy, and those in whom the risks of intensive glycemic control appears to outweigh the benefits, a less stringent target HbA_{1c} concentration such as 8% is appropriate. An even less stringent target HbA_{1c} concentration (i.e., less than 8.5%) may be considered in geriatric patients in very poor health and with a limited life expectancy. Hyperglycemia leading to symptoms or risk of acute hyperglycemic complications should be avoided in all geriatric patients.

In children and adolescents with type 1 diabetes mellitus, ADA recommends target preprandial and bedtime/overnight plasma glucose concentrations of 90–130 and 90–150 mg/dL, respectively, and HbA_{1c} concentrations of less than 7.5% (a lower goal of less than 7% may be reasonable if it can be achieved without excessive hypoglycemia). Special consideration should be given to the risk of hypoglycemia in young children (younger than 6 years of age) who may be unable to recognize, articulate, and/or manage hypoglycemia. However, some data indicate that young children can achieve target HbA_{1c} concentrations without increased risk of severe hypoglycemia. In children and adolescents with type 2 diabetes mellitus, ADA recommends a target HbA_{1c} concentration of less than 7% in those patients treated with oral antidiabetic agents alone; more stringent targets (i.e., less than 6.5%) may be appropriate for certain individuals who can achieve this concentration without substantial hypoglycemia or other adverse effects. Treatment goals should be individualized and the benefits of achieving a lower HbA_{1c} concentration should be weighed against the risks of hypoglycemia and the developmental burdens of intensive antidiabetic regimens in children and adolescents.

■ **Gestational Diabetes Mellitus** Gestational diabetes mellitus is a condition in which a woman without clearly overt diabetes mellitus prior to pregnancy develops glucose intolerance (i.e., elevated blood glucose concentrations) during pregnancy. (See Insulin Use during Pregnancy under Dosage and Administration: Dosage.) Gestational diabetes mellitus may be associated with macrosomia, birth complications, and an increased risk of maternal type

2 diabetes mellitus after pregnancy. (See Cautions: Pregnancy.) ADA states that insulin therapy is preferred in patients with gestational diabetes who, despite dietary management (medical nutrition therapy [MNT]), have fasting blood glucose concentrations of 95 mg/dL or higher, 1-hour postprandial blood glucose concentrations of 140 mg/dL or higher, or 2-hour postprandial blood glucose concentrations of 120 mg/dL or higher. Long-acting and intermediate-acting insulins used in gestational diabetes mellitus include NPH insulin, insulin glargine, and insulin detemir. When short-acting insulins are used, insulin lispro and insulin aspart are preferred over regular human insulin because of the former drugs' rapid onset of action. Oral antidiabetic agents (e.g., glyburide, metformin) are not recommended as first-line therapy because these drugs are able to cross the placenta and data on the safety of these drugs in offspring are lacking.

Women with gestational diabetes should be evaluated for prediabetes or persistent diabetes mellitus at least 4–12 weeks postpartum using a 75-g, 2-hour oral glucose tolerance test. Follow-up should be performed every 1–3 years thereafter if the results of the postpartum glucose tolerance test at 4–12 weeks are normal. Women with impaired glucose tolerance in the postpartum period should attempt lifestyle changes to prevent or delay the progression to diabetes mellitus; initiating therapy with metformin also may be considered. Subsequent pregnancies should be planned to ensure optimal glycemic control throughout pregnancy.

■ **Critical Illness** Moderate glycemic control has been shown to reduce morbidity and mortality in hospitalized patients with critical illness† requiring intensive care. Randomized, clinical studies and meta-analyses of studies in surgical patients have indicated lower rates of mortality and stroke with a perioperative blood glucose target of less than 180 mg/dL compared with a target of less than 200 mg/dL; no substantial additional benefit was found with more stringent glycemic control (i.e., blood glucose concentration less than 140 mg/dL). Some experts recommend a blood glucose target of 140–180 mg/dL in most hospitalized patients; more stringent goals (i.e., 110–140 mg/dL) may be appropriate in selected patients if substantial hypoglycemia can be avoided. While some experts recommend initiating insulin therapy when blood glucose concentrations reach 180 mg/dL or higher, other clinicians recommend initiating therapy at lower blood glucose concentrations (e.g., 150 mg/dL or higher). When insulin is used in critically ill patients, most experts recommend that insulin be administered by continuous IV infusion.

■ **Acute Myocardial Infarction** Data from several clinical trials in patients with ST-segment-elevation myocardial infarction (STEMI) suggest that blood glucose concentrations are positively correlated with mortality. Current data suggest that high-dose regular insulin in combination with IV potassium chloride and dextrose (D-glucose) (referred to as glucose-insulin-potassium or GIK therapy) is *not* beneficial in reducing mortality following ST-segment-elevation myocardial infarction (STEMI) and may even be harmful. The American College of Cardiology Foundation (ACCF) and American Heart Association (AHA) state that blood glucose levels should be maintained below 180 mg/dL if possible while avoiding hypoglycemia and that there is no established role for GIK infusions in patients with STEMI.

■ **Hyperalimentation Adjunct** Regular insulin has been added to IV hyperalimentation solutions to assure proper utilization of glucose and reduce glycosuria in diabetic patients. Addition of insulin also may be beneficial in nondiabetic patients whose glycosuria cannot be controlled by adjustment of the infusion flow rate. Because not all nondiabetic patients receiving hyperalimentation therapy require insulin and because of variable adsorption of insulin to the IV infusion system, there is debate over the value of adding insulin to hyperalimentation solutions. If insulin is required in patients receiving hyperalimentation therapy, some clinicians prefer subcutaneous or direct IV injection. Since insulin requirements may vary abruptly in patients receiving hyperalimentation, insulin dosage must be carefully adjusted based on frequent determinations of blood and urine glucose concentrations.

■ **Growth Hormone Reserve Test** IV injection of regular insulin is used as a provocative test for growth hormone secretion.

■ **Hyperkalemia** Regular insulin has also been added to IV dextrose infusions to facilitate an intracellular shift of potassium in the treatment of severe hyperkalemia.

Dosage and Administration

■ **Administration** Insulin usually is administered by subcutaneous injection. The subcutaneous route is preferred to IM administration because it provides more prolonged absorption and is less painful. Regular insulin may be given IV or IM under medical supervision with close monitoring of blood glucose and potassium concentrations to avoid hypoglycemia and hypokalemia. Regular insulin also may be administered IV for general perioperative use and during the postoperative period following cardiac surgery or organ transplantation; in patients with diabetic ketoacidosis, nonketotic hyperosmolar state, cardiogenic shock, critical illness, or exacerbated hyperglycemia during high-dose corticosteroid therapy, or in those who are not eating; and to facilitate determination of optimal dosage prior to initiating or reinitiating subcutaneous insulin therapy in patients with type 1 or type 2 diabetes mellitus. Rapid-acting insulins (e.g., insulin lispro, insulin glulisine, insulin aspart) have been used IV, but such use offers no advantage over regular insulin (insulin human).

Subcutaneous administration of insulin has been made into the thighs, upper arms, buttocks, or abdomen using a 25- to 28-gauge needle 1.3–1.6 cm in length. With the availability of smaller 30- and 31-gauge needles, the needle tip may become bent to form a hook, which can lacerate tissue or break off to leave needle fragments within the skin. The medical consequences of these needle fragments are unknown but may increase the risk of lipodystrophy or other adverse effects. *It is essential to use only syringes calibrated for the particular concentration of insulin administered.* To avoid painful injections, patients should inject insulin that is at room temperature. To prevent air bubbles in an insulin pen, the injection pen should be primed with 2 units of insulin before injection; patients should avoid leaving a needle in the pen between injections. In most individuals, a fold of the skin is grasped lightly with the fingers at least 7.6 cm apart and the needle inserted at a 90° angle; thin individuals or children may need to pinch the skin and inject at a 45° angle to avoid IM injection of the dose, especially in the thigh area. Routine aspiration (to check for inadvertent intravascular injection as indicated by the presence of blood in the syringe) after subcutaneous injection of insulin generally is not necessary. The insulin should be injected over a period of at least 6 seconds; presence of air bubbles could interfere with accurate dosing. The push button of the insulin injection pen or other compatible insulin delivery device should continue to be depressed during drug delivery until the needle is withdrawn from the skin to ensure that the full dose has been delivered. Preparations of insulin suspensions that are injected slowly may clog the tip of the needle, preventing completion of the injection. The injection site should be pressed lightly for a few seconds after the needle is withdrawn but should not be rubbed. A planned rotation of sites within one area should be followed so that any one site is not injected more than once every 1–2 weeks. Rotating injection sites within one anatomic region (e.g., rotating injections systematically in the abdominal area) rather than selecting a different anatomic region is recommended to decrease day-to-day variability in insulin absorption. Variability in insulin absorption by injection site is reduced with insulin lispro compared with that with insulin human.

The American Diabetes Association (ADA) states that if an insulin injection seems particularly painful or if blood or clear fluid is observed after withdrawing the needle, patients should be instructed to apply pressure to the injection site for 5–8 seconds without rubbing and perform blood glucose monitoring more frequently that day. If the patient suspects that an appreciable portion of the insulin dose was not administered, blood glucose should be checked within a few hours after the injection and supplemental insulin administered if necessary. (See Dosage and Administration: Administration.)

Although most insulin syringes have been designed to eliminate dead-space volume, dosage errors attributable to the dead-space volume within some insulin syringes may result when 2 types of insulin are mixed in the syringes. Patients stabilized on a particular order of mixing and using a particular brand and design of syringe should not change these factors without first consulting their physician.

Alternatively, specialized delivery devices (e.g., subcutaneous controlled-infusion devices [pumps], insulin pens) have been used to administer insulins, and the manufacturers' instructions should be consulted for proper methods of assembly, administration (including dosage calibration), and care. For information on subcutaneous controlled-infusion devices, see Dosage and Administration: Administration, in Insulin Aspart 68:20.08/04 and also see Dosage and Administration: Administration, in Insulin Lispro 68:20.08.04.

■ **Dosage** Dosage of insulin injection is always expressed in USP units. The number of units in a given volume varies with the strength of the preparation employed. Commercially available insulin human (regular insulin) preparations contain 100 (U-100) or 500 (U-500) units per mL. All commercially available preparations have standardized label colors to facilitate identification. Concentrated (U-500) insulin human injection is indicated in diabetic patients with daily insulin requirements exceeding 200 units, so that a large dose may be administered subcutaneously in a relatively small volume.

Insulin Regimens Both conventional and intensive insulin treatment regimens have been used in patients with type 1 or type 2 diabetes mellitus. (See Glycemic Control and Microvascular Complications under Uses: Diabetes Mellitus.) Conventional therapy generally consists of 1 or 2 subcutaneous doses of insulin per day (e.g., at breakfast and/or dinner), usually with a mixture of intermediate-acting and rapid- or short-acting insulin; blood glucose concentrations generally are monitored 1–4 times daily. Commercially available premixed insulin combinations may be used if the insulin ratio is appropriate to the patient's insulin requirements; these preparations may be especially useful in patients with type 2 diabetes mellitus who eat small lunches, geriatric patients, those unable to use more complex regimens, and those with visual impairment. Premixed insulins offer little flexibility for meal size and time, particularly in patients with severe insulin deficiency (i.e., most patients with type 1 diabetes mellitus), since such mixtures of insulins may not provide enough insulin for lunchtime needs.

The selection of a particular insulin treatment program is dependent on a number of factors including the age of the patient, the nature of the disease (ketoacidosis-prone or ketoacidosis-resistant), the presence or absence of symptoms of hyperglycemia, and the experience and judgment of the clinician. Initial total daily insulin dosages in adults and children with type 1 diabetes mellitus generally range from 0.4–1 units/kg; basal insulin requirements with an intermediate-acting or long-acting insulin usually comprise 40–60% of the total daily insulin dosage, with the remainder given preprandially as rapid- or short-acting insulin. Alternatively, some manufacturers recommend that basal insulin comprise approximately one-third to one-half of the total daily insulin dosage in insulin-naive patients with type 1 diabetes mellitus, with the remainder of the daily dosage given preprandially as rapid- or short-acting insulin.

To initiate therapy in patients with severe symptomatic diabetes, unstable type 1 diabetes, severe metabolic dysfunction, or diabetes with complications, hospitalization and the use of regular insulin may be advisable. Some clinicians suggest that in general, insulin therapy in adults of normal weight may be initiated with 15–20 units daily of an intermediate-acting (e.g., insulin human isophane [NPH]) or long-acting (e.g., insulin glargine, insulin detemir) insulin given subcutaneously before breakfast, dinner, or bedtime; obese patients, because of associated insulin resistance, may initially be given 25–30 units daily. Use of rapid- or short-acting insulin alone before meals may rarely be sufficient in newly diagnosed patients with diabetes mellitus who have some residual basal endogenous insulin secretion.

In patients with type 2 diabetes mellitus who have secondary failure to oral antidiabetic agent(s), an intermediate-acting or long-acting insulin may be added to the existing oral antidiabetic regimen; premixed insulin combinations containing insulin human isophane (NPH) may be given once daily with the evening meal in such patients. Initial dosage of a basal insulin (e.g., intermediate-acting insulin at bedtime, long-acting insulin at bedtime or morning) in patients with type 2 diabetes mellitus inadequately controlled on oral antidiabetic agent(s) generally is 0.1–0.2 units/kg daily or 10 units daily. Patients should be advised that initial insulin dosages are approximations and that frequent dosage adjustments will be required over the next few weeks. ADA recommends the use of an evidence-based insulin dosage titration algorithm (i.e., increase of 2 units every 3 days to achieve target fasting plasma glucose concentration).

Virtually all patients with type 1 diabetes mellitus and many with type 2 diabetes mellitus will require 2 or more insulin injections daily with intermediate-acting and/or rapid- or short-acting insulins to maintain adequate control of blood glucose throughout the night while avoiding daytime hypoglycemia. ADA currently recommends the same blood glucose and HbA_{1c} concentration goals for all nonpregnant adults with type 1 or type 2 diabetes mellitus but states that less stringent treatment goals may be appropriate for certain patients. (See Treatment Goals under Uses: Diabetes Mellitus.) If a patient's HbA_{1c} remains above target despite the use of adequately titrated basal insulin or daily basal insulin dosages exceeding 0.7–1 unit/kg, or despite achieving target fasting plasma glucose concentrations, prandial insulin should be initiated. Prandial insulin should be given with the largest meal of the day or the meal associated with the greatest postprandial plasma glucose concentration. More prandial insulin may be added in a stepwise manner (i.e., 2, then 3 additional injections) to a patient's regimen as needed. The recommended starting dose of prandial insulin in patients with type 2 diabetes mellitus is either 4 units or 10% of the basal dose at each meal.

Intensive insulin therapy generally refers to regimens consisting of 3 or more doses of insulin per day administered by subcutaneous injection or continuous subcutaneous infusion of insulin via an insulin pump, with dosage adjustments made according to the results of frequent (e.g., at least 3–4 times daily) self-monitored blood glucose determinations and anticipated dietary intake and exercise. Since patients receiving intensive insulin therapy generally will achieve greater postprandial glycemic control than those receiving conventional therapy because of increased use of rapid- or short-acting insulin, patients receiving conventional insulin regimens generally will require a smaller total daily insulin dosage when switched to an intensive insulin regimen.

In patients with type 1 diabetes mellitus who have been receiving conventional insulin therapy (e.g., twice-daily doses of intermediate-acting and rapid- or short-acting insulin given before breakfast and the evening meal), intensive insulin therapy may be initiated with a stepwise approach in which the number of insulin injections per day is gradually increased until near-normal postprandial and basal glycemic control is attained. Alternatively, a dose of long-acting insulin (e.g., insulin glargine) may be administered in the evening in conjunction with doses of a rapid-acting (e.g., insulin lispro, insulin aspart, insulin glulisine) or short-acting (e.g., regular) insulin before each meal. Because of insulin degludec's very long duration of action (e.g., 42 hours) and low variability in insulin concentrations over the dosing interval, it can be administered at any time of day in adults, which may provide greater dosing flexibility than other basal insulins such as insulin detemir or insulin glargine.

A subcutaneous insulin regimen in hospitalized patients is comprised of regularly scheduled subcutaneous injections (basal and prandial) and correctional (supplemental) injections as an adjunct to regularly scheduled insulin to meet nutritional needs. Premixed insulin regimens are not routinely recommended for in-hospital use. Daily insulin dose requirements can be met by various types of insulin, depending on the particular clinical situation. Since insulin human has a longer duration of action than more rapid-acting analogues, use of correctional insulin for premeal or between-meal hyperglycemia before previously administered regular insulin has reached a peak effect may lead to hypoglycemia.

IV insulin is considered the standard of care for management of hyperglycemia in critically ill patients. IV infusion of regular insulin may be used in hospitalized patients with diabetic ketoacidosis, nonketotic hyperosmolar states, cardiogenic shock, exacerbated hyperglycemia during high-dose corticosteroid therapy, poorly controlled diabetes mellitus and widely fluctuating blood glucose concentrations, severe insulin resistance, or as a dose-finding strategy prior to initiation or reinitiation of subcutaneous insulin therapy. IV administration of regular insulin also is recommended during general perioperative care and the postoperative period following cardiac surgery or organ transplantation or when a prolonged postoperative period with no oral intake is anticipated (e.g., cardiothoracic, major abdominal, CNS surgery). The initial perioperative maintenance insulin infusion rate in patients undergoing major surgery is 0.2 units/kg per hour. When regular insulin is administered by continuous IV infusion, bedside glucose testing should be performed every hour until blood glucose concentrations are stable for 6–8 hours; the frequency of testing can then be reduced to every 2–3 hours. Dosing algorithms should achieve correction of hyperglycemia in a timely manner, provide a method to adjust the insulin infusion rate required to maintain blood glucose concentrations within a defined target range, and allow for the adjustment of insulin infusion maintenance rate as patient's insulin sensitivity or carbohydrate intake changes.

When normoglycemia has been reached after IV insulin infusion in hospitalized patients, some patients will require subcutaneous insulin maintenance therapy and some patients with type 2 diabetes mellitus will have therapy transferred to oral antidiabetic agents. For those who require subcutaneous insulin, basal insulin should be administered 2–4 hours prior to discontinuance of the IV insulin infusion. Converting to basal insulin at 60–80% of the daily IV insulin infusion dose has been shown to be effective.

Data indicate that continuous subcutaneous insulin injection (i.e., insulin pump) may provide a slight advantage in reducing HbA_{1c} and the risk of severe hypoglycemia compared with multiple daily insulin injections. ADA recommends that most adults, children, and adolescents with type 1 diabetes mellitus should be treated with intensive insulin therapy with multiple daily insulin injections or an insulin pump. ADA also states that an insulin pump may be considered in all children and adolescents requiring insulin therapy, especially those younger than 7 years of age.

Any change of insulin preparation or dosage regimen should be made with caution and only under medical supervision. Should a brand of insulin become unavailable temporarily, the same insulin formulation from another manufacturer may be substituted. Although it is not possible to clearly identify which patients will require a change in dosage when therapy with a different preparation is started, it is known that a limited number of patients will require such a change. Adjustments may be needed with the first dose or may occur over a period of several weeks. In general, the usual initial dosage reduction in these patients is about 10–20%.

Considerations in Monitoring Insulin Therapy Patients receiving intensive insulin regimens should self-monitor blood glucose concentrations prior to meals and snacks, at bedtime, occasionally postprandially, prior to exercise, when low blood glucose is suspected, after treating low blood glucose (until normoglycemic), and prior to critical tasks (e.g., driving); this may require patients to test up to 6–10 times daily. Patients not receiving intensive insulin regimens, such as those receiving basal insulin only, should at least assess fasting blood glucose concentrations in order to facilitate dosage adjustments; data regarding the exact number of times a patient should ideally check their blood glucose concentrations are lacking in this patient population. Blood glucose concentrations may be influenced by food consumption, exercise, stress, hormonal changes, illness, travel, insulin absorption rates, and insulin sensitivity.

If preprandial blood glucose concentrations consistently exceed 300 mg/dL, patients should be instructed to monitor for ketones in urine or blood (β-hydroxybutyric acid). The presence of ketones in urine or blood may indicate insulin deficiency or insulin resistance; in such cases, clinicians should consider possible causes of insulin deficiency, such as a missed insulin dose or illness, and supplement the dosage of insulin as appropriate. (See Diabetic Ketoacidosis and Hyperosmolar Hyperglycemic States under Dosage and Administration: Dosage, in Insulin Human 68:20.08.08.)

If blood glucose concentrations are unexpectedly high, additional doses of short- or rapid-acting insulin (e.g., up to 15% of the regular dose) may be necessary to reestablish glycemic control. Blood glucose concentrations should be reassessed approximately 4 hours after additional doses have been given. If blood glucose concentrations are still high, another dose of insulin (e.g., 5% of the regular dose) may be given to achieve glycemic control. Records of self-monitored blood glucose concentrations should be compared with clinician-obtained values for evidence of faulty injection technique or patient noncompliance. Patients should contact their clinician if extra insulin fails to reduce high blood glucose concentrations and/or ketonuria or ketonemia.

Insulin Use During Pregnancy Insulin requirements generally increase, sometimes dramatically, in pregnant patients with diabetes. In addition, pregnancy may induce a temporary state of diabetes in patients not previously known to be diabetic (i.e., gestational diabetes mellitus). (See Uses: Gestational Diabetes Mellitus.) The increased need for insulin generally begins in the second trimester, and an insulin regimen should be established during preconception care visits. In high-risk pregnancies, hospitalization may be required to ensure an appropriate insulin regimen. Since the renal threshold for glucose may be decreased during pregnancy, blood glucose determinations are needed to ascertain the effectiveness of therapy.

In patients with gestational diabetes mellitus requiring insulin therapy, the usual initial total daily dosage is 0.7–1 units/kg, given in divided doses. In women with gestational diabetes, if fasting and postprandial hyperglycemia are present, an insulin regimen consisting of long-acting or intermediate-acting insulin in conjunction with short-acting insulin is recommended. In women with gestational diabetes mellitus who have only isolated high blood glucose concentrations at specific times of the day, an insulin regimen which focuses on the times when hyperglycemia occurs is preferred (e.g., administering short-acting insulin prior to certain meals of the day).

Maternal blood glucose monitoring in women with gestational diabetes mellitus should be instituted to assess glycemic control. Self-monitoring of fasting and postprandial blood glucose concentrations are recommended in women with gestational diabetes mellitus and pre-existing diabetes mellitus. Additionally, pregnant women who are using an insulin pump or basal-bolus insulin therapy should also test preprandial blood glucose concentrations in order to facilitate insulin dosage adjustments.

Cautions

■ **Endocrine and Metabolic Effects** ***Hypoglycemia*** Hypoglycemia is the most common adverse effect of insulins, and monitoring of blood glucose concentrations is recommended for all patients with diabetes. The timing of hypoglycemia depends on the time of peak action of insulin in relation to food intake (absorption) and/or exercise. The risk of hypoglycemia is increased in patients with unstable type 1 diabetes, autonomic neuropathy, or irregular eating patterns and in patients receiving intensive insulin therapy or who exercise without making appropriate insulin dosage adjustments or ingesting extra food. Hypoglycemia also may result from increased insulin absorption rates (e.g., increased skin temperature resulting from sunbathing or exposure to hot water). Hypoglycemic reactions also have been reported in patients who were transferred from beef to pork insulin or mixed beef-pork preparations or from pork insulin (no longer commercially available in the US) to insulin human; however, preparations containing beef insulin alone or in combination with pork insulin are no longer commercially available in the US. Hypoglycemia also may occur in association with increased insulin sensitivity that accompanies secondary adrenocortical insufficiency or Addison's disease.

Symptoms of hypoglycemia usually are manifested when the administered insulin reaches its peak action and may include hunger, pallor, fatigue, mild or profuse perspiration, headache, nausea, palpitation, numbness of the mouth, tingling in the fingers, tremors, muscle weakness, blurred or double vision, hypothermia, uncontrolled yawning, nervousness, irritability or agitation, difficulty in concentrating, mental confusion, aggressiveness, drowsiness, tachycardia, shallow breathing, seizures, and loss of consciousness. Insulin overdosage may result in psychic disturbances such as aphasia, personality changes, or maniacal behavior. Homeostatic responses to hypoglycemia include cessation of insulin release and mobilization of counterregulatory hormones such as glucagon, epinephrine, and less acutely, growth hormone and cortisol. These responses become defective, and early warning signs of hypoglycemia may be diminished or absent, in patients with long-standing type 1 diabetes mellitus diabetic neuropathy, and/or those receiving drugs such as β-adrenergic blocking agents that mask catecholamine-induced manifestations of hypoglycemia (e.g., tremors, palpitations) or intensive insulin therapy. If untreated, severe prolonged hypoglycemia can result in irreversible brain damage.

Hypoglycemic reactions in geriatric diabetic patients may mimic a cerebrovascular accident. In addition, because of an increased incidence of macrovascular disease in geriatric patients with type 2 diabetes mellitus, such patients may be more vulnerable to serious consequences of hypoglycemia, including fainting, seizures, falls, stroke, silent ischemia, myocardial infarction, or sudden death.

The more vigorous the attempt to achieve euglycemia, the greater the risk of hypoglycemia. In the Diabetes Control and Complications Trial (DCCT), the incidence of severe hypoglycemia, including multiple episodes in some patients, was 3 times higher in patients receiving intensive insulin treatment (3 or more insulin injections daily with dosage adjusted according to results of at least 4 daily blood glucose determinations, dietary intake, and anticipated exercise) than in those receiving conventional treatment (1 or 2 insulin injections daily, self-monitoring of blood or urine glucose values, education about diet and exercise). In the Action to Control Cardiovascular Risk in Diabetes (ACCORD) trial in patients with type 2 diabetes mellitus, the incidence of severe hypoglycemia (episodes requiring medical assistance) was 10.5 or 3.5% in patients receiving intensive (median achieved HbA_{1c} concentrations: 6.4%) or conventional (median achieved HbA_{1c} concentrations: 7.5%) treatment, respectively. Hypoglycemia is the major risk that must be considered against the benefits of intensive insulin therapy. An increased rate of mortality was noted among patients in the ACCORD trial receiving intensive treatment; preliminary exploratory analyses evaluating numerous variables, including hypoglycemia, were unable to identify an explanation for increased mortality in the intensive therapy group. However, in DCCT, there was no increase in mortality or permanent neuropsychologic morbidity associated with the increased rate of severe hypoglycemia in that study. Since symptoms of hypoglycemia may develop suddenly, diabetic patients should be instructed to carry a ready source of carbohydrate as well as some form of diabetic identification. Episodes of late postprandial hypoglycemia (i.e., 4–6 hours after a meal) observed with the use of short-acting insulin before meals occur as a consequence of hyperinsulinemia present when the meal has been almost totally absorbed. The potential for late postprandial hypoglycemia observed with short-acting insulin may be reduced by altering the timing, frequency, and content of meals, altering exercise patterns, frequently monitoring blood glucose concentrations, adjusting insulin dosage, and/or switching to a more rapid-acting insulin (e.g., insulin lispro, insulin glulisine).

Rebound Hyperglycemia Hyperglycemia that occurs as a result of excessive counterregulatory hormone responses to hypoglycemia (Somogyi effect, posthypoglycemic hyperglycemia) appears to occur principally in patients with type 1 diabetes mellitus. While the exact mechanism of this effect is unknown and there is controversy regarding whether it even exists, it has been suggested that excessive doses of an intermediate-acting (e.g., isophane [NPH]) insulin in the evening lead to nocturnal hypoglycemia and a compensatory release of counterregulatory hormones (e.g., epinephrine, growth hormone, cortisol, glucagon), resulting in increased hepatic glucose production and rebound hyperglycemia the following morning. The existence of such "rebound" hyperglycemia and/or the frequency with which it occurs has been questioned since the effect often has not been reproducible in clinical studies (particularly in adults), and neuroendocrine counterregulatory responses to hypoglycemia are known to be reduced in patients with long-standing diabetes mellitus. Some clinicians suggest that morning hyperglycemia occurring after an episode of nocturnal hypoglycemia results principally from overzealous intake of carbohydrate in an attempt to correct the hypoglycemia; other proposed mechanisms for this effect include the waning action of the insulin that caused the hypoglycemia and hypoglycemia-induced insulin resistance.

Manifestations suggesting an excessive insulin dosage in patients with hyperglycemia include excessive appetite and weight gain, nocturnal hypoglycemia, extreme variations in glucose concentrations, and frequent ketosis (especially in the absence of glycosuria), with worsening of these manifestations when insulin dosage is increased. The Somogyi effect must be differentiated from the "dawn phenomenon," which is characterized by early morning hyperglycemia that appears related to nocturnal growth hormone release and the patient's inability to compensate for increased blood glucose concentrations with an increase in endogenous insulin secretion; differentiation of the Somogyi effect and the dawn phenomenon may be accomplished by monitoring blood glucose at 3 a.m. Recommended treatment for the Somogyi effect, if it is suspected, is gradual *reduction* of the evening intermediate-acting insulin dosage or addition of/increase in the size of the nighttime snack (with a slowly absorbable carbohydrate) in conjunction with continuous blood glucose monitoring. (See Dosage and Administration: Dosage.) The dawn phenomenon reflects a relative deficiency of insulin and is treated by *increasing* the evening intermediate-acting insulin dose and/or later administration of that dose (i.e., at bedtime rather than at dinner).

Potassium Effects Hypokalemia may occur with insulin therapy since insulin promotes an intracellular shift of potassium as a result of stimulating cell membrane Na+- K+-ATPase. Untreated hypokalemia may result in respiratory paralysis, ventricular arrhythmia, and death.

■ **Dermatologic and Sensitivity Reactions** Localized allergic reactions such as pruritus, erythema, swelling, stinging or warmth at the site of injection may develop in patients receiving insulin. Localized allergic reactions may occur within 1–3 weeks after initiating insulin therapy, are relatively minor, and usually disappear within a few days to weeks. Poor injection technique may contribute to localized injection site reactions.

Manifestations of immediate hypersensitivity commonly occur within 30–120 minutes after the injection, may last for several hours or days, and usually subside spontaneously. True insulin allergy is rare and is characterized by generalized urticaria or bullae, dyspnea, wheezing, hypotension, tachycardia, diaphoresis, angioedema, and anaphylaxis. These reactions may represent a secondary anamnestic response and occur most frequently after intermittent insulin therapy or in patients with increased circulating insulin antibodies. Severe cases of generalized insulin allergy may be life-threatening. (See Cautions: Precautions and Contraindications.) There is some evidence that the incidence of allergic reactions has decreased with the availability of more purified insulin (e.g., insulin human, insulin lispro). In addition, several studies have shown insulin human and insulin lispro to be less immunogenic than animal-source insulin (i.e., purified pork insulin, beef insulin). Preparations containing beef or pork insulin are no longer commercially available in the US. (See Cautions: Immunogenicity, in Insulin Human 68:20.08.08 and Insulin Lispro 68:20.08.04.)

Atrophy or hypertrophy of subcutaneous fat tissue may occur at sites of frequent insulin injections. (See Cautions: Precautions and Contraindications.) Lipoatrophy is thought to be the result of an immune reaction to some contaminant of insulin.

■ **Insulin Resistance** Resistance to insulin in patients with type 1 diabetes mellitus occurs infrequently and may be caused by either immune or nonimmune factors. Patients with insulin resistance usually require more than 200 units of insulin daily; in comparison, data from a small number of patients who had undergone pancreatectomy indicate that 10–44 units of insulin daily were required to control secondary diabetes mellitus.

Insulin resistance in patients with type 2 diabetes mellitus is frequently associated with obesity. This type of resistance results from tissue insensitivity to insulin, which may be caused by a decrease in the number of insulin receptors or a decreased affinity of insulin for the receptors. The principal treatment for obesity-related insulin resistance is weight reduction.

Acute insulin resistance may develop in diabetic patients with infections, surgical or other trauma, emotional disturbances, or additional endocrine disorders (e.g., hyperthyroidism, acromegaly, Cushing's syndrome); therapy is aimed at relieving the intercurrent medical illness. Insulin requirements usually increase during pregnancy. (See Insulin Use during Pregnancy under Dosage and Administration: Dosage.)

Chronic insulin resistance resulting from immunity may occur when insulin therapy is reinstituted after a period of withdrawal. Most patients with chronic insulin resistance have been found to have markedly elevated concentrations of circulating insulin antibodies. Chronic insulin resistance resulting from immunity has been decreased by changing from beef (no longer commercially available in the US) to pork insulin (since some patients have selective resistance to beef insulin) or by changing to a purified insulin preparation (e.g., insulin human). Animal insulins are no longer commercially available in the US. Insulin lispro also has been effective in establishing glycemic control in patients with insulin resistance. (See Uses, in Insulin Lispro 68:20.08.04.) Patients with insulin immune resistance who are switched to another type of insulin should be started at a lower dosage because their dosage requirements may be greatly decreased. Although administration of corticosteroids has been associated with induction of diabetes mellitus and insulin resistance, these drugs have been used with limited success in the treatment of immune-mediated insulin resistance. Sulfated insulin (not commercially available in the US) has been used in patients with immune-mediated insulin resistance in whom other methods had failed.

■ **Ocular Effects** Transient presbyopia or blurred vision may occur in diabetic patients given insulin whose blood glucose concentrations have been uncontrolled for an extended period of time or in newly diagnosed diabetic patients in whom rapid glycemic control has been achieved. Patients with proliferative retinopathy who have hemoglobin A_{1c} (HbA_{1c}) concentrations exceeding 10% are at highest risk of worsening retinopathy. When blood glucose concentration is lowered in these patients, the osmotic equilibrium between the lens and ocular fluids occurs slowly but visual acuity will stabilize eventually. Some clinicians recommend that HbA_{1c} concentrations be reduced slowly (2% per year) in such patients and that frequent ophthalmologic examinations (e.g., every 6 months or when symptoms appear) be performed to ensure aggressive treatment of progressive retinopathy. New eyeglasses should not be prescribed for these patients until vision has stabilized.

■ **Heart Failure** Peroxisome proliferator-activated receptor (PPAR)-γ agonists (e.g., thiazolidinediones) can cause dose-related fluid retention, particularly when used in combination with insulin. Fluid retention may lead to or exacerbate heart failure. Patients receiving insulin and a PPAR-γ agonist should be observed for manifestations of heart failure (e.g., excessive/rapid weight gain, shortness of breath, edema). If heart failure develops, it should be managed according to current standards of care, and discontinuance of the PPAR-γ agonist or reduction of the dosage must be considered. Concomitant use of rosiglitazone and insulin therapy is not recommended.

■ **Precautions and Contraindications** ***Formulation Considerations*** Any change in insulin should be made cautiously and only under medical supervision. Patients should be informed of the reasons for any change in the insulin regimen and the potential need for additional glucose monitoring. Changes in insulin strength, manufacturer, type (e.g., regular, NPH), or method of manufacture may necessitate a change in dosage. Patients receiving insulin should be monitored with regular laboratory evaluations, including blood glucose determinations and glycosylated hemoglobin (hemoglobin A_{1c} [HbA_{1c}]) concentrations, to determine the minimum effective dosage of insulin when used alone, with other insulins, or in combination with an oral antidiabetic agent.

Hypoglycemia and Hypokalemia As hypoglycemia and hypokalemia may occur with insulin therapy, care should be taken in patients who are most at risk for the development of these effects, including patients who are fasting, those with defective counterregulatory responses (e.g., patients with autonomic neuropathy, adrenal or pituitary insufficiency, those receiving β-adrenergic blocking agents) or patients who are receiving potassium-lowering drugs. Insulin human is contraindicated during episodes of hypoglycemia. As IV insulin has a rapid onset of action, increased attention to hypoglycemia and hypokalemia is necessary. Blood glucose and potassium concentrations should be monitored closely when insulin is administered IV. Rapid changes in serum glucose concentrations may precipitate manifestations of hypoglycemia, regardless of glucose concentration. The potential for late postprandial hypoglycemia observed with short-acting insulin may be reduced by altering the timing, frequency, and content of meals, altering exercise patterns, frequently monitoring blood glucose concentrations, adjusting insulin dosage, and/or switching to a more rapid-acting insulin (e.g., insulin lispro, insulin glulisine). Patients with a history of hypoglycemic unawareness or recurrent, severe hypoglycemic episodes should be particularly vigilant in monitoring their blood glucose concentrations frequently, especially before activities such as driving; intensive insulin therapy should be used with caution in these patients. Maintenance of higher target blood glucose concentrations for at least several weeks is advisable in patients with a history of hypoglycemic unawareness or one or more episodes of severe hypoglycemia to avoid further hypoglycemia, partially reverse hypoglycemic unawareness, and reduce the risk of future episodes. Severe or frequent hypoglycemia is an absolute indication for the modification of treatment regimens, including setting higher glycemic goals. All adolescents with diabetes mellitus should monitor their blood glucose concentrations before driving and take corrective action to avoid hypoglycemia and cognitive-motor impairments. Such adolescents should carry a source of glucose in the car and should cease driving immediately should symptoms of hypoglycemia occur.

Management of Hypoglycemia. Oral administration of 15–20 g of dextrose is the preferred treatment for mild hypoglycemia, although any form of carbohydrate that contains glucose may be used, such as orange or other fruit juice, sugar, hard candy, regular nondiet soda, or dextrose gel or chewable tablets. The dose may be repeated in 15 minutes if blood glucose concentrations remain below 70 mg/dL (as determined by self-monitoring of blood glucose concentrations) or if symptoms of hypoglycemia are still present. Once blood glucose concentrations return to normal, ADA suggests that patients eat a meal or snack to prevent the recurrence of hypoglycemia.

In children and adolescents, administration of 15 g of an easily-absorbed carbohydrate followed by a protein-containing snack is sufficient for mild hypoglycemia; younger children may require about 10 g of carbohydrate to alleviate symptoms. Adjustments in the carbohydrate amounts should be based on blood glucose concentrations. Treatment of moderate hypoglycemia requires that someone other than the child or adolescent administer treatment, usually 20–30 g of glucose to restore blood glucose concentrations to greater than 80 mg/dL. Severe hypoglycemia (associated with altered states of consciousness, including coma and seizures) requires treatment with glucagon or IV dextrose solutions. (See Acute Toxicity: Treatment.)

Following a hypoglycemic reaction, patients should review the probable cause (e.g., excessive exercise, insufficient food intake, inappropriate insulin dosage) with their clinician and take action to prevent further such reactions. Alterations in snack patterns and adjustment in timing and/or dosage of insulin relative to activity levels should be discussed. (See Acute Toxicity.)

Sensitivity Reactions Patients who have had severe allergic reactions to insulin (i.e., generalized rash, swelling, or breathing difficulty) should be skin-tested with *any new* insulin preparation before it is initiated. Desensitization may be required in patients with a potential for allergic reaction. Because patients may have selective allergic reactions to pork or beef insulin, or to protamine or proteins, further allergic reactions may be prevented by substitution of an insulin that contains less protein (i.e., purified insulins, including insulin human) or that does not contain protamine. Pure beef and mixed beef-pork insulins are no longer commercially available in the US.

Patient Instructions It is important that the patient receive careful instruction in the importance of proper mixing and storage of insulin, timing of insulin dosing, adherence to meal planning, regular physical exercise, periodic HbA_{1c} concentration testing, recognition and management of hypoglycemia and hyperglycemic reactions, and periodic assessment of diabetic complications.

Patients and their families should be informed of the potential risks and advantages of conventional and intensive insulin therapy. While an intensive insulin regimen consisting of multiple insulin injections daily may not be advisable clinically in certain patient populations, such a regimen also may be problematic in noncompliant patients (e.g., substance abusers, psychiatric patients) or patients who not capable of adjusting their insulin requirements based on frequent self-monitoring of blood glucose concentrations.

Patients should be aware of the need for possible changes in the dosage of insulin and the need for additional monitoring of blood glucose concentrations during an illness, emotional disturbances or stress, or travel. Adjustment of insulin dosage may be needed if patients change their physical activity or usual meal plan.

Patients should be aware of symptoms of diabetic ketoacidosis and should monitor blood ketones if preprandial blood glucose concentrations repeatedly exceed 250–300 mg/dL or if they have an acute illness. Patients should be advised about sick-day procedures to assist in managing their diabetes during acute illness. Patients should contact their physician if results of self-monitored blood glucose concentrations are consistently abnormal.

Administration Considerations. Careful instruction about insulin administration technique and periodic reevaluation can minimize the likelihood of local adverse effects associated with faulty technique (e.g., lipoatrophy, lipohypertrophy). (See Dosage and Administration: Administration.) Subcutaneous injection sites should be rotated to prevent tissue damage that can occur with repeated subcutaneous injections of insulin into the same site. Direct injection of insulin into the outside edge of the atrophied area may result in improvement or complete disappearance of the atrophy in some patients. Rotating injection sites within one anatomical region (e.g., rotating injections systematically in the abdominal area) rather than selecting a different anatomical region is recommended to decrease day-to-day variability in insulin absorption. Variability in insulin absorption by injection site is reduced with insulin lispro compared with that with insulin human. Patients should be instructed to contact their clinician if lipoatrophy, lipohypertrophy, or local adverse effects (e.g., burning, itching, swelling) occur at the site of injection. Direct injection of insulin into the outside edge of the atrophied area may result in improvement or complete disappearance of the atrophy in some patients.

■ **Pediatric Precautions** In young patients (i.e., those younger than 6 years of age) who may be unable to recognize, articulate, and/or manage hypoglycemia, the risk of hypoglycemia should be considered when setting glycemic targets. However, some data indicate that lower HbA_{1c} targets can be achieved in young children without increased risk of severe hypoglycemia. The risks of hypoglycemia and the developmental burdens of intensive insulin regimens in children and adolescents should be weighed against the long-term health benefits associated with achieving a lower HbA_{1c}.

ADA generally recommends that all children and adolescents with type 1 diabetes mellitus be treated with intensive insulin regimens; all children and adolescents should self-monitor blood glucose concentrations multiple times daily (up to 6–10 times per day), including premeal and prebedtime determinations, as needed for safety (e.g., prior to exercise or driving), or during the presence of hypoglycemic symptoms. Continuous glucose monitoring should be considered in all children and adolescents with type 1 diabetes mellitus.

■ **Geriatric Precautions** Long-term studies conducted in geriatric patients with diabetes mellitus demonstrating the benefits of tight glycemic, blood pressure, and lipid control are lacking. Older adults are at an increased risk of developing hypoglycemia due to multiple factors such as renal insufficiency and cognitive deficits. It is important to prevent hypoglycemia in older adults to reduce the risk of cognitive decline and other adverse effects. Treatment goals for older patients should be individualized and should take into consideration multiple patient specific factors (e.g., comorbidities, cognitive function, functional status, life expectancy). Although control of hyperglycemia is important in geriatric patients with diabetes mellitus, greater reductions in morbidity and mortality may result from control of all cardiovascular risk factors. However, intensive management of diabetes mellitus and coexisting conditions may not be feasible in a proportion of geriatric patients, and clinicians may have to prioritize reduction of some of these risks. In frail geriatric patients with appreciable comorbid conditions, short life expectancy, cognitive or functional impairment, or noncompliance with treatment recommendations, clinicians may choose to enact treatment goals that enhance the quality of life and to treat symptoms or related conditions associated with diabetes mellitus.

■ **Pregnancy** Diabetic pregnancy is a high-risk state for both mother and fetus/infant. Women with diabetes mellitus who are pregnant or planning pregnancy require tight glycemic control. In women with preexisting diabetes mellitus or gestational diabetes mellitus, the ADA currently recommends a target fasting blood glucose concentrations of less than 95 mg/dL, a 1-hour postprandial blood glucose concentrations of less than 140 mg/dL, a 2-hour postprandial blood glucose concentration of less than 120 mg/dL, and a target HbA_{1c} concentration of less than 6% in such women. If women cannot achieve these glycemic targets without substantial hypoglycemia, less stringent targets may be appropriate and should be individualized.

Patients with diabetes mellitus should inform their physician if they are pregnant or intend to become pregnant; preconception glycemic control is crucial in preventing congenital malformations and reducing the risk of other complications, Many experts recommend institution of strict glycemic control, including use of intensive insulin regimens as needed, before conception and throughout pregnancy in patients with diabetes. (See Insulin Use During Pregnancy under Dosage and Administration: Dosage.) Experts recommend the use of insulin for the management of both type 1 and type 2 diabetes mellitus in pregnant women. Newer rapid-acting insulin analogs have been used increasingly in pregnant women, and based on current evidence, insulin lispro and insulin aspart are not teratogenic. These rapid-acting insulin analogs have been shown to be safe and effective during pregnancy and may provide better postprandial glycemic control with less hypoglycemia than regular insulin. In an open-label clinical study of pregnant women with type 1 diabetes mellitus, insulin detemir therapy did not increase the risk of fetal abnormalities. Additionally, there was no difference in pregnancy outcomes or the health of the fetus and newborn with insulin detemir use. Experience with insulin degludec and insulin glargine in pregnant women is limited.

Maintenance of normal glycemia during pregnancy appears to reduce the risk of congenital malformations, fetal macrosomia and other neonatal morbidities (e.g., hypoglycemia, hypocalcemia, polycythemia, hyperbilirubinemia) as well as perinatal mortality (e.g., miscarriage, intrauterine death, stillbirth). Diabetic women of childbearing age should be informed about the risks of unplanned pregnancy and the appropriate use of contraception until glycemic control is achieved.

Drug Interactions

■ **Drugs That May Have a Variable Effect on Glycemic Control** Anabolic steroids, lithium salts, pentamidine, clonidine, and β-adrenergic blocking agents have variable effects on glucose metabolism as such agents may impair glucose tolerance or increase the frequency or severity of hypoglycemia. In addition, β-adrenergic blocking agents may suppress hypoglycemia-induced tachycardia but not hypoglycemic sweating, which may actually be increased; delay the rate of recovery of blood glucose concentration following drug-induced hypoglycemia; alter the hemodynamic response to hypoglycemia, possibly resulting in an exaggerated hypertensive response; and possibly impair peripheral circulation.

Nonselective β-adrenergic blocking agents (e.g., propranolol, nadolol) without intrinsic sympathomimetic activity are more likely to affect glucose metabolism than more selective β-adrenergic blocking agents (e.g., metoprolol, atenolol) or those with intrinsic sympathomimetic activity (e.g., acebutolol, pindolol). Signs of hypoglycemia (e.g., tachycardia, blood pressure changes, tremor, feelings of anxiety) mediated by catecholamines may be masked by either nonselective or selective β-adrenergic blockade or by other sympatholytic agents such as centrally acting α-adrenergic blocking agents (e.g., clonidine) or reserpine. These drugs should be used with caution in patients with diabetes mellitus, especially in those with labile disease or in those prone to hypoglycemia. Use of low-dose, selective β_1-adrenergic blockers (e.g., metoprolol, atenolol) or β-adrenergic blocking agents with intrinsic sympathomimetic activity in patients receiving insulin may theoretically decrease the risk of affecting glycemic control. When insulin and a β-adrenergic blocking agent are used concomitantly, the patient should be advised about and monitored closely for altered glycemic control.

■ **Other Drugs Affecting Glycemic Control** The hypoglycemic activity of insulin may be potentiated by concomitant administration of alcohol, α-adrenergic blocking agents, certain antidepressants (e.g., monoamine oxidase inhibitors), glucagon-like peptide-1 (GLP-1) receptor agonists, guanethidine (no longer commercially available in the US), oral hypoglycemic agents, pramlintide, salicylates, sulfa antibiotics, certain angiotensin-converting enzyme inhibitors, angiotensin II receptor antagonists, and inhibitors of pancreatic function (e.g., octreotide). When such drugs are added to or withdrawn from therapy in patients receiving insulin, patients should be observed closely for evidence of altered glycemic control and possibly decreased insulin requirements.

Drugs with hyperglycemic activity that may antagonize the activity of insulin and exacerbate glycemic control in patients with diabetes mellitus include asparaginase, calcium-channel blocking agents, diazoxide, certain antilipemic agents (e.g., niacin), corticosteroids, danazol, estrogens,oral contraceptives, isoniazid, phenothiazines, sympathomimetics (e.g., epinephrine, albuterol, terbutaline), thiazide diuretics, furosemide, ethacrynic acid, and thyroid hormones. When such drugs are added to or withdrawn from therapy in patients receiving insulin, patients should be observed closely for evidence of altered glycemic control and possibly increased insulin requirements.

Acute Toxicity

■ **Pathogenesis** Acute hypoglycemia may result from excessive insulin dosage relative to food intake and/or energy expenditure, and numerous conditions may predispose to the development of insulin-induced hypoglycemia (e.g., defective counterregulatory response, hypoglycemic unawareness, insulin dosage errors, excessive alcohol intake, diabetic nephropathy, adrenal insufficiency, gastroparesis). (See Cautions: Precautions and Contraindications.) Hypoglycemia may result from overinsulinization, irregular eating patterns, increased physical activity, and/or decreased carbohydrate content of meals.

■ **Manifestations** Hypoglycemia, which may be severe, is the principal manifestation of acute insulin overdosage. Symptoms of moderate hypoglycemia include aggressiveness, drowsiness, confusion, and autonomic symptoms. Severe hypoglycemia is associated with altered states of consciousness, including coma and seizures. Severe hypoglycemia may result in loss of consciousness and seizures, with resultant neurologic sequelae (e.g., cerebral damage, seizures); fatalities have been reported following severe, insulin-induced hypoglycemia Other complications reported with insulin overdosage include hypokalemia, respiratory insufficiency/failure, pulmonary edema, congestive heart failure, hypertension, and cerebral edema.

■ **Treatment** Mild hypoglycemia (symptoms of sweating, pallor, palpitations, tremors, headache, behavioral changes) may be relieved by oral administration of carbohydrate-containing food or drink (e.g., orange or other fruit juice, lump sugar, candy). (See Management of Hypoglycemia under Precautions and Contraindications: Hypoglycemia and Hypokalemia, in Cautions.)

Severe hypoglycemia (associated with altered states of consciousness, including coma and seizures) requires treatment with glucagon or IV dextrose solutions. Severe insulin-induced hypoglycemia occurs infrequently but constitutes a medical emergency requiring immediate treatment. Adults with severe hypoglycemia (e.g., symptoms of lethargy, headache, confusion, sweating, agitation, seizures) or who are comatose from insulin overdosage and have adequate liver glycogen stores should receive 1 unit (1 mg) of subcutaneous, IM, or IV glucagon; patients should have a vial of glucagon available for family members to administer in emergency situations. Family members should be instructed in the proper administration of glucagon and the indications for its use. Patients unresponsive to or unable to receive glucagon should be given approximately 10–25 g of glucose as 20–50 mL of 50% dextrose injection IV. Higher or repeated doses of IV dextrose may be required in severe cases (e.g., intentional overdosage), and subsequent continuous IV infusion of glucose at 5–10 g/hour may be necessary to maintain adequate blood glucose concentrations until the patient is conscious and able to eat. The patient should be monitored closely until complete recovery is assured as hypoglycemia may recur. To prevent late or recurrent hypoglycemic reactions, oral carbohydrate should be given as soon as the comatose patient awakens.

In children and adolescents with severe hypoglycemia, glucagon at a dose of 30 mcg/kg subcutaneously up to a maximum of 1 mg (1 unit) will increase blood glucose concentrations within 5–15 minutes but may be associated with nausea and vomiting. A lower glucagon dose of 10 mcg/kg results in a lower glycemic response but is associated with less nausea. Repeated episodes of hypoglycemia or longstanding diabetes mellitus may result in defective glucose counterregulation and hypoglycemia unawareness. In such patients, blood glucose should be monitored frequently to avoid recurrent episodes.

Pharmacology

Exogenous insulin elicits all the pharmacologic responses usually produced by endogenous insulin.

Insulin stimulates carbohydrate metabolism in skeletal and cardiac muscle and adipose tissue by facilitating transport of glucose into these cells. Nerve tissues, erythrocytes, and cells of the intestines, liver, and kidney tubules do not require insulin for transfer of glucose. In the liver, insulin facilitates phosphorylation of glucose to glucose-6-phosphate which is converted to glycogen or further metabolized.

Insulin also has a direct effect on fat and protein metabolism. The hormone stimulates lipogenesis and inhibits lipolysis and release of free fatty acids from adipose cells. Insulin also stimulates protein synthesis.

Administration of suitable doses of insulin to patients with type 1 (insulin-dependent) diabetes mellitus temporarily restores their ability to metabolize carbohydrates, fats, and proteins; to store glucose in the liver; and to convert glycogen to fat. When insulin is given in suitable doses at regular intervals to a patient with diabetes mellitus, blood glucose is maintained at a reasonable concentration, the urine remains relatively free of glucose and ketone bodies, and diabetic acidosis and coma are prevented. The action of insulin is antagonized by somatotropin (growth hormone), epinephrine, glucagon, adrenocortical hormones, thyroid hormones, and estrogens.

Insulin promotes an intracellular shift of potassium and magnesium and thereby appears to temporarily decrease elevated blood concentrations of these ions.

Pharmacokinetics

■ **Absorption** Because of its protein nature, insulin is destroyed in the GI tract and usually is administered parenterally; however, regular insulin also has been administered via oral inhalation. Regular insulin also has been administered intranasally† or transdermally† in a limited number of patients. Following subcutaneous or IM administration, insulin is absorbed directly into the blood. Rate of absorption depends on many factors including route of administration, site of injection, volume and concentration of the injection, and type of insulin. One study in lean, healthy, fasting adults indicates that regular insulin is absorbed more rapidly following IM administration than when it is given subcutaneously. Absorption may be delayed and/or decreased by the presence of insulin-binding antibodies, which develop in all patients after 2–3 months of insulin treatment. Absorption of regular insulin following intranasal or transdermal administration generally has been variable and incomplete, and absorption enhancers (e.g., bile salts) have been used to facilitate delivery of insulin given by these routes. Some data suggest that intrapulmonary absorption of insulin and other peptides may be enhanced in cigarette smokers.

Commercially available insulin preparations differ mainly in their onset, peak, and duration of action following *subcutaneous* administration. Currently available insulin preparations are classified as rapid-acting, short-acting, intermediate-acting, or long-acting. The values for onset, peak, and duration of action of insulin injections shown in Table 1 are only approximate; substantial interindividual and intraindividual variation in these values may occur based on site of injection, injection technique, tissue blood supply, temperature, presence of insulin antibodies, exercise, excipients in insulin formulations, and/or interindividual and intraindividual differences in response. In addition, human insulins may have a more rapid onset and shorter duration of action than porcine insulins (no longer commercially available in the US) in patients with diabetes. (See Pharmacokinetics, in Insulin Human 68:20.08.08.) Similarly, insulin aspart has a more rapid onset and shorter duration of effect than insulin human; differences in pharmacodynamics between the 2 types of insulins are not associated with differences in overall glycemic control.

Table 1.

	Onset (hours)	Peak (hours)	Duration (hours)
Rapid-Acting			
Insulin Aspart Injection	0.17–0.33	1–3	3–5
Insulin Glulisine Injection	0.41	0.75–0.8	4–5.3
Insulin Lispro Injection	0.25–0.5	0.5–2.5	3–6.5
Short-Acting			
Insulin Human Injection	0.5–1	1–5	6–10
Intermediate-Acting			
Insulin Human Isophane (NPH) Injection	1–2	6–14	16–24+
Long-Acting			
Insulin Degludec Injection (100 or 200 units/mL)	0.5–1.5	No pronounced peak	42+
Insulin Detemir Injection	1.1–2	No pronounced peak	5.7–24
Insulin Glargine Injection (100 units/mL)	1.1	No pronounced peak	24
Insulin Glargine Injection (300 units/mL)	6	No pronounced peak	36

The hypoglycemic effect of commercially available mixtures containing insulin human isophane (NPH) 70 units/mL and insulin human 30 units/mL (Novolin® 70/30, Humulin® 70/30) usually occurs within 30 minutes, peaks within 1.5–12 hours, and persists for up to 24 hours. The hypoglycemic effect of the commercially available mixture containing insulin human isophane (NPH) 50 units/mL and insulin human 50 units/mL usually occurs within 0.5–1 hour, peaks within 1.5–4.5 hours, and persists for 7.5–24 hours. The addition of insulin lispro protamine 75 units/mL to insulin lispro 25 units/mL in the commercially available mixture (Humalog® 75/25) or 50 units/mL of insulin lispro protamine to insulin lispro 50 units/mL in the commercially available mixture (Humalog® 50/50) does not affect the onset of hypoglycemic effect compared with that with insulin lispro alone, which usually occurs within 0.25–0.5 hours, peaks within 2 hours, and persists for more than 22 hours. The hypoglycemic effect of the commercially available mixture containing insulin aspart protamine 70 units/mL and insulin aspart 30 units/mL usually occurs within 10–20 minutes, peaks within 1–4 hours, and persists for up to 24 hours. When administered in fixed combination with insulin aspart protamine, rapid absorption of the insulin aspart component is preserved, and absorption of insulin aspart protamine component is prolonged.

■ **Distribution** Insulin is rapidly distributed throughout extracellular fluids. It is not known whether insulin aspart is distributed into milk. Insulin aspart is minimally bound to plasma proteins (0–9%).

■ **Elimination** Insulin has a plasma half-life of a few minutes in healthy individuals; however, the biologic half-life may be prolonged in diabetic patients, probably as a result of binding of the hormone to antibodies, and in patients with renal impairment as a result of altered degradation/decreased clearance. Following subcutaneous administration, the half-life of insulin aspart averages 81 minutes. The half-life of insulin aspart in fixed combination with insulin aspart protamine is about 8–9 hours. Data from a pharmacokinetic study in patients with a wide range of body mass index, indicate that clearance of insulin aspart is reduced by 28% in obese patients with type 1 diabetes mellitus compared with that in leaner patients.

Insulin is rapidly metabolized mainly in the liver by the enzyme glutathione insulin transhydrogenase and to a lesser extent in the kidneys and muscle tissue. In the kidneys, insulin is filtered at the glomerulus and almost completely (98%) reabsorbed in the proximal tubule. About 40% of this reabsorbed insulin is returned to venous blood and 60% is metabolized in the cells lining the proximal convoluted tubule. In normal patients, only a small amount (less than 2%) of a filtered insulin dose is excreted unchanged in the urine.

In a pharmacokinetic study in a limited number of patients receiving an IV infusion (1.5 milliunits/kg per minute for 120 minutes) of either insulin aspart or insulin human, the mean insulin clearance was similar for the 2 types of insulins (1.22–1.24 L/hour per kg).

Chemistry and Stability

■ **Chemistry** Insulin is a hormone secreted by the beta cells of the pancreatic islets of Langerhans. Insulin is a protein with a molecular weight of about 6000 and is composed of 2 chains (A and B chains) of amino acids connected by disulfide linkages.

The potency of insulin is standardized according to its ability to lower blood glucose concentrations of normal fasting rabbits as compared to the USP Insulin Reference Standard. Potency is expressed in USP units per mL.

Insulin Aspart Insulin aspart is a rapid-acting, biosynthetic (recombinant DNA origin) insulin human analog that is structurally identical to insulin human except for the replacement of aspartic acid with proline at position 28 on the B chain of the molecule.

Insulin Degludec Insulin degludec is a long-acting, biosynthetic (recombinant DNA origin) insulin human analog that is prepared using a process that includes expression of recombinant DNA in *Saccharomyces cerevisiae* followed by chemical modification. Insulin degludec differs structurally from insulin human by the deletion of threonine at position 30 on the B chain and by the acylation of lysine at position 29 on the B chain with hexadecandioic acid, a 16-carbon fatty acid, via a glutamic acid spacer.

Insulin Detemir Insulin detemir is a long-acting, biosynthetic (recombinant DNA origin) insulin human analog that is prepared using a process that includes expression of recombinant DNA in *Saccharomyces cerevisiae* followed by chemical modification. Insulin detemir differs structurally from insulin human by the deletion of threonine at position 30 on the B chain and by the acylation of lysine at position 29 on the B chain with myristic acid, a 14-carbon fatty acid.

Insulin Glargine Insulin glargine is a long-acting, biosynthetic (recombinant DNA origin) insulin human analog that is prepared using special laboratory strains of nonpathogenic *E. coli*, insulin glargine that differs structurally from insulin human by the replacement of asparagine with glycine at position 21 of the A chain and the addition of 2 arginine groups to the C-terminus of the B chain.

Insulin Glulisine Insulin glulisine is a rapid-acting, biosynthetic (recombinant DNA origin) insulin human analog that is structurally identical to insulin human except for the replacement of asparagine at position 3 on the B chain with lysine and by replacement of lysine at position 29 on the B chain with glutamic acid.

Insulin Human Commercially available insulin human (regular insulin) is structurally identical to human insulin. Insulin human is *not* extracted from the human pancreas but rather is prepared biosynthetically using recombinant DNA technology and special laboratory strains of *Escherichia coli* or *Saccharomyces cerevisiae*. Biosynthetic insulin human isophane (NPH insulin) is an intermediate-acting, sterile suspension of zinc insulin crystals and protamine sulfate in buffered water for injection. (See Chemistry and Stability: Chemistry, in Insulin Human 68:20.08.08.)

Insulin Lispro Insulin lispro is a rapid-acting, biosynthetic (recombinant DNA origin) insulin human analog that is structurally identical to insulin human except for transposition of the natural sequence of lysine and proline on the B chain of the molecule. (See Chemistry and Stability: Chemistry, in Insulin Lispro 68:20.08.04.)

■ **Stability** ***Insulin Human*** Regular insulin (insulin human) injection may be mixed with other insulin preparations that have an approximately neutral pH (e.g., insulin human isophane [NPH]). Whenever regular insulin is mixed with other insulin preparations, regular insulin should be drawn into the syringe first in order to avoid transfer of the modified insulin preparation into the regular insulin vial.

When regular insulin is mixed with NPH insulin, binding of added regular insulin occurs in vitro because of excess protamine in the formulation of NPH. In vitro binding of regular insulin by NPH insulin is rapid and marked, occurring within about 5–15 minutes after mixing; however, these chemical changes appear to have no clinical importance since the onset and duration of action of mixtures containing regular and NPH insulins are similar to those observed when these insulins are administered separately.

Mixtures containing regular insulin and NPH insulin appear to be stable for at least 1 month when stored at room temperature or 3 months when stored at 2–8°C; however, the possibility of microbial contamination should be considered. Fixed combinations that contain 30 units/mL of insulin human injection and 70 units/mL of insulin human isophane (NPH) suspension (Humulin® 70/30, Novolin® 70/30), 25 units/mL of insulin lispro and 75 units/mL of insulin lispro protamine suspension (Humalog® mix 75/25), 30 units/mL of insulin aspart and 70 units/mL of insulin aspart protamine (Novolog® mix 70/30), 50 units/mL of insulin lispro and 50 units/mL of insulin lispro protamine (Humalog® mix 50/50), and those that contain 50 units/mL of insulin human injection and 50 units/mL of insulin human isophane (NPH) suspension (Humulin® 50/50) are commercially available. (See Insulin Human, Insulin Lispro, and Insulin Aspart 68:20.08.04.)

Regular insulin may be mixed in any proportion with water for injection or 0.9% sodium chloride injection for use in an insulin subcutaneous infusion pump. However, the mixtures should be used within 24 hours after preparation, since changes in pH and dilution of buffer may affect stability. Insulins are physically and chemically compatible with Lilly's insulin diluting fluids, and may be mixed in any proportion for use in an infusion pump. The mixtures using Lilly's insulin diluting fluids are stable for up to 4 weeks when stored at room temperature. Lilly's insulin diluting fluids are not commercially available; the preparations and specific information about their use should be obtained from the manufacturer. Regular insulin may form crystal deposits on the tubing of insulin infusion pumps.

Studies indicate that the addition of regular insulin to an IV infusion solution may result in adsorption of insulin to the container and tubing. The amount of an insulin dose lost by adsorption to an IV infusion system is highly variable and depends on the concentration of insulin, the type and surface area of the infusion system, the duration of contact time, and the flow rate of the infusion. The lesser the concentration of insulin in solution or the slower the rate of flow of solution, the greater the percentage of adsorption. Adding more insulin to the solution may saturate binding sites of the infusion system. Alternatively, insulin injection may be administered from a syringe directly into a vein or IV tubing with no significant loss due to adsorption. Insulin adsorption is decreased by the presence of negatively charged proteins, such as normal serum albumin. In one study, addition of 7 mL of 25% normal human serum albumin to 500 mL of 0.9% sodium chloride injection with 5, 10, 20, or 40 units of insulin prevented significant insulin adsorption.

Insulin Aspart, Insulin Glulisine, and Insulin Lispro When a rapid-acting insulin is mixed with a longer-acting insulin (i.e., insulin human isophane [NPH]), the rapid onset of action of the rapid-acting insulin (i.e., insulin lispro, insulin aspart) is not affected; therefore, such insulins can be mixed. A slight decrease in absorption rate but not total bioavailability is seen when rapid-acting insulin and insulin human isophane (NPH) are mixed. In clinical trials, postprandial glycemic control was similar when a rapid-acting insulin was mixed with either insulin human isophane (NPH) or extended insulin human zinc (Ultralente®, no longer commercially available in the US). Insulin lispro has been administered with a longer-acting insulin (insulin human isophane [Humulin N®]) in the same syringe. Mixing of insulin lispro with other insulins may be associated with physicochemical changes (either immediately or over time) that could alter the physiologic response to the insulins. For additional information on the stability of insulin lispro or insulin mixtures containing insulin lispro, see Chemistry and Stability: Stability, in Insulin Lispro 68:20.08.04. Insulin aspart or insulin glulisine may be mixed with insulin human isophane (NPH). Although some attenuation of peak serum insulin aspart or insulin glulisine concentrations was observed when administered concomitantly with insulin human isophane (NPH) in the same syringe, the time to peak concentration and total bioavailability of insulin aspart were not substantially affected. If insulin aspart or insulin glulisine is mixed with insulin human isophane (NPH), insulin aspart should be drawn into the syringe first and the mixture administered immediately after mixing. The manufacturer states that the effect of mixing insulin aspart with insulins of animal origin (no longer commercially available in the US), insulins produced by other manufacturers, or crystalline insulin zinc formulations has not been studied. The manufacturer of insulin glulisine states that the effects of mixing insulin glulisine in the same syringe with insulins other than insulin human isophane (NPH), or mixing insulin glulisine with diluents or other insulins when used in external subcutaneous infusion pumps have not been studied.

Unopened insulin aspart alone or in fixed combination with insulin aspart protamine should be stored at 2–8°C until the expiration date and protected from light. Insulin aspart alone or in fixed combination with insulin aspart protamine should not be subjected to freezing; do not use insulin aspart if freezing has occurred or if exposed to temperatures exceeding 37°C. In-use vials, cartridges, or injection pens containing insulin aspart alone should be stored at temperatures below 30°C for up to 28 days. In-use vials containing insulin aspart in fixed combination with insulin aspart protamine vials may be stored at temperatures below 30°C for up to 28 days, provided such vials are kept as cool as possible and away from direct heat and light. Opened insulin aspart should not be exposed to excessive heat or sunlight; do not use the drug if exposure to temperatures exceeding 37°C has occurred. Opened vials of insulin aspart may be refrigerated. Cartridges of insulin aspart assembled into an injection pen or other compatible insulin delivery device should not be refrigerated. Punctured cartridges containing insulin aspart in fixed combination with insulin aspart protamine or Novolog® Mix 70/30 FlexPen® are stable for up to 14 days if stored at temperatures below 30°C; do not refrigerate and keep away from direct heat and sunlight. Infusion bags containing insulin aspart or insulin human regular are stable at room temperature for 24 hours. A certain amount of insulin will be adsorbed initially to material of the infusion bag. The infusion set (tubing, reservoirs, catheters, needle) and the drug in the reservoir should be discarded at least every 48 hours or after exposure to temperatures exceeding 37°C.

When insulin aspart, insulin lispro, or insulin glulisine is used in an external subcutaneous insulin infusion pump, the drug should not be diluted or mixed with any other insulin. Malfunctioning of the external infusion pump or infusion set (e.g., infusion set occlusion, leakage, disconnection or kinking) or insulin degradation can lead to hyperglycemia or ketosis within a short time period because of the small subcutaneous depot of insulin with continuous infusion administration and the rapid onset and short duration of action of insulin aspart, insulin lispro, or insulin glulisine. Prompt identification and correction of the cause of hyperglycemia or ketosis is necessary. If these problems cannot be corrected promptly, patients should resume therapy with subcutaneous injections of insulin and contact their clinician. Patients who are switching from multiple-injection therapy or infusion with buffered regular insulin to subcutaneous infusion with insulin aspart may be particularly susceptible to hyperglycemia or ketosis, and interim therapy with subcutaneous injections with insulin aspart may be required.

In vitro studies have shown that pump malfunction, loss of cresol, and insulin degradation may occur with the use of insulin aspart or insulin glulisine for more than 2 days at 37°C. Insulin aspart, insulin glulisine, and insulin lispro should not be exposed to temperatures exceeding 37°C during administration. The temperature of insulin aspart or insulin glulisine may exceed ambient temperature when the pump housing, cover, tubing, or sport case is exposed to sunlight or radiant heat. Insulin aspart or insulin glulisine exposed to higher than recommended temperatures should be discarded. To avoid insulin degradation, infusion set occlusion, and loss of preservative (cresol), infusions sets (reservoir syringe, tubing, and catheter) and insulin aspart, insulin lispro, or insulin glulisine in the reservoir should be replaced and a new infusion site selected at least every 48 hours. The 3-mL insulin lispro cartridge used in the Disetronic®D-TRON® or Disetronic®D-TRON plus insulin infusion device should be discarded after 7 days, even if some drug still remains in the reservoir.

Insulin Degludec The manufacturer states that insulin degludec must not be mixed with any other insulin or solution.

Insulin Detemir The manufacturer states that insulin detemir must not be diluted or mixed with any other insulin or solution. Such dilution or mixing of insulin detemir may result in unpredictable alterations in the pharmacokinetic and/or pharmacodynamic characteristics (e.g., onset of action, time to peak effect) of insulin detemir and/or the mixed insulin.

Insulin Glargine The manufacturer states that insulin glargine must not be diluted or mixed with any other insulin or solution. Such dilution or mixing of insulin glargine may result in clouding of the solution and unpredictable alterations in the pharmacokinetic and/or pharmacodynamic characteristics (e.g., onset of action, time to peak effect) of insulin glargine and/or the mixed insulin.

For the dosage of regular insulin in the treatment of severe diabetic ketoacidosis and coma, see Insulin Human 68:20.08.08. For further information on the chemistry and stability, uses, and dosage and administration of specific insulin preparations, see the individual monographs in 68:20.08.

†Use is not currently included in the labeling approved by the US Food and Drug Administration

RAPID-ACTING INSULINS 68:20.08.04

Insulin Aspart

■ Insulin aspart (rDNA origin) is a biosynthetic, rapid-acting human insulin analog that is prepared using recombinant DNA technology and genetically modified *Saccharomyces cerevisiae*.

Uses

■ **Diabetes Mellitus** Insulin aspart is used to control hyperglycemia in the management of diabetes mellitus. When administered subcutaneously, insulin aspart has a more rapid onset and shorter duration of action compared with insulin human (regular); therefore, insulin aspart is associated with greater relative reductions in postprandial blood glucose concentrations and may provide greater patient convenience in terms of the timing of insulin injections in relation to meals in patients with type 1 (insulin-dependent) and type 2 (non-insulin-dependent) diabetes mellitus. Because of its short onset and duration of action, insulin aspart usually is used in regimens that include an intermediate-acting (e.g., isophane [NPH] insulin) or long-acting insulin.

Safety and efficacy of insulin aspart administered immediately before meals has been demonstrated by comparison with insulin human (regular) administered 30 minutes before meals in open, clinical studies of 6 months' duration in adults with type 1 or type 2 diabetes mellitus; patients in these studies also received NPH insulin as the basal insulin supplement. Glycemic control (as determined by glycosylated hemoglobin [hemoglobin A_{1c}, HbA_{1c}]) was comparable or slightly improved in patients receiving insulin aspart compared with those receiving insulin human. Patients receiving insulin aspart required slightly higher total daily dosages of insulin (1–3 units daily), principally due to altered basal insulin requirements.

Insulin aspart also is administered by continuous subcutaneous infusion using an external controlled-infusion pump (e.g., Minimed® model 500 series, Disetronic H-TRON series or other equivalent pumps) in patients with type 1 or type 2 diabetes mellitus.Available data in patients with type 1 diabetes mellitus suggest that continuous subcutaneous administration of insulin aspart provides glycemic control (as measured by glycosylated hemoglobin) that is similar to that provided by continuous subcutaneous administration of buffered human insulin or insulin lispro† therapy. In an open-label, short-term trial (16 weeks) in patients with type 2 diabetes mellitus, glycemic control was similar during therapy with insulin aspart administered via an external subcutaneous continuous infusion pump or with preprandial injections of insulin aspart in conjunction with basal isophane insulin injections. These data indicate a similar incidence of hypoglycemia among patients receiving any type of study insulin via external infusion pumps versus a regimen of multiple daily injections.

Insulin aspart has been administered as an IV infusion in a limited number of patients with diabetes mellitus, but The American Diabetes Association (ADA) states that insulin aspart offers no advantage over regular crystalline insulin in patients who require IV insulin.

For additional information on the management of diabetes mellitus, see Uses in the Insulins General Statement 68:20.08.

Dosage and Administration

■ **General** Dosage of insulin aspart alone (Novolog®) or in fixed combination with insulin aspart protamine (Novolog® Mix 70/30) must be individualized and should be regularly adjusted based on the results of blood glucose determinations. Whenever possible, patients should self-monitor blood glucose concentrations. Glucose monitoring is particularly important for patients receiving insulin via an external infusion pump. Patients previously receiving insulin may require a change in dosage if insulin therapy is changed to insulin aspart.

■ **Administration** Insulin aspart alone or in fixed combination with insulin aspart protamine is administered by subcutaneous injection using a conventional insulin syringe, an insulin injection pen (e.g., NovoPen® 3 PenMate, Novolog® FlexPen®), or a compatible insulin delivery device (Innovo®, InDuo®). The manufacturer states that NovoLog® or Novolog Mix 70/30 PenFill® cartridges are intended for use with NovoPen® 3 PenMate® or a compatible insulin delivery device (Innovo®, InDuo®).

Insulin aspart also is administered by continuous subcutaneous infusion using an external controlled-infusion device (e.g., Minimed® model 500 series, Disetronic H-TRON series or other equivalent pump). Insulin aspart is recommended for use in any reservoir and infusion sets that are compatible with insulin and the specific pump. Insulin aspart in fixed combination with insulin aspart protamine should not be used in insulin infusion pumps. For information on the stability of insulin aspart in external infusion pumps, see Insulin Aspart and Insulin Lispro under Chemistry and Stability: Stability, in the Insulins General Statement 68:20.08.

Because of its short duration of action, insulin aspart is used concomitantly with a longer-acting insulin (e.g., isophane [NPH] insulin human, insulin aspart protamine) to meet basal insulin needs in patients with diabetes mellitus and to provide more optimal glycemic control. Insulin aspart may be mixed with isophane insulin human. Although some attenuation of peak serum insulin aspart concentrations was observed when administered concomitantly with isophane insulin human in the same syringe, the time to peak concentration and total bioavailability of insulin aspart were not substantially affected. Whenever insulin aspart is mixed with isophane insulin human, insulin aspart should be drawn into the syringe first in order to avoid transfer of isophane insulin human into the insulin vial. The mixture should be administered immediately after mixing, and such mixtures should not be administered IV. The manufacturer states that the effect of mixing insulin aspart with insulins of animal origin, insulins produced by other manufacturers, or crystalline insulin zinc formulations has not been studied.

The manufacturer states that insulin aspart in fixed combination with insulin aspart protamine suspension (Novolog® Mix 70/30) is intended only for subcutaneous administration and should not be given IV. To resuspend the mixture in a vial immediately before use, the vial should be rolled gently between the hands 10 times until the suspension appears to be uniformly white and cloudy.

Before inserting the Novolog® PenFill® cartridge into a compatible delivery device, the cartridge should be rolled between the palms 10 times. The cartridge should then be turned upside down so that the glass ball inside the cartridge moves the length of the cartridge. This rolling and turning of the cartridge should be repeated at least 10 times or until the suspension appears to be uniformly white and cloudy. The dose should be injected immediately after resuspension, and the rolling and turning of the cartridge should be repeated before each subsequent injection.

Similarly, if using the Novolog® FlexPen®, the pen should be rolled between the palms 10 times. The injection pen should then be turned upside down so that the glass ball inside the pen moves from one end of the reservoir to the other. This rolling and turning procedure should be repeated at least 10 times or until the suspension appears uniformly white and cloudy. The dose should be injected immediately after resuspension, and the rolling and turning of the FlexPen® should be repeated before each subsequent injection.

Insulin aspart is administered immediately (within 5–10 minutes) before a meal. Insulin aspart in fixed combination with insulin aspart protamine (Novolog® Mix 70/30) generally is administered twice daily, 15 minutes before the morning and evening meals, with each dose intended to optimize glycemic control during 2 meals or a meal and a snack. Insulin aspart can be administered by subcutaneous injection into the abdominal wall, thigh, or upper arm. A planned rotation of injection sites within an area should be followed.

Insulin aspart may be administered by IV infusion under proper medical supervision in a clinical setting. For IV infusion in polypropylene infusion bags, insulin aspart is usually diluted to a concentration of 0.05–1 units/mL in 0.9% sodium chloride, 5% dextrose, or 10% dextrose injection with 40 mEq/L of potassium chloride.

Dispensing and Administration Precautions Because of the similarity in names and product packaging between Novolog® (insulin aspart) and Novolog® Mix 70/30 (insulin aspart 30 units/mL with insulin aspart protamine 70 units/mL), the manufacturer has recently implemented color-branded labeling to help prevent dispensing errors. The current packaging for NovoLog® Mix 70/30 is very similar to the previous packaging and remains white with a blue band along the left side of the package. The previous packaging for NovoLog® was also white with a blue band. The current packaging for Novolog® is now white with an orange band along the left side of the package. Although color differentiation can help with product recognition, color should not be relied upon as the sole means of identification of the correct drug. Pharmacists should also use the drug name and NDC number and other measures to carefully distinguish between insulin formulations when dispensing. (See Dispensing and Administration Precautions under Warnings/Precautions: General Precautions, in Cautions.)

■ **Dosage** Because of its short duration of action, insulin aspart is used concomitantly with a longer-acting insulin (e.g., isophane [NPH] insulin human, insulin aspart protamine) to meet basal insulin needs in patients with diabetes mellitus and to provide more optimal glycemic control. Initial *total* daily insulin requirements may vary and generally range from 0.5–1 units/kg. When used in a meal-related subcutaneous injection regimen, 50–70% of the *total* daily insulin requirement may be provided by insulin aspart and the remainder by an intermediate-acting or long-acting insulin. Because of the comparatively rapid onset and short duration of activity of insulin aspart, some patients may require more basal insulin and more total daily insulin to prevent pre-meal hyperglycemia than when using insulin human (regular).

When insulin aspart is used in external infusion pumps, the initial dosage is based on the total daily insulin dosage of the previous regimen. Approximately 50% of the total dosage is given as meal-related injections and the remainder as a basal infusion. Adjustments in basal insulin injections or higher basal infusion rates may be necessary.

When insulin aspart in fixed combination with insulin aspart protamine is used as monotherapy in patients with type 1 or 2 diabetes mellitus, an initial total daily dosage of 0.4–0.6 units/kg given in 2 doses (before the morning and evening meal) has been recommended, with subsequent dosage titrated in increments of 2–4 units every 3–4 days to achieve the target fasting plasma glucose. When the fixed combination of insulin aspart and insulin aspart protamine is given in combination with oral antidiabetic agents, an initial total daily dosage of 0.2–0.3 units/kg has been recommended, with subsequent dosage titration to target glycemic goals. (See Treatment Goals under Uses: Diabetes Mellitus, in the Insulins General Statement 68:20.08.) Because of diurnal variation in insulin resistance and endogenous insulin secretion, variability in the time and content of meals, and variability in the time and extent of exercise, fixed-ratio insulin mixtures may not provide optimal glycemic control for all patients. The dose of the insulin mixture required to provide adequate glycemic control for one of the meals may result in hypoglycemia or hyperglycemia for the other meal. The pharmacodynamic profile of insulin aspart in fixed combination with insulin aspart protamine also may be inadequate for patients who require more frequent meals (e.g., pregnant women).

When the fixed combination of insulin aspart and insulin aspart protamine is used to replace isophane insulin alone or a biphasic insulin product (e.g., premixed isophane and regular insulin) in patients with adequate glycemic control, the initial dosage of insulin aspart in fixed combination with insulin aspart protamine should be identical to the previous insulin dosage, with subsequent adjustment of dosage as required. Patients inadequately controlled on isophane insulin may require increases of 10–20% in the dosage of the fixed combination of insulin aspart and insulin aspart protamine during the first week. In patients transferring from a multiple-daily-dose regimen consisting of an intermediate-acting (e.g., isophane) insulin and a rapid- or short-acting insulin at mealtimes, the initial dosage of the insulin aspart protamine component of the fixed combination should be same as the dosage of the previously used intermediate-acting insulin. Adjustments in the dosage or type of insulin may be needed during illness, emotional or physiologic stress, or changes in meals and exercise.

■ **Special Populations** In a pharmacokinetic study in a limited number of patients with or without renal impairment (creatinine clearance ranging from normal to less than 30 mL/minute but not requiring hemodialysis) who received a single subcutaneous dose of insulin aspart, peak serum drug concentrations and AUC were not affected; however, only 2 patients with severe renal impairment were studied. Similarly, coexisting hepatic impairment (Child-Pugh score 12 or less) did not affect the pharmacokinetics of insulin aspart. However, since increased circulating concentrations of insulin have been observed in patients with renal or hepatic failure who were receiving insulin human, careful monitoring of blood glucose and adjustment of insulin aspart dosage may be necessary in such patients. Dosage requirements for insulin aspart may be reduced in patients with hepatic or renal impairment.

Because of the greater frequency of decreased hepatic, renal, and/or cardiac function and of concomitant disease and drug therapy in geriatric patients, the manufacturer suggests that patients in this age group receive initial dosages of insulin aspart at the lower end of the usual range.

Cautions

■ **Contraindications** Known hypersensitivity to insulin aspart or any ingredient in the formulation. Contraindicated during episodes of hypoglycemia.

■ **Warnings/Precautions** ***Warnings*** **Formulation Considerations.** Because insulin aspart has a more rapid onset and shorter duration of action than insulin human (regular), administration of insulin aspart should be *immediately* followed by a meal. In addition, a longer-acting insulin is required to maintain adequate glycemic control in patients with type 1 diabetes mellitus. Any change in insulin should be made cautiously and only under medical supervision. Insulin aspart in fixed combination with insulin aspart protamine should not be mixed with any other insulin. Patients previously receiving insulin may require a change in dosage if insulin therapy is changed to insulin aspart.

Hypoglycemia. Hypoglycemia is the most common adverse effect of insulins, including insulin aspart, and monitoring of blood glucose concentrations is recommended for all patients with diabetes mellitus.

Insulin Pumps. Pump or infusion set malfunction or insulin degradation may lead to hyperglycemia and ketosis in a short time period because of the small subcutaneous depot of insulin. Because of rapid absorption and short duration of action, such effects may occur when patients are switched from multiple injection therapy or infusion with buffered regular insulin. Prompt indentification and correction of hyperglycemia or ketosis is necessary; interim therapy with intermittent subcutaneous injections may be required.

Sensitivity Reactions **Dermatologic and Sensitivity Reactions.** Localized allergic reactions (e.g., pruritus, erythema, swelling) at the injection site may develop in patients receiving insulins, including insulin aspart alone or in fixed combination with insulin aspart protamine. These reactions are relatively minor and usually resolve within a few days to a few weeks but occasionally may require discontinuance of insulin aspart. Poor injection technique or irritants in skin cleansing agents may contribute to localized injection site reactions. As with any insulin, atrophy or hypertrophy of subcutaneous fat tissue may occur at sites of frequent insulin injection. Injection site rotation within an area may reduce or prevent these effects.

Generalized hypersensitivity to insulin characterized by rash, pruritus, shortness of breath, wheezing, hypotension, tachycardia, and diaphoresis has occurred less frequently than localized reactions. Severe cases of generalized insulin allergy with anaphylaxis may be life-threatening. In several clinical studies in patients with type 1 and 2 diabetes mellitus receiving insulin human or insulin aspart alone or in fixed combination with insulin aspart protamine, formation of insulin aspart-specific or insulin human-specific antibodies was low in patients receiving either insulin, but among patients receiving insulin aspart-containing regimens, concentrations of cross-reactive antibodies increased after 3–6 months of therapy before returning to near-baseline levels at 12 months. It was not necessary to increase the dosage of insulin aspart in patients experiencing increased cross-reactive antibodies, and the manufacturer states that the clinical importance of these findings is unknown. No consistent relationship between antibody formation and glycemic control (as measured by HbA_{1c}) was observed, and dosage adjustments were not necessary to maintain glycemic control.

Localized reactions and generalized myalgias have been reported with the use of cresol, which is included in the NovoLog® (insulin aspart) and Novolog® Mix 70/30 formulations as an excipient.

General Precautions **Hypoglycemia and Hypokalemia.** As hypoglycemia and hypokalemia may occur with insulin therapy, care should be taken in patients who are most at risk for the development of these effects, including patients who are fasting, patients with autonomic neuropathy, or patients who are receiving potassium-lowering drugs or drug therapy that may be affected by altered serum potassium concentrations. Untreated hypokalemia may cause respiratory paralysis, ventricular arrhythmia, and death. Since IV insulin aspart has a rapid onset of action, increased attention to hypoglycemia and hypokalemia is necessary. Serum glucose and potassium concentrations must be monitored closely when insulin aspart or any other insulin is administered IV.

Dispensing and Administration Precautions. Because of the similarity in names and product packaging between Humalog® and Humalog® 75/25, medication errors with these 2 drugs have been noted. The manufacturer of Novolog® Mix 70/30 and Novolog® has recently implemented color-branded labeling to help prevent dispensing errors. The current packaging for NovoLog® Mix 70/30 is very similar to the previous packaging and remains white with a blue band along the left side of the package. The packaging for NovoLog® previously was also white with a blue band. The current packaging of Novolog® is now white with an orange band along the left side of the package. Although color differentiation can help with product recognition, color should not be relied upon as the sole means of identification of the correct agent. Pharmacists should also use the drug name and NDC number and other measures (e.g., matching product name on the prescription to the pharmacy-issued label, separating agents with similar names on pharmacy shelves, counseling patients) to carefully distinguish between insulin formulations when dispensing. This recent packaging change will not help prevent name confusion errors involving these 2 agents (Novolog® and Novolog® Mix 70/30) or other insulin products (e.g., Novolog® Mix 70/30 and Novolin® 70/30, or Novolog® and Novolin®).

Dispensing errors involving Novolog® or Novolog® Mix 70/30 should be reported to the manufacturer (800-727-6500), the USP Medication Errors Reporting Program (800-233-7767), or the FDA MedWATCH program by phone (800-FDA-1088, 800-FDA-0178 [fax]) or online at http://www.fda.gov/Safety/MedWatch/default.htm.

Specific Populations **Pregnancy.** Category C. (See Users' Guide.)

Lactation. It is unknown whether insulin aspart is distributed into milk; caution is advised if used in nursing women.

Pediatric Use. Safety and efficacy of insulin aspart in fixed combination with insulin aspart protamine not established in children. The comparative safety and efficacy of insulin aspart and insulin human (regular) have been demonstrated in a 24-week clinical study in children and adolescents 6–18 years of age with type 1 diabetes mellitus; children also received isophane insulin as the basal insulin supplement. Glycemic control (as determined by glycosylated hemoglobin [hemoglobin A_{1c}, HbA_{1c}]) was comparable in patients receiving insulin aspart or insulin human. In addition, safety and efficacy of insulin aspart were comparable with insulin human in another clinical study in adolescents 12–17 years of age with type 1 diabetes mellitus. In comparative study in a limited number of children 2–6 years of age, glycemic control (as measured by HbA_{1c}, fructosamine) was comparable in children receiving insulin aspart or insulin human. As observed in the 6- to 18-year age group, the rates of hypoglycemia in children 2-6 years of age were similar with insulin aspart or insulin human. In one pharmacokinetic study, insulin aspart had a more rapid onset and a shorter duration of action when compared with insulin human in a limited number of children and adolescents 6–17 years of age; such effects are similar to those observed in adults.

Geriatric Use. Experience in those 65 years of age and older insufficient to determine whether safety differs from younger adults. Efficacy of insulin aspart (as measured by HbA_{1c}) as compared to insulin human appears to be similar in geriatric and younger patients, particularly in patients with type 2 diabetes mellitus.

■ **Common Adverse Effects** Hypoglycemia, hypersensitivity reactions, lipodystrophy, pruritus, rash, and injection site reactions have been reported with insulin aspart monotherapy. In clinical studies, small but persistent elevations in alkaline phosphatase were observed in some patients with type 1 diabetes mellitus who received insulin aspart. However, the clinical importance, if any, of these findings has not been established. Injection site reactions have been reported in 7% of patients receiving insulin aspart in fixed combination with insulin aspart protamine. Data from comparative clinical trials evaluating insulin aspart in fixed combination with insulin aspart protamine (Novolog® Mix 70/30) and insulin human (regular) injection in fixed combination with isophane insulin human (Novolin® 70/30) did not reveal differences in the frequency of adverse effects between the 2 preparations.

Drug Interactions

■ **Drugs Affecting Glycemic Control** ***Drugs that May Potentiate Hypoglycemic Effects*** Angiotensin-converting enzyme (ACE) inhibitors, disopyramide, fibrate derivatives, fluoxetine, monoamine oxidase (MAO) inhibitors, oral antidiabetic agents, propoxyphene, salicylates, somatostatin derivatives (e.g., octreotide), sulfonamide anti-infectives.

Drugs that May Antagonize Hypoglycemic Effects Corticosteroids, danazol, diuretics, estrogens and progestins (e.g., oral contraceptives), isoniazid, niacin, phenothiazines, somatropin, sympathomimetic agents (e.g., albuterol, epinephrine, terbutaline), thyroid hormones.

Drugs that May Have a Variable Effect of Glycemic Control Alcohol, β-adrenergic blocking agents, clonidine, lithium salts, pentamidine.

Sympatholytic Agents May decrease or eliminate the signs of hypoglycemia in patients receiving insulin aspart concomitantly with these drugs (e.g., β-adrenergic blocking agents, clonidine, guanethidine, reserpine).

Description

Insulin aspart (rDNA origin) is a biosynthetic, rapid-acting human insulin analog that is prepared using recombinant DNA technology and genetically modified *Saccharomyces cerevisiae*. Insulin aspart differs structurally from insulin human by the replacement of proline at position B28 with aspartic acid. This structural modification results in decreased tendency to form hexamers, more rapid absorption and onset of action, and a shorter duration of action compared with insulin human when given subcutaneously to patients with type 1 diabetes mellitus. Interindividual and intraindividual variation in rate of absorption and consequently, the onset of action of insulins, including insulin aspart alone or in fixed combination with insulin aspart protamine, may occur based on site of injection, tissue blood supply, temperature, and physical activity.

Advice to Patients

Provide information regarding the potential risks and advantages of insulin aspart-containing therapy.

Provide instructions to patient regarding use of subcutaneous insulin infusion devices (e.g., infusion pumps and accessories) and intensive insulin therapy with multiple injections.

Provide instructions regarding self-monitoring of blood glucose, insulin storage and injection technique, adherence to meal planning, regular physical exercise, periodic hemoglobin A_{1c} (HbA_{1c}) monitoring, and management of hypoglycemia or hyperglycemia.

Importance of *not* mixing insulin aspart with crystalline zinc insulin preparations, insulins of animal source, or preparations produced by other manufacturers. Importance of using insulin aspart only if solution is clear and colorless with no particles visible; resuspended insulin aspart in fixed combination with insulin aspart protamine must appear uniformly white and cloudy.

Importance of *not* mixing insulin aspart with other insulins or diluent when used in external subcutaneous infusion pumps.

Importance of administering insulin aspart or the fixed combination of insulin aspart and insulin aspart protamine within 5–10 minutes or within 15 minutes, respectively, of the start of a meal.

Discuss potential for alterations in insulin requirements in special situations (e.g., illness, emotional disturbances or other stresses).

Importance of informing clinicians of the development of skin reactions (erythema, pruritus, thickened skin) at infusion sites in patients using insulin infusion pumps. Importance of selection of a new infusion site, as continued infusion may increase skin reactions and/or alter the absorption of insulin aspart.

Importance of resumption of subcutaneous insulin injection therapy and of contacting a clinician if pump malfunctions occur and cannot be corrected promptly.

Importance of informing clinicians of existing or contemplated concomitant therapy, including prescription and OTC drugs. Importance of women informing clinicians if they are or plan to become pregnant or breast-feed.

Importance of informing patients of other important precautionary information. (See Cautions.)

Overview (see Users Guide). For additional information until a more detailed monograph is developed and published, the manufacturer's labeling should be consulted. It is *essential* that the manufacturer's labeling be consulted for more detailed information on usual cautions, precautions, contraindications, potential drug interactions, laboratory test interferences, and acute toxicity.

Preparations

Excipients in commercially available drug preparations may have clinically important effects in some individuals; consult specific product labeling for details.

Insulin Aspart (Recombinant DNA Origin)

Parenteral		
Injection for subcutaneous use	100 units/mL (U-100)	**NovoLOG®**, Novo Nordisk **NovoLOG® FlexPen®** (available as a 3 mL prefilled syringe preassembled into pen), Novo Nordisk
Injection, for use with NovoPen® 3 PenMate® or other compatible devices	100 units/mL (300 units)	**NovoLOG® Penfill®**, Novo Nordisk

Insulin Aspart Combinations (Recombinant DNA Origin)

Parenteral		
Injectable Suspension	Insulin Aspart 30 units/mL with Insulin Aspart Protamine 70 units/mL	**NovoLOG® Mix 70/30**, Novo Nordisk **NovoLOG® Mix 70/30 FlexPen®** (available as a 3 mL prefilled syringe preassembled into pen), Novo Nordisk
Injectable Suspension, for use with NovoPen® 3 PenMate® or other compatible devices	100 units/mL (300 units)	**NovoLOG® Mix 70/30 Penfill®**, Novo Nordisk

†Use is not currently included in the labeling approved by the US Food and Drug Administration

Insulin Lispro

■ Insulin lispro is a rapid-acting biosynthetic human insulin analog that is structurally identical to insulin human except for reversal of the sequence of lysine and proline on the B chain of the molecule; in insulin lispro, lysine and proline occur at positions 28 and 29, respectively, of the B chain.

Uses

■ **Diabetes Mellitus** Insulin lispro is a rapid-acting insulin analog that is used to control hyperglycemia in the management of diabetes mellitus. In patients with type 1 diabetes mellitus, insulin lispro generally is used in conjunction with a longer-acting insulin (except when administered via an external insulin infusion device [pump]); in patients with type 2 diabetes mellitus, insulin lispro may be used without a longer-acting insulin when given with an oral sulfonylurea antidiabetic agent. (See Combination Therapy under Uses: Diabetes Mellitus, in the Insulins General Statement 68:20.08.) When administered subcutaneously, insulin lispro has a more rapid onset and shorter duration of action compared with insulin human (regular); therefore, insulin lispro is associated with greater relative reductions in postprandial blood glucose concentrations and may provide greater patient convenience in terms of the timing of insulin injections in relation to meals in patients with type 1 and type 2 diabetes mellitus. Because of its short onset and duration of action, insulin lispro usually is used in regimens that include a longer-acting insulin (i.e., isophane [NPH] insulin human, insulin lisproprotamine [as the fixed combination Humalog® Mix75/25®, Humalog® Mix50/50®], insulin glargine) in an attempt to provide more physiologic insulin levels throughout the day.

Insulin lispro also is administered by continuous subcutaneous infusion using selected external controlled-infusion devices (pumps) in patients with diabetes mellitus. Limited data in patients with type 1 diabetes mellitus suggest that continuous subcutaneous administration of insulin lispro provides greater glycemic control (as measured by glycosylated hemoglobin) than that provided by continuous subcutaneous administration of buffered human insulin or regular human insulin. These data indicate a similar incidence of hypoglycemia among patients receiving insulin lispro or regular or buffered human insulin via external infusion pumps. Available data suggest that continuous subcutaneous administration of insulin provides glycemic control similar to that provided by intensive, multiple-daily-dose insulin therapy. Insulin lispro administration via external controlled-infusion devices has not been studied in patients with type 2 diabetes mellitus.

The American Diabetes Association (ADA) currently classifies diabetes mellitus as type 1 (immune mediated or idiopathic), type 2 (predominantly insulin resistance with relative insulin deficiency to predominantly an insulin secretory defect with insulin resistance), gestational diabetes mellitus, or that associated with certain conditions or syndromes (e.g., drug- or chemical-induced, hormonal, that associated with pancreatic disease, infections, specific genetic defects or syndromes). Type 1 diabetes mellitus previously was described as juvenile-onset (JOD) diabetes mellitus, since it usually occurs during youth. Type 2 diabetes mellitus previously was described as adult-onset (AODM) diabetes mellitus. However, type 1 or type 2 diabetes mellitus can occur at any age, and the current classification is based on pathogenesis (e.g., autoimmune destruction of pancreatic β cells, insulin resistance) and clinical presentation rather than on age of onset. Many patients' diabetes mellitus does not easily fit into a single classification. Epidemiologic data indicate that the incidence of type 2 diabetes mellitus is increasing in children and adolescents such that 8–45% of children with newly diagnosed diabetes have nonimmune-mediated diabetes mellitus.

Comparative clinical studies in patients with type 1 or type 2 diabetes mellitus who received insulin lispro or insulin human (regular) indicate that insulin lispro is associated with improved control of postprandial blood glucose concentrations. However, while therapy with insulin lispro was associated with reduced postprandial (e.g., post-breakfast) blood glucose excursions in these patients, overall glycemic control (as measured by hemoglobin A_{1c} values) did not differ appreciably from that in patients receiving insulin human (regular). The clinical importance of increased glycemic control of postprandial glucose excursions in nonpregnant diabetic patients with similar glycosylated hemoglobin (hemoglobin A_{1c} [HbA_{1c}]) values has not been established. Most comparative studies of insulin lispro and insulin human (regular) were of open, crossover design in which patients received either insulin lispro within approximately 15 minutes before a meal or insulin human (regular) 20–45 minutes before a meal in addition to an intermediate-acting (e.g., NPH insulin) or long-acting (Ultralente®) insulin as the basal insulin supplement. Main efficacy end points were 1–2 hour-postprandial blood glucose concentrations, glycosylated hemoglobin concentrations, frequency of hypoglycemia, and quality-of-life measures. However, in most of the larger studies conducted to date, patients were evaluated for only 3 months, which some clinicians state may not have been a sufficient period in which to assess changes in glycosylated hemoglobin. Since the duration of action of insulin lispro is brief, some clinicians have suggested that basal (e.g., intermediate-acting) insulin dosage be optimized to reflect the short duration of action of insulin lispro. The dosage or frequency of administration of the longer-acting insulin may be increased or the evening dose of longer-acting insulin may be delayed until bedtime; continuous subcutaneous infusion of insulin also may be used to manage increased preprandial and nighttime glucose concentrations (as compared with insulin human [regular]) observed with insulin lispro.

Some clinicians suggest that patient-related factors such as motivation and knowledge of the disease may be more important in determining glycemic control than the type of insulin or insulin regimen used, and that patients who are well-controlled on conventional short-acting insulin preparations without frequent hypoglycemia should not be routinely switched to insulin lispro. Patients likely to benefit from insulin lispro therapy include type 1 diabetics who would appreciate the more flexible injection schedule associated with insulin lispro's shorter onset and duration of activity, those with low glycosylated hemoglobin values who are at high risk for hypoglycemic episodes, and patients with recent-onset type 1 diabetes mellitus who have some residual β-cell function to provide basal insulin levels between meals.

Insulin lispro therapy generally has been associated with a reduced frequency of hypoglycemic episodes compared with insulin human (regular) in patients with type 1 diabetes mellitus and no change in hypoglycemic episodes in type 2 diabetics. In parallel-group clinical trials of insulin lispro and insulin human (regular) in patients with type 1 or type 2 diabetes mellitus, the overall incidence of hypoglycemia was not significantly different among patients receiving either of the 2 insulin preparations; however, patients with type 1 diabetes receiving insulin lispro had fewer late hypoglycemic episodes (i.e., between 12 midnight and 6 a.m.) than those receiving insulin human (regular), possibly because of higher nocturnal blood glucose concentrations (as reflected by a small increase in fasting blood glucose concentrations).

Limited evidence suggests that insulin lispro also may be effective in establishing glycemic control in patients with resistance to insulin human. Transfer from insulin human (regular) to insulin lispro resulted in a reduction in insulin requirements in a patient with excessive insulin antibodies whose response was refractory to insulin human (regular). Further study and experience are needed to determine whether insulin lispro has clinical advantages over regular insulin for the long-term management of diabetes mellitus.

For further information on indications for insulin therapy and considerations in selecting and monitoring such therapy in patients with diabetes mellitus, see the Insulins General Statement 68:20.08.

Dosage and Administration

■ **Administration** Insulin lispro is administered by subcutaneous injection using a conventional insulin syringe or an injection pen (e.g., Humalog® Pen, Owen Mumford Autopen®). Whenever possible, insulin should be self-administered by the patient. Patients should be instructed regarding proper administration and dosage of insulin lispro and given a copy of the patient information provided by the manufacturer. To improve accuracy of dosing in pediatric patients, insulin lispro may be diluted to a ratio of 1:10 or 1:2 with the sterile diluent supplied by the manufacturer. Use of injection pens may improve accuracy of insulin delivery and be more convenient in patients who are visually or neurologically impaired or who are receiving multiple daily injections of insulin. When a compatible delivery device is used for subcutaneous injection of insulin lispro, the labeling accompanying the delivery device should be consulted for proper methods of assembly, administration (including dose calibration), and care.

The manufacturer states that insulin lispro in fixed combination with insulin lispro protamine suspension (Humalog® Mix50/50®, Humalog Mix75/25®) is intended only for subcutaneous administration and should not be given IV. Before injecting the fixed combination of insulin lispro and insulin lispro protamine suspension using the injection pen, the pen should be rolled between the palms 10 times. The pen should then be turned upside down so that the glass ball inside the pen moves the length of the pen. This rolling and turning of the pen should be repeated at least 10 times or until the suspension appears to be uniformly white and cloudy.

Insulin lispro also is administered by continuous subcutaneous infusion using selected external controlled-infusion devices (pumps). The pumps deliver rapid- or short-acting insulin at a basal rate continuously throughout the day, with patient-initiated increased delivery of insulin prior to meals. The manufacturer states that insulin lispro is recommended for use in Disetronic H-TRON®plus V100 (with Disetronic 3.15-mL insulin reservoir), Disetronic D-TRON®, or Disetronic D-TRON®plus external infusion pumps with Disetronic Rapid® Infusion sets and in MiniMed model 506, 507, or 508 pumps with MiniMed Polyfin® infusion sets.

The safety and efficacy of insulin lispro following IV administration†, such as in the treatment of diabetic ketoacidosis, has not been adequately evaluated to date. Insulin lispro's favorable pharmacokinetic profile compared with insulin human (regular) is based on its more rapid subcutaneous absorption rather than on more rapid post-absorptive uptake to insulin receptor sites, and no clinical advantage of IV insulin lispro compared with IV insulin human (regular) has been identified. While insulin lispro and insulin human have similar hypoglycemic effects when given IV†, the manufacturer states that insulin lispro is intended for subcutaneous administration and that insulin human (regular) should be used when IV administration of insulin is required. Some clinicians suggest that insulin lispro should not be used IV, especially in patients with diabetic ketoacidosis, as data are limited concerning the IV use of insulin lispro.

The manufacturer states that the safety and efficacy of insulin lispro following IM† administration has not been evaluated in clinical trials.

For additional information concerning insulin administration, see Dosage and Administration: Administration, in the Insulins General Statement 68:20.08.

When used as a mealtime insulin alone or in fixed combination with isophane insulin human to control postprandial hyperglycemia, insulin lispro should be administered within 15 minutes prior to a meal. Because of its short duration of action, insulin lispro is used concomitantly with, but not necessarily administered at the same time as, a longer-acting insulin (e.g., isophane [NPH] insulin human) to meet basal insulin needs in patients with type 1 diabetes mellitus and to provide more optimal glycemic control. Insulin lispro alone or in fixed combination with isophane insulin human can be administered by subcutaneous injection into the abdominal wall, thigh, or upper arm. A planned rotation of injection sites within an area (injections should be spaced at least 0.5 inch from a previous injection site) should be followed.

Conflicting data have been reported regarding the effects of mixing insulin lispro and a longer-acting insulin on the pharmacodynamic effects of insulin lispro. Some data in healthy individuals indicate that mixing insulin lispro (Humalog®) and NPH insulin human (i.e., Humulin N®) in the same syringe results in a decreased rate of absorption, but no change in total bioavailability, of insulin lispro; this finding may be attributable to adsorption of insulin lispro to excess protamine in the NPH insulin formulation. Clinical studies in patients with type 1 diabetes mellitus indicate that mixtures of insulin lispro (Humalog®) and NPH insulin human (i.e., Humulin N®) either improve or produce similar effects on postprandial glycemic control compared with separate injection of these insulins. Concomitant administration of insulin lispro and Ultralente® (no longer commercially available in the US) insulin human in the same syringe reportedly did not affect the absorption of insulin lispro in healthy individuals who received these insulins immediately after mixing. The manufacturer states that the effect of mixing Humalog® (insulin lispro) with insulins of animal origin (no longer commercially available in the US) or human insulins produced by other manufacturers (i.e., other than Lilly) has not been studied. When insulin lispro is mixed with a longer-acting insulin preparation, insulin lispro should be drawn into the syringe first in order to prevent precipitation or turbidity of the insulin lispro solution by the longer-acting insulin. Insulin mixtures should not be administered IV.

■ **Dosage** Dosage of insulin lispro, which is always expressed in USP units, must be based on the results of blood glucose determinations and carefully individualized to attain optimum therapeutic effects. (*Glucose concentrations in plasma generally are 10–15% higher than those in whole blood; glucose concentrations also may vary according to the method and laboratory used for these determinations.*) Patients should be monitored with regular laboratory evaluations, including fasting blood (or plasma) glucose determinations, to assess therapeutic response and obtain the minimum effective dosage of insulin lispro. Whenever possible, patients should self-monitor blood glucose concentrations. Urine glucose concentrations correlate poorly with blood glucose; therefore, urine glucose determinations should be used only when patients cannot or will not test blood glucose concentrations. Glucose monitoring is particularly important for patients receiving insulin lispro via an external infusion pump. Following initiation of insulin lispro therapy and dosage titration, determination of glycosylated hemoglobin (hemoglobin A_{1c} [HbA_{1c}]) concentrations at intervals of approximately 3 months is useful for assessing the patient's continued response to therapy.

For additional information on monitoring and management of insulin therapy, see Dosage: Considerations in Monitoring Insulin Therapy, in Dosage and Administration in the Insulins General Statement 68:20.08.

Both conventional and intensive insulin treatment regimens have been used in patients with type 1 or severe type 2 diabetes mellitus. (See Glycemic Control and Microvascular Complications of Diabetes Mellitus, in Uses in the Insulins General Statement 68:20.08.) Insulin lispro generally is administered in multiple daily doses in regimens that also include an intermediate- or long-acting insulin (e.g., NPH, Lente, Ultralente®) given in the morning and/or evening to provide basal insulin needs. Insulin lispro in fixed combination with insulin lispro protamine (Humalog® Mix75/25®) generally is administered twice daily with the morning and evening meal. Dosage of insulin lispro alone or in fixed combination with insulin lispro protamine must be based on the results of blood glucose determinations and carefully individualized to obtain optimum therapeutic effect. While absorption of insulin lispro is more rapid, and duration of action slightly shorter, when administered in abdominal compared with deltoid or thigh sites, variations in absorption related to site of administration are smaller with insulin lispro than with regular insulin when insulin lispro is not mixed with other insulins in the same syringe.

Transferring from Therapy with Other Insulins Any change in insulin preparation or dosage regimen should be made with caution and only under medical supervision. When insulin lispro replaces insulin human (regular) in regimens consisting of multiple daily insulin doses, the initial dosage of insulin lispro can be identical to the previous insulin (regular) dosage with subsequent adjustment as required. However, patients in whom insulin lispro is initiated should be carefully advised regarding the difference in action profiles between insulin lispro and insulin human (regular); adjustments in the consumption and/or timing of snacks or exercise relative to that with the use of insulin (regular) may be necessary to avoid hypoglycemic episodes and/or prevent preprandial hyperglycemia. While pharmacokinetic and pharmacodynamic studies indicate that insulin lispro and insulin human are equipotent on a unit-for-unit basis with regard to glucose-lowering activity, changes in insulin purity, strength, brand, type, and/or species source or method of manufacture may necessitate a change in insulin dosage. Although it is not possible to clearly identify which patients will require a change in dosage when therapy with a different preparation is initiated, it is known that a limited number of patients will require such a change. Adjustments may be needed with the first dose or over a period of several weeks.

When insulin lispro is substituted for insulin human (regular) in patients receiving combination therapy with insulin human (regular) and a longer-acting insulin, adjustment of the dosage of the longer-acting insulin may be required because of the shorter duration of action of insulin lispro. Patients receiving intensive insulin therapy will achieve greater postprandial glycemic control than those receiving conventional therapy because of the increased use of rapid- or short-acting insulin; patients who previously were poorly controlled on conventional insulin therapy generally will require a smaller total daily insulin dosage when switched to an intensive insulin regimen.

■ **Dosage in Renal and Hepatic Impairment** Results from clinical trials in a limited number of patients with type 2 diabetes mellitus and renal or hepatic impairment who were receiving either insulin lispro or insulin human indicate that the pharmacokinetic differences between the 2 types of insulin generally were maintained. The presence of hepatic impairment does not affect the absorption or distribution of insulin lispro in patients with type 2 diabetes mellitus. However, increased circulating concentrations of insulin have been observed in patients with renal or hepatic impairment who were receiving insulin human; therefore, insulin lispro requirements may be reduced in these patients. Careful monitoring of blood glucose and adjustment of insulin lispro (alone or in fixed combination with isophane insulin human) dosage may be necessary in such patients.

For further information on the chemistry and stability, uses, and dosage and administration of specific insulin preparations, see the individual monographs in 68:20.08.

Cautions

Insulin lispro shares the toxic potential of other insulins, and the usual precautions of insulin therapy should be observed with insulin lispro. (See Cautions in the Insulins General Statement 68:20.08.) The overall frequency and severity of adverse reactions to insulin lispro appear to be similar to those associated with insulin human (regular).

■ **Hypoglycemia** In comparative studies in patients with type 1 or type 2 diabetes mellitus, the overall rate of hypoglycemic reactions with insulin lispro was similar or somewhat less than that with insulin human; the frequency of nocturnal hypoglycemic reactions in patients with type 1 diabetes mellitus is less among those receiving insulin lispro. The lower rate of hypoglycemia observed with insulin lispro may be related to its shorter duration of action, resulting in a slightly greater degree of fasting hyperglycemia compared with insulin human.

■ **Immunogenicity** Several studies have shown that insulin lispro is no more immunogenic than insulin human. In one study in patients with type 1 or type 2 diabetes mellitus receiving insulin lispro or insulin human for 12 months, insulin specific antibody titers at endpoint were no different for each of the 2 insulin preparations. In large clinical trials, formation of insulin lispro-specific antibodies was low in patients receiving insulin lispro, but cross-reactive antibodies were observed in patients receiving insulin human or insulin lispro. The largest increase in antibody levels during year-long trials was observed in patients with type 1 diabetes mellitus who were receiving insulin therapy for the first time. In one study in rhesus monkeys, insulin antibody titers (IgG type) were found in 1 of 4 monkeys immunized with 6 weekly injections of insulin lispro (up to 100 mcg) prepared in Freund's adjuvant and in none of the monkeys receiving insulin human or purified pork insulin in Freund's adjuvant; none of the monkeys developed elevated insulin antibody titers of IgE type. As insulin allergies are mediated primarily by IgE insulin antibodies, use of insulin lispro is not expected to pose an increased risk for the development of insulin allergies.

■ **Other Effects** Localized reactions and generalized myalgias have been reported with the use of *m*-cresol, which is included in the Humalog®, Humalog® Mix75/25®, or Humalog® Mix50/50® (insulin lispro) formulations as an excipient.

■ **Precautions and Contraindications** Insulin lispro has a more rapid onset and shorter duration of action than insulin human (regular). Clinicians who prescribe rapid-acting insulins should be familiar with the indications, limitations, and patient-selection criteria for therapy with insulin to ensure appropriate patient management. Because insulin lispro has a short duration of action, patients with type 1 diabetes also require a longer-acting insulin to maintain adequate nighttime and preprandial blood glucose control.

Patients should read carefully and follow instructions regarding use of subcutaneous insulin infusion devices (e.g., infusion pumps and accessories) and intensive insulin therapy with multiple injections. Patients using insulin infusion devices should inform clinicians of the development of skin reactions (erythema, pruritus, thickened skin) at infusion sites. If such reactions occur, a new infusion site should be selected. Malfunctioning of the external-controlled infusion device or infusion set or insulin degradation can lead to hyperglycemia or ketosis within a short time period. If such symptoms occur, prompt identification and correction of the cause is necessary. Interim therapy with subcutaneous injections with insulin may be required if the cause of the symptoms cannot be promptly determined. (See Insulin Regimens under Dosage and Administration: Dosage, in the Insulins General Statement 68:20.08.) Complications such as undetected interruptions in insulin delivery may result in more frequent and more rapid ketotic episodes or unexplained hyperglycemia compared with multiple daily injections.

Any change in insulin should be made cautiously and only under medical supervision. Changes in insulin strength, manufacturer, type (e.g., regular, NPH), species, (animal, human), or method of manufacture (rDNA versus animal-source insulin) may necessitate a change in dosage.

The manufacturer states that insulin lispro alone or in fixed combination with isophane insulin human (Humalog® Mix50/50®, Humalog® Mix75/25®) is contraindicated during episodes of hypoglycemia and in patients with hypersensitivity to the drug or any of its excipients. Patients with a history of hypersensitivity to *other* insulins should be given insulin lispro only if the clinician has determined that the possible benefits outweigh the potential adverse effects. (See Cautions: Dermatologic and Sensitivity Reactions, in the Insulins General Statement 68:20.08.) Patients should seek immediate medical assistance if they experience a generalized allergic reaction after injection of insulin lispro.

■ **Pediatric Precautions** The safety and efficacy of insulin lispro in fixed combination with insulin lispro protamine in children younger than 18 years of age have not been established. However, clinical trials with insulin lispro are ongoing in children aged 3–18 years of age with type 1 diabetes mellitus, and preliminary data suggest no unusual effects of insulin lispro therapy in adolescents receiving the drug. In several long-term (e.g., 8–9 months) comparative studies evaluating insulin lispro and insulin human in children and adolescents with diabetes mellitus, insulin lispro (given either immediately before or after meals) was as effective as insulin human (given 30–45 minutes before a meal) in improving glycemic control as determined by glycosylated hemoglobin (hemoglobin A_{1c} [HbA_{1c}]) concentrations. Adjustment of basal insulin dosage may be required in these children. (See Cautions: Pediatric Precautions, in the Insulins General Statement 68:20.08.)

■ **Geriatric Precautions** In clinical trials, the efficacy (as measured by HbA_{1c}values) of insulin lispro or incidence of hypoglycemia did not differ by age. Pharmacokinetic/pharmacodynamic studies to assess the effect of age on the onset of action of insulin lispro have not been performed. Subgroup analyses of large clinical trials have not revealed evidence of altered effectiveness of insulin lispro compared with insulin human based on age. However, some evidence suggests an increased risk of cardiovascular morbidity associated with hypoglycemia in geriatric patients receiving intensive insulin therapy. (See Cautions: Geriatric Precautions, in the Insulins General Statement 68:20.08.)

With insulin lispro in fixed combination with isophane insulin human, experience in those 65 years of age or older is insufficient to determine whether they respond differently from younger adults. However, dosage of insulin lispro in fixed combination with isophane insulin human should be selected carefully in geriatric patients, and the greater frequency of decreased hepatic, renal, and/or cardiac function and of concomitant disease and drug therapy observed in the elderly also should be considered.

■ **Mutagenicity and Carcinogenicity** No evidence of mutagenicity or chromosomal damage with insulin lispro was observed in vivo in a micronucleus test or chromosome aberration test or in in vitro test systems, including microbial (bacterial mutation tests) and mammalian (mouse lymphoma) assays. There was no increase in DNA repair when insulin lispro was tested in an unscheduled DNA synthesis test.. In addition, no evidence of carcinogenicity was observed in a study in rats receiving up to 200 units/kg daily of insulin lispro subcutaneously for 12 months.

■ **Pregnancy, Fertility, and Lactation** Insulin lispro has been evaluated in a limited number of pregnant women with gestational diabetes. The American Diabetes Association (ADA) suggests that continuous subcutaneous insulin infusion with insulin lispro may improve glycemic control during pregnancy. Congenital abnormalities (including kidney dysplasia) have been reported in at least 2 infants of patients with type 1 diabetes mellitus who received insulin lispro and other insulins during pregnancy; a causal relationship to insulin lispro has not been established. Abnormal maternal blood glucose concentrations during pregnancy have been associated with a higher incidence of congenital abnormalities. Although glycemic control reportedly was well maintained during pregnancy in these women, optimization of glycemic control before conception and throughout pregnancy does not completely eliminate the risk of congenital anomalies. The manufacturer states that insulin lispro alone or in fixed combination with isophane insulin human should be used in pregnant women only when clearly needed.

Reproduction studies of insulin lispro in pregnant rats and rabbits using parenteral dosages of up to 4 or 0.3 times, respectively, the average human dosage (40 units daily) have not revealed evidence of fetal malformations. Modest decreases in food consumption and weight gain, and occasional instances of severe hypoglycemia and death, were noted when insulin lispro was administered subcutaneously at a dosage of 20 units/kg daily to male rats prior to cohabitation through two consecutive matings and to female rats prior to cohabitation and through gestational day 19; these effects were expected based on the pharmacologic effects of the drug. Transient decreases in fetal and newborn pup weights and an increased incidence of fetal runts per litter suggested a marginal effect on in utero growth at an insulin lispro dosage of 20 units/kg daily; however, no effects on pup growth were observed with dosages of 1–5 units/kg daily.

Reproduction studies evaluating the effect of insulin lispro on fertility have not been conducted. Reproduction studies in male rats receiving subcutaneous injections of insulin lispro at doses up to 20 units/kg daily have not revealed evidence of impaired reproductive performance, testicular histopathology, or impaired fertility in the parental generation or in the untreated successive generation.

Insulin lispro alone or in fixed combination with isophane insulin human should be used with caution in nursing women, since it is not known whether the drug is distributed into milk in humans. However, other insulins (e.g., insulin human) are distributed into milk. Patients with diabetes who are lactating may require adjustments in insulin lispro (alone or in fixed combination with isophane insulin human) dosage, meal plans, or both.

For additional information on the use of insulin in gestational diabetes mellitus and during the perinatal period, see Uses: Gestational Diabetes Mellitus and see Dosage: Insulin Use during Pregnancy, in the Insulins General Statement 68:20.20.

Pharmacology

Studies in animals, healthy adults, and patients with type 1 (insulin-dependent) diabetes mellitus indicate that insulin lispro has pharmacologic effects comparable to those of insulin human. The fixed combination of insulin lispro and insulin lispro protamine (Humalog® Mix75/25®) has glucose-lowering effects similar to those of the fixed combination of insulin human (regular) and isophane insulin human (Humulin® 70/30) on a unit-for-unit basis.

The potency of insulin lispro, with respect to its efficacy for replacement therapy in patients with type 1 diabetes mellitus, is similar to that of insulin human. Short-term, in vitro receptor-binding studies demonstrate that insulin lispro and insulin human have similar affinity for insulin receptor binding sites. However, the number and affinity of insulin receptors on circulating monocytes in a limited number of patients with type 1 diabetes mellitus increased to levels similar to those in healthy individuals following 3 months of therapy with insulin lispro, while patients receiving insulin human (regular) had a decrease in insulin receptor affinity and binding capacity. It has been suggested that the improvement in insulin receptor status during prolonged therapy with insulin lispro may be related to its more physiologic pharmacokinetic profile relative to that of regular insulin.

Insulin lispro and insulin human have similar short-term hypoglycemic effects when given IV. In patients with type 1 diabetes mellitus in whom hypoglycemia was induced experimentally, the counterregulatory hormone response to hypoglycemia was similar with insulin lispro and insulin human; similar counterregulatory hormone responses to ingestion of a meal have been reported in other studies. Limited data suggest that insulin lispro suppresses hepatic glucose production and promotes peripheral glucose utilization to a greater extent than does insulin human when the drugs are given subcutaneously. In patients with type 1 diabetes mellitus who received insulin lispro or insulin human (regular) by continuous subcutaneous infusion for 3 months, glycosylated hemoglobin (hemoglobin A_{1c} [HbA_{1c}]) values and postprandial blood glucose concentrations were lower with insulin lispro therapy; however, timing of insulin human administration was not optimized since both insulin human and insulin lispro were administered within 5 minutes before meals. (See Insulin Regimens, under Dosage and Administration: Dosage in the Insulins General Statement 68:20.08.) The incidence of hypoglycemic episodes was lower than baseline levels and similar for both drugs.

For further information on the pharmacology of insulin, see the Insulins General Statement 68:20.08.

Pharmacokinetics

■ **Absorption** Insulin lispro is more rapidly absorbed than soluble preparations of insulin human or insulins of animal origin following subcutaneous administration because of its ability to dissociate faster from the insulin hexamer in solution. Absorption of other insulins (e.g., insulin human) from subcutaneous sites is delayed by the time required for dissociation of insulin hexamers into dimers and monomers that can diffuse into the systemic circulation. Therefore, insulin lispro has a faster onset and shorter duration of action than other insulins and, when administered subcutaneously 15 minutes before a meal, more closely mimics the endogenous postprandial insulin response. After subcutaneous administration of 0.1–0.4 units/kg of insulin lispro or insulin human in healthy individuals or patients with type 1 diabetes mellitus, peak plasma insulin concentrations are higher and occur earlier with insulin lispro (at 30–90 minutes) than with insulin human (at 50–120 minutes). Addition of zinc to the commercially available formulation of insulin lispro reduces peak serum concentrations somewhat compared with an insulin lispro formulation without zinc (not commercially available in the US) but does not appreciably alter the time to peak concentration. Unlike with insulin human, the time to peak serum concentration following subcutaneous administration of insulin lispro does not increase with increasing doses. Serum concentrations of insulin lispro also exhibit less intraindividual and interindividual variability than those of insulin human, possibly because of differences in the intrinsic properties of these insulins.

The fixed combination of insulin lispro and insulin lispro protamine (Humalog® Mix75/25®, Humalog® Mix50/50®) exhibits 2 phases of absorption. The early phase represents insulin lispro and its rapid onset of action; the late phase represents the prolonged action of insulin lispro protamine suspension. In a limited number of nondiabetic individuals, peak serum insulin concentrations were observed 30–240 minutes (median: 60 minutes) following subcutaneous administration of the fixed combination (0.3 units/kg) of insulin lispro and insulin lispro protamine (Humalog® Mix75/25®); results were identical in diabetic patients. In patients with type 1 diabetes mellitus, peak serum (immunoreactive) insulin concentrations were observed at 45–120 minutes (median: 60 minutes) following administration of the Humalog® Mix50/50® fixed combination. The fixed combinations of insulin lispro and insulin lispro protamine (Humalog® Mix75/25®, Humalog® Mix50/50®) are absorbed more rapidly than the fixed combination of insulin human (regular) and isophane insulin human (Humulin® 70/30®, Humulin® 50/50), including in patients with type 1 diabetes mellitus. The duration of action of Humalog® Mix75/25® and Humalog® Mix50/50® also is similar to that of Humulin® 70/30® and Humulin® 50/50®.

The pharmacokinetics and pharmacodynamics of insulin human and insulin lispro are similar following IV administration in healthy individuals; however, the safety and efficacy of IV insulin lispro have not been evaluated in clinical trials in patients with diabetes mellitus. Following single IV doses of 0.1–0.2 units/kg, the absolute bioavailabilities of insulin lispro and insulin human were similar, ranging from 55–77%.

The onset of glycemic response following subcutaneous injection of insulin lispro in healthy individuals or in patients with type 1 or 2 diabetes mellitus generally ranges from 0.25–0.5 hours versus 0.5–1 hours for insulin human; peak glycemic response for insulin lispro or insulin human occurs at 0.5–2.5 or 1–5 hours, respectively. Following subcutaneous administration in these individuals or patients, the duration of hypoglycemic action of insulin lispro is 3–6.5 hours compared with 6–10 hours for insulin human. Many factors can affect the onset, degree, and duration of insulin activity, including injection technique, presence of insulin antibodies, site of injection, tissue blood supply, temperature, excipients in insulin formulations, and interindividual and intraindividual differences in response. After subcutaneous administration, onset of action of insulin lispro from abdominal, deltoid, and thigh sites is similar, and variations in absorption related to site of administration are smaller than those observed with regular insulin. However, the effects of age, obesity, gender, and type of diabetes mellitus on glycemic response do not appear to differ in patients receiving insulin lispro versus insulin human.

■ **Distribution** The volume of distribution of insulin lispro reportedly is identical to that of insulin human and ranges from 0.26–0.36 L/kg. Distribution of insulin lispro when given in the fixed-combination formulation containing protamine sulfate (Humalog® Mix75/25®) has not been determined. It is not known whether insulin lispro is distributed into human milk; however, other insulins (e.g., insulin human) are distributed into milk. In a study in a limited number of pregnant women with gestational diabetes, the drug did not appear to cross the placenta.

■ **Elimination** In healthy adults, the half-life of subcutaneously administered insulin lispro or insulin human is 1 or 1.5 hours, respectively, while systemic clearance of insulin lispro and insulin human is similar. Following IV administration, insulin lispro and insulin human reportedly exhibit identical dose-dependent elimination, with half-lives of 26 or 52 minutes at doses of 0.1 or 0.2 units/kg, respectively.

The metabolic fate of insulin lispro alone or in fixed combination with insulin lispro protamine has not been determined in humans; however, in animals, metabolism of insulin lispro is identical to that of insulin human.

Some studies with insulin human have shown increased circulating insulin concentrations in patients with renal or hepatic failure; information on the use of insulin lispro in such patients is limited. In a study in a limited number of patients with type 2 diabetes mellitus and various degrees of renal function, sensitivity to insulin lispro increased as renal function declined. (See Cautions: Precautions and Contraindications and see Dosage and Administration: Dosage in Renal and Hepatic Impairment.)

Chemistry and Stability

■ **Chemistry** Insulin lispro is a biosynthetic human insulin analog that is structurally identical to insulin human except for reversal of the sequence of lysine and proline on the B chain of the molecule; in insulin lispro, lysine and proline occur at positions 28 and 29, respectively, of the B chain. The inversion of lysine and proline in the amino acid sequence eliminates hydrophobic interactions and weakens some of the hydrogen bonds that contribute to the stability of dimer subunits composing the hexameric form of insulin lispro. Endogenous insulin is stored in the pancreas as a stable, zinc-containing hexamer; stabilization of insulin lispro in the commercial formulation is accomplished by addition of zinc and *m*-cresol. The hexamers formed with zinc and insulin lispro are weak compared with those of human insulin and dissociate rapidly into monomers of the insulin analog that are absorbed through vascular endothelial cells. Consequently, insulin lispro has a more rapid onset of action than insulin human when given subcutaneously while retaining the conformation of critical sites necessary for binding to and activating the insulin receptor.

Biosynthetic insulin lispro (Humalog®) is prepared using recombinant DNA technology and special laboratory strains of nonpathogenic *E. coli*. The *E. coli* bacteria have been genetically modified by the addition of plasmids that incorporate genes for the lispro form of human proinsulin.

Commercially available biosynthetic insulin lispro injection consists of zinc insulin lispro crystals that are prepared by precipitating insulin lispro in the presence of zinc oxide and dissolving the crystals in water for injection, resulting in a clear aqueous solution. Each mL contains 100 USP units of biosynthetic insulin lispro solution and 19.7 mcg of zinc. Each mL of insulin lispro also contains dibasic sodium phosphate 1.88 mg, glycerin 16 mg, *m*-cresol 3.15 mg, and trace amounts of phenol. Sodium hydroxide and/or hydrochloric acid may be added during manufacture of biosynthetic insulin lispro zinc injection to adjust pH to 7–7.8.

Insulin lispro also is commercially available in fixed combination with insulin lispro protamine (neutral protamine lispro [NPL]), an intermediate-acting insulin. Insulin lispro protamine is prepared by crystallizing insulin lispro with protamine sulfate to produce a suspension with similar pharmacokinetics as isophane (NPH) insulin human. Each mL of the fixed combination of insulin lispro and insulin lispro protamine suspension (Humalog® Mix75/25®) contains

100 USP units of insulin lispro, 25 mcg of zinc (as zinc oxide), and 0.28 mg of protamine sulfate. Each mL of Humalog® Mix75/25® also contains dibasic sodium phosphate 3.78 mg, glycerin 16 mg, cresol 1.76 mg, and phenol 0.715 mg. Sodium hydroxide and/or hydrochloric acid may be added during manufacture of Humalog® Mix75/25® or Humalog® Mix50/50® injection to adjust pH to 7–7.8. Each mL of Humalog® Mix50/50® contains 100 units of insulin lispro, 0.03 mg of zinc ion (as zinc oxide), and 0.19 mg of protamine sulfate. Each mL of Humalog® Mix50/50® also contains dibasic sodium phosphate 3.78 mg, glycerin 16 mg, m-cresol 2.2 mg, and phenol 0.89 mg.

■ **Stability** Insulin lispro injection should be dispensed in the original, unopened, multiple-dose vial, disposable injection pen, or injection cartridge supplied by the manufacturer. When stored as directed, the vials and cartridges have an expiration date of not later than 2 years after the date of manufacture. Unopened vials or disposable injection pens of insulin lispro alone or in fixed combination with insulin lispro protamine or cartridges of the drug that have not been placed in a delivery device should be stored at 2–8°C and should not be subjected to freezing; the drug vial or cartridge should be discarded if it is frozen. Vials or cartridges of insulin lispro that cannot be refrigerated or vials and disposable injection pens that are in use may be stored at room temperature not exceeding 30°C for up to 28 days; exposure to extremes in temperature or direct sunlight should be avoided. Disposable injection pens of insulin lispro in fixed combination with insulin lispro protamine (Humalog® Mix75/25® Pen, Humalog® Mix50/50® Pen) that are in use may be stored at room temperature (below 30°C) for up to 10 days; exposure to extremely hot temperatures or direct light should be avoided. The manufacturer states that, once assembled by placement in the injectable pen (Owen Mumford Autopen®), insulin lispro cartridges and the injection device should be stored at room temperature and should *not* be refrigerated *nor* exposed to extremely hot temperatures or direct sunlight. Any unused insulin lispro in unrefrigerated vials, disposable injection pens, or cartridges should be discarded after 28 days. With the fixed combination of insulin lispro and insulin lispro protamine in disposable injection pens (Humalog® Mix75/25® Pen, Humalog® Mix50/50® Pen) or in vials, any unused portion should be discarded after 10 or 28 days, respectively.

When insulin lispro is diluted with the sterile diluent supplied by the manufacturer for improved accuracy in preparing pediatric dosages (see Dosage and Administration: Administration), the diluted solution should be discarded after 28 days when stored at 5°C or after 14 days when stored at 30°C.

Insulin lispro injection should be inspected visually prior to administration whenever the solution and the container permit. If the solution exhibits discoloration, turbidity, or unusual viscosity, the vial or cartridge should be discarded, since these changes indicate deterioration or contamination. Insulin lispro in fixed combination with insulin lispro protamine should be not be used if resuspension cannot be achieved (suspension should appear uniformly cloudy). (See Dosage and Administration: Administration.)Patients observing unexplained increases in blood glucose concentrations during insulin therapy should be particularly vigilant for any indications of loss of insulin potency and should contact a clinician if insulin requirements change markedly.

The compatibility of insulin lispro injection with other drugs depends on several factors (e.g., pH of the injection, concentration of the drugs, specific diluents used, temperature, resulting pH); specialized references should be consulted for specific compatibility information. For convenience, insulin lispro has been administered with a longer-acting insulin (e.g., isophane [NPH] insulin human) in the same syringe. Mixing of insulin lispro with other insulins may be associated with physicochemical changes that could alter the physiologic response to the insulins. When insulin lispro (Humalog®) was mixed with isophane (NPH) insulin human (Humulin N®), binding of insulin lispro with stabilizers/excipients (e.g., zinc, protamine) in the NPH insulin decreased the absorption rate and the peak concentration, but not the total bioavailability, of insulin lispro. (See Dosage and Administration: Administration.) Mixtures of insulin lispro and a longer-acting insulin (e.g., NPH insulin human should be given within 5 minutes after mixing; insulin mixtures should not be given IV. The manufacturer states that the effect of mixing Humalog® with insulins of animal origin (no longer commercially available in the US) or human insulins produced by other manufacturers has not been studied. Whenever insulin lispro is mixed with a longer-acting insulin preparation, insulin lispro should be drawn into the syringe first in order to prevent precipitation or turbidity of the insulin lispro solution by the longer-acting insulin.

When insulin lispro is administered via an external subcutaneous controlled-infusion device (pump), the drug should not be diluted or mixed with any other insulin. Insulin lispro in the external infusion device should not be exposed to temperatures exceeding 37°C during administration. Infusions sets (reservoir syringe, tubing, and catheter), the Disetronic® D-TRON® or Disetronic® D-TRON®plus cartridge adapter, and insulin lispro in the pump reservoir should be replaced and a new infusion site selected at least every 48 hours. The 3-mL cartridges used in the Disetronic® D-TRON® or Disetronic® D-TRON®plus insulin pumps should be discarded after 7 days, even if some drug remains in the reservoir.

Simulated administration of insulin lispro by continuous subcutaneous infusion in several external infusion pump systems (i.e., Disetronic H-Tron, MiniMed Model 504 pumps) revealed no changes in the potency, purity, or physical stability of insulin lispro when stored within each of these devices for 48 hours. However, precipitation of insulin lispro on infusion catheters (i.e., Silhouette, Soft-Set catheters) has been noted in several patients who were receiving insulin lispro via one of several external pump systems (i.e., Disetronic H-Tron V-100, MiniMed 507C pumps).

Preparations

Excipients in commercially available drug preparations may have clinically important effects in some individuals; consult specific product labeling for details.

Insulin Lispro (Recombinant DNA Origin)

Parenteral		
Injection	100 units/mL	**HumaLOG®** (available as 3-mL cartridge, 3-mL disposable delivery device, and 10-mL vial), Lilly

Insulin Lispro Combinations (Recombinant DNA Origin)

Parenteral		
Injectable Suspension	Insulin Lispro 25 units/mL with Insulin Lispro Protamine 75 units/mL	**HumaLOG® Mix75/25** (available as 3-mL delivery device and 10-mL vial), Lilly
	Insulin Lispro 50 units/mL with Insulin Lispro Protamine 50 units/mL	**HumaLOG® Mix50/50** (available as 3-mL delivery device), Lilly

†Use is not currently included in the labeling approved by the US Food and Drug Administration

SHORT-ACTING INSULINS 68:20.08.08

Insulin Human

Human Insulin

■ Insulin human is a biosynthetic protein that is structurally identical to endogenous insulin secreted by the beta cells of the human pancreas; commercially available insulin human preparations are classified as short-acting or intermediate-acting.

REMS

FDA approved a REMS for insulin human to ensure that the benefits outweigh the risks. The REMS may apply to one or more preparations of insulin human and consists of the following: communication plan. See the FDA REMS page (https://www.accessdata.fda.gov/scripts/cder/rems/index.cfm).

Uses

■ **Diabetes Mellitus** Insulin human is used as replacement therapy for the management of diabetes mellitus, including in the emergency treatment of diabetic ketoacidosis or hyperosmolar hyperglycemic states when rapid control of hyperglycemia is required. (See Diabetic Ketoacidosis and Hyperosmolar Hyperglycemic States under Dosage: Diabetes Mellitus, in Dosage and Administration.) Insulin human may be used in all patients with type 1 (insulin-dependent) diabetes mellitus, including all newly diagnosed patients requiring insulin therapy. In patients with type 1 diabetes mellitus, insulin human generally should be used in conjunction with a longer-acting insulin. In patients with type 2 diabetes mellitus, insulin human may be used in combination with oral antidiabetic agents and/or longer-acting insulins. (See Combination Therapy with Other Antidiabetic Agents under Uses: Diabetes Mellitus, in the Insulins General Statement 68:20.08.) Human insulin manufactured using recombinant DNA technology has replaced animal-source insulin (no longer commercially available in the US).

Safety and efficacy of insulin human injection have been established during short-term and long-term use.

Concentrated (U-500) insulin human (regular) is used in patients with marked insulin resistance (daily insulin requirements exceeding 200 units) so that a large dose may be administered subcutaneously in a reasonable volume.

The American Diabetes Association (ADA) states that human insulin is preferred for use in pregnant women, women considering pregnancy, individuals with allergies or immune resistance to animal-derived insulins, those initiating insulin therapy, and those expected to use insulin only intermittently. Use of insulin human has been associated with a reduction in insulin requirements in some diabetic patients with excessive insulin antibodies whose response was refractory to purified pork insulin (no longer commercially available in US).

Gestational Diabetes Mellitus ADA recommends that insulin therapy (using insulin human) be considered in patients with gestational diabetes who, despite dietary management, have fasting plasma glucose concentrations exceeding 105 mg/dL or 2-hour postprandial plasma glucose concentrations exceeding 130 mg/dL.

■ **Hospitalized Patients** IV administration of regular crystalline insulin provides the greatest flexibility in dosing and is used in preference to subcutaneous administration in hospitalized patients with hyperglycemia (e.g., unrecognized diabetes mellitus, hospital-related hyperglycemia), diabetic ketoacidosis, nonketotic hyperosmolar states, poorly controlled diabetes mellitus and widely fluctuating blood glucose concentrations, or severe insulin resistance. Other situations that may require IV infusion of insulin include use in diabetic or hyperglycemic hospitalized patients who are not eating and those with hyperkalemia or critical illness requiring intensive care. (See Uses: Critical Illness, in the Insulins General Statement 68:20.08.) IV insulin infusion also is used in general preoperative, intraoperative, and postoperative care, including heart or solid organ transplantation or surgery, or surgical patients requiring mechanical ventilation.

■ **Cardiovascular Disease** While insulin human (regular) has been used in combination with IV potassium chloride and dextrose (D-glucose) (referred to as glucose-insulin-potassium or GIK therapy) early in the course of suspected acute ST-segment-elevation myocardial infarction† (STEMI) for metabolic modulation and potential beneficial effects on morbidity and mortality, current data from a large randomized trial suggest that high-dose GIK therapy is not beneficial in reducing mortality following acute STEMI. For additional details, see Uses: Acute Myocardial Infarction, in the Insulins General Statement 60:20.08.

IV infusion of insulin also may be required in diabetic hospitalized patients with cardiogenic shock or hemodynamic instability.

■ **Acute Stroke** Insulin injection (e.g., insulin human) also has been used IV in combination with IV potassium chloride and dextrose (i.e., GIK therapy) in a limited number of patients with acute stroke† and mild to moderate hyperglycemia. Pending completion of randomized trials, some experts suggest the use of insulin and fluids (but not IV dextrose-containing solutions) to lower markedly elevated blood glucose concentrations to less than 300 mg/dL in such patients.

Dosage and Administration

■ **Administration** ***Insulin Human (Regular)*** Insulin human (regular) injection is usually administered by subcutaneous injection. Insulin human (regular) also may be administered IV or IM† under medical supervision with close monitoring of blood glucose and potassium concentrations to avoid hypoglycemia or hypokalemia.

Parenteral Administration. Excessive agitation of the vial prior to withdrawing the insulin dose should be avoided since loss of potency, clumping, frosting, or precipitation may occur. Warming refrigerated insulin to room temperature prior to use will limit local irritation at the injection site.

For IV infusion, insulin human (regular) injection is usually diluted to a concentration of 0.05–1 unit/mL in 0.9% sodium chloride or 5 or 10% dextrose injection with 40 mEq/L of potassium chloride in polypropylene infusion bags.

The manufacturer of Novolin® R states that the injection should not be used in continuous infusion pumps, as such use may result in adsorption onto pump catheters.

When concentrated (U-500) insulin human (regular) injection is used in patients with marked insulin resistance (i.e., daily insulin requirements exceeding 200 units), extreme caution must be exercised in dosage measurement because inadvertent overdosage may result in irreversible insulin shock. The manufacturer further warns that serious consequences may result if this concentrated injection were used other than under constant medical supervision.

Isophane Insulin Human **Parenteral Administration.** Isophane insulin human suspension is usually administered subcutaneously; this form of insulin must *not* be administered IV. Since the active ingredient in isophane insulin suspensions is in the precipitate and not in the clear supernatant liquid, the vial should be gently agitated to assure a homogeneous mixture for accurate measurement of each dose. This may be done by slowly rotating and inverting or *carefully* shaking the vial several times before withdrawal of each dose. Vigorous shaking should be avoided since this causes frothing, which interferes with correct measurement of a dose.

Preparations of isophane insulin suspensions that are slowly injected subcutaneously may clog the tip of the needle, resulting in an inability to complete the injection. Since this is less likely to occur when the insulin is injected subcutaneously more rapidly, the dose should be injected over a period of less than 5 seconds.

When a compatible delivery device is used for subcutaneous injection of isophane insulin human suspension (e.g., Humulin® N pen) or the fixed combination containing insulin human (regular) injection and isophane insulin human suspension (Humulin® 70/30 Pen®), the accompanying labeling should be consulted for proper methods of assembly, administration, and care.

■ **Dosage** ***Diabetes Mellitus*** Any change in insulin preparation or dosage regimen should be made with caution and only under medical supervision. Changes in strength, brand, type, and/or method of manufacture may necessitate a change in dosage. Illness, particularly nausea and vomiting, and changes in eating patterns may alter insulin requirements. Although it is not possible to clearly identify which patients will require a change in dosage when therapy with a different preparation is initiated, it is known that a limited number of patients will require such a change. Adjustments may be needed with the first dose or may occur over a period of several weeks.

Parenteral Dosage. Dosage of insulin human as the injection is always expressed in USP units. Dosage of insulin must be based on the results of blood and urine glucose determinations and must be carefully individualized to attain optimum therapeutic effect.

Initial total daily insulin dosages in adults and children with type 1 diabetes mellitus range from 0.2–1 units/kg. Children with newly diagnosed type 1 diabetes usually require an initial total daily dosage of approximately 0.5–1 units/kg; the dosage requirement can be much lower during the period of partial remission. In severe insulin resistance (e.g., puberty, obesity), the daily insulin dosage may be substantially higher. In patients with type 2 diabetes mellitus, the initial total daily insulin dosage ranges from 0.2–0.4 units/kg.

Diabetic Ketoacidosis and Hyperosmolar Hyperglycemic States Because it has a relatively rapid onset of action and can be administered IV, regular insulin (e.g., insulin human [regular]) is the insulin of choice in the treatment of diabetic emergencies such as diabetic ketoacidosis or hyperosmolar hyperglycemic coma. Prompt correction of hyperglycemia with adequate doses of insulin, correction of dehydration and electrolyte imbalances with IV fluid and electrolyte therapy, and frequent monitoring of clinical and laboratory data are essential to successful treatment of these hyperglycemic crises. Hydration status should be carefully monitored in patients with diabetic ketoacidosis or hyperosmolar hyperglycemia, and 0.9% sodium chloride injection generally should be infused IV (in the absence of cardiac compromise) if serum sodium concentrations (corrected for the effect of hyperglycemia) are low; 0.45% sodium chloride injection may be used if serum sodium concentrations are normal or elevated. Since diabetic ketoacidosis often is associated with hypokalemia, the possibility of potassium imbalance should be evaluated and, if present, corrected before administration of insulin as long as adequate renal function is assured. Blood pH should be determined, and if acidosis is severe (blood pH less than 7), patients should receive IV sodium bicarbonate until blood pH exceeds 7.

Adults. For the treatment of *moderate to severe* diabetic ketoacidosis (plasma glucose exceeding 250 mg/dL with arterial pH of 7–7.24 or less and serum bicarbonate of 10–15 mEq/L or less) or hyperosmolar hyperglycemia in adults, the American Diabetes Association (ADA) recommends a loading dose of 0.15 units/kg of regular insulin by direct IV injection, followed by continuous IV infusion of 0.1 units/kg per hour. Plasma glucose should decrease at a rate of 50–75 mg/dL per hour. If plasma glucose concentrations do not fall by 50 mg/dL within the first hour of insulin therapy, the insulin infusion rate may be doubled every hour, provided the patient is adequately hydrated, until plasma glucose decreases steadily by 50–75 mg/dL per hour. When a plasma glucose concentration of 250 or 300 mg/dL is achieved in patients with diabetic ketoacidosis or hyperosmolar hyperglycemia, respectively, the insulin infusion rate may be decreased to 0.05–0.1 units/kg per hour. Once these target glucose concentrations have been achieved, infusion with 0.9% sodium chloride injection may be changed to dextrose 5% with 0.45% sodium chloride solution and administered with insulin to maintain serum glucose concentrations between 150–200 mg/dL in patients with diabetic ketoacidosis or 250–300 mg/dL in those with hyperosmolar hyperglycemia. Serum determinations of electrolytes, BUN, creatinine, osmolality, and glucose should be made every 2–4 hours until the patient is stable; monitoring of serum osmolality and cardiac, renal, and mental status is particularly important in patients with renal or cardiac compromise to avoid iatrogenic fluid overload. The rate of insulin administration or the concentration of dextrose may need to be adjusted to maintain glucose concentration until resolution of diabetic ketoacidosis (i.e., serum glucose less than 200 mg/dL, venous pH exceeding 7.3, serum bicarbonate of at least 18 mEq/L) or hyperosmolar hyperglycemia (i.e., patient mentally alert, serum osmolality of 315 mOsm/kg or less).

For the treatment of *mild* diabetic ketoacidosis (plasma glucose exceeding 250 mg/dL with an arterial pH of 7.25–7.3 and serum bicarbonate of 15–18 mEq/L), ADA states that regular insulin given subcutaneously or IM† every hour is as effective as IV insulin administration in reducing hyperglycemia and ketonemia. A loading dose of regular insulin 0.4–0.6 units/kg may be administered in 2 doses, with 50% given by direct IV injection and 50% by subcutaneous or IM† injection. After the loading dose, 0.1 units/kg per hour of regular insulin may be given subcutaneously or IM†.

After resolution of diabetic ketoacidosis (i.e., plasma glucose less than 200 mg/dL, venous pH exceeding 7.3, serum bicarbonate of 18 mEq/L or greater) or hyperosmolar hyperglycemia in patients who are unable to eat, IV insulin and fluid replacement is continued, and subcutaneous regular insulin may be given as needed every 4 hours. Regular insulin may be given subcutaneously in 5-unit increments for every 50 mg/dL increase in blood glucose concentrations above 150 mg/dL, to a dose of up to 20 units of insulin for a blood glucose of 300 mg/dL or higher. When the patient is able to eat, a multiple-dose, subcutaneous insulin regimen consisting of a short- or rapid-acting insulin and an intermediate- or long-acting insulin is initiated. Regular insulin is continued IV for 1–2 hours after initiation of the subcutaneous insulin regimen to ensure adequate plasma insulin concentrations during the transition from IV to subcutaneous insulin; otherwise, abrupt discontinuance of IV insulin with the institution of delayed-onset subcutaneous insulin may lead to worsened glycemic control. Patients with known diabetes mellitus may reinstitute the insulin regimen they were receiving before the onset of diabetic ketoacidosis or hyperosmolar hyperglycemia, and the regimen may then be adjusted further as needed for adequate glycemic control.

Patients with newly diagnosed diabetes mellitus should receive a total insulin dosage of 0.5–1 units/kg daily as part of a multiple-dose regimen of short- and long-acting insulin until an optimal dosage is established. Some patients with newly diagnosed type 2 diabetes mellitus may be managed with diet therapy and oral antidiabetic agents following resolution of hyperglycemic crises.

Pediatric Patients. In pediatric patients (younger than 20 years of age) with diabetic ketoacidosis or hyperosmolar hyperglycemia, ADA recommends initiation of insulin therapy with an IV infusion of regular insulin at a rate of 0.1 units/kg per hour; an initial direct IV injection of insulin is *not* recommended in pediatric patients. If IV access is unavailable, insulin may be given IM in an initial dose of 0.1 units/kg, followed by 0.1 units/kg per hour subcutaneously or IM until acidosis is resolved (i.e., venous pH exceeds 7.3, serum bicarbonate concentration exceeds 15 mEq/L). Upon resolution, the insulin infusion rate should be decreased to 0.05 units/kg per hour until subcutaneous replacement insulin therapy (using a multiple-dose regimen of short- and intermediate-acting insulins) is initiated. When a serum glucose concentration of 250 mg/dL is achieved in pediatric patients with diabetic ketoacidosis or hyperosmolar hyperglycemia, dextrose 5–10% with 0.45–0.75% sodium chloride injection is administered to complete rehydration in 48 hours and maintain serum glucose concentrations between 150–250 mg/dL. Serum electrolyte and glucose concentrations should be determined every 2–4 hours until the patient is stable. After diabetic ketoacidosis in pediatric patients has resolved, subcutaneous insulin may be initiated at a dosage of 0.5–1 units/kg daily in divided doses (⅔ of the daily dosage in the morning [⅓ as short-acting insulin, ⅔ as intermediate-acting insulin] and ⅓ in the evening [½ as short-acting insulin, ½ as intermediate-acting insulin]). In pediatric patients with newly diagnosed diabetes mellitus, regular insulin 0.1–0.25 units/kg may be given every 6–8 hours during the first 24 hours to determine insulin requirements.

Cautions

Insulin human shares the toxic potentials of other insulins, and the usual precautions of insulin therapy should be observed with insulin human. (See Cautions in the Insulins General Statement 68:20.08.)

Frequency and severity of adverse reactions to insulin human appear to be similar to those associated with purified pork insulin (no longer commercially available in the US).

■ **Immunogenicity** Several studies have shown parenteral insulin human to be less immunogenic than purified pork insulin (no longer commercially available in the US). Data from several studies in patients with diabetes mellitus have shown that insulin antibodies (IgE type) develop less frequently following administration of insulin human than following purified animal insulins (no longer commercially available in the US). Although a few patients in these studies developed elevated insulin antibody titers (IgE type) following administration of insulin human, they did not develop any signs or symptoms of insulin allergy or adverse reactions to insulin human. In one study in patients with diabetes mellitus who had not previously received insulin therapy, insulin human was associated with relatively weaker immunogenicity than purified pork insulin as determined by fasting insulin antibody levels.

Insulin human is contraindicated in patients who are hypersensitive to insulin human or to any ingredient in the formulation.

Pharmacology

Studies in animals, healthy adults, and patients with type 1 (insulin-dependent) diabetes mellitus have shown insulin human to have essentially identical pharmacologic effects compared with purified pork insulin (no longer commercially available in the US). Potency of insulin human, with respect to its efficacy for replacement therapy in patients with type 1 diabetes mellitus, is similar to that of purified pork insulin. For further information on the pharmacology of insulin human, see the Insulins General Statement 68:20.08.

Pharmacokinetics

The pharmacokinetic profile of insulin human has been shown to be essentially identical to that of purified pork insulin (no longer commercially available in the US). No clinically important differences in total body clearance rates, plasma half-lives, apparent volume of distribution, or effect on blood glucose concentration have been observed following administration of insulin human or purified pork insulin. In vitro studies have shown that the binding affinities for human erythrocyte receptors and for receptors on porcine hepatocytes are similar for insulin human and purified pork insulin.

Chemistry and Stability

■ **Chemistry** Insulin human is a biosynthetic protein that is structurally identical to endogenous insulin secreted by the beta cells of the human pancreas. Although structurally identical to endogenous human insulin, commercially available insulin human is *not* extracted from the human pancreas, but is prepared biosynthetically from cultures of genetically modified *Escherichia coli* or *Saccharomyces cerevisiae*.

Biosynthetic insulin human (Humulin®) is prepared using recombinant DNA technology and special laboratory strains of nonpathogenic *E. coli*; the A and B chains of human insulin are synthesized by different strains of *E. coli*. The bacteria have been genetically modified by the addition of plasmids that incorporate genes for human insulin synthesis. Biosynthetic insulin human (Novolin® [formerly available as semisynthetic insulin]) is prepared using recombinant DNA technology and strains of *Saccharomyces cerevisiae*. The bacteria have been genetically modified by the addition of plasmids that incorporate genes for human insulin synthesis. Unlike the process used for the production of animal insulins (no longer commercially available in the US), the commercial process using recombinant DNA technology to produce insulin human avoids contamination with glucagon, somatostatin, and proinsulin. Although a possible theoretical source of protein contamination (i.e., *E. coli* polypeptides [ECPs]) of certain biosynthetic insulin human (i.e., Humulin®) could be derived from the *E. coli* organism used in its manufacture, this commercially available biosynthetic insulin human contains less than 4 ppm of immunoreactive ECPs.

Each mg of insulin human has a biologic potency of not less than 27.5 USP insulin human units calculated on a dried basis.

Insulin (Regular) **Biosynthetic.** Biosynthetic insulin human (regular) injection consists of zinc insulin crystals that are prepared by precipitating insulin in the presence of zinc chloride. Commercially available insulin human (regular) injections containing 100 units/mL are clear and colorless. Each 100 USP units of biosynthetic insulin human (regular) contains 10–40 mcg of zinc. However, Novolin® R contains approximately 7 mcg/mL of zinc chloride. Humulin® R also contains 1.4–1.8% glycerin and 0.225–0.275% cresol and has a pH of 7–7.8. Novolin® R also contains 16 mg/mL of glycerin and 3 mg/mL of metacresol and has a pH of 7.4.

Insulin, Isophane **Biosynthetic.** Biosynthetic isophane insulin human is an intermediate-acting, sterile suspension of zinc insulin crystals and protamine sulfate in buffered water for injection, combined in a manner such that the solid phase of the suspension consists of crystals composed of insulin, protamine, and zinc. Biosynthetic isophane insulin human suspension is a cloudy or milky suspension of rod-shaped crystals free from large aggregates of crystals following moderate agitation. When examined microscopically, the insoluble material in biosynthetic isophane insulin human suspension (Humulin® N) is crystalline and contains not more than trace amounts of amorphous material. Each 100 USP units of biosynthetic isophane insulin human (Humulin® N) contains 10–40 mcg of zinc and 0.15–0.25% dibasic sodium phosphate. In addition, it contains 1.4–1.8% glycerin, 0.15–0.175% cresol, and 0.05–0.07% phenol. Biosynthetic isophane insulin human (Humulin® N) suspension has a pH of 7.1–7.4. Biosynthetic isophane insulin human (Novolin® N) has a pH of 7–7.8 and contains unspecified amounts of zinc, dibasic sodium phosphate, glycerin, cresol, and phenol.

■ **Stability** Insulin human injections and suspensions should be dispensed in the original, unopened, multiple-dose containers supplied by the manufacturers and have an expiration date of not later than 24–36 months, depending on the specific preparation, after the vial was filled. Unopened vials of insulin human injections, prefilled syringes, and suspensions should be stored at 2–8°C and should not be subjected to freezing or exposed to heat and sunlight; freezing will cause isophane insulin human to resuspend improperly, preventing accurate measurement of a dose. Unopened solutions and suspensions that have been frozen should be discarded. In addition, agglomeration of particles may occur, altering absorption from the injection site. The insulin vial in use may be kept at room temperature for up to 1 month; exposure to extremes in temperature (less than 2 °C or greater than 30 °C) or direct sunlight should be avoided. Insulin vials in use and stored in the refrigerator may be used beyond 30 days. Length of storage of refrigerated insulin vials is dependent on light, agitation, and technique used for dose preparation. (See Dosage and Administration: Administration.) Warming refrigerated insulin to room temperature prior to use will limit local irritation at the injection site. Because of possible microbial contamination, a partially empty vial should be discarded if it has not been used for several weeks. Insulin human (regular) injection exhibiting discoloration, turbidity, or unusual viscosity should be discarded, since these changes indicate deterioration or contamination. Isophane insulin human suspension alone or in combination with insulin human should be discarded if the suspension is clear and remains clear after the vial is rotated or if the precipitate has become clumped or granular in appearance or has formed a deposit of solid particles on the wall of the vial.

The individual manufacturer's labeling should be consulted for instructions regarding storage of specific disposable insulin pens or other insulin delivery systems preassembled with cartridges (e.g., Humulin® N Pen, Humulin® 70/30 Pen).

Infusion bags containing insulin human (regular) are stable at room temperature for 24 hours. A certain amount of insulin will initially be adsorbed onto the walls of the infusion bag.

The compatibility of insulin human (regular) injection with other drugs depends on several factors (e.g., pH of the insulin injection used, concentration of the drugs, specific diluents used, temperature, resulting pH); specialized references should be consulted for specific compatibility information.

For further information on chemistry and stability, compatibility of insulin mixtures, pharmacology, pharmacokinetics, uses, cautions, drug interactions, and dosage and administration of insulin human, see the Insulins General Statement 68:20.08.

Preparations

Excipients in commercially available drug preparations may have clinically important effects in some individuals; consult specific product labeling for details.

Insulin Human (Regular) (Recombinant DNA Origin)

Parenteral		
Injection	100 units/mL	**HumuLIN® R**, Lilly
		NovoLIN® R, Novo Nordisk
	500 units/mL	**HumuLIN® R** (concentrated U-500), Lilly

Isophane Insulin Human (Recombinant DNA Origin)

Parenteral		
Injectable Suspension	100 units/mL	**HumuLIN® N**, Lilly
		HumuLIN® N Pen (available as prefilled cartridge preassembled into pen), Lilly
		NovoLIN® N, Novo Nordisk

Insulin Human Combinations (Recombinant DNA Origin)

Parenteral		
Injectable Suspension	Insulin Human (Regular) 30 units/mL with Isophane Insulin Human 70 units/mL	**HumuLIN® 70/30**, Lilly
		HumuLIN® 70/30 Pen (available as cartridge preassembled into pen), Lilly
		NovoLIN® 70/30, Novo Nordisk

†Use is not currently included in the labeling approved by the US Food and Drug Administration

LONG-ACTING INSULINS 68:20.08.16

Insulin Degludec

■ Insulin degludec is a biosynthetic (rDNA origin), long-acting human insulin analog.

Uses

■ **Diabetes Mellitus** Insulin degludec is used to improve glycemic control in the management of type 1 or type 2 diabetes mellitus in patients who require a long-acting insulin. Insulin degludec also is commercially available in fixed combination with liraglutide (Xultophy®); the fixed combination is used as an adjunct to diet and exercise to improve glycemic control in adults with type 2 diabetes mellitus.

Insulin degludec is *not* indicated for the treatment of diabetic ketoacidosis; a short-acting insulin (e.g., insulin human) is the preferred agent. Insulin degludec also is not recommended for use in pediatric patients who require less than 5 units of insulin degludec daily.

Insulin Degludec Insulin degludec appears to be at least as effective for glycemic control as insulin glargine or insulin detemir (as determined by glycosylated hemoglobin [hemoglobin A_{1c}, HbA_{1c}]) in adult and pediatric (1 year and older) patients with type 1 or type 2 diabetes mellitus and is more effective in adults with type 2 diabetes mellitus than the oral antidiabetic agent, sitagliptin. Current evidence suggests that the prolonged duration of action and low variability in insulin degludec concentrations over the dosing interval may contribute to potentially lower rates of hypoglycemia (particularly nocturnal hypoglycemia) compared with other basal insulins. The peakless pharmacokinetic profile of insulin degludec allows for the timing of a once-daily injection to be varied from day to day in adults (when required) without increasing the risk of hypoglycemia (see Description); this flexibility in dosing may make insulin therapy less demanding and more acceptable to some patients, potentially improving patient compliance and glycemic control. Some clinicians suggest that insulin degludec may be a more suitable option than other basal insulins (i.e., insulin detemir, insulin glargine) in individuals who are prone to hypoglycemia and in those who require twice-daily administration of a basal insulin for adequate glycemic control, as well as in patients who experience variability in glycemic control with other basal insulins.

Type 1 Diabetes Mellitus. Safety and efficacy of insulin degludec for the treatment of type 1 diabetes mellitus has been demonstrated in comparisons with insulin detemir or insulin glargine in 3 randomized, open-label, noninferiority phase 3 trials of 26 or 52 weeks' duration in adults and a study in pediatric patients 1–17 years of age; patients also received mealtime insulin aspart during these trials. In a phase 3 trial in adults with type 1 diabetes mellitus who had been treated with basal and rapid-acting ("bolus") insulins for at least 1 year, patients received insulin degludec once daily with the evening meal or insulin glargine once daily at the same time each day, both in conjunction with mealtime insulin aspart. Basal insulin dosages were titrated based upon fasting plasma glucose concentrations. After 52 weeks of therapy, the decrease in HbA_{1c} from baseline was similar between treatment groups (average reduction in HbA_{1c} of 0.36 and 0.34% for insulin degludec and insulin glargine, respectively). The rate of nocturnal hypoglycemia (per patient-year of exposure) with insulin degludec in this trial was 25% lower than that with insulin glargine; however, the rate of severe hypoglycemic episodes did not differ substantially between the treatment groups. In another similar phase 3 trial, adults with type 1 diabetes mellitus received insulin degludec or insulin detemir once daily between the evening meal and bedtime, both in conjunction with mealtime insulin aspart. Patients who received insulin detemir were eligible to receive a second dose daily if there was inadequate glycemic control after at least 8 weeks of therapy. Basal insulin dosages were titrated based upon fasting blood glucose concentrations. After 26 weeks of therapy, the decrease in HbA_{1c} from baseline was similar between treatment groups (average reduction in HbA_{1c} of 0.71 and 0.61% for insulin degludec and insulin detemir treatment groups, respectively). Treatment with insulin degludec was associated with a substantially lower rate of nocturnal hypoglycemia than insulin detemir. In a third phase 3 trial, adults with type 1 diabetes mellitus received insulin degludec once daily (at the same time each day or at alternating times daily [minimum of 8 and maximum of 40 hours between doses]) or insulin glargine once daily, all in conjunction with mealtime insulin aspart. Basal insulin dosages were titrated based upon fasting plasma glucose concentrations. After 26 weeks of therapy, the treatment group that received insulin degludec at varying times of the day had similar reductions in HbA_{1c} as those patients who received insulin degludec or insulin glargine injections at the same time every day (average reduction in HbA_{1c} of 0.41, 0.4, and 0.57% for insulin degludec administered at the same time each day, insulin degludec administered at varying times, and insulin glargine treatment groups, respectively). The treatment group receiving insulin degludec at varying times of the day had lower rates of nocturnal hypoglycemia than the insulin glargine treatment group.

In another study, pediatric patients 1–17 years of age (mean age: 10 years) with type 1 diabetes mellitus received insulin degludec once daily or insulin detemir once or twice daily, all in conjunction with mealtime insulin aspart. After 26 weeks of therapy, the mean decrease in HbA_{1c} from baseline did not differ substantially between treatment groups (reduction in HbA_{1c} of 0.19 and 0.34% for insulin degludec and insulin detemir treatment groups, respectively). At the conclusion of the additional 26-week extension period of this study, the observed mean decrease in HbA_{1c} remained similar between the 2 treatment groups; no substantial difference in the rates of hypoglycemia between groups was observed.

Type 2 Diabetes Mellitus. Safety and efficacy of insulin degludec administered once daily in adults with type 2 diabetes mellitus have been established in 6 open-label, randomized clinical trials of 26 or 52 weeks' duration that compared insulin degludec with sitagliptin or with other basal insulins (i.e., insulin detemir or insulin glargine) in conjunction with oral antidiabetic agents or mealtime insulin. In a noninferiority trial in insulin-naive patients with type 2 diabetes mellitus who were inadequately controlled with oral antidiabetic therapy, once-daily therapy with insulin degludec or insulin glargine was added to existing therapy with metformin with or without a dipeptidyl peptidase-4 (DPP-4) inhibitor. Insulin degludec and insulin glargine provided similar improvements in glycemic control (as measured by HbA_{1c}, the primary clinical end point) in this trial. The proportion of patients attaining target HbA_{1c} values of less than 7% at trial end point was similar across treatment groups. The risk of nocturnal hypoglycemia was lower with insulin degludec compared with that observed with insulin glargine.

In another noninferiority trial in insulin-naive Asian patients with type 2 diabetes mellitus who were inadequately controlled with oral antidiabetic therapy, once-daily therapy with insulin degludec or insulin glargine was added to existing therapy with 1 or more oral antidiabetic agents (metformin, a sulfonylurea, a meglitinide, or an alpha-glucosidase inhibitor). Patients receiving a glucagon-like peptide-1 (GLP-1) receptor agonist (exenatide or liraglutide) or a thiazolidinedione within 3 months of trial screening were excluded from the trial. All patients received an initial insulin degludec or insulin glargine dosage of 10 units subcutaneously once daily. Insulin dosages were titrated once weekly based on fasting plasma glucose concentrations. After 26 weeks of treatment, the observed mean HbA_{1c} and fasting plasma glucose concentrations were similar for insulin degludec and insulin glargine. Additionally, there was no substantial difference in the proportion of patients achieving an HbA_{1c} less than 7%.

In a trial evaluating the safety and efficacy of varying the daily injection time of insulin degludec, adults with type 2 diabetes mellitus inadequately controlled on basal insulin, oral antidiabetic agents, or a combination of these agents received insulin degludec once daily with the evening meal, insulin degludec once daily at varying times, or insulin glargine once daily. Patients who received insulin degludec at varying times were given alternating morning and evening injections (minimum of 8 hours and maximum of 40 hours maintained between injections). Patients receiving once-daily basal insulin prior to the study were transitioned to insulin degludec or insulin glargine on a unit-for-unit basis. Insulin dosages were titrated individually once a week throughout the trial based upon fasting plasma glucose concentrations. Patients receiving oral antidiabetic agents were allowed to continue treatment with up to 3 oral antidiabetic agents (metformin, a sulfonylurea, a meglitinide, or a thiazolidinedione) during the trial. Overall, insulin degludec given at variable dosing intervals resulted in similar glycemic control, hypoglycemic risk, and weight gain compared with either insulin glargine or insulin degludec given at fixed dosing intervals. There was no substantial difference in HbA_{1c} between patients who received insulin degludec once daily, insulin degludec once daily at varying administration times, or insulin glargine once daily.

In a noninferiority trial in adults with type 2 diabetes mellitus inadequately controlled on insulin and/or oral antidiabetic agents, no difference in overall glycemic control (as assessed by HbA_{1c}) was observed in patients receiving therapy with insulin degludec or insulin glargine; however, insulin degludec therapy was associated with a lower risk of hypoglycemia than insulin glargine. In this trial, patients received once-daily insulin degludec or once-daily insulin glargine, both in combination with mealtime insulin aspart, with or without oral antidiabetic agents (metformin, pioglitazone, or both). After 52 weeks of treatment, HbA_{1c} decreased by 1.1 and 1.2% in the insulin degludec and insulin glargine treatment groups, respectively. Rates of overall, nocturnal, and diurnal hypoglycemia were substantially lower in patients treated with insulin degludec versus insulin glargine.

In a trial comparing the efficacy of insulin degludec with sitagliptin in insulin-naive adults with type 2 diabetes mellitus, insulin degludec improved glycemic control and was superior to sitagliptin in terms of lowering HbA_{1c}. Patients in this trial received add-on treatment with subcutaneous insulin degludec once daily at any time of the day (minimum of 8 hours and maximum of 40 hours between injections) or sitagliptin 100 mg orally once daily; all patients were receiving stable therapy with 1–2 oral antidiabetic agents (metformin, a meglitinide, a sulfonylurea, or pioglitazone) at baseline. The starting dosage of insulin degludec was 10 units once daily, which was titrated weekly based upon fasting plasma glucose concentrations. Sitagliptin was administered at a dosage of 100 mg orally once daily. After 26 weeks of treatment, HbA_{1c} was reduced by 1.52 and 1.09% in patients receiving insulin degludec and sitagliptin therapy, respectively. Patients receiving insulin degludec therapy also had a lower fasting blood glucose after 26 weeks of treatment compared with those receiving sitagliptin therapy (mean fasting glucose 112 versus 154 mg/dL, respectively).

Insulin Degludec/Liraglutide Fixed-combination Therapy Current data indicate that the fixed combination of insulin degludec and liraglutide is more effective than either drug (as add-on therapy to one or more oral antidiabetic agents) in improving glycemic control (as determined by reductions in HbA_{1c}) in patients with type 2 diabetes mellitus. Safety and efficacy of insulin degludec and liraglutide in fixed combination for the treatment of type 2 diabetes mellitus have been established in 5 parallel, randomized, active- or placebo-controlled phase 3 clinical trials of 26 weeks' duration in adults with type 2 diabetes mellitus.

In 2 clinical studies, the use of the fixed combination of insulin degludec and liraglutide substantially improved glycemic control in adults with type 2 diabetes mellitus who had inadequate glycemic control with oral antidiabetic agents and who were naive to therapy with a basal insulin or GLP-1 receptor agonist. In the first study, all patients continued on prestudy treatment with metformin with or without pioglitazone. In addition to the prestudy treatment, patients also received insulin degludec and liraglutide in fixed combination (initially 10 units of insulin degludec and 0.36 mg liraglutide), liraglutide (initially 0.6 mg), or insulin degludec (initially 10 units) subcutaneously once daily. Patients in the fixed-combination group or the insulin degludec treatment group had their dosages titrated twice weekly towards a target fasting plasma glucose concentration of 72–90 mg/dL. Patients in the liraglutide treatment group followed a fixed-escalation scheme with weekly dosage increases of 0.6 mg until the maintenance dosage of 1.8 mg once daily was achieved. After 26 weeks, the reduction in HbA_{1c} from baseline was 1.81, 1.35, or 1.21% in patients treated with the fixed combination of insulin degludec and liraglutide, insulin degludec, or liraglutide, respectively. In the second study, all patients continued on prestudy treatment with a sulfonylurea with or without metformin. In addition to the prestudy treatment, patients also received insulin degludec and liraglutide in fixed combination (initially 10 units of insulin degludec and 0.36 mg liraglutide) or placebo once daily. Patients in the fixed-combination group had their dosage titrated twice weekly towards a target fasting plasma glucose concentration of 72–108 mg/dL. After 26 weeks, the reduction in HbA_{1c} from baseline was 1.42 or 0.62% in patients treated with the fixed combination of insulin degludec and liraglutide or placebo, respectively.

In another trial, insulin-naive adults with type 2 diabetes mellitus who were inadequately controlled on metformin alone or in combination with pioglitazone and/or a sulfonylurea plus maximum-dose (or maximally tolerated) liraglutide (mean daily dosage at baseline: 1.7 mg) continued to receive their pretrial therapy or had their therapy converted from liraglutide to the fixed combination of insulin degludec and liraglutide. Oral antidiabetic agents were continued at pretrial dosages throughout the trial in both treatment groups. The starting dosage of the fixed combination was insulin degludec 16 units and liraglutide 0.58 mg once daily; dosage adjustments were performed twice weekly based on fasting blood glucose concentrations (end-of-trial dosage of the fixed combination: insulin degludec 44 units and liraglutide 1.58 mg daily). After 26 weeks, the reduction in HbA_{1c} from baseline was 1.31 or 0.36% with the fixed combination of insulin degludec and liraglutide versus liraglutide, respectively. A mean weight gain from baseline of 2 kg was observed in patients receiving the fixed combination of insulin degludec and liraglutide compared with a weight loss of 0.8 kg in those receiving liraglutide. A higher rate of hypoglycemia was observed in the fixed-combination treatment group.

In another trial comparing the fixed combination of insulin degludec and liraglutide with insulin degludec therapy in adults with type 2 diabetes mellitus who were inadequately controlled with basal insulin and metformin with or without a sulfonylurea or a meglitinide, patients who received the fixed combination at equivalent insulin dosages achieved superior glycemic control. In this trial, all basal insulins and oral antidiabetic drugs except for metformin hydrochloride (mean daily dosage: 1984 mg) were discontinued at randomization; patients received a starting insulin degludec dosage of 16 units (given separately or in fixed combination with liraglutide 0.58 mg) once daily, which was titrated biweekly based on fasting plasma glucose concentrations. After 26 weeks, the mean daily dosage of insulin degludec was 46 units (with liraglutide 1.66 mg in the fixed combination) in both treatment groups. The reductions in HbA_{1c} from baseline were superior with the fixed combination of insulin degludec and liraglutide compared with insulin degludec treatment (reduction of 1.94 versus 1.05%, respectively). There was no substantial difference between the 2 treatment groups with regard to hypoglycemia.

In another trial comparing the fixed combination of insulin degludec and liraglutide with insulin glargine therapy in adults with type 2 diabetes mellitus inadequately controlled on insulin glargine and metformin, patients who received the fixed combination of insulin degludec and liraglutide achieved substantially greater reductions in HbA_{1c} compared with those who received insulin glargine. Patients in this trial either continued treatment with insulin glargine or were switched to the fixed combination of insulin degludec and liraglutide, both in conjunction with metformin. The starting insulin degludec dosage was 16 units daily (with liraglutide 0.58 mg in the fixed combination), irrespective of the patient's previous daily dosage of insulin glargine (mean insulin glargine pretrial dosage: 31 units daily). Patients whose therapy was switched from insulin glargine to the fixed combination of insulin degludec and liraglutide showed no worsening of blood glucose control immediately following the switch, despite the initial reduction in insulin dosage for patients who received the fixed combination. Each treatment was titrated biweekly based on fasting blood glucose concentrations with no upper dosing limit in the insulin glargine group and a maximum daily dosage of 50 units of insulin degludec in the fixed-combination treatment group. The mean dosage of the fixed combination of insulin degludec and liraglutide or insulin glargine was 41 units insulin degludec and 1.48 mg liraglutide or 66 units of insulin glargine daily, respectively. The reductions in HbA_{1c} from baseline were substantially greater with the fixed combination of insulin degludec and liraglutide compared with insulin glargine (reduction of 1.67 versus 1.16 %, respectively).

Insulin degludec and liraglutide in fixed combination should not be used for the treatment of diabetic ketoacidosis or for the treatment of type 1 diabetes mellitus. The fixed combination also should not be used with any other preparation containing liraglutide or another GLP-1 receptor agonist. Data are lacking on the use of the fixed combination of insulin degludec and liraglutide with prandial insulin.

Dosage and Administration

■ **General** The dosage of insulin degludec is expressed in units. Each mL of insulin degludec injection contains 100 or 200 units of insulin degludec. Each mL of the fixed combination of insulin degludec and liraglutide contains 100 units of insulin degludec and 3.6 mg of liraglutide.

Dosage of insulin degludec should be carefully individualized to obtain optimum therapeutic effect based on the patient's metabolic needs, blood glucose determinations, and glycemic control goals. Glucose monitoring is recommended for all patients with diabetes mellitus.

Dosage adjustments of insulin degludec or the fixed combination of insulin degludec and liraglutide may be needed when used with other drugs or with intercurrent conditions (e.g., illness, stress, emotional disturbances), changes in physical activity, changes in meal patterns (i.e., macronutrient content or timing of food intake), or changes in weight or renal or hepatic function.

The 100-units/mL and 200-units/mL formulations of insulin degludec are pharmacodynamically and pharmacokinetically bioequivalent and have shown similar effects on glycemic control at equivalent dosages in clinical trials. Dose conversions between the insulin degludec 100- and 200-units/mL FlexTouch® injection pens based on differences in insulin concentration are not necessary and should *not* be performed. The dose window for the insulin degludec 100- and 200-units/mL FlexTouch® injection pens displays the number of insulin degludec units to be delivered independent of insulin concentration, and no conversion is needed to calculate the dose using either injection pen.

■ **Administration** Insulin degludec is administered by subcutaneous injection once daily using a FlexTouch® injection pen. Because of its delayed absorption and long duration of action, insulin degludec may be administered at any time of the day in adults. However, in pediatric patients, the drug should be administered once daily at the same time every day.

The fixed combination of insulin degludec and liraglutide is administered by subcutaneous injection once daily at the same time each day without regard to meals in adults; the injection is administered using the Xultophy® injection pen.

Insulin degludec or the fixed combination of insulin degludec and liraglutide should *not* be given IV or IM, nor should it be given via an insulin infusion pump. (See Description.) Insulin degludec or the fixed combination with liraglutide should not be mixed with any other insulin preparations or solutions.

Insulin degludec or the fixed combination of insulin degludec and liraglutide is administered subcutaneously into the thigh, abdomen, or upper arm. A planned rotation of sites within an area should be followed to reduce the risk of lipodystrophy.

The accompanying labeling should be consulted for proper methods of administration and care of the FlexTouch® or Xultophy® injection pen. These injection pens are used with NovoFine® or NovoTwist® needles. Insulin degludec should *not* be transferred from the FlexTouch® injection pen into a syringe for administration. (See Hypoglycemia: Hypoglycemia Due to Medication Errors under Warnings/Precautions, in Cautions.)

For adults who miss a dose of insulin degludec, the missed dose should be injected as soon as remembered during waking hours if at least 8 hours have elapsed between consecutive doses. If a pediatric patient misses a dose of insulin degludec, the patient or a parent or caregiver should be instructed to contact the child's clinician for guidance about dosing and monitoring blood glucose concentrations more frequently until the next scheduled insulin degludec dose. Patients who miss a dose of the fixed combination of insulin degludec and liraglutide should be instructed to resume the once-daily regimen as prescribed with the next scheduled dose; however, if more than 3 days have elapsed since the last dose, the fixed combination of insulin degludec and liraglutide should be reinitiated at the starting dose to mitigate GI symptoms related to the liraglutide component.

Unopened injection pens containing insulin degludec or the fixed combination of insulin degludec and liraglutide should be stored at 2–8°C until the expiration date. Alternatively, unopened insulin degludec injection pens may be stored at room temperature (up to 30°C) for up to 56 days. Injection pens containing insulin degludec or the fixed combination of insulin degludec and liraglutide should not be subjected to freezing; if freezing has occurred, the pen should not be used. In-use insulin degludec pens may be stored at room temperature (up to 30°C) or under refrigeration (2–8°C) away from direct heat and light for up to 56 days. In-use pens containing the fixed combination of insulin degludec and liraglutide may be stored at room temperature (15–30°C) or under refrigeration (2–8°C) away from heat or light for up to 21 days.

■ **Dosage** ***Insulin Degludec Therapy*** Dosage of insulin degludec may be increased every 3–4 days as needed.

Insulin-Naive Patients. In patients with type 1 diabetes mellitus, insulin degludec should be administered once daily concomitantly with a prandial, shorter-acting ("bolus") insulin to provide more optimal postprandial glycemic control. In patients with type 2 diabetes mellitus, insulin degludec can be administered alone or concomitantly with oral antidiabetic agents or with a shorter-acting insulin. When used in a meal-related subcutaneous insulin regimen in patients with type 1 diabetes mellitus, an initial insulin degludec dosage usually comprises one-third to one-half of the total daily insulin dosage, with the remainder given preprandially in divided doses as a rapid- or short-acting insulin. An initial *total* daily dosage of insulin (total combined dosages of basal and rapid- or short-acting insulins) of 0.2–0.4 units/kg generally is recommended for insulin-naive patients with type 1 diabetes mellitus. The dosage of insulin degludec should be titrated based upon the patient's metabolic needs, blood glucose monitoring results, and glycemic control goal.

In insulin-naive adult and pediatric patients with type 2 diabetes mellitus, the recommended initial dosage of insulin degludec is 10 units once daily, with subsequent dosage adjustments to achieve glycemic goals.

Transferring from Therapy with Other Insulins. When insulin degludec is substituted for another intermediate- or long-acting insulin in adults with type 1 or type 2 diabetes mellitus, the manufacturer states that the initial dosage of insulin degludec for adults can be identical (on a unit-for-unit basis) to the total daily dosage of the previous longer-acting insulin. The dosage and timing of concurrent short- or rapid-acting insulins or other concomitant antidiabetic agents may need to be adjusted with the initiation of insulin degludec therapy.

For pediatric patients 1 year of age and older with type 1 or type 2 diabetes mellitus, the manufacturer recommends initiating insulin degludec at 80% of the previous total daily intermediate- or long-acting insulin dose to reduce the risk of hypoglycemia. The dosage of insulin degludec should then be adjusted according to blood glucose determinations to achieve glycemic goals. Close monitoring of blood glucose concentrations is recommended during the transition to insulin degludec from other insulin therapies. Additionally, adjustments to the dose and timing of concurrent short- or rapid-acting insulin or other glucose-lowering treatments (e.g., oral antidiabetic agents) may also be required.

For additional information on monitoring and management of insulin therapy, see Dosage: Considerations in Monitoring Insulin Therapy, in Dosage and Administration in the Insulins General Statement 68:20.08.

Insulin Degludec/Liraglutide Fixed-combination Therapy In adults with type 2 diabetes mellitus who are naive to basal insulin or a glucagon-like peptide-1 (GLP-1) receptor agonist, the recommended initial dosage of the fixed combination of insulin degludec and liraglutide (Xultophy®) is 10 units (10 units of insulin degludec and 0.36 mg of liraglutide) once daily.

In adults with type 2 diabetes mellitus who are currently receiving basal insulin or a GLP-1 receptor agonist (e.g., liraglutide), such therapy must be discontinued prior to initiation of the fixed combination of insulin degludec and liraglutide. The recommended initial dosage of the fixed combination in these patients is 16 units (16 units of insulin degludec and 0.58 mg of liraglutide) once daily.

Dosage of insulin degludec in the fixed combination with liraglutide may be increased or decreased by 2 units (2 units of insulin degludec and 0.072 mg of liraglutide) every 3–4 days as needed. The fixed combination of insulin degludec and liraglutide should not be administered more than once daily. Adjustments in concomitant oral antidiabetic therapy may be needed.

The maximum daily dosage of insulin degludec in fixed combination with liraglutide is 50 units (50 units of insulin degludec and 1.8 mg of liraglutide).

■ **Special Populations** ***Hepatic Impairment*** As with all insulin preparations, glucose monitoring should be intensified and the dosage of insulin degludec adjusted on an individual basis in patients with hepatic impairment. Safety and efficacy of the fixed combination of insulin degludec and liraglutide have not been established in patients with hepatic impairment.

Renal Impairment As with all insulin preparations (including combination preparations), glucose monitoring should be intensified and the dosage of insulin degludec adjusted on an individual basis in patients with renal impairment. Safety and efficacy of the fixed combination of insulin degludec and liraglutide have not been established in patients with renal impairment.

Geriatric Patients In geriatric patients, the initial dosage, dose increments, and maintenance dosage of insulin degludec or the fixed combination of insulin degludec and liraglutide should be conservative in order to avoid hypoglycemia.

Cautions

■ **Contraindications** Insulin degludec alone or in fixed combination with liraglutide is contraindicated in patients with known hypersensitivity to insulin degludec or to any ingredient in the formulation. Insulin degludec alone or in fixed combination with liraglutide also is contraindicated during episodes of hypoglycemia.

The fixed combination of insulin degludec and liraglutide is contraindicated in patients with a personal or family history of medullary thyroid carcinoma (MTC) or in patients with multiple endocrine neoplasia type 2 (MEN 2).

■ **Warnings/Precautions** ***Use of Fixed Combinations*** When insulin degludec is used in fixed combination with liraglutide or other drugs, the cautions, precautions, contraindications, and interactions associated with the concomitant agent(s) should be considered in addition to those associated with insulin degludec.

Hypoglycemia Hypoglycemia is the most common adverse effect of insulins, including insulin degludec, and monitoring of blood glucose concentrations is recommended for all patients with diabetes mellitus. Severe hypoglycemia can cause seizures, may be life-threatening, or cause death. The onset of hypoglycemia depends on the action profile of the insulin used and may change when the treatment regimen or timing of dosing of the insulin is changed. (See Transferring from Therapy with Other Insulins under Dosage: Insulin Degludec Therapy, in Dosage and Administration.) As with all insulin preparations, the time course of the glucose-lowering effect of insulin degludec or the fixed combination of insulin degludec and liraglutide may vary among different individuals or at different times in the same individual and depends on many conditions (e.g., the area of injection, the injection site blood supply and temperature). The risk of hypoglycemia generally increases with the intensity of glycemic control. Other factors that may increase a patient's risk of hypoglycemia include changes in meal patterns, changes in level of physical activity, or changes to concomitant drug therapy. Patients with renal or hepatic impairment may be at higher risk of hypoglycemia. (See Renal Impairment and also see Hepatic Impairment under Dosage and Administration: Special Populations.) Some evidence suggests that insulin degludec may be associated with a lower risk of hypoglycemia, particularly nocturnal hypoglycemia, than insulin glargine and insulin detemir. (For more information on the symptoms associated with hypoglycemia, see Hypoglycemia under Cautions: Endocrine and Metabolic Effects, in the Insulins General Statement 68:20.08.)

Hypoglycemia Due to Medication Errors. Confusion between basal insulin preparations and other insulins, particularly rapid-acting insulins, has caused medication errors. To avoid such errors, patients should be advised to check the label on all insulin preparations to confirm the correct formulation and strength prior to administration. Insulin degludec should *not* be transferred from the FlexTouch® injection pen into an insulin syringe; the insulin syringe will not measure the dose correctly, and may cause an overdose and severe hypoglycemia.

Formulation Considerations Any change in insulin should be made cautiously and only under medical supervision. Insulin degludec should not be diluted or mixed with any other insulins or solutions. Changes in insulin type, manufacturer, and/or method of administration may predispose patients to hypoglycemia or hyperglycemia. The frequency of blood glucose monitoring should be increased when changing a patient's insulin regimen. Adjustments to the dosage and timing of concurrent short- or rapid-acting insulin or other glucose-lowering treatments (e.g., oral antidiabetic agents) may be required. (See Transferring from Therapy with Other Insulins under Dosage: Insulin Degludec Therapy, in Dosage and Administration.)

Sharing of Injection Pens Injection pens containing insulin degludec or the fixed combination of insulin degludec and liraglutide must never be shared among patients, even if the needle has been changed. Sharing of injection pens poses a risk for transmission of blood-borne pathogens.

Hypokalemia All insulin preparations, including insulin degludec, cause a shift in potassium from the extracellular to intracellular space, possibly leading to hypokalemia. Untreated hypokalemia may cause respiratory paralysis, ventricular arrhythmia, and death. Serum potassium concentrations should be monitored in patients at risk for hypokalemia (e.g., patients receiving potassium-lowering drugs, patients taking drugs with effects sensitive to serum potassium concentrations).

Metabolic Effects Insulin therapy may cause sodium retention and edema. Insulin therapy, including insulin degludec, also may cause weight gain attributable to the anabolic effects of insulin.

Heart Failure Peroxisome proliferator-activated receptor (PPAR)-γ agonists (e.g., thiazolidinediones) can cause dose-related fluid retention, particularly when used in combination with insulin. Fluid retention may lead to or exacerbate heart failure. Patients treated with insulins, including insulin degludec, and a PPAR-γ agonist should be observed for manifestations of heart failure (e.g., excessive/rapid weight gain, shortness of breath, edema). If heart failure develops, it should be managed according to current standards of care and discontinuance or reduction of the dosage of the PPAR-γ agonist must be considered. Concomitant use of rosiglitazone and insulin therapy is not recommended.

Immunogenicity As with all therapeutic proteins, there is a potential for immunogenicity with insulin degludec or the fixed combination of insulin degludec and liraglutide. In studies in patients with type 1 and type 2 diabetes mellitus, anti-insulin antibodies were detected in patients receiving insulin degludec therapy, including some patients who had anti-insulin antibodies at baseline. The presence of antibodies that affect clinical efficacy may require dosage adjustments to correct for tendencies toward hyperglycemia or hypoglycemia. The incidence of anti-insulin degludec antibodies has not been established.

Antiliraglutide antibodies have been found in patients who received the fixed combination of insulin degludec and liraglutide; however, this antibody formation has not been associated with reduced efficacy of the fixed combination.

Sensitivity Reactions **Dermatologic and Hypersensitivity Reactions.** As with any insulin therapy, lipodystrophy may occur at sites of insulin injections and may affect insulin absorption. Injection site rotation may reduce the risk of lipodystrophy. Localized allergic reactions (e.g., pruritus, erythema, swelling) at the injection site may develop in patients receiving insulin, including insulin degludec. Pain, hematoma, hemorrhage, discoloration, warmth, injection site mass, and nodules at the injection site of insulin degludec or the fixed combination of insulin degludec and liraglutide also have been reported.

Severe, life-threatening, generalized allergic reactions, including anaphylaxis, angioedema, bronchospasm, hypotension, and shock, may occur with insulin preparations, including insulin degludec. If hypersensitivity reactions occur, insulin degludec therapy or the fixed combination of insulin degludec and liraglutide should be discontinued and appropriate treatment initiated; patients should be monitored until the hypersensitivity reaction resolves.

Specific Populations **Pregnancy.** Data are lacking on the use of insulin degludec in pregnant women. In reproduction studies in animals, insulin degludec caused pre- and post-implantation loss and visceral/skeletal abnormalities in the offspring of pregnant rats and rabbits at maternal plasma concentrations 5–10 times higher than those achieved with a subcutaneous human dosage of 0.75 units/kg per day. The manufacturer states that these effects are probably secondary to maternal hypoglycemia. Insulin degludec should be used during pregnancy only if the potential benefit justifies the potential risk to the fetus.

Data are lacking on the use of the fixed combination of insulin degludec and liraglutide in pregnant women. Animal studies suggest that there may be risks to the fetus from exposure to liraglutide during pregnancy. The fixed combination of insulin degludec and liraglutide should be used during pregnancy only if the potential benefit justifies the potential risk to the fetus.

Lactation. Insulin degludec is distributed into milk in rats; it is not known whether the drug is distributed into human milk. The benefits of breast-feeding and the importance of insulin degludec to the woman should be considered along with any potential adverse effects on the breast-fed infant from the drug or from the underlying maternal condition.

Pediatric Use. Safety and efficacy of insulin degludec have not been established in pediatric patients younger than 1 year of age. Insulin degludec is not recommended for pediatric patients who require less than 5 units of insulin degludec daily; in clinical trials, pediatric patients receiving less than 5 units daily had their dosages titrated in 0.5-unit increments, which cannot be measured accurately with the commercially available FlexTouch® injection pen. In pediatric patients whose therapy is being transferred from another long- or intermediate-acting insulin to insulin degludec, the drug should be initiated at a reduced dosage to minimize the risk of hypoglycemia. (See Transferring from Therapy with Other Insulins under Dosage: Insulin Degludec Therapy, in Dosage and Administration.)

Safety and efficacy of insulin degludec in pediatric patients 1 year of age and older are based on a noninferiority clinical study of 12 months' duration in patients 1–17 years of age with type 1 diabetes mellitus, a pharmacokinetic study that included approximately 200 patients 1–17 years of age with type 1 diabetes mellitus, and data from clinical trials conducted in adults with type 2 diabetes mellitus. In the noninferiority study, insulin degludec and insulin detemir provided similar glycemic control (as determined by glycosylated hemoglobin [hemoglobin A_{1c}, HbA_{1c}]). Adverse effects reported in pediatric patients with type 1 diabetes mellitus who were receiving insulin degludec therapy were similar to those reported in adults.

Safety and efficacy of the fixed combination of insulin degludec and liraglutide have not been established in pediatric patients.

Geriatric Use. No substantial differences in safety and efficacy of insulin degludec or the fixed combination of insulin degludec and liraglutide have been observed in geriatric patients relative to younger patients; however, increased sensitivity of some older patients cannot be ruled out. Data indicate that the pharmacokinetic and pharmacodynamic properties of insulin degludec at steady sate are similar in younger adults and geriatric patients; however, greater variability has been observed among geriatric patients. Initial dosage, dose increments, and maintenance dosage should be conservative to avoid hypoglycemia. Hypoglycemia may be difficult to recognize in geriatric patients.

Renal Impairment. In a pharmacokinetic study in patients with or without renal impairment (including some patients with end-stage renal disease) who received a single subcutaneous dose of insulin degludec, there was no clinically relevant difference in the pharmacokinetic parameters in the renally impaired patients compared with healthy individuals. Blood glucose concentrations should be monitored closely; adjustment of insulin degludec dosage may be necessary.

Experience with the fixed combination of insulin degludec and liraglutide in patients with mild, moderate, or severe renal impairment is limited; the drug should be used with caution in such patients. (See Dosage and Administration: Special Populations.)

Hepatic Impairment. In a pharmacokinetic study in patients with or without hepatic impairment (mild to severe hepatic impairment) who received a single subcutaneous dose of insulin degludec, there was no clinically relevant difference in the pharmacokinetic parameters in the hepatically impaired patients compared with healthy individuals. Blood glucose concentrations should be monitored closely; adjustment of insulin degludec dosage may be necessary.

Experience with the fixed combination of insulin degludec and liraglutide in patients with mild, moderate, or severe hepatic impairment is lacking. (See Dosage and Administration: Special Populations.)

■ **Common Adverse Effects** Common adverse effects associated with insulin degludec during clinical trials include hypoglycemia, allergic reactions, injection site reactions, lipodystrophy, pruritus, rash, edema, and weight gain. Adverse effects occurring in at least 5% of patients with type 1 or type 2 diabetes mellitus who received insulin degludec during clinical trials include nasopharyngitis, headache, and upper respiratory tract infection. Sinusitis and gastroenteritis also were reported in at least 5% of patients with type 1 diabetes mellitus who received insulin degludec during clinical trials. Diarrhea was reported in at least 5% of patients with type 2 diabetes mellitus who received insulin degludec during clinical trials.

Adverse effects occurring in at least 5% of patients with type 2 diabetes mellitus who received the fixed combination of insulin degludec and liraglutide include nasopharyngitis, headache, nausea, diarrhea, increased lipase concentrations, and upper respiratory tract infection.

Drug Interactions

■ **Drugs Affecting Glycemic Control** ***Drugs that May Potentiate Hypoglycemic Effects*** Angiotensin-converting enzyme (ACE) inhibitors, angiotensin II receptor antagonists, antidiabetic agents, dipeptidyl peptidase-4 (DPP-4) inhibitors, disopyramide, fibrate derivatives, fluoxetine, glucagon-like peptide-1 (GLP-1) receptor agonists, monoamine oxidase (MAO) inhibitors, pentoxifylline, pramlintide, propoxyphene (no longer commercially available in US), salicylates, sodium-glucose cotransporter 2 (SGLT2) inhibitors, somatostatin analogs (e.g., octreotide), sulfonamide anti-infectives. Dosage reductions and increased frequency of glucose monitoring may be required if insulin degludec or the fixed combination of insulin degludec and liraglutide is used concomitantly with these drugs.

Drugs that May Antagonize Hypoglycemic Effects Atypical antipsychotics (e.g., olanzapine, clozapine), corticosteroids, danazol, diuretics (e.g., thiazides), estrogens or progestins (e.g., oral contraceptives), glucagon, niacin, phenothiazines, protease inhibitors, somatropin, sympathomimetic agents (e.g., albuterol, epinephrine, terbutaline), thyroid hormones. Insulin degludec dosage increases and increased frequency of glucose monitoring may be required if insulin degludec is used concomitantly with these drugs.

Drugs With a Variable Effect on Glycemic Control Alcohol, β-adrenergic blocking agents (β-blockers), clonidine, lithium salts, pentamidine. Adjustments of insulin degludec dosage and increased frequency of glucose monitoring may be required if insulin degludec is used concomitantly with these drugs.

Sympatholytic Agents May decrease or eliminate the signs and symptoms of hypoglycemia in patients receiving insulin degludec concomitantly with these drugs (e.g., β-blockers, clonidine, guanethidine, reserpine). Increased frequency of glucose monitoring may be required if insulin degludec is used concomitantly with these drugs.

■ **Peroxisome Proliferator-activated Receptor-γ Agonists** Peroxisome proliferator-activated receptor (PPAR)-γ agonists (e.g., thiazolidinediones) can cause dose related fluid retention, particularly when used in combination with insulin. Fluid retention may lead to or exacerbate heart failure. Patients treated with insulin, including insulin degludec, and a PPAR-γ agonist should be observed for manifestations of heart failure (e.g., excessive/rapid weight gain, shortness of breath, edema). (See Heart Failure under Cautions: Warnings/Precautions.) Concomitant use of rosiglitazone and insulin therapy is not recommended.

■ **Protein-bound Drugs** No clinically relevant interaction suggested by in vitro binding studies with other protein-bound drugs.

Description

Insulin degludec is a biosynthetic (rDNA origin), long-acting insulin human analog that is prepared using a process that includes expression of recombinant DNA in *Saccharomyces cerevisiae* followed by chemical modification. Insulin degludec differs structurally from insulin human by the deletion of threonine at position 30 on the B chain and by the acylation of lysine at position 29 on the B chain with hexadecandioic acid, a 16-carbon fatty acid, via a glutamic acid spacer.

Insulin degludec has pharmacologic effects comparable to those of insulin human. (See the Insulins General Statement 68:20.08.) The prolonged duration of action of insulin degludec is dependent in part on slow systemic absorption, predominantly due to the formation of a depot of soluble multihexamer chains after subcutaneous injection and to a lesser extent due to binding of insulin degludec to circulating albumin. The fatty acid side chain modification of insulin degludec favors the formation of stable dihexamers while in solution at a neutral pH in the presence of phenol and zinc. After subcutaneous injection, these dihexamers assemble into long multihexamers; the large molecular weight of these multihexamers slows absorption, which creates a subcutaneous depot of insulin degludec from which monomers slowly dissociate in circulation. Insulin degludec has a long, flat, stable glucose lowering-profile, with a duration of action exceeding 42 hours and a terminal elimination half-life of approximately 25 hours. Due to the prolonged pharmacodynamics of insulin degludec, under steady state conditions the overlapping effect of daily injections results in less variability in glucose-lowering effect. Total exposure (in terms of area under the concentration-time curve [AUC]) and glucose-lowering effect of insulin degludec have been shown to be more evenly distributed than other basal insulins across a 24-hour dosing interval (i.e., peakless) in patients with type 1 or type 2 diabetes mellitus. Insulin degludec has a longer duration of action than insulin detemir and insulin glargine, and insulin degludec therapy is associated with less pharmacodynamic variability than other basal insulins. Insulin degludec has been associated with a fourfold lower within-patient day-to-day variability with regard to total glucose lowering effect compared to insulin glargine.

Advice to Patients

When insulin degludec is used in fixed combination with other drugs, importance of informing patients of important cautionary information about the concomitant agents.

Importance of providing patient a copy of manufacturer's patient information. Importance of advising patient to read the manufacturer's medication guide before beginning treatment with insulin degludec in fixed combination with liraglutide and of reviewing this information each time the prescription is refilled.

Importance of instructing patients not to administer the fixed combination of insulin degludec and liraglutide concurrently with other glucagon-like peptide-1 (GLP-1) receptor agonists. Importance of advising patients that dosages of insulin degludec exceeding 50 units daily given as the fixed combination with liraglutide can result in an overdose of the liraglutide component.

Importance of informing patients that serious hypersensitivity reactions have been reported with insulin degludec or the fixed combination of insulin degludec and liraglutide; importance of instructing patients to stop taking insulin degludec or the fixed combination and seek prompt medical attention if such adverse reactions occur.

Importance of advising patients to refer to patient information for additional information about the potential side effects of insulin therapy, including lipodystrophy (and the need to rotate injection sites within the same body region), weight gain, allergic reactions, and hypoglycemia.

Importance of informing patients that they should never share an injection pen containing insulin degludec or the fixed combination of insulin degludec and liraglutide with another person, even if the needle is changed; sharing of the pen may pose a risk of transmission of infection.

Importance of informing patients that hypoglycemia is the most common adverse effect of insulin. Importance of informing patients of the symptoms of hypoglycemia; the ability to concentrate and react may be impaired as a result of hypoglycemia, which may pose a risk in situations where these abilities are especially important (e.g., driving, operating machinery). Importance of advising patients who experience frequent hypoglycemia or reduced or absent warning signs of hypoglycemia to use caution when driving or operating machinery.

Importance of advising patients that changes in insulin regimen can predispose to hyperglycemia or hypoglycemia. Importance of changing insulin dosage with caution and only under medical supervision.

Discuss potential for alterations in insulin requirements in special situations (e.g., illness, emotional disturbances, other stresses). Discuss potential for alterations in insulin requirements as a result of inadequate or skipped doses, or inadvertent administration of an incorrect dose.

Importance of advising patients regarding what to do in the event of missed or delayed doses. (See Dosage and Administration: Administration.)

Importance of *not* mixing insulin degludec or the fixed combination of insulin degludec and liraglutide with other insulins or solutions. Importance of using insulin degludec or the fixed combination of insulin degludec and liraglutide only if the solution is clear and colorless with no visible particles.

Importance of informing patients to always check the insulin label prior to each injection; insulin degludec is available in concentrations of 100 and 200 units/mL. Importance of informing patients that the dose window of the insulin degludec FlexTouch® injection pen displays the number of units to be injected independent of insulin concentration; no recalculation of the dose is required to convert between different concentrations of insulin degludec. Importance of informing patients that the dose window of the injection pen containing the fixed combination of insulin degludec and liraglutide shows the number of units of insulin degludec to be injected; with each unit of insulin degludec, the pen also delivers 0.036 mg of liraglutide.

Provide instructions regarding self-management procedures including glucose monitoring, proper injection technique, and management of hypoglycemia and hyperglycemia.

Provide instructions to patient regarding use of the subcutaneous injection devices containing insulin degludec or the fixed combination of insulin degludec and liraglutide. Patients should be cautioned against reuse of needles. Importance of advising patients to never use a syringe to remove insulin degludec from the FlexTouch® injection pen.

Importance of informing clinicians of existing or contemplated concomitant therapy, including prescription and OTC drugs.

Importance of women informing clinicians if they are or plan to become pregnant or plan to breast-feed.

Importance of informing patients of other important precautionary information. (See Cautions.)

Overview® (see Users Guide). For additional information on this drug until a more detailed monograph is developed and published, the manufacturer's labeling should be consulted. It is *essential* that the manufacturer's labeling be consulted for more detailed information on usual cautions, precautions, contraindications, potential drug interactions, laboratory test interferences, and acute toxicity.

Preparations

Excipients in commercially available drug preparations may have clinically important effects in some individuals; consult specific product labeling for details.

Insulin Degludec (Recombinant DNA Origin)

Parenteral		
Injection, for subcutaneous use	100 units/mL	**Tresiba®** (available as FlexTouch® prefilled pens), Novo Nordisk
	200 units/mL	**Tresiba®** (available as FlexTouch® prefilled pens), Novo Nordisk

Insulin Degludec (Recombinant DNA Origin) Combinations

Parenteral		
Injection, for subcutaneous use	100 units/mL with Liraglutide 3.6 mg/mL	**Xultophy®** (available as prefilled injection pens), Novo Nordisk

Selected Revisions November 2019,

Insulin Detemir

■ Insulin detemir is a biosynthetic (rDNA origin), long-acting human insulin analog that is prepared using a process that includes expression of recombinant DNA in *Saccharomyces cerevisiae* followed by chemical modification.

Uses

■ **Diabetes Mellitus** Insulin detemir is used to improve glycemic control in the management of type 1 or type 2 diabetes mellitus in patients who require a long-acting insulin. Insulin detemir appears to be at least as effective for glycemic control in adults with diabetes mellitus as isophane (NPH) insulin or insulin glargine (as determined by glycosylated hemoglobin [hemoglobin A_{1c}, HbA_{1c}] and fasting plasma glucose values). Current evidence suggests that insulin detemir may be associated with less interindividual variability in fasting blood glucose concentrations and a lower risk of hypoglycemia and weight gain than isophane insulin. Less variability in the pharmacodynamic effects of insulin detemir may facilitate more optimal adjustment of basal insulin dosage without an increased risk of hypoglycemia. Insulin detemir may provide advantages over isophane insulin in patients with diabetes mellitus who have had difficulty achieving adequate glycemic control without frequent hypoglycemic episodes and/or those at high risk of hypoglycemia, particularly nocturnal hypoglycemia.

Safety and efficacy of insulin detemir compared with isophane insulin human for the treatment of type 1 diabetes mellitus have been demonstrated in several randomized, open-label, noninferiority studies of up to 26 weeks' duration in adults. In these studies, patients received basal insulin once or twice daily in conjunction with insulin human (regular) or insulin aspart as premeal insulin. A preliminary report suggests that glycemic control with insulin detemir is maintained at 24 months in adults with type 1 diabetes mellitus. Safety and efficacy of insulin detemir compared with isophane insulin human in pediatric patients 2–17 years of age with type 1 diabetes mellitus also have been demonstrated in 2 randomized, open-label studies of 26 or 52 weeks' duration in which the basal insulins were administered once or twice daily with premeal insulin aspart. (See Pediatric Use under Warnings/Precautions: Special Populations, in Cautions.) In the 26-week study, therapy with insulin detemir generally resulted in similar reductions in HbA_{1c} as isophane insulin but was associated with less weight gain and a lower risk of nocturnal hypoglycemia. Fasting plasma glucose concentrations with insulin detemir therapy were similar to or lower than those achieved with isophane insulin; however, target fasting blood glucose concentrations (e.g., 72–126 mg/dL) were not achieved in some studies, possibly because of insufficient titration of basal insulin dosage. In the 52-week study, insulin detemir was noninferior to isophane insulin human in terms of glycemic control (as determined by HbA_{1c}); however, a slight increase in HbA_{1c} was observed in both treatment groups. The observed increase in HbA_{1c} was principally attributable to the suboptimal glycemic control in the subgroup of patients 13–16 years of age. This increase may be explained in part by the difficulties of treating children for whom many factors (e.g., hormonal changes and growth, social status, variable lifestyles, fear of hypoglycemia) influence glycemic control. Therapy with insulin detemir also was associated with less weight gain and a lower risk of 24-hour and nocturnal hypoglycemia.

Some evidence also indicates similar glycemic control with insulin detemir and insulin glargine in adults with type 1 diabetes mellitus. In a randomized, open-label, noninferiority study, reductions in HbA_{1c} at 26 weeks were similar in adults with type I diabetes mellitus who received either twice-daily (morning and bedtime) insulin detemir or once-daily (bedtime) insulin glargine as basal insulin therapy in conjunction with premeal insulin aspart therapy. Target prebreakfast (fasting) plasma glucose concentrations (less than 132 mg/dL) were achieved more often with insulin glargine than with insulin detemir in this study, probably because of the effects of the entire daily insulin glargine dose being administered at bedtime. Body weight gain was similar in both treatment groups. Overall, the risk of hypoglycemia was similar in both treatment groups, but the risk of severe and nocturnal hypoglycemia was lower with insulin detemir than with insulin glargine.

Safety and efficacy of insulin detemir administered once or twice daily in adults with type 2 diabetes mellitus have been established in 2 open-label, randomized clinical studies of 22 or 24 weeks' duration that compared insulin detemir with isophane insulin human administered once or twice daily. In a noninferiority study in insulin-naive patients with type 2 diabetes mellitus who were inadequately controlled with oral antidiabetic therapy, twice-daily therapy with insulin detemir or isophane insulin human was added to existing therapy with 1 or 2 oral antidiabetic agents (metformin, insulin secretagogue, and/or α-glucosidase inhibitor). Insulin detemir and isophane insulin human provided similar improvements in glycemic control (as measured by HbA_{1c}, the primary clinical end point) in this study. The proportion of patients attaining target HbA_{1c} values of 7% or less at study end point was similar across treatment groups. Basal insulin doses were titrated to achieve prebreakfast and predinner target blood glucose concentrations; an increased dosage of insulin detemir (0.77 units/kg) compared with that of insulin isophane human (0.52 units/kg) was required to achieve similar glycemic control. The risk of hypoglycemia, particularly nocturnal hypoglycemia, was reduced with insulin detemir compared with that observed with isophane insulin human; less weight gain was observed with insulin detemir than with isophane insulin human. In another comparative study in patients with type 2 diabetes mellitus previously receiving insulin or a combination of oral antidiabetic agents and insulin, insulin detemir and isophane insulin human provided similar glycemic control (as measured by HbA_{1c}). Insulin aspart or insulin human (regular) was given as the mealtime insulin in patients treated with insulin detemir or isophane insulin human, respectively. Basal insulin was given once or twice daily, based on the patient's prestudy insulin regimen (basal and preprandial insulin, biphasic insulin, or insulin and oral antidiabetic agents); oral antidiabetic agents were discontinued at study entry. Basal and mealtime insulin doses were titrated to achieve fasting, preprandial, and postprandial target plasma glucose concentrations of less than 107 mg/dL, 90–125 mg/dL, and 161 mg/dL or less, respectively; if these target plasma glucose concentrations were not met with a once-daily basal insulin regimen, patients were transferred to a twice-daily basal insulin regimen. (See Transferring from Therapy with Other Insulins under Dosage: Diabetes Mellitus, in Dosage and Administration.)

When given as add-on therapy to metformin and liraglutide in a clinical study, insulin detemir further improved glycemic control as determined by HbA_{1c} and fasting plasma glucose concentrations. Efficacy and safety of insulin detemir as add-on therapy with liraglutide and metformin were established in a 26-week, open-label study in patients with inadequate glycemic control while receiving metformin alone or in combination with a sulfonylurea. In this study, all patients entered a 12-week run-in period during which patients continued metformin therapy and received add-on therapy with liraglutide titrated to 1.8 mg once daily. Therapy with sulfonylureas was discontinued at the start of the run-in period. At the end of the run-in period, approximately 50% of patients had achieved the target HbA_{1c} of less than 7%. Compared with patients who did not reach the target HbA_{1c} during the run-in period, those who did reach the target HbA_{1c} had a shorter duration of type 2 diabetes mellitus, lower initial HbA_{1c} and fasting plasma glucose concentrations, and more had been treated with only metformin before study enrollment. Patients with HbA_{1c} values of 7% or greater (excluding those who withdrew from the study) received 26 weeks of once-daily insulin detemir administered in the evening as add-on therapy or continued unchanged treatment with liraglutide and metformin. The addition of insulin detemir to liraglutide and metformin therapy resulted in clinically relevant further reductions of HbA_{1c} compared with continued, unchanged treatment with liraglutide and metformin alone (reduction of 0.5 versus 0%, respectively, in HbA_{1c}). Mean fasting blood glucose concentrations decreased more in the insulin detemir add-on therapy group than with metformin and liraglutide alone (decrease of 38 and 7 mg/dL, respectively). Additionally, a greater percentage of patients in the add-on therapy insulin detemir treatment group achieved an HbA_{1c} of less than 7% compared with the liraglutide and metformin alone treatment group (43 versus 17% of patients, respectively). There was a mean weight reduction of 0.3 or 1.1 kg in the patients who received insulin detemir add-on therapy or unchanged treatment with liraglutide and metformin alone, respectively. Patients who received add-on therapy with insulin detemir maintained the substantial weight reduction achieved during the liraglutide run-in period rather than gaining weight as typically occurs with insulin therapy.

Insulin detemir, a long-acting basal insulin, is not indicated for the treatment of diabetic ketoacidosis; a short-acting insulin (e.g., regular insulin) is the preferred agent.

Dosage and Administration

■ General Dosage of insulin detemir is expressed in units. Each unit of insulin detemir is approximately equal to 0.142 mg of the drug.

Dosage of insulin detemir based on the results of blood glucose determinations and carefully individualized to obtain optimum therapeutic effect. Glucose monitoring is recommended for all patients with diabetes mellitus.

■ Administration Insulin detemir is administered by subcutaneous injection once or twice daily using a conventional insulin syringe or FlexTouch® injection pen.

The prolonged duration of action of soluble insulin detemir is dependent in part on slow systemic absorption (e.g., secondary to albumin binding). (See Description.) Insulin detemir should *not* be given IV or IM, nor should it be given via an insulin infusion pump. Insulin detemir is absorbed more rapidly and more extensively following IM or IV administration than when it is given subcutaneously. IV administration of the usual subcutaneous dosage of insulin detemir could result in severe hypoglycemia. Insulin detemir is administered by subcutaneous injection into the thigh, abdominal wall, or upper arm. A planned rotation of sites within an area should be followed. Insulin detemir should not be mixed with any other insulin or solution, as such mixing may result in unpredictable alterations in the pharmacokinetic and/or pharmacodynamic characteristics (e.g., onset of action, time to peak effect) of insulin detemir and/or the mixed insulin.

When the FlexTouch® injection pen is used for subcutaneous injection of insulin detemir, the accompanying labeling should be consulted for proper methods of administration and care. The FlexTouch® injection pen is used with NovoFine®, NovoFine Plus®, or NovoTwist® needles.

When insulin detemir is given once daily, the daily dose should be administered with the evening meal or at bedtime. However, insulin detemir also has been administered once daily in the morning† in patients with type 2 diabetes mellitus. For patients who require twice-daily doses of insulin detemir (i.e., predinner blood glucose concentrations above the target blood glucose concentration), the first dose may be administered in the morning and the second dose may be administered after the evening meal, at bedtime, or 12 hours after the morning dose.

When insulin detemir is used in conjunction with a glucagon-like peptide-1 (GLP-1) receptor agonist, the drugs should be administered as separate injections; these injections should *not* be mixed. Insulin detemir and the GLP-1 receptor agonist may be injected into the same body region; however, the injections should not be adjacent to each other.

Unopened insulin detemir injection pens and vials should be protected from light and stored in the original carton at 2–8°C until the expiration date; the drug should *not* be frozen. Insulin detemir should not be stored directly adjacent to the refrigerator cooling element; insulin detemir should not be used if freezing has occurred. Alternatively, if refrigeration is not possible, unopened insulin detemir injection pens and vials may be stored at room temperature and away from direct heat and light for up to 42 days. Opened (in-use) insulin detemir *vials* should be stored at 2–8°C. Alternatively, if refrigeration is not possible, in-use insulin detemir vials may be stored at room temperature away from direct heat and light for up to 42 days. In-use insulin detemir injection *pens* should be stored at room temperature away from heat and direct light for up to 42 days; in-use injection pens should *not* be refrigerated or stored with the needle attached.

■ Dosage ***Diabetes Mellitus*** Because of its long duration of action, insulin detemir is used alone as a basal insulin (e.g., insulin-naive patients) or concomitantly with a shorter-acting ("bolus") insulin (e.g., insulin aspart, insulin human) to provide more optimal postprandial glycemic control. When used in a meal-related subcutaneous insulin regimen, the initial insulin detemir dosage should be approximately one-third of the total daily insulin dosage, with the remainder given preprandially as a rapid- or short-acting insulin. Initial total daily insulin dosages in adults and children with type 1 diabetes mellitus generally range from 0.2–1 unit/kg. The dosage of insulin detemir should be increased until the desired fasting plasma glucose concentrations are achieved.

In comparative clinical studies of short duration (16 weeks to 6 months) in adults with type 1 diabetes mellitus, the mean total daily dosage of insulin detemir or isophane insulin human at the completion of the study was 0.27–0.45 units/kg or 0.33–0.38 units/kg, respectively.

In a comparative clinical study in pediatric patients 6–17 years of age with type 1 diabetes mellitus, the mean total daily dosage of insulin detemir or isophane insulin human at completion of the study was 0.67 or 0.64 units/kg, respectively, and the total daily dosage of insulin aspart given preprandially was 0.52 units/kg.

In insulin-naive adults with type 2 diabetes mellitus who are inadequately controlled with oral antidiabetic agents, the recommended initial dosage of insulin detemir is 10 units (or 0.1–0.2 units/kg) given once daily in the evening or divided into a twice-daily regimen, with subsequent dosage adjusted to achieve glycemic goals. Close monitoring of blood glucose concentrations is recommended during the transition to insulin detemir and in the initial weeks thereafter.

In adults with type 2 diabetes mellitus with inadequate glycemic control while receiving a glucagon-like peptide-1 (GLP-1) receptor agonist, the recommended initial dosage of insulin detemir is 10 units given once daily in the evening, with subsequent dosage adjustments to achieve glycemic goals. When a GLP-1 receptor agonist is used in conjunction with insulin detemir, a reduction in the dosage of insulin detemir, or more conservative titration, may be required to minimize the risk of hypoglycemia.

The dosage and timing of concurrent short- or rapid-acting insulins or other concomitant antidiabetic agents may need to be adjusted. Insulin requirements may be altered during illness, emotional disturbances, or other stresses.

Transferring from Therapy with Other Insulins. When insulin detemir is substituted for another intermediate- or long-acting insulin in patients with diabetes mellitus receiving combination therapy with a short- or rapid-acting insulin and a longer-acting insulin, the initial dosage of insulin detemir can be identical (on a unit-for-unit basis) to the dosage of the previous longer-acting insulin. The dosage of insulin detemir should then be adjusted according to blood glucose determinations to achieve glycemic goals. In patients currently receiving a basal insulin only, insulin detemir may be substituted on a unit-for-unit basis for the basal insulin currently in use. Some patients with type 2 diabetes mellitus who are switched from isophane insulin human may require a higher dosage of insulin detemir. Close monitoring of blood glucose concentrations is recommended during the transition to insulin detemir and in the initial weeks thereafter. The dosage and timing of concurrent short- or rapid-acting insulin or other concomitant antidiabetic agents may need to be adjusted.

■ Special Populations In a pharmacokinetic study in patients with or without renal impairment (mild to severe renal impairment, some patients requiring hemodialysis) who received a single subcutaneous dose of insulin detemir, the pharmacokinetic parameters in renally impaired patients were no different that those in healthy individuals. However, since clearance of insulin human has been decreased in patients with renal impairment, blood glucose concentrations should be monitored carefully, and adjustment of insulin detemir dosage may be necessary in such patients.

In patients with hepatic impairment, the area under the concentration-time curve (AUC) of insulin detemir decreased with increasing degrees of hepatic impairment. However, some studies conducted with human insulin in patients with hepatic impairment have shown increased circulating levels of insulin. Blood glucose concentrations should be monitored carefully, and adjustment of insulin detemir dosage may be necessary in such patients.

In geriatric patients, the initial dosage, dose increments, and maintenance dosage should be conservative in order to avoid hypoglycemia.

Based on preliminary data, dosage adjustments in children or adolescents based solely on age do not appear to be necessary.

Cautions

■ **Contraindications** Known hypersensitivity to insulin detemir or any ingredient in the formulation.

■ **Warnings/Precautions** ***Hypoglycemia*** Hypoglycemia is the most common adverse effect of insulins, including insulin detemir, and monitoring of blood glucose concentrations is recommended for all patients with diabetes mellitus. The prolonged effect of subcutaneous insulin detemir may delay recovery from hypoglycemia. Severe hypoglycemia requiring the assistance of another person, IV glucose infusions, or glucagon administration has occurred with insulin therapy, including insulin detemir. As with all insulin preparations, the time course of the glucose-lowering effect of insulin detemir may vary among different individuals or at different times in the same individual and depends on many conditions (e.g., area of injection, injection site blood supply and temperature). The risk of hypoglycemia generally increases with the intensity of glycemic control. Other factors that may increase a patient's risk of hypoglycemia include changes in meal patterns, level of physical activity, or coadministered drugs. The onset of hypoglycemia depends on the action profile of the insulins used and may change when the treatment regimen or timing of dosing of the insulins is changed. (See Transferring from Therapy with Other Insulins under Dosage and Administration: Dosage.) Some evidence suggests that insulin detemir may be associated with a lower risk of hypoglycemia, particularly nocturnal hypoglycemia, than isophane insulin. In comparative studies, the incidence of severe hypoglycemic reactions with insulin detemir was similar to that with isophane insulin human. In a comparative study with insulin glargine, the incidence of severe and nocturnal hypoglycemia was lower with insulin detemir. (For more information on the symptoms associated with hypoglycemia, See Hypoglycemia under Cautions: Endocrine and Metabolic Effects, in the Insulins General Statement 68:20.08.)

Formulation Considerations Any change in insulin should be made cautiously and only under medical supervision. Insulin detemir should not be diluted or mixed with any other insulin. Patients previously receiving insulin may require a change in dosage if insulin therapy is changed to insulin detemir. Likewise, adjustment of oral antidiabetic dosage may be necessary in patients receiving concomitant therapy with insulin detemir. Changes in insulin strength, manufacturer, timing of dosing, type, and/or method of manufacture may necessitate a change in insulin dosage. (See Transferring from Therapy with Other Insulins under Dosage and Administration: Dosage.)

Sharing of Injection Pens Insulin detemir injection pens must never be shared among patients, even if the needle has been changed. Sharing of injection pens poses a risk for transmission of blood-borne pathogens.

Metabolic Effects Insulin may cause sodium retention and edema, particularly if metabolic control is improved by intensive insulin therapy. Insulin therapy, including insulin detemir, also may cause weight gain attributable to the anabolic effects of insulin and the decrease in glucosuria.

Heart Failure Peroxisome proliferator-activated receptor (PPAR)-γ agonists (e.g., thiazolidinediones) can cause dose-related fluid retention, particularly when used in combination with insulin. Fluid retention may lead to or exacerbate heart failure. Patients treated with insulin, including insulin detemir, and a PPAR-γ agonist should be observed for manifestations of heart failure (e.g., excessive/rapid weight gain, shortness of breath, edema). If heart failure develops, it should be managed according to current standards of care and discontinuance or dose reduction of the PPAR-γ agonist must be considered. Concomitant use of rosiglitazone and insulin therapy is not recommended.

Immunogenicity As with all therapeutic proteins, there is a potential for immunogenicity with insulin detemir. Insulin antibodies may increase or decrease the efficacy of insulin and insulin dosage adjustments may be required. During phase 3 clinical trials of insulin detemir, antibody development has been observed with no apparent impact on glycemic control.

Sensitivity Reactions **Dermatologic and Sensitivity Reactions.** As with any insulin therapy, lipodystrophy may occur at sites of insulin injections and may delay insulin absorption. Localized allergic reactions (e.g., pruritus, erythema, swelling, urticaria) at the injection site may develop in patients receiving insulins, including insulin detemir. Pain, inflammation, and subcutaneous nodules at the injection site also have been reported. These reactions generally are relatively minor and usually resolve within a few days to a few weeks but rarely may be severe and require discontinuance of insulin detemir. Poor injection technique or irritants in skin cleansing agents may contribute to localized injection site reactions; it also has been theorized that the myristic acid moiety of insulin detemir may be allergenic in some patients. Injection site rotation within an area may reduce or prevent these effects in some but not all cases.

Generalized hypersensitivity to insulin, characterized by whole-body rash, pruritus, shortness of breath, wheezing, hypotension, tachycardia, and diaphoresis, has occurred less frequently than localized reactions. Severe cases of generalized insulin allergy with anaphylaxis may be life-threatening.

Specific Populations **Pregnancy.** Category B. (See Users Guide.)

In an open-label clinical study of pregnant women with type 1 diabetes mellitus, insulin detemir therapy did not increase the risk of fetal abnormalities compared with isophane (NPH) insulin human. Additionally, there was no difference in pregnancy outcomes or the health of the fetus and newborn with insulin detemir use. Studies in rats and rabbits indicate that insulin detemir and human insulin have similar embryotoxic and teratogenic effects, which may be attributable to maternal hypoglycemia.

Lactation. Not known whether insulin detemir is distributed into milk. Caution is advised if used in nursing women. Diabetic women who are lactating may require adjustments in insulin detemir dosage, meal plans, or both.

Pediatric Use. The safety and efficacy of insulin detemir compared with isophane insulin human have been demonstrated in 2 randomized, open-label studies of 26 or 52 weeks' duration in children and adolescents 2–17 years of age with type 1 diabetes mellitus; children also received insulin aspart as the preprandial insulin. Insulin detemir and isophane insulin human provided similar glycemic control (as determined by glycosylated hemoglobin [hemoglobin A_{1c}, HbA_{1c}]) in these studies. Safety and efficacy of insulin detemir in pediatric patients with type 2 diabetes mellitus have not been established.

Geriatric Use. No substantial differences in safety and efficacy relative to younger adults, but increased sensitivity cannot be ruled out. Pharmacokinetic data indicate a higher exposure (increased area under the concentration-time curve) for insulin detemir among geriatric patients compared with young adults, as a result of decreased clearance of the drug. Initial dosage, dose increments, and maintenance dosage should be conservative to avoid hypoglycemia. Hypoglycemia may be difficult to recognize in geriatric patients.

Hepatic Impairment. Blood glucose concentrations should be monitored closely; adjustment of insulin detemir dosage may be necessary. (See Dosage and Administration: Special Populations.)

Renal Impairment. Blood glucose concentrations should be monitored closely; adjustment of insulin detemir dosage may be necessary. (See Dosage and Administration: Special Populations.)

■ **Common Adverse Effects** Common adverse effects associated with insulin detemir include hypoglycemia, allergic reactions, pruritus, rash, injection site reactions, lipodystrophy, peripheral edema, and weight gain. Additional adverse effects occurring in at least 5% of adults receiving insulin detemir for the management of type 1 or type 2 diabetes mellitus in clinical trials of 16–26 weeks' duration include upper respiratory tract infection, headache, pharyngitis, influenza-like illness, abdominal pain, back pain, gastroenteritis, and bronchitis.

Adverse effects occurring in at least 5% of pregnant women receiving insulin detemir for the management of type 1 diabetes mellitus include anemia, diarrhea, preeclampsia, urinary tract infection, gastroenteritis, upper abdominal pain, vomiting, spontaneous abortion, abdominal pain, and oropharyngeal pain.

Adverse effects occurring in at least 5% of children and adolescents receiving insulin detemir for the management of type 1 diabetes mellitus in a clinical trial of 26 weeks' duration include upper respiratory tract infection, headache, pharyngitis, gastroenteritis, influenza-like illness, abdominal pain, pyrexia, cough, viral infection, nausea, rhinitis, and vomiting.

Drug Interactions

■ **Drugs Affecting Glycemic Control** ***Drugs that May Potentiate Hypoglycemic Effects*** Angiotensin-converting enzyme (ACE) inhibitors, disopyramide, fibrate derivatives, fluoxetine, monoamine oxidase (MAO) inhibitors, oral antidiabetic agents, pentoxifylline, pramlintide, propoxyphene, salicylates, somatostatin analogs (e.g., octreotide), sulfonamide anti-infectives.

Drugs that May Antagonize Hypoglycemic Effects Atypical antipsychotics (e.g., olanzapine, clozapine), corticosteroids, danazol, diuretics, estrogens or progestins (e.g., oral contraceptives), glucagon, isoniazid, niacin, phenothiazines, protease inhibitors, somatropin, sympathomimetic agents (e.g., albuterol, epinephrine, terbutaline), thyroid hormones.

Drugs that May Have a Variable Effect of Glycemic Control Alcohol, β-adrenergic blocking agents, clonidine, lithium salts, pentamidine.

Sympatholytic Agents May decrease or eliminate the signs of hypoglycemia in patients receiving insulin detemir concomitantly with these drugs (e.g., β-adrenergic blocking agents, clonidine, guanethidine, reserpine).

■ **Glucagon-like Peptide 1 Receptor Agonists** No pharmacokinetic interaction was observed following administration of single-dose subcutaneous injections of insulin detemir (0.5 units/kg) during steady-state liraglutide therapy (titrated to a 1.8-mg daily dosage over 3 weeks) in patients with type 2 diabetes mellitus. However, an additive glucose-lowering effect was observed. When a GLP-1 receptor agonist (e.g., liraglutide) is used concomitantly with insulin detemir, a reduction in the dosage of insulin detemir, or more conservative dosage titration, may be required to minimize the risk of hypoglycemia.

■ **Peroxisome Proliferator-activated Receptor-γ Agonists** Peroxisome proliferator-activated receptor (PPAR)-γ agonists (e.g., thiazolidinediones) can cause dose-related fluid retention, particularly when used in conjunction with insulin. Fluid retention may lead to or exacerbate heart failure. Patients treated with insulin, including insulin detemir, and a PPAR-γ agonist should be observed for manifestations of heart failure (e.g., excessive/rapid weight gain, shortness of breath, edema). (See Heart Failure under Cautions: Warnings/Precautions.)

■ **Protein-bound Drugs** No clinically relevant in vivo or in vitro interaction with other protein-bound drugs.

Description

Insulin detemir is a biosynthetic (rDNA origin), long-acting insulin human analog that is prepared using a process that includes expression of recombinant DNA in *Saccharomyces cerevisiae* followed by chemical modification. Insulin detemir differs structurally from insulin human by the deletion of threonine at position 30 on the B chain and by the acylation of lysine at position 29 on the B chain with myristic acid, a 14-carbon fatty acid. The prolonged (up to 24 hours) duration of action of insulin detemir appears to result from slow systemic absorption of the drug from the injection site and delayed distribution to target tissues. The fatty acid side chain modification of insulin detemir increases self-association of the drug molecules and reversible binding to albumin at the injection site. Once absorbed systemically, insulin detemir also is strongly (greater than 98%) bound to circulating albumin, which delays the distribution of the drug to target tissues and prolongs its action. Insulin detemir is soluble at neutral pH and the subcutaneous depot of the drug remains liquid; therefore, absorption of the drug is expected to occur with less variability than with other basal insulins. Insulin detemir has a longer duration of action than isophane insulin human, and insulin detemir therapy is associated with less intrapatient variability in blood glucose concentrations than therapy with isophane insulin human.

Interindividual and intraindividual variation in rate of absorption and consequently, the onset of action of insulins, including insulin detemir, may occur based on site of injection, tissue blood supply, temperature, and physical activity.

Advice to Patients

Provide copy of manufacturer's information for patients.

Importance of informing patients that they should never share an insulin detemir injection pen with another person, even if the needle is changed; sharing of the pen may pose a risk of transmission of infection.

Importance of informing patients that changes to insulin regimens should be made cautiously and only under medical supervision.

Advise patients of the potential adverse effects of insulin therapy (e.g., hypoglycemia, weight gain, lipodystrophy [and the need to rotate injection sites], allergic reactions).

Inform patients that the ability to concentrate and react may be impaired as a result of hypoglycemia, which may pose a risk in situations where these abilities are especially important (e.g., driving, operating machinery). Advise patients who experience frequent hypoglycemia or reduced or absent warning signs of hypoglycemia to use caution when driving or operating machinery.

Inform patients to always check the insulin container label prior to each injection; medication errors involving confusion between insulin detemir and other insulins (e.g., short-acting insulins) have occurred.

Provide instructions regarding self-monitoring of blood glucose concentrations, injection technique, and management of hypoglycemia or hyperglycemia.

Importance of *not* mixing insulin detemir with other insulins or solutions. Importance of using insulin detemir only if solution is clear and colorless with no visible particles.

Discuss potential for alterations in insulin requirements in special situations (e.g., illness, emotional disturbances, or other stresses). Discuss potential for alterations in insulin requirements as a result of inadequate or skipped doses, inadvertent administration of an incorrect dose, inadequate food intake, or skipped meals.

Importance of informing clinicians of existing or contemplated concomitant therapy, including prescription and OTC drugs.

Importance of women informing clinicians if they are or plan to become pregnant or plan to breast-feed.

Importance of informing patients of other important precautionary information. (See Cautions.)

Overview® (see Users Guide). For additional information on this drug until a more detailed monograph is developed and published, the manufacturer's labeling should be consulted. It is *essential* that the manufacturer's labeling be consulted for more detailed information on usual cautions, precautions, contraindications, potential drug interactions, laboratory test interferences, and acute toxicity.

Preparations

Excipients in commercially available drug preparations may have clinically important effects in some individuals; consult specific product labeling for details.

Insulin Detemir (Recombinant DNA Origin)

Parenteral

Injection, for subcutaneous use	100 units/mL	**Levemir®** (available as FlexTouch® prefilled pens and 10-mL vials), Novo Nordisk

†Use is not currently included in the labeling approved by the US Food and Drug Administration

Insulin Glargine

■ Insulin glargine is a biosynthetic (rDNA origin), long-acting human insulin analog.

Uses

Insulin glargine is commercially available as Lantus® (100 units/mL), a "follow-on" preparation (Basaglar®; 100 units/mL), and a concentrated preparation (Toujeo®; 300 units/mL).

Lantus® and Basaglar® are structurally and pharmacologically similar drugs that contain a related drug substance. Basaglar® was licensed by the US Food and Drug Administration (FDA) through an abbreviated approval pathway [505(b)(2)] that relies in part on FDA's finding of safety and effectiveness for Lantus®. Comparative studies have found no substantial differences between the pharmacokinetics, immunogenicity, or toxicity of Lantus® and Basaglar®. Although Basaglar® is highly similar to Lantus® in terms of composition, strength, presentation, structure, and physicochemical and biological properties, it was *not* approved as a biosimilar or an interchangeable biologic product. Insulin is classified by FDA as a chemical, not a biologic product, so there is no biologic reference product for insulin glargine; thus, biosimilarity to insulin glargine cannot be established. Instead, Basaglar® is referred to as a "follow-on" insulin glargine preparation; FDA determined that there was no need to use a different nonproprietary name (insulin glargine) for Basaglar® at this time.

■ **Diabetes Mellitus** Insulin glargine 100-unit/mL preparations (Basaglar® and Lantus®) are used for the treatment of type 1 diabetes mellitus in adults and pediatric patients or type 2 diabetes mellitus in adults who require long-acting insulin for control of hyperglycemia. The 300-unit/mL preparation of insulin glargine (Toujeo®) is used for the treatment of type 1 or type 2 diabetes mellitus in adults who require long-acting insulin for control of hyperglycemia.

Insulin glargine in fixed combination with lixisenatide (Soliqua® 100/33) is used as an adjunct to diet and exercise to improve glycemic control in adults with type 2 diabetes mellitus inadequately controlled on lixisenatide or on less than 60 units daily of basal insulin.

For additional information on the management of diabetes mellitus, see Uses in the Insulins General Statement 68:20.08.

Insulin Glargine Efficacy of insulin glargine administered once daily at bedtime (as Lantus®) in patients with type 1 diabetes mellitus has been demonstrated in comparisons with isophane (NPH) insulin human administered once or twice daily in 3 open-label, randomized studies of up to 28 weeks' duration in adults and one study in pediatric patients 6–15 years of age; patients also received regular insulin or insulin lispro before meals during these studies. Glycemic control (as determined by glycosylated hemoglobin [hemoglobin A_{1c}, HbA_{1c}]) was similar in patients receiving insulin glargine or isophane insulin human.

Efficacy of insulin glargine administered once daily at bedtime (as Lantus®) in adults with type 2 diabetes mellitus has been established in 2 open-label, randomized clinical studies comparing insulin glargine with isophane insulin human administered once or twice daily; patients continued to receive regular insulin or oral antidiabetic agents during these studies. Insulin glargine achieved a level of glycemic control similar to that of isophane insulin human as measured by HbA_{1c}.

Glycemic control with insulin glargine appears to be similar regardless of which meal it is administered before during the day. In a 24-week, open-label, randomized clinical study in adults with type 1 diabetes mellitus, insulin glargine (as Lantus®) was administered prior to breakfast, dinner, or bedtime; patients received supplemental insulin lispro at mealtimes. Glycemic control (as determined by HbA_{1c} values at the end of the study, the primary end point) was not significantly different among the 3 treatment groups; only minor reductions in HbA_{1c} occurred. Symptomatic and documented nocturnal hypoglycemia occurred in fewer patients receiving insulin glargine before breakfast than in the other 2 groups. However, 5% of patients in the before-breakfast group discontinued treatment because of lack of efficacy.

In another open-label, randomized, 24-week clinical study in patients with type 2 diabetes mellitus poorly controlled on oral antidiabetic agents, insulin glargine (as Lantus®) given prior to breakfast was more effective in reducing HbA_{1c} than insulin glargine or isophane (NPH) insulin human given at bedtime. All patients were switched to or continued to receive glimepiride (3 mg daily in the morning) for 4 weeks prior to the addition of insulin therapy, and glimepiride therapy was continued throughout the remainder of the study. The incidence of hypoglycemia (primary safety end point) was similar across all treatment groups.

In an open-label study of 5 years' duration comparing therapy with once-daily insulin glargine (as Lantus®) to twice-daily NPH insulin in patients with type 2 diabetes mellitus, the progression of diabetic retinopathy was similar between the 2 treatment groups.

In a study evaluating the cardiovascular safety of insulin glargine (Outcome Reduction with Initial Glargine Intervention [ORIGIN]), the early use of insulin glargine to achieve normal plasma glucose concentrations in patients with dysglycemia neither reduced nor increased adverse cardiovascular outcomes as compared with guideline-suggested glycemic control. In this study, approximately 12,500 adults with cardiovascular risk factors in addition to impaired fasting glucose, impaired glucose tolerance, or type 2 diabetes mellitus received treatment with insulin glargine (as Lantus®, median dosage: 0.45 units/kg daily) or standard care (antidiabetic drugs other than insulin glargine in patients with a diagnosis of type 2 diabetes mellitus) for a median duration of 6 years. Patients who received standard care were not able to receive insulin therapy until maximal dosages of 2 different oral antidiabetic drugs had been used. There were 2 coprimary composite end points in this study: the composite of death from cardiovascular causes, nonfatal myocardial infarction [MI], and nonfatal stroke, and a composite of any of the previously mentioned cardiovascular adverse events, a revascularization procedure, or hospitalization due to heart failure. At a median follow-up of 6.2 years, there was no substantial difference between the 2 treatment groups in terms of major adverse cardiovascular outcomes or all-cause mortality. Additionally, the incidence of cancer or death from cancer was similar between treatment groups. Therapy with insulin glargine reduced the incidence of diabetes mellitus; however, the long-term clinical benefits of this reduction is unknown.

Safety and efficacy of the "follow-on" 100-unit/mL preparation of insulin glargine (Basaglar®) have been established by studies demonstrating its similarity to Lantus® and by the clinical trials that established the safety and efficacy of Lantus®, as well as by 2 clinical trials conducted using Basaglar® in patients with type 1 or type 2 diabetes mellitus. In these studies, Basaglar® was deemed sufficiently similar to Lantus® in terms of pharmacokinetics, toxicity, and immunogenicity and provided comparable glycemic control.

Safety and efficacy of the 300-unit/mL preparation of insulin glargine (Toujeo®) administered once daily in adults with type 1 or type 2 diabetes mellitus have been established in 4 open-label, controlled trials comparing a 100-unit/mL insulin glargine preparation (Lantus®) to Toujeo®. In these trials, the 300-unit/mL preparation of insulin glargine provided similar glycemic control as the 100-unit/mL preparation (as assessed by reductions in HbA_{1c}). Patients treated with insulin glargine 300 unit/mL required approximately 11–17.5% higher insulin dosages after 6 months of therapy compared with those receiving the 100-unit/mL preparation. Additionally, there were no clinically important differences in weight gain between the 2 insulin groups.

Insulin glargine is *not* the insulin of choice for treatment of diabetic ketoacidosis; a short-acting insulin (e.g., insulin regular) is the preferred agent.

Insulin Glargine/Lixisenatide Fixed-combination Therapy Current data indicate that treatment with the fixed combination of insulin glargine and lixisenatide (insulin glargine/lixisenatide) is more effective than monotherapy with either drug in improving glycemic control (as determined by reductions in HbA_{1c}) in patients with type 2 diabetes mellitus. Additionally, therapy with insulin glargine/lixisenatide was associated with weight loss while weight gain was observed with insulin glargine monotherapy. Safety and efficacy of insulin glargine/lixisenatide have been established in an open-label trial in approximately 740 patients with type 2 diabetes mellitus inadequately controlled on basal insulin (e.g., insulin glargine, NPH insulin, insulin detemir) alone or in conjunction with 1 or 2 oral antidiabetic agents (e.g., metformin, a sulfonylurea, a meglitinide, a sodium-glucose cotransporter 2 [SGLT2] inhibitor, a dipeptidyl peptidase-4 [DPP-4] inhibitor). Patients underwent a 6-week run-in period in which all oral antidiabetic drugs (except metformin) were discontinued and therapy with insulin glargine was initiated and titrated prior to randomization. Patients then received treatment with insulin glargine/lixisenatide or continued insulin glargine therapy. The dosages of insulin glargine or insulin glargine/lixisenatide were titrated once weekly based upon fasting plasma glucose concentrations (mean final dosages of insulin glargine/lixisenatide or insulin glargine were equivalent at week 30 [46.7 units]). At week 30, there was a substantially greater reduction in HbA_{1c} with insulin glargine/lixisenatide than with insulin glargine alone (reduction of 1.1 versus 0.6%, respectively). Patients receiving insulin glargine/lixisenatide had an average weight loss of 0.7 kg while those receiving insulin glargine monotherapy gained an average of 0.7 kg.

In another open-label trial of 30 weeks' duration, approximately 1170 patients with type 2 diabetes mellitus inadequately controlled on metformin with or without another antidiabetic agent (e.g., a sulfonylurea, a meglitinide, an SGLT2 inhibitor, a DPP-4 inhibitor) received therapy with insulin glargine/lixisenatide, insulin glargine, or lixisenatide, all in conjunction with metformin. Greater reductions in HbA_{1c} were observed with insulin glargine/lixisenatide than with either component alone (reduction of 1.6, 1.3, or 0.9% with insulin glargine/lixisenatide, insulin glargine, or lixisenatide therapy, respectively). Mean body weight was reduced by 0.3 or 2.3 kg in patients receiving insulin glargine/lixisenatide or lixisenatide, respectively. Mean body weight was increased by 1.1 kg in patients receiving insulin glargine monotherapy.

The manufacturer states that insulin glargine/lixisenatide should not be used in patients with type 1 diabetes mellitus or for the treatment of diabetic ketoacidosis. The safety and efficacy of insulin glargine/lixisenatide in conjunction with short-acting (e.g., prandial) insulin have not been established, and such concomitant use is not recommended. Insulin glargine/lixisenatide is not recommended for use with any other drug preparations containing lixisenatide or another glucagon-like peptide-1 (GLP-1) receptor agonist.

Dosage and Administration

■ General The dosage of insulin glargine is expressed in units. Each unit of insulin glargine is approximately equal to 0.036 mg of the drug. The dosage of the fixed combination of insulin glargine and lixisenatide (insulin glargine/lixisenatide) has been expressed in terms of the insulin glargine component; however, each mL of insulin glargine/lixisenatide contains 100 units of insulin glargine *and* 33 mcg of lixisenatide.

Therapy with lixisenatide or basal insulin should be discontinued prior to initiating therapy with insulin glargine/lixisenatide.

■ Administration Insulin glargine is administered by subcutaneous injection once daily into the abdomen, thigh, or upper arm at the same time each day using a conventional insulin syringe or the appropriate injection pen (e.g., SoloStar®, KwikPen®).

Insulin glargine/lixisenatide is administered by subcutaneous injection once daily using a prefilled injection pen. Insulin glargine/lixisenatide should be administered within 1 hour *before* the first meal of the day. If a dose of insulin glargine/lixisenatide is missed, the patient should resume the once-daily regimen with the next scheduled dose.

Insulin glargine or insulin glargine/lixisenatide should *not* be administered IV, IM, or via an infusion pump. A planned rotation of sites within an area should be followed so that any one site is not injected more than once every 1–2 weeks to reduce the risk of lipodystrophy. Clinical studies have not indicated important differences in absorption of insulin glargine from the various injection areas (e.g., abdomen, thigh, upper arm). It is *not* necessary to shake the vial of insulin glargine prior to measuring the dosage. Insulin glargine or insulin glargine/lixisenatide should not be mixed with other insulins, other drugs, or diluted with other solutions.

Insulin glargine injection should be inspected visually for particulate matter and discoloration before administration whenever solution and container permit. Insulin glargine or insulin glargine/lixisenatide should be administered only if the solution is clear, colorless, and without particulates.

Unopened injection pens and vials containing insulin glargine 100 units/mL should be stored at 2–8°C and protected from direct heat and light until the expiration date; the drug should *not* be frozen. Alternatively, unopened injection pens and vials containing insulin glargine 100 units/mL may be stored at room temperature (below 30°C) and away from direct heat and light for up to 28 days. Opened (in-use) *vials* containing insulin glargine 100 units/mL should be stored at 2–8°C for up to 28 days. Alternatively, such in-use *vials* may be stored at room temperature away from direct heat and light for up to 28 days. In-use *injection pens* of insulin glargine 100 units/mL (Kwikpen®, SoloStar®) should be stored at room temperature away from heat and direct light for up to 28 days; in-use *injection pens* should *not* be refrigerated.

Unopened injection pens of insulin glargine 300 units/mL (Toujeo®) should be stored at 2–8°C and protected from light until the expiration date; the drug should *not* be frozen. In-use injection pens of insulin glargine 300 units/mL should be stored at room temperature away from heat and direct light for up to 42 days; such in-use injection pens should *not* be refrigerated.

Injection pens containing insulin glargine/lixisenatide should be stored at 2–8°C in the original carton and protected from light before first use; after first use, the injection pens should be stored at room temperature below 25°C. The injection pens should not be frozen; they should not be used if freezing has occurred. Injection pens of insulin glargine/lixisenatide should be discarded 28 days after first use, even if some drug remains in the pen.

The accompanying labeling should be consulted for additional details about the administration of insulin glargine or insulin glargine/lixisenatide.

■ Dosage ***Insulin Glargine Therapy*** In patients with type 1 diabetes mellitus, insulin glargine must be used concomitantly with short-acting (e.g., prandial) insulin. In general, an initial total daily insulin dosage of 0.2–0.4 units/kg may be used in insulin-naive patients with type 1 diabetes mellitus. When used in conjunction with short-acting insulin, the manufacturers state that an initial insulin glargine dosage should be approximately one-third or one-third to one-half of the total daily insulin dosage for the 100- or 300-unit/mL preparations, respectively. The remainder of the daily insulin dosage should be given preprandially as rapid- or short-acting insulin.

In insulin-naive patients with type 2 diabetes mellitus, the recommended initial dosage of the 100-unit/mL preparation of insulin glargine is 0.2 unit/kg or up to 10 units given once daily. The recommended initial dosage of the 300-unit/mL preparation of insulin glargine in insulin-naive patients with type 2 diabetes mellitus is 0.2 units/kg once daily. The dosage of insulin glargine should be titrated based upon a patient's metabolic needs, blood glucose concentrations, and glycemic control goal.

The dosage of the 300-unit/mL preparation of insulin glargine should be increased no more frequently than every 3–4 days to minimize the risk of hypoglycemia. The maximum glucose-lowering effect of a dose of insulin glargine 300 units/mL may take 5 days to fully manifest, and the first dose of the 300-unit/mL preparation may not be able to fulfill the metabolic needs of the patient in the first 24 hours of use. Therefore, blood glucose concentrations should be monitored and dosages of coadministered antidiabetic drugs should be adjusted per the standard of care.

The dosage and timing of concurrent short- or rapid-acting insulins or other concomitant antidiabetic agents may need to be adjusted in patients receiving insulin glargine. Insulin requirements may be altered with changes in physical activity, changes in meal patterns (i.e., macronutrient content or timing of food intake), or during illness, emotional disturbances, or other stresses.

Transferring from Therapy with Other Insulins. When insulin glargine is substituted for another intermediate- or long-acting insulin in patients with diabetes mellitus, a change in the dosage of the basal insulin may be required. The dosage and timing of concurrent short- or rapid-acting insulin or other concomitant antidiabetic agents may also need to be adjusted.

In patients transferring from another 100-unit/mL preparation of insulin glargine (e.g., Lantus®) to Basaglar®, the dosage of Basaglar® should be the same as the other preparation, and the administration time should be determined by the clinician. In patients currently receiving once-daily isophane (NPH) insulin, the 100-unit/mL preparation of insulin glargine administered once daily may be substituted on a unit-for-unit basis for NPH insulin. In patients currently receiving twice-daily NPH insulin, the recommended initial dosage of the 100-unit/mL preparation of insulin glargine once daily is 80% of the total daily NPH insulin dosage that is being discontinued. For patients transferring from the 300-unit/mL preparation of insulin glargine to the 100-unit/mL preparation of insulin glargine, the recommended initial dosage of the 100-unit/mL insulin glargine preparation is 80% of the insulin glargine 300-unit/mL preparation dosage.

On a unit-for-unit basis, the 300-unit/mL preparation of insulin glargine has less of a glucose-lowering effect than the 100-unit/mL preparation. In patients currently receiving once-daily insulin glargine (100 units/mL) or an intermediate-acting insulin preparation, the recommended initial dosage of the 300-unit/mL preparation of insulin glargine is the same as the current long-acting insulin dosage. For patients controlled on the 100-unit/mL preparation of insulin glargine, a higher daily dose of the 300-unit/mL preparation of insulin glargine will be needed to maintain the current level of glycemic control. Patients transferring from other basal insulins to the 300-unit/mL preparation of insulin glargine may experience higher average fasting plasma glucose concentrations during the first weeks of therapy. In patients currently receiving twice-daily NPH insulin, the recommended initial dosage of the 300-unit/mL preparation of insulin glargine once daily is 80% of the total daily NPH insulin dosage that is being discontinued. Close monitoring of blood glucose concentrations is recommended during the transition to insulin glargine and in the initial weeks thereafter.

For patients with type 1 diabetes mellitus transitioning from IV insulin to the 300-unit/mL preparation of insulin glargine, the longer onset of action of the 300-unit/mL preparation of insulin glargine (onset of action develops over 6 hours) should be considered before stopping IV insulin. The full glucose-lowering effect of the 300-unit/mL preparation of insulin glargine may not be apparent for at least 5 days.

Insulin Glargine/Lixisenatide Fixed-combination Therapy The recommended initial dosage of insulin glargine/lixisenatide for patients with type 2 diabetes mellitus inadequately controlled on less than 30 units of basal insulin or on lixisenatide is 15 units (15 units insulin glargine/5 mcg lixisenatide) subcutaneously once daily. For patients inadequately controlled on 30–60 units of basal insulin, the recommended initial dosage of insulin glargine/lixisenatide is 30 units (30 units insulin glargine/10 mcg lixisenatide) subcutaneously once daily. The dosage should be titrated by 2–4 units every week based on the patient's metabolic needs, blood glucose concentrations, and glycemic control goal. The recommended daily dosage of insulin glargine/lixisenatide is 15–60 units (15–60 units insulin glargine/5–20 mcg lixisenatide) once daily. Alternative antidiabetic therapy should be used if the patient requires a daily dosage of insulin glargine/lixisenatide of less than 15 units (15 units insulin glargine/5 mcg lixisenatide) or exceeding 60 units (60 units insulin glargine/20 mcg lixisenatide) daily.

■ **Special Populations** ***Hepatic Impairment*** Data regarding the effects of hepatic impairment on the pharmacokinetics of insulin glargine in patients with diabetes mellitus are lacking. Careful monitoring of blood glucose and adjustment of insulin glargine or insulin glargine/lixisenatide dosage may be necessary in such patients.

Renal Impairment Data regarding the effects of renal impairment on the pharmacokinetics of insulin glargine in patients with diabetes mellitus are lacking. However, increased circulating concentrations of insulin have been observed in patients with renal impairment who were receiving insulin human; therefore, insulin glargine requirements may be reduced in these patients. Careful monitoring of blood glucose and adjustment of insulin glargine or insulin glargine/lixisenatide dosage may be necessary in such patients. Safety and efficacy of insulin glargine/lixisenatide have not been established in patients with end-stage renal disease (estimated glomerular filtration rate [eGFR] less than 15 mL/minute per 1.73 m^2); the fixed combination is not recommended for use in such patients.

Geriatric Patients In geriatric patients, the initial dosage, dose increments, and maintenance dosage of insulin glargine or insulin glargine/lixisenatide should be conservative in order to avoid hypoglycemia.

Cautions

■ **Contraindications** Known hypersensitivity to insulin glargine or any ingredient in the preparation. Contraindicated during episodes of hypoglycemia.

■ **Warnings/Precautions** ***Hypoglycemia*** Hypoglycemia is the most common adverse effect of insulins, including insulin glargine, and monitoring of blood glucose concentrations is recommended for all patients with diabetes mellitus. The prolonged effect of subcutaneous insulin glargine may delay recovery from hypoglycemia. Severe hypoglycemia requiring the assistance of another person, IV glucose infusions, or glucagon administration has occurred with insulin therapy, including insulin glargine. As with all insulin preparations, the time course of the glucose-lowering effect of insulin glargine or insulin glargine/lixisenatide may vary among different individuals or at different times in the same individual and depends on many factors (e.g., area of injection, injection site blood supply, temperature). The risk of hypoglycemia generally increases with the intensity of glycemic control. Other factors that may increase a patient's risk of hypoglycemia include changes in meal patterns (e.g., macronutrient content, timing of meals), level of physical activity, and concomitant drug therapy. Patients with renal or hepatic impairment may be at a higher risk of hypoglycemia. In comparative studies, the overall rate of hypoglycemic reactions with insulin glargine was similar to that with isophane insulin human. For more information on the symptoms associated with hypoglycemia, See Hypoglycemia under Cautions: Endocrine and Metabolic Effects, in the Insulins General Statement 68:20.08.

Hypoglycemia Due to Medication Errors. Confusion between basal insulin preparations and other insulins, particularly rapid-acting insulins, has caused medication errors. To avoid such errors, patients should be advised to check the label on all insulin preparations to confirm the correct preparation and strength prior to administration.

Formulation Considerations Any change in insulin should be made cautiously and only under medical supervision. Insulin glargine should not be diluted or mixed with any other insulin. Patients previously receiving insulin may require a change in dosage if insulin therapy is changed to insulin glargine. Likewise, adjustment of oral antidiabetic dosage may be necessary in patients receiving concomitant therapy with insulin glargine. Changes in insulin strength, manufacturer, type, and/or method of administration may necessitate a change in insulin dosage.

On a unit-for-unit basis, the 300-unit/mL preparation of insulin glargine has less of a glucose lowering effect than the 100-unit/mL preparation. To minimize the risk of hyperglycemia when initiating insulin glargine 300 unit/mL, blood glucose concentrations should be monitored daily, the dosage of the 300-unit/mL insulin glargine preparation should be titrated appropriately, and dosage of coadministered antidiabetic drugs should be adjusted per the standard of care. (See Transferring from Therapy with Other Insulins under Dosage: Insulin Glargine Therapy, in Dosage and Administration.)

Sharing of Injection Pens Injection pens containing insulin glargine or insulin glargine/lixisenatide must never be shared among patients, even if the needle has been changed. Sharing of injection pens poses a risk for transmission of blood-borne pathogens.

Hypokalemia All insulin preparations, including insulin glargine, cause a shift in potassium from the extracellular to the intracellular space, possibly leading to hypokalemia. Untreated hypokalemia can lead to respiratory paralysis, ventricular arrhythmias, and death. Serum potassium concentrations should be monitored in patients at risk for hypokalemia (e.g., patients receiving potassium-lowering drugs, patients taking drugs with effects sensitive to serum potassium concentrations).

Metabolic Effects Insulin may cause sodium retention and edema, particularly if metabolic control is improved by intensive insulin therapy. Insulin therapy, including insulin glargine, also may cause weight gain attributable to the anabolic effects of insulin and the decrease in glucosuria.

Heart Failure Peroxisome proliferator-activated receptor (PPAR)-γ agonists (e.g., thiazolidinediones) can cause dose-related fluid retention, particularly when used in conjunction with insulin. Fluid retention may lead to or exacerbate heart failure. Patients treated with insulin, including insulin glargine, and a PPAR-γ agonist should be observed for manifestations of heart failure (e.g., excessive/rapid weight gain, shortness of breath, edema). If heart failure develops, it should be managed according to current standards of care, and discontinuance or reduction of the dosage of the PPAR-γ agonist must be considered. Concomitant use of rosiglitazone and insulin therapy is not recommended.

Immunogenicity As with all therapeutic proteins, there is a potential for immunogenicity with insulin glargine or insulin glargine/lixisenatide. Insulin antibodies may increase or decrease the efficacy of insulin, and insulin dosage adjustments may be required. During phase 3 clinical trials of insulin glargine (as Lantus®), the incidence of insulin antibody development with insulin glargine therapy was similar to the incidence observed with isophane (NPH) insulin. Insulin antibodies have also been detected in patients receiving other insulin glargine preparations (Basaglar® or Toujeo®).

Potential Carcinogenicity FDA has notified healthcare professionals and patients about the results of several observational studies suggesting an increased risk of cancer in patients with diabetes receiving insulin glargine; however, upon further analysis, FDA states that the results of these studies are inconclusive due to limitations in how the studies were designed and carried out and in the data available for analysis. At this time, FDA states that it has *not* concluded that insulin glargine increases the risk of cancer.

In a health insurance database cohort of over 127,000 diabetic patients in Germany, a positive, dose-related association was found between diagnosis of a malignant neoplasm and use of insulin human or an insulin analog (insulin glargine, insulin aspart, insulin lispro) over a mean follow-up period of 1.63 years. After adjusting for insulin dosage, patients who had received insulin glargine dosages of 10, 30, or 50 units daily had a 9, 19, or 31% increase, respectively, in cancer risk compared with that for insulin human; no such increased risk was found for insulin aspart or insulin lispro. The results of this study prompted similar reviews of patient databases in Sweden and Scotland, both of which also suggested a positive association between cancer (e.g., of the breast) and use of insulin glargine. Review of a third database of patients in the United Kingdom and post hoc analysis of data from a controlled trial in patients with type 2 diabetes mellitus receiving insulin glargine or isophane (NPH) insulin human for a mean cumulative period exceeding 4 years did not reveal such an association. Potentially confounding factors (e.g., patient age, blood pressure, weight, concomitant antidiabetic therapy) and other limitations of retrospective analyses prevent firm conclusions based on these data. However, in vitro studies indicating that insulin promotes the growth of cancer cells and that insulin glargine is more mitogenic than insulin human support the concerns raised by these observations. and additional epidemiologic analyses worldwide have been called for to further examine any association between insulin analogs such as insulin glargine and cancer. In a study evaluating the cardiovascular safety of insulin glargine (Outcomes Reduction with Initial Glargine Intervention [ORIGIN]), the overall incidence of cancer or death from cancer was similar among patients who received insulin glargine and those who received other antidiabetic drugs (e.g., oral antidiabetic agents, insulin other than insulin glargine).

Based on currently available data, FDA recommends that patients *not* stop taking their insulin therapy without consulting a clinician, since uncontrolled hyperglycemia can have both immediate and long-term serious adverse effects. Some clinicians suggest that use of a long-acting human insulin (e.g., isophane [NPH] insulin human) or a combination of a long- and short-acting insulin twice daily may be considered as an alternative to insulin glargine therapy. FDA is continuing to evaluate the long-term risk, if any, for cancer associated with the use of insulin glargine. FDA encourages both healthcare professionals and patients to report adverse effects with the use of insulin glargine to the FDA's MedWatch Adverse Event Reporting Program (http://www.fda.gov/Safety/MedWatch/default.htm).

Use of Fixed Combinations When insulin glargine is used in fixed combination with lixisenatide or other drugs, the cautions, precautions, contraindications, and interactions associated with the concomitant agent(s) should be considered in addition to those associated with insulin glargine.

Sensitivity Reactions **Dermatologic and Sensitivity Reactions.** As with any insulin therapy, lipodystrophy may occur at sites of insulin injections and may affect insulin absorption. Injection site rotation within an area may reduce or prevent these effects. Pain at the injection site was reported among 2.7% of patients receiving insulin glargine (as Lantus®) compared with 0.7% of those receiving isophane insulin human in clinical studies. Other adverse local reactions reported with insulin glargine include redness, itching, urticaria, edema, and inflammation.

Hypersensitivity characterized by generalized skin reactions, angioedema, anaphylaxis, bronchospasm, hypotension, or shock may occur with insulin glargine therapy and may be life-threatening. If hypersensitivity reactions occur, insulin glargine or insulin glargine/lixisenatide should be discontinued and the patient should be treated per standard of care until hypersensitivity manifestations resolve.

Specific Populations **Pregnancy.** Data are lacking on the use of insulin glargine or insulin glargine/lixisenatide in pregnant women. In animal reproduction studies in rats and rabbits, insulin glargine (100 units/mL) administered during pregnancy at dosages 2–7 times the human dose of 10 units daily did not cause any effects different than those seen with insulin human (regular). However, dilation of the cerebral ventricles was observed in some rabbit fetuses. Insulin glargine or insulin glargine/lixisenatide should be used during pregnancy only if the potential benefit justifies the potential risk to the fetus.

Lactation. It is unknown whether insulin glargine is distributed into milk; caution is advised if used in nursing women. Use of insulin glargine is compatible with breast-feeding; however, women who are lactating may require adjustments of their insulin dose.

Pediatric Use. Safety and efficacy of the 100-unit/mL preparations of insulin glargine (Lantus®, Basaglar®) have not been established in children younger than 6 years of age with type 1 diabetes mellitus or in pediatric patients with type 2 diabetes mellitus. Safety and efficacy of the 300-unit/mL preparation of insulin glargine (Toujeo®) or of insulin glargine/lixisenatide have not been established in pediatric patients.

Geriatric Use. Initial dosage, dose increments, and maintenance dosage of insulin glargine or insulin glargine/lixisenatide should be conservative to avoid hypoglycemia.

■ **Common Adverse Effects** Common adverse effects associated with insulin glargine therapy during clinical trials include hypoglycemia, allergic reactions, injection site reactions, lipodystrophy, pruritus, rash, edema, and weight gain.

Adverse effects occurring in at least 5% patients receiving insulin glargine/lixisenatide in clinical trials include hypoglycemia, nausea, nasopharyngitis, diarrhea, upper respiratory tract infection, and headache.

Drug Interactions

■ **Drugs Affecting Glycemic Control** ***Drugs That May Potentiate Hypoglycemic Effects*** Drug interactions are possible with drugs that may potentiate hypoglycemic effects of insulin glargine (e.g., angiotensin-converting enzyme [ACE] inhibitors, angiotensin II receptor antagonists, disopyramide, fibrate derivatives, fluoxetine, monoamine oxidase [MAO] inhibitors, oral antidiabetic agents, pentoxifylline, pramlintide, propoxyphene [no longer commercially available in the US], salicylates, somatostatin derivatives [e.g., octreotide], sulfonamide anti-infectives). Dosage reductions and increased frequency of glucose monitoring may be required if insulin glargine is used concomitantly with these drugs.

Drugs That May Antagonize Hypoglycemic Effects Drug interactions are possible with drugs that may antagonize hypoglycemic effects such as atypical antipsychotics (e.g., olanzapine, clozapine), corticosteroids, danazol, diuretics, estrogens and progestins (e.g., oral contraceptives), glucagon, isoniazid, niacin, phenothiazines, protease inhibitors, somatropin, sympathomimetic agents (e.g., albuterol, epinephrine, terbutaline), and thyroid hormones. Dosage increases and increased frequency of glucose monitoring may be required if insulin glargine is used concomitantly with these drugs.

Drugs That May Have a Variable Effect on Glycemic Control Drug interactions are possible with drugs that may have a variable effect on glycemic control (e.g., alcohol, β-adrenergic blocking agents, clonidine, lithium salts, pentamidine). Dosage adjustments and increased frequency of glucose monitoring may be required if insulin glargine is used concomitantly with these drugs.

Sympatholytic Agents Sympatholytic agents (e.g., β-adrenergic blocking agents, clonidine, guanethidine, reserpine) may decrease or eliminate the signs of hypoglycemia. Increased frequency of glucose monitoring may be required when insulin glargine is used concomitantly with these drugs.

Description

Insulin glargine is a biosynthetic (rDNA origin), long-acting human insulin analog that is prepared using recombinant DNA technology and a special laboratory strain of nonpathogenic *Escherichia coli* (K12). Insulin glargine differs structurally from insulin human by the replacement of asparagine at position A21 with glycine and the addition of 2 arginines to the C-terminus of the B-chain. Insulin glargine has pharmacologic effects comparable to those of insulin human. (See the Insulins General Statement 68:20.08.) In clinical studies, the glucose-lowering effect of the 100-unit/mL preparation of insulin glargine was approximately the same as insulin human on a molar basis.

Insulin glargine is commercially available as an acidic solution with a pH of approximately 4. Neutralization of the acidic insulin glargine solution following injection into subcutaneous tissue results in the formation of microprecipitates of the drug from which small amounts of insulin glargine are slowly released. This results in a relatively constant concentration-time profile over 24–36 hours (dependent upon insulin concentration) with no pronounced peak. Compared with the 100-unit/mL preparation of insulin glargine, the pharmacokinetic and pharmacodynamic profiles of the 300-unit/mL preparation of insulin glargine demonstrate a less variable response and a longer duration of action (36 versus 24 hours).

Advice to Patients

Provide copy of manufacturer's patient information.

Importance of *not* mixing or diluting insulin glargine or the fixed combination of insulin glargine and lixisenatide (insulin glargine/lixisenatide) with any other insulin or solution. Importance of using insulin glargine or insulin glargine/lixisenatide only if solution is clear and colorless with no particles visible.

Provide instructions regarding proper glucose monitoring, injection technique, and management of hyperglycemia or hypoglycemia. Discuss insulin requirements in special situations such as intercurrent conditions (illness, stress, emotional disturbances), missed doses, or inadvertent administration of incorrect doses. Risk of inadequate, or variable timing of, food intake.

Importance of advising patients to refer to patient information for additional information about the potential adverse effects of insulin therapy, including lipodystrophy (and the need to rotate injection sites within the same body region), weight gain, allergic reactions, and hypoglycemia.

Provide instructions to patient regarding use of the subcutaneous insulin glargine devices. Patients should be cautioned against reuse of needles. Importance of advising patients to never use a syringe to remove insulin glargine from the SoloStar® injection pen.

Importance of informing patients that they should never share injection pens containing insulin glargine or insulin glargine/lixisenatide with another person, even if the needle has been changed; sharing of the pen may pose a risk of transmission of infection.

Importance of informing patients that changes to insulin regimens should be made cautiously and only under medical supervision. Importance of advising patients that changes in insulin regimen can predispose to hyperglycemia or hypoglycemia.

Importance of informing patients that their ability to concentrate and react may be impaired as a result of hypoglycemia, which may pose a risk in situations where these abilities are especially important (e.g., driving, operating machinery). Importance of advising patients who experience frequent hypoglycemia or reduced or absent warning signs of hypoglycemia to use caution when driving or operating machinery.

Importance of advising patients to always check the insulin label prior to each injection; medication errors involving confusion between insulins, particularly long- and short-acting insulins, have occurred.

Importance of informing patients that the 300-unit/mL preparation of insulin glargine (Toujeo®) contains 3 times as much insulin in 1 mL as standard insulin preparations (100 units/mL).

Importance of informing patients that the dose counter of the Toujeo® SoloStar® injection pen displays the number of units to be injected; no recalculation of the dose is required to convert between different concentrations of insulin glargine.

Importance of informing patients that if they are transitioned to the 300-unit/mL preparation of insulin glargine (Toujeo®) from other basal insulins, they may experience higher average fasting plasma glucose concentrations during the first weeks of therapy. Importance of advising patients to monitor glucose concentrations daily when initiating insulin glargine.

Importance of informing clinicians of existing or contemplated concomitant therapy, including prescription and OTC drugs.

Importance of women informing clinicians if they are or plan to become pregnant or breast-feed.

Importance of informing patients of other important precautionary information. (See Cautions.)

Overview (see Users Guide). For additional information until a more detailed monograph is developed and published, the manufacturer's labeling should be consulted. It is *essential* that the manufacturer's labeling be consulted for more detailed information on usual cautions, precautions, contraindications, potential drug interactions, laboratory test interferences, and acute toxicity.

Preparations

Excipients in commercially available drug preparations may have clinically important effects in some individuals; consult specific product labeling for details.

Insulin Glargine (Recombinant DNA Origin)

Parenteral

Injection, for subcutaneous use only	100 units/mL (U-100)	**Basaglar®** (in prefilled KwikPen® pens), Lilly
		Lantus® (in vials and prefilled SoloStar® pens), Sanofi-Aventis
	300 units/mL (U-300)	**Toujeo®** (in prefilled SoloStar® pens), Sanofi-Aventis

Insulin Glargine (Recombinant DNA Origin) Combinations

Parenteral

Injection, for subcutaneous use	100 units/mL with Lixisenatide 33 mcg/mL	**Soliqua® 100/33** (available as prefilled injection pens), Sanofi-Aventis

SODIUM-GLUCOSE COTRANSPORTER 2 (SGLT2) INHIBITORS 68:20.18

Canagliflozin

■ Canagliflozin, a sodium-glucose cotransporter 2 (SGLT2) inhibitor, is an antidiabetic agent.

Uses

■ **Type 2 Diabetes Mellitus** Canagliflozin is used as monotherapy as an adjunct to diet and exercise to improve glycemic control in patients with type 2 diabetes mellitus. Canagliflozin also is used to reduce the risk of major cardiovascular events (e.g., cardiovascular death, nonfatal myocardial infarction [MI], nonfatal stroke) in patients with type 2 diabetes mellitus and established cardiovascular disease. Canagliflozin is commercially available in fixed combination with immediate- or extended-release metformin hydrochloride (Invokamet® or Invokamet® XR); the fixed combination is used when treatment with both drugs is appropriate. The manufacturer states that the effectiveness of the fixed combination of canagliflozin and immediate- or extended-release metformin hydrochloride in reducing the risk of major cardiovascular events in patients with type 2 diabetes mellitus and cardiovascular disease has not been established. Canagliflozin also is used in combination with other antidiabetic agents (e.g., metformin, a sulfonylurea, a peroxisome proliferator-activated receptor$_\gamma$ [PPAR$_\gamma$] agonist [thiazolidinedione]) or insulin as an adjunct to diet and exercise in patients with type 2 diabetes mellitus who have not achieved adequate glycemic control.

Current guidelines for the treatment of type 2 diabetes mellitus generally recommend metformin as first-line therapy in addition to lifestyle modifications because of its well-established safety and efficacy (e.g., beneficial effects on glycosylated hemoglobin [hemoglobin A_{1c}; HbA_{1c}], weight, and cardiovascular mortality) in patients with recent-onset or newly diagnosed type 2 diabetes mellitus or mild hyperglycemia. Because of the progressive nature of the disease, patients initially receiving an oral antidiabetic agent will eventually require multiple oral and/or injectable antidiabetic agents of different therapeutic classes and/or insulin for adequate glycemic control. Patients with inadequate glycemic control with metformin monotherapy should receive treatment with additional antidiabetic agents; data suggest that the addition of each noninsulin agent to initial therapy lowers HbA_{1c} by approximately 0.7–1%. Some experts recommend initiating antidiabetic therapy with 2 agents (metformin plus another agent) in patients whose HbA_{1c} is 7.5% or higher, while other experts recommend initiating such dual therapy in patients whose HbA_{1c} is at least 1.5% above the target level. When the greater glucose-lowering effect of an injectable drug is needed, some experts currently suggest that glucagon-like peptide-1 (GLP-1) receptor agonists are preferred over insulin because of a lower risk of hypoglycemia and beneficial effects on body weight, although adverse GI effects may diminish tolerability. Early introduction of insulin therapy should be considered when hyperglycemia is severe (e.g., blood glucose of at least 300 mg/dL, HbA_{1c} of at least 10%), especially in the presence of catabolic manifestations (e.g., weight loss, hypertriglyceridemia, ketosis), or if symptoms of hyperglycemia are present. For additional information regarding the initiation of insulin therapy, see Uses: Diabetes Mellitus, in the Insulins General Statement 68:20.08.

Experts state that a patient's comorbidities should be considered when selecting additional (in addition to metformin) antidiabetic agents. Patients with type 2 diabetes mellitus who have established atherosclerotic cardiovascular disease (ASCVD) should receive a drug with demonstrated cardiovascular disease benefit (e.g., GLP-1 receptor agonist [e.g., liraglutide], sodium-glucose cotransporter 2 [SGLT2] inhibitor [e.g., canagliflozin, empagliflozin]). In patients with ASCVD and heart failure or with an increased risk of heart failure, an SGLT2 inhibitor with demonstrated cardiovascular benefit may be preferred. An SGLT2 inhibitor or GLP-1 receptor agonist shown to reduce the risk of chronic kidney disease (CKD) progression, cardiovascular events, or both (e.g., canagliflozin, empagliflozin, liraglutide) should be considered in patients with type 2 diabetes mellitus and CKD. Experts state that SGLT2 inhibitors may be a good choice for patients at high risk of CKD progression (i.e., patients with albuminuria or a history of estimated glomerular filtration rate [eGFR] decline) because they may have a beneficial effect on the incidence of CKD; however, adequate renal function is required for their use. Some GLP-1 receptor agonists may be used in patients with lower eGFR and may provide greater benefits for reduction of ASCVD than for CKD progression or heart failure. In patients without ASCVD, heart failure, or CKD, the decision regarding the addition of other antidiabetic agents (e.g., sulfonylurea, thiazolidinedione, dipeptidyl peptidase-4 [DPP-4] inhibitor, SGLT2 inhibitor, GLP-1 receptor agonist, basal insulin) should be based on drug-specific effects and individual patient factors.

Canagliflozin should not be used in patients with type 1 diabetes mellitus or for the treatment of diabetic ketoacidosis.

Canagliflozin Monotherapy When given as monotherapy for the management of type 2 diabetes mellitus, canagliflozin improves glycemic control compared with placebo as evidenced by reductions in glycosylated hemoglobin HbA_{1c} and in fasting and 2-hour postprandial plasma glucose concentrations. Efficacy of canagliflozin as monotherapy for the management of type 2 diabetes mellitus has been established in a double-blind, placebo-controlled study of 26 weeks' duration. Canagliflozin (100 or 300 mg once daily) improved glycemic control as evidenced by reductions in HbA_{1c} and fasting and 2-hour postprandial plasma glucose concentrations. HbA_{1c} was reduced by 0.77 or 1% in patients receiving canagliflozin 100 or 300 mg once daily, respectively, compared with an increase of 0.1% in those receiving placebo. Patients receiving canagliflozin 100 or 300 mg once daily also lost substantially more body weight (2.8 or 3.9%, respectively) than those receiving placebo (0.6%).

Combination Therapy When given in combination with one or more oral antidiabetic agents or insulin, canagliflozin improves glycemic control compared with monotherapy with these drugs and generally is associated with reductions in body weight. Canagliflozin generally is well tolerated, although genital mycotic infections appear to be more common with canagliflozin than with other antidiabetic agents. (See Genital Mycotic Infections under Cautions: Warnings/Precautions.)

Efficacy of canagliflozin in combination with metformin, a sulfonylurea, and/or a thiazolidinedione for the management of type 2 diabetes mellitus (in patients inadequately controlled with metformin, a sulfonylurea, and/or a thiazolidinedione monotherapy) is supported by results from several long-term, randomized, active- or placebo-controlled trials. In these trials, the addition of canagliflozin (100 or 300 mg once daily) to existing therapy improved glycemic control as evidenced by reductions in HbA_{1c}, fasting plasma glucose, 2-hour postprandial plasma glucose concentrations, and/or body weight compared with placebo. In a 26-week study in patients receiving metformin hydrochloride therapy (dosage of at least 1.5 g daily), the addition of canagliflozin resulted in a reduction of 0.8–0.9% in HbA_{1c}, while HbA_{1c} was increased by 0.1% with add-on placebo. In a 52-week study in patients receiving metformin hydrochloride therapy (dosage of at least 1.5 g daily), canagliflozin 100 mg once daily was noninferior to glimepiride (titrated to 6 or 8 mg once daily), and canagliflozin 300 mg once daily was superior to glimepiride, in reducing HbA_{1c}; patients achieved reductions of 0.8, 0.9, or 0.8% in HbA_{1c} with canagliflozin 100 mg, canagliflozin 300 mg, or glimepiride, respectively. In an 18-week trial in patients receiving a sulfonylurea (generally glimepiride, glyburide [glibenclamide], or gliclazide [not commercially available in the US]), add-on therapy with canagliflozin 100 or 300 mg once daily resulted in a reduction in HbA_{1c} of 0.74 or 0.83%, respectively, compared with placebo.

Efficacy and safety of the combination of canagliflozin and metformin as initial therapy in patients with type 2 diabetes mellitus inadequately controlled with diet and exercise is supported by results of a 26-week, randomized, double-blind trial. In this trial, concurrent therapy with canagliflozin (100 or 300 mg once daily) and metformin hydrochloride extended-release (dosage of at least 1.5 g daily; 90% of patients achieved a dosage of 2 g daily) substantially improved glycemic control (as evidenced by reductions in HbA_{1c}) compared with canagliflozin or metformin hydrochloride monotherapy. Reductions in

HbA_{1c} were 1.77 or 1.78% with canagliflozin 100 or 300 mg once daily, respectively, plus metformin hydrochloride; 1.37 or 1.42% with canagliflozin 100 or 300 mg once daily, respectively; and 1.3% with metformin hydrochloride monotherapy. Additionally, a greater percentage of patients achieved an HbA_{1c} of less than 7% with canagliflozin and metformin combination therapy compared with canagliflozin or metformin hydrochloride monotherapy.

In a 26-week trial in patients receiving metformin hydrochloride (dosage of at least 1.5 g daily) and a sulfonylurea (sulfonylurea not specified), addition of canagliflozin 100 or 300 mg once daily resulted in a reduction in HbA_{1c} of 0.85 or 1.06%, respectively, compared with a 0.13% reduction in HbA_{1c} with placebo. In a 52-week study in patients receiving metformin hydrochloride (dosage of at least 1.5 g daily) and a sulfonylurea (generally glipizide, glyburide [glibenclamide], or gliclazide [not commercially available in the US]), addition of canagliflozin 300 mg or sitagliptin 100 mg resulted in a reduction in HbA_{1c} of 1 or 0.6%, respectively. Canagliflozin was noninferior to sitagliptin and demonstrated superiority to sitagliptin in reducing HbA_{1c} in subsequent analyses. In a 26-week trial in patients inadequately controlled on metformin hydrochloride (dosage of at least 1.5 g daily) and sitagliptin (100 mg daily), the addition of canagliflozin (100 mg daily titrated to 300 mg daily) resulted in a substantial reduction in HbA_{1c} from baseline at 26 weeks compared with the addition of placebo (reduction of 0.83 versus 0.03%, respectively).

In a 26-week trial in patients receiving metformin hydrochloride (dosage of at least 1.5 g daily) and pioglitazone (30 or 45 mg daily), addition of canagliflozin 100 or 300 mg once daily or placebo resulted in a reduction in HbA_{1c} of approximately 0.9, 1, or 0.3%, respectively.

Efficacy of canagliflozin in combination with insulin in the management of type 2 diabetes mellitus in patients who have inadequate glycemic control with insulin is supported by results of an 18-week, randomized, placebo-controlled trial. In this trial, addition of canagliflozin (100 or 300 mg daily) to existing insulin therapy resulted in improvements in HbA_{1c}, fasting plasma glucose, and body weight. In patients who received canagliflozin 100 or 300 mg as add-on therapy to insulin, 20 or 25%, respectively, had HbA_{1c} reductions to less than 7%, compared with 8% of patients receiving add-on placebo.

Macrovascular Outcomes and Cardiovascular Risk Reduction Some SGLT2 inhibitors such as canagliflozin have demonstrated the ability to reduce the risk of cardiovascular events in patients with type 2 diabetes mellitus and established cardiovascular disease. In addition to lowering blood glucose, SGLT2 inhibitors appear to modify several nonglycemic cardiovascular risk factors such as blood pressure, body weight, adiposity, and arterial stiffness. When canagliflozin is used for the management of type 2 diabetes mellitus in patients at an increased risk for cardiovascular events, canagliflozin reduces the risk of cardiovascular and renal outcomes, although with an increased risk of lower extremity amputations. The Canagliflozin Cardiovascular Assessment Studies (CANVAS and CANVAS-R) were designed to assess the cardiovascular safety and efficacy of canagliflozin in patients with type 2 diabetes mellitus. In CANVAS and CANVAS-R, adults (mean age: 63.3 years) with type 2 diabetes mellitus and established cardiovascular disease (i.e., secondary prevention treatment group) or at high risk for cardiovascular disease (i.e., primary prevention treatment group [at least 50 years of age with at least 2 risk factors for cardiovascular disease]) received canagliflozin (100 or 300 mg) once daily or placebo for a mean of 149 weeks. During the studies, antidiabetic and cardiovascular therapies were modified to achieve standard-of-care treatment targets with respect to blood glucose, lipids, and blood pressure. Concomitant use of other standard-of-care treatments for diabetes mellitus and atherosclerotic cardiovascular disease (renin-angiotensin system inhibitors [80%], β-blockers [53%], loop diuretics [36%], statins [75%], antiplatelet agents [74%]) was permitted. The primary outcome was the composite of death from cardiovascular causes, nonfatal MI, or nonfatal stroke. In these studies, patients who received treatment with canagliflozin had substantially lower rates of the primary cardiovascular outcome compared with those who received placebo (event rate 9.2 versus 10.4%).

Beneficial Effects on Renal Function In several cardiovascular outcomes trials involving the use of SGLT2 inhibitors (e.g., canagliflozin, dapagliflozin, empagliflozin) in patients with type 2 diabetes mellitus at high risk for cardiovascular disease or with existing cardiovascular disease, beneficial effects on renal function have been observed as a secondary outcome. Experts state that the risk-benefit balance of SGLT2 inhibitor treatment appears to be favorable for most patients with type 2 diabetes mellitus and CKD. In the CANVAS trials (see Macrovascular Outcomes and Cardiovascular Risk Reduction under Uses: Type 2 Diabetes Mellitus), canagliflozin therapy was associated with a 27% reduction of the risk of progression of albuminuria; in addition, regression of albuminuria occurred more frequently among those receiving canagliflozin than placebo. The composite outcome of a sustained 40% reduction in eGFR, the need for renal replacement therapy, or death from renal causes also occurred less frequently among those receiving canagliflozin than placebo.

The effects of canagliflozin on renal outcomes also have been evaluated in a randomized, double-blind, placebo-controlled study (CREDENCE) in approximately 4400 patients with type 2 diabetes mellitus and albuminuria (urine albumin:creatinine ratio exceeding 300 but less than 5000 mg/g) chronic kidney disease (eGFR 30–89 mL/minute per 1.73 m²; mean: 56.2 mL/minute per 1.73 m²). In this study, patients received canagliflozin 100 mg orally or placebo once daily in conjunction with the standard of care for glycemic control. Patients also had to have been receiving a stable dosage of an angiotensin-converting enzyme (ACE) inhibitor or an angiotensin II receptor antagonist for at least 4 weeks prior to randomization. The primary outcome was the composite of end-stage kidney disease, doubling of serum creatinine concentrations from baseline, or death from renal or cardiovascular disease. The study was stopped early after a planned interim analysis (median follow-up: 2.6 years) at which the relative risk of the primary outcomes was found to be 30% lower in the canagliflozin group than in the placebo group. These outcomes were observed despite very small differences in blood glucose control, weight, and blood pressure between the canagliflozin and placebo groups. These findings suggest that the beneficial renal effects of SGLT2 inhibitors may be independent of glucose homeostasis and may be related to other mechanisms, such as a reduction in intraglomerular pressure.

Dosage and Administration

■ **Administration** Canagliflozin should be administered orally once daily, before the first meal of the day. The fixed combination of canagliflozin and immediate-release metformin hydrochloride should be administered twice daily with meals. The fixed combination of canagliflozin and extended-release metformin hydrochloride should be administered once daily with the morning meal; the tablet should be swallowed whole and should not be crushed, chewed, or cut.

If a dose is missed, the missed dose should be taken as soon as it is remembered followed by resumption of the regular schedule. If the missed dose is not remembered until the time of the next dose, the missed dose should be skipped and the regular schedule resumed; the dose should not be doubled to replace a missed dose.

■ **Dosage** ***Type 2 Diabetes Mellitus*** **Canagliflozin Monotherapy.** Dosage of canagliflozin is expressed in terms of anhydrous canagliflozin.

The recommended initial dosage of canagliflozin for the management of type 2 diabetes mellitus is 100 mg once daily, taken before the first meal of the day. If well tolerated, the dosage may be increased to 300 mg once daily in patients with an estimated glomerular filtration rate (eGFR) of at least 60 mL/minute per 1.73 m² who require additional glycemic control.

In patients with an eGFR of at least 60 mL/minute per 1.73 m² who are receiving concurrent therapy with a uridine diphosphate-glucuronosyltransferase (UGT) enzyme inducer (e.g., phenobarbital, phenytoin, rifampin, ritonavir), consideration should be given to increasing the dosage of canagliflozin to 300 mg once daily in patients who are tolerating a dosage of 100 mg once daily and require additional glycemic control. (See Drug Interactions: Uridine Diphosphate-glucuronosyltransferase Enzyme Inducers.)

Patients with volume depletion should have this condition corrected before initiation of canagliflozin therapy.

Canagliflozin/Metformin Hydrochloride Fixed-combination Therapy. Dosage of canagliflozin in fixed combination with metformin hydrochloride should be individualized based on the patient's current antidiabetic regimen. In patients with an eGFR of at least 60 mL/minute per 1.73 m², the dosage of the fixed-combination preparation may be increased gradually based on effectiveness and tolerability up to a maximum of 300 mg of canagliflozin and 2 g of metformin hydrochloride daily.

In patients *not* currently receiving treatment with either canagliflozin or metformin hydrochloride, the recommended initial dosage of the fixed combination of canagliflozin and *immediate-release* metformin hydrochloride (Invokamet®) is 50 mg of canagliflozin and 500 mg of metformin hydrochloride twice daily; the recommended initial dosage of the fixed combination of canagliflozin and *extended-release* metformin hydrochloride (Invokamet® XR) is 100 mg of canagliflozin and 1 g of metformin hydrochloride once daily.

In patients currently receiving metformin hydrochloride, the recommended initial total daily dosage of the fixed combination is 100 mg of canagliflozin and a metformin hydrochloride dosage similar to the patient's existing total daily dosage, administered in 2 divided doses (when given as the fixed combination containing *immediate-release* metformin hydrochloride) or once daily (when given as the fixed combination containing *extended-release* metformin hydrochloride). Patients who are currently receiving an evening dose of extended-release metformin hydrochloride should skip their last dose prior to initiating therapy with the fixed combination of canagliflozin and metformin hydrochloride the following morning.

In patients currently receiving canagliflozin, the recommended initial total daily dosage of the fixed combination is the same daily dosage of canagliflozin and 1 g of metformin hydrochloride, administered in 2 divided doses (when given as the fixed combination containing *immediate-release* metformin hydrochloride) or once daily (when given as the fixed combination containing *extended-release* metformin hydrochloride).

In patients currently receiving both canagliflozin and metformin hydrochloride as separate components, the recommended initial total daily dosage of the fixed combination is the same daily dosage of canagliflozin and a metformin hydrochloride dosage similar to the patient's existing total daily dosage, administered in 2 divided doses (when given as the fixed combination containing *immediate-release* metformin hydrochloride) or once daily (when given as the fixed combination containing *extended-release* metformin hydrochloride).

In patients with an eGFR of at least 60 mL/minute per 1.73 m² who are receiving concurrent therapy with a UGT enzyme inducer (e.g., phenobarbital, phenytoin, rifampin, ritonavir), consideration should be given to increasing the dosage of canagliflozin to 300 mg once daily in patients who are tolerating a dosage of 100 mg once daily and require additional glycemic control. (See Drug Interactions: Uridine Diphosphate-glucuronosyltransferase Enzyme Inducers.)

■ **Special Populations** ***Hepatic Impairment*** **Canagliflozin Monotherapy.** No dosage adjustment is necessary in patients with mild or moderate hepatic impairment. Data are lacking on use of canagliflozin in patients with severe hepatic impairment, and the manufacturer states that such use is not recommended.

Canagliflozin/Metformin Hydrochloride Fixed-combination Therapy. Use of the fixed-combination preparations of canagliflozin and metformin hydrochloride is not recommended in patients with hepatic impairment.

Renal Impairment **Canagliflozin Monotherapy.** No dosage adjustment is necessary in patients with mild renal impairment (eGFR of at least 60 mL/minute per 1.73 m^2). In patients with moderate renal impairment (eGFR of 45 to less than 60 mL/minute per 1.73 m^2), the dosage of canagliflozin should not exceed 100 mg daily. Initiation of canagliflozin is not recommended in patients with an eGFR of less than 45 mL/minute per 1.73 m^2. Continued use of canagliflozin is not recommended in patients with an eGFR persistently less than 45 mL/minute per 1.73 m^2; the drug is contraindicated in patients with an eGFR less than 30 mL/minute per 1.73 m^2.

Therapy with another antidiabetic agent should be considered in patients with an eGFR of 45 to less than 60 mL/minute per 1.73 m^2 who are receiving concurrent therapy with a UGT enzyme inducer. (See Drug Interactions: Uridine Diphosphate-glucuronosyltransferase Enzyme Inducers.)

Canagliflozin/Metformin Hydrochloride Fixed-combination Therapy. In patients with moderate renal impairment (eGFR 45 to less than 60 mL/minute per 1.73 m^2), the dosage of the canagliflozin component should not exceed 100 mg daily. Use of the fixed-combination preparation of canagliflozin and metformin hydrochloride is contraindicated in patients with an eGFR of less than 45 mL/minute per 1.73 m^2.

Therapy with another antidiabetic agent should be considered in patients with an eGFR of 45 to less than 60 mL/minute per 1.73 m^2 who are receiving concurrent therapy with a UGT enzyme inducer. (See Drug Interactions: Uridine Diphosphate-glucuronosyltransferase Enzyme Inducers.)

Geriatric Patients **Canagliflozin Monotherapy.** The manufacturer makes no specific dosage recommendations for geriatric patients.

Canagliflozin/Metformin Hydrochloride Fixed-combination Therapy. Renal function should be monitored frequently after initiating the fixed-combination preparation; the dosage should be adjusted according to the patient's renal function. (See Renal Impairment under Dosage and Administration: Special Populations.)

Cautions

■ **Contraindications** History of serious hypersensitivity reactions (e.g., anaphylaxis, angioedema) to canagliflozin.

Severe renal impairment (estimated glomerular filtration rate [eGFR] less than 30 mL/minute per 1.73 m^2), end-stage renal disease, or on hemodialysis.

■ **Warnings/Precautions** ***Warnings*** **Lower Limb Amputation.** In 2 randomized, placebo-controlled studies (Canagliflozin Cardiovascular Assessment Study [CANVAS] and CANVAS-R) evaluating the effects of canagliflozin on the risk of cardiovascular disease and the overall safety and tolerability of the drug, canagliflozin-treated patients had a twofold increased risk of lower limb (leg and foot) amputations (mostly affecting the toes and midfoot) compared with placebo. In the CANVAS study, canagliflozin- or placebo-treated patients had 5.9 or 2.8 amputations per 1000 patients per year, respectively; the amputation rate in the CANVAS-R trial was 7.5 or 4.2 per 1000 patients per year with canagliflozin or placebo, respectively. Amputations below and above the knee also occurred, and some patients had more than one amputation (some involving both lower limbs). The increased risk of lower limb amputation was observed with both the 100- and 300-mg daily dosage regimens. Patients with a baseline history of prior amputation, peripheral vascular disease, or neuropathy were at greatest risk for amputation. The most common precipitating medical events leading to an amputation were lower limb infections, gangrene, diabetic foot ulcers, and ischemia.

Prior to initiating therapy with canagliflozin, clinicians should consider patient factors that may predispose them to the need for amputation, such as a history of amputation, peripheral vascular disease, neuropathy, or diabetic foot ulcers. Clinicians should monitor patients receiving canagliflozin for the presence of infection (including osteomyelitis), new pain or tenderness, and sores or ulcers involving the lower limbs; canagliflozin should be discontinued if such complications occur. Patients should also be counseled on the importance of routine preventative foot care.

Sensitivity Reactions Hypersensitivity reactions (e.g., generalized urticaria), some serious, have been reported with canagliflozin treatment. These reactions generally occurred within hours to days of canagliflozin initiation. If a hypersensitivity reaction occurs, the drug should be discontinued, appropriate treatment instituted, and the patient monitored until signs and symptoms resolve.

Other Warnings/Precautions **Use of Fixed Combinations.** When canagliflozin is used in fixed combination with other drugs (e.g., metformin), the cautions, precautions, contraindications, and interactions associated with the concomitant agent(s) must be considered in addition to those associated with canagliflozin.

Ketoacidosis. Use of sodium glucose cotransporter 2 (SGLT2) inhibitors (canagliflozin, dapagliflozin, empagliflozin) in patients with type 2 diabetes mellitus may lead to ketoacidosis requiring hospitalization. Ketoacidosis associated with use of SGLT2 inhibitors may be present without markedly elevated blood glucose concentrations (e.g., less than 250 mg/dL).

FDA identified 73 cases of acidosis (reported as diabetic ketoacidosis [DKA], ketoacidosis, or ketosis) associated with SGLT2 inhibitor use in the FDA Adverse Event Reporting System (FAERS) between March 2013 and May 2015. DKA had an atypical presentation in most of the reported cases in that type 2 diabetes mellitus was noted as the indication for the drug, and glucose concentrations were only slightly elevated (median: 211 mg/dL); type 1 diabetes mellitus was named as the indication in a few cases, and in some reports the indication was not specified. The median time to onset of symptoms of acidosis following initiation or increase in dosage of the SGLT2 inhibitor was 43 days (range: 1–365 days). No trend demonstrating a relationship between the dosage of an SGLT2 inhibitor and the risk of ketoacidosis was identified. In all reported episodes, a diagnosis of DKA or ketoacidosis was made by the clinician and hospitalization or treatment in an emergency department was warranted. In most cases, at least 1 diagnostic laboratory criterion suggestive of ketoacidosis (e.g., high anion gap metabolic acidosis, ketonemia, reduced serum bicarbonate) was reported. Most cases of ketoacidosis were associated with a concurrent event, most commonly dehydration, infection, or change in insulin dosage. Potential factors for development of ketoacidosis with SGLT2 inhibitor therapy identified in the 73 cases included infection, low carbohydrate diet or reduced caloric intake (due to illness or surgery), pancreatic disorders suggesting insulin deficiency (e.g., type 1 diabetes mellitus, history of pancreatitis, pancreatic surgery), reduced dosage or discontinuance of insulin, discontinuance of an oral insulin secretagogue, and alcohol use.

Prior to initiating therapy with an SGLT2 inhibitor, clinicians should consider patient factors that may predispose the patient to ketoacidosis, such as pancreatic insulin deficiency from any cause, reduced caloric intake, and alcohol abuse. Clinicians should evaluate for the presence of acidosis, including ketoacidosis, in patients experiencing signs or symptoms of acidosis while receiving SGLT2 inhibitors, regardless of the patient's blood glucose concentration. Additionally, clinicians should consider monitoring for ketoacidosis and temporarily discontinuing therapy with an SGLT2 inhibitor in clinical situations known to predispose individuals to ketoacidosis (e.g., prolonged fasting due to acute illness or surgery). If acidosis is confirmed, the SGLT2 inhibitor should be discontinued and appropriate treatment initiated to correct the acidosis; glucose concentrations should be monitored appropriately. In addition, supportive medical treatment should be instituted to treat and correct factors that may have precipitated or contributed to the metabolic acidosis. Euglycemic DKA associated with SGLT2 inhibitors may be detected and potentially prevented by having patients monitor urine and/or plasma ketone levels if they feel unwell, regardless of ambient glucose concentrations. Clinicians should inform patients and caregivers of the signs and symptoms of ketoacidosis (e.g., tachypnea or hyperventilation, anorexia, abdominal pain, nausea, vomiting, lethargy, mental status changes) and instruct patients to discontinue the SGLT2 inhibitor and immediately seek medical attention should they experience such signs or symptoms.

Hypotension. Canagliflozin may cause intravascular volume contraction. Following initiation of canagliflozin, symptomatic hypotension can occur, particularly in patients with impaired renal function (eGFR less than 60 mL/minute per 1.73 m^2), geriatric patients, patients receiving diuretics or drugs that interfere with the renin-angiotensin-aldosterone system (e.g., angiotensin-converting enzyme [ACE] inhibitors, angiotensin II receptor antagonists), or patients with low systolic blood pressure. (See Drug Interactions: Drugs Affecting the Renin-Angiotensin System, and also see Drug Interactions: Diuretics.) Prior to initiating canagliflozin in such patients, intravascular volume should be assessed and corrected. Patients should be monitored for signs and symptoms of hypotension after initiating canagliflozin therapy.

Renal Effects. Canagliflozin causes intravascular volume contraction and can cause renal impairment. Canagliflozin may increase serum creatinine concentration and decrease eGFR; patients with hypovolemia may be more susceptible to these changes. Abnormalities in renal function can occur following initiation of the drug. Patients should be monitored for acute kidney injury, and more frequent monitoring is recommended for patients with an eGFR less than 60 mL/minute per 1.73 m^2. If acute kidney injury occurs during canagliflozin therapy, the drug should be discontinued and appropriate treatment initiated.

FDA identified 101 cases of acute kidney injury associated with canagliflozin or dapagliflozin therapy in FAERS between March 2013 and October 2015. Hospitalization for evaluation and management of kidney injury was warranted in most cases, and some cases required admission to an intensive care unit and initiation of dialysis. In approximately half of the cases, onset of acute kidney injury occurred within 1 month or less of initiating canagliflozin or dapagliflozin therapy, and most patients' kidney function improved after stopping the drug. However, kidney injury may not be fully reversible in some situations and has led to death in some patients.

Prior to initiating canagliflozin therapy, clinicians should consider patient factors that may predispose the patient to acute kidney injury, including hypovolemia, chronic renal insufficiency, heart failure, and concomitant drug therapy (e.g., diuretics, angiotensin converting enzyme [ACE] inhibitors, angiotensin II receptor antagonists, nonsteroidal anti-inflammatory agents [NSAIAs]). Clinicians should consider temporarily discontinuing canagliflozin in any setting of reduced oral intake (e.g., acute illness, fasting) or fluid losses (e.g., GI illness, excessive heat exposure).

Concomitant Therapy with Hypoglycemic Agents. When canagliflozin is added to therapy with an insulin secretagogue (e.g., a sulfonylurea) or insulin, the risk of hypoglycemia is increased compared with sulfonylurea or insulin monotherapy. Therefore, patients receiving canagliflozin may require a reduced dosage of the concomitant insulin secretagogue or insulin to reduce the risk of hypoglycemia. (See Drug Interactions: Antidiabetic Agents.)

Fournier Gangrene. Fournier gangrene (necrotizing fasciitis of the perineum), a rare but serious or life-threatening bacterial infection requiring urgent surgical intervention, has been reported during postmarketing surveillance in men and women with type 2 diabetes mellitus receiving an SGLT2 inhibitor, including canagliflozin. Permanent disfigurement, prolonged hospitalization, disability, and complications from sepsis all may be associated with Fournier gangrene. Although diabetes mellitus is a risk factor for developing Fournier gangrene, this condition is still rare among patients with diabetes mellitus.

FDA identified 12 cases of Fournier gangrene in patients taking an SGLT2 inhibitor reported in FAERS and the medical literature between March 2013 and May 2018. Since FDA's review, additional cases of Fournier gangrene have been reported. In the initial cases reviewed by FDA, the average time to onset of infection was 9.2 months (range 7 days to 25 months) after initiation of therapy with an SGLT2 inhibitor. Some experts speculate that the variation in time to diagnosis of Fournier gangrene might be due to fluctuating glycemic control, microvascular complications, or an inciting event associated with SGLT2 inhibitors (e.g., urinary tract infection, mycotic infection, skin or mucosal breakdown due to pruritus). In all reported cases, hospitalization and surgery were required. Among these cases, some patients required multiple disfiguring surgeries, some developed complications (e.g., diabetic ketoacidosis, acute kidney injury, septic shock), and 1 patient died. In a review of other antidiabetic drugs (e.g., insulin, biguanides, sulfonylureas, dipeptidyl peptidase-4 inhibitors) over a period of more than 30 years, only 6 cases of Fournier gangrene were identified; all of theses cases occurred in men.

Patients receiving canagliflozin who develop pain or tenderness, erythema, or swelling in the genital or perineal area, in addition to fever or malaise, should be assessed for necrotizing fasciitis. If Fournier gangrene is suspected, canagliflozin should be discontinued and treatment should be initiated with broad-spectrum antibiotics; surgical debridement should be performed if necessary. Blood glucose concentrations should be closely monitored; alternative antidiabetic agents should be initiated to maintain glycemic control.

Genital Mycotic Infections. Canagliflozin may increase the risk of genital mycotic infections in males (e.g., balanoposthitis, candidal balanitis) and females (e.g., vulvovaginal candidiasis, vulvovaginal mycotic infection, vulvovaginitis). In clinical trials, patients with a history of genital mycotic infections and uncircumcised males were more likely to develop such infections. Patients should be monitored for genital mycotic infections and appropriate treatment should be instituted if these infections occur.

Urosepsis and Pyelonephritis. Treatment with an SGLT2 inhibitor (e.g., canagliflozin) increases the risk for serious urinary tract infections.

Cases of serious urinary tract infections, including urosepsis and pyelonephritis, have been reported in patients receiving an SGLT2 inhibitor. FDA identified 19 cases of urosepsis and pyelonephritis, which began as urinary tract infections associated with SGLT2 inhibitor use, in FAERS between March 2013 and October 2014. In all cases reported, hospitalization was warranted and some patients required admission to an intensive care unit or dialysis for treatment. The median time to onset of infection following initiation of the SGLT2 inhibitor was 45 days (range: 2–270 days).

Prior to initiating therapy with an SGLT2 inhibitor, clinicians should consider patient factors that may predispose them to serious urinary tract infections, such as a history of difficulty urinating or infections of the bladder, kidneys, or urinary tract. Patients should be monitored for urinary tract infections and treatment instituted if indicated.

Risk of Bone Fracture. In the CANVAS study, an increased risk of bone fracture was observed in patients receiving canagliflozin 100 or 300 mg once daily. Fractures were observed as early as 12 weeks after initiation of treatment and were more likely to affect the distal portion of upper and lower extremities and be associated with minor trauma (e.g., falls from no greater than standing height). Dose-related decreases in bone mineral density (e.g., hip and lumbar spine) also have been observed in older adults (mean age: 64 years) receiving canagliflozin therapy over a period of 2 years. Clinicians should consider factors that contribute to fracture risk and counsel patients about such factors prior to initiating canagliflozin therapy. (See Advice to Patients.)

Effects on Lipoproteins. Dose-related increases in low-density lipoprotein (LDL)-cholesterol have been observed during canagliflozin therapy. Serum LDL-cholesterol concentrations should be monitored during treatment with canagliflozin and such lipid elevations treated if appropriate.

Laboratory Test Interferences. SGLT2 inhibitors such as canagliflozin increase urinary glucose excretion and will result in false-positive urine glucose tests. In addition, the manufacturer states that the 1,5-anhydroglucitol assay is unreliable for monitoring glycemic control in patients taking SGLT2 inhibitors. Alternative methods of monitoring glycemic control should be used in patients receiving SGLT2 inhibitors.

Specific Populations **Pregnancy.** Based on the results of reproductive and developmental toxicity studies in animals, canagliflozin use during pregnancy may affect renal development and maturation, especially during the second and third trimesters of pregnancy. Limited data with canagliflozin in pregnant women are not sufficient to determine a drug-associated risk for major birth defects or miscarriage, and poorly controlled diabetes mellitus during pregnancy carries risks to the mother and fetus; however, canagliflozin therapy is not recommended in pregnant women during the second and third trimesters of pregnancy.

Lactation. Canagliflozin is distributed into milk in rats; it is not known whether the drug is distributed into human milk. Because many drugs are distributed into human milk and because of the potential for serious adverse reactions in nursing infants from canagliflozin, use of the drug is not recommended while breastfeeding.

Pediatric Use. Safety and efficacy of canagliflozin have not been established in pediatric patients younger than 18 years of age.

Geriatric Use. Among patients in 13 clinical trials, 2294 were 65 years of age or older and 351 were 75 years of age or older, including one trial in patients 55 to 80 years of age. Geriatric patients experienced reduced efficacy of canagliflozin compared with younger patients, which may be related to decreased renal function in geriatric patients. Geriatric patients also were more likely to experience certain adverse effects related to reduced intravascular volume (e.g., hypotension, postural dizziness, orthostatic hypotension, syncope, dehydration) with canagliflozin, particularly those receiving 300 mg daily.

Hepatic Impairment. Compared with values in individuals with normal hepatic function, canagliflozin area under the concentration-time curve (AUC) and peak plasma concentrations were increased by 10 and 7%, respectively (based on geometric mean ratios), in patients with mild hepatic impairment (Child-Pugh class A) following a single 300-mg dose of the drug; canagliflozin AUC was increased by 11% and peak plasma concentration was decreased by 4% in patients with moderate hepatic impairment (Child-Pugh class B). These differences were not considered clinically important.

Data are lacking on the use of canagliflozin in patients with severe hepatic impairment (Child-Pugh class C), and such use is not recommended.

Renal Impairment. Safety and efficacy of canagliflozin were evaluated in a study that included 269 patients with moderate renal impairment (eGFR 30 to less than 50 mL/minute per 1.73 m^2) and type 2 diabetes mellitus. These patients experienced less overall improvement in glycemic control and had higher rates of adverse effects related to reduced intravascular volume, renal-related adverse effects, and decreases in eGFR compared with those who had mild renal impairment or normal renal function. Patients receiving canagliflozin 300 mg were more likely to experience increases in serum potassium concentrations.

Renal impairment did not affect peak plasma concentrations of canagliflozin. In patients with mild (eGFR 60 to less than 90 mL/minute per 1.73 m^2), moderate (eGFR 30 to less than 60 mL/minute per 1.73 m^2), or severe renal impairment (eGFR less than 30 mL/minute per 1.73 m^2), canagliflozin AUC was increased by 15, 29, or 53%, respectively, compared with that in healthy individuals following a single 200-mg dose of the drug.

Renal function should be assessed prior to initiation of therapy and periodically thereafter.

■ **Common Adverse Effects** Adverse effects reported in at least 2% of patients receiving canagliflozin in clinical trials and more frequently than with placebo include female genital mycotic infections, urinary tract infection, increased urination, male genital mycotic infections, vulvovaginal pruritus, thirst, constipation, and nausea.

Drug Interactions

The major metabolic elimination pathway for canagliflozin is *O*-glucuronidation; the drug is mainly glucuronidated by uridine diphosphate-glucuronosyltransferase (UGT) isoenzymes UGT1A9 and UGT2B4.

Canagliflozin is a P-glycoprotein substrate and weakly inhibits P-glycoprotein. Canagliflozin also is a substrate of MRP2.

■ **Drugs Affecting or Metabolized by Hepatic Microsomal Enzymes** Canagliflozin did not induce cytochrome P-450 (CYP) isoenzymes 3A4, 2C9, 2C19, 2B6, or 1A2 in cultured human hepatocytes. Canagliflozin also does not inhibit CYP isoenzymes 1A2, 2A6, 2C19, 2D6, or 2E1 but weakly inhibits CYP2B6, 2C8, 2C9, and 3A4 in human hepatic microsomes.

■ **Drugs Affecting the Renin-Angiotensin System** Concomitant use of canagliflozin with drugs that interfere with the renin-angiotensin-aldosterone system, including angiotensin-converting enzyme (ACE) inhibitors or angiotensin II receptor antagonists, may increase the incidence of symptomatic hypotension. Prior to initiating canagliflozin in such patients, intravascular volume should be assessed and corrected; patients should be monitored for signs and symptoms of hypotension after initiating therapy. (See Hypotension under Cautions: Warnings/Precautions.) These drugs also may cause hyperkalemia in patients with moderate renal impairment. Serum potassium concentrations should be monitored periodically following initiation of canagliflozin in patients predisposed to hyperkalemia due to drug therapy. (See Hyperkalemia under Cautions: Warnings/Precautions.)

■ **Uridine Diphosphate-glucuronosyltransferase Enzyme Inducers** Concomitant use of canagliflozin with an inducer of UGT enzymes may decrease the efficacy of canagliflozin. When a single dose of canagliflozin (300 mg) was administered to patients receiving rifampin (600 mg once daily for 8 days), a nonselective inducer of UGT isoenzymes 1A9 and 2B4, canagliflozin area under the concentration-time curve (AUC) was decreased by 51% and peak plasma concentration was reduced by 28% (based on geometric mean ratios). If concomitant use of a UGT enzyme inducer (e.g., rifampin, phenytoin, phenobarbital, ritonavir) and canagliflozin cannot be avoided, increasing the daily dosage of canagliflozin to 300 mg once daily should be considered in patients with an estimated glomerular filtration rate (eGFR) exceeding 60 mL/minute per 1.73 m^2 who are currently tolerating canagliflozin 100 mg once daily and require additional glycemic control. In patients with an eGFR of 45 to less than 60 mL/minute per 1.73 m^2 who are receiving concomitant therapy with a UGT enzyme inducer and require additional glycemic control, an alternative antidiabetic agent should be considered.

■ **Acetaminophen** Administration of a single dose of acetaminophen (1 g) to individuals receiving canagliflozin (300 mg twice daily for 25 days) had no effect on peak plasma acetaminophen concentration; acetaminophen AUC increased by 6% (based on geometric mean ratios). No adjustment of concomitant acetaminophen dosage is necessary.

■ **Antidiabetic Agents** When canagliflozin is added to therapy with an insulin secretagogue (e.g., a sulfonylurea) or insulin, the incidence of hypoglycemia is increased compared with sulfonylurea or insulin monotherapy. Patients receiving canagliflozin may require a reduced dosage of the concomitant insulin secretagogue or insulin to reduce the risk of hypoglycemia.

Administration of a single dose of glyburide (1.25 mg) to individuals receiving canagliflozin (200 mg once daily for 6 days) increased glyburide AUC by 2% (based on geometric mean ratios) and decreased peak plasma concentrations by 7% (based on geometric mean ratios). No adjustment of glyburide dosage is necessary with concomitant canagliflozin.

■ **Cyclosporine** Administration of a single dose of cyclosporine (400 mg) to individuals receiving canagliflozin (300 mg once daily for 8 days) increased canagliflozin AUC and peak plasma concentrations by 23 and 1%, respectively (based on geometric mean ratios). No adjustment of canagliflozin dosage is necessary with concomitant cyclosporine.

■ **Digoxin** Concomitant use of canagliflozin (300 mg once daily for 7 days) and digoxin (0.5 mg once daily for one day, then 0.25 mg once daily for 6 days) increased AUC and mean peak plasma concentration of digoxin by 20 and 36%, respectively (based on geometric mean ratios). Patients should be monitored appropriately when receiving canagliflozin and digoxin concomitantly.

■ **Diuretics** Concomitant use of canagliflozin with diuretics may increase the incidence of symptomatic hypotension. Prior to initiation of canagliflozin, volume status should be assessed and corrected in patients receiving diuretics. Patients should be monitored for signs and symptoms of symptomatic hypotension following initiation of canagliflozin therapy.

Patients with moderate renal impairment receiving potassium-sparing diuretics are more likely to develop hyperkalemia. Serum potassium concentrations should be monitored periodically following initiation of canagliflozin in patients predisposed to hyperkalemia due to drug therapy.

■ **Hormonal Contraceptives** Administration of a single dose of ethinyl estradiol (0.03 mg) and levonorgestrel (0.15 mg) to individuals receiving canagliflozin (200 mg once daily for 6 days) increased ethinyl estradiol and levonorgestrel AUC (7 and 6%, respectively, based on geometric mean ratios) and peak plasma concentration (22% for both drugs, based on geometric mean ratios) and decreased canagliflozin AUC and peak plasma concentration (9 and 8%, respectively, based on geometric mean ratios). No dosage adjustment is necessary for any of the drugs.

■ **Hydrochlorothiazide** Concurrent use of hydrochlorothiazide (25 mg once daily for 35 days) and canagliflozin (300 mg once daily for 7 days) increased canagliflozin AUC and peak plasma concentrations (12 and 15%, respectively, based on geometric mean ratios) and decreased hydrochlorothiazide AUC and peak plasma concentrations (1 and 6%, respectively, based on geometric mean ratios). No dosage adjustment is necessary for either drug. (See also Drug Interactions: Diuretics.)

■ **Metformin** In individuals receiving canagliflozin (300 mg once daily for 8 days), a single dose of metformin hydrochloride (2 g) increased canagliflozin and metformin AUCs (10 and 20%, respectively, based on geometric mean ratios) and peak plasma concentrations (5 and 6%, respectively, based on geometric mean ratios). No dosage adjustment is necessary for either drug.

■ **Probenecid** Concomitant use of probenecid (500 mg twice daily for 3 days) and canagliflozin (300 mg once daily for 17 days) increased canagliflozin AUC and peak plasma concentration by 21 and 13%, respectively (based on geometric mean ratios). No adjustment of canagliflozin dosage is necessary.

■ **Simvastatin** Administration of a single dose of simvastatin (40 mg) in individuals receiving canagliflozin (300 mg once daily for 7 days) increased simvastatin AUC and peak plasma concentration by 12 and 9%, respectively (based on geometric mean ratios). No simvastatin dosage adjustment is necessary.

■ **Warfarin** Administration of a single dose of warfarin (30 mg) in individuals receiving canagliflozin (300 mg once daily for 12 days) slightly increased *R*- and *S*-warfarin AUC (1 and 6%, respectively, based on geometric mean ratios) and peak plasma concentrations (3 and 1%, respectively, based on geometric mean ratios). No warfarin dosage adjustment is necessary.

Description

Canagliflozin inhibits sodium-glucose cotransporter 2 (SGLT2), a transporter that is expressed in the proximal renal tubules and is responsible for most of the reabsorption of filtered glucose from the tubular lumen. Through inhibition of SGLT2, canagliflozin reduces reabsorption of filtered glucose and lowers the renal threshold for glucose in a dose-dependent manner, leading to increased urinary glucose excretion; increased glucose excretion is independent of insulin secretion. Canagliflozin also may delay oral glucose absorption through transient inhibition of SGLT1 in the intestinal lumen.

Following oral administration of a single dose of canagliflozin, the median time to peak plasma concentration was 1–2 hours; mean absolute oral bioavailability of the drug is 65%. Administration of canagliflozin with a high-fat meal had no effect on the pharmacokinetics of the drug; canagliflozin may be administered with or without food. However, based on the potential of the drug to reduce postprandial plasma glucose excursions due to delayed intestinal glucose absorption, the manufacturer recommends that canagliflozin be taken with the first meal of the day. Following administration of a radiolabeled dose of canagliflozin, the dose was recovered in feces as unchanged drug (41.5%), a hydroxylated metabolite (7%), and an *O*-glucuronide metabolite (3.2%) and in urine as the *O*-glucuronide metabolites (30.5%) and unchanged drug (less than 1%). Terminal elimination half-life of canagliflozin was 10.6 and 13.1 hours for single doses of 100 and 300 mg, respectively.

The fixed combination of canagliflozin and extended-release metformin hydrochloride (Invokamet® XR) contains immediate-release canagliflozin and extended-release metformin hydrochloride. Results of a bioequivalence study indicate that the fixed-combination tablets containing canagliflozin and immediate-release metformin hydrochloride (Invokamet®) are bioequivalent to individual tablets of canagliflozin and metformin hydrochloride administered concomitantly in equivalent doses under fed conditions.

Advice to Patients

When canagliflozin is used in fixed combination with other drugs, importance of informing patients of important cautionary information about the concomitant agent(s).

Importance of patient reading medication guide before initiating therapy and each time the drug is dispensed.

Importance of informing patients of the potential risks and benefits of canagliflozin and of alternative therapies. Importance of *not* using canagliflozin in patients with type 1 diabetes mellitus or diabetic ketoacidosis.

Importance of informing patients that if a dose of canagliflozin or the fixed combination of canagliflozin and metformin hydrochloride is missed, it should be taken as soon as it is remembered; if it is almost time for the next dose, the patient should skip the missed dose and take the drug at the next regularly scheduled time. Advise patients not to take 2 doses of the drug at the same time.

Importance of informing patients that ketoacidosis, which can be a life-threatening condition, has been reported with canagliflozin therapy. Importance of informing patients receiving canagliflozin and their caregivers about the signs and symptoms of ketoacidosis (e.g., tachypnea or hyperventilation, anorexia, abdominal pain, nausea, vomiting, lethargy, mental status changes) and of instructing patients to discontinue canagliflozin and seek medical attention immediately should they experience any such signs or symptoms. Advise patients to use a ketone dipstick to check for ketones in their urine (when possible) if symptoms of ketoacidosis occur, even if blood glucose is not elevated (i.e., less than 250 mg/dL).

Importance of informing patients that canagliflozin therapy is associated with an increased risk of requiring lower limb amputations; risk may be higher in some patients, including those with peripheral vascular disease, neuropathy, diabetic foot ulcers, or a history of amputation. Importance of counseling patients on the importance of routine preventative foot care. Advise patients to monitor for new pain or tenderness, sores or ulcers, or infections involving the leg or foot and to seek medical attention immediately should they experience such signs or symptoms.

Importance of informing patients that symptomatic hypotension may occur with canagliflozin and to report such symptoms to their clinicians. Inform patients that canagliflozin-induced dehydration may increase the risk of hypotension and that patients should maintain adequate fluid intake.

Importance of informing patients that acute kidney injury has been reported with canagliflozin therapy. Advise patients to seek medical attention immediately if they experience decreased urine output, or swelling of the legs or feet. Advise patients to seek medical advice immediately if they have reduced oral intake (such as due to acute illness or fasting) or increased fluid losses (such as due to vomiting, diarrhea, or excessive heat exposure), as it may be appropriate to temporarily discontinue canagliflozin in those settings.

Importance of informing patients that yeast infection may occur (e.g., vulvovaginitis, balanitis, balanoposthitis). Importance of informing female patients of the signs and symptoms of vaginal yeast infections (e.g., vaginal discharge, odor, itching) and male patients of the signs and symptoms of balanitis or balanoposthitis (e.g., rash or redness of the glans or foreskin of the penis). Advise patients of treatment options and when to seek medical advice.

Importance of informing patients of the potential for urinary tract infections, which may be serious, with canagliflozin therapy. Advise patients of the signs and symptoms of urinary tract infection and the need to contact a clinician promptly if such signs and symptoms occur.

Importance of informing patients that necrotizing infections of the perineum (Fournier gangrene) have occurred with canagliflozin therapy. Advise patients to seek prompt medical attention if they experience any symptoms of tenderness, redness, or swelling of the genitals or the area from the genitals back to the rectum, occurring with a fever above 38°C or malaise.

Importance of informing patients that due to the mechanism of action of canagliflozin, patients taking the drug will test positive for glucose in urine.

Importance of not using urine glucose tests to monitor glycemic status while taking canagliflozin. (See Laboratory Test Interferences under Cautions: Warnings/Precautions.)

Risk of serious hypersensitivity reactions, such as rash, urticaria, and swelling of the face, lips, tongue, and throat that may result in difficulty breathing or swallowing. If signs or symptoms of such a reaction or anaphylaxis or angioedema occur, importance of discontinuing canagliflozin and informing clinician promptly.

Importance of informing patients about the potential for bone fractures (e.g., hip, lumbar spine) with canagliflozin therapy and of providing them with information about factors contributing to fracture risk.

Importance of informing patients about the importance of adherence to dietary instructions, regular physical activity, periodic blood glucose monitoring and glycosylated hemoglobin (hemoglobin A_{1c}; HbA_{1c}) testing, recognition and management of hypoglycemia and hyperglycemia, and assessment of diabetes complications.

Importance of seeking medical advice promptly during periods of stress such as fever, trauma, infection, or surgery as drug dosage requirements may change.

Importance of taking canagliflozin exactly as directed by clinician. Importance of advising patients not to discontinue canagliflozin without first discussing it with the prescribing clinician.

Importance of women informing their clinicians if they are or plan to become pregnant or plan to breast-feed. Advise pregnant women and women of childbearing potential of the possible risk to the fetus with canagliflozin therapy. Advise women that breastfeeding is not recommended during canagliflozin therapy.

Importance of informing clinicians of existing or contemplated concomitant therapy, including prescription (e.g., diuretics, rifampin, phenytoin, phenobarbital, ritonavir, digoxin) and OTC drugs and dietary or herbal supplements, as well as any concomitant illnesses.

Importance of informing patients of other important precautionary information. (See Cautions.)

Overview® (see Users Guide). For additional information on this drug until a more detailed monograph is developed and published, the manufacturer's labeling should be consulted. It is *essential* that the manufacturer's labeling be consulted for more detailed information on usual cautions, precautions, contraindications, potential drug interactions, laboratory test interferences, and acute toxicity.

Preparations

Excipients in commercially available drug preparations may have clinically important effects in some individuals; consult specific product labeling for details.

Canagliflozin

Oral

Tablet, film-coated	100 mg (of anhydrous canagliflozin)	**Invokana®**, Janssen
	300 mg (of anhydrous canagliflozin)	**Invokana®**, Janssen

Canagliflozin Combinations

Oral

Tablets, extended-release	50 mg (of anhydrous canagliflozin) with Extended-release Metformin Hydrochloride 500 mg	**Invokamet® XR**, Janssen
	50 mg (of anhydrous canagliflozin) with Extended-release Metformin Hydrochloride 1 g	**Invokamet® XR**, Janssen
	150 mg (of anhydrous canagliflozin) with Extended-release Metformin Hydrochloride 500 mg	**Invokamet® XR**, Janssen
	150 mg (of anhydrous canagliflozin) with Extended-release Metformin Hydrochloride 1 g	**Invokamet® XR**, Janssen
Tablets, film-coated	50 mg (of anhydrous canagliflozin) with Metformin Hydrochloride 500 mg	**Invokamet®**, Janssen
	50 mg (of anhydrous canagliflozin) with Metformin Hydrochloride 1 g	**Invokamet®**, Janssen
	150 mg (of anhydrous canagliflozin) with Metformin Hydrochloride 500 mg	**Invokamet®**, Janssen
	150 mg (of anhydrous canagliflozin) with Metformin Hydrochloride 1 g	**Invokamet®**, Janssen

Dapagliflozin Propanediol

■ Dapagliflozin propanediol, a sodium-glucose cotransporter 2 (SGLT2) inhibitor, is an antidiabetic agent.

Uses

■ **Type 2 Diabetes Mellitus** Dapagliflozin propanediol is used as monotherapy as an adjunct to diet and exercise to improve glycemic control in patients with type 2 diabetes mellitus. Dapagliflozin also is commercially available in fixed combination with extended-release metformin hydrochloride (Xigduo® XR) or saxagliptin (Qtern®). The fixed combination of dapagliflozin and extended-release metformin hydrochloride is used as an adjunct to diet and exercise to improve glycemic control in patients with type 2 diabetes mellitus when treatment with both drugs is appropriate. The fixed combination of dapagliflozin and saxagliptin is used as an adjunct to diet and exercise to improve glycemic control in patients with type 2 diabetes mellitus. Dapagliflozin also is used in combination with other antidiabetic agents (e.g., metformin, a sulfonylurea, a peroxisome proliferator-activated $receptor_\gamma$ [$PPAR_\gamma$] agonist [thiazolidinedione], a dipeptidyl peptidase-4 [DPP-4] inhibitor, a glucagon-like peptide [GLP-1] receptor agonist) or insulin as an adjunct to diet and exercise in patients with type 2 diabetes mellitus who have not achieved adequate glycemic control.

Current guidelines for the treatment of type 2 diabetes mellitus generally recommend metformin as first-line therapy in addition to lifestyle modifications because of its well-established safety and efficacy (e.g., beneficial effects on glycosylated hemoglobin [hemoglobin A_{1c}; HbA_{1c}], weight, and cardiovascular mortality) in patients with recent-onset or newly diagnosed type 2 diabetes mellitus or mild hyperglycemia. Because of the progressive nature of the disease, patients initially receiving an oral antidiabetic agent will eventually require multiple oral and/or injectable antidiabetic agents of different therapeutic classes and/or insulin for adequate glycemic control. Patients with inadequate glycemic control with metformin monotherapy should receive treatment with additional antidiabetic agents; data suggest that the addition of each noninsulin agent to initial therapy lowers HbA_{1c} by approximately 0.7–1%. Some experts recommend initiating antidiabetic therapy with 2 agents (metformin plus another agent) in patients whose HbA_{1c} is 7.5% or higher, while other experts recommend initiating such dual therapy in patients whose HbA_{1c} is at least 1.5% above the target level. When the greater glucose-lowering effect of an injectable drug is needed, some experts currently suggest that GLP-1 receptor agonists are preferred over insulin because of a lower risk of hypoglycemia and beneficial effects on body weight, although adverse GI effects may diminish tolerability. Early introduction of insulin therapy should be considered when hyperglycemia is severe (e.g., blood glucose of at least 300 mg/dL, HbA_{1c} of at least 10%), especially in the presence of catabolic manifestations (e.g., weight loss, hypertriglyceridemia, ketosis), or if symptoms of hyperglycemia are present. For additional information regarding the initiation of insulin therapy, see Uses: Diabetes Mellitus, in the Insulins General Statement 68:20.08.

Experts state that a patient's comorbidities should be considered when selecting additional (in addition to metformin) antidiabetic agents. Patients with type 2 diabetes mellitus who have established atherosclerotic cardiovascular disease (ASCVD) should receive a drug with demonstrated cardiovascular disease benefit (e.g., GLP-1 receptor agonist [e.g., liraglutide], sodium-glucose cotransporter 2 [SGLT2] inhibitor [e.g., empagliflozin]). In patients with ASCVD and heart failure or with an increased risk of heart failure, an SGLT2 inhibitor with demonstrated cardiovascular benefit may be preferred. An SGLT2 inhibitor or GLP-1 receptor agonist shown to reduce the risk of chronic kidney disease (CKD) progression, cardiovascular events, or both (e.g., canagliflozin, empagliflozin, liraglutide) should be considered in patients with type 2 diabetes mellitus and CKD. Experts state that SGLT2 inhibitors may be a good choice for patients at high risk of CKD progression (i.e., patients with albuminuria or a history of estimated glomerular filtration rate [eGFR] decline) because they may have a beneficial effect on the incidence of CKD; however, adequate renal function is required for their use. Some GLP-1 receptor agonists may be used in patients with lower eGFR and may provide greater benefits for reduction of ASCVD than for CKD progression or heart failure. In patients without ASCVD, heart failure, or CKD, the decision regarding the addition of other antidiabetic agents (e.g., sulfonylurea, thiazolidinedione, dipeptidyl peptidase-4 [DPP-4] inhibitor, SGLT2 inhibitor, GLP-1 receptor agonist, basal insulin) should be based on drug-specific effects and individual patient factors.

Dapagliflozin or the fixed combinations of dapagliflozin and extended-release metformin hydrochloride or saxagliptin should not be used in patients with type 1 diabetes mellitus or for the treatment of diabetic ketoacidosis.

Dapagliflozin Monotherapy When given as monotherapy for the management of type 2 diabetes mellitus, dapagliflozin improves glycemic control compared with placebo as evidenced by reductions in glycosylated hemoglobin (hemoglobin A_{1c}; HbA_{1c}) and in fasting and 2-hour postprandial plasma glucose concentrations. Efficacy of dapagliflozin as monotherapy has been established in 2 double-blind, placebo-controlled studies of 24-weeks' duration in 840 treatment-naive patients with type 2 diabetes mellitus and baseline HbA_{1c} concentrations of 7–10%. In the first study, HbA_{1c} was reduced by 0.8 or 0.9% in patients receiving dapagliflozin 5 or 10 mg once daily, respectively, compared with a decrease of 0.2% in those receiving placebo. In patients who received dapagliflozin 5 or 10 mg, approximately 44 or 51%, respectively, had HbA_{1c} reductions to less than 7%, compared with approximately 32% of patients receiving placebo. In the second study, mean HbA_{1c} reduction at week 24 was 0.68, 0.72, or 0.82% in patients receiving 1, 2.5, or 5 mg of dapagliflozin, respectively, compared with an increase of 0.02% in those receiving placebo.

Combination Therapy Clinical trials evaluating the safety and efficacy of the fixed combination of dapagliflozin and extended-release metformin hydrochloride (Xigduo® XR) in reducing HbA_{1c} have not been conducted; unless otherwise specified, clinical trials of dapagliflozin in combination with metformin discussed in this monograph were conducted using concomitantly administered dapagliflozin and immediate- or extended-release metformin hydrochloride. Bioequivalence between the fixed combination of dapagliflozin and extended-release metformin hydrochloride and each agent (dapagliflozin and extended-release metformin hydrochloride) given concurrently as separate tablets has been demonstrated. (See Description.) Safety and efficacy of the fixed combination of dapagliflozin and saxagliptin (Qtern®) have been established by clinical studies evaluating treatment with saxagliptin as add-on therapy to treatment with dapagliflozin and metformin hydrochloride or with dapagliflozin and saxagliptin as add-on therapy to treatment with metformin.

When given in combination with one or more oral antidiabetic agents (e.g., metformin, a sulfonylurea, a thiazolidinedione, a DPP-4 inhibitor) and/or insulin or a GLP-1 receptor agonist (e.g., exenatide), dapagliflozin improves glycemic control compared with monotherapy with these drugs and generally is associated with reductions in body weight and systolic blood pressure. Dapagliflozin generally is well tolerated, although genital mycotic infections appear to be more common with dapagliflozin than with other antidiabetic therapy.

Efficacy of dapagliflozin in combination with other antidiabetic agents for the management of type 2 diabetes mellitus is supported by results from several randomized, active- or placebo-controlled studies in patients receiving dapagliflozin with metformin, a sulfonylurea, metformin and a sulfonylurea, a thiazolidinedione, a DPP-4 inhibitor, a GLP-1 receptor agonist, or insulin. In these studies, initial combined therapy with dapagliflozin (5 or 10 mg once daily) and one or more antidiabetic drugs or addition of dapagliflozin to existing therapy improved glycemic control as evidenced by reductions in HbA_{1c}, fasting plasma glucose, and 2-hour postprandial plasma glucose concentrations; combined therapy also had beneficial effects on weight reduction and blood pressure compared with placebo and/or monotherapy.

In two 24-week studies in treatment-naive patients with baseline mean HbA_{1c} concentrations of 9–9.2%, the combination of extended-release metformin hydrochloride (up to 2 g daily) and dapagliflozin 5 or 10 mg once daily resulted in a reduction of 2.1 or 2%, respectively, in HbA_{1c} compared with a reduction of 1.5, 1.2 or 1.4% in HbA_{1c} with dapagliflozin 10 mg, dapagliflozin 5 mg, or extended-release metformin hydrochloride alone, respectively. Dapagliflozin 10 mg once daily was noninferior to metformin in reducing HbA_{1c}, and superior in reducing fasting plasma glucose; dapagliflozin in this dosage also was associated with substantially greater weight loss than metformin monotherapy.

In a 24-week study in patients with HbA_{1c} concentrations of 7–10% while receiving metformin hydrochloride (dosage of at least 1.5 g daily), the addition of dapagliflozin 5 or 10 mg resulted in a reduction of 0.7 or 0.8%, respectively, in HbA_{1c} compared with a 0.3% HbA_{1c} reduction with placebo. In these patients, add-on therapy with dapagliflozin 5 or 10 mg resulted in HbA_{1c} reductions to less than 7% in 37.5 or 40.6% of patients, respectively, compared with 25.9% of patients receiving add-on placebo. In a 78-week extension of this study, add-on dapagliflozin was associated with sustained reductions in HbA_{1c}, fasting plasma glucose, and body weight.

In a study in patients with HbA_{1c} concentrations of approximately 6.5–10% while receiving metformin hydrochloride (dosage of at least 1.5 g daily), add-on therapy with dapagliflozin (titrated to 10 mg once daily) was noninferior to add-on glipizide (titrated to 20 mg once daily) in reducing HbA_{1c} after 52 weeks of therapy. In addition, weight loss with add-on dapagliflozin therapy (3.2 kg) was superior to that with add-on glipizide therapy (1.4 kg).

In a 24-week study in patients who had inadequate glycemic control (HbA_{1c} concentration of 7–10%) while receiving a sulfonylurea antidiabetic agent (glimepiride), add-on therapy with dapagliflozin 2.5, 5, or 10 mg once daily resulted in a reduction of approximately 0.6, 0.6, or 0.8%, respectively, in HbA_{1c} compared with a reduction of approximately 0.1% with add-on placebo. In a 24-week study in patients who had inadequate glycemic control (HbA_{1c} concentration of 7–10.5%) on pioglitazone (30 or 45 mg daily), the addition of dapagliflozin 5 or 10 mg resulted in a reduction of 0.8 or 1%, respectively, in HbA_{1c} compared with a reduction of 0.4% with add-on placebo. Dapagliflozin also improved postprandial and fasting plasma glucose concentrations as well as reducing body weight and systolic blood pressure. In a 24-week study in patients who were treatment naive or who had inadequate glycemic control (HbA_{1c} concentration of 7–10%) while receiving sitagliptin (100 mg once daily) with or without metformin hydrochloride (dosage of at least 1.5 g daily), addition of dapagliflozin 10 mg once daily reduced HbA_{1c} by 0.45%, while patients receiving add-on placebo experienced no appreciable change. Patients receiving dapagliflozin add-on therapy also showed improved fasting plasma glucose and reduced body weight.

In a 24-week study in patients who had inadequate glycemic control (HbA_{1c} concentration 7–10.5%) while receiving immediate- or extended-release metformin hydrochloride (at least 1.5 g daily) plus a sulfonylurea antidiabetic agent at the maximum tolerated dosage (and at least 50% of the maximum dosage), add-on therapy with dapagliflozin 10 mg once daily was associated with a 0.7% reduction in HbA_{1c} compared with add-on placebo at 24 weeks. Add-on dapagliflozin therapy also was associated with reductions in fasting plasma glucose and body weight at week 24, and systolic blood pressure at week 8 compared with placebo.

In a 24-week study examining the effects of dapagliflozin on total body weight in patients with inadequate glycemic control on metformin hydrochloride, addition of dapagliflozin 10 mg once daily reduced total body weight by 2.96 kg compared with a reduction of 0.88 kg in those receiving add-on placebo.

Efficacy of dapagliflozin as add-on therapy to insulin in the management of type 2 diabetes mellitus in patients who have inadequate glycemic control (HbA_{1c} concentration of 7.5–10.5%) with insulin is supported by results of a 24-week, randomized, placebo-controlled study. In this study, addition of dapagliflozin (5 or 10 mg daily) to existing stable therapy with insulin (mean daily dosage of at least 30 units) with or without up to 2 additional oral antidiabetic agents resulted in improvements in HbA_{1c}, fasting plasma glucose, 2-hour postprandial plasma glucose concentrations, and body weight. In patients who received dapagliflozin 5 or 10 mg as add-on to insulin therapy with or without 1 or 2 additional antidiabetic agents, addition of dapagliflozin 5 or 10 mg reduced HbA_{1c} by 0.8 or 0.9%, respectively, compared with a 0.3% reduction in those receiving add-on placebo. During extended treatment and follow-up in this study, reductions in HbA_{1c}, body weight, and insulin dosage were maintained for 104 weeks with dapagliflozin therapy.

In a 12-week randomized, double-blind study in patients receiving insulin with or without up to 2 oral antidiabetic agents, HbA_{1c} was reduced by 0.7 or 0.78% with addition of dapagliflozin 10 or 20 mg once daily, respectively, to existing therapy compared with addition of placebo. The mean change from baseline in body weight at the end of the study was 4.5, 4.3, or 1.9 kg with dapagliflozin 10 mg, 20 mg, or placebo, respectively. Patients receiving add-on dapagliflozin 10 or 20 mg had mean *reductions* in insulin dosage from baseline of 1.4 and 0.8 units, respectively, at the end of the study compared with a mean *increase* from baseline of 1.7 units in those receiving add-on placebo.

Efficacy of the combination of dapagliflozin and saxagliptin with metformin hydrochloride for the management of type 2 diabetes mellitus is supported by several randomized, controlled clinical studies. In a 24-week study in patients with inadequate glycemic control (HbA_{1c} concentration of 7.5–10%) despite treatment with metformin hydrochloride, the addition of dapagliflozin and saxagliptin to existing therapy with metformin hydrochloride substantially improved glycemic control. Patients who received triple therapy with dapagliflozin, saxagliptin, and metformin hydrochloride had an HbA_{1c} reduction of 1.02% compared with a reduction of 0.62 or 0.69% in those who received dual therapy with dapagliflozin and metformin hydrochloride or saxagliptin and metformin hydrochloride, respectively. Additionally, a larger proportion of patients who received triple therapy achieved HbA_{1c} below 7% compared with those who received dual therapy.

In another clinical study of 24 weeks' duration, adults with type 2 diabetes mellitus who had inadequate glycemic control on metformin alone (HbA_{1c} 8–12%) received add-on therapy with 10 mg of dapagliflozin and 5 mg of saxagliptin, 10 mg of dapagliflozin, or 5 mg of saxagliptin. After 24 weeks, concomitant therapy with dapagliflozin and saxagliptin resulted in substantial decreases in HbA_{1c}, and a greater proportion of patients receiving this therapy achieved an HbA_{1c} below 7% compared with those receiving add-on therapy with dapagliflozin or saxagliptin.

In a clinical study evaluating the efficacy of add-on therapy with saxagliptin in adults (mean age: 54.6 years, 52.7% female, 87.9% Caucasian) with type 2 diabetes mellitus (mean HbA_{1c}: 7.9%) already receiving concomitant dapagliflozin and metformin therapy, the addition of saxagliptin resulted in substantial reductions in HbA_{1c}. The combination of the 3 agents was well tolerated, and patients receiving therapy with all 3 agents had a reduction in HbA_{1c} of 0.5% compared with a reduction of 0.2% in patients receiving dapagliflozin and metformin therapy.

Efficacy of dapagliflozin in conjunction with extended-release exenatide as add-on therapy to metformin hydrochloride in the management of type 2 diabetes mellitus in patients who have inadequate glycemic control (HbA_{1c} concentration of 8 to less than 12%) with metformin hydrochloride is supported by results of a 28-week, randomized, active-controlled study. In this study, addition of dapagliflozin (10 mg daily) and extended-release exenatide (2 mg subcutaneously every week) to existing stable therapy with metformin hydrochloride (at least 1.5 g daily) resulted in substantially greater improvements in HbA_{1c} and fasting plasma glucose compared with dapagliflozin or extended-release exenatide alone. In patients who received dapagliflozin 10 mg once daily and extended-release exenatide 2 mg once weekly as add-on to metformin hydrochloride therapy, addition of dapagliflozin and extended-release exenatide reduced HbA_{1c} by 1.8% compared with a 1.3 or 1.4% reduction in those receiving add-on therapy with dapagliflozin or extended-release exenatide alone, respectively. More weight loss and greater reductions in systolic blood pressure also were observed among those who received add-on therapy with dapagliflozin and extended-release exenatide compared with add-on therapy with either drug alone.

Macrovascular Outcomes and Cardiovascular Risk Reduction Some SGLT2 inhibitors have demonstrated the ability to reduce the risk of cardiovascular events in patients with type 2 diabetes mellitus and established cardiovascular disease. In addition to lowering blood glucose, SGLT2 inhibitors appear to modify several nonglycemic cardiovascular risk factors such as blood pressure, body weight, adiposity, and arterial stiffness.

Based on the findings of the TIMI-58 study, dapagliflozin appears to have a beneficial cardiovascular effect specifically related to heart failure; a lower rate of major adverse cardiovascular events compared with placebo was not observed. In the TIMI-58 study, patients 40 years of age or older with type 2 diabetes mellitus who had or were at risk for ASCVD received dapagliflozin 10 mg once daily or placebo for a median of 4.2 years. The use of other antidiabetic agents was at the discretion of the treating clinician. Approximately 59% of the patients had multiple risk factors for ASCVD (not *established* ASCVD); 10% of patients had a history of heart failure. The primary efficacy outcomes were major adverse cardiovascular events (e.g., cardiovascular death, myocardial infarction [MI], ischemic stroke) and the composite of cardiovascular death or hospitalization for heart failure. No difference between dapagliflozin and placebo with regards to major adverse cardiovascular effects was observed (event rate: 8.8 versus 9.4%, respectively). A lower rate of hospitalization for heart failure was observed in the dapagliflozin treatment group compared with placebo (event rate: 2.5 versus 3.3%, respectively); however, there was no difference between placebo and dapagliflozin with regards to the rate of cardiovascular death.

Beneficial Effects on Renal Function In several cardiovascular outcomes trials involving the use of SGLT2 inhibitors (e.g., canagliflozin, dapagliflozin, empagliflozin) in patients with type 2 diabetes mellitus at high risk for cardiovascular disease or with existing cardiovascular disease, beneficial effects on renal function have been observed as a secondary outcome. Experts state that the risk-benefit balance of SGLT2 inhibitor treatment appears to be favorable for most patients with type 2 diabetes mellitus and CKD. In the TIMI-58 study (see Macrovascular Outcomes and Cardiovascular Risk Reduction under Uses: Type 2 Diabetes Mellitus), dapagliflozin use was associated with a lower incidence of the composite renal outcome (at least a 40% decrease in eGFR to less than 60 mL/minute per 1.73 m^2, end-stage renal disease, or death from renal or cardiovascular causes).

Dosage and Administration

■ General Volume depletion should be corrected before initiating dapagliflozin. In addition, renal function should be assessed prior to treatment and periodically thereafter. (See Dosage and Administration: Special Populations.)

■ Administration Dapagliflozin or the fixed combination of dapagliflozin and saxagliptin is administered orally once daily in the morning, with or without food. The fixed combination of dapagliflozin and extended-release metformin hydrochloride is administered once daily in the morning with food to reduce the adverse GI effects of the metformin hydrochloride component.

The fixed-combination tablets of dapagliflozin and metformin hydrochloride or saxagliptin should be swallowed whole; tablets should not be split or cut.

If a dose of dapagliflozin, the fixed combination of dapagliflozin and extended-release metformin hydrochloride, or the fixed-combination of dapagliflozin and saxagliptin is missed, the missed dose should be taken as soon as it is remembered followed by resumption of the regular schedule. If the missed dose is not remembered until it is almost time for the next dose, the missed dose should be skipped and the regular schedule resumed; the dose should not be doubled to replace a missed dose.

■ Dosage ***Type 2 Diabetes Mellitus*** Dosage of dapagliflozin propanediol is expressed in terms of dapagliflozin.

Dapagliflozin Monotherapy. The recommended initial dosage of dapagliflozin for the management of type 2 diabetes mellitus in adults is 5 mg once daily. If well tolerated, the dosage may be increased to 10 mg once daily in patients who require additional glycemic control.

Dapagliflozin/Extended-Release Metformin Hydrochloride Fixed-Combination Therapy. When the commercially available fixed-combination preparation containing dapagliflozin and extended-release metformin hydrochloride (Xigduo® XR) is used in patients with type 2 diabetes mellitus, the recommended initial dosage is based on the patient's current regimen of dapagliflozin and/or metformin hydrochloride. For patients *not* currently receiving dapagliflozin, the recommended initial dosage of the dapagliflozin component is 5 mg once daily. Dosage should be titrated gradually based on effectiveness and tolerability, up to a maximum daily dosage of 10 mg of dapagliflozin and 2 g of extended-release metformin hydrochloride. Patients who are already receiving extended-release metformin hydrochloride in the evening and are switching to the fixed combination of dapagliflozin and metformin hydrochloride should skip their last dose of metformin hydrochloride before initiating therapy with the fixed combination the following morning.

Dapagliflozin/Saxagliptin Fixed-Combination Therapy. In patients *not* already receiving dapagliflozin therapy, the recommended initial dosage of the fixed combination of dapagliflozin and saxagliptin (Qtern®) is 5 mg of dapagliflozin and 5 mg of saxagliptin once daily in the morning. In patients who tolerate the initial dosage and require additional glycemic control, the dosage of the fixed combination may be increased to 10 mg of dapagliflozin and 5 mg of saxagliptin once daily in the morning.

The fixed combination of dapagliflozin and saxagliptin should not be used in patients receiving concomitant therapy with a potent cytochrome P-450 (CYP) 3A4/5 inhibitor (e.g., atazanavir, clarithromycin, indinavir, itraconazole, ketoconazole, nefazodone, nelfinavir, ritonavir, saquinavir, telithromycin). (See Drug Interactions: Drugs Affecting or Metabolized by Hepatic Microsomal Enzymes, in Saxagliptin 68:20.05.)

■ Special Populations Dosage adjustments for dapagliflozin or the fixed combination of dapagliflozin and saxagliptin are not necessary in patients with mild, moderate, or severe hepatic impairment. The use of the fixed-combination preparation containing dapagliflozin and extended-release metformin hydrochloride is not recommended in patients with hepatic impairment.

Dosage adjustments for dapagliflozin, the fixed combination of dapagliflozin and extended-release metformin hydrochloride, or the fixed combination of dapagliflozin and saxagliptin are not necessary in patients with an estimated glomerular filtration rate (eGFR) of at least 45 mL/minute per 1.73 m^2.

Dapagliflozin or the fixed combination of dapagliflozin and metformin hydrochloride should not be used in patients with an eGFR of less than 45 mL/minute per 1.73 m^2. (See Renal Impairment under Warnings/Precautions: Specific Populations, in Cautions.) Use of dapagliflozin or the fixed combination of dapagliflozin and metformin hydrochloride is contraindicated in patients with an eGFR of less than 30 mL/minute per 1.73 m^2. The fixed combination of dapagliflozin and saxagliptin is contraindicated in patients with an eGFR of less than 45 mL/minute per 1.73 m^2.

No dosage adjustment for dapagliflozin is necessary based solely on age. In addition, dosage adjustment is not recommended based on gender, race, or body weight.

Cautions

■ Contraindications History of serious hypersensitivity reaction to dapagliflozin or any ingredient in the formulation.

Dapagliflozin is contraindicated in patients with severe renal impairment (estimated glomerular filtration rate [eGFR] less than 30 mL/minute per 1.73 m^2), end-stage renal disease, or on dialysis.

■ Warnings/Precautions ***Ketoacidosis*** Use of sodium glucose cotransporter 2 (SGLT2) inhibitors in patients with type 2 diabetes mellitus may lead to ketoacidosis requiring hospitalization. Fatal cases of ketoacidosis have been reported in patients receiving dapagliflozin. Ketoacidosis associated with use of SGLT2 inhibitors may be present without markedly elevated blood glucose concentrations (e.g., less than 250 mg/dL).

FDA identified 73 cases of acidosis (reported as diabetic ketoacidosis [DKA], ketoacidosis, or ketosis) associated with SGLT2 inhibitor use in the FDA Adverse Event Reporting System (FAERS) between March 2013 and May 2015. DKA had an atypical presentation in most of the reported cases in that type 2 diabetes mellitus was noted as the indication for the drug, and glucose concentrations were only slightly elevated (median: 211 mg/dL); type 1 diabetes mellitus was named as the indication in a few cases, and in some reports the indication was not specified. The median time to onset of symptoms of acidosis following initiation or increase in dosage of the SGLT2 inhibitor was 43 days (range: 1–365 days). No trend demonstrating a relationship between the dosage of an SGLT2 inhibitor and the risk of ketoacidosis was identified. In all reported episodes, a diagnosis of DKA or ketoacidosis was made by the clinician and hospitalization or treatment in an emergency department was warranted. In most cases, at least 1 diagnostic laboratory criterion suggestive of ketoacidosis (e.g., high anion gap metabolic acidosis, ketonemia, reduced serum bicarbonate) was reported. Potential factors for the development of ketoacidosis with SGLT2 inhibitor therapy identified in the 73 cases included infection, low carbohydrate diet or reduced caloric intake (due to illness or surgery), pancreatic disorders suggesting insulin deficiency (e.g., type 1 diabetes mellitus, history of pancreatitis, pancreatic surgery), reduced dosage or discontinuance of insulin, discontinuance of an oral insulin secretagogue, and alcohol use.

Prior to initiating therapy with an SGLT2 inhibitor, clinicians should consider patient factors that may predispose the patient to ketoacidosis such as pancreatic insulin deficiency from any cause, reduced caloric intake, and alcohol abuse. Clinicians should evaluate for the presence of acidosis, including ketoacidosis, in patients experiencing signs or symptoms of acidosis while receiving SGLT2 inhibitors, regardless of the patient's blood glucose concentration. Additionally, clinicians should consider monitoring for ketoacidosis and temporarily discontinuing therapy with an SGLT2 inhibitor in clinical situations known to predispose individuals to ketoacidosis (e.g., prolonged fasting due to acute illness or surgery). If acidosis is confirmed, the SGLT2 inhibitor should be discontinued and appropriate treatment initiated to correct the acidosis; glucose concentrations should be monitored appropriately. In addition, supportive medical treatment should be instituted to treat and correct factors that may have precipitated or contributed to the metabolic acidosis. Euglycemic DKA associated with SGLT2 inhibitors may be detected and potentially prevented by having patients monitor urine and/or plasma ketone levels if they feel unwell, regardless of ambient glucose concentrations. Clinicians should inform patients and caregivers of the signs and symptoms of ketoacidosis (e.g., tachypnea or hyperventilation, anorexia, abdominal pain, nausea, vomiting, lethargy, mental status changes) and instruct patients to discontinue the SGLT2 inhibitor and immediately seek medical attention should they experience such signs or symptoms.

Hypotension Dapagliflozin may cause intravascular volume contraction. Following initiation of dapagliflozin, symptomatic hypotension can occur, particularly in patients with impaired renal function (eGFR less than 60 mL/minute per 1.73 m^2), geriatric patients, or patients receiving loop diuretics. (See Drug Interactions: Diuretics.) Prior to initiating dapagliflozin in such patients, intravascular volume status should be assessed and corrected. Patients should be monitored for signs and symptoms of hypotension after initiating dapagliflozin therapy.

Renal Effects Dapagliflozin causes intravascular volume contraction and can cause renal impairment. Dapagliflozin may increase serum creatinine concentration and decrease eGFR; geriatric patients and patients with impaired renal function may be more susceptible to these changes. Adverse reactions related to renal function can occur following initiation of the drug. Renal function should be evaluated prior to initiation of dapagliflozin and periodically thereafter.

FDA identified 101 cases of acute kidney injury associated with canagliflozin or dapagliflozin therapy in FAERS between March 2013 and October 2015. Hospitalization for evaluation and management of kidney injury was warranted in most cases, and some cases required admission to an intensive care unit and dialysis. In approximately half of the cases, onset of acute kidney injury occurred within 1 month or less of initiating canagliflozin or dapagliflozin therapy, and most patients' kidney function improved after stopping the drug. However, kidney injury may not be fully reversible in some situations and has led to death in some patients.

Prior to initiating dapagliflozin therapy, clinicians should consider patient factors that may predispose the patient to acute kidney injury, including hypovolemia, chronic renal insufficiency, heart failure, and concomitant medications (e.g., diuretics, angiotensin converting enzyme [ACE] inhibitors, angiotensin II receptor antagonists, nonsteroidal anti-inflammatory agents [NSAIAs]). Clinicians should consider temporarily discontinuing dapagliflozin in any setting of reduced oral intake (e.g., acute illness, fasting) or fluid losses (e.g., GI illness, excessive heat exposure). Patients should be monitored for acute kidney injury and the drug should be discontinued and appropriate treatment should be initiated if such injury occurs.

Concomitant Therapy with Hypoglycemic Agents When dapagliflozin is added to therapy with an insulin secretagogue (e.g., a sulfonylurea) or insulin, the incidence of hypoglycemia is increased compared with sulfonylurea or insulin monotherapy. Therefore, patients receiving dapagliflozin may require a reduced dosage of the concomitant insulin secretagogue or insulin to reduce the risk of hypoglycemia. (See Drug Interactions: Antidiabetic Agents.)

Fournier Gangrene Fournier gangrene (necrotizing fasciitis of the perineum), a rare but serious or life-threatening bacterial infection requiring urgent surgical intervention, has been reported during postmarketing surveillance in men and women with type 2 diabetes mellitus receiving an SGLT2 inhibitor, including dapagliflozin. Permanent disfigurement, prolonged hospitalization, disability, and complications from sepsis all may be associated with Fournier gangrene. Although diabetes mellitus is a risk factor for developing Fournier gangrene, this condition is still rare among patients with diabetes mellitus.

FDA identified 12 cases of Fournier gangrene in patients taking an SGLT2 inhibitor reported in FAERS and the medical literature between March 2013 and May 2018. Since FDA's review, additional cases of Fournier gangrene have been reported. In the initial cases reviewed by FDA, the average time to onset of infection was 9.2 months (range 7 days to 25 months) after initiation of therapy with an SGLT2 inhibitor. Some experts speculate that the variation in time to diagnosis of Fournier gangrene might be due to fluctuating glycemic control, microvascular complications, or an inciting event associated with SGLT2 inhibitors (e.g., urinary tract infection, mycotic infection, skin or mucosal breakdown due to pruritus). In all reported cases, hospitalization and surgery were required. Among these cases, some patients required multiple disfiguring surgeries, some developed complications (e.g., diabetic ketoacidosis, acute kidney injury, septic shock), and 1 patient died. In a review of other antidiabetic drugs (e.g., insulin, biguanides, sulfonylureas, dipeptidyl peptidase-4 inhibitors) over a period of more than 30 years, only 6 cases of Fournier gangrene were identified; all of theses cases occurred in men.

Patients receiving dapagliflozin who develop pain or tenderness, erythema, or swelling in the genital or perineal area, in addition to fever or malaise, should be assessed for necrotizing fasciitis. If Fournier gangrene is suspected, dapagliflozin should be discontinued and treatment should be initiated with broad-spectrum antibiotics; surgical debridement should be performed if necessary. Blood glucose concentrations should be closely monitored; alternative antidiabetic agents should be initiated to maintain glycemic control.

Genital Mycotic Infections Dapagliflozin may increase the risk of genital mycotic infections in males (e.g., balanitis) and females (e.g., vulvovaginal mycotic infection). In clinical trials, patients with a history of genital mycotic infections were more likely to develop such infections. Patients should be monitored for genital mycotic infections and appropriate treatment should be instituted if these infections occur.

Urosepsis and Pyelonephritis Dapagliflozin may increase the risk of serious urinary tract infections.

FDA identified 19 cases of urosepsis and pyelonephritis, which began as urinary tract infections associated with SGLT2 inhibitor use, in FAERS between March 2013 and October 2014. In all cases reported, hospitalization was warranted and some patients required admission to an intensive care unit or dialysis for treatment. The median time to onset of infection following initiation of the SGLT2 inhibitor was 45 days (range: 2–270 days).

Prior to initiating therapy with an SGLT2 inhibitor, clinicians should consider patient factors that may predispose the patient to serious urinary tract infections such as a history of difficulty urinating or infections of the bladder, kidneys, or urinary tract. Patients should be monitored for urinary tract infections and treatment instituted if indicated.

Risk of Bone Fracture An increased risk of bone fracture, along with dose-related decreases in bone mineral density in older adults, has been observed in patients receiving another drug in the SGLT2 inhibitor class (canagliflozin). (See Risk of Bone Fracture under Cautions: Warnings/Precautions, in Canagliflozin 68:20.18.) In a clinical trial, bone fractures were reported more frequently than with placebo in patients with moderate renal impairment (eGFR 30 to less than 60 mL/minute per 1.73 m^2) receiving dapagliflozin for up to 104 weeks; most fractures occurred within 52 weeks of initiating therapy. FDA is continuing to evaluate the risk of bone fracture with SGLT2 inhibitors.

Effects on Lipoproteins Increases in low-density lipoprotein (LDL)-cholesterol can occur during dapagliflozin therapy. Serum LDL-cholesterol concentrations should be monitored during treatment with dapagliflozin and such lipid elevations treated according to the standard of care.

Bladder Cancer In clinical studies, newly diagnosed cases of bladder cancer were reported in 0.17% of 6045 patients receiving dapagliflozin and 0.03% of 3512 patients receiving placebo or comparator drugs. In patients receiving the study drug for at least one year, there were 4 cases of bladder cancer with dapagliflozin and none with placebo or comparator drugs. There were too few cases to determine whether the emergence of these events is related to dapagliflozin; there are insufficient data to determine whether dapagliflozin has an effect on pre-existing bladder tumors.

The manufacturer states that dapagliflozin should not be used in patients with active bladder cancer. In patients with a history of bladder cancer, the benefits of glycemic control versus unknown risks for cancer recurrence with dapagliflozin should be considered.

Laboratory Test Interferences SGLT2 inhibitors such as dapagliflozin increase urinary glucose excretion and will result in false-positive urine glucose tests. In addition, the manufacturer states that the 1,5-anhydroglucitol assay is unreliable for monitoring glycemic control in patients taking SGLT2 inhibitors. Alternative methods of monitoring glycemic control should be used in patients receiving SGLT2 inhibitors.

Use of Fixed Combinations When dapagliflozin is used in fixed combination with metformin hydrochloride, saxagliptin, or other drugs, the cautions, precautions, contraindications, and interactions associated with the concomitant agent(s) must be considered in addition to those associated with dapagliflozin.

Sensitivity Reactions Hypersensitivity reactions (e.g., angioedema, urticaria, hypersensitivity), some serious, have been reported with dapagliflozin treatment. If a hypersensitivity reaction occurs, the drug should be discontinued, appropriate treatment instituted, and the patient monitored until signs and symptoms resolve.

Specific Populations **Pregnancy.** Data are lacking on the use of dapagliflozin in pregnant women. Based on the results of reproductive and developmental toxicity studies in animals, dapagliflozin use during pregnancy may affect renal development and maturation, especially during the second and third trimesters of pregnancy. The manufacturer states that dapagliflozin therapy is not recommended in pregnant women during the second and third trimesters of pregnancy.

Lactation. Dapagliflozin is distributed into milk in rats; it is not known whether the drug is distributed into human milk. Since human kidney maturation occurs in utero and during the first 2 years of life when lactational exposure may occur, there may be risk to the developing human kidney. Use of dapagliflozin in women who are breast-feeding is not recommended.

Pediatric Use. Safety and efficacy of dapagliflozin have not been established in pediatric patients younger than 18 years of age.

Geriatric Use. Among patients in 21 clinical trials, 1424 (24%) were 65 years of age or older and 207 (3.5%) were 75 years of age or older. Efficacy of dapagliflozin was similar for patients younger than 65 years of age and those 65 years of age or older after controlling for renal function (eGFR). Geriatric patients receiving dapagliflozin were more likely to experience certain adverse reactions related to volume depletion and renal impairment or failure compared with patients treated with placebo.

Hepatic Impairment. No dosage adjustment for dapagliflozin is recommended for patients with mild, moderate, or severe hepatic impairment. However, the benefits versus risks of using dapagliflozin in patients with severe hepatic impairment should be individually assessed since the safety and efficacy of dapagliflozin have not been established in this population.

Compared with values in healthy individuals, values for peak plasma dapagliflozin concentration were increased by 40% in patients with severe hepatic impairment (Child-Pugh Class C) following a single 10-mg dose of the drug. The area under the concentration-time curve (AUC) of dapagliflozin was increased by 67% in patients with severe hepatic impairment compared with that in healthy individuals. Differences in peak plasma concentration and AUC in patients with mild or moderate hepatic impairment were not considered clinically important.

Renal Impairment. Safety and efficacy of dapagliflozin were evaluated in 2 randomized, placebo-controlled studies that included patients with moderate renal impairment (eGFR of 45 to less than 60 mL/minute per 1.73 m^2 or eGFR of 30 to less than 60 mL/minute per 1.73 m^2). Patients with an eGFR of 45 to less than 60 mL/minute per 1.73 m^2 experienced adverse effects similar to those observed in patients without renal impairment. Additionally, these patients also experienced a substantial reduction in glycosylated hemoglobin (hemoglobin A_{1c}; HbA_{1c}) compared with placebo. Patients in this study who received dapagliflozin therapy had a greater reduction in eGFR compared with those who received placebo; however, renal function generally increased back to baseline values after discontinuing treatment with dapagliflozin. Patients with an eGFR of 30 to less than 60 mL/minute per 1.73 m^2 who received dapagliflozin had a greater incidence of bone fractures compared with those who were receiving placebo. (See Cautions: Contraindications.)

In patients with type 2 diabetes mellitus with mild, moderate, or severe renal impairment, geometric mean systemic exposures of dapagliflozin at steady state (20 mg once daily for 7 days) were 45%, 2.04-fold, or 3.03-fold higher, respectively, compared with patients with type 2 diabetes mellitus and normal renal function. Higher systemic exposure of dapagliflozin did not result in a correspondingly higher 24-hour urinary glucose excretion.

The impact of hemodialysis on dapagliflozin exposure is not known. (See Cautions: Contraindications.)

Renal function should be assessed prior to initiation of therapy and periodically thereafter.

■ **Common Adverse Effects** Adverse effects reported in at least 2% of patients receiving dapagliflozin in clinical trials and more commonly than with placebo include female genital mycotic infection, nasopharyngitis, urinary tract infection, back pain, increased urination, male genital mycotic infection, nausea, dyslipidemia, constipation, discomfort with urination, and pain in extremity.

Adverse effects reported in at least 2% of patients receiving dapagliflozin in combination with metformin hydrochloride and more commonly than with placebo in combination with metformin hydrochloride include female genital mycotic infection, nasopharyngitis, urinary tract infection, diarrhea, headache, male genital mycotic infection, influenza, nausea, back pain, dizziness, cough, constipation, dyslipidemia, pharyngitis, increased urination, and discomfort with urination.

Adverse effects reported in at least 2% of patients receiving dapagliflozin in combination with saxagliptin and metformin hydrochloride include upper respiratory tract infection, urinary tract infection, dyslipidemia, headache, diarrhea, back pain, genital infection, and arthralgia.

Drug Interactions

The metabolism of dapagliflozin is primarily mediated by uridine diphosphate-glucuronosyltransferase (UGT) isoenzyme 1A9.

■ **Drugs Affecting or Metabolized by Hepatic Microsomal Enzymes** Dapagliflozin and dapagliflozin 3-*O*-glucuronide, an inactive metabolite of dapagliflozin, did not inhibit cytochrome P-450 (CYP) isoenzymes 1A2, 2A6, 2B6, 2C8, 2C9, 2C19, 2D6 or 3A4 in in vitro studies. Dapagliflozin also does not induce CYP isoenzymes 1A2, 2B6, or 3A4 in vitro.

■ **Drugs Affected by Organic Anion Transporter** Dapagliflozin 3-*O*-glucuronide is a substrate of organic anion transport (OAT) 3. Dapagliflozin and dapagliflozin 3-*O*-glucuronide did not meaningfully inhibit OAT1 or OAT3 active transporters; pharmacokinetic interactions are unlikely with substrates of OAT1 or OAT3.

■ **Drugs Affected by Organic Cation Transporter** Dapagliflozin and dapagliflozin 3-*O*-glucuronide did not meaningfully inhibit organic cation transporter (OCT) 2; pharmacokinetic interactions are unlikely with substrates of OCT2.

■ **Drugs Affected by P-glycoprotein Transport** Dapagliflozin is a weak P-glycoprotein substrate, but does not meaningfully inhibit P-glycoprotein. The manufacturer states that dapagliflozin is unlikely to affect the pharmacokinetics of concurrently administered P-glycoprotein substrates.

■ **Antidiabetic Agents** When dapagliflozin is added to therapy with an insulin secretagogue (e.g., a sulfonylurea) or insulin, the incidence of hypoglycemia is increased compared with sulfonylurea or insulin monotherapy. Patients receiving dapagliflozin may require a reduced dosage of the concomitant insulin secretagogue or insulin to reduce the risk of hypoglycemia.

■ **Diuretics** Concomitant use of dapagliflozin with loop diuretics may increase the incidence of symptomatic hypotension. Prior to initiation of dapagliflozin, volume status should be assessed and corrected in patients receiving diuretics. Patients should be monitored for signs and symptoms of symptomatic hypotension following initiation of dapagliflozin therapy.

■ **Bumetanide** Administration of a single dose of bumetanide (1 mg) to individuals receiving dapagliflozin (10 mg once daily for 7 days) increased bumetanide area under the concentration-time curve (AUC) and peak plasma concentrations by 13%. The manufacturer states that no dosage adjustment of dapagliflozin or bumetanide is necessary. (See also Drug Interactions: Diuretics.)

■ **Digoxin** Administration of a single dose of digoxin (0.25 mg) with dapagliflozin (20 mg loading dose, then 10 mg once daily for 7 days) did not have a clinically meaningful effect on the AUC or peak plasma concentration of digoxin. The manufacturer states that no dosage adjustment of digoxin is necessary.

■ **Glimepiride** Administration of a single dose of glimepiride (4 mg) with a single dose of dapagliflozin (20 mg) increased glimepiride AUC by 13%; no dosage adjustment of either drug is necessary.

■ **Hydrochlorothiazide** Administration of a single dose of hydrochlorothiazide (25 mg) with a single dose of dapagliflozin (50 mg) did not have a clinically important effect on the pharmacokinetics of hydrochlorothiazide or dapagliflozin. The manufacturer states that no dosage adjustment of dapagliflozin or hydrochlorothiazide is necessary. (See also Drug Interactions: Diuretics.)

■ **Mefenamic Acid** Concurrent use of mefenamic acid (loading dose of 500 mg, then 250 mg every 6 hours for 14 doses) and a single dose of dapagliflozin (10 mg) increased dapagliflozin peak plasma concentration and AUC by 13 and 51%, respectively. No dosage adjustment of dapagliflozin is necessary.

■ **Metformin** Administration of a single dose of metformin (1 g) with a single dose of dapagliflozin (20 mg) did not have a clinically meaningful effect on the pharmacokinetics of dapagliflozin or metformin. No dosage adjustment of either drug is necessary.

■ **Pioglitazone** Administration of a single dose of pioglitazone (45 mg) with a single dose of dapagliflozin (50 mg) decreased pioglitazone peak plasma concentration by 7%. No dosage adjustment of either drug is necessary.

■ **Rifampin** Administration of rifampin (600 mg once daily for 6 days) with a single dose of dapagliflozin (10 mg) decreased dapagliflozin peak plasma concentration and AUC by 7 and 22%, respectively. No dosage adjustment of dapagliflozin is necessary.

■ **Simvastatin** Administration of a single dose of simvastatin (40 mg) with a single dose of dapagliflozin (20 mg) increased simvastatin AUC by 19%. The manufacturer states that no dosage adjustment of dapagliflozin or simvastatin is necessary.

■ **Sitagliptin** Administration of a single dose of sitagliptin (100 mg) with a single dose of dapagliflozin (20 mg) did not have a clinically meaningful effect on the pharmacokinetics of dapagliflozin or sitagliptin. No dosage adjustment of either drug is necessary.

■ **Valsartan** Administration of a single dose of valsartan (320 mg) with a single dose of dapagliflozin (20 mg) decreased peak plasma concentrations of valsartan and dapagliflozin by 6 and 12%, respectively, and increased valsartan AUC by 5%. The manufacturer states that no dosage adjustment of dapagliflozin or valsartan is necessary.

■ **Voglibose** Concomitant administration of voglibose (0.2 mg three times daily; not commercially available in the US) with a single dose of dapagliflozin (10 mg) did not have a clinically meaningful effect on the pharmacokinetics of dapagliflozin.

■ **Warfarin** Administration of a single dose of warfarin (25 mg) in individuals receiving dapagliflozin (20 mg loading dose, then 10 mg once daily for 7 days) did not have a clinically meaningful effect on the pharmacokinetics or pharmacodynamics of warfarin. No warfarin dosage adjustment is necessary.

Description

Dapagliflozin propanediol is a potent, competitive, reversible and highly selective inhibitor of sodium-glucose cotransporter 2 (SGLT2), a transporter that is expressed in the proximal renal tubules and is responsible for most of the reabsorption of filtered glucose from the tubular lumen. Through inhibition of SGLT2, dapagliflozin reduces reabsorption of filtered glucose and lowers the renal threshold for glucose in a dose-dependent manner, leading to increased urinary glucose excretion; increased glucose excretion is independent of insulin secretion. Reduction of plasma glucose with dapagliflozin to induce glucosuria improves sensitivity of muscle to insulin; however, glucosuria induction appears to be associated with a paradoxical increase in endogenous glucose production. Following dapagliflozin treatment, endogenous glucose production increased, accompanied by an increase in fasting plasma glucagon concentration.

Following oral administration of dapagliflozin in the fasting state, peak plasma concentration is usually attained within 2 hours. Following administration of a 10-mg dose, the absolute oral bioavailability of the drug is 78%. Administration of dapagliflozin with a high-fat meal decreased peak plasma concentration by up to 50% and prolonged time to peak plasma concentration by approximately 1 hour, but did not alter the area under the concentration-time curve (AUC). These changes are not considered clinically meaningful and dapagliflozin can be administered with or without food. Dapagliflozin is approximately 91% protein bound. Following administration of a single 50-mg radiolabeled dose of dapagliflozin, 75% and 21% total radioactivity is excreted in urine and feces, respectively, with less than 2% in urine as parent drug and approximately 15% in feces as parent drug. The mean terminal elimination half-life of dapagliflozin was approximately 12.9 hours following a single oral 10-mg dose.

Bioequivalence between the fixed combination of dapagliflozin and extended-release metformin hydrochloride (Xigduo® XR) and each agent (dapagliflozin and extended-release metformin hydrochloride) given concurrently as separate tablets has been demonstrated; however, the relative bioavailability of the fixed combination of dapagliflozin and extended-release metformin hydrochloride (Xigduo® XR) and concomitantly administered dapagliflozin and immediate-release metformin hydrochloride has not been established. Metformin hydrochloride immediate-release and extended-release tablets have a similar extent of absorption (AUC), but peak plasma concentrations of metformin following administration of the drug as extended-release tablets are approximately 20% lower than peak concentrations following administration of the same dose as immediate-release tablets.

Advice to Patients

Importance of patient reading medication guide before initiating therapy and each time the drug is dispensed.

When dapagliflozin is used in fixed combination with other drugs, importance of informing patients of important cautionary information about the concomitant agent(s).

Importance of informing patients of the potential risks and benefits of dapagliflozin and of alternative therapies. Importance of *not* using dapagliflozin in patients with type 1 diabetes mellitus or diabetic ketoacidosis.

Importance of informing patients that ketoacidosis, which can be a life-threatening condition, has been reported with dapagliflozin therapy. Importance of informing patients receiving dapagliflozin and their caregivers of the signs and symptoms of ketoacidosis (e.g., tachypnea or hyperventilation, anorexia, abdominal pain, nausea, vomiting, lethargy, mental status changes) and of instructing patients to discontinue dapagliflozin and seek medical attention immediately should they experience any such signs or symptoms. Advise patients to use a ketone dipstick to check for ketones in their urine (when possible) if symptoms of ketoacidosis occur, even if blood glucose is not elevated (e.g., less than 250 mg/dL).

Importance of informing patients that symptomatic hypotension may occur with dapagliflozin and advising patients to report such symptoms to their clinician. Inform patients that dapagliflozin-induced dehydration may increase the risk of hypotension and that patients should maintain adequate fluid intake.

Importance of informing patients that acute kidney injury has been reported with dapagliflozin therapy. Advise patients to seek medical attention immediately if they experience decreased urine output, or swelling of the legs or feet. Advise patients to seek medical advice immediately if they have reduced oral intake (such as due to acute illness or fasting) or increased fluid losses (such as due to vomiting, diarrhea, or excessive heat exposure), as it may be appropriate to temporarily discontinue dapagliflozin in those settings.

Importance of informing patients that necrotizing infections of the perineum (Fournier gangrene) have occurred with sodium-glucose cotransporter 2 (SGLT2) inhibitor therapy. Advise patients to promptly seek medical attention if they develop pain or tenderness, redness, or swelling of the genitals or the area from the genitals back to the rectum, in addition to fever (above 38°C) or malaise.

Importance of informing patients that yeast infection may occur (e.g., vulvovaginitis, balanitis, balanoposthitis). Importance of informing female patients of the signs and symptoms of vaginal yeast infections (e.g., vaginal discharge, odor, itching) and male patients of the signs and symptoms of balanitis or balanoposthitis (e.g., rash or redness of the glans or foreskin of the penis). Advise patients of treatment options and when to seek medical advice.

Importance of informing patients of the potential for urinary tract infections, which may be serious, with dapagliflozin therapy. Advise patients of the signs and symptoms of urinary tract infection and the need to contact a clinician if such signs and symptoms occur.

Importance of informing patients that due to the mechanism of action of dapagliflozin, patients taking the drug will test positive for glucose in their urine. Importance of not using urine glucose tests to monitor glycemic status while taking dapagliflozin. (See Laboratory Test Interferences under Cautions: Warnings/Precautions.)

Risk of serious hypersensitivity reactions, such as urticaria and angioedema. If signs or symptoms of such a reaction or angioedema occur, importance of discontinuing dapagliflozin and promptly informing clinician.

Importance of informing patients to promptly report any signs of macroscopic hematuria or other symptoms potentially indicative of bladder cancer.

Importance of informing patients about the importance of adherence to dietary instructions, regular physical activity, periodic blood glucose monitoring and glycosylated hemoglobin (hemoglobin A_{1c}; HbA_{1c}) testing, recognition and management of hypoglycemia and hyperglycemia, and assessment of diabetes complications.

Importance of promptly seeking medical advice during periods of stress such as fever, trauma, infection, or surgery as medication requirements may change.

Importance of taking dapagliflozin exactly as directed by clinician. (See Dosage and Administration: Administration.)

Importance of women informing their clinicians immediately if they are or plan to become pregnant or plan to breast-feed.

Importance of informing clinicians of existing or contemplated concomitant therapy, including prescription and OTC drugs and dietary or herbal supplements, as well as any concomitant illnesses.

Importance of informing patients of other important precautionary information. (See Cautions.)

Overview® (see Users Guide). For additional information on this drug until a more detailed monograph is developed and published, the manufacturer's labeling should be consulted. It is *essential* that the manufacturer's labeling be consulted for more detailed information on usual cautions, precautions, contraindications, potential drug interactions, laboratory test interferences, and acute toxicity.

Preparations

Excipients in commercially available drug preparations may have clinically important effects in some individuals; consult specific product labeling for details.

Dapagliflozin Propanediol

Oral		
Tablets, film-coated	5 mg (of dapagliflozin)	**Farxiga®**, AstraZeneca
	10 mg (of dapagliflozin)	**Farxiga®**, AstraZeneca

Dapagliflozin Propanediol Combinations

Oral		
Tablets, extended-release	2.5 mg (of dapagliflozin) with Extended-release Metformin Hydrochloride 1 g	**Xigduo® XR**, AstraZeneca
	5 mg (of dapagliflozin) with Extended-release Metformin Hydrochloride 500 mg	**Xigduo® XR**, AstraZeneca
	5 mg (of dapagliflozin) with Extended-release Metformin Hydrochloride 1 g	**Xigduo® XR**, AstraZeneca
	10 mg (of dapagliflozin) with Extended-release Metformin Hydrochloride 500 mg	**Xigduo® XR**, AstraZeneca
	10 mg (of dapagliflozin) with Extended-release Metformin Hydrochloride 1 g	**Xigduo® XR**, AstraZeneca
Tablets, film-coated	5 mg (of dapagliflozin) with Saxagliptin 5 mg	**Qtern®**, AstraZeneca
	10 mg (of dapagliflozin) with Saxagliptin 5 mg	**Qtern®**, AstraZeneca

Empagliflozin

■ Empagliflozin, a sodium-glucose cotransporter 2 (SGLT2) inhibitor, is an antidiabetic agent.

Uses

■ **Type 2 Diabetes Mellitus** Empagliflozin is used as monotherapy as an adjunct to diet and exercise to improve glycemic control in patients with type 2 diabetes mellitus. Empagliflozin also is used to reduce the risk of cardiovascular death in patients with type 2 diabetes mellitus and established cardiovascular disease. Empagliflozin is commercially available in fixed combination with immediate- or extended-release metformin hydrochloride (Synjardy® or Synjardy® XR, respectively) or linagliptin (Glyxambi®); the fixed-combination preparations are used as an adjunct to diet and exercise to improve glycemic control in patients with type 2 diabetes mellitus when treatment with both drugs is appropriate. The manufacturer states that the effectiveness of the fixed combination of empagliflozin and immediate- or extended-release metformin hydrochloride or linagliptin in reducing the risk of cardiovascular death in patients with type 2 diabetes mellitus and cardiovascular disease has not been established. Empagliflozin also is used in combination with other antidiabetic agents (e.g., metformin, a sulfonylurea, a peroxisome proliferator-activated receptor$_\gamma$ [PPAR$_\gamma$] agonist [thiazolidinedione], a dipeptidylpeptidase-4 [DPP-4] inhibitor) or insulin as an adjunct to diet and exercise in patients with type 2 diabetes mellitus who have not achieved adequate glycemic control.

Current guidelines for the treatment of type 2 diabetes mellitus generally recommend metformin as first-line therapy in addition to lifestyle modifications because of its well-established safety and efficacy (e.g., beneficial effects on glycosylated hemoglobin [hemoglobin A_{1c}; HbA_{1c}], weight, and cardiovascular mortality) in patients with recent-onset or newly diagnosed type 2 diabetes mellitus or mild hyperglycemia. Because of the progressive nature of the disease, patients initially receiving an oral antidiabetic agent will eventually require multiple oral and/or injectable antidiabetic agents of different therapeutic classes and/or insulin for adequate glycemic control. Patients with inadequate glycemic control with metformin monotherapy should receive treatment with additional antidiabetic agents; data suggest that the addition of each noninsulin agent to initial therapy lowers HbA_{1c} by approximately 0.7–1%. Some experts recommend initiating antidiabetic therapy with 2 agents (metformin plus another agent) in patients whose HbA_{1c} is 7.5% or higher, while other experts recommend initiating such dual therapy in patients whose HbA_{1c} is at least 1.5% above the target level. When the greater glucose-lowering effect of an injectable drug is needed, some experts currently suggest that glucagon-like peptide-1 (GLP-1) receptor agonists are preferred over insulin because of a lower risk of hypoglycemia and beneficial effects on body weight, although adverse GI effects may diminish tolerability. Early introduction of insulin therapy should be considered when hyperglycemia is severe (e.g., blood glucose of at least 300 mg/dL, HbA_{1c} of at least 10%), especially in the presence of catabolic manifestations (e.g., weight loss, hypertriglyceridemia, ketosis), or if symptoms of hyperglycemia are present. For additional information regarding the initiation of insulin therapy, see Uses: Diabetes Mellitus, in the Insulins General Statement 68:20.08.

Experts state that a patient's comorbidities should be considered when selecting additional (in addition to metformin) antidiabetic agents. Patients with type 2 diabetes mellitus who have established atherosclerotic cardiovascular disease (ASCVD) should receive a drug with demonstrated cardiovascular disease benefit (e.g., GLP-1 receptor agonist [e.g., liraglutide], sodium-glucose cotransporter 2 [SGLT2] inhibitor [e.g., empagliflozin]). In patients with ASCVD and heart failure or with an increased risk of heart failure, an SGLT2 inhibitor with demonstrated cardiovascular benefit may be preferred. An SGLT2 inhibitor or GLP-1 receptor agonist shown to reduce the risk of chronic kidney disease (CKD) progression, cardiovascular events, or both (e.g., canagliflozin, empagliflozin, liraglutide) should be considered in patients with type 2 diabetes mellitus and CKD. Experts state that SGLT2 inhibitors may be a good choice for patients at high risk of CKD progression (i.e., patients with albuminuria or a history of estimated glomerular filtration rate [eGFR] decline) because they may have a beneficial effect on the incidence of CKD; however, adequate renal function is required for their use. Some GLP-1 receptor agonists may be used in patients with lower eGFR and may provide greater benefits for reduction of ASCVD than for CKD progression or heart failure. In patients without ASCVD, heart failure, or CKD, the decision regarding the addition of other antidiabetic agents (e.g., sulfonylurea, thiazolidinedione, DPP-4 inhibitor, SGLT2 inhibitor, GLP-1 receptor agonist, basal insulin) should be based on drug-specific effects and individual patient factors.

Empagliflozin should not be used in patients with type 1 diabetes mellitus or for the treatment of diabetic ketoacidosis.

Empagliflozin Monotherapy When given as monotherapy for the management of type 2 diabetes mellitus, empagliflozin improves glycemic control compared with placebo as evidenced by reductions in glycosylated hemoglobin (hemoglobin A_{1c} [HbA_{1c}]) and fasting plasma glucose concentrations, and also reduces body weight. Efficacy of empagliflozin as monotherapy for the management of type 2 diabetes mellitus has been established in a phase 3, double-blind, placebo-controlled study of 24 weeks' duration in 986 adults with previously untreated type 2 diabetes mellitus (defined as receiving no oral or injected antidiabetic agents for 12 weeks prior to randomization or initiation of open-label treatment). Empagliflozin (10 mg or 25 mg once daily) improved glycemic control as evidenced by reductions in HbA_{1c}, fasting plasma glucose concentrations, and body weight. Patients with HbA_{1c} concentrations exceeding 10% were assigned open-label treatment with empagliflozin 25 mg once daily with no placebo run-in phase. Patients with HbA_{1c} concentrations of 7–10% entered a placebo run-in period for 2 weeks, and those who remained inadequately controlled received empagliflozin 10 mg once daily, empagliflozin 25 mg once daily, sitagliptin 100 mg once daily, or placebo. The primary end point of the study was change from baseline in HbA_{1c} at week 24. At 24 weeks, reductions (adjusted mean) in HbA_{1c} were 0.7, 0.8, or 0.7% in patients who received empagliflozin 10 mg, empagliflozin 25 mg, or sitagliptin 100 mg once daily, respectively; an increase (adjusted mean) in HbA_{1c} of 0.1% was observed in patients who received placebo. Also, at 24 weeks, the reduction (adjusted mean) in fasting plasma glucose concentrations was 19 or 25 mg/dL in patients who received empagliflozin 10 or 25 mg once daily, respectively, compared with an increase of 12 mg/dL in those receiving placebo. Patients who received empagliflozin 10 mg, empagliflozin 25 mg, or placebo once daily had reductions (adjusted mean) in body weight of 2.8, 3.2, or 0.4%, respectively, at week 24; systolic blood pressure was reduced by 2.6 mm Hg in patients who received empagliflozin 10 mg once daily and by 3.4 mm Hg in those who received empagliflozin 25 mg once daily compared with that in placebo recipients.

Combination Therapy When given in combination with one or more oral antidiabetic agents (e.g., metformin, a sulfonylurea, a thiazolidinedione, a DPP-4 inhibitor) or insulin, empagliflozin improves glycemic control compared with monotherapy with these drugs and generally is associated with reductions in body weight and systolic blood pressure. In a 24-week phase 3, randomized, double-blind, placebo-controlled study in 637 adults with inadequately controlled type 2 diabetes mellitus who were receiving metformin hydrochloride (at least 1.5 g daily, or maximum tolerated dosage, or maximum labeled dosage), addition of empagliflozin 10 or 25 mg once daily resulted in reductions of HbA_{1c} compared with placebo. Patients with HbA_{1c} concentrations exceeding 10% were assigned open-label treatment with empagliflozin 25 mg once daily without a placebo run-in phase. Patients with HbA_{1c} concentrations of 7–10% entered a placebo run-in period for 2 weeks, and those who remained inadequately controlled following the run-in phase received empagliflozin 10 mg, empagliflozin 25 mg, or placebo once daily for 24 weeks. The primary end point of the study was change from baseline in HbA_{1c} at week 24. Following 24 weeks of therapy, the addition of empagliflozin to current metformin treatment resulted in reductions (adjusted mean) in HbA_{1c} of 0.7, 0.8, and 0.1% in patients who received empagliflozin 10 mg once daily, empagliflozin 25 mg once daily, and placebo, respectively. In addition, at 24 weeks, the reduction (adjusted mean) in fasting plasma glucose concentration was 20 or 22 mg/dL in patients who received empagliflozin 10 or 25 mg once daily, respectively, compared with an increase of 6 mg/dL in those receiving placebo. Patients who received empagliflozin 10 mg, empagliflozin 25 mg, or placebo experienced reductions (adjusted mean) in body weight of 2.5, 2.9, or 0.5%, respectively, at week 24; systolic blood pressure was reduced compared with placebo by 4.1 mm Hg in patients who received empagliflozin 10 mg and by 4.8 mm Hg in those who received empagliflozin 25 mg.

Efficacy and safety of the combination of empagliflozin and metformin hydrochloride as initial therapy in treatment-naive patients with type 2 diabetes mellitus is supported by results of a 24-week, randomized, double-blind trial. In this trial, concurrent therapy with empagliflozin (10 or 25 mg once daily) and metformin hydrochloride (1 or 2 g daily) substantially improved glycemic control (as evidenced by reductions in HbA_{1c}), compared with empagliflozin or metformin hydrochloride monotherapy. Reductions in HbA_{1c} were 2 or 2.1% with 1 or 2 g daily, respectively, of metformin hydrochloride plus empagliflozin 10 mg once daily; 1.9 or 2.1% with 1 or 2 g daily, respectively, of metformin hydrochloride plus empagliflozin 25 mg once daily; 1.2 or 1.8% with 1 or 2 g daily, respectively, of metformin hydrochloride; and 1.4% with empagliflozin 10 or 25 mg once daily.

Efficacy of empagliflozin 10 or 25 mg once daily in combination with metformin hydrochloride (dosage of at least 1.5 g daily, or maximum tolerated dosage, or maximum labeled dosage) plus a sulfonylurea was established in 666 adults with type 2 diabetes mellitus in an international 24-week, phase 3, randomized, double-blind, placebo-controlled study. Patients with HbA_{1c} concentrations exceeding 10% were assigned open-label treatment with empagliflozin 25 mg. Patients with HbA_{1c} concentrations of 7–10% entered a placebo run-in period for 2 weeks, and those who remained inadequately controlled received empagliflozin 10 mg, empagliflozin 25 mg, or placebo once daily. The primary end point of the study was change from baseline in HbA_{1c} at week 24. Following 24 weeks of therapy, add-on therapy with empagliflozin reduced HbA_{1c} by 0.8, 0.8, or 0.2% (adjusted mean values) in patients who received empagliflozin 10 mg, empagliflozin 25 mg, or placebo once daily, respectively. Also, at 24 weeks, the reduction (adjusted mean) in fasting plasma glucose concentrations was 23 mg/dL in patients who received empagliflozin 10 or 25 mg once daily, compared with an increase of 6 mg/dL in those receiving placebo. Patients who received empagliflozin 10 mg, empagliflozin 25 mg, or placebo once daily had reductions (adjusted mean) in body weight of 2.9, 3.2, or 0.5%, respectively, at week 24.

Efficacy of empagliflozin 25 mg in combination with metformin hydrochloride (dosage of at least 1.5 g daily, or maximum tolerated dosage, or maximum labeled dosage) in an international phase 3, randomized, double-blind study was established in 1545 adults with type 2 diabetes mellitus. Patients with inadequately controlled type 2 diabetes mellitus (HbA_{1c} concentration of 7–10%) received empagliflozin 25 mg once daily or glimepiride 1–4 mg once daily (mean daily dosage of 2.7 mg) following a 2-week run-in period. The primary end point was change from baseline in HbA_{1c} concentrations at weeks 52 and 104. At week 52, add-on therapy with empagliflozin 25 mg or glimepiride 1–4 mg in patients receiving metformin resulted in a reduction in HbA_{1c} concentration of 0.7% for both drugs. At week 52, add-on therapy with empagliflozin 25 mg or glimepiride 1–4 mg reduced fasting plasma glucose concentrations by 19 or 9 mg/dL, respectively. Body weight was reduced by 3.9 or increased by 2% in those who received empagliflozin 25 mg or glimepiride 1–4 mg, respectively, plus metformin at week 52. At week 52, the reduction in systolic blood pressure in patients who received empagliflozin (3.6 mm Hg) was not appreciably different from that in patients who received glimepiride (2.2 mm Hg). Empagliflozin demonstrated noninferiority to glimepiride in glycemic control at weeks 52 and 104; the reduction (adjusted mean) in HbA_{1c} with empagliflozin was 0.11% greater than that with glimepiride at week 104.

In a 24-week, double-blind, placebo-controlled study in 498 adults with type 2 diabetes mellitus receiving pioglitazone (dosage of at least 30 mg daily, or maximum tolerated dosage, or maximum labeled dosage) with or without metformin hydrochloride (dosage of at least 1.5 g daily, or maximum tolerated dosage, or maximum labeled dosage), addition of empagliflozin 10 or 25 mg once daily reduced HbA_{1c}, fasting plasma glucose concentrations, and body weight. Following an open-label placebo run-in period of 2 weeks, patients with inadequate glycemic control (HbA_{1c} concentrations of 7–10%) received empagliflozin 10 mg, empagliflozin 25 mg, or placebo once daily, in addition to existing antidiabetic therapy with pioglitazone with or without metformin. The primary end point was change from baseline in HbA_{1c} concentrations at week 24. Addition of empagliflozin 10 or 25 mg to existing antidiabetic therapy resulted in reductions (adjusted mean) in HbA_{1c} of 0.6 or 0.7%, respectively, at week 24 compared with a reduction of 0.1% in patients receiving placebo. Patients receiving empagliflozin 10 or 25 mg had reductions (adjusted mean) in fasting plasma glucose concentrations of 17 or 22 mg/dL, respectively, at week 24 compared with an increase of 7 mg/dL with placebo. Reductions in body weight were 2.0, 1.8, or 0.6% in patients who received empagliflozin 10 mg, empagliflozin 25 mg, or placebo once daily, respectively.

In an international, phase 3, randomized, double-blind trial, add-on therapy with empagliflozin and linagliptin in fixed combination was more effective in reducing HbA_{1c} and fasting plasma glucose concentrations than add-on empagliflozin or linagliptin monotherapy in 686 adults with type 2 diabetes mellitus inadequately controlled with metformin hydrochloride (dosage of at least 1.5 g daily, or maximum tolerated dosage, or maximum labeled dosage). At 24 weeks, reduction in mean HbA_{1c} from baseline was 1.19% with empagliflozin 25 mg/linagliptin 5 mg, 1.08% with empagliflozin 10 mg/linagliptin 5 mg, 0.62% with empagliflozin 25 mg, 0.66% with empagliflozin 10 mg, and 0.7% with linagliptin 5 mg. Glycemic efficacy (HbA_{1c} reductions) with the fixed combinations of empagliflozin/linagliptin was maintained at week 52. The fixed combinations of empagliflozin and linagliptin also were associated with reductions from baseline in systolic blood pressure compared with linagliptin monotherapy. Body weight was reduced in patients receiving the fixed combinations of empagliflozin/linagliptin compared with linagliptin but not empagliflozin monotherapy.

In a double-blind, placebo-controlled study in 494 adults with inadequately controlled type 2 diabetes mellitus while receiving insulin with or without metformin and/or a sulfonylurea, add-on therapy with empagliflozin 10 or 25 mg once daily reduced HbA_{1c}, fasting plasma glucose concentrations, and body weight after 18 and 78 weeks of treatment. Following a 2-week placebo run-in period on basal insulin (e.g., insulin glargine, insulin detemir, or NPH insulin) with or without metformin and/or sulfonylurea therapy, patients received empagliflozin 10 or 25 mg or placebo once daily in addition to existing antidiabetic therapy. Patients were maintained on a stable dose of insulin prior to enrollment, during the run-in period, and during the first 18 weeks of treatment; for the remaining 60 weeks, adjustment of insulin dosage was permitted. Mean total daily insulin dosages at baseline for patients receiving empagliflozin 10 mg, empagliflozin 25 mg, or placebo were 45, 48, or 48 units, respectively. At 18 weeks, add-on therapy with empagliflozin 10 or 25 mg reduced HbA_{1c} concentration by 0.6 or 0.7% (adjusted mean values), respectively, compared with no change in HbA_{1c} concentration in patients who received placebo. Also, at 78 weeks, addition of empagliflozin 10 or 25 mg reduced HbA_{1c} concentration by 0.4 or 0.6% (adjusted mean values), respectively, compared with an increase of 0.1% in patients who received placebo. Following 18 weeks of treatment, the reduction in fasting plasma glucose concentrations in patients who received empagliflozin 10 or 25 mg plus existing antidiabetic therapy was 17.9 or 19.1 mg/dL, compared with an increase of 10.4 mg/dL in those who received placebo; at 78 weeks, the reduction in fasting plasma glucose concentrations in patients who received empagliflozin 10 or 25 mg was 10.1 or 15.2 mg/dL, compared with an increase of 2.8 mg/dL in those receiving placebo. Furthermore, reductions in body weight at 18 weeks in patients who received empagliflozin 10 mg, empagliflozin 25 mg, or placebo were 1.8, 1.4, or 0.1%, respectively; at 78 weeks, patients who received empagliflozin 10 or 25 mg had reductions of 2.4% in body weight, while those receiving placebo had an increase of 0.7% in body weight.

In a randomized, double-blind, placebo-controlled, international study in 563 obese patients (body mass index [BMI] of 30–45 kg/m^2) with inadequately controlled type 2 diabetes mellitus (HbA_{1c} concentrations 7.5–10%) despite multiple daily injections of insulin with or without metformin, add-on therapy with empagliflozin reduced HbA_{1c} and body weight. Following a 2-week, open-label, placebo run-in period, patients received empagliflozin 10 or 25 mg or placebo once daily as add-on therapy to insulin, with or without metformin hydrochloride (dosage of at least 1.5 g daily, maximum tolerated dosage, or maximum labeled dosage), for 52 weeks. The total daily dosage of insulin was adjusted to achieve a preprandial glucose target of less than 100 mg/dL and a postprandial glucose target of less than 140 mg/dL, except during the first 18 weeks (adjusted to be within 10% of prescribed dosage at randomization) and during weeks 41–52 (adjusted to be within 10% of the prescribed dosage at week 40 except for safety reasons). Metformin hydrochloride dosage was not adjusted during the study, although rescue therapy (e.g., metformin, insulin) could be initiated at any time during treatment if patients experienced clinically important hyperglycemia. The primary end point of the study was change from baseline in HbA_{1c} at week 18. At week 18, the reduction in HbA_{1c} was 0.94 or 1.02% in patients who received empagliflozin 10 or 25 mg once daily, respectively, as add-on therapy, compared with a reduction of 0.5% in patients who received placebo. At week 52, insulin titration resulted in additional reductions in HbA_{1c} of 1.18, 1.27, or 0.81% in those who received empagliflozin 10 mg, empagliflozin 25 mg, or placebo once daily, respectively. Also, at week 52, patients who received empagliflozin 10 or 25 mg once daily experienced reductions in body weight of 1.95 or 2.04 kg, respectively, compared with an increase in body weight of 0.44 kg in patients receiving placebo.

Efficacy and safety of empagliflozin in 738 adults with inadequately controlled type 2 diabetes mellitus (HbA_{1c} concentrations of 7–10%) and renal impairment were established in a phase 3, randomized, double-blind, placebo-controlled study. Patients with an estimated glomerular filtration rate (eGFR) of 60–89 mL/minute per 1.73 m^2 (mild renal impairment) received empagliflozin 10 or 25 mg or placebo once daily in addition to existing antidiabetic therapy. Patients with an eGFR of 30–59 mL/minute per 1.73 m^2 (moderate renal impairment) or 15–29 mL/minute per 1.73 m^2 (severe renal impairment) received empagliflozin 25 mg once daily or placebo. The primary end point was change from baseline in HbA_{1c} at week 24. At 24 weeks, empagliflozin 25 mg reduced HbA_{1c} concentration by 0.5% in the combined group of patients with mild or moderate renal impairment. Empagliflozin 25 mg also reduced HbA_{1c} concentration in patients with either mild (0.7% reduction) or moderate (0.4% reduction) renal impairment, and empagliflozin 10 mg reduced HbA_{1c} concentration by 0.5% in patients with mild renal impairment. Antihyperglycemic efficacy of empagliflozin 25 mg was reduced with decreasing level of renal function in the mild to moderate range. Mean reductions in HbA_{1c} at 24 weeks were 0.6, 0.5, and 0.2% for those with a baseline eGFR of 60–89 mL/minute per 1.73 m^2, 45–59 mL/minute per 1.73 m^2, and 30–44 mL/minute per 1.73 m^2 , respectively, for patients receiving empagliflozin 25 mg. In contrast, mean HbA_{1c} at 24 weeks increased by 0.1 or 0.2% in patients with a baseline eGFR of 60–89 mL/minute per 1.73 m^2 or 30–44 mL/minute per 1.73 m^2, respectively, and decreased by 0.1% in patients with a baseline eGFR of 45–59 mL/minute per 1.73 m^2 for patients receiving placebo. For patients with severe renal impairment, the analyses of changes in HbA_{1c} and fasting plasma glucose concentrations showed no discernible treatment effect of empagliflozin 25 mg compared with placebo.

Macrovascular Outcomes and Cardiovascular Risk Reduction

Some SGLT2 inhibitors such as empagliflozin have demonstrated the ability to reduce the risk of cardiovascular events in patients with type 2 diabetes mellitus and established cardiovascular disease. In addition to lowering blood glucose, SGLT2 inhibitors appear to modify several nonglycemic cardiovascular risk factors such as blood pressure, body weight, adiposity, and arterial stiffness. When empagliflozin is used for the management of type 2 diabetes mellitus in patients with established cardiovascular disease, empagliflozin reduces the risk of cardiovascular death, although with an increased risk of genital infections.

In the EMPA-REG OUTCOME study, adults (mean age: 63 years; 72% Caucasian) with type 2 diabetes mellitus and established, stable ASCVD (documented history of coronary artery disease [76%], stroke [23%], or peripheral artery disease [21%]) received empagliflozin (10 or 25 mg) once daily or placebo for a median duration of 2.6 years. During the study, additional antidiabetic agents and cardiovascular therapies were modified to achieve standard-of-care treatment targets with respect to blood glucose, lipids, and blood pressure. Concomitant use of other standard-of-care treatments for diabetes mellitus and ASCVD (renin-angiotensin system inhibitors [81%], β-blockers [65%], diuretics [43%], statins or ezetimibe [77%], antiplatelet agents [86%]) was permitted. A greater proportion of patients in the placebo group received additional antidiabetic agents (e.g., sulfonylurea, insulin), antihypertensive agents (e.g., diuretics), and anticoagulants during the study than those in the empagliflozin group. The primary outcome was the composite of death from cardiovascular causes, nonfatal myocardial infarction, or nonfatal stroke. In this study, patients who received empagliflozin had substantially lower rates of the primary cardiovascular outcome compared with those who received placebo (event rate 10.5 versus 12.1%, respectively). The lower rate of the composite outcome was driven by the substantial reduction in death from cardiovascular causes; there was no substantial difference between groups with regard to myocardial infarction or stroke.

Beneficial Effects on Renal Function In several cardiovascular outcomes trials involving the use of SGLT2 inhibitors (e.g., canagliflozin, dapagliflozin, empagliflozin) in patients with type 2 diabetes mellitus at high risk for cardiovascular disease or with existing cardiovascular disease, beneficial effects on renal function have been observed as a secondary outcome. Experts state that the risk-benefit balance of SGLT2 inhibitor treatment appears to be favorable for most patients with type 2 diabetes mellitus and CKD. In the EMPA-REG OUTCOME study (see Macrovascular Outcomes and Cardiovascular Risk Reduction under Uses: Type 2 Diabetes Mellitus), empagliflozin therapy was associated with slower progression of kidney disease and lower rates of renal events. Compared with placebo, empagliflozin reduced the risk of incident or worsening nephropathy (composite of urine:creatinine ratio exceeding 300 mg/dL, doubling of serum creatinine, end-stage renal disease, or death from end-stage renal disease) by 39%.

Dosage and Administration

■ **General** Volume depletion should be corrected before initiating empagliflozin. In addition, renal function should be assessed prior to treatment and periodically thereafter. (See Special Populations under Dosage and Administration: Dosage.)

■ **Administration** Empagliflozin or the fixed combination of empagliflozin and linagliptin is administered orally once daily in the morning, with or without food. The fixed combination of empagliflozin and immediate-release metformin hydrochloride should be administered twice daily with meals. The fixed combination of empagliflozin and extended-release metformin hydrochloride should be administered once daily with the morning meal; the tablet should be swallowed whole and should not be crushed, chewed, or cut.

If a dose is missed, the missed dose should be taken as soon as it is remembered followed by resumption of the regular schedule. If the missed dose is not remembered until it is almost time for the next dose, the missed dose should be skipped and the regular schedule resumed; the dose should not be doubled to replace a missed dose.

■ **Dosage** ***Type 2 Diabetes Mellitus*** **Empagliflozin Monotherapy.** The recommended initial dosage of empagliflozin for the management of type 2 diabetes mellitus in adults is 10 mg once daily in the morning. If this dosage is well tolerated, the dosage may be increased to 25 mg once daily in patients who require additional glycemic control.

Empagliflozin/Linagliptin Fixed-combination Therapy. The recommended initial dosage of the fixed-combination preparation is 10 mg of empagliflozin and 5 mg of linagliptin once daily in the morning. If this dosage is well tolerated, the dosage may be increased to 25 mg of empagliflozin and 5 mg of linagliptin once daily.

Empagliflozin/Metformin Hydrochloride Fixed-combination Therapy. The dosage of empagliflozin in fixed combination with metformin hydrochloride should be individualized based on the patient's current antidiabetic regimen. The dosage of the fixed-combination preparation may be increased gradually based on effectiveness and tolerability up to a maximum of 25 mg of empagliflozin and 2 g of metformin hydrochloride daily.

In patients currently receiving metformin hydrochloride, the recommended initial total daily dosage of the fixed combination is 10 mg of empagliflozin and a metformin hydrochloride dosage similar to the patient's existing total daily dosage, administered in 2 divided doses (when given as the fixed combination containing *immediate-release* metformin hydrochloride) or once daily (when given as the fixed combination containing *extended-release* metformin hydrochloride).

In patients currently receiving empagliflozin, the recommended initial total daily dosage of the fixed combination is the same daily dosage of empagliflozin and 1 g metformin hydrochloride, administered in 2 divided doses (when given as the fixed combination containing *immediate-release* metformin hydrochloride) or once daily (when given as the fixed combination containing *extended-release* metformin hydrochloride).

In patients currently receiving both empagliflozin and metformin hydrochloride, the recommended initial total daily dosage of the fixed combination is the same daily dosage of empagliflozin and a metformin hydrochloride dosage similar to the patient's total daily existing dosage, administered in 2 divided doses (when given as the fixed combination containing *immediate-release* metformin hydrochloride) or once daily (when given as the fixed combination containing *extended-release* metformin hydrochloride).

■ **Special Populations** Body mass index, gender, and race do not have a clinically meaningful effect on the pharmacokinetics of empagliflozin.

Hepatic Impairment **Empagliflozin Monotherapy.** Empagliflozin may be used in patients with hepatic impairment. No dosage adjustment is necessary in patients with mild, moderate, or severe hepatic impairment.

Empagliflozin/Linagliptin Fixed-combination Therapy. The fixed combination of empagliflozin and linagliptin may be used in patients with hepatic impairment.

Empagliflozin/Metformin Hydrochloride Fixed-combination Therapy. Use of the fixed-combination preparation of empagliflozin and immediate- or extended-release metformin hydrochloride is not recommended in patients with hepatic impairment.

Renal Impairment **Empagliflozin Monotherapy.** No dosage adjustment is necessary in patients with an estimated glomerular filtration rate (eGFR) of at least 45 mL/minute per 1.73 m^2. Empagliflozin should not be initiated in patients with an eGFR of less than 45 mL/minute per 1.73 m^2. (See Renal Impairment under Warnings/Precautions: Specific Populations, in Cautions.) The drug should be discontinued if the eGFR is persistently less than 45 mL/minute per 1.73 m^2. Renal function should be assessed before initiating empagliflozin and during therapy. More frequent monitoring is recommended in patients with eGFR less than 60 mL/minute per 1.73 m^2.

Empagliflozin/Linagliptin Fixed-combination Therapy. No dosage adjustment is necessary in patients with an eGFR of at least 45 mL/minute per 1.73 m^2. The fixed combination should not be initiated in patients with an eGFR less than 45 mL/minute per 1.73 m^2. The fixed-combination preparation should be discontinued if the eGFR is persistently less than 45 mL/minute per 1.73 m^2.

Empagliflozin/Metformin Hydrochloride Fixed-combination Therapy. No dosage adjustment is necessary in patients with an eGFR of at least 45 mL/minute per 1.73 m^2. Use of the fixed-combination preparation of empagliflozin and immediate- or extended-release metformin hydrochloride is contraindicated in patients with an eGFR less than 45 mL/minute per 1.73 m^2.

Geriatric Patients **Empagliflozin Monotherapy.** No dosage adjustment is necessary based solely on age.

Empagliflozin/Metformin Hydrochloride Fixed-combination Therapy. Renal function should be monitored frequently after initiating the fixed-combination preparation of empagliflozin and immediate- or extended-release metformin hydrochloride.

Cautions

■ **Contraindications** History of serious hypersensitivity reaction to empagliflozin or any ingredient in the formulation.

Severe renal impairment (estimated glomerular filtration rate [eGFR] less than 30 mL/minute per 1.73 m^2, end-stage renal disease, or dialysis.

■ **Warnings/Precautions** ***Ketoacidosis*** Use of sodium glucose cotransporter 2 (SGLT2) inhibitors (canagliflozin, dapagliflozin, empagliflozin) in patients with type 2 diabetes mellitus may lead to ketoacidosis requiring hospitalization. Ketoacidosis associated with use of SGLT2 inhibitors may be present without markedly elevated blood glucose concentrations (e.g., less than 250 mg/dL).

FDA identified 73 cases of acidosis (reported as diabetic ketoacidosis [DKA], ketoacidosis, or ketosis) associated with SGLT2 inhibitor use in the FDA Adverse Event Reporting System (FAERS) between March 2013 and May 2015 . DKA had an atypical presentation in most of the reported cases in that type 2 diabetes mellitus was noted as the indication for the drug, and glucose concentrations were only slightly elevated (median: 211 mg/dL); type 1 diabetes mellitus was named as the indication in a few cases, and in some reports the indication was not specified. The median time to onset of symptoms of acidosis following initiation or increase in dosage of the SGLT2 inhibitor was 43 days (range: 1–365 days). No trend demonstrating a relationship between the dosage of an SGLT2 inhibitor and the risk of ketoacidosis was identified. In all reported episodes, a diagnosis of DKA or ketoacidosis was made by the clinician and hospitalization or treatment in an emergency department was warranted. In most cases, at least 1 diagnostic laboratory criterion suggestive of ketoacidosis (e.g., high anion gap metabolic acidosis, ketonemia, reduced serum bicarbonate) was reported. Most cases of ketoacidosis were associated with a concurrent event, most commonly dehydration, infection, or change in insulin dosage. Potential factors for the development of ketoacidosis with SGLT2 inhibitor therapy identified in the 73 cases included infection, low carbohydrate diet or reduced caloric intake (due to illness or surgery), pancreatic disorders suggesting insulin deficiency (e.g., type 1 diabetes mellitus, history of pancreatitis, pancreatic surgery), reduced dosage or discontinuance of insulin, discontinuance of an oral insulin secretagogue, and alcohol use.

Prior to initiating therapy with an SGLT2 inhibitor, clinicians should consider patient factors that may predispose the patient to ketoacidosis such as pancreatic insulin deficiency from any cause, reduced caloric intake, and alcohol abuse. Clinicians should evaluate for the presence of acidosis, including ketoacidosis, in patients experiencing signs or symptoms of acidosis while receiving SGLT2 inhibitors, regardless of the patient's blood glucose concentration. Additionally, clinicians should consider monitoring for ketoacidosis and temporarily discontinuing therapy with an SGLT2 inhibitor in clinical situations known to predispose individuals to ketoacidosis (e.g., prolonged fasting due to acute illness or surgery). If acidosis is confirmed, the SGLT2 inhibitor should be discontinued and appropriate treatment initiated to correct the acidosis; glucose concentrations should be monitored appropriately. In addition, supportive medical treatment should be instituted to treat and correct factors that may have precipitated or contributed to the metabolic acidosis. Some clinicians suggest that euglycemic DKA associated with SGLT2 inhibitors may be detected and potentially prevented by having patients monitor urine and/or plasma ketone levels if they feel unwell, regardless of ambient glucose concentrations. Clinicians should inform patients and caregivers of the signs and symptoms of ketoacidosis (e.g., tachypnea or hyperventilation, anorexia, abdominal pain, nausea, vomiting, lethargy, mental status changes) and instruct patients to discontinue the SGLT2 inhibitor and immediately seek medical attention should they experience such signs or symptoms.

Hypotension Empagliflozin causes intravascular volume contraction. Following initiation of empagliflozin, symptomatic hypotension may occur, particularly in patients with impaired renal function, geriatric patients, patients with low systolic blood pressure, or patients receiving diuretics. (See Drug Interactions: Diuretics.) Prior to initiating empagliflozin, intravascular volume should be assessed and corrected if necessary. Patients should be monitored for signs and symptoms of hypotension after initiating therapy; monitoring should be increased in clinical situations in which volume contraction is expected.

Renal Effects Empagliflozin causes intravascular volume contraction and can cause renal impairment. Empagliflozin may increase serum creatinine concentration and decrease eGFR; patients with hypovolemia may be more susceptible to these changes. Abnormalities in renal function can occur following initiation of the drug. Patients should be monitored for acute kidney injury, and more frequent monitoring is recommended for patients with an eGFR less than 60 mL/minute per 1.73 m^2. If acute kidney injury occurs during empagliflozin therapy, the drug should be discontinued and appropriate therapy initiated.

There have been postmarketing reports of acute kidney injury in patients receiving SGLT2 inhibitors, including empagliflozin. FDA identified 101 cases of acute kidney injury associated with canagliflozin or dapagliflozin therapy in FAERS between March 2013 and October 2015. Hospitalization for evaluation and management of kidney injury was warranted in most cases, and in some cases required admission to an intensive care unit and initiation of dialysis. In approximately half of the cases, onset of acute kidney injury occurred within 1 month or less of initiating canagliflozin or dapagliflozin therapy, and most patients' kidney function improved after stopping the drug.

Prior to initiating empagliflozin therapy, clinicians should consider patient factors that may predispose the patient to acute kidney injury, including hypovolemia, chronic renal insufficiency, heart failure, and concomitant drug therapy (e.g., diuretics, angiotensin-converting enzyme [ACE] inhibitors, angiotensin II receptor antagonists, nonsteroidal anti-inflammatory agents [NSAIAs]). Clinicians should consider temporarily discontinuing empagliflozin in any setting of reduced oral intake (e.g., acute illness, fasting) or fluid losses (e.g., GI illness, excessive heat exposure).

Concomitant Therapy with Hypoglycemic Agents When empagliflozin is added to therapy with an insulin secretagogue (e.g., a sulfonylurea) or insulin, the risk of hypoglycemia is increased compared with sulfonylurea or insulin monotherapy. Therefore, patients receiving empagliflozin may require a reduced dosage of the concomitant insulin secretagogue or insulin to reduce the risk of hypoglycemia.

Fournier Gangrene Fournier gangrene (necrotizing fasciitis of the perineum), a rare but serious or life-threatening bacterial infection requiring urgent surgical intervention, has been reported during postmarketing surveillance in men and women with type 2 diabetes mellitus receiving an SGLT2 inhibitor, including empagliflozin. Permanent disfigurement, prolonged hospitalization, disability, and complications from sepsis all may be associated with Fournier gangrene. Although diabetes mellitus is a risk factor for developing Fournier gangrene, this condition is still rare among patients with diabetes mellitus.

FDA identified 12 cases of Fournier gangrene in patients taking an SGLT2 inhibitor reported in FAERS and the medical literature between March 2013 and May 2018. Since FDA's review, additional cases of Fournier gangrene have been reported. In the initial cases reviewed by FDA, the average time to onset of infection was 9.2 months (range 7 days to 25 months) after initiation of therapy with an SGLT2 inhibitor. Some experts speculate that the variation in time to diagnosis of Fournier gangrene might be due to fluctuating glycemic control, microvascular complications, or an inciting event associated with SGLT2 inhibitors (e.g., urinary tract infection, mycotic infection, skin or mucosal breakdown due to pruritus). In all reported cases, hospitalization and surgery were required. Among these cases, some patients required multiple disfiguring surgeries, some developed complications (e.g., diabetic ketoacidosis, acute kidney injury, septic shock), and 1 patient died. In a review of other antidiabetic drugs (e.g., insulin, biguanides, sulfonylureas, dipeptidyl peptidase-4 inhibitors) over a period of more than 30 years, only 6 cases of Fournier gangrene were identified; all of theses cases occurred in men.

Patients receiving empagliflozin who develop pain or tenderness, erythema, or swelling in the genital or perineal area, in addition to fever or malaise, should be assessed for necrotizing fasciitis. If Fournier gangrene is suspected, empagliflozin should be discontinued and treatment should be initiated with broad-spectrum antibiotics; surgical debridement should be performed if necessary. Blood glucose concentrations should be closely monitored; alternative antidiabetic agents should be initiated to maintain glycemic control.

Genital Mycotic Infections Empagliflozin may increase the risk of genital mycotic infections (e.g., vaginal mycotic infection, vaginal infection, genital fungal infection, vulvovaginal candidiasis, fungal vulvitis). In clinical trials, patients with a history of chronic or recurrent genital mycotic infections were more likely to develop such infections. Genital mycotic infections also occurred more frequently in female than male patients. Patients should be monitored for genital mycotic infections and appropriate treatment should be instituted if these infections occur.

Urosepsis and Pyelonephritis Empagliflozin may increase the risk of serious urinary tract infections.

FDA identified 19 cases of urosepsis and pyelonephritis, which began as urinary tract infections associated with SGLT2 inhibitor use, in FAERS between March 2013 and October 2014. In all cases reported, hospitalization was warranted and some patients required admission to an intensive care unit or dialysis for treatment. The median time to onset of infection following initiation of the SGLT2 inhibitor was 45 days (range: 2–270 days). In clinical studies of empagliflozin, urinary tract infections occurred more frequently in female patients compared with male patients, and risk of urinary tract infections increased in patients 75 years of age or older. Patients with a history of chronic or recurrent urinary tract infections were also more likely to develop such infections.

Prior to initiating therapy with an SGLT2 inhibitor, clinicians should consider patient factors that may predispose the patient to serious urinary tract infections such as a history of difficulty urinating; or infections of the bladder, kidneys, or urinary tract. Patients should be monitored for urinary tract infections and treatment instituted if indicated.

Effects on Lipoproteins Dose-related increases in low-density lipoprotein (LDL)-cholesterol concentration have been observed during empagliflozin therapy. Serum LDL-cholesterol concentrations should be monitored during treatment with empagliflozin and such lipid elevations should be treated according to the standard of care.

Potential Risk of Bone Fracture An increased risk of bone fracture, along with dose-related decreases in bone mineral density in older adults, has been observed in patients receiving another drug in the SGLT2 inhibitor class (canagliflozin). (See Risk of Bone Fracture under Cautions: Warnings/Precautions, in Canagliflozin.) FDA is continuing to evaluate the risk of bone fracture with SGLT2 inhibitors.

Laboratory Test Interferences SGLT2 inhibitors such as empagliflozin increase urinary glucose excretion and will result in false-positive urine glucose tests. In addition, the manufacturer states that the 1,5-anhydroglucitol assay is unreliable for monitoring glycemic control in patients taking SGLT2 inhibitors. Alternative methods of monitoring glycemic control should be used in patients receiving SGLT2 inhibitors.

Use of Fixed Combinations When empagliflozin is used in fixed combination with metformin hydrochloride, linagliptin, or other drugs, the cautions, precautions, contraindications, and interactions associated with the concomitant agent(s) must be considered in addition to those associated with empagliflozin.

Sensitivity Reactions Serious hypersensitivity reactions (e.g., angioedema, urticaria) have been reported with empagliflozin treatment. If a hypersensitivity reaction occurs, the drug should be discontinued, appropriate treatment instituted, and the patient monitored until signs and symptoms resolve. Empagliflozin is contraindicated in patients with a previous serious hypersensitivity reaction to empagliflozin or any excipient in the drug formulation.

Specific Populations **Pregnancy.** Data on the use of empagliflozin in pregnant women are lacking. Based on the results of reproductive and developmental toxicity studies in animals, empagliflozin use during pregnancy may affect renal development and maturation, especially during the second and third trimesters of pregnancy. Limited data with empagliflozin in pregnant women are not sufficient to determine a drug-associated risk for major birth defects or miscarriage, and poorly controlled diabetes mellitus during pregnancy carries risks to the mother and fetus; however, empagliflozin therapy is not recommended in pregnant women during the second and third trimesters of pregnancy.

Lactation. Empagliflozin is distributed into milk in rats; it is not known whether the drug is distributed into human milk. Because many drugs are distributed into human milk and because of the potential for serious adverse reactions in nursing infants from empagliflozin, a decision should be made whether to discontinue nursing or the drug, taking into account the importance of the drug to the woman.

Pediatric Use. Safety and efficacy of empagliflozin have not been established in pediatric patients younger than 18 years of age.

Geriatric Use. In clinical studies, 2721 (32%) patients treated with empagliflozin were 65 years of age or older and 491 (6%) were 75 years of age or older. Geriatric patients with renal impairment are expected to experience reduced efficacy when treated with empagliflozin. The risk of volume depletion-related adverse effects and urinary tract infections is increased in patients 75 years of age or older.

Hepatic Impairment. Empagliflozin may be used in patients with hepatic impairment. Compared with values in individuals with normal hepatic function, empagliflozin area under the concentration-time curve (AUC) was increased by approximately 23, 47, or 75% in patients with mild, moderate, or severe (Child-Pugh class A, B, or C) hepatic impairment, respectively; peak plasma concentrations of the drug in patients with mild, moderate, or severe hepatic function were increased by approximately 4, 23, or 48%, respectively.

Renal Impairment. Safety and efficacy of empagliflozin were evaluated in a study that included patients with mild or moderate renal impairment. Of those who received empagliflozin, 195 patients had an eGFR of 60–90 mL/minute per 1.73 m^2, 91 patients had an eGFR of 45–60 mL/minute per 1.73 m^2, and 97 patients had an eGFR of 30–45 mL/minute per 1.73 m^2. The glucose-lowering effect of empagliflozin 25 mg was reduced in patients with worsening renal function. In addition, the risk of renal impairment and of adverse effects related to volume depletion, and urinary tract infection increased with worsening renal function.

In patients with mild (eGFR 60 to less than 90 mL/minute per 1.73 m^2), moderate (eGFR 30 to less than 60 mL/minute per 1.73 m^2), or severe (eGFR less than 30 mL/minute per 1.73 m^2) renal impairment, and in patients with renal failure/end-stage renal disease, AUC of empagliflozin increased by approximately 18, 20, 66, and 48%, respectively, compared with those with normal renal function. Peak plasma concentrations of empagliflozin were similar in patients with moderate renal impairment or renal failure/end-stage renal disease compared with those with normal renal function; however, peak plasma concentrations of empagliflozin were approximately 20% higher in patients with mild or severe renal impairment compared with such concentrations in individuals with normal renal function.

Population pharmacokinetic studies demonstrated that the apparent oral clearance of empagliflozin was reduced, with a reduction in eGFR resulting in an increase in drug exposure. However, the fraction of empagliflozin excreted unchanged in urine and urinary glucose excretion declined with decrease in eGFR.

Efficacy and safety of empagliflozin have not been established in patients with severe renal impairment or end-stage renal disease, or in those receiving dialysis; empagliflozin is not expected to be effective in these patients.

■ **Common Adverse Effects** Adverse effects reported in at least 2% of patients receiving empagliflozin in clinical trials and more commonly than with placebo include urinary tract infection, female genital mycotic infections, upper respiratory tract infection, increased urination, dyslipidemia, arthralgia, male genital mycotic infections, and nausea.

Adverse effects reported in at least 5% of patients receiving empagliflozin and linagliptin in clinical trials include urinary tract infection, nasopharyngitis, and upper respiratory tract infection.

Adverse effects reported in at least 5% of patients receiving empagliflozin concomitantly with metformin and a sulfonylurea include hypoglycemia, urinary tract infection, and nasopharyngitis.

Drug Interactions

The major metabolic pathway for empagliflozin is glucuronidation; the drug is principally glucuronidated by uridine diphosphate-glucuronosyltransferase (UGT) isoenzymes 2B7, 1A3, 1A8, and 1A9.

■ **Drugs Affecting or Metabolized by Hepatic Microsomal Enzymes** Empagliflozin did not inhibit, inactivate, or induce cytochrome P-450 (CYP) isoforms in vitro; no effect of empagliflozin is expected on concomitantly administered drugs that are substrates of the major CYP isoforms.

■ **Drugs Affecting or Affected by Organic Anion Transporters** Empagliflozin is a substrate of organic anion transporter (OAT) 3 and organic anion transport proteins (OATP) 1B1 and 1B3. Empagliflozin is not a substrate of OAT1. Empagliflozin does not inhibit any of these transporters at clinically relevant plasma concentrations, and no effect of empagliflozin is expected on concomitantly administered drugs that are substrates of these uptake transporters.

■ **Drugs Affecting or Affected by Organic Cation Transporters** Empagliflozin is not a substrate of organic cation transporter (OCT) 2, nor does it inhibit OCT2 at clinically relevant plasma concentrations; no effect of empagliflozin is expected on concomitantly administered drugs that are substrates of this uptake transporter.

■ **Drugs Affecting or Metabolized by Uridine Diphosphate-glucuronosyltransferase** Empagliflozin does not inhibit UGT isoenzymes 1A1, 1A3, 1A8, 1A9, or 2B7, and no effect of empagliflozin is expected on concomitantly administered drugs that are substrates of these UGT isoenzymes. The manufacturer states the effect of UGT induction on empagliflozin exposure has not been established.

■ **Drugs Affecting or Affected by P-glycoprotein Transport** Empagliflozin is a substrate of P-glycoprotein (P-gp), but it does not inhibit P-gp at therapeutic doses. Empagliflozin is considered unlikely to cause interactions with drugs that are P-gp substrates based on in vitro studies.

■ **Drugs Affecting or Affected by Breast Cancer Resistance Protein** Empagliflozin is a substrate of breast cancer resistance protein (BCRP), but it does not inhibit BCRP at therapeutic doses.

■ **Antidiabetic Agents** Concomitant use of empagliflozin with insulin or insulin secretagogues increases the risk for hypoglycemia. Patients receiving empagliflozin may require a reduced dosage of the concomitant insulin secretagogue or insulin to reduce the risk of hypoglycemia.

■ **Digoxin** Administration of a single dose of digoxin (0.5 mg) in healthy individuals receiving empagliflozin 25 mg once daily did not have a clinically relevant effect on the pharmacokinetics of digoxin. No adjustment of digoxin dosage is necessary.

■ **Diuretics** Concomitant use of empagliflozin with diuretics may increase urine volume and frequency of urination, which may increase the risk of volume depletion. Patients should be assessed for volume contraction, and volume status should be corrected if indicated before initiating empagliflozin. Patients should be monitored for signs and symptoms of hypotension after initiating therapy, and monitoring should be increased in clinical situations where volume contraction is expected.

■ **Gemfibrozil** Concomitant administration of gemfibrozil 600 mg twice daily and a single dose of empagliflozin 25 mg resulted in an increase in area under the concentration-time curve (AUC) of empagliflozin, although this effect was not considered clinically relevant. No adjustment of empagliflozin dosage is necessary when administered with gemfibrozil.

■ **Glimepiride** Administration of a single dose of glimepiride (1 mg) in healthy individuals receiving empagliflozin 50 mg once daily did not have a clinically relevant effect on the pharmacokinetics of glimepiride or empagliflozin. No adjustment in either drug's dosage is necessary.

■ **Hormonal Contraceptives** Administration of 30 mcg of ethinyl estradiol once daily in healthy individuals receiving empagliflozin 25 mg once daily did not have a clinically relevant effect on the pharmacokinetics of ethinyl estradiol. Also, concomitant administration of levonorgestrel 150 mcg once daily and empagliflozin 25 mg once daily had no clinically relevant effect on the pharmacokinetics of levonorgestrel. No adjustment of ethinyl estradiol or levonorgestrel dosage is necessary when administered concomitantly with empagliflozin.

■ **Hydrochlorothiazide** Administration of hydrochlorothiazide 25 mg once daily in healthy individuals receiving empagliflozin 25 mg once daily did not have a clinically relevant effect on the pharmacokinetics of hydrochlorothiazide or empagliflozin. No adjustment in either drug's dosage is necessary. (See also Drug Interactions: Diuretics.)

■ **Linagliptin** Administration of linagliptin 5 mg once daily in healthy individuals receiving empagliflozin 50 mg once daily did not have a clinically relevant effect on the pharmacokinetics of linagliptin or empagliflozin. No adjustment in either drug's dosage is necessary.

■ **Metformin** Administration of metformin hydrochloride 1 g twice daily in healthy individuals receiving empagliflozin 50 mg once daily did not have a clinically relevant effect on the pharmacokinetics of metformin or empagliflozin. No adjustment in either drug's dosage is necessary.

■ **Pioglitazone** Concomitant use of pioglitazone 45 mg once daily in healthy individuals receiving empagliflozin 50 mg once daily did not have a clinically relevant effect on the pharmacokinetics of empagliflozin. Similarly, administration of pioglitazone 45 mg once daily in patients receiving empagliflozin 25 mg once daily did not have a clinically relevant effect on the pharmacokinetics of pioglitazone. No adjustment of empagliflozin dosage is necessary.

■ **Probenecid** Concomitant use of probenecid 500 mg twice daily in healthy individuals receiving a single dose of empagliflozin 10 mg resulted in an increase in AUC of empagliflozin. However, this effect was not clinically relevant. No adjustment of empagliflozin dosage is necessary when administered with probenecid. In patients with normal renal function, concomitant use of empagliflozin with probenecid resulted in a 30% decrease in the fraction of empagliflozin excreted in urine without any effect on 24-hour urinary glucose excretion. The manufacturer states that the relevance of this observation to patients with renal impairment is not known.

■ **Ramipril** Concomitant use of ramipril 5 mg once daily in healthy individuals receiving empagliflozin 25 mg once daily did not have a clinically relevant effect on the pharmacokinetics of ramipril or its active metabolite ramiprilat, or on empagliflozin pharmacokinetics. No adjustment of ramipril or empagliflozin dosage is necessary.

■ **Rifampin** Administration of a single dose of rifampin 600 mg in healthy individuals also receiving a single dose of empagliflozin 10 mg resulted in an increase in AUC of empagliflozin. However, this effect was not clinically relevant. No adjustment of empagliflozin dosage is necessary when administered with rifampin.

■ **Simvastatin** Administration of a single dose of simvastatin 40 mg in healthy individuals also receiving a single dose of empagliflozin 25 mg did not have a clinically relevant effect on the pharmacokinetics of simvastatin or its active metabolite simvastatin acid, or on empagliflozin pharmacokinetics. No adjustment of simvastatin or empagliflozin dosage is necessary.

■ **Sitagliptin** Concomitant administration of sitagliptin 100 mg once daily in healthy individuals receiving empagliflozin 50 mg once daily did not have a clinically relevant effect on the pharmacokinetics of sitagliptin or empagliflozin. No adjustment in either drug's dosage is necessary.

■ **Torsemide** Concomitant use of torsemide 5 mg once daily in healthy individuals receiving empagliflozin 25 mg once daily did not have a clinically relevant effect on the pharmacokinetics of torsemide or empagliflozin. No adjustment in either drug's dosage is necessary.

■ **Verapamil** Administration of a single dose of verapamil 120 mg in healthy individuals also receiving a single dose of empagliflozin 25 mg did not have a clinically relevant effect on the pharmacokinetics of empagliflozin. No adjustment of verapamil dosage is necessary.

■ **Warfarin** Administration of a single dose (25 mg) of warfarin sodium in healthy individuals also receiving empagliflozin 25 mg once daily did not have a clinically relevant effect on the pharmacokinetics of *R*- or *S*-warfarin or on the pharmacokinetics of empagliflozin. No adjustment in either drug's dosage is necessary.

Description

Empagliflozin is an orally active inhibitor of sodium-glucose cotransporter 2 (SGLT2), the transporter principally responsible for the reabsorption of glucose from the glomerular filtrate back into the circulation. Through inhibition of SGLT2, empagliflozin reduces renal reabsorption of filtered glucose and lowers the renal threshold for glucose, thereby increasing urinary glucose excretion and reducing blood glucose concentrations, independent of insulin secretion.

Following oral administration of empagliflozin 10 or 25 mg under fasting conditions, empagliflozin is rapidly absorbed; median time to peak plasma concentration of the drug was 1 hour for both doses. Empagliflozin exposure increased in proportion to the dose. Administration of empagliflozin 25 mg following intake of a high-fat and high-calorie meal resulted in slightly lower exposure. Peak concentration and area under the concentration-time curve decreased by approximately 37 and 16%, respectively, compared with fasting conditions. Effect of food on empagliflozin pharmacokinetics was not considered clinically relevant, and empagliflozin can be administered with or without food. Empagliflozin is 86.2% bound to plasma proteins. The apparent terminal elimination half-life of empagliflozin is approximately 12.4 hours. Following administration of a radiolabeled dose of empagliflozin, 41.2% of the administered dose was eliminated in feces and 54.4% was eliminated in urine.

Results of bioequivalence studies indicate that the fixed-combination tablets containing empagliflozin and immediate-release metformin hydrochloride or empagliflozin and linagliptin are bioequivalent to corresponding doses of empagliflozin, metformin hydrochloride, or linagliptin given concurrently as individual tablets.

Advice to Patients

When empagliflozin is used in fixed combination with other drugs, importance of informing patients of important cautionary information about the concomitant agent(s).

Importance of patient reading medication guide before initiating therapy and each time the drug is dispensed.

Importance of informing patients of the potential risks and benefits of empagliflozin and of alternative therapies. Importance of informing patients that use of empagliflozin with other antidiabetic agents may increase risk of hypoglycemia. Importance of *not* using empagliflozin in patients with type 1 diabetes mellitus or diabetic ketoacidosis.

Importance of informing patients that ketoacidosis, which can be a life-threatening condition, has been reported with empagliflozin therapy. Importance of informing patients receiving empagliflozin and their caregivers of the signs and symptoms of ketoacidosis (e.g., tachypnea or hyperventilation, anorexia, abdominal pain, nausea, vomiting, lethargy, mental status changes). If signs or symptoms of acidosis occur, importance of discontinuing empagliflozin and seeking medical attention immediately. Advise patients to use a ketone dipstick to check for ketones in their urine (when possible) if symptoms of ketoacidosis occur, even if blood glucose is not elevated (e.g., less than 250 mg/dL).

Importance of informing patients that hypotension may occur with empagliflozin and to report such symptoms to their clinicians. Inform patients that empagliflozin-induced dehydration may increase the risk of hypotension and that patients should maintain adequate fluid intake.

Importance of informing patients that acute kidney injury has been reported with empagliflozin therapy. Advise patients to seek medical advice immediately if they have reduced oral intake (such as due to acute illness or fasting) or increased fluid losses (such as due to vomiting, diarrhea, or excessive heat exposure), as it may be appropriate to temporarily discontinue empagliflozin in those situations.

Importance of informing female patients that vaginal yeast infections (e.g., vulvovaginitis) may occur. Importance of informing male patients that yeast infections may occur (e.g., balanitis, balanoposthitis), especially in uncircumcised males. Importance of informing patients that yeast infections occur more frequently in females and in patients with chronic and recurrent infections. Importance of informing female patients of the signs and symptoms of vaginal yeast infections (e.g., vaginal discharge, odor, itching) and male patients of the signs and symptoms of balanitis or balanoposthitis (e.g. rash or redness of the glans or foreskin of the penis, foul-smelling discharge from the penis, pain in skin around penis). Advise patients of treatment options and when to seek medical advice.

Importance of informing patients of the potential for urinary tract infections, which may be serious, with empagliflozin therapy. Advise patients of the signs and symptoms of urinary tract infection (e.g., dysuria, cloudy urine, pelvic or back pain) and the need to contact a clinician if such signs and symptoms occur.

Importance of informing patients that necrotizing infections of the perineum (Fournier gangrene) have occurred with empagliflozin therapy. Advise patients to seek prompt medical attention if they experience any symptoms of tenderness, redness, or swelling of the genitals or the area from the genitals back to the rectum, occurring with a fever above 38°C or malaise.

Risk of serious hypersensitivity reactions, such as urticaria and angioedema. If signs or symptoms of such reactions occur, importance of discontinuing empagliflozin and informing clinician promptly.

Importance of informing patients that due to the mechanism of action of empagliflozin, patients taking the drug will test positive for glucose in urine. Importance of not using urine glucose tests to monitor glycemic status while taking empagliflozin. (See Laboratory Test Interferences under Cautions: Warnings/Precautions.)

Importance of informing patients about the importance of adherence to dietary instructions, regular physical activity, periodic blood glucose monitoring and glycosylated hemoglobin (hemoglobin A_{1c} [HbA_{1c}]) testing, recognition and management of hypoglycemia and hyperglycemia, and assessment of diabetes complications.

Importance of seeking medical advice promptly during periods of stress such as fever, trauma, infection, or surgery as drug dosage requirements may change.

Importance of informing patient *not* to take empagliflozin if allergic to the drug or any ingredients in the formulation.

Importance of taking empagliflozin exactly as directed by clinician. Importance of informing patients that if a dose is missed, it should be taken as soon as remembered; the dose should not be doubled to make up for the missed dose. (See Dosage and Administration: Administration.)

Importance of informing patients that renal function should be assessed prior to initiation of empagliflozin and monitored periodically thereafter.

Importance of women informing their clinicians if they are or plan to become pregnant or plan to breast-feed.

Importance of informing clinicians of existing or contemplated concomitant therapy, including prescription and OTC drugs and dietary or herbal supplements, as well as any concomitant illnesses.

Importance of informing patients of other important precautionary information. (See Cautions.)

Overview® (see Users Guide). For additional information on this drug until a more detailed monograph is developed and published, the manufacturer's labeling should be consulted. It is *essential* that the manufacturer's labeling be consulted for more detailed information on usual cautions, precautions, contraindications, potential drug interactions, laboratory test interferences, and acute toxicity.

Preparations

Excipients in commercially available drug preparations may have clinically important effects in some individuals; consult specific product labeling for details.

Empagliflozin

Oral		
Tablets, film-coated	10 mg	**Jardiance®**, Boehringer Ingelheim
	25 mg	**Jardiance®**, Boehringer Ingelheim

Empagliflozin Combinations

Oral		
Tablets, extended-release	5 mg with Extended-release Metformin Hydrochloride 1 g	**Synjardy® XR**, Boehringer Ingelheim
	10 mg with Extended-release Metformin Hydrochloride 1 g	**Synjardy® XR**, Boehringer Ingelheim
	12.5 mg with Extended-release Metformin Hydrochloride 1 g	**Synjardy® XR**, Boehringer Ingelheim
	25 mg with Extended-release Metformin Hydrochloride 1 g	**Synjardy® XR**, Boehringer Ingelheim
Tablets, film-coated	5 mg with Metformin Hydrochloride 500 mg	**Synjardy®**, Boehringer Ingelheim
	5 mg with Metformin Hydrochloride 1 g	**Synjardy®**, Boehringer Ingelheim
	10 mg with Linagliptin 5 mg	**Glyxambi®**, Boehringer Ingelheim
	12.5 mg with Metformin Hydrochloride 500 mg	**Synjardy®**, Boehringer Ingelheim
	12.5 mg with Metformin Hydrochloride 1 g	**Synjardy®**, Boehringer Ingelheim
	25 mg with Linagliptin 5 mg	**Glyxambi®**, Boehringer Ingelheim

Ertugliflozin L-pyroglutamic Acid

■ Ertugliflozin L-pyroglutamic acid, a sodium-glucose cotransporter 2 (SGLT2) inhibitor, is an antidiabetic agent.

Uses

■ **Type 2 Diabetes Mellitus** Ertugliflozin is used as monotherapy as an adjunct to diet and exercise to improve glycemic control in patients with type 2 diabetes mellitus. Ertugliflozin also is used in combination with other antidiabetic agents (e.g., metformin, sitagliptin) as an adjunct to diet and exercise in patients with type 2 diabetes mellitus who have not achieved adequate glycemic control. Ertugliflozin is commercially available in fixed combination with metformin hydrochloride (Segluromet®) or sitagliptin (Steglujan®). The fixed combination of ertugliflozin and metformin hydrochloride is used as an adjunct to diet and exercise to improve glycemic control in patients with type 2 diabetes mellitus who are not adequately controlled with ertugliflozin or metformin monotherapy, or in patients who are already receiving therapy with both drugs. The fixed combination of ertugliflozin and sitagliptin is used as an adjunct to diet and exercise to improve glycemic control in patients with type 2 diabetes mellitus when treatment with both drugs is appropriate.

Current guidelines for the treatment of type 2 diabetes mellitus generally recommend metformin as first-line therapy in addition to lifestyle modifications because of its well-established safety and efficacy (e.g., beneficial effects on glycosylated hemoglobin [hemoglobin A_{1c}; HbA_{1c}], weight, and cardiovascular mortality) in patients with recent-onset or newly diagnosed type 2 diabetes mellitus or mild hyperglycemia. Because of the progressive nature of the disease, patients initially receiving an oral antidiabetic agent will eventually require multiple oral and/or injectable antidiabetic agents of different therapeutic classes and/or insulin for adequate glycemic control. Patients with inadequate glycemic control with metformin monotherapy should receive treatment with additional antidiabetic agents; data suggest that the addition of each noninsulin agent added to initial therapy lowers HbA_{1c} by approximately 0.7–1%. Some experts recommend initiating antidiabetic therapy with 2 agents (metformin plus another agent) in patients whose HbA_{1c} is 7.5% or higher, while other experts recommend initiating such dual therapy in patients whose HbA_{1c} is at least 1.5% above the target level. When the greater glucose-lowering effect of an injectable drug is needed, some experts suggest that glucagon-like peptide-1 (GLP-1) receptor agonists are preferred over insulin because of a lower risk of hypoglycemia and beneficial effects on body weight, although adverse GI effects may diminish tolerability. Early initiation of insulin therapy should be considered when hyperglycemia is severe (e.g., blood glucose of at least 300 mg/dL, HbA_{1c} of at least 10%), especially in the presence of catabolic manifestations (e.g., weight loss, hypertriglyceridemia, ketosis), or if symptoms of hyperglycemia are present. For additional information regarding the initiation of insulin therapy, see Uses: Diabetes Mellitus, in the Insulins General Statement 68:20.08.

Experts state that a patient's comorbidities should be considered when selecting additional (in addition to metformin) antidiabetic agents. Patients with type 2 diabetes mellitus who have established atherosclerotic cardiovascular disease (ASCVD) should receive a drug with demonstrated cardiovascular disease benefit (e.g., GLP-1 receptor agonist [e.g., liraglutide], sodium-glucose cotransporter 2 [SGLT2] inhibitor [e.g., canagliflozin, empagliflozin]). In patients with ASCVD and heart failure or with an increased risk of heart failure, an SGLT2 inhibitor with demonstrated cardiovascular benefit may be preferred. An SGLT2 inhibitor or GLP-1 receptor agonist shown to reduce the risk of chronic kidney disease (CKD) progression, cardiovascular events, or both (e.g., canagliflozin, empagliflozin, liraglutide) should be considered in patients with type 2 diabetes mellitus and CKD. Experts state that SGLT2 inhibitors may be a good choice for patients at high risk of CKD progression (i.e., patients with albuminuria or a history of estimated glomerular filtration rate [eGFR] decline) because they may have a beneficial effect on the incidence of CKD; however, adequate renal function is required for their use. Some GLP-1 receptor agonists may be used in patients with lower eGFR and may provide greater benefits for reduction of ASCVD than for CKD progression or heart failure. In patients without ASCVD, heart failure, or CKD, the decision regarding the addition of other antidiabetic agents (e.g., sulfonylurea, thiazolidinedione, dipeptidyl peptidase-4 [DPP-4] inhibitor, SGLT2 inhibitor, GLP-1 receptor agonist, basal insulin) should be based on drug-specific effects and individual patient factors.

Ertugliflozin should not be used in patients with type 1 diabetes mellitus or for the treatment of diabetic ketoacidosis.

Ertugliflozin Monotherapy When given as monotherapy for the management of type 2 diabetes mellitus, ertugliflozin improves glycemic control compared with placebo as evidenced by reductions in HbA_{1c} and in fasting and 2-hour postprandial plasma glucose concentrations. Efficacy of ertugliflozin as monotherapy has been established in a double-blind, placebo-controlled trial of 26-weeks' duration in approximately 460 patients with type 2 diabetes mellitus and a mean baseline HbA_{1c} of 8.21%. Patients were either treatment naive or were not receiving any antidiabetic agents for at least 8 weeks prior to trial screening. Ertugliflozin (5 or 15 mg once daily) improved glycemic control as evidenced by reductions in HbA_{1c} and fasting and 2-hour postprandial plasma glucose concentrations. HbA_{1c} was reduced by 0.7 or 0.8% in patients receiving ertugliflozin 5 or 15 mg once daily, respectively, compared with a reduction of 0.2% in those receiving placebo. In patients who received ertugliflozin 5 or 15 mg, approximately 30 or 39%, respectively, had HbA_{1c} reductions to less than 7% compared with approximately 17% of patients receiving placebo. Patients receiving ertugliflozin 5 or 15 mg once daily also lost substantially more body weight (reduction of 3 or 3.1 kg, respectively) than those receiving placebo (reduction of 1 kg).

Combination Therapy When given in combination with one or more oral antidiabetic agents, ertugliflozin improves glycemic control compared with monotherapy with these drugs and generally is associated with reductions in body weight and systolic blood pressure. Ertugliflozin generally is well tolerated, although genital mycotic infections appear to be more common with SGLT2 inhibitors such as ertugliflozin than with other classes of antidiabetic drugs.

Efficacy of ertugliflozin in combination with other antidiabetic agents for the management of type 2 diabetes mellitus is supported by results from several randomized, active- or placebo-controlled trials in patients receiving ertugliflozin with metformin, sitagliptin, or metformin and sitagliptin. In these trials, initial combined therapy with ertugliflozin (5 or 15 mg once daily) and one or more antidiabetic drugs or addition of ertugliflozin to existing therapy improved glycemic control as evidenced by reductions in HbA_{1c}, fasting plasma glucose, and 2-hour postprandial plasma glucose concentrations; combined therapy also had beneficial effects on weight reduction and blood pressure compared with placebo and/or monotherapy.

In a 26-week, randomized, double-blind trial in patients with type 2 diabetes mellitus inadequately controlled with metformin monotherapy, concomitant therapy with ertugliflozin (5 or 15 mg once daily) and existing metformin hydrochloride therapy (dosage of at least 1.5 g daily) substantially improved glycemic control (as evidenced by reductions in HbA_{1c}) compared with metformin monotherapy. Reductions in HbA_{1c} were 0.7 or 0.9% with ertugliflozin 5 or 15 mg once daily, respectively, plus metformin and 0.2% with existing metformin hydrochloride monotherapy. In patients who received metformin in conjunction with ertugliflozin 5 or 15 mg, approximately 36 or 43%, respectively, had HbA_{1c} reductions to less than 7%, compared with approximately 18% of patients receiving metformin monotherapy. The addition of ertugliflozin to existing metformin therapy also was associated with greater reductions in fasting plasma glucose, body weight, and blood pressure.

In a noninferiority trial of 52 weeks' duration in patients with type 2 diabetes mellitus who were inadequately controlled with metformin hydrochloride monotherapy (dosage of at least 1.5 g daily), once-daily therapy with ertugliflozin (5 or 15 mg) or glimepiride (mean daily dose 3 mg) was added to existing therapy with metformin. Ertugliflozin and glimepiride provided similar improvements in glycemic control (as measured by HbA_{1c}) and ertugliflozin 15 mg once daily was noninferior to glimepiride therapy. At week 52, approximately 48, 40, and 42% of patients in the glimepiride, ertugliflozin 5 mg, and ertugliflozin 15 mg treatment groups, respectively, had an HbA_{1c} of less than 7%. Greater reductions in body weight and systolic blood pressure from baseline also were observed in those patients who received ertugliflozin.

In a trial evaluating the safety and efficacy of ertugliflozin in combination with sitagliptin in adults with type 2 diabetes mellitus inadequately controlled with metformin hydrochloride monotherapy (dosage of at least 1.5 g daily), the addition of ertugliflozin and sitagliptin combination therapy to existing metformin therapy substantially improved glycemic control compared with the addition of either ertugliflozin or sitagliptin alone. In this trial, patients received ertugliflozin 5 mg, ertugliflozin 15 mg, sitagliptin 100 mg, ertugliflozin 5 mg and sitagliptin 100 mg, or ertugliflozin 15 mg and sitagliptin 100 mg once daily. At week 26, patients who received concomitant therapy with ertugliflozin 5 or 15 mg and sitagliptin 100 mg had greater reductions in HbA_{1c} (reduction of 1.4%) compared with those receiving ertugliflozin or sitagliptin alone (reduction of 1%). Additionally, a higher proportion of patients who received ertugliflozin 5 or 15 mg and sitagliptin 100 mg as an add-on to existing metformin therapy achieved an HbA_{1c} of less than 7% (53 or 51%, respectively) compared with those who received ertugliflozin 5 or 15 mg or sitagliptin 100 mg alone (29, 34, or 39%, respectively).

In a 26-week trial in patients receiving metformin hydrochloride (dosage of at least 1.5 g daily) and sitagliptin (100 mg once daily), the addition of ertugliflozin 5 or 15 mg once daily resulted in a reduction in HbA_{1c} of 0.7 or 0.8%, respectively, compared with a 0.2% reduction in HbA_{1c} with placebo. Approximately 35 or 42% of patients who received ertugliflozin 5 or 15 mg, respectively, had HbA_{1c} reductions to less than 7%, compared with approximately 20% of patients receiving placebo. Patients receiving ertugliflozin 5 or 15 mg once daily also had greater reductions in fasting plasma glucose, body weight, and systolic blood pressure than those receiving placebo.

Efficacy and safety of the combination of ertugliflozin and sitagliptin as initial therapy in patients with type 2 diabetes mellitus inadequately controlled with diet and exercise are supported by results of a 26-week, randomized, double-blind, placebo-controlled trial. In this trial, concomitant therapy with ertugliflozin (5 or 15 mg once daily) and sitagliptin (100 mg daily) substantially improved glycemic control (as evidenced by reductions in HbA_{1c}) compared with placebo. Reductions in HbA_{1c} were 1.6 or 1.7% with ertugliflozin 5 or 15 mg once daily, respectively, plus sitagliptin and 0.4% with placebo. Additionally, a greater proportion of patients receiving ertugliflozin and sitagliptin combination therapy achieved an HbA_{1c} of less than 7%, and greater reductions in fasting plasma glucose were observed with ertugliflozin and sitagliptin combination therapy compared with placebo.

Macrovascular Outcomes and Cardiovascular Risk Reduction Some SGLT2 inhibitors (e.g., canagliflozin, empagliflozin) have demonstrated the ability to reduce the risk of cardiovascular events in patients with type 2 diabetes mellitus and established cardiovascular disease. In addition to lowering blood glucose, SGLT2 inhibitors appear to modify several nonglycemic cardiovascular risk factors such as blood pressure, body weight, adiposity, and arterial stiffness.

The manufacturer states that data on the use of ertugliflozin for macrovascular risk reduction are lacking. For further discussion on the use of SGLT2 inhibitors for cardiovascular risk reduction, see Macrovascular Outcomes and Cardiovascular Risk Reduction under Uses: Type 2 Diabetes Mellitus, in Canagliflozin 68:20.18 and in Empagliflozin 68:20.18.

Beneficial Effects on Renal Function In several cardiovascular outcomes trials involving the use of SGLT2 inhibitors (e.g., canagliflozin, dapagliflozin, empagliflozin) in patients with type 2 diabetes mellitus at high risk for cardiovascular disease or with existing cardiovascular disease, beneficial effects on renal function were observed as a secondary outcome. Experts state that the risk-benefit balance of SGLT2 inhibitor treatment appears to be favorable for most patients with type 2 diabetes mellitus and CKD. For further discussion of the beneficial effects on renal function of SGLT2 inhibitors, see Beneficial Effects on Renal Function under Uses: Type 2 Diabetes Mellitus, in Empagliflozin 68:20.18.

Dosage and Administration

■ **General** Volume depletion should be corrected before initiating ertugliflozin. In addition, renal function should be assessed prior to treatment and periodically thereafter. (See Renal Impairment under Dosage and Administration: Special Populations.)

■ **Administration** Ertugliflozin or the fixed combination of ertugliflozin and sitagliptin is administered orally once daily in the morning, with or without food.

The fixed combination of ertugliflozin and metformin hydrochloride is administered orally twice daily with meals to reduce the adverse GI effects of the metformin hydrochloride component.

If a dose of ertugliflozin, the fixed combination of ertugliflozin and metformin hydrochloride, or the fixed combination of ertugliflozin and sitagliptin is missed, the missed dose should be taken as soon as it is remembered followed by resumption of the regular schedule. If the missed dose is not remembered until it is almost time for the next dose, the missed dose should be skipped and the regular schedule resumed; the dose should not be doubled to replace a missed dose.

■ **Dosage** ***Type 2 Diabetes Mellitus*** Dosage of ertugliflozin L-pyroglutamic acid is expressed in terms of ertugliflozin.

Ertugliflozin Monotherapy. The recommended initial dosage of ertugliflozin for the management of type 2 diabetes mellitus in adults is 5 mg once daily. If well tolerated, the dosage may be increased to 15 mg once daily in patients who require additional glycemic control.

Ertugliflozin/Metformin Hydrochloride Fixed-combination Therapy. When the commercially available fixed-combination preparation containing ertugliflozin and immediate-release metformin hydrochloride (Segluromet®) is used in patients with type 2 diabetes mellitus, the recommended initial dosage is based on the patient's current regimen of ertugliflozin and/or metformin hydrochloride. The dosage of the fixed combination may be increased gradually based on effectiveness and tolerability. The total dosage of the drugs in the fixed combination should not exceed 15 mg of ertugliflozin and 2 g of metformin hydrochloride daily.

For patients currently receiving metformin hydrochloride, the recommended initial total daily dosage of the fixed combination is 5 mg of ertugliflozin (using the fixed-combination tablets containing 2.5 mg of ertugliflozin) and a metformin hydrochloride dosage similar to the patient's existing total daily dosage, administered in 2 divided doses.

For patients currently receiving ertugliflozin, the recommended initial total daily dosage of the fixed combination is 1 g of metformin hydrochloride and an ertugliflozin dosage similar to the patient's existing total daily dosage, administered in 2 divided doses.

For patients currently receiving both ertugliflozin and metformin hydrochloride as separate components, the initial total daily dosage of the fixed combination is the same daily dosage of ertugliflozin and a metformin hydrochloride dosage similar to the patient's existing total daily dosage, administered in 2 divided doses.

Ertugliflozin/Sitagliptin Fixed-combination Therapy. The recommended initial dosage of the fixed combination of ertugliflozin and sitagliptin is 5 mg of ertugliflozin and 100 mg of sitagliptin once daily in the morning without regard to meals. If tolerated, the dosage may be increased to a dosage of 15 mg of ertugliflozin and 100 mg of sitagliptin in patients who require additional glycemic control. In patients currently receiving ertugliflozin and switching to the fixed combination of ertugliflozin and sitagliptin therapy, the current dosage of ertugliflozin can be maintained.

■ **Special Populations** ***Hepatic Impairment*** Dosage adjustments of ertugliflozin or the fixed combination of ertugliflozin and sitagliptin are not necessary in patients with mild or moderate hepatic impairment. Data are lacking on use of ertugliflozin or the fixed combination of ertugliflozin and sitagliptin in patients with severe hepatic impairment, and the manufacturer states that such use is not recommended. The manufacturer states that the use of the fixed combination of ertugliflozin and metformin hydrochloride is not recommended in patients with hepatic impairment.

Renal Impairment Dosage adjustments of ertugliflozin or the fixed combinations of ertugliflozin and metformin hydrochloride or ertugliflozin and sitagliptin are not necessary in patients with mild renal impairment (estimated glomerular filtration rate [eGFR] 60–89 mL/minute per 1.73 m^2). Initiation of ertugliflozin or the fixed combinations of ertugliflozin and metformin hydrochloride or ertugliflozin and sitagliptin is not recommended in patients with an eGFR of 30 to less than 60 mL/minute per 1.73 m^2. Continued use of ertugliflozin or the fixed combinations of ertugliflozin and metformin hydrochloride or ertugliflozin and sitagliptin is not recommended in patients with an eGFR persistently between 30 and less than 60 mL/minute per 1.73 m^2. The use of ertugliflozin or the fixed combinations of ertugliflozin and metformin hydrochloride or ertugliflozin and sitagliptin is contraindicated in patients with an eGFR less than 30 mL/minute per 1.73 m^2. (See Renal Impairment under Warnings/Precautions: Specific Populations, in Cautions.)

Cautions

■ **Contraindications** History of serious hypersensitivity reaction to ertugliflozin or any ingredient in the formulation.

Severe renal impairment (estimated glomerular filtration rate [eGFR] less than 30 mL/minute per 1.73 m^2), end-stage renal disease (ESRD), or on dialysis.

■ **Warnings/Precautions** ***Hypotension*** Ertugliflozin may cause intravascular volume contraction. Following initiation of ertugliflozin, symptomatic hypotension can occur, particularly in patients with impaired renal function (eGFR less than 60 mL/minute per 1.73 m^2), geriatric patients, patients with low systolic blood pressure, or patients receiving diuretics. (See Drug Interactions: Diuretics.) Prior to initiating ertugliflozin in such patients, intravascular volume status should be assessed and corrected. Patients should be monitored for signs and symptoms of hypotension after initiating ertugliflozin therapy.

Ketoacidosis Use of sodium glucose cotransporter 2 (SGLT2) inhibitors in patients with type 1 or 2 diabetes mellitus may lead to ketoacidosis requiring hospitalization. In clinical studies, ketoacidosis was reported in 0.1% of patients who received ertugliflozin; ketoacidosis was not reported in any of the comparator-treated patients. Ketoacidosis associated with use of SGLT2 inhibitors may be present without markedly elevated blood glucose concentrations (e.g., less than 250 mg/dL).

FDA identified 73 cases of acidosis (reported as diabetic ketoacidosis [DKA], ketoacidosis, or ketosis) associated with SGLT2 inhibitor use in the FDA Adverse Event Reporting System (FAERS) between March 2013 and May 2015. DKA had an atypical presentation in most of the reported cases in that type 2 diabetes mellitus was noted as the indication for the drug, and glucose concentrations were only slightly elevated (median: 211 mg/dL); type 1 diabetes mellitus was named as the indication in a few cases, and in some reports the indication was not specified. The median time to onset of symptoms of acidosis following initiation or increase in dosage of the SGLT2 inhibitor was 43 days (range: 1–365 days). No trend demonstrating a relationship between the dosage of an SGLT2 inhibitor and the risk of ketoacidosis was identified. In all reported episodes, a diagnosis of DKA or ketoacidosis was made by the clinician and hospitalization or treatment in an emergency department was warranted. In most cases, at least 1 diagnostic laboratory criterion suggestive of ketoacidosis (e.g., high anion gap metabolic acidosis, ketonemia, reduced serum bicarbonate) was reported. Potential factors for the development of ketoacidosis with SGLT2 inhibitor therapy identified in the 73 cases included infection, low carbohydrate diet or reduced caloric intake (due to illness or surgery), pancreatic disorders suggesting insulin deficiency (e.g., type 1 diabetes mellitus, history of pancreatitis, pancreatic surgery), reduced dosage or discontinuance of insulin, discontinuance of an oral insulin secretagogue, and alcohol use.

Prior to initiating therapy with an SGLT2 inhibitor, clinicians should consider patient factors that may predispose the patient to ketoacidosis such as pancreatic insulin deficiency from any cause, reduced caloric intake, and alcohol abuse. Clinicians should evaluate for the presence of acidosis, including ketoacidosis, in patients experiencing signs or symptoms of acidosis while receiving SGLT2 inhibitors, regardless of the patient's blood glucose concentration. Additionally, clinicians should consider monitoring for ketoacidosis and temporarily discontinuing therapy with an SGLT2 inhibitor in clinical situations known to predispose individuals to ketoacidosis (e.g., prolonged fasting due to acute illness or surgery). If acidosis is confirmed, the SGLT2 inhibitor should be discontinued and appropriate treatment initiated to correct the acidosis; glucose concentrations should be monitored appropriately. In addition, supportive medical treatment should be instituted to treat and correct factors that may have precipitated or contributed to the metabolic acidosis. Euglycemic DKA associated with SGLT2 inhibitors may be detected and potentially prevented by having patients monitor urine and/or plasma ketone levels if they feel unwell, regardless of ambient glucose concentrations. Clinicians should inform patients and caregivers of the signs and symptoms of ketoacidosis (e.g., tachypnea or hyperventilation, anorexia, abdominal pain, nausea, vomiting, lethargy, mental status changes) and instruct patients to discontinue the SGLT2 inhibitor and immediately seek medical attention should they experience such signs or symptoms.

Renal Effects Ertugliflozin causes intravascular volume contraction and can cause renal impairment. Ertugliflozin increases serum creatinine concentrations and decreases eGFR; patients with impaired renal function may be more susceptible to these changes. Adverse effects related to renal function can occur following initiation of the drug. Renal function should be evaluated prior to initiation of ertugliflozin and periodically thereafter.

FDA identified 101 cases of acute kidney injury associated with canagliflozin or dapagliflozin therapy in FAERS between March 2013 and October 2015. Hospitalization for evaluation and management of kidney injury was warranted in most cases, and some cases required admission to an intensive care unit and dialysis. In approximately half of the cases, onset of acute kidney injury occurred within 1 month or less of initiating canagliflozin or dapagliflozin therapy, and most patients' kidney function improved after stopping the drug. However, kidney injury may not be fully reversible in some situations and has led to death in some patients.

Prior to initiating ertugliflozin therapy, clinicians should consider patient factors that may predispose the patient to acute kidney injury, including hypovolemia, chronic renal insufficiency, heart failure, and concomitant medications (e.g., diuretics, angiotensin-converting enzyme [ACE] inhibitors, angiotensin II receptor antagonists, nonsteroidal anti-inflammatory agents [NSAIAs]). Clinicians should consider temporarily discontinuing ertugliflozin in any setting of reduced oral intake (e.g., acute illness, fasting) or fluid losses (e.g., GI illness, excessive heat exposure). Patients should be monitored for acute kidney injury and the drug should be discontinued and appropriate treatment should be initiated if such injury occurs.

Urosepsis and Pyelonephritis Treatment with an SGLT2 inhibitor increases the risk for urinary tract infections.

Cases of serious urinary tract infections, including urosepsis and pyelonephritis, have been reported in patients receiving an SGLT2 inhibitor. FDA identified 19 cases of urosepsis and pyelonephritis, which began as urinary tract infections associated with SGLT2 inhibitor use, in FAERS between March 2013 and October 2014. In all cases reported, hospitalization was warranted and some patients required admission to an intensive care unit or dialysis for treatment. The median time to onset of infection following initiation of the SGLT2 inhibitor was 45 days (range: 2–270 days).

Prior to initiating therapy with an SGLT2 inhibitor, clinicians should consider patient factors that may predispose the patient to serious urinary tract infections such as a history of difficulty urinating or infections of the bladder, kidneys, or urinary tract. Patients should be monitored for urinary tract infections and treatment instituted if indicated.

Lower Limb Amputation In 2 randomized, placebo-controlled studies evaluating the effects of another drug in the SGLT2 inhibitor class (canagliflozin) on the risk of cardiovascular disease and the overall safety and tolerability of the drug, canagliflozin-treated patients had a twofold increased risk of lower limb (leg and foot) amputations (mostly affecting the toes and midfoot) compared with placebo recipients. (See Lower Limb Amputation under Warnings/Precautions: Warnings, in Cautions, in Canagliflozin 68:20.18.) In clinical trials conducted with ertugliflozin, nontraumatic lower limb amputations were reported in 0.2 or 0.5% of patients receiving ertugliflozin 5 or 15 mg daily, respectively, compared with 0.1% of patients receiving a comparator drug. A causal association between ertugliflozin and lower limb amputation has not been established. Prior to initiating therapy with ertugliflozin, clinicians should consider patient factors that may predispose them to the need for amputation, such as a history of amputation, peripheral vascular disease, neuropathy, or diabetic foot ulcers. Clinicians should monitor patients receiving ertugliflozin for the presence of infection (including osteomyelitis), new pain or tenderness, and sores or ulcers involving the lower limbs; ertugliflozin should be discontinued if such complications occur. Patients should also be counseled on the importance of routine preventative foot care.

Concomitant Therapy with Hypoglycemic Agents When ertugliflozin is added to therapy with an insulin secretagogue (e.g., a sulfonylurea) or insulin, the incidence of hypoglycemia is increased compared with sulfonylurea or insulin monotherapy. Therefore, patients receiving ertugliflozin may require a reduced dosage of the concomitant insulin secretagogue or insulin to reduce the risk of hypoglycemia.

Fournier Gangrene Fournier gangrene (necrotizing fasciitis of the perineum), a rare but serious or life-threatening bacterial infection requiring urgent surgical intervention, has been reported during postmarketing surveillance in men and women with type 2 diabetes mellitus receiving an SGLT2 inhibitor. Permanent disfigurement, prolonged hospitalization, disability, and complications from sepsis all may be caused by Fournier gangrene. Although diabetes mellitus is a risk factor for developing Fournier gangrene, this condition is still rare among patients with diabetes mellitus.

FDA identified 12 cases of Fournier gangrene in patients taking an SGLT2 inhibitor reported in FAERS and medical literature between March 2013 and May 2018. Since FDA's review, additional cases of Fournier gangrene have been reported. In the initial cases reviewed by FDA, the average time to onset of infection was 9.2 months (range 7 days to 25 months) after initiating therapy with an SGLT2 inhibitor. Some experts speculate that the variation in time to diagnosis of Fournier gangrene might be due to fluctuating glycemic control, microvascular complications, or an inciting event associated with SGLT2 inhibitors (e.g., urinary tract infection, mycotic infection, skin or mucosal breakdown due to pruritus). In all cases reported, hospitalization and surgery were required. Among these cases, some patients required multiple disfiguring surgeries, some developed complications (e.g., diabetic ketoacidosis, acute kidney injury, septic shock), and 1 patient died. In a review of other antidiabetic drugs (e.g., insulin, biguanides, sulfonylureas, dipeptidyl peptidase-4 inhibitors) over a period of more than 30 years, only 6 cases of Fournier gangrene were identified; all of theses cases occurred in men.

Patients receiving ertugliflozin who develop pain or tenderness, erythema, or swelling in the genital or perineal area, in addition to fever or malaise, should be assessed for necrotizing fasciitis. If Fournier gangrene is suspected, ertugliflozin should be discontinued and treatment should be initiated with broad-spectrum antibiotics; surgical debridement should be performed if necessary. Blood glucose concentrations should be closely monitored; alternative antidiabetic agents should be initiated to maintain glycemic control.

Genital Mycotic Infections Ertugliflozin increases the risk of genital mycotic infections in males (e.g., balanitis) and females (e.g., vulvovaginal mycotic infection). Patients with a history of genital mycotic infections and uncircumcised males are at an increased risk for developing genital mycotic infections. Patients should be monitored for genital mycotic infections and appropriate treatment should be instituted if these infections occur.

Risk of Bone Fracture An increased risk of bone fracture, along with dose-related decreases in bone mineral density in older adults, has been observed in patients receiving another drug in the SGLT2 inhibitor class (canagliflozin). (See Risk of Bone Fracture under Warnings/Precautions: Other Warnings/Precautions, in Cautions, in Canagliflozin 68:20.18.) FDA is continuing to evaluate the risk of bone fracture with SGLT2 inhibitors.

Effects on Lipoproteins Increases in low-density lipoprotein (LDL)-cholesterol can occur during ertugliflozin therapy. Serum LDL-cholesterol concentrations should be monitored during treatment with ertugliflozin and such lipid elevations treated according to the standard of care.

Laboratory Test Interferences SGLT2 inhibitors such as ertugliflozin increase urinary glucose excretion and will result in false-positive urine glucose tests. In addition, the manufacturer states that the 1,5-anhydroglucitol assay is unreliable for monitoring glycemic control in patients taking SGLT2 inhibitors. Alternative methods of monitoring glycemic control should be used in patients receiving SGLT2 inhibitors.

Use of Fixed Combinations When ertugliflozin is used in fixed combination with metformin, sitagliptin, or other drugs, the cautions, precautions, contraindications, and interactions associated with the concomitant agent(s) should be considered in addition to those associated with ertugliflozin.

Specific Populations **Pregnancy.** Based on the results of reproductive and developmental toxicity studies in animals, ertugliflozin use during pregnancy may affect renal development and maturation, especially during the second and third trimesters of pregnancy. Limited data with ertugliflozin in pregnant women are not sufficient to determine a drug-associated risk for major birth defects or miscarriage, and poorly controlled diabetes mellitus during pregnancy carries risks to the mother and fetus; however, ertugliflozin therapy is not recommended in pregnant women during the second and third trimesters of pregnancy.

Lactation. Ertugliflozin is distributed into milk in rats; it is not known whether the drug is distributed into human milk. Because many drugs are distributed into human milk and because of the potential for serious adverse reactions in nursing infants from ertugliflozin, a decision should be made whether to discontinue nursing or the drug, taking into account the importance of the drug to the woman.

Pediatric Use. Safety and efficacy of ertugliflozin have not been established in pediatric patients younger than 18 years of age.

Geriatric Use. In clinical trials, 25.7% of patients were 65 years of age or older and 4.5% were 75 years of age or older. Geriatric patients receiving ertugliflozin were more likely to experience certain adverse reactions related to volume depletion compared with younger patients. Ertugliflozin is expected to have diminished efficacy in geriatric patients with renal impairment.

Hepatic Impairment. Compared with values in individuals with normal hepatic function, ertugliflozin area under the concentration-time curve (AUC) and peak plasma concentrations were decreased by 13 and 21%, respectively, in patients with moderate hepatic impairment (Child-Pugh class B); however, these decreases are not considered clinically meaningful. The plasma protein binding of ertugliflozin is unaffected in patients with moderate hepatic impairment. Data are lacking on the use of ertugliflozin in patients with severe hepatic impairment (Child-Pugh class C), and such use is not recommended.

Renal Impairment. Renal function should be assessed prior to initiation of ertugliflozin therapy and periodically thereafter.

Safety and efficacy of ertugliflozin have not been established in patients with moderate renal impairment (estimated glomerular filtration rate [eGFR] 30–59 mL/minute per 1.73 m^2). The safety and efficacy of ertugliflozin were evaluated in adults with moderate renal impairment (mean eGFR: 47 mL/minute per 1.73 m^2) and type 2 diabetes mellitus inadequately controlled on diet and exercise with or without other antidiabetic agents (a biguanide [24.6%], a dipeptidyl peptidase-4 [DPP-4] inhibitor [13.5%], a glucagon-like peptide-1 [GLP-1] receptor agonist [2.8%], insulin [55.9%], a sulfonylurea [40.3%], other [5.4%]). The addition of ertugliflozin 5 or 15 mg administered once daily to background antidiabetic agents did not improve glycemic control compared with placebo. Additionally, patients who received ertugliflozin had an increased risk of renal impairment, renal-related adverse effects, and adverse effects related to volume depletion compared with placebo-treated patients.

Ertugliflozin is not expected to be effective in patients with severe renal impairment (including those with end-stage renal disease [ESRD]) or those undergoing dialysis; the drug is contraindicated in such patients. (See Contraindications.)

In patients with mild (eGFR 60–89 mL/minute per 1.73 m^2), moderate (eGFR 30–59 mL/minute per 1.73 m^2), or severe (eGFR less than 30 mL/minute per 1.73 m^2) renal impairment, AUC of ertugliflozin was increased by 1.6-, 1.7-, or 1.6-fold, respectively, compared with those with normal renal function. However, these increases are not considered clinically important. In patients receiving ertugliflozin, 24-hour urinary glucose excretion declined with increasing severity of renal impairment. Plasma protein binding of ertugliflozin was unaffected in patients with renal impairment.

■ **Common Adverse Effects** Adverse effects reported in at least 2% of patients receiving ertugliflozin in clinical trials and more commonly than with placebo include female genital mycotic infection, male genital mycotic infection, urinary tract infection, headache, vaginal pruritus, increased urination, nasopharyngitis, back pain, decreased weight, and thirst.

Drug Interactions

The major metabolic pathway for ertugliflozin is glucuronidation; the drug is principally glucuronidated by uridine diphosphate-glucuronosyltransferase (UGT) isoenzymes 1A9 and 2B7.

■ **Drugs Affecting or Metabolized by Hepatic Microsomal Enzymes** Ertugliflozin in minimally metabolized by cytochrome P-450 (CYP) isoenzymes. Ertugliflozin and ertugliflozin glucuronides (clinically inactive metabolites) did not inhibit CYP isoenzymes 1A2, 2B6, 2C9, 2C19, 2C8, 2D6, or 3A4 and did not induce CYP isoenzymes 1A2, or 3A4 in vitro. Additionally, the drug is not a time-dependent inhibitor of CYP3A in vitro. Pharmacokinetic interactions are unlikely with drugs that are metabolized by these CYP isoenzymes.

■ **Drugs Affecting or Affected by Organic Anion Transporters** Ertugliflozin is not a substrate of organic anion transporter (OAT) 1 or OAT3. Ertugliflozin and ertugliflozin glucuronides did not meaningfully inhibit OAT1 or OAT3; pharmacokinetic interactions are unlikely with substrates of OAT1 or OAT3.

■ **Drugs Affecting or Affected by Organic Cation Transporters** Ertugliflozin is not a substrate of organic cation transporter (OCT) 1 or OCT2. Ertugliflozin and ertugliflozin glucuronides did not meaningfully inhibit OCT2; pharmacokinetic interactions are unlikely with substrates of OCT2.

■ **Drugs Affecting or Affected by P-glycoprotein Transport** Ertugliflozin is a P-glycoprotein (P-gp) substrate. Ertugliflozin and ertugliflozin glucuronides did not meaningfully inhibit P-gp. Ertugliflozin is unlikely to affect the pharmacokinetics of concomitantly administered P-gp substrates.

■ **Drugs Affected by Uridine Diphosphate-glucuronosyltransferase** Ertugliflozin did not inhibit UGT isoenzymes 1A6, 1A9, or 2B7 in vitro and was a weak inhibitor of UGT1A1 and 1A4. Ertugliflozin glucuronides did not inhibit UGT1A1, 1A4, 1A6, 1A9, or 2B7 in vitro. Pharmacokinetic interactions are unlikely with drugs that are metabolized by these enzymes.

■ **Drugs Affecting Breast Cancer Resistance Protein** Ertugliflozin is a substrate of breast cancer resistance protein (BCRP).

■ **Drugs Affecting or Affected by Organic Anion Transport Polypeptides** Ertugliflozin is not a substrate of organic anion transport polypeptides (OATP) 1B1 or 1B3. Ertugliflozin and ertugliflozin glucuronides did not meaningfully inhibit OATP1B1 or OATP1B3; pharmacokinetic interactions are unlikely with substrates of OATP1B1 or OATP1B3.

■ **Diuretics** Concomitant use of ertugliflozin with diuretics may increase the incidence of symptomatic hypotension. Prior to initiation of ertugliflozin, volume status should be assessed and corrected in patients receiving diuretics. Patients should be monitored for signs and symptoms of symptomatic hypotension following initiation of ertugliflozin therapy.

■ **Mefenamic Acid** Concomitant use of mefenamic acid, a UGT inhibitor, and ertugliflozin increased ertugliflozin peak plasma concentration and area under the concentration-time curve (AUC) by 1.51- and 1.19-fold, respectively. These increases are not considered to be clinically relevant.

■ **Metformin** Administration of a single dose of metformin hydrochloride (1 g) with a single dose of ertugliflozin (15 mg) did not have a clinically meaningful effect on the pharmacokinetics of ertugliflozin or metformin. No adjustment of ertugliflozin dosage is necessary when used concomitantly with metformin.

■ **Rifampin** Administration of rifampin (600 mg once daily) with a single dose of ertugliflozin (15 mg) decreased ertugliflozin peak plasma concentration and AUC by 15 and 39%, respectively. No adjustment of ertugliflozin dosage is necessary when used concomitantly with rifampin.

■ **Simvastatin** Administration of a single dose of simvastatin (40 mg) with a single dose of ertugliflozin (15 mg) did not have a clinically meaningful effect on the pharmacokinetics of ertugliflozin or simvastatin. No adjustment of ertugliflozin dosage is necessary when used concomitantly with simvastatin.

■ **Sitagliptin** Administration of a single dose of sitagliptin (100 mg) with a single dose of ertugliflozin (15 mg) did not have a clinically meaningful effect on the pharmacokinetics of ertugliflozin or sitagliptin. No adjustment of ertugliflozin dosage is necessary when used concomitantly with sitagliptin.

■ **Sulfonylureas or Insulin** When ertugliflozin is added to therapy with an insulin secretagogue (e.g., a sulfonylurea) or insulin, the incidence of hypoglycemia is increased compared with sulfonylurea or insulin monotherapy. Patients receiving ertugliflozin may require a reduced dosage of the concomitant insulin secretagogue or insulin to reduce the risk of hypoglycemia.

Glimepiride Administration of a single dose of glimepiride (1 mg) with a single dose of ertugliflozin (15 mg) did not have a clinically important effect on the pharmacokinetics of glimepiride or ertugliflozin.

Description

Ertugliflozin is a reversible and highly selective inhibitor of sodium-glucose cotransporter 2 (SGLT2), a transporter that is expressed in the proximal renal tubules and is responsible for most of the reabsorption of filtered glucose from the tubular lumen. Through inhibition of SGLT2, ertugliflozin reduces reabsorption of filtered glucose and lowers the renal threshold for glucose in a dose-dependent manner, leading to increased urinary glucose excretion; increased glucose excretion is independent of insulin secretion.

Following oral administration of ertugliflozin in the fasting state, peak plasma concentration is attained in 1 hour. Following oral administration of a 15-mg dose of ertugliflozin, the absolute oral bioavailability of the drug is 100%. Administration of ertugliflozin with a high-fat, high-calorie meal decreased peak plasma ertugliflozin concentration by 29% and prolonged time to peak plasma concentration by 1 hour, but did not alter the area under the concentration-time curve (AUC). These changes are not considered clinically meaningful and ertugliflozin can be administered with or without food. Ertugliflozin is 93.6% protein bound. Renal or hepatic impairment does not meaningfully alter plasma protein binding. Ertugliflozin is principally metabolized by uridine diphosphate-glucuronosyltransferase (UGT) 1A9 and UGT2B7 to inactive metabolites. Following oral administration of a radiolabeled 25-mg dose of ertugliflozin, 41% of the total radioactivity was excreted in urine and 50% was excreted in feces, with 1.5 or approximately 33.8% of the administered dose recovered as parent drug in urine or feces, respectively. The mean elimination half-life of ertugliflozin is approximately 16.6 hours.

Advice to Patients

When ertugliflozin is used in fixed combination with other drugs, importance of informing patients of important cautionary information about the concomitant agent(s).

Importance of patient reading medication guide before initiating therapy and each time the drug is dispensed.

Importance of informing patients of the potential risks and benefits of ertugliflozin-containing therapy and of alternative therapies.

Importance of informing patients about the importance of adherence to dietary instructions, regular physical activity, periodic blood glucose monitoring and glycosylated hemoglobin (hemoglobin A_{1c}; HbA_{1c}) testing, recognition and management of hypoglycemia and hyperglycemia, and assessment of diabetes mellitus complications.

Importance of promptly seeking medical advice during periods of stress such as fever, trauma, infection, or surgery as medication requirements may change.

Importance of taking ertugliflozin exactly as directed by the clinician. Importance of advising patients about what to do if a dose of ertugliflozin is missed. (See Dosage and Administration: Administration.)

Importance of informing patients that the incidence of hypoglycemia may be increased if ertugliflozin is used concomitantly with insulin and/or an insulin secretagogue. Importance of informing patients that a lower dosage of insulin or insulin secretagogue may be required to reduce the risk of hypoglycemia if used concomitantly with ertugliflozin.

Importance of informing patients that symptomatic hypotension may occur with ertugliflozin and advising patients to report such symptoms to their clinician. Inform patients that ertugliflozin-induced dehydration may increase the risk of hypotension and that patients should maintain adequate fluid intake.

Importance of informing patients that ketoacidosis, which can be a life-threatening condition, has been reported with ertugliflozin therapy. Importance of informing patients receiving ertugliflozin and their caregivers of the signs and symptoms of ketoacidosis (e.g., tachypnea or hyperventilation, anorexia, abdominal pain, nausea, vomiting, lethargy, mental status changes) and importance of instructing patients to discontinue ertugliflozin and seek medical attention immediately should they experience any such signs or symptoms. Advise patients to use a ketone dipstick to check for ketones in their urine (when possible) if symptoms of ketoacidosis occur, even if blood glucose is not elevated (e.g., less than 250 mg/dL).

Importance of informing patients that acute kidney injury has been reported with ertugliflozin therapy. Advise patients to seek medical advice immediately if they have reduced oral intake (such as due to acute illness or fasting) or increased fluid losses (such as due to vomiting, diarrhea, or excessive heat exposure), as it may be appropriate to temporarily discontinue ertugliflozin in those settings. Importance of regular renal function testing during ertugliflozin therapy.

Importance of informing patients receiving ertugliflozin of the potential for urinary tract infections, which may be serious. Advise patients of the signs and symptoms of urinary tract infection and the need to contact a clinician if such signs and symptoms occur.

Importance of informing patients of the potentially increased risk of amputation with ertugliflozin therapy. Advise patients of the importance of routine preventative foot care. Advise patients to monitor for new pain, tenderness, sores or ulcers, or infections involving the leg or foot, and to seek prompt medical advice if such signs or symptoms develop.

Importance of informing patients that necrotizing infections of the perineum (Fournier gangrene) have occurred with sodium-glucose cotransporter 2 (SGLT2) inhibitor therapy. Advise patients to promptly seek medical attention if they develop pain or tenderness, redness, or swelling of the genitals or the area from the genitals back to the rectum, in addition to fever (above 38°C) or malaise.

Importance of informing patients that yeast infection may occur (e.g., vulvovaginitis, balanitis, balanoposthitis). Importance of informing female patients of the signs and symptoms of vaginal yeast infections (e.g., vaginal discharge, odor, itching) and male patients of the signs and symptoms of balanitis or balanoposthitis (e.g., rash or redness of the glans or foreskin of the penis). Advise patients of treatment options and when to seek medical advice.

Importance of informing patients that due to the mechanism of action of ertugliflozin, patients taking the drug will test positive for glucose in their urine. Importance of not using urine glucose tests to monitor glycemic status while taking ertugliflozin. (See Laboratory Test Interferences under Cautions: Warnings/Precautions.)

Importance of women informing their clinicians immediately if they are or plan to become pregnant or plan to breast-feed. Advise patients that ertugliflozin use is not recommended while breast-feeding. Importance of advising pregnant women about the potential risks to the fetus if ertugliflozin is used during pregnancy. All women of childbearing potential should be advised to report pregnancy to their clinician as soon as possible. (See Specific Populations under Cautions: Warnings/Precautions.)

Importance of informing clinicians of existing or contemplated concomitant therapy, including prescription and OTC drugs and dietary or herbal supplements, as well as any concomitant illnesses.

Importance of informing patients of other important precautionary information. (See Cautions.)

Overview® (see Users Guide). For additional information on this drug until a more detailed monograph is developed and published, the manufacturer's labeling should be consulted. It is *essential* that the manufacturer's labeling be consulted for more detailed information on usual cautions, precautions, contraindications, potential drug interactions, laboratory test interferences, and acute toxicity.

Preparations

Excipients in commercially available drug preparations may have clinically important effects in some individuals; consult specific product labeling for details.

Ertugliflozin L-pyroglutamic Acid

Oral		
Tablets, film-coated	5 mg (of ertugliflozin)	**Steglatro®**, Merck
	15 mg (of ertugliflozin)	**Steglatro®**, Merck

Ertugliflozin L-pyroglutamic Acid Combinations

Oral		
Tablets, film-coated	2.5 mg (of ertugliflozin) with Metformin Hydrochloride 500 mg	**Segluromet®**, Merck
	2.5 mg (of ertugliflozin) with Metformin Hydrochloride 1 g	**Segluromet®**, Merck
	5 mg (of ertugliflozin) with Sitagliptin Phosphate 100 mg (of sitagliptin)	**Steglujan®**, Merck
	7.5 mg (of ertugliflozin) with Metformin Hydrochloride 500 mg	**Segluromet®**, Merck
	7.5 mg (of ertugliflozin) with Metformin Hydrochloride 1 g	**Segluromet®**, Merck
	15 mg (of ertugliflozin) with Sitagliptin Phosphate 100 mg (of sitagliptin)	**Steglujan®**, Merck

SULFONYLUREAS 68:20.20

glipiZIDE

Glydiazinamide

■ Glipizide is a sulfonylurea antidiabetic agent.

Uses

■ **Diabetes Mellitus** Glipizide is used as an adjunct to diet for the management of type 2 diabetes mellitus in patients whose hyperglycemia cannot be controlled by diet and exercise alone. Sulfonylureas, including glipizide, may be used in combination with one or more other oral antidiabetic agents (e.g., metformin, thiazolidinedione derivatives, α-glucosidase inhibitors) or insulin as an adjunct to diet and exercise for the management of type 2 diabetes mellitus in patients who do not achieve adequate glycemic control with diet, exercise, and oral antidiabetic agent monotherapy. Glipizide is commercially available in fixed combination with metformin for use as initial therapy in patients with type 2 diabetes mellitus whose hyperglycemia cannot be controlled by diet and exercise alone and as second-line therapy in patients with type 2 diabetes who are inadequately controlled with either sulfonylurea or metformin monotherapy.

The American Diabetes Association (ADA) currently classifies diabetes mellitus as type 1 immune mediated or idiopathic), type 2 (predominantly insulin resistance with relative insulin deficiency to predominantly an insulin secretory defect with insulin resistance), gestational diabetes mellitus, or that associated with certain conditions or syndromes (e.g., drug- or chemical-induced, hormonal, that associated with pancreatic disease, infections, specific genetic defects or syndromes). Type 1 diabetes mellitus was previously described as juvenile-onset (JOD) diabetes mellitus, since it usually occurs during youth. Type 2 diabetes mellitus was previously described as adult-onset (AODM) diabetes mellitus. However, type 1 or type 2 diabetes mellitus can occur at any age, and the current classification is based on pathogenesis (e.g., autoimmune destruction of pancreatic β cells, insulin resistance) and clinical presentation rather than on age of onset. Epidemiologic data indicate that the incidence of type 2 diabetes mellitus is increasing in children and adolescents such that 8–45% of children with newly diagnosed diabetes have nonimmune-mediated diabetes mellitus; most of these individuals have type 2 diabetes mellitus, although other types, including idiopathic or nonimmune-mediated type 1 diabetes mellitus, also have been reported.

Patients with type 2 diabetes mellitus have insulin resistance and usually have relative (rather than absolute) insulin deficiency. Most patients with type 2 diabetes mellitus (about 80–90%) are overweight or obese; obesity itself also contributes to the insulin resistance and glucose intolerance observed in these patients. Patients with type 2 diabetes mellitus who are not obese may have an increased percentage of abdominal fat, which is an indicator of increased cardiometabolic risk. While children with immune-mediated type 1 diabetes generally are not overweight, the incidence of obesity in children with this form of diabetes is increasing with the increasing incidence of obesity in the US population. Distinguishing between type 1 and type 2 diabetes in children may be difficult since obesity may occur with either type of diabetes mellitus, and autoantigens and ketosis may be present in a substantial number of children with features of type 2 diabetes mellitus (e.g., obesity, acanthosis nigricans).

Oral antidiabetic agents are *not* effective as sole therapy in patients with type 1 diabetes mellitus; insulin is necessary in these patients. Sulfonylurea antidiabetic agents are not routinely recommended in hospitalized patients with diabetes mellitus. Because of their long duration of action (24 hours with glipizide), sulfonylureas do not allow rapid dosage adjustments to meet changing needs of hospitalized patients. In addition, the risk of hypoglycemia during sulfonylurea therapy is increased in such patients with irregular eating patterns.

Patients with type 2 diabetes mellitus are *not* dependent initially on insulin (although many patients eventually require insulin for glycemic control) nor are they prone to ketosis; however, insulin may occasionally be required for correction of symptomatic or persistent hyperglycemia that is not controlled by dietary regulation or oral antidiabetic agents (e.g., sulfonylureas), and ketosis occasionally may develop during periods of severe stress (e.g., acute infections, trauma, surgery). Type 2 diabetes mellitus is a heterogeneous subclass of the disease, and subclassification criteria (e.g., basal and stimulated plasma insulin concentrations, insulin resistance) remain to be clearly established. Endogenous insulin is present in type 2 diabetic patients, although plasma insulin concentrations may be decreased, increased, or normal. In type 2 diabetic patients, glucose-stimulated secretion of endogenous insulin is frequently, but not always, reduced and decreased peripheral sensitivity to insulin is almost always associated with glucose intolerance.

Glycemic Control and Microvascular Complications Current evidence from epidemiologic and clinical studies supports an association between chronic hyperglycemia and the pathogenesis of microvascular complications in patients with diabetes mellitus, and results of randomized, controlled studies in patients with type 1 or type 2 diabetes mellitus indicate that intensive management of hyperglycemia with near-normalization of blood glucose and glycosylated hemoglobin (hemoglobin A_{1c} [HbA_{1c}]) concentrations provides substantial benefits in terms of reducing chronic microvascular (e.g., retinopathy, nephropathy, neuropathy) complications associated with the disease. HbA_{1c} concentration reflects the glycosylation of other proteins throughout the body as a result of recent hyperglycemia and is used as a predictor of risk for development of diabetic microvascular complications. Microvascular complications of diabetes are the principal causes of blindness and renal failure in developed countries and are more closely associated with hyperglycemia than are macrovascular complications.

In the Diabetes Control and Complications Trial (DCCT), the reduction in risk of microvascular complications in patients with type 1 diabetes mellitus correlated continuously with the reduction in HbA_{1c} concentration produced by intensive insulin treatment (e.g., a 40% reduction in risk of microvascular disease for each 10% reduction in HbA_{1c}). These data imply that any decrease in HbA_{1c} levels is beneficial and that complete normalization of blood glucose concentrations may prevent diabetic complications. Data from the largest United Kingdom Prospective Diabetes Study (UKPDS) and other smaller studies in patients with type 2 diabetes mellitus generally are consistent with the same benefits on microvascular complications as those observed with type 1 diabetes mellitus in the DCCT study.

Data from long-term follow-up (over 10 years) of UKPDS patients with type 2 diabetes mellitus who received initial therapy with conventional (diet and oral antidiabetic agents or insulin to achieve fasting plasma glucose concentrations below 270 mg/dL without symptoms of hyperglycemia) antidiabetic treatment or intensive (stepwise introduction of a sulfonylurea [i.e., chlorpropamide, glyburide], then insulin, or an oral sulfonylurea and insulin, or insulin alone to achieve fasting plasma glucose concentrations of 108 mg/dL) antidiabetic regimens indicate that intensive treatment with monotherapy generally is not capable of maintaining strict glycemic control (i.e., maintenance of blood glucose concentrations of 108 mg/dL or normal values) over time and that combination therapy eventually becomes necessary in most patients to attain target glycemic levels in the long term; in UKPDS, intensive treatment that eventually required combination therapy in most patients resulted in median HbA_{1c} concentrations of 7%. Because of the benefits of strict glycemic control, the goal of therapy for type 2 diabetes mellitus is to lower blood glucose to as close to normal as possible, which generally requires aggressive management efforts (e.g., mixing therapy with various antidiabetic agents including sulfonylureas, metformin, insulin, and/or possibly others) over time. For additional information on clinical studies demonstrating the benefits of strict glycemic control on microvascular complications in patients with type 1 or 2 diabetes mellitus, see Glycemic Control and Microvascular Complications under Uses: Diabetes Mellitus, in Metformin 68:20.04.

Glycemic Control and Macrovascular Complications Current evidence indicates that appropriate management of dyslipidemia, blood pressure, and vascular thrombosis provides substantial benefits in terms of reducing macrovascular complications associated with diabetes mellitus; intensive glycemic control generally has not been associated with appreciable reductions in macrovascular outcomes in controlled trials. Reduction in blood pressure to a mean of 144/82 mm Hg ("tight blood pressure control") in patients with diabetes mellitus and uncomplicated mild to moderate hypertension in UKPDS substantially reduced the incidence of virtually all macrovascular (e.g., stroke, heart failure) and microvascular (e.g., retinopathy, vitreous hemorrhage, renal failure) outcomes and diabetes-related mortality; blood pressure and glycemic control were additive in their beneficial effects on these end points. While intensive antidiabetic therapy titrated with the goal of reducing HbA_{1c} to near-normal concentrations (6–6.5% or less) has not been associated with appreciable reductions in cardiovascular events during the randomized portion of controlled trials examining such outcomes, results of long-term follow-up (10–11 years) from DCCT and UKPDS indicate a delayed cardiovascular benefit in patients treated with intensive antidiabetic therapy early in the course of type 1 or type 2 diabetes mellitus. For additional details regarding the effects of intensive antidiabetic therapy on macrovascular outcomes, see Glycemic Control and Macrovascular Complications, under Uses: Diabetes Mellitus, in Metformin 68:20.04.

Treatment Goals The ADA currently states that it is reasonable to attempt to achieve in patients with type 2 diabetes mellitus the same blood glucose and HbA_{1c} goals recommended for patients with type 1 diabetes mellitus. Based on target values for blood glucose and HbA_{1c} used in clinical trials (e.g., DCCT) for type 1 diabetic patients, modified somewhat to reduce the risk of severe hypoglycemia, ADA currently recommends target preprandial (fasting) and peak postprandial (1–2 hours after the *beginning* of a meal) *plasma* glucose concentrations of 70–130 and less than 180 mg/dL, respectively, and HbA_{1c} concentrations of less than 7% (based on a nondiabetic range of 4–6%) *in general* in patients with type 1 or type 2 diabetes mellitus who are not pregnant. HbA_{1c} concentrations of 7% or greater should prompt clinicians to initiate or adjust antidiabetic therapy in nonpregnant patients with the goal of achieving HbA_{1c} concentrations of less than 7%. Patients with diabetes mellitus who have elevated HbA_{1c} concentrations despite having adequate preprandial glucose concentrations should monitor glucose concentrations 1–2 hours after the start of a meal. Treatment with agents (e.g., α-glucosidase inhibitors, exenatide, pramlintide) that principally lower postprandial glucose concentrations to within target ranges also should reduce HbA_{1c}.

More stringent treatment goals (i.e., an HbA_{1c} less than 6%) may be considered in selected patients. An *individualized* HbA_{1c} concentration goal that is closer to normal without risking substantial hypoglycemia is reasonable in patients with a short duration of diabetes mellitus, no appreciable cardiovascular disease, and a long life expectancy. Less stringent treatment goals may be appropriate in patients with long-standing diabetes mellitus in whom the general HbA_{1c} concentration goal of less than 7% is difficult to obtain despite adequate education on self-management of the disease, appropriate glucose monitoring, and effective dosages of multiple antidiabetic agents, including insulin. Achievement of HbA_{1c} values of less than 7% is not appropriate or practical for some patients, and clinical judgment should be used in designing a treatment regimen based on the potential benefits and risks (e.g., hypoglycemia) of more intensified therapy. For additional details on individualizing treatment in patients with diabetes mellitus, see Treatment Goals under Uses: Diabetes Mellitus, in Metformin 68:20.04.

Considerations in Initiating and Maintaining Antidiabetic Therapy When initiating therapy for patients with type 2 diabetes mellitus who do not have severe symptoms, most clinicians recommend that diet be emphasized as the primary form of treatment; caloric restriction and weight reduction are essential in obese patients. Although appropriate dietary management and weight reduction alone may be effective in controlling blood glucose concentration and symptoms of hyperglycemia, many patients receiving dietary advice fail to achieve and maintain adequate glycemic control with dietary modification alone.

Recognizing that lifestyle interventions often fail to achieve or maintain the target glycemic goal within the first year of initiation of such interventions, ADA currently suggests initiation of metformin concurrently with lifestyle interventions at the time of diagnosis of type 2 diabetes mellitus. Other experts suggest concurrent initiation of lifestyle interventions and antidiabetic agents only when HbA_{1c} levels of 9% or greater are present at the time of diagnosis of type 2 diabetes mellitus. ADA and other clinicians state that lifestyle interventions should remain a principal consideration in the management of diabetes even after pharmacologic therapy is initiated. The manufacturer states that patients and clinicians should recognize that dietary management is the principal consideration in the management of diabetes mellitus and that antidiabetic therapy is used only as an adjunct to, and not as a substitute for or a convenient means to avoid, proper dietary management. In addition, loss of blood glucose control on diet alone may be temporary in some patients, requiring only short-term management with drug therapy. The importance of regular physical activity should be emphasized, and cardiovascular risk factors should be identified and corrective measures employed when feasible.

If lifestyle interventions alone are initiated and these interventions fail to reduce symptoms and/or blood glucose concentration, initiation of monotherapy with an oral antidiabetic agent (e.g., sulfonylurea, metformin, acarbose) or insulin should be considered. For more information on the stepwise approach to the management of type 2 diabetes mellitus, See Uses: Diabetes Mellitus, in Metformin 68:20.04.

Several large, long-term studies have evaluated the cardiovascular risks associated with the use of oral sulfonylurea antidiabetic agents. For information on these studies and associated recommendations, see Cautions: Precautions and Contraindications, in Glyburide 68:20.20. The ADA currently considers the beneficial effects of intensive glycemic control with insulin or sulfonylureas and blood pressure control in diabetic patients to outweigh the risks overall.

Glipizide Monotherapy Clinical studies indicate that glipizide is as effective as chlorpropamide, glyburide, tolazamide, or tolbutamide for the management of type 2 diabetes mellitus. A relative advantage of glipizide compared with other sulfonylurea antidiabetic agents has not been clearly established. Although the glipizide-induced increase in glucose- or meal-stimulated secretion of endogenous insulin appears to be sustained during long-term therapy, the clinical importance of this effect in the long-term efficacy of the drug and any resultant therapeutic difference compared with other sulfonylureas remain to be determined. Reversal of basement-membrane thickening of muscle capillaries in asymptomatic individuals with impaired glucose tolerance (chemical diabetes) treated with glipizide has been reported, suggesting that early drug therapy to improve control of blood glucose concentration might reverse or delay microangiopathy, but this finding requires further evaluation.

Clinical trial data indicate that sulfonylureas are as effective as metformin in managing hyperglycemia (approximately 1.5% average reduction in HbA_{1c} values), but sulfonylurea use is associated with hypoglycemia and weight gain. ADA generally recommends metformin as initial oral antidiabetic therapy because of the absence of weight gain or hypoglycemia, relatively low expense, and generally low adverse effect profile compared with other oral antidiabetic agents. (See Uses: Diabetes Mellitus, in Metformin 68:20.04)

Glipizide may be useful in some patients with type 2 diabetes mellitus who have primary or secondary failure to other sulfonylurea antidiabetic agents; however, primary or secondary failure to glipizide also may occur. Adequate adjustment of dosage and adherence to diet should be assessed before determining if secondary failure to glipizide has occurred. If primary or secondary failure to glipizide extended-release tablets has occurred, another oral antidiabetic agent may be added to glipizide therapy. Patients with secondary failure to one oral antidiabetic agent occasionally may respond to another agent.

Secondary failure to sulfonylurea antidiabetic agents is characterized by progressively decreasing diabetic control following 1 month to several years of good control. Interim data from a substudy (UKPD 26) of the UKPD study in newly diagnosed type 2 diabetic patients receiving intensive therapy (maintenance of fasting plasma glucose below 108 mg/dL by increasing doses of either a sulfonylurea [i.e., glyburide or chlorpropamide] to maximum recommended dosage) showed that secondary failure (defined as fasting plasma glucose exceeding 270 mg/dL or symptoms of hyperglycemia despite maximum recommended daily dosage of 20 mg of glyburide or 500 mg of chlorpropamide) occurred overall at about 7% per year. The failure rate at 6 years was 48% among patients receiving glyburide and about 40% among patients receiving chlorpropamide. In the UKPD studies, stepwise addition of insulin or metformin to therapy with maximal dosage of a sulfonylurea was required periodically over time to improve glycemic control. In another substudy (UKPD 49), progressive deterioration in diabetes control was such that monotherapy was effective in only about 50% of patients after 3 years and in only about 25% of patients after 9 years; thus, most patients require multiple-drug antidiabetic therapy over time to maintain such target levels of disease control. At diagnosis, risk factors predisposing toward sulfonylurea failure included higher fasting plasma glucose concentrations, younger age, and lower pancreatic β-cell reserve.

In some type 2 diabetic patients who are being treated with insulin, glipizide alone may be effective alternative therapy. However, glipizide is *not* effective as sole therapy in patients with diabetes mellitus complicated by acidosis, ketosis, or coma; management of these conditions requires the use of insulin.

Combination Therapy with Metformin or Other Oral Antidiabetic Agents Sulfonylureas may be used in combination with one or more other oral antidiabetic agents (e.g., metformin, thiazolidinedione derivatives, α-glucosidase inhibitors) as an adjunct to diet and exercise for the management of type 2 diabetes mellitus in patients who do not achieve adequate glycemic control with diet, exercise, and oral antidiabetic agent monotherapy. Combined therapy with metformin or other oral antidiabetic agents generally is used in patients with longstanding type 2 diabetes mellitus who have poor glycemic control with monotherapy.

The sequence in which metformin or a sulfonylurea is used at initiation of therapy does not appear to alter the effectiveness of combined therapy with the drugs. However, ADA and other clinicians currently recommend initiating therapy with metformin and adding another antidiabetic agent, such as a sulfonylurea, insulin, or a thiazolidinedione, if patients fail to achieve or maintain target HbA_{1c} goals. Optimal benefit generally is obtained by addition of a second antidiabetic agent as soon as monotherapy with metformin at the maximum tolerated dosage no longer provides adequate glycemic control (i.e., when the target glycemic goal is not achieved within 2–3 months of initiation of therapy with metformin or at any other time when the HbA_{1c} goal is not achieved).

A major factor in choosing additional therapy is the degree of glycemic control obtained during metformin monotherapy. In patients with a HbA_{1c} exceeding 8.5% or symptoms secondary to hyperglycemia despite metformin monotherapy, ADA states that consideration should be given to adding insulin. When glycemic control is closer to the target HbA_{1c} goal with metformin monotherapy (e.g., HbA_{1c} less than 7.5%), agents with a lesser potential to lower hyperglycemia and/or slower onset of action may be considered (e.g., sulfonylurea, thiazolidinedione) as additional therapy to metformin. ADA states that other antidiabetic agents such as α-glucosidase inhibitors, meglitinides, exenatide, and pramlintide generally are less effective, less well studied, and/or more expensive than recommended therapies (i.e., metformin, sulfonylurea, thiazolidinedione, insulin). However, these agents may be appropriate for treatment of type 2 diabetes mellitus in selected patients.

Glipizide is used in fixed combination with metformin as initial therapy in the management of patients with type 2 diabetes mellitus whose hyperglycemia cannot be controlled by diet and exercise alone. In a comparative study in such patients, therapy with the fixed combination of glipizide and metformin was more effective in improving glycemic control (as determined by HbA_{1c} values, fasting plasma glucose concentrations) than monotherapy with either component. A greater percentage of patients receiving the fixed combination achieved strict glycemic control (HbA_{1c} values below 7%) than did those receiving metformin or glipizide monotherapy.

Glipizide also is used in fixed combination with metformin as second-line therapy in patients with type 2 diabetes whose hyperglycemia is inadequately controlled with either sulfonylurea or metformin monotherapy. In a comparative study, greater glycemic control (as determined by HbA_{1c} values and fasting plasma glucose concentrations) was achieved with the fixed combination of glipizide and metformin than with either drug as monotherapy. Strict glycemic control (e.g., HbA_{1c} values less than 7%) also was achieved in a greater percentage of patients receiving the fixed combination of glipizide and metformin.

When lifestyle interventions, metformin, and a second oral antidiabetic agent are not effective in maintaining the target glycemic goal in patients with type 2 diabetes mellitus, ADA and other clinicians generally recommend the addition of insulin therapy. In patients whose HbA_{1c} is close to the target level (less than 8%) on metformin and a second oral antidiabetic agent, addition of a third oral antidiabetic agent instead of insulin may be considered. However, ADA states that triple combination oral antidiabetic therapy is more costly and potentially not as effective as adding insulin therapy to dual combination oral antidiabetic therapy.

Combination Therapy with Insulin Combined therapy with insulin and oral antidiabetic agents may be useful in some patients with type 2 diabetes mellitus whose blood glucose concentrations are not adequately controlled with maximal dosages of the oral agent and/or as a means of providing increased flexibility with respect to timing of meals and amount of food ingested. Concomitant therapy with insulin (e.g., given as intermediate- or long-acting insulin at bedtime or rapid-acting insulin at meal times) and one or more oral antidiabetic agents appears to improve glycemic control with lower dosages of insulin than would be required with insulin alone and may decrease the potential for body weight gain associated with insulin therapy. Oral antidiabetic therapy combined with insulin therapy may delay progression to either intensive insulin monotherapy or to a second daytime injection of insulin combined with oral antidiabetic agents. Preliminary data indicate that combination therapy with glipizide and insulin may be useful in some type 2 diabetic patients. However, combined therapy may increase the risk of hypoglycemic reactions.

ADA and other clinicians state that combined therapy with insulin and metformin with or without other oral antidiabetic agents is one of several options for the management of hyperglycemia in patients not responding adequately to oral monotherapy with metformin, the preferred initial oral antidiabetic agent. In patients with a HbA_{1c} exceeding 8.5% or symptoms secondary to hyperglycemia despite metformin monotherapy, ADA states that consideration should be given to adding insulin. When patients are not controlled with metformin with or without other oral antidiabetic agents (i.e., sulfonylurea, thiazolidinedione) and basal insulin (e.g., given as intermediate- or long-acting insulin at bedtime or in the morning), therapy with insulin should be intensified by adding additional short-acting or rapid-acting insulin injections at mealtimes. Therapy with insulin secretagogues (i.e., sulfonylureas, meglitinides) should be tapered and discontinued when intensive insulin therapy is initiated, as insulin secretagogues do not appear to be synergistic with such insulin therapy.

For additional information on combination therapy with sulfonylureas and other oral antidiabetic agents, see the sections on combination therapy in Uses in the individual monographs in 68:20.

Dosage and Administration

■ **Administration** Glipizide is administered orally. The extended-release tablets should be swallowed whole and should *not* be divided, chewed, or crushed. Patients receiving the extended-release tablets become alarmed if they notice a tablet-like substance in their stools; this is normal since the tablet containing the drug is designed to remain intact and slowly release the drug from a nonabsorbable shell during passage through the GI tract.

Extended-release tablets of glipizide are administered once daily, generally with breakfast. Conventional tablets of the drug usually are administered as a single daily dose given each morning before breakfast. It is generally recommended that glipizide be administered approximately 30 minutes before a meal(s) to achieve the maximum reduction in postprandial blood glucose concentration. Once-daily dosing of glipizide at dosages up to 15–20 mg daily provides adequate control of blood glucose concentration throughout the day in most patients with usual meal patterns; however, some patients may have a more satisfactory response when the drug is administered in 2 or 3 divided doses daily as conventional tablets. When glipizide dosage exceeds 15–20 mg daily as conventional tablets, the drug should usually be administered in divided doses before meals of sufficient caloric content. The maximum once-daily dose as conventional tablets recommended by the manufacturer is 15 mg. When a divided-dosing regimen as conventional tablets is employed in patients receiving more than 15 mg of glipizide daily, the doses and schedule of administration should be individualized according to the patient's meal pattern and response. Dosages greater than 30 mg daily have been given safely in twice-daily dosing regimens for prolonged periods.

■ **Dosage** Dosage of glipizide must be based on blood and urine glucose determinations and must be carefully individualized to obtain optimum therapeutic effect. Patients must be closely monitored (i.e., glycosylated hemoglobin [hemoglobin A_{1c}, HbA_{1c}], fasting blood glucose concentrations) to determine the minimum effective glipizide dosage and to detect primary or secondary failure to the drug. Self-monitoring of blood glucose concentrations may provide useful information to the patient and their clinician. *If appropriate glipizide dosage regimens are not followed, hypoglycemia may be precipitated.*

Patients receiving glipizide should be monitored carefully to determine the need for continued therapy and to ensure that the drug continues to be effective; if adequate lowering of blood glucose concentration is no longer achieved during maintenance therapy, the drug should be discontinued. Following initiation of glipizide therapy and dosage titration, determination of HbA_{1c} concentrations at intervals of approximately 3 months is the preferred method for assessing the patient's continued response to therapy. While fasting blood glucose concentrations generally reach steady-state following initiation or change in glipizide dosage, a single fasting blood glucose determination may not accurately assess glycemic response. If fasting blood glucose concentrations are used to assess the need for dosage adjustments, 2 consecutive determinations of similar value should be obtained 7 or more days after the previous dosage adjustment. Patients who do not adhere to their prescribed dietary and drug regimens are more likely to have an unsatisfactory response to therapy. In patients usually well controlled by dietary management alone, short-term therapy with glipizide may be sufficient during periods of transient loss of diabetic control.

Initial Dosage in Previously Untreated Patients For the management of type 2 diabetes mellitus in patients not previously receiving insulin or sulfonylurea antidiabetic agents, the recommended initial adult dosage of glipizide is 5 mg daily as conventional or extended-release tablets; in geriatric patients or those with hepatic disease, an initial dosage of 2.5 or 5 mg daily as conventional or extended-release tablets, respectively, may be used. Initial glipizide dosage should be conservative in debilitated, malnourished, or geriatric patients, patients with impaired renal or hepatic function, or those who may otherwise be more sensitive to oral hypoglycemic agents because of an increased risk of hypoglycemia in these patients. (See Cautions: Precautions and Contraindications.) Subsequent dosage should be adjusted according to the patient's tolerance and therapeutic response; dosage adjustments in increments of 2.5–5 mg daily at intervals of at least several days (usually 3–7 days) are recommended when conventional tablets are used. The manufacturer of extended-release glipizide tablets states that if fasting plasma glucose determinations are used to monitor response, dosage adjustment should be based on at least 2 similar consecutive values obtained at least 7 days after the previous dose adjustment.

Initial Dosage in Patients Transferred from Conventional to Extended-release Tablets Based on results of a randomized crossover study, patients receiving conventional glipizide tablets may be switched safely to extended-release glipizide tablets by giving the nearest equivalent total daily dose once daily. Alternatively, dosage can be titrated beginning with an initial dosage of 5 mg once daily as extended-release tablets. The decision to switch to the nearest equivalent dosage versus re-titration should be individualized using clinical judgment.

Initial Dosage in Patients Transferred from Other Antidiabetic Agents A transition period generally is not required when transferring from other sulfonylurea antidiabetic agents to glipizide, and administration of the other agent may be abruptly discontinued. Because of the prolonged elimination half-life of chlorpropamide, an exaggerated hypoglycemic response may occur in some patients during the transition from chlorpropamide to glipizide, and patients being transferred from chlorpropamide should be closely monitored for the occurrence of hypoglycemia during the initial 2 weeks of the transition period with conventional glipizide tablets or 1–2 weeks with extended-release glipizide tablets. A drug-free interval of 2–3 days may be advisable before glipizide therapy is initiated as conventional tablets in patients being transferred from chlorpropamide, particularly if blood glucose concentration was adequately controlled with chlorpropamide. An initial or loading dose of glipizide is *not* necessary when transferring from other sulfonylurea antidiabetic agents to glipizide. The transfer should be performed conservatively.

For the management of type 2 diabetes mellitus in patients previously receiving other sulfonylurea antidiabetic agents, the usual initial dosage of glipizide is 5–10 mg daily, but the initial dosage is variable and must be carefully individualized. Subsequent dosage is adjusted according to the patient's tolerance and therapeutic response. Although an exact dosage relationship between glipizide and other sulfonylurea antidiabetic agents does not exist, approximate dosage equivalencies have been estimated. (See Pharmacology: Antidiabetic Effect.)

In general, patients who were previously maintained on insulin dosages up to 20 units daily may be transferred directly to the usual recommended initial dosage of glipizide, and administration of insulin may be abruptly discontinued. In patients requiring insulin dosages greater than 20 units daily, the usual recommended initial dosage of glipizide should be started and insulin dosage reduced by 50%. Subsequently, insulin is withdrawn gradually and dosage of glipizide is adjusted in increments of 2.5–5 mg daily at intervals of at least several days, according to the patient's tolerance and therapeutic response. During the period of insulin withdrawal, patients should test their urine at least 3 times daily for glucose and ketones, and should be instructed to report the results to their physician so that appropriate adjustments in therapy may be made, if necessary; when feasible, patient or laboratory monitoring of blood glucose concentration is preferable. The presence of persistent ketonuria with glycosuria, ketosis, and/or inadequate lowering or persistent elevation of blood glucose concentration indicates that the patient requires insulin therapy. In some patients, especially those requiring greater than 40 units of insulin daily, the manufacturer suggests that it may be advisable to consider hospitalization during the transition from insulin to glipizide; however, some clinicians believe that hospitalization should rarely be necessary.

Maintenance Dosage The adult maintenance dosage of glipizide for the management of type 2 diabetes mellitus varies considerably, ranging from 2.5–40 mg daily. Most patients appear to require 5–25 mg daily as conventional tablets or 5–10 mg daily as extended-release tablets, but some clinicians report that higher dosages may be necessary in many patients. Dosage adjustments in patients receiving glipizide extended-release tablets may be made at approximately 3-month intervals, based on HbA_{1c} measurements. In patients receiving an initial dosage of 5 mg daily of extended-release glipizide tablets, dosage may be increased to 10 mg daily after 3 months if glycemic response is inadequate, based on a HbA_{1c} measurement. Subsequent dosage should be adjusted according to patient's therapeutic response, using the lowest possible effective dosage. If an enhanced glycemic response is not observed after 3 months at a higher dosage, the dosage should be decreased to the previous equally effective dosage.

Maintenance dosage of glipizide should be conservative in debilitated, malnourished, or geriatric patients or patients with impaired renal or hepatic function because of an increased risk of hypoglycemia in these patients. (See Cautions: Precautions and Contraindications.) The maximum recommended dosage is 40 mg daily as conventional tablets or 20 mg daily as extended-release tablets. While glycemic control may improve with glipizide extended-release tablets in certain patients receiving dosages exceeding 10 mg daily, clinical studies to date have not demonstrated an additional group average reduction in HbA_{1c} beyond what was achieved with the 10-mg daily dosage. Dosages up to 50 mg daily have been employed in some patients. Although the mechanism(s) has not been elucidated and further documentation is needed, some clinicians have reported that an increase in glipizide maintenance dosage actually resulted in a worsening of diabetic control in a few patients.

Combination Therapy with Other Oral Antidiabetic Agents Glipizide may be used in combination with other oral antidiabetic agents if glycemic control is inadequate with glipizide, either upon initiation of therapy or after a period of effectiveness. The second oral antidiabetic agent should be added to glipizide at the lowest recommended dosage, and patients should be observed carefully. Titration of the additional oral antidiabetic agent should be based on clinical judgment.

When glipizide is added to therapy with other antidiabetic agents, glipizide extended-release tablets may be initiated at a dosage of 5 mg daily. Initiation of therapy with glipizide extended-release tablets at a lower dosage may be appropriate in patients who may be more sensitive to oral hypoglycemic agents. Titration of glipizide as add-on therapy to another oral antidiabetic agent should be based on clinical judgment.

If the fixed combination of glipizide and metformin is used as initial therapy, the recommended initial dosage is 2.5 mg of glipizide and 250 mg of metformin hydrochloride once daily with a meal. In patients with more severe hyperglycemia (i.e., fasting plasma glucose concentrations of 280–320 mg/dL), an initial dosage of 2.5 mg of glipizide and 500 mg of metformin hydrochloride twice daily may be considered. Dosage may be increased in increments of one tablet (using the tablet strength at which therapy was initiated, either 2.5 mg glipizide/250 mg metformin hydrochloride or 2.5 mg glipizide/500 mg metformin hydrochloride) daily every 2 weeks until the minimum effective dosage required to achieve adequate glycemic control or a maximum daily dosage of 10 mg of glipizide and 2 g of metformin hydrochloride given in divided doses is reached. A total daily dosage exceeding 10 mg of glipizide and 2 g of metformin hydrochloride has not been evaluated in clinical trials in patients receiving the fixed-combination preparation as initial therapy. The efficacy of glipizide in fixed combination with metformin hydrochloride has not been established in patients with fasting plasma glucose concentrations exceeding 320 mg/dL.

When the commercially available fixed-combination preparation is used as second-line therapy in patients with type 2 diabetes mellitus whose blood glucose is not adequately controlled by therapy with a sulfonylurea antidiabetic agent or metformin alone, the recommended initial dosage in previously treated patients is 2.5 or 5 mg of glipizide and 500 mg of metformin hydrochloride twice daily with the morning and evening meals. In order to minimize the risk of hypoglycemia, the initial dosage of glipizide and metformin hydrochloride in fixed combination should not exceed the daily dosage of glipizide or metformin hydrochloride previously received. The dosage of glipizide and metformin hydrochloride in fixed combination should be titrated upward in increments not exceeding 5 mg of glipizide and 500 mg of metformin hydrochloride until adequate glycemic control or a maximum daily dosage of 20 mg of glipizide and 2 g of metformin hydrochloride is reached.

For patients being switched from combination therapy using separate preparations of glipizide (or another sulfonylurea antidiabetic agent) and metformin, the initial dosage of the fixed-combination preparation should not exceed the daily dosages of glipizide (or equivalent dosage of another sulfonylurea) and metformin hydrochloride currently being taken. Such patients should be monitored for signs and symptoms of hypoglycemia following the switch. In the transfer from previous antidiabetic therapy to the fixed combination of glipizide and metformin hydrochloride, the decision to switch to the nearest equivalent dosage or to titrate dosage is based on clinical judgment. Hypoglycemia or hyperglycemia are possible in such patients, and any change in the therapy of type 2 diabetic patients should be undertaken with appropriate monitoring. The safety and efficacy of switching from combined therapy with separate preparations of glipizide (or another sulfonylurea antidiabetic agent) and metformin hydrochloride to the fixed-combination preparation containing these drugs have not been established in clinical studies.

Cautions

When glipizide is used in fixed combination with metformin, the cautions, precautions, and contraindications associated with metformin must be considered in addition to those associated with glipizide.

■ **Hypoglycemia** Hypoglycemia may occur in patients receiving glipizide alone or in fixed combination with metformin. Hypoglycemia (defined as blood glucose of less than 60 mg/dL or symptoms associated with hypoglycemia) occurred in 3.4% of patients receiving glipizide extended-release tablets in clinical trials. *Appropriate patient selection and careful attention to dosage are important to avoid glipizide-induced hypoglycemia.* (See Cautions: Precautions and Contraindications.) Hypoglycemia may occur as a result of excessive glipizide dosage; however, since the development of hypoglycemia is a function of many factors, including diet, or exercise without adequate caloric supplementation, this effect may occur in some patients receiving usual dosages of the drug. Although glipizide-induced hypoglycemia has been reported infrequently and has usually been mild, severe hypoglycemia has occurred, principally in patients with predisposing conditions (e.g., impaired renal and/or hepatic function).

Management of glipizide-induced hypoglycemia depends on the severity of the reaction; patients with severe reactions require immediate hospitalization and treatment and observation until complete recovery is assured. Because of glipizide's elimination characteristics, the risk of prolonged hypoglycemia is likely to be low. Hypoglycemia is usually, but not always, readily controlled by administration of glucose. If hypoglycemia occurs during therapy with the drug, immediate reevaluation and adjustment of glipizide dosage and/or the patient's meal pattern are necessary.

For further discussion of the pathogenesis, manifestations, and treatment of glipizide-induced hypoglycemia, see Acute Toxicity.

■ **Other Endocrine and Metabolic Effects** Therapy with sulfonylureas, including glipizide, may be associated with weight gain. Although the exact mechanisms associated with such alterations in weight have not been established, suggested mechanisms include an increase in insulin secretion (which may increase appetite), stimulation of lipogenesis in fat tissue, or an increase in blood leptin concentrations. Data from the United Kingdom Prospective Diabetes (UKPD) study in patients receiving long-term therapy (over 10 years) with glyburide and other antidiabetic agents indicate that weight gain was greatest in those receiving intensive therapy (stepwise introduction of a sulfonylurea then insulin or an oral sulfonylurea and insulin, or insulin alone to achieve fasting glucose concentrations of 108 mg/dL) than conventional therapy (diet and oral antidiabetic agents or insulin to achieve fasting plasma glucose concentrations less than 270 mg/dL without symptoms of hyperglycemia), and weight gain was greatest in those initially receiving insulin or chlorpropamide compared with those receiving glyburide.

■ **GI Effects** Adverse GI effects such as nausea, anorexia, vomiting, pyrosis, gastralgia, diarrhea, and constipation are the most common adverse reactions to glipizide conventional tablets, occurring in about 1–2% of patients. Diarrhea or flatulence occurred in 5 or 3%, respectively, of patients receiving extended-release glipizide tablets in controlled clinical trials. Diarrhea was reported in 2.3–5.2 or 8.5% of patients receiving the fixed combination of glipizide and metformin or metformin monotherapy, respectively, as initial therapy for type 2 diabetes mellitus, and in 18.4 or 17.3% of patients receiving the fixed combination of glipizide and metformin or metformin monotherapy, respectively, as second-line therapy. Abdominal pain occurred in 5.7 or 6.7% of patients receiving the fixed combination of glipizide and metformin or metformin monotherapy, respectively, in clinical trials as second-line therapy for type 2 diabetes mellitus. Nausea, dyspepsia, constipation, or vomiting occurred in less than 3% of patients receiving extended-release glipizide tablets in clinical trials. Anorexia, thirst, or trace blood in the stool has been reported in less than 1% of patients receiving extended-release glipizide in clinical trials. Nausea or vomiting was reported in 0.6–1.7 or 5.1% of patients receiving the fixed combination of glipizide and metformin or metformin monotherapy, respectively, as initial therapy for type 2 diabetes mellitus, and in 8% of patients receiving either the fixed combination of glipizide and metformin or metformin monotherapy as second-line therapy. Glipizide-induced adverse GI effects appear to be dose related and may subside following a reduction in dosage or administration of the drug in divided doses.

■ **Dermatologic Effects** Allergic skin reactions including pruritus, erythema, eczema, urticaria, and morbilliform or maculopapular eruptions occur in about 1.5% of patients receiving glipizide conventional tablets. Rash or urticaria has been reported in less than 1% of patients receiving extended-release glipizide tablets in clinical trials. Glipizide-induced adverse dermatologic effects may be transient and disappear despite continued therapy; however, if adverse dermatologic effects persist with continued glipizide therapy, the drug should be discontinued. Photosensitivity reactions and porphyria cutanea tarda have been reported with other sulfonylurea antidiabetic agents.

■ **Hepatic Effects** One case of glipizide-associated jaundice has been reported. Cholestatic jaundice has occurred with other sulfonylureas and is an indication for discontinuing glipizide. Although a causal relationship has not been established, mild to moderate increases in serum LDH, AST (SGOT), and alkaline phosphatase concentration have occurred occasionally in patients receiving glipizide. Exacerbation of hepatic porphyria has been reported with other sulfonylurea antidiabetic agents, but has not been reported to date with glipizide.

■ **Hematologic Effects** Like other sulfonylurea antidiabetic agents, glipizide may rarely cause leukopenia, thrombocytopenia, pancytopenia, agranulocytosis, aplastic anemia, and hemolytic anemia.

■ **Nervous System Effects** Dizziness, drowsiness, and headache have been reported in about 2% of patients receiving glipizide conventional tablets, usually as manifestations of mild hypoglycemia. Asthenia, headache, dizziness, nervousness, pain, or tremor has been reported in 10, 9, 7, or 4% of patients receiving glipizide extended-release tablets in controlled clinical trials. Headache has been reported in 12.6 or 5.3% of patients receiving the fixed combination of glipizide and metformin or metformin monotherapy, respectively, as second-line therapy for type 2 diabetes mellitus. Dizziness has been reported in 1.7–5.2 or 1.1% of patients receiving the fixed combination of glipizide and metformin or metformin monotherapy, respectively, in clinical trials as initial therapy for type 2 diabetes mellitus. Insomnia, paresthesia, anxiety, depression, and hypesthesia have been reported in less than 3% of patients receiving glipizide extended-release tablets in clinical trials. Chills, hypertonia, confusion, vertigo, somnolence, or gait abnormality has been reported in less than 1% of patients receiving extended-release glipizide in clinical trials.

■ **Other Adverse Effects** Arthralgia, leg cramps, or myalgia has been reported in less than 3% of patients receiving extended-release glipizide in clinical trials. Musculoskeletal pain has been reported in 8 or 6.7% of patients receiving the fixed combination of glipizide and metformin or metformin monotherapy, respectively, as second-line therapy for type 2 diabetes mellitus. Syncope has been reported in less than 3%, and arrhythmia, migraine, flushing, hypertension, or edema has been reported less than 1% of patients receiving extended-release glipizide tablets in clinical trials. Hypertension has been reported in 2.9–3.5 or 5.6 % of patients receiving glipizide in fixed combination with metformin or metformin alone, respectively, as initial therapy for type 2 diabetes mellitus. Rhinitis has reported in less than 3%, and pharyngitis or dyspnea has been reported in than 1% of patients receiving extended-release glipizide tablets in clinical trials. Upper respiratory tract infection was reported in 8.1–9.9 or 8.5% of patients receiving the fixed combination of glipizide and metformin or metformin monotherapy, respectively, as initial therapy for type 2 diabetes mellitus, and in 10.3 or 10.7% of patients receiving the fixed combination of glipizide and metformin or metformin monotherapy, respectively, as second-line therapy. Blurred vision has been reported in less than 3%, and ocular pain, conjunctivitis, or retinal hemorrhage has been reported in less than 1% of patients receiving extended-release glipizide tablets in clinical trials. Although a causal relationship has not been established, mild to moderate increases in BUN and serum creatinine concentration have occurred occasionally in patients receiving glipizide. Urinary tract infection has been reported in 1.1 or 8% of patients receiving the fixed combination of glipizide and metformin or metformin monotherapy, respectively, as second-line therapy for type 2 diabetes mellitus. Decreased libido or polyuria has been reported in less than 3%, and dysuria has been reported in less than 1% of patients receiving extended-release glipizide tablets in clinical trials.

Like other sulfonylureas, hyponatremia and the syndrome of inappropriate secretion of antidiuretic hormone (SIADH) have occurred in patients receiving glipizide.

■ Precautions and Contraindications Glipizide shares the toxic potentials of other sulfonylurea antidiabetic agents, and the usual precautions associated with their use should be observed. The diagnostic and therapeutic measures for managing diabetes mellitus that are necessary to ensure optimum control of the disease with insulin generally are necessary with glipizide. Glipizide should only be prescribed for carefully selected patients by clinicians who are familiar with the indications, limitations, and patient-selection criteria for therapy with oral sulfonylurea antidiabetic agents.

Patients receiving glipizide should be monitored with regular clinical and laboratory evaluations, including blood and urine glucose determinations, to determine the minimum effective dosage and to detect primary failure (inadequate lowering of blood glucose concentration at the maximum recommended dosage) or secondary failure (loss of control of blood glucose concentration following an initial period of effectiveness) to the drug. Glycosylated hemoglobin (hemoglobin A_{1c} [HbA_{1c}]) measurements may also be useful for monitoring the patient's response to glipizide therapy. During the withdrawal period in patients in whom glipizide is replacing insulin, patients should be instructed to test their urine for glucose and ketones at least 3 times daily, and to report the results to their physician; when feasible, patient or laboratory monitoring of blood glucose concentration is preferable. Care should be taken to avoid ketosis, acidosis, and coma during the withdrawal period in patients being switched from insulin to glipizide. If adequate lowering of blood glucose concentration is no longer achieved during maintenance therapy with glipizide, the drug should be discontinued. When use of glipizide in asymptomatic type 2 diabetic patients is being considered, it should be recognized that control of blood glucose concentration in these patients has not been definitely established as effective for prevention of long-term cardiovascular or nervous system complications of the disease. There is limited evidence that sulfonylureas may reverse basement-membrane thickening of muscle capillaries in asymptomatic individuals with impaired glucose tolerance (chemical diabetes) and possibly reverse or retard the progression of microangiopathy in type 2 diabetic patients, but these findings require further evaluation.

Several large, long-term studies have evaluated the cardiovascular risks associated with the use of oral sulfonylurea antidiabetic agents. In 1970, the University Group Diabetes Program (UGDP) reported that administration of oral antidiabetic agents (i.e., tolbutamide or phenformin) was associated with increased cardiovascular mortality as compared to treatment with dietary regulation alone or with dietary regulation and insulin. The UGDP reported that type 2 diabetic patients who were treated for 5–8 years with dietary regulation and a fixed dose of tolbutamide (1.5 g daily) had a cardiovascular mortality rate approximately 2.5 times that of patients treated with dietary regulation alone; although a substantial increase in total mortality was not observed, the use of tolbutamide was discontinued because of the increase in cardiovascular mortality, thereby limiting the ability of the study to show an increase in total mortality. The results of the UGDP study have been exhaustively analyzed, and there has been general disagreement in the scientific and medical communities regarding the study's validity and clinical importance. However, recent results from the United Kingdom Prospective Diabetes (UKPD) study, a large, long-term (over 10 years) study in newly diagnosed type 2 diabetic patients, did not confirm an increase in cardiovascular events or mortality in the group treated intensively with sulfonylureas, insulin, or combination therapy compared with less intensive conventional antidiabetic therapy.

In the UKPD study, the overall aggregate rates of death from macrovascular diseases such as myocardial infarction, sudden death, stroke, or peripheral vascular disease were not appreciably different among either intensive therapies (stepwise introduction of a sulfonylurea [i.e., chlorpropamide, glyburide] then insulin, or an oral sulfonylurea and insulin, or insulin alone to achieve fasting plasma glucose concentrations of 108 mg/dL) or less intensive conventional therapy (diet and oral antidiabetic agents or insulin to achieve fasting plasma glucose concentrations below 270 mg/dL without symptoms of hyperglycemia). However, a trend in reduction in fatal and nonfatal myocardial infarction with intensive therapy was noted with sulfonylurea or insulin, and epidemiologic analysis of the data indicate that each 1% decrease in HbA_{1c} was associated with an 18% reduction of fatal and nonfatal myocardial infarction. Among the single end points, the incidence of angina increased among patients receiving chlorpropamide, and blood pressure also was higher with chlorpropamide compared with glyburide or insulin intensive therapies. As a result of these and other findings (e.g., beneficial effects on microvascular [retinopathy, nephropathy, and possibly neuropathy] complications, confirmation of the beneficial effects of concomitant antihypertensive therapy and blood pressure lowering) of the UKDP study, the American Diabetes Association (ADA) currently considers the beneficial effects of intensive glycemic control with insulin or sulfonylureas and blood pressure control in diabetic patients to outweigh the risks overall.

Patients should be fully and completely advised about the nature of diabetes mellitus, what they must do to prevent and detect complications, and how to control their condition. *Patients should be informed of the potential risks and advantages of glipizide therapy and alternative forms of treatment.* Patients should be instructed that dietary regulation is the principal consideration in the management of diabetes, and that glipizide therapy is only used as an adjunct to, and not a substitute for or a convenient means to avoid, proper dietary regulation. Patients should also be advised that they should not neglect dietary restrictions, develop a careless attitude about their condition, or disregard instructions about body-weight control, exercise, hygiene, and avoidance of infection. Primary and secondary failure to oral sulfonylurea antidiabetic agents should also be explained to patients.

Patients and responsible family members should be informed of the risks of hypoglycemia, the symptoms and treatment of hypoglycemic reactions, and conditions that predispose to the development of hypoglycemic reactions, since these reactions may occasionally occur during therapy with glipizide. *Appropriate patient selection and careful attention to dosage are important to avoid glipizide-induced hypoglycemia.* Debilitated, malnourished, or geriatric patients and patients with impaired hepatic or renal function should be carefully monitored and dosage of glipizide should be carefully adjusted in these patients, since they may be predisposed to developing hypoglycemia (sometimes severe). Renal or hepatic insufficiency may cause increased serum concentrations of glipizide and hepatic insufficiency may also diminish gluconeogenic capacity, both of which increase the risk of severe hypoglycemic reactions. Alcohol ingestion, severe or prolonged exercise, deficient caloric intake, use of more than one antidiabetic agent, and adrenal or pituitary insufficiency may also predispose patients to the development of hypoglycemia. Hypoglycemia may be difficult to recognize in geriatric patients or in patients receiving β-adrenergic blocking agents. Intensive treatment (e.g., IV dextrose) and close medical supervision may be required in some patients who develop severe hypoglycemia during glipizide therapy. (See Acute Toxicity: Treatment.)

To maintain control of diabetes during periods of stress (e.g., fever of any cause, trauma, infection, surgery), temporary discontinuance of glipizide and administration of insulin may be required.

As with other nondeformable material, extended-release glipizide tablets should be used with caution in patients with severe preexisting GI narrowing, since obstruction may occur. The inert portion of glipizide extended-release tablets is not absorbed and is excreted in feces where it may be noticeable. If cholestatic jaundice occurs or if adverse dermatologic effects occur and persist during glipizide therapy, the drug should be discontinued. Glipizide is contraindicated as sole therapy in patients with type 1 diabetes mellitus or in those with diabetes complicated by ketosis, acidosis, or diabetic coma. Like other sulfonylureas, glipizide is generally contraindicated in patients with severe renal or hepatic impairment. Glipizide is also contraindicated in patients with known hypersensitivity or allergy to the drug.

■ Pediatric Precautions The manufacturer states that safety and efficacy of glipizide alone or in fixed combination with metformin in children have not been established. However, the American Diabetes Association (ADA) states that most pediatric diabetologists use oral antidiabetic agents in children with type 2 diabetes mellitus because of greater patient compliance and convenience for the patient's family and a lack of evidence demonstrating better efficacy of insulin as initial therapy for type 2 diabetes mellitus.

■ Geriatric Precautions Safety and efficacy of glipizide extended-release tablets in geriatric patients have not been specifically studied to date; however, in clinical studies of the drug, approximately 33% of patients were 65 years of age or older. It has not been determined whether clinical trials of glipizide conventional tablets did not include sufficient numbers of patients 65 years and older to determine whether they respond differently than younger adults. Although no overall differences in safety or efficacy were observed between geriatric and younger patients in clinical studies of glipizide extended-release tablets, the possibility that some older patients may exhibit increased sensitivity cannot be ruled out. Because of the greater frequency of decreased hepatic, renal, and/or cardiac function and of concomitant disease and drug therapy in geriatric patients, the manufacturer suggests that patients in this age group receive initial dosages of the drug in the lower end of the usual range. Geriatric patients should be carefully monitored and dosage of glipizide should be carefully adjusted in these patients, since they may be predisposed to developing hypoglycemia (sometimes severe).

■ Mutagenicity and Carcinogenicity It is not known if glipizide is mutagenic or carcinogenic in humans. The drug did not exhibit mutagenic activity in the Ames microbial mutagen test or in vivo in animal tests. Evidence of carcinogenicity was not observed in rats or mice receiving up to 75 times the maximum human dosage of glipizide daily for 20 or 18 months, respectively.

■ **Pregnancy, Fertility, and Lactation** Although there are no adequate and controlled studies to date in humans, glipizide has been shown to be mildly fetotoxic in rats when given at doses of 5–50 mg/kg; the fetotoxic effect is perinatal and similar to that of some other sulfonylureas, and is believed to be directly related to the hypoglycemic effect of the drug. No teratogenic effects were observed in reproduction studies in rats or rabbits. Since abnormal maternal blood glucose concentrations during pregnancy may be associated with a higher incidence of congenital abnormalities, many experts recommend that insulin be used during pregnancy to maintain optimum control of blood glucose concentration. Use of glipizide in pregnant women is generally *not* recommended, and the drug should be used during pregnancy only when clearly necessary (e.g., when insulin therapy is infeasible). Prolonged, severe hypoglycemia lasting 4–10 days has been reported in some neonates born to women who were receiving other sulfonylurea antidiabetic agents up to the time of delivery; this effect has been reported more frequently with the use of those agents having prolonged elimination half-lives. To minimize the risk of neonatal hypoglycemia if glipizide is used during pregnancy, the manufacturer recommends that the drug be discontinued at least 1 month before the expected delivery date.

Reproduction studies in rats using glipizide doses up to 75 times the usual human dose have not revealed evidence of impaired fertility.

Although it is not known whether glipizide is distributed into milk in humans, some sulfonylurea antidiabetic agents are distributed into milk. Because of the potential for hypoglycemia in nursing infants, a decision should be made whether to discontinue nursing or the drug, taking into account the importance of the drug to the woman. If glipizide is discontinued, and if dietary management alone is inadequate for controlling blood glucose concentration, administration of insulin should be considered.

Drug Interactions

■ **Protein-bound Drugs** Because glipizide is highly protein bound, it theoretically could be displaced from binding sites by, or could displace from binding sites, other protein-bound drugs such as oral anticoagulants, hydantoins, salicylate and other nonsteroidal anti-inflammatory agents, and sulfonamides. However, unlike the protein binding of some other sulfonylurea antidiabetic agents (e.g., acetohexamide, chlorpropamide, tolazamide, tolbutamide) and like that of glyburide, the protein binding of glipizide is principally nonionic; in addition, glipizide appears to bind to different but closely related sites on serum albumin than does tolbutamide. Consequently, glipizide may be less likely to be displaced from binding sites by, or displace from binding sites, other highly protein-bound drugs whose protein binding is ionic in nature. In vitro studies indicate that glipizide does not displace dicumarol or salicylate from plasma proteins. Whether any differences in protein binding demonstrated in vitro will result in fewer clinically important drug interactions in vivo has not been established. There appears to be no clinically important interaction between indoprofen and glipizide. Patients receiving highly protein-bound drugs should be observed for adverse effects when glipizide therapy is initiated or discontinued and vice versa.

■ **Cimetidine** Preliminary data indicate that cimetidine may potentiate the hypoglycemic effects of glipizide. The exact mechanism(s) of this interaction is not known, but cimetidine may inhibit hepatic metabolism of the sulfonylurea. Oral cimetidine has been shown to substantially increase the area under the plasma glipizide concentration-time curve and was associated with a substantial reduction in the postprandial increase in blood glucose concentration in diabetic patients receiving the drugs concomitantly. If cimetidine is administered concomitantly with glipizide, the patient should be closely monitored for signs and symptoms of hypoglycemia; dosage adjustment of glipizide may be necessary when cimetidine therapy is initiated or discontinued.

■ **Thiazide Diuretics** Thiazide diuretics may exacerbate diabetes mellitus, resulting in increased requirements of sulfonylurea antidiabetic agents, temporary loss of diabetic control, or secondary failure to the antidiabetic agent. When thiazide diuretics are administered concomitantly with sulfonylurea antidiabetic agents, caution should be used.

■ **Alcohol** Disulfiram-like reactions have occurred very rarely following the concomitant use of alcohol and glipizide.

■ **β-Adrenergic Blocking Agents** Several potential interactions between β-adrenergic blocking agents and sulfonylurea antidiabetic agents exist. β-Adrenergic blocking agents may impair glucose tolerance; increase the frequency or severity of hypoglycemia; block hypoglycemia-induced tachycardia, but not hypoglycemic sweating which may actually be increased; delay the rate of recovery of blood glucose concentration following drug-induced hypoglycemiater the hemodynamic response to hypoglycemia, possibly resulting in an exaggerated hypertensive response; and possibly impair peripheral circulation. There is some evidence that many of these effects may be minimized by use of a β_1-selective adrenergic blocking agent rather than a nonselective β-adrenergic blocking agent. In one study in type 2 diabetic patients, tolbutamide-induced insulin secretion was not affected by short-term propranolol therapy, but the hypoglycemic action of a single dose of glipizide in conjunction with an oral glucose load appeared to be slightly reduced. It generally is recommended that concomitant use of β-adrenergic blocking agents and sulfonylurea antidiabetic agents be avoided when possible; if concomitant therapy is necessary, use of a β_1-selective adrenergic blocking agent may be preferred. When glipizide and a β-adrenergic blocking agent are used concomitantly, the patient should be monitored closely for altered antidiabetic response.

■ **Antifungal Antibiotics** Concomitant use of certain antifungal antibiotics (i.e., miconazole, fluconazole) and oral antidiabetic agents has resulted in increased plasma concentrations of glipizide and/or hypoglycemia. In a study in healthy individuals, the area under the plasma concentration-time curve (AUC) of glipizide increased by 57% following concomitant administration with fluconazole (100 mg daily for 7 days). Clinically important hypoglycemia may be precipitated by concomitant use of oral hypoglycemic agents and fluconazole, and at least one fatality has been reported from hypoglycemia in a patient receiving glyburide and fluconazole concomitantly. (See Drug Interactions: Sulfonylurea Antidiabetic Agents in Fluconazole in 8:14.08).

■ **Other Drugs** Drugs that may enhance the hypoglycemic effect of sulfonylurea antidiabetic agents, including glipizide, include chloramphenicol, monoamine oxidase inhibitors, and probenecid. When these drugs are administered or discontinued in patients receiving glipizide, the patient should be observed closely for hypoglycemia or loss of diabetic control, respectively. When glipizide was administered to counter the hyperglycemic effect of diazoxide in several severely hypertensive nondiabetic patients with impaired renal function, hypoglycemic reactions resulted, prompting some clinicians to recommend that the drugs not be used concomitantly in such circumstances.

Drugs that may decrease the hypoglycemic effect of sulfonylurea antidiabetic agents, including glipizide, include nonthiazide diuretics (e.g., furosemide), corticosteroids, phenothiazines, thyroid agents, estrogens, oral contraceptives, phenytoin,nicotinic acid, sympathomimetic agents, calcium-channel blocking agents, rifampin, and isoniazid. When these drugs are administered or discontinued in patients receiving glipizide, the patient should be observed closely for loss of diabetic control or hypoglycemia, respectively.

Preliminary data suggest that glipizide may reduce the rate and/or extent of absorption of concomitantly administered oral xylose in type 2 diabetic patients.

Acute Toxicity

■ **Pathogenesis** There is no well documented experience to date with glipizide overdosage. The oral LD_{50} of the drug was greater than 4 g/kg in all animal species tested. Acute glipizide toxicity may result from excessive dosage, and numerous conditions may predispose patients to the development of glipizide-induced hypoglycemia. (See Cautions: Precautions and Contraindications.) Severe glipizide-induced hypoglycemia has reportedly occurred almost exclusively in patients with predisposing conditions (e.g., impaired renal and/or hepatic function).

■ **Manifestations** Acute glipizide overdosage is manifested principally as hypoglycemia, which is usually mild but occasionally may be severe. Severe sulfonylurea-induced hypoglycemia may result in loss of consciousness and seizures, with resultant neurologic sequelae. Because of glipizide's elimination characteristics, the risk of prolonged hypoglycemia is likely to be low. In some cases, hypoglycemia may persist despite continuous IV administration of dextrose.

■ **Treatment** Treatment of acute glipizide overdosage consists principally of administration of glucose and supportive therapy. *The patient should be monitored closely until complete recovery is assured.*

Patients with mild hypoglycemic symptoms without loss of consciousness or adverse neurologic effects should be treated aggressively with orally administered glucose, and glipizide dosage and/or the patient's meal pattern should be appropriately adjusted. Severe glipizide-induced hypoglycemia with coma, seizures, or other neurologic impairment occurs infrequently, but constitutes a medical emergency requiring immediate hospitalization and treatment. If hypoglycemic coma is diagnosed or suspected, 50% dextrose injection (e.g., 50 mL) should be administered IV rapidly, followed immediately by a continuous IV infusion of 10% dextrose injection at a rate sufficient to maintain a blood glucose concentration greater than 100 mg/dL. In some patients, subsequent administration of IV glucagon and/or corticosteroids may also be necessary. Blood glucose concentrations should be monitored at least every 3 hours during the first 24 hours and as often as necessary thereafter. Care should be taken to avoid inducing excessive hyperglycemia. Other symptomatic therapy (e.g., anticonvulsants) should be administered as necessary. Glipizide is effectively adsorbed by activated charcoal in vitro. Experimental studies using chlorpropamide suggest that if sulfonylurea overdosage is the result of an acute ingestion, administration of activated charcoal within several hours of the ingestion may be effective in reducing sulfonylurea absorption. Because glipizide is highly protein bound, dialysis is not likely to enhance elimination of the drug. Since hypoglycemia may occur after apparent clinical recovery, patients must be closely monitored for *at least* 24–48 hours; in patients with substantial renal or hepatic dysfunction, longer periods of monitoring may be necessary.

Pharmacology

■ **Antidiabetic Effect** Like other sulfonylurea antidiabetic agents, glipizide lowers blood glucose concentration in diabetic and nondiabetic individuals. Although the hypoglycemic action of the various sulfonylureas is generally similar, the drugs may differ quantitatively and/or possibly qualitatively in the extent to which they produce specific effects, and the effects may vary as a function of duration of treatment. On a weight basis, glipizide is one of the most potent of the sulfonylurea antidiabetic agents; although an exact dosage relationship does not exist, a daily glipizide dose of 5 mg controls blood glucose concentration to approximately the same degree as daily doses of acetohexamide 500 mg, chlorpropamide or tolazamide 250 mg, glyburide 2.5–5 mg, or tolbutamide 0.5–1 g.

The precise mechanism(s) of hypoglycemic action of sulfonylurea antidiabetic agents has not been clearly established, but the drugs, including glipizide, initially appear to lower blood glucose concentration principally by stimulating secretion of endogenous insulin from the beta cells of the pancreas. Glipizide also appears to enhance peripheral insulin action at postreceptor (probably intracellular) site(s) during short-term therapy. Like other sulfonylureas, glipizide alone is ineffective in the absence of functioning beta cells.

The mechanism(s) of action of glipizide during prolonged administration has not been fully established. The glipizide-induced increase in glucose- or meal-stimulated secretion of endogenous insulin appears to be sustained during prolonged administration and has persisted in most diabetic patients for up to at least 2 years. The prolonged effect of glipizide on secretion of endogenous insulin is unlike that of most other sulfonylureas, but its clinical importance in the long-term efficacy of the drug remains to be clearly determined; while this effect likely contributes to the improvement in glucose tolerance in many patients during prolonged glipizide therapy, it alone does not appear to be sufficient for a long-term, effective response to the drug and glucose tolerance can improve in some patients without an increase in insulin secretion. Fasting plasma insulin concentrations are usually not increased during prolonged glipizide therapy but have been reported to be slightly increased in some patients. The drug generally does not appear to alter glucagon secretion. During prolonged administration of sulfonylureas, including glipizide, extrapancreatic effects appear to substantially contribute to the hypoglycemic action of the drugs. Many extrapancreatic effects of the drugs have been proposed and/or studied, but the principal effects appear to include enhanced peripheral sensitivity to insulin and reduction of basal hepatic glucose production; however, the nature of the long-term hypoglycemic effect and the mechanism(s) involved remain to be fully elucidated. There is evidence that glipizide enhances the peripheral action of insulin at postreceptor (probably intracellular) site(s) during long-term administration, and this appears to be a principal mechanism of action during prolonged therapy. An increase in insulin binding in erythrocytes obtained from diabetic patients receiving long-term therapy with the drug has also been reported.

■ **Other Effects** In patients with type 2 diabetes mellitus, glipizide-induced improvement in plasma glucose concentration is associated with a reduction in plasma total and very low-density lipoprotein (VLDL) triglyceride concentrations and plasma low-density lipoprotein (LDL) cholesterol concentration; mean serum or plasma total, LDL, and high-density lipoprotein (HDL) cholesterol concentrations generally do not appear to be changed during therapy with the drug, but the ratio of plasma HDL cholesterol to total cholesterol may be slightly increased. The effects of glipizide on plasma lipids are apparently secondary to improved control of plasma glucose concentration.

Glipizide has been reported to slightly enhance renal free water clearance in healthy individuals, possibly by increasing electrolyte reabsorption in the loop of Henle.

In vitro, glipizide reportedly inhibits platelet aggregation induced by collagen or adenosine diphosphate (ADP). The effect, if any, of the drug on platelet aggregation in vivo has not been determined to date.

Pharmacokinetics

■ **Absorption** Glipizide is rapidly and essentially completely absorbed from the GI tract. First-pass metabolism of glipizide appears to be minimal, and the absolute oral bioavailability of the drug is reported to be 80–100%. Food delays the absorption of glipizide but does not affect peak serum concentrations achieved or the extent of absorption of the drug.

Following oral administration of a single 5-mg dose of glipizide as conventional tablets in fasting and nonfasting individuals, the drug appears in plasma or serum within 15–30 minutes and average peak plasma or serum concentrations of approximately 310–450 ng/mL usually are attained within 1–3 hours (range: 1–6 hours). Peak serum concentrations generally are delayed 20–40 minutes in the nonfasting state compared with the fasting state. A few reports indicate that biphasic peak serum concentrations may occur in some patients, suggesting that the drug may undergo enterohepatic circulation. The area under the serum concentration-time curve (AUC) for glipizide increases in proportion to increasing doses. Time to reach steady-state plasma glipizide concentrations following administration of glipizide extended-release tablets was delayed by 1–2 days in geriatric patients compared with younger patients.

Following administration of glipizide extended-release tablets in men with type 2 diabetes mellitus and patients younger than 65 years of age, steady-state plasma glipizide concentrations were achieved by at least the fifth day of dosing.

Following single oral doses of glipizide as conventional tablets in nonfasting diabetic or healthy individuals, plasma insulin concentration generally begins to increase within 10–30 minutes and is maximal within 0.5–2 hours; increased plasma insulin concentrations generally do not persist beyond the time of the meal challenge. Following single oral doses in fasting healthy individuals, the hypoglycemic action of glipizide generally begins within 15–30 minutes and is maximal within 1–2 hours. In nonfasting diabetic patients, the hypoglycemic action of a single morning dose of the drug may persist for up to 24 hours. Although a correlation between the plasma concentration of glipizide and its hypoglycemic effect has not been established, plasma insulin concentration was increased only when the plasma glipizide concentration was 200 ng/mL or higher in one study.

■ **Distribution** Distribution of glipizide into human body tissues and fluids has not been fully characterized. Following IV administration of glipizide in mice, highest concentrations of the drug were attained in the liver and blood, with lower concentrations in the lungs, kidneys, adrenals, myocardium, salivary glands, and retroscapular fat; the drug was not detected in the brain or spinal cord. In humans, small amounts of glipizide are apparently distributed into bile and very small amounts are distributed into erythrocytes and saliva. Although glipizide apparently did not cross the placenta in mice in one study, the drug was detected in the fetuses of pregnant rats given the drug. It is not known if glipizide is distributed into milk in humans.

Following IV administration in humans, glipizide undergoes rapid distribution. Following IV administration of the drug, the volumes of distribution in the central compartment and at steady-state average 4.2–4.6 L (range: 3.5–13.2 L) and 10.2–11.7 L (range: 4.6–15.1 L), respectively, suggesting that the drug is distributed principally within extracellular fluid. Although pharmacokinetic data from one single-dose study suggest that glipizide might accumulate in a deep tissue compartment, data from other single-dose studies suggest that the drug does not accumulate in tissue depots.

At a concentration of 9–612 ng/mL, glipizide is approximately 92–99% bound to plasma proteins. Glipizide has a lower affinity for binding to serum albumin than does glyburide. Unlike the protein binding of some other sulfonylurea antidiabetic agents (e.g., acetohexamide, chlorpropamide, tolazamide, tolbutamide) and like that of glyburide, the protein binding of glipizide appears to be principally nonionic; consequently, glipizide may be less likely to be displaced from binding sites by, or displace from binding sites, other highly protein-bound drugs whose protein binding is ionic in nature. (See Drug Interactions: Protein-Bound Drugs.)

■ **Elimination** Following IV administration, serum concentrations of glipizide decline in a biphasic manner. Following IV administration of glipizide in healthy individuals or diabetic patients with normal renal and hepatic function, the half-life of the drug averages 8.4–36 minutes (range: 4–36 minutes) in the initial phase and 2.1–3.6 hours (range: 1.1–3.7 hours) in the terminal phase. Following oral administration in healthy individuals or diabetic patients with normal renal and hepatic function, the terminal elimination half-life of glipizide averages 3–4.7 hours (range: 2–7.3 hours). The terminal elimination half-life of total glipizide metabolites reportedly ranges from 2–6 hours in patients with normal renal and hepatic function. Serum glipizide concentrations may be increased in patients with renal or hepatic insufficiency. Data are limited, but the terminal elimination half-life of unchanged glipizide does not appear to be substantially increased in patients with impaired renal function. The terminal elimination half-life of total glipizide metabolites may be prolonged to greater than 20 hours in patients with impaired renal function; however, since glipizide metabolites are considered essentially inactive, this is probably of little clinical importance, at least in patients with moderate renal impairment.

Glipizide is almost completely metabolized, mainly in the liver. The drug is metabolized principally at the cyclohexyl ring to 4-*trans*-hydroxyglipizide; the drug is also metabolized to the 3-*cis*-hydroxy derivative, *N*-(2-acetylaminoethylphenylsulfonyl)-*N*′-cyclohexyl urea (DCDA), and at least 2 unidentified metabolites.

Glipizide and its metabolites are excreted principally in urine. The drug and its metabolites are also excreted in feces, apparently almost completely via biliary elimination; only small amounts may be excreted in feces as unabsorbed drug following oral administration. Most urinary excretion occurs within the first 6–24 hours after oral administration of the drug. Following oral administration of a single 5-mg dose of glipizide in individuals with normal renal and hepatic function, approximately 60–90% of the dose is excreted in urine as unchanged drug and metabolites within 24–72 hours and about 5–20% is excreted in feces within 24–96 hours; less than 10% of a dose is excreted in urine as unchanged drug within 24 hours, about 20–60% as the 4-*trans*-hydroxy metabolite, 10–15% as the 3-*cis*-hydroxy metabolite, 1–2% as DCDA, and the remainder as unidentified metabolites.

Total plasma or serum clearance of glipizide reportedly averages 21–38 mL/hour per kg in individuals with normal renal and hepatic function. Renal clearance of unchanged glipizide increases substantially with increasing urinary pH, but is only about 5% of total plasma clearance at urinary pH of 5–6; the low renal clearance indicates that the drug undergoes renal tubular reabsorption. The effects have not been fully evaluated, but elimination of glipizide may be reduced in patients with impaired renal and/or hepatic function. Limited data indicate that renal excretion and terminal elimination half-life of glipizide metabolites are substantially decreased and increased, respectively, in patients with severe renal impairment.

Chemistry and Stability

■ **Chemistry** Glipizide is a sulfonylurea antidiabetic agent. The drug is structurally similar to acetohexamide and glyburide. Glipizide occurs as a whitish powder and is practically insoluble in water and in alcohol. The drug has a pK_a of 5.9.

■ **Stability** Glipizide tablets should be stored in tight, light-resistant containers at a temperature less than 30°C. Glipizide extended-release tablets should be stored at controlled room temperatures of 15–30°C and protected from moisture and humidity.

Preparations

Excipients in commercially available drug preparations may have clinically important effects in some individuals; consult specific product labeling for details.

glipiZIDE

Oral		
Tablets	5 mg*	**glipiZIDE Tablets**
		Glucotrol® (scored), Pfizer
	10 mg*	**glipiZIDE Tablets**
		Glucotrol® (scored), Pfizer
Tablets, extended-release	2.5 mg*	**glipiZIDE Tablets ER**
		Glucotrol XL®, Pfizer
	5 mg*	**glipiZIDE Tablets ER**
		Glucotrol XL®, Pfizer
	10 mg*	**glipiZIDE Tablets ER**
		Glucotrol XL®, Pfizer

*available from one or more manufacturer, distributor, and/or repackager by generic (nonproprietary) name

glipiZIDE Combinations

Oral		
Tablets, film-coated	2.5 mg with 250 mg Metformin Hydrochloride*	**glipiZIDE with Metformin Hydrochloride Tablets**
		Metaglip®, Bristol-Myers Squibb
	2.5 mg with 500 mg Metformin Hydrochloride*	**glipiZIDE with Metformin Hydrochloride Tablets**
		Metaglip®, Bristol-Myers Squibb
	5 mg with 500 mg Metformin Hydrochloride*	**glipiZIDE with Metformin Hydrochloride Tablets**
		Metaglip®, Bristol-Myers Squibb

*available from one or more manufacturer, distributor, and/or repackager by generic (nonproprietary) name

glyBURIDE

Glibenclamide, Glybenclamide, Glybenzcyclamide

■ Glyburide is a sulfonylurea antidiabetic agent.

Uses

■ **Diabetes Mellitus** Glyburide alone or in fixed combination with metformin hydrochloride is used as initial therapy as an adjunct to diet and exercise for the management of type 2 diabetes mellitus in patients whose hyperglycemia cannot be controlled by diet alone. Glyburide also may be used in combination with metformin as second-line therapy as an adjunct to diet and exercise for the management of type 2 diabetes mellitus in patients whose hyperglycemia cannot be controlled with glyburide or metformin monotherapy, diet, and exercise. Sulfonylureas, including glyburide, also may be used in combination with one or more other oral antidiabetic agents or insulin as an adjunct to diet and exercise for the management of type 2 diabetes mellitus in patients who do not achieve adequate glycemic control with diet, exercise, and oral antidiabetic agent monotherapy. A thiazolidinedione antidiabetic agent (e.g., rosiglitazone) has been added to therapy with the fixed combination of glyburide and metformin hydrochloride to improve glycemic control in patients not responding adequately to the fixed combination.

The American Diabetes Association (ADA) currently classifies diabetes mellitus into several subclasses including type 1 (immune mediated or idiopathic), type 2 (predominantly insulin resistance with relative insulin deficiency to predominantly an insulin secretory defect with insulin resistance), gestational diabetes mellitus, or that associated with certain conditions or syndromes (e.g., drug induced, hormonal, that associated with pancreatic disease, infections, specific genetic defects or syndromes). Type 1 diabetes mellitus was previously described as juvenile-onset (JOD) diabetes mellitus, since it usually occurs during youth. Type 2 diabetes mellitus was previously described as adult-onset (AODM) diabetes mellitus. However, type 1 or type 2 diabetes mellitus can occur at any age, and the current classification is based on pathogenesis (e.g., autoimmune destruction of pancreatic β cells, insulin resistance) and clinical presentation rather than on the age of onset. Many patients' diabetes mellitus does not easily fit into a single classification. Epidemiologic data indicate that the incidence of type 2 diabetes mellitus is increasing in children and adolescents such that 8–45% of children with newly diagnosed diabetes have nonimmune-mediated diabetes mellitus; most of these individuals have type 2 diabetes mellitus, although other types, including idiopathic or nonimmune-mediated type 1 diabetes mellitus, also have been reported.

Patients with type 2 diabetes mellitus have insulin resistance and usually have relative (rather than absolute) insulin deficiency. Most patients with type 2 diabetes mellitus (about 80–90%) are overweight or obese; obesity itself also contributes to the insulin resistance and glucose intolerance observed in these patients. Patients with type 2 diabetes mellitus who are not obese may have an increased percentage of abdominal fat, which is an indicator of increased cardiometabolic risk. While children with immune-mediated type 1 diabetes generally are not overweight, the incidence of obesity in children with this form of diabetes is increasing with the increasing incidence of obesity in the US population. Distinguishing between type 1 and type 2 diabetes in children may be difficult since obesity may occur with either type of diabetes mellitus, and autoantigens and ketosis may be present in a substantial number of children with features of type 2 diabetes mellitus (e.g., obesity, acanthosis nigricans).

Oral antidiabetic agents are *not* effective as sole therapy for patients with type 1 diabetes mellitus; insulin is necessary in these patients. Sulfonylurea antidiabetic agents are not routinely recommended in hospitalized patients with diabetes mellitus. Because of their long duration of action (24 hours with glyburide), sulfonylureas do not allow rapid dosage adjustments to meet changing needs of hospitalized patients. In addition, the risk of hypoglycemia during sulfonylurea therapy is increased in such patients with irregular eating patterns.

Patients with type 2 diabetes mellitus are *not* dependent initially on insulin (although many patients eventually require insulin for glycemic control) nor are they prone to ketosis; however, insulin may occasionally be required for correction of symptomatic or persistent hyperglycemia that is not controlled by dietary regulation or oral antidiabetic agents (e.g., sulfonylureas), and ketosis may occasionally develop during periods of severe stress (e.g., acute infections, trauma, surgery). Type 2 diabetes mellitus is a heterogeneous subclass of the disease, and subclassification criteria (e.g., basal and stimulated plasma insulin concentrations, insulin resistance) remain to be clearly established. Endogenous insulin is present in type 2 diabetic patients, although plasma insulin concentrations may be decreased, increased, or normal. In type 2 diabetic patients, glucose-stimulated secretion of endogenous insulin is frequently, but not always, reduced and decreased peripheral sensitivity to insulin is almost always associated with glucose intolerance.

Glycemic Control and Microvascular Complications Current evidence from epidemiologic and clinical studies supports an association between chronic hyperglycemia and the pathogenesis of microvascular complications in patients with diabetes mellitus, and results of randomized, controlled studies in patients with type 1 or type 2 diabetes mellitus indicate that intensive management of hyperglycemia with near-normalization of blood glucose and glycosylated hemoglobin (hemoglobin A_{1c} [HbA_{1c}]) concentrations provides substantial benefits in terms of reducing chronic microvascular (e.g., retinopathy, nephropathy, neuropathy) complications associated with the disease. HbA_{1c} concentration reflects the glycosylation of other proteins throughout the body as a result of recent hyperglycemia and is used as a predictor of risk for development of diabetic microvascular complications. Microvascular complications of diabetes are the principal causes of blindness and renal failure in developed countries and are more closely associated with hyperglycemia than are macrovascular complications.

In the Diabetes Control and Complications Trial (DCCT), the reduction in risk of microvascular complications in patients with type 1 diabetes mellitus correlated continuously with the reduction in HbA_{1c} concentration produced by intensive insulin treatment (e.g., a 40% reduction in risk of microvascular disease for each 10% reduction in HbA_{1c}. These data imply that any decrease in HbA_{1c} levels is beneficial and that complete normalization of blood glucose concentrations may prevent diabetic complications. Data from the largest United Kingdom Prospective Diabetes Study (UKPDS) and other smaller studies in patients with type 2 diabetes mellitus are generally consistent with the same benefits on microvascular complications as those observed with type 1 diabetes mellitus in the DCCT study.

Data from long-term follow-up (over 10 years) of UKPDS patients with type 2 diabetes mellitus who received initial therapy with conventional (diet and oral antidiabetic agents or insulin to achieve fasting plasma glucose concentrations below 270 mg/dL without symptoms of hyperglycemia) antidiabetic treatment or intensive (stepwise introduction of a sulfonylurea [i.e., chlorpropamide, glyburide], then insulin, or an oral sulfonylurea and insulin, or insulin alone to achieve fasting plasma glucose concentrations of 108 mg/dL) antidiabetic regimens indicate that intensive treatment with monotherapy generally is not capable of maintaining strict glycemic control (i.e., maintenance of blood glucose concentrations of 108 mg/dL or normal values) over time and that combination therapy eventually becomes necessary in most patients to attain target glucose concentrations in the long term; in UKPDS, intensive treatment that eventually required combination therapy in most patients resulted in median HbA_{1c} concentrations of 7%. Because of the benefits of strict glycemic control, the goal of therapy for type 2 diabetes mellitus is to lower blood glucose to as close to normal as possible, which generally requires aggressive management efforts (e.g., mixing therapy with various antidiabetic agents including sulfonylureas, metformin, insulin, and/or possibly others) over time. For additional information on clinical studies demonstrating the benefits of strict glycemic control on microvascular complications in patients with type 1 or 2 diabetes mellitus, see Glycemic Control and Microvascular Complications under Uses: Diabetes Mellitus, in Metformin 68:20.04.

Glycemic Control and Macrovascular Complications Current evidence indicates that appropriate management of dyslipidemia, blood pressure, and vascular thrombosis provides substantial benefits in terms of reducing macrovascular complications associated with diabetes mellitus; intensive glycemic control generally has not been associated with appreciable reductions in macrovascular outcomes in controlled trials. Reduction in blood pressure to a mean of 144/82 mm Hg ("tight blood pressure control") in patients with diabetes mellitus and uncomplicated mild to moderate hypertension in UKPDS substantially reduced the incidence of virtually all macrovascular (e.g., stroke, heart failure) and microvascular (e.g., retinopathy, vitreous hemorrhage, renal failure) outcomes and diabetes-related mortality; blood pressure and glycemic control were additive in their beneficial effects on these end points. While intensive antidiabetic therapy titrated with the goal of reducing HbA_{1c} to near-normal concentrations (6–6.5% or less) has not been associated with appreciable reductions in cardiovascular events during the randomized portion of controlled trials examining such outcomes, results of long-term follow-up (10–11 years) from DCCT and UKPDS indicate a delayed cardiovascular benefit in patients treated with intensive antidiabetic therapy early in the course of type 1 or type 2 diabetes mellitus. For additional details regarding the effects of intensive antidiabetic therapy on macrovascular outcomes, see Glycemic Control and Macrovascular Complications, under Uses: Diabetes Mellitus, in Metformin 68:20.04.

Treatment Goals The ADA currently states that it is reasonable to attempt to achieve in patients with type 2 diabetes mellitus the same blood glucose and HbA_{1c} goals recommended for patients with type 1 diabetes mellitus. Based on target values for blood glucose and HbA_{1c} used in clinical trials (e.g., DCCT) for type 1 diabetic patients, modified somewhat to reduce the risk of severe hypoglycemia, ADA currently recommends target preprandial (fasting) and peak postprandial (1–2 hours after the *beginning* of a meal) *plasma* glucose concentrations of 70–130 and less than 180 mg/dL, respectively, and HbA_{1c} concentrations of less than 7% (based on a nondiabetic range of 4–6%) *in general* in patients with type 1 or type 2 diabetes mellitus who are not pregnant. HbA_{1c} concentrations of 7% or greater should prompt clinicians to initiate or adjust antidiabetic therapy in nonpregnant patients with the goal of achieving HbA_{1c} concentrations of less than 7%. Patients with diabetes mellitus who have elevated HbA_{1c} concentrations despite having adequate preprandial glucose concentrations should monitor glucose concentrations 1–2 hours after the start of a meal. Treatment with agents (e.g., α-glucosidase inhibitors, exenatide, pramlintide) that principally lower postprandial glucose concentrations to within target ranges also should reduce HbA_{1c}.

More stringent treatment goals (i.e., an HbA_{1c} concentration less than 6%) may be considered in selected patients. An *individualized* HbA_{1c} goal that is closer to normal without risking substantial hypoglycemia is reasonable in patients with short duration of diabetes mellitus, no appreciable cardiovascular disease, and a long life expectancy. Achievement of HbA_{1c} values of less than 7% is not appropriate or practical for some patients, and clinical judgment should be used in designing a treatment regimen based on the potential benefits and risks (e.g., hypoglycemia) of more intensified therapy. For additional details on individualizing treatment in patients with diabetes mellitus, see Treatment Goals under Uses: Diabetes Mellitus, in Metformin 68:20.04.

Considerations in Initiating and Maintaining Antidiabetic Therapy When initiating therapy for type 2 diabetes mellitus who do not have severe symptoms, most clinicians recommend that diet be emphasized as the primary form of treatment; caloric restriction and weight reduction are essential in obese patients. Although appropriate dietary management and weight reduction alone may be effective in controlling blood glucose concentration and symptoms of hyperglycemia, many patients receiving dietary advice fail to achieve and maintain adequate glycemic control with dietary modification alone.

Recognizing that lifestyle interventions often fail to achieve or maintain the target glycemic goal within the first year of initiation of such interventions, ADA currently suggests initiation of metformin concurrently with lifestyle interventions at the time of diagnosis of type 2 diabetes mellitus. Other experts suggest concurrent initiation of lifestyle interventions and antidiabetic agents only when HbA_{1c} values of 9% or greater are present at the time of diagnosis of type 2 diabetes mellitus. ADA and other clinicians state that lifestyle interventions should remain a principal consideration in the management of diabetes even after pharmacologic therapy is initiated. The manufacturer states that patients and clinicians should recognize that dietary management is the principal consideration in the management of diabetes mellitus and that antidiabetic therapy is used only as an adjunct to, and not as a substitute for or a convenient means to avoid, proper dietary management. In addition, loss of blood glucose control on diet alone may be temporary in some patients, requiring only short-term management with drug therapy. The importance of regular physical activity should also be emphasized, and cardiovascular risk factors should be identified and corrective measures employed when feasible. If lifestyle interventions alone are initiated and these interventions fail to reduce symptoms and/or blood glucose concentration, initiation of monotherapy with an oral antidiabetic agent (e.g., metformin, sulfonylurea, acarbose) or insulin should be considered.

Several large, long-term studies have evaluated the cardiovascular risks associated with the use of oral sulfonylurea antidiabetic agents. (See Cautions: Precautions and Contraindications.) The ADA currently considers the beneficial effects of intensive glycemic control with insulin or sulfonylureas and blood pressure control (e.g., concomitant antihypertensive therapy) in diabetic patients to outweigh the risks overall.

Glyburide Monotherapy Clinical studies indicate that glyburide is as effective as chlorpropamide, glipizide, tolazamide, or tolbutamide for the management of type 2 diabetes mellitus. A relative advantage compared with other sulfonylurea antidiabetic agents has not been clearly established. Some clinicians have suggested that, because of its diuretic action, glyburide may be particularly useful in patients with conditions associated with abnormal fluid retention. In some type 2 diabetic patients who are being treated with insulin, glyburide alone may be effective alternative therapy.

Clinical trial data indicate that sulfonylureas are as effective as metformin in lowering HbA_{1c} (approximately 1.5% decrease) values, but such use is associated with hypoglycemia and weight gain. ADA generally recommends metformin as initial antidiabetic therapy because of the absence of weight gain or hypoglycemia, relatively low expense, and generally low adverse effect profile. (See Uses: Diabetes Mellitus, in Metformin 68:20.04.)

Glyburide may be useful in some patients with type 2 diabetes mellitus who have primary or secondary failure to other sulfonylurea antidiabetic agents; however, primary or secondary failure to glyburide may also occur.

Secondary failure to sulfonylurea drugs is characterized by progressively decreasing diabetic control following 1 month to several years of good control. Interim data from a substudy (UKPDS 26) of UKPDS in newly diagnosed type 2 diabetic patients receiving intensive therapy (maintenance of fasting plasma glucose below 108 mg/dL by increasing doses of either a sulfonylurea [i.e., glyburide or chlorpropamide] to maximum recommended dosage) showed that secondary failure (defined as fasting plasma glucose exceeding 270 mg/dL or symptoms of hyperglycemia despite maximum recommended daily dosage of 20 mg of glyburide or 500 mg of chlorpropamide) occurred overall at about 7% per year. The failure rate at 6 years was 48% among patients receiving glyburide and about 40% among patients receiving chlorpropamide. In the UKPD studies, stepwise addition of insulin or metformin to therapy with maximal dosage of a sulfonylurea was required periodically over time to improve glycemic control. In another substudy (UKPDS 49), progressive deterioration in diabetes control was such that monotherapy was effective in only about 50% of patients after 3 years and in only about 25% of patients after 9 years; thus, most patients require multiple-drug antidiabetic therapy over time to maintain such target levels of disease control. At diagnosis, risk factors predisposing toward sulfonylurea failure included higher fasting plasma glucose concentrations, younger age, and lower pancreatic β-cell reserve.

Glyburide is *not* effective as sole therapy in patients with diabetes mellitus complicated by acidosis, ketosis, or coma; management of these conditions requires the use of insulin.

Combination Therapy with Metformin or Other Oral Antidiabetic Agents Sulfonylureas, including glyburide, may be used in combination with one or more other oral antidiabetic agents (e.g., metformin, thiazolidinedione derivatives, α-glucosidase inhibitors) as an adjunct to diet and exercise for the management of type 2 diabetes mellitus in patients who do not achieve adequate glycemic control with diet, exercise, and oral antidiabetic agent monotherapy. Combined therapy with metformin or other oral antidiabetic agents generally is used in patients with longstanding type 2 diabetes mellitus who have poor glycemic control with monotherapy.

ADA and other clinicians recommend initiating therapy with metformin and adding another antidiabetic agent, such as a sulfonylurea, insulin, or a thiazolidinedione if patients fail to achieve or sustain target HbA_{1c} goals. Optimal benefit generally is obtained by addition of a second antidiabetic agent as soon as monotherapy with metformin at the maximum tolerated dosage no longer provides adequate glycemic control (i.e., when the target glycemic goal is not achieved within 2–3 months of initiation of therapy with metformin or at any other time when the target HbA_{1c} goal is not achieved).

A major factor in choosing additional therapy is the degree of glycemic control obtained during metformin monotherapy. In patients with an HbA_{1c} concentration exceeding 8.5% or symptoms secondary to hyperglycemia despite metformin monotherapy, ADA states that consideration should be given to adding insulin. When glycemic control is closer to the target HbA_{1c} goal with metformin monotherapy (e.g., HbA_{1c} less than 7.5%), agents with a lesser potential to lower hyperglycemia and/or slower onset of action may be considered (e.g., sulfonylurea, thiazolidinedione) as additional therapy to metformin. Other antidiabetic agents such as α-glucosidase inhibitors, meglitinides, exenatide, and pramlintide generally are less effective, less well studied, and/or more expensive than recommended therapies (i.e., metformin, sulfonylurea, thiazolidinedione, insulin). However, these agents may be appropriate for treatment of type 2 diabetes mellitus in selected patients.

Glyburide may be used concomitantly with metformin as initial therapy in the management of patients with type 2 diabetes mellitus whose hyperglycemia cannot be controlled by diet and exercise alone. In a 20-week, double-blind, randomized trial in drug-naive patients with type 2 diabetes mellitus whose hyperglycemia was inadequately controlled (baseline HbA_{1c} values between 7 and 11%) by diet and exercise, treatment was initiated with either placebo, glyburide 2.5 mg, metformin hydrochloride 500 mg, or the fixed combination of glyburide 1.25 mg/metformin hydrochloride 250 mg or glyburide 2.5 mg/metformin hydrochloride 500 mg daily. The dosage of each therapy was progressively increased during weeks 4–8 to achieve a target fasting plasma glucose concentration of 126 mg/dL or to a maximum of 4 tablets daily. Patients receiving the fixed combination of glyburide and metformin had greater reductions in HbA_{1c} and fasting plasma glucose concentrations than those receiving glyburide, metformin, or placebo; at the end of the study, strict glycemic control (e.g., HbA_{1c} values less than 7%) was achieved in 59.9, 50.4, 66.4, or 71.7% of patients receiving mean dosages of glyburide 5.3 mg, metformin hydrochloride 1.32 g, glyburide 2.78 mg/metformin hydrochloride 557 mg, or glyburide 4.1 mg/metformin hydrochloride 824 mg, respectively.

In a comparative clinical trial in pediatric patients (9–16 years of age) with type 2 diabetes mellitus, therapy with glyburide in fixed combination with metformin hydrochloride (titrated to a final mean daily dosage of 3.1 mg of glyburide and 623 mg of metformin hydrochloride) was no more effective in improving glycemic control (as determined by reductions in HbA_{1c}) than monotherapy with either component (titrated to a final mean daily dosage of 6.5 mg of glyburide or 1.5 g of metformin hydrochloride).

Glyburide also may be used concomitantly with metformin as second-line therapy in patients who do not achieve adequate control of hyperglycemia despite diet, exercise, and monotherapy with either glyburide (or another sulfonylurea antidiabetic agent) or metformin. In a double-blind, randomized study, patients with type 2 diabetes mellitus whose hyperglycemia was inadequately controlled (mean baseline HbA_{1c} values: 9.5%, mean baseline fasting plasma glucose: 213 mg/dL) with oral sulfonylurea therapy at a dosage at least 50% of the maximum recommended daily dosage (e.g., glyburide 10 mg daily, glipizide 20 mg daily) received therapy with glyburide 20 mg (fixed dosage), metformin hydrochloride 500 mg, or the fixed combination of glyburide 2.5 mg/metformin hydrochloride 500 mg or glyburide 5 mg/metformin hydrochloride 500 mg daily. The dosages of metformin and the fixed-combination preparations were titrated to achieve a target fasting plasma glucose concentration of less than 140 mg/dL or to a maximum of 4 tablets daily. At 16 weeks, patients receiving the fixed combination of glyburide and metformin hydrochloride in daily dosages of up to 20 mg of glyburide and 2 g of metformin hydrochloride had lower HbA_{1c}, fasting plasma glucose, and postprandial plasma glucose concentrations than patients receiving monotherapy with glyburide or metformin, who had no appreciable change in HbA_{1c} values.

In a 24-week double-blind, randomized study, addition of rosiglitazone to therapy in patients not adequately controlled with the fixed combination of glyburide and metformin produced additional improvement in fasting plasma glucose concentrations and HbA_{1c} values compared with the fixed-combination regimen. Strict glycemic control (e.g., HbA_{1c} values less than 7%) was achieved in 42.4% of patients receiving the 3-drug combination regimen compared with 13.5% of those receiving the fixed combination of glyburide and metformin.

For additional information on combination therapy with sulfonylureas and other oral antidiabetic agents, see the sections on combination therapy in Uses in the individual monographs in 68:20.

When lifestyle interventions, metformin, and a second oral antidiabetic agent are not effective in maintaining the target glycemic goal in patients with type 2 diabetes mellitus, ADA and other clinicians generally recommend the addition of insulin therapy. In patients whose HbA_{1c} is close to the target value (less than 8%) on metformin and a second oral antidiabetic agent, addition of a third oral antidiabetic agent instead of insulin may be considered. However, triple combination oral antidiabetic therapy is more costly and potentially not as effective as adding insulin therapy to dual combination oral antidiabetic therapy.

Combination Therapy with Insulin Combined therapy with insulin and oral antidiabetic agents may be useful in some patients with type 2 diabetes mellitus whose blood glucose concentrations are not adequately controlled with maximal dosages of the oral agent and/or as a means of providing increased flexibility with respect to timing of meals and amount of food ingested. Concomitant therapy with insulin (e.g., given as intermediate- or long-acting insulin at bedtime or rapid-acting insulin at meal times) and one or more oral antidiabetic agents appears to improve glycemic control with lower dosages of insulin than would be required with insulin alone and may decrease the potential for body weight gain associated with insulin therapy. Oral antidiabetic therapy combined with insulin therapy may delay progression to either intensive insulin monotherapy or to a second daytime injection of insulin combined with oral antidiabetic therapy. However, combined therapy may increase the risk of hypoglycemic reactions.

ADA and other clinicians state that combined therapy with insulin and metformin with or without other oral antidiabetic agents is one of several options for the management of hyperglycemia in patients not responding adequately to oral monotherapy with metformin, the preferred initial oral antidiabetic agent. In patients with an HbA_{1c} concentration exceeding 8.5% or symptoms secondary to hyperglycemia despite metformin monotherapy, ADA states that consideration should be given to adding insulin. When patients are not controlled with metformin with or without other oral antidiabetic agents (i.e., sulfonylurea, thiazolidinedione) and basal insulin (e.g., given as intermediate- or long-acting insulin at bedtime or in the morning), therapy with insulin should be intensified by adding additional short-acting or rapid-acting insulin injections at mealtimes. Therapy with insulin secretagogues (i.e., sulfonylureas, meglitinides) should be tapered and discontinued when intensive insulin therapy is initiated, as insulin secretagogues do not appear to be synergistic with such insulin therapy.

Misuse and Abuse **Dietary Supplements.** Some herbal dietary supplements promoted for the treatment of diabetes mellitus and purported to contain only natural Chinese herbal ingredients have been found to contain glyburide and phenformin (a biguanide similar to metformin but no longer commercially available in the US). Adulteration of these dietary supplements was discovered after use of one of the glyburide- and phenformin-containing dietary supplements by a patient with diabetes mellitus resulted in several episodes of hypoglycemia, from which the patient fully recovered. Restrictions on the importation and sale of these dietary supplements have been initiated by FDA.

Dosage and Administration

Administration Glyburide is administered orally. The drug is usually administered as a single daily dose given each morning with breakfast, or with the first main meal. Once-daily dosing of glyburide provides adequate control of blood glucose concentration throughout the day in most patients with usual meal patterns; however, some patients, particularly those who require more than 10 mg of the drug daily, may have a more satisfactory response when glyburide is administered in 2 divided doses daily. When a twice-daily dosing regimen is employed in patients receiving more than 10 mg of glyburide daily, the doses and schedule of administration should be individualized according to the patient's meal pattern and response. There is some evidence that, when a divided-dosing regimen is used, blood glucose concentration following breakfast may be better controlled when the morning dose is administered 30 minutes before rather than with the meal; a similar tendency has been observed following the midday meal, but not the evening meal, when the remaining portions of the equally divided daily dose were administered 30 minutes before rather than with these meals.

Dosage Dosage of glyburide must be based on periodic fasting blood glucose and glycosylated hemoglobin (hemoglobin A_{1c} [HbA_{1c}]) determinations and must be carefully individualized to obtain optimum therapeutic effect. The goal of therapy should be to reduce fasting plasma glucose, postprandial plasma glucose, and HbA_{1c} values to normal or near normal using the lowest effective dosage of glyburide-containing therapy. (*Glucose concentrations in plasma generally are 10–15% higher than those in whole blood; glucose concentrations also may vary according to the method and laboratory used for these determinations.*) Periodic HbA_{1c} determinations are better indicators of long-term glycemic control than fasting plasma glucose concentrations alone. Following initiation of glyburide-containing therapy, determination of HbA_{1c} concentrations at intervals of approximately 3 months is useful for assessing the patient's continued response to therapy. Patients must be closely monitored to determine the minimum effective glyburide dosage and to detect primary or secondary failure to the drug.*If appropriate glyburide dosage regimens are not followed, hypoglycemia may be precipitated.*

Formulations of micronized glyburide (Glynase® PresTab®, Pfizer, Glycron®, Zoetica, and micronized tablets available by nonproprietary name) contain smaller particles of the drug than those contained in conventional formulations (e.g., DiaBeta®, Micronase®). As a result, micronized formulations of glyburide are not bioequivalent with conventional formulations, and dosage should be retitrated when transferring patients from micronized to conventional formulations or vice versa. In general, initial dosages of micronized glyburide range from 1.5–3 mg daily, although it may be necessary to initiate micronized therapy with 0.75 mg daily in patients who are sensitive to the hypoglycemic effects of sulfonylureas (e.g., geriatric, debilitated, or malnourished patients); the manufacturer recommends that the initial dosage not exceed 3 mg daily regardless of the dosage of other sulfonylurea employed at transfer. Maintenance dosage of the micronized formulation should be individualized according to glycemic control but usually ranges from 0.75–12 mg daily. The manufacturers' labeling should be consulted for additional information on the use of micronized glyburide, including associated precautions and detailed information on dosage titration.

Glyburide therapy should be discontinued at least annually and blood glucose concentration monitored carefully to ensure that the drug continues to be effective. If adequate lowering of blood glucose concentration is no longer achieved during maintenance therapy, the drug should be discontinued. Patients who do not adhere to their prescribed dietary and drug regimens are more likely to have an unsatisfactory response to therapy. In patients usually well controlled by dietary management alone, short-term therapy with glyburide may be sufficient during periods of transient loss of diabetic control.

Initial Dosage in Previously Untreated Patients For the management of type 2 diabetes mellitus in patients not previously receiving insulin or sulfonylurea antidiabetic agents, the usual initial adult dosage of glyburide is 2.5–5 mg daily; in debilitated, malnourished, or geriatric patients, or other patients at increased risk of hypoglycemia (See Cautions: Precautions and Contraindications), the initial dosage of glyburide should be 1.25 mg daily. The manufacturers also recommend an initial dosage of 1.25 mg daily in patients with impaired renal or hepatic function. (See Cautions: Precautions and Contraindications.) Subsequent dosage should be adjusted according to the patient's tolerance and therapeutic response; increases in dosage should be made in increments of *no more than* 2.5 mg daily at weekly intervals.

Initial Dosage in Patients Transferred from Other Antidiabetic Agents A transition period generally is not required when transferring from most other sulfonylurea antidiabetic agents to glyburide, and administration of the other agent may be abruptly discontinued. Because of the prolonged elimination half-life of chlorpropamide, an exaggerated hypoglycemic response may occur in some patients during the transition from chlorpropamide to glyburide, and patients being transferred from chlorpropamide should be closely monitored for the occurrence of hypoglycemia during the initial 2 weeks of the transition period. A drug-free interval of 2–3 days may be advisable before glyburide therapy is initiated in patients being transferred from chlorpropamide, particularly if blood glucose concentration was adequately controlled with chlorpropamide. An initial or loading dose of glyburide is *not* necessary when transferring from other sulfonylurea antidiabetic agents to glyburide. The transfer should be performed conservatively.

For the management of type 2 diabetes mellitus in patients previously receiving other sulfonylurea antidiabetic agents, the initial dosage of glyburide should be 2.5–5 mg daily. Although patients may be transferred from the maximum dosage of other sulfonylurea antidiabetic agents, the initial dosage of glyburide should *not* exceed 5 mg daily. Subsequent dosage is adjusted according to the patient's tolerance and therapeutic response. Although an exact dosage relationship between glyburide and other sulfonylurea antidiabetic agents does not exist, approximate dosage equivalencies have been estimated. (See Pharmacology: Antidiabetic Effect.)

In general, patients who were previously maintained on insulin dosages not exceeding 40 units daily may be transferred directly to glyburide, and administration of insulin may be abruptly discontinued; the initial glyburide dosage is 2.5–5 mg daily in patients whose insulin dosage was less than 20 units daily and 5 mg daily in patients whose insulin dosage was 20–40 units daily. In patients requiring insulin dosages exceeding 40 units daily, an initial glyburide dosage of 5 mg daily should be started and insulin dosage reduced by 50%. Subsequently, insulin is withdrawn gradually and dosage of glyburide is increased in increments of 1.25–2.5 mg daily every 2–10 days, according to the patient's tolerance and therapeutic response. During the period of insulin withdrawal, patients should test their blood for glucose and their urine for glucose and/or ketones at least 3 times daily, and should be instructed to report the results to their physician so that appropriate adjustments in therapy may be made, if necessary. The presence of persistent ketonuria with glycosuria, ketosis, and/or inadequate lowering or persistent elevation of blood glucose concentration indicates that the patient requires insulin therapy. During the period of insulin withdrawal, hypoglycemia may rarely occur. In some patients, hospitalization may be necessary during the transition from insulin to glyburide.

Maintenance Dosage The adult maintenance dosage of glyburide for the management of type 2 diabetes mellitus ranges from 1.25–20 mg daily. Most patients require 2.5–10 mg daily and some may require up to 15 mg daily; only a few patients will benefit from dosages exceeding 15 mg daily. Maintenance dosage of glyburide should be conservative in debilitated, malnourished, or geriatric patients or patients with impaired renal or hepatic function because of an increased risk of hypoglycemia in these patients. (See Cautions: Precautions and Contraindications.)The maximum recommended dosage is 20 mg daily.

Concomitant Glyburide and Metformin Therapy Combination therapy with glyburide and metformin may be used in patients who do not respond adequately to diet and exercise alone, and in those who do not respond adequately to either glyburide (or another sulfonylurea antidiabetic agent) or metformin monotherapy, diet, and exercise. When glyburide and metformin are administered concomitantly, dosage of each drug should be adjusted upward until adequate glycemic control is achieved, and patients should be monitored periodically (e.g., determination of blood glucose concentrations) to determine the minimum effective dosage of each drug. Glyburide should be added gradually to the existing dosage regimen of patients not responding adequately to 4 weeks of metformin monotherapy at maximum dosage. When glyburide is administered concomitantly with metformin, the risk of hypoglycemia may be increased. (See Cautions: Precautions and Contraindications.)

The commercially available preparation containing glyburide in fixed combination with metformin hydrochloride may be used as initial therapy in patients with type 2 diabetes mellitus whose blood glucose is not adequately controlled with diet and exercise alone, or as second-line therapy in those in whom glycemic control with a sulfonylurea antidiabetic agent (e.g., glyburide) or metformin monotherapy is not adequate. If the fixed-combination preparation of glyburide and metformin hydrochloride is used as initial therapy, the recommended initial dosage is 1.25 mg of glyburide and 250 mg of metformin hydrochloride daily with a meal. Patients with more severe hyperglycemia (as determined by HbA_{1c} exceeding 9% or fasting plasma glucose concentrations exceeding 200 mg/dL) may receive an initial dosage of 1.25 mg of glyburide and 250 mg of metformin hydrochloride twice daily with the morning and evening meals. Dosage may be titrated in increments of 1.25 mg of glyburide and 250 mg of metformin hydrochloride daily at 2-week intervals until the minimum effective dosage required to achieve adequate blood glucose control is reached. A total daily dosage exceeding 10 mg of glyburide and 2 g of metformin hydrochloride has not been evaluated in clinical trials in patients receiving the fixed-combination preparation as initial therapy. The manufacturer states that the fixed-combination preparation containing 5 mg of glyburide and 500 mg of metformin hydrochloride should not be used as initial therapy in treatment-naïve patients because of the increased risk for hypoglycemia.

The commercially available preparation containing glyburide in fixed combination with metformin hydrochloride also may be initiated as second-line therapy in patients whose blood glucose concentrations are not adequately controlled by either glyburide (or another sulfonylurea antidiabetic agent) or metformin alone. The recommended initial dosage of the commercially available fixed-combination preparation in previously treated patients is 2.5 or 5 mg of glyburide with 500 mg of metformin hydrochloride twice daily with morning and evening meals. In order to minimize the risk of hypoglycemia, the initial dosage of glyburide and metformin hydrochloride in fixed combination should not exceed the daily dosage of glyburide or metformin given separately. The dosage of the fixed combination of glyburide and metformin should be titrated upward in increments not exceeding 5 mg of glyburide and 500 mg of metformin hydrochloride until adequate control of blood glucose is achieved or a maximum daily dosage of 20 mg of glyburide and 2 g of metformin hydrochloride is reached.

For patients being switched from combined therapy with separate preparations, the initial dosage of the fixed-combination preparation of glyburide and metformin should not exceed the daily dosage of glyburide (or equivalent dosage of another sulfonylurea antidiabetic agent) *and* metformin currently being taken. Such patients should be monitored for signs and symptoms of hypoglycemia following the switch. Hypoglycemia and hyperglycemia are possible in such patients, and any change in the therapy of type 2 diabetic patients should be undertaken with caution and appropriate monitoring. The safety and efficacy of switching from combined therapy with separate preparations of glyburide (or another sulfonylurea antidiabetic agent) and metformin to the fixed-combination preparation have not been established in clinical studies.

Glyburide alone or in fixed combination with metformin should be used with caution in geriatric patients, since aging is associated with reduced renal function. The initial and maintenance dosages of glyburide alone or in fixed combination with metformin should be conservative and should be titrated carefully in such patients. Renal function should be assessed with initial dosage selection and with each dosage adjustment in geriatric patients. To minimize the risk of hypoglycemia, maintenance dosage of the fixed combination of glyburide and metformin hydrochloride in geriatric, debilitated, or malnourished patients should *not* be titrated to the maximum dosage recommended for other patients.

Concomitant Glyburide, Metformin, and Thiazolidinedione Therapy For patients whose hyperglycemia is not adequately controlled on therapy with the fixed combination of glyburide and metformin, a thiazolidinedione (e.g., pioglitazone, rosiglitazone) may be added at its recommended initial dosage and the dosage of the fixed combination may be continued unchanged. In patients requiring further glycemic control, the dosage of the thiazolidinedione may be titrated upward, based on the dosage regimen recommended by the manufacturer. Triple therapy with glyburide, metformin, and a thiazolidinedione may increase the potential for hypoglycemia at any time of day. If hypoglycemia develops with such triple therapy, consideration should be given to reducing the dosage of the glyburide component; adjustment of the dosage of the other components of the antidiabetic regimen also should be considered as clinically indicated.

Cautions

■ **Hypoglycemia** Hypoglycemia, which may be severe and has occasionally been fatal, may occur in patients receiving glyburide alone or combined with other antidiabetic agents. In a controlled clinical trial in patients receiving initial therapy, symptoms of hypoglycemia (e.g., dizziness, shakiness, sweating, hunger) occurred in 21.3, 3.1, 11.4, or 37.7% of patients receiving glyburide (mean daily dosage: 5.3 mg), metformin hydrochloride (mean daily dosage: 1317 mg), glyburide in fixed combination with metformin hydrochloride (mean daily dosage: 2.78 mg of glyburide/557 mg of metformin hydrochloride), or glyburide in fixed combination with a higher dosage of metformin hydrochloride (mean daily dosage: 4.1 mg of glyburide/824 mg of metformin hydrochloride). Approximately 6.8% of patients experienced hypoglycemic symptoms while receiving the fixed combination of glyburide and metformin hydrochloride as second-line therapy following inadequate control with sulfonylurea monotherapy. Self-monitored blood glucose measurements of 50 mg/dL or less were reported by 22% of patients receiving the fixed combination of glyburide and metformin hydrochloride plus rosiglitazone compared with 3.3% of patients receiving the fixed combination of glyburide and metformin hydrochloride plus placebo. *Appropriate patient selection and careful attention to dosage are important to avoid glyburide-induced hypoglycemia.* (See Cautions: Precautions and Contraindications.)

Although not clearly established, it has been suggested that glyburide may be more likely than other sulfonylurea antidiabetic agents to produce severe hypoglycemia. In some clinical studies, hypoglycemia was the most frequent adverse effect of the drug. Hypoglycemia may occur as a result of excessive glyburide dosage; however, since the development of hypoglycemia is a function of many factors, including diet, or exercise without adequate caloric supplementation, this effect may occur in some patients receiving usual dosages of the drug. Severe hypoglycemia, sometimes fatal, has occurred in some patients receiving as little as 2.5–5 mg of glyburide daily. The risk of hypoglycemia is increased during concurrent use of other antidiabetic agents, certain other agents, or alcohol. (See: Drug Interactions.) In patients receiving glyburide in fixed combination with metformin, renal or hepatic insufficiency may increase the serum concentrations of both agents, and hepatic insufficiency may diminish gluconeogenic capacity; both of these conditions increase the risk of hypoglycemia. Debilitated, malnourished, or geriatric patients may be particularly susceptible to glyburide-induced hypoglycemia; this condition may be difficult to recognize in geriatric patients or in those receiving β-adrenergic blocking agents. (See Drug Interactions: β-Adrenergic Blocking Agents.) Glyburide-induced hypoglycemia may also occur in nontherapeutic situations (e.g., inadvertent or intentional ingestion).

Management of glyburide-induced hypoglycemia depends on the severity of the reaction; patients with severe reactions require immediate hospitalization and treatment and observation until complete recovery is assured. Hypoglycemia is usually, but not always, readily controlled by administration of glucose. If hypoglycemia occurs during therapy with the drug, immediate reevaluation and adjustment of glyburide dosage and/or the patient's meal pattern are necessary.

For further discussion of the pathogenesis, manifestations, and treatment of glyburide-induced hypoglycemia, see Acute Toxicity.

Other Endocrine and Metabolic Effects Therapy with sulfonylureas, including glyburide, may be associated with weight gain. Weight gain observed in patients receiving rosiglitazone in addition to the fixed combination of glyburide and metformin in a controlled clinical trial was similar to that reported with rosiglitazone monotherapy. Although the exact mechanisms associated with such alterations in weight have not been established, suggested mechanisms include an increase in insulin secretion (which may increase appetite), stimulation of lipogenesis in fat tissue, or an increase in blood leptin concentrations. Data from the United Kingdom Prospective Diabetes Study (UKPDS) in patients receiving long-term (over 10 years) therapy with glyburide and other antidiabetic agents indicate that weight gain was greatest in those receiving intensive therapy (stepwise introduction of a sulfonylurea then insulin or an oral sulfonylurea and insulin, or insulin alone to achieve fasting glucose concentrations of 108 mg/dL) than conventional therapy (diet and oral antidiabetic agents or insulin to achieve fasting plasma glucose concentrations less than 270 mg/dL without symptoms of hyperglycemia), and weight gain was greatest in those initially receiving insulin or chlorpropamide compared with that in those receiving glyburide.

Like other sulfonylureas, hyponatremia and the syndrome of inappropriate secretion of antidiuretic hormone (SIADH) have occurred in patients receiving glyburide. Hyponatremia appears to occur more often in patients who concurrently are receiving other medications or have medical conditions known to cause hyponatremia or an increased release of vasopressin.

■ **GI Effects** Adverse GI effects such as nausea, epigastric fullness, and heartburn are the most common adverse reactions to glyburide, occurring in about 1–2% of patients. Glyburide-induced adverse GI effects appear to be dose related and may subside following a reduction in dosage.

■ **Hepatic Effects** Cholestatic jaundice may occur rarely in patients receiving glyburide and is an indication for discontinuing the drug. Glyburide-induced cholestatic jaundice has occurred rarely in conjunction with other severe systemic adverse effects (e.g., visceral arteritis, cutaneous bullae). Liver function test abnormalities, including elevations in serum aminotransferase concentrations (which may subside with continued therapy), have been reported in patients receiving glyburide. Exacerbation of hepatic porphyria has been reported with other sulfonylurea antidiabetic agents, but has not been reported to date with glyburide.

■ **Dermatologic and Sensitivity Reactions** Allergic skin reactions including pruritus, erythema, urticaria, and morbilliform or maculopapular eruptions occur in about 1.5% of patients receiving glyburide. Glyburide-induced adverse dermatologic effects generally subside rapidly following discontinuance of the drug, but may also disappear despite continued treatment; however, if adverse dermatologic effects persist with continued glyburide therapy, the drug should be discontinued. Cutaneous bullae occurred in conjunction with cholestatic jaundice in one patient receiving glyburide. Photosensitivity reactions have also been reported with glyburide, and porphyria cutanea tarda has been reported with other sulfonylurea antidiabetic agents.

Nondermatologic allergic reactions to glyburide have included angioedema, arthralgia, myalgia, and vasculitis. A generalized hypersensitivity reaction with toxic erythema, cholestatic jaundice, eosinophilia, and visceral arteritis, resulting in death, has also been reported in one patient receiving the drug.

■ **Hematologic Effects** Like other sulfonylurea antidiabetic agents, glyburide may rarely cause leukopenia, thrombocytopenia, pancytopenia, agranulocytosis, aplastic anemia, and hemolytic anemia. Thrombocytopenic purpura has been reported in one patient receiving glyburide.

■ **Other Adverse Effects** Although a causal relationship has not been established, paresthesia, joint pain, and nocturia have been reported in patients receiving glyburide. Changes in accommodation and/or blurred vision have been reported in patients receiving glyburide or other sulfonylureas and are thought to be related to fluctuations in blood glucose concentrations. Edema has been reported in 2.2% of patients receiving the fixed combination of glyburide and metformin versus 7.7% of those receiving combined glyburide, metformin, and rosiglitazone therapy in a controlled clinical trial.

■ **Precautions and Contraindications** When glyburide is used in fixed combination with metformin, the cautions, precautions, and contraindications associated with metformin must be considered in addition to those associated with glyburide.

Glyburide shares the toxic potentials of other sulfonylurea antidiabetic agents, and the usual precautions associated with their use should be observed. The diagnostic and therapeutic measures for managing diabetes mellitus that are necessary to ensure optimum control of the disease with insulin generally are necessary with glyburide. Glyburide should only be prescribed for carefully selected patients by clinicians who are familiar with the indications, limitations, and patient-selection criteria for therapy with oral sulfonylurea antidiabetic agents.

Patients receiving glyburide should be monitored with regular clinical and laboratory evaluations, including urine and/or fasting blood glucose determinations, to determine the minimum effective dosage and to detect primary failure (inadequate lowering of blood glucose concentration at the maximum recommended dosage) or secondary failure (loss of control of blood glucose concentration following an initial period of effectiveness) to the drug. Glycosylated hemoglobin (hemoglobin A_{1c} [HbA_{1c}]) measurements should also be performed periodically to monitor the patient's response to glyburide therapy. During the withdrawal period in patients in whom glyburide is replacing insulin, patients should be instructed to test their blood for glucose and their urine for glucose and/or ketones at least 3 times daily, and to report the results to their physician. Renal function should be evaluated prior to initiation of therapy with glyburide in fixed combination with metformin and at least annually thereafter. Care should be taken to avoid ketosis, acidosis, and coma during the withdrawal period in patients being switched from insulin to glyburide. If adequate lowering of blood glucose concentration is no longer achieved during maintenance therapy with glyburide, the drug should be discontinued. Alternatively, combined therapy with glyburide and metformin may be used in patients who do not have an adequate glycemic response to glyburide or metformin monotherapy. However, adequate adjustment of dosage and adherence to diet should be assessed before considering that secondary failure to oral antidiabetic therapy has occurred. When use of glyburide in asymptomatic type 2 diabetic patients is being considered, it should be recognized that control of blood glucose concentration in these patients has not been definitely established as effective for prevention of long-term cardiovascular or nervous system complications of the disease. There is limited evidence that sulfonylureas may reverse basement-membrane thickening of muscle capillaries in asymptomatic individuals with impaired glucose tolerance (chemical diabetes) and possibly reverse or retard the progression of microangiopathy in type 2 diabetic patients, but these findings require further evaluation.

Several large, long-term studies have evaluated the cardiovascular risks associated withy the use of oral sulfonylurea antidiabetic agents. In 1970, the University Group Diabetes Program (UGDP) reported that administration of oral antidiabetic agents (i.e., tolbutamide or phenformin) was associated with increased cardiovascular mortality as compared to treatment with dietary regulation alone or with dietary regulation and insulin. The UGDP reported that type 2 diabetic patients who were treated for 5–8 years with dietary regulation and a fixed dose of tolbutamide (1.5 g daily) had a cardiovascular mortality rate approximately 2.5 times that of patients treated with dietary regulation alone; although a substantial increase in total mortality was not observed, the use of tolbutamide was discontinued because of the increase in cardiovascular mortality, thereby limiting the ability of the study to show an increase in total mortality. The results of the UGDP study have been exhaustively analyzed, and there has been general disagreement in the scientific and medical communities regarding the study's validity and clinical importance. However, recent results from the United Kingdom Prospective Diabetes Study (UKPDS), a large, long-term (over 10 years) study in newly diagnosed type 2 diabetic patients, did not confirm an increase in cardiovascular events or mortality in the group treated intensively with sulfonylureas, insulin, or combination therapy compared with that in the group treated with less intensive conventional antidiabetic therapy.

In the UKDP study, the overall aggregate rates of death from macrovascular diseases such as myocardial infarction, sudden death, stroke, or peripheral vascular disease were not appreciably different among either intensive therapies (stepwise introduction of a sulfonylurea [i.e., chlorpropamide, glyburide] then insulin, or an oral sulfonylurea and insulin, or insulin alone to achieve fasting plasma glucose concentrations of 108 mg/dL) or less intensive conventional therapy (diet and oral antidiabetic agents or insulin to achieve fasting plasma glucose concentrations below 270 mg/dL without symptoms of hyperglycemia). However, a trend in reduction in fatal and nonfatal myocardial infarction with intensive therapy was noted with sulfonylurea or insulin, and epidemiologic analysis of the data indicate that each 1% decrease in HbA_{1c} was associated with an 18% reduction of fatal and nonfatal myocardial infarction. Among the single end points, the incidence of angina increased among patients receiving chlorpropamide, and blood pressure also was higher with chlorpropamide compared with glyburide or insulin intensive therapies. As a result of these and other findings (e.g., beneficial effects on microvascular [retinopathy, nephropathy, and possibly neuropathy] complications, confirmation of the beneficial effects of concomitant antihypertensive therapy and blood pressure lowering) of the UKDP study, the American Diabetes Association (ADA) currently considers the beneficial effects of intensive glycemic control with insulin or sulfonylureas and blood pressure control in diabetic patients to outweigh the risks overall. The ADA also recommends that clinicians continue to emphasize dietary management and weight reduction as the principal therapy for the management of type 2 diabetes mellitus, and that oral sulfonylurea antidiabetic agents or insulin be used only after these measures have failed; the decision to use sulfonylurea or insulin should be made by the clinician in consultation with the patient.

Patients should be fully and completely advised about the nature of diabetes mellitus, what they must do to prevent and detect complications, and how to control their condition. *Patients should be informed of the potential risks and advantages of glyburide therapy and alternative forms of treatment.* Patients should be instructed that dietary regulation is the principal consideration in the management of diabetes, and that glyburide therapy is only used as an adjunct to, and not a substitute for or a convenient means to avoid, proper dietary regulation. Patients should also be advised that they should not neglect dietary restrictions, develop a careless attitude about their condition, or disregard instructions about body-weight control, exercise, hygiene, and avoidance of infection. Primary and secondary failure to oral sulfonylurea antidiabetic agents should also be explained to patients.

Patients and responsible family members should be informed of the risks of hypoglycemia, the symptoms and treatment of hypoglycemic reactions, and conditions that predispose to the development of hypoglycemic reactions, since these reactions may occur during therapy with glyburide. *Appropriate patient selection and careful attention to dosage are important to avoid glyburide-induced hypoglycemia.* Debilitated, malnourished, or geriatric patients and patients with mild disease or impaired hepatic or renal function should be carefully monitored and dosage of glyburide should be carefully adjusted in these patients, since they may be predisposed to developing hypoglycemia (sometimes severe). Renal or hepatic insufficiency may cause increased serum concentrations of glyburide and hepatic insufficiency may also diminish glyconeogenic capacity, both of which increase the risk of severe hypoglycemic reactions. Some clinicians recommend that glyburide generally *not* be used in patients with renal or hepatic impairment. Alcohol ingestion, severe or prolonged exercise, deficient caloric intake, use of more than one antidiabetic agent (e.g., glyburide and metformin), severe endocrine disorders, and adrenal or pituitary insufficiency may also predispose patients to the development of hypoglycemia. Hypoglycemia may be difficult to recognize in geriatric patients or in patients receiving β-adrenergic blocking agents. Intensive treatment (e.g., IV dextrose) and close medical supervision may be required in some patients who develop severe hypoglycemia during glyburide therapy. (See Acute Toxicity: Treatment.) Renal or hepatic insufficiency in patients receiving glyburide in fixed combination with metformin may elevate blood concentrations of both drugs and hepatic insufficiency may diminish gluconeogenic capacity, both of which increase the risk of hypoglycemic reactions.

To maintain control of diabetes during periods of stress (e.g., fever of any cause, trauma, infection, surgery), temporary discontinuance of glyburide and administration of insulin may be required.

Although initial batches of Diaβeta® 5-mg tablets contained the dye tartrazine (FD&C yellow No. 5), which may cause allergic reactions including bronchial asthma in susceptible individuals, currently distributed tablets have been reformulated and do not contain this dye. The incidence of tartrazine sensitivity is low, but tartrazine sensitivity frequently occurs in patients who are sensitive to aspirin.

If cholestatic jaundice occurs or if adverse dermatologic effects occur and persist during glyburide therapy, the drug should be discontinued. Glyburide is contraindicated as sole therapy in patients with type 1 diabetes mellitus; glyburide alone or in fixed combination with metformin is contraindicated in those with diabetes complicated by ketosis, acidosis, or diabetic coma. Diabetic ketoacidosis should be treated with insulin. Like other sulfonylureas, glyburide is generally contraindicated in patients with severe renal or hepatic impairment.

Glyburide is also contraindicated in patients with known hypersensitivity or allergy to any ingredient in the respective formulations.

■ **Pediatric Precautions** Safety and efficacy of glyburide in children have not been established. The manufacturer states that the drug is not recommended for use in this age group. Data from a comparative trial evaluating the safety and efficacy of glyburide in fixed combination with metformin compared with monotherapy with each agent in pediatric patients (9–16 years of age) with type 2 diabetes mellitus indicate no unexpected safety concerns with such combination therapy. (See Combination Therapy with Metformin or Other Oral Antidiabetic Agents under Uses: Diabetes Mellitus.) The American Diabetes Association (ADA) states that most pediatric diabetologists use oral antidiabetic agents in children with type 2 diabetes mellitus because of greater patient compliance and convenience for the patient's family and a lack of evidence demonstrating better efficacy of insulin as initial therapy for type 2 diabetes mellitus.

■ **Mutagenicity and Carcinogenicity** It is not known if glyburide is mutagenic or carcinogenic in humans. The drug did not exhibit mutagenic activity in the Ames microbial mutagen test or the DNA damage/alkaline elution assay. Evidence of carcinogenicity was not observed in studies in rats receiving up to 300 mg/kg of glyburide daily for 18 months or in mice receiving the drug for 2 years.

■ **Pregnancy, Fertility, and Lactation** When a glyburide dosage 6250 times the maximum recommended human dosage was given to rats, a shortening of long bones (humerus and femur) in rat pups was noted. These effects were observed during the period of lactation and not during organogenesis. Since abnormal maternal blood glucose concentrations during pregnancy may be associated with a higher incidence of congenital abnormalities, many experts recommend that insulin be used during pregnancy to maintain optimum control of blood glucose concentration. Use of glyburide in pregnant women is generally *not* recommended, and the drug should be used during pregnancy only when clearly necessary (e.g., when insulin therapy is infeasible) or when the potential benefit justifies the possible risks to the fetus. Glyburide has been used in some pregnant women without unusual adverse effects. In a prospective, comparative clinical trial in women with gestational diabetes, treatment with glyburide (mean daily dosage 9 mg, range 2.5–20 mg) initiated in the second trimester (11–33 weeks gestation) and continued until delivery resulted in similar degrees of glycemic control and perinatal outcomes as treatment with insulin human (mean daily dosage: 85 units). The incidence of hypoglycemia in neonates whose mothers received either insulin or glyburide therapy also was similar. Additional studies in a larger number of patients are needed to establish the safety of glyburide in gestational diabetes. In a retrospective study, hypoglycemia occurred and persisted for up to 2 days or longer in a few neonates whose mothers had received glyburide up to the time of delivery. Prolonged, severe hypoglycemia lasting 4–10 days has been reported in some neonates born to women who were receiving other sulfonylurea antidiabetic agents up to the time of delivery; this effect has been reported more frequently with the use of those agents having prolonged elimination half-lives. To minimize the risk of neonatal hypoglycemia if glyburide is used during pregnancy, the manufacturers recommend that the drug be discontinued at least 2 weeks before the expected delivery date.

Reproduction studies in rats and rabbits using glyburide doses up to 500 times the usual human dose have not revealed evidence of impaired fertility or harm to the fetus.

Although it is not known whether glyburide is distributed into milk, some sulfonylurea antidiabetic agents are distributed into milk. Because of the potential for hypoglycemia in nursing infants, a decision should be made whether to discontinue nursing or the drug, taking into account the importance of the drug to the woman. If glyburide is discontinued, and if dietary management alone is inadequate for controlling blood glucose concentration, administration of insulin should be considered.

Drug Interactions

■ **Protein-bound Drugs** Because glyburide is highly protein bound, it theoretically could be displaced from binding sites by, or could displace from binding sites, other protein-bound drugs such as oral anticoagulants, hydantoins, salicylate and other nonsteroidal anti-inflammatory agents, and sulfonamides. However, unlike the protein binding of some other sulfonylurea antidiabetic agents (e.g., acetohexamide, chlorpropamide, tolazamide, tolbutamide) and like that of glipizide, the protein binding of glyburide is principally nonionic; in addition, glyburide appears to bind to different but closely related sites on serum albumin and with a greater affinity than acetohexamide, chlorpropamide, or tolbutamide. Consequently, glyburide may be less likely to be displaced from binding sites by, or displace from binding sites, other highly protein-bound drugs whose protein binding is ionic in nature. In vitro studies indicate that glyburide is less susceptible to displacement from serum albumin by acidic drugs (e.g., phenylbutazone, salicylate, warfarin) than is chlorpropamide or tolbutamide. Whether this difference in protein binding demonstrated in vitro will result in fewer clinically important drug interactions in vivo has not been established. There appears to be no clinically important interaction between tolmetin and glyburide. Patients receiving highly protein-bound drugs should be observed for adverse effects when glyburide therapy is initiated or discontinued and vice versa.

■ **Phenylbutazone** Phenylbutazone may potentiate the hypoglycemic effects of glyburide. The exact mechanism(s) of this interaction is not known. Phenylbutazone has been shown to decrease the renal excretion of glyburide metabolites without affecting metabolism of the sulfonylurea. If phenylbutazone is administered concomitantly with glyburide, the patient should be closely monitored for signs and symptoms of hypoglycemia; dosage adjustment of glyburide may be necessary when phenylbutazone therapy is initiated or discontinued.

■ **Thiazide Diuretics** Thiazide diuretics may exacerbate diabetes mellitus, resulting in increased requirements of sulfonylurea antidiabetic agents, temporary loss of diabetic control, or secondary failure to the antidiabetic agent. When thiazide diuretics are administered concomitantly with sulfonylurea antidiabetic agents, caution should be used.

■ **Alcohol** Disulfiram-like reactions have occurred very rarely following the concomitant use of alcohol and glyburide.

■ **Bosentan** An increased risk of elevated serum aminotransferase concentrations has been observed in patients receiving glyburide and bosentan concomitantly. The manufacturer of bosentan states that concomitant use of glyburide and bosentan is contraindicated.

■ **β-Adrenergic Blocking Agents** Several potential interactions between β-adrenergic blocking agents and sulfonylurea antidiabetic agents exist. β-Adrenergic blocking agents may impair glucose tolerance; increase the frequency or severity of hypoglycemia; block hypoglycemia-induced tachycardia, but not hypoglycemic sweating which may actually be increased; delay the rate of recovery of blood glucose concentration following drug-induced hypoglycemia; alter the hemodynamic response to hypoglycemia, possibly resulting in an exaggerated hypertensive response; and possibly impair peripheral circulation. There is some evidence that many of these effects may be minimized by use of a β_1-selective adrenergic blocking agent rather than a nonselective β-adrenergic blocking agent. Acebutolol and propranolol have been shown to decrease the hypoglycemic action of glyburide in type 2 diabetic patients, presumably by decreasing insulin secretion. In another study in type 2 diabetic patients, insulin secretion during short-term atenolol therapy was reduced, but the hypoglycemic action of glyburide was not altered during short- or long-term atenolol administration. It generally is recommended that concomitant use of β-adrenergic blocking agents and sulfonylurea antidiabetic agents be avoided when possible; if concomitant therapy is necessary, use of a β_1-selective adrenergic blocking agent may be preferred. When glyburide and a β-adrenergic blocking agent are used concomitantly, the patient should be monitored closely for altered antidiabetic response.

■ **Antifungal Antibiotics** Concomitant use of certain antifungal antibiotics (i.e., miconazole, fluconazole) and oral antidiabetic agents has resulted in increased plasma concentrations of the oral antidiabetic agent and/or hypoglycemia. Clinically important hypoglycemia may be precipitated by concomitant use of oral hypoglycemic agents and fluconazole, and at least one fatality has been reported from hypoglycemia in a patient receiving glyburide and fluconazole concomitantly. (See Drug Interactions: Sulfonylurea Antidiabetic Agents, in Fluconazole 8:14.08.)

■ **Other Drugs** Drugs that may enhance the hypoglycemic effect of sulfonylurea antidiabetic agents, including glyburide, include chloramphenicol, monoamine oxidase inhibitors, fluoroquinolone antibiotics (e.g., ciprofloxacin), and probenecid. When these drugs are administered or discontinued in patients receiving glyburide, the patient should be observed closely for hypoglycemia or loss of diabetic control, respectively.

Drugs that may decrease the hypoglycemic effect of sulfonylurea antidiabetic agents, including glyburide, include nonthiazide diuretics (e.g., furosemide), corticosteroids, phenothiazines, thyroid agents, estrogens, oral contraceptives, phenytoin, nicotinic acid, sympathomimetic agents, calcium-channel blocking agents, rifampin, and isoniazid. When these drugs are administered or discontinued in patients receiving glyburide, the patient should be observed closely for loss of diabetic control or hypoglycemia, respectively.

Acute Toxicity

■ **Pathogenesis** Acute glyburide toxicity may result from excessive dosage, and numerous conditions may predispose patients to the development of glyburide-induced hypoglycemia. (See Cautions: Precautions and Contraindications.) Acute glyburide toxicity may also result from inadvertent or intentional (e.g., attempted suicide) ingestion of the drug; glyburide, like other sulfonylurea antidiabetic agents, has also been used by some nondiabetic individuals to produce factitious hypoglycemia. Adults have survived intentional ingestions of up to 200 mg of glyburide, but death has occurred in some adults following severe hypoglycemia induced by as little as 2.5–5 mg of the drug.

■ **Manifestations** Acute glyburide overdosage is manifested principally as hypoglycemia, which may be severe and has occasionally been fatal. Severe hypoglycemia may result in loss of consciousness and seizures, with resultant neurologic sequelae. In 2 children 11 and 30 months of age who inadvertently ingested unknown amounts of glyburide, hypoglycemia occurred with seizures and apparently resulted in permanent cerebral damage; mental retardation could not be excluded. In another child 22 months of age who inadvertently ingested 10–15 mg of the drug, atrophy of the optic nerve with cerebral symptoms was reported. Severe hypoglycemic coma has been reported in one 79-year-old nondiabetic woman who inadvertently received a single 5-mg dose of glyburide. Although glyburide-induced hypoglycemia is generally not prolonged, hypoglycemia and/or loss of consciousness have persisted for up to 3–5 days in some cases (e.g., in geriatric patients). In some patients, hypoglycemia may persist despite continuous IV administration of dextrose, and in some fatalities, loss of consciousness persisted despite correction of hypoglycemia. Glyburide-induced hypoglycemia may be more severe and/or protracted in patients with renal and/or hepatic impairment.

■ **Treatment** Treatment of acute glyburide overdosage consists principally of administration of glucose and supportive therapy. *The patient should be monitored closely until complete recovery is assured.*

Patients with mild hypoglycemic symptoms without loss of consciousness or adverse neurologic effects should be treated aggressively with orally administered glucose, and glyburide dosage and/or the patient's meal pattern should be appropriately adjusted. Severe glyburide-induced hypoglycemia with coma, seizures, or other neurologic impairment occurs infrequently, but constitutes a medical emergency requiring immediate hospitalization and treatment. If hypoglycemic coma is diagnosed or suspected, 50% dextrose injection (e.g., 50 mL) should be administered IV rapidly, followed immediately by a continuous IV infusion of 10% dextrose injection at a rate sufficient to maintain a blood glucose concentration exceeding 100 mg/dL. In some patients, subsequent administration of IV glucagon and/or corticosteroids may also be necessary. Blood glucose concentrations should be monitored at least every 3 hours during the first 24 hours and as often as necessary thereafter. Care should be taken to avoid inducing excessive hyperglycemia. Other symptomatic therapy (e.g., anticonvulsants) should be administered as necessary. Glyburide is effectively adsorbed by activated charcoal in vitro. Experimental studies using chlorpropamide suggest that if sulfonylurea overdosage is the result of an acute ingestion, administration of activated charcoal within several hours of the ingestion may be effective in reducing sulfonylurea absorption. Since hypoglycemia may occur after apparent clinical recovery, patients must be closely monitored for *at least* 24–72 hours; glyburide-induced hypoglycemia has persisted for longer periods in some patients, and recurring hypoglycemia after apparently successful treatment has resulted in death in at least one patient.

Pharmacology

■ **Antidiabetic Effect** Like other sulfonylurea antidiabetic agents, glyburide lowers blood glucose concentration in diabetic and nondiabetic individuals. Although the hypoglycemic action of the various sulfonylureas is generally similar, the drugs may differ quantitatively and/or possibly qualitatively in the extent to which they produce specific effects, and the effects may vary as a function of duration of treatment. On a weight basis, glyburide is one of the most potent of the sulfonylurea antidiabetic agents; although an exact dosage relationship does not exist, a daily glyburide dose of 5 mg controls blood glucose concentration to approximately the same degree as daily doses of acetohexamide 500–750 mg, chlorpropamide or tolazamide 250–375 mg, glipizide 5–10 mg, or tolbutamide 1–1.5 g.

The precise mechanism(s) of hypoglycemic action of sulfonylurea antidiabetic agents has not been clearly established, but the drugs, including glyburide, initially appear to lower blood glucose concentration principally by stimulating secretion of endogenous insulin from the beta cells of the pancreas. Other mechanisms of the hypoglycemic action associated with short-term glyburide therapy appear to include reduction of basal hepatic glucose production and enhancement of peripheral insulin action at postreceptor (probably intracellular) site(s). Following short-term administration of glyburide, an increase in insulin binding has been demonstrated in monocytes obtained from healthy individuals, but not in adipocytes obtained from diabetic patients. Like other sulfonylureas, glyburide alone is ineffective in the absence of functioning beta cells.

The mechanism(s) of action of glyburide during prolonged administration has not been fully established. Glyburide-induced improvement in glucose tolerance during long-term therapy persists despite a gradual decline in glucose- or meal-stimulated secretion of endogenous insulin towards pretreatment levels. During prolonged administration of sulfonylureas, including glyburide, extrapancreatic effects appear to substantially contribute to the hypoglycemic action of the drugs. Many extrapancreatic effects of the drugs have been proposed and/or studied, but the principal effects appear to include enhanced peripheral sensitivity to insulin and reduction of basal hepatic glucose production; however, the nature of the long-term hypoglycemic effect and the mechanism(s) involved remain to be fully elucidated. There is evidence that glyburide enhances the peripheral action of insulin at postreceptor (probably intracellular) site(s) and reduces basal hepatic glucose production during long-term administration. An increase in insulin binding and/or number of insulin receptors has also been demonstrated in monocytes and adipocytes obtained from diabetic patients receiving long-term therapy with the drug.

■ **Other Effects** Glyburide produces a mild diuresis by enhancing renal free water clearance. The diuretic effect has been demonstrated in healthy individuals, diabetic patients, and patients with neurohypophyseal diabetes insipidus; the drug apparently has no diuretic effect in patients with nephrogenic diabetes insipidus. Glyburide has been shown to reduce the duration of antidiuresis induced by IV desmopressin in patients with neurohypophyseal diabetes insipidus; IV desmopressin inhibits the diuretic effect of glyburide in these patients. The exact mechanism by which glyburide enhances renal free water clearance is not known. The diuretic action apparently is not mediated through an effect on the release of vasopressin (antidiuretic hormone) from the posterior pituitary or on the action of vasopressin at the renal collecting ducts. It has been suggested that glyburide inhibits reabsorption of sodium in the proximal renal tubule or nonvasopressin-dependent reabsorption of water in the distal renal tubule.

Glyburide has been reported to inhibit in vitro platelet aggregation induced by epinephrine or collagen and to normalize in vitro platelet aggregation induced by adenosine diphosphate (ADP) in individuals with type 2 diabetes mellitus; however, conflicting results have also been reported, and further evaluation is needed to determine the effect of glyburide on platelet function.

Pharmacokinetics

■ **Absorption** Currently available tablet formulations of glyburide appear to be reliably and almost completely absorbed following oral administration; however, studies to determine the absolute bioavailability are generally lacking. Initial pharmacokinetic studies using other tablet formulations suggested that the drug was variably and incompletely absorbed. Food apparently does not affect the rate or extent of absorption of glyburide.

Following oral administration of a single 5-mg dose of glyburide, the drug appears in plasma or serum within 15–60 minutes and average peak plasma or serum concentrations of approximately 140–350 ng/mL usually are attained within 2–4 hours (range: 2–8 hours). The area under the serum concentration-time curve (AUC) for glyburide increases in proportion to increasing doses. Substantial interindividual variations in steady-state serum concentration have been reported in diabetic patients receiving the same dosage of glyburide.

Following single oral doses of glyburide in nonfasting diabetic or healthy individuals, plasma insulin concentration generally begins to increase within 15–60 minutes and is maximal within 1–2 hours; in diabetic patients, increases in plasma insulin concentration may persist for up to 24 hours. Following single oral doses of the drug in fasting healthy individuals, the degree and duration of lowering of blood glucose concentration are proportional to the dose administered and the AUC; the hypoglycemic action generally begins within 45–60 minutes and is maximal within 1.5–3 hours. In nonfasting diabetic patients, the hypoglycemic action of a single morning dose of glyburide may persist for up to 24 hours. There is some evidence that a serum glyburide concentration of approximately 30–50 ng/mL is required to lower blood glucose concentration. A correlation between blood concentrations of the drug and fasting blood glucose concentration in diabetic patients receiving long-term glyburide therapy has not been established.

■ **Distribution** Distribution of glyburide into human body tissues and fluids has not been fully characterized. Following oral or IV administration in animals, highest concentrations of the drug are attained in the liver, kidneys, and small and large intestines, with lower concentrations in the stomach, pancreas, spleen, mesenteric lymph nodes, mesenteric and retroperitoneal fat, heart, lungs, gonads, skeletal muscle, and brain. In humans, glyburide is distributed in substantial amounts into bile. Glyburide appears to cross the placenta, since prolonged hypoglycemia has occurred in neonates born to women who received the drug up to the time of delivery. It is not known if the drug is distributed into milk.

In healthy adults, the volume of distribution of glyburide during the elimination phase averages 0.155 L/kg and the apparent steady-state volume of distribution averages 0.125 L/kg. Serum glyburide concentration-time curves in diabetic individuals receiving multiple doses of the drug have been shown to be similar to those following single doses, suggesting that glyburide does not accumulate in tissue depots; however, other pharmacokinetic data have suggested that the drug may accumulate in a deep tissue compartment following continuous administration.

At a concentration of 0.05–10 mcg/mL in vitro, glyburide is more than 99% bound to serum proteins and its major metabolite, 4-*trans*-hydroxyglyburide, is more than 97% bound to serum proteins. Glyburide has a higher affinity for binding to serum albumin than does acetohexamide, chlorpropamide, glipizide, or tolbutamide. Unlike the protein binding of some other sulfonylurea antidiabetic agents (e.g., acetohexamide, chlorpropamide, tolazamide, tolbutamide) and like that of glipizide, the protein binding of glyburide is principally nonionic; consequently, glyburide may be less likely to be displaced from binding sites by, or displace from binding sites, other highly protein-bound drugs whose protein binding is ionic in nature. (See Drug Interactions: Protein-Bound Drugs.)

■ **Elimination** Serum concentrations of glyburide appear to decline in a biphasic manner. In studies in healthy adults using assays relatively specific for unchanged glyburide, the terminal elimination half-life has reportedly averaged 1.4–1.8 hours (range: 0.7–3 hours); when assays that also measured metabolites of the drug were used, the terminal elimination half-life has averaged about 10 hours (range: 5–26 hours). Serum glyburide concentrations may be increased in patients with renal or hepatic insufficiency. Data are limited, but the half-life may be prolonged in patients with severe renal impairment. In one study in patients with normal hepatic function and impaired renal function given a single oral dose of radiolabeled glyburide, the plasma half-life of total radioactivity was 2–5 hours in those with creatinine clearances of 29–131 mL/minute per 1.73 m^2 and 11 hours in one patient with a creatinine clearance of 5 mL/minute per 1.73 m^2; in those patients with creatinine clearances of 29–131 mL/minute per 1.73 m^2, no relationship between plasma half-life and creatinine clearance was observed.

Glyburide appears to be completely metabolized, probably in the liver. The drug is metabolized at the cyclohexyl ring principally to 4-*trans*-hydroxyglyburide; the 4-*trans*-hydroxy metabolite has only 0.25% of the hypoglycemic activity of glyburide following oral administration in rabbits, but has about 15% of the hypoglycemic activity of the parent compound following intraperitoneal administration in rats. Glyburide is also metabolized to the 3-*cis*-hydroxy derivative and to another unidentified metabolite; the 3-*cis*-hydroxy metabolite has 2.5% of the hypoglycemic activity of glyburide following oral administration in rabbits. The hypoglycemic activity of glyburide metabolites is generally considered clinically unimportant; however, results of studies in rats indicate that retention of the 4-*trans*-hydroxy metabolite in the presence of renal insufficiency may enhance and prolong the hypoglycemic effect of the drug.

Unlike other currently available sulfonylurea antidiabetic agents which are excreted principally in urine, glyburide is excreted as metabolites in urine and feces in approximately equal proportions. Fecal excretion appears to occur almost completely via biliary elimination; only small amounts may be excreted in feces as unabsorbed drug following oral administration. Most urinary excretion occurs within the first 6–24 hours after oral administration of the drug. Following oral administration of a single 5-mg dose of glyburide in healthy individuals, approximately 30–50% of the dose is excreted in urine as metabolites within 24 hours; about 80% of the urinary excretion occurs as the 4-*trans*-hydroxy metabolite, 15% as the 3-*cis*-hydroxy metabolite, and 5% as an unidentified metabolite. Fecal excretion occurs more slowly, but a single oral dose of the drug is completely excreted in urine and feces within 3–5 days in healthy individuals.

Total plasma clearance of glyburide reportedly averages 78 mL/hour per kg in healthy adults. The effects of renal impairment on the elimination of glyburide and its metabolites have *not* been fully evaluated. Limited data indicate that renal excretion of glyburide metabolites and plasma clearance of glyburide may be substantially decreased in patients with severe renal impairment.

Glyburide appears to be only minimally removed by hemodialysis.

Chemistry and Stability

■ **Chemistry** Glyburide is a sulfonylurea antidiabetic agent. The drug is structurally similar to acetohexamide and glipizide. Although chemically related to sulfonamides, glyburide has no antibacterial activity. Glyburide also is commercially available alone and in fixed combination with metformin hydrochloride.

Glyburide occurs as a white or almost white, odorless or almost odorless, crystalline powder. The solubility of glyburide in water increases with increasing pH; the solubility of the drug in water is approximately 4 mcg/mL at pH 4 and 600 mcg/mL at pH 9. Glyburide has a solubility of approximately 3 mg/mL in alcohol. The drug has a pK_a of 6.8.

■ **Stability** Glyburide tablets should be stored in well-closed containers at 15–30 or 20–25°C, depending on the specific preparation. Fixed-combination preparations containing glyburide and metformin hydrochloride should be stored in light-resistant containers at a controlled room temperature up to 25°C.

Preparations

Excipients in commercially available drug preparations may have clinically important effects in some individuals; consult specific product labeling for details.

glyBURIDE

Oral		
Tablets	1.25 mg*	**DiaBeta**® (scored), Sanofi-Aventis
		Glyburide Tablets
		Micronase® (scored), Pfizer
	2.5 mg*	**DiaBeta**® (scored), Sanofi-Aventis
		Glyburide Tablets
		Micronase® (scored), Pfizer
	5 mg*	**DiaBeta**® (scored), Sanofi-Aventis
		Glyburide Tablets
		Micronase® (scored), Pfizer
Tablets (micronized)	1.5 mg*	**Glyburide Micronized Tablets**
		Glycron® (scored), Zoetica
		Glynase® PresTab® (scored), Pfizer
	3 mg*	**Glyburide Micronized Tablets**
		Glycron® (scored), Zoetica
		Glynase® PresTab® (scored), Pfizer
	4.5 mg*	**Glycron**® (scored), Zoetica
	6 mg*	**Glyburide Micronized Tablets**
		Glycron® (scored), Zoetica
		Glynase® PresTab® (scored), Pfizer

*available from one or more manufacturer, distributor, and/or repackager by generic (nonproprietary) name

glyBURIDE Combinations

Oral		
Tablets, film-coated	1.25 mg with Metformin Hydrochloride 250 mg*	**Glucovance**® (with povidone), Bristol-Myers Squibb
		Glyburide with Metformin Hydrochloride Tablets
	2.5 mg with Metformin Hydrochloride 500 mg*	**Glucovance**® (with povidone), Bristol-Myers Squibb
		Glyburide with Metformin Hydrochloride Tablets
	5 mg with Metformin Hydrochloride 500 mg*	**Glucovance**® (with povidone), Bristol-Myers Squibb
		Glyburide with Metformin Hydrochloride Tablets

*available from one or more manufacturer, distributor, and/or repackager by generic (nonproprietary) name

THIAZOLIDINEDIONES 68:20.28

Pioglitazone Hydrochloride

■ Pioglitazone is a thiazolidinedione (glitazone) antidiabetic agent that is structurally and pharmacologically related to troglitazone and rosiglitazone.

Uses

■ **Diabetes Mellitus** Pioglitazone is used alone (monotherapy) or in combination with a sulfonylurea antidiabetic agent, metformin (either as a fixed-combination preparation or as individual drugs given concurrently), or insulin as an adjunct to diet and exercise to improve glycemic control in patients with type 2 diabetes mellitus. Pioglitazone also is used in fixed combination with glimepiride in patients with type 2 diabetes mellitus who are already receiving a thiazolidinedione and a sulfonylurea separately or who are inadequately controlled on a sulfonylurea or a thiazolidinedione alone. In patients whose hyperglycemia cannot be controlled with these other antidiabetic agents, pioglitazone should be added to, not substituted for, such antidiabetic therapy.

The American Diabetes Association (ADA) currently classifies diabetes mellitus as type 1 (immune mediated or idiopathic), type 2 (predominantly insulin resistance with relative insulin deficiency to predominantly an insulin secretory defect with insulin resistance), gestational diabetes mellitus, or that associated with certain conditions or syndromes (e.g., drug- or chemical-induced, hormonal, that associated with pancreatic disease, infections, specific genetic defects or syndromes). Type 1 diabetes mellitus was previously described as juvenile-onset (JOD) diabetes mellitus, since it usually occurs during youth. Type 2 diabetes mellitus was previously described as adult-onset (AODM) diabetes mellitus. However, type 1 or type 2 diabetes mellitus can occur at any age, and the current classification is based on pathogenesis (e.g., autoimmune destruction of pancreatic β cells, insulin resistance) and clinical presentation rather than on age of onset. Many patients' diabetes mellitus does not easily fit into a single classification. Epidemiologic data indicate that the incidence of type 2 diabetes mellitus is increasing in children and adolescents such that 8–45% of children with newly diagnosed diabetes have nonimmune-mediated diabetes mellitus; most of these individuals have type 2 diabetes mellitus, although other types, including idiopathic or nonimmune-mediated type 1 diabetes mellitus, also have been reported.

Patients with type 2 diabetes mellitus have insulin resistance and usually have relative (rather than absolute) insulin deficiency. Most patients with type 2 diabetes mellitus are overweight or obese; obesity itself also contributes to the insulin resistance and glucose intolerance observed in these patients. Patients with type 2 diabetes mellitus who are not obese may have an increased percentage of abdominal fat, which is an indicator of increased cardiometabolic risk. While children with immune-mediated type 1 diabetes mellitus generally are not overweight, the incidence of obesity in children with this form of diabetes is increasing with the increasing incidence of obesity in the US population. Distinguishing between type 1 and type 2 diabetes mellitus in children may be difficult since obesity may occur with either type of diabetes mellitus, and autoantigens and ketosis may be present in a substantial number of children with features of type 2 diabetes mellitus (e.g., obesity, acanthosis nigricans). For additional details on the clinical classification, complications, and management of diabetes mellitus, see Uses in Metformin 68:20.04.

A thiazolidinedione (i.e., pioglitazone or rosiglitazone) generally is considered one of several second-line agents (e.g., including insulin and sulfonylureas) used for the management of hyperglycemia in patients with type 2 diabetes mellitus not responding adequately to oral monotherapy with metformin, the preferred initial oral antidiabetic therapy.

Some data suggest a possible protective effect of pioglitazone with regard to certain cardiovascular outcomes (e.g., death, myocardial infarction, stroke) in patients with type 2 diabetes mellitus. In a randomized, controlled study in over 5000 patients with type 2 diabetes mellitus who were at high risk for macrovascular complications, addition of pioglitazone to existing antidiabetic therapy was associated with a reduction in the secondary composite end point of all-cause mortality, nonfatal myocardial infarction, and stroke compared with placebo; no difference between the study groups was observed with respect to the primary composite study end point (all-cause mortality, nonfatal myocardial infarction, stroke, acute coronary syndrome, endovascular or surgical intervention on the coronary or leg arteries, or above-the-ankle amputation). Results of a meta-analysis of data from randomized, placebo- or active-controlled trials in over 16,000 patients indicated an 18% lower risk of the primary composite end point of death, myocardial infarction, or stroke with pioglitazone therapy. The incidence of serious heart failure was increased with pioglitazone therapy but without an associated increase in mortality. While an increased risk of myocardial ischemic events has not been documented to date with pioglitazone therapy in patients with type 2 diabetes mellitus, both pioglitazone and rosiglitazone, alone or in combination with other antidiabetic agents, can cause fluid retention and other cardiovascular effects that may lead to or exacerbate heart failure. Therefore, the potential risks and benefits of thiazolidinediones versus other second-line antidiabetic agents (sulfonylureas, insulin) should be carefully considered. (See Heart Failure under Warnings/Precautions: Warnings, in Cautions.) For information on the effects of intensive glycemic control on microvascular and macrovascular complications in patients with diabetes mellitus, see Uses in Metformin 68:20.04.

Pioglitazone Monotherapy Efficacy as monotherapy for the management of type 2 diabetes mellitus was established in 3 controlled studies of 16–26 weeks' duration. Pioglitazone improved glycemic control as measured by fasting glucose and glycosylated hemoglobin (HbA_{1c}) concentrations.

Combination Therapy Efficacy of pioglitazone in combination with a sulfonylurea antidiabetic agent, metformin, or insulin in patients whose type 2 diabetes mellitus was inadequately controlled by therapy with one or more of these agents was established in several controlled studies in which combined therapy improved glycemic control regardless of the dosage of the other antidiabetic agent(s). A thiazolidinedione such as pioglitazone also may be added to therapy with the fixed combination of glyburide and metformin in patients whose hyperglycemia is not adequately controlled with the fixed combination. A thiazolidinedione antidiabetic agent also may be used concomitantly with repaglinide in patients whose hyperglycemia is inadequately controlled with diet, exercise, and monotherapy with metformin, a sulfonylurea, repaglinide, or a thiazolidinedione antidiabetic agent. In a clinical trial in patients with type 2 diabetes mellitus poorly controlled (as determined by HbA_{1c} concentrations exceeding 7%) by metformin or sulfonylurea monotherapy, the combination of repaglinide and pioglitazone reduced fasting plasma glucose and HbA_{1c} concentrations compared with pioglitazone or repaglinide monotherapy. Greater glycemic control was achieved with the combination of pioglitazone (fixed dosage: 30 mg daily) and repaglinide at a lower daily dosage of repaglinide (final median dosage: 6 mg daily) than with repaglinide monotherapy (final median dosage: 10 mg daily).

Pioglitazone also is used in fixed combination with metformin in patients with type 2 diabetes mellitus who have inadequate glycemic control with pioglitazone or metformin monotherapy or in those who are already receiving pioglitazone and metformin concurrently as separate components. Efficacy and safety of pioglitazone in fixed combination with metformin were established in a 24-week, randomized clinical study in 600 patients with type 2 diabetes mellitus (mean baseline HbA_{1c} 8.7%) inadequately controlled with diet and exercise. Substantial improvements in fasting plasma glucose and HbA_{1c} were observed in patients receiving the fixed combination of pioglitazone and metformin compared with each individual component alone. Efficacy and safety of the fixed combination also have been established based on concurrent administration of the 2 agents given separately and extrapolations from clinical trials evaluating pioglitazone as add-on therapy to metformin. Bioequivalence has been demonstrated between the fixed combination of pioglitazone and metformin and each agent given concurrently.

Pioglitazone also is used in fixed combination with glimepiride in patients with type 2 diabetes mellitus who are already receiving a thiazolidinedione and a sulfonylurea separately or who are inadequately controlled on a sulfonylurea or a thiazolidinedione alone. No clinical trials have been conducted evaluating the fixed combination of pioglitazone and glimepiride as second-line therapy in patients who are inadequately controlled on monotherapy with a sulfonylurea. Safety and efficacy of the fixed combination of pioglitazone and glimepiride in patients with type 2 diabetes mellitus who are inadequately controlled on a sulfonylurea alone have been extrapolated from clinical trials evaluating pioglitazone as add-on therapy to a sulfonylurea.

Because pioglitazone requires insulin for activity, it would not be effective and should not be used in patients with type 1 diabetes mellitus or ketoacidosis.

Dosage and Administration

■ **General** Dosage should be carefully individualized based on patient response and tolerance. Following initiation of pioglitazone therapy or dosage increase, patients should be monitored for adverse effects related to fluid retention. (See Heart Failure under Warnings/Precautions: Warnings, in Cautions.) Fasting plasma glucose (FPG) concentrations should be monitored periodically to determine the patient's response. Periodic glycosylated hemoglobin (hemoglobin A_{1c} [HbA_{1c}]) determinations also should be performed; HbA_{1c} is a better indicator of long-term glycemic control than fasting plasma glucose concentrations alone.

Administration Pioglitazone hydrochloride is administered orally once daily and can be taken without regard to meals. Pioglitazone in fixed combination with immediate- or extended-release metformin hydrochloride (ActoPlus Met® or ActoPlus Met® XR) is administered once or twice daily with meals to reduce the GI effects of the metformin hydrochloride component. Pioglitazone in fixed combination with glimepiride is administered once daily with the first main meal.

Dosage Dosage of pioglitazone hydrochloride is expressed in terms of pioglitazone. Bioequivalence has been demonstrated between the fixed combination of immediate-release pioglitazone and immediate-release metformin hydrochloride (ActoPlus® Met) and each agent given concurrently as separate tablets at the currently approved dosage strengths (500 or 850 mg of metformin hydrochloride and 15 mg of pioglitazone), and between the fixed combination of immediate-release pioglitazone and extended-release metformin hydrochloride (ActoPlus® Met XR) and each agent given concurrently as separate tablets at the currently approved dosage strengths (1 g of metformin hydrochloride and 15 or 30 mg of pioglitazone). Bioequivalence also has been demonstrated between the fixed combination of pioglitazone and glimepiride (Duetact®) and each agent given concurrently as separate tablets at the currently approved dosage strengths (2 or 4 mg of glimepiride and 30 mg of pioglitazone).

Pioglitazone Monotherapy. The initial dosage of pioglitazone as monotherapy is 15 or 30 mg once daily. If the response is inadequate, dosage may be increased gradually up to a maximum recommended dosage of 45 mg daily.

Combination Therapy with Other Oral Antidiabetic Agents. The usual initial dosage of pioglitazone in combination with a sulfonylurea antidiabetic agent, metformin hydrochloride, or insulin (as separate components) is 15 or 30 mg once daily. Pioglitazone dosage should not exceed 45 mg daily.

Should hypoglycemia occur during combination therapy with an insulin secretagogue (e.g., sulfonylurea), the dosage of the insulin secretagogue should be decreased. If hypoglycemia occurs with concomitant pioglitazone and insulin therapy, the dosage of insulin should be reduced by 10–25%; further adjustments to insulin dosage should be individualized according to glycemic response. (See Hypoglycemia under Warnings/Precautions: Other Warnings/Precautions, in Cautions.)

When the commercially available fixed-combination preparations containing immediate-release pioglitazone and immediate-release metformin hydrochloride (ActoPlus Met®) or immediate-release pioglitazone and extended-release metformin hydrochloride (ActoPlus Met® XR) are used, dosage of the fixed combinations is based on the patient's existing dosages of pioglitazone and/or metformin hydrochloride and on usual initial dosages of these drugs, effectiveness, and tolerability. When the fixed combination is used to replace therapy with separate tablets given concurrently, the dosage of the fixed combination is based on the patient's existing dosage of metformin and pioglitazone. Metformin hydrochloride doses exceeding 2 g may be better tolerated when administered three times daily.

The usual initial dosage of the fixed combination containing pioglitazone and immediate-release metformin hydrochloride is pioglitazone 15 mg/metformin hydrochloride 500 mg twice daily or pioglitazone 15 mg/metformin hydrochloride 850 mg once daily. When the commercially available preparation containing pioglitazone in fixed combination with immediate-release metformin hydrochloride is used to replace metformin monotherapy, the usual initial dosage is pioglitazone 15 mg/metformin hydrochloride 500 mg twice daily or pioglitazone 15 mg/metformin hydrochloride 850 mg once or twice daily depending on the patient's existing metformin hydrochloride dosage. The usual initial dosage of the fixed combination in patients currently receiving pioglitazone monotherapy is pioglitazone 15 mg/metformin hydrochloride 500 mg twice daily or pioglitazone 15 mg/metformin hydrochloride 850 mg once daily. Dosage should be titrated gradually after assessing therapeutic response, up to a maximum daily dosage of 45 mg of pioglitazone and 2.55 g of immediate-release metformin hydrochloride.

The usual initial dosage of the fixed combination containing pioglitazone and extended-release metformin hydrochloride is pioglitazone 15 mg/metformin hydrochloride 1 g or pioglitazone 30 mg/metformin hydrochloride 1 g once daily. When the commercially available preparation containing pioglitazone in fixed combination with extended-release metformin hydrochloride is used to replace metformin monotherapy, the usual initial dosage is pioglitazone 15 mg/metformin hydrochloride 1 g twice daily or pioglitazone 30 mg/metformin hydrochloride 1 g once daily depending on the patient's existing metformin hydrochloride dosage. The usual initial dosage of the fixed combination in patients currently receiving pioglitazone monotherapy is pioglitazone 15 mg/metformin hydrochloride 1 g twice daily or pioglitazone 30 mg/metformin hydrochloride 1 g once daily. Dosage should be titrated gradually after assessing therapeutic response, up to a maximum daily dosage of 45 mg of pioglitazone and 2 g of extended-release metformin hydrochloride.

The safety and efficacy of transferring from therapy with other oral antidiabetic agents to the fixed combination of pioglitazone and metformin hydrochloride have not been established in clinical studies. Any change in the therapy of type 2 diabetic patients should be undertaken with caution and appropriate monitoring, as changes in glycemic control can occur.

The initial dosage of pioglitazone in fixed combination with glimepiride should be based on the patient's existing regimen with pioglitazone and/or a sulfonylurea. When the commercially available preparation containing pioglitazone in fixed combination with glimepiride is used in to replace glimepiride monotherapy, the usual initial dosage of the fixed combination is 30 mg of pioglitazone and 2 or 4 mg of glimepiride once daily with the first main meal. The usual initial dosage of the fixed combination in patients currently receiving pioglitazone monotherapy is 30 mg of pioglitazone and 2 mg of glimepiride once daily. When the fixed combination is used to replace concurrent therapy as separate tablets, the dosage of the fixed combination is based on the patient's existing dosage of glimepiride and pioglitazone. Therapy may be initiated with 2 or 4 mg of glimepiride and 30 mg of pioglitazone once daily. Following initiation of therapy with the fixed combination in patients previously receiving monotherapy with pioglitazone or a sulfonylurea or combination therapy with each component given separately, subsequent dosage should be adjusted according to the patient's therapeutic response. For patients transferring from monotherapy with a sulfonylurea other than glimepiride or from combination therapy with pioglitazone and a sulfonylurea other than glimepiride, the usual initial dosage of the fixed combination is 30 mg of pioglitazone and 2 mg of glimepiride once daily. Because an exaggerated hypoglycemic response may occur in some patients during the transition from a sulfonylurea antidiabetic agent with a prolonged half-life (e.g., chlorpropamide) to glimepiride in fixed combination with pioglitazone, patients being transferred from such agents should be monitored closely for the occurrence of hypoglycemia during the initial 1–2 weeks of the transition period.

If additional glycemic control is needed, dosage may be increased to a maximum total daily dosage of 8 mg of glimepiride and 45 mg of pioglitazone.

Concomitant Therapy with Potent CYP2C8 Inhibitors or Inducers. Because concomitant use of pioglitazone and potent inhibitors of cytochrome P-450 (CYP) isoenzyme 2C8 (e.g., gemfibrozil) increases exposure to pioglitazone, the maximum recommended dosage of pioglitazone in patients taking potent CYP2C8 inhibitors is 15 mg once daily. Patients receiving pioglitazone in fixed combination with glimepiride and a potent CYP2C8 inhibitor should be switched to therapy with the individual drug components administered separately because the minimum dose of pioglitazone in the fixed-combination preparation exceeds 15 mg. The maximum recommended dosage of pioglitazone in fixed combination with immediate-release metformin hydrochloride is pioglitazone 15 mg/metformin hydrochloride 850 mg once daily when used in combination with a potent CYP2C8 inhibitor. The maximum recommended dosage of pioglitazone in fixed combination with extended-release metformin hydrochloride is pioglitazone 15 mg/metformin hydrochloride 1 g once daily when used in combination with a potent CYP2C8 inhibitor.

If treatment with a CYP2C8 inducer (e.g., rifampin) is initiated or discontinued during pioglitazone therapy, changes in antidiabetic therapy may be required based on clinical response; however, the dosage of pioglitazone should not exceed the maximum recommended dosage of 45 mg daily. (See Drug Interactions: Drugs Affecting Hepatic Microsomal Enzymes.)

■ **Special Populations** ***Hepatic Impairment*** Pioglitazone dosage adjustment is not necessary in patients with hepatic impairment when the drug is given as monotherapy. Pioglitazone should be initiated with caution in patients with hepatic impairment. If the fixed combination of glimepiride and pioglitazone is considered for use in patients with hepatic impairment, the drug should be initiated and dosage increased with caution. Patients with hepatic impairment should be closely monitored for hypoglycemia during initiation and subsequent dosage adjustment of such combination therapy. The use of the fixed combination of metformin hydrochloride and pioglitazone is not recommended in patients with hepatic impairment.

Renal Impairment Pioglitazone dosage adjustment is not necessary in patients with renal impairment. Due to the risk of lactic acidosis with metformin hydrochloride therapy, the manufacturers state that the initiation of pioglitazone in fixed combination with metformin hydrochloride is not recommended in patients with an estimated glomerular filtration rate (eGFR) of 30–45 mL/minute per 1.73 m^2; the benefits and risks of continuing the drug should be assessed in those with an eGFR in this range who are already receiving the drug. The manufacturers state that pioglitazone in fixed combination with metformin hydrochloride should not be used in patients with an eGFR of less than 30 mL/minute per 1.73 m^2. If the fixed combination of glimepiride and pioglitazone is considered for use in patients with renal impairment, the initial dosage, dose increments, and maintenance dosage of the drug should be conservative. Patients with renal impairment should be closely monitored for hypoglycemia during initiation and subsequent dosage adjustment of such combination therapy.

Geriatric Patients Pioglitazone dosage adjustment is not necessary for geriatric patients solely because of age. Pioglitazone in fixed combination with metformin hydrochloride should be used with caution in geriatric patients since aging is associated with reduced renal function. Initial and maintenance dosages of the fixed combination should be conservative and should be titrated carefully.

As geriatric patients are particularly susceptible to hypoglycemia, the initial and maintenance dosages of pioglitazone in fixed combination with glimepiride should be conservative. Blood glucose concentrations of such patients should be closely monitored prior to and after initiation of therapy to avoid hypoglycemia.

Debilitated or Malnourished Patients Caution should be used when initiating and increasing the dosage of pioglitazone in fixed combination with glimepiride in patients who are debilitated or malnourished and in those with adrenal, pituitary, or hepatic impairment. Such patients are particularly susceptible to the hypoglycemic effect of glucose-lowering drugs.

Heart Failure The recommended initial dosage of pioglitazone in patients with New York Heart Association (NYHA) class I or II heart failure is 15 mg once daily. If subsequent dosage escalation is necessary, the dosage should be increased gradually in increments of 15 mg up to a maximum dosage of 45 mg daily according to glycemic response based on HbA_{1c}. For patients with NYHA class I or II heart failure, the recommended initial dosage of the fixed combination containing pioglitazone and immediate-release metformin hydrochloride is pioglitazone 15 mg/metformin hydrochloride 500 mg or pioglitazone 15 mg/metformin hydrochloride 850 mg once daily. For patients with NYHA class I or II heart failure, the recommended initial dosage of the fixed combination containing pioglitazone and extended-release metformin hydrochloride is pioglitazone 15 mg/metformin hydrochloride 1 g or pioglitazone 30 mg/metformin hydrochloride 1 g once daily. Following initiation of pioglitazone and any increase in dosage, patients should be monitored carefully for weight gain, edema, and manifestations of congestive heart failure (CHF). Initiation of pioglitazone therapy in patients with more severe heart failure (NYHA class III or IV) is contraindicated. (See Heart Failure under Warnings/Precautions: Warnings, in Cautions and see Cautions: Contraindications.)

Before receiving therapy with the fixed-combination preparation containing glimepiride 2 mg and pioglitazone 30 mg, patients with diabetes mellitus and systolic dysfunction should receive pioglitazone 15 mg once daily as monotherapy and should safely tolerate dosage titration to 30 mg once daily as monotherapy. If subsequent dosage adjustment is necessary with the fixed-combination preparation, patients should be closely monitored for weight gain, edema, or other signs or symptoms of exacerbation of CHF.

Cautions

■ **Contraindications** Known serious hypersensitivity reaction to pioglitazone or any ingredient in the formulation.

Initiation of therapy with pioglitazone is contraindicated in patients with New York Heart Association (NYHA) class III or IV heart failure. (See Heart Failure under Warnings/Precautions: Warnings, in Cautions.)

■ **Warnings/Precautions** ***Warnings*** **Heart Failure.** Thiazolidinediones, including pioglitazone, alone or in combination with other antidiabetic agents, can cause fluid retention, which may lead to or exacerbate heart failure. Use of thiazolidinediones is associated with an approximately twofold increased risk of heart failure. (See Edema under Warnings/Precautions: Warnings, in Cautions.) Use of pioglitazone in combination with insulin or in patients with NYHA class I or II heart failure may increase the risk. Patients should be observed for signs and symptoms of heart failure (e.g., dyspnea, rapid weight gain, edema, unexplained cough or fatigue), especially during initiation of therapy and dosage titration. If signs and symptoms of heart failure develop, the disorder should be managed according to current standards of care. In addition, a decrease in the dosage or discontinuance of pioglitazone must be considered in such patients.

Patients with NYHA class III or IV cardiac status with or without congestive heart failure (CHF) or with an acute coronary event were not studied in clinical trials of pioglitazone; initiation of therapy with the drug is contraindicated in patients with NYHA class III or IV heart failure. Use of pioglitazone is *not* recommended in patients with symptomatic heart failure. Caution should be exercised in patients with edema and in those who are at risk for heart failure. Thiazolidinedione therapy should not be initiated in hospitalized patients with diabetes mellitus because of the delayed onset of action and because possible drug-related increases in vascular volume and CHF may complicate care of patients with hemodynamic changes induced by coexisting conditions or in-hospital interventions.

Findings from a meta-analysis of randomized controlled studies that assessed the risk of development of CHF and death from cardiovascular causes in patients receiving thiazolidinediones indicate that the risk of CHF is higher in patients receiving thiazolidinediones (relative risk of 1.72; 95% confidence interval: 1.21–2.42) than in controls (individuals receiving other antidiabetic agents or placebo). The relative risk for CHF was increased across a wide background of cardiovascular risk (i.e., patients with prediabetes, with type 2 diabetes mellitus without cardiovascular disease, with type 2 diabetes mellitus and cardiovascular disease other than CHF, or with type 2 diabetes mellitus and CHF [NYHA class I and II] and ejection fraction less than 40%). In contrast to the increased risk for CHF observed in thiazolidinedione-treated patients, the risk of cardiovascular death was not increased in patients receiving these agents.

In a 16-week, controlled study in patients with type 2 diabetes mellitus, CHF was reported in 1.1% of patients receiving combined therapy with pioglitazone and insulin and in none of the patients receiving insulin therapy alone; all patients who experienced CHF had a history of cardiac disease (e.g., coronary artery disease, previous coronary artery bypass graft procedures, myocardial infarction).

CHF has been reported during postmarketing experience in pioglitazone-treated patients who did or did not have previously known heart disease and who did or did not receive concomitant insulin therapy. In a 24-week postmarketing safety study in patients with NYHA class II and III heart failure and poorly controlled diabetes despite use of pioglitazone or glyburide, a higher incidence of CHF requiring hospitalization was observed in those receiving pioglitazone (9.9% of patients) than in those receiving glyburide (4.7% of patients). Patients who were older than 64 years of age or receiving insulin at study entry were particularly susceptible to this adverse event. No differences in cardiovascular mortality were noted between pioglitazone and glyburide therapy.

Data from a long-term (34.5 months) cardiovascular outcomes study (PROspective pioglitAzone Clinical Trial In macroVascular Events [PROACTIVE]) in patients with a history of macrovascular disease (those with NYHA class II–IV heart failure were excluded) receiving pioglitazone or placebo in addition to existing antidiabetic therapy (e.g., insulin, metformin, sulfonylureas) and cardiovascular agents indicated a higher incidence of serious heart failure (e.g., requiring hospitalization or prolonging hospital stay, fatal or life-threatening, resulting in substantial disability) in patients receiving pioglitazone than in those receiving placebo. Serious heart failure occurred in 5.7 or 4.1% of patients receiving pioglitazone or placebo, respectively; mortality rates from heart failure did not differ between pioglitazone or placebo recipients.

Edema. Fluid retention can occur and may lead to or exacerbate CHF in patients receiving a thiazolidinedione, including pioglitazone, alone or in combination with other antidiabetic agents, including insulin. Diuretic therapy may be necessary for management of fluid retention. Caution should be exercised in patients with edema and those at risk for CHF. (See Heart Failure under Warnings/Precautions: Warnings, in Cautions.)

All patients receiving thiazolidinedione therapy (e.g., rosiglitazone, pioglitazone) should be advised to monitor for weight gain and edema. Other potential causes of edema should be excluded. Pioglitazone-induced edema is reversible when the drug is discontinued. Hospitalization for edema usually is not required unless there is coexisting CHF.

Weight Gain. Dose-related weight gain, probably involving a combination of fluid retention and fat accumulation, has been observed during therapy with pioglitazone alone or in combination with other antidiabetic agents (e.g., metformin, sulfonylureas, insulin). Unusually rapid increases in weight and increases in excess of that usually observed in clinical trials have been reported during postmarketing experience. Patients who experience rapid or excessive weight gain should be assessed for fluid accumulation and volume-related events such as excessive edema and CHF.

Other Warnings/Precautions

Hepatic Effects. No evidence of hepatotoxicity has been noted with pioglitazone in clinical studies to date. However, hepatitis, liver function test abnormalities (i.e., elevations in hepatic enzymes to at least 3 times the upper limit of normal), mixed hepatocellular-cholestatic liver injury, and liver failure with or without fatalities have been reported during postmarketing experience with the drug. Patients with type 2 diabetes mellitus may have fatty liver disease or cardiac disease with episodic CHF, both of which may cause liver test abnormalities; such patients also may have other forms of liver disease, many of which can be treated or managed. Liver function tests (serum ALT and AST, alkaline phosphatase, total bilirubin) should be obtained prior to initiation of pioglitazone therapy. If results of such tests are abnormal, the probable cause should be investigated, treated (if possible), and monitored appropriately. Pioglitazone should be initiated with caution in patients with abnormal liver function test results. The manufacturer states that routine periodic monitoring of liver function tests during pioglitazone treatment is not recommended in patients without liver disease.

Development of manifestations suggestive of hepatic dysfunction (e.g., unexplained nausea, vomiting, abdominal pain, fatigue, anorexia, dark urine) should lead to prompt rechecking of liver function. If such symptoms are accompanied by serum ALT increases exceeding 3 times the upper limit of normal, pioglitazone therapy should be interrupted and investigation done to establish the probable cause of the abnormal test results. Patients receiving pioglitazone who have serum ALT concentrations exceeding 3 times the reference range and serum total bilirubin concentrations exceeding twice the reference range without alternative explanations are at risk for severe drug-induced liver injury; the drug should not be restarted in such patients. The manufacturer states that pioglitazone may be used with caution in patients with lesser elevations of serum ALT or bilirubin who have an alternative probable cause for such elevations.

Musculoskeletal Effects. Thiazolidinedione use is associated with bone loss and fractures in women and possibly in men with type 2 diabetes mellitus. In a long-term (34.5 months of follow-up) cardiovascular outcomes study (PROACTIVE) in patients with type 2 diabetes mellitus (mean duration of diabetes: 9.5 years), 5.1 or 2.5% of women receiving pioglitazone or placebo, respectively, experienced a fracture. Such effects were noted after the first year of treatment and persisted throughout the study. The majority of fractures observed in female patients receiving pioglitazone were nonvertebral, occurring in a distal upper limb (i.e., forearm, hand, wrist) or distal lower limb (i.e., foot, ankle, fibula, tibia). In an observational study in the United Kingdom in men and women (mean age: 60.7 years) with diabetes mellitus, use of pioglitazone or rosiglitazone for approximately 12–18 months (as estimated from prescription records) was associated with a twofold to threefold increase in fractures, particularly of the hip and wrist. The overall risk of fracture was similar among men and women and was independent of body mass index, comorbid conditions, diabetic complications, duration of diabetes mellitus, and use of other oral antidiabetic drugs.

Risk of fracture should be considered when initiating or continuing thiazolidinedione therapy, particularly in female patients. Bone health should be assessed and maintained according to current standards of care.

Risk of Bladder Cancer. Although the results of various clinical studies evaluating the association of pioglitazone use and bladder cancer have varied, overall findings from studies in animals and humans suggest that pioglitazone therapy may be associated with an increased risk of bladder cancer. There are insufficient data to determine whether pioglitazone is a tumor promoter for urinary bladder tumors.

In preclinical carcinogenicity studies of pioglitazone, bladder tumors were observed in male rats receiving doses of pioglitazone that produced blood concentrations of pioglitazone approximately equivalent to those resulting from the maximum recommended clinical dose in humans. In addition, results from two 3-year controlled clinical studies of pioglitazone (the PROACTIVE study and a liver safety study) demonstrated a higher percentage of bladder cancer cases in patients receiving pioglitazone versus comparator drugs. However, an increased risk of bladder cancer was not observed when patients who completed the PROACTIVE study were observed for an additional 10 years, with minimal exposure to pioglitazone.

A 10-year epidemiologic study conducted by the manufacturer concluded that there was no statistically significant association overall between pioglitazone exposure and bladder cancer. However, there was a slight trend towards higher risk of bladder cancer with increasing duration of pioglitazone use. The median duration of therapy among pioglitazone-treated patients in this study was 2.8 years (range 0.2–13.2 years). In addition, results of a retrospective cohort (nested case-control design) study involving more than 115,000 patients in a United Kingdom general practice database found a statistically significant 83% increase in the rate of bladder cancer with ever use of pioglitazone, but no increased risk with rosiglitazone therapy. This cohort study found a dose-response relationship for cumulative duration of pioglitazone use, with the highest risk observed in patients who received the drug for more than 24 months. Similarly, another retrospective cohort study involving more than 145,000 patients found a 63% increase in the rate of bladder cancer with pioglitazone therapy and no increased risk with rosiglitazone therapy. A duration-response and dose-response relationship also was evident in this study; substantial increases in the risk of bladder cancer were observed with increasing cumulative duration of use and cumulative dose of pioglitazone.

The manufacturer and FDA state that pioglitazone should not be used in patients with active bladder cancer; in addition, the drug should be used with caution in patients who have a history of bladder cancer, weighing the benefits of glycemic control against the unknown risks of cancer recurrence with pioglitazone therapy. Patients who are concerned about the possible risks associated with using pioglitazone should be advised to consult their healthcare professional.

Hypoglycemia. Concomitant therapy with pioglitazone and insulin or other antidiabetic drugs (particularly insulin secretagogues such as sulfonylureas) increases the risk for hypoglycemia. A reduced dosage of the concomitant antidiabetic agent may be needed to decrease the risk of hypoglycemia. (See Combination Therapy with Other Oral Antidiabetic Agents under Dosage and Administration: Dosage.)

Ocular Effects. During postmarketing experience, rare cases of new-onset or worsening (diabetic) macular edema with decreased visual acuity have been reported with pioglitazone or another thiazolidinedione; such patients frequently reported concurrent peripheral edema. Some patients with macular edema presented with symptoms of blurred vision or decreased visual acuity, but other cases were detected by routine ophthalmologic examination. Symptoms improved in some patients following discontinuance of pioglitazone. Patients with diabetes mellitus should have regular eye examinations by an ophthalmologist. Patients receiving pioglitazone who report any visual symptoms should be referred promptly to an ophthalmologist, regardless of the presence of other concurrent therapy or physical findings.

Ovulatory Effects. Like other thiazolidinediones, pioglitazone may promote ovulation in some premenopausal anovulatory women. Premenopausal women receiving pioglitazone should be advised of the potential for an unintended pregnancy.

Macrovascular Outcomes. Evidence of macrovascular risk reduction with pioglitazone or any other antidiabetic agent has not been conclusively demonstrated in controlled clinical trials.

Laboratory Abnormalities. Dose-related decreases in hemoglobin and hematocrit usually becomes evident 4–12 weeks after initiation of therapy and values remain stable thereafter. These effects may be related to plasma volume expansion and have rarely been associated with clinically important hematologic manifestations.

Isolated elevations in serum creatine kinase (CK, creatine phosphokinase, CPK) exceeding 10 times the upper limit of normal were noted rarely during protocol-specified measurements in clinical trials. Such elevations resolved in most patients without apparent sequelae despite continued therapy; any relationship to pioglitazone therapy is unknown.

Use of Fixed Combinations. When pioglitazone is used in fixed combination with other drugs (e.g., metformin, glimepiride), the cautions, precautions, and contraindications associated with those drugs must be considered in addition to those associated with pioglitazone.

Specific Populations **Pregnancy.** Data are lacking on the use of pioglitazone in pregnant women. Blood glucose abnormalities during pregnancy are associated with an increased incidence of congenital anomalies and neonatal morbidity and mortality. In reproduction studies in rats and rabbits, pioglitazone administered during organogenesis at exposures up to 5 and 35 times the maximum recommended human dose, respectively, was not associated with adverse developmental effects. However, delayed parturition and reduced embryofetal viability were observed with pioglitazone dosages at least 9 times the maximum recommended human dose. Offspring of pregnant rats who were administered pioglitazone at dosages at least 2 times the maximum recommended human dose during late gestation and lactation had delayed postnatal development attributed to decreased body weight.

Lactation. Pioglitazone is distributed into milk in rats; it is unknown whether pioglitazone is distributed into human milk. The benefits of breastfeeding should be weighed against the potential risk of adverse effects on the breast-fed infant from pioglitazone.

Pediatric Use. Safety and efficacy of pioglitazone have not been established in children or adolescents younger than 18 years of age; use in this age group currently is not recommended by the manufacturer because of adverse effects observed in adults (e.g., fluid retention and heart failure, fractures, urinary bladder tumors). However, the American Diabetes Association (ADA) states that most pediatric diabetologists use oral antidiabetic agents in children with type 2 diabetes mellitus because of greater patient compliance with therapy and convenience for the patient's family and a lack of evidence demonstrating better efficacy of insulin as initial therapy for type 2 diabetes mellitus.

Geriatric Use. Pharmacokinetic, efficacy, and adverse effect profiles in geriatric patients are similar to those in younger adults, although small sample sizes in studies of patients 75 years or older limit conclusions. While pioglitazone area under the concentration-time curve (AUC) is about 21% higher in healthy geriatric individuals than in younger individuals and mean terminal half-life is also prolonged (10 hours versus 7 hours, respectively), these changes are not considered clinically relevant.

Hepatic Impairment. Pioglitazone therapy should be initiated with caution in patients with abnormal liver function test results. Pioglitazone therapy should be interrupted if ALT exceeds 3 times the upper limit of normal and the cause of liver test abnormalities should be investigated. (See Hepatic Effects under Warnings/Precautions: Other Warnings/Precautions, in Cautions.)

■ **Common Adverse Effects** Adverse effects (not dose related) occurring in at least 5% of patients receiving pioglitazone and more frequently than with placebo include upper respiratory tract infection, headache, sinusitis, myalgia, pharyngitis, and edema. Adverse effects generally were similar with pioglitazone monotherapy versus combined therapy with sulfonylureas, metformin, or insulin; however, edema was more common during pioglitazone monotherapy and during all combined therapies than with placebo. Pioglitazone-induced reductions in hyperglycemia are associated with mild weight gain.

Drug Interactions

■ **Drugs Affecting Hepatic Microsomal Enzymes** ***Inhibitors or Inducers of CYP3A4*** Potential pharmacokinetic interaction with inhibitors or inducers of cytochrome P-450 (CYP) isoenzyme 3A4.

Concomitant use of pioglitazone (45 mg daily for 7 days) and ketoconazole (200 mg twice daily for 7 days), an inhibitor of CYP3A4, increased peak plasma concentration and area under the concentration-time curve (AUC) of pioglitazone by 14 and 34%, respectively.

Concomitant use of ranitidine (150 mg twice daily for 4 days), a relatively weak CYP3A4 inhibitor, and pioglitazone (45 mg daily for 7 days) reduced pioglitazone AUC and peak plasma concentration by 13 and 16%, respectively; pioglitazone had a negligible effect on ranitidine pharmacokinetics.

CYP3A4 Substrates Pioglitazone is a weak inducer of CYP3A4. Potential pharmacokinetic interaction (reduction in peak plasma concentration and AUC) with CYP3A4 substrates (e.g., atorvastatin, midazolam, ethinyl estradiol, nifedipine).

Concomitant use of pioglitazone (45 mg daily for 7 days) and atorvastatin (80 mg daily for 7 days) resulted in reductions of 14 and 23% in atorvastatin AUC and peak plasma concentration, respectively; pioglitazone AUC and peak plasma concentration were reduced by 24 and 31%, respectively.

Administration of pioglitazone (45 mg daily for 7 days) and midazolam (single dose of 7.5 mg on day 15) reduced midazolam AUC and peak plasma concentration each by 26%.

Administration of pioglitazone (45 mg daily for 4 days) with extended-release nifedipine (30 mg daily for 4 days) reduced nifedipine AUC and peak plasma concentration by 13 and 17%, respectively; pioglitazone AUC and peak plasma concentration were increased by 5 and 4%, respectively, with concomitant use of pioglitazone (45 mg daily for 7 days) and extended-release nifedipine (30 mg daily for 7 days).

Concomitant use of an estrogen-progestin contraceptive (ethinyl estradiol 0.035 mg with norethindrone 1 mg daily for 21 days) and pioglitazone (45 mg daily for 21 days) resulted in small decreases in peak plasma concentration (13%) and AUC (11%) of ethinyl estradiol. The clinical importance of these changes is unknown.

Inhibitors or Inducers of CYP2C8 Pioglitazone is a CYP2C8 substrate; potential pharmacokinetic interaction with inhibitors (e.g., gemfibrozil) or inducers (e.g., rifampin) of CYP2C8. Adjustments in pioglitazone dosage may be needed during initiation or discontinuance of an inhibitor or inducer of CYP2C8. (See Concomitant Therapy with Potent CYP2C8 Inhibitors or Inducers under Dosage and Administration: Dosage.)

Concomitant use of pioglitazone (single 30-mg dose) and gemfibrozil (600 mg twice daily for 2 days) resulted in a 3.4-fold increase in AUC of pioglitazone and a 6% increase in pioglitazone peak plasma concentration; half-life of pioglitazone also increased from 6.5 to 15.1 hours.

Concomitant use of pioglitazone (single 30-mg dose) and rifampin (600 mg daily for 5 days) resulted in a 54% decrease in AUC and a 5% decrease in peak plasma concentration of pioglitazone.

CYP2C9 or CYP1A2 Substrates Pharmacokinetic interaction is unlikely with CYP2C9 substrates (e.g., warfarin). Concomitant therapy with warfarin sodium (dosage adjusted to achieve therapeutic anticoagulation [Quick's prothrombin value of 35 ± 5%]) and pioglitazone (45 mg daily for 7 days) resulted in changes of 3% or less in AUC and peak plasma concentration of *R*- or *S*-warfarin.

Pharmacokinetic interaction is unlikely with theophylline, a CYP1A2 substrate. Concomitant use of pioglitazone (45 mg daily for 7 days) and theophylline (400 mg twice daily for 7 days) did not appreciably alter (i.e., 5% or less change) AUC and peak plasma concentration of pioglitazone or theophylline.

■ **Antidiabetic Agents** Potential pharmacodynamic interaction (risk of hypoglycemia) with insulin or oral hypoglycemic agents; reduction in the dose of the concomitant agent may be necessary.

Pharmacokinetic interaction with metformin or glipizide is unlikely. With concomitant use of pioglitazone (45 mg daily for 7 days) and glipizide (5 mg daily for 7 days), glipizide AUC and peak plasma concentration were reduced by 3 and 8%, respectively. Concomitant administration of pioglitazone (45 mg daily for 8 days) and metformin hydrochloride (single 1-g dose on day 8) resulted in reductions of 3 and 5% in metformin AUC and peak plasma concentration, respectively.

■ **Digoxin** Concomitant therapy with digoxin (0.2 mg for 2 doses as a loading dose, then 0.25 mg daily for 7 days) and pioglitazone (45 mg daily for 7 days) resulted in increases of 15 and 17% in digoxin AUC and peak plasma concentration, respectively.

■ **Fexofenadine** Concomitant administration of pioglitazone (45 mg daily for 7 days) and fexofenadine hydrochloride (60 mg twice daily for 7 days) resulted in an increase of 30 and 37% in fexofenadine AUC and peak plasma concentration, respectively; fexofenadine had no appreciable effect on pioglitazone pharmacokinetics.

Description

Pioglitazone is a thiazolidinedione (glitazone) antidiabetic agent that is structurally and pharmacologically related to troglitazone and rosiglitazone but unrelated to other antidiabetic agents, including sulfonylureas, biguanides, and α-glucosidase inhibitors.

Pioglitazone acts principally by increasing insulin sensitivity in target tissues, as well as decreasing hepatic gluconeogenesis. Pioglitazone is a peroxisome proliferator-activated receptor$_\gamma$ (PPAR$_\gamma$) agonist that increases transcription of insulin-responsive genes and increases insulin sensitivity. Pioglitazone, like other thiazolidinediones, ameliorates insulin resistance associated with type 2 diabetes mellitus without stimulating insulin release from pancreatic β cells, thus avoiding the risk of hypoglycemia. Because pioglitazone does not lower glucose concentrations below euglycemia, the drug is appropriately referred to as an antidiabetic agent rather than a hypoglycemic agent. Some evidence suggests that the glucoregulatory effects of thiazolidinediones are mediated in part via enhanced hepatic and peripheral glucose uptake and reduced systemic and tissue lipid availability.

Pioglitazone is extensively metabolized, principally via the cytochrome P-450 (CYP) 2C8 and CYP3A4 isoenzymes, with involvement of several other isoforms, including CYP1A1 (mainly an extrahepatic isoenzyme).

Advice to Patients

When pioglitazone is used in fixed combination with other drugs, importance of informing patients of important cautionary information about the concomitant agent(s).

Importance of reading medication guide provided by the manufacturer before starting pioglitazone and each time prescription is refilled.

Importance of informing patients of potential risks and advantages of therapy and of alternative therapies.

Discuss potential for alterations in dosage requirements during periods of stress (e.g., fever, trauma, infection, surgery); importance of contacting a clinician promptly.

Importance of informing patients that pioglitazone must not be used in patients with severe heart failure (NYHA class III or IV). Importance of identifying and reporting to clinicians potential symptoms of heart failure, such as unusually rapid increase in weight, edema (especially in ankles or legs), unusual fatigue, trouble breathing, or shortness of breath (especially when lying down).

Importance of immediate reporting of potential manifestations of hepatotoxicity (e.g., unexplained nausea or vomiting, abdominal pain, fatigue, loss of appetite, or dark urine, yellowing of skin or whites of eyes).

Increased risk of bladder cancer with pioglitazone therapy. Importance of patient not taking pioglitazone if receiving treatment for bladder cancer. Importance of patient reporting any sign of macroscopic hematuria or symptoms such as dysuria or urinary urgency that develop or increase during pioglitazone treatment.

Importance of taking exactly as prescribed. If a dose is missed on one day, take the next dose as prescribed unless otherwise instructed by your clinician; do not double the dose to make up for the missed dose. Importance of changing dosage only under medical supervision. Importance of immediately contacting a clinician if accidental overdosage occurs.

Importance of advising patient not to chew, cut, or crush the combination preparation containing pioglitazone and extended-release metformin hydrochloride (ActoPlus Met® XR); this dosage form must be swallowed whole. Patients should be aware that the biologically inert components of the extended-release combination tablet may occasionally be eliminated in the feces as a soft mass that may resemble the original tablet.

Risk of hypoglycemia in patients receiving concomitant insulin or other antidiabetic therapy. Provide instructions regarding management of hypoglycemia, including recognition of symptoms, predisposing conditions, and treatment.

Risk of pregnancy in premenopausal anovulatory women.

Importance of diet and exercise regimen adherence. Importance of regular monitoring (preferably self-monitoring) of blood glucose and of glycosylated hemoglobin (HbA_{1c}) concentrations.

Risk of fractures (e.g., hand, upper arm, foot) in women.

Importance of regular eye examinations. Importance of reporting changes in vision.

Importance of informing clinicians of existing or contemplated concomitant therapy, including prescription and OTC drugs, as well as any concomitant illnesses.

Importance of women informing their clinician if they are or plan to become pregnant or plan to breast-feed.

Importance of informing patients of other important precautionary information. (See Cautions.)

Overview (see Users Guide). For additional information until a more detailed monograph is developed and published, the manufacturer's labeling should be consulted. It is *essential* that the manufacturer's labeling be consulted for more detailed information on usual cautions, precautions, contraindications, potential drug interactions, laboratory test interferences, and acute toxicity.

Preparations

Excipients in commercially available drug preparations may have clinically important effects in some individuals; consult specific product labeling for details.

Pioglitazone Hydrochloride

Oral		
Tablets, film-coated	15 mg (of pioglitazone)	**Actos®**, Takeda
	30 mg (of pioglitazone)	**Actos®**, Takeda
	45 mg (of pioglitazone)	**Actos®**, Takeda

Pioglitazone Hydrochloride Combinations

Oral		
Tablets	15 mg (of pioglitazone) with Metformin Hydrochloride 500 mg	**Actoplus Met®**, Takeda
	15 mg (of pioglitazone) with Metformin Hydrochloride 850 mg	**Actoplus Met®**, Takeda
	30 mg (of pioglitazone) with Glimepiride 2 mg	**Duetact®**, Takeda
	30 mg (of pioglitazone) with Glimepiride 4 mg	**Duetact®**, Takeda
Oral		
Tablets, extended-release (metformin hydrochloride core)	15 mg (of pioglitazone) with Metformin Hydrochloride 1 g	**Actoplus Met® XR**, Takeda
	30 mg (of pioglitazone) with Metformin Hydrochloride 1 g	**Actoplus Met® XR**, Takeda

Rosiglitazone Maleate

■ Rosiglitazone is a thiazolidinedione (glitazone) antidiabetic agent that is structurally and pharmacologically related to pioglitazone and troglitazone.

REMS

FDA approved a REMS for rosiglitazone maleate to ensure that the benefits outweigh the risks. However, FDA later rescinded REMS requirements. See the FDA REMS page (https://www.accessdata.fda.gov/scripts/cder/rems/index.cfm).

Uses

■ **Diabetes Mellitus** Rosiglitazone is used as monotherapy or in combination with a sulfonylurea, metformin hydrochloride, or a sulfonylurea and metformin as an adjunct to diet and exercise to improve glycemic control in patients with type 2 diabetes mellitus.

Rosiglitazone in fixed combination with metformin hydrochloride is used as an adjunct to diet and exercise to improve glycemic control in patients with type 2 diabetes mellitus. Rosiglitazone also is used in fixed combination with glimepiride as an adjunct to diet and exercise for the management of type 2 diabetes mellitus.

Rosiglitazone may be added to therapy with the fixed combination of glyburide and metformin hydrochloride in patients whose hyperglycemia is not adequately controlled on therapy with the fixed combination. (See Concomitant Glyburide, Metformin, and Thiazolidinedione Therapy under Dosage and Administration: Dosage, in Glyburide 68:20.20.) A thiazolidinedione such as rosiglitazone also may be used with repaglinide in patients who have inadequate glycemic control with repaglinide monotherapy. (See Uses: Diabetes Mellitus, in Repaglinide 68:20.16.)

The American Diabetes Association (ADA) currently classifies diabetes mellitus as type 1 (immune mediated or idiopathic), type 2 (predominantly insulin resistance with relative insulin deficiency to predominantly an insulin secretory defect with insulin resistance), gestational diabetes mellitus, or that associated with certain conditions or syndromes (e.g., drug- or chemical-induced, hormonal, that associated with pancreatic disease, infections, specific genetic defects or syndromes). Type 1 diabetes mellitus was previously described as juvenile-onset (JOD) diabetes mellitus, since it usually occurs during youth. Type 2 diabetes mellitus previously was described as maturity-onset (MOD) or adult-onset (AODM) diabetes mellitus, since it usually occurs in patients older than 40 years of age. However, type 1 or type 2 diabetes mellitus can occur at any age, and the current classification is based on pathogenesis (e.g., autoimmune destruction of pancreatic β cells, insulin resistance) and clinical presentation rather than on age of onset. Many patients' diabetes mellitus does not easily fit into a single classification. Epidemiologic data indicate that the incidence of type 2 diabetes mellitus is increasing in children and adolescents such that 8–45% of children with newly diagnosed diabetes have nonimmune-mediated diabetes mellitus; most of these individuals have type 2 diabetes mellitus, although other types, including idiopathic or nonimmune-mediated type 1 diabetes mellitus, also have been reported.

Patients with type 2 diabetes mellitus have insulin resistance and usually have relative (rather than absolute) insulin deficiency. Most individuals with type 2 diabetes mellitus (about 80–90%) are overweight or obese; obesity itself also contributes to the insulin resistance and glucose intolerance observed in these patients. Patients with type 2 diabetes mellitus who are not obese may have an increased percentage of abdominal fat, which is an indicator of increased cardiometabolic risk. While children with immune-mediated type 1 diabetes generally are not overweight, the incidence of obesity in children with this form of diabetes is increasing with the increasing incidence of obesity in the US population. Distinguishing between type 1 and type 2 diabetes mellitus in children may be difficult since obesity may occur with either type of diabetes mellitus, and autoantigens and ketosis may be present in a substantial number of children with features of type 2 diabetes mellitus (e.g., obesity, acanthosis nigricans).

Current evidence from epidemiologic and clinical studies supports an association between chronic hyperglycemia and the pathogenesis of microvascular complications in patients with diabetes mellitus, and results of randomized, controlled studies in patients with type 1 diabetes mellitus indicate that intensive management of hyperglycemia with near-normalization of blood glucose and glycosylated hemoglobin (hemoglobin A_{1c} [HbA_{1c}]) concentrations provides substantial benefits in terms of reducing chronic microvascular (e.g., neuropathy, retinopathy, nephropathy) complications associated with the disease. HbA_{1c} reflects the nonenzymatic glycosylation of other proteins throughout the body as a result of recent (e.g., previous 6–8 weeks) hyperglycemia; this measure is used as an indicator of chronically elevated blood glucose concentrations and as a predictor of risk for the development of diabetic microvascular complications (e.g., neuropathy, retinopathy, nephropathy). Microvascular complications of diabetes are the principal causes of blindness and renal failure in developed countries and are more closely associated with hyperglycemia than are macrovascular complications. For additional details on the clinical classification, microvascular and macrovascular complications, and management of diabetes mellitus, see Uses: Diabetes Mellitus, in Metformin 68:20.04.

Rosiglitazone Monotherapy Efficacy of rosiglitazone as monotherapy for the management of type 2 diabetes mellitus was established in 6 controlled studies of 8–52 weeks' duration. Rosiglitazone improved glycemic control as measured by fasting glucose and HbA_{1c} concentrations. Some evidence suggests that rosiglitazone has a more durable glycemic effect than sulfonylureas or metformin. In a long-term (4–6 years' duration) randomized, controlled clinical trial (A Diabetes Outcome Progression Trial [ADOPT]) evaluating the duration of glycemic control after initiation of monotherapy with rosiglitazone, metformin, or glyburide, the cumulative incidence of treatment failure (i.e., defined as confirmed fasting plasma glucose concentrations exceeding 180 mg/dL on consecutive testing after at least 6 weeks of treatment at the maximum dictated or tolerated dosage of the study drug) at 5 years was 15, 21, and 34%, respectively; this represents a risk reduction with rosiglitazone monotherapy of 32% or 63% compared with metformin or glyburide monotherapy, respectively. However, the use of fasting glucose concentrations as a measure of treatment failure rather than HbA_{1c} concentration, which correlates more closely with diabetic complications, has been criticized; also, differences among the treatment groups in mean HbA_{1c} concentration at 4 years were less pronounced, particularly between rosiglitazone and metformin.

Combination Therapy Data from a number of comparative trials evaluating combination therapy with rosiglitazone and metformin or a sulfonylurea agent indicate that such combination therapy may result in an additive effect on glycemic control. Efficacy of the combination of rosiglitazone and metformin in patients whose type 2 diabetes mellitus was inadequately controlled with metformin alone was established in several controlled studies of 26 weeks' duration in which combined therapy improved glycemic control without affecting serum insulin concentrations. In patients inadequately controlled with sulfonylurea (e.g., glyburide, glipizide, glimepiride) monotherapy, the combination of rosiglitazone and a sulfonylurea reduced fasting glucose and HbA_{1c} concentrations compared with monotherapy with a sulfonylurea alone.

Rosiglitazone in fixed combination with metformin is used in patients with type 2 diabetes mellitus who require treatment with both rosiglitazone and metformin. Although the fixed-combination preparation has not been specifically studied in patients previously receiving metformin monotherapy, clinical trials have evaluated rosiglitazone 4 or 8 mg once daily as add-on therapy in patients who had inadequate glycemic control with metformin (2.5 g once daily). In these studies, substantial improvements in fasting plasma glucose and HbA_{1c} concentrations were observed in patients receiving concurrent rosiglitazone and metformin therapy compared with those receiving metformin alone. In a dose-ranging trial evaluating rosiglitazone 4 or 8 mg as add-on therapy to the maximum daily dosage of metformin hydrochloride, 28.1% of patients receiving the higher dosage of rosiglitazone concurrently with metformin achieved HbA_{1c} values not exceeding 7%.

In patients inadequately controlled with sulfonylurea (e.g., glyburide, glipizide, glimepiride) monotherapy, the combination of rosiglitazone and a sulfonylurea reduced fasting glucose and HbA_{1c} concentrations compared with monotherapy with a sulfonylurea alone. In a 2-year study in geriatric patients (59–89 years of age) who were inadequately controlled on glipizide at half the maximum recommended dosage (10 mg twice daily), the addition of rosiglitazone (4–8 mg daily) was more effective in preventing loss of glycemic control (defined as fasting plasma glucose concentrations of at least 180 mg/dL, the primary clinical end point) than continued upward titration of glipizide (maximum of 20 mg twice daily).

Rosiglitazone in fixed combination with glimepiride is used in patients with type 2 diabetes mellitus who require treatment with both rosiglitazone and glimepiride. No clinical trials have been conducted specifically evaluating the *fixed combination* of glimepiride and rosiglitazone in patients who are inadequately controlled with sulfonylurea or rosiglitazone monotherapy. Safety and efficacy of the fixed combination of glimepiride and rosiglitazone in patients with type 2 diabetes mellitus who are inadequately controlled on a sulfonylurea alone are extrapolated from clinical trials evaluating rosiglitazone as add-on therapy to a sulfonylurea (e.g., glyburide, glipizide).

Because rosiglitazone requires endogenous insulin for activity, it should not be used in patients with type 1 diabetes mellitus or diabetic ketoacidosis.

Dosage and Administration

■ **General** Following initiation of rosiglitazone therapy or dosage increases, patients should be monitored for adverse effects related to fluid retention. (See Congestive Heart Failure under Warnings/Precautions: Warnings, in Cautions.) Fasting blood glucose (FPG) and glycosylated hemoglobin (hemoglobin A_{1c} [HbA_{1c}]) concentrations should be monitored periodically to determine the patient's response to therapy.

Following initiation of rosiglitazone therapy or dosage increases, sufficient time should be allowed to assess therapeutic response to rosiglitazone (8–12 weeks using FPG concentrations). Similarly, in patients receiving fixed-combination preparations containing rosiglitazone, sufficient time (8–12 weeks) should be allowed to assess therapeutic response after an increase in dosage of the rosiglitazone component.

■ **Administration** Rosiglitazone maleate is administered orally once daily or in divided doses twice daily, without regard to meals. If the patient misses a dose of rosiglitazone, the missed dose should be taken as soon as it is remembered. If the missed dose is remembered at the time of the next dose, the regularly scheduled dose should be taken; a double dose should *not* be taken to make up for the missed dose.

Rosiglitazone in fixed combination with glimepiride should be administered once daily with the first meal of the day. If the patient misses a dose of the fixed-combination tablet, the dose should be taken as soon as it is remembered. If the missed tablet is remembered at the time of the next dose, the regularly scheduled dose should be taken; a double dose should not be taken to make up for the missed dose.

Rosiglitazone in fixed combination with metformin hydrochloride generally is administered in divided doses (i.e., twice daily) with meals.

■ **Dosage** Dosage of rosiglitazone maleate is expressed in terms of the base. Bioequivalence has been demonstrated between the fixed combination of rosiglitazone and metformin hydrochloride and each agent given concurrently as separate tablets.

Rosiglitazone Monotherapy The recommended initial dosage of rosiglitazone is 4 mg once daily or 2 mg twice daily. If the response is inadequate after 8–12 weeks, dosage may be increased to 8 mg daily as a single dose or 2 divided doses daily. The maximum recommended dosage is 8 mg daily; studies suggest no additional benefit from 12-mg daily dosages.

Combination Therapy with Other Oral Antidiabetic Agents When the commercially available fixed-combination preparation containing rosiglitazone and glimepiride (Avandaryl®) is used in patients with type 2 diabetes mellitus, the recommended initial dosage is 4 mg of rosiglitazone and 1 mg of glimepiride once daily. An initial dosage of 4 mg of rosiglitazone and 2 mg of glimepiride once daily may be considered in those already receiving rosiglitazone or a sulfonylurea. In patients previously receiving rosiglitazone monotherapy, sufficient time (approximately 1–2 weeks) should be allowed to assess therapeutic response; dosage titration of the glimepiride component is recommended if adequate glycemic control is not achieved after this time. If additional glycemic control is needed, the manufacturer recommends that the dosage of the glimepiride component be increased in increments not exceeding 2 mg. Therapeutic response to an increase in the glimepiride component should be assessed after 1–2 weeks to determine the need for further dosage adjustment.

In patients previously receiving sulfonylurea monotherapy who are switched to the fixed combination of glimepiride and rosiglitazone, 2 weeks may be required to observe a reduction in blood glucose concentrations and 2–3 months to observe full therapeutic response to the rosiglitazone component. If additional glycemic control is needed after 8–12 weeks, an increase in dosage of the rosiglitazone component is recommended. Further dosage titration of the fixed combination is recommended if therapeutic response is not achieved 2–3 months after an increase in dosage of the rosiglitazone component. Because an exaggerated hypoglycemic response may occur in some patients during transition from a long-acting sulfonylurea antidiabetic agent (e.g., chlorpropamide) to rosiglitazone in fixed combination with glimepiride, close monitoring for the occurrence of hypoglycemia may be necessary for 1–2 weeks after switching to the fixed combination. If hypoglycemia occurs, dosage of the glimepiride component of the fixed combination should be reduced. The maximum recommended total daily dose is 4 mg of glimepiride and 8 mg of rosiglitazone.

When the commercially available preparation containing rosiglitazone in fixed combination with metformin hydrochloride (Avandamet®) is used in patients with type 2 diabetes mellitus, selection of the fixed combination dosage should be based on the patient's current dosages of the individual drugs. (See Table 1.)

In patients currently receiving metformin hydrochloride monotherapy, the usual initial dosage of rosiglitazone (in fixed combination with metformin hydrochloride) is 4 mg daily plus the patient's existing daily dosage of metformin hydrochloride, given in 2 divided doses. In patients currently receiving rosiglitazone monotherapy, the usual initial dosage of metformin hydrochloride (in fixed combination with rosiglitazone) is 1 g daily plus the patient's existing daily dosage of rosiglitazone, given in 2 divided doses.

Table 1. Initial Dosage of the Fixed Combination of Rosiglitazone and Metformin Hydrochloride (Avandamet®)

Prior Therapy	Usual Initial Dosage of Avandamet®	
Total Daily Dosage	Tablet strength	Number of tablets
Metformin Hydrochloride		
1 g	2 mg/500 mg	1 tablet twice daily
2 g	2 mg/1 g	1 tablet twice daily
Rosiglitazone		
4 mg	2 mg/500 mg	1 tablet twice daily
8 mg	4 mg/500 mg	1 tablet twice daily

Therapy should be individualized in those patients already receiving metformin hydrochloride in doses not available in the fixed combination (i.e., doses other than 1 or 2 g). The manufacturer states that dosage recommendations cannot be made for rosiglitazone in fixed combination with metformin hydrochloride in patients currently receiving metformin hydrochloride in dosages lower than 1 g daily.

For patients switching from combined therapy with separate preparations of rosiglitazone and metformin hydrochloride, the initial dosage of the fixed-combination preparation of rosiglitazone and metformin hydrochloride should be the same as the daily dosage of rosiglitazone and metformin hydrochloride currently being taken.

If additional glycemic control is needed, the dosage of the fixed combination of rosiglitazone and metformin hydrochloride may be titrated upward in increments of 4 mg of rosiglitazone and/or 500 mg of metformin hydrochloride until adequate glycemic control is achieved or a maximum daily dosage of 8 mg of rosiglitazone and 2 g of metformin hydrochloride is reached. If the metformin component is increased, therapeutic response should be assessed after 1–2 weeks; dosage of the fixed combination should be further titrated if adequate glycemic control is not achieved. If the rosiglitazone component is increased, therapeutic response should be assessed after 8–12 weeks; dosage of the fixed combination should be further titrated if adequate glycemic control is not achieved.

A thiazolidinedione such as rosiglitazone may be added to the antidiabetic regimen in patients who have inadequate glycemic control with repaglinide monotherapy. Conversely, if glycemic control with thiazolidinedione monotherapy is inadequate, repaglinide may be added to the antidiabetic regimen. (See Diabetes Mellitus: Concomitant Therapy with Repaglinide and Metformin or a Thiazolidinedione under Dosage and Administration: Dosage, in Repaglinide 68:20.16.) To minimize the risk of hypoglycemia, the dosage of each agent should be carefully adjusted to determine the minimal dosage required to achieve glycemic control.

For patients who have inadequate glycemic control on the fixed combination of glyburide and metformin hydrochloride, a thiazolidinedione such as rosiglitazone may be added at its recommended initial dosage and the dosage of the fixed combination may be continued unchanged. In patients requiring further glycemic control, the dosage of rosiglitazone may be titrated upward according to the manufacturer's recommendations. Triple therapy with glyburide, metformin hydrochloride, and a thiazolidinedione may increase the potential for hypoglycemia at any time of day. If hypoglycemia develops with such triple therapy, consideration should be given to reducing the dosage of the glyburide component; adjustment of the dosage of the other components of the antidiabetic regimen also should be considered as clinically indicated.

■ Special Populations Rosiglitazone maleate should be initiated (or continued) with caution in patients with mild hepatic enzyme elevations (ALT not exceeding 2.5 times the upper limit of normal) but no evidence of active liver disease. Therapy with rosiglitazone should not be initiated in patients with baseline ALT concentrations exceeding 3 times the upper limit of normal. (See Hepatic Effects under Warnings/Precautions: General Precautions, in Cautions.) When the fixed combination of rosiglitazone and glimepiride is used in patients with mild hepatic impairment, initial dosage, dosage increments, and maintenance dosage should be conservative to avoid hypoglycemic reactions; these individuals may be particularly sensitive to the hypoglycemic effects of glimepiride. If hypoglycemia occurs, dosage of the glimepiride component should be reduced.

Adjustment of rosiglitazone dosage is *not* necessary for patients with renal impairment *nor* for geriatric patients. However, therapy with the fixed combination of rosiglitazone and metformin hydrochloride should be used with caution in geriatric patients, since aging is associated with reduced renal function. When the fixed combination of rosiglitazone and metformin hydrochloride is used in geriatric patients, the initial and maintenance dosage should be conservative. Renal function should be assessed with initial dosage selection and with each dosage adjustment, particularly in geriatric patients, to minimize the risk of lactic acidosis. To minimize the risk of hypoglycemia, maintenance dosage of the fixed combination of rosiglitazone and metformin hydrochloride in geriatric, debilitated, or malnourished patients should *not* be titrated to the maximum dosage recommended for other patients.

When the fixed combination of rosiglitazone and glimepiride is used in geriatric patients, debilitated or malnourished patients, and patients with renal, hepatic, or adrenal impairment, initial dosage, dosage increments, and maintenance dosage should be conservative to avoid hypoglycemic reactions. If hypoglycemia occurs, dosage of the glimepiride component of the fixed combination should be reduced; geriatric patients, debilitated or malnourished patients, and patients with renal, hepatic, or adrenal impairment may be particularly sensitive to the hypoglycemic effects of glimepiride.

Cautions

■ Contraindications Initiation of therapy with rosiglitazone is contraindicated in patients with New York Heart Association (NYHA) class III or IV heart failure. (See Congestive Heart Failure under Warnings/Precautions: Warnings, in Cautions.) Rosiglitazone is contraindicated in patients with a history of hypersensitivity to the drug or to any ingredient in the formulation.

When rosiglitazone is used in fixed combination with other drugs (e.g., metformin, glimepiride), the cautions, precautions, and contraindications associated with those drugs must be considered in addition to those associated with rosiglitazone.

■ Warnings/Precautions ***Warnings*** Congestive Heart Failure. Thiazolidinediones, including rosiglitazone, alone or in combination with other antidiabetic agents, can cause fluid retention and may lead to or exacerbate congestive heart failure (CHF). Use of thiazolidinediones is associated with an approximately twofold increased risk of CHF. (See Edema under Warnings/Precautions: General Precautions, in Cautions.) Patients should be observed for signs and symptoms of CHF (e.g., dyspnea, rapid weight gain, edema, unexplained cough or fatigue), especially during initiation of therapy and dosage titration. If signs and symptoms of CHF develop, the disorder should be managed according to current standards of care. In addition, a decrease in the dosage of rosiglitazone or discontinuance of the drug should be considered.

Initiation of therapy with rosiglitazone is contraindicated in patients with NYHA class III or IV heart failure. Patients with NYHA class III or IV cardiac status with or without CHF or with acute coronary syndromes were not studied in clinical trials of rosiglitazone; use of rosiglitazone is *not* recommended in these patients. If an acute coronary event occurs, the manufacturer states that discontinuance of rosiglitazone should be considered during the acute phase of a coronary event, as such patients are at risk for development of CHF. In addition, use of rosiglitazone is *not* recommended in patients with symptomatic heart failure. Caution should be exercised in patients with edema and in those who are at risk for CHF. Thiazolidinedione therapy should not be initiated in hospitalized patients with diabetes mellitus because of the delayed onset of action and because possible drug-related increases in vascular volume and CHF may complicate care of patients with hemodynamic changes induced by coexisting conditions or in-hospital interventions.

Findings from a meta-analysis of randomized controlled studies that assessed the risk of development of CHF and death from cardiovascular causes in patients receiving thiazolidinediones indicate that the risk of CHF is higher in patients receiving thiazolidinediones (relative risk of 1.72; 95% confidence interval: 1.21–2.42) than in controls (individuals receiving other antidiabetic agents or placebo). The relative risk for CHF was increased across a wide background of cardiovascular risk (i.e., patients with prediabetes, with type 2 diabetes mellitus without cardiovascular disease, with type 2 diabetes mellitus and cardiovascular disease other than CHF, or with type 2 diabetes mellitus and CHF [NYHA class I or II] and ejection fraction less than 40%). In contrast to the increased risk for CHF observed in thiazolidinedione-treated patients, the risk of cardiovascular death was not increased in patients receiving these agents.

In a placebo-controlled echocardiographic study in patients with type 2 diabetes mellitus and NYHA class I or II heart failure receiving rosiglitazone in addition to other antidiabetic and CHF therapy, an increased incidence of adverse cardiovascular events (e.g., edema, need for additional CHF therapy) was reported in patients receiving rosiglitazone compared with patients receiving placebo. Changes in the left ventricular ejection fraction from baseline did not differ among rosiglitazone- or placebo-treated patients. In a long-term, cardiovascular outcomes trial in patients with type 2 diabetes mellitus, heart failure was reported in 2.7% of patients receiving rosiglitazone compared with 1.3% of those receiving active control (metformin plus a sulfonylurea).

An increased incidence of CHF has been observed in a number of clinical trials (duration of 16–26 weeks) in patients receiving rosiglitazone as add-on therapy to insulin compared with that in patients receiving insulin monotherapy. These trials included patients with long-standing diabetes mellitus (median duration: 12 years) and a high prevalence of preexisting medical conditions, including peripheral neuropathy, retinopathy, ischemic heart disease, vascular disease, and CHF. The incidence of emergent symptomatic heart failure was at least twofold higher with concurrent rosiglitazone and insulin therapy compared with that observed with insulin therapy alone. The manufacturer states that concurrent administration of rosiglitazone and insulin therapy is *not* recommended.

Some observational studies have indicated a substantially increased risk of heart failure requiring hospitalization in geriatric patients 65 years of age or older receiving rosiglitazone compared with another thiazolidinedione antidiabetic agent (pioglitazone).

General Precautions Other Cardiovascular Effects. The cardiovascular safety of rosiglitazone has been an area of ongoing concern and study. Findings from several meta-analyses of principally short-term trials and observational studies suggested that rosiglitazone may be associated with an increased risk of myocardial infarction (MI) and other adverse cardiovascular events. In one such meta-analysis of 52 randomized, double-blind trials (mean duration: 6 months), a substantially increased risk of MI was observed with rosiglitazone versus placebo; in addition, major adverse cardiovascular events (MACE) occurred more frequently in patients receiving rosiglitazone than in those receiving comparator agents, although the difference was not statistically significant. As a result of these findings, the US Food and Drug Administration (FDA) restricted use of rosiglitazone in 2010 to patients who were unable to achieve glycemic control with other antidiabetic agents. However, evidence regarding the cardiovascular risk of rosiglitazone has been conflicting, and the findings observed in previous meta-analyses have not been confirmed in long-term (greater than 3 years' duration), prospective randomized studies. These studies, which include a dedicated cardiovascular outcomes trial in patients with type 2 diabetes mellitus (the Rosiglitazone Evaluated for Cardiac Outcomes and Regulation of Glycemia in Diabetes [RECORD] study), generally have found no evidence of an increased risk of mortality or MACE with rosiglitazone compared with metformin and/or a sulfonylurea. In the RECORD study, rosiglitazone was noninferior to the combination of metformin and a sulfonylurea with respect to the primary composite end point of cardiovascular hospitalization or cardiovascular death. During the course of FDA's original review of the RECORD study, important questions arose about potential bias in the identification of cardiovascular events, prompting FDA to commission outside experts to perform an independent readjudication of the data. Results of this comprehensive reanalysis confirmed the original findings that failed to show an increased risk of MI with rosiglitazone versus metformin and a sulfonylurea. While some component end points appeared to favor rosiglitazone (i.e., cardiovascular deaths, nonfatal strokes, all-cause mortality) or metformin/sulfonylurea (i.e., nonfatal MI), these findings were not statistically significant. Results of 2 other long-term, prospective randomized studies also showed no statistically significant differences in MACE or its individual components between rosiglitazone and placebo (the Diabetes Reduction Assessment with Ramipril and Rosiglitazone Medication [DREAM] trial in patients with impaired glucose tolerance) or between rosiglitazone and metformin or a sulfonylurea (the Diabetes Outcome Progression Trial [ADOPT] in patients with type 2 diabetes mellitus who were initiating oral antidiabetic monotherapy).

Although some uncertainty remains regarding the cardiovascular risk of rosiglitazone, FDA states that concerns have been substantially reduced in light of the readjudicated findings of the RECORD study. FDA has therefore removed previous prescribing and dispensing restrictions for the drug. Despite some limitations, the RECORD trial is considered to represent a higher level of evidence regarding cardiovascular risk than meta-analyses and observational studies, and therefore provides some reassurance that rosiglitazone does not increase the risk of MI or other adverse cardiovascular effects compared with other antidiabetic agents.

Edema. Fluid retention can occur and may lead to or exacerbate heart failure in patients receiving a thiazolidinedione, including rosiglitazone, alone or in combination with other antidiabetic agents, including insulin. Patients with ongoing edema are more likely to have adverse events associated with edema if therapy with rosiglitazone in combination with insulin is initiated. Diuretic therapy may be necessary for management of fluid retention. Weight gain possibly associated with fluid retention and fat accumulation has been observed during therapy with rosiglitazone alone or in combination with other antidiabetic agents (e.g., metformin, sulfonylureas, insulin). Caution should be exercised in patients with edema and those at risk for CHF. (See Congestive Heart Failure under Warnings/Precautions: Warnings, in Cautions.)

All patients receiving thiazolidinedione therapy (e.g., rosiglitazone, pioglitazone) should be advised to monitor for weight gain and edema. Any patient developing edema within the first few months of therapy should be evaluated for possible CHF. Other potential causes of edema should be excluded.

Musculoskeletal Effects. Thiazolidinedione use is associated with bone loss and fractures in women and possibly in men with type 2 diabetes mellitus. In long-term comparative clinical trials in patients with type 2 diabetes mellitus, the incidence of bone fracture was increased in patients (particularly women) receiving rosiglitazone versus comparator agents (glyburide and/or metformin). Such effects were noted after the first year of treatment and persisted throughout the study. The majority of fractures observed in patients taking thiazolidinediones were in a distal upper limb (i.e., forearm, hand, wrist) or distal lower limb (i.e., foot, ankle, fibula, tibia). In an observational study in the United Kingdom in men and women (mean age: 60.7 years) with diabetes mellitus, use of pioglitazone or rosiglitazone for approximately 12–18 months (as estimated from prescription records) was associated with a twofold to threefold increase in fractures, particularly of the hip and wrist. The overall risk of fracture was similar among men and women and was independent of body mass index, comorbid conditions, diabetic complications, duration of diabetes mellitus, and use of other oral antidiabetic drugs.

Risk of fractures should be considered when initiating or continuing thiazolidinedione therapy in female patients with type 2 diabetes mellitus. Bone health should be assessed and maintained according to current standards of care. Although increased risk of fracture may also apply to men, the risk appears to be higher among women than men.

Ovulatory Effects. Risk for pregnancy unless contraceptive measures initiated; anovulatory premenopausal women with insulin resistance may resume ovulation during therapy. The frequency of resumption of ovulation with rosiglitazone therapy has not been evaluated in clinical studies, and, therefore, is unknown. If menstrual dysfunction occurs, weigh risks versus benefits of continued rosiglitazone.

Hepatic Effects. No evidence of hepatotoxicity has been noted with rosiglitazone in clinical studies to date, including a long-term (4–6 years) study (ADOPT) in patients with recently diagnosed type 2 diabetes mellitus. In the ADOPT study, the incidence of ALT elevation exceeding 3 times the upper limit of normal was similar in patients receiving rosiglitazone or active comparators (i.e., glyburide or metformin). However, hepatitis, elevations in hepatic enzymes to at least 3 times the upper limit of normal, and liver failure with or without fatalities have been reported during postmarketing experience with rosiglitazone.

Liver function tests are recommended in patients receiving rosiglitazone (prior to therapy, then periodically according to clinician judgment). Therapy with rosiglitazone should not be initiated if baseline ALT concentrations exceed 2.5 times the upper limit of normal. Patients with mildly elevated liver enzymes (e.g., ALT not exceeding 2.5 times the upper limit of normal) prior to or during therapy should be evaluated to determine the cause of the elevation; rosiglitazone should be initiated or continued in such patients with caution and close clinical monitoring.

If ALT increases to more than 3 times the upper limit of normal at any time during therapy, liver function tests should be rechecked as soon as possible. Development of manifestations suggestive of hepatic dysfunction (e.g., unexplained nausea, vomiting, abdominal pain, fatigue, anorexia, dark urine) also should prompt rechecking of liver function. The decision whether to continue therapy should be guided by clinical judgment pending laboratory evaluation. If ALT increases to 3 times the upper limit of normal during therapy and remains elevated, or if jaundice develops, rosiglitazone should be discontinued.

Hematologic Effects. Dose-related decreases in hemoglobin (not exceeding 1 g/dL) and hematocrit (not exceeding 3.3%) usually become evident within the first 3 months after initiation of therapy with rosiglitazone alone and in combination with other antidiabetic agents. Slight decreases in leukocyte counts have been observed in patients receiving rosiglitazone. These effects may be related to plasma volume expansion.

Ocular Effects. During postmarketing experience, rare cases of new-onset or worsening (diabetic) macular edema with decreased visual acuity have been reported with rosiglitazone or another thiazolidinedione; such patients frequently reported concurrent peripheral edema. Some patients with macular edema presented with symptoms of blurred vision or decreased visual acuity, but other cases were detected by routine ophthalmologic examination. Symptoms improved in some patients following discontinuance of rosiglitazone or, rarely, after dosage reduction. Patients with diabetes mellitus should have regular eye examinations by an ophthalmologist. Patients receiving rosiglitazone who report any visual symptoms should be referred promptly to an ophthalmologist, regardless of the presence of other concurrent therapy or physical findings.

Specific Populations

Pregnancy. Category C. The background risk of birth defects, pregnancy loss, or other adverse outcomes is increased in pregnancies complicated by hyperglycemia and may be decreased with good glycemic control. Most clinicians recommend use of insulin monotherapy for maintenance of optimum blood glucose concentrations during pregnancy. Women with diabetes mellitus or a history of gestational diabetes who are pregnant or planning pregnancy require excellent blood glucose control before conception and throughout pregnancy. Careful monitoring of blood glucose concentration is essential in such patients. Rosiglitazone should be used during pregnancy only when the potential benefits justify the possible risk to the fetus.

Lactation. Rosiglitazone-related material is distributed into milk in rats; it is not known whether the drug is distributed into human milk. Because many drugs are distributed into human milk, a decision should be made whether to discontinue nursing or the drug, taking into account the importance of the drug to the woman.

Pediatric Use. Rosiglitazone has been studied in children and adolescents 10–17 years of age; data are insufficient to recommend use in pediatric patients younger than 18 years of age. Safety and efficacy of rosiglitazone in fixed combination with glimepiride have not been established in pediatric patients younger than 18 years of age. The manufacturer states that safety and efficacy of rosiglitazone alone or in fixed combination with metformin have not been established in pediatric patients. However, the American Diabetes Association (ADA) states that most pediatric diabetologists use oral antidiabetic agents in children with type 2 diabetes mellitus because of greater patient compliance with therapy and convenience for the patient's family and a lack of evidence demonstrating better efficacy of insulin as initial therapy for type 2 diabetes mellitus.

Geriatric Use. Pharmacokinetic and adverse effect profiles of rosiglitazone similar to those in younger adults. Dosage adjustment based solely on age is not necessary in geriatric patients receiving rosiglitazone alone. Caution with the use of rosiglitazone in fixed combination with metformin hydrochloride in geriatric patients since aging is associated with reduced renal function, which increases the risk of serious adverse reactions with metformin. (See Cautions: Geriatric Precautions, in Metformin 68:20.04.)

Data from several observational studies suggest that the risk of all-cause mortality may be increased in geriatric diabetic patients 65 years of age or older receiving rosiglitazone versus another thiazolidinedione antidiabetic agent (pioglitazone).

Hepatic Impairment. Rosiglitazone should be used with caution in patients with mild hepatic impairment; use is not recommended in moderate to severe hepatic impairment (ALT exceeding 2.5 times upper limit of normal, or active liver disease). (See Hepatic Effects under Warnings/Precautions: General Precautions, in Cautions.)

■ Common Adverse Effects

Adverse effects of rosiglitazone occurring in at least 2% of patients include upper respiratory tract infection, injury, headache, edema, back pain, hyperglycemia, fatigue, sinusitis, and diarrhea. Anemia and edema generally were mild to moderate and usually did not require discontinuance. Rosiglitazone-induced reductions in hyperglycemia are associated with mild weight gain. Increased total, low-density lipoprotein (LDL)-, and high-density lipoprotein (HDL)-cholesterol; LDL/HDL-cholesterol ratio generally decreases after initial increase.

Adverse effects generally were similar with rosiglitazone monotherapy versus combined therapy with metformin; however, anemia was more common during combined therapy (7.1 versus 1.9%) with metformin compared with that in patients receiving rosiglitazone monotherapy or combination therapy with a sulfonylurea. Hypoglycemia occurs infrequently with rosiglitazone therapy. However, hypoglycemia was more common during combined therapy with rosiglitazone and metformin, a sulfonylurea, or insulin. In addition, self-monitored blood glucose measurements of 50 mg/dL or less were reported by 22% of patients receiving the fixed combination of glyburide and metformin hydrochloride plus rosiglitazone compared with 3.3% of patients receiving the fixed combination of glyburide and metformin hydrochloride. Hypoglycemia, confirmed by capillary blood glucose concentrations of 50 mg/dL or less, was reported by 12 or 14% of patients receiving combination therapy with insulin and rosiglitazone at dosages of 4 or 8 mg, respectively, compared with 6% of patients receiving insulin alone.

Drug Interactions

■ **Drugs Affecting Hepatic Microsomal Enzymes** Inhibitors (e.g., gemfibrozil) or inducers (e.g., rifampin) of cytochrome P-450 (CYP) isoenzyme 2C8; potential pharmacokinetic interaction. With concurrent gemfibrozil, potential pharmacokinetic interaction (increased area under the concentration-time curve [AUC] for rosiglitazone). With concurrent rifampin, potential pharmacokinetic interaction (decreased AUC for rosiglitazone). Adjustments in rosiglitazone dosage may be needed during initiation or discontinuance of an inhibitor or inducer of CYP2C8.

Because rosiglitazone does *not* affect CYP3A4, pharmacokinetic interactions unlikely with drugs metabolized mainly via this isoenzyme (e.g., nifedipine, estrogen-progestin combination contraceptives).

■ **Antidiabetic Agents** Additive glycemic control with metformin; no pharmacokinetic interaction.

Additive glycemic control with glimepiride; no pharmacokinetic interaction.

Acarbose reduced extent of absorption and prolonged half-life, but not considered clinically important; effect of combined rosiglitazone and acarbose on glycemic control remains to be established.

Although the manufacturer states that glyburide-induced reductions in blood glucose are unaltered by short-term (7 days) rosiglitazone in patients stabilized on the sulfonylurea, rosiglitazone can improve glycemic control during long-term combined therapy. With concurrent glyburide in Caucasian individuals, potential pharmacokinetic interaction (decreased glyburide concentrations). With concurrent glyburide in Japanese individuals, potential pharmacokinetic interaction (slightly increased glyburide concentrations).

Increased risk of congestive heart failure (CHF) with concomitant insulin therapy. Concomitant use of rosiglitazone and insulin therapy is not recommended. (See Congestive Heart Failure under Warnings/Precautions: Warnings, in Cautions.)

■ **Alcohol** Rosiglitazone-exacerbated hypoglycemia unlikely.

■ **Digoxin** Pharmacokinetic interaction unlikely.

■ **Ranitidine** Pharmacokinetic interaction unlikely.

■ **Warfarin** Pharmacokinetic interaction unlikely.

■ **Other Drugs** Pharmacodynamic interaction (hyperglycemia and potential loss of glycemic control) with thiazide and other diuretics, corticosteroids, phenothiazines, thyroid agents, estrogens, oral contraceptives, phenytoin, nicotinic acid, sympathomimetics, calcium channel blocking agents, and isoniazid.

Description

Rosiglitazone is a thiazolidinedione (glitazone) antidiabetic agent that is structurally and pharmacologically related to pioglitazone and troglitazone but unrelated to other antidiabetic agents, including sulfonylureas, biguanides, and α-glucosidase inhibitors.

Rosiglitazone acts principally by increasing insulin sensitivity in target tissues, as well as decreasing hepatic gluconeogenesis. Rosiglitazone is a peroxisome proliferator-activated receptor$_\gamma$ (PPAR$_\gamma$) agonist that increases transcription of insulin-responsive genes and increases insulin sensitivity. Rosiglitazone, like other thiazolidinediones, ameliorates insulin resistance associated with type 2 diabetes mellitus without stimulating insulin release from pancreatic β cells, thus avoiding the risk of hypoglycemia. Because rosiglitazone does not lower glucose concentrations below euglycemia, the drug is appropriately referred to as an antidiabetic agent rather than a hypoglycemic agent. Some evidence suggests that the glucoregulatory effects of thiazolidinediones are mediated in part via reduced systemic and tissue lipid availability. Circulating concentrations of insulin and C-peptide are reduced during rosiglitazone therapy. Rosiglitazone is extensively metabolized, principally via the cytochrome P-450 (CYP) 2C8 isoenzyme; unlike troglitazone, rosiglitazone does not induce CYP3A4-mediated metabolism. Because of the delayed onset of action of rosiglitazone (2 weeks) and other thiazolidinediones and potential adverse effects, therapy with the drugs should not be initiated in hospitalized patients with diabetes mellitus. (See Congestive Heart Failure under Warnings/Precautions: Warnings, in Cautions.)

Advice to Patients

Importance of patient reading medication guide before starting rosiglitazone and each time the prescription is refilled.

Importance of informing patients of the current state of knowledge regarding the cardiovascular risks of rosiglitazone, and that although there is some evidence suggesting an increased risk of myocardial infarction compared with placebo, data from long-term clinical trials, including a cardiovascular outcomes trial, generally have not confirmed these findings. (See General Precautions: Other Cardiovascular Effects, under Warnings/Precautions in Cautions.)

Importance of informing patients that rosiglitazone is not recommended for patients with symptomatic heart failure. Importance of identifying and reporting to clinicians potential symptoms of congestive heart failure (CHF), such as unusually rapid increase in weight, edema, unusual fatigue, or shortness of breath.

Importance of patients not taking rosiglitazone if they are allergic to the drug or any ingredients in the tablet. Signs and symptoms of a severe allergic reaction to rosiglitazone include swelling of the face, lips, tongue, or throat; problems breathing or swallowing; rash, itching, or hives; blisters on the skin or in the mouth, nose, or eyes; skin peeling; faintness or dizziness; rapid heartbeat.

Importance of taking exactly as prescribed. Importance of taking a missed dose as soon as possible, unless it is almost time for next dose. Do not double dose to make up for the missed dose. Importance of immediately contacting a clinician or a poison control center if accidental overdosage occurs.

Importance of continuing rosiglitazone therapy even if response is not evident within 2 weeks; full therapeutic response may not be evident for 2–3 months after initiation of therapy.

Risk of pregnancy in premenopausal anovulatory women with insulin resistance. Advise patients regarding use of effective contraception during therapy.

Importance of diet and exercise regimen adherence. Importance of regular monitoring (preferably self-monitoring) of blood glucose and glycosylated hemoglobin (HbA_{1c}) concentrations.

Importance of informing patients that rosiglitazone is not recommended in patients taking insulin due to potentially increased risk of CHF.

Risk of hypoglycemia in patients receiving concomitant antidiabetic agent therapy. Provide instructions regarding management of hypoglycemia, including recognition of symptoms, predisposing conditions, and treatment.

Importance of liver function test monitoring and immediate reporting of potential manifestations of hepatotoxicity (e.g., nausea or vomiting, abdominal pain, unusual fatigue, loss of appetite, dark urine, yellowing of skin or whites of eyes).

Risk of fractures (e.g., hand, upper arm, foot) in women.

Importance of regular eye examinations. Importance of reporting changes in vision to clinician.

Importance of informing clinicians of existing or contemplated concomitant therapy, including prescription (e.g., drugs that affect blood glucose concentrations; nitrates; antihypertensive agents; antilipemic agents; agents for CHF or prevention of coronary heart disease or stroke) and dietary or herbal supplements, as well as any concomitant illnesses (e.g., CHF or other cardiac disease, type 1 diabetes mellitus, history of diabetic ketoacidosis, macular edema, liver disease, history of liver disease associated with troglitazone, irregular menstrual periods).

Importance of women informing their clinician if they are or plan to become pregnant or plan to breast-feed.

Importance of informing patients of other important precautionary information. (See Cautions.)

Overview (see Users Guide). For additional information until a more detailed monograph is developed and published, the manufacturer's labeling should be consulted. It is *essential* that the manufacturer's labeling be consulted for more detailed information on usual cautions, precautions, contraindications, potential drug interactions, laboratory test interferences, and acute toxicity.

Preparations

Excipients in commercially available drug preparations may have clinically important effects in some individuals; consult specific product labeling for details.

Rosiglitazone Maleate

Oral		
Tablets, film-coated	2 mg (of rosiglitazone)	**Avandia**®, GlaxoSmithKline
	4 mg (of rosiglitazone)	**Avandia**®, GlaxoSmithKline
	8 mg (of rosiglitazone)	**Avandia**®, GlaxoSmithKline

Rosiglitazone Maleate Combinations

Oral		
Tablets, film-coated	1 mg (of rosiglitazone) with 500 mg Metformin Hydrochloride	**Avandamet**®, GlaxoSmithKline
	2 mg (of rosiglitazone) with 500 mg Metformin Hydrochloride	**Avandamet**®, GlaxoSmithKline
	2 mg (rosiglitazone) with 1 g Metformin Hydrochloride	**Avandamet**®, GlaxoSmithKline
	4 mg of (rosiglitazone) with Glimepiride 1 mg	**Avandaryl**®, GlaxoSmithKline
	4 mg of (rosiglitazone) with Glimepiride 2 mg	**Avandaryl**®, GlaxoSmithKline
	4 mg of (rosiglitazone) with Glimepiride 4 mg	**Avandaryl**®, GlaxoSmithKline

4 mg (of rosiglitazone) with 500 mg Metformin, Hydrochloride	**Avandamet®**, GlaxoSmithKline
4 mg (of rosiglitazone) with 1 g Metformin Hydrochloride	**Avandamet®**, GlaxoSmithKline

ANTIHYPOGLYCEMIC AGENTS 68:22

GLYCOGENOLYTIC AGENTS 68:22.12

Glucagon

■ Glucagon, an antihypoglycemic agent, is a hormone synthesized and secreted by the α_2 cells of the pancreatic islets of Langerhans that increases blood glucose concentration by stimulating hepatic glycogenolysis.

Uses

■ **Hypoglycemia** Glucagon is used for the emergency treatment of severe hypoglycemia. Glucagon is only effective in patients with hypoglycemia if liver glycogen is available; the drug is of little or no value in patients with chronic hypoglycemia or in those with hypoglycemia associated with starvation or adrenal insufficiency. The increase in blood glucose concentration produced by glucagon is not as great in patients with type 1 diabetes mellitus as compared to those with type 2 diabetes mellitus; supplemental carbohydrate should be administered as soon as possible, especially to pediatric patients. The hyperglycemic response produced by glucagon may be reduced in emaciated or undernourished patients or in those with uremia or hepatic disease. Unlike IV dextrose, parenteral administration of glucagon results in a smooth, gradual termination of insulin coma. Glucagon is convenient for use in emergency situations when dextrose cannot be administered IV.

Depending on the stage of coma and the route of administration, patients usually become conscious within 5–20 minutes following parenteral administration of glucagon. After the patient responds, supplemental carbohydrate should be administered to restore liver glycogen and prevent secondary hypoglycemia. In patients in very deep coma, IV dextrose should be administered in addition to glucagon. If an unconscious diabetic patient suspected of being in insulin coma does not awaken following administration of glucagon, an additional dose of glucagon can be administered; emergency assistance should be sought. Other causes of coma should be considered. Failure of glucagon to relieve the coma may be caused by marked depletion of hepatic glycogen stores or irreversible brain damage resulting from prolonged hypoglycemia. In emergency situations in which hypoglycemia is suspected but not established, glucagon should *not* be substituted for IV dextrose.

■ **Radiographic Examination of the GI Tract** Glucagon is used as a diagnostic aid in the radiographic examination of the stomach, duodenum, small intestine, and colon when a hypotonic state would be advantageous. Glucagon appears to be as effective as antimuscarinics for this purpose and is associated with fewer adverse effects. Concomitant administration of glucagon and an antimuscarinic agent may result in increased adverse effects.

■ **Other Uses** Glucagon has been used with some success as a cardiac stimulant for the management of cardiac manifestations (e.g., bradycardia, hypotension, myocardial depression) associated with severe β-adrenergic blocking agent overdosage† or calcium-channel blocking agent overdosage†. Glucagon has successfully reversed such manifestations in patients unresponsive to other drugs (e.g., atropine, epinephrine, dopamine, dobutamine), and should be administered early in the management of severe β-blocker overdosage. Experience in calcium-channel blocker overdosage is more limited, but glucagon (combined with inamrinone in at least one case) has been similarly effective in some patients.

Dosage and Administration

■ **Reconstitution and Administration** Glucagon and glucagon hydrochloride may be administered by subcutaneous, IM, or IV injection.

Glucagon (rDNA origin) for injection (Lilly) is reconstituted by adding 1 mL of sterile diluent to a vial labeled as containing 1 mg of the drug to provide a solution containing 1 mg of glucagon per mL. Concentrations greater than 1 mg/mL should not be used. Only the diluent provided by the manufacturer (Lilly) should be used to reconstitute glucagon, and the diluent should not be used to reconstitute other drugs.

Glucagon (rDNA origin) for injection (GlucaGen®) is reconstituted by adding 1 mL of sterile water for injection to a vial labeled as containing 1 mg of glucagon to provide a solution containing approximately 1 mg of glucagon per mL.

Reconstituted solutions of glucagon should be used immediately; any unused portion should be discarded.

■ **Dosage** Dosage of glucagon hydrochloride (GlucaGen®) is expressed in terms of glucagon.

Hypoglycemia For the emergency treatment of severe hypoglycemia in adults and children weighing more than 20 kg, the usual subcutaneous, IM, or IV dose of glucagon (rDNA origin, Lilly) is 1 mg. The usual subcutaneous, IM, or IV dose of glucagon (rDNA origin, Lilly) in children weighing less than 20 kg is 0.5 mg; alternatively, a dose of 20–30 mcg/kg can be administered in children weighing less than 20 kg.

For the emergency treatment of severe hypoglycemia in adults and children weighing 25 kg or more, the usual subcutaneous, IM, or IV dose of glucagon (rDNA origin, GlucaGen®) is 1 mg. The usual subcutaneous, IM, or IV dose of glucagon (rDNA origin, GlucaGen®) in children weighing less than 25 kg or younger than 6–8 years of age is 0.5 mg. After the patient responds, supplemental carbohydrate should be administered to restore liver glycogen and prevent secondary hypoglycemia.

If the patient does not awaken within 15 minutes following administration of the drug, an additional dose may be administered; however, because of the potential serious adverse effects associated with prolonged cerebral hypoglycemia emergency aid should be sought so that parenteral dextrose can be given. *If the patient fails to respond to glucagon, IV dextrose must be given.*

Radiographic Examination of the GI Tract When glucagon (rDNA) is used as a diagnostic aid in the radiographic examination of the stomach, duodenum, and small intestine in adults, 1 or 2 mg may be given IM or 0.25–2 mg may be given IV, depending on the onset of action and duration of effect required for the specific examination. (See Pharmacokinetics: Absorption.) Since the stomach is less sensitive to the effect of glucagon, the manufacturer (Lilly) recommends that doses of 0.5 mg IV or 2 mg IM be used when relaxation of the stomach is desired.

To facilitate a more satisfactory radiographic examination of the colon, a dose of 2 mg may be given as a single IM injection approximately 10 minutes prior to initiation of the procedure.

Other Uses For the management of cardiac manifestations of β-blocker or calcium-channel blocker overdosage†, glucagon has been administered as an initial IV dose of 50 mcg/kg over 1–2 minutes; higher doses may be needed if this is ineffective, and up to 10 mg may be needed in some adults. In many cases, the initial dose(s) may be followed by a continuous IV infusion at a rate of 2–5 mg/hour (maximum: 10 mg/hour) diluted in 5% dextrose injection; the infusion rate can then be tapered downward according to response.

Cautions

■ **Adverse Effects** Glucagon is generally well tolerated, and adverse effects occur only rarely following administration of usual dosages of the drug for short periods of time. The most frequent adverse effects of glucagon are nausea and vomiting, which are dose related; however, these adverse effects may be caused by hypoglycemia rather than the drug. Allergic reactions, including rash, urticaria, and rarely, hypotension and anaphylactic shock with respiratory distress have been reported in patients receiving glucagon. Anaphylactic reactions generally have occurred in patients undergoing endoscopic examination who received glucagon as well as contrast media and local anesthetics.

■ **Precautions** Glucagon should be used with caution in patients with a history of insulinoma and/or pheochromocytoma. Although IV administration of glucagon produces an initial increase in blood glucose concentration in patients with insulinoma, hypoglycemia may subsequently develop as a result of glucagon's insulin-releasing effect. Exogenous administration of glucagon stimulates the release of catecholamines, which may cause a marked increase in blood pressure in patients with pheochromocytoma.

When glucagon is used for the treatment of hypoglycemic shock, liver glycogen must be available. Administration of dextrose by IV injection or by gavage should be considered in patients with hypoglycemia.

Patients with diabetes mellitus should be fully and completely advised about the nature of the disease, what they must do to prevent and detect complications, and how to control their condition. Patients should be instructed that dietary regulation is the principal consideration in the management of diabetes, and that antidiabetic therapy is only used as an adjunct to, and not a substitute for, proper dietary regulation. Patients should also be advised that they cannot neglect dietary restrictions, develop a careless attitude about their condition, or disregard instructions about body weight control, exercise, hygiene, and avoidance of infection. Patients should be properly instructed in the early detection and treatment of hypoglycemia, and should be advised to routinely carry sugar, candy, or other readily absorbable carbohydrate so that it may be taken at the first sign of a developing hypoglycemic reaction; if patients are unaware of the symptoms of hypoglycemia, they may lapse into insulin shock. Patients (and their families) should be properly instructed in the technique of preparing and administering glucagon for injection before an emergency situation occurs. Although glucagon may be used for the treatment of hypoglycemia by the patient during an emergency, patients should be instructed to notify their physician when hypoglycemic reactions occur so that appropriate adjustment of insulin dosage can be made.

Since glucagon is a protein, the possibility of hypersensitivity reactions should be considered. In a 3-month study in individuals receiving either animal-source glucagon or biosynthetic glucagon (rDNA origin), glucagon-specific antibodies were not detected in either treatment group.

■ **Pediatric Precautions** Glucagon has been used safely and effectively for the treatment of hypoglycemia in children. Safety and efficacy of glucagon in diagnostic procedures in children have not been established.

Pharmacology

Exogenous glucagon elicits all the pharmacologic responses usually produced by endogenous glucagon.

Glucagon is an antyhypoglycemic agent that increases blood glucose concentration by stimulating hepatic glycogenolysis. Some of the metabolic effects produced by glucagon in various tissues (e.g., liver, adipose tissue) are similar to those of epinephrine. Glucagon stimulates the formation of adenylate cyclase, which catalyzes the conversion of ATP to cAMP, particularly in the liver and in adipose tissue. Formation of cAMP initiates a series of intracellular reactions including activation of phosphorylase, which promote the degradation of glycogen to glucose. The increase in blood glucose concentration occurs within minutes. Endogenous secretion of glucagon is stimulated when blood glucose concentration is low or when serum insulin concentration is increased. In general, the actions of glucagon are antagonistic to those of insulin; however, glucagon has been reported to stimulate insulin secretion in healthy individuals and in patients with type 2 diabetes mellitus. Glucagon also has been reported to enhance peripheral utilization of glucose. The intensity of the hyperglycemic effect of glucagon depends on hepatic glycogen reserve and the presence of phosphorylases. The action of glucagon is not blocked by sympatholytic agents such as dihydroergotamine. The hyperglycemic effect of glucagon is increased and prolonged by concomitant administration of epinephrine.

Glucagon produces extrahepatic effects that are independent of its hyperglycemic action. Although the exact mechanism(s) of action has not been conclusively determined, glucagon produces relaxation of smooth muscle of the stomach, duodenum, small intestine, and colon. The drug has also been shown to inhibit gastric and pancreatic secretions.

Glucagon has a positive inotropic and chronotropic effect. Following rapid IV administration in anesthetized animals, glucagon causes a decrease in blood pressure. Glucagon has also been shown to decrease plasma amino nitrogen concentration; enhance renal excretion of electrolytes; decrease synthesis of protein and fat; increase the metabolic rate; and, following prolonged administration, to produce a diabetic effect, which may persist for several days.

Pharmacokinetics

■ **Absorption** Because of its polypeptide nature, glucagon is destroyed in the GI tract, and therefore must be administered parenterally.

Following parenteral administration of glucagon, maximum plasma or blood glucose concentrations occur within 30 minutes; hyperglycemic activity persists for 60–90 minutes. Following IV administration of a single 0.25- to 0.5-mg or 2-mg dose of the drug, relaxation of GI smooth muscle occurs within 1 minute and persists for 9–17 or 22–25 minutes, respectively. Following IM administration of a single 1-mg dose of the drug, relaxation of GI smooth muscle occurs within 8–10 minutes and persists for 12–27 minutes; after a single 2-mg IM dose, relaxation of GI smooth muscle occurs within 4–7 minutes and persists for 21–32 minutes.

■ **Elimination** Following IV administration, glucagon has a plasma half-life of about 8–18 minutes. Following IM administration, a mean apparent half-life of 45 minutes has been reported. Although the exact metabolic fate of glucagon is not clearly established, the drug is extensively degraded in the plasma, liver, and kidneys.

Chemistry and Stability

■ **Chemistry** Glucagon is a hormone synthesized and secreted by the α_2 cells of the pancreatic islets of Langerhans. Glucagon is a straight-chain polypeptide with a molecular weight of 3483 and contains 29 amino acids; histidine is the N-terminal acid and threonine is the C-terminal residue of the molecule. Glucagon is *not* chemically or structurally related to insulin; unlike insulin, glucagon does not contain cysteine and has no disulfide linkages. Although structurally identical to endogenous human glucagon, commercially available glucagon is prepared using recombinant DNA technology and special laboratory strains of nonpathogenic *Escherichia coli* or *Saccharomyces cerevisiae*. One mg of glucagon is equivalent to 1 International Unit (IU, unit).

Glucagon occurs as a fine, white or off-white, crystalline powder, is practically odorless and tasteless, and is practically insoluble in water and soluble in dilute alkali and acid solutions. Commercially available glucagon (rDNA origin) for injection (Lilly) is a mixture of the drug and lactose; hydrochloric acid may be added to adjust the pH of glucagon. Glucagon (rDNA origin) for injection (Lilly) is a sterile, white, lyophilized powder; a sterile diluent containing glycerin, hydrochloric acid, and sterile water for injection is provided by the manufacturer for reconstitution. Commercially available glucagon (rDNA origin) for injection (GlucaGen®) is a mixture of the hydrochloride salt of the drug and lactose and occurs as a sterile, white, lyophilized powder. Sterile water for injection is provided by the manufacturer for reconstitution.

■ **Stability** Glucagon (rDNA origin) for injection (Lilly) should be stored at a controlled room temperature of 20–25°C. Glucagon (rDNA origin) for injection (GlucaGen®) is stable for at least 24 months following the date of manufacture when stored in light-resistant containers at 2–8°C; freezing should be avoided. Glucagon (rDNA origin) for injection (GlucaGen®) may be stored at 20–25°C for up to 12 months. Following reconstitution of glucagon (rDNA origin) for injection (Lilly) and glucagon (rDNA origin) for injection (GlucaGen®), solutions of glucagon should be used immediately.

Preparations

Excipients in commercially available drug preparations may have clinically important effects in some individuals; consult specific product labeling for details.

Glucagon (Recombinant DNA origin)

Parenteral		
For injection	1 mg (1 unit)	**Glucagon Diagnostic Kit** (with 1 mL diluent available in Hyporet® disposable syringe), Lilly
		Glucagon Emergency Kit (with 1 mL diluent available in Hyporet® disposable syringe), Lilly

Glucagon Hydrochloride (Recombinant DNA origin)

Parenteral		
For injection	1 mg (1 unit) (of glucagon)	**GlucaGen® Diagnostic Kit** (with 1 mL sterile water for injection diluent), Bedford

†Use is not currently included in the labeling approved by the US Food and Drug Administration

PITUITARY 68:28

Desmopressin Acetate

■ Desmopressin, a synthetic polypeptide structurally related to arginine vasopressin (antidiuretic hormone), the natural human posterior pituitary hormone, elicits a greater antidiuretic response, on a weight basis, than does arginine vasopressin, and, among other pharmacologic effects, causes a dose-dependent increase in plasma factor VIII (antihemophilic factor) activity.

Uses

■ **Polyuria and Polydipsia** Desmopressin is used intranasally, orally, or parenterally to prevent or control polydipsia, polyuria, and dehydration in patients with diabetes insipidus caused by a deficiency of endogenous posterior pituitary vasopressin (antidiuretic hormone) (neurohypophyseal diabetes insipidus) and to manage temporary polyuria and polydipsia associated with trauma or surgery in the pituitary region. Because of its relatively long duration of action and relative lack of adverse effects, many experts consider intranasal desmopressin the drug of choice for chronic treatment in patients with mild to severe neurohypophyseal diabetes insipidus. In children, intranasal desmopressin is preferred to vasopressin injection and to oral antidiuretic agents such as chlorpropamide because of the frequency of adverse effects of these agents in pediatric patients. Although intranasal administration of the drug is preferred for chronic therapy, parenteral administration of the drug may be useful when factors that can make nasal insufflation ineffective or inappropriate are present; these include poor intranasal absorption, nasal congestion and blockage, nasal discharge, atrophy of nasal mucosa, and severe atrophic rhinitis. In addition, parenteral administration of the drug may be preferred when the patient has an impaired level of consciousness. Parenteral administration of the drug also may be necessary during recovery from surgery or when nasal packing is present in patients who have undergone cranial surgical procedures such as transsphenoidal hypophysectomy.

Desmopressin is not effective in controlling polyuria caused by renal disease, nephrogenic diabetes insipidus, hypokalemia, or hypercalcemia. In uncontrolled studies, desmopressin had variable effectiveness in controlling polyuria secondary to administration of lithium.

■ **Primary Nocturnal Enuresis** Desmopressin is used orally for the management of primary nocturnal enuresis. It may be used alone or as an adjunct to behavioral therapy and/or other nondrug measures, and has been shown to be effective in some cases refractory to standard therapies (e.g., imipramine, enuresis alarms).

Some desmopressin intranasal preparations (i.e., nasal solutions containing 0.1 mg of desmopressin acetate per mL) initially received approval from the US Food and Drug Administration (FDA) for the treatment of primary nocturnal enuresis. However in late 2007, FDA withdrew its prior approval for the treatment of primary nocturnal enuresis due to the risk of serious hyponatremia that may result in seizures and death, particularly in children, following a review of 61 postmarketing cases of hyponatremia-related seizures associated with the use of desmopressin. FDA requested that prescribing information for desmopressin be revised to include information about the risk of severe hyponatremia and seizures and the safe use of desmopressin, and to state that these desmopressin intranasal preparations are no longer indicated for the treatment of primary nocturnal enuresis. FDA states that the status of all other approved indications for the individual desmopressin intranasal preparations has not changed. (See Cautions: Adverse Effects and Precautions and Contraindications.)

The etiology of nocturnal enuresis is not precisely known, but appears to be related to delayed maturation of the cortical mechanisms that allow voluntary control of the micturition reflex. The condition is characterized by nocturnal incontinence without overt daytime voiding symptoms and is usually 3 times more common in boys than in girls. Primary nocturnal enuresis is diagnosed when a child never has experienced a period of consistent nighttime continence; the condition is considered secondary when nocturnal enuresis occurs in a formerly "dry" child, and usually is associated with an emotionally disruptive event. Treatment is not usually indicated until a child reaches the age of 6; the condition will then spontaneously remit in 15% of patients every year thereafter. The frequency of this condition in adults is less than 1%. Other possible etiologies for nocturnal enuresis (e.g., neurologic and/or spinal abnormalities, diabetes insipidus or diabetes mellitus, chronic renal failure, bacteriuria [especially in girls]) should be ruled out before initiation of drug therapy.

Controlled studies of oral desmopressin in doses of 0.2–0.6 mg daily for 2 weeks in patients 5–17 years of age with primary nocturnal enuresis indicated that patients experienced about 27–40% fewer nights of incontinence while receiving the drug versus placebo; a greater response was observed with increasing dosages up to 0.6 mg daily. In an open-label extension study of 6 months' duration in patients completing the placebo-controlled studies, 11% of patients receiving desmopressin achieved a complete or near complete response (no more than 2 nights of incontinence/2 weeks) and did not require titration to the 0. 6-mg daily dose. The majority of patients (86%) were titrated to the 0. 6-mg daily dose. When all dosage arms were combined (0.2–0.6 mg daily), 56% of patients receiving desmopressin experienced at least a 50% reduction in the number of nights of incontinence/2 weeks, while 38% of patients achieved a complete or near complete response. Although limited data demonstrate that desmopressin is effective for the control of primary nocturnal enuresis, the relapse rate after cessation of desmopressin therapy is high (with rates of nocturnal incontinence sometimes approaching incontinence rates before treatment); enuresis alarms have been observed to be the most effective treatment for nocturnal enuresis.

■ **Hemophilia A** Desmopressin acetate is used intranasally or parenterally for the management of spontaneous or trauma-induced bleeding episodes such as hemarthrosis, intramuscular hematoma, or mucosal bleeding in patients with mild hemophilia A. The drug is designated an orphan drug by the US Food and Drug Administration (FDA) for use in this condition. Desmopressin acetate also is used parenterally or intranasally to maintain hemostasis during surgical procedures and postoperatively in patients with hemophilia A. The drug is not indicated for patients with hemophilia B or those with factor VIII antibodies. Desmopressin acetate generally is indicated in patients with hemophilia A whose plasma factor VIII activity is greater than 5%. Although use of desmopressin may be justified in certain clinical situations in patients with hemophilia A whose factor VIII activity is between 2–5%, these patients should be carefully monitored if the drug is used. Desmopressin is ineffective in patients with severe hemophilia A.

The National Hemophilia Foundation's Medical and Scientific Advisory Council (MASAC) currently recommends that parenteral or intranasal desmopressin be used whenever possible for the treatment of mild hemophilia A. When desmopressin does not provide adequate treatment, patients should be treated with antihemophilic factor (recombinant) or antihemophilic factor (human). MASAC states that cryoprecipitate is not recommended as a treatment alternative for the management of hemophilia A. Despite the fact the donor units used to prepare cryoprecipitate are screened for antibody to HIV-1, HIV-2, hepatitis C virus, and hepatitis B surface antigen (HBsAg), cryoprecipitate may still be infectious for several reasons, including the several months' delay in seroconversion after HIV or hepatitis C infection.

■ **von Willebrand Disease** Desmopressin acetate is used intranasally or parenterally for the management of spontaneous or trauma-induced bleeding episodes in patients with mild to moderate type 1 von Willebrand disease. The drug is designated an orphan drug by the FDA for use in this condition. The drug also is used parenterally to maintain hemostasis during surgical procedures and postoperatively in these patients. MASAC and other experts state that desmopressin acetate is the treatment of choice for the management of mild to moderate type 1 von Willebrand disease, especially those whose plasma factor VIII activity is greater than 5%. Patients least likely to respond to the drug are those with severe homozygous von Willebrand disease whose factor VIII and factor VIII/von Willebrand factor activities are less than 1%; the response of other patients may be variable depending on the type of molecular defect associated with their disease. Desmopressin acetate is not indicated for patients with severe type 1 von Willebrand disease or when there is evidence of an abnormal molecular form of factor VIII antigen. Bleeding time, factor VIII and ristocetin cofactor activities, and von Willebrand factor antigen should be monitored during desmopressin therapy to ensure that an adequate response is being achieved. If individuals with type 1 disease become transiently unresponsive to desmopressin acetate, many experts recommend use of antihemophilic factor (human) preparations rich in von Willebrand factor (i.e., Alphanate®, Humate-P®, Koate®-DVI).

Desmopressin acetate may be effective for the management of bleeding in some, but not all, individuals with type 2A, 2M, or 2N von Willebrand disease†. Although desmopressin acetate reportedly has been used effectively in some patients with type 2B von Willebrand disease, the drug usually is not used in these individuals because of an increased risk of thromboembolic events. Desmopressin acetate is ineffective for the management of bleeding in individuals with type 3 von Willebrand disease. Experts generally recommend use of antihemophilic factor (human) preparations rich in von Willebrand factor if prevention or control of bleeding is necessary in individuals with type 2A, 2M, or 2N von Willebrand disease who do not respond to desmopressin acetate or when prevention or control of bleeding is considered necessary in those with type 2B or type 3 von Willebrand disease (e.g., in surgical situations). These antihemophilic factor (human) preparations are particularly useful for the management of von Willebrand disease in pediatric patients who are too young to receive desmopressin acetate. (See Cautions: Pediatric Precautions.) Cryoprecipitate should not be used in the management of von Willebrand disease except in emergency, life- or limb-threatening situations when desmopressin acetate or appropriate preparations of antihemophilic factor (human) are not available.

■ **Other Uses** Intranasal desmopressin has been used in adults and children to evaluate the ability of the kidneys to concentrate urine†. Use of the drug for this purpose is easier and more rapid but may be less accurate than the Mosenthal concentrating test.

Intranasal desmopressin has been used in a small number of patients with sickle cell anemia to induce hyponatremia for the prevention and treatment of sickle cell crisis†; however, further studies are needed to establish the safety and efficacy of the drug for this condition. In a few patients, chronic hyponatremia induced by desmopressin reduced the frequency of painful crises, and acutely induced hyponatremia shortened the duration of crises; however, successful therapy requires strict dietary regulation and patient supervision. Because of the need for further studies and the potential complications of hyponatremia (e.g., seizures), use of intranasal desmopressin for the management of patients with sickle cell disease should be limited to severely afflicted patients who can be treated and evaluated in a strictly supervised setting.

In one randomized, placebo-controlled study in uremic patients† with prolonged bleeding times and hemorrhagic tendencies, IV desmopressin increased factor VIII activity and reduced bleeding time; in some additional uremic patients who received IV desmopressin before surgery or renal biopsy, bleeding time was reduced and associated with normal hemostasis.

Dosage and Administration

■ **Administration** Desmopressin acetate is administered intranasally, orally, by subcutaneous injection, direct IV injection, or slow IV infusion.

Intranasal Administration Desmopressin acetate intranasal preparations should be administered in children under adult supervision in order to monitor the dose and fluid intake.

Desmopressin acetate nasal solutions containing 0.1 mg of the drug per mL are used for the treatment of diabetes insipidus; desmopressin acetate nasal solution containing 1.5 mg of the drug per mL is used for the treatment of hemophilia A or von Willebrand disease. Desmopressin acetate nasal solutions containing 0.1 or 1.5 mg/mL are administered using the spray pump supplied by the manufacturers; alternatively, desmopressin acetate nasal solutions containing 0.1 mg/mL can be administered using a calibrated nasal tube supplied by the manufacturers.

The intranasal spray pump provided by the manufacturers delivers 0.1 mL of solution per actuation. When the nasal solution containing 0.1 mg/mL is administered using the spray pump, each 0.1-mL spray delivers a dose of 10 mcg of desmopressin acetate; if a dose other than a multiple of 10 mcg is required, the solution should be administered using a nasal tube. The nasal tube has 4 graduation markings that measure 0.05, 0.1, 0.15, or 0.2 mL and can be used to administer 5, 10, 15, or 20 mcg, respectively. When the nasal solution containing 1.5 mg/mL is administered using the spray pump, each 0.1-mL spray delivers a dose of 150 mcg of desmopressin acetate; if a dose other than a multiple of 150 mcg is required, parenteral desmopressin acetate therapy should be used.

Desmopressin acetate nasal solution should be administered intranasally according to the manufacturer's instructions to ensure that the drug is deposited high in the nasal cavity and does not pass down the throat. The patient must be carefully instructed in the proper use of the nasal tube or spray pump in order to obtain optimum results. Desmopressin generally should not be administered intranasally when changes in the nasal mucosa such as scarring, edema, or other condition may cause erratic, unreliable absorption of the drug. The drug should not be administered intranasally when nasal congestion and blockage, nasal discharge, atrophy of nasal mucosa, or severe atrophic rhinitis is present. Intranasal therapy also may be inappropriate when the patient has impaired consciousness. In addition, cranial surgical procedures, such as transphenoidal hypophysectomy, create situations in which an alternative route of administration is needed as in cases of nasal packing or recovery from surgery.

Parenteral Administration For IV infusion, the appropriate dose of desmopressin acetate should be diluted in 10 or 50 mL of 0.9% sodium chloride injection for administration in children weighing 10 kg or less or in adults and children weighing more than 10 kg, respectively; the solution is then infused IV slowly over 15–30 minutes. Blood pressure and pulse should be monitored during infusion of the drug.

■ **Dosage** ***Polyuria and Polydipsia*** The intranasal, oral, or parenteral dose of desmopressin acetate required for antidiuresis is variable and must be adjusted according to the patient's requirements and response. Morning and evening doses must be adjusted separately for an adequate diurnal rhythm of water turnover. Response is generally estimated by duration of sleep and adequate, not excessive, turnover of water.

Intranasal Dosage. For the management of neurohypophyseal diabetes insipidus, the usual adult maintenance dosage of desmopressin acetate recommended by the manufacturer is 10–40 mcg (0.1–0.4 mL or 1–4 sprays from the spray pump of a solution containing 0.1 mg/mL) given intranasally in 1–3 divided doses daily. Some clinicians have recommended an adult desmopressin acetate maintenance dosage of 5–40 mcg (0.05–0.4 mL of a solution containing 0.1 mg/mL). Most adults require 20 mcg daily administered in 2 divided doses in the morning and the evening. In children 3 months to 12 years of age, the initial dose of desmopressin acetate is 5 mcg or less (0.05 mL of a solution containing 0.1 mg/mL) administered intranasally in the evening. In children 3 months to 12 years of age, the usual intranasal dosage is 5–30 mcg (0.05–0.3 mL of a solution containing 0.1 mg/mL) daily in a single evening dose or divided in 2 doses. About 25–33% of adults and children can be controlled with a single daily dose. The lowest effective dosage should be used. Fluid intake should be restricted. (See Cautions: Precautions and Contraindications.)

Parenteral Dosage. If the drug is administered by subcutaneous or direct IV injection in adults or children 12 years of age or older for the management of diabetes insipidus, the usual maintenance dosage is 2–4 mcg daily given in 2 divided doses. The parenteral dosage for the management of diabetes insipidus in children younger than 12 years of age has not been established. (See Cautions: Pediatric Precautions.) Patients with diabetes insipidus being switched from intranasal to subcutaneous or IV administration of the drug should generally receive one-tenth their maintenance intranasal dosage parenterally. The lowest effective parenteral dosage should be given. During long-term use, patients rarely may develop tolerance to the drug and require cautious increase in dosage to achieve an adequate therapeutic response. Fluid intake should be restricted. (See Cautions: Precautions and Contraindications.)

Oral Dosage. If oral desmopressin acetate is used for the management of diabetes insipidus in patients who previously received the drug intranasally, oral therapy should be initiated 12 hours after the last intranasal dose. The usual initial oral dosage of desmopressin acetate for adults and pediatric patients is 0.05 mg twice daily, and subsequent dosage should be adjusted according to response. In clinical studies, the optimal dosage range for most patients was 0.1–0.8 mg daily given in divided doses. Each dose should be adjusted separately for an adequate diurnal rhythm of water turnover. Total oral daily dosage should be increased or decreased in the range of 0.1–1.2 mg divided into 2 or 3 daily doses as needed to obtain adequate antidiuresis. Fluid intake should be restricted. (See Cautions: Precautions and Contraindications.)

Primary Nocturnal Enuresis If oral desmopressin acetate is used for the treatment of primary nocturnal enuresis in patients who previously received the drug intranasally, oral therapy should be initiated the night following (24 hours after) the last intranasal dose. The usual initial oral dose of desmopressin acetate for adults and pediatric patients 6 years of age or older is 0.2 mg at bedtime. The dose may be titrated up to 0.6 mg to achieve the desired response. Duration of desmopressin therapy has not been established in pediatric patients responding to therapy; some experts have suggested that it is reasonable to continue therapy for 3–6 months; after 3–6 months, therapy can be withdrawn and the patient reevaluated.

Fluid restriction should be in effect for a minimum of 1 hour before desmopressin administration and continued until the next morning or at least 8 hours after desmopressin administration. Some experts recommend that not more than 240 mL of fluid should be consumed on any night when desmopressin is used. Desmopressin therapy should be interrupted during episodes of fluid and/or electrolyte imbalance (e.g., systemic infections, fever, recurrent vomiting or diarrhea) and under conditions associated with increased water intake (e.g., extremely hot weather, vigorous exercise). (See Cautions: Precautions and Contraindications.)

Hemophilia A and von Willebrand Disease For the management of bleeding in patients with hemophilia A or mild to moderate type 1 von Willebrand disease, dosage of desmopressin acetate should be adjusted according to response. Factor VIII and factor VIII/ristocetin cofactor activities, factor VIII antigen levels, and activated partial thromboplastin activity should be monitored in patients with hemophilia A, and factor VIII and factor VIII/ristocetin cofactor activities and factor VIII/von Willebrand factor antigen levels should be monitored in patients with von Willebrand disease. Determination of bleeding time may also be useful in monitoring therapy in patients with von Willebrand disease.

The usual parenteral dose for adults and children 3 months of age and older with hemophilia A or type 1 von Willebrand disease is 0.3 mcg/kg given by slow IV infusion; if the dose is administered preoperatively, the drug should be injected 30 minutes prior to the scheduled procedure. Fluid intake should be restricted. (See Cautions: Precautions and Contraindications.)

The usual intranasal dosage of desmopressin acetate for the management of hemophilia A or type 1 von Willebrand disease is 300 mcg (0.1 mL or 1 spray from the spray pump into each nostril of a solution containing 1.5 mg/mL). A dosage of 150 mcg (0.1 mL or 1 spray from the spray pump into a single nostril of a solution containing 1.5 mg/mL) may be sufficient in patients who weigh less than 50 kg. If intranasal desmopressin acetate is used preoperatively, the drug should be administered 2 hours prior to surgery.

The need for additional doses of the desmopressin acetate or use of blood products for hemostasis should be determined by the clinical response of the patient and the response as determined by appropriate laboratory tests. The tendency toward tachyphylaxis (decreasing responsiveness) when doses of desmopressin are repeated more frequently than every 48 hours should be considered. When desmopressin acetate is used for the management of von Willebrand disease, the National Hemophilia Foundation' Medical and Scientific Advisory Council (MASAC) recommends that the drug be administered no more frequently than once every 24 hours and used for no more than 3 consecutive days unless such therapy is recommended by a clinician with expertise in the treatment of the disease.

Other Uses To evaluate the urine concentrating ability of the kidneys†, fasting or nonfasting adults have been given 10–40 mcg (0.1–0.4 mL of 0.01% solution or 1–4 sprays from the spray pump) intranasally; nonfasting children 2–15 years of age have been given 20 mcg (0.2 mL of 0.01% solution); and nonfasting infants 1–12 weeks of age have been given 10 mcg (0.1 mL of 0.01% solution or 1 spray from the spray pump) intranasally. Then, a urine sample is collected in 1–5 hours and specific gravity of the urine is determined. Under test conditions, the average individual should concentrate the urine to a specific gravity of at least 1.020.

Cautions

■ **Adverse Effects** In late 2007, the US Food and Drug Administration (FDA) reported the results of a review of 61 postmarketing cases of hyponatremia-related seizures associated with the use of desmopressin. In 55 cases, sodium concentrations ranged from 104–130 mEq/L during the seizure event. Two of these 55 cases were fatal; although both patients experienced hyponatremia and seizures, the direct contribution of desmopressin to the fatalities is not clear. Intranasal formulations were used in 36 cases; 25 of these cases involved pediatric patients (i.e., patients younger than 17 years of age). The most commonly reported indication for use of desmopressin in the 25 pediatric patients was nocturnal enuresis. In 39 of the 61 cases, the patient received at least one concomitant drug or had diseases associated with hyponatremia and/or seizures. As a result, FDA withdrew its prior approval for the treatment of primary nocturnal enuresis from desmopressin *intranasal* preparations; there is no change in the other approved indications for the individual intranasal preparations. (See Cautions: Precautions and Contraindications.)

Intranasal Administration Adverse effects reported with intranasal desmopressin have been infrequent and mild. Rarely, conjunctivitis, ocular edema, lacrimation disorder, transient headache, dizziness, asthenia, chills, nasal congestion, nostril pain, rhinitis, epistaxis, sore throat, cough, upper respiratory infection, flushing, nausea, vomiting, mild abdominal cramps or pain, GI disorder, somnolence, insomnia, pain, chest pain, palpitations, tachycardia, agitation, balanitis, and vulval pain have occurred with usual intranasal doses. Unlike vasopressin and lypressin, usual doses of desmopressin do not cause skin pallor or severe smooth muscle or abdominal cramps. With large intranasal doses, blood pressure may increase. Severe hyponatremia was reported in one patient with neurohypophyseal diabetes insipidus who abused intranasal desmopressin and in one pediatric patient receiving the drug for primary nocturnal enuresis; the pediatric patient also experienced a single tonic-clonic seizure. Hyponatremia, convulsion, and coma were reported in a 13-year-old patient with cystic fibrosis also receiving the drug for primary nocturnal enuresis. Adverse effects with intranasal desmopressin usually disappear when the dose or the frequency of administration is decreased but, rarely, necessitate discontinuance of the drug.

Oral Administration Desmopressin acetate generally is well tolerated when administered orally. In patients with diabetes insipidus who received desmopressin acetate tablets for up to 44 months, transient increases in AST (SGOT) (up to 1.5 times the normal upper limit) occurred occasionally but returned to the normal range despite continued administration of the drug. In clinical studies evaluating use of oral desmopressin for the treatment of primary nocturnal enuresis, the only adverse effect reported in 3% or more of patients that was probably, possibly, or remotely related to the drug was headache (4% in those receiving desmopressin acetate and 3% in those receiving placebo). Abnormal thinking, diarrhea, and edema-weight gain have been reported in patients receiving oral desmopressin acetate but a causal relationship has not been established.

Parenteral Administration Adverse effects following parenteral administration of desmopressin have generally been infrequent and mild; however, there have been rare reports of thrombotic events (e.g., acute cerebrovascular thrombosis, acute myocardial infarction) following injection of the drug in patients predisposed to such events. Other reported adverse effects include transient headache, nausea, mild abdominal cramps, and vulval pain; these symptoms usually disappear with a reduction in dosage. Local erythema, swelling, and burning pain have been reported occasionally at the site of injection. Severe pain along the injected vein has been reported with large IV doses. Facial flushing has been reported occasionally following parenteral administration of the drug and slight increases in blood pressure, which disappeared with a reduction in dosage or slight decreases in blood pressure (with compensatory increases in heart rate), have been reported infrequently. With large IV doses of desmopressin, tachycardia, hypotension, and facial flushing have been reported. Water intoxication and hyponatremia are possible in patients who do not require vasopressin for its antidiuretic effect. (See Cautions: Precautions and Contraindications.) Excessive water retention occurred in a hemophiliac patient who received an IV dose of desmopressin acetate of 0.5 mcg/kg for bleeding.

Severe allergic reactions, including anaphylaxis, have been reported rarely with parenteral and intranasal desmopressin acetate. In addition, fatal anaphylaxis has been reported in patients receiving parenteral desmopressin.

■ **Precautions and Contraindications** Desmopressin acetate intranasal preparations should be reserved for situations in which oral therapy is not feasible.

All desmopressin preparations should be used cautiously in patients at risk for water intoxication with hyponatremia. Hyponatremia has been reported very rarely during international postmarketing surveillance in patients receiving desmopressin acetate. (See Cautions: Adverse Effects.) Desmopressin is a potent antidiuretic; use of desmopressin may result in water intoxication and/or hyponatremia, and hyponatremia may be fatal unless properly diagnosed and treated. Therefore, fluid restriction is recommended and should be discussed with the patient and/or guardian; careful medical supervision is required. The patient should promptly contact the clinician if water intake changes.

Fluid intake should be carefully restricted, particularly in pediatric and geriatric patients, to reduce the risk of potential water intoxication and hyponatremia. All patients receiving desmopressin therapy should be observed for signs and symptoms associated with hyponatremia (i.e., headache, nausea/vomiting, decreased serum sodium, weight gain, restlessness, fatigue, lethargy, disorientation, depressed reflexes, appetite loss, irritability, muscle weakness, spasms or cramps, abnormal mental status [e.g., hallucinations, decreased consciousness, confusion]); severe symptoms may include seizure, coma, and/or respiratory arrest. An extreme decrease in plasma osmolality that may result in seizures, which may lead to coma, has occurred rarely, and this possibility should be considered.

Desmopressin should be used with caution in patients with habitual or psychogenic polydipsia and in patients who are receiving certain drugs (e.g., tricyclic antidepressants, selective serotonin-reuptake inhibitors [SSRIs]) as these patients may be more likely to drink excessive amounts of water resulting in an increased risk for hyponatremia. (See Drug Interactions.)

Desmopressin should be used with caution in patients with conditions associated with fluid and electrolyte imbalances (e.g., cystic fibrosis, heart failure, renal disorders); these patients are prone to hyponatremia.

When fluid intake is not excessive, there is little danger of water intoxication and hyponatremia with usual intranasal or parenteral doses of desmopressin used to control diabetes insipidus. When the drug is used for its hemostatic effect in patients who do not require exogenous vasopressin for its antidiuretic effect, the risk of potential water intoxication and hyponatremia may be increased and these patients should be cautioned to ingest only enough fluid to satisfy their thirst. Water retention can usually be controlled by decreasing the dosage of desmopressin; severe water retention caused by overdosage may be treated with a diuretic such as furosemide.

Although vasoactive effects are minimal or absent with usual intranasal antidiuretic doses of desmopressin and also are minimal and infrequent and usually respond to dosage reduction when usual parenteral hemostatic doses of the drug are used, caution should be exercised in patients with coronary artery insufficiency and/or hypertensive cardiovascular disease. Desmopressin also should be used with caution in these patients and in patients predisposed to thrombotic events because of the drug's potential prothrombotic effect; although a causal relationship to the drug has not been determined, thrombotic events have been reported rarely in patients predisposed to thrombus formation.

In patients with diabetes insipidus or polyuria and polydipsia associated with head surgery or trauma, urine volume and osmolality and, in some cases, plasma osmolality should be monitored periodically during desmopressin therapy. In otherwise healthy patients with primary nocturnal enuresis, serum electrolytes should be checked at least once if therapy is continued beyond 7 days.

In patients with hemophilia A, factor VIII and factor VIII/ristocetin cofactor (von Willebrand factor) activities, factor VIII antigen levels, and activated partial thromboplastin time should be monitored during desmopressin therapy. Factor VIII activity should be determined prior to initiating desmopressin therapy for hemostasis; desmopressin therapy should not be relied on in patients with a factor VIII activity less than 5% of normal.

In patients with von Willebrand disease, factor VIII and factor VIII/ristocetin cofactor activities and factor VIII/von Willebrand factor antigen levels should be monitored during desmopressin therapy. Determination of bleeding time may also be useful in monitoring therapy in these patients.

Desmopressin is contraindicated in patients with hypersensitivity to the drug or any ingredient in the formulation. Desmopressin also is contraindicated in patients with moderate to severe renal impairment (creatinine clearance less than 50 mL/minute) and in patients with hyponatremia or a history of hyponatremia. Because of the risk of platelet aggregation and thrombocytopenia, the drug also should not be used in patients with type 2B or platelet-type (pseudo) von Willebrand disease. (See Pharmacology.)

■ **Pediatric Precautions** Fluid intake should be carefully restricted in pediatric patients to prevent possible hyponatremia and water intoxication; fluid restriction should be discussed with the patient and/or guardian. (See Cautions: Precautions and Contraindications.)

Desmopressin acetate nasal solutions containing 0.1 mg of desmopressin acetate per mL have been used in children with diabetes insipidus. However, pediatric dosage must be carefully adjusted according to individual patient needs and tolerance, with particular attention to the risk of an extreme decrease in plasma osmolality and resulting seizures in young children. There have been occasional reports of a change in response to desmopressin therapy over time, usually after periods exceeding 6 months. Some patients show a decreased responsiveness to the drug, while others show a shortened duration of effect. There is no evidence that this change in responsiveness results from the development of binding antibodies, but it may result from a local inactivation of the peptide.

Desmopressin acetate nasal solution containing 1.5 mg of desmopressin acetate per mL can be used for the treatment of hemophilia A or von Willebrand disease in children 11 months of age or older; however, safety and efficacy of the nasal solution have not been established in children younger than 11 months of age.

Desmopressin acetate tablets have been used safely for up to 44 months in pediatric patients 4 years of age or older with diabetes insipidus. In younger patients, dosage adjustment of oral desmopressin should be individualized to prevent an excessive decrease in plasma osmolality leading to hyponatremia and possible seizures.

Desmopressin acetate tablets have been used safely for up to 6 months in pediatric patients 6 years of age and older with primary nocturnal enuresis. In patients with primary nocturnal enuresis, desmopressin therapy should be interrupted during acute intercurrent illness characterized by fluid and/or electrolyte imbalance (e.g., systemic infections, fever, recurrent vomiting or diarrhea) and under conditions associated with increased water intake (e.g., extremely hot weather, vigorous exercise). (See Cautions: Precautions and Contraindications.)

Safety and efficacy of *parenteral* desmopressin for the management of *diabetes insipidus* in children younger than 12 years of age have not been established.

The manufacturers state that desmopressin acetate injection should not be used in the management of hemophilia A or von Willebrand disease in children younger than 3 months of age.

■ **Geriatric Precautions** Fluid intake should be carefully restricted in geriatric patients to prevent possible hyponatremia and water intoxication; fluid restriction should be discussed with the patient. (See Cautions: Precautions and Contraindications.)

Clinical studies of desmopressin did not include sufficient numbers of patients 65 years of age and older to determine whether geriatric patients respond differently than younger patients. While other clinical experience has not revealed age-related differences in response, drug dosage generally should be titrated carefully in geriatric patients, usually initiating therapy at the low end of the dosage range. The greater frequency of decreased hepatic, renal, and/or cardiac function and of concomitant disease and drug therapy observed in the elderly also should be considered. Desmopressin is known to be substantially excreted by the kidney and the risk of severe adverse reactions to the drug may be increased in patients with impaired renal function. Because geriatric patients may have decreased renal function, renal function should be monitored and dosage adjusted accordingly.

■ **Pregnancy and Lactation** Safe use of desmopressin during pregnancy or lactation has not been established. Reproduction studies in rats and rabbits using desmopressin dosages up to 12.5 times the usual human hemostatic dosage or 125 times the usual human antidiuretic dosage have not revealed evidence of harm to the fetus. There are no adequate and controlled studies to date using desmopressin in pregnant women; however, the drug has been used throughout pregnancy without adverse effect to mother or fetus and has been used during lactation without adverse effect to the lactating woman or nursing infant. Although published reports state that desmopressin, unlike preparations containing the natural hormones, has no uterotonic effect at usual antidiuretic doses, the physician must weigh the potential therapeutic benefits against the possible risks. Because it is not known whether desmopressin is distributed into milk, the drug should be used with caution in nursing women.

Drug Interactions

Although drug interactions have been reported with vasopressin, few specific interactions have been reported with desmopressin. Desmopressin should be used cautiously in patients who are receiving lithium, large doses of epinephrine, demeclocycline, heparin, or alcohol, because the antidiuretic response to desmopressin may be decreased; drugs such as chlorpropamide, urea, or fludrocortisone may potentiate the antidiuretic response. Concurrent administration of clofibrate with desmopressin reportedly potentiates and prolongs the antidiuretic effect of desmopressin. In one patient, prior administration of carbamazepine decreased the duration of action of desmopressin. Patients receiving large doses of desmopressin (e.g., 0.3 mcg/kg) should be carefully monitored if the drug is administered concurrently with other vasopressor agents. Desmopressin has been used with aminocaproic acid without adverse effects.

Concomitant use of drugs that may increase the risk of water intoxication with hyponatremia (e.g., tricyclic antidepressants, selective serotonin-reuptake inhibitors [SSRIs], chlorpromazine, opiates, nonsteroidal anti-inflammatory agents [NSAIAs], lamotrigine, carbamazepine) with desmopressin should be undertaken with caution. Hyponatremic seizures have been reported rarely in patients receiving desmopressin and imipramine or oxybutynin during postmarketing surveillance.

Pharmacology

Desmopressin elicits a greater antidiuretic response, on a weight basis, than does arginine vasopressin. One important physiologic role of vasopressin is to maintain serum osmolality within a normal range. The antidiuretic potency of IV desmopressin is about 10 times that following intranasal administration of the drug. Vasopressin increases reabsorption of water by the collecting ducts in the kidneys resulting in increased urine osmolality and decreased urinary flow rate. In patients with neurohypophyseal diabetes insipidus, desmopressin has the same effects on water reabsorption as does vasopressin. Therapeutic doses of desmopressin do not directly affect urinary sodium or potassium excretion, or serum sodium, potassium, or creatinine concentrations.

Structural modifications of vasopressin present in desmopressin result in reduced smooth muscle contracting and vasopressor properties compared with vasopressin and lypressin. Intranasal doses of 20 mcg of desmopressin acetate have no effect on blood pressure or pulse rate, but mean arterial pressure may increase as much as 15 mm Hg with doses of 40 mcg or more. Desmopressin has not been reported to stimulate uterine contractions.

Desmopressin, unlike vasopressin, does not stimulate adrenocorticotropic hormone release or increase plasma cortisol concentrations. In children, intranasal administration of desmopressin has no effect on growth hormone, prolactin, or luteinizing hormone concentrations.

Desmopressin causes a dose-dependent increase in plasma factor VIII (antihemophilic factor), plasminogen activator, and, to a smaller degree, factor VIII-related antigen and ristocetin cofactor activities. Large IV doses of desmopressin acetate (0.2–0.5 mcg/kg) increase factor VIII activity in healthy individuals, in patients with mild to moderate hemophilia A and B, in patients with certain types of von Willebrand disease, and in patients with uremia. Desmopressin elicits a greater increase in plasma factor VIII activity, on a weight basis, than does arginine vasopressin in patients with hemophilia or type I von Willebrand's disease. The percentage increase in plasma factor VIII activity in patients with mild hemophilia A or type 1 von Willebrand disease is reportedly similar to that in healthy individuals following IV infusion of a 0.3-mcg/kg dose of the drug over 10 minutes. A gradual diminution in the magnitude of the desmopressin-induced increase in plasma factor VIII activity generally occurs when administration of the drug is repeated every 12–24 hours, but the magnitude is usually the same as the initial response when a period of 2–3 days elapses between administration. Patients with moderate, rather than mild, hemophilia A may or may not respond with an adequate increase in factor VIII to ensure clotting, and patients with type 1 von Willebrand disease may respond better than those with type 2 disease. Patients with severe hemophilia or severe von Willebrand disease are unresponsive to desmopressin. Following intranasal (2–4 mcg/kg) or IV (0.2 mcg/kg) administration of single doses of desmopressin in one study, 3/3 healthy individuals, 27/31 patients with mild or moderate von Willebrand disease, and 6/7 patients with mild to moderate hemophilia A had a greater than 200% increase in plasma factor VIII activity; a lesser but substantial increase in factor VIII-related antigen and ristocetin cofactor also occurred. In this study, 2 patients with severe von Willebrand disease were unresponsive to desmopressin. Although plasminogen activator activity increases rapidly after desmopressin administration, clinically important fibrinolysis has not been reported to date in patients being treated with the drug.

In patients with type 2B von Willebrand disease, desmopressin has been reported to induce platelet aggregation and thrombocytopenia; it was suggested that platelet aggregation resulted from desmopression-induced release of the larger multimers of factor VIII/von Willebrand factor which subsequently were adsorbed to platelets. The drug has also been reported to induce platelet aggregation and thrombocytopenia in patients with platelet-type (pseudo) von Willebrand disease; however, the specific mechanism of this effect may be different in these patients.

Desmopressin has also reportedly increased factor VIII activity and, to a lesser extent, factor VIII-related antigen and ristocetin cofactor in patients with uremia; these changes were accompanied by a shortening of bleeding time. In addition, the drug induced the release into plasma of the larger multimers of factor VIII/von Willebrand factor in these patients.

In a few patients with sickle cell anemia, hyponatremia induced by intranasal desmopressin has resulted in decreased mean corpuscular hemoglobin concentration and a decreased degree of sickling.

Pharmacokinetics

■ **Absorption** Following intranasal administration of desmopressin acetate as directed by the manufacturer, approximately 10–20% of a dose is absorbed through the nasal mucosa. The manufacturer states that nasal congestion does not interfere with the effectiveness of the drug; however, investigators have reported that patients with nasal congestion may require an increased dosage. Following intranasal administration of usual doses of desmopressin acetate in patients with neurohypophyseal diabetes insipidus, antidiuretic effects occur within 15–60 minutes, peak in 1–5 hours, persist 5–21 hours, and then abruptly end over a period of 60–90 minutes. Duration of action varies among individuals with a specific dose. The relatively prolonged duration of action of desmopressin may result from slower enzymatic inactivation of desmopressin than vasopressin or from sequestration of desmopressin in a membrane compartment. Studies using the nasal solution containing 1.5 mg of desmopressin acetate per mL indicate that bioavailability of the drug is 3.3–4.1% and peak plasma concentrations are attained 40–45 minutes after a dose. Following intranasal administration of 150–450 mcg of desmopressin acetate (1–3 sprays of a solution containing 1.5 mg/mL), increases in plasma concentrations of factor VIII and von Willebrand factor are evident within 30 minutes and peak at about 1.5 hours.

Following oral administration of desmopressin acetate tablets, the drug is only minimally absorbed from the GI tract, and bioavailability is about 5% compared with intranasal administration and about 0.16% compared with IV administration of the drug. Peak plasma concentrations of desmopressin acetate are attained 0.9 or 1.5 hours following oral or intranasal administration, respectively. Antidiuretic effects occur at about 1 hour and peak at about 4–7 hours after an oral dose of the drug.

Following IV infusion of desmopressin, the increase in plasma factor VIII activity occurs within 15–30 minutes and peaks between 90 minutes and 2 hours after administration; the increase in factor VIII activity is dose dependent, with a 300–400% maximum increase reportedly occurring after IV infusion of a 0.4-mcg/kg dose.

■ **Distribution** Distribution of desmopressin has not been fully characterized. It is not known if desmopressin crosses the placenta. The drug is distributed into milk.

■ **Elimination** Desmopressin is excreted principally in the urine.

Following intranasal administration of 150–450 mcg of desmopressin acetate (1–3 sprays of a solution containing 1.5 mg/mL), half-life of the drug is 3.3–3.5 hours.

Following oral administration, half-life of desmopressin acetate is independent of dosage and averages 1.5–2.5 hours.

After IV administration of 2–3 mcg of desmopressin acetate in patients with neurohypophyseal diabetes insipidus, plasma concentrations decline in a biphasic manner with a mean initial plasma half-life of 7.8 minutes and a mean terminal plasma half-life of 75.5 minutes (range: 0.4–4 hours).

The metabolic fate of desmopressin is unknown. Unlike vasopressin, desmopressin apparently is not degraded by aminopeptidases or other peptidases that cleave oxytocin and endogenous vasopressin in the plasma during late pregnancy.

Renal clearance of desmopressin decreases with decreasing renal function. Following administration of a single IV dose of 2 mcg of desmopressin acetate in individuals with normal renal function (average creatinine clearance of 103 mL/minute), mild renal impairment (average creatinine clearance of 72 mL/minute), moderate renal impairment (average creatinine clearance of 37 mL/minute), or severe renal impairment (average creatinine clearance of 16 mL/minute; not on dialysis), terminal half-lives of desmopressin averaged 3.7, 4.8, 7.2, or 10 hours, respectively.

Chemistry and Stability

■ **Chemistry** Desmopressin is a synthetic polypeptide structurally related to arginine vasopressin (antidiuretic hormone), the natural human posterior pituitary hormone. Desmopressin acetate is commercially available as nasal solutions for intranasal administration, tablets for oral administration, and injections for parenteral administration.

Desmopressin acetate nasal solutions are aqueous solutions of the drug. For the treatment of central cranial diabetes insipidus, desmopressin acetate is commercially available as nasal solutions containing 0.1 mg of the drug per mL with 0.75 or 0.9% sodium chloride for administration via a spray pump or nasal tube; for the treatment of hemophilia A or von Willebrand disease, desmopressin acetate is commercially available as a nasal solution containing 1.5 mg of the drug per mL with 0.75% sodium chloride for administration via a spray pump. These nasal solutions contain either benzalkonium chloride or chlorobutanol as preservatives.

Desmopressin acetate injection is a sterile, aqueous solution containing 4 mcg of the drug per mL with 0.9% sodium chloride. Hydrochloric acid is added during the manufacture of the injection to adjust the pH to approximately 4; the injection also may contain chlorobutanol as a preservative.

■ **Stability** Commercially available nasal solutions of desmopressin acetate preserved with benzalkonium chloride should be stored at controlled room temperature (20–25°C, not to exceed 25°C). Commercially available nasal solutions containing 1.5 mg of the drug per mL should be discarded 6 months after opening. Commercially available nasal solutions of desmopressin acetate preserved with chlorobutanol should be refrigerated at 2–8°C; when traveling, closed bottles are stable for 3 weeks at controlled room temperature (20–25°C).

Desmopressin acetate tablets should be stored at 20–25°C; exposure to excessive heat or light should be avoided.

Commercially available desmopressin acetate injection should be refrigerated at 2–8°C; freezing should be avoided.

Preparations

Excipients in commercially available drug preparations may have clinically important effects in some individuals; consult specific product labeling for details.

Desmopressin Acetate

Nasal

Solution*	0.1 mg/mL*	**DDAVP® Nasal Spray** (with spray pump), Sanofi-Aventis
		DDAVP® Rhinal Tube (with 2 calibrated nasal tubes; refrigerate), Sanofi-Aventis
		Desmopressin Acetate Nasal Spray, Apotex, Bausch & Lomb
		Desmopressin Acetate Rhinal Tube (with 2 calibrated nasal tubes; refrigerate), Ferring
		Minirin®, Ferring

	1.5 mg/mL*	**Desmopressin Acetate Nasal Spray**
		Stimate® Nasal Spray (with spray pump), CSL Behring
Oral		
Tablets	0.1 mg*	**DDAVP®**, Sanofi-Aventis
		Desmopressin Acetate Tablets
	0.2 mg*	**DDAVP®**, Sanofi-Aventis
		Desmopressin Acetate Tablets
Parenteral		
Injection	4 mcg/mL*	**DDAVP®**, Sanofi-Aventis
		Desmopressin Acetate Injection

*available from one or more manufacturer, distributor, and/or repackager by generic (nonproprietary) name

†Use is not currently included in the labeling approved by the US Food and Drug Administration

Vasopressin

Antidiuretic Hormone, ADH

■ Vasopressin (antidiuretic hormone) is a polypeptide hormone secreted by the neurons of the supraoptic and paraventricular nuclei of the hypothalamus and stored in the posterior pituitary (neurohypophysis) in mammals; the primary physiologic role of vasopressin is to maintain serum osmolality within a normal range, but the hormone also causes vasoconstriction.

Uses

■ **Vasodilatory Shock** Vasopressin is used for its vasoconstrictive effects to increase blood pressure in patients with vasodilatory shock (e.g., postcardiotomy shock, septic shock); the drug is considered a second-line therapy in patients who remain hypotensive despite adequate fluid resuscitation and treatment with catecholamines (e.g., norepinephrine).

Evidence supporting the use of vasopressin in the management of vasodilatory shock is based principally on studies from the published literature, including 7 studies in adults with septic shock and 8 studies in adults with vasodilatory shock after cardiac surgery (i.e., postcardiotomy shock). While these studies had some limitations, vasopressin (administered in doses of 0.01 to 0.1 units/minute by continuous IV infusion) was shown to consistently increase mean arterial pressure (MAP) in patients with these hypotensive states. Although vasopressin appears to have a catecholamine-sparing effect, the effect of the drug on mortality remains unclear. In a randomized double-blind study comparing the effects of vasopressin (0.01–0.03 units/minute) and norepinephrine (5–10 mcg/minute) in patients with septic shock, no substantial difference in 28-day mortality was observed between the vasopressors. Large studies comparing vasopressin to other vasopressors for the treatment of septic shock generally are lacking.

The Surviving Sepsis Campaign International Guidelines for Management of Sepsis and Septic Shock recommend norepinephrine as the first-line vasopressor of choice in adults with septic shock. Vasopressin may be added if further increase in MAP is required or to reduce dosage requirements of norepinephrine. The guidelines recommend that vasopressin be used with caution in patients who are not euvolemic. Because of the risk of ischemic complications, use of vasopressin dosages greater than 0.03 units/minute should be reserved for situations in which alternative vasopressors have failed.

■ **Advanced Cardiovascular Life Support** Vasopressin has been used for its vasopressor effects as a nonadrenergic peripheral vasoconstrictor in patients with cardiac arrest†.

High-quality cardiopulmonary resuscitation (CPR) and defibrillation are integral components of advanced cardiovascular life support (ACLS) and the only proven interventions to increase survival to hospital discharge. Other resuscitative efforts, including drug therapy, are considered secondary and should be performed without compromising the quality and timely delivery of chest compressions and defibrillation. The principal goal of pharmacologic therapy during cardiac arrest is to facilitate return of spontaneous circulation (ROSC), and epinephrine is considered the drug of choice for this use. In previous ACLS guidelines, vasopressin was recommended as a substitute for epinephrine, with one dose of vasopressin (40 units by IV or intraosseous [IO] injection) replacing either the first or second dose of epinephrine, in the treatment of adult cardiac arrest. While some clinicians have suggested that vasopressin may be more effective than epinephrine in asystolic arrest because of underlying differences in the mechanism of action and cardiovascular effects of the drugs (e.g., epinephrine consumes oxygen whereas vasopressin increases coronary blood flow), current evidence indicates that vasopressin offers no advantage compared with epinephrine in patients with cardiac arrest. Results of several randomized controlled studies demonstrated no difference in outcomes (ROSC, survival to discharge or neurologic outcome) when vasopressin (used alone or in combination with epinephrine) was compared with epinephrine alone. In one of these studies in patients with out-of-hospital ventricular fibrillation, a larger proportion of patients initially treated with vasopressin (40 units IV) were suc-

cessfully resuscitated and survived 24 hours compared with those treated with epinephrine (1 mg IV); however, there was no difference in survival to hospital discharge. In another large (1186 patients), multinational, European study in adults with out-of-hospital cardiac arrest, vasopressin (up to 2 initial 40-unit IV doses) and epinephrine (up to 2 initial 1-mg IV doses) were comparably effective in the primary end point of survival to hospital admission as well as the secondary end point of survival to hospital discharge in patients with ventricular fibrillation (patients who responded successfully to electrical defibrillation were excluded) or pulseless electrical activity. Although a post-hoc analysis found that vasopressin was more effective than epinephrine for survival to hospital admission as well as hospital discharge in patients with asystolic cardiac arrest, vasopressin did not improve neurologically intact survival. Because of the equivalence of effect of vasopressin and epinephrine and efforts to simplify the management approach when therapies are found to be equivalent, vasopressin has been removed from the current ACLS treatment algorithm for adult cardiac arrest. (See Uses: Advanced Cardiovascular Life Support and Arrhythmias, in Epinephrine 12:12.12.) There is insufficient evidence to recommend for or against routine use of vasopressin during cardiac arrest in pediatric patients.

Vasopressin has been used in the treatment of drug-induced distributive shock† associated with drug-induced cardiovascular emergencies or altered vital signs.

Vasopressin also has been used in severely hypotensive patients with anaphylaxis† as a potential therapy to prevent cardiopulmonary arrest.

■ **Diabetes Insipidus** Vasopressin has been used in the management of central diabetes insipidus†, a disorder caused by a deficiency of endogenous vasopressin, to control symptoms of polydypsia, polyuria, and dehydration. However, desmopressin, a synthetic analog of vasopressin that has a longer duration of action and lower incidence of adverse effects, is considered the drug of choice for this use. Although vasopressin injection may be used in the initial or emergency treatment of the disease, chronic therapy with the drug is impractical because of its short duration of action. Vasopressin is not effective in controlling polyuria caused by renal disease, nephrogenic diabetes insipidus, hypokalemia or hypercalcemia, or polyuria secondary to the administration of demeclocycline or lithium carbonate.

■ **Abdominal Distention and Abdominal Radiographic Procedures** Vasopressin injection has been used to stimulate peristalsis in the prevention or treatment of intestinal paresis†, postoperative abdominal distention†, and distention complicating pneumonias or toxemias†. In addition, the drug has been used prior to abdominal radiographic procedures† including IV urography, cholecystography, and kidney biopsy to dispel interfering gas shadows and/or to concentrate the contrast media.

■ **Diagnostic Uses** Vasopressin injection has been used in the past as a provocative test for pituitary release of growth hormone and corticotropin†; however, other diagnostic tests (e.g., insulin tolerance test) are considered more reliable diagnostic indicators of growth hormone reserve.

■ **GI Hemorrhage** Vasopressin has been administered IV or intra-arterially† into the superior mesenteric artery as an adjunct in the treatment of acute, massive GI hemorrhage† caused by various conditions including esophageal varices, inflammatory bowel disease, peptic ulcer disease, esophagogastritis, esophageal laceration, acute gastritis, colitis associated with Behcet's disease, colonic diverticulosis, Mallory-Weiss syndrome, and intestinal perforation. The drug also has been infused into the mesenteric artery prior to and during portosystemic shunt surgery for esophageal varices. Use of vasopressin in such situations is a temporary measure, intended to decrease portal venous pressure and increase clotting and hemostasis. There is no evidence that the drug substantially improves overall survival. Although vasopressin is a potent splanchnic vasoconstrictor that may provide effective control of bleeding, the clinical usefulness of the drug is limited because of its adverse effects. In addition, there is a high recurrence of bleeding when the drug is discontinued. Current management of acute GI hemorrhage usually includes endoscopic therapy or a combination of endoscopy and pharmacologic therapy with a splanchnic vasoconstrictor (e.g., most commonly octreotide because of its longer duration of action and favorable adverse effect profile).

Dosage and Administration

■ **Administration** Vasopressin is administered by IV infusion for the management of vasodilatory shock. The drug also has been administered by IM† or subcutaneous† injection for other uses (e.g., postoperative abdominal distention, diabetes insipidus).

Vasopressin also has been applied topically† to the nasal mucosa (e.g., with a cotton pledget, nasal spray, or dropper) in the treatment of diabetes insipidus.

Vasopressin has been administered by intraosseous (IO)† injection for advanced cardiovascular life support (ACLS)†, generally when IV access is not readily available; onset of action and systemic concentrations of the drug are comparable to those achieved with venous administration. Vasopressin also has been administered endotracheally† when vascular (IV or IO) access cannot be established during cardiac arrest; however, IV or IO administration is preferred whenever possible because of more predictable drug delivery and pharmacologic effect.

In addition, the drug has been administered by intra-arterial infusion† in the management of GI hemorrhage†. Intra-arterial infusion of the drug requires specialized techniques, including angiographic placement of the catheter, and should only be performed by clinicians familiar with this method of administration and the management of potential complications. (See Cautions: Adverse Effects.)

IV Administration For IV administration, vasopressin is commercially available as a 20-units/mL injection that should be further diluted with 0.9% sodium chloride or 5% dextrose injection prior to administration. The manufacturer recommends dilution to a final concentration of 0.1 or 1 unit/mL depending on the patient's fluid status. In patients who are not fluid restricted, a concentration of 0.1 units/mL may be prepared by mixing 50 units (2.5 mL) of vasopressin injection with 500 mL of diluent. In patients who are fluid restricted, a more concentrated solution of 1 unit/mL may be prepared by mixing 100 units (5 mL) of vasopressin injection with 100 mL of diluent.

Unused portions of the diluted solution should be discarded after 18 hours at room temperature or 24 hours under refrigeration. Vasopressin solutions should be inspected visually for particulate matter and discoloration prior to administration.

■ **Dosage** Vasopressin dosage requirements are variable and must be adjusted according to patient response. In order to avoid adverse effects, it is desirable to give doses that are just sufficient to elicit the desired response.

Vasodilatory Shock The manufacturer states that dosage of vasopressin is empiric for the management of vasodilatory shock; in general, dosage should be titrated to the lowest dose compatible with a clinically acceptable response. The goal of therapy is to optimize and maintain perfusion to critical organs without causing ischemic complications.

The manufacturer recommends an initial vasopressin dosage of 0.03 units/minute in adults with postcardiotomy shock and 0.01 units/minute in adults with septic shock. If target blood pressure response is not achieved, the infusion rate may be increased by 0.005 units/minute at intervals of 10–15 minutes to a maximum dosage of 0.1 units/minute for postcardiotomy shock or 0.07 units/minute for septic shock. Some experts recommend that infusion rates higher than 0.03 units/minute be used with caution because of the risk of cardiac and peripheral ischemia. After target blood pressure has been maintained for 8 hours without the use of catecholamines, the vasopressin infusion rate should be tapered by 0.005 units/minute every hour as tolerated to maintain target blood pressure.

Advanced Cardiovascular Life Support For advanced cardiovascular life support (ACLS) in patients with cardiac arrest†, vasopressin has been given in a single dose of 40 units by IV or IO† injection as a replacement for the first or second dose of epinephrine. (See Uses: Advanced Cardiovascular Life Support.)

Diabetes Insipidus For the treatment of central diabetes insipidus†, vasopressin has been given in an adult dosage of 5–10 units 2–3 times daily as needed by IM or subcutaneous injection. Dosage has ranged from 5–60 units daily. In children, vasopressin has been given in proportionately reduced doses of 2.5–10 units by IM or subcutaneous injection 2–4 times daily. For the treatment of diabetes insipidus, vasopressin also has been administered intranasally at individualized dosages.

Abdominal Distention and Abdominal Radiographic Procedures For the management of postoperative abdominal distention† in adults, vasopressin has been administered at an initial dose of 5 units by IM injection. Subsequent injections have been given every 3–4 hours with doses increased to 10 units if necessary. In children, proportionately reduced doses have been used.

For use in abdominal roentgenography†, it has been suggested that two 10-unit IM or subcutaneous injections of vasopressin be administered, the first injection at 2 hours and the second injection at 30 minutes, prior to exposure of the radiograph; many clinicians recommend giving an enema prior to the first dose of vasopressin.

Diagnostic Uses When used as a provocative test for growth hormone and corticotropin release†, vasopressin injection has been given IM in a dose of 10 units for adults and 0.3 units/kg for children.

GI Hemorrhage For the management of GI hemorrhage†, vasopressin has been administered by continuous IV or intra-arterial infusion after dilution with 0.9% sodium chloride or 5% dextrose injection to a concentration of 0.1–1 unit/mL. Continuous IV rather than intra-arterial infusion of the drug is preferred. (See Uses: GI Hemorrhage.)

For IV infusion in patients with GI hemorrhage, vasopressin has been infused into a peripheral vein via a controlled infusion device. For continuous intra-arterial infusion in patients with esophageal varices or upper GI bleeding, the drug has been infused into the superior or inferior mesenteric artery via a controlled infusion device.

For the management of GI bleeding†, dosage of vasopressin is empiric and must be individualized according to the response and tolerance of the patient. Because many of the adverse effects of vasopressin are dose related, the lowest possible effective dosage should be used. Some experts recommend continuous use of vasopressin for no longer than 24 hours. IV dosage generally has been initiated at 0.2–0.4 units/minute and progressively increased to a maximum of 0.6–0.9 units/minute if necessary based on individual patient response. To minimize adverse effects, some experts recommend concomitant use of IV nitroglycerin (initiated at 40 mcg/minute, increased to a maximum of 400 mcg/minute). When vasopressin is administered by intra-arterial infusion, a dosage of 0.1–0.5 units/minute has been used.

■ **Dosage in Hepatic and Renal Impairment** There is limited information regarding exposure of vasopressin in patients with hepatic impairment and no specific dosage recommendations are available for such patients; dosage should be titrated to effect.

There is limited information regarding exposure of vasopressin in patients with renal impairment and no specific dosage recommendations are available for such patients; dosage should be titrated to effect.

Cautions

■ **Adverse Effects** Adverse effects associated with low doses of vasopressin are infrequent and mild, but increase in frequency and severity with high doses. Reported adverse effects include circumoral pallor, sweating, tremor, pounding in the head, abdominal cramps, passage of gas, vertigo, nausea, vomiting, and eructation. In addition, diarrhea, intestinal hyperactivity, and uterine cramps may occur. Some manufacturers state that blanching of the skin, abdominal cramps, and nausea that may occur following subcutaneous or IM injection of the drug can be minimized by drinking 1 or 2 glasses of water at the time of vasopressin administration. Vasopressin may also increase plasma cortisol concentrations and serum concentrations of growth hormone.

In large doses, vasopressin may produce increased blood pressure, bradycardia, minor arrhythmias, premature atrial contraction, heart block, peripheral vascular constriction or collapse, coronary insufficiency, decreased cardiac output, myocardial ischemia, or myocardial infarction. In patients with vascular disease (especially of the coronary arteries), even small doses of the drug can precipitate angina. Coronary vasodilators (e.g., nitroglycerin) may be used to treat angina if it occurs. An ECG should be used to monitor the hormone's cardiac effects during IV or intra-arterial therapy.

Adverse effects reported in the published literature with IV vasopressin in patients with vasodilatory shock include hemorrhagic shock, decreased platelets, intractable bleeding, right heart failure, atrial fibrillation, bradycardia, myocardial ischemia, mesenteric ischemia, increased bilirubin levels, acute renal insufficiency, distal limb ischemia, hyponatremia, and ischemic lesions.

When fluid intake is not excessive, there is little danger involved in the use of small antidiuretic doses of vasopressin to control diabetes insipidus. Overhydration was more likely to occur with the long-acting suspension of vasopressin tannate (no longer commercially available in the US) than with vasopressin injection; infants and children are often much more susceptible to such volume disturbances than are adults. If water intoxication occurs, some experts have recommended that vasopressin be discontinued and fluid intake restricted until the specific gravity of the urine decreases to less than 1.015 and polyuria occurs. In severe overhydration, osmotic diuresis with mannitol, hypertonic dextrose, or urea, alone or in conjunction with furosemide, is often effective in rapidly decreasing fluid overload. Hypertonic saline solutions are not indicated unless immediate correction of hyponatremia is required.

Hypersensitivity reactions characterized by urticaria, angioedema, bronchoconstriction, fever, rash, wheezing, dyspnea, circulatory collapse, cardiac arrest, and anaphylaxis have been reported with vasopressin administration. Appropriate agents for the treatment of hypersensitivity reactions should be readily available.

Coronary thrombosis, mesenteric infarction, venous thrombosis, infarction and necrosis of the small bowel, and peripheral emboli resulting from intra-arterial catheterization have been reported following infusion of vasopressin injection into the superior mesenteric artery. In one patient, intra-arterial injection of vasopressin produced mottling and cyanosis of the left foot. Several patients reportedly developed signs of cutaneous gangrene proximal to the site of IV infusion of the drug. Bilateral nipple necrosis, which gradually resolved over 10–14 days after discontinuance of the drug, has occurred in at least 2 patients during IV infusion of the drug. Reversible ischemic colitis has been reported in a patient receiving IV infusion of the drug for the management of variceal hemorrhage.

■ **Precautions and Contraindications** Vasopressin should be used cautiously in preoperative and postoperative polyuric patients, since hormone requirements in these patients may be considerably less than normal. Fluid intake and output should be monitored closely, especially in comatose or semicomatose patients. Electrolyte balance also should be monitored periodically. Patients receiving vasopressin should be observed for early signs of water intoxication such as drowsiness, listlessness, headache, confusion, anuria, and weight gain in order to prevent ensuing seizures, coma, and death.

Vasopressin should be used cautiously in patients with seizure disorders, migraine, asthma, heart failure, vascular disease (especially of the coronary arteries), angina pectoris, coronary thrombosis, renal disease, goiter with cardiac complications, arteriosclerosis, or any other disease in which rapid addition to extracellular fluids may be hazardous. ECG monitoring should be performed periodically during therapy with the drug. Patients with impaired cardiac response may experience worsening cardiac output.

Aggressive treatment with vasopressin in patients with vasodilatory shock can compromise perfusion of organs, including those of the GI tract, whose function is difficult to monitor. Dosage should be titrated to the lowest dose compatible with a clinically acceptable response.

Geriatric patients and children are particularly sensitive to the effects of vasopressin; therefore, the drug should be used cautiously in these patients.

Vasopressin is contraindicated in patients with known allergy or hypersensitivity (e.g., anaphylaxis) to synthetic vasopressin (8-L-arginine vasopressin) or chlorobutanol (a preservative in the formulation). Some manufacturers have stated that the drug is also contraindicated in patients with chronic nephritis accompanied by nitrogen retention and should not be used until reasonable nitrogen concentrations are attained.

■ **Pediatric Precautions** The manufacturer states that safety and efficacy of vasopressin in pediatric patients with vasodilatory shock have not been established. Although the drug has been evaluated in several studies for the treatment of pediatric vasodilatory shock, inconclusive results were reported and a wide range of doses were employed.

■ **Geriatric Precautions** Clinical studies of vasopressin did not include sufficient numbers of patients 65 years of age and older to determine whether geriatric patients respond differently than younger patients. Clinical experience to date has not identified any differences in response between geriatric and younger patients. In general, dosage selection in geriatric patients should be cautious, usually starting at the low end of the dosage range, since renal, hepatic, and cardiovascular dysfunction and concomitant disease or other drug therapy are more common in this age group.

■ **Pregnancy and Lactation** There are no adequate or well-controlled studies of vasopressin in pregnant women, and animal reproduction studies with the drug have not been conducted. It is not known whether vasopressin can cause fetal harm when administered to pregnant women or can affect reproduction capacity; the drug should be used during pregnancy only if the potential benefits justify the potential risks to a fetus.

Vasopressin may produce tonic uterine contractions that could threaten the continuation of pregnancy.

Clearance of vasopressin is increased in the second and third trimester of pregnancy; dosages exceeding 0.1 units/minute may be required in patients with postcardiotomy shock and dosages exceeding 0.07 units/minute may be required in patients with septic shock.

It is not known whether vasopressin is distributed into human milk. Some manufacturers recommend that the drug be used with caution in nursing women.

Oral absorption of vasopressin in a nursing infant is considered unlikely since the drug is rapidly destroyed in the GI tract. Consideration may be given to advising a lactating woman to pump and discard her breast milk for 1.5 hours after receiving vasopressin to minimize potential exposure to the infant.

Drug Interactions

■ **Alcohol** Alcohol may decrease the antidiuretic effects of vasopressin.

■ **Catecholamines** Concomitant use of catecholamines and vasopressin is expected to result in additive effects on mean arterial blood pressure and other hemodynamic parameters.

■ **Drugs Causing Diabetes Insipidus** Drugs suspected of causing diabetes insipidus (e.g., demeclocycline, lithium, foscarnet, clozapine) may decrease the pressor effect and antidiuretic activity of vasopressin.

■ **Drugs Causing Syndrome of Inappropriate Secretion of Antidiuretic Hormone** Drugs suspected of causing syndrome of inappropriate secretion of antidiuretic hormone (SIADH) (e.g., selective serotonin-reuptake inhibitors [SSRIs], tricyclic antidepressants, haloperidol, chlorpropamide, enalapril, methyldopa, pentamidine, vincristine, cyclophosphamide, ifosfamide, felbamate) may increase the pressor effect and antidiuretic activity of vasopressin.

■ **Furosemide** Furosemide increases the effect of vasopressin on osmolar clearance and urine flow. Furosemide increased osmolar clearance and urine flow by 4 and 9 times, respectively, in healthy subjects receiving vasopressin.

■ **Ganglionic Blocking Agents** Ganglionic blocking agents may markedly increase sensitivity to the pressor effects of vasopressin. In healthy individuals, administration of tetra-ethylammonium (a ganglionic blocking agent) increased the pressor effect of vasopressin by 20%.

■ **Heparin** Heparin may decrease the antidiuretic effects of vasopressin.

■ **Indomethacin** Indomethacin may prolong the effects of vasopressin on peripheral vascular resistance and cardiac output.

■ **Norepinephrine** Norepinephrine may decrease the antidiuretic effects of vasopressin.

Pharmacology

Exogenous vasopressin elicits all the pharmacologic responses usually produced by endogenous vasopressin (antidiuretic hormone). The primary physiologic role of vasopressin is to maintain serum osmolality within a normal range. The hormone produces relatively concentrated urine by increasing reabsorption of water by the renal tubules. Its action in regulating body fluid balance is mediated by renal vasopressin V_2 receptors, which are coupled to adenyl cyclase and the generation of cyclic AMP. At the tubular level, vasopressin stimulates adenyl cyclase activity, leading to increases in cyclic adenosine monophosphate (AMP). Cyclic AMP increases water permeability at the luminal surface of the distal convoluted tubule and collecting duct, resulting in increased urine osmolality and decreased urinary flow rate. The antidiuretic activity of vasopressin conserves up to 90% of the water that might otherwise be excreted in the urine. Vasopressin also increases reabsorption of urea by the collecting ducts. Although solute diuresis does not generally occur, increased sodium and decreased potassium reabsorption have been induced by vasopressin. Vasopressin, however, plays no etiologic role in edema formation.

In doses greater than those required for antidiuretic effects, vasopressin directly stimulates contraction of smooth muscle V_1 receptors. The vasoconstrictive action of vasopressin is mediated by vascular V_1 receptors; the vascular receptors are coupled to phospholipase C, resulting in release of calcium from sarcoplasmic reticulum in smooth muscle cells, leading to vasoconstriction. The hormone exhibits relatively little vasoconstrictor effect in hemodynamically normal individuals, but is an important endogenous vasopressor when arterial pressure is threatened. Vasopressin causes vasoconstriction, particularly of capillaries and of small arterioles, resulting in decreased blood flow to the splanchnic, coronary, GI, pancreatic, skin, and muscular systems. At therapeutic doses, vasopressin elicits a vasoconstrictive effect in most vascular beds, including the splanchnic, renal, and cutaneous circulation. When administered into the celiac or superior mesenteric arteries, vasopressin constricts gastroduodenal, left gastric, superior mesenteric, and splenic arteries; however, hepatic arteries are not constricted and, instead, hepatic blood flow often increases. When used to produce antidiuresis, vasopressin has little effect on blood pressure. The drug indirectly decreases coronary blood flow and may precipitate myocardial infarction. In addition, the hormone can decrease heart rate and cardiac output and increase pulmonary arterial pressure and blood pressure.

Patients with septic shock or postcardiotomy shock appear to have a relative deficiency of endogenous vasopressin, which can contribute to the vasodilatory hypotension observed in these shock states. When administered in therapeutic doses to patients with vasodilatory shock, vasopressin increases systemic vascular resistance and mean arterial blood pressure. In addition, the drug tends to decrease heart rate and cardiac output. The pressor effect of vasopressin is proportional to the infusion rate of the drug. No evidence of tachyphylaxis or tolerance to the pressor effect of vasopressin has been observed.

Endogenous vasopressin concentrations in patients undergoing cardiopulmonary resuscitation (CPR) are higher in those who survive than in those who do not have return to spontaneous circulation (ROSC). This finding suggested that exogenous vasopressin might be beneficial during cardiac arrest. (See Uses: Advanced Cardiovascular Life Support.) After ventricular fibrillation of short duration, administration of vasopressin during CPR has increased coronary perfusion pressure, vital organ blood flow, ventricular fibrillation median frequency, and cerebral oxygen delivery. Similar findings have been reported with prolonged cardiac arrest and pulseless electrical activity. The hormone did not result in bradycardia after ROSC. Interaction of vasopressin with V_1 receptors during CPR causes intense peripheral vasoconstriction of skin, skeletal muscle, intestine, and fat with relatively less vasoconstriction of coronary and renal vascular beds and vasodilatation of cerebral vasculature. Vasopressin does not exhibit β-adrenergic activity and therefore does not produce skeletal muscle vasodilatation or increased myocardial oxygen consumption during CPR.

At pressor doses, vasopressin triggers contraction of smooth muscles in the GI tract mediated by muscular V_1 receptors and release of prolactin and ACTH via V_3 receptors. In the intestinal tract, vasopressin increases peristaltic activity, particularly of the large bowel. Vasopressin also causes an increase in GI sphincter pressure and a decrease in gastric secretion but has no effect on gastric acid concentration.

The oxytocic properties of vasopressin are minimal, but in large doses the drug may stimulate uterine contraction. The hormone also possesses slight milk ejecting properties but its role during lactation is negligible.

In addition to its peripheral effects, vasopressin causes release of corticotropin, growth hormone, and follicle-stimulating hormone.

Pharmacokinetics

■ **Absorption** Vasopressin is destroyed by trypsin, which is found in the GI tract, and, therefore, must be administered parenterally or intranasally. Absorption of vasopressin through the nasal mucosa is relatively poor. Following subcutaneous or IM administration of vasopressin injection, the duration of antidiuretic activity is variable but effects are usually maintained for 2–8 hours. Urine isotonicity is maintained when plasma concentrations of vasopressin are approximately 1 microunit/mL, while plasma concentrations of 4.5–6 microunits/mL produce maximum concentration of urine. Following IV infusion of vasopressin in patients with vasodilatory shock, onset of the pressor effect is rapid, with peak effects occurring within 15 minutes. Pressor effects fade within 20 minutes following discontinuance of infusion.

■ **Distribution** Vasopressin is distributed throughout the extracellular fluid; there is no evidence of plasma protein binding.

It is not known whether vasopressin is distributed into human milk.

■ **Elimination** Vasopressin is predominantly metabolized by the liver and kidneys. The drug is cleaved by serine protease, carboxipeptidase, and disulfide oxidoreductase at relevant sites for its pharmacologic activity; resulting metabolites are not expected to be pharmacologically active. Vasopressin has a plasma half-life of about 10–20 minutes. When administered by IV infusion at usual rates for vasodilatory shock (e.g., 0.1–1 units/minute), the apparent half-life is 10 minutes or less. Oxytocinase, a circulating enzyme produced early in pregnancy, is capable of cleaving the polypeptide; otherwise, plasma inactivation of vasopressin is negligible. Approximately 5% of a subcutaneous dose of vasopressin is excreted in urine unchanged after 4 hours, and following IV administration, 5–15% of the total vasopressin dosage appears in urine.

Chemistry and Stability

■ **Chemistry** Vasopressin is a polypeptide hormone secreted by the neurons of the supraoptic and paraventricular nuclei of the hypothalamus and stored in the posterior pituitary (neurohypophysis) in mammals. In humans and most other mammals, the natural hormone is arginine vasopressin. Commercially available vasopressin injection is an aqueous solution of synthetic arginine vasopressin. The potency of vasopressin (arginine) is standardized according to its pressor activity in rats and is expressed in USP Posterior Pituitary (pressor) Units. Antidiuretic activity of the commercially available preparations may be variable.

Vasopressin is soluble in water. Vasopressin injection for IV infusion contains a sodium acetate buffer to adjust the pH to 3.8. Vasopressin injection solution contains chlorobutanol (anhydrous) as a preservative; glacial acetic acid and/or sodium hydroxide may be added during manufacture to adjust the pH to 2.5–4.5.

■ **Stability** Vasopressin injection for IV infusion should be stored at 2–8°C and should not be frozen. Unopened vials may be stored at room temperature (20–25°C) for up to 12 months or up to the manufacturer's labeled expiration date (whichever comes first); once removed from the refrigerator, the vials should be marked to indicate the revised 12-month expiration date (if it occurs before the manufacturer's labeled expiration date). Unused diluted solutions should be discarded after 18 hours at room temperature or after 24 hours under refrigeration.

Preparations

Excipients in commercially available drug preparations may have clinically important effects in some individuals; consult specific product labeling for details.

Vasopressin

Parenteral		
Injection, for IV infusion	20 units/mL	**Vasostrict®**, Par

†Use is not currently included in the labeling approved by the US Food and Drug Administration

Selected Revisions December 2017, © Copyright, May 1977, American Society of Health-System Pharmacists, Inc.

PROGESTINS 68:32

Progestins General Statement

■ Progestins elicit, to varying degrees, all the pharmacologic responses usually produced by progesterone.

Uses

Progesterone is used to support embryo implantation and early pregnancy by supplementing corpus luteal function as part of assisted reproductive technology (ART) treatment of infertile women.

Progestins are used in the treatment of functional uterine bleeding caused by hormonal imbalance and involving a hyperplastic nonsecretory endometrium and the absence of underlying organic pathology such as fibroids or uterine cancer, and for the treatment of primary and secondary amenorrhea in the presence of estrogen. Medroxyprogesterone also is used in the adjunctive and palliative treatment of some cancers. (See the individual monographs in 68:32.) Some progestins are used alone or in combination with estrogens for the prevention of conception. (See Progestins 68:12 and Estrogen-Progestin Combinations 68:12.) Medroxyprogesterone prevents follicular maturation and ovulation following IM administration, and the drug has been used parenterally for contraception. (See Uses: Contraception in Females in Medroxyprogesterone Acetate 68:32.)

Progestins (e.g., drospirenone, medroxyprogesterone, norethindrone acetate, norgestimate, progesterone) are used to reduce the incidence of endometrial hyperplasia and the attendant risk of endometrial carcinoma in postmenopausal women receiving estrogen replacement therapy. (See Uses: Prevention of Endometrial Changes Associated with Estrogens in Medroxyprogesterone Acetate 68:32.) Morphologic and biochemical studies of the endometrium suggest that 10–13 days of progestin are needed to provide maximum maturation of the endometrium and to eliminate any hyperplastic changes.

For other uses of progestins, see Uses in Medroxyprogesterone Acetate 68:32.

Although progestins have been used beginning in the first trimester of pregnancy to prevent habitual abortion or to treat threatened abortion, there is no adequate evidence from well-controlled studies to substantiate the efficacy of progestins for these uses; however, there is evidence of potential adverse effects on the fetus when these drugs are administered during the first 4 months of pregnancy. (See Cautions: Pregnancy and Lactation.) Although some progestins were previously used to induce withdrawal bleeding as a test for pregnancy when laboratory tests were not readily available, progestins are currently *contraindicated* for this use.

Cautions

■ **Adverse Effects** Progestins may cause breakthrough bleeding, spotting, changes in menstrual flow, amenorrhea, changes in cervical erosion and secretions, edema, weight gain or loss, nausea, cholestatic jaundice, allergic rash with or without pruritus, anaphylactoid reactions and anaphylaxis, melasma or chloasma, pyrexia, somnolence or insomnia, and mental depression.

An association between pulmonary embolism and cerebral thrombosis and embolism and use of estrogen-progestin combination preparations has been shown. (See Thromboembolic Disorders in Cautions: Cardiovascular Effects, in Estrogen-Progestin Combinations 68:12.) The possibility that thromboembolic disorders may occur in patients receiving progestins should be considered and patients should be carefully observed for these effects during therapy with the drugs. (See Cautions: Precautions and Contraindications.)

Although available evidence suggests that an association exists between neuro-ocular lesions such as optic neuritis or retinal thrombosis and use of estrogen-progestin combination preparations, such a relationship has been neither confirmed nor refuted. Increased blood pressure in susceptible individuals, premenstrual-like syndrome, changes in libido or appetite, cystitis-like syndrome, headache, nervousness, dizziness, fatigue, backache, hirsutism, loss of scalp hair, erythema multiforme or nodosum, hemorrhagic skin eruption, and itching have occurred in patients receiving estrogen-progestin combination preparations. Use of estrogen-progestin combinations has also been associated with increased levels of coagulation factors VII, VIII, IX, and X. The possibility that these effects may occur in patients receiving progestins should be considered and patients should be carefully observed for these effects during therapy with the drugs.

Because drospirenone has antimineralocorticoid activity, the potential exists for hyperkalemia to occur in high-risk patients (e.g., those with renal or hepatic impairment, adrenal insufficiency) receiving this progestin.

■ **Precautions and Contraindications** Because oral contraceptive combinations contain progestins, the precautions associated with oral contraceptives should generally be considered in patients receiving progestins. (See Cautions in Estrogen-Progestin Combinations 68:12.) Prior to initiation of therapy with progestins in women, a physical examination should be performed, including special attention to the breasts and pelvic organs and a Papanicolaou test (Pap smear). Women receiving progestins should be given a copy of the patient labeling for the drugs.

Progestins should be used with caution, and only with careful monitoring, in patients with conditions that might be aggravated by fluid retention (e.g., asthma, seizure disorders, migraine, or cardiac or renal dysfunction). Progestins should also be used with caution in patients with a history of mental depression; the drugs should be discontinued if depression recurs to a serious degree during progestin therapy.

When breakthrough bleeding or irregular vaginal bleeding occurs during progestin therapy, nonfunctional causes should be considered. Adequate diagnostic procedures should be performed in patients with undiagnosed vaginal bleeding.

The effect of long-term progestin therapy on pituitary, ovarian, adrenal, hepatic, or uterine function has not been determined. Diabetic patients should be carefully monitored during progestin therapy, since decreased glucose tolerance has been observed in women receiving estrogen-progestin combinations. Progestins may mask the onset of climacteric in women.

The clinician and the patient using progestins should be alert to the earliest signs and symptoms of thromboembolic and thrombotic disorders (e.g., thrombophlebitis, pulmonary embolism, cerebrovascular insufficiency, coronary occlusion, retinal thrombosis, mesenteric thrombosis). Progestins should be discontinued immediately when any of these disorders occurs or is suspected.

A safety review conducted by the US Food and Drug Administration (FDA) indicates that use of combination oral contraceptives containing the progestin drospirenone may be associated with an increased risk of venous thromboembolism (VTE) compared with that of oral contraceptives containing levonorgestrel or other progestins. This conclusion was based on results of several epidemiologic studies evaluating the risk of VTE in women using oral contraceptives containing drospirenone. These studies reported that the risk of VTE in such women ranged from no increase to a threefold increase in risk. The FDA's safety review was prompted by results of 2 recent case-control studies that showed a twofold to threefold increased risk of VTE (including deep-vein thrombosis and pulmonary embolism) in patients receiving oral contraceptives containing drospirenone compared with those receiving oral contraceptives containing the progestin levonorgestrel. These studies evaluated cases of idiopathic VTE occurring in women 15–44 years of age who were current users of oral contraceptives containing 30 mcg of estrogen with either drospirenone or levonorgestrel; women with risk factors for VTE were excluded from the studies. The FDA has also reviewed data from a large US retrospective cohort study in more than 800,000 women evaluating thrombotic and thromboembolic risks (including VTE) associated with hormonal contraceptives. Final results from this study suggest an increased risk of VTE (hazard ratio greater than 1) in women using oral contraceptives containing drospirenone compared with women using other hormonal contraceptives.

Given the conflicting results of the previous epidemiologic studies and the recent findings, the FDA held a joint meeting of the Reproductive Health Drugs Advisory Committee and the Drug Safety and Risk Management Advisory Committee on December 8, 2011, to review the risks and benefits of such therapy and specifically to discuss the risk of VTE associated with drospirenone-containing hormonal contraceptives. The studies reviewed by the FDA did not provide consistent data for the comparative risk of thromboembolic events between oral contraceptives that contain drospirenone and those that do not. In addition, the studies did not account for important known and unknown patient characteristics that may influence prescribing patterns and may affect risk of VTE. For these reasons, the FDA states that it is unclear whether the increased risk of thromboembolic events observed in these epidemiologic studies actually resulted from use of drospirenone-containing oral contraceptives. At this time, the FDA has concluded that the risk of VTE may be higher for such oral contraceptives and will continue to communicate any new safety information as it becomes available.

Oral contraceptive combinations containing drospirenone should be discontinued if an arterial or venous thrombotic event occurs during therapy. The risk of VTE is highest during the first year of oral contraceptive use. Results from a large, prospective cohort safety study of various estrogen-progestin oral contraceptives suggest that this increased risk is highest during the first 6 months of use compared with that in nonusers. Data from this safety study indicate that the highest risk of VTE occurs after initiation of estrogen-progestin oral contraceptive therapy or resumption of therapy (following a 4-week or longer drug-free interval) with the same or a different oral contraceptive combination. Before initiating use of an estrogen-progestin combination containing drospirenone in a new user or in a woman who is switching from an oral contraceptive not containing drospirenone, clinicians should consider the risks and benefits of drospirenone-containing oral contraceptives, including risk for developing VTE, specific to that woman.

Women currently receiving an oral contraceptive combination containing drospirenone should be informed of the potential risk of thromboembolic events. Patients also should be advised about the current information available regarding the risk of VTE with oral contraceptives containing drospirenone compared with those containing levonorgestrel. Patients should contact a clinician if they experience any signs or symptoms of VTE (e.g., persistent leg pain, severe chest pain, sudden shortness of breath). Known risk factors for development of VTE include smoking, obesity, family history, and other factors that contraindicate the use of oral contraceptive combinations. Patients should discuss their risk of VTE with their clinician before deciding which contraceptive method or hormonal contraceptive to use. The risk of thromboembolic disease associated with oral contraceptive use gradually disappears after such therapy is discontinued. However, the FDA states that patients should not discontinue oral contraceptives containing drospirenone without consulting a clinician.

If unexplained, sudden or gradual, partial or complete loss of vision; proptosis or diplopia; papilledema; retinal vascular lesions; or migraine occur during therapy with progestins, the drugs should be discontinued and appropriate diagnostic and therapeutic measures instituted. Because steroidal hormones are metabolized in the liver, progestins should be used with caution in patients with impaired liver function.

Drospirenone should not be used in patients who are predisposed to developing hyperkalemia (e.g., those with renal or hepatic impairment or adrenal insufficiency). If drospirenone is used in women receiving daily, long-term therapy with agents that may increase serum potassium concentrations (e.g., angiotensin-converting enzyme (ACE) inhibitors, angiotensin II type 1 (AT_1) receptor antagonists, potassium-sparing diuretics, potassium supplements, heparin, aldosterone antagonists [spironolactone], nonsteroidal anti-inflammatory agents [NSAIAs]), the serum potassium concentration should be determined during the first treatment cycle.

Progestins are contraindicated in patients with thrombophlebitis, thromboembolic disorders, cerebral apoplexy, or a history of these conditions. The drugs are also contraindicated in patients with undiagnosed vaginal bleeding, missed abortion, known sensitivity to the drug or any ingredient in the formulation, markedly impaired liver function or liver disease, or carcinoma of the breast or for use as a pregnancy test.

■ **Mutagenicity and Carcinogenicity** The carcinogenic and mutagenic potentials of progestins have not been fully determined.

Administration of medroxyprogesterone to beagles has been associated with the development of mammary nodules, some of which were malignant. Although nodules occasionally occurred in control beagles, they were intermittent in nature; nodules in drug-treated beagles were larger, more numerous, persistent, and occasionally malignant with metastases. The clinical relevance of these findings to humans has not been established. For additional information on the carcinogenic potential of progestins, see Cautions: Mutagenicity and Carcinogenicity, in Medroxyprogesterone Acetate 68:32.

■ **Pregnancy and Lactation** Progesterone is used to support embryo implantation and maintain pregnancy as a component of assisted reproductive technology (ART) treatment in infertile women. Such use is associated with increased ongoing pregnancy rates.

Although progestins have been used beginning in the first trimester of pregnancy to prevent habitual abortion or to treat threatened abortion, there is no adequate evidence from well-controlled studies to substantiate the efficacy of progestins for these uses; however, there is evidence of potential adverse effects on the fetus when these drugs are administered during the first 4 months of pregnancy. In addition, in most women, the cause of abortion is a defective ovum, which progestins could not be expected to influence. Because of their uterine-relaxant effects, progestins may delay spontaneous abortion of fertilized defective ova. Masculinization of the female fetus has reportedly occurred when progestins were used during pregnancy. Clitoral hypertrophy and fusion of the labia have been reported in a few female neonates born to women who had received medroxyprogesterone during pregnancy; hypospadias in male neonates born to women receiving progestational agents occurs at approximately twice the rate of occurrence in male neonates born to women not receiving the drugs. An association between intrauterine exposure to female sex hormones and congenital anomalies, including cardiovascular and limb defects, has been suggested. (See Cautions: Pregnancy, Fertility, and Lactation, in Estrogen-Progestin Combinations 68:12.) Use of progestins generally is not recommended during the first 4 months of pregnancy. If a woman becomes pregnant while receiving progestins or is inadvertently exposed to the drugs during the first 4 months of pregnancy, she should be advised of the potential risks to the fetus.

Progestins should *not* be used to induce withdrawal bleeding as a test for pregnancy.

Progestins are reportedly distributed into milk. The possible effects of progestins in milk on nursing infants have not been determined.

Laboratory Test Interferences

Estrogen-progestin combinations have caused abnormal thyroid function test results. (See Effects on Thyroid in Cautions: Endocrine and Metabolic Effects, in Estrogen-Progestin Combinations 68:12.) Estrogen-progestin combinations have altered the metyrapone test (see Laboratory Test Interferences in Estrogen-Progestin Combinations 68:12) and liver function test results (see Cautions: Hepatic Effects, in Estrogen-Progestin Combinations 68:12). These combinations have also caused decreased pregnanediol excretion.

The pathologist should be advised of progestin use when relevant specimens from a patient exposed to the drug are submitted.

Pharmacology

Progestins elicit, to varying degrees, all the pharmacologic responses usually produced by progesterone: induction of secretory changes in the endometrium, increase in basal body temperature (thermogenic action), production of histologic changes in vaginal epithelium, relaxation of uterine smooth muscle, stimulation of mammary alveolar tissue growth, pituitary inhibition, and production of withdrawal bleeding in the presence of estrogen. For further discussion on the pharmacologic effects of progestins, see Progesterone and the other individual monographs in 68:32.

Chemistry

The use of progesterone, a hormone secreted by the corpus luteum, is well established in medicine. Its relative inactivity following oral administration and the local reactions and pain sometimes produced upon injection have led to the synthesis of chemical derivatives that are effective orally, are more potent, more specific in action, or have a longer duration of action.

Ethisterone was the first synthetic progestin developed; the drug is not currently available. 19-Nor,17-acetoxy, and 6-methyl derivatives, which exhibit interesting structural-pharmacologic relationships, have been synthesized. Some estrogenic or androgenic activity, anabolic effects, nitrogen retention, and weight gain are exhibited by the 19-nor derivatives. The 17-hydroxy or acetoxy compounds, on the other hand, elicit responses more nearly resembling those of progesterone. They have little or no estrogenic or androgenic activity and may produce catabolic and slight diuretic effects. The 19-nor derivatives are more effective in postponing the normal menstrual period.

For further information on chemistry and stability, pharmacology, uses, cautions, and dosage and administration of progestins, see the individual monographs in 68:32 and the monographs on Estrogen-Progestin Combinations and Progestins in 68:12.

HYDROXYprogesterone Caproate

■ Hydroxyprogesterone caproate is a synthetic progestin.

Uses

■ **Preterm Birth Risk Reduction** Hydroxyprogesterone caproate is used to reduce the risk of preterm birth in women with a singleton pregnancy who have a history of singleton spontaneous preterm birth. Hydroxyprogesterone caproate has been designated an orphan drug by the US Food and Drug Administration (FDA) for this use. Efficacy of the drug for this use is based on improvement in the proportion of women who delivered at less than 37 weeks of gestation; direct clinical benefit (e.g., improvement in neonatal morbidity and mortality) has not been established. While there are many risk factors for preterm birth, safety and efficacy of hydroxyprogesterone caproate have been demonstrated only in women with a prior spontaneous singleton birth; hydroxyprogesterone is not intended for use in women with multiple gestations or other risk factors for preterm birth. The American College of Obstetricians and Gynecologists (ACOG) recommends that progesterone supplementation for the prevention of recurrent preterm birth be offered to women with a singleton pregnancy and a prior spontaneous preterm birth at less than 37 weeks of gestation due to spontaneous preterm labor or premature rupture of membranes.

Safety and efficacy of hydroxyprogesterone caproate for risk reduction of spontaneous preterm birth have been evaluated in a multicenter, randomized, double-blind, placebo-controlled study in 463 women 16–43 years of age with a singleton pregnancy who had a documented history of singleton spontaneous preterm birth (defined as delivery at less than 37 weeks of gestation following spontaneous preterm labor or premature rupture of membranes). Patients were randomized to receive weekly IM injections of either hydroxyprogesterone caproate 250 mg or placebo starting between 16 weeks, 0 days and 20 weeks, 6 days of gestation and continuing until 37 weeks of gestation or delivery, whichever occurred first. The proportion of women who delivered preterm at less than 37 weeks of gestation, the primary end point, was lower in patients receiving hydroxyprogesterone caproate compared with those receiving placebo (37.1 versus 54.9%). The proportion of women delivering at less than 35 and 32 weeks of gestation also was lower in patients receiving hydroxyprogesterone caproate (21.3 and 11.9%, respectively) compared with those receiving placebo (30.7 and 19.6%, respectively). After adjusting for time in the study, 7.5% of patients receiving hydroxyprogesterone caproate delivered prior to 25 weeks of gestation compared with 4.7% of those receiving placebo. Miscarriages at less than 20 weeks of gestation and stillbirths were reported in 2.4 and 2%, respectively, of patients receiving hydroxyprogesterone caproate compared with 0 and 1.3%, respectively, of those receiving placebo; neonatal deaths were reported in 2.6% of patients receiving hydroxyprogesterone caproate compared with 5.9% of those receiving placebo. Because of the higher incidence of miscarriages and stillbirths in patients receiving hydroxyprogesterone caproate, no overall survival difference was observed. Although the proportion of neonates who experienced one or more events in a composite neonatal morbidity and mortality index (based on number of neonatal deaths, respiratory distress syndrome, bronchopulmonary dysplasia, grade 3 or 4 intraventricular hemorrhage, proven sepsis, necrotizing enterocolitis) was lower in the hydroxyprogesterone caproate group compared with the placebo group (11.9 versus 17.2%), the number of adverse outcomes was limited and the difference between groups was not statistically significant.

In a follow-up safety study, neurodevelopmental and other health outcomes of 278 surviving infants (mean age: 48 months) born to women enrolled in the randomized, double-blind, placebo-controlled study were evaluated to assess whether there were adverse effects of hydroxyprogesterone caproate evident after in utero exposure. The proportion of children whose scores met the screening threshold for developmental delay in each developmental domain of the Ages and Stages Questionnaire (i.e., communication, gross motor, fine motor, problem solving, and personal/social parameters) was similar in both the hydroxyprogesterone caproate and placebo groups. In addition, no substantial differences were observed in health status (e.g., type or incidence of diagnoses, caregivers' assessment of child's health); physical examination (e.g., physical abnormalities including genital anomalies, height, weight, head circumference, blood pressure, physical growth); or scores for gender-specific roles (as measured by the Preschool Activities Inventory) in both groups.

Dosage and Administration

■ Administration Hydroxyprogesterone caproate is administered by slow IM injection (over one minute or longer) by a clinician. Hydroxyprogesterone caproate should not be self-administered by the patient. The appropriate dose of hydroxyprogesterone caproate should be withdrawn from the vial using a 3-mL syringe with an 18-gauge needle; prior to administration, the 18-gauge needle should be replaced with a 21-gauge, 1.5-inch needle. After preparing the skin, hydroxyprogesterone caproate should be injected into the upper outer quadrant of the gluteus maximus. Bruising and swelling may be minimized by applying pressure to the injection site. Hydroxyprogesterone caproate injection is a clear, yellow, viscous, and oily solution; the drug should be discarded if the solution is cloudy or solid particles appear. Any unused portions of hydroxyprogesterone caproate should be discarded 5 weeks after first use. Hydroxyprogesterone caproate injection should be stored upright at 15–30°C in the original carton and protected from light.

Prior to the commercial availability of hydroxyprogesterone caproate injection (Makena®), another formulation containing the active ingredient was available to patients whose clinicians requested the drug from pharmacists who compounded the injection. To support access to hydroxyprogesterone caproate at this time and under this unique situation, the US Food and Drug Administration (FDA) does not intend to take enforcement action against pharmacies that compound hydroxyprogesterone caproate based on a valid prescription for an individually identified patient unless the compounded products are unsafe, of substandard quality, or are not being compounded in accordance with appropriate standards for compounding sterile products. The FDA may reconsider a decision to exercise enforcement discretion at any time.

■ Dosage The recommended adult dosage of hydroxyprogesterone caproate to reduce the risk of preterm birth in women with a singleton pregnancy who have a history of singleton spontaneous preterm birth is 250 mg once weekly (every 7 days) by slow IM injection. Treatment should begin between 16 weeks, 0 days and 20 weeks, 6 days of gestation, and continue once weekly until week 37 (through 36 weeks, 6 days) of gestation or delivery, whichever occurs first.

■ Special Populations The manufacturer makes no specific dosage recommendations at this time.

Cautions

■ Contraindications Current thrombosis or thromboembolic disorders or history of these conditions. (See Thromboembolic Disorders under Cautions: Warnings/Precautions.)

Known or suspected breast cancer, other hormone-sensitive cancer, or history of these conditions.

Undiagnosed abnormal vaginal bleeding unrelated to pregnancy.

Cholestatic jaundice of pregnancy. (See Jaundice under Cautions: Warnings/Precautions.)

Liver tumors (benign or malignant) or active liver disease.

Uncontrolled hypertension. (See Hypertension under Cautions: Warnings/Precautions.)

■ Warnings/Precautions ***Thromboembolic Disorders*** Hydroxyprogesterone caproate should be discontinued if an arterial or deep venous thrombotic or thromboembolic event occurs. Hydroxyprogesterone caproate is contraindicated in patients with current thrombosis or thromboembolic disorders or a history of these conditions.

Sensitivity Reactions Allergic reactions, including urticaria, pruritus, and angioedema, have been reported with hydroxyprogesterone caproate and other products containing castor oil. Discontinuance of hydroxyprogesterone caproate should be considered if such reactions occur.

Decreased Glucose Tolerance Decreased glucose tolerance has been observed in some patients receiving progestin therapy. The mechanism of this decrease is unknown. Patients with prediabetes or diabetes should be carefully monitored during hydroxyprogesterone caproate therapy.

Fluid Retention Because progestational agents may cause some degree of fluid retention, patients with conditions that may be aggravated by fluid retention (e.g., preeclampsia, epilepsy, migraine, asthma, cardiac or renal dysfunction) should be carefully monitored.

Depression Patients with a history of clinical depression should be monitored during therapy with hydroxyprogesterone caproate. Hydroxyprogesterone caproate should be discontinued if clinical depression recurs.

Jaundice Patients receiving hydroxyprogesterone caproate who develop jaundice should be carefully monitored, and clinicians should consider whether the benefit of hydroxyprogesterone use warrants continuation of therapy. Hydroxyprogesterone caproate is contraindicated in cholestatic jaundice of pregnancy.

Hypertension Patients receiving hydroxyprogesterone caproate who develop hypertension should be carefully monitored, and clinicians should consider whether the benefit of hydroxyprogesterone use warrants continuation of therapy. Hydroxyprogesterone caproate is contraindicated in patients with uncontrolled hypertension.

Specific Populations **Pregnancy.** Category B. (See Users Guide.) There are no adequate and well-controlled studies of hydroxyprogesterone caproate use in women during the first trimester of pregnancy. Data from a placebo-controlled study of pregnant women receiving hydroxyprogesterone caproate (250 mg weekly by IM injection) during their second and third trimesters, as well as a long-term (2–5 years) follow-up safety study of their infants, did not demonstrate any teratogenic risks to infants from in utero exposure to hydroxyprogesterone caproate. (See Uses: Preterm Birth Risk Reduction.)

Hydroxyprogesterone caproate is not intended for use to stop active preterm labor. The effect of hydroxyprogesterone caproate in active preterm labor is unknown.

Lactation. Detectable amounts of progestins have been identified in the milk of women receiving progestin therapy. Many studies have found no adverse effects of progestins on breast-feeding performance or on the health, growth, or development of the infant. However, hydroxyprogesterone caproate should be discontinued at 37 weeks of gestation or upon delivery.

Pediatric Use. Hydroxyprogesterone caproate is not indicated for use in pediatric patients. Safety and efficacy of hydroxyprogesterone caproate in pediatric patients younger than 16 years of age have not been established. A limited number of women younger than 18 years of age have been studied; safety and efficacy are expected to be the same in women 16 years of age or older compared with those 18 years of age or older.

Geriatric Use. Hydroxyprogesterone caproate has not been evaluated in women 65 years of age or older and is not intended for use in postmenopausal women. Safety and efficacy of hydroxyprogesterone caproate in postmenopausal women have not been established.

Hepatic Impairment. The effect of hepatic impairment on the pharmacokinetics of hydroxyprogesterone caproate has not been evaluated. Hydroxyprogesterone caproate is extensively metabolized and hepatic impairment may reduce elimination of the drug. Hydroxyprogesterone caproate is contraindicated in patients with liver tumors (benign or malignant) or active liver disease.

Renal Impairment. The effect of renal impairment on the pharmacokinetics of hydroxyprogesterone caproate has not been evaluated.

■ Common Adverse Effects Adverse effects reported in 2% or more of patients receiving hydroxyprogesterone caproate include injection site reactions (pain, swelling, pruritus, nodule), urticaria, pruritus, nausea, and diarrhea. Other adverse effects reported include miscarriage, stillbirth, admission for preterm labor (other than delivery), preeclampsia or gestational hypertension, oligohydramnios, pulmonary embolus, and injection site cellulitis.

Drug Interactions

No formal drug interaction studies have been performed to date with hydroxyprogesterone caproate.

■ **Drugs Affecting or Metabolized by Hepatic Microsomal Enzymes** Hydroxyprogesterone caproate is metabolized principally by cytochrome P-450 (CYP) isoenzymes 3A4 and 3A5.

An in vitro study indicated that hydroxyprogesterone caproate increased the metabolic rate of CYP isoenzymes 1A2, 2A6, and 2B6 by approximately 80, 150, and 80%, respectively. The clinical importance of this in vitro metabolic acceleration has not been fully elucidated. The metabolic induction potential of hydroxyprogesterone caproate has not been evaluated. The metabolism of drugs metabolized by CYP1A2 (e.g., clozapine, theophylline, tizanidine), CYP2A6 (e.g., acetaminophen, halothane, nicotine), and CYP2B6 (e.g., bupropion, efavirenz, methadone) may be increased during hydroxyprogesterone caproate therapy.

In vitro data indicate that therapeutic concentrations of hydroxyprogesterone caproate are unlikely to inhibit the activity of CYP isoenzymes 2C8, 2C9, 2C19, 2D6, 2E1, and 3A4.

Description

Hydroxyprogesterone caproate is a synthetic progestin produced by esterification of 17α-hydroxyprogesterone, a naturally occurring metabolite of progesterone, with caproic acid. Hydroxyprogesterone caproate injection is commercially available as a sterile solution of the drug in castor oil and benzyl benzoate with benzyl alcohol as a preservative. Hydroxyprogesterone caproate has strong progestogenic activity, and appears to produce a longer lasting and more potent progestational effect on the endometrium than progesterone. Hydroxyprogesterone caproate does not appear to have androgenic, antiandrogenic, estrogenic, or glucocorticoid activity. Although progesterone is known to have many actions beneficial to the maintenance of pregnancy, the mechanism of action of hydroxyprogesterone caproate in reducing the risk of recurrent preterm birth is not known.

In vitro, hydroxyprogesterone caproate can be metabolized by human hepatocytes via both phase I and II reactions. In vitro data indicate that metabolism of hydroxyprogesterone caproate is mediated principally by cytochrome P-450 (CYP) isoenzymes 3A4 and 3A5, and that the caproic acid group remains intact during metabolism. Hydroxyprogesterone caproate undergoes extensive reduction, hydroxylation, and conjugation. The conjugated metabolites include sulfated, glucuronidated, and acetylated products. The drug is excreted in urine and feces principally as conjugated metabolites and also as free steroids. Following IM administration in pregnant women at 10–12 weeks of gestation, approximately 50 and 30% of a dose was recovered in feces and urine, respectively. The elimination half-life of hydroxyprogesterone caproate is 7.8 days.

Advice to Patients

Importance of patients reading the manufacturer's patient information prior to initiation of therapy.

Risk of pain, soreness, swelling, itching, or bruising with injections of hydroxyprogesterone caproate. Importance of informing clinicians if increased discomfort, oozing of blood or fluid, or inflammatory reaction at the injection site occurs.

Importance of women informing clinicians if they are breast-feeding or plan to breast-feed.

Importance of informing clinicians of existing or contemplated concomitant therapy, including prescription and OTC drugs, vitamins, and herbal supplements, as well as any concomitant illnesses.

Importance of informing patients of other important precautionary information. (See Cautions.)

Overview® (see Users Guide). For additional information on this drug until a more detailed monograph is developed and published, the manufacturer's labeling should be consulted. It is *essential* that the manufacturer's labeling be consulted for more detailed information on usual cautions, precautions, contraindications, potential drug interactions, laboratory test interferences, and acute toxicity.

Preparations

Prior to the commercial availability of hydroxyprogesterone caproate injection (Makena®), another formulation containing the active ingredient was available to patients whose clinicians requested the drug from pharmacists who compounded the injection. (See Dosage and Administration: Administration.)

Excipients in commercially available drug preparations may have clinically important effects in some individuals; consult specific product labeling for details.

HYDROXYprogesterone Caproate

Parenteral

Injection, for IM use	250 mg/mL	**Makena®**, Ther-Rx

medroxyPROGESTERone Acetate

Acetoxymethylprogesterone, Methylacetoxyprogesterone

■ Medroxyprogesterone acetate is a synthetic progestin.

Uses

■ **Prevention of Endometrial Changes Associated with Estrogens** Medroxyprogesterone acetate is used orally to reduce the incidence of endometrial hyperplasia and the attendant risk of endometrial carcinoma in postmenopausal women receiving estrogen replacement therapy. When estrogens are used in combination with progestins, such therapy usually is referred to as hormone replacement therapy (HRT) or postmenopausal replacement therapy. Evidence from the Women's Health Initiative (WHI) study indicates that combined estrogen (conjugated estrogens 0.625 mg daily) and medroxyprogesterone acetate (2.5 mg daily) therapy in postmenopausal women is associated with increased risks of myocardial infarction, stroke, invasive breast cancer, pulmonary emboli, and deep-vein thrombosis. The risks identified in this study should be assumed to be similar with other hormonal regimens, including different dosages of these drugs as well as other estrogen/progestin combinations not studied in WHI, in the absence of comparable data to the contrary. If HRT is used, it should be prescribed in the lowest effective dosage and for the shortest duration consistent with treatment goals and risks for the individual women. (See Uses: Estrogen Replacement Therapy in the Estrogens General Statement 68:16.04.)

While there appears to be no increased risk of endometrial carcinoma in postmenopausal women receiving estrogen therapy for less than 1 year, prolonged estrogen therapy may be associated with an increased risk of such carcinoma. The risk of endometrial cancer reportedly is increased 2- to 12-fold in postmenopausal women receiving unopposed estrogen therapy compared with those not receiving estrogens; such increased risk may depend on dosage and duration of estrogen therapy and may be increased 15- to 24-fold in women receiving long-term (5 years or more) estrogen therapy. Limited data indicate that a substantial increased risk of endometrial carcinoma may persist for up to 15 years following discontinuance of estrogen therapy. Results of several studies indicate that addition of a progestin (e.g., medroxyprogesterone acetate) to estrogen replacement therapy reduces the incidence of endometrial hyperplasia and risk of endometrial carcinoma in women with an intact uterus. In a randomized, double-blind, controlled, multicenter study in postmenopausal women, endometrial hyperplasia occurred in 20 or 1% or less of women receiving conjugated estrogens alone or in conjunction with medroxyprogesterone acetate, respectively. Although estrogen-associated risk of endometrial carcinoma is substantially reduced when estrogens are administered concomitantly with progestins, a risk still exists. Therefore, clinical evaluation of all menopausal women receiving estrogen therapy in conjunction with a progestin is essential. Existing data do not support addition of a progestin in women who have undergone hysterectomy and are receiving estrogen replacement therapy.

Clinical studies indicate that use of a progestin in conjunction with estrogen replacement therapy does not interfere with the efficacy of the estrogen in the management of vasomotor symptoms associated with menopause, treatment of vulvar and vaginal atrophy, or prevention of osteoporosis. However, addition of a progestin to estrogen therapy may adversely affect some metabolic effects associated with long-term estrogen therapy and potential risks of concomitant therapy may include adverse effects on lipid metabolism and glucose tolerance. Results of several clinical studies in postmenopausal women indicate that replacement therapy with unopposed conjugated estrogens may reduce LDL-cholesterol and increase HDL-cholesterol by about 8–15%; concomitant progestin therapy may blunt some of the favorable effects of estrogens on the lipid profile of menopausal women. (See Pharmacology in the Estrogens General Statement 68:16.04.) Data from several studies suggest that administration of a progestin concomitantly with estrogen therapy is associated with an increased risk of breast cancer beyond that associated with estrogen alone. (See Carcinogenicity in the Estrogens General Statement 68:16.04.)

■ **Contraception in Females** Medroxyprogesterone acetate (alone or in fixed combination with estradiol cypionate) is used parenterally as a long-acting contraceptive in women.

Medroxyprogesterone acetate (e.g., Depo-Provera® Contraceptive, depo-subQ provera 104®) is used parenterally for the prevention of conception. However, long-term use of parenteral medroxyprogesterone is associated with loss in bone mineral density (BMD). The loss of BMD in women of all ages and the possible impact on peak bone mass in adolescents should be considered when assessing the risks versus benefits of this contraceptive method. Parenteral medroxyprogesterone should be used as a long-term contraceptive method (e.g., longer than 2 years) *only* if other contraceptive methods are inadequate and the benefits are expected to outweigh the risks. (See Cautions: Precautions and Contraindications). Contraceptive measures other than parenteral medroxyprogesterone should be considered in women at risk for osteoporosis. When used according to the prescribed regimen (once every 3 months), parenteral medroxyprogesterone used alone provides almost completely effective contraception. The pregnancy rate in women using the drug alone generally is reported as less than 1 pregnancy per 100 women-years of use (as calculated via the Pearl index method) or as ranging from 0–0.7% during the first year of use (as calculated via life-table analysis). Compared with common contraceptive methods (e.g., estrogen-progestin combinations, condoms) other than intrauterine devices, implants, and sterilization, for which efficacy depends in large part on the reliability of appropriate use (patient compliance), contraceptive efficacy of parenteral medroxyprogesterone monotherapy depends on substantially less frequent patient-initiated actions (i.e., compliance with receipt of the injection only once every 3 months).

Medroxyprogesterone has been used extensively and effectively worldwide for many years as a contraceptive and has been recommended for this use by the World Health Organization (WHO) and the International Planned Parenthood Federation (IPPF); contraceptive use of medroxyprogesterone was added to the labeling approved by the US Food and Drug Administration (FDA) in the early 1990s. FDA's delay of approval of medroxyprogesterone for use as a contraceptive was based on questions of safety raised by studies in beagles in which the drug was associated with an increased incidence of mammary tumors; the availability of safer alternate methods for contraception and the lack of clear evidence that a substantial patient population in need of the drug exists in the US; the possibility that increased drug-induced bleeding disturbances may necessitate concomitant administration of an estrogen, imposing an additional risk and decreasing the benefits of progestin-only contraception; the possibility that exposure (possibly prolonged) of the fetus to the drug, if contraception fails, poses a risk of congenital malformation; and concerns that postmarketing surveillance for breast and cervical carcinoma might not provide meaningful data. Subsequently, the WHO Toxicology Review Panel, the IPPF, and several scientific advisory panels concluded that available evidence does not indicate a risk of adverse effects associated with parenteral medroxyprogesterone that would preclude its use as a contraceptive. These conclusions generally have been confirmed by various epidemiologic studies, including those conducted by WHO regarding the risk of various neoplasms and contraceptive steroid use. (See Cautions: Mutagenicity and Carcinogenicity and also see Pregnancy, Fertility, and Lactation.)

Medroxyprogesterone in a fixed combination with estradiol is used parenterally for the prevention of conception. In clinical trials with the fixed combination containing medroxyprogesterone acetate and estradiol cypionate (Lunelle®), the 12-month pregnancy rate reportedly was less than 0.2%. Because of limitations of the available data (e.g., loss to follow-up, lack of pregnancy testing, use of barrier contraceptives, concomitant drug therapy), it is not possible to estimate precisely the contraceptive failure rate, but the failure rate is likely to range from 0.1–1%. As with other estrogen-progestin contraceptives, the efficacy of medroxyprogesterone acetate in fixed combination with estradiol cypionate depends largely on adherence to the recommended dosage schedule. To ensure that the fixed combination of medroxyprogesterone acetate and estradiol cypionate is not inadvertently administered to a pregnant woman, the first injection should be given during the first 5 days of a normal menstrual period. (See Pregnancy, Fertility, and Lactation: Pregnancy, in Cautions.)

■ **Endometriosis** Medroxyprogesterone acetate (depo-subQ provera 104®) is used parenterally in the management of pain associated with endometriosis. In controlled clinical studies, medroxyprogesterone acetate (104 mg administered subcutaneously every 3 months for 6 months) was effective in relieving clinical symptoms (e.g., dysmenorrhea, dyspareunia, pelvic pain) and signs (e.g., pelvic tenderness, pelvic induration) of endometriosis. Long-term use of parenteral medroxyprogesterone is associated with loss in bone mineral density (BMD). The loss of BMD in women of all ages and the possible impact on peak bone mass in adolescents should be considered when assessing the risks versus benefits of therapy with medroxyprogesterone. (See Cautions: Precautions and Contraindications).

■ **Amenorrhea and Uterine Bleeding** Medroxyprogesterone acetate is used orally for the treatment of secondary amenorrhea and for the treatment of abnormal uterine bleeding caused by hormonal imbalance in patients without underlying organic pathology such as fibroids or uterine cancer.

■ **Endometrial or Renal Carcinoma** Medroxyprogesterone acetate is used parenterally as adjunctive and palliative therapy for the treatment of inoperable, recurrent, and metastatic endometrial carcinoma. The initial treatment of the early stages (I and II) of endometrial carcinoma is surgery, sometimes combined with radiation therapy. In advanced endometrial carcinoma that is no longer amenable to surgery or radiation, hormonal therapy with progestins or chemotherapy should be considered.

Although medroxyprogesterone has been used in the treatment of metastatic renal cell carcinoma, other agents are considered more effective for the systemic treatment of this cancer. (See Interferon Alfa 10:00 and Aldesleukin 10:00.)

■ **Paraphilia in Males** Medroxyprogesterone acetate has been used parenterally (e.g., 100–500 mg IM weekly) for the management of paraphilia (e.g., homosexual, heterosexual, or bisexual pedophilia; heterosexual voyeurism, sexual sadism, or exhibitionism; transvestism) in males†. The drug has been shown to decrease the frequency of erotic imagery and the intensity of erotic cravings in most of these males. Sexual deviance generally returns following discontinuance of the drug.

■ **Other Uses** Medroxyprogesterone acetate has been used for the management of both GnRH-dependent (central) and -independent (peripheral) forms of precocious puberty† and was the most widely used drug for the management of various forms of precocity. However, use of medroxyprogesterone in the management of central (true) precocious puberty† generally has been supplanted by GnRH analogs (e.g., leuprolide) because of the improved pharmacologic specificity and adverse effect profile of these latter drugs; occasionally, medroxyprogesterone continues to be used for central precocity in patients who do not tolerate GnRH analog therapy. The optimum therapeutic regimen for the management of familial male precocious puberty† (testotoxicosis) or for McCune-Albright syndrome†, both GnRH-independent forms of precocity, remains to be established, and medroxyprogesterone is one of several therapeutic regimens (e.g., medroxyprogesterone, testolactone/spironolactone, testolactone/flutamide, or ketoconazole for familial male precocity; medroxyprogesterone or testolactone for McCune-Albright syndrome) currently being employed. While comparative safety and efficacy have not been established by controlled studies, medroxyprogesterone may be less likely than other regimens to favorably affect growth rate and skeletal maturation and more likely to adversely affect adrenocortical function.

Medroxyprogesterone acetate also has been used in the management of postmenopausal symptoms in females†, obesity-hypoventilation syndrome† (Pickwickian syndrome), obstructive sleep apnea syndrome and hypersomnolence in adults†, hirsutism† and homozygous sickle-cell disease†.

Dosage and Administration

■ **Administration** Medroxyprogesterone acetate (alone or in fixed combination with estrogens [i.e., conjugated estrogens, estradiol cypionate]) is administered orally, subcutaneously, or IM. When used as a contraceptive in females, medroxyprogesterone acetate is administered subcutaneously or IM; the drug is administered subcutaneously for the management of pain associated with endometriosis. Medroxyprogesterone acetate is administered IM in the treatment of cancer or male sexual deviance† (paraphilia). Because of the prolonged action, parenteral administration of the drug is not recommended for the treatment of secondary amenorrhea or abnormal uterine bleeding.

Medroxyprogesterone acetate injectable suspension (containing medroxyprogesterone acetate alone or in fixed combination with estradiol cypionate) must be vigorously shaken immediately before each use to ensure complete suspension of the drug(s). IM injection of medroxyprogesterone acetate alone (Depo-Provera® Contraceptive, Depo-Provera®, Medroxyprogesterone Acetate Contraceptive) or in combination with estradiol cypionate (Lunelle® Monthly Contraceptive) should be made deep into the gluteal, deltoid, or anterior thigh muscle. Subcutaneous injection of medroxyprogesterone acetate (depo-subQ provera 104®) is made into the anterior thigh or abdomen; the preparation for subcutaneous administration should not be administered IM.

Oral dosage preparations containing medroxyprogesterone acetate in combination with conjugated estrogens as monophasic or biphasic regimens are commercially available in a mnemonic dispensing package that is designed to aid the user in complying with the prescribed dosage schedule. The monophasic combination (Prempro®) is available in a 28-day dosage preparation that contains 28 tablets of conjugated estrogens (0.625 mg) in fixed combination with medroxyprogesterone acetate (2.5 or 5 mg). The monophasic combination (Prempro®) also is available in a 28-day dosage preparation that contains 28 tablets of conjugated estrogens USP (0.3 or 0.45 mg) in fixed combination with medroxyprogesterone acetate (1.5 mg). The biphasic combination (Premphase®) also is available in a 28-day dosage preparation that contains 14 tablets of conjugated estrogens (0.625 mg) and 14 tablets of conjugated estrogens (0.625 mg) in fixed combination with medroxyprogesterone acetate (5 mg).

■ **Dosage** ***Prevention of Endometrial Changes Associated with Estrogens*** When medroxyprogesterone acetate is used in conjunction with estrogen replacement therapy, medroxyprogesterone may be administered in a monophasic (Prempro®) or biphasic (Premphase®) manner. In the monophasic regimen, oral conjugated estrogens is administered in a daily dosage of 0.3 mg in conjunction with oral medroxyprogesterone acetate in a daily dosage of 1.5 mg. Alternatively, conjugated estrogens is administered in a daily dosage of 0.45 mg in conjunction with medroxyprogesterone acetate in a daily dosage of 1.5 mg, or conjugated estrogens is administered in a daily dosage of 0.625 mg in conjunction with medroxyprogesterone acetate in a daily dosage of 2.5 or 5 mg. In the biphasic regimen (Premphase®) oral conjugated estrogens is administered in a daily dosage of 0.625 mg, while oral medroxyprogesterone acetate is administered in a dosage of 5 mg daily on days 15–28 of the cycle.

Contraception in Females When medroxyprogesterone acetate injectable suspension (Depo-Provera® Contraceptive, Medroxyprogesterone Acetate Contraceptive) is used for the prevention of conception in women, the recommended dosage of medroxyprogesterone acetate is 150 mg IM every 3 months. The possibility of pregnancy should be excluded prior to administering the first dose of medroxyprogesterone and whenever more than 13 weeks has elapsed since the previous dose. To avoid inadvertent administration of the contraceptive to a pregnant woman, the initial injection should be given during the first 5 days of a normal menstrual cycle, within 5 days postpartum in those who do not breast-feed, or during the sixth postpartum week in women who breast-feed. (See Pregnancy, Fertility, and Lactation: Pregnancy, in Cautions.) Parenteral medroxyprogesterone should be used as a long-term contraceptive method (e.g., longer than 2 years) *only* if other contraceptive methods are inadequate and the benefits are expected to outweigh the risks. (See Cautions: Precautions and Contraindications.)

When medroxyprogesterone acetate injectable suspension (depo-subQ provera 104®) is used for the prevention of conception in women, the recommended dosage of medroxyprogesterone acetate is 104 mg administered subcutaneously every 3 months (12–14 weeks). The possibility of pregnancy should be excluded prior to administering the first dose of medroxyprogesterone and whenever more than 14 weeks has elapsed since the previous dose.

To avoid inadvertent administration of the contraceptive to a pregnant woman, the initial injection should be given during the first 5 days of a normal menstrual cycle. In addition, the initial injection should be given no earlier than 6 weeks postpartum in women who breast-feed. (See Pregnancy, Fertility, and Lactation: Pregnancy, in Cautions.) When switching from other contraceptive methods, the manufacturer recommends that therapy with medroxyprogesterone acetate (depo-subQ provera 104®) be initiated in a manner that ensures continuous contraceptive coverage based on the mechanism of action of both methods (e.g., patients switching from combined estrogen-progestin contraceptives should be given an initial injection within 7 days after taking the last hormonally active tablet or removal of a transdermal patch or vaginal ring; patients switching from IM injections of medroxyprogesterone acetate [Depo-Provera® Contraceptive] to depo-subQ provera 104® should be given an initial injection of depo-subQ provera 104® within the dosing period recommended for the IM contraceptive preparation). Parenteral medroxyprogesterone should be used as a long-term contraceptive method (e.g., longer than 2 years) *only* if other contraceptive methods are inadequate and the benefits are expected to outweigh the risks. (See Cautions: Precautions and Contraindications.)

When Lunelle® is used for the prevention of conception in women, the usual dosage of medroxyprogesterone acetate is 25 mg (in fixed combination with 5 mg of estradiol cypionate per 0.5 mL) IM monthly. To avoid inadvertent administration of the contraceptive to a pregnant woman, the initial injection should be given during the first 5 days of a normal menstrual cycle or within 5 days of a complete first-trimester abortion. In addition, the initial injection should be given no earlier than 6 weeks postpartum in women who breast-feed and no earlier than 4 weeks postpartum in those who do not breast-feed. Subsequent injections should be given monthly (every 28–30 days, but no more than 33 days after the previous injection); the dosage schedule should be determined by the number of days between injections and not by bleeding episodes. If the patient has not adhered to the prescribed administration schedule (i.e., if more than 33 days have elapsed since the previous injection), an alternative (i.e., barrier) method of contraception should be instituted, and pregnancy ruled out, prior to continuation of Lunelle® (medroxyprogesterone acetate-estradiol cypionate) therapy. It should be noted that shortening of the injection interval may result in a change in menstrual pattern. When switching from other contraceptive methods, the manufacturer recommends that therapy with the fixed combination of medroxyprogesterone acetate and estradiol cypionate be initiated in a manner that ensures continuous contraceptive coverage based on the mechanism of action of both methods (e.g., patients switching from oral contraceptives should be given an initial injection within 7 days after taking the last hormonally active tablet).

Endometriosis When medroxyprogesterone acetate injectable suspension (depo-subQ provera 104®) is used for the management of pain associated with endometriosis, the recommended dosage of medroxyprogesterone acetate is 104 mg administered subcutaneously every 3 months (12–14 weeks). The possibility of pregnancy should be excluded prior to administering the first dose of medroxyprogesterone and whenever more than 14 weeks has elapsed since the previous dose. To avoid inadvertent administration of the drug to a pregnant woman, the initial injection should be given during the first 5 days of a normal menstrual cycle. In addition, the initial injection should be given no earlier than 6 weeks postpartum in women who breast-feed. Efficacy of medroxyprogesterone acetate (depo-subQ provera 104®) for the management of pain associated with endometriosis was established in studies of 6 months' duration; data establishing continued efficacy with use beyond 6 months are lacking. Therapy with the drug for longer than 2 years is not recommended because of concerns about the potential long-term effects on bone density. If retreatment is considered following recurrence of endometriosis, bone density should be assessed. (See Effects on Bone under Cautions: Adverse Effects in Women.)

Amenorrhea and Uterine Bleeding For the treatment of secondary amenorrhea, the usual oral dosage of medroxyprogesterone acetate is 5–10 mg daily for 5–10 days; although one manufacturer states that therapy may be initiated at any time, the drug is usually started during the assumed latter half (e.g., 16th to 21st day) of the menstrual cycle. In patients with a poorly developed endometrium, conventional estrogen therapy may be used in conjunction with medroxyprogesterone acetate. To induce optimum secretory transformation of an endometrium that has been adequately primed with endogenous or exogenous estrogen, one manufacturer recommends an oral dosage of 10 mg daily for 10 days. Progestin-induced withdrawal bleeding usually occurs within 3–7 days after discontinuing therapy with the drug.

For the treatment of abnormal uterine bleeding, 5–10 mg of medroxyprogesterone acetate may be given orally for 5–10 days beginning on the assumed or calculated 16th or 21st day of the menstrual cycle. When bleeding is caused by a deficiency of estrogen and progestin, as indicated by a poorly proliferative endometrium, estrogens should be used in conjunction with medroxyprogesterone acetate; if bleeding is controlled satisfactorily, 2 subsequent cycles of combined therapy should be given. To induce optimum secretory transformation of an endometrium that has been adequately primed with endogenous or exogenous estrogen, one manufacturer recommends that 10 mg of the drug may be given orally for 10 days beginning on the calculated 16th day of the cycle. Progestin-induced withdrawal bleeding usually occurs within 3–7 days after discontinuing therapy with the drug. Patients with a history of recurrent episodes of abnormal uterine bleeding may benefit from planned menstrual cycling with medroxyprogesterone acetate.

Endometrial or Renal Carcinoma For the adjunctive and palliative treatment of advanced, inoperable endometrial or renal carcinoma, an initial IM medroxyprogesterone acetate dosage of 400–1000 mg/week has been recommended. If improvement is noted within a few weeks or months and the disease appears to have stabilized, it may be possible to maintain response with as little as 400 mg/month. Medroxyprogesterone acetate is not recommended as primary therapy, but as adjunctive and palliative therapy in advanced inoperable cases including those with recurrent or metastatic disease.

Paraphilia in Males For the management of paraphilia in males†, initial IM dosages of 200 mg 2 or 3 times daily or 500 mg weekly have been used. Dosage is generally adjusted according to patient response and tolerance and/or plasma testosterone concentration. Generally, the dose and/or frequency of administration is decreased to an effective maintenance level. In one study, maintenance dosages ranged from 100 mg once weekly to once monthly. Published protocols should be consulted for more specific dosage information in these males.

Cautions

■ **Adverse Effects in Women** ***Genitourinary Effects*** In women receiving parenteral medroxyprogesterone for contraception (alone or in fixed combination with estradiol cypionate) or the management of pain associated with endometriosis, the most common adverse effects are menstrual abnormalities. Irregular and unpredictable menstrual bleeding pattern, including spotting, occurs frequently during the first months of therapy with the drug. In women receiving IM medroxyprogesterone acetate in fixed combination with estradiol cypionate, about 59% experienced alterations in menstrual bleeding pattern (e.g., amenorrhea; frequent, irregular, prolonged, or infrequent bleeding) after 1 year of use; the incidence of irregular bleeding remained relatively constant at approximately 30% throughout the first year of use. If abnormal bleeding persists or is severe, appropriate steps to investigate the possibility of organic pathology should be undertaken, and appropriate therapy instituted as necessary.

Amenorrhea also occurs frequently in women receiving the drug for contraception or the management of pain associated with endometriosis, and as the duration of therapy increases the likelihood of intermenstrual bleeding decreases and that of amenorrhea increases; up to about 60 and 70% of women reportedly have amenorrhea after 1 and 2 years, respectively, of contraceptive therapy with medroxyprogesterone.

Although concomitant use of low doses of estrogens has been suggested to treat medroxyprogesterone-induced menstrual disturbances, the evidence for efficacy of this therapy is equivocal. Contraceptive use of the drug should be discontinued in women who do not tolerate irregular and unpredictable bleeding or amenorrhea.

Heavy or continuous vaginal bleeding may occur in some women receiving medroxyprogesterone, but rarely requires estrogen therapy. Impaired fertility persists long after discontinuance of the drug. (See Cautions: Pregnancy, Fertility, and Lactation.)

Effects on Bone Use of parenteral medroxyprogesterone acetate (e.g., Depo-Provera® Contraceptive, depo-subQ provera 104®) reduces serum estrogen concentrations and is associated with loss of bone mineral density (BMD) as bone metabolism adjusts to lower serum estrogen concentrations. Bone loss is greater with increasing duration of medroxyprogesterone therapy and may not be completely reversible following discontinuance. In one clinical study, adult women receiving parenteral medroxyprogesterone (Depo-Provera® Contraceptive) for up to 5 years experienced a 5–6% loss in BMD of lumbar spine, total hip, and femoral neck; clinically important changes in BMD were not observed in a control group of women not receiving a hormonal contraceptive. The decline in BMD was more pronounced during the first 2 years of use of medroxyprogesterone; smaller declines were observed in subsequent years. Bone loss during the first 2 years of therapy with depo-subQ provera 104® is similar to that observed during the first 2 years of therapy with Depo-Provera® Contraceptive. In one comparative study, women receiving depo-subQ provera 104® for the management of endometriosis experienced a loss in BMD of lumbar spine and total hip of 0.03–1.2% over 6 months of therapy compared with a loss in BMD of 1.8–4.1% in women receiving leuprolide for the same period of time.

Evaluation of BMD 2 years after discontinuance of medroxyprogesterone indicates that BMD increases toward baseline values over this time period. However, longer duration of medroxyprogesterone therapy is associated with less complete recovery of BMD over the 2-year period after discontinuance of the drug. In an ongoing, open-label, self-selected, non-randomized study in adolescent females 12–18 years of age, use of parenteral medroxyprogesterone (Depo-Provera® Contraceptive) was associated with decreased bone density at the lumbar spine, total hip, and femoral neck; adolescents usually increase BMD during growth following menarche. Limited data indicate that BMD increases following discontinuance of medroxyprogesterone in these females. However, loss of BMD is of particular concern during adolescence and early adulthood.

It remains to be determined whether use of parenteral medroxyprogesterone in younger women will reduce peak bone mass and increase the risk of fractures secondary to osteoporosis later in life. Osteoporosis, including osteoporotic fractures, rarely has been reported during postmarketing surveillance of patients receiving IM medroxyprogesterone for contraception. (For information on women at risk for osteoporosis, see Cautions: Precautions and Contraindications.) The effect of BMD changes in women receiving medroxyprogesterone acetate in fixed combination with estradiol cypionate remains to be determined.

Effects on Body Weight Weight changes (e.g., gain) also occur commonly during use of parenteral medroxyprogesterone (Depo Provera® Contraceptive, depo-subQ provera 104®). From an initial body weight averaging 61.8 kg, average weight gains of 2.45, 3.68, 6.27, and 7.5 kg occur after completion of 1, 2, 4, and 6 years of contraceptive use, respectively. In several large studies, 2–6% of women discontinued therapy with medroxyprogesterone alone or in fixed combination with estradiol cypionate because of excessive weight gain.

Other Adverse Effects Medroxyprogesterone, like other progestins, may cause cholestatic jaundice, melasma or chloasma, and mental depression. Breast tenderness or galactorrhea has occasionally occurred. Alopecia, acne, and hirsutism have been reported rarely. Adverse CNS effects including nervousness, insomnia, somnolence, fatigue, and dizziness have occasionally occurred. Rarely, headache, hyperpyrexia, nausea, or jaundice, including neonatal jaundice, has been reported. Hypersensitivity reactions including urticaria, pruritus, angioedema, generalized rash (with or without pruritus), and anaphylactoid reactions and anaphylaxis have occasionally occurred in patients receiving the drug. Adverse local effects at the site of injection include residual lump, skin discoloration, and sterile abscess.

Other adverse effects reported during contraceptive use of medroxyprogesterone alone or in fixed combination with estradiol cypionate include abdominal pain or discomfort (e.g., bloating, enlarged abdomen), changes in mood or libido, emotional lability, anorgasmia, asthenia (weakness or fatigue), hot flushes (flashes), edema, absent hair growth, leukorrhea, vaginitis (e.g., candidiasis), vulvovaginal disorder, pelvic pain, breast pain, leg cramps, and backache. Infrequent (in less than 1% of patients) adverse effects associated with contraceptive use of medroxyprogesterone include seizures, appetite changes, GI disturbances, genitourinary infections, vaginal cysts, dyspareunia, paresthesia, chest pain, pulmonary embolus, anemia, and drowsiness. Other infrequent adverse effects associated with such use include syncope, dyspnea and asthma, tachycardia, fever, excessive sweating or body odor, dry skin, chills, increased or decreased libido, excessive thirst, hoarseness, pain at the injection site, blood dyscrasia, rectal bleeding, changes in breast size, breast lumps or nipple bleeding, axillary swelling, breast cancer, prevention of lactation, sensation of pregnancy, lack of return to fertility, accidental pregnancy, uterine hyperplasia, cervical cancer, thrombophlebitis, deep vein thrombosis, varicose veins, dysmenorrhea, paralysis, scleroderma, and osteoporosis.

Other adverse effects reported with noncontraceptive use of estrogen-progestin combination preparations include increased blood pressure in susceptible individuals, premenstrual-like syndrome, changes in libido or appetite, cystitis-like syndrome, backache, loss of scalp hair, erythema multiforme or nodosum, hemorrhagic skin eruption, and itching.

Allergic reactions reported with the injectable fixed combination of medroxyprogesterone acetate and estradiol cypionate (Lunelle®) have been principally dermatologic rather than respiratory in nature. If an anaphylactic reaction occurs, appropriate measures should be instituted; serious anaphylactic reactions require emergency medical treatment.

Cholecystitis and cholelithiasis have been reported in women receiving the fixed combination of medroxyprogesterone acetate and estradiol cypionate for up to 15 months. Other adverse effects reported with IM medroxyprogesterone acetate in fixed combination with estradiol cypionate generally are similar to those reported with estrogen-progestin oral contraceptives. For additional information on adverse effects associated with such combinations, see Cautions in Estrogen-Progestin Combinations 68:12.

Thromboembolic disorders including thrombophlebitis and pulmonary embolism have occurred in patients receiving medroxyprogesterone. An association between thrombophlebitis, pulmonary embolism, and cerebral thrombosis and embolism and use of estrogen-progestin combination preparations has been shown. (See Thromboembolic Disorders in Cautions: Cardiovascular Effects, in the Estrogen-Progestin Combinations 68:12.) The possibility that thromboembolic disorders may occur in patients receiving medroxyprogesterone should be considered and patients should be carefully observed for these effects during therapy with the drug.

Although available evidence suggests that an association exists between neuro-ocular lesions such as optic neuritis or retinal thrombosis and use of estrogen-progestin combination preparations, such a relationship has been neither confirmed nor refuted.

Use of estrogen-progestin combinations has also been associated with increased levels of coagulation factors VII, VIII, IX, and X. The possibility that these effects may occur in patients receiving medroxyprogesterone should be considered and patients should be carefully observed for these effects during therapy with the drug.

■ **Adverse Effects in Males** In males receiving parenteral medroxyprogesterone for the management of paraphilia, fatigue and weight gain occur commonly. Plasma testosterone concentrations decrease in most patients receiving the drug, and the decrease is generally associated with a diminution in the frequency and quality of erection and ejaculation; in one study, impotence generally occurred when plasma testosterone concentration decreased to one-fourth the pretreatment concentration. The drug is reportedly nonfeminizing in these males. Other adverse effects reported in these males include hot and cold flashes, headache, insomnia, nausea, and phlebitis.

■ **Precautions and Contraindications** Medroxyprogesterone acetate shares the toxic potentials of progestins, and the usual precautions of progestin therapy should be observed. Because oral contraceptive combinations contain progestins, the precautions associated with oral contraceptives should generally be considered in patients receiving progestins. (See Cautions in Estrogen-Progestin Combinations 68:12.) In addition, when medroxyprogesterone is used in conjunction with estrogens (i.e., conjugated estrogens, estradiol cypionate), the cautions, precautions, and contraindications associated with estrogens must be considered in addition to those associated with medroxyprogesterone.

Prior to initiation of therapy with medroxyprogesterone-containing preparations in women and annually thereafter during continued use (e.g., as a contraceptive, for the management of endometriosis, in conjunction with estrogen replacement therapy), a history should be obtained and physical examination performed, including special attention to the breasts and pelvic organs and a Papanicolaou test (Pap smear). Women receiving medroxyprogesterone-containing preparations should be given a copy of the patient labeling for the drug. In addition, women receiving the drug alone or in fixed combination with estradiol cypionate for contraceptive purposes or for management of endometriosis should be advised of anticipated effects on menstruation (e.g., initial irregular and unpredictable bleeding pattern), with the eventual development of amenorrhea in a large proportion of such women as use of the drug continues, and of the likelihood of weight gain during such use. (See Cautions: Adverse Effects Associated with Contraceptive Use in Women.) Women receiving parenteral medroxyprogesterone acetate alone or in fixed combination with estradiol cypionate for contraceptive purposes also should be advised that the contraceptive efficacy of such therapy depends on adherence to the recommended dosage schedule. Women with a family history of breast cancer or who have breast nodules should be monitored with particular care, and appropriate diagnostic measures to rule out malignancy should be employed if abnormal vaginal bleeding persists or recurs during therapy with the drug. In addition, women also should be advised that the contraceptive effect of parenteral medroxyprogesterone is prolonged, persisting long after the last dose of the drug. (See Pregnancy, Fertility, and Lactation: Fertility, in Cautions.) When medroxyprogesterone is to be used in conjunction with estrogen replacement therapy, potential risks may include adverse effects on lipid metabolism and glucose tolerance; addition of a progestin may adversely affect some beneficial metabolic effects associated with long-term estrogen therapy. Addition of medroxyprogesterone to estrogen replacement therapy appears to increase the risk of breast cancer beyond that associated with estrogen alone. (See Carcinogenicity in the Estrogens General Statement 68:16.04.) In addition, it should be considered that although estrogen-associated risk of endometrial carcinoma is substantially reduced when estrogens are administered concomitantly with progestins, such risk still exists, therefore, clinical evaluation of all menopausal women receiving estrogen therapy in conjunction with a progestin is essential. Diagnostic tests, including endometrial sampling when indicated, should be performed in all women who have undiagnosed, persistent, or abnormal vaginal bleeding.

Long-term use of parenteral medroxyprogesterone is associated with loss of bone mineral density (BMD). Parenteral medroxyprogesterone should be used as a long-term contraceptive method (e.g., longer than 2 years) *only* if other contraceptive methods are inadequate and the benefits are expected to outweigh the risks. Use of medroxyprogesterone (depo-subQ provera 104®) for the management of endometriosis for longer than 2 years is not recommended. BMD should be evaluated periodically when medroxyprogesterone is used long term; the patient's age (adult or adolescent) and skeletal maturity should be considered when evaluating BMD results. If retreatment with medroxyprogesterone is considered following recurrence of endometriosis, bone density should be assessed.Therapies other than parenteral medroxyprogesterone should be considered in women with preexisting risk factors for osteoporosis; use of medroxyprogesterone may be an additional risk in women at risk for osteoporosis. Risk factors for osteoporosis include metabolic bone disease, drinking excessive amounts of alcohol, cigarette smoking, anorexia nervosa, a family history of osteoporosis, and long-term use of drugs that can reduce BMD (e.g., anticonvulsants, corticosteroids). Whether supplemental calcium and vitamin D can reduce BMD loss that occurs in women using long-term medroxyprogesterone remains to be determined; all women should have adequate intake of calcium and vitamin D.

If medroxyprogesterone is to be used for the treatment of cancer, patients should be referred to physicians who are actively engaged in investigation of the disease and are therefore familiar with the latest and most advantageous forms of therapy.

Medroxyprogesterone should be used with caution, and only with careful monitoring, in patients with conditions that might be aggravated by fluid retention (e.g., asthma, seizure disorders, migraine, or cardiac or renal dysfunction). The drug should also be used with caution in patients with a history of mental depression; medroxyprogesterone should be discontinued if depression recurs to a serious degree during therapy with the drug. While a causal relationship to the drug and the possible contribution of a preexisting condition remain unclear, the possibility of seizures during medroxyprogesterone use should be considered.

When breakthrough bleeding or irregular vaginal bleeding occurs during medroxyprogesterone therapy, nonfunctional causes should be considered. Adequate diagnostic procedures should be performed in patients with undiagnosed vaginal bleeding.

The manufacturers caution that the effect of long-term medroxyprogesterone therapy on pituitary, ovarian, adrenal, hepatic, or uterine function has not been determined. Diabetic patients should be carefully monitored during medroxyprogesterone therapy, since decreased glucose tolerance has been observed in women receiving estrogen-progestin combinations. Medroxyprogesterone may mask the onset of climacteric in women.

The clinician and the patient using medroxyprogesterone should be alert to the earliest signs and symptoms of thromboembolic and thrombotic disorders (e.g., thrombophlebitis, pulmonary embolism, cerebrovascular insufficiency, coronary occlusion, retinal thrombosis, mesenteric thrombosis). The drug should be discontinued immediately when any of these disorders occurs or is suspected. The clinician and patient also should be alert to the earliest manifestations of hepatic dysfunction (e.g., jaundice) during use of the drug. The drug should be discontinued and the patient's status reevaluated if such manifestations occur or are suspected. The manufacturer states that medroxyprogesterone acetate in fixed combination with estradiol cypionate (Lunelle®) should not be readministered to women in whom thromboembolic or thrombotic disorders have occurred or are suspected.

If unexplained, sudden or gradual, partial or complete loss of vision; proptosis or diplopia; papilledema; retinal vascular lesions; or migraine occur during therapy with medroxyprogesterone, the drug should be discontinued and appropriate diagnostic and therapeutic measures instituted. If ocular examination reveals evidence of papilledema or retinal vascular lesions, medroxyprogesterone therapy should *not* be reinitiated.

The onset or exacerbation of migraine or development of headache with a new pattern that is recurrent, persistent, or severe requires evaluation of the cause before further administration of medroxyprogesterone acetate in fixed combination with estradiol cypionate for contraceptive purposes.

Medroxyprogesterone is contraindicated in patients with active thrombophlebitis or a current or past history of thromboembolic disorders or of cerebral vascular disease or apoplexy. The drug is also contraindicated in patients with undiagnosed vaginal bleeding, missed abortion, liver dysfunction or disease or with known or suspected malignancy of the genital organs, known sensitivity to the drug or any ingredient in the formulation, or known or suspected pregnancy or carcinoma of the breast, or for use as a pregnancy test. The manufacturer states that use of medroxyprogesterone acetate in combination with estradiol cypionate for contraceptive purposes also is contraindicated in patients with carcinoma of the endometrium, severe hypertension, diabetes mellitus with vascular involvement, headaches with focal neurologic symptoms, valvular heart disease with complications, and those 35 years of age or older who smoke 15 cigarettes or more daily. Women receiving medroxyprogesterone acetate in fixed combination with estradiol cypionate should be strongly advised not to smoke.

■ **Mutagenicity and Carcinogenicity** Administration of medroxyprogesterone to beagles has been associated with the development of mammary nodules, some of which were malignant. Although nodules occasionally occurred in control beagles, they were intermittent in nature; nodules in drug-treated beagles were larger, more numerous, persistent, and occasionally malignant with metastases. The clinical relevance of these findings to humans has not been established. In addition, there is evidence of species differences in the response of beagles and humans to medroxyprogesterone; because of these species differences, some experts state that it is not possible to draw conclusions from the observations in beagles. In long-term (10 years) toxicology studies in monkeys, 2 of the animals developed undifferentiated carcinoma of the uterus following administration of 150 mg/kg every 90 days. The relevance of this finding has been questioned since progestins are thought to protect against the development of endometrial cancer and because of the unusual nature of the cancer in these monkeys; additional study is needed to determine the relevance to humans. Transient mammary nodules occurred in control monkeys and those receiving 3 or 30 mg/kg every 90 days, but not in those receiving 150 mg/kg. At sacrifice, nodules still existed in 3 monkeys; histopathologic examination showed the nodules to be hyperplastic. No evidence of uterine or breast abnormalities was revealed in rats.

Analysis of worldwide epidemiologic evidence on the relationship between the risk of breast cancer and postmenopausal hormone replacement therapy and results of most, but not all, studies indicate that prolonged use of postmenopausal hormone replacement therapy is associated with an increased risk of breast cancer in current or recent recipients. In the Women's Health Initiative (WHI) study evaluating estrogen/progestin therapy, there was a small increase in the risk of breast cancer in postmenopausal women receiving hormone replacement therapy (i.e., conjugated estrogens 0.625 mg in conjunction with medroxyprogesterone acetate 2.5 mg daily) compared with those receiving placebo. (See Cautions: Mutagenicity and Carcinogenicity, in the Estrogens General Statement 68:16.04.) The increase in breast cancer risk was apparent after 4 years of estrogen/progestin therapy, and the risk appeared to be cumulative. Results of a large (involving more than 100,000 women) prospective cohort study (the Nurses' Health Study) in postmenopausal women who received conjugated estrogens indicated that while there appears to be no increased risk of breast cancer in postmenopausal women with prior or relatively short-term use of estrogens, long-term (exceeding 5 years) estrogen therapy may be associated with an increased risk of such carcinoma, especially in women 55 years and older. Addition of progestins to estrogen replacement therapy appears to increase the risk of breast cancer beyond that associated with estrogen alone. (See: Carcinogenicity in the Estrogens General Statement 68:16.04.)

In one retrospective study in black women who received sterile medroxyprogesterone acetate suspension for contraception, there was no evidence of an increased risk of developing cancer of the breast, uterine corpus, or ovary. Although the study indicated that there was no strong association between medroxyprogesterone and these cancers, limitations of the study included inability to detect a weak carcinogenic effect of the drug or a carcinogenic effect that would become evident only after a long latent period.

Long-term case-controlled studies conducted by the World Health Organization (WHO) in other users of medroxyprogesterone contraception have revealed slight or no evidence of increased overall risk of breast cancer and no evidence of increased overall risk of ovarian or cervical cancer. While there also was no evidence of an increased overall risk of liver cancer among users in populations in which hepatitis B infection was endemic, the relevance of these findings to populations in which this infection is not endemic currently is not known since relative risks of live cancer associated with use of oral estrogen-progestin combinations have been estimated to be lower among populations in which this infection is endemic compared with nonendemic populations. In the case-control study assessing the risk of breast cancer, there was evidence of an increased risk of breast cancer within the first 4 years of initial exposure to medroxyprogesterone, principally among those younger than 35 years of age. The relative risk estimated for users whose first exposure to the drug was within the previous 4 years was 2.19 times that in nonusers; this would represent an increase in the annual risk of breast cancer from 26.7 cases per 100,000 women among nonusers to 58.5 cases per 100,000 women among medroxyprogesterone users. Thus, the attributable annual risk for breast cancer among users in the US is 3.18 per 10,000 women. In the case-control study assessing the risk of cervical cancer, while there was no evidence of an increased overall risk of this cancer among medroxyprogesterone users (even after more than 12 years since initial use), there was a statistically insignificant increase in the relative risk (to 1.22–1.28) of invasive squamous cell carcinoma among users who were first exposed to the drug before age 35; however, no trends in risk with duration of use or times since initial or most recent use were observed.

There also is evidence from a long-term case-control study conducted by WHO in users of medroxyprogesterone contraception of a prolonged (e.g., for at least 8 years after discontinuance of the drug) protective effect manifested as a reduced risk of endometrial cancer among users; however, this possible protective effect of medroxyprogesterone may be reduced by concomitant estrogen use.

■ **Pregnancy, Fertility, and Lactation** ***Pregnancy*** Although progestins have been used beginning in the first trimester of pregnancy to prevent habitual abortion or to treat threatened abortion, there is no adequate evidence from well-controlled studies to substantiate the efficacy of progestins for these uses; however, there is evidence of potential adverse effects on the fetus when these drugs are administered within the first 4 months of pregnancy. In addition, in most women, the cause of abortion is a defective ovum, which progestins could not be expected to influence. Because of their uterine-relaxant effects, progestins may delay spontaneous abortion of fertilized defective ova. Masculinization of the female fetus has reportedly occurred when progestins were used during pregnancy. Clitoral hypertrophy and fusion of the labia have been reported in a few female neonates born to women who had received medroxyprogesterone during pregnancy; hypospadias in male neonates born to women receiving progestational agents occurs at approximately twice the rate of occurrence in male neonates born to women not receiving the drugs. Postpartum bleeding, postabortal bleeding, and missed abortion have been reported in women who received the drug during pregnancy. An association between intrauterine exposure to female sex hormones and congenital anomalies, including cardiovascular and limb defects, has been suggested. (See Cautions: Pregnancy, Fertility, and Lactation, in Estrogen-Progestin Combinations 68:12.) Use of progestins, including medroxyprogesterone, is not recommended during the first 4 months of pregnancy. If a woman becomes pregnant while receiving medroxyprogesterone or is inadvertently exposed to the drug during the first 4 months of pregnancy, she should be advised of the potential risks to the fetus. To increase ensurance that the drug is not administered inadvertently to a pregnant woman, it is important that use of the drug be initiated only during the first 5 days after onset of normal menses, within 5 days postpartum if the woman is not lactating, or at the sixth postpartum week if she is. If more than 13–14 weeks has elapsed since the last dose of medroxyprogesterone, appropriate assessment should be performed to ensure that the woman is not pregnant prior to administering a dose.

When medroxyprogesterone is used as a contraceptive, unintended pregnancies that occur within 1–2 months after IM injection of the drug may be characterized by impaired fetal growth as evidenced by low birthweights, which theoretically could result in an increased risk of neonatal death. However, the attributable risk of this adverse effect is low because such pregnancies are unlikely. The risk of low birthweight was particularly evident when conception was estimated to occur within 4 weeks of medroxyprogesterone injection. While an increase in polysyndactyly, particularly among offspring of women younger than 30 years of age, and chromosomal anomalies also have been observed in neonates born to women who received IM medroxyprogesterone contraception, the unrelated nature of these effects, the lack of confirmation from other studies, the prolonged period of time between use of the drug and conception in many cases, and chance effects resulting from the multiple statistical comparisons applied make an association between these effects and the drug unlikely.

The possibility of ectopic pregnancy should be considered in any women using medroxyprogesterone contraception if pregnancy occurs or the woman develops complaints of severe abdominal pain.

Medroxyprogesterone should *not* be used to induce withdrawal bleeding as a test for pregnancy.

Fertility Impairment of fertility persists for prolonged periods after the last dose of parenteral medroxyprogesterone in women receiving the drug for contraception or the management of endometriosis. Life-table analysis of data from one study in which follow-up was available in 61% of participants who received IM medroxyprogesterone indicated that, in women who intend to become pregnant following discontinuance of the drug, 68, 83, and 93% of women who successfully conceive are likely to do so within 12, 15, and 18 months, respectively, after the last dose. The median time to conception for those who do conceive is 10 months (range: 4–31 months) after the last dose and is unrelated to the duration of contraceptive medroxyprogesterone use. However, pregnancy (e.g., unintended) can occur rarely within 4 weeks after a dose of the drug. The median time to ovulation in women who received several doses of depo-subQ provera 104® was 10 months after the last injection; 80% of women ovulated within 1 year after the last injection. Ovulation may occur as early as 14 weeks after a single dose of depo-subQ provera 104®.

Lactation Progestins reportedly are distributed into milk, and detectable amounts of medroxyprogesterone have been identified in milk of lactating women receiving the drug IM. Milk composition, quality, and volume are not affected adversely by medroxyprogesterone use. While the manufacturers warn that the possible effects of progestins in milk on nursing infants have not been determined, study of infants exposed to the drug via breast milk has revealed no evidence of adverse developmental or behavioral effects through puberty.

The effects of combined medroxyprogesterone acetate and estradiol cypionate therapy on lactation and nursing infants have not been established. However, because adverse effects such as jaundice and breast enlargement have been reported in nursing infants of women receiving estrogen-progestin combination oral contraceptives, the usual cautions and precautions associated with estrogens must be considered in lactating women receiving IM medroxyprogesterone acetate in fixed combination with estradiol cypionate. The manufacturer states that use of estrogen-progestin combination contraceptives should be deferred until 6 weeks postpartum. For additional information, see Cautions: Pregnancy, Fertility, and Lactation, in Estrogen-Progestin Combinations 68:12.

Laboratory Test Interferences

The manufacturers caution that estrogen-progestin combinations have caused abnormal thyroid function test results. (See Effects on Thyroid in Cautions: Endocrine and Metabolic Effects, in Estrogen-Progestin Combinations 68:12.) The manufacturers also caution that estrogen-progestin combinations have altered the metyrapone test (see Laboratory Test Interferences in Estrogen-Progestin Combinations 68:12), and that these combinations have altered liver function test results (see Cautions: Hepatic Effects, in Estrogen-Progestin Combinations 68:12). These combinations have also caused decreased pregnanediol excretion.

The manufacturers state that the pathologist should be advised of medroxyprogesterone use when relevant specimens from a patient exposed to the drug are submitted.

Pharmacology

Medroxyprogesterone shares the pharmacologic actions of the progestins. In women with adequate endogenous estrogen, medroxyprogesterone transforms a proliferative endometrium into a secretory one. Medroxyprogesterone has been shown to have slight androgenic activity in animals. Anabolic effects have also been reported, but the drug apparently lacks appreciable estrogenic activity in humans. In animals, the drug exhibits pronounced adrenocorticoid activity, but a clinically important effect has not been observed in humans. Medroxyprogesterone inhibits the secretion of pituitary gonadotropins following usual IM or subcutaneous dosages (e.g., 150 or 104 mg every 3 months), thus preventing follicular maturation and ovulation and resulting in endometrial thinning; these effects result in contraceptive activity. Available evidence indicates that these effects do not occur following oral administration of usual dosages (i.e., 5–10 mg daily as single daily doses) of the drug. High doses of medroxyprogesterone inhibit pituitary secretion of luteinizing hormone (LH) and follicle-stimulating hormone (FSH), and will prevent cyclic gonadotropin surges that occur during the normal menstrual cycle. It has been suggested that the drug acts at the hypothalamus since it does not suppress the release of LH and FSH following administration of gonadotropin-releasing hormone and since basal concentrations of LH and FSH remain within the low normal range when the drug is used as a contraceptive. Although the mechanism of action has not been determined, medroxyprogesterone has antineoplastic activity against some cancers (e.g., endometrial carcinoma, renal carcinoma).

Chemistry and Stability

■ **Chemistry** Medroxyprogesterone acetate is a synthetic progestin. Medroxyprogesterone acetate is a derivative of 17 α-hydroxyprogesterone that differs structurally by the addition of a 6 α-methyl group and a 17 α-acetate group.

Medroxyprogesterone acetate occurs as a white to off-white, odorless, crystalline powder and is insoluble in water and sparingly soluble in alcohol. Medroxyprogesterone acetate is commercially available alone and in fixed combination with estrogens (i.e., conjugated estrogens, estradiol cypionate). Medroxyprogesterone acetate suspension is a sterile suspension of the drug in a suitable aqueous medium. The commercially available medroxyprogesterone acetate injectable suspension containing 150 mg/mL also contains polyethylene glycol 3350, polysorbate 80, sodium chloride, and parabens as a preservative; the sterile suspension containing 400 mg/mL also contains polyethylene glycol 3350, sodium sulfate, and myristyl-gamma-picolinium chloride as a preservative. The commercially available medroxyprogesterone acetate injectable suspension containing 104 mg/0.65 mL contains polyethylene glycol, sodium chloride, povidone, polysorbate 80, parabens as a preservative, methionine, and phosphate buffers. The commercially available injection containing medroxyprogesterone acetate in fixed combination with estradiol cypionate is available as a sterile aqueous suspension; the injection also contains polyethylene glycol, polysorbate (Tween®) 80, sodium chloride, and parabens as preservatives. Sodium hydroxide and/or hydrochloric acid may be added during the manufacture of the sterile suspensions to adjust the pH to 3–7.

■ **Stability** Sterile medroxyprogesterone acetate suspensions should be stored at 20–25°C. The sterile injectable suspension containing medroxyprogesterone acetate in fixed combination with estradiol cypionate should be stored at 25°C, but may be exposed to temperatures ranging from 15–30°C. Medroxyprogesterone acetate tablets should be stored in well-closed containers at 20–25°C.

Preparations

Excipients in commercially available drug preparations may have clinically important effects in some individuals; consult specific product labeling for details.

medroxyPROGESTERone Acetate

Oral		
Tablets	2.5 mg*	**Medroxyprogesterone Acetate Tablets**
		Provera® (scored), Pfizer
	5 mg*	**Medroxyprogesterone Acetate Tablets**
		Provera® (scored), Pfizer
	10 mg*	**Medroxyprogesterone Acetate Tablets**
		Provera® (scored), Pfizer
Parenteral		
Injectable suspension	104 mg/0.65 mL	**depo-subQ provera 104®** (available in prefilled syringes with UltraSafe Passive® needle guard), Pfizer
	150 mg/mL*	**Depo-Provera® Contraceptive,** Pfizer
		Medroxyprogesterone Acetate Contraceptive
	400 mg/mL	**Depo-Provera®**, Pfizer

*available from one or more manufacturer, distributor, and/or repackager by generic (nonproprietary) name

medroxyPROGESTERone Acetate Combinations

Oral		
Tablets, monophasic regimen	1.5 mg with Conjugated Estrogens 0.3 mg (28 tablets)	**Prempro®**, Wyeth
	1.5 mg with Conjugated Estrogens 0.45 mg (28 tablets)	**Prempro®**, Wyeth
	2.5 mg with Conjugated Estrogens 0.625 mg (28 tablets)	**Prempro®**, Wyeth
	5 mg with Conjugated Estrogens 0.625 mg (28 tablets)	**Prempro®**, Wyeth
Tablets, biphasic regimen	5 mg with Conjugated Estrogens 0.625 mg (14 tablets) and Conjugated Estrogens 0.625 mg (14 tablets)	**Premphase®**, Wyeth
Parenteral		
Injectable suspension	25 mg/0.5 mL with Estradiol Cypionate 5 mg/0.5 mL	**Lunelle® Monthly Contraceptive Injection,** Pfizer

†Use is not currently included in the labeling approved by the US Food and Drug Administration

Norethindrone Acetate

Norethisterone Acetate

■ Norethindrone acetate is a synthetic progestin.

Uses

Norethindrone acetate is used for the treatment of secondary amenorrhea and for the treatment of abnormal uterine bleeding caused by hormonal imbalance in patients without underlying organic pathology such as fibroids or uterine cancer. The drug also is used for the treatment of endometriosis.

For the use of low-dose norethindrone as a progestin-only oral contraceptive, see Progestins 68:12. For the use of norethindrone or norethindrone acetate in combination with estrogens as an oral contraceptive, see Estrogen-Progestin Combinations 68:12.

Dosage and Administration

■ **Administration** Norethindrone acetate is administered orally.

■ **Dosage** ***Amenorrhea and Uterine Bleeding*** In establishing the dosage cycle for the treatment of secondary amenorrhea or abnormal uterine bleeding, the menstrual cycle is considered to be 28 days. The first day of bleeding is counted as the first day of the cycle. For the treatment of secondary amenorrhea or abnormal uterine bleeding, the usual oral dosage of norethindrone acetate is 2.5–10 mg daily for 5–10 days, beginning during the assumed latter half of the menstrual cycle to produce an optimum secretory transformation of an endometrium that has been adequately primed with endogenous or exogenous estrogen. Progestin-induced withdrawal bleeding usually occurs within 3–7 days after discontinuing therapy with the drug. Patients with a history of recurrent episodes of uterine bleeding may benefit from planned cycling with the drug.

Endometriosis For the treatment of endometriosis, the usual initial oral dosage of norethindrone acetate is 5 mg daily for 14 consecutive days. Norethindrone acetate therapy may be increased by 2.5 mg daily at 14-day intervals until a maximum dosage of 15 mg daily is reached. Daily therapy may then be continued consecutively (*no* cyclic drug-free periods) for 6–9 months; if annoying breakthrough bleeding occurs, therapy should be temporarily discontinued.

Cautions

■ **Adverse Effects** Norethindrone, like other progestins, may cause breakthrough bleeding, spotting, changes in menstrual flow, amenorrhea, changes in cervical erosion and secretions, edema, weight gain or loss, cholestatic jaundice, allergic rash with or without pruritus, melasma or chloasma, and mental depression.

An association between thrombophlebitis, pulmonary embolism, and cerebral thrombosis and embolism and use of estrogen-progestin combination preparations has been shown. (See Thromboembolic Disorders in Cautions: Cardiovascular Effects, in Estrogen-Progestin Combinations 68:12.) The possibility that thromboembolic disorders may occur in patients receiving norethindrone should be considered and patients should be carefully observed for these effects during therapy with the drug. Although available evidence suggests that an association exists between neuro-ocular lesions such as optic neuritis or retinal thrombosis and use of estrogen-progestin combination preparations, such a relationship has been neither confirmed nor refuted. Increased blood pressure in susceptible individuals, premenstrual-like syndrome, changes in libido or appetite, cystitis-like syndrome, headache, nervousness, dizziness, fatigue, backache, hirsutism, loss of scalp hair, erythema multiforme or nodosum, hemorrhagic skin eruption, and itching have occurred in patients receiving estrogen-progestin combination preparations. Use of estrogen-progestin combinations has also been associated with increased levels of coagulation factors VII, VIII, IX, and X. The possibility that these effects may occur in patients receiving norethindrone should be considered and patients should be carefully observed for these effects during therapy with the drug.

■ **Precautions and Contraindications** Norethindrone shares the toxic potentials of progestins, and the usual precautions of progestin therapy should be observed. Because oral contraceptive combinations contain progestins, the precautions associated with oral contraceptives should generally be considered in patients receiving progestins. (See Cautions in Estrogen-Progestin Combinations 68:12.) Prior to initiation of therapy with norethindrone in women, a physical examination should be performed, including special attention to the breasts and pelvic organs and a Papanicolaou test (Pap smear). Women receiving norethindrone should be given a copy of the patient labeling for the drug.

Norethindrone should be used with caution, and only with careful monitoring, in patients with conditions that might be aggravated by fluid retention (e.g., asthma, seizure disorders, migraine, or cardiac or renal dysfunction). The drug should also be used with caution in patients with a history of mental depression; norethindrone should be discontinued if depression recurs to a serious degree during therapy with the drug.

When breakthrough bleeding or irregular vaginal bleeding occurs during norethindrone therapy, nonfunctional causes should be considered. Adequate diagnostic procedures should be performed in patients with undiagnosed vaginal bleeding.

The manufacturers caution that the effect of long-term norethindrone therapy on pituitary, ovarian, adrenal, hepatic, or uterine function has not been determined. Diabetic patients should be carefully monitored during norethindrone therapy, since decreased glucose tolerance has been observed in women receiving estrogen-progestin combinations. Norethindrone may mask the onset of climacteric in women.

The clinician and the patient using norethindrone should be alert to the earliest signs and symptoms of thromboembolic and thrombotic disorders (e.g., thrombophlebitis, pulmonary embolism, cerebrovascular insufficiency, coronary occlusion, retinal thrombosis, mesenteric thrombosis). The drug should be discontinued immediately when any of these disorders occurs or is suspected.

If unexplained, sudden or gradual, partial or complete loss of vision; proptosis or diplopia; papilledema; retinal vascular lesions; or migraine occur during therapy with norethindrone, the drug should be discontinued and appropriate diagnostic and therapeutic measures instituted. Because steroidal hormones are metabolized in the liver, norethindrone should be used with caution in patients with impaired liver function.

Norethindrone is contraindicated in patients with thrombophlebitis, thromboembolic disorders, cerebral apoplexy, or a history of these conditions. The drug is also contraindicated in patients with undiagnosed vaginal bleeding, missed abortion, known sensitivity to the drug or any ingredient in the formulation, markedly impaired liver function or liver disease, or carcinoma of the breast or for use as a pregnancy test.

■ **Mutagenicity and Carcinogenicity** The carcinogenic and mutagenic potentials of norethindrone have not been specifically determined.

Administration of medroxyprogesterone to beagles has been associated with the development of mammary nodules, some of which were malignant. Although nodules occasionally occurred in control beagles, they were intermittent in nature; nodules in drug-treated beagles were larger, more numerous, persistent, and occasionally malignant with metastases. The clinical relevance of these findings to humans has not been established. For additional information on the carcinogenic potential of progestins, see Cautions: Mutagenicity and Carcinogenicity, in Medroxyprogesterone Acetate 68:32.

■ **Pregnancy and Lactation** Although progestins have been used beginning in the first trimester of pregnancy to prevent habitual abortion or to treat threatened abortion, there is no adequate evidence from well-controlled studies to substantiate the efficacy of progestins for these uses; however, there is evidence of potential adverse effects on the fetus when these drugs are administered during the first 4 months of pregnancy. In addition, in most women, the cause of abortion is a defective ovum, which progestins could not be expected to influence. Because of their uterine-relaxant effects, progestins may delay spontaneous abortion of fertilized defective ova. Masculinization of the female fetus has reportedly occurred when progestins were used during pregnancy. Clitoral hypertrophy and fusion of the labia have been reported in a few female neonates born to women who had received medroxyprogesterone during pregnancy; hypospadias in male neonates born to women receiving progestational agents occurs at approximately twice the rate of occurrence in male neonates born to women not receiving the drugs. An association between intrauterine exposure to female sex hormones and congenital anomalies, including cardiovascular and limb defects, has been suggested. (See Cautions: Pregnancy, Fertility, and Lactation, in Estrogen-Progestin Combinations 68:12.) Use of progestins, including norethindrone, is not recommended during the first 4 months of pregnancy. If a woman becomes pregnant while receiving norethindrone or is inadvertently exposed to the drug during the first 4 months of pregnancy, she should be advised of the potential risks to the fetus.

Norethindrone should *not* be used to induce withdrawal bleeding as a test for pregnancy.

Progestins are reportedly distributed into milk. The manufacturers warn that the possible effects of progestins in milk on nursing infants have not been determined.

Pharmacology

Norethindrone shares the pharmacologic actions of the progestins. In women with adequate endogenous estrogen, norethindrone transforms a proliferative endometrium into a secretory one. Norethindrone has been shown to have some estrogenic, androgenic, and anabolic activity. The drug inhibits the secretion of pituitary gonadotropins at usual dosages and thus prevents follicular maturation and ovulation.

Chemistry and Stability

■ **Chemistry** Norethindrone is a synthetic progestin. The drug is the 17α-ethinyl derivative of 19-nortestosterone which differs structurally from norethynodrel only in the position of the double bond in the A ring of the steroid. Norethindrone acetate is the acetic acid ester of norethindrone.

Norethindrone acetate occurs as a white to creamy white, odorless, crystalline powder and is practically insoluble in water and soluble in alcohol. Norethindrone acetate is about twice as potent as norethindrone.

■ **Stability** Norethindrone acetate tablets should be stored in well-closed containers at room temperature (approximately 25°C).

Preparations

Excipients in commercially available drug preparations may have clinically important effects in some individuals; consult specific product labeling for details.

Norethindrone Acetate

Oral		
Tablets	5 mg*	Aygestin® (scored), Duramed
		Norethindrone Acetate Tablets (scored)

*available from one or more manufacturer, distributor, and/or repackager by generic (nonproprietary) name

Progesterone

Pregnenedione, Progestin

■ Progesterone is a naturally occurring progestin secreted by the corpus luteum and is the prototype of the progestins.

Uses

Progesterone is used orally to reduce the incidence of endometrial hyperplasia in postmenopausal women receiving estrogen replacement therapy.

Progesterone is used orally or intravaginally for the management of secondary amenorrhea.

Progesterone is used intravaginally to support embryo implantation and early pregnancy by supplementing corpus luteal function as part of assisted reproductive technology (ART) treatment of infertile women. Efficacy of progesterone vaginal insert for this indication has not been established in women 35 years of age or older.

Progesterone is used parenterally for the treatment of amenorrhea and for the treatment of abnormal uterine bleeding caused by hormonal imbalance in patients without underlying organic pathology such as fibroids or uterine cancer. Progesterone also is used parenterally to support embryo implantation and early pregnancy by supplementing corpus luteal function as part of ART treatment† of infertile women.

Dosage and Administration

■ **Administration** Progesterone is administered by orally, intravaginally, and by IM injection.

Progesterone capsules are administered orally once daily at bedtime. Women who have difficulty swallowing the capsules should be advised to swallow progesterone capsules while in an upright position and with adequate amounts of fluid (e.g., a glass of water). Administration at bedtime may alleviate some of the adverse effects (e.g., dizziness, blurred vision) associated with the drug.

Progesterone vaginal gel should *not* be administered concurrently with other intravaginal preparations. If therapy with another agent administered intravaginally is needed, such therapy should be administered 6 hours before or 6 hours after progesterone vaginal gel.

Concomitant use of progesterone vaginal inserts with other preparations that are administered intravaginally is *not* recommended. Although specific studies have not been undertaken, the possibility exists that concomitant administration of a progesterone vaginal insert with another preparation administered intravaginally may alter the release and absorption of progesterone from the vaginal insert.

■ **Dosage** ***Amenorrhea*** When progesterone capsules are used in the management of secondary amenorrhea, the recommended dosage of progesterone is 400 mg once daily at bedtime for 10 days.

When progesterone vaginal gel is used for the management of secondary amenorrhea, the contents of one prefilled applicator of progesterone 4% vaginal gel (approximately 1.125 g of gel containing 45 mg of progesterone) should be inserted intravaginally every other day for a total of 6 doses. Women who do not respond to the 4% gel may be given progesterone 8% vaginal gel. For these women, the contents of one prefilled applicator of the 8% vaginal gel (approximately 1.125 g of gel containing 90 mg of progesterone) should be inserted intravaginally every other day for a total of 6 doses. Women who require the higher dose should receive the 8% vaginal gel; increasing the volume of the 4% gel will not achieve the same progesterone concentrations as administration of the 8% gel.

When parenteral progesterone is used for the treatment of amenorrhea, the usual dosage of progesterone is 5–10 mg administered IM daily for 6–8 days. When sufficient ovarian activity is present to produce a proliferative endometrium, withdrawal bleeding will usually occur within 48–72 hours after discontinuing therapy with the drug. Spontaneous normal cycles may occur in some patients after a single course of therapy.

Assisted Reproductive Technology Treatment When progesterone vaginal gel is used as part of an assisted reproductive technology (ART) treatment regimen in women who require progesterone supplementation, the contents of one prefilled applicator of progesterone 8% vaginal gel (approximately 1.125 g of gel containing 90 mg of progesterone) should be inserted intravaginally once daily. When progesterone vaginal gel is used in women with partial or complete ovarian failure who require progesterone replacement, the contents of one prefilled applicator of progesterone 8% vaginal gel (approximately 1.125 g of gel containing 90 mg of progesterone) should be inserted intravaginally twice daily. If pregnancy occurs, treatment with progesterone gel may be continued until placental autonomy is achieved, up to 10–12 weeks.

When progesterone vaginal inserts are used as part of an ART treatment regimen in women younger than 35 years of age, one vaginal insert containing 100 mg of progesterone is inserted intravaginally 2 or 3 times daily, starting at oocyte retrieval. Therapy may be continued for up to 10 weeks. The appropriate dosage for women 35 years of age or older has not been established.

Prevention of Endometrial Changes Associated with Estrogens When progesterone capsules are used in conjunction with estrogen replacement therapy, progesterone is administered in a dosage of 200 mg once daily at bedtime for 12 consecutive days (e.g., days 17–28) of the 28-day cycle.

Uterine Bleeding When parenteral progesterone is used for the treatment of abnormal uterine bleeding, the usual dosage of progesterone is 5–10 mg administered IM daily for 6 days. When estrogen therapy is used concomitantly with progesterone, progesterone therapy is usually initiated after 2 weeks of estrogen therapy. Therapy with progesterone is usually discontinued if menses occurs during the series of injections.

Cautions

■ **Adverse Effects** Adverse effects reported in patients receiving oral progesterone include dizziness, breast pain, headache, abdominal pain, fatigue, viral infection, abdominal distention, musculoskeletal pain, emotional lability, irritability, and upper respiratory tract infection. Extreme dizziness and/or drowsiness, blurred vision, slurred speech, difficulty walking, loss of consciousness, vertigo, confusion, disorientation, and shortness of breath have been reported in a few women receiving the drug. Hypotension and syncope have occurred rarely in women receiving progesterone capsules.

Adverse effects reported in patients receiving progesterone vaginal gel include breast pain/enlargement, somnolence, constipation, nausea, headache, and perineal pain.

Adverse effects reported in patients receiving progesterone vaginal insert include abdominal pain, nausea, and ovarian hyperstimulation syndrome.

Adverse effects reported in patients receiving IM progesterone include breakthrough bleeding, spotting, changes in menstrual flow, amenorrhea, changes in cervical erosion and secretions, edema, weight gain or loss, cholestatic jaundice, allergic rash with or without pruritus, breast tenderness, galactorrhea, alopecia, hirsutism, pyrexia, sleep disturbances, nausea, and mental depression. Pain and swelling at the site of injection may occur following IM administration of progesterone. Large doses (50–100 mg daily) of progesterone may cause a moderate catabolic effect and a transient increase in sodium and chloride excretion.

An association between pulmonary embolism and cerebral thrombosis and embolism and use of estrogen-progestin combination preparations has been shown. (See Thromboembolic Disorders in Cautions: Cardiovascular Effects, in Estrogen-Progestin Combinations 68:12.) The possibility that thromboembolic disorders may occur in patients receiving progesterone should be considered and patients should be carefully observed for these effects during therapy with the drug. Although available evidence suggests that an association exists between neuro-ocular lesions such as optic neuritis or retinal thrombosis and use of estrogen-progestin combination preparations, such a relationship has been neither confirmed nor refuted.

■ **Precautions and Contraindications** Progesterone shares the toxic potentials of progestins, and the usual precautions of progestin therapy should be observed. Prior to initiation of therapy with progesterone in women, a physical examination should be performed, including special attention to the breasts and pelvic organs and a Papanicolaou test (Pap smear). Women receiving progesterone should be given a copy of the patient labeling for the drug.

Progesterone should be used with caution, and only with careful monitoring, in patients with conditions that might be aggravated by fluid retention (e.g., asthma, seizure disorders, migraine, or cardiac or renal dysfunction). The drug should also be used with caution in patients with a history of mental depression; progesterone should be discontinued if depression recurs to a serious degree during therapy with the drug.

When breakthrough bleeding or irregular vaginal bleeding occurs during progesterone therapy, nonfunctional causes should be considered. Adequate diagnostic procedures should be performed in patients with undiagnosed vaginal bleeding.

Diabetic patients should be carefully monitored during progesterone therapy, since decreased glucose tolerance has been observed in women receiving estrogen-progestin combinations. Progesterone may mask the onset of climacteric in women.

The clinician and the patient using progesterone should be alert to the earliest signs and symptoms of myocardial infarction, cerebrovascular disorders, thromboembolism (e.g., venous thromboembolism, pulmonary embolism), thrombophlebitis, or retinal thrombosis. The drug should be discontinued immediately when any of these disorders occurs or is suspected.

If unexplained, sudden or gradual, partial or complete loss of vision; proptosis or diplopia; papilledema; retinal vascular lesions; or migraine occur during therapy with progesterone, the drug should be discontinued and appropriate diagnostic and therapeutic measures instituted.

Because dizziness has been reported during therapy with oral progesterone, patients receiving such therapy should be advised to use caution while driving or operating machinery.

Progesterone is contraindicated in patients with thrombophlebitis, thromboembolic disorders, cerebral apoplexy, or a history of these conditions. The drug is also contraindicated in patients with undiagnosed vaginal bleeding, missed abortion, known sensitivity to the drug or any ingredient in the formulation, markedly impaired liver function or liver disease, or carcinoma of the breast or for use as a pregnancy test.

Progesterone capsules are contraindicated in individuals with known hypersensitivity to peanuts because the capsules contain peanut oil.

■ **Mutagenicity and Carcinogenicity** The carcinogenic and mutagenic potentials of progesterone have not been specifically determined.

Administration of medroxyprogesterone to beagles has been associated with the development of mammary nodules, some of which were malignant. Although nodules occasionally occurred in control beagles, they were intermittent in nature; nodules in drug-treated beagles were larger, more numerous, persistent, and occasionally malignant with metastases. The clinical relevance of these findings to humans has not been established. For additional information on the carcinogenic potential of progestins, see Cautions: Mutagenicity and Carcinogenicity, in Medroxyprogesterone Acetate 68:32.

■ **Pregnancy and Lactation** Progesterone is used to support embryo implantation and maintain pregnancy as a component of assisted reproductive technology (ART) treatment in infertile women. Such use is associated with increased ongoing pregnancy rates.

Although progestins have been used beginning in the first trimester of pregnancy to prevent habitual abortion or to treat threatened abortion, there is no adequate evidence from well-controlled studies to substantiate the efficacy of progestins for these uses; however, there is evidence of potential adverse effects on the fetus when these drugs are administered during the first 4 months of pregnancy. In addition, in most women, the cause of abortion is a defective ovum, which progestins could not be expected to influence. Because of their uterine-relaxant effects, progestins may delay spontaneous abortion of fertilized defective ova. Masculinization of the female fetus has reportedly occurred when progestins were used during pregnancy. Clitoral hypertrophy has been reported in a few female neonates born to women who had received medroxyprogesterone during pregnancy. An association between intrauterine exposure to female sex hormones and congenital anomalies, including cardiovascular and limb defects, has been suggested. (See Cautions: Pregnancy, Fertility, and Lactation, in Estrogen-Progestin Combinations 68:12.) Use of progestins generally is not recommended during the first 4 months of pregnancy.

Progesterone should *not* be used to induce withdrawal bleeding as a test for pregnancy.

Progestins are reportedly distributed into milk. The manufacturers warn that the possible effects of progestins in milk on nursing infants have not been determined.

Laboratory Test Interferences

The manufacturers caution that estrogen-progestin combinations have caused abnormal thyroid function test results. (See Effects on Thyroid in Cautions: Endocrine and Metabolic Effects, in Estrogen-Progestin Combinations 68:12.) The manufacturers also caution that estrogen-progestin combinations have altered the metyrapone test (see Laboratory Test Interferences in Estrogen-Progestin Combinations 68:12), and that these combinations have altered liver function test results (see Cautions: Hepatic Effects, in Estrogen-Progestin Combinations 68:12). These combinations have also caused decreased pregnanediol excretion.

The manufacturers state that the pathologist should be advised of progesterone use when relevant specimens from a patient exposed to the drug are submitted.

Pharmacology

Progesterone is a progestinic hormone secreted mainly from the corpus luteum of the ovary during the latter half of the menstrual cycle. Progesterone is formed from steroid precursors in the ovary, testis, adrenal cortex, and placenta. Luteinizing hormone (LH) stimulates the synthesis and secretion of progesterone from the corpus luteum. Progesterone is necessary for nidation (implantation) of the ovum and for maintenance of pregnancy. Although the hormone is secreted mainly during the luteal phase of the menstrual cycle, small amounts of progesterone are also secreted during the follicular phase. High concentrations of the hormone are secreted during the latter part of pregnancy. Amounts comparable to those secreted in women during the follicular phase have been shown to be secreted in males.

Progesterone shares the pharmacologic actions of the progestins. In women with adequate endogenous estrogen, progesterone transforms a proliferative endometrium into a secretory one. The abrupt decline in the secretion of progesterone at the end of the menstrual cycle is principally responsible for the onset of menstruation. Progesterone also stimulates the growth of mammary alveolar tissue and relaxes uterine smooth muscle. Progesterone has minimal estrogenic and androgenic activity.

Progesterone has a short plasma half-life of several minutes. The hormone is reduced to pregnanediol in the liver and conjugated with glucuronic acid, and then excreted mainly in urine.

Chemistry and Stability

■ **Chemistry** Progesterone is a naturally occurring progestin secreted by the corpus luteum. Progesterone is the prototype of the progestins. The drug may be obtained from animal ovaries but is usually prepared synthetically from stigmasterol or from diosgenin (extracted from *Dioscorea mexicana*, a Mexican yam).

Progesterone occurs as a white or creamy white, crystalline powder and is practically insoluble in water, soluble in alcohol, and sparingly soluble in vegetable oils. Progesterone injection is a sterile solution of the drug in a suitable solvent.

■ **Stability** Progesterone is stable when exposed to air. The drug should be stored in tight, light-resistant containers. Parenteral progesterone preparations, progesterone capsules, progesterone vaginal inserts, and progesterone vaginal gel should be stored at 15–30°C.

Preparations

Excipients in commercially available drug preparations may have clinically important effects in some individuals; consult specific product labeling for details.

Progesterone

Powder		**Progesterone Powder Micronized or Microcrystalline for Prescription Compounding**
Oral		
Capsules	100 mg	**Prometrium®**, Abbott
	200 mg	**Prometrium®**, Abbott
Parenteral		
Injection	50 mg/mL*	**Progesterone Injection**
Vaginal		
Gel	4%	**Crinone®** (available in prefilled, disposable applicators), Watson
	8%	**Crinone®** (available in prefilled, disposable applicators), Watson
Insert	100 mg	**Endometrin®** (with disposable applicators), Ferring Pharmaceuticals

*available from one or more manufacturer, distributor, and/or repackager by generic (nonproprietary) name

†Use is not currently included in the labeling approved by the US Food and Drug Administration

THYROID AND ANTITHYROID AGENTS 68:36

THYROID AGENTS 68:36.04

Thyroid Agents General Statement

■ Thyroid agents are natural or synthetic preparations containing tetraiodothyronine (thyroxine, T_4) and/or triiodothyronine (T_3).

Uses

■ **Hypothyroidism** Thyroid agents are used for supplementation or replacement of diminished or absent thyroid function resulting from primary causes including functional deficiency, primary atrophy, or partial or complete absence of the gland, or from the effects of surgery, radiation, or antithyroid agents; the drugs are not used for the management of transient hypothyroidism during the recovery phase of subacute thyroiditis. Thyroid agents also are used for replacement or supplemental therapy in patients with secondary (pituitary) or tertiary (hypothalamic) hypothyroidism and subclinical hypothyroidism. Therapy must be maintained continuously to control the symptoms of hypothyroidism. Levothyroxine sodium generally is the preferred thyroid agent for replacement therapy because its hormonal content is standardized and its effect is therefore predictable. Levothyroxine sodium also is considered the thyroid agent of choice for the treatment of congenital hypothyroidism (cretinism); however, other thyroid agents have been used. The earlier replacement therapy is initiated in congenital hypothyroidism, the greater is the potential for normal growth and development. (See Cautions: Pediatric Precautions.)

Levothyroxine sodium IV injection is used in the treatment of myxedema coma. Levothyroxine sodium injection has been used in other conditions when rapid thyroid replacement is required†; however, this is not an FDA-labeled use for the currently available injection.

■ **Pituitary TSH Suppression** Thyroid agents may be beneficial in the management or prevention of various types of euthyroid goiters, including thyroid nodules, subacute or chronic lymphocytic thyroiditis (Hashimoto's thyroiditis), and multinodular goiter. In these conditions, thyroid agents act as replacement therapy and may cause a reduction in goiter size by suppressing the secretion of thyrotropin.

Thyroid agents also may be used in conjunction with surgery and radioactive iodine therapy in the management of thyrotropin-dependent well-differentiated, papillary or follicular carcinoma of the thyroid.

■ **Other Uses** Thyroid agents may be used in combination with antithyroid agents in the treatment of thyrotoxicosis to prevent goitrogenesis and hypothyroidism. While administration of thyroid agents may occasionally be useful to prevent antithyroid agent-induced hypothyroidism in the management of thyrotoxicosis during pregnancy, combination therapy generally is considered unnecessary since it may increase the requirement for antithyroid agents and therefore the risk of fetal hypothyroidism, which is not amenable to exogenous thyroid agent therapy.

Thyroid agents may be used diagnostically in suppression tests to differentiate suspected hyperthyroidism from euthyroidism in patients with clinical signs and symptoms compatible with mild hyperthyroidism in whom baseline laboratory tests do not confirm the diagnosis, or to determine thyroid gland autonomy in patients with eye changes compatible with Graves' ophthalmology who are clinically and biochemically euthyroid and in whom demonstration of thyroid gland autonomy would support the diagnosis.

The use of thyroid agents, alone or in combination with other drugs, in the treatment of obesity and for weight loss is unjustified and has been shown to be ineffective. (See Cautions: Precautions and Contraindications.) The use of thyroid agents for the treatment of male or female infertility also is not justified unless the condition is accompanied by hypothyroidism.

Dosage and Administration

■ **Administration** Thyroid agents usually are administered orally. Levothyroxine sodium (and occasionally liothyronine sodium) may be given by IV injection. Levothyroxine sodium also has been administered by IM injection†, however, the IV route is preferred since absorption may be variable following IM administration. IM administration is not an FDA-labeled route of administration for the currently available levothyroxine sodium injection. Oral therapy should replace parenteral therapy as soon as possible.

■ **Dosage** Dosage of thyroid agents must be carefully adjusted according to individual requirements and response. (See Cautions: Precautions and Contraindications.) The age and general physical condition of the patient and the severity and duration of hypothyroid symptoms determine the initial dosage and the rate at which dosage may be increased to the eventual maintenance dosage. Dosage should be initiated at a lower level in geriatric patients; in patients with long-standing disease, other endocrinopathies, or functional or ECG evidence of cardiovascular disease; and in patients with severe hypothyroidism. Adjustment of thyroid replacement therapy should be determined mainly by the patient's clinical response and confirmed by appropriate laboratory tests.

In infants and children, it is essential to achieve rapid and complete thyroid replacement because of the critical importance of thyroid hormone in sustaining growth and maturation. In general, despite the smaller body size of children, the dosage (on a weight basis) required to sustain a full rate of growth, development, and general thriving is higher in children than in adults.

■ **Laboratory Monitoring** Thyroid function status must be assessed periodically in patients receiving thyroid agents as a guide to therapy. Various laboratory tests are available to monitor thyroid function, and clinicians should consult specialized references for information on specific tests and their use and interpretation. Selection of appropriate tests for the diagnosis and management of hypothyroidism or hyperthyroidism depends on patient-specific variables (e.g., signs and symptoms of thyroid disease, pregnancy, concomitant administration of drugs). A combination of sensitive thyrotropin (thyroid-stimulating hormone, TSH) assay *plus* free thyroxine (T_4) and/or total or free triiodothyronine (T_3) assay usually is recommended to confirm a diagnosis of thyroid disease. TSH assay alone may be used initially to screen for thyroid disease and to monitor during drug therapy. Other thyroid function tests that may be used include total serum concentrations of T_4 triiodothyronine resin uptake, free T_4 index (the product of total serum T_4 multiplied by the percentage of serum T_3 resin uptake), and thyrotropin-releasing hormone (TRH) stimulation test.

Cautions

Adverse reactions to thyroid agents result principally from overdosage. (See Toxicity.)

■ **Toxicity** ***Manifestations*** Adverse reactions to thyroid agents result from overdosage and are manifested principally as signs and symptoms of hyperthyroidism including fatigue, weight loss, increased appetite, palpitations, nervousness, hyperactivity, anxiety, irritability, emotional lability, diarrhea, abdominal cramps, vomiting, elevated liver transaminase concentrations, sweating, tachycardia, increased pulse and blood pressures, angina pectoris, cardiac arrhythmias, tremors, muscle weakness, headache, insomnia, intolerance to heat, fever, hair loss, flushing, decreased bone mineral density, impaired fertility, and menstrual irregularities. Complications of severe overdosage may include cardiac decompensation, cardiac failure, myocardial infarction, cardiac arrest, and possibly death secondary to cardiac arrhythmia or failure. Seizures have been reported rarely with levothyroxine therapy. The effects of levothyroxine sodium, thyroid, or thyroglobulin may not appear for 1–3 weeks following initiation of therapy or an increase in dosage, but may appear within 24–72 hours after initiation of therapy or an increase in dosage with liothyronine sodium.

Treatment Manifestations of overdosage are usually readily reversible following temporary discontinuance of therapy and are obviated by a reduction in dosage. If manifestations of overdosage appear with levothyroxine sodium, thyroid, or thyroglobulin, the drug should be discontinued for 2–7 days, and for 2–3 days in the case of liothyronine sodium, and then resumed at a lower dosage. For information on the treatment of acute overdosage of thyroid agents, see Acute Toxicity: Treatment.

■ **Other Adverse Effects** Hypersensitivity reactions to excipients in formulations of thyroid agents have been reported rarely. Manifestations include urticaria, pruritus, skin rash, flushing, angioedema, various GI symptoms (e.g., abdominal pain, nausea, vomiting, diarrhea), fever, arthralgia, serum sickness, and wheezing. Thyroid also may rarely cause GI intolerance in patients highly sensitive to pork. One manufacturer states that GI intolerance may also rarely occur in patients highly sensitive to corn.

■ **Precautions and Contraindications** Because thyroid agents have a narrow therapeutic index, dosage must be carefully adjusted to avoid the consequences of under or over treatment, including adverse effects on growth and development in pediatric patients, cardiovascular function, bone metabolism, reproductive function, cognitive function, emotional state, GI function, and glucose and lipid metabolism.

Patients receiving thyroid agents must be closely monitored and thyroid function status must be periodically assessed by appropriate laboratory studies. (See Dosage and Administration: Laboratory Monitoring.) Since hypothyroid patients, especially those with myxedema, are particularly sensitive to thyroid agents, replacement therapy should be initiated with low doses and subsequent dosage should be gradually increased in such patients.

Thyroid agents should be used with extreme caution and in reduced dosage in patients with angina pectoris or other cardiovascular disease, including hypertension. If chest pain or other aggravation of cardiovascular disease occurs in patients receiving thyroid agents, dosage should be reduced or temporarily withheld and reinstituted at a lower dosage. Overtreatment with thyroid agents may result in adverse cardiovascular effects (e.g., increased heart rate, cardiac wall thickness, cardiac contractility) and may precipitate angina pectoris or arrhythmias. Because the possibility of precipitating cardiac arrhythmias may be greater in patients receiving thyroid agents, patients with coronary artery disease should be closely monitored during surgery. Thyroid agents should be used with caution in geriatric patients since occult cardiac disease may be present.

Morphologic hypogonadism and nephroses should be ruled out before thyroid agents are administered. In patients whose hypothyroidism is secondary to hypopituitarism, adrenal insufficiency is likely to be present. When adrenal insufficiency and hypothyroidism exist concomitantly, adrenal insufficiency must be corrected by administration of corticosteroids before therapy with thyroid agents is initiated. Initiation of thyroid hormone therapy without prior treatment with corticosteroids may result in increased metabolic clearance of corticosteroids and, thus, may precipitate an acute adrenal crisis. Hypopituitarism, adrenal insufficiency, and other endocrine disorders such as diabetes mellitus and diabetes insipidus are characterized by signs and symptoms which may be diminished in severity or obscured by hypothyroidism. Thyroid agents may aggravate the intensity of previously obscured symptoms in patients with endocrine disorders, and appropriate adjustment of therapy for these concomitant disorders may be required.

Except in patients with transient hypothyroidism or in those receiving a therapeutic trial with an agent, patients should be advised that replacement therapy with a thyroid agent must be maintained continuously to control the symptoms of hypothyroidism and that clinical improvement may not occur until after several weeks of therapy. Patients should be instructed to immediately report any signs or symptoms of thyroid toxicity (hyperthyroidism) (e.g., chest pain, increased pulse rate, palpitations, excessive sweating, heat intolerance, nervousness) or any unusual event which occurs during therapy with a thyroid agent. (See Cautions: Toxicity and Other Adverse Effects.) Because dosage of antidiabetic agents (i.e., insulin, sulfonylureas) may require adjustment during thyroid agent replacement therapy, patients with diabetes mellitus receiving an antidiabetic agent concomitantly should be advised to closely monitor urinary and/or blood glucose concentrations during concomitant therapy. Hypoglycemia may occur in these patients if therapy with a thyroid agent is stopped. Patients should be advised that partial loss of hair may occur during the first few months of therapy, but this effect is usually transient and subsequent regrowth usually occurs. When surgery is required, patients should be advised to inform the attending clinician (e.g., physician, dentist) that they are receiving thyroid hormone therapy.

Although thyroid agents have been used alone and in combination with other drugs for the treatment of obesity, dosages of thyroid agents within the usual range of daily requirements are *ineffective* for weight reduction in euthyroid individuals. Higher dosages may produce serious and even life-threatening manifestations of toxicity, especially when given in conjunction with sympathomimetic agents (e.g., amphetamines) used for their anorectic effect. The use of thyroid agents for the treatment of obesity or for weight loss is unjustified and contraindicated.

Thyroid agents are generally contraindicated in the presence of thyrotoxicosis and in acute myocardial infarction uncomplicated by hypothyroidism. When hypothyroidism is a complicating or causative factor in myocardial infarction, judicious use of small doses of thyroid agents may be considered. Thyroid agents are contraindicated in patients with uncorrected adrenal insufficiency because the drugs increase tissue demands for adrenal hormones and may precipitate an acute adrenal crisis in these patients. Although there is no well-documented evidence of true allergic or idiosyncratic reactions to thyroid agents, a particular agent should not be used in patients with apparent hypersensitivity to that agent or any ingredient in the formulation.

■ **Pediatric Precautions** Little, if any, maternal thyroid hormone is distributed to the fetus. The incidence of congenital hypothyroidism is relatively high (1:4000) and the hypothyroid fetus probably does not derive any benefit from the small amounts of thyroid hormones that may cross the placental barrier. Routine determination of serum thyroxine and/or thyrotropin (thyroid-stimulating hormone, TSH) concentrations is strongly advised in neonates because of the deleterious effects of thyroid deficiency on growth and development. Normal adult ranges for serum thyroxine concentrations must *not* be used to evaluate neonatal thyroid function, since failure to diagnose the condition may occur and result in disastrous effects on the prognosis. The Committee on Drugs of the American Academy of Pediatrics (AAP) recommends that physicians caring for children participate in state or regional screening programs for hypothyroidism and maintain a high level of clinical suspicion to assure the earliest possible diagnosis of congenital hypothyroidism. Signs and symptoms of congenital hypothyroidism include lethargy, hypothermia, feeding problems, failure to gain weight, dry skin, skin mottling, thick tongue, hoarse cry, umbilical hernia, persistence of mild jaundice, respiratory problems, and a large anterior and posterior fontanel.

Treatment, preferably with levothyroxine sodium, should be initiated immediately upon diagnosis, and maintained for life, unless transient hypothyroidism is suspected. If receipt of laboratory results will be delayed for several days or weeks, thyroid agent therapy may be initiated in neonates with suspected hypothyroidism pending the results of confirmative tests. The earlier replacement therapy is initiated in congenital hypothyroidism, the greater the potential for normal growth and development. If a positive diagnosis cannot be made on the basis of laboratory findings but there is a strong clinical suspicion of congenital hypothyroidism, a conservative approach would be to ensure euthyroidism with replacement therapy until the child is 1–2 years of age. Thyroid agent therapy can then be discontinued while diagnostic tests are carried out, and reinstituted if indicated; this treatment approach avoids the potential risk of the infant incurring serious, permanent brain damage. When transient hypothyroidism is suspected, therapy may be interrupted (or dosage of the thyroid agent reduced by half in suspected severe hypothyroidism) for 4–8 weeks to reassess the condition when the child is older than 3 years of age. If the diagnosis of permanent hypothyroidism is confirmed, full replacement therapy should be reinstituted. However, if serum concentrations of T_4 and TSH are normal, thyroid agent therapy may be discontinued, and the patient should be carefully monitored; thyroid function tests should be repeated if manifestations of hypothyroidism develop.

During the first 2 weeks of thyroid agent therapy, infants should be closely monitored for cardiac overload, arrhythmias, and aspiration resulting from avid suckling. Evaluation of the infant's clinical response to thyroid agent therapy should be performed about 6 weeks after initiation of therapy; additional examinations should be performed at least at 6 and 12 months of age and yearly thereafter. Achievement of normal serum thyrotropin concentration must *not* be used as the sole criterion of the adequacy of the dose in children with congenital hypothyroidism, since thyrotropin concentrations may remain elevated for several months during replacement therapy using proper or even excessive dosages of the thyroid agent. The goal of replacement therapy in these children is to maintain the serum thyroxine concentration at levels appropriate for age throughout infancy and childhood and to achieve and maintain normal intellectual and physical growth and development. Patients should be monitored closely to avoid undertreatment or overtreatment. Undertreatment may result in poor school performance (due to impaired concentration and slowed mentation) and reduced adult height. Overtreatment may result in craniosynostosis in infants and accelerate the aging of bones, resulting in premature epiphyseal closure and compromised adult stature.

Treated children may manifest a period of catch-up growth, which may be adequate in some cases to achieve normal adult height. In children with severe or long-standing hypothyroidism, catch-up growth may not be adequate to achieve normal adult height.

Pseudotumor cerebri and slipped capital femoral epiphysis have been reported in children receiving thyroid agent therapy.

■ **Mutagenicity and Carcinogenicity** Animal studies to determine the mutagenic or carcinogenic potential of thyroid agents have not been performed. Although an apparent association between prolonged thyroid therapy and breast cancer has been reported, the validity of the report has been seriously questioned. Patients receiving thyroid agents for established indications should not discontinue therapy.

■ **Pregnancy and Lactation** Thyroid agents do not readily cross the placenta, and clinical experience does not indicate any adverse effect on the fetus when thyroid agents are administered during pregnancy. Thyroid agent replacement therapy for hypothyroidism should be continued throughout pregnancy, and if hypothyroidism is diagnosed during pregnancy, treatment should be initiated. Serum thyroxine concentrations are lower than normal during pregnancy, and the diagnosis should be confirmed by determination of serum thyrotropin concentration. In pregnant women dependent on thyroid replacement therapy, increased dosage may be required.

If myxedema coma develops during pregnancy, patients should be treated with IV levothyroxine sodium. Although the manufacturer states that there are no reports of levothyroxine sodium injection use in pregnant women with myxedema, nontreatment is associated with a high probability of maternal or fetal morbidity or mortality.

Although only minimal amounts of thyroid hormones are distributed into milk, thyroid agents should be used with caution in nursing women.

Lactating women who develop myxedema coma should be treated with IV levothyroxine sodium. Although the manufacturer states that there are no reports of levothyroxine sodium injection use in lactating women with myxedema coma, nontreatment is associated with a high probability of maternal morbidity or mortality.

Acute Toxicity

■ **Manifestations** In general, acute overdosage of thyroid agents may be expected to produce signs and symptoms of hyperthyroidism. (See Toxicity.) Cerebral embolism, shock, coma, and death have been reported. In addition, confusion and disorientation may occur. Seizures have occurred in a child who ingested approximately 18 mg of levothyroxine; manifestations of toxicity may not necessarily be evident or may not appear until several days after ingestion of levothyroxine sodium.

■ **Treatment** In the treatment of acute thyroid agent overdosage, symptomatic and supportive therapy should be instituted immediately. Treatment consists principally of reducing GI absorption of the drugs and counteracting central and peripheral effects, mainly those of increased sympathetic activity. Initially, the stomach should be emptied immediately by inducing emesis or by gastric lavage; activated charcoal or cholestyramine resin also may be used to decrease absorption. If the patient is comatose, having seizures, or lacks the gag reflex, gastric lavage may be performed if an endotracheal tube with cuff inflated is in place to prevent aspiration of gastric contents. Oxygen may be administered and ventilation maintained. If congestive heart failure develops, cardiac glycosides may be administered. Measures to control arrhythmia, fever, hypoglycemia, or fluid loss should be initiated as necessary. β-Adrenergic blocking agents (e.g., propranolol) are useful to counteract many of the effects of increased sympathetic activity. Large doses of antithyroid drugs (e.g., methimazole, propylthiouracil) followed in 1–2 hours by large doses of iodine may be administered to inhibit synthesis and release of thyroid hormones. Corticosteroids may be given to inhibit the conversion of T_4 to triiodothyronine (T_3). Plasmapheresis, charcoal hemoperfusion, and exchange transfusion have been reserved for cases in which continued clinical deterioration occurs despite conventional therapy. Because T_4 is highly protein bound, very little drug will be removed by dialysis.

Drug Interactions

In addition to the drug interactions described in this section, some drugs can interfere with thyroid function test results and their interpretation. (See Laboratory Test Interferences.)

■ **Oral Anticoagulants** Thyroid agents may potentiate the hypoprothrombinemic effect of warfarin and other oral anticoagulants, apparently by increasing catabolism of vitamin K-dependent clotting factors. When thyroid agents are administered to patients receiving oral anticoagulants, the prothrombin time should be determined frequently and anticoagulant dosage adjusted accordingly, and patients should be observed closely for adverse effects. It has been suggested that the dosage of the oral anticoagulant be reduced by one-third when thyroid therapy is started. No special precautions appear to be necessary when oral anticoagulant therapy is initiated in patients already stabilized on maintenance thyroid replacement therapy.

■ **Antidepressants** Concomitant use of tricyclic (e.g., amitriptyline) or tetracyclic (e.g., maprotiline) antidepressants and levothyroxine may increase the therapeutic and toxic effects (e.g., increased risk of cardiac arrhythmias and CNS stimulation) of both classes of drugs, possibly secondary to increased receptor sensitivity to catecholamines; onset of action of tricyclic antidepressants may be accelerated. Concomitant use of selective serotonin-reuptake inhibitors (SSRIs, e.g., sertraline) in patients stabilized on levothyroxine may result in increased levothyroxine requirements.

■ **Antidiabetic Agents** Hypothyroidism may reduce the severity of diabetes mellitus, resulting in decreased requirements of insulin or oral antidiabetic agents (e.g., sulfonylureas). Administration of thyroid agents to patients with diabetes mellitus may cause an increase in the required dosage of insulin or oral antidiabetic agents. When therapy with thyroid agents is initiated or discontinued or when dosage of a thyroid agent is adjusted in diabetic patients receiving insulin or an oral antidiabetic agent, patients should be closely monitored and appropriate adjustments in dosage of insulin or the oral antidiabetic agent made accordingly if necessary.

■ **Sympathomimetic Agents** Parenteral administration of sympathomimetic agents (e.g., epinephrine) to patients with coronary artery disease may precipitate an episode of coronary insufficiency. Because this reaction may be enhanced in patients receiving thyroid agents, patients with coronary artery disease who are receiving thyroid agents should be carefully observed when catecholamines are administered.

■ **Bile Acid Sequestrants** Bile acid sequestrants (e.g., cholestyramine resin, colestipol) bind thyroid agents in the GI tract and substantially impair their absorption. In vitro studies indicate that the binding is not readily reversible. To minimize or prevent this interaction, these agents should be administered at least 4 hours apart when the drugs must be used concurrently.

■ **GI Drugs** Antacids (e.g., aluminum hydroxide, magnesium hydroxide, calcium carbonate), simethicone, and sucralfate bind thyroid agents in the GI tract and delay or prevent their absorption. Calcium carbonate may form an insoluble chelate with levothyroxine, resulting in decreased levothyroxine absorption and increased serum thyrotropin concentrations; in vitro studies indicate that levothyroxine binds to calcium carbonate at acidic pH levels. To minimize or prevent this interaction, some clinicians recommend that these agents be administered approximately 4 hours apart when the drugs must be used concurrently with thyroid agents.

■ **Drugs Affecting Hepatic Microsomal Enzymes** Drugs that induce hepatic microsomal enzymes (e.g., carbamazepine, phenytoin, phenobarbital, rifampin) may accelerate metabolism of thyroid agents, resulting in increased thyroid agent dosage requirements. Phenytoin and carbamazepine also reduce serum protein binding of levothyroxine, and total- and free-T_4 may be reduced by 20–40%, but most patients have normal serum concentrations of thyrotropin (thyroid-stimulating hormone, TSH) and are clinically euthyroid.

■ **Cardiac Glycosides** Serum concentrations of digitalis glycosides may be decreased in patients with hyperthyroidism or in patients with hypothyroidism in whom a euthyroid state has been achieved. Thus, therapeutic effects of digitalis glycosides may be reduced in these patients.

■ **Growth Hormones** Excessive use of thyroid agents with growth hormones (e.g., somatropin) may accelerate epiphyseal closure. However, untreated hypothyroidism may interfere with growth response to growth hormone.

■ **Xanthine Derivatives** Decreased clearance of xanthine derivatives (e.g., theophylline) may occur in hypothyroid patients; clearance returns to normal when the euthyroid state is achieved.

■ **Other Drugs** Cation-exchange resins (e.g., sodium polystyrene sulfonate) and ferrous sulfate bind thyroid agents in the GI tract and delay or prevent their absorption. To minimize or prevent this interaction, thyroid agents should be administered at least 4 hours apart from these drugs.

Concomitant use of ketamine with thyroid agents may produce marked hypertension and tachycardia; caution is advised when the drug is administered in patients receiving thyroid hormone therapy.

Laboratory Test Interferences

■ **Drugs Affecting Thyroid Function or Thyroid Function Tests** Certain drugs and various pathologic and physiologic conditions can interfere with thyroid function tests and their interpretation, and the resultant effects must be considered.

Use of dopamine hydrochloride (at dosages of 1 mcg/kg per minute or greater), corticosteroids (at hydrocortisone-equivalent dosages of 100 mg daily or greater), or octreotide (at dosages exceeding 100 mcg daily) may result in a transient reduction in thyrotropin (thyroid-stimulating hormone, TSH) secretion. However, because these effects are transient, hypothyroidism is not expected to occur.

Drugs that may decrease thyroid hormone secretion (e.g., aminoglutethimide, amiodarone, iodide [including iodine-containing radiographic contrast agents], lithium, sulfonamides, tolbutamide) may be associated with hypothyroidism. Long-term lithium therapy can result in goiter in up to 50% of patients, and in subclinical or overt hypothyroidism, each in up to 20% of patients. The fetus, neonates, geriatric patients, and euthyroid patients with underlying thyroid disease (e.g., Hashimoto's thyroiditis, Grave's disease previously treated with radioiodine or surgery) are particularly susceptible to iodine-induced hypothyroidism. Oral cholecystographic agents and amiodarone are excreted slowly, producing more prolonged hypothyroidism than parenterally administered iodinated contrast agents. Long-term aminoglutethimide therapy may minimally decrease concentrations of T_4 and triiodothyronine (T_3) and increase concentrations of thyrotropin, although all values remain within normal limits in most patients.

Iodide (including iodine-containing radiographic contrast agents) and drugs that contain pharmacologic amounts of iodide may cause hyperthyroidism in euthyroid patients with Grave's disease previously treated with antithyroid drugs or in euthyroid patients with thyroid autonomy (e.g., multinodular goiter or hyperfunctioning thyroid adenoma). Hyperthyroidism may develop over several weeks and may persist for several months following discontinuance of therapy. Amiodarone may induce hyperthyroidism by causing thyroiditis.

Pregnancy, estrogens, estrogen-containing oral contraceptives, methadone, fluorouracil, mitotane, and tamoxifen increase serum concentrations of thyroxine-binding globulin; in patients with normal thyroid function only a transient decrease in free serum thyroxine concentration results, but in patients receiving thyroid replacement therapy, an increase in thyroid agent dosage may be necessary. Chronic active hepatitis, neonatal state, acute intermittent porphyria, and genetic factors also may increase thyroxine-binding globulin concentrations. Androgens, usual doses of corticosteroids, asparaginase, and sustained release niacin decrease serum concentrations of thyroxine-binding globulin; decreases in serum concentrations of thyroxine-binding globulin also occur in nephrosis, cirrhosis, and acromegaly. Some drugs (e.g., phenylbutazone [no longer commercially available in the US], salicylates) competitively bind to thyroxine-binding globulin and/or thyroxine-binding prealbumin. Familial hyper- or hypo-thyroxine-binding-globulinemias also have been reported.

Concomitant use of levothyroxine sodium with furosemide (at IV dosages exceeding 80 mg), heparin, hydantoins, nonsteroidal anti-inflammatory agents (NSAIAs, e.g., fenamates, phenylbutazone), or salicylates (at dosages exceeding 2 g daily) results in an initial transient increase in concentrations of free T_4. Continued administration results in a decrease in serum T_4 and normal free T_4 and TSH concentrations; therefore, patients are clinically euthyroid. Salicylates inhibit binding of T_4 and T_3 to thyroxine-binding globulin (TBG) and transthyretin. An initial increase in serum free T_4 is followed by return of free T_4 to normal levels with sustained therapeutic serum salicylate concentrations, although total T_4 concentrations may decrease by as much as 30%.

Concomitant use of thyroid agents with amiodarone, β-adrenergic blocking agents (e.g., propranolol hydrochloride at dosages exceeding 160 mg daily), or corticosteroids (e.g., dexamethasone at dosages of 4 mg daily or greater) decreases peripheral conversion of T_4 to T_3, resulting in decreased T_3 concentrations. However, serum T_4 concentrations usually remain within normal range but may occasionally be slightly increased. In patients treated with large doses of propranolol hydrochloride (i.e., exceeding 160 mg/day), T_3 and T_4 concentrations change slightly, TSH levels remain normal, and patients are clinically euthyroid. It should be noted that actions of particular β-adrenergic blocking agents may be impaired when the hypothyroid patient is converted to the euthyroid state. Short-term administration of large doses of corticosteroids may decrease serum T_3 concentrations by 30% with minimal change in serum T_4 levels. However, long-term corticosteroid therapy may result in slightly decreased T_3 and T_4 concentrations because of decreased TBG production.

Therapy with interferon alfa has been associated with the development of antithyroid microsomal antibodies in 20% of patients, and some experience transient hypothyroidism, hyperthyroidism, or both. Patients who have antithyroid antibodies prior to treatment with thyroid agents are at higher risk for thyroid dysfunction during treatment. Interleukin 2 (e.g., aldesleukin) has been associated with transient painless thyroiditis in 20% of patients. Interferon beta and gamma have not been reported to cause thyroid dysfunction.

Other agents that have been associated with alterations in thyroid hormone and/or TSH concentrations include chloral hydrate, diazepam, ethionamide, lovastatin, metoclopramide, mercaptopurine, nitroprusside, aminosalicylate sodium, perphenazine, resorcinol (excessive topical use), and thiazide diuretics.

■ **Other Laboratory Test Interferences** Radioactive iodine uptake tests used in evaluating thyroid function can be interfered with by dietary sources of iodine or iodine- or iodide-containing medications (e.g., potassium iodide).

Thyroid hormones may reduce the uptake of ^{123}I, ^{131}I, and ^{99m}Tc.

Pharmacology

■ **Thyroid Hormone Synthesis and Regulation** The extracts of the thyroid gland and hormones secreted by the gland or prepared synthetically are essential hormones that affect the rate of many physiologic processes. The amounts of thyroxine and triiodothyronine released into the circulation from the normally functioning thyroid gland are regulated by thyrotropin (thyroid-stimulating hormone, TSH), which is secreted by the anterior pituitary. Secretion of thyrotropin is in turn controlled by a feedback mechanism effected by concentrations of circulating thyroid hormones and by secretion of thyrotropin-releasing hormone (TRH) from the hypothalamus. Endogenous thyroid hormone secretion is suppressed when exogenous thyroid hormones are administered to euthyroid individuals in excess of the gland's normal secretion.

Tetraiodothyronine (thyroxine, T_4) and triiodothyronine (T_3) are produced in the thyroid gland by the iodination and coupling of the amino acid tyrosine. Iodine is an essential component of thyroid hormones, thyroxine and triiodothyronine, comprising 65 and 59% of the weights, respectively. Thyroid hormones and thus iodine are essential for human life. The hormones regulate many key biochemical reactions, especially protein synthesis and enzymatic activity, and target the developing brain, muscle, heart, pituitary, and kidneys.

The thyroid gland selectively concentrates iodide in amounts required for adequate thyroid hormone synthesis, with most of the remaining iodide being excreted renally. A sodium/iodide transporter in the thyroidal basal membrane is responsible for iodine concentration in the gland, transferring iodide from systemic circulation into the thyroid gland at a concentration gradient of 20–50 times that of plasma to ensure that the gland receives adequate amounts of iodine for hormone synthesis. During iodine deficiency, the thyroid gland concentrates most of the iodine available from plasma. Iodide participates in a complex series of reactions in the thyroid gland to produce thyroid hormones. Thyroglobulin is synthesized in thyroid cells and serves as an iodination vehicle. Thyroperoxidase and hydrogen peroxide promote the oxidation of iodide and its attachment to tyrosyl residues within the thyroglobulin molecule to produce the hormone precursors diiodotyrosine and monoiodotyrosine. Thyroperoxidase further catalyzes intramolecular coupling of 2 molecules of diiodotyrosine to produce thyroxine (T_4) and coupling of a molecule of diiodotyrosine and a molecule of monoiodotyrosine to produce triiodothyronine (T_3). The average adult thyroid gland in individuals residing in an iodine-sufficient geographic region contains about 15 mg of iodine. Iodine is not released into systemic circulation but instead is stored principally in diiodo and monoiodo tyrosine precursors, removed from the tyrosine moiety by a specific deiodinase, and then recycled within the thyroid gland as a mechanism of iodine conservation.

Once in systemic circulation, thyroxine and triiodothyronine attach to several binding proteins (e.g., thyronine-binding globulin, transthyretin, albumin), which then migrate to target tissues where thyroxine is deiodinated to triiodothyronine, the metabolically active form of thyroid hormone. The iodine that is removed from thyroxine returns to the serum iodine pool and follows the usual iodine cycle or is excreted renally. Thyrotropin is the major thyroid function regulator. Thyrotropin affects several sites within thyrocytes, the principal actions of which are to increase thyroidal uptake of iodine and to break down thyroglobulin to release thyroid hormone into systemic circulation. An elevated serum thyrotropin concentration indicates primary hypothyroidism and a decreased serum concentration indicates hyperthyroidism. The normal thyroid gland takes up the amount of systemically circulating iodine necessary to make the amount of thyroid hormone for the body's needs. In iodine deficiency, the thyroid gland will concentrate more iodine, and the gland will concentrate less in iodine excess. When iodine equilibrium is present, the mean daily thyroid iodine accumulation and release are similar.

■ **Pharmacologic Effects of Exogenous Thyroid Hormones** The principal pharmacologic effect of exogenous thyroid hormones is to increase the metabolic rate of body tissues. Thyroid hormones affect protein and carbohydrate metabolism, promoting gluconeogenesis, increasing the utilization and mobilization of glycogen stores, and stimulating protein synthesis. Thyroid hormones affect lipid metabolism by decreasing hepatic and serum cholesterol concentrations. Thyroid hormones are also involved in the regulation of cell growth and differentiation. The hormones aid in the development of the brain and CNS (particularly axonal and dendritic networks and myelination), and are involved with somatotropin in the development of bones and teeth and in the broad aspect of growth.

Although the exact mechanism of action by which thyroid hormones affect metabolism and cellular growth and differentiation is not clearly established, it is known that these physiologic effects are mediated at the cellular level, principally via triiodothyronine. A major portion of triiodothyronine (approximately 70–90%) is derived from thyroxine by deiodination in peripheral tissues; approximately 35% of secreted thyroxine is monodeiodinated peripherally to triiodothyronine. Thyroxine is the major component of normal secretions of the thyroid gland and is therefore the principal determinant of normal thyroid function. In normal human thyroid tissue, the thyroxine:triiodothyronine ratio is 10:1 to 15:1; in hyperthyroid patients with Graves' disease, the ratio is decreased to about 5:1.

Thyroid hormones also exhibit a cardiostimulatory effect which may be the result of a direct action on the heart. Thyroid hormones also may increase the sensitivity of the heart to catecholamines and/or increase the number of myocardial β-adrenergic receptors. Thyroid hormones increase cardiac output, in part, secondary to increased peripheral oxygen consumption. Thyroid hormones may increase renal blood flow and glomerular filtration rate in hypothyroid patients, resulting in a diuresis within 24 hours following administration.

Thyroid hormones will reverse the signs and symptoms of hypothyroidism and myxedema; in hypothyroid children, the hormones increase epiphyseal growth and bone ossification. For thyroid hormones to prevent the developmental abnormalities associated with congenital hypothyroidism (e.g., mental and growth retardation), the condition must be diagnosed and therapy initiated early.

Pharmacokinetics

■ **Absorption** Levothyroxine sodium is variably absorbed from the GI tract (range 40–80%) following oral administration. The extent of absorption is increased in the fasting state and decreased in malabsorption states. Liothyronine sodium is almost completely absorbed from the GI tract (about 95%) following oral administration. The absorption of hormones contained in the natural thyroid agent preparations is similar to that of the synthetic hormones. Absorption of levothyroxine sodium or liothyronine sodium following IM administration may be variable and poor. Thyroxine apparently undergoes enterohepatic circulation.

In healthy individuals, total serum thyroxine (endogenous) concentrations range from about 5–12 mcg/dL, and free (unbound) serum thyroxine concentrations range from about 1–3 ng/dL (about 0.02% of total). Total serum triiodothyronine (endogenous) concentrations range from 70–200 ng/dL (considerable interlaboratory variation) in healthy individuals, and free serum triiodothyronine concentrations range from 0.2–0.4 ng/dL (about 0.2% of total). Total serum reverse triiodothyronine (See Pharmacokinetics: Elimination) concentrations range from 10–60 ng/dL, and free serum reverse triiodothyronine concentrations range from about 0.05–0.15 ng/dL (about 0.5% of total). Serum triiodothyronine concentrations appear to decline slightly with age, are slightly increased in obese individuals, and are decreased in the fetus and neonates. Serum reverse triiodothyronine concentrations appear to be increased in healthy individuals older than 70 years of age and markedly increased in the fetus and neonates. Age-adjusted normal range values for serum thyroid hormone concentrations may be required for proper interpretation of such measurements. Although the normal range for endogenous thyroid hormones is the therapeutic range for exogenously administered hormones in hypothyroid patients, free hormone concentrations are often not easily measured and other measures of thyroid function (e.g., resin triiodothyronine uptake, free thyroxine index) are generally used to monitor thyroid hormone replacement therapy.

The maximum effects of liothyronine sodium are apparent within 24–72 hours following initiation of oral therapy and persist for up to 72 hours following discontinuance of the drug. Levothyroxine sodium, thyroid, and thyroglobulin have a much slower onset and longer duration of action than liothyronine sodium. The full effects of levothyroxine sodium, thyroid, and thyroglobulin do not occur for 1–3 weeks following initiation of oral therapy, and effects are maintained for a similar period of time following discontinuance of the drugs.

■ **Distribution** Distribution of thyroid hormones into human body tissues and fluids has not been fully characterized. Thyroxine is distributed into most body tissues and fluids with highest concentrations in the liver and kidneys. Thyroid hormones do not readily cross the placenta. Placental transfer of thyroid hormones is slow and the importance has not been precisely determined; the mother provides little, if any, thyroid hormone to the developing fetus. Minimal amounts of thyroid hormones are distributed into milk.

Thyroxine and triiodothyronine are more than 99% bound to serum proteins, principally thyronine-binding globulin (thyroxine-binding globulin, TBG) and transthyretin (thyroxine-binding prealbumin, TBPA) (and to a small extent albumin), whose capacities and affinities for the hormones vary. Thyroxine is more extensively and firmly bound than is triiodothyronine. The high affinity of thyroxine for TBG and TBPA is responsible for thyroxine's high serum concentration and slow metabolic clearance. Certain drugs and various pathologic and physiologic conditions can alter the binding of thyroid hormones to serum proteins and/or the concentrations of the serum proteins that bind the hormones; these effects must be considered when interpreting the results of thyroid function tests. (See Laboratory Test Interferences.)

■ **Elimination** The usual plasma half-lives of thyroxine and triiodothyronine are approximately 6–8 and 1–2 days, respectively. The plasma half-lives of thyroxine and triiodothyronine are decreased in patients with hyperthyroidism and increased in those with hypothyroidism.

In humans, endogenous thyroglobulin within the thyroid gland is proteolytically hydrolyzed, resulting in the release of thyroxine and triiodothyronine into the circulation. Thyroxine is conjugated with glucuronic and sulfuric acids in the liver and distributed into bile; a portion is then hydrolyzed in the intestine and reabsorbed, and a portion reaches the colon unchanged, where it is then hydrolyzed and eliminated unchanged in the feces. About 20–40% of thyroxine is eliminated in feces. About 35% of secreted thyroxine is monodeiodinated at the 5′ position of the phenolic (outer) ring in peripheral tissues, principally liver and kidney, to form triiodothyronine; this accounts for about 80% of the total daily production of triiodothyronine. Thyroxine also undergoes peripheral monodeiodination at the 5 position of the tyrosyl (inner) ring to form reverse triiodothyronine (reverse T_3, rT_3), which is calorigenically inactive. About 85% of thyroxine metabolized daily is deiodinated. Deiodination is apparently an enzymatic process, and probably involves separate iodothyronine 5′- and 5-deiodinases which have a high capacity and are probably subject to some form(s) of regulation. The metabolic fate of triiodothyronine is not clearly established. Triiodothyronine and reverse triiodothyronine undergo peripheral monodeiodination to form 3,3′-diiodothyronine. Additional thyroid hormone metabolites in which the diphenyl ether linkage is either intact or broken have also been detected. Iodine liberated by deiodination reactions is utilized by the thyroid gland for hormone synthesis or is excreted in feces via bile or in urine.

Chemistry

Thyroid agents are natural or synthetic preparations containing tetraiodothyronine (thyroxine, T_4) and/or triiodothyronine (T_3). Thyroxine and triiodothyronine are produced in the human thyroid gland; the commercially available synthetic preparations of these hormones, levothyroxine sodium and liothyronine sodium, respectively, are the sodium salts of the L-isomers of the hormones. Thyroxine and triiodothyronine are produced in the thyroid gland by the iodination and coupling of the amino acid tyrosine. Thyroxine contains 4 iodine atoms and is formed by the coupling of 2 molecules of diiodotyrosine. Triiodothyronine contains 3 iodine atoms and is formed by the coupling of one molecule of diiodotyrosine with one molecule of monoiodotyrosine. Thyroxine and triiodothyronine are stored in the thyroid colloid as thyroglobulin.

Natural thyroid agent preparations, which are derived from animal thyroid, include thyroid and thyroglobulin. USP previously required that thyroid and thyroglobulin be standardized only by their iodine content which is only an indirect indicator of true hormonal biologic activity. Some manufacturers of thyroid perform bioassays of their preparations to assure batch-to-batch reproducibility of metabolic potency, and the manufacturer of thyroglobulin standardizes the levothyroxine and liothyronine contents of the preparation by chromatographic analysis; however, the concentrations of levothyroxine and liothyronine and the ratio of these hormones in these commercially available preparations may vary considerably. Even preparations that are standardized for metabolic potency via a bioassay may differ from other bioassay preparations in the ratio of levothyroxine:liothyronine concentration. Current USP standards specify the measurable amounts of levothyroxine and liothyronine in each 65 mg of thyroid or thyroglobulin; however, because of difficulty in measuring the actual hormonal content of thyroid USP or thyroglobulin USP, these measurable amounts may be less than the clinical equivalent. In guiding dosage adjustment, the clinical equivalent and not the measurable amount should be used.

Synthetic thyroid agent preparations include levothyroxine sodium, liothyronine sodium, and liotrix, a combination preparation containing a ratio of levothyroxine sodium to liothyronine sodium of 4:1 by weight; however, current USP standards do not specify the ratio of levothyroxine sodium and liothyronine sodium in liotrix.

Because some thyroid agent preparations currently may not be standardized by their levothyroxine and/or liothyronine contents and because the measurable amounts of these drugs in thyroid and thyroglobulin may be less than the clinical equivalent, thyroid agent preparations are not necessarily directly comparable; however, the following equivalencies have been suggested based on clinical response:

Thyroid Agent	Approximate Equivalent Dosage
Levothyroxine Sodium	100 mcg or less
Liothyronine Sodium	25 mcg
Liotrix (Levothyroxine Sodium/Liothyronine Sodium)	50 mcg/12.5 mcg (Thyrolar®)
Thyroglobulin	65 mg
Thyroid	60–65 mg (1 grain)

These approximate clinical equivalents should be used in guiding dosage adjustment; following a change from one type of thyroid hormone preparation to another, patients still may require fine adjustment of dosage since the equivalents are only estimates.

For further information on chemistry and stability, pharmacology, pharmacokinetics, uses, cautions, and dosage and administration of thyroid agents, see the individual monographs in 68:36.04.

†Use is not currently included in the labeling approved by the US Food and Drug Administration

Levothyroxine Sodium

L-Thyroxine Sodium, T4 Thyroxine Sodium

■ Levothyroxine sodium, the sodium salt of the L-isomer of thyroxine, is a thyroid agent.

Uses

■ **Hypothyroidism** Levothyroxine sodium is used as replacement or supplemental therapy in congenital or acquired hypothyroidism of any etiology, except transient hypothyroidism during the recovery phase of subacute thyroiditis. Levothyroxine sodium is specifically indicated for use in the management of subclinical hypothyroidism and primary (thyroidal), secondary (pituitary), and tertiary (hypothalamic) hypothyroidism. Primary hypothyroidism may result from functional deficiency, primary atrophy, partial or complete absence of the thyroid gland, or from the effects of surgery, radiation, or antithyroid agents, with or without the presence of goiter.

Replacement therapy with levothyroxine sodium must be maintained continuously to control the symptoms of hypothyroidism. Levothyroxine sodium generally is the preferred thyroid agent for replacement therapy because its hormonal content is standardized and its effect is therefore predictable.

Levothyroxine sodium also is considered the drug of choice for the treatment of congenital hypothyroidism (cretinism). For a discussion on the use of levothyroxine in the treatment of congenital hypothyroidism, see Cautions: Pediatric Precautions, in the Thyroid Agents General Statement 68:36.04.

Levothyroxine sodium IV injection is used in the treatment of myxedema coma. Levothyroxine sodium injection has been used in other conditions when rapid thyroid replacement is required†; however, this is not an FDA-labeled use for the currently available injection.

Levothyroxine sodium may be used with antithyroid agents in the treatment of thyrotoxicosis to prevent goitrogenesis and hypothyroidism. While administration of levothyroxine occasionally may be useful to prevent antithyroid agent-induced hypothyroidism in the management of thyrotoxicosis during pregnancy, combination therapy generally is considered unnecessary since it may increase the requirement for antithyroid agents and therefore the risk of fetal hypothyroidism, which is not amenable to exogenous thyroid agent therapy.

■ **Pituitary TSH Suppression** Levothyroxine sodium may be used to suppress the secretion of thyrotropin (thyroid-stimulating hormone, TSH) in the treatment or prevention of various types of euthyroid goiters, including thyroid nodules, subacute or chronic lymphocytic thyroiditis (Hashimoto's thyroiditis), and multinodular goiter. Levothyroxine sodium also is used as an adjunct to surgery and radioiodine therapy in the management of thyrotropin-dependent well-differentiated (papillary and follicular) thyroid cancer.

Dosage and Administration

■ **Reconstitution and Administration** Levothyroxine sodium is administered orally or by IV injection. The drug also has been administered by IM injection†; however, the IV route is preferred since absorption may be variable following IM administration. IM administration is not an FDA-labeled route of administration for the currently available levothyroxine sodium injection.

Oral Administration Levothyroxine sodium usually is administered orally on an empty stomach, preferably one-half to one hour before breakfast or the first food of the day. Because Levoxyl® tablets may rapidly swell and disintegrate following oral administration (resulting in choking, gagging, or difficulty in swallowing), the manufacturer states that Levoxyl® tablets should be taken with a full glass of water.

In individuals who are unable to swallow the intact tablets (e.g., pediatric patients), the appropriate dose of levothyroxine tablets may be crushed and placed in a small amount (5–10 mL) of water; the resultant suspension should be administered by spoon or dropper immediately and should not be stored.

Foods that decrease absorption of levothyroxine (e.g., soybean infant formula, soybean flour, cotton seed meal) should not be used for administering levothyroxine. (See Pharmacokinetics: Absorption.) Oral levothyroxine sodium should be administered at least 4 hours apart from drugs that are known to interfere with its absorption (e.g., antacids, bile acid sequestrants, cation-exchange resins, ferrous sulfate, sucralfate, simethicone, calcium carbonate). See Drug Interactions in the Thyroid Agents General Statement 68:36.04.

IV Administration Levothyroxine sodium also is administered by IV injection.

Levothyroxine sodium powder for injection should be reconstituted by adding 5 mL of 0.9% sodium chloride injection to a vial labeled as containing 100, 200, or 500 mcg of the drug, and shaking the vial to mix completely. The resultant solutions contain approximately 20, 40, or 100 mcg/mL, respectively, of levothyroxine sodium. Prior to administration, the reconstituted solution should be inspected visually for particulate matter and discoloration whenever solution and container permit. Reconstituted solutions of levothyroxine sodium should be used immediately and any unused portions discarded; the solutions should *not* be admixed with IV infusion solutions. (See Chemistry and Stability: Stability.)

■ **Dosage** The FDA states that all approved levothyroxine sodium preparations should be considered therapeutically *in*equivalent unless equivalence has been established and noted in FDA's *Approved Drug Products with Therapeutic Equivalence Evaluations* (Orange Book). Theoretically, such preparations can be used interchangeably, and in some cases, pharmacists may be able to substitute generic for proprietary (brand) preparations without notifying the prescriber. However, because of the narrow therapeutic index of the drug, the American Thyroid Association (ATA) and the American Association of Clinical Endocrinologists (AACE) state that levothyroxine sodium preparations generally should *not* be used interchangeably. If a patient switches levothyroxine sodium preparations (e.g., from brand to generic), pharmacists are encouraged to notify the patient and prescriber of the switch. In addition, serum thyrotropin (thyroid-stimulating hormone, TSH) concentration should be measured about 4–8 weeks after starting the new preparation and the levothyroxine dosage adjusted if needed.

Dosage of levothyroxine sodium must be carefully adjusted according to individual requirements and response. The age, body weight, and general physical condition of the patient and the severity and duration of hypothyroid symptoms determine the initial dosage and rate at which dosage may be increased to the eventual maintenance dosage. Under- or over-treatment, which may result in adverse effects on growth and development in pediatric patients, cardiovascular function, bone metabolism, reproductive function, cognitive function, emotional state, GI function, and glucose and lipid metabolism, should be avoided.

Dosage should be initiated at a lower level in geriatric patients, in patients with functional or ECG evidence of cardiovascular disease, and in patients with severe, long-standing hypothyroidism, since an abrupt increase in metabolic rate and demand for increased cardiac output associated with levothyroxine therapy may precipitate angina pectoris, myocardial infarction, congestive heart failure, arrhythmias, or sudden cardiac death in such patients. In patients with severe, long-standing hypothyroidism in whom pituitary and adrenal function may be secondarily decreased, rapid replacement therapy with levothyroxine sodium also may precipitate adrenal insufficiency; in addition, psychosis or agitation occasionally may develop during initiation of levothyroxine therapy, necessitating a lower initial dosage in these patients. Adjustment of thyroid replacement therapy should be determined mainly by the patient's clinical response and confirmed by appropriate laboratory tests.

The manufacturer of levothyroxine sodium for injection states that caution should be used when switching patients from oral to IV levothyroxine sodium since the relative bioavailability and an accurate dosing conversion between the oral and IV preparations have not been established. Relative bioavailability between oral and IV administration has been estimated to range from 48–74%.

Hypothyroidism **Adult Dosage.** For the management of hypothyroidism in otherwise healthy individuals younger than 50 years of age and in those older than 50 years of age who have been recently treated for hyperthyroidism or who have been hypothyroid for only a short time (i.e., several months), the usual initial oral dosage (full replacement dosage) of levothyroxine sodium is 1.7 mcg/kg daily (e.g., 100–125 mcg daily for a 70-kg adult) given as a single dose. Older patients may require less than 1 mcg/kg daily. In one study, the usual maintenance dosage for geriatric patients was about 25% less than that for younger and heavier adults. Some manufacturers state that levothyroxine sodium dosages greater than 200 mcg daily are seldom required, and that failure to respond adequately to oral dosages of 300 mcg daily or greater is rare and should prompt reevaluation of the diagnosis, or suggest the presence of malabsorption, patient noncompliance, and/or drug interactions.

Patients should be evaluated initially about every 6–8 weeks to monitor the response to therapy. Once normalization of thyroid function and serum thyrotropin (thyroid-stimulating hormone, TSH) concentrations has been achieved, patients may be evaluated less frequently (i.e., every 6–12 months). However, if the dosage of levothyroxine sodium tablets is changed, serum TSH concentrations should be measured after 8–12 weeks or 4–8 weeks after switching from one levothyroxine sodium preparation to another.

For most patients older than 50 years of age or in patients younger than 50 years of age with underlying cardiovascular disease, the usual initial oral dosage of levothyroxine sodium is 25–50 mcg daily given as a single dose; dosage may be increased at intervals of 6–8 weeks. The usual initial dosage in geriatric patients with underlying cardiovascular disease is 12.5–25 mcg daily, with gradual dosage increments at intervals of 4–6 weeks. Dosage may be increased by increments of 12.5–25 mcg at recommended intervals until the patient becomes euthyroid and serum TSH concentrations return to normal.

For the management of severe, long-standing hypothyroidism in adults, the usual initial oral dosage of levothyroxine sodium is 12.5–25 mcg daily given as a single dose. Although the manufacturers state that dosage may be increased by increments of 25 mcg at intervals of 2–4 weeks until serum TSH concentrations return to normal, some clinicians suggest that dosage may be adjusted at intervals of 4–8 weeks.

If treatment is considered necessary in patients with subclinical hypothyroidism, the manufacturers state that lower initial levothyroxine dosages (e.g., 1 mcg/kg daily) may be adequate to normalize TSH concentrations. If levothyroxine replacement therapy is not initiated, patients still should be monitored annually for changes in clinical status and thyroid laboratory parameters.

Although the average full replacement dosage of levothyroxine sodium is about 1.6–1.7 mcg/kg daily, some patients (e.g., younger pediatric patients, pregnant women) may require higher dosages.

Pediatric Dosage. Despite the smaller body size of pediatric patients, the dosage of levothyroxine sodium (on a weight basis) required to sustain a full rate of growth, development, and general thriving is higher in these patients than in adults. In general, levothyroxine sodium therapy should be initiated at full replacement dosages in pediatric patients as soon as possible after diagnosis of hypothyroidism to prevent deleterious effects on intellectual and physical growth and development; however, dosage should be initiated at a lower level in children with long-standing or severe hypothyroidism.

For the treatment of congenital hypothyroidism (cretinism) or acquired hypothyroidism in pediatric patients, levothyroxine sodium therapy usually is initiated at full replacement dosages; daily dose per body weight decreases with age. The following dosages have been recommended:

Age	Daily Dose
0–3 months	10–15 mcg/kg
3–6 months	25–50 mcg or 8–10 mcg/kg
6–12 months	50–75 mcg or 6–8 mcg/kg
1–5 years	75–100 mcg or 5–6 mcg/kg
6–12 years	100–150 mcg or 4–5 mcg/kg
Older than 12 years	> 150 mcg or 2–3 mcg/kg
Growth and puberty complete	1.6–1.7 mcg/kg

The usual initial oral dosage of levothyroxine sodium in otherwise healthy, full-term neonates is 10–15 mcg/kg daily given as a single dose. A lower initial dosage (e.g., 25 mcg daily) should be considered in neonates at risk of cardiac failure; dosage may be increased at intervals of 4–6 weeks as needed based on clinical and laboratory response to treatment. In neonates with very low (less than 5 mcg/dL) or undetectable serum thyroxine (T_4) concentrations, the usual initial dosage is 50 mcg daily.

The manufacturers state that hyperactivity in an older child may be minimized by initiating therapy at a dosage approximately one-fourth of the recommended full replacement dosage; the dosage may then be increased by an amount equal to one-fourth the full recommended replacement dosage at weekly intervals until the full recommended replacement dosage is reached.

For the treatment of severe, long-standing hypothyroidism in pediatric patients, the usual initial oral dosage of levothyroxine sodium is 25 mcg daily. Dosage may be increased in increments of 25 mcg at intervals of 2–4 weeks until the desired response is obtained.

Myxedema Coma For the treatment of myxedema coma, levothyroxine sodium is given by IV injection; oral administration is not recommended because absorption of the drug from the GI tract is unpredictable in such patients.

Initial and maintenance dosages of IV levothyroxine sodium should be selected after taking into account the age, general physical condition, and cardiac risk factors of the patient, as well as the clinical severity and duration of myxedema symptoms. The manufacturer states that the initial adult IV loading dose for the treatment of myxedema coma is 300–500 mcg; however, some clinicians recommend an initial dose of 100–500 mcg. Lower IV maintenance dosages of 50–100 mcg once daily should be administered thereafter as clinically indicated until the patient's condition is stabilized and the drug can be given orally.

In the geriatric population and in patients with underlying cardiovascular disease, administration of IV levothyroxine sodium, especially loading doses exceeding 500 mcg, may precipitate severe adverse cardiovascular effects (e.g., arrhythmias, tachycardia, myocardial ischemia or infarction, worsening of heart failure, death). The manufacturer states that cautious use (e.g., dosages in the lower end of the recommended range) of IV levothyroxine sodium may be warranted in geriatric patients and in those with known cardiac risk factors.

Pituitary TSH Suppression Some manufacturers caution that the target level for TSH suppression in the management of well-differentiated thyroid cancer and thyroid nodules has not been established. In addition, the efficacy of TSH suppression for benign nodular disease remains controversial. Therefore, dosage of levothyroxine sodium used for TSH suppression should be individualized based on patient characteristics and the nature of the disease.

For the management of thyrotropin-dependent well-differentiated (papillary and follicular) thyroid cancer, an oral levothyroxine sodium replacement dosage of greater than 2 mcg/kg daily given as a single dose has been recommended to suppress TSH concentrations to less than 0.1 mU/L. In patients with high-risk tumors, the target level for TSH suppression may be less than 0.01 mU/L.

For the management of benign nodules and nontoxic multinodular goiter, TSH concentrations generally are suppressed to a higher target (e.g., 0.1–0.5 mU/L for nodules and 0.5–1 mU/L for multinodular goiter) than that used for the treatment of thyroid cancer.

Cautions

Levothyroxine sodium shares the toxic potentials of other thyroid agents and the usual precautions of thyroid agent therapy should be observed. (See Cautions in the Thyroid Agents General Statement 68:36.04.) Adverse reactions to levothyroxine sodium result from overdosage and are manifested principally as signs and symptoms of hyperthyroidism (e.g., chest pain, palpitations, cardiac arrhythmias, difficulty in sleeping). Hyperthyroidism is a risk factor for osteoporosis. Evidence from several studies in premenopausal women receiving levothyroxine sodium for replacement or suppressive therapy suggests that subclinical hyperthyroidism is associated with bone loss. Therefore, to minimize the risk of osteoporosis, dosage of levothyroxine sodium should be titrated to the lowest possible effective level. (See Dosage and Administration: Dosage.) In addition, hypothyroidism manifested by severe depression, fatigue, weight gain, constipation, cold intolerance, edema, and difficulty in concentration may occur in patients receiving levothyroxine sodium preparations with inadequate potency.

Choking, gagging, dysphagia, or lodging of a tablet in the throat has been reported with Levoxyl®, particularly when the tablets were not administered with water. Therefore, the manufacturer states that Levoxyl® tablets should be taken with a full glass of water.

Patients with a history of lactose intolerance may be sensitive to Levothroid®, Synthroid®, and Unithroid® tablets, since lactose is used in the manufacture of the tablets.

Pharmacology

The principal pharmacologic effect of exogenous thyroid hormones is to increase the metabolic rate of body tissues. Thyroid hormones are also involved in the regulation of cell growth and differentiation. Although the precise mechanism of action by which thyroid hormones affect metabolism and cellular growth and differentiation is not clearly established, it is known that these physiologic effects are mediated at the cellular level, principally via triiodothyronine; a major portion of triiodothyronine is derived from thyroxine by deiodination in peripheral tissues. Thyroxine is the major component of normal secretions of the thyroid gland and is therefore the principal determinant of normal thyroid function. For further information, see Pharmacology in the Thyroid Agents General Statement 68:36.04.

Pharmacokinetics

■ **Absorption** Levothyroxine is variably absorbed from the GI tract (range: 40–80%). In animals, levothyroxine is absorbed in the proximal and middle jejunum; the drug is not absorbed from the stomach or distal colon and little, if any, absorption occurs in the duodenum. Studies in humans indicate that levothyroxine is absorbed from the jejunum and ileum and some absorption also occurs in the duodenum. The degree of absorption of levothyroxine from the GI tract depends on the product formulation and type of intestinal contents, including plasma protein and soluble dietary factors that may bind thyroid hormone and make it unavailable for diffusion. In addition, concurrent oral administration of infant soybean formula, soybean flour, cotton seed meal, walnuts, foods containing large amounts of fiber, ferrous sulfate, antacids, sucralfate, calcium carbonate, cation-exchange resins (e.g., sodium polystyrene sulfonate), simethicone, or bile acid sequestrants may decrease absorption of levothyroxine. The extent of levothyroxine absorption is increased in the fasting state and decreased in malabsorption states (e.g., sprue); absorption also may decrease with age.

The absorption of levothyroxine is variable following IM administration (not an FDA-labeled route of administration for the currently available levothyroxine sodium injection).

In the past, results of studies evaluating the bioequivalence and interchangeability of various commercially available oral preparations of levothyroxine have been conflicting. Results of several early studies indicated that various commercially available levothyroxine sodium tablets (i.e., Levothroid®, Synthroid® [formulation available prior to 1982], several nonproprietary [generic] preparations) were not bioequivalent based on measurements of thyroxine content in the tablets and of thyroid function in patients receiving the preparations. Potency of oral levothyroxine sodium preparations manufactured in the US after 1985 reportedly was more uniform since USP required all manufacturers of the drug to monitor levothyroxine content and ensure tablet potency. Several reports published after 1984 indicated that the drug content of various levothyroxine preparations (Synthroid®, Levothroid®, Levoxine®, and certain nonproprietary preparations) was within FDA specifications (i.e., no less than 90% and no more than 110% of labeled potency). However, the FDA concluded in 1997 that stability problems with oral levothyroxine sodium preparations commercially available at that time continued to result in unpredictable drug potency and announced that orally administered levothyroxine sodium products are considered new drugs; manufacturers wishing to market levothyroxine preparations were required to submit a new drug application (NDA) to the FDA. (See Chemistry and Stability: Stability.) Results of one single-blind, randomized, 4-way cross-over study in women with hypothyroidism who were clinically and chemically euthyroid and who received levothyroxine sodium 100 or 150 mcg daily for a minimum of 3 months prior to study entry suggested that the commercially available levothyroxine sodium tablets tested in this study (i.e., Levoxyl® [formerly Levoxine®], Synthroid®, 2 nonproprietary preparations) were bioequivalent and interchangeable in the majority of patients receiving such preparations, based on measurements of levothyroxine sodium content in the tablets and of patient thyroid function. However, the FDA states that all approved levothyroxine sodium preparations should be considered therapeutically *in*equivalent unless equivalency has been established and noted in FDA's *Approved Drug Products with Therapeutic Equivalency Evaluations* (Orange Book). (See Dosage and Administration: Dosage.)

■ **Distribution** Because thyroxine is more highly and firmly protein bound than triiodothyronine, levothyroxine has a much slower onset of pharmacologic action and a longer duration of action than liothyronine.

■ **Elimination** The usual plasma half-lives of thyroxine and triiodothyronine are 6–7 days and approximately 1–2 days, respectively. The plasma half-lives of thyroxine and triiodothyronine are decreased in patients with hyperthyroidism and increased in those with hypothyroidism.

Chemistry and Stability

■ **Chemistry** Levothyroxine sodium is commercially available as tablets for oral administration and as a lyophilized powder for injection for IV administration.

Levothyroxine sodium is the monosodium salt of the *levo* isomer of thyroxine, the principal secretion of the thyroid gland. The commercially available drug is prepared synthetically. Structurally, levothyroxine sodium differs from liothyronine sodium only in the presence of an iodine atom in the 5′ position.

Levothyroxine sodium occurs as a light yellow to buff-colored, odorless, tasteless, hygroscopic powder and is very slightly soluble in water and slightly soluble in alcohol.

■ **Stability** Levothyroxine sodium is stable in dry air but may acquire a slight pink color upon exposure to light. Commercially available preparations of levothyroxine sodium should be stored in tight, light-resistant containers. Levothyroxine sodium is unstable in the presence of light, heat, air, and humidity. The manufacturers' labeling should be consulted for recommended storage temperatures, which can vary depending on the specific manufacturer and preparation. In some cases, tablets of the drug have been unstable even at room temperature, and storage at temperatures of 8–15°C were required to maintain potency.

In 1997, the FDA determined that important stability and potency problems existed for oral levothyroxine sodium preparations, and such problems potentially could result in serious health consequences because of inconsistent drug potency. It appeared that many oral levothyroxine sodium preparations that were commercially available at that time failed to maintain potency throughout their customary 2-year shelf-life even when stored as directed, and it was suggested that this shelf-life might not be appropriate for these preparations because of accelerated degradation secondary to a variety of factors (e.g., light, temperature, air, humidity). In addition, some excipients contained in oral levothyroxine sodium preparations might hasten such degradation. Results of some stability studies indicate that levothyroxine sodium exhibits biphasic, first-order degradation with an initial fast degradation rate (which is temperature dependent), followed by a slower terminal phase. To compensate for the initial fast degradation rate, some manufacturers used excessive amounts of active ingredient, which could result in superpotency. It appeared that oral levothyroxine sodium preparations failed to maintain potency throughout their shelf-life, and the amount of active ingredient varied from lot to lot in identical-strength tablets supplied by the same manufacturer. As a result of stability problems and manufacturing practices used to compensate for instability of the drug, potency of a given preparation could not be ensured, even when the same brand of oral levothyroxine sodium preparation was used.

Levothyroxine sodium was introduced into the US market before 1962 without an approved new drug application (NDA), apparently with the belief that it was not a new drug. In patients with diminished or absent thyroid function, uniform potency and bioavailability of levothyroxine sodium tablets are very important since hypothyroidism or hyperthyroidism may result from administration of preparations with less or more than the specified potency and bioavailability, respectively. (See Cautions.) Between 1987 and 1994, the FDA received 58 reports of adverse drug reactions (e.g., manifestations of hypothyroidism or hyperthyroidism) apparently associated with irregular potency, mainly subpotency but also superpotency, of levothyroxine sodium preparations. Some of these adverse effects occurred following a switch in the brand of levothyroxine sodium, while others may have occurred secondary to inconsistent stability, potency, and bioavailability of a given preparation supplied by the same manufacturer. Since levothyroxine sodium preparations were marketed without an approved NDA, manufacturers were required to report only unexpected and severe adverse drug reactions to FDA; therefore, it is believed that this reported incidence of adverse effects secondary to potency problems may be conservative because of underreporting of such effects. In addition, since manufacturers were not required to obtain FDA approval to reformulate preparations containing levothyroxine sodium, preparations with substantially increased potency and associated severe adverse effects occasionally were marketed.

Because of reported potency and stability problems, the FDA announced in 1997 that oral preparations containing levothyroxine sodium were considered new drugs. Manufacturers who wished to continue marketing oral preparations containing levothyroxine sodium were required to submit an NDA to the FDA by August 14, 2000. Oral levothyroxine sodium preparations commercially available in the US after August 14, 2003 have been approved by the FDA and are considered to be safe and effective for their intended uses. The current edition of FDA's *Approved Drug Products with Therapeutic Equivalence Evaluations* (Orange Book; http://www.accessdata.fda.gov/scripts/cder/ob/default.cfm) should be consulted to determine which levothyroxine sodium preparations the FDA has evaluated and deemed as being therapeutically equivalent (i.e., as bioequivalent and expected to have the same clinical effect and safety profile when administered appropriately). (See Dosage and Administration: Dosage.)

Levothyroxine sodium powder for injection should be stored at 20–25°C and protected from light. Following reconstitution, the drug is stable for 4 hours; however, the manufacturer states that reconstituted solutions of levothyroxine sodium should be used immediately and should not be added to other IV fluids. Any unused portion should be discarded.

For further information on chemistry, pharmacology, pharmacokinetics, uses, toxicity, cautions, acute toxicity, drug interactions, laboratory test interferences, and dosage and administration of levothyroxine sodium, see the Thyroid Agents General Statement 68:36.04.

Preparations

Excipients in commercially available drug preparations may have clinically important effects in some individuals; consult specific product labeling for details.

Levothyroxine Sodium

Oral

Tablets	25 mcg*	**Levothroid®**, Forest
		Levothyroxine Sodium Tablets
		Levoxyl® (scored), Jones
		Synthroid® (scored), Abbott
		Unithroid®, Watson
	50 mcg*	**Levothroid®**, Forest
		Levothyroxine Sodium Tablets
		Levoxyl® (scored), Jones
		Synthroid® (scored), Abbott
		Unithroid®, Watson
	75 mcg*	**Levothroid®**, Forest
		Levothyroxine Sodium Tablets
		Levoxyl® (scored), Jones
		Synthroid® (scored), Abbott
		Unithroid®, Watson
	88 mcg*	**Levothroid®**, Forest
		Levothyroxine Sodium Tablets
		Levoxyl® (scored), Jones
		Synthroid® (scored), Abbott
		Unithroid®, Watson
	100 mcg*	**Levothroid®**, Forest
		Levothyroxine Sodium Tablets
		Levoxyl® (scored), Jones
		Synthroid® (scored), Abbott
		Unithroid®, Watson
	112 mcg*	**Levothroid®**, Forest
		Levothyroxine Sodium Tablets
		Levoxyl® (scored), Jones
		Synthroid® (scored), Abbott
		Unithroid®, Watson
	125 mcg*	**Levothroid®**, Forest
		Levothyroxine Sodium Tablets
		Levoxyl® (scored), Jones
		Synthroid® (scored), Abbott
		Unithroid®, Watson

	137 mcg*	**Levothroid®**, Forest
		Levothyroxine Sodium Tablets
		Levoxyl® (scored), Jones
		Synthroid® (scored), Abbott
	150 mcg*	**Levothroid®**, Forest
		Levothyroxine Sodium Tablets
		Levoxyl® (scored), Jones
		Synthroid® (scored), Abbott
		Unithroid®, Watson
	175 mcg*	**Levothroid®**, Forest
		Levothyroxine Sodium Tablets
		Levoxyl® (scored), Jones
		Synthroid® (scored), Abbott
		Unithroid®, Watson
	200 mcg*	**Levothroid®**, Forest
		Levothyroxine Sodium Tablets
		Levoxyl® (scored), Jones
		Synthroid® (scored), Abbott
		Unithroid®, Watson
	300 mcg*	**Levothroid®**, Forest
		Levothyroxine Sodium Tablets
		Levoxyl® (scored), Jones
		Synthroid® (scored), Abbott
		Unithroid®, Watson
Parenteral		
For injection	100 mcg*	**Levothyroxine Sodium for Injection**
	200 mcg*	**Levothyroxine Sodium for Injection**
	500 mcg*	**Levothyroxine Sodium for Injection**

*available from one or more manufacturer, distributor, and/or repackager by generic (nonproprietary) name

†Use is not currently included in the labeling approved by the US Food and Drug Administration

Liothyronine Sodium

Sodium L-Triiodothyronine, L-Triiodothyronine, T3 Thyronine Sodium

■ Liothyronine sodium, the sodium salt of the L-isomer of 3,3′,5-triiodothyronine, is a thyroid agent.

Uses

Liothyronine sodium may be used for replacement or substitution of diminished or absent thyroid function resulting from primary causes including functional deficiency, primary atrophy, or partial or complete absence of the gland or the effects of surgery, radiation, or antithyroid agents; however, levothyroxine sodium is generally preferred for long-term therapy in these conditions. Liothyronine sodium also may be used for replacement or supplemental therapy in patients with secondary (pituitary) or tertiary (hypothalamic) hypothyroidism. Therapy must be maintained continuously to control the symptoms of hypothyroidism. Because liothyronine sodium has a rapid onset and short duration of action, some clinicians prefer its use to levothyroxine sodium when a rapid effect or rapidly reversible effect is desired (e.g., diagnostic procedures requiring short-term thyrotropin suppression, myxedema coma); however, the fact that liothyronine produces wide swings in serum triiodothyronine concentrations and the possibility of more pronounced adverse cardiovascular effects generally make the drug unsatisfactory for long-term use. Liothyronine sodium may be useful when absorption of levothyroxine sodium is questionable or impairment of peripheral conversion of thyroxine to triiodothyronine is suspected.

Liothyronine sodium may also be used therapeutically in patients with simple (nontoxic) goiter to reduce the size of the goiter.

Liothyronine sodium is used IV in the treatment of myxedema coma or precoma. Simultaneous administration of corticosteroids is required. Myxedema coma should be considered a medical emergency, and therapy should be directed at the correction of electrolyte disturbances, possible infection, or other intercurrent illness in addition to the administration of IV liothyronine sodium.

Liothyronine sodium is used principally in the T_3 suppression test to differentiate suspected hyperthyroidism from euthyroidism in patients with I 131 thyroid uptake values in the borderline-high range.

Dosage and Administration

■ **Administration** Liothyronine sodium is administered orally. The drug also is administered by IV injection in the treatment of myxedema coma or precoma. The manufacturer states that liothyronine sodium injection should *not* be administered IM or subcutaneously.

■ **Dosage** Dosage of liothyronine sodium is expressed in terms of liothyronine. Dosage of liothyronine must be carefully adjusted according to individual requirements and response. The age and general physical condition of the patient and the severity and duration of hypothyroid symptoms determine the initial dosage and the rate at which dosage may be increased to the eventual maintenance dosage. Dosage should be initiated at a lower level in geriatric patients; in patients with long-standing disease, other endocrinopathies, or functional or ECG evidence of cardiovascular disease; and in patients with severe hypothyroidism. Adjustment of thyroid replacement therapy should be determined mainly by the patient's clinical response and confirmed by appropriate laboratory tests.

Prompt administration of an adequate dose of IV liothyronine sodium is important in determining clinical outcome of myxedema coma. Initial and subsequent doses of liothyronine sodium should be based on continuous monitoring of the patient's clinical status and response to therapy. Myxedematous patients are very sensitive to the effects of thyroid hormones; therefore, dosage in such patients should be initiated at a low level and increased gradually since acute changes may precipitate adverse cardiovascular events.

For the management of mild hypothyroidism in adults, the usual initial oral dosage of liothyronine is 25 mcg daily given as a single dose; dosage is increased by increments of 12.5 or 25 mcg daily at intervals of 1–2 weeks until the desired response is obtained. The usual maintenance dosage is 25–75 mcg daily; some patients may require higher or lower dosages. For the management of severe hypothyroidism in adults, the usual initial oral dosage is 5 mcg daily given as a single dose; dosage is increased by increments of 5–10 mcg daily at intervals of 1–2 weeks until the desired response is obtained. The usual maintenance dosage is 50–100 mcg daily. For geriatric patients with hypothyroidism, the usual initial oral dosage of liothyronine is 5 mcg daily given as a single dose; dosage is increased by increments of 5 mcg daily at intervals of 1–2 weeks until the desired response is obtained.

In infants and children, it is essential to achieve rapid and complete thyroid replacement because of the critical importance of thyroid hormone in sustaining growth and maturation. In general, despite the smaller body size, the dosage (on a weight basis) required to sustain a full rate of growth, development, and general thriving is higher in children than in adults. Although levothyroxine sodium is considered the drug of choice for the treatment of congenital hypothyroidism (cretinism), liothyronine has been used. The initial oral dosage of liothyronine recommended by the manufacturer for the treatment of congenital hypothyroidism is 5 mcg daily given as a single dose; dosage is increased by increments of 5 mcg daily at intervals of 3–4 days until the desired response is obtained. For additional information on the use of thyroid agents in the treatment of congenital hypothyroidism, see Cautions: Pediatric Precautions, in the Thyroid Agents General Statement 68:36.04.

For the management of simple (nontoxic) goiter in adults, the usual initial oral dosage of liothyronine is 5 mcg daily; dosage is increased by increments of 5–10 mcg daily at intervals of 1–2 weeks until a dosage of 25 mcg daily is reached. Thereafter, dosage may be increased by increments of 12.5 or 25 mcg daily at intervals of 1–2 weeks until the desired response is obtained. The usual maintenance dosage is 75 mcg daily.

When a patient is transferred from another thyroid preparation to liothyronine, the other thyroid preparation should be discontinued and liothyronine therapy initiated at a low dosage. Liothyronine dosage may be increased in small increments after residual effects of the previous thyroid preparation have subsided. When a patient is transferred from liothyronine to another thyroid preparation, it must be kept in mind that the onset and dissipation of effects of liothyronine are relatively rapid, and, to avoid relapse, it is necessary to start therapy with the replacement thyroid preparation several days before complete withdrawal of liothyronine.

Although levothyroxine sodium is generally considered the drug of choice in the treatment of myxedema coma, some clinicians prefer liothyronine because of its rapid onset of action. Liothyronine has been given orally via a nasogastric tube, but the IV route of administration is preferred. The usual initial adult IV dose of liothyronine recommended by the manufacturer for the emergency treatment of myxedema coma or precoma is 25–50 mcg. In patients with known or suspected cardiovascular disease, the manufacturer suggests an initial dose of 10–20 mcg of liothyronine. The manufacturer states that additional doses of liothyronine should be administered at least 4 hours after the initial dose to allow for adequate assessment of therapeutic response, but no more than 12 hours should elapse between doses to avoid fluctuations in hormone levels. However, both the initial and subsequent doses of the drug should be determined based on continuous monitoring of the patient's clinical condition and response to liothyronine sodium therapy. Administration of at least 65 mcg daily of IV liothyronine in the initial days of therapy reportedly has been associated with lower mortality. However, clinical experience with liothyronine dosages exceeding 100 mcg daily is limited. Oral therapy with thyroid hormones should be resumed as soon as the patient's condition stabilizes and the drug can be given orally. Oral therapy with liothyronine sodium should be initiated at a low dosage following discontinuance of the IV drug, and dosage should be increased gradually according to the patient's response. If levothyroxine sodium rather than liothyronine sodium is used in initiating oral therapy, the clinician should consider the delay in onset of activity of levothyroxine sodium and IV liothyronine sodium should be discontinued gradually.

When used in the T_3 suppression test to differentiate suspected hyperthyroidism from euthyroidism, liothyronine is given in a dosage of 75–100 mcg daily for 7 days. Radioactive I 131 uptake test is performed before and after administration of the 7-day course of liothyronine. In patients with hyperthyroidism, the radioactive iodine thyroid uptake will not be substantially affected, while in the euthyroid patient, it will decrease to less than 20% of the baseline value.

For further information on chemistry, pharmacology, pharmacokinetics, uses, toxicity, cautions, acute toxicity, drug interactions, laboratory test interferences, and dosage and administration of liothyronine sodium, see the Thyroid Agents General Statement 68:36.04.

Cautions

Liothyronine sodium shares the toxic potentials of other thyroid agents, and the usual precautions of thyroid agent therapy should be observed. (See Toxicity and Cautions in the Thyroid Agents General Statement 68:36.04). Adverse reactions to liothyronine sodium result from overdosage and are manifested principally as signs and symptoms of hyperthyroidism.

The manufacturer states that there is limited clinical experience with liothyronine sodium injection in children and that safety and efficacy of this preparation have not been established in children.

Pharmacology

The principal pharmacologic effect of exogenous thyroid hormones is to increase the metabolic rate of body tissues. Thyroid hormones are also involved in the regulation of cell growth and differentiation. Although the precise mechanism of action by which thyroid hormones affect metabolism and cellular growth and differentiation is not clearly established, it is known that these physiologic effects are mediated at the cellular level, principally via triiodothyronine; a major portion of triiodothyronine is derived from thyroxine by deiodination in peripheral tissues.

Pharmacokinetics

Liothyronine sodium is almost completely absorbed from the GI tract (about 95%) following oral administration. Because triiodothyronine is not highly or firmly protein bound, liothyronine has a more rapid onset of pharmacologic action and a shorter duration of action than levothyroxine. The usual plasma half-lives of triiodothyronine and thyroxine are approximately 1–2 days and 6–7 days, respectively. The plasma half-lives of thyroxine and triiodothyronine are decreased in patients with hyperthyroidism and increased in those with hypothyroidism.

Following a single IV dose of liothyronine sodium, a detectable metabolic response occurs within as little as 2–4 hours, with a maximum therapeutic response within 2 days.

Chemistry and Stability

■ **Chemistry** Liothyronine sodium is the sodium salt of the L-isomer of 3,3′,5-triiodothyronine. Liothyronine sodium is prepared synthetically. Structurally, liothyronine sodium differs from levothyroxine sodium only in the absence of an iodine atom in the 5′ position. Each 25 mcg of liothyronine sodium is approximately clinically equivalent to 60–65 mg of thyroid or thyroglobulin or 100 mcg or less of levothyroxine sodium.

Liothyronine sodium occurs as a light tan, odorless, crystalline powder and is very slightly soluble in water and slightly soluble in alcohol.

■ **Stability** Commercially available liothyronine sodium tablets should be stored in tight containers at a temperature less than 40°C, preferably between 15–30°C. Commercially available liothyronine sodium injection should be stored at 2–8°C.

Preparations

Excipients in commercially available drug preparations may have clinically important effects in some individuals; consult specific product labeling for details.

Liothyronine Sodium

Oral		
Tablets	5 mcg (of liothyronine)	**Cytomel®**, King
	25 mcg (of liothyronine)	**Cytomel®** (scored), King
	50 mcg (of liothyronine)	**Cytomel®** (scored), King
Parenteral		
Injection, for IV use only	10 mcg (of liothyronine) per mL*	**Liothyronine Sodium Injection**
		Triostat®, Jones

*available from one or more manufacturer, distributor, and/or repackager by generic (nonproprietary) name

ANTITHYROID AGENTS 68:36.08

methIMAzole

Thiamazole

■ Methimazole is a thioimidazole-derivative antithyroid agent.

Uses

■ **Hyperthyroidism** Methimazole is used in patients with Graves' disease with hyperthyroidism or toxic multinodular goiter for whom surgery or radioactive iodine therapy is not an appropriate treatment option. The drug also is used to ameliorate symptoms of hyperthyroidism in preparation for thyroidectomy or radioactive iodine therapy.

Some clinicians state that methimazole should be used in virtually every patient who chooses antithyroid drug therapy for the treatment of Graves' disease, except during the first trimester of pregnancy when propylthiouracil is preferred (see Pregnancy under Cautions: Pregnancy and Lactation), in the treatment of thyroid storm (see Thyrotoxic Crisis under Uses: Hyperthyroidism), and in patients with minor adverse reactions to methimazole who refuse radioactive iodine therapy or surgery.

Because of postmarketing reports of severe liver injury in pediatric patients receiving propylthiouracil, methimazole is the preferred agent when an antithyroid drug is required for a pediatric patient. (See Cautions: Pediatric Precautions.)

Thioamide antithyroid agents (e.g., methimazole, propylthiouracil) are used to control the symptoms of hyperthyroidism associated with Graves' disease and maintain the patient in a euthyroid state for a period of several years (generally 1–2 years) until a spontaneous remission occurs. Thioamide antithyroid agents do not affect the underlying cause of hyperthyroidism. Spontaneous remission does not occur in all patients receiving therapy with thioamide antithyroid agents, and most patients eventually require ablative therapy (i.e., surgery, radioactive iodine). The minimum duration of thioamide therapy necessary before assessing whether spontaneous remission has occurred is not clearly established. However, some clinicians state that if methimazole is chosen as the primary therapy for Graves' disease, the drug should be continued for approximately 12–18 months in adults or 1–2 years in children, then tapered or discontinued if thyrotropin (thyroid stimulating hormone, TSH) concentrations return to normal at that time. If adults or children with Graves' disease remain hyperthyroid after completing a course of methimazole, treatment with radioactive iodine or thyroidectomy should be considered. Some clinicians state that treatment with low-dose methimazole for longer than 12–18 months in adults may be considered in patients not in remission who prefer this pharmacologic approach. Methimazole therapy also may be continued in children until the child is considered old enough for radioactive iodine therapy or surgery.

Methimazole is used to return the hyperthyroid patient to a normal metabolic state prior to thyroidectomy and to control the thyrotoxic crisis that may accompany thyroidectomy. (See Thyrotoxic Crisis under Uses: Hyperthyroidism.) Some clinicians recommend that, whenever possible, adults or children with Graves' disease undergoing thyroidectomy or adults with toxic adenoma† or toxic multinodular goiter undergoing surgery be rendered euthyroid with methimazole prior to the procedure.

Methimazole is used as an adjunct to radioactive iodine therapy in patients who require control of symptoms of hyperthyroidism prior to and after administration of radioactive iodine until the ablative effects of the iodine occur. However, the beneficial and detrimental effects and optimal sequencing of antithyroid drugs before or after radioactive iodine therapy have not been clearly established. Some clinicians recommend that pretreatment with methimazole prior to radioactive iodine therapy for Graves' disease, toxic adenoma†, or toxic multinodular goiter be considered in adults who are at increased risk for complications due to worsening of hyperthyroidism (e.g., geriatric patients, patients with severe hyperthyroidism [e.g., extremely symptomatic, free thyroxine (T_4) estimates 2–3 times the upper limit of normal] or substantial comorbidities [e.g., cardiovascular disease]). However, conflicting opinions exist, and other clinicians state that pretreatment with methimazole prior to radioactive iodine therapy is not necessary because there is insufficient evidence to indicate that radioactive iodine worsens the clinical or biochemical aspects of hyperthyroidism, and that pretreatment with methimazole will only delay treatment with radioactive iodine. In addition, some evidence indicates that pretreatment with methimazole may reduce the efficacy of subsequent radioactive iodine therapy. In children with Graves' disease having total T_4 concentrations exceeding 20 mcg/dL or free T_4 estimates exceeding 5 ng/dL who are to receive radioactive iodine therapy, some clinicians suggest pretreatment with methimazole and β-adrenergic blockade until total T_4 and/or free T_4 estimates normalize before proceeding with radioactive iodine.

Antithyroid agents do not induce remission in patients with nodular thyroid disease (i.e., toxic adenoma†, toxic multinodular goiter), and discontinuance of therapy results in relapse. Therefore, some clinicians suggest that adults with overt toxic adenoma or toxic multinodular goiter be treated with either radioactive iodine therapy or thyroidectomy, and that long-term methimazole therapy be avoided. However, these clinicians state that long-term (life-long) antithyroid drug therapy may be the best choice for some geriatric or otherwise ill patients with limited longevity and increased surgical risk who can be monitored regularly (e.g., residents of nursing homes or other care facilities where compliance with radiation safety regulations may be difficult) or for patients who prefer this pharmacologic approach.

Thyrotoxic Crisis In the management of thyrotoxic crisis, thioamide antithyroid agents are used to inhibit thyroid hormone synthesis. Because propylthiouracil also blocks the peripheral conversion of thyroxine to triiodothyronine, it theoretically may be more useful than methimazole or carbimazole (not commercially available in the US) in the management of thyrotoxic crisis. Iodides (e.g., potassium iodide, strong iodine solution) are given to inhibit the release of thyroid hormone from the gland but may subsequently be used as a substrate for thyroid hormone synthesis; therefore, treatment with a thioamide antithyroid agent is usually initiated before iodide therapy. A β-adrenergic blocking agent (e.g., propranolol) is also usually given concomitantly to manage peripheral signs and symptoms of hyperthyroidism, particularly cardiovascular effects (e.g., tachycardia).

Dosage and Administration

■ **Administration** Methimazole is administered orally. The manufacturer states that the total daily dosage is usually given in 3 equally divided doses at approximately 8-hour intervals. Alternatively, some clinicians state that methimazole may be administered as a single daily dose.

■ **Dosage** ***Adult Dosage*** The manufacturer states that the initial adult dosage of methimazole is 15, 30–40, or 60 mg daily for the treatment of mild, moderately severe, or severe hyperthyroidism, respectively. Alternatively, for the treatment of Graves' disease, some clinicians recommend an initial adult methimazole dosage of 10–20 mg daily to restore euthyroidism. In general, most patients improve considerably or achieve normal thyroid function following 4–12 weeks of therapy, after which dosage may be decreased while maintaining normal thyroid function. Subsequent dosage should be carefully adjusted according to the patient's tolerance and therapeutic response. The manufacturer states that the adult maintenance dosage is 5–15 mg daily. Alternatively, for the treatment of Graves' disease, some clinicians generally recommend an adult maintenance dosage of 5–10 mg daily. (See Cautions: Precautions and Contraindications.)

If methimazole is used during pregnancy for the management of hyperthyroidism, the manufacturer states that a sufficient, but not excessive, dosage of methimazole is necessary; the lowest possible dosage of methimazole to control the maternal disease should be used. The manufacturer states that because thyroid dysfunction diminishes in many women as the pregnancy proceeds, a reduction in dosage of antithyroid therapy may be possible, and, in some patients, use of antithyroid therapy can be discontinued 2–3 weeks before delivery. (See Pregnancy under Cautions: Pregnancy and Lactation.)

For the treatment of thyrotoxic crisis (i.e., thyroid storm) in adults, some clinicians recommend a methimazole dosage of 60–80 mg daily.

The optimum duration of antithyroid therapy remains to be clearly established. However, some clinicians state that if methimazole is chosen as the primary therapy for Graves' disease in adults, the drug should be continued for approximately 12–18 months, then tapered or discontinued if thyrotropin (thyroid stimulating hormone, TSH) concentrations return to normal at that time. If a patient with Graves' disease remains hyperthyroid after completing a course of methimazole, treatment with radioactive iodine or thyroidectomy should be considered. However, treatment with low-dose methimazole for longer than 12–18 months may be considered in adult patients not in remission who prefer this pharmacologic approach.

If methimazole is used prior to thyroidectomy or surgery to render adults euthyroid, the drug should be discontinued at the time of the procedure.

If methimazole is used as pretreatment prior to radioactive iodine therapy, some clinicians recommend that methimazole be discontinued 2–7 days before administration of radioactive iodine, restarted 3–7 days after radioactive iodine, and generally tapered over 4–6 weeks as thyroid function normalizes and radioactive iodine becomes effective.

Pediatric Dosage For the treatment of hyperthyroidism in children, the manufacturer states that the initial dosage of methimazole is 0.4 mg/kg daily. The manufacturer states that the maintenance dosage in children is approximately one-half of the initial dosage. Alternatively, for the treatment of Graves' disease, some clinicians state that the usual dosage of methimazole in children is 0.2–0.5 mg/kg daily, with a range of 0.1–1 mg/kg daily. These clinicians also suggest the following general dosages, calculated based on the patient's age and rounded to the nearest quarter-, half-, or whole-tablet dosage strengths: 1.25 mg daily for infants; 2.5–5 mg daily for children 1–5 years of age; 5–10 mg daily for children 5–10 years of age; and 10–20 mg daily for children 10–18 years of age. Patients with severe clinical or biochemical hyperthyroidism may receive methimazole dosages that are 50–100% higher than those usually recommended for the treatment of Graves' disease. When thyroid hormone concentrations normalize, these clinicians state that methimazole dosages may be reduced by 50% or more to maintain a euthyroid state.

The optimum duration of antithyroid therapy remains to be clearly established. However, some clinicians state that if methimazole is chosen as first-line therapy for Graves' disease in children, the drug should be continued for 1–2 years and then discontinued, or dosage reduced, to assess whether the patient is in remission. If the patient is not in remission following 1–2 years of methimazole therapy, treatment with radioactive iodine or thyroidectomy should be considered, depending on the age of the patient. Alternatively, methimazole may be continued for extended periods as long as adverse effects do not occur and hyperthyroidism is controlled; this approach may be used as a bridge to radioactive iodine therapy or surgery at a later age if remission still has not occurred. Low-dose methimazole may be continued in selected situations in which radioactive iodine therapy or surgery may not be suitable or possible.

If methimazole is used prior to thyroidectomy to render children with Graves' disease euthyroid, some clinicians state that methimazole is usually administered for 1–2 months in preparation for the procedure.

If methimazole is used as pretreatment prior to radioactive iodine therapy in children with Graves' disease, some clinicians recommend that methimazole be discontinued 3–5 days before administration of radioactive iodine. Although some clinicians restart antithyroid drugs after radioactive iodine therapy, other clinicians state that this practice is seldom required in children.

Cautions

■ **Adverse Effects** Adverse dermatologic effects are most commonly reported. Minor adverse effects of methimazole include rash, urticaria, pruritus, abnormal hair loss, skin pigmentation, edema, nausea, vomiting, epigastric distress, loss of taste, arthralgia, myalgia, paresthesia, and headache. Drowsiness, neuritis, vertigo, jaundice, sialadenopathy, and lymphadenopathy also have occurred in patients receiving the drug. (See Cautions: Hepatic Effects.) In one patient, peripheral neuritis occurred during long-term (23 months) therapy with methimazole but disappeared following discontinuance of the drug.

Although reported much less frequently, severe adverse effects of methimazole include inhibition of myelopoieses (agranulocytosis [see Cautions: Agranulocytosis], granulocytopenia, thrombocytopenia, and aplastic anemia); drug fever; lupus-like syndrome; insulin autoimmune syndrome (which can result in hypoglycemic coma); hepatitis (see Cautions: Hepatic Effects); periarteritis; and hypoprothrombinemia. Nephritis occurs very rarely in patients receiving methimazole.

■ **Agranulocytosis** Agranulocytosis is a potentially life-threatening adverse effect of methimazole therapy. Most cases of agranulocytosis appear to occur within the first 2 months of therapy, but rarely may occur after 4 months of therapy. Although methimazole-induced agranulocytosis may be dose related (possibly occurring more frequently with higher dosages of the drug), agranulocytosis may occur irrespective of dosage, length of treatment, or previous exposure to the antithyroid drug, and may occur more frequently in geriatric patients. The mechanism(s) of methimazole-induced agranulocytosis has not been determined, but antigranulocyte antibodies have been reported in some patients with thioamide-induced agranulocytosis; a direct toxic effect of these drugs on bone marrow has not been excluded as an additional possible cause.

■ **Hepatic Effects** Although there have been reports of hepatotoxicity (including acute liver failure) associated with methimazole, the risk of hepatotoxicity appears to be lower with methimazole than with propylthiouracil, especially in pediatric patients. (See Cautions: Pediatric Precautions.) Jaundice associated with methimazole-induced hepatitis may persist for several weeks after discontinuance of the drug.

■ **Hypothyroidism** Methimazole may cause hypothyroidism necessitating routine monitoring of thyrotropin (thyroid stimulating hormone, TSH) and free thyroxine (T_4) concentrations; dosage should be adjusted to maintain a euthyroid state. (See Cautions: Precautions and Contraindications.) Because methimazole readily crosses the placenta, the drug can cause fetal goiter and cretinism when administered to a pregnant woman. (See Pregnancy under Cautions: Pregnancy and Lactation.)

■ **Precautions and Contraindications** Some clinicians suggest that a baseline complete blood count, including white count with differential, be performed prior to initiating antithyroid drug therapy in patients with Graves' disease. Patients receiving methimazole should be closely monitored and should be instructed to contact their clinician immediately if signs or symptoms of illness, particularly sore throat, skin eruptions, fever, chills, headache, or general malaise, occur; it is particularly important to carefully monitor for these signs and symptoms during the early stages of methimazole therapy since methimazole-induced agranulocytosis usually occurs during the first several months of therapy. Leukopenia, thrombocytopenia, and/or aplastic anemia (pancytopenia) also may occur. Leukocyte and differential counts should be performed in patients who develop fever or sore throat or other signs or symptoms of illness while receiving the drug. Methimazole should be used with extreme caution in patients receiving other drugs known to cause agranulocytosis. The manufacturer states that methimazole should be discontinued in the presence of agranulocytosis, aplastic anemia (pancytopenia), ANCA-positive vasculitis, hepatitis, or exfoliative dermatitis, and the patient's bone marrow indices should be monitored. Some clinicians state that patients should be informed of the adverse effects associated with methimazole (e.g., agranulocytosis) and advised to immediately discontinue the drug and promptly contact their clinician if fever or pharyngitis occurs. In a patient who develops agranulocytosis or other serious adverse effects while receiving either methimazole or propylthiouracil, some clinicians state that use of the other drug also is contraindicated because of the risk of cross-sensitivity between the two drugs. Because methimazole may cause hypoprothrombinemia and bleeding, prothrombin time should be monitored during therapy, particularly prior to surgery (see Drug Interactions: Anticoagulants).

Some clinicians suggest that liver function tests, including alkaline phosphatase, aminotransferase, and bilirubin, be performed prior to initiating antithyroid drug therapy in patients with Graves' disease. Patients should be informed of the adverse hepatic effects associated with methimazole and advised to immediately discontinue the drug and promptly contact their clinician if pruritic rash, jaundice, acholic stools, dark urine, arthralgias, abdominal pain, nausea, or fatigue occurs. Patients with symptoms suggestive of hepatic dysfunction (e.g., anorexia, pruritus, right upper-quadrant pain) should have prompt evaluation of their liver function (alkaline phosphatase, bilirubin) and hepatocellular integrity (ALT, AST). If there is evidence of a clinically important liver abnormality, including hepatic aminotransferase concentrations exceeding 3 times the upper limit of normal, the manufacturer states that the drug should be discontinued promptly.

Thyroid function should be monitored periodically in patients receiving methimazole. In patients with Graves' disease, some clinicians state that thyroid function (e.g., serum free T_4, serum free or total triiodothyronine [T_3], TSH) should be monitored before initiating therapy and then every 4–8 weeks thereafter (with subsequent dosage adjustments as needed) until thyroid function is stable or the patient is euthyroid; once the patient is euthyroid, thyroid function may be monitored every 2–3 months. Early in the course of antithyroid therapy, serum TSH concentration is not a reliable parameter to monitor because it may remain suppressed for several months after initiation of therapy despite normalization of free T_4 concentrations. The finding of a suppressed TSH concentration during this period, therefore, does not indicate a need for a dosage increase. However, once clinical evidence of resolution of hyperthyroidism occurs, the finding of an elevated serum TSH concentration indicates that a lower maintenance dosage of methimazole should be employed. Monitoring serum T_3 concentrations may sometimes be useful for dosage adjustment; in patients in whom total or free T_3 concentrations remain elevated despite low, normal, or reduced free T_4 concentrations, an increase in antithyroid dosage may be necessary. When methimazole is discontinued in patients with Graves' disease, thyroid function should be monitored every 1–3 months for 6–12 months to diagnose relapse early, and patients should be advised to contact clinicians if symptoms of hyperthyroidism occur.

Methimazole is contraindicated in patients who are hypersensitive to the drug or any ingredient in the formulation. Cross-sensitivity between thioamides may occur (i.e., in approximately 50% of patients switched from one thioamide agent to the other). In patients who develop agranulocytosis or other serious adverse effects while receiving either methimazole or propylthiouracil, some clinicians state that use of the other drug also is contraindicated because of the risk of cross-sensitivity between the two drugs. In patients experiencing serious allergic reactions to methimazole, some clinicians state that using the alternative antithyroid drug (i.e., propylthiouracil) is not recommended.

■ Pediatric Precautions Because of postmarketing reports of severe liver injury in pediatric patients receiving propylthiouracil, methimazole is preferred over propylthiouracil when an antithyroid drug is required for a pediatric patient. (See Uses: Hyperthyroidism.) During postmarketing experience, cases of severe liver injury, including hepatic failure requiring liver transplantation or resulting in death, have been reported in pediatric patients receiving propylthiouracil; however, no such cases have been reported in pediatric patients treated with methimazole. (See Cautions: Precautions and Contraindications.)

■ Pregnancy and Lactation ***Pregnancy*** Methimazole readily crosses the placental membranes and may cause fetal harm, particularly when administered in the first trimester of pregnancy. The drug can also cause fetal goiter and hypothyroidism (cretinism) when administered to a pregnant woman.

In April 2010, the US Food and Drug Administration (FDA) reported a review of postmarketing data analyzing the potential for birth defects associated with use of propylthiouracil or methimazole during pregnancy. FDA found that congenital malformations were reported approximately 3 times more often with prenatal exposure to methimazole compared with propylthiouracil (29 cases with methimazole; 9 cases with propylthiouracil). In addition, there was a distinct and consistent pattern of congenital malformations associated with the use of methimazole that was not found with propylthiouracil. Approximately 90% of the congenital malformations with methimazole were craniofacial malformations (e.g., scalp epidermal aplasia [aplasia cutis], facial dysmorphism, choanal atresia). In most of the cases, there were multiple malformations that frequently included a combination of craniofacial defects and GI atresia or aplasia. These specific birth defects were associated with the use of methimazole during the first trimester of pregnancy but were not found when the drug was administered later in pregnancy. In contrast, FDA did not find a consistent pattern of birth defects associated with the use of propylthiouracil and concluded that there is no convincing evidence of an association between propylthiouracil use and congenital malformations, even with use during the first trimester.

Despite the potential fetal hazard, antithyroid agents are still considered the therapy of choice for the management of hyperthyroidism during pregnancy. Since methimazole may be associated with the rare development of fetal abnormalities, such as aplasia cutis, craniofacial malformations (facial dysmorphism, choanal atresia), and GI malformations (esophageal atresia with or without tracheoesophageal fistula, umbilical abnormalities), propylthiouracil is the preferred agent when an antithyroid drug is indicated during organogenesis in the first trimester of pregnancy or just prior to the first trimester of pregnancy. Patients receiving methimazole should be switched to propylthiouracil if pregnancy is confirmed in the first trimester. Because of the potential adverse maternal effects of propylthiouracil (e.g., hepatotoxicity), however, it may be preferable to switch from propylthiouracil to methimazole for the second and third trimesters (i.e., after the first trimester). If the patient is switching from propylthiouracil to methimazole, thyroid function should be assessed after 2 weeks and then every 2–4 weeks thereafter. It is not known if the risk of methimazole-induced aplasia cutis or embryopathy outweighs the risk of propylthiouracil-induced hepatotoxicity.

If methimazole is used during pregnancy for the management of hyperthyroidism, the manufacturer states that a sufficient, but not excessive, dosage of methimazole is necessary; the lowest possible dosage of methimazole to control the maternal disease should be used. Some clinicians state that antithyroid drug therapy should be initiated or adjusted to maintain maternal free thyroxine (T_4) concentrations at or just above the upper limit of normal (ULN) of the nonpregnant reference range, or to maintain total T_4 concentrations at 1.5 times the ULN or the free T_4 index in the ULN, while using the lowest possible dosage of antithyroid drugs. In women receiving antithyroid drugs during pregnancy, free T_4 and TSH concentrations should be monitored approximately every 2–6 weeks. The manufacturer states that because thyroid dysfunction diminishes in many women as pregnancy proceeds, a reduction in dosage of antithyroid therapy may be possible, and, in some patients, use of antithyroid therapy can be discontinued 2–3 weeks before delivery.

Patients should be advised to contact their clinician immediately about their therapy if they are or plan to become pregnant while receiving an antithyroid drug. If methimazole is used during pregnancy or if the patient becomes pregnant while receiving the drug, the patient should be advised of the potential hazard to the fetus; in addition, when considering antithyroid drug use during pregnancy, the patient should be informed of the risks of methimazole-associated fetal malformations, as well as the risks of propylthiouracil-associated hepatotoxicity.

Lactation Methimazole is distributed into milk. However, several studies found no effect on clinical status in nursing infants of women receiving methimazole, particularly if thyroid function is monitored at frequent (weekly or biweekly) intervals. A long-term study of 139 thyrotoxic lactating women and their infants failed to demonstrate toxicity in infants who are breast-fed by women receiving methimazole.

Methimazole generally is compatible with breast-feeding, and moderate dosages of the drug (i.e., 20–30 mg daily) appear to be safe during breast-feeding. Because of concerns regarding severe hepatotoxicity (i.e., hepatic necrosis in either woman or child) associated with maternal use of propylthiouracil, some clinicians consider methimazole to be the preferred antithyroid drug in nursing women. If an antithyroid drug is used in nursing women, some clinicians recommend that the drug be administered *after* a feeding and in divided doses, and that thyroid function be monitored in nursing infants.

Drug Interactions

■ Drugs Known to Cause Agranulocytosis Methimazole should be used with extreme caution in patients receiving other drugs known to cause agranulocytosis. (See Cautions: Agranulocytosis and also see Cautions: Precautions and Contraindications.)

■ Anticoagulants Because of the potential inhibition of vitamin K activity by methimazole, the activity of oral anticoagulants (e.g., warfarin) may be increased. However, methimazole also may decrease the anticoagulant effect of warfarin. Additional monitoring of prothrombin time (PT)/international normalized ratio (INR) should be considered, particularly prior to surgery. Dosage adjustment of warfarin may be necessary.

■ β-Adrenergic Blocking Agents Hyperthyroidism may cause an increased clearance of β-adrenergic blocking agents with a high extraction ratio. Dosage reduction of the β-adrenergic blocking agent may be needed when a hyperthyroid patient becomes euthyroid.

■ Digitalis Glycosides Serum digitalis concentrations may be increased when hyperthyroid patients receiving a stable digitalis glycoside regimen become euthyroid; dosage reduction of the digitalis glycoside may be needed.

■ Theophylline Theophylline clearance may decrease when hyperthyroid patients receiving a stable theophylline regimen become euthyroid; dosage reduction of theophylline may be needed.

Acute Toxicity

■ Manifestations In general, overdosage of methimazole may be expected to produce effects that are extensions of common adverse reactions. Symptoms may include nausea, vomiting, epigastric distress, headache, fever, joint pain, pruritus, and edema. Aplastic anemia (pancytopenia) or agranulocytosis may be manifested in hours to days. Agranulocytosis is the most serious effect associated with methimazole overdosage. Less frequent adverse effects include exfoliative dermatitis, hepatitis, nephrotic syndrome, neuropathies, and CNS stimulation or depression. No data are available on the median lethal dose of methimazole or the concentration of drug in biologic fluids associated with toxicity and/or death.

■ Treatment Treatment of methimazole overdosage generally involves appropriate supportive care as dictated by the patient's medical status. Clinicians should consider consulting a poison control center for the most current information on the management of methimazole overdosage.

Pharmacology

Methimazole inhibits the synthesis of thyroid hormones by interfering with the incorporation of iodine into tyrosyl residues of thyroglobulin; the drug also inhibits the coupling of these iodotyrosyl residues to form iodothyronine. Although the exact mechanism(s) has not been fully elucidated, methimazole may interfere with the oxidation of iodide ion and iodotyrosyl groups. Based on limited evidence, it appears that the coupling reaction is more sensitive to antithyroid agents than the iodination reaction. Methimazole does not inhibit the action of thyroid hormones already formed and present in the thyroid gland or circulation nor does the drug interfere with the effectiveness of exogenously administered thyroid hormones. Patients whose thyroid gland contains a relatively high concentration of iodine (e.g., from prior ingestion or from administration during diagnostic radiologic procedures) may respond relatively slowly to antithyroid agents. Unlike propylthiouracil, methimazole does not inhibit the peripheral deiodination of thyroxine to triiodothyronine.

Pharmacokinetics

Methimazole is rapidly absorbed from the GI tract following oral administration with peak plasma concentrations occurring within about 1 hour. Methimazole readily crosses the placenta and is distributed into milk in concentrations approximately equal to those in maternal serum. Methimazole is metabolized in the liver. The elimination half-life of methimazole reportedly ranges from about 5–13 hours. The drug is excreted in urine. In one study, about 12% of a dose was excreted in urine within 24 hours.

Chemistry and Stability

■ **Chemistry** Methimazole is a thioimidazole-derivative antithyroid agent. The drug differs chemically and structurally from propylthiouracil and other thiouracil derivatives in that methimazole has a 5-membered ring instead of a 6-membered ring. Although presence of a thioamide group appears to be sufficient for antithyroid activity, methimazole, like propylthiouracil and carbimazole, contains the thioureylene moiety.

Methimazole occurs as a white, crystalline substance and is freely soluble in water.

■ **Stability** Commercially available methimazole tablets should be stored at controlled room temperature (15–30°C).

Preparations

Excipients in commercially available drug preparations may have clinically important effects in some individuals; consult specific product labeling for details.

methIMAzole

Oral		
Tablets	5 mg*	**methIMAzole Tablets**
		Tapazole® (scored), King
	10 mg*	**methIMAzole Tablets**
		Tapazole® (scored), King

*available from one or more manufacturer, distributor, and/or repackager by generic (nonproprietary) name

†Use is not currently included in the labeling approved by the US Food and Drug Administration

Potassium Iodide

KISSKI

■ Potassium iodide is an antithyroid agent, antisporotrichotic agent, and expectorant.

Uses

■ **Hyperthyroidism** Oral potassium iodide is used in the preoperative management of hyperthyroidism in patients with Graves' disease undergoing thyroidectomy†, usually as an adjunct to other antithyroid agents (e.g., methimazole, propylthiouracil) and/or β-adrenergic blocking agents (e.g., propranolol). The American Thyroid Association (ATA), American Association of Clinical Endocrinologists (AACE), and others recommend that patients with Graves' disease scheduled for thyroidectomy be rendered euthyroid using other antithyroid agents (preferably methimazole) and then receive oral potassium iodide for 7–14 days (usually 10 days) in the immediate preoperative period. In exceptional circumstances when the euthyroid state cannot be achieved prior to thyroidectomy (e.g., urgent need for surgery, allergy to antithyroid drugs), these experts recommend that oral potassium iodide and a β-adrenergic blocking agent (e.g., propranolol) be administered in the immediate preoperative period. Preoperative potassium iodide has traditionally been used in Graves' disease patients undergoing surgery in an attempt to decrease thyroid blood flow, vascularity, and intraoperative blood loss; however, the necessity and benefits of this strategy have been questioned. Because of the risk of exacerbating hyperthyroidism, preoperative potassium iodide is not indicated in patients with toxic multinodular goiter or toxic adenoma undergoing thyroidectomy.

Oral potassium iodide also is used in the management of severe, life-threatening thyrotoxicosis† (thyroid storm, thyrotoxicosis crisis) in conjunction with other antithyroid agents (e.g., methimazole, propylthiouracil), β-adrenergic blocking agents (e.g., propranolol), corticosteroids (hydrocortisone, dexamethasone), treatment of hyperpyrexia, and appropriate fluid, electrolyte, and respiratory support. Other antithyroid agents (e.g., methimazole, propylthiouracil) are initiated first to block thyroid hormone synthesis and conversion of tetraiodothyronine (thyroxine, T_4) to triiodothyronine (T_3); potassium iodide is initiated 1 hour after the other antithyroid agents and is used to block new hormone synthesis and thyroid hormone release.

■ **Radiation Emergency** Oral potassium iodide is used during a radiation emergency to block thyroidal uptake of radioactive isotopes of iodine (e.g., I 131) that may be released into the environment (e.g., from a nuclear power plant) and thus minimize the risk of radiation-induced thyroid neoplasms related to *internal* exposures to radioiodines (inhaled or ingested). *Although potassium iodide provides protection for the thyroid from radioiodines, the drug has no impact on body uptake of other radioactive materials and does not provide protection against external irradiation of any kind.*

The extent of protection that oral potassium iodide can provide against inhaled or ingested radioiodines depends on several factors, including how quickly the drug is initiated and the total dose of radioactivity involved in the exposure. Thyroidal uptake of radioiodine can be reduced by more than 90–99% by oral intake of 130 mg of potassium iodide daily initiated shortly before or within 1–2 hours after acute exposure. Potassium iodide may still provide substantial protection if taken 3–4 hours after exposure; however, although some data indicate that the drug may be about 40% effective if taken 8 hours after exposure, it may offer little protection if taken 12 hours or more after exposure. The thyroid-blocking effect of a single 130-mg dose of potassium iodide persists for about 24 hours. If the exposure lasts longer than 24 hours and involves continuing or ongoing contamination, additional doses may be necessary until the risk of significant exposure to radioiodines no longer exists.

The US Food and Drug Administration (FDA) issued updated recommendations in December 2001 on the use of potassium iodide in the event of a radiation emergency involving the release of radioactive iodine. These recommendations provide guidance to other federal agencies, including the Environmental Protection Agency (EPA) and Nuclear Regulatory Commission (NRC), and to state and local governments on safe and effective dosages of potassium iodide as an adjunct to other protective measures (e.g., evacuation, sheltering, assurance of uncontaminated milk and food). FDA recommendations issued in 1978 and 1982 were based on studies that estimated *external* thyroid exposure to radiation resulting from nuclear detonations in Hiroshima and Nagasaki and analogous studies in children who received therapeutic radiation to the head and neck. The 2001 recommendations were derived from much more comprehensive and reliable data relating *internal* radioiodine exposure (e.g., through inhalation or ingestion) to thyroid cancer risk following the 1986 Chernobyl nuclear reactor accident. Data from the Chernobyl incident indicated that the risk of thyroid cancer following a radiation emergency (e.g., nuclear reactor accident) is inversely related to age and that exposure to relatively small doses of radioiodine may lead to dramatic increases in thyroid cancer among exposed children. The revised FDA guidelines therefore recommend potassium iodide prophylaxis at predicted radiation exposures that are lower than previously recommended (particularly for children) and, to reduce the risk of hypothyroidism, lower dosage of potassium iodide for neonates, infants, and children compared with previous FDA recommendations. In addition, FDA no longer recommends emergency use of potassium iodide in adults over 40 years of age, unless a large internal radiation dose (e.g., at least 500 centigrays [cGy]) is anticipated. Potassium iodide is used as an adjunct to other protective measures (e.g., evacuation, sheltering, assurance of uncontaminated milk and food). The FDA recommends that individuals who are intolerant of potassium iodide and those for whom repeat doses of the drug are a concern (e.g., neonates 1 month of age or younger, pregnant or lactating women) be given priority with regard to these other protective measures.

If a radiation emergency related to a US nuclear power plant occurs, decisions to recommend use of protective measures for public health and safety (including use of potassium iodide for thyroidal blockade) reside with state and/or local government authorities responsible for radiological emergency planning and response. These authorities should inform the public of the nature of the radiation hazard and potential benefits and adverse effects of potassium iodide. For use in radiation emergencies, potassium iodide is commercially available in appropriate dosage forms (see Radiation Emergency under Dosage and Administration: Dosage) and may also be retained in state or local stockpiles.

■ **Exposure to Radiopharmaceuticals** Oral potassium iodide is used for protection of the thyroid during diagnostic or therapeutic use of radiopharmaceuticals or drugs that have radioactive components† (e.g., iodine I 131 tositumomab; no longer commercially available in the US). Potassium iodide treatment is initiated prior to use of the radiolabeled diagnostic or therapeutic agent to saturate the thyroid and protect it from uptake of radioiodide and is continued until the estimated activity of the radiolabeled agent has decreased to acceptable levels after the procedure or treatment has been completed. In some cases, oral potassium iodide has been used in conjunction with other thyroid protective agents (e.g., methimazole, thyroxine).

■ **Sporotrichosis** Oral potassium iodide is used for the treatment of cutaneous sporotrichosis† (localized to skin; also known as fixed cutaneous sporotrichosis) and lymphocutaneous sporotrichosis† (involves skin, subcutaneous tissues, regional lymphatics) caused by *Sporothrix schenckii*. Since it is inexpensive and generally has been effective, potassium iodide (oral solution containing 1 g/mL; also known as saturated solution of potassium iodide [SSKI®]) has historically been considered a standard of care for the treatment of cutaneous and lymphocutaneous sporotrichosis and continues to be a drug of first choice for these infections in some resource-limited settings and countries where the disease is endemic. However, compliance with the long-term treatment regimen can be a problem since the drug is associated with a substantial number of adverse effects (e.g., nausea, rash, fever, bitter or metallic taste, salivary gland enlargement, risk of iodism or potassium toxicity with prolonged use). In addition, safety and efficacy of oral potassium iodide for the treatment of cutaneous or lymphocutaneous sporotrichosis have not been established in randomized, controlled clinical studies and efficacy of the drug compared with that of other antifungals used for the treatment of these infections (e.g., itraconazole, terbinafine, fluconazole) has not been established.

The Infectious Diseases Society of America (IDSA) and other experts state that oral itraconazole is the drug of choice for the treatment of cutaneous and lymphocutaneous sporotrichosis and oral terbinafine and potassium iodide (oral solution containing 1 g/mL; also known as saturated solution of potassium iodide [SSKI®]) are the preferred alternatives. For the treatment of cutaneous sporotrichosis, local hyperthermia (i.e., direct application of heat using a pocket warmer, infrared or far-infrared heater, or similar device that warms tissue to 42–43°C) is another alternative that can be used when antifungal agents or potassium iodide cannot be used (e.g., pregnant or nursing women).

Oral potassium iodide is not effective for and should not be used for the treatment of extracutaneous sporotrichosis† (osteoarticular, pulmonary, meningeal) or disseminated sporotrichosis†. IV amphotericin B and oral itraconazole are the drugs of choice for these forms of sporotrichosis.

■ **Cough** Oral potassium iodide (oral solution containing 1 g/mL; also known as saturated solution of potassium iodide [SSKI®]) has been used as an expectorant in the symptomatic management of chronic pulmonary diseases where tenacious mucus complicates the condition (e.g., bronchial asthma, bronchitis, pulmonary emphysema); however, the drug has generally been replaced by more effective and safer expectorants. Although there is limited evidence that saline expectorants like potassium iodide can increase respiratory tract secretions, possibly as a reflex response to drug-induced gastric irritation, such evidence is sparse and inconclusive. In addition, there currently is insufficient evidence from well-designed studies to support the efficacy of potassium iodide as an expectorant.

Dosage and Administration

■ **Administration** Potassium iodide is administered orally.

For use during a radiation emergency, potassium iodide is commercially available as tablets containing 65 or 130 mg of the drug and as an oral solution containing 65 mg/mL. If the oral solution containing 65 mg/mL is used, the dose should be administered undiluted using the calibrated dropper provided by the manufacturer.

For other indications, an oral solution of potassium iodide containing 1 g/mL (also known as saturated solution of potassium iodide [SSKI®]) also is available. If this oral solution is used, the dose should be administered in a glassful of water, fruit juice, or milk. To minimize GI irritation, the dose should be taken with food or milk. A calibrated dropper marked to deliver 300 mg (0.3 mL) or 600 mg (0.6 mL) of the drug is provided by the manufacturer. If a dose of the oral solution containing 1 g/mL is administered using a standard medicinal dropper, each drop (0.05 mL) contains 50 mg of potassium iodide.

Potassium iodide may be available as strong iodine solution (also known as Lugol's solution), an oral solution containing 50 mg of iodine and 100 mg of potassium iodide per mL; this preparation may be commercially available but is not approved by the US Food and Drug Administration (FDA). Doses of strong iodine solution should be diluted in water or juice. If a dose of strong iodine solution is administered using a standard medicinal dropper, each drop contains 8 mg of iodide.

Extemporaneous Oral Solutions For use during a radiation emergency in infants, small children, and others who cannot swallow tablets, oral solutions (liquid mixtures) of potassium iodide can be prepared extemporaneously using 65- or 130-mg tablets of the drug.

To prepare an oral solution containing 8.125 mg/5 mL (8.125 mg/teaspoon), the manufacturers state that a single 65-mg tablet of potassium iodide should be pulverized in a small bowl using the back of a teaspoon; 4 teaspoons (20 mL) of water should then be added to the bowl and mixed until the tablet dissolves. This potassium iodide mixture should then be added to 4 teaspoons (20 mL) of milk (low-fat white or chocolate), orange juice, flat soda, raspberry syrup, or infant formula.

To prepare an oral solution containing 16.25 mg/5 mL (16.25 mg/teaspoon), the manufacturers state that a single 130-mg tablet of potassium iodide should be pulverized in a small bowl using the back of a teaspoon; 4 teaspoons (20 mL) of water should then be added to the bowl and mixed until the tablet dissolves. This potassium iodide mixture should then be added to 4 teaspoons (20 mL) of milk (low-fat white or chocolate), orange juice, flat soda, raspberry syrup, or infant formula.

Alternatively, the FDA states that an oral solution containing 16.25 mg/5 mL (16.25 mg/teaspoon) can be prepared by putting two 65-mg tablets or one 130-mg tablet in a small bowl and adding 4 teaspoons (20 mL) of water to the bowl. After soaking in the water for 1 minute, the tablet(s) should be crushed using the back of the teaspoon until no large pieces remain. This potassium iodide mixture should then be added to 4 teaspoons (20 mL) of milk (white or chocolate), orange juice, soda (e.g., cola), infant formula, raspberry syrup, or water.

These extemporaneous oral solutions of potassium iodide should be stored in a refrigerator and used within 7 days.

■ **Dosage** ***Hyperthyroidism*** When oral potassium iodide is used in the preoperative management of hyperthyroidism in patients with Graves' disease undergoing thyroidectomy†, the drug is administered for 7–14 days (usually 10 days) in the immediate preoperative period (see Uses: Hyperthyroidism). If the potassium iodide oral solution containing 1 g/mL (also known as saturated solution of potassium iodide [SSKI®]) is used, the recommended dosage is 50–100 mg (1–2 drops or 0.05–0.1 mL) 3 times daily in adults or 150–350 mg (3–7 drops or 0.15–0.35 mL) 3 times daily in children. Alternatively, if strong iodine solution (also known as Lugol's solution; commercially available but not FDA approved) is used, the recommended dosage in adults is 5–7 drops (0.25–0.35 mL) 3 times daily.

When oral potassium iodide is used in the management of severe, life-threatening thyrotoxicosis† (thyroid storm, thyrotoxicosis crisis), the drug is initiated 1 hour after the initial dose of other antithyroid agents (see Uses: Hyperthyroidism). If the potassium iodide oral solution containing 1 g/mL (also known as saturated solution of potassium iodide [SSKI®]) is used, the recommended adult dosage is 250 mg (5 drops or 0.25 mL) every 6 hours. For the treatment of thyrotoxicosis in children, some experts recommend that the oral solution containing 1 g/mL (also known as saturated solution of potassium iodide [SSKI®]) be administered in a dosage of 50–250 mg (1–5 drops or 0.05–0.25 mL) 3 times daily.

Radiation Emergency The dosage and duration of potassium iodide recommended during a radiation emergency and potential *internal* (inhalation or ingestion) exposure to radioiodines is based on predicted thyroid exposure, age and/or weight, and pregnancy and lactation status.

For use during a radiation emergency, potassium iodide is available as 65- or 130-mg tablets or as a solution containing 65 mg/mL. If necessary in an emergency situation for an infant, small child, or other individual who cannot swallow tablets, the manufacturers and FDA have provided instructions on how to prepare extemporaneous oral solutions (liquid mixtures) using potassium iodide tablets. (See Extemporaneous Oral Solutions under Dosage and Administration: Administration.)

For optimal protection against inhaled radioiodines, oral potassium iodide should be administered before or immediately coincident with passage of a radioactive cloud; potassium iodide may still have a substantial protective effect if administered 3–4 hours after exposure. The protective effect of potassium iodide persists for about 24 hours.

Potassium iodide should be administered once daily until a risk of substantial exposure to inhaled or ingested radioiodines no longer exists. However, to minimize the risk of hypothyroidism during a period of critical brain development, repeat administration of potassium iodide should be avoided in neonates 1 month of age or younger, unless other protective measures are not available. (See Cautions: Pediatric Precautions.) In addition, repeat administration of the drug should be avoided in pregnant and lactating women, unless other protective measures are not available. (See Cautions: Pregnancy and Lactation.)

Adult Dosage. The recommended adult dosage of oral potassium iodide for a radiation emergency is 130 mg once daily (one 130-mg tablet or two 65-mg tablets once daily). If the commercially available oral solution containing 65 mg/mL is used, adults should receive 130 mg once daily (2 mL once daily). Alternatively, if an extemporaneous oral solution containing 16.25 mg/5 mL (16.25 mg/teaspoon) is used, adults should receive a dosage of 130 mg once daily (40 mL or 8 teaspoons once daily).

During a radiation emergency, the FDA recommends use of potassium iodide in adults 19 through 40 years of age if predicted thyroid exposure is 10 centigrays (cGy) or more and in pregnant or lactating women if predicted thyroid exposure is 5 cGy or more. Because of the risk of hypothyroidism, the FDA recommends potassium iodide in adults older than 40 years of age only if predicted thyroid exposure is 500 cGy or more.

Pediatric Dosage. For a radiation emergency, adolescents older than 12 through 18 years of age should receive oral potassium iodide in a dosage of 130 mg once daily if they weigh 70 kg (150 lbs) or more or a dosage of 65 mg once daily if they weigh less than 70 kg (150 lbs). (See Table 1 and Table 2.) The FDA recommends use of potassium iodide in adolescents if predicted thyroid exposure is 5 cGy or more.

For a radiation emergency, neonates and children through 12 years of age should receive potassium iodide in a dosage based on age. (See Table 1 and Table 2.) The FDA recommends use of potassium iodide in neonates and children 12 years of age or younger if predicted thyroid exposure is 5 cGy or more.

Table 1. Recommended Pediatric Dosage of Potassium Iodide for Radiation Emergency (65- or 130-mg Tablets or Oral Solution Containing 65 mg/mL)

Age and Weight	Potassium Iodide Tablets (Iosat®, ThyroSafe®)	Potassium Iodide Oral Solution Containing 65 mg/mL (Thyroshield®)
Birth to 1 month	(See Table 2)	16.25 mg once daily (0.25 mL)
>1 month to 3 years	(See Table 2)	32.5 mg once daily (0.5 mL)
>3 through 12 years	65 mg once daily (one 65-mg tablet or ½ of 130-mg tablet)	65 mg once daily (1 mL)
>12 through 18 years weighing <70 kg (150 lbs)	65 mg once daily (one 65-mg tablet or ½ of 130-mg tablet)	65 mg once daily (1 mL)
>12 through 18 years weighing ≥70 kg (150 lbs)	130 mg once daily (two 65-mg tablets or one 130-mg tablet)	130 mg once daily (2 mL)

Table 2. Recommended Pediatric Dosage of Potassium Iodide for Radiation Emergency (Extemporaneous Oral Solutions)

Age and Weight	Extemporaneous Oral Solution Containing 8.125 mg/5 mL (8.125 mg/teaspoon)	Extemporaneous Oral Solution Containing 16.25 mg/5 mL (16.25 mg/teaspoon)
Birth to 1 month	16.25 mg once daily (10 mL or 2 teaspoons)	16.25 mg once daily (5 mL or 1 teaspoon)
>1 month to 3 years	32.5 mg once daily (20 mL or 4 teaspoons)	32.5 mg once daily (10 mL or 2 teaspoons)
>3 through 12 years	65 mg once daily (40 mL or 8 teaspoons)	65 mg once daily (20 mL or 4 teaspoons)
>12 through 18 years weighing <70 kg (150 lbs)	65 mg once daily (40 mL or 8 teaspoons)	65 mg once daily (20 mL or 4 teaspoons)
>12 through 18 years weighing ≥70 kg (150 lbs)	Use alternative preparation	130 mg once daily (40 mL or 8 teaspoons)

Sporotrichosis For the treatment of cutaneous or lymphocutaneous sporotrichosis† caused by *Sporothrix schenckii*, the Infectious Diseases Society of America (IDSA) and other clinicians state that the usual initial dosage of potassium iodide oral solution containing 1 g/mL (also known as saturated solution of potassium iodide [SSKI®]) in adults is 250 mg (5 drops or 0.25 mL) 3 times daily; dosage may then be increased gradually as tolerated to a maximum of 2–2.5 g (40–50 drops or 2–2.5 mL) 3 times daily. For the treatment of cutaneous or lymphocutaneous sporotrichosis in children, some experts recommend that the oral solution containing 1 g/mL (also known as saturated solution of potassium iodide [SSKI®]) be given in an initial dosage of 50 mg (1 drop or 0.05 mL) 3 times daily; dosage may then be increased gradually as tolerated. The IDSA states that the maximum pediatric dosage of the oral solution containing 1 g/mL is 1 drop/kg 3 times daily or 2–2.5 g (40–50 drops or 2–2.5 mL) 3 times daily, whichever is lowest.

The usual duration of oral potassium iodide therapy for the treatment of cutaneous or lymphocutaneous sporotrichosis† is 3–6 months. The IDSA recommends that potassium iodide be continued for 2–4 weeks after cutaneous lesions resolve; other experts recommend that the drug be continued for 4–6 weeks after cutaneous lesions resolve.

Cough If the potassium iodide oral solution containing 1 g/mL (also known as saturated solution of potassium iodide [SSKI®]) is used as an expectorant, the usual adult dosage is 300 or 600 mg (0.3 or 0.6 mL) 3 or 4 times daily.

Cautions

■ Adverse Effects Hypersensitivity reactions to iodides may occur and may be manifested by angioedema, cutaneous and mucosal hemorrhage, and signs and symptoms resembling serum sickness, such as fever, arthralgia, lymph node enlargement, and eosinophilia. Urticaria, thrombotic thrombocytopenic purpura, and fatal periarteritis have also been attributed to iodide hypersensitivity. Hypocomplementemic vasculitis in some patients with chronic urticaria or systemic lupus erythematosus has been associated with iodide sensitivity, and some clinicians caution that potassium iodide may precipitate severe systemic illness in such patients. Jodbasedow or iodine-induced thyrotoxicosis may occur with low doses of iodides (i.e., less than 25 mg of iodine daily); this effect is uncommon in the US but more frequent in areas with endemic iodine deficiency.

Manifestations of iodism (chronic iodine poisoning) may occur when potassium iodide is given in large doses or over extended periods of time. Iodism is usually manifested as a metallic taste, burning in the mouth and throat, soreness of the teeth and gums, increased salivation, coryza, sneezing, and irritation of the eyes with swelling of the eyelids. Severe headache, productive cough, pulmonary edema, dyspnea, bronchospasm, and swelling and tenderness of the parotid and submaxillary glands may occur. The throat, pharynx, larynx, and tonsils may become inflamed. Mild acneiform eruptions may occur, usually in seborrheic areas; rarely, severe and sometimes fatal eruptions (ioderma) may occur. Gastric irritation is common and diarrhea, sometimes bloody, may also occur. Signs and symptoms of iodism generally subside spontaneously within a few days of discontinuing the drug; symptomatic and supportive therapy, including abundant fluid and salt intake to help eliminate iodide, may be necessary.

Prolonged use of iodides or excessive doses may result in thyroid gland hyperplasia, thyroid adenoma, goiter, and severe hypothyroidism. Prolonged use of iodides may also induce hyperthyroidism, particularly in older individuals, patients with preexisting nontoxic nodular goiter, and patients residing in areas with endemic iodine deficiency.

■ Precautions and Contraindications Potassium iodide is contraindicated in individuals with known sensitivity to iodides or any ingredient in the formulation.

Potassium iodide also is contraindicated in patients with dermatitis herpetiformis, hypocomplementemic vasculitis, or nodular thyroid disease (e.g., multinodular goiter) *with* heart disease.

Since some individuals are markedly sensitive to iodides, initial potassium iodide doses should be administered with caution. Patients at risk for iodine-induced adverse effects (e.g., hyperthyroidism, thyrotoxicosis) include older patients and those with goiter or autoimmune thyroid disease. Potassium iodide, especially when indicated for more than a few days, should be used with caution in patients with multinodular goiter, Graves' disease, or autoimmune thyroiditis.

In the event of a radiation emergency, potassium iodide should be used with caution and as directed by public authorities. For radiation emergencies, potassium iodide may be used in patients with preexisting thyroid diseases if they do not have nodular thyroid conditions *with* heart disease; however, careful supervision by clinicians is recommended if therapy must be administered for more than a few days.

Vesication and desquamation may occur if strong iodine solution (also known as Lugol's solution; commercially available but not approved by the US Food and Drug Administration [FDA]) is allowed to pool in contact with skin. If accidental contact of strong iodine solution with skin or eyes occurs, the skin or eyes should be flushed with copious amounts of water for 15 minutes.

■ Pediatric Precautions Safety and efficacy of potassium iodide oral solution containing 1 g/mL (also known as saturated solution of potassium iodide [SSKI®]) have not been established in children. Potassium iodide oral solution containing 1 g/mL has been used for the treatment of cutaneous and lymphocutaneous sporotrichosis in children† and is recommended by the Infectious Disease Society of America (IDSA) as an alternative for the treatment of these infections in children. (See Uses: Sporotrichosis.)

Children are more susceptible to the dangerous effects of radioactive iodide than adults and the benefits of potassium iodide during a radiation emergency exceed the risks. However, to minimize the risk of hypothyroidism during a period of critical brain development, repeat administration of potassium iodide should be avoided in neonates 1 month of age or younger, unless other protective measures are not available. If potassium iodide is used in a neonate 1 month of age or younger, the neonate should be monitored for the potential development of hypothyroidism by measuring thyrotropin (thyroid-stimulating hormone, TSH) and, if indicated, free thyroxine (free T_4) and thyroid replacement therapy should be instituted if hypothyroidism occurs.

In a radiation emergency, children and neonates unable to tolerate potassium iodide and neonates in whom repeat administration of the drug is a concern should be given priority with regard to other protective measures (e.g., evacuation, sheltering, assurance of uncontaminated milk and food).

■ Pregnancy and Lactation ***Pregnancy*** Iodides readily cross the placenta and may result in abnormal thyroid function and/or goiter in the neonate. Fetal thyroid may be most susceptible to the effects of excess iodine at the end of gestation.

Some experts state that potassium iodide is contraindicated in pregnant women. The American Academy of Pediatrics (AAP) states that use of potassium iodide as an expectorant is contraindicated during pregnancy.

There is no evidence that short-term use (e.g., 10 days) of potassium iodide for preoperative management of hyperthyroidism in pregnant women with Graves' disease undergoing thyroidectomy† is harmful to the fetus. If thyroidectomy is necessary for the treatment of hyperthyroidism during pregnancy, the American Thyroid Association (ATA) and American Association of Clinical Endocrinologists (AACE) recommend that the surgery be performed during the second trimester.

The FDA recommends that pregnant women receive potassium iodide during a radiation emergency for their own protection and that of the fetus; however, repeat administration should be avoided during pregnancy, unless other protective measures are not available. When repeat administration is indicated in a pregnant woman, consultation with a clinician is recommended and thyroid function monitoring may be indicated in the neonate.

If potassium iodide is used during pregnancy or if the patient becomes pregnant while receiving the drug, the patient should be informed of the potential risks to the fetus.

Lactation Potassium iodide is distributed into milk and may cause rash and thyroid suppression in nursing infants.

The AAP considers potassium iodide to be compatible with breast-feeding. In a radiation emergency, the FDA recommends that lactating women receive potassium iodide for their own protection. However, repeat administration should be avoided in lactating women unless other protective measures are not available. If repeat administration is indicated in a nursing woman, consultation with a clinician is recommended; thyroid function monitoring may be indicated in a breast-fed neonate.

Because radioactive iodine is distributed into milk, some experts (including the AAP) recommend that lactating women temporarily *not* breast-feed after a radiation emergency, unless no alternative is available. Breast-feeding can then be resumed when public authorities declare it safe to do so. The fact that administration of potassium iodide to lactating women potentially can reduce the radioiodine content of milk should be considered.

Drug Interactions

Concomitant use of lithium salts and iodides may result in additive or synergistic hypothyroid effects. Hypothyroidism has been reported in several patients who received the drugs concomitantly. A lithium salt and potassium iodide generally should not be used concomitantly; if the drugs are used together, the patient should be monitored closely for signs and symptoms of hypothyroidism.

Concomitant use of antithyroid agents (e.g., methimazole) and potassium iodide may result in additive hypothyroid and goitrogenic effects.

Concomitant use of potassium iodide and potassium-containing drugs, potassium-sparing diuretics, or angiotensin-converting enzyme (ACE) inhibitors may be associated with hyperkalemia, which may result in cardiac arrhythmias or cardiac arrest.

Pharmacology

■ **Thyroid Hormone Synthesis and Regulation** Iodine is an essential component of thyroid hormones, tetraiodothyronine (thyroxine, T_4) and triiodothyronine (T_3), comprising 65 and 59% of the weights, respectively. Thyroxine and triiodothyronine are produced in the thyroid gland by the iodination and coupling of the amino acid tyrosine. (See Chemistry in the Thyroid Agents General Statement.) Thyroid hormones and thus iodine are essential for human life. The hormones regulate many key biochemical reactions, especially protein synthesis and enzymatic activity, and target the developing brain, muscle, heart, pituitary, and kidneys.

Iodine is ingested in a variety of chemical forms, but because its content in most food sources is low, iodine present in iodized salt or in processed foods from the addition of iodized salt or other additives (potassium iodate, calcium iodate, cuprous iodide) is its principal source in humans in developed countries. Iodine also is available in dietary supplements and from other sources (e.g., drugs such as thyroid agents [hormones] and amiodarone). Most ingested iodine is reduced in the GI tract and absorbed almost completely. Under normal conditions, the absorption of dietary iodine exceeds 90%. Once absorbed systemically, iodide is removed principally by the thyroid gland and kidneys. The thyroid gland selectively concentrates iodide in amounts required for adequate thyroid hormone synthesis, with most of the remaining iodide being excreted renally. Salivary glands, breast, choroid plexus, and gastric mucosa also can concentrate iodide; however, other than the lactating breast, these tissues are minor pathways of uncertain importance.

A sodium/iodide transporter in the thyroidal basal membrane is responsible for iodine concentration in the gland, transferring iodide from systemic circulation into the thyroid gland at a concentration gradient of 20–50 times that of plasma to ensure that the gland receives adequate amounts of iodine for hormone synthesis. During iodine deficiency, the thyroid gland concentrates most of the iodine available from plasma. Iodide participates in a complex series of reactions in the thyroid gland to produce thyroid hormones. Thyroglobulin is synthesized in thyroid cells and serves as an iodination vehicle. Thyroperoxidase and hydrogen peroxide promote the oxidation of iodide and its attachment to tyrosyl residues within the thyroglobulin molecule to produce the hormone precursors diiodotyrosine and monoiodotyrosine. Thyroperoxidase further catalyzes intramolecular coupling of 2 molecules of diiodotyrosine to produce T_4 and coupling of a molecule of diiodotyrosine and a molecule of monoiodotyrosine to produce T_3. The average adult thyroid gland in individuals residing in an iodine-sufficient geographic region contains about 15 mg of iodine. Iodine is not released into systemic circulation but instead is stored principally in diiodo and monoiodo tyrosine precursors, removed from the tyrosine moiety by a specific deiodinase, and then recycled within the thyroid gland as a mechanism of iodine conservation.

Once in systemic circulation, thyroxine and triiodothyronine attach to several binding proteins (e.g., thyronine-binding globulin, transthyretin, albumin), which then migrate to target tissues where thyroxine is deiodinated to triiodothyronine, the metabolically active form of thyroid hormone. The iodine that is removed from thyroxine returns to the serum iodine pool and follows the usual iodine cycle or is excreted renally. Thyrotropin (TSH) is the major thyroid function regulator. Thyrotropin affects several sites within thyrocytes, the principal actions of which are to increase thyroidal uptake of iodine and to break down thyroglobulin to release thyroid hormone into systemic circulation. An elevated serum thyrotropin concentration indicates primary hypothyroidism and a decreased serum concentration indicates hyperthyroidism.

The normal thyroid gland takes up the amount of systemically circulating iodine necessary to make the necessary amount of thyroid hormone for the body's needs. In iodine deficiency, the thyroid gland will concentrate more radioactive iodine, and the gland will concentrate less in iodine excess. However, other factors can influence radioactive iodine uptake, including thyroidal overproduction of hormone (hyperthyroidism), hypothyroidism, subacute thyroiditis, and many chemical and medicinal products. When iodine equilibrium is present, the mean daily thyroid iodine accumulation and release are similar.

■ **Effects in Hyperthyroidism** In patients with hyperthyroidism, iodide rapidly inhibits the release of thyroid hormones via a direct effect on the thyroid gland and inhibits the synthesis of thyroid hormones. Iodide apparently attenuates the effects of thyrotropin that are mediated via cAMP. The vascularity of the thyroid gland is reduced, the gland becomes much firmer, the cells become smaller, colloid reaccumulates in the follicles, and the quantity of bound iodine increases. The effects of potassium iodide on thyroid function are usually observed within 24 hours and are maximal after 10–15 days of continuous therapy; however, the drug does not completely control the manifestations of hyperthyroidism, and after a variable period of time the salutary effects subside.

■ **Effects in Radiation Emergencies** In the event of a radiation emergency, isotopes of iodine may be released into the environment. Radioactive iodine is taken up and stored in the thyroid gland in the same manner as stable iodine. (See Pharmacology: Thyroid Hormone Synthesis and Regulation.) The selective and rapid concentration and storage of radioactive iodine in the thyroid gland results in internal radiation exposure to the thyroid and increased risk of thyroid cancer and benign nodules and, at high doses, hypothyroidism. Administration of stable iodine (potassium iodide) before or promptly after intake of radioactive iodine blocks or reduces accumulation of radioactive iodine in the thyroid gland.

■ **Antifungal Effects** The mechanism of action of potassium iodide in the treatment of cutaneous or lymphocutaneous sporotrichosis† caused by *Sporothrix schenckii* has not been determined. In vitro, potassium iodide does not appear to increase monocyte or neutrophil killing of *S. schenckii*. However, exposure of the yeast form of *S. schenckii* to various concentrations of iodine (iodine and potassium iodide solution) in vitro has resulted in rapid cell destruction.

■ **Effects on Respiratory Tract Secretions** Potassium iodide is thought to act as an expectorant by increasing respiratory tract secretions and thereby decreasing the viscosity of mucus; however, this remains to be clearly established.

Chemistry and Stability

■ **Chemistry** Potassium iodide occurs as hexahedral crystals, either transparent and colorless or somewhat opaque and white, or as a white, granular powder. The drug is slightly hygroscopic. Potassium iodide is very soluble in water and soluble in alcohol. Each gram of potassium iodide contains about 6 mEq of potassium.

Potassium iodide is commercially available as tablets containing 65 or 130 mg of the drug and as an oral solution containing 65 mg/mL in a black raspberry-flavored solution. An aqueous oral solution of potassium iodide containing 1 g/mL also is commercially available; this preparation is known as saturated solution of potassium iodide (SSKI®).

Potassium iodide may be available as strong iodine solution (also known as Lugol's solution), a solution containing 50 mg of iodine and 100 mg of potassium iodide per mL. Strong iodine solutions may be commercially available for oral or topical administration, but these preparations are not approved by the US Food and Drug Administration (FDA).

■ **Stability** Potassium iodide tablets should be stored at 20–25°C in their original foil pack and protected from moisture.

Potassium iodide oral solution containing 65 mg/mL should be stored at 25°C, but may be exposed to 15–30°C; the solution should be stored in a tight container and protected from light.

Potassium iodide oral solution containing 1 g/mL (also known as saturated solution of potassium iodide [SSKI®]) should be stored at 15–30°C in a tight container and protected from light. The oral solution may crystallize if exposed to cold temperatures; however, crystals will dissolve if the solution is warmed and shaken. The solution should be discarded if it turns brownish-yellow in color.

Oral solutions of potassium iodide prepared extemporaneously using 65- or 130-mg tablets (see Extemporaneous Oral Solutions under Dosage and Administration: Administration) should be stored in the refrigerator and any unused solution discarded after 7 days.

Preparations

Excipients in commercially available drug preparations may have clinically important effects in some individuals; consult specific product labeling for details.

Potassium Iodide

Oral		
Solution	65 mg/mL	**ThyroShield®**, Fleming
	1 g/mL	**SSKI®**, Upsher-Smith
Tablets	65 mg	**Iosat®** (scored), Anbex
		ThyroSafe® (scored), Recipharm
	130 mg	**Iosat®** (scored), Anbex

Strong Iodine Solution

Oral		
Solution	Iodine 50 mg/mL and Potassium Iodide 100 mg/mL	**Strong Iodine Solution** **Lugol's Solution**

†Use is not currently included in the labeling approved by the US Food and Drug Administration

Propylthiouracil

PTU

■ Propylthiouracil is a thiourea-derivative antithyroid agent.

Uses

■ **Hyperthyroidism** Propylthiouracil is used in patients with Graves' disease with hyperthyroidism or toxic multinodular goiter who are intolerant of methimazole and for whom surgery or radioactive iodine therapy is not an appropriate treatment option. The drug also is used to ameliorate symptoms of hyperthyroidism in preparation for thyroidectomy or radioactive iodine therapy in patients who are intolerant of methimazole.

Because use of propylthiouracil is associated with a higher risk of clinically serious or fatal liver injury in adult and pediatric patients compared with methimazole, propylthiouracil should be reserved for patients who cannot tolerate methimazole and for whom radioactive iodine therapy or surgery are not appropriate for the management of hyperthyroidism. (See Cautions: Hepatic Effects and also see Cautions: Precautions and Contraindications.) Propylthiouracil is not recommended for use in pediatric patients except in rare instances in which methimazole is not well tolerated and surgery or radioactive iodine therapy are not appropriate therapies. (See Cautions: Hepatic Effects and also see Cautions: Pediatric Precautions.)

Because of the risk of fetal abnormalities associated with methimazole, propylthiouracil is the preferred agent when an antithyroid drug is indicated during or just prior to the first trimester of pregnancy (during organogenesis). However, it may be preferable to switch from propylthiouracil to methimazole for the second and third trimesters (i.e., after the first trimester) because of the risk of maternal adverse effects associated with propylthiouracil (e.g., hepatotoxicity). (See Pregnancy under Cautions: Pregnancy and Lactation.)

Thioamide antithyroid agents (e.g., propylthiouracil, methimazole) are used to control the symptoms of hyperthyroidism associated with Graves' disease and maintain the patient in a euthyroid state for a period of several years (generally 1–2 years) until a spontaneous remission occurs. Thioamide antithyroid agents do not affect the underlying cause of hyperthyroidism. Spontaneous remission does not occur in all patients receiving therapy with thioamide antithyroid agents, and most patients eventually require ablative therapy (i.e., surgery, radioactive iodine). The minimum duration of thioamide therapy necessary before assessing whether spontaneous remission has occurred is not clearly established. However, some clinicians suggest that the optimum duration of antithyroid drug therapy in patients with Graves' disease generally is 12–18 months.

Propylthiouracil returns the hyperthyroid patient to a normal metabolic state prior to thyroidectomy and controls the thyrotoxic crisis that may accompany thyroidectomy. (See Thyrotoxic Crisis under Uses: Hyperthyroidism.)

Propylthiouracil also controls symptoms of hyperthyroidism prior to and after administration of radioactive iodine until the ablative effects of the iodine occur. However, the beneficial and detrimental effects and optimal sequencing of antithyroid drugs before or after radioactive iodine therapy have not been clearly established. In addition, pretreatment with propylthiouracil may increase the radioresistance of the thyroid and the risk of radioactive iodine treatment failure.

Antithyroid agents do not induce remission in patients with nodular thyroid disease (i.e., toxic adenoma†, toxic multinodular goiter), and discontinuance of therapy results in relapse. Therefore, some clinicians suggest that adults with overt toxic adenoma or toxic multinodular goiter be treated with either radioactive iodine therapy or thyroidectomy.

Thyrotoxic Crisis In the management of thyrotoxic crisis, thioamide antithyroid agents are used to inhibit thyroid hormone synthesis. Because propylthiouracil also blocks the peripheral conversion of thyroxine to triiodothyronine, it theoretically may be more useful than methimazole or carbimazole (not commercially available in the US) in the management of thyrotoxic crisis. Iodides (e.g., potassium iodide, strong iodine solution) are given to inhibit the release of thyroid hormone from the gland but may subsequently be used as a substrate for thyroid hormone synthesis; therefore, treatment with a thioamide antithyroid agent is usually initiated before iodide therapy. A β-adrenergic blocking agent (e.g., propranolol) is also usually given concomitantly to manage peripheral signs and symptoms of hyperthyroidism, particularly cardiovascular effects (e.g., tachycardia).

■ **Alcoholic Liver Disease** Propylthiouracil has been studied in patients with alcoholic liver disease†. However, analysis of data from 6 randomized clinical trials with propylthiouracil found that no substantial benefit has been demonstrated on any clinically important outcomes of alcoholic liver disease (e.g., all-cause mortality, liver-related mortality, complications associated with the liver disease, liver histology) and that the currently available evidence does not support its use outside of randomized clinical studies. Additional research (e.g., large clinical trials with adequate methodology, several years of treatment, independent and close monitoring of efficacy and safety) is needed to determine the safety and efficacy of propylthiouracil in patients with alcoholic liver disease.

Dosage and Administration

■ **Administration** Propylthiouracil is administered orally; daily dosage is usually given in 3 equally divided doses at approximately 8-hour intervals. In some cases, more frequent administration (e.g., at 4- or 6-hour intervals) may be necessary.

■ **Dosage** ***Adult Dosage*** For the treatment of hyperthyroidism, the manufacturer states that the usual initial adult dosage of propylthiouracil is 300 mg daily, usually given in 3 equally divided doses at approximately 8-hour intervals. The manufacturer also states that in patients with severe hyperthyroidism and/or very large goiters, the initial dosage may be increased to 400 mg daily; however, initial dosages of 600–900 mg daily occasionally may be required. Alternatively, for the treatment of Graves' disease, some clinicians recommend an initial adult dosage of 50–150 mg 3 times daily, depending on the severity of the hyperthyroidism. In general, most patients improve considerably or achieve normal thyroid function following 4–12 weeks of therapy, after which dosage may be decreased while maintaining normal thyroid function. Subsequent dosage should be carefully adjusted according to the patient's tolerance and therapeutic response. The manufacturer states that the usual adult maintenance dosage is 100–150 mg daily, given in 3 equally divided doses at approximately 8-hour intervals. Alternatively, as the clinical findings and thyroid function tests return to normal, some clinicians state that reducing the maintenance dosage to 50 mg 2 or 3 times daily is usually possible for treatment of Graves' disease. (See Cautions: Precautions and Contraindications and also see Cautions: Adverse Effects.) The optimum duration of antithyroid therapy remains to be clearly established. However, some clinicians suggest that the optimum duration of antithyroid drug therapy in patients with Graves' disease generally is 12–18 months.

If propylthiouracil is used during pregnancy for the management of hyperthyroidism, the manufacturer states that a sufficient, but not excessive, dosage of propylthiouracil is necessary. The manufacturer states that because thyroid dysfunction diminishes in many women as pregnancy proceeds, a reduction in dosage may be possible, and, in some patients, propylthiouracil can be discontinued several weeks or months before delivery. (See Pregnancy under Cautions: Pregnancy and Lactation.)

Dosage of propylthiouracil should be selected with caution in geriatric patients because of the greater frequency of decreased hepatic, renal, and/or cardiac function and of concomitant disease and drug therapy. (See Cautions: Geriatric Precautions.)

For the treatment of thyrotoxic crisis (i.e., thyroid storm) in adults, some clinicians recommend a propylthiouracil loading dose of 500 mg to 1 g, followed by 250 mg every 4 hours.

If propylthiouracil is used prior to thyroidectomy to render adults euthyroid, propylthiouracil should be discontinued at the time of the procedure.

If propylthiouracil is used as pretreatment prior to radioactive iodine therapy in adults, some clinicians recommend that propylthiouracil be discontinued 2–7 days before administration of radioactive iodine, restarted 3–7 days after radioactive iodine, and discontinued once thyroid function has normalized.

Pediatric Dosage Propylthiouracil generally is not recommended for use in pediatric patients except in rare instances in which alternative therapies are not appropriate options. The manufacturer states that studies evaluating appropriate dosage regimens have not been conducted in the pediatric population, although general practice would suggest initiation of therapy in children 6 years of age or older at a dosage of 50 mg daily with careful upward titration based on clinical response and evaluation of thyrotropin (thyroid stimulating hormone, TSH) and free thyroxine (T_4) concentrations. Although cases of severe liver injury have been reported with dosages as low as 50 mg daily, most cases were associated with dosages of 300 mg daily and higher. (See Cautions: Pediatric Precautions and also see Cautions: Hepatic Effects.)

Cautions

■ **Adverse Effects** Minor adverse effects of propylthiouracil include rash, urticaria, pruritus, abnormal hair loss, skin pigmentation, edema, nausea, vomiting, epigastric distress, loss of taste, taste perversion, arthralgia, myalgia, paresthesia, and headache. Drowsiness, neuritis, vertigo, sialadenopathy, lymphadenopathy, and jaundice also have occurred in patients receiving the drug. (See Cautions: Hepatic Effects.)

Although reported much less frequently, severe adverse effects of propylthiouracil include liver injury (resulting in hepatitis, liver failure, a need for liver transplantation, or death [see Cautions: Hepatic Effects]); inhibition of myelopoiesis with resultant agranulocytosis (see Cautions: Agranulocytosis), granulocytopenia, and thrombocytopenia; aplastic anemia; drug fever; lupus-like syndrome (including splenomegaly and vasculitis); hepatitis; periarteritis; and hypoprothrombinemia and bleeding. Nephritis, glomerulonephritis, interstitial pneumonitis, exfoliative dermatitis, and erythema nodosum also have been reported.

A vasculitic syndrome associated with the presence of antineutrophil cytoplasmic antibodies (ANCA) has been reported. Manifestations of ANCA-positive vasculitis may include rapidly progressive glomerulonephritis (crescentic and pauci-immune necrotizing glomerulonephritis), sometimes resulting in acute renal failure; pulmonary infiltrates or alveolar hemorrhage; skin ulcers; and leukocytoclastic vasculitis. Cutaneous vasculitis, which may manifest as purpuric and/or bullous hemorrhagic lesions or erythema nodosum, and possibly may progress to necrotic ulcerations, and polymyositis also have occurred.

■ **Hepatic Effects** Liver injury (including severe liver injury) resulting in hepatitis, liver failure (including acute liver failure), liver transplantation, or death has been reported with propylthiouracil therapy in adult and pediatric patients. An analysis of adverse event reports received by the US Food and Drug Administration (FDA) found that, while severe propylthiouracil-associated hepatotoxicity has been reported among patients in all age groups, the reports and signals of hepatotoxicity were highest among those younger than 17 years of age. No cases of liver failure have been reported with the use of methimazole, another antithyroid drug, in pediatric patients. For this reason, propylthiouracil is not recommended for use in pediatric patients except in rare instances in which methimazole is not well tolerated and surgery or radioactive iodine therapy are not appropriate therapies. (See Cautions: Pediatric Precautions.)

Cases of liver injury, including liver failure and death, have been reported in women receiving propylthiouracil during pregnancy. Two cases of in utero exposure to the drug with liver failure and death of a newborn have been reported. The use of an alternative antithyroid drug (e.g., methimazole) may be advisable after the first trimester of pregnancy. (See Pregnancy under Cautions: Pregnancy and Lactation.)

The extent of propylthiouracil-induced hepatitis and the true incidence of severe liver injury in patients receiving propylthiouracil is not known. The total annual number of cases of propylthiouracil-induced hepatitis in the United States has been estimated to be approximately 40–50 (31 adults, 4–8 pregnant women, 4 children) based on a 0.1% incidence of severe hepatitis; the total number of annual cases could range from 20–100 depending on the frequency of propylthiouracil-induced hepatitis and the prevalence of propylthiouracil use. In addition, propylthiouracil-induced acute liver failure has been estimated to occur in approximately 0.01% of adults and 0.025–0.05% of children receiving the drug. Between 1969 and June 2009, a total of 34 cases (23 adult and 11 pediatric) of serious liver injury associated with propylthiouracil use was reported to the FDA Adverse Event Reporting System (AERS). Among the 23 adult cases, 13 resulted in death and 5 resulted in liver transplantation; among the 11 pediatric cases, 2 resulted in death and 7 resulted in liver transplantation (one patient died while awaiting transplantation). In contrast, 5 AERS cases of serious liver injury were identified for methimazole; all cases were in adults and 3 resulted in death. Based on these results and a review of the medical literature, FDA has concluded that use of propylthiouracil is associated with a higher risk for clinically serious or fatal liver injury compared with methimazole in both adult and pediatric patients. According to the United Network for Organ Sharing (UNOS) and the Organ Procurement and Transplantation Network (OPTN), liver transplantation was performed in 16 adults and 7 children between 1990 and 2007 as a result of propylthiouracil-induced liver failure; no liver transplantation attributed to methimazole toxicity occurred during this same time period.

Propylthiouracil-induced liver failure may occur at any time during therapy with a sudden onset, rapid progression, and a low chance of reversibility. According to data from the AERS database, liver failure occurred after 6–450 days of propylthiouracil therapy (median: 120 days). Although the effect of dosage on the risk of hepatotoxicity has not been clearly elucidated, the reported average daily dosage of propylthiouracil associated with liver failure in the AERS database was approximately 300 mg in both children and adults. Biochemical monitoring of liver function (bilirubin, alkaline phosphatase) and hepatocellular integrity (ALT, AST) is not expected to attenuate the risk of severe liver injury due to its rapid and unpredictable onset. (See Cautions: Precautions and Contraindications.)

■ **Agranulocytosis** Agranulocytosis occurs in approximately 0.2–0.5% of patients receiving propylthiouracil and is a potentially life-threatening adverse effect of the drug. Agranulocytosis typically occurs within the first 3 months of therapy, but rarely may occur after 4 months of therapy. Agranulocytosis may occur irrespective of dosage, length of treatment, or previous exposure to the antithyroid drug, and may occur more frequently in geriatric patients. Although the mechanism(s) of propylthiouracil-induced agranulocytosis has not been determined, antigranulocyte antibodies have been reported in some patients with thioamide-induced agranulocytosis; a direct toxic effect of these drugs on bone marrow has not been excluded as an additional possible cause.

■ **Hypothyroidism** Propylthiouracil may cause hypothyroidism necessitating routine monitoring of thyrotropin (thyroid stimulating hormone, TSH) and free thyroxine (T_4) concentrations; dosage should be adjusted to maintain a euthyroid state. (See Cautions: Precautions and Contraindications.) Because propylthiouracil readily crosses the placenta, the drug can cause fetal goiter and cretinism when administered to a pregnant woman. (See Pregnancy under Cautions: Pregnancy and Lactation.)

■ **Precautions and Contraindications** Some clinicians suggest that liver function tests, including alkaline phosphatase, aminotransferase, and bilirubin, be performed prior to initiating antithyroid drug therapy in patients with Graves' disease. Patients receiving propylthiouracil should be closely monitored for signs and symptoms of liver injury, particularly during the first 6 months following initiation of therapy. (See Cautions: Hepatic Effects.) Routine biochemical monitoring of liver function (bilirubin, alkaline phosphatase) and hepatocellular integrity (ALT, AST) may not be effective in identifying patients at risk of developing propylthiouracil-induced liver failure and is not expected to attenuate the risk of severe liver injury because of its rapid and unpredictable onset; however, such tests should be performed in symptomatic patients. Patients should be informed of the risk of liver failure associated with propylthiouracil and advised to immediately discontinue the drug and promptly contact their clinician if signs and symptoms of liver injury or hepatic dysfunction (e.g., fatigue, weakness, vague abdominal pain, right upper quadrant pain, anorexia, pruritus, easy bruising, jaundice, pruritic rash, light-colored stool, dark urine, joint pain, bloating, nausea) occur, particularly in the first 6 months of therapy. Propylthiouracil should be discontinued immediately if a patient develops these symptoms, and the patient should be promptly evaluated for evidence of liver injury, including evaluation of liver function (bilirubin, alkaline phosphatase) and hepatocellular integrity (ALT, AST), and should be provided supportive care. Some clinicians state that propylthiouracil should be discontinued if aminotransferase concentrations (whether elevated at initiation of therapy, found incidentally, or measured as clinically indicated) increase to 2–3 times the upper limit of normal and fail to improve within 1 week with repeat testing. Following discontinuance of the drug, liver function (i.e., alkaline phosphatase, bilirubin, transaminases) should be monitored weekly until there is evidence of resolution. If resolution is not evident, prompt referral to a gastroenterologist or hepatologist is warranted.

Some clinicians suggest that a baseline complete blood count, including white count with differential, should be performed prior to initiating antithyroid drug therapy in patients with Graves' disease. Patients receiving propylthiouracil should be closely monitored and should be instructed to contact their clinician immediately if signs or symptoms of illness, particularly sore throat, skin eruptions, fever, chills, headache, or general malaise, occur; it is particularly important to carefully monitor for these signs and symptoms during the early stages of propylthiouracil therapy since propylthiouracil-induced agranulocytosis usually occurs during the first several months of therapy. Leukopenia, thrombocytopenia, and/or aplastic anemia (pancytopenia) also may occur. Leukocyte and differential counts should be performed in patients who develop fever or sore throat or other signs or symptoms of illness while receiving the drug. Leukopenia (i.e., leukocyte count less than 4000/mm^3) occurs in 10% of untreated hyperthyroid patients and often is associated with relative granulocytopenia; this should be considered when evaluating the patient's myelopoietic response to the drug. Propylthiouracil should be used with extreme caution in patients receiving concomitant drugs known to be associated with agranulocytosis. The manufacturer states that propylthiouracil should be discontinued if agranulocytosis, aplastic anemia (pancytopenia), ANCA-positive vasculitis, hepatitis, interstitial pneumonitis, fever, or exfoliative dermatitis is suspected, and the patient's bone marrow indices should be obtained. Some clinicians state that patients should be informed of the adverse effects associated with propylthiouracil (e.g., agranulocytosis) and advised to immediately discontinue the drug and promptly contact their clinician if fever or pharyngitis occurs. In a patient who develops agranulocytosis or other serious adverse effects while receiving either methimazole or propylthiouracil, some clinicians state that use of the other drug also is contraindicated because of the risk of cross-sensitivity between the two drugs.

Because propylthiouracil may cause hypoprothrombinemia and bleeding, monitoring of prothrombin time should be considered during therapy with the drug, particularly prior to surgery (see Drug Interactions: Anticoagulants).

Thyroid function should be monitored periodically in patients receiving propylthiouracil. In patients with Graves' disease, some clinicians state that thyroid function (e.g., serum free T_4, serum free or total triiodothyronine [T_3], TSH) should be monitored before initiating therapy and then every 4–8 weeks thereafter (with subsequent dosage adjustments as needed) until thyroid function is stable or the patient is euthyroid; once the patient is euthyroid, thyroid function may be monitored every 2–3 months. Early in the course of antithyroid therapy, serum TSH concentration is not a reliable parameter to monitor because it may remain suppressed for several months after initiation of therapy despite normalization of free T_4 concentrations. The finding of a suppressed TSH concentration during this period, therefore, does not indicate a need for a dosage increase. However, once clinical evidence of resolution of hyperthyroidism occurs, the finding of an elevated serum TSH concentration indicates that a lower maintenance dosage of propylthiouracil should be employed. Monitoring serum T_3 concentrations may sometimes be useful for dosage adjustment; in patients in whom total or free T_3 concentrations remain elevated despite low, normal, or reduced free T_4 concentrations, an increase in antithyroid dosage may be necessary.

Patients should inform clinicians of existing or contemplated concomitant therapy, including prescription and OTC drugs, as well as any concomitant illnesses. Patients also should be advised not to discontinue propylthiouracil therapy unless instructed to do so by their clinician.

Propylthiouracil is contraindicated in patients who are hypersensitive to the drug or any ingredient in the formulation. Cross-sensitivity between thioamides may occur (i.e., in approximately 50% of patients switched from one thioamide agent to the other). In patients who develop agranulocytosis or other serious adverse effects while receiving either propylthiouracil or methimazole, some clinicians state that use of the other drug also is contraindicated because of the risk of cross-sensitivity between the two drugs. In patients experiencing serious allergic reactions to propylthiouracil, some clinicians state that using the alternative antithyroid drug (i.e., methimazole) is not recommended.

■ **Pediatric Precautions** During postmarketing experience, cases of severe liver injury, including hepatic failure requiring liver transplantation or resulting in death, have been reported in pediatric patients receiving propylthiouracil; however, no such cases have been reported in pediatric patients treated with methimazole. Therefore, propylthiouracil is not recommended for use in pediatric patients except in rare instances in which methimazole is not well tolerated and surgery or radioactive iodine therapy are not appropriate therapies. In addition, some experts state that alternative therapy should be considered for children who are currently receiving propylthiouracil and that it is reasonable and prudent to discontinue propylthiouracil use in children receiving this drug for the treatment of Graves' disease. When propylthiouracil is used in children, parents and patients should be informed of the risk of liver failure. If patients receiving propylthiouracil develop tiredness, nausea, anorexia, fever, pharyngitis, or malaise, propylthiouracil should be discontinued immediately, a clinician should be contacted, and a leukocyte count, liver function tests, and transaminase concentrations obtained. (See Cautions: Hepatic Effects and also see Cautions: Precautions and Contraindications.)

■ **Geriatric Precautions** Clinical studies of propylthiouracil did not include sufficient numbers of patients 65 years of age and older to determine whether geriatric patients respond differently than younger patients. Other reported clinical experience has not identified differences in responses between geriatric and younger patients. Dosage of propylthiouracil generally should be selected with caution in geriatric patients because of the greater frequency of decreased hepatic, renal, and/or cardiac function and of concomitant disease and drug therapy.

■ **Pregnancy and Lactation** ***Pregnancy*** Propylthiouracil crosses the placenta and may cause fetal harm when administered to pregnant women; the drug can induce goiter and hypothyroidism (cretinism) in the developing fetus. In April 2010, FDA reported a review of postmarketing data analyzing the potential for birth defects associated with use of propylthiouracil or methimazole during pregnancy. FDA found that congenital malformations were reported approximately 3 times more often with prenatal exposure to methimazole compared with propylthiouracil (29 cases with methimazole; 9 cases with propylthiouracil). In addition, there was a distinct and consistent pattern of congenital malformations associated with the use of methimazole that was not found with propylthiouracil. Approximately 90% of the congenital malformations with methimazole were craniofacial malformations (e.g., scalp epidermal aplasia [aplasia cutis], facial dysmorphism, choanal atresia). In most of the cases, there were multiple malformations that frequently included a combination of craniofacial defects and GI atresia or aplasia. These specific birth defects were associated with the use of methimazole during the first trimester of pregnancy but were not found when the drug was administered later in pregnancy. In contrast, FDA did not find a consistent pattern of birth defects associated with the use of propylthiouracil and concluded that there is no convincing evidence of an association between propylthiouracil use and congenital malformations, even with use during the first trimester.

Despite the potential fetal hazard, antithyroid agents are still considered the therapy of choice for the management of hyperthyroidism during pregnancy. Since methimazole may be associated with the rare development of fetal abnormalities, such as aplasia cutis and choanal atresia, propylthiouracil is the preferred agent when an antithyroid drug is indicated during organogenesis in the first trimester of pregnancy or just prior to the first trimester of pregnancy. Patients receiving methimazole should be switched to propylthiouracil if pregnancy is confirmed in the first trimester. Because of the potential adverse maternal effects of propylthiouracil (e.g., hepatotoxicity), however, it may be preferable to switch from propylthiouracil to methimazole for the second and third trimesters (i.e., after the first trimester). If the patient is switching from propylthiouracil to methimazole, thyroid function should be assessed after 2 weeks and then every 2–4 weeks thereafter. It is not known if the risk of methimazole-induced aplasia cutis or embryopathy outweighs the risk of propylthiouracil-induced hepatotoxicity.

If propylthiouracil is used during pregnancy for the management of hyperthyroidism, the manufacturer states that a sufficient, but not excessive, dosage of propylthiouracil is necessary. Some clinicians state that antithyroid drug therapy should be initiated or adjusted to maintain maternal free thyroxine (T_4) concentrations at or just above the upper limit of normal (ULN) of the nonpregnant reference range, or to maintain total T_4 concentrations at 1.5 times the ULN or the free T_4 index in the ULN, while using the lowest possible dosage of antithyroid drugs. In women receiving antithyroid drugs during pregnancy, free T_4 and TSH concentrations should be monitored approximately every 2–6 weeks. The manufacturer states that because thyroid dysfunction diminishes in many women as pregnancy proceeds, a reduction in dosage may be possible, and, in some patients, propylthiouracil can be discontinued several weeks or months before delivery.

Patients should be advised to contact their clinician immediately about their therapy if they are or plan to become pregnant while receiving an antithyroid drug. If propylthiouracil is used during pregnancy or if the patient becomes pregnant while receiving the drug, the patient should be advised of the rare potential hazard of liver damage in the mother and fetus; in addition, when considering antithyroid drug use during pregnancy, the patient should be informed of this potential risk, as well as the risks of methimazole-associated fetal malformations. Although liver toxicity may appear abruptly, some clinicians state that it is reasonable to monitor liver function every 3–4 weeks in pregnant women receiving propylthiouracil and to encourage patients to promptly report any new symptoms. (See Cautions: Hepatic Effects and also see Cautions: Precautions and Contraindications.)

Lactation The manufacturer and some clinicians state that propylthiouracil is distributed into milk to a small extent and, therefore, is unlikely to result in clinically important doses in the nursing infant. In one study in 9 lactating women who received a single 400-mg dose of propylthiouracil orally, the mean amount of propylthiouracil distributed into milk during 4 hours following drug administration was 0.025% (range: 0.007–0.077%) of the administered dose.

Propylthiouracil generally is compatible with breast-feeding, and moderate dosages of the drug (i.e., less than 300 mg daily) appear to be safe during breast-feeding. However, some clinicians consider propylthiouracil to be a second-line agent in nursing women because of concerns regarding severe hepatotoxicity (i.e., hepatic necrosis in either woman or child) following maternal use of the drug; these clinicians state that methimazole is the preferred antithyroid drug in nursing women. If an antithyroid drug is used in nursing women, some clinicians recommend that the drug be administered *after* a feeding and in divided doses, and that thyroid function be monitored in nursing infants.

Drug Interactions

■ **Drugs Known to be Associated with Agranulocytosis** Propylthiouracil should be used with extreme caution in patients receiving concomitant treatment with drugs known to be associated with agranulocytosis. (See Cautions: Agranulocytosis and also see Cautions: Precautions and Contraindications.)

■ **Anticoagulants** Because of the potential inhibition of vitamin K activity by propylthiouracil, the activity of oral anticoagulants (e.g., warfarin) may be increased. However, propylthiouracil also may decrease the anticoagulant effect of warfarin. Additional monitoring of prothrombin time (PT)/international normalized ratio (INR) should be considered, particularly prior to surgery. Adjustment of warfarin dosage may be necessary.

■ **β-Adrenergic Blocking Agents** Hyperthyroidism may cause an increased clearance of β-adrenergic blocking agents with a high extraction ratio. Dosage reduction of the β-adrenergic blocking agent may be needed when a hyperthyroid patient becomes euthyroid.

■ **Digitalis Glycosides** Serum digitalis concentrations may be increased when hyperthyroid patients receiving a stable digitalis glycoside regimen become euthyroid; dosage reduction of the digitalis glycoside may be needed.

■ **Theophylline** Theophylline clearance may decrease when hyperthyroid patients receiving a stable theophylline regimen become euthyroid; dosage reduction of theophylline may be needed.

Acute Toxicity

■ **Manifestations** In general, overdosage of propylthiouracil may be expected to produce effects that are extensions of common adverse reactions. Nausea, vomiting, epigastric distress, headache, fever, arthralgia, pruritus, edema, and pancytopenia have been reported. Agranulocytosis is the most serious adverse effect associated with propylthiouracil overdosage. Exfoliative dermatitis, hepatitis, neuropathies, or CNS stimulation or depression may occur rarely.

■ **Treatment** Treatment of propylthiouracil overdosage generally involves appropriate supportive care as dictated by the patient's medical status. Clinicians should consider consulting a poison control center for the most current information on the management of propylthiouracil overdosage.

Pharmacology

Propylthiouracil inhibits the synthesis of thyroid hormones by interfering with the incorporation of iodine into tyrosyl residues of thyroglobulin; the drug also inhibits the coupling of these iodotyrosyl residues to form iodothyronine. Although the exact mechanism(s) has not been fully elucidated, propylthiouracil may interfere with the oxidation of iodide ion and iodotyrosyl groups. Based on limited evidence it appears that the coupling reaction is more sensitive to antithyroid agents than the iodination reaction. Propylthiouracil does not inhibit the action of thyroid hormones already formed and present in the thyroid gland or circulation nor does the drug interfere with the effectiveness of exogenously administered thyroid hormones. Patients whose thyroid gland contains relatively high concentration of iodine (e.g., from prior ingestion or from administration during diagnostic radiologic procedures) may respond relatively slowly to antithyroid agents. Unlike methimazole, propylthiouracil inhibits the peripheral deiodination of thyroxine to triiodothyronine. Although the importance of this inhibition has not been established, propylthiouracil has a theoretical advantage compared with methimazole or carbimazole in patients with thyrotoxic crisis, since a decreased rate of conversion of circulating thyroxine to triiodothyronine may be clinically beneficial in these patients.

Pharmacokinetics

■ **Absorption** Propylthiouracil is rapidly and readily absorbed from the GI tract following oral administration with peak plasma concentrations of about

6–9 mcg/mL occurring within 1–1.5 hours after a single dose of 200–400 mg. In one study in which the drug was administered orally and IV, about 75% of the oral dose was absorbed. Plasma concentrations of the drug do not appear to correlate with the therapeutic effects.

■ **Distribution** Although distribution of propylthiouracil into human body tissues and fluids has not been fully characterized, the drug appears to be concentrated in the thyroid gland. Propylthiouracil readily crosses the placenta. The manufacturer states that propylthiouracil is distributed into milk to a small extent; one study indicated that the extent of distribution is about 0.007–0.077% of a single dose. (See Cautions: Pregnancy and Lactation.)

■ **Elimination** The elimination half-life of propylthiouracil has generally been reported to be about 1–2 hours.

Although the exact metabolic fate of propylthiouracil has not been fully established, the drug is extensively metabolized to its glucuronide conjugate and other minor metabolites. The drug and its metabolites are excreted in urine, with about 35% of a dose excreted within 24 hours.

Chemistry and Stability

■ **Chemistry** Propylthiouracil is a thiourea-derivative antithyroid agent. The drug differs chemically and structurally from methimazole in that propylthiouracil has a 6-membered ring instead of a 5-membered ring. Although presence of a thioamide group appears to be sufficient for antithyroid activity, propylthiouracil, like methimazole and carbimazole, contains the thioureylene moiety.

Propylthiouracil is a white, crystalline substance with a bitter taste. The drug is very slightly soluble in water.

■ **Stability** Commercially available propylthiouracil tablets should be stored in well-closed containers at 25°C but may be exposed to temperatures ranging from 15–30°C.

Preparations

Excipients in commercially available drug preparations may have clinically important effects in some individuals; consult specific product labeling for details.

Propylthiouracil

Oral

Tablets	50 mg*	**Propylthiouracil Tablets**

*available from one or more manufacturer, distributor, and/or repackager by generic (nonproprietary) name

†Use is not currently included in the labeling approved by the US Food and Drug Administration

LEPTINS 68:40

Metreleptin

■ Metreleptin is a recombinant analog of human leptin.

REMS

FDA approved a REMS for metreleptin to ensure that the benefits outweigh the risks. The REMS may apply to one or more preparations of metreleptin and consists of the following: communication plan, elements to assure safe use and implementation system. See the FDA REMS page (https://www.accessdata.fda.gov/scripts/cder/rems/index.cfm).

Uses

■ **Generalized Lipodystrophy** Metreleptin is used as replacement therapy as an adjunct to diet to treat the complications of leptin deficiency in patients with congenital or acquired generalized lipodystrophy. Metreleptin has been designated an orphan drug by FDA for treatment of metabolic disorders secondary to lipodystrophy.

Lipodystrophy, also called lipoatrophy, is a heterogeneous group of rare disorders characterized by loss of adipose tissue. Lipodystrophies can be classified as congenital or acquired and by the extent of adipose tissue loss (i.e., generalized or partial). Congenital lipodystrophies may be apparent at birth and have been linked to several genetic mutations, although not all are known. Acquired lipodystrophies may occur in childhood or adulthood and have been associated with autoimmune disorders or may occur following acute viral illness. Generalized lipodystrophy, whether congenital or acquired, is characterized by adipocyte loss from nearly the entire body, with increased circulating triglycerides and accumulation of fat in non-adipose tissues such as muscle and liver. Loss of adipose tissue results in deficiency of leptin, a hormone secreted by adipocytes that plays a crucial role in energy homeostasis, appetite and satiety, and metabolic regulation. Leptin deficiency leads to metabolic abnormalities such as insulin resistance, diabetes mellitus, steatosis, and hypertriglyceridemia. In addition, leptin deficiency results in increased appetite and hyperphagia; excessive caloric intake exacerbates metabolic abnormalities. Complications of generalized lipodystrophy include acute pancreatitis due to severe hypertriglyceridemia, steatosis leading to steatohepatitis and cirrhosis, and chronic complications related to diabetes mellitus. Although no standard therapy for generalized lipodystrophy has been established, management of metabolic abnormalities includes attention to diet, increased physical activity, antilipemic agents (e.g., fibrates) and/or medium-chain fatty acid supplementation for hypertriglyceridemia, and oral antidiabetic agents (e.g., metformin) and/or insulin for insulin resistance and diabetes mellitus.

Efficacy of metreleptin for the treatment of metabolic complications in patients with generalized lipodystrophy is based principally on the results of an open-label, single-arm trial conducted at the National Institutes of Health (NIH) in 48 patients with generalized lipodystrophy (67% congenital, 33% acquired) and diabetes mellitus, hypertriglyceridemia, and/or hyperinsulinemia. In this study, metreleptin therapy given subcutaneously once or twice daily was associated with reductions in glycosylated hemoglobin (HbA_{1c}), fasting glucose, and fasting triglyceride concentrations at 1 year. The median duration of metreleptin therapy was 2.7 years (range: 3.6 months to 10.9 years). The weighted average daily metreleptin dosage (i.e., average dosage considering treatment duration at various dosages) during the first year of therapy for patients weighing more than 40 kg was 2.6 or 4.6 mg for male or female patients, respectively, and 3.2 or 6.3 mg, respectively, over the entire study period; the average daily dosage for patients weighing less than 40 kg was 0.06–0.11 mg/kg (0.8–4.3 mg) over the entire study period. Dosages of concomitant antidiabetic and antilipemic agents were adjusted or the drugs were discontinued (e.g., insulin) as necessary during the study period. Among 28 patients with a baseline HbA_{1c} of 7% or greater for whom data were available at 12 months, the mean baseline HbA_{1c} was 9.3% and the mean reduction in HbA_{1c} was 2.4%. Among 12 patients who had a baseline triglyceride concentration of 500 mg/dL or greater and for whom data were available at 12 months, the median baseline triglyceride concentration was 1527 mg/dL and the median reduction in triglyceride concentration was 1117 mg/dL.

In another open-label, single-arm study in 28 patients with partial or generalized lipodystrophy, 23 of whom had partial lipodystrophy, changes in metabolic parameters were not substantially improved overall. However, in the 5 patients with generalized lipodystrophy, improvements in HbA_{1c}, fasting glucose, and fasting triglycerides were similar to those reported in the NIH principal efficacy study. Efficacy and safety of metreleptin for the treatment of complications of *partial* lipodystrophy have not been established.

■ **Other Uses** The manufacturer states that safety and efficacy of metreleptin for the treatment of liver disease, including nonalcoholic steatohepatitis (NASH), have not been established. The manufacturer also states that the drug is *not* indicated for use in patients with HIV-related lipodystrophy, or in patients with general obesity or metabolic disease (e.g., diabetes mellitus, hypertriglyceridemia) who do not have concurrent evidence of congenital or acquired generalized lipodystrophy. (See Cautions: Contraindications.)

Dosage and Administration

■ **General** Patients taking drugs known to cause hypoglycemia (e.g., insulin or insulin secretagogues, including sulfonylureas) may require dosage reductions of those agents during metreleptin therapy. Blood glucose should be closely monitored in patients receiving concomitant insulin or insulin secretagogues. (See Hypoglycemia with Concomitant Use of Insulin or Insulin Secretagogues under Warnings/Precautions: Other Warnings and Precautions, in Cautions.)

When discontinuing metreleptin in patients with risk factors for pancreatitis (e.g., history of pancreatitis, severe hypertriglyceridemia), dosage should be reduced gradually over a one-week period. During tapering, serum triglyceride concentrations should be measured and the patient should be monitored for signs and symptoms of pancreatitis; initiation or dosage adjustment of antilipemic agents may be necessary.

Restricted Distribution Program Because of the risks associated with the development of anti-metreleptin antibodies that neutralize endogenous leptin and/or metreleptin, the risk of lymphoma (see Antibody Formation and see Lymphoma under Warnings/Precautions: Warnings, in Cautions), and to ensure use in appropriate patients, metreleptin can be obtained only through a restricted distribution program called the Myalept® Risk Evaluation and Mitigation Strategy (REMS) Program. (See REMS.) Clinicians must be enrolled in the program and complete training before they can prescribe metreleptin. In addition, clinicians must complete a prescription authorization form for each new metreleptin prescription and submit it to the REMS program for certification. Only certified pharmacies may dispense metreleptin to patients after receipt of the completed prescription authorization form.

Additional information about the Myalept® REMS Program is available by calling 855-6MYALEPT (855-669-2537) or at http://www.myaleptrems.com.

■ **Administration** Metreleptin is administered by subcutaneous injection after reconstitution; the drug should *not* be administered IV or IM. Recommended sites of injection include the abdomen, thigh, or upper arm. The same area of the body may be used for daily injections; however, injection sites should be rotated with each dose. Metreleptin should not be administered into the same injection site with other drugs and should not be mixed with insulin in the same syringe or vial. Doses exceeding 1 mL can be administered as 2 injections to minimize potential injection-site discomfort due to injection volume. Metreleptin may be self-administered by the patient or caregiver after appropriate training on dose preparation and subcutaneous injection technique;

patients should self-administer their first dose under the supervision of a clinician.

Metreleptin is administered once daily at the same time each day without regard to meals. If a dose is missed, the missed dose should be administered as soon as it is remembered, followed by resumption of the regular schedule the next day; dose should not be doubled or increased to replace a missed dose.

Reconstitution Metreleptin lyophilized powder for injection must be reconstituted with either bacteriostatic water for injection or preservative-free sterile water for injection prior to administration. For neonates and infants, preservative-free sterile water for injection should be used for reconstitution. (See Pediatric Use under Warnings/Precautions: Specific Populations, in Cautions.) Prior to use, the vial should be removed from the refrigerator and allowed to reach room temperature (10–15 minutes). The vial should not be left at room temperature for longer than 4 hours. Upon visual inspection of the vial, the cake of lyophilized powder should be intact and white in color; the vial should be discarded if the powder is discolored. A vial containing 11.3 mg of metreleptin should be reconstituted by adding 2.2 mL of bacteriostatic or preservative-free sterile water for injection to provide a solution containing 5 mg/mL of metreleptin. The contents of the vial should be mixed gently and should not be shaken. The reconstituted solution should be clear; vials containing discolored or cloudy solution or particulate matter should be discarded. After reconstitution, metreleptin solution should not be frozen or shaken vigorously.

When reconstituted with bacteriostatic water for injection, metreleptin solution should be stored at 2–8°C and protected from light; the solution may be used for multiple doses within 3 days of reconstitution. When reconstituted with preservative-free sterile water for injection, the dose should be administered immediately upon reconstitution and any unused solution should be discarded.

Unopened vials of metreleptin for injection should be protected from light and stored in the original carton at 2–8°C until use; vials should not be frozen.

■ **Dosage** ***Generalized Lipodystrophy*** Dosage of metreleptin should be individualized based on clinical response and tolerability. For the treatment of complications of leptin deficiency in patients with generalized lipodystrophy, the recommended dosage of metreleptin is based on weight and/or gender. For male and female patients weighing 40 kg or less at baseline, dosage is based on weight; for patients weighing more than 40 kg at baseline, dosage is based on gender. (See Table 1.)

Table 1. Metreleptin Recommended Dosage.

Baseline Body Weight	Initial Daily Dosage (Injection Volume)	Dosage Adjustments (Injection Volume)	Maximum Daily Dosage (Injection Volume)
≤40 kg (males and females)	0.06 mg/kg (0.012 mL/kg)	0.02 mg/kg (0.004 mL/kg)	0.13 mg/kg (0.026 mL/kg)
Males >40 kg	2.5 mg (0.5 mL)	1.25–2.5 mg (0.25–0.5 mL)	10 mg (2 mL)
Females >40 kg	5 mg (1 mL)	1.25–2.5 mg (0.25–0.5 mL)	10 mg (2 mL)

■ **Special Populations** The manufacturer makes no specific dosage recommendations for geriatric patients or patients with hepatic or renal impairment.

Cautions

■ **Contraindications** General obesity not associated with congenital leptin deficiency; metreleptin is not effective in treating general obesity and patients may develop anti-metreleptin antibodies with neutralizing activity. (See Antibody Formation under Warnings/Precautions: Warnings, in Cautions.)

Hypersensitivity to metreleptin or any ingredient in the formulation.

■ **Warnings/Precautions** ***Warnings*** **Antibody Formation.** Anti-metreleptin antibodies with in vitro neutralizing activity to leptin have been identified in patients treated with metreleptin. Clinical implications of anti-metreleptin antibodies with neutralizing activity are not known but such antibodies may lead to loss of metreleptin efficacy and/or loss of endogenous leptin activity. Anti-metreleptin antibodies with neutralizing activity associated with adverse events consistent with loss of endogenous leptin activity and/or loss of metreleptin efficacy have been observed in clinical trials in 2 of 33 patients with generalized lipodystrophy (severe infection and/or worsening metabolic control) and 3 of 579 patients with obesity (excessive weight gain, development of glucose intolerance or diabetes mellitus). Metreleptin is contraindicated in patients with general obesity. (See Contraindications in Cautions.)

Patients who develop severe infections or who show signs suggesting loss of metreleptin efficacy during therapy should be tested for anti-metreleptin antibodies. The manufacturer should be contacted at 866-216-1526 for information about neutralizing antibody testing of clinical samples.

Lymphoma. T-cell lymphoma has been reported in a few patients with acquired generalized lipodystrophy treated with metreleptin; some of these patients had evidence of lymphoma and/or bone marrow abnormalities prior to therapy with metreleptin. A causal relationship between metreleptin therapy and the development or progression of lymphoma has not been established. Acquired lipodystrophies are associated with autoimmune disorders, which are associated with an increased risk of malignancies, including lymphoma. Clinicians should carefully consider the potential risks and benefits of metreleptin therapy in patients with acquired generalized lipodystrophy and/or serious hematologic abnormalities (including leukopenia, neutropenia, bone marrow abnormalities, lymphoma, and/or lymphadenopathy).

Sensitivity Reactions Anaphylaxis, urticaria, and generalized rash have been reported. (See Cautions: Contraindications.)

Other Warnings and Precautions **Hypoglycemia with Concomitant Use of Insulin or Insulin Secretagogues.** Patients receiving metreleptin concomitantly with insulin or insulin secretagogues (e.g., sulfonylureas) may have an increased risk of hypoglycemia. Blood glucose should be closely monitored in patients receiving concomitant insulin therapy, especially in patients taking high dosages, or in those taking insulin secretagogues. Dosage adjustments, including possibly large reductions of insulin or insulin secretagogue dosage, may be necessary in some patients.

Autoimmunity. Leptin is involved in immune system homeostasis, and acquired lipodystrophies are associated with autoimmune disorders, including autoimmune hepatitis and membranoproliferative glomerulonephritis. Progression of autoimmune hepatitis and membranoproliferative glomerulonephritis (associated with massive proteinuria and renal failure) has been reported in some patients with acquired generalized lipodystrophy treated with metreleptin. A causal relationship between metreleptin therapy and the development and/or progression of autoimmune diseases has not been established; however, the potential risk should be carefully considered in patients with autoimmune disease.

Benzyl Alcohol Toxicity. Metreleptin for injection contains benzyl alcohol when reconstituted with bacteriostatic water for injection. Benzyl alcohol has been associated with serious adverse events and death in pediatric patients, particularly in neonates and premature infants. When prepared for use in neonates and infants, the manufacturer recommends reconstituting metreleptin with preservative-free sterile water for injection. (See Pediatric Use under Warnings/Precautions: Specific Populations, in Cautions and also see Reconstitution under Dosage and Administration: Administration.)

Immunogenicity. As with all therapeutic proteins, there is a potential for immunogenicity with metreleptin therapy. Anti-metreleptin antibodies were found in 84% of patients in generalized lipodystrophy clinical trials. (See Antibody Formation under Warnings/Precautions: Warnings, in Cautions.)

Specific Populations **Pregnancy.** Category C. (See Users Guide.)

Although there are no adequate and controlled studies to date in humans, metreleptin has been shown to cause prolonged gestation and dystocia in mice resulting in maternal death and decreased survival of offspring when given in dosages approximately equivalent to the maximum recommended human dosage. In an in vitro study, exposure to recombinant leptin caused inhibition of contractility in human myometrial tissue. No developmental abnormalities were seen in mice exposed during the period of organogenesis to metreleptin at dosages over 7 times the maximum recommended human dosage.

The manufacturer has established a program that monitors outcomes in women exposed to metreleptin during pregnancy. Women who become pregnant during metreleptin therapy are encouraged to enroll in the program by calling 855-6MYALEPT (855-669-2537).

Lactation. It is not known whether metreleptin is distributed into human milk. Endogenous leptin is distributed into human milk. Because of the potential for serious adverse reactions to metreleptin in nursing infants and because of the possibility of anti-metreleptin antibodies distributing into milk, a decision should be made whether to discontinue nursing or the drug, taking into account the importance of the drug to the woman.

Pediatric Use. In the principal clinical trial of metreleptin in patients with generalized lipodystrophy, 73% of the patients were younger than 18 years of age (range: 1–17 years). The median age of all patients in the study at baseline was 15 years. No overall differences in safety or efficacy were observed between these pediatric patients and adult patients.

Metreleptin contains benzyl alcohol when reconstituted with bacteriostatic water for injection. When reconstituted with 2.2 mL of bacteriostatic water for injection, metreleptin contains 1.76 mg of benzyl alcohol per mg of metreleptin or 9 mg of benzyl alcohol per mL of reconstituted solution. Although a causal relationship has not been established, administration of injections preserved with benzyl alcohol has been associated with toxicity in neonates and low-birth-weight infants. Toxicity appears to have resulted from administration of large amounts (i.e., 100–400 mg/kg daily) of benzyl alcohol in these neonates. The manufacturer states that usual therapeutic doses of metreleptin deliver substantially lower amounts of benzyl alcohol than those associated with toxicity; however, the minimum amount of benzyl alcohol at which toxicity may occur is not known. Clinicians should consider the combined daily dose of benzyl alcohol from all sources.

When prepared for use in neonates and infants, the manufacturer recommends that metreleptin be reconstituted with preservative-free sterile water for injection. (See Reconstitution under Dosage and Administration: Administration.)

Geriatric Use. Clinical studies of metreleptin did not include sufficient numbers of patients 65 years of age or older to determine whether geriatric patients respond differently than younger adults. In general, dosage of metreleptin in geriatric patients should be initiated at the low end of the dosage range because of the greater frequency of age-related decreases in hepatic, renal, and/or cardiac function and of concomitant disease or other drug therapy.

Hepatic Impairment. Data are lacking on the pharmacokinetics of metreleptin in patients with hepatic impairment.

Renal Impairment. Formal pharmacokinetic studies of metreleptin are lacking in patients with renal impairment. Nonclinical data indicate that renal excretion is the major route of metreleptin elimination; the manufacturer warns that the pharmacokinetics of metreleptin may be altered in patients with renal impairment.

■ **Common Adverse Effects** Adverse effects reported in at least 5% of patients receiving metreleptin in the principal clinical trial include headache, hypoglycemia, decreased weight, abdominal pain, arthralgia, dizziness, ear infection, fatigue, nausea, ovarian cyst, upper respiratory tract infection, anemia, back pain, diarrhea, paresthesia, proteinuria, and pyrexia.

Drug Interactions

No formal drug interaction studies have been conducted with metreleptin to date.

Description

Metreleptin is a recombinant analog of human leptin. The drug is produced in *Escherichia coli* using recombinant DNA technology and differs from native human leptin by the addition of a single methionine residue at its amino terminus.

Generalized lipodystrophy is characterized by a deficiency of leptin resulting from loss of adipose tissue. Metreleptin exerts its effects by binding to and activating leptin receptors located throughout the CNS, particularly in the hypothalamus, and in several peripheral tissues. In the hypothalamus, leptin regulates energy homeostasis and neuroendocrine function. In patients with leptin deficiency, leptin replacement therapy increases insulin sensitivity, improves lipid metabolism, and reduces caloric intake.

Formal pharmacokinetic studies of metreleptin are lacking. Peak serum leptin concentrations occur approximately 4 hours (range: 2–8 hours) after subcutaneous administration in patients with lipodystrophy. Nonclinical data indicate that renal excretion is the major route of metreleptin elimination, with no apparent contribution of systemic metabolism or degradation. Elimination half-life of metreleptin is 3.8–4.7 hours in healthy individuals.

Advice to Patients

Importance of reading the manufacturer's medication guide and instructions for use prior to beginning metreleptin therapy and each time the prescription is refilled.

If a dose is missed, the missed dose should be administered as soon as it is remembered, followed by resumption of the regular schedule the next day. The regular daily dose should not be exceeded; the dose should not be doubled or increased to replace a missed dose.

Risk of loss of endogenous leptin activity and/or metreleptin efficacy due to neutralizing antibodies. Importance of promptly informing clinician of symptoms that warrant antibody testing (e.g., infection, increased blood glucose or triglycerides).

Possible increased risk of lymphoma. Importance of routine laboratory assessments and monitoring for signs and symptoms that indicate changes in hematologic status.

Increased risk of hypoglycemia in patients taking concomitant insulin and/or insulin secretagogues (e.g., sulfonylureas). Importance of reviewing signs and symptoms of hypoglycemia. Dosage adjustment of insulin and/or insulin secretagogues may be required.

Importance of informing patients that worsening of autoimmune disease has been reported with metreleptin. Importance of routine monitoring of patients with autoimmune disease to detect symptoms that may warrant additional tests.

Importance of informing patients that hypersensitivity reactions (e.g., anaphylaxis, urticaria, generalized rash) have been reported with metreleptin. Importance of informing clinician if hypersensitivity reactions occur.

Importance of women informing their clinician if they are or plan to become pregnant or plan to breast-feed. Women who become pregnant during metreleptin therapy should be encouraged to enroll in the pregnancy monitoring program by calling 855-6MYALEPT (855-669-2537).

Importance of clinicians instructing patients on how to prepare and administer the correct dosage of metreleptin prior to self-administration. The first dose of metreleptin should be administered by the patient or caregiver under the supervision of a clinician.

Importance of reviewing proper injection technique, dosing regimen, and proper storage of metreleptin; care should be taken to avoid IM injection, especially in patients with minimal subcutaneous adipose tissue. (See Reconstitution under Dosage and Administration: Administration.)

Importance of informing patients with a history of pancreatitis and/or severe hypertriglyceridemia that metreleptin should not be suddenly stopped. When discontinuing metreleptin in patients at risk for pancreatitis, the dosage should be gradually tapered over 1 week. Additional monitoring of triglyceride concentrations and/or initiation or dosage adjustment of lipid-lowering drugs may be needed.

Importance of informing clinicians of existing or contemplated concomitant therapy, including prescription and OTC drugs and dietary or herbal supplements, as well as any concomitant illnesses.

Importance of informing patients of other important precautionary information. (See Cautions.)

Overview® (see Users Guide). For additional information on this drug until a more detailed monograph is developed and published, the manufacturer's labeling should be consulted. It is *essential* that the manufacturer's labeling be consulted for more detailed information on usual cautions, precautions, contraindications, potential drug interactions, laboratory test interferences, and acute toxicity.

Preparations

Excipients in commercially available drug preparations may have clinically important effects in some individuals; consult specific product labeling for details.

Metreleptin

Parenteral

For Injection, for subcutaneous use	11.3 mg (delivers 5 mg/mL)	**Myalept®**, Aegerion

RENIN-ANGIOTENSIN-ALDOSTERONE SYSTEM 68:44

Angiotensin II Acetate

Human angiotensin II

■ Angiotensin II acetate is a synthetic form of endogenous angiotensin II, a peptide hormone of the renin-angiotensin-aldosterone system (RAAS) that causes vasoconstriction and increased blood pressure.

Uses

■ **Shock** Angiotensin II acetate is used for its vasoconstrictive effects to increase blood pressure in patients with septic or other forms of distributive shock.

Vasopressors are used as standard therapy in the management of septic shock when fluid resuscitation alone fails to restore blood pressure. Current treatment guidelines recommend norepinephrine as the first-line vasopressor of choice in adults with septic shock. Angiotensin II may provide an additional treatment option for patients who do not respond adequately to traditional vasopressors.

In a randomized, double-blind, placebo-controlled study (Angiotensin II for the Treatment of High-Output Shock [ATHOS-3]), angiotensin II substantially increased mean arterial pressure (MAP) in patients with distributive shock (91% of cases caused by sepsis) who remained hypotensive (MAP of 55–70 mm Hg) despite fluid and vasopressor therapy. A total of 321 adults who were receiving more than 0.2 mcg/kg per minute of norepinephrine or an equivalent dosage of another vasopressor for at least 6 hours but no longer than 48 hours were enrolled in the study and received an IV infusion of angiotensin II (initial dosage of 20 ng/kg per minute) or placebo. During the first 3 hours of treatment, dosage of angiotensin II was titrated to achieve a target MAP of at least 75 mm Hg, while dosages of other vasopressors were maintained; in the subsequent 3 to 48 hours, dosage of angiotensin II was titrated to maintain MAP of 65–70 mm Hg, while dosages of other vasopressors were reduced or discontinued. The primary end point was MAP response (defined as a MAP of at least 75 mm Hg or an increase in MAP from baseline of at least 10 mm Hg, without an increase in baseline vasopressor therapy) at 3 hours. The primary end point was achieved in 70% of patients receiving angiotensin II compared with 23% of patients receiving placebo. The median time to reach target MAP with angiotensin II was approximately 5 minutes. The rapid treatment effect permitted reductions in both the dosage of angiotensin II and dosages of concomitant vasopressors. At 30 minutes, the median dosage of angiotensin II was 10 ng/kg per minute. Patients who received angiotensin II had lower catecholamine requirements compared with those who received placebo. In addition, there was a trend toward a 28-day mortality benefit with angiotensin II compared with placebo (mortality rate of 46 versus 54%, respectively); however, the difference was not statistically significant.

Additional studies are needed to further elucidate the role of angiotensin II in the management of shock, particularly in regard to the patient populations that are most likely to benefit, the optimal timing of administration, long-term benefits and harm, and comparative efficacy with other vasopressors.

Dosage and Administration

■ **Administration** Angiotensin II acetate is administered by continuous IV infusion. It is recommended that the drug be infused through a central venous line.

Prior to administration, the commercially available injection concentrate must be diluted in 0.9% sodium chloride injection to a final concentration of 5000 or 10,000 ng/mL depending on the patient's fluid status. In patients who are not fluid restricted, a concentration of 5000 ng/mL may be prepared by adding 1 mL (2.5 mg) of the injection concentrate to an infusion bag containing 500 mL of 0.9% sodium chloride injection. In patients who are fluid restricted, a concentration of 10,000 ng/mL may be prepared by adding 1 mL (2.5 mg) of the injection concentrate to an infusion bag containing 250 mL of 0.9% sodium chloride injection. Diluted solutions may be stored at room temperature or under refrigeration for up to 24 hours.

Solutions of angiotensin II should be inspected visually for particulate matter and discoloration prior to administration.

■ **Dosage** Dosage of angiotensin II acetate is expressed in terms of angiotensin II.

Shock The recommended initial dosage of angiotensin II in adults with septic or other distributive shock is 20 ng/kg per minute by continuous IV infusion. Dosage should be titrated based on blood pressure response. The infusion rate may be increased by increments of up to 15 ng/kg per minute as frequently as every 5 minutes as needed to achieve or maintain the target blood pressure. During the first 3 hours of treatment, dosage should not exceed 80 ng/kg per minute. Once the underlying shock has sufficiently improved, the infusion rate should be titrated downward by decrements of up to 15 ng/kg per minute every 5 to 15 minutes as tolerated to maintain target blood pressure. During maintenance therapy, dosage should not exceed 40 ng/kg per minute. Dosages as low as 1.25 ng/kg per minute may be used.

In the ATHOS-3 study, mean arterial pressure (MAP) increased rapidly following administration of angiotensin II, allowing for rapid down-titration of the initial dosage of 20 ng/kg per minute in 67% of the patients within 30 minutes; the median dosage at 30 minutes was 10 ng/kg per minute.

■ **Special Populations** The manufacturer makes no special population dosage recommendations at this time.

Cautions

■ **Contraindications** The manufacturer states that there are no known contraindications to the use of angiotensin II acetate.

■ **Warnings/Precautions** ***Thromboembolic Risk*** An increased incidence of arterial and venous thromboembolic events, particularly deep venous thrombosis (DVT), was reported in patients receiving angiotensin II compared with those receiving placebo in the ATHOS-3 study (13 versus 5%, respectively). DVT occurred in 7 (4.3%) patients who received angiotensin II compared with none of the patients who received placebo. Preclinical studies and studies in healthy individuals also have demonstrated prothrombotic effects of the drug.

Concurrent use of venous thromboembolism (VTE) prophylaxis is recommended during angiotensin II therapy.

Specific Populations **Pregnancy.** There are insufficient data in pregnant women to determine whether angiotensin II is associated with a risk of adverse developmental effects. Animal reproduction studies have not been conducted with the drug.

Septic or other distributive shock is a medical emergency that can be fatal if untreated; a delay in treatment in pregnant women with hypotension associated with shock is likely to increase the risk of maternal and fetal morbidity and mortality.

Lactation. It is not known whether angiotensin II is distributed into human milk or if the drug has any effects on the nursing infant or on milk production.

Pediatric Use. Safety and efficacy of angiotensin II have not been established in pediatric patients.

Geriatric Use. In the ATHOS-3 study, 48% of the total patient population was 65 years of age or older. No substantial differences in safety or efficacy of angiotensin II have been observed between geriatric patients (65 years of age or older) and younger adults.

Hepatic Impairment. The pharmacokinetics of angiotensin II are not expected to be altered by hepatic impairment.

Renal Impairment. The pharmacokinetics of angiotensin II are not expected to be altered by renal impairment.

■ **Common Adverse Effects** Adverse reactions reported in 4% or more of patients receiving angiotensin II in clinical studies include thromboembolic events (e.g., DVT), thrombocytopenia, tachycardia, fungal infection, delirium, acidosis, hyperglycemia, and peripheral ischemia.

Drug Interactions

No drug interaction studies have been performed to date with angiotensin II acetate. Concomitant use of angiotensin-converting enzyme (ACE) inhibitors may increase the response to angiotensin II and concomitant use of angiotensin II receptor antagonists (ARBs) may decrease the response to angiotensin II.

Description

Angiotensin II acetate is a synthetic preparation of endogenous human angiotensin II, a peptide hormone of the renin-angiotensin-aldosterone system (RAAS) that plays an essential role in blood pressure regulation. The drug is a potent vasoconstrictor that is used to increase blood pressure in patients with septic or other forms of distributive shock.

In patients with septic shock, a variety of physiologic responses are activated to restore effective circulating volume, vascular resistance, and arterial pressure, including activation of RAAS and production of angiotensin II. There is some evidence suggesting that patients with septic shock may have a relative deficiency of angiotensin II that may be reversed with exogenous administration of angiotensin II. Angiotensin II increases blood pressure through direct vasoconstriction of the peripheral vasculature in addition to other mechanisms (e.g., aldosterone secretion, vasopressin release, activation of the sympathetic nervous system). The physiologic effects of angiotensin II are mediated by specific G protein-coupled receptors located in the kidneys, vascular smooth muscle, lung, heart, brain, adrenal gland, pituitary gland, and liver. The angiotensin II receptor type 1 (AT1 receptor) is responsible for the vasoconstrictive effects of angiotensin II; activation of the receptor stimulates calcium/calmodulin-dependent phosphorylation of myosin and causes smooth muscle contraction. Angiotensin II also has been shown to have cardiac remodeling properties and preferential vasoconstrictive effects on renal efferent arterioles.

Following IV infusion, angiotensin II is rapidly metabolized by aminopeptidase A to angiotensin 2-8 (angiotensin III) and by angiotensin-converting enzyme 2 to angiotensin 1-7 in plasma, erythrocytes, and many other major organs (e.g., intestine, kidney, liver, lungs). Angiotensin III retains approximately 40% of the activity of angiotensin II, while angiotensin 1-7 exhibits opposing actions to angiotensin II and causes vasodilation, natriuresis, and reduced blood pressure. The plasma half-life of angiotensin II is less than 1 minute. Elimination of the drug is not dependent on renal or hepatic routes.

Advice to Patients

Importance of informing clinicians of existing or contemplated concomitant therapy, including prescription and OTC drugs as well as any concomitant illnesses.

Importance of women informing clinicians if they are or plan to become pregnant or plan to breast-feed.

Importance of informing patients of other important precautionary information. (See Cautions.)

Overview® (see Users Guide). For additional information on this drug until a more detailed monograph is developed and published, the manufacturer's labeling should be consulted. It is *essential* that the manufacturer's labeling be consulted for more detailed information on usual cautions, precautions, contraindications, potential drug interactions, laboratory test interferences, and acute toxicity.

Preparations

Excipients in commercially available drug preparations may have clinically important effects in some individuals; consult specific product labeling for details.

Angiotensin II Acetate

Parenteral

Concentrate for injection, for IV infusion	2.5 mg/mL (of angiotensin II)	**Giapreza®**, La Jolla

72:00 LOCAL ANESTHETICS

see also:
Antipruritics and Local Anesthetics 84:08
Local Anesthetics 52:16

§ Omitted from the print version of *AHFS Drug Information*® because of space limitations. This monograph is available on the *AHFS Drug Information*® website, http://ahfsdruginformation.com. Username: ahfs2020; Password: ASHP94498.

LOCAL ANESTHETICS 72:00

Local Anesthetics, Parenteral, General Statement

■ Local anesthetics are drugs that reversibly block nerve conduction near their site of application or injection and thus produce temporary loss of feeling or sensation in a limited area of the body.

Uses

Parenteral local anesthetics are used for infiltration and nerve block anesthesia. Because of differences in systemic absorption and toxicity, not all of these drugs are indicated for all types of local anesthesia and the concentration of the drug used depends on the anesthetic procedure. For indications of each parenteral local anesthetic and concentrations used for various procedures, see the individual monographs in 72:00.

Infiltration anesthesia, which is frequently used in minor surgical and dental procedures, is achieved by injecting the local anesthetic solution intradermally, subcutaneously, or submucosally across the path of nerves supplying the area to be anesthetized. Field block technique, in which the local anesthetic is infiltrated subcutaneously in a circular pattern around the operative field, is a common type of infiltration anesthesia. Infiltration anesthesia has occasionally been used for cesarean section, but epidural or spinal anesthesia is generally preferred.

Nerve block (regional) anesthesia, used in surgical, dental, and diagnostic procedures and in therapeutic management of pain, is achieved by injecting a local anesthetic solution into or around nerve trunks or ganglia supplying the area to be anesthetized. Nerve block procedures require a high degree of specialization and should be performed only by clinicians experienced in local anesthetic procedures. Peripheral nerve blocks (e.g., paracervical blocks, pudendal blocks, brachial plexus nerve blocks, ulnar nerve blocks, and intercostal blocks) and sympathetic nerve blocks (e.g., stellate ganglion blocks) involve a variety of nerves. Spinal (subarachnoid, intrathecal) and epidural (extradural, peridural) blocks are special forms of nerve block anesthesia. Spinal anesthesia is achieved by injecting local anesthetic solutions intrathecally into the subarachnoid space at the lumbar level, and epidural anesthesia is produced by injecting the drug into the epidural space. Caudal (sacral) anesthesia is a type of epidural anesthesia in which the injection is made through the sacral hiatus.

Several nerve block procedures such as epidural (including caudal), paracervical, pudendal, and low spinal (saddle) blocks are used in obstetrics; high spinal anesthesia using high or medium drug doses should not be used for normal vaginal deliveries because undue ascent of the anesthetic may result from variations in CSF pressure during labor. Local anesthetics should not be given until the cervix is well dilated and labor is progressing normally. In spinal anesthetic procedures, the drugs should not be injected during uterine contractions since undesired ascent of the anesthetic may occur.

Vasoconstrictors (e.g., epinephrine), when added to solutions of some local anesthetics, may decrease the rate of vascular absorption of the anesthetic, thereby localizing anesthesia and prolonging the duration of anesthesia; systemic toxicity of the local anesthetic is also decreased. When infiltration anesthesia is used, vasoconstrictors may also decrease bleeding in the operative field. Epinephrine appears to be the most effective vasoconstrictor. Mepivacaine and prilocaine produce little or no vasodilation and, therefore, administration of a vasoconstrictor with these drugs is usually not necessary. Epinephrine also does not appear to affect time of onset or duration of ropivacaine anesthesia. The optimal concentration of vasoconstrictors varies with the vascularity of the injection site and with the individual anesthetic agent. In general, 0.1 mg of epinephrine (20 mL of a 1:200,000 solution) is used and up to 0.2 mg of epinephrine (20 mL of a 1:100,000 solution) is generally well tolerated by normal patients. If the therapeutic benefit of epinephrine administration is considered to outweigh the possible risks in high-risk patients, a lower maximum dose of 0.02–0.05 mg (2–5 mL of a 1:100,000 solution) may be considered.

Local anesthetics should be used as a component of multimodal analgesia (i.e., simultaneous use of a combination of analgesic agents and techniques that target different mechanisms of action in the peripheral and central nervous systems) in the management of postoperative pain. Studies have demonstrated that multimodal pain management strategies are associated with superior pain relief and decreased need for opiates. Experts recommend that clinicians consider the use of local anesthetic infiltration or site-specific regional analgesic techniques as part of a multimodal approach to the management of postoperative pain.

Parenteral local anesthetics (e.g., lidocaine hydrochloride) have been used to produce regional anesthesia by injecting the drug IV (Bier Block) into a limb in which circulation has been interrupted by application of a tourniquet. However, this route of administration is not recommended with some local anesthetics (e.g., bupivacaine, ropivacaine); cardiac arrest and death have been reported when bupivacaine was administered using this technique. Procaine and lidocaine have also been administered IV as systemic analgesics; however, use of these drugs for analgesia is of doubtful value and may result in serious toxic reactions. Lidocaine hydrochloride is used IV to treat acute ventricular arrhythmias (see 24:04.04.08).

For information on topical local anesthetics, see 52:16 and 84:08.

Dosage and Administration

■ **Administration** Parenteral local anesthetics may be administered by local infiltration or by epidural (including caudal), spinal (subarachnoid, intrathecal), retrobulbar, dental, peripheral, or sympathetic block. The drugs may be given by single injection or continuous block techniques in which repeat injections are given through a catheter inserted into the area being anesthetized. Local anesthetics have been administered by continuous intra-articular infusion† using elastomeric infusion devices (e.g., for control of postoperative pain); however, such use has been associated with chondrolysis. (See Cautions: Musculoskeletal Effects.)

Local anesthetic solutions containing preservatives should *not* be used for spinal or epidural (including caudal) anesthesia. Partially used bottles of solutions which do not contain preservatives should be discarded.

Because of the risk of hypotension, the patient's blood pressure should be monitored during spinal anesthesia.

Resuscitative equipment, oxygen, drugs, and personnel required for treatment of adverse reactions should be immediately available when local anesthetics are used. (See Cautions: Precautions and Contraindications.) Proper positioning of the patient is extremely important in spinal anesthesia. For specific procedures and techniques of administration, specialized references should be consulted.

Local anesthetics should be administered slowly in incremental doses to reduce the risk of adverse effects (e.g., local anesthetic systemic toxicity). Frequent aspirations for blood or cerebrospinal fluid (when applicable) should be performed to avoid intravascular administration and to either confirm entry into the subarachnoid space (for spinal anesthesia) or avoid inadvertent subarachnoid injection.

■ **Dosage** Generally, lower concentrations of local anesthetics are used for infiltration and peripheral or sympathetic nerve block anesthesia than for epidural anesthesia; highest concentrations (but small doses) are used in spinal anesthesia. Dosage varies with the anesthetic procedure, the degree of anesthesia required, and individual patient response. The smallest dose and concentration required to produce the desired effect should be used, especially in obstetrics. Reduced dosage is indicated in debilitated or acutely ill patients, in very young children or geriatric patients, and in patients with liver disease, arteriosclerosis, or occlusive arterial disease.

Cautions

Adverse effects of local anesthetics usually result from high plasma concentrations of the drug caused by inadvertent intravascular injection, excessive dosage, excessive rate of injection, slow metabolic degradation, or injection into highly vascular tissue. Local anesthetic systemic toxicity occurs rarely, but is associated with serious adverse effects, principally involving the CNS and cardiovascular systems.

■ **CNS and Cardiovascular Effects** High plasma concentrations of local anesthetics affect the CNS and cardiovascular system. Generally, high plasma concentrations of the drugs initially produce CNS stimulatory effects manifested by anxiety, apprehension, restlessness, nervousness, disorientation, confusion, dizziness, blurred vision, tremors, twitching, shivering, and seizures, followed by CNS depression manifested by drowsiness, unconsciousness, and respiratory arrest. Nausea, vomiting, chills, miosis, and tinnitus also may occur. In some patients, especially those receiving lidocaine or other amides, symptoms of CNS stimulation may be transient or absent, and initial CNS effects are depressant in nature.

Adverse cardiovascular effects are depressant and include myocardial depression, bradycardia, cardiac arrhythmias, hypotension, cardiovascular collapse, and cardiac arrest. Although adverse cardiovascular effects usually occur only with high plasma concentrations of local anesthetic, in rare instances small doses of the drugs used for infiltration have caused cardiovascular collapse. Clinicians should consider that anesthesia itself, especially when the drugs are administered by epidural or subarachnoid routes, can affect the cardiovascular and respiratory systems.

Adverse reactions resulting from administration of epinephrine-containing solutions include anxiety, palpitation, dizziness, headache, restlessness, tremors, tachycardia, anginal pain, and hypertension. In extreme cases, pulmonary edema and ventricular fibrillation may occur. Norepinephrine is less likely to cause cardiac arrhythmias but instead may cause reflex bradycardia.

In the treatment of CNS and cardiovascular reactions, general physiologic supportive measures such as maintenance of adequate airway, oxygen uptake, and carbon dioxide removal should be instituted immediately. Administration of oxygen and assisted respiration may be sufficient to control anoxia in patients with seizures and avoids the hazards associated with administration of CNS depressant drugs. For control of severe seizures, slow IV infusion of diazepam, an ultra-short acting barbiturate, or, if these are not available, a short-acting barbiturate has been recommended. CNS depressants should not be used when asystole, coma, respiratory failure, or hypotension are present. Administration of a short-acting skeletal muscle relaxant (e.g., succinylcholine) in conjunction with artificial respiration has been recommended to block peripheral manifestations of seizures. Some clinicians, however, have questioned the value of skeletal muscle relaxants for treatment of local anesthetic-induced seizures. In the treatment of cardiovascular collapse, assisted respiration is of utmost importance. IV fluids and vasopressor drugs, preferably those that stimulate the myocardium, have been used to treat hypotension and circulatory collapse. The value of vasopressors in the treatment of cardiogenic shock is controversial, however. Cardiac massage should be used if necessary.

■ **Musculoskeletal Effects** Chondrolysis, a condition characterized by necrosis and destruction of articular cartilage, has been reported in patients receiving continuous intra-articular infusions of local anesthetics for treatment of postoperative pain. Approximately 35 such cases of chondrolysis were reported to the FDA between 2006 and 2008 and have resulted in substantial injury to otherwise healthy young adults and adolescents. In most of the reported cases, chondrolysis occurred in the shoulder joint following arthroscopic or other shoulder surgery. While most (91%) of the affected patients received bupivacaine with or without epinephrine as the infused drug, several patients received other local anesthetics. The local anesthetics were infused directly into the intra-articular space using an elastomeric infusion device for periods of 48–72 hours postoperatively. Symptoms of cartilage damage (e.g., joint pain, stiffness, loss of motion) were reported as early as 2 months following administration of the infusions. It is not known whether the drug, device materials, other factors, or a combination of factors contributed to the development of chondrolysis. Additional cases of chondrolysis following intra-articular infusions of local anesthetics have been described in the medical literature. Although a causal relationship could not be established, use of continuous infusion devices to deliver the local anesthetic intra-articularly appeared to be associated with the development of chondrolysis in these cases. There currently is no effective treatment for chondrolysis; patients who develop the condition often require additional intervention, including debridement and/or corrective surgical measures (e.g., arthroplasty). Neither local anesthetics nor elastomeric infusion devices are approved for use for continuous intra-articular infusion therapy.

■ **Respiratory Effects** Respiratory paralysis or underventilation can occur following spinal anesthesia (due to cephaled extension of the motor level of anesthesia).

■ **Sensitivity Reactions** Hypersensitivity or allergic reactions occur rarely in patients receiving local anesthetics. These reactions may be manifested by dermatologic reactions, edema, status asthmaticus, or anaphylactoid reactions, which may result in death. There is probably no cross-sensitivity between local anesthetics of the amide type and those of the ester type; however, cross-sensitivity within each type does exist. Although some investigators and manufacturers have recommended skin testing in patients with suspected drug sensitivity, the value of this procedure in predicting sensitivity is controversial.

■ **Other Adverse Effects** A transient burning sensation may occur at the site of injection of local anesthetics. Rarely, prolonged burning, pain, skin discoloration, tissue irritation, swelling, neuritis, neurolysis, tissue necrosis, and sloughing may occur.

Methemoglobinemia may occur in patients receiving some parenteral local anesthetics (e.g., prilocaine hydrochloride). (See Prilocaine Hydrochloride 72:00).

Aseptic meningitis, occasionally resulting in permanent and sometimes fatal paralysis, has occurred in patients undergoing spinal anesthesia and has been attributed to injection of irritating antiseptics or detergents in which the ampuls or syringes may have been stored or cleaned. If stability of the local anesthetic solution permits, ampuls of local anesthetics should be sterilized by autoclaving. Antiseptic or detergent solutions should not be used on the glass surface of ampuls because undetectable cracks may permit leakage of irritants into the local anesthetic solution. If ampuls are stored in antiseptic or detergent solutions, a dye should be added to the solution to facilitate detection of ampul leakage.

■ **Precautions and Contraindications** Accidental intravascular injection of local anesthetics may result in seizures, CNS or cardiorespiratory depression, coma, and/or respiratory arrest. Local anesthetics should be used only by clinicians who are sufficiently knowledgeable in the diagnosis and management of dose-related toxicity and other acute emergencies that might arise from the type of anesthetic block to be used. Patients should be carefully and constantly monitored for possible cardiovascular, respiratory, or CNS complications during and after administration of local anesthetics. Resuscitative equipment, oxygen, drugs, and personnel required for treatment of adverse reactions must be immediately available whenever the drugs are used. Delay in appropriate management of dose-related toxicity, underventilation from any cause, and/or altered sensitivity may lead to the development of acidosis, cardiac arrest, and possibly death. For information on the management of severe CNS or cardiovascular reactions, see Cautions: CNS and Cardiovascular Effects.

Proper technique is inherent to safe use of local anesthetics. The drugs should be injected slowly and with frequent aspiration to guard against intravascular injection. The injection should be terminated if toxic effects appear. In intercostal and supraclavicular brachial plexus block, care should be taken to avoid puncture of the pleura. Care should be exercised in performing epidural (including caudal) anesthesia to prevent intravascular or subarachnoid injection of the large dose of local anesthetic. In epidural anesthesia, a test dose of anesthetic solution (usually 2 mL or 20% of the total dose—whichever is less) should be injected at least 5 minutes prior to administering the total dose; whenever clinical conditions permit, use of a test dose solution that contains epinephrine should be considered. If inadvertent subarachnoid injection has occurred, the patient should be resuscitated with oxygen; vasopressor drugs may be administered if necessary for control of blood pressure. In obstetric patients undergoing local anesthetic procedures, care must be taken to prevent accidental injection of the drug directly into the fetus. In spinal anesthesia, proper positioning of the patient and administration techniques are required to minimize spinal fluid leakage and subsequent headaches and to prevent mechanical injury to nerve tissue. Injections into the head and neck area (e.g., retrobulbar, dental, or stellate ganglion blocks) require particular caution since serious adverse effects due to complications of the anesthetic technique (e.g., inadvertent intra-arterial administration with resultant retrograde flow to the cerebral circulation, inadvertent puncture of the dural sheath of the optic nerve) have been reported.

Since *p*-aminobenzoic acid may antagonize the activity of aminosalicylic acid and sulfonamides, some clinicians have suggested that local anesthetics of the ester type which are hydrolyzed in vivo to aminobenzoic acid derivatives (procaine and tetracaine) should not be given concomitantly with these drugs. In anesthetized individuals, the neuromuscular blocking effect of succinylcholine has been reported to be increased by IV administration of lidocaine or procaine following succinylcholine; however, this effect appears to be important only following high IV doses of the anesthetics.

Some commercially available formulations of articaine, bupivacaine, lidocaine, prilocaine, procaine, and tetracaine contain sulfites that may cause allergic-type reactions, including anaphylaxis and life-threatening or less severe asthmatic episodes, in certain susceptible individuals. The overall prevalence of sulfite sensitivity in the general population is unknown but probably low; such sensitivity appears to occur more frequently in asthmatic than in nonasthmatic individuals.

It has been suggested that patients with cardiac disease, hyperthyroidism, or other endocrine diseases may be particularly susceptible to toxic effects of local anesthetics. The drugs should be used with caution in severely debilitated patients and in those with liver disease. Ester-type local anesthetics should be used with extreme caution, if at all, in patients with low plasma pseudocholinesterase concentrations. Local anesthetics are contraindicated in patients with known hypersensitivity to the particular drug or group of local anesthetics (i.e., ester type or amide type) or any ingredient in the formulation (i.e., sulfites) and should be used cautiously in individuals with a history of allergic reactions. Local anesthetics should not be used in patients with myasthenia gravis, severe shock, or impaired cardiac conduction. The drugs are contraindicated by any route when the area or site of injection is infected or inflamed and should be used with extreme caution in patients with skin infections anywhere on the body.

Contraindications to epidural (including caudal) and spinal anesthesia include serious diseases of the CNS or of the spinal cord such as meningitis, spinal fluid block, cranial or spinal hemorrhage, tumors, poliomyelitis, syphilis, tuberculosis, or metastatic lesions of the spinal cord. Although CNS disease is generally a contraindication to spinal or epidural anesthesia, it is not a contraindication to peripheral nerve block. The following conditions are generally considered contraindications to epidural, caudal, or spinal anesthesia, but the therapeutic benefits to the patient should be weighed against the potential risks: spinal deformities that make epidural or spinal puncture inadvisable or difficult; bleeding resulting from traumatic lumbar puncture; arteriosclerosis; occlusive arterial disease; pernicious anemia with spinal cord involvement; severe anemia, cachexia, or moribund condition; septicemia; bowel obstruction; chronic backache; preoperative headaches of long duration or history of migraine; extreme age or youth; high or low blood pressure; and emotional instability, hysteria, or nervous tension. Blood pressure should be closely monitored during spinal anesthesia. Spinal anesthesia is generally contraindicated in patients with septicemia, severe hemorrhage, severe hypotension or shock, and complete heart block or other arrhythmias that severely restrict cardiac output. Spinal and epidural anesthesia may be contraindicated in patients with an abnormality of the blood clotting mechanism as in those with a bleeding tendency, those with hypofibrinogenemia, or those receiving anticoagulant therapy. Spinal or epidural puncture in these patients may cause subarachnoid or epidural hemorrhage which could result in neurologic sequelae. Patients on prolonged therapy with chlorpromazine or other antipsychotic agents that interfere with vasomotor control or patients with preexisting vasomotor instability should generally not receive spinal or epidural anesthesia, especially if anesthesia of the upper spinal cord is required. Viral disease, whether local or generalized, is usually a contraindication to spinal anesthesia.

Local anesthetic solutions containing a vasoconstrictor such as epinephrine should be used with caution, if at all, in geriatric patients and in patients with cardiovascular diseases including hypertension, peripheral vascular diseases, diabetes, hyperthyroidism, or Graves' disease. In addition, vasoconstrictors should not be used in conjunction with anesthesia of the digits, ears, nose, or penis. During labor, vasoconstriction of uterine blood vessels may occur and decrease placental circulation and intensity of uterine contractions, thereby prolonging labor. It should be kept in mind that oxytocic drugs of the ergot type may cause severe persistent hypertension and even rupture of a cerebral blood vessel in postpartum patients who have received local anesthetics containing a vasoconstrictor. Vasoconstrictors should not be used when potent inhalation anesthetics are administered, since severe cardiac arrhythmias may occur. Local anesthetic solutions containing vasoconstrictors should be used with extreme caution, if at all, in patients receiving monoamine oxidase inhibitors or tricyclic antidepressants because prolonged hypertension may result.

Life-threatening adverse effects (e.g., irregular heart beat, seizures, breathing difficulties, coma, death) may occur when topical anesthetics are applied to a large area of skin, when the area of application is covered with an occlusive dressing, if a large amount of topical anesthetic is applied, if the anesthetic is applied to irritated or broken skin, or if the skin temperature increases (from exercise or use of a heating pad). Serious adverse effects (e.g., seizures, coma, irregular heart beat, respiratory depression) have been reported following topical application of local anesthetics to the skin. These events have occurred following application of extemporaneously prepared topical preparations containing high concentrations of anesthetics for cosmetic procedures and following use for indications approved by the FDA. When a topical anesthetic is needed for a procedure, use of a preparation approved by the FDA has been recommended. A preparation containing the lowest concentration of anesthetic likely to be effective should be used; a small amount of topical anesthetic should be applied to the affected area for the shortest period necessary for the desired effect. The patient should apply the topical preparation as directed by a clinician, and should not apply the topical preparation to broken or irritated skin. Patients should speak with their clinician if they are considering using a topical anesthetic before obtaining a mammogram.

■ **Pediatric Precautions** Some local anesthetics are not recommended for use in pediatric patients until more experience is gained. Some manufacturers state that dosage of local anesthetics (e.g., articaine, lidocaine) in pediatric patients should be reduced in proportion to age, weight, and physical condition. For specific recommendations regarding the use of local anesthetics in pediatric patients, see the individual monographs on local anesthetics in 72:00.

■ **Geriatric Precautions** Most manufacturers provide no specific guidance regarding safety and efficacy of local anesthetics in geriatric patients relative to younger adults. Although no overall differences in safety or efficacy were observed between geriatric and younger patients in clinical studies of articaine, the possibility that some older patients may exhibit increased sensitivity to the drug cannot be ruled out. The manufacturers generally state that local anesthetics should be used in reduced dosages in geriatric patients.

■ **Mutagenicity and Carcinogenicity** Long-term studies in animals to evaluate the mutagenic and carcinogenic potential of most local anesthetics have not been conducted to date. However, results of standard in vitro and in vivo tests using articaine hydrochloride showed no evidence of mutagenic activity. Limited data from reproductive studies in rats using high doses (approximately 2 times the human dose) of various local anesthetics (i.e., articaine) have not revealed evidence of impaired fertility.

■ **Pregnancy** Local anesthetics generally cross the placenta rapidly, and when used for epidural, paracervical, pudendal, or caudal block anesthesia, can cause varying degrees of maternal, fetal, and neonatal toxicity. The incidence and degree of toxicity depend on the procedure performed, the type and amount of drug used, and the technique of drug administration. Adverse reactions in the parturient, fetus, and neonate involve alterations of the CNS, peripheral vascular tone, and cardiac function.

Maternal hypotension has resulted from regional anesthesia. Elevating the patient's legs and positioning her on her left side may help prevent hypotension. Fetal heart rate should be monitored continuously, especially during paracervical block, and electronic fetal monitoring is advisable.

Epidural, spinal, paracervical, or pudendal anesthesia may alter the forces of parturition through changes in uterine contractility or maternal expulsive efforts. Use of obstetric anesthesia may increase the need for forceps assistance during delivery.

Administration of local anesthetics by paracervical nerve block during labor has been associated with a high incidence of fetal acidosis and bradycardia and has occasionally resulted in perinatal death. Fetal bradycardia may occur in 20–30% of patients receiving paracervical block anesthesia with the amide-type local anesthetics and may be associated with fetal acidosis. The risk of fetal bradycardia appears to be increased with prematurity, toxemia of pregnancy, and fetal distress. Changes in fetal heart rate and blood pH have been reported following epidural anesthesia. Use of bupivacaine for obstetrical paracervical block anesthesia is contraindicated.

Possible inadvertent intracranial injection of local anesthetic solution into the fetus has reportedly occurred following attempted paracervical and/or pudendal block. Such inadvertent injection has resulted in unexplained neonatal depression at birth which was associated with high serum concentration of the anesthetic; seizures usually occurred within 6 hours after birth. Prompt use of supportive measures and forced urinary excretion of the local anesthetic has reportedly been effective for managing this complication.

Systemic absorption of some local anesthetics during paracervical block in early pregnancy (anesthesia for elective abortion) may be rapid, since maternal seizures and cardiovascular collapse have occurred under these conditions. Therefore, the recommended maximum dose of the drug should not be exceeded and injection should be made slowly and with frequent aspiration, allowing a 5-minute interval between sides.

In obstetrics, low spinal (saddle block) and caudal anesthesia are contraindicated in psychologically unsuited patients and in those with pelvic disproportion, abruptio placentae, unengaged or floating fetal head and placenta praevia, unless cesarean section is contemplated after induction of caudal anesthesia. In addition, these anesthetic procedures should not be used when intrauterine manipulations are required.

Safe use of local anesthetics during pregnancy prior to labor has not been established with respect to adverse effects on fetal development. Careful consideration should be given to this fact before administering these drugs in pregnant women.

Pharmacology

Local anesthetics are drugs which reversibly block nerve conduction near their site of application or injection and thus produce temporary loss of feeling or sensation in a limited area of the body. A wide variety of drugs have local anesthetic properties. Many of these drugs, however, are used only as topical anesthetics or antipruritics (see 52:16 and 84:08) or for other therapeutic purposes (e.g., Antihistamines 4:00). Although local anesthetics that are administered parenterally differ in quantitative and even in some qualitative effects, the similarity of their pharmacologic and therapeutic properties permits their discussion as a class.

Local anesthetics block the generation and conduction of impulses through all nerve fibers—sensory, motor, and autonomic. Local anesthetics appear to block conduction of nerve impulses by decreasing permeability of the nerve cell membrane to sodium ions, thereby decreasing the rate of depolarization of the nerve membrane, increasing the threshold for electrical excitability, and preventing propagation of the action potential. A current theory is that local anesthetics reduce nerve cell membrane permeability by competing with calcium for the membrane binding sites that control membrane permeability to sodium.

Small nerve fibers are generally more susceptible to the effects of local anesthetics than are large ones. In general, autonomic activity is affected first, followed by loss of pain and other sensory functions and, finally, loss of motor activity; regression of anesthesia usually occurs in the reverse order.

The various anesthetics produce different degrees of vasoactivity. Sympathetic blockade resulting from spinal anesthesia produces cardiovascular effects, including decreased stroke volume, cardiac output, and peripheral resistance, which may lead to hypotension. Circulatory changes associated with epidural anesthesia also result, in part, from sympathetic blockade. When epinephrine is administered with a local anesthetic, the pharmacologic effects of absorbed epinephrine may also affect the cardiovascular system.

Sympathetic blockade, whether from spinal or epidural anesthesia, results in contraction of the bowel and relaxation of sphincters. The vagus is not blocked, however, and visceral manipulation can cause pain or discomfort and precipitate nausea and vomiting. Spinal and epidural anesthesia, especially high spinal anesthesia, may interfere with normal respiratory function. Medullary depression and death may result from upward diffusion of large doses of local anesthetics. Circulatory and respiratory difficulties from local anesthesia develop more readily in pregnant women than in nonpregnant patients as a result of compression of the vena cava by the gravid uterus.

Tachyphylaxis to local anesthetic agents may develop and occurs most frequently after repeated administration of the drug into areas with limited buffer capacity such as the subarachnoid or epidural space. Although the precise cause of local anesthetic tachyphylaxis has not been determined, it appears that repeated administration of acidic injections lowers pH at the site of injection, thereby decreasing the amount of the free base available for diffusion through the epineurium to the receptor site. It has been suggested that development of tachyphylaxis may be retarded by the following measures: administration of a local anesthetic with a comparatively long duration of action and a high pK_a value; addition of epinephrine to the local anesthetic solution to prolong the duration of action; and use of a buffer to increase pH within the epidural or subarachnoid space.

Since local anesthetics exert a generalized effect on all excitable membranes, systemic absorption of these drugs may affect the cardiovascular and central nervous system. High blood concentrations of local anesthetics produce peripheral vasodilatation initially, followed by decreased myocardial contractility which can lead to hypotension and cardiovascular collapse. Toxic blood concentrations of the drugs depress cardiac conduction which can lead to atrioventricular dissociation and ultimately cardiac arrest. High blood concentrations of local anesthetics also produce CNS depression. Initially this is manifested by central excitation, which ultimately leads to seizures resulting from blockade of inhibitory cortical synapses. Generalized CNS depression leading to respiratory depression and finally respiratory arrest may occur.

Other pharmacologic effects including ganglionic blocking activity, neuromuscular blocking activity, anticholinergic activity, antihistaminic activity, and antibacterial action have been attributed to local anesthetics; however, these effects do not appear to be clinically important when the drugs are used alone.

Pharmacokinetics

■ Absorption Absorption of local anesthetics into the blood is influenced by the pharmacologic properties of the specific drug including its vasoactivity, the total dose of the drug administered, and the site of injection. Duration of anesthesia depends on the time during which the drug is in contact with nerve tissue. In general, the greater the degree of vasodilation produced by the local anesthetic, the faster the rate of absorption and shorter the duration of action. Procaine and chloroprocaine have relatively short durations of action; articaine, lidocaine, mepivacaine, propoxycaine (no longer commercially available in the US), and prilocaine have intermediate durations of action; and bupivacaine, etidocaine (no longer commercially available in the US), levobupivacaine (no longer commercially available in the US), ropivacaine, and tetracaine have long durations of action. Addition of a vasoconstrictor such as epinephrine to solutions of some local anesthetics decreases the rate of absorption and consequently prolongs the duration of action. (See Uses.)

■ Distribution Following systemic absorption, local anesthetics are distributed into all body tissues. Individual drugs vary in the rate and degree to which they are distributed into various tissues and organs. Local anesthetics pass the blood-brain barrier in varying degrees. Distribution of local anesthetics in the CSF following epidural administration appears to parallel the degree of vascular absorption. Some direct diffusion across the dura mater may occur. Individual local anesthetics differ in the degree to which they are bound to plasma proteins. Local anesthetics cross the placental barrier in varying degrees. Because they are more rapidly degraded, it has been reported that ester-type local anesthetics are less likely to produce toxic plasma concentrations in the fetus. Drugs with the highest protein-binding capacity (e.g., bupivacaine) appear to have the lowest degree of placental transfer. When used in paracervical block procedures, local anesthetics may reach especially high concentrations in fetal plasma.

To produce anesthesia, local anesthetics must penetrate through surrounding tissue to the nerve cell membrane. The free base form of the local anesthetic has a high oil/water distribution coefficient which produces optimal penetration. Because the relative alkalinity of extracellular fluid favors formation of the free base, penetration in the extracellular space is usually adequate unless inflammation (which results in an unusually low pH) is present. After penetration to the nerve cell membrane, a new equilibrium between the free base and the cation is established. There has been considerable controversy as to whether the cation or the free base of the local anesthetic is active at the nerve membrane. The free base of procaine appears to be its more active form, whereas the cation appears to be essential for activity in most other local anesthetics. Some investigators have suggested, however, that the aromatic lipophilic portion of the molecule is responsible for anesthetic properties and that the cationic portion merely intensifies nerve-blocking effects.

Hyaluronidase has been added to local anesthetic solutions to facilitate penetration of the drug, particularly with nerve block and infiltration anesthesia. Because spread of anesthesia is undesirable in certain blocks and there is an increased incidence of systemic reactions to the local anesthetic when hyaluronidase is used, the enzyme is now used infrequently.

In spinal anesthesia, upward diffusion of the drug in the subarachnoid space depends on many factors including the concentration of the drug, the volume and specific gravity of the solution administered, the rate of injection, the position of the patient, the curvature of the patient's spine, movements of the patient, and the size of the subarachnoid space. In conjunction with appropriate positioning of the patient, hypobaric local anesthetic solutions rise in the subarachnoid space and produce anesthesia at levels higher than the site of injection; isobaric solutions of local anesthetics act at about the level of subarachnoid injection; and hyperbaric local anesthetic solutions exert their effects at levels below the site of injection. Following epidural administration of local anesthetics, leakage of the drug through the intervertegral foramina results in a multiple paravertebral block; uptake of the drug by dura-covered nerve roots within the epidural space results in spinal root blockade, and diffusion of the drug across the dura mater to the subarachnoid nerve roots and the spinal cord produces spinal cord blockade. The relative contribution of each of these factors to epidural anesthesia has not been determined. Since diffusion of the drug through the epidural space and to the above mentioned sites is a slow process, complete onset of action with epidural anesthesia is about 15–30 minutes after administration. Onset of action with spinal anesthesia is considerably shorter (average 5–12 minutes), since the epineurium is the only diffusion barrier in the subarachnoid space.

■ Elimination Ester-type local anesthetics are hydrolyzed mainly in plasma by pseudocholinesterases and also by esterases in the liver. Patients with impaired renal function or hepatic disease and neonates with undeveloped renal or hepatic function have decreased serum pseudocholinesterase concentrations and, therefore, hydrolyze ester-type anesthetics more slowly than do other patients. Most local anesthetics with an amide linkage are metabolized principally in the liver by microsomal enzymes. Animal studies suggest that some local anesthetics may undergo enterohepatic circulation. Both ester- and amide-type local anesthetics are excreted mainly in urine as metabolites and small amounts of unchanged drug. Urinary excretion of lidocaine, prilocaine, bupivacaine, and possibly other local anesthetics may be enhanced by acidification of urine; however, the degree of increased urinary excretion is not clinically important.

Chemistry and Stability

■ Chemistry Parenteral local anesthetics are synthetic drugs that structurally consist of a secondary or tertiary amino group connected to an aromatic residue by an intermediate group. The aromatic residue is connected to the intermediate group by an ester or amide linkage. Parenteral local anesthetics can be classified by the type of linkage that they possess:

ESTER TYPE

*benzocaine	procaine hydrochloride
chloroprocaine hydrochloride	*proparacaine hydrochloride
*cocaine	tetracaine hydrochloride

* *used only for topical anesthesia (see 52:16 and 84:08)*

AMIDE TYPE

articaine hydrochloride	lidocaine hydrochloride
bupivacaine hydrochloride	mepivacaine hydrochloride
liposomal bupivacaine	prilocaine hydrochloride
*dibucaine	ropivacaine hydrochloride

* *used only for topical anesthesia (see 52:16 and 84:08)*

The type of linkage appears to affect principally the site of metabolism and metabolic pathway of the drug. The aromatic portion of the local anesthetic determines its lipophilic properties, and the amine portion is responsible for its hydrophilic properties. Variations in these portions of the molecule affect the lipid-water distribution coefficient, protein-binding characteristics, and the ability of the drug to penetrate tissues. These and other structural changes in the molecule alter anesthetic potency, duration of action, rate of metabolism, and toxicity.

Because most of the free bases are poorly soluble in water and unstable in solution, parenteral local anesthetics are generally marketed as water-soluble hydrochloride salts. A liposomal formulation of bupivacaine containing the free base drug in an aqueous suspension of multivesicular liposomes is commercially available. Local anesthetics are weak bases, and solutions of their hydrochloride salts are usually acidic, a condition that enhances their stability. In solution, the local anesthetic salt is present as the uncharged free amine and as the positively charged ion in a ratio dependent on the pH of the solution and the pK_a of the drug. Equilibrium shifts toward the charged cation form as pH decreases or toward the free-base form as pH increases. The pK_a of most local anesthetics is in the range of 7.5–9.

■ Stability Local anesthetics of the ester type are generally less stable in solution than are the amide-type anesthetics and, therefore, should not be subjected to repeated autoclaving. Chloroprocaine is very unstable, and solutions of this drug should not be autoclaved. Local anesthetic solutions that are cloudy, discolored, or contain crystals should be discarded.

For specific dosages and additional information on chemistry and stability, pharmacokinetics, uses, and cautions of the parenteral local anesthetics, see the individual monographs in 72:00.

†Use is not currently included in the labeling approved by the US Food and Drug Administration

Bupivacaine

■ Bupivacaine hydrochloride is a long-acting local anesthetic of the amide type.

Uses

Bupivacaine is used for local or regional anesthesia or analgesia in surgical, obstetrical, dental, diagnostic, and therapeutic procedures. The drug is commercially available as conventional bupivacaine hydrochloride preparations with or without epinephrine or as a liposomal injection containing bupivacaine in an aqueous suspension of multivesicular liposomes (Exparel®).

Conventional bupivacaine hydrochloride preparations are used for local infiltration anesthesia and for nerve block techniques including peripheral, sympathetic, epidural (including caudal), retrobulbar, and dental block anesthesia. The concentration used (0.25, 0.5 or 0.75%) is dependent on the anesthetic technique and degree of muscle relaxation desired. The 0.75% concentration of bupivacaine hydrochloride produces complete motor block and should be reserved for procedures that require a high degree of muscle relaxation and prolonged anesthetic effect (e.g., epidural block in abdominal surgeries, retrobulbar block). Use of bupivacaine hydrochloride 0.75% is not recommended for obstetrical anesthesia since such use has resulted in cardiac arrest and death, presumably from systemic toxicity following inadvertent intravascular injection. A hyperbaric solution containing 0.75% bupivacaine hydrochloride in 8.25% dextrose is used for spinal anesthesia.

Bupivacaine liposomal injection (Exparel®) is used for local infiltration or interscalene brachial plexus nerve block in the management of postoperative pain. Because liposomal encapsulation or incorporation into a lipid complex can substantially alter the physiochemical and functional properties of a drug, liposomal bupivacaine should *not* be used interchangeably with other bupivacaine-containing preparations. Efficacy of liposomal bupivacaine for local infiltration analgesia is based principally on 2 randomized, double-blind, placebo-controlled studies in adults undergoing bunionectomy or hemorrhoidectomy. In these studies, liposomal bupivacaine (administered directly into the surgical site at the conclusion of surgery) was substantially more effective than placebo in reducing postoperative pain; however, the treatment effect was apparent mainly during the first 12–24 hours after the drug was administered. Efficacy of liposomal bupivacaine as a brachial plexus nerve block was demonstrated in a randomized, double-blind, placebo-controlled study in patients undergoing total shoulder arthroplasty or rotator cuff repair. In this study, patients receiving liposomal bupivacaine (administered as a brachial plexus nerve block via interscalene approach) had substantially reduced cumulative pain scores through 48 hours compared with those receiving placebo. Use of liposomal bupivacaine was associated with a small reduction in opiate requirements relative to placebo in some of these studies; however, the clinical benefits of these findings are not known. Although liposomal bupivacaine has been evaluated for other regional nerve block techniques, the manufacturer states that the current data are insufficient to support use of the drug for nerve blocks other than interscalene brachial plexus nerve block because of safety concerns (e.g., risk of falls when used as a femoral nerve block) and/or lack of efficacy (e.g., when used as an intercostal nerve block).

Local anesthetics such as bupivacaine should be used as a component of multimodal analgesia (i.e., simultaneous use of a combination of analgesic agents and techniques that target different mechanisms) in the management of postoperative pain. (See Uses in the Local Anesthetics, Parenteral, General Statement 72:00.) Studies comparing the relative efficacy of liposomal bupivacaine and conventional bupivacaine hydrochloride for postsurgical analgesia have shown variable results; some studies demonstrated improved pain relief and reduced opiate requirements with the liposomal formulation, while other studies demonstrated only minimal or no substantial differences between the formulations.

Bupivacaine should *not* be used for obstetric paracervical block.

Bupivacaine hydrochloride has been used for IV regional anesthesia† in various orthopedic and general surgical procedures; however, high plasma concentrations of the drug may occur following tourniquet release, and cardiac arrest and death have resulted. Bupivacaine therefore should *not* be used for IV regional anesthesia.

Dosage and Administration

■ **Administration** Conventional bupivacaine hydrochloride preparations may be administered by local infiltration or by lumbar epidural (including caudal), peripheral, retrobulbar, sympathetic, or dental block. For spinal anesthesia, 0.75% bupivacaine hydrochloride in 8.25% dextrose is administered by subarachnoid injection. Bupivacaine liposomal injection (Exparel®) is administered by local infiltration or interscalene brachial plexus nerve block; the liposomal formulation should not be administered by epidural or intrathecal routes, and should not be used for other regional nerve blocks.

Local anesthetics, including bupivacaine, have been administered by continuous intra-articular infusion† (e.g., for control of postoperative pain); however, such use has been associated with chondrolysis. (See Cautions: Musculoskeletal Effects in the Local Anesthetics, Parenteral, General Statement 72:00.) Bupivacaine should not be administered using the Bier block technique (IV regional anesthesia) due to the risk of cardiac arrest and death.

Bupivacaine solutions containing preservatives should *not* be used for epidural or caudal block. Partially used solutions that do not contain preservatives should be discarded.

The liposomal formulation is not bioequivalent to and should not be used interchangeably with other bupivacaine formulations.

Liposomal Bupivacaine Bupivacaine liposomal injection (Exparel®) is commercially available in a 10- or 20-mL vial containing 13.3 mg/mL of bupivacaine in an aqueous suspension of multivesicular liposomes. The liposomal injection may be administered undiluted or diluted (if an increased volume of drug is necessary to cover a larger surgical area). If dilution is desired, the drug should be diluted with preservative-free 0.9% sodium chloride injection or lactated Ringer's injection up to a final concentration of 0.89 mg/mL (1:14 dilution by volume); sterile water for injection or other hypotonic solutions should not be used since disruption of the liposomal particles may occur. The diluted suspension should be used within 4 hours of preparation in a syringe. Any unused portions of the drug should be discarded.

Vials of liposomal bupivacaine should be inverted multiple times to resuspend the particles immediately prior to drug withdrawal. Liposomal bupivacaine should be administered using a 25-gauge or larger bore needle. The drug should not be filtered.

When liposomal bupivacaine is administered concomitantly with lidocaine (or other non-bupivacaine local anesthetic), immediate release of free (unencapsulated) bupivacaine may occur, potentially resulting in toxic plasma concentrations. Administration of liposomal bupivacaine should be delayed for at least 20 minutes after administration of lidocaine. The compatibility of liposomal bupivacaine and conventional bupivacaine hydrochloride is concentration dependent. The manufacturer states that bupivacaine hydrochloride and liposomal bupivacaine may be administered simultaneously in the same syringe, and bupivacaine hydrochloride may be injected immediately before liposomal bupivacaine as long as the ratio (based on mg dose) of conventional to liposomal drug does not exceed 1:2. The potential for additive toxic effects should be considered whenever these drugs are used concomitantly. Additional administration of local anesthetics should be avoided for at least 96 hours after liposomal bupivacaine is administered.

The manufacturer states that liposomal bupivacaine should not be allowed to come into contact with topical antiseptics (e.g., povidone iodine); the topical antiseptic should be allowed to dry before liposomal bupivacaine is administered.

Dispensing and Administration Precautions Local anesthetics should only be administered by clinicians experienced in the use and complications of these agents. Resuscitative equipment, oxygen, drugs, and personnel required for treatment of adverse reactions should be immediately available whenever bupivacaine is administered. For specific procedures and techniques of administration, specialized references should be consulted.

Bupivacaine should be administered slowly in incremental doses to reduce the risk of adverse effects (e.g., local anesthetic systemic toxicity). Frequent aspirations to check for blood or cerebrospinal fluid (when applicable) should be performed to avoid inadvertent intravascular administration and to either confirm entry into the subarachnoid space (for spinal anesthesia) or avoid inadvertent subarachnoid injection; however, a negative aspiration does not ensure protection against inadvertent intravascular or subarachnoid injection. During major regional nerve blocks, IV fluids should be administered via an indwelling catheter to ensure a functioning IV pathway. Injections into the head and neck area (e.g., retrobulbar, dental, or stellate ganglion blocks) require particular care since serious adverse effects have been reported due to complications from the anesthetic technique.

Because of similarity in appearance (milky white suspension) and use in similar healthcare settings, the potential exists for confusion between liposomal bupivacaine and propofol. If liposomal bupivacaine is mistaken for propofol, accidental IV administration of liposomal bupivacaine may occur, potentially causing substantial patient harm (e.g., cardiac arrhythmias and arrest). The Institute for Safe Medication Practices (ISMP) recommends that special precautions (e.g., proper labeling of syringes, storage segregation, routine double-checks) be taken to ensure that such confusion and "wrong route" administration errors do not occur. Instructions for the treatment of bupivacaine toxicity should be readily available in all surgical areas where liposomal bupivacaine is used.

■ **Dosage** Dosage of bupivacaine varies with the anesthetic procedure, degree of anesthesia required, surgical site, and individual patient response. The usual dosages should generally be reduced in geriatric, debilitated, or acutely ill patients and in patients with cardiac and/or hepatic disease. The lowest effective dose should be used.

Conventional Bupivacaine Conventional bupivacaine hydrochloride is commercially available in concentrations of 0.25, 0.5, or 0.75% with or without epinephrine. The appropriate concentration should be used based on the anesthetic technique and degree of muscle relaxation desired. Most experience to date with conventional bupivacaine hydrochloride is with single doses up to 175 mg without epinephrine or up to 225 mg with epinephrine 1:200,000, but individual patients and procedures may require more or less of the drug. Doses should not be repeated more frequently than every 3 hours and a maximum dose of 400 mg should not be exceeded in any 24-hour period; clinical experience with higher dosages is lacking. For most indications, a single dose is usually sufficient. Dosage recommendations given by the manufacturer are based on use of the drug in the average adult.

For infiltration anesthesia, 0.25% bupivacaine hydrochloride with or without epinephrine may be used.

Solutions of 0.25 or 0.5% bupivacaine hydrochloride with or without epinephrine and *containing no preservatives* are used for epidural or caudal anesthesia. For caudal block, the usual adult dose of bupivacaine hydrochloride is 15–30 mL of a 0.25 or 0.5% solution (37.5–150 mg). For epidural block (other than caudal block), the usual adult dose of bupivacaine hydrochloride is 10–20 mL of a 0.25 or 0.5% solution (25–100 mg); in obstetrics, incremental doses of 3–5 mL of the 0.5% solution, not exceeding 50–100 mg at any dosing interval, are recommended. To prevent intravascular or subarachnoid injection of a large epidural dose of bupivacaine hydrochloride, a test dose of anesthetic solution should be injected prior to administering the full dose and the patient should be monitored (e.g., pulse rate, blood pressure, signs of spinal block); when a continuous catheter technique is used, a test dose should be administered prior to each dose to ensure that the catheter has not been displaced. Each test dose should contain 10–15 mg of bupivacaine hydrochloride (or an equivalent dose of another local anesthetic) to detect inadvertent subarachnoid injection and, when clinical conditions permit, epinephrine (e.g., 10–15 mcg) to detect inadvertent intravascular injection. Solutions of 0.75% bupivacaine hydrochloride with or without epinephrine should be used for single dose epidural (but not caudal) anesthesia and may be given in a dose of 10–20 mL (75–150 mg) in adults; the 0.75% solution should *not* be used for obstetric anesthesia (see Cautions) and should be reserved for surgical procedures in which a high degree of muscle relaxation and prolonged effect are necessary. During epidural administration, the 0.5 and 0.75% solutions should be administered in incremental doses of 3–5 mL, with sufficient time between doses to detect toxic manifestations of inadvertent intravascular or intrathecal injection. Epidural injections should be made slowly with frequent aspirations.

For peripheral nerve block, bupivacaine hydrochloride 0.25 or 0.5% with or without epinephrine may be given in a dose of 5 mL (12.5–25 mg) up to a maximum of 400 mg in 24 hours in adults. For sympathetic nerve block, the usual adult dose of bupivacaine hydrochloride is 20–50 mL of a 0.25% solution (50–125 mg).

For retrobulbar anesthesia, the usual adult dose of bupivacaine hydrochloride with or without epinephrine is 2–4 mL of a 0.75% solution (15–30 mg).

Local injections into the head and neck area should be performed carefully and dosage recommendations should not be exceeded to minimize the risk of complications from the anesthetic technique.

For anesthesia in the maxillary and mandibular area when a longer duration of local anesthesia is desired (e.g., for oral surgery procedures generally associated with substantial postoperative pain), the usual adult dose of bupivacaine hydrochloride with epinephrine is 1.8 mL of a 0.5% solution (9 mg) per injection site; occasionally, a second dose of 1.8 mL (9 mg) per injection site may be necessary. Injections should be made slowly with frequent aspirations. The total dose of 0.5% bupivacaine hydrochloride solution for all injection sites spread out over a single dental sitting usually should not exceed 18 mL (90 mg) in healthy adults.

If the hyperbaric solution containing 0.75% bupivacaine hydrochloride in 8.25% dextrose is used for spinal anesthesia, an adult dose of 1 mL (7.5 mg) is generally sufficient for lower extremity and perineal procedures. For lower abdominal procedures, a dose of 1.6 mL (12 mg) may be used. For obstetrical spinal anesthesia in vaginal deliveries, doses as low as 0.8 mL (6 mg) have been used. For spinal anesthesia in cesarean section, doses of 1–1.4 mL (7.5–10.5 mg) have been used. Complete sensory and motor blockade are generally achieved with recommended doses of bupivacaine hydrochloride in dextrose injection for spinal anesthesia.

Liposomal Bupivacaine A single dose of up to 266 mg of liposomal bupivacaine is recommended in adults for local infiltration analgesia; the dose should be individualized based on the surgical site, volume of drug required to cover the area, and individual patient factors (e.g., physical status, presence of renal or hepatic impairment). In the bunionectomy study, a total dose of 106 mg (8 mL) was administered, with 7 mL infiltrated into the tissues surrounding the osteotomy and 1 mL infiltrated throughout the subcutaneous tissue. In the hemorrhoidectomy study, a single dose of 266 mg (20 mL of drug diluted with 10 mL of 0.9% sodium chloride injection) was administered; the total volume of 30 mL was divided into 5-mL increments and infiltrated into 6 sites in the perianal tissue using a standard anal block procedure with moving-needle technique.

If liposomal bupivacaine is used for interscalene brachial plexus nerve block, the recommended adult dose based on the study in patients undergoing total shoulder arthroplasty or rotator cuff repair is 133 mg (10 mL).

Cautions

■ **Precautions** Bupivacaine shares the toxic potentials of the local anesthetics, and the usual precautions of local anesthetic therapy should be observed. (See Cautions in the Local Anesthetics, Parenteral, General Statement 72:00.)

Adverse effects of bupivacaine generally are limited when administered locally at the recommended dosages and routes. However, excessive plasma concentrations can lead to systemic toxicity manifesting principally as CNS and cardiovascular effects.

The 0.75% solution of bupivacaine hydrochloride is not recommended for obstetric anesthesia since use of this concentration for epidural anesthesia in obstetric patients has been associated with cardiac arrest with difficult resuscitation or death. Cardiac arrest has occurred after seizures resulting from systemic toxicity, apparently following inadvertent intravascular injection.

Some commercially available formulations of bupivacaine hydrochloride contain sodium metabisulfite, a sulfite that may cause allergic-type reactions, including anaphylaxis and life-threatening or less severe asthmatic episodes, in certain susceptible individuals. The overall prevalence of sulfite sensitivity in the general population is unknown but probably low; such sensitivity appears to occur more frequently in asthmatic than in nonasthmatic individuals.

■ **Pediatric Precautions** Pending accumulation of further data on the use of the drug in pediatric patients, bupivacaine hydrochloride with or without epinephrine should not be used in children younger than 12 years of age and the hyperbaric bupivacaine hydrochloride in dextrose solution for spinal anesthesia should not be used in children younger than 18 years of age. Efficacy and safety of bupivacaine liposomal injection have not been established in pediatric patients.

Continuous infusions of bupivacaine in children have resulted in high plasma concentrations and seizures; high plasma concentrations also may be associated with adverse cardiovascular effects.

Pharmacokinetics

■ **Absorption** Bupivacaine has a long duration of action. Onset of anesthesia following administration of 0.5% solutions of bupivacaine hydrochloride for dental anesthesia occurs in about 2–10 minutes and duration of action is up to 7 hours in many patients. Onset of anesthesia following administration of 0.25 or 0.5% solutions of bupivacaine hydrochloride in epidural, including caudal block, and peripheral or sympathetic nerve block occurs in about 4–17 minutes and duration of action ranges from 3–7 hours. In epidural block, 0.75% solutions of bupivacaine hydrochloride produce a slightly shorter onset of action; duration of action may be from 6–9 hours. Although 0.25 and 0.5% solutions provide adequate sensory blockade in single doses, they do not produce complete muscle relaxation. If given by the continuous block method, however, repeat doses will increase the degree of motor block. The first repeat dose of 0.5% bupivacaine hydrochloride may give complete motor block. Single-dose epidural block with usual doses of 0.75% bupivacaine hydrochloride or single-dose intercostal nerve block with usual doses of a 0.25% solution may produce complete motor blockade which is necessary for abdominal surgery. In spinal anesthesia, a 0.75% solution of bupivacaine hydrochloride in 8.25% dextrose has an onset of sensory blockade within 1 minute and motor blockade and dermatome level are usually maximal within 15 minutes; the duration of sensory blockade averages 2 hours and complete return of motor ability averages 3.5 hours following a 12-mg dose. Epinephrine may prolong the duration of action of bupivacaine. The onset of action of liposomal bupivacaine is less than 2 minutes, which appears to be similar to conventional bupivacaine hydrochloride, and the duration of analgesic effect based on the principal efficacy studies appears to be no more than 24 hours.

Systemic absorption of bupivacaine (administered either as the conventional or liposomal formulation) is dependent on the total dose administered, route of administration, vascularity at the site of administration, and presence or absence of epinephrine in the formulation. After epidural or caudal administration of 125 or 150 mg of bupivacaine hydrochloride, peak plasma concentrations of 0.45–1.25 mcg/mL have been demonstrated. After administration of bupivacaine hydrochloride for caudal, epidural, or peripheral nerve block, peak blood bupivacaine concentrations occur within 30–45 minutes. Accumulation of the drug occurs with multiple doses; however, the long duration of bupivacaine hydrochloride anesthesia reduces the need for repeated doses. Following local infiltration of liposomal bupivacaine in patients undergoing bunionectomy or hemorrhoidectomy, peak plasma concentrations were 0.17 or 0.87 mcg/mL, respectively; following administration as an interscalene brachial plexus nerve block, peak plasma concentration was 0.21 mcg/mL. Systemic concentrations of liposomal bupivacaine can persist for up to 96 hours after local infiltration or up to 120 hours after interscalene brachial plexus nerve block; however, systemic concentrations are not correlated with local efficacy.

■ **Distribution** After absorption into the blood, bupivacaine hydrochloride is more highly bound to plasma proteins than are any other local anesthetics; bupivacaine is reportedly 82–96% bound. Bupivacaine hydrochloride has the lowest degree of placental transmission of parenteral local anesthetics and may cause the least fetal depression.

Distribution of liposomal bupivacaine is expected to be similar to that of other bupivacaine formulations after bupivacaine is released from the multivesicular liposome.

■ **Elimination** The elimination half-life of bupivacaine hydrochloride is 1.5–5.5 hours in adults and 8.1 hours in neonates. Bupivacaine hydrochloride is principally metabolized to pipecolylxylidine (PPX) by *N*-dealkylation, probably in the liver. Bupivacaine is excreted in urine as small amounts of PPX, unchanged drug (5%), and other metabolites as yet unidentified.

Elimination of liposomal bupivacaine is expected to be similar to that of other bupivacaine formulations after bupivacaine is released from the multivesicular liposome.

Chemistry and Stability

■ **Chemistry** Bupivacaine occurs as a 50:50 racemic mixture of the *R*- and *S*-enantiomers. Bupivacaine is a local anesthetic of the amide type with a long duration of action. The drug is commercially available as a conventional bupivacaine hydrochloride formulation or a liposomal formulation containing bupivacaine (as the free base) in a white to off-white preservative-free aqueous suspension of multivesicular liposomes. A hyperbaric solution of 0.75% bupivacaine hydrochloride in 8.25% dextrose injection also is commercially available for spinal anesthesia. Bupivacaine hydrochloride differs structurally from mepivacaine hydrochloride only in the substitution of a butyl group for the *N*-methyl group. Bupivacaine hydrochloride occurs as a white, odorless, crystalline powder and is freely soluble in water and in alcohol. The pK_a of bupivacaine hydrochloride is 8.1.

Commercially available solutions of bupivacaine hydrochloride have a pH of 4–6.5. Bupivacaine hydrochloride solutions that contain epinephrine bitartrate have a pH of 3.3–5.5. Bupivacaine hydrochloride solutions, with or without epinephrine, in multiple-dose vials may contain methylparaben 0.1% as a preservative. A hyperbaric solution for spinal anesthesia is commercially available and contains 0.75% bupivacaine hydrochloride in 8.25% dextrose. The hyperbaric solution has a pH of 4–6.5 and a specific gravity of 1.030–1.035 at 25°C and 1.03 at 37°C. Bupivacaine liposomal injection has a pH of 5.8–7.4.

■ **Stability** Bupivacaine hydrochloride solutions should be stored at 20–25°C; solutions containing epinephrine should be protected from light. Bupivacaine hydrochloride solutions should not be used if their color is pinkish or darker than slightly yellow or if a precipitate is present.

Bupivacaine hydrochloride solutions that do not contain epinephrine may be autoclaved at 15 PSI at 121°C for 15 minutes; solutions containing epinephrine should not be autoclaved. Hyperbaric solutions for spinal anesthesia should not be resterilized more than once. Liposomal bupivacaine should not be autoclaved.

Bupivacaine liposomal injection should be stored at 2–8°C prior to use; the drug should not be frozen or exposed to high temperatures (exceeding 40°C). Alternatively, intact vials of liposomal bupivacaine may be stored at room temperature (20–25°C) for up to 30 days; the drug should not be re-refrigerated once it has been stored at room temperature.

For further information on chemistry and stability, pharmacology, pharmacokinetics, uses, cautions, and dosage and administration of bupivacaine hydrochloride, see the Local Anesthetics, Parenteral, General Statement 72:00.

Preparations

Excipients in commercially available drug preparations may have clinically important effects in some individuals; consult specific product labeling for details.

Bupivacaine Hydrochloride

Parenteral		
Injection	0.25%*	**Bupivacaine Hydrochloride Injection**
		Marcaine®, Hospira
		Sensorcaine®, Fresenius Kabi
		Sensorcaine®-MPF, Fresenius Kabi
	0.5%*	**Bupivacaine Hydrochloride Injection**
		Marcaine®, Hospira
		Sensorcaine®, Fresenius Kabi
		Sensorcaine®-MPF, Fresenius Kabi
	0.75%*	**Bupivacaine Hydrochloride Injection**
		Marcaine®, Hospira
		Sensorcaine®-MPF, Fresenius Kabi

*available from one or more manufacturer, distributor, and/or repackager by generic (nonproprietary) name

Bupivacaine Hydrochloride in Dextrose

Parenteral		
Injection	0.75% in 8.25% Dextrose*	**Bupivacaine Hydrochloride in 8.25% Dextrose Injection Spinal**
		Marcaine® Spinal, Hospira

*available from one or more manufacturer, distributor, and/or repackager by generic (nonproprietary) name

Bupivacaine Liposomal

Parenteral		
Injectable suspension	13.3 mg (of bupivacaine) per mL (133 or 266 mg)	**Exparel®**, Pacira

Bupivacaine Hydrochloride Combinations

Parenteral		
Injection	0.25% with Epinephrine Bitartrate 1:200,000 (of epinephrine)*	**Bupivacaine Hydrochloride and Epinephrine Injection**
		Marcaine® with Epinephrine, Hospira
		Sensorcaine® with Epinephrine, Fresenius Kabi
		Sensorcaine®-MPF with Epinephrine, Fresenius Kabi
	0.5% with Epinephrine Bitartrate 1:200,000 (of epinephrine)*	**Bupivacaine Hydrochloride and Epinephrine Injection**
		Marcaine® with Epinephrine, Hospira
		Sensorcaine® with Epinephrine, Fresenius Kabi
		Sensorcaine®-MPF with Epinephrine, Fresenius Kabi
	0.75% with Epinephrine Bitartrate 1:200,000 (of epinephrine)	**Sensorcaine®-MPF with Epinephrine**, Fresenius Kabi

*available from one or more manufacturer, distributor, and/or repackager by generic (nonproprietary) name

†Use is not currently included in the labeling approved by the US Food and Drug Administration

Lidocaine Hydrochloride

Lignocaine Hydrochloride

■ Lidocaine hydochloride is an intermediate-acting local anesthetic of the amide type.

Uses

Lidocaine hydrochloride is used for infiltration anesthesia and for nerve block techniques including peripheral, sympathetic, epidural (including caudal), and spinal block anesthesia. Lidocaine has been administered intraperitoneally† for anesthesia of the peritoneum and pelvic viscera.

For use of lidocaine hydrochloride as an antiarrhythmic agent, see 24:04.04.

Dosage and Administration

■ **Administration** Lidocaine hydrochloride may be administered by infiltration or by epidural (including caudal) block, peripheral or sympathetic nerve block, and subarachnoid block. The manufacturers state that only the preservative-free, epinephrine-free 0.5% lidocaine injection should be used for IV regional anesthesia. Local anesthetics, including lidocaine hydrochloride, have been administered by continuous intra-articular infusion† (e.g., for control of postoperative pain); however, such use has been associated with chondrolysis.(See Cautions: Musculoskeletal Effects in the Local Anesthetics, Parenteral, General Statement 72:00.) Lidocaine hydrochloride solutions containing preservatives should *not* be used for spinal or epidural (including caudal) block. Partially used bottles of solutions that do not contain preservatives should be discarded.

Aspiration for blood should be performed prior to injection of lidocaine hydrochloride to avoid inadvertent intravascular administration; however, a negative aspiration does not ensure protection against inadvertent intravascular injection.

Local anesthetics should only be administered by clinicians who are experienced in the diagnosis and management of dose-related toxicities and other acute emergencies associated with these agents. Resuscitative equipment, oxygen, drugs, and personnel required for treatment of adverse reactions should be immediately available when lidocaine is administered. Proper positioning of the patient is extremely important in spinal anesthesia. For specific procedures and techniques of administration, specialized references should be consulted.

■ **Dosage** Dosage of lidocaine hydrochloride varies with the anesthetic procedure, the degree of anesthesia required, and individual patient response. The usual dosages should generally be reduced in children, geriatric patients, debilitated or acutely ill patients, and patients with cardiac and/or hepatic disease. The smallest dose and lowest concentration required to produce the desired effect should be used. Use of dilute solutions (i.e., 0.25–0.5%) and total dosages not to exceed 3 mg/kg are recommended for induction of IV regional anesthesia in children.

Single doses of lidocaine hydrochloride (for anesthesia other than spinal) should not exceed 4.5 mg/kg (or 300 mg) in healthy adults or 4.5 mg/kg in children younger than 10 years of age. When administered with epinephrine, lidocaine hydrochloride doses should not exceed 7 mg/kg (or 500 mg) in healthy adults or 7 mg/kg in children younger than 10 years of age. For spinal anesthesia, up to 100 mg of the drug may be given. For continuous epidural or caudal anesthesia, the maximum dose should not be repeated at intervals of less than 1.5 hours. When continuous lumbar or caudal epidural anesthesia is used for nonobstetric procedures, additional drug may be administered if necessary to attain adequate anesthesia. For paracervical block for nonobstetric and obstetric analgesia (including abortion), the maximum recommended dosage (200 mg) should not be repeated at intervals of less than 1.5 hours. For IV regional anesthesia in adults using a 0.5% solution without epinephrine, the dose administered should not exceed 4 mg/kg.

Solutions of 1–2% lidocaine hydrochloride with or without epinephrine and *containing no preservatives* are used for epidural or caudal anesthesia. To prevent intravascular or subarachnoid injection of a large epidural dose of lidocaine, a test dose (e.g., 2–3 mL of a 1.5% solution) of anesthetic solution should be injected at least 5 minutes prior to administering the total dose. When clinical conditions permit, use of a test dose solution that contains epinephrine (e.g., 10–15 mcg) should be considered to detect inadvertent intravascular injection. The test dose should be repeated if the patient is moved such that the epidural catheter may have been displaced. Rapid injection of a large, single dose through a catheter should be avoided; instead, the drug should be administered, when feasible, in fractional doses. In epidural anesthesia, 2–3 mL of the indicated solution is usually required for each dermatome to be anesthetized. In caudal block for production of obstetric analgesia or in epidural thoracic block, 20–30 mL of a 1% solution (200–300 mg) of the drug may be used. For surgical anesthesia with caudal block, 15–20 mL of a 1.5% solution (225–300 mg) is given. For epidural lumbar analgesia, the dose is 25–30 mL (250–300 mg) of a 1% solution, and for epidural lumbar anesthesia, the recommended dose is 15–20 mL of a 1.5% solution (225–300 mg) or 10–15 mL of a 2% solution (200–300 mg).

A solution of 5% lidocaine hydrochloride with 7.5% dextrose is used for spinal anesthesia in adults and adolescents 16 years of age or older. For obstetric low spinal or saddle-block anesthesia in a normal vaginal delivery, the dose is approximately 1 mL (50 mg). For cesarean section or deliveries which require intrauterine manipulations, 1.5 mL of the 5% solution (75 mg) may be given. For surgical anesthesia, 1.5–2 mL of the 5% solution (75–100 mg) may be administered.

The following doses of lidocaine hydrochloride have been suggested for various nerve blocks: brachial nerve block, 15–20 mL of a 1.5% solution (225–300 mg); dental nerve block, 1–5 mL of a 2% solution (20–100 mg); intercostal nerve block, 3 mL of a 1% solution (30 mg); paravertebral nerve block, 3–5 mL of a 1% solution (30–50 mg); pudendal nerve block (each side), 10 mL of a 1% solution (100 mg); and paracervical nerve block (each side) for obstetric analgesia, 10 mL of a 1% solution (100 mg). For sympathetic nerve blocks, the following doses may be used: cervical (stellate ganglion) nerve block, 5 mL of a 1% solution (50 mg), and lumbar nerve block, 5–10 mL of a 1% solution (50–100 mg). For percutaneous infiltration anesthesia, the dose of lidocaine hydrochloride is 1–60 mL of a 0.5 or 1% solution (5–300 mg). For IV regional anesthesia, 10–60 mL of a 0.5% solution (50–300 mg) may be employed.

For retrobulbar injection, 3–5 mL of a 4% sterile solution (120–200 mg) or 1.7–3 mg/kg is suggested; a portion of the dose is injected retrobulbarly and the remainder may be used to block the facial nerve.

For transtracheal injection, 2–3 mL of a 4% solution (80–120 mg) is administered rapidly. When both transtracheal injection and topical application (oropharyngeal spray) of a 4% solution are needed to achieve complete analgesia, the combined total dose of lidocaine hydrochloride administered by injection and by oropharyngeal spray should not exceed 5 mL of a 4% solution (200 mg) or 3 mg/kg.

Lidocaine hydrochloride with or without epinephrine is used for various dental procedures by infiltration injection or nerve block. In oral infiltration and/or mandibular block, initial doses of 1–5 mL of 2% lidocaine hydrochloride (20–100 mg) with epinephrine 1:100,000 are usually effective. If greater hemostasis is required, epinephrine 1:50,000 may be used. In children younger than 10 years of age, 0.9–1 mL of 2% lidocaine hydrochloride (18–20 mg) is adequate for a procedure involving 1 tooth (local infiltration), 2–3 teeth (maxillary infiltration), or teeth in an entire quadrant (mandibular block).

Cautions

Lidocaine hydrochloride shares the toxic potentials of local anesthetics, and the usual precautions of local anesthetic therapy should be observed. (See Cautions in the Local Anesthetics, Parenteral, General Statement 72:00.)

Some commercially available formulations of lidocaine hydrochloride contain sodium metabisulfite, a sulfite that may cause allergic-type reactions, including anaphylaxis and life-threatening or less severe asthmatic episodes, in certain susceptible individuals. The overall prevalence of sulfite sensitivity in the general population is unknown but probably low; such sensitivity appears to occur more frequently in asthmatic than in nonasthmatic individuals.

Serious adverse effects (e.g., seizures, coma, irregular heart beat, respiratory depression) have been reported following topical application of local anesthetics to the skin. These events have occurred following application of extemporaneously prepared topical preparations containing high concentrations of anesthetics for cosmetic procedures and following use for indications approved by the US Food and Drug Administration (FDA).

Life-threatening adverse effects (e.g., irregular heart beat, seizures, breathing difficulties, coma, death) may occur when topical anesthetics are applied to a large area of skin, when the area of application is covered with an occlusive dressing, if a large amount of topical anesthetic is applied, if the anesthetic is applied to irritated or broken skin, or if the skin temperature increases (from exercise or use of a heating pad). When applied in such a manner, the amount of anesthetic that is absorbed systemically is unpredictable and the plasma concentrations achieved may be high enough to cause life-threatening adverse effects.

Topical application of lidocaine 4% gel has been investigated to reduce discomfort during mammography. In this study, up to 30 g of lidocaine 4% gel was applied to a wide area of the chest (from the clavicles to the inferior costal margins and laterally to the midaxillary lines) and covered with an occlusive dressing; the gel was left on the skin for an average of 48 minutes and was removed 30–65 minutes before the first mammographic film. No serious adverse effects were reported in this study; however, the study was not large enough to evaluate whether uncommon but serious reactions could occur with such use. Patients should speak with their clinician if they are considering using a topical anesthetic before obtaining a mammogram.

When a topical anesthetic is needed for a procedure, use of a preparation approved by the FDA has been recommended. A preparation containing the lowest concentration of anesthetic likely to be effective should be used; a small amount of topical anesthetic should be applied to the affected area for the shortest period necessary for the desired effect. The patient should apply the topical preparation as directed by a clinician, and should not apply the topical preparation to broken or irritated skin.

Pharmacokinetics

When used for block or infiltration anesthesia without epinephrine, the onset of anesthesia of lidocaine hydrochloride is more rapid and the duration of action is longer than that of an equal dose of procaine hydrochloride. When used for lumbar epidural block, the duration of action of a 2% solution of lidocaine hydrochloride is about 100 minutes. In caudal block, the duration of a 1 or 2% solution of the drug is about 75–135 minutes. When used for spinal anesthesia, 1 mL of 5% lidocaine hydrochloride solution provides motor anesthesia for about 100 minutes and sensory anesthesia for an additional 40 minutes. Administration of 1.5–2 mL of 5% lidocaine hydrochloride solution provides spinal anesthesia for 2 hours. Lidocaine produces some vasodilation and epinephrine 1:200,000 to 1:100,000 may be added to slow vascular absorption and prolong duration of action of the anesthetic.

For information on absorption, distribution, and elimination of lidocaine hydrochloride, see Pharmacokinetics in Lidocaine Hydrochloride 24:04.04.

Chemistry and Stability

■ **Chemistry** Lidocaine hydochloride is a local anesthetic of the amide type with an intermediate duration of action. Lidocaine hydrochloride occurs as a white, odorless, crystalline powder having a slightly bitter taste. The drug is very soluble in water and in alcohol. The pK_a of lidocaine hydrochloride is 7.86.

Commercially available solutions of lidocaine hydrochloride have a pH of 5–7; sodium hydroxide and/or hydrochloric acid may have been added during manufacture of the solutions to adjust pH. Solutions containing epinephrine have a pH of 3.3–5.5 and may contain sodium metabisulfite as an antioxidant. Hyperbaric solutions for spinal anesthesia are commercially available and contain lidocaine hydrochloride 5% with dextrose 7.5%. Hyperbaric solutions containing lidocaine hydrochloride 5% have a pH of 5.5–7 and a specific gravity of 1.030–1.035.

■ **Stability** Lidocaine hydrochloride injections should be stored at a 20–25°C; solutions containing epinephrine should be protected from light.

Lidocaine hydrochloride solutions are highly resistant to acid or alkaline hydrolysis and can be autoclaved repeatedly; dental cartridges, however, should not be autoclaved because the closures used in the cartridges will not withstand autoclaving. Epinephrine-containing solutions are not stable to autoclaving. Since lidocaine solutions for spinal anesthesia contain dextrose, caramelization may occur with prolonged heating or, in some instances, with prolonged storage. The solutions for spinal anesthesia may be autoclaved at 15 PSI and 121°C for 15 minutes; these solutions should not be resterilized more than once. The solutions for spinal anesthesia should not be allowed to remain in the sterilizer any longer than necessary; solutions containing a precipitate should not be used.

For further information on chemistry and stability, pharmacology, pharmacokinetics, uses, cautions, and dosage and administration of lidocaine hydrochloride, see the Local Anesthetics, Parenteral, General Statement 72:00.

Preparations

Excipients in commercially available drug preparations may have clinically important effects in some individuals; consult specific product labeling for details.

Lidocaine Hydrochloride

Parenteral		
Injection	0.5%*	**Lidocaine Hydrochloride Injection**
		Xylocaine®, APP Pharmaceuticals
		Xylocaine®-MPF, APP Pharmaceuticals
	1%*	**Lidocaine Hydrochloride Injection**
		Xylocaine®, APP Pharmaceuticals
		Xylocaine®-MPF, APP Pharmaceuticals
	1.5%*	**Lidocaine Hydrochloride Injection**
		Xylocaine®-MPF, APP Pharmaceuticals
	2%*	**Lidocaine Hydrochloride Injection**
		Xylocaine®, APP Pharmaceuticals
		Xylocaine® Dental (available as dental cartridge), Dentsply
		Xylocaine®-MPF, APP Pharmaceuticals
	4%*	**Lidocaine Hydrochloride Injection**
		Xylocaine®-MPF Sterile Solution, APP Pharmaceuticals

*available from one or more manufacturer, distributor, and/or repackager by generic (nonproprietary) name

Lidocaine Hydrochloride in Dextrose

Parenteral		
Injection	5% Lidocaine Hydrochloride in 7.5% Dextrose*	**Lidocaine Hydrochloride Injection in Dextrose**

*available from one or more manufacturer, distributor, and/or repackager by generic (nonproprietary) name

Lidocaine Hydrochloride Combinations

Parenteral		
Injection	0.5% with Epinephrine 1:200,000*	**Lidocaine Hydrochloride and Epinephrine Injection**
		Xylocaine® with Epinephrine, APP Pharmaceuticals
	1% with Epinephrine 1:100,000*	**Lidocaine Hydrochloride and Epinephrine Injection**
		Xylocaine® with Epinephrine, APP Pharmaceuticals
	1% with Epinephrine 1:200,000	**Xylocaine®-MPF with Epinephrine**, APP Pharmaceuticals
	1.5% with Epinephrine 1:200,000*	**Lidocaine Hydrochloride and Epinephrine Injection**
		Xylocaine®-MPF with Epinephrine, APP Pharmaceuticals
	2% with Epinephrine 1:100,000*	**Lidocaine Hydrochloride and Epinephrine Injection**
		Xylocaine® with Epinephrine, APP Pharmaceuticals
	2% with Epinephrine 1:200,000*	**Lidocaine Hydrochloride and Epinephrine Injection**
		Xylocaine®-MPF with Epinephrine, APP Pharmaceuticals
	2% with Epinephrine Bitartrate 1:50,000 (of epinephrine)*	**Lidocaine Hydrochloride and Epinephrine Injection** (available as dental cartridge)
		Xylocaine® Dental (available as dental cartridge), Dentsply
	2% with Epinephrine Bitartrate 1:100,000 (of epinephrine)*	**Lidocaine Hydrochloride and Epinephrine Injection** (available as dental cartridge)
		Xylocaine® Dental (available as dental cartridge), Dentsply

*available from one or more manufacturer, distributor, and/or repackager by generic (nonproprietary) name

†Use is not currently included in the labeling approved by the US Food and Drug Administration

Ropivacaine Hydrochloride

■ Ropivacaine hydrochloride is a long-acting local anesthetic of the amide type.

Uses

■ **Local or Regional Anesthesia and Analgesia** Ropivacaine hydrochloride is used to produce local or regional anesthesia for surgery (including cesarean section) and for the management of acute pain (e.g., postoperative pain, labor pain). When used for postoperative pain, ropivacaine should be administered as a component of multimodal analgesia (i.e., simultaneous use of a combination of analgesic agents and techniques that target different mechanisms). (See Uses in the Local Anesthetics, Parenteral, General Statement 72:00.)

Efficacy of ropivacaine for surgical anesthesia has been evaluated in numerous studies in which the drug was administered as an epidural block for general surgery or cesarean section, or as a peripheral nerve block (e.g., brachial plexus block). Studies in patients undergoing general surgery demonstrated that epidural administration of ropivacaine hydrochloride in doses of 100–200 mg was effective in producing T10 sensory blockade with an onset of 5–13 minutes and duration of 3–5 hours; in general, higher doses produced a more profound block with a greater duration of effect. Studies in patients undergoing cesarean section demonstrated that epidural administration of ropivacaine hydrochloride 0.5% was effective in producing T6 sensory blockade with an onset of 11–26 minutes and duration of 1.7–3.2 hours; adequate muscle relaxation also was achieved during surgery. In several active-controlled studies using epidural ropivacaine hydrochloride 0.75% for cesarean section, median onset of a T6 block was 4–15 minutes. When used for brachial plexus block, the anesthetic efficacy of ropivacaine hydrochloride appeared to vary based on the concentration (0.5 or 0.75%) and anesthetic technique (e.g., supraclavicular versus axillary block) used.

Efficacy of ropivacaine hydrochloride for acute pain management has been evaluated in several studies using 0.2 or 0.25% concentrations of the drug in patients with labor pain or postoperative pain (after abdominal or orthopedic surgeries). When administered epidurally as a continuous infusion or intermittent injections for labor pain, ropivacaine provided adequate relief of pain and had a similar effect on neonatal outcomes as bupivacaine. When used to control postoperative pain after abdominal or orthopedic surgery, continuous epidural infusion of ropivacaine hydrochloride 0.2% for up to 72 hours produced adequate analgesia with only slight and nonprogressive motor blockade; in addition, a reduction in the need for rescue analgesics (e.g., morphine) was observed.

Efficacy of ropivacaine hydrochloride for local infiltration has been evaluated in studies using the 0.5% concentration of the drug to provide surgical anesthesia or postoperative analgesia; in these studies, use of ropivacaine resulted in lower pain scores and a reduction in analgesic consumption.

Compared with bupivacaine, ropivacaine generally has a similar onset and duration of sensory block, but a lower intensity and shorter duration of motor block. Ropivacaine appears to have a lower potential for CNS and cardiovascular toxicity than bupivacaine. (See Description.)

Ropivacaine should *not* be used for obstetrical paracervical block, retrobulbar block for ophthalmic surgery, or spinal anesthesia (subarachnoid block) because of insufficient data to support such uses. Ropivacaine also should *not* be used for IV regional anesthesia (Bier block) because of the lack of clinical experience and risk of toxicity.

Dosage and Administration

■ **Administration** Ropivacaine hydrochloride may be administered by epidural block, peripheral nerve block (e.g., brachial plexus block), or local infiltration. The manufacturer states that ropivacaine should *not* be used for obstetrical paracervical block, retrobulbar block, or spinal anesthesia (subarachnoid block), and should not be administered using the Bier block technique (IV regional anesthesia).

Local anesthetics, including ropivacaine, have been administered by continuous intra-articular infusion† (e.g., for control of postoperative pain); however, such use has been associated with chondrolysis. (See Cautions: Musculoskeletal Effects in the Local Anesthetics, Parenteral, General Statement 72:00.)

To prevent intravascular or subarachnoid injection of a large epidural dose of ropivacaine hydrochloride, a test dose (e.g., 3–5 mL of a short-acting local anesthetic solution containing epinephrine) should be injected prior to administering the total dose. When clinical conditions permit, use of a test dose solution that contains epinephrine should be considered to detect inadvertent intravascular injection. The test dose should be repeated if the epidural catheter is displaced. An adequate time for onset of anesthesia should be allowed following administration of each test dose.

Dispensing and Administration Precautions Local anesthetics should only be administered by clinicians who are experienced in the diagnosis and management of dose-related toxicities and other acute emergencies associated with these agents. Resuscitative equipment, oxygen, drugs, and personnel required for the treatment of adverse reactions should be immediately available whenever ropivacaine is administered. For specific procedures and techniques of administration, specialized references should be consulted.

Ropivacaine should be administered slowly in incremental doses to reduce the risk of adverse effects (e.g., local anesthetic systemic toxicity). Inadvertent administration of large volumes of local anesthetic into highly vascularized areas can result in high plasma concentrations and increase the potential for systemic toxicity. Frequent aspirations for blood or cerebrospinal fluid (when applicable) should be performed to avoid intravascular administration or inadvertent subarachnoid injection; however, a negative aspiration does not ensure protection against inadvertent intravascular or subarachnoid injection.

Patients should have a functioning IV line prior to receiving a major regional nerve block.

Injections into the head and neck area require particular care since serious adverse effects have been reported due to complications from the anesthetic technique.

■ **Dosage** Dosage of ropivacaine hydrochloride is expressed in terms of ropivacaine hydrochloride. Dosage of ropivacaine hydrochloride varies with the anesthetic procedure, degree of anesthesia required, surgical site, and individual patient response. The smallest dose and lowest concentration required to produce the desired effect should be used. Rapid administration of a large single dose should be avoided. The manufacturer's dosage recommendations are based on the expected average dosage range necessary to produce a successful block in adults and should be used as a general guideline.

Surgical Anesthesia For lumbar epidural anesthesia in general surgery, the recommended adult dose of ropivacaine hydrochloride is 15–30 mL of a 0.5% solution (75–150 mg), 15–25 mL of a 0.75% solution (113–188 mg), or 15–20 mL of a 1% solution (150–200 mg); onset of anesthesia is approximately 10–30 minutes and duration is approximately 2–6 hours depending on the dose administered. For thoracic epidural anesthesia in general surgery, the recommended adult dose of ropivacaine hydrochloride is 5–15 mL of a 0.5 or 0.75% solution (25–113 mg); onset of anesthesia is about 10–20 minutes depending on the dose administered.

For lumbar epidural anesthesia in cesarean section, the recommended adult dose of ropivacaine hydrochloride is 20–30 mL of a 0.5% solution (100–150 mg) or 15–20 mL of a 0.75% solution (113–150 mg); onset of anesthesia is approximately 10–25 minutes and duration is approximately 2–5 hours depending on the dose administered.

For major nerve blocks (e.g., brachial plexus block), the recommended adult dose of ropivacaine hydrochloride is 35–50 mL of a 0.5% solution (175–250 mg) or 10–40 mL of a 0.75% solution (75–300 mg); onset of anesthesia is approximately 10–30 minutes and duration is approximately 5–10 hours depending on the dose administered. Doses given for major nerve blocks must be adjusted based on the site of administration and patient status. A ropivacaine hydrochloride dose of 300 mg for brachial plexus block may result in plasma concentrations that approach the threshold for CNS toxicity and should be administered with caution. Supraclavicular brachial plexus blocks may be associated with a higher frequency of serious adverse reactions regardless of the local anesthetic used.

For production of a field block (e.g., minor nerve blocks and infiltration), the recommended adult dose of ropivacaine hydrochloride is 1–40 mL of a 0.5% solution (5–200 mg); onset of anesthesia is approximately 1–15 minutes and duration is approximately 2–6 hours depending on the dose administered.

Acute Pain Management For the management of labor pain, an initial lumbar epidural injection of 20–40 mg (10–20 mL of a 0.2% solution) is recommended in adults, followed by a continuous epidural infusion of 12–28 mg/hour (6–14 mL/hour of a 0.2% solution) or incremental epidural injections (top-ups) of 20–30 mg/hour (10–15 mL/hour of a 0.2% solution). Following administration of the initial dose, onset of anesthesia is approximately 10–15 minutes and duration is approximately 0.5–1.5 hours.

For the management of postoperative pain in adults, a continuous lumbar or thoracic epidural infusion of ropivacaine hydrochloride at a rate of 12–28 mg/hour (6–14 mL/hour of a 0.2% solution) is recommended. In clinical studies, epidural infusions of the drug were administered for up to 72 hours. For local infiltration analgesia (e.g., minor nerve block) in the management of postoperative pain, the recommended adult dose of ropivacaine hydrochloride is 1–100 mL of a 0.2% solution (2–200 mg) or 1–40 mL of a 0.5% solution (5–200 mg). Onset of analgesia is approximately 1–5 minutes and duration is approximately 2–6 hours depending on the dose administered.

■ **Special Populations** The possibility of increased toxicity should be considered in patients with severe hepatic or renal impairment, and dosage of ropivacaine hydrochloride should be adjusted accordingly.

The usual dosages of ropivacaine hydrochloride generally should be reduced in geriatric, debilitated, or acutely ill patients. Caution should be exercised when the drug is administered for prolonged periods (e.g., greater than 70 hours) in debilitated patients because of the risk of reaching a toxic plasma concentration or inducing local neural injury. (See Geriatric Use under Warnings/Precautions: Specific Populations, in Cautions.)

Cautions

■ **Contraindications** Known hypersensitivity to ropivacaine hydrochloride or other local anesthetics of the amide type.

■ **Warnings/Precautions** ***Warnings*** Ropivacaine hydrochloride shares the toxic potentials of the local anesthetics, and the usual precautions of local anesthetic therapy should be observed. (See Cautions in the Local Anesthetics, Parenteral, General Statement 72:00.)

Administration Precautions. Because of the potential for serious adverse effects, special precautions should be taken during administration of ropivacaine. (See Dosage and Administration: Administration.) Oxygen, resuscitative equipment, drugs, and personnel required for the treatment of adverse reactions should be immediately available. A delay in the proper management of dose-related toxicities may result in acidosis, cardiac arrest, and possibly death.

Risk of Chondrolysis Associated with Intra-articular Infusions of Local Anesthetics. Chondrolysis (necrosis and destruction of articular cartilage) has been reported in patients receiving continuous intra-articular infusions of local anesthetics for treatment of postoperative pain. In most reported cases, chondrolysis occurred in the shoulder joint following arthroscopic or other shoulder surgery. (See Cautions in the Local Anesthetics, Parenteral, General Statement 72:00.)

Accidental Injection. Accidental intravascular or subarachnoid injection of ropivacaine may cause cardiac and CNS toxicity. Cardiac arrests have been reported rarely following unintentional accidental intravascular administration of the drug and were observed mostly in geriatric patients and in those with concomitant heart disease. (See Cardiovascular Effects and also see CNS Effects under Warnings/Precautions: Other Warnings and Precautions, in Cautions.) Clinical pharmacology studies and animal studies suggest that the cardiotoxic potential of ropivacaine is less than that of bupivacaine, although both drugs are substantially more toxic than lidocaine. Serious adverse effects were not observed in clinical studies that were performed to evaluate the safety of ropivacaine injected into the subarachnoid space.

Aspiration should be performed prior to administration of ropivacaine to avoid intravascular or subarachnoid injection; however, a negative aspiration does not ensure against an intravascular or subarachnoid injection.

Sensitivity Reactions Although rare, allergic-type reactions have been reported with ropivacaine and may include manifestations such as urticaria, pruritus, erythema, angioedema (including laryngeal edema), tachycardia, sneezing, nausea, vomiting, dizziness, syncope, excessive sweating, elevated temperature, and possibly anaphylactoid symptoms (including severe hypotension).

Cross-hypersensitivity between ropivacaine and other amide-type local anesthetics has been reported. (See Cautions: Contraindications.)

Other Warnings and Precautions **CNS Effects.** Ropivacaine can cause adverse CNS effects if absorbed systemically. (See Cautions in the Local Anesthetics, Parenteral, General Statement 72:00.) Restlessness, anxiety, incoherent speech, lightheadedness, numbness and tingling of the mouth and lips, metallic taste, tinnitus, dizziness, blurred vision, tremors, twitching, depression, or drowsiness may be early warning signs of CNS toxicity. Prolonged blocks can increase the risk of toxic plasma concentrations or induce local neural injury. Administration of 300 mg of ropivacaine hydrochloride for brachial plexus block may increase the risk of CNS toxicity.

Patients should be carefully monitored for possible CNS toxicity after administration of ropivacaine.

Cardiovascular Effects. Ropivacaine can cause adverse cardiovascular effects (e.g., decreased cardiac output, arrhythmias, reduced myocardial contractility and conductivity) if absorbed systemically. (See Cautions in the Local Anesthetics, Parenteral, General Statement 72:00.)

Patients should be carefully monitored for possible cardiovascular toxicity and vital signs should be obtained after administration of the local anesthetic. If cardiac arrest occurs, prolonged resuscitative efforts may be required. Ropivacaine should be used with caution in patients with impaired cardiovascular function, hypotension, hypovolemia, or heart block.

Familial Malignant Hyperthermia. Many drugs used during the conduct of anesthesia may trigger familial malignant hyperthermia, but it is not known whether amide-type local anesthetics such as ropivacaine can trigger this reaction. Therefore, a standard protocol for familial malignant hyperthermia management should be available.

Specific Populations **Pregnancy.** Category B.

There are no adequate and well-controlled studies of ropivacaine in pregnant women. Animal reproductive studies have not shown any evidence of teratogenicity or adverse developmental effects; however, maternal toxicity has been observed. Local anesthetics rapidly cross the placenta during epidural administration and can cause varying degrees of maternal, fetal, and neonatal toxicity. Ropivacaine should be used during pregnancy only if the benefits outweigh the risks.

Maternal hypotension has occurred with the use of ropivacaine for obstetrical pain relief. (See Cautions in the Local Anesthetics, Parenteral, General Statement 72:00.)

Lactation. Ropivacaine is distributed into milk in rats; it is not known whether the drug or its metabolites are distributed into human milk. Based on the milk to plasma concentration ratio and estimated exposures in rats, infant exposure to ropivacaine from breastfeeding is expected to be far less than the exposure in utero. Ropivacaine should be used with caution in nursing women.

Pediatric Use. The manufacturer states that efficacy and safety of ropivacaine have not been established in pediatric patients; however, the drug has been used in children for postoperative analgesia.

Geriatric Use. In clinical studies of ropivacaine, 27% of patients receiving the drug were 65 years of age or older and 4% were 75 years of age or older. The drug was found to be safe and effective in these patients.

Differences in various pharmacodynamic measures of ropivacaine have been observed with increasing age. In one clinical study, the upper level of analgesia increased with age, the maximum decrease of mean arterial pressure declined with age for the first hour following epidural administration, and the intensity of motor blockade increased with age.

Because ropivacaine and its metabolites are substantially excreted by the kidneys, the risk of toxic reactions to the drug may be greater in patients with renal impairment. Dosage should therefore be selected with caution in geriatric patients, usually starting at the lower end of the dosage range, since such patients are more likely to have decreased hepatic, renal, and/or cardiac function as well as concomitant illnesses. The manufacturer states that it may be useful to monitor renal function in geriatric patients.

Hepatic Impairment. Ropivacaine is extensively metabolized in the liver and should be used with caution in patients with hepatic impairment, particularly in those receiving repeat doses of the drug. Patients with severe hepatic impairment are at greater risk of developing toxic plasma concentrations.

Renal Impairment. Ropivacaine and its metabolites are eliminated by the kidneys; therefore, patients with renal impairment may be at increased risk of drug-related toxicity.

■ **Common Adverse Effects** Adverse effects reported in 5% or more of patients receiving ropivacaine hydrochloride in clinical studies include hypotension, nausea, vomiting, bradycardia, fever, pain, postoperative complications, anemia, paresthesia, headache, pruritus, and back pain.

Drug Interactions

No formal drug interaction studies have been performed to date with ropivacaine hydrochloride.

■ **Drugs Affecting or Affected by Hepatic Microsomal Enzymes** Ropivacaine is metabolized to its major metabolite (3-hydroxyropivacaine) by cytochrome P-450 (CYP) isoenzyme 1A2. Potent inhibitors of CYP1A2, such as fluvoxamine, can increase plasma ropivacaine concentrations when administered concomitantly. When ropivacaine was coadministered with fluvoxamine (25 mg twice daily for 2 days), plasma clearance of ropivacaine was reduced by 70%. Caution should be exercised when ropivacaine is administered concomitantly with CYP1A2 inhibitors. There also is a possibility that drugs known to be metabolized by CYP1A2 (e.g., theophylline, imipramine) can interact with ropivacaine via competitive inhibition.

When ropivacaine was administered 1 hour after ketoconazole (100 mg twice daily for 2 days), a selective and potent inhibitor of CYP3A4, a 15% reduction in plasma clearance of ropivacaine was observed; however, the effect was not clinically important. When ropivacaine was coadministered with rifampin, an inducer of CYP3A4, plasma clearance of ropivacaine was increased by 93%.

■ **Antiarrhythmic Agents** Concomitant use of class III antiarrhythmic agents (e.g., amiodarone) with ropivacaine has not been studied, but may result in additive cardiac effects; the manufacturer recommends close surveillance and to consider ECG monitoring.

■ **Local Anesthetics** Caution is advised when ropivacaine is used with other local anesthetics or drugs that are structurally related to amide-type local anesthetics because the toxic effects of these drugs are additive.

Description

Ropivacaine hydrochloride is a long-acting local anesthetic of the amino amide class. Local anesthetics block the generation and conduction of nerve impulses possibly by increasing the threshold for electrical excitation, slowing the propagation of the nerve impulse, and reducing the rate of rise of the action potential. Progression of anesthesia is related to the diameter, myelination, and conduction velocity of affected nerve fibers. Unlike most other local anesthetics, the addition of epinephrine has no substantial effect on the onset time or duration of ropivacaine. The onset, depth, and duration of sensory block with ropivacaine are generally similar to bupivacaine; however, the depth and duration of motor block are less than bupivacaine.

Ropivacaine is structurally related to bupivacaine; however, unlike bupivacaine, which exists in its racemic form, ropivacaine is an *S*-enantiomer. Ropivacaine is less lipophilic and less likely to penetrate large myelinated nerve fibers than bupivacaine. These physiochemical and stereoselective differences are thought to contribute to the lower cardiac and CNS toxicity of ropivacaine compared with bupivacaine.

Advice to Patients

Importance of advising patients of the possibility of temporary loss of sensation and motor activity following lumbar epidural anesthesia.

Importance of informing clinicians of existing or contemplated therapy, including prescription and OTC drugs, as well as any concomitant illnesses (e.g., cardiovascular disease).

Importance of women informing clinicians if they are or plan to become pregnant or plan to breast-feed.

Importance of informing patients of other important precautionary information. (See Cautions.)

Overview® (see Users Guide). For additional information on this drug until a more detailed monograph is developed and published, the manufacturer's labeling should be consulted. It is *essential* that the manufacturer's labeling be consulted for more detailed information on usual cautions, precautions, contraindications, potential drug interactions, laboratory test interferences, and acute toxicity.

Preparations

Excipients in commercially available drug preparations may have clinically important effects in some individuals; consult specific product labeling for details.

Ropivacaine Hydrochloride

Parenteral		
Injection	0.2%*	**Naropin®**, Fresenius Kabi **Ropivacaine Hydrochloride Injection**
	0.5%*	**Naropin®**, Fresenius Kabi **Ropivacaine Hydrochloride Injection**
	0.75%*	**Naropin®**, Fresenius Kabi **Ropivacaine Hydrochloride Injection**
	1%*	**Naropin®**, Fresenius Kabi **Ropivacaine Hydrochloride Injection**

*available from one or more manufacturer, distributor, and/or repackager by generic (nonproprietary) name

†Use is not currently included in the labeling approved by the US Food and Drug Administration

76:00 OXYTOCICS

§ Omitted from the print version of *AHFS Drug Information®* because of space limitations. This monograph is available on the *AHFS Drug Information®* website, http://ahfsdruginformation.com. Username: ahfs2020; Password: ASHP94498.

OXYTOCICS 76:00

Oxytocin

■ Oxytocin, a nonapeptide hormone secreted by the neurons of the supraoptic and paraventricular nuclei of the hypothalamus and stored in the posterior pituitary (neurohypophysis) in mammals, indirectly stimulates contraction of uterine smooth muscle.

Uses

■ **Antepartum Uses** IV infusion of dilute solutions of oxytocin is the method of choice for inducing labor at term and stimulating uterine contractions during the first and second stages of labor.

Induction of Labor Induction of labor with oxytocin infusion is indicated in term or near-term pregnancies associated with hypertension (e.g., preeclampsia, eclampsia, cardiovascular-renal disease), erythroblastosis fetalis, maternal or gestational diabetes mellitus, antepartum bleeding, or preterm, premature rupture of the membranes in which spontaneous labor does not ensue. Routine induction of labor with oxytocin may be indicated in prolonged pregnancies (greater than 42 weeks' gestation). *Elective induction of labor merely for physician or patient convenience is not a valid indication for oxytocin use.* In patients with eclampsia, if delivery is not imminent within 12 hours following an initial oxytocin infusion, some clinicians recommend cesarean section be done rather than continue administration of oxytocin.

Induction of labor also may be indicated in cases of uterine fetal death, fetal growth retardation, or static or decreasing maternal weight. However, in cases of missed abortion, intrauterine fetal death in late pregnancy, benign hydatidiform mole, or fetuses with anencephaly or erythroblastosis fetalis with hydrops or other congenital abnormalities incompatible with life, some clinicians recommend intravaginal dinoprostone because oxytocin may be relatively ineffective.

Pelvic adequacy and other maternal and fetal conditions (including fetal lung maturity) must be evaluated carefully whenever induction of labor is considered. Oxytocin should not be used to induce labor when the benefit-to-risk ratio for the mother or child favors surgical intervention. Induction of labor is contraindicated in cases of cephalopelvic disproportion, unfavorable fetal position or presentation (e.g., transverse lies), uterine or cervical scarring from previous cesarean section or major cervical or uterine surgery, fetal distress when delivery is not imminent, unengaged fetal head, when vaginal delivery is contraindicated (e.g., total placenta previa, vasa previa, cord presentation or prolapse, active genital herpes infection), or when uterine activity fails to progress adequately. Except in unusual circumstances requiring the clinician's judgment, the manufacturers warn that labor generally should not be induced with oxytocin when pregnancy is complicated by fetal distress, hydramnios, partial placenta previa, prematurity, borderline cephalopelvic disproportion, previous major surgery of the cervix or uterus (including cesarean section), overdistension of the uterus, grand multiparity, invasive cervical carcinoma, or history of uterine sepsis or traumatic delivery. Oxytocin should not be administered for prolonged periods in cases of severe toxemia.

Augmentation of Labor During the first and second stages of labor, IV oxytocin infusion may be used to augment contractions if labor is prolonged or if dysfunctional uterine inertia occurs. Use of oxytocin is not recommended when labor is progressing normally during the first and second stages or when hypertonic patterns of labor occur, especially since response to the drug may be accentuated during the second stage of labor. In cases of uterine inertia, the drug should not be administered for prolonged periods (usually not more than 6–8 hours). Oxytocin should not be used to augment labor when vaginal delivery is contraindicated (e.g., total placenta previa).

■ **Postpartum Uses** Oxytocin infusions have been used to shorten the third stage of labor immediately following delivery of the infant (when the absence of additional fetuses is established), but some clinicians warn that oxytocics may inhibit, rather than assist in, expulsion of the placenta and increase the risk of hemorrhage and infection. If an oxytocic is used for this purpose, however, most clinicians recommend oxytocin.

Infusion of oxytocin is routinely used postpartum or following cesarean section to stimulate immediate contractions of the uterus and to control uterine bleeding. However, for the management of postpartum hemorrhage and uterine atony, most clinicians prefer ergonovine or methylergonovine to oxytocin unless an immediate contractile response is desired, because the amine ergot alkaloids produce more sustained contractions and higher uterine tonus than does oxytocin. Some clinicians prefer to manage postpartum bleeding with dilute IV oxytocin followed by an amine ergot alkaloid administered IM.

■ **Other Uses of Parenteral Oxytocin** Oxytocin infusion has been used following prostaglandin or hypertonic abortifacients to shorten the induction-to-abortion time when these abortifacients are being used to induce second trimester abortions, to induce abortion when a patient has failed to respond to the abortifacient, or to induce abortion after membranes have ruptured. Oxytocin also has been used as an adjunct in cases of incomplete abortion when the placenta fails to abort spontaneously within 1 hour after abortion of the fetus; however, some clinicians maintain that oxytocin may hinder rather than assist in expulsion of the placenta. Because concurrent use of oxytocin with abortifacients may produce uterine contractions of such intensity that uterine rupture or cervical laceration may be more likely to occur, oxytocin usually should not be administered until the oxytocic effect of the abortifacient has subsided, and patients should be carefully monitored. Oxytocin, however, is routinely used in conjunction with hypertonic urea- and dinoprostone-induced abortions.

Oxytocin infusion has been used with success to evaluate the adequacy of fetal respiratory capabilities in high-risk pregnancies of greater than 31 weeks gestation†. By inducing uterine contractions, oxytocin transiently impedes uterine blood flow. If placental reserve is low, a late deceleration in fetal heart rate may occur following oxytocin administration, indicating chronic hypoxia (positive response). If fetal heart rate is unchanged (negative response) by the oxytocin challenge, adequate placental support is probably available. The test should be repeated in 1 week to reassess fetal response. A positive response indicates that there may be fetal distress and may be an indication for termination of pregnancy, especially if a lecithin-sphingomyelin ratio of greater than 1.5 can be demonstrated.

Dosage and Administration

■ **Administration** As an oxytocic, oxytocin should be given by IV infusion using a controlled-infusion device. Although oxytocin has been given IM, most clinicians believe this route of administration should *not* be used for augmentation or induction of labor because the effects it produces are unpredictable and difficult to control.

Prior to IV administration, the commercially available injection *must* be diluted. Generally, oxytocin infusions containing 10 milliunits/mL are used for induction or augmentation of labor. This solution may be prepared by adding 10 units (1 mL of the commercially available injection) to 1 L of 0.9% sodium chloride, lactated Ringer's, or 5% dextrose injection. Except under unusual circumstances, a physiologic electrolyte solution preferably should be used for preparing IV infusions of the drug intended for use in the induction or augmentation of labor. Infusions containing 20 milliunits/mL are used to produce intense uterine contractions and reduce postpartum bleeding, and as adjuncts to prostaglandin or hypertonic abortifacients. This solution may be prepared by adding 10 units (1 mL of the commercially available injection) to 500 mL of one of the above IV infusion solutions.

■ **Dosage** ***Antepartum Uses*** Oxytocin dosage and rate of infusion are determined by uterine response. The drug should be discontinued if prolonged uterine contractions (greater than 90 seconds in duration) or rising intrauterine pressure occur or if uterine motility interferes with fetal heart rate; in addition, oxygen should be administered to the mother, who preferably should be in the lateral position, and other appropriate measures taken as necessary. For induction of labor, oxytocin usually is infused at an initial rate of

0.5–1 milliunit/minute. The infusion rate generally is increased in 1- to 2-milliunit/minute increments at 30- to 60-minute intervals until a response is observed. When the desired frequency of contractions is established (a uterine pattern comparable to spontaneous labor), without evidence of fetal distress, and labor has progressed to 5–6 cm dilation, the rate of oxytocin infusion may be reduced by similar increments. IV infusion rates up to 6 milliunits/minute have been shown to produce oxytocin concentrations in maternal plasma comparable to those associated with spontaneous labor. At term, higher rates of infusion should be employed with caution, and rates exceeding 9–10 milliunits/minute rarely are required. Before term, when uterine sensitivity to oxytocin is reduced secondary to decreased oxytocin receptors, higher infusion rates may be necessary.

Postpartum Uses To produce intense uterine contractions and reduce postpartum bleeding after expulsion of the placenta, a total of 10 units of oxytocin may be infused at a rate of 20–40 milliunits/minute after delivery of the infant(s) (when the absence of additional fetuses is established); rate is adjusted to maintain uterine contraction and control uterine atony. Most clinicians recommend that oxytocin not be given until after delivery of the placenta.

Other Uses of Parenteral Oxytocin When used to shorten the induction-to-abortion time, to induce abortion in patients who have failed to abort following administration of second trimester abortifacients, or to induce abortion after membranes have ruptured, IV oxytocin infusions of 10–100 milliunits/minute have been used. However, it is recommended that cumulative dose in a 12-hour period not exceed 30 units because of the risk of water intoxication.

To evaluate fetal distress† using the oxytocin challenge test, 5–10 units of oxytocin (0.5–1.0 mL of the commercially available injection) is diluted with 1 L of 5% dextrose injection; the resultant solution contains 5–10 milliunits/mL. Initially the drug is infused IV in the mother at a rate of 0.5 milliunits/minute. The infusion rate may be gradually increased at 15- to 30-minute intervals to a maximum of 20 milliunits/minute. Fetal heart rate and uterine contractions should be monitored immediately before and during the oxytocin infusion. When 3 moderate uterine contractions occur within one 10-minute interval, the infusion should be discontinued and baseline and oxytocin-induced fetal heart rates should be compared. If no change in fetal heart rate occurs, the test should be repeated in 1 week. If a late deceleration in fetal heart rate occurs, termination of the pregnancy may be indicated.

Cautions

■ Adverse Effects When oxytocin is administered in excessive dosage, with abortifacients or to sensitive patients, hyperstimulation of the uterus, with strong (hypertonic) and/or prolonged (tetanic) contractions, or a resting uterine tone of 15–20 mm H_2O between contractions may occur, possibly resulting in uterine rupture, cervical and vaginal lacerations, postpartum hemorrhage, abruptio placentae, impaired uterine blood flow, amniotic fluid embolism, and fetal trauma including intracranial hemorrhage. Increased uterine motility also may cause adverse fetal effects, including sinus bradycardia, tachycardia, premature ventricular complexes and other arrhythmias, permanent CNS or brain damage, and death secondary to asphyxia. Excessive maternal dosage or administration of the drug to sensitive women also can cause uteroplacental hypoperfusion and variable deceleration of fetal heart rate, fetal hypoxia, perinatal hepatic necrosis, and fetal hypercapnia. Rare incidents of pelvic hematoma have been reported, but these were probably also related to the high incidence of operative vaginal deliveries in primiparas, the fragility of engorged pelvic veins (especially if varicosed), and faulty episiotomy repair.

When large amounts of oxytocin are administered, severe decreases in maternal systolic and diastolic blood pressure, increases in heart rate, systemic venous return and cardiac output, and arrhythmia may occur; these effects may be particularly hazardous to patients with valvular heart disease and those receiving spinal and epidural anesthesia.

Postpartum bleeding may be increased by administration of oxytocin; this effect may be related to reports of oxytocin-induced thrombocytopenia, afibrinogenemia, and hypoprothrombinemia. By carefully controlling delivery, the incidence of postpartum bleeding may be minimized.

Nausea, vomiting, maternal sinus bradycardia, and premature ventricular complexes reported in patients receiving oxytocin are probably related to labor and not the drug. The risk of neonatal hyperbilirubinemia appears to be about 1.6 times greater following oxytocin-induced labor than that following spontaneous labor, and neonatal jaundice has occurred. Other adverse neonatal effects from oxytocin-induced labor include retinal hemorrhage and low Apgar scores at 5 minutes.

Severe water intoxication with seizures, coma, and death has been reported following prolonged IV infusion of oxytocin with an excessive volume of fluid. Neonatal seizures also have been reported. Injudicious use of oxytocin has also resulted in maternal deaths secondary to hypertensive episodes and subarachnoid hemorrhage.

Anaphylactic and other allergic reactions have occurred in patients receiving oxytocin and may rarely be fatal.

■ Precautions and Contraindications Parenteral oxytocin should be used only by qualified professional personnel in a hospital where intensive care and surgical facilities are immediately available. During administration of oxytocin, uterine contractions, fetal and maternal heart rate, maternal blood pressure, and, if possible, intrauterine pressure should be continuously monitored to avoid complications. If uterine hyperactivity occurs, oxytocin administration should be immediately discontinued; oxytocin-induced stimulation of uterine contractions usually decreases soon after discontinuance of the drug. Electronic monitoring of the fetus is the best method for early detection of oxytocin overdosage. However, accurate measurement of intrauterine pressure during contractions requires intrauterine pressure recording. Determination of fetal heart rate via a fetal scalp electrode is more dependable than via external monitoring.

Since oxytocin may produce some antidiuretic effects, some clinicians recommend restricting fluid intake, avoiding administration of low-sodium infusion fluids and high oxytocin doses for prolonged periods, and monitoring fluid intake and output during administration of the drug.

Oxytocin should not be given simultaneously by more than one route of administration. Oxytocin is contraindicated in patients with a history of hypersensitivity to the drug. *For additional discussion on the precautions and contraindications associated with oxytocin, see Uses.*

■ Mutagenicity and Carcinogenicity The mutagenic and carcinogenic potentials of oxytocin have not been determined.

■ Pregnancy, Fertility, and Lactation Animal reproduction studies have not been performed with oxytocin; however, the manufacturers state that the drug is not indicated for use during the first or second trimester of pregnancy other than in relation to spontaneous or induced abortion. Based on wide experience with oxytocin and on its chemical and pharmacologic properties, the drug would not be expected to cause fetal abnormalities when used as indicated. Oxytocin can, however, cause nonteratogenic adverse effects. (See Cautions: Adverse Effects.)

It is not known whether oxytocin affects fertility.

Oxytocin may be distributed in small quantities into milk. If oxytocin therapy is required postpartum (e.g., to control severe bleeding), commencement of nursing should be delayed for at least 1 day after the drug has been discontinued.

Drug Interactions

Severe hypertension has been reported when oxytocin was given 3–4 hours following prophylactic administration of a vasoconstrictor in conjunction with caudal block anesthesia. Cyclopropane anesthesia may modify oxytocin's cardiovascular effects, producing less pronounced tachycardia but more severe hypotension than occurs with oxytocin alone; maternal sinus bradycardia with abnormal atrioventricular rhythms has been noted when oxytocin was used concomitantly with cyclopropane anesthesia. Oxytocin reportedly has delayed induction of thiopental (no longer commercially available in the US) anesthesia by producing venous spasm that caused peripheral pooling of thiopental; however, this interaction has not been conclusively established.

Pharmacology

Exogenous oxytocin elicits all the pharmacologic responses usually produced by endogenous oxytocin.

Oxytocin indirectly stimulates contraction of uterine smooth muscle by increasing the sodium permeability of uterine myofibrils. High estrogen concentrations lower the threshold for uterine response to oxytocin. Uterine response to oxytocin increases with the duration of pregnancy and is greater in patients who are in labor than those not in labor; only very large doses elicit contractions in early pregnancy. Contractions produced in the term uterus by oxytocin are similar to those occurring during spontaneous labor. In the term uterus, oxytocin increases the amplitude and frequency of uterine contractions which in turn tend to decrease cervical activity producing dilation and effacement of the cervix and to transiently impede uterine blood flow.

Oxytocin contracts myoepithelial cells surrounding the alveoli of the breasts, forcing milk from the alveoli into the larger ducts and thus facilitating milk ejection. The drug possesses no galactopoietic properties.

Oxytocin produces vasodilation of vascular smooth muscle, increasing renal, coronary, and cerebral blood flow. Blood pressure is usually unchanged, but following IV administration of very large doses or undiluted solutions, blood pressure may decrease transiently, and tachycardia and an increase in cardiac output may be reflexly induced. Any initial fall in blood pressure is usually followed by a small but sustained increase in blood pressure.

In contrast to vasopressin, oxytocin has minimal antidiuretic effects; however, water intoxication may occur when oxytocin is administered with an excessive volume of electrolyte-free IV fluids and/or at too rapid a rate.

Pharmacokinetics

■ Absorption Oxytocin is destroyed by chymotrypsin in the GI tract. Uterine response occurs almost immediately and subsides within 1 hour following IV administration of oxytocin. Following IM injection of the drug, uterine response occurs within 3–5 minutes and persists for 2–3 hours. Following intranasal application of 10–20 units of oxytocin (nasal preparations are no longer commercially available in the US), contractions of myoepithelial tissue surrounding the alveoli of the breasts begin within a few minutes and continue for 20 minutes; IV oxytocin produces the same effect with a dose of 100–200 milliunits.

■ Distribution Like vasopressin, oxytocin is distributed throughout the extracellular fluid. Small amounts of oxytocin probably reach the fetal circulation.

■ Elimination Oxytocin has a plasma half-life of about 3–5 minutes. Most of the drug is rapidly destroyed in the liver and kidneys. Oxytocinase, a circulating enzyme produced early in pregnancy, is also capable of inactivating the polypeptide. Only small amounts of oxytocin are excreted in urine unchanged.

Chemistry and Stability

■ **Chemistry** Oxytocin is a nonapeptide hormone secreted by the neurons of the supraoptic and paraventricular nuclei of the hypothalamus and stored in the posterior pituitary (neurohypophysis) in mammals. Commercially available oxytocin preparations are prepared synthetically. Although the highly purified synthetic preparations are substantially free from the pressor and antidiuretic principles of the posterior pituitary, even these preparations may contain some impurities with inherent pressor and antidiuretic properties which may be manifested following administration of large doses. The potency of oxytocin is standardized according to its vasodepressor activity in chickens (which closely parallels oxytocic activity) and is expressed in USP Posterior Pituitary units. Each unit is equivalent to about 2–2.2 mcg of the pure hormone.

Oxytocin occurs as a white powder and is soluble in water. During manufacture, the pH of commercially available oxytocin injection is adjusted to 2.5–4.5 with acetic acid.

■ **Stability** Oxytocin injection should be stored at temperatures less than 15–25°C but should not be frozen. Pitocin® should be refrigerated at 2–8°C but may be exposed to temperatures ranging from 15–25°C for up to 30 days; Pitocin® exposed to this latter temperature range for longer periods should be discarded.

Oxytocin injection appears to be compatible with most IV infusion fluids but is reported to be physically incompatible with fibrinolysin, norepinephrine bitartrate, prochlorperazine edisylate, and warfarin sodium. Oxytocin injection has also been reported to be incompatible with various other drugs, but the compatibility depends on several factors (e.g., the concentration of the drugs, resulting pH, temperature). Specialized references should be consulted for more specific compatibility information.

Preparations

Excipients in commercially available drug preparations may have clinically important effects in some individuals; consult specific product labeling for details.

Oxytocin

Parenteral		
Injection	10 units/mL*	**Oxytocin Injection**
		Pitocin®, Monarch

*available from one or more manufacturer, distributor, and/or repackager by generic (nonproprietary) name

†Use is not currently included in the labeling approved by the US Food and Drug Administration

80:00 ANTITOXINS, IMMUNE GLOBULINS, TOXOIDS, AND VACCINES

80:02 Allergenic Extracts*

80:04 Antitoxins and Immune Globulins

80:08 Toxoids

80:12 Vaccines

§ Omitted from the print version of *AHFS Drug Information®* because of space limitations. This monograph is available on the *AHFS Drug Information®* website, http://ahfsdruginformation.com. Username: ahfs2020; Password: ASHP94498.
* Please see the full *AHFS Pharmacologic-Therapeutic Classification©* on p. viii. Not all classes are used in the printed edition.

ANTITOXINS, IMMUNE GLOBULINS, TOXOIDS, AND VACCINES 80:00

Immunobiologic Agents Available from CDC

General

The US Centers for Disease Control and Prevention (CDC) distributes the immunobiologic agents (antitoxins, vaccines) listed below to clinicians in the US through the Drug Service, Division of Scientific Resources, and the Division of Global Migration and Quarantine. These products are not commercially available in the US and FDA has granted permission to CDC to distribute them to qualifying US clinicians for patients residing in the US. Some of these immunobiologic agents are licensed by FDA and some are made available under investigational new drug (IND) status. These products can only be dispensed to licensed US physicians who register as clinical sub-investigators by completing form FDA-1572.

For information on how to obtain these immunobiologic agents, clinicians should contact the CDC Drug Service at 404-639-3670 (during working hours) or 770-488-7100 (emergency operations center at any time). Some products (e.g., botulism antitoxin, diphtheria antitoxin) are stored at CDC quarantine stations located in major US airports to ensure delivery to any location in the US within hours. Additional information is available at the CDC Drug Service website (http://www.cdc.gov/laboratory/drugservice) or by email (drugservice@cdc.gov).

Immunobiologics	Uses
Anthrax Vaccine Adsorbed	Active immunization against anthrax (*Bacillus anthracis* infection) in individuals at high risk
Botulism Antitoxin Heptavalent (Equine), Types A–G	Treatment of symptomatic botulism following documented or suspected exposure to botulinum neurotoxin
Diphtheria Antitoxin (Equine)	Treatment or prevention of actual or suspected cases of diphtheria caused by *Corynebacterium diphtheriae*
Vaccinia (Smallpox) Vaccine	Active immunization against smallpox in individuals at high risk

Immunization Schedules, US

Recommended US Immunization Schedules

Recommended US immunization schedules for infants, children, and adolescents from birth through 18 years of age and adults 19 years of age and older are updated annually and interim changes or additional recommendations are issued whenever necessary.

The US childhood and adolescent immunization schedules include recommendations for routine immunization of children and adolescents 18 years of age or younger and catch-up immunization of children and adolescents 4 months through 18 years of age. The childhood and adolescent immunization schedules are approved by the US Public Health Service Advisory Committee on Immunization Practices (ACIP), American Academy of Pediatrics (AAP), American Academy of Family Physicians (AAFP), and American College of Obstetricians and Gynecologists (ACOG).

The US adult immunization schedules include recommendations for routine immunization of adults 19 years of age or older based on age and recommendations for immunization of adults based on medical and other indications. The adult immunization schedules are approved by the ACIP, Centers for Disease Control and Prevention (CDC), AAFP, ACOG, American College of Physicians (ACP), and American College of Nurse-Midwives (ACNM).

The current annual US immunization schedules for children and adolescents18 years of age or younger and adults 19 years of age or older and information about any changes or additional recommendations that are issued before the next annual schedules are released may be obtained at the CDC immunization website at http://www.cdc.gov/vaccines.

For specific information about the vaccines included in the US immunization schedules (e.g., dosage and administration, precautions and contraindications, drug interactions), see the individual monographs in 80:00.

Clinically important adverse effects that occur following immunization should be reported to the Vaccine Adverse Event Reporting System (VAERS) at http://www.vaers.hhs.gov or 800-822-7967.

ANTITOXINS AND IMMUNE GLOBULINS 80:04

Hepatitis B Immune Globulin

Hepatitis B Immune Globulin, HBIG, Hepatitis B Immune Globulin IV, HBIG IV

■ Hepatitis B immune globulin (HBIG) is a specific immune globulin (hyperimmune globulin). HBIG contains antibody to hepatitis B surface antigen (anti-HBs) prepared from plasma of donors with high titers of anti-HBs and is used to provide temporary passive immunity to hepatitis B virus (HBV).

Uses

Hepatitis B immune globulin (HBIG) is used to provide passive immunity to hepatitis B virus (HBV) infection for prevention of perinatal HBV infection in neonates born to hepatitis B surface antigen-positive (HBsAg-positive) mothers, for postexposure prophylaxis in susceptible individuals exposed to HBV or HBsAg-positive materials (e.g., blood, plasma, serum), and for prevention of HBV recurrence in liver transplant recipients who are HBsAg-positive.

A combined regimen that includes *passive* immunization with HBIG and *active* immunization with hepatitis B vaccine is used for prevention of perinatal HBV infection. (See Uses: Prevention of Perinatal Hepatitis B Virus [HBV] Infection.) Depending on the exposure circumstances, a combined regimen of *passive* immunization with HBIG and *active* immunization with hepatitis B vaccine also may be indicated for postexposure prophylaxis of HBV infection in individuals exposed to HBV or HBsAg-positive materials (e.g., health-care personnel, sexual or intimate contacts of individuals with acute or chronic HBV infection) since it provides both short- and long-term protection. (See Uses: Postexposure Prophylaxis of Hepatitis B Virus [HBV] Infection.)

HBIG is *not* indicated in the treatment of acute or chronic HBV infection.

■ Risks of Exposure and Infection HBV is transmitted by percutaneous or mucosal exposure to HBsAg-positive blood, serum, plasma, semen, or saliva from individuals who have acute HBV infection or individuals who are carriers of the virus. The principal sources of HBV are blood (plasma or serum) and serous fluids. Lower concentrations are found in saliva, semen, vaginal secretions, and wound exudates. Although saliva can be a vehicle of HBV transmission through bites, other types of exposure to saliva (e.g., kissing) are unlikely modes of transmission. Transmission of HBV does not appear to occur via tears, sweat, urine, feces, or droplet nuclei and the virus is not transmitted via the fecal-oral route.

HBV can be transmitted perinatally from mother to infant at birth, usually as the result of blood exposures during labor and delivery. In utero transmission of HBV is rare. Without postexposure HBV prophylaxis in the neonate, the risk for perinatal transmission of the virus and chronic infection is 5–20% if the mother is HBsAg-positive and hepatitis B e antigen-negative (HBeAg-negative) and about 70–90% if the mother is positive for both HBsAg and HBeAg. Up to 90% of infants who become infected perinatally will become HBV carriers.

In the US, the primary risk factors for HBV infection in adults and adolescents are unprotected sex with an infected partner, unprotected sex with more than one partner, men who have sex with men, history of other sexually transmitted diseases (STDs), and illicit injection drug use. The US Centers for Disease Control and Prevention (CDC) states that individuals considered at high risk of exposure to HBsAg-positive material include immigrants or refugees from areas of high HBV endemicity, residents in institutions for the developmentally disabled, users of illicit parenteral drugs, homosexually active men, hemodialysis patients, and household contacts of HBV carriers. Those considered at intermediate risk include male prisoners, health-care workers who have frequent blood contact, staff of institutions for the developmentally disabled, and heterosexuals with multiple partners.

Presence of HBeAg indicates a high degree of infectivity of body fluids. Individuals exposed to body fluids that are positive for HBsAg, HBeAg, and HBV-specific DNA polymerase are more likely to develop HBV infection than individuals exposed to body fluids that are positive for HBsAg and anti-HBe but negative for HBeAg and DNA polymerase. The development of the HBV carrier state generally is associated with high serum titers of HBsAg and persistent, high serum titers of antibody to hepatitis B core antigen (anti-HBc); HBeAg also may be present.

Acute HBV infection may be self-limited resulting in production of antibody to HBsAg (anti-HBs) and immunity against reinfection; however, it also may progress to chronic HBV infection (especially in infants or young children, immunocompromised individuals, patients with diabetes) or to fatal, fulminant hepatitis. The case fatality rate is 0.5–1.5% among those with acute HBV infection, and the highest fatality rates are in adults older than 60 years of age. Chronic HBV infection develops in 90% or more of infants infected perinatally, 25–50% of children infected at 1–5 years of age, and less than 5% of those infected at 5 years of age or older. Chronic infection is associated with persistent HBV replication in the liver and may result in liver cirrhosis, liver cancer, liver failure, and death. Data from 2006 indicate that approximately 800,000–1.4 million people in the US have chronic HBV infection.

■ Prevention of Perinatal Hepatitis B Virus (HBV) Infection

A regimen that includes *active* immunization with hepatitis B vaccine and *passive* immunization with HBIG is used to prevent perinatal HBV infection in neonates born to HBsAg-*positive* women. This regimen is 85–95% effective in preventing acute and chronic HBV infection in infants born to women positive for both HBsAg and HBeAg.

HBIG has been used alone for prevention of perinatal HBV infection in neonates born to HBsAg-positive women, but use of passive immunization alone no longer is recommended since a regimen that includes both HBIG and hepatitis B vaccine is more effective.

The ACIP and AAP recommend routine serologic screening of *all* pregnant women during an early prenatal visit (e.g., first trimester) to determine their HBsAg status, even if they were tested previously or already have been vaccinated against HBV. Pregnant women who were not tested prenatally, those who engage in behaviors that put them at high risk for HBV (e.g., more than one sex partner in the previous 6 months, HBsAg-positive sex partner, evaluation or treatment for STDs, recent or current injection drug abuse), and those with clinical hepatitis should be tested for HBsAg status when admitted to the hospital for delivery.

To prevent perinatal HBV infection, ACIP and AAP recommend that *all* neonates born to HBsAg-positive women receive a dose of HBIG and a dose of hepatitis B vaccine as soon as possible after birth (within 12 hours of birth), regardless of gestational age or birthweight.

If maternal HBsAg status is unknown at birth, the neonate should receive the first dose of hepatitis B vaccine (within 12 hours of birth) and the mother's HBsAg status should be determined as quickly as possible; if positive, the infant should receive a dose of HBIG as soon as possible (no later than 7 days of age). For neonates weighing less than 2 kg, if the mother's HBsAg status cannot be determined within 12 hours of birth, a dose of HBIG should be given as soon as possible (within 12 hours of birth), and the birth vaccine dose should not be counted toward completion of the hepatitis B vaccine series; the usual 3-dose vaccine series should begin when the infant is 1 month of age.

■ Postexposure Prophylaxis of Hepatitis B Virus (HBV) Infection

HBV postexposure prophylaxis is recommended in certain individuals exposed to HBV or HBsAg-positive materials (e.g., health-care personnel, sexual or intimate contacts of individuals with acute or chronic HBV infection). Depending on the exposure circumstances, a postexposure prophylaxis regimen may include combined *passive* immunization with HBIG and *active* immunization with hepatitis B vaccine to provide both short- and long-term protection. Although HBIG alone may effectively prevent HBV transmission, it typically is used as an adjunct to hepatitis B vaccine following occupational or nonoccupational exposures to HBV.

Although a 2-dose regimen of HBIG alone (first dose at the time of exposure and second dose 1 month later) is reported to be about 75% effective in preventing HBV infection following percutaneous exposure, there is evidence that combined passive and active immunization is more effective than HBIG alone following perinatal HBV exposure. Therefore, although there are no prospective studies directly determining the efficacy of combined passive and active immunization in preventing HBV infection following percutaneous, permucosal, or peroral exposure to HBsAg-positive material, combined active and passive immunization is preferred for postexposure prophylaxis following an exposure to HBsAg-positive material. Combined passive and active immunization will provide both short-term protection and prolonged immunity to subsequent exposures and may increase efficacy in preventing HBV infection in such postexposure situations.

The major determinant of postexposure prophylaxis effectiveness is early administration of the initial dose of hepatitis B vaccine with or without HBIG; postexposure prophylaxis is less effective depending on how long it has been since the exposure. Studies are limited regarding the maximum interval after exposure during which HBV postexposure prophylaxis is effective, but such prophylaxis is unlikely to be effective if initiated 7 days or longer after percutaneous (e.g., needlestick) exposures.

HBV postexposure prophylaxis is *not* necessary in individuals who previously received primary immunization with hepatitis B vaccine and have serologic evidence of adequate levels of anti-HBs (10 mIU/mL or greater). In addition, HBV postexposure prophylaxis is *not* necessary in individuals previously infected with HBV since such individuals are immune to reinfection.

The ACIP recommends that exposure to HBV infection and to body fluids that may be HBsAg-positive be evaluated individually according to the identity and HBsAg serologic status of the source and the hepatitis B vaccination status of the exposed individual. The US Public Health Service (USPHS), ACIP, and the Hospital Infection Control Practices Advisory Committee (HICPAC) recommend routine use of hepatitis B vaccine in certain individuals, including all health-care personnel who, because of their occupation and work environment, are at risk of exposure to blood, blood-contaminated body fluids, other body fluids, and/or needles that might be contaminated with HBsAg. Such health-care personnel should undergo serologic testing 1–2 months after completing the 3-dose vaccine series to confirm an anti-HBs response. (See Healthcare Personnel under Uses: Preexposure Vaccination in High-Risk Groups, in Hepatitis B Vaccine 80:12.) Nonresponders to vaccination who are HBsAg-negative should be considered susceptible to HBV infection and should be counseled regarding precautions to prevent HBV infection and the need for HBIG postexposure prophylaxis for any known or probable parenteral exposure to HBsAg-positive blood. An exposure-control plan should be established by health-care organizations that includes protocols for prompt reporting, evaluation, counseling, treatment, and follow-up of occupational exposures, as well as appropriate reporting of occupational exposure to blood-borne pathogens as required by standards established by the Occupational Safety and Health Administration. Working health-care personnel should always have convenient access to clinicians who can provide timely postexposure prophylaxis with HBIG and/or hepatitis B vaccine.

Exposure to Materials with Known or Potential HBsAg-Positivity Following percutaneous (e.g., needlestick, laceration) exposure to, direct mucous membrane contact (e.g., oral, ophthalmic) with, or ingestion of material containing HBV or a HBsAg-positive source of known identity or following a bite from a human carrier of HBsAg which penetrates the skin, the ACIP and USPHS state that immunization routinely should consist of combined passive immunization with HBIG and active immunization with hepatitis B vaccine for individuals incompletely or not previously vaccinated. HBIG should be administered as soon as possible, routinely within 24 hours but not later than 7 days after exposure, and hepatitis B vaccine should be administered in a recommended primary immunization regimen. (See Dosage and Administration: Dosage, in Hepatitis B Vaccine 80:12.)

For those not previously vaccinated, the first dose of hepatitis B vaccine is administered concurrently with HBIG (at a separate site) not later than 7 days after exposure; subsequent doses of the vaccine should be given according to the recommended schedule to complete primary immunization. For those incompletely vaccinated at the time of exposure, a dose of HBIG should be given immediately and the usual recommended regimen for primary immunization with the vaccine should be completed as previously scheduled.

For individuals exposed to HBsAg-positive material and who previously completed primary immunization with the vaccine, the need for combined passive and active versus just passive or active immunization depends on the anti-HBs response of the individual. For those known to have exhibited an adequate anti-HBs response (i.e., an anti-HBs titer of 10 mIU/mL or greater), no treatment is necessary. For those whose response is not known, anti-HBs testing should be performed and the need for immunization based on this determination. No treatment is necessary when the antibody level is adequate; however, if an anti-HBs titer is determined to be less than 10 mIU/mL, the individual should receive a booster dose of hepatitis B vaccine and a single dose of HBIG administered concurrently but at separate sites. For those known to be nonresponders to completed primary immunization with the vaccine, a single dose of HBIG and the initial dose of the 3-dose vaccine series should be given as soon as possible after exposure; alternately, 2 doses of HBIG should be given, one as soon as possible after exposure and the second 1 month later. This latter 2-dose HBIG regimen is preferred for those who have failed to respond to 2 complete 3-dose series of vaccine or refuse to receive hepatitis B vaccine.

Following exposure to a source of known identity but unknown HBsAg status, a decision regarding the need for HBsAg serologic testing and appropriate immunization must be made based on the likelihood that the source is HBsAg-positive or HBsAg-negative and on the hepatitis B vaccination status of the exposed individual. Individuals considered at high risk of exposure to HBsAg-positive material are considered likely HBsAg-positive sources. If HBsAg testing of the source is positive, postexposure immunization is undertaken as described above for exposure to HBsAg-positive materials. If HBsAg testing of the source is negative, postexposure active immunization need only be undertaken in those incompletely or not previously vaccinated. Such previously unvaccinated individuals should receive the first dose of vaccine as soon as possible, preferably within 24 hours (with subsequent doses given according to the recommended schedule to complete primary immunization), and those incompletely vaccinated should simply complete the previously scheduled primary immunization regimen with the vaccine. Likewise, previously unvaccinated or incompletely vaccinated individuals exposed to an unknown source or one that is unavailable for testing should receive such active immunization with the vaccine. Individuals exposed to HBsAg-negative materials and who have completed primary immunization with the vaccine need not receive any further immunization at the time of such exposure, regardless of their response to such previous primary immunization. When the source of exposure is unavailable for testing or unknown in vaccinated individuals with a known anti-HBs response, those with an adequate response need receive no further immunization, but nonresponders exposed to a high-risk source can be immunized as described above for nonresponders exposed to HBsAg-positive materials. Vaccinees exposed to an unknown source or one that is unavailable for testing and in whom the anti-HBs response is unknown should undergo antibody testing and, if adequate, no further immunization is necessary but, if inadequate, a single booster dose of the vaccine should be given. (See Table 1.)

Table 1. Postexposure Prophylaxis of HBV following Occupational (Percutaneous or Mucosal) Exposure to Blood

	Treatment when Source Is:		
Vaccination and Antibody Status of Exposed Individual	**HBsAg-positive**	**HBsAg-negative**	**Source Unknown or Not Available for Testing**
Unvaccinated	Single HBIG dose (within 24 hours) and initiate hepatitis B vaccine series (within 24 hours)	Initiate hepatitis B vaccine series	Initiate hepatitis B vaccine series
Previously vaccinated			
Known responder (anti-HBs 10 mIU/mL or greater)	No treatment	No treatment	No treatment
Known nonresponder (anti-HBs less than 10 mIU/mL)	Single HBIG dose and initiate hepatitis B revaccination series or 2 HBIG doses (first dose as soon as possible; second dose 1 month later)	No treatment	If known high-risk source, *treat as if source were HBsAg-positive*
Antibody response unknown	Test exposed individual for anti-HBs 1. If inadequate, single dose of HBIG and a booster dose of hepatitis B vaccine 2. If adequate, no treatment	No treatment	Test exposed individual for anti-HBs 1. If inadequate, give a booster dose of hepatitis B vaccine and recheck titer in 1–2 months 2. If adequate, no treatment

Sexual Assault Victims ACIP and CDC recommend postexposure prophylaxis with hepatitis B vaccine with or without HBIG for victims of sexual assault (adult, adolescent, child) who are susceptible to HBV. Postexposure prophylaxis after a sexual assault is not necessary in those who previously received the complete hepatitis B vaccine series. If the victim is unvaccinated or incompletely vaccinated and the perpetrator is HBsAg-positive, the victim should receive a dose of HBIG within 14 days of the assault (preferably within 24 hours) and the hepatitis B vaccine series should be initiated or completed.

Contacts of Individuals with Acute HBV Infection Sexual or intimate contacts of individuals with acute HBV infection are at increased risk of acquiring HBV infection; therefore, postexposure prophylaxis is recommended in these contacts. The ACIP and CDC recommend that all susceptible individuals whose sexual or intimate contact has active HBV infection, contracts HBV, or is a chronic carrier receive postexposure prophylaxis with a single dose of HBIG and initiation of a primary immunization series of hepatitis B vaccine if such prophylaxis can be started within 14 days of the last such contact or if ongoing sexual or intimate contact with an infected individual is likely. This combined immunization strategy could potentially improve the efficacy of postexposure therapy compared with HBIG alone and can confer prolonged protection in this population. HBIG is most effective when administered as soon as possible after exposure (preferably within 24 hours) and may be ineffective if administered more than 14 days after a sexual exposure. Screening sexual or intimate contacts of individuals with acute HBV infection is recommended if it will not delay HBIG administration beyond 14 days after exposure.

Data regarding the use of HBIG in children are mainly limited to its administration to neonates born to HBsAg-positive women. However, the AAP recommends that postexposure prophylaxis in children follow the ACIP guidelines for adults. In addition, because infants have a high risk of becoming chronic HBV carriers following acute infection, unvaccinated infants younger than 12 months of age who have close contact with a primary caregiver or family member with acute HBV infection should receive combined passive immunization with HBIG and active immunization with hepatitis B vaccine. If the infant has previously received a single dose of hepatitis B vaccine, the second vaccine dose should be administered if the interval is appropriate or, if it is too soon to give a vaccine dose, the infant should receive a dose of HBIG. HBIG is not required if, at the time of exposure, the infant has already received at least 2 doses of hepatitis B vaccine.

Because of the potential risks from exposure to HBV infection and the potential for development of chronic infection in neonates, pregnancy is not considered a contraindication to the use of HBIG when clearly needed. (See Cautions: Pregnancy, Fertility, and Lactation.)

Household contacts of individuals with acute HBV infection, other than those described elsewhere as being at risk (e.g., infants, sexual or intimate contacts), generally do not require HBIG prophylaxis unless they have had identifiable blood exposure (e.g., sharing toothbrushes or razors) to the index patient. However, all household contacts of individuals with acute HBV infection should be encouraged to complete primary immunization with hepatitis B vaccine.

Contacts of Individuals with Chronic HBV Infection Sexual or needle-sharing partners and nonsexual household contacts of individuals with chronic HBV infection are at risk for HBV infection through percutaneous or mucosal exposures to blood or infectious body fluids (e.g., sharing a toothbrush or razor, contact with exudates from dermatologic lesions, contact with HBsAg-contaminated surfaces). Therefore, the ACIP recommends postexposure vaccination with hepatitis B vaccine for such individuals. A dose of HBIG also may be indicated for postexposure prophylaxis if the most recent sexual exposure to an HBsAg-positive individual occurred within the last 14 days.

Individuals Wounded in Mass Casualty Settings The CDC recommends that individuals wounded in bombings or other mass casualty settings who have not previously received hepatitis B vaccine or have an uncertain vaccination history receive postexposure vaccination with hepatitis B vaccine. (See Individuals Wounded in Mass Casualty Settings in Uses: Postexposure Prophylaxis, in Hepatitis B Vaccine 80:12.) In addition, the CDC recommends that responders and other personnel in mass casualty settings be managed using postexposure prophylaxis regimens recommended for occupational exposures to HBV. (See Table 1.)

■ **Prevention of Hepatitis B Virus (HBV) Recurrence in Liver Transplant Recipients** HBIG is used to prevent HBV recurrence in liver transplant recipients who are HBsAg-positive.

HBIG has been used alone or in conjunction with an antiviral agent active against HBV (e.g., lamivudine, adefovir) to suppress HBV replication and prevent recurrence of HBV infection in patients with chronic HBV infection undergoing liver transplantation. Optimum regimens for such prophylaxis (i.e., dosage, route, and duration of HBIG; specific antiviral for a combined regimen) have not been established.

HepaGam B® given by IV infusion is labeled by the Food and Drug Administration (FDA) for prevention of HBV recurrence in liver transplant recipients based on interim results of a clinical study in HBsAg-positive, HBeAg-negative transplant recipients who had only low or undetectable levels of HBV replication at the time of transplant. Although other HBIG preparations have been administered IM or IV for prevention of HBV recurrence in liver transplant recipients† and have been used alone or in conjunction with an antiviral active against HBV, safety and efficacy of these preparations have not been established for this use.

Dosage and Administration

■ **Administration** Hepatitis B immune globulin (HBIG) is administered by IM injection for prevention of perinatal hepatitis B virus (HBV) infection or for postexposure prophylaxis of HBV infection. HBIG is administered by IV infusion for prevention of HBV recurrence in liver transplant recipients

Prior to administration, HBIG should be inspected visually for particulate matter and discoloration. HBIG should be administered undiluted and should *not* be mixed with any other drug or solution.

IM Administration HyperHEP B®, Nabi-HB®, and HepaGam B® are administered by IM injection for prevention of perinatal HBV infection or for postexposure prophylaxis of HBV infection. *HBIG should* **not** *be administered by IV infusion for these indications.*

In adults and children, IM injections of HBIG preferably should be made into the deltoid muscle or anterolateral aspect of the thigh. In neonates and infants 12 months of age or younger, IM injections of HBIG preferably should be made into the anterolateral aspect of the thigh. In children 1–2 years of age, IM injections should preferably be administered into the anterolateral thigh; the deltoid muscle is an alternative if muscle mass is adequate. For children and adolescents 3–18 years of age and adults, the deltoid muscle is preferred, although the anterolateral thigh is an alternative.

To ensure delivery into muscle, IM injections should be made at a 90° angle to the skin using a needle length appropriate for the individual's age and body mass, the thickness of adipose tissue and muscle at the injection site, and the injection technique.

Because of the risk of injury to the sciatic nerves, the upper, outer quadrant of the gluteal muscle should be used for IM injection of HBIG *only* if a large volume is indicated in an adult or if a large dose must be divided into multiple injection sites. If use of the gluteal area is considered necessary, use *only* the upper, outer quadrant and avoid the central gluteal region.

Although some manufacturers recommend that aspiration (i.e., pulling back on the syringe plunger after needle insertion and before injection) should be performed to ensure that a blood vessel has not been entered, the US Public Health Service Advisory Committee on Immunization Practices (ACIP) and the American Academy of Pediatrics (AAP) state that this procedure is not required because large blood vessels are not present at recommended IM injection sites.

HBIG may be given simultaneously with hepatitis B vaccine (using different syringes and different injection sites) when *passive* immunization is considered necessary in addition to *active* immunization with the vaccine (e.g., in neonates born to HBsAg-positive women, postexposure prophylaxis regimen in certain individuals exposed to HBV or HBsAg-positive materials).

IV Administration HepaGam B® is given by IV infusion for prevention of HBV recurrence in liver transplant recipients. Other HBIG preparations also have been administered by IV infusion† for prevention of HBV recurrence in liver transplant recipients, but are not labeled by the US Food and Drug Administration (FDA) for this use.

Vials of HepaGam B® should *not* be shaken to avoid foaming.

HepaGam B® should be administered IV using a separate IV line and an IV infusion pump.

Rate of Administration. HepaGam B® should be administered by IV infusion at a rate of 2 mL/minute. If the patient develops discomfort or infusion-related adverse effects or if there is concern about the rate of infusion, the rate of administration should be decreased to 1 mL/minute or less.

■ **Dosage** ***Prevention of Perinatal HBV Infection*** **Neonates Born to HBsAg-positive Women.** Neonates born to HBsAg-*positive* women, including those infected with human immunodeficiency virus (HIV), should receive combined *passive* immunization with HBIG and *active* immunization with hepatitis B vaccine to prevent perinatal HBV infection.

The usual dose of HBIG in neonates born to HBsAg-positive women is 0.5 mL given IM within 12 hours of birth. These neonates also should receive a dose of monovalent hepatitis B vaccine within 12 hours of birth (using a different syringe and different injection site).

If the first dose of hepatitis B vaccine is delayed for 3 months or longer, the manufacturer of HyperHEP B® recommends that a second 0.5-mL dose of HBIG be given IM at 3 months of age. In addition, if hepatitis B vaccine is contraindicated or not available, this manufacturer recommends that second and third 0.5-mL doses of HBIG be given IM at 3 and 6 months of age, respectively.

All infants born to HBsAg-positive women should undergo serologic testing at 9–18 months of age to document whether the combined regimen of active immunization with hepatitis B vaccines and passive immunization with HBIG prevented perinatal HBV infection. (See Uses: Pre- and Postvaccination Serologic Testing, in Hepatitis B Vaccine 80:12.)

Neonates Born the Women with Unknown HBsAg Status. Neonates born to women with *unknown* HBsAg status should receive *active* immunization with hepatitis B vaccine and, depending on the circumstances (e.g., HBsAg status of the mother), *passive* immunization with HBIG also may be indicated.

All neonates born to women with *unknown* HBsAg status should receive a dose of monovalent hepatitis B vaccine within 12 hours of birth, and the HBsAg status of the mother should be determined as soon as possible. If the mother of a full-term neonate or preterm neonate weighing more than 2 kg at birth is subsequently found to be HBsAg-positive, these neonates should receive a 0.5-mL dose of HBIG as soon as possible (no later than 1 week of age). If the neonate was preterm and weighed less than 2 kg at birth, the neonate should receive a 0.5 mL dose of HBIG within 12 hours of birth if mother is found to be HBsAg-positive or if results are not available.

Postexposure Prophylaxis of HBV Infection The ACIP recommends that exposure to HBV infection or body fluids that might be HBsAg-positive should be evaluated individually according to the identity and HBsAg serologic status of the source and the hepatitis B vaccination status of the exposed individual to determine the need for postexposure prophylaxis. (See Uses: Postexposure Prophylaxis of Hepatitis B Virus [HBV] Infection.)

Known Source with HBsAg-positive Status. Following exposure to a HBsAg-positive source of known identity in an individual who has not previously received primary immunization with hepatitis B vaccine, the usual adult dose of HBIG is 0.06 mL/kg. A dose of hepatitis B vaccine should be administered concurrently (at a separate site) and the recommended primary immunization schedule for the vaccine should be completed; alternatively, the first dose of vaccine may be administered up to 7 days after percutaneous exposure. In individuals who have begun but not completed primary immunization with hepatitis B vaccine at the time of exposure, the usual dose of HBIG should be given immediately and the recommended primary immunization schedule for the vaccine completed as scheduled. Because immunoglobulins are most effective if given immediately after exposure, HBIG should be administered as soon as possible after exposure, preferably within 24 hours; the value of administering immunoglobulins later than 7 days after exposure is not known. Individuals who elect not to receive hepatitis B vaccine should receive the usual dose of HBIG as soon as possible (but within 24 hours after exposure) and a second dose of HBIG should be administered 1 month later.

If the source is known to be HBsAg-positive and the exposed individual is unvaccinated or a known nonresponder to hepatitis B vaccine (anti-HBs is less than 10 mIU/mL), combined active immunization with hepatitis B vaccine and passive immunization with HBIG is indicated. (See Table 1 under Uses.)

Known Source with HBsAg-negative Status. Administration of HBIG is unnecessary following exposure to an HBsAg-negative source in vaccinated individuals. However, hepatitis B vaccine is indicated in previously unvaccinated or incompletely vaccinated individuals following such exposures. (See Hepatitis B Vaccine 80:12.)

Known Source with Unknown HBsAg Status or Unknown Source. Following exposure to a source of known identity but unknown HBsAg status (i.e., not tested) or an unknown source, previously unvaccinated individuals should receive a complete series of primary immunization with hepatitis B vaccine, initiated within 7 days of exposure and completed according to the usual schedule. Incompletely vaccinated individuals should simply complete the previously scheduled primary vaccine series. Administration of HBIG is unnecessary in either incompletely or not previously vaccinated individuals. Previously vaccinated individuals whose response in the past was adequate need receive no further immunization at the time of exposure. Those who were nonresponders and now are exposed to a source that is likely to be HBsAg-positive can receive 0.06 mL/kg of HBIG immediately along with a booster dose of hepatitis B vaccine. Alternatively, such nonresponders can receive 2 doses (0.06 mL/kg each) of HBIG, one administered immediately and the second 1 month later; this regimen is preferred for those who have failed to respond to at least 4 doses of vaccine.

Unvaccinated or Incompletely Vaccinated Sexual Assault Victims. Active immunization with hepatitis B vaccine is indicated and passive immunization with HBIG also may be indicated following a sexual assault.

If the victim is unvaccinated or incompletely vaccinated and the perpetrator is HBsAg-positive, the victim should receive 0.06 mL/kg of HBIG within 14 days of the assault (preferably within 24 hours). In addition, primary immunization with hepatitis B vaccine should be initiated or completed in unvaccinated or incompletely vaccinated sexual assault victims.

Contacts of Individuals with Acute HBV Infection. Active immunization with hepatitis B vaccine is indicated and passive immunization with HBIG also may be indicated following sexual or intimate exposure to individuals with acute HBV infection.

Following sexual or intimate exposure to individuals with acute HBV infection, 0.06 mL/kg of HBIG should be given within 14 days of the last sexual or intimate exposure. In addition, primary immunization with hepatitis B vaccine should be initiated or completed in unvaccinated or incompletely vaccinated sexual assault victims.

For unvaccinated or incompletely vaccinated infants younger than 12 months of age whose mother or other primary caregiver has acute HBV infection, a 0.5-mL dose of HBIG should be administered and primary immunization with hepatitis B vaccine should be initiated and completed. HBIG is unnecessary if the infant has already received 2 or more doses of hepatitis B vaccine.

Prevention of HBV Recurrence in Liver Transplant Recipients (HepaGam B®) For prevention of HBV recurrence following liver transplantation in HBsAg-positive liver transplant recipients, HepaGam B® is administered by IV infusion in a dosage designed to provide anti-HBs serum levels greater then 500 international units/L.

The manufacturer states that an initial IV dose of 20,000 international units of HepaGam B® should be given concurrently with the grafting of the transplanted liver (anhepatic phase). Then, 20,000 international units should be given once daily on postoperative days 1–7, 20,000 international units should be given once every 2 weeks during postoperative weeks 2–12, and 20,000 international units should be given once monthly beginning at postoperative month 4.

The treatment response should be tracked by monitoring serum HBsAg and anti-HBs antibody levels using a quantitative assay. The dosage of HepaGam B® should be adjusted if anti-HBs levels do not increase to 500 international units/L or more within the first postoperative week. In such cases, dosage can be increased to 10,000 international units every 6 hours until the target anti-HBs level is reached. Individuals with surgical bleeding or abdominal fluid drainage (greater than 500 mL) and those undergoing plasmapheresis are particularly susceptible to extensive loss of circulating anti-HBs.

Cautions

■ Local Reactions

Following IM administration of hepatitis B immune globulin (HBIG), local pain, tenderness, swelling, and erythema may occur at the injection site.

■ Systemic Effects

Following IM administration of HBIG, urticaria, angioedema, nausea, vomiting, myalgia, headache, flu or cold symptoms, lightheadedness/fainting, and malaise have been reported. Elevated serum alkaline phosphatase, AST (SGPT), and creatinine concentrations and ecchymosis, joint stiffness, and decreased leukocyte counts also have been reported.

The most common adverse effects reported with IV immune globulins are chills, fever, headache, vomiting, allergic reactions, nausea, arthralgia, and moderate low back pain. In a clinical study evaluating IV administration of HBIG (HepaGam B®) for prevention of hepatitis B recurrence in liver transplant patients, interim analysis indicated that the only adverse effects attributed to HBIG given by IV infusion were tremor and hypotension. Other adverse events reported in more than 10% of liver transplant patients in this study (including events assessed as unrelated to HBIG) include splenomegaly, presbyopia, aphthous stomatitis, diarrhea, dyspepsia, gingival hyperplasia, fatigue, peripheral edema, pyrexia, hepatobiliary disease, liver transplant rejection, infectious diarrhea, pneumonia, sepsis, hyperglycemia, back pain, amnesia, essential tremor, headache, agitation, nocturia, pleural effusion, pruritus, rash, hypertension, and hypotension.

■ Precautions and Contraindications

HepaGam B® and Nabi-HB® are contraindicated in individuals with a history of anaphylactic or severe systemic reactions to parenteral human immune globulin. The manufacturer of HyperHEP B® states that there are no known contraindications to use of this preparation of immune globulin, but the preparation should be used with caution in individuals who have exhibited previous systemic allergic reactions to immune globulin.

Sensitivity Reactions Although anaphylactic reactions have not been reported to date with HBIG, anaphylaxis has been reported rarely following administration of human immune globulins.

Epinephrine should be readily available in case anaphylaxis occurs. If hypotension or a hypersensitivity reaction (e.g., anaphylaxis) occurs, HBIG should immediately be discontinued and appropriate therapy initiated as indicated.

Selective IgA Deficiency HBIG should be used with caution in individuals with specific IgA deficiency since these individuals may have serum antibodies to IgA or may develop such antibodies and anaphylaxis could result following administration of blood products containing IgA.

HepaGam B® contains less than 40 mcg/mL and Nabi-HB® contains less than 100 mcg/mL of IgA. If these preparations are used, the potential benefits should be weighed against the potential for a hypersensitivity reaction.

Individuals with Bleeding Disorders HBIG should be administered IM with caution in patients with thrombocytopenia or bleeding disorders since bleeding may occur following IM injections (probably because of injury from injection). HBIG should be administered IM in these patients only if the expected benefits outweigh the potential risks.

The US Public Health Service Advisory Committee on Immunization Practices (ACIP) states that IM injections can be used in individuals who have bleeding disorders or are receiving anticoagulant therapy if a clinician familiar with the patient's bleeding risk determines that the injection can be administered with reasonable safety. In these cases, a fine needle (23 gauge) should be used to administer the dose and firm pressure applied to the injection site (without rubbing) for at least 2 minutes. If the patient is receiving antihemophilia therapy, the IM dose should be administered shortly after a scheduled dose of such therapy. The patient and/or their family should be advised about the risk of hematoma from IM injections.

Risk of Transmissible Agents in Plasma-derived Preparations Because HBIG is prepared from pooled human plasma, it is a potential vehicle for transmission of human viruses, including the causative agents of viral hepatitis and human immunodeficiency virus (HIV) infection, and theoretically may carry a risk of transmitting the causative agent of Creutzfeldt-Jakob disease (CJD) or variant CJD (vCJD). The manufacturing process for HBIG includes a chemical (solvent/detergent) treatment procedure and filtration procedures that reduce the viral infectious potential of the preparations. Solvent/detergent inactivation processes apparently can inactivate lipid-enveloped viruses (e.g., hepatitis B virus [HBV], hepatitis C virus [HCV], human immunodeficiency virus [HIV] type 1 and type 2 [HIV-1 and HIV-2]) but are less effective against viruses that do not have a lipid envelope (e.g., hepatitis A virus [HAV], parvovirus B-19). Certain filtering procedures are effective in reducing levels of some enveloped and non-enveloped viruses.

Improved donor screening, viral-inactivation procedures (e.g., solvent/detergent treatment), and/or filtration procedures have reduced, but not completely eliminated, risk of pathogen transmission with plasma-derived preparations. Because no purification method has been shown to be totally effective in removing the risk of viral infectivity from plasma-derived preparations and because new blood-borne viruses or other disease agents may emerge which may not be inactivated by the manufacturing process or the chemical (solvent/detergent) treatment procedures currently used, HBIG should be administered only when a benefit is expected. Any infection believed to have been transmitted by HBIG should be reported to the manufacturer.

Epidemiologic and laboratory evidence to date indicate that preparations of HBIG do not have a discernible risk of transmitting HIV infection. In addition to the screening of all donor units for antibody to HIV and rejection of all repeatedly reactive units, the manufacturing process of HBIG includes purification steps that provide an extremely high margin of safety in removal of HIV infectivity. Although some HBIG produced in 1982–1985 may have contained antibody to HIV, all HBIG produced since April 1985 should be free of the antibody.

For further information on precautions related to transmissible agents in plasma-derived preparations, see Risk of Transmissible Agents in Plasma-derived Preparations under Cautions: Precautions and Contraindications, in Antihemophilic Factor (Human) 20:12.16.

Individuals with Altered Immunocompetence HBIG may be administered to individuals immunosuppressed as the result of disease or immunosuppressive therapy.

Recommendations regarding the use of HBIG in HIV-infected individuals or use in neonates born to HIV-infected women are the same as those for individuals who are not infected with HIV.

Infusion Reactions HyperHEP B® administered by IV infusion may be associated with certain adverse effects related to the rate of infusion. Therefore, the recommended infusion rate (2 mL/minute) should not be exceeded. In addition, the patient should be monitored closely during and immediately following the infusion.

■ Pediatric Precautions

HepaGam B® is labeled by the US Food and Drug Administration (FDA) for use in neonates and children.

Although the manufacturers of HyperHEP B® and Nabi-HB® state that safety and efficacy of these preparations have not been established in infants and children, safety and efficacy of similar HBIG preparations have been demonstrated in infants and children.

HBIG is used in conjunction with hepatitis B vaccine for prevention of perinatal HBV infection in neonates born to HBsAg-positive mothers and for postexposure prophylaxis in unvaccinated children younger than 12 months of age whose mother or primary caregiver has acute HBV infection. (See Uses.)

■ **Geriatric Precautions** The manufacturer of Nabi-HB® states that clinical studies of HBIG did not include sufficient numbers of adults 65 years of age and older to determine whether geriatric adults respond differently than younger individuals. Other reported clinical experience has not identified differences in responses between geriatric and younger individuals.

■ **Pregnancy, Fertility, and Lactation** Because of the potential risks to the neonate from exposure to HBV infection, pregnancy and lactation are not considered a contraindications to the use of HBIG when clearly needed. Animal reproduction studies have not been performed with HBIG and it is not known whether HBIG can cause fetal harm when administered to pregnant women. The manufacturers state that HBIG should be given to pregnant women only when clearly needed. The ACIP states there are no known risks associated with use of immune globulins for passive immunization in pregnant women.

It is not known if HBIG affects fertility.

Information on the distribution of HBIG into milk is not available; it is not known if transmission of HBIG to a nursing infant presents any unusual risk. HBIG should be administered with caution to nursing women.

Drug Interactions

■ **Immunosuppressive Agents** Recommendations for use of immune globulins, including hepatitis B immune globulin (HBIG), in patients receiving immunosuppressive agents (e.g., alkylating agents, antimetabolites, corticosteroids, radiation) are the same as those for patients not receiving such agents.

■ **Inactivated Vaccines and Toxoids** The US Public Health Service Advisory Committee on Immunization Practices (ACIP), American Academy of Pediatrics (AAP), and American Academy of Family Physicians (AAFP) state that immune globulins (including HBIG) are not expected to have a clinically important effect on the immune response to inactivated vaccines and toxoids. Therefore, inactivated vaccines, recombinant vaccines, polysaccharide vaccines, or toxoids may be administered simultaneously with (using different syringes and injection sites) or at any interval before or after administration of HBIG.

Neonates born to hepatitis B surface antigen-positive (HBsAg-positive) women who receive combined *passive* immunization with HBIG and *active* immunization with hepatitis B vaccine at birth can receive immunization with other age-appropriate vaccines (e.g., diphtheria and tetanus toxoids and acellular pertussis vaccine adsorbed [DTaP], poliovirus vaccine inactivated [IPV], haemophilus b [Hib] conjugate vaccine) according to the usual childhood immunization schedule.

Hepatitis B Vaccine Passively acquired antibody to hepatitis B surface antigen (anti-HBs), which is present in HBIG, does not appear to interfere with the active immune response to hepatitis B vaccine. When combined *active* immunization with hepatitis B vaccine and *passive* immunization with HBIG is indicated, the first dose of vaccine should be administered simultaneously with HBIG (using different syringes and injection sites).

The manufacturer of HepaGam B® states that this preparation may be administered concurrently with (at a different site) or up to 1 month preceding hepatitis B vaccine without impairing the active immune response to the vaccine.

Influenza Vaccine HBIG is not expected to interfere with the immune response to parenteral trivalent influenza virus vaccine inactivated (TIV); therefore, the parenteral vaccine may be given simultaneously with HBIG (using different syringes and injection sites) or at any time before or after HBIG.

Typhoid Vaccine Because parenteral typhoid Vi polysaccharide vaccine (Typhim Vi®) is an inactivated vaccine, HBIG is not expected to interfere with the immune response to the vaccine; therefore, the parenteral vaccine may be given simultaneously with HBIG (using different syringes and injection sites) or at any time before or after HBIG.

■ **Live Vaccines** Antibodies present in immune globulins, including HBIG, may interfere with the immune response to certain live virus vaccines, including measles virus vaccine live, mumps virus vaccine live, rubella virus vaccine live, rotavirus vaccine live oral, and varicella virus vaccine live, and these vaccines should not be administered simultaneously with or for specified intervals before or after administration of HBIG.

There is no evidence that immune globulin preparations interfere with the immune response to yellow fever virus vaccine live, typhoid vaccine live oral (Vivotif®), influenza virus vaccine live intranasal (LAIV; Flumist®), or poliovirus vaccine live oral (OPV; no longer commercially available in the US), and these live vaccines may be administered simultaneously with or at any time before or after administration of HBIG.

Measles, Mumps, Rubella, and Varicella Vaccines Antibodies contained in HBIG may interfere with the immune response to measles virus vaccine live and rubella virus vaccine live. The duration of possible interference between immune globulin preparations and live viral vaccines appears to depend on the dosage of the immune globulin and there is evidence that high doses of certain immune globulin preparations can inhibit the immune response to measles virus vaccine live and rubella virus vaccine live for more than 3 months. Although specific information regarding the effect of immune globulin preparations on the immune response to mumps virus vaccine live and varicella virus vaccine live are not available, there is potential for similar interference since immune globulin preparations contain antibodies to these viruses.

Measles, mumps, and rubella virus vaccine live (MMR) or varicella virus vaccine live should not be administered simultaneously with or within 3 months before or after HBIG. If a dose of a vaccine containing live measles, mumps, rubella, or varicella virus is deemed necessary (e.g., because of imminent exposure to the disease) and is administered simultaneously with (at a separate site) or within 6 months after HBIG administration, the ACIP and AAFP recommend that a repeat dose of the vaccine be given at least 3 months after the HBIG dose, unless serologic testing is feasible and indicates an adequate immune response to the vaccine. In addition, the fact that revaccination may be necessary in individuals who receive HBIG shortly after a live virus vaccine also should be considered. In general, vaccine virus replication and stimulation of immunity occur within 7–14 days after administration of a live virus vaccine. Therefore, if HBIG must be administered within 14 days after receipt of a vaccine containing live measles, mumps, rubella, or varicella virus, revaccination is necessary at least 3 months after administration of HBIG, unless there is serologic evidence of an adequate immune response to the vaccine.

Rotavirus Vaccine Safety and efficacy data are not available regarding the use of rotavirus vaccine live oral in infants who have received an immune globulin within 42 days. Therefore, if possible, the dose of rotavirus vaccine should be deferred until 42 days (6 weeks) after the immune globulin; alternatively, if the 42-day deferral would result in the first dose of rotavirus vaccine being scheduled at 13 weeks of age or older, a shorter interval may be used.

Laboratory Test Interferences

■ **Immunohematology Tests** The manufacturer states that antibodies present in HepaGam B® may interfere with some serologic tests. Administration of immune globulins similar to HepaGam B® result in transitory increases of passively transferred antibodies in patient blood and may result in misleading positive results in serologic tests (e.g. direct antiglobulin [Coombs'] test).

■ **Tests for anti-HBs** Antibodies specific to hepatitis B surface antigen (HBsAg) (anti-HBs) are present in serum for 2–6 months following a dose of hepatitis B immune globulin (HBIG) and may result in positive tests for anti-HBs that reflect passively-acquired antibody rather than an immune response to hepatitis B vaccine.

In neonates who receive a combined regimen of HBIG and hepatitis B vaccine for prevention of perinatal hepatitis B virus (HBV) infection (i.e., neonates born to HBsAg-positive mothers), postvaccination testing for anti-HBs to confirm an immunologic response to the vaccine should not be performed until the child is 9 months of age or older to avoid detecting passively-acquired antibody from HBIG.

If a combined regimen of HBIG and hepatitis B vaccine is used for post-exposure prophylaxis following exposure to HBV or HBsAg-positive materials, postvaccination testing for anti-HBs should not be performed until 3–4 months after the HBIG dose.

■ **Tests for Glucose** HepaGam B® contains maltose, which may interfere with blood glucose monitoring systems based on glucose dehydrogenase pyrroloquinequinone (GDH-PQQ) and cause falsely elevated blood glucose results. This may result in inappropriate insulin administration and life-threatening hypoglycemia or may mask true hypoglycemia. Only glucose-specific test methods not affected by maltose (e.g., glucose dehydrogenase nicotine adenine dinucleotide [GDH-NAD], glucose oxidase, glucose hexokinase) should be used in patients receiving HepaGam B®.

Product information for the blood glucose testing meter and test strips should be reviewed to determine if the testing system is appropriate for patients receiving HepaGam B®; If any uncertainty exists, the manufacturer of the glucose testing system should be contacted to determine whether the system will provide accurate blood glucose determinations in patients receiving HepaGam B®.

Acute Toxicity

Data are not available regarding overdosage of hepatitis B immune globulin (HBIG). The manufacturers state that clinical experience with other IM immunoglobulin preparations suggests that the only manifestations of overdosage would be pain and tenderness at the injection site.

Pharmacology

Hepatitis B immune globulin (HBIG) is used to provide temporary passive immunity to hepatitis B virus (HBV) infection in the postexposure prophylaxis of individuals exposed to HBV or hepatitis B surface antigen-positive (HBsAg-positive) materials (e.g., blood, plasma, serum). Antibody to HBsAg (anti-HBs) present in HBIG combines with HBsAg and neutralizes circulating HBV so that its infective or pathogenic properties are inhibited.

HBIG administered to HBsAg-positive individuals undergoing liver transplantation may protect the new liver from HBV reinfection. Reinfection in such individuals may occur immediately at the time of liver reperfusion because of circulating HBV or may occur at a later time because of HBV retained in extrahepatic sites. The mechanism by which HBIG protects the transplanted liver against HBV reinfection has not been fully determined. HBIG may protect naive hepatocytes against infection by blocking an HBV receptor. Alternatively, HBIG may neutralize circulating HBV through immune precipitation and immune complex formation or may trigger an antibody-dependent cell-mediated cytotoxicity response resulting in target cell lysis. There is evidence that HBIG binds to hepatocytes and interacts with HBsAg within cells.

■ **Hepatitis B Virus and Infection** HBV is a DNA virus from the family Hepadnaviridae consisting of antigenically distinct surface and core components. The presence of HBsAg in serum indicates active HBV infection (either acute or chronic). HBsAg also may be found in other body fluids and tissues. (See Uses: Risks of Exposure and Infection, in Hepatitis B Vaccine 80:12.) The HBV viral core consists of DNA, DNA polymerase, hepatitis B core antigen (HBcAg), and hepatitis B e antigen (HBeAg). The presence of HBeAg and HBV DNA in serum generally indicates high levels of viral replication and suggests that the serum is highly infectious.

The incubation period from exposure to HBV to onset of symptoms of HBV infection is 6 weeks to 6 months (average: 90–150 days). Serologic markers of HBV infection (i.e., HBsAg, HBeAg, antibody to hepatitis B core antigen [anti-HBc], antibody to hepatitis B e antigen [anti-HBe], anti-HBs) are used to define the clinical status of those exposed to HBV infection or virus. HBsAg appears in the serum about 30 days (range 6–60 days) after exposure and indicates an ongoing HBV infection. HBsAg persists during an acute infection and usually disappears as the acute infection resolves; however, the presence of HBsAg in the serum for 6 months or longer generally indicates chronic infection. Anti-HBs develops during convalescence after an acute HBV infection (usually within 3–4 months). The presence of anti-HBs indicates recovery from and immunity to further HBV infection.

Acute HBV infection may be self-limited resulting in production of anti-HBs and immunity against reinfection; however, it also may progress to chronic HBV infection (especially in infants or young children, immunocompromised individuals, patients with diabetes) or to fatal, fulminant hepatitis. The case fatality rate is 0.5–1.5% among those with acute HBV infection and the highest fatality rates are in adults older than 60 years of age. Chronic HBV infection develops in 90% or more of infants infected perinatally, 25–50% of children infected at 1–5 years of age, and less than 5% of those infected at 5 years of age or older. Chronic infection is associated with continuing viral replication in the liver and persistent viremia and may result in liver cirrhosis, liver cancer, liver failure, and death. Data from 2006 indicate that approximately 800,000–1.4 million people in the US have chronic HBV infection. HBV is transmitted by percutaneous or mucosal exposure to HBsAg-positive blood, serum, plasma, semen, or saliva and can be transmitted perinatally from mother to infant at birth, usually from blood exposures during labor and delivery.

■ **Response to HBIG** Once HBV infection becomes clinically apparent and/or serologic testing indicates the presence of HBsAg, it does *not* appear that the virus can be neutralized by HBIG, although HBIG may modify or ameliorate the infection.

A single HBIG dose provides passive immunity against HBV for about 3–6 months. In some patients, postexposure administration of HBIG may delay the development of HBV infection. Since the virus may be established in the individual at the time of HBIG administration, clinical symptoms of the disease may appear as passively acquired anti-HBs decreases. Alternatively, delay in development of infection may result from a second exposure to the virus several months after HBIG administration when circulating levels of passively acquired anti-HBs have decreased.

When HBIG is administered concomitantly with hepatitis B vaccine at separate sites, it does not appear to suppress the active immune to the vaccine. (See Hepatitis B Vaccine under Drug Interactions: Inactivated Vaccines and Toxoids.)

Pharmacokinetics

■ **Absorption** Hepatitis B immune globulin (HBIG) is slowly absorbed following IM administration. Following IM administration of HBIG, serum concentrations of anti-HBs usually peak within 3–7 days and persist for about 2–6 months. In a study using HepaGam B®, mean peak concentrations occurred 4–5 days after an IM dose of 0.06 mL/kg.

■ **Distribution** Although specific information is not available, it is likely that HBIG crosses the placenta since other immunoglobulins cross the placenta. Virtually all transplacental passage of immunoglobulins occurs during the last 4 weeks of pregnancy.

Information on the distribution of HBIG into milk is not available; HBIG may be distributed into milk since immunoglobulins (e.g., IgA, IgM, IgG) are present in the colostrum.

The volume of distribution of HepaGam B® or Nabi-HB® is approximately 7.5 L or11.2 L, respectively.

■ **Elimination** Following IM administration, the mean half-life of HepaGam B®, HyperHEP B®, or Nabi-HB® is 22–25 days, 17.5–25 days, or 23 days, respectively.

The clearance rate of HepaGam B® or Nabi-HB® is 0.21–0.24 L/day or 0.35 L/day, respectively.

Chemistry and Stability

■ **Chemistry** Hepatitis B immune globulin (HBIG) is a sterile solution prepared from plasma of healthy individuals with high titers of antibody to hepatitis B surface antigen (anti-HBs) and whose plasma does not show serologic evidence of hepatitis B surface antigen (HBsAg).

Commercially available HBIG meets standards established by the Center for Biologics Evaluation and Research of the US Food and Drug Administration and contains an anti-HBs titer equivalent to or greater than that contained in a US reference HBIG. Plasma donors and plasma used in the preparation of HBIG have been screened and tested for certain viruses and shown to be negative. In addition, the manufacturing process used for HBIG includes purification steps and a chemical (solvent/detergent) inactivation process that reduce the risk for transmission of bloodborne viruses. However, these steps may not completely eliminate the risk of pathogen transmission with plasma-derived preparations. (See Risk of Transmissible Agents in Plasma-derived Preparations under Cautions: Precautions and Contraindications.)

HBIG is commercially available as HepaGam B®, HyperHEP B® S/D, and Nabi-HB®. HepaGam B® occurs as a clear to opalescent liquid, contains 5% protein with 10% maltose and 0.03% polysorbate 80, and has a pH of 5.6. HyperHEP B® S/D contains 15–18% protein stabilized in 0.21–0.32 *M* glycine, and has a pH of 6.4–7.2. Nabi-HB® contains 4–6% protein in 0.075 *M* sodium chloride, 0.15 *M* glycine, and 0.01% polysorbate; has a pH of 6.2; and occurs as a clear to opalescent, nonturbid liquid.

HepaGam B®, HyperHEP B® S/D, and Nabi-HB® do not contain thimerosal or any other preservatives.

■ **Stability** HyperHEP B®, Nabi-HB®, and HepaGam B® should be refrigerated at 2–8°C; freezing should be avoided.

Single-dose vials of HBIG should be used within 6 hours after the vial has been entered, and any unused portion should be discarded.

Preparations

Excipients in commercially available drug preparations may have clinically important effects in some individuals; consult specific product labeling for details.

Hepatitis B Immune Globulin

Parenteral	
Injection, for IM use	**HyperHEP B® S/D** (solvent/detergent treated), Talecris
	Nabi-HB® (solvent/detergent treated), Nabi

Hepatitis B Immune Globulin Intravenous

Parenteral	
Injection, for IV or IM use	**HepaGam B®** (solvent/detergent treated), Cangene

†Use is not currently included in the labeling approved by the US Food and Drug Administration

Immune Globulin Immune Serum Globulin, Gamma Globulin, IG
Immune Globulin IM Immune Globulin IM, IGIM
Immune Globulin IV, IGIV
Immune Globulin Subcutaneous, IGSC Immune Globulin Sub-Q

■ Immune globulin IM (IGIM), immune globulin IV (IGIV), and immune globulin subcutaneous are sterile, nonpyrogenic preparations of globulins containing many antibodies normally present in adult human blood.

Uses

■ **Immune Globulin IM (IGIM)** ***Hepatitis A Virus Infection*** IGIM is used to provide passive immunity to hepatitis A virus (HAV) infection for *preexposure* or *postexposure* prophylaxis in susceptible individuals who are at risk of or have been exposed to the virus. IGIM is used for short-term protection against HAV in unvaccinated individuals who have been recently exposed to HAV and for individuals who cannot receive hepatitis A virus vaccine inactivated (hepatitis A vaccine) (e.g., infants younger than 12 months of age†, individuals hypersensitive to vaccine components). Because active immunization with hepatitis A vaccine provides long-term protection, combined passive immunization with IGIM and active immunization with hepatitis A vaccine can be used in unvaccinated individuals with recent HAV exposure in whom long-term protection is indicated. Combined passive immunization with IGIM and active immunization with hepatitis A virus vaccine also may be indicated in certain individuals to ensure preexposure protection against HAV when exposure may occur before protection is provided by the vaccine (e.g., travelers whose departure is imminent). The choice of *active* immunization with hepatitis A vaccine and/or *passive* immunization with IGIM should take into account the magnitude of risk associated with the exposure and characteristics of the patient that may be associated with more severe manifestations of HAV (e.g., older age, chronic liver disease). For information regarding recommendations for vaccination against HAV infection, see Uses in Hepatitis A Virus Vaccine Inactivated 80:12.

HAV usually is transmitted via the fecal-oral route either by person-to-person contact or ingestion of contaminated food or water. Transmission is facilitated by poor personal hygiene, poor sanitation, and intimate contact (e.g., household or sexual exposure). Common-source infections from contaminated food and water also occur. Illicit drug use is another common source of HAV infection. The incubation period for HAV infection following exposure to the virus ranges from 15–50 days and averages 28 days. For further information on types of exposure, risk of exposure, and management of exposure, see Uses in Hepatitis A Virus Vaccine Inactivated 80:12.

For preexposure prophylaxis against HAV, IGIM is considered protective immediately after administration. To be effective for postexposure prophylaxis of HAV in susceptible individuals, IGIM should be administered within 2 weeks after exposure to HAV and is not indicated in individuals with clinical symptoms of HAV infection or in those exposed to the virus more than 2 weeks previously. When given within 2 weeks after exposure, IGIM is about 80–90% effective in preventing symptomatic HAV; efficacy is greatest when IGIM is administered early in the incubation period and the immune globulin may only attenuate clinical HAV infection if given later in the incubation period. Because HAV infection cannot be reliably diagnosed on clinical presentation alone, serologic confirmation of HAV infection in the index case is recommended before postexposure treatment of contacts. However, routine screening of contacts for serologic markers of HAV infection prior to administration of postexposure prophylaxis is not recommended because such screening would delay prophylaxis.

For HAV postexposure prophylaxis in healthy individuals 12 months through 40 years of age, the US Public Health Service (USPHS) Advisory Committee on Immunization Practices (ACIP) and American Academy of Pediatrics (AAP) prefer use of monovalent hepatitis A vaccine. There is some evidence that monovalent hepatitis A vaccine administered within 2 weeks of exposure may be as effective as IGIM in healthy individuals 1–40 years of age. Hepatitis A vaccine also offers certain advantages over IGIM (e.g., induces active immunity and longer protection, more readily available, easier to administer, greater patient acceptance).

For HAV postexposure prophylaxis in adults older than 40 years of age, ACIP prefers use of IGIM since data are not available to date regarding efficacy of the vaccine for postexposure prophylaxis in this age group and these individuals are at risk for more severe manifestations of HAV. The vaccine can be used in these individuals if IGIM cannot be obtained. IGIM also is preferred for HAV postexposure prophylaxis in infants younger than 12 months of age†, immunocompromised individuals, individuals with chronic liver disease, and whenever the vaccine is contraindicated.

For individuals in whom IGIM is preferred for HAV postexposure prophylaxis, a dose of hepatitis A vaccine should also be administered simultaneously (using different syringes and different injection sites) if the vaccine is indicated for other reasons (e.g., catch-up vaccination, preexposure vaccination in high-risk groups) and is not contraindicated. If a dose of hepatitis A vaccine is used with or without IGIM for HAV postexposure prophylaxis, an additional (booster) dose of the vaccine should be administered according to the usually recommended schedule to ensure long-term protection.

Household or Sexual Contacts. Postexposure prophylaxis of HAV is recommended for *all* previously unvaccinated individuals who had household or sexual (heterosexual or homosexual) contact (within the past 2 weeks) with an individual with serologically confirmed HAV infection. Consideration also should be given to providing HAV postexposure prophylaxis to other individuals (e.g., regular babysitter) with ongoing, close personal contact with an individual with HAV infection.

Illicit Drug Users. Individuals who have shared illicit drugs (within the past 2 weeks) with an individual who has serologically confirmed HAV infection should receive HAV postexposure prophylaxis (hepatitis A vaccine with or without IGIM).

Unvaccinated Staff and Attendees of Child-care Facilities and Schools. If HAV infection occurs in one or more employees or attendees of a child-care facility that cares for children in diapers or in household contacts of 2 or more of the attendees (within the past 2 weeks), ACIP and AAP recommend HAV postexposure prophylaxis for all previously unvaccinated staff and attendees. If an outbreak of HAV (cases in 3 or more families) occurs or if recognition of the outbreak is delayed by 3 or more weeks from the onset of the index case, the infection is likely to have already spread widely and in these circumstances HAV postexposure prophylaxis also should be considered for all members of households whose diapered children attend. Children and adults with acute HAV infection should be excluded from the center until 1 week after onset of the illness and until the HAV prophylaxis program has been initiated or until directed by the responsible health department. During the 6 weeks after the last case of HAV is identified, unvaccinated new employees and new attendees also should receive prophylaxis.

If HAV infection is identified in an employee or attendee in a child-care facility in which all children are toilet trained, HAV postexposure prophylaxis is recommended only for previously unvaccinated employees in contact with the index case and for unvaccinated children in the same classroom as the index case.

HAV outbreaks involving student-to-student transmission in primary and secondary schools are rare in developed countries, but outbreaks have been documented. Routine HAV postexposure prophylaxis is not indicated for pupils and teachers in contact with a single primary or secondary school student with HAV infection; however, postexposure prophylaxis is recommended for close personal contacts of these children when epidemiologic evidence clearly shows the existence of a school- or classroom-centered outbreak of the disease.

Residents and Staff of Institutions for Custodial Care. Postexposure prophylaxis is indicated in institutions for custodial care, including prisons and facilities for the developmentally disabled, which favor transmission of HAV. When outbreaks occur in these institutions, HAV postexposure prophylaxis in residents and staff who have close contact with HAV-infected inmates or patients may reduce spread of the disease and is recommended.

ACIP states that routine HAV postexposure prophylaxis is not indicated when a single case of HAV occurs in usual office or other work situations.

Food Handlers. If HAV infection is diagnosed in an individual who handles food and common-source transmission of the disease is likely, HAV postexposure prophylaxis is recommended (within 2 weeks) for coworkers of the food handler. Because common-source transmission is unlikely, administration of postexposure prophylaxis to patrons usually is not indicated, but may be considered if, during the time the food handler was likely to be infectious, the food handler handled (without gloves) uncooked or cooked foods and the food handler had diarrhea or poor hygienic practices and patrons can be identified and given prophylaxis within 2 weeks of exposure. In settings in which repeated exposures to HAV may have occurred (e.g., institutional cafeterias), stronger consideration of HAV postexposure prophylaxis is warranted. In the event of a common-source outbreak, HAV postexposure prophylaxis should not be administered to exposed individuals after cases have begun to occur because the 2-week period during which IGIM is effective will have been exceeded.

Health-care Personnel. Health-care personnel, including those exposed to sewage, are not considered to be at increased risk for HAV infection as the result of occupational exposures. Nosocomial HAV transmission is rare. HAV outbreaks caused by transmission from adult patients to health-care personnel usually are associated with fecally incontinent patients; however, the majority of patients hospitalized with HAV infection are admitted after onset of jaundice when they are beyond the point of peak infectivity.

ACIP and AAP state that routine use of HAV postexposure prophylaxis is not indicated for health-care personnel providing care for patients with HAV. Instead, hygienic practices should be emphasized and health-care personnel should be made aware of the risk of exposure to HAV and precautions regarding direct contact with potentially infective materials (e.g., handwashing). If an epidemiologic investigation indicates that HAV transmission has occurred among hospital patients and/or hospital staff, ACIP recommends postexposure prophylaxis against HAV only in individuals in close contact with index patients.

Travelers. HAV is one of the most common vaccine-preventable diseases acquired during travel. IGIM is used for preexposure or postexposure prophylaxis of HAV infection in susceptible individuals (including pregnant women) traveling to foreign countries when there is a risk of exposure to HAV or HAV infection or if an exposure has occurred.

The risk of acquiring HAV for US citizens traveling abroad varies with living conditions, length of stay, and incidence of HAV infection in areas visited. The risk increases with the duration of travel and is highest for those living in or visiting rural areas, trekking in back country, or eating or drinking frequently in settings with poor sanitation. However, cases of travel-related HAV can occur in travelers to developing countries with "standard" tourist itineraries, accommodations, and food and beverage consumption behaviors. ACIP, US Centers for Disease Control and Prevention (CDC), and other experts state that the best way to prevent HAV and other enteric diseases when traveling to developing countries is to avoid potentially contaminated water and food. The CDC website (http://wwwnc.cdc.gov/travel) should be consulted for information regarding which countries have high or intermediate levels of HAV endemicity.

ACIP and CDC recommend preexposure prophylaxis with hepatitis A vaccine and/or IGIM in *all* susceptible individuals traveling for any purpose, frequency, or duration to areas where the risk of exposure to HAV is intermediate or high. Some experts advise individuals traveling outside the US to consider preexposure prophylaxis with hepatitis A vaccine regardless of their travel destination.

Primary immunization with a complete age-appropriate schedule of hepatitis A vaccine is preferred for HAV preexposure prophylaxis in adults, adolescents, children, and infants 12 months of age or older since active immunization provides long-term protection. Active immunization is particularly important for individuals planning to travel repeatedly to or reside for long periods in areas with intermediate or high levels of endemic HAV infection. IGIM should be used for HAV preexposure prophylaxis when the vaccine is unavailable or cannot be used (e.g., in infants younger than 12 months of age†, individuals hypersensitive to vaccine components) or when the traveler chooses not to receive the vaccine, provided that only short-term protection is required. Although additional doses of IGIM can be given every 6 months if the traveler remains in a high-risk setting, primary immunization with hepatitis A vaccine should be encouraged if the vaccine is not contraindicated.

For adults and children with imminent departure dates (e.g., in less than 4 weeks) who require both immediate and long-term protection against HAV, IGIM and hepatitis A vaccine may be administered simultaneously at separate sites; if only short-term protection is required, IGIM can be used alone.

ACIP states that if the complete age-appropriate immunization schedule cannot be administered prior to travel, 1 dose of single-antigen hepatitis A vaccine administered any time before departure can provide adequate protection in most healthy individuals 12 months through 40 years of age. However, for optimal protection in travelers at greatest risk for HAV (older adults or individuals with altered immunocompetence, chronic liver disease, or other chronic medical condition) who plan to depart within 2 weeks, ACIP and CDC recommend that a single dose of IGIM be given for preexposure prophylaxis concurrently with the first dose of hepatitis A vaccine (using different syringes and different injection sites).

Recommendations for HAV postexposure prophylaxis in travelers are the same as those for other individuals. Hepatitis A vaccine is recommended for HAV postexposure prophylaxis in unvaccinated travelers 12 months through 40 years of age. IGIM is preferred for HAV postexposure prophylaxis in travelers older than 40 years of age, but the vaccine can be used in these individuals if IGIM cannot be obtained. IGIM also is preferred for HAV postexposure prophylaxis in infants younger than 12 months of age†, immunocompromised individuals, individuals with chronic liver disease, and whenever the vaccine is contraindicated.

ACIP and CDC suggest that screening for total anti-HAV antibodies before travel may be useful in some circumstances to determine susceptibility to HAV and eliminate unnecessary vaccination or IGIM prophylaxis in individuals who are already immune. Such serologic screening may be indicated for travelers who are likely to have had prior HAV infection, including those older than 40 years of age, those who were born in or lived for extensive periods of time in parts of the world with intermediate or high HAV endemicity, and those in certain groups with a high prevalence of infections (e.g., those who inject illicit drugs). However, serologic testing to evaluate susceptibility to HAV should be considered only if it will not interfere with subsequent receipt of the vaccine or IGIM and if the cost of screening is less than the cost of vaccination or IGIM prophylaxis.

Measles IGIM and IGIV are used for postexposure prophylaxis to prevent or modify symptoms of measles (rubeola) in susceptible individuals exposed to the disease less than 6 days previously. Immune globulin should not be used in an attempt to control measles outbreaks.

Individuals born before 1957 and individuals with documentation of adequate vaccination against measles at 12 months of age or older, laboratory evidence of measles immunity, or laboratory confirmation of prior measles infection have acceptable presumptive evidence of measles immunity. Other individuals should be considered susceptible to measles.

Because administration of vaccine containing measles virus vaccine live (e.g., measles, mumps, and rubella virus vaccine live; MMR) within 72 hours of initial measles exposure may provide some protection against infection or modify the clinical course of measles and also provides future protection in individuals who do not contract the disease, ACIP and AAP recommend that susceptible individuals receive postexposure vaccination with a vaccine containing measles virus vaccine live within 72 hours after exposure, unless the vaccine is contraindicated. Postexposure vaccination is preferred to postexposure prophylaxis with immune globulin for most susceptible individuals 12 months of age or older who are exposed to measles in most settings (e.g., day-care facilities, schools, colleges, health-care facilities), provided the vaccine can be administered within 72 hours of the exposure and is not contraindicated.

Postexposure prophylaxis with immune globulin administered within 6 days of measles exposure is recommended in certain individuals at risk for severe disease and complications from measles, including infants younger than 12 months of age, pregnant women without evidence of measles immunity, and severely immunocompromised patients. ACIP and AAP recommend that IGIM be used for such prophylaxis in infants younger than 12 months of age† and that IGIV be used for such prophylaxis in susceptible pregnant women and severely immunocompromised individuals.

Although infants usually are immune to measles at birth because of passively acquired maternal antibodies, the duration of immunity depends on the amount of maternal antibody transferred to the infant. Most women of child-bearing age in the US have vaccine-derived immunity to measles, which results in lower antibody titers compared with women who have had measles, and epidemiologic data indicate that 7% of infants born in the US do not have anti-measles antibodies and up to 90% may be seronegative for such antibodies by 6 months of age. Because infants are at higher risk for severe measles and complications and are susceptible to measles if mothers are nonimmune or have low antibody titers, ACIP states that infants younger than 12 months of age† should receive IGIM following exposure to measles. Alternatively, infants 6 through 11 months of age can receive postexposure vaccination with MMR, provided the vaccine can be administered within 72 hours of exposure.

Pregnant women are at increased risk for severe measles and complications, and ACIP and AAP state that those without evidence of measles immunity should receive postexposure prophylaxis with immune globulin (preferably IGIV) within 6 days following exposure to measles. (See Measles under Uses: Immune Globulin IV [IGIV].)

Severely immunocompromised patients are at increased risk for severe measles and complications, and ACIP and AAP state that such individuals should receive postexposure prophylaxis with immune globulin (preferably IGIV) within 6 days following exposure to measles, regardless of immunologic or vaccination status. (See Measles under Uses: Immune Globulin IV [IGIV].)

Because passive immunity to measles following administration of immune globulin is temporary (unless modified or typical measles occurs), individuals who receive immune globulin for postexposure prophylaxis should receive immunization with a vaccine containing measles virus vaccine live (e.g., MMR) initiated at least 6 months after IGIM or at least 8 months after IGIV, providing the individual is at least 12 months of age and there are no contraindications to the vaccine. Immune globulin should *not* be given concurrently with a vaccine containing measles virus vaccine live. (See Measles, Mumps, Rubella, and Varicella Vaccines under Drug Interactions: Live Vaccines.)

Mumps IGIM is *not* effective for and should *not* be used for postexposure prophylaxis or treatment of mumps.

Poliomyelitis IGIM is *not* indicated for and should *not* be used for prophylaxis or treatment of poliomyelitis.

Rubella IGIM is *not* indicated for and should *not* be used for routine prophylaxis or treatment of rubella.

Although there is some evidence that use of IGIM for postexposure prophylaxis in susceptible women exposed to rubella during the first trimester of pregnancy may lessen the likelihood of rubella infection and associated adverse fetal effects, ACIP and AAP state that use of IGIM after exposure to rubella will not prevent infection or viremia but may modify or suppress symptoms and can create an unwarranted sense of security. Infants with congenital rubella have been born to women who received IGIM shortly after exposure to the disease.

ACIP and AAP state that IGIM should *not* be used routinely for postexposure prophylaxis of rubella in early pregnancy or any other circumstance. The only instance in which IGIM might be considered for postexposure prophylaxis of rubella is in a susceptible pregnant woman who is exposed to a confirmed case of rubella early in the pregnancy and who will not consider terminating the pregnancy under any circumstances. In such cases, administration of IGIM within 72 hours of rubella exposure might reduce, but will not eliminate, the risk for rubella.

Varicella IGIM is *not* indicated for and should *not* be used for routine prophylaxis or treatment of varicella (chickenpox).

Although the manufacturer states that IGIM may be considered for postexposure prophylaxis of varicella in susceptible individuals who are immunocompromised if varicella-zoster immune globulin (VZIG) is unavailable, IGIV (not IGIM) is recommended when VZIG is unavailable. (See Varicella under Uses: Immune Globulin IV [IGIV].)

■ **Immune Globulin IV (IGIV)** ***Primary Immunodeficiency Diseases*** IGIV (i.e., Bivigam® 10%, Carimune® NF, Flebogamma® 5% DIF, Flebogamma® 10% DIF, Gammagard® S/D, Gammagard® S/D [IgA less than 1 mcg/mL], Gammagard® 10%, Gammaked® 10%, Gammaplex® 5%, Gamunex®-C 10%, Octagam® 5%, Privigen® 10%) is used for replacement therapy in patients with primary humoral immunodeficiency who are unable to produce sufficient amounts of IgG antibodies. This includes, but is not limited to, patients with common variable immunodeficiency (CVID), X-linked agammaglobulinemia, congenital agammaglobulinemia, Wiskott-Aldrich syndrome, and severe combined immunodeficiencies.

IGIV is contraindicated in IgA-deficient individuals with antibodies against IgA and a history of hypersensitivity. (See Cautions: Precautions and Contraindications and see IgA Deficiency under Precautions and Contraindications: Sensitivity Reactions, in Cautions.)

Safety and efficacy of IGIV for replacement therapy in patients with primary immunodeficiency diseases has been established in various clinical trials in adults and children who received IGIV once every 3 or 4 weeks for 12 months. The primary efficacy end point in these studies generally was the rate of serious acute bacterial infections (e.g., pneumonia, bacteremia/sepsis, osteomyelitis/septic arthritis, bacterial meningitis, and visceral abscess) per patient per year. Results indicated that the annual rate of serious acute bacterial infections in patients receiving IGIV was substantially less than 1 infection per patient year (0–0.2 infections per patient year).

Idiopathic Thrombocytopenic Purpura IGIV (i.e., Carimune® NF, Flebogamma® 10% DIF, Gammagard® S/D, Gammagard® S/D [IgA less than 1 mcg/mL], Gammaked® 10%, Gammaplex® 5%, Gamunex®-C 10%, Octagam® 10%, Privigen® 10%) is used in the management of idiopathic thrombocytopenic purpura (ITP; also known as immune thrombocytopenic purpura or immune thrombocytopenia).

IGIV is used to increase platelet counts to prevent and/or control bleeding in patients with ITP or to allow a patient with ITP to undergo surgery.

Safety and efficacy of IGIV in adults and pediatric patients with chronic ITP (ITP of more than 6 months' duration) have been evaluated in various clinical trials and results indicate that a temporary increase in platelet counts can be obtained in patients who respond to the immune globulin. In many of these studies, the primary efficacy end point was the percentage of patients with an increase in platelet count to 50,000/mm³ or greater within 7–9 days after the first IGIV infusion (responders) and results indicated that 81–90% of patients with chronic ITP responded to IGIV. The median duration of response in patients who responded to IGIV with an increase in platelet count to 50,000/mm³ or greater was 10–15 days (range: 1–82 days or longer).

Results of a clinical study evaluating Carimune® in children with acute ITP (ITP of less than 6 months' duration) indicate that sequential platelet counts of 30,000, 100,000, and 150,000/mm³ are attained faster with the immune globulin than with corticosteroid therapy. However, many cases of acute ITP in children resolve spontaneously within weeks to months. Carimune® also has been used with good results in the treatment of acute ITP in adults. In a study in 10 adults with ITP of less than 16 weeks' duration, platelet counts increased to within the normal range after a 5-day course of Carimune® and this effect lasted a mean of greater than 173 days (range: 30–372 days).

Individuals with B-cell Chronic Lymphocytic Leukemia IGIV (i.e., Gammagard® S/D, Gammagard® S/D [IgA less than 1 mcg/mL]) is used for the prevention of bacterial infections in patients with hypogammaglobulinemia and/or recurrent bacterial infections associated with B-cell chronic lymphocytic leukemia (CLL).

Efficacy and safety of Gammagard® S/D in reducing bacterial infections in patients with B-cell CLL were evaluated in a double-blind, placebo-controlled trial. Patients received Gammagard® S/D (400 mg/kg) or placebo (saline solution) once every 3 weeks for a year (total of 17 infusions). The frequency of bacterial infections was 56% in patients receiving IGIV and 105% in those receiving placebo; the mean time to first bacterial infection was more than 365 days in patients receiving IGIV compared with 192 days in those receiving placebo. Patients receiving IGIV had fewer infections caused by *Streptococcus pneumoniae* and *Haemophilus influenzae* than those receiving placebo, but the incidence of other gram-negative infections was similar in both groups.

Kawasaki Disease IGIV (i.e., Gammagard® S/D, Gammagard® S/D [IgA less than 1 mcg/mL]) is used in conjunction with aspirin therapy for initial treatment of the acute phase of Kawasaki disease.

Concomitant use of IGIV and high-dose aspirin therapy initiated within 10 days of onset of fever is more effective than aspirin alone in preventing or reducing the occurrence of coronary artery abnormalities associated with Kawasaki disease and may result in more rapid resolution of fever and other clinical and laboratory indicators of acute inflammation.

AAP, American Heart Association (AHA), and American College of Chest Physicians (ACCP) state that combined therapy with IGIV and aspirin should be administered as soon as possible after Kawasaki disease is diagnosed or strongly suspected (optimally within 7–10 days of disease onset). In those with a delayed diagnosis (i.e., more than 10 days after disease onset), AAP and AHA suggest that combined therapy with IGIV and aspirin should be initiated if the patient has unexplained persistent fever or aneurysms and manifestations of ongoing systemic inflammation (e.g., elevated erythrocyte sedimentation rate [ESR] or C-reactive protein [CRP]) or evolving coronary artery disease.

Approximately 10% or more of patients with Kawasaki disease fail to respond to initial treatment with IGIV and aspirin therapy and have persistent fever or recurrence of fever after an initial afebrile period. Retreatment with IGIV (within 24–48 hours of persistent or recrudescent fever) and continued aspirin therapy usually is recommended for these patients.

In one study in patients with Kawasaki disease, coronary artery abnormalities were observed in 9% of those who received a single infusion of IGIV (2 g/kg) given in conjunction with high-dose aspirin therapy (100 mg/kg daily) compared with 23% of a historical control group that received only high-dose aspirin therapy. When patients with coronary artery abnormalities at study enrollment were excluded, such abnormalities were reported in 5% of patients treated with a single infusion of IGIV (2 g/kg) given in conjunction with high-dose aspirin therapy compared to 20% of a historical control group treated with only high-dose aspirin therapy.

In a controlled, multicenter, clinical study in patients with Kawasaki disease randomized to receive a single infusion of IGIV (2 g/kg over 8–12 hours) given in conjunction with aspirin (80–100 mg/kg daily) or a 4-day regimen of IGIV infusions (400 mg/kg over 2 hours for 4 days) given in conjunction with aspirin (80–100 mg/kg daily), the single infusion of IGIV was at least as effective in preventing coronary artery abnormalities as a 4-day regimen of IGIV. Coronary artery abnormalities were detected 2 weeks after treatment was initiated in 5 or 9% of patients receiving a single infusion of IGIV or a 4-day regimen of IGIV, respectively, and at 7 weeks such abnormalities were detected in 4 and 7% of patients, respectively. In addition, patients receiving a single infusion of IGIV experienced more rapid defervescence, shorter duration of fever, and a more rapid return to normal of clinical measures of inflammation than those receiving the 4-day regimen of IGIV.

Coronary artery abnormalities develop in 15–25% of children with Kawasaki disease if they are not treated within 10 days of fever onset; approximately 4% of patients develop coronary artery abnormalities despite prompt treatment with IGIV and aspirin. Long-term management of those who develop coronary abnormalities depends on the severity of coronary involvement and may include low-dose aspirin (with or without clopidogrel or dipyridamole), anticoagulant therapy with warfarin or low molecular weight heparin, or a combination of antiplatelet and anticoagulant therapy (usually low-dose aspirin and warfarin).

For additional information on long-term management of Kawasaki disease in individuals with coronary abnormalities, specialized references should be consulted.

Neurologic and Neuromuscular Disorders **Chronic Inflammatory Demyelinating Polyneuropathy.** IGIV (i.e., Gammaked® 10%, Gamunex®-C 10%) is used in the treatment of chronic inflammatory demyelinating polyneuropathy (CIDP) in adults to improve neuromuscular disability and impairment and for maintenance therapy to prevent relapse. Some clinicians consider IGIV the preferred treatment for CIDP, especially in children†, patients with poor venous access that precludes the use of plasma exchange, and in those susceptible to complications of long-term corticosteroid therapy.

Safety and efficacy of Gammaked® 10% IGIV for the treatment of CIDP were evaluated in a multicenter, randomized, double-blind, placebo-controlled trial in adults. The study included IGIV-naive and IGIV-experienced patients who were randomized to receive Gammaked® 10% (loading dose of 2 g/kg given by IV infusion over 2–4 consecutive days, then maintenance dosage of 1 g/kg given by IV infusion once every 3 weeks) or an equal volume of placebo. The study design included a 24-week efficacy period with crossover (rescue) where patients who did not improve and maintain improvement over the 24-week efficacy period were switched to the alternative treatment. Response was measured by the Inflammatory Neuropathy Cause and Treatment (INCAT) score used to assess functional disability of both upper and lower extremities in demyelinating polyneuropathy, and responders were defined as those who had at least 1-point improvement from baseline in the adjusted INCAT score that was maintained through the 24-week efficacy period. The response rate in patients treated with Gammaked® 10% was 47.5% compared with 22.4% in those treated with placebo.

Safety and efficacy of Gamunex®-C 10% IGIV for treatment of CIDP were evaluated in a multicenter, randomized, double-blind, placebo-controlled study in adults with CIDP who had progressive or relapsing motor and sensory dysfunction over the 2 months before study entry and substantial disability (defined as INCAT score of 2–9) (study 100538; ICE study). The study included IGIV-naive and IGIV-experienced patients. Patients were randomized to receive Gamunex®-C 10% (loading dose of 2 g/kg given by IV infusion over 2–4 consecutive days, then maintenance dosage of 1 g/kg given by IV infusion over 1–2 days once every 3 weeks) or placebo (0.1% albumin given in an equivalent volume). The study design included a 24-week efficacy period with response-conditional crossover (rescue) where patients who did not improve and maintain improvement over the 24-week efficacy period were switched to the alternative treatment; patients were withdrawn from the study if they failed to improve by week 3 after crossover or improved but then returned to baseline or lower. The response rate was measured by an adjusted INCAT disability score on day 16 and every 3 weeks for up to 24 weeks; responders were defined as those who had at least 1-point improvement from baseline in the adjusted INCAT score. In the intent-to-treat population, the response rate in the 24-week efficacy period was 47.5% in those who received Gamunex®-C 10% (43.6% in IGIV-naive and 55% in IGIV-experienced patients) compared with 22.4% in those who received placebo (28.3% in IGIV-naive and 0% in IGIV-experienced patients). After the 24-week efficacy period, patients who responded to Gamunex®-C 10% were entered into a randomized, double-blind, 24-week extension phase and either continued to receive Gamunex®-C 10% (1 g/kg over 1–2 days once every 3 weeks) or were reassigned to placebo. The time to relapse (relapse defined as 1 point or more decrease in adjusted INCAT score compared with baseline score at start of extension phase) was longer in those who continued to receive Gamunex®-C 10%; the probability of relapse was 13% in those who continued to receive the drug compared with 45% in those who received placebo during the extension phase.

Multifocal Motor Neuropathy. IGIV (i.e., Gammagard® Liquid 10%) is used for maintenance therapy to improve muscle strength and disability in adults with multifocal motor neuropathy (MMN). Some clinicians recommend IGIV as a treatment of choice for MMN when disability is severe enough to warrant treatment.

Safety and efficacy of Gammagard® Liquid 10% for maintenance therapy of MMN were evaluated in a randomized, double-blind, placebo-controlled, cross-over, withdrawal study in 44 adults with MMN already receiving IGIV at the time of study enrollment. The study protocol included 5 study periods consisting of three 12-week clinical stabilization phases, a 12-week double-blind withdrawal phase, and a 12-week double-blind cross-over period. Patients were evaluated for grip strength in the more affected hand (measured with dynamometer) and Guy's Neurological Disability Scale (GNDS) for the upper limbs. Results of this study indicate that a relative decline of 30% or more in grip strength in the more affected hand occurred in approximately 43% of patients during the placebo period but not during treatment with Gammagard® Liquid 10%, whereas approximately 5% of patients experienced a 30% or greater decline during treatment with Gammagard® Liquid 10%, but not during treatment with placebo. As determined by GNDS scores for the upper limbs, approximately 36% of patients deteriorated while receiving placebo but not during treatment with the immune globulin whereas approximately 12% of patients deteriorated during treatment with the immune globulin but not during the placebo period. The Overall Disability Sum Score (ODSS) changed by −7.14% during treatment with placebo (indicating worsening of disability) and by −1.11% during treatment with Gammagard® Liquid 10% (indicating minimal change in disability).

Other Neurologic and Neuromuscular Disorders. IGIV is used in the treatment of Guillain-Barré syndrome† (GBS). Although safety and efficacy have not been definitely established, IGIV initiated within 2 weeks of symptom onset appears to be as effective as plasma exchange and is recommended by some clinicians as a treatment of choice for GBS in adults and children, especially if disease is severe. Additional study is needed to determine whether IGIV is beneficial in patients with mild GBS or Miller Fischer syndrome.

IGIV has been used in the management of multiple sclerosis† (MS) and has provided benefits (e.g., reduced exacerbations, reduced disability scores) in some patients with relapsing-remitting MS. However, subsequent studies did not confirm these findings. Although some clinicians suggest that IGIV can be considered as second- or third-line treatment in patients with relapsing-remitting MS, others state that IGIV is not recommended for the treatment of relapsing-remitting or secondary progressive MS or the treatment of chronic symptoms of MS.

Although further study is needed, IGIV has been used with some success in the treatment of myasthenia gravis† and Lambert-Eaton myasthenic syndrome† (LEMS). It has been suggested that IGIV may be beneficial for second-line or adjunctive treatment of severe or worsening myasthenia gravis when other treatments have been unsuccessful or are not tolerated and also can be considered for second-line treatment of LEMS. Although there is some evidence that IGIV may be beneficial in patients with severe myasthenia gravis exacerbation, data are insufficient regarding use of the drug (either alone or in conjunction with other agents) in those with stable or chronic myasthenia gravis.

There is evidence that IGIV may provide some benefits in the management of Stiff-person syndrome† (Moersch-Woltmann syndrome). Although safety and efficacy have not been established, some clinicians recommend use of IGIV as second-line treatment when other treatments have been unsuccessful or cannot be used.

IGIV has been used in a limited number of children with intractable epilepsy†. Although there is some evidence that IGIV may be beneficial in some patients with Lennox-Gastaut syndrome† or Rasmussen syndrome†, further study is needed to evaluate efficacy of IGIV in the treatment of these conditions. Some clinicians suggest that IGIV can be considered in children with intractable epilepsy if they have not responded to antiepileptic agents and corticosteroids, especially if they are otherwise candidates for surgical resection.

Infections in Immunocompromised Individuals **HIV-infected Individuals.** IGIV has been used in an attempt to control or prevent infections and improve immunologic parameters in children with symptomatic human immunodeficiency virus (HIV) infection† who are immunosuppressed in association with acquired immunodeficiency syndrome (AIDS) or AIDS-related complex (ARC). IGIV also has been used in an attempt to control or prevent infections in HIV-infected adults†. Results of studies in adults and children with symptomatic HIV infection indicate that IGIV, used in dosages similar to those used for replacement therapy in patients with primary immunodeficiencies, reduces the incidence of recurrent bacterial infections and sepsis, including upper respiratory tract infections.

ACIP, AAP, CDC, National Institutes of Health (NIH), and other experts state that HIV-infected infants and children who have hypogammaglobulinemia (IgG less than 400 mg/dL) should receive IGIV (400 mg/kg once every 2–4 weeks) to prevent serious bacterial infections (e.g., those caused by *S. pneumoniae*). These experts state that use of IGIV for is no longer recommended for *routine* primary prophylaxis of serious bacterial infections in HIV-infected infants or children and that IGIV should be used for primary prophylaxis of infections *only* if hypogammaglobulinemia is present or functional antibody deficiency is demonstrated by either poor specific antibody titers or recurrent bacterial infections.

Efficacy of IGIV in preventing serious bacterial infections in symptomatic HIV-infected children was evaluated in several studies done prior to the availability of highly active antiretroviral therapy (HAART). Results of a randomized, double-blind, controlled comparison of IGIV (400 mg/kg administered every 28 days) and placebo (albumin human) for prevention of serious bacterial infections in immunologically or clinically symptomatic HIV-infected children younger than 13 years of age sponsored by the National Institute of Child Health and Human Development (NICHD) indicated that IGIV was effective in prolonging infection-free time in immunologically or clinically symptomatic HIV-infected children with $CD4^+$ T-cell counts of 200 cells/mm^3 or greater. Efficacy in prolonging infection-free time was not evident in children with $CD4^+$ T-cell counts less than 200 cells/mm^3. This study did not include children with hemophilia, and 78% of those studied were younger than 5 years of age; 91% of those studied had acquired HIV infection perinatally. In a double-blind study in infants and children 3 months to 12 years of age with AIDS or ARC who were receiving zidovudine monotherapy, prophylactic administration of IGIV decreased the risk of serious bacterial infections over the 2-year study period, but there was no effect on survival. In this study, children receiving co-trimoxazole prophylaxis for *Pneumocystis carinii* pneumonia did not appear to benefit from IGIV prophylaxis.

Bone Marrow Transplant Recipients. IGIV has been used in adults and children undergoing bone marrow transplantation† (BMT) to decrease the risk of septicemia and other infections, interstitial pneumonia of infectious or idiopathic etiologies, and acute graft-versus-host disease (GVHD). However, the effect of IGIV on the incidence of cytomegalovirus (CMV) infection, other infections, or GVHD in patients undergoing allogeneic BMT is unclear. IGIV prophylaxis in BMT patients does not appear to affect survival or risk of cancer relapse, and the long-term effects of such therapy remain to be determined.

In a controlled study in adults who underwent BMT with or without IGIV prophylaxis, there was a clinically important decrease in the incidence of acute GVHD and associated interstitial pneumonia and septicemia during the first 100 days following the procedure in patients who received IGIV; a beneficial effect was not evident in patients younger than 20 years of age. Other studies failed to demonstrate decreased rates of GVHD or infection when IGIV was used in patients undergoing unrelated allogeneic BMT. In a study in patients at risk for developing CMV (i.e., patients who were CMV-seropositive prior to transplantation or CMV-negative patients who received a transplant from a CMV-positive donor), administration of IGIV resulted in a substantial decrease in the incidence of CMV pneumonitis, but this effect did not occur in other studies.

Although efficacy and safety in BMT patients have not been established, some clinicians suggest that IGIV be used for prophylaxis in all allogeneic BMT patients, especially those who are CMV-positive or have received a transplant from a CMV-positive donor.

Some clinicians suggest that, although there is a perceived benefit of IGIV prophylaxis in infants with severe combined immunodeficiency or other primary immunodeficiency diseases undergoing BMT, the effect of IGIV in these children is difficult to study since they generally are receiving IGIV for replacement therapy. These clinicians also state that use of IGIV appears to offer little benefit in patients with malignancies undergoing HLA-identical sibling BMT and that additional study is needed to determine whether the drug is beneficial in those undergoing HLA-matched unrelated BMT or cord blood transplants.

Hematopoietic Stem Cell Transplant Recipients. Individuals who undergo hematopoietic stem cell transplant (HSCT) are at risk for a variety of opportunistic infections during the period prior to engraftment and subsequent immune system recovery. CDC, Infectious Diseases Society of America (IDSA), and American Society of Blood and Marrow Transplantation (ASBMT) have established guidelines for preventing opportunistic infections in HSCT recipients that include recommendations regarding certain vaccinations and prophylactic regimens. These guidelines state that, although routine administration of IGIV for prophylaxis is *not* recommended for autologous HSCT recipients, some clinicians recommend use of IGIV to prevent bacterial infections (e.g., *S. pneumoniae* sinopulmonary infections) in adult, adolescent, or pediatric allogeneic HSCT recipients† who experience severe hypogammaglobulinemia (IgG less than 400 mg/dL) within the first 100 days after transplant. If IGIV is used in hypogammaglobulinemic allogeneic HSCT recipients, the fact that the pharmacokinetics of IGIV in these individuals may differ from that in healthy adults should be considered. It is recommended that trough serum IgG concentrations be monitored regularly (e.g., approximately every 2 weeks) in HSCT recipients and that IGIV dosage adjusted to maintain trough serum IgG concentrations exceeding 400–500 mg/dL. Routine administration of IGIV in HSCT recipients more than 90 days after HSCT is not recommended in the absence of severe hypogammaglobulinemia.

The guidelines for preventing opportunistic infections among HSCT recipients published by CDC, IDSA, and ASBMT should be consulted for additional information on preventing opportunistic infections in these patients (including vaccinations) and for information on hospital infection control, strategies for safe living after transplantation, and hematopoietic stem cell safety.

Other Individuals. IGIV has been used alone or in conjunction with appropriate anti-infective therapy to prevent or modify acute bacterial or viral infections (e.g., cytomegalovirus infections) in patients with iatrogenically induced or disease-associated immunosuppression†, such as patients undergoing major surgery (e.g., cardiac transplants) or patients with hematologic malignancies, extensive burns, or collagen-vascular diseases.

Infections in Low-birthweight Neonates IGIV has been used for prophylaxis and treatment of infections in certain high-risk, preterm, low-birthweight neonates†. Preterm neonates generally have low serum IgG concentrations at birth since the bulk of transplacental transfer of IgG to the fetus occurs at 32 weeks of gestation or later. Although the role of low neonatal IgG concentrations in the pathogenesis of nosocomial bacterial infections in preterm, low-birthweight infants has not been elucidated, some clinicians have suggested that IGIV therapy may be used to prevent or modify systemic bacterial infections in these infants by maintaining therapeutic concentrations of IgG. However, use of IGIV for prophylaxis of infections in high-risk neonates is controversial. AAP does *not* recommend routine use of IGIV for prophylaxis of infections in preterm neonates. Results of several controlled and uncontrolled studies indicate that administration of IGIV to preterm, low-birthweight neonates beginning shortly after birth reduces the incidence of nosocomial sepsis (including infections caused by *S. agalactiae* [group B streptococci]) in these infants; administration of IGIV appeared to have a negligible influence on mortality in some studies. Results of other studies have failed to show that IGIV therapy resulted in any clinically important reduction in the incidence of sepsis and/or mortality due to sepsis in the neonatal period. In one prospective, controlled study sponsored by the NICHD Neonatal Research Network, use of prophylactic IGIV in low-birthweight neonates had no clinically important effect on nosocomial infections.Septicemia, meningitis, or urinary tract infections occurred in 17% of neonates receiving IGIV and 19% of neonates receiving placebo. Until results of other studies are available and until further studies are done to evaluate safety of IGIV therapy in neonates, IGIV should not be used routinely for prophylaxis or treatment of nosocomial infections in preterm, low-birthweight infants.

Autoimmune Neutropenia and Autoimmune Hemolytic Anemia IGIV has been used with some success in a limited number of adults and children for the treatment of autoimmune neutropenia†. Although there is some evidence that IGIV may be beneficial in patients with autoimmune neutropenia, it is unclear whether IGIV offers any advantages over corticosteroid therapy.

IGIV has been used with variable results in patients with autoimmune hemolytic anemia†. A few patients with autoimmune hemolytic anemia appeared to respond to IGIV, but the drug either had no effect or potentiated hemolysis in other patients. Some clinicians state that IGIV should be used in the management of autoimmune hemolytic anemia only in patients who fail to respond to other treatment options.

Dermatomyositis and Polymyositis IGIV has been used in the treatment of dermatomyositis† and polymyositis†. In a limited number of patients with biopsy-proven, treatment-resistant dermatomyositis, IGIV therapy resulted in improvements in muscle strength and neuromuscular symptoms within about 2 weeks after the first dose; some patients had marked clearance of rash and scaling. Although efficacy and safety have not been established, it has been suggested that IGIV (usually in conjunction with corticosteroids) may be beneficial as second-line therapy in patients with dermatomyositis when other therapies are unsuccessful or cannot be used.

Graves' Ophthalmopathy Although further study is needed, there is some evidence that IGIV may be beneficial in the management of Graves' ophthalmopathy†. Some patients treated with IGIV had improvements in diplopia, proptosis, visual acuity, and intraocular pressure; the response rate appeared to be similar to that obtained with corticosteroid treatment.

Measles IGIV is used for postexposure prophylaxis to prevent or modify symptoms of measles† (rubeola) in susceptible individuals exposed to the disease less than 6 days previously. Immune globulin should not be used in an attempt to control measles outbreaks.

Individuals born before 1957 and individuals with documentation of adequate vaccination against measles at 12 months of age or older, laboratory evidence of measles immunity, or laboratory confirmation of prior measles infection have acceptable presumptive evidence of measles immunity. Other individuals should be considered susceptible to measles.

Postexposure prophylaxis with immune globulin administered within 6 days of measles exposure is recommended in certain individuals at risk for severe disease and complications from measles, including infants younger than 12 months of age†, pregnant women without evidence of measles immunity, and severely immunocompromised patients. ACIP and AAP recommend that IGIM be used for such prophylaxis in infants younger than 12 months of age† and that IGIV be used for such prophylaxis in susceptible pregnant women and severely immunocompromised individuals.

Because infants are at higher risk for severe measles and complications and are susceptible to measles if mothers are nonimmune or have low antibody titers, ACIP states that infants younger than 12 months of age should receive immune globulin (preferably IGIM) following exposure to measles. Alternatively, infants 6 through 11 months of age can receive postexposure vaccination with MMR, provided the vaccine can be administered within 72 hours of exposure. (See Measles under Uses: Immune Globulin IM [IGIM].)

Pregnant women are at increased risk for severe measles and complications, and ACIP and AAP state that pregnant women without evidence of measles immunity should receive postexposure prophylaxis with immune globulin (preferably IGIV) within 6 days following exposure to measles. IGIV is recommended instead of IGIM in pregnant women to ensure protective levels of measles antibody titers.

Severely immunocompromised patients are at increased risk for severe measles and complications, and ACIP and AAP state that such individuals should receive postexposure prophylaxis with immune globulin (preferably IGIV) within 6 days following exposure to measles, regardless of immunologic or vaccination status. Severely immunocompromised individuals who should receive postexposure prophylaxis with immune globulin include those with severe primary immunodeficiency; bone marrow transplant recipients (until at least 12 months after completion of immunosuppressive treatment or even longer in those with graft-versus-host disease); patients being treated for acute lymphocytic leukemia (until at least 6 months after completion of immunosuppressive chemotherapy); and HIV-infected patients with AIDS or other HIV-infected individuals with severe immunosuppression (defined as $CD4^+$ T-cell percentage less than 15% [all ages] or $CD4^+$ T-cell count less than 200/mm^3 [older than 5 years of age]). Postexposure prophylaxis with immune globulin also is recommended for HIV-infected individuals who have not received a dose of MMR since effective antiretroviral therapy was initiated and for those without laboratory evidence of measles immunity.

Because passive immunity to measles following administration of immune globulin is temporary (unless modified or typical measles occurs), individuals who receive immune globulin for postexposure prophylaxis should receive immunization with a vaccine containing measles virus vaccine live (e.g., MMR) initiated at least 8 months after IGIV was given or at least 6 months after IGIM was given, providing the individual is at least 12 months of age and there are no contraindications to the vaccine. Immune globulin should *not* be given concurrently with a vaccine containing measles virus vaccine live. (See Measles, Mumps, Rubella, and Varicella Vaccines under Drug Interactions: Live Vaccines.)

Systemic Lupus Erythematosus IGIV has been used with some success in the treatment of systemic lupus erythematosus† (SLE); however, efficacy and safety have not been established and additional study is needed to evaluate use of IGIV in patients with SLE. Some clinicians suggest that IGIV can be considered in patients with severe active SLE when other drugs have been ineffective or not tolerated; other clinicians recommend caution.

Tetanus Although tetanus immune globulin (TIG) is the immune globulin of choice, IGIV is recommended as an alternative for the treatment of tetanus† when TIG is unavailable.

IGIV also has been recommended as an alternative for postexposure prophylaxis of tetanus† in individuals with tetanus-prone wounds when TIG is unavailable.

Toxic Shock Syndrome IGIV has been used as an adjunct to anti-infectives and surgical intervention in the treatment of staphylococcal or streptococcal toxic shock syndrome† or necrotizing fasciitis† in severely ill patients.

Although data are limited and efficacy and safety have not been established, AAP and others suggest that use of IGIV may be considered as an adjunct in the management of severe staphylococcal or streptococcal toxic shock syndrome† or necrotizing fasciitis† (e.g., when the infection is refractory to several hours of aggressive therapy, an undrainable focus is present, the patient has persistent oliguria with pulmonary edema). IGIV is most likely to be beneficial if initiated early in the course of the disease. The mechanism of action of IGIV in toxic shock syndrome is unclear, but may be related to neutralization of circulating bacterial toxins.

Varicella IGIV has been used and is recommended as an alternative to VZIG for postexposure prophylaxis of varicella† in susceptible individuals when VZIG is unavailable. Although VZIG or IGIV given shortly after exposure to varicella zoster virus can prevent or modify the course of the disease, immune globulin preparations are not effective once disease is established.

VZIG is the preferred immune globulin for postexposure prophylaxis of varicella in patients who do not have evidence of immunity (i.e., without a history of varicella or varicella vaccination) and are at high risk for severe disease and complications (e.g., HIV-infected or other immunocompromised patients, pregnant women). Clinical data demonstrating effectiveness of IGIV for postexposure prophylaxis of varicella are not available and, although commercially available IGIV preparations are known to contain anti-varicella antibody titers, the titer of any specific lot of IGIV is uncertain since IGIV is not routinely tested for anti-varicella antibodies.

ACIP, AAP, CDC, NIH, and other experts state that HIV-infected adults, adolescents, or children or other individuals who are receiving IGIV replacement therapy (400 mg/kg or greater given at regular intervals) and received a dose of IGIV within 3 weeks prior to exposure to wild-type varicella zoster virus should be protected and should not require postexposure prophylaxis with VZIG or IGIV.

■ **Immune Globulin Subcutaneous** ***Primary Immunodeficiency Diseases*** Immune globulin subcutaneous (Cuvitru® 20%, Gammagard® Liquid 10%, Gammaked® 10%, Gamunex®-C 10%, Hizentra® 20%) and immune globulin subcutaneous in conjunction with recombinant human hyaluronidase (Hyqvia®; immune globulin subcutaneous 10% copackaged with recombinant human hyaluronidase) are used for replacement therapy in patients with primary humoral immunodeficiency. This includes, but is not limited to, patients with CVID, X-linked agammaglobulinemia, congenital agammaglobulinemia, Wiskott-Aldrich syndrome, and severe combined immunodeficiencies.

Immune globulin subcutaneous is contraindicated in IgA-deficient individuals with antibodies against IgA and a history of hypersensitivity. (See IgA Deficiency under Precautions and Contraindications: Sensitivity Reactions, in Cautions.)

Safety and efficacy of Cuvitru® 20% administered subcutaneously for replacement therapy in patients with primary immunodeficiency were evaluated in an open-label, prospective study that included 77 adults and children 2 years of age and older. All patients received a regimen of IGIV initially (IGIV 10% given once every 3 or 4 weeks for 13 weeks) before being switched to subcutaneous Cuvitru® 20% (once weekly for 12 weeks at an adjusted dose of 145% of the IGIV dose). The mean dose of subcutaneous Cuvitru® 20% was 222 mg/kg once weekly and the median duration of treatment was 380.5 days (range: 30–629 days). The annual rate of acute serious bacterial infections during Cuvitru® 20% treatment was lower than 1 infection per patient per year and the annual rate of any infection was 2.41 infections per patient per year.

Safety and efficacy of Gammagard® Liquid 10% administered subcutaneously for replacement therapy in adults and children with primary immunodeficiency were evaluated in an open-label, prospective, multicenter US study in 49 adult and pediatric patients, including those who had been receiving IGIV or another subcutaneous immune globulin preparation. All patients (regardless of their prior regimen) received an initial IV regimen of Gammagard® Liquid 10% (IV once every 3 or 4 weeks for 12 weeks) before being switched to subcutaneous Gammagard® Liquid 10%. The median duration of subcutaneous Gammagard® Liquid 10% therapy was 379 days (range: 57–477 days). The annual rate of acute serious bacterial infections while patients were receiving subcutaneous Gammagard® Liquid 10% was 0.067 infections per patient per year and the annual rate of any infection (including viral and fungal infections) was 4.1 infections per patient per year.

Safety and efficacy of Hizentra® 20% immune globulin subcutaneous for replacement therapy in patients with primary immune deficiency were evaluated in an open-label, prospective, multicenter US study that included 49 adult and pediatric patients who were previously receiving a once-monthly regimen of IGIV and were switched to a once-weekly regimen of subcutaneous Hizentra® 20% given. After a 3-month wash-in/wash-out period, the dose of Hizentra® 20% was adjusted individually to achieve an IgG area under the concentration-time curve (AUC) that was equivalent to that attained with their previous IGIV therapy and the next 12 months of therapy was considered the efficacy period. In the modified intention-to-treat (MITT) population (38 patients who completed the 3-month wash-in/wash-out period and received at least 1 subcutaneous infusion of Hizentra® 20%), there were no serious bacterial infections (defined as bacterial pneumonia, bacteremia/septicemia, osteomyelitis/septic arthritis, bacterial meningitis, or visceral abscess) and the annual rate of any infection was 2.76 infections per patient per year. Safety and efficacy of Hizentra® 20% immune globulin subcutaneous also have been evaluated in an open-label, prospective, multicenter study in Europe that included 51 adult and pediatric patients with primary immunodeficiency who were previously receiving once-monthly IGIV (31 patients) or once-weekly immune globulin subcutaneous (20 patients) and were switched to once-weekly Hizentra® 20%. During the efficacy period, there were no serious bacterial infections and the annual rate of any infection was 5.18 infections per patient per year.

Safety and efficacy of immune globulin subcutaneous 10% with recombinant human hyaluronidase (Hyqvia®) for replacement therapy in patients with primary immunodeficiency were evaluated in an open-label, uncontrolled, prospective, multicenter US trial that included 83 adult and pediatric patients switched from a regimen of IGIV or another subcutaneous immune globulin preparation to Hyqvia®. For each dose, the recombinant human hyaluronidase component (acts locally to temporarily increase permeability of subcutaneous tissue to increase dispersion and absorption of the immune globulin) was administered first and the immune globulin subcutaneous 10% component was administered within approximately 10 minutes at the same site. All patients (regardless of prior regimen) received Hyqvia® in an initial dose ramp-up period that allowed them to adjust to the large volumes required for a full 3- to 4-week treatment regimen, after which Hyqvia® was administered once every 3 or 4 weeks for the remainder of the trial. After 3 doses at full volume, dosage of the immune globulin component of Hyqvia® was individually adjusted to achieve serum IgG levels comparable to those attained with their previous immune globulin therapy. During the 12 months of treatment after the ramp-up period, patients were assessed for several outcomes, including rate of infections. The overall rate of infections in patients treated with Hyqvia® was 2.97 infections per patient per year. There were 2 acute serious bacterial infections during the 12-month efficacy period and, based on this, the annualized rate of acute serious bacterial infections was 0.025 infections per patient per year.

Dosage and Administration

■ **Reconstitution and Administration** ***Immune Globulin IM (IGIM)*** Immune globulin IM (GamaSTAN® S/D) is administered by IM injection. IGIM should not be administered IV or subcutaneously because of the risk of serious reactions (e.g., renal dysfunction, acute renal failure, hemolysis, transfusion-related acute lung injury).

In adults and children, IM injection with IGIM preferably should be made into the deltoid muscle or anterolateral aspect of the thigh. Because of the risk of injury to sciatic nerves, the gluteal muscle should not be routinely used for IM injections.

When the dose of IGIM is greater than 10 mL, the dose should be divided and injected into several muscle sites to reduce local pain and discomfort. IM administration of a total dose exceeding 20 mL (even in adults) should be avoided.

Prior to administration, IGIM solutions should be inspected visually for particulate matter and discoloration whenever solution and container permit. The plunger of the syringe should be drawn back before injection of IGIM to ensure that the needle is not in a blood vessel.

Patients should be adequately hydrated prior to administration of IGIM.

The recommended dosage of IGIM should not be exceeded in patients at increased risk of thrombosis (e.g., those with multiple cardiovascular risk factors, advanced age, prolonged periods of immobilization, hypercoagulable disorders, previous thrombotic or thromboembolic event, concomitant use of estrogen-containing preparations, indwelling central vascular catheters, and/or known or suspected hyperviscosity).

Immune Globulin IV (IGIV) Immune globulin IV (Bivigam® 10%, Carimune® NF, Flebogamma® 5% DIF, Flebogamma® 10% DIF, Gammagard® Liquid 10%, Gammagard® S/D, Gammagard® S/D [IgA less than 1 mcg/mL], Gammaked® 10%, Gammaplex® 5%, Gamunex®-C 10%, Octagam® 5%, Octagam® 10%, Privigen® 10%) is administered by IV infusion. Certain IGIV preparations can be administered by IV infusion *or* subcutaneous infusion for the treatment of primary humoral immunodeficiency (Gammagard® Liquid 10%, Gammaked® 10%, Gamunex®-C 10%); all other IGIV preparations should *only* be administered by IV infusion.

IGIV should be administered IV using a separate line and should not be mixed with other drugs or IV infusion fluids. In addition, different IGIV preparations should not be admixed.

Prior to administration, IGIV solutions should be inspected visually for particulate matter and discoloration whenever solution and container permit and should not be used if discolored or turbid or if particulate matter is present.

The rate of infusion of IGIV should be individualized based on the preparation used and individual patient requirements. In general, IGIV infusions in patients receiving initial doses or switching from one IGIV preparation to another should be initiated at the lower end of the range of recommended rates; if the first few infusions are tolerated, the rate of infusion for subsequent infusions may be slowly increased to the maximum recommended rate.

If adverse reactions occur during infusion of IGIV, the rate of infusion should be decreased or the infusion stopped until adverse reactions subside. In some cases when symptoms subside promptly, the infusion may then be resumed at a rate that is tolerated by the individual. A rapid infusion rate should *not* be used in patients with or at risk for renal dysfunction or thrombosis.

Prior to initiation of the IGIV infusion, clinicians should ensure that patients are not volume depleted and are adequately hydrated.

Bivigam® 10%. Bivigam® 10% is administered *only* by IV infusion.

Bivigam® 10% is administered undiluted and should not be mixed with other drugs, IV infusion fluids, or other IGIV preparations.

Vials are for single use only.

When large doses are to be administered, the contents of several vials of Bivigam® 10% may be pooled into an empty, sterile IV infusion bag using aseptic technique. Partially used vials should be discarded.

Bivigam® 10% should be at room temperature during IV infusion.

IV infusions of Bivigam® 10% should be initiated at a rate of 0.5 mg/kg per minute (0.005 mL/kg per minute). If this rate is well tolerated for the first 10 minutes, the rate may be gradually increased every 20 minutes by 0.8 mg/kg per minute up to a maximum of 6 mg/kg per minute. If adverse effects related to the rate of infusion occur, the IV infusion should be stopped or slowed. If symptoms subside promptly, the IV infusion may be resumed at a lower rate that is comfortable for the patient.

In patients at increased risk of thrombosis or renal dysfunction (including those 65 years of age or older), Bivigam® 10% should be infused at the minimum IV infusion rate practicable. If renal function deteriorates, discontinuance of Bivigam® 10% should be considered.

Carimune® NF. Carimune® NF is administered *only* by IV infusion.

Carimune® NF should be reconstituted according to the manufacturer's directions with 0.9% sodium chloride, 5% dextrose injection, or sterile water for injection to prepare a solution containing 30, 60, 90, or 120 mg of protein per mL (3, 6, 9, or 12% solution, respectively). The patient's fluid, electrolyte, and caloric requirements should be considered when selecting an appropriate diluent and concentration. After the diluent is added, vials should be swirled vigorously to dissolve the drug, but should not be shaken since this may cause foaming. Carimune® NF generally dissolve within a few minutes, although in exceptional cases it may take up to 20 minutes for complete dissolution.

The manufacturer of Carimune® NF states that, although the drug may be filtered, filtering is not required. If a filter is used, filters with pore sizes of 15 μm or larger are less likely to slow the infusion, especially when higher concentrations of the drugs are administered; antibacterial filters (0.2 μm) may be used.

If Carimune® NF is reconstituted outside of sterile laminar airflow conditions, reconstituted solutions should be administered promptly and any partially used vials discarded. If the drug is reconstituted in a sterile laminar flow hood using aseptic technique and the reconstituted solution is stored under refrigeration, the IV infusion should be initiated within 24 hours after reconstitution.

Prior to administration, solutions should be clear and at approximately room temperature. If large doses of Carimune® NF are to be administered, the contents of several reconstituted vials of the identical concentration and diluent may be pooled into an empty, sterile glass or plastic IV infusion container using aseptic technique.

Reconstituted Carimune® NF should be administered through a separate IV line and should not be mixed with other drugs, IV infusion fluids, or other IGIV preparations.

When Carimune® NF is used for the treatment of primary immunodeficiency in individuals with previously untreated agammaglobulinemia or hypogammaglobulinemia, a solution containing 30 mg/mL should be used for the initial dose and given at an initial IV infusion rate of 0.5 mg/kg per minute. After 30 minutes, the infusion rate may be increased to 1 mg/kg per minute for the next 30 minutes; thereafter, the infusion rate may be gradually increased in a stepwise manner up to a maximum of 3 mg/kg per minute as tolerated. If the initial IV infusion was well tolerated, higher concentrations may be used for subsequent infusions. (For information on concentrations of Carimune® NF and corresponding infusion rates, see Table 1.) Use of an initial infusion rate exceeding 2 mg/kg per minute in patients with agammaglobulinemia or hypogammaglobulinemia who had not previously received IGIV or had not received a dose within the last 8 weeks has resulted in inflammatory reactions. (See Infusion Reactions under Cautions: Immune Globulin IV [IGIV].)

When Carimune® NF is used for the treatment of idiopathic thrombocytopenic purpura (ITP; also known as immune thrombocytopenic purpura or immune thrombocytopenia), a solution containing 60 mg/mL is recommended. The recommended initial IV infusion rate in patients with ITP is 0.5 mg/kg per minute. After 30 minutes, the infusion rate may be increased to 1 mg/kg per minute for the next 30 minutes; thereafter, the infusion rate may be gradually increased in a stepwise manner up to a maximum of 3 mg/kg per minute as tolerated. (See Table 1.)

In patients at risk of developing renal dysfunction (e.g., adults older than 65 years of age; individuals receiving nephrotoxic drugs; individuals with diabetes mellitus, volume depletion, paraproteinemia, or sepsis), Carimune® NF should be infused at a rate less than 2 mg/kg per minute.

In patients at increased risk of thrombosis (e.g., those with cardiovascular risk factors, advanced age, prolonged periods of immobilization, hypercoagulable disorders, history of venous or arterial thrombosis, concomitant use of estrogen-containing preparations, indwelling central vascular catheters, and/or hyperviscosity), Carimune® NF should be infused at a rate less than 2 mg/kg per minute.

Table 1. Carimune® NF Concentrations and IV Infusion Rates

Concentration	Initial Infusion Rate: 0.5 mg/kg per minute	1 mg/kg per minute	2 mg/kg per minute[a]	3 mg/kg per minute[b]
3%	0.0167 mL/kg per minute	0.033 mL/kg per minute	0.067 mL/kg per minute	0.10 mL/kg per minute
6%	0.008 mL/kg per minute	0.0167 mL/kg per minute	0.033 mL/kg per minute	0.05 mL/kg per minute
9%	0.006 mL/kg per minute	0.011 mL/kg per minute	0.022 mL/kg per minute	0.033 mL/kg per minute
12%	0.004 mL/kg per minute	0.008 mL/kg per minute	0.016 mL/kg per minute	0.025 mL/kg per minute

[a] Maximum IV infusion rate for patients at risk of renal dysfunction or thromboembolic events.

[b] Maximum IV infusion rate for patients *not* at risk of renal dysfunction or thromboembolic events.

Flebogamma® 5% DIF. Flebogamma® 5% DIF is administered *only* by IV infusion.

Flebogamma® 5% DIF is administered undiluted and should *not* be mixed with other drugs, IV infusion fluids, or other IGIV preparations.

If large doses are indicated, several vials of Flebogamma® 5% DIF may be pooled into an empty, sterile IV container using aseptic technique. Partially used vials and administration sets should be discarded after use.

IV infusions of Flebogamma® 5% DIF should be initiated at a rate of 0.01 mL/kg per minute (0.5 mg/kg per minute). If tolerated during the first 30 minutes, the rate of infusion may be gradually increased to a maximum of 0.1 mL/kg per minute (5 mg/kg per minute).

For individuals 65 years of age or older or at increased risk for renal dysfunction or thrombosis, the minimum infusion rate practicable should be used. The maximum IV infusion rate for Flebogamma® 5% DIF in geriatric patients is less than 0.06 mL/kg per minute (less than 3 mg/kg per minute).

Flebogamma® 10% DIF. Flebogamma® 10% DIF is administered *only* by IV infusion.

Flebogamma® 10% DIF is administered undiluted and should not be mixed with other drugs, IV infusion fluids, or other IGIV preparations.

Vials of Flebogamma® 10% DIF are for single use only.

When large doses are to be administered, the contents of several vials of Flebogamma® 10% DIF may be pooled into an empty, sterile IV container using aseptic technique. Partially used vials and administration sets should be discarded.

IV infusions of Flebogamma® 10% DIF should be initiated at a rate of 0.01 mL/kg per minute (1 mg/kg per minute). If no adverse reactions occur during the first 30 minutes, the rate of infusion may be gradually increased to 0.04 mL/kg per minute (4 mg/kg per minute). If tolerated, the infusion rate may then be gradually increased to a maximum of 0.08 mL/kg per minute (8 mg/kg per minute).

For individuals 65 years of age or older or at risk for renal dysfunction or thrombosis, the minimum infusion rate practicable should be used. The maximum IV infusion rate for Flebogamma® 10% DIF in geriatric patients is less than 0.04 mL/kg per minute (less than 4 mg/kg per minute).

Gammagard® Liquid 10%. Gammagard® Liquid 10% is administered by IV infusion. Alternatively, Gammagard® Liquid 10% may be administered by subcutaneous infusion for the treatment of primary humoral immunodeficiency (see Gammagard Liquid 10% under Reconstitution and Administration: Immune Globulin Subcutaneous, in Dosage and Administration).

If necessary, Gammagard® Liquid 10% may be diluted with 5% dextrose injection; 0.9% sodium chloride should *not* be used as a diluent.

Gammagard® Liquid 10% should not be mixed with other drugs or other IGIV preparations.

Gammagard® Liquid 10% should not be shaken.

Use of an in-line filter is optional. The IV infusion line may be flushed with 0.9% sodium chloride injection.

Gammagard® Liquid 10% should be at room temperature during IV infusion; it should not be warmed in a microwave.

Vials are for single use only.

For the treatment of primary humoral immunodeficiency, IV infusions of Gammagard® Liquid 10% should be given at an initial infusion rate of 0.5 mL/kg per hour (0.8 mg/kg per minute) for 30 minutes. The infusion rate may then be increased every 30 minutes (if tolerated) up to a maximum of 5 mL/kg per hour (8 mg/kg per minute).

For maintenance therapy of multifocal motor neuropathy (MMN), IV infusions of Gammagard® Liquid 10% should be given at an initial infusion rate of 0.5 mL/kg per hour (0.8 mg/kg per minute). The IV infusion rate may then be increased (if tolerated) up to a maximum of 5.4 mL/kg per hour (9 mg/kg per minute).

For individuals older than 65 years of age or at risk for renal dysfunction or thrombosis, the minimum infusion rate practicable should be used. In such patients, the maximum IV infusion rate should be less than 2 mL/kg per hour (less than 3.3 mg/kg per minute).

Gammagard® S/D. Gammagard® S/D and Gammagard® S/D (IgA less than 1 mcg/mL) are administered *only* by IV infusion.

Gammagard® S/D and Gammagard® S/D (IgA less than 1 mcg/mL) should be reconstituted according to the manufacturer's directions with the sterile water for injection diluent and transfer device provided to prepare a solution containing 50 mg of protein per mL (5%) or 100 mg of protein per mL (10%). Prior to reconstitution, the powder for injection and sterile water for injection diluent should be warmed to room temperature. After the diluent is added, the vial should be gently rotated to dissolve the drug; to avoid foaming, the vial should not be shaken.

If Gammagard® S/D or Gammagard® S/D (IgA less than 1 mcg/mL) was reconstituted outside of sterile laminar airflow conditions, the IV infusion should be initiated within 2 hours after reconstitution (preferably as soon as possible). If the drug was reconstituted in a sterile laminar flow hood using aseptic technique and the reconstituted solution is stored under constant refrigeration (2–8° C), the reconstituted solution should be administered within 24 hours after reconstitution (preferably as soon as possible).

When large doses are to be administered, the contents of several vials of Gammagard® S/D or Gammagard® S/D (IgA less than 1 mcg/mL) may be pooled into an empty, sterile IV container using aseptic technique. Partially used vials should be discarded.

Gammagard® S/D or Gammagard® S/D (IgA less than 1 mcg/mL) should be infused with the administration set provided by the manufacturer which contains an integral airway and a filter with a pore size of 15 μm; if this administration set is not used, a similar filter must be used.

The antecubital vein should be used for IV infusions of Gammagard® S/D or Gammagard® S/D (IgA less than 1 mcg/mL) whenever possible, especially when a 10% solution is used; this may reduce discomfort at the infusion site.

IV infusions of Gammagard® S/D 5% or Gammagard® S/D 5% (IgA less than 1 mcg/mL) should be initiated using a 5% solution at a rate of 0.5 mL/kg per hour and, if tolerated, the rate of IV infusion may be increased gradually to a maximum of 4 mL/kg per hour. Patients who tolerate the 5% solution at this maximum rate can be transferred to a 10% solution, initiated at an IV infusion rate of 0.5 mL/kg per hour. If tolerated, the infusion rate for the 10% solution may be increased gradually to a maximum of 8 mL/kg per hour. In general, it is recommended that the rate of IV infusion in patients beginning therapy with IGIV or switching from one IGIV product to another should be started at a slow rate and the rate increased to the maximum IV infusion rate only after the patient has tolerated several infusions at intermediate rates of infusion.

For patients at risk of renal dysfunction (e.g., adults older than 65 years of age; individuals receiving nephrotoxic drugs; individuals with diabetes mellitus, volume depletion, paraproteinemia, or sepsis) or patients at risk of thrombosis, Gammagard® S/D and Gammagard® S/D (IgA less than 1 mcg/mL) should be administered at the minimum IV infusion rate practicable and the rate gradually titrated up to a reduced maximum rate of less than 3.3 mg/kg per minute (e.g., less than 4 mL/kg per hour as a 5% solution and less than 2 mL/kg per hour as a 10% solution). (See Cautions: Precautions and Contraindications.)

Gammaked® 10%. Gammaked® 10% is administered by IV infusion. Alternatively, Gammaked® 10% may be administered by subcutaneous infusion for the treatment of primary humoral immunodeficiency (see Gammaked® 10% under Reconstitution and Administration: Immune Globulin Subcutaneous, in Dosage and Administration).

Prior to administration, Gammaked® 10% should be allowed to come to room temperature (this may take 60 minutes or longer); the solution should be clear to opalescent and colorless to pale yellow.

If necessary, Gammaked® 10% may be diluted with 5% dextrose injection; however, saline solutions are not compatible with the drug and should not be used as diluents.

Gammaked® 10% vials are for single use only and should not be shaken. When the 10-mL vial of Gammaked® 10% (containing 1 g of protein) is used, the vial stopper should be penetrated only with an 18-gauge needle; when 25-, 50-, 100-, or 200-mL vials (containing 2.5, 5, 10, or 20 g of protein, respectively) are used, the vial stopper should be penetrated only with a 16-gauge needle or dispensing pin. Any vial that has been entered should be used promptly; partially used vials should be discarded. However, the manufacturer states that the contents of full vials may be pooled under aseptic conditions into sterile infusion bags and infused within 8 hours after pooling.

The infusion line can be flushed with either 0.9% sodium chloride injection or 5% dextrose injection. The infusion line should *not* be flushed with heparin because of the potential for incompatibility between Gammaked® 10% and heparin.

For primary humoral immunodeficiency or ITP, IV infusions of Gammaked® 10% should be initiated at a rate of 1 mg/kg per minute (0.01 mL/kg per minute) for the first 30 minutes. If well tolerated, the IV infusion rate may be gradually increased to a maximum of 8 mg/kg per minute (0.08 mL/kg per minute). If adverse effects related to the rate of IV infusion occur, symptoms may disappear if the infusion is stopped or slowed.

For treatment of chronic inflammatory demyelinating polyneuropathy (CIDP), IV infusions of Gammaked® 10% should be initiated at a rate of 2 mg/kg per minute (0.02 mL/kg per minute) for the first 30 minutes. If well tolerated, the IV infusion rate may be gradually increased to a maximum rate of 8 mg/kg per minute (0.08 mL/kg per minute). If adverse effects related to the rate of IV infusion occur, symptoms may disappear if the infusion is stopped or slowed.

In patients at increased risk for renal dysfunction or thrombosis, IV infusions of Gammaked® 10% should be administered at the minimum infusion rate practicable (less than 8 mg/kg per minute [less than 0.08 mL/kg per minute]).

Gammaplex® 5%. Gammaplex® 5% is administered *only* by IV infusion.

Prior to administration, Gammaplex® 5% should be clear or slightly opalescent and at room temperature (up to 25° C).

If large doses of Gammaplex® 5% are to be administered, several bottles may be pooled using aseptic technique; the IV infusion should be started within 2 hours after pooling.

Gammaplex® 5% should not be shaken prior to administration.

An infusion pump may be used to control the rate of administration.

The solution should be used promptly after the single-use bottle has been entered; partially used bottles should be discarded.

For the treatment of primary humoral immunodeficiency or ITP, the recommended initial IV infusion rate of Gammaplex® 5% is 0.5 mg/kg per minute (0.01 mL/kg per minute). If this rate is well tolerated for the first 15 minutes, the rate may be gradually increased every 15 minutes to a maximum of 4 mg/kg per minute (0.08 mL/kg per minute).

In patients at risk for renal dysfunction or thrombosis, Gammaplex® 5% should be administered using the minimum IV infusion rate practicable. Gammaplex® 5% should be discontinued if renal function deteriorates.

Gamunex®-C 10%. Gamunex®-C 10% is administered by IV infusion. Alternatively, Gamunex®-C 10% may be administered by subcutaneous infusion for the treatment of primary humoral immunodeficiency (see Gamunex®-C 10% under Reconstitution and Administration: Immune Globulin Subcutaneous, in Dosage and Administration).

Gamunex®-C 10% should be administered at room temperature. If necessary, Gamunex®-C 10% may be diluted with 5% dextrose injection; however, saline solutions are not compatible with the drug and should not be used as diluents.

Gamunex®-C 10% vials are for single use only. When the 10-mL vial of Gamunex®-C 10% (containing 1 g of protein) is used, the vial stopper should be penetrated only with an 18-gauge needle; when 25-, 50-, 100-, 200, or 400-mL vials (containing 2.5, 5, 10, 20, or 40 g of protein, respectively) are used, the vial stopper should be penetrated only with a 16-gauge needle or dispensing pin. Any vial that has been entered should be used promptly; partially used vials should be discarded. However, the manufacturer states that the contents of full vials may be pooled under aseptic conditions into sterile infusion bags and infused within 8 hours after pooling.

The infusion line may be flushed with either 0.9% sodium chloride injection or 5% dextrose injection. The infusion line should *not* be flushed with heparin because of the potential for incompatibility between Gamunex®-C 10% and heparin.

For primary humoral immunodeficiency or ITP, IV infusions of Gamunex®-C 10% should be initiated at a rate of 1 mg/kg per minute (0.01 mL/kg per minute) for the first 30 minutes. If tolerated, the IV infusion rate may be gradually increased to a maximum rate of 8 mg/kg per minute (0.08 mL/kg per minute). If adverse effects related to the rate of IV infusion occur, symptoms may disappear if the infusion is stopped or slowed.

For treatment of CIDP, IV infusions of Gamunex®-C 10% should be initiated at a rate of 2 mg/kg per minute (0.02 mL/kg per minute) for the first 30 minutes. If tolerated, the IV infusion rate may be gradually increased to a maximum rate of 8 mg/kg per minute (0.08 mL/kg per minute). If adverse effects related to the rate of IV infusion occur, symptoms may disappear if the infusion is stopped or slowed.

In patients at increased risk for renal dysfunction or thrombosis, IV infusions of Gamunex®-C 10% should be administered at the minimum IV infusion rate practicable (less than 8 mg/kg per minute [less than 0.08 mL/kg per minute]).

Octagam® 5%. Octagam® 5% is administered *only* by IV infusion.

Octagam® 5% should not be diluted or mixed with other drugs, IV infusion fluids, or other IGIV preparations.

Octagam® 5% should be at room temperature during administration.

The stopper of the single-use bottle of Octagam® 5% should be penetrated with a 16-gauge or smaller needle; the needles should be inserted only once. The solution should be used promptly after the single-use bottle has been entered; partially used bottles should be discarded.

If necessary, the contents of several single-use bottles of Octagam® 5% may be pooled using aseptic technique; the solution should be infused within 8 hours after pooling.

An infusion set is not provided with Octagam® 5%; if an infusion set is used (not mandatory), the filter pore size must be 0.2–200 μm.

The IV infusion line may be flushed with either 0.9% sodium chloride injection or 5% dextrose injection before or after administration of Octagam® 5%.

IV infusions of Octagam® 5% should be given at a rate of 30 mg/kg per hour (0.5 mg/kg per minute or 0.01 mL/kg per minute) for the first 30 minutes. If tolerated, the rate of infusion may be increased to 60 mg/kg per hour (1 mg/kg per minute or 0.02 mL/kg per minute) for the second 30 minutes and, if further tolerated, increased to 120 mg/kg per hour (2 mg/kg per minute or 0.04 mL/kg per minute) for the third 30 minutes. The maximum IV infusion rate is 200 mg/kg per hour (maximum 3.33 mg/kg per minute or 0.07 mL/kg per minute).

In patients at risk for renal dysfunction or thrombosis, IV infusions of Octagam® 5% should be administered using the minimum infusion rate practicable. The maximum IV infusion rate in patients at risk for renal dysfunction is 200 mg/kg per hour (3.33 mg/kg per minute or 0.07 mL/kg per minute). Octagam® 5% should be discontinued if renal function deteriorates.

Octagam® 10%. Octagam® 10% is administered *only* by IV infusion.

Octagam® 10% should not be diluted or mixed with other drugs, IV infusion fluids, or other IGIV preparations.

Octagam® 10% should be at room temperature during IV infusion.

The stopper of the single-use bottle of Octagam® 10% should be penetrated with a 16-gauge or smaller needle; the needles should be inserted only once. The solution should be used promptly after the single-use bottle has been entered; partially used bottles should be discarded.

If necessary, the contents of several single-use bottles of Octagam® 10% may be pooled using aseptic technique; the solution should be infused within 8 hours after pooling.

An infusion set is not provided with Octagam® 10%; if an infusion set is used (not mandatory), the filter pore size should be 0.2–200 μm.

The IV infusion line may be flushed with either 0.9% sodium chloride injection or 5% dextrose injection before and after administration of Octagam® 10%.

IV infusions of Octagam® 10% should be given at a rate of 60 mg/kg per hour (1 mg/kg per minute or 0.01 mL/kg per minute) for the first 30 minutes. If no adverse reactions occur, the rate of infusion may be increased to 120 mg/kg per hour (2 mg/kg per minute or 0.02 mL/kg per minute) for the second 30 minutes; if tolerated, the rate of infusion may be further increased to 240 mg/kg per hour (4 mg/kg per minute or 0.04 mL/kg per minute) for the third 30 minutes; and if further tolerated, increased to 480 mg/kg per hour (8 mg/kg per minute or 0.08 mL/kg per minute) for the fourth 30 minutes. The maximum IV infusion rate is 720 mg/kg per hour (maximum 12 mg/kg per minute or 0.12 mL/kg per minute).

In patients at risk for renal dysfunction or thrombosis, IV infusions of Octagam® 10% should be administered using the minimum infusion rate practicable. The maximum IV infusion rate in patients at risk for renal dysfunction or thrombosis is 200 mg/kg per hour (maximum 3.33 mg/kg per minute or 0.03 mL/kg per minute). Octagam® 10% should be discontinued if renal function deteriorates.

Privigen® 10%. Privigen® 10% is administered *only* by IV infusion.

Privigen® 10% should be administered at room temperature (up to 25°C). The solution should be used promptly after the vial has been entered; partially used vials should be discarded.

If necessary, Privigen® 10% may be diluted with dextrose injection.

If large doses are to be administered, several vials of Privigen® 10% may be pooled using aseptic technique; the IV infusion should be started within 8 hours after pooling.

Privigen® 10% should not be shaken prior to administration.

The IV infusion line may be flushed with either 0.9% sodium chloride injection or 5% dextrose injection.

An infusion pump may be used to control the rate of administration.

For the treatment of primary humoral immunodeficiency, the recommended initial IV infusion rate of Privigen® 10% is 0.5 mg/kg per minute (0.005 mL/kg per minute). If tolerated, the rate may be gradually increased to a maximum of 8 mg/kg per minute (0.08 mL/kg per minute).

For the treatment of chronic ITP, the recommended initial IV infusion rate of Privigen® 10% is 0.5 mg/kg per minute (0.005 mL/kg per minute). If no adverse reactions occur, the IV infusion rate may be gradually increased to a maximum of 4 mg/kg per minute (0.04 mL/kg per minute).

Patients who have not previously received Privigen® 10% (or another immune globulin preparation), patients who have not received the drug within the past 8 weeks, and patients switching from another immune globulin preparation to Privigen® 10% may be at risk of developing inflammatory reactions if a rapid IV infusion rate (e.g., greater than 4 mg/kg per minute [greater than 0.04 mL/kg per minute]) is used. In such patients, Privigen® 10% should be initiated using a slow IV infusion rate (e.g., 0.5 mg/kg per minute or slower [0.005 mL/kg per minute or slower]) and the rate gradually increased to the maximum IV infusion rate tolerated.

In patients at risk of renal dysfunction or thrombosis, IV infusions of Privigen® 10% should be administered using the minimum IV infusion rate practicable. Privigen® 10% should be discontinued if renal function deteriorates.

Immune Globulin Subcutaneous **Cuvitru® 20%.** Cuvitru® 20% is administered *only* by subcutaneous infusion.

Cuvitru® 20% may be *self-administered* in the home or other appropriate setting if the clinician determines that the patient and/or their caregiver is competent to safely administer the drug subcutaneously after appropriate training and with medical follow-up as necessary.

Cuvitru® 20% is administered undiluted and should not be mixed with other drugs, IV infusion fluids, or other immune globulin preparations.

Vials of Cuvitru® 20% are for single use only.

Subcutaneous infusions of Cuvitru® 20% should be made into the abdomen, thighs, upper arms, or lateral hip; bony areas, visible blood vessels, scars, and any areas with inflammation (irritation) or infection should be avoided.

The dose may be divided and infused simultaneously in up to 4 different sites that are at least 4 inches apart; a multi-needle administration set can be used to facilitate simultaneous subcutaneous infusion at multiple sites. The number of sites to be used depends on the volume of the dose and can be calculated by dividing the total volume to be infused by the maximum volume per site. For the first 2 subcutaneous infusions, the maximum volume per site is 20 mL in those weighing less than 40 kg or 60 mL in those weighing 40 kg or more; for subsequent infusions, the maximum volume per site is 60 mL regardless of weight. Subcutaneous infusion sites should be rotated for each subsequent dose.

For the treatment of primary humoral immunodeficiency, the first 2 subcutaneous infusions of Cuvitru® 20% should be given at a rate of 10–20 mL/hour at each infusion site. For subsequent subcutaneous infusions, the infusion rate may be increased as tolerated to a maximum of 60 mL/hour at each infusion site.

The manufacturer's instructions provided with Cuvitru® 20% and with the infusion pump should be consulted for specific information regarding subcutaneous administration.

Gammagard Liquid 10%. Gammagard® Liquid 10% may be administered by subcutaneous infusion in patients with primary humoral immunodeficiency. Gammagard® Liquid 10% also may be administered by IV infusion (see Gammagard Liquid 10% under Reconstitution and Administration: Immune Globulin IV [IGIV], in Dosage and Administration).

Gammagard® Liquid 10% may be *self-administered* in the home or other appropriate setting if the clinician determines that the patient and/or their caregiver is competent to safely administer the drug subcutaneously after appropriate training and with medical follow-up as necessary.

Subcutaneous infusions of Gammagard® Liquid 10% should be made into the abdomen, thighs, upper arms, and/or lower back using an infusion pump; bony prominences should be avoided.

To determine the number of subcutaneous infusion sites needed, the weekly dose (in mL) should be divided by 30 or 20 (i.e., divide by recommended volume per site based on patient weight). Infusion sites should be located at least 2 inches apart and should be changed for each weekly dose. A maximum of 8 simultaneous infusion sites should be used.

In patients weighing 40 kg or more, initial subcutaneous infusions should be given using a volume of 30 mL per infusion site and an infusion rate of 20 mL/hour per site. For maintenance doses in these patients, a volume of 30 mL per site and a subcutaneous infusion rate of 20–30 mL/hour per site should be used.

In patients weighing less than 40 kg, initial subcutaneous infusions should be given using a volume of 20 mL per infusion site and an infusion rate of 15 mL/

hour per site. For maintenance doses in these patients, a volume of 20 mL per site and a subcutaneous infusion rate of 15–20 mL/hour per site should be used.

The manufacturer's instructions provided with Gammagard® Liquid 10% and with the infusion pump should be consulted for specific information regarding subcutaneous administration.

Gammaked® 10%. Gammaked® 10% may be administered by subcutaneous infusion in patients with primary humoral immunodeficiency. Gammaked® 10% also may be administered by IV infusion (see Gammaked® 10% under Reconstitution and Administration: Immune Globulin IV [IGIV], in Dosage and Administration).

Gammaked® 10% may be *self-administered* in the home or other appropriate setting if the clinician determines that the patient and/or their caregiver is competent to safely administer the drug subcutaneously after appropriate training and with medical follow-up as necessary.

Prior to administration, Gammaked® 10% should be allowed to come to room temperature (this may take 60 minutes or longer); the solution should be clear to opalescent and colorless to pale yellow.

Vials are for single use only and should not be shaken.

The solution should be used promptly after the vial has been entered; any partially used vials should be discarded.

Subcutaneous infusions of Gammaked® 10% should be made into the abdomen, thighs, upper arms, and/or lateral hip using an infusion pump.

Depending on the total volume required, each subcutaneous dose of Gammaked® 10% may be divided and infused into multiple sites. A maximum of 8 different infusion sites may be used simultaneously in adults (4 infusion sites used simultaneously in most adults) and a maximum of 6 different infusion sites may be used simultaneously in children. Infusion sites should be located at least 2 inches apart.

For the treatment of primary humoral immunodeficiency in adults, subcutaneous infusions of Gammaked® 10% should be given at a rate of 20 mL/hour at each infusion site.

For the treatment of primary humoral immunodeficiency in pediatric patients 2 years of age or older weighing 25 kg or more, subcutaneous infusions of Gammaked® 10% should be initiated at a rate of 15 mL/hour at each infusion site. The subcutaneous infusion rate may then be increased up to 20 mL/hour at each infusion site.

For the treatment of primary humoral immunodeficiency in pediatric patients 2 years of age or older weighing less than 25 kg, subcutaneous infusions of Gammaked® 10% should be given at a rate of 10 mL/hour at each infusion site.

The manufacturer's instructions provided with Gammaked® 10% and with the infusion pump should be consulted for specific information regarding subcutaneous administration.

Gamunex®-C 10%. Gamunex®-C 10% may be administered by subcutaneous infusion in patients with primary humoral immunodeficiency. Gamunex®-C 10% also may be administered by IV infusion (see Gamunex®-C 10% under Reconstitution and Administration: Immune Globulin IV [IGIV], in Dosage and Administration).

Gamunex®-C 10% may be *self-administered* in the home or other appropriate setting if the clinician determines that the patient and/or their caregiver is competent to safely administer the drug subcutaneously after appropriate training and with medical follow-up as necessary.

Prior to administration, Gamunex®-C 10% should be at room temperature. The solution should not be shaken prior to administration.

Subcutaneous infusions of Gamunex®-C 10% should be made into the abdomen, thighs, upper arms, and/or lateral hip using an infusion pump.

Depending on the total volume required, each subcutaneous dose of Gamunex®-C 10% may be divided and infused into multiple sites. A maximum of 8 different infusion sites may be used simultaneously in adults (4 infusion sites used simultaneously in most adults) and a maximum of 6 different infusion sites may be used simultaneously in children. Infusion sites should be located at least 2 inches apart.

For the treatment of primary humoral immunodeficiency in adults, subcutaneous infusions of Gamunex®-C 10% should be given at a rate of 20 mL/hour at each infusion site.

For the treatment of primary humoral immunodeficiency in pediatric patients 2 years of age or older weighing 25 kg or more, subcutaneous infusions of Gamunex®-C 10% should be initiated at a rate of 15 mL/hour at each infusion site. The subcutaneous infusion rate may then be increased up to 20 mL/hour at each infusion site.

For the treatment of primary humoral immunodeficiency in pediatric patients 2 years of age or older weighing less than 25 kg, subcutaneous infusions of Gamunex®-C 10% should be given at a rate of 10 mL/hour at each infusion site.

The manufacturer's instructions provided with Gamunex®-C 10% and with the infusion pump should be consulted for specific information regarding subcutaneous administration.

Hizentra® 20%. Hizentra® 20% is administered *only* by subcutaneous infusion.

Hizentra® 20% may be *self-administered* in the home or other appropriate setting if the clinician determines that the patient and/or their caregiver is competent to safely administer the drug subcutaneously after appropriate training and with medical follow-up as necessary.

Subcutaneous infusions of Hizentra® 20% should be made in the abdomen, thighs, upper arms, and/or lateral hips using an infusion pump.

Depending on the total volume required, each subcutaneous dose of Hizentra® 20% may be divided and infused into multiple sites. A maximum of 4 different administration sites may be used simultaneously; however, if more sites are needed for the full weekly dose, a maximum of 12 sites can be used consecutively for each infusion. Administration sites should be located at least 2 inches apart and should be changed for each weekly dose.

For the treatment of primary humoral immunodeficiency, subcutaneous infusions of Hizentra® 20% should be initiated using a maximum volume of 15 mL and a maximum infusion rate of 15 mL/hour at each administration site. For subsequent infusions, the subcutaneous infusion rate may be increased to a maximum of 25 mL/hour per site as tolerated. After the fourth infusion, the volume may be increased to 20 mL at each infusion site and then increased to a maximum volume of 25 mL per site as tolerated.

The manufacturer's instructions provided with Hizentra® 20% and with the infusion pump should be consulted for specific information regarding subcutaneous administration.

Hyqvia® (Immune Globulin Subcutaneous 10% with Recombinant Human Hyaluronidase). Immune globulin subcutaneous 10% with recombinant human hyaluronidase (Hyqvia®) is commercially available as a kit that contains a vial of immune globulin subcutaneous 10% copackaged with a vial of recombinant human hyaluronidase. Both components are administered *only* by subcutaneous infusion and are administered *sequentially* at the same infusion site.

The recombinant human hyaluronidase component and the immune globulin subcutaneous 10% component should *not* be mixed together in the same container; the individual components should *not* be mixed with or administered with other drugs or infusion fluids.

Subcutaneous infusions of the Hyqvia® components should be made using an appropriate infusion pump and subcutaneous needle set. *The manufacturer's instructions provided with Hyqvia® and with the infusion pump should be consulted for specific information regarding subcutaneous administration.*

For each dose of Hyqvia®, the recombinant human hyaluronidase component (acts locally to temporarily increase permeability of subcutaneous tissue to increase dispersion and absorption of the immune globulin component) must be administered first. Within approximately 10 minutes after completion of the subcutaneous infusion of the recombinant human hyaluronidase component, the appropriate dose of the immune globulin subcutaneous 10% component should then be administered using the same subcutaneous infusion site and the same needle set.

Hyqvia® may be *self-administered* in the home or other appropriate setting if the clinician determines that the patient and/or their caregiver is competent to safely administer the components by subcutaneous infusion after appropriate training and with medical follow-up as necessary.

Subcutaneous infusions of Hyqvia® should be made in the abdomen or thigh; bony prominences or scarred, infected, or inflamed areas should be avoided. Administration sites should be rotated on opposite sides of the body between successive infusions.

A maximum volume of 600 mL may be administered at each subcutaneous infusion site in patients weighing 40 kg or more, or a maximum volume of 300 mL may be administered at each subcutaneous infusion site in those weighing less than 40 kg.

If necessary because of the total volume required and/or tolerability, the immune globulin subcutaneous 10% dose may be divided and administered using 2 infusion sites on opposite sides of the body. When 2 administration sites are used, the dose of recombinant human hyaluronidase must be divided and half administered at each site prior to the immune globulin component.

Subcutaneous infusions of the recombinant human hyaluronidase component of Hyqvia® should be initiated at a rate approximately 1–2 mL/minute at each administration site or as tolerated.

Subcutaneous infusions of the immune globulin 10% component of Hyqvia® should be administered using variable rates for the first 4 or 5 infusions (ramp-up period). Time intervals and number of rate changes should be adjusted as needed.

The manufacturer's literature should be consulted for specific information on recommended infusion rates and time intervals for subcutaneous administration of Hyqvia® during the ramp-up period.

■ Dosage for Immune Globulin IM (IGIM)

Hepatitis A Virus Infection If IGIM is used for *preexposure* prophylaxis of hepatitis A virus (HAV) infection in adults or children† who plan to travel to countries with intermediate or high levels of endemic HAV, the manufacturer and the US Public Health Service (USPHS) Advisory Committee on Immunization Practices (ACIP) recommend a single dose of 0.1 or 0.2 mL/kg of IGIM in those who will be staying in such areas for up to 1 or 2 months, respectively. If the period of exposure to HAV infection in such areas will be 2 months or longer, 0.2 mL/kg of IGIM should be administered once every 2 months. Ideally, preexposure vaccination with the age-appropriate schedule of hepatitis A virus vaccine inactivated (hepatitis A vaccine) before an expected exposure to HAV should be used to ensure the highest level of protection. (See Hepatitis A Virus Infection under Uses: Immune Globulin IM [IGIM].)

If IGIM is used for *postexposure* prophylaxis of HAV infection in adults older than 40 years of age, infants younger than 12 months of age†, immunocompromised individuals, individuals with chronic liver disease, or whenever preexposure vaccination with hepatitis A vaccine is contraindicated, the manufacturer and ACIP recommend a single dose of 0.1 mL/kg of IGIM administered as soon as possible after exposure (ideally within 2 weeks). Data are not available regarding efficacy of IGIM for HAV postexposure prophylaxis if administered more than 2 weeks after exposure. Individuals who have received at least 1 dose of hepatitis A vaccine given at least 1 month prior to the current HAV exposure do not need to receive postexposure prophylaxis with IGIM. (See Hepatitis A Virus Infection under Uses: Immune Globulin IM [IGIM].)

Healthcare professionals should consider that IGIM dosages currently recommended for *preexposure* or *postexposure* prophylaxis of HAV are higher than those previously recommended. A change in dosage recommendations was made in 2017 based on data indicating that HAV immunoglobulin G antibody (anti-HAV IgG) potency of IGIM commercially available in the US is lower than in the past, most likely because decreasing prevalence of previous HAV infection among plasma donors resulted in lower anti-HAV antibody levels in donor plasma used to prepare IGIM.

If combined active and passive immunization is used for preexposure prophylaxis or postexposure prophylaxis to provide long-term protection against HAV, the first dose of hepatitis A vaccine may be administered concurrently with the dose of IGIM at a separate site using a separate syringe. (See Dosage and Administration in Hepatitis A Virus Vaccine Inactivated 80:12.)

Measles If IGIM is used for postexposure prophylaxis of measles in susceptible individuals, the manufacturer recommends that most individuals receive a single dose of 0.25 mL/kg administered within 6 days after exposure. If a susceptible child who is immunocompromised is exposed to measles, the manufacturer recommends that IGIM be given as a single dose of 0.5 mL/kg (up to 15 mL) immediately after the exposure.

Whenever IGIM is indicated for postexposure prophylaxis of measles, ACIP and the American Academy of Pediatrics (AAP) recommend a single dose of 0.5 mL/kg (up to 15 mL) given within 6 days after exposure. ACIP states that the optimal dose of IGIM needed to provide protection against measles infection is unknown.

Active immunization with a vaccine containing measles virus vaccine live (e.g., measles, mumps, and rubella virus vaccine live; MMR) should then be initiated at least 6 months after administration of IGIM in individuals 12 months of age or older, unless the vaccine is contraindicated (see Measles, Mumps, Rubella, and Varicella Vaccines under Drug Interactions: Live Vaccines).

Individuals currently receiving immune globulin therapy who received IGIV (400 mg/kg or greater) within 3 weeks prior to measles exposure or received immune globulin subcutaneous (200 mg/kg) for 2 consecutive weeks prior to measles exposure should be sufficiently protected and do not need IGIM for postexposure prophylaxis of measles.

Rubella If IGIM is used for postexposure prophylaxis of rubella in susceptible pregnant women exposed to the disease, 0.55 mL/kg is administered as a single dose. However, routine use of IGIM is not recommended. (See Rubella under Uses: Immune Globulin IM [IGIM].)

Varicella If IGIM is used as an alternative to varicella-zoster immune globulin (VZIG) for postexposure prophylaxis of varicella infection, the manufacturer recommends that 0.6–1.2 mL/kg be administered as a single dose and states that the lower range of dosage should be used in patients at risk of thrombosis.

IGIV (not IGIM) usually is recommended for postexposure prophylaxis when VZIG is unavailable. (See Varicella under Dosage: Dosage for Immune Globulin IV [IGIV], in Dosage and Administration.)

■ **Dosage for Immune Globulin IV (IGIV)** ***Primary Immunodeficiency Diseases*** The minimum serum concentration of IgG necessary for protection in patients with primary humoral immunodeficiency varies among patients and has not been established in controlled clinical studies. Clinical response should be monitored and dosage of IGIV should be individualized since there are interindividual differences in the half-life of IgG among patients with primary immunodeficiencies. Dosage should be adjusted to achieve the desired trough serum IgG concentrations and/or clinical responses.

Bivigam® 10%. The usual IV dosage of Bivigam® 10% for replacement therapy in adults and children 6 years of age or older with primary humoral immunodeficiency is 300–800 mg/kg given by IV infusion once every 3–4 weeks.

Starting with the second IV infusion, dosage of Bivigam® 10% should be adjusted over time to achieve and maintain trough serum IgG concentrations exceeding 600 mg/dL. In patients who fail to maintain trough serum IgG concentrations at least 500 mg/dL, dosage should be adjusted to achieve a target trough serum IgG concentration of 600 mg/dL.

Carimune® NF. The usual IV dosage of Carimune® NF for replacement therapy in adults and children with primary immunodeficiency is 400–800 mg/kg given by IV infusion once every 3–4 weeks.

Flebogamma® 5% DIF. The usual IV dosage of Flebogamma® 5% DIF for replacement therapy in adults and children 2 years of age or older with primary humoral immunodeficiency is 300–600 mg/kg given by IV infusion once every 3–4 weeks.

Dosage should be adjusted over time to achieve desired trough serum IgG concentrations and clinical responses. The manufacturer states that data are not available to date from randomized, controlled studies to determine an optimum target trough serum IgG concentration.

Flebogamma® 10% DIF. The usual IV dosage of Flebogamma® 10% DIF for replacement therapy in adults with primary immunodeficiency is 300–600 mg/kg given by IV infusion once every 3–4 weeks.

Dosage should be adjusted over time to achieve desired trough serum IgG concentrations and clinical responses. The manufacturer states that data are not available to date from randomized, controlled studies to determine an optimum target trough serum IgG concentration.

Gammagard® Liquid 10%. The usual IV dosage of Gammagard® Liquid 10% for replacement therapy in adults and children 2 years of age or older with primary humoral immunodeficiency is 300–600 mg/kg given by IV infusion once every 3–4 weeks.

Dosage should be adjusted over time to achieve desired trough serum IgG concentrations and clinical responses. The manufacturer states that data are not available to date from randomized, controlled studies to determine an optimum target trough serum IgG concentration.

Gammagard® S/D. The recommended IV dosage of Gammagard® S/D or Gammagard® S/D (IgA less than 1 mcg/mL) for the treatment of primary immunodeficiency in adults and children 2 years of age or older is 300–600 mg/kg given by IV infusion once every 3–4 weeks.

Dosage should be adjusted over time based on clinical responses. The manufacturer states that data are not available to date from randomized, controlled studies to determine an optimum target trough serum IgG concentration.

Gammaked® 10%. The recommended IV dosage of Gammaked® 10% for replacement therapy in adults and pediatric patients 2 years of age or older with primary humoral immunodeficiency is 300–600 mg/kg (3–6 mL/kg) given by IV infusion once every 3–4 weeks. Dosage may be adjusted over time to achieve the desired trough serum IgG concentrations and clinical responses.

If a patient receiving Gammaked® 10% IV in a dosage less than 400 mg/kg once every 3–4 weeks is at risk of measles exposure (i.e., susceptible traveler to measles endemic area), a dose of at least 400 mg/kg (4 mL/kg) should be administered just prior to the expected measles exposure. If a susceptible patient has been exposed to measles, a dose of 400 mg/kg (4 mL/kg) should be administered as soon as possible after the exposure.

Gammaplex® 5%. The recommended IV dosage of Gammaplex® 5% for replacement therapy in adults and children 2 years of age or older with primary humoral immunodeficiency is 300–800 mg/kg (6–16 mL/kg) given by IV infusion once every 3–4 weeks. Dosage should be adjusted over time to achieve the desired trough serum IgG concentration and clinical response.

If a patient misses a dose, the missed dose should be given as soon as possible and scheduled doses should be resumed every 3 or 4 weeks as applicable.

Gamunex®-C 10%. The recommended IV dosage of Gamunex®-C 10% for replacement therapy in adults and pediatric patients 2 years of age or older with primary humoral immunodeficiency is 300–600 mg/kg (3–6 mL/kg) given by IV infusion once every 3–4 weeks. Dosage may be adjusted over time to achieve the desired trough serum IgG concentrations and clinical response.

If a patient receiving IV Gamunex®-C 10% in a dosage less than 400 mg/kg once every 3–4 weeks is at risk of measles exposure (i.e., susceptible traveler to measles endemic area), a dose of at least 400 mg/kg (4 mL/kg) should be administered just prior to the expected measles exposure. If a susceptible patient has been exposed to measles, a dose of 400 mg/kg (4 mL/kg) should be administered as soon as possible after the exposure.

Octagam® 5%. The recommended IV dosage of Octagam® 5% for replacement therapy in adults and pediatric patients with primary humoral immunodeficiency disease is 300–600 mg/kg (6–12 mL/kg) given by IV infusion once every 3–4 weeks. Dosage may be adjusted over time to achieve desired trough IgG concentrations and clinical responses. If a patient misses a dose, missed dose should be given as soon as possible and scheduled doses should be resumed every 3 or 4 weeks as applicable.

If a patient receiving IV Octagam® 5% in a dosage less than 400 mg/kg once every 3–4 weeks is at risk of measles exposure (i.e., susceptible traveler to an area outside the US where measles is endemic, measles outbreak in US), Octagam® 5% dosage should be increased to at least 400 mg/kg. If the patient has been exposed to measles, a dose of at least 400 mg/kg should be administered as soon as possible after the exposure.

Privigen® 10%. The recommended IV dosage of Privigen® 10% for replacement therapy in adults and children 3 years of age and older with primary humoral immunodeficiency disease is 200–800 mg/kg (2–8 mL/kg) given by IV infusion once every 3–4 weeks. Dosage should be adjusted over time to achieve the desired trough serum IgG concentrations and clinical responses. There are no data from randomized, controlled studies to date to determine an optimum target trough IgG concentration.

If a patient misses a dose, the missed dose should be given as soon as possible and scheduled doses should be resumed every 3 or 4 weeks as applicable.

Idiopathic Thrombocytopenic Purpura **Carimune® NF.** The usual IV dosage of Carimune® NF for initial induction therapy in adults and children with idiopathic thrombocytopenic purpura (ITP; also known as immune thrombocytopenic purpura or immune thrombocytopenia) is 400 mg/kg given by IV infusion once daily for 2–5 consecutive days.

In the treatment of acute ITP of childhood, if an initial platelet count response to the first 2 doses is adequate (30,000–50,000/mm³), therapy may be discontinued after the second day of the 5-day regimen.

In the treatment of chronic ITP in adults and children, if the platelet count decreases to less than 30,000/mm³ and/or clinically important bleeding becomes apparent following initial induction therapy with Carimune® NF, a maintenance dose of 400 mg/kg may be given as a single infusion. If an adequate response does not occur, the maintenance dose may be increased to 800–1000 mg/kg given as a single infusion.

Flebogamma® 10% DIF. The recommended IV dosage of Flebogamma® 10% DIF for treatment of chronic ITP in adults and children 2 years of age or older is 1 g/kg given by IV infusion once daily for 2 consecutive days.

Gammagard® S/D. The usual IV dosage of Gammagard® S/D or Gammagard® S/D (IgA less than 1 mcg/mL) for the treatment of chronic ITP in adults is 1 g/kg given by IV infusion as a single dose. The need for additional doses can be determined by clinical response and platelet count. If required, up to 3 doses may be given on alternate days.

Gammaked® 10%. The usual IV dosage of Gammaked® 10% for the treatment of ITP in adults and pediatric patients is 1 g/kg (10 mL/kg) given by IV infusion once daily on 2 consecutive days (total dose of 2 g/kg); if an adequate increase in platelet count is obtained at 24 hours after the initial dose of 1 g/kg (10 mL/kg) of the 2-dose regimen, the second 1-g/kg dose may be withheld. Alternatively, 400 mg/kg (4 mL/kg) may be given by IV infusion once daily for 5 consecutive days (total dose of 2 g/kg).

The high-dose regimen of Gammaked® 10% (1 g/kg given on 2 consecutive days) is not recommended in patients with expanded fluid volumes or when fluid volume may be a concern.

Gammaplex® 5%. The usual IV dosage of Gammaplex® 5% in adults with ITP is 1 g/kg (20 mL/kg) given by IV infusion once daily on 2 consecutive days (total dosage of 2 g/kg). The risks and benefits of this high-dose regimen should be carefully considered before using it in patients at increased risk of thrombosis, hemolysis, acute kidney injury, or volume overload.

Adequate data are not available regarding the platelet response to a lower-dose regimen of Gammaplex® 5% (i.e., 400 mg/kg per day for 5 consecutive days).

Gamunex®-C 10%. The usual IV dosage of Gamunex®-C 10% for the treatment of ITP in adults and pediatric patients is 1 g/kg (10 mL/kg) given by IV infusion on 2 consecutive days (total dose of 2 g/kg); if an adequate increase in platelet count is obtained at 24 hours after the initial dose of 1 g/kg (10 mL/kg) of the 2-dose regimen, the second 1-g/kg dose may be withheld. Alternatively, 400 mg/kg (4 mL/kg) may be given by IV infusion once daily for 5 consecutive days (total dose of 2 g/kg).

The high-dose regimen of Gamunex®-C 10% (1 g/kg given on 2 consecutive days) is not recommended in patients with expanded fluid volumes or when fluid volume may be a concern.

Octagam® 10%. The usual IV dosage of Octagam® 10% in adults with chronic ITP is 1 g/kg (10 mL/kg) given by IV infusion once daily for 2 consecutive days (total dose of 2 g/kg).

Privigen® 10%. The recommended IV dosage of Privigen® 10% in adults and adolescents 15 years of age and older with chronic ITP is 1 g/kg (10 mL/kg) given by IV infusion once daily for 2 consecutive days (total dose of 2 g/kg). The risks and benefits of this high-dose regimen should be carefully considered before using it in patients at increased risk of thrombosis, hemolysis, acute kidney injury, or volume overload.

Individuals with B-cell Chronic Lymphocytic Leukemia The usual IV dosage of Gammagard® S/D or Gammagard® S/D (IgA less than 1 mcg/mL) for adults with hypogammaglobulinemia and/or recurrent bacterial infections secondary to B-cell chronic lymphocytic leukemia (CLL) is 400 mg/kg given by IV infusion once every 3–4 weeks.

Kawasaki Disease For initial treatment of the acute phase of Kawasaki disease, AAP, American Heart Association (AHA), and American College of Chest Physicians (ACCP) recommend that a single dose of 2 g/kg of IGIV be given in conjunction with aspirin (80–100 mg/kg daily for up to 14 days, then 1–5 mg/kg daily for 6–8 weeks) beginning as soon as possible after the disease is diagnosed or strongly suspected (optimally within 7–10 days of disease onset). If there is no response (i.e., fever persists or recurs 36 hours or longer after the initial IGIV dose), retreatment with another single dose of 2 g/kg of IGIV (given within 24–48 hours of persistent or recrudescent fever) and continued aspirin therapy is recommended.

Gammagard® S/D. For initial treatment of Kawasaki disease in adults or pediatric patients, the manufacturer recommends that Gammagard® S/D or Gammagard® S/D (IgA less than 1 mcg/mL) be given by IV infusion as a single dose of 1 g/kg or, alternatively, in a dosage of 400 mg/kg once daily for 4 consecutive days beginning within 7 days of fever onset.

Chronic Inflammatory Demyelinating Polyneuropathy **Gammaked® 10%.** For the treatment of chronic inflammatory demyelinating polyneuropathy (CIDP) in adults, a loading dose of Gammaked® 10% of 2 g/kg (20 mL/kg) should be given by IV infusion in divided doses over 2–4 consecutive days. Then, a maintenance dosage of 1 g/kg (10 mL/kg) may be given as a single IV infusion once every 3 weeks or, alternatively, as 2 doses of 0.5 g/kg (5 mL/kg) given by IV infusion on 2 consecutive days once every 3 weeks.

Gamunex®-C 10%. For the treatment of CIDP in adults, a loading dose of Gamunex®-C 10% of 2 g/kg (20 mL/kg) should be given by IV infusion in divided doses over 2–4 consecutive days. Then, a maintenance dosage of 1 g/kg (10 mL/kg) may be given as a single IV infusion once every 3 weeks or, alternatively, as 2 doses of 0.5 g/kg (5 mL/kg) given by IV infusion on 2 consecutive days once every 3 weeks. In clinical studies in patients with CIDP, Gamunex®-C 10% has been continued for up to 48 weeks.

Multifocal Motor Neuropathy Although optimum dosage of IGIV has not been established for use in patients with multifocal motor neuropathy (MMN) when disability is severe enough to warrant treatment, the European Federation of Neurological Societies (EFNS) and the Peripheral Nerve Society (PNS) suggest an initial dosage of 2 g/kg given in divided doses over 2–5 consecutive days. If the initial regimen is effective, these clinicians state that maintenance therapy can be considered using an IGIV dosage of 1 g/kg once every 2–4 weeks or 2 g/kg once every 1–2 months. The frequency of IGIV maintenance therapy should be guided by response.

Gammagard® Liquid 10%. The manufacturer states that the usual maintenance dosage of Gammagard® Liquid 10% for adults with MMN ranges from 500 mg/kg to 2.4 g/kg given by IV infusion once every month. Dosage adjustment may be required to achieve the desired clinical response and avoid worsening of muscle weakness. In a clinical trial, 9% of patients experienced neurologic decompensation that required an increase in dosage.

Guillain-Barré Syndrome Although safety and efficacy and optimum dosage of IGIV for the treatment of Guillain-Barré syndrome† (GBS) have not been established, EFNS and others recommend a dosage of 0.4 g/kg daily for 5 days. It is unclear whether IGIV is effective when initiated more than 2 weeks after symptom onset.

If relapse of GBS† occurs after an initial response, EFNS states that retreatment with an IGIV dosage of 2 g/kg given in divided doses over 2–5 consecutive days can be considered. Retreatment also can be considered in those who do not respond to the initial regimen; however, other clinicians state that it is unclear whether retreatment is beneficial in such patients.

Infections in HIV-infected Individuals If IGIV is used for prevention of serious bacterial infections in HIV-infected infants and children† who have hypogammaglobulinemia (IgG less than 400 mg/dL), ACIP, AAP, US Centers for Disease Control and Prevention (CDC), National Institutes of Health (NIH), and other experts recommend that IGIV be given in a dosage of 400 mg/kg once every 2–4 weeks.

Infections in Hematopoietic Stem Cell Transplant Recipients If IGIV is used to prevent bacterial infections (e.g., *Streptococcus pneumoniae* sinopulmonary infections) in allogeneic hematopoietic stem cell transplant (HSCT) recipients† who experience severe hypogammaglobulinemia (IgG less than 400 mg/dL) within the first 100 days after transplant, some clinicians recommend that adults and adolescents receive 500 mg/kg once weekly and that pediatric patients receive 400 mg/kg once monthly. However, whenever IGIV is used for prophylaxis in hypogammaglobulinemic allogeneic HSCT recipients, it is recommended that dosage be individualized to maintain trough serum IgG concentrations exceeding 400–500 mg/dL and that trough serum IgG concentrations be monitored regularly (e.g., approximately every 2 weeks).

Measles If IGIV is used for postexposure prophylaxis of measles† in susceptible individuals, ACIP and AAP recommend 400 mg/kg administered as a single dose within 6 days after exposure.

Individuals receiving immune globulin replacement therapy who received IGIV (400 mg/kg or greater) within 3 weeks prior to measles exposure or immune globulin subcutaneous (200 mg/kg) for 2 consecutive weeks prior to measles exposure should be sufficiently protected and do not need additional IGIV for postexposure prophylaxis of measles. Those receiving IGIV in a dosage less than 400 mg/kg once every 3–4 weeks should receive an additional IGIV dose of 400 mg/kg as soon as possible after measles exposure.

Active immunization with a vaccine containing measles virus vaccine live (e.g., MMR) should then be initiated at least 8 months after administration of IGIV in individuals 12 months of age or older, unless the vaccine is contraindicated (see Measles, Mumps, Rubella, and Varicella Vaccines under Drug Interactions: Live Vaccines).

Tetanus If IGIV is used as an alternative to tetanus immune globulin (TIG) for the treatment of tetanus† when TIG is unavailable, a dosage of 200–400 mg/kg has been recommended.

Toxic Shock Syndrome When used as an adjunct in the treatment of staphylococcal or streptococcal toxic shock syndrome†, IGIV has been given in dosages of 150–400 mg/kg once daily for 5 days or, alternatively, a single dose of 1–2 g/kg has been used. Because the half-life of IGIV may be shortened in these patients, some clinicians suggest that more than a single dose may be needed. However, the optimal dosage regimen of IGIV in patients with toxic shock syndrome has not been identified.

Varicella If IGIV is used as an alternative to VZIG for postexposure prophylaxis of varicella infection† in individuals who do not have evidence of immunity and are at high risk for severe disease and complications, the recommended dosage is 400 mg/kg administered as a single dose (ideally within 96 hours after varicella exposure). IGIV may not be necessary in patients receiving replacement therapy with IGIV (i.e., 400 mg/kg or greater given at regular intervals) if the last dose was administered within 3 weeks prior to varicella exposure. IGIV should be considered only when VZIG is unavailable.

■ **Dosage for Immune Globulin Subcutaneous** ***Primary Immunodeficiency Diseases*** **Cuvitru® 20%.** For replacement therapy in adults and children 2 years of age or older with primary humoral immunodeficiency disease, Cuvitru® 20% is administered subcutaneously at regular intervals ranging from once daily up to once every 2 weeks (biweekly).

In patients switching from IGIV or immune globulin subcutaneous 10% with recombinant human hyaluronidase (Hyqvia®), the first dose of Cuvitru® 20% should be given 1 week after the last dose of the other immune globulin.

The initial dose of Cuvitru® 20% can be calculated based on the monthly dose of the prior immune globulin regimen.

The manufacturer's literature should be consulted for specific information regarding initial and subsequent dosage of Cuvitru® 20%.

Gammagard® Liquid 10%. For replacement therapy in adults and children 2 years of age or older with primary humoral immunodeficiency disease, Gammagard® Liquid 10% is administered subcutaneously once weekly.

The initial weekly subcutaneous dose of Gammagard® Liquid 10% should be given approximately 1 week after the last IGIV dose. The initial dose is calculated by dividing the patient's previous IGIV dose (in g) by the number of weeks between IGIV doses (i.e., divide by 3 or 4 depending on whether the patient was receiving IGIV every 3 or 4 weeks), then multiplying this value by a dose adjustment factor of 1.37.

The maintenance weekly subcutaneous dose of Gammagard® Liquid 10% is based on clinical response and target trough IgG concentrations.

The manufacturer's literature should be consulted for specific information on how to adjust dosage of Gammagard® Liquid 10% based on trough serum IgG concentrations.

Gammaked® 10%. For replacement therapy in adults and pediatric patients 2 years of age or older with primary humoral immunodeficiency disease, Gammaked® 10% is administered subcutaneously once weekly.

The initial weekly subcutaneous dose of Gammaked® 10% should be given 1 week after the last IGIV dose. The initial dose is calculated by dividing the patient's previous IGIV dose (in g) by the number of weeks between IGIV doses (i.e., divide by 3 or 4 depending on whether the patient was receiving IGIV every 3 or 4 weeks), then multiplying this value by a dose adjustment factor of 1.37. This dose can be converted to mL by multiplying the calculated dose (in g) by 10.

The weekly dose of Gammaked® 10% may be adjusted over time to achieve the desired trough serum IgG concentrations and clinical response.

The manufacturer's literature should be consulted for specific information on how to adjust dosage of Gammaked® 10% based on trough serum IgG concentrations and for specific information regarding dosage requirements for patients switching from another immune globulin subcutaneous preparation to Gammaked® 10%.

Gamunex®-C 10%. For replacement therapy in adults and pediatric patients 2 years of age or older with primary humoral immunodeficiency disease, Gamunex®-C 10% is administered subcutaneously once weekly.

The initial weekly subcutaneous dose of Gamunex®-C 10% should be given 1 week after the last IGIV dose. The initial dose is calculated by dividing the patient's previous IGIV dose (in g) by the number of weeks between IGIV doses (i.e., divide by 3 or 4 depending on whether the patient was receiving IGIV every 3 or 4 weeks), then multiplying this value by a dose adjustment factor of 1.37. This dose can be converted to mL by multiplying the calculated dose (in g) by 10.

Adjustment of the weekly dose of Gamunex®-C 10% may be required over time to achieve the desired trough serum IgG concentrations and clinical response.

The manufacturer's literature should be consulted for specific information on how to adjust dosage of Gamunex®-C 10% based on trough serum IgG concentrations and for specific information regarding dosage requirements for patients switching from another immune globulin subcutaneous preparation to Gamunex®-C 10%.

Hizentra® 20%. For replacement therapy in adults and children 2 years of age or older with primary humoral immunodeficiency disease, Hizentra® 20% is administered subcutaneously at regular intervals ranging from once daily up to once every 2 weeks (biweekly).

Patients should have been receiving IGIV for at least 3 months before being switched to Hizentra® 20%. The initial dose of Hizentra® 20% should be given 1 week after the last IGIV dose. The initial weekly dose of Hizentra® 20% should be calculated by dividing the patient's previous IGIV dose (in g) by the number of weeks between IGIV doses (e.g., divide by 3 or 4 depending on whether the patient was receiving IGIV every 3 or 4 weeks), then multiplying this value by a dose adjustment factor of 1.37.

The manufacturer's literature should be consulted for specific information regarding initial and subsequent dosage of Hizentra® 20%.

If a patient receiving Hizentra® 20% is at risk of measles exposure (i.e., susceptible traveler to an area outside the US where measles is endemic, measles outbreak in US), the minimum weekly dosage of Hizentra® 20% should be at least 200 mg/kg for 2 consecutive weeks; if the patient is receiving a biweekly regimen, a single dose of at least 400 mg/kg should be given. If the patient has been exposed to measles, a single dose of at least 400 mg/kg should be administered as soon as possible after the exposure.

Hyqvia® (Immune Globulin Subcutaneous 10% with Recombinant Human Hyaluronidase). Immune globulin subcutaneous 10% with recombinant human hyaluronidase (Hyqvia®) is commercially available as a kit that contains a vial of immune globulin subcutaneous 10% copackaged with a vial of recombinant human hyaluronidase. Although dosage of the recombinant human hyaluronidase component is the same for all patients, dosage of the immune globulin subcutaneous 10% component must be individualized.

For replacement therapy in adults with primary immunodeficiency, Hyqvia® is administered subcutaneously once every 3 to 4 weeks *after* an initial ramp-up period that incrementally changes the dosage regimen from a 1-week regimen to a 3- or 4-week regimen and allows the patient to become accustomed to the large volumes required for a full monthly dose.

For each dose of Hyqvia®, the *entire* contents of the vial containing recombinant human hyaluronidase (2.5 mL containing 160 units/mL) should be administered first. The appropriate dose of the immune globulin subcutaneous 10% component should then be administered within approximately 10 minutes at the same subcutaneous infusion site using the same needle set. (See Hyqvia® [Immune Globulin Subcutaneous 10% with Recombinant Human Hyaluronidase] under Reconstitution and Administration: Immune Globulin Subcutaneous, in Dosage and Administration.)

In patients already receiving an immune globulin preparation, the first dose of Hyqvia® for the ramp-up period should be administered approximately 1 week after the last dose of the previous immune globulin preparation. The target dose of the immune globulin subcutaneous 10% component of Hyqvia® *after* the ramp-up period should be the same as the immune globulin dose the patient was previously receiving.

In patients who are immune globulin naive or have been receiving a different immune globulin subcutaneous preparation, the target dose of the immune globulin subcutaneous 10% component of Hyqvia® *after* the initial dose ramp-up period should be 300–600 mg/kg once every 3–4 weeks.

Dosage adjustment of the immune globulin 10% component may be required over time to achieve the desired clinical response and trough serum IgG concentrations.

The manufacturer's literature should be consulted for specific information on the ramp-up schedule, including dosage of the immune globulin 10% component and dosing intervals. The manufacturer's literature also should be consulted for specific information on how to adjust dosage of the immune globulin 10% component based on trough serum IgG concentrations.

Cautions

■ **Immune Globulin IM (IGIM)** Pain and tenderness may occur at the immune globulin IM (IGIM) injection site. Urticaria and angioedema may also occur. Headache, malaise, fever, arthralgia, and nephrotic syndrome have also been reported.

Severe local and systemic reactions, including anaphylactic reactions, have been reported in patients hypersensitive to IGIM. (See Sensitivity Reactions under Cautions: Precautions and Contraindications.)

Thrombosis Thrombosis may occur following treatment with immune globulin, including IGIM.

Risk factors for thrombosis in patients receiving IGIM may include advanced age, prolonged immobilization, hypercoagulable conditions, history of venous or arterial thrombosis, use of estrogen-containing preparations, indwelling central vascular catheters, hyperviscosity, and cardiovascular risk factors. Thrombosis may occur in the absence of known risk factors. (See Thrombosis Precautions under Cautions: Precautions and Contraindications.)

■ **Immune Globulin IV (IGIV)** Adverse reactions to immune globulin IV (IGIV) have been reported in 10% or less of individuals receiving the drug. Adverse reactions to IGIV generally occur in less than 1% of patients who are not immunodeficient; however, adverse systemic effects may occur in agammaglobulinemic or hypogammaglobulinemic patients who have not previously received IGIV or who have not received the drug within the preceding 8 weeks. Certain severe adverse reactions to IGIV appear to be related to the rate of administration rather than the dose and may be relieved by decreasing the rate of administration or by temporarily stopping the infusion.

Infusion site reactions (pain, irritation); mild chest, hip, joint, or back pain; leg cramps; arthralgia or myalgia; diarrhea; nausea; vomiting; chills; fever; asthenia; malaise; fatigue; insomnia; dizziness; lightheadedness; headache; immediate anaphylactoid and hypersensitivity reactions; allergic and cutaneous reactions such as rash, erythema, pruritus, urticaria, eczema, or dermatitis; flushing; hypertension or changes in blood pressure; palpitations; tachycardia; increased liver function test results; asthma; wheezing; otic pain; upper respiratory tract infection; cough (increased or productive); bronchitis; rhinitis/nasal congestion; sinusitis; and pharyngitis have been reported following administration of IGIV. Reversible increases in liver function test results also have been reported.

In clinical studies using IGIV in adults and children with idiopathic thrombocytopenic purpura (ITP; also known as immune thrombocytopenic purpura or immune thrombocytopenia), the most frequent adverse effect occurring during or following IV infusions was headache (usually mild). In ITP patients receiving high doses of IGIV (0.4 g/kg daily or greater), adverse reactions have been reported with 2.9% of infusions. Oral antihistamines and analgesics may alleviate these headaches and have been used for pretreatment in those patients who had posttransfusion headaches following induction therapy for ITP and required additional IGIV therapy.

Infusion Reactions Occasionally, IGIV causes a precipitous fall in blood pressure and clinical manifestations of anaphylaxis, even in patients without a history of sensitivity to immune globulin. These reactions generally appear 30 minutes to 1 hour after initiation of the infusion and include flushing of the face, tightness in the chest, chills, fever, dizziness, nausea, vomiting, diaphoresis, and hypotension or hypertension. These reactions appear to be related to the rate of administration of IGIV. Individuals receiving IGIV for the first time or restarting IGIV after a treatment hiatus of more than 8 weeks may be at higher risk for the development of fever, chills, nausea, and vomiting. (See Administration Precautions under Cautions: Precautions and Contraindications.)

Thrombosis Thrombotic events, including some fatalities, have been reported in patients receiving IGIV and include chest pain, myocardial infarction, congestive heart failure, cerebral vascular accident or infarction, ischemic encephalopathy, severe headache requiring hospitalization, pulmonary embolism, retinal vein occlusion, and peripheral deep-vein thrombosis. Although the precise etiology of these events has not been fully elucidated, immune globulin-induced alterations of blood rheology (e.g., activation of platelets, increases in blood viscosity, elevated levels of activated coagulation factor XI [XIa]) and infusion-related hypertensive effects appear to contribute to the development of such thrombotic complications.

Patients at risk for thrombotic events may include those with a history of atherosclerosis, cardiovascular risk factors, impaired cardiac output, coagulation or hypercoagulable disorders (e.g., factor V Leiden), prolonged periods of immobilization, advanced age, acquired or inherited thrombotic disorder, previous thrombotic or thromboembolic event, known or suspected hyperviscosity, indwelling central vascular catheters, and/or those receiving estrogen-containing preparations. The risk of such complications also appears to be increased in patients with a history of cardiovascular disease and/or thrombosis who receive IGIV by rapid IV infusion. Thrombosis may occur in patients without known risk factors. (See Thrombosis Precautions under Cautions: Precautions and Contraindications.)

Renal Effects Renal dysfunction, acute renal failure, osmotic nephrosis, and death have been reported in patients receiving IGIV. In some patients with IGIV-associated acute renal failure, renal histopathology findings suggested osmotic injury to the proximal renal tubules (acute tubular necrosis, vacuolar degeneration, osmotic nephrosis). Increases in serum creatinine and BUN have occurred as soon as 1–2 days following infusion of IGIV, predominately with preparations stabilized with sucrose. Progression to oliguria or anuria (requiring dialysis) has been observed, although some patients have improved spontaneously following discontinuance of IGIV. Many of the reported fatalities related to nephrotoxicity occurred in patients with serious underlying conditions.

Approximately 55% of reported cases of renal dysfunction have involved patients receiving IGIV for the treatment of ITP; less than 5% involved patients receiving the drug for primary immunodeficiency diseases. The increased rate of renal dysfunction among patients with ITP may be related to the fact that IGIV is administered in higher dosages and is given for several consecutive days for the treatment of ITP instead of the intermittent dosing regimen usually used for primary immunodeficiency diseases. Further study is needed to determine if other factors (e.g., age, baseline glomerular filtration rate) are associated with the increased rate of renal dysfunction reported in patients receiving IGIV for ITP.

There is some evidence that IGIV preparations stabilized with sucrose (e.g., Carimune® NF), are associated with a greater risk of developing IGIV-associated renal dysfunction since approximately 88% of reports of such adverse effects in the US have involved use of these preparations. The degree of risk may depend on the amount of sucrose contained in the formulation and hyperosmolality after reconstitution.

To reduce the risk of acute renal failure in patients receiving IGIV, patients should be adequately hydrated prior to administration of the drug, recommended dosage and rate of IV infusion should not be exceeded, and renal function should be monitored. In addition, if the drug is used in patients considered at risk of acute renal failure (e.g., adults older than 65 years of age, individuals with any degree of preexisting renal insufficiency, individuals receiving nephrotoxic drugs, individuals with diabetes mellitus, volume depletion, paraproteinemia, or sepsis), a reduction in dose, concentration, and/or rate of administration should be considered. (See Renal Precautions under Cautions: Precautions and Contraindications.)

Hyperproteinemia, Increased Viscosity, and Hyponatremia Hyperproteinemia, increased serum viscosity, and hyponatremia may occur in patients receiving IGIV. The hyponatremia is likely to be pseudohyponatremia, as demonstrated by a decreased calculated serum osmolality or elevated osmolar gap.

If hyponatremia occurs, it is critical to distinguish true hyponatremia from pseudohyponatremia. Treatment aimed at decreasing serum free water in patients with pseudohyponatremia may lead to volume depletion, a further increase in serum viscosity, and may predispose to thromboembolic events.

Aseptic Meningitis Syndrome Aseptic meningitis syndrome has been reported in patients receiving IGIV therapy. The syndrome, which may occur more frequently in patients receiving high doses (e.g., 2 g/kg) and/or rapid infusion of immune globulin, usually is evident within several hours to 2 days after administration and is characterized by severe headache (including migraine), nuchal rigidity, drowsiness, lethargy, fever, photophobia, painful eye movements, and nausea and vomiting. Aseptic meningitis syndrome may occur more frequently in female patients. In addition, although information is limited, patients with a history of migraine may be more susceptible to aseptic meningitis syndrome and may have severe symptoms requiring additional hospitalization and treatment with opiate analgesics. The cause of aseptic meningitis syndrome in patients receiving immune globulin is not known. It has been suggested that the syndrome may result from an allergic hypersensitivity reaction associated with distribution of components of the preparation into the CSF; alternatively, IgG antibodies present in immune globulin, which are allogeneic, may accumulate in the CNS and initiate reactions resulting in aseptic meningitis. The syndrome has been reported with various commercially available preparations and does not appear to be related to a specific formulation.

Patients with signs and symptoms of aseptic meningitis should receive a thorough neurologic examination, including CSF analysis, to rule out other causes of meningitis. CSF analysis frequently reveals protein levels (up to several hundred mg/dL) and pleocytosis (up to several thousand cells per mm^3), predominantly from the granulocytic series, but negative culture results.

In most reported cases, discontinuation of immune globulin results in resolution of aseptic meningitis syndrome within several days (3–5 days) without sequelae.

Hemolysis IGIV may contain blood group antibodies which can act as hemolysins and induce in vivo coating of erythrocytes with immunoglobulin, causing a positive direct antiglobulin reaction and, rarely, hemolysis. Acute intravascular hemolysis has been reported and delayed hemolytic anemia can develop subsequent to IGIV therapy due to enhanced erythrocyte sequestration and/or intravascular erythrocyte destruction. (See Other Precautions and Contraindications under Cautions: Precautions and Contraindications.)

Transfusion-related Acute Lung Injury Transfusion-related acute lung injury (noncardiogenic pulmonary edema) has been reported in patients receiving IGIV. This typically occurs within 1–6 hours after infusion and is characterized by severe respiratory distress, pulmonary edema, hypoxemia, normal left ventricular function, and fever. Patients should be managed using oxygen therapy with adequate ventilatory support. (See Other Precautions and Contraindications under Cautions: Precautions and Contraindications.)

■ **Immune Globulin Subcutaneous** The most frequent adverse effects reported with immune globulin subcutaneous (Cuvitru® 20%, Gammagard® Liquid 10%, Gammaked® 10%, Gamunex®-C 10%, Hizentra® 20%, Hyqvia®) are infusion site reactions (erythema, pain, swelling, pruritus, heat), headache, migraine headache, fever, GI effects (nausea, vomiting, diarrhea, upper abdominal pain), increased heart rate, increased systolic blood pressure, fatigue, pain (back pain, extremity pain), arthralgia, cough, rash, and pruritus.

Aseptic meningitis syndrome has been reported with immune globulin subcutaneous. The syndrome, which may occur more frequently in patients receiving high doses (e.g., 2 g/kg) and/or rapid infusion of immune globulin, usually is evident within several hours to 2 days after administration and is characterized by severe headache (including migraine), nuchal rigidity, drowsiness, lethargy, fever, photophobia, painful eye movements, and nausea and vomiting. (See Aseptic Meningitis Syndrome under Immune Globulin IV [IGIV], in Cautions.)

Other serious adverse effects reported with IGIV (e.g., anaphylactic and hypersensitivity reactions, infusion reactions, renal dysfunction or acute renal failure, hemolysis, transfusion-related acute lung injury) may occur with immune globulin subcutaneous. (See Cautions: Immune Globulin IV [IGIV].)

Thrombosis Thrombotic events have been reported in patients receiving immune globulin products, including immune globulin subcutaneous, and have included chest pain, myocardial infarction, congestive heart failure, cerebral vascular accident or infarction, ischemic encephalopathy, severe headache requiring hospitalization, pulmonary embolism, retinal vein occlusion, and peripheral deep-vein thrombosis. Although the precise etiology of these events has not been fully elucidated, immune globulin-induced alterations of blood rheology (e.g., activation of platelets, increases in blood viscosity) and infusion-related hypertensive effects appear to contribute to the development of such thrombotic complications.

Patients at risk for thrombotic events may include those with multiple cardiovascular risk factors, coagulation or hypercoagulable disorders, prolonged periods of immobilization, advanced age, previous thrombotic or thromboembolic event, known or suspected hyperviscosity, indwelling central vascular catheters, and/or those receiving estrogen-containing preparations. Thrombotic events may also occur in the absence of known risk factors. (See Thrombosis Precautions under Cautions: Precautions and Contraindications.)

Immunogenicity of Recombinant Human Hyaluronidase In clinical studies evaluating immune globulin subcutaneous 10% with recombinant human hyaluronidase (Hyqvia®), 18% of patients developed nonneutralizing antibodies to the recombinant human hyaluronidase component. The clinical importance of these anti-recombinant human hyaluronidase antibodies is not known. Animal studies indicate that antibodies to recombinant human hyaluronidase cross the placenta and are transferred to offspring during lactation. There also is the potential for these antibodies to cross-react with endogenous human hyaluronidase, which is expressed in adult male testes, epididymis, and sperm. (See Cautions: Pregnancy, Fertility, and Lactation.)

■ **Precautions and Contraindications** IGIM, IGIV, and immune globulin subcutaneous are contraindicated in individuals with a history of anaphylactic or severe systemic hypersensitivity reactions to immune globulin or any ingredient in the formulation.

IGIM, IGIV, and immune globulin subcutaneous also are contraindicated in IgA-deficient individuals with antibodies against IgA and a history of hypersensitivity. (See IgA Deficiency under Precautions and Contraindications: Sensitivity Reactions, in Cautions.)

Flebogamma® 10% DIF is contraindicated in patients with hereditary fructose intolerance since it contains sorbitol, which presents a risk to individuals with hereditary fructose intolerance. Hereditary fructose intolerance is typically suspected based on dietary history, especially in young children who become symptomatic after breast-feeding.

Gammaplex® 5% is contraindicated in patients with hereditary fructose intolerance and in neonates and infants for whom sucrose or fructose tolerance has not been established.

Hizentra® 20% and Privigen 10% contain L-proline as a stabilizer and these preparations are contraindicated in individuals with hyperprolinemia (type I or II).

Hyqvia® (immune globulin subcutaneous 10% with recombinant human hyaluronidase) is contraindicated in patients with known systemic hypersensitivity to hyaluronidase, including recombinant human hyaluronidase.

Octagam® 5% is contraindicated in individuals with acute hypersensitivity reactions to corn. (See Corn Allergy under Precautions and Contraindications: Sensitivity Reactions, in Cautions.)

Administration Precautions IGIV occasionally causes a precipitous fall in blood pressure and the clinical manifestations of anaphylaxis, even in patients who previously tolerated IGIV. Some severe reactions appear to be related to the rate of administration of the drug; the recommended rate of infusion should not be exceeded. If flushing, changes in blood pressure or pulse, or other infusion reactions occur, the infusion should be slowed or temporarily stopped. If symptoms subside, the infusion may be resumed at a rate that is comfortable for the patient.

Patients who have not previously received IGIM, IGIV, or immune globulin subcutaneous, who are being switched from another preparation of immune globulin, or who have not received immune globulin within the preceding 8 weeks are at risk of developing reactions including fever, chills, nausea, and vomiting.

The manufacturer states that IGIM should not be used in individuals with severe thrombocytopenia or any coagulation disorder that would contraindicate IM injections. The US Public Health Service Advisory Committee on Immunization Practices (ACIP) states that vaccines may be given IM to individuals who have bleeding disorders or are receiving anticoagulant therapy if a clinician familiar with the patient's bleeding risk determines that the preparation can be administered with reasonable safety. In these cases, a fine needle (23 gauge or smaller) should be used to administer the vaccine and firm pressure should be applied to the injection site (without rubbing) for at least 2 minutes. If IGIM is used in individuals with a bleeding disorder who is receiving antihemophilic factor or other similar therapy, the IM dose should be given shortly after a scheduled dose of such therapy to minimize the risk of bleeding. The individual and/or their family should be instructed concerning the risk of hematoma from the injection.

Thrombosis Precautions The fact that thrombotic events, including chest pain, myocardial infarction, congestive heart failure, cerebral vascular accident or infarction, ischemic encephalopathy, severe headache requiring hospitalization, pulmonary embolism, retinal vein occlusion, and peripheral deep-vein thrombosis, have been reported in patients receiving immune globulin should be considered. (See Thrombosis under Cautions: Immune Globulin IV [IGIV].)

Prior to immune globulin therapy, all patients with risk factors for thrombosis should be carefully evaluated. This includes those with a history of atherosclerosis, cardiovascular risk factors, impaired cardiac output, coagulation or hypercoagulable disorders (e.g., factor V Leiden), prolonged periods of immobilization, advanced age, acquired or inherited thrombotic disorder, history of venous or arterial thrombosis, known or suspected hyperviscosity, indwelling central vascular catheters, and/or treatment with estrogen-containing preparations. However, thrombosis may occur in patients with no known risk factors.

For all patients, the potential risks and benefits of immune globulin should be weighed against those of alternative therapies.

When immune globulin is used in patients at risk for thrombosis, the minimum dose and minimum infusion rate practicable should be used and patients should be monitored closely for signs and symptoms of thrombosis. In addition, all patients should be adequately hydrated prior to administration of immune globulin.

Because of the possible increased risk of thrombosis, baseline assessment of blood viscosity should be considered in patients at risk for hyperviscosity, including those with cryoglobulins, fasting chylomicronemia/markedly high triacylglycerols (triglycerides), or monoclonal gammopathies.

Patients receiving immune globulin should be advised to immediately inform a clinician if symptoms of thrombosis occur, including pain and/or swelling of an arm or leg with warmth over the affected area, discoloration of an arm or leg, unexplained shortness of breath, unexplained rapid pulse, chest pain or discomfort that worsens on deep breathing, numbness or weakness on one side of the body, changes in mental status/confusion, numbness in the face or extremities, weakness or paralysis, severe headache, and/or visual disturbances.

Renal Precautions Because renal dysfunction, acute renal failure, osmotic nephrosis, and death have been reported in patients receiving IGIV, urine output and renal function (BUN and serum creatinine concentrations) should be assessed prior to and at appropriate intervals during therapy with IGIV or immune globulin subcutaneous, especially in patients considered at increased risk of acute renal failure. In addition, all patients should be adequately hydrated prior to administration of immune globulin.

Patients considered at increased risk of developing acute renal failure include, but are not limited to, those with any degree of preexisting renal insufficiency, diabetes mellitus, hypovolemia, volume depletion, sepsis, or paraproteinemia; those receiving concomitant nephrotoxic drugs; and/or those older than 65 years of age. Particular caution should be observed if immune globulin is administered to patients considered at increased risk of developing acute renal failure, and reduction in dosage, concentration, and/or rate of administration should be considered in such patients.

When immune globulin is used in patients at risk for renal dysfunction, the minimum dose and minimum infusion rate practicable should be used and patients should be monitored closely for signs and symptoms of renal dysfunction. (See Dosage and Administration: Reconstitution and Administration.) If renal function deteriorates, immune globulin therapy should be discontinued.

Because renal dysfunction has been reported more frequently with IGIV preparations stabilized with sucrose (Carimune® NF) than with other IGIV preparations, the benefits of such preparations should be carefully weighed against the potential risk of IGIV-associated renal dysfunction. If a sucrose-containing IGIV preparation is used, it has been recommended that the rate of infusion of these preparations not exceed 3 mg of sucrose/kg per minute (maximum infusion rate that will deliver 2 mg IgG/kg per minute for Carimune® NF).

Patients should be instructed to immediately report symptoms of decreased urine output, sudden weight gain, fluid retention/edema, and/or shortness of breath (which may suggest renal damage) to their clinician.

Sensitivity Reactions Severe hypersensitivity reactions, including anaphylaxis, may occur rarely following administration of IGIV, IGIM, or immune globulin subcutaneous in patients hypersensitive to immune globulin or some component of the preparation.

IgA-deficient individuals with antibodies against IgA may be at increased risk of severe hypersensitivity and anaphylactoid reactions if they receive immune globulin. (See IgA Deficiency under Precautions and Contraindications: Sensitivity Reactions, in Cautions.)

If a severe hypersensitivity reaction occurs, the immune globulin should be discontinued immediately and appropriate therapy should be instituted as indicated. Epinephrine and antihistamines should be readily available in case anaphylaxis or an anaphylactoid reaction occurs.

Patients should be advised about the early signs of hypersensitivity (e.g., hives, generalized urticaria, chest tightness, wheezing, hypotension, anaphylaxis) and the importance of immediately contacting a clinician if allergic symptoms occur.

IGIM should be used with caution in patients with a history of systemic allergic reactions to immune globulin preparations. The manufacturer of IGIM states that intradermal sensitivity testing should not be performed because intradermal injection of concentrated buffered immune globulin solution causes a localized area of inflammation in most patients because of chemical irritation and this may be misinterpreted as evidence of hypersensitivity. Such misinterpretation may result in beneficial therapy being withheld from a patient who is not hypersensitive to immune globulin.

IgA Deficiency. IGIM, IGIV, and immune globulin subcutaneous should not be used in IgA-deficient individuals with antibodies against IgA and a history of hypersensitivity.

Individuals with selective IgA deficiency or individuals in whom IgA deficiency exists as a component of an immunodeficiency disease may have serum antibodies to IgA or may develop such antibodies following administration of immune globulin or other blood products containing IgA. Severe hypersensitivity reactions (e.g., anaphylaxis) could result following administration of immune globulin in individuals with antibodies to IgA.

All commercially available preparations of IGIV and immune globulin subcutaneous contain trace amounts of IgA, but the amount varies among the different preparations. In a limited number of patients who reacted to IGIV preparations containing higher IgA concentrations, IGIV preparations depleted of IgA (0.4–2.9 mcg/mL of IgA) were better tolerated. However, the concentration of IgA that will not provoke a reaction to IgA is not known. Therefore, all IGIV preparations carry the risk of inducing an anaphylactic reaction to IgA and a risk of anaphylaxis may exist despite the use of preparations containing only trace amounts of IgA.

Bivigam® 10% contains less than 200 mcg/mL of IgA.

Carimune® NF contains trace amounts of IgA.

Cuvitru® 20% contains an average of 80 mcg/mL of IgA.

Flebogamma® 5% DIF contains less than 50 mcg/mL of IgA.

Flebogamma® 10% DIF contains less than 32 mcg/mL of IgA.

Gammagard® Liquid 10% contains an average of 37 mcg/mL of IgA.

Gammagard® S/D is available in a formulation containing 2.2 mcg/mL or less of IgA and a formulation containing less than 1 mcg/mL of IgA.

Gammaked® 10% contains an average of 46 mcg/mL of IgA.

Gammaplex® 5% contains trace amounts of IgA (less than 10 mcg/mL).

Gamunex®-C 10% contains an average of 46 mcg/mL of IgA.

Hizentra® 20% contains 50 mcg/mL or less of IgA.

The immune globulin component of Hyqvia® contains an average of 37 mcg/mL of IgA.

Octagam® 5% contains 200 mcg/mL or less of IgA.

Octagam® 10% contains an average of 106 mcg/mL of IgA.

Privigen® 10% contains 25 mcg/mL or less of IgA.

Corn Allergy. Some IGIV preparations (i.e., Octagam® 5%, Octagam® 10%) contain maltose, a disaccharide sugar derived from corn. Hypersensitivity reactions may occur if these preparations are used in patients with corn allergy. The manufacturer states that Octagam® 5% should be avoided in patients with known corn allergies and is contraindicated in those with acute hypersensitivity reactions to corn.

Risk of Transmissible Agents in Plasma-derived Preparations Because IGIM, IGIV, and immune globulin subcutaneous are prepared from pooled human plasma, they are potential vehicles for transmission of human viruses (e.g., hepatitis A virus [HAV], hepatitis B virus [HBV], hepatitis C virus [HCV], human immunodeficiency virus [HIV]) and theoretically may carry a risk of transmitting the causative agents of Creutzfeldt-Jakob disease (CJD) or variant CJD (vCJD).

Although donor plasma used to prepare immune globulin is screened for certain viruses (e.g., HBV, HIV type 1 and type 2 [HIV-1, HIV-2], HCV) and the manufacturing process for the various immune globulin preparations includes different procedures (e.g., cold ethanol precipitation, column chromatography, solvent/detergent [S/D] treatment, pasteurization/heat treatment, incubation at low pH, octanoic acid fractionation, caprylate precipitation, caprylate incubation, filtration) that further reduce the risk of transmission of infectious agents, a potential for transmission of infectious agents still remains.

Any infections that possibly may have been transmitted by immune globulin preparations should be reported to the appropriate manufacturer.

Risk of Hepatitis and Human Immunodeficiency Virus Infection. Although HCV infection was reported in a few individuals who received immune globulin preparations prepared outside the US and a US IGIV preparation (subsequently removed from the market) was implicated in the transmission of the virus, donors and/or donor units are now screened for HCV and commercially available preparations of immune globulin undergo various procedures during manufacture to reduce the risk of transmission of viral infection.

Epidemiologic and laboratory evidence indicate that commercially available preparations of IGIM, IGIV, and immune globulin subcutaneous do not have a discernible risk of transmitting HIV infection. In addition to the screening of all donor units for antibody to HIV and rejection of all repeatedly reactive units, the manufacturing processes for immune globulin include purification steps that provide an extremely high margin of safety in removal of HIV infectivity. Although some IGIM or IGIV produced in 1982–1985 may have contained antibody to HIV, all immune globulin produced since April 1985 should be free of the antibody.

Risk of Creutzfeldt-Jakob Disease or Variant Creutzfeldt-Jakob Disease. Because IGIM, IGIV, and immune globulin subcutaneous are prepared from human blood, they theoretically may carry a risk of transmitting the causative agent of CJD or vCJD. Although no cases of transmission of CJD or vCJD through plasma-derived preparations have been documented to date, an ongoing epidemiologic review being conducted in the United Kingdom identified several probable cases of vCJD acquired through transfusion of non-leukoreduced human red blood cell (RBC) concentrate. Tests are being developed to detect CJD and vCJD infection in blood and plasma donors. Until such donor screening tests are available for the disease, the FDA has recommended interim preventive measures based on the available scientific data and evolving state of knowledge regarding these diseases. These interim recommendations include specific guidelines for deferral of blood and plasma donors at increased risk of CJD and vCJD and specific guidelines for withdrawal, retrieval, quarantine, and disposition of blood and plasma products when post-donation information reveals that donors had CJD or vCJD or risk factors for these diseases. For further information on CJD and vCJD, see Risk of Creutzfeldt-Jakob Disease and Variant Creutzfeldt-Jakob Disease under Cautions: Precautions and Contraindications, in Albumin Human 16:00.

Other Precautions and Contraindications Whenever use of immune globulin is being considered, the potential risks and benefits should be weighed against those of alternative therapies and discussed with the patient.

Because aseptic meningitis syndrome has been reported rarely, patients receiving immune globulin should be instructed to immediately inform their clinician if signs or symptoms of aseptic meningitis occur (e.g., severe headache, neck stiffness, drowsiness, fever, sensitivity to light, painful eye movements, nausea and vomiting). Patients with signs and symptoms of aseptic meningitis should receive a thorough neurologic examination, including CSF analysis, to rule out other causes of meningitis. (See Aseptic Meningitis Syndrome under Cautions: Immune Globulin IV [IGIV].)

Because hemolysis has been reported rarely (see Hemolysis under Cautions: Immune Globulin IV [IGIV]), patients receiving immune globulin should be monitored for clinical signs and symptoms of hemolysis (e.g., increased heart rate, swelling, fatigue, difficulty breathing, yellowing of skin or eyes, dark-colored urine) and appropriate confirmatory laboratory tests should be performed if necessary. Patients should be instructed to immediately inform their clinician if signs or symptoms of hemolysis occur (e.g., increased heart rate, fatigue, yellowing of skin or eyes, dark-colored urine). If a blood transfusion is indicated for a patient who developed hemolysis with clinically compromising anemia after receiving immune globulin, adequate cross-matching should be performed to avoid exacerbating on-going hemolysis.

Because transfusion-related acute lung injury (noncardiogenic pulmonary edema) has been reported (see Transfusion-related Acute Lung Injury under Cautions: Immune Globulin IV [IGIV]), patients receiving immune globulin should be monitored for adverse pulmonary reactions. Patients should be instructed to immediately inform their clinician if signs or symptoms of transfusion-related acute lung injury occur (e.g., difficulty breathing, severe respiratory distress, chest pain, pulmonary edema, hypoxia, blue lips or extremities, fever) and advised that such effects typically occur within 1–6 hours following infusion of immune globulin. If transfusion-related acute lung injury is suspected, appropriate tests should be performed for the presence of antineutrophil antibodies and anti-human leukocyte antigen (HLA) antibodies in the product and in patient serum. Patients should be managed using oxygen therapy with adequate ventilatory support.

Because of the risk of volume overload, the manufacturers of Gammaplex 5% and Privigen® 10% state that the relative risks and benefits of the high-dose IGIV regimens (1 g/kg daily for 1–2 days) used for treatment of chronic ITP should be carefully considered before these preparations are used in individuals at increased risk of volume overload. The manufacturers of Gammaked® 10% and Gamunex®-C 10% state that high-dose regimens for treatment of ITP should *not* be used in patients with expanded fluid volumes or when fluid volume may be a concern.

Patients should be advised that immune globulin may interfere with the immune response to certain live viral vaccines (e.g., measles, mumps and rubella virus vaccine live [MMR], fixed-combination vaccine containing MMR and varicella virus vaccine live [MMRV], varicella virus vaccine live) and instructed to inform clinicians administering vaccines about any current or recent immune globulin therapy. (See Drug Interactions: Live Vaccines.)

The fact that IGIV preparations that contain maltose (e.g., Octagam® 5%, Octagam® 10%) may cause falsely elevated results in blood glucose determinations that use nonspecific methods based on glucose dehydrogenase pyrroloquinolinequinone (GDH-PQQ) or glucose-dye oxidoreductase should be considered if blood glucose testing is indicated in a patient receiving one of these preparations. Falsely elevated glucose determinations in patients receiving parenteral products containing maltose have resulted in inappropriate administration of insulin and life-threatening hypoglycemia and there also is a risk that such falsely elevated glucose determinations may mask true hypoglycemic states. (See Laboratory Test Interferences: Tests for Glucose.)

Gammagard® S/D and Gammagard® S/D (IgA less than 1 mcg/mL) contain approximately 8.5 mg of sodium chloride per mL. The amount of sodium in these preparations should be considered when determining dietary sodium in patients on a low-sodium diet since hypernatremia may occur.

■ **Pediatric Precautions** ***Immune Globulin IM*** Safety and efficacy of IGIM have not been established in pediatric patients; however, passive immunization with IGIM is recommended by the ACIP and American Academy of Pediatrics (AAP) in pediatric patients under certain circumstances. (See Uses: Immune Globulin IM [IGIM].)

Immune Globulin IV Safety and efficacy of Bivigam® 10% have not been established in pediatric patients younger than 6 years of age. Only limited data are available regarding the safety and efficacy of Bivigam® 10% in pediatric patients.

Studies using high doses of Carimune® NF in pediatric patients with acute or chronic ITP did not reveal any specific differences in safety in pediatric patients versus adults.

Flebogamma® 5% DIF has been evaluated for the treatment of primary immunodeficiency in pediatric patients 2 years of age or older; pediatric-specific dosage was not required to achieve desired serum IgG concentrations. Safety and efficacy of Flebogamma® 5% DIF have not been established in pediatric patients younger than 2 years of age.

Safety and efficacy of Flebogamma® 10% DIF have not been established for the treatment of primary immunodeficiency in pediatric patients. Flebogamma® 10% DIF has been evaluated in a limited number of children and adolescents with chronic ITP; treatment-emergent adverse effects were reported more frequently in pediatric patients than in adults. Safety and efficacy of Flebogamma® 10% DIF have not been established for the treatment of ITP in pediatric patients younger than 2 years of age.

Safety and efficacy of Gammagard® Liquid 10% for the treatment of primary immunodeficiency have not been established in pediatric patients younger than 2 years of age. Clinical studies evaluating Gammagard® Liquid 10% administered by IV infusion for replacement therapy in patients with primary immunodeficiency included pediatric patients 2 years to less than 16 years of age; safety and efficacy profiles in these pediatric patients were similar to those reported in adults and pediatric-specific dosage was not required to achieve desired serum IgG concentrations. Safety and efficacy of Gammagard® Liquid 10% have not been established for the treatment of multifocal motor neuropathy (MMN) in pediatric patients.

Clinical studies evaluating Gammagard® S/D and Gammagard® S/D (IgA less than 1 mcg/mL) for the treatment of primary immunodeficiency did not include sufficient numbers of pediatric patients 16 years of age or younger to determine whether they respond differently than adults. Safety and efficacy of Gammagard® S/D and Gammagard® S/D (IgA less than 1 mcg/mL) for the treatment of ITP in pediatric patients have not been established. Safety and efficacy of Gammagard® S/D and Gammagard® S/D (IgA less than 1 mcg/mL) for the treatment of Kawasaki disease in pediatric patients have been established; the majority of patients in clinical studies were younger than 5 years of age.

Gammaked® 10% administered by IV infusion can be used for the treatment of primary immunodeficiency or ITP in pediatric patients; pediatric-specific dosage is not necessary to achieve desired serum IgG concentrations. Safety and efficacy of Gammaked® 10% have not been established for the treatment of chronic inflammatory demyelinating polyneuropathy (CIDP) in pediatric patients.

Safety and efficacy of Gammaplex® 5% for the treatment of primary humoral immunodeficiency have not been established in pediatric patients younger than 2 years of age. In pediatric patients 2–16 years of age, safety and efficacy have been established in those with primary humoral immunodeficiency; pediatric-specific dosage was not required to achieve desired serum IgG concentrations in this age group. Gammaplex® 5% has been evaluated for the treatment of ITP in only a limited number of pediatric patients; data were insufficient to determine whether efficacy for treatment of ITP in pediatric patients differs from that in adults.

Safety and efficacy of Gamunex®-C 10% given by IV infusion were evaluated in a limited number of children and adolescents with primary immunodeficiency or chronic ITP. The pharmacokinetics, efficacy, and safety were similar to that reported in adults (except vomiting and fever were reported more frequently in pediatric patients); no pediatric-specific dosage requirements were necessary to achieve desired serum IgG concentrations. Safety and efficacy of Gamunex®-C 10% given by IV infusion have not been established for the treatment of CIDP in pediatric patients.

Octagam® 5% was evaluated in a limited number of children 6–16 years of age. There were no obvious differences in pharmacokinetics, efficacy, or safety between pediatric patients and adults and no pediatric-specific dosage requirements were necessary to achieve desired serum IgG concentrations.

Safety and efficacy of Octagam® 10% have not been established for the treatment of ITP in pediatric patients.

Safety and efficacy of Privigen® 10% for the treatment of primary humoral immunodeficiency have not been established in pediatric patients younger than 3 years of age. Privigen® 10% has been evaluated in a limited number of children and adolescents with primary immunodeficiency. There were no apparent differences in safety and efficacy compared with adults and no pediatric-specific dosage requirements were necessary to achieve desired serum IgG concentrations. Safety and efficacy of Privigen® 10% have not been established for the treatment of ITP in pediatric patients younger than 15 years of age.

Immune Globulin Subcutaneous Cuvitru® 20% can be used for the treatment of primary immunodeficiency in pediatric patients 2 years of age or older; in clinical studies, safety and efficacy profiles in this age group were similar to those reported in adults and pediatric-specific dosage was not necessary to achieve desired serum IgG concentrations. Safety and efficacy of Cuvitru® 20% have not been established in pediatric patients younger than 2 years of age.

Safety and efficacy of Gammagard® Liquid 10% for the treatment of primary immunodeficiency have not been established in pediatric patients younger than 2 years of age. Clinical studies evaluating Gammagard® Liquid 10% administered by subcutaneous infusion for replacement therapy in patients with primary immunodeficiency included pediatric patients 2 years to less than 16 years of age; safety and efficacy profiles in these pediatric patients were similar to those reported in adults and pediatric-specific dosage was not required to achieve desired serum IgG concentrations.

Safety and efficacy of Gammaked® 10% administered by subcutaneous infusion have not been established for the treatment of primary immunodeficiency in pediatric patients younger than 2 years of age. Safety and efficacy of Gammaked® 10% administered subcutaneously have not been established for the treatment of ITP or CIDP in pediatric patients.

Safety and efficacy of Gamunex®-C 10% administered by subcutaneous infusion have not been established for the treatment of primary humoral immunodeficiency in pediatric patients younger than 2 years of age. Safety and efficacy of Gamunex®-C 10% administered subcutaneously have not been established for the treatment of ITP or CIDP in pediatric patients.

Safety and efficacy of Hizentra® 20% have not been established in pediatric patients younger than 2 years of age. In pediatric patients 2–16 years of age, safety and efficacy have been established for the treatment of primary immunodeficiency. In clinical studies evaluating Hizentra® 20%, there were no differences in safety and efficacy profiles in pediatric patients compared with adults; pediatric-specific dosage was not required to achieve desired serum IgG concentrations.

Safety of Hyqvia® (immune globulin subcutaneous 10% with recombinant human hyaluronidase) has not been established in pediatric patients.

■ **Geriatric Precautions** Geriatric patients older than 65 years of age receiving immune globulin are at increased risk of acute renal failure or thrombotic events.

Immune globulin should be used with caution in patients 65 years of age or older. Recommended dosage should not be exceeded and the minimum practicable infusion rate should be used for IGIV or immune globulin subcutaneous. (See Dosage and Administration: Reconstitution and Administration.)

Clinical studies of IGIV did not include a sufficient number of patients 65 years of age or older to determine whether geriatric individuals respond differently than younger patients.

Clinical studies evaluating safety and efficacy of immune globulin subcutaneous (Cuvitru® 20%, Gammagard® Liquid 10%, Hizentra® 20%, Hyqvia®) included only a limited number of patients 65 years of age or older; no overall differences in safety or efficacy were observed in these patients compared with younger patients.

■ **Pregnancy, Fertility, and Lactation** Animal reproduction studies have not been performed with IGIM, IGIV, or immune globulin subcutaneous and it is not known whether these immune globulins can cause fetal harm when administered to pregnant women. The manufacturers state that IGIM, IGIV, or immune globulin subcutaneous should be used during pregnancy only when clearly needed.

ACIP states that there are no known risks associated with use of immune globulins for passive immunization in pregnant women and pregnancy is not generally considered a contraindication to the use of immune globulin.

Intact immune globulins such as those contained in IGIV cross the placenta in increasing amounts after 30 weeks of gestation. Results of studies in pregnant women with ITP who received IGIV prior to delivery indicate that the platelet response and clinical effects of IGIV were similar in the mother and neonate.

Animal reproduction studies have been performed with the recombinant human hyaluronidase component of immune globulin subcutaneous 10% with recombinant human hyaluronidase (Hyqvia®). In mice and rabbits, antibodies to recombinant human hyaluronidase that developed in the mother were shown to cross the placenta. It is not known whether anti-recombinant human hyaluronidase antibodies that develop in women cause fetal harm. If the patient becomes pregnant while receiving Hyqvia®, the patient should be encouraged to enroll in the Hyqvia® Pregnancy Registry (866-424-6724).

Fertility It is not known if IGIM, IGIV, or immune globulin subcutaneous affects fertility.

Some patients receiving immune globulin subcutaneous 10% with recombinant human hyaluronidase (Hyqvia®) have developed antibodies to recombinant human hyaluronidase and these antibodies potentially could cross-react with endogenous human hyaluronidase, which is expressed in adult male testes, epididymis, and sperm. It is not known whether these anti-recombinant human hyaluronidase antibodies interfere with fertilization in humans.

Lactation IGIV and immune globulin subcutaneous have not been evaluated in nursing women.

It is not known whether immune globulin is distributed into milk following IM, IV, or subcutaneous administration, affects milk production, or affects the breast-fed infant.

Immune globulin should be used with caution in nursing women. The benefits of breast-feeding and the importance of immune globulin to the woman should be considered along with the potential adverse effects on the breast-fed infant from the drug or from the underlying maternal condition.

The manufacturer of immune globulin subcutaneous 10% with recombinant human hyaluronidase (Hyqvia®) states that the drug should be used in nursing women only when clearly needed. In lactating animals, maternal antibodies bound to recombinant human hyaluronidase were transferred to offspring during lactation and the possible effects of these antibodies to recombinant human hyaluronidase that may be transferred to infants are unknown.

Drug Interactions

■ **Live Vaccines** Antibodies present in immune globulin may interfere with the immune response to certain live virus vaccine, including measles, mumps, and rubella virus vaccine live (MMR) and varicella virus vaccine live. These vaccines should not be administered simultaneously with or for specified intervals before or after administration of immune globulin.

There is no evidence that immune globulin preparations interfere with the immune response to influenza virus vaccine live intranasal, yellow fever vaccine, typhoid vaccine live oral, rotavirus vaccine live oral, zoster vaccine live, or poliovirus vaccine live oral (OPV; no longer commercially available in the US), and these live vaccines may be given simultaneously with or at any interval before or after immune globulin.

Measles, Mumps, Rubella, and Varicella Vaccines Antibodies present in immune globulin can interfere with the immune response to measles and rubella antigens contained in MMR and measles, mumps, rubella, and varicella virus vaccine live (MMRV) for at least 3 months or longer. Although specific information regarding the effect of immune globulin preparations on the immune response to mumps antigen contained in MMR or MMRV or varicella antigen contained in varicella virus vaccine live or MMRV are not available, there is potential for similar interference since immune globulin preparations contain antibodies to these viruses. The duration of interference with the immune response to vaccines containing measles, mumps, rubella, and/or varicella antigens following administration of immune globulin depends on the amount of antigen-specific antibody contained in the immune globulin preparation. Based on the assumption that passively acquired antibody has an estimated half-life of 30 days and data indicating that a 80-mg/kg dose of IgG interferes with the immune response to measles virus vaccine live for 5 months, the US Public Health Service Advisory Committee on Immunization Practices (ACIP) and American Academy of Pediatrics (AAP) have made the following recommendations concerning administration of live viral vaccines.

Administration of vaccines containing measles or varicella antigens (MMR, MMRV, or varicella virus vaccine live) should be deferred for 3 months following administration of immune globulin IM (IGIM) used for preexposure or postexposure prophylaxis of hepatitis A virus (HAV) infection; for 5 months following administration of IGIM used for measles prophylaxis in immunocompetent individuals; for 6 months following use of IGIM for measles prophylaxis in immunodeficient individuals; for 8 months following administration of immune globulin IV (IGIV) for replacement therapy of immunodeficiencies or for postexposure prophylaxis against varicella; for 8–10 months following administration of IGIV for the treatment of idiopathic thrombocytopenic purpura (ITP; also known as immune thrombocytopenic purpura or immune thrombocytopenia); and for 11 months following administration of IGIV for Kawasaki disease.

Immune globulin and MMR, MMRV, or varicella virus vaccine live should not be administered simultaneously. If simultaneous administration (at a separate site) is deemed necessary (e.g., because of imminent exposure to measles) or if a dose of MMR, MMRV, or varicella virus vaccine live is given after immune globulin at an interval shorter than that recommended, ACIP and AAP state that the vaccine dose should be repeated after the recommended interval, unless serologic testing is feasible and indicates an adequate antibody response to the live virus vaccine. In general, vaccine virus replication and stimulation of immunity occur within 1–2 weeks after administration of a live virus vaccine. Therefore, if immune globulin is administered less than 14 days after MMR, MMRV, or varicella virus vaccine live, an additional dose of vaccine should be given after the recommended interval previously specified, unless there is serologic evidence of an adequate antibody response to the vaccine.

Rotavirus Vaccine A decreased antibody response to rotavirus vaccine live oral potentially could occur in infants who recently received immune globulin. Safety and efficacy data are not available from clinical trials regarding the use of rotavirus vaccine live oral in infants who have received immune globulin within the last 42 days. However, ACIP and AAP state that rotavirus vaccine live oral may be administered simultaneously with or at any time before or after antibody-containing blood products.

■ **Inactivated Vaccines and Toxoids** ACIP and AAP state that administration of inactivated vaccines and toxoids simultaneously with (at different sites) or at any interval before or after administration of immune globulin preparations should not have a clinically important effect on the immune response to the vaccines or toxoids.

Hepatitis A Virus Vaccine Inactivated Hepatitis A virus vaccine inactivated (hepatitis A vaccine) may be administered simultaneously with immune globulin at a separate site using a different syringe. Although antibody to hepatitis A virus (anti-HAV) passively acquired from immune globulin may decrease the active immune response stimulated by hepatitis A vaccine, the reduced immunogenicity caused by the presence of passively acquired antibody does not appear to be clinically important since seroconversion rates are not affected. In studies in healthy adults who received 3-dose regimens of hepatitis A vaccine, geometric mean titers of antibody after the second and third vaccine doses were lower in those who received a single dose of IGIM at the same time as the initial vaccine dose; however, the seroconversion rate was similar in both groups.

Laboratory Test Interferences

■ **Immunohematology and Serologic Tests** Because immune globulin can contain blood group antibodies (e.g., anti-A, anti-B, anti-D), positive direct antiglobulin (Coombs') test results may occur in patients receiving the drug. This reaction may interfere with hematologic studies or transfusion cross-matching procedures.

Patients receiving immune globulin may have transitory increases in various passively acquired antibodies that could cause false-positive serologic test results and misinterpretation of these test results.

■ **Tests for Fungus** False-positive readings in assays used for the diagnosis of fungal infections may occur in patients receiving immune globulin if the tests depend on detection of beta-D-glucans. Interference with these assays may persist during the weeks following infusion of immune globulin.

■ **Tests for Glucose** Immune globulin IV (IGIV) preparations that contain maltose (e.g., Octagam® 5%, Octagam® 10%) may cause falsely elevated results in blood glucose determinations that use nonspecific methods based on glucose dehydrogenase pyrroloquinolinequinone (GDH-PQQ) or glucose-dye oxidoreductase. Such falsely elevated glucose determinations in patients receiving parenteral products containing maltose have resulted in inappropriate administration of insulin and life-threatening hypoglycemia. In addition, there is a risk that true cases of hypoglycemia may go untreated if a hypoglycemic state is masked by falsely elevated blood glucose determinations. Therefore, only glucose-specific test methods that are not affected by maltose (e.g., methods that use glucose dehydrogenase nicotine adenine dinucleotide [GDH-NAD], glucose oxidase, glucose hexokinase) should be used to measure blood glucose concentrations in patients receiving IGIV preparations that contain maltose. If blood glucose determinations are indicated in a patient receiving an IGIV preparation that contains maltose (e.g., Octagam® 5%), the product information for the blood glucose testing system (including glucose test strips) should be carefully reviewed to determine if the testing system is appropriate. If any uncertainty exists, the manufacturer of the glucose testing system should be contacted to determine if the system will provide accurate blood glucose determinations in this situation.

Pharmacology

Immune globulin IM (IGIM), immune globulin IV (IGIV), and immune globulin subcutaneous provide a broad spectrum of opsonic and neutralizing IgG antibodies against a wide variety of bacterial and viral agents. These IgG antibodies are used to provide passive immunity by increasing an individual's antibody titer and antigen-antibody reaction potential and prevent or modify certain infectious diseases in susceptible individuals. The mechanism of action of immune globulin in the treatment of primary humoral immunodeficiency has not been fully elucidated.

The mechanism by which IGIV increases platelet counts in the treatment of idiopathic thrombocytopenic purpura (ITP; also known as immune thrombocytopenic purpura or immune thrombocytopenia) has not been fully elucidated. It has been suggested that IGIV may saturate Fc (crystallizable fragment) receptors on cells of the reticuloendothelial system, resulting in a decrease in Fc-mediated phagocytosis of antibody-coated cells. This Fc-receptor blockade may occur in bone marrow, spleen, and other parts of the reticuloendothelial system and may occur through competition for Fc receptors by increased serum concentrations of IgG or by circulating immune complexes. Altered Fc-receptor affinity for IgG or suppression of antiplatelet antibody production may also be involved.

The mechanism of action of IGIV in the treatment of Kawasaki disease is not known, but possibly may include modulation of cytokine production, neutralization of bacterial superantigens or other etiologic agents, augmentation of T-cell suppressor activity, suppression of antibody synthesis, and provision of anti-idiotypic antibodies. IGIV and aspirin appear to have additive anti-inflammatory effects in the treatment of Kawasaki disease.

The mechanism of action of IGIV in the treatment of chronic inflammatory demyelinating polyneuropathy (CIDP) has not been fully elucidated.

Pharmacokinetics

Following IM administration of immune globulin IM (IGIM), serum concentrations of IgG peak within 2 days. IgG present in IGIM is rapidly and evenly distributed between intravascular and extravascular spaces.

Following IV infusion of immune globulin IV (IGIV), there is an immediate post-infusion peak in serum IgG concentrations followed by a biphasic decline. There is an initial rapid decline in serum IgG concentrations associated with equilibration between plasma and extravascular fluid compartments that is followed by a second phase characterized by a slower and constant rate of elimination.

Peak serum concentrations of IgG attained with immune globulin subcutaneous are lower than those attained with IGIV, but trough IgG concentrations generally are higher than those attained with IGIV. In addition, in contrast to the biphasic IgG concentrations reported with IGIV, once-weekly administration of immune globulin subcutaneous results in relatively stable IgG concentrations. Peak serum IgG concentrations in patients receiving once-weekly immune globulin subcutaneous occur approximately 3 days (range: 0–7 days) after a dose.

In studies evaluating immune globulin subcutaneous 10% with recombinant human hyaluronidase (Hyqvia®), peak serum concentrations of IgG were lower but trough IgG concentrations generally were comparable to those attained with IGIV. In addition, the area under the plasma concentration-time curve (AUC) of IgG was 20% higher than that attained with immune globulin subcutaneous administered without recombinant human hyaluronidase. Peak serum IgG concentrations in patients receiving Hyqvia® occurred 5 days (range: 3.3–5.1 days) after a dose.

The half-life of IgG in individuals with normal serum IgG concentrations is reportedly about 18–25 days. The half-life of IGIV preparations in patients with immunodeficiencies has been reported to range from 12–59 days. High IgG concentrations and hypermetabolism associated with fever and infection have been reported to coincide with a shortened IgG half-life. Following IV administration of IGIV once every 3 or 4 weeks in patients with primary humoral immunodeficiency, the elimination half-life of IgG was approximately 35 days.

Immune globulins can cross the placenta in increasing amounts after 30 weeks' gestation. It is not known whether IGIM or IGIV is distributed into milk.

Chemistry and Stability

■ **Chemistry** Immune globulin is a sterile, nonpyrogenic preparation of globulins containing many antibodies normally present in adult human blood. Immune globulin is commercially available for IM administration as immune globulin IM (IGIM), for IV administration as immune globulin IV (IGIV), and for subcutaneous administration as immune globulin subcutaneous.

IGIM, IGIV, and immune globulin subcutaneous meet standards established by the Center for Biologics Evaluation and Research of the US Food and Drug Administration (FDA). IGIM and IGIV are prepared by cold alcohol fractionation of pooled plasma from venous blood of at least 1000 individuals. Plasma donors and plasma used in the preparation of commercially available immune globulin have been tested and shown to be negative for certain human blood-borne viruses and all commercially available preparations of IGIM, IGIV, and immune globulin subcutaneous undergo at least one heat-treatment, filtration, and/or chemical (solvent/detergent) procedure during the manufacturing process to reduce virus infectious potential. (See Risk of Transmissible Agents in Plasma-derived Preparations under Cautions: Precautions and Contraindications.)

Immune Globulin IM Immune globulin IM (IGIM) is commercially available as GamaSTAN® S/D.

GamaSTAN® S/D. GamaSTAN® S/D is a sterile solution containing 15–18% protein stabilized in 0.21–0.32 *M* glycine. GamaSTAN® S/D occurs as a colorless to pale yellow or pink solution, has a pH of 6.4–7.2, and does not contain thimerosal or any other preservative. GamaSTAN® S/D has been purified using precipitation, filtration, ultrafiltration, and diafiltration and undergoes a chemical (solvent/detergent) procedure designed to reduce the viral infectious potential of the preparation.

Immune Globulin IV Immune globulin IV (IGIV) is commercially available as Bivigam® 10%, Carimune® NF, Flebogamma® 5% DIF, Flebogamma® 10% DIF, Gammagard® Liquid 10%, Gammagard® S/D, Gammaked® 10%, Gammaplex® 5%, Gamunex®-C 10%, Octagam® 5%, Octagam® 10%, and Privigen® 10%. The various manufacturers of IGIV use different methods to isolate and purify immune globulin after cold alcohol fractionation and different methods to reduce the viral infectious potential of the preparations.

Bivigam® 10%. Bivigam® 10% is a sterile solution containing 10% protein, of which not less 96% is IgG. The preparation contains less than 200 mcg/mL of IgA. During manufacture, Bivigam® 10% undergoes cold alcohol fractionation, solvent-detergent treatment, nanofiltration, and low pH incubation to reduce the virus infectious potential of the preparation.

Bivigam® 10% is a clear or slightly opalescent, colorless to pale yellow solution with a pH of 4–4.6. Bivigam® 10% contains 0.2–0.29 *M* glycine, 0.15–0.25% polysorbate 80, and 0.1–0.14 *M* sodium chloride, but does not contain preservatives or sucrose.

Carimune® NF. Carimune® NF is a sterile, lyophilized preparation of immune globulin that has been modified at acid pH in the presence of trace amounts of pepsin to make it suitable for IV administration. Carimune® NF contains not less than 96% IgG; the distribution of the IgG subclasses corresponds to that of normal serum. Most immunoglobulins contained in the preparation are monomeric (7S) IgG and the remainder are dimeric IgG, small amounts of polymeric IgG, traces of IgA and IgM, and immunoglobulin fragments. Carimune® NF contains 1.67 g of sucrose as a stabilizing agent and also contains small amounts (less than 20 mg) of sodium chloride per gram of protein. Carimune® NF undergoes filtration procedures during manufacturer to reduce the risk of transmission of viral infections. The manufacturing process also includes nanofiltration (removing viruses via size-exclusion); this is performed prior to the viral inactivation step in order to reduce the potential viral load before inactivation is performed. Treatment with pepsin at pH 4 rapidly inactivates enveloped viruses.

Following reconstitution as directed with a neutral unbuffered diluent, Carimune® NF solutions have a pH of 6.4–6.8. Carimune® NF that has been reconstituted to a concentration of 30–120 mg of protein per mL with 0.9% sodium chloride injection, 5% dextrose injection, or sterile water for injection has a calculated osmolality of 498–1074, 444–1020, or 192–768 mOsm/kg, respectively.

Flebogamma® 5% DIF. Flebogamma® 5% DIF contains at least 97% IgG and trace amounts of IgA (typically less than 50 mcg/mL) and IgM. The distribution of IgG subclasses is approximately 66.6% IgG_1, 28.5% IgG_2, 2.7% IgG_3, and 2.2% IgG_4. Flebogamma® 5% DIF undergoes several procedures during manufacture to reduce the risk of transmission of viral infections. The manufacturing process includes cold alcohol fractionation, polyethylene glycol precipitation, ion exchange chromatography, pasteurization, solvent-detergent treatment, and double sequential nanofiltration.

Flebogamma® 5% DIF is a clear or slightly opalescent and colorless to pale yellow liquid. The pH of Flebogamma® 5% DIF is 5–6 and the osmolality is 240–370 mOsm/kg. Flebogamma® 5% DIF contains sorbitol as a stabilizing agent, polyethylene glycol, and trace amounts of sodium, but does not contain preservatives or sucrose.

Flebogamma® 10% DIF. Flebogamma® 10% DIF contains at least 97% IgG and trace amounts of IgA (typically less than 32 mcg/mL) and IgM. The distribution of IgG subclasses is approximately 66.6% IgG_1, 27.9% IgG_2, 3.0% IgG_3, and 2.5% IgG_4. Flebogamma® 10% DIF undergoes several procedures during manufacture to reduce the risk of transmission of viral infections. The manufacturing process includes cold alcohol fractionation, polyethylene glycol precipitation, ion exchange chromatography, low pH treatment, pasteurization, solvent-detergent treatment, and nanofiltration.

Flebogamma® 10% DIF occurs as a clear or slightly opalescent and colorless to pale yellow solution with a pH of 5–6 and an osmolarity of 240–370 mOsm/L. Flebogamma® 10% DIF contains sorbitol as a stabilizing agent, polyethylene glycol, and trace amounts of sodium, but does not contain preservatives or sucrose.

Gammagard® Liquid 10%. Gammagard® Liquid 10% is a sterile solution of IgG. At least 98% is IgG; the distribution of the IgG subclasses corresponds to that of normal serum and the Fc and Fab functions are maintained. The average IgA concentration in this preparation is 37 mcg/mL and IgM is present in only trace amounts. During manufacture, Gammagard® Liquid 10% undergoes a chemical (solvent/detergent) procedure, nanofiltration, and low pH incubation at elevated temperatures to reduce the virus infectious potential of the preparation.

Gammagard® Liquid 10% is a clear or slightly opalescent and colorless or pale yellow solution with a pH of 4.6–5.1. The solution has an osmolality of 240–300 mOsm/kg, which is similar to physiologic osmolality (285–295 mOsm/kg). Gammagard® Liquid 10% contains 0.25 *M* glycine as a stabilizing and buffering agent, but does not contain preservatives, sodium, or sucrose.

Gammagard® S/D. Gammagard® S/D is a sterile, lyophilized preparation of immune globulin that has been purified using ultrafiltration and ion exchange adsorption. In addition, this preparation undergoes a chemical (solvent/detergent) procedure during manufacture to reduce the risk of transmission of viral infection.

Following reconstitution as directed, Gammagard® S/D contains approximately 50 mg of protein per mL, of which not less than 90% is IgG. The distribution of the IgG subclasses on average corresponds to that of normal serum. Gammagard® S/D is commercially available as a formulation that contains no more than 2.2 mcg/mL of IgA and as a formulation that contains less than 1 mcg/mL of IgA.

The manufacturing process for Gammagard® S/D isolates IgG without additional chemical or enzymatic modification and the Fc portion is maintained intact. This preparation also contains glycine, dextrose, polyethylene glycol, and human albumin as stabilizing agents.

Reconstituted solutions of Gammagard® S/D contain approximately 8.5 mg of sodium chloride per mL and have a pH of 6.4–7.2. The reconstituted solution is clear to slightly opalescent and colorless to pale yellow. Gammagard® S/D does not contain preservatives or sucrose.

Gammaked® 10%. Gammaked® 10% is a sterile solution containing 9–11% protein stabilized in 0.16–0.24 *M* glycine. Not less than 98% of the protein content of Gammaked® 10% has the electrophoretic mobility of IgG. The distribution of the IgG subclasses in Gammaked® 10% is similar to that of normal serum; the preparation contains trace amounts of fragments, IgA (average 46 mcg/mL), and IgM. Gammaked® 10% has been purified using caprylate precipitation and filtration and anion-exchange chromatography. Various steps used in the manufacturing process (caprylate precipitation/cloth filtration, caprylate incubation, depth filtration, column chromatography, incubation in the final container at pH 4–4.3) reduce the risk of transmission of viral infections.

Gammaked® 10% is a clear to opalescent and colorless to pale yellow solution and has a pH of 4–4.5. Gammaked® 10% has a buffering capacity of 35 mEq/L and an osmolality of 258 mOsm/kg of solvent. Gammaked® 10% does not contain preservatives or sucrose.

Gammaplex® 5%. Gammaplex® 5% is a sterile solution of polyclonal human IgG for IV administration. Gammaplex® 5% is prepared from large pools of human plasma by a combination of cold ethanol fractionation and ion exchange chromatography. The manufacturing process for Gammaplex® 5% includes several steps (solvent/detergent treatment, filtration steps, terminal low pH incubation) to reduce the risk of transmission of viral infections.

Gammaplex® 5% has a purity of at least 95% IgG and contains less than 10 mcg/mL of IgA. The IgG subclass distribution is approximately 64%IgG_1, 30% IgG_2, 5% IgG_3, and 1% IgG_4. Gammaplex® 5% has an osmolality of not less than 240 mOsm/kg (typically 420–500 mOsm/kg) and a pH of 4.8–5.1. This preparation contains sorbitol, glycine, and polysorbate 80 as stabilizers. Gammaplex® 5% does not contain any carbohydrate stabilizers (e.g., sucrose, maltose) or preservatives.

Gamunex®-C 10%. Gamunex®-C 10% is a sterile solution containing 9–11% protein stabilized in 0.16–0.24 M glycine. Not less than 98% of the protein content of Gamunex®-C 10% has the electrophoretic mobility of IgG. The distribution of the IgG subclasses in Gamunex®-C 10% is similar to that of normal serum; it contains trace amounts of fragments and IgA (average 46 mcg/mL) and IgM. Gamunex®-C 10% does not contain preservatives or sucrose. Gamunex®-C 10% has been purified using caprylate precipitation and filtration and anion-exchange chromatography; the protein has not been modified using heat, chemical, or enzymatic modification steps. Various steps used in the manufacturing process (caprylate precipitation/cloth filtration, caprylate incubation, depth filtration, column chromatography, incubation in the final container at low pH [pH 4–4.3 for at least 21 days at 23–27°C]) reduce the risk of transmission of viral infections. The pH of Gamunex®-C 10% is 4–4.5. Gamunex®-C 10% has a buffering capacity of 35 mEq/L and an osmolality of 258 mOsm/kg of solvent.

Octagam® 5%. Octagam® 5% is a sterile solution containing 5% protein stabilized with 10% maltose. Octagam® 5% contains approximately 50 mg of protein per mL, of which not less than 96% is IgG, and contains aggregates (3% or less), monomers and dimers (90% or greater), and fragments (3 % or less). The distribution of the IgG subclasses in Octagam® 5% is approximately 65% IgG_1, 30% IgG_2, 3% IgG_3, and 2% IgG_4, which is similar to that of normal serum; only trace amounts of IgA (no more than 200 mcg/mL) and IgM are present. In addition, the Fc portion is maintained intact. Octagam® 5% is prepared using cold ethanol fractionation and is purified using ultrafiltration and chromatography; the protein has not been chemically or enzymatically modified. Octagam® 5% undergoes a chemical (solvent/detergent) procedure during manufacture to reduce the risk of transmission of viral infections.

The pH of Octagam® 5% is 5.1–6 and the osmolality is 310–380 mOsm/kg. Octagam® 5% does not contain preservatives or sucrose.

Octagam® 10%. Octagam® 10% is a sterile solution containing 10% protein stabilized with 9% maltose. Octagam® 10% contains approximately 100 mg of protein per mL, of which not less than 96% is IgG, and contains aggregates (3% or less), monomers and dimers (94% or greater), and fragments (3% or less). The distribution of the IgG subclasses in Octagam® 10% is approximately 65% IgG_1, 30% IgG_2, 3% IgG_3, and 2% IgG_4, which is similar to that of normal serum; the preparation contains only trace amounts of IgA (average 106 mcg/mL) and IgM. In addition, the Fc portion is maintained intact. Octagam® 10% is prepared using cold ethanol fractionation and is purified using ultrafiltration and chromatography; the protein has not been chemically or enzymatically modified. Octagam® 10% undergoes a chemical (solvent/detergent) procedure during manufacture to reduce the risk of transmission of viral infections.

The pH of Octagam® 10% is 4.5–5 and the osmolality is 310–380 mOsm/kg. Octagam® 10% does not contain preservatives or sucrose.

Privigen® 10%. Privigen® 10% is a sterile, solution of polyvalent human IgG for IV administration. Privigen® 10% is prepared from large pools of human plasma by a combination of cold ethanol fractionation, octanoic acid fractionation, and anion exchange chromatography. The IgG proteins are not subjected to heating or to chemical or enzymatic modification. The Fc and Fab functions of the IgG molecule are retained. Privigen® 10% does not activate the complement system or prekallikrein in an unspecific manner. The manufacturing process for Privigen® 10% includes several steps (incubation at pH 4, filtration steps) to reduce the risk of transmission of viral infections.

Privigen® 10% has a purity of at least 98% IgG, consisting primarily of monomers. Privigen® 10% contains IgA (not exceeding 25 mcg/mL). The IgG subclass distribution (approximate mean values) is IgG_1 67.8%, IgG_2 28.7%, IgG_3 2.3%, and IgG_4 1.2%. Privigen® 10% has an osmolality of approximately 320 mOsm/kg (range: 240–440) and a pH of 4.8 (range: 4.6–5). Privigen® 10% contains approximately 250 mmol/L (range: 210–290) of L-proline (a nonessential amino acid) as a stabilizer and trace amounts of sodium. Privigen® 10% does not contain any carbohydrate stabilizers (e.g., sucrose, maltose) or preservatives.

Immune Globulin Subcutaneous Immune globulin subcutaneous is commercially available as Cuvitru® 20% and Hizentra® 20%, and also is commercially available as immune globulin subcutaneous 10% with recombinant human hyaluronidase (Hyqvia®). In addition, certain IGIV preparations also can be administered subcutaneously (i.e., Gammagard® Liquid 10%, Gammaked® 10%, Gamunex®-C 10%).

Cuvitru® 20%. Cuvitru® 20% is a sterile solution containing 20% protein, of which not less than 98% is IgG. The distribution of the IgG subclasses is similar to that of normal plasma; the Fc and Fab functions are maintained. The preparation contains trace amounts of IgA (average 80 mcg/mL). The manufacturing process includes several procedures, including cold ethanol fractionation, cation and anion exchange chromatography, solvent/detergent treatment, incubation at low pH, and nanofiltration, to reduce the risk of transmission of infective agents.

Cuvitru® 20% is a clear and colorless or pale yellow or light brown solution and has a pH of 4.6–5.1 and an osmolality of 280–292 mOsm/kg. Cuvitru® 20% contains glycine as a stabilizing and buffering agent, but does not contain any preservatives, sodium, or sucrose.

Hizentra® 20%. Hizentra® 20% is a sterile solution containing 20% protein, of which not less than 98% is IgG. The preparation contains trace amounts of IgA (50 mcg/mL or less). The manufacturing process for Hizentra® 20% includes cold alcohol fractionation, octanoic acid fractionation, and anion exchange chromatography. The Fc and Fab functions of the IgG molecule are retained since the process does not include heating or chemical or enzymatic modification. The manufacturing process includes steps to reduce the risk of virus transmission, including incubation at pH 4, virus filtration based on size exclusion, and depth filtration. Several of the manufacturing processes (e.g., octanoic acid fractionation, depth filtration, virus filtration) have been shown to decrease the infectivity of an experimental agent of transmissible spongiform encephalopathy (TSE).

Hizentra® 20% occurs as a clear, pale yellow to light brown solution and has a pH of 4.6–5.2. The preparation contains approximately 250 mmol/L (range: 210–290 mmol/L) of L-proline (a nonessential amino acid) as a stabilizer, polysorbate 80 (8–30 mg/L), and trace amounts of sodium. Hizentra® 20% does not contain any carbohydrate stabilizers (e.g., sucrose, maltose) or preservatives.

Hyqvia® (Immune Globulin Subcutaneous 10% with Recombinant Human Hyaluronidase). Immune globulin subcutaneous 10% with recombinant human hyaluronidase (Hyqvia®) is commercially available as a kit that contains a vial of immune globulin subcutaneous 10% copackaged with a vial of recombinant human hyaluronidase. The recombinant human hyaluronidase component is administered prior to the immune globulin component and acts locally to temporarily increase permeability of subcutaneous tissue to increase dispersion and absorption of the immune globulin.

The immune globulin subcutaneous 10% component of Hyqvia® is a sterile preparation of highly purified and concentrated IgG antibodies (not less than 98% IgG) with a distribution of IgG subclasses similar to that of normal serum; Fc and Fab portions are maintained intact and prekallikrein activator activity is not detectable. The preparation contains an average of 37 mcg/mL of IgA and trace amounts of IgM. The immune globulin is prepared from large pools of human plasma by a combination of cold ethanol fractionation and cation and anion exchange chromatography and undergoes solvent/detergent treatment, nanofiltration, and low pH incubation at elevated temperatures to reduce the risk of transmission of viral infections. The immune globulin subcutaneous 10% component of Hyqvia® is a clear or slightly opalescent and colorless or pale yellow solution with a pH of 4.6–5.1 and an osmolality of 240–300 mOsm/kg. The immune globulin component contains glycine as a stabilizing and buffering agent, but does not contain preservatives, sodium, or sucrose.

The recombinant human hyaluronidase component of Hyqvia® is prepared from mammalian cells using recombinant DNA technology. It is a clear and colorless solution with a pH of 7.4 and an osmolality of 290–350 mOsm/kg. Each vial contains 160 units/mL of recombinant human hyaluronidase and also contains sodium chloride, sodium phosphate dibasic dihydrate, human albumin, edentate disodium dihydrate, and calcium chloride dihydrate; sodium hydroxide is added to adjust pH. The solution does not contain preservatives.

■ Stability

Immune Globulin IM IGIM (GamaSTAN® S/D) should be refrigerated at 2–8°C and should not be frozen.

Immune Globulin IV Partially used vials or bottles of IGIV preparations should be discarded.

Because of the potential for incompatibility, the commercially available lyophilized preparations of IGIV (Carimune® NF, Gammagard® S/D) should be reconstituted only with the diluent provided or specified by the manufacturers. Although certain immune globulin preparations may be diluted with compatible infusion fluids specified by the manufacturer (Gammagard® Liquid 10%, Gammaked® 10%, Gamunex®-C 10%, Privigen® 10%), other immune globulin preparations should not be diluted. IGIV should not be admixed with other drugs.

Bivigam® 10%. Bivigam® 10% should be stored at 2–8°C. Bivigam® 10% should not be frozen or heated and should be discarded if it has been frozen or heated. Vials are for single use only; partially used vials should be discarded.

Carimune® NF. Carimune® NF lyophilized powder for injection should be stored at room temperature not exceeding 30°C. Carimune® NF solutions should be administered promptly if the drug is reconstituted outside of sterile laminar airflow conditions. If the drug is reconstituted in a sterile laminar flow hood using aseptic technique, reconstituted solutions may be stored for up to 24 hours under refrigeration. Carimune® NF solutions should not be frozen.

Flebogamma® 5% DIF. Flebogamma® 5% DIF should be stored at 2–25°C and is stable for up to 24 months as indicated by the expiration date on the outer carton and container label. Flebogamma® 5% DIF should not be frozen and should be discarded if frozen. Any partially used vials should be discarded. To protect Flebogamma® 5% from light, it should be stored in the original carton until used.

Flebogamma® 10% DIF. Flebogamma® 10% DIF should be stored at 2–25°C and is stable for up to 24 months as indicated by the expiration date on the outer carton and container label. Flebogamma® 10% DIF should not be frozen and should be discarded if frozen. Vials are for single use only; partially used vials should be discarded. To protect Flebogamma® 10% from light, it should be stored in the original carton until used.

Gammagard® Liquid 10%. Gammagard® Liquid 10% may be stored at 2–8°C for up to 36 months as indicated by the expiration date on the outer carton and container label. Alternatively, Gammagard® Liquid 10% may be stored at room temperature (up to 25°C) for up to 24 months as indicated by the expiration date on the outer carton and container label. Gammagard® Liquid 10% should not be frozen.

Gammagard® Liquid 10% vials are for single use only; any partially used vials should be discarded.

Gammagard® S/D. Prior to reconstitution, Gammagard® S/D lyophilized powder for injection and Gammagard® S/D (IgA less than 1 mcg/mL) lyophilized powder for injection should be stored at a temperature not exceeding 25°C and should not be frozen. Following reconstitution, Gammagard® S/D solution should be administered promptly. If reconstitution is performed outside of sterile laminar airflow conditions, administration should begin within 2 hours of reconstitution. If reconstitution is performed in a sterile laminar flow hood using aseptic technique, the manufacturers state that the reconstituted solutions may be stored in the original glass container or in Viaflex IV bags for up to 24 hours at 2–8°C. Partially used vials of Gammagard® S/D and Gammagard® S/D (IgA less than 1 mcg/mL) should be discarded.

Gammaked® 10%. Gammaked® 10% may be stored at 2–8°C for 36 months after the date of manufacture. The drug also may be stored at room temperature (up to 25°C) for up to 6 months at any time during the 36 months, but then must be used immediately or discarded. Gammaked® 10% should not be frozen and should be discarded if frozen.

Vials of Gammaked® 10% that have been entered should be promptly used; partially used vials should be discarded. If the contents of full vials are pooled under aseptic conditions, the solution should be used within 8 hours of pooling.

Gammaplex® 5%. Gammaplex® 5% should be stored at 2–25°C for up to 36 months after the date of manufacture. Gammaplex® 5% should not be frozen and should be discarded if frozen. To protect Gammaplex® 5% from light, it should be stored in the original carton until used.

Bottles of Gammaplex® 5% that have been entered should be promptly used; partially used bottles should be discarded. If the contents of bottles are pooled under aseptic conditions, the IV infusion should be started within 2 hours of pooling.

Gamunex®-C 10%. Gamunex®-C 10% may be stored at 2–8°C for 36 months after the date of manufacture. The drug also may be stored at room temperature (up to 25°C) for up to 6 months at any time during the 36 months, but then must be used immediately or discarded. Gamunex®-C 10% should not be frozen.

Vials of Gamunex®-C 10% that have been entered should be promptly used; partially used vials should be discarded. If the contents of full vials are pooled under aseptic conditions, the solution should be used within 8 hours of pooling.

Octagam® 5%. Octagam® 5% may be stored at 2–25°C for 24 months after the date of manufacture. Octagam® 5% should not be frozen and should be discarded if frozen.

Octagam® 5% single-use bottles that have been entered should be used promptly; partially used bottles should be discarded.

Octagam® 10%. Octagam® 10% may be stored at 2–8°C for 24 months after the date of manufacture. Within the first 12 months from the date of manufacture, Octagam® 10% may be stored for up to 9 months at room temperature (up to 25°C), but then must be used immediately or discarded. Octagam® 10% should not be frozen and should be discarded if frozen.

Octagam® 10% single-use bottles that have been entered should be used promptly; partially used bottles should be discarded.

Privigen® 10%. Privigen® 10% is stable for up to 36 months when stored at room temperature (up to 25°C) as indicated by the expiration date on the outer carton and vial label. Privigen® 10% should not be frozen and should be discarded if it has been frozen. Privigen® 10% should be protected from light.

Immune Globulin Subcutaneous **Cuvitru® 20%.** Cuvitru® 20% should be stored at 2–8°C and is stable for up to 36 months. Alternatively, Cuvitru® 20% can be stored at room temperature (up to 25°C) for up to 12 months, but should not be returned to refrigeration. Cuvitru® 20% should not be frozen. To protect Cuvitru® 20% from light, it should be stored in the original carton until used.

Cuvitru® 20% vials are for single use only; any partially used vials should be discarded.

Hizentra® 20%. Hizentra® 20% should be stored at room temperature (up to 25°C) and is stable for up to 30 months as indicated by the expiration date on the outer carton and vial label. Hizentra® 20% should not be frozen and should be discarded if it has been frozen. To protect Hizentra® 20% from light, it should be stored in the original carton until used.

Partially used vials of Hizentra® 20% should be discarded.

Hyqvia® (Immune Globulin Subcutaneous 10% with Recombinant Human Hyaluronidase). The kit containing immune globulin subcutaneous 10% with recombinant human hyaluronidase (Hyqvia®; vial of immune globulin subcutaneous 10% copackaged with a vial of recombinant human hyaluronidase) can be stored at 2–8°C for up to 36 months. Alternatively, the kit can be stored at room temperature (up to 25°C) for up to 3 months during the first 24 months from the date of manufacture printed on the carton. If the kit is removed from refrigeration and subsequently stored at room temperature (up to 25°C), it should be used within 3 months after removal to room temperature (but within the expiration date on the carton and vial labels) and should not be returned to refrigeration. The vials of immune globulin subcutaneous 10% and vials of recombinant human hyaluronidase should be stored in the original carton to protect from light and should not be frozen.

Preparations

Excipients in commercially available drug preparations may have clinically important effects in some individuals; consult specific product labeling for details.

Immune Globulin IM

Parenteral		
Injection, for IM use	150–180 mg (of protein) per mL	**GamaSTAN® S/D,** Grifols

Immune Globulin IV

Parenteral		
For injection, for IV infusion	2.5 g (of protein)	**Gammagard® S/D,** Baxalta
	5 g (of protein)	**Gammagard® S/D,** Baxalta
		Gammagard® S/D (IgA less than 1 mcg/mL), Baxalta
	6 g (of protein)	**Carimune® NF,** CSL Behring
	10 g (of protein)	**Gammagard® S/D,** Baxalta
		Gammagard® S/D (IgA less than 1 mcg/mL), Baxalta
	12 g (of protein)	**Carimune® NF,** CSL Behring
Injection, for IV infusion	50 mg (of protein) per mL	**Flebogamma® 5% DIF,** Grifols
		Gammaplex® 5%, Bio Products
		Octagam® 5%, Octapharma
	100 mg (of protein) per mL	**Bivigam® 10%,** BioTest
		Flebogamma® 10% DIF, Grifols
		Octagam® 10%, Octapharma
		Privigen® 10%, CSL Behring
Injection, for IV or subcutaneous infusion	100 mg (of protein) per mL	**Gammagard® Liquid 10%,** Baxalta
		Gammaked® 10%, Kedrion
		Gamunex®-C 10%, Grifols

Immune Globulin Subcutaneous

Parenteral		
Injection, for subcutaneous infusion	200 mg (of protein) per mL	**Cuvitru® 20%,** Baxalta
		Hizentra® 20%, CSL Behring

Immune Globulin Subcutaneous with Hyaluronidase (Human Recombinant)

Parenteral		
Kit	100 mg (of protein) per mL, Injection, for subcutaneous infusion	**Hyqvia®,** Baxalta
	160 units recombinant human hyaluronidase per mL, Injection, for subcutaneous infusion	

†Use is not currently included in the labeling approved by the US Food and Drug Administration

Tetanus Immune Globulin TIG

■ Tetanus immune globulin (TIG) is a specific immune globulin (hyperimmune globulin) that contains tetanus antitoxin and is used to provide temporary passive immunity to tetanus. TIG commercially available in the US is prepared from plasma of donors immunized with tetanus toxoid; other tetanus antitoxin preparations (e.g., equine tetanus antitoxin) may be available in other countries.

Uses

■ **Tetanus** Tetanus immune globulin (TIG) is used to provide passive immunity to tetanus as part of a postexposure prophylaxis regimen following a tetanus-prone wound and also is used in the treatment of tetanus.

Postexposure Prophylaxis *Passive* immunization with TIG is used in conjunction with *active* immunization with a preparation containing tetanus toxoid adsorbed for postexposure prophylaxis of tetanus in individuals with tetanus-prone wounds who are inadequately vaccinated against tetanus or whose tetanus immunization history is unknown or uncertain. The US Public Health Service Advisory Committee on Immunization Practices (ACIP) and American Academy of Pediatrics (AAP) state that TIG is not necessary for postexposure prophylaxis in patients with clean, minor wounds (regardless of their immunization status) or for patients with tetanus-prone wounds who have previously received 3 or more doses of a preparation containing tetanus toxoid adsorbed or tetanus toxoid fluid (no longer commercially available in the US). Any individual whose tetanus immunization status is unknown or uncertain should be considered to have had no previous doses of tetanus toxoid adsorbed or tetanus toxoid fluid.

In the event of injury and possible exposure to tetanus, the need for *active* immunization with a preparation containing tetanus toxoid adsorbed with or without *passive* immunization with TIG depends on the individual's vaccination status and the likelihood of contamination with tetanus bacilli (e.g., condition of wound, source of contamination). Tetanus-prone wounds include, but are not limited to, wounds contaminated with dirt, feces, soil, or saliva; puncture wounds; avulsions; and wounds resulting from crushing, burns, or frostbite. Tetanus also has been associated with apparently clean, superficial wounds, surgical procedures, insect bites, animal bites, dental infections, chronic sores and infections, and IV drug abuse. Tetanus is not transmitted person-to-person.

Table 1 summarizes the ACIP guidelines for active and passive immunization against tetanus in routine wound management.

Table 1. Summary Guide to Tetanus Prophylaxis in Routine Wound Management

Previous Doses of Tetanus Toxoid Adsorbed Received	Clean, Minor Wounds		All Other Wounds	
	Tdap[a] or Td[b]	TIG	Tdap[a] or Td[b]	TIG
Unknown or less than 3 doses	Yes	No	Yes	Yes
3 or more doses[c]	No[d]	No	No[e]	No

[a] Tetanus toxoid, reduced diphtheria toxoid and acellular pertussis vaccine adsorbed (Tdap). A dose of Tdap is preferred to a dose of Td in adolescents and adults 11 through 64 years of age who have not previously received a dose of Tdap. Use Td in individuals in this age group who previously received a dose of Tdap.

[b] Tetanus and diphtheria toxoids adsorbed (Td). Td is used in adults, adolescents, and children 7 years of age and older. For children 6 weeks through 6 years of age, diphtheria and tetanus toxoids and acellular pertussis vaccine adsorbed (DTaP) usually is indicated, but diphtheria and tetanus toxoids adsorbed (DT) can be used in this age group if pertussis antigens are contraindicated. Monovalent tetanus toxoid adsorbed generally is used only when preparations containing tetanus and diphtheria antigens and preparations containing tetanus, diphtheria, and pertussis antigens are contraindicated or unavailable.

[c] If only 3 doses of tetanus toxoid fluid (no longer commercially available in the US) have been received previously, a fourth dose should be given as a preparation containing tetanus toxoid adsorbed.

[d] Yes, if it has been 10 or more years since last dose of tetanus toxoid-containing preparation.

[e] Yes, if it has been 5 or more years since last dose of tetanus toxoid-containing preparation; more frequent booster doses not needed and can accentuate adverse effects.

Adapted from ACIP recommendations for prevention of diphtheria, tetanus, and pertussis published in *MMWR Recomm Rep.* 1991; 40(RR-10):1-28, *MMWR Recomm Rep.* 2006; 55(RR-3):1-43, and *MMWR Recomm Rep.* 2006; 55(RR-17):1-37.

When passive immunization against tetanus is indicated for postexposure prophylaxis, TIG is the preferred form of tetanus immunoglobulin for postexposure prophylaxis. Tetanus antitoxin (equine) (no longer commercially available in the US but may be used in other countries) provides a shorter duration of protection than TIG and is associated with a high risk of adverse reactions (e.g., serum sickness). Tetanus antitoxin (equine) should only be used when TIG is not available and only after appropriate sensitivity testing and, if necessary, desensitization.

Administration of a prophylactic dose of TIG should not be considered a substitute for active immunization with a preparation containing tetanus toxoid adsorbed, nor a substitute for adequate medical and surgical care of contaminated or potentially contaminated wounds. Wound care is an essential part of postexposure prophylaxis or treatment of tetanus and is necessary regardless of vaccination status. Cleansing of the wound and removal of necrotic tissue and foreign material should be performed, especially if dirt or necrotic tissue is present. Anti-infectives are not indicated for tetanus postexposure prophylaxis.

The ACIP states that recommendations concerning use of TIG in patients with altered immunocompetence, including those with human immunodeficiency virus (HIV) infection or those who are severely immunocompromised because of congenital immunodeficiency, leukemia, lymphoma, aplastic anemia, generalized malignancy, or therapy with alkylating agents, antimetabolites, radiation, or corticosteroids, are the same as those for patients who are not immunocompromised. The AAP states that TIG should be used in the management of tetanus prone wounds in all HIV-infected individuals, regardless of their tetanus immunization history.

For additional information on tetanus-prone wounds and associated risks of tetanus and recommendations for postexposure prophylaxis of tetanus, see Uses in Diphtheria and Tetanus Toxoids Adsorbed/Tetanus and Diphtheria Toxoids Adsorbed 80:08.

Treatment TIG is used for the treatment of tetanus in conjunction with anti-infective agents active against *Clostridium tetani* (e.g., metronidazole, penicillin G), sedatives, and muscle relaxants. TIG has been used in conjunction with anti-infective therapy (e.g., penicillin G) for the treatment of neonatal tetanus†. Evidence of effectiveness of TIG in the treatment of active tetanus infection is limited and the optimum therapeutic dosage of TIG for treatment of tetanus infection has not been established. Although TIG can neutralize unbound exotoxin, it does *not* affect toxin already bound to nerve endings.

TIG is the preferred form of tetanus immunoglobulin for the treatment of active tetanus. Immune globulin IV (IGIV) contains tetanus antitoxin and may be used if TIG is unavailable. Tetanus antitoxin (equine) (no longer commercially available in the US but may be used in other countries) should only be used when TIG is not available and only after appropriate sensitivity testing and, if necessary, desensitization. Intrathecal TIG or tetanus antitoxin (equine) is *not* of proven benefit in the treatment of tetanus.

Recovery from tetanus does *not* result in naturally acquired tetanus immunity. As soon as possible, active immunization against tetanus should be initiated or completed using a preparation containing tetanus toxoid adsorbed. (See Diphtheria and Tetanus Toxoids Adsorbed/Tetanus and Diphtheria Toxoids Adsorbed 80:08.)

Dosage and Administration

■ **Administration** Tetanus immune globulin (TIG) is administered by deep IM injection. TIG should *not* be administered IV or intrathecally. In the treatment of tetanus, some clinicians recommend infiltration of part of the TIG dose locally around the wound; however, efficacy of this approach has not been proven.

IM injections of TIG preferably should be made into the anterolateral aspect of the thigh or the deltoid muscle. Because of the risk of injury to the sciatic nerve, the gluteal muscle should be *not* be used as an injection site. Although the manufacturer recommends that aspiration (i.e., pulling back on the syringe plunger after needle insertion and before injection) be performed to ensure that a blood vessel has not been entered, the US Public Health Service Advisory Committee on Immunization Practices (ACIP) states that this procedure is not required because large blood vessels are not present at recommended IM injection sites.

When *passive* immunization with TIG is indicated in addition to *active* immunization with a preparation containing tetanus toxoid adsorbed for postexposure prophylaxis of tetanus, TIG may be given simultaneously with the tetanus toxoid adsorbed preparation using different syringes and different injection sites.

■ **Dosage** ***Postexposure Prophylaxis of Tetanus*** The usual dosage of TIG for postexposure prophylaxis of tetanus in adults is 250 units as a single dose.

Although safety and efficacy have not been definitely established in children†, the manufacturer states that the usual dosage of TIG in children 7 years of age or older for postexposure prophylaxis of tetanus is 250 units as a single dose. For children younger than 7 years of age, the manufacturer states that the dosage for routine prophylaxis may be calculated using body weight (4 units/kg); however, it may be advisable to administer 250 units regardless of the child's size since theoretically the amount of toxin produced by *Clostridium tetani* in a child's body would be the same as that produced in an adult's body.

Treatment of Tetanus For the treatment of tetanus in adults, a TIG dosage of 3000–6000 units usually is recommended. However, the optimum therapeutic dosage of TIG for the treatment of active tetanus has not been established, and the manufacturer states that dosage should be adjusted according to the severity of the infection.

Although safety and efficacy have not been definitely established in children†, a TIG dosage of 3000–6000 units usually is recommended.

Some clinicians suggest that a portion of the TIG dose be infiltrated locally around the wound, although efficacy of this approach has not been established.

In the treatment of neonatal tetanus†, neonates have received 500 units of TIG in conjunction with anti-infective therapy (e.g., a 10-day regimen of penicillin G).

Cautions

■ **Adverse Effects** Adverse effects reported with tetanus immune globulin (TIG) include slight soreness at the site of injection and low-grade fever.

Sensitization to repeated injections of human immune globulin occurs rarely, and there have been isolated occurrences of angioneurotic edema, nephrotic syndrome, and anaphylactic shock.

■ **Precautions and Contraindications** The manufacturer states that there are no known contraindications to TIG.

Hypersensitivity Reactions TIG should be administered with caution to individuals who have exhibited previous systemic allergic reactions to immune globulin preparations. Use of skin testing (i.e., intradermal injection of concentrated IgG solutions) to evaluate possible hypersensitivity is unreliable since localized areas of inflammation may occur as the result of localized tissue irritation and can be misinterpreted as a positive allergy reaction.

Although systemic reactions to human immune globulin preparations are rare, epinephrine and other appropriate agents should be readily available in case anaphylaxis or other serious allergic reaction occurs.

Risk of Transmissible Agents in Plasma-derived Preparations Because TIG is prepared from pooled human plasma, it is a potential vehicle for transmission of human viruses, including the causative agents of viral hepatitis and human immunodeficiency virus (HIV) infection, and theoretically may carry a risk of transmitting the causative agent of Creutzfeldt-Jakob disease (CJD) or variant CJD (vCJD). The risk for transmission of recognized blood-borne viruses is considered to be low because plasma donors are screened for certain viruses (hepatitis B virus [HBV], hepatitis C virus [HCV], HIV) and because of the viral inactivation and removal properties inherent in the Cohn cold ethanol precipitation method used for purification of immune globulin products. In addition, TIG undergoes chemical (solvent/detergent) and/or heat-treatment procedures to reduce viral infectious potential. Improved donor screening, viral-inactivation procedures (e.g., solvent/detergent treatment), and/or filtration procedures have reduced, but not completely eliminated, the risk of pathogen transmission with plasma-derived preparations. However, because no purification method has been shown to be totally effective in removing the risk of viral infectivity from plasma-derived products and because new blood-borne viruses may emerge which may not be inactivated by the manufacturing process or the chemical (solvent/detergent) treatment procedure currently used, patients should be advised of the risks and benefits of TIG. Any infection believed to have been transmitted by TIG should be reported to the manufacturer at 800-520-2807.

For further information on precautions related to transmissible agents in plasma-derived preparations, see Risk of Transmissible Agents in Plasma-derived Preparations under Cautions: Precautions and Contraindications, in Albumin Human 16:00.

Individuals with Altered Immunocompetence Recommendations regarding the use of TIG in individuals with altered immunocompetence are the same as those for individuals who are not immunocompromised.

The US Public Health Service Advisory Committee on Immunization Practices (ACIP) states that recommendations concerning use of TIG in individuals with altered immunocompetence, including HIV-infected individuals or those severely immunocompromised because of congenital immunodeficiency, leukemia, lymphoma, aplastic anemia, generalized malignancy, or therapy with alkylating agents, antimetabolites, radiation, or corticosteroids, are the same as those for patients who are not immunocompromised.

Administration Precautions TIG should *not* be administered in the same syringe or at the same injection site as tetanus toxoid adsorbed. (See Drug Interactions: Inactivated Vaccines and Toxoids.)

Serious systemic reactions (e.g., precipitous decrease in blood pressure) have occurred following IV administration of immune globulin intended for IM administration; therefore, inadvertent IV administration of TIG should be avoided.

Individuals with Bleeding Disorders Because bleeding may occur following IM administration in individuals with thrombocytopenia or a bleeding disorder (e.g., hemophilia) or in those receiving anticoagulant therapy, TIG should be used in such individuals only if benefits outweigh risks.

The ACIP states that IM injections can be used in individuals who have bleeding disorders or are receiving anticoagulant therapy if a clinician familiar with the patient's bleeding risk determines that the injection can be administered with reasonable safety. In these cases, a fine needle (23 gauge) should be used to administer the dose and firm pressure applied to the injection site (without rubbing) for at least 2 minutes. If patient is receiving antihemophilia therapy, the IM dose should be administered shortly after a scheduled dose of such therapy. In addition, the individual and/or their family should be advised about the risk of hematoma from IM injections.

Duration of Immunity TIG provides only short-term protection against tetanus. Therefore, active immunization against tetanus using a preparation containing tetanus toxoid adsorbed should be initiated or completed as soon as possible.

■ **Pediatric Precautions** Safety and efficacy of TIG have not been established in children. However, recommendations regarding use of TIG in children (including for postexposure prophylaxis of tetanus) usually are the same as those for adults.

■ **Pregnancy** Animal reproduction studies have not been performed with TIG and it is not known whether TIG can cause harm when administered to pregnant women. TIG should be used during pregnancy only when clearly needed.

The ACIP states that pregnancy is not generally considered a contraindication to the use of TIG for treatment or postexposure prophylaxis of tetanus.

Drug Interactions

■ **Inactivated Vaccines and Toxoids** Immune globulins, including tetanus immune globulin (TIG), are not expected to have a clinically important effect on the immune response to inactivated vaccines or toxoids; therefore, inactivated vaccines (e.g., parenteral inactivated influenza vaccine, parenteral inactivated typhoid vaccine [Typhim Vi®]), recombinant vaccines, polysaccharide vaccines, and toxoids may be administered simultaneously with (using different syringes and different injection sites) or at any interval before or after administration of TIG.

Tetanus Toxoid Adsorbed If indicated, active immunization against tetanus should be initiated at the same time as passive immunization with TIG; however, TIG and the preparation containing tetanus toxoid adsorbed should be given at separate sites using different syringes.

■ **Live Vaccines** Antibodies present in immune globulin preparations, including TIG, may interfere with the immune response to certain live virus vaccines (e.g., measles, mumps, and rubella virus vaccine live [MMR], rotavirus vaccine live oral, varicella virus vaccine live).

There is no evidence that immune globulin preparations interfere with the immune response to yellow fever virus vaccine live, typhoid vaccine live oral, influenza virus vaccine live intranasal, or poliovirus vaccine live oral (OPV; no longer commercially available in the US) and these vaccines may be administered simultaneously with or at any time before or after administration of TIG.

Measles, Mumps, and Rubella Vaccine Immune globulin preparations, including TIG, may interfere with the immune response to measles and rubella antigens contained in MMR; the effect of TIG on the immune response to mumps antigen is unknown. The US Public Health Service Advisory Committee on Immunization Practices (ACIP) states that MMR should not be administered simultaneously with or within 3 months before or after TIG.

In general, vaccine virus replication and stimulation of active immunity occur within 1–2 weeks after administration of a live virus vaccine. Therefore, if TIG is administered less than 14 days after MMR, revaccination is necessary at least 3 months after the TIG dose, unless serologic testing indicates that there was an adequate antibody response to all 3 antigens contained in MMR.

Rotavirus Vaccine TIG may interfere with the immune response to rotavirus vaccine. Safety and efficacy data are not available regarding use of rotavirus vaccine live oral in infants who have received an immune globulin within 42 days. Although there is potential for decreased antibody response to rotavirus vaccine, the ACIP and American Academy of Pediatrics (AAP) state that the vaccine may be administered simultaneously with or at any time before or after administration of blood or antibody-containing preparations.

Varicella Vaccine TIG may interfere with the immune response to varicella virus vaccine live. Varicella vaccine should not be administered simultaneously with or within 3 months before or after TIG.

In general, vaccine virus replication and stimulation of active immunity occur within 1–2 weeks after administration of a live virus vaccine. Therefore, if TIG is administered less than 14 days after varicella virus vaccine live, revaccination is necessary at least 3 months after the TIG dose, unless serologic testing indicates that there was an adequate antibody response to the vaccine.

Pharmacology

Tetanus immune globulin (TIG) is used to provide passive immunity to tetanus. TIG contains tetanus antitoxin antibodies which neutralize the exotoxin produced by *Clostridium tetani*, the causative organism of tetanus. TIG can only neutralize unbound exotoxin; it does *not* affect toxin already bound to nerve endings. The half-life of TIG is approximately 28 days.

■ **Tetanus Infection** Tetanus is a potentially fatal disease caused by a neurotoxic exotoxin (tetanospasmin) produced by *C. tetani*. *C. tetani* spores are ubiquitous in the environment and are found in soil and in animal (e.g., horses, sheep, cattle, dogs, cats, rats, guinea pigs, chickens) and human intestinal tracts. The spores can contaminate open wounds, especially puncture wounds or those with devitalized tissue; anaerobic wound conditions allow the spores to germinate and produce exotoxins that disseminate through the blood and lymphatic system. Following infection of a wound, the incubation period for tetanus is usually 8–10 days (range 3–21 days).

Tetanus occurs worldwide, almost exclusively in individuals who are unvaccinated or inadequately vaccinated against the disease. An average of 31 cases was reported each year in the US from 2000 through 2007 (case fatality rate 10%); a low of 20 cases was reported in 2003. Most cases of tetanus in the US occur following acute injuries or wounds (puncture wounds, lacerations, abrasions) and usually occur in adults 40 years of age or older; however, an increase in the disease recently has been reported in younger adults (e.g., heroin abusers).

The most common form of tetanus is generalized tetanus characterized by rigidity and convulsive muscle spasms that usually involve the jaw (lockjaw) and neck and then become generalized. Neonatal tetanus (tetanus neonatorum) occurs in infants born under nonsterile conditions to women inadequately vaccinated against tetanus; infection usually involves a contaminated umbilical stump and occurs because the infant does not have passively acquired maternal antibodies against tetanus. Symptoms of neonatal tetanus usually occur during the first 2 weeks of life. Obstetric tetanus occurs within 6 weeks after delivery or termination of pregnancy because of contaminated wounds or abrasions or unclean deliveries or abortions.

Chemistry and Stability

■ **Chemistry** Tetanus immune globulin (TIG) is a sterile, concentrated, nonpyrogenic solution of immunoglobulins prepared by cold alcohol fractionation from plasma of adults hyperimmunized with tetanus toxoid. TIG contains 15–18% protein. Commercially available TIG meets standards established by the Center for Biologics Evaluation and Research of the US Food and Drug Administration, and contains not less than 250 tetanus antitoxin units per dose.

TIG has a pH of 6.4–7.2 and undergoes a chemical (solvent/detergent) procedure during manufacture to reduce the risk of transmission of viral infection. TIG contains glycine as a stabilizing agent, but does not contain thimerosal or any other preservative.

■ **Stability** TIG should be refrigerated at 2–8°C; freezing should be avoided. TIG that has been frozen should not be used.

Preparations

Excipients in commercially available drug preparations may have clinically important effects in some individuals; consult specific product labeling for details.

Tetanus Immune Globulin

Parenteral		
Injection, for IM use	≥250 units	**HyperTET® S/D** (solvent/detergent treated), Talecris

†Use is not currently included in the labeling approved by the US Food and Drug Administration

Selected Revisions September 2010, © Copyright, September 1969, American Society of Health-System Pharmacists, Inc.

TOXOIDS 80:08

Diphtheria and Tetanus Toxoids Adsorbed

Diphtheria and Tetanus Toxoids Adsorbed for Pediatric Use, DT

Tetanus and Diphtheria Toxoids Adsorbed

Tetanus and Diphtheria Toxoids Adsorbed for Adult Use, Td

■ Diphtheria and tetanus toxoids adsorbed (DT) and tetanus and diphtheria toxoids adsorbed (Td) are fixed-combination preparations contain tetanus and diphtheria toxins (toxoids) adsorbed onto an aluminum adjuvant and are used to stimulate active immunity to diphtheria and tetanus. DT contains a higher dose of diphtheria toxoid than Td.

Uses

Diphtheria and tetanus toxoids adsorbed (DT) is used to stimulate active immunity to diphtheria and tetanus in infants and children 6 weeks through 6 years of age; tetanus and diphtheria toxoids adsorbed (Td) is used to stimulate active immunity to diphtheria and tetanus in adults, adolescents, and children 7 years of age or older.

The US Public Health Service Advisory Committee on Immunization Practices (ACIP), American Academy of Pediatrics (AAP), American Academy of Family Physicians (AAFP), and other experts recommend that *all* individuals receive *routine* immunization against diphtheria, tetanus, and pertussis. Use of a combination vaccine generally is preferred over separate injections of the equivalent component vaccines; considerations should include provider assessment (e.g., number of injections, vaccine availability, likelihood of improved coverage, likelihood of patient return, storage requirements, cost), patient preference, and potential for adverse effects. Therefore, a fixed-combination preparation that contains antigens for all 3 diseases (diphtheria and tetanus toxoids and acellular pertussis vaccine adsorbed; DTaP) is preferred for primary and booster immunization against these diseases in infants and children 6 weeks through 6 years of age unless pertussis antigens are contraindicated or should not be used. DT should be used for primary or booster immunization against diphtheria and tetanus *only* when DTaP cannot be used. (See Diphtheria and Tetanus Toxoids and Acellular Pertussis Vaccine Adsorbed/Tetanus Toxoid, Reduced Diphtheria Toxoid and Acellular Pertussis Vaccine Adsorbed 80:08.)

Td usually is the preparation of choice for primary and booster immunization against diphtheria and tetanus in adults, adolescents, and children 7 years of age or older. However, to reduce the morbidity associated with pertussis, ACIP, AAP, and other experts recommend that a *single* dose of a fixed-combination preparation that also contains pertussis antigens (tetanus toxoid and reduced diphtheria toxoid and acellular pertussis vaccine adsorbed [Tdap]) be used in place of a required primary or booster dose of Td in individuals 7 years of age or older who have *not* previously received Tdap, unless pertussis antigens are contraindicated or should not be used. Individuals in this age group who previously received a dose of Tdap should then receive Td for subsequent primary or booster doses. (See Diphtheria and Tetanus Toxoids and Acellular Pertussis Vaccine Adsorbed/Tetanus Toxoid, Reduced Diphtheria Toxoid and Acellular Pertussis Vaccine Adsorbed 80:08.)

DT or Td may be indicated for postexposure vaccination against diphtheria in addition to anti-infective postexposure prophylaxis in unvaccinated or inadequately vaccinated household and other close contacts of an individual with diphtheria. (See Uses: Postexposure Prophylaxis of Diphtheria.)

DT or Td may be indicated in conjunction with passive immunization with tetanus immune globulin (TIG) for postexposure prophylaxis against tetanus in individuals with tetanus-prone wounds who are inadequately immunized against tetanus or whose tetanus immunization history is unknown or uncertain. (See Uses: Postexposure Prophylaxis of Tetanus.)

DT and Td are *not* indicated for *treatment* of diphtheria or *treatment* of tetanus infection. However, because diphtheria and tetanus infections do not necessarily confer immunity, initiation or completion of active immunization against these diseases is indicated at the time of recovery in any previously unvaccinated or incompletely vaccinated individual.

■ Risks of Diphtheria and Tetanus Exposure and Infection

Diphtheria Diphtheria is caused by toxigenic strains of *Corynebacterium diphtheriae* or, rarely, toxigenic strains of *C. ulcerans*. Diphtheria occurs worldwide, particularly in tropical countries. Although diphtheria occurs rarely in the US, *C. diphtheriae* continues to circulate in the US in areas where diphtheria previously was endemic.

Before widespread immunization against diphtheria was initiated in the 1940s, diphtheria was a major cause of morbidity and mortality among children. During the 1920s, there were approximately 100,000–200,000 cases of diphtheria and 13,000–15,000 diphtheria-related deaths each year in the US. From 1980 through 2011, 55 cases of diphtheria were reported in the US with an average of 1–2 per year (range: 0–5 cases per year). In 1996, toxigenic *C. diphtheriae* was isolated from residents of a Native American community in South Dakota and toxigenic *C. ulcerans* was isolated from an individual in Indiana with respiratory diphtheria. In 2003, fatal respiratory diphtheria occurred in an unvaccinated Pennsylvania resident who had returned from a trip to rural Haiti (a country where diphtheria is endemic).

Most cases of diphtheria occur in individuals who are unvaccinated or incompletely vaccinated against the disease.

Diphtheria is endemic in many countries in Asia, the South Pacific, the Middle East, and Eastern Europe and also is endemic in Haiti and the Dominican Republic. Since 2011, large outbreaks of diphtheria have occurred in Indonesia, Thailand, and Laos. Individuals who are unvaccinated or inadequately vaccinated against diphtheria, especially travelers who will live or work with local populations in countries where diphtheria is endemic, are at risk.

The US Centers for Disease Control and Prevention (CDC) Travelers' Health website (http://wwwnc.cdc.gov/travel) should be consulted for information regarding where diphtheria is endemic.

Tetanus Tetanus is a potentially fatal disease caused by a neurotoxic exotoxin (tetanospasmin) produced by *Clostridium tetani*. Tetanus occurs worldwide, but is reported most frequently in densely populated regions in hot, damp climates with soil rich in organic matter.

In the US, a marked decrease in mortality from tetanus occurred from the early 1900s to the late 1940s when immunization against tetanus became part of routine childhood immunization. From 2001 through 2008, 233 cases of tetanus were reported in the US (average of 29 per year) with a case fatality rate of 13%. From 2009 through 2012, an average of 29 cases of tetanus per year were reported in the US.

Tetanus is not transmitted person-to-person. *C. tetani* usually enters the body through a wound. Any open wound can become contaminated with *C. tetani*, including tetanus-prone wounds (wounds contaminated with dirt, feces, soil, or saliva; deep wounds; burns; crush injuries; wounds containing devitalized or necrotic tissue) and apparently clean, superficial wounds (wounds from surgical procedures, insect bites, animal bites, dental infections, compound fractures, chronic sores and infections, IV drug use). Heroin users, particularly those who inject themselves subcutaneously, appear to be at high risk for tetanus. Most cases of tetanus in the US occur following an acute wound, usually a puncture or contaminated, infected, or devitalized wound considered tetanus-prone.

Almost all reported cases of tetanus occur in individuals who are unvaccinated or inadequately vaccinated against the disease (i.e., received an incomplete primary immunization series or received a complete primary series but did not receive recommended booster doses).

Because *C. tetani* spores are ubiquitous in the environment worldwide, travelers can acquire tetanus anywhere in the world if they are unvaccinated or incompletely vaccinated against the disease. Tetanus is more common in rural and agricultural regions, areas where contact with soil or animal excreta is more likely, and areas where immunization rates are inadequate.

■ Primary and Booster Immunization with Diphtheria and Tetanus Toxoids Adsorbed (DT)

Infants and Children 6 Weeks Through 6 Years of Age DT is used for primary and booster immunization against diphtheria and tetanus in infants and children 6 weeks through 6 years of age when initiation or continuation of immunization with DTaP is contraindicated because of the pertussis component. (See Diphtheria and Tetanus Toxoids and Acellular Pertussis Vaccine Adsorbed/Tetanus Toxoid, Reduced Diphtheria Toxoid and Acellular Pertussis Vaccine Adsorbed 80:08.)

When DT is used in infants and children 6 weeks through 6 years of age (i.e., when DTaP cannot be used), primary immunization consists of a series of 4 or 5 doses. ACIP, AAP, and other experts recommend that the first 3 doses be given at 2, 4, and 6 months of age and a fourth dose be given at 15–18 months of age. In those who received 4 doses before their fourth birthday, a fifth dose is recommended at 4 through 6 years of age (usually just prior to entry into kindergarten or elementary school). This dose is not necessary if the last dose of the primary series was given on or after the fourth birthday.

Primary immunization against diphtheria and tetanus may be integrated with primary immunization against pertussis, hepatitis A, hepatitis B, *Haemophilus influenzae* type b (Hib), influenza, poliomyelitis, measles, meningococcal disease, mumps, rubella, rotavirus, varicella, and pneumococcal disease. (See Drug Interactions: Vaccines.)

■ Primary and Booster Immunization with Tetanus and Diphtheria Toxoids Adsorbed (Td)

Primary Immunization in Children 7 through 10 Years of Age Td is used for primary immunization against diphtheria and tetanus in children 7 through 10 years of age.

Children 7 through 10 years of age who did not receive primary immunization against diphtheria and tetanus with DTaP, DT, or diphtheria and tetanus toxoids and whole cell pertussis vaccine (DTP; not commercially available in the US) in early childhood according to the recommended childhood immunization schedule (see Immunization Schedules, US 80:00) and those who previously received fewer than the total recommended doses of DTaP, DT, Td, or DTP should receive catch-up immunization against these diseases.

For catch-up vaccination in children 7 through 10 years of age, ACIP, AAP, and other experts recommend 3 doses of a preparation containing tetanus and diphtheria toxoids adsorbed. The preferred primary immunization schedule in previously unvaccinated or incompletely vaccinated children 7 through 10 years of age is a *single* dose of Tdap followed by a dose of Td given 1–2 months after the Tdap dose and a second dose of Td given 6–12 months after the first dose of Td; however, the Tdap dose may be substituted for any 1 of the 3 doses of Td. These children should *not* receive the booster dose of Tdap usually recommended at 11 through 12 years of age. (See Diphtheria and Tetanus Toxoids and Acellular Pertussis Vaccine Adsorbed/Tetanus Toxoid, Reduced Diphtheria Toxoid and Acellular Pertussis Vaccine Adsorbed 80:08.)

Booster Immunization in Adolescents 11 through 18 Years of Age ACIP, AAP, and other experts recommend that *all* adolescents who received primary immunization with DTaP, DT, Td, or DTP (not commercially available in the US) receive a booster dose of a preparation containing diphtheria and tetanus toxoids adsorbed at 11 through 18 years of age (preferably at 11 through 12 years of age). Because adolescents also may be at risk for pertussis, these experts recommend that a *single* dose of Tdap be used (instead of Td) for the adolescent booster dose at 11 through 18 years of age (preferably at 11 through 12 years of age), unless pertussis antigens are contraindicated or should not be used. If Tdap is unavailable or was administered previously, Td should be used for this adolescent booster dose. (See Diphtheria and Tetanus Toxoids and Acellular Pertussis Vaccine Adsorbed/Tetanus Toxoid, Reduced Diphtheria Toxoid and Acellular Pertussis Vaccine Adsorbed 80:08.)

Primary and Booster Immunization in Adults 19 Years of Age or Older Td is used for primary and booster immunization against diphtheria and tetanus in adults 19 years of age or older.

Adults with an incomplete or uncertain history of primary immunization against diphtheria and tetanus should receive primary immunization with 3 doses of Td. However, because adults may also be susceptible to pertussis, ACIP recommends that primary immunization against diphtheria and tetanus in previously unvaccinated adults 19 years of age or older (including those 65 years of age or older) include a *single* dose of Tdap, unless pertussis antigens are contraindicated or should not be used. The preferred primary immunization schedule in previously unvaccinated adults 19 years of age or older is a *single* dose of Tdap followed by a dose of Td given at least 4 weeks after the Tdap dose and a second dose of Td given 6–12 months after the first dose of Td; however, the Tdap dose may be substituted for any 1 of the 3 doses of Td. This Tdap booster dose should only be used in those who have *not* previously received a dose of Tdap. (See Diphtheria and Tetanus Toxoids and Acellular Pertussis Vaccine Adsorbed/Tetanus Toxoid, Reduced Diphtheria Toxoid and Acellular Pertussis Vaccine Adsorbed 80:08.) If Tdap is not available or was administered previously, Td should be used.

Adults who have received primary immunization against diphtheria and tetanus should receive routine booster doses of Td every 10 years. In addition, an emergency booster dose of Td may be indicated in the event of injury and possible exposure to tetanus infection. (See Uses: Postexposure Prophylaxis of Tetanus.) Although Td usually is recommended for these booster doses, adults also may be at risk for pertussis and ACIP recommends that a *single* dose of Tdap be used (instead of Td) when a booster dose is needed in adults 19 years of age or older (including those 65 years of age or older). Although a 10-year interval between the last dose of a preparation containing tetanus and diphtheria toxoids and the booster dose of Tdap has been recommended to reduce the risk of local and systemic reactions, ACIP states that the Tdap dose should be given when indicated (regardless of the interval between doses) since this ensures protection against pertussis. (See Diphtheria and Tetanus Toxoids and Acellular Pertussis Vaccines Adsorbed/Tetanus Toxoid, Reduced Diphtheria Toxoid and Acellular Pertussis Vaccine Adsorbed 80:08.) If Tdap is not available or was administered previously, Td should be given.

Pregnant Women Unless contraindicated, all women of childbearing potential should be adequately immunized against tetanus and diphtheria. Pregnant women who are immune to these diseases can confer protection to their infants through transplacental transfer of maternal antibody. Obstetric and neonatal tetanus and obstetric and neonatal diphtheria are prevented if protective levels of tetanus and diphtheria antitoxin (i.e., at least 0.1 international units when tested using enzyme-linked immunosorbent assay [ELISA]) are present in the mother. (See Pharmacology.)

Ideally, primary immunization against diphtheria and tetanus should be completed prior to pregnancy. However, because of the risks associated with diphtheria and tetanus, ACIP, AAP, and other experts state that pregnancy is not considered a contraindication for preparations containing diphtheria and tetanus toxoids.

Pregnant women who have *not* received primary immunization with DTaP, DTP (not commercially available in the US), DT, Td, or single-antigen tetanus toxoid adsorbed (not commercially available in the US) and those whose tetanus immunization history is unknown or uncertain should receive a primary series of 3 doses of vaccine containing diphtheria and tetanus antigens beginning during pregnancy. Because of the risks of pertussis, ACIP and other experts recommend that a dose of Tdap be substituted for one of the required Td doses, preferably during the third trimester (optimally between 27 and 36 weeks of gestation). In addition, to ensure protection against pertussis, these experts recommend that a dose of Tdap be administered during *each* pregnancy, irrespective of the woman's prior vaccination history. (See Diphtheria and Tetanus Toxoids and Acellular Pertussis Vaccine Adsorbed/Tetanus Toxoid, Reduced Diphtheria Toxoid and Acellular Pertussis Vaccine Adsorbed 80:08.)

If feasible, the primary vaccination series should be completed in those who previously received only 1 or 2 doses of a preparation containing tetanus and diphtheria antigens. Two doses of a preparation containing tetanus toxoid adsorbed given at least 4–6 weeks before delivery stimulate antitoxin levels that are sufficient to protect the mother and cross the placenta to protect the neonate against tetanus.

When a pregnant woman's history of tetanus vaccination is uncertain, serologic testing can be done to determine whether she has protective levels of antitoxin. Those who have never been vaccinated against tetanus or have levels of tetanus antitoxin that are not protective should be vaccinated during pregnancy to ensure protection against maternal and neonatal tetanus. Because diphtheria is rare in the US, serologic testing for diphtheria antitoxin is not usually necessary in pregnant women.

Pregnant women who were previously vaccinated but received the most recent dose of a preparation containing tetanus and diphtheria antigens 10 or more years previously should receive a booster dose of a preparation containing diphtheria and tetanus toxoids during the second or third trimester of pregnancy (and before 36 weeks of gestation). This dose is important if the woman does not have sufficient tetanus immunity to protect against maternal and neonatal tetanus or if protection against diphtheria is needed (e.g., for travel to an area where diphtheria is endemic). ACIP recommends that Tdap be used (instead of Td) when a booster dose is indicated in a pregnant woman.

If postexposure prophylaxis of tetanus is indicated as part of wound management in a pregnant women, the usual recommendations regarding emergency booster doses should be followed. (See Uses: Postexposure Prophylaxis of Tetanus.) If 5 or more years have elapsed since she received a preparation containing tetanus antigen, a booster dose of a preparation containing tetanus toxoid be administered. ACIP recommends that Tdap be used (instead of Td) when a booster dose is indicated for postexposure prophylaxis of tetanus in a pregnant woman.

HIV-infected Individuals ACIP, AAP, and other experts state that recommendations regarding primary or booster immunization against tetanus and diphtheria in individuals with human immunodeficiency virus (HIV) infection are the same as those for individuals who are not HIV-infected. However, immunization may be less effective in HIV-infected individuals than in immunocompetent individuals.

Health-care Personnel Health-care personnel should have documentation of age-appropriate primary immunization with a preparation containing diphtheria and tetanus toxoids and a booster dose of Td every 10 years. In addition, ACIP recommends that *all* health-care personnel (regardless of age) receive a *single* dose of Tdap if they have *not* previously received a dose.

Health-care personnel who do not have documentation of primary immunization against tetanus and diphtheria should receive a 3-dose vaccination series using Tdap for the first dose and Td for subsequent primary and booster doses. Previously vaccinated health-care personnel who have *not* received a dose of Tdap should receive a dose as soon as feasible, regardless of the interval since the last dose of vaccine containing diphtheria or tetanus toxoids (e.g., Td). (See Diphtheria and Tetanus Toxoids and Acellular Pertussis Vaccine Adsorbed/Tetanus Toxoid, Reduced Diphtheria Toxoid and Acellular Pertussis Vaccine Adsorbed 80:08.) Td should be used for subsequent booster doses.

Travelers Tetanus, diphtheria, and pertussis occur worldwide, and travelers are at risk if they are unvaccinated or incompletely vaccinated against these diseases. (See Uses: Risks of Diphtheria and Tetanus Exposure and Infection.)

CDC recommends that all travelers, including children, be adequately immunized against diphtheria, tetanus, and pertussis before leaving the US.

Because children 6 weeks through 6 years of age also should be immunized against pertussis, travelers in this age group who are unvaccinated or incompletely vaccinated should receive the remaining required doses of DTaP or, if the pertussis component is contraindicated, the remaining required doses of DT prior to travel. If necessary to complete the vaccination series before departure, an accelerated immunization schedule using the age-appropriate minimum intervals between doses can be used. (See Dosage and Administration: Dosage.)

Adults, adolescents, and children 7 years of age or older who are unvaccinated or incompletely vaccinated should receive a *single* dose of Tdap (unless pertussis antigens are contraindicated or should not be used) followed by the remaining recommended doses of Td prior to travel.

Because immunity from childhood vaccination and natural disease wanes with time and to provide protection against pertussis in travelers, previously vaccinated adults and adolescents 11 years of age or older who have *not* received a dose of Tdap should receive a *single* booster dose of Tdap. (See Diphtheria and Tetanus Toxoids and Acellular Pertussis Vaccine Adsorbed/Tetanus Toxoid, Reduced Diphtheria Toxoid and Acellular Pertussis Vaccine Adsorbed 80:08.) Individuals who have previously received Tdap should receive a booster dose of Td if indicated.

■ Postexposure Prophylaxis of Diphtheria Postexposure vaccination with a preparation containing diphtheria toxoid adsorbed may be indicated in addition to anti-infective postexposure prophylaxis in unvaccinated or inadequately vaccinated household and other close contacts of an individual with diphtheria.

Regardless of vaccination status, ACIP, AAP, and CDC recommend that *all* household and other close contacts of an individual with culture-confirmed or suspected diphtheria promptly receive anti-infective postexposure prophylaxis (single IM dose of penicillin G benzathine or oral erythromycin given for 7–10 days). Samples for cultures should be taken prior to initiating anti-infective therapy and the individual should be observed for 7 days for evidence of diphtheria.

Individuals exposed to diphtheria who previously received less than 3 doses of a preparation containing diphtheria toxoid adsorbed or whose vaccination status is unknown or uncertain should receive an immediate dose of an age-appropriate preparation containing diphtheria toxoid adsorbed, and the primary vaccination series should be completed. In addition, close contacts who previously completed the primary vaccination series against diphtheria should receive a booster dose of an age-appropriate preparation containing diphtheria toxoid adsorbed if it has been 5 years or longer since their last booster dose.

Diphtheria carriers should receive an anti-infective regimen active against *C. diphtheriae*. Vaccination does not eliminate carriage of *C. diphtheriae*. However, diphtheria carriers who are unvaccinated or inadequately vaccinated should receive immunization using an age-appropriate preparation containing diphtheria toxoid adsorbed and those who are vaccinated but have not received a dose of a preparation containing diphtheria toxoid adsorbed within the last 5 years should receive a booster dose.

Because diphtheria infection does not necessarily confer immunity, the primary vaccination series using an age-appropriate preparation of diphtheria toxoid adsorbed should be initiated or completed during convalescence.

Diphtheria antitoxin (equine) (available in the US only from CDC under an investigational new drug [IND] protocol) is no longer routinely recommended for postexposure prophylaxis of diphtheria in contacts, but may be recommended in *exceptional* circumstances for postexposure prophylaxis in individuals with known or suspected exposure to toxigenic *Corynebacterium*. (See Diphtheria Antitoxin (Equine) 80:04.) To obtain diphtheria antitoxin (equine), clinicians should contact the CDC at 404-639-8257 from 8:00 a.m. to 4:30 p.m. EST Monday–Friday or the CDC Emergency Operations Center at 770-488-7100 after hours, on weekends, and holidays.

■ Postexposure Prophylaxis of Tetanus Td is used in individuals 7 years of age or older requiring primary or booster immunization against tetanus for routine wound management. When active immunization against tetanus is indicated for routine wound management in children younger than 7 years of age, use of DTaP is preferred; DT should be used only if pertussis antigens are contraindicated or should not be used.

In the event of injury and possible exposure to tetanus infection, the need for *active* immunization against tetanus (with a preparation containing tetanus toxoid adsorbed) with or without *passive* immunization against tetanus (with tetanus immune globulin [TIG]) depends on the individual's history of tetanus immunizations and the likelihood of contamination with tetanus bacilli (e.g., condition of the wound, source of contamination). A thorough attempt must be made to determine whether the individual has previously received a full primary series of tetanus vaccination and any required booster doses. Because of the very small amount of tetanus toxin required to produce illness, there is no natural immunity to tetanus and individuals who recover will not be immune to future tetanus disease. Therefore, individuals recovering from tetanus should begin or complete active immunization against tetanus during convalescence.

Wounds generally are characterized as being tetanus prone or as clean, minor wounds. Tetanus-prone wounds include, but are not limited to, wounds contaminated with dirt, feces, soil, or saliva, deep wounds, burns, crush injuries, and wounds containing devitalized or necrotic tissue. Tetanus also has been associated with apparently clean, superficial wounds, surgical procedures, insect bites, animal bites, dental infections, compounds fractures, chronic sores and infections, and IV drug abuse. Wound care is an essential part of postexposure prophylaxis of tetanus and is necessary regardless of vaccination status. Wounds should be properly cleaned and debrided, especially if dirt or necrotic tissue is present and all necrotic tissue and foreign material should be removed.

Any individual whose tetanus immunization status is unknown or uncertain should be considered to have had no previous doses of tetanus toxoid adsorbed. An emergency booster dose of a preparation containing tetanus toxoid adsorbed is unnecessary if the wound is clean and minor (not tetanus prone) and the patient has previously received the complete primary vaccination series against tetanus and any indicated booster doses within the last 10 years. However, an emergency booster dose of a tetanus toxoid-containing preparation is necessary in individuals with a clean, minor wound if fewer than 3 doses were administered in the past (incompletely immunized) or if 10 or more years have elapsed since primary immunization or the last booster dose. If the wound is tetanus prone, an emergency booster dose of a tetanus toxoid-containing preparation should be given if fewer than 3 doses were administered in the past (incompletely immunized) or if 5 or more years have elapsed since primary immunization or the last booster dose. In addition, a dose of TIG should be administered concomitantly with the tetanus toxoid-containing preparation at a separate site if the wound is tetanus prone and if the patient received fewer than 3 doses of a tetanus toxoid-containing preparation in the past (incompletely immunized).

ACIP, AAP, and other experts recommend that a *single* dose of Tdap be used in place of a dose of Td for postexposure prophylaxis of tetanus in adults and adolescents 11 years of age or older (including adults 65 years of age or older) who have *not* previously received a dose of Tdap, unless pertussis antigens are contraindicated or should not be used. If Tdap is unavailable or was administered previously, Td should be used for postexposure prophylaxis.

Table 1 summarizes ACIP guidelines for active and passive immunization against tetanus in routine wound management.

Table 1. Summary Guide to Tetanus Prophylaxis in Routine Wound Management

Previous Doses of Tetanus Toxoid Adsorbed Received	Clean, Minor Wounds		All Other Wounds	
	Tdap[a] or Td[b]	TIG	Tdap[a] or Td[b]	TIG
Unknown or less than 3 doses	Yes	No	Yes	Yes
3 or more doses[c]	No[d]	No	No[e]	No

[a] Tetanus toxoid, reduced diphtheria toxoid and acellular pertussis vaccine adsorbed (Tdap). A dose of Tdap is preferred instead of a dose of Td in adults and adolescents 11 years of age or older who have not previously received a dose of Tdap. Use Td in individuals in this age group who previously received a dose of Tdap.

[b] Tetanus and diphtheria toxoids adsorbed for adults use (Td). Td is used in adults, adolescents, and children 7 years of age or older. For children 6 weeks through 6 years of age, diphtheria and tetanus toxoids and acellular pertussis vaccine adsorbed (DTaP) usually is indicated, but diphtheria and tetanus toxoids adsorbed (DT) can be used in this age group if pertussis antigens are contraindicated. Single-antigen tetanus toxoid adsorbed is not commercially available in the US.

[c] If only 3 doses of tetanus toxoid fluid (no longer commercially available in the US) have been received previously, a fourth dose should be given as a preparation containing tetanus toxoid adsorbed.

[d] Yes, if it has been 10 or more years since last dose of tetanus toxoid-containing preparation.

[e] Yes, if it has been 5 or more years since last dose of tetanus toxoid-containing preparation; more frequent booster doses not needed and can accentuate adverse effects.

Adapted from ACIP recommendations for prevention of diphtheria, tetanus, and pertussis published in *MMWR Recomm Rep.* 2006; 55(RR-3):1-43 and *MMWR Recomm Rep.* 2006; 55(RR-17):1-37.

Anti-infectives are not indicated for tetanus postexposure prophylaxis since anti-infectives do not neutralize exotoxin already formed and cannot eradicate *C. tetani* spores, which may revert to toxin-producing vegetative forms.

Dosage and Administration

■ **Administration** Diphtheria and tetanus toxoids adsorbed (DT) and tetanus and diphtheria toxoids adsorbed (Td) are administered *only* by IM injection.

To ensure delivery into muscle, IM injections should be made at a 90° angle to the skin using a needle length appropriate for the individual's age and body mass, thickness of adipose tissue and muscle at the injection site, and the injection technique.

Depending on patient age, IM injections of DT or Td should be made into the anterolateral muscles of the thigh or deltoid muscle of the arm. In adults, adolescents, and children 3 years of age or older, IM injections should preferably be made in the deltoid muscle. In infants and children 6 weeks to 2 years of age, IM injections should preferably be made into the anterolateral thigh; alternatively, the deltoid muscle can be used in those 1–2 years of age if muscle mass is adequate.

The gluteal area or areas where there may be a major nerve trunk should be avoided. If the gluteal muscle is chosen for infants younger than 12 months of age because of special circumstances (e.g., physical obstruction of other sites), it is *essential* that the clinician identify anatomic landmarks prior to injection.

DT and Td should be inspected visually for particulate matter and discoloration prior to administration. To ensure a uniform suspension of antigens, single-dose vials of DT or single-dose vials or single-dose prefilled syringes of Td should be shaken well prior to use. After shaking, a uniform, white, cloudy suspension should result; the vaccine should be discarded if it contains particulate matter, is discolored, or cannot be resuspended.

Syncope (vasovagal or vasodepressor reaction; fainting) may occur following vaccination; such reactions may be accompanied by transient neurologic signs (e.g., visual disturbance, paresthesia, tonic-clonic limb movements). Syncope occurs most frequently in adolescents and young adults. Procedures should be in place to avoid falling injury and to restore cerebral perfusion following syncope. Syncope and secondary injuries may be averted if vaccinees sit or lie down during and for 15 minutes after vaccination. If syncope occurs, the patient should be observed until symptoms resolve.

DT and Td should not be diluted and should not be mixed with any other vaccine or solution.

When *passive* immunization with tetanus immune globulin (TIG) is indicated in addition to *active* immunization with a preparation containing tetanus toxoid adsorbed for postexposure prophylaxis of tetanus, DT or Td may be given simultaneously with TIG using different syringes and different injection sites. (See Uses: Postexposure Prophylaxis of Tetanus.)

DT or Td may be given simultaneously with other age-appropriate vaccines. When multiple vaccines are administered during a single health-care visit, each parenteral vaccine should be given with a different syringe and at different injection sites. Injection sites should be separated by at least 1 inch (if anatomically feasible) to allow appropriate attribution of any local adverse effects that may occur.

■ **Dosage** DT and Td are administered in 0.5-mL doses.

Each 0.5 mL of DT contains 25 flocculation units (Lf) units of diphtheria toxoid adsorbed and 5 Lf units of tetanus toxoid adsorbed.

Each 0.5 mL of Td contains 2 Lf units of diphtheria toxoid adsorbed and, depending on the manufacturer, either 2 or 5 Lf units of tetanus toxoid adsorbed.

The dosing schedule (i.e., number of doses) and specific preparation (i.e., DT, Td) for primary and/or booster immunization varies depending on age. The age-appropriate recommendations for the specific preparation used should be followed.

DT is used *only* in infants and children 6 weeks through 6 years of age and *only* when diphtheria and tetanus toxoids and acellular pertussis vaccine adsorbed (DTaP) cannot be used (i.e., when pertussis antigens are contraindicated or should not be used).

Td is used *only* in adults, adolescents, and children 7 years of age or older.

The complete primary vaccination series and recommended booster doses must be administered to ensure optimal protection against diphtheria and tetanus. Interruption of the primary immunization series resulting in intervals between doses longer than recommended do not interfere with the final immunity achieved; therefore, it is not necessary to give additional doses or to start the series over.

If an accelerated immunization schedule is necessary in infants and children 6 weeks through 6 years of age (e.g., for catch-up immunization, immunization prior to travel), the minimum intervals between the first, second, and third doses of DT are 4 weeks and the minimum intervals between the third, fourth, and fifth doses are 6 months. In adults, adolescents, and children 7 years of age or older, the minimum interval between the first and second dose of Td is 4 weeks and the minimum interval between second and third dose is 6 months.

Primary and Booster Immunization **Infants and Children 6 Weeks Through 6 Years of Age (DT).** For primary immunization in infants and children 6 weeks through 6 years of age when DTaP cannot be used (i.e., when pertussis antigens are contraindicated or should not be used), the manufacturer, ACIP, American Academy of Pediatrics (AAP), and other experts recommend that DT be given in a series of 4 doses with or without a fifth (booster) dose. The first 3 doses are given 4–8 weeks apart (usually at 2, 4, and 6 months of age) and the fourth dose is given approximately 6–12 months after the third dose (usually at 15–18 months of age). The fourth dose may be administered as early as 12 months of age, provided at least 6 months have elapsed since the third dose.

At 4 through 6 years of age (usually just prior to entry into kindergarten or elementary school), children who received primary immunization with DT before their fourth birthday should receive a fifth (booster) dose of the preparation. The fifth dose is not necessary if the last dose of the primary series was given on or after the fourth birthday.

Previously Unvaccinated Children 7 through 10 Years of Age (Td). For primary immunization in children 7 through 10 years of age who were not vaccinated at a younger age, Td is given in a series of 3 doses; the second dose is given 4–8 weeks after the first dose, and the third dose is given 6–12 months after the second dose.

The preferred primary immunization schedule recommended by ACIP, AAP, and other experts for catch-up vaccination in previously unvaccinated children 7 through 10 years of age is a *single* dose of Tdap (unless pertussis antigens are contraindicated or should not be used) followed by a dose of Td given 1–2 months after the Tdap dose and a second Td dose given 6–12 months after the first Td dose. Alternatively, Tdap may be substituted for any 1 of the Td doses. Children who receive a dose of Tdap at 7 through 10 years of age should *not* receive a Tdap booster dose at 11 through 12 years of age. (See Diphtheria and Tetanus Toxoids and Acellular Pertussis Vaccine Adsorbed/Tetanus Toxoid, Reduced Diphtheria Toxoid and Acellular Pertussis Vaccine Adsorbed 80:08.)

Previously Unvaccinated Adolescents 11 through 18 years (Td). For primary immunization in adolescents 11 through 18 years of age who were not vaccinated at a younger age, Td is given in a series of 3 doses; the second dose is given 4–8 weeks after the first dose, and the third dose is given 6–12 months after the second dose.

The preferred primary immunization schedule recommended by ACIP, AAP, and other experts for previously unvaccinated adolescents 11 through 18 years of age is a *single* dose of Tdap (unless pertussis antigens are contraindicated or should not be used) followed by a Td dose given at least 4 weeks after the Tdap dose and a second dose of Td given 6–12 months after the Td dose. Alternatively, the Tdap dose may be substituted for any 1 of the 3 doses of Td. (See Diphtheria and Tetanus Toxoids and Acellular Pertussis Vaccine

Adsorbed/Tetanus Toxoid, Reduced Diphtheria Toxoid and Acellular Pertussis Vaccine Adsorbed 80:08.) Td should be used for all subsequent booster doses.

Booster Doses in Adolescents 11 through 18 Years of Age (Td). All individuals who received primary immunization with DTaP, diphtheria and tetanus toxoids adsorbed and whole-cell pertussis vaccine (DTP; not commercially available in the US), DT, or Td should receive a booster dose of a preparation containing diphtheria and tetanus toxoids adsorbed at 11 through 18 years of age (preferably at 11 through 12 years of age) and routine booster doses of Td every 10 years to maintain adequate immunity against diphtheria and tetanus.

Because adolescents also may be at risk for pertussis, ACIP, AAP, and other experts recommend that a *single* dose of Tdap be used (instead of Td) for the adolescent booster dose given at 11 through 18 years of age (preferably at 11 through 12 years of age), unless Tdap has already been given or pertussis antigens are contraindicated or should not be used. If Tdap is unavailable or was administered previously, a dose of Td should be used for this adolescent booster dose. (See Diphtheria and Tetanus Toxoids and Acellular Pertussis Vaccine Adsorbed/Tetanus Toxoid, Reduced Diphtheria Toxoid and Acellular Pertussis Vaccine Adsorbed 80:08.)

Previously Unvaccinated Adults 19 Years of Age or Older (Td). For primary immunization in previously unvaccinated adults and adults with an uncertain history of immunization against diphtheria and tetanus, ACIP and other experts recommend that Td be given in a series of 3 doses; the second dose is given 4–8 weeks after the first dose and the third dose is given 6–12 months after the second dose.

The preferred primary immunization schedule recommended by ACIP and other experts for previously unvaccinated adults 19 years of age or older (including those 65 years of age or older) is a *single* dose of Tdap (unless pertussis antigens are contraindicated or should not be used) followed by a dose of Td given at least 4 weeks after the Tdap dose and a second dose of Td given 6–12 months after the first dose of Td. Alternatively, the Tdap dose may be substituted for any 1 of the 3 doses of Td. If Tdap is not available or was administered previously, Td may be given. (See Diphtheria and Tetanus Toxoids and Acellular Pertussis Vaccine Adsorbed/Tetanus Toxoid, Reduced Diphtheria Toxoid and Acellular Pertussis Vaccine Adsorbed 80:08.)

Booster Doses in Adults 19 Years of Age or Older (Td). All adults who received primary immunization against diphtheria and tetanus should receive routine booster doses of Td every 10 years. In addition, an emergency booster dose of Td may be indicated in the event of injury and possible exposure to tetanus infection. (See Uses: Postexposure Prophylaxis of Tetanus.)

ACIP and other experts recommend that a *single* dose of Tdap should be used (instead of Td) when a booster dose is needed in adults 19 years of age or older (including those 65 years of age or older), unless pertussis antigens are contraindicated or should not be used. Thereafter, Td should be used whenever a booster dose is indicated.

Postexposure Prophylaxis of Tetanus For postexposure prophylaxis of tetanus, an emergency dose of a preparation containing tetanus toxoid adsorbed may be indicated with or without a dose of TIG. (See Table 1 in Uses: Postexposure Prophylaxis of Tetanus.)

Wound care is an essential part of postexposure prophylaxis of tetanus and wound care is necessary regardless of vaccination status. Wounds should be properly cleaned and debrided, especially if dirt or necrotic tissue is present and all necrotic tissue and foreign material should be removed.

In the event of injury and possible exposure to tetanus infection in adults, adolescents, and children 7 years of age or older, an emergency booster dose of Td should be given as soon as possible if the individual has previously received less than 3 doses of any tetanus toxoid-containing preparation or if their immunization history is unknown or uncertain. If the injury is a clean, minor wound (not tetanus prone), the booster dose of a preparation containing tetanus toxoid adsorbed is given without passive immunization with TIG. However, for all other types of wounds (tetanus-prone wounds), a dose of TIG should be given in addition to the preparation of tetanus toxoid adsorbed. After the emergency booster dose, the primary vaccination series should be completed using a preparation containing tetanus toxoid adsorbed.

In the event of injury and possible exposure to tetanus infection in adults, adolescents, and children 7 years of age or older who previously received 3 doses or more of a preparation containing tetanus toxoid adsorbed, an emergency booster dose of Td should be given if the injury is a clean, minor wound (not tetanus prone) and it has been 10 or more years since primary immunization against tetanus or the last booster dose of a preparation containing tetanus toxoid adsorbed. If the injury is a tetanus-prone wound, an emergency booster dose of Td should be given if it has been 5 or more years since primary immunization against tetanus or the last booster dose of a preparation containing tetanus toxoid adsorbed. In addition, those with tetanus-prone wounds should receive a dose of TIG.

If the individual previously received only 3 doses of tetanus toxoid fluid (no longer commercially available in the US), a booster dose of a preparation containing tetanus toxoid adsorbed should be given.

ACIP and other experts recommend that a *single* dose of Tdap should be used (instead of Td) in individuals 11 years of age or older (including those 65 years of age or older) who have *not* previously received a dose of Tdap, unless pertussis antigens are contraindicated or should not be used. If Tdap is not available or was administered previously, Td should be used. (See Diphtheria and Tetanus Toxoids and Acellular Pertussis Vaccine Adsorbed/Tetanus Toxoid, Reduced Diphtheria Toxoid and Acellular Pertussis Vaccine Adsorbed 80:08.)

Postexposure Prophylaxis of Diphtheria For postexposure prophylaxis of diphtheria, a dose of a preparation containing diphtheria toxoid adsorbed may be indicated in conjunction with anti-infective prophylaxis. (See Uses: Postexposure Prophylaxis of Diphtheria.)

All household and other close contacts of an individual with known or suspected diphtheria should receive an immediate dose of an age-appropriate preparation containing diphtheria toxoid adsorbed (DT or Td) if their vaccination status is unknown or they previously received less than 3 doses and the primary vaccination series should then be completed. Individuals who previously completed the primary vaccination series against diphtheria but have not received a dose of a preparation containing diphtheria toxoid adsorbed within the last 5 years should receive an immediate booster dose of an age-appropriate preparation (DT or Td).

Cautions

Adverse reactions to tetanus and diphtheria toxoids adsorbed (Td), especially Arthus-type hypersensitivity reactions, occur most frequently in individuals who have received a large number of booster doses of preparations containing diphtheria and/or tetanus toxoids.

■ Local Effects

The most frequent adverse effects of preparations containing diphtheria and tetanus toxoids adsorbed are mild to moderate local reactions at the injection site that may persist for several days. These local effects include erythema, warmth, swelling, edema, induration, pain, tenderness, cellulitis, pruritus, urticaria, and rash. A nodule may be palpable at the injection site for several weeks. Sterile abscesses or subcutaneous atrophy have also been reported rarely.

Rarely, extensive local reactions manifested by erythema and boggy edema (Arthus-type hypersensitivity reactions) occur after injection of preparations containing tetanus toxoid. These reactions generally begin 2–12 hours after administration and are a local inflammatory reaction (vasculitis) that can include severe pain, swelling, induration, edema, hemorrhage, and necrosis. In some cases, painful swelling may extend from the shoulder to the elbow. Arthus reactions usually resolve without sequelae. The reactions occur most frequently in individuals who have received multiple prior booster doses of preparations containing tetanus toxoid adsorbed or tetanus toxoid fluid (no longer commercially available in the US).

Local reactions to preparations containing adsorbed diphtheria and tetanus toxoids (without other severe adverse effects) do not preclude future use of the toxoid. However, individuals who experienced an Arthus-type hypersensitivity reaction usually have high serum tetanus antitoxin levels and should not be given emergency doses of a tetanus toxoid-containing preparation any more frequently than every 10 years, even if they have a wound that is neither clean nor minor.

■ Systemic Effects

Rarely, systemic reactions including fever, chills, malaise, fatigue, myalgia, arthralgia or generalized aches and pains, nausea and vomiting, erythema multiforme or other rash, flushing, generalized urticaria or pruritus, tachycardia, dizziness, and hypotension have been reported following administration of preparations containing diphtheria and tetanus toxoids adsorbed. Fever may be immediate (occurring within 1–3 hours) or delayed. Such reactions generally are self-limited and can be managed effectively with symptomatic treatment.

Rarely, severe anaphylactic or anaphylactoid reactions, characterized by urticaria and angioedema, difficulty breathing, hypotension, and/or shock, have been reported following administration of preparations containing tetanus and/or diphtheria antigens. In one study, 94 of 95 individuals with a history of anaphylactoid manifestations following a previous dose of tetanus toxoid were nonreactive following intradermal testing and tolerated further full immunizing doses of adsorbed diphtheria and tetanus toxoids. Deaths have been reported in temporal association with the administration of tetanus toxoid adsorbed.

Guillain-Barré syndrome (GBS) has been reported in temporal association with tetanus toxoid. A review by the Institute of Medicine (IOM) found evidence of a causal relationship between tetanus toxoid and brachial neuritis and GBS. Analysis of active surveillance data collected during 1991 failed to demonstrate an increased risk of GBS in children or adults within 6 weeks following vaccination with a preparation containing tetanus toxoid adsorbed. (See Guillain-Barré Syndrome and Other Neurologic Disorders under Cautions: Precautions and Contraindications.)

■ Precautions and Contraindications

DT and Td are contraindicated in individuals who have had a severe allergic reaction (e.g., anaphylaxis) after a previous dose of the vaccine, any vaccine component, or any other preparation containing diphtheria or tetanus toxoids. (See Sensitivity Reactions under Cautions: Precautions and Contraindications.)

To determine whether there are any contraindications to administration of DT or Td and to accurately assess the benefits and risks of the vaccines for each patient, the patient and/or the patient's parent or guardian should be questioned about the health status of the patient and the occurrence of sensitivity or any adverse events after previous doses.

The patient and/or the patient's parent or guardian should be informed of the benefits and risks of immunization with DT or Td and should be provided with a copy of the appropriate Vaccine Information Statement (available at CDC website http://www.cdc.gov/vaccines/pubs/vis/default.htm). Patient and/or the patient's parent or guardian also should be advised of the importance of completing the primary immunization series and receiving recommended booster doses to ensure the highest level of protection against tetanus and diphtheria.

Patients and/or the patient's parent or guardian should be instructed to report any severe or unusual adverse reactions to their health-care provider. Clinicians or individuals can report any adverse reactions that occur following vaccination to VAERS at 800-822-7967 or http://vaers.hhs.gov.

If a contraindication to tetanus toxoid-containing preparations exists in an individual who has previously received less than 3 doses, only passive immunization with tetanus immune globulin (TIG) should be considered when postexposure prophylaxis of tetanus is indicated.

Sensitivity Reactions Prior to administration of DT or Td, the clinician should review the patient's health status and history regarding possible sensitivity or any other adverse reactions after previous doses and should take all precautions known for prevention of allergic or any other adverse effects. Epinephrine and other appropriate agents and equipment should be available for immediate use in case an anaphylactic reaction occurs.

Some manufacturers suggest that individuals who have a history of severe allergic reaction to a previous dose may be referred to an allergist for evaluation if further doses are being considered (e.g., for tetanus postexposure prophylaxis). Although skin testing has been suggested to help determine whether additional doses of a tetanus toxoid-containing preparation can be used in an individuals who developed a systemic reaction to the toxoid, utility of skin testing has been questioned since mild, nonspecific skin-test reactivity to tetanus toxoid commonly occurs, particularly when the preparation is used undiluted.

Arthus-type Hypersensitivity Reactions. Individuals who experience Arthus-type hypersensitivity reactions or fever greater than 39.4°C after administration of tetanus toxoid adsorbed (see Cautions: Local Effects) usually have very high serum tetanus antitoxin levels and usually should not receive additional routine or emergency booster doses of a preparation containing tetanus toxoid adsorbed more frequently than every 10 years, even if postexposure prophylaxis of tetanus is indicated.

Latex Sensitivity. Some packaging components of Td (Tenivac®) single-dose prefilled syringes (i.e., tip caps) contain dry natural latex. Because some individuals may be hypersensitive to natural latex proteins, appropriate precautions should be taken if this preparation is administered to individuals with a history of latex sensitivity.

ACIP states that vaccines supplied in vials or syringes containing dry natural rubber or natural rubber latex may be administered to individuals with latex allergies other than anaphylactic allergies (e.g., history of contact allergy to latex gloves), but should *not* be used in those with a history of severe (anaphylactic) allergy to latex, unless the benefits of vaccination outweigh the risk of a potential allergic reaction. Contact-type allergy is the most common type of latex sensitivity.

Precautions Related to Booster Doses Booster doses of Td should only be administered when indicated. Booster doses given more frequently than recommended are associated with an increased incidence and severity of adverse effects.

Routine booster doses of Td should be administered once every 10 years. Emergency booster doses are not usually indicated unless at least 5 years have elapsed since the last dose. If a booster dose is given earlier than 10 years after a previous dose, the next routine booster dose should not be given for 10 years.

Guillain-Barré Syndrome and Other Neurologic Disorders The risk of developing GBS may be increased in individuals with a history of GBS within 6 weeks after receiving a prior dose of any preparation containing tetanus toxoid. Some manufacturers state that a decision to administer a preparation containing tetanus toxoid adsorbed to an individual with a history of GBS within 6 weeks after receiving a prior dose of any preparation containing tetanus toxoid should be based on careful consideration of the potential benefits and possible risks.

ACIP states that a history of GBS occurring within 6 weeks after a previous dose of a preparation containing tetanus toxoid adsorbed should be considered a precaution for subsequent doses of such preparations.

ACIP does not consider brachial neuritis a precaution or contraindication for further doses.

Individuals with Altered Immunocompetence If DT or Td is administered to individuals immunosuppressed as the result of disease or immunosuppressive therapy, the possibility that the immune response to the vaccine and efficacy may be reduced should be considered.

Recommendations regarding use of tetanus and diphtheria toxoids in individuals with human immunodeficiency virus (HIV) infection are the same as those for individuals who are not HIV-infected. However, immunization may be less effective in individuals with HIV infection than in immunocompetent individuals.

Thimerosal Precautions Although there is no convincing evidence that the low concentrations of thimerosal (a mercury-containing preservative) contained in some vaccines is harmful to vaccine recipients, efforts to eliminate or reduce the thimerosal content in vaccines is recommended as a prudent measure to reduce mercury exposure in infants and children and part of an overall strategy to reduce mercury exposures from all sources, including food and drugs.

It was suggested that thimerosal in vaccines theoretically could have adverse effects in vaccine recipients; however, there is no conclusive evidence that the low levels of thimerosal contained in vaccines cause harm in vaccine recipients.

Td (manufactured by MassBiologics) contains trace amounts of thimerosal from the manufacturing process (no more than 0.3 mcg of mercury per 0.5-mL dose). The US Food and Drug Administration (FDA) states that trace amounts of thimerosal from the manufacturing process are not considered clinically important.

DT and Td (Tenivac®) do not contain thimerosal or any other preservatives.

For additional information on thimerosal in vaccines, see Thimerosal Precautions under Cautions: Precautions and Contraindications, in Influenza Virus Vaccine Inactivated 80:12.

Concomitant Illnesses A decision to administer or delay vaccination in an individual with a current or recent febrile illness depends on the severity of symptoms and etiology of the illness. Minor acute illness, such as mild diarrhea or mild upper respiratory tract infection (with or without fever) generally does not preclude vaccination, but defer vaccination in individuals with moderate or severe acute illness (with or without fever).

Limitations of Vaccine Effectiveness DT and Td may not protect all individuals from diphtheria and tetanus.

Optimum protection against diphtheria and tetanus is achieved with a primary series of 3 doses of preparations containing diphtheria and tetanus toxoids adsorbed.

Duration of Immunity Following primary immunization, the duration of protection against diphtheria is approximately 10 years.

Following primary immunization, the duration of protection against tetanus is approximately 10 years. Although some individuals may be protected for life, antitoxin levels decrease over time and only approach the minimal protective level in most individuals 10 years after the last dose. The antitoxin response induced by tetanus toxoid adsorbed has a longer duration than that induced by tetanus toxoid fluid (no longer commercially available in the US).

Pre- and Postvaccination Serologic Testing Routine *prevaccination* serologic testing is not recommended.

When postexposure prophylaxis against tetanus or preexposure vaccination in high-risk groups (e.g., travelers) is indicated, individuals with an unknown or uncertain history of vaccination generally should be considered unvaccinated and should receive the complete primary vaccination series.

To avoid unnecessary vaccination, ACIP states that *prevaccination* serologic testing for tetanus and diphtheria antitoxin antibodies can be considered in adults, adolescents, or children 7 years of age or older who probably were vaccinated but cannot produce vaccination records. If levels of tetanus and diphtheria antitoxin are both at least 0.1 international units/mL, previous vaccination with diphtheria and tetanus toxoids adsorbed can be assumed.

Improper Storage or Handling Improper storage or handling of vaccines may reduce vaccine potency and can result in reduced or inadequate immune responses in vaccinees.

All vaccines should be inspected upon delivery and monitored during storage to ensure that the appropriate temperature is maintained. (See Chemistry and Stability: Stability.)

DT or Td that has been mishandled or has not been stored at the recommended temperature should not be administered.

If there are concerns about mishandling, the manufacturer or state or local immunization or health departments should be contacted for guidance on whether the vaccine is usable.

■ **Pediatric Precautions** Safety and efficacy of DT have not been established in infants younger than 6 weeks of age or in children 7 years of age or older. DT contains a higher dose of diphtheria toxoid (25 Lf units) than Td (2 Lf units). Because individuals 7 years of age and older have an increased incidence of adverse reactions to preparations containing more than 2 Lf units of diphtheria toxoid, DT should *not* be used in individuals 7 years of age or older.

Safety and efficacy of Td have not been established in children younger than 7 years of age.

The most common adverse effects following administration of DT in infants and children 2 months through 6 years of age are crying, fever, loss of appetite, and local reactions (pain, tenderness, swelling, erythema).

Apnea has been reported following IM administration of vaccines in some infants born prematurely. Decisions regarding when to administer an IM vaccine in infants born prematurely should be based on consideration of the individual infant's medical status and potential benefits and possible risks of vaccination.

■ **Geriatric Precautions** In a clinical study that included 449 adults 65 years of age or older (including 192 adults 75 years of age or older), the proportion of those 65 years of age or older who had seroprotective antibody levels following a dose of Td (Tenivac®) was marginally lower for tetanus and lower for diphtheria compared with younger individuals. The rate of solicited adverse events in those 65 years of age and older generally was similar to the rate in younger adults.

■ **Mutagenicity and Carcinogenicity** Studies have not been performed to date to evaluate the mutagenic or carcinogenic potential of DT or Td.

■ **Pregnancy and Lactation** ***Pregnancy*** Animal reproduction studies have not been performed with Td. It is not known whether the toxoids can cause fetal harm, and they should be used during pregnancy only when clearly needed. Tetanus toxoids have been administered to pregnant women to prevent tetanus in neonates considered to be at high risk for the disease.

Because of the risks associated with tetanus and diphtheria infection, ACIP, American Academy of Pediatrics (AAP), and other experts state that preparations containing diphtheria and tetanus antigens are not contraindicated during pregnancy. Although there is no evidence that diphtheria and tetanus toxoids are teratogenic, waiting until the second or third trimester of pregnancy (and before 36 weeks of gestation) to administer Td is recommended.

Ideally, primary immunization against tetanus and diphtheria should be completed prior to pregnancy. Pregnant women who have not received primary immunization with DTaP, DTP (not commercially available in the US), DT, Td, or single-antigen tetanus toxoid adsorbed (not commercially available in the US) and those whose tetanus immunization history is unknown or uncertain should receive a primary series of 3 doses of vaccine containing diphtheria and tetanus toxoids beginning during pregnancy.

Although Td generally is the preferred preparation for primary immunization against diphtheria and tetanus during pregnancy, ACIP, AAP, and other experts state that a dose of Tdap should be substituted for one of the required primary Td doses, preferably in the third trimester (optimally between 27 and 36 weeks of gestation) in previously unvaccinated or incompletely vaccinated pregnant women. In addition, to ensure protection against pertussis, these experts recommend that a dose of Tdap be administered during *each* pregnancy, regardless of the woman's prior vaccination history. To maximize maternal antibody response and passive antibody transfer to the infant, optimal timing for the Tdap dose is between 27 and 36 weeks of gestation. (See Pregnant Women under Uses: Primary and Booster Immunization with Tetanus and Diphtheria Toxoids Adsorbed [Td].)

When a pregnant woman's history of tetanus vaccination is uncertain, serologic testing can be done to determine whether she has protective levels of tetanus antitoxin (i.e., at least 0.1 international units when tested using enzyme-linked immunosorbent assay [ELISA]). Those who have never been vaccinated against tetanus or have levels of tetanus antitoxin that are not protective should be vaccinated during pregnancy to ensure protection against maternal and neonatal tetanus. Because diphtheria is rare in the US, serologic testing for diphtheria antitoxin is not usually necessary in pregnant women. Two doses of a preparation containing tetanus toxoid adsorbed given at least 4–6 weeks before delivery stimulates tetanus antitoxin levels that protect the mother and readily cross the placenta to protect the neonate against tetanus. (See Pregnant Women under Uses: Primary and Booster Immunization with Tetanus and Diphtheria Toxoids Adsorbed [Td].)

Sufficient tetanus protection is likely if the pregnant woman is younger than 31 years of age and received the complete childhood tetanus and diphtheria vaccination series and a booster dose of Td during adolescence or received the complete adult vaccination series of 3 doses of Td or single-antigen tetanus toxoid adsorbed (not commercially available in the US). Sufficient tetanus protection may also be present if the pregnant woman is 31 years of age or older and received the complete childhood vaccination series and at least 2 booster doses of Td; if the pregnant woman received a primary vaccination series consisting of 3 doses of Td or single-antigen tetanus toxoid adsorbed during adolescence or as an adult; or if serologic testing indicates protective levels of serum tetanus antitoxin.

If postexposure prophylaxis of tetanus is indicated as part of wound management in a pregnant woman, the usual recommendations regarding emergency booster doses should be followed. (See Uses: Postexposure Prophylaxis of Tetanus.) Tdap should be used for the booster dose (instead of Td).

Lactation It is not known whether diphtheria or tetanus toxoids are distributed into milk. The manufacturers state that Td for adult use should be used with caution in nursing women.

ACIP states that breastfeeding is not considered a contraindication for diphtheria and tetanus toxoids adsorbed.

Drug Interactions

■ **Diphtheria Antitoxin (Equine)** If both diphtheria antitoxin (equine) (available in the US only from CDC under an investigational new drug [IND] protocol) and a dose of diphtheria and tetanus toxoids adsorbed (DT) or tetanus and diphtheria toxoids adsorbed (Td) are required, they should be given at separate sites using different syringes. Although specific studies are not available, diphtheria antitoxin (equine) is unlikely to impair the immune response to diphtheria toxoid adsorbed.

■ **Immune Globulins** DT or Td may be administered simultaneously with (using different syringes and injection sites) or at any time before or after immune globulin (e.g., immune globulin IM [IGIM], immune globulin IV [IGIV]) or specific immune globulin (e.g., hepatitis B immune globulin [HBIG], rabies immune globulin [RIG], tetanus immune globulin [TIG], varicella zoster immune globulin [VZIG]).

When passive immunization with TIG is indicated in addition to active immunization with a preparation containing tetanus toxoid adsorbed for postexposure prophylaxis of tetanus (see Uses: Postexposure Prophylaxis of Tetanus), TIG and the preparation containing tetanus toxoid adsorbed may be given simultaneously at separate sites using different syringes.

■ **Immunosuppressive Agents** Individuals receiving immunosuppressive agents (e.g., alkylating agents, antimetabolites, corticosteroids, radiation therapy) may have a diminished immunologic response to DT or Td. Short-term (less than 2 weeks), low- to moderate-dose systemic corticosteroid therapy; long-term, alternate-day, systemic corticosteroid therapy using low to moderate doses of short-acting drugs; topical corticosteroid therapy (e.g., nasal, cutaneous, ophthalmic); or intra-articular, bursal, or tendon injections with corticosteroids should not be immunosuppressive in usual dosages. There is some evidence that children receiving immunosuppressive therapy, including those with malignancies receiving maintenance chemotherapy, may have adequate antibody responses to diphtheria and tetanus toxoids adsorbed. Therefore, it has been suggested that these children receive the usual recommended doses of these toxoids at the usual intervals.

■ **Vaccines** Although specific data are not available regarding concurrent administration of DT or Td with all other available vaccines, the US Public Health Service Advisory Committee on Immunization Practices (ACIP), American Academy of Pediatrics (AAP), and other experts state that primary immunization against diphtheria and tetanus can be integrated with primary immunization against pertussis, *Haemophilus influenzae* type b (Hib), hepatitis A, hepatitis B, human papillomavirus (HPV), influenza, measles, mumps, rubella, meningococcal disease, pneumococcal disease, poliomyelitis, rotavirus, and varicella. However, unless combination vaccines appropriate for the age and vaccination status of the recipient are used, each parenteral vaccine should be administered using a different syringe and different injection site.

DT or Td may be administered simultaneously with or at any interval before or after live viral vaccines, including measles, mumps, and rubella virus vaccine live (MMR). In addition, DT or Td may be administered simultaneously with or at any interval before or after inactivated vaccines, including Hib vaccine, hepatitis B vaccine, meningococcal vaccine, and poliovirus vaccine inactivated (IPV).

Meningococcal Vaccine Td has been administered concomitantly with meningococcal (groups A, C, Y and W-135) polysaccharide diphtheria toxoid conjugate vaccine (MCV4; Menactra®) at a different site in adolescents 11 through 17 years of age without a decrease in antibody responses to either vaccine or a clinically important increase in adverse effects. Although antibody responses to some meningococcal antigens (serogroups C, Y, W-135) were higher when MCV4 (Menactra®) was administered concurrently with Td than when MCV4 (Menactra®) was given 1 month after Td, the clinical importance of these findings has not been determined. Antibody responses to tetanus and diphtheria antigens were similar in both study groups.

ACIP states that Td may be administered simultaneously with (using different syringes and different injection sites) or at any interval before or after MCV4 (Menactra®, Menveo®) or meningococcal polysaccharide vaccine, groups A, C, Y and W-135 combined (MPSV4; Menomune®).

Pharmacology

Diphtheria and tetanus toxoids adsorbed (DT) and tetanus and diphtheria toxoids adsorbed (Td) stimulate active immunity to diphtheria and tetanus by inducing production of specific antitoxin antibodies.

The diphtheria toxoid adsorbed component provides protection against the exotoxin elucidated by *Corynebacterium diphtheriae*. Primary immunization against diphtheria reduces the risk of developing diphtheria and the severity of clinical illness, but does not prevent or eliminate colonization or carriage of *C. diphtheriae* in the pharynx, nose, or skin of vaccinees. A complete primary immunization series with the age-appropriate preparation is needed to induce optimum levels of antitoxin that provide protection. Protective levels of diphtheria antitoxin (defined as at least 0.1 international units/mL) are attained at least 95% of individuals after the primary vaccination series. Following primary immunization, protective levels of diphtheria antitoxin levels may persist for about 10 years.

Tetanus toxoid adsorbed induces production of specific antitoxin antibodies that neutralize exotoxin produced by *Clostridium tetani*. A complete primary series of a preparation containing tetanus toxoid adsorbed results in protective levels of tetanus antitoxin that persist for approximately 10 years. Protective levels of tetanus antitoxin were previously defined as at least 0.01 international units/mL when measured by in vivo neutralization assay, but are currently defined as at least 0.1 international units/mL when measured by enzyme-linked immunosorbent assay (ELISA) or other methods. Although some individuals may be protected against tetanus for life following primary immunization with a preparation containing tetanus toxoid adsorbed, antitoxin levels decrease over time and only approach the minimal protective level in most individuals 10 years after the last dose of tetanus toxoid adsorbed. The antitoxin response induced by tetanus toxoid adsorbed has a longer duration than that induced by tetanus toxoid fluid (no longer commercially available in the US).

■ **Diphtheria Infection** Diphtheria is caused by toxigenic strains of *Corynebacterium diphtheriae* or, rarely, toxigenic strains of *C. ulcerans*. Toxigenic strains of *Corynebacterium* produce an exotoxin that can affect the mucous membranes of the respiratory tract (respiratory diphtheria [nasal, pharyngeal, tonsillar, laryngeal]), the skin (cutaneous diphtheria), and occasionally mucous membranes at other sites (conjunctival, otic, or vulvovaginal diphtheria). The toxin interferes with enzymes necessary for protein synthesis, leading to cell damage and death. The toxin causes local tissue destruction and membrane formation and can be absorbed into the bloodstream from the site of infection and distributed throughout the body resulting in serious complications (e.g., myocarditis, neuritis, thrombocytopenia, renal dysfunction or failure).

Humans are the only known reservoir of *C. diphtheriae*. Diphtheria is transmitted to close contacts by oral or respiratory droplets or by direct contact with discharge from skin lesions or, rarely, contact with items soiled with such discharge (fomites). Raw milk or unpasteurized dairy products also have been reported to transmit toxigenic *C. ulcerans*. Diphtheria can be acquired from carriers (i.e., asymptomatic individuals colonized with toxin-producing *C. diphtheriae*).

Following infection, the incubation period usually is 2–5 days (range 1–10 days). Although systemic complications of diphtheria can occur during the first week of illness, they usually occur later in the disease process (e.g., myocarditis usually occurs 1–2 weeks and neuritis usually occurs 2–8 weeks after disease onset). Most cases of diphtheria occur in individuals who are unvaccinated or incompletely vaccinated against the disease. The overall case-fatality rate for diphtheria is 5–10% with higher death rates (up to 20%) among individuals younger than 5 years of age and older than 40 years of age.

■ **Tetanus Infection** Tetanus is a potentially fatal disease caused by a neurotoxic exotoxin (tetanospasmin) produced by *C. tetani. C. tetani* spores are ubiquitous in the environment and are found in soil and in animal (e.g., horses, sheep, cattle, dogs, cats, rats, guinea pigs, chickens) and human intestinal tracts. The spores can contaminate open wounds, especially puncture wounds or those with devitalized tissue; anaerobic wound conditions allow the spores to germinate and produce exotoxins that disseminate through the blood and lymphatic system. Following infection of a wound, the incubation period for tetanus is 8–10 days (range 3–21 days).

The most common form of tetanus is generalized tetanus characterized by rigidity and convulsive muscle spasms that usually involve the jaw (lockjaw) and neck and then become generalized. Neonatal tetanus (tetanus neonatorum) occurs in infants born under nonsterile conditions to women inadequately vaccinated against tetanus; infection usually involves a contaminated umbilical stump and occurs because the infant does not have passively acquired maternal antibodies against tetanus. Obstetric tetanus occurs within 6 weeks after delivery or termination of pregnancy because of contaminated wounds or abrasions or unclean deliveries or abortions.

Chemistry and Stability

■ **Chemistry** Diphtheria and tetanus toxoids adsorbed (DT) and tetanus and diphtheria toxoids adsorbed (Td) are sterile suspensions prepared by mixing suitable quantities of diphtheria and tetanus toxoids that have been formaldehyde-treated, purified, and adsorbed onto an aluminum adjuvant.

DT and Td meet standards established by the Center for Biologics Evaluation and Research of the US Food and Drug Administration. The antigen content of the toxoids is expressed in terms of flocculation units (Lf).

DT appears as a uniform, white, cloudy suspension after shaking. Each 0.5 mL of DT contains 25 Lf units of diphtheria toxoid, 5 Lf units of tetanus toxoid, 1.5 mg of aluminum phosphate adjuvant, and less than 100 mcg of residual formaldehyde. Commercially available single-dose vials of DT do not contain thimerosal or any other preservative;

Td appears as a uniform, white, cloudy suspension after shaking. Each 0.5 mL of Td (Tenivac®) contains 2 Lf units of diphtheria toxoid, 5 Lf units of tetanus toxoid, 1.5 mg of aluminum phosphate (0.33 mg of aluminum) adjuvant, and no more than 5 mcg of residual formaldehyde. Td (Tenivac®) commercially available in single-dose vials or single-dose prefilled syringes does not contain thimerosal or any other preservative. Each 0.5 mL of Td (manufactured by MassBiologics) contains 2 Lf units of diphtheria toxoid, 2 Lf units of tetanus toxoid, no more than 0.53 mg of aluminum adjuvant, and less than 100 mcg of residual formaldehyde. Td (manufactured by MassBiologics) commercially available in single-dose vials does not contain preservatives, but does contain trace amounts of thimerosal from the manufacturing process (no more than 0.3 mcg of mercury per 0.5-mL dose).

■ **Stability** DT and Td should be stored at 2–8°C and should not be frozen. DT or Td that has been frozen should be discarded.

Preparations

Excipients in commercially available drug preparations may have clinically important effects in some individuals; consult specific product labeling for details.

Diphtheria and Tetanus Toxoids Adsorbed (DT)

Parenteral

Injectable suspension, for IM use	Diphtheria Toxoid 25 Lf units and Tetanus Toxoid 5 Lf units per 0.5 mL	**Diphtheria and Tetanus Toxoids Adsorbed,** Sanofi Pasteur

Tetanus and Diphtheria Toxoids Adsorbed (Td)

Parenteral

Injectable suspension, for IM use	Tetanus Toxoid 2 Lf units and Diphtheria Toxoid 2 Lf units per 0.5 mL	**Tetanus and Diphtheria Toxoids Adsorbed,** MassBiologics
	Tetanus Toxoid 5 Lf units and Diphtheria Toxoid 2 Lf units per 0.5 mL	**Tenivac®**, Sanofi Pasteur

Diphtheria and Tetanus Toxoids and Acellular Pertussis Vaccine Adsorbed
Tetanus Toxoid, Reduced Diphtheria Toxoid and Acellular Pertussis Vaccine Adsorbed

DTaP, Tdap

■ Diphtheria and tetanus toxoids and acellular pertussis vaccine adsorbed (DTaP; Daptacel®, Infanrix®) and tetanus toxoid, reduced diphtheria toxoid and acellular pertussis vaccine adsorbed (Tdap; Adacel®, Boostrix®) are fixed-combination preparations containing tetanus and diphtheria toxins (toxoids) and acellular pertussis vaccine adsorbed onto an aluminum adjuvant and are used to stimulate active immunity to diphtheria, tetanus, and pertussis. Antigen potency varies depending on the manufacturer. DTaP also is commercially available in fixed-combination vaccines containing diphtheria, tetanus, pertussis, and poliovirus antigens (DTaP-IPV; Kinrix®, Quadracel®), a fixed-combination vaccine containing diphtheria, tetanus, pertussis, hepatitis B, and poliovirus antigens (DTaP-HepB-IPV; Pediarix®), and a combination vaccine containing diphtheria, tetanus, pertussis, poliovirus, and Hib antigens (DTaP-IPV/Hib; Pentacel®). Although no longer available in the US, diphtheria and tetanus toxoids and whole-cell pertussis vaccine adsorbed (DTP, also referred to as DTwP) may still be used in other countries.

Uses

Diphtheria and tetanus toxoids and acellular pertussis vaccine adsorbed (DTaP) and tetanus toxoid, reduced diphtheria toxoid and acellular pertussis vaccine adsorbed (Tdap) are used to stimulate active immunity to diphtheria, tetanus, and pertussis. The appropriate vaccine containing diphtheria, tetanus, and pertussis antigens is selected based on age and whether primary or booster immunization is indicated. (See Uses: Choice of Vaccines Containing Diphtheria, Tetanus, and Pertussis Antigens.)

DTaP or Tdap may be indicated for postexposure vaccination against diphtheria in addition to anti-infective postexposure prophylaxis in unvaccinated or inadequately vaccinated household and other close contacts of an individual with diphtheria. (See Uses: Postexposure Prophylaxis of Diphtheria.)

DTaP or Tdap may be indicated in conjunction with passive immunization with tetanus immune globulin (TIG) for postexposure prophylaxis against tetanus in individuals with tetanus-prone wounds who are inadequately immunized against tetanus or whose tetanus immunization history is unknown or uncertain. (See Uses: Postexposure Prophylaxis of Tetanus.)

DTaP may be indicated for postexposure prophylaxis against pertussis in infants and children who are unvaccinated or incompletely vaccinated against pertussis. (See Uses: Postexposure Prophylaxis of Pertussis.)

DTaP and Tdap are *not* indicated for *treatment* of diphtheria, tetanus, or pertussis. However, because diphtheria and tetanus infections do not necessarily confer immunity, initiation or completion of active immunization against these diseases is indicated at the time of recovery in any previously unvaccinated or incompletely vaccinated individual. In addition, although pertussis is likely to confer short-term immunity, the duration of immunity is uncertain (waning may begin as early as 5–7 years after infection) and initiation or completion of active immunization against pertussis is indicated at the time of recovery.

■ **Choice of Vaccines Containing Diphtheria, Tetanus, and Pertussis Antigens** DTaP (Daptacel®, Infanrix®) is used for primary and booster immunization against diphtheria, tetanus, and pertussis in infants and children 6 weeks through 6 years of age. DTaP can be used to complete the remaining required doses in the vaccination series in children through 6 years of age who received DTP (not commercially available in the US) for initial doses (e.g., children vaccinated in countries where DTP is still used). DTaP should *not* be used in individuals 7 years of age or older.

There are no data to date indicating that any one DTaP preparation is preferred over any other DTaP preparation in terms of safety or efficacy for primary or booster immunization. The US Public Health Service Advisory Committee on Immunization Practices (ACIP) recommends that the same DTaP preparation used for the initial dose be used to complete the primary and booster immunization series since only limited data are available regarding use of different DTaP preparations interchangeably in the primary and booster vaccination series. However, these and other experts state that any age-appropriate commercially available DTaP vaccine should be used to complete the vaccination series if the particular DTaP vaccine used previously is not known or not available. (See Dosage and Administration: Dosage.)

DTaP also is commercially available in a fixed-combination vaccine with poliovirus antigens (DTaP-IPV; Kinrix®, Quadracel), in a fixed-combination vaccine with poliovirus and hepatitis B antigens (DTaP-HepB-IPV; Pediarix®), and in a combination vaccine with poliovirus and Hib antigens (DTaP-IPV/Hib; Pentacel®). (See Combination Vaccines Containing DTaP and Other Antigens under Uses: Choice of Vaccines Containing Diphtheria, Tetanus, and Pertussis Antigens.)

Tdap (Adacel®, Boostrix®) is used for booster immunization in adults and adolescents 10 years of age or older. Tdap (Adacel®) is labeled by the US Food and Drug Administration (FDA) for booster immunization in adolescents 10 years of age or older and adults 19 through 64 years of age; Tdap (Boostrix®) is labeled by FDA for booster immunization in adolescents 10 years of age or older and adults 19 years of age or older. For adults 65 years of age or older, ACIP states that Tdap (Boostrix®) should be used when feasible, but that Tdap (Adacel®) would provide protection when used for booster immunization in this age group and can be used in adults 65 years of age or older† if Tdap (Boostrix®) is not available. (See Uses: Primary and Booster Immunization with Tetanus Toxoid, Reduced Diphtheria Toxoid and Acellular Pertussis Vaccine Adsorbed [Tdap].)

Although safety and efficacy of Tdap for primary immunization have not been established, ACIP, the American Academy of Pediatrics (AAP), and other experts recommend that a *single* dose of Tdap be included in the vaccination series when adults, adolescents, or children as young as 7 years of age† require primary immunization† against diphtheria and tetanus, unless pertussis antigens are contraindicated or should not be used. (See Uses: Primary and Booster Immunization with Tetanus Toxoid, Reduced Diphtheria Toxoid and Acellular Pertussis Vaccine Adsorbed [Tdap].)

Combination Vaccines Containing DTaP and Other Antigens When indicated based on the age and vaccination status of the child and when there are no contraindications to any of the individual components, combination vaccines containing DTaP and other antigens can be used instead of separate injections. ACIP, AAP, and other experts state that a combination vaccine generally is preferred over separate injections of the equivalent component vaccines; considerations include provider assessment (e.g., number of injections, vaccine availability, likelihood of improved coverage, likelihood of patient return, storage requirements, cost), patient preference, and potential for adverse effects.

When there are no contraindications to any of the individual components, the commercially available fixed-combination vaccine containing diphtheria, tetanus, pertussis, and poliovirus antigens (DTaP-IPV; Kinrix®) can be used in children 4 through 6 years of age to provide the fifth dose of the DTaP vaccination series and the fourth dose of the IPV vaccination series in those receiving primary immunization with Infanrix® (DTaP) and/or Pediarix® (DTaP-HepB-IPV). Alternatively, the commercially available fixed-combination vaccine containing diphtheria, tetanus, pertussis, and poliovirus antigens (DTaP-IPV; Quadracel®) can be used in children 4 through 6 years of age to provide the fifth dose of the DTaP vaccination series and the fourth or fifth dose of the IPV vaccination series in those receiving primary immunization with Daptacel® (DTaP) and/or Pentacel® (DTaP-IPV/Hib). (For information on Kinrix® and Quadracel®, see Poliovirus Vaccine Inactivated 80:12.)

The commercially available fixed-combination vaccine containing diphtheria, tetanus, pertussis, hepatitis B, and poliovirus antigens (DTaP-HepB-IPV; Pediarix®) can be used for a 3-dose immunization series in infants and children 6 weeks through 6 years of age if there are no contraindications to any of the individual components. For the prevention of diphtheria, tetanus, and pertussis in infants and children 6 weeks through 6 years of age, Pediarix® may be used for the initial 3 doses in the DTaP series or may be used to complete the first 3 doses of the DTaP series in children who have received 1 or 2 doses of Infanrix® DTaP; data are not available regarding the safety and efficacy of Pediarix® used following 1 or more doses of a DTaP vaccine from a different manufacturer. Children who have received a 3-dose series of Pediarix® should complete the DTaP and IPV series according to the recommended childhood immunization schedule. To complete the DTaP series, the manufacturer recommends that Infanrix® be used for the fourth dose of DTaP and either Infanrix® DTaP or DTaP-IPV (Kinrix®) be used as the fifth dose of DTaP since these vaccines contain the same pertussis antigens as Pediarix®. (For information on Pediarix®, see Poliovirus Vaccine Inactivated 80:12 and see Hepatitis B Vaccine 80:12.)

The combination vaccine containing diphtheria, tetanus, pertussis, poliovirus, and Hib antigens (DTaP-IPV/Hib; Pentacel®) can be used as a 4-dose series for immunization in infants and children 6 weeks through 4 years of age when doses of DTaP, IPV, and Hib vaccine are indicated and there are no contraindications to any of the individual components. For prevention of diphtheria, tetanus, and pertussis, Pentacel® may be used for the initial 4 doses in the DTaP series at 2, 4, 6, and 15 through 18 months of age and a dose of Daptacel® should be given at 4 through 6 years of age to provide the fifth dose of DTaP. Pentacel® also may be used in infants and children 6 weeks through 4 years of age who have received 1 or more doses of Daptacel® DTaP. However, data are not available on the safety and immunogenicity of mixed sequences of Pentacel® and Daptacel® for successive doses in the DTaP series or mixed sequences of Pentacel® and DTaP from other manufacturers. (For information on Pentacel®, see Poliovirus Vaccine Inactivated 80:12 and see Haemophilus b Vaccine 80:12.)

■ Risks of Diphtheria, Tetanus, and Pertussis Exposure and Infection

Diphtheria Diphtheria is caused by toxigenic strains of *Corynebacterium diphtheriae* or, rarely, toxigenic strains of *C. ulcerans*. Diphtheria occurs worldwide, particularly in tropical countries. Although diphtheria occurs rarely in the US, *C. diphtheriae* continues to circulate in the US in areas where diphtheria previously was endemic.

Before widespread immunization against the disease, diphtheria was a major cause of morbidity and mortality among children. During the 1920s, there were approximately 100,000–200,000 cases of diphtheria and 13,000–15,000 diphtheria-related deaths each year in the US. From 1980 through 2011, 55 cases of diphtheria were reported in the US with an average of 1–2 per year (range: 0–5 cases per year). In 1996, toxigenic *C. diphtheriae* was isolated from residents of a Native American community in South Dakota and toxigenic *C. ulcerans* was isolated from an individual in Indiana with respiratory diphtheria. In 1999, a resident of Washington died from an illness clinically consistent with respiratory diphtheria and toxigenic *C. ulcerans* was isolated from a throat swab. In 2003, fatal respiratory diphtheria occurred in an unvaccinated Pennsylvania resident who had returned from a trip to rural Haiti (a country where diphtheria is endemic).

Most cases of diphtheria occur in individuals who are unvaccinated or incompletely vaccinated against the disease.

Diphtheria is endemic in many countries in Asia, the South Pacific, the Middle East, and Eastern Europe and also is endemic in Haiti and the Dominican Republic. Since 2011, large outbreaks of diphtheria have occurred in Indonesia, Thailand, and Laos. Individuals who are unvaccinated or inadequately vaccinated against diphtheria, especially travelers who will live or work with local populations in countries where diphtheria is endemic, are at risk.

The US Centers for Disease Control and Prevention (CDC) Travelers' Health website (http://wwwnc.cdc.gov/travel) should be consulted for information regarding where diphtheria is endemic.

Tetanus Tetanus is a potentially fatal disease caused by a neurotoxic exotoxin (tetanospasmin) produced by *Clostridium tetani*. Tetanus occurs worldwide, but is reported most frequently in densely populated regions in hot, damp climates with soil rich in organic matter.

In the US, a marked decrease in mortality from tetanus occurred from the early 1900s to the late 1940s when immunization against tetanus became part of routine childhood immunization. From 2001 through 2008, 233 cases of tetanus were reported in the US (average of 29 per year) with a case fatality rate of 13%.

Tetanus is not transmitted person-to-person. *C. tetani* usually enters the body through a wound. Any open wound can become contaminated with *C. tetani*, including tetanus-prone wounds (wounds contaminated with dirt, feces, soil, or saliva; deep wounds; burns; crush injuries; wounds containing devitalized or necrotic tissue) and apparently clean, superficial wounds (wounds from surgical procedures, insect bites, animal bites, dental infections, compound fractures, chronic sores and infections, IV drug abuse). Heroin users, particularly those who inject themselves subcutaneously, appear to be at high risk for tetanus. Most cases of tetanus in the US occur following an acute wound, usually a puncture or contaminated, infected, or devitalized wound considered tetanus-prone.

Almost all reported cases of tetanus occur in individuals who are unvaccinated or inadequately vaccinated against the disease (i.e., received an incomplete primary immunization series or received a complete primary series but did not receive recommended booster doses).

Because *C. tetani* spores are ubiquitous in the environment worldwide, travelers can acquire tetanus anywhere in the world if they are unvaccinated or incompletely vaccinated against the disease. Tetanus is more common in rural and agricultural regions, areas where contact with soil or animal excreta is more likely, and areas where immunization rates are inadequate.

Pertussis Pertussis (whooping cough) is an acute respiratory tract infection caused by *Bordetella pertussis*. Pertussis remains endemic worldwide (even in areas with high vaccination rates); the incidence is highest in young children in developing countries and other countries where routine immunization against pertussis is not widely practiced. Before widespread immunization against the disease, pertussis was one of the most common childhood diseases and a major cause of morbidity and mortality among children in the US. There were more than 1 million cases of pertussis reported in the US from 1940 through 1945 (average of 175,000 cases per year). After pertussis immunization was introduced, the incidence of the disease gradually declined and the average number of cases reported per year in the US during 1980–1990 was 2900. However, pertussis incidence has been gradually increasing since the early 1980s. During 2010, there were 27,550 cases of pertussis and 27 pertussis-related deaths reported in the US. The risk for severe pertussis and death is highest among infants younger than 1 year of age (especially those younger than 6 months of age). In recent years, adolescents 11 years of age or older and adults have accounted for an increasing proportion of pertussis cases. *B. pertussis* infection in adults and adolescents may be asymptomatic or range from mild to severe. Outbreaks involving adolescents have occurred in various settings (e.g., middle and high schools, residence facilities for disabled individuals, entire communities). Adults and older siblings (including adolescents) with asymptomatic or mild pertussis are important sources of pertussis in unvaccinated or incompletely vaccinated infants and young children.

Pertussis is highly communicable and 80–90% of nonimmune or unvaccinated household contacts acquire the disease. Transmission occurs via large respiratory droplets generated by coughing or sneezing or direct contact with respiratory secretions. Communicability is most likely during the catarrhal stage or early paroxysmal phase and untreated patients (especially infants) may remain infectious for 6 weeks or longer. Older children and adults with a history of previous pertussis infection or vaccination who develop pertussis may remain infectious for up to 14–21 days. Anti-infective therapy may limit the communicability of pertussis and also may ameliorate the disease if given in the catarrhal stage.

■ Primary and Booster Immunization with Diphtheria and Tetanus Toxoids and Acellular Pertussis Vaccine Adsorbed (DTaP)

Infants and Children 6 Weeks through 6 Years of Age ACIP, AAP, and other experts recommend that *all* infants receive primary immunization against diphtheria, tetanus, and pertussis. Therefore, a fixed-combination preparation that contains antigens for all 3 diseases (DTaP) is preferred for primary and booster immunization in infants and children 6 weeks through 6 years of age, unless a component is contraindicated or should not be used.

The complete vaccination series against diphtheria, tetanus, and pertussis in children younger than 7 years of age generally requires 5 doses of DTaP. ACIP, AAP, and other experts state that DTaP doses preferably should be administered at 2, 4, 6, 15 through 18 months of age, and 4 through 6 years of age. The fourth DTaP dose (booster dose) may be given as early as 12 months of age, provided at least 6 months have elapsed since the third dose. The fifth dose (booster dose) is not necessary if the fourth dose was administered at 4 years of age or older. (See Dosage and Administration: Dosage.)

Preterm infants generally should receive primary immunization with usual doses of DTaP at the usual chronologic age (even if the child still is in the hospital). (See Cautions: Pediatric Precautions.)

Immunization of infants younger than 6 weeks of age against diphtheria, tetanus, and pertussis generally should not be attempted because most infants have maternal antibodies that may prevent a satisfactory immunologic response to DTaP. However, ACIP states that individual circumstances may warrant administration of the first 3 doses of vaccine at 6, 10, and 14 weeks of age to provide protection as early as possible, especially during pertussis outbreaks. In addition, AAP states that if pertussis is prevalent in the community, the first dose of vaccine can be given as early as 6 weeks of age, with subsequent doses given as frequently as 4 weeks apart.

Primary immunization against diphtheria, tetanus, and pertussis can be integrated with primary immunization against *Haemophilus influenzae* type b (Hib), hepatitis A, hepatitis B, human papillomavirus (HPV), influenza, measles, mumps, rubella, meningococcal disease, pneumococcal disease, poliomyelitis, rotavirus, and varicella. (See Drug Interactions: Vaccines.)

If initiation or continuation of primary or booster immunization with DTaP is contraindicated because of the pertussis component, infants and children 6 weeks through 6 years of age should receive the fixed-combination preparation containing only diphtheria and tetanus toxoids (diphtheria and tetanus toxoids adsorbed [DT]). (See Diphtheria and Tetanus Toxoids Adsorbed/Tetanus and Diphtheria Toxoids Adsorbed 80:08.)

Children with Altered Immunocompetence ACIP states that DTaP and other toxoids can be administered safely to individuals with altered immunocompetence and the usual doses and immunization schedules are recommended. However, effectiveness of immunizations may be suboptimal in such patients. (See Drug Interactions: Immunosuppressive Agents.)

ACIP, AAP, CDC, National Institutes of Health (NIH), HIV Medicine Association of the Infectious Diseases Society of America (IDSA), Pediatric Infectious Diseases Society, and other experts recommend that children with asymptomatic or symptomatic human immunodeficiency virus (HIV) infection, including those who are immunosuppressed in association with acquired immunodeficiency syndrome (AIDS) or other clinical manifestations of HIV infection, receive primary and booster immunization against diphtheria, tetanus, and pertussis according to the usual recommended schedules. However, immunization may be less effective in HIV-infected individuals than in immunocompetent individuals.

Internationally Adopted Children and Other Immigrants The number of children adopted from outside the US has increased substantially in recent years and the immune status of such children may be difficult to determine base on country of origin and medical records. Children adopted from other countries whose immune status is uncertain should be vaccinated according to the US Recommended Childhood and Adolescent Immunization Schedules. (See Immunization Schedules, US 80:00.) The fact that immunization schedules of other countries may differ from US schedules (e.g., different recommended vaccines, recommended ages of administration, and/or number and timing of vaccine doses) should be considered. Vaccines administered outside the US can generally be accepted as valid if the administration schedule was similar to that recommended in the US childhood and adolescent immunization schedules. Only written vaccination records should be considered as evidence of previous vaccination since such records are more likely to accurately predict protection if the vaccines administered, intervals between doses, and child's age at the time of vaccination are similar to US recommendations; however, the extent to which an internationally adopted child's immunization record reflects their protection against disease is unclear and it is possible there may be transcription errors in such records (e.g., single-antigen vaccine may have been administered although a multiple-antigen vaccine was recorded). Although vaccines with inadequate potency have been produced in other countries, most of vaccines used worldwide are immunogenic and produced with adequate quality control standards.

When the immune status of an internationally adopted child is uncertain, ACIP recommends that health-care providers either repeat vaccinations (since this usually is safe and avoids the need to obtain and interpret serologic tests) and/or use selective serologic testing to determine the need for immunizations (helps avoid unnecessary injections). Regarding DTaP vaccination, ACIP states that health-care providers may revaccinate a child with DTaP without regard to the child's prior vaccination record; however, there is concern about this approach since data indicate increased rates of local adverse reactions after the fourth and fifth doses of DTP or DTaP (see Cautions: Local Effects). If a child adopted from another country is revaccinated with DTaP and experiences a severe local reaction, serologic tests for specific IgG antibody to tetanus and diphtheria toxins (if available) can be done prior to administration of additional doses. If protective levels of antibody are detected (defined as 0.1 international units per mL or higher for diphtheria and 0.1 international units/mL or higher for tetanus; a correlate of protection for pertussis has not been established), further DTaP doses are unnecessary and subsequent age-appropriate vaccination can occur.

An internationally adopted child whose vaccine record indicates that 3 or more doses of DTP or DTaP have been administered may be tested for serologic evidence of IgG antibody to diphtheria and tetanus toxins to determine the need for additional DTaP doses. If the child has protective concentrations of diphtheria and tetanus antibodies, their prior recorded immunization record may be considered valid and the DTaP vaccination series may be completed as age-appropriate. Children with indeterminate antibody concentrations may have immunologic memory but waning immunity; in this situation, unnecessary revaccination with a full series may be avoided if a booster dose of DTaP is given followed by repeat serologic testing. If a child's vaccination record indicates that 3 or more doses of DTP or DTaP have been administered, a single booster of DTaP can be given followed 1 month later by serologic testing for specific IgG antibody to diphtheria and tetanus toxins. If the child has antibody concentrations considered protective, their prior recorded immunization record can be considered valid. Children with indeterminate antibody concentration after a booster dose should be revaccinated with the complete DTaP series.

Travelers Tetanus, diphtheria, and pertussis occur worldwide, and travelers are at risk if they are unvaccinated or incompletely vaccinated against these diseases. (See Uses: Risks of Diphtheria, Tetanus, and Pertussis Exposure and Infection.)

CDC recommends that all travelers, including children, be adequately immunized against diphtheria, tetanus, and pertussis before leaving the US. If necessary to complete the vaccination series before departure, an accelerated immunization schedule using the age-appropriate minimum intervals between doses can be used. (See Dosage and Administration: Dosage.)

■ **Primary and Booster Immunization with Tetanus Toxoid, Reduced Diphtheria Toxoid and Acellular Pertussis Vaccine Adsorbed (Tdap)** ***Primary Immunization in Children 7 through 10 Years of Age*** Although safety and efficacy of Tdap have not been established for primary immunization or for use in children younger than 10 years of age, ACIP, AAP and other experts recommend that a *single* dose of Tdap be included in the vaccination series when primary immunization† is indicated in children 7 through 10 years of age† who are unvaccinated or incompletely vaccinated against diphtheria, tetanus, and pertussis, unless pertussis antigens are contraindicated or should not be used. Children are considered fully vaccinated if they have received 5 doses of DTaP or have received 4 doses of DTaP with the fourth dose administered on or after the fourth birthday.

The preferred primary immunization schedule in previously unvaccinated or incompletely vaccinated children 7 through 10 years of age† is a *single* dose of Tdap followed by the remaining required doses of Td; however, the Tdap dose may be substituted for any of the required doses of Td. These children should *not* receive the booster dose of Tdap usually recommended at 11 through 12 years of age.

Primary Immunization in Adolescents and Adults 11 through 64 Years of Age Although safety and efficacy of Tdap for primary immunization† have not been established, ACIP and AAP recommend that a *single* dose of Tdap be included in the vaccination series when primary immunization against diphtheria and tetanus is indicated in previously unvaccinated adolescents and adults 11 through 64 years of age.

Adolescents and adults with an incomplete or uncertain history of primary immunization against diphtheria and tetanus should receive primary immunization with 3 doses of a preparation containing diphtheria and tetanus toxoids. Because such individuals also may be susceptible to pertussis, ACIP, AAP, and other experts recommend that primary immunization† against diphtheria and tetanus in previously unvaccinated adolescents and adults 11 through 64 years of age include a *single* dose of Tdap, unless pertussis antigens are contraindicated or should not be used. The preferred primary immunization schedule in previously unvaccinated adolescents and adults 11 through 64 years of age is a *single* dose of Tdap followed by a dose of Td given at least 4 weeks after the Tdap dose and a second dose of Td given 6–12 months after the first dose of Td; however, the Tdap dose may be substituted for any 1 of the 3 doses of Td. Individuals who previously received Tdap should receive Td for all subsequent primary or booster doses.

Booster Immunization in Adolescents 10 through 18 Years of Age Tdap (Adacel®, Boostrix®) is used for booster immunization against tetanus, diphtheria, and pertussis in adolescents 10 through 18 years of age.

ACIP, AAP, and other experts recommend that *all* adolescents who received primary immunization with DTaP, DTP (not commercially available in the US), DT, or Td receive a booster dose of a preparation containing diphtheria and tetanus toxoids at 11 through 18 years of age (preferably at 11 through 12 years of age). Because adolescents also may be at risk for pertussis, ACIP, AAP, and other experts recommend that a *single* dose of Tdap (Adacel®, Boostrix®) be used (instead of Td) for the adolescent booster dose at 11 through 18 years of age (preferably at 11 through 12 years of age), unless pertussis antigens are contraindicated or should not be used. If Tdap is unavailable or was administered previously, Td should be used for this adolescent booster dose.

Booster Immunization in Adults 19 Years of Age or Older Tdap (Adacel®, Boostrix®) is used for booster immunization against tetanus, diphtheria, and pertussis in adults. Tdap (Adacel®) is labeled by FDA for use in adults 19 through 64 years of age; Tdap (Boostrix®) is labeled by FDA for use in adults 19 years of age or older (including those 65 years of age or older).

Adults who received primary immunization against diphtheria and tetanus should receive routine booster doses of Td every 10 years. In addition, an emergency booster dose of Td may be indicated in the event of injury and possible exposure to tetanus infection. (See Uses: Postexposure Prophylaxis of Tetanus.) Because adults also may be at risk for pertussis, ACIP and other experts recommend that *all* adults (including those 65 years of age or older) receive a *single* dose of Tdap (instead of Td) when a booster dose is needed in those who have *not* previously received a dose of Tdap, unless pertussis antigens are contraindicated or should not be used. The Tdap booster dose can be administered regardless of the interval since the last dose of vaccine containing tetanus or diphtheria toxoids (e.g., Td). Although a long interval between Td and Tdap may decrease the occurrence of local reactions and an interval of at least 5 years usually has been recommended between the last dose of any vaccine containing diphtheria, tetanus, or pertussis antigens and Tdap, ACIP states that the benefits of protection against pertussis outweigh the potential risk for adverse effects. If Tdap is not available or was administered previously, Td should be used for booster doses.

A *single* Tdap dose is recommend for *all* adult 65 years of age or older who have *not* previously received a dose. Because only Tdap (Boostrix®) is labeled by FDA for booster immunization in adults 65 years of age or older, Tdap (Boostrix®) should be used when feasible. However, ACIP states that both Tdap (Adacel®) and Tdap (Boostrix®) are immunogenic and either Tdap vaccine would provide protection when used for booster immunization in this age group. Because any opportunity to administer Tdap to adults 65 years of age or older should not be missed, ACIP states that providers may administer the Tdap (Adacel®, Boostrix®) that is available.

Adolescents and Adults in Contact with Infants ACIP and AAP recommend that adolescents and adults who have or anticipate having close contact with an infant younger than 12 months of age (e.g., parents, siblings, grandparents, childcare providers, health-care personnel) who have *not* previously received Tdap receive a *single* booster dose of Tdap to provide protection against pertussis and reduce the likelihood of pertussis transmission to the infant. Ideally, the Tdap dose should be given at least 2 weeks prior to beginning close contact with the infant. If indicated for pertussis vaccination, Tdap should be administered regardless of the interval since the last dose of vaccine containing diphtheria or tetanus toxoids (e.g., Td).

Pregnant Women Unless contraindicated, all women of childbearing potential should be adequately immunized against tetanus, diphtheria, and pertussis. Pregnant women who are immune to these diseases can confer protection to their infants through transplacental transfer of maternal antibody.

Obstetric and neonatal tetanus and obstetric and neonatal diphtheria are prevented if protective levels of tetanus and diphtheria antitoxin (i.e., at least 0.1 international units when tested using enzyme-linked immunosorbent assay [ELISA]) are present in the mother. Although the effectiveness and optimal concentration of maternal antipertussis antibodies that would provide protection is not known, high levels of maternal antibodies in neonates during the first few weeks after birth are likely to confer protection and might prevent or modify severity of the disease.

Because of the risks associated with diphtheria, tetanus, and pertussis, ACIP, AAP, and other experts state that pregnancy is not considered a contraindication for preparations containing diphtheria and tetanus toxoids, including Tdap.

Ideally, primary immunization against tetanus and diphtheria should be completed prior to pregnancy. If primary immunization against these diseases is initiated in previously unvaccinated or incompletely vaccinated pregnant women, ACIP and others recommend that a dose of Tdap be substituted for one of the required Td doses, preferably during the third trimester (optimally between 27 and 36 weeks of gestation). In addition, to ensure protection against pertussis, ACIP and other experts recommend that a dose of Tdap be administered during *each* pregnancy, regardless of the woman's prior vaccination history. Although Tdap can be administered any time during the pregnancy, the optimal time that maximizes maternal antibody response and passive antibody transfer to the infant is between 27 and 36 weeks of gestation. (See Pregnancy under Cautions: Pregnancy and Lactation.)

Health-care Personnel Health-care personnel should have documentation of age-appropriate primary immunization with a preparation containing diphtheria and tetanus toxoids and booster doses of Td every 10 years. In addition, ACIP recommends that *all* health-care personnel (regardless of age) receive a *single* dose of Tdap if they have *not* previously received a dose. Vaccinating health-care personnel with Tdap protects them against pertussis and also is expected to reduce transmission of pertussis to patients. Priority should be given to those who have direct contact with infants younger than 12 months of age.

Health-care personnel who do not have documentation of primary immunization against diphtheria and tetanus should received a 3-dose vaccination series using Tdap for the first dose and Td for subsequent primary and booster doses. Previously vaccinated health-care personnel who have *not* received a dose of Tdap should receive a dose as soon as feasible, regardless of the interval since the last dose of vaccine containing diphtheria or tetanus toxoids (e.g., Td). Td should be used for subsequent booster doses.

Hospitals and ambulatory care facilities should provide Tdap for health-care personnel and should use approaches that maximize vaccination rates (e.g., education regarding the benefits of vaccination, convenient access, provision of Tdap at no charge).

Travelers Tetanus, diphtheria, and pertussis occur worldwide, and travelers are at risk if they are unvaccinated or incompletely vaccinated against these diseases. (See Uses: Risks of Diphtheria, Tetanus, and Pertussis Exposure and Infection.)

CDC recommends that all travelers, including adolescents and adults, be adequately immunized against diphtheria, tetanus, and pertussis before leaving the US.

Adults, adolescents, and children 7 through 10 years of age† who are unvaccinated or incompletely vaccinated should receive a *single* dose of Tdap (unless the pertussis antigens are contraindicated or should not be used) followed by the recommended doses of Td according to the usual age-appropriate catch-up vaccination schedule. If necessary to complete the vaccination series before departure, an accelerated immunization schedule using the age-appropriate minimum intervals between doses can be used. (See Dosage and Administration: Dosage.)

Because immunity from childhood vaccination and natural disease wanes with time, previously vaccinated adults and adolescents 11 years of age or older who have *not* previously received a dose of Tdap should receive a *single* booster dose of Tdap. Individuals who have previously received Tdap should receive a booster dose of Td if indicated.

■ **Postexposure Prophylaxis of Diphtheria** Postexposure vaccination with a preparation containing diphtheria toxoid adsorbed may be indicated in addition to anti-infective postexposure prophylaxis in unvaccinated or inadequately vaccinated household and other close contacts of an individual with diphtheria.

Regardless of vaccination status, ACIP, AAP, and CDC recommend that all household and other close contacts of an individual with culture-confirmed or suspected diphtheria promptly receive anti-infective postexposure prophylaxis (single IM dose of penicillin G benzathine or oral erythromycin given for 7–10 days). Samples for cultures should be taken prior to initiating anti-infective therapy and the individual should be observed for 7 days for evidence of diphtheria.

Individuals exposed to diphtheria who previously received less than 3 doses of a preparation containing diphtheria toxoid adsorbed or whose vaccination status is unknown or uncertain should receive an immediate dose of an age-appropriate preparation containing diphtheria toxoid adsorbed, and the primary vaccination series should be completed. In addition, close contacts who previously completed the primary vaccination series against diphtheria should receive a booster dose of an age-appropriate preparation containing diphtheria toxoid adsorbed if it has been 5 years or longer since their last booster dose.

Diphtheria carriers should receive an anti-infective regimen active against *C. diphtheriae*. Vaccination does not eliminate carriage of *C. diphtheriae*. However, diphtheria carriers who are unvaccinated or inadequately vaccinated should receive immunization using an age-appropriate preparation containing diphtheria toxoid adsorbed and those who are vaccinated but have not received a dose of a preparation containing diphtheria toxoid adsorbed within the last 5 years should receive a booster dose.

Because diphtheria infection does not necessarily confer immunity, the primary vaccination series using an age-appropriate preparation of diphtheria toxoid adsorbed should be initiated or completed during convalescence.

Diphtheria antitoxin (equine) (available in the US only from the CDC under an investigational new drug [IND] protocol) is no longer routinely recommended for postexposure prophylaxis of diphtheria in contacts, but may be recommended in *exceptional* circumstances for postexposure prophylaxis in individuals with known or suspected exposure to toxigenic *Corynebacterium*. (See Diphtheria Antitoxin (Equine) 80:04.) To obtain diphtheria antitoxin (equine), clinicians should contact the CDC at 404-639-8257 from 8:00 a.m. to 4:30 p.m. EST Monday–Friday or the CDC Emergency Operations Center at 770-488-7100 after hours, on weekends, and holidays.

■ **Postexposure Prophylaxis of Tetanus** When active immunization against tetanus is indicated as part of postexposure prophylaxis after injury and possible exposure to tetanus infection in infants and children 6 weeks through 6 years of age, use of DTaP is preferred; however, DT should be used in this age group if the pertussis antigen is contraindicated.

Although Td usually is recommended in individuals 7 years of age or older requiring primary or booster immunization against tetanus as part of postexposure prophylaxis and wound management, a *single* dose of Tdap should be used instead of Td in adults and adolescents 11 years of age or older (including pregnant women and adults 65 years of age or older) who have *not* previously received a dose of Tdap, unless pertussis antigens are contraindicated or should not be used. If Tdap is not available or was administered previously, Td should be used for postexposure prophylaxis.

For information on tetanus-prone wounds and associated risks of tetanus and ACIP recommendations for postexposure prophylaxis of tetanus, see Uses: Postexposure Prophylaxis of Tetanus in Diphtheria and Tetanus Toxoids Adsorbed/Tetanus and Diphtheria Toxoids Adsorbed 80:08.

■ **Postexposure Prophylaxis of Pertussis** Postexposure vaccination with DTaP or Tdap may be indicated in addition to anti-infective postexposure prophylaxis in household and other close contacts of an individual with pertussis.

Regardless of vaccination status or age, ACIP, AAP, and CDC recommend that all household and other close contacts of an individual with suspected pertussis receive prophylaxis with an anti-infective active against *B. pertussis* (usually azithromycin, clarithromycin, erythromycin; alternatively, co-trimoxazole). In addition, all close contacts younger than 7 years of age who have not completed primary immunization with DTaP should complete the vaccination series with minimal intervals between doses. Those who received their third dose of DTaP 6 months or longer before the exposure should receive a fourth dose.

ACIP and AAP state that *all* individuals 7 years of age or older at increased risk of pertussis during pertussis outbreaks or because they are close contacts of an individual with pertussis (e.g., in a family, residential facility, school, school-related activity) should receive a *single* dose of Tdap if they have *not* previously received a dose. This includes children 7 through 10 years of age† who did not complete the DTaP vaccination series.

Dosage and Administration

■ **Administration** Diphtheria and tetanus toxoids and acellular pertussis vaccine adsorbed (DTaP) and tetanus toxoid, reduced diphtheria toxoid and acellular pertussis vaccine adsorbed (Tdap) are administered *only* by IM injection. DTaP and Tdap should *not* be administered subcutaneously, intradermally, or IV.

To ensure delivery into muscle, IM injections should be made at a 90° angle to the skin using a needle length appropriate for the individual's age and body mass, thickness of adipose tissue and muscle at the injection site, and the injection technique.

Depending on patient age, IM injections of DTaP or Tdap should be made into the anterolateral muscles of the thigh or deltoid muscle of the arm. In adults, adolescents, and children 3 years of age or older, IM injections should preferably be made in the region of the deltoid muscle. In infants and children 6 weeks through 2 years of age, IM injections should preferably be made into the anterolateral thigh; alternatively, the deltoid muscle can be used in those 1 through 2 years of age if muscle mass is adequate.

DTaP and Tdap should *not* be injected into the gluteal area or any area where there may be a major nerve trunk. If the gluteal muscle is chosen for infants younger than 12 months of age because of special circumstances (e.g., physical obstruction of other sites), it is *essential* that the clinician identify anatomic landmarks prior to injection.

DTaP and Tdap should be inspected visually for particulate matter and discoloration prior to administration. Prior to use, vials or prefilled syringes of DTaP or Tdap should be shaken vigorously until a uniform, turbid, white suspension results. DTaP and Tdap should not be used if the vaccines cannot be resuspended.

Syncope (vasovagal or vasodepressor reaction; fainting) may occur following vaccination; such reactions may be accompanied by transient neurologic signs (e.g., visual disturbance, paresthesia, tonic-clonic limb movements). Syncope occurs most frequently in adolescents and young adults. Procedures should be in place to avoid falling injury and to restore cerebral perfusion following syncope. Syncope and secondary injuries may be averted if vaccinees sit or lie down during and for 15 minutes after vaccination. If syncope occurs, the patient should be observed until symptoms resolve.

DTaP or Tdap should *not* be mixed with any other vaccine or solution. Although DTaP is commercially available in a kit containing DTaP and inactivated poliovirus vaccine (DTaP-IPV) and Haemophilus b (Hib) vaccine to provide a combination vaccine containing DTaP, poliovirus, and Hib antigens (DTaP-IPV/Hib; Pentacel®), extemporaneous vaccine combinations of DTaP or Tdap and other commercially available vaccines should *not* be prepared by admixing the vaccines.

When *passive* immunization with tetanus immune globulin (TIG) is indicated in addition to *active* immunization with a preparation containing tetanus toxoid adsorbed for postexposure prophylaxis of tetanus, DTaP or Tdap may be given simultaneously with TIG using different syringes and different injection sites.

DTaP or Tdap may be given simultaneously with other age-appropriate vaccines. (See Drug Interactions: Vaccines.) When multiple vaccines are administered during a single health-care visit, each parenteral vaccine should be given with a different syringe and at different injection sites. Injection sites should be separated by at least 1 inch (if anatomically feasible) to allow appropriate attribution of any local adverse effects that may occur.

■ **Dosage** The dosing schedule (i.e., number of doses) and specific preparation for primary and/or booster immunization (i.e., DTaP, Tdap) varies depending on age. *The age-appropriate recommendations for the specific preparation used should be followed.*

DTaP (Daptacel®, Infanrix®) is used *only* in infants and children 6 weeks through 6 years of age.

Tdap (Adacel®) is labeled by the US Food and Drug Administration (FDA) for booster immunization in adolescents 10 years of age or older and adults 19 through 64 years of age; Tdap (Boostrix®) is labeled by FDA for booster immunization in adolescents 10 years of age or older and adults 19 years of age or older. Although safety and efficacy of Tdap for primary immunization or for use in children younger than 10 years of age have not been established, ACIP recommends Tdap (Adacel®, Boostrix®) in catch-up primary immunization† regimens in children 7 through 10 years of age†. In addition, although only Tdap (Boostrix®) is labeled by FDA for use in adults 65 years of age or older, ACIP states that either Tdap (Adacel®) or Tdap (Boostrix®) can be used when booster immunization is indicated in this age group.

ACIP recommends that the same DTaP preparation used for the initial dose be used to complete the primary and booster immunization series since data is limited regarding safety, efficacy, or immunogenicity of the different DTaP vaccine preparations administered interchangeably in the primary or booster immunization series. However, if the particular DTaP vaccine used previously is not known or not available, any age-appropriate commercially available DTaP vaccine should be used to complete the vaccination series.

The complete primary vaccination series and recommended booster doses must be administered to ensure optimal protection against diphtheria and tetanus. Interruption of the recommended primary immunization schedule, regardless of length of time between doses, does not interfere with the final immunity achieved; it is not necessary to give additional doses or start the vaccine series over.

Diphtheria and Tetanus Toxoids and Acellular Pertussis Vaccine Adsorbed (DTaP) DTaP (Daptacel®, Infanrix®) is administered in 0.5-mL doses.

Each 0.5-mL dose of Daptacel® contains 15 Lf units of diphtheria toxoid, 5 Lf units of tetanus toxoid, and pertussis antigens consisting of 10 mcg of detoxified pertussis toxoid, 5 mcg of filamentous hemagglutinin (FHA), 3 mcg of pertactin, and 5 mcg of fimbriae types 2 and 3.

Each 0.5 mL of Infanrix® contains 25 Lf units of diphtheria toxoid, 10 Lf units of tetanus toxoid, and pertussis antigens consisting of 25 mcg of inactivated pertussis toxin, 25 mcg of FHA, and 8 mcg of pertactin.

Primary and Booster Immunization in Infants and Children 6 Weeks through 6 Years of Age. For primary immunization in infants and children 6 weeks through 6 years of age, ACIP, AAP, and other experts recommend that DTaP be given in a series of 3 primary doses and 1 or 2 booster doses. The first 3 doses of DTaP should be given at 4- to 8-week intervals (usually at 2, 4, and 6 months of age) and the fourth dose (booster dose) given approximately 6–12 months after the third dose (usually at 15 through 18 months of age). The fourth dose may be administered as early as 12 months of age, provided at least 6 months have elapsed since the third dose. Some manufacturers recommend that this dose be given at 15–20 months.

At 4 through 6 years of age (usually just prior to entry into school), children who received the fourth dose of the DTaP vaccination series at younger than 4 years of age should receive a fifth dose (booster dose). The fifth dose is not necessary if the fourth dose was given at 4 years of age or older.

For accelerated vaccination (e.g., for catch-up or prior to travel) in children 6 weeks to 6 years of age who did not receive DTaP at the usually recommended time in early infancy, a dose of DTaP should be given at the first visit and the second and third doses given at 4-week intervals after first dose. The fourth and fifth of DTaP doses should then be given at 6-month intervals after third dose. A fifth dose is not necessary if the fourth dose was given at 4 years of age or older.

Deferral of Pertussis Vaccination in Children 6 Weeks through 6 Years of Age. When initiation or continuation of DTaP vaccination is contraindicated because of the pertussis component of the vaccine (see Cautions: Precautions and Contraindications), children younger than 7 years of age should receive diphtheria and tetanus toxoids adsorbed (DT) to complete the vaccination series. If DTaP administration is deferred (e.g., while the neurologic status of the child is evaluated) and it is subsequently decided to proceed with the vaccination series following individual assessment in these children, there is no need to restart the series regardless of the time elapsed between doses.

Tetanus Toxoid, Reduced Diphtheria Toxoid and Acellular Pertussis Vaccine Adsorbed (Tdap) Tdap (Adacel®, Boostrix®) is administered in a 0.5-mL dose.

Each 0.5-mL dose of Tdap (Adacel®) contains 5 Lf units of tetanus toxoid, 2 Lf units of diphtheria toxoid, and pertussis antigens consisting of 2.5 mcg of detoxified pertussis toxin, 5 mcg of FHA, 3 mcg of pertactin, and 5 mcg of fimbriae types 2 and 3.

Each 0.5 mL of Tdap (Boostrix®) contains 5 Lf of tetanus toxoid, 2.5 Lf units of diphtheria toxoid, and pertussis antigens consisting of 8 mcg of detoxified pertussis toxin, 2.5 mcg of FHA, and 2.5 mcg of pertactin.

Primary Immunization in Children 7 through 10 Years of Age. Although safety and efficacy of Tdap have not been established for primary immunization or for use in children younger than 10 years of age, ACIP, AAP, and other experts recommend that primary immunization† against diphtheria, tetanus, and pertussis in previously unvaccinated or incompletely vaccinated children 7 through 10 years of age† include a *single* dose of Tdap, unless pertussis antigens are contraindicated or should not be used.

The preferred primary immunization schedule recommended by ACIP, AAP, and other experts for catch-up vaccination in children 7 through 10 years of age is a *single* dose of Tdap followed by a dose of Td given 1–2 months after the Tdap dose and a second Td dose given 6–12 months after the first Td dose. Alternatively, Tdap may be substituted for any 1 of the Td doses. Children who receive a dose of Tdap at 7 through 10 years of age† should *not* receive a Tdap booster dose at 11 through 12 years of age.

Primary Immunization in Adolescents and Adults 11 through 64 Years of Age. Although safety and efficacy of Tdap for primary immunization have not been established, ACIP recommends that primary immunization† against diphtheria and tetanus in previously unvaccinated or incompletely vaccinated adolescents and adults 11 through 64 years of age include a *single* dose of Tdap, unless pertussis antigens are contraindicated or should not be used.

The preferred primary immunization schedule recommended by ACIP, AAP, and other experts for previously unvaccinated adolescents and adults 11 through 64 years of age is a *single* dose of Tdap followed by a dose of Td given at least 4 weeks after the Tdap dose and a second dose of Td given 6–12 months after the first Td dose. Alternatively, the Tdap dose may be substituted for any 1 of the 3 doses of Td. Td should be used for all subsequent booster doses.

Booster Doses in Adolescents 10 through 18 Years of Age. All individuals who received primary immunization with DTaP, DTP (not commercially available in the US), DT, or Td receive a booster dose of a preparation containing diphtheria and tetanus toxoids at 11 through 18 years of age (preferably at 11 through 12 years of age) and routine booster dose of Td every 10 years to maintain adequate immunity against diphtheria and tetanus.

Because adolescents also may be at risk for pertussis, ACIP, AAP, and other experts recommend that a *single* dose of Tdap (Adacel®, Boostrix®) be used (instead of Td) for the adolescent booster dose at 11 through 18 years of age (preferably at 11 through 12 years of age), unless Tdap has already been given or the pertussis antigens are contraindicated or should not be used. If Tdap is unavailable or was administered previously, Td should be used for this adolescent booster dose.

Booster Doses in Adults 19 through 64 Years of Age. Adults who have received primary immunization against diphtheria and tetanus should receive routine booster doses of Td every 10 years. In addition, an emergency booster dose of Td may be indicated in the event of injury and possible exposure to tetanus infection. Because adults may be at risk for pertussis, ACIP and other experts recommend that a *single* dose of Tdap be used (instead of Td) when a booster dose is needed in adults 19 through 64 years of age who have *not* previously received Tdap, unless pertussis antigens are contraindicated or should not be used. If Tdap is not available or was administered previously, Td should be used for booster doses.

Booster Doses in Adults 65 Years of Age or Older. A *single* dose of Tdap should be used (instead of Td) when a booster dose of vaccine containing tetanus and diphtheria toxoids is needed in adults 65 years of age or older who have *not* previously received Tdap. Although only Tdap (Boostrix®) is labeled for use in adults 65 years of age or older, ACIP states that either Tdap (Adacel®) or Tdap (Boostrix®) can be used when a dose of Tdap is indicated in this age group. If Tdap was administered previously, Td should be used for subsequent booster doses. (See Uses: Primary and Booster Immunization with Tetanus Toxoid, Reduced Diphtheria Toxoid and Acellular Pertussis Vaccine Adsorbed [Tdap].)

Combination Vaccines Containing DTaP and Other Antigens
For information on dosage and administration of the fixed-combination vaccines containing DTaP and poliovirus antigens (DTaP-IPV; Kinrix®, Quadracel), see Poliovirus Vaccine Inactivated 80:12.

For information on dosage and administration of the fixed-combination vaccine containing DTaP and hepatitis B and poliovirus antigens (DTaP-HepB-IPV; Pediarix®), see Poliovirus Vaccine Inactivated 80:12 and see Hepatitis B Vaccine 80:12.

For information on dosage and administration of the combination vaccine containing DTaP and poliovirus and Hib antigens (DTaP-IPV/Hib; Pentacel®), see Poliovirus Vaccine Inactivated 80:12 and see Haemophilus b Vaccine 80:12.

Cautions

Diphtheria and tetanus toxoids and acellular pertussis vaccine adsorbed (DTaP) is associated with a lower incidence of adverse local reactions and a lower incidence of adverse systemic effects (including severe adverse effects) than diphtheria and tetanus toxoids and whole-cell pertussis vaccine adsorbed (DTP, also referred to as DTwP; not commercially available in the US).

The incidence and severity of adverse reactions reported to date with use of a single dose of tetanus toxoid, reduced diphtheria toxoid and acellular pertussis vaccine adsorbed (Tdap) in adolescents and adults have been similar to that reported with use of tetanus and diphtheria toxoids adsorbed (Td) in this age group.

■ Diphtheria and Tetanus Toxoids and Acellular Pertussis Vaccine Adsorbed (DTaP) ***Local Effects*** Local adverse effects, including pain or tenderness, erythema, and swelling, have been reported following administration of DTaP. Adverse local effects are reported more frequently and are more severe following booster doses of DTaP (fourth and fifth doses) than following the initial 3 doses in the vaccination series. This increased incidence of adverse effects with the fourth and fifth doses has been reported with all commercially available DTaP vaccines. Although additional safety data are needed to determine the frequency and severity of adverse events after a fifth dose of Daptacel® in children who have previously received 4 doses of the DTaP vaccine, data from studies evaluating Infanrix® indicate that higher rates of local injection site reactions (redness, swelling, pain) and larger local reactions occur following a fifth dose of the vaccine compared with the fourth dose. Adverse local reactions usually occur within 1–3 days after vaccination and resolve within about 5–7 days without sequelae.

In one study in infants and children who received Daptacel® at 2, 4, 6, and 17–18 months of age, the incidence of tenderness, erythema, or swelling was 4.3–12.7% after the first dose, 4.3–20.6% after the second dose, 4.7%–22.2% after the third dose, and 18.6–36.5% after the fourth dose.

In one study in US infants and children who received primary immunization with Infanrix® at 2, 4, and 6 months of age, the incidence of pain, erythema, or swelling at the injection site was 9.6–31.9% after the first dose, 20.4–32.8% after the second dose, and 24.8–39% after the third dose. When a booster dose of Infanrix® was given at 15–18 months of age in a US study in children who previously received 3 doses of the vaccine, 32.8–48.2% had pain, erythema, or swelling at the injection site and 33.2% had an increase in mid-thigh circumference on the leg where the dose was given. When the fifth consecutive dose of Infanrix® (booster dose) was given at 4–6 years of age, 27–53.3% had pain, erythema, or swelling at the injection site and 37.8% had an increase in arm circumference on the arm where the dose was given.

Edematous swelling, sometimes involving the entire injected thigh or upper arm has been reported following booster doses of DTaP (fourth or fifth doses). In US studies evaluating local reactions to the fourth and fifth consecutive doses of Infanrix®, 2.3% of infants 15–18 months of age had large swelling reactions (defined as swelling more than 50 mm in diameter, more than a 50 mm increase in thigh circumference, and/or any diffuse swelling that interfered with or prevented daily activities) occurring within 4 days of the fourth dose and 1% of children 4–6 years of age had large swelling reactions (defined as involving more than 50% of the upper arm length and associated with more than a 30 mm increase in mid-upper arm circumference) occurring within 4 days of the fifth dose.

The pathogenesis of these substantial local reactions and limb swelling is unknown. Analysis of data from one study indicated that swelling that increased limb circumference more than 5 cm after the fourth dose was associated with the pertussis toxoid content of the vaccine administered; swelling after the fifth dose was associated with the aluminum content of the vaccine; and entire thigh swelling after the fourth dose was associated with the diphtheria toxoid content of the vaccine. Prevaccination antibody titers to diphtheria, tetanus, or pertussis toxins were not predictive of these reactions. The inconsistent pattern of associations of vaccine content and swelling possibly could indicate that the associations were a statistical artifact attributable to a limited sample size or to differential reporting of entire thigh swelling among the DTaP vaccine groups. Whether children who experience entire limb swelling after a fourth dose of DTaP are at increased risk for this reaction after the fifth dose is unknown.

Systemic Effects Mild to moderate fever (38–40.4°), fretfulness or irritability, and drowsiness, have been reported following administration of DTaP. These systemic effects have been reported in 8.9–61.6% of children receiving the first 4 doses of Infanrix® and 7.7–43.2% of children receiving the first 4 doses of Daptacel®. Anorexia and vomiting have been reported in 4.3–11.2% of children receiving the first 3 doses of Daptacel®. Data are limited to date regarding the incidence of adverse systemic effects following the fifth dose of DTaP. In a study in US children, fever (37.5°C or greater), drowsiness, or loss of appetite was reported in14.8–17.5% after the fifth dose of Infanrix®.

Severe adverse effects, including fever (40°C or higher); unusual or persistent crying (lasting 3 hours or longer), seizures (febrile or nonfebrile), or hypotonic-hyporesponsive episodes, have been reported only rarely to date with DTaP. The incidence of these adverse effects appears to be substantially lower than that reported for DTP. In one large German study in which 22,505 infants received 66,867 doses of Infanrix®, severe adverse effects (in rates per 1000 doses) occurring within 8 days (including events interpreted by investigators as related as well as those interpreted as unrelated to vaccination) were unusual crying (0.09), febrile seizures (0.0), afebrile seizures (0.13), and hypotonic/hyporesponsive episodes (0.01). In a study in which 2587 infants received Daptacel® at 2, 4, and 6 months, serious adverse effects (rate per 1000 doses at 2, 4, and 6 months) reported were fever of 40°C or higher within 48 hours of vaccination (0.39), persistent crying 3 hours or longer within 24 hours of vaccination (0.39–1.16), seizures within 72 hours of vaccination (0), and hypotonic/hyporesponsive episodes occurring within 24 hours of vaccination (0.39).

■ Tetanus Toxoid, Reduced Diphtheria Toxoid and Acellular Pertussis Vaccine Adsorbed (Tdap) ***Local Effects*** In adolescents and adults 11 through 64 years of age who received a single dose of Tdap (Adacel®), pain at the injection site occurred in 66–78% and was the most frequently reported adverse effect. In addition, erythema occurred in 21–25% and injection site swelling occurred in 21%. Following a single dose of Tdap (Adacel®), rates of adverse effects at the injection site reported in adolescents 10 to less than 11 years of age are similar to rates reported in adolescents 11 to less than 12 years of age.

The most common local effects reported in adolescents and adults 10 through 64 years of age who received a single dose of Tdap (Boostrix®) were pain (61–75%), erythema (21–48%), swelling (18–39%), and increase in arm circumference of the injected arm (28%). In adults 65 years of age or older who received a single dose of Tdap (Boostrix®), pain, erythema, and swelling at the injection site were reported in 21.5, 10.8, and 7.5%, respectively.

Systemic Effects In adolescents and adults 11 through 64 years of age who received a single dose of Tdap (Adacel®), headache occurred in 34–44%, body ache or muscle weakness occurred in 22–30%, fatigue occurred in 24–30%, sore and swollen joints occurred in 9–11%, GI effects (nausea, diarrhea, vomiting) occurred in 3–13%, chills occurred in 8–15%, fever (38°C or higher) occurred in 1–5%, and rash occurred in 2–3%. Serious adverse events were reported in 1.5% of vaccine recipients, including neuropathic events such as severe migraine with unilateral facial paralysis and nerve compression in neck and left arm. Following a single dose of Tdap (Adacel®), rates of adverse systemic effects reported in adolescents 10 to less than 11 years of age are similar to rates reported in adolescents 11 to less than 12 years of age.

The most common systemic effects reported in adolescents and adults 10 through 64 years of age who received a single dose of Tdap (Boostrix®) were headache (30–43%), fatigue (28–37%), GI symptoms such as nausea, vomiting, diarrhea, and abdominal pain (16–26%), and fever (6–14%). In adults 65 years of age or older who received a single dose of Tdap (Boostrix®), fatigue, headache, GI symptoms, and fever occurred in 2–12.5%.

■ Precautions and Contraindications DTaP and Tdap are contraindicated in individuals who have had severe allergic reactions (e.g., anaphylaxis) after a previous dose of DTaP, any vaccine component, or any vaccine containing tetanus, diphtheria, or pertussis antigens. (See Sensitivity Reactions under Cautions: Precautions and Contraindications.)

DTaP and Tdap are contraindicated in individuals who have had encephalopathy (e.g., coma, decreased level of consciousness, prolonged seizures) within 7 days of a previous dose of a vaccine containing pertussis antigens that could not be attributable to another identifiable cause. The vaccines also are contraindicated in individuals with progressive neurologic disorder, including infantile spasms, uncontrolled epilepsy, or progressive encephalopathy. (See Precautions Related to Pertussis Components under Cautions: Precautions and Contraindications.)

To determine whether any contraindications to administration of DTaP or Tdap exist and to accurately assess the benefits and risks of the vaccines for each patient, the patient and/or the patient's parent or guardian should be questioned about the health status of the patient and questioned regarding the occurrence of any adverse effect after a previous dose.

The patient and/or the patient's parent or guardian should be informed of the benefits and risks of immunization with DTaP and Tdap and the importance of completing the primary immunization series and receiving recommended booster doses (unless there is a contraindication to further doses). The patients and/or the patient's parent or guardian should be provided with a copy of the appropriate Vaccine Information Statement (available at the CDC website http://www.cdc.gov/vaccines/pubs/vis/default.htm). Patients and/or the patient's parent or guardian also should be instructed to report any adverse reactions to their health-care provider. Clinicians or individuals can report any adverse reactions that occur following vaccination to VAERS at 800-822-7967 or http://vaers.hhs.gov.

When further doses of preparations containing pertussis antigens are contraindicated, DT should be used to complete the vaccination series in infants and children 6 weeks through 6 years of age and Td should be used in adults, adolescents, and children 7 years of age or older.

Precautions Related to Pertussis Components The pertussis components (antigens) contained in DTaP and Tdap are prepared from inactivated acellular pertussis and appear to be less reactogenic than the pertussis antigens prepared from inactivated or disrupted whole cells of *Bordetella pertussis* that are contained in DTP (no longer commercially available in the US).

Encephalopathy. ACIP, AAP, and the manufacturers state that encephalopathy (not due to another identifiable cause) that occurs within 7 days following a dose of any preparation that contains pertussis antigens (e.g., DTaP, Tdap, DTP) is a *contraindication* to doses of DTaP or Tdap, regardless of whether causation is established. Encephalopathy is defined as an acute, severe CNS disorder which may be manifested by coma or major alterations in consciousness or generalized or focal seizures that persist more than a few hours without recovery within 24 hours.

Progressive or Unstable Neurologic Disorders. ACIP, AAP, and the manufacturers state that DTaP and Tdap are contraindicated in individuals with progressive neurologic disorder, including infantile spasms, uncontrolled epilepsy, or progressive encephalopathy. DTaP and Tdap should be deferred in individuals with progressive or unstable neurologic conditions (e.g., cerebrovascular event, acute encephalopathic condition). It is not known whether administration to individuals with an unstable or progressive neurologic disorder might hasten manifestations of the disorder or affect the prognosis; administration in such individuals may result in diagnostic confusion between manifestations of the underlying illness and possible adverse effects of vaccination.

AAP states that pertussis immunization should be deferred (possibly permanently) in infants and children with progressive neurologic disorders characterized by developmental delay or neurologic findings (e.g., infantile spasms, other epilepsies beginning in infancy). Administration of DTaP in infancy may coincide with or hasten the recognition of inevitable manifestations of the disorder, with resulting confusion over causation. Such disorders should be differentiated from those that are nonprogressive with symptoms that may change as the child matures.

Stable neurologic conditions (e.g., cerebral palsy, well-controlled seizure disorder, developmental delay) are not considered contraindications for DTaP or Tdap.

Unexplained Fever, Collapse, or Crying. ACIP, AAP, and the manufacturers state that the following adverse reactions reported in temporal relation to previous doses of a preparation containing pertussis antigens (e.g., DTaP, Tdap, DTP) should be considered *precautions* for, rather than absolute contraindications to, doses of DTaP or Tdap: a temperature of 40.5°C or greater within 48 hours of a dose that is unexplained by another cause; collapse or a shock-like state (i.e., a hypotonic-hyporesponsive episode) within 48 hours of a dose; or persistent, severe, inconsolable screaming or crying lasting 3 hours or more occurring within 48 hours of a dose. Although many of these adverse effects previously were considered contraindications for pertussis vaccine, they are now considered precautions because they have not been proven to cause permanent sequelae.

The risks of giving subsequent doses of a pertussis vaccine to a child who has had one of these events are unknown; the possibility of another reaction of similar or greater severity may justify discontinuing pertussis immunization. However, in certain circumstances (e.g., during a community pertussis outbreak), the potential benefits of vaccination may outweigh the risks of another reaction. Whenever one of these adverse effects occurs in temporal relation to administration of a dose of DTaP, the decision to administer subsequent doses of DTaP or a dose of Tdap should be based on the clinical assessment of the prior reaction, the likelihood of pertussis exposure in the child's community, and the potential benefits and risks of pertussis vaccine.

Personal or Family History of Seizures. ACIP, AAP, and the manufacturers state that a seizure (with or without fever) occurring within 3 days of a dose of a preparation containing pertussis antigens (e.g., DTaP, Tdap, DTP) is considered a precaution (not a contraindication) for doses of DTaP or Tdap. Available data to date provide no convincing evidence that seizures alone, temporally associated with DTP administration, result in permanent brain damage, cause epilepsy, aggravate neurologic disorders, or affect the prognosis for children with underlying disorders.

Although there are uncertainties in reported studies, data suggest that infants and young children with a personal seizure history (whether febrile or not) appear to be more likely to have a seizure following administration of a pertussis-containing vaccine than those without such history. A seizure occurring within 3 days of DTP administration in a child with a seizure history may result from vaccine-induced fever (in children prone to febrile seizures), may be related to the pertussis component of the vaccine, or may be unrelated to the vaccine.

ACIP states that the decision whether and, if so, when to vaccinate children with a history of seizures must be decided on an individual basis. AAP states that because the risk of a postimmunization seizure is increased, pertussis immunization of children with recent seizures should be deferred until a progressive neurologic disorder is excluded; DTaP may be used in infants and children with well-controlled seizures or those in whom a seizure is unlikely to recur.

ACIP and AAP state that a family history of seizures in parents or siblings is not a contraindication or precaution for preparations containing pertussis antigens and that children with such family histories should receive DTaP according to the usual recommended schedule. AAP states that, although the risk of seizures in children with a family history of seizures may be increased, these seizures are usually febrile in origin and generally benign, and a family history of seizure disorders or a severe reaction following receipt of a pertussis-containing vaccine in another family member is not a contraindication. This recommendation is based on the risks of pertussis disease, the large number of children with a family history of seizures (5–7%), the clustering of these children within families, and the low risk of seizures following pertussis vaccination.

AAP states that prematurity is not believed to increase the risk of seizures following immunization, but the risk associated with certain types of prematurity (e.g., that with intracranial bleeding of varying severity) has not been fully determined. ACIP states that a history of prematurity generally is not a reason to defer immunization.

Although it is not known whether prophylactic use of antipyretics following administration of preparations containing pertussis antigens can decrease the risk of febrile seizures, some manufacturers state that acetaminophen or other appropriate antipyretic can be given at the time of DTaP vaccination and then every 4 hours for 24 hours after the dose to reduce the possibility of postvaccination fever. ACIP states that use of antipyretics in children with previous febrile seizures does not appear to be effective in preventing febrile seizures. Although evidence does not support use of antipyretics before or at the time of vaccination, antipyretics can be used for the treatment of fever or local discomfort that might occur following vaccination. Fever that does not begin until 24 hours or longer after vaccination or that persists for more than 24 hours following vaccination should not be assumed to be caused by vaccination; other causes for such new or persistent fever should be sought so that treatment is not delayed for serious conditions such as otitis media or meningitis.

Sensitivity Reactions Anaphylactic or anaphylactoid reactions, characterized by urticaria and angioedema, difficulty breathing, hypotension, and/or shock, have been reported following administration of preparations containing tetanus and/or diphtheria toxoids.

Prior to administration of DTaP or Tdap, the clinician should review the patient's history regarding possible sensitivity and any previous adverse reactions and should take all precautions known for prevention of allergic or any other adverse effects. Epinephrine and other appropriate agents and equipment should be available for immediate use in case an anaphylactic reaction occurs.

DTaP and Tdap are *contraindicated* in individuals hypersensitive to any ingredient in the formulations.

DTaP and Tdap are contraindicated in any individual who has had a severe allergic reaction (e.g., anaphylaxis) temporally associated with a dose of any preparation containing tetanus, diphtheria, or pertussis antigens. Because of the uncertainty as to which component might be responsible for the sensitivity reaction, no further doses of diphtheria, tetanus, or pertussis antigens should be administered. Alternatively, such individuals may be referred to an allergist for evaluation if further doses are being considered.

Arthus-type Hypersensitivity Reactions. Rarely, extensive local reactions (Arthus-type hypersensitivity reactions) may occur after injection of preparations containing tetanus toxoid. These reactions generally begin 2–12 hours after administration and are a local inflammatory reaction (vasculitis) that can include severe pain, swelling, induration, edema, hemorrhage, and necrosis. (See Cautions: Local Effects in Diphtheria and Tetanus Toxoids Adsorbed/Tetanus and Diphtheria Toxoids Adsorbed 80:08.)

Individuals who experience Arthus-type hypersensitivity reactions or fever greater than 39.4°C after administration of a preparation containing tetanus toxoid adsorbed usually have very high serum tetanus antitoxin levels and usually should not receive additional routine or emergency booster doses of a preparation containing tetanus toxoid adsorbed more frequently than every 10 years, even if postexposure prophylaxis of tetanus is indicated.

Latex Sensitivity. Some components (i.e., tip caps) of the single-dose prefilled syringes of DTaP (Infanrix®) Tdap (Adacel®, Boostrix®), DTaP-IPV (Kinrix®), and DTaP-HepB-IPV (Pediarix®) may contain natural rubber latex which may cause sensitivity reactions in susceptible individuals.

ACIP states that vaccines supplied in vials or syringes containing dry natural rubber or natural rubber latex may be administered to individuals with latex allergies other than anaphylactic allergies (e.g., history of contact allergy to latex gloves), but should *not* be used in those with a history of severe (anaphylactic) allergy to latex, unless the benefits of vaccination outweigh the risk of a potential allergic reaction. Contact-type allergy is the most common type of latex sensitivity.

Precautions Related to Booster Doses Parents or caregivers of children receiving booster doses of DTaP (fourth or fifth doses) should be informed that increases in reactogenicity have been reported with these doses compared with the first 3 doses of the vaccination series. Parents also should be informed that edematous swelling involving the entire thigh or upper arm has been reported. Whether children who experience entire limb swelling after a fourth dose of DTaP are at increased risk for this reaction after the fifth dose is unknown. However, because reports to date indicate that the reactions are self-limited and resolve without sequelae and because of the benefits provided by the preschool booster dose of DTaP (fifth dose), ACIP states that a history of extensive swelling after the fourth dose should not be considered a contraindication for receipt of the fifth dose of DTaP. The fact that these reactions may be clinically indistinguishable from other conditions (e.g., cellulitis) that require treatment should be considered. Therefore, ACIP recommends that providers make decisions regarding evaluation and management of children with suspected reactions to DTaP on a case-by-case basis.

Individuals with Altered Immunocompetence DTaP and Tdap may be administered to individuals immunosuppressed as the result of disease or immunosuppressive therapy. However, the possibility that the immune response to the vaccine and efficacy may be reduced in these individuals should be considered. (See Drug Interactions: Immunosuppressive Agents.)

Recommendations regarding use of DTaP or Tdap in adults, adolescents, or children with human immunodeficiency virus (HIV) infection are the same as those for individuals who are not HIV-infected. However, immunization may be less effective in HIV-infected individuals than in immunocompetent individuals.

Guillain-Barré Syndrome and Brachial Neuritis If Guillain-Barré syndrome (GBS) occurs within 6 weeks after receipt of a vaccine containing tetanus toxoid, the risk for GBS may be increased following a dose of DTaP or Tdap. Some manufacturers state that a decision to administer subsequent doses of DTaP, Tdap, or any vaccine containing tetanus toxoid in such patients should be based on careful consideration of the potential benefits and possible risks.

A review by the Institute of Medicine (IOM) found evidence of a causal relationship between tetanus toxoid and brachial neuritis and GBS. Analysis of active surveillance data collected during 1991 failed to demonstrate an increased risk of GBS in children or adults within 6 weeks following vaccination with a preparation containing tetanus toxoid adsorbed.

ACIP states that a history of GBS occurring within 6 weeks after a previous dose of a preparation containing tetanus toxoid adsorbed should be considered a precaution for subsequent doses of such preparations.

ACIP does not consider brachial neuritis a precaution or contraindication for further doses of preparations containing tetanus toxoid adsorbed.

Concomitant Illnesses A decision to administer or delay vaccination in an individual with a current or recent febrile illness depends on the severity of symptoms and etiology of the illness.

Minor acute illness, such as mild diarrhea or mild upper respiratory tract infection (with or without fever), generally does not preclude vaccination, but vaccination should be deferred in individuals with moderate or severe acute illness (with or without fever).

Limitations of Vaccine Effectiveness DTaP or Tdap may not protect all individuals from diphtheria, tetanus, and pertussis.

Optimum protection against diphtheria and tetanus is achieved with a primary series of 3 doses of preparations containing diphtheria and tetanus toxoids adsorbed.

Duration of Immunity Following primary immunization, the duration of protection against diphtheria is approximately 10 years.

Following primary immunization, the duration of protection against tetanus is approximately 10 years. Although some individuals may be protected for life, antitoxin levels decrease over time and only approach the minimal protective level in most individuals 10 years after last dose.

The duration of immunity against pertussis is estimated to be about 5–10 years or longer, but protection wanes over time. (See Pharmacology.)

Pre- and Postvaccination Serologic Testing Routine *prevaccination* serologic testing is not recommended prior to administration of DTaP or Tdap.

When postexposure prophylaxis against tetanus or preexposure vaccination in high-risk groups (e.g., travelers) is indicated, individuals with an unknown or uncertain history of vaccination generally should be considered unvaccinated and should receive the complete primary vaccination series.

To avoid unnecessary vaccination, ACIP states that *prevaccination* serologic testing for tetanus and diphtheria antitoxin antibodies can be considered in adults, adolescents, or children 7 years of age or older who probably were vaccinated but cannot produce vaccination records. If levels of tetanus and diphtheria antitoxin are both at least 0.1 international units/mL, previous vaccination with diphtheria and tetanus toxoids adsorbed can be assumed.

Use of Fixed Combinations When a fixed-combination vaccine containing diphtheria, tetanus, pertussis, and poliovirus antigens (DTaP-IPV; Kinrix®, Quadracel) is used, the cautions, precautions, and contraindications associated with each antigen should be considered. (See Poliovirus Vaccine Inactivated 80:12.)

When the fixed-combination vaccine containing diphtheria, tetanus, pertussis, hepatitis B virus, and poliovirus antigens (DTaP-HepB-IPV; Pediarix®) is used, the cautions, precautions, and contraindications associated with each antigen should be considered. (See Poliovirus Vaccine Inactivated 80:12 and see Hepatitis B Vaccine 80:12.)

When the combination vaccine containing diphtheria, tetanus, pertussis, poliovirus, and *Haemophilus* b (Hib) antigens (DTaP-IPV/Hib; Pentacel®) is used, the cautions, precautions, and contraindications associated with each antigen should be considered. (See Poliovirus Vaccine Inactivated 80:12 and see Haemophilus b Vaccine 80:12.)

Improper Storage and Handling Improper storage or handling of vaccines may reduce vaccine potency and can result in reduced or inadequate immune responses in vaccinees.

All vaccines should be inspected upon delivery and monitored during storage to ensure that the appropriate temperature is maintained. (See Chemistry and Stability: Stability.)

DTaP or Tdap that has been mishandled or has not been stored at the recommended temperature should not be administered.

If there are concerns about mishandling, the manufacturer or state or local immunization or health departments should be contacted for guidance on whether the vaccine is usable.

■ **Pediatric Precautions** Safety and efficacy of DTaP (Daptacel®, Infanrix®) in children younger than 6 weeks of age or in children 7 years of age or older have not been established.

Safety and efficacy of Tdap (Adacel®, Boostrix®) in children younger than 10 years of age have not been established.

Apnea has been reported following IM administration of vaccines in some infants born prematurely. Decisions regarding when to administer an IM vaccine in infants born prematurely should be based on consideration of the individual infant's medical status and potential benefits and possible risks of vaccination.

■ **Geriatric Precautions** Clinical studies evaluating the safety and efficacy of Tdap (Boostrix®) included adults 65 years of age or older, and this preparation is labeled by the US Food and Drug Administration (FDA) for booster immunization in geriatric adults.

Safety and efficacy of Tdap (Adacel®) have not been established in adults 65 years of age or older. Although Tdap (Adacel®) is not labeled by FDA for use in adults 65 years of age or older, ACIP states the vaccine can be used in this age group if it is the only Tdap vaccine available. (See Booster Immunization in Adults 19 Years of Age or Older under Uses: Primary and Booster Immunization with Tetanus Toxoid, Reduced Diphtheria Toxoid and Acellular Pertussis Vaccine Adsorbed [Tdap].)

■ **Mutagenicity and Carcinogenicity** Studies have not been performed to date to evaluate the mutagenic or carcinogenic potential of DTaP (Infanrix®) or Tdap (Adacel®, Boostrix®).

■ **Pregnancy and Lactation** ***Pregnancy*** Animal reproduction studies have not been performed with Tdap (Adacel®). A developmental toxicity study in female rats using Tdap (Boostrix®) at a dose approximately 40 times the human dose (on a mL/kg basis) did not reveal evidence of harm to the fetus. Animal fertility studies have not been conducted with Tdap (Adacel®, Boostrix®).

There are no adequate and well-controlled studies using Tdap in pregnant women, and it is not known whether the vaccine can cause fetal harm when administered to a pregnant woman or can affect reproductive capacity. The manufacturers state that Tdap should be used during pregnancy only when clearly needed.

ACIP and AAP state that pregnancy is not generally considered a contraindication to Tdap if a dose is indicated to provide protection against pertussis. ACIP states that available data do not suggest any elevated frequency or unusual patterns of adverse events in pregnant women who received Tdap and the few serious adverse events reported were unlikely to have been caused by the vaccine. These experts state that the potential benefit of preventing pertussis morbidity and mortality in infants outweighs theoretical concerns of possible severe adverse events.

Ideally, primary immunization against tetanus and diphtheria should be completed prior to pregnancy. Pregnant women who have not received primary immunization with DTaP, DTP (not commercially available in the US), DT, Td, or single-antigen tetanus toxoid adsorbed and those with unknown or incomplete tetanus immunization should receive a primary series of 3 doses of vaccine containing diphtheria and tetanus toxoids beginning during pregnancy. Although Td usually is the preferred preparation for primary or booster immunization against diphtheria and tetanus in adults, ACIP, AAP, and other experts state that *all* pregnant women should receive a dose of Tdap, regardless of prior vaccination.

When primary or booster immunization against diphtheria and tetanus is indicated during pregnancy in previously unvaccinated or incompletely vaccinated pregnant women, ACIP and other experts state that a dose of Tdap should be substituted for one of the required Td doses, preferably during the third trimester (optimally between 27 and 36 weeks of gestation). In addition, to ensure protection against pertussis, these experts recommend that a dose of Tdap be administered during *each* pregnancy, regardless of the woman's prior vaccination history. To maximize the maternal antibody response and passive antibody transfer to the infant, the optimal timing for the Tdap dose is between 27 and 36 weeks of gestation.

Pregnant women who were previously vaccinated but received the most recent dose of a preparation containing tetanus and diphtheria toxoids 10 or more years previously should receive a booster dose of a preparation containing tetanus toxoid during the second or third trimester of pregnancy (and before

36 weeks of gestation). This dose is important if the woman does not have sufficient tetanus immunity to protect against maternal and neonatal tetanus or if protection against diphtheria is needed (e.g., for travel to an area where diphtheria is endemic). ACIP and other experts state that Tdap should be used for the booster dose (instead of Td).

If postexposure prophylaxis of tetanus is indicated as part of wound management in a pregnant woman, the usual recommendations regarding emergency booster doses should be followed. (See Uses: Postexposure Prophylaxis of Tetanus.) Tdap should be used for the booster dose (instead of Td).

Clinicians are encouraged to register pregnant women who receive Tdap with the manufacturer's pregnancy registry at 800-822-2463 (Adacel®) or 888-452-9622 (Boostrix®).

Lactation It is not known whether Tdap (Adacel®, Boostrix®) is distributed into milk. The manufacturers state that Tdap should be used with caution in nursing women.

ACIP states that breast-feeding is not a contraindication for Tdap and women, including those who are breastfeeding, should receive a *single* dose of Tdap during the immediate postpartum period if they have *not* previously received a dose.

Drug Interactions

■ **Diphtheria Antitoxin (Equine)** If both diphtheria antitoxin (equine) (available in the US only from the US Centers for Disease Control and Prevention (CDC) under an investigational new drug [IND] protocol) and a dose of diphtheria and tetanus toxoids and acellular pertussis vaccine adsorbed (DTaP) or tetanus toxoid, reduced diphtheria toxoid and acellular pertussis vaccine adsorbed (Tdap) are required, they should be given at separate sites using different syringes. Although specific studies are not available, diphtheria antitoxin (equine) is unlikely to impair the immune response to diphtheria toxoid adsorbed.

■ **Immune Globulins** DTaP or Tdap may be administered simultaneously with (using different syringes and injection sites) or at any time before or after immune globulin (e.g., immune globulin IM [IGIM], immune globulin IV [IGIV]) or specific hyperimmune globulin (e.g., hepatitis B immune globulin [HBIG], rabies immune globulin [RIG], tetanus immune globulin [TIG], varicella zoster immune globulin [VZIG]).

When both active and passive immunization against tetanus is indicated, DTaP or Tdap may be administered concomitantly with TIG at a different site using a separate syringe.

■ **Immunosuppressive Agents** Individuals receiving immunosuppressive agents (e.g., corticotropin, corticosteroids, alkylating agents, antimetabolites, radiation therapy) may have a diminished immunologic response to DTaP and Tdap. Short-term (less than 2 weeks), low- to moderate-dose systemic corticosteroid therapy; long-term, alternate-day, systemic corticosteroid therapy using low to moderate doses of short-acting drugs; topical corticosteroid therapy (e.g., nasal, cutaneous, ophthalmic); or intra-articular, bursal, or tendon injections with corticosteroids should not be immunosuppressive. If immunosuppressive therapy is to be discontinued shortly, it is reasonable to defer routine DTaP vaccination until 1 month after the immunosuppressive agent is discontinued. If immunosuppressive therapy is likely to continue, routine vaccination should be initiated.

■ **Vaccines** Although specific data are not available regarding concurrent administration of DTaP or Tdap with all other available vaccines, the US Public Health Service Advisory Committee on Immunization Practices (ACIP), American Academy of Pediatrics (AAP), and American Academy of Family Physicians (AAFP) state that primary immunization against diphtheria, tetanus, and pertussis can be integrated with primary immunization against *Haemophilus influenzae* type b (Hib), hepatitis A, hepatitis B, human papillomavirus (HPV), influenza, measles, mumps, rubella, meningococcal disease, pneumococcal disease, poliomyelitis, rotavirus, and varicella. However, unless combination vaccines appropriate for the age and vaccination status of the recipient are used, each parenteral vaccine should be administered using a different syringe and different injection site.

Haemophilus b Vaccines DTaP can be administered concurrently with haemophilus b (Hib) conjugate (meningococcal protein conjugate) vaccine (PRP-OMP; PedvaxHIB®) or Hib conjugate (tetanus toxoid conjugate) vaccine (PRP-T; ActHIB®) at a different site using different syringes without a decrease in the antibody response or an increase in adverse reactions to either vaccine. Alternatively, depending on the age and vaccination status of the child and if there are no contraindications to any of the individual components, commercially available combination vaccines that contain DTaP and Hib antigens can be used instead of separate injections.

Alternatively, the combination vaccine containing DTaP and Hib and poliovirus antigens (DTaP-IPV/Hib; Pentacel®) can be used for primary or booster immunization in infants and children 6 weeks through 4 years of age when doses of DTaP, poliovirus vaccine inactivated (IPV), and Hib vaccine are indicated and there are no contraindications to any of the individual components. (For information on Pentacel®, see Poliovirus Vaccine Inactivated 80:12 and see Haemophilus b Vaccine 80:12.)

There is some evidence that extemporaneous combinations of Hib vaccine and other vaccines administered to infants 2–6 months of age may result in suboptimal immune responses to the Hib vaccine. Therefore, other commercially available DTaP and Hib vaccines should not be mixed extemporaneously.

Although an increase in serum concentrations of tetanus antitoxin may occur following administration of PRP-T, this Hib conjugate vaccine is not considered an immunizing agent against tetanus.

Hepatitis B Vaccine DTaP or Tdap may be given concurrently with hepatitis B vaccine using different syringes and different injection sites. Alternatively, depending on the age and vaccination status of the child and if there are no contraindications to any of the individual components, the commercially available fixed-combination vaccine containing DTaP and hepatitis B and poliovirus antigens (DTaP-HepB-IPV; Pediarix®) can be used instead of separate injections for primary immunization in infants and children 6 weeks through 6 years of age. (For information on Pediarix®, see Poliovirus Vaccine Inactivated 80:12 and see Hepatitis B Vaccine 80:12.)

Tdap (Adacel®) has been administered concurrently with hepatitis B vaccine in adolescents 11 through 14 years of age without a decrease in the antibody response to any of the antigens. Although the incidence of fever and injection site pain were similar when the vaccines were given concurrently or 4–6 weeks apart, the incidence of injection site erythema and swelling and swollen and/or sore joints and generalized body aches were slightly higher with concurrent administration.

Human Papillomavirus Vaccine Tdap (Adacel®) may be administered concurrently with human papillomavirus (HPV) vaccine using different syringes and different injection sites.

Human Papillomavirus Quadrivalent Vaccine (4vHPV; Gardasil®). Tdap (Adacel®) was administered concurrently with 4vHPV (Gardasil®) and meningococcal polysaccharide (serogroups A, C, Y and W-135) diphtheria toxoid conjugate vaccine (MCV4; Menactra®) in an open-label, randomized controlled study in 1040 boys and girls 11 through 17 years of age (mean age 12.6 years). Concurrent administration of these 3 vaccines at different injection sites did not interfere with the antibody response to any of the vaccine antigens compared with administration of 4vHPV (Gardasil®) alone followed by administration of Tdap (Adacel®) and MCV4 (Menactra®) concurrently at different sites 1 month after the 4vHPV (Gardasil®) dose. Although the overall incidence of adverse injection site and systemic reactions in those who received all 3 vaccines concurrently at different sites was similar to that reported when 4vHPV (Gardasil®) was given alone followed by Tdap (Adacel®) and MCV4 (Menactra®) 1 month later, concurrent administration was associated with an increased incidence of swelling at the 4vHPV (Gardasil®) injection site and an increased incidence of bruising or pain at the other injection sites.

Human Papillomavirus 9-valent Vaccine (9vHPV; Gardasil® 9). Tdap (Adacel®) was administered concurrently with human papillomavirus 9-valent vaccine, recombinant (9vHPV; Gardasil® 9) and MCV4 (Menactra®) in a randomized study in 1237 boys and girls 11 through 15 years of age. These adolescents received 9vHPV (Gardasil® 9) in one limb concurrently with Tdap (Adacel®) and MCV4 (Menactra®) given at different sites in the opposite limb or received 9vHPV (Gardasil® 9) in one limb followed 1 month later by Tdap (Adacel®) and MCV4 (Menactra®) given concurrently at different sites in the opposite limb. Although overall rates of adverse reactions at the injection sites in those who received all 3 vaccines on the same day (at separate sites) were similar to the overall rates reported when 9vHPV (Gardasil® 9) was given 1 month before the other 2 vaccines, an increased rate of swelling at the 9vHPV (Gardasil® 9) injection site occurred when all 3 vaccines were administered concurrently compared with administration of 9vHPV (Gardasil® 9) alone. Concurrent administration of all 3 vaccines did not interfere with antibody responses to 9vHPV (Gardasil® 9) or the other vaccines compared with administration 1 month apart.

Influenza Vaccine DTaP or Tdap may be given concurrently with influenza virus vaccine inactivated using a different syringe and different injection site.

Tdap (Adacel®) has been administered concurrently with influenza virus vaccine inactivated (Fluzone®) in adults 19 through 64 years of age without a clinically important decrease in the antibody response to tetanus, diphtheria, and influenza antigens. There was a lower antibody response to pertactin when Tdap (Adacel®) was administered concurrently with influenza virus vaccine inactivated, but responses to the other pertussis antigens (detoxified pertussis toxin, fimbriae types 2 and 3, filamentous hemagglutinin) were not affected. Although the booster response to the tetanus antigen was lower in those receiving Tdap and influenza vaccine concurrently compared with those who received the vaccines 4–6 weeks apart, at least 98% of individuals in both groups achieved seroprotective levels of tetanus antitoxin. The incidence of fever and injection site erythema and swelling were similar when the vaccines were given concurrently or 4–6 weeks apart; however, the incidence of injection site pain and swollen and/or sore joints were slightly higher with concurrent administration.

Concurrent administration of Tdap (Boostrix®) and influenza virus vaccine inactivated (Fluarix®) was evaluated in adults 19 through 64 years of age randomized to receive the vaccines concurrently (at different injection sites) or 1 month apart. The immune responses to the diphtheria, tetanus, and influenza antigens and the pertussis toxin antigen were noninferior following concurrent administration. However, the immune responses to the pertussis filamentous hemagglutinin (FHA) and pertactin antigens (measured as geometric mean antibody concentrations [GMCs] of anti-FHA and anti-pertactin) were lower when Tdap (Boostrix®) was administered concurrently with Fluarix® compared with administration 1 month apart; however, it is not known whether efficacy of the vaccine is affected by the reduced response to these pertussis antigens.

Measles, Mumps, Rubella, and Varicella Vaccines DTaP may be administered simultaneously with measles, mumps, and rubella virus vaccine live (MMR) and varicella virus vaccine live (using different syringes and different injection sites) or at any interval before or after the live viral vaccines.

Meningococcal Vaccine ACIP and AAP state that Tdap may be administered concurrently with MCV4 (Menactra®) using different syringes and different injection sites. If not given concurrently, ACIP states that the meningococcal vaccine may be given at any interval before or after Tdap; however, AAP states that the vaccines should be given at least 1 month apart if not given concurrently.

Tdap (Adacel®) was administered concurrently with MCV4 (Menactra®) and either 4vHPV (Gardasil®) or 9vHPV (Gardasil® 9) in randomized studies in adolescent boys and girls. Concurrent administration of the 3 vaccines at different injection sites did not interfere with the antibody response to any of the vaccine antigens. Although the overall incidence of adverse reactions in those who received all 3 vaccines concurrently at different sites was similar to that reported when 4vHPV (Gardasil®) or 9vHPV (Gardasil® 9) was given alone followed by Tdap (Adacel®) and MCV4 (Menactra®) 1 month later, concurrent administration was associated with an increased incidence of adverse local reactions at the 4vHPV (Gardasil®) or 9vHPV (Gardasil® 9) injection sites. (See Human Papillomavirus Vaccine under Drug Interactions: Vaccines.)

Concurrent administration of Tdap (Boostrix®) and MCV4 (Menactra®) was evaluated in a study in adolescents 11–18 years of age randomized to receive the vaccines concurrently (at different injection sites) or 1 month apart. The immune responses to the diphtheria, tetanus, and meningococcal antigens were noninferior following concurrent administration. However, the immune response to the pertactin pertussis antigen (measured as GMCs of anti-pertactin) was lower when Tdap (Boostrix®) was administered concurrently with MCV4; however, it is not known whether efficacy of the vaccine is affected by the reduced response to pertactin.

Concurrent administration of MCV4 (Menveo®) and Tdap (Boostrix®) and 4vHPV (Gardasil®) in adolescents 11 through 18 years of age did not interfere with the immune response to the meningococcal antigens. Although the clinical importance is unclear, the antibody response to some pertussis antigens was decreased when MCV4 (Menveo®), Tdap (Boostrix®), and 4vHPV (Gardasil®) were administered concurrently compared with Tdap (Boostrix®) alone. Systemic adverse reactions were more frequent in those receiving all 3 vaccines concurrently compared with administration of MCV4 (Menveo®) alone.

Pneumococcal Vaccine **Pneumococcal 13-valent Conjugate Vaccine.** DTaP may be administered concurrently with pneumococcal 13-valent conjugate vaccine (diphtheria CRM_{197} protein) (PCV13; Prevnar® 13) using different syringes and different injection sites.

Pneumococcal 23-valent Vaccine. Concurrent administration of DTaP and pneumococcal vaccine, polyvalent (pneumococcal 23-valent vaccine; PPSV23; Pneumovax® 23) does not increase the severity of adverse reactions or diminish the antibody responses to the vaccines. DTaP may be administered concurrently with PPSV23 (Pneumovax® 23) using different syringes and different injection sites.

Poliovirus Vaccine Inactivated DTaP may be administered concurrently with IPV using different syringes and different injection sites. Alternatively, depending on the age and vaccination status of the child and if there are no contraindications to any of the individual components, a commercially available fixed-combination vaccine containing DTaP and IPV (DTaP-IPV; Kinrix®, Quadracel®), the fixed-combination vaccine containing DTaP, IPV, and hepatitis B virus antigens (DTaP-HepB-IPV; Pediarix®), or the combination vaccine containing DTaP, IPV, and Hib antigens (DTaP-IPV/Hib; Pentacel®) can be used instead of separate injections. (For information on Kinrix® and Quadracel, see Poliovirus Vaccine Inactivated 80:12; for information on Pediarix®, see Poliovirus Vaccine Inactivated 80:12 and see Hepatitis B Vaccine 80:12; for information on Pentacel®, see Poliovirus Vaccine Inactivated 80:12 and see Haemophilus b Vaccine 80:12.)

Although data regarding the immunologic response are not available, IPV has been safely administered concurrently (at a separate site) with DTaP (Infanrix®).

Pharmacology

■ Response to Diphtheria and Tetanus Toxoids and Acellular Pertussis Vaccines Adsorbed (DTaP)

Diphtheria and tetanus toxoids and acellular pertussis vaccine adsorbed (DTaP) stimulates active immunity to diphtheria, tetanus, and pertussis by inducing production of specific antitoxins and antibodies. A complete primary immunization series with the age-appropriate preparations is needed to induce optimum levels of antitoxin antibodies that provide protection.

The diphtheria toxoid adsorbed component provides protection against the exotoxin elucidated by *Corynebacterium diphtheriae*. Primary immunization against diphtheria reduces the risk of developing diphtheria and the severity of clinical illness, but does not prevent or eliminate colonization or carriage of *C. diphtheriae* in the pharynx, nose, or skin of vaccinees. Protective levels of diphtheria antitoxin (defined as at least 0.1 international units/mL) are attained in at least 95% of individuals after the primary vaccination series. Following primary immunization, protective levels of diphtheria antitoxin levels may persist for about 10 years.

Tetanus toxoid adsorbed induces production of specific antitoxin antibodies that neutralize exotoxin produced by *Clostridium tetani*. A complete primary series of a preparation containing tetanus toxoid adsorbed results in protective levels of tetanus antitoxin that persist for approximately 10 years. Protective levels of tetanus antitoxin were previously defined as at least 0.01 international units/mL when measured by in vivo neutralization assay, but are currently defined as at least 0.1 international units/mL when measured by enzyme-linked immunosorbent assay (ELISA) or other methods. Although some individuals may be protected against tetanus for life following primary immunization with a preparation containing tetanus toxoid adsorbed, antitoxin levels decrease over time and only approach the minimal protective level in most individuals 10 years after the last dose of tetanus toxoid adsorbed. The antitoxin response induced by tetanus toxoid adsorbed has a longer duration than that induced by tetanus toxoid fluid (no longer commercially available in the US).

The acellular pertussis vaccine component includes several pertussis antigens and induces production of specific anti-pertussis antibodies; however, the mechanism of protection against the disease has not been fully determined. There is no accepted serologic or laboratory correlation of protection against pertussis. The duration of immunity following primary immunization against pertussis is estimated to be 5–10 years or longer, but protection wanes over time and vaccinated individuals may become susceptible to infection or reinfection. Residual immunity from previous infection or vaccination can lessen the severity of *B. pertussis* infection.

■ Response to Tetanus Toxoid, Reduced Diphtheria Toxoid and Acellular Pertussis Vaccine Adsorbed (Tdap)

Adolescents and Adults 10 through 64 Years of Age The immunologic response to a booster dose of Tdap (Adacel®) has been evaluated in adolescents and adults 11 through 64 years of age who were randomized to receive a dose of Tdap or tetanus and diphtheria toxoids adsorbed (Td); participants had not received a preparation containing diphtheria or tetanus toxoid within the last 5 years. One month after the booster dose, antibody responses to the tetanus and diphtheria antigens in individuals who received Tdap were similar to that in individuals who received Td. In addition, the antibody response to the pertussis antigens in Tdap was similar to that reported in infants who receive a 3-dose primary immunization series of DTaP (Daptacel®).

The immunologic response to a booster dose of Tdap (Boostrix®) has been evaluated in adolescents 10–18 years of age who were randomized to receive a dose of Tdap or Td; 98% had received the recommended series of 4 or 5 doses of DTaP and/or DTP (not commercially available in the US) in childhood. One month after the booster dose of Tdap, antibody responses to the tetanus and diphtheria antigens were similar in both groups and there also was an acceptable booster response to the pertussis antigens in Tdap (i.e., the response was similar to that reported in infants who receive a 3-dose primary immunization series of DTaP [Infanrix®]). In adults 19 through 64 years of age who had not received a dose of a preparation containing diphtheria and tetanus toxoids adsorbed within the last 5 years, a single booster dose of Tdap (Boostrix®) resulted in tetanus and diphtheria antitoxin levels 1 month after the dose that were seroprotective (i.e., at least 0.1 international units/mL) in 95.9 and 85.2% of patients, respectively. There also was an acceptable booster response to the pertussis antigens.

Adults 65 Years of Age or Older Based on prespecified criteria, administration of a dose of Tdap (Adacel®) in adults 65 years of age or older† was associated with lower geometric mean antibody concentrations (GMCs) to the pertussis antigens (pertussis toxin, filamentous hemagglutinin, pertactin) compared with GMCs reported in infants who received a primary immunization series of DTaP (Daptacel®).

In a randomized study in adults 65 years of age or older who had not received a dose of Td within 5 years, immune responses to the tetanus and diphtheria antigens measured 1 month after a single dose of Tdap (Boostrix®) were comparable to those attained in those who received a dose of Td. In addition, the GMCs to the pertussis antigens 1 month following a single dose of Tdap (Boostrix®) in adults 65 years of age or older were noninferior to those reported in infants following a primary immunization series of DTaP (Infanrix®).

Chemistry and Stability

■ Chemistry

Diphtheria and tetanus toxoids and acellular pertussis vaccine adsorbed (DTaP) and tetanus toxoid, reduced diphtheria toxoid and acellular pertussis vaccine adsorbed (Tdap) contain diphtheria and tetanus toxoids and a pertussis vaccine component that is prepared from inactivated acellular pertussis. In contrast to the many pertussis antigens present in the pertussis component of diphtheria and tetanus toxoids and whole-cell pertussis vaccine adsorbed (DTP, also referred to as DTwP; no longer commercially available in the US), only several biologically active components of *B. pertussis* are present in DTaP or Tdap. DTaP and Tdap, therefore, contain less endotoxin relative to DTP and, although immunogenic, are less reactogenic than DTP.

Diphtheria and Tetanus Toxoids and Acellular Pertussis Vaccine Adsorbed (DTaP) DTaP is a sterile suspension prepared by mixing suitable quantities of the two toxoids and acellular pertussis vaccine that have been adsorbed onto an aluminum adjuvant. There are 2 different DTaP preparations commercially available in the US. These preparations contain similar diphtheria and tetanus toxoids but slightly different acellular pertussis vaccine components. DTaP (Daptacel®) contains 5 distinct acellular antigens derived from *B. pertussis*; DTaP (Infanrix®) contains 3 distinct acellular antigens derived from *B. pertussis*.

DTaP (Daptacel®). DTaP (Daptacel®) contains diphtheria and tetanus toxoids prepared from toxins that are detoxified with formalin and purified by ammonium sulfate fractionation and diafiltration. The acellular pertussis vaccine component of DTaP (Daptacel®) contains 5 acellular pertussis antigens isolated from *B. pertussis* grown in modified Stainer-Scholte liquid media. The fimbriae types 2 and 3 are extracted from the bacterial cells and the pertussis toxin (PT), filamentous hemagglutinin (FHA), and pertactin (PRN) are prepared from the supernatant. The pertussis antigens are then purified using sequential filtration, salt-precipitation, ultrafiltration and chromatography. PT is detoxified with glutaraldehyde and FHA is treated with formaldehyde. Potency of the pertussis component is evaluated by measurement of the antibody response to PT, FHA, PRN, and fimbriae types 2 and 3 in immunized mice using ELISA; the diphtheria and tetanus toxoids are measured in a guinea pig potency test. The diphtheria, tetanus, and pertussis antigens are individually adsorbed onto aluminum phosphate.

After shaking, DTaP (Daptacel®) occurs as a homogeneous, white, cloudy suspension. Each 0.5 mL of DTaP (Daptacel®) contains 15 Lf units of diphtheria toxoid, 5 Lf units of tetanus toxoid, 23 mcg of pertussis antigens (10 mcg of detoxified PT, 5 mcg of FHA, 3 mcg of PRN, 5 mcg of fimbriae types 2 and 3) and 1.5 mg of aluminum phosphate adjuvant (0.33 mg of aluminum). Each 0.5 mL also contains not more than 5 mcg of residual formaldehyde, less than 0.05 mcg of residual glutaraldehyde, and 3.3 mg of 2-phenoxyethanol (not as a preservative). DTaP (Daptacel®) does not contain thimerosal.

DTaP (Infanrix®) DTaP (Infanrix®) contains diphtheria and tetanus toxoids that are concentrated by ultrafiltration, purified by precipitation, sterile filtration, and dialysis, and detoxified using formaldehyde. Any bovine materials used in preparation of the diphtheria and tetanus toxoids are obtained from countries which the US Department of Agriculture (USDA) has determined do not have and are not at risk of bovine spongiform encephalopathy (BSE). The acellular pertussis vaccine component of Infanrix® contains 3 acellular pertussis antigens isolated from *B. pertussis* grown in modified Stainer-Scholte liquid media. PT and FHA are extracted from the fermentation broth and PRN is extracted by heat treatment and flocculation. The pertussis antigens are then purified using successive chromatography steps. PT is detoxified using formaldehyde and glutaraldehyde; FHA and PRN are treated with formaldehyde. Potency of the pertussis component is evaluated by measurement of the antibody response to PT, FHA, and PRN in immunized mice using ELISA. The diphtheria, tetanus, and pertussis antigens are individually adsorbed onto aluminum hydroxide.

After shaking, DTaP (Infanrix®) occurs as a homogeneous, turbid, white suspension. Each 0.5 mL of DTaP (Infanrix®) contains 25 Lf units of diphtheria toxoid, 10 Lf units of tetanus toxoid, and 58 mcg of pertussis antigens (25 mcg of inactivated PT, 25 mcg of FHA, 8 mcg of PRN) and aluminum hydroxide adjuvant (not more than 0.625 mg of aluminum). Each 0.5 mL also contains 4.5 mg sodium chloride, not more than 100 mcg of residual formaldehyde, and not more than 100 mcg of polysorbate 80. Infanrix® does not contain thimerosal or any other preservatives.

Tetanus Toxoid, Reduced Diphtheria Toxoid and Acellular Pertussis Vaccine Adsorbed (Tdap) Tdap is a sterile suspension prepared by mixing suitable quantities of tetanus toxoid, diphtheria toxoid, and acellular pertussis vaccine that have been adsorbed onto an aluminum adjuvant. Tdap contains a lower content of diphtheria and pertussis antigens than that contained in DTaP. There are 2 different Tdap preparations commercially available in the US: Adacel® and Boostrix®.

Tdap (Adacel®). Tdap (Adacel®) contains the same tetanus toxoid, diphtheria toxoid, and acellular pertussis antigens as DTaP (Daptacel®); however, Adacel® contains a lower content of the diphtheria and pertussis antigens compared with Daptacel®.

After shaking, Tdap (Adacel®) occurs as a homogeneous white cloudy suspension. Each 0.5 mL of Tdap (Adacel®) contains 5 Lf units of tetanus toxoid, 2 Lf units of diphtheria toxoid, 15.5 mcg of pertussis antigens (2.5 mcg of detoxified PT, 5 mcg of FHA, 3 mcg of PRN, 5 mcg of fimbriae types 2 and 3) and 1.5 mg of aluminum phosphate adjuvant (0.33 mg of aluminum). Each 0.5 mL also contains not more than 5 mcg of residual formaldehyde, less than 0.05 mcg of residual glutaraldehyde, and 3.3 mg of 2-phenoxyethanol (not as a preservative). Tdap (Adacel®) does not contain thimerosal or any other preservatives.

Tdap (Boostrix®) Tdap (Boostrix®) contains the same tetanus toxoid, diphtheria toxoid, and acellular pertussis antigens as DTaP (Infanrix®); however, Boostrix® contains a lower content of all 3 antigens compared with Infanrix®.

After shaking, Tdap (Boostrix®) occurs as a homogeneous white turbid suspension. Each 0.5 mL of Tdap (Boostrix®) contains 5 Lf units of tetanus toxoid, 2.5 Lf units of diphtheria toxoid, 18.5 mcg of pertussis antigens (8 mcg of detoxified PT, 8 mcg of FHA, 2.5 mcg of PRN) and aluminum hydroxide adjuvant (not more than 0.39 mg of aluminum). Each 0.5 mL also contains 4.5 mg of sodium chloride, not more than 100 mcg of residual formaldehyde, and not more than 100 mcg of polysorbate 80. Tdap (Boostrix®) does not contain thimerosal or any other preservatives.

■ **Stability** DTaP (Daptacel®, Infanrix®) and Tdap (Adacel®, Boostrix®) should be stored at 2–8°C and should not be frozen. Any DTaP or Tdap vaccine that has been frozen should be discarded.

Preparations

Excipients in commercially available drug preparations may have clinically important effects in some individuals; consult specific product labeling for details.

Diphtheria and Tetanus Toxoids and Acellular Pertussis Vaccine Adsorbed (DTaP)

Parenteral

Injectable suspension, for IM use	Diphtheria Toxoid 15 Lf units, Tetanus Toxoid 5 Lf units, and Acellular Pertussis Vaccine 23 mcg (of pertussis antigens) per 0.5 mL	**Daptacel®**, Sanofi Pasteur
	Diphtheria Toxoid 25 Lf units, Tetanus Toxoid 10 Lf units, and Acellular Pertussis Vaccine 58 mcg (of pertussis antigens) per 0.5 mL	**Infanrix®**, GlaxoSmithKline

Tetanus Toxoid, Reduced Diphtheria Toxoid and Acellular Pertussis Vaccine Adsorbed (Tdap)

Parenteral

Injectable suspension, for IM use	Tetanus Toxoid 5 Lf units, Diphtheria Toxoid 2 Lf units, and Acellular Pertussis Vaccine 15.5 mcg (of pertussis antigens) per 0.5 mL	**Adacel®**, Sanofi Pasteur
	Tetanus Toxoid 5 Lf units, Diphtheria Toxoid 2.5 Lf units, and Acellular Pertussis Vaccine 18.5 mcg (of pertussis antigens) per 0.5 mL	**Boostrix®**, GlaxoSmithKline

Diphtheria and Tetanus Toxoids and Acellular Pertussis Adsorbed and Inactivated Poliovirus Vaccine (DTaP-IPV)

Parenteral

For injection, for IM use	Diphtheria Toxoid 15 Lf units, Tetanus Toxoid 5 Lf units, Acellular Pertussis Vaccine 48 mcg (of pertussis antigen) and Poliovirus Type 1 40 DU, Poliovirus Type 2 8 DU, and Poliovirus Type 3 32 DU per 0.5 mL	**Quadracel®**, Sanofi Pasteur
	Diphtheria Toxoid 25 Lf units, Tetanus Toxoid 10 Lf units, Acellular Pertussis Vaccine 58 mcg (of pertussis antigen) and Poliovirus Type 1 40 DU, Poliovirus Type 2 8 DU, and Poliovirus Type 3 32 DU per 0.5 mL	**Kinrix®**, GlaxoSmithKline

Diphtheria and Tetanus Toxoids and Acellular Pertussis Adsorbed, Hepatitis B (Recombinant) and Inactivated Poliovirus Vaccine Combined (DTaP-HepB-IPV)

Parenteral

Injectable suspension, for IM use	Diphtheria Toxoid 25 Lf units, Tetanus Toxoid 10 Lf units, Acellular Pertussis Vaccine 58 mcg (of pertussis antigen), Hepatitis B Surface Antigen 10 mcg, Poliovirus Type 1 40 DU, Poliovirus Type 2 8 DU, and Poliovirus Type 3 32 DU per 0.5 mL	**Pediarix®**, GlaxoSmithKline

Diphtheria and Tetanus Toxoids and Acellular Pertussis Adsorbed, Inactivated Poliovirus and Haemophilus b Conjugate (Tetanus Toxoid Conjugate) Vaccine (DTaP-IPV/Hib)

Parenteral

Kit, for IM use	Injection, for IM use, Diphtheria Toxoid 15 Lf units, Tetanus Toxoid 5 Lf units, Acellular Pertussis Vaccine 48 mcg (of pertussis antigen), Poliovirus Type 1 40 DU, Poliovirus Type 2 8 DU, and Poliovirus Type 3 32 DU per 0.5 mL	**Pentacel®**, Sanofi Pasteur
	For injectable suspension, for IM use, Haemophilus b Polysaccharide 10 mcg, Tetanus Toxoid 24 mcg per 0.5 mL, ActHIB®	

†Use is not currently included in the labeling approved by the US Food and Drug Administration

VACCINES 80:12

Haemophilus b Vaccine

Hib Polysaccharide Conjugate (Meningococcal Protein Conjugate Vaccine), Hib (PRP-OMP), PRP-OMPHib Polysaccharide Conjugate (Tetanus Toxoid Conjugate) Vaccine, PRP-T, DTaP-IPV/Hib

■ Haemophilus b (Hib) vaccine is an inactivated (polysaccharide) vaccine that is commercially available in the US as 2 different vaccine types: Hib conjugate vaccine (meningococcal protein conjugate) (PRP-OMP; PedvaxHIB®) and Hib conjugate vaccine (tetanus toxoid conjugate) (PRP-T; ActHIB®, Hiberix®). PRP-T also is commercially available in a combination vaccine containing diphtheria, tetanus, pertussis, poliovirus, and Hib antigens (DTaP-IPV/Hib; Pentacel®).

Uses

Haemophilus b (Hib) conjugate vaccine (meningococcal protein conjugate) (PRP-OMP; PedvaxHIB®) and Hib conjugate vaccine (tetanus toxoid conjugate) (PRP-T; ActHIB®, Hiberix®) are used to stimulate active immunity to invasive disease caused by *Haemophilus influenzae* type b (Hib). Hib vaccines will *not* provide protection against other types of *H. influenzae* (e.g., nonencapsulated [nontypeable] strains) or against other microorganisms that cause meningitis, septicemia, or other invasive infections.

The US Public Health Service Advisory Committee on Immunization Practices (ACIP), American Academy of Pediatrics (AAP), and other experts recommend *routine* primary and booster immunization against Hib infection in *all* infants and children 2 through 59 months of age. ACIP, AAP, and other experts also recommend use of Hib vaccine in certain individuals 5 years of age and older† at increased risk for invasive Hib disease because of certain medical conditions. (See Uses: Primary and Booster Immunization.)

■ Risks of Exposure and Infection Hib is a gram-negative bacterium that causes meningitis and other serious infections (e.g., pneumonia, epiglottitis, sepsis, cellulitis, septic arthritis, osteomyelitis, endocarditis, purulent pericarditis), principally in infants and children younger than 5 years of age.

Prior to the availability of Hib vaccine, Hib was the most common cause of bacterial meningitis and other invasive bacterial disease in young children worldwide and there were approximately 20,000 cases of invasive Hib disease (including approximately 12,000 cases of Hib meningitis) reported annually in the US, principally in infants and children younger than 5 years of age. The case fatality rate was 3–6% despite appropriate anti-infective treatment and 15–30% of meningitis survivors had hearing loss or neurologic sequelae. After Hib vaccine became available, the incidence of invasive Hib disease in the US decreased by 99% to fewer than 1 case per 100,000 children younger than 5 years of age. Most cases now occur in infants and children who are unvaccinated or incompletely vaccinated, including infants younger than 6 months of age who are too young to have received a complete vaccination series. During 2012, there were only 30 cases of invasive Hib disease reported in US children younger 5 years of age. Nontypeable *H. influenzae* is now the leading cause of invasive *H. influenzae* disease in all age groups.

Unvaccinated children younger than 5 years of age are at increased risk of invasive Hib disease, especially if they are household contacts of a child with invasive Hib disease. Some factors associated with an increased risk of invasive Hib infection include functional or anatomic asplenia, sickle cell disease, antibody deficiency syndromes, human immunodeficiency virus (HIV) infection, other immunodeficiency syndromes, and Hodgkin's disease or other malignancies (especially during chemotherapy or radiation therapy). Historically, invasive Hib disease was more common in American Indians (e.g., Apache and Navajo tribes), Alaskan natives, Hispanics, blacks, boys, daycare attendees, children living in crowded conditions, and children who were not breastfed.

Outbreaks or direct secondary transmission of invasive Hib disease can occur under certain circumstances, particularly when unvaccinated or incompletely vaccinated infants and children younger than 4 years of age are exposed through close contact with an index patient in household, child-care, or institutional settings. Attack rates vary substantially with age, and have been reported to be about 4% among susceptible contacts 2 years of age and younger and 0% among contacts 6 years of age or older. A secondary attack rate of 0.3% has been reported among household contacts in the month following onset of the index case (about 600 times higher than the risk for the general population). Most secondary cases in households occur during the first week after hospitalization of the index case. Data are conflicting regarding the risk of secondary transmission among child-care contacts, and secondary attack rates of 0–2.7% have been reported. Most studies suggest that child-care contacts are at relatively low risk for secondary transmission of Hib disease, particularly if contacts have received age-appropriate vaccination with Hib vaccine. Rifampin prophylaxis may be indicated to decrease the risk of secondary systemic Hib disease in exposed contacts. (See Uses: Postexposure Prophylaxis.)

■ Choice of Hib Vaccines ***Monovalent Hib Conjugate Vaccines*** There are 2 different types of monovalent Hib conjugate vaccine commercially available in the US for active immunization against invasive disease caused by Hib: PRP-OMP (PedvaxHIB®) and PRP-T (ActHIB®, Hiberix®).

ACIP and AAP state that PRP-OMP is preferred for primary immunization against invasive Hib disease in American Indian and Alaskan native children 6 weeks of age and older. The peak incidence of Hib meningitis in these populations occurs at a younger age (4–6 months) than in other US infants and there is evidence that vaccines containing PRP-OMP can induce protective antibody levels after the first dose and provide earlier protection than vaccines containing PRP-T. After primary immunization with PRP-OMP, American Indian and Alaskan native children can receive any commercially available age-appropriate Hib vaccine (PRP-OMP or PRP-T) for the booster dose given at 12 through 15 months of age.

In all other infants and children, ACIP and AAP do not state a preference for the type of Hib vaccine and state that all age-appropriate monovalent Hib vaccines (PRP-OMP or PRP-T) are considered interchangeable for primary and booster doses. However, the dosing schedule (i.e., number and timing of doses) differs depending on which vaccine type is used. (See Dosage and Administration: Dosage.)

Combination Vaccines Containing Hib Vaccine and Other Antigens PRP-T Hib vaccine also is commercially available in a combination vaccine that contains diphtheria, tetanus, pertussis, poliovirus, and Hib antigens (DTaP-IPV/Hib; Pentacel®). DTaP-IPV/Hib can be used when doses of diphtheria and tetanus toxoids and acellular pertussis vaccine adsorbed (DTaP), poliovirus vaccine inactivated (IPV), and Hib vaccine are indicated in infants and children 6 weeks through 4 years of age and there are no contraindications to any of the individual components. For prevention of Hib, ACIP states that DTaP-IPV/Hib may be used for the primary immunization doses and the booster dose at 12 through 15 months of age.

Data are not available regarding the interchangeability of DTaP-IPV/Hib and monovalent Hib vaccines.

■ Primary and Booster Immunization ACIP, AAP, and other experts recommend that *all* infants receive primary and booster immunization against Hib disease initiated at 2 months of age (minimum age 6 weeks) with an appropriate Hib vaccine. These experts also recommend catch-up vaccination for *all* children younger than 5 years of age who are unvaccinated or incompletely vaccinated against Hib disease.

Although Hib vaccine is *not* usually recommended in adults, adolescents, or children 5 years of age or older, it may be considered in certain individuals 5 years of age and older† at increased risk for invasive Hib disease because of certain medical conditions. (See Adults and Children 5 Years of Age or Older under Uses: Primary and Booster Immunization.)

Primary immunization against Hib infection can be integrated with age-appropriate primary immunization against diphtheria, tetanus, pertussis, hepatitis B, influenza, pneumococcal disease, poliomyelitis, rotavirus, measles, mumps, rubella, and varicella. (See Drug Interactions: Vaccines.)

Children 2 through 15 Months of Age ACIP, AAP, and other experts recommend that *all* children receive primary and booster immunization against Hib infection beginning at 2 months of age (minimum age 6 weeks). Catch-up vaccination with an age-appropriate Hib vaccine is recommended if primary immunization was not initiated at 2 months of age.

If *monovalent* Hib vaccine containing PRP-OMP (PedvaxHIB®) is used for active immunization against Hib disease in infants, 2 primary doses are given at 2 and 4 months of age and 1 booster dose is given at 12 through 15 months of age. If *monovalent* Hib vaccine containing PRP-T (ActHIB®, Hiberix®) is used, 3 primary doses are given at 2, 4, and 6 months of age and 1 booster dose is given at 12 through 18 months of age. Alternatively, if the *combination* vaccine DTaP-IPV/Hib (Pentacel®) is used for primary and booster immunization in infants, 3 primary doses are given at 2, 4, and 6 months of age and 1 booster dose is given at 12 through 18 months of age.

ACIP, AAP, and other experts recommend that the booster dose be given at 12 through 15 months of age and at least 2 months (8 weeks) after the last primary dose and state that any age-appropriate Hib vaccine (monovalent or combination vaccine) may be used for the booster dose.

PRP-OMP is preferred for primary immunization against invasive Hib disease in American Indian and Alaskan native infants. (See Uses: Choice of Hib Vaccines.)

Medically stable preterm infants generally should receive primary immunization against Hib infection at the usual chronologic age. (See Cautions: Pediatric Precautions.)

Children 15 through 59 Months of Age ACIP, AAP, and other experts recommend that all children who are 15 through 59 months of age and have not yet received primary immunization against Hib infection receive a single dose of an age-appropriate Hib vaccine. Additional or booster doses of Hib vaccine (monovalent or combination vaccine) are not usually recommended for children who received a first dose at 15 months of age or older.

Adults and Children 5 Years of Age or Older PRP-OMP (PedvaxHIB®) and PRP-T (ActHIB®) are labeled by FDA for use in children through 5 years of age (prior to sixth birthday); PRP-T (Hiberix®) and DTaP-IPV/Hib (Pentacel®) are labeled by FDA for use in children through 4 years of age (prior to fifth birthday). Efficacy and safety of Hib vaccines have not been established in older children or adults.

Although ACIP, AAP, and other experts do *not* recommend *routine* use of Hib vaccine in individuals 5 years of age or older, these experts state that certain adults† and children 5 years of age or older† at increased risk for invasive Hib disease should receive the vaccine. (See Individuals at Increased Risk Because of Certain Medical Conditions under Uses: Primary and Booster Immunization.)

Individuals at Increased Risk Because of Certain Medical Conditions Individuals with certain immunocompromising conditions are considered at increased risk of invasive Hib disease. This includes individuals with functional or anatomic asplenia, sickle cell disease, immunoglobulin deficiency (including IgG_2 deficiency), early component complement deficiency, or HIV infection and those who have undergone hematopoietic stem cell transplantation (HSCT) or are receiving chemotherapy or radiation therapy for malignant neoplasms.

Children 12 through 59 months of age who are at increased risk for Hib disease and are unvaccinated or incompletely vaccinated should receive Hib vaccine according to age-specific recommendations. Children at high risk who have received no doses or only 1 dose of Hib vaccine before 12 months of age should receive 2 doses of any age-appropriate Hib vaccine given 2 months (8 weeks) apart; those who received 2 or more doses of Hib vaccine before 12 months of age should receive 1 additional dose given at least 8 weeks after the last dose. Although it is unclear whether children at increased risk of invasive Hib disease (e.g., those with HIV infection, IgG_2 deficiency, early component complement deficiency) would benefit from additional doses of Hib vaccine after completion of the usual age-appropriate vaccination regimen, ACIP and AAP state that no additional doses are necessary in those who received the complete primary immunization series of Hib vaccine followed by a booster dose given at 12 months of age or older.

Previously unvaccinated children 5 years of age or older† with underlying disease predisposing to Hib disease should receive a single dose of Hib vaccine.

Hib vaccine also is recommended in certain adults† with medical conditions that increase the risk of invasive Hib disease.

The fact that the immune response to Hib vaccine may be reduced in immunocompromised individuals should be considered. (See Individuals with Altered Immunocompetence under Cautions: Precautions and Contraindications.)

Anatomic or Functional Asplenia and Sickle Cell Disease. Children 12 through 59 months of age with decreased or absent splenic function who received a primary immunization series in early infancy followed by a booster dose at 12 months of age or older do not need further doses of Hib vaccine. Those who received a complete age-appropriate primary and booster immunization series of Hib vaccine but are scheduled for splenectomy (e.g., for Hodgkin's disease, spherocytosis, immune thrombocytopenia, hypersplenism) may benefit from an additional dose of Hib vaccine given at least 14 days prior to the procedure.

Adults†, adolescents†, and children 5 years of age or older† who have anatomic or functional asplenia or sickle cell disease and are unvaccinated (i.e., did not receive a primary series and a booster dose of Hib vaccine in early infancy or at least 1 dose of Hib vaccine after 14 months of age) should receive a single dose of Hib vaccine.

Unvaccinated adults†, adolescents†, and children 15 months of age or older (including children 5 years of age or older†) undergoing splenectomy should receive a single dose of Hib vaccine administered at least 14 days before surgery. Some experts suggest administering a dose of Hib vaccine at least 14 days before splenectomy regardless of prior vaccination history. If Hib vaccine was not administered before splenectomy, the dose should be administered as soon as possible at least 2 weeks after surgery when the patient's condition is stable.

HIV-infected Individuals. ACIP, AAP, Centers for Disease Control and Prevention (CDC), National Institutes of Health (NIH), HIV Medicine Association of the Infectious Diseases Society of America (IDSA), and AAP state that recommendations regarding use of Hib vaccine in HIV-infected infants and children up to 5 years of age are the same as those for individuals who are not infected with HIV. It is unclear whether HIV-infected children would benefit from additional doses of Hib vaccine after completion of the usually recommended primary and booster immunization series.

HIV-infected children and adolescents 5 through 18 years of age† who are unvaccinated or incompletely vaccinated against Hib should receive a single dose of Hib vaccine.

Because the incidence of Hib infection in HIV-infected adults is low, Hib vaccine is not usually recommended in HIV-infected adults, unless they also have anatomic or functional asplenia.

Immunization may be less effective in individuals with HIV infection than in immunocompetent individuals since the antibody response to vaccines may be reduced and may be inversely correlated with severity of the disease.

Hematopoietic Stem Cell Transplant Recipients. Adults†, adolescents†, and children (including children 5 years of age or older†) who have undergone HSCT should be considered unvaccinated, regardless of any prior doses of Hib vaccine. ACIP, AAP, and other experts state that, starting 6–12 months after successful transplant, *all* HSCT recipients should receive 3 doses of Hib vaccine given at least 1 month (4 weeks) apart.

Individuals undergoing Chemotherapy or Radiation Therapy. Hib vaccination generally should be avoided during chemotherapy or radiation therapy because of possible suboptimal response. If Hib vaccine is indicated in an individual who will be receiving immunosuppressive therapy, the vaccine should be administered at least 2 weeks prior to initiation of such therapy if possible. Children younger than 5 years of age who received Hib vaccine within 14 days prior to initiation of immunosuppressive therapy or while receiving immunosuppressive therapy should be considered unimmunized, and vaccine doses should be repeated beginning at least 3 months after such therapy is discontinued. In patients receiving treatment with anti-B-cell antibodies (e.g., rituximab), Hib vaccination should be deferred until at least 6 months after such therapy is discontinued. (See Drug Interactions: Immunosuppressive Agents.)

Individuals Vaccinated Outside the US The immune status of individuals vaccinated outside the US (e.g., children adopted from other countries, immigrants) may be difficult to determine based on country of origin and medical records. Such individuals whose immune status is uncertain should be vaccinated according to the US recommended immunization schedules. (See Immunization Schedules, US 80:00.) The fact that immunization schedules of other countries may differ from US schedules (e.g., different recommended vaccines, recommended ages of administration, and/or number and timing of vaccine doses) should be considered. Vaccines administered outside the US can generally be accepted as valid if there is documentation and the administration schedule was similar to that recommended in the US immunization schedules. Only written vaccination records should be considered as evidence of previous vaccination since such records are more likely to accurately predict protection if the specific vaccines administered, intervals between doses, and individual's age at the time of vaccination are similar to US recommendations; however, the extent to which an internationally adopted child's immunization record reflects their protection against disease is unclear and it is possible there may be transcription errors in such records (e.g., single-antigen vaccine may have been administered although a multiple-antigen vaccine was recorded). Although vaccines with inadequate potency have been produced in other countries, the majority of vaccines used worldwide are immunogenic and produced with adequate quality control standards.

When the immune status of an internationally adopted child is uncertain, ACIP recommends that health-care providers either repeat vaccinations (since this usually is safe and avoids the need to obtain and interpret serologic tests) and/or use selective serologic testing to determine the need for immunizations (helps avoid unnecessary injections). However, interpretation of serologic tests used to verify whether a child vaccinated more than 2 months previously is protected against Hib can be difficult. Therefore, because the required number of doses needed for protection against Hib decreases with age and because adverse effects reported with Hib vaccines are rare, ACIP recommends age-appropriate revaccination.

Children Younger than 24 Months of Age with Invasive Hib Infection Children younger than 24 months of age who develop systemic Hib infection may be at risk of developing a second episode of the disease since most children in this age group fail to develop adequate immunity following natural infection. Such children should be considered unvaccinated, regardless of prior doses of Hib vaccine, and should receive age-appropriate primary immunization as if they had received no previous doses of Hib vaccine; the immunization series should be initiated 1 month (4 weeks) after disease onset or as soon as possible thereafter.

■ **Postexposure Prophylaxis** Data are insufficient to determine whether Hib vaccine administered immediately after exposure to natural Hib would prevent illness. Whenever a case of invasive Hib disease is identified, unvaccinated or incompletely vaccinated children 2 through 59 months of age who are household or day-care contacts of the infected individual should receive a dose of Hib vaccine and be scheduled to complete the recommended age-specific Hib vaccination schedule.

If a case of Hib is diagnosed, rifampin postexposure prophylaxis is recommended for all household contacts (regardless of age) in households with children younger than 4 years of age who are unvaccinated or incompletely vaccinated against Hib and for all household contacts in households with an immunocompromised individual younger than 18 years of age. In childcare settings, rifampin postexposure prophylaxis is recommended for all attendees and all childcare providers if 2 or more cases of invasive Hib disease have occurred within 60 days and unvaccinated or incompletely vaccinated children attend the facility. Rifampin eradicates nasopharyngeal carriage of Hib in approximately 95% of carriers and decreases the risk of secondary invasive disease in exposed household contacts. (See Uses: Prevention of Haemophilus influenzae type b Infection, in Rifampin 8:16.04.)

Dosage and Administration

■ **Reconstitution and Administration** Haemophilus b (Hib) conjugate vaccine (meningococcal protein conjugate) (PRP-OMP; PedvaxHIB®) and Hib conjugate vaccine (tetanus toxoid conjugate) (PRP-T; ActHIB®, Hiberix®) are administered by IM injection.

The combination vaccine containing diphtheria and tetanus toxoids and acellular pertussis vaccine adsorbed (DTaP), poliovirus vaccine inactivated (IPV), and Hib conjugate vaccine (DTaP-IPV/Hib; Pentacel®) is administered by IM injection.

Monovalent Hib vaccine and combination vaccine containing Hib and other antigens should *not* be given IV, subcutaneously, or intradermally.

Syncope (vasovagal or vasodepressor reaction; fainting) may occur following vaccination; such reactions may be accompanied by transient neurologic signs (e.g., visual disturbance, paresthesia, tonic-clonic limb movements). Syncope occurs most frequently in adolescents and young adults. Procedures should be in place to avoid falling injury and to restore cerebral perfusion following syncope. Syncope and secondary injuries may be averted if vaccinees sit or lie down during and for 15 minutes after vaccination. If syncope occurs, the patient should be observed until symptoms resolve.

Hib vaccine may be given concurrently with other age-appropriate vaccines. When multiple vaccines are administered during a single health-care visit, each parenteral vaccine should be given using separate syringes and different injection sites. The injection sites should be separated by at least 1 inch (if anatomically feasible) to allow appropriate attribution of any local adverse effects that may occur.

IM Administration Depending on patient age, IM injections should be made into the anterolateral muscles of the thigh or deltoid muscle of the arm.

In infants younger than 12 months of age, IM injections should preferably be made into the anterolateral thigh; in certain circumstances (e.g., physical obstruction at other sites and no reasonable indication to defer the vaccine dose), IM injections can be made into the gluteal muscle using care to identify anatomical landmarks prior to injection.

In infants and children 1 through 2 years of age, the anterolateral thigh is preferred; alternatively, IM injections can be made into the deltoid muscle if muscle mass is adequate.

In adults, adolescents, and children 3 years of age or older, IM injections should preferably be made into the deltoid muscle; IM injections also can be made into the anterolateral thigh.

To ensure delivery into muscle, IM injections should be made at a 90° angle to the skin using a needle length appropriate for the individual's age and body mass, the thickness of adipose tissue and muscle at the injection site, and the injection technique. Anatomic variability, especially in the deltoid, should be considered and clinical judgment should be used to avoid inadvertent under-penetration or overpenetration of muscle.

Some manufacturers state that Hib vaccine should *not* be injected into the gluteal area or any area where there may be a major nerve trunk.

PRP-OMP (PedvaxHIB®). PRP-OMP (PedvaxHIB®) is administered undiluted.

Single-dose vials of PRP-OMP should be shaken well prior to withdrawing the dose. Thorough agitation is necessary to maintain a suspension; the vaccine should appear as a slightly opaque white suspension.

PRP-T (ActHIB®). Single-dose vials of lyophilized PRP-T (ActHIB®) should be reconstituted by adding 0.6 mL of the 0.4% sodium chloride diluent supplied by the manufacturer. The vial should be agitated thoroughly to ensure complete reconstitution; the reconstituted vaccine should appear clear and colorless. The manufacturer's labeling should be consulted for additional information regarding reconstitution of PRP-T.

PRP-T should be administered promptly after reconstitution or may be stored at 2–8°C and administered within 24 hours after reconstitution. The reconstituted vaccine should be shaken well prior to use.

PRP-T should not be mixed with any other vaccine or solution.

PRP-T (Hiberix®). Single-dose vials of lyophilized PRP-T (Hiberix®) should be reconstituted by adding the entire amount of 0.9% sodium chloride diluent supplied by the manufacturer. The vial should be agitated thoroughly to ensure complete reconstitution. The manufacturer's labeling should be consulted for additional information regarding reconstitution of PRP-T.

PRP-T should be administered promptly after reconstitution or may be stored at 2–8°C and administered within 24 hours after reconstitution. The reconstituted vaccine should be shaken well prior to use.

PRP-T should not be mixed with any other vaccine or solution.

DTaP-IPV/Hib (Pentacel®). DTaP-IPV/Hib (Pentacel®) is commercially available as a kit containing a single-dose vial of a fixed-combination vaccine containing diphtheria, tetanus, pertussis, and poliovirus antigens (DTaP-IPV vaccine) and a single-dose vial of lyophilized Hib vaccine (PRP-T; ActHIB®).

Prior to administration, the vial of lyophilized PRP-T vaccine from the kit should be reconstituted by adding the entire contents of the vial of the DTaP-IPV vaccine from the kit according to manufacturer's instructions to provide a combination vaccine containing diphtheria, tetanus, pertussis, IPV, and Hib antigens. The vial should be gently swirled until a cloudy, uniform, white to off-white (yellow tinge) suspension is obtained.

DTaP-IPV/Hib should be administered immediately after reconstitution.

■ Dosage

The dosage schedule (i.e., number of doses) recommended for primary immunization against Hib infection varies according to the specific Hib vaccine administered and the age at which vaccination is started. *The age-appropriate recommendations for the specific preparation used should be followed.*

Monovalent PRP-OMP and monovalent PRP-T are considered interchangeable for both primary and booster immunization. If the primary immunization series included both PRP-OMP and PRP-T or if there is uncertainty about which vaccine type was administered previously, 3 primary doses and a booster dose are needed to complete the series.

The US Public Health Service Advisory Committee on Immunization Practices (ACIP) and American Academy of Pediatrics (AAP) state that PRP-OMP is preferred for primary immunization in American Indian and Alaskan native children. (See Uses: Choice of Hib Vaccines.)

Medically stable preterm infants should be vaccinated at the usual chronologic age using usual dosage. (See Cautions: Pediatric Precautions.)

If interruptions or delays result in an interval between Hib vaccine doses longer than recommended, it is not necessary to administer additional doses or start the vaccination series over. Such interruptions should not reduce the final level of antibodies produced or interfere with final immunity achieved, although protection may not be attained until all recommended doses have been administered.

PRP-OMP (PedvaxHIB®) PRP-OMP (PedvaxHIB®) is administered IM in 0.5-mL doses.

PRP-OMP is labeled by FDA for use in infants and children 2 through 71 months of age.

Routine primary immunization in early infancy using PRP-OMP consists of a series of 2 doses and a booster dose. The manufacturer, ACIP, AAP, and other experts recommend that doses be given at 2, 4, and 12 through 15 months of age. The initial dose may be given as early as 6 weeks of age. The minimum interval between the first and second doses is 2 months (8 weeks). A third dose (booster dose) of PRP-OMP should be given no earlier than 2 months after the second dose and is necessary only if the second dose of PRP-OMP was administered before 12 months of age.

For catch-up immunization in infants who receive the first dose of Hib vaccine at 7 through 11 months of age, ACIP, AAP, and other experts recommend that a second dose be given at least 4 weeks after the first dose and that a third dose be given at 12 through 15 months of age or 8 weeks after the second dose, whichever is later.

For catch-up immunization in previously unvaccinated infants 12 through 14 months of age, ACIP, AAP, and other experts recommend that 2 doses be given; the first dose should be given immediately and a second dose should be given 8 weeks after the first dose. A third dose is not necessary.

In previously unvaccinated infants and children 15 through 59 months of age, ACIP, AAP, and other experts recommend that a single dose of Hib vaccine be given.

PRP-T (ActHIB®) PRP-T (ActHIB®) is administered IM in 0.5-mL doses. This PRP-T vaccine is labeled by FDA for use in infants and children 2 months through 5 years of age.

Routine primary immunization in early infancy using PRP-T consists of a series of 3 doses and a booster dose. ACIP, AAP, and other experts recommend that doses be given at 2, 4, 6, and 12 through 15 months of age. The manufacturer recommends that doses be given at 2, 4, 6, and 15 through 18 months of age. The initial dose may be given as early as 6 weeks of age.

For catch-up immunization in infants who receive the first dose of Hib vaccine at 7 through 11 months of age, ACIP, AAP, and other experts recommend that a second dose be given at least 4 weeks after the first dose and that a third dose be given at 12 through 15 months of age or 8 weeks after the second dose, whichever is later.

For catch-up immunization in previously unvaccinated infants 12 through 14 months of age, ACIP, AAP, and other experts recommend that 2 doses be given; the first dose should be given immediately and a second dose should be given 8 weeks after the first dose. A third dose is not necessary.

In previously unvaccinated infants and children 15 through 59 months of age, ACIP, AAP, and other experts recommend that a single dose of Hib vaccine be given.

PRP-T (Hiberix®) PRP-T (Hiberix®) is administered IM in 0.5-mL doses. This PRP-T is labeled by FDA for use in infants and children 6 weeks through 4 years of age.

Routine primary immunization in early infancy using PRP-T consists of a series of 3 doses and a booster dose. ACIP, AAP, and other experts recommend that doses be given at 2, 4, 6, and 12 through 15 months of age. The manufacturer recommends that doses be given at 2, 4, 6, and 15 through 18 months of age. The initial dose may be given as early as 6 weeks of age.

For catch-up immunization in infants who receive the first dose of Hib vaccine at 7 through 11 months of age, ACIP, AAP, and other experts recommend that a second dose be given at least 4 weeks after the first dose and that a third dose be given at 12 through 15 months of age or 8 weeks after the second dose, whichever is later.

For catch-up immunization in previously unvaccinated infants 12 through 14 months of age, ACIP, AAP, and other experts recommend that 2 doses be given; the first dose should be given immediately and a second dose should be given 8 weeks after the first dose. A third dose is not necessary.

In previously unvaccinated infants and children 15 through 59 months of age, ACIP, AAP, and other experts recommend that a single dose of Hib vaccine be given.

DTaP-IPV/Hib (Pentacel®) DTaP-IPV/Hib (Pentacel®) is administered IM in 0.5-mL doses.

DTaP-IPV/Hib is labeled by FDA for use in infants and children 6 weeks through 4 years of age.

In previously unvaccinated infants or children 6 weeks through 4 years of age, DTaP-IPV/Hib is given in a series of 4 doses. ACIP, AAP, and other experts recommend that doses be given at 2, 4, 6, and 12 through 15 months of age. The manufacturer recommends that doses be given at 2, 4, 6, and 15 through 18 months of age. The initial dose usually is given at 2 months of age, but may be given as early as 6 weeks of age.

In infants or children 6 weeks through 4 years of age who previously received 1 or more doses of Hib vaccine, DTaP-IPV/Hib can be used to complete the Hib vaccination series when doses of IPV and DTaP also are indicated and there are no contraindications to any of the individual components.

To complete the recommended primary and booster vaccination series against diphtheria, tetanus, and pertussis, children who received the 4-dose series of DTaP-IPV/Hib (Pentacel®) should receive a fifth dose of DTaP (Daptacel®) at 4 through 6 years of age. DTaP-IPV/Hib should not be used for the booster dose of DTaP indicated at 4 through 6 years of age; however, if a dose of DTaP-IPV/Hib is inadvertently given to a child 5 years of age or older, ACIP states the dose may be counted as a valid dose.

To complete vaccination against poliovirus in children who received the 4-dose series of DTaP-IPV/Hib at 2, 4, 6, and 15 through 18 months of age, an additional booster dose of age-appropriate vaccine containing IPV (IPOL® or Kinrix®) should be given at 4 through 6 years of age.

Cautions

Adverse reactions generally are mild and transient following administration of haemophilus b (Hib) vaccines and rarely persist longer than 24–48 hours.

■ **PRP-OMP (PedvaxHIB®)** In infants 2–6 months of age who received haemophilus b (Hib) conjugate vaccine (meningococcal protein conjugate) (PRP-OMP; PedvaxHIB®), adverse local effects included erythema (exceeding 2.5 cm in diameter) in 0.4–2% of vaccinees within 6–48 hours after the first or second dose and swelling/induration (exceeding 2.5 cm in diameter) in 1–3% within 6–48 hours after the first dose and in 1% within 6–48 hours after the second dose. Similar adverse effects have been reported when a third dose is given at 12–15 months of age. Urticaria, pain, soreness, and sterile abscess at the injection site have been reported rarely with PRP-OMP.

In infants 2–6 months of age who received PRP-OMP (PedvaxHIB®), fever (exceeding 38.3°C) occurred in 0.5–18% within 6–48 hours after the first dose and in 3–14% within 6–24 hours after the second dose. Although a causal relationship was not established, urticaria, tracheitis, thrombocytopenia, lymphadenopathy, angioedema, and seizures have been reported rarely in infants or children who received PRP-OMP.

■ **PRP-T (ActHIB®)** In a study in US children who received Hib conjugate vaccine (tetanus toxoid conjugate) (PRP-T; ActHIB®) at 2, 4, 6, and 15–16 months of age concurrently with various other vaccines containing diphtheria, tetanus, pertussis, poliovirus, pneumococcal, or hepatitis B antigens administered at different injection sites, solicited systemic adverse effects occurring within 3 days after a dose included fussiness/irritability (54–76%), decreased activity/lethargy (24–51%), inconsolable crying (36–59%), and fever (9–16%).

Other adverse effects reported during postmarketing experience in children who received this PRP-T include anaphylaxis, other hypersensitivity reactions (e.g., rash, pruritus, urticaria, angioedema), seizures, extensive limb swelling, and peripheral edema.

■ **PRP-T (Hiberix®)** Adverse effects reported in at least 20% of children who received PRP-T (Hiberix®) in clinical studies were pain and redness at the injection site, irritability, drowsiness, fever, loss of appetite, fussiness, and restlessness.

In a clinical study in US children who received this PRP-T at 2, 4, and 6 months of age concurrently with various other vaccines containing diphtheria, tetanus, pertussis, hepatitis B, pneumococcal, poliovirus, and rotavirus antigens, solicited adverse effects occurring within 4 days after each dose were local effects, including pain (43–49%), redness (19–29%), and swelling (13–19%), and systemic effects, including irritability (67–70%), drowsiness (49–60%), loss of appetite (28–29%), and fever (14–19%).

In a clinical study in US children who received primary immunization with a 3-dose series of this PRP-T given at 2, 4, and 6 months of age and then received a booster dose of the vaccine at 15–18 months of age administered concurrently with diphtheria and tetanus toxoids and acellular pertussis vaccine adsorbed (DTaP) at a different injection site, solicited adverse effects occurring within 4 days after the booster dose were local effects, including pain (41%), redness (30%), and swelling (18%), and systemic effects, including irritability (58%), drowsiness (39%), loss of appetite (28%), and fever (15%).

In an open-label, multicenter study in infants (mean age 16 months) who received a booster dose of this PRP-T concurrently with a combination vaccine containing diphtheria, tetanus, pertussis, hepatitis B, and poliovirus antigens (DTaP-HBV-IPV) administered at a different injection site, solicited adverse effects occurring within 4 days of vaccination were local effects, including redness (25%), pain (21%), and swelling (15%), and systemic effects, including fever (35%), fussiness (26%), loss of appetite (23%), restlessness (22%), sleepiness (20%), diarrhea (15%), and vomiting (5%).

Other adverse effects that have been reported to have a plausible causal connection to this PRP-T include local effects (extensive swelling of the vaccinated limb, injection site induration), hypersensitivity reactions (anaphylaxis, anaphylactoid reaction, angioedema, rash, urticaria), nervous system effects (seizures with or without fever, hypotonic-hyporesponsive episode, somnolence, syncope or vasovagal response to the injection), and apnea.

■ **DTaP-IPV/Hib (Pentacel®)** In a clinical study in infants who received a 4-dose primary immunization series (at 2, 4, 6, and 15–16 months of age) of either the combination vaccine containing diphtheria, tetanus, pertussis, poliovirus, and Hib antigens (DTaP-IPV/Hib; Pentacel®) or control vaccines (IPV, DTaP [Daptacel®], and Hib [ActHIB®] at 2, 4, and 6 months and Daptacel® and ActHIB® at 15–16 months) administered concurrently at separate injection sites, adverse effects occurring within 3 days of vaccination were solicited from parents and included local injection site reactions (redness, swelling, tenderness, increase in arm circumference) and systemic effects (fever, decreased activity/lethargy, inconsolable crying, fussiness/irritability). All infants also received hepatitis B vaccine (at 2 and 6 months) and pneumococcal 7-valent conjugate vaccine (at 2, 4, and 6 months) concurrently at different injection sites.

The incidence of swelling or tenderness at the injection site in those who received DTaP-IPV/Hib was 5–10 or 39–56%, respectively, and was similar to that reported with DTaP vaccine alone (4–10 or 38–51%, respectively).

The incidence of fever (38°C or higher) after the first, second, and third dose was 6, 11, and 16%, respectively, after the fixed-combination vaccine and 9, 16, and 16%, respectively, when the doses of DTaP, IPV, and Hib vaccines were given separately at different injection sites. The incidence of inconsolable crying or fussiness/irritability was 47–59 or 68–77%, respectively, after the fixed-combination vaccine compared with 48–59 or 67–76%, respectively, when the doses of DTaP, IPV, and Hib vaccine were given separately at different injection sites.

■ **Precautions and Contraindications** Prior to administration of monovalent Hib vaccine containing PRP-OMP, monovalent Hib vaccine containing PRP-T, or combination Hib vaccine containing PRP-T, all known precautions should be taken to prevent adverse reactions, including a review of the patient's history with respect to health status and possible sensitivity to the vaccine or similar vaccines. (See Sensitivity Reactions under Cautions: Precautions and Contraindications.)

The patient and/or the patient's parent or guardian should be informed of the benefits and risks of immunization with Hib vaccine and should be provided with a copy of the appropriate Vaccine Information Statement (available at the CDC website https://www.cdc.gov/vaccines/hcp/vis/index.html). Patients and/or the patient's parent or guardian also should be instructed to report any severe or unusual adverse reactions to their health-care provider. Clinicians or individuals can report any adverse reactions that occur following vaccination to VAERS at 800-822-7967 or http://www.vaers.hhs.gov.

PRP-OMP (PedvaxHIB®) is contraindicated in individuals hypersensitive to any vaccine component.

PRP-T (ActHIB®, Hiberix®) is contraindicated in individuals who have had a severe allergic reaction (e.g., anaphylaxis) after a dose of any Hib vaccine, a dose of any vaccine containing tetanus toxoid, or any component in PRP-T.

DTaP-IPV/Hib (Pentacel®) is contraindicated in individuals with severe allergic reaction (e.g., anaphylaxis) to any ingredient in the vaccine or after a previous dose of the vaccine or any vaccine containing diphtheria, tetanus, pertussis, poliovirus, or Hib antigens. In addition, because of the pertussis antigen, DTaP-IPV/Hib (Pentacel®) is contraindicated in individuals who had encephalopathy (e.g., coma, decreased consciousness, prolonged seizures) within 7 days of a dose of pertussis-containing vaccine and in individuals with progressive neurologic disorder, including infantile spasms, uncontrolled epilepsy, or progressive encephalopathy.

Although PRP-OMP contains Hib antigen conjugated to the outer membrane protein complex (OMPC) of *Neisseria meningitidis* and antibodies to OMPC have been demonstrated in patients who received the vaccine, the clinical relevance of these antibodies has not been established. PRP-OMP (PedvaxHIB®) should *not* be considered an immunizing agent against meningococcal disease.

Although PRP-T contains Hib antigen conjugated to tetanus toxoid, PRP-T vaccines are *not* a substitute for routine immunization against tetanus.

Sensitivity Reactions Prior to administration of Hib vaccine, clinicians should review the patient's history regarding possible sensitivity and any previous adverse reactions and should take all precautions known for prevention of allergic or any other adverse effects.

Epinephrine and other appropriate agents and equipment should be available for immediate treatment if an anaphylactic or other serious allergic reaction occurs.

Latex Sensitivity. Some packaging components of PRP-OMP (PedvaxHIB®) (i.e., vial stoppers) contain natural rubber latex which may cause sensitivity reactions in susceptible individuals. Delayed-type (cell-mediated) allergic contact dermatitis is the most common type of latex hypersensitivity; however, immediate-type allergic reactions have been reported rarely.

The US Public Health Service Advisory Committee on Immunization Practices (ACIP) states that vaccines supplied in vials or syringes that contain dry natural rubber or natural rubber latex may be administered to individuals with a history of contact allergy to latex. However, vaccines supplied in vials or syringes that contain natural rubber latex should be avoided, if possible, in individuals with a history of severe (anaphylactic) latex allergy; if used in such individuals, appropriate agents and equipment should be available to treat anaphylaxis or other immediate allergic reaction to latex.

Neomycin and/or Polymyxin B Allergy. DTaP-IPV/Hib (Pentacel®) contains trace amounts of neomycin sulfate (no more than 4 pg per 0.5-mL dose) and polymyxin B (no more than 4 pg per 0.5-mL dose).

Neomycin hypersensitivity usually manifests as a delayed-type (cell-mediated) contact dermatitis.

ACIP states that a history of delayed-type allergic reaction to neomycin is not a contraindication for administration of vaccines containing trace amounts of neomycin; however, individuals with a history of anaphylactic reaction to neomycin should be evaluated by an allergist before receiving a neomycin-containing vaccine.

Individuals with Altered Immunocompetence Like other inactivated vaccines, Hib vaccines may be administered to individuals immunosuppressed as a result of disease or medical therapy; however, immune responses to vaccines and efficacy may be reduced in individuals with altered immunocompetence.

The manufacturer of PRP-T (Hiberix®) monovalent Hib vaccine states that safety and efficacy of the vaccine have not been evaluated in immunosuppressed children.

Immune responses have been obtained following administration of Hib vaccine in patients with sickle disease, leukemia, or HIV infection, and in those who have undergone splenectomies; immune responses in HIV-infected individuals vary with the degree of immunocompromise.

ACIP, American Academy of Pediatrics (AAP), US Centers for Disease Control and Prevention (CDC), National Institutes of Health (NIH), HIV Medicine Association of the Infectious Diseases Society of America (IDSA), and other experts state that recommendations regarding use of Hib vaccine in HIV-infected children are the same as those for children who are not infected with HIV. (See HIV-infected Individuals under Primary and Booster Immunization: Individuals at Increased Risk Because of Certain Medical Conditions, in Uses.)

AAP states that children who have received the usual age-appropriate regimen of Hib vaccine (primary and booster doses) and have decreased or absent splenic function do not need additional doses of Hib vaccine; however, those who are scheduled for splenectomy (e.g., for Hodgkin's disease, spherocytosis, immune thrombocytopenia, hypersplenism) may benefit from an additional dose of any Hib vaccine given at least 14 days before surgery. (See Anatomic or Functional Asplenia and Sickle Cell Disease under Primary and Booster Immunization: Individuals at Increased Risk Because of Certain Medical Conditions, in Uses.)

Inactivated vaccines generally should be administered prior to initiation of immunosuppressive therapy or deferred until immunosuppressive therapy is discontinued. (See Drug Interactions: Immunosuppressive Agents.)

Concomitant Illness A decision to administer or delay vaccination in an individual with a current or recent acute illness depends on the severity of symptoms and etiology of the illness.

ACIP states that mild acute illness generally does not preclude vaccination. However, moderate or severe acute illness (with or without fever) is a precaution for vaccination and vaccines should be deferred until the individual has recovered from the acute phase of the illness. This precaution avoids superimposing adverse effects of the vaccine on the underlying illness or mistakenly concluding that a manifestation of the underlying illness resulted from administration of the vaccine.

Guillain-Barré Syndrome If Guillain-Barré syndrome (GBS) occurred within 6 weeks of receipt of a vaccine containing tetanus toxoid, the manufacturers state that a decision to administer a dose of PRP-T (ActHIB®, Hiberix®) should be based on careful consideration of potential benefits and possible risks.

Individuals with Bleeding Disorders Individuals who have bleeding disorders or are receiving anticoagulant therapy and/or their family members should be advised about the risk of hematoma from IM injections.

ACIP states that IM vaccines may be given to individuals who have bleeding disorders or are receiving anticoagulant therapy if a clinician familiar with the patient's bleeding risk determines that the vaccine can be administered IM with reasonable safety. In these cases, a fine needle (23 gauge or smaller) should be used to administer the vaccine and firm pressure should be applied to the injection site (without rubbing) for at least 2 minutes. In individuals receiving therapy for hemophilia, IM vaccines can be scheduled for shortly after a dose of such therapy.

Use of Combination Vaccines When the combination vaccine containing diphtheria, tetanus, pertussis, poliovirus, and Hib antigens (DTaP-IPV/Hib; Pentacel®) is used, the cautions, precautions, and contraindications associated with each antigen should be considered. (See Cautions in Poliovirus Vaccine Inactivated 80:12 and see Cautions in Diphtheria and Tetanus Toxoids and Acellular Pertussis Vaccine Adsorbed/Tetanus Toxoid and Reduced Diphtheria Toxoid and Acellular Pertussis Vaccine Adsorbed 80:08.)

Limitations of Vaccine Effectiveness Hib vaccines may not protect all vaccine recipients against invasive *Haemophilus influenzae* type b (Hib) disease.

Hib vaccines will not provide protection against other types of *H. influenzae* (e.g., nonencapsulated [nontypeable] strains) or against other pathogens that cause meningitis, septicemia, or other invasive disease.

Hib vaccine does not result in protective antibodies immediately following vaccination.

There is some evidence that vaccines containing PRP-OMP (PedvaxHIB®) result in more rapid seroconversion to protective antibody concentrations within the first 6 months of life compared with vaccines containing PRP-T (ActHIB®, Hiberix®). This is particularly important in American Indian and Alaskan native children because these children are at increased risk for Hib disease during the first 6 months of life. (See Uses: Choice of Hib Vaccines.)

Although PRP-OMP contains Hib antigen conjugated to outer membrane protein complex (OMPC) of *Neisseria meningitidis* and antibodies to OMPC have been demonstrated in individuals who received the vaccine, the clinical relevance of these antibodies not established. PRP-OMP is *not* an immunizing agent against meningococcal disease.

Although PRP-T contains Hib antigen conjugated to tetanus toxoid, the vaccine is *not* a substitute for routine immunization against tetanus.

Improper Storage and Handling Improper storage or handling of vaccines may reduce vaccine potency resulting in reduced or inadequate immune responses in vaccinees.

All vaccines should be inspected upon delivery and monitored during storage to ensure that the appropriate temperature is maintained. (See Chemistry and Stability: Stability.)

Monovalent Hib vaccines or combination vaccines containing Hib and other antigens that have been mishandled or have not been stored at the recommended temperature should not be administered.

If there are concerns about mishandling, the manufacturer or state or local immunization or health departments should be contacted for guidance on whether the vaccine is usable.

■ **Pediatric Precautions** PRP-OMP (PedvaxHIB®): Safety and efficacy have not been established in infants younger than 6 weeks of age or in children 6 years of age or older. The manufacturer states that administration of PRP-OMP before 6 weeks of age may result in immunologic tolerance to the vaccine (i.e., impaired ability to respond to subsequent exposure to PRP antigen).

PRP-T (ActHIB®): Safety and efficacy have not been established in infants younger than 6 weeks of age.

PRP-T (Hiberix®): Safety and efficacy have not been established in infants younger than 6 weeks of age or in children and adolescents 5–16 years of age.

DTaP-IPV/Hib (Pentacel®): Safety and efficacy have not been established in infants younger than 6 weeks of age or in children 5–16 years of age.

ACIP and AAP state that immunization against Hib infection using an age-appropriate vaccine can be initiated as early as 6 weeks of age. Hib vaccines should *not* be administered to infants younger than 6 weeks of age.

Apnea has been reported following IM administration of vaccines in some infants born prematurely. Decisions regarding when to administer an IM vaccine in infants born prematurely should be based on consideration of the individual infant's medical status and potential benefits and possible risks of vaccination.

■ **Geriatric Precautions** Safety and efficacy of Hib vaccines have not been established in adults, including geriatric adults, and these vaccines are not usually used in this age group. (See Adults and Children 5 Years of Age or Older under Uses: Primary and Booster Immunization.)

■ **Mutagenicity and Carcinogenicity** Studies have not been performed to date to evaluate the mutagenic or carcinogenic potential of Hib vaccines.

■ **Pregnancy, Fertility, and Lactation** ***Pregnancy*** Hib vaccines are not labeled by FDA for use in adolescents or adults, and these vaccines are not usually used in this age group. (See Adults and Children 5 Years of Age or Older under Uses: Primary and Booster Immunization.)

Animal reproduction studies have not been performed with Hib vaccines. It is not known whether the vaccines can cause fetal harm when administered to pregnant women or whether they can affect fertility.

It is not known whether Hib capsular antigens contained in Hib vaccines cross the placenta. In one study, neonates born to women who received unconjugated Hib vaccine (no longer commercially available in the US) at 34–36 weeks' gestation had approximately 100-fold increases in cord blood anticapsular antibody levels compared with neonates born to women who did not receive the vaccine. Anticapsular antibody levels remained elevated for 12 months in the infants whose mothers were vaccinated during pregnancy. Serum Hib anticapsular antibody levels in these neonates were approximately 30% of levels reported in the mother.

ACIP states that there is no evidence of risk to the fetus if inactivated vaccines are administered during pregnancy.

Lactation Hib vaccines are not labeled by FDA for use in adolescents or adults, and these vaccines are not usually used in this age group. (See Adults and Children 5 Years of Age or Older under Uses: Primary and Booster Immunization.)

It is not known whether antigens contained in Hib vaccines are distributed into milk, affect human milk production, or affect the breast-fed infant.

In one study, Hib anticapsular antibody was distributed into milk of lactating women who received unconjugated Hib vaccine (no longer commercially available in the US) during the third trimester of pregnancy; anticapsular antibody levels in the milk of these women were 20 times higher than levels in the milk of women who received the vaccine prior to or following pregnancy. Antibodies to Hib capsular polysaccharide have been detected in the milk of nursing women who have natural immunity to Hib disease.

ACIP states that administration of an inactivated vaccine to a woman who is breast-feeding does not pose any safety concerns for the woman or the breast-fed infant.

Drug Interactions

■ **Immune Globulins** Immune globulin (immune globulin IM [IGIM], immune globulin IV [IGIV], immune globulin subcutaneous) or specific hyperimmune globulin (hepatitis B immune globulin [HBIG], rabies immune globulin [RIG], tetanus immune globulin [TIG], varicella zoster immune globulin [VZIG]) should not substantially impair the immune response to inactivated vaccines. The US Public Health Service Advisory Committee on Immunization Practices (ACIP) states that inactivated vaccines such as haemophilus b (Hib) vaccine may be given concurrently with (using separate syringes and different injection sites) or at any interval before or after immune globulin preparations.

■ **Immunosuppressive Agents** Individuals receiving immunosuppressive therapy (e.g., alkylating agents, antimetabolites, certain biologic response modifiers, corticosteroids, cytotoxic drugs, radiation therapy) may have reduced immune responses to vaccines, including Hib vaccine.

Inactivated vaccines generally should be administered at least 2 weeks prior to initiation of immunosuppressive therapy and, because of possible suboptimal response, should not be administered during and for certain periods of time after immunosuppressive therapy is discontinued. Because the intervals between discontinuance of immunosuppressive therapy and restoration of immune competence vary depending on the type and intensity of immunosuppressive therapy, underlying disease, and other factors, optimal timing for vaccine administration following discontinuance of immunosuppressive therapy has not been identified for every situation.

ACIP and the Infectious Diseases Society of America (IDSA) recommend that inactivated vaccines be administered at least 2 weeks before initiation of chemotherapy or radiation therapy, if possible, and avoided during such therapy. If Hib vaccine was administered to children younger than 5 years of age during or within 14 days of starting chemotherapy or radiation therapy, the child should be considered unimmunized and Hib vaccine doses should be repeated beginning at least 3 months following completion of such therapy if immune competence has been restored. Although administration of inactivated vaccines can be considered in children receiving maintenance chemotherapy, vaccine doses administered during such therapy should *not* be considered valid unless there is documentation of a protective antibody response. Individuals who received Hib vaccine more than 14 days prior to initiation of chemotherapy do not require revaccination.

Inactivated vaccines should be administered at least 2 weeks prior to treatment with anti-B-cell antibodies (e.g., rituximab). The optimal time to administer vaccines in patients who have received treatment with anti-B-cell antibodies is unclear. Some experts state that administration of inactivated vaccines should be deferred until at least 6 months after treatment with anti-B-cell antibodies has been discontinued.

Inactivated vaccines should be administered at least 2 weeks prior to initiation of therapy with certain other immunosuppressive biologic response modifiers (e.g., colony-stimulating factors, interleukins, tumor necrosis factor-α inhibitors). Some experts state that, if an inactivated vaccine is indicated in a patient with a chronic inflammatory illness who is receiving maintenance therapy with a biologic response modifier, the vaccine should not be withheld because of concern about exacerbation of the inflammatory illness.

Corticosteroids given in greater than physiologic doses may reduce immune responses to vaccines, including Hib vaccine. ACIP and the American Academy of Pediatrics (AAP) state that inactivated vaccines preferably should be administered at least 2 weeks prior to initiation of corticosteroid therapy that is considered immunosuppressive; however, if this is not feasible in patients receiving long-term corticosteroid therapy for inflammatory or autoimmune diseases, inactivated vaccines can be administered during such therapy. IDSA states that, although it may be reasonable to delay administration of inactivated vaccines in patients treated with high-dose corticosteroid therapy because of possible reduced immune responses, recommendations for use of Hib vaccine in individuals receiving corticosteroid therapy, including high-dose corticosteroid therapy, generally are the same as those for other individuals.

■ Vaccines

Although specific studies may not be available evaluating concurrent administration of Hib vaccine with each antigen, concurrent administration with other age-appropriate vaccines, including live virus vaccines, toxoids, or inactivated or recombinant vaccines, during the same health-care visit is not expected to affect immunologic responses or adverse reactions to any of the preparations.

Immunization with Hib vaccine can be integrated with immunization against diphtheria, tetanus, pertussis, hepatitis A, hepatitis B, influenza, measles, mumps, rubella, meningococcal disease, pneumococcal disease, poliovirus, rotavirus, and varicella. However, unless combination vaccines appropriate for the age and vaccination status of the recipient are used, each parenteral vaccine should be administered using separate syringes and different injection sites.

Inactivated Vaccines and Toxoids

Diphtheria and Tetanus Toxoids and Pertussis Vaccines. Monovalent Hib conjugate vaccine (meningococcal protein conjugate) (PRP-OMP; PedvaxHIB®) and monovalent Hib conjugate vaccine (tetanus toxoid conjugate) (PRP-T; ActHIB®, Hiberix®) can be administered concurrently with diphtheria and tetanus toxoids and acellular pertussis vaccine adsorbed (DTaP) using separate syringes and different injection sites without a decrease in the antibody response or an increase in adverse reactions to either vaccine. Alternatively, Hib vaccine is commercially available in a combination vaccine with DTaP, poliovirus vaccine inactivated (IPV), and Hib vaccine (DTaP-IPV/Hib; Pentacel®). Depending on the age and vaccination status of the child, this combination vaccine can be used instead of separate injections of Hib vaccine and DTaP vaccine when indicated and if there are no contraindications to any of the individual components. (See Combination Vaccines Containing Hib Vaccine and Other Antigens under Uses: Choice of Hib Vaccines.)

PRP-T (Hiberix®) has been administered concurrently with the fixed-combination vaccine containing diphtheria, tetanus, pertussis, hepatitis B, and poliovirus antigens (DTaP-HepB-IPV; Pediarix®) and pneumococcal 13-valent conjugate vaccine (PCV13; Prevnar® 13) in infants 2, 4, and 6 months of age without a reduced antibody response to DTaP or any of the other antigens. Concurrent administration of a booster dose of PRP-T (Hiberix®) and DTaP at different injection sites in children 15–18 months of age did not affect antibody responses to DTaP.

Hepatitis A Vaccine. In clinical studies in children 15 months of age who received hepatitis A virus vaccine inactivated (Havrix®, Vaqta®) and Hib vaccine concurrently at different injection sites (with or without other concurrent vaccines), immune responses and adverse effects were similar to those reported when the vaccines were administered at different times.

Hepatitis B Vaccine. Although specific data are not available, monovalent Hib vaccine may be given concurrently with hepatitis B vaccine (using separate syringes and different injection sites). Extemporaneous vaccine combinations of Hib vaccine and hepatitis B vaccine should *not* be prepared by admixing commercially available monovalent Hib vaccine and monovalent hepatitis B vaccine.

Pneumococcal Vaccines. Hib vaccine has been administered concurrently with PCV13; (Prevnar 13®) using a separate syringe at a different injection site.

Hib vaccine may be administered concurrently with pneumococcal 23-valent polysaccharide vaccine (PPSV23; Pneumovax®) using separate syringes and different injection sites.

Poliovirus Vaccine. Monovalent PRP-OMP or monovalent PRP-T may be administered concurrently with IPV using separate syringes and different injection sites. Alternatively, Hib vaccine is commercially available in combination with DTaP and IPV (DTaP-IPV/Hib; Pentacel®). Depending on the age and vaccination status of the child, this combination vaccine can be used instead of separate injections of Hib vaccine and IPV vaccine when indicated and if there are no contraindications to any of the individual components. (See Combination Vaccines Containing Hib Vaccine and Other Antigens under Uses: Choice of Hib Vaccines.)

Live Vaccines

Measles, Mumps, and Rubella Virus Vaccine Live. Concurrent administration of measles, mumps, and rubella virus vaccine live (MMR) and Hib vaccine does not interfere with the immune response or increase adverse effects of either vaccine. Hib vaccine and MMR vaccine may be administered concurrently (using separate syringes and different injection sites).

Rotavirus Vaccines. Rotavirus vaccine (Rotarix®, RotaTeq®) has been administered concurrently with Hib vaccines without a decrease in immune response to either vaccine.

Varicella Virus Vaccine Live. Although specific studies are not available, ACIP and AAP state that Hib vaccine may be administered concurrently with varicella virus vaccine live. Results of a retrospective cohort study that used data from the Vaccine Safety Datalink (VSD) project and included children 12 months of age or older who were vaccinated during January 1995 to December 1999 indicate that administration of varicella virus vaccine live concurrently with or less than 30 days after Hib vaccine did not increase the risk of breakthrough varicella infections.

Laboratory Test Interferences

Haemophilus b (Hib) vaccines potentially may interfere with interpretation of antigen detection tests such as latex agglutination and countercurrent immunoelectrophoresis that are used for diagnosis of systemic Hib disease. Antigenuria resulting from administration of unconjugated Hib vaccine (no longer commercially available in the US) in one child produced positive urinary latex agglutination tests for 7 days following immunization and initially obscured a diagnosis of aseptic meningitis in this patient. Hib capsular polysaccharide has also been detected in urine following administration of Hib conjugate vaccine. Therefore, urine antigen detection may not have diagnostic value in evaluating suspected Hib disease in children if performed within 1–2 weeks following administration of a Hib vaccine. Antigen testing of urine and serum specimens is no longer recommended for diagnosis of Hib infection.

Pharmacology

Haemophilus b conjugate (meningococcal protein conjugate) vaccine (PRP-OMP) and haemophilus b conjugate (tetanus toxoid conjugate) vaccine (PRP-T) are used to stimulate active immunity to *Haemophilus influenzae* type b (Hib) infection by inducing production of specific antibodies. Hib capsular polysaccharide present in the vaccines promotes the production of Hib anticapsular antibody; evidence indicates that this antibody provides protection against infection with *H. influenzae* type b.

■ Haemophilus influenzae Type b Infection

H. influenzae type b causes bacterial meningitis and other serious bacterial infections (e.g., pneumonia, epiglottitis, sepsis, cellulitis, septic arthritis, osteomyelitis, endocarditis, purulent pericarditis), especially in infants and children younger than 5 years of age. Nonencapsulated (nontypeable) strains of *H. influenzae* can also cause invasive disease, but usually cause mucosal infections such as otitis media, conjunctivitis, sinusitis, or bronchitis.

Hib disease occurs worldwide. Prior to the availability of Hib vaccine, a child's cumulative risk of developing systemic Hib infection in the US during the first 5 years of life was about 0.5%. The peak incidence of invasive Hib infections occurs between 6 and 18 months of age. Children younger than 3–6 months of age may have protection against Hib disease, possibly as a result of passively acquired maternal antibodies and/or antibodies acquired from breast milk.

Hib is transmitted from person to person, presumably by inhalation of respiratory tract droplets or by direct contact with respiratory tract secretions. Hib transiently colonizes the nasopharynx in some individuals without causing symptoms (asymptomatic carrier). In other individuals, Hib causes an invasive infection. Appropriate anti-infective therapy reduces the mortality from Hib meningitis, but long-term neurologic sequelae (e.g., mental retardation, deafness, blindness, seizure disorders, behavioral disorders, decreased school performance) occur in some survivors.

■ **Response to Conjugated Haemophilus b Vaccines** Hib capsular polysaccharide contained in Hib vaccines promotes the formation of Hib anticapsular antibody. All currently available Hib vaccines contain Hib capsular polysaccharide covalently bound to carrier protein antigens (tetanus toxoid or *Neisseria meningitidis* outer membrane protein complex [OMP]). These conjugated Hib vaccines induce an enhanced antibody response against Hib infection compared with that induced by unconjugated Hib vaccine (no longer commercially available in the US). This increased immunogenicity occurs because the carrier protein antigens (tetanus toxoid or OMP) confer T-lymphocyte-dependent (T-dependent) features to the polysaccharide antigen. T-dependent antigens induce an immune response that is predominantly IgG and potentially boostable following repeat doses.

Studies using unconjugated Hib vaccines (no longer commercially available in the US) indicate that antibody titers to *H. influenzae* capsular polysaccharide (anti-PRP) of 1 mcg/mL or greater after vaccination correlate with long-term protection against invasive Hib disease.

Twofold or greater increases in Hib anticapsular antibody levels compared with prevaccination levels have been observed in children 2–17 months of age following administration of 1–3 doses of various conjugated Hib vaccines. Booster responses have been observed following administration of a dose of conjugated Hib vaccine in children 15 through 18 months of age who previously received primary immunization with a Hib capsular polysaccharide/protein antigen combination.

In a clinical study using PRP-OMP (PedvaxHIB®), 80% of infants developed protective antibody levels (anti-PRP greater than 1 mcg/mL) after a primary series of 2 doses initiated at 2–3 months of age and 95% had protective antibody levels approximately 1 month after a booster dose given at 12–15 months of age.

In clinical studies using PRP-T (ActHIB®, Hiberix®), 81–97% of infants developed protective antibody levels (anti-PRP 1 mcg/mL or greater) after a primary immunization series of 3 doses given at 2, 4, and 6 months of age and 98–100% had protective antibody levels 1 month after a booster dose given at 15–23 months of age.

When a complete vaccination series is administered as recommended, regimens that include PRP-OMP or PRP-T are considered equivalent. However, there is some evidence that vaccines containing PRP-OMP result in more rapid seroconversion to protective antibody concentrations within the first 6 months of life compared with vaccines containing PRP-T. This is particularly important in American Indian and Alaskan native children because these children are at increased risk for Hib disease during the first 6 months of life. (See Uses: Choice of Hib Vaccines.)

Chemistry and Stability

■ **Chemistry** Haemophilus b (Hib) conjugate vaccines are noninfectious, bacteria-derived vaccines containing antigenic capsular polysaccharide extracted from *Haemophilus influenzae* type b. The vaccine capsular polysaccharides are derived from polyribosylribitol phosphate (PRP), a major Hib virulence factor. Hib conjugate vaccines are commercially available as the polysaccharide conjugate of *Neisseria meningitidis* outer membrane protein complex (PRP-OMP; PedvaxHIB®) or as the polysaccharide conjugate of tetanus toxoid (PRP-T; ActHIB®) (PRP-T; Hiberix®). These conjugated vaccines differ in the protein carrier, polysaccharide size, and method of conjugation, including use of a spacer (linking moiety) between the PRP and protein carrier.

Hib Conjugate Vaccine (Meningococcal Protein Conjugate) (PRP-OMP; PedvaxHIB®) Hib conjugate vaccine (meningococcal protein conjugate) (PRP-OMP) is a lyophilized preparation containing Hib capsular polysaccharide covalently bound to outer membrane protein complex (OMPC) of the B11 strain of *N. meningitidis* serogroup B. The capsular polysaccharide used in the preparation is PRP extracted from the Ross strain of Hib.

PRP-OMP is commercially available as PedvaxHIB®. PRP-OMP occurs as a slightly opaque, white suspension. Each 0.5-mL dose of PRP-OMP contains 7.5 mcg of purified Hib capsular polysaccharide, 125 mcg of *N. meningitidis* OMPC, and 225 mcg of aluminum as aluminum hydroxide in 0.9% sodium chloride. The vaccine does not contain thimerosal or any other preservative.

Hib Conjugate Vaccine (Tetanus Toxoid Conjugate) (PRP-T; ActHIB®) Hib conjugate vaccine (tetanus toxoid conjugate) (PRP-T; ActHIB®) is a lyophilized preparation containing Hib capsular polysaccharide covalently bound to tetanus toxoid.

The capsular polysaccharide contained in this PRP-T is prepared from Hib strain 1482; the tetanus toxoid conjugate is prepared by extraction, ammonium sulfate purification, and formalin inactivation of toxin from cultures of *Clostridium tetani* (Harvard strain) and is filter-sterilized prior to the conjugation process.

Following reconstitution of this PRP-T with the 0.4% sodium chloride diluent provided by the manufacturer, the vaccine is clear and colorless and each 0.5-mL dose contains 10 mcg of purified Hib capsular polysaccharide, 24 mcg of tetanus toxoid, and 8.5% sucrose. PRP-T reconstituted with 0.4% sodium chloride diluent does not contain thimerosal or any other preservative.

Hib Conjugate Vaccine (Tetanus Toxoid Conjugate) (PRP-T; Hiberix®) Hib conjugate vaccine (tetanus toxoid conjugate) (PRP-T; Hiberix®) is a lyophilized preparation containing Hib capsular polysaccharide covalently bound to tetanus toxoid.

The capsular polysaccharide contained in this PRP-T (Hiberix®) is prepared from Hib strain 20,752; the tetanus toxoid conjugate is prepared from cultures of *C. tetani* that are detoxified with formaldehyde and purified.

Following reconstitution of this PRP-T with the 0.9% sodium chloride diluent provided by the manufacturer, the vaccine is clear and colorless and each 0.5-mL dose contains 10 mcg of purified Hib capsular polysaccharide, 25 mcg of tetanus toxoid, 12.6 mg of lactose, and 0.5 mcg or less of residual formaldehyde. PRP-T reconstituted with 0.9% sodium chloride diluent does not contain thimerosal or any other preservative.

DTaP-IPV/Hib (Pentacel®) A combination vaccine containing diphtheria, tetanus, pertussis, poliovirus, and Hib antigens (DTaP-IPV/Hib; Pentacel®) is commercially available as a kit containing a fixed-combination liquid vaccine containing diphtheria, tetanus, pertussis, and poliovirus antigens (DTaP-IPV) and lyophilized Hib tetanus toxoid conjugate vaccine (PRP-T; ActHIB®). The DTaP-IPV vaccine from the kit is used to reconstitute the PRP-T vaccine from the kit to provide a single vaccine containing antigens for all 5 diseases. The diphtheria, tetanus, and pertussis antigens are identical to those contained in Daptacel® (DTaP) vaccine: however, the amounts of pertussis toxin (PT) and filamentous hemagglutinin (FHA) antigens in DTaP-IPV/Hib (Pentacel®) are twofold and fourfold higher, respectively, than those contained in Daptacel®. For information on these DTaP antigens, see Cautions in Diphtheria and Tetanus Toxoids and Acellular Pertussis Vaccine Adsorbed/Tetanus Toxoid and Reduced Diphtheria Toxoid and Acellular Pertussis Vaccine Adsorbed 80:08. For information on the poliovirus antigens, see Poliovirus Vaccine Inactivated 80:12.

Following reconstitution, each 0.5-mL dose of DTaP-IPV/Hib (Pentacel®) contains 15 Lf of diphtheria toxoid, 5 Lf of tetanus toxoid, 48 mcg of pertussis antigens, 40 D antigen units (DU) of poliovirus type 1, 8 DU of poliovirus type 2, 32 DU of poliovirus type 3, and 10 mcg of Hib antigen. Each 0.5 mL of DTaP-IPV/Hib also contains 0.33 mg of aluminum adjuvant, approximately 10 ppm of polysorbate 80, less than 50 ng of residual glutaraldehyde, not more than 50 ng of residual bovine serum albumin, not more than 5 mcg of residual formaldehyde, and 3.3 mg of 2-phenoxyethanol. Although neomycin sulfate and polymyxin B are used in the manufacturing process of the poliovirus antigen component, DTaP-IPV/Hib contains less than 4 pg of each anti-infective per dose.

■ **Stability** ***Hib Conjugate Vaccine (Meningococcal Protein Conjugate) (PRP-OMP; PedvaxHIB®)*** PRP-OMP (PedvaxHIB®) should be refrigerated at 2–8°C and should not be frozen.

Hib Conjugate Vaccine (Tetanus Toxoid Conjugate) (PRP-T; ActHIB®) Lyophilized PRP-T (ActHIB®) and the 0.4% sodium chloride diluent provided by the manufacturer should be refrigerated at 2–8°C and should not be frozen. The vaccine contains no preservatives.

Following reconstitution with the sodium chloride diluent, this PRP-T should be used promptly. Alternatively, the reconstituted vaccine may be stored at 2–8°C and used within 24 hours after reconstitution.

Hib Conjugate Vaccine (Tetanus Toxoid Conjugate) (PRP-T; Hiberix®) Lyophilized PRP-T (Hiberix®) should be stored at 2–8°C and protected from light. The 0.9% sodium chloride diluent supplied by the manufacturer should be stored at 2–8°C or at room temperature up to 25°C. The diluent should not be frozen and should be discarded if freezing occurs.

Following reconstitution with the diluent provided by the manufacturer, this PRP-T should be stored at 2–8°C, used within 24 hours, and protected from freezing. The reconstituted vaccine should be discarded if it has been frozen or has not been used within 24 hours.

DTaP-IPV/Hib (Pentacel®) The commercially available kit containing a fixed-combination DTaP-IPV vaccine and lyophilized PRP-T (ActHIB®) vaccine (DTaP-IPV/Hib; Pentacel®) should be stored at 2–8°C and should not be frozen. If freezing occurs, the vaccines should be discarded.

DTaP-IPV/Hib should be used immediately after reconstitution.

Preparations

Excipients in commercially available drug preparations may have clinically important effects in some individuals; consult specific product labeling for details.

Haemophilus b Conjugate Vaccine (Meningococcal Protein Conjugate) (PRP-OMP)

Parenteral

Injectable suspension, for IM use	7.5 mcg of Haemophilus b capsular polysaccharide conjugated to 125 mcg of *Neisseria meningitidis* OMPC protein carrier per 0.5 mL	**PedvaxHIB® Liquid,** Merck

Haemophilus b Conjugate Vaccine (Tetanus Toxoid Conjugate) (PRP-T)

Parenteral

For injectable suspension, for IM use	10 mcg of Haemophilus b capsular polysaccharide conjugated to 24 mcg of tetanus toxoid protein carrier per 0.5 mL	**ActHIB®,** Sanofi Pasteur

For injection, for IM use	10 mcg of Haemophilus b capsular polysaccharide conjugated to 25 mcg of tetanus toxoid protein carrier per 0.5 mL	Hiberix®, GlaxoSmithKline

Diphtheria and Tetanus Toxoids and Acellular Pertussis Adsorbed, Inactivated Poliovirus and Haemophilus b Conjugate (Tetanus Toxoid Conjugate) Vaccine (DTaP-IPV/Hib)

Parenteral		
Kit, for IM use	Injection, for IM use, Diphtheria Toxoid 15 Lf units, Tetanus Toxoid 5 Lf units, Acellular Pertussis Vaccine 48 mcg (of pertussis antigen), Poliovirus Type 1 40 DU, Poliovirus Type 2 8 DU, and Poliovirus Type 3 32 DU per 0.5 mL	Pentacel®, Sanofi Pasteur
	For injectable suspension, for IM use, 10 mcg of Haemophilus b polysaccharide conjugated to 25 mcg of tetanus toxoid protein carrier per 0.5 mL, ActHIB®	

†Use is not currently included in the labeling approved by the US Food and Drug Administration

Hepatitis A Virus Vaccine Inactivated

HAV Vaccine Inactivated, HepA, HepA-HepB

■ Hepatitis A virus vaccine is an inactivated vaccine that contains cell culture-adapted, attenuated hepatitis A virus (HAV) and is used to stimulate active immunity to HAV infection. Hepatitis A virus vaccine is commercially available in the US as monovalent vaccines (Havrix®, Vaqta®) and in a fixed-combination vaccine with hepatitis B vaccine (HepA-HepB; Twinrix®).

Uses

Hepatitis A virus vaccine inactivated (hepatitis A vaccine) is used to stimulate active immunity to hepatitis A virus (HAV) infection in individuals 12 months of age and older.

The US Public Health Service Advisory Committee on Immunization Practices (ACIP), American Academy of Pediatrics (AAP), and American Academy of Family Physicians (AAFP) recommend *routine* vaccination with hepatitis A vaccine for *all* children at 1 year of age (i.e., at 12 through 23 months of age), unless the vaccine is contraindicated. In addition, the ACIP, AAP, and AAFP recommend preexposure vaccination for previously unvaccinated children, adolescents, or adults who are at high risk of exposure to HAV and for any other unvaccinated individual desiring protection from HAV infection. Hepatitis A vaccine also is used alone or in conjunction with passive immunization with immune globulin IM (IGIM) for postexposure prophylaxis† in susceptible individuals with recent (within 2 weeks) exposure to HAV. (See Uses: Postexposure Prophylaxis.)

Hepatitis A vaccine will not prevent hepatitis caused by other infectious agents (e.g., hepatitis B virus [HBV], hepatitis C virus [HCV], hepatitis E virus [HEV]).

When vaccination against both HAV and HBV is indicated in adults 18 years of age or older, the commercially available fixed-combination vaccine containing hepatitis A vaccine and hepatitis B vaccine (HepA-HepB; Twinrix®) can be used. The ACIP, AAP, and AAFP state that use of a combination vaccine generally is preferred over separate injections of the equivalent component vaccines; considerations should include provider assessment (e.g., number of injections, vaccine availability, likelihood of improved coverage, likelihood of patient return, storage and cost considerations), patient preference, and potential for adverse effects. However, the HepA-HepB (Twinrix®) fixed-combination vaccine should *not* be used for HAV *postexposure* prophylaxis. (See Use of Fixed Combinations under Cautions: Precautions and Contraindications.)

■ Past and Current Considerations Regarding Hepatitis A Vaccine Recommendations Prior to the availability of hepatitis A vaccine, the principal means of preventing HAV infection involved hygienic and sanitary measures and prophylaxis with IGIM. From 1995–2005 after the vaccine became available, the strategy for HAV prevention and reduction in the overall incidence of the disease in the US consisted of selective vaccination of individuals in high-risk groups and in children residing in areas with consistently elevated rates of HAV infection. This limited strategy of selective vaccination in areas with consistently elevated rates of HAV infection reduced the overall incidence of the disease in the US to the lowest level ever recorded. The largest decreases occurred in areas where children received routine vaccination against HAV. Infection rates became more equally distributed in the US, with the highest rates reported in children who lived in areas of the country where selective vaccination had not been implemented.

Therefore, in late 2005, the ACIP expanded their recommendations regarding vaccination against HAV to include universal vaccination of all children in the US at 1 year of age. Since the continued implementation of the previous selective immunization strategy was unlikely to further reduce the overall incidence of HAV infection in the US, the new recommendations were developed by the ACIP to achieve more widespread routine vaccination of children to prevent infection in this age group and eventually among older individuals and thereby achieve a sustained reduction in HAV infection rates with the goal of total elimination of HAV transmission in the US. It is expected that universal childhood immunization against HAV will substantially lower disease incidence and potentially may eliminate indigenous transmission of HAV infection in the US.

Despite the relatively mild nature of HAV infection in most patients, the infection results in substantial morbidity and associated health-care and work-loss costs. Surveillance data indicate that 11–22% of individuals with clinical HAV infection will require hospitalization; the estimated duration of work loss is 33.2 days for adults with clinical illness requiring hospitalization and 15.5 days for those whose illness does not require hospitalization. The overall case fatality rate for HAV in the US is 0.3–0.6%, but increases to about 2% in patients older than 40 years of age. Epidemiologic changes in HAV during the past several decades are resulting in an increasingly larger proportion of older Americans who are susceptible to the disease (i.e., at an age when the risk of fulminant hepatitis is increased).

Available data regarding use of hepatitis A vaccine indicate that the observed reductions in HAV infection rates among children appear to have been achieved with modest levels of vaccine coverage, which suggests a strong herd immunity effect associated with use of the vaccine. Observed reductions in HAV infection rates among adults also suggest that use of hepatitis A vaccine among children may reduce HAV transmission among other age groups through herd immunity. Similar observations supporting the effect of herd immunity associated with routine hepatitis A vaccination of infants or children have been reported from other countries (e.g., Israel, Spain). Models evaluating the association between HAV infection rates and HAV vaccine coverage also indicate a strong herd immunity effect which may be responsible for preventing 33% of the estimated number of HAV cases prevented by vaccination in the US.

■ Types of Exposure HAV infection is highly contagious with the principal mode of transmission being enteric (i.e., through fecal contamination and oral ingestion), most commonly from person to person, particularly from children to adults. HAV is shed in feces and is highly resistant to degradation by environmental conditions, which is a major factor in maintenance and common-source spread of HAV within populations. Depending on conditions, the virus may be environmentally stable for months; heating foods and beverages to temperatures exceeding 85°C for 1 minute or disinfecting surfaces with a 1:100 dilution of household bleach (sodium hypochlorite) is required for inactivation. Because HAV is so environmentally stable, transmission can occur by ingestion of contaminated water or food. While there is evidence from studies in non-human primates that the virus can be isolated from saliva during the incubation period, epidemiologic studies have not revealed evidence of transmission of HAV via saliva in humans.

Prior to the availability of hepatitis A vaccine, most HAV infections within the US resulted from person-to-person transmission of HAV during community-wide outbreaks and the most common reported sources of infection were contact (household or sexual) with an HAV-infected individual (12–26% of cases), contact with children attending or employees of child-care centers (particularly those with inadequately toilet-trained children) or with a child-care-related case (14–16% of cases), international travel (4–6% of cases), or being part of a recognized common-source (food or waterborne) outbreak (2–3% of cases). Among international travelers who developed HAV during this period, about 36% of cases were reported in children and 84% of cases involved travel to Mexico. Although the number of international travel-related cases of HAV has remained relatively constant following the availability of hepatitis A vaccine, recently the overall incidence of such HAV cases has declined. During 2006, international travel was the identified risk factor for 15% of HAV infections. Illicit drug use remains another common source of HAV infection.

In approximately 45–50% of reported cases of HAV prior to widespread HAV vaccination, no specific risk factor was identified, but children played a major role in HAV transmission, and approximately 52% of households of such reported HAV cases contained a child younger than 6 years of age. About 33% of reported cases of HAV infection in the US occurred in children younger than 15 years of age, and many more pediatric cases presumably went unrecognized because of the increased likelihood of asymptomatic HAV infection in this age group. In addition, studies of household contacts of adults with HAV and in whom no source of infection is known indicate that 25–40% of contacts younger than 6 years of age had serologic evidence of acute HAV infection (i.e., immunoglobulin M [IgM] anti-HAV). Therefore, children serve as a major source of infection for members of the household. However, in recent years only about 9% of individuals with HAV infection report exposure to child-care centers.

Person-to-person contact via the fecal-oral route is thought to be the principal source of HAV outbreaks among parenteral and nonparenteral illicit drug users and among homosexual and bisexual men. In addition, HAV transmission among parenteral drug users occurs by the percutaneous route through shared needles and other drug paraphernalia. Cyclic outbreaks continue to be reported among parenteral and nonparenteral illicit drug users and among men who have sex with men; before HAV vaccine was available, up to 15% of cases reported in the US involved individuals who reported one or more of these behaviors. Over the last couple of decades, the frequency of HAV outbreaks has been increasing among illicit drug users in the US; up to 48% of reported cases during such outbreaks involved illicit use of methamphetamine (injected or noninjected). HAV outbreaks continue to be reported among homosexual and bisexual men in the US.

While HAV principally is spread enterically between close contacts, the virus also can be spread by infected food handlers, by a breakdown in usual sanitary conditions (e.g., sewage-contaminated drinking water), by raw or undercooked shellfish (e.g., clams, mussels, oysters) from contaminated waters, by contaminated foods (e.g. fruits, vegetables) that are eaten uncooked, by poor hygienic conditions during travel to certain areas of the world, by closed living conditions (e.g., among institutionalized children and adults), in health-care settings, and by parenteral transmission (e.g., transfusions of blood or plasma-derived preparations, sharing needles with infected individuals).

A chronic carrier state has not been identified in individuals with HAV infection; however, relapse of clinical infection occurs in up to 15% of patients, and fecal viral shedding can recur at this time. During the convalescent phase of the disease, immunoglobulin G (IgG) anti-HAV can be detected in the patient's serum and generally remains present for the life of the patient, conferring lifelong immunity to HAV and presumably protection from reinfection.

■ Risks of Exposure and Infection

Hepatitis A Epidemiology Prior to Availability of Hepatitis A Vaccine The epidemiology of HAV infection in the US was fundamentally changed by the availability of hepatitis A vaccine and subsequent implementation of ACIP recommendations for use of the vaccine. The incidence of HAV infection in the US had been cyclic, with nationwide epidemics occurring every 10–15 years; the last reported nationwide increase in HAV morbidity was in 1995.

The incidence of HAV infection was highest among children 5–14 years of age and approximately 33% of reported cases involved children younger than 15 years of age. Incidence models indicate that during 1980–1999, most HAV infections occurred among children younger than 10 years of age and the highest incidence was among those younger than 4 years of age. Before hepatitis A vaccine was available, the rate of HAV infection among Native Americans and Alaskans was 5 times the rate reported in other racial/ethnic populations, and the rate among Hispanics was approximately 3 times higher than rates among non-Hispanics.

During the several decades prior to the availability of hepatitis A vaccine, the highest rates of HAV infection occurred in a limited number of states and counties in the US, especially in the western and southwestern US, including Arizona, Alaska, Oregon, New Mexico, Utah, Washington, Oklahoma, South Dakota, Idaho, Nevada, and California. Although annual infection rates in these states fluctuated, 50% (annual average) of reported cases during the period from 1987–1997 were from these states, where average disease rates exceed 20 cases per 100,000 during 1987–1997 (twice the national average rate); however, the combined population in these states is only about 22% of the US population. During this period, an additional 18% of cases were from states with average annual HAV infection rates that were higher than the national average but less than twice the national average (e.g., Missouri, Texas, Colorado, Arkansas, Montana, Wyoming).

Seroepidemiologic studies indicated that the likelihood of prior HAV infection in the US was related to age, household size, and ethnic/socioeconomic status. During 1988–1994, the Third National Health and Nutrition Examination Survey (NHANES-III) indicated that approximately 31–33% of the US population had serologic evidence of previous HAV infection. Serologic evidence of exposure was present in 9% of Americans 6–11 years of age, in 19% of those 20–29 years of age, in 33% of those 40–49 years of age, and in 75% by age 70. Age-adjusted anti-HAV serologic prevalence was considerably higher among Mexican-American (70%) compared with black (39%) and white (23%) individuals, and among foreign-born (69%) compared with US-born (25%) individuals.

Hepatitis A Epidemiology Following Availability of Hepatitis A Vaccine Following US Food and Drug Administration (FDA) approval of hepatitis A vaccine in 1995, the rate of HAV infection declined sharply in the US, especially after ACIP recommendations in 1999 regarding routine vaccination of children living in areas with consistently elevated rates of HAV infection. In 2004, a total of 5683 cases of HAV infection (rate: 1.9 cases per 100,000 population) were reported; considering underreporting, the actual number of cases of acute HAV that year is estimated to be approximately 24,000. This is the lowest rate of HAV infection ever reported in the US and is 79% lower than the previously reported low rate in 1992.

The recent decline in the rate of HAV infection is also reflected in other fundamental changes in the epidemiology of HAV infection. Since age-specific rates of HAV declined more rapidly among children than adults during the past decade, rates have become similar across all age groups. In addition, differences in HAV rates among racial/ethnic populations have also narrowed following the availability of hepatitis A vaccine. Recent HAV rates among Native Americans and Alaskans have decreased by 99% compared with rates before the vaccine was available; the rates in these populations are now approximately the same as or lower than those of other racial/ethnic populations. Although the rate of HAV infection remains higher among Hispanics than among non-Hispanics, the rates among Hispanics did decline 87% during this period, from 20.6 cases per 100,000 during 1990–1997 to 2.7 per 100,000 in 2004.

Previous geographic differences in incidence rates have also been eliminated; since 2001, the incidence of HAV in states with vaccination programs is similar to that in the rest of the US. Recently, counties with higher rates have varied annually and have been distributed throughout the entire US. Following implementation of the 1999 ACIP recommendations for routine vaccination in children in areas with a high prevalence of HAV infection, the incidence of HAV decreased sharply in states with previously consistently elevated rates. As a result, the majority of HAV infections during recent years have been reported from states with previously low rates where routine use of hepatitis A vaccine of children has not been widely implemented. In addition, the decrease or elimination of differences in age, race/ethnicity, and state-specific rates in the US can be attributed largely to changes that occurred in the states with programs for routine vaccination of children. Approximately 66% of the 6000 cases of HAV reported in 2004 were from states where the ACIP did not recommend routine childhood vaccination. The rate of HAV among all Hispanics in these states in 2004 remained 4 times higher than among non-Hispanics and was 7 times higher among Hispanic children compared with non-Hispanic children. The highest rate of HAV infection reported in any demographic subgroup was among Hispanic children in states that did not have routine childhood HAV vaccination programs.

Individuals Considered at Risk **Household and Sexual Contacts.** Household and sexual contacts of individuals with confirmed HAV infection are at high risk of exposure to HAV. Approximately 13% of reported cases in the US during 2002–2004 were attributable to such contact. Cyclic outbreaks of HAV have been reported frequently in male homosexuals and bisexuals in urban areas of the US, Canada, Europe, and Australia, and the likelihood of prior HAV infection is related to the nature and duration of homosexual activity and number of sexual partners.

Travelers. HAV infection remains one of the most commonly reported vaccine-preventable diseases in travelers. HAV infection is common (high or intermediate endemicity) in developing countries, and travelers to these countries are at risk and should be vaccinated against the disease. Travelers to countries with low HAV endemicity (e.g., Australia, Canada, western Europe, Japan, New Zealand) are at no greater risk for infection than individuals living or traveling in the US. The risk of acquiring HAV while traveling varies with living conditions, length of stay, and incidence of HAV infection in the area visited. Many cases of HAV occur in travelers to developing countries with standard tourist itineraries, accommodations, and food consumption behaviors. The Centers for Disease Control and Prevention (CDC) website (http://www.cdc.gov/travel) should be consulted for information regarding which countries have high or intermediate levels of HAV endemicity.

Occupational Risk. Individuals at high risk of occupational exposure to HAV in the US include those working with HAV-susceptible nonhuman primates and those working with the live virus in a research laboratory setting. Nonhuman primates (i.e., great apes, several species of old- and new-world monkeys) are susceptible to HAV infection, and outbreaks of HAV have occurred in workers handling such animals.

The risk of occupational exposure to HAV has not been shown to be increased in other occupational groups in the US, including health-care workers, those working in a child-care setting, or food handlers. When proper infection control practices are followed, nosocomial HAV transmission is rare and occupational exposure generally does not increase the risk of infection for health-care personnel. Although some epidemiologic evidence from abroad suggests that workers with sewage exposure may be at high risk of HAV exposure, the quality of the evidence has been questioned (e.g., other risk factors such as socioeconomic status were not controlled for). In addition, data from 3 serologic surveys of US wastewater workers with appropriate control populations indicate that there is no substantial or consistent increase in the serologic prevalence of anti-HAV among wastewater workers and no work-related cases of HAV transmission or outbreaks among such workers have been reported to date in the US.

Others Considered at Risk. Other individuals considered at high risk of exposure to HAV include individuals engaging in high-risk sexual activity (e.g., homosexually and bisexually active adolescent and adult males); users of illicit injectable or noninjectable drugs; and residents of a community that is experiencing an outbreak of HAV. Although not at increased risk of HAV infection, individuals with chronic liver disease, including those with alcoholic cirrhosis, chronic HBV or HCV infection, autoimmune hepatitis, or primary biliary cirrhosis and those awaiting or having received liver transplants are at increased risk of developing severe consequences of HAV infection, including fatal fulminant hepatitis and hepatic failure.

Because blood products (e.g., whole blood, packed red blood cells, plasma) and plasma-derived preparations (e.g., albumin human, antihemophilic factor [human], anti-inhibitor coagulant complex, factor IX [human], factor IX complex) are potential vehicles for transmission of human viruses, including HAV, individuals who receive frequent and/or large-volume transfusions of blood products or plasma-derived preparations (e.g., individuals with hemophilia or thalassemia) may be at increased risk for HAV. (See Recipients of Blood Products and Plasma-derived Preparations, under Uses: Preexposure Vaccination in High-risk Groups.)

The epidemiology of HAV infection does not permit identification of other specific populations at high risk of disease, but outbreaks of HAV infection or exposure to HAV have been described in a variety of populations in which hepatitis A vaccine may be useful, such as certain institutional workers (e.g., caretakers for the developmentally disabled), employees of child-care centers, and individuals exposed to HAV. Additional study is needed to define the benefit, if any, of hepatitis A vaccine if an outbreak occurs in such settings.

Settings Associated with Risk of Transmission In addition to populations considered at high risk for HAV infection, certain settings are associated with a high risk of outbreaks of the virus. Such settings include child-care centers, institutions for the developmentally disabled, health-care settings, correctional facilities, and areas of common-source outbreaks.

Child-care Centers. HAV outbreaks in children attending child-care centers and in child-care employees have been reported since 1970; however, the frequency of such outbreaks has decreased with the recent decline in HAV prevalence in children. Lack of hygienic practices among diapered children in addition to changing and handling of diapers by staff contribute to the spread of HAV in child-care centers. Outbreaks rarely occur in centers that serve only nondiapered children. Because pediatric HAV infection usually is mild or asymptomatic, outbreaks in child-care centers often go unrecognized until an adult contact (usually a parent) becomes symptomatic. Although outbreaks among children and employees of child-care centers may be the source of larger outbreaks in certain communities, HAV infection in child-care centers more often is indicative of extended transmission from the community. Despite the occurrence of such outbreaks, child-care center staff and children and adolescents with a history of child-care center attendance do not exhibit an increased rate of HAV seropositivity.

Institutions for the Developmentally Disabled. HAV historically was endemic in institutions for the developmentally disabled. While the incidence and prevalence of HAV infection in these institutions has declined secondary to declining censuses and improvements in living conditions, sporadic outbreaks continue to occur in this setting.

Correctional Facilities. The AAP recommends that hepatitis A vaccine be given to incarcerated adolescents in correctional facilities located in states with existing programs for hepatitis A immunization of adolescents. Because of the likelihood that adolescents in the juvenile correctional system have indications for the vaccine, other correctional facilities also should consider routine hepatitis A immunization of all adolescents under their care. Incarcerated adolescents with signs or symptoms of hepatitis should be tested for acute HAV, HBV, and HCV infection. Those with HAV should be reported to the local health department and appropriate postexposure prophylaxis with hepatitis A vaccine should be given to susceptible exposed residents.

Schools. Transmission of HAV between children within primary and secondary schools is uncommon in developed countries, but outbreaks can occur. In developing countries, transmission of HAV between children within primary schools is more common.

Cases of HAV infection in primary or secondary schools in the US generally indicate community disease transmission. Child-to-child disease transmission in the school setting is uncommon; however, if multiple cases of HAV occur among children at a particular school, common-source infection should be excluded by epidemiologic investigation.

Health-care Settings. Nosocomial transmission of HAV in health-care settings is rare. Occasional outbreaks have occurred in neonatal intensive-care settings secondary to transmission by staff exposed to a neonate who acquired the infection from transfused blood products. Outbreaks in health-care settings also can occur secondary to staff handling of infected adults who are fecally incontinent, although most hospitalized patients with HAV infection are admitted subsequent to jaundice onset, at which time peak infectivity has passed. Epidemiologic evidence from many types of US and European health-care workers has not revealed any evidence of an increased rate of HAV seropositivity compared with that in other workers.

Food Service Establishments. Common-source foodborne HAV outbreaks, although relatively uncommon in the US, appear to be on the increase and require intensive public health intervention when they occur. Foodborne outbreaks in the US often result from contamination of food during preparation by an HAV-infected food handler, although contamination of uncooked produce or fruit (e.g., green onions, lettuce, raspberries, strawberries), shellfish, and sandwiches prior to arrival at the food service establishment has been reported with increasing frequency. In contrast to the relatively low risk in the US, contaminated food (e.g., fruit, shellfish, uncooked vegetables or other foods) is a common source of HAV transmission during international travel.

Other Settings. Common-source waterborne outbreaks are infrequent in the US and other developed countries and usually are related to sewage contamination of drinking water or inadequately treated water. In contrast, water is a common source of HAV transmission during international travel.

Communitywide Risk Prior to the availability of hepatitis A vaccine, most HAV infections within the US resulted from person-to-person transmission of HAV in households and extended family settings during communitywide outbreaks. These outbreaks often spread throughout the community; a single risk factor or group generally was not identified. Such communitywide outbreaks often persisted for 1–2 years and were difficult to control. HAV infection in children often is asymptomatic or not recognized; therefore children played a key role in sustaining HAV transmission during these outbreaks. Since the implementation of selective childhood hepatitis A vaccination programs, large communitywide HAV outbreaks have decreased considerably. It is expected that universal childhood vaccination against HAV will substantially lower disease incidence and may potentially eliminate indigenous transmission of HAV infection in the US.

Although there has been some interest in the use of hepatitis A vaccine to interrupt ongoing communitywide epidemics by vaccinating children in affected populations, such vaccine programs have been difficult to implement. First-dose vaccine coverage during such programs has generally been low (20–45%) and the benefit of HAV vaccination was limited to vaccinated age groups that were not representative of groups reporting high rates of HAV infection. Sustained efforts to implement routine childhood vaccination with hepatitis A vaccine to maintain high levels of immunity are expected to prevent future epidemics.

■ **Primary Immunization** ***Children 12 Months of Age and Older*** The ACIP, AAP, and AAFP recommend that *all* children 1 year of age (i.e., 12 through 23 months) receive primary immunization against HAV infection using hepatitis A vaccine, unless the vaccine is contraindicated. Children who are not vaccinated by 2 years of age may be vaccinated at subsequent visits. The ACIP also recommends that states, counties, and communities with existing selective preexposure hepatitis A vaccination programs for children 2 through 18 years of age maintain these programs. (See Uses: Preexposure Vaccination in High-risk Groups.) In such areas, new efforts focused on routine vaccination of children at 1 year of age should enhance, not replace, ongoing programs directed at a broader population of children In areas without existing selective preexposure hepatitis A vaccination programs, catch-up vaccination of unvaccinated children 2 through 18 years of age may be considered. Catch-up vaccination programs may be warranted in the context of rising incidence or ongoing outbreaks of HAV among children or adolescents.

Infants Younger than 12 Months of Age Safety and efficacy of hepatitis A vaccine have not been established in children younger than 12 months of age. Data regarding the use of the vaccine in neonates and infants younger than 12 months of age are limited; the optimal dose and vaccination schedule in this age group as well as the effect of passively acquired maternal antibody on vaccine immunogenicity remain to be more fully elucidated. (See Cautions: Pediatric Precautions.)

Internationally Adopted Children and Other Immigrants Individuals seeking an immigrant visa for permanent US residency must provide proof of age-appropriate vaccination according to the US Recommended Childhood and Adolescent Immunization Schedules or the US Recommended Adult Schedule (see Immunization Schedules, US 80:00). Although this vaccination requirement applies to all immigrant infants and children entering the US, internationally adopted children younger than 11 years of age are exempt from the overseas vaccination requirements; however, adoptive parents are required to sign a waiver indicating their intention to comply with the vaccination requirements within 30 days after the infant or child arrives in the US. The CDC states that more than 90% of newly arrived internationally adopted children need catch-up vaccinations to meet the US Recommended Immunization Schedules.

The fact that immunization schedules of other countries may differ from US schedules (e.g., different recommended vaccines, recommended ages of administration, and/or number and timing of vaccine doses) should be considered. Vaccines administered outside the US can generally be accepted as valid if the administration schedule was similar to that recommended in the US childhood and adolescent immunization schedules. Only written vaccination records should be considered as evidence of previous vaccination since such records are more likely to accurately predict protection if the vaccines administered, intervals between doses, and child's age at the time of vaccination are similar to US recommendations; however, the extent to which an internationally adopted child's immunization record reflects their protection against disease is unclear and it is possible there may be transcription errors in such records (e.g., single-antigen vaccine may have been administered although a multiple-antigen vaccine was recorded). Although vaccines with inadequate potency have been produced in other countries, most vaccines used worldwide are immunogenic and produced with adequate quality control standards.

For internationally adopted children whose immune status is uncertain, vaccinations can be repeated or serologic tests performed to confirm immunity. For hepatitis A vaccine, the ACIP states that the simplest approach is to revaccinate according to the US recommended immunization schedule in children 12 months of age or older. Alternatively, test for serologic evidence of susceptibility to HAV.

When a child is being adopted from a country with high or intermediate HAV endemicity, the ACIP states that all previously unvaccinated individuals who anticipate close personal contact with the adoptee during the child's initial 60 days in the US (e.g., household members, regular babysitters) should receive routine vaccination with hepatitis A vaccine, with the first dose given as soon as adoption is planned (ideally at least 2 weeks before the child's arrival). The CDC website (http://www.cdc.gov/travel) should be consulted for information regarding which countries have high or intermediate levels of HAV endemicity.

■ **Preexposure Vaccination in High-risk Groups** The ACIP, AAP, and AAFP recommend preexposure vaccination for previously unvaccinated children, adolescents, or adults who are at high risk of exposure to HAV and for any other unvaccinated individual desiring protection from HAV infection. Hepatitis A vaccine is used for selective immunization of previously unvaccinated children 12 months of age or older who reside in states, counties, or communities where the rate of HAV infection is high and for preexposure vaccination in unvaccinated individuals who are or will be at high risk of exposure to HAV, including travelers, populations with a high risk of infection, individuals at risk because of their sexual practices, individuals with potential occupational exposure, military personnel, and other individuals at risk of exposure. Preexposure vaccination also is recommended for unvaccinated individuals with chronic liver disease because of the potentially serious consequences of HAV infection if it were to occur.

IGIM generally is used for preexposure passive immunoprophylaxis in situations when hepatitis A vaccine cannot be used for preexposure vaccination (e.g., when the vaccine is contraindicated, unavailable, or is cost prohibitive) and when short-term protection is required.

Children Who Reside in High-risk Areas The ACIP, AAP, and AAFP recommend routine vaccination of previously unvaccinated children who reside in states, counties, and communities where the rate of HAV infection is high. The strategy of routine primary immunization against HAV in *all* children at 1 year of age (i.e., 12 through 23 months of age) is expected to eventually eliminate transmission of HAV in the US. (See Children 12 Months of Age and Older under Uses: Primary Immunization.) The ACIP recommends that states, counties, and communities with existing selective preexposure hepatitis A vaccination programs for children 2 through 18 years of age maintain these programs. In such areas, new efforts focused on routine vaccination of children at 1 year of age should enhance, not replace, ongoing programs directed at a broader population of children. In areas without existing selective vaccination programs, catch-up vaccination of unvaccinated children 2 through 18 years of age may be considered. Catch-up vaccination programs may especially be warranted in the context of rising incidence or ongoing outbreaks of HAV among children or adolescents.

HIV-infected Individuals Because hepatitis A vaccine is an inactivated vaccine, it can be used safely in immunocompromised individuals, including individuals with human immunodeficiency virus (HIV) infection; however, the fact that the vaccine may be less immunogenic in immunocompromised individuals than in immunocompetent individuals should be considered. (See Pharmacology: Response to Hepatitis A Virus Vaccine Inactivated.)

Recommendations for use of hepatitis A vaccine in HIV-infected individuals are the same as those for individuals without HIV infection. HIV-infected individuals with chronic liver disease (including those coinfected with HBV or HCV) are at risk of fulminant hepatic failure if they acquire HAV. The ACIP, AAP, CDC, National Institutes of Health (NIH), Infectious Diseases Society of America (IDSA), Pediatric Infectious Diseases Society, and others recommend that HAV-susceptible, HIV-infected adults, adolescents, and children receive hepatitis A vaccine. Because the response to the vaccine may be reduced in those with $CD4^+$ T-cell counts less than 200 cells/mm^3, some experts suggest delaying vaccination until the patient is receiving antiretroviral therapy and the $CD4^+$ T-cell count is greater than 200 cells/mm^3.

Travelers Travelers to areas with intermediate to high levels of endemic HAV are at risk of exposure to the disease. (See Travelers, under Uses: Risks of Exposure and Infection.) Clinicians should be alert to opportunities to provide vaccination for all travelers whose plans might include travel at some time in the future to an area of high or intermediate HAV endemicity, including those whose current medical evaluation is for travel to an area where hepatitis A vaccination is not recommended.

The ACIP, CDC, World Health Organization (WHO), and other clinicians state that all susceptible individuals traveling to or working in areas with intermediate to high levels of endemic HAV should receive preexposure vaccination with hepatitis A vaccine or, alternatively, preexposure prophylaxis with IGIM prior to departure. A complete schedule of HAV vaccination at the age-appropriate dose is preferable to prophylaxis with IGIM in children 12 months of age and older, adolescents, and adults because of the longer duration of immunity conferred by the vaccine, especially for individuals planning to travel repeatedly to, or reside for long periods in, areas with intermediate or high levels of endemic HAV infection. Travelers who are allergic to a vaccine component or younger than 12 months of age and travelers electing not to receive the vaccine should receive preexposure prophylaxis with IGIM since it provides protection for up to 3 months; if travel will be more prolonged, a high dose of IGIM should be given initially or repeated (if travel will exceed 5 months) during travel.

Administration of a primary and second (booster) dose of hepatitis A vaccine prior to possible HAV exposure ensures the highest antibody titers. Unvaccinated individuals should receive the first dose of hepatitis A vaccine as soon as travel to countries with high or intermediate HAV endemicity is considered. Protection can be assumed if a single vaccine dose is administered at least 4 weeks prior to possible exposure to HAV. Although the degree of protection provided 2–4 weeks after an initial dose of hepatitis A virus vaccine is unknown, data from a study that evaluated the relative efficacy of a single dose of monovalent hepatitis A vaccine or a single dose of IGIM for postexposure prophylaxis in susceptible individuals 12 months to 40 years of age (see Clinical Experience under Uses: Postexposure Prophylaxis) suggest that a single vaccine dose administered at any time before departure can provide adequate protection for most healthy individuals 12 months to 40 years of age.

For optimal protection in travelers at greatest risk for HAV (older adults or individuals with altered immunocompetence, chronic liver disease, or other chronic medical condition) who are planning to depart to an area of HAV risk within 2 weeks should receive the initial dose of hepatitis A vaccine and also should receive simultaneously (at a different site) a dose of IGIM. Completion of the recommended vaccine series is necessary for long-term protection.

Whenever the vaccine is contraindicated or cannot be used (e.g., in travelers younger than 12 months of age) or when travelers elect not to receive the vaccine, a single dose of IGIM should be administered prior to travel since it provides effective protection against HAV for up to 3 months.

Data are not available regarding the possible efficacy of the fixed-combination vaccine containing hepatitis A vaccine and hepatitis B vaccine (HepA-HepB; Twinrix®) for preexposure vaccination of travelers who will depart prior to 2 weeks after receipt of the vaccine. The ACIP states that the fixed-combination vaccine should not be used in such situations. (See Use of Fixed Combinations under Cautions: Precautions and Contraindications.)

Individuals who receive a dose of hepatitis A vaccine within 2 weeks of departure and who do not receive IGIM (e.g., by choice or because of limited availability) will be at lower risk for infection than those who do not receive the vaccine or IGIM. Although at least 80% of healthy adults develop protective levels of anti-HAV within 15 days of a single 1440-unit dose of Havrix® vaccine, and 69% of healthy adults develop protective levels of anti-HAV within 2 weeks of a single 50-unit dose of Vaqta®, a second dose 6–12 months later is necessary for long-term protection. In addition, other data indicate that up to 50% of vaccinees may not be protected at 14 days after receiving an initial dose of vaccine. (See Pharmacology: Response to Hepatitis A Virus Vaccine Inactivated.) For individuals with imminent departure dates (e.g. less than 4 weeks after the initial vaccine dose) who require both immediate and long-term protection, the vaccine and IGIM can be administered simultaneously at different sites; if only short-term protection is required, IGIM can be used alone.

For travelers older than 40 years of age, adult travelers who were born in or resided for extensive periods in geographic areas with a high or intermediate level of endemic hepatitis A, and certain older adolescent and adult travelers (e.g., those from certain high-risk populations such as Native Americans and Alaskans, Hispanics), prevaccination serologic testing for susceptibility to HAV can be considered. (See Uses: Serologic Testing.)

Individuals at Risk of Exposure Because of Their Sexual Practices Male homosexuals and bisexuals are at high risk of exposure to HAV infection secondary to their sexual practices. Therefore, the ACIP, CDC, and manufacturers recommend that all sexually active male adolescents and adults who have sex with men (homosexual, bisexual) receive preexposure vaccination with hepatitis A vaccine. Primary-care clinicians and those in specialty medical settings should offer hepatitis A vaccine to male adolescents and adults who have sex with men; strategies to increase coverage (e.g., use of standing orders) should be considered. Prevaccination serologic testing for susceptibility to HAV may be cost effective in certain men who have sex with men since the prevalence of HAV infection is likely to be high. The ACIP recommends that prevaccination serologic testing be considered for older adults of this group, but may not be indicated for adolescents.

Illicit Drug Users Individuals who illicitly use injectable or noninjectable drugs may be at increased risk of exposure to HAV infection. (See Uses: Types of Exposure.) The ACIP and CDC recommend preexposure vaccination with hepatitis A vaccine for illicit users of injectable or noninjectable drugs. Prevaccination serologic testing for HAV susceptibility may be considered for adults in this group, but testing is not indicated for adolescents. In addition, the need for prevaccination serologic testing may also depend on the specific characteristics of a particular population of drug users (e.g., type and duration of drug use). Clinicians should obtain a complete history to identify individuals who might benefit from hepatitis A vaccination (e.g., those who use illicit drugs or who are at increased risk for such drug use). Clinicians should consider implementing strategies to increase vaccine coverage in these patients (e.g., use of standing orders).

Recipients of Blood Products and Plasma-derived Preparations The extent to which recipients of blood products (e.g., whole blood, packed red blood cells, plasma) and plasma-derived preparations (e.g., albumin human, antihemophilic factor [human], anti-inhibitor coagulant complex, factor IX [human], factor IX complex) may be at high risk of HAV exposure is unclear, but certain populations (e.g., individuals with hemophilia receiving solvent/detergent-treated plasma-derived preparations) appear to be at increased risk of exposure to the virus via such preparations. Several outbreaks of HAV infection have been reported in Europe in individuals with hemophilia receiving chemically (solvent/detergent) treated antihemophilic factor (human) preparations that presumably were contaminated from plasma of donors who were incubating HAV at the time of donation. Data from one serologic study in the US suggest that individuals with hemophilia may be at increased risk for HAV infection. In addition, HAV seroconversion has been reported in a few recipients of similar plasma-derived preparations marketed in the US and in at least one patient who received a factor IX (human) product inactivated by a chemical (solvent/detergent) process. However, more effective viral inactivation procedures, high HAV vaccine coverage, and improved donor screening have decreased the risk for HAV transmission from clotting factors. Analysis of serosurveillance data from 140 participating hemophilia treatment centers obtained during May 1998 through July 2002, indicates that there were no new cases of HAV infection attributable to blood products during this period. Because HAV can be transmitted via blood products and plasma-derived products including antihemophilic factor (human), the ACIP recommends that all susceptible individuals receiving plasma-derived clotting-factor concentrates receive preexposure vaccination with the vaccine. The National Hemophilia Foundation's Medical and Scientific Advisory Council (MASAC) recommends that all individuals with hemophilia or other congenital bleeding who are HAV-seronegative should receive age-appropriate preexposure vaccination with hepatitis A vaccine. This is especially important for those who have HCV infection. Although postvaccination serologic testing to confirm immunity is not usually indicated because of the high rate of vaccine response, MASAC strongly recommends such testing following HAV vaccination in adults and children with hemophilia. (See Cautions: Precautions and Contraindications.)

Individuals with Occupational Risk ACIP recommends preexposure vaccination with hepatitis A vaccine in workers handling HAV-infected nonhuman primates (born in the wild) and workers in contact with live HAV in a research laboratory setting. *Routine* immunization with the vaccine currently is not recommended for other occupational groups in the US. (See Occupational Risk, under Uses: Risks of Exposure and Infection.)

The ACIP and the Hospital Infection Control Practices Advisory Committee (HICPAC) state that routine preexposure vaccination with hepatitis A vaccine or routine use of IGIM in health-care personnel providing care to patients with HAV infection is not indicated. Instead, hygienic practices should be emphasized and health-care personnel should be made aware of the risk of exposure to HAV and precautions regarding direct contact with potentially infective materials. In documented outbreaks of HAV infection, postexposure prophylaxis with IGIM may be indicated in health-care workers and others who have close contact with the infected individuals. (See Hepatitis A Virus Infection under Uses: Immune Globulin IM, in Immune Globulin 80:04.) The usefulness of hepatitis A vaccine in controlling outbreaks in health-care settings has not been investigated.

Individuals with Chronic Liver Disease Although individuals with chronic liver disease are not at increased risk of acquiring HAV infection, data indicate that such individuals are at increased risk of severe consequences of HAV infection, including fatal fulminant hepatitis and hepatic failure. The ACIP and AAP recommend that susceptible individuals with chronic liver disease and those who are awaiting or have undergone liver transplantation receive preexposure vaccination with hepatitis A vaccine.

Although some clinicians have recommended that hepatitis A vaccine be used for preexposure vaccination in susceptible individuals with HBV or HCV infection, autoimmune hepatitis, or primary biliary cirrhosis, the ACIP states that data do not support routine vaccination of individuals with chronic HBV or HCV infection who do not have evidence of chronic liver disease.

Food Handlers Individuals employed as food handlers can become infected with HAV and may possibly transmit HAV to patrons. Food-source outbreaks often are associated with contamination of food during preparation by an HAV-infected food handler; a single infected food handler can transmit HAV to numerous, possibly hundreds of patrons through contaminated food. However, analysis of US economic data indicates that routine use of hepatitis A vaccine in all food handlers is not economically feasible from a societal or food industry perspective. However, HAV vaccination of restaurant employees may be considered in areas where the state and local health authorities or private employers have determined that such vaccination is indicated to decrease the frequency of evaluations of food handlers for HAV and the need for postexposure prophylaxis of restaurant patrons. Under these circumstances, a record of HAV vaccination should be provided to vaccinated food handlers and those not vaccinated should be informed of the signs and symptoms of HAV infection. In addition, all food handlers should receive instruction on food preparation practices that reduce the risk for fecal contamination. Occasionally, vaccination of foodhandlers may be considered during a community outbreak.

Outbreak Control Prior to widespread use of hepatitis A vaccine, HAV infection was transmitted from direct contact through the fecal-oral route within households and extended family settings during communitywide epidemics. Such HAV epidemics often persisted for 1–2 years, were difficult to control, typically spread throughout the community, and could not generally be attributed to a single risk factor or group. Children played a key role in sustaining HAV transmission during these epidemics since they often have asymptomatic or undiagnosed infections. In the context of increasing HAV incidence or ongoing outbreaks among children or adolescents in areas without existing hepatitis A vaccination programs, catch-up vaccination of unvaccinated children 2 through 18 years of age should be considered.

The frequency of large communitywide outbreaks has decreased considerably following implementation of recommended childhood hepatitis A vaccination programs. Universal childhood vaccination with hepatitis A vaccine for all children should further reduce the occurrence of outbreaks. In the event of a communitywide outbreak, accelerated vaccination programs may be considered as an additional control measure. The decision to initiate an outbreak-control vaccination program should take into account the feasibility of rapidly vaccinating the target population of children, adolescents, or young adults, and the costs associated with such a program. Routine vaccination of children in affected communities should continue in order to maintain high levels of immunity and prevent future epidemics. Prevaccination serologic testing for HAV susceptibility generally is not indicated for routine or "catch-up" vaccination of children in such populations. (See Children Who Reside in High-Risk Areas under Uses: Preexposure Vaccination in High-risk Groups.)

Limited HAV outbreaks, especially those involving adults at increased risk (e.g., illicit drug users, men who have sex with men) continue to occur and may be expected until higher rates of vaccination are achieved in these populations. Vaccination programs in these risk groups to control such outbreaks have been difficult to implement. Some success in vaccine coverage has been achieved in programs to control HAV outbreaks among illicit drug users (e.g., methamphetamine users) that focused on vaccination in county jails and judicial diversion programs. Efforts to control and prevent HAV outbreaks among adults in such populations at increased risk should generally focus on initiating and maintaining routine vaccination programs in these individuals.

Child-care center outbreaks have decreased considerably since the implementation of childhood hepatitis A vaccination programs and further decreases are expected now that universal childhood vaccination against HAV is recommended. ACIP does *not* recommend *routine* preexposure vaccination with hepatitis A vaccine for personnel in child-care centers. However, postexposure prophylaxis is recommended in all previously unvaccinated staff and attendees of child-care centers or homes if one or more cases of HAV are recognized in children or employees or if HAV is recognized in 2 or more households of center attendees. If an outbreak occurs in a child-care center (i.e., HAV in 3 or more families), postexposure prophylaxis should also be considered for members of households that have diapered children attending the center. (See Uses: Postexposure Prophylaxis.)

ACIP does *not* recommend *routine* preexposure vaccination with hepatitis A vaccine in hospitals, schools, and institutions for the developmentally disabled because the frequency of outbreaks in these institutions is not high enough to warrant such recommendations. Outbreaks involving student-to-student transmission in primary and secondary schools are rare in developed countries, but outbreaks have been documented; in developing countries, outbreaks among children in primary schools is more common. If an epidemiologic investigation indicates HAV transmission has occurred among students in a school or among patients or between patients and staff in a hospital, postexposure prophylaxis should be administered to individuals who have close contact with index patients. (See Uses: Postexposure Prophylaxis.)

■ **Postexposure Prophylaxis** Hepatitis A vaccine is used for HAV postexposure prophylaxis†. Unvaccinated individuals with recent (within 2 weeks) exposure to HAV should receive postexposure prophylaxis with a single dose of hepatitis A vaccine and/or a dose of IGIM as soon as possible. The choice of active immunization with the vaccine or passive immunization with IGIM should take into account the magnitude of risk associated with the exposure and characteristics of the patient that are associated with more severe manifestations of HAV (e.g., older age, chronic liver disease). Although IGIM was traditionally the recommended regimen for postexposure prophylaxis of HAV since it is 80–90% effective in preventing clinical HAV if administered within 2 weeks of exposure (see Uses: Hepatitis A Virus Infection, in Immune Globulin 80:04), there is limited evidence that hepatitis A vaccine administered within 2 weeks of exposure may be as effective as IGIM in healthy individuals 1–40 years of age. Because the vaccine offers certain advantages over IGIM (induces active immunity and longer protection, more readily available, easier to administer, greater patient acceptance), the ACIP updated their recommendations regarding postexposure prophylaxis of HAV in June 2007 to include use of the vaccine for postexposure prophylaxis in certain individuals.

When HAV postexposure prophylaxis is indicated in healthy individuals 12 months to 40 years of age, the ACIP states that an age-appropriate dose of monovalent hepatitis A vaccine should be used and is preferred to IGIM. In adults older than 40 years of age, the ACIP states that IGIM is preferred for HAV postexposure prophylaxis since data are not available to date regarding efficacy of the vaccine for prophylaxis in this age group and because these individuals are at risk of more severe manifestations of HAV; however, the vaccine can be used if IGIM cannot be obtained. IGIM should be used for postexposure prophylaxis in children younger than 12 months of age, in immunocompromised individuals, individuals with chronic liver disease, and whenever the vaccine is contraindicated.

When HAV postexposure prophylaxis is indicated, it should be administered as soon as possible. Data are not available regarding efficacy of hepatitis A vaccine or IGIM for postexposure prophylaxis of HAV if administered more than 2 weeks after exposure.

Whenever hepatitis A vaccine is used for postexposure prophylaxis†, a monovalent vaccine (Havrix®, Vaqta®) should be used. The fixed-combination vaccine containing hepatitis A vaccine and hepatitis B vaccine (HepA-HepB; Twinrix®) should *not* be used for HAV postexposure prophylaxis. (See Use of Fixed Combinations under Cautions: Precautions and Contraindications.)

Combined active immunization with hepatitis A vaccine and passive immunization with IGIM (using different syringes and different injection sites) is recommended by the ACIP for individuals with recent HAV exposure in whom providing long-term protection is indicated. If a dose of hepatitis A vaccine is used with or without IGIM for HAV postexposure prophylaxis, a second (booster) dose of the vaccine should be administered according to the usually recommended schedule to ensure long-term protection.

Routine screening of contacts for serologic markers of HAV infection prior to administration of HAV postexposure prophylaxis is not recommended. However, because HAV infection cannot be diagnosed reliably by clinical presentation alone, serologic confirmation of HAV in the index case is recommended before treatment of contacts. (See Uses: Serologic Testing.)

Postexposure Prophylaxis in Close Personal Contacts HAV postexposure prophylaxis with hepatitis A vaccine or IGIM should be administered within 2 weeks to all previously unvaccinated household and sexual contacts of individuals with serologically confirmed HAV. Consideration also should be given to administering postexposure prophylaxis with the vaccine or IGIM to individuals with other types of ongoing, close personal contact (e.g., regular babysitting) with a person with HAV.

Contacts who have shared illicit drugs with an individual with serologically confirmed HAV within the last 2 weeks should receive postexposure prophylaxis with the hepatitis A vaccine or with both the vaccine and IGIM administered simultaneously (at separate sites).

Postexposure Prophylaxis in Child-care Centers HAV postexposure prophylaxis with hepatitis A vaccine or IGIM should be administered to all previously unvaccinated staff and attendees of child-care centers or homes if one or more cases of HAV are recognized in children or employees or if HAV is recognized in 2 or more households of center attendees within the last 2 weeks. In centers that do not provide care to children who wear diapers, postexposure prophylaxis with the vaccine or IGIM needs to be administered only to classroom contacts of the index patient.

When an outbreak occurs (i.e., HAV in 3 or more families), postexposure prophylaxis with hepatitis A vaccine or IGIM should also be considered for members of households that have diapered children attending the center.

Postexposure Prophylaxis in Common-source Exposures If HAV is diagnosed in a food handler, the ACIP recommends postexposure prophylaxis with hepatitis A vaccine or IGIM within 2 weeks for other food handlers at the same establishment. Postexposure prophylaxis for patrons typically is not indicated since common-source transmission to patrons is unlikely. However, postexposure prophylaxis for patrons may be considered if the food handler directly handled uncooked or cooked foods and had diarrhea or poor hygienic practices during the time when they were likely to be infectious and if patrons can be identified and treated within 2 weeks after the exposure. Settings where repeated HAV exposure might have occurred (e.g., institutional cafeterias) warrant stronger consideration of postexposure prophylaxis for patrons.

If a common-source outbreak of HAV occurs, the ACIP states that postexposure prophylaxis should not be provided to exposed individuals after cases have begun to occur because the 2-week period after exposure during which the vaccine or IGIM is known to be effective will have been exceeded.

Postexposure Prophylaxis in Schools, Hospitals, and Work Settings The ACIP states that routine HAV postexposure prophylaxis is not indicated when a single HAV case occurs in an elementary or secondary school or an office or other work setting if the source case is outside the school or work setting.

When an individual with HAV is admitted to a hospital, staff members do not need to receive routine postexposure prophylaxis; careful hygienic practices should be emphasized in such situations.

If an epidemiologic investigation indicates that HAV transmission has occurred among students in a school or among patients or between patients and staff members in a hospital, the ACIP recommends that postexposure prophylaxis with hepatitis A vaccine or IGIM should be administered in individuals who have close contact with index patients.

Clinical Experience Efficacy of hepatitis A vaccine for postexposure prophylaxis† of HAV has been evaluated in a randomized, double-blind, noninferiority trial in susceptible individuals 2–40 years of age who were household or child-care center contacts of index patients with HAV (study NCT00139139). Individuals were randomized to receive a single dose of monovalent hepatitis A vaccine (age-appropriate dose of Vaqta®) or IGIM (0.02 mL/kg) within 14 days after exposure to a laboratory-confirmed index case of HAV. The primary end point was laboratory-confirmed symptomatic HAV occurring between 15–56 days after exposure. In the per-protocol analyses, HAV was confirmed in 4.4% of those who received the vaccine and 3.3% of those who received IGIM. The relative risk of HAV among vaccine recipients was noninferior to that reported for IGIM recipients.

In a study in Naples, Italy where HAV infection is endemic, hepatitis A vaccine (Havrix®) was administered to family contacts of individuals with primary HAV infection (index cases) for postexposure prophylaxis†. The vaccine was administered to family contacts who were 1–40 years of age (1440-unit dose in adolescents and adults and 720-unit dose in children 1–11 years of age) and was given within 8 days of symptom onset in the index cases. During 45 days of follow-up, secondary cases of HAV infection occurred in 13.3% of households in the unvaccinated group and 2.8% of households in the vaccinated group; the protective efficacy of the vaccine was 79%.

■ **Serologic Testing** HAV infection confers lifelong immunity to HAV and presumably against subsequent reinfection. Although high rates of HAV seropositivity are present in some populations for whom HAV vaccination is recommended, vaccination of an individual with preexisting immunity is not associated with any unusual risk. Therefore, prevaccination testing for susceptibility to HAV generally is not indicated unless such testing would be less costly than unnecessarily vaccinating an individual who is already immune. If prevaccination testing is indicated, commercially available tests that measure total anti-HAV (i.e., both IgG and IgM anti-HAV) should be used. A positive result indicates that the individual is immune to HAV as the result of past infection or vaccination.

The ACIP and AAP state that prevaccination serologic testing is not recommended in children because of their expected low prevalence of prior infection. For adults, the possibility of prior infection and resultant immunity is the basis for considering testing. Factors to consider include the cost of vaccination versus the cost of serologic testing (including the cost of an additional visit), the expected prevalence of immune individuals, and the likelihood that prevaccination testing will not interfere with completion of the vaccine series if vaccination is indicated. For example, if the cost of screening (including laboratory and office visit costs) is one-third the cost of the vaccine series, then screening of potential recipients from populations with a prevalence of HAV infection of 33% should be cost-effective.

The ACIP also states that populations for whom prevaccination serologic testing is likely to be most cost-effective include adults who were born or lived for extensive periods in geographic areas with high endemicity for HAV infection, older adolescents and adults in certain groups with a high prevalence of infection (e.g., Native Americans, Alaska Natives, Hispanics), adults over 40 years of age, adult men who have sex with men, and adults who illicitly use injectable or noninjectable drugs.

Based on epidemiologic evidence from the National Health and Nutrition Examination Survey (NHANES), the anti-HAV prevalence among adults older than 40 years of age in the US generally exceeds 33% regardless of race/ethnicity or income level. Therefore, prevaccination serologic testing for any adult older than 40 years of age is likely to be cost-effective, assuming that the cost of screening is one-third the cost of the vaccination series.

Prevaccination serologic testing before routine or "catch-up" vaccination of children, including adolescents, generally is not indicated. Prevaccination testing also is not routinely indicated for adolescent homosexual or bisexual males nor for adolescent illicit drug users, although it may be warranted for older adults. However, prevaccination testing in populations that have expected high rates of HAV infection may be cost-effective. (See Uses: Preexposure Vaccination in High-Risk Groups.)

Serologic testing of contacts of an HAV-infected individual for possible preexisting immunity prior to administration of postexposure prophylaxis with IGIM is not recommended since screening is more costly than IGIM and would delay its administration, thus potentially compromising prophylactic efficacy. However, because HAV infection cannot be diagnosed reliably by clinical presentation alone, serologic confirmation of HAV in the index case is recommended before HAV postexposure prophylaxis is initiated in contacts.

Postvaccination serologic testing is not recommended because of the high rate of vaccine response among adults and children and the lack of an approved, commercially available assay in the US with sensitivity to detect low anti-HAV concentrations. (See Pharmacology.) However, the National Hemophilia Foundation's Medical and Scientific Advisory Council (MASAC) strongly recommends such testing following hepatitis A vaccination in adults and children with hemophilia.

Dosage and Administration

■ **Administration** Hepatitis A virus vaccine inactivated (hepatitis A vaccine) is administered by IM injection. The fixed-combination vaccine containing hepatitis A vaccine and hepatitis B vaccine (HepA-HepB; Twinrix®) also is administered by IM injection. These vaccines should *not* be administered IV, intradermally, or subcutaneously.

To ensure delivery of vaccine into the muscle, IM injections of hepatitis A vaccine should be made at a 90-degree angle to the skin using a needle size that is appropriate for the individual's age and body mass, thickness of adipose tissue and muscle at the injection site, and injection technique. Anatomic variability, especially in the deltoid, should be considered and clinical judgment should be used to avoid inadvertent underpenetration or overpenetration of muscle. Depending on the age of the patient, the IM injection should be made into the deltoid muscle or anterolateral thigh.

For toddlers 1–2 years of age, the IM injection should preferably be administered into the anterolateral thigh; the deltoid muscle is an alternative if the muscle mass is adequate. For children 3 years of age or older, adolescents, and adults, the deltoid muscle is preferred, although the anterolateral thigh is an alternative for those 3–18 years of age.

Generally, muscles of the buttock should not be used for administration of vaccines in children because of the well-documented potential for injection-associated injury to the sciatic nerve. In addition, studies in adults indicate that a suboptimal response may occur when hepatitis A vaccine is injected into the gluteal rather than the deltoid muscle; therefore, the deltoid region is the preferred site for IM injection of the vaccine in adults.

Although some experts state that aspiration (i.e., pulling back on the syringe plunger after needle insertion and before injection) can be performed to ensure that a blood vessel has not been entered, the US Public Health Service Advisory Committee on Immunization Practices (ACIP) and American Academy of Pediatrics (AAP) state that this procedure is not required because large blood vessels are not present at the recommended IM injection sites.

When multiple vaccines are administered during a single visit, administration of each preparation at a different anatomic site is preferred. In younger children, the thigh is the preferred injection site when more than 2 vaccines must be administered into a single limb. Injection sites should be separated by at least 1 inch (if anatomically feasible) to allow appropriate attribution of any local adverse effects that may occur. The deltoid muscle may be used in older children and adults when more than one vaccine must be administered.

Before withdrawing a dose of monovalent hepatitis A vaccine or the fixed-combination vaccine containing hepatitis A vaccine and hepatitis B vaccine, the vial should be shaken well to obtain a uniform, slightly turbid, white suspension; the vaccine should be discarded if a homogenous suspension does not result.

Since syncope may occur following vaccination, vaccinees should be observed for approximately 15 minutes after the vaccine dose is administered. If syncope occurs, the patient should be observed until symptoms resolve. Syncope after vaccination occurs most frequently in adolescents and young adults.

Hepatitis A vaccine may be given simultaneously with other age-appropriate vaccines during the same health-care visit (using different syringes and different injection sites). (See Drug Interactions: Vaccines.) In addition, hepatitis A vaccine may be given simultaneously with immune globulin IM (IGIM), using different syringes and different injection sites, when *passive* immunization is considered necessary in addition to *active* immunization with the vaccine (e.g., in travelers who will depart within 2 weeks).

■ **Dosage** The recommended dose and dosing schedule for hepatitis A vaccine vary according to the individual's age and specific vaccine administered (Havrix® or Vaqta® monovalent vaccines or Twinrix® fixed-combination vaccine). Dosage recommendations for the specific preparation used should be followed.

Whenever possible, the monovalent vaccine chosen for the initial dose should be used for subsequent doses in the same individual. However, because there is evidence from several studies in adults that vaccination schedules that alternated doses of both monovalent formulations of hepatitis A vaccine resulted in protective antibody levels similar to those attained with a dosage schedule that used a single vaccine formulation, the ACIP and AAP state that the commercially available formulations of monovalent hepatitis A vaccine may be considered interchangeable.

When vaccination against both hepatitis A virus (HAV) and hepatitis B virus (HBV) infection is indicated in adults 18 years of age or older, the commercially available fixed-combination vaccine containing hepatitis A vaccine and hepatitis B vaccine(HepA-HepB; Twinrix®) can be used.

Primary Immunization against Hepatitis A Virus Infection

Havrix®. If Havrix® is used for primary immunization, an initial dose of the age-appropriate preparation should be given followed by a second (booster) dose 6–12 months after the initial dose. Children and adolescents 12 months through 18 years of age should receive 720-unit doses and adults 19 years of age or older should receive 1440-unit doses.

The ACIP, AAP, and the American Academy of Family Physicians (AAFP) recommend that the initial dose be given routinely to all children at 1 year of age (i.e., 12 through 23 months of age) and that the second dose be given at least 6 months after the initial dose. Children not fully vaccinated by 2 years of age can be vaccinated at subsequent health-care visits. Catch-up vaccination should be considered for children 2 through 18 years of age in areas without existing selective preexposure hepatitis A vaccination programs.

If a different hepatitis A vaccine (e.g., Vaqta®) was used for the initial dose, a second (booster) dose of Havrix® may be given 6–18 months after the initial dose of the other vaccine; however, whenever possible, the formulation chosen for the initial dose should be used for subsequent doses in the same individual.

The need for subsequent doses after the initial and additional (booster) dose has not been fully determined. Subsequent booster doses are not recommended.

Vaqta®. If Vaqta® is used for primary immunization, an initial dose of the age-appropriate preparation should be given followed by a second (booster) dose 6–12 months after the initial dose. Children and adolescents 12 months through 18 years of age should receive 25-unit doses and adults 19 years of age or older should receive 50-unit doses.

The ACIP, AAP, and AAFP recommend that the initial dose be given routinely to all children at 1 year of age (i.e., 12 through 23 months of age) and that the second dose be given at least 6 months after the initial dose. Children not fully vaccinated by 2 years of age can be vaccinated at subsequent health-care visits. Catch-up vaccination should be considered for children 2 through 18 years of age in areas without existing selective preexposure hepatitis A vaccination programs.

If a different hepatitis A vaccine (e.g., Havrix®) was used for the initial dose, a second (booster) dose of Vaqta® may be given 6–12 months after the initial dose of the other vaccine; however, whenever possible, the formulation chosen for the initial dose should be used for subsequent doses in the same individual.

The need for subsequent doses after the initial and second (booster) dose has not been fully determined. Subsequent booster doses are not recommended.

HepA-HepB (Twinrix®). If the fixed-combination vaccine containing hepatitis A vaccine and hepatitis B vaccine (HepA-HepB; Twinrix®) is used for primary immunization in adults 18 years of age or older, three 1-mL doses, administered at 0, 1, and 6 months, should be given. Alternatively, if an accelerated dosing schedule is needed, three 1-mL doses, administered at 0, 7, and 21–30 days, may be given, followed by a booster dose given at 12 months. Each 1-mL dose of the fixed-combination vaccine contains 720 units of hepatitis A viral antigen and 20 mcg of hepatitis B surface antigen (HBsAg). Safety and efficacy of the fixed-combination vaccine in children younger than 18 years of age have not been established.

Preexposure Vaccination and Outbreak Control When hepatitis A vaccine is indicated for preexposure vaccination in individuals who are or will be at high risk of exposure to HAV (e.g., international travelers, individuals at risk because of their sexual practices, individuals with potential occupational exposure, military personnel, illicit drug users, recipients of blood products, individuals with chronic liver disease) and any other unvaccinated individual desiring protection from HAV infection or to prevent or control HAV outbreaks in certain populations that have high or intermediate rates of infection, the recommended vaccine regimens are the same as the age-specific regimens recommended for primary immunization. Administration of the recommended initial and second (booster) dose before an expected exposure to HAV ensures the highest level of protection. However, individuals who have received at least 1 dose of hepatitis A vaccine 1 month prior to an exposure probably will be protected. (See Pharmacology: Response to Hepatitis A Virus Vaccine Inactivated.)

For individuals who plan to travel or work in areas with intermediate to high levels of endemic HAV, the first dose of hepatitis A vaccine should be given as soon as travel is considered. For most healthy children, adolescents, and adults 40 years of age and younger, a single dose will provide adequate protection regardless of the scheduled departure date. To ensure protection in adults older than 40 years of age, immunocompromised individuals, or those with chronic liver disease or other chronic medical conditions who plan to depart within 2 weeks, the ACIP recommends that a single dose of IGIM (0.02 mL/kg) be given concurrently with the initial vaccine dose using a different syringe and different injection site.

Postexposure Prophylaxis For postexposure prophylaxis† of HAV in unvaccinated healthy individuals 12 months to 40 years of age, a single dose of age-appropriate hepatitis A vaccine can be given alone or in conjunction with IGIM (0.02 mL/kg). Although IGIM is preferred for postexposure prophylaxis in unvaccinated individuals older than 40 years of age, a single age-appropriate dose of hepatitis A vaccine can be used if IGIM cannot be obtained. Efficacy of HAV postexposure prophylaxis has not been established if given more than 2 weeks after exposure.

If hepatitis A vaccine is administered in conjunction with IGIM for postexposure prophylaxis in previously unvaccinated individuals to provide long-term protection against HAV, the recommended vaccine regimens are the same as the age-specific regimens recommended for primary immunization. The first dose of vaccine can be administered simultaneously with IGIM but at a separate anatomic site using different syringes. (See Dosage and Administration: Dosage, in Immune Globulin 80:04.) IGIM should be administered as soon as possible after confirmed HAV exposure, but preferably no later than 2 weeks after exposure. Administration of IGIM later than 2 weeks after HAV exposure may only attenuate rather than prevent clinical manifestations of HAV infection. Individuals who have received at least 1 dose of hepatitis A vaccine at least 1 month prior to the HAV exposure do not need to receive postexposure prophylaxis with IGIM.

Confirmation of Immunity Serologic confirmation of immunity against HAV following vaccination with hepatitis A vaccine is not necessary in most individuals because of the high rate of vaccine response among adults and children and because of the lack of an approved, commercially available test with the sensitivity to detect the anti-HAV levels necessary for protection.

Duration of Response The duration of protection and the need for subsequent doses after primary and additional (booster) doses of hepatitis A vaccine has not been fully determined. Antibodies induced by hepatitis A vaccine decline steadily with time and geometric mean antibody titers (GMTs) generally decrease by 50% in 48 months in adult vaccinees receiving three 720-unit doses of Havrix® hepatitis A vaccine at 0, 1, and 6 months, although anti-HAV levels considered protective were still maintained 8 years after the first dose. In a small study in adults who received three 720-unit doses of Havrix® hepatitis A vaccine at 0, 1, and 6 months, vaccinees maintained anti-HAV levels greater than 15 mIU/mL 12 years after the first dose. All the adults in a larger study who received two 1440-unit doses of Havrix® hepatitis A vaccine maintained anti-HAV levels considered protective 10 years after vaccination. Of children who received Vaqta® hepatitis A vaccine, 99% maintained anti-HAV levels considered protective 5–6 years after vaccination. In addition, there were no cases of HAV infection reported from surveillance data in children who were followed 9 years after vaccination. Some estimates based on kinetic modeling suggest that protective antibody levels may persist for 25 years or longer in adults and 14–20 years or longer in children (see Pharmacology: Response to Hepatitis A Virus Vaccine Inactivated); however, the ACIP states that the long-term protective efficacy of hepatitis A vaccine must be determined in ongoing postvaccination studies and future postmarketing surveillance before recommendations can be made regarding the need, if any, for additional booster doses of the vaccine.

Cautions

Hepatitis A virus vaccine inactivated (hepatitis A vaccine) generally is well tolerated, and reported adverse reactions to the vaccine have been infrequent, mild, and transient. No serious adverse effects have been definitely attributed to the commercially available preparations of hepatitis A vaccine. In a postmarketing safety study involving 42,110 children, adolescents, and adults who received 1 or 2 doses of Vaqta®, there were no serious vaccine-related adverse events and diarrhea/gastroenteritis requiring an outpatient visit to a health-care provider was determined to be the only vaccine-related nonserious adverse event. There were no vaccine-related adverse effects identified in this postmarketing study that had not been reported in earlier clinical studies of the vaccine. In 2 other postlicensure studies of Vaqta®, one involving 11,417 children and 25,023 adults and the other involving 2000 children and adults, there were no serious vaccine-related adverse effects reported.

Of 6136 adverse effects reported to the Vaccine Adverse Event Reporting System (VAERS) in hepatitis A vaccine recipients (with or without the concurrent use of other vaccines) since FDA approval, the most frequently reported effects included fever, injection-site reaction, rash, and headache; serious adverse effects reported in 871 vaccinees included Guillain-Barré syndrome, transaminitis, idiopathic thrombocytopenic purpura, and seizures (among children). The safety of hepatitis A vaccine will continue to be evaluated through ongoing monitoring of data from VAERS and other surveillance systems; it is possible that increased clinical use of hepatitis A vaccine may reveal rare, unreported adverse effects.

Among adults, the most common adverse effects of hepatitis A vaccine occurring within 3 days of vaccination for Havrix® or 5 days for Vaqta® are local effects at the site of injection (soreness for Havrix® and tenderness, pain, and warmth for Vaqta®) and headache. With the exception of fever, the frequency and severity of adverse effects tend to decrease with successive doses of hepatitis A vaccine. Among children, the most frequently reported adverse effects of Havrix® were soreness at the injection site, feeding problems, headache, and induration at the injection site, and of Vaqta® were local pain, tenderness, and warmth. Adverse effects appear to be similar for Havrix® and Vaqta®.

The fixed-combination vaccine containing hepatitis A vaccine and hepatitis B vaccine (HepA-HepB; Twinrix®) generally is well tolerated and adverse effects reported with the vaccine have been mild and transient (usually persisting for no longer than 48 hours). In adults, adverse effects reported with the fixed-combination vaccine were similar to those reported when monovalent hepatitis A vaccine and monovalent hepatitis B vaccine were administered alone or concurrently at different sites. No increase in the frequency of adverse effects has been reported with successive doses of the fixed-combination vaccine. In addition, adverse effects reported with an accelerated vaccination regimen of Twinrix® (doses at 0, 7, and 21–30 days and a booster dose at 12 months) have been similar to those reported with the usual 3-dose regimen (doses at 0, 1, and 6 months).

■ **Local Effects** Local reactions are the most common adverse effects with either formulation of monovalent hepatitis A vaccine, with soreness/pain at the injection site being reported in 56% of adults (1440-unit doses) and 21% of children (720-unit doses) receiving primary immunization with the Havrix® vaccine and in 6.4% of children (25-unit dose) receiving primary immunization with Vaqta® vaccine. In adults or children receiving one or more doses of Vaqta®, pain was reported in 51 or 19% of vaccines, respectively. However, of those individuals reporting soreness, less than 0.5% described it as severe.

Adverse local effects at the injection site following administration of hepatitis A vaccine that occur with 1–10% of doses include induration, erythema, warmth, and swelling. Although tenderness also was reported in 1–10% of doses of Havrix®, it was reported in up to 53% of adults receiving Vaqta® and in up to 17% of children receiving this vaccine. Hematoma or ecchymosis was reported at the injection site with less than 2% of doses of the vaccine. With Vaqta® vaccine, adverse local effects were reported more commonly in adults than in children.

In children 11–25 months of age who received Havrix® hepatitis A vaccine, local effects reported within 4 days after the initial or booster dose included pain in 15–21%, erythema in 16–22%, and swelling in 8%. In children 11–25 months of age who received Vaqta® hepatitis A vaccine (with or without other routine childhood immunizations administered concurrently at a different site), local effects reported within 5 days after the initial or booster dose included pain, tenderness, and/or soreness in 3.1–3.5%, erythema in 1.3–1.6%, swelling in 1.3–1.6%, ecchymosis in 1%, and warmth in 0.8–0.9%.

Adverse local reactions reported in adults receiving the fixed-combination vaccine containing hepatitis A vaccine and hepatitis B vaccine (HepA-HepB; Twinrix®) include soreness (37–41%), erythema (8–11%), and swelling (4–6%).

■ **Systemic Effects** Adverse dermatologic effects have been reported with less than 1% of hepatitis A vaccine doses and include urticaria, pruritus, and rash. Erythema multiforme also has been reported with Havrix® and generalized erythema and dermatitis have been reported with Vaqta®, but these effects have not been directly attributed to the vaccine.

Mild adverse systemic effects have been reported in about 14% of patients receiving primary immunization with Havrix® hepatitis A vaccine. Headache, the most frequently reported adverse systemic effect with Havrix®, occurred in 14% of adults and less than 9% of children receiving primary immunization with the vaccine; headache was reported in 16% of adults and in up to 2.3% of children receiving Vaqta®.

In children 11–25 months of age who received Havrix® hepatitis A vaccine, adverse systemic effects reported within 4 days after the initial or booster dose included irritability in 24–36%, loss of appetite in 16–19%, drowsiness in 15–17%, and fever (exceeding 39.5°C) in up to 2%. In children 11–25 months of age who received Vaqta® hepatitis A vaccine (with or without other routine childhood vaccines given concurrently at a different site), adverse systemic effects reported within 14 days after the initial or booster dose included irritability in 10.8%, crying in 1.8%, rash in 4.5% (measles-like, rubella-like, or varicella-like in about 1%), fever (exceeding 38°C) in 9.1–11.3%, fever (exceeding 38.9°C) in 3.1–3.8%, diarrhea in 5.9%, vomiting in 4%, and anorexia in 1.2%.

Adverse systemic effects occurring with up to 10% of Havrix® doses or Vaqta® vaccinees in adults and children include fatigue/asthenia, feeding problems, fussiness, lethargy, fever (37.5°C or higher, low-grade fever lasting 1 day), malaise, anorexia, and nausea. The frequency of fever does not appear to diminish with successive doses of the vaccine. Other adverse systemic effects occurring occasionally with hepatitis A vaccine include pharyngitis, upper respiratory tract infection, nasal congestion, abdominal pain, diarrhea, vomiting, arthralgia, elevation of creatine kinase (CK, creatine phosphokinase, CPK), elevation of liver enzymes, myalgia, arm or back pain, stiffness, lymphadenopathy, hypertonia, insomnia, menstrual disorder, ocular irritation or itching, photophobia, and vertigo.

Somnolence, syncope, thrombocytopenia, possible vasculitis, idiopathic thrombocytopenic purpura, purpura, Kawasaki disease, autoimmune hemolytic anemia, jaundice, hepatitis, diabetes mellitus, pancreatitis, transient hypertension, pericarditis, rhabdomyolysis, hyperhidrosis, angioedema, dyspnea, encephalitis, seizures, febrile seizure in a child 18 months of age, cerebellar ataxia, encephalopathy, dizziness, neuropathy (brachial plexus), myelitis (transverse), paresthesia, Guillain-Barré syndrome, multiple sclerosis, congenital abnormality and death have been reported rarely in individuals receiving Havrix® or Vaqta® hepatitis A vaccine. Most of these rare effects have been postlicensure reports in adults from over 1.3 million vaccinees who received Havrix® in Europe and Asia, and about one-third of cases have occurred in individuals receiving other vaccines concurrently or in adults or children who received Havrix® or Vaqta® in the US or outside the US, and about 40% of cases have occurred in those receiving at least one other vaccine concurrently; therefore, a definite causal relationship to hepatitis A vaccine has not been established. In addition, for serious adverse effects for which background incidences are known (e.g., Guillain-Barré syndrome, brachial plexus neuropathy), the rates among vaccinees are no higher than would be expected among an unvaccinated population.

In the US, more than 6.5 million doses of hepatitis A vaccine were administered from 1995–1998, including over 2.3 million pediatric doses. During this period, 247 adverse events were reported in individuals receiving hepatitis A vaccine, including 80 in children and adults younger than 19 years old and 167 in adults; of these events, approximately 33% occurred in individuals receiving at least one other vaccine concurrently. Serious adverse events, including neurologic, hematologic, and autoimmune syndromes were reported in 13 children (0.6/100,000 vaccine doses distributed) and 85 adults (1.4/100,000 vaccine doses distributed); however, these serious events could not be definitively attributed to hepatitis A virus (HAV) vaccination and the rates of these serious adverse events were not higher than reported background rates for which incidence data are available. For example, published background incidence rates for Guillain-Barré syndrome have ranged from 0.5–2.4 cases per 100,000 person-years. The 5 Guillain-Barré cases among adult recipients of hepatitis A vaccine represent an estimated incidence of 0.2 cases per 100,000 person-years.

While the risk of sensitivity reactions to hepatitis A vaccine appears to be low, anaphylaxis and anaphylactoid manifestations have been reported rarely in patients receiving the vaccine. Bronchoconstriction, asthma, and wheezing have been reported in less than 1% of vaccinees. Additional data and experience are needed to define more precisely the frequencies of uncommon reactions. If a hypersensitivity reaction occurs, it should be treated appropriately and additional doses of the vaccine should *not* be administered.

■ **Precautions and Contraindications** Hepatitis A vaccine is contraindicated in individuals who are hypersensitive to any ingredient in the respective formulation, including neomycin. The vaccine also is contraindicated in individuals with previous hypersensitivity or severe allergic reactions (e.g., anaphylaxis) to any hepatitis A vaccine.

The fixed-combination vaccine containing hepatitis A vaccine and hepatitis B vaccine (HepA-HepB; Twinrix®) is contraindicated in individuals hypersensitive to any ingredient in the vaccine, including the hepatitis A vaccine component (Havrix®), the hepatitis B vaccine component (Engerix-B®), yeast, or neomycin. The vaccine is contraindicated in individuals with previous hypersensitivity reactions to Twinrix® or monovalent hepatitis A or hepatitis B vaccines.

Prior to vaccine administration, the patient and/or the patient's parent or guardian should be informed of benefits and risks of immunization and should be provided with a copy of the appropriate Vaccine Information Statement (available at the CDC website http://www.cdc.gov/vaccines/pubs/vis/default.htm). Patients and/or patient's parent or guardian also should be instructed to report any severe or unusual adverse reactions to their healthcare provider. Clinicians or individuals can report any adverse reactions that occur following vaccination to the Vaccine Adverse Event Reporting System (VAERS) at 800-822-7967 or http://www.vaers.hhs.gov.

Sensitivity Reactions Prior to administration of monovalent hepatitis A vaccine (Havrix®, Vaqta®) or the fixed-combination vaccine containing hepatitis A vaccine and hepatitis B vaccine (HepA-HepB; Twinrix®) all known precautions should be taken to prevent adverse reactions, including a review of the patient's history with respect to possible hypersensitivity to the vaccine or to similar vaccines; epinephrine and other appropriate agents should be readily available for immediate treatment of anaphylaxis or an anaphylactoid reaction if such a reaction should occur. Patients experiencing hypersensitivity reactions after a vaccine dose should not receive further injections of the vaccine.

Both the monovalent hepatitis A vaccine (Havrix®) and the fixed-combination vaccine containing hepatitis A vaccine and hepatitis B vaccine (HepA-HepB; Twinrix®) contain trace amounts of neomycin sulfate. Manufacturers state that these vaccines are contraindicated in individuals hypersensitive to neomycin. Neomycin allergy usually results in delayed-type (cell-mediated) hypersensitivity reactions manifested as contact dermatitis. The US Public Health Service Advisory Committee on Immunization Practices (ACIP) and the American Academy of Pediatrics (AAP) state that vaccines containing trace amounts of neomycin should not be used in individuals with a history of anaphylactic reaction to neomycin, but use of such vaccines may be considered in those with a history of delayed-type neomycin hypersensitivity if benefits of vaccination outweigh risks.

Some packaging components (e.g., needle cover, syringe plunger) of the single-dose prefilled syringes of Havrix® contain dry natural latex; the stopper on the vial of Havrix® does not contain latex. In addition, some packaging components (e.g., vial stopper, syringe plunger) of Vaqta® contain dry natural latex. Some individuals may be hypersensitive to natural latex proteins found in a wide range of medical devices, including such packaging components, and the level of sensitivity may vary depending on the form of natural rubber present; rarely, hypersensitivity reactions to natural latex proteins have been fatal. Health-care professionals should take appropriate precautions if these preparations are administered to individuals with a history of latex sensitivity. Preparations packaged with components containing dry natural latex should not be administered to individuals with a history of serious hypersensitivity reaction (anaphylaxis) to latex, unless the benefit of vaccination outweighs the risk for a potential severe hypersensitivity reaction.

Individuals with Altered Immunocompetence Hepatitis A vaccine may be administered to individuals immunosuppressed as the result of disease or immunosuppressive therapy. However, active immunization against HAV may be less effective in immunocompromised individuals and in individuals receiving immunosuppressive therapy since the immune response to the vaccine may be decreased.

Recommendations regarding use of hepatitis A vaccine in individuals with human immunodeficiency virus (HIV) infection are the same as those for individuals who are not infected with HIV. Because HIV-infected individuals with chronic liver disease (including those coinfected with hepatitis B virus [HBV] or hepatitis C virus [HCV]) are at risk of fulminant hepatic failure if they acquire HAV, the US Centers for Disease Control and Prevention (CDC), the National Institutes of Health (NIH), and the Infectious Diseases Society of America (IDSA) recommend that such individuals be vaccinated against HAV. Because the response to the vaccine may be reduced in those with $CD4^+$ T-cell counts less than 200 cells/mm^3, some experts suggest delaying vaccination until the patient is receiving antiretroviral therapy and the $CD4^+$ T-cell count is greater than 200 cells/mm^3. These experts also recommend that the antibody response to the vaccine be assesed 1 month after vaccination and that nonresponders be revaccinated.

Concomitant Illness The decision whether to administer or delay administration of hepatitis A vaccine or the fixed-combination vaccine containing hepatitis A vaccine and hepatitis B vaccine in an individual with a current or recent acute illness depends largely on the severity of symptoms and etiology of the illness. The ACIP states that minor acute illness, such as mild upper respiratory infection (with or without fever) or mild diarrhea, usually does not preclude vaccination. However, vaccination of individuals with moderate or severe acute illness generally should be delayed until they have recovered from the acute phase of the illness. This precaution avoids superimposing adverse effects of the vaccine on the underlying illness or mistakenly concluding that a manifestation of the underlying illness resulted from vaccination. The manufacturer states that hepatitis A vaccine may be given to individuals with acute infection or febrile illness if withholding the vaccine poses greater risk to the patient.

Individuals with Bleeding Disorders Hepatitis A vaccine and the fixed-combination vaccine containing hepatitis A vaccine and hepatitis B vaccine should be administered with caution to individuals with thrombocytopenia or a bleeding disorder (e.g., hemophilia) or individuals receiving anticoagulant therapy, since bleeding may occur following IM administration of the vaccines in such individuals. The ACIP and the National Hemophilia Foundation's Medical and Scientific Advisory Council (MASAC) state that a vaccine may be given IM to individuals who have bleeding disorders or are receiving anticoagulant therapy if a clinician familiar with the patient's bleeding risk determines that the vaccine can be administered with reasonable safety. In these cases, a fine needle (23 gauge or smaller) should be used to administer the vaccine and firm pressure should be applied to the injection site (without rubbing) for at least 2 minutes. In individuals with a bleeding disorder who are receiving antihemophilic factor or other similar therapy, IM vaccination can be scheduled shortly after a dose of such therapy to minimize the risk of bleeding. The individual and/or their family should be instructed concerning the risk of hematoma from the injection.

Use of Fixed Combinations Whenever the fixed-combination vaccine containing hepatitis A vaccine and hepatitis B vaccine (HepA-HepB; Twinrix®) is used, the contraindications and precautions related to both antigens should be considered.

Although an accelerated dosing schedule of the fixed-combination vaccine containing hepatitis A vaccine and hepatitis B vaccine (HepA-HepB; Twinrix®) can be used when necessary (e.g., for travelers), a booster dose of the vaccine is necessary 1 year later. The ACIP states that this fixed-combination vaccine should *not* be used for *preexposure* vaccination of travelers who will depart within 2 weeks after receipt of the vaccine since this vaccine contains less HAV antigen and data are not available regarding efficacy in this situation.

The fixed-combination vaccine containing hepatitis A vaccine and hepatitis B vaccine (HepA-HepB; Twinrix®) should *not* be used for HAV *postexposure* prophylaxis since this vaccine contains less HAV antigen and data are not available regarding efficacy in this situation.

Limitations of Vaccine Effectiveness The possibility that unrecognized HAV infection may be present in some individuals at the time of vaccination (since the infection has a long incubation period of 15–50 days) and that hepatitis A vaccine may not prevent infection in such individuals should be considered. In addition, the possibility that hepatitis A vaccine may not prevent infection in any individual who does not achieve protective antibody titers should be considered, although the lowest titer needed to confer protection has not been established.

The monovalent hepatitis A vaccines (Havrix® or Vaqta®) provide protection only against HAV. The fixed-combination vaccine containing hepatitis A vaccine and hepatitis B vaccine (HepA-HepB; Twinrix®) provides protection only against HAV and HBV. These vaccines do not provide protection against other infectious agents (e.g., HCV, HEV).

Passively acquired anti-HAV (e.g., acquired from IGIM administration or from maternal transfer) may interfere with the active antibody response to hepatitis A vaccine. Reduced titers have been observed in adults receiving concurrent IGIM and primary immunization with the vaccine, and vaccine immunogenicity also is reduced in infants with anti-HAV passively acquired through maternal transfer. However, the clinical importance of the reduced immunogenicity is yet to be determined, since seroconversion levels are greater than levels considered to be protective. When concomitant administration of other vaccines or IGIM is required, they should be given with different syringes and at different injection sites.

Following the initial dose, immunogenicity of hepatitis A vaccine (Havrix®) in adults with chronic liver disease of various etiologies (e.g., chronic HBV, chronic HCV, moderate chronic liver disease, alcoholic cirrhosis, autoimmune hepatitis, chronic hepatitis/cryptogenic cirrhosis, hemochromatosis, primary biliary cirrhosis, primary sclerosing cholangitis) was lower than in healthy subjects. However, 1 month after the second (booster) dose at month 6, seroconversion rates were similar among both groups. Relevance of these data to the duration of protection afforded by hepatitis A vaccine (Havrix®) is unknown.

Travelers to areas with intermediate to high levels of endemic HAV who are 40 years of age or older, immunocompromised, or have chronic liver disease or other chronic medical conditions who receive *preexposure* vaccination with a dose of monovalent hepatitis A vaccine given within 2 weeks of departure also should receive *passive* immunization with a dose of IGIM to ensure optimal protection.

The fixed-combination vaccine containing hepatitis A vaccine and hepatitis B vaccine (HepA-HepB; Twinrix®) should *not* be used for preexposure vaccination in travelers who will depart within 2 weeks and should *not* be used for postexposure prophylaxis against HAV. (See Use of Fixed Combinations under Cautions: Precautions and Contraindications.)

Improper Storage and Handling Improper storage or handling of vaccines may result in loss of vaccine potency and reduced immune response in vaccinees.

Single antigen hepatitis A vaccine (Havrix®, Vaqta®) or fixed-combination vaccine containing hepatitis A vaccine and hepatitis B vaccine (HepA-HepB; Twinrix®) that has been mishandled or has not been stored at the recommended temperature should not be administered. (See Chemistry and Stability: Stability.)

All vaccines should be inspected upon delivery and monitored during storage to ensure that the appropriate temperature is maintained. If there are concerns about mishandling, the manufacturer or state or local health departments should be contacted for guidance on whether the vaccine is usable.

■ **Pediatric Precautions** Safety and efficacy of hepatitis A vaccine have not been established in infants younger than 12 months of age. In young infants, passively-acquired maternal anti-HAV antibody may interfere with the active immune response to hepatitis A vaccine. Passively-acquired antibody declines to undetectable levels in most infants by 1 year of age, and the vaccine is highly immunogenic in children who begin the vaccine series after 1 year of age (regardless of maternal anti-HAV status). Data regarding the use of the vaccine in neonates and infants younger than 12 months of age are limited; the optimal dose and vaccination schedule in this age group as well as the effect of passively acquired maternal antibody on vaccine immunogenicity remain to be more fully elucidated. (See Infants Younger than 12 Months of Age under Pharmacology: Response to Hepatitis A Virus Vaccine Inactivated.)

Safety and efficacy of the fixed-combination vaccine containing hepatitis A vaccine and hepatitis B vaccine (HepA-HepB; Twinrix®) have not been established in children younger than 18 years of age.

■ **Geriatric Precautions** Clinical studies of Havrix® hepatitis A vaccine did not include sufficient numbers of patients 65 years of age or older to determine whether geriatric patients respond differently from younger patients; however, other clinical experience has revealed no evidence of age-related differences.

Clinical studies to date evaluating Vaqta® hepatitis A vaccine have included 68 vaccinees 65 years of age or older and 10 of these were 75 years of age or older. In addition, postmarketing safety studies have included 4769 individuals 65 years of age or older, including 1073 who were 75 years of age or older. Although no overall differences in immunogenicity or safety were observed between geriatric and younger patients, and other clinical experience revealed no evidence of age-related differences, the possibility that some older patients may exhibit increased sensitivity to the vaccine cannot be ruled out.

Clinical studies of the fixed-combination vaccine containing hepatitis A vaccine and hepatitis B vaccine (HepA-HepB; Twinrix®) did not include sufficient numbers of individuals 65 years of age or older to determine whether geriatric individuals respond differently than younger adults.

■ **Mutagenicity and Carcinogenicity** Studies have not been performed to date to evaluate the mutagenic or carcinogenic potential of hepatitis A vaccine or the fixed-combination vaccine containing hepatitis A vaccine and hepatitis B vaccine (HepA-HepB; Twinrix®).

■ **Pregnancy, Fertility, and Lactation** Animal reproduction studies have not been performed with hepatitis A vaccine or the fixed-combination vaccine containing hepatitis A vaccine and hepatitis B vaccine (HepA-HepB; Twinrix®), and it is not known whether the vaccines can cause fetal harm when administered to pregnant women or can affect reproductive capacity. The vaccines should be used during pregnancy only if clearly needed.

Because hepatitis A vaccine is produced from inactivated HAV, the theoretical risk to the fetus is expected to be low. The ACIP, AAP, American Academy of Family Physicians (AAFP), American College of Obstetricians and Gynecologists (ACOG), and the American College of Physicians (ACP) state that the vaccine may be used in pregnant women when indicated for preexposure vaccination in high-risk groups (including travelers) or for postexposure prophylaxis. However, if only short-term protection against HAV infection is needed during pregnancy, *passive* immunization with IGIM should be considered as an alternative to *active* immunization with hepatitis A vaccine.

Hepatitis A vaccine and the fixed-combination vaccine containing hepatitis A vaccine and hepatitis B vaccine should be used in pregnant women only when clearly needed, weighing the risk of vaccination against the risk of infection. Clinicians are encouraged to register pregnant women who receive the fixed-combination vaccine with the manufacturer's vaccination pregnancy registry at 888-452-9622.

It is not known whether hepatitis A vaccine or the fixed-combination vaccine containing hepatitis A vaccine and hepatitis B vaccine (HepA-HepB; Twinrix®) affect fertility.

Hepatitis A vaccine and the fixed-combination vaccine containing hepatitis A vaccine and hepatitis B vaccine should be used with caution, but are not contraindicated, in nursing women. Because inactivated vaccines do not multiply within the body, they should not pose any unusual problems for lactating women or their infants.

Drug Interactions

■ **Anti-infective Agents** Concurrent use of anti-infective agents generally does not affect the immune response to inactivated vaccines, including hepatitis A virus vaccine inactivated (hepatitis A vaccine) or the fixed-combination vaccine containing hepatitis A vaccine and hepatitis B vaccine (HepA-HepB; Twinrix®).

■ **Immune Globulin** Passively acquired antibody to hepatitis A virus (anti-HAV) from administration of immune globulin IM (IGIM) appears to interfere with the active immune response produced by hepatitis A vaccine; however, because vaccine-induced titers generally are so much higher than antibody levels considered protective, the reduced immunogenicity associated with passively acquired antibody may not be clinically important. Adults receiving IGIM concurrently with the initial dose of hepatitis A vaccine developed the same rate of protective antibodies as adults who received the vaccine alone; however, geometric mean titers were lower (2488 versus 3614 mIU/mL, respectively) 1 month after three 720-unit doses of Havrix® vaccine were administered. The effect of reduced geometric mean titers on long-term protection has not been determined following concurrent use of IGIM and the initial dose of hepatitis A vaccine. Since adequate antibody levels are achieved when hepatitis A vaccine and IGIM are administered concomitantly, the 2 can be given simultaneously but in different syringes and at separate injection sites.

The US Public Health Service Advisory Committee on Immunization Practices (ACIP) states that the development of a protective antibody response to hepatitis A vaccine should not be impaired when used concurrently or at any interval before or after administration of an antibody-containing preparation. If combined *active* immunization with hepatitis A vaccine and *passive* immunization with IGIM is used (e.g., for postexposure prophylaxis), the first dose of vaccine should be administered concurrently with IGIM (using different syringes and different injection sites).

■ **Immunosuppressive Agents** Individuals receiving immunosuppressive therapy (e.g., alkylating agents, antimetabolites, corticosteroids, cytotoxic agents, radiation) may require additional doses of hepatitis A vaccine to develop circulating HAV antibody levels considered protective. Vaccines generally should be administered 2 weeks prior to initiation of immunosuppressive therapy or deferred until at least 3 months after such therapy is discontinued.

■ **Vaccines** Since hepatitis A vaccine is a noninfectious, inactivated preparation, concurrent use of hepatitis A vaccine and other killed or live vaccines is not likely to cause interference with the immune response to these vaccines. Studies conducted in infants 18 months of age or younger indicate that concurrent use of hepatitis A vaccine with diphtheria and tetanus toxoids and acellular pertussis vaccine adsorbed (DTaP), Haemophilus influenzae type b (Hib) vaccine, hepatitis B vaccine, measles, mumps, and rubella virus vaccine live (MMR), or inactivated poliovirus (IPV) vaccine does not affect the immunogenicity and reactogenicity of these vaccines. The ACIP, American Academy of Pediatrics (AAP), and American Academy of Family Physicians (AAFP) state that primary immunization with hepatitis A vaccine can be integrated with primary immunization against diphtheria, tetanus, pertussis, *Haemophilus influenzae* type b (Hib), hepatitis B, influenza, measles, mumps, rubella, meningococcal disease, pneumococcal disease, poliomyelitis, and varicella. However, hepatitis A vaccine should be administered at a different site using a separate syringe.

Diphtheria and Tetanus Toxoids and Pertussis Vaccines Hepatitis A vaccine may be given concurrently with DTaP using different syringes and different injection sites.

In one study in children who received Havrix® hepatitis A vaccine at 15–18 months of age concurrently with diphtheria and tetanus toxoids and acellular pertussis vaccine adsorbed (DTaP; Infanrix®) and Hib polysaccharide conjugate (tetanus toxoid conjugate) vaccine (PRP-T; OmniHIB® [not commercially available in the US]) at different sites, the immune response to Havrix® was the same as that reported when Havrix® is given alone. However, there was a higher incidence of some adverse effects (e.g., irritability, drowsiness, loss of appetite) in those who received Havrix® concurrently with DTaP and PRP-T than in those who received Havrix® alone. In addition, the manufacturer of Havrix® states that data are insufficient to date to assess the immune response to a fourth dose of DTaP when the dose is administered concurrently with Havrix®.

Vaqta® hepatitis A vaccine has been administered in children 18 months of age concomitantly with DTaP (Tripedia®) at different sites without a decrease in the antibody response to hepatitis A vaccine; however, immunogenicity data were insufficient to assess the antibody response to DTaP in these children.

Haemophilus b Vaccine Hepatitis A vaccine may be given concurrently with Hib vaccine using different syringes and different injection sites.

In one study in children who received Havrix® hepatitis A vaccine at 15–18 months of age concurrently with Hib polysaccharide conjugate (tetanus toxoid conjugate) vaccine (PRP-T; OmniHIB® [not commercially available in the US]) and DTaP at different sites, the immune response to Havrix® and the immune response to the Hib vaccine was the same as that reported when the vaccines are given alone. However, there was a higher incidence of some adverse effects (e.g., irritability, drowsiness, loss of appetite) in those who received Havrix® concurrently with PRP-T and DTaP than in those who received Havrix® alone.

The manufacturer of Vaqta® hepatitis A vaccine states that data are not available to date regarding concurrent administration of the vaccine and Hib conjugate vaccines.

Hepatitis B Vaccine Studies have shown that monovalent hepatitis A vaccine and monovalent hepatitis B vaccine can be administered simultaneously at different sites using separate syringes without interfering with the immune response or increasing the frequency of adverse effects to either vaccine. In addition, studies in adults indicate that immune responses and adverse effects reported in individuals who received a 3-dose series of the fixed-combination vaccine containing hepatitis A vaccine and hepatitis B vaccine (HepA-HepB; Twinrix®) are similar to those reported in individuals who received a 2-dose series of monovalent hepatitis A vaccine (Havrix®) and a 3-dose series of monovalent hepatitis B vaccine (Engerix-B®) given concurrently in opposite arms. Data are not available to date regarding concomitant administration of Twinrix® and other vaccines.

Measles, Mumps, and Rubella Virus Vaccine Live Hepatitis A vaccine can be administered concurrently at a separate site with measles, mumps, and rubella virus vaccine live (MMR).

Pneumococcal Vaccine Hepatitis A vaccine may be given concurrently with pneumococcal vaccine using different syringes and different injection sites.

Concomitant administration of pneumococcal 7-valent conjugate vaccine (PCV7; Prevnar®) and Havrix® hepatitis A vaccine in children 15 months of age did not affect the immune response to either vaccine.

Varicella Virus Vaccine Live Vaqta® hepatitis A vaccine has been administered concurrently with varicella virus vaccine live at a different site without a decrease in the antibody response to the hepatitis A vaccine; however, immunogenicity data to date are insufficient to assess the response to the varicella vaccine.

Typhoid and Yellow Fever Vaccines The ACIP states that hepatitis A vaccine may be given concomitantly (using different syringes and different injection sites) with yellow fever vaccine.

The manufacturer of Vaqta® hepatitis A vaccines states that the vaccine may be administered concurrently with typhoid and yellow fever vaccines. Although lower anti-HAV geometric mean antibody titers (GMTs) were observed in vaccinees who received Vaqta® concurrently with typhoid and yellow fever vaccines compared with those who received Vaqta® alone, similar anti-HAV GMTs were observed in vaccinees after a booster dose of Vaqta® was administered.

Limited data indicate that the concurrent administration of hepatitis A vaccine with typhoid (IM or oral) or yellow fever vaccines at different sites in adults does not affect the immunogenicity or adverse effect profile of the vaccines. In one study, hepatitis A vaccine did not appear to affect the immune response or adverse reactions to parenteral inactivated typhoid vaccine (Typhim Vi®). In another study, hepatitis A vaccine was administered concurrently on the same day or within the 4-week period before administration of typhoid or yellow fever vaccines without evidence of impaired antibody response to any of the vaccines.

Other Vaccines Limited data from adults indicate that the concurrent administration of hepatitis A vaccine with cholera vaccine (not commercially available in the US), Japanese encephalitis virus vaccine, IPV or poliovirus vaccine live oral (OPV; no longer commercially available in the US), or rabies vaccines does not affect the immunogenicity or adverse effect profile of the vaccines. Hepatitis A vaccine has been administered concurrently on the same day or within the 4-week period before administration of various other vaccines used in travelers, including vaccines against Japanese encephalitis, poliovirus, and rabies. There was no evidence that concurrent administration of any of these vaccines impaired the antibody response to hepatitis A vaccine. In addition, there was a 100% response rate to vaccines against Japanese encephalitis and rabies.

In individuals initially seronegative who received one dose of OPV (no longer commercially available in the US) concurrently with hepatitis A vaccine, the seroconversion rate was lower for poliovirus type 3 (39%) than for poliovirus types 1 or 2 (67%).

Laboratory Test Interferences

■ **Serologic Tests Used in the Diagnosis of Hepatitis A Virus Infection** Individuals who have received hepatitis A virus vaccine inactivated (hepatitis A vaccine) and who are being evaluated for suspected hepatitis A virus (HAV) infection by serology to detect immunoglobulin M (IgM) anti-HAV to confirm a specific diagnosis of HAV infection may have a positive test result in the absence of infection, especially if the test is performed soon after vaccine administration. In adults who received a single dose of hepatitis A vaccine, IgM anti-HAV was detected 2–3 weeks after vaccine administration; however, only 1% of vaccinees had detectable IgM anti-HAV 1 month after vaccination.

Pharmacology

Hepatitis A virus vaccine inactivated (hepatitis A vaccine) stimulates active immunity to hepatitis A virus (HAV) infection by inducing production of HAV-specific immunoglobulin G (IgG) and M (IgM) antibodies (anti-HAV), resulting in humoral immunity. Protection is provided only against HAV and not against other infectious agents (e.g., hepatitis B virus [HBV]; hepatitis C virus [HCV], hepatitis E virus [HEV]).

Protection against HAV infection is virtually complete in individuals who develop adequate antibody levels after immunization with hepatitis A vaccine. Because HAV infection does not induce a chronic carrier state and no known animal reservoir exists, high levels of population immunization with hepatitis A vaccine should reduce substantially the incidence of infection. The US Public Health Service Advisory Committee on Immunization Practices (ACIP) does not recommend postvaccination testing for serologic response because vaccine immunogenicity has been very high in clinical studies, the absolute lower limit of antibody required to prevent HAV infection has not been defined, and the lack of an approved, commercially available assay with the sensitivity to detect the anti-HAV concentrations associated with protection (although modifications of these assays successfully have measured low levels of antibodies under research conditions [e.g., lower detection limits of 10–12 mIU/mL]). In most clinical trials, seroconversion levels of anti-HAV of 20 mIU/mL or greater, or in more recent clinical trials, 33 mIU/mL or greater, measured by modified enzyme immunoassays have been used to define a protective antibody response for Havrix® vaccine and levels of 10 mIU/mL or greater measured by modified radioimmunoassay have been used for Vaqta® vaccine. Clinical trial data regarding the minimum protective level of anti-HAV have been limited because of high vaccine-induced levels of anti-HAV following vaccination and the fact that diagnosis of HAV infection in vaccinees has been uncommon. Because the lower detection limit of unmodified (standard) immunoassays currently is approximately 100 mIU/mL, ACIP states that detection by such assays of any level of anti-HAV (i.e., seropositivity) after immunoprophylaxis indicates protection with either vaccine; likewise, individuals who are anti-HAV negative by such assays may still have protective levels of anti-HAV since the lower detection limit exceeds levels considered protective. Evidence from primate studies indicates that while antibody levels less than 10 mIU/mL may not prevent infection by the virus, they do prevent the development of clinical hepatitis and viral shedding.

Hepatitis A vaccine has been shown to be effective in preventing infection when employed for preexposure vaccination. Unlike immune globulin IM (IGIM), hepatitis A vaccine is not approved for use in postexposure prophylaxis. Primate studies suggest that administration of hepatitis A vaccine soon after HAV exposure may prevent HAV infection. In addition, the fact that HAV infection was not reported 17 days or more following vaccination during a clinical trial also suggests possible postexposure benefit since the incubation period of HAV infection can be as long as 50 days. While administration of the vaccine during the incubation period of infection (i.e., after exposure to HAV but prior to onset of clinical manifestations such as jaundice) also may prevent HAV infection if given shortly after exposure, definitive studies have not been conducted to compare the postexposure efficacy of hepatitis A vaccine with that of IGIM to determine if hepatitis A vaccine without IGIM can provide effective postexposure protection.

The active immune response produced by hepatitis A vaccine appears to be decreased by IGIM when administered concomitantly at a separate site. Reduced titers have been observed in adults receiving concurrent IGIM and primary immunization with either monovalent formulation of hepatitis A vaccine, but the degree of interference by IGIM generally does not affect the rate of seroprotection (i.e., antibody levels still generally exceed those considered protective by several fold) and therefore is unlikely to be clinically important. (See Drug Interactions: Immune Globulin.) The active immune response to hepatitis A vaccine may be reduced in infants with maternally acquired antibody. (See Pharmacology: Response to Hepatitis A Virus Vaccine Inactivated.) Immunogenicity of the vaccine also may be reduced in individuals with human immunodeficiency virus (HIV) infection, resulting in decreased protection rates and geometric mean antibody titers (GMTs). It remains to be determined whether other factors (e.g., age, obesity, smoking) associated with decreased response with other vaccines also may be associated with decreased responses to hepatitis A vaccine. Limited data indicate that the immunogenicity of hepatitis A vaccine may be reduced in older individuals; although the rates of protection in adults older than 40 years of age were similar to those in younger vaccinees, GMTs were lower.

■ **Hepatitis A Virus and Infection** Hepatitis A virus (HAV) is an RNA virus that is classified as a member of the Hepatovirus genus within the Picornaviridae family. Only one serotype of HAV among the various human strains isolated worldwide has been described. While minor differences in monoclonal antibody-binding patterns exist between human and simian HAV strains, they appear to elicit cross-protective immunity. Neither nucleotide similarity nor serologic cross-reactivity has been observed between HAV and non-A viruses causing hepatitis.

HAV replicates mainly in the liver and is shed in feces via biliary excretion. The incubation period for HAV infection following exposure to the virus is shorter than that following exposure to hepatitis B, ranging from 15–50 days and averaging about 1 month for HAV regardless of the route of infection; however, the greater the inoculum of virus the shorter the incubation period. The illness associated with HAV infection typically has an abrupt onset that can include fever, malaise, anorexia, nausea, abdominal discomfort, dark urine, and jaundice. The likelihood of symptomatic infection is age related, with about 70% of children younger than 6 years of age experiencing asymptomatic infection and, even when symptomatic, usually is not accompanied by jaundice. HAV infection usually is symptomatic in older children and adults, with jaundice occurring in greater than 70% of patients. Manifestations usually persist for less than 2 months, although 10–15% of patients develop prolonged or relapsing disease persisting up to 6 months. While a chronic carrier state does not exist for HAV, illness may be prolonged, and relapse of clinical illness with fecal viral shedding has been described. Data from individuals with HAV infection reported to the National Notifiable Diseases Surveillance System indicate that the overall case-fatality rate is approximately 0.3–0.6% and may be as high as 1.8% among adults older than 50 years of age; infected individuals with chronic liver disease are at increased risk for acute liver failure.

The initial antibody response to HAV infection is detectable by the time clinical manifestations develop (e.g., anorexia, abdominal discomfort, dark urine, fever, malaise, nausea, elevated serum ALT [SGPT], jaundice) and consists of IgM, IgG, and immunoglobulin A (IgA), with 7S (IgA or IgG) antibodies generally being detectable as early as 2 days after the onset of illness. Peak viral shedding of HAV in feces of, and peak viremia in, infected individuals occurs during the 2-week period prior to the onset of clinical manifestations (e.g., jaundice); thus, patients are asymptomatic during the period of greatest infectivity. At the time the infection becomes symptomatic, anti-HAV almost always is present; in rare cases when it is not, interferon gamma is detectable before seroconversion. In adults, fecal excretion of the virus usually declines following the development of jaundice, but children may excrete the virus for longer periods (e.g., 10 weeks after the onset of symptoms). In one nosocomial outbreak, infants infected as neonates shed HAV for up to 6 months. With conventional assays, IgM anti-HAV usually becomes detectable 5–10 days before clinical manifestations are observed and remains detectable for up to 6 months after symptomatic disease subsides in most patients; however, the antibody occasionally may be detected in serum by sensitive immunoassay for 1 year or longer after acute hepatitis. In addition, there have been reports of false-positive test results in individuals without evidence of recent HAV infection. HAV infection cannot be differentiated from other types of viral hepatitis based on clinical or epidemiologic characteristics alone. HAV RNA is detectable in the blood and stool of most patients during the acute phase of infection by using nucleic acid amplification methods, and nucleic acid sequencing has been used in epidemiologic investigations to determine the relatedness of HAV isolates; however, only a limited number of research laboratories have the capacity to use these methods. Although sensitive saliva tests for IgM and IgG anti-HAV have been developed, they are not commercially available in the US. Therefore, serologic detection of IgM anti-HAV generally is required to confirm a specific diagnosis of HAV.

There are 2 serologic tests commercially available in the US for the detection of antibodies to HAV; one measures IgM anti-HAV and the other measures total anti-HAV (i.e., IgM and IgG anti-HAV). Measurement of total anti-HAV is used in epidemiologic studies to determine the prevalence of previous HAV infection or by clinicians to determine whether an individual in whom preexposure prophylaxis is being considered is already immune.

During convalescence, the major class of antibody to HAV detectable in serum is IgG, and evidence indicates that anti-HAV IgG is the principal defense against reinfection, generally remaining detectable for the life of the individual and conferring lifelong immunity to illness from HAV and presumably against subsequent HAV infection. Detection of total anti-HAV (IgG and IgM) in serum is of limited value in diagnosing acute HAV infection because of the high seroprevalence rate in many populations (e.g., 31% of the US population has serologic evidence of prior HAV infection).

■ **Response to Hepatitis A Virus Vaccine Inactivated** Hepatitis A vaccine appears to be highly immunogenic in most individuals. The HAV epitopes that stimulate the formation of protective antibodies include 2 capsid polypeptides (VP_1 and VP_3). The presence of antibodies to HAV (anti-HAV) confers protection against HAV infection; however, the lowest titer conferring protection has not been established. Clinical trials evaluating Havrix® vaccine generally have defined a protective anti-HAV response as 20 mIU/mL or greater as measured by modified enzyme immunoassays (recent studies have defined a protective response as greater than 33 mIU/mL) and clinical trials evaluating Vaqta® vaccine generally have defined a protective anti-HAV response as 10 mIU/mL or greater as measured by radioimmunoassay. ACIP states that any level of anti-HAV detected by commercially available (i.e., unmodified) enzyme or radioimmunoassay can be considered protective since the lower antibody detection limits of such assays (i.e., about 100 mIU/mL) greatly exceed defined levels of protections; however, individuals who are anti-HAV negative by such assays may still have protective levels of anti-HAV.

The protective efficacy of Havrix® hepatitis A vaccine has been demonstrated in a double-blind, randomized controlled study in school children 1–16 years of age living in villages in Thailand with high endemic rates of HAV and thus considered at high risk of infection. Children receiving hepatitis A vaccine at 0, 1, and 12 months were observed after day 138 of the study for 8 months for protocol-defined manifestations of HAV infection (2 days or more absence from school, serum ALT concentration exceeding 45 U/mL, and a positive enzyme-linked immunosorbent assay [ELISA] test result). In the control group, 32 cases of HAV infection were demonstrated, while in the group receiving hepatitis A vaccine, 2 cases of HAV infection were positively identified and 3 additional illnesses that could neither be proven nor disproven to be caused by HAV were observed. The calculated efficacy rate for prevention of clinical HAV infection ranges from 84–94%, depending on inclusion or exclusion of the 3 unproven illnesses. In a double-blind, randomized controlled study in children 2–16 years of age residing in a New York community with a high rate of HAV, the protective efficacy of Vaqta® hepatitis A vaccine in preventing clinical HAV infection was 100% of vaccinees beginning 18 days after a single dose.

The protective efficacy of hepatitis A vaccine has also been evaluated in demonstration projects and through analysis of surveillance and vaccine coverage data that focused on communities with the highest historical rates of HAV infection (e.g., Native American and Alaskan communities). Such data indicate that when relatively high vaccination coverage is achieved and sustained, ongoing epidemics are interrupted and reduced HAV infection rates are sustained. A communitywide HAV epidemic in 1992–1993 among Native Alaskans in a rural community ended within 4–8 weeks of HAV vaccination of approximately 80% of children and young adults in the community. Following the ACIP recommendations for routine HAV vaccination of children in these high-risk areas in 1996, surveys indicated that vaccine coverage among preschool- and school-aged Native American and Alaskan children was 50–80%; the incidence of HAV infection among these populations by 2000 had decreased 97% compared with the beginning of the decade and was lower than the overall US rate of HAV infection. Such low rates of HAV infection continue to be maintained; the 2004 rate of HAV infection among Native Americans and Alaskans was 0.1 case per 100,000 population, the lowest rate of any US racial/ethnic population. Considerable reductions in the overall incidence of HAV infection have also been achieved in populations with consistently elevated rates of HAV infection following implementation of an ongoing routine childhood vaccination program that achieved fairly modest coverage (i.e., receipt of at least a single dose of hepatitis A vaccine in 66% of the approximately 45,000 eligible children older than 2 years of age). During this 6-year project, a 94% decline in HAV infection was observed in the population, and the number of cases reported during the final year of the project was the lowest number reported since HAV surveillance began in 1966.

The most comprehensive evidence of the protective efficacy of hepatitis A vaccine is derived from analysis of trends in HAV infection rates following the implementation of the 1999 ACIP recommendations for selective routine vaccination of children residing in 17 states with consistently elevated rates of HAV infection. Rates of HAV infection in these states decreased approximately 88% from the baseline prevaccine period rate of 21.1 cases per 100,000 population to the 2003 rate of 2.5 cases per 100,000 population. US rates of HAV infection are similar among regions with and without statewide recommendations for routine childhood HAV vaccination. Compared with HAV infection rates during 1990–1997, rates decreased most dramatically among children 2–18 years of age; rates among children decreased from 35 to 19%. However, because the incidence of HAV infection has been cyclic in the US, the precise contribution of routine childhood vaccination to the observed decrease in HAV infection rates has been difficult to measure. Modeling studies also suggest that during 1995–2001, an estimated 97,800 cases of HAV infection were prevented because of the direct effects of HAV immunization and resultant herd immunity.

Infants Younger than 12 Months of Age Few data are available evaluating the use of hepatitis A vaccine in infants younger than 12 months of age. Administration of hepatitis A vaccine to infants with passively acquired antibody (because of previous maternal HAV infection) appears to be associated with reduced vaccine immunogenicity. In most studies, all vaccinated infants developed protective anti-HAV levels, but the final geometric mean titers (GMT) were approximately 10–33% of that observed in infants vaccinated by the same schedule and born to mothers negative for anti-HAV. Infants with passively acquired antibody who received hepatitis A vaccine developed substantially lower levels of anti-HAV 6 years later compared with vaccinated infants with no passively acquired antibody. Despite lower antibody levels after the primary series, the majority of infants with passively acquired antibody had an anamnestic response to a booster dose administered 1–6 years later. Passively acquired antibody declines to undetectable levels in most infants by 1 year of age. Hepatitis A vaccine is highly immunogenic in children who begin the vaccine series after 1 year of age, regardless of maternal anti-HAV status.

The immunologic response to a 2-dose regimen of Havrix® (720-unit doses given at 5 and 11 months of age) was evaluated in healthy infants with and without maternal anti-HAV. One month after the primary dose, all infants born to anti-HAV-negative mothers had seroconverted and the GMT was 171 mIU/mL; the GMT in these infants increased to 3021 mIU/mL one month after the booster dose. In the group of infants with maternal anti-HAV (prevaccination GMT of 409 mIU/mL), 96% had seroconverted and the GMT was 225 mIU/mL one month after the primary dose; however, the GMT in these infants decreased to 62 mIU/mL prior to the booster dose and then increased to 399 mIU/mL one month after the booster dose.

Children 1 through 2 Years of Age In clinical studies evaluating the immunogenicity of a 2-dose regimen of Havrix® hepatitis A vaccine (720 units given 6 months apart) in children 11–13 months of age, 15–18 months of age, and 23–25 months of age, similar vaccine response rates (99–100%) and GMTs (1461–1911 mIU/mL) were obtained among these age groups when the response was assessed 1 month after the second dose. Vaccine response was defined as seroconversion in children initially seronegative or maintenance of at least the prevaccination anti-HAV concentration in initially seropositive children.

Vaqta® hepatitis A vaccine also has been highly immunogenic when administered in a 2-dose regimen (25 units each dose) to initially seronegative children 12–23 months of age (with or without concurrent administration of other routine childhood vaccines) with 96% seroconverting 1 month after the first dose with a GMT of 48 mIU/mL and 100% seroconverting after the second dose with a GMT of 6920 mIU/mL.

Older Children and Adolescents Hepatitis A vaccine (Havrix® and Vaqta®) is highly immunogenic when administered to children and adolescents by various schedules; 97–100% of individuals 2–18 years of age develop protective levels of antibody 1 month after receiving the initial dose and 100% develop levels of antibodies well above protective levels 1 month after the second dose.After receiving the vaccine, children with Down syndrome developed levels of protective antibody that were similar to those observed in children without the syndrome.

In clinical studies evaluating the immunogenicity of 360-unit doses of Havrix® hepatitis A vaccine (Havrix® preparations containing 360 units/0.5 mL are no longer commercially available in the US) in children and adolescents 1–18 years of age, essentially all children developed protective antibody levels (GMT of 433 [range: 197–660] mIU/mL) within 2 months after a second dose (360 units each at 0 and 1 month) of vaccine. One month after a third dose of 360 units of Havrix® vaccine (administered at 6 months), the GMT increased to 3831 (range: 3388–4643) mIU/mL. At 12 months (6 months after the third dose), protective levels persisted in all children, although the GMT had declined to 1069 mIU/mL. In children and adolescents 2–18 years of age who received two 720-unit doses at 0 and 6 months, protective antibody levels developed in 99% of such children 1 month after the first dose and in all such children 1 month after the second dose (i.e., 7 months after the initial dose), with GMTs of 253 or 2576 mIU/mL at 1 or 7 months, respectively.

When administered to children and adolescents 2–18 years of age in a variety of 2-dose schedules (25-units/dose), Vaqta® also has been highly immunogenic, with 97–100% developing protective antibody levels 1 month after the first dose and 100% developing such levels after a second dose administered at 6, 12, or 18 months. In clinical studies evaluating the immunogenicity of Vaqta® in this age group, 97% of such children seroconverted with a GMT of 43 mIU/mL within 1 month of a single 25-unit IM dose; seroconversion has persisted for up to 18 months after a single dose in vaccinees. After a second 25-unit dose of Vaqta® administered at 18 months in children and adolescents who were still seropositive at this time (35 out of 39 vaccinees), an anamnestic response developed in 95% of these vaccinees. In children and adolescents who received a 25-unit booster dose at 6, 12, or 18 months after the primary dose, seroconversion was 100% and GMT was 10,433 mIU/mL 1 month after the 6-month booster, 100% and 12,308 mIU/mL, respectively, 1 month after the 12-month booster, and 100% and 9591 mIU/mL, respectively, 1 month after the 18-month booster.

Adults Hepatitis A vaccine (Havrix® and Vaqta®) is highly immunogenic when administered to adults by the recommended schedules; 94–100% of adults developed protective levels of antibody 1 month after receiving the initial dose and 100% had protective levels following the second dose. Limited data indicate that 54–62% or 94–100% of vaccinees who were evaluated developed serum neutralizing antibodies by 14 days or 1 month, respectively, after the initial dose.

Data from several clinical studies show that at least 80% (range: 80–98%) of healthy adults develop protective levels of anti-HAV (GMT range: 264–339 mIU/mL) by day 15 after a single 1440-unit dose of Havrix® hepatitis A vaccine. One month after vaccination with Havrix®, the rate of protective antibody levels was 99% and the GMT increased to a range of 335–637 mIU/mL, and at 6 months approximately 95% of vaccinees had seroconverted with a GMT of 208 mIU/mL. The geometric mean serum titers of anti-HAV attained after 4 doses of Havrix® hepatitis A vaccine (administered at 0, 1, 2, and 12 months) are 100- to 300-fold higher than those attained after passive immunization with immune globulin IM (IGIM) and are similar to levels after natural infection. The manufacturer of Havrix® states that the GMTs of serum anti-HAV obtained after a single dose of hepatitis A vaccine are at least several times higher than those observed following administration of 2.5–5 times the standard dose of IGIM (standard dose = 0.02–0.06 mL/kg); the GMTs in individuals receiving such doses of IGIM were 146, 77, and 63 mIU/mL after 5 days, 1 month, and 2 months, respectively. Similar immunogenicity is provided in adults by Vaqta® hepatitis A vaccine. One month after vaccination with a single 50-unit IM dose of Vaqta® in clinical studies in adults, 95% of vaccinees had seroconverted with a GMT of 37 mIU/mL; seroconversion has persisted for up to 18 months after a single dose of Vaqta® in adults. An amnestic response occurred in children and adolescents who received a booster dose 6–18 months after the initial dose and in adults who received a booster dose 6 or 12 months after the initial dose. After a second 50-unit dose of Vaqta® administered at 6 months in adults, seroconversion was 98%, and had increased to 100% and 5987 mIU/mL, respectively, 1 month later. After a second 25-unit dose of Vaqta® administered at 6 months in children and adolescents, seroconversion was 97% and

GMT was 107 mIU/mL after the second dose, and had increased to 100% and 10,433 mIU/mL, respectively, 1 month later. Similar seroconversion rates and increases in GMT were observed in adults who received a second 50-unit dose 12 months after the initial dose and in children, and adolescents who received a second 25-unit dose 12 or 18 months after the initial dose.

In adults receiving both an initial dose (1440 units) of Havrix® hepatitis A vaccine and an additional (booster) dose (1440 units) 6 months later, protective antibody levels (defined as a serum anti-HAV level of at least 20 mIU/mL) developed in all vaccinees (GMT of 4383 [range: 3318–5925] mIU/mL) 1 month after the second dose (i.e., 7 months after the initial dose). The initial dose resulted in protective levels in 88% (GMT: 293 mIU/mL) of these adults at 15 days and in 99% (GMT: 466 mIU/mL) at 1 month after this dose. The second dose of Havrix® hepatitis A vaccine induced an anti-HAV titer similar to levels seen several years after natural infection.

Limited data from 3 small studies involving children and adults indicate that interruption of the recommended vaccination schedule and a delay in administration of the second dose of hepatitis A vaccine may result in an immune response similar to that attained in those who receive the vaccine according to the usually recommended schedule. In one study, 97% of adults 18 years of age or older had protective levels of anti-HAV 18 months after the first 50-unit dose of Vaqta® and final antibody concentrations attained after the second dose were similar to those reported in vaccinees who were vaccinated according to the usual schedule. In another study, 27 months after receiving one dose of the age-appropriate dose of Havrix®, 84% of individuals 1 month to 64 years of age had protective levels of anti-HAV and practically all vaccinees developed a marked increase in concentrations of anti-HAV after receiving the second vaccine dose. In a third study, 72% of adults developed anti-HAV levels of 10 mIU/mL or greater following an initial dose of hepatitis A vaccine (Havrix®; 1440 units in adults) and all vaccinees experienced a substantial increase in anti-HAV levels following a second dose 4–8 years following the initial dose.

Limited data indicate that the immune response to hepatitis A vaccine may be decreased in older individuals. In several efficacy studies, the proportion of individuals older than 40 years of age who developed a protective antibody response after receiving the vaccine was similar to that of individuals 40 years of age or younger, but final anti-HAV concentrations were lower in the older age group.

Although adults or children with chronic liver disease of viral or nonviral etiology appear to develop similar rates of protection after receiving hepatitis A vaccine compared with those observed in healthy adults, final anti-HAV concentrations may be lower in patients with chronic liver disease.

Additional factors associated with decreased immunogenicity to other vaccines (e.g., smoking and obesity) have not been evaluated with the commercially available formulations of hepatitis A vaccine. Data are not available to date regarding response rates following revaccination with hepatitis A vaccine in individuals who failed to respond to the primary vaccine series.

HIV-infected Individuals The usual recommended dosage and schedule of hepatitis A vaccine is immunogenic in certain HIV-infected children and adults. The immune response observed in adults with $CD4^+$ T-cell counts of at least 300 cells/mm^3 is similar to that observed in healthy adults; however, adults with lower $CD4^+$ T-cell counts are less likely to acquire protective levels of anti-HAV antibodies. Protective levels of antibody were observed in 61–87% of HIV-infected adults and in 100% of HIV-infected children following vaccination with hepatitis A vaccine. At the time of vaccination, a low $CD4^+$ T-cell count (not the $CD4^+$ T-cell count nadir) was associated with a lack of immune response to the vaccine; this observation suggests that immunologic reconstitution with highly active antiretroviral therapy may restore the immune system's ability to respond to vaccination.

The antibody response and GMTs achieved with hepatitis A vaccine in individuals with HIV infection may be decreased compared with that in noninfected individuals. In a limited number of HIV-infected or noninfected individuals who received three 720-unit doses of Havrix® vaccine, the seroconversion rate was 77 or 100%, respectively, and the GMT was 636 or 1687 mIU/mL, respectively. In a study in HIV-infected adults who received 2 doses of hepatitis A vaccine, the seroconversion rate was 68% in those with $CD4^+$ T-cell counts of 200/mm^3 or greater but was only 9% in those with lower $CD4^+$ T-cell counts. The vaccine was well tolerated in these HIV-infected patients and there was no evidence that the vaccine had any adverse effects on the course of HIV infection or plasma HIV RNA levels.

Individuals with Chronic Liver Disease In a study evaluating the immunogenicity of hepatitis A vaccine (Havrix®) in adults with chronic liver disease of various etiologies (e.g., chronic HBV, chronic HCV, alcoholic cirrhosis, autoimmune hepatitis, chronic hepatitis/cryptogenic cirrhosis, hemochromatosis, primary biliary cirrhosis, primary sclerosing cholangitis), the GMT response and seroconversion rates to the initial 1440-unit dose of vaccine were lower in those with chronic liver disease than in healthy subjects. However, the seroconversion rates were similar in both groups 1 month after a second 1440-unit dose (booster dose) given 6 months after the initial dose. The relevance of these results to the duration of protection afforded by hepatitis A vaccine (Havrix®) is unknown.

Transplant Recipients Conflicting data have been reported regarding immunogenicity of hepatitis A vaccine in liver transplant recipients. In one small study of 8 liver transplant patients, none responded to hepatitis A vaccine. In another study, only 26% of 23 liver transplant patients responded to hepatitis A vaccine. In a larger controlled study evaluating the immunogenicity of a 2-dose regimen of Havrix® (1400-unit doses given 6 months apart) in liver and renal transplant patients, the seroconversion rate after the initial vaccine dose was low in both the liver and renal transplant patients (41 and 24%, respectively) compared with that attained in healthy controls (90%). However, the seroconversion rate one month after the second vaccine dose was 97% in those who received liver transplants, 72% in those who received renal transplants, and 100% in healthy controls. This study included transplant recipients 18 years of age or older who were seronegative for anti-HAV and also seronegative for HIV. The mean time interval since transplantation was 40 months among the liver transplant patients (41% had undergone transplantation because of chronic HBV or HCV infection) and 96 months among the renal transplant patients (10% had serologic evidence of chronic HBV infection and 28% had serologic evidence of chronic HCV infection). Most liver transplant patients were receiving either tacrolimus or cyclosporine; all renal transplant patients were receiving 2 or more immunosuppressive agents which possibly may have contributed to the lower seroconversion rate in these patients. Follow-up of these transplant recipients indicated that anti-HAV levels may decline more rapidly for both liver and kidney transplant recipients compared with observed rates of antibody decline in healthy individuals.

■ **Response to Hepatitis A Virus Vaccine Inactivated and Hepatitis B Vaccine (Recombinant)** Data from several studies in healthy adults (17–70 years of age) indicate that the immunogenicity of a 3-dose series (at 0, 1, and 6 months) of the fixed-combination vaccine (HepA-HepB; Twinrix®) that contains the antigens of hepatitis A vaccine (Havrix®) and hepatitis B vaccine (Engerix-B®) is similar to that of a 2-dose series (at 0 and 6 months) of the monovalent hepatitis A vaccine (Havrix®) and a 3-dose series (at 0, 1, and 6 months) of the monovalent hepatitis B vaccine (Engerix-B®) administered concurrently at separate sites or administered alone. In adults who received a 3-dose series of the fixed-combination vaccine, 99.9% developed anti-HAV titers of at least 20 mIU/mL and 98.5% developed anti-HBsAg titers of at least 10 mIU/mL 1 month after completion of the vaccine series. In one US study in adults 18–70 years of age, serum anti-HAV titers of at least 20 mIU/mL and anti-HBsAg titers of at least 10 mIU/mL were observed in 99.6 or 95.1% of vaccinees, respectively, who received a 3-dose series (at 0, 1, 6 months) of the fixed-combination vaccine compared with 99.3 or 92.2%, respectively, of vaccinees who received the separate monovalent hepatitis A vaccine and monovalent hepatitis B vaccine concurrently. The GMT of anti-HAV measured 1 month after completion of the vaccine series was 4756 mIU/mL in vaccinees who received the fixed-combination vaccine versus 2948 mIU/mL in vaccinees who received both monovalent vaccines; this difference is not considered clinically important and has been attributed to the differences in the hepatitis A viral antigen content in the 2 regimens (3 doses of 720 units in the regimen compared to 2 doses of 1440 units in the monovalent regimen). The average GMTs of anti-HBsAg measured 1 month after completion of the vaccine series was 2099 mIU/mL in vaccinees who received the fixed-combination vaccine versus 1871 mIU/mL in vaccinees who received both monovalent vaccines.

When an accelerated dosage regimen of the fixed-combination vaccine (HepA-HepB; Twinrix®) was used (doses at 0, 7, and 21–30 days and a booster dose at 12 months) in healthy adults, the seroprotection rate for HBV and seroconversion rate for HAV at month 13 was noninferior to the rates reported with monovalent hepatitis A vaccine (Havrix®) and monovalent hepatitis B vaccine (Engerix-B®) administered at separate sites (i.e., Havrix® at 1 and 12 months and Engerix-B® at 0, 1, 2, and 12 months). On day 37 (after 3 doses of Twinrix®), the seroprotection rate for HBV was 63.2% compared with 43.5% in the control group who had received 2 doses of Engerix-B®; the HAV seroconversion rates were similar in both groups (98.5 or 98.6%, respectively). On day 90, the seroprotection rate for HBV was 83.2% in the Twinrix® group and 76.7% in the control group; the HAV seroconversion rate was 100 or 95.6%, respectively. At month 12 (before the booster dose of Twinrix®), the seroprotection rate for HBV was 82.1% in the Twinrix® group and 77.8% in the control group; HAV seroconversion rates were 96.9 or 86.9%, respectively.

■ **Duration of Immunity** The duration of protection from HAV infection following administration of either commercially available monovalent formulation of hepatitis A vaccine and the need for additional booster doses have not been fully defined. All 31 adults who received three 720-unit doses (at 0, 1, and 6 months) of Havrix® hepatitis A vaccine maintained anti-HAV levels of 15 mIU/mL or greater at 12 years following the first dose. After receiving two 1440-unit doses of Havrix® hepatitis A vaccine, all 307 adults maintained anti-HAV levels exceeding 20 mIU/mL at 10 years following vaccination. Of 549 children who received Vaqta® hepatitis A vaccine, 99% maintained protective levels of anti-HAV at 5–6 years following vaccination.

In one study of antibody persistence in healthy adults, anti-HAV levels were maintained at a GMT of approximately 1500 mIU/mL 3 years after administration of a series of three 720-unit doses (at 0, 1, and 6 months) of Havrix® hepatitis A vaccine. In one study in healthy adults who received a primary dose of Havrix® followed by a booster dose given 6 or 12 months after the first dose, more than 99% of vaccinees still had detectable levels of anti-HAV antibodies 4 years after the second dose. In another study, the rate of decrease in anti-HAV titers calculated from the antibody decrease between months 6 and 12 and between months 13 and 18 in individuals vaccinated with 4 doses of hepatitis A vaccine suggests the duration of anti-HAV levels of at least 10 mIU/mL to be at least 10 years. After 18 months, anti-HAV titers were approximately 1200–8000 mIU/mL in this study; however, the rate of disappearance of protective antibodies was independent of the absolute titer, vaccine dose or strain, or vaccination schedule. Experience with Vaqta® vaccine in vaccinees who were observed for 36 months also indicates that anti-HAV levels decline over time; however, protective levels persisted in 100% of vaccinees during this period. Studies have been initiated to evaluate persistence of immunity in healthy children, adolescents, and adults who have been vaccinated with Vaqta® and to determine if additional booster doses will be required.

In 2 studies evaluating antibody persistence in healthy adults following a 3-dose series (at 0, 1, and 6 months) of the fixed-combination vaccine (HepA-HepB; Twinrix®) containing hepatitis A vaccine (Havrix®) and hepatitis B vaccine (Engerix-B®), anti-HAV and anti-HBsAg levels were maintained for at least 4 years.

Estimates of antibody persistence derived from kinetic models of decline suggest that protective levels of anti-HAV may persist for 25 years or longer in adults and 14–20 years or longer in children. However, it has been suggested that the duration of antiviral protection induced by the vaccine may exceed persistence of measurable antibodies. For example, cellular memory (anamnestic antiviral response) may contribute to long-term protection. Additional long-term study and experience are needed and ongoing to elucidate more fully the duration of protective efficacy of currently recommended regimens of hepatitis A vaccine and the possible need for booster doses. Surveillance data and population-based studies are ongoing and data to date indicate that no cases of HAV infection have been detected among children followed for 9 years after receiving hepatitis A vaccine.

Chemistry and Stability

■ Chemistry

Hepatitis A Virus Vaccine Inactivated Hepatitis A virus vaccine inactivated (hepatitis A vaccine) is a noninfectious, sterile suspension of a cell culture-adapted, attenuated strain of hepatitis A virus (HAV). Hepatitis A vaccine is prepared from attenuated strains of the virus that have been propagated in MRC-5 human diploid fibroblasts, harvested and purified from cell lysates using a combination of physical (e.g., ultrafiltration) and chromatographic (e.g., exclusion gel chromatography, high-performance liquid chromatography [HPLC]) techniques, inactivated with formaldehyde, and then adsorbed onto an aluminum adjuvant. Hepatitis A vaccine commercially available in the US is prepared using either the attenuated virus strain HM175 (Havrix®) or the attenuated virus strain CR326F′ (Vaqta®). Havrix® and Vaqta® do not contain thimerosal or any other preservatives.

Commercially available hepatitis A vaccine meets standards established by the Center for Biologics Evaluation and Research of the US Food and Drug Administration (FDA) and purity requirements of the World Health Organization (WHO) for vaccines prepared in human diploid cells. Viral antigen activity of hepatitis A vaccine prepared from the HM175 strain (Havrix®) is referenced to a standard using an enzyme-linked immunosorbent assay (ELISA), and therefore is expressed in terms of ELISA units (ELU). This calibration reflects the presence of antigenic sites recognizable by neutralizing antibodies. Viral antigen activity of the vaccine prepared from the CR326F′ strain (Vaqta®) is referenced to a standard confirmed by amino acid analysis in which 1 unit (U) approximately equals 1 ng of viral protein antigen; therefore, potency of Vaqta® is expressed in units (U) of HAV antigen.

Each 0.5-mL pediatric or 1-mL adult dose of Havrix® vaccine containing at least 720 or 1440 units of viral antigen, respectively, also contains 0.25 or 0.5 mg of aluminum (as aluminum hydroxide). Havrix® also contains an amino acid supplement (0.3 mg/mL) in a phosphate-buffered saline solution, and polysorbate (Tween®) 20 (0.05 mg/mL). Residual MRC-5 cellular proteins (not exceeding 5 mcg/mL), which represent 95% of the total protein in the vaccine, and trace amounts of formalin (not exceeding 0.1 mg/mL) also are present. Trace amounts (not exceeding 40 ng/mL) of neomycin may be present in Havrix® since the aminoglycoside is included in the cell growth media used in the manufacture of the vaccine and trace amounts may remain following purification. Following thorough agitation, the vaccine is a uniform, slightly turbid, white suspension. The suspension has a pH of 6.8–7.5.

Each 1-mL adult dose of Vaqta® vaccine contains approximately 50 units of viral antigen, 0.45 mg of aluminum (as amorphous aluminum hydroxyphosphate sulfate), and 70 mcg of sodium borate as a pH stabilizer, in 0.9% sodium chloride. Each 0.5-mL pediatric dose of Vaqta® vaccine contains approximately 25 units of viral antigen, 0.225 mg of aluminum (as amorphous aluminum hydroxyphosphate sulfate), and 35 mcg of sodium borate, in 0.9% sodium chloride. Within the limits of assay variability, each 1-mL of vaccine (50 units) also contains less than 0.1 mcg of nonviral protein, less than 4×10^{-6} mcg of DNA, less than 10^{-4} mcg of bovine albumin, and less than 0.8 mcg of formaldehyde. Other chemical residuals from the manufacturing process are present in a concentration of less than 10 parts per billion. Following thorough agitation, the vaccine appears as a slightly opaque, white suspension. The suspension has a pH of 5.5–7.5.

Live attenuated hepatitis A virus vaccines (currently not commercially available in the US) also have been developed and tested in nonhuman primate models of HAV infection and human immunogenicity trials. In addition, a live attenuated hepatitis A vaccine (based on the H2 strain) has been tested in the People's Republic of China and is in use in that country. However, these vaccines have not been shown to offer distinct advantages over inactivated vaccines, and the US Public Health Service Advisory Committee on Immunization Practices (ACIP) states that only inactivated hepatitis A virus vaccines have been evaluated in controlled clinical efficacy trials.

Hepatitis A Virus Vaccine Inactivated and Hepatitis B Vaccine (Recombinant) Hepatitis A virus vaccine inactivated and hepatitis B vaccine (recombinant) is a fixed-combination vaccine that contains both HAV and hepatitis B virus (HBV) antigens. The commercially available fixed-combination vaccine (HepA-HepB; Twinrix®) is a sterile suspension containing the antigenic components used to produce Havrix® hepatitis A vaccine and Engerix-B® hepatitis B vaccine. Each antigenic component is adsorbed separately onto aluminum phosphate or aluminum hydroxide and then pooled to form the fixed-combination preparation.

Each 1-mL dose of Twinrix® contains 720 units of hepatitis A viral antigen and 20 mcg of hepatitis B surface antigen (HBsAg) and also contains 0.45 mg of aluminum (as aluminum hydroxide and aluminum phosphate). Each 1-mL dose of the vaccine also contains residual MRC-5 cellular (not exceeding 2.5 mcg), yeast proteins (not exceeding 50 mg), trace amounts of formaldehyde (not exceeding 0.1 mg), trace amounts of neomycin sulfate (not exceeding 0.02 mcg), and amino acids in a phosphate-buffered saline solution with polysorbate (Tween®) 20. Twinrix® does not contain any preservatives. The vaccine has a pH of 5.8–6.6. Following thorough agitation, Twinrix® appears as a homogeneous, turbid, white suspension.

■ Stability

Hepatitis A Virus Vaccine Inactivated Hepatitis A vaccine should be refrigerated at 2–8°C and should not be frozen; if freezing occurs, the vaccine should be discarded. When stored as recommended, Havrix® has an expiration date of 3 years after the date of manufacture. While refrigeration is the recommended storage and shipping condition for Havrix® and Vaqta® vaccines, the vaccines are reported to be thermally stable. Reactogenicity and immunogenicity of Havrix® stored at 37°C for up to 1 week and Vaqta® stored at 37°C for 12 months or longer does not differ from that reported for these vaccines when stored at 2–8°C.

Hepatitis A Virus Vaccine Inactivated and Hepatitis B Vaccine (Recombinant) The fixed-combination vaccine containing hepatitis A vaccine and hepatitis B vaccine (HepA-HepB; Twinrix®) should be refrigerated at 2–8°C and should not be frozen; if freezing occurs, the vaccine should be discarded. When stored as recommended, the vaccine has an expiration date of 3 years after the date of manufacture.

Preparations

Excipients in commercially available drug preparations may have clinically important effects in some individuals; consult specific product labeling for details.

Hepatitis A Virus Vaccine Inactivated

Parenteral

Injectable suspension, for IM use	25 units (of viral antigen) per 0.5 mL	**Vaqta® Pediatric/Adolescent,** Merck
	50 units (of viral antigen) per mL	**Vaqta® Adult,** Merck
	720 ELISA units (of viral antigen) per 0.5 mL	**Havrix® Pediatric,** GlaxoSmithKline
	1440 ELISA units (of viral antigen) per mL	**Havrix® Adult,** GlaxoSmithKline

Hepatitis A Inactivated and Hepatitis B (Recombinant) Vaccine (HepA-HepB)

Parenteral

Injectable suspension, for IM use	Hepatitis A Virus Vaccine Inactivated 720 ELISA units (of viral antigen) and Hepatitis B Vaccine (Recombinant) 20 mcg (of hepatitis B surface antigen) per mL	**Twinrix®**, GlaxoSmithKline

†Use is not currently included in the labeling approved by the US Food and Drug Administration

Hepatitis B Vaccine

Hepatitis B Vaccine (Recombinant)
HepA-HepB

■ Hepatitis B vaccine is an inactivated (recombinant) vaccine containing hepatitis B surface antigen (HBsAg) and is used to stimulate active immunity to hepatitis B virus (HBV) infection. Hepatitis B vaccine is commercially available in the US as monovalent vaccines (Engerix-B®, Recombivax HB®). Hepatitis B vaccine also is commercially available in a fixed-combination vaccine with *Haemophilus influenzae* type b (Hib) vaccine (Hib-HepB; Comvax®), in a fixed-combination vaccine with hepatitis A virus vaccine (HepA-HepB; Twinrix®), and in a fixed-combination vaccine that contains diphtheria, tetanus, pertussis, hepatitis B, and poliovirus antigens (DTaP-HepB-IPV; Pediarix®).

Uses

Hepatitis B vaccine (recombinant) is used to stimulate active immunity to hepatitis B virus (HBV) for prevention of HBV infection in susceptible individuals, including those considered at risk of potential exposure to HBV or hepatitis B surface antigen-positive (HBsAg-positive) materials (e.g., blood, plasma, serum).

The US Public Health Service Advisory Committee on Immunization Practices (ACIP), American Academy of Pediatrics (AAP), and American Academy of Family Physicians (AAFP) recommend that *all* neonates and infants and *all* previously unvaccinated children and adolescents through 18 years of age receive *routine* primary immunization against HBV infection with hepatitis B vaccine, unless contraindicated. In addition, the ACIP, AAFP, American College of Obstetricians and Gynecologists (ACOG), and American College of Physicians (ACP) recommend preexposure vaccination with hepatitis B vaccine for *all* susceptible adults with medical, occupational, behavioral, or other factors that put them at risk for HBV infection and for any other susceptible adult requesting protection from HBV.

Postexposure prophylaxis using combined *active* immunization with hepatitis B vaccine and *passive* immunization with hepatitis B immune globulin (HBIG) is used to prevent perinatal HBV infection in neonates born to HBsAg-positive women and also is used to prevent HBV infection in certain susceptible individuals exposed to HBV or HBsAg-positive material (e.g., blood, plasma, serum). (See Uses: Postexposure Prophylaxis.)

Successful prevention of HBV infection, either by primary or preexposure vaccination with hepatitis B vaccine or postexposure prophylaxis with hepatitis B vaccine and HBIG, generally will also prevent hepatitis D virus (HDV) infection (delta virus infection). HDV infection occurs only as a coinfection or superinfection in patients with HBV infection. HDV is dependent on HBV for replication; therefore, individuals immune to HBV also should be immune to HDV infection. Routes of transmission of HDV are similar to those for HBV, and HDV infection in the US most commonly affects individuals at high risk for HBV, particularly parenteral drug abusers and individuals receiving plasma-derived clotting factor concentrates. Individuals who are carriers of HBsAg are at risk of HDV infection, especially if they are at high risk of repeated exposure to HBV (e.g., parenteral drug abusers, homosexuals); however, there currently is no effective means for preexposure or postexposure prophylaxis of HDV infection in HBsAg carriers.

With the exception of HDV, monovalent hepatitis B vaccine will not prevent hepatitis caused by other viruses known to infect the liver, including hepatitis A virus (HAV), hepatitis C virus (HCV), or hepatitis E virus (HEV).

Primary immunization against HBV can be integrated with age-appropriate primary immunization against diphtheria, tetanus, pertussis, hepatitis A, *Haemophilus influenzae* type b (Hib), human papillomavirus (HPV), influenza, measles, mumps, rubella, pneumococcal disease, meningococcal disease, poliomyelitis, rotavirus, and varicella. (See Drug Interactions: Vaccines.)

■ Combination Vaccines Containing Hepatitis B Vaccine and Other Antigens Hepatitis B vaccine is commercially available in a fixed-combination vaccine with *Haemophilus influenzae* type b (Hib) vaccine (Hib-HepB; Comvax®), in a fixed-combination vaccine with hepatitis A virus vaccine (HepA-HepB; Twinrix®), and in a fixed-combination vaccine containing diphtheria, tetanus, pertussis, hepatitis B, and poliovirus antigens (DTaP-HepB-IPV; Pediarix®). When indicated based on the age and vaccination status of the individual and when there are no contraindications to any of the individual components, these combination vaccines can be used instead of separate injections.

The commercially available fixed-combination vaccine containing diphtheria, tetanus, pertussis, hepatitis B, and poliovirus antigens (DTaP-HepB-IPV; Pediarix®) can be used in infants and children 6 weeks through 6 years of age born to HBsAg-negative women when doses of poliovirus vaccine inactivated (IPV), diphtheria and tetanus toxoids adsorbed and acellular pertussis vaccine adsorbed (DTaP), and hepatitis B vaccine are indicated and there are not contraindications to any of the individual components. The ACIP states that this fixed-combination vaccine also may be used to complete the hepatitis B vaccine series in infants 6 weeks of age or older born to HBsAg-*positive* women†. Pediarix® should *not* be used for the initial dose of hepatitis B vaccine that is indicated in neonates. (See Neonates and Infants under Uses: Primary Immunization.)

The commercially available fixed-combination vaccine containing *Haemophilus influenzae* type b (Hib) and hepatitis B vaccine (Hib-HepB; Comvax®) can be used whenever a dose of Hib vaccine and a dose of hepatitis B vaccine are both indicated in an infant 6 weeks to 15 months of age born to an HBsAg-negative woman. The ACIP states that this fixed-combination vaccine also may be used to complete the hepatitis B vaccine series in infants 6 weeks to 15 months of age born to HBsAg-positive women†. Comvax® should *not* be used for the initial dose of hepatitis B vaccine that is indicated in neonates. (See Neonates and Infants under Uses: Primary Immunization.)

When vaccination against both hepatitis A and hepatitis B infection is indicated in adults 18 years of age or older, the commercially available fixed-combination vaccine containing hepatitis A and hepatitis B antigens (HepA-HepB; Twinrix®) can be used.

■ Past and Current Considerations Regarding Hepatitis B Vaccine Recommendations Hepatitis B vaccines have been available in the US since 1981.Although early hepatitis B vaccines were plasma-derived vaccines (no longer commercially available in the US), vaccines produced using recombinant DNA technology became available in 1986. Initially (from 1981–1991), the strategy for HBV prevention in the US consisted of selective vaccination of individuals in high-risk groups and serologic screening of all pregnant women for HBsAg with vaccination of neonates born to HBsAg-positive mothers. This limited strategy was successful only in reducing the risk of acquiring infection through occupational exposure, a group that accounts for only approximately 4% of cases of HBV infection, and failed to effectively target the majority of high-risk groups. In addition, it became evident that screening pregnant women for HBsAg and active and passive immunization of their neonates prevented only a small percentage of HBV infections that occurred annually in the US and had little impact on the control of HBV and its sequelae.

Therefore, the ACIP and AAP expanded their recommendations in 1991 and 1992 to include *universal* primary immunization of all neonates (regardless of the HBsAg status of the mother). This recommendation was based on the belief that universal immunization of all neonates has an immediate impact on reducing vertical transmission of HBV infection from mothers to neonates and would diminish or eliminate horizontal transmission between preschool-age children within 5 years. In 1995, a comprehensive vaccination strategy was adopted by the ACIP, AAP, and AAFP that included *universal* immunization for all adolescents not vaccinated previously. This expansion of recommendations to include immunization of older children was based on the fact that most individuals infected with HBV in the US acquired their infection while they were adolescents or young adults and efforts aimed at universal immunization of neonates were not likely to substantially affect the incidence of acute disease in the US for 20–30 years. Therefore, targeting neonates and adolescents was expected to result in a more rapid decline in the incidence of HBV infection. To encourage vaccination of children and adolescents, the ACIP, AAP, and AAFP beginning in 1999 recommended that all children and adolescents through 18 years of age who had not previously received hepatitis B vaccine begin the primary immunization series during any routine health care visit.

As a result of these strategies, the incidence of acute HBV reported in the US declined 78% during 1990–2005 and the greatest decline (96%) occurred among children and adolescents younger than 19 years of age. As of 2004, more than 92% of US children 19–35 months of age had received 3 doses of hepatitis B vaccine and data from 2003 indicate the vaccine coverage rate is 50–60% among adolescents 13–15 years of age.

The vaccination rate among adults, however, has remained low and adults accounted for approximately 95% of new HBV infections reported in 2005. Although the incidence of acute HBV infection among adults decreased 35% during 2002–2005, the highest incidence of acute HBV infection occurred among adults 25–45 years of age. Data indicate that ongoing HBV transmission occurs principally among unvaccinated adults with risk behaviors for HBV transmission and among household contacts and sexual partners of individuals with chronic HBV infection. Therefore, in 2006, the ACIP updated guidelines regarding hepatitis B vaccination in adults in an attempt to increase vaccination coverage in this age group. The ACIP now recommends hepatitis B vaccine (inactivated) for *all* unvaccinated adults at risk for HBV infection and for *all* unvaccinated adults who request protection from HBV. It is hoped that expanded use of the vaccine in adults in conjunction with routine use of the vaccine in neonates, children, and adolescents will ultimately result in the elimination of HBV transmission in the US.

■ Risks of Exposure and Infection HBV is transmitted by percutaneous or mucosal exposure to hepatitis B surface antigen-positive (HBsAg-positive) blood, serum, plasma, semen, or saliva from individuals who have acute HBV infection or individuals who are carriers of the virus. The principal sources of HBV are blood (plasma or serum) and serous fluids. Lower concentrations are found in saliva, semen, vaginal secretions, and wound exudates. Although saliva can be a vehicle of HBV transmission through bites, other types of exposure to saliva (e.g., kissing) are unlikely modes of transmission. Transmission of HBV does not appear to occur via tears, sweat, urine, feces, or droplet nuclei and the virus is not transmitted via the fecal-oral route.

HBV can be transmitted perinatally from mother to infant at birth, usually as the result of blood exposures during labor and delivery. In utero transmission of HBV is rare. Without postexposure HBV prophylaxis in the neonate, the risk for perinatal transmission of the virus and chronic infection is 5–20% if the mother is HBsAg-positive and hepatitis B e antigen-negative (HBeAg-negative) and about 70–90% if the mother is positive for both HBsAg and HBeAg. Up to 90% of infants who become infected perinatally will become HBV carriers.

In the US, the primary risk factors for HBV infection in adults and adolescents are unprotected sex with an infected partner, unprotected sex with more than one partner, men who have sex with men, history of other sexually transmitted diseases (STDs), and illicit injection drug use. The US Centers for Disease Control and Prevention (CDC) states that individuals considered at high risk of exposure to HBsAg-positive material include immigrants or refugees from areas of high HBV endemicity, residents in institutions for the developmentally disabled, users of illicit parenteral drugs, homosexually active men, hemodialysis patients, and household contacts of HBV carriers. Those considered at intermediate risk include male prisoners, health-care workers who have frequent blood contact, staff of institutions for the developmentally disabled, and heterosexuals with multiple partners.

Transmission from infected health-care personnel to patients is uncommon, but has been documented during certain invasive, exposure-prone procedures (e.g., certain oral, cardiothoracic, colorectal, or obstetric/gynecologic surgery). HBsAg-positive health-care personnel need not be restricted from patient contact unless they have been associated epidemiologically with transmission of HBV; adherence to recommended surgical and dental techniques, compliance with universal precautions for the prevention of blood-borne pathogens in health-care settings, and recommendations for sterilization/disinfection minimize the risk of transmission. However, health-care personnel who are HBeAg-positive should not perform *exposure-prone* procedures unless they have sought the advice and guidance of experts and have a clear understanding of the risks, associated precautions, and circumstances under which such procedures can continue to be performed.

Presence of HBeAg indicates a high degree of infectivity of body fluids. Individuals exposed to body fluids that are positive for HBsAg, HBeAg, and HBV-specific DNA polymerase are more likely to develop HBV infection than individuals exposed to body fluids that are positive for HBsAg and anti-HBe but negative for HBeAg and DNA polymerase. The development of the HBV carrier state generally is associated with high serum titers of HBsAg and persistent, high serum titers of antibody to hepatitis core antigen (anti-HBc); HBeAg may also be present.

Acute HBV infection may be self-limited resulting in production of antibody to HBsAg (anti-HBs) and immunity against reinfection; however, it may also progress to chronic HBV infection (especially in infants or young children, immunocompromised individuals, patients with diabetes). The case fatality rate is 0.5–1.5% among those with acute HBV infection, and the highest fatality rates are in adults older than 60 years of age. Chronic HBV infection develops in 90% or more of infants infected perinatally, 25–50% of children infected at 1–5 years of age, and less than 5% of those infected at 5 years of age or older. Chronic infection is associated with persistent HBV replication in the liver and may result in liver cirrhosis, liver cancer, liver failure, and death. Data from 2006 indicate that approximately 800,000–1.4 million people in the US have chronic HBV infection.

The risk of HBV infection for international travelers generally is low, except for certain travelers in countries with intermediate or high HBV endemicity (i.e., prevalence of HBsAg 2% or greater). The prevalence of chronic HBV infection is low (less than 2%) in the general populations of the US, Canada, Northern and Western Europe, Australia, New Zealand, Mexico, and southern South America. The prevalence of chronic HBV infection is intermediate (2–7%) in South Central and Southwest Asia, Israel, Japan, Eastern and Southern Europe, Russia, and most areas surrounding the Amazon River basin, Honduras, and Guatemala. However, the prevalence of chronic HBV infection is high (8% or more) in all socioeconomic groups in certain areas, including all of Africa; Southeast Asia, including China, Korea, Indonesia, and the Philippines; the Middle East, except Israel; southern and western Pacific islands; the interior Amazon Basin; and certain parts of the Caribbean, such as Haiti and the Dominican Republic. In China, Southeast Asia, most of Africa, most Pacific islands, parts of the Middle East, and the Amazon Basin, most individuals acquire the disease at birth or during childhood, and 8–15% of the population is chronically infected.

■ Primary Immunization

Neonates and Infants Hepatitis B vaccine is used to stimulate active immunity to HBV in neonates and infants. The ACIP, AAP, and AAFP recommend that *all* neonates and infants receive primary immunization against HBV with hepatitis B vaccine regardless of the HBsAg status of the mother. Special efforts should be made to ensure that infants in populations with current or previously high rates of childhood HBV infection (e.g., native Alaskans, Asian-Pacific Islanders, infants who reside in households of first-generation immigrants from Asia, Africa, or other regions with intermediate or high endemic rates of HBV) are completely vaccinated by 6–12 months of age.

Medically stable neonates weighing 2 kg or more at birth should receive the first dose of hepatitis B vaccine at birth, prior to discharge from the hospital; only monovalent hepatitis B vaccine should be used for this dose. On a case-by-case basis and only in rare circumstances, administration of the first dose may be delayed until hospital discharge in neonates weighing 2 kg or more provided the mother is HBsAg-*negative*. If the first dose is not given before hospital discharge to infants born to HBsAg-*negative* mothers, it should be administered no later than 2 months of age.

Neonates born to women who are HBsAg *positive* should receive the first dose of hepatitis B vaccine within 12 hours of birth (in conjunction with passive immunization with HBIG), regardless of gestational age or birthweight, and the second and third doses of vaccine at 1–2 and 6 months, respectively. (See Prevention of Perinatal Hepatitis B Virus Infection, in Uses.)

For neonates born to HBsAg-*negative* women, the first dose optimally should be administered at birth (but may be given at birth to 2 months of age); the second dose optimally should be administered at 1–2 months of age (but may be given at 1–4 months of age or at least 4 weeks after the first dose); and the third dose should be given at 6–18 months of age.

If the mother's HBsAg status is unknown at the time of delivery, the neonate or infant should receive the dosage of hepatitis B vaccine recommended for those born to HBsAg-positive women within 12 hours of birth and the mother should be screened for HBsAg as soon as possible to determine the subsequent management of the infant, including the need to administer HBIG. If it is unlikely that the HBsAg status of the mother can be determined within the first 12 hours, the AAP recommends that preterm neonates weighing less than 2 kg receive a dose of HBIG (in addition to a dose of vaccine) within 12 hours of birth since the vaccine may be less immunogenic in these infants. (See Premature and Low-birthweight Neonates under Primary Immunization: Neonates and Infants, in Uses.) If the mother of a full-term neonate or preterm neonate weighing more than 2 kg at birth is subsequently found to be HBsAg-positive, these infants should receive a dose of HBIG as soon as possible, but within 7 days of birth.

The ACIP and AAP recommend routine serologic screening of *all* pregnant women during an early prenatal visit (e.g., first trimester) to determine their HBsAg status, even if they have previously been tested or received hepatitis B vaccine. Women who are not tested prenatally, those who engage in behaviors that put them at high risk for HBV (e.g., more than one sex partner in the previous 6 months, an HBsAg-positive sex partner, evaluation or treatment for a STD, recent or current injection drug abuse), and those with clinical hepatitis should be tested at the time of admission to the hospital for delivery. Routine serologic testing to confirm the immune response to the vaccine is not necessary in infants born to HBsAg-*negative* women. However, all infants born to HBsAg-*positive* women should undergo serologic testing 9–18 months after completion of the vaccine series (usually at the next well-child visit). (See Uses: Pre-and Postvaccination Serologic Testing.)

Premature and Low-birthweight Neonates. There is some evidence that the seroconversion rate is lower in low-birthweight neonates when the initial dose of hepatitis B vaccine is administered shortly after birth than when it is administered when the neonate is older or weighs more than 2 kg. By 1 month of age, medically stable preterm infants (regardless of initial birthweight or gestational age) have a response to vaccination that is comparable to that of full-term neonates.

The ACIP and AAP recommend that neonates born to HBsAg-positive women receive a dose of hepatitis B vaccine and HBIG as soon as possible after birth (within 12 hours of birth), regardless of gestational age or birthweight. However, for neonates weighing less than 2 kg, this dose should not be counted toward completion of the vaccine series; the usual 3-dose series should be initiated when the infant is 1 month of age.

If the maternal HBsAg status is unknown at birth, preterm infants should receive the first dose of hepatitis B vaccine within 12 hours of birth. The mother's HBsAg status should be determined as quickly as possible and, if positive, HBIG should be administered as soon as possible, but within 7 days of birth. For neonates weighing less than 2 kg, if the mother's HBsAg status cannot be determined within 12 hours of birth, HBIG should be given within 12 hours of birth, and the birth dose of vaccine should not be counted toward completion of the vaccine series.

For premature neonates born to HBsAg-negative women, the AAP recommends that those weighing less than 2 kg at birth receive the first dose of hepatitis B vaccine at 1 month of age. However, those with low birthweight who are medically stable and showing consistent weight gain when discharged from the hospital before 1 month of age may receive the first vaccine dose at the time of discharge.

Children and Adolescents The ACIP, AAP, and AAFP recommend that all previously unvaccinated children and adolescents through 18 years of age receive primary immunization with hepatitis B vaccine.

For most children in the US, the risk of HBV infection is low until adolescence, and immunization before or as these children approach adolescence will provide age-appropriate protection against infection. However, younger children of certain population groups with high rates of childhood HBV infection (e.g., native Alaskans, Asian-Pacific Islanders, children of immigrants from countries in which HBV infection is endemic) are at high risk of infection from person-to-person transmission. Because of the high risk of chronic HBV infection during the first 5 years of life, vaccination of this age group in these populations should be a high priority. Children in institutions for the developmentally disabled also are at high risk of HBV infection and should be vaccinated.

As a strategy to ensure immunization of adolescents, the ACIP, AAP, AAFP, and other clinicians recommend that hepatitis B vaccination be initiated or completed at a routine preadolescent preventive health-care visit at 11–12 years of age. This routine health-care visit provides an opportunity to initiate protection against HBV before the adolescent begins high-risk behaviors and facilitates administration of other vaccines recommended at this age (e.g., measles, mumps, and rubella virus vaccine live (MMR), human papillomavirus [HPV] vaccine, varicella virus vaccine live, meningococcal vaccine).

Hepatitis B vaccine should be administered to *all* children and adolescents 13 through 18 years of age or older (without regard to degree of risk) if they have not previously received the vaccine. The ACIP and AAP state that HBV immunization should be emphasized for adolescents with the major risk factors for acquisition of HBV infection. This includes adolescents who have multiple sexual partners (more than one in 6 months) or STDs; are sexually active homosexual or bisexual males; sexual or regular household contacts of individuals positive for HBsAg; IV drug abusers; employees, volunteers, or trainees in jobs that involve contact with blood or blood-contaminated body fluids; residents of institutions for the developmentally disabled; recipients of clotting factors; or living in areas with increased rates of parenteral drug abuse, teenage pregnancy, and/or STD. Adolescents can be vaccinated against HBV in various settings, including school-based clinics, community health centers, family planning clinics, clinics for the treatment of STDs, and special adolescent clinics.

Internationally Adopted Children and Other Immigrants The number of children adopted from outside the US has increased substantially in recent years and the immune status of such children may be difficult to determine based on country of origin and medical records. To complete an international adoption and bring an infant or a child to the US, prospective parents must fulfill requirements of the Bureau of Citizenship and Immigration Services (BICS), the foreign country in which the infant or child resides, and, possibly, the state of residence of the adoptive parents. Individuals seeking an immigrant visa for permanent US residency must provide proof of age-appropriate vaccination according to the US Recommended Childhood and Adolescent Immunization Schedule or the US Recommended Adult Immunization Schedule (see Immunization Schedules, US 80:00). Although this vaccination requirement applies to all immigrant infants and children entering the US, internationally adopted children younger than 11 years of age are exempt from the overseas vaccination requirements; however, adoptive parents are required to sign a waiver indicating their intention to comply with the vaccination requirements within 30 days after the infant or child arrives in the US.

The fact that immunization schedules of other countries may differ from US schedules (e.g., different recommended vaccines, recommended ages of administration, and/or number and timing of vaccine doses) also should be considered. Vaccines administered outside the US can generally be accepted as valid if the administration schedule was similar to that recommended in the US childhood and adolescent immunization schedule. Only written vaccination records should be considered as evidence of previous vaccination since such records are more likely to accurately predict protection if the vaccines administered, intervals between doses, and child's age at the time of vaccination are similar to US recommendations; however, the extent to which an internationally adopted child's immunization record reflects their protection against disease is unclear and it is possible there may be transcription errors in such records (e.g., single-antigen vaccine may have been administered although a multiple-antigen vaccine was recorded). Although vaccines with inadequate potency have been produced in other countries, most vaccines used worldwide are immunogenic and produced with adequate quality control standards.

When the immune status of an internationally adopted child is uncertain, the ACIP and the AAFP recommend that health-care providers either repeat vaccinations (since this usually is safe and avoids the need to obtain and interpret serologic tests) and/or use selective serologic testing to determine the need for immunizations (helps avoid unnecessary injections). Internationally adopted children should be tested for HBsAg and those found to be HBsAg-positive should be monitored for the development of liver disease. Regardless of vaccination status, individuals born in Asia, Pacific Islands, Africa, or other regions where HBV is highly endemic should be tested for HBsAg. The ACIP states that the age-appropriate hepatitis B vaccine series should be initiated or completed if the child's vaccination history is uncertain or less than 3 vaccine doses were given previously. If a child's prior vaccination record indicates receipt of 3 or more doses of hepatitis B vaccine, additional vaccine doses are not necessary provided at least 1 of the prior doses were administered at 6 months of age or older; however, if the child's vaccination record indicates that the last dose of the hepatitis B vaccine series was given when the child was younger than 6 months of age, the ACIP recommends that an additional vaccine dose should be given when the child is at least 6 months of age. The AAP recommends that serologic testing for HBsAg be performed in *all* internationally adopted children and that the hepatitis B vaccine series should be given if such testing is not available and vaccination history is uncertain.

Adults The ACIP recommends that *all* unvaccinated adults at risk for HBV infection receive primary immunization with hepatitis B vaccine and states that any unvaccinated adult who requests protection from HBV can receive primary immunization with the vaccine.

In settings in which a high proportion of individuals are likely to be at risk for HBV, ACIP recommends *universal* vaccination for all adults who have not completed the vaccine series. Standing orders should be implemented to administer hepatitis B vaccine as part of routine services to all susceptible individuals who visit these settings. This includes facilities that test and treat STDs and human immunodeficiency virus (HIV), drug abuse treatment and prevention facilities, health-care settings targeting services for injection drug abusers, health-care settings targeting men who have sex with men, correctional facilities, end-stage renal disease programs, facilities for chronic hemodialysis patients, and institutions and nonresidential daycare facilities for persons with developmental disabilities. In addition, because not all adults with HBV risk factors visit these settings, ACIP recommends that primary care and specialty medical settings (e.g., physicians' offices, community health centers, family planning clinics, liver disease clinics, travel clinics) also implement standing orders to identify susceptible adults and provide hepatitis B vaccine whenever indicated or requested as part of regular preventive care. (See Uses: Preexposure Vaccination in High-risk Groups.)

Individuals with Altered Immunocompetence Recommendations regarding use of hepatitis B vaccine in individuals with altered immunocompetence generally are the same as those for individuals who are not immunocompromised. Therefore, if indicated, hepatitis B vaccine may be used in HIV-infected individuals; individuals severely immunocompromised because of congenital immunodeficiency, leukemia, lymphoma, generalized malignancy, or therapy with alkylating agents, antimetabolites, radiation, or corticosteroids; individuals with solid organ transplants or receiving chronic immunosuppressive therapy; or those with asplenia, renal failure, diabetes, alcoholism, or alcoholic cirrhosis. However, the immunologic response to the vaccine may be lower in immunocompromised patients, including HIV-infected patients, than in immunocompetent individuals.

HIV-infected Individuals. The ACIP, AAP, CDC, National Institutes of Health (NIH), HIV Medicine Association of the Infectious Diseases Society of America (IDSA), Pediatric Infectious Diseases Society, and others state that recommendations for use of hepatitis B vaccine in HIV-infected individuals are the same as those for individuals who are not HIV-infected. Therefore, all HIV-infected neonates, children, adolescents, and adults should receive hepatitis B vaccine according to the usually recommended childhood and adult immunization schedules.

Some HIV-infected individuals may not have a satisfactory response to hepatitis B vaccine. Lower antibody responses to the vaccine may occur in HIV-infected children, especially older children or those with $CD4^+$ T-cell counts less than 200/mm^3. Following vaccination with hepatitis B vaccine, the seroconversion rate in HIV-infected adults is 18–72% compared with 90% or greater in healthy adults who are not infected with HIV. In addition, mean antibody titers are lower and decline faster in HIV-infected individuals than in those who are not infected with HIV. There is some evidence that doses of hepatitis B vaccine twice the usual dose may result in higher seroconversion rates in HIV-infected individuals with $CD4^+$ T-cell counts greater than 350/mm^3. Administration of an additional vaccine dose in HIV-infected individuals also may result in a higher antibody response or higher seroconversion rate. However, the ACIP, AAP, CDC, NIH, and other experts state that data are insufficient to make recommendations regarding use of higher or additional doses of hepatitis B vaccine in HIV-infected children or adults.

Because there is some evidence that the immunologic response to hepatitis B vaccine may be better in adults with $CD4^+$ T-cell counts greater than 350/mm^3, the ACIP, AAP, CDC, NIH, and others recommend early use of the vaccine in HIV-infected patients before the $CD4^+$ T-cell counts decreases to less than 350/mm^3. However, vaccination should not be deferred until the $CD4^+$ T-cell count increases to greater than 350/mm^3.

Because HIV-infected individuals (especially children with $CD4^+$ T-cell counts less than 200/mm^3 or adults with $CD4^+$ T-cell counts less than 350/mm^3) may have an inadequate response to hepatitis B vaccine, postvaccination serologic testing should be done 1–2 month after the vaccine series is completed to determine whether an adequate anti-HBs response was attained. (See Postvaccination Serologic Testing under Uses: Pre- and Postvaccination Serologic Testing.) If there is no response to the initial vaccine series, revaccination should be considered. Some clinicians might delay revaccination until the patient has had a sustained increase in $CD4^+$ T-cell count in response to antiretroviral therapy.

Although transient increases in HIV RNA concentrations have been reported following use of hepatitis B vaccine in HIV-infected individuals, this does not appear to be clinically important and there is no evidence of accelerated HIV disease progression in vaccinated individuals.

■ **Preexposure Vaccination Against Hepatitis B Virus (HBV) Infection in High-risk Groups** Hepatitis B vaccine is used for preexposure vaccination in previously unvaccinated children, adolescents, or adults at risk of exposure to HBsAg-positive materials (e.g., blood, plasma, serum). The ACIP recommends preexposure vaccination for *all* unvaccinated adults in settings in which a high proportion of individuals are likely to be at risk for HBV infection. This includes health-care personnel, selected patients and patient contacts, populations with high risk of infection, individuals at risk because of their sexual practices, military personnel identified as being at increased risk, and other individuals at risk of exposure (e.g., injection drug abusers).

In settings in which a high proportion of individuals are likely to be at risk for HBV, the ACIP recommends *universal* vaccination for *all* adults who have not completed the vaccine series and suggests standing orders to administer hepatitis vaccine as part of routine services to all susceptible individuals who visit these settings. This includes facilities that test and treat sexually transmitted diseases (STDs) and HIV facilities that provide drug abuse treatment and prevention, health-care facilities targeting services for injection drug abusers or men who have sex with men, and correctional facilities.

Health-care Personnel HBV infection is a major infectious occupational hazard for health-care personnel. Health-care personnel at risk of exposure to blood, blood-contaminated body fluids, other body fluids, and/or needles that might be contaminated with HBsAg are at risk of HBV infection and should be vaccinated against HBV. Among susceptible health-care personnel, the risk for HBV infection after a needlestick injury involving an HBV-positive source is 23–62%. Many HBV infections that occurred before widespread vaccination of health-care personnel probably resulted from unapparent exposures (e.g., inoculation into cutaneous scratches, lesions, or mucosal surfaces). Generally, regardless of institutional experience and institutional differences, individuals (e.g., health-care personnel and public-safety workers) exposed to blood, blood products, body fluids or tissues are at substantial risk of exposure to HBV infection, and the risk of acquiring HBV infection from occupational exposure depends on the frequency of percutaneous or permucosal exposures.

The ACIP and the Hospital Infection Control Practices Advisory Committee (HICPAC) recommend use of hepatitis B vaccine in all health-care personnel who, because of their occupation and work environment, are at risk of exposure to blood, blood-contaminated body fluids, other body fluids, and/or needles that might be contaminated with HBsAg. This includes individuals who provide health-care to patients or work in institutions that provide patient care (e.g., clinicians, nurses, emergency medical personnel, dental professionals and students, medical and nursing students, phlebotomists, medical and laboratory technicians, hospital volunteers, and administrative and support staff in health-care institutions). Hepatitis B vaccine should be administered to health-care personnel, including students, prior to beginning work in a high-risk environment. Because risks for health-care professionals vary during the training and working career of each individual but often are highest during professional training, ACIP and HICPAC recommend that vaccination be completed during training in schools of medicine, dentistry, nursing, laboratory technology, and other allied health professions before exposure to a high-risk environment.

Prevaccination serologic screening for previous infection is not indicated for individuals being vaccinated because of occupational risk, unless the health-care facility considers such screening cost-effective. However, ACIP and HICPAC recommend postvaccination testing to confirm an anti-HBs response in health-care personnel who have blood or patient contact and are at ongoing risk for percutaneous or mucosal exposure to blood or body fluids (e.g., physicians or physician assistants, nurses or nurse practitioners, dentists or dental hygienists, phlebotomists, emergency medical technicians, first responders, laboratory technologists or technicians, acupuncturists, and students of these professions). Most experts recommend postvaccination testing to document a response 1–2 months after completion of the primary vaccine series and consider additional periodic testing and booster vaccination of health-care workers unnecessary in those who responded to the primary series.

Recipients of Blood Products and Plasma-derived Preparations Because blood products (e.g., whole blood, packed red blood cells, plasma) and plasma-derived preparations (e.g., albumin human, antihemophilic factor [human], anti-inhibitor coagulant complex, factor IX [human], factor IX complex) are potential vehicles for transmission of human viruses, including HBV, the manufacturers, the ACIP, and the National Hemophilia Foundation's Medical and Scientific Advisory Council (MASAC) recommend that all seronegative individuals who receive frequent and/or large volume transfusions of blood, blood products, or plasma-derived preparations (e.g., individuals with hemophilia or thalassemia) be vaccinated with hepatitis B vaccine. The risk for transmission of recognized blood-borne viruses in blood and plasma-derived preparations is considered to be low because donors are screened for HBV. In addition, most commercially available plasma-derived preparations undergo heat-treatment, filtration, and/or chemical (solvent/detergent) procedures to reduce viral infectious potential. Studies using plasma-derived coagulation factor preparations indicate that improved donor screening practices and viral inactivation procedures have resulted in plasma-derived preparations with greatly reduced risk for transmission of HBV. However, the possibility of transmission of HBV with available viral-inactivated, plasma-derived products still remains. For further information on precautions related to transmissible agents in plasma-derived preparations, see Risk of Transmissible Agents in Plasma-derived Preparations under Cautions: Precautions and Contraindications, in Antihemophilic Factor (Human) 20:12.16.

MASAC considers immunization against HBV essential for all seronegative patients with hemophilia or other congenital bleeding disorders. If immunization against HBV was not initiated at birth, it should be initiated at the time of diagnosis of hemophilia or other congenital bleeding disorder. Although *postvaccination* serologic testing to confirm immunity is not usually indicated after routine vaccination of infants, children, or adolescents, MASAC recommends that such testing be performed following completion of the hepatitis B vaccine series (see Uses: Pre- and Postvaccination Serologic Testing) in individuals with hemophilia and that nonresponders receive 1 or more additional doses of the vaccine. MASAC states that subsequent booster doses or additional serologic testing to assess antibody levels is not necessary in immunocompetent children and adults.

Certain Patients and Patient Contacts Patients and staff of hemodialysis, organ transplant, or oncology wards are at high risk of exposure to HBsAg-positive material and should be vaccinated against HBV. Although a decrease in the rate of HBV infection in hemodialysis wards can occur with environmental control measures alone (e.g., serologic screening of staff and patients, segregation of carriers, environmental hygiene), the manufacturers and the ACIP recommend use of hepatitis B vaccine in these individuals. While seroconversion rates and anti-HBs titers induced are lower in patients undergoing hemodialysis than in healthy individuals, for those patients who do respond, vaccination will provide protection against HBV infection and reduce the need for frequent serologic screening. In addition, the ACIP recommends that potential candidates for hepatitis B vaccination be identified as early as possible in the course of their renal disease since there is some evidence that higher seroconversion rates and antibody titers can be achieved in uremic patients when they are vaccinated before requiring dialysis.

Residents and staff of institutions for the developmentally disabled, including those in small (group) residential settings, are at high risk of exposure to HBsAg-positive material and should be vaccinated. Risk of exposure to HBsAg-positive material in these institutions is associated not only with exposure to blood or blood products, but commonly results from bites or contact with open skin lesions (e.g., those due to impetigo, scabies, or scratched insect bites), saliva, or other infective secretions or excretions. Therefore, the manufacturers and ACIP recommend use of hepatitis B vaccine in susceptible residents and staff of institutions for the developmentally disabled. Residents and staff who live or work in smaller (group) residential settings with known HBsAg carriers also should be vaccinated. In addition, residents discharged from residential institutions into community settings should be screened for HBsAg so that appropriate measures can be taken to prevent transmission in the community; such measures include both environmental controls and appropriate vaccination.

Classroom contacts (principally teachers but also classmates) of aggressive, deinstitutionalized developmentally disabled individuals are at high risk of exposure to HBsAg-positive material. Use of hepatitis B vaccine in classroom contacts of these individuals may be necessary. Vaccination of classroom contacts of a HBsAg carrier is strongly encouraged when the carrier is aggressive or has special medical problems that increase the risk of exposure to their blood or serous secretions. In addition, staff of nonresidential day-care programs (e.g., schools, sheltered workshops for the developmentally disabled) attended by known HBsAg carriers have a risk of infection comparable to that among health-care personnel and therefore should be vaccinated. Vaccination of other enrollees in such day-care programs also should be considered.

Spouses and nonsexual household and sexual contacts of HBsAg carriers are at high risk of exposure to HBsAg-positive material; however, sexual contacts appear to be at the greatest risk of exposure to HBV infection or virus. When carriers are identified through routine screening of donated blood, diagnostic testing in hospitals, prenatal screening, screening of refugees from certain areas, or other screening programs, they should be notified of their HBsAg status. Although some unvaccinated spouses and nonsexual household and sexual contacts of HBsAg carriers may develop immunity against HBV infection during continuous, long-term exposure, all such contacts be tested and those who are susceptible should receive hepatitis B vaccine.

Prisoners Prisoners may be at high risk of exposure to HBV and should be vaccinated against HBV. In addition, initiation of vaccination programs in prisoners provides an opportunity to potentially affect transmission of HBV in the parenteral drug abuser population.

Populations with High Endemicity of Infection Individuals of certain US population groups (e.g., native Alaskans, Pacific Islanders, refugees from HBV-endemic areas) have high rates of infection with HBV (high endemicity) and should be vaccinated against HBV. Initiation of the hepatitis B vaccine series at birth and completion of the series by 6–12 months of age is particularly important in these population groups since transmission occurs principally during childhood in such populations. In addition, more extensive vaccination programs of other pediatric age-groups in these populations should be considered if resources are available, so that reductions in transmission can be achieved more rapidly.

Prevaccination serologic testing is recommended for all foreign-born individuals (e.g., immigrants, refugees, asylum seekers, internationally adopted children) born in areas with high endemicity of HBV (e.g., Africa, Asia, the Pacific Islands). All susceptible household contacts of HBsAg carriers identified by such screening should be vaccinated. Because of the high rate of interfamily transmission among children in these populations, vaccination also is indicated for all susceptible children and adolescents who have at least one parent who was born in a highly endemic area.

Individuals at Risk of Exposure Because of Their Sexual Practices Individuals at high risk of HBV because of their sexual practices include men who have sex with men, individuals with more than 1 sexual partner in the previous 6 months, sexual partners of HBsAg-positive individuals, female prostitutes, and individuals seeking evaluation or treatment for a STD. All such individuals should be vaccinated against HBV. Hepatitis B vaccine is recommended in all susceptible adolescent and adult men who have sex with men (homosexual, bisexual), regardless of their age or duration of such sexual practices. Because of the prevalence of HBV infection in this population, serologic screening prior to vaccination may be cost effective, depending on the relative costs of laboratory testing and vaccine.

Military Personnel at Increased Risk of Exposure Military personnel identified as being at increased risk of exposure to HBV should be vaccinated with hepatitis B vaccine. (See Individuals Wounded in Mass Casualty Settings under Uses: Postexposure Prophylaxis.)

Travelers Travelers to areas with levels of endemic HBV that are intermediate (2–7%) or high (8% or greater) are at risk of exposure to the disease. The ACIP, CDC, and others state that hepatitis B vaccine is indicated for previously unvaccinated travelers (neonates, infants, adolescents, adults) who are traveling to areas where the prevalence of chronic HBV infection is intermediate or high. (See Uses: Risks of Exposure and Infection.) This includes individuals who anticipate sexual contact with the local population, those who will live in rural areas and/or have daily physical contact with the local population, and those who are likely to seek medical, dental, or other treatment at local facilities during their stay in these areas. Individuals, including infants and young children, who will stay for 6 months or longer in areas highly endemic for HBV infection may be at risk of direct exposure to blood from the local population because of continuous close contact with local inhabitants who have open skin lesions (impetigo, scabies, scratched insect bites), exposure to unsterilized needles (or other medical or dental equipment) in local health facilities or tattoo parlors, or receipt of blood transfusions not screened for HBsAg. In addition, travelers should be advised not to use IV drugs, share needles for any purpose, or receive medications from multidose vials that may have been contaminated by used needles. Previously unvaccinated health-care workers who plan to work in health-care fields (e.g., medical, dental, laboratory) for any duration in areas with intermediate or high levels of endemic HBV are strongly advised to receive hepatitis B vaccine prior to travel.

Ideally, vaccination should begin 6 months prior to travel in order to complete the full primary series of 3 doses. Although optimal protection is conferred by the complete 3-dose vaccine series, a partial series will offer some protection against HBV infection and the vaccine series should be initiated even if it cannot be completed before travel. Alternatively, the CDC suggests that travelers who will depart before the usual primary 3-dose series can be completed may receive an optional accelerated schedule† (doses given at 0, 7, and 21 days and a booster dose at least 1 year after the start of the series). (See Dosage and Administration: Dosage.)

Other Individuals at Risk of Exposure Morticians and embalmers are at high risk of exposure to HBsAg-positive material, and the manufacturers recommend use of hepatitis B vaccine in these individuals.

Public-safety personnel (e.g., police, fire department personnel) also may be at risk for occupational exposure to HBV, depending on the tasks performed; if contact with blood or blood-contaminated body fluids is involved, such personnel should be vaccinated.

Individuals with chronic hepatitis C virus (HCV) infection may be at increased risk for HBV exposure and should receive hepatitis B vaccine. However, the optimal vaccination regimen for this group has not been determined since individuals with chronic HCV infection may have a reduced response to hepatitis B vaccine. (See Individuals with Hepatitis C Virus Infection under Pharmacology: Response to Hepatitis B Vaccine [Recombinant].)

Individuals addicted to parenterally administered drugs are at high risk of exposure to HBsAg-positive material. Hepatitis B vaccine should be used in these individuals as soon as possible after their drug use is identified.

Individuals in casual contact with HBsAg carriers in settings such as schools, offices, and business environments are at minimal risk of exposure to HBV infection or virus; therefore, the ACIP does not recommend routine use of hepatitis B vaccine in these individuals. At child-care centers (other than those for the developmentally disabled), HBV transmission between children or between children and staff has rarely been documented. Unless special circumstances (e.g., behavior problems such as biting or scratching, medical conditions such as severe skin disease) that might facilitate transmission exist, the ACIP states that vaccination of contacts of carriers in child care is not necessary.

■ Prevention of Perinatal Hepatitis B Virus (HBV) Infection

A regimen that includes *active* immunization with hepatitis B vaccine and *passive* immunization with HBIG is used to prevent perinatal HBV infection in neonates born to HBsAg-*positive* women. This regimen is 85–95% effective in preventing acute and chronic HBV infection in infants born to women positive for both HBsAg and HBeAg.

The ACIP and AAP recommend routine serologic screening of *all* pregnant women during an early prenatal visit (e.g., first trimester) to determine their HBsAg status, even if they were tested previously or have already been vaccinated against HBV. (See Neonates and Infants under Uses: Primary Immunization.)

To prevent perinatal HBV infection, the ACIP and AAP recommend that *all* neonates born to HBsAg-*positive* women receive a dose of hepatitis B vaccine and a dose of HBIG as soon as possible after birth (within 12 hours of birth), regardless of gestational age or birthweight, followed by a second and third dose of hepatitis B vaccine given at 1–2 and 6 months, respectively.

If maternal HBsAg status is unknown at birth, the neonate should receive the first dose of hepatitis B vaccine (within 12 hours of birth) and the mother's HBsAg status should be determined as quickly as possible and, if positive, the infant should receive a dose of HBIG as soon as possible (no later than 7 days of age). (See Neonates and Infants under Uses: Primary Immunization.)

■ Postexposure Prophylaxis of Hepatitis B Virus (HBV) Infection

Hepatitis B vaccine is used for postexposure prophylaxis in certain individuals exposed to HBV or HBsAg-positive materials (e.g., health-care personnel, sexual assault victims, sexual or intimate contacts of HBsAg-positive individuals). Depending on the exposure circumstances, the postexposure prophylaxis regimen may include combined *active* immunization with the vaccine and *passive* immunization with HBIG. Active immunization with hepatitis B vaccine in conjunction with passive HBIG immunization can provide both short- and long-term protection. Recommendations concerning postexposure prophylaxis are based on available efficacy data and on the likelihood of future exposure to HBV in the individual requiring postexposure therapy. For further information on the use of hepatitis B vaccine in conjunction with HBIG for postexposure prophylaxis (see Uses: Postexposure Prophylaxis of Hepatitis B Virus [HBV] Infection, in Hepatitis B Immune Globulin 80:04).

Postexposure prophylaxis is *not* necessary in individuals who previously received primary immunization with hepatitis B vaccine and have serologic evidence of adequate levels of anti-HBs (10 mIU/mL or greater). In addition, postexposure prophylaxis is *not* necessary in individuals previously infected with HBV; such individuals are immune to reinfection.

The major determinant of postexposure prophylaxis effectiveness is early administration of the initial dose of hepatitis B vaccine or HBIG; postexposure prophylaxis is less effective depending on how long it has been since the exposure. Studies are limited regarding the maximum interval after exposure during which postexposure prophylaxis is effective, but postexposure prophylaxis is unlikely to be effective if initiated 7 days or longer after percutaneous (e.g., needlestick) exposures.

Health-care Personnel Following Occupational Exposure Hepatitis B vaccine is used in susceptible, unvaccinated health-care personnel following occupational exposures to blood and other body fluids that might contain HBV. All health-care personnel at risk of exposure to blood, blood-contaminated body fluids, other body fluids, and/or needles that might be contaminated with HBsAg should receive preexposure vaccination against HBV infection. (See Health-care Personnel under Uses: Preexposure Vaccination in High-risk Groups.) In addition, vaccination may be indicated as part of postexposure prophylaxis in individuals who have not previously received the vaccine or in individuals who have an inadequate or unknown antibody response to the vaccine. (See Table 1.) When both HBIG and hepatitis B vaccine are required for postexposure prophylaxis, they can be given simultaneously at separate sites.

If an occupational exposure to HBV occurs, the vaccination status and vaccine-response status (if known) of the exposed individual and the HBsAg status of the source should be reviewed. If the exposed individual was not previously vaccinated, the hepatitis B vaccine series should be initiated as soon as possible (preferably within 24 hours). In addition, if the source is found to be HBsAg-positive, a single dose of HBIG should be given as soon as possible (preferably within 24 hours); HBIG is unnecessary if the source is found to be HBsAg-negative or the source is unknown or not available for testing.

If the exposed individual was previously vaccinated and is a known responder (serum anti-HBs 10 mIU/mL or greater), no postexposure prophylaxis is necessary.

If the exposed individual was previously vaccinated but is a known nonresponder (serum anti-HBs less than 10 mIU/mL), no postexposure prophylaxis is necessary if the source is HBsAg-negative. However, if the source is HBsAg-positive or the source is known to be high-risk for HBV, a single dose of HBIG should be given and a second hepatitis B vaccine series should be reinitiated with the first vaccine dose given as soon as possible after exposure. A 2-dose regimen of HBIG (without the vaccine) is preferred in individuals who already previously failed to respond to a second vaccine series.

If the immune status of the exposed individual is unknown, they should be tested for anti-HBs prior to initiation of postexposure prophylaxis. If the exposed individual is found to be a responder, no treatment is necessary. If they are found to be a nonresponder (serum anti-HBs less than 10 mIU/mL) and the source is HBsAg-positive, a single dose of HBIG and a booster dose of hepatitis B vaccine should be administered. If they are found to be a nonresponder and the source is unknown or not available for testing, a booster dose of hepatitis B vaccine should be given and the antibody titer rechecked in 1–2 months.

Table 1. Postexposure Prophylaxis of HBV following Occupational (Percutaneous or Mucosal) Exposure to Blood

	Treatment when Source Is:		
Vaccination and Antibody Status of Exposed Individual	**HBsAg-positive**	**HBsAg-negative**	**Source Unknown or Not Available for Testing**
Unvaccinated	Single HBIG dose (within 24 hours) and initiate hepatitis B vaccine series (within 24 hours)	Initiate hepatitis B vaccine series	Initiate hepatitis B vaccine series
Previously vaccinated			
Known responder (anti-HBs 10 mIU/mL or greater)	No treatment	No treatment	No treatment
Known nonresponder (anti-HBs less than 10 mIU/mL)	Single HBIG dose and initiate hepatitis B revaccination series or 2 HBIG doses (first dose as soon as possible; second dose 1 month later)	No treatment	If known high-risk source, *treat as if source were HBsAg-positive*
Antibody response unknown	Test exposed individual for anti-HBs 1. If inadequate, single dose of HBIG and a booster dose of hepatitis B vaccine 2. If adequate, no treatment	No treatment	Test exposed individual for anti-HBs 1. If inadequate, give a booster dose of hepatitis B vaccine and recheck titer in 1–2 months 2. If adequate, no treatment

Sexual Assault Victims The CDC and ACIP recommend postexposure vaccination with hepatitis B vaccine in susceptible adult, adolescent, and child victims of sexual assault. Trichomoniasis, genital chlamydial infection, gonorrhea, and bacterial vaginosis are the STDs most commonly diagnosed in women following sexual assault, and many experts recommend routine empiric anti-infective prophylaxis (i.e., a 3-drug regimen of IM ceftriaxone, oral metronidazole, and either oral azithromycin or oral doxycycline) in adult and adolescent victims of sexual assault. In addition, postexposure hepatitis B vaccination (without HBIG) is recommended. Unless the offender is HBsAg-positive, HBIG is not required. Individuals who have previously received the complete vaccine series are fully protected and do not need further doses of hepatitis B vaccine after a sexual assault; those who have received some, but not all, doses of the vaccine series should receive the remaining required doses as scheduled. If the victim is unvaccinated or incompletely vaccinated and the perpetrator is HBsAg-positive, a single dose of HBIG should be given within 14 days of the assault (preferably within 24 hours) and the hepatitis B vaccine series should be initiated or completed. For further information on anti-infective prophylaxis in sexual assault victims, see Uses: Prophylaxis in Sexual Assault Victims, in Ceftriaxone 8:12.06.12.

Contacts of Individuals with Acute HBV Infection The ACIP and CDC recommend that previously unvaccinated sexual partners of individuals with acute HBV infection receive postexposure prophylaxis with both HBIG and hepatitis B vaccine as soon as possible, preferably within less than 24 hours. Studies are limited on the maximum interval after exposure during which postexposure prophylaxis is effective, but the interval is unlikely to exceed 14 days for sexual exposures. Completion of the hepatitis B vaccine series confers long-term protection in case the individual with acute HBV infection becomes chronically infected. Prevaccination serologic testing (anti-HBc) of sexual partners can be considered as long as it does not delay postexposure vaccination beyond 14 days.

The AAP recommends that postexposure prophylaxis in children follow the ACIP guidelines for adults. In addition, because infants have a high risk of becoming chronic HBV carriers following acute infection, unvaccinated infants younger than 12 months of age who have close contact with a primary caregiver or family member with acute HBV infection should receive combined passive immunization with HBIG and active immunization with hepatitis B vaccine. If the infant has previously received a single dose of hepatitis B vaccine, the second vaccine dose should be administered if the interval is appropriate or, if it is too early to give a vaccine dose, the infant should receive a dose of HBIG. HBIG is not required if, at the time of exposure, the infant has already received at least 2 doses of hepatitis B vaccine.

Other nonsexual household contacts of individuals with acute HBV infection are not at increased risk for infection unless they have other risk factors or are exposed to the blood of the infected patient (e.g., by sharing a toothbrush or razor). However, all household contacts of patients with acute HBV infection should be encouraged to complete primary immunization with hepatitis B vaccine. If the patient with acute HBV infection becomes chronically infected (i.e., remains HBsAg-positive after 6 months), all household contacts should be vaccinated with hepatitis B vaccine.

Contacts of Individuals with Chronic HBV Infection Sexual or needle-sharing partners and nonsexual household contacts of individuals with chronic HBV infection are at risk for HBV infection through percutaneous or mucosal exposures to blood or infectious body fluids (e.g., sharing a toothbrush or razor, contact with exudates from dermatologic lesions, contact with HBsAg-contaminated surfaces). The ACIP states that postexposure vaccination with hepatitis B vaccine is recommended for such individuals. A dose of HBIG also may be indicated if the most recent sexual exposure to an HBsAg-positive individual occurred within the last 14 days.

Although efficacy of postexposure vaccination has not been evaluated for contacts of chronic HBV patients, such vaccination is expected to provide protection based on efficacy demonstrated in perinatal postexposure prophylaxis. The ACIP state that postvaccination serologic testing (anti-HBs) should be considered in sexual contacts of individuals with chronic HBV infection. Although most are expected to respond to vaccination, nonresponders should receive a second complete vaccine series. Those who do not respond to a second vaccine series should be counseled about abstinence and use of other methods to protect themselves from HBV via sexual transmission.

Individuals Wounded in Mass Casualty Settings Postexposure vaccination with hepatitis B vaccine (without HBIG) may be indicated after bombings or other mass casualty situations because of the high concentration of HBV in the blood of infected individuals, the durability of HBV in the environment, and the efficacy and relative ease of administration of the vaccine.

In a mass casualty setting, the CDC states that use of hepatitis B vaccine generally is warranted in individuals who are unvaccinated or have an uncertain vaccination history if they have wounds (penetrating injuries), nonintact skin, or mucous membranes that may have been exposed to blood or body fluids from other individuals. In these situations, failure to provide hepatitis B vaccination could result in preventable illness, whereas unnecessary vaccination is unlikely to cause harm. If postexposure vaccination with hepatitis B vaccine is indicated in a mass casualty setting, a vaccine dose should be given as soon as possible (preferably within 24 hours) and not later than 7 days after the event, unless contraindicated. The age-appropriate vaccine series should then be completed at the time of discharge or during follow-up health-care visits. If the vaccine is in short supply, the fact that children younger than 17 years of age and health-care personnel are more likely to have previously received the vaccine than other individuals should be considered.

Responders and other personnel in mass casualty settings should be managed using HBV postexposure prophylaxis regimens recommended for occupational exposures to HBV. (See Table 1.)

■ **Pre- and Postvaccination Serologic Testing** ***Prevaccination Serologic Testing*** Prevaccination testing for serologic markers of HBV infection are not usually necessary for individuals in populations with low prevalence of HBV serologic markers, including infants, children, or adolescents receiving routine vaccination or health-care personnel undergoing vaccination during their training years. However, prevaccination serologic testing is recommended for all foreign-born individuals (e.g., immigrants, refugees, asylum seekers, internationally adopted children) born in Africa, Asia, the Pacific Islands, or other regions with high HBV endemicity (i.e., prevalence of HBsAg 8% or greater). In addition, prevaccination serologic screening is recommended for individuals in risk groups with high rates of HBV infection, including HIV-infected individuals, injection drug abusers, incarcerated individuals, men who have sex with men, individuals born in countries with intermediate HBV endemicity (i.e., prevalence of HBsAg 2–7%), and household, sexual, and needle-sharing contacts of HBsAg-positive individuals.

A decision to use prevaccination serologic testing to determine whether an individual was previously infected with HBV generally is based on whether such testing is less costly than unnecessarily vaccinating an individual who already is immune. For routine testing, a single test (anti-hepatitis core antigen; anti-HBc) or a panel of tests (HBsAg and anti-HBs) should be used. Anti-HBc identifies individuals with previous HBV infection, including those with chronic HBV infection. Individuals who are anti-HBc-negative are susceptible and should be vaccinated against HBV. In addition, anti-HBc-positive individuals should be tested for HBsAg.

Postvaccination Serologic Testing Postvaccination serologic testing to confirm an adequate anti-HBs response following the hepatitis B vaccine series is not necessary in most individuals because of the high rate of immunologic response among children, adolescents, and adults. However, postvaccination serologic testing is recommended in health-care personnel who have blood or patient contact and are at ongoing risk for percutaneous or mucosal exposure to blood or body fluids (e.g., physicians or physician assistants, nurses or nurse practitioners, dentists or dental hygienists, phlebotomists, emergency medical technicians, first responders, laboratory technologists or technicians, acupuncturists, and students of these professions). Postvaccination serologic testing also is recommended in infants born to HBsAg-*positive* women, chronic hemodialysis patients, HIV-infected individuals or other immunocompromised individuals, individuals with hemophilia, and sexual or needle-sharing partners of HBsAg-positive individuals.

All infants born to HBsAg-*positive* women should undergo serologic testing at 9–18 months of age (usually at the next well-child visit) to document whether the combined regimen of active immunization with hepatitis B vaccine and passive immunization with HBIG prevented perinatal HBV infection. Infants should not be tested before 9 months of age to avoid detecting anti-HBs passively acquired from the HBIG dose administered at birth and to maximize the likelihood of detecting late HBV infections. Serologic testing is *not* necessary in infants born to HBsAg-*negative* women.

When postvaccination serologic testing is indicated in adults, adolescents, and children (not neonates), including HIV-infected individuals, it usually is done 1–2 months after completion of the hepatitis B vaccine series. Individuals who received a combined regimen of *active* immunization with hepatitis B vaccine and *passive* immunization with HBIG may have passively acquired anti-HBs present in serum for several months and this may interfere with postvaccination serologic tests that measure anti-HBs.

A repeat hepatitis B vaccine series should be given to individuals who had an inadequate response to the initial vaccine series (i.e., anti-HBs less than 10 mIU/mL). Those who do not respond to the second series (i.e., total of 6 doses) are unlikely to respond to additional vaccine doses.

Dosage and Administration

■ **Administration** Monovalent hepatitis B vaccine (recombinant) (Engerix-B®, Recombivax HB®) usually is administered by IM injection. Hepatitis B vaccine may be administered by subcutaneous injection, but only when necessary in individuals at risk of hemorrhage following IM injections (e.g., patients with thrombocytopenia or a bleeding disorder such as hemophilia). (See Individuals with Bleeding Disorders under Cautions: Precautions and Contraindications.) The vaccine should *not* be administered IV or intradermally; there is evidence that intradermal administration may be associated with reduced immunogenicity.

The fixed-combination vaccine containing *Haemophilus influenzae* type b (Hib) and hepatitis B antigens (Hib-HepB; Comvax®), the fixed-combination vaccine containing hepatitis A and hepatitis B antigens (HepA-HepB; Twinrix®), and the fixed-combination vaccine containing diphtheria, tetanus, pertussis, hepatitis B, and poliovirus antigens (DTaP-HepB-IPV; Pediarix®) are administered by IM injection. These fixed-combination vaccines should *not* be given IV, intradermally, or subcutaneously.

Prior to administration, the vaccine should be inspected visually for particulate matter and discoloration. The vaccine should be shaken well immediately prior to administration and should not be used if it contains particulates, appears discolored, or cannot be resuspended with thorough agitation.

Monovalent hepatitis B vaccine or fixed-combination vaccines containing hepatitis B vaccine should *not* be diluted and should *not* be mixed with any other vaccine or solution.

Depending on the age of the patient, the IM injection should be made into the deltoid or anterolateral thigh. To ensure delivery of vaccine into the muscle, IM injections should be made at a 90° angle to the skin using a needle size that is appropriate for the individual's age and body mass, the thickness of adipose tissue and muscle at the injection site, and the injection technique.

In neonates and young children (up to 12 months of age), IM injections should be made into the anterolateral thigh. For children 1–2 years of age, IM injections should preferably be administered into the anterolateral thigh; the deltoid muscle is an alternative if the muscle mass is adequate. For adults, adolescents, and children 3 years of age or older, the deltoid is preferred, although the anterolateral thigh is an alternative.

Generally, muscles of the buttock should not be used for administration of vaccines in children because of the well-documented potential for injection-associated injury to the sciatic nerve. In addition, studies in adults indicate that the seroconversion rate may be lower when the vaccine is given into the buttocks rather than the deltoid. The vaccine should *not* be injected into or near blood vessels.

Although some experts state that aspiration (i.e., pulling back on the syringe plunger after needle insertion and before injection) can be performed to ensure that a blood vessel has not been entered, the US Public Health Service Advisory Committee on Immunization Practices (ACIP) and American Academy of Pediatrics (AAP) state that this procedure is not required because large blood vessels are not present at the recommended IM injection sites.

Since syncope may occur following vaccination, vaccinees should be observed for approximately 15 minutes after the vaccine dose is administered. If syncope occurs, the patient should be observed until symptoms resolve. Syncope after vaccination occurs most frequently in adolescents and young adults.

Monovalent hepatitis B vaccine (Engerix-B®, Recombivax HB®) may be given simultaneously with hepatitis B immune globulin (HBIG) (using different syringes and different injection sites) when *passive* immunization is considered necessary in addition to *active* immunization with the vaccine (e.g., in neonates born to hepatitis B surface antigen-positive [HBsAg-positive] women, postexposure prophylaxis in certain individuals exposed to hepatitis B virus (HBV) or HBsAg-positive materials). Hepatitis B vaccine and HBIG should *not* be given in the same syringe and should *not* be injected at the same site.

Hepatitis B vaccine may be given simultaneously with other age-appropriate vaccines during the same health-care visit (using different syringes and different injection sites). (See Drug Interactions: Vaccines.)

When multiple vaccines are administered during a single visit, administration of each preparation at a different anatomic site is preferred. In younger children, the thigh is the preferred injection site when more than 2 vaccines must be administered into a single limb. Injection sites should be separated by at least 1 inch (if anatomically feasible) to allow appropriate attribution of any local adverse effects that may occur. The deltoid may be used in older children and adults when more than one vaccine must be administered.

■ Dosage

Dosage recommendations for hepatitis B vaccine vary depending on the specific preparation used, the recipient's age, the HBsAg status of the mother (for neonates), and the presence of underlying disease.

Because the recommended doses for Recombivax HB® and Engerix-B® are different, dosage recommendations for the specific preparation used should be followed.

Monovalent hepatitis B vaccines (Engerix-B®, Recombivax HB®) generally are considered interchangeable; therefore, if the hepatitis B vaccine series is started with one monovalent vaccine, it may be completed using a different vaccine given in the dosage recommended for that specific preparation.

Only monovalent hepatitis B vaccine (Engerix-B®, Recombivax HB®) should be used for the initial (birth) dose in neonates or infants younger than 6 weeks of age. However, the vaccine series can be completed using either a monovalent hepatitis B vaccine or an age-appropriate fixed-combination vaccine containing hepatitis B vaccine.

The complete hepatitis B vaccine series must be administered to ensure optimal protection. Interruptions resulting in an interval between doses longer than recommended should not interfere with the final immunity achieved. In addition, it is not necessary to give additional doses or start the vaccination series over.

If the hepatitis B vaccination series is interrupted after the initial dose, the second dose should be given as soon as possible (minimum interval between first and second dose is 4 weeks) and the third dose should be given at least 8 weeks after the second dose (minimum interval between first and third dose is 16 weeks). If only the third dose is delayed, it should be administered as soon as possible. Infants should receive the final dose at 24 weeks of age or older.

Hepatitis B Vaccine (Engerix-B®)

Neonates and Infants. When Engerix-B® is used in neonates and infants, primary immunization consists of 3 doses of the pediatric/adolescent formulation containing 10 mcg/0.5 mL.

The manufacturer of Engerix-B® recommends that 10-mcg doses be given at 0, 1, and 6 months of age. Alternatively, the manufacturer states that a 4-dose regimen consisting of 10-mcg doses given at 0, 1, 2, and 12 months can be used.

The US Public Health Service Advisory Committee on Immunization Practices (ACIP), American Academy of Pediatrics (AAP), and American Academy of Family Physicians (AAFP) recommend that full-term neonates born to HBsAg-*positive* women or women with unknown HBsAg status receive the initial 10-mcg dose of Engerix-B® as soon as possible after birth (within 12 hours of birth) and the second and third 10-mcg doses at 1–2 and 6 months of age, respectively. The third dose should be given no earlier than 24 weeks of age. If the mother is known or found to be HBsAg-positive, the neonate also should receive a dose of HBIG as soon as possible after birth (within 12 hours of birth). (See Neonates and Infants under Uses: Primary Immunization.)

The ACIP, AAP, and AAFP recommend that full-term neonates born to HBsAg-*negative* women receive the initial 10-mcg dose of Engerix-B® at birth (before hospital discharge) and the second and third 10-mcg doses at 1–2 and 6–18 months of age, respectively. If the vaccine is not given before hospital discharge, the initial dose should be given no later than 2 months of age. The third dose should be given no earlier than 24 weeks of age.

Preterm neonates weighing less than 2 kg born to HBsAg-*positive* women or women with unknown HBsAg status should receive a dose of hepatitis B vaccine and a dose of HBIG as soon as possible after birth (within 12 hours of birth). This birth dose of hepatitis B vaccine should not be counted toward completion of the vaccine series; the usual 3-dose vaccine series should be initiated when the infant is 1 month of age.

Preterm neonates weighing less than 2 kg born to HBsAg-*negative* women should be given the initial dose of hepatitis B vaccine at 1 month of age; however, the initial dose may be given at the time of hospital discharge (before 1 month of age) if the infant is medically stable and showing consistent weight gain. After the initial dose, the second and third doses of hepatitis B vaccine should be given at 1–2 and 6–18 months, respectively.

Children 10 Years of Age or Younger. When Engerix-B® is used in children 10 years of age or younger, primary immunization (including catch-up vaccination) usually consists of 3 doses of the pediatric/adolescent formulation containing 10 mcg/0.5 mL.

The initial dose of 10 mcg should be given on a selected date and the second and third 10-mcg doses should be given at 1 and 6 months, respectively, after the initial dose. Alternatively, the manufacturer states that children 5–10 years of age can receive a 3-dose regimen consisting of 10-mcg doses given on a selected date and at 12 and 24 months after the initial dose or children 10 years of age or younger can receive a 4-dose regimen consisting of 10-mcg doses given on a selected dated and at 1, 2, and 12 months after the initial dose.

Adolescents 11–19 Years of Age. When Engerix-B® is used in adolescents 11–19 years of age, primary immunization (including catch-up vaccination) usually consists of 3 doses of either the pediatric/adolescent formulation containing 10 mcg/0.5 mL or the adult formulation containing 20 mcg/mL.

If the pediatric/adolescent formulation is used, the initial dose of 10 mcg should be given on a selected date and the second and third 10-mcg doses should be given at 1 and 6 months, respectively, after the initial dose. Alternatively, in those 11–16 years of age, the manufacturer states that 10-mcg doses can be given on a selected date and at 12 and 24 months after the initial dose.

If the adult formulation is used, the initial dose of 20 mcg should be given on a selected date and the second and third 20-mcg doses should be given at 1 and 6 months, respectively, after the initial dose. Alternatively, the manufacturer states that adolescents 11–19 years of age can receive a 4-dose regimen consisting of 20-mcg doses given on a selected date and at 1, 2, and 12 months after the initial dose.

Adults 20 Years of Age or Older. When Engerix-B® is used in adults 20 years of age or older, primary immunization consists of 3 doses of the adult formulation containing 20 mcg/mL.

The initial dose of 20 mcg should be given on a selected date and the second and third 20-mcg doses should be given at 1–2 and 4–6 months, respectively, after the initial dose. Alternatively, a 4-dose regimen can be used consisting of 20-mcg doses given on a selected date and at 1, 2, and 12 months after the initial dose.

Adults Undergoing Hemodialysis. When Engerix-B® is used in adult hemodialysis patients, primary immunization consists of four 40-mcg doses using the adult formulation containing 20 mcg/mL. Each 40-mcg dose may be given using 1 or 2 injections.

An initial 40-mcg dose should be given on a selected date followed by additional 40-mcg doses at 1, 2, and 6 months after the initial dose.

Hepatitis B Vaccine (Recombivax HB®)

Neonates and Infants. When Recombivax HB® is used in neonates and infants, primary immunization consists of 3 doses of the pediatric/adolescent formulation containing 5 mcg/0.5 mL.

The manufacturer of Recombivax HB® recommends that 5-mcg doses be given at 0, 1, and 6 months of age.

ACIP, AAP, and AAFP recommend that full-term neonates born to HBsAg-*positive* women or women with unknown HBsAg status receive the initial 5-mcg dose of Recombivax HB® as soon as possible after birth (within 12 hours of birth) and the second and third 5-mcg doses at 1–2 and 6 months of age, respectively. The third dose should be given no earlier than 24 weeks of age. If the mother is known or found to be HBsAg-positive, the neonate also should receive a dose of HBIG as soon as possible after birth (within 12 hours of birth). (See Neonates and Infants under Uses: Primary Immunization.)

The ACIP, AAP, and AAFP recommend that full-term neonates born to HBsAg-*negative* women receive the initial 5-mcg dose of Recombivax HB® at birth (before hospital discharge) and the second and third 5-mcg doses at 1–2 and 6–18 months of age, respectively. If the vaccine is not given before hospital discharge, the initial dose should be given no later than 2 months of age. The third dose should be given no earlier than 24 weeks of age.

Preterm neonates weighing less than 2 kg born to HBsAg-*positive* women or women with unknown HBsAg status should receive a dose of hepatitis B vaccine and a dose of HBIG as soon as possible after birth (within 12 hours of birth). This birth dose of hepatitis B vaccine should not be counted toward completion of the vaccination series; the usual 3-dose vaccination series should be initiated when the infant is 1 month of age.

Preterm neonates weighing less than 2 kg born to HBsAg-*negative* women should be given the initial dose of hepatitis B vaccine at 1 month of age; however, the initial dose may be given at the time of hospital discharge (before 1 month of age) if the infant is medically stable and showing consistent weight gain. After the initial dose, the second and third doses of hepatitis B vaccine should be given at 1–2 and 6–18 months, respectively.

Children 10 Years of Age or Younger. When Recombivax HB® is used in children 10 years of age or younger, primary immunization (including catch-up vaccination) consists of 3 doses of the pediatric/adolescent formulation containing 5 mcg/0.5 mL.

The manufacturer recommends that the initial 5-mcg dose be given on a selected date and the second and third 5-mcg doses given at 1 and 6 months, respectively, after the initial dose.

Adolescents 11–19 Years of Age. When Recombivax HB® is used in adolescents 11–19 years of age, primary immunization (including catch-up vaccination) usually consists of 3 doses of the pediatric/adolescent formulation containing 5 mcg/0.5 mL. Alternatively, the manufacturer states that 2 doses of the adult formulation containing 10 mcg/mL can be used for primary immunization in adolescents 11–15 years of age.

If the pediatric/adolescent formulation is used, the manufacturer recommends that the initial 5-mcg dose be given on a selected date and the second and third 5-mcg doses be given at 1 and 6 months, respectively, after the initial dose.

If the adult formulation is used in adolescents 11–15 years of age, a 10-mcg dose should be given on a selected date and a second 10-mcg dose given 4–6 months later.

Adults 20 Years of Age or Older. When Recombivax HB® is used in adults 20 years of age or older, primary immunization consists of 3 doses of the adult formulation containing 10 mcg/mL.

The initial dose of 10 mcg should be given on a selected date and the second and third 10-mcg doses should be given at 1–2 and 4–6 months, respectively, after the initial dose.

Adults Undergoing Hemodialysis. When Recombivax HB® is used in predialysis/dialysis patients, primary immunization consists of 3 doses of the dialysis formulation containing 40 mcg/mL.

The initial 40-mcg should be given on a selected date and the second and third 40-mcg doses should be given at 1 and 6 months, respectively, after the initial dose.

Preexposure Vaccination in High-risk Groups **Travelers.** Individuals requiring primary immunization against HBV prior to travel to areas with intermediate or high levels of endemic HBV (see Travelers under Uses: Preexposure Vaccination in High-risk Groups) should receive an initial dose of the vaccine on a selected date and a second and third dose 1 and 6 months, respectively, after the initial dose. To ensure completion of the 3-dose hepatitis B vaccine series and to provide optimal protection against HBV, the vaccine series should be initiated 6 months prior to travel. Because a partial series offers some protection, the series should be initiated even if it cannot be completed before travel.

Alternatively, the CDC states that international travelers with time constraints that preclude completion of the usual 3-dose vaccination regimen may receive an optional accelerated schedule† with doses given at 0, 7, and 21 days. The US Food and Drug Administration (FDA) has approved this accelerated schedule for the fixed-combination vaccine containing hepatitis A and hepatitis B antigens (HepA-HepB; Twinrix®), but not for the monovalent hepatitis B vaccines (Engerix-B®, Recombivax HB®). Individuals who receive hepatitis B vaccine using the optional accelerated schedule also should receive a booster dose at 1 year after the initial dose of the series to promote long-term immunity.

Alternatively, a 4-dose regimen can be used. The initial dose should be given on a selected date and the other 3 doses given at 1, 2, and 12 months after the initial dose. This regimen induces immunity more rapidly than the usual 3-dose regimen and may be useful when there are time constraints; the first 3 doses should be administered before travel (i.e., at 0, 1, and 2 months).

Prevention of Perinatal HBV Infection **Neonates Born to HBsAg-positive Women.** Combined *passive* immunization with HBIG and *active* immunization with hepatitis B vaccine is indicated to prevent perinatal HBV infection in neonates born to HBsAg-*positive* women.

Neonates born to HBsAg-*positive* women should receive the first dose of hepatitis B vaccine within 12 hours of birth in conjunction with a dose of HBIG using different syringes and different injection sites. Only monovalent hepatitis B vaccine should be used for the birth dose. The hepatitis B vaccine series should then be completed by giving second and third doses of hepatitis B vaccine at 1–2 and 6 months (24 weeks) of age, respectively. The final dose of the vaccine series should be given at 24 weeks of age or older.

For preterm neonates weighing less than 2 kg at birth, the initial (birth) dose of hepatitis B vaccine should not be counted as part of the 3-dose vaccine series. In addition to the birth dose, 3 vaccine doses beginning at 1 month of age (total of 4 doses) should be given.

After completion of the hepatitis B vaccine series, these neonates should undergo serologic testing at 9–18 months of age (usually at the next well-child visit) to evaluate the success or failure of postexposure prophylaxis. (See Postvaccination Serologic Testing under Uses: Pre- and Postvaccination Serologic Testing.) If HBsAg is not detected and anti-HB levels are at least 10 mIU/mL, the child is protected and does not need additional doses of hepatitis B vaccine. If the child has anti-HBs concentrations less than 10 mIU/ mL and is HBsAg-negative, the ACIP and AAP state that a second 3-dose series of hepatitis B vaccine should be administered (initial dose on a selected date and a second and third dose at 1–2 and 6 months, respectively, after the initial dose).

If the mother's HBsAg status is unknown at the time of delivery, the neonate or infant should receive a dose of monovalent hepatitis B vaccine within 12 hours of birth. In addition, the mother should be screened for HBsAg as soon as possible to determine the subsequent management of the infant, including the need to administer HBIG. If the mother of a full-term neonate or preterm neonate weighing more than 2 kg at birth is subsequently found to be HBsAg-positive, the infant should receive a dose of HBIG as soon as possible, but within 7 days of birth. If it is unlikely that the HBsAg status of the mother can be determined within the first 12 hours, the AAP recommends that preterm neonates weighing less than 2 kg receive a dose of HBIG (in addition to a dose of vaccine) within 12 hours of birth since the vaccine may be less immunogenic in these infants.

Postexposure Prophylaxis of HBV Infection Depending on the exposure circumstances, combined *active* immunization with hepatitis B vaccine and *passive* immunization with HBIG may be indicated for postexposure prophylaxis of HBV infection. When hepatitis B vaccine is indicated for postexposure prophylaxis in certain susceptible exposed individuals, including health-care personnel, sexual assault victims, or contacts of individuals with acute HBV infection (see Uses: Postexposure Prophylaxis), the usual 3-dose vaccine series should be used. If the hepatitis B vaccine series was initiated prior to the exposure, the remaining required doses should be administered as originally scheduled.

Occupational Exposure in Susceptible Health-care Personnel. For postexposure prophylaxis of HBV infection in susceptible health-care workers following occupational exposures to blood and other body fluids that might contain HBV, combined *active* immunization with hepatitis B vaccine and *passive* immunization with HBIG may be indicated. (See Table 1 under Uses.)

If hepatitis B vaccine is indicated following occupational exposure to HBV in susceptible health-care personnel, the first dose should be administered as soon as possible (preferably within 24 hours) and the second and third doses administered 1 and 6 months, respectively, after the first dose. If the hepatitis B vaccine series was initiated prior to the exposure, the remaining required doses should be given as originally scheduled.

Unvaccinated or Incompletely Vaccinated Sexual Assault Victims. For postexposure prophylaxis of HBV infection in susceptible victims of sexual assault, the hepatitis B vaccine series should be initiated or completed. The CDC recommends that the first dose of hepatitis B vaccine should be given at the time of the initial examination within 14 days of the assault (preferably within 24 hours) and the second and third doses given at 1–2 and 4–6 months, respectively, after the initial dose. If the perpetrator is HBsAg-positive, the sexual assault victim also should receive a dose of HBIG within 14 days of the assault (preferably within 24 hours).

Unvaccinated or Incompletely Vaccinated Contacts of Individuals with Acute Hepatitis B Virus Infection. For postexposure prophylaxis in unvaccinated or incompletely vaccinated infants younger than 12 months of age exposed to acute HBV infection, *active* immunization with hepatitis B vaccine is indicated and *passive* immunization with HBIG also may be indicated. If the mother or other primary caregiver has acute HBV infection, a dose of HBIG should be given and primary immunization with hepatitis B vaccine should be initiated or completed. However, HBIG is not necessary if the infant already received 2 or more doses of hepatitis B vaccine.

Previously unvaccinated sexual partners of individuals with acute HBV infection should receive postexposure prophylaxis with a dose of hepatitis B vaccine and a dose of HBIG as soon as possible, preferably within less than 24 hours. The hepatitis B vaccine series should then be completed. If the hepatitis B vaccine series was initiated prior to exposure, the remaining required doses should be given as originally scheduled.

Individuals Wounded in Mass Casualty Settings. When HBV vaccine is indicated in a mass casualty setting for individuals who are unvaccinated or have an uncertain vaccination history (see Individuals Wounded in Mass Casualty Settings under Uses: Postexposure Prophylaxis), a dose of hepatitis B vaccine should be given as soon as possible (preferably within 24 hours) and not later than 7 days after the event. The age-appropriate hepatitis B vaccine series should then be completed at the time of discharge or during follow-up health-care visits.

Revaccination or Booster Doses The duration of protection and the need for booster doses after primary immunization with hepatitis B vaccine has not been fully determined.

Antibodies induced by hepatitis B vaccine decline steadily with time and between 30–50% of vaccinees who develop an adequate antibody response to a 3-dose primary series will lose detectable antibody within 7 years, but protection against viremic infection and clinical disease appears to persist in adults and children despite declining antibodies. (See Pharmacology: Duration of Immunity.) Therefore, ACIP states that booster doses are not routinely recommended in immunocompetent individuals who were vaccinated as infants, children, adolescents, or adults and routine serologic testing to assess antibody levels in these individuals are only necessary in certain circumstances.

The ACIP and AAP state that routine annual serologic testing to monitor anti-HBs levels and determine the need for booster doses is indicated in hemodialysis patients since the immunologic response in these individuals is usually less and of shorter duration than that in healthy individuals, and protection may persist only as long as the anti-HBs level is at least 10 mIU/mL. The ACIP and AAP state that hemodialysis patients should receive a booster dose of vaccine when anti-HBs levels decline to less than 10 mIU/mL.

For other immunocompromised individuals (e.g., HIV-infected individuals, hematopoietic stem-cell transplant recipients, individuals receiving chemotherapy or immunosuppressive therapy), the need for booster doses has not been determined. The ACIP and other experts recommend that annual anti-HBs testing be done in such individuals and that booster doses of the vaccine be considered when anti-HBs levels decline to less than 10 mIU/mL.

Combination Vaccines Containing Hepatitis B Vaccine and Other Antigens **Hib-HepB (Comvax®).** The commercially available fixed-combination vaccine containing Hib and hepatitis B antigens (Hib-HepB; Comvax®) is used *only* for primary immunization in infants 6 weeks to 15 months of age.

Comvax® is administered in 0.5-mL doses.

For primary immunization in infants born to HBsAg-*negative* women, Comvax® is given in a series of 3 doses, ideally at 2, 4, and 12–15 months of age. If the recommended schedule cannot be followed exactly, the interval between the first 2 doses should be at least 6 weeks and the interval between the second and third dose should be as close as possible to 8–11 months.

Infants who received a dose of monovalent hepatitis B vaccine at or shortly after birth may receive primary immunization with Comvax® doses given at 2, 4, and 12–15 months of age. There are no data to support the use of a 3-dose series of Comvax® in infants who previously received more than one dose of monovalent hepatitis B vaccine. However, Comvax® may be administered to children otherwise scheduled to receive a dose of hepatitis B vaccine and a dose of Hib conjugate vaccine (PedvaxHIB®).

When primary immunization is initiated in older infants (in the age range of 15 months of age or younger), the immunization schedule for Comvax® should be considered on an individual basis since the number of doses of PedvaxHIB® required for primary immunization depends on the age of the child. The manufacturer's recommendations should be consulted if use of Comvax® is being considered for infants who have not been immunized in early infancy according to the recommended primary immunization schedule.

DTaP-HepB-IPV (Pediarix®). The fixed-combination vaccine containing diphtheria, tetanus, pertussis, hepatitis B, and poliovirus antigens (DTaP-HepB-IPV; Pediarix®) is used *only* in infants and children 6 weeks of age through 6 years of age.

Pediarix® is administered in 0.5-mL doses.

For primary immunization, Pediarix® is given in a series of 3 doses at 6- to 8-week intervals (preferably 8 weeks). The initial dose usually is given at 2 months of age, but may be given as early as 6 weeks of age.

Pediarix® may be used to complete the diphtheria and tetanus toxoids and acellular pertussis vaccine adsorbed (DTaP) vaccine series in infants and children younger than 7 years of age who are scheduled to receive the other components of the vaccine.

Pediarix® may be used to complete the hepatitis B vaccine series or the IPV vaccine series in infants and children younger than 7 years of age who are scheduled to receive the other components of the vaccine.

The manufacturer states that Pediarix® is indicated only in infants born to HBsAg-*negative* women. The ACIP states that Pediarix® also may be used to complete the hepatitis B vaccination series in infants born to HBsAg-*positive* women†.

To complete the DTaP and poliovirus primary vaccine series in children who received a 3-dose primary series of Pediarix®, a dose of Infanrix® (DTaP) should be given at 15–18 months of age and a dose of monovalent IPV (IPOL®) should be given at 4–6 years of age.

HepA-HepB (Twinrix®). The fixed-combination vaccine containing hepatitis A and hepatitis B antigens (HepA-HepB; Twinrix®) is used *only* for primary immunization in adults 18 years of age or older. Twinrix® is not indicated in infants, children, or adolescents younger than 18 years of age.

Twinrix® is given in 1-ml doses.

For primary immunization, adults 18 years of age or older should receive a series of 3 doses of Twinrix® given at 0, 1, and 6 months. Alternatively, if an accelerated dosing schedule is needed, a series of 3 doses may be given on days 0, 7, and 21–30 and a booster dose given at 12 months.

Cautions

■ Hepatitis B Vaccine

Hepatitis B vaccine (recombinant) generally is well tolerated. Adverse reactions to the vaccine are infrequent, mild, and transient. The most common adverse effects are local effects at the site of injection.

Local Effects Adverse local effects, including soreness, pain, induration, tenderness, pruritus, erythema, ecchymosis, swelling, warmth, burning, and nodule formation, have been reported in 10–29% of individuals who received monovalent hepatitis B vaccine.

Systemic Effects Mild systemic adverse effects have been reported in about 15% of patients who received monovalent hepatitis B vaccine. The most frequently reported systemic effects are fatigue, weakness, headache, fever (i.e., 37.8°C or higher), vertigo/dizziness, and malaise; these effects have been reported in at least 1% of patients who received the vaccine. Nausea, diarrhea, pharyngitis, and symptoms of upper respiratory illnesses have also been reported in at least 1% of individuals who received hepatitis B vaccine.

Sweating, achiness, sensation of warmth, lightheadedness, chills, flushing, somnolence, disturbed sleep (e.g., insomnia), irritability, agitation, arthralgia (including monoarticular), myalgia, and pain/stiffness in the back, neck, arm, and/or shoulder have been reported in less than 1% of individuals who received hepatitis B vaccine. Other adverse effects that have been reported with a frequency of less than 1% include vomiting, GI disturbances, constipation, abdominal pains/cramps, dyspepsia, anorexia/diminished appetite, pruritus, rash, lupus-like syndrome, vasculitis, polyarteritis nodosa, alopecia, arthritis, pain in the extremities, petechiae, eczema, erythema, urticaria, rhinitis, influenza-like symptoms,cough, lymphadenopathy, nosebleed, earache, dysuria, tachycardia/palpitations, and hypotension.

Peripheral neuropathy (including Bell's palsy and hypoesthesia), muscle weakness, paresthesia, Guillain-Barré syndrome, transverse myelitis, migraine, syncope, paresis, tinnitus, conjunctivitis, keratitis, visual disturbances, optic neuritis, and multiple sclerosis have been reported in individuals who received hepatitis B vaccine; however, a definite causal relationship was not established. Although a possible association between Guillain-Barré syndrome and administration of the first dose of plasma-derived vaccine (no longer commercially available in the US) was observed during postmarketing surveillance, a causal relationship was not definitely established. In addition, use of the recombinant vaccine in an estimated 2.5 million adults between 1986-1990 has revealed no evidence of an association between receipt of this vaccine and Guillain-Barré syndrome. Other infrequent adverse effects reported with the recombinant vaccine include thrombocytopenia, liver function test abnormalities, eczema, purpura, increased erythrocyte sedimentation rate, and herpes zoster.

Anaphylaxis and symptoms of immediate hypersensitivity, including rash, pruritus, urticaria, edema, angioedema, dyspnea, chest discomfort, bronchospasm (including asthma-like symptoms), palpitation, or symptoms consistent with a hypotensive episode, have been reported within the first few hours after administration of hepatitis B vaccine. Based on data from the Vaccine Adverse Events Reporting System (VAERS), the incidence rate for anaphylaxis with hepatitis B vaccine appears to be low (i.e., approximately one case per 600,000 doses distributed), and only 2 of the cases were in children. In British Columbia, only one case of anaphylaxis was reported among 100,763 children 10–11 years of age who received the recombinant vaccine, and no cases were reported among 166,757 children in New Zealand who received the plasma-derived vaccine (no longer commercially available in the US). Although none of these cases was fatal, the vaccine can cause life-threatening hypersensitivity reactions. (See Sensitivity Reactions under Cautions: Precautions and Contraindications.)

An apparent serum-sickness reaction with delayed onset has been reported days to weeks after administration hepatitis B vaccine; this reaction consists of arthralgia and/or arthritis (usually transient), fever, and dermatologic reactions such as urticaria, erythema multiforme (including Stevens-Johnson syndrome), ecchymoses, and erythema nodosum. There is no evidence to date that use of the vaccine causes adverse effects related to changes in titers of antibodies to yeast-derived antigens. However, up to 5% of the protein contained in hepatitis B vaccine is yeast-derived, and further clinical experience is needed to confirm that sensitization to yeast proteins does not occur following administration of the vaccine.

■ DTaP-HepB-IPV (Pediarix®)

The most common adverse effects reported to date with the fixed-combination vaccine containing diphtheria, tetanus, pertussis, hepatitis B, and poliovirus antigens (DTaP-HepB-IPV; Pediarix®) are local reactions at the injection site (pain, erythema, swelling), loss of appetite, drowsiness, fever, and fussiness.

In a US clinical study in infants who received a 3-dose primary series (at 2, 4, and 6 months of age) of either the fixed-combination vaccine (DTaP-HepB-IPV; Pediarix®) or control vaccines (IPV, DTaP [Infanrix®], and hepatitis B vaccine [Engerix-B®] administered concomitantly at separate sites), adverse effects occurring within 4 days of vaccination were solicited from parents and included local injection site reactions (pain, redness, swelling) and systemic effects (fever, drowsiness, irritability/fussiness, loss of appetite). All infants also received *Haemophilus influenzae* type b (Hib) vaccine and pneumococcal 7-valent conjugate vaccine concomitantly at separate sites. There was a higher incidence of redness and swelling with the fixed-combination vaccine compared with concomitant administration of all the individual components of the vaccine at separate sites. There also was a higher incidence of fever (38°C or higher) after each of the 3 doses of the fixed-combination vaccine compared with when the vaccines were given separately.

■ Hib-HepB (Comvax®)

In clinical studies in healthy infants 6 weeks to 15 months of age, the fixed-combination vaccine containing Hib and hepatitis B antigens (Hib-HepB; Comvax®) generally was well tolerated and adverse effects were similar in type and frequency to those reported in infants who received monovalent Hib vaccine (PedvaxHIB®) and monovalent hepatitis B vaccine (Recombivax HB®) concomitantly at separate sites.

In infants who received Hib-HepB (Comvax®), local effects at the injection site occurring within 5 days after a vaccine dose included pain/soreness in 23.9–34.5%, erythema in 22.4–27.2%, and swelling/induration in 27.2–30.4%.

In infants who received Hib-HepB (Comvax®), systemic effects occurring within 5 days after a dose included irritability in 32.2–57%, somnolence in 21.1–49.5%, crying (unusual, high-pitched) in 2.9–10.6%, and fever (38.3–39°C) in 10.5–14.2%.

■ HepA-HepB (Twinrix®)

The fixed-combination vaccine containing hepatitis A and hepatitis B antigens (HepA-HepB; Twinrix®) generally is well tolerated in adults and adverse effects reported with the vaccine have been mild and transient (usually persisting for no longer than 48 hours). Adverse effects reported with the fixed-combination vaccine were similar to those reported when monovalent hepatitis A virus vaccine inactivated (Havrix®) and monovalent hepatitis B vaccine (Engerix-B®) were administered simultaneously at different sites. No increase in the frequency of adverse effects has been reported with successive doses of the fixed-combination vaccine. In addition, adverse effects reported with an accelerated vaccination regimen of Twinrix® (doses at 0, 7, and 21–30 days and a booster dose at 12 months) have been similar to those reported with the usual 3-dose regimen (doses at 0, 1, and 6 months).

Adverse local reactions reported in adults receiving HepA-HepB (Twinrix®) include soreness (35–41%), erythema (8–11%), and swelling (4–6%).

Adverse systemic reactions reported in adults receiving HepA-HepB (Twinrix®) include upper respiratory tract infections, sweating, weakness, flushing, influenza-like symptoms, headache, fatigue, diarrhea, nausea, fever, vomiting, syncope, abdominal pain, anorexia, arthralgia, myalgia, back pain, migraine, paresthesia, vertigo, somnolence, insomnia, irritability, agitation, and dizziness.

■ Precautions and Contraindications

Monovalent hepatitis B vaccine (Engerix-B®, Recombivax HB®) is contraindicated in individuals hypersensitive to any ingredient in the vaccine, including yeast. Hepatitis B vaccine also is contraindicated in individuals with a history of previous hypersensitivity to any hepatitis B vaccine.

The fixed-combination vaccine containing Hib and hepatitis B antigens (Hib-HepB; Comvax®) is contraindicated in individuals hypersensitive to any vaccine component, including yeast.

The fixed-combination vaccine containing diphtheria, tetanus, pertussis, hepatitis B, and poliovirus antigens (DTaP-HepB-IPV; Pediarix®) is contraindicated in individuals with a history of hypersensitivity to any ingredient in the vaccine (e.g., yeast, neomycin, polymyxin B) or a history of serious allergic reaction (e.g., anaphylaxis) temporally associated with a previous dose of the vaccine or any vaccine component. In addition, the vaccine is contraindicated (because of the pertussis antigen) in individuals with encephalopathy (e.g., coma, decreased consciousness, prolonged seizures) within 7 days of a previous dose of vaccine containing pertussis antigens that could not be attributed to another identifiable cause and in individuals with progressive neurologic disorder, including infantile spasms, uncontrolled epilepsy, or progressive encephalopathy.

The fixed-combination vaccine containing hepatitis A and hepatitis B antigens (HepA-HepB; Twinrix®) is contraindicated in individuals hypersensitive to any ingredient in the vaccine, including the hepatitis A virus vaccine inactivated component (Havrix®), the hepatitis B vaccine component (Engerix-B®), yeast, or neomycin. The vaccine also is contraindicated in individuals with previous hypersensitivity reactions to Twinrix® or monovalent hepatitis A or hepatitis B vaccines.

Sensitivity Reactions Prior to administration of hepatitis B vaccine or fixed-combination vaccines containing hepatitis B vaccine, all known precautions should be taken to prevent adverse reactions, including a review of the patient's history with respect to possible sensitivity to the vaccine or to similar vaccines.

Anaphylaxis and symptoms of immediate hypersensitivity have been reported with hepatitis B vaccine. (See Systemic Effects under Cautions: Hepatitis B Vaccine.)

Epinephrine and other appropriate agents should be available for immediate treatment of an anaphylactoid reaction if it occurs. Individuals with symptoms of hypersensitivity after a previous dose should not receive additional vaccine doses.

Yeast Allergy. The manufacturing process for hepatitis B vaccine involves baker's yeast (*Saccharomyces cerevisiae*) and monovalent hepatitis B vaccine and fixed-combination vaccines containing hepatitis B vaccine contain up to 5% yeast protein.

The manufacturers state that monovalent and fixed-combination vaccines containing hepatitis B vaccine should not be used in individuals with yeast allergy. There is a theoretical risk of an allergic reaction in individuals allergic to yeast, but there is no evidence to date that such reactions have occurred when hepatitis B vaccine was used in such individuals.

Allergy to Neomycin or Other Anti-infectives. The fixed-combination vaccine containing diphtheria, tetanus, pertussis, hepatitis B, and poliovirus antigens (DTaP-HepB-IPV; Pediarix®) contains trace amounts of neomycin sulfate (not exceeding 0.05 ng) and polymyxin B (not exceeding 0.01 ng). The fixed-combination vaccine containing hepatitis A and hepatitis B antigens (HepA-HepB; Twinrix®) contains trace amounts of neomycin sulfate (not exceeding 20 ng). The manufacturers state that Pediarix® and Twinrix® are contraindicated in individuals hypersensitive to these anti-infectives.

Neomycin allergy usually results in delayed-type (cell-mediated) hypersensitivity reactions manifested as contact dermatitis. The ACIP and AAP state that vaccines containing trace amounts of neomycin should *not* be used in individuals with a history of anaphylactic reaction to neomycin, but use of such vaccines may be considered in those with a history of a delayed-type hypersensitivity reaction to neomycin if benefits of vaccination outweigh risks.

Latex Allergy. Some packaging components (e.g., needle cover, syringe plunger) of the single-dose prefilled syringes of Engerix-B® or single-dose prefilled syringes of DTaP-HepB-IPV (Pediarix®) contain dry natural latex. The stopper on vials of Comvax® contains natural rubber latex.

Some individuals may be hypersensitive to natural latex proteins found in a wide range of medical devices, including such packaging components, and the level of sensitivity may vary depending on the form of natural rubber present; rarely, hypersensitivity reactions to natural latex proteins have been fatal.

The ACIP states that vaccines supplied in vials or syringes containing dry natural rubber or natural rubber latex may be administered to individuals with latex allergies other than anaphylactic allergies (e.g., history of contact allergy to latex gloves), but should *not* be used in those with a history of severe (anaphylactic) allergy to latex, unless the benefits of vaccination outweigh the risk of a potential allergic reaction.

Individuals with Altered Immunocompetence The recommendations regarding use of hepatitis B vaccine in individuals with altered immunocompetence generally are the same as those for individuals who are not immunocompromised. Hepatitis B vaccine may be used in immunocompromised individuals, including those who have human immunodeficiency virus (HIV) infection or immunocompromised because of congenital immunodeficiency, leukemia, lymphoma, generalized malignancy, or therapy with alkylating agents, antimetabolites, radiation, or corticosteroids. The vaccine also may be used in solid organ or hematopoietic stem cell transplant recipients, patients with asplenia, renal failure, diabetes, alcoholism, or alcoholic cirrhosis. The possibility that the immune response to the vaccine may be reduced in these individuals should be considered.

Recommendations regarding the use of hepatitis B vaccine in HIV-infected individuals are the same as those for individuals who are not HIV-infected. Some HIV-infected individuals may not have a satisfactory response to hepatitis B vaccine and anti-HBs may persist for shorter periods of time in HIV-infected individuals. Immunogenicity of higher than usual vaccine doses or additional vaccine doses in HIV-infected individuals have not been fully evaluated; therefore, firm recommendations cannot be made regarding use of such doses in these individuals. (See Individuals with Altered Immunocompetence under Uses: Primary Immunization.)

The anti-HBs response generally is lower and persists for shorter periods in hemodialysis patients than in healthy adults. Only 50–86% of hemodialysis patients reportedly develop protective levels of anti-HBs after receiving a 3-dose vaccine series consisting of 40-mcg doses of hepatitis B vaccine (i.e., 10 mIU/mL or greater measured 1–2 months after completion of the hepatitis B vaccine series). Therefore, larger vaccine doses (e.g., 2–4 times the usual adult dose) are required to induce protective antibody levels in a large proportion of patients undergoing hemodialysis. (See Dosage and Administration: Dosage.)

Concomitant Illness The decision whether to administer or delay administration of hepatitis B vaccine in an individual with a current or recent acute illness depends largely on the severity of symptoms and etiology of the illness. The ACIP states that a minor acute illness, such as mild diarrhea or mild upper respiratory tract infection (with or without fever), generally does not preclude vaccination, but vaccination should be deferred in individuals with moderate or severe acute illness (with or without fever). Some manufacturers state that the vaccine may be given to individuals with acute infection or febrile illness if withholding the vaccine poses a greater risk to the patient.

The manufacturer of hepatitis B vaccine (Recombivax HB®) recommends that the vaccine be used with caution and appropriate care in individuals with severely compromised cardiopulmonary status or in others in whom a febrile or systemic reaction could pose a significant risk.

Exacerbation of multiple sclerosis has been reported following administration of hepatitis B vaccine or other vaccines; however, a causal relationship has not been established. One manufacturer states that the benefits of hepatitis B vaccination should be weighed against the risk of exacerbation of multiple sclerosis.

Individuals with Bleeding Disorders Hepatitis B vaccine and fixed-combination vaccines containing hepatitis B vaccine should be administered IM with caution to individuals with thrombocytopenia or a bleeding disorder (e.g., hemophilia) or in those receiving anticoagulant therapy, since bleeding may occur following IM administration in these individuals.

The manufacturers of monovalent hepatitis B vaccine (Engerix-B®, Recombivax HB®) state that the vaccine can be administered by subcutaneous rather than IM injection in individuals at risk of hemorrhage (e.g., hemophilia patients). However, subcutaneous administration of hepatitis B vaccine has been associated with reduced antibody response. In addition, an increased incidence of local reactions, including subcutaneous nodules, has been reported following subcutaneous administration of other aluminum-adsorbed vaccines; therefore, hepatitis B vaccine should be administered by subcutaneous injection only in individuals at risk for hemorrhage following IM administration.

The ACIP states that vaccines may be given IM to individuals who have bleeding disorders or are receiving anticoagulant therapy if a clinician familiar with the patient's bleeding risk determines that the vaccine can be administered with reasonable safety. In these cases, a fine needle (23 gauge) should be used to administer the vaccine and firm pressure should be applied to the injection site (without rubbing) for at least 2 minutes. If IM administration is used in individuals with a bleeding disorder who are receiving antihemophilic factor or other similar therapy, the IM dose can be scheduled shortly after a dose of such therapy to minimize the risk of bleeding. The individual and/or their family should be instructed concerning the risk of hematoma from the injection.

Use of Combination Vaccines When the fixed-combination vaccine containing diphtheria, tetanus, pertussis, hepatitis B, and poliovirus antigens (DTaP-HepB-IPV; Pediarix®), the fixed-combination vaccine containing Hib and hepatitis antigens (Hib-HepB; Comvax®), or the fixed-combination vaccine containing hepatitis A and hepatitis B antigens (HepA-HepB; Twinrix®) is used, the adverse effects, precautions, and contraindications associated with each antigen should be considered.

For more complete information regarding the adverse effects, precautions, and contraindications associated with use of vaccines that contain diphtheria, tetanus, and pertussis antigens, see Cautions in Diphtheria and Tetanus Toxoids and Acellular Pertussis Vaccine Adsorbed/Tetanus Toxoid and Reduced Diphtheria Toxoid and Acellular Pertussis Vaccine Adsorbed 80:08.

For more complete information regarding the adverse effects, precautions, and contraindications associated with use of vaccines that contain Hib antigens, see Cautions in Haemophilus b Vaccine 80:12.

For more complete information regarding the adverse effects, precautions, and contraindications associated with use of vaccines that contain poliovirus antigens, see Cautions in Poliovirus Vaccine Inactivated 80:12.

For more complete information regarding the adverse effects, precautions, and contraindications associated with use of vaccines that contain hepatitis A antigens, see Cautions in Hepatitis A Virus Vaccine Inactivated 80:12.

Limitations of Vaccine Effectiveness Hepatitis B vaccine may not protect all vaccine recipients against HBV infection, especially individuals who have not achieved protective titers of anti-HBs (i.e., 10 mIU/mL or greater measured 1–2 months after completion of the hepatitis B vaccine series).

Unrecognized HBV infection may be present in some individuals at the time of vaccination since the infection has an incubation period of 6 weeks to 6 months and hepatitis B vaccine may not prevent infection in such individuals.

Monovalent hepatitis B vaccine (Engerix-B®, Recombivax HB®) provides protection only against HBV. The fixed-combination vaccine containing hepatitis A virus vaccine and hepatitis B vaccine (Twinrix®) provides protection only against hepatitis A virus (HAV) and HBV. Monovalent hepatitis B vaccine and fixed-combination vaccines containing hepatitis B vaccine generally will also prevent hepatitis D virus (HDV) infection since HDV occurs only as a coinfection or superinfection in patients with HBV infection. These vaccines do not provide protection against other hepatitis viruses (e.g., hepatitis C virus [HCV], hepatitis E virus [HEV]).

Improper Storage and Handling Improper storage or handling of vaccines may result in loss of vaccine potency and a reduced immune response in vaccinees. Hepatitis B vaccine should not be administered if it has been mishandled or has not been stored at the recommended temperature. (See Chemistry and Stability: Stability.)

All vaccines should be inspected upon delivery and monitored during storage to ensure that the appropriate temperature is maintained. If there are concerns about mishandling, the manufacturer or state or local health departments should be contacted for guidance on whether the vaccine is usable.

■ **Pediatric Precautions** Monovalent hepatitis B vaccine (Engerix-B®, Recombivax HB®) is highly immunogenic in infants and children. In neonates, passively acquired maternal anti-HBs antibodies do not appear to interfere with the active immune response to hepatitis B vaccine. However, there is some evidence that the seroconversion rate is lower in low-birthweight infants when the initial dose of hepatitis B vaccine is administered shortly after birth than when it is administered when the infant is older or weighs more than 2 kg.

Safety and efficacy of Recombivax® HB Dialysis Formulation have not been established in children.

Safety and efficacy of Hib-HepB (Comvax®) have not been established in infants younger than 6 weeks of age or in infants or children older than 15 months of age.

Safety and efficacy of DTaP-HepB-IPV (Pediarix®) have not been established in infants younger than 6 weeks of age or in children 7 years of age or older.

Safety and efficacy of HepA-HepB (Twinrix®) have not been established in children younger than 18 years of age.

■ **Geriatric Precautions** Clinical studies of monovalent hepatitis B vaccine (Engerix-B®, Recombivax HB®) did not include sufficient numbers of individuals 65 years of age or older to determine whether these individuals respond differently than younger individuals. Other reported clinical experience indicates that hepatitis B vaccine may be less immunogenic in individuals 65 years of age or older than in younger individuals. No overall differences in safety have been reported between geriatric individuals and younger adults.

Clinical studies of HepA-HepB (Twinrix®) did not include sufficient numbers of individuals 65 years of age or older to determine whether geriatric individuals respond differently than younger adults.

Hib-HepB (Comvax®) and DTaP-HepB-IPV (Pediarix®) are *not* indicated for use in adults, including geriatric adults.

■ **Mutagenicity and Carcinogenicity** Studies have not been performed to date to evaluate the mutagenic or carcinogenic potential of hepatitis B vaccine or fixed-combination vaccines containing hepatitis B vaccine.

■ **Pregnancy, Fertility, and Lactation** ***Pregnancy*** Animal reproduction studies have not been performed with hepatitis B vaccine. It is not known whether the vaccine can cause fetal harm when administered to a pregnant woman. Hepatitis B vaccine should be used during pregnancy only when clearly needed.

Because of the potential risks from exposure to HBV infection in a pregnant woman and the potential for development of chronic infection in the neonate, pregnancy is not considered a contraindication to use of hepatitis B vaccine when clearly needed. Since hepatitis B vaccine contains only noninfectious hepatitis B surface antigen (HBsAg) particles, the US Public Health Service Advisory Committee on Immunization Practices (ACIP) states that the theoretical risk to the fetus from the vaccine should be negligible.

HepA-HepB (Twinrix®) should be used during pregnancy only when clearly needed. Clinicians are encouraged to register pregnant women who receive Twinrix® with the manufacturer's vaccination pregnancy registry at 888-452-9622.

Hib-HepB (Comvax®) and DTaP-HepB-IPV (Pediarix®) are not indicated for use in women of childbearing age.

Fertility It is not known whether hepatitis B vaccine or fixed-combination vaccines containing hepatitis B vaccine affect fertility.

Lactation It is not known whether the antigens contained in hepatitis B vaccine are distributed into milk. The manufacturers state that hepatitis B vaccine (Engerix-B®, Recombivax HB®) and HepA-HepB (Twinrix®) should be used with caution in nursing women.

Although specific data are not available, the ACIP, CDC, and AAP state that breast-feeding is not a contraindication to administration of hepatitis B vaccine and lactating women should receive the vaccine as recommended for other adults.

Drug Interactions

■ **Anti-infective Agents** Concurrent use of anti-infective agents generally does not affect the immune response to inactivated vaccines, including hepatitis B vaccine (recombinant).

■ **Blood Products** Hepatitis B vaccine does not need to be deferred in individuals who have received a blood transfusion or other blood products.

■ **Immune Globulins** There is no evidence that immune globulin (immune globulin IM [IGIM], immune globulin IV [IGIV]) or specific immune globulin (hepatitis B immune globulin [HBIG], rabies immune globulin [RIG], tetanus immune globulin [TIG], varicella zoster immune globulin [VZIG]) interferes with the immune response to inactivated vaccines. The US Public Health Service Advisory Committee on Immunization Practices (ACIP) states that inactivated vaccines such as hepatitis B vaccine may be given simultaneously with (using different syringes and different injection sites) or at any interval before or after immune globulin preparations.

Hepatitis B Immune Globulin Passively acquired antibody to hepatitis B surface antigen (anti-HBs), which is present in HBIG, does not appear to interfere with the active immune response stimulated by hepatitis B vaccine. Clinical studies in neonates indicate that the immune response to hepatitis B vaccine is not altered by concomitant use of HBIG.

When combined *active* immunization with hepatitis B vaccine and *passive* immunization with HBIG is indicated, the first dose of vaccine should be administered simultaneously with HBIG (using different syringes and different injection sites). The manufacturer of HepaGam B® states that HBIG administered simultaneously with or up to 1 month before hepatitis B vaccine does not appear to impair the active immune response to the vaccine.

■ **Immunosuppressive Agents** Individuals receiving immunosuppressive therapy (e.g., corticotropin, corticosteroids, alkylating agents, antimetabolites, radiation) may have a reduced response to hepatitis B vaccine. The ACIP recommends that vaccines generally be administered 2 weeks prior to initiation of immunosuppressive therapy or deferred until at least 3 months after such therapy is discontinued. Individuals receiving immunosuppressive therapy may require larger than usual doses of hepatitis B vaccine in order to develop adequate circulating antibody levels. (See Dosage and Administration: Dosage.)

■ **Vaccines** Although specific studies may not be available evaluating concurrent administration of hepatitis B vaccine with each antigen, simultaneous administration with other age-appropriate vaccines, including live virus vaccines, toxoids, or inactivated or recombinant vaccines, during the same health-care visit is not expected to affect immunologic responses or adverse reactions to any of the preparations.

Immunization with hepatitis B vaccine can be integrated with immunization against diphtheria, tetanus, pertussis, *Haemophilus influenzae* type b (Hib), hepatitis A, human papillomavirus (HPV), influenza, poliovirus, measles, mumps, rubella, rotavirus, meningococcal disease, pneumococcal disease, and varicella. However, unless combination vaccines appropriate for the age and vaccination status of the recipient are used, each parenteral vaccine should be administered using a different syringe and different injection site.

Inactivated Vaccines and Toxoids Since hepatitis B vaccine is a noninfectious inactivated preparation, concomitant administration with killed vaccines is not likely to cause interference with the immune response to these vaccines. However, hepatitis B vaccine should not be mixed in the same syringe with any other vaccine since compatibility between products has not been demonstrated and injections should preferably be given at different sites.

Diphtheria and Tetanus Toxoids and Pertussis Vaccines. Hepatitis B vaccine may be administered concomitantly (at a different site) with diphtheria and tetanus toxoids and acellular pertussis vaccine adsorbed (DTaP). Alternatively, hepatitis B vaccine is commercially available in a fixed-combination vaccine containing DTaP, hepatitis B vaccine, and poliovirus vaccine inactivated (IPV) (DTaP-HepB-IPV; Pediarix®). Depending on the age and vaccination status of the child, this combination vaccine can be used instead of separate injections of DTaP and hepatitis B vaccine when indicated and if there are no contraindications to any of the individual components. (See Uses: Combination Vaccines Containing Hepatitis B Vaccine and Other Antigens.) Extemporaneous preparations of hepatitis B vaccine mixed with commercially available monovalent vaccines containing these antigens should not be prepared since compatibility between these preparations has not been demonstrated.

Concomitant administration of tetanus toxoid and reduced diphtheria toxoid and acellular pertussis vaccine adsorbed (Tdap) (Adacel®) and hepatitis B vaccine (Recombivax HB®) did not result in reduced antibody responses to either vaccine. Therefore, Tdap may be administered simultaneously with (using different syringes and injection sites) or at any time before or after hepatitis B vaccine.

Haemophilus b Vaccines. Monovalent hepatitis B vaccine may be administered concomitantly with monovalent Hib vaccine; however, the vaccines should be administered at different sites using separate syringes. Alternatively, hepatitis B vaccine is commercially available in a fixed-combination vaccine that contains Hib vaccine and hepatitis B vaccine (Hib-HepB; Comvax®) and this combination vaccine can be used whenever a dose of hepatitis B vaccine and a dose of Hib vaccine are both indicated in an infant 6 weeks to 15 months of age. (See Uses: Combination Vaccines Containing Hepatitis B Vaccine and Other Antigens.) However, extemporaneous vaccine combinations of hepatitis B vaccine and Hib vaccine should *not* be prepared by admixing commercially available monovalent hepatitis B vaccine and monovalent Hib vaccine.

Hepatitis A Vaccine. Studies have shown that monovalent hepatitis A virus vaccine inactivated and monovalent hepatitis B vaccine can be administered simultaneously at different sites using separate syringes without interfering with the immune response to either vaccine. Alternatively, hepatitis B vaccine and hepatitis A virus vaccine inactivated may be given simultaneously as the commercially available fixed-combination vaccine (HepA-HepB; Twinrix®). (See Uses: Combination Vaccines Containing Hepatitis B Vaccine and Other Antigens.)

Human Papillomavirus Virus Vaccine. Concomitant administration of the complete primary immunization series (3 doses each) of quadrivalent HPV vaccine (HPV4) and hepatitis B vaccine (at different injection sites) during the same health-care visit in women 16–23 years of age did not decrease the antibody response to either vaccine and did not increase the incidence of clinically important adverse effects compared with administration during separate visits. Therefore, HPV vaccine and hepatitis B vaccine may be administered concomitantly using different syringes and different injection sites.

Influenza Virus Vaccine. Hepatitis B vaccine may be administered concurrently with influenza virus vaccine inactivated (TIV) at a different site using a separate syringe.

Pneumococcal Vaccines. Hepatitis B vaccine should not interfere with the response to pneumococcal 23-valent polysaccharide vaccine (PPSV23).

Hepatitis B vaccine may be administered concurrently with pneumococcal 7-valent conjugate vaccine (PCV13) at a different site using a separate syringe.

Live Vaccines Although specific studies evaluating simultaneous administration of hepatitis B vaccine and measles, mumps, and rubella virus vaccine live (MMR) or varicella virus vaccine live are not available, these vaccines may be administered concomitantly. However, hepatitis B vaccine should not be mixed in the same syringe with any other vaccine since compatibility between products has not been demonstrated and injections should preferably be given at different sites. If hepatitis B vaccine is administered simultaneously with another vaccine and if injections are administered into the same anterolateral thigh or deltoid, the injections must be given one or more inches apart.

Hepatitis B vaccine can be given concurrently with yellow fever vaccine using different syringes and different injection sites without affecting safety or immunogenicity.

Pharmacology

Hepatitis B vaccine (recombinant) stimulates active immunity to hepatitis B virus (HBV) infection. Hepatitis B surface antigen (HBsAg), which is present in hepatitis B vaccine, promotes the production of antibody to HBsAg (anti-HBs); anti-HBs neutralizes HBV so that its infective or pathogenic properties are inhibited.

Protection against HBV infection is virtually complete in immunocompetent individuals who develop adequate antibody levels after immunization with hepatitis B vaccine. The US Public Health Service Advisory Committee on Immunization Practices (ACIP) defines a protective level of anti-HBs as 10 mIU/mL or greater measured 1–2 months after completion of the hepatitis B vaccine series. While only anti-HBs levels expressed in mIU/mL and determined against the World Health Organization (WHO) anti-HBs reference preparation have been standardized, the ACIP in 1987 suggested that the minimum anti-HBs level of 10 mIU/mL is approximately equivalent to 10 sample ratio units (SRU) determined by radioimmunoassay (RIA) or a positive enzyme immunoassay (EIA) because of similarities in the degree of immunogenicity represented by such determinations. The SRU value of 10 was based on results of routine screening and hepatitis B vaccine efficacy studies conducted in the early 1980s and the EIA indicator was based on the manufacturers' recommended positive threshold for such immunoassays. More recently, the Centers for Disease Control and Prevention (CDC) compared the predictive level of these latter tests relative to the WHO standard measure in several hundred public safety workers vaccinated 1–6 months prior to testing. Results of this comparison indicated the predictive value of currently available RIA and EIA tests in indicating an anti-HBs titer of at least 10 mIU/mL as being 99.2 and 97.6%, respectively. Thus, while these tests are highly predictive, a small number of individuals tested since March 1986 and reported as having a protective antibody level based *only* (i.e., who did not also have a WHO-standardized quantitative determination of anti-HBs) on an RIA determination of at least 10 SRU and/or positivity by RIA may *not* actually have developed an adequate response to the vaccine (i.e., falsely positive immunity determinations secondary to oversensitivity of these assays). Therefore, the CDC states that any such individual who subsequently is exposed to an HBsAg-positive source without having had a quantitative determination of anti-HBs (based on a value of at least 10 mIU/mL) should be considered as having an unknown response to the vaccine when making decisions regarding the possible need for postexposure prophylaxis.

Administration of hepatitis B vaccine during the incubation period of infection (i.e., after exposure to HBV but prior to onset of clinical symptoms) may only modify or ameliorate, rather than prevent, infection.

The active immune response produced by hepatitis B vaccine does not appear to be suppressed by hepatitis B immune globulin (HBIG) when HBIG is administered concomitantly at a separate site. (See Drug Interactions.)

■ **Hepatitis B Virus and Infection** HBV is a DNA virus from the family Hepadnaviridae consisting of antigenically distinct surface and core components. The presence of HBsAg in serum indicates the presence of active HBV infection (either acute or chronic). HBsAg may also be found in other body fluids and tissues. (See Uses: Risks of Exposure and Infection.) The HBV viral core consists of DNA, DNA polymerase, hepatitis B core antigen (HBcAg), and hepatitis B e antigen (HBeAg). All HBsAg-positive individuals are infectious and those that are positive for HBeAg will also have high HBV titers and are considered highly infectious. The presence of HBeAg and HBV DNA in serum generally indicates high levels of viral replication and suggests that the serum is highly infectious.

The incubation period from exposure to HBV to onset of symptoms of HBV infection is 6 weeks to 6 months (average: 90–150 days). Serologic markers of HBV infection (i.e., HBsAg, HBeAg, antibody to hepatitis B core antigen [anti-HBc], antibody to hepatitis B e antigen [anti-HBe], anti-HBs) are used to define clinical status of those exposed to HBV infection or virus. HBsAg appears in the serum about 30 days (range 6–60 days) after exposure and indicates an ongoing HBV infection. HBsAg persists during an acute infection and usually disappears as the acute infection resolves; however, the presence of HBsAg in the serum for 6 months or longer generally indicates chronic infection. Anti-HBs develops during convalescence after an acute HBV infection (usually within 3–4 months). The presence of anti-HBs indicates recovery from and immunity to further HBV infection.

Acute HBV infection may be self-limited resulting in production of antibody to HBsAg (anti-HBs) and immunity against reinfection; however, it may also progress to chronic HBV infection (especially in infants or young children, immunocompromised individuals, patients with diabetes) or to fatal, fulminant hepatitis. The case fatality rate is 0.5–1.5% among those with acute HBV infection and the highest fatality rates are in adults older than 60 years of age. Chronic HBV infection develops in 90% or more of infants infected perinatally, 25–50% of children infected at 1–5 years of age, and less than 5% of those infected at 5 years of age or older. Chronic infection is associated with persistent HBV replication in the liver and may result in liver cirrhosis, liver cancer, liver failure, and death. Data from 2006 indicate that approximately 800,000–1.4 million people in the US have chronic HBV infection. HBV is transmitted by percutaneous or mucosal exposure to HBsAg-positive blood, serum, plasma, semen, or saliva and can be transmitted perinatally from mother to infant at birth, usually from blood exposures during labor and delivery.

■ **Response to Hepatitis B Vaccine (Recombinant)** ***Neonates and Infants 18 Months of Age or Younger*** Studies evaluating immunogenicity of hepatitis B vaccine administered to neonates in various dosage schedules beginning at birth or 2 months of age indicate that protective levels of anti-HBs generally are attained in more than 95% of infants following 3 doses of vaccine. However, geometric mean titers (GMTs) of antibody achieved generally are lower when accelerated dosing schedules are used. The effect of higher antibody levels on long-term disease protection currently is not known, but achievement of high titers ensures longer persistence of antibody.

In a study using Engerix-B® in healthy neonates born to healthy HBsAg-*negative* women, administration of 10-mcg doses at birth and 1 and 2 months of age or at birth and 1 and 6 months of age induced protective levels of anti-HBs in about 96% of infants at 6–7 months; GMTs of antibody in seroconverters at 7 months were 420 mIU/mL in those who received the accelerated schedule and 3142 mIU/mL in those who received the other schedule. In a study using Recombivax HB® in healthy infants born to HBsAg-*negative* women, GMTs of antibody (1 month after the third dose) were 1358 mIU/mL in those who received 2.5-mcg doses at 2, 4, and 12 months of age and 3424 mIU/mL in those who received 2.5-mcg doses at 2, 4, and 15 months of age.

Adults and Adolescents In several studies, at least 90% of healthy young adults and teenagers developed protective levels of anti-HBs after a series of three 10-mcg doses of hepatitis B vaccine given IM into the deltoid. The seroconversion rate following administration of hepatitis B vaccine may be lower in men than in women and appears to vary with age. The seroconversion rate following administration of 3 doses of hepatitis B vaccine in infants and children 19 years of age or younger is 96–100%, but is 94–99% in adults 20–39 years of age and 88–91% in adults 40 years of age or older. After 40 years of age, the proportion of adults who have a protective antibody response after a 3-dose vaccination regimen declines below 90%, and by 60 years of age, protective antibody levels occur in only 75% of those vaccinated.

Results of an open, randomized, multicenter study in adolescents 11–15 years of age indicate that the immunogenicity of a 2-dose regimen of 10-mcg doses of Recombivax HB® (second dose given 4–6 months after the first dose) is similar to that of a 3-dose regimen of 5-mcg doses of Recombivax HB® (second and third doses given 1 and 6 months, respectively, after the first dose) and that both regimens are equally well tolerated. At one month after the last dose, 99% of those who received the 2-dose regimen and 98% of those who received the 3-dose regimen had protective levels of antibody. Short-term follow-up data indicate that the rate of decline in antibody levels for the 2-dose regimen is similar to that of the 3-dose regimen; however, data are not available to assess long-term protection (beyond 2 years) or immunologic memory following vaccination with the 2-dose regimen and it is not known whether booster doses of vaccine will be required.

Individuals with Altered Immunocompetence The anti-HBs response in hemodialysis patients and immunocompromised patients generally is less than that in immunocompetent individuals, and adequate levels generally persist for shorter periods.

Only 50–86% of hemodialysis patients reportedly develop protective levels of anti-HBs after receiving three 40-mcg doses of hepatitis B vaccine. Larger vaccine doses (e.g., 2–4 times the usual adult dose) or an increased number of doses (4 doses) are required to induce protective antibody levels in a large proportion of patients undergoing hemodialysis.

Larger vaccine doses (e.g., 2–4 times the usual adult dose) or an increased number of doses (4 doses) in the hepatitis B vaccine series may be necessary to induce protective antibody levels in other immunocompromised individuals, including those receiving immunosuppressive therapy or with human immunodeficiency virus (HIV) infection. HIV-infected children (especially older children or those with CD4$^+$ T-cell counts less than 200/mm^3) may have lower antibody responses to hepatitis B vaccine than those who do not have HIV infection. The seroconversion rate in HIV-infected adults is 18–72% following vaccination with hepatitis B vaccine and is lower than that reported in healthy adults. In addition, mean antibody titers are lower and decline faster in HIV-infected individuals than in those who are not infected with HIV. (See HIV-infected Individuals under Primary Immunization: Individuals with Altered Immunocompetence, in Uses.)

Immunogenicity of hepatitis B vaccine may be reduced in parenteral drug abusers, possibly secondary to altered immunity in these individuals.

Individuals with Hepatitis C Virus Infection The immunologic response to hepatitis B vaccine may be decreased in patients with hepatitis C virus (HCV) infection and may be adversely affected by HCV viral load. In one study that used an accelerated 3-dose vaccination schedule of hepatitis B vaccine (doses given at 0, 1, and 2 months), a protective antibody response was attained in 63.6% of adults with chronic HCV infection compared with 93.9% of healthy adults. Among the HCV patients, nonresponders had higher viral loads of HCV than those who responded to the vaccine. There was no evidence that vaccination with hepatitis B vaccine affected the HCV viral load during or after vaccination. In another study that used the usual 3-dose vaccination schedule (Engerix B® doses of 20 mcg given at 0, 1, and 6 months), a protective antibody response was attained in 72.9% of adults with chronic HCV infection (without cirrhosis) compared with 90.9% of healthy adults. In addition, although the clinical importance is unclear, only 34.1% of the HCV patients still had seroprotective titers of anti-HBs 1 year after completion of the vaccine regimen compared with 90% of the healthy controls.

■ **Response to Combination Vaccines Containing Hepatitis B Vaccine and Other Antigens** ***Hib-HepB (Comvax®)*** Results of a randomized, open-label study in 882 infants approximately 2 months of age who had not previously received any doses of haemophilus b (Hib) vaccine or hepatitis B vaccine indicate that a 3-dose regimen of the fixed-combination vaccine containing Hib and hepatitis B antigens (Hib-HepB; Comvax®) results in an immunologic response rate similar to that attained when monovalent Hib vaccine (PedvaxHIB®) and monovalent hepatitis B vaccine (Recombivax HB®) are given concurrently at different sites. In this study, vaccine doses were given at approximately 2, 4, and 12–15 months of age. The PRP antibody response (anti-PRP) after the second dose of Comvax® (72.4% had levels exceeding 1 mcg/mL with a GMT of 2.5 mcg/mL) was comparable to that in infants who received the monovalent Hib vaccine (76.2% with a GMT of 2.8 mcg/mL). Therefore, efficacy of Comvax® in preventing invasive Hib disease is expected to be similar to that reported with monovalent PedvaxHIB®. The anti-HBs response after the third dose of Comvax® (98.4% had levels 10 mIU/mL or greater with a GMT of 4467.5) was slightly lower than that in infants who received the monovalent hepatitis B vaccine (100% with a GMT of 6943.9). Although this difference in GMT may result in differences in the duration of anti-HBs response after a number of years, this probably is not clinically important because of immunologic memory. In addition, the anti-HBs response to Comvax® is considered protective. Therefore, because the HBsAg component of Comvax® induces an antibody response comparable to that obtained with Recombivax HB®, efficacy of the fixed-combination vaccine in providing protection against HBV infection is expected to be similar.

HepA-HepB (Twinrix®) Data from several studies in healthy adults 17–70 years of age indicate that the immunogenicity of a 3-dose series (at 0, 1, and 6 months) of the fixed combination vaccine containing hepatitis A and hepatitis B antigens (HepA-HepB; Twinrix®) is similar to that of a 2-dose series (at 0 and 6 months) of the monovalent hepatitis A virus vaccine inactivated (Havrix®) and a 3-dose series (at 0, 1, and 6 months) of the monovalent hepatitis B vaccine (Engerix-B®) administered concurrently at separate sites or administered alone.

In adults who received a 3-dose series of the fixed-combination vaccine, 99.9% developed anti-hepatitis A virus (anti-HAV) titers of at least 20 mIU/mL and 98.5% developed anti-HBsAg titers of at least 10 mIU/mL 1 month after completion of the vaccine series. In one US study in adults 18–70 years of age, serum anti-HAV titers of at least 20 mIU/mL and anti-HBsAg titers of at least 10 mIU/mL were observed in 99.6 or 95.1% of vaccinees, respectively, who received a 3-dose series (at 0, 1, 6 months) of the fixed-combination vaccine compared with 99.3 or 92.2%, respectively, of vaccinees who received the separate monovalent hepatitis A virus vaccine inactivated and monovalent hepatitis B vaccine concurrently. The GMT of anti-HAV measured 1 month after completion of the vaccine series was 4756 mIU/mL in vaccinees who received the fixed-combination vaccine versus 2948 mIU/mL in vaccinees who received both monovalent vaccines; this difference is not considered clinically important and has been attributed to the differences in the hepatitis A viral antigen content in the 2 regimens (3 doses of 720 units in the regimen compared to 2 doses of 1440 units in the monovalent regimen). The average GMTs of anti-HBsAg measured 1 month after completion of the vaccine series was 2099 mIU/mL in vaccinees who received the fixed-combination vaccine versus 1871 mIU/mL in vaccinees who received both monovalent vaccines.

When an accelerated dosage regimen of Twinrix® was used (doses at 0, 7, and 21–30 days and a booster dose at 12 months) in healthy adults, the seroprotection rate for HBV and seroconversion rate for HAV at month 13 was noninferior to the rates reported with monovalent hepatitis A virus vaccine inactivated (Havrix®) and monovalent hepatitis B vaccine (Engerix-B®) administered at separate sites (i.e., Havrix® at 1 and 12 months and Engerix-B® at 0, 1, 2, and 12 months). On day 37 (after 3 doses of Twinrix®), the seroprotection rate for HBV was 63.2% compared with 43.5% in the control group who had received 2 doses of Engerix-B®; the HAV seroconversion rates were similar in both groups (98.5 or 98.6%, respectively). On day 90, the seroprotection rate for HBV was 83.2% in the Twinrix® group and 76.7% in the control group; the HAV seroconversion rate was 100 or 95.6%, respectively. At month 12 (before the booster dose of Twinrix®), the seroprotection rate for HBV was 82.1% in the Twinrix® group and 77.8% in the control group; HAV seroconversion rates were 96.9 or 86.9%, respectively.

DTaP-HepB-IPV (Pediarix®) Following a 3-dose series of the fixed-combination vaccine containing diphtheria, tetanus, pertussis, hepatitis B, and poliovirus antigens (DTaP-HepB-IPV; Pediarix®), the immunologic response generally is similar to that reported following 3 primary doses of separately administered Infanrix®, Engerix-B®, and inactivated poliovirus vaccine (IPV).

■ **Duration of Immunity** The duration of protection from HBV infection following administration of hepatitis B vaccine and the need for additional booster doses of the vaccine have not yet been fully defined. In one study in adults, anti-HBs levels 1.5 years after administration of a series of 3 doses of hepatitis B vaccine reportedly had decreased to less than the minimum protective level in 24% of those who received 20-mcg doses and 48% of those who received 10-mcg doses of the vaccine.

There is some evidence from long-term follow-up of vaccine recipients that immunologic memory may persist for at least 10–20 years in individuals who respond to hepatitis B vaccine, and that maintenance of detectable anti-HBs levels may not be necessary to protect these individuals against clinically important breakthrough infections. Because immunologic memory may confer protection, it has been suggested that booster doses of vaccine may not be necessary in immunocompetent individuals even if antibody titers decline after vaccination. Subsequent exposure to HBV results in an anamnestic anti-HBs response that prevents clinically important HBV infection.

In 2 studies evaluating antibody persistence in healthy adults following a 3-dose series (at 0, 1, and 6 months) of the fixed-combination vaccine (Twinrix®) containing hepatitis A virus vaccine inactivated (Havrix®) and hepatitis B vaccine (Engerix-B®), anti-HAV and anti-HBsAg levels were maintained for at least 4 years.

Chemistry and Stability

■ **Chemistry**

Hepatitis B Vaccine (Recombinant) Monovalent hepatitis B vaccine is commercially available in the US as Recombivax HB® and Engerix-B®. Both Recombivax HB® and Engerix-B® contain hepatitis B surface antigen (HBsAg) prepared using yeast cells (*Saccharomyces cerevisiae*) and recombinant DNA technology. These vaccines are available in several formulations containing different concentrations of HBsAg.

Each 1-mL dose of Engerix-B® Adult contains 20 mcg of HBsAg adsorbed onto 0.5 mg of aluminum (as aluminum hydroxide) and each 0.5-mL dose of Engerix-B® Pediatric/Adolescent contains 10 mcg of HBsAg adsorbed onto 0.25 mg of aluminum (as aluminum hydroxide). Engerix-B® Adult and Engerix-B® Pediatric/Adolescent are formulated without preservatives. Before shaking, Engerix-B® may occur as a fine white deposit with a clear colorless supernatant; after shaking, the vaccine occurs as a slightly turbid white suspension.

Each 1-mL dose of Recombivax HB® Adult Formulation contains 10 mcg of HBsAg; each 0.5-mL dose of Recombivax HB® Pediatric/Adolescent Formulation contains 5 mcg of HBsAg; and each 1-mL dose of Recombivax HB® Dialysis Formulation contains 40 mcg of HBsAg. In each formulation, the antigen is adsorbed onto approximately 0.5 mg of aluminum (as amorphous aluminum hydroxyphosphate sulfate) per mL of vaccine. Recombivax HB® preparations do not contain thimerosal or any other preservative. After shaking, Recombivax HB® occurs as a slightly opaque white suspension.

Combination Vaccines Containing Hepatitis B Vaccine and Other Antigens **DTaP-HepB-IPV (Pediarix®).** DTaP-HepB-IPV (Pediarix®) is a fixed-combination vaccine containing diphtheria, tetanus, pertussis, hepatitis B, and poliovirus antigens.

The hepatitis B antigen contained in Pediarix® is identical to that contained in Engerix-B® monovalent hepatitis B vaccine. The diphtheria, tetanus, and pertussis antigens are identical to those contained in Infanrix® (DTaP) vaccine. For information on these DTaP antigens, see Diphtheria and Tetanus Toxoids and Acellular Pertussis Vaccine Adsorbed/Tetanus Toxoid and Reduced Diphtheria Toxoid and Acellular Pertussis Vaccine Adsorbed 80:08. The poliovirus antigens contained in Pediarix® are similar to those contained in the commercially available monovalent IPV vaccine. For information on the poliovirus antigens, see Poliovirus Vaccine Inactivated 80:12.

After vigorous shaking, Pediarix® appears as a homogeneous, turbid, white suspension. Each 0.5-mL dose of Pediarix® is formulated to contain 25 Lf of diphtheria toxoid, 10 Lf of tetanus toxoid, 58 mcg of pertussis antigens, 10 mcg of HBsAg, 40 D-antigen units (DU) of Type 1 poliovirus, 8 DU of Type 2 poliovirus, and 32 DU of Type 3 poliovirus. Each 0.5 mL of Pediarix® contains 4.5 mg of sodium chloride, not more than 0.85 mg of aluminum adjuvant, not more than 100 mcg of polysorbate 80, and not more than 100 mcg of residual formaldehyde. Although neomycin sulfate and polymyxin B are used in the manufacturing process of the poliovirus antigen component, Pediarix® contains no more than 0.05 and 0.01 ng, respectively, of these anti-infectives per dose. No more than 5% yeast protein may be present in Pediarix® as part of the hepatitis B antigen component. Pediarix® does not contain thimerosal or any other preservatives.

Hib-HepB (Comvax®) Hib-HepB (Comvax®) is a fixed-combination vaccine containing Hib and hepatitis B antigens.

The antigens used to produce Comvax® are the same as those used to produce PedvaxHIB® monovalent Hib vaccine and Recombivax HB® monovalent hepatitis B vaccine. Each antigenic component is prepared separately and then pooled to form the fixed-combination vaccine. After thorough agitation, the vaccine appears as a slightly opaque, white suspension.

Each 0.5-mL dose of Comvax® contains 7.5 mcg of purified Hib capsular polysaccharide conjugated to approximately 125 mcg of *Neisseria meningitidis* outer membrane protein complex (OMPC), 5 mcg of HBsAg), approximately 225 mcg of aluminum (as amorphous aluminum hydroxyphosphate sulfate), and 35 mcg sodium borate (decahydrate) as a pH stabilizer in 0.9% sodium chloride. Comvax® does not contain thimerosal or any other preservative.

HepA-HepB (Twinrix®) HepA-HepB (Twinrix®) is a fixed-combination vaccine that contains both hepatitis A and hepatitis B antigens. Twinrix® is a sterile suspension containing the antigenic components used to produce Havrix® monovalent hepatitis A virus vaccine inactivated and Engerix-B® monovalent hepatitis B vaccine. Each antigenic component is adsorbed separately onto aluminum phosphate or aluminum hydroxide and then pooled to form the fixed-combination vaccine.

Following thorough agitation, Twinrix® appears as a homogeneous, turbid, white suspension. Each 1-mL dose of Twinrix® contains 720 units of hepatitis A viral antigen and 20 mcg of HBsAg and also contains 0.45 mg of aluminum (as aluminum hydroxide and aluminum phosphate). Each 1-mL dose of the vaccine also contains residual MRC-5 cellular (not exceeding 2.5 mcg), yeast proteins (not exceeding 50 mg), trace amounts of formaldehyde (not exceeding 0.1 mg), trace amounts of neomycin sulfate (not exceeding 0.02 mcg), and amino acids in a phosphate-buffered saline solution with polysorbate (Tween®) 20. Twinrix® does not contain thimerosal or any other preservatives. The vaccine has a pH of 5.8–6.6.

■ **Stability** ***Hepatitis B Vaccine (Recombinant)*** Monovalent hepatitis B vaccine (Engerix-B®, Recombivax HB®) should be refrigerated at 2–8°C; storage above or below this temperature may reduce potency. Freezing of the vaccine results in a substantial decrease in potency and must be avoided. If freezing occurs, the vaccine should be discarded.

Combination Vaccines Containing Hepatitis B Vaccine and Other Antigens **DTaP-HepB-Hib (Pediarix®).** DTaP-HepB-Hib (Pediarix®) should be refrigerated at 2–8°C and should not be frozen. If freezing occurs, the vaccine should be discarded. Improper storage may result in formation of a gel-like substance and the vaccine should be discarded if this occurs.

Hib-HepB (Comvax®) Hib-HepB (Comvax®) should be refrigerated at 2–8°C and should not be frozen.

HepA-HepB (Twinrix®) HepA-HepB (Twinrix®) should be refrigerated at 2–8°C and should not be frozen; if freezing occurs, the vaccine should be discarded. When stored as recommended, the vaccine has an expiration date of 3 years after the date of manufacture.

Preparations

Excipients in commercially available drug preparations may have clinically important effects in some individuals; consult specific product labeling for details.

Hepatitis B Vaccine (Recombinant)

Parenteral		
Injectable suspension	5 mcg (of hepatitis B surface antigen) per 0.5 mL	**Recombivax HB® Pediatric/ Adolescent Formulation,** Merck
	10 mcg (of hepatitis B surface antigen) per mL	**Recombivax HB® Adult Formulation,** Merck
	10 mcg (of hepatitis B surface antigen) per 0.5 mL	**Engerix-B® Pediatric/ Adolescent Formulation,** GlaxoSmithKline
	20 mcg (of hepatitis B surface antigen) per mL	**Engerix-B® Adult Formulation,** GlaxoSmithKline
	40 mcg (of hepatitis B surface antigen) per mL	**Recombivax HB® Dialysis Formulation,** Merck

Diphtheria and Tetanus Toxoids and Acellular Pertussis Adsorbed, Hepatitis B (Recombinant) and Inactivated Poliovirus Vaccine Combined (DTaP-HepB-IPV)

Parenteral		
Injectable suspension, for IM use	Diphtheria Toxoid 25 Lf units, Tetanus Toxoid 10 Lf units, Acellular Pertussis Vaccine 58 mcg (of pertussis antigen), Hepatitis B Surface Antigen 10 mcg, Poliovirus Type 1 40 DU, Poliovirus Type 2 8 DU, and Poliovirus type 3 32 DU per 0.5 mL	**Pediarix®,** GlaxoSmithKline

Haemophilus b Conjugate (Meningococcal Protein Conjugate) and Hepatitis B (Recombinant) Vaccine (Hib-HepB)

Parenteral		
Injectable suspension, for IM use	Haemophilus b Capsular Polysaccharide 7.5 mcg/0.5 mL, *Neisseria meningitidis* OMPC 125 mcg/0.5 mL, and Hepatitis B Vaccine 5 mcg (of hepatitis B surface antigen) per 0.5 mL	**Comvax®,** Merck

Hepatitis A Inactivated and Hepatitis B (Recombinant) Vaccine (HepA-HepB)

Parenteral		
Injectable suspension, for IM use	Hepatitis A Virus Vaccine Inactivated 720 ELISA units (of viral antigen) and Hepatitis B Vaccine (Recombinant) 20 mcg (of hepatitis B surface antigen) per mL	**Twinrix®,** GlaxoSmithKline

†Use is not currently included in the labeling approved by the US Food and Drug Administration

Human Papillomavirus Vaccine

HPV Nonavalent Recombinant Vaccine, HPV Vaccine, Human Papillomavirus Vaccine (9-valent), Human Papillomavirus Vaccine (Nonavalent), 9-valent Human Papillomavirus (Types 6, 11, 16, 18, 31, 33, 45, 52, 58) Recombinant Vaccine, 9vHPV

■ Human papillomavirus (HPV) vaccine is an inactivated (recombinant) virus vaccine containing virus-like particles (VLPs) of the major capsid (L1) proteins of certain HPV types and is used to stimulate active immunity to the HPV serotypes represented in the vaccine. HPV vaccine is commercially available in the US as human papillomavirus 9-valent vaccine recombinant (9vHPV) containing VLPs of HPV types 6, 11, 16, 18, 31, 33, 45, 52, and 58. Other HPV vaccines (human papillomavirus quadrivalent vaccine [4vHPV], human papillomavirus bivalent vaccine [2vHPV]) are no longer available in the US.

Uses

■ **Prevention of Disease Caused by Human Papillomavirus (HPV)** Human papillomavirus 9-valent vaccine recombinant (9vHPV) is used in individuals 9 through 45 years of age to prevent disease caused by HPV types represented in the vaccine.

Anogenital HPV is the most common sexually transmitted infection in the US. Approximately 79 million individuals in the US are already infected with anogenital HPV, and approximately 14 million more become infected each year (about 50% of these cases are occurring in adolescents and young adults 15 through 24 years of age). More than 150 HPV types have been identified and about 40 of these can cause anogenital infections. Although most HPV infections are asymptomatic and resolve spontaneously within 1–2 years without causing clinical disease or complications, some HPV types cause anogenital warts (condyloma acuminata) and benign or low-grade cervical cell abnormalities and other HPV types are associated with persistent anogenital infections, dysplastic lesions, and development of cervical and other anogenital cancers. HPV types have been categorized according to their epidemiologic association with cervical cancer. Low-risk (nononcogenic) types (e.g., HPV types 6 and 11) can cause genital warts, benign or low-grade cervical cell changes, recurrent respiratory papillomatosis, and conjunctival papillomas. High-risk (oncogenic) types (e.g., HPV types 16, 18, 31, 33, 35, 39, 45, 51, 52, 56, 58, 59, 66, 68) have the potential to act as carcinogens and can cause low-grade cervical cell abnormalities or high-grade cervical cell abnormalities that are precursors to cervical cancer and other anogenital cancers, including cancer of the vulva, vagina, penis, and anus, and cancer of the oropharynx. Essentially all cervical cancers are caused by high-risk HPV types, and the majority of these cancers (about 70%) are caused by HPV types 16 and 18.

9vHPV contains antigens representing 7 high-risk (oncogenic) types (HPV types 16, 18, 31, 33, 45, 52, and 58) and 2 low-risk types (HPV 6 and 11). 9vHPV is used in *females* 9 through 45 years of age to prevent cervical, vulvar, vaginal, and anal cancer caused by HPV types 16, 18, 31, 33, 45, 52, and 58 and to prevent precancerous or dysplastic lesions caused by HPV types 6, 11, 16, 18, 31, 33, 45, 52, and 58, including cervical intraepithelial neoplasia (CIN) grades 1 and 2/3, cervical adenocarcinoma in situ (AIS), vulvar intraepithelial neoplasia (VIN) grades 2 and 3, vaginal intraepithelial neoplasia (VaIN) grades 2 and 3, and anal intraepithelial neoplasia (AIN) grades 1, 2, and 3. In *males* 9 through 45 years of age, 9vHPV is used to prevent anal cancer caused by HPV types 16, 18, 31, 33, 45, 52, and 58 and to prevent precancerous or dysplastic lesions caused by HPV types 6, 11, 16, 18, 31, 33, 45, 52, and 58, including AIN grades 1, 2, and 3. In addition, 9vHPV is used in *females* and *males* 9 through 45 years of age to prevent genital warts (condyloma acuminata) caused by HPV types 6 and 11.

HPV vaccine does *not* prevent infection or disease caused by HPV types not represented in the vaccine and will *not* prevent non-HPV related cervical disease.

HPV vaccine does *not* prevent disease caused by HPV types that vaccinees already are infected with (i.e., polymerase chain reaction [PCR] positive and/or seropositive prior to vaccination), but may prevent certain diseases caused by the vaccine HPV types that vaccinees have not already acquired.

HPV vaccine is *not* used for the *treatment* of active genital warts and is *not* used for the *treatment* of precancerous or dysplastic genital lesions (i.e., AIN, CIN, VIN, VaIN) or cervical, vulvar, vaginal, or anal cancer. There is no evidence that HPV vaccination provides any therapeutic effect for existing HPV infections, HPV-associated precancerous lesions, cancer, or anogenital warts.

The US Centers for Disease Control and Prevention (CDC) Advisory Committee on Immunization Practices (ACIP), American Academy of Pediatrics (AAP), American Academy of Family Physicians (AAFP), American College of Obstetricians and Gynecologists (ACOG), and other experts recommend that all *females* and *males* 9 through 26 years of age receive *routine* and catch-up immunization with 9vHPV.

ACIP states that *routine* and catch-up vaccination with 9vHPV is recommended for *females* and *males* 9 through 26 years of age with primary or secondary immunocompromising conditions that might reduce cell-mediated or humoral immunity (e.g., B-lymphocyte antibody deficiencies, T-lymphocyte complete or partial defects, human immunodeficiency virus [HIV] infection, malignant neoplasms, transplantation, autoimmune disease, immunosuppressive therapy).

ACIP states that decisions regarding use of 9vHPV in *females* and *males* 27 through 45 years of age should be based on shared clinical decision-making and discussion between the patient and clinician regarding the benefits and risks of the vaccine.

The first dose of HPV vaccine usually should be given at 11 through 12 years of age, although the first dose can be given to individuals as young as 9 years of age. ACIP and other experts recommend *routine* immunization in individuals as young as 9 years of age when sexual abuse or sexual assault is suspected. Ideally, HPV vaccination should be completed before potential exposure to HPV occurs through sexual activity; however, age-appropriate individuals who are sexually active and may have already been exposed to HPV should still be vaccinated when indicated. Although sexually active individuals who have not been infected with any of the HPV types contained in the vaccine receive the full benefit of vaccination, vaccination may still be beneficial for those who have already been infected with one or more of the vaccine HPV types.

When routine or catch-up vaccination is initiated in immunocompetent individuals 9 through 14 years of age, ACIP, AAP, and other experts recommend a 2-dose regimen of 9vHPV. When primary or catch-up vaccination is initiated in immunocompetent individuals 15 through 26 years of age, these experts recommend a 3-dose regimen of 9vHPV. Because response to vaccination may be reduced in immunocompromised individuals, a 3-dose regimen of 9vHPV should be used for routine or catch-up vaccination in such individuals, regardless of age. (See Dosage and Administration: Dosage.)

9vHPV can be used to continue or complete the HPV vaccination series in individuals who previously received 1 or more doses of an HPV vaccine that is no longer available in the US (human papillomavirus quadrivalent vaccine [4vHPV], human papillomavirus bivalent vaccine [2vHPV]). ACIP states that individuals who initiated HPV vaccination prior to 15 years of age and received 2 doses of *any* HPV vaccine administered at the recommended dosage schedule (i.e., 0 and 6–12 months) or received 3 doses of *any* HPV vaccine administered at the recommended dosage schedule (i.e., 0, 1–2, and 6 months) are considered adequately vaccinated. Individuals who initiated HPV vaccination at 15 years of age or older and received 3 doses of *any* HPV vaccine administered at the recommended dosage schedule (i.e., 0, 1–2, and 6 months) also are considered adequately vaccinated. ACIP has made no recommendations to date regarding additional vaccination with 9vHPV in individuals considered adequately vaccinated with 4vHPV or 2vHPV.

Prevaccination HPV testing or screening (e.g., Papanicolaou [Pap] testing or screening for high-risk HPV DNA, type-specific HPV DNA tests, HPV antibody test) is *not* needed and is *not* recommended in any individuals. HPV vaccine can be administered regardless of history of anogenital warts, abnormal Pap or HPV tests, or anogenital precancer.

HPV vaccination does not eliminate the necessity for routine cervical cancer screening. Women vaccinated against HPV should continue to receive routine cervical cancer screening according to current guidelines for such testing and men and women vaccinated against HPV should continue to receive anal cancer screening if recommended by their health-care provider. In addition, all vaccine recipients should continue to adhere to behaviors that help avoid HPV exposures (e.g., sexual abstinence, monogamy, limited number of sexual partners, use of condoms).

Clinical Experience **Females and Males 9 through 14 Years of Age (2-Dose Regimen).** Efficacy of 9vHPV given in a 2-dose series in individuals 9 through 14 years of age is inferred from immunogenicity data. In a randomized, parallel-group study, immunogenicity of 9vHPV given in a 2-dose series (second dose given at 6 or 12 months after the first dose) to females and males 9 through 14 years of age was compared with immunogenicity of 9vHPV given in a 3-dose series (second and third doses given 2 and 6 months, respectively, after the first dose) in females 16 through 26 years of age. For all 9 HPV types contained in the vaccine, the immune response 1 month after the last dose in females and males 9 through 14 years of age who received 2 doses of the vaccine was noninferior to that in females 16 through 26 years of age who received 3 doses of the vaccine. More than 98% of individuals enrolled in the study had an antibody response (seroconversion) to each of the 9 HPV types contained in the vaccine by 1 month after completion of the 2- or 3-dose vaccination series. In addition, geometric mean titers (GMTs) of antibodies to the 9 HPV vaccine types that were attained in individuals who received the 2-dose vaccination series were noninferior to GMTs attained in those who received the 3-dose vaccination series.

Females 9 through 15 Years of Age (3-Dose Regimen). Efficacy of 9vHPV given in a 3-dose series in females 9 through 15 years of age is inferred from immunogenicity data. In one study, 600 females 9 through 15 years of age were randomized to receive 9vHPV or 4vHPV (no longer available in the US). Results from this study indicate that 99.7% of females 9 through 15 years of age who received a 3-dose regimen of 9vHPV became seropositive for antibodies to HPV types 6, 11, 16, and 18 by 1 month after dose 3 and GMTs of these antibodies attained in this age group were noninferior to those attained in females 9 through 15 years of age who received 4vHPV. In another immunogenicity study, females 9 through 15 years of age who received a 3-dose regimen of 9vHPV became seropositive for antibodies to HPV types 6, 11, 16, 18, 31, 33, 45, 52, and 58 by 1 month after dose 3 and GMTs of these antibodies attained in this age group were noninferior to those attained in females 16–26 years of age for which positive efficacy data exist (i.e., immunogenicity bridging). Results from this study indicate that GMTs of these antibodies 1 month after the third vaccine dose range from approximately 708–6934 mMU/mL in those 9 through 15 years of age, and results of immunogenicity studies in females 16–26 years of age indicate that GMTs of these antibodies range from approximately 272–3523 mMU/mL in this older group.

Males 9 through 15 Years of Age (3-Dose Regimen). Efficacy of 9vHPV given in a 3-dose series in males 9 through 15 years of age is inferred based on evidence that more than 99% of males 9 through 15 years of age became seropositive for antibodies to HPV types 6, 11, 16, 18, 31, 33, 45, 52, and 58 by 1 month after the third vaccine dose and GMTs of these antibodies attained in this age group are noninferior to those attained in females 16 through 26 years of age for which positive efficacy data exist (i.e., immunogenicity bridging). Immunogenicity studies in males 9 through 15 years of age indicate that GMTs of these antibodies 1 month after the third vaccine dose range from 912–8683 mMU/mL in this age group.

Females 16 through 26 Years of Age (3-Dose Regimen). Safety and efficacy of 9vHPV for the prevention of disease caused by HPV types 6, 11, 16, 18, 31, 33, 45, 52, and 58 have been evaluated in a double-blind, randomized, active comparator-controlled study in 14,204 women 16 through 26 years of age at the time of enrollment (mean: 19.4–24.4 years of age) in the US and other countries. Study participants were randomized to receive a 3-dose series of either 9vHPV or 4vHPV (no longer available in the US). The second and third vaccine doses were given 2 and 6 months, respectively, after the first dose and the median duration of follow-up was 3.3 years. The prophylactic efficacy analysis was based on clinical endpoints including CIN (any grade including 2/3), AIS, VIN (any grade), VaIN (any grade), cervical carcinoma, vulvar cancer, or vaginal cancer related to HPV types 31, 33, 45, 52, and 58. The per-protocol efficacy (PPE) population consisted of those who completed the 3-dose vaccine series within 1 year of enrollment, did not have major study protocol deviations, and were naive (seronegative and cervicovaginal specimens PCR negative) to the relevant vaccine HPV types when tested prior to the first vaccine dose and at 1 month after the third dose.

Results from the efficacy analysis indicate that 9vHPV was effective in preventing HPV disease caused by HPV types 31, 33, 45, 52, and 58 in individuals who were seronegative and PCR negative to these HPV types at baseline. In the PPE population, the vaccine was 96.7% effective in preventing CIN 2/3, AIS, VIN 2/3, VaIN 2/3, cervical cancer, vulvar cancer, or vaginal cancer related to HPV types 31, 33, 45, 52, and 58 and 98.6% effective in preventing CIN 1 related to HPV types 31, 33, 45, 52, and 58.

Efficacy of 9vHPV for the prevention of disease caused by HPV types 6, 11, 16, and 18, including genital warts, CIN (any grade including 2/3), AIS, VIN (any grade), and VaIN (any grade), is inferred from immunogenicity data. Efficacy of the vaccine is based on evidence that 99.7% of females 16 through 26 years of age who received 9vHPV become seropositive for antibodies to HPV types 6, 11, 16, and 18 by 1 month after dose 3 and the GMTs of these antibodies attained in this age group were noninferior to those attained in females 16 through 26 years of age who received 4vHPV and for which positive efficacy data exist (i.e., immunogenicity bridging).

Data indicate that 9vHPV was effective only against the HPV types represented in the vaccine and only when given prior to infection by these types. Women already infected with one or more vaccine-related HPV types prior to vaccination were protected from disease caused by the remaining vaccine HPV types to which they were naive (PCR negative and seronegative).

Efficacy of 9vHPV for the prevention of anal HPV infection, AIN, and anal cancer was not studied in women, but efficacy of the vaccine against anal disease caused by HPV types 6, 11, 16, and 18 is inferred from data in males.

Males 16 through 26 Years of Age (3-Dose Regimen). Efficacy of 9vHPV for the prevention of disease caused by HPV types 6, 11, 16, 18, 31, 33, 45, 52, and 58 in males 16 through 26 years of age is inferred based on evidence from an open-label study that included males and females 16 through 26 years of age who received 9vHPV in a 3-dose series (second and third dose given 2 and 6 months, respectively, after first dose). Results from this study demonstrated that the immune response observed in males 16 through 26 years of age after the third vaccine dose was noninferior to that observed in females 16 through 26 years of age for which positive efficacy data exist (i.e., immunogenicity bridging). More than 99% of males and females 16 through 26 years of age became seropositive for antibodies to HPV types 6, 11, 16, 18, 31, 33, 45, 52, and 58.

Females 27 through 45 Years of Age (3-Dose Regimen). Efficacy and safety of 4vHPV in females 27 through 45 years of age are relevant to use of 9vHPV in females in this age group. Efficacy of 4vHPV for the prevention of HPV disease in females 27 through 45 years of age has been evaluated in a clinical trial that included a base study and a long-term study extension. A total of 3253 females in this age group were randomized 1:1 to receive 4vHPV or the preformed aluminum-containing adjuvant used in the vaccine (amorphous aluminum hydroxyphosphate sulfate [AAHS]) given in a 3-dose series. Efficacy was based on a combined end point of persistent HPV type 6, 11, 16, or 18 infection, genital warts, vulvar and vaginal dysplastic lesions of any grade, CIN of any grade, AIS, and cervical cancer. The PPE population consisted of those who completed the 3-dose series of 4vHPV within 1 year of enrollment, did not have major deviations from the study protocol, and were naive (PCR negative and seronegative) to HPV types 6, 11, 16, and 18 prior to the first vaccine dose through month 7 (1 month after the third dose).

In the base study (median follow-up duration of 3.5 years after the third vaccine dose), efficacy of 4vHPV against the combined incidence of HPV 6-, 11-, 16-, and 18-related persistent infection, genital warts, VIN, VaIN, vulvar cancer, vaginal cancer, cervical dysplasia (any grade CIN), AIS, and cervical cancer was 87.7% in the PPE population. The efficacy estimate for the combined end point was driven principally by prevention of persistent infection. Efficacy of 4vHPV against the combined incidence of HPV 6-, 11-, 16-, and 18-related genital warts or cervical dysplasia was 95% in the PPE population. Data from the base study did not demonstrate statistically significant efficacy of 4vHPV for the prevention of CIN 2/3, AIS, or cervical cancer related to HPV types 16 and 18; however, CIN 2/3 was observed in 1 individual in the 4vHPV group (tested positive by PCR for HPV 16 and HPV 51) compared with 5 cases in the placebo group.

In the long-term extension of this study (median follow-up duration of 8.9 years after the third vaccine dose), 600 study participants who had been randomized to receive 4vHPV in the base study were monitored for HPV 6-, 11-, 16-, and 18-related genital warts or cervical dysplasia. No cases of HPV 6-, 11-, 16-, or 18-related CIN (any grade) or genital warts were observed in the PPE population during the long-term extension phase.

Males 27 through 45 Years of Age (3-Dose Regimen). Efficacy and safety of 4vHPV in males 27 through 45 years of age are relevant to use of 9vHPV in males in this age group. Efficacy of 4vHPV for the prevention of HPV disease in males 27 through 45 years of age is inferred from efficacy data from the clinical trial in females 27 through 45 years of age and is supported by immunogenicity data from a clinical trial that included 150 males 27 through 45 years of age who received a 3-dose regimen of 4vHPV (second and third doses given 2 and 6 months, respectively, after the first dose). In addition, results of a cross-study analysis of per-protocol immunogenicity populations that compared HPV 6, 11, 16, and 18 GMTs at month 7 in males 27 through 45 years of age (study A) to GMTs in males 16 through 26 years of age in whom efficacy of 4vHPV had been established (study B) indicated that GMT ratios (study A/study B) for antibodies to HPV 6, 11, 16, and 18 were 0.82, 0.79, 0.91, and 0.74, respectively.

Dosage and Administration

■ Administration

Human papillomavirus 9-valent vaccine recombinant (9vHPV) is administered by IM injection. The vaccine should *not* be administered IV, subcutaneously, or intradermally.

Syncope (vasovagal or vasodepressor reaction; fainting) may occur following vaccination; such reactions may be accompanied by transient neurologic signs (e.g., tonic-clonic limb movements). Syncope occurs most frequently in adolescents and young adults. Procedures should be in place to avoid falling injury and to restore cerebral perfusion following syncope. Syncope and secondary injuries may be averted if vaccinees sit or lie down during and for 15 minutes after vaccination. If syncope occurs, the patient should be observed until symptoms resolve.

9vHPV may be given simultaneously with other age-appropriate vaccines. (See Drug Interactions: Vaccines.) When multiple vaccines are administered during a single health-care visit, each parenteral vaccine should be given using separate syringes and different injection sites. Injection sites should be separated by at least 1 inch (if anatomically feasible) to allow appropriate attribution of any local adverse effects that may occur.

IM Administration

IM injections of 9vHPV should be made in the deltoid region of the upper arm or anterolateral aspect of the upper thigh.

To ensure delivery of vaccine into muscle, IM injections should be made at a 90° angle to the skin using a needle length appropriate for the individual's age and body mass, thickness of adipose tissue and muscle at the injection site, and injection technique. Anatomic variability, especially in the deltoid, should be considered and clinical judgment should be used to avoid inadvertent underpenetration or overpenetration of muscle.

Immediately prior to administration, 9vHPV should be shaken well to obtain a uniform, cloudy, white suspension. The vaccine should be discarded if it contains particulates, appears discolored, or cannot be resuspended with thorough agitation.

9vHPV should *not* be diluted and should *not* be mixed with any other vaccine or solution.

9vHPV is provided in 0.5-mL single-dose vials or single-dose prefilled syringes. The vaccine does not contain thimerosal or any other preservatives.

9vHPV should be stored at 2–8°C and protected from light and freezing. The vaccine should be administered as soon as possible after removal from refrigeration, but can be used if kept at temperatures between 8–25°C for no more than 72 hours.

■ Dosage

The dosage schedule (i.e., number of doses) for 9vHPV is based on age at the time the first dose is administered and the immunocompetence of the vaccinee. The manufacturer recommends a 2- or 3-dose series if HPV vaccination is initiated at 9 through 14 years of age and a 3-dose series if HPV vaccination is initiated at 15 through 45 years of age. The US Centers for Disease Control and Prevention (CDC) Advisory Committee on Immunization Practices (ACIP), American Academy of Pediatrics (AAP), and other experts recommend a 2-dose series if initiated at 9 through 14 years of age and a 3-dose series if initiated at 15 through 45 years of age; these experts recommend that a 3-dose series of HPV vaccine be used in all immunocompromised individuals 9 years of age or older.

If interruptions occur resulting in an interval between doses longer than recommended, there is no need to start the vaccination series over.

An accelerated schedule for the HPV vaccination series (i.e., using intervals between doses shorter than recommended) should *not* be used.

Pediatric Dosage

Females and Males 9 through 14 Years of Age. 9vHPV is administered IM in 0.5-mL doses.

If a 2-dose regimen of 9vHPV is used for routine or catch-up immunization in individuals 9 through 14 years of age, the manufacturer recommends that the second dose be given 6–12 months after the first dose (i.e., 0 and 6–12 months); if the second dose is given earlier than 5 months after the first dose, a third dose should be given at least 4 months after the second dose. If a 3-dose regimen is used in this age group, the manufacturer recommends that the second dose be given 2 months after the first dose and that the third dose be given 6 months after the first dose (i.e., 0, 2, and 6 months).

For routine or catch-up vaccination in *immunocompetent* individuals 9 through 14 years of age, ACIP, AAP, and other experts recommend that a 2-dose regimen of 9vHPV be used. These experts recommend that the first dose be given at 11 through 12 years of age (but may be given as early as 9 years of age) and that the second dose be given 6–12 months after the first dose (i.e., 0 and 6–12 months). The minimum interval between the first and second doses is 5 months; if the second dose is given earlier than 5 months after the first dose, ACIP, AAP, and other experts recommend that a third dose be given at least 12 weeks after the second dose and at least 5 months after the first dose.

For routine or catch-up vaccination in *immunocompromised* individuals 9 through 14 years of age, ACIP, AAP, and other experts recommend that a 3-dose regimen of 9vHPV be used. The second dose should be given 1–2 months after the first dose and the third dose should be given 6 months after the first dose (i.e., 0, 1–2, and 6 months). The minimum interval between the first and second doses is 4 weeks; the minimum intervals for the third dose are 12 weeks after the second dose and 5 months after the first dose.

9vHPV can be used to continue or complete the vaccination series in individuals who previously received 1 or more doses of an HPV vaccine that is no longer available in the US (human papillomavirus quadrivalent vaccine [4vHPV], human papillomavirus bivalent vaccine [2vHPV]). ACIP states that individuals are considered adequately vaccinated if the HPV series was initiated prior to 15 years of age and a 2- or 3-dose regimen of *any* HPV vaccine (9vHPV, 4vHPV, or 2vHPV) was given using recommended dosage schedules.

Females and Males 15 through 18 Years of Age. 9vHPV is administered IM in 0.5-mL doses.

For routine or catch-up vaccination in *immunocompetent* or *immunocompromised* individuals 15 through 18 years of age, the manufacturer, ACIP, AAP, and other experts recommend a 3-dose regimen of 9vHPV. The second dose should be given 1–2 months after the first dose and the third dose should be given 6 months after the first dose (i.e., 0, 1–2, and 6 months). The minimum interval between the first and second doses is 4 weeks; the minimum intervals for the third dose are 12 weeks after the second dose and 5 months after the first dose.

9vHPV can be used to continue or complete the vaccination series in individuals who previously received 1 or more doses of an HPV vaccine that is no longer available in the US (4vHPV, 2vHPV). ACIP states that individuals are considered adequately vaccinated if the HPV series was initiated at 15 years of age or older and a 3-dose regimen of *any* HPV vaccine (9vHPV, 4vHPV, or 2vHPV) was given using recommended dosage schedules.

Adult Dosage

Females and Males 19 through 45 Years of age. 9vHPV is administered IM in 0.5-mL doses.

For routine or catch-up vaccination in *immunocompetent* or *immunocompromised* individuals 19 through 45 years of age, a 3-dose regimen of 9vHPV is recommended. The second dose should be given 1–2 months after the first dose and the third dose should be given 6 months after the first dose (i.e., 0, 1–2, and 6 months). The minimum interval between the first and second doses is 4 weeks; the minimum intervals for the third dose are 12 weeks after the second dose and 5 months after the first dose.

9vHPV can be used to continue or complete the vaccination series in individuals who previously received 1 or more doses of an HPV vaccine that is no longer available in the US (4vHPV, 2vHPV). ACIP states that individuals are considered adequately vaccinated if the HPV series was initiated at 15 years of age or older and a 3-dose regimen of *any* HPV vaccine (9vHPV, 4vHPV, or 2vHPV) was given using recommended dosage schedules.

Cautions

■ Contraindications

Human papillomavirus 9-valent vaccine recombinant (9vHPV) is contraindicated in individuals with hypersensitivity to any vaccine component (including severe allergic reactions to yeast) or hypersensitivity following a previous dose of HPV vaccine.

■ Warnings/Precautions

Sensitivity Reactions

Hypersensitivity Reactions. There have been postmarketing reports of hypersensitivity reactions (e.g., anaphylactic/anaphylactoid reactions, bronchospasm, urticaria, angioedema, generalized rash, erythema multiforme) after administration of HPV vaccine.

Most reported cases of anaphylaxis occurred following the first dose in the HPV vaccination series. In an Australian vaccination program in adolescents and women 12–26 years of age, the rate of anaphylaxis following HPV vaccination was 2.6 cases per 100,000 doses.

The cause of hypersensitivity reactions following administration of HPV vaccine is unclear. When sensitivity tests were performed in individuals who had suspected anaphylaxis following a dose of HPV vaccine, skin prick or intradermal tests using the vaccine, yeast, or polysorbate 80 generally were negative. However, at least one patient had a positive intradermal test that was consistent with IgE-mediated hypersensitivity.

Appropriate medical treatment should be readily available in case an anaphylactic reaction occurs following administration of HPV vaccine.

Yeast Allergy. 9vHPV is manufactured using fermentation cultures of a recombinant strain of *Saccharomyces cerevisiae* (yeast); each dose contains less than 7 mcg of yeast protein.

Data from the Vaccine Adverse Event Reporting System (VAERS) indicate that recombinant yeast-derived vaccines pose a minimal risk for anaphylactic reactions in individuals with a history of allergic reactions to yeast.

Syncope Syncope, sometimes associated with tonic-clonic movements and other seizure-like activity, has been reported following vaccination with HPV vaccine. Tonic-clonic movements are transient and typically respond to restoration of cerebral perfusion by maintaining vaccinee in a supine or Trendelenburg position. Syncope also has been reported with other vaccines and occurs most frequently in adolescents and young adults.

The vaccinee should be observed for 15 minutes following vaccination and procedures should be in place to avoid falling injury and restore cerebral perfusion if syncope occurs. (See Dosage and Administration: Administration.)

Individuals with Altered Immunocompetence Like other inactivated vaccines, HPV vaccine may be administered to individuals immunosuppressed as a result of disease (e.g., congenital immunodeficiency, human immunodeficiency virus [HIV] infection, hematologic or generalized malignancy, solid organ transplantation) or medical therapy. However, the immune response to the vaccine and efficacy may be reduced in these patients. (See Drug Interactions: Immunosuppressive Agents.) Immunosuppressed individuals should receive a 3-dose HPV vaccination series. (See Dosage and Administration: Dosage.)

Although data are not available regarding safety, efficacy, and immunogenicity in individuals with HIV infection, the US Centers for Disease Control and Prevention (CDC) Advisory Committee on Immunization Practices (ACIP), American Academy of Pediatrics (AAP), National Institutes of Health (NIH), HIV Medicine Association of the Infectious Diseases Society of America (IDSA), and other experts state that recommendations regarding use of HPV vaccine in HIV-infected individuals are the same as those for individuals who are not infected with HIV. However, HIV-infected individuals 9 through 26 years of age should receive a 3-dose HPV vaccination series.

Inactivated vaccines generally should be administered prior to initiation of immunosuppressive therapy or deferred until immunosuppressive therapy is discontinued. (See Drug Interactions: Immunosuppressive Agents.)

Concomitant Illness The decision whether to administer or delay vaccination in an individual with a current or recent acute illness depends on the severity of symptoms and etiology of the illness.

ACIP states that mild acute illness generally does not preclude vaccination. However, moderate or severe acute illness (with or without fever) is a precaution for vaccination and vaccines should be deferred until the individual has recovered from the acute phase of the illness. This precaution avoids superimposing adverse effects of the vaccine on the underlying illness or mistakenly concluding that a manifestation of the underlying illness resulted from vaccination.

Individuals with Bleeding Disorders Individuals who have bleeding disorders or are receiving anticoagulant therapy and/or their family members should be advised about the risk of hematoma from IM injections.

ACIP states that IM vaccines may be given to individuals who have bleeding disorders or are receiving anticoagulant therapy if a clinician familiar with the patient's bleeding risk determines that the vaccine can be administered IM with reasonable safety. In these cases, a fine needle (23 gauge or smaller) should be used to administer the vaccine, and firm pressure applied to the injection site (without rubbing) for at least 2 minutes. In individuals receiving therapy for hemophilia, IM vaccines can be scheduled for administration shortly after a dose of such therapy.

Limitations of Vaccine Effectiveness HPV vaccine may not protect all vaccine recipients against HPV infection.

Vaccination with HPV vaccine does not substitute for routine cervical cancer screening. Female recipients of HPV vaccine should continue to undergo cervical cancer screening (e.g., Papanicolaou [Pap] tests) according to current recommendations for such screening.

Male and female recipients of HPV vaccine should continue to undergo anal cancer screening if recommended by their health-care professional.

HPV vaccine does not provide protection against disease due to HPV types not represented in the vaccine and does not provide protection from vaccine and nonvaccine HPV types an individual has previously been exposed to through sexual activity.

HPV vaccine may be used in patients who have already become infected with HPV (including HPV types represented in the vaccine). Although the vaccine will not provide any beneficial effects in regard to preexisting HPV infections, it will provide protection against the vaccine HPV types that the vaccinee has not already acquired.

HPV vaccine is *not* used for *treatment* of active genital warts.

HPV vaccine is *not* used for *treatment* of precancerous or dysplastic lesions (e.g., anal intraepithelial neoplasia [AIN], cervical intraepithelial neoplasia [CIN], vulvar intraepithelial neoplasia [VIN], vaginal intraepithelial neoplasia [VaIN]) or cervical, vulvar, vaginal, or anal cancer.

Duration of Immunity The duration of immunity following a 2- or 3-dose vaccination series of HPV vaccine has not been fully determined.

Data to date suggest that a 3-dose regimen of HPV vaccine induces anti-HPV antibody levels that provide protection against HPV types represented in the vaccine for at least 10 years. A similar duration of protection is expected when a 2-dose regimen of HPV vaccine is used.

Improper Storage and Handling Improper storage or handling of vaccines may reduce vaccine potency resulting in reduced or inadequate immune response in vaccinees.

All vaccines should be inspected upon delivery and monitored during storage to ensure that the appropriate temperature is maintained. (See Dosage and Administration: Administration.)

Vaccine that has been mishandled or has not been stored at the recommended temperature should *not* be administered.

If there are concerns about mishandling, the manufacturer or state or local immunization or health departments should be contacted for guidance on whether the vaccine is usable.

Specific Populations **Pregnancy.** There are no adequate and well-controlled studies using 9vHPV in pregnant women. The manufacturer states that human data to date have not demonstrated any vaccine-associated risk of major birth defects and miscarriages when 9vHPV is administered during pregnancy.

ACIP, AAP, American College of Obstetricians and Gynecologists (ACOG), and other experts state that HPV vaccine is *not* recommended for use in pregnant women.

Although pregnancy testing is not needed before initiation of the HPV vaccination series, health-care providers should question sexually active individuals about the possibility of pregnancy. HPV vaccination should be deferred until pregnancy is completed. If a woman is found to be pregnant after the HPV vaccine series is initiated, ACIP, AAP, ACOG, and other experts state that no intervention is needed, but any remaining doses of the series should be deferred until after completion of the pregnancy.

To monitor pregnancy outcomes in women who receive 9vHPV during pregnancy, the manufacturer has established a pregnancy registry. Any exposure to 9vHPV that occurs around the time of conception or during pregnancy can be reported to the pregnancy registry at 800-986-8999.

Lactation. Data are insufficient to assess the effects of 9vHPV on the breast-fed infant or on milk production/excretion.

The manufacturer of 9vHPV states that the benefits of breast-feeding and the importance of the vaccine to the woman should be considered along with the potential adverse effects on the breast-fed child from the vaccine or from the underlying maternal condition (i.e., susceptibility to HPV infection).

ACIP states that inactivated vaccines do not pose any unusual risks for the mother or her breast-fed infant. These and other experts state that HPV vaccine may be administered to women who are breast-feeding.

Pediatric Use. Safety and efficacy of 9vHPV have not been established in females or males younger than 9 years of age.

Adults 27 through 64 Years of Age. Safety of 9vHPV in adults 27 through 45 years of age is inferred from safety data for human papillomavirus quadrivalent vaccine (4vHPV; no longer available in the US) in individuals 9 through 45 years of age and safety data for 9vHPV in individuals 9 through 26 years of age.

Safety and efficacy of 9vHPV have not been established in females or males 46 years of age or older.

Geriatric Use. Safety and efficacy of 9vHPV have not been established in females or males 65 years of age or older.

■ Common Adverse Effects

In *females* 9 through 26 years of age, the most common adverse reactions to 9vHPV are injection site reactions, including pain (89–90%), swelling (40–48%), erythema (34%), pruritus (4–6%), and hematoma (1–4%), and systemic reactions, including headache (11–15%), fever (5–7%), nausea (3–4%), dizziness (1–3%), fatigue (2%), and oropharyngeal pain (1–3%).

In *males* 9 through 26 years of age, the most common adverse reactions to 9vHPV are injection site reactions, including pain (63–72%), swelling (20–27%), erythema (21–25%), and hematoma (1%), and systemic reactions, including headache (7–9%), fever (2–9%), nausea (1%), dizziness (1%), and fatigue (1%).

Drug Interactions

■ Estrogens or Progestins

HPV vaccine has been used in women receiving hormonal contraceptives. The manufacturer of human papillomavirus 9-valent vaccine recombinant (9vHPV) states that use of hormonal contraceptives in women in clinical studies did not alter the immunologic response to the vaccine.

■ Immunosuppressive Agents

Individuals receiving immunosuppressive therapy (e.g., alkylating agents, antimetabolites, corticosteroids, radiation therapy) may have a diminished response to HPV vaccine.

The US Centers for Disease Control and Prevention (CDC) Advisory Committee on Immunization Practices (ACIP) and other experts state that age-appropriate patients who are immunocompromised either from disease or drug therapy may receive HPV vaccine; however, the immune response to the vaccine and vaccine efficacy may be decreased compared with that observed in immunocompetent vaccinees.

Inactivated vaccines generally should be administered at least 2 weeks prior to initiation of immunosuppressive therapy and, because of possible suboptimal response, should not be administered during immunosuppressive therapy and for certain periods of time after such therapy is discontinued. Because the intervals between discontinuance of immunosuppressive therapy and restoration of immune competence vary depending on the type and intensity of immunosuppressive therapy, underlying disease, and other factors, optimal timing for vaccine administration following discontinuance of immunosuppressive therapy has not been identified for every situation.

ACIP and the Infectious Diseases Society of America (IDSA) recommend that inactivated vaccines be administered at least 2 weeks before initiation of cancer chemotherapy or radiation therapy, if possible, and avoided during such therapy. Individuals vaccinated during or within 14 days of starting chemotherapy or radiation therapy should be considered unimmunized and should be revaccinated at least 3 months after such therapy is discontinued if immunocompetence has been restored.

Inactivated vaccines should be administered at least 2 weeks prior to treatment with anti-B-cell antibodies (e.g., rituximab). The optimal time to administer vaccines in patients who have received treatment with anti-B-cell antibodies is unclear. Some experts state that administration of inactivated vaccines should be deferred until at least 6 months after treatment with anti-B-cell antibodies has been discontinued.

Inactivated vaccines should be administered at least 2 weeks prior to initiation of therapy with certain other immunosuppressive biologic response modifiers (e.g., colony-stimulating factors, interleukins, tumor necrosis factor [TNF; TNF-α] blocking agents). Some experts state that, if an inactivated vaccine is indicated in a patient with a chronic inflammatory illness who is receiving maintenance therapy with a biologic response modifier, the vaccine should not be withheld because of concern about exacerbation of the inflammatory illness.

Corticosteroids given in greater than physiologic doses may reduce immune responses to vaccines. ACIP and the American Academy of Pediatrics (AAP) state that inactivated vaccines preferably should be administered at least 2 weeks prior to initiation of corticosteroid therapy that is considered immunosuppressive; however, if this is not feasible in patients receiving long-term corticosteroid therapy for inflammatory or autoimmune diseases, inactivated vaccines can be administered during such therapy.

■ **Vaccines** Limited data are available to date to evaluate the concomitant use of HPV vaccine with other vaccines. Although specific studies may not be available evaluating concurrent administration with each antigen, simultaneous administration with other age-appropriate vaccines, including live virus vaccines, toxoids, or inactivated or recombinant vaccines, during the same health-care visit is not expected to affect immunologic responses or adverse reactions to any of the preparations. However, each parenteral vaccine should be administered using separate syringes and different injection sites.

Diphtheria and Tetanus Toxoids and Pertussis Vaccine HPV vaccine may be administered concurrently with tetanus toxoid and reduced diphtheria toxoid and acellular pertussis vaccine adsorbed (Tdap) using different syringes and different injection sites.

Tdap (Adacel®) was administered concurrently with human papillomavirus quadrivalent vaccine (4vHPV; no longer available in the US) and meningococcal polysaccharide (serogroups A, C, Y and W-135) diphtheria toxoid conjugate vaccine (MenACWY-D; Menactra®) in an open-label, randomized controlled study in 1040 boys and girls 11 through 17 years of age (mean age 12.6 years). Concurrent administration of these 3 vaccines at different injection sites did not interfere with the antibody response to any of the vaccine antigens compared with administration of 4vHPV alone followed by administration of Tdap (Adacel®) and MenACWY-D (Menactra®) concurrently at different sites 1 month after the 4vHPV dose. Although the overall incidence of adverse injection site and systemic reactions in those who received all 3 vaccines concurrently at different sites was similar to that reported when 4vHPV was given alone followed by Tdap (Adacel®) and MenACWY-D (Menactra®) 1 month later, concurrent administration was associated with an increased incidence of swelling at the HPV vaccine injection site and an increased incidence of bruising or pain at the other injection sites.

Tdap (Adacel®) was administered concurrently with 9vHPV and MenACWY-D (Menactra®) in a randomized study in 1237 boys and girls 11 through 15 years of age. These adolescents received 9vHPV in one limb concurrently with Tdap (Adacel®) and MenACWY-D (Menactra®) given at different sites in the opposite limb or received 9vHPV followed 1 month later by Tdap (Adacel®) and MenACWY-D (Menactra®) given concurrently at different sites. Although overall rates of adverse reactions at the injection sites in those who received all 3 vaccines on the same day (at separate sites) were similar to the overall rates reported when 9vHPV was given 1 month before the other 2 vaccines, an increased rate of swelling at the HPV vaccine injection site occurred when all 3 vaccines were administered concurrently compared with administration of HPV vaccine alone. Concurrent administration of all 3 vaccines did not interfere with antibody responses to HPV vaccine or the other vaccines compared with administration 1 month apart.

Hepatitis B Vaccine HPV vaccine (4vHPV; no longer available in the US) has been administered concurrently with hepatitis B vaccine (Recombivax HB®) at a different site in women 16–23 years of age without a decrease in antibody response to either vaccine or a clinically important increase in adverse effects compared with administration during separate visits. Hepatitis B vaccine (Recombivax HB®) may be administered currently with HPV vaccine using different syringes and different injection sites.

Meningococcal Vaccines **Meningococcal Groups A, C, Y, and W-135 Vaccine.** HPV vaccine may be administered concurrently with meningococcal (groups A, C, Y and W-135) polysaccharide diphtheria toxoid conjugate vaccine (MenACWY-D; Menactra®) using different syringes and different injection sites.

MenACWY-D (Menactra®) has been administered concurrently with Tdap (Adacel®) and either 9vHPV or 4vHPV (no longer available in the US) in randomized studies in adolescent boys and girls. Concurrent administration of the 3 vaccines at different injection sites did not interfere with the antibody response to any of the vaccine antigens. Although the overall incidence of adverse reactions in those who received all 3 vaccines concurrently at different sites was similar to that reported when 9vHPV or 4vHPV was given alone followed by MenACWY-D (Menactra®) and Tdap (Adacel®) 1 month later, concurrent administration was associated with an increased incidence of swelling at the HPV vaccine injection sites compared with administration of the HPV vaccine alone. (See Diphtheria and Tetanus Toxoids and Pertussis Vaccine under Drug Interactions: Vaccines.)

HPV vaccine (4vHPV; no longer available in the US) has been administered concurrently with meningococcal (groups A, C, Y and W-135) oligosaccharide diphtheria CRM_{197} conjugate vaccine (MenACWY-CRM; Menveo®) and Tdap (Boostrix®) in a study in healthy adolescents 11 through 18 years of age. There was no interference with the immune response to the meningococcal antigens compared with administration of MenACWY-CRM (Menveo®) alone. Systemic adverse reactions (e.g., headache, malaise, myalgia, arthralgia) were reported more frequently in the those who received HPV vaccine, Tdap (Boostrix®), and MenACWY-CRM (Menveo®) concurrently compared with those who received MenACWY-CRM (Menveo®) alone.

Meningococcal Group B Vaccine. Meningococcal group B vaccine (MenB-FHbp; Trumenba®) has been administered concurrently with 4vHPV (no longer available in the US) in adolescents 11 to less than 18 years of age without a decrease in antibody response to the meningococcal serogroup B antigens and without a decrease in antibody response to 3 of the 4 HPV antigens (i.e., HPV types 6, 11, 16); at 1 month after the third dose of 4vHPV, the antibody response to HPV type 18 was decreased, but at least 99% of vaccinees achieved seroconversion for all 4 HPV antigens.

Description

Human papillomavirus (HPV) vaccine is an inactivated (recombinant) virus vaccine containing virus-like particles (VLPs) of the major capsid (L1) proteins of certain HPV types associated with anogenital infections. Some HPV types are classified as high-risk (oncogenic) types and can cause low-grade cervical cell abnormalities or high-grade cervical cell abnormalities that are precursors to cancer; other HPV types are classified as low-risk types and can cause genital warts, benign or low-grade cervical cell changes, and recurrent respiratory papillomatosis. HPV vaccine is used to stimulate active immunity to the HPV types represented in the vaccine. VLPs contained in HPV vaccine are produced using recombinant DNA technology and are structurally indiscernible from native HPV virions; the VLPs are noninfectious because they do not contain DNA.

HPV vaccine is commercially available in the US as a 9-valent vaccine (9vHPV) that contains the purified VLPs of the L1 proteins of 9 HPV types (types 6, 11, 16, 18, 31, 33, 45, 52, and 58). The vaccine includes HPV VLPs representing the 4 HPV types contained in the previously available quadrivalent HPV vaccine (4vHPV) and 5 additional high-risk (oncogenic) HPV types. The type-specific L1 proteins are prepared by separate fermentations in recombinant *S. cerevisiae* and self-assemble into VLPs. The VLPs are released from the yeast cells by cell disruption; purified by a series of chemical and physical methods; and adsorbed onto preformed aluminum-containing adjuvant (amorphous aluminum hydroxyphosphate sulfate). In addition to the 9 HPV type-specific VLPs, each 0.5 mL dose of 9vHPV contains approximately 500 mcg of aluminum (provided as amorphous aluminum hydroxyphosphate sulfate), 9.56 mg of sodium chloride, 0.78 mg of L-histidine, 50 mcg of polysorbate 80, 35 mcg of sodium borate, less than 7 mcg of yeast protein, and water for injection.

Administration of a 3-dose vaccination series of 9vHPV can prevent disease caused by HPV types 6, 11, 16, 18, 31, 33, 45, 52, and 58, including genital warts caused by HPV types 6 and 11; cervical, vulvar, vaginal, and anal cancer caused by HPV types 16, 18, 31, 33, 45, 52, and 58; and precancerous anal and genital lesions caused by HPV types 6, 11, 16, 18, 31, 33, 45, 52, and 58. Data indicate that at least 99.5% of all female and male vaccine recipients 9 through 26 years of age develop antibodies to HPV types 6, 11, 16, 18, 31, 33, 45, 52, and 58 by 1 month following the third dose of 9vHPV. The immune response to a 2-dose regimen of 9vHPV administered to females and males 9 through 14 years of age is noninferior to that reported with a 3-dose regimen of 9vHPV administered to females 16 through 26 years of age. The minimum titer of anti-HPV antibody that provides protection against disease caused by HPV types 6, 11, 16, 18, 31, 33, 45, 52, and 58 and the duration of immunity following vaccination with 9vHPV have not been established to date.

Advice to Patients

Prior to administration of each vaccine dose, provide a copy of manufacturer's patient information to the patient and/or patient's parent or guardian. Also provide a copy of the appropriate Centers for Disease Control and Prevention (CDC) Vaccine Information Statement (VIS) to the patient or patient's legal representative (VISs are available at http://www.cdc.gov/vaccines/hcp/vis/index.html).

Advise the patient and/or patient's parent or legal guardian of the risks and benefits of vaccination with human papillomavirus (HPV) vaccine.

Advise the patient and/or patient's parent or guardian that vaccination with HPV vaccine does not provide protection against disease from vaccine and nonvaccine HPV types that an individual has previously been exposed to through sexual activity.

Advise the patient and/or patient's parent or legal guardian that vaccination with HPV vaccine is not a substitute for routine cervical cancer screening. Vaccine recipients should continue to receive routine cervical cancer screening (e.g., Papanicolaou [Pap] tests) according to current guidelines for such testing.

Advise vaccine recipients not to discontinue anal cancer screening that has been recommended by a health-care provider.

Advise vaccine recipients to continue to practice behaviors that limit the risk of exposure to HPV (e.g., sexual abstinence, monogamy, limited number of sexual partners, use of condoms).

Importance of completing the vaccination series of HPV vaccine, unless contraindicated.

Advise the patient and/or patient's parent or guardian that fainting, sometimes resulting in falling with injury, has been reported following vaccination with HPV vaccine and that the patient should be observed for 15 minutes after the dose.

Importance of contacting clinicians if a hypersensitivity reaction (difficulty breathing, wheezing, hives, rash, swollen glands [neck, armpit, or groin], joint pain, weakness, chest pain) occurs following a vaccine dose. Clinicians or individuals can report any adverse reactions that occur following vaccination to the Vaccine Adverse Event Reporting System (VAERS) at 800-822-7967 or http://www.vaers.hhs.gov/.

Importance of informing clinicians of existing or contemplated concomitant therapy, including prescription and OTC drugs, and any concomitant illnesses.

Importance of women informing clinicians if they are or plan to become pregnant or plan to breast-feed. Advise vaccine recipients that HPV vaccine is *not* recommended for use in pregnant women or women planning on becoming pregnant during the 3-dose vaccination series. If any exposure to HPV vaccine occurs around the time of conception or during pregnancy, vaccinees and their clinicians are encouraged to contact the pregnancy registry at 800-986-8999.

Importance of informing patients of other important precautionary information. (See Cautions.)

Overview® (see Users Guide). For additional information on this drug until a more detailed monograph is developed and published, the manufacturer's labeling should be consulted. It is *essential* that the manufacturer's labeling be consulted for more detailed information on usual cautions, precautions, contraindications, potential drug interactions, laboratory test interferences, and acute toxicity.

Preparations

Excipients in commercially available drug preparations may have clinically important effects in some individuals; consult specific product labeling for details.

Human Papillomavirus 9-valent (Types 6, 11, 16, 18, 31, 33, 45, 52, 58) Vaccine, Recombinant

Parenteral		
Injectable suspension, for IM use	30 mcg of HPV type 6 L1, 40 mcg of HPV type 11 L1, 60 mcg of HPV type 16 L1, 40 mcg of HPV type 18 L1, 20 mcg of HPV type 31 L1, 20 mcg of HPV type 33 L1, 20 mcg of HPV type 45 L1, 20 mcg of HPV type 52 L1, and 20 mcg of HPV type 58 L1 protein per 0.5 mL	**Gardasil® 9**, Merck

Measles Virus Vaccine Live

MMR

■ Measles virus vaccine live is a preparation of live, attenuated measles virus that stimulates active immunity to measles infection. Measles virus vaccine live is commercially available as a fixed-combination vaccine containing measles, mumps, and rubella antigens (MMR; M-M-R® II) and a fixed-combination vaccine containing measles, mumps, rubella, and varicella antigens (MMRV; ProQuad®). For information on MMRV, see Varicella Virus Vaccine Live 80:12.

Uses

Measles virus vaccine live is used to stimulate active immunity to measles (rubeola). Monovalent measles virus vaccine live (Attenuvax®) is no longer commercially available in the US. Measles virus vaccine live is commercially available in the US as a fixed-combination vaccine containing measles, mumps, and rubella antigens (MMR; M-M-R® II) for use in adults, adolescents, and children 12 months of age or older and as a fixed-combination vaccine containing measles, mumps, rubella, and varicella antigens (MMRV; ProQuad®) for use in children 12 months through 12 years of age.

The US Public Health Service Advisory Committee on Immunization Practices (ACIP), the American Academy of Pediatrics (AAP), the American Academy of Family Physicians (AAFP), and the National Vaccine Advisory Committee (NVAC) recommend *universal* immunization against measles for all susceptible children, adolescents, and adults, unless measles virus vaccine live is contraindicated. (See Cautions: Precautions and Contraindications.)

Most individuals born before 1957 are likely to have been infected naturally with measles and generally can be considered immune. Individuals born in 1957 or later should be considered immune to measles only if there is documentation of adequate immunization against measles (2 doses of MMR or measles-containing vaccine for school aged-children in grades K-12, college students, health-care personnel, international travelers), natural measles infection diagnosed by a health-care provider, or serologic evidence of measles immunity. Individuals who lack adequate documentation of immunity should be considered susceptible to measles and should be vaccinated, unless measles virus vaccine live is contraindicated. A parental report of measles vaccination, by itself, is not considered adequate documentation of immunization. Clinicians should not provide documentation of immunization for a patient unless they administered the vaccine to the patient or have seen a record documenting vaccination.

Previously, individuals who received a single dose of any live measles virus vaccine when 12 months of age or older were considered to be adequately immunized against measles. In 1989, because of increased measles outbreaks in school-aged children in the US, the ACIP and AAP revised their recommendations to specify that routine primary immunization against measles generally should consist of 2 doses of measles virus vaccine live given at least 1 month (i.e., at least 28 days) apart. This recommendation was made because primary vaccine failure was considered to be a principal contributing factor to these measles outbreaks, and it was further strengthened in 1998 to unequivocally recommend that a 2-dose primary immunization series be completed prior to entry into kindergarten or first grade (i.e., by 4 through 6 years of age).

The ACIP, AAP, AAFP, and NVAC state that MMR is preferred over monovalent measles virus vaccine live (no longer commercially available in the US) for both primary immunization and revaccination to assure immunity to all 3 diseases. Alternatively, in children 12 months through 12 years of age when a dose of MMR and a dose of varicella virus vaccine live are indicated for primary immunization, use of the fixed-combination vaccine containing MMR and varicella virus vaccine live (MMRV; ProQuad®) can be considered. For information on MMRV, see Varicella Virus Vaccine Live 80:12.

■ **Primary Immunization** ***Infants and Children 12 Months through 12 Years of Age*** For routine primary immunization in children, the ACIP, AAP, and AAFP recommend that the first dose of MMR be given at 12 through 15 months of age. Initiation of immunization with MMR at 12 months of age is recommended for children residing in areas at high risk for measles transmission among preschool-age children, especially large urban areas. (See Infants and Children in High-Risk Areas under Uses: Primary Immunization.) The second dose of MMR preferably should be given at 4 through 6 years of age (just prior to entry into kindergarten or first grade), but may be given earlier during any routine visit provided at least 4 weeks have elapsed since the first dose and both the first and second doses are administered beginning at or after 12 months of age. Those who have not previously received the second MMR dose should complete the schedule by 11–12 years of age (just prior to entry into middle or junior high school). Children who do not have adequate documentation of immunity against measles, mumps, and rubella should be admitted to kindergarten or first grade only after receiving at least one dose of a measles virus-containing vaccine.

The ACIP, AAP, and AAFP state that primary immunization against measles, mumps, and rubella can be integrated with primary immunization against diphtheria, tetanus, pertussis, *Haemophilus influenzae* type b (Hib), hepatitis B, influenza, pneumococcal disease, poliomyelitis, and varicella. In general, simultaneous administration (on the same day) of the most widely used vaccines, including diphtheria and tetanus toxoids and acellular pertussis vaccine adsorbed (DTaP), hepatitis B vaccine, Hib conjugate vaccine, MMR, poliovirus vaccine inactivated (IPV), and varicella virus vaccine live, has resulted in seroconversion rates and adverse effects similar to those observed when the vaccines were administered separately. Therefore, the ACIP, AAP, and AAFP recommend simultaneous administration of all vaccines appropriate for the age and previous vaccination status of the recipient, including DTaP, Hib conjugate vaccine, hepatitis B vaccine, influenza vaccine, MMR, IPV, pneumococcal vaccine, and varicella virus vaccine live, especially if an individual is unlikely to return for further vaccination. (See Drug Interactions.)

Infants and Children in High-Risk Areas During the late 1980s and early 1990s, the incidence of measles in the US increased. At that time, measles outbreaks occurred among unvaccinated preschool-aged children, including those younger than the recommended age for routine vaccination, and also occurred among vaccinated school-aged children. In 1986, 39.2% of measles patients were younger than 5 years of age and children 16 months to 4 years of age accounted for 44.7% of the total preventable cases of measles (i.e., cases in unvaccinated individuals). In 1990, 48.1% of measles patients were younger than 5 years of age; this was the first time since detailed age-related reporting started in 1973 that the proportion of measles cases in this age group exceeded that in school-aged children. In these outbreaks, up to 88% of cases in children 16 months to 4 years of age were unvaccinated. Children in this age group may not yet be enrolled in institutions such as day-care facilities or schools with immunization requirements for enrollment. The ACIP and AAP recommend that increased emphasis be placed on vaccinating preschoolers before they encounter measles in day-care facilities or other environments where young children cluster. In addition, unique measles vaccination strategies may be needed in areas of the US with large numbers of Hispanic individuals who are recent immigrants, preschool-age children, or undocumented residents. Vaccination programs offered at churches and workplaces might reach undocumented residents; however, any strategy should account for the reluctance of such residents to have contact with government agencies.

The ACIP and AAP recommend that all children be vaccinated against measles using a 2-dose regimen of MMR beginning at 12 through 15 months of age in order to achieve maximal seroconversion, unless contraindicated; vaccination of younger children generally has been discouraged because most infants have maternal antibodies that may prevent an adequate immunologic response to the vaccine. In order to improve immunity levels in children younger than 15 months of age living in areas in the US with recurrent measles transmission, the ACIP and AAP recommend that routine measles immunization be initiated at 12 months of age for children residing in areas where the risk of measles is high, especially large urban areas. High-risk areas are defined as counties with more than 5 reported measles cases among preschool-aged children during each of the last 5 years, counties with a recent outbreak among unvaccinated preschool-aged children, or counties with large inner-city urban populations. This recommendation can be implemented for the entire county or only within defined areas of the county. Although there is a slightly lower rate of seroconversion among children vaccinated with a measles virus-containing vaccine at 12–14 months of age than among those vaccinated at 15 months of age or older, the benefit of preventing measles cases among children 12 through 15 months of age is assumed to outweigh the slightly reduced efficacy.

The risk of complications from measles is high among children younger than 12 months of age. Therefore, considering the benefits and risks, the ACIP and AAP recommend that children 6 through 11 months of age be vaccinated against measles when exposure to natural measles is considered likely (e.g., during an outbreak, during international travel). Although monovalent measles virus vaccine live is preferred in such children since benefit from exposure to other antigens included in MMR may be low secondary to persisting maternal antibodies that interfere with seroconversion in this young age group, monovalent measles virus vaccine live is no longer commercially available in the US and MMR should be used when protection against measles is indicated in children 6 through 11 months of age. Regardless of which measles virus-containing vaccine is administered, children vaccinated before 12 months of age have a substantially lower rate of seroconversion than those vaccinated at an older age and should be considered unvaccinated against measles, mumps, and rubella for the purposes of determining the need for further vaccination; such children should be revaccinated with the usual 2-dose regimen of MMR. These children should receive a dose of MMR when they are 12 through 15 months of age (12 months of age for those remaining in a high-risk area) and a second dose at least 1 month (i.e., at least 28 days) later, usually at 4 through 6 years of age (just prior to entry into kindergarten or first grade). The AAP states that, alternatively, immunocompetent infants 6 through 11 months of age who are at high risk of exposure to natural measles virus may be given a dose of immune globulin immediately, and then be given MMR at least 5–6 months after the dose of immune globulin, provided the child is at least 12 months of age. (See Drug Interactions: Immune Globulins.)

Internationally Adopted Children and Other Immigrants Individuals seeking an immigrant visa for permanent US residency must provide proof of age-appropriate vaccination according to the US Recommended Childhood and Adolescent Immunization Schedule or the US Recommended Adult Schedule (see Immunization Schedules, US 80:00). Although this vaccination requirement applies to all immigrant infants and children entering the US, internationally adopted children less than 11 years of age are exempt from the overseas vaccination requirements; however, adoptive parents are required to sign a waiver indicating their intention to comply with the vaccination requirements within 30 days after the infant or child arrives in the US. The CDC states that more than 90% of newly arrived internationally adopted children need catch-up vaccinations to meet the US Recommended Immunization Schedules.

The fact that immunization schedules of other countries may differ from US schedules (e.g., different recommended vaccines, recommended ages of administration, and/or number and timing of vaccine doses) also should be considered. Only written vaccination records should be considered as evidence of previous vaccination since such records are more likely to accurately predict protection if the vaccines administered, intervals between doses, and child's age at the time of vaccination are similar to US recommendations; however, the extent to which an internationally adopted child's immunization record reflects their protection against disease is unclear and it is possible there may be transcription errors in such records (e.g., single-antigen vaccine may have been administered although a multiple-antigen vaccine was recorded). Although vaccines with inadequate potency have been produced in other countries, most vaccines used worldwide are immunogenic and produced with adequate quality control standards.

When the immune status of an internationally adopted child is uncertain, health-care providers can either repeat vaccinations (since this usually is safe and avoids the need to obtain and interpret serologic tests) and/or use selective serologic testing to determine the need for immunizations (helps avoid unnecessary injections). The child may have received monovalent measles virus vaccine live in their country of origin, but MMR is not used in most countries. Therefore, although serologic testing is available to verify immunization status in children 12 months of age or older, the CDC states that administration of MMR is preferable to serologic testing unless there is documentation that the child has had mumps and rubella. The ACIP states that the recommended approach is to revaccinate an internationally adopted child with 1 or 2 doses of MMR (depending on the child's age) without regard to the child's prior vaccination record since serious adverse effects after MMR vaccination are rare and there is no evidence that administration of MMR increases the risk for adverse reactions among individuals already immune to measles, mumps, or rubella.

Adolescents and Adults In 1986 and 1990, 10 and 23%, respectively, of measles patients whose ages were reported were 20 years of age or older. During 1990–1994, 47% of reported measles cases occurred in children 10 years of age and older. Measles outbreaks continue to occur at secondary schools, universities and colleges, and other places where young adults congregate. Therefore, the ACIP and AAP state that greater emphasis needs to be placed on vaccinating young adults and recommends that educational institutions require evidence of measles immunity as a criterion for enrollment. The American College Health Association also recommends that colleges and universities implement a prematriculation immunization requirement for measles.

Adolescents 11–12 Years of Age. Because the recommendation for a second dose of MMR was made in 1989, many adolescents born before 1985 (and some born after 1985) may not have received the second vaccine dose. The ACIP, AAP, and AAFP recommend that any adolescent who has not previously received a second dose of MMR receive the dose during a routine preadolescent preventive health-care visit at 11–12 years of age. This routine health-care visit provides an opportunity to administer "catch-up" vaccines that were missed at an earlier age, administer vaccines routinely recommended at 11–12 years of age, administer vaccines recommended for certain high-risk adolescents, schedule future appointments that may be necessary to complete recommended immunization schedules, and provide adolescents with other recommended preventive health services such as guidance on health behaviors and screening for biomedical, behavioral, and emotional conditions. During the health-care visit at 11–12 years of age, the vaccination history of the adolescent should be assessed. If the adolescent does not have information regarding their vaccination history, the healthcare provider should attempt to obtain such information through documentation from the parent, previous providers, or school records. When documentation of an adolescent's vaccination status is not available at the time of the preventive health-care visit, an assumption can be made that the adolescent has received those vaccines required by state laws and regulations that have been in effect for some time (e.g., those required on entry to kindergarten) and these vaccines can be withheld while awaiting documentation. However, vaccine doses recommended for adolescents that were not included in previous laws and recommendations should be administered.

Ideally, all vaccines routinely indicated at 11–12 years of age should be administered during the initial adolescent visit (MMR, hepatitis B vaccine, tetanus toxoid and reduced diphtheria toxoid and acellular pertussis vaccine adsorbed (Tdap), varicella virus vaccine live). However, since multiple doses of some vaccines are required to complete primary immunization and because simultaneous administration of a large number of vaccines may be indicated in some adolescents, providers may need to be flexible in determining which vaccines to administer during the initial visit and which to schedule for return visits. While specific studies evaluating the safety and efficacy of simultaneous administration of vaccines in adolescents are not available, there is extensive evidence from clinical studies and experience in infants and children that simultaneous administration of the most widely used vaccines does not decrease the antibody response or increase adverse reactions to these vaccines. In circumstances where multiple vaccines (i.e., 4 or more) are indicated in adolescents 11–12 years of age, the provider may choose to defer some vaccines for administration during one or more future visits; however, the vaccines should be prioritized based on which require multiple doses, which diseases pose an immediate threat to the adolescent, and whether the adolescent is likely to return for scheduled visits. During any subsequent visits, the adolescent's vaccination status should be rechecked and any deficiencies corrected.

Adults. Adults who received a measles vaccine in 1968 or later generally do not need to be revaccinated routinely, provided they received the vaccine at 12 months of age or older without concurrent immune globulin; however, such individuals should receive a dose of MMR if they are entering college, beginning employment in a health-care facility, or planning international travel. Some, but not all, studies have demonstrated lower vaccine efficacy and higher attack rates in individuals who received measles vaccine at 12–14 months of age. In 1965–1976, the recommended age for measles vaccination in the US was 12 months of age; therefore, a large proportion of individuals who were 15–26 years of age in 1992 are likely to have been vaccinated when they were 12–14 months of age. The ACIP states that routine revaccination of individuals who received measles vaccine at 12–14 months of age is not recommended, but should be considered during selected measles outbreaks, particularly those in junior and senior high schools.

HIV-infected Individuals Individuals with human immunodeficiency virus (HIV) infection are at increased risk for severe complications if infected with measles. MMR can be used in HIV-infected children, adolescents, or adults who do not have evidence of *severe* immunosuppression.

The ACIP, AAP, US Centers for Disease Control and Prevention (CDC), National Institutes of Health (NIH), Infectious Diseases Society of America (IDSA), Pediatric Infectious Diseases Society, and others state that all *asymptomatic* HIV-infected children, adolescents, and adults should receive MMR according to the usually recommended immunization schedules. In addition, MMR should be considered for all symptomatic HIV-infected individuals who do *not* have evidence of severe immunosuppression and who otherwise would be eligible for vaccination. Because the immunologic response to vaccines may decrease as HIV disease progresses, vaccination early in the course of HIV infection may be more likely to induce an immune response; in addition, approximately 5% of HIV-infected infants born in the US will be severely immunocompromised at 12 months of age. Therefore, the ACIP and other experts recommend that HIV-infected infants who are not severely immunocompromised receive MMR as soon as possible upon reaching their first birthday (i.e., at 12 months of age) and consideration should be given to administering the second dose of MMR as soon as 1 month (minimum 28 days) after the first dose rather than waiting until 4 through 6 years of age. If there is an increased risk of exposure to measles, such as during an outbreak, ACIP states that children with HIV infection who are not severely immunosuppressed should receive immunization at an earlier age. At such times, children 6 through 11 months of age should receive MMR and should be revaccinated with MMR as soon as possible upon reaching their first birthday, provided at least 1 month has elapsed since administration of the previous dose of measles virus-containing vaccine, and again as early as 1 month after the second dose but no later than on entry into school.

MMR is contraindicated in HIV-infected individuals with *severe immunosuppression* (i.e., children younger than 12 months of age with CD4+ T-cell count less than 750/mm^3; children 1 through 5 years of age with CD4+ T-cell count less than 500/mm^3; children 6 years of age or older, adolescents, and adults with CD4+ T-cell count less than 200/mm^3; children younger than 13 years of age with CD4+ T-cell percentage less than 15%). Such individuals should receive immune globulin IM (IGIM) if protection against measles is needed (e.g., in travelers, following exposure to measles). There has been a report of progressive pneumonitis in an individual with advanced acquired immunodeficiency syndrome (AIDS) who received MMR. (See Individuals with Altered Immunocompetence under Cautions: Precautions and Contraindications.)

The serologic response to vaccines (including MMR) may be reduced in some HIV-infected patients and may be inversely correlated with the severity of the disease. AAP and ACIP state that HIV-infected individuals should receive immune globulin IM (IGIM) following exposure to measles, regardless of their prior vaccination status. (See Measles under Uses: Immune Globulin IM, in Immune Globulin 80:04.) In addition, the fact that MMR may be ineffective in HIV-infected patients who have received high-dose IV immune globulin therapy (e.g., for the prevention of serious bacterial infections) within the 6 months preceding vaccination should be considered. (See Drug Interactions: Immune Globulins.)

MMR may be given to any family member residing in the household or any other close contact of an HIV-infected patient since extensive experience has shown that live, attenuated MMR vaccine viruses are not transmitted from vaccinated individuals to others.

Health-care Personnel Health-care personnel are at increased risk for acquiring measles and transmitting the disease to susceptible patients, and the ACIP and the Hospital Infection Control Practices Advisory Committee (HICPAC) recommend that all health-care facilities (i.e., inpatient and outpatient, public and private) ensure that all workers (i.e., medical or nonmedical, paid or volunteer, full- or part-time, student or nonstudent, with or without patient-care responsibilities) have adequate documentation of measles vaccination or immunity (i.e., 2 doses of measles virus-containing vaccine with the first dose given on or after 12 months of age and the second dose given at least 28 days after the first dose, laboratory evidence of immunity, or laboratory confirmation of disease). Facilities that provide care exclusively to geriatric patients who are at minimal risk for measles and complications of the disease are possible exceptions to this recommendation. Health-care workers have a responsibility to avoid transmitting measles to patients and thereby causing them harm.

Although birth before 1957 generally is considered acceptable evidence of measles immunity, health-care facilities should consider recommending 2 doses of MMR to unvaccinated workers born before 1957 who do not have laboratory evidence of measles immunity or laboratory confirmation of disease. Serologic screening prior to measles vaccination is not necessary unless the health-care facility considers it cost-effective.

Travelers Because the risk of acquiring measles outside the US is greater than the risk incurred in the US and because an increasing proportion of measles cases in the US results from exposure to the disease in foreign countries, the ACIP, AAP, and many clinicians recommend that travelers be immune to measles before leaving the US. Unless a live measles virus-containing vaccine is contraindicated, individuals who travel or reside abroad and who do not have adequate evidence of measles, mumps, and rubella immunity should be vaccinated with MMR.

The optimum age for vaccinating children against measles is 12 through 15 months of age (see Infants and Children under Uses: Primary Immunization) and children 12 months of age or older who will be traveling or residing abroad should receive 2 doses of MMR prior to departure with the doses given 1 month apart (i.e., at least 28 days apart). Children 6 through 11 months of age should receive at least 1 dose of MMR prior to departure. Although monovalent measles virus vaccine live is preferred in those 6 through 11 months of age since the risk of serious disease from mumps or rubella infection is relatively low in infants and benefit from exposure to other antigens included in MMR may be low secondary to persisting maternal antibodies that interfere with seroconversion in this young age group, monovalent measles virus vaccine live is no longer commercially available in the US. Any child who received MMR before 12 months of age should be revaccinated using 2 doses of MMR beginning at 12 through 15 months of age (12 months of age for those remaining in a high-risk area); the second dose of MMR should be given at least 28 days later, usually when the child enters school. Virtually all children younger than 6 months of age are protected against measles because of maternally derived antibodies and usually do not need to receive the vaccine prior to international travel unless the mother is diagnosed with measles.

■ **Postexposure Vaccination** There is some evidence that a measles virus-containing vaccine, if given within 72 hours of exposure to natural measles virus, may provide protection in some cases. Postexposure vaccination also provides future protection to individuals who do not contract the disease. For most susceptible individuals 12 months of age or older who are exposed to measles in most settings (e.g., day-care facilities, schools, colleges, health-care facilities), administration of MMR or other measles virus-containing vaccine within 72 hours of exposure is preferable to using immune globulin IM (IGIM) for postexposure prophylaxis. If MMR is contraindicated (e.g., infants less than 6 months of age, pregnant women, immunocompromised individuals), susceptible individuals may receive an immediate dose of IGIM. For susceptible individuals 6 months of age or older, without contraindications, who are exposed to measles in the home setting, postexposure prophylaxis within 72 hours using the vaccine also is acceptable. However, measles often is not recognized as such until longer than 72 hours has elapsed since initial exposure. Therefore, if more than 72 hours but less than 6 days have elapsed since exposure to natural measles virus, susceptible individuals may receive an immediate dose of IGIM followed by MMR 5–6 months later. Immune globulin should not be given concurrently with a measles virus-containing vaccine. (See Drug Interactions: Immune Globulins.) Any immunity conferred by immune globulin is only temporary unless modified or typical measles occurs despite administration of the globulin.

The use of a measles virus-containing vaccine (MMR) within 72 hours of the exposure is generally preferable to use of immune globulin in individuals 12 months of age or older; immune globulin is principally indicated when the vaccine is contraindicated or more than 72 hours since initial exposure has elapsed. Immune globulin may be especially indicated for susceptible household contacts for whom the risk of complications from measles is high (e.g., contacts who are younger than 12 months of age, pregnant women, immunocompromised individuals). Immune globulin should not be used in an attempt to control measles outbreaks. Severely immunocompromised individuals with HIV infection are at increased risk of serious complications from measles infection and should receive a dose of immune globulin following exposure to measles, regardless of their immunization status. (See HIV-infected Individuals under Uses: Primary Immunization.) Some clinicians administer full replacement doses of immune globulin on a 2- to 4-week schedule to children with AIDS and other clinical manifestations of HIV infection; such therapy may provide protection against measles if the last dose was administered within 3 weeks of the measles exposure.

■ **Outbreak Control** If a measles outbreak occurs in a child-care facility, school (elementary, middle, junior high, senior high), college, university, or other secondary educational institution, the ACIP and AAP recommend that all students (and their siblings) and all school personnel born in 1957 or later be vaccinated against measles, unless they can provide documentation that they received 2 doses of a measles virus-containing vaccine at 12 months of age or older or other evidence of measles immunity. Individuals revaccinated, as well as unvaccinated individuals receiving their first dose of MMR as part of the outbreak control program, may be immediately readmitted to school. Mass revaccination of entire communities is unnecessary. Individuals who have been exempted from measles immunization for medical, religious, or other reasons should be excluded from the outbreak area until at least 2 weeks after the onset of rash in the last case of measles. During measles outbreaks, children as young as 6 months of age also should be vaccinated if exposure to natural measles is considered likely. (See Infants and Children in High-Risk Areas under Uses: Primary Immunization.)

Dosage and Administration

■ **Reconstitution and Administration** The fixed-combination vaccine containing measles, mumps, and rubella antigens (MMR; M-M-R® II) is administered by subcutaneous injection. The vaccine should *not* be given IV.

For information on reconstitution and administration of the fixed-combination vaccine containing MMR and varicella virus vaccine live (MMRV; ProQuad®), see Varicella Virus Vaccine Live 80:12.

MMR is reconstituted by adding the entire amount of diluent supplied by the manufacturer to the vial of lyophilized vaccine and agitating the vial. Only the diluent provided by the manufacturer should be used. The preparation should be discarded if the lyophilized vaccine does not dissolve completely.

Reconstituted MMR should be inspected visually for particulate matter and discoloration prior to administration. The vaccine should be reconstituted and administered using sterile syringes and needles that are free of preservatives, antiseptics, and detergents, since these substances may inactivate live virus vaccines.

To minimize loss of potency and ensure an adequate immunizing dose, MMR should be administered immediately following reconstitution. (See Chemistry and Stability: Stability.)

The preferred site for subcutaneous injection of MMR is the upper-outer triceps area; injections also can be given into the anterolateral thigh. For children 1 year of age and older, adolescents, and adults, the upper-outer triceps area usually is preferred. To ensure appropriate delivery, subcutaneous injections should be made at a 45° angle using a 5/8-inch, 23- to 25-gauge needle.

Since syncope may occur following vaccination, vaccinees should be observed for approximately 15 minutes after the vaccine dose is administered. If syncope occurs, the patient should be observed until symptoms resolve. Syncope after vaccination occurs most frequently in adolescents and young adults.

When multiple vaccines are administered during a single health-care visit, each vaccine should be given with a different syringe and at different injection sites. Injection sites should be separated by at least 1 inch (if anatomically feasible) to allow appropriate attribution of any local adverse effects that may occur.

■ **Dosage** The usual dose of MMR is 0.5 mL and is the same for all individuals. When reconstituted as specified, each 0.5-mL dose of MMR contains not less than 1000 $TCID_{50}$ of measles virus, 12,500 $TCID_{50}$ of mumps virus, and 1000 $TCID_{50}$ of rubella virus. The entire volume of reconstituted solution in the single-dose vial should be administered.

For information regarding dosage of the fixed-combination vaccine containing MMR and varicella virus vaccine live (MMRV; ProQuad®), see Varicella Virus Vaccine Live 80:12.

Infants 6 through 11 Months of Age When protection against measles is considered necessary (e.g., for outbreak control, for children traveling to or residing in areas outside the US with an increased risk of measles) in infants 6 through 11 months of age, who are considered too young to receive routine primary immunization, a single 0.5-mL dose of MMR should be given. Such children should be considered inadequately immunized and should be revaccinated with the usual 2-dose MMR regimen with the first dose given at 12 through 15 months of age and the second dose usually given prior to elementary school entry (4 through 6 years of age).

Infants and Children 12 Months through 6 Years of Age For primary immunization against measles in infants and children, a 2-dose regimen of MMR is recommended and the first dose generally is administered at 12 through 15 months of age. For routine childhood immunization, the ACIP, AAP, and AAFP recommend that the first dose of MMR be given at 12 through 15 months of age and the second dose be routinely given at 4 through 6 years of age (just prior to entry into kindergarten or first grade). The second dose may be given earlier during any routine visit, provided at least 4 weeks (i.e., at least 28 days) have elapsed since the first dose and both the first and second doses are administered beginning at or after 12 months of age.

Children who received a dose of monovalent measles virus vaccine live (no longer commercially available in the US) or MMR prior to 12 months of age should be considered inadequately immunized and should be revaccinated with a 2-dose MMR regimen beginning as soon as possible after they reach their first birthday. (See Infants 6 through 11 Months of Age under Dosage and Administration: Dosage.)

Children and Adolescents 7 through 18 Years of Age A 2-dose regimen is recommended when MMR is indicated in previously unvaccinated children and adolescents 7 through 18 years of age. A preadolescent preventive health-care visit at 11–12 years of age provides an opportunity to complete the 2-dose vaccination series in adolescents who have not previously received the second vaccine dose or to initiate the series in those who have not yet received the vaccine. The minimum interval between doses of MMR should be 4 weeks (i.e., at least 28 days).

Individuals who received monovalent measles virus vaccine live (no longer commercially available in the US) when younger than 12 months of age should be considered susceptible to measles and therefore should be revaccinated with a 2-dose regimen of MMR.

Adults For adults 19 years of age and older, primary immunization consists of 1 or 2 doses of MMR. The minimum interval between doses is 4 weeks (i.e., at least 28 days).

Cautions

■ **Systemic Effects** Serious reactions associated with measles virus vaccine live occur very rarely. Limited data indicate that reactions to the vaccine are not age-related. In addition, adverse reactions following revaccination with the vaccine generally should be expected to occur only among the small proportion of vaccinees who failed to respond to the first dose.

The National Academy of Sciences Institute of Medicine determined that a causal relationship exists between measles, mumps, and rubella virus vaccine live (MMR) vaccination and anaphylaxis, thrombocytopenia, febrile seizures, and acute arthritis. Although vasculitis, otitis media, conjunctivitis, optic neuritis, ocular palsies, Guillain-Barré, and ataxia also have been reported after administration of MMR or its component vaccines and are included in the manufacturers' labeling, a causal relationship between MMR and these effects has not been established.

Fever and Rash Moderate fever (38.3–39.4°C) occurs occasionally during the month following vaccination. High fever (39.4°C or higher) has been reported in 5–15% of vaccinees who received monovalent measles virus vaccine live (no longer commercially available in the US). Transient rash also occurs in approximately 5% of vaccinees, is usually minimal, and occurs without generalized distribution. Fever and/or rash, if they occur, generally begin 7–12 and 7–10 days, respectively, following vaccination and are transient, with fever generally persisting for 1–2 days. Most individuals with fever are otherwise asymptomatic. Erythema multiforme, Stevens-Johnson syndrome, and urticaria have been reported rarely.

Seizures Febrile seizures have occurred rarely in children following administration of measles virus vaccine live, and they can occur in children without known risk factors. Children with a personal or family (i.e., in first-degree family members [siblings or parents]) history of seizures may be at increased risk of seizures following vaccination with measles virus vaccine live; although the precise risk of seizures in such children currently is unknown, it appears to be low. (See Seizures under Cautions: Precautions and Contraindications.) In addition, while children with a personal or family seizure history are at increased risk of developing idiopathic epilepsy, febrile seizures following vaccination do not in themselves increase the probability of subsequent epilepsy or other neurologic disorders.

Most seizures following measles vaccination resemble febrile seizures typical of any agent that can produce fever since they usually are associated with fever, occurring 5–11 days after vaccination when febrile reactions to the vaccine are most common, and are rarely associated with any sequelae. Studies conducted to date have not established an association between measles vaccination and the development of a residual seizure disorder. Rarely, afebrile convulsions and seizures have occurred following administration of measles virus vaccine live.

Antipyretics can prevent febrile seizures associated with measles vaccination if administered before the onset of fever and continued for 5–7 days. However, such antipyretic prophylaxis is difficult because the onset of fever often is sudden and occurs unpredictably. Seizures can occur early in the course of fever. Parents and caregivers should be vigilant for fever that occurs subsequent to vaccination and should be advised regarding appropriate treatment; because of the risk of Reye's syndrome, aspirin generally should *not* be used to prevent or control fever among children and adolescents.

Sensitivity Reactions Hypersensitivity reactions, including anaphylaxis and anaphylactoid reactions as well as related phenomena such as angioedema (including peripheral or facial edema) and bronchial spasm, have been reported rarely following administration of MMR in individuals with or without an allergic history. Most hypersensitivity reactions have been minor, consisting of a wheal and flare or urticaria at the injection site. Immediate, anaphylactic reactions to measles virus vaccine live or MMR are extremely rare. Although more than 70 million doses of measles-containing vaccines (MMR) have been distributed in the US since the Vaccine Adverse Events Reporting System (VAERS) was implemented in 1990, only 33 cases of anaphylactic reactions have been reported after MMR vaccination. In addition, only 11 of these cases occurred immediately after vaccination with manifestations consistent with anaphylaxis.

Immediate allergic reactions (i.e., breathing difficulty, hypotension), which may be life threatening, have occurred following administration of monovalent measles virus vaccine live (no longer commercially available in the US) in several children with a history of anaphylactoid reactions to egg ingestion. However, it has been suggested that measles virus vaccine live does not contain enough egg protein to cause a severe reaction in most egg-allergic children, and evidence from recent studies and reports of anaphylactic reactions to the vaccine in individuals who had no evidence of egg allergy suggest that hypersensitivity reactions to the vaccine may be related to some other, as yet undefined, component. Measles virus vaccine live generally has been administered safely to children who had egg allergies that were not anaphylactoid in nature and also has been administered safely to children with a history of immediate reactions to eggs. Some clinicians have suggested that skin testing with MMR be used in children with a history of severe allergic reactions to eggs (e.g., generalized urticaria, shock, manifestations of upper or lower airway obstruction) to identify those who may be at risk for severe reactions to the vaccine and that desensitization procedures be used prior to administration of the vaccine in those with positive skin test results. However, the American Academy of Pediatrics (AAP) and other experts question the predictive value and necessity of such testing since anaphylactic reactions may be unrelated to egg protein and the risk of serious reactions to the vaccine in egg-sensitive individuals appears to be extremely low. (See Allergy to Egg-related Antigens under Cautions: Sensitivity Reactions, in Precautions and Contraindications.)

MMR contains hydrolyzed gelatin as a stabilizer, which rarely may stimulate hypersensitivity reactions in some individuals. An anaphylactic reaction following MMR vaccination has been reported in the US in at least one individual with IgE-mediated anaphylactic sensitivity to gelatin, and similar cases have been reported elsewhere. (See Gelatin Allergy under Cautions: Sensitivity Reactions, in Precautions and Contraindications.)

CNS Effects A causal relationship has not been definitely established, but a few cases of encephalitis and encephalopathy have been reported rarely after measles vaccination. However, the risk of serious neurologic disorders following vaccination with a measles virus-containing vaccine is considerably less than the risk of encephalitis and encephalopathy associated with wild-type measles infection. Ocular palsies, Guillain-Barré syndrome, measles inclusion body encephalitis (MIBE), aseptic meningitis, seizures, polyneuritis, polyneuropathy, paresthesia, and ataxia have occurred after administration of vaccines containing live, attenuated measles virus.

Rarely, subacute sclerosing panencephalitis (SSPE) has been reported in children who did not have a history of natural measles infection but did receive measles virus vaccine live. Some of these cases may have resulted from unrecognized measles in the first year of life or possibly from the measles vaccination. However, by protecting against natural measles infection, widespread vaccination with measles virus vaccine live has been associated with near elimination of subacute sclerosing panencephalitis overall, indicating that the vaccine substantially reduces the likelihood of developing this encephalitis. Administration of measles virus vaccine live does not increase the risk for developing subacute sclerosing panencephalitis, regardless of whether the vaccinee previously had natural measles infection or has received the vaccine before.

Hematologic Effects Surveillance of adverse effects in the US and elsewhere indicates that measles virus-containing vaccines (e.g., MMR) rarely can cause clinically evident thrombocytopenia (e.g., purpura) within 2 months after vaccination. In prospective studies, the reported incidence of clinically evident thrombocytopenia after MMR vaccination ranged from 1 per 30,000 to 1 per 40,000 vaccinated children, with a temporal clustering of cases occurring 2–3 weeks after vaccination. With passive surveillance, the reported incidence ranged from 1 per 100,000 to 1 per million distributed doses. Results of one retrospective study confirmed that a causal relation exists between receipt of MMR and idiopathic thrombocytopenic purpura and indicated that the absolute risk within 6 weeks of vaccination was 1 in 22,300 doses with 2 out of 3 cases occurring in the 6-week post-vaccination period being caused by MMR. However, the incidence of thrombocytopenia with natural measles or rubella infection is substantially greater than that with vaccination, being reported as 1 per 3000 children during one measles epidemic. Evidence from case reports suggests that the risk of vaccine-induced thrombocytopenia may be increased in individuals with a history of idiopathic (immune) thrombocytopenic purpura, particularly for those who developed it with a previous dose of the vaccine; however, results of one retrospective study indicate that children with a history of idiopathic thrombocytopenic purpura prior to the first dose of MMR are not at increased risk of vaccine-associated idiopathic thrombocytopenic purpura. In most cases, vaccine-associated thrombocytopenic purpura usually has been transient and benign, although hemorrhage occurred rarely.

Ocular Effects Ocular palsies generally occurred approximately 3–24 days following measles vaccination; however, a causal relationship has not been definitely established. Forms of optic neuritis, including retrobulbar neuritis, papillitis, and retinitis, occur rarely following viral infections, and have been reported to occur 1–3 weeks following administration of some live virus vaccines.

Other Adverse Systemic Effects Mild lymphadenopathy is uncommon, and headache, cough, rhinitis, eye pain, generalized malaise, diarrhea, nausea, vomiting, and vasculitis have been reported rarely following measles virus vaccine live. Syncope also has been reported.

Although it has been suggested that administration of measles virus vaccine live is associated with an increased risk of Crohn's disease, concerns have been raised about the methods used in epidemiologic studies that suggested such an association, and evidence does not support a causal association between the vaccine and risk for Crohn's or any other inflammatory bowel disease.

Measles inclusion body encephalitis (MIBE), pneumonitis, and death related to disseminated measles vaccine virus infection have been reported in immunocompromised individuals (e.g., those with acquired immunodeficiency syndrome [AIDS]) who received measles-containing vaccines.

■ **Local Effects** Burning and/or stinging of short duration may occur at the injection site because of the slightly acidic pH (6.2–6.6) of the vaccine. Allergic reactions such as wheal and flare at the injection site or urticaria have been reported rarely.

Local reactions characterized by marked swelling, induration, erythema, vesiculation, and edema at the injection site, with or without fever and lymphadenopathy, have occurred following administration of measles virus vaccine live in 4–55% of patients who previously received inactivated measles vaccine. Rarely, more severe reactions that may require hospitalization, including prolonged, high fevers and extensive local reactions, have been reported. These reactions are considerably milder than atypical measles syndrome, an illness which may occur when individuals who previously received inactivated measles vaccine are exposed to natural measles. There is no evidence that individuals who are already immune to measles, either from vaccination with a live measles vaccine or natural disease, are at increased risk of adverse effects following administration of measles virus vaccine live.

■ **Precautions and Contraindications** MMR is contraindicated in individuals who are hypersensitive to the vaccine or any component in the formulation, including gelatin. (See Gelatin Allergy under Cautions: Sensitivity Reactions, in Precautions and Contraindications.) In addition, MMR is contraindicated in those with a history of anaphylactic or anaphylactoid reaction to neomycin. (See Neomycin Allergy under Cautions: Sensitivity Reactions, in Precautions and Contraindications.)

MMR also is contraindicated in certain other individuals. (See Individuals with Altered Immunocompetence under Cautions: Precautions and Contraindications and see Cautions: Pregnancy, Fertility, and Lactation.)

Sensitivity Reactions Prior to administration, the recipient and/or parent or guardian should be questioned concerning reactions to previous doses of measles virus-containing vaccine or MMR. Individuals who have a hypersensitivity reaction to the first dose of MMR should be tested for immunity to measles; if results indicate immunity, a second dose is not necessary. Any individual with an anaphylactic reaction to a previous dose should not receive another dose, regardless of results of serologic testing.

Epinephrine should be readily available for immediate treatment of an anaphylactic reaction if such a reaction should occur.

Allergy to Egg-related Antigens. MMR is produced in chick embryo cell culture; individuals with a history of anaphylactic, anaphylactoid, or other immediate reaction (e.g., hives, swelling of the mouth or throat, difficulty breathing, hypotension, shock) to egg ingestion may be at increased risk of immediate-type hypersensitivity reactions after receiving vaccines containing traces of chick embryo antigen. The manufacturer states that the potential benefits and risks should be carefully evaluated before considering administration of MMR to individuals with a history of immediate hypersensitivity reactions to egg ingestion, and recommends that such individuals be vaccinated with extreme caution and with adequate treatment readily available should a reaction occur.

The US Public Health Service Advisory Committee on Immunization Practices (ACIP) and others *previously* recommended that, since MMR is produced in chick embryo fibroblasts, administration of the vaccine in these individuals be deferred until after appropriate skin testing and desensitization procedures had been performed and that the vaccine be administered to these individuals *only* with extreme caution (in a setting where an immediate allergic reaction can be detected and treated). However, the predictive value and necessity of such testing have been questioned by most experts since measles virus vaccine live has been administered safely to some children with histories of immediate reactions to eggs and most anaphylactic reactions to the vaccine are not associated with egg allergy but to other vaccine components. Therefore, ACIP states that skin testing and use of special protocols are not required when administering a measles virus-containing vaccine in individuals with a history of anaphylactic-like reactions after egg ingestion. A reasonable precaution for individuals with a history of immediate reactions to eggs is to administer MMR in a supervised setting where appropriate emergency treatment material is available.

Evidence indicates that individuals are *not* at increased risk of hypersensitivity reactions to measles virus-containing vaccine if they have egg allergies that are *not* anaphylactoid in nature, and administration of MMR to these individuals should follow the usually recommendations. There is no evidence that individuals with allergies to chickens or feathers are at increased risk of allergic reactions to the vaccine.

Neomycin Allergy. Because MMR contain trace amounts of neomycin, the vaccine is contraindicated in individuals who have had an anaphylactic reaction to topically or systemically administered neomycin.

Neomycin allergy usually is characterized by a delayed-type (cell-mediated) hypersensitivity reaction, such as contact dermatitis, rather than an anaphylactic reaction. Following administration of measles virus vaccine live to individuals who have had a delayed-type hypersensitivity reaction to neomycin, the typical adverse reaction, if any, is a contact dermatitis (e.g., an erythematous, pruritic nodule or papule) occurring within 48–96 hours.

The ACIP and the American Academy of Pediatrics (AAP) state that vaccines containing trace amounts of neomycin should *not* be used in individuals with a history of anaphylactic reaction to neomycin, but use of such vaccines may be considered in those with a history of delayed-type hypersensitivity reaction to neomycin if benefits of vaccination outweigh risks.

Gelatin Allergy. The possibility of allergic reactions to hydrolyzed gelatin, which is present in MMR as a stabilizer, should be considered since anaphylactic reactions to the vaccine have been reported rarely in individuals with anaphylactic sensitivity to gelatin. MMR should not be administered to individuals with a history of anaphylactic reactions to gelatin or gelatin-containing products. Although skin testing for gelatin sensitivity before administering a gelatin-containing vaccine such as MMR can be considered, there are no specific protocols for this purpose. Because gelatin used in vaccines manufactured in the US usually is derived from porcine sources and food gelatin may be derived solely from bovine sources, a negative food history does not exclude the possibility of a reaction to the gelatin contained in the vaccines.

Individuals with Altered Immunocompetence MMR generally is contraindicated in individuals with primary immunodeficiencies (e.g., cellular immune deficiency, hypogammaglobulinemia, dysgammaglobulinemia) and in individuals with suppressed immune responses resulting from AIDS or other clinical manifestations of human immunodeficiency virus (HIV) infection, blood dyscrasias, leukemia, lymphomas of any type, or any other malignant neoplasms affecting the bone marrow or lymphatic systems.

Because replication of measles vaccine virus may be potentiated in individuals with primary immunodeficiencies (e.g., cellular immune deficiency, hypogammaglobulinemia, dysgammaglobulinemia) or with suppressed immune response resulting from leukemia, lymphoma, other malignancies affecting the bone marrow or lymphatic system, or blood dyscrasias, concern exists about the potential risk of administering any live virus vaccine to such individuals. Evidence based on case reports has linked measles virus-containing vaccine and measles infection to subsequent death in some severely immunocompromised children. Of the more than 200 million doses of measles virus-containing vaccine administered in the US, fewer than 5 such deaths have been reported. Because of this potentially fatal association, the ACIP states that, with the exception of most HIV-infected individuals, immunocompromised individuals should not receive a measles virus-containing vaccine. MMR should not be given to an individual with a family history of congenital or hereditary immunodeficiency until the immunocompetence of the individual has been documented. There are no case reports linking MMR or other mumps or rubella virus-containing vaccines to clinically important infection caused by the mumps or rubella component in immunocompromised vaccinees.

Severe immunosuppression may be caused by many disease conditions (e.g., congenital immunodeficiency, HIV infection, hematologic or generalized malignancy) and by immunosuppressive therapy. For some conditions, all affected individuals are severely immunocompromised, whereas for other conditions, the degree of immune compromise depends on the severity of the condition, which in turn depends on the disease and treatment stage. MMR generally is contraindicated in individuals receiving immunosuppressive therapy (e.g., corticotropin, corticosteroids [at immunosuppressive dosages], alkylating agents, antimetabolites, radiation therapy), although the manufacturer states that the vaccine is not contraindicated in individuals receiving corticosteroids as replacement therapy (e.g., for Addison's disease). (See Drug Interactions: Immunosuppressive Agents.) Ultimately, the patient's clinician must assume responsibility for determining whether the patient is severely immunocompromised based on clinical and laboratory assessment. Measles virus-containing vaccine should *not* be administered to *severely* immunocompromised individuals.

The ACIP states that use of live virus vaccines can be considered in patients with leukemia, lymphoma, or other malignancies if the disease is in remission and chemotherapy was terminated at least 3 months prior to vaccination.

Antibody responses to MMR and efficacy may be decreased in immunocompromised individuals.

HIV-infected Individuals. Because of the risk of severe measles in symptomatic HIV-infected individuals and because limited studies and experience with measles, mumps, and rubella immunization in patients with HIV infection have not documented serious or unusual adverse effects, the ACIP, AAP, US Centers for Disease Control and Prevention (CDC), National Institutes of Health (NIH), Infectious Diseases Society of America (IDSA), Pediatric Infectious Diseases Society, and others state that MMR should be administered to all *asymptomatic* HIV-infected individuals according to the usually recommended immunization schedules and should be considered for all symptomatic HIV-infected individuals who do *not* have evidence of severe immunosuppression and who otherwise would be eligible for measles vaccination. The presence of immunocompromised or HIV-infected individuals in a household does not preclude administration of MMR to other household members.

Because of a reported case of progressive pneumonitis in a measles vaccinee who had advanced AIDS and because of other evidence indicating that the antibody response to measles vaccine is diminished in severely immunocompromised individuals, MMR is contraindicated in HIV-infected individuals with *severe immunosuppression*. (See HIV-Infected Individuals under Uses: Primary Immunization.)

The reported case of pneumonitis occurred in a 20-year-old HIV-infected man with hemophilia A who received a dose of MMR to fulfill a college prematriculation vaccination requirement; a previous dose of measles-containing vaccine had been administered during infancy. At the time of vaccination, the individual was asymptomatic for HIV but immunosuppressed and was not receiving antiretroviral or antipneumocystis therapy. Approximately 13 months after the MMR dose, symptoms of measles pneumonitis developed, and a presumptive diagnosis was made and then confirmed by measles virus culture from a lung biopsy. One month later the patient was rehospitalized for presumptive *Mycobacterium avium* complex (MAC) disease and then discharged, but subsequently was readmitted and died with a presumptive diagnosis of cytomegalovirus (CMV) encephalitis, with pulmonary measles and MAC as contributing factors; no autopsy was performed. Postmortem testing of the measles virus isolate recovered before the patient's death showed a high degree of similarity to the Moraten measles virus vaccine strain, and the vaccine strain as the source of the patient's lung isolate was confirmed.

Fever or Febrile Seizures Febrile seizures have occurred rarely following administration of a measles virus-containing vaccine. Fever (39.4°C or greater) has been reported. Following administration of MMR, patients should be monitored for temperature elevations.

Caution should be used in individuals with a history of cerebral injury, individual or family history of seizures, or any other condition in which fever-induced stress should be avoided.

Risk of Transmissible Agents in Preparations Containing Albumin MMR contains *recombinant* human albumin.

Monovalent measles virus vaccine live (no longer commercially available in the US) and the fixed-combination vaccine containing measles, mumps, rubella, and varicella antigens (MMRV; ProQuad®) contain albumin human. Since albumin human is prepared from pooled human plasma, it is a potential vehicle for transmission of human viruses, and theoretically may carry the risk of transmitting the causative agent of Creutzfeldt-Jakob disease (CJD).

For further information on precautions related to transmissible agents in plasma-derived preparations, see Risk of Transmissible Agents in Plasma-derived Preparations under Cautions: Precautions and Contraindications, in Albumin Human 16:00.

Concomitant Illness The decision whether to administer or delay administration of MMR in an individual with a current or recent acute illness depends largely on the severity of symptoms and etiology of the illness. The manufacturer states that MMR is contraindicated in patients with any febrile respiratory illness or other active febrile infections. The ACIP and AAP state that minor acute illness, such as mild upper respiratory infection (with or without fever) or mild diarrhea, usually does not preclude vaccination. However, vaccination of individuals with moderate or severe acute illness (with or without fever) generally should be deferred until they have recovered from the acute phase of the illness. This precaution avoids superimposing adverse effects of the vaccine on the underlying illness or mistakenly concluding that a manifestation of the underlying illness resulted from vaccination. Data generally are not available on the safety and immunogenicity of measles, mumps, and rubella virus-containing vaccines in individuals with moderate or severe febrile illness. Based on preliminary evidence, the possibility that immune response occasionally may be suppressed by concurrent mild upper respiratory infection (possibly secondary to viral infection-induced interferon formation) should be considered when vaccination is undertaken in such individuals; additional study is needed to confirm these findings, but they do not change current recommendations concerning vaccination of individuals with minor concurrent illness.

Thrombocytopenia Individuals with a history of thrombocytopenic purpura or thrombocytopenia may be at increased risk of developing clinically apparent thrombocytopenia after vaccination. Thrombocytopenia has worsened in those with preexisting thrombocytopenia and may worsen with subsequent doses. The decision to vaccinate such individuals should depend on the benefits of immunity and the risks of recurrence or exacerbation of thrombocytopenia after vaccination or during natural infection with viruses. Although thrombocytopenia can be life-threatening, no deaths have been reported to date as a direct consequence of vaccine-induced thrombocytopenia. Because the benefits of vaccination usually exceed the risks, ACIP states that vaccination with a measles- and/or rubella-containing vaccine is justified in such individuals, particularly considering the even greater risk of thrombocytopenia associated with natural infection with these viruses. However, avoiding a subsequent dose might be prudent if the previous episode of thrombocytopenia occurred in close temporal proximity to (i.e., within 6 weeks after) the previous dose. Serologic evidence of measles immunity may be obtained in lieu of vaccination.

Risk of Neurodevelopmental Disorders Although it has been theorized that there is a link between the antigens contained in MMR and neurodevelopmental disorders in children (autism), evidence has been insufficient to support an association between neurodevelopmental disorders and MMR. In 2004, the Immunization Safety Review Committee of the Institute of Medicine (IOM) examined the hypothesis that MMR is causally associated with autism and concluded that the evidence favors rejection of a causal relationship between MMR and autism.

Tuberculosis Vaccination with a measles virus-containing vaccine is not recommended for individuals with untreated, active tuberculosis. Vaccination in these individuals should be deferred until antituberculosis therapy has been initiated. Administration of live, attenuated vaccines is not contraindicated in individuals with a positive tuberculin skin test who do not have active tuberculosis infection. Tuberculin testing is not a prerequisite for administration of MMR.

Transmission of Vaccine Virus MMR contains live, attenuated virus; there is a theoretical risk that transmission of vaccine virus could occur between vaccinees and susceptible contacts.

Transmission of live, attenuated measles from vaccinees to susceptible contacts has not been reported.

Limitations of Vaccine Effectiveness MMR may not protect all individuals from measles.

Safety and efficacy of MMR have not been established for postexposure prophylaxis following exposure to measles. (See Uses: Postexposure Vaccination.)

Improper Storage and Handling Improper storage or handling of vaccines may result in loss of vaccine potency and reduced immune response in vaccinees.

MMR that has been mishandled or has not been stored at the recommended temperature should not be administered. (See Chemistry and Stability: Stability.)

Lyophilized and reconstituted vaccine should be protected from light at all times because exposure to light may inactivate the vaccine virus.

Freezing or exposing the diluent supplied by the manufacturer to freezing temperatures should be avoided; the diluent may be refrigerated or stored at room temperature.

All vaccines should be inspected upon delivery and monitored during storage to ensure that the appropriate temperature is maintained.

■ **Pediatric Precautions** Safety and efficacy of MMR in children younger than 6 months of age have not been established, and use of the vaccine in this age group is not recommended.

Routine immunization against measles is initiated at 12 through 15 months of age. Infants 6 through 11 months of age may receive measles vaccine if protection against measles is considered necessary (e.g., for measles outbreak control, for travelers). Although monovalent measles virus vaccine live is preferred instead of MMR in infants 6 through 11 months of age since the risk of serious disease from mumps or rubella infection is relatively low in infants and benefit from exposure to the mumps or rubella antigens may be low secondary to persisting maternal antibodies that may interfere with seroconversion in this young age group, monovalent measles virus vaccine is no longer commercially available in the US and such infants should receive MMR.

There is some evidence that infants born to mothers who had wild-type measles may not develop sustained antibody levels if vaccinated at less than 12 months of age and later revaccinated.

■ **Geriatric Precautions** Clinical studies of MMR did not include sufficient numbers of seronegative individuals 65 years of age or older to determine whether these individuals respond differently than younger individuals. Other reported clinical experience has not identified differences in responses between geriatric and younger individuals.

■ **Mutagenicity and Carcinogenicity** The mutagenic or carcinogenic potential of MMR have not been evaluated.

■ **Pregnancy, Fertility, and Lactation** ***Pregnancy*** Measles virus-containing vaccine should not be administered to pregnant women, and pregnancy should be avoided for 1–3 months following vaccination with. Although the ACIP and AAP state that measles virus-containing vaccine is contraindicated during pregnancy and that pregnancy should be avoided for 4 weeks after vaccination, the manufacturer states that pregnancy should be avoided for 3 months after vaccination. This precaution is based on the theoretical risk of fetal infection from a live virus vaccine; however, there is no evidence substantiating such risk with measles virus vaccine live.

Natural measles infection during pregnancy increases the risk of spontaneous abortion, stillbirth, congenital defects, and prematurity. Animal reproduction studies have not been performed with MMR. It is not known if the vaccine can cause fetal harm when administered to pregnant women or affect reproductive capacity. There are no adequate studies of the effects of measles virus vaccine live on fetal development; however, there is a theoretical risk of adverse effects for up to 3 months following vaccination. These theoretical risks should be weighed against the risks associated with natural measles infection in unimmunized adolescents or adults.

Reasonable precautions should be taken to preclude vaccination of pregnant women, including asking women if they are pregnant, excluding those who state that they are, and informing the others of the theoretical risks. If a pregnant woman is vaccinated or became pregnant within 1–3 months after vaccination, she should be counseled about the theoretical risks to the fetus; measles, mumps, and/or rubella vaccination during pregnancy should not usually be a reason to consider termination of pregnancy. (See also Cautions: Pregnancy, Fertility, and Lactation, in Rubella Virus Vaccine Live 80:12). If exposure to measles occurs during pregnancy, the possibility of providing temporary passive immunity with immune globulin should be considered.

Lactation It is not known whether MMR is distributed into milk. The manufacturer states that MMR should be administered with caution to nursing women. The ACIP states that breastfeeding generally is not a contraindication to administration of measles virus-containing vaccine since live vaccines appear to pose no special problems for the mother or her nursing infant.

Drug Interactions

■ **Blood Products** Blood products (e.g., whole blood, packed red blood cells, plasma) may interfere with the immune response to certain live virus vaccines, including measles, mumps, and rubella virus vaccine live (MMR; M-M-R® II); therefore, MMR should not be administered simultaneously with or for specified intervals before or after administration of blood products.

Administration of MMR should be deferred for at least 3 months following administration of red blood cells (with adenine-saline added); for at least 6 months following administration of packed red blood cells or whole blood; and for at least 7 months following administration of plasma or platelet products.

After receiving MMR, vaccinees should avoid blood products for 2 weeks; if use of a blood product is considered necessary during this period, a repeat vaccine dose should be given after the recommended interval unless serologic testing is feasible and indicates a response to the vaccine was attained.

■ **Immunosuppressive Agents** Individuals receiving immunosuppressive agents (e.g., alkylating agents, antimetabolites, corticotropin, corticosteroids [at immunosuppressive dosages], radiation therapy) may have a diminished response to measles virus-containing vaccine and replication of the virus may be potentiated. Vaccination with MMR should be deferred until the immunosuppressive agent is discontinued; the manufacturer states that individuals receiving corticosteroids as replacement therapy (e.g., those with Addison's disease) generally may receive the vaccine. The exact interval between discontinuance of immunosuppressive therapy and regaining the ability to respond to live virus vaccines is not known, but live viral vaccines generally should not be administered for at least 3 months after discontinuance of immunosuppressive therapy. Individuals with leukemia in remission who have not received chemotherapy for at least 3 months may receive a live virus vaccine. The precise amount and duration of systemically absorbed corticosteroid therapy needed to suppress the immune system of an otherwise healthy individual are not well defined. Although of recent theoretical concern, there is no evidence of increased severe reactions to live vaccines in individuals receiving corticosteroid aerosol therapy, and such therapy is not in itself a reason to delay vaccination. Most experts, including the US Public Health Service Advisory Committee on Immunization Practices (ACIP) and American Academy of Pediatrics (AAP) agree that short-term (less than 2 weeks), low- to moderate-dose systemic corticosteroid therapy; long-term, alternate-day, systemic corticosteroid therapy using low to moderate doses of short-acting drugs; topical corticosteroid therapy (e.g., nasal, cutaneous, ophthalmic); aerosol corticosteroid therapy; or intra-articular, bursal, or tendon injections with corticosteroids should not be immunosuppressive in usual dosages and do not necessarily contraindicate vaccination with live virus vaccines. Although the immunosuppressive effects of corticosteroid therapy vary, many clinicians consider a dose equivalent to 2 mg/kg or 20 mg total of prednisone daily for 2 weeks or longer as sufficiently immunosuppressive to raise concerns about the safety of vaccination with live virus vaccines.

■ **Immune Globulins** Antibodies contained in immune globulin preparations (e.g., immune globulin IM [IGIM], immune globulin IV [IGIV], hepatitis B immune globulin [HBIG], rabies immune globulin [RIG], tetanus immune globulin [TIG], varicella-zoster immune globulin [VZIG]) may interfere with the immune response to certain live virus vaccines, including measles virus-containing vaccines. The duration of possible interference appears to depend on the dosage of the immune globulin preparation. It was previously suggested that vaccines containing measles virus vaccine live (e.g., MMR) could be administered as early as 6 weeks to 3 months after immune globulin preparations; however, this recommendation was based on data from individuals who received low doses of immune globulin. Recent evidence suggests that high doses of immune globulin preparations can inhibit the immune response to measles virus vaccine live for 3 months or longer.

The ACIP and AAP have made the following recommendations concerning administration of measles virus-containing vaccines in patients who have received immune globulins: MMR should be deferred for at least 3 months following administration of TIG, HBIG, IGIM used for prophylaxis of tetanus, hepatitis B virus (HBV), or hepatitis A virus (HAV); for at least 4 months following administration of RIG; for at least 5 months following administration of VZIG for varicella prophylaxis or IGIM used for measles prophylaxis in immunocompetent individuals; for at least 6 months following use of cytomegalovirus immune globulin IV (CMV-IGIV) or IGIM used for measles prophylaxis in immunocompromised individuals; for at least 8 months following administration of IGIV for replacement therapy of immunodeficiencies or VZIG or IGIV used for postexposure prophylaxis of severe varicella; for at least 8–10 months following administration of IGIV for the treatment of idiopathic thrombocytopenic purpura (ITP); or for at least 11 months following administration of IGIV for Kawasaki syndrome.

If simultaneous administration of a measles virus-containing vaccine and one of these immune globulin preparations or administration at less than the recommended interval is deemed necessary (e.g., because of imminent exposure to disease), the fact that vaccine-induced immunity may be compromised should be considered and, unless there is serologic evidence of an adequate antibody response to the live virus vaccine, an additional dose of vaccine should be administered at the specified interval. If administered simultaneously, the live virus vaccine and immune globulin should be administered at separate sites anatomically remote from one another.

The fact that revaccination may be necessary in individuals who receive an immune globulin preparation shortly after a measles virus-containing vaccine also should be considered. In general, vaccine virus replication and stimulation of immunity occur within 7–14 days after administration of a live virus vaccine. Therefore, if the interval between administration of a measles virus-containing vaccine and subsequent administration of one of these preparations is less than 14 days, an additional dose of vaccine should be given after the appropriate interval previously specified, unless serologic testing indicates that an adequate antibody response to the vaccine occurred. An additional dose of vaccine generally is unnecessary if the interval between vaccination and administration of the immune globulin or blood product is longer than 2 weeks.

■ **Live Vaccines** ***Measles, Mumps, Rubella, and Varicella Vaccines*** Measles virus vaccine live may be administered concurrently with mumps virus vaccine live, rubella virus vaccine live, and varicella virus vaccine live.

Measles virus vaccine live is commercially available in a fixed-combination vaccine containing mumps virus vaccine live and rubella virus vaccine live (MMR) to facilitate concomitant administration of all 3 antigens. Administration of MMR results in immunologic responses similar to those obtained with administration of the 3 antigens at separate sites.

MMR may be administered concurrently with monovalent varicella virus vaccine live (Varivax®) at a different site using a separate syringe. Results of studies in healthy children 12–36 months of age indicate that seroconversion rates, antibody responses, and adverse effects reported with simultaneous administration of the vaccines are similar to those reported when the vaccines are administered 6 weeks apart. Because there is a theoretical concern that the immune response to one live viral vaccine may be impaired if administered within 1 month of another, if MMR and varicella virus vaccine live are not administered simultaneously then they should be administered at least 1 month apart. There is some evidence that administration of varicella virus vaccine live less than 30 days after MMR decreases the effectiveness of the varicella vaccine. Results of a retrospective cohort study that used data from the Vaccine Safety Datalink (VSD) project and included children 12 months of age or older who were vaccinated during January 1995 to December 1999 indicate that administration of varicella virus vaccine live less than 30 days after MMR results in a 2.5-fold increase in the incidence of breakthrough varicella infections. However, when the vaccines were administered concurrently, there was no increase in the risk for breakthrough infections.

Measles virus vaccine live also is commercially available in a fixed-combination vaccine containing MMR and varicella virus vaccine live (MMRV; ProQuad®). This fixed-combination vaccine is safe and effective in healthy children 12 months through 12 years of age. Studies using MMRV (ProQuad®) in healthy children 1–6 years of age indicate that the antibody response to measles, mumps, rubella, and varicella antigens following a single dose of the fixed-combination vaccine are similar to those obtained after a single dose of MMR and a single dose of varicella virus vaccine live (Varivax®). However, there is some evidence that the relative risk for febrile seizures in infants may be higher with the fixed-combination vaccine MMRV than that reported when a dose of single-antigen varicella virus vaccine live (Varivax®) and a dose of MMR are given concomitantly. For information on the fixed-combination vaccine containing MMR and varicella virus vaccine live (MMRV; ProQuad®), see Varicella Virus Vaccine Live 80:12.

Influenza Vaccine Live Intranasal Because of theoretical concerns that the immune response to one live virus vaccine might be impaired if given within 30 days of another live virus vaccine, if MMR and influenza virus vaccine live intranasal are not administered on the same day, they should be administered at least 4 weeks apart.

Other Live Vaccines Some oral live vaccines (e.g., rotavirus vaccine live oral, typhoid vaccine live oral) can be administered concomitantly with or at any interval before or after MMR.

Because of theoretical concerns that the immune response to other live virus vaccines might be impaired if given within 30 days of another live virus vaccine, if MMR and yellow fever vaccine are not administered on the same day, they should be administered at least 4 weeks apart.

■ **Inactivated Vaccines and Toxoids** MMR may be administered concurrently with (using different syringes and different injection sites) or at any interval before or after inactivated vaccines, recombinant vaccines, polysaccharide vaccines, or toxoids.

Haemophilus b Conjugate Vaccines MMR and *Haemophilus influenzae* type b (Hib) conjugate vaccines may be given concomitantly at a different site using a separate syringe. Concomitant administration of MMR and Hib vaccine does not interfere with the immune response or increase adverse effects of either vaccine.

Influenza Vaccines MMR may be given concomitantly with parenteral inactivated influenza vaccines (using different syringes and different injection sites) or at any interval before or after administration of inactivated influenza vaccines.

Pneumococcal Vaccines MMR may be administered concurrently with pneumococcal vaccine, including pneumococcal conjugate vaccine (PCV) or pneumococcal 23-valent polysaccharide vaccine (PPSV23), at a different site using a separate syringe.

Hepatitis B Vaccine Although data are limited concerning simultaneous administration of MMR and hepatitis B vaccine, MMR may be administered concomitantly (using different syringes and different injection sites) or at any interval before or after hepatitis B vaccine.

Diphtheria and Tetanus Toxoids and Pertussis Vaccines Although data are limited concerning simultaneous administration of MMR and diphtheria and tetanus toxoids and acellular pertussis vaccine adsorbed (DTaP), or tetanus toxoid and reduced diphtheria toxoid and acellular pertussis vaccine adsorbed (Tdap), MMR may be administered concomitantly (using different syringes and different injection sites) or at any interval before or after DTaP or Tdap.

Laboratory Test Interferences

■ **Tuberculin** Live attenuated measles, mumps, and rubella virus vaccines have been reported to temporarily suppress tuberculin skin sensitivity; therefore, tuberculin tests (if required) should be administered simultaneously with or 4–6 weeks after administration of measles, mumps, and rubella virus vaccine live (MMR; M-M-R® II). The US Public Health Service Advisory Committee on Immunization Practices (ACIP) states that simultaneous administration of tuberculin and MMR is the preferred option since this does not interfere with reading the tuberculin test result at 48–72 hours and ensures that the individual has been vaccinated against measles, mumps, and rubella. Although tuberculin testing can be performed and read before administering the vaccine, the ACIP states that this option is the least favored since it will delay vaccination.

Pharmacology

Monovalent measles virus vaccine live (no longer commercially available in the US) and the fixed-combination vaccine containing measles, mumps, and rubella antigens (measles, mumps, and rubella virus vaccine live [MMR; M-M-R® II]) stimulate active immunity to measles by inducing production of measles-specific immunoglobulin G (IgG) and M (IgM) antibodies (humoral immunity). Studies using monovalent measles virus vaccine live indicate that the antibody response to initial vaccination (primary response) resembles that caused by primary natural measles infection, with an initial transient increase in serum IgM titers and a subsequent increase in serum IgG titers, although the titers achieved with vaccination are lower. As with natural infection, IgG antibody titers decline slowly over time, but immunity is thought to persist for many years and possibly lifelong in most vaccinees. Individuals who experience initial antigenic stimulation from either natural infection or vaccine generally exhibit an anamnestic (secondary) response to subsequent revaccination or exposure to natural measles. This anamnestic response generally is characterized by a rapid but often transient increase in serum IgG titers but little or no detectable IgM production; however, with more sensitive assays, IgM titers may be detected more frequently, albeit still in low proportion to IgG.

While measurement of measles-specific antibody and assessment of immunity most commonly have been determined using the hemagglutination-inhibition (HI) assay, other more sensitive assays, including enzyme-linked immunosorbent (ELISA), plaque reduction neutralization (PRN), and antihemolysin (AH) assays, are available and being employed. The US Public Health Service Advisory Committee on Immunization Practices (ACIP) states that individuals with serologic evidence of measles-specific antibody, determined by any of the available assays, is considered immune. However, a minimum protective antibody titer has not been established, and some evidence suggests that relatively low titers determined by highly sensitive assays (e.g., PRN titers of 120 or less) may not be protective.

If MMR is administered at 9 months of age or older, a single dose is approximately 85% effective in preventing measles. If MMR is administered at 12 months of age or older, the vaccine is 95% effective after a single dose and 99% effective after 2 doses.

The duration of immunity following vaccination with measles virus-containing vaccine has not yet been established and can only be determined by continued long-term observation. There is serologic and epidemiologic evidence that vaccine-induced immunity to measles persists at least 13–23 years and probably life-long in most vaccinees. Titers of vaccine-induced HI antibodies slowly decline and are lower than those following natural measles infection. However, vaccine failure secondary to waning immunity after initially successful immunization appears to occur in only a small percentage of vaccinees, but evidence of such waning is limited.

Chemistry and Stability

■ **Chemistry** Measles virus vaccine live is a preparation of live, attenuated measles virus. Monovalent measles virus vaccine live (Attenuvax®) is no longer commercially available in the US. Measles virus vaccine live is commercially available in the US in a fixed-combination vaccine with mumps virus vaccine live and rubella virus vaccine live (MMR; M-M-R® II) and in a fixed-combination vaccine containing MMR and varicella virus vaccine live (MMRV; ProQuad®). For information on the fixed-combination vaccine containing MMR and varicella virus vaccine live, see Varicella Virus Vaccine Live 80:12.

Vaccines containing measles virus vaccine live, including MMR, meet standards established by the Center for Biologics Evaluation and Research of the US Food and Drug Administration. Measles virus-containing vaccines commercially available in the US contain the more attenuated Enders' line of measles virus derived from attenuated Edmonston strain and propagated in chick embryo cell cultures. The potency of MMR is expressed in terms of the amount of virus estimated to infect 50% of a number of standardized tissue culture preparations under specified conditions (Tissue Culture Infective Dose 50% or $TCID_{50}$). Following reconstitution with the diluent provided by the manufacturer, each 0.5-mL dose of MMR contains not less than 1000 $TCID_{50}$ of measles virus, 12,500 $TCID_{50}$ of mumps virus, and 1000 $TCID_{50}$ of rubella virus.Each 0.5-mL dose of MMR contains sorbitol (14.5 mg), sodium phosphate, sucrose (1.9 mg), sodium chloride, hydrolyzed gelatin (14.5 mg), recombinant albumin human (up to 0.3 mg), fetal bovine serum (less than 1 part per million), and approximately 25 mcg of neomycin. The cells, virus pools, fetal bovine serum, and albumin human used in preparation of MMR are screened for the absence of adventitious agents; the albumin human is processed using the Cohn cold alcohol fractionation procedure.

Lyophilized MMR occurs as a light yellow compact crystalline plug and the reconstituted vaccine occurs as a clear, yellow solution. MMR do not contain thimerosal or any other preservative.

■ **Stability** In lyophilized form, MMR should be refrigerated at 2–8°C but may be frozen. The vials containing diluent provided by the manufacturer may be refrigerated at 2–8°C or stored at room temperature. During shipping, MMR must be stored at 10°C or less and may be packed in solid carbon dioxide (dry ice). If the vaccine is shipped with dry ice, the diluent must be shipped separately.

Following reconstitution with the diluent provided by the manufacturer, MMR should be refrigerated at 2–8°C and discarded if not used within 8 hours. Both the lyophilized and reconstituted vaccine should be protected from light, which may inactivate the vaccine.

Preparations

Excipients in commercially available drug preparations may have clinically important effects in some individuals; consult specific product labeling for details.

Measles, Mumps, and Rubella Virus Vaccine Live (MMR)

Parenteral

For injection, for subcutaneous use	Measles Virus Vaccine Live (More Attenuated Enders' Line) 1000 $TCID_{50}$, Mumps Virus Vaccine Live (Jeryl Lynn [B level] Strain) 12,500 $TCID_{50}$, and Rubella Virus Vaccine Live (Wistar RA 27/3 Strain) 1000 $TCID_{50}$ per 0.5 mL	**M-M-R® II**, Merck

Measles, Mumps, Rubella and Varicella Virus Vaccine Live (MMRV)

Parenteral

For injection, for subcutaneous use	Measles Virus Vaccine Live (More Attenuated Enders' Line) ≥3 log $_{10}$ tissue culture infective dose 50% ($TCID_{50}$), Mumps Virus Vaccine Live (Jeryl Lynn [B level] Strain) ≥4.3 log $_{10}$ $TCID_{50}$, Rubella Virus Vaccine Live (Wistar RA 27/3 Strain) ≥3 log $_{10}$ $TCID_{50}$, and Varicella Virus Vaccine Live (Oka/Merck Strain) ≥3.99 log $_{10}$ plaque-forming units (PFU) per 0.5 mL	**ProQuad®**, Merck

Meningococcal Group B Vaccine

Serogroup B Meningococcal Vaccine, Serogroup B Bivalent rLP2086 Vaccine, MenB, MenB-FHbp, MenB-4C, 4CMenB

■ Meningococcal group B (MenB) vaccine is an inactivated (recombinant) vaccine that is commercially available in the US as 2 different vaccines containing antigens derived from *Neisseria meningitidis* serogroup B. MenB-4C (Bexsero®) contains 3 recombinant cell surface proteins (neisserial adhesion A [NadA], neisserial heparin-binding antigen [NHBA], factor H-binding protein [FHbp]) and outer membrane vesicles (OMV) containing outer membrane protein PorA (serosubtype P1.4) derived from *N. meningitidis* serogroup B. MenB-FHbp (Trumenba®) contains 2 FHbp variants, one from FHbp subfamily A (A05) and one from FHbp subfamily B (B01), derived from *N. meningitidis* serogroup B. MenB vaccine is used to stimulate active immunity to infection caused by *N. meningitidis* serogroup B.

Uses

■ **Prevention of Meningococcal Group B Infection** Meningococcal group B (MenB) vaccine is used to stimulate active immunity to infection caused by *Neisseria meningitidis* serogroup B in adults, adolescents, and children 10 through 25 years of age. MenB vaccine also is recommend in certain adults 26 years of age or older† at increased risk for meningococcal infection caused by *N. meningitidis* serogroup B.

N. meningitidis can cause invasive meningococcal disease that usually presents as acute, severe and potentially life-threatening meningitis and/or meningococcemia with abrupt onset. Less frequently, *N. meningitidis* infection results in focal disease (e.g., pneumonia, arthritis, otitis media, epiglottitis). Based on chemical differences in the antigenic capsular polysaccharide, at least 13 different serogroups of *N. meningitidis* have been identified. In the US, serogroups B, C, and Y cause most cases of meningococcal disease and serogroup W-135 causes a small percentage of cases. The proportion of cases caused by each serogroup has changed over time and varies based on geographic location and age group. Although the overall incidence of meningococcal disease in the US has been historically low during the last 10–15 years, the overall case fatality rate for invasive meningococcal disease has remained at 10–15% (even with anti-infective treatment) and the fatality rate may be as high as 40% in those with meningococcemia. In addition, long-term sequelae (e.g., hearing loss, neurologic disability, digit or limb amputations) has been reported in 11–20% of patients. Serogroup B causes approximately 60% of cases of meningococcal disease reported in the US in infants and children younger than 5 years of age. The incidence of meningococcal disease caused by serogroup B in the US in adults and adolescents 11–23 years of age is low (approximately 50–60 cases and 5–10 fatalities reported annually); however, more than 80% of these cases are reported in older adolescents and adults 16–23 years of age and outbreaks of meningococcal serogroup B disease have occurred on college campuses during recent years.

Although the risk of exposure to meningococcal disease is considered to be low in the general US population, the risk is increased in individuals who have certain underlying chronic medical conditions that make them more susceptible to severe and/or recurrent invasive meningococcal disease. Individuals with complement component deficiencies (e.g., C3, C5–C9, properdin, factor H, or factor D) are more susceptible to *N. meningitidis* infection than complement-sufficient individuals, and individuals with functional or anatomic asplenia appear to be at increased risk for severe meningococcal disease. Individuals with other conditions associated with immunosuppression, including individuals with human immunodeficiency virus (HIV) infection and hematopoietic cell transplant recipients, also may be at increased risk for meningococcal disease. In addition, individuals receiving eculizumab are at increased risk for meningococcal disease because the drug binds to C5 and inhibits terminal complement activation. The risk of meningococcal disease also is increased in certain age groups, including infants and children 5 years of age or younger, adolescents and young adults 16 through 21 years of age (especially first-year college students living in dormitories), and geriatric adults 65 years of age or older, and in certain health-care and laboratory personnel, military recruits, and individuals who travel to or reside in areas outside the US where meningococcal disease is highly endemic or epidemic.

The US Public Health Service Advisory Committee on Immunization Practices (ACIP), American Academy of Pediatrics (AAP), and other experts recommend *routine* immunization against meningococcal serogroup B infection in *selected* adults, adolescents, and children 10 through 25 years of age at increased risk for the disease because of certain chronic medical conditions (e.g., persistent complement component deficiencies in C3, C5–C9, properdin, factor H, or factor D; anatomic or functional asplenia, including sickle cell disease; individuals taking eculizumab). These experts also recommend *routine* immunization against meningococcal serogroup B infection in adults, adolescents, and children 10 through 25 years of age at increased risk because of potential exposure to *N. meningitidis* serogroup B (e.g., laboratory personnel routinely exposed to *N. meningitidis*, community or institutional outbreaks of *N. meningitidis* serogroup B disease).

ACIP, AAP, and others state that data are insufficient to recommend *routine* vaccination against *N. meningitidis* serogroup B in *all* adolescents, but use of MenB vaccine may be considered in otherwise healthy adolescents and young adults 16 through 23 years of age to provide short-term protection against *N. meningitidis* serogroup B. When MenB vaccine is used in adolescents, ACIP, AAP, and others state that the preferred age for vaccination is 16 through 18 years of age since this maximizes the likelihood that protection will last into the highest age-related risk period in young adults (i.e., 18 through 23 years of age). Unlike meningococcal groups A, C, Y, and W-135 vaccine (MenACWY vaccine), *routine* use of MenB vaccine is *not* currently recommended in college freshmen who plan to live in dormitories.

Although safety and efficacy of MenB vaccine have *not* been established in adults 26 years of age or older, ACIP recommends *routine* immunization against meningococcal serogroup B infection in *selected* adults 26 years of age or older† at increased risk because of certain chronic medical conditions (e.g., persistent complement component deficiencies in C3, C5–C9, properdin, factor H, or factor D; anatomic or functional asplenia, including sickle cell disease; individuals taking eculizumab). Routine immunization also is recommended in adults 26 years of age or older† at increased risk because of potential exposure to *N. meningitidis* serogroup B (e.g., laboratory personnel routinely exposed to *N. meningitidis*, community or institutional outbreaks of *N. meningitidis* serogroup B). ACIP states that there is no theoretical difference in the safety of MenB vaccine in adults in this age group compared with individuals 10 through 25 years of age.

MenB vaccine is *not* recommended in infants and children younger than 10 years of age†.

ACIP, AAP, and other experts state that *routine* immunization against *N. meningitidis* serogroup B is *not* recommended in military recruits.

ACIP, AAP, and other experts state that *routine* immunization against *N. meningitidis* serogroup B is *not* recommended in individuals who will be traveling to or residing in areas where *N. meningitidis* is highly endemic or epidemic (e.g., sub-Saharan Africa in area known as the "meningitis belt") because meningococcal disease in these areas is usually caused by serogroups A, C, X, or W-135 and is not generally caused by serogroup B.

Choice of Meningococcal Group B Vaccines There are 2 different inactivated (recombinant) vaccines available in the US for immunization against meningococcal serogroup B infection: MenB-4C (Bexsero®) and MenB-FHbp (Trumenba®). MenB-4C and MenB-FHbp are both labeled by FDA for use in adults and adolescents 10 through 25 years of age and have also been recommended for certain adults 26 years of age or older†.

Both vaccines contain recombinant meningococcal serogroup B antigens and stimulate active immunity to infection caused by *N. meningitidis* serogroup B. Current clinical data suggest that both MenB-4C and MenB-FHbp provide protection against disease caused by several strains of meningococcal serogroup B circulating in the US. However, effectiveness of the vaccines against diverse serogroup B strains has not been confirmed and neither vaccine is expected to provide protection again all meningococcal serogroup B strains.

When vaccination against meningococcal serogroup B infection is indicated in adolescents and adults, ACIP, AAP, and other experts state that either MenB-4C or MenB-FHbp may be used. Data are not available to date regarding the interchangeability of MenB-4C and MenB-FHbp in the vaccinations series. ACIP, AAP, and other experts state that the vaccines are *not* interchangeable and that the same MenB vaccine should be used for the entire vaccination series.

Clinical Experience with MenB-4C (Bexsero®) Efficacy of MenB-4C (Bexsero®) is inferred based on immune response to the vaccine as demonstrated by serum bactericidal activity with human complement (hSBA). In clinical studies, hSBA assays were performed using 3 strains of *N. meningitidis* serogroup B, each selected to measure response to 1 of 3 vaccine antigens (i.e., neisserial adhesion A [NadA], factor H-binding protein [FHbp], outer membrane protein PorA [serosubtype P1.4]). Studies assessed the proportion of vaccinees with a fourfold or greater increase in hSBA titer for each of the 3 strains and the proportion of vaccinees with an antibody titer greater than or equal to the lower limit of quantitation of the assay for all 3 strains (composite response).

Adolescents and Adults 10 through 25 Years of Age. In a randomized controlled study that included 299 adolescents 11 through 17 years of age in Canada and Australia who received 2 doses of MenB-4C given 1 month apart (evaluable immunogenicity population), 98, 99, and 39% of vaccine recipients had a fourfold or greater antibody response to FHbp, NadA, and PorA P1.4, respectively, at 1 month after the second dose; 63% of these individuals had a composite response at 1 month after the second dose. In a randomized, controlled extension study involving adolescents 11 through 17 years of age in Chile who received 2 doses of MenB-4C given 1, 2, or 6 months apart, 90–94% had an antibody response to all 3 *N. meningitidis* serogroup B strains tested (composite response) at 1 month after the second dose and 77–94% had an hSBA titer of 1:4 or greater against all 3 strains tested at 18–24 months after the second dose.

In a randomized, controlled study evaluating MenB-4C in 148 adult university students 18 through 24 years of age in the United Kingdom who received 2 doses of MenB-4C given 1 month apart (evaluable immunogenicity population), 78, 94, and 67% of vaccine recipients had a fourfold or greater antibody response to FHbp, NadA, and PorA P1.4, respectively, at 1 month after the second dose; 24% already had a composite response prior to vaccination (baseline antibody response), 88% had a composite response at 1 month after the second dose, and 66% had a composite response 11 months after the second dose.

Adults 26 Years of Age or Older. MenB-4C has been used for prevention of meningococcal serogroup B infection in healthy adults 26 years of age or older†. In an open-label study in laboratory personnel routinely exposed to *N. meningitidis* isolates, adults 18 through 25 years of age and adults 26 through 50 years of age† received a 2-dose regimen of MenB-4C and 83% had an antibody response to at least 1 of the 3 serogroup B antigens tested at 1 month after the second dose.

In other studies that included laboratory personnel 26–65 years of age† at risk of occupational exposure to meningococci, 2 or 3 doses of MenB-4C were administered in conjunction with meningococcal (groups A, C, Y and W-135) oligosaccharide diphtheria CRM_{197} conjugate vaccine (MenACWY-CRM). (See Meningococcal Vaccine under Vaccines: Inactivated Vaccines and Toxoids, under Drug Interactions.)

Clinical Experience with MenB-FHbp (Trumenba®) Efficacy of MenB-FHbp (Trumenba®) is inferred based on immune response to the vaccine as demonstrated by hSBA. In clinical studies, hSBA assays were performed using 4 meningococcal serogroup B strains that express 4 different FHbp variants (A22, A56, B24, B44) and the proportion of vaccinees with a fourfold or greater increase in hSBA titer for each of the 4 strains of *N. meningitidis* serogroup B and the proportion of vaccinees with a titer greater than or equal to the lower limit of quantitation of the assay for all 4 strains (composite response) was assessed.

Adolescents and Adults 10 through 25 Years of Age. In a randomized, controlled study in adolescents 11 through 17 years of age, a 3-dose series of MenB-FHbp was used (second and third dose given 2 and 6 months, respectively, after the first dose) and study participants were randomized to also receive a dose of saline or a dose of human papillomavirus quadrivalent (types 6, 11, 16, 18) vaccine recombinant (v4HPV; Gardasil®) concomitantly at a separate site. Approximately 53% of vaccinees who received MenB-FHbp administered concomitantly with saline had an antibody response to all 4 serogroup B antigens tested (composite antibody response) by 1 month after the second dose and 84% had a composite response by 1 month after the third dose. In the group that received each dose of MenB-FHbp concomitantly with a dose of 4vHPV, 50% of vaccinees had a composite antibody response to the meningococcal serogroup B vaccine by 1 month after the second dose and 81% had a composite antibody response to the vaccine by 1 month after the third dose.

In another randomized study in adolescents 11 through 18 years of age, a 2-dose regimen of MenB-FHbp (second dose given 6 months after the first dose) or a 3-dose regimen of MenB-FHbp (second dose given either 2 or 3 months after the first dose and third dose given 6 months after the first dose) was used. In those who received the 2-dose regimen, 73% of vaccinees had a composite response 1 month after the second dose. In those who received the 3-dose regimen, 52% had a composite response after the second dose and 80–82% had a composite response at 1 month after the third dose.

Adults 26 Years of Age or Older. MenB-FHbp has been used for prevention of meningococcal serogroup B infection in healthy adults 26 years of age or older†. In a study that included 7 laboratory personnel 24–62 years of age† who received 3 doses of MenB-FHbp (second dose 2 months after the first dose and third dose 6 months after the first dose), the 6 evaluable vaccinees had hSBA titers equal to or greater than the lower limit of quantitation against 3 of the 4 *N. meningitidis* serogroup B strains tested and 3 of these individuals achieved titers equal to or greater than the lower limit of quantitation for all 4 strains.

Dosage and Administration

■ Administration

Meningococcal group B (MenB) vaccine is administered as MenB-4C (Bexsero®) or MenB-FHbp (Trumenba®).

MenB-4C and MenB-FHbp are administered *only* by IM injection.

Syncope (vasovagal or vasodepressor reaction; fainting) may occur following vaccination. Syncope occurs most frequently in adolescents and young adults. Procedures should be in place to avoid falling injury and to restore cerebral perfusion following syncope. Syncope and secondary injuries may be averted if vaccinees sit or lie down during and for 15 minutes after vaccination. If syncope occurs, the patient should be observed until symptoms resolve.

MenB vaccine may be given simultaneously with other age-appropriate vaccines. When multiple vaccines are administered during a single health-care visit, each parenteral vaccine should be given with a different syringe and at different injection sites. Injection sites should be separated by at least 1 inch (if anatomically feasible) to allow appropriate attribution of any local adverse effects that may occur.

IM Administration IM injections of MenB vaccine should be made in the deltoid region of the upper arm.

To ensure delivery of vaccine into muscle, IM injections should be made at a 90° angle to the skin using a needle length appropriate for the individual's age and body mass, thickness of adipose tissue and muscle at the injection site, and injection technique. Anatomic variability, especially in the deltoid, should be considered and clinical judgment should be used to avoid inadvertent underpenetration or overpenetration of muscle.

MenB-4C (Bexsero®). Immediately prior to administration, the single-dose prefilled syringe containing MenB-4C should be shaken well to obtain a homogeneous suspension. The vaccine should appear as a white, opalescent suspension and should be discarded if it contains particulates, appears discolored, or cannot be resuspended.

MenB-4C should be stored at 2–8°C and protected from light. The vaccine should be protected from freezing and should be discarded if it has been frozen.

MenB-FHbp (Trumenba®). Immediately prior to administration, the single-dose prefilled syringe containing MenB-FHbp should be shaken well to obtain a homogeneous white suspension. The vaccine should be discarded if it contains particulates, appears discolored, or cannot be resuspended with thorough agitation.

MenB-FHbp should *not* be mixed with any other vaccine.

MenB-FHbp should be stored horizontally (flat on a shelf) at 2–8°C; horizontal storage is recommended to minimize redispersion time. The vaccine should be protected from freezing and should be discarded if it has been frozen.

■ Dosage

The dosing schedule (i.e., number and timing of doses) differ between MenB-4C (Bexsero®) and MenB-FHbp (Trumenba®) and may depend on the individual's risk of exposure and susceptibility to *Neisseria meningitidis* serogroup B. *Recommendations for the specific vaccine used should be followed.*

The manufacturers state that data available to date are insufficient regarding the interchangeability of MenB-4C and MenB-FHbp. The US Public Health Service Advisory Committee on Immunization Practices (ACIP) and American Academy of Pediatrics (AAP) state that MenB-4C and MenB-FHbp are *not* interchangeable and recommend that the MenB vaccine used for the initial dose should be used to complete the vaccination series.

MenB-4C (Bexsero®) MenB-4C (Bexsero®) is given in a series of 2 doses. Each dose consists of the entire contents (0.5 mL) of the commercially available single-dose prefilled syringe containing the vaccine.

Children and Adolescents 10 through 18 Years of Age. For primary immunization in children and adolescents 10 through 18 years of age at increased risk for meningococcal serogroup B disease because of certain chronic medical conditions (e.g., persistent complement component deficiencies, anatomic or functional asplenia) or because of potential exposure to meningococcal infection (e.g., community or institutional outbreaks of *N. meningitidis* serogroup B disease), 2 doses of MenB-4C (Bexsero®) should be administered at least 1 month apart.

If MenB-4C is used in otherwise healthy adolescents to provide short-term protection against *N. meningitidis* serogroup B, 2 doses should be administered at least 1 month apart. ACIP, AAP, and others state that the preferred age for vaccination in otherwise healthy adolescents is 16 through 18 years of age.

Adults 19 through 25 Years of Age. For primary immunization in adults 19 through 25 years of age at increased risk for meningococcal serogroup B disease because of certain medical conditions (e.g., persistent complement component deficiencies, anatomic or functional asplenia) or because of potential exposure to meningococcal infection (e.g., laboratory personnel routinely exposed to *N. meningitidis*, community or institutional outbreaks of *N. meningitidis* serogroup B disease), 2 doses of MenB-4C (Bexsero®) should be administered at least 1 month apart.

If MenB-4C is used in otherwise healthy adults 19 through 23 years of age to provide short-term protection against *N. meningitidis* serogroup B, 2 doses should be administered at least 1 month apart.

Adults 26 Years of Age or Older. If MenB-4C (Bexsero®) is used for primary immunization in adults 26 years of age or older† at increased risk for meningococcal serogroup B disease because of certain chronic medical conditions (e.g., persistent complement component deficiencies, anatomic or functional asplenia) or because of potential exposure to meningococcal infection (e.g., laboratory personnel routinely exposed to *N. meningitidis*, community or institutional outbreaks of *N. meningitidis* serogroup B disease), 2 doses should be administered at least 1 month apart.

MenB-FHbp (Trumenba®) MenB-FHbp (Trumenba®) is given in a series of 2 or 3 doses. Each dose consists of the entire contents (0.5 mL) of the commercially available single-dose prefilled syringe containing the vaccine.

ACIP and AAP state that the 3-dose regimen of MenB-FHbp should be used for primary immunization in individuals at increased risk for meningococcal serogroup B disease and when vaccination is indicated during outbreaks of meningococcal serogroup B. These experts state that a 2-dose regimen of MenB-FHbp can be used for primary immunization in otherwise healthy individuals not at increased risk.

Children and Adolescents 10 through 18 Years of Age. For primary immunization in children and adolescents 10 through 18 years of age at increased risk for meningococcal serogroup B disease because of certain chronic medical conditions (e.g., persistent complement component deficiencies, anatomic or functional asplenia) or because of potential exposure to meningococcal infection (e.g., community or institutional outbreaks of *N. meningitidis* serogroup B disease), MenB-FHbp (Trumenba®) should be given in a series of 3 doses; the second dose should be given 1–2 months after the first dose and the third dose should be given 6 months after the first dose. If a 2-dose regimen of MenB-FHbp is used in such patients, the second dose should be given 6 months after the first dose.

If MenB-FHbp is used in otherwise healthy adolescents to provide short-term protection against *N. meningitidis* serogroup B, a 2-dose regimen should be used and the second dose should be given 6 months after the first dose. ACIP, AAP, and others state that the preferred age for vaccination in otherwise healthy adolescents is 16 through 18 years of age.

Adults 19 through 25 Years of Age. For primary immunization in adults 19 through 25 years of age at increased risk for meningococcal serogroup B disease because of certain medical conditions (e.g., persistent complement component deficiencies, anatomic or functional asplenia) or because of potential exposure to meningococcal infection (e.g., laboratory personnel routinely exposed to *N. meningitidis*, community or institutional outbreaks of *N. meningitidis* serogroup B disease), MenB-FHbp (Trumenba®) should be given in a series of 3 doses; the second dose should be given 1–2 months after the first dose and the third dose should be given 6 months after the first dose. If a 2-dose regimen of MenB-FHbp is used in such patients, the second dose should be given 6 months after the first dose.

If MenB-FHbp is used in otherwise healthy adults 19 through 23 years of age to provide short-term protection against *N. meningitidis* serogroup B, a 2-dose regimen should be used and the second dose should be given 6 months after the first dose.

Adults 26 Years of Age or Older. If MenB-FHbp (Trumenba®) is used for primary immunization in adults 26 years of age or older† at increased risk for meningococcal serogroup B disease because of certain medical conditions (e.g., persistent complement component deficiencies, anatomic or functional asplenia) or because of potential exposure to meningococcal infection (e.g., laboratory personnel routinely exposed to *N. meningitidis*, community or institutional outbreaks of *N. meningitidis* serogroup B disease), MenB-FHbp should be given in a series of 3 doses; the second dose should be given 1–2 months after the first dose and the third dose should be given 6 months after the first dose.

Cautions

■ Contraindications

Meningococcal group B vaccine (MenB-4C; Bexsero®) is contraindicated in individuals with hypersensitivity, including severe allergic reactions, to any component of the vaccine or a previous dose of the vaccine.

Meningococcal group B vaccine (MenB-FHbp; Trumenba®) is contraindicated in individuals with severe allergic reaction following a previous dose of the vaccine.

■ Warnings/Precautions

Sensitivity Reactions **Hypersensitivity Reactions.** Hypersensitivity reactions (e.g., anaphylaxis, rash, eye swelling) have been reported after administration of MenB-4C.

Appropriate medical treatment (e.g., epinephrine) should be readily available in case an anaphylactic reaction occurs following administration of MenB-4C or MenB-FHbp.

Latex Sensitivity. Some packaging components of single-dose prefilled syringes (i.e., tip cap) of MenB-4C (Bexsero®) contain natural rubber latex. Some individuals may be hypersensitive to natural latex proteins and these packaging components may cause allergic reactions in such individuals.

The US Public Health Service Advisory Committee on Immunization Practices (ACIP) states that vaccines supplied in vials or syringes containing dry natural rubber or natural rubber latex may be administered to individuals with latex allergies other than anaphylactic allergies (e.g., history of contact allergy to latex gloves), but should not be used in those with a history of severe (anaphylactic) allergy to latex unless the benefits of vaccination outweigh the risk of a potential allergic reaction. Contact-type allergy is the most common type of latex sensitivity.

Syncope Syncope (vasovagal reaction; fainting) has been reported following administration of vaccines, including MenB-4C. Syncope following vaccination occurs most frequently in adolescents and young adults.

The vaccinee should be observed for 15 minutes following vaccination and procedures should be in place to avoid falling injury and restore cerebral perfusion if syncope occurs. (See Dosage and Administration: Administration.)

Individuals with Altered Immunocompetence Like other inactivated vaccines, MenB-4C or MenB-FHbp may be administered to individuals immunosuppressed as a result of disease or medical therapy; however, the possibility that such individuals may have a reduced immune response to the vaccine should be considered.

Limitations of Vaccine Effectiveness MenB vaccine (MenB-4C, MenB-FHbp) may not protect all vaccine recipients against meningococcal serogroup B infection.

MenB-4C and MenB-FHbp contain antigens representing several strains of meningococcal serogroup B circulating in the US. However, effectiveness of the vaccines against diverse serogroup B strains has not been confirmed and neither vaccine is expected to provide protection against all meningococcal serogroup B strains.

Although *N. meningitidis* protein antigens used to produce MenB vaccines (e.g., factor H binding protein [FHbp]) may be shared across other meningococcal serotypes, additional study is needed to determine whether MenB vaccines can provide any cross protection against other *N. meningitidis* serotypes (e.g., serogroups A, C, Y, W-135).

Duration of Immunity In a study evaluating a 2-dose regimen of MenB-4C in adolescents 11 through 17 years of age (doses given 1, 2, or 6 months apart), 90–94% of vaccinees had a composite response to all 3 *N. meningitidis* serogroup B strains tested at 1 month after the second dose; 77–94% had a serum bactericidal activity with human complement (hSBA) titer of 1:4 or greater against all 3 strains tested at 18–24 months after the second dose.

In a study evaluating a 3-dose regimen of MenB-FHbp, data indicate that there is an initial rapid decline in antibodies after vaccination, followed by a flattening out of the antibody curve at approximately 6 months after the third dose. At 48 months, more than 50% of vaccinees still had hSBA titers greater than or equal to the lower limit of quantification against 3 of the 4 *N. meningitidis* serogroup B strains tested.

Improper Storage and Handling Improper storage or handling of vaccines may reduce vaccine potency resulting in reduced or inadequate immune response in vaccinees.

All vaccines should be inspected upon delivery and monitored during storage to ensure that the appropriate temperature is maintained. (See Dosage and Administration: Administration.)

Vaccine that has been mishandled or has not been stored at the recommended temperature should *not* be administered.

If there are concerns about mishandling, the manufacturer or state or local immunization or health departments should be contacted for guidance on whether the vaccine is usable.

Specific Populations **Pregnancy.** MenB-4C and MenB-FHbp: Category B. (See Users Guide.)

The manufacturers state that there are no adequate and well-controlled studies using MenB vaccine (MenB-4C, MenB-FHbp) in pregnant women, and the vaccine should be used during pregnancy only if clearly needed.

ACIP state that administration of MenB vaccine should be deferred in pregnant women, unless the woman is at increased risk for meningococcal serogroup B disease and benefits of vaccination outweigh potential risks.

If any exposure to MenB-4C vaccine occurs during pregnancy, vaccinees and their clinicians are encouraged to contact the manufacturer at 877-413-4759.

Any exposure to MenB vaccine (MenB-4C, MenB-FHbp) that occurs during pregnancy can be reported to the Vaccine Adverse Event Reporting System (VAERS) at 800-822-7967 or http:// www.vaers.hhs.gov/.

Lactation. It is not known whether MenB vaccine is distributed into milk. The manufacturers state that MenB vaccine (MenB-4C, MenB-FHbp) should be used with caution in nursing women.

ACIP states that administration of MenB vaccine should be deferred in nursing women, unless the woman is at increased risk for meningococcal serogroup B disease and benefits of vaccination outweigh potential risks.

Pediatric Use. MenB-4C (Bexsero®): Safety and efficacy have not been established in infants and children younger than 10 years of age.

MenB-FHbp (Trumenba®): Safety and efficacy have not been established in infants and children younger than 10 years of age. In a clinical study in infants younger than 12 months of age† who received a reduced dosage of MenB-FHbp, fever occurred in 90% of vaccinees.

Geriatric Use. MenB-4C and MenB-FHbp: Safety and efficacy have not been established in adults 65 years of age or older.

■ Common Adverse Effects

MenB-4C: The most common adverse reactions in children and adults 10 through 25 years of age are injection site reactions, including pain (83–90%), induration (28–32%), and erythema (45–50%), and systemic reactions, including fatigue (35–37%), headache (33–34%), nausea (18–19%), myalgia (48–49%), arthralgia (13–16%), and fever (1–5%).

MenB-FHbp: The most common adverse reactions in children and adolescents 11 through 17 years of age are injection site reactions, including pain (85–93%), swelling (20–22%), and erythema (16–20%), and systemic reactions, including fatigue (40–62%), headache (35–55%), vomiting (2–7%), diarrhea (9–15%), myalgia (30–42%), arthralgia (15–22%), chills (16–29%), and fever (1–6%).

Drug Interactions

■ Immune Globulins

There is no evidence that immune globulin (immune globulin IM [IGIM], immune globulin IV [IGIV]) or specific immune globulin (hepatitis B immune globulin [HBIG], rabies immune globulin [RIG], tetanus immune globulin [TIG], varicella zoster immune globulin [VZIG]) interferes with the immune response to inactivated vaccines. The US Public Health Service Advisory Committee on Immunization Practices (ACIP) states that inactivated vaccines such as meningococcal vaccines may be given simultaneously with (using different syringes and different injection sites) or at any interval before or after immune globulin preparations.

■ Immunosuppressive Agents

While specific information regarding use of meningococcal group B (MenB) vaccine in individuals receiving immunosuppressive agents or radiation therapy is not available, immune responses to MenB vaccine may be reduced in such patients.

ACIP states that inactivated vaccines generally can be administered safely to individuals with altered immunocompetence. However, if possible, vaccination should be avoided during chemotherapy or radiation therapy. Patients vaccinated within 14 days before starting immunosuppressive therapy or while receiving immunosuppressive therapy should be considered unimmunized and should be revaccinated at least 3 months after such therapy is discontinued if immunocompetence has been restored.

■ Vaccines

The manufacturers state that available data are insufficient to date to evaluate concurrent use of MenB vaccine (MenB-4C, MenB-FHbp) with other vaccines. Although specific studies may not be available evaluating concurrent administration with each antigen, ACIP and AAP state that MenB vaccine may be administered simultaneously with other age-appropriate vaccines. However, each parenteral vaccine should be administered using a different syringe and different injection site.

Inactivated Vaccines and Toxoids **Diphtheria and Tetanus Toxoids and Pertussis Vaccines.** Although the manufacturer of MenB-FHbp states that data are insufficient to assess safety and immunogenicity of concurrent administration of the vaccine with tetanus toxoid, reduced diphtheria toxoid and acellular pertussis vaccine adsorbed (Tdap), MenB-FHbp has been administered concurrently with Tdap (Adacel®) without a decrease in antibody responses to either vaccine.

MenB-FHbp (Trumenba®) also has been administered concurrently with a fixed-combination vaccine containing diphtheria, tetanus, pertussis, and poliovirus antigens (Tdap/IPV) in healthy adolescents 11 to younger than 19 years of age without a decrease in antibody responses to Tdap/IPV.

Human Papillomavirus Vaccine. MenB-FHbp (Trumenba®) has been administered concurrently with human papillomavirus quadrivalent (types 6, 11, 16, 18) vaccine recombinant (4vHPV; Gardasil®) in adolescents 11 to less than 18 years of age without a decrease in antibody response to the meningococcal serogroup B antigens and without a decrease in antibody response to 3 of the 4 HPV antigens (i.e., HPV types 6, 11, 16); at 1 month after the third dose of 4vHPV, the antibody response to HPV type 18 was decreased, but at least 99% of vaccinees achieved seroconversion for all 4 HPV antigens.

Meningococcal Vaccine. ACIP and others state that MenB vaccine (MenB-4C, MenB-FHbp) may be administered concurrently with meningococcal groups A, C, Y, and W-135 vaccine (MenACWY vaccine) using separate syringes and separate injection sites.

MenB-4C (Bexsero®) has been administered concurrently or sequentially with meningococcal (groups A, C, Y and W-135) oligosaccharide diphtheria CRM_{197} conjugate vaccine (MenACWY-CRM) in laboratory personnel 18–65 years of age at risk for meningococcal disease because of exposure to *Neisseria meningitidis* in the laboratory environment. In one study in healthy adults 18–50 years of age routinely exposed to *N. meningitidis* in a laboratory setting, 3 doses of MenB-4C (second dose 2 months after the first dose and third dose 6 months after the first dose) were administered followed by a single dose of MenACWY-CRM (Menveo®) given 1 month later. Among study participants with baseline serum bactericidal activity with human complement (hSBA) titers less than 4 against 1 or more *N. meningitidis* serogroup B strains, at least 89% had hSBA titers of 4 or greater after the second dose and at least 90% had hSBA titers of 4 or greater after the third dose of MenB-4C. At 1 month after the single dose of MenACWY-CRM, the majority of study participants had hSBA titers of 8 or greater against *N. meningitidis* serogroups A, C, Y, and W-135. In another study in laboratory personnel 18–65 years of age, the first dose of MenB-4C was administered concurrently with MenACWY-CRM, followed by a second and third dose of MenB-4C given 3 and 6 months later, without any unusual adverse effects.

Although the manufacturer of MenB-FHbp (Trumenba®) states that data are insufficient to assess safety and immunogenicity of concurrent administration of the vaccine with MenACWY vaccine, MenB-FHbp has been administered concurrently with meningococcal (groups A, C, Y, and W-135) polysaccharide diphtheria toxoid conjugate vaccine (MenACWY-D; Menactra®) without a decrease in antibody responses to the meningococcal antigens in either vaccine.

Description

Meningococcal group B (MenB) vaccine is commercially available in the US as 2 different inactivated (recombinant) vaccines containing antigens derived from immunogenic proteins found on the cell surface of *Neisseria meningitidis* serogroup B: MenB-4C and MenB-FHbp. The antigens contained in MenB vaccine promote production of specific antibodies that activate complement-mediated killing of meningococci to provide protection against infection by strains of *N. meningitidis* serogroup B represented in the vaccine.

MenB-4C (Bexsero®) is a white, opalescent suspension that contains 3 recombinant *N. meningitidis* serogroup B surface proteins (neisserial adhesion A [NadA], neisserial heparin-binding antigen [NHBA], factor H-binding protein [FHbp]) and also contains outer membrane vesicles (OMV) containing outer membrane protein PorA (serosubtype P1.4). The 3 surface protein components (NadA, NHBA, FHbp) are produced using recombinant DNA technology in *Escherichia coli* and purified by column chromatography. The OMV protein component (PorA P1.4) is produced by fermentation of a strain of *N. meningitidis* that expresses PorA P1.4 and inactivated using deoxycholate. The antigens are then adsorbed onto aluminum hydroxide. In addition to these antigens, each 0.5-mL dose of MenB-4C contains aluminum hydroxide (1.5 mg), sodium chloride (3.125 mg), histidine (0.776 mg), sucrose (10 mg), and kanamycin (no more than 0.01 mcg).

MenB-FHbp (Trumenba®) is a suspension that contains 2 recombinant lipidated FHbp antigens, one from FHbp subfamily A (A05) and one from FHbp subfamily B (B01). The 2 outer membrane protein components (FHbp A05 and FHbp B01) are produced using recombinant DNA technology in *E. coli* and purified by column chromatography. In addition to these antigens, each 0.5-mL dose of MenB-FHbp contains 0.25 mg of aluminum (provided as aluminum phosphate) and 18 mcg of polysorbate 80 in 10mM histidine-buffered saline.

Following IM administration of MenB vaccine (MenB-4C or MenB-FHbp), complement-mediated antibody response to the antigens contained in the vaccine is measured as serum bactericidal activity with human complement (hSBA). An hSBA titer of at least 4 (serum dilution of 1:4) in response to the MenB vaccine antigens is generally accepted as correlating with protection against *N. meningitidis* serogroup B. However, susceptibility of *N. meningitidis* serogroup B to complement-mediated antibody-dependent killing following vaccination with a 2-dose regimen of MenB-4C or a 2- or 3-dose regimen of MenB-FHbp depends on the degree of similarity between the vaccine antigens and the invading strain of *N. meningitidis* serogroup B and the amount of antigen expressed on the surface of the invading strain.

Advice to Patients

Prior to administration of each vaccine dose, provide a copy of the appropriate Centers for Disease Control and Prevention (CDC) Vaccine Information Statement (VIS) to the patient or patient's parent or guardian (VISs are available at http://www.cdc.gov/vaccines/hcp/vis/index.html).

Advise patient and/or patient's parent or guardian of the risks and benefits of vaccination with meningococcal group B (MenB) vaccine.

Importance of completing the vaccination series using the recommended number of doses of MenB-4C or MenB-FHbp, unless contraindicated.

Advise patient and/or patient's parent or guardian that MenB vaccine may not provide protection in all vaccinees.

Advise patient and/or patient's parent or guardian that fainting (sometimes resulting in falling with injury) has been reported following vaccination, especially in adolescents and young adults, and that patients should sit or lie down during and for 15 minutes after vaccine administration.

Importance of informing clinicians of a history of allergic reactions to MenB vaccine, any vaccine component, or packaging component (e.g., latex).

Importance of contacting clinician if any adverse reactions (including allergic reactions) occur with MenB vaccine. Clinicians or individuals can report any adverse reactions that occur following vaccination to the Vaccine Adverse Event Reporting System (VAERS) at 800-822-7967 or http://vaers.hhs.gov/index.

Importance of informing clinicians of existing or contemplated concomitant therapy, including prescription and OTC drugs, and any concomitant illnesses.

Importance of women informing clinicians if they are or plan to become pregnant or plan to breast-feed.

Importance of informing patients of other important precautionary information. (See Cautions.)

Overview® (see Users Guide). For additional information on this drug until a more detailed monograph is developed and published, the manufacturer's labeling should be consulted. It is *essential* that the manufacturer's labeling be consulted for more detailed information on usual cautions, precautions, contraindications, potential drug interactions, laboratory test interferences, and acute toxicity.

Preparations

Excipients in commercially available drug preparations may have clinically important effects in some individuals; consult specific product labeling for details.

Meningococcal Group B Vaccine

Parenteral

Injection, for IM use	50 mcg of meningococcal B NadA protein, 50 mcg of meningococcal B NHBA fusion protein, 50 mcg of meningococcal B FHbp fusion protein, and 25 mcg of meningococcal B outer membrane vesicle per 0.5 mL	**Bexsero®**, GlaxoSmithKline
	60 mcg of meningococcal B FHbp A05 protein and 60 mcg of meningococcal B FHbp B01 protein per 0.5 mL	**Trumenba®**, Pfizer

†Use is not currently included in the labeling approved by the US Food and Drug Administration

Meningococcal Groups A, C, Y, and W-135 Vaccine

Quadrivalent Meningococcal Conjugate Vaccine, MCV4, MCV4-CRM, MenACWY, MenACWY-CRM, MenACWY-CRM_{197}Quadrivalent Meningococcal Conjugate Vaccine, MenACWY-D, MCV4

■ Meningococcal groups A, C, Y, and W-135 vaccine is an inactivated (polysaccharide) vaccine that is commercially available in the US as 2 different quadrivalent conjugated vaccines: meningococcal (groups A, C, Y and W-135) polysaccharide diphtheria toxoid conjugate vaccine (MenACWY-D; Menactra®) and meningococcal (groups A, C, Y and W-135) oligosaccharide diphtheria CRM_{197} conjugate vaccine (MenACWY-CRM; Menveo®). Both conjugated vaccines contain A, C, Y, and W-135 capsular polysaccharide antigens extracted from *Neisseria meningitidis* linked to a carrier protein and are used to stimulate active immunity to meningococcal infection caused by serogroups A, C, Y, and W-135. The previously available meningococcal groups A, C, Y, and W-135 vaccine containing unconjugated capsular polysaccharide antigens (MPSV4; Menomune®) is no longer commercially available in the US.

Uses

Meningococcal (groups A, C, Y and W-135) polysaccharide diphtheria toxoid conjugate vaccine (MenACWY-D; Menactra®) and meningococcal (groups A, C, Y and W-135) oligosaccharide diphtheria CRM_{197} conjugate vaccine (MenACWY-CRM; Menveo®) are quadrivalent conjugated meningococcal groups A, C, Y, and W-135 (MenACWY) vaccines used to stimulate active immunity to infection caused by *Neisseria meningitidis* serogroups A, C, Y, and W-135.

MenACWY vaccines are used for primary and booster immunization against infection caused by the *N. meningitidis* serogroups represented in the vaccines (i.e., serogroups A, C, Y, and W-135). (See Uses: Primary and Booster Immunization.) MenACWY vaccines also may be used as an adjunct to anti-infective prophylaxis in household and other contacts of individuals with invasive meningococcal disease when cluster cases or outbreaks are caused by *N. meningitidis* serogroups represented in the vaccines. (See Uses: Outbreak Control.)

MenACWY vaccines will *not* stimulate immunity to meningococcal infection caused by *N. meningitidis* serogroups not represented in the vaccines (e.g., serogroup B) or to infections caused by other pathogens.

The US Public Health Service Advisory Committee on Immunization Practices (ACIP), American Academy of Pediatrics (AAP), and other experts recommend *routine* primary immunization against meningococcal serogroups A, C, Y, and W-135 infection in *all* adolescents using MenACWY vaccine (MenACWY-D or MenACWY-CRM), preferably at 11 through 12 years of age, followed by a booster dose at 16 years of age. These experts recommend catch-up vaccination with MenACWY vaccine (MenACWY-D or MenACWY-CRM) at 13 through 18 years of age for those not previously vaccinated against meningococcal serogroups A, C, Y, and W-135 infection. (See Adolescents 11 through 18 Years of Age under Uses: Primary and Booster Immunization.) Catch-up vaccination with MenACWY vaccine also is recommended for *all* first-year college students through 21 years of age living in residence halls if they did not receive a dose of the vaccine on or after their 16th birthday. (See Adults under Uses: Primary and Booster Immunization.)

ACIP, AAP, and other experts also recommend *routine* primary and booster immunization against meningococcal serogroups A, C, Y, and W-135 infection using MenACWY vaccine in *selected* adults, adolescents, children, and infants 2 months of age or older at increased risk for the disease because of certain chronic medical conditions (e.g., persistent complement component deficiencies, anatomic or functional asplenia, human immunodeficiency virus [HIV] infection) or because they will be traveling to or residing in areas with hyperendemic or epidemic meningococcal disease caused by serogroups represented in the vaccine. Primary and booster immunization with MenACWY vaccine also is recommended for some other individuals at increased risk for meningococcal disease (e.g., certain health-care and laboratory personnel, military recruits). (See Uses: Primary and Booster Immunization.)

■ **Risks of Exposure and Infection** *N. meningitis* can cause invasive meningococcal disease that usually presents as acute, severe and potentially life-threatening meningitis and/or meningococcemia with abrupt onset. Less frequently, *N. meningitidis* infection results in focal disease (e.g., pneumonia, arthritis, otitis media, epiglottitis). Based on chemical differences in the antigenic capsular polysaccharide, at least 13 different serogroups of *N. meningitidis* have been identified. In the US, serogroups B, C, and Y cause most cases of meningococcal disease and serogroup W-135 causes a small percentage of cases. The proportion of cases caused by each serogroup has changed over time and varies based on geographic location and age group. Serogroup B causes approximately 60% of cases of meningococcal disease reported in the US in infants and children younger than 5 years of age. Serogroups C, Y, or W-135 cause approximately 67% of cases of meningococcal disease reported in the US in adults and adolescents 11 years of age or older. (See Pharmacology: Neisseria meningitidis and Infection.)

The overall annual incidence of meningococcal disease in the US was 1.1 cases per 100,000 population in 1996, but decreased to 0.4 cases per 100,000 population by 2005. During 2005–2011, an estimated 800–1200 cases of meningococcal disease occurred annually in the US. In 2016, there were about 370 cases of meningococcal disease reported to the US Centers for Disease Control and Prevention (CDC) (0.12 cases per 100,000). Although the overall incidence of meningococcal disease in the US has been historically low during the last 10–15 years, the overall case fatality rate for invasive meningococcal disease has remained at 10–15% (even with appropriate anti-infective treatment) and the fatality rate may be as high as 40% in those with meningococcemia. In addition, meningococcal infection can result in substantial morbidity; long-term sequelae (e.g., hearing loss, neurologic disability, digit or limb amputations) have been reported in 11–20% of patients.

Although the risk of exposure to meningococcal disease is considered to be low in the general US population, the risk is increased in individuals who have certain underlying chronic medical conditions that make them more susceptible to severe and/or recurrent invasive meningococcal disease. The risk of meningococcal disease also is increased in certain age groups, including infants and children 5 years of age or younger, adolescents and young adults 16 through 23 years of age (especially first-year college students living in dormitories), and geriatric adults 65 years of age or older, and in certain health-care and laboratory personnel, military recruits, and individuals who travel to or reside in areas outside the US where meningococcal disease is highly endemic or epidemic.

Individuals with complement component deficiencies (e.g., C3, C5–C9, properdin, factor H, factor D) are more susceptible to *N. meningitidis* infection, particularly serogroup Y, than complement-sufficient individuals, and it has been estimated that the risk of infection is 10,000 times greater in such individuals. In addition, complement component-deficient individuals frequently experience recurrent meningococcal disease since their immune response to natural infection may be less complete than that of complement-sufficient individuals. Individuals receiving eculizumab also are at increased risk for meningococcal disease. (See Individuals with Complement Deficiency, Properdin Deficiency, or Asplenia under Uses: Primary and Booster Immunization.)

Individuals with functional or anatomic asplenia appear to be at increased risk for severe meningococcal disease, possibly because they may not be able to effectively clear encapsulated bacteria from the bloodstream. (See Individuals with Complement Deficiency, Properdin Deficiency, or Asplenia under Uses: Primary and Booster Immunization.)

Individuals with other conditions associated with immunosuppression, including individuals with HIV infection, and hematopoietic cell transplant recipients also may be at increased risk for meningococcal disease. (See HIV-infected Individuals under Uses: Primary and Booster Immunization.)

While the incidence of meningococcal disease in college students appears to be similar to or somewhat lower than that reported for the general population of individuals 18–22 years of age, there is some evidence that first-year college students who reside on campus in dormitory housing are at higher risk of the disease than other students.

Health-care personnel who have close contact with nasopharyngeal secretions from a patient with invasive meningococcal disease (e.g., unprotected mouth-to-mouth resuscitation, unprotected contact during endotracheal intubation or endotracheal tube management) during the 7 days before onset of disease in the patient or before anti-infective therapy is initiated in the patient are at increased risk of infection. Research, industrial, and clinical laboratory personnel (e.g., microbiologists) exposed to isolates of *N. meningitidis* or solutions containing the organism that may be aerosolized also are at increased risk of infection.

N. meningitidis is transmitted person to person by the respiratory route and the principal type of exposure that places an individual at increased risk of meningococcal infection is close personal contact (household or child-care or nursery school contact) with an individual with invasive meningococcal disease or direct exposure to nasopharyngeal secretions from an infected individual. However, many cases of meningococcal disease in the US occur in individuals who have had no known exposure to an individual with invasive disease and presumably acquire infection from an asymptomatic carrier. *N. meningitidis* can be introduced into a household by an individual who is an asymptomatic *N. meningitidis* carrier; the infection then spreads to one or more susceptible household contacts by exposure to oropharyngeal secretions through close intimate contact (kissing) or sharing toothbrushes or eating or drinking utensils. The rate of infection in household contacts exposed to an individual with sporadic meningococcal disease has been estimated to be 4 cases per 1000 population or 500–800 times greater than that for the general population. Casual contacts who have no history of direct exposure to an index case's oropharyngeal secretions (e.g., school or work mates) and individuals who had only indirect contact with the index case (only contact was with a high-risk contact of the index case) are not at increased risk of infection. The infection risk in household or close personal contacts following exposure to an index case is inversely related to the age of the contact, and young children are at greatest risk of infection. The attack rate after household or other close contact is highest immediately after onset of the disease in the index case, and the majority of secondary cases occur within 2 weeks after contact and infection in susceptible individuals.

■ **Choice of Meningococcal Groups A, C, Y, and W-135 Vaccines** There are 2 different conjugated MenACWY vaccines commercially available in the US for active immunization against meningococcal disease caused by serogroups A, C, Y, and W-135: MenACWY-D and MenACWY-CRM.

Both vaccines contain A, C, Y, and W-135 capsular polysaccharide antigens extracted from *N. meningitidis* and stimulate active immunity to infection caused by the serotypes represented in the vaccines. The capsular polysaccharide antigens contained in MenACWY-D are conjugated to diphtheria toxoid protein and the capsular polysaccharide antigens contained in MenACWY-CRM are conjugated to diphtheria CRM_{197} protein. Conjugation of meningococcal capsular polysaccharide antigens to protein carriers with T-cell epitopes changes the immune response to the vaccine polysaccharides from T-cell-independent to T-cell-dependent, resulting in an improved primary response to the antigens and a strong anamnestic response after re-exposure to the antigens. Unconjugated meningococcal capsular polysaccharide antigens do not induce long-lasting immunity or an anamnestic response after subsequent exposure to the same antigen. (See Pharmacology: Response to Meningococcal Vaccines.)

MenACWY-D is labeled by FDA for use in infants and children 9 months through 10 years of age, adolescents 11 through 18 years of age, and adults 19 through 55 years of age for prevention of invasive meningococcal disease caused by *N. meningitidis* serogroups A, C, Y, and W-135.

MenACWY-CRM is labeled by FDA for use in infants and children 2 months through 10 years of age, adolescents 11 through 18 years of age, and adults 19 through 55 years of age for prevention of invasive meningococcal disease caused by *N. meningitidis* serogroups A, C, Y, and W-135.

ACIP and AAP do not state a preference for MenACWY-D or MenACWY-CRM and state that either age-appropriate MenACWY vaccine can be used for primary immunization and/or revaccination or booster doses. However, the dosage schedules (i.e., number and timing of doses for primary immunization) differ depending on which vaccine is used. (See Dosage and Administration: Dosage.)

■ **Primary and Booster Immunization** ***Infants 2 through 23 Months of Age*** ACIP, AAP, and other experts recommend *routine* primary immunization against meningococcal serogroups A, C, Y, and W-135 disease in *selected* infants 2 months through 23 months of age at increased risk for meningococcal disease because of certain chronic medical conditions (e.g., persistent complement component deficiencies, anatomic or functional asplenia, HIV infection) or because they will be traveling to or residing in areas with hyperendemic or epidemic meningococcal disease and for outbreak control.

ACIP and AAP state that *routine* primary immunization against meningococcal serogroups A, C, Y, and W-135 disease is *not* recommended in infants who are *not* at increased risk.

For primary immunization against meningococcal disease in infants, MenACWY-CRM is labeled for use in infants 2 months of age or older and MenACWY-D is labeled for use in infants 9 months of age or older.

Children 2 through 10 Years of Age ACIP, AAP, and other experts recommend *routine* primary immunization against meningococcal serogroups A, C, Y, and W-135 disease in *selected* children 2 through 10 years of age at increased risk for meningococcal disease because of certain chronic medical conditions (e.g., persistent complement component deficiencies, anatomic or functional asplenia, HIV infection) or because they will be traveling to or residing in areas with hyperendemic or epidemic meningococcal disease.

ACIP and AAP state that *routine* primary immunization against meningococcal serogroups A, C, Y, and W-135 disease is *not* recommended in children 2 through 10 years who are *not* at increased risk for meningococcal disease. However, *routine* primary immunization is indicated in *all* young adolescents 11 through 12 years of age. (See Adolescents 11 through 18 Years of Age under Uses: Primary and Booster Immunization.)

Adolescents 11 through 18 Years of Age ACIP, AAP, and other experts recommend *routine* primary immunization against meningococcal serogroups A, C, Y, and W-135 disease in *all* young adolescents with a primary dose of MenACWY vaccine (MenACWY-D or MenACWY-CRM) at 11 through 12 years of age, followed by a booster dose at 16 years of age. The booster dose is considered necessary because immunologic data indicate waning effectiveness against meningococcal disease and there is evidence that many adolescents are not protected 5 years following vaccination. Those who receive a single dose of MenACWY vaccine at the recommended 11 through 12 years of age are unlikely to be protected at 16 through 21 years of age, an age when the risk of meningococcal disease is increased.

Catch-up immunization against meningococcal serogroups A, C, Y, and W-135 disease with MenACWY vaccine (MenACWY-D or MenACWY-CRM) is recommended at the first opportunity for *all* older adolescents 13 through 18 years of age who were not vaccinated at 11 through 12 years of age. Adolescents who receive their first dose of MenACWY vaccine at 13 through 15 years of age should receive a booster dose at 16 through 18 years of age. A booster dose is not needed in those who receive the first dose at 16 years of age or older.

Adults **College Students.** ACIP, AAP, and other experts recommend that *all* first-year college students through 21 years of age who plan to live in dormitories receive primary immunization with MenACWY vaccine (MenACWY-D or MenACWY-CRM) if they did not receive a dose of the vaccine at 16 years of age or older.

Beginning in 2000, ACIP and AAP recommended that colleges, public health agencies, and providers of medical care to incoming and current college freshmen inform these students and their parents about meningococcal disease and the benefits of vaccination since college freshmen (particularly those who reside in dormitory housing) are at increased risk for meningococcal disease compared with other individuals the same age. At that time, ACIP and AAP also recommended that meningococcal vaccine be provided or made easily available to those college freshmen who wanted to reduce their risk for meningococcal disease. In May 2005, ACIP strengthened their recommendations regarding vaccination against meningococcal disease for college students by recommending universal immunization against *N. meningitidis* serogroups A, C, Y, and W-135 infection for *all* college freshmen who plan to live in dormitories.

Other Adults. ACIP, AAP, and other experts recommend *routine* primary immunization against meningococcal serogroups A, C, Y, and W-135 disease in *selected* adults at increased risk for meningococcal disease because of certain chronic medical conditions (e.g., persistent complement component deficiencies, anatomic or functional asplenia, HIV infection) or because they will be traveling to or residing in areas with hyperendemic or epidemic meningococcal disease. Primary immunization against meningococcal serogroups A, C, Y, and W-135 disease also is recommended in other adults at increased risk (e.g., health-care and laboratory personnel, military recruits).

Although a 2-dose series of MenACWY vaccine (MenACWY-D or MenACWY-CRM) is recommended for primary immunization in adults at increased risk for meningococcal infection because of persistent complement component deficiencies, anatomic or functional asplenia, or HIV infection, a single dose is adequate for primary immunization in other adults at increased risk. Booster doses of MenACWY vaccine generally are recommended every 5 years in individuals who received primary immunization with MenACWY vaccine or the previously available unconjugated meningococcal vaccine (MPSV4; Menomune®) and remain at prolonged increased risk.

MenACWY-D and MenACWY-CRM are both labeled by FDA for use in adults 19 through 55 years of age. However, ACIP states that MenACWY vaccine (MenACWY-D or MenACWY-CRM) can be used in adults 56 years of age or older† for primary immunization or when revaccination or booster doses are indicated in those at continued increased risk of meningococcal groups A, C, Y, and W-135 disease (e.g., those with certain chronic medical conditions, health-care and laboratory personnel, travelers).

Individuals with Complement Deficiency, Properdin Deficiency, or Asplenia Because individuals with persistent complement component deficiencies (e.g., inherited or chronic deficiencies in C3, C5–C9, properdin, factor D, factor H) or anatomic or functional asplenia (e.g., sickle cell disease) and those receiving treatment with eculizumab are at increased risk for meningococcal disease, ACIP, AAP, and other experts recommend *routine* age-appropriate primary and booster immunization against meningococcal serogroups A, C, Y, and W-135 disease in these individuals. Those who received primary immunization with MenACWY vaccine or the previously available unconjugated meningococcal vaccine (MPSV4) generally should receive a booster dose of MenACWY vaccine every 5 years.

If not previously vaccinated, patients scheduled to undergo elective splenectomy should be vaccinated against meningococcal disease at least 14 days prior to surgery whenever possible. If not administered before surgery, MenACWY vaccine should be administered as soon as possible after the procedure when the patient's condition is stable.

HIV-infected Individuals HIV-infected individuals are at increased risk for meningococcal disease, especially those with low CD4+ T-cell counts or high HIV viral loads. ACIP, AAP, US Centers for Disease Control and Prevention (CDC), National Institutes of Health (NIH), HIV Medicine Association of the Infectious Diseases Society of America (IDSA), and other experts recommend that all HIV-infected adults, adolescents, children, and infants 2 months of age or older receive *routine* age-appropriate primary and booster immunization against meningococcal serogroups A, C, Y, and W-135 using MenACWY vaccine.

Because HIV-infected individuals may not respond optimally to a single dose, all HIV-infected individuals 2 years of age or older should receive a 2-dose primary series of MenACWY vaccine. ACIP states that HIV-infected individuals 2 years of age or older who previously received only a single dose for primary immunization should receive a booster dose of MenACWY vaccine at the earliest opportunity, provided it is at least 8 weeks after the previous dose. HIV-infected infants 2 months to less than 2 years of age should receive the usually recommended age-appropriate multiple-dose primary series of MenACWY vaccine.

Studies using MenACWY-D indicate that the vaccine is safe and immunogenic in HIV-infected children, adolescents, and adults. (See HIV-infected Individuals under Response to Meningococcal Vaccines: Conjugated Meningococcal Vaccines, in Pharmacology.) However, the possibility that vaccines may be less immunogenic in HIV-infected individuals should be considered. (See Individuals with Altered Immunocompetence under Cautions: Precautions and Contraindications.)

HIV-infected individuals immunized with MenACWY vaccine or the previously available unconjugated meningococcal vaccine (MPSV4) should receive a booster dose of MenACWY vaccine every 5 years.

Health-care and Laboratory Personnel ACIP and Healthcare Infection Control Practices Advisory Committee (HICPAC) state that *routine* immunization against meningococcal serogroups A, C, Y, and W-135 disease is *not* recommended in health-care personnel. However, health-care personnel with certain chronic medical conditions that put them at increased risk of meningococcal disease (e.g., persistent complement component deficiencies, anatomic or functional asplenia, HIV infection) should receive a 2-dose primary immunization series of MenACWY vaccine (MenACWY-D or MenACWY-CRM). In addition, primary immunization with a single dose of the vaccine is recommended for laboratory personnel who may be routinely exposed to isolates of *N. meningitidis* and for health-care personnel who will be traveling to areas where meningococcal disease is hyperendemic or epidemic.

ACIP and HICPAC state that health-care and laboratory personnel who received primary immunization against meningococcal serogroups A, C, Y, and W-135 disease and remain at prolonged increased risk should receive a booster dose of MenACWY vaccine every 5 years.

In the setting of a community or institutional outbreak of meningococcal disease, MenACWY vaccine may be indicated for health-care personnel if the outbreak is caused by a meningococcal serogroup represented in the vaccine.

Regardless of vaccination status, postexposure anti-infective prophylaxis against meningococcal infection (i.e., 2-day regimen of oral rifampin or single dose of IM ceftriaxone, oral ciprofloxacin, or oral azithromycin) is recommended for *all* health-care personnel who have had unprotected (i.e., without wearing a mask) intensive contact (i.e., mouth-to-mouth resuscitation, endotracheal intubation or endotracheal tube management) with an infected patient.

Military Recruits Because the risk of meningococcal serogroups A, C, Y, and W-135 disease is increased among military recruits, *all* US military recruits *routinely* receive primary immunization with a single dose of MenACWY vaccine.

Travelers Travelers to or residents of areas where *N. meningitidis* is highly endemic or epidemic are at risk of exposure and should receive primary immunization against meningococcal serogroups A, C, Y, and W-135 disease. Although *N. meningitidis* is found worldwide, the highest incidence of meningococcal disease occurs in that portion of sub-Saharan Africa known as the "meningitis belt," which extends from Senegal and Guinea eastward to Ethiopia. Meningococcal disease is hyperendemic in this region with epidemics occurring periodically during the dry season (i.e., December through June). Historically, meningococcal disease outbreaks in the meningitis belt were caused by serogroup A; however, recent outbreaks have primarily been caused by serogroups C and W, although serogroup X outbreaks also have been reported.

ACIP, AAP, CDC, and other experts recommend age-appropriate primary immunization against meningococcal serogroups A, C, Y, and W-135 disease with MenACWY vaccine prior to travel for individuals 2 months of age and older who will be traveling to or residing in hyperendemic or epidemic areas, including the meningitis belt of sub-Saharan Africa during the dry season (i.e., December through June), especially if prolonged contact with local populations is expected.

ACIP recommends that international travelers who previously received primary immunization receive a booster dose of MenACWY vaccine if 5 or more years have elapsed since the last dose of meningococcal groups A, C, Y, and W-135 vaccine.

The Hajj pilgrimage to Saudi Arabia has been associated with outbreaks of meningococcal disease in returning pilgrims and their contacts. Officials in Saudi Arabia require that individuals traveling to their country for the annual Hajj and Umrah pilgrimage or for seasonal work in Hajj and Umrah zones must have a valid vaccination certificate indicating vaccination against meningococcal serogroups A, C, Y, and W-135 administered not less than 10 days and not more than 3 years (unconjugated polysaccharide vaccine) or 5 years (conjugated polysaccharide vaccine) prior to arrival in Saudi Arabia.

Advisories for US travelers are issued whenever epidemics of meningococcal disease caused by vaccine-preventable serogroups are reported in other countries. The most recent information concerning geographic areas for which vaccination against meningococcal disease is recommended can be obtained from international health clinics for travelers, state health departments, the CDC international travelers' hotline at 877-394-8747, or the CDC Travelers' Health website (http://wwwnc.cdc.gov/travel).

Household and Other Close Contacts of Individuals with Invasive Meningococcal Disease Whenever a case of invasive meningococcal disease occurs, anti-infective prophylaxis (i.e., 2-day regimen of oral rifampin or single dose of IM ceftriaxone, oral ciprofloxacin, or oral azithromycin) is indicated for close contacts of the index case (i.e., household contacts; day-care center contacts; individuals exposed to the index case's oropharyngeal secretions through kissing, sharing toothbrushes or eating or drinking utensils, mouth-to-mouth resuscitation, endotracheal intubation or management). For travelers, anti-infective prophylaxis should be considered for any passenger who had direct contact with respiratory secretions from an index case or for anyone seated directly next to an index case on a prolonged flight (i.e., one lasting longer than 8 hours). Anti-infective prophylaxis is the principal means of preventing secondary cases of meningococcal disease in contacts.

Because protective levels of anticapsular antibodies are not achieved until 7–14 days following administration of meningococcal groups A, C, Y, and W-135 vaccines, vaccination cannot prevent early-onset disease in contacts and usually is not recommended following sporadic cases of invasive meningococcal disease. However, vaccination is a possible adjunct to anti-infective prophylaxis when an outbreak is caused by a meningococcal serogroup represented in the vaccine. If cluster cases of invasive disease occur, there may be ongoing risk of infection and in these situations public health professionals (e.g., epidemiologists in state and local health departments) may recommend that MenACWY vaccine be administered to close contacts in addition to anti-infective prophylaxis. Vaccine administered to close contacts at the time meningococcal disease is diagnosed in the index case may provide protection against secondary disease occurring several weeks or later in the event that there are additional exposures or if exposure occurs after the period of time during which anti-infective prophylaxis provides protection.

■ **Outbreak Control** MenACWY vaccine may be recommended when an outbreak of meningococcal disease occurs in the US and the outbreak is caused by a *N. meningitidis* serogroup represented in the vaccine (i.e., serogroups A, C, Y, W-135).

While the vast majority (98%) of cases of meningococcal disease in the US are sporadic, localized outbreaks of meningococcal disease do occur. Organization-based outbreaks of meningococcal disease have occurred in elementary and junior high schools, universities, and correctional institutions; community-based outbreaks have occurred in towns, cities, and counties. An outbreak is defined as the occurrence of 3 or more confirmed or probable primary cases of meningococcal disease caused by the same serogroup during a period of 3 months or less, with a resulting primary attack rate of at least 10 cases per 100,000 population. This threshold is calculated using population-based rates, not age-specific attack rates. Recent meningococcal outbreaks in the US have been caused by serogroups B and C.

Whenever sporadic or cluster cases or outbreaks of meningococcal disease occur in the US, anti-infective prophylaxis (i.e., 2-day regimen of oral rifampin or single dose of IM ceftriaxone, oral ciprofloxacin, or oral azithromycin) is the principal means of preventing secondary cases in household and other close contacts of individuals with invasive disease. Adjunctive use of MenACWY vaccine may be indicated in situations where there is an ongoing risk of exposure (e.g., when cluster cases or outbreaks occur) and when a meningococcal serogroup represented in the vaccine is involved.

Large-scale, mass vaccination programs may be indicated in some meningococcal outbreaks. The decision to implement a mass vaccination campaign to prevent meningococcal disease depends on whether the occurrence of more than one case represents an outbreak or an unusual clustering of endemic disease. Although mass vaccination campaigns are expensive, require a massive public health effort, and can create unwarranted concern among the public, such campaigns might offer an opportunity to increase coverage in otherwise hard-to-reach populations (e.g., adolescents who have dropped out of school). When a suspected outbreak of meningococcal disease occurs in the US, public health authorities will then determine whether mass vaccinations (with or without mass anti-infective prophylaxis) is indicated and delineate the target population to be vaccinated based on risk assessment.

MenACWY vaccine (MenACWY-D or MenACWY-CRM) does not stimulate immunity to meningococcal infection caused by serogroup B, and is *not* indicated when outbreaks are caused by meningococcal serogroup B.

Dosage and Administration

■ **Reconstitution and Administration** Meningococcal (groups A, C, Y and W-135) polysaccharide diphtheria toxoid conjugate vaccine (MenACWY-D; Menactra®) and meningococcal (groups A, C, Y and W-135) oligosaccharide diphtheria CRM_{197} conjugate vaccine (MenACWY-CRM; Menveo®) are administered *only* by IM injection. These vaccines should *not* be administered subcutaneously, IV, or intradermally.

Syncope (vasovagal or vasodepressor reaction; fainting) may occur following vaccination. Syncope occurs most frequently in adolescents and young adults. Procedures should be in place to avoid falling injury and to restore cerebral perfusion following syncope. Syncope and secondary injuries may be averted if vaccinees sit or lie down during and for 15 minutes after vaccination. If syncope occurs, the patient should be observed until symptoms resolve.

MenACWY vaccine (MenACWY-D or MenACWY-CRM) usually can be given concurrently with other age-appropriate vaccines; however, MenACWY-D should *not* be given concurrently with pneumococcal 13-valent conjugate vaccine (PCV13) in infants and children with anatomic or functional asplenia (see Pneumococcal Vaccines under Vaccines: Inactivated Vaccines and Toxoids, in Drug Interactions). When multiple vaccines are administered during a single health-care visit, each parenteral vaccine should be given using separates syringes and different injection sites. Injection sites should be separated by at least 1 inch (if anatomically feasible) to allow appropriate attribution of any local adverse effects that may occur.

IM Administration Depending on patient age, IM injections should be made into the anterolateral muscles of the thigh or deltoid muscle of the arm.

In infants younger than 12 months of age, IM injections should preferably be made into the anterolateral thigh. In certain circumstances (e.g., physical obstruction at other sites and no reasonable indication to defer the vaccine dose), IM injections can be made into the gluteal muscle using care to identify anatomical landmarks prior to injection.

In infants and children 1 through 2 years of age, the anterolateral thigh is the preferred site for IM injections; alternatively, IM injections can be made into the deltoid muscle if muscle mass is adequate.

In adults, adolescents, and children 3 years of age or older, IM injections should preferably be made into the deltoid muscle; alternatively, IM injections can be made into the anterolateral thigh.

To ensure delivery into muscle, IM injections should be made at a 90° angle to the skin using a needle length appropriate for the individual's age and body mass, thickness of adipose tissue and muscle at the injection site, and injection technique. Anatomic variability, especially in the deltoid, should be considered and clinical judgment should be used to avoid inadvertent underpenetration or overpenetration of muscle.

Meningococcal (Groups A, C, Y and W-135) Polysaccharide Diphtheria Toxoid Conjugate Vaccine (MenACWY-D; Menactra®). MenACWY-D is administered *only* by IM injection.

MenACWY-D is administered undiluted. The vaccine should be shaken well prior to use and should appear as a clear to slightly turbid liquid. The vaccine should be discarded if it contains particulate matter, appears discolored, or cannot be resuspended with thorough agitation.

MenACWY-D should not be mixed with any other vaccine.

Meningococcal (Groups A, C, Y and W-135) Oligosaccharide Diphtheria CRM_{197} Conjugate Vaccine (MenACWY-CRM; Menveo®). MenACWY-CRM is administered *only* by IM injection.

MenACWY-CRM is supplied by the manufacturer as 2 components that must be combined prior to administration: a single-dose vial containing the meningococcal A conjugate component (MenA) in lyophilized form and a single-dose vial containing the meningococcal C, Y, and W-135 conjugate component (MenCYW-135) as a liquid. The entire contents of the vial containing the MenCYW-135 liquid component should be withdrawn into a syringe and injected into the vial containing the lyophilized MenA component. The vial should be inverted and shaken well until the vaccine is completely dissolved.

Reconstituted MenACWY-CRM should be a clear, colorless solution and should not be used if it contains particulate matter or appears discolored.

MenACWY-CRM should be administered immediately after reconstitution, but may be stored for up to 8 hours at 25°C or lower.

MenACWY-CRM or its individual components should not be mixed with any other vaccine or diluent.

■ **Dosage** The dosage schedule (i.e., number and timing of doses for primary immunization) and specific MenACWY vaccine administered (MenACWY-D or MenACWY-CRM) depend on the individual's age, immunization status, and risk factors. *The age-appropriate recommendations for the specific preparation used should be followed.*

Limited data suggest that MenACWY-D and MenACWY-CRM can be used interchangeably, including use in an age-appropriate multiple-dose primary immunization series or for booster doses after primary immunization. The US Public Health Service Advisory Committee on Immunization Practices (ACIP) states that if the same MenACWY vaccine used previously is not available or not known, any age-appropriate MenACWY vaccine can be administered for subsequent doses.

If interruptions or delays result in an interval between vaccine doses longer than recommended, ACIP states that it is not necessary to administer additional doses or start the vaccination series over.

Meningococcal (Groups A, C, Y and W-135) Polysaccharide Diphtheria Toxoid Conjugate Vaccine (MenACWY-D; Menactra®) MenACWY-D is administered IM in 0.5-mL doses.

MenACWY-D is labeled by FDA for use in infants and children 9 months through 10 years of age, adolescents 11 through 18 years of age, and adults 19 through 55 years of age.

Infants 9 through 23 Months of Age. For primary immunization in infants 9 through 23 months of age at increased risk for meningococcal serogroups A, C, Y, and W-135 disease because of certain chronic medical conditions (e.g., persistent complement component deficiencies, anatomic or functional asplenia, human immunodeficiency virus [HIV] infection) or travel to areas with hyperendemic or epidemic meningococcal disease, the manufacturer, ACIP, American Academy of Pediatrics (AAP), and other experts recommend that 2 doses of MenACWY-D be administered 3 months apart (minimum 12 weeks apart). If necessary (e.g., before travel), ACIP and AAP state that the doses may be given 2 months (8 weeks) apart.

For those who remain at prolonged increased risk for meningococcal disease, ACIP and AAP recommend a booster dose of MenACWY vaccine at 3 years after completion of the primary immunization series and every 5 years thereafter.

Children 2 through 10 Years of Age. For primary immunization in children 2 through 10 years of age at increased risk for meningococcal serogroups A, C, Y, and W-135 disease because of certain chronic medical conditions (e.g., persistent complement component deficiencies, anatomic or functional asplenia, HIV infection), ACIP, AAP, and other experts recommend that 2 doses of MenACWY-D be administered 2–3 months apart (minimum 8 weeks apart).

For primary immunization in children 2 through 10 years of age at increased risk for meningococcal serogroups A, C, Y, and W-135 disease because they are travelers to or residents of areas with hyperendemic or epidemic meningococcal disease, ACIP and AAP recommend a single dose of MenACWY-D.

ACIP and AAP recommend that children who received primary immunization at 2 through 6 years of age and remain at prolonged increased risk for meningococcal disease should receive a booster dose of MenACWY vaccine at 3 years after completion of the primary immunization series and every 5 years thereafter. Those who received primary immunization at 7 years of age or older and remain at prolonged increased risk for meningococcal disease should receive a booster dose of MenACWY vaccine at 5 years after completion of the primary immunization series and every 5 years thereafter.

The manufacturer states that a single dose of MenACWY-D can be used for primary immunization in children 2 through 10 years of age.

Adolescents 11 through 18 Years of Age. For *routine* primary immunization against meningococcal serogroups A, C, Y, and W-135 disease in adolescents, ACIP, AAP, and other experts recommend that a primary dose of MenACWY-D be given at 11 through 12 years of age, followed by a booster dose at 16 years of age.

Catch-up vaccination with MenACWY-D is recommended at the first opportunity for *all* adolescents 13 through 18 years of age who were not vaccinated at 11 through 12 years of age. Adolescents who receive their first dose of MenACWY vaccine at 13 through 15 years of age should receive a booster dose at 16 through 18 years of age given at least 8 weeks after the first dose. A booster dose is not needed if the first dose was given at 16 years of age or older.

For primary immunization in adolescents 11 through 18 years of age at increased risk for meningococcal serogroups A, C, Y, and W-135 disease because of certain chronic medical conditions (e.g., persistent complement component deficiencies, anatomic or functional asplenia, HIV infection), ACIP, AAP, and other experts recommend that 2 doses of MenACWY-D be administered 2–3 months apart (minimum 8 weeks apart). ACIP and other experts state that those who remain at increased risk for meningococcal disease should receive a booster dose of MenACWY vaccine every 5 years.

The manufacturer states that a single dose of MenACWY-D can be used for primary immunization in adolescents 11 through 18 years of age.

Adults 19 Years of Age or Older. For primary immunization in adults 19 through 55 years of age at increased risk for meningococcal serogroups A, C, Y, and W-135 disease because of certain chronic medical conditions (e.g., persistent complement component deficiencies, anatomic or functional asplenia, HIV infection), ACIP, AAP, and other experts recommend that 2 doses of MenACWY-D be administered 2–3 months apart (minimum 8 weeks apart).

For primary immunization in adults 19 through 55 years of age at increased risk for meningococcal serogroups A, C, Y, and W-135 disease because they are health-care or laboratory personnel, military recruits, or travelers to or residents of areas with hyperendemic or epidemic meningococcal disease, ACIP and other experts recommend a single dose of MenACWY-D.

The manufacturer states that a single dose of MenACWY-D can be used for primary immunization in adults 19 through 55 years of age.

Although safety and efficacy of MenACWY-D have not been established in adults 56 years of age or older, ACIP states that MenACWY vaccine can be used in adults 56 years of age or older† when primary immunization or revaccination or booster doses are indicated in this age group. (See Adults under Uses: Primary and Booster Immunization.)

ACIP and other experts state that adults who remain at prolonged increased risk for meningococcal disease should receive a booster dose of MenACWY vaccine every 5 years.

Meningococcal (Groups A, C, Y and W-135) Oligosaccharide Diphtheria CRM_{197} Conjugate Vaccine (MenACWY-CRM; Menveo®) MenACWY-CRM is administered IM in 0.5-mL doses.

MenACWY-CRM is labeled by FDA for use in children 2 months through 10 years of age, adolescents 11 through 18 years of age, and adults 19 through 55 years of age.

Infants 2 through 23 Months of Age. If primary immunization with MenACWY-CRM is initiated in infants 2 months of age at increased risk for meningococcal serogroups A, C, Y, and W-135 disease because of certain chronic medical conditions (e.g., persistent complement component deficiencies, anatomic or functional asplenia, HIV infection) or travel to areas with hyperendemic or epidemic meningococcal disease, a series of 4 doses should be used. The doses should be given at 2, 4, 6, and 12 months of age.

If primary immunization with MenACWY-CRM is initiated in infants 7 through 23 months of age at increased risk for meningococcal serogroups A, C, Y, and W-135 disease because of certain chronic medical conditions (e.g., persistent complement component deficiencies, anatomic or functional asplenia, HIV infection) or travel to areas with hyperendemic or epidemic meningococcal disease, a 2-dose regimen should be used. The second dose should be administered after the first birthday and at least 3 months (12 weeks) after the first dose.

For those who remain at prolonged increased risk for meningococcal disease, ACIP and AAP recommend a booster dose of MenACWY vaccine at 3 years after completion of the primary immunization series and every 5 years thereafter.

Children 2 through 10 Years of Age. For primary immunization in children 2 through 10 years of age at increased risk for meningococcal serogroups A, C, Y, and W-135 disease because of certain chronic medical conditions (e.g., persistent complement component deficiencies, anatomic or functional asplenia, HIV infection), ACIP, AAP, and other experts recommend that 2 doses of MenACWY-CRM be administered 2 months apart (minimum 8 weeks apart).

For primary immunization in children 2 through 10 years of age at increased risk for meningococcal disease because they are travelers to or residents of areas with hyperendemic or epidemic meningococcal disease, ACIP and AAP recommend a single dose of MenACWY-CRM.

ACIP and AAP recommend that children who received primary immunization at 2 through 6 years of age and remain at prolonged increased risk for meningococcal disease should receive a booster dose of MenACWY vaccine at 3 years after completion of the primary immunization series and every 5 years thereafter. Those who received primary immunization at 7 years of age or older and remain at prolonged increased risk for meningococcal disease should receive a booster dose of MenACWY vaccine at 5 years after completion of the primary immunization series and every 5 years thereafter.

The manufacturer states that a single dose of MenACWY-CRM can be used for primary immunization in children 2 through 10 years of age at increased risk for meningococcal serogroups A, C, Y, and W-135 disease and that a second dose of the vaccine may be administered 2 months after the first dose in children 2 through 5 years of age at increased risk for meningococcal disease.

Adolescents 11 through 18 Years of Age. For *routine* primary immunization against meningococcal serogroups A, C, Y, and W-135 disease in adolescents, ACIP, AAP, and other experts recommend that a primary dose of MenACWY-CRM be given at 11 through 12 years of age, followed by a booster dose at 16 years of age.

Catch-up vaccination with MenACWY-CRM is recommended at the first opportunity for *all* adolescents 13 through 18 years of age who were not vaccinated at 11 through 12 years of age. Adolescents who receive their first dose of MenACWY-CRM at 13 through 15 years of age should receive a booster dose at 16 through 18 years of age given at least 8 weeks after the first dose. A booster dose is not needed if the first dose was given at 16 years of age or older.

For primary immunization in adolescents 11 through 18 years of age at increased risk for meningococcal serogroups A, C, Y, and W-135 disease because of certain chronic medical conditions (e.g., persistent complement component deficiencies, anatomic or functional asplenia, HIV infection), ACIP, AAP, and other experts recommend that 2 doses of MenACWY-CRM be administered 2–3 months apart (minimum 8 weeks apart). ACIP and other experts state that those who remain at prolonged increased risk for meningococcal disease should receive a booster dose of MenACWY vaccine every 5 years.

The manufacturer states that a single dose of MenACWY-CRM can be used for primary immunization in adolescents 11 through 18 years of age.

Adults 19 Years of Age or Older. For primary immunization in adults at increased risk for meningococcal serogroups A, C, Y, and W-135 disease because of certain chronic medical conditions (e.g., persistent complement component deficiencies, anatomic or functional asplenia, HIV infection), ACIP, AAP, and other experts recommend 2 doses of MenACWY-CRM administered 2–3 months apart (minimum 8 weeks apart).

For primary immunization in adults 19 through 55 years of age at increased risk for meningococcal serogroups A, C, Y, and W-135 disease because they are health-care or laboratory personnel, military recruits, or travelers to or residents of areas with hyperendemic or epidemic meningococcal disease, ACIP and other experts recommend a single dose of MenACWY-CRM.

The manufacturer states that a single dose of MenACWY-CRM can be used for primary immunization in adults 19 through 55 years of age.

Although safety and efficacy of MenACWY-CRM have not been established in adults 56 years of age or older, ACIP states that MenACWY vaccine can be used in adults 56 years of age or older† when primary immunization or revaccination or booster doses are indicated in this age group. (See Adults under Uses: Primary and Booster Immunization.)

ACIP and other experts recommend that adults who remain at prolonged increased risk for meningococcal disease should receive a booster dose of MenACWY vaccine every 5 years.

Revaccination and Booster Doses The duration of immunity after primary immunization with MenACWY vaccine (MenACWY-D or MenACWY-CRM) or the previously available unconjugated meningococcal vaccine (MPSV4) has not been fully determined. (See Pharmacology: Duration of Immunity.)

Revaccination or booster doses of MenACWY vaccine may be necessary in individuals who previously received MenACWY-D, MenACWY-CRM, or MPSV4 and continue to be at prolonged increased risk for meningococcal disease. This includes individuals with increased susceptibility because of certain chronic medical conditions (e.g., complement component deficiencies, anatomic or functional asplenia, HIV infection) and those who have prolonged exposure (e.g., microbiologists routinely working with *Neisseria meningitidis*, travelers to or residents of areas where meningococcal disease is hyperendemic or epidemic).

Cautions

■ Meningococcal (Groups A, C, Y and W-135) Polysaccharide Diphtheria Toxoid Conjugate Vaccine (MenACWY-D; Menactra®)

Information on the safety of meningococcal (groups A, C, Y and W-135) polysaccharide diphtheria toxoid conjugate vaccine (MenACWY-D) has been obtained principally from 8 clinical studies in which 10,057 individuals 2–55 years of age received the vaccine. In the 3 primary safety studies, individuals were randomized to receive MenACWY-D or unconjugated meningococcal polysaccharide vaccine, groups A, C, Y and W-135 combined (MPSV4; no longer commercially available in the US). In 2 of the safety studies, MenACWY-D was administered concurrently with typhoid Vi polysaccharide vaccine or with tetanus and diphtheria toxoids adsorbed (Td). (See Drug Interactions: Vaccines.)

Adverse effects reported most frequently when MenACWY-D was used in children 2 through 10 years of age were local effects at the injection site (e.g., pain) and irritability. Diarrhea, drowsiness, and anorexia were also common in this age group.

The most common adverse effects reported in adolescents and adults 11 through 55 years of age following a single dose of MenACWY-D were local effects at the site of injection (e.g., pain), headache, and fatigue.

Local Effects Adverse local effects, including pain, induration, erythema, and swelling, have been reported in 17–45% of children 2 through 10 years of age, 11–59% of adolescents 11 through 18 years of age, and 13–54% of adults 19 through 55 years of age who received MenACWY-D.

Systemic Effects The most frequently reported systemic adverse effects in children 2 through 10 years of age who received MenACWY-D were irritability, diarrhea, drowsiness, anorexia, arthralgia, fever, vomiting, and rash. While irritability, drowsiness, and diarrhea were reported in 11–12% of these children, arthralgia, fever, vomiting, and rash were reported in 3–8%. The most frequently reported systemic effects in adolescents and adults 11 through 55 years of age following a single dose of MenACWY-D were headache, fatigue, malaise, arthralgia, diarrhea, anorexia, chills, fever, vomiting, and rash. While headache, fatigue, malaise, and arthralgia were reported in 17–41%, GI effects, chills, fever, and rash were reported in only 1–16%.

In clinical studies comparing safety and efficacy of MenACWY-D in children, adolescents, and adults 2 through 55 years of age, fever (39.5°C or higher) was reported in 5% of adolescents who received MenACWY-D. The overall rate of severe systemic adverse effects reported within 6 months of vaccination was about 1% in adolescents and adults and was less than 1% in children 2 through 10 years of age following administration of the conjugated meningococcal vaccine.

Although a causal relationship to MenACWY-D has not been established, vasovagal syncope, facial palsy, transverse myelitis, acute disseminated encephalomyelitis, myalgia, and lymphadenopathy have been reported during postmarketing surveillance.

Hypersensitivity reactions (e.g., anaphylactic/anaphylactoid reaction, wheezing, difficulty breathing, upper airway swelling, urticaria, erythema, pruritus, hypotension, erythema multiforme) have been reported rarely in patients who received MenACWY-D.

Guillain-Barré Syndrome. There have been postmarketing reports of Guillain-Barré syndrome (GBS) temporally associated with administration of MenACWY-D. Reported cases of GBS generally involved individuals 11 through 19 years of age at the time of vaccination with onset of symptoms within 6 weeks of the vaccine dose. One individual had experienced previous episodes of GBS at 2 and 5 years of age after receiving routine childhood vaccinations and another had no personal history of GBS but had a mother with a history of GBS.

GBS is a serious neurologic disorder involving inflammatory demyelination of peripheral nerves and may occur spontaneously or after certain antecedent events such as infections. The disorder is characterized by subacute onset of progressive, symmetrical weakness in the legs and arms, with loss of reflexes. Sensory abnormalities, cranial nerve involvement, and paralysis of respiratory muscles may also develop. GBS is sometimes fatal and 20% of hospitalized patients may have prolonged disability.

Because of these initial reports, FDA, the US Centers for Disease Control and Prevention (CDC), and others began investigating the possible relationship between administration of MenACWY-D and the occurrence of GBS. In one postmarketing retrospective safety study that evaluated the risk of GBS following administration of MenACWY-D, claims data from over 9 million individuals 11 through 18 years of age was analyzed (15% of these individuals had received the vaccine). Based on 72 chart-confirmed cases of GBS in this population, none had received MenACWY-D within 42 days of symptom onset. An additional 129 potential cases of GBS could not be confirmed or excluded using chart review. An analysis taking into account the missing data estimated that the attributable risk of GBS ranged from 0–5 additional cases per 1 million vaccinees within the 6-week period following vaccination. In another retrospective, cohort study involving 12.6 million individuals 11–21 years of age, more than 1.4 million doses of MenACWY-D had been administered and there were 99 confirmed cases of GBS (5.4 cases per 1 million vaccinees); none of these occurred within 6 weeks following vaccination.

Because of the known risk for meningococcal exposure and the limited data indicating an association between MenACWY-D vaccination and GBS, CDC continues to recommend routine vaccination with MenACWY-D for adolescents, first-year college students living in dormitories, and other populations at increased risk for meningococcal serogroups A, C, Y, and W-135 infection. (See Guillain-Barré Syndrome under Cautions: Precautions and Contraindications.)

■ Meningococcal (Groups A, C, Y and W-135) Oligosaccharide Diphtheria CRM_{197} Conjugate Vaccine (MenACWY-CRM; Menveo®)

Information on the safety of meningococcal (groups A, C, Y and W-135) oligosaccharide diphtheria CRM_{197} conjugate vaccine (MenACWY-CRM) has been obtained from clinical studies in infants 2 through 23 months of age, children 2 through 10 years of age, and adolescents and adults 11 through 55 years of age. In 4 safety studies conducted in children 2 through 10 years of age, individuals were randomized to receive MenACWY-CRM or a comparator vaccine (MenACWY-D or MPSV4 [no longer commercially available in the US]). In 5 safety studies in adolescents and adults 11 through 55 years of age, 5286 individuals received MenACWY-CRM alone, 899 individuals received MenACWY-CRM concomitantly with other vaccines (i.e., tetanus toxoid, reduced diphtheria toxoid and acellular pertussis vaccine adsorbed [Tdap; Boostrix®] with or without human papillomavirus quadrivalent [types 6, 11, 16, 18] vaccine, recombinant [4vHPV; no longer commercially available in the US). (See Drug Interactions: Vaccines.) The remaining individuals were randomized to receive a comparator vaccine (MenACWY-D or MPSV4 [no longer commercially available in the US).

Adverse effects reported most frequently in infants 2 through 23 months of age who received a 4-dose regimen of MenACWY-CRM administered concurrently with other routine infant vaccines were tenderness (24–41%) and erythema (11–15%) at the injection site, irritability (42–57%), sleepiness (29–50%), persistent crying (21–41%), change in eating habits (17–23%), vomiting (5–11%), and diarrhea (8–16%). The rates of solicited local and systemic adverse effects in these infants were comparable to rates among those who received the routine infant vaccines without MenACWY-CRM.

Adverse effects reported most frequently when MenACWY-CRM was used in children 2 through 10 years of age were injection site pain (31%), erythema (23%), irritability (18%), induration (16%), sleepiness (14%), malaise (12%), and headache (11%).

Among adolescents and adults 11 through 55 years of age, the most frequently reported adverse effects were injection site pain (41%), headache (30%), myalgia (18%), malaise (16%), and nausea (10%).

Local Effects Adverse local effects (pain, erythema, induration) were reported in 18–33% of children 2 through 5 years of age, 17–39% of children 6 through 10 years of age, 12–44% of adolescents 11 through 18 years of age, and 13–38% of adults 19 through 55 years of age who received a single dose of MenACWY-CRM. These local effects were considered moderate in 2–8% and severe in up to 1% of children 2 through 10 years of age, and were considered moderate in 1–9% and severe in up to 1% of individuals 11 through 55 years of age.

Systemic Effects Adverse systemic effects, including irritability, sleepiness, change in eating, diarrhea, headache, rash, arthralgia, vomiting, and fever, have been reported in children 2 through 5 years of age who received a single dose of MenACWY-CRM in clinical studies. While irritability, sleepiness, and change in eating were reported in 9–21% of these children, diarrhea, headache, rash, arthralgia, vomiting, and fever occurred in 2–7%.

In children 6 through 10 years of age who received a single dose of MenACWY-CRM in clinical studies, headache, malaise, myalgia, nausea, arthralgia, chills, rash, and fever have been reported. While headache, malaise, and myalgia were reported in 10–18% of these children, nausea, arthralgia, chills, rash, and fever were reported in 2–8%.

The most frequently reported systemic effects in adolescents and adults 11 through 55 years of age who received a single dose of MenACWY-CRM in clinical studies were headache, myalgia, nausea, malaise, chills, arthralgia, rash, and fever. While headache, myalgia, nausea, and malaise were reported in 11–29% of adolescents 11 through 18 years of age, chills, arthralgia, rash, and fever were reported in 1–8% of these adolescents. Headache, myalgia, and malaise were reported in 10–25% and nausea, arthralgia, chills, rash, and fever were reported in 1–7% of adults 19 through 55 years of age who received a single dose of MenACWY-CRM.

There have been postmarketing reports of Bell's palsy in temporal association with administration of a dose of MenACWY-CRM in adolescents and young adults 11–21 years of age. Symptoms of Bell's palsy resolved in all reported cases to date. In 6 of 8 cases that occurred within 84 days after vaccination, MenACWY-CRM had been administered concomitantly with at least 1 other vaccine (i.e., HPV vaccine, Tdap, influenza vaccine).

Ear and eye disorders (e.g., impaired hearing, ear pain, vertigo, vestibular disorder, eyelid ptosis), vaccination site cellulitis, nervous system disorders (e.g., dizziness, syncope, tonic convulsions, facial paresis, balance disorder), oropharyngeal pain, arthralgia, bone pain, and skin exfoliation have been reported during postmarketing surveillance. A causal relationship to MenACWY-CRM has not been established.

Hypersensitivity reactions have been reported in patients who received MenACWY-CRM.

■ Precautions and Contraindications

Prior to administration of MenACWY vaccine (MenACWY-D or MenACWY-CRM), all known precautions should be taken to prevent adverse reactions, including a review of the patient's history with respect to health status and possible sensitivity to the vaccine, similar vaccines, or vaccine components. Epinephrine and other appropriate agents and equipment should be available for immediate treatment if an anaphylactic or other serious allergic reaction occurs.

The patient and/or the patient's parent or guardian should be informed of the benefits and risks of immunization with MenACWY-D and MenACWY-CRM and should be provided with a copy of the appropriate Vaccine Information Statement (available at CDC website at http://www.cdc.gov/vaccines/pubs/vis/default.htm). Patients and/or the patient's parent or guardian also should be instructed to report any severe or unusual adverse reactions to their healthcare provider. Clinicians or individuals can report any adverse reactions that occur following vaccination to VAERS at 800-822-7967 or http://www.vaers.hhs.gov.

Meningococcal (Groups A, C, Y and W-135) Polysaccharide Diphtheria Toxoid Conjugate Vaccine (MenACWY-D; Menactra®) MenACWY-D is contraindicated in individuals with a history of severe allergic reaction (e.g., anaphylaxis) after a previous dose of the vaccine, any vaccine component, or any vaccine containing meningococcal capsular polysaccharide, diphtheria toxoid, or diphtheria CRM_{197}.

Meningococcal (Groups A, C, Y and W-135) Oligosaccharide Diphtheria CRM_{197} Conjugate Vaccine (MenACWY-CRM; Menveo®) MenACWY-CRM is contraindicated in individuals with a history of severe allergic reaction (e.g., anaphylaxis) after a previous dose of the vaccine or any vaccine containing meningococcal antigens, diphtheria toxoid, or diphtheria CRM_{197}.

Individuals with Altered Immunocompetence Like other inactivated vaccines, MenACWY vaccine may be administered to individuals immunosuppressed as a result of disease or medical therapy; however, immune responses to vaccines and efficacy may be reduced in individuals with altered immunocompetence.

The manufacturers state that immunogenicity of MenACWY-D and MenACWY-CRM has not been specifically studied in immunocompromised individuals.

The US Public Health Service Advisory Committee on Immunization Practices (ACIP), American Academy of Pediatrics (AAP), Centers for Disease Control and Prevention (CDC), National Institutes of Health (NIH), HIV Medicine Association of the Infectious Diseases Society of America (IDSA), and other experts recommend that adults, adolescents, children, and infants 2 months of age or older with human immunodeficiency virus (HIV) infection receive age-appropriate MenACWY vaccine for primary and booster immunization against meningococcal serogroups A, C, Y, and W-135 infection. (See HIV-infected Individuals under Uses: Primary and Booster Immunization.)

Individuals with functional or anatomic asplenia (including sickle cell disease) are at increased risk for meningococcal disease and should receive age-appropriate immunization against meningococcal serogroups A, C, Y, and W-135. (See Individuals with Complement Deficiency, Properdin Deficiency, or Asplenia under Uses: Primary and Booster Immunization.) When planning immunization against meningococcal disease and pneumococcal disease in infants and children with anatomic or functional asplenia, clinicians should consider that MenACWY-D should *not* be administered concomitantly with or within 4 weeks after pneumococcal 13-valent conjugate vaccine (PCV13) (see Pneumococcal Vaccines under Vaccines: Inactivated Vaccines and Toxoids, in Drug Interactions).

In patients scheduled for elective splenectomy, MenACWY vaccine should be administered at least 14 days prior to surgery; if not administered prior to surgery, MenACWY vaccine should be administered as soon as possible 2 weeks or longer following the procedure when the patient's condition is stable.

Individuals with persistent complement component deficiency, including those receiving treatment that inhibits terminal complement activation (e.g., eculizumab), are at increased risk for invasive disease caused by meningococcal serogroups A, C, Y, and W-135, even if they develop antibodies following vaccination with MenACWY vaccine. Because life-threatening and fatal meningococcal infections have occurred in patients receiving eculizumab, meningococcal vaccines should be administered at least 2 weeks prior to the first dose of eculizumab, unless the risks of delaying initiation of the drug outweigh the risks of meningococcal infection.

Inactivated vaccines generally should be administered prior to initiation of immunosuppressive therapy or deferred until immunosuppressive therapy is discontinued. (See Drug Interactions: Immunosuppressive Agents.)

Concomitant Illness A decision to administer or delay vaccination in an individual with a current or recent acute illness depends on the severity of symptoms and etiology of the illness.

ACIP states that mild acute illness generally does not preclude vaccination. However, moderate or severe acute illness (with or without fever) is a precaution for vaccination and vaccines should be deferred until the individual has recovered from the acute phase of the illness. This precaution avoids superimposing adverse effects of the vaccine on the underlying illness or mistakenly concluding that a manifestation of the underlying illness resulted from vaccination.

Guillain-Barré Syndrome Because there have been postmarketing reports of GBS temporally associated with MenACWY-D, the manufacturer states that individuals with a history of GBS may be at increased risk of GBS following administration of the vaccine and the decision to administer MenACWY-D in such individuals should take into account the potential benefits and risks of immunization.

The manufacturer of MenACWY-CRM states that, because GBS has been reported in temporal relationship following administration of another US quadrivalent polysaccharide meningococcal conjugate vaccine, a decision to administer MenACWY-CRM in an individual with a history of GBS should take into account the potential benefits and risks.

After reviewing available safety data, ACIP concluded that the benefits of meningococcal vaccination outweigh the risks of GBS recurrence in individuals with a history of GBS.

Clinicians should remain alert to the possibility of vaccine-associated GBS and report any suspected cases to VAERS at 800-822-7967 or http://www.vaers.hhs.gov.

Individuals with Bleeding Disorders Individuals who have bleeding disorders or are receiving anticoagulant therapy and/or their family members should be advised about the risk of hematoma from IM injections.

ACIP states that IM vaccines may be given to individuals who have bleeding disorders or are receiving anticoagulant therapy if a clinician familiar with the patient's bleeding risk determines that the vaccine can be administered IM with reasonable safety. In these cases, a fine needle (23 gauge or smaller) should be used to administer the vaccine and firm pressure should be applied to the injection site (without rubbing) for at least 2 minutes. In individuals receiving therapy for hemophilia, IM vaccines can be scheduled for shortly after a dose of such therapy.

Limitations of Vaccine Effectiveness MenACWY vaccine (MenACWY-D or MenACWY-CRM) may not protect all vaccine recipients against meningococcal serogroups A, C, Y, and W-135 infection. In addition, these quadrivalent meningococcal vaccines provide protection only against those serogroups represented in the vaccine (i.e., groups A, C, Y, W-135). MenACWY vaccine will *not* prevent meningococcal infection caused by *N. meningitidis* serogroups not represented in the vaccine (e.g., serogroup B) and will *not* prevent infections caused by other pathogens.

The possibility that MenACWY vaccine may not prevent infection in individuals who do not achieve protective antibody titers should be considered since the minimum titer of serum anticapsular antibody needed to confer immunity against *N. meningitidis* serogroups A, C, Y, or W-135 has not been established. However, studies evaluating serogroup A and C meningococcal disease indicate that anticapsular antibody levels of 2 mcg/mL or greater may be protective.

While there is evidence that meningococcal vaccines can stimulate antibody responses in individuals with inherited complement deficiencies and individuals whose spleens have been removed, efficacy has not been fully established in these individuals and the vaccines may not provide complete protection. (See Individuals with Complement Deficiency, Properdin Deficiency, or Asplenia under Uses: Primary and Booster Immunization.)

Duration of Immunity Duration of protection following primary immunization with conjugated MenACWY vaccine (MenACWY-D or MenACWY-CRM) or the previously available unconjugated meningococcal vaccine (MPSV4) has not been fully determined. (See Pharmacology: Duration of Immunity.)

Meningococcal antigens in MenACWY-D and MenACWY-CRM are conjugated to a diphtheria toxoid or CRM_{197} protein carrier, respectively. These T-cell epitopes may result in an improved primary response to the meningococcal antigens and a strong anamnestic response after re-exposure to the antigens. MenACWY-D and MenACWY-CRM are expected to provide a longer duration of protection than the previously available unconjugated meningococcal vaccine (MPSV4).

Because of waning immunity, a single dose of MenACWY vaccine (MenACWY-D or MenACWY-CRM) administered to adolescents at 11 through 12 years of age is unlikely to provide continued protection against meningococcal serogroups A, C, Y, and W-135 in these individuals at 16 through 21 years of age. The duration of protective antibody after a booster dose of MenACWY vaccine given at 16 through 18 years of age is not known, but is expected to last at least through 21 years of age.

Revaccination or booster doses of MenACWY vaccine may be necessary in individuals who previously received MenACWY vaccine or MPSV4 vaccine (no longer commercially available in the US) and continue to be at prolonged increased risk of exposure to meningococcal infection. (See Dosage and Administration: Dosage.)

Improper Storage and Handling Improper storage or handling of vaccines may reduce vaccine potency resulting in reduced or inadequate immune response in vaccinees.

All vaccines should be inspected upon delivery and monitored during storage to ensure that the appropriate temperature is maintained. (See Chemistry and Stability: Stability.)

Meningococcal vaccine that has been mishandled or has not been stored at the recommended temperature should not be administered.

If there are concerns about mishandling, the manufacturer or state or local immunization or health departments should be contacted for guidance on whether the vaccine is usable.

■ **Pediatric Precautions** Safety and efficacy of MenACWY-D have not been established in infants younger than 9 months of age.

Safety and efficacy of MenACWY-CRM have not been established in children younger than 2 months of age.

Apnea has been reported following IM administration of vaccines in some infants born prematurely. Decisions regarding when to administer an IM vaccine in infants born prematurely should be based on consideration of the individual infant's medical status and potential benefits and possible risks of vaccination.

■ **Geriatric Precautions** Safety and efficacy of MenACWY-D and MenACWY-CRM have not been established in adults 56 years of age or older†, including geriatric adults. However, ACIP recommends use of MenACWY vaccine in certain adults in this age group. (See Adults under Uses: Primary and Booster Immunization.)

■ **Mutagenicity and Carcinogenicity** The mutagenic and carcinogenic potential of MenACWY vaccine (MenACWY-D or MenACWY-CRM) has not been evaluated.

■ **Pregnancy, Fertility, and Lactation** ***Pregnancy*** Animal reproduction studies performed in pregnant mice using 0.1 mL of MenACWY-D administered 14 days prior to mating and on days 6 and 18 of gestation did not reveal any vaccine-related fetal malformations or variations and no adverse effects on postnatal development. There are no adequate and well-controlled studies in pregnant women. The manufacturer states that data from a pregnancy registry indicate there were 2 major birth defects and 6 miscarriages among 87 prospectively followed pregnancies of women who received MenACWY-D within 30 days before or at any time during pregnancy. Clinicians are encouraged to report any exposure to MenACWY-D that occurs during pregnancy to the manufacturer's vaccination pregnancy registry at 800-822-2463.

Animal reproduction studies performed in female rabbits using MenACWY-CRM at a dosage approximately 20 times the human dose (calculated on a mg/kg basis) did not reveal evidence of harm to the fetus. However, there are no adequate and well-controlled studies in pregnant women. Although data are limited regarding the safety of MenACWY-CRM in pregnant women, this vaccine was administered to 37 women enrolled in clinical studies who were found to be pregnant during the 6-month follow-up period after vaccination. There was no evidence of congenital anomalies, but 7 cases of spontaneous abortion occurred in these pregnant women. The manufacturer states that MenACWY-CRM should be used in pregnant women only when clearly needed. Clinicians are encouraged to report any exposure to MenACWY-CRM that occurs during pregnancy to the manufacturer's vaccination pregnancy registry at 877-413-4759.

VAERS reports of exposure to MenACWY vaccine during pregnancy have not identified adverse effects among pregnant women or infants born to women vaccinated during pregnancy.

ACIP and AAP state that MenACWY vaccine (MenACWY-D or MenACWY-CRM) may be used during pregnancy if indicated in a woman at increased risk of meningococcal disease. ACIP states that there is no evidence of risk to the fetus if inactivated vaccines are administered during pregnancy.

Analysis of anticapsular antibody levels in maternal and cord blood samples obtained at the time of delivery from women who received unconjugated capsular polysaccharide antigens from *N. meningitidis* serogroups A and C (not commercially available in the US) indicate that pregnant women have a good antibody response to antigens from both serogroup A and C, and these antibodies cross the placenta. The extent of placental transfer of group A and C antibodies shows considerable interindividual variation; the ratio of cord blood anticapsular antibody levels to maternal anticapsular antibody levels has ranged from 0.1–1.1 (mean: 0.3–0.6). Levels of maternal group A and C antibodies in the child decline over the first few months after birth; by 4–8 months of age, children born to mothers who were vaccinated during pregnancy have anticapsular antibody levels similar to those in children born to unvaccinated mothers. There was no evidence that administration of bivalent meningococcal vaccines containing capsular polysaccharide antigens from serogroups A and C to pregnant women had any effect on the antibody response in the child following subsequent vaccination with a meningococcal polysaccharide vaccine.

Fertility Animal reproduction studies performed in pregnant mice using MenACWY-D did not reveal any effects on fertility.

Animal reproduction studies performed in rabbits using a dose of MenACWY-CRM approximately 20 times the human dose (calculated on a mg/kg basis) did not reveal any evidence of impaired fertility.

Lactation It is not known whether antigens contained in MenACWY vaccine (MenACWY-D or MenACWY-CRM) are distributed into milk. The manufacturers state that MenACWY vaccine should be used with caution in nursing women.

ACIP states that administration of inactivated vaccines to a woman who is breast-feeding does not pose any safety concerns for the woman or the breast-fed infant.

Drug Interactions

■ **Immune Globulins** There is no evidence that immune globulin (immune globulin IM [IGIM], immune globulin IV [IGIV], immune globulin subcutaneous) or specific hyperimmune globulin (hepatitis B immune globulin [HBIG], rabies immune globulin [RIG], tetanus immune globulin [TIG], varicella zoster immune globulin [VZIG]) interferes with the immune response to inactivated vaccines. The US Public Health Service Advisory Committee on Immunization Practices (ACIP) states that inactivated vaccines such as meningococcal groups A, C, Y, and W-135 vaccine (MenACWY vaccine) may be given concurrently with (using separate syringes and different injection sites) or at any interval before or after immune globulin preparations.

■ **Immunosuppressive Agents** Individuals receiving immunosuppressive therapy (e.g., alkylating agents, antimetabolites, certain biologic response modifiers, corticosteroids, cytotoxic drugs, radiation) may have reduced immune responses to vaccines, including meningococcal (groups A, C, Y and W-135) polysaccharide diphtheria toxoid conjugate vaccine (MenACWY-D; Menactra®) and meningococcal (groups A, C, Y and W-135) oligosaccharide diphtheria CRM_{197} conjugate vaccine (MenACWY-CRM; Menveo®).

Inactivated vaccines generally should be administered at least 2 weeks prior to initiation of immunosuppressive therapy and, because of possible suboptimal response, should not be administered during and for certain periods of time after immunosuppressive therapy is discontinued. Because the intervals between discontinuance of immunosuppressive therapy and restoration of immune competence vary depending on the type and intensity of immunosuppressive therapy, underlying disease, and other factors, optimal timing for vaccine administration following discontinuance of immunosuppressive therapy has not been identified for every situation.

ACIP and the Infectious Diseases Society of America (IDSA) recommend that inactivated vaccines be administered at least 2 weeks before initiation of chemotherapy or radiation therapy, if possible, and avoided during such therapy. Individuals vaccinated during or within 14 days of starting chemotherapy or radiation therapy should be considered unimmunized and should be revaccinated at least 3 months after such therapy is discontinued if immunocompetence has been restored.

Inactivated vaccines should be administered at least 2 weeks prior to treatment with anti-B-cell antibodies (e.g., rituximab). The optimal time to administer vaccines in patients who have received treatment with anti-B-cell antibodies is unclear. Some experts state that administration of inactivated vaccines should be deferred until at least 6 months after treatment with anti-B-cell antibodies has been discontinued.

Inactivated vaccines should be administered at least 2 weeks prior to initiation of therapy with certain other immunosuppressive biologic response modifiers (e.g., colony-stimulating factors, interleukins, tumor necrosis factor-α inhibitors). Some experts states that, if an inactivated vaccine is indicated in a patient with a chronic inflammatory illness who is receiving maintenance therapy with an immunosuppressive agent, the vaccine should not be withheld because of concerns about exacerbation of the inflammatory illness.

Corticosteroids given in greater than physiologic doses may reduce immune responses to vaccines. ACIP and the American Academy of Pediatrics (AAP) state that inactivated vaccines preferably should be administered at least 2 weeks prior to initiation of corticosteroid therapy that is considered immunosuppressive; however, if this is not feasible in patients receiving long-term corticosteroid therapy for inflammatory or autoimmune diseases, inactivated vaccines can be administered during such therapy. IDSA states that, although it may be reasonable to delay administration of inactivated vaccines in patients treated with high-dose corticosteroid therapy because of possible reduced immune responses, recommendations for use of MenACWY vaccine in individuals receiving corticosteroid therapy, including high-dose corticosteroid therapy, generally are the same as those for other individuals.

■ **Vaccines** Although specific studies may not be available evaluating concurrent administration with each antigen, concurrent administration of MenACWY vaccine (MenACWY-D or MenACWY-CRM) with other age-appropriate vaccines, including live virus vaccines, toxoids, or inactivated or recombinant vaccines, during the same health-care visit usually is not expected to affect immunologic responses or adverse reactions to any of the preparations. (See Pneumococcal Vaccines under Vaccines: Inactivated Vaccines and Toxoids, in Drug Interactions.)

Immunization with MenACWY vaccine can be integrated with immunization against diphtheria, tetanus, pertussis, *Haemophilus influenzae* type b (Hib), hepatitis A, hepatitis B, human papillomavirus (HPV), influenza, measles, mumps, rubella, pneumococcal disease, poliomyelitis, and varicella. However, each parenteral vaccine should be administered using separate syringes and different injection sites.

Inactivated Vaccines and Toxoids **Tetanus and Diphtheria Toxoids Adsorbed.** In a double-blind, randomized study in adolescents 11 through 17 years of age, MenACWY-D (Menactra®) was administered concomitantly with or 1 month after tetanus and diphtheria toxoids adsorbed (Td). Antibody responses to some meningococcal antigens (i.e., serogroups C, Y, W-135) were higher when MenACWY-D and Td were administered concomitantly than when MenACWY-D was administered 1 month after Td; antibody responses to the tetanus and diphtheria antigens were similar in both study groups. The overall rate of systemic adverse effects was higher when the vaccines were administered concomitantly.

Diphtheria and Tetanus Toxoids and Pertussis Vaccines. ACIP states that MenACWY-D may be administered concurrently with diphtheria and tetanus toxoids and acellular pertussis vaccine adsorbed (DTaP) using separate syringes and different injection sites. If the vaccines are not administered concurrently, ACIP states that MenACWY-D should be given before DTaP (during a different health-care visit) or more than 6 months after DTaP in children 2 through 6 years of age. This recommendation is based on some limited data suggesting interference with the immunologic response to meningococcal antigens (immunologic blunting) if MenACWY-D is administered following DTaP. If the MenACWY-D dose is inadvertently given within 6 months after DTaP, ACIP states that the MenACWY-D dose does not need to be repeated. In addition, if a child will be traveling to an area with high risk of meningococcal disease or is at risk during a community outbreak of meningococcal disease, ACIP does not recommend waiting 6 months after DTaP to administer MenACWY-D, even if blunting may occur.

ACIP states that MenACWY-CRM may be administered concurrently with or at any interval before or after DTaP.

Concurrent administration of MenACWY-D and tetanus toxoid, reduced diphtheria toxoid and acellular pertussis vaccine adsorbed (Tdap; Boostrix®) was evaluated in a study in adolescents 11–18 years of age randomized to receive the vaccines concurrently (at different injection sites) or 1 month apart. The immune responses to the diphtheria, tetanus, and meningococcal antigens obtained following concurrent administration were noninferior to those reported when the vaccines were given 1 month apart. Although the immune response to the pertactin pertussis antigen (measured as geometric mean antibody concentration [GMC] of anti-pertactin) was lower when Tdap (Boostrix®) was administered concurrently with MenACWY-D, it is not known whether efficacy of Tdap is affected by the reduced response to pertactin.

MenACWY-D has been administered concurrently with Tdap (Adacel®) and human papillomavirus 9-valent vaccine, recombinant (9vHPV; Gardasil® 9) in a randomized controlled study in adolescents 11 through 15 years of age. Concurrent administration of these 3 vaccines at different injection sites did not interfere with the antibody response to any of the vaccine antigens. (See Human Papillomavirus Vaccine under Vaccines: Inactivated Vaccines and Toxoids, in Drug Interactions.)

In a randomized, controlled study in adolescents and young adults 11–25 years of age, concomitant administration of MenACWY-CRM and Tdap (Boostrix®) did not affect the immune responses to the diphtheria, tetanus, and meningococcal antigens. However, immune responses to the pertussis antigens were lower when MenACWY-CRM and Tdap were administered concurrently compared with administration of Tdap alone.

MenACWY-CRM has been administered concurrently with Tdap or with Tdap and human papillomavirus vaccine in a study in healthy adolescents 11 through 18 years of age. There was no interference with the immune response to the meningococcal antigens compared with administration of MenACWY-CRM alone. Although lower geometric mean antibody concentrations to the pertussis antigens were observed when MenACWY-CRM was administered concomitantly with Tdap and HPV vaccine compared with administration of Tdap alone, the clinical implications of the lower antibody response to the pertussis antigen in this study are not known. Systemic adverse reactions (e.g., headache, malaise, myalgia, arthralgia) were reported more frequently in those who received MenACWY-CRM, Tdap, and HPV vaccine concurrently compared with those who received MenACWY-CRM alone.

Human Papillomavirus Vaccine. MenACWY-D has been administered concurrently with Tdap (Adacel®) and 9vHPV (Gardasil® 9) in adolescents 11 through 15 years of age. Concurrent administration of the 3 vaccines at different injection sites did not interfere with the antibody response to any of the vaccine antigens. Although the overall incidence of adverse reactions in those who received all 3 vaccines concurrently at different sites was similar to that reported when 9vHPV was given alone followed by MenACWY-D and Tdap 1 month later, concurrent administration of all 3 vaccines was associated with an increased incidence of swelling at the 9vHPV injection site compared with administration of the HPV vaccine alone.

MenACWY-CRM has been administered concurrently with human papillomavirus quadrivalent (types 6, 11, 16, 18) vaccine, recombinant (4vHPV; no longer commercially available in the US) and Tdap in adolescents 11 through 18 years of age. There was no interference with immune responses to the meningococcal antigens compared with administration of MenACWY-CRM alone. Systemic adverse reactions (e.g., headache, malaise, myalgia, arthralgia) were reported more frequently in the those who received 4vHPV, Tdap, and MenACWY-CRM concurrently compared with those who received MenACWY-CRM alone.

Meningococcal Vaccines. ACIP and others state that MenACWY vaccine may be administered concurrently with meningococcal group B (MenB) vaccine (MenB-4C [Bexsero®] or MenB-FHbp [Trumenba®]) using separate syringes and different injection sites.

MenACWY-D has been administered concurrently with MenB-FHbp (Trumenba®) without a decrease in immune responses to the meningococcal antigens in either vaccine.

Pneumococcal Vaccines. Concurrent administration of pneumococcal 7-valent conjugate vaccine (PCV7; no longer commercially available in the US) with the second dose of MenACWY-D in infants at 12 months of age resulted in a decreased immune response to PCV7 (i.e., noninferiority criteria were not met for 3 of the 7 pneumococcal vaccine serotypes compared with administration of PCV7 without MenACWY-D).

Concurrent administration of MenACWY-CRM and PCV7 in infants at 2, 4, 6, and 12 months of age resulted in possible interference with the antibody response to 2 of the pneumococcal vaccine serotypes at 1 month after the third dose, but no evidence of interference with immune response to any pneumococcal vaccine serotypes after the fourth dose.

The manufacturer of pneumococcal 13-valent conjugate vaccine (PCV13; Prevnar 13®) states that data are insufficient to assess concomitant administration with MenACWY vaccine in children and adolescents.

To avoid possible interference with the immune response to PCV13 in infants and children with anatomic or functional asplenia, ACIP and AAP state that MenACWY-D and PCV13 should *not* be administered concurrently and that the PCV13 immunization series should be completed first; MenACWY-D immunization should be initiated at least 4 weeks later.

Pneumococcal 23-valent polysaccharide vaccine (PPSV23; Pneumovax® 23) may be administered concomitantly with MenACWY vaccine using separate syringes and different injection sites.

Typhoid Vaccine. MenACWY-D and parenteral inactivated typhoid Vi polysaccharide vaccine (Typhim Vi®) have been administered concomitantly at different sites in adults 18 through 55 years of age without a reduced immune response to either vaccine and without a clinically important increase in adverse effects compared with administration alone. Because both vaccines are inactivated vaccines, parenteral inactivated typhoid vaccine (Typhim Vi®) may be administered simultaneously with MenACWY vaccine (using separate syringes and different injection sites) or at any interval before or after the meningococcal vaccine.

Results of a study in healthy adults who received a bivalent vaccine containing unconjugated meningococcal capsular polysaccharide antigens from serogroups A and C (not commercially available in the US) given concurrently with or 3–6 weeks before or after typhoid Vi capsular polysaccharide vaccine (Typhim Vi®) indicate that concomitant administration of the vaccines does not affect the incidence of adverse effects or the antibody response to any of the antigens.

Live Vaccines **Measles, Mumps, Rubella, and Varicella Vaccines.** When MenACWY-D was administered with measles, mumps, and rubella virus vaccine live (MMR) and varicella virus vaccine live (VAR) (or the fixed-combination vaccine containing measles, mumps, rubella, and varicella antigens [MMRV]) and PCV7 (no longer commercially available in the US) in infants 12 months of age, antibody responses to the measles, mumps, rubella, and varicella antigens approximately 30 days later were comparable to those reported in children who received MMRV (or MMR and VAR) and PCV7 without MenACWY-D.

When MenACWY-CRM was administered concurrently with MMRV in infants 12 months of age, antibody responses to the measles, mumps, rubella, and varicella antigens measured 6 weeks after vaccination were comparable to those reported in infants who received MMRV alone. In addition, concurrent administration of MenACWY-CRM and MMRV in these infants did not increase the rate of solicited local or systemic adverse effects compared with administration of either vaccine alone.

Typhoid Vaccine. ACIP states that oral live typhoid vaccine may be administered concurrently with or at any interval before or after MenACWY vaccine (MenACWY-D or MenACWY-CRM) since the meningococcal vaccines are inactivated vaccines.

Yellow Fever Vaccine. Yellow fever vaccine has been administered concomitantly with a previously available unconjugated meningococcal vaccine (MPSV4; Menomune®) without evidence of reduced antibody response to either vaccine and without any unusual adverse effects.

Pharmacology

Meningococcal groups A, C, Y, and W-135 vaccines are inactivated (polysaccharide) vaccines that stimulate active immunity to infections caused by the *Neisseria meningitidis* serotypes represented in the vaccines (i.e., groups A, C, Y, and W-135). The antibody response to each of the antigens contained in quadrivalent meningococcal groups A, C, Y, and W-135 vaccines occurs independently of the response to the other antigens. These vaccines will *not* stimulate immunity to infection caused by meningococcal serogroups not represented in the vaccines (e.g., serogroup B) or to infection caused by other pathogens.

Although a meningococcal groups A, C, Y, and W-135 polysaccharide vaccine containing unconjugated meningococcal antigens (MPSV4; Menomune®) was previously available in the US, unconjugated meningococcal vaccines are no longer commercially available the US. There currently are 2 different conjugated meningococcal groups A, C, Y, and W-135 (MenACWY) vaccines available in the US: meningococcal (groups A, C, Y and W-135) polysaccharide diphtheria toxoid conjugate vaccine (MenACWY-D; Menactra®) and meningococcal (groups A, C, Y and W-135) oligosaccharide diphtheria CRM_{197} conjugate vaccine (MenACWY-CRM; Menveo®). Both vaccines contain capsular polysaccharide antigens extracted from 4 serotypes of *N. meningitidis* (A, C, Y, and W-135); however, the meningococcal antigens contained in MenACWY-D are conjugated to diphtheria toxoid protein and the antigens contained in MenACWY-CRM are conjugated to diphtheria CRM_{197} protein.

■ Neisseria meningitidis and Infection

N. meningitidis is a gram-negative diplococcus that causes both endemic and epidemic disease. Based on chemical differences in the antigenic capsular polysaccharide of the organism, at least 13 different serogroups of *N. meningitidis* have been recognized (serogroups A, B, C, D, X, Y, Z, 29E, W-135, H, I, K, L). Serogroups involved in human disease include serogroups A, B, C, X, Y, Z, W-135, and L, with serogroups A, B, C, Y, and W-135 being responsible for the majority of cases worldwide.

The proportion of cases caused by the *N. meningitidis* serotypes varies geographically and has changed over time. In the past 30 years, serogroups B and C have been responsible for the vast majority of cases of meningococcal disease in the Americas and Europe. Serogroup A and, to a lesser extent, serogroup C have been responsible for most meningococcal cases in Africa and in some areas of Asia.

In the US, serogroups B, C, and Y are the major causes of meningococcal disease; each serogroup is responsible for approximately one-third of cases. The proportion of cases of meningococcal disease caused by each serogroup varies by age. In the US, approximately 60% of cases of meningococcal disease reported in infants and children younger than 5 years of age are caused by serogroup B and approximately 75% of cases in adults and adolescents 11 years of age or older are caused by serogroups C, Y, or W-135.

N. meningitidis frequently colonizes the upper respiratory tract, particularly the nasopharynx, without causing any symptoms. Asymptomatic nasopharyngeal carriage of the organism usually is transient and resolves within several weeks; however, a chronic carrier state can persist for up to 2 years. Up to 10% of adolescents and adults are asymptomatic carriers of *N. meningitidis*, although most of these individuals carry strains that are not pathogenic. The meningococcal carrier state is an immunizing process in most individuals and stimulates immunity against future infections caused by the serogroup involved. However, in some individuals, invasive *N. meningitidis* disease occurs resulting in potentially fatal meningococcemia and/or meningitis. In addition, asymptomatic *N. meningitidis* carriers may transmit the organism to others via respiratory secretions. Antecedent viral infection or concomitant respiratory infections, including those caused by influenza viruses or *Mycoplasma*, appear to enhance the spread of meningococcal infection, and such coincident infection, chronic underlying illness and active and passive smoking may contribute to the development of invasive disease in some patients. Overcrowding (e.g., close living conditions), bar or nightclub patronage, and alcohol use have been suggested as possible risk factors in the spread of meningococcal infection.

As a result of control of *Haemophilus influenzae* type b infections through immunization efforts launched over a decade ago, *N. meningitidis* has become one of the leading causes of bacterial meningitis in children and young adults in the US and remains an important cause of septicemia. Despite improvements in supportive care and the use of anti-infective agents, the overall case fatality rate associated with invasive meningococcal disease in the US is 9–15% and the fatality rate may be as high as 40% in those with meningococcal sepsis (meningococcemia). Serious, long-term sequelae (e.g., neurologic disability, digit or limb loss, hearing loss) occurs in 11–20% of surviving patients.

Susceptibility to invasive meningococcal disease appears to be related to low or absent levels of bactericidal antibodies against the infecting pathogenic serogroup. However, other antibodies (including those involved in opsonization or directed against noncapsular antigens) also may contribute to protection against meningococcal disease. Bactericidal antibodies formed in response to *N. meningitidis* infection or administration of meningococcal polysaccharide vaccine consist of IgG, IgM, and IgA antibodies. The relative importance of each type of antibody in providing initial and long-term bactericidal protection against *N. meningitidis* has not been determined. While the clinical importance is unclear, there is some evidence that IgA produced locally actually may impair the bactericidal activity of IgG and IgM.

■ Response to Meningococcal Vaccines

Unconjugated Meningococcal Vaccines The group-specific capsular polysaccharides contained in the previously available unconjugated meningococcal groups A, C, Y, and W-135 polysaccharide vaccine (MPSV4) were T-cell-independent antigens that stimulated a primary antibody response following subcutaneous administration and could not induce long-lasting immunity or an anamnestic response after subsequent exposure to the same antigens. Anticapsular antibodies formed in response to unconjugated meningococcal polysaccharide vaccines generally appear in serum within 7 days and peak within 14 days. Levels of serum anticapsular antibody necessary to provide protection against *N. meningitidis* serogroups A, C, Y, or W-135 are not known; however, studies evaluating serogroup A and C meningococcal disease indicate that anticapsular antibody levels of 2 mcg/mL or greater may be protective.

The immunologic response to a specific unconjugated meningococcal capsular polysaccharide antigen is the same regardless of whether the antigen is administered as a component of a monovalent, bivalent, or quadrivalent meningococcal vaccine. The antibody response to each antigen is independent of and does not appear to affect the response to the other antigens. The magnitude of response to each specific antigen generally is inversely related to group-specific antibody levels present prior to vaccination. In addition, the extent and duration of the immunologic response to unconjugated meningococcal polysaccharide vaccines vary depending on the age of the recipient; the vaccines are less immunogenic in children younger than 2 years of age than in older children and adults.

In a study in healthy children 2–12 years of age who received a single dose of unconjugated meningococcal polysaccharide vaccine (MPSV4 [Menomune®]; no longer commercially available in the US), the seroconversion rate (twofold or greater increase in titers of IgG anticapsular antibody) against serogroups A, C, and Y was 100%; however, the seroconversion rate against serogroup W-135 was only 21%. A single dose of the quadrivalent unconjugated meningococcal vaccine in children 2–12 years of age resulted in a seroconversion rate (based on bactericidal antibody) of 72, 58, 90, and 82% for serogroups A, C, Y, and W-135, respectively, and a seroconversion rate (based on anticapsular antibody) of 99, 99, 97, and 89% for serogroups A, C, Y, and W-135, respectively.

In studies in healthy adults 18–54 years of age who received a single dose of a quadrivalent unconjugated meningococcal polysaccharide vaccine containing 50 mcg each of capsular polysaccharide antigens from serogroups A, C, Y, and W-135, the seroconversion rate (fourfold or greater increase in bactericidal antibody titer) against each serogroup 4 weeks after vaccination was 92–100, 93–100, 87–100, and 90–100%, respectively. Seroconversion occurred most frequently in adults with low or absent levels of bactericidal antibodies prior to vaccination.

In a limited study in individuals with late complement component-deficiency and in healthy complement-sufficient individuals, the antibody response to a quadrivalent unconjugated meningococcal polysaccharide vaccine was similar in both groups; however, antibody levels declined more rapidly in those who were complement-deficient. In a study that involved administration of a quadrivalent meningococcal polysaccharide vaccine to 57 children and adolescents 2–20 years of age with sickle cell disease and 42 age-matched controls without sickle cell disease, the immune response to the serogroup C component of the vaccine was similar in both groups.

There is evidence that the immunologic response to unconjugated meningococcal polysaccharide vaccines may be reduced in individuals who have undergone splenectomy because of trauma and in individuals with lymphoid or nonlymphoid tumors or idiopathic thrombocytopenic purpura. In one study, seroconversion (defined as a change in titer from undetectable to detectable concentrations, or a 50% or greater increase in convalescent titers) of IgG, IgA, and IgM antibodies to polysaccharide group A occurred in 88, 100, and 63% of patients with trauma; 63, 75, and 0% of patients with lymphoid tumors; 60, 80 and 20% of patients with nonlymphoid tumors; and 100, 100, and 0% of patients with idiopathic thrombocytopenic purpura, respectively. Seroconversion of IgG, IgA, and IgM antibodies to polysaccharide group C occurred in 100, 100, and 75% of patients with trauma; 75, 38, and 13% of patients with lymphoid tumors; 80, 80, and 40% of patients with nonlymphoid tumors; and 100% of patients with idiopathic thrombocytopenic purpura, respectively.

In a study in individuals with Hodgkin's disease who had received treatment (radiation and/or chemotherapy) at least 2 years prior to the study, the antibody response to the group A meningococcal capsular polysaccharide component of a quadrivalent unconjugated meningococcal vaccine was similar to that in healthy controls. At 3–6 weeks after vaccination, there was a 5.4- or 8.4-fold increase in geometric mean concentrations of IgG antibody against serogroup A in individuals with the Hodgkin's disease or healthy controls, respectively. The response to the other antigens contained in the vaccine was not evaluated in this study.

Conjugated Meningococcal Vaccines The capsular polysaccharide antigens contained in MenACWY-D are conjugated to diphtheria toxoid protein and the capsular polysaccharide antigens contained in MenACWY-CRM are conjugated to CRM_{197} protein. Conjugation of meningococcal capsular polysaccharide antigens to protein carriers with T-cell epitopes changes the immune response to the vaccine polysaccharides from T-cell-independent to T-cell-dependent, resulting in an improved primary response to the antigens and a stronger anamnestic response (i.e., immunologic memory) at re-exposure to the antigens.

Infants 2 through 23 Months of Age. The effectiveness of MenACWY-CRM for primary immunization against meningococcal serogroups A, C, Y, and W-135 infection in infants was evaluated in a randomized, controlled, multicenter study. In this study, infants received MenACWY-CRM at 2, 4, 6, and 12 months of age and immunogenicity was assessed using predefined criteria based on serum bactericidal antibodies measured using human complement (hSBA). At 1 month following the third dose (7 months of age), the proportion of infants with hSBA at least 1:8 was 94–98% for serogroups C, W-135, and Y and 76% for serogroup A. At 1 month after the fourth dose, the predefined criteria for immunogenicity were met for all 4 serogroups.

The effectiveness of a 2-dose regimen of MenACWY-CRM for primary immunization against meningococcal serogroups A, C, Y, and W-135 infection in infants 7 months of age and older was evaluated in a randomized, controlled, multicenter study. In this study, infants received MenACWY-CRM at 7–9 and 12 months of age. In the per protocol population who received both vaccine doses, the proportion of infants with hSBA at least 1:8 for serogroups A, C, W-135, and Y was 88, 100, 98, and 96%, respectively.

Adults, Adolescents, and Children, 2 Years of Age or Older. In a limited study in healthy children 2 through 10 years of age, the immunologic response to a single dose of MenACWY-D was similar to that obtained with a single dose of unconjugated MPSV4 (no longer commercially available in the US). In a study in adolescents and young adults 11 through 18 years of age who were randomized to receive a single dose of MenACWY-D or MPSV4 (no longer commercially available in the US), the immune response to both vaccines was similar for all 4 *N. meningitidis* serotypes (i.e., A, C, Y, W-135). At 28 days after vaccination, the seroconversion rate (defined as 4-fold or greater increase in serum bactericidal antibody) to the 4 serotypes was 82–97% in those who received the conjugated vaccine and 80–95% in those who received the unconjugated vaccine. In a similar study in adults 18 through 55 years of age, the seroconversion rate at 28 days after a single dose was 74–89% in those who received the conjugated vaccine and 79–94% in those who received the unconjugated vaccine.

The immune response to a single dose of MenACWY-CRM in individuals 2 through 55 years of age is similar to that reported with a single dose of MenACWY-D. Results of a randomized, multicenter, active-controlled study in adolescents 11 through 18 years of age and adults 19 through 55 years of age indicate that seroresponses to all 4 *N. meningitidis* serotypes at 28 days after a single dose of MenACWY-CRM are noninferior to seroresponses obtained with a single dose of MenACWY-D. In a similar study that compared seroresponses at 28 days after a single dose of MenACWY-CRM or MenACWY-D in children 2 through 10 years of age, the response to MenACWY-CRM was noninferior to that obtained with MenACWY-D for serogroups C, Y, and W-135; however, the noninferiority criterion was not met for serogroup A. In a separate group of children 2 through 5 years of age randomized to receive 2 doses of MenACWY-CRM administered 2 months apart, seroresponse rates 1 month after the second dose were 91% for serogroup A, 98% for serogroup C, 95% for serogroup Y, and 89% for serogroup W-135.

In an open-label trial conducted in the US, 834 individuals who had previously received a dose of MenACWY-D received a booster dose of the vaccine 4–6 years after the prior dose (median age at the time of the booster dose was 17.1 years). Prior to revaccination (booster dose), approximately 65, 44, 39, and 69% of 781 trial participants had hSBA titers of at least 1:8 for meningococcal serogroups A, C, Y, and W-135, respectively. At day 28 after the booster dose, more than 99% of trial participants had hSBA titers of at least 1:8 for each of the meningococcal serogroups. In a subset of 112 trial participants for whom hSBA responses were assessed at day 6 after the booster dose, approximately 87, 91, 95, and 92% achieved at least a fourfold increase in hSBA titer for meningococcal serogroups A, C, Y, and W-135, respectively. Data for all 781 trial participants indicated that by day 28 after the booster dose, 95, 95, 97, and 96% had achieved at least a fourfold increase in hSBA titer for meningococcal serogroups A, C, Y, and W-135, respectively.

In adolescents who had received primary immunization with a single dose of either MenACWY-D or MenACWY-CRM at 11 through 18 years of age, revaccination with MenACWY-CRM given 3 years later resulted in protective antibody titers in 99% or more of these individuals. Data are not available to date regarding revaccination with MenACWY-D following primary immunization with MenACWY-CRM.

Asplenic Individuals. Asplenic individuals may have a lower response rate to conjugated meningococcal vaccines than healthy individuals and there is some evidence that a 2-dose primary series may be more effective in these individuals. In one study in asplenic individuals who received a dose of a meningococcal group C conjugate vaccine (not commercially available in the US), 20% of these individuals did not achieve serum bactericidal titers measured using rabbit complement (rSBA) of at least 1:8. When these nonresponders received a second dose of the meningococcal group C conjugate vaccine 2 months later, only 7% were still considered nonresponders.

HIV-infected Individuals. Studies in adolescents and adults 11 through 24 years of age with human immunodeficiency virus (HIV) infection indicate that a single dose of MenACWY-D is safe and immunogenic in such individuals, but the response rate is lower than the response rate reported in healthy individuals in this age group. A second dose of MenACWY-D administered 6 months after the first dose substantially improved response rates in HIV-infected individuals 11 through 24 years of age with $CD4^+$ T-cell percentages of 15% or greater. Individuals with $CD4^+$ T-cell percentages less than 15% at study entry had lower response rates despite 2 doses of MenACWY-D. In another study in HIV-infected children 2 through 10 years of age with $CD4^+$ T-cell percentages greater than 25%, 2 doses of MenACWY-D administered 6 months apart were safe and immunogenic. Most HIV-infected children who did not respond to the first dose did respond to the second dose.

■ **Duration of Immunity** Duration of immunity following primary immunization with the previously available unconjugated meningococcal vaccines (MPSV4) or the currently available conjugated meningococcal vaccines (MenACWY-D, MenACWY-CRM) is not known.

Unconjugated Meningococcal Vaccines Bactericidal antibodies formed in response to unconjugated group A, C, Y, and W-135 meningococcal capsular polysaccharide antigens decline markedly during the first 2–3 years after vaccination. However, there is considerable interindividual variation, and the decline occurs more rapidly in infants and young children than in adults. In school-aged children and adults, some level of anticapsular antibody is likely to persist for 3–5 years or longer after vaccination with unconjugated meningococcal vaccine. Results of a retrospective study of US military recruits who received a quadrivalent unconjugated meningococcal vaccine indicate that anticapsular antibody and bactericidal titers against serogroups A and C can remain above prevaccination levels for up to 10 years after vaccination. In a study in healthy children who received a dose of MPSV4 (no longer commercially available in the US) at 2–8 years of age, bactericidal titers of antibody for group A were detected in 12% and bactericidal titers of antibody for groups C, Y, and W-135 were detected in 25–30% of vaccinees 1 year after vaccination. Studies using a divalent vaccine containing unconjugated groups A and C capsular polysaccharide antigens indicate that protective levels of antibody are present at 3 years after vaccination in 67% of children who received the vaccine at older than 4 years of age; however, these levels are still present in less than 10% of those who received the vaccine at younger than 4 years of age.

Booster responses to second doses of unconjugated meningococcal polysaccharide vaccines generally are poor and unpredictable. In individuals who previously received a dose of unconjugated meningococcal polysaccharide vaccine containing serogroup A and/or C antigens, administration of a second dose of vaccine containing these antigens generally results in an antibody response that is similar to or slightly less than that obtained with the initial dose.

Conjugated Meningococcal Vaccines There is evidence that adolescents who receive a single dose of MenACWY vaccine containing conjugated meningococcal antigens (MenACWY-D or MenACWY-CRM) at 11 through 12 years of age may have waning immunity 5 years after the dose and may have decreased protection against meningococcal disease by 16 through 21 years of age. Studies using MenACWY-D indicate that a booster dose in adolescents administered at 3–5 years after the primary dose elicits higher antibody responses than those elicited by the primary dose. The duration of protective antibody after a booster dose of conjugated meningococcal vaccine given at 16 through 18 years of age is not known, but is expected to last through at least 21 years of age.

Chemistry and Stability

■ **Chemistry** Meningococcal groups A, C, Y, and W-135 vaccine is commercially available in the US as 2 different conjugated vaccines: meningococcal (groups A, C, Y and W-135) polysaccharide diphtheria toxoid conjugate vaccine (MenACWY-D; Menactra®) and meningococcal (groups A, C, Y and W-135) oligosaccharide diphtheria CRM_{197} conjugate vaccine (MenACWY-CRM; Menveo®). Both vaccines contain A, C, Y, and W-135 capsular polysaccharide antigens extracted from *Neisseria meningitidis*, but these antigens are covalently linked to different T-cell dependent carrier proteins depending on the specific vaccine.

Meningococcal (Groups A, C, Y and W-135) Polysaccharide Diphtheria Toxoid Conjugate Vaccine (MenACWY-D; Menactra®) MenACWY-D is a sterile solution containing purified capsular polysaccharide antigens A, C, Y, and W-135 extracted from *N. meningitidis* and conjugated to diphtheria toxoid protein. Each serotype of *N. meningitidis* is cultured and grown on suitable media and the individual polysaccharides are extracted and purified using centrifugation, alcohol and detergent precipitation, solvent extraction, and diafiltration. The polysaccharides are depolymerized, derivatized, and purified by diafiltration to prepare them for conjugation and the derivatized polysaccharides are then each individually covalently linked to diphtheria toxoid protein and purified by serial diafiltration to form the serogroup-specific glycoconjugates. Potency of MenACWY-D is determined by quantification of each of the polysaccharide antigens conjugated to diphtheria toxoid protein and the unconjugated polysaccharide antigens present.

MenACWY-D commercially available in the US occurs as a clear to slightly turbid liquid. Each 0.5-mL dose of MenACWY-D contains 4 mcg of each polysaccharide for *N. meningitidis* serotypes A, C, Y, and W-135, approximately 48 mcg of diphtheria toxoid carrier protein, and not more than 2.66 mcg of residual formaldehyde. MenACWY-D does not contain thimerosal or any other preservative.

Meningococcal (Groups A, C, Y and W-135) Oligosaccharide Diphtheria CRM_{197} Conjugate Vaccine (MenACWY-CRM; Menveo®) MenACWY-CRM contains purified capsular oligosaccharide antigens A, C, Y, and W-135 extracted from *N. meningitidis* and conjugated to *Corynebacterium diphtheriae* CRM_{197} protein. Each serotype of *N. meningitidis* is cultured and grown on suitable media and treated with formaldehyde. The meningococcal polysaccharide antigens A, Y, and W-135 are purified by several extraction and precipitation steps; the meningococcal polysaccharide antigen C is purified by a combination of chromatography and precipitation. The oligosaccharides are prepared for conjugation from purified polysaccharides by hydrolysis, sizing, and reductive amination. After activation, each oligosaccharide is then individually covalently linked to the diphtheria CRM_{197} protein and purified to form the serogroup-specific glycoconjugates.

MenACWY-CRM commercially available in the US is supplied as 2 components that must be combined prior to administration: a lyophilized component containing meningococcal oligosaccharide antigen A (MenA) and a liquid component containing meningococcal oligosaccharide antigens C, Y, and W-135 (MenCYW-135). When the lyophilized component is reconstituted with the liquid component as directed, each 0.5-mL dose of MenACWY-CRM contains 10 mcg of *N. meningitidis* oligosaccharide serotype A, 5 mcg each of *N. meningitidis* oligosaccharide serotypes C, Y, and W-135, and 32.7–64.1 mcg of diphtheria CRM_{197} protein. Each 0.5-mL dose is estimated to contain not more than 0.3 mcg of residual formaldehyde from the manufacturing process. The reconstituted vaccine occurs as a clear, colorless solution. MenACWY-CRM does not contain thimerosal or any other preservative.

■ **Stability** ***Meningococcal (Groups A, C, Y and W-135) Polysaccharide Diphtheria Toxoid Conjugate Vaccine (MenACWY-D; Menactra®)*** MenACWY-D should be refrigerated at 2–8°C and should not be frozen. If freezing occurs, the vaccine should be discarded. The vaccine should be protected from light.

Meningococcal (Groups A, C, Y and W-135) Oligosaccharide Diphtheria CRM_{197} Conjugate Vaccine (MenACWY-CRM; Menveo®) Prior to reconstitution, both the lyophilized and liquid components of MenACWY-CRM should be refrigerated at 2–8°C and should not be frozen. If the vaccine components or reconstituted vaccine is frozen, they should be discarded. The vaccine components and reconstituted vaccine should be protected from light. MenACWY-CRM components must be maintained at 2–8°C during transport.

MenACWY-CRM should be used immediately after reconstitution, but may be stored at or below 25°C for up to 8 hours.

Preparations

Excipients in commercially available drug preparations may have clinically important effects in some individuals; consult specific product labeling for details.

Meningococcal (Groups A, C, Y and W-135) Polysaccharide Diphtheria Toxoid Conjugate Vaccine (MenACWY-D)

Parenteral		
Injection, for IM use	4 mcg each of meningococcal A, C, Y, W-135 capsular polysaccharides conjugated to approximately 48 mcg of diphtheria toxoid protein carrier per 0.5 mL	Menactra®, Sanofi Pasteur

Meningococcal (Groups A, C, Y and W-135) Oligosaccharide Diphtheria CRM_{197} Conjugate Vaccine (MenACWY-CRM)

Parenteral		
For injection, for IM use	10 mcg of meningococcal A capsular polysaccharide and 5 mcg each of meningococcal C, Y, W-135 capsular oligosaccharides conjugated to 32.7–64.1 mcg of diphtheria CRM_{197} protein carrier per 0.5 mL	Menveo®, GlaxoSmithKline

†Use is not currently included in the labeling approved by the US Food and Drug Administration

Mumps Virus Vaccine Live

MMR

■ Mumps virus vaccine live is a preparation of live, attenuated organisms of the Jeryl Lynn (B level) strain of mumps virus that stimulates active immunity to mumps infection. Mumps virus vaccine live is commercially available as a fixed-combination vaccine containing mumps, measles, and rubella antigens (MMR; M-M-R® II) and as a fixed-combination vaccine containing mumps, measles, rubella, and varicella antigens (MMRV; ProQuad®). For information on MMRV, see Varicella Virus Vaccine Live 80:12.

Uses

Mumps virus vaccine live is used to stimulate active immunity to mumps. Monovalent mumps virus vaccine live (Mumpsvax®) is no longer commercially available in the US. Mumps virus vaccine live is commercially available in the US as a fixed-combination vaccine containing measles, mumps, and rubella antigens (MMR; M-M-R® II) for use in adults, adolescents, and children 12 months of age or older and as a fixed-combination vaccine containing measles, mumps, rubella, and varicella antigens (MMRV; ProQuad®) for use in children 12 months through 12 years of age.

The US Public Health Service Advisory Committee on Immunization Practices (ACIP), the American Academy of Pediatrics (AAP), and the American Academy of Family Physicians (AAFP) recommend *universal* immunization against mumps for all susceptible children, adolescents, and adults, unless mumps virus vaccine live is contraindicated. (See Cautions: Precautions and Contraindications.)

The ACIP, AAP, and AAFP state that the fixed-combination vaccine containing measles, mumps, and rubella vaccine live (MMR) is preferred over monovalent mumps virus vaccine live (no longer commercially available in the US) for both primary immunization and revaccination to assure immunity to all 3 diseases. Alternatively, in children 12 months through 12 years of age when a dose of MMR and a dose of varicella virus vaccine live are indicated for primary immunization, use of the fixed-combination vaccine containing MMR and varicella virus vaccine live (MMRV; ProQuad®) can be considered. For information on MMRV, see Varicella Virus Vaccine Live 80:12.

A killed mumps virus vaccine was available in the US from 1950–1978, and while this vaccine induced antibody to the mumps virus, the resultant mumps immunity was transient. Therefore, individuals who previously received killed mumps virus vaccine may benefit from revaccination with MMR.

Adults born before 1957 are likely to have been infected naturally with mumps and generally can be considered immune, even if they did not have clinically recognizable disease. Other individuals can be considered immune to mumps if there is documentation of adequate immunization against mumps (2 doses of MMR or mumps virus-containing vaccine for school aged-children in grades K-12, college students, health-care personnel, international travelers; at least 1 dose in preschool-aged children, adults not at high risk), physician-diagnosed natural mumps infection, or serologic evidence of mumps immunity. Adults born in 1957 or later who lack adequate documentation of immunity should receive 1 dose of MMR to provide immunity against mumps, unless MMR is contraindicated.

Individuals with an equivocal serologic test should be considered susceptible to mumps unless they have other evidence of mumps immunity or a subsequent serologic test indicates mumps immunity. The demonstration of mumps immunoglobulin G (IgG) by any commonly used serologic assay is acceptable evidence of mumps immunity. It is not necessary to test for susceptibility prior to administration of MMR since there is no evidence that individuals already immune because of previous vaccination or natural disease are at any unusual risk of local or systemic reactions to the vaccine. Any individual who is unsure about their mumps disease history and/or mumps vaccination history should be vaccinated with MMR.

■ **Primary Immunization** ***Infants and Children 12 Months through 12 Years of Age*** For routine primary immunization in children, the ACIP, AAP, and AAFP recommend that the first dose of MMR be given at 12 through 15 months of age. The vaccine should not be administered to children younger than 12 months of age solely for mumps protection, because most infants have maternal antibodies which may prevent a satisfactory immunologic response to the vaccine; however, vaccination with MMR aimed at preventing measles occasionally may be warranted in children as young as 6 months of age in certain situations associated with increased risk of exposure to measles virus (e.g., during measles outbreaks, travel to areas with increased risk of measles). (See Uses in Measles Virus Vaccine Live 80:12.) If a live mumps virus-containing vaccine was administered to a child younger than 12 months of age, the child may benefit from revaccination with MMR after reaching 12 months of age.

To improve control of measles, mumps, and rubella, a second dose of MMR is recommended for routine immunization in children. The second dose preferably should be given at 4 through 6 years of age (just prior to entry into kindergarten or first grade), but may be given earlier during any routine visit provided at least 4 weeks (i.e., at lest 28 days) have elapsed since the first dose and both the first and second doses are administered beginning at or after 12 months of age. Those who have not previously received the second MMR dose should complete the vaccination schedule by 11–12 years of age (just prior to entry into middle or junior high school). (See Primary Immunization: Infants and Children 12 Months through 12 Years of Age, under Uses in Measles Virus Vaccine Live 80:12.) If MMR is administered to infants before their first birthday, they should be considered unimmunized for the purposes of determining the need for further vaccination; they should be revaccinated with a 2-dose regimen of MMR initiated at 12 months of age.

The ACIP, AAP, and AAFP state that primary immunization against mumps, measles, and rubella can be integrated with primary immunization against diphtheria, tetanus, pertussis, *Haemophilus influenzae* type b (Hib), hepatitis A, hepatitis B, influenza, pneumococcal disease, poliomyelitis, and varicella. In general, simultaneous administration (on the same day) of the most widely used vaccines, including diphtheria and tetanus toxoids and acellular pertussis vaccine adsorbed (DTaP), Hib conjugate vaccine, MMR, poliovirus vaccine inactivated (IPV), and varicella virus vaccine live, has resulted in seroconversion rates and adverse effects similar to those observed when the vaccines were administered separately. Therefore, the ACIP, AAP, and AAFP recommend simultaneous administration of all vaccines appropriate for the age and previous vaccination status of the recipient, including DTaP, Hib conjugate vaccine, hepatitis A vaccine, hepatitis B vaccine, influenza vaccine, MMR, pneumococcal vaccine, IPV, and varicella virus vaccine live, especially if an individual is unlikely to return for further vaccination. (See Drug Interactions: Vaccines.)

Internationally Adopted Children and Other Immigrants Individuals seeking an immigrant visa for permanent US residency must provide proof of age-appropriate vaccination according to the US Recommended Childhood and Adolescent Immunization Schedules or the US Recommended Adult Immunization Schedule (see Immunization Schedules, US 80:00). Although this vaccination requirement applies to all immigrant infants and children entering the US, internationally adopted children younger than 11 years of age are exempt from the overseas vaccination requirements; however, adoptive parents are required to sign a waiver indicating their intention to comply with the vaccination requirements within 30 days after the infant or child arrives in the US. The CDC states that more than 90% of newly arrived internationally adopted children need catch-up vaccinations to meet the US Recommended Immunization Schedules.

The fact that immunization schedules of other countries may differ from US schedules (e.g., different recommended vaccines, recommended ages of administration, and/or number and timing of vaccine doses) should be considered. Vaccines administered outside the US can generally be accepted as valid if the administration schedule was similar to that recommended in the US childhood and adolescent immunization schedules. Only written vaccination records should be considered as evidence of previous vaccination since such records are more likely to accurately predict protection if the vaccines administered, intervals between doses, and child's age at the time of vaccination are similar to US recommendations; however, the extent to which an internationally adopted child's immunization record reflects their protection against disease is unclear and it is possible there may be transcription errors in such records (e.g., single-antigen vaccine may have been administered although a multiple-antigen vaccine was recorded). Although vaccines with inadequate potency have been produced in other countries, most vaccines used worldwide are immunogenic and produced with adequate quality control standards.

When the immune status of an internationally adopted child is uncertain, the ACIP recommends that health-care providers either repeat vaccinations (since this usually is safe and avoids the need to obtain and interpret serologic tests) and/or use selective serologic testing to determine the need for immunizations (helps avoid unnecessary injections). MMR is not used in most countries. Therefore, although serologic testing is available to verify immunization status in children 12 months of age or older, the CDC states that administration of MMR is preferable to serologic testing unless there is documentation that the child has had mumps. The ACIP states that the recommended approach is to revaccinate an internationally adopted child with 1 or 2 doses of MMR (depending on the child's age) without regard to the child's prior vaccination record since serious adverse effects after MMR vaccination are rare and there is no evidence that administration of MMR increases the risk for adverse reactions among individuals already immune to measles, mumps, or rubella.

Adolescents and Adults During the late 1980s, there was in increase in the reported prevalence of mumps in unvaccinated middle and high school students and mumps outbreaks were reported at universities and colleges and other places where young adults congregate. In addition, data from the late 1980s and early 1990s indicate that mumps outbreaks were occurring in schools with extremely high (more than 95%) vaccination coverage, suggesting that a single dose of mumps virus vaccine live or MMR was not sufficient to prevent mumps outbreaks in school settings. Therefore, the ACIP now states that adequate immunization of adults at high risk (e.g., health-care personnel, international travelers, students at college or other post-high school educational institutions) is defined as 2 doses of a mumps virus-containing vaccine. Mumps infection during adulthood is likely to produce more severe disease, including orchitis. Although fatalities related to mumps are rare, death resulting from mumps and its complications occurs most often in adults.

Adolescents 11–12 Years of Age. The ACIP, AAP, and AAFP recommend that any adolescent who has not previously received a second dose of MMR receive the dose during a routine preadolescent preventive health-care visit at 11–12 years of age. This routine health-care visit provides an opportunity to administer "catch-up" vaccines that were missed at an earlier age, administer vaccines routinely recommended at 11–12 years of age, administer vaccines recommended for certain high-risk adolescents, schedule future appointments that may be necessary to complete recommended immunization schedules, and provide adolescents with other recommended preventive health services such as guidance on health behaviors and screening for biomedical, behavioral, and emotional conditions. During the health-care visit at 11–12 years of age, the vaccination history of the adolescent should be assessed. If the adolescent does not have information regarding their vaccination history, the health-care provider should attempt to obtain such information through documentation from the parent, previous providers, or school records. When documentation of an adolescent's vaccination status is not available at the time of the preventive health-care visit, an assumption can be made that the adolescent has received those vaccines required by state laws and regulations that have been in effect for some time (e.g., those required on entry to kindergarten) and these vaccines can be withheld while awaiting documentation. However, vaccine doses recommended for adolescents that were not included in previous laws and recommendations should be administered.

Ideally, all vaccines routinely indicated at 11–12 years of age should be administered during the initial adolescent visit (MMR, hepatitis B vaccine, tetanus toxoid and reduced diphtheria toxoid and acellular pertussis vaccine adsorbed (Tdap), varicella virus vaccine live). However, since multiple doses of some vaccines are required to complete primary immunization and because simultaneous administration of a large number of vaccines may be indicated in some adolescents, providers may need to be flexible in determining which vaccines to administer during the initial visit and which to schedule for return visits. While specific studies evaluating the safety and efficacy of simultaneous administration of vaccines in adolescents are not available, there is extensive evidence from clinical studies and experience in infants and children that simultaneous administration of the most widely used vaccines does not decrease the antibody response or increase adverse reactions to these vaccines. In circumstances where multiple vaccines (i.e., 4 or more) are indicated in adolescents 11–12 years of age, the provider may choose to defer some vaccines for administration during one or more future visits; however, the vaccines should be prioritized based on which require multiple doses, which diseases pose an immediate threat to the adolescent, and whether the adolescent is likely to return for scheduled visits. During any subsequent visits, the adolescent's vaccination status should be rechecked and any deficiencies corrected.

HIV-infected Individuals MMR can be used in adults, adolescents, or children with human immunodeficiency virus (HIV) infection who do not have evidence of *severe* immunosuppression.

The ACIP, AAP, US Centers for Disease Control and Prevention (CDC), National Institutes of Health (NIH), Infectious Diseases Society of America (IDSA), Pediatric Infectious Diseases Society, and others state that all *asymptomatic* HIV-infected children, adolescents, and adults should receive MMR according to the usually recommended immunization schedules. In addition, MMR should be considered for all symptomatic HIV-infected individuals who do *not* have evidence of severe immunosuppression and who otherwise would be eligible for vaccination. Because the immunologic response to vaccines may decrease as HIV disease progresses, vaccination early in the course of HIV infection may be more likely to induce an immune response; in addition, approximately 5% of HIV-infected infants born in the US will be severely immunocompromised at 12 months of age. Therefore, the ACIP and other experts recommend that HIV-infected infants who are not severely immunocompromised receive MMR as soon as possible upon reaching their first birthday (i.e., at 12 months of age) and consideration should be given to administering the second dose of MMR as soon as 1 month (i.e., at least 28 days) after the first dose.

MMR is contraindicated in HIV-infected individuals with *severe immunosuppression* (i.e., children younger than 12 months of age with $CD4^+$ T-cell count less than 750/mm^3; children 1 through 5 years of age with $CD4^+$ T-cell count less than 500/mm^3; children 6 years of age or older, adolescents, and adults with $CD4^+$ T-cell count less than 200/mm^3; children younger than 13 years of age with $CD4^+$ T-cell percentage less than 15%). (See Individuals with Altered Immunocompetence under Cautions: Precautions and Contraindications.)

The serologic response to vaccines (including MMR) may be reduced in some HIV-infected patients and may be inversely correlated with the severity of the disease. In addition, MMR may be ineffective in HIV-infected individuals who have received high-dose IV immune globulin therapy (e.g., for the prevention of serious bacterial infections) within the 3 months preceding administration of the vaccine. (See Drug Interactions: Immune Globulins.)

MMR may be given to any family member residing in the household or any close contact of an HIV-infected patient since extensive experience has shown that live, attenuated MMR vaccine viruses are not transmitted from vaccinated individuals to others.

Health-care Personnel Because transmission of mumps has occurred in medical settings, the ACIP recommends that all individuals who work in health-care facilities have adequate documentation of mumps vaccination or immunity (i.e., documentation of vaccination with 2 doses of mumps virus-containing vaccine with the first dose given on or after 12 months of age and the second dose given at least 28 days after the first dose, laboratory evidence of immunity, or laboratory confirmation of disease). Those who have received only 1 dose of a mumps virus-containing vaccine should receive a dose of MMR (provided it has been at least 4 weeks [i.e., at least 28 days] since the first dose).

Although birth before 1957 generally is considered acceptable evidence of mumps immunity, health-care facilities should consider recommending 2 doses of MMR to unvaccinated workers born before 1957 who do not have laboratory evidence of mumps immunity or laboratory confirmation of disease.

Sporadic nosocomial cases of mumps have occurred in long-term care facilities housing adolescents and young adults. Mumps virus is less transmissible than measles or other respiratory viruses, and low levels of mumps transmission in the community result in a low risk of introduction of the disease into health-care facilities. Nonetheless, an effective routine MMR vaccination program for health-care workers is the best approach for preventing nosocomial transmission since mumps virus is shed by infected individuals before clinical symptoms become evident and many infected individuals remain asymptomatic.

Travelers Although vaccination against mumps is not a requirement for entry into any country, susceptible individuals, particularly children approaching puberty, adolescents, and adults, traveling or living abroad should be immunized against the disease, unless the vaccine is contraindicated. The risk for exposure to mumps outside the US is high. Mumps virus is endemic in many countries throughout the world; mumps vaccine is used in only 57% of World Health Organization (WHO) member countries.

The ACIP and CDC state that adequate vaccination against mumps for international travelers is defined as 2 doses of a vaccine containing mumps virus vaccine live. Because the risk of serious disease from natural mumps infection is small in infants, administration of MMR to travelers younger than 12 months of age is unnecessary unless protection against measles is indicated.

■ **Postexposure Vaccination** In individuals who have been exposed to natural mumps virus, there is no evidence that administration of a mumps virus-containing vaccine would prevent infection; however, if exposure did *not* result in infection, postexposure vaccination may be given to provide protection against subsequent infection. There is no increased risk associated with administration of a mumps virus-containing vaccine during the incubation period of the disease. Because about 90% of adults who have no knowledge of past infection are immune by serologic testing, postexposure vaccination is not routinely indicated for individuals born prior to 1957 unless they are known to be seronegative; however, vaccination of such individuals also is not precluded and can be undertaken in outbreak settings.

During a mumps outbreak, the ACIP recommends that consideration be given to administering a second dose of MMR to children 1–4 years of age and to adults at low risk (provided it has been at least 28 days since they received the first dose). In addition, in an outbreak setting, the ACIP states that health-care facilities should strongly consider recommending 2 doses of MMR to unvaccinated personnel born before 1957 unless they have laboratory evidence of immunity or laboratory confirmation of disease.

Dosage and Administration

■ **Reconstitution and Administration** The fixed-combination vaccine containing measles, mumps, and rubella antigens (MMR; M-M-R® II) is administered by subcutaneous injection. The vaccine should *not* be administered IV.

For information on reconstitution and administration of the fixed-combination vaccine containing MMR and varicella virus vaccine live (MMRV; ProQuad®), see Varicella Virus Vaccine Live 80:12.

MMR is reconstituted by adding the entire amount of diluent supplied by the manufacturer to the vial of lyophilized vaccine and agitating the vial. Only the diluent provided by the manufacturer should be used. The preparation should be discarded if the lyophilized vaccine does not dissolve completely.

Reconstituted MMR should be inspected visually for particulate matter and discoloration prior to administration. The vaccine should be reconstituted and administered using sterile syringes and needles that are free of preservatives, antiseptics, and detergents, since these substances may inactivate live virus vaccines.

To minimize loss of potency and ensure an adequate immunizing dose, MMR should be administered immediately following reconstitution. (See Chemistry and Stability: Stability.)

The preferred site for subcutaneous injection of MMR is the upper-outer triceps area; injections also can be given into the anterolateral thigh. For children 1 year of age and older, adolescents, and adults, the upper-outer triceps area usually is preferred. To ensure appropriate delivery, subcutaneous injections should be made at a 45° angle using a 5/8-inch, 23- to 25-gauge needle.

Since syncope may occur following vaccination, vaccinees should be observed for approximately 15 minutes after the vaccine dose is administered. If syncope occurs, the patient should be observed until symptoms resolve. Syncope after vaccination occurs most frequently in adolescents and young adults.

When multiple vaccines are administered during a single health-care visit, each vaccine should be given with a different syringe and at different injection sites. Separate injection sites by at least 1 inch (if anatomically feasible) to allow appropriate attribution of any local adverse effects that may occur.

■ **Dosage** The usual dose of MMR is 0.5 mL and is the same for all individuals. When reconstituted as specified, each 0.5-mL dose of MMR contains not less than 1000 $TCID_{50}$ of measles virus, 12,500 $TCID_{50}$ of mumps virus, and 1000 $TCID_{50}$ of rubella virus. The entire volume of reconstituted solution in the single-dose vial should be administered.

For information regarding dosage of the fixed-combination vaccine containing MMR and varicella virus vaccine live (MMRV; ProQuad®), see Varicella Virus Vaccine Live 80:12.

Infants and Children 12 Months through 12 Years of Age For primary immunization against mumps in infants and children, a 2-dose regimen of MMR is recommended and the first dose generally is administered at 12 through 15 months of age. For routine childhood immunization, the ACIP, AAP, and AAFP recommend that the first dose of MMR be given at 12 through 15 months of age and the second dose be routinely given at 4 through 6 years of age (just prior to entry into kindergarten or first grade). The second dose may be given earlier during any routine visit, provided at least 4 weeks (i.e., at least 28 days) have elapsed since the first dose and both the first and second doses are administered beginning at or after 12 months of age.

Children who received a dose of monovalent mumps virus vaccine live (no longer commercially available in the US) or MMR before 12 months of age should be considered susceptible to mumps and should be revaccinated with a 2-dose MMR regimen beginning as soon as possible after they reach their first birthday.

During a mumps outbreak, a dose of MMR should be considered for children 1–4 years of age who have only received 1 dose of a mumps virus-containing vaccine.

Adolescents 13 through 18 Years of Age For primary immunization against mumps in previously unvaccinated adolescents 13 through 18 years of age, a 2-dose regimen of MMR is recommended. The second dose should be administered at least 4 weeks (i.e., at least 28 days) after the initial dose.

Adults For adults 19 years of age and older, primary immunization consists of 1 or 2 doses of MMR. The minimum interval between doses is 4 weeks (i.e., at least 28 days).

During a mumps outbreak, a dose of MMR should be considered for adults who have only received 1 dose of a mumps virus-containing vaccine.

Cautions

■ **Systemic Effects** ***Subclinical Vaccine Virus Infection*** The most common systemic effects associated with administration of monovalent mumps virus vaccine live (no longer commercially available in the US) have been low-grade fever and episodes of parotitis. However, in field trials with the vaccine prior to licensure, these and other effects did not occur more frequently in vaccinees compared with unvaccinated controls. Mild fever occurs occasionally; fever exceeding 39.4°C is uncommon.

Subclinical infection induced by monovalent mumps virus vaccine live has not been shown to be contagious. Rarely, parotitis or orchitis has been reported in vaccinees; however, a causal relationship to the vaccine has not been definitely established and, in most instances, these effects were probably caused by natural mumps infection. Mild lymphadenopathy, cough, and rhinitis also have been reported.

Encephalitis and Aseptic Meningitis Although a causal relationship was not definitely established, meningoencephalitis caused by mumps virus has been reported in a few children about 2.5 weeks after they received the fixed-combination vaccine containing measles, mumps, and rubella virus vaccines live (MMR; M-M-R® II). The reported occurrence of encephalitis within 30 days of mumps vaccination (0.4 per million doses) does not exceed the observed background incidence of CNS dysfunction in the normal population.

Aseptic meningitis has been associated epidemiologically with receipt of mumps virus vaccine live containing the *Urabe strain* of the virus but not with formulations currently available in the US, which contains the *Jeryl Lynn strain*. During 1988–1992, 15 sentinel surveillance laboratories in the United Kingdom (UK) identified 13 cases of aseptic meningitis that had occurred within 15–35 days after vaccination with the Urabe strain of the virus (91 cases per million doses distributed). However, no additional cases of mumps vaccine-associated meningitis have been reported in the UK since 1992, when only mumps virus vaccine live formulated with the Jeryl Lynn strain has been used.

Other Nervous System Effects CNS reactions, including febrile seizures, unilateral nerve deafness, and visual disturbances, have been reported very rarely within 30 days after administration of mumps virus vaccine live; however, no deaths have been reported among patients with such reactions, and almost all have fully recovered. A causal relationship between CNS reactions and the vaccine has not been definitely established, and CNS reactions do not appear to occur any more frequently in individuals receiving a mumps-containing vaccine than in the normal background population used in calculating incidence risk. In addition, there is no evidence that febrile seizures associated with mumps vaccination result in any residual seizure disorder.

Although sensorineural deafness has been reported rarely following mumps vaccination, data are inadequate to distinguish between vaccine and nonvaccine causation. Forms of optic neuritis, including retrobulbar neuritis, papillitis, and retinitis, occur rarely following viral infections, and have been reported following administration of some live virus vaccines.

There have been isolated cases of Guillain-Barré following administration of vaccines containing mumps virus live; however, the National Academy of Sciences Institute of Medicine concluded that evidence is insufficient to accept or reject a causal relationship.

Sensitivity Reactions Allergic reactions such as rash, urticaria, and pruritus have occurred rarely in vaccinees, but usually are mild and of brief duration. More serious hypersensitivity reactions, including anaphylaxis and anaphylactoid reactions as well as related phenomena such as angioneurotic edema (including peripheral or facial edema) and bronchial spasm, have been reported rarely following administration of mumps virus vaccine live or MMR in individuals with or without an allergic history. Most hypersensitivity reactions have been minor, consisting of a wheal and flare or urticaria at the injection site. Immediate, anaphylactic reactions to mumps virus vaccine live or MMR are extremely rare. Although more than 70 million doses of mumps virus-containing vaccines (MMR) have been distributed in the US since the Vaccine Adverse Events Reporting System (VAERS) was implemented in 1990, only 33 cases of anaphylactic reactions have been reported after MMR vaccination. In addition, only 11 of these cases occurred immediately after vaccination with manifestations consistent with anaphylaxis.

MMR contains hydrolyzed gelatin as a stabilizer, which rarely may stimulate hypersensitivity reactions is some individuals. An anaphylactic reaction following MMR vaccination has been reported in the US in at least one individual with IgE-mediated anaphylactic sensitivity to gelatin, and similar cases have been reported elsewhere. (See Gelatin Allergy under Cautions: Sensitivity Reactions, in Precautions and Contraindications.) Erythema multiforme and Stevens-Johnson syndrome have been reported rarely with mumps virus vaccine live.

Hematologic Effects Surveillance of adverse effects in the US and elsewhere indicates that mumps virus-containing vaccines (e.g., MMR) rarely can cause clinically evident thrombocytopenia (e.g., purpura) within 2 months after vaccination. (See Cautions: Hematologic Effects, in Measles Virus Vaccine Live 80:12.)

Endocrine Effects Natural mumps virus infection can precipitate the onset of diabetes mellitus. However, an association between vaccination with mumps virus vaccine live or MMR and pancreatic toxicity or subsequent development of diabetes mellitus has not been established.

Other Adverse Systemic Effects Syncope, vasculitis, and pancreatitis have been reported in patients receiving mumps virus vaccine live. Diarrhea also has been reported.

■ **Local Effects** Local reactions, including soreness, burning, and stinging, may occur at the site of injection following administration of mumps virus vaccine live. These local reactions are usually of short duration and may occur because of the slightly acidic pH of the vaccine. Purpura and allergic reactions (e.g., wheal and flare) at the injection site have been reported very rarely.

■ **Precautions and Contraindications** MMR is contraindicated in individuals who are hypersensitive to the vaccine or any component in the formulation, including gelatin. (See Gelatin Allergy under Cautions: Sensitivity Reactions, in Precautions and Contraindications.) In addition, MMR is contraindicated in those with a history of anaphylactic or anaphylactoid reaction to neomycin. (See Neomycin Allergy under Cautions: Sensitivity Reactions, in Precautions and Contraindications.)

MMR is contraindicated in certain other individuals. (See Individuals with Altered Immunocompetence under Cautions: Precautions and Contraindications and Cautions: Pregnancy, Fertility, and Lactation.)

Sensitivity Reactions Prior to administration, the recipient and/or parent or guardian should be questioned concerning reactions to previous doses of mumps virus-containing vaccine or MMR.

Epinephrine should be available for immediate treatment of an anaphylactic reaction if such a reaction occurs.

Allergy to Egg-related Antigens. MMR is produced in chick embryo cell culture; individuals with a history of anaphylactic, anaphylactoid, or other immediate reaction (e.g., urticaria, swelling of the mouth and throat, difficulty in breathing, hypotension, shock) following ingestion of eggs may be at increased risk of immediate-type hypersensitivity reactions after receiving vaccines containing traces of chick embryo antigen. The manufacturer states that the benefits and risks should be carefully evaluated before considering vaccination in individuals with a history of immediate-type hypersensitivity following ingestion of eggs and such individuals should be vaccinated with extreme caution and with adequate treatment on hand should a reaction occur.

The US Public Health Service Advisory Committee on Immunization Practices (ACIP) and others *previously* recommended that, since mumps virus vaccine live is produced in chick embryo fibroblasts, vaccination with mumps virus vaccine live in individuals with a history of anaphylactoid reactions to egg ingestion be deferred until after appropriate skin testing and desensitization procedures had been performed and that the vaccine be administered *only* with extreme caution (in a setting where an immediate allergic reaction can be detected and treated). However, the predictive value and necessity of such testing have been questioned by most experts since mumps virus vaccine live has been administered safely to some children with histories of immediate reactions to eggs and most anaphylactic reactions to the vaccine are not associated with egg allergy but with other vaccine components. Therefore, ACIP states that skin testing and use of special protocols are not required when administering a mumps virus-containing vaccine in individuals with a history of anaphylactic-like reactions after egg ingestion. In addition, skin testing unnecessarily delays administration of the vaccine. A reasonable precaution for individuals with a history of immediate reactions to eggs is to administer MMR in a supervised setting where appropriate emergency treatment material is available.

Evidence indicates that individuals are *not* at increased risk of hypersensitivity reactions to MMR if they have egg allergies that are *not* anaphylactic or anaphylactoid in nature and administration of the vaccine to these individuals should follow the usually recommendations. (See Uses.) There is no evidence that individuals with allergies to chickens or feathers are at increased risk of allergic reactions to the vaccine.

Neomycin Allergy. Because MMR contains trace amounts of neomycin, the vaccine is contraindicated in individuals who have had an anaphylactic reaction to topically or systemically administered neomycin.

Neomycin allergy usually is characterized by a delayed-type (cell-mediated) hypersensitivity reaction, such as contact dermatitis, rather than an anaphylactic reaction. Following administration of mumps virus vaccine live to individuals who have had a delayed-type hypersensitivity reaction to neomycin, the typical adverse reaction, if any, is a contact dermatitis (e.g., characterized by an erythematous, pruritic nodule or papule) occurring within 48–96 hours.

The ACIP and the American Academy of Pediatrics (AAP) state that vaccines containing trace amounts of neomycin should *not* be used in individuals with a history of anaphylactic reaction to neomycin, but use of such vaccines may be considered in those with a history of delayed-type hypersensitivity reaction to neomycin if benefits of vaccination outweigh risks.

Gelatin Allergy. The possibility of allergic reactions to hydrolyzed gelatin, which is present in MMR as a stabilizer, should be considered since anaphylactic reactions to the vaccine have been reported rarely in individuals with anaphylactic sensitivity to gelatin. MMR should not be administered to individuals with a history of anaphylactic reactions to gelatin or gelatin-containing products. Although skin testing for gelatin sensitivity before administering the vaccine to such individuals can be considered, there are no specific protocols for this purpose. Because gelatin used in vaccines manufactured in the US usually is derived from porcine sources and because food gelatin may be derived solely from bovine sources, a negative food history does not exclude the possibility of a reaction to the gelatin contained in the vaccine.

Individuals with Altered Immunocompetence MMR generally is contraindicated in individuals with primary immunodeficiencies (e.g., cellular immune deficiency, hypogammaglobulinemia, dysgammaglobulinemia) and in individuals with suppressed immune responses resulting from acquired immunodeficiency syndrome (AIDS) or other clinical manifestations of human immunodeficiency virus (HIV) infection, blood dyscrasias, leukemia, lymphomas of any type, or any other malignant neoplasms affecting the bone marrow or lymphatic systems.

Because replication of mumps vaccine virus may be potentiated in individuals with primary immunodeficiencies (e.g., cellular immune deficiency, hypogammaglobulinemia, dysgammaglobulinemia) or with suppressed immune response resulting from leukemia, lymphoma, other malignancies affecting the bone marrow or lymphatic system, or blood dyscrasias, concern exists about the potential risk of administering any live virus vaccine to such individuals. Severe immunosuppression may be caused by many disease conditions (e.g., congenital immunodeficiency, HIV infection, hematologic or generalized malignancy) and by immunosuppressive therapy. For some conditions, all infected individuals are severely immunocompromised, whereas for other conditions, the degree of immune compromise depends on the severity of the condition, which in turn depends on the disease and treatment stage. Although there is no evidence that mumps virus-containing vaccine causes serious illness in immunocompromised individuals, concern exists about the potential risk of administering any live vaccine to such individuals. Therefore, with the exception of individuals with HIV infection, immunocompromised individuals should not receive a mumps virus-containing vaccine, especially those who are severely immunosuppressed. Ultimately, the patient's clinician must assume responsibility for determining whether the patient is severely immunocompromised based on clinical and laboratory assessment. MMR should not be given to an individual with a family history of congenital or hereditary immunodeficiency until the immunocompetence of the individual has been documented. Because mumps vaccinees do not transmit mumps vaccine virus, the risk of mumps exposure in such immunocompromised individuals may be reduced by vaccinating their close susceptible contacts against mumps. The greatest risk associated with administering a live mumps virus-containing vaccine in immunosuppressed patients appears to be with vaccines that also include live measles virus as a component. (See Cautions: Precautions and Contraindications in Measles Virus Vaccine Live 80:12.)

MMR generally is contraindicated in individuals receiving immunosuppressive therapy (e.g., corticotropin, corticosteroids [at immunosuppressive dosages], alkylating agents, antimetabolites, radiation therapy), although the manufacturer states that the vaccine is not contraindicated in individuals receiving corticosteroids as replacement therapy (e.g., for Addison's disease). (See Drug Interactions: Immunosuppressive Agents.)

The ACIP states that use of live virus vaccines can be considered in patients with leukemia, lymphoma, or other malignancies if the disease is in remission and chemotherapy was terminated at least 3 months prior to vaccination.

Antibody responses to MMR and efficacy may be decreased in immunocompromised individuals.

HIV-infected Individuals. The ACIP, AAP, US Centers for Disease Control and Prevention (CDC), National Institutes of Health (NIH), Infectious Diseases Society of America (IDSA), Pediatric Infectious Diseases Society, and others state that MMR should be administered to all *asymptomatic* HIV-infected individuals according to the usually recommended immunization schedules and should be considered for all symptomatic HIV-infected individuals who do *not* have evidence of severe immunosuppression and who otherwise would be eligible for such vaccination. The presence of immunocompromised or HIV-infected individuals in a household does not preclude administration of MMR to other household members.

MMR is contraindicated in HIV-infected individuals with *severe immunosuppression*. (See HIV-Infected Individuals under Uses: Primary Immunization.)

Fever Following vaccination, patients should be monitored for temperature elevations.

Risk of Transmissible Agents in Preparations Containing Albumin MMR contains *recombinant* human albumin.

Monovalent mumps virus vaccine live (no longer commercially available in the US) and the fixed-combination vaccine containing measles, mumps, rubella, and varicella antigens (MMRV; ProQuad®) contain albumin human. Since albumin human is prepared from pooled human plasma, it is a potential vehicle for transmission of human viruses, and theoretically may carry a risk of transmitting the causative agent of Creutzfeldt-Jakob disease (CJD).

For further information on precautions related to transmissible agents in plasma-derived preparations, see Risk of Transmissible Agents in Plasma-derived Preparations under Cautions: Precautions and Contraindications, in Albumin Human 16:00.

Concomitant Illness The decision whether to administer or delay administration of MMR in an individual with a current or recent acute illness depends largely on the severity of symptoms and etiology of the illness. The manufacturer states that MMR is contraindicated in patients with any febrile respiratory illness or other active febrile infections. The ACIP and AAP state that minor acute illness, such as diarrhea or mild upper respiratory infection (with or without fever), does not preclude vaccination. However, vaccination of individuals with moderate or severe acute illness (with or without fever) generally should be deferred until they have recovered from the acute phase of the illness. This precaution avoids superimposing adverse effects of the vaccine on the underlying illness or mistakenly concluding that a manifestation of the underlying illness resulted from vaccination. However, data generally are not available on the safety and immunogenicity of measles, mumps, and rubella virus-containing vaccines in individuals with moderate or severe febrile illness.

Thrombocytopenia Individuals with a history of thrombocytopenic purpura or thrombocytopenia may be at increased risk of developing clinically apparent thrombocytopenia after vaccination. Thrombocytopenia has worsened in those with preexisting thrombocytopenia and may worsen with subsequent doses. Serologic evidence of immunity may be obtained in lieu of vaccination. The decision to vaccinate such individuals should depend on the benefits of immunity and the risks of recurrence or exacerbation of thrombocytopenia after vaccination or during natural infection with viruses.

Risk of Neurodevelopmental Disorders Although it has been theorized that there is a link between the antigens contained in MMR and neurodevelopmental disorders in children (autism), evidence has been insufficient to support an association between neurodevelopmental disorders and MMR. In 2004, the Immunization Safety Review Committee of the Institute of Medicine (IOM) examined the hypothesis that MMR is causally associated with autism and concluded that the evidence favors rejection of a causal relationship between MMR and autism.

Tuberculosis Vaccination is not recommended for individuals with untreated, active tuberculosis. Defer vaccination in these individuals until antituberculosis therapy has been initiated. Administration of live, attenuated vaccines is not contraindicated in individuals with a positive tuberculin skin test who do not have active tuberculosis infection. Tuberculin testing is not a prerequisite for administration of mumps virus vaccine live or MMR.

Transmission of Vaccine Virus MMR contains live, attenuated virus; there is a theoretical risk that transmission of vaccine virus could occur between vaccinees and susceptible contacts.

Transmission of live, attenuated mumps from vaccinees to susceptible contacts has not been reported.

Limitations of Vaccine Effectiveness MMR may not protect all individuals from mumps.

Safety and efficacy of MMR have not been established for postexposure prophylaxis following exposure to mumps. (See Uses: Postexposure Vaccination.)

Improper Storage and Handling Improper storage or handling of vaccines may result in loss of vaccine potency and reduced immune response in vaccinees.

MMR that has been mishandled or has not been stored at the recommended temperature should not be administered. (See Chemistry and Stability: Stability.)

Lyophilized and reconstituted vaccine should be protected from light at all times because exposure to light may inactivate the vaccine virus.

Freezing or exposing the diluent supplied by the manufacturer to freezing temperatures should be avoided; the diluent may be refrigerated or stored at room temperature.

Inspect all vaccines upon delivery and monitor during storage to ensure that the appropriate temperature is maintained.

■ Pediatric Precautions Safety and efficacy of MMR in children younger than 6 months of age have not been established, and use of the vaccine in this age group is not recommended.

■ Geriatric Precautions Clinical studies of MMR did not include sufficient numbers of seronegative individuals 65 years of age or older to determine whether these individuals respond differently than younger individuals. Other reported clinical experience has not identified differences in responses between geriatric and younger individuals.

■ Mutagenicity and Carcinogenicity The mutagenic or carcinogenic potential of MMR have not been evaluated.

■ Pregnancy, Fertility, and Lactation ***Pregnancy*** The effect of MMR on fetal development is not known. Mumps virus vaccine live has been shown to distribute into the placenta and fetus, but there is no evidence that vaccines containing mumps virus can cause congenital malformations in humans. Because of the theoretical risk of harm to the fetus, the ACIP and AAP state that it is prudent to avoid administering mumps virus-containing vaccine to pregnant women. Although the manufacturer states that MMR should not be administered to pregnant women and that appropriate steps be taken to prevent conception for 3 months following vaccination, the ACIP and AAP state that women who receive MMR should avoid becoming pregnant for 4 weeks (i.e., 28 days) after vaccination.

Lactation It is not known whether MMR is distributed into milk. The manufacturer states that MMR should be administered with caution to nursing women. The ACIP states that breastfeeding generally is not a contraindication to administration of mumps virus-containing vaccine since live vaccines appear to pose no special problems for the mother or her nursing infant.

Drug Interactions

■ Blood Products Blood products (e.g., whole blood, packed red blood cells, plasma) may interfere with the immune response to certain live virus vaccines, including measles, mumps, and rubella virus vaccine live (MMR; M-M-R® II); therefore, MMR should not be administered simultaneously with or for specified intervals before or after administration of blood products.

Administration of MMR should be deferred for at least 3 months following administration of red blood cells (with adenine-saline added); for at least 6 months following administration of packed red blood cells or whole blood; and for at least 7 months following administration of plasma or platelet products.

After receiving MMR, vaccinees should avoid blood products for 2 weeks; if use of a blood product is considered necessary during this period, a repeat vaccine dose should be given after the recommended interval unless serologic testing is feasible and indicates a response to the vaccine was attained.

■ Immunosuppressive Agents Individuals receiving immunosuppressive agents (e.g., alkylating agents, antimetabolites, corticotropin, corticosteroids [at immunosuppressive dosages], radiation therapy) may have a diminished response to mumps virus-containing vaccine and replication of the virus may be potentiated. Vaccination with MMR should be deferred until the immunosuppressive agent is discontinued; the manufacturer states that individuals receiving corticosteroids as replacement therapy (e.g., those with Addison's disease) generally may receive the vaccine. The exact interval between discontinuance of immunosuppressive therapy and regaining the ability to respond to live virus vaccines is not known, but live viral vaccines generally should not be administered for at least 3 months after discontinuance of immunosuppressive therapy. Individuals with leukemia in remission who have not received chemotherapy for at least 3 months may receive a live virus vaccine. The precise amount and duration of systemically absorbed corticosteroid therapy needed to suppress the immune system of an otherwise healthy individual are not well defined. Although of recent theoretical concern, there is no evidence of increased severe reactions to live vaccines in individuals receiving corticosteroid aerosol therapy, and such therapy is not in itself a reason to delay vaccination. Most experts, including the US Public Health Service Advisory Committee on Immunization Practices (ACIP) and American Academy of Pediatrics (AAP), agree that short-term (less than 2 weeks), low- to moderate-dose systemic corticosteroid therapy; long-term, alternate-day, systemic corticosteroid therapy using low to moderate doses of short-acting drugs; topical corticosteroid therapy (e.g., nasal, cutaneous, ophthalmic); aerosol corticosteroid therapy; or intra-articular, bursal, or tendon injections with corticosteroids should not be immunosuppressive in usual dosages and do not necessarily contraindicate vaccination with live virus vaccines. Although the immunosuppressive effects of corticosteroid therapy vary, many clinicians consider a dose equivalent to 2 mg/kg or 20 mg total of prednisone daily for 2 weeks or longer as sufficiently immunosuppressive to raise concerns about the safety of vaccination with live virus vaccines.

■ Immune Globulins Antibodies contained in immune globulin preparations (e.g., immune globulin IM [IGIM], immune globulin IV [IGIV], hepatitis B immune globulin [HBIG], rabies immune globulin [RIG], tetanus immune globulin [TIG], varicella-zoster immune globulin [VZIG]) may interfere with the immune response to certain live virus vaccines, including mumps virus-containing vaccine. The manufacturer, ACIP, and AAP state that, since passively acquired antibody may interfere with the response to live attenuated virus vaccines, administration of MMR should be given at least 2 weeks before or deferred for at least 3 months after administration of an immune globulin. The effect of immune globulin on the response to MMR has not been fully determined. The ACIP states that if simultaneous administration of an immune globulin preparation and mumps virus-containing vaccine becomes necessary because of imminent exposure to disease, vaccine-induced immunity may be compromised. If simultaneous vaccination is deemed necessary, the live virus vaccine should be administered at a separate site remote from that of the immune globulin and, unless there is serologic evidence of an adequate antibody response to the live virus vaccine, an additional dose of vaccine should be administered 3 months later. If a vaccine containing mumps in combination with measles virus vaccine live (MMR) is used, a longer interval (up to at least 11 months) may be required to ensure an adequate immune response to the vaccine. (See Drug Interactions: Immune Globulins, in Measles Virus Vaccine Live 80:12.) In addition, an immune globulin should not be administered until at least 2 weeks after vaccination if possible. If an immune globulin must be administered within 14 days after administration of a mumps virus-containing vaccine, an additional dose of the vaccine should be given 3 months after the immune globulin unless serologic testing, indicates that an adequate antibody response to the vaccine occurred; an additional dose of the vaccine is generally unnecessary if the interval between vaccination and administration of the immune globulin is longer than 14 days.

■ Live Vaccines ***Measles, Mumps, Rubella, and Varicella Vaccines*** Mumps virus vaccine live may be administered concurrently with rubella virus vaccine live, measles virus vaccine live, and varicella virus vaccine live.

Mumps virus vaccine live is commercially available in a fixed-combination vaccine containing measles virus vaccine live and rubella virus vaccine live (MMR) to facilitate concomitant administration of all 3 antigens. Administration of MMR results in immunologic responses similar to those obtained with concurrent administration of the 3 antigens at separate sites.

MMR may be administered concurrently with monovalent varicella virus vaccine live (Varivax®) at a different site using a separate syringe. Results of studies in healthy children 12–36 months of age indicate that seroconversion rates, antibody responses, and adverse effects reported with simultaneous administration of the vaccines are similar to those reported when the vaccines are administered 6 weeks apart. Because there is a theoretical concern that the immune response to one live viral vaccine may be impaired if administered within 1 month of another, if MMR and varicella virus vaccine live are not administered simultaneously then they should be administered at least 1 month apart. There is some evidence that administration of varicella virus vaccine live less than 30 days after MMR decreases the effectiveness of the varicella vaccine. Results of a retrospective cohort study that used data from the Vaccine Safety Datalink (VSD) project and included children 12 months of age or older who were vaccinated during January 1995 to December 1999 indicate that administration of varicella virus vaccine live less than 30 days after MMR results in a 2.5-fold increase in the incidence of breakthrough varicella infections. However, when the vaccines were administered concurrently, there was no increase in the risk for breakthrough infections.

Mumps virus vaccine live also is commercially available in a fixed-combination vaccine containing MMR and varicella virus vaccine live (MMRV; ProQuad®). This fixed-combination vaccine is safe and effective in healthy children 12 months through 12 years of age. Studies using MMRV (ProQuad®) in healthy children 1–6 years of age indicate that the antibody responses against measles, mumps, rubella, and varicella antigens following a single dose of ProQuad® are similar to those obtained after a single dose of MMR and a single dose of varicella virus vaccine live (Varivax®). However, there is some evidence that the relative risk for febrile seizures in infants may be higher with the fixed-combination vaccine MMRV than that reported when a dose of single-antigen varicella virus vaccine live (Varivax®) and a dose of MMR are given concomitantly. For information on the fixed-combination vaccine containing MMR and varicella virus vaccine live (MMRV; ProQuad®), see Varicella Virus Vaccine Live 80:12.

Influenza Vaccine Live Intranasal Because of theoretical concerns that the immune response to one live virus vaccine might be impaired if given within 30 days of another live virus vaccine, if MMR and influenza virus vaccine live intranasal are not administered on the same day, they should be administered at least 4 weeks apart.

Other Live Vaccines Some oral live vaccines (e.g., rotavirus vaccine live oral, typhoid vaccine live oral) can be administered concomitantly with or at any interval before or after MMR.

Because of theoretical concerns that the immune response to other live virus vaccines might be impaired if given within 30 days of another live virus vaccine, if MMR and yellow fever vaccine are not administered on the same day, they should be administered at least 4 weeks apart.

■ Inactivated Vaccines and Toxoids MMR may be administered concurrently with (using different syringes and different injection sites) or at any interval before or after inactivated vaccines, recombinant vaccines, polysaccharide vaccines, or toxoids.

MMR may be given concurrently with *Haemophilus influenzae* type b (Hib) conjugate vaccines at a different site using a separate syringe.

Although specific studies evaluating simultaneous administration of MMR and hepatitis A vaccine, hepatitis B vaccine, diphtheria and tetanus toxoids and acellular pertussis vaccine adsorbed (DTaP) or tetanus toxoid and reduced diphtheria toxoid and acellular pertussis vaccine adsorbed (Tdap) are not available, these vaccines may be administered concomitantly.

MMR may be given concomitantly with parenteral inactivated influenza vaccines (using different syringes and different injection sites) or at any interval before or after administration of inactivated influenza vaccines.

MMR may be administered concurrently with pneumococcal vaccine, including pneumococcal conjugate vaccine (PCV) or pneumococcal 23-valent polysaccharide vaccine (PPSV23), at a different site using a separate syringe.

Laboratory Test Interferences

■ **Tuberculin** Live attenuated measles, mumps, and rubella virus vaccines have been reported to temporarily suppress tuberculin skin sensitivity; therefore, tuberculin skin tests (if required) should be done before, simultaneously with, or at least 4–6 weeks or longer after administration of measles, mumps, and rubella virus vaccine live (MMR; M-M-R® II).

Pharmacology

Monovalent mumps virus vaccine live (no longer commercially available in the US) and the fixed-combination vaccine containing measles, mumps, and rubella antigens (measles, mumps, and rubella virus vaccine live [MMR; M-M-R® II]) stimulate active immunity to mumps by inducing production of specific antibodies. Studies using monovalent mumps virus vaccine live indicate that a single subcutaneous dose produces a serologic response in about 97% of susceptible children older than 12 months of age and about 93% of susceptible adults; however, a small percentage (1–5%) of vaccinees may fail to seroconvert after the primary dose. Studies in the US have reported that 1 dose of mumps virus vaccine live was 78–91% effective in preventing clinical mumps with parotitis. Although vaccine-induced antibody titers are generally lower than those stimulated by natural mumps infection, observations from 30 years of use of the live vaccine indicate the persistence of antibody and continuing protection against infection. The duration of immunity following administration of mumps virus-containing vaccine is believed to be greater than 25 years, and is probably lifelong in most vaccine recipients. Clinical efficacy of the vaccine reportedly ranges from 75–95%. The killed mumps virus vaccine (available in the US from 1950 through 1978) induced antibody, but the resulting immunity was transient.

Chemistry and Stability

■ **Chemistry** Mumps virus vaccine live is a preparation of live, attenuated organisms of the Jeryl Lynn (B level) strain of mumps virus. Monovalent mumps virus vaccine live (Mumpsvax®) is no longer commercially available in the US. Mumps virus vaccine live is commercially available in the US in a fixed-combination vaccine with measles virus vaccine live and rubella virus vaccine live (MMR; M-M-R® II) and in a fixed-combination vaccine containing MMR and varicella virus vaccine live (MMRV; ProQuad®). For information on the fixed-combination vaccine containing MMR and varicella virus vaccine live, see Varicella Virus Vaccine Live 80:12.

Vaccines containing mumps virus vaccine live meet standards established by the Center for Biologics Evaluation and Research of the US Food and Drug Administration. The mumps virus used in production of these vaccines is propagated and attenuated by serial passage in chick embryo tissue culture. The potency of MMR is expressed in terms of the amount of virus estimated to infect 50% of a number of standardized tissue culture preparations under specified conditions (tissue culture infective dose 50% or $TCID_{50}$). Following reconstitution with the diluent provided by the manufacturer, each 0.5-mL dose of reconstituted MMR contains not less than 1000 $TCID_{50}$ of measles virus, 12,500 $TCID_{50}$ of mumps virus, and 1000 $TCID_{50}$ of rubella virus. Each 0.5-mL dose of MMR also contains sorbitol (14.5 mg), sodium phosphate, sucrose (1.9 mg), sodium chloride, hydrolyzed gelatin (14.5 mg), recombinant albumin human (up to 0.3 mg), fetal bovine serum (less than 1 part per million), and approximately 25 mcg of neomycin. The cells, virus pools, fetal bovine serum, and albumin human used in preparation of MMR are screened for the absence of adventitious agents; the albumin human is processed using the Cohn cold alcohol fractionation procedure.

Lyophilized MMR occurs as light yellow compact crystalline plugs and the reconstituted vaccine occurs as a clear yellow solution. MMR does not contain thimerosal or any other preservative.

■ **Stability** In lyophilized form, MMR should be refrigerated at 2–8°C but may be frozen. The vials containing diluent provided by the manufacturer may be stored in the refrigerator at 2–8°C or at room temperature. During shipping, MMR must be stored at 10°C or less and may be packed in solid carbon dioxide (dry ice). If the vaccine is shipped with dry ice, the diluent must be shipped separately.

Following reconstitution with the diluent provided by the manufacturer, MMR should be refrigerated at 2–8°C and discarded if not used within 8 hours. Both the lyophilized and reconstituted vaccine should be protected from light, which may inactivate the virus.

Preparations

Excipients in commercially available drug preparations may have clinically important effects in some individuals; consult specific product labeling for details.

Measles, Mumps, and Rubella Virus Vaccine Live (MMR)

Parenteral

For injection, for subcutaneous use	Measles Virus Vaccine Live (More Attenuated Enders' Line) 1000 $TCID_{50}$, Mumps Virus Vaccine Live (Jeryl Lynn [B level] Strain) 12,500 $TCID_{50}$, and Rubella Virus Vaccine Live (Wistar RA 27/3 Strain) 1000 $TCID_{50}$ per 0.5 mL	**M-M-R® II,** Merck

Measles, Mumps, Rubella and Varicella Virus Vaccine Live (MMRV)

Parenteral

For injection, for subcutaneous use	Measles Virus Vaccine Live (More Attenuated Enders' Line) ≥3 $\log_{10}$ tissue culture infective dose 50% ($TCID_{50}$), Mumps Virus Vaccine Live (Jeryl Lynn [B level] Strain) ≥4.3 $\log_{10}$ $TCID_{50}$, Rubella Virus Vaccine Live (Wistar RA 27/3 Strain) ≥3 $\log_{10}$ $TCID_{50}$, and Varicella Virus Vaccine Live (Oka/Merck Strain) ≥3.99 $\log_{10}$ plaque-forming units (PFU) per 0.5 mL	**ProQuad®,** Merck

Selected Revisions January 2010,

Pneumococcal Vaccine

PCV, PCV13Pneumococcal 23-valent Polysaccharide Vaccine, Pneumococcal 23-valent Vaccine, PPSV, PPV, PPSV23

■ Pneumococcal vaccine is an inactivated (polysaccharide) vaccine that is commercially available in the US as 2 different vaccine types: pneumococcal 13-valent conjugate vaccine (diphtheria CRM_{197} protein) (PCV13; Prevnar 13®) and pneumococcal vaccine, polyvalent (pneumococcal 23-valent vaccine; PPSV23; Pneumovax® 23). Both vaccines contain capsular antigens extracted from *Streptococcus pneumoniae* and are used to stimulate active immunity to pneumococcal infection. Various other pneumococcal vaccines are being investigated or may be available in other countries.

Uses

Pneumococcal 13-valent conjugate vaccine (diphtheria CRM_{197} protein) (PCV13; Prevnar 13®) and pneumococcal vaccine, polyvalent (pneumococcal 23-valent vaccine; PPSV23; Pneumovax® 23) are used to stimulate active immunity to infection caused by *Streptococcus pneumoniae* serotypes contained in the vaccines. Pneumococcal vaccines are used for prevention of invasive disease caused by *S. pneumoniae*, including pneumonia, meningitis, and bacteremia. PCV13 (Prevnar 13®) also is used for prevention of acute otitis media (AOM) caused by certain serotypes of *S. pneumoniae* contained in the vaccine.

Pneumococcal vaccines will *not* prevent pneumococcal infection caused by *S. pneumoniae* serotypes not represented in the vaccines.

S. pneumoniae is a major cause of serious or invasive illness and death worldwide. In the US, pneumococcal pneumonia results in an estimated 175,000 hospitalizations each year (case fatality rate 5–7%) and there are more than 50,000 cases of pneumococcal bacteremia (case fatality rate about 20%) and 3000–6000 cases of pneumococcal meningitis (case fatality rate about 30%) reported annually. Case fatality rates for pneumococcal disease are higher in the elderly, and have been reported to be 60–80% when pneumococcal bacteremia or meningitis occurs in this age group. In children younger than 5 years of age, *S. pneumoniae* has been a leading cause of bacterial meningitis. However, the epidemiology of pneumococcal disease in the US has changed substantially since routine infant and childhood vaccination against pneumococcal disease was initiated in 2000. Data indicate that the overall incidence of invasive pneumococcal disease in children younger than 5 years of age has decreased from approximately 99 cases per 100,000 population in 1998–1999 to 21 cases per 100,000 population in 2008. There also is evidence that routine infant and childhood vaccination against pneumococcal disease has reduced the incidence of invasive pneumococcal disease among unvaccinated individuals of all ages, including infants too young to be vaccinated and the elderly. Data from 1998–1999 and 2008 indicate that the overall rates of invasive pneumococcal disease in individuals 18–49, 50–64, and 65 years of age or older have decreased 34, 14, and 37%, respectively.

■ **Choice of Pneumococcal Vaccines** There are 2 different types of pneumococcal vaccine commercially available in the US for active immunization against pneumococcal disease: PCV13 (Prevnar 13®) and PPSV23 (Pneumovax® 23). Although both vaccines contain capsular antigens extracted from *S. pneumoniae*, the vaccines contain different numbers and forms of these antigens. PCV13 (Prevnar 13®) contains capsular antigens from 13 different serotypes of *S. pneumoniae* (i.e., serotypes 1, 3, 4, 5, 6A, 6B, 7F, 9V, 14, 18C, 19A, 19F,

23F), which are conjugated to a T-cell dependent carrier protein (diphtheria CRM_{197} protein). PPSV23 (Pneumovax® 23) contains capsular antigens from 23 different serotypes of *S. pneumoniae* (i.e., serotypes 1, 2, 3, 4, 5, 6B, 7F, 8, 9N, 9V, 10A, 11A, 12F, 14, 15B, 17F, 18C, 19F, 19A, 20, 22F, 23F, 33F); these antigens are unconjugated. (See Chemistry and Stability: Chemistry.)

Surveillance data from 2008 indicated that the 13 serotypes contained in PCV13 (Prevnar 13®) accounted for approximately 61% of US cases of invasive pneumococcal disease occurring in children younger than 5 years of age, with serotype 19A accounting for 43% of cases. In immunocompromised children and adolescents 6 through 18 years of age, surveillance data from 2007–2009 indicated that 49% of cases of invasive pneumococcal disease in this population were caused by serotypes contained in PCV13 (Prevnar 13®) and an additional 23% of cases were caused by serotypes contained in PPSV23 (Pneumovax® 23). Surveillance data from 2008 regarding adults 18–49, 50–64, and 65 years of age or older indicated that the 13 serotypes contained in PCV13 (Prevnar 13®) accounted for 53, 49, and 44% of invasive pneumococcal disease reported in these age groups, respectively; the 23 serotypes contained in PPSV23 (Pneumovax® 23) accounted for 78, 76, and 66% of invasive pneumococcal disease reported in these age groups, respectively. Data from 2010 indicated that 50% of cases of invasive pneumococcal disease in immunocompromised adults were caused by serotypes contained in PCV13 (Prevnar 13®) and an additional 21% of cases were caused by serotypes contained in PPSV23 (Pneumovax® 23).

PCV13 (Prevnar 13®) is labeled by the US Food and Drug Administration (FDA) for use in infants and children 6 weeks through 17 years of age and in adults 50 years of age or older. The US Public Health Service Advisory Committee on Immunization Practices (ACIP), American Academy of Pediatrics (AAP), and other experts recommend that *all* infants 2 through 23 months of age and healthy children 2 through 5 years of age receive *routine* primary and catch-up vaccination with PCV13 (Prevnar 13®). These experts also recommend use of PCV13 (Prevnar 13®) in children and adolescents 2 through 18 years of age who are unvaccinated or incompletely vaccinated and have certain underlying medical conditions that put them at increased risk for pneumococcal disease. ACIP and other experts also recommend use of PCV13 (Prevnar 13®) in adults 19 years of age or older who have certain underlying medical conditions that put them at increased risk for pneumococcal disease† and *routine* use of PCV13 (Prevnar 13®) in *all* adults 65 years of age or older. (See Uses: Pneumococcal 13-valent Conjugate Vaccine [PCV13; Prevnar 13®].)

PPSV23 (Pneumovax® 23) is labeled by FDA for use in children 2 years of age or older at increased risk for pneumococcal disease and in adults 50 years of age or older. ACIP, AAP, and other experts recommend vaccination with PPSV23 (Pneumovax® 23) in children and adolescents 2 through 18 years of age who have certain underlying medical conditions that put them at increased risk for pneumococcal disease. ACIP and other experts also recommend use of PPSV23 (Pneumovax® 23) in adults 19 years of age or older who have certain medical conditions or behaviors that put them at increased risk for pneumococcal disease and *routine* use of PPSV23 (Pneumovax® 23) in *all* adults 65 years of age or older. (See Uses: Pneumococcal 23-valent Vaccine [PPSV23; Pneumovax® 23].)

Pneumococcal 7-valent conjugate vaccine (diphtheria CRM_{197} protein) (PCV7; Prevnar®; no longer commercially available in the US) was the first conjugated vaccine to become commercially available in the US for prevention of pneumococcal disease in infants and children. PCV7 (Prevnar®) contained conjugated saccharide antigens representing 7 serotypes (i.e., 4, 6B, 9V, 14, 18C, 19F, 23F) and was available in the US from February 2000 until September 2010. PCV13 (Prevnar 13®) was approved by the FDA in February 2010 and *replaced* PCV7 (Prevnar®) for primary and catch-up vaccination in infants and children. PCV13 (Prevnar 13®) contains all 7 of the conjugated antigens that were in the previously available 7-valent vaccine (PCV7; Prevnar®) and also contains 6 additional conjugated antigens representing 6 more *S. pneumoniae* serotypes associated with invasive pneumococcal disease. Since PCV13 (Prevnar 13®) contains additional antigens not contained in PCV7 (Prevnar®), ACIP, AAP, and other experts state that individuals who previously received age-appropriate vaccination or incomplete vaccination with PCV7 (Prevnar®) should receive PCV13 (Prevnar 13®). (See Uses: Pneumococcal 13-valent Conjugate Vaccine [PCV13; Prevnar 13®].)

Because the conjugated antigens in PCV13 (Prevnar 13®) are more immunogenic in infants and young children than the unconjugated antigens in PPSV23 (Pneumovax® 23), ACIP, AAP, and other experts state that PCV13 (Prevnar 13®) is the preferred pneumococcal vaccine for primary vaccination in infants 2 through 23 months of age and catch-up vaccination in healthy children 2 through 5 years of age. However, because PPSV23 (Pneumovax® 23) contains 11 additional antigens not contained in PCV13 (Prevnar 13®) and use of both vaccines provides benefits in terms of immunity against a broader range of serotypes, ACIP, AAP, and other experts recommend sequential use of PCV13 (Prevnar 13®) *and* PPSV23 (Pneumovax® 23) in children and adolescents 2 through 18 years of age with certain medical conditions that put them at increased risk for pneumococcal disease. Sequential vaccination with PCV13 (Prevnar 13®) *and* PPSV23 (Pneumovax® 23) also is recommended in adults 19 years of age or older with certain medical conditions that put them at increased risk for pneumococcal disease and in *all* adults 65 years of age or older. When both vaccines are indicated, all required doses of PCV13 (Prevnar 13®) should be administered *before* PPSV23 (Pneumovax® 23) vaccination, if possible. PCV13 (Prevnar 13®) and PPSV23 (Pneumovax® 23) should *not* be administered concurrently since safety and efficacy of concurrent administration have not been studied. (See Dosage and Administration.)

■ **Pneumococcal 13-valent Conjugate Vaccine (PCV13; Prevnar 13®)** PCV13 (Prevnar 13®) is used in infants and children 6 weeks and older, adolescents, and adults for prevention of invasive pneumococcal disease caused by the 13 *S. pneumoniae* serotypes contained in the vaccine (i.e., serotypes 1, 3, 4, 5, 6A, 6B, 7F, 9V, 14, 18C, 19A, 19F, 23F). PCV13 (Prevnar 13®) also is used in infants and children 6 weeks through 5 years of age for prevention of AOM caused by certain serotypes of *S. pneumoniae* (i.e., serotypes 4, 6B, 9V, 14, 18C, 19F, 23F). (See Prevention of Acute Otitis Media under Uses: Pneumococcal 13-valent Conjugate Vaccine [PCV13; Prevnar 13®].)

ACIP, AAP, and other experts recommend *routine* primary and catch-up vaccination with PCV13 (Prevnar 13®) in *all* previously unvaccinated or incompletely vaccinated infants 2 through 23 months of age and healthy children 2 through 5 years of age. These experts also recommend use of the vaccine in previously unvaccinated or incompletely vaccinated children 2 through 18 years of age with certain underlying medical conditions that put them at increased risk for pneumococcal disease. In addition, ACIP and other experts recommend vaccination with PCV13 (Prevnar 13®) in adults 19 years of age or older with certain medical conditions that put them at increased risk for pneumococcal disease† and *routine* vaccination with PCV13 (Prevnar 13®) in *all* adults 65 years of age or older.

Although PCV13 (Prevnar 13®) is labeled by FDA for prevention of pneumococcal disease in children 6 through 17 years of age and adults 50 years of age or older, ACIP, AAP, and other experts do *not* recommend *routine* use of PCV13 (Prevnar 13®) in healthy children and adolescents 6 through 17 years of age or *routine* use of the vaccine in healthy adults 18 through 64 years of age who do not have medical conditions that put them at increased risk for pneumococcal disease.

Primary immunization with PCV13 (Prevnar 13®) can be integrated with primary immunization against diphtheria, tetanus, pertussis, *Haemophilus influenzae* type b (Hib), hepatitis A, hepatitis B, human papillomavirus (HPV), influenza, measles, mumps, rubella, meningococcal disease, poliomyelitis, rotavirus, and varicella. (See Drug Interactions: Vaccines.)

Infants 2 through 23 Months of Age Infants 2 through 23 months of age are at increased risk for invasive pneumococcal disease. Therefore, ACIP, AAP, and other experts recommend that *all* infants 2 through 23 months of age (minimum age 6 weeks) receive *routine* primary immunization against pneumococcal disease using PCV13 (Prevnar 13®). For routine childhood immunization initiated in early infancy, ACIP, AAP, and other experts recommend a 4-dose regimen of PCV13 (Prevnar 13®) with doses given at 2, 4, 6, and 12 through 15 months of age. All infants 2 through 23 months of age who are unvaccinated or incompletely vaccinated against pneumococcal disease should receive catch-up vaccination using the age-appropriate number of doses of PCV13 (Prevnar 13®). (See PCV13 [Prevnar 13®] under Dosage: Infants 2 through 23 Months of Age, in Dosage and Administration.)

Infants 14 through 23 months of age who received age-appropriate vaccination with the previously available 7-valent vaccine (PCV7; Prevnar®) should receive a single supplemental dose of PCV13 (Prevnar 13®) since this may provide additional protection.

Healthy Children 2 through 5 Years of Age ACIP, AAP, and other experts recommend that *all* otherwise healthy children 2 through 5 years of age who are unvaccinated or incompletely vaccinated against pneumococcal disease for their age group should receive catch-up vaccination with a single dose of PCV13 (Prevnar 13®). (See PCV13 [Prevnar 13®] under Dosage: Healthy Children 2 through 5 Years of Age, in Dosage and Administration.)

Children 2 through 5 years of age who received age-appropriate vaccination with the previously available 7-valent vaccine (PCV7; Prevnar®) should receive a single supplemental dose of PCV13 (Prevnar 13®) since this may provide additional protection.

Children 2 through 5 Years of Age at Increased Risk for Pneumococcal Disease ACIP, AAP, and other experts recommend PCV13 (Prevnar 13®) in all previously unvaccinated or incompletely vaccinated children 2 through 5 years of age who are at increased risk for pneumococcal disease because of functional or anatomic asplenia (including sickle cell disease or other hemoglobinopathies, congenital or acquired asplenia), immunocompromising medical conditions (congenital or acquired immunodeficiency, human immunodeficiency virus [HIV] infection, chronic renal failure, nephrotic syndrome, malignant neoplasms, leukemia, lymphoma, Hodgkin's disease, solid organ transplantation), or certain other medical conditions (chronic heart disease [especially cyanotic congenital heart disease and cardiac failure], chronic lung disease [including asthma if treated with high-dose oral corticosteroid therapy], diabetes mellitus, CSF leaks, cochlear implants).

Children 2 through 5 years of age with these medical conditions who previously received fewer than 3 doses of PCV13 (Prevnar 13®) or received fewer than 3 doses of the previously available 7-valent vaccine (PCV7; Prevnar®) should receive catch-up vaccination with 2 doses of PCV13 (Prevnar 13®) given at least 8 weeks apart. A single dose of PCV13 (Prevnar 13®) is recommended in children 2 through 5 years of age with these medical conditions if they previously received a total of 3 doses of PCV given as PCV13 (Prevnar 13®) and/or PCV7 (Prevnar®) or received 4 doses or other age-appropriate vaccination series of PCV7 (Prevnar®).

PPSV23 (Pneumovax® 23) also is recommended in children 2 through 5 years of age or older who are at increased risk for pneumococcal disease because of certain medical conditions. (See Children 2 through 5 Years of Age at Increased Risk for Pneumococcal Disease under Uses: Pneumococcal 23-valent Vaccine [PPSV23; Pneumovax® 23].)

Children and Adolescents 6 through 18 Years of Age at Increased Risk for Pneumococcal Disease ACIP, AAP, and other experts recommend PCV13 (Prevnar 13®) in children and adolescents 6 through 18 years who are at increased risk for pneumococcal disease because of functional or anatomic asplenia (including sickle cell disease or other hemoglobinopathies, congenital or acquired asplenia), immunocompromising medical conditions (congenital or acquired immunodeficiency, HIV infection, chronic renal failure, nephrotic syndrome, malignant neoplasms, leukemia, lymphoma, Hodgkin's disease, generalized malignancy, solid organ transplantation, multiple myeloma), or certain other medical conditions (CSF leaks, cochlear implants). AAP states that PCV13 (Prevnar 13®) also can be considered in children and adolescents 6 through 18 years who are at increased risk for pneumococcal disease because of chronic heart disease (especially cyanotic congenital heart disease and cardiac failure), chronic lung disease (including asthma if treated with prolonged high-dose oral corticosteroids), or diabetes mellitus.

Children and adolescents 6 through 18 years of age with these medical conditions who have not previously received PCV13 (Prevnar 13®) should receive a single dose of the vaccine. The dose of PCV13 (Prevnar 13®) is indicated in these children and adolescents even if they were vaccinated with the previously available 7-valent vaccine (PCV7; Prevnar®).

PPSV23 (Pneumovax® 23) also is recommended in children and adolescents 6 through 18 years of age who are at increased risk for pneumococcal disease because of certain medical conditions. (See Children and Adolescents 6 through 18 Years of Age at Increased Risk for Pneumococcal Disease under Uses: Pneumococcal 23-valent Vaccine [PPSV23; Pneumovax® 23].)

Adults 19 Years of Age or Older at Increased Risk for Pneumococcal Disease ACIP and other experts recommend PCV13 (Prevnar 13®) in adults 19 years of age or older who are at increased risk for pneumococcal disease because of functional or anatomic asplenia (including sickle cell disease or other hemoglobinopathies, congenital or acquired asplenia, splenic dysfunction, splenectomy), immunocompromising medical conditions (congenital or acquired immunodeficiency, HIV infection, chronic renal failure, nephrotic syndrome, leukemia, lymphoma, Hodgkin's disease, generalized malignancy, solid organ transplantation, multiple myeloma), iatrogenic immunosuppression (including long-term systemic corticosteroid therapy or radiation therapy), or other medical conditions (CSF leaks, cochlear implants). Adults 19 years of age or older with these medical conditions who have not previously received PCV13 (Prevnar 13®) or have unknown vaccination status should receive a single dose of the vaccine. PCV13 (Prevnar 13®) is not usually recommended in adults 19 years of age or older who are at increased risk for pneumococcal disease because of chronic heart disease (including congestive heart failure and cardiomyopathies [excluding hypertension]), chronic lung disease (chronic obstructive pulmonary disease, emphysema, asthma), diabetes mellitus, alcoholism, chronic liver disease, or cirrhosis or because they smoke cigarettes.

PPSV23 (Pneumovax® 23) also is recommended in adults 19 years of age or older who are at increased risk for pneumococcal disease because of certain medical conditions. (See Adults 19 Years of Age or Older at Increased Risk for Pneumococcal Disease under Uses: Pneumococcal 23-valent Vaccine [PPSV23; Pneumovax® 23].)

Healthy Adults 50 through 64 Years of Age Although PCV13 (Prevnar 13®) is labeled by FDA for prevention of pneumonia and invasive pneumococcal disease in adults as young as 50 years of age, ACIP and other experts do not recommend *routine* vaccination with PCV13 (Prevnar 13®) in healthy adults 50 through 64 years of age who do not have medical conditions that increase the risk for pneumococcal disease.

Adults 65 Years of Age or Older ACIP and other experts recommend *routine* vaccination with a single dose of PCV13 (Prevnar 13®) in *all* adults 65 years of age or older who are unvaccinated or have unknown vaccination status.

PPSV23 (Pneumovax® 23) also is recommended *routinely* in *all* adults 65 years of age or older. (See Adults 65 Years of Age or Older under Uses: Pneumococcal 23-valent Vaccine [PPSV23; Pneumovax® 23].)

HIV-infected Individuals Because HIV-infected individuals are at high risk for invasive or recurrent pneumococcal infection compared with those who are not infected with HIV, the ACIP, AAP, US Centers for Disease Control and Prevention (CDC), National Institutes of Health (NIH), HIV Medicine Association of the Infectious Diseases Society of America (IDSA), Pediatric Infectious Diseases Society, and others recommend that *all* HIV-infected infants and children 2 months of age or older, adolescents, and adults receive vaccination against pneumococcal disease.

HIV-infected infants and children 2 months through 5 years of age should receive PCV13 (Prevnar 13®) according to the usual primary and catch-up immunization schedules recommended for infants and children in this age group.

HIV-infected children and adolescents 6 through 18 years of age who have not previously received PCV13 (Prevnar 13®) should receive a single dose of the vaccine. The dose of PCV13 (Prevnar 13®) is indicated in these children and adolescents even if they were vaccinated with the previously available 7-valent vaccine (PCV7; Prevnar®).

HIV-infected adults 19 years of age or older who have not previously received PCV13 (Prevnar 13®) or have an unknown vaccination status should receive a single dose of PCV13 (Prevnar 13®), regardless of CD4+ T-cell count.

PPSV23 (Pneumovax® 23) also is recommended in HIV-infected children 2 years of age or older, adolescents, and adults 19 years of age or older. (See HIV-infected Individuals under Uses: Pneumococcal 23-valent Vaccine [PPSV23; Pneumovax® 23].)

Cochlear Implant Recipients Because cochlear implant recipients are at substantially increased risk for pneumococcal meningitis, AAP, ACIP, CDC, and other experts recommend that *all* individuals with cochlear implants receive age-appropriate vaccination against pneumococcal disease.

The incidence of bacterial meningitis, particularly pneumococcal meningitis, is higher among children with cochlear implants than children in the general population, and *S. pneumoniae* is the most common pathogen causing bacterial meningitis in cochlear implant recipients of all ages with meningitis of known etiology. In May 2003, CDC and FDA announced that they were aware of 118 cases of bacterial meningitis reported worldwide among cochlear implant recipients 13 months to 81 years of age (55 cases in the US and 63 cases in foreign countries); at least 17 fatalities related to meningitis had been reported in cochlear implant recipients at that time. Most of the US cases involved children 5 years of age or younger, while cases reported in non-US patients were distributed equally among children and adults. Aside from the risks of the implant or the implantation procedure, many of the 118 patients had certain preexisting risk factors for meningitis, including a history of preimplant meningitis, congenital inner ear deformity, and basilar skull fracture; cochlear implants with electrode positioners were associated with a greater risk of developing meningitis than those without positioners. In the US patients, the onset of meningitis symptoms ranged from less than 24 hours to greater than 6 years after implant; 32 of the US patients developed meningitis within 1 year following implantation, and many of these cases occurred within the first few weeks of surgery. Subsequent data indicated that children with cochlear implants with positioners (implant models voluntarily recalled in the US in 2002) were at greater risk for meningitis than those with cochlear implants without positioners and that the risk for meningitis in those with positioners continued beyond 24 months after implantation.

Health-care providers should review vaccination records of all cochlear implant recipients and all cochlear implant candidates to ensure that they have received age-appropriate vaccination against pneumococcal disease. Depending on the patient's vaccination history, doses of PCV13 (Prevnar 13®) and/or PPSV23 (Pneumovax® 23) may be indicated. When cochlear implant placement is being planned for an individual who is unvaccinated or incompletely vaccinated against pneumococcal disease, ACIP, CDC, and AAP recommend that age-appropriate vaccination be completed at least 2 weeks prior to surgery.

All cases of meningitis occurring in cochlear implant recipients should be reported to the device manufacturer, state health departments (according to state requirements), or the FDA MedWatch program (by phone [800-FDA-1088], by fax [800-FDA-0178], by the internet [http://www.fda.gov/Safety/MedWatch], or by mail [MedWatch, HF-2, FDA, 5600 Fishers Lane, Rockville, MD 20857]). Because information about *S. pneumoniae* serotypes causing pneumococcal meningitis in cochlear implant recipients is limited, health-care providers are encouraged to send isolates to their state health department (by contacting the CDC's National Center for Infectious Diseases at 404-639-2215), which can forward isolates to CDC, where serotyping can be performed to determine whether the type is included in the vaccines.

Internationally Adopted Infants and Children The number of children adopted from outside the US has increased substantially in recent years and the immune status of such children may be difficult to determine based on country of origin and medical records. Children adopted from other countries whose immune status is uncertain should be vaccinated according to the US recommended Childhood and Adolescent Immunization Schedules. (See Immunization Schedules, US 80:00.) The fact that immunization schedules of other countries may differ from US schedules (e.g., different recommended vaccines, recommended ages of administration, and/or number and timing of vaccine doses) should be considered. Vaccines administered outside the US can generally be accepted as valid if the administration schedule was similar to that recommended in the US Childhood and Adolescent Immunization Schedules. Only written vaccination records should be considered as evidence of previous vaccination since such records are more likely to accurately predict protection if the vaccines administered, intervals between doses, and child's age at the time of vaccination are similar to US recommendations; however, the extent to which an internationally adopted child's immunization record reflects their protection against disease is unclear and it is possible there may be transcription errors in such records (e.g., single-antigen vaccine may have been administered although a multiple-antigen vaccine was recorded). Although vaccines with inadequate potency have been produced in other countries, the majority of vaccines used worldwide are immunogenic and produced with adequate quality control standards.

When the immune status of an internationally adopted child is uncertain, ACIP recommends that health-care providers either repeat vaccinations (since this usually is safe and avoids the need to obtain and interpret serologic tests) and/or use selective serologic testing to determine the need for immunizations (helps avoid unnecessary injections). Although pneumococcal vaccine is recommended in many countries, the fact that the vaccine may not be routinely administered should be considered. ACIP recommends that PCV13 (Prevnar 13®) and PPSV23 (Pneumovax® 23) be administered to internationally adopted children as age-appropriate and as indicated by the presence of underlying medical conditions that put them at risk for pneumococcal disease.

Travelers Travelers at highest risk for pneumococcal disease include young children, the elderly, and individuals of any age with chronic medical conditions or immunosuppression. Although pneumococcal disease occurs worldwide, CDC makes no specific recommendations regarding pneumococcal vaccination in travelers.

Prevention of Acute Otitis Media PCV13 (Prevnar 13®) is used for prevention of AOM caused by *S. pneumoniae* serotypes 4, 6B, 9V, 14, 18C, 19F, and 23F. This indication is based on efficacy studies that evaluated use of the previously available 7-valent vaccine (PCV7; Prevnar®) for prevention of AOM caused by these serotypes. Efficacy data are not available to date regarding use of PCV13 (Prevnar 13®) for prevention of AOM caused by the other *S. pneumoniae* serotypes contained in the vaccine (i.e., serotypes 1, 3, 5, 6A, 7F, 19A).

Efficacy of PCV7 (Prevnar®) for prevention of AOM was evaluated in 2 controlled clinical trials. In a prospective, double-blind study involving children in Finland, 1662 infants were randomized to receive PCV7 (Prevnar®) or a control vaccine (hepatitis B virus vaccine) at approximately 2, 4, 6, and 12–15 months of age; all infants also received immunization against diphtheria, tetanus, pertussis, and *Haemophilus influenzae* type b (Hib) at 2, 4, and 6 months of age and immunization against poliovirus at 7 and 12 months of age. Tympanocentesis was performed and the middle ear fluid cultured if AOM was diagnosed in any of these infants (defined as visually abnormal tympanic membrane suggesting middle ear effusion with at least one of the following symptoms: fever, earache, irritability, diarrhea, vomiting, acute otorrhea not caused by otitis externa, or other symptoms of respiratory infection); if *S. pneumoniae* was isolated, the strain was serotyped. The primary end point was efficacy against AOM episodes caused by vaccine serotypes in the per protocol population; the per protocol analysis included AOM episodes that occurred at least 14 days after the third vaccine dose. There were a total of 107 episodes of AOM caused by vaccine serotypes of *S. pneumoniae* in vaccine recipients compared with 250 such episodes in the control group, and this corresponds to a point estimate for vaccine efficacy of 57% in the per protocol population. Vaccine recipients also had a 51% reduction in the frequency of AOM episodes caused by *S. pneumoniae* serotypes that cross-react with serotypes contained in the vaccine; however, these children had a 33% increase in the incidence of AOM caused by all other pneumococcal serotypes compared with children who did not receive the vaccine. Other studies have reported similar changes in carriage of pneumococcal serotypes after vaccination with PCV7 (Prevnar®) (i.e., a decrease in carriage of serotypes contained in the vaccine and an increase in serotypes not contained in the vaccine). Although use of PCV7 (Prevnar®) was associated with only a 6% decrease in the overall incidence of AOM episodes from any cause, additional analysis of the per protocol data indicated that the risk of recurrent AOM (at least 3 episodes within 6 months or 4 or more episodes within 12 months) was reduced by 16% in vaccine recipients.

In a US study evaluating efficacy of PCV7 (Prevnar®) for prevention of invasive disease in children, efficacy of the vaccine in reducing the incidence of AOM also was assessed. Long-term follow-up of children included in this study (up to 3.5 years of age) indicates that use of PCV7 (Prevnar®) reduced the overall incidence of AOM by 7.8% in the per protocol population. There was evidence that, although 2 doses of the vaccine provided protection against AOM, this protection was not sustained through the first year of life without the third vaccine dose of the primary series. Results of this study also indicated that PCV7 (Prevnar®) reduced the incidence of recurrent AOM in the per protocol population and also resulted in a 24% decrease in the placement of tympanostomy tubes in this population.

Although data are limited regarding use of PCV7 (Prevnar®) in older children, results of one study in the Netherlands indicate that use of pneumococcal vaccine in previously unvaccinated children 1–7 years of age with a history of recurrent AOM may not be effective in preventing future episodes of AOM. In this study, 383 children 1–7 years of age with a history of 2 or more episodes of AOM in the year prior to study entry were randomized to receive PCV7 (Prevnar®) (2 doses given 1 month apart for those 12–24 months of age and 1 dose for those 25–84 months of age) followed by PPSV23 (Pneumovax® 23) (a single dose given 6–7 months after the last dose of the 7-valent vaccine) or control vaccines (hepatitis B and hepatitis A virus vaccines). The primary end point was the efficacy of pneumococcal vaccination against clinical episodes of AOM during an 18-month follow-up period beginning 1 month after completion of the vaccine schedule. In the per protocol population, the rate ratio of recurrence of AOM in the pneumococcal vaccine group versus the control group was 1.29. Subgroup analysis suggested a slightly higher rate ratio of recurrence of AOM in the pneumococcal vaccine group than in controls in children who were older than 2 years of age at the time vaccination was initiated compared with the group of children who were 1–2 years of age at the time of initiation of vaccination. There was no clinically important difference in the duration of AOM episodes or in the number of children requiring tympanostomy tube insertion between the group that received pneumococcal vaccine and the group that did not. Because pneumococcal vaccine does not appear to prevent AOM in previously unvaccinated children who have already had recurrent episodes of AOM prior to vaccination, it has been suggested that use of pneumococcal vaccine is not indicated in the management of recurrent AOM in children older than 1 year of age.

■ Pneumococcal 23-valent Vaccine (PPSV23; Pneumovax® 23)

PPSV23 (Pneumovax® 23) is used in children 2 years of age or older and adults 50 years of age or older for prevention of invasive pneumococcal disease caused by the 23 *S. pneumoniae* serotypes contained in the vaccine (i.e., serotypes 1, 2, 3, 4, 5, 6B, 7F, 8, 9N, 9V, 10A, 11A, 12F, 14, 15B, 17F, 18C, 19F, 19A, 20, 22F, 23F, 33F).

ACIP and other experts recommend use of PPSV23 (Pneumovax® 23) in children 2 through 18 years of age with certain underlying medical conditions that put them at increased risk for pneumococcal disease. In addition, ACIP and other experts recommend vaccination with PPSV23 (Pneumovax® 23) in adults 19 years of age or older with certain medical conditions that put them at increased risk for pneumococcal disease and *routine* vaccination with PCV13 (Prevnar 13®) in *all* adults 65 years of age or older.

Children 2 through 5 Years of Age at Increased Risk for Pneumococcal Disease ACIP, AAP, and other experts recommend PPSV23 (Pneumovax® 23) in children 2 through 5 years of age who are at increased risk for pneumococcal disease because of functional or anatomic asplenia (including sickle cell disease or other hemoglobinopathies, congenital or acquired asplenia), immunocompromising medical conditions (congenital or acquired immunodeficiency, HIV infection, chronic renal failure, nephrotic syndrome, malignant neoplasms, leukemia, lymphoma, Hodgkin's disease, solid organ transplantation), or certain other medical conditions (chronic heart disease [especially cyanotic congenital heart disease and cardiac failure], chronic lung disease [including asthma if treated with prolonged high-dose oral corticosteroids], diabetes mellitus, CSF leaks, cochlear implants).

Children 2 through 5 years of age with these medical conditions who have not previously received PPSV23 (Pneumovax® 23) should receive a single dose of the vaccine.

PCV13 (Prevnar 13®) also is recommended in children 2 through 5 years of age who are at increased risk for pneumococcal disease because of certain medical conditions. (See Children 2 through 5 Years of Age at Increased Risk for Pneumococcal Disease under Uses: Pneumococcal 13-valent Conjugate Vaccine [PCV13; Prevnar 13®].)

Children and Adolescents 6 through 18 Years of Age at Increased Risk for Pneumococcal Disease ACIP, AAP, and other experts recommend PPSV23 (Pneumovax® 23) in children and adolescents 6 through 18 years of age who are at increased risk for pneumococcal disease because of functional or anatomic asplenia (including sickle cell disease or other hemoglobinopathies, congenital or acquired asplenia), immunocompromising medical conditions (congenital or acquired immunodeficiency, HIV infection, chronic renal failure, nephrotic syndrome, malignant neoplasms, leukemia, lymphoma, Hodgkin's disease, generalized malignancy, solid organ transplantation, multiple myeloma), or certain other medical conditions (chronic heart disease [especially cyanotic congenital heart disease and cardiac failure], chronic lung disease [including asthma if treated with prolonged high-dose oral corticosteroids], diabetes mellitus, CSF leaks, cochlear implants, alcoholism, or chronic liver disease or because they smoke cigarettes).

Children and adolescents 6 through 18 years of age with these medical conditions who have not previously received PPSV23 (Pneumovax® 23) should receive a single dose of the vaccine. In addition, ACIP and other experts recommend that those with functional or anatomic asplenia and those with immunocompromising conditions receive revaccination with a second dose of PPSV23 (Pneumovax® 23) 5 years after the first dose.

PCV13 (Prevnar 13®) also is recommended in children and adolescents 6 through 18 years of age who are at increased risk for pneumococcal disease because of certain medical conditions. (See Children and Adolescents 6 through 18 Years of Age at Increased Risk for Pneumococcal Disease under Uses: Pneumococcal 13-valent Conjugate Vaccine [PCV13; Prevnar 13®].)

Adults 19 Years of Age or Older at Increased Risk for Pneumococcal Disease ACIP and other experts recommend PPSV23 (Pneumovax® 23) in previously unvaccinated adults 19 years of age or older who are at increased risk for pneumococcal disease because of functional or anatomic asplenia (including sickle cell disease or other hemoglobinopathies, congenital or acquired asplenia, splenic dysfunction, splenectomy), immunocompromising medical conditions (congenital or acquired immunodeficiency, HIV infection, chronic renal failure, nephrotic syndrome, leukemia, lymphoma, Hodgkin's disease, generalized malignancy, solid organ transplantation, multiple myeloma), iatrogenic immunosuppression (including long-term systemic corticosteroid therapy or radiation therapy), or other medical conditions (chronic heart disease [including congestive heart failure and cardiomyopathies, excluding hypertension], chronic lung disease [including chronic obstructive pulmonary disease, emphysema, asthma], diabetes mellitus, CSF leaks, cochlear implants, alcoholism, chronic liver disease, or cirrhosis or because they smoke cigarettes).

Adults 19 years of age or older with these medical conditions who have not previously received PPSV23 (Pneumovax® 23) should receive a single dose of PPSV23 (Pneumovax® 23). In addition, ACIP and other experts recommend that those with functional or anatomic asplenia or immunocompromising conditions receive revaccination with a second dose of PPSV23 (Pneumovax® 23) 5 years after the first dose.

PCV13 (Prevnar 13®) also is recommended in adults 19 years of age or older who are at increased risk for pneumococcal disease because of certain medical conditions. (See Adults 19 Years of Age or Older at Increased Risk for Pneumococcal Disease under Uses: Pneumococcal 13-valent Conjugate Vaccine [PCV13; Prevnar 13®].)

Healthy Adults 50 through 64 Years of Age Although PPSV23 (Pneumovax® 23) is labeled by FDA for prevention of pneumococcal disease in adults as young as 50 years of age, ACIP and other experts do not recommend *routine* vaccination with PPSV23 (Pneumovax® 23) in healthy adults 50 through 64 years of age who do not have medical conditions that increase the risk for pneumococcal disease.

Adults 65 Years of Age or Older ACIP and other experts recommend *routine* vaccination with PPSV23 (Pneumovax® 23) in *all* adults 65 years of age or older who are unvaccinated or have unknown vaccination status.

Adults 65 years of age or older who received a dose of PPSV23 (Pneumovax® 23) when they were younger than 65 years of age should be revaccinated with a dose of PPSV23 (Pneumovax® 23) at least 5 years after the previous dose.

PCV13 (Prevnar 13®) also is recommended *routinely* in *all* adults 65 years of age or older. (See Adults 65 Years of Age or Older, under Uses: Pneumococcal 13-valent Conjugate Vaccine [PCV13; Prevnar 13®].)

HIV-infected Individuals Because HIV-infected individuals are at high risk for invasive and recurrent pneumococcal disease compared with those who are not infected with HIV, the ACIP, AAP, CDC, NIH, IDSA, and other experts recommend that all HIV-infected individuals receive vaccination against pneumococcal disease.

HIV-infected children 2 years of age and older, adolescents, and adults who have not previously received PPSV23 (Pneumovax® 23) or have an unknown vaccination status should receive the vaccine. Although ACIP and other experts state that PPSV23 (Pneumovax® 23) can be used in HIV-infected adults regardless of CD4+ T-cell count, some experts state that it may be preferable to defer administration of PPSV23 (Pneumovax® 23) in HIV-infected adults and adolescents until CD4+ T-cell counts increase to greater than 200 cells/mm^3 in response to antiretroviral therapy.

ACIP and other experts state that HIV-infected individuals should be revaccinated with a second dose of PPSV23 (Pneumovax® 23) at least 5 years after the first dose. Some experts recommend a third dose of PPSV23 (Pneumovax® 23) in HIV-infected individuals at 65 years of age or later, as long as 5 years have elapsed since the previous dose. No more than 3 lifetime doses of PPSV23 (Pneumovax® 23) are recommended.

PCV13 (Prevnar 13®) also is recommended in HIV-infected children, adolescents, and adults. (See HIV-infected Individuals under Uses: Pneumococcal 13-valent Conjugate Vaccine [PCV13; Prevnar 13®].)

Cochlear Implant Recipients Because cochlear implant recipients are at substantially increased risk for pneumococcal meningitis, ACIP, AAP, CDC, and other experts recommend that all individuals with cochlear implants receive age-appropriate vaccination against pneumococcal disease.

Health-care providers should review vaccination records of all cochlear implant recipients and all cochlear implant candidates to ensure that they have received age-appropriate vaccination against pneumococcal disease. Depending on the patient's vaccination history, doses of PCV13 (Prevnar 13®) and/or PPSV23 (Pneumovax® 23) may be indicated. When cochlear implant placement is being planned for an individual who is unvaccinated or incompletely vaccinated against pneumococcal disease, ACIP, CDC, and AAP recommend that age-appropriate vaccination be completed at least 2 weeks prior to surgery. (See Cochlear Implant Recipients under Uses: Pneumococcal 13-valent Conjugate Vaccine [PCV13; Prevnar 13®].)

Cigarette Smokers Individuals who smoke cigarettes are at substantially increased risk for invasive pneumococcal disease. Unvaccinated individuals who smoke cigarettes should receive a dose of PPSV23 (Pneumovax® 23) and smoking cessation counseling.

Internationally Adopted Infants and Children When the immune status of an internationally adopted child is uncertain, ACIP recommends that health-care providers either repeat vaccinations (since this usually is safe and avoids the need to obtain and interpret serologic tests) and/or use selective serologic testing to determine the need for immunizations (helps avoid unnecessary injections). Although pneumococcal vaccine is recommended in many countries, the fact that the vaccine may not be routinely administered should be considered. ACIP recommends that PPSV23 (Pneumovax® 23) be administered to internationally adopted children as age-appropriate and as indicated by the presence of underlying medical conditions that put them at risk for pneumococcal disease. (See Internationally Adopted Infants and Children under Uses: Pneumococcal 13-valent Conjugate Vaccine [PCV13; Prevnar 13®].)

Travelers Travelers at highest risk for pneumococcal disease include young children, the elderly, and individuals of any age with chronic medical conditions or immunosuppression. Although pneumococcal disease occurs worldwide, CDC makes no specific recommendations regarding pneumococcal vaccination in travelers.

Dosage and Administration

■ **Administration** Pneumococcal 13-valent conjugate vaccine (diphtheria CRM$_{197}$ protein) (PCV13; Prevnar 13®) is administered *only* by IM injection.

Pneumococcal vaccine, polyvalent (pneumococcal 23-valent vaccine; PPSV23; Pneumovax® 23) is administered *only* by IM or subcutaneous injection.

PCV13 (Prevnar 13®) and PPSV23 (Pneumovax® 23) should *not* be diluted or mixed with any other vaccine or solution.

PCV13 (Prevnar 13®) should *not* be administered concomitantly with PPSV23 (Pneumovax® 23). When both vaccines are indicated, PPSV23 (Pneumovax® 23) should be administered sequentially *after* the recommended age-appropriate regimen of PCV13 (Prevnar 13®), if possible.

PCV13 (Prevnar 13®) or PPSV23 (Pneumovax® 23) may be given simultaneously with other age-appropriate vaccines during the same health-care visit. (See Drug Interactions: Vaccines.) When multiple vaccines are administered during a single health-care visit, each parenteral vaccine should be given with a different syringe and at different injection sites, and injection sites should be separated by at least 1 inch (if anatomically feasible) to allow appropriate attribution of any local adverse effects that may occur.

Syncope (vasovagal or vasodepressor reaction; fainting) may occur following vaccination; such reactions occur most frequently in adolescents and young adults. Syncope and secondary injuries may be averted if vaccinees sit or lie down during and for 15 minutes after the vaccination. If syncope occurs, the patient should be observed until symptoms resolve.

IM Administration Depending on patient age, IM injections should be made into the anterolateral muscles of the thigh or deltoid muscle of the arm. In infants and children 6 weeks to 2 years of age, IM injections should preferably be made into the anterolateral thigh; alternatively, the deltoid muscle can be used in those 1 through 2 years of age if muscle mass is adequate. In adults, adolescents, and children 3 years of age or older, IM injections should preferably be made into the deltoid muscle.

To ensure delivery into muscle, IM injections should be made at a 90° angle to the skin using a needle length appropriate for the individual's age and body mass, thickness of adipose tissue and muscle at the injection site, and injection technique.

IM injections should *not* be made into the gluteal area or any area where there may be a major nerve trunk. If the gluteal muscle is chosen for infants younger than 12 months of age because of special circumstances (e.g., physical obstruction of other sites), it is *essential* that the clinician identify anatomic landmarks prior to injection.

Pneumococcal 13-valent Conjugate Vaccine (PCV13; Prevnar 13®). PCV13 (Prevnar 13®) is administered *only* by IM injection. The vaccine should *not* be administered subcutaneously or intradermally since it contains an aluminum adjuvant.

PCV13 (Prevnar 13®) is commercially available in single-dose prefilled syringes. After attaching a sterile needle, the entire contents of the prefilled syringe should be administered IM.

PCV13 (Prevnar 13®) must be shaken vigorously immediately prior to administration to obtain a uniform, white suspension. The vaccine should be discarded if it cannot be resuspended or if particulate matter or discoloration are present.

Pneumococcal 23-valent Vaccine (PPSV23; Pneumovax® 23). PPSV23 (Pneumovax® 23) is administered by IM or, alternatively, by subcutaneous injection. (See Subcutaneous Administration under Dosage and Administration: Administration.) The vaccine should *not* be administered IV or intradermally.

PPSV23 (Pneumovax® 23) is commercially available in single-dose prefilled syringes and in single- or multiple-dose vials. If a single-dose prefilled syringe is used, a sterile needle should be attached to the syringe according to the manufacturer's instructions and the entire contents of the prefilled syringe administered IM. If a single- or multiple-dose vial is used, 0.5 mL of the vaccine should be withdrawn from the vial using a sterile needle and syringe free of preservatives, antiseptics, and detergents and then administered IM.

PPSV23 (Pneumovax® 23) should be inspected visually for particulate matter and discoloration prior to administration. The vaccine should be a clear colorless solution and should not be administered if it contains particulates or appears discolored.

Subcutaneous Administration Subcutaneous injections should be made at a 45° angle using a 5/8 inch, 23- to 25-gauge needle.

Subcutaneous injections should be made into the upper-outer triceps area or anterolateral thigh. In adults, adolescents, and children 2 years of age or older, subcutaneous injections should be made into the upper-outer triceps area.

Pneumococcal 23-valent Vaccine (PPSV23; Pneumovax® 23). PPSV23 (Pneumovax® 23) is administered by subcutaneous or, alternatively, by IM injection. (See IM Administration under Dosage and Administration: Administration.) The vaccine should *not* be administered IV or intradermally.

PPSV23 (Pneumovax® 23) is commercially available in single-dose prefilled syringes and in single- or multiple-dose vials. If a single-dose prefilled syringe is used, a sterile needle should be attached to the syringe according to the manufacturer's instructions and the entire contents of the prefilled syringe administered subcutaneously. If a single- or multiple-dose vial is used, 0.5 mL of the vaccine should be withdrawn from the vial using a sterile needle and syringe free of preservatives, antiseptics, and detergents and then administered by subcutaneous injection.

PPSV23 (Pneumovax® 23) should be inspected visually for particulate matter and discoloration prior to administration. The vaccine should be discarded if it contains particulates or appears discolored.

■ **Dosage** The dosage schedule (i.e., number of doses) and specific pneumococcal vaccine administered (PCV13 [Prevnar 13®] and/or PPSV23 [Pneumovax® 23]) vary depending on age, immunization status, and presence of medical conditions that increase the risk of pneumococcal disease. *The age-appropriate recommendations for the specific preparation used should be followed.*

Medically stable preterm infants (i.e., gestational age less than 37 weeks), regardless of birthweight, should be vaccinated at the usual chronologic age using the usual dosage and dosage schedules.

Interruptions resulting in an interval between doses longer than recommended should not interfere with the final immunity achieved; there is no need to administer additional doses or start the vaccination series over.

Each IM dose of PCV13 (Prevnar 13®) in infants and children 6 weeks of age or older, adolescents, and adults consists of the entire contents (0.5 mL) of the commercially available single-dose prefilled syringe.

Each IM or subcutaneous dose of PPSV23 (Pneumovax® 23) in children 2 years of age or older, adolescents, and adults consists of the entire contents (0.5 mL) of the commercially available single-dose prefilled syringe or 0.5 mL from a single- or multiple-dose vial.

Infants 2 through 23 Months of Age **PCV13 (Prevnar 13®).** For *routine* primary immunization initiated in early infancy, PCV13 (Prevnar 13®) is given in a series of 4 doses. The US Public Health Service Advisory Committee on Immunization Practices (ACIP), American Academy of Pediatrics (AAP), and other experts recommend that PCV13 (Prevnar 13®) be given at 2, 4, 6, and 12 through 15 months of age. Although the first dose of PCV13 (Prevnar 13®) usually is given at 2 months of age, the first dose can be given as early as 6 weeks of age. The first 3 doses of PCV13 (Prevnar 13®) should be given at approximately 4- to 8-week intervals and the fourth dose should be given at least 8 weeks (2 months) after the third dose.

For catch-up vaccination in infants 7 through 23 months of age who did not receive PCV13 (Prevnar 13®) at the usually recommended time in early infancy, the recommended number of doses of PCV13 (Prevnar 13®) varies depending on the age of the child when the first dose is given. Infants who are 7 through 11 months of age when they receive the first dose of PCV13 (Prevnar 13®) should receive 2 doses given at least 4 weeks apart and a third dose given after 12 months of age and at least 8 weeks (2 months) after the second dose; a fourth dose is not necessary in healthy infants unless all previous doses were given before 12 months of age. Infants who are 12 through 23 months of age when they receive the first dose of PCV13 (Prevnar 13®) should receive 2 doses given at least 8 weeks (2 months) apart; a third dose is not necessary if the second dose was given at 24 months of age or older.

Infants 14 through 23 months of age who previously received age-appropriate vaccination with the previously available 7-valent vaccine (PCV7; Prevnar®) should receive a single supplemental dose of PCV13 (Prevnar 13®).

Healthy Children 2 through 5 Years of Age **PCV13 (Prevnar 13®).** For catch-up vaccination in otherwise healthy children 2 through 5 years of age who are unvaccinated and have not received *any* doses of PCV13 (Prevnar 13®), ACIP, AAP, and other experts recommend a single dose of PCV13 (Prevnar 13®). Additional doses are not necessary in healthy children if the PCV13 (Prevnar 13®) dose is given at 2 years of age or older.

For catch-up vaccination in otherwise healthy children 2 through 5 years of age who are incompletely vaccinated for their age and have not received the total recommended age-appropriate number of doses of PCV13 (Prevnar 13®) and/or PCV7 (Prevnar®), ACIP, AAP, and other experts recommend a single dose of PCV13 (Prevnar 13®) given at least 8 weeks after the most recent dose of PCV13 (Prevnar 13®) or PCV7 (Prevnar®).

Children 2 through 5 years of age who received age-appropriate vaccination with the previously available 7-valent vaccine (PCV7; Prevnar®) but have not received any doses of PCV13 (Prevnar 13®) should receive a single supplemental dose of PCV13 (Prevnar 13®) since this may provide additional protection.

Children 2 through 5 Years of Age at Increased Risk for Pneumococcal Disease **PCV13 (Prevnar 13®).** Children 2 through 5 years of age with certain medical conditions that put them at increased risk for pneumococcal disease (see Children 2 through 5 Years of Age at Increased Risk for Pneumococcal Disease under Uses: Pneumococcal 13-valent Conjugate Vaccine [PCV13; Prevnar 13®]) who previously received fewer than 3 doses of PCV13 (Prevnar 13®) or received fewer than 3 doses of the previously available 7-valent vaccine (PCV7; Prevnar®) should receive 2 doses of PCV13 (Prevnar 13®) given at least 8 weeks apart. Children 2 through 5 years of age with these medical conditions who previously received a total of 3 doses of PCV given as PCV13 (Prevnar 13®) and/or PCV7 (Prevnar®) or received 4 doses or other age-appropriate vaccination series of PCV7 (Prevnar®) should receiving a single dose of PCV13 (Prevnar 13®).

PPSV23 (Pneumovax® 23). Children 2 through 5 years of age with certain medical conditions that put them at increased risk for pneumococcal disease (see Children 2 through 5 Years of Age at Increased Risk for Pneumococcal Disease, under Uses: Pneumococcal 23-valent Vaccine [PPSV23; Pneumovax® 23]) who have *not* previously received PPSV23 (Pneumovax® 23) should receive a single dose of the vaccine.

Sequential Administration. When both PCV13 (Prevnar 13®) *and* PPSV23 (Pneumovax® 23) are indicated in a child 2 through 5 years of age at increased risk for pneumococcal disease, PCV13 (Prevnar 13®) should be given first and PPSV23 (Pneumovax® 23) should be given at least 8 weeks after the most recent dose of PCV13 (Prevnar 13®).

In those who have *not* previously received PCV13 (Prevnar 13®) but have previously received PPSV23 (Pneumovax® 23), PCV13 (Prevnar 13®) should be given at least 8 weeks after the most recent dose of PPSV23 (Pneumovax® 23).

PCV13 (Prevnar 13®) and PPSV23 (Pneumovax® 23) should *not* be given concurrently.

Children and Adolescents 6 through 18 Years of Age at Increased Risk for Pneumococcal Disease **PCV13 (Prevnar 13®).** Children and adolescents 6 through 18 years of age with certain medical conditions that put them at increased risk for pneumococcal disease (see Children and Adolescents 6 through 18 Years of Age at Increased Risk for Pneumococcal Disease under Uses: Pneumococcal 13-valent Conjugate Vaccine [PCV13; Prevnar 13®]) who have *not* previously received PCV13 (Prevnar 13®) should receive a single dose of the vaccine.

PPSV23 (Pneumovax® 23). Children and adolescents 6 through 18 years of age with certain medical conditions that put them at increased risk for pneumococcal disease (see Children and Adolescents 6 through 18 Years of Age at Increased Risk for Pneumococcal Disease, under Uses: Pneumococcal 23-valent Vaccine [PPSV23; Pneumovax® 23]) who have *not* previously received PPSV23 (Pneumovax® 23) should receive a single dose of the vaccine. In addition, those with functional or anatomic asplenia or immunocompromising conditions should be revaccinated with a second dose of PPSV23 (Pneumovax® 23) 5 years after the first dose.

Sequential Administration. When both PCV13 (Prevnar 13®) *and* PPSV23 (Pneumovax® 23) are indicated in a child or adolescent 6 through 18 years of age at increased risk for pneumococcal disease, PCV13 (Prevnar 13®) should be given first and PPSV23 (Pneumovax® 23) should be given at least 8 weeks after the most recent dose of PCV13 (Prevnar 13®).

If a child or adolescent 6 through 18 years of age at increased risk for pneumococcal disease has *not* previously received PCV13 (Prevnar 13®) but has previously received PPSV23 (Pneumovax® 23), PCV13 (Prevnar 13®) should be given at least 8 weeks after the most recent dose of PPSV23 (Pneumovax® 23).

When a second dose of PPSV23 (Pneumovax® 23) is indicated, it should be given at least 8 weeks after PCV13 (Prevnar 13®) and at least 5 years after the previous PPSV23 (Pneumovax® 23) dose.

PCV13 (Prevnar 13®) and PPSV23 (Pneumovax® 23) should *not* be given concurrently.

Adults 19 Years of Age or Older at Increased Risk for Pneumococcal Disease **PCV13 (Prevnar 13®).** Adults 19 years of age or older with certain medical conditions that put them at increased risk for pneumococcal disease† (see Adults 19 Years of Age or Older at Increased Risk for Pneumococcal Disease under Uses: Pneumococcal 13-valent Conjugate Vaccine [PCV13; Prevnar 13®]) who have *not* previously received PCV13 (Prevnar 13®) should receive a single dose of the vaccine.

PPSV23 (Pneumovax® 23). Adults 19 years of age or older with certain medical conditions that put them at increased risk for pneumococcal disease (see Adults 19 Years of Age or Older at Increased Risk for Pneumococcal Disease under Uses: Pneumococcal 23-valent Vaccine [PPSV23; Pneumovax® 23]) who have *not* previously received PPSV23 (Pneumovax® 23) should receive a dose of the vaccine. In addition, those with functional or anatomic asplenia or immunocompromising conditions should be revaccinated with a second dose of PPSV23 (Pneumovax® 23) 5 years after the first dose.

Sequential Administration. When both PCV13 (Prevnar 13®) *and* PPSV23 (Pneumovax® 23) are indicated in an adult 19 years of age or older at increased risk for pneumococcal disease, PCV13 (Prevnar 13®) should be given first and PPSV23 (Pneumovax® 23) should be given at least 8 weeks after the most recent dose of PCV13 (Prevnar 13®).

If an adult 19 years of age or older at increased risk has *not* previously received PCV13 (Prevnar 13®) but previously received PPSV23 (Pneumovax® 23), PCV13 (Prevnar 13®) should be given at least 1 year after the most recent dose of PPSV23 (Pneumovax® 23).

If an adult 19 years of age or older at increased risk has previously received PCV13 (Prevnar 13®) but has *not* previously received PPSV23 (Pneumovax® 23), PPSV23 (Pneumovax® 23) should be given at least 8 weeks after PCV13 (Prevnar 13®).

When a second dose of PPSV23 (Pneumovax® 23) is indicated, it should be given at least 8 weeks after PCV13 (Prevnar 13®) and at least 5 years after the previous PPSV23 (Pneumovax® 23) dose.

PCV13 (Prevnar 13®) and PPSV23 (Pneumovax® 23) should *not* be given concurrently.

Healthy Adults 50 through 64 Years of Age **PCV13 (Prevnar 13®).** The manufacturer recommends a single dose of PCV13 (Prevnar 13®) in adults 50 through 64 years of age.

Although PCV13 (Prevnar 13®) is labeled by FDA for use in adults as young as 50 years of age, ACIP and other experts do not recommend *routine* vaccination with PCV13 (Prevnar 13®) in healthy adults 50 through 64 years of age who do not have medical conditions that increase the risk for pneumococcal disease.

PPSV23 (Pneumovax® 23). The manufacturer recommends a single dose of PPSV23 (Pneumovax® 23) in adults 50 through 64 years of age.

Although PPSV23 (Pneumovax® 23) is labeled by FDA for use in adults as young as 50 years of age, ACIP and other experts do not recommend *routine* vaccination with PPSV23 (Pneumovax® 23) in healthy adults 50 through 64 years of age who do not have medical conditions that increase the risk for pneumococcal disease.

Adults 65 Years of Age or Older **PCV13 (Prevnar 13®).** Adults 65 years of age or older who are unvaccinated or have unknown vaccination status should receive a single dose of PCV13 (Prevnar 13®).

PPSV23 (Pneumovax® 23). Adults 65 years of age or older who are unvaccinated or have unknown vaccination status should receive a single dose of PPSV23 (Pneumovax® 23).

Those who received a dose of PPSV23 (Pneumovax® 23) before 65 years of age for any indication should be revaccinated with another dose of the vaccine at 65 years of age, provided it has been at least 5 years since the previous dose.

Sequential Administration. When both PCV13 (Prevnar 13®) *and* PPSV23 (Pneumovax® 23) are indicated in an adult 65 years of age or older who is unvaccinated or has unknown vaccination status, PCV13 (Prevnar 13®) should be given first and PPSV23 (Pneumovax® 23) should be given at least 1 year after the PCV13 (Prevnar 13®) dose.

If an adult 65 years of age or older has *not* previously received PCV13 (Prevnar 13®) but previously received PPSV23 (Pneumovax® 23) at less than 65 years of age, the PCV13 (Prevnar 13®) dose should be given at least 1 year after the most recent PPSV23 (Pneumovax® 23) dose. Then, another dose of PPSV23 (Pneumovax® 23) should be given at least 1 year after the PCV13 (Prevnar 13®) dose and at least 5 years after the most recent PPSV23 (Pneumovax® 23) dose.

If an adult 65 years of age or older has *not* previously received PCV13 (Prevnar 13®) but previously received PPSV23 (Pneumovax® 23) at 65 years of age or older, the PCV13 (Prevnar 13®) dose should be given at least 1 year after the most recent dose of PPSV23 (Pneumovax® 23).

If an adult 65 years of age or older previously received PCV13 (Prevnar 13®) at less than 65 years of age but has *not* previously received PPSV23 (Pneumovax® 23), the PPSV23 (Pneumovax® 23) dose should be given at least 1 year after the PCV13 (Prevnar 13®) dose.

If an adult 65 years of age or older previously received PCV13 (Prevnar 13®) and PPSV23 (Pneumovax® 23) at less than 65 years of age, another dose of PPSV23 (Pneumovax® 23) should be given at least 1 year after the PCV13 (Prevnar 13®) dose and at least 5 years after the most recent PPSV23 (Pneumovax® 23) dose.

PCV13 (Prevnar 13®) and PPSV23 (Pneumovax® 23) should *not* be given concurrently.

To facilitate completion of pneumococcal vaccination in immunocompetent adults 65 years of age or older, ACIP recommends an interval of at least 1 year between PCV13 (Prevnar 13®) and PPSV23 (Pneumovax® 23), regardless of the order in which the vaccines are given. If a dose of PPSV23 (Pneumovax® 23) is inadvertently given earlier than 1 year after PCV13 (Prevnar 13®), the dose does not need to repeated. The minimum interval between PCV13 (Prevnar 13®) and PPSV23 (Pneumovax® 23) is 8 weeks.

HIV-infected Individuals **PCV13 (Prevnar 13®).** HIV-infected infants and children 2 through 23 months of age should receive 4 doses of PCV13 (Prevnar 13®) given at 2, 4, 6, and 12 through 15 months of age according to the usually recommended primary immunization schedule. Unvaccinated or incompletely vaccinated HIV-infected infants 7 through 23 years of age should receive catch-up vaccination with the age-appropriate number of doses of PCV13 (Prevnar 13®) according to the usually recommended catch-up schedules. (See PCV13 [Prevnar 13®] under Dosage: Infants 2 through 23 Months of Age, in Dosage and Administration.)

HIV-infected children 2 through 5 years of age who are incompletely vaccinated should receive PCV13 (Prevnar 13®) according to the usually recommended catch-up immunization schedules. (See PCV13 [Prevnar 13®] under Dosage: Healthy Children 2 through 5 Years of Age, in Dosage and Administration.)

HIV-infected children and adolescents 6 through 18 years of age who have *not* previously received PCV13 (Prevnar 13®) or have unknown vaccination status should receive a single dose of PCV13 (Prevnar 13®).

HIV-infected adults 19 years of age or older who have *not* previously received PCV13 (Prevnar 13®) or have unknown vaccination status should receive a single dose of PCV13 (Prevnar 13®), regardless of CD4+ T-cell count.

PPSV23 (Pneumovax® 23). HIV-infected children 2 years of age and older, adolescents, and adults who have *not* previously received PPSV23 (Pneumovax® 23) or have an unknown vaccination status should receive a single dose of the vaccine. In addition, HIV-infected individuals should be revaccinated with a second dose of PPSV23 (Pneumovax® 23) 5 years after the first dose. Some experts recommend that HIV-infected individuals receive a third dose of PPSV23 (Pneumovax® 23) at 65 years of age or later, provided it has been at least 5 years since the previous dose. No more than 3 lifetime doses of PPSV23 (Pneumovax® 23) are recommended.

Revaccination and Booster Doses **PCV13 (Prevnar 13®).** The duration of protection after administration of PCV13 (Prevnar 13®) is not known.

Revaccination with PCV13 (Prevnar 13®) after age-appropriate vaccination is not currently recommended.

PPSV23 (Pneumovax® 23). The duration of protection after administration of PPSV23 (Pneumovax® 23) has not been fully determined. (See Duration of Immunity under Pharmacology: Response to Pneumococcal 23-valent Vaccine [PPSV23; Pneumovax® 23].)

Routine revaccination with PPSV23 (Pneumovax® 23) in immunocompetent individuals is not recommended. However, ACIP, AAP, and other experts recommend that individuals at increased risk of pneumococcal disease who have certain medical conditions (i.e., functional or anatomic asplenia or immunocompromising conditions) should be revaccinated with a second dose of PPSV23 (Pneumovax® 23) 5 years after the first dose. Revaccination with a second dose of PPSV23 (Pneumovax® 23) also is recommended in adults 65 years of age or older who received the initial dose when they were younger than 65 years of age, provided at least 5 years have elapsed since the initial dose. Some experts recommend a third dose of PPSV23 (Pneumovax® 23) in HIV-infected adults when they reach 65 years of age, provided at least 5 years have elapsed since the previous dose.

Cautions

■ Pneumococcal 13-valent Conjugate Vaccine (PCV13; Prevnar 13®)

The safety of pneumococcal 13-valent conjugate vaccine (diphtheria CRM_{197} protein) (PCV13; Prevnar 13®) in infants 6 weeks though 15 months of age was evaluated in 13 clinical studies in which 4729 infants received at least 1 dose of PCV13 (Prevnar 13®) compared with 2760 infants who received the active control consisting of at least 1 dose of the previously available 7-valent conjugate vaccine (PCV7; Prevnar®). Three US studies evaluated the safety of a 4-dose immunization series of PCV13 (Prevnar 13®) in conjunction with other routine childhood vaccines. Adverse local or systemic effects were solicited from and recorded daily by parents/guardians using an electronic diary for 7 consecutive days after each dose of PCV13 (Prevnar 13®). Study subjects also were monitored for unsolicited adverse events from the time of the first vaccine dose until 1 month after administration of the third dose and for 1 month after the fourth dose. Information regarding unsolicited and serious adverse events, newly diagnosed chronic medical conditions, and hospitalizations was collected during the clinic visit following the fourth dose and during a scripted telephone interview 6 months after the fourth dose.

A US study evaluated safety of PCV13 (Prevnar 13®) in 596 children 15 through 59 months of age who had been vaccinated with 3 or 4 doses of the previously available 7-valent vaccine (PCV7; Prevnar®) in early infancy. Children 15 through 23 months of age received 2 doses of PCV13 (Prevnar 13®) and those 24 through 59 months of age received a single dose of PCV13 (Prevnar 13®). Adverse local or systemic effects occurring within 7 days after administration of PCV13 (Prevnar 13®) were solicited.

The safety of PCV13 (Prevnar 13®) in children 5 through 17 years of age who previously received at least 1 dose of the previously available 7-valent vaccine (PCV7; Prevnar®) was evaluated in a US study that included 592 children (54.5% had received 4 doses of PCV7 [Prevnar®]). Adverse local or systemic effects occurring within 7 days after administration of PCV13 (Prevnar 13®) were solicited.

The safety of PCV13 (Prevnar 13®) in adults was evaluated in 6 clinical studies in the US and Europe that included 5667 individuals 50 through 95 years of age who received a dose of PCV13 (Prevnar 13®). Data from 4 of these studies evaluated the safety of PCV13 (Prevnar 13®) given alone in 3751 previously unvaccinated adults (had not previously received PPSV23 [Pneumovax® 23]) or in 1916 previously vaccinated adults (had received PPSV23 [Pneumovax® 23] at least 3–5 years prior to study enrollment). Adverse local or systemic effects were solicited from and recorded daily by vaccinees using an electronic diary for 14 consecutive days following the dose of PCV13 (Prevnar 13®). These individuals also were monitored for unsolicited serious and nonserious adverse events for 1 month following the vaccine dose. Information regarding serious adverse events was collected for an additional 5 months after vaccination during a telephone interview 6 months after the vaccine dose.

Local Effects The most common adverse effects reported with PCV13 (Prevnar 13®) are local reactions at the injection site, including pain/tenderness, redness, and swelling.

In infants who received a 4-dose immunization series of PCV13 (Prevnar 13®) at 2, 4, 6, and 12–15 months of age in 3 US safety studies, tenderness at the injection site was reported in 59–65% of infants after each of the first 3 vaccine doses and in 58% after the fourth dose; tenderness interfered with limb movement in 8–10% and 7% of these infants, respectively. Redness was reported in 24–37% of infants after the first 3 vaccine doses and in 42% after the fourth dose. Swelling at the injection site was reported in 20–27% of infants after the first 3 vaccine doses and in 32% after the fourth dose.

In children who had been vaccinated with 3 or 4 doses of the previously available 7-valent vaccine (PCV7; Prevnar®) in early infancy and received a dose of PCV13 (Prevnar 13®) at 15 through 59 months of age, tenderness at the injection site was reported in 47–49% of children who received PCV13 (Prevnar 13®) at 15 through 23 months of age and in 63% of those who received the vaccine at 24 through 59 months of age; 6 and 11% of these children, respectively had tenderness that interfered with limb movement. Redness and swelling were reported after the PCV13 (Prevnar 13®) dose in 26–28% and 20–24%, respectively, of children who received PCV13 (Prevnar 13®) at 15 through 23 months of age and in 35 or 21%, respectively, of those who received the vaccine at 24 through 59 months of age.

When a dose of PCV13 (Prevnar 13®) was administered to children 5 through 9 years of age who had received at least 1 dose of the previously available 7-valent vaccine (PCV7; Prevnar®) or to children 10 through 17 years of age who had not received any pneumococcal vaccine previously, tenderness at the injection site was reported in 87 or 89%, respectively. Redness was reported in 43 or 30%, respectively, and swelling was reported in 38 or 37%, respectively.

When a dose of PCV13 (Prevnar 13®) was administered to adults 50–64 years of age who were previously unvaccinated (had not received PPSV23 [Pneumovax® 23]), local reactions at the injection site, including pain (69–89%), redness (12–20%), and swelling (10–22%), were commonly reported and limitation of arm movement was reported in 24–41%. When a dose of PCV13 (Prevnar 13®) was administered to previously vaccinated adults 68 years of age or older (had received PPSV23 [Pneumovax® 23] at least 3–5 years prior to study enrollment), pain, redness, swelling, and limitation of arm movement were reported in 51–52%, 11–14%, 10–13%, and 11–16%, respectively.

Dermatitis, urticaria, and pruritus at the injection site were reported during postmarketing experience with PCV13 (Prevnar 13®).

Systemic Effects In infants who received a 4-dose immunization series of PCV13 (Prevnar 13®) at 2, 4, 6, and 12–15 months of age in 3 US safety studies, fever (38°C or greater) occurred in 24–37% of infants after each of the first 3 doses; fever was reported in 32% after the fourth dose. Irritability was reported in 80–86%, increased sleep in 58–72%, and decreased sleep in 43–

47% of infants after each of the first 3 doses; after the fourth dose, these effects were reported in 80, 49, and 45%, respectively. Decreased appetite was reported in 48% of infants after each of the first 3 doses of PCV13 (Prevnar 13®) and in 51% after the fourth dose. Diarrhea, vomiting, and rash have been reported in greater than 1% of infants and children receiving PCV13 (Prevnar 13®) in clinical studies. Adverse reactions occurring in less than 1% of infants and children receiving the vaccine included crying, hypersensitivity reaction (e.g., facial edema, dyspnea, bronchospasm), seizures (e.g., febrile seizures), and urticaria or urticaria-like rash.

In children who had been vaccinated with 3 or 4 doses of the previously available 7-valent vaccine (PCV7; Prevnar®) in early infancy and received a dose of PCV13 (Prevnar 13®) at 15 through 59 months of age, fever (38°C or greater) occurred after the PCV13 (Prevnar 13®) dose in 19–20% of children who received PCV13 (Prevnar 13®) at 15 through 23 months of age and in 8% of those who received the vaccine at 24 through 59 months of age. Irritability, increased sleep, decreased sleep, and decreased appetite occurred in 65–73, 35, 25–30, and 39–44%, respectively, of those who received PCV13 (Prevnar 13®) at 15 through 23 months of age and in 46, 19, 15, and 28%, respectively, of those who received the vaccine at 24 through 59 months of age.

When a dose of PCV13 (Prevnar 13®) was administered to children 5 through 9 years of age who had received at least 1 dose of the previously available 7-valent vaccine (PCV7; Prevnar®) or to children 10 through 17 years of age who had not received any pneumococcal vaccine previously, fever (38°C or greater) occurred in 6%. Irritability, increased sleep, decreased sleep, and decreased appetite occurred in 6–31% of these children. In addition, urticaria was reported in 1–2%.

When a dose of PCV13 (Prevnar 13®) was administered to adults 50–64 years of age who were previously unvaccinated (had not received PPSV23 [Pneumovax® 23]), fatigue occurred in 51–63%, headache in 50–66%, chills in 20–24%, muscle pain in 22–62%, joint pain in 14–32%, rash in 9–17%, decreased appetite in 15–25%, vomiting in 3–7%, and fever in 2–4%. When a dose of PCV13 (Prevnar 13®) was administered to previously vaccinated adults 68 years of age and older (had received PPSV23 [Pneumovax® 23] at least 3–5 years prior to study enrollment), fatigue occurred in 34%, headache in 24–26%, chills in 8%, muscle pain in 12–37%, joint pain in 10–13%, rash in 7–8%, decreased appetite in 10–11%, vomiting in 1–2%, and fever in 1%.

Lymphadenopathy in the region of the injection site, cyanosis, pallor, hypotonia, anaphylactic/anaphylactoid reactions (including shock), angioedema, erythema multiforme, and apnea were reported during postmarketing experience with PCV13 (Prevnar 13®).

■ Pneumococcal 23-valent Vaccine (PPSV23; Pneumovax® 23)

Local Effects The most common adverse effects reported after initial vaccination with PPSV23 (Pneumovax® 23) are local reactions at the injection site, including pain/soreness/tenderness (60%), swelling/induration (20%), and erythema (16%). Following revaccination with PPSV23 (Pneumovax® 23) approximately 3–5 years after the initial vaccine dose, the most common local adverse effects are pain/soreness/tenderness (77%), swelling (40%), and erythema (35%). Injection site reactions generally resolve within 5 days after vaccination.

Data from one study in adults indicate that the incidence of adverse effects at the injection site in those 50–64 years of age is similar following initial vaccination (73%) and revaccination (80%). However, the incidence of injection site reactions is higher following revaccination than following initial vaccination in those 65 years of age or older. (See Geriatric Precautions under Cautions: Precautions and Contraindications.)

There have been postmarketing reports of cellulitis or cellulitis-like reactions, warmth at the injection site, decreased limb mobility, and peripheral edema in the injected extremity following administration of PPSV23 (Pneumovax® 23).

Systemic Effects The most common systemic adverse effects reported after initial vaccination with PPSV23 (Pneumovax® 23) are headache (18%), asthenia/fatigue (13%), and myalgia (12%). Following revaccination with PPSV23 (Pneumovax® 23) approximately 3–5 years after the initial vaccine dose, the most common systemic adverse effects are headache (18%), asthenia/fatigue (18%), and myalgia (17%).

Rash, urticaria, and erythema multiforme have been reported following vaccination with PPSV23 (Pneumovax® 23). Anaphylactoid reactions, serum sickness, and angioedema also have been reported.

Other systemic reactions reported following vaccination with PPSV23 (Pneumovax® 23) during clinical studies or postmarketing include fever, chills, arthralgia, arthritis, malaise, diarrhea, dyspepsia, nausea, and vomiting.

There have been postmarketing reports of lymphadenitis, lymphadenopathy, thrombocytopenia (in patients with stabilized idiopathic thrombocytopenic purpura), hemolytic anemia (in patients who have had other hematologic disorders), and leukocytosis. There also have been postmarketing reports of adverse nervous system effects, including paresthesia, radiculoneuropathy, Guillain-Barré syndrome, and febrile seizures.

Data from one study in adults indicate that the incidence of systemic adverse effects in those 50–64 years of age is similar following initial vaccination (36%) and revaccination (38%). However, the incidence of systemic reactions is higher following revaccination than following initial vaccination in those 65 years of age or older. (See Geriatric Precautions under Cautions: Precautions and Contraindications.)

■ Precautions and Contraindications

PCV13 (Prevnar 13®) is contraindicated in individuals who have had a severe allergic reaction (e.g., anaphylaxis) to any ingredient in the formulation or to any vaccine containing diphtheria toxoid.

PPSV23 (Pneumovax® 23) is contraindicated in individuals with a history of anaphylactic/anaphylactoid reactions or severe allergic reaction to any ingredient in the formulation.

Prior to administration of PCV13 (Prevnar 13®) or PPSV23 (Pneumovax® 23), all known precautions should be taken to prevent adverse reactions, including a review of the patient's history with respect to health status, possible sensitivity to the vaccine, and similar vaccines.

Allergic reactions, including anaphylactic/anaphylactoid reactions, rash, urticaria, bronchospasm, serum sickness, erythema multiforme, and angioedema, have been reported with pneumococcal vaccines. Epinephrine and other appropriate agents and equipment should be available for immediate treatment if an anaphylactic or other serious allergic reaction occurs following vaccination.

The patient and/or the patient's parent or guardian should be informed of the benefits and risks of immunization with PCV13 (Prevnar 13®) or PPSV23 (Pneumovax® 23) and should be provided with a copy of the appropriate Vaccine Information Statement (available at the CDC website http://www.cdc.gov/vaccines/pubs/vis/default.htm). Patients and/or the patient's parent or guardian also should be instructed to report any severe or unusual adverse reactions to their health-care provider. Clinicians or individuals can report any adverse reactions that occur following vaccination to VAERS at 800-822-7967 or http://vaers.hhs.gov/index.

Individuals with Altered Immunocompetence Like other inactivated vaccines, PCV13 (Prevnar 13®) and PPSV23 (Pneumovax® 23) may be administered to individuals immunosuppressed as a result of disease or immunosuppressive therapy; however, immune responses to the vaccines may be diminished or suboptimal in these individuals.

If possible, PCV13 (Prevnar 13®) or PPSV23 (Pneumovax® 23) should be administered at least 2 weeks prior to initiation of immunosuppressive therapy or deferred until at least 3 months after immunosuppressive therapy is discontinued. (See Drug Interactions: Immunosuppressive Agents.)

Since antibody response may be impaired after splenectomy, the US Public Health Service Advisory Committee on Immunization Practices (ACIP) and American Academy of Pediatrics (AAP) recommend that vaccination with PCV13 (Prevnar 13®) and/or PPSV23 (Pneumovax® 23) be completed at least 2 weeks prior to elective splenectomy, if possible.

Concomitant Illnesses The decision to administer or delay vaccination in an individual with a current or recent acute illness depends on the severity of symptoms and etiology of the illness.

ACIP, AAP, and other experts state that minor acute illness, such as mild diarrhea or mild upper respiratory infection (with or without fever), usually does not preclude vaccination. However, vaccination of individuals with moderate or severe acute illness (with or without fever) generally should be deferred until they have recovered from the acute phase of the illness. This precaution avoids superimposing adverse effects of the vaccine on the underlying illness or mistakenly concluding that a manifestation of the underlying illness resulted from vaccination.

The manufacturer of PPSV23 (Pneumovax® 23) states that vaccination should be deferred in individuals with moderate or severe acute illness.

The manufacturer of PPSV23 (Pneumovax® 23) states that the vaccine should be administered with caution in individuals with severely compromised cardiovascular and/or pulmonary function in whom a systemic reaction could pose a substantial risk.

Limitations of Vaccine Effectiveness PCV13 (Prevnar 13®) and PPSV23 (Pneumovax® 23) may not protect all vaccine recipients against pneumococcal disease.

Pneumococcal vaccines will *not* prevent pneumococcal infection caused by *Streptococcus pneumoniae* serotypes not represented in the vaccines.

Primary immunization with the usually recommended age-appropriate vaccination regimen before an expected exposure to pneumococcal infection ensures the highest level of protection.

The manufacturer of PCV13 (Prevnar 13®) states that effectiveness of the vaccine administered less than 5 years after PPSV23 (Pneumovax® 23) is not known.

The possibility that pneumococcal vaccines may not prevent infection in individuals who do not achieve protective antibody titers should be considered, although the minimum antibody titer needed to confer protection has not been established.

The manufacturer of PCV13 (Prevnar 13®) states that effectiveness of the vaccine has not been established in children with sickle cell disease or in adults with HIV infection.

Vaccination with PCV13 (Prevnar 13®) and/or PPSV23 (Pneumovax® 23) does not replace prophylaxis with penicillin (or other appropriate anti-infectives) for prevention of pneumococcal disease in patients with functional or anatomic asplenia (e.g., sickle cell disease). If such prophylaxis is indicated, it should be continued regardless of vaccination status.

Although ACIP and AAP recommend use of PPSV23 (Pneumovax® 23) in individuals with CSF leaks, the manufacturer of PPSV23 (Pneumovax® 23) states that the vaccine may not be effective in preventing pneumococcal meningitis in patients who have chronic CSF leakage resulting from congenital lesions, skull fractures, or neurosurgical procedures.

Antigens in PCV13 (Prevnar 13®) are conjugated to a carrier protein and conjugated antigens are more immunogenic in infants and young children than the unconjugated antigens in PPSV23 (Pneumovax® 23). (See Pharmacology.)

Duration of Immunity Duration of protection after age-appropriate vaccination with PCV13 (Prevnar 13®) is not known. Because the capsular antigens contained in PCV13 (Prevnar 13®) are conjugated to a T-cell dependent carrier protein (diphtheria CRM_{197} protein), this may result in improved primary responses to the antigens. Revaccination with PCV13 (Prevnar 13®) after age-appropriate vaccination is not currently recommended.

Duration of protection after administration of PPSV23 (Pneumovax® 23) has not been fully determined. Because PPSV23 (Pneumovax® 23) is an unconjugated vaccine, the vaccine antigens do not induce long-lasting immunity or an anamnestic response after subsequent exposure to the same antigens. Although *routine* revaccination of immunocompetent individuals who previously received a dose of PPSV23 (Pneumovax® 23) is not recommended, revaccination may be indicated in individuals with certain medical conditions that put them at increased risk for pneumococcal disease. Revaccination with PPSV23 (Pneumovax® 23) also is recommended in adults 65 years of age or older who received a dose of the vaccine at a younger age, provided at least 5 years have elapsed since the previous dose. (See PPSV23 [Pneumovax® 23] under Dosage: Revaccination and Booster Doses, in Dosage and Administration.)

Improper Storage and Handling Improper storage or handling of vaccines may reduce vaccine potency resulting in reduced or inadequate immune responses in vaccinees.

All vaccines should be inspected upon delivery and monitored during storage to ensure that the appropriate temperature is maintained. (See Chemistry and Stability: Stability.)

Vaccine that has been mishandled or has not been stored at the recommended temperature should not be administered. If there are concerns about mishandling, the manufacturer or state or local immunization or health departments should be contacted for guidance on whether the vaccine is usable.

■ **Pediatric Precautions** Safety and efficacy of PCV13 (Prevnar 13®) have not been established in infants younger than 6 weeks of age.

The manufacturer of PCV13 (Prevnar 13®) states that the immune response to the vaccine in preterm infants has not been adequately studied to date. Although the vaccination schedule differed from the US recommended schedule, there is some evidence from a study in preterm infants (gestational age less than 37 weeks) that immunoglobulin G (IgG) antibody responses to some of the pneumococcal vaccine serotypes were lower after the third and fourth vaccine dose compared with responses in term infants (gestational age 37 weeks or greater). Because apnea has been reported following IM vaccination in some infants born prematurely, decisions regarding use of IM vaccines in such infants should be based on consideration of the individual infant's medical status and potential benefits and possible risks of vaccination.

Safety and efficacy of PPSV23 (Pneumovax® 23) have not been established in children younger than 2 years of age. Children younger than 2 years of age may not have a satisfactory antibody response to PPSV23 (Pneumovax® 23).

■ **Geriatric Precautions** Antibody responses to PCV13 (Prevnar 13®) in adults 65 years of age or older are lower compared with antibody responses in adults 50 through 59 years of age. There are no overall differences in safety outcomes in adults 65 years of age or older compared with adults 50 through 59 years of age.

Several clinical studies evaluating PPSV23 (Pneumovax® 23) included individuals 65 years of age or older. In one study, the rate of vaccine-related systemic adverse effects was similar following primary vaccination and revaccination in adults 50–64 years of age, but was higher following revaccination than primary vaccination in those 65 years of age or older. The possibility that some older adults may exhibit a higher frequency and/or greater severity of adverse reactions to the vaccine cannot be ruled out.

■ **Pregnancy and Lactation** *Pregnancy* Animal developmental and reproduction studies in female rabbits using PCV13 (Prevnar 13®) at doses 20 times the human dose based on body weight did not reveal evidence of fetal harm or impaired female fertility. There are no adequate and well-controlled studies using PCV13 (Prevnar 13®) in pregnant women, and the vaccine should be used during pregnancy only when clearly needed.

Animal reproduction studies have not been conducted with PPSV23 (Pneumovax® 23). It is not known whether PPSV23 (Pneumovax® 23) can cause fetal harm when administered to a pregnant woman or can affect reproductive capacity. PPSV23 (Pneumovax® 23) should be administered during pregnancy only when clearly needed.

ACIP, AAP, and other experts state that PPSV23 (Pneumovax® 23) may be used when indicated in pregnant women at increased risk for pneumococcal disease.

AAP states that pneumococcal vaccination generally should be deferred during pregnancy, but the risk of severe pneumococcal disease in a pregnant woman who has not received PPSV23 (Pneumovax® 23) within the previous 5 years and has an underlying medical condition that increases the risk of invasive pneumococcal disease should prompt immunization with PPSV23 (Pneumovax® 23).

Lactation It is not known if antigens contained in PCV13 (Prevnar 13®) or PPSV23 (Pneumovax® 23) are distributed into milk. The vaccines should be used with caution in nursing women.

ACIP states that, because inactivated vaccines do not multiply within the body, they should not pose any unusual problems for lactating women or their infants.

Drug Interactions

■ **Acetaminophen** In infants receiving vaccination with pneumococcal 13-valent conjugate vaccine (PCV13; Prevnar 13®), acetaminophen for prophylaxis (first dose given at the time of each vaccine dose and additional doses given every 6–8 hours) reduced the antibody response to some pneumococcal vaccine serotypes following the third dose of PCV13 (Prevnar 13®) compared with antibody responses in infants who received antipyretics only as needed for treatment. Reduced antibody responses were not observed after the fourth dose of PCV13 (Prevnar 13®) in those receiving acetaminophen prophylactically.

ACIP states that evidence does not support the use of antipyretics before or at the time of vaccination; however, antipyretics can be used for treatment of fever and local discomfort that might occur following vaccination.

■ **Immune Globulins** There is no evidence that immune globulin (immune globulin IM [IGIM], immune globulin IV [IGIV]) or specific hyperimmune globulin (hepatitis B immune globulin [HBIG], rabies immune globulin [RIG], tetanus immune globulin [TIG], varicella zoster immune globulin [VZIG]) interferes with the immune response to inactivated vaccines. The US Public Health Service Advisory Committee on Immunization Practices (ACIP) states that inactivated vaccines such as pneumococcal vaccines may be given simultaneously with (using different syringes and different injection sites) or at any interval before or after immune globulin or specific hyperimmune globulin preparations.

■ **Immunosuppressive Agents** Individuals receiving immunosuppressive therapy (e.g., alkylating agents, antimetabolites, corticosteroids, radiation) may have diminished or suboptimal antibody responses to PCV13 (Prevnar 13®) or pneumococcal 23-valent vaccine (PPSV23; Pneumovax® 23). Pneumococcal vaccination during chemotherapy or radiation therapy should be avoided. If possible, PCV13 (Prevnar 13®) or PPSV23 (Pneumovax® 23) should be administered at least 2 weeks prior to initiation of immunosuppressive therapy or should be deferred until at least 3 months after immunosuppressive therapy is discontinued. If administered during chemotherapy, the patient should be revaccinated after immune competence is regained.

■ **Vaccines** Although specific studies may not be available regarding concurrent administration with each antigen, simultaneous administration of PCV13 (Prevnar 13®) or PPSV23 (Pneumovax® 23) with other age-appropriate vaccines, including live virus vaccines, toxoids, or inactivated or recombinant vaccines, during the same health-care visit generally is not expected to affect immunologic responses or adverse reactions to any of the preparations. Immunization with pneumococcal vaccines can be integrated with immunization against diphtheria, tetanus, pertussis, *Haemophilus influenzae* type b (Hib), hepatitis A, hepatitis B, human papillomavirus (HPV), influenza, measles, mumps, rubella, meningococcal disease, poliomyelitis, rotavirus, and varicella. However, each parenteral vaccine should be administered using a different syringe and different injection site.

Diphtheria and Tetanus Toxoids and Pertussis Vaccines PCV13 (Prevnar 13®) or PPSV23 (Pneumovax® 23) may be administered concurrently with diphtheria and tetanus toxoids and acellular pertussis vaccine adsorbed (DTaP) using different syringes and different injection sites.

In clinical studies evaluating PCV13 (Prevnar 13®) in infants, the pneumococcal vaccine was administered concurrently with the first 3 doses of a fixed-combination vaccine containing DTaP (DTaP-HepB-IPV; Pediarix®) at 2, 4, and 6 months of age.

Haemophilus b Vaccines PCV13 (Prevnar 13®) or PPSV23 (Pneumovax® 23) may be administered concurrently with haemophilus b (Hib) conjugate vaccine at a different site using a separate syringe.

In clinical studies evaluating PCV13 (Prevnar 13®) in infants, the pneumococcal vaccine was administered concurrently with the first 3 doses of Hib at 2, 4, and 6 months of age.

ACIP states that the fixed-combination vaccine containing Hib conjugate vaccine and meningococcal polysaccharide groups C and Y vaccine (Hib-MenCY; MenHibrix®) may be administered concurrently with PCV13 (Prevnar 13®) in infants 2 through 18 months of age at a different site using a different syringe.

Hepatitis A Vaccine PCV13 (Prevnar 13®) or PPSV23 (Pneumovax® 23) may be administered concomitantly with hepatitis A virus vaccine inactivated using different syringes and different injection sites.

In clinical studies, hepatitis A virus vaccine inactivated was administered concurrently with the fourth dose of PCV13 (Prevnar 13®) in infants 12–15 months of age. In a study evaluating concomitant administration of hepatitis A vaccine (Havrix®) and the previously available 7-valent vaccine (PCV7; Prevnar®) in infants 15 months of age, there was no evidence of decreased immune response to any of the serotypes contained in PCV7 (Prevnar®).

Hepatitis B Vaccine PCV13 (Prevnar 13®) or PPSV23 (Pneumovax® 23) may be administered concurrently with hepatitis B virus vaccine inactivated using different syringes and different injection sites.

In clinical studies evaluating PCV13 (Prevnar 13®) in infants, the pneumococcal vaccine was administered concurrently with the first 3 doses of a fixed-combination vaccine containing hepatitis B virus vaccine (DTaP-HepB-IPV; Pediarix®) at 2, 4, and 6 months of age.

Influenza Virus Vaccine **Influenza Virus Vaccine Inactivated.** PCV13 (Prevnar 13®) or PPSV23 (Pneumovax® 23) may be administered concurrently with parenteral influenza virus vaccine inactivated using different syringes and different injection sites.

Concomitant administration of PCV13 (Prevnar 13®) and parenteral influenza virus vaccine inactivated (using different syringes and different injection sites) in adults 50 years of age or older resulted in similar frequencies of local reactions at the injection site compared with administration of PCV13 (Prevnar 13®) alone. However, there was an increase in some solicited systemic reactions when PCV13 (Prevnar 13®) and parenteral influenza virus vaccine inactivated were administered concomitantly compared with administration of the influenza vaccine alone (headache, chills, rash, decreased appetite, muscle and joint pain) or the pneumococcal vaccine alone (fatigue, headache, chills, decreased appetite, joint pain).

There have been some reports of an increased incidence of adverse local and systemic effects when PPSV23 (Pneumovax® 23) was administered concomitantly with influenza virus vaccine inactivated (at a different injection site) compared with administration of influenza virus vaccine inactivated alone, but these reactions generally were mild and well tolerated and do not preclude simultaneous administration of the vaccines at different sites. ACIP states that concomitant administration of PPSV23 (Pneumovax® 23) and parenteral influenza virus vaccine inactivated results in satisfactory antibody responses without increasing the incidence or severity of adverse reactions.

Influenza Vaccine Live Intranasal. Concomitant administration of pneumococcal vaccines and influenza vaccine live intranasal has not been specifically studied. ACIP states that, in the absence of specific data indicating interference, inactivated vaccines can be administered simultaneously with or at any interval before or after influenza vaccine live intranasal.

Measles, Mumps, Rubella, and Varicella Vaccines PCV13 (Prevnar 13®) or PPSV23 (Pneumovax® 23) and measles, mumps, and rubella virus vaccine live (MMR) or varicella virus vaccine live may be administered concurrently (using different syringes and different injection sites).

In clinical studies evaluating PCV13 (Prevnar 13®) in infants, MMR and varicella virus vaccine live or, alternatively, the fixed-combination vaccine containing MMR and varicella virus vaccine live (MMRV; ProQuad®) was administered concurrently with the fourth dose of PCV13 (Prevnar 13®) in infants 12–15 months of age.

Meningococcal Vaccines The manufacturer of PCV13 (Prevnar 13®) states that data are insufficient to assess concomitant administration with meningococcal (groups A, C, Y and W-135) polysaccharide diphtheria toxoid conjugate vaccine (MCV4-D, MenACWY-D; Menactra®) or meningococcal (groups A, C, Y and W-135) oligosaccharide diphtheria CRM_{197} conjugate vaccine (MCV4-CRM, MenACWY-CRM; Menveo®) in children and adolescents.

Concurrent administration of pneumococcal 7-valent conjugate vaccine (PCV7; Prevnar®; no longer commercially available in the US) with the second dose of MCV4-D (Menactra®) in infants 12 months of age resulted in a decreased immune response to PCV7 (i.e., noninferiority criteria were not met for 3 of the 7 pneumococcal vaccine serotypes compared with administration of PCV7 without MCV4-D).

When PCV7 (Prevnar®) was administered concurrently with MCV4-CRM (Menveo®) in infants at 2, 4, 6, and 12 months of age, there was some evidence of interference with the antibody response to 2 of the pneumococcal vaccine serotypes at 1 month after the third dose, but there was no evidence of immune interference to any of the pneumococcal vaccine serotypes after the fourth dose.

ACIP and AAP state that MCV4-D (Menactra®) should not be administered concurrently with or within 4 weeks after PCV13 (Prevnar 13®). To avoid possible interference with the immune response to PCV13 in infants and children with anatomic or functional asplenia, the PCV13 immunization series should be completed first and MCV4-D (Menactra®) administered at least 4 weeks later.

PPSV23 (Pneumovax® 23) can be administered concurrently with MCV4 (Menactra®, Menveo®) or MPSV4 (Menomune®) at a different site using a different syringe.

ACIP states that the fixed-combination vaccine containing meningococcal polysaccharide groups C and Y vaccine and Hib conjugate vaccine (Hib-MenCY; MenHibrix®) may be administered concurrently with PCV13 (Prevnar 13®) in infants 2 through 18 months of age at a different site using a different syringe.

Poliovirus Vaccine Inactivated PCV13 (Prevnar 13®) or PPSV23 (Pneumovax® 23) may be given concurrently with poliovirus vaccine inactivated (IPV) using different syringes and different injection sites.

In clinical studies evaluating PCV13 (Prevnar 13®) in infants, the pneumococcal vaccine was administered concurrently with the first 3 doses of a fixed-combination vaccine containing IPV (DTaP-HepB-IPV; Pediarix®) at 2, 4, and 6 months of age.

Rotavirus Vaccines PCV13 (Prevnar 13®) may be given concurrently with rotavirus vaccine live oral (Rotarix®, RotaTeq®).

Rotavirus vaccine live oral (Rotarix®, RotaTeq®) has been administered concomitantly with the previously available 7-valent vaccine (PCV7; Prevnar®) without a decrease in immune response to either vaccine.

Zoster Vaccine The manufacturer of zoster vaccine live and PPSV23 (Pneumovax® 23) states that consideration should be given to administering these 2 vaccines at least 4 weeks apart.

Data from a randomized, double-blind, controlled study in adults 60 years of age or older indicate that concurrent administration of zoster vaccine live and PPSV23 (Pneumovax® 23) resulted in reduced antibody response to zoster vaccine live compared with that reported when the vaccines were administered 4 weeks apart. When assessed using representative pneumococcal serotypes (3, 14, 19A, 22F), the antibody response to PPSV23 (Pneumovax® 23) following concomitant administration was similar to that reported when the vaccines were administered 4 weeks apart. Concurrent administration of zoster vaccine live and PPSV23 (Pneumovax® 23) did not result in a clinically important increase in adverse effects compared with administration during separate visits (4 weeks apart).

Pharmacology

Pneumococcal 13-valent conjugate vaccine (PCV13; Prevnar 13®) and pneumococcal vaccine, polyvalent (pneumococcal 23-valent vaccine; PPSV23; Pneumovax® 23) are used to stimulate active immunity to infection caused by the serotypes of *Streptococcus pneumoniae* contained in the vaccines.

S. pneumoniae is a common cause of acute otitis media (AOM), sinusitis, and pneumonia and can cause invasive disease, including bacteremia and meningitis. In the US, infection with *S. pneumoniae* has been a leading cause of bacterial meningitis among children younger than 5 years of age. The principal mode of transmission of pneumococcal infection is the respiratory route, most commonly through close personal contact with an individual with invasive pneumococcal disease or direct exposure to nasopharyngeal secretions from an infected individual or by autoinoculation in persons carrying the bacteria in their upper respiratory tract. Onset of pneumonia usually is sudden with signs and symptoms including fever, chills, pleuritic chest pain, productive cough, dyspnea, tachypnea, hypoxia, tachycardia, malaise, and weakness; headache, nausea, and vomiting occur less frequently.

■ Response to Pneumococcal 13-valent Conjugate Vaccine (PCV13; Prevnar 13®) The capsular saccharides present in PCV13 (Prevnar 13®) promote production of antibody specific for each pneumococcal capsular type in the vaccine. PCV13 (Prevnar 13®) elicits a T-cell dependent immune response. Protein carrier-specific T-cells provide the signals needed for maturation of the B-cell response. Antibodies produced in response to pneumococcal conjugate vaccines enhance opsonization, phagocytosis, and killing of *S. pneumoniae* by leukocytes and other phagocytic cells.

Nonclinical and clinical data support opsonophagocytic activity, as measured by opsonophagocytic activity (OPA) antibody assay, as a contributor to protection against pneumococcal disease. The OPA antibody assay provides an in vitro measurement of the ability of serum antibodies to eliminate pneumococci by promoting complement-mediated phagocytosis and is believed to reflect relevant in vivo mechanisms of protection against pneumococcal disease. In infants who receive PCV13 (Prevnar 13®), opsonophagocytic activity correlates well with serotype specific anticapsular polysaccharide immunoglobulin G (IgG) levels as measured by enzyme-linked immunosorbent assay (ELISA). A serum anticapsular polysaccharide antibody concentration of at least 0.35 mcg/mL as measured by ELISA 1 month after the third dose of a single antibody reference concentration has been used to estimate the effectiveness of PCV13 (Prevnar 13®) against invasive pneumococcal disease in infants and children. An antipolysaccharide binding antibody IgG level to predict protection against invasive pneumococcal disease or nonbacteremic pneumonia has not been defined in adults.

In a US noninferiority study that evaluated the response to PCV13 (Prevnar 13®) and PCV7 (Prevnar®) in healthy infants who received a 4-dose vaccination series (3 primary doses given at 2, 4, and 6 months of age and a fourth dose given at 12–15 months of age), responses to 10 of the 13 serotypes in PCV13 (Prevnar 13®) measured 1 month after the third dose met the primary endpoint criterion. Approximately 87–98% of the infants had anticapsular IgG antibody concentrations of at least 0.35 mcg/mL for 12 of the 13 pneumococcal serotypes in the vaccine; only 63.5% of the infants achieved an antibody concentration of at least 0.35 mcg/mL against serotype 3. When determined 1 month after the third dose of PCV13 (Prevnar 13®), functional antibody responses as measures by OPA were reported for all 13 vaccine serotypes. These immunologic parameters generally indicated that PCV13 (Prevnar 13®) induced antibody concentrations comparable to those induced by PCV7 (Prevnar®) and protective against invasive pneumococcal disease. When the immune response 1 month after the fourth dose of PCV13 (Prevnar 13®) was compared with the response 1 month after the third primary dose, geometric mean concentrations (GMCs) of anticapsular IgG antibody were higher for all 13 serotypes and geometric mean titers (GMTs) of functional antibody were greater for all 13 serotypes. After the fourth dose of vaccine, antibody responses to 12 of the 13 serotypes met the primary endpoint criterion; the response to serotype 3 did not meet this criterion.

The response to a single dose of PCV13 (Prevnar 13®) in children 5 through 17 years of age was evaluated in a US open-label study. In children 5 through 9 years of age who had previously received at least 1 dose of PCV7 (Prevnar®), serotype-specific IgG concentrations measured 1 month after the PCV13 (Prevnar 13®) dose were noninferior to the response reported in toddlers 1 month after a fourth dose of pneumococcal vaccine (after the fourth dose of PCV7 (Prevnar®) for the 7 common serotypes and after the fourth dose of PCV13 (Prevnar 13®) for the 6 additional serotypes). In children 10 through 17 years of age who had not previously received any pneumococcal vaccine, OPA GMTs 1 month after the PCV13 (Prevnar 13®) dose were noninferior to functional OPA antibody responses reported in children 5 through 9 years of age for 12 of 13 serotypes, but not for serotype 3.

Immunogenicity of PCV13 (Prevnar 13®) in adults has been evaluated in various studies that included healthy adults and immunocompetent adults with stable underlying medical conditions or behaviors known to increase the risk of serious pneumococcal pneumonia and invasive pneumococcal disease (e.g., chronic cardiovascular disease, chronic pulmonary disease, renal disorders, diabetes mellitus, chronic liver disease, alcoholism, smoking). In 2 noninferiority trials, the immune response to a single dose of PCV13 (Prevnar 13®) was compared with the immune response to PPSV23 (Pneumovax® 23) in previously unvaccinated adults 50 through 64 years of age or in adults 70 years of age or older who had received at least 1 dose of PPSV23 (Pneumovax® 23) at least 5 years previously. PCV13 (Prevnar 13®) elicited functional OPA antibody responses in adults 60 through 64 years of age that were noninferior to those induced by PPSV23 (Pneumovax® 23) for the 12 serotypes in common to both vaccines; PCV13 also elicited functional OPA antibody GMTs in adults 50 through 59 years of age that were noninferior to the corresponding functional OPA antibody GMTs elicited by PCV13 (Prevnar 13®) in adults 60 through 64 years of age. In adults 70 years of age who had received PPSV23 (Pneumovax® 23) at least 5 years previously, vaccination with PCV13 (Prevnar 13®) elicited immune responses that were noninferior to those elicited by revaccination with PPSV23 (Pneumovax® 23).

Data are limited to date regarding the immunogenicity of PCV13 (Prevnar 13®) in children and adults at increased risk of pneumococcal disease, including those with sickle cell disease, asplenia, or human immunodeficiency virus (HIV) infection.

Duration of Immunity The duration of protection following administration of PCV13 (Prevnar 13®) is not known.

The extent and duration of immunologic response may vary depending on age and immunocompetence of the vaccinee. Antigens in PCV13 (Prevnar 13®) are conjugated to a carrier protein and are more immunogenic in infants and young children than the unconjugated antigens in PPSV23 (Pneumovax® 23).

■ **Response to Pneumococcal 23-valent Vaccine (PPSV23; Pneumovax® 23)** The capsular polysaccharides present in PPSV23 (Pneumovax® 23) promote production of antibody specific for each pneumococcal capsular type in the vaccine. These antibodies enhance opsonization, phagocytosis, and killing of *S. pneumoniae* by leukocytes and other phagocytic cells. Although the immune response to PPSV23 (Pneumovax® 23) generally has been evaluated using quantitative measurements of antibodies, antibody levels that correlate with protections against pneumococcal disease have not been clearly defined.

Following administration of a single dose of PPSV23 (Pneumovax® 23) in healthy adults, more than 80% develop antibodies specific for the pneumococcal capsular types present in the vaccine, usually within 2–3 weeks. The antibody response to the pneumococcal capsular polysaccharides contained in PPSV23 (Pneumovax® 23) generally is poor or inconsistent in infants younger than 2 years of age.

A retrospective cohort analysis study based on US Centers for Disease Control and Prevention (CDC) pneumococcal surveillance data indicated that the overall protective effectiveness of PPSV23 (Pneumovax® 23) against invasive pneumococcal infection caused by serotypes included in the vaccine was 57% in individuals 6 years of age or older, 65–84% among specific patient groups (e.g., those with diabetes mellitus, coronary vascular disease, congestive heart failure, chronic pulmonary disease, and anatomic asplenia), and 75% in immunocompetent adults 65 years of age or older.

Individuals with immunodeficiency diseases (e.g., hypogammaglobulinemia, leukemia, lymphoma, multiple myeloma), individuals receiving immunosuppressive therapy (see Drug Interactions: Immunosuppressive Agents), and individuals with Hodgkin's disease who have received extensive chemotherapy, radiation therapy, and splenectomy may have diminished or suboptimal antibody responses to PPSV23 (Pneumovax® 23).

Duration of Immunity The duration of protection following administration of PPSV23 (Pneumovax® 23) is not known.

Following administration of PPSV23 (Pneumovax® 23) in healthy adults, antibodies formed in response to the vaccine remain elevated for at least 5 years, but antibody levels decline after 5–10 years. Antibody levels decline more rapidly in individuals with certain underlying illnesses, including those who have undergone splenectomy following trauma and those with sickle cell disease or nephrotic syndrome.

Antigens contained in PPSV23 (Pneumovax® 23) cannot induce long-lasting immunity, since they do not induce T-cell-dependent responses associated with immunologic memory.

Chemistry and Stability

■ **Chemistry** Pneumococcal vaccine is commercially available in the US as 2 different vaccine types: pneumococcal 13-valent conjugate vaccine (PCV13; Prevnar 13®) and pneumococcal vaccine, polyvalent (pneumococcal 23-valent vaccine; PPSV23; Pneumovax® 23). Although both vaccines contain capsular antigens extracted from *Streptococcus pneumoniae*, the vaccines contain different numbers and forms of these antigens. PPSV23 (Pneumovax® 23) contains purified capsular polysaccharides from 23 different serotypes of *S. pneumoniae*. PCV13 (Prevnar 13®) contains purified capsular saccharide antigens from 13 different serotypes of the organism and these antigens are conjugated to a T-cell dependent carrier protein (diphtheria CRM_{197} protein). Pneumococcal capsular antigens conjugated to a carrier protein are more immunogenic in infants and young children than the unconjugated capsular antigens contained in PPSV23 (Pneumovax® 23).

Pneumococcal 13-valent Conjugate Vaccine (PCV13; Prevnar 13®) PCV13 (Prevnar 13®) is a sterile suspension containing purified capsular saccharide antigens extracted from 13 serotypes of *S. pneumoniae* and individually conjugated to diphtheria CRM_{197}. PCV13 (Prevnar 13®) contains the following 13 capsular saccharide serotypes: 1, 3, 4, 5, 6A, 6B, 7F, 9V, 14, 18C, 19A, 19F, and 23F. Each serotype of *S. pneumoniae* is cultured in soy peptone broth and the individual polysaccharides are purified using centrifugation, precipitation, ultrafiltration, and column chromatography. The polysaccharides are chemically inactivated to make saccharides and these are directly conjugated by reductive amination to the protein carrier (diphtheria CRM_{197}) to form the glycoconjugate. Potency of the vaccine is determined by quantification of each of the saccharide antigens and by the saccharide to protein ratios in the individual glycoconjugates. After shaking, PCV13 (Prevnar 13®) occurs as a homogeneous white suspension.

Pneumococcal 23-valent Vaccine (PPSV23; Pneumovax® 23) PPSV23 (Pneumovax® 23) is a sterile solution containing purified capsular polysaccharide antigens extracted from 23 different serotypes of *S. pneumoniae*. PPSV23 (Pneumovax® 23) contains the following 23 capsular polysaccharide serotypes: 1, 2, 3, 4, 5, 6B, 7F, 8, 9N, 9V, 10A, 11A, 12F, 14, 15B, 17F, 18C, 19F, 19A, 20, 22F, 23F, and 33F. PPSV23 (Pneumovax® 23) occurs as a clear, colorless solution.

Each 0.5-mL dose of PPSV23 (Pneumovax® 23) contains 25 mcg of each type of capsular polysaccharide antigen in 0.9% sodium chloride injection. The vaccine does not contain thimerosal, but does contain phenol as a preservative.

■ **Stability** ***Pneumococcal 13-valent Conjugate Vaccine (PCV13; Prevnar 13®)*** PCV13 (Prevnar 13®) should be stored at 2–8°C; after shipping, the vaccine may arrive at temperatures ranging from 2–25°C.

PCV13 (Prevnar 13®) should not be frozen. Since the vaccine contains an aluminum adjuvant, exposure to freezing temperatures causes irreversible loss of vaccine potency.

Pneumococcal 23-valent Vaccine (PPSV23; Pneumovax® 23) PPSV23 (Pneumovax® 23) should be stored at 2–8°C.

Preparations

Excipients in commercially available drug preparations may have clinically important effects in some individuals; consult specific product labeling for details.

Pneumococcal 13-valent Conjugate Vaccine (Diphtheria CRM_{197} Protein) (PCV13)

Parenteral	
Injection	**Prevnar 13®**, Wyeth

Pneumococcal Vaccine, Polyvalent (PPSV23)

Parenteral	
Injection	**Pneumovax® 23**, Merck

†Use is not currently included in the labeling approved by the US Food and Drug Administration

Rotavirus Vaccine Live Oral

■ Rotavirus vaccine is commercially available in the US as a monovalent live, attenuated virus vaccine derived from a human rotavirus strain (Rotarix®; RV1) and as a pentavalent live virus vaccine containing 5 live, reassortant rotaviruses derived from human and bovine hosts (RotaTeq®; RV5). Some other rotavirus vaccines (e.g., other monovalent or multivalent human-animal reassortant vaccines) are being investigated or may be available in other countries.

Uses

■ **Prevention of Rotavirus Gastroenteritis** Rotavirus vaccine live oral (Rotarix®; RV1) is used to prevent gastroenteritis caused by rotavirus type G1 and non-G1 types (G3, G4, G9).

Rotavirus vaccine live oral pentavalent (RotaTeq®; RV5) is used to prevent gastroenteritis caused by rotavirus types G1, G2, G3, G4, and G9.

Prior to widespread use of rotavirus vaccines, rotavirus was the most common cause of severe gastroenteritis in infants and young children, the most common cause of healthcare-associated diarrhea in young children, and an important cause of acute gastroenteritis in children attending child-care centers. Worldwide, rotavirus gastroenteritis was the cause of approximately 500,000 deaths each year in children younger than 5 years of age. In the US, rotavirus gastroenteritis was estimated to cause up to 70,000 hospitalizations and up to 60–70 deaths each year in children younger than 5 years of age.

After rotavirus vaccine (RotaTeq®) was licensed in the US in 2006, there was a marked decrease in the incidence of rotavirus disease and substantial changes in the epidemiology of the disease. A second rotavirus vaccine (Rotarix®) was licensed in the US in 2008. Surveillance data collected by the US Centers for Disease Control and Prevention (CDC) National Respiratory and Enteric Virus Surveillance System (NREVSS) indicated that the 2007–2008 and 2008–2009 rotavirus seasons were shorter, had a later onset, and had substantially fewer reports of positive rotavirus test results compared with the 2000–2006 seasons. Additional NREVSS data indicated that the national decline in rotavirus detection ranged from 58–90% in each of the 7 postvaccine years (2007–2014) compared with all 7 prevaccine years (2000–2006) combined and there was a biennial pattern of rotavirus activity with alternating years of lower or greater activity. Although onset of rotavirus season and duration of the season varied in different regions of the US, most seasons within each region were of shorter duration with decreased rotavirus activity compared with prevaccine years. There also is some evidence that rotavirus vaccination may provide clinical benefits to both vaccinated and unvaccinated individuals by reducing overall rotavirus transmission (i.e., herd immunity).

The US Public Health Service Advisory Committee on Immunization Practices (ACIP) and American Academy of Pediatrics (AAP) recommend that *all* infants be vaccinated against rotavirus gastroenteritis beginning at 6 weeks of age, unless contraindicated. These experts state that the first dose of the rotavirus vaccination series should be given at 6 through 14 weeks of age (no later than 14 weeks 6 days of age) and the vaccination series should be completed by 8 months 0 days of age.

ACIP and AAP do not state a preference for Rotarix® or RotaTeq® vaccine for primary immunization in infants. There is evidence that efficacy and safety of the vaccines are similar. However, dosage and dosing schedule (i.e., number and timing of doses) differ depending on which vaccine is used. (See Dosage and Administration: Dosage.)

Data are not available regarding efficacy and safety of rotavirus vaccine for postexposure prophylaxis following exposure to natural rotavirus.

Clinical Experience **Rotavirus Vaccine Live Oral (Rotarix®).** Safety and efficacy of Rotarix® for prevention of rotavirus gastroenteritis have been evaluated in several randomized, placebo-controlled, multinational studies that included healthy infants from Europe and Latin America. These infants received a 2-dose series of Rotarix® (initial dose given at 6–14 weeks of age, second dose given at least 4 weeks after the first dose) that was generally completed by 24 weeks of age.

In a European study that involved 3994 infants, efficacy of Rotarix® in preventing rotavirus gastroenteritis (any grade of severity) from 2 weeks following vaccination through the first rotavirus season was 87%, and efficacy in preventing severe rotavirus gastroenteritis through the first rotavirus season was 96%. In a Latin American study that involved more than 15,000 infants, efficacy of Rotarix® in preventing severe rotavirus gastroenteritis from 2 weeks following vaccination up to 1 year of age was 83%. There was a 100% reduction in hospitalizations for rotavirus gastroenteritis in the European infants through the first rotavirus season, and an 85% reduction in hospitalizations for this infection in the Latin American infants up to 1 year of age.

In the European study, Rotarix® was 79% effective in preventing rotavirus gastroenteritis (any grade of severity) from 2 weeks following vaccination through the second rotavirus season. In the Latin American study, vaccine efficacy was 80.5% in preventing severe rotavirus gastroenteritis from the time of the first dose up to 2 years of age. Efficacy of Rotarix® beyond the second rotavirus season following vaccination has not been evaluated to date.

Efficacy of Rotarix® in preventing any grade of severity and severe rotavirus gastroenteritis based on the specific type (i.e., G1, G3, G4, G9, and combined non-G1) was statistically significant compared with placebo through 1 year following vaccination. In addition, efficacy against any grade of severity and severe rotavirus gastroenteritis caused by G1, G2, G3, G4, G9, and combined non-G1 types was statistically significant compared with placebo through 2 years following vaccination.

Rotavirus Vaccine Live Oral Pentavalent (RotaTeq®). RotaTeq® has been evaluated in 4 placebo-controlled, phase 3 studies that included 73,086 infants. Efficacy of the vaccine for preventing rotavirus gastroenteritis was demonstrated in 7,744 infants who were enrolled in 3 of these studies (Rotavirus Efficacy and Safety Trial [REST; study 006]; study 007; study 029). An additional placebo-controlled, phase 3 trial (study 009) contributed data to the overall safety evaluation of RotaTeq®.

Study 006 and study 007 included 6983 healthy infants in the US and Finland who received a 3-dose series of RotaTeq® (initial dose given at 6–12 weeks of age, second and third doses given at 4- to 10-week intervals with the third dose given by 32 weeks of age). Efficacy of the vaccine in preventing rotavirus gastroenteritis caused by naturally occurring types G1, G2, G3, or G4 (any grade of severity occurring at least 14 days after the third vaccine dose through the first rotavirus season following vaccination) was 74% in study 006 and 72.5% in study 007. Vaccine efficacy in preventing severe rotavirus gastroenteritis caused by these types (occurring through the first rotavirus season following vaccination) in study 006 and study 007 was 98 and 100%, respectively. In study 006, vaccine efficacy was 62.6% against any grade of severity of rotavirus gastroenteritis caused by these types during the second rotavirus season after vaccination and there was a 95.8% reduction in hospitalizations for severe rotavirus gastroenteritis caused by types G1, G2, G3, and G4 during the first 2 years following the final dose of RotaTeq®. Vaccine efficacy beyond the second rotavirus season after vaccination has not been fully evaluated to date.

Dosage and Administration

■ **Reconstitution and Administration** Rotavirus vaccine live oral (Rotarix®; RV1) and rotavirus vaccine live oral pentavalent (RotaTeq®; RV5) are administered orally.

The vaccines are for oral use only and should *not* be given by IM, IV, or subcutaneous injection.

Rotavirus vaccine should *not* be mixed with any other vaccine or solution.

There is no need to restrict food or liquid intake, including breast milk, either before or after administration of rotavirus vaccine.

Rotavirus vaccine may be given simultaneously with other age-appropriate vaccines during the same health-care visit. (See Drug Interactions: Vaccines.)

Rotavirus Vaccine Live Oral (Rotarix®; RV1) Rotarix® lyophilized vaccine should be reconstituted using the diluent and transfer adapter provided by the manufacturer. Reconstituted Rotarix® is a white, turbid suspension.

Following reconstitution, Rotarix® is administered orally directly into the infant's mouth from the oral applicator supplied by the manufacturer.

If an incomplete dose is given (e.g., infant spits or regurgitates during or after vaccine dose), the manufacturer states that a single replacement dose may be considered at the same vaccination visit. However, the US Public Health Service Advisory Committee on Immunization Practices (ACIP) and American Academy of Pediatrics (AAP) do *not* recommend a replacement dose if an incomplete dose is given since data are not available on the benefits or risks associated with readministration. The infant should receive the remaining dose in the recommended 2-dose series at the usually recommended interval (minimum interval 4 weeks between doses).

Single-dose vials of lyophilized Rotarix® for oral suspension should be stored at 2–8°C and protected from light. The diluent supplied by the manufacturer should be stored at 2–8°C or at room temperature (up to 25°C); the diluent should be protected from freezing and should be discarded if frozen. Reconstituted Rotarix® may be stored for up to 24 hours at 2–8°C or at room temperature (up to 25°C). The reconstituted vaccine should be discarded if exposed to freezing temperatures or if not used within 24 hours.

Rotarix® does not contain thimerosal or any other preservatives.

Rotavirus Vaccine Live Oral Pentavalent (RotaTeq®; RV5) RotaTeq® is administered orally directly from the single-dose tubing supplied by the manufacturer. The dose should be administered by gently squeezing the entire contents of the tubing into the infant's mouth toward the inner cheek. A residual drop may remain in the tip of the dosing tube.

If an incomplete dose is administered (e.g., infant spits or regurgitates during or after vaccine dose), a replacement dose is *not* recommended by the manufacturer, ACIP, or AAP since data are not available on the benefits or risks associated with readministration. The infant should continue to receive any remaining doses in the recommended 3-dose series at usually recommended intervals (minimum interval 4 weeks between doses).

RotaTeq® oral solution is a pale yellow, clear liquid that may have a pink tint. The vaccine should be stored at 2–8°C and protected from light. To minimize loss of potency and ensure an adequate immunizing dose, the vaccine should be administered as soon as possible following removal from refrigeration.

RotaTeq® does not contain thimerosal or any other preservatives.

■ **Dosage** Dosage and dosing schedule (i.e., number and timing of doses) differ depending on the specific vaccine (Rotarix® or RotaTeq®) administered. *Dosage recommendations for the specific vaccine used should be followed.*

Data not available regarding interchangeability of rotavirus vaccines. The specific rotavirus vaccine (Rotarix® or RotaTeq®) used for the initial dose should be used to complete the vaccination series, whenever possible. If the specific rotavirus vaccine used for previous doses is unknown or unavailable, the vaccination series should be continued or completed with the currently available rotavirus vaccine; vaccination should not be deferred.

If RotaTeq® or an unknown rotavirus vaccine was administered for any dose in the vaccination series, a total of 3 primary doses should be administered to complete the series.

ACIP and AAP state that the first dose of rotavirus vaccine should be given at 6 weeks through 14 weeks of age (up to 14 weeks 6 days of age). Because of insufficient data, ACIP and AAP state that the vaccination series should *not* be initiated in infants who are 15 weeks of age or older. If the first dose of rotavirus vaccine is inadvertently administered to an infant 15 weeks of age or older, the remainder of the series should be completed according to the usually recommended vaccination schedule since timing of the first vaccine dose should not affect the safety and efficacy of subsequent doses.

Preterm infants who are medically stable should receive rotavirus vaccine at the usual chronologic age using the usual dosage, provided the vaccine is administered to the age-eligible infant after or at the time of discharge from the neonatal intensive care unit (NICU) or hospital nursery. Possible risk of transmission of rotavirus vaccine virus to other hospitalized infants outweigh benefits of vaccination in age-eligible infants who will remain in the NICU or hospital nursery after the dose. (See Pediatric Use under Warnings/Precautions: Specific Populations, in Cautions.)

Because natural rotavirus infection frequently provides only partial immunity, ACIP and AAP recommend that the rotavirus vaccination series be initiated or completed in infants who had rotavirus gastroenteritis before receiving the complete series.

Prevention of Rotavirus Gastroenteritis **Infants 6–24 Weeks of Age (Rotarix®; RV1).** Rotarix® is given in a series of 2 doses. Each dose consists of the entire contents of the reconstituted single-dose vial.

The manufacturer recommends that the initial dose of Rotarix® be given at 6 weeks of age and the second dose given at least 4 weeks after the first dose. In addition, the manufacturer recommends that the 2-dose vaccination series be completed by 6 months (24 weeks) of age.

ACIP and AAP recommend that infants receive a dose of Rotarix® at 2 and 4 months of age with a minimum interval of 4 weeks between doses. These experts state that the maximum age for the final dose in the 2-dose vaccination series is 8 months 0 days of age.

Infants 6–32 Weeks of Age (RotaTeq®; RV5). RotaTeq® is given orally in a series of 3 doses. Each dose consists of the entire contents of the commercially available single-dose tubing containing the vaccine.

The manufacturer recommends that the initial dose of RotaTeq® be given at 6–12 weeks of age and the remaining 2 doses given at 4- to 10-week intervals. In addition, the manufacturer states that the third dose should *not* be given after 32 weeks of age.

ACIP and AAP recommend that infants receive a dose of RotaTeq® at 2, 4, and 6 months of age with a minimum interval of 4 weeks between doses. These experts state that the maximum age for the final dose in the 3-dose vaccination series is 8 months 0 days of age.

Specific Populations

■ **Dosage in Hepatic Impairment** No specific dosage recommendations.

■ **Dosage in Renal Impairment** No specific dosage recommendations.

Geriatric Patients Not indicated in adults, including geriatric adults.

Cautions

■ **Contraindications** Rotavirus vaccine live oral (Rotarix®; RV1) is contraindicated in infants with known hypersensitivity to the vaccine or any vaccine component (e.g., latex). Rotarix® also is contraindicated in infants with a history of intussusception (a type of bowel obstruction that occurs when the bowel folds in on itself) or with a history of uncorrected congenital malformation of the GI tract (e.g., Meckel's diverticulum) that would predispose an infant to intussusception. In addition, the vaccine is contraindicated in infants with severe combined immunodeficiency disease (SCID).

Rotavirus vaccine live oral pentavalent (RotaTeq®; RV5) is contraindicated in infants with known hypersensitivity to the vaccine or any vaccine component. RotaTeq® also is contraindicated in infants with a history of intussusception. In addition, the vaccine is contraindicated in infants with SCID.

■ **Warnings/Precautions** ***Sensitivity Reactions*** **Hypersensitivity Reactions.** Anaphylactic reactions have been reported following administration of rotavirus vaccine (RotaTeq®). Urticaria and angioedema also have been reported.

Prior to administration of rotavirus vaccine, the clinician should review the infant's immunization history to determine whether there is a history of hypersensitivity or other reactions to any vaccine components.

Infants who develop symptoms suggestive of hypersensitivity after receiving a dose of rotavirus vaccine should *not* receive any further doses of the vaccine.

Appropriate medical treatment and supervision must be available to manage possible anaphylactic reactions following administration of rotavirus vaccine.

Latex Sensitivity. A packaging component of Rotarix® (i.e., tip cap of the oral applicator containing diluent) contains natural rubber latex, which may cause hypersensitivity reactions in susceptible individuals. Rotarix® vial stoppers are *not* made with natural rubber latex.

The US Public Health Service Advisory Committee on Immunization Practices (ACIP) states that vaccines supplied in vials or syringes containing dry natural rubber or natural rubber latex may be administered to individuals with latex allergies other than anaphylactic allergies (e.g., history of contact allergy to latex gloves), but should *not* be used in those with a history of severe (anaphylactic) allergy to latex, unless the benefits of vaccination outweigh the risk of a potential allergic reaction.

Use of RotaTeq® (which is latex-free) should be considered as an alternative to Rotarix® in infants with severe allergy to latex. Some experts prefer that infants with spina bifida or bladder exstrophy, who are at high risk for acquiring latex allergy, receive RotaTeq® as an alternative to Rotarix® to minimize latex exposure. However, ACIP and the American Academy of Pediatrics (AAP) state that Rotarix® should be administered if it is the only rotavirus vaccine available since the benefits of rotavirus vaccination are considered to be greater than the risk for latex sensitization.

Individuals with Altered Immunocompetence Safety and efficacy of Rotarix® or RotaTeq® have *not* been established in immunocompromised or potentially immunocompromised infants. Examples of such infants include those with blood dyscrasias, leukemia, lymphomas of any type, or other malignant neoplasms affecting the bone marrow or lymphatic system; those receiving immunosuppressive therapy (see Drug Interactions: Immunosuppressive Agents); those with primary and acquired immunodeficiency states such as human immunodeficiency virus (HIV) infection, cellular immune deficiencies, or hypogammaglobulinemic and dysgammaglobulinemic states; and those of indeterminate HIV status born to HIV-infected mothers (HIV-exposed).

There have been postmarketing reports of vaccine-acquired rotavirus gastroenteritis, including severe diarrhea and prolonged shedding of vaccine virus, in infants who received Rotarix® or RotaTeq® and were subsequently diagnosed with SCID. Some of these infants continued to shed vaccine virus for 5–12 months. Rotarix® and RotaTeq® are contraindicated in infants with SCID.

The potential risks and benefits of administering rotavirus vaccine to infants with known or suspected altered immunocompetence should be considered. Consultation with an immunologist or infectious diseases specialist is advised.

ACIP, AAP, US Centers for Disease Control and Prevention (CDC), National Institutes of Health (NIH), HIV Medicine Association of the Infectious Diseases Society of America (IDSA), and Pediatric Infectious Diseases Society state that use of rotavirus vaccine in HIV-infected or HIV-exposed infants is supported since HIV diagnosis in infants born to HIV-infected mothers may not be established before the recommended age for the first dose of the vaccine, only 1.5–3% of HIV-exposed infants in the US will eventually be determined to be HIV infected, and the rotavirus strains used in the vaccines are considerably attenuated. Limited data to date indicate that the safety profile of rotavirus vaccine reported in clinically asymptomatic or mildly symptomatic HIV-infected infants is similar to that in infants without HIV infection.

Intussusception Cases of intussusception, including some fatalities, have been reported rarely in infants who received Rotarix® or RotaTeq®. Although data from initial clinical trials of these 2 vaccines did not suggest an increased risk of intussusception relative to placebo, there is postmarketing evidence that rotavirus vaccines are associated with an increased risk of intussusception, particularly during the first week after the first vaccine dose.

In a postmarketing observational study in Mexico, cases of intussusception were observed in temporal association (within 31 days) following the first dose of Rotarix®, with a clustering of cases in the first 7 days. Other postmarketing observational studies in Brazil and Australia also suggest an increased risk of intussusception within the first 7 days following the second dose of Rotarix®. (See Rotarix® [RV1] under Warnings/Precautions: Intussusception, in Cautions.)

In a postmarketing observational study in the US, cases of intussusception were observed in temporal association (within 21 days) following the first dose of RotaTeq®, with a clustering of cases in the first 7 days. Cases of intussusception in temporal association with RotaTeq® also were reported in worldwide passive postmarketing experience. (See RotaTeq® [RV5] under Warnings/Precautions: Intussusception, in Cautions.)

A previously available rotavirus vaccine live oral containing tetravalent human-rhesus reassortant rotaviruses (RotaShield®; Wyeth) was voluntarily withdrawn from the US market in October 1999 following postmarketing reports of intussusception in infants who received the vaccine. Data indicated that the period of highest risk of intussusception associated with RotaShield® was the first 42 days following the initial vaccine dose.

Infants receiving rotavirus vaccine should be closely monitored for intussusception, particularly during the first week following vaccination. Any cases of intussusception or other serious events possibly associated with the vaccine should be reported to VAERS at 800-822-7967 or http://www.vaers.hhs.gov/.

Rotarix® and RotaTeq® are contraindicated in infants with a history of intussusception. During postmarketing experience, intussusception resulting in death was reported when a second dose of Rotarix® was given to an infant with a history of intussusception after the first dose.

Rotarix® (RV1). In a randomized study conducted in Latin America and Finland, 63,225 infants received a 2-dose regimen of Rotarix® or placebo and were monitored for intussusception for 31 days after each dose and for a median duration of 100 days after the first dose. There were 6 cases of confirmed intussusception in vaccine recipients and 7 cases in placebo recipients within 31 days following administration of either dose. After the 31-day observation period, there were 3 additional cases of intussusception in those who received the vaccine and 9 cases in those who received placebo. There were no confirmed cases of intussusception in vaccine recipients within the first 14 days after the initial vaccine dose. In a subset of infants followed for up to 1 year after the first vaccine dose, there were 4 cases of intussusception in vaccine recipients compared with 14 cases in placebo recipients. All infants in the study who developed intussusception recovered without sequelae.

The temporal association between vaccination with Rotarix® and intussusception was evaluated in a hospital-based active surveillance study that identified infants with intussusception at participating hospitals in Mexico. Using a self-controlled case series method, the incidence of intussusception during the first 7 days after a dose of Rotarix® and during the 31-day period after the dose was compared with a control period. The control period was from birth to 1 year, excluding the predefined risk period (first 7 days or first 31 days after the vaccine dose). Over a 2-year period, participating hospitals provided health services to approximately 1 million infants younger than 1 year of age. Among 750 infants with intussusception, the relative incidence of intussusception in the 31-day period after the first dose of Rotarix® compared with the control period was 1.96; the relative incidence of intussusception in the first 7 days after the first dose of Rotarix® compared with the control period was 6.07. This study did not take into account all medical conditions that may predispose infants to intussusception and results may not be generalizable to US infants who have a lower background rate of intussusception than Mexican infants. However, if a temporal increase in the risk for intussusception following Rotarix® similar in magnitude to that observed in the Mexico study does exist in US infants, it is estimated that approximately 1–3 additional cases of intussusception hospitalizations would occur per 100,000 vaccinated infants in the US within 7 days following the first dose of Rotarix®. In the first year of life, the background rate of intussusception hospitalizations in the US has been estimated to be approximately 34 per 100,000 infants.

RotaTeq® (RV5). Infants who received RotaTeq® (34,837) or placebo (34,788) in the Rotavirus Efficacy and Safety Trial (REST; study 006) were monitored by active surveillance for intussusception at 7, 14, and 42 days after each dose and then every 6 weeks for a period of 1 year after the initial dose. A total of 13 vaccine recipients and 15 placebo recipients developed confirmed cases of intussusception within 1 year of the first dose. There were 6 or 5 confirmed cases of intussusception that occurred within 42 days of any dose in those who received vaccine or placebo, respectively; there were no confirmed cases of intussusception reported within the first 42 days following the initial dose of RotaTeq®. All infants in the study who developed intussusception recovered without sequelae, except a male 9 months of age who developed intussusception 98 days after the third vaccine dose and died of postoperative sepsis. Intussusception was not reported in other initial phase 3 clinical studies (study 007 and 009).

Postmarketing surveillance has identified some cases of intussusception (including a death) in temporal association with RotaTeq® administration. A total of 160 confirmed cases of intussusception, but no related fatalities, were reported to VAERS during the first 19 months of postmarketing surveillance (February 1, 2006 to September 25, 2007). Of these 160 cases, 47 occurred in infants within 21 days following vaccination with RotaTeq®, including 27 cases that occurred within the first 7 days. Twenty-two of these infants required surgery; intussusception in the other 25 infants resolved through use of enema reduction. Among these intussusception cases reported to VAERS, more cases occurred within 7 days than within 14 or 21 days following the first dose of RotaTeq®.

The temporal association between vaccination with RotaTeq® and intussusception was evaluated in the Post-licensure Rapid Immunization Safety Monitoring (PRISM) program, an electronic active surveillance program comprised of 3 US health insurance plans. PRISM evaluated more than 1.2 million RotaTeq vaccinations (507,000 first doses) administered to infants 5 through 36 weeks of age. From 2004 through 2011, potential cases of intussusception in either inpatient or emergency department settings and vaccine exposures were identified through electronic procedure and diagnosis codes. Medical records were reviewed to confirm intussusception and rotavirus vaccination status. Intussusception was observed in temporal association within 21 days following the first dose of RotaTeq®, with a clustering of cases in the first 7 days. Based on these results, approximately 1–1.5 excess cases of intussusception occur per 100,000 vaccinated US infants within 21 days following the first dose of RotaTeq®. In the first year of life, the background rate of hospitalizations in the US related to intussusception is estimated to be approximately 34 per 100,000 infants.

Other GI Disorders or Illnesses Safety and efficacy of Rotarix® have not been evaluated in infants with chronic GI disorders, and administration of the vaccine should be delayed in infants with acute diarrhea or vomiting.

RotaTeq® should be used with caution in infants with a history of GI disorders (e.g., active acute GI illness, chronic diarrhea and failure to thrive, history of congenital abdominal disorders, abdominal surgery) since safety and efficacy data are not available regarding use of the vaccine in such infants. The manufacturer states that clinical study data are available that support use of RotaTeq® in infants with controlled gastroesophageal reflux disease (GERD).

Although safety and efficacy of rotavirus vaccine have not been evaluated in infants with preexisting chronic GI disorders, ACIP and AAP state that benefits outweigh theoretical risks in those with certain preexisting GI tract conditions (e.g., congenital malabsorption syndrome, Hirschsprung disease, short-gut syndrome) if they are not receiving immunosuppressive therapy.

Use of rotavirus vaccine has not been studied in infants with concurrent acute gastroenteritis, and ACIP and AAP state that immunogenicity and efficacy of rotavirus vaccine may be compromised in these infants. These experts state that the vaccine should not be administered to infants with acute, moderate-to-severe gastroenteritis until improvement of the condition is noted. However, infants with mild acute gastroenteritis can be vaccinated, particularly if the delay in vaccination is substantial and may result in the child becoming ineligible to receive the vaccine based on age at first dose.

Hematochezia (passage of blood in feces) occurring within 42 days of a vaccine dose has been reported as an adverse effect in 0.6% of infants receiving RotaTeq®; this was similar to the incidence of hematochezia observed in those receiving placebo in clinical trials. Postmarketing surveillance data also include reports of hematochezia in infants following immunization with Rotarix® or RotaTeq®. A causal relationship between the administration of rotavirus vaccine and the occurrence of hematochezia has not been established.

Transmission of Vaccine Virus Rotarix® contains live, attenuated rotavirus and RotaTeq® contains live, reassortant rotaviruses. Viral shedding can occur in vaccine recipients and the vaccine virus has been transmitted between vaccinees and susceptible contacts.

After a dose of Rotarix®, peak shedding occurs approximately 7 days after the dose. In a prospective, randomized, double-blind, placebo-controlled study, healthy twins 6–14 weeks of age were randomized so that 1 twin in each household received Rotarix® and the other twin received placebo. Transmission of vaccine virus from the vaccinated twin to the twin who received placebo was reported in 19% of the pairs; GI symptoms related to transmitted virus were not reported. The median duration of vaccine virus shedding was 10 days in twins who received Rotarix® compared with 4 days in the twin sibling who received placebo, but acquired the vaccine virus.

In a clinical study evaluating safety and efficacy of RotaTeq® (REST; study 006), shedding of vaccine virus was assessed among a subset of infants 4–6 days after each vaccine dose and among all study participants who submitted a stool sample that was positive for rotavirus antigen at any time. The RotaTeq® vaccine virus was shed in the stools of 9% of vaccine recipients tested after dose 1 and in 0 or 0.3% of vaccine recipients tested after dose 2 or 3, respectively. In phase 3 studies evaluating RotaTeq®, viral shedding was observed as early as 1 day and as late as 15 days after a dose. Transmission of the vaccine virus to susceptible contacts was not evaluated in phase 3 studies, but there have been postmarketing reports of such transmission.

Caution is advised when considering whether to administer rotavirus vaccine to infants with close contacts who are immunocompromised (e.g., individuals who have malignancies or are otherwise immunocompromised, individuals with primary immunodeficiencies, or individuals receiving immunosuppressive therapy). The manufacturers state that the risk of possible transmission of the vaccine virus should be weighed against the risk of the infant developing natural rotavirus infection that could be transmitted to susceptible contacts.

ACIP and AAP state that infants living in households with individuals who are immunocompromised should receive rotavirus vaccine when indicated. Protection of immunocompromised household contacts afforded by rotavirus vaccination of infants in the household and prevention of wild-type rotavirus disease outweighs the small risk of transmitting vaccine virus to the immunocompromised individual and any subsequent theoretical risk of vaccine virus-associated disease.

To minimize potential virus transmission from the vaccinee, all household contacts should be advised to use hygienic measures (e.g., good hand washing) following contact with the feces of a vaccinated infant (e.g., diaper changing) for at least 1 week after each vaccine dose.

If an infant recently vaccinated with rotavirus vaccine is hospitalized for any reason, no special cautionary measures (other than standard precautions) are necessary to prevent the spread of vaccine virus in the hospital setting. Because of the possible risk of transmission of rotavirus vaccine virus to other hospitalized infants, if a preterm infant previously vaccinated with rotavirus vaccine requires readmission to the neonatal intensive care unit (NICU) or hospital nursery within 2 weeks following a dose of the vaccine, contact precautions should be initiated for the preterm infant and should be maintained for 2–3 weeks following the dose. (See Pediatric Use under Warnings/Precautions: Specific Populations, in Cautions.)

Kawasaki Disease Kawasaki disease was reported during phase 3 clinical trials of Rotarix® and RotaTeq®. Kawasaki disease is a serious, but rare illness in children that is poorly understood, and is characterized by high fever and inflammation of the blood vessels affecting the lymph nodes, skin, mouth, and heart. The cause of Kawasaki disease has not been determined.

In 16 completed or ongoing clinical studies evaluating Rotarix®, Kawasaki disease was reported in 18 infants who received the vaccine (0.035%) compared with 9 infants who received placebo (0.021%). Of these 27 cases, 5 occurred following a dose of Rotarix® in clinical trials that were either not placebo controlled or 1:1 randomized. In placebo-controlled trials evaluating Rotarix®, Kawasaki disease was reported in 17 vaccine recipients and 9 placebo recipients (relative risk of 1.71). Among recipients of the vaccine, the time of onset of Kawasaki disease after the dose ranged from 3 days to 19 months.

During phase 3 testing of RotaTeq®, there were 5 cases of Kawasaki disease reported in the 36,150 infants who received the vaccine and 1 case reported in the 35,536 infants who received placebo. In addition, there were 3 cases of Kawasaki disease reported to VAERS in infants who received RotaTeq® and one unconfirmed case occurring within 30 days of vaccination was identified through the CDC Vaccine Safety Datalink (VSD) project.

A causal relationship between rotavirus vaccine (or any vaccine) and the occurrence of Kawasaki disease has not been established. The number of reported cases of Kawasaki disease occurring in association with use of RotaTeq® to date does not exceed the number of expected cases occurring randomly in this population. Postmarketing surveillance data to date do not indicate that RotaTeq® is associated with an increased risk of Kawasaki disease.

Any cases of Kawasaki disease that occur following administration of rotavirus vaccine (or any other vaccine) should be reported to VAERS at 1-800-822-7967 or http://www.vaers.hhs.gov/.

Concomitant Illness A decision to administer or delay administration of rotavirus vaccine in an infant with a current or recent febrile illness depends on the severity of symptoms and etiology of the illness. The manufacturer of RotaTeq® states that the presence of low-grade fever (temperature less than 38.1°C) or mild upper respiratory infection does not preclude vaccination.

ACIP and AAP state that rotavirus vaccine may be administered to infants with transient, mild illnesses (with or without low-grade fever). However, vaccination of individuals with moderate or severe acute illness generally should be deferred until they have recovered from the acute phase of the illness.

Risk of Adventitious Agents Porcine-derived materials are used in the manufacture of Rotarix® and Rotateq®, and DNA from porcine circoviruses is present in the vaccines.

In March 2010, after becoming aware that DNA from porcine circovirus type 1 (PCV1) had been detected in Rotarix®, FDA advised that use of the vaccine be temporarily suspended as a safety precaution pending further investigation. In May 2010, the FDA provided additional information that DNA fragments from PCV1 and porcine circovirus type 2 (PCV2) were detected in RotaTeq®. After careful evaluation, the FDA decided that it was appropriate to resume the use of Rotarix® and to continue the use of RotaTeq® for prevention of rotavirus infection in infants.

FDA states that there is no evidence to date that PCV1 or PCV2 can cause clinical infection or disease in humans or that either virus poses a safety risk in humans. Because available evidence supports the safety record of Rotarix® and RotaTeq® in infants, the FDA states that the clinical benefits of vaccination against rotavirus infection outweigh any theoretical risks from the presence of PCV1 or PCV2 in rotavirus vaccines. The FDA and the manufacturers will continue to investigate the presence of porcine virus DNA in Rotarix® and RotaTeq® and evaluate safety data from ongoing studies.

Limitations of Vaccine Efficacy Rotavirus vaccine may not protect all vaccine recipients against rotavirus infection.

Data are not available to determine the level of protection provided against rotavirus infection in infants who have not received the complete vaccination series (i.e., have received only a single dose of Rotarix® or only 1 or 2 doses of RotaTeq®).

Duration of Immunity Duration of protection against rotavirus gastroenteritis following the 2-dose vaccination series of Rotarix® or following the 3-dose vaccination series of RotaTeq® has not been fully determined.

There is evidence from clinical trials that the complete vaccination series of either Rotarix® or RotaTeq® generally provides protection against rotavirus infection through the second rotavirus season after vaccination or up to 2 years of age. There is some evidence that RotaTeq® reduces emergency department visits or hospitalizations related to rotavirus gastroenteritis through the first 3 years of life. Efficacy of Rotarix® beyond the second rotavirus season after vaccination has not been fully evaluated to date.

Improper Storage and Handling Improper storage or handling of vaccines may reduce vaccine potency resulting in reduced or inadequate immune response in vaccinees.

All vaccines should be inspected upon delivery and monitored during storage to ensure that the appropriate temperature is maintained. (See Dosage and Administration: Administration.)

Vaccine that has been mishandled or has not been stored at the recommended temperature should *not* be administered.

If there are concerns about mishandling, the manufacturer or state or local immunization or health departments should be contacted for guidance on whether the vaccine is usable.

Specific Populations **Pregnancy.** Rotavirus vaccine is not indicated for use in adults, including pregnant women.

ACIP and AAP state that infants living in households with pregnant women may receive rotavirus vaccine. Most women of childbearing age would be expected to have preexisting immunity to rotavirus. Most experts agree that the risk of acquiring rotavirus infection from potential exposure to the vaccine virus is very low. In addition, there is no evidence that infection with rotavirus during pregnancy poses any risk to the fetus. Furthermore, vaccination of infants against rotavirus avoids potential exposure of pregnant women to natural rotavirus from unvaccinated infants with rotavirus gastroenteritis.

Lactation. Rotavirus vaccine is not indicated for use in adults, including nursing women.

ACIP and AAP state that nursing infants may receive rotavirus vaccine, since efficacy of the vaccine in breast-feeding infants is similar to that in infants not breast-feeding.

Pediatric Use. Rotarix®: Safety and efficacy have *not* been established in infants younger than 6 weeks or older than 24 weeks of age. The manufacturer states that efficacy in preterm infants has not been established. Safety data to date in preterm infants indicate serious adverse events in 5.2% of vaccine recipients compared with 5% in placebo recipients; deaths or cases of intussusception have not been reported in this patient population to date.

RotaTeq®: Safety and efficacy have *not* been established in infants younger than 6 weeks or older than 32 weeks of age. The manufacturer states that RotaTeq® has been studied in preterm infants (i.e., gestational age 25–36 weeks), and clinical study data support use of the vaccine in such infants according to their age in weeks since birth. Safety data in preterm infants indicate serious adverse events in 5.5% of vaccine recipients compared with 5.8% of placebo recipients; there were 2 deaths among vaccine recipients and no cases of intussusception.

Pending additional data, ACIP and AAP state that the benefits of routine vaccination with rotavirus vaccine outweigh the theoretical risks in medically stable preterm infants. These experts state that clinically stable preterm infants who meet the age requirements (at least 6 weeks and not greater than 14 weeks 6 days of age) may receive the first dose of rotavirus vaccine after or at the time of discharge from the NICU or hospital nursery. However, the possible risk of transmission of rotavirus vaccine virus to other hospitalized infants outweigh the benefits of vaccination in age-eligible infants who will remain in the NICU or nursery after the dose. In addition, if a preterm infant who previously received rotavirus vaccine requires readmission to the NICU or hospital nursery within 2 weeks following a dose of the vaccine, contact precautions should be initiated for the preterm infant and should be maintained for 2–3 weeks following the vaccine dose.

ACIP and AAP state that a replacement dose of rotavirus vaccine is *not* recommended if an infant receives an incomplete vaccine dose (e.g., infant spits or regurgitates the dose). (See Dosage and Administration: Reconstitution and Administration.) In limited postmarketing experience of reported overdosage of RotaTeq® (e.g., as the result of more than 1 dose or a replacement dose after regurgitation), adverse events reported after incorrect administration of higher than recommended doses of the vaccine were similar to adverse events reported with the recommended dosage and dosing schedule.

Geriatric Use. Rotavirus vaccine is not recommended for use in adults, including geriatric adults.

■ **Common Adverse Effects** Rotarix®: Adverse events reported within 8 days following the first dose of vaccine include fussiness/irritability (52%), cough/runny nose (28%), fever (25%), loss of appetite (25%), vomiting (13%), and diarrhea (4%). Frequency of adverse events within 8 days following the second dose of vaccine is similar and includes fussiness/irritability (42%), cough/runny nose (31%), fever (28%), loss of appetite (21%), vomiting (8%), and diarrhea (3%). The incidence of adverse events in the week following the first and second doses of vaccine was similar to that occurring with placebo.

RotaTeq®: Fever has occurred in 42.6% of infants within 42 days of any dose of the vaccine; this was similar to the incidence reported with placebo. Adverse events reported within 42 days following any dose of the vaccine and reported more frequently than with placebo include diarrhea (24.1%), vomiting (15.2%), otitis media (14.5%), nasopharyngitis (6.9%), and bronchospasm (1.1%).

Drug Interactions

■ **Immune Globulins and Blood Products** Safety and efficacy data are not available regarding use of Rotarix® (RV1) or RotaTeq® (RV5) in infants who have received blood transfusions or blood products (including immunoglobulins). The US Public Health Service Advisory Committee on Immunization Practices (ACIP) and American Academy of Pediatrics (AAP) state that immune globulin preparations are not expected to affect the immune response to rotavirus vaccine; therefore, rotavirus vaccine may be administered simultaneously with or at any time before or after administration of blood or antibody-containing products.

■ **Immunosuppressive Agents** Individuals receiving immunosuppressive therapy (e.g., alkylating agents, antimetabolites, corticosteroids, cytotoxic agents, radiation) may have a diminished antibody response to vaccines, including rotavirus vaccine.

Rotarix®: Safety and efficacy of the vaccine in infants receiving immunosuppressive therapy have not been established.

RotaTeq®: Safety and efficacy data are not available regarding use of the vaccine in infants receiving immunosuppressive therapy (e.g., systemic corticosteroid therapy at greater than physiologic dosages); however, the manufacturer states that the vaccine may be administered to infants receiving topical or inhaled corticosteroids.

■ **Vaccines** Although specific studies may not be available evaluating concurrent administration of rotavirus vaccine with each antigen, simultaneous administration with other age-appropriate vaccines, including live virus vaccines, toxoids, or inactivated or recombinant vaccines, during the same health-care visit is not expected to affect immunologic responses or adverse reactions to any of the preparations.

Immunization with rotavirus vaccine can be integrated with immunization against diphtheria, tetanus, pertussis, haemophilus influenza type b (Hib), hepatitis B, influenza, poliovirus, measles, mumps, rubella, pneumococcal disease, and varicella.

Inactivated Vaccines or Toxoids Rotavirus vaccine may be administered concomitantly with or at any interval before or after inactivated vaccines (e.g., Hib vaccine, poliovirus vaccine inactivated [IPV], hepatitis B vaccine, influenza virus vaccines, pneumococcal vaccine) indicated in infants.

Studies using Rotarix® indicate that concomitant administration with pneumococcal 7-valent conjugate vaccine (PCV7; no longer commercially available in the US) or Hib vaccine does not affect the immune response to any of these antigens. Studies using Rotateq® indicate that concomitant administration with Hib vaccine, IPV, hepatitis B vaccine, and pneumococcal conjugate vaccine does not affect the immune response to the vaccines.

Although the immune response resulting from concomitant administration of rotavirus vaccine and inactivated influenza virus vaccines in infants 6 months of age has not been studied, ACIP and AAP state that inactivated vaccines (e.g., influenza virus vaccines) may be administered simultaneously with or at any time before or after a live vaccine (e.g., rotavirus vaccine).

Rotavirus vaccine may be administered concomitantly with or at any interval before or after toxoids (e.g., diphtheria and tetanus toxoids and acellular pertussis vaccine adsorbed [DTaP]) routinely recommended in infants. Studies using Rotarix® indicate that concomitant administration with a fixed-combination vaccine containing DTaP, hepatitis B vaccine, and IPV did not affect the immune response to any of the antigens. Studies using RotaTeq® indicate that concomitant administration with DTaP does not reduce the antibody response to the diphtheria or tetanus antigens, but data are insufficient to date to determine whether there is any interference with the immune response to the pertussis antigens.

Live Vaccines RotaTeq® may be administered concomitantly with or at any interval before or after other live vaccines recommended in infants. There is no evidence to date that the vaccine interferes with live vaccines administered parenterally or intranasally.

Concomitant administration of poliovirus vaccine live oral (OPV; not commercially available in the US) was not permitted during clinical studies of rotavirus vaccine.

Description

Rotavirus vaccine live oral (Rotarix®; RV1) is a lyophilized vaccine containing live, attenuated rotavirus derived from a human strain (89-12) belonging to type G1P[8] type.

Rotavirus vaccine live oral pentavalent (RotaTeq®; RV5) is a solution containing 5 live, reassortant rotaviruses that represent the G types responsible for most cases of rotavirus gastroenteritis worldwide (G1, G2, G3, G4, and G9) and the most common P type associated with these strains (P1A; genotype P[8]).

Porcine-derived materials are used during the manufacture of Rotarix® and RotaTeq®; DNA from porcine circovirus type 1 (PCV1) has been detected in Rotarix® and DNA from PCV1 and porcine circovirus type 2 (PCV2) has been detected in RotaTeq®. (See Risk of Adventitious Agents under Cautions: Warnings/Precautions.)

Following vaccination, the live, attenuated virus in Rotarix® or the live, reassortant rotaviruses in RotaTeq® replicate in the small intestine and induce active immunity to rotavirus types represented in the vaccine.

Rotaviruses have 2 outer capsid proteins termed VP7 (G protein) and VP4 (P protein) and generally are classified according to their G and P types. Reassortant human-animal rotaviruses are produced using parent strains isolated from human and animal hosts and contain genes that code for the outer capsid proteins of human rotaviruses. RotaTeq® contains reassortant rotaviruses produced using human parent strains and a parent bovine strain (Wistar calf 3 [WC3]).

The exact immunologic mechanism by which rotavirus vaccine protects against rotavirus gastroenteritis has not been determined. A correlation between antibody response to rotavirus vaccine and protection against rotavirus gastroenteritis has not been established to date. Data from studies of wild-type rotavirus infection suggest that serum neutralizing antibodies, fecal anti-rotavirus immunoglobulin A (IgA), and serum anti-rotavirus IgA may correlate with protection against rotavirus gastroenteritis and infection. Studies using Rotarix® indicate that 76.8–86.5% of vaccine recipients seroconvert after 2 doses. Seroconversion in these studies was defined as appearance of anti-rotavirus IgA antibody in infants previously negative for rotavirus. Studies using RotaTeq® indicate that a threefold or greater increase in serum anti-rotavirus IgA concentrations occurred in 93–100% of those who received a 3-dose vaccination series compared with 12–20% of those who received placebo.

Because Rotarix® contains live, attenuated rotavirus and RotaTeq® contains live, reassortant rotaviruses, vaccine virus can be shed in the stools of vaccinees and transmitted between vaccinees and susceptible contacts. (See Transmission of Vaccine Virus under Cautions: Warnings/Precautions.)

Advice to Patients

Prior to administration of each vaccine dose, provide copy of manufacturer's patient information to the patient's parent or guardian. Also provide a copy of the appropriate CDC Vaccine Information Statement (VIS) to the patient's parent or legal representative (VISs are available at https://www.cdc.gov/vaccines/hcp/vis/index.html).

Advise the patient's parent or legal guardian of the risks and benefits of vaccination with rotavirus vaccine.

Advise the patient's parent or legal guardian that porcine circoviruses (or fragments of the viruses) have been found in rotavirus vaccines, and that there is no evidence to date that these viruses cause infection or disease in humans or pose a safety risk. (See Risk of Adventitious Agents under Cautions: Warnings/Precautions.)

Advise the patient's parent or legal guardian that rotavirus vaccine may not provide complete protection in all vaccinees. In addition, the vaccine will not protect against disease due to rotavirus strains not represented in the vaccine.

Advise the patient's parent or legal guardian of the possible risk of transmitting the vaccine virus to rotavirus-susceptible individuals, including household or other close contacts with a weakened immune system (e.g., individual with cancer or one who is receiving immunosuppressive therapy) or pregnant women who have not had rotavirus infection.

Importance of informing clinicians if a child has any illness with fever, diarrhea, or vomiting; has failure to gain weight or is not growing as expected; has a blood disorder, any type of cancer, a weakened immune system (e.g., human immunodeficiency virus [HIV] infection, severe combined immunodeficiency disease [SCID]), or a history of GI problems (e.g., intussusception, blockage, abdominal surgery); or receives treatment that may weaken the immune system (e.g., high-dose corticosteroids).

For infants receiving Rotarix® (2-dose vaccination series) or RotaTeq® (3-dose vaccination series), advise the patient's parent or legal guardian of the importance of completing the vaccination series by the time the infant is 8 months 0 days of age, unless contraindicated.

Importance of informing clinicians if any adverse reactions (including allergic reactions) occur. Clinicians or individuals can report any adverse reactions that occur following vaccination to VAERS at 800-822-7967 or http://www.vaers.hhs.gov/.

Advise the patient's parent or legal guardian that rotavirus vaccine should not be administered to children who have an allergic reaction following a dose of the vaccine or in those who are allergic to any components of the vaccine.

Importance of informing clinicians immediately if a child has any signs and/or symptoms of intussusception, including vomiting, diarrhea, severe stomach pain, blood in their stools, or high fever. The clinician should be contacted if a child has any of these symptoms following vaccination, especially if symptoms occur within 7 days following the first dose of vaccine, but even if they occur several weeks following the last vaccine dose.

Importance of informing clinicians of existing or contemplated concomitant therapy, including prescription and OTC drugs, and any concomitant illnesses.

Importance of informing patients of other important precautionary information. (See Cautions.)

Overview® (see Users Guide). For additional information on this drug until a more detailed monograph is developed and published, the manufacturer's labeling should be consulted. It is *essential* that the manufacturer's labeling be consulted for more detailed information on usual cautions, precautions, contraindications, potential drug interactions, laboratory test interferences, and acute toxicity.

Preparations

Excipients in commercially available drug preparations may have clinically important effects in some individuals; consult specific product labeling for details.

Rotavirus Vaccine Live Oral

Oral		
For Suspension	Live attenuated rotavirus content: ≥1 x 10^6 median cell culture infective dose of G1P[8] per 1 mL	**Rotarix®**, GlaxoSmithKline

Rotavirus Vaccine Live Oral Pentavalent

Oral		
Solution	Live human-bovine reassortant rotavirus content: ≥ 2.2 x 10^6 infectious units of G1, 2.8 x 10^6 infectious units of G2, 2.2 x 10^6 infectious units of G3, 2 x 10^6 infectious units of G4, and 2.3 x 10^6 infectious units of P1A (P[8]) per 2 mL	**RotaTeq®**, Merck

Selected Revisions December 2017.

Rubella Virus Vaccine Live

MMR

■ Rubella virus vaccine live is a preparation of live, attenuated rubella virus that stimulates active immunity to rubella infection. Rubella virus vaccine live is commercially available as a fixed-combination vaccine containing measles, mumps, and rubella antigens (MMR; M-M-R® II) and as a fixed-combination vaccine containing measles, mumps, rubella, and varicella antigens (MMRV; ProQuad®). For information on MMRV, see Varicella Virus Vaccine Live 80:12.

Uses

Rubella virus vaccine live is used to stimulate active immunity to rubella (German measles). Monovalent rubella virus vaccine live (Meruvax® II) is no longer commercially available in the US. Rubella virus vaccine live is commercially available in the US as a fixed-combination vaccine containing measles, mumps, and rubella antigens (MMR; M-M-R® II) for use in adults, adolescents, and children 12 months of age or older and as a fixed-combination vaccine containing measles, mumps, rubella, and varicella antigens (MMRV; ProQuad®) for use in children 12 months through 12 years of age.

The major objective of rubella immunization is to prevent rubella infection during pregnancy and resultant congenital rubella infection and congenital rubella syndrome (CRS). Congenital rubella infection may cause miscarriage, abortion, stillbirth, fetal anomalies, or asymptomatic infection in the infant. (See Pharmacology: Rubella Virus and Infection.) Because many countries do not have rubella vaccination programs or have only recently implemented such programs, many adults throughout the world remain susceptible. Adults in the US who were born in countries where routine rubella vaccination was not offered are at higher risk for contracting rubella and having infants with CRS compared with adults born in the US.

The US Public Health Service Advisory Committee on Immunization Practices (ACIP), the American Academy of Pediatrics (AAP), and the American Academy of Family Physicians (AAFP) recommend *universal* immunization against rubella for all susceptible children, adolescents, and adults, unless rubella virus vaccine live is contraindicated. (See Cautions: Precautions and Contraindications.)

The ACIP, AAP, and AAFP state that the fixed-combination vaccine containing measles, mumps, and rubella vaccine live (MMR) is preferred over monovalent rubella virus vaccine live (no longer commercially available in the US) for both primary immunization and revaccination to assure immunity to all 3 diseases. Alternatively, in children 12 months through 12 years of age when a dose of MMR and a dose of varicella virus vaccine live are indicated for primary immunization, use of the fixed-combination vaccine containing

MMR and varicella virus vaccine live (MMRV; ProQuad®) can be considered. For information on MMRV, see Varicella Virus Vaccine Live 80:12.

Individuals generally can be considered immune to rubella if they have serologic (i.e., laboratory) evidence of rubella immunity, documentation of adequate immunization with at least one dose of live rubella virus-containing vaccine at 12 months of age or older, or were born before 1957 (except women of childbearing potential). Birth before 1957 is not acceptable for evidence of immunity in women who may become pregnant because it provides only presumptive evidence of rubella immunity and does not guarantee that an individual is immune. Rubella infection can occur in some unvaccinated individuals born before 1957 and congenital rubella and CRS can occur among offspring of women infected with rubella during pregnancy. Individuals with an equivocal serologic test should be considered susceptible to rubella unless they have adequate evidence of vaccination or a subsequent serologic test result indicates rubella immunity. Although only one dose of live rubella virus-containing vaccine is required as acceptable evidence of rubella immunity, recommendations for routine childhood immunization include a 2-dose regimen of MMR. The ACIP states that clinical diagnosis of rubella is unreliable and should not be considered in assessing immunity to the disease. Because many rash illnesses may mimic rubella and many rubella infections are unrecognized, the only reliable evidence of previous rubella infection is the presence of serum rubella immunoglobulin G (IgG). Although tests for immunoglobulin (IgM) antibody have been used to diagnose acute and recent rubella infection, IgM tests should *not* be used to determine rubella immunity since false-positive results can occur. Laboratories that regularly perform antibody testing generally provide the most reliable results because their reagents and procedures are more likely to be strictly standardized. There is no conclusive evidence that individuals who are already immune to rubella when vaccinated are at any increased risk of vaccine-associated adverse effects, and therefore there is no need to test for susceptibility to rubella infection before administering the vaccine. Although routine serologic testing for rubella antibody in women of childbearing potential during clinic visits for routine health care, premarital evaluation, family planning, or diagnosis and treatment of sexually transmitted diseases may identify women who are not immune to rubella before they become pregnant, such testing is not useful unless it is linked to timely follow-up and vaccination of women who are susceptible.

Hemagglutination-inhibiting (HI) antibody testing formerly was the method most frequently used to screen for rubella antibodies. However, this method has been replaced by other assays of equal or greater sensitivity. Enzyme immunoassays (EIAs) are the most commonly used of the newer commercial assays, but latex agglutination, immunofluorescence assay (IFA), passive hemagglutination, hemolysis-in-gel, and virus neutralization tests also are available. Any antibody level above the standard positive cutoff value for the specific assay method can be considered acceptable evidence of immunity. Occasionally, individuals with documented histories of rubella vaccination have serum rubella IgG levels that are not clearly positive by enzyme-linked immunosorbent assay (ELISA); such individuals can be given another dose of MMR and need not be retested for serologic evidence of rubella immunity.

Efforts to vaccinate rubella-susceptible, postpubertal individuals, especially women of childbearing age, should be intensified, particularly among women who emigrated from areas outside the US where routine rubella vaccination may have been unlikely. Therefore, in addition to immunization of children, the following strategies should be followed to hasten the elimination of rubella and CRS in the US: making the general public and health-care providers more aware of the dangers of rubella infection; ensuring that patients are vaccinated as part of routine medical and gynecologic care; ensuring vaccination of all women visiting family planning clinics; ensuring vaccination of unimmunized women immediately after undergoing childbirth, miscarriage, or abortion; vaccinating susceptible women identified during occasions when their children undergo routine examinations or vaccinations; vaccinating susceptible women identified by premarital serology; routinely vaccinating susceptible women before discharge from hospitals, birthing centers, or other medical facilities, unless a specific contraindication exists; requiring proof of immunity (i.e., positive serologic evidence or documented rubella vaccination) for college entry; and requiring proof of immunity for all hospital personnel who might be exposed to patients with rubella or who might be in contact with pregnant patients.

The number of cases of rubella reported in the US has decreased 99% since the licensure of rubella vaccine in 1969 (57,686 cases in 1969 and fewer than 25 cases in 2001); however, the epidemiology of the disease has changed. Since the beginning of the 1990s, most reported cases of rubella in the US have occurred among adults (86% of cases in 1999) and most have involved foreign-born individuals, especially those from Mexico and South America. Although the number of cases of CRS in the US also has declined, CRS now disproportionately affects infants born to foreign-born women (92% of infants with CRS during 1997–1999 had foreign-born mothers). Before the mid-1990s, rubella outbreaks in the US generally occurred among children and adults in religious communities that did not accept vaccination and in unvaccinated individuals in schools, jails, and other closed environments. Rubella outbreaks in several areas of the US (e.g., California, Massachusetts, Connecticut, North Carolina) have occurred principally in Hispanic women, and the risk for both rubella and CRS is increased in this ethnic group, particularly those born outside the US where routine rubella vaccination may not occur. Outbreaks also have been reported in workplaces that employ large numbers of foreign-born workers (e.g., poultry and meat processing plants). An average of 5 CRS cases per year was reported in the US between 1995 and 2000; since 2001, an average of one CRS case per year has been reported. In 2004, a panel of experts stated that rubella is no longer endemic in the US.

■ **Primary Immunization** ***Infants and Children 12 Months through 12 Years of Age*** For routine primary immunization in children, the ACIP, AAP, and AAFP recommend that the first dose of MMR be given at 12 through 15 months of age. Vaccination of younger children solely for rubella protection generally should not be attempted because most infants have maternal antibodies which may prevent a satisfactory immunologic response to the vaccine; however, vaccination with MMR aimed at preventing measles occasionally may be warranted in children as young as 6 months of age in certain situations associated with increased risk of exposure to measles virus (e.g., during measles outbreaks, travel to areas with increased risk of measles). (See Uses in Measles Virus Vaccine Live 80:12.) A history of rubella illness or immunization when younger than 12 months of age is not a reliable indicator of immunity and should not be used to exclude children from vaccination. Previously unimmunized children of rubella-susceptible pregnant women should be vaccinated with MMR to minimize the risk of exposing the woman to natural rubella infection.

To improve control of measles, mumps, and rubella, a second dose of MMR is recommended for routine immunization in children. The second dose preferably should be given at 4 through 6 years of age (just prior to entry into kindergarten or first grade), but may be given earlier during any routine visit provided at least 4 weeks (i.e., at least 28 days) have elapsed since the first dose and both the first and second doses are administered beginning at or after 12 months of age. Those who have not previously received the second MMR dose should complete the vaccination schedule by 11–12 years of age (just prior to entry into middle or junior high school). (See Primary Immunization: Infants and Children 12 Months through 12 Years of Age, under Uses in Measles Virus Vaccine Live 80:12.) If MMR is administered to infants before their first birthday, they should be considered unimmunized for the purposes of determining the need for further vaccination; they should be revaccinated with a 2-dose regimen of MMR initiated at 12 months of age. Although available data indicate that one dose of rubella virus vaccine live confers long-term, probably life-long, immunity in more than 90% of vaccinees, the potential consequences of rubella vaccine failure are substantial (e.g., congenital rubella) and the additional dose currently recommended provides an added safeguard against such failures.

The ACIP, AAP, and AAFP state that primary immunization against measles, mumps, and rubella can be integrated with primary immunization against diphtheria, tetanus, pertussis, *Haemophilus influenzae* type b (Hib), hepatitis B, influenza, pneumococcal disease, poliomyelitis, and varicella. In general, simultaneous administration (on the same day) of the most widely used vaccines, including diphtheria and tetanus toxoids and acellular pertussis vaccine adsorbed (DTaP), Hib conjugate vaccine, MMR, poliovirus vaccine inactivated (IPV), and varicella virus vaccine live, has resulted in seroconversion rates and adverse effects similar to those observed when the vaccines were administered separately. Therefore, the ACIP, AAP, and AAFP recommend simultaneous administration of all vaccines appropriate for the age and previous vaccination status of the recipient, including DTaP, Hib conjugate vaccine, hepatitis B vaccine, influenza vaccine, MMR, IPV, pneumococcal vaccine, and varicella virus vaccine live, especially if an individual is unlikely to return for further vaccination. (See Drug Interactions.)

Internationally Adopted Children and Other Immigrants Individuals seeking an immigrant visa for permanent US residency must provide proof of age-appropriate vaccination according to the US Recommended Childhood and Adolescent Immunization Schedule or the US Adult Schedule (see Immunization Schedules, US 80:00). Although this vaccination requirement applies to all immigrant infants and children entering the US, internationally adopted children younger than 11 years of age are exempt from the overseas vaccination requirements; however, adoptive parents are required to sign a waiver indicating their intention to comply with the vaccination requirements within 30 days after the infant or child arrives in the US. The CDC states that more than 90% of newly arrived internationally adopted children need catch-up vaccinations to meet the US Recommended Immunization Schedules.

The fact that immunization schedules of other countries may differ from US schedules (e.g., different recommended vaccines, recommended ages of administration, and/or number and timing of vaccine doses) also should be considered. Only written vaccination records should be considered as evidence of previous vaccination since such records are more likely to accurately predict protection if the vaccines administered, intervals between doses, and child's age at the time of vaccination are similar to US recommendations; however, the extent to which an internationally adopted child's immunization record reflects their protection against disease is unclear and it is possible there may be transcription errors in such records (e.g., single-antigen vaccine may have been administered although a multiple-antigen vaccine was recorded). Although vaccines with inadequate potency have been produced in other countries, most vaccines used worldwide are immunogenic and produced with adequate quality control standards.

When the immune status of an internationally adopted child is uncertain, the ACIP recommends that health-care providers either repeat vaccinations (since this usually is safe and avoids the need to obtain and interpret serologic tests) and/or use selective serologic testing to determine the need for immunizations (helps avoid unnecessary injections). MMR is not used in most countries. Therefore, although serologic testing is available to verify immunization status in children 12 months of age or older, the CDC states that administration of MMR is preferable to serologic testing unless there is documentation that the child has had rubella. The ACIP states that the recommended approach is to revaccinate an internationally adopted child with 1 or 2 doses of MMR (depending on the child's age) without regard to the child's prior vaccination record since serious adverse effects after MMR vaccination are rare and there is no evidence that administration of MMR increases the risk for adverse reactions among individuals already immune to measles, mumps, or rubella.

Adolescents and Adults Most cases of rubella occur in adolescents and young adults, and about 15–20% of adolescent girls and young women (including some who were vaccinated as children) have no detectable rubella antibodies. Therefore, the ACIP and AAP recommend administration of MMR to susceptible prepubertal girls and nonpregnant women of childbearing potential.

Adolescents 11–12 Years of Age. The ACIP, AAP, and AAFP recommend that adolescents who have not previously received a second dose of MMR receive the dose during a routine preadolescent preventive health-care visit at 11–12 years of age. This routine health-care visit provides an opportunity to administer "catch-up" vaccines that were missed at an earlier age, administer vaccines routinely recommended at 11–12 years of age, administer vaccines recommended for certain high-risk adolescents, schedule future appointments that may be necessary to complete recommended immunization schedules, and provide adolescents with other recommended preventive health services such as guidance on health behaviors and screening for biomedical, behavioral, and emotional conditions. During the health-care visit at 11–12 years of age, the vaccination history of the adolescent should be assessed. If the adolescent does not have information regarding their vaccination history, the healthcare provider should attempt to obtain such information through documentation from the parent, previous providers, or school records. When documentation of an adolescent's vaccination status is not available at the time of the preventive health-care visit, an assumption can be made that the adolescent has received those vaccines required by state laws and regulations that have been in effect for some time (e.g., those required on entry to kindergarten) and these vaccines can be withheld while awaiting documentation. However, vaccine doses currently recommended for adolescents that were not included in previous laws and recommendations should be administered.

Ideally, all vaccines routinely indicated at 11–12 years of age should be administered during the initial adolescent visit (MMR, hepatitis B vaccine, tetanus toxoid and reduced diphtheria toxoid and acellular pertussis vaccine adsorbed (Tdap), varicella virus vaccine live). However, since multiple doses of some vaccines are required to complete primary immunization and because simultaneous administration of a large number of vaccines may be indicated in some adolescents, providers may need to be flexible in determining which vaccines to administer during the initial visit and which to schedule for return visits. While specific studies evaluating the safety and efficacy of simultaneous administration of vaccines in adolescents are not available, there is extensive evidence from clinical studies and experience in infants and children that simultaneous administration of the most widely used vaccines does not decrease the antibody response or increase adverse reactions to these vaccines. In circumstances where multiple vaccines (i.e., 4 or more) are indicated in adolescents 11–12 years of age, the provider may choose to defer some vaccines for administration during one or more future visits; however, the vaccines should be prioritized based on which require multiple doses, which diseases pose an immediate threat to the adolescent, and whether the adolescent is likely to return for scheduled visits. During any subsequent visits, the adolescent's vaccination status should be rechecked and any deficiencies corrected.

Adults. Vaccinating rubella-susceptible, postpubertal, nonpregnant women of childbearing potential confers individual protection against rubella-induced fetal injury. Ideally, rubella antibody levels should be determined in all adolescent girls and women of childbearing potential and those without evidence of immunity should receive MMR *if they are not pregnant and understand they should not become pregnant for a specified length of time.* (See Cautions: Pregnancy and Lactation.) Lack of serologic tests should not be a deterrent to immunization. Asking these women if they are pregnant, excluding those who are, and informing the others of the theoretical risks are reasonable precautions in a rubella immunization program.

The ACIP recommends that educational and training institutions (e.g., colleges, military bases) seek proof of rubella immunity (positive serologic test results or documentation of rubella vaccination) from all women students and employees of childbearing age and that nonpregnant women who lack proof of immunity be vaccinated unless the vaccine is contraindicated. Premarital serologic tests also are useful to identify rubella-susceptible women prior to their first pregnancy. Pregnant women should be tested for rubella susceptibility and susceptible women should receive the vaccine *postpartum* before they leave the hospital; seroconversion should be confirmed 6–8 weeks after vaccination in women who received blood products or $Rh_o(D)$ immune globulin. (See Drug Interactions.) There is no evidence that administration of a rubella virus-containing vaccine to a pregnant woman presents any fetal risk, although such a risk cannot be excluded on theoretical grounds. (See Cautions: Pregnancy and Lactation.) Unless contraindicated, vaccination of susceptible women of childbearing age should be part of routine general medical and gynecologic outpatient care; take place in all family-planning settings; and be provided routinely prior to discharge from a hospital, birthing center, or other medical facilities.

Immunization of adult males also may help reduce the spread of rubella. Immunization of adolescent or adult males working in medical facilities that provide care for women of childbearing age and those in settings where young adult males and females congregate has been recommended by the ACIP and CDC. All rubella-susceptible military recruits are required to receive MMR.

Adults in the US who were born in countries where routine rubella vaccination was not offered are at high risk for contracting rubella and having infants with CRS. Vaccinating foreign-born susceptible adults can be challenging since they might have little or no contact with the US health-care system. Health-care providers who treat foreign-born adults should document their rubella immunity with a written record of a rubella virus-containing vaccine or by serologic testing.

HIV-infected Individuals MMR can be used in individuals with human immunodeficiency virus (HIV) infection who do not have evidence of *severe* immunosuppression.

The ACIP, AAP, US Centers for Disease Control and Prevention (CDC), National Institutes of Health (NIH), Infectious Diseases Society of America (IDSA), Pediatric Infectious Diseases Society, and others state that all *asymptomatic* HIV-infected children, adolescents, and adults should receive MMR according to the usually recommended immunization schedules. In addition, MMR should be considered for all symptomatic HIV-infected individuals who do *not* have evidence of severe immunosuppression and who otherwise would be eligible for such vaccination. Asymptomatic individuals do not need to be evaluated and tested for HIV before decisions concerning immunization are made; such individuals in need of MMR but without evidence of severe immunosuppression should receive the vaccine. Because the immunologic response to vaccines may decrease as HIV disease progresses, vaccination early in the course of HIV infection may be more likely to induce an immune response; in addition, approximately 5% of HIV-infected infants born in the US will be severely immunocompromised at 12 months of age. Therefore, the ACIP and other experts recommend that HIV-infected infants without severe immunosuppression should receive MMR as soon as possible upon reaching their first birthday (i.e., at 12 months of age) and consideration should be given to administering the second dose of MMR as soon as 1 month (i.e., at least 28 days) after the first dose.

MMR is contraindicated in HIV-infected individuals with *severe immunosuppression* (i.e., children younger than 12 months of age with $CD4^+$ T-cell count less than 750/mm^3; children 1 through 5 years of age with $CD4^+$ T-cell count less than 500/mm^3; children 6 years of age or older, adolescents, and adults with $CD4^+$ T-cell count less than 200/mm^3; children younger than 13 years of age with $CD4^+$ T-cell percentage less than 15%). (See Individuals with Altered Immunocompetence under Cautions: Precautions and Contraindications.)

The serologic response to vaccines (including MMR) may be reduced in some HIV-infected patients and may be inversely correlated with the severity of the disease. In addition, MMR may be ineffective in HIV-infected patients who have received high-dose IV immune globulin therapy (e.g., for the prevention of serious bacterial infections) within the 3 months preceding administration of the vaccine. (See Drug Interactions: Immune Globulins.)

MMR may be given to any family member residing in the household or any other close contact of an HIV-infected patient since extensive experience has shown that live, attenuated MMR vaccine viruses are not transmitted from vaccinated individuals to others.

Health-care Personnel Health-care personnel are at increased risk for acquiring rubella and transmitting the disease to susceptible patients, and the ACIP and the Hospital Infection Control Practices Advisory Committee (HICPAC) recommend that all health-care facilities (i.e., inpatient and outpatient, public and private) ensure that all workers (i.e., medical or nonmedical, paid or volunteer, full- or part-time, student or nonstudent, with or without direct patient-care responsibilities) have adequate documentation of rubella vaccination or immunity (i.e., documentation of vaccination with a dose of rubella virus-containing vaccine given on or after 12 months of age, laboratory evidence of immunity, or laboratory confirmation of disease). Facilities that provide care exclusively to geriatric patients who are at minimal risk for rubella and complications of the disease may be possible exceptions to this recommendation. Health-care workers have a responsibility to avoid transmitting rubella to patients and thereby causing them harm.

Although birth before 1957 generally is considered acceptable evidence of rubella immunity, health-care facilities should consider recommending a dose of MMR to unvaccinated workers born before 1957 who do not have laboratory evidence of rubella immunity or laboratory confirmation of disease. Serologic surveys of hospital workers indicate that 5–9% of those born before 1957 do not have detectable measles antibody and about 6% do not have detectable rubella antibody.

To avoid rubella outbreaks in medical facilities, the CDC recommends that health-care facilities providing care for women of childbearing potential ensure that all personnel (both male and female), volunteer workers, and those frequently using the medical facility for training purposes are immune to rubella. Proof of rubella immunity (i.e., documentation of a dose of rubella virus-containing vaccine, laboratory evidence of rubella immunity, or laboratory confirmation of disease) should be a prerequisite to employment in such facilities. Routine prevaccination serologic tests are not necessary but may be desirable in some cases. Susceptible pregnant personnel and personnel in whom use of the vaccine is contraindicated should not be vaccinated; however, susceptible pregnant personnel should be vaccinated immediately postpartum. Susceptible personnel who work with female patients of childbearing age should be educated about the importance of compliance with rubella vaccination; personnel who still refuse immunization should be transferred to another area of the hospital or termination of their employment should be considered.

Travelers Rubella occurs worldwide and the risk of exposure to the disease outside the US may be high. Individuals who are not immune and travel outside the US may acquire and import the infection into the US. Vaccination against rubella is not a requirement for entry into any country; all travelers (especially women of childbearing potential) should be immune to rubella.

■ Postexposure Vaccination In individuals who have been exposed to natural rubella virus, there is no evidence that administration of a rubella virus-containing vaccine would prevent illness; however, a single exposure may not cause infection. Because postexposure vaccination provides future protection to individuals who do not contract the disease and because there is *no* evidence that administering a rubella virus-containing vaccine to an individual who is incubating rubella would be harmful, vaccination is recommended by the ACIP and AAP, unless otherwise contraindicated.

■ Outbreak Control Rubella outbreak control is essential for eliminating indigenous rubella and preventing congenital rubella infection and CRS. Because the incidence of rubella is low in the US, the CDC states that even a single case of rubella should be considered a potential outbreak. Suspected cases of rubella, CRS, or congenital rubella infection should be reported to local health departments within 24 hours, and such reports should not be delayed while waiting for laboratory confirmation. Control measures should be implemented as soon as a case of rubella is identified; maintaining control measures is essential when pregnant women are possible contacts of patients with rubella.

During a rubella outbreak, patients should be isolated for 5–7 days after rash onset and susceptible contacts should be identified and vaccinated (unless the vaccine is contraindicated). Pregnant women who were exposed to rubella and do not have adequate proof of immunity should be tested for serologic evidence of the disease. Susceptible pregnant women should be counseled regarding the risks for intrauterine rubella infection and should be advised to restrict contact with individuals with confirmed, probable, or suspected rubella for at least 6 weeks after rash onset in the last identified patient and also to avoid activities where they might be exposed to rubella for 6 weeks after the onset of symptoms of rubella in the last patient for whom rubella cannot be ruled out.

If a rubella outbreak occurs in a congregate environment (e.g., household, jail, day-care center, military setting, school, place of worship, athletic event, other social gathering), exposed individuals without adequate proof of rubella immunity should be vaccinated. If an outbreak occurs in a health-care setting (e.g., hospital, doctor's office, clinic, nursing home, other facility where patients receive subacute or extended care), health-care workers without adequate evidence of immunity should be excluded from work and vaccinated (especially in setting where pregnant women could be exposed). Despite subsequent vaccination, exposed health-care workers should be excluded from direct patient care for 23 days after the last exposure to rubella. Because birth before 1957 does not guarantee immunity, health-care facilities should recommend 2 doses of MMR to workers born before 1957 who do not have laboratory evidence of immunity or laboratory evidence of disease. If a community-wide outbreak occurs, any person exposed to a patient with rubella or CRS who cannot demonstrate proof of immunity should be vaccinated or restricted from contact with patients with rubella or CRS.

The CDC's recommendations for evaluation and management of suspected rubella outbreaks should be consulted for additional information, including information on criteria for rubella case classification (suspected, probable, confirmed, asymptomatic confirmed), criteria for case classification of CRS (suspected, probable, confirmed, infection only), laboratory diagnosis of rubella and CRS, surveillance and control measures, and outreach activities to prevent future rubella outbreaks.

Dosage and Administration

■ Reconstitution and Administration The fixed-combination vaccine containing measles, mumps, and rubella antigens (MMR; M-M-R® II) is administered by subcutaneous injection. The vaccine should *not* be administered IV.

For information on reconstitution and administration of the fixed-combination vaccine containing MMR and varicella virus vaccine live (MMRV; ProQuad®), see Varicella Virus Vaccine Live 80:12.

MMR is reconstituted by adding the entire amount of diluent supplied by the manufacturer to the vial of lyophilized vaccine and agitating the vial. Only the diluent provided by the manufacturer should be used for reconstitution. Discard the preparation if the lyophilized vaccine does not dissolve completely.

Reconstituted MMR should be inspected visually for particulate matter and discoloration prior to administration. The vaccine should be reconstituted and administered using sterile syringes and needles that are free of preservatives, antiseptics, and detergents, since these substances may inactivate live virus vaccines.

To minimize loss of potency and ensure an adequate immunizing dose, MMR should be administered immediately following reconstitution. (See Chemistry and Stability: Stability.)

The preferred site for subcutaneous injection of MMR is the upper-outer triceps area; injections also can be given into the anterolateral thigh. For children 1 year of age and older, adolescents, and adults, the upper-outer triceps area usually is preferred. To ensure appropriate delivery, subcutaneous injections should be made at a 45° angle using a 5/8-inch, 23- to 25-gauge needle. Prior to injection, care should be taken to ensure that the needle is not in a blood vessel.

Since syncope may occur following vaccination, vaccinees should be observed for approximately 15 minutes after the vaccine dose is administered. If syncope occurs, the patient should be observed until symptoms resolve. Syncope after vaccination occurs most frequently in adolescents and young adults.

When multiple vaccines are administered during a single health-care visit, each vaccine should be given with a different syringe and at different injection sites. Separate injection sites by at least 1 inch (if anatomically feasible) to allow appropriate attribution of any local adverse effects that may occur.

■ Dosage The usual dose of MMR is 0.5 mL and is the same for all individuals. When reconstituted as specified, each 0.5-mL dose of MMR contains not less than 1000 $TCID_{50}$ of measles virus, 12,500 $TCID_{50}$ of mumps virus, and 1000 $TCID_{50}$ of rubella virus. The entire volume of reconstituted solution in the single-dose vial should be administered.

Although a single dose of MMR may provide long-term (probably lifelong) immunity against rubella, 2 doses of MMR administered at least 1 month (i.e., at least 28 days) apart are recommended.

For information on dosage of the fixed-combination vaccine containing MMR and varicella virus vaccine live (MMRV; ProQuad®), see Varicella Virus Vaccine Live 80:12.

Infants and Children 12 Months through 12 Years of Age For primary immunization against rubella in infants and children, a 2-dose regimen of MMR is recommended and the first dose generally is administered at 12 through 15 months of age. For routine childhood immunization, the ACIP, AAP, and AAFP recommend that the first dose of MMR be given at 12 through 15 months of age and the second MMR dose be routinely given at 4 through 6 years of age (just prior to entry into kindergarten or first grade). The second dose may be given earlier during any routine visit, provided at least 4 weeks (i.e., at least 28 days) have elapsed since the first dose and both the first and second doses are administered beginning at or after 12 months of age.

Adolescents 13 through 18 Years of Age For primary immunization against rubella in previously unvaccinated adolescents 13 through 18 years of age, a 2-dose regimen of MMR is recommended. The second dose should be administered at least 4 weeks (i.e., at least 28 days) after the initial dose.

Adults For adults 19 years of age and older, primary immunization consists of 1 or 2 doses of MMR. The minimum interval between doses is 4 weeks (i.e., at least 28 days).

Cautions

The incidence of adverse effects of monovalent rubella virus vaccine live (no longer commercially available in the US) appears to increase with the age of the vaccinee, particularly in postpubertal females. Vaccine-induced adverse effects generally have only been reported in rubella-susceptible vaccinees. There is no conclusive evidence that individuals who are already immune when vaccinated are at any increased risk of vaccine-associated adverse effects.

■ Systemic Effects Symptoms associated with natural rubella infection, including mild regional lymphadenopathy, rash, urticaria, fever, malaise, sore throat, dizziness, headache, nausea, vomiting, diarrhea, general aches, and polyneuritis (e.g., paresthesia and pain in the arms and legs), occur occasionally in vaccinees. Rubella-like symptoms may occur 11–20 days after vaccination and usually are mild and transient, generally persisting 1–5 days.

Musculoskeletal and Associated Effects Arthralgia and, rarely, transient arthritis may occur following administration of rubella virus vaccine live. Joint symptoms are infrequent and generally of brief duration in children but occur in up to about 12–26% of susceptible postpubertal women who receive the vaccine; the incidence of these reactions in adolescent girls appears to be greater than that in children but less than that in adult women. About 10% of postpubertal females develop arthritis-like manifestations. The US Public Health Service Advisory Committee in Immunization Practices (ACIP) states that in large-scale field trials up to 40% of vaccinees developed joint pain, usually of the small peripheral joints, but frank arthritis reportedly occurred in less than 2% of vaccinees.

Acute joint reactions associated with rubella vaccination generally are mild and occur 1–3 weeks after vaccination, usually persist 1 day to several weeks, and rarely recur. Infrequently and principally in adult women, these arthralgic symptoms have been reported to be chronic and recurrent, continuing for months or years; occasionally arthralgic symptoms are accompanied by arthritis and/or neurologic symptoms (e.g., paresthesia, blurred vision, carpal tunnel syndrome). Such symptoms usually are evident within 1 month after initial vaccination and may be associated with prolonged rubella viremia. While the frequency of chronic joint symptoms has been reported to be as high as 5–11% in adult females, other experience from the US and other countries using vaccines containing the RA 27/3 rubella strain suggest that such symptoms occur only rarely.

Although the Institute of Medicine reported in 1991 that some data were consistent with a causal relationship between RA 27/3 rubella vaccine and chronic arthritis in adult women, the evidence was limited in scope and confined to reports from a single institution. Results of a large, retrospective cohort study of women 15–59 years of age did not reveal evidence of an increased risk of new onset chronic arthropathies or neurologic conditions within 1 year following receipt of the currently available rubella virus vaccine live. Several other recent studies also found no evidence of increased risk for new onset of chronic arthropathies among women vaccinated with the RA 27/3 rubella vaccine. Chronic arthritis has been associated with natural rubella infection and has been related to persistent virus and/or viral antigen isolated from body tissues. The frequency of chronic joint complaints is substantially higher following natural infection than following vaccination.

Joint symptoms associated with rubella vaccination tend to be more severe in susceptible women than in children, but adults who develop such symptoms usually have tolerated them well and have not had to disrupt normal (e.g., work) activities. Rarely, however, the symptoms are severe enough to disrupt normal activities. Destruction of the joint has been reported rarely.

Although transient peripheral neuritic complaints have occurred rarely, a causal relationship between the RA 27/3 rubella vaccine and peripheral neuropathies has not been established. Such pain and/or paresthesias may not be associated with specific joints, but they generally follow the same time course for onset and duration and the frequency of recurrence of acute joint symptoms. Myalgia has also been reported rarely following administration of rubella virus vaccine live.

The mechanism of joint abnormalities following administration of rubella virus vaccine live is unclear. It has been suggested that persistence of virus in peripheral blood lymphocytes may occur in a substantial number of affected individuals. It also has been suggested that defective immunity resulting from partial antibody may facilitate persistence of the virus. There is no conclusive evidence that immune complexes contribute to disease pathogenesis. While rubella virus has been isolated from both peripheral blood lymphocytes and synovial cells of children with chronic (primary juvenile) arthritis, a causal relationship has not been established.

Sensitivity Reactions Allergic reactions have been reported rarely in individuals receiving rubella virus vaccine live. Most hypersensitivity reactions have been minor, consisting of a wheal and flare or urticaria at the injection site. However, more serious hypersensitivity reactions, including anaphylaxis and anaphylactoid reactions as well as related phenomena such as angioneurotic edema (including peripheral or facial edema) and bronchial spasm, have been reported rarely following administration of rubella virus vaccine live or measles, mumps, and rubella virus vaccine live (MMR) in individuals with or without an allergic history. Immediate, anaphylactic reactions to rubella virus vaccine live or MMR are extremely rare. Although more than 70 million doses of rubella virus-containing vaccines (MMR) have been distributed in the US since the Vaccine Adverse Events Reporting System (VAERS) was implemented in 1990, only 33 cases of anaphylactic reactions have been reported after MMR vaccination. In addition, only 11 of these cases occurred immediately after vaccination with manifestations consistent with anaphylaxis. .

MMR contains hydrolyzed gelatin as a stabilizer, which rarely may stimulate hypersensitivity reactions in some individuals. An anaphylactic reaction following MMR vaccination has been reported in the US in at least one individual with IgE-mediated anaphylactic sensitivity to gelatin, and similar cases have been reported elsewhere. (See Cautions: Precautions and Contraindications.) Erythema multiforme, Stevens-Johnson syndrome, rash, urticaria, and vasculitis have been reported rarely with rubella virus vaccine live.

Hematologic Effects Surveillance of adverse effects in the US and elsewhere indicates that rubella virus-containing vaccines (e.g., MMR) rarely can cause clinically evident thrombocytopenia (e.g., purpura) within 2 months after vaccination. In prospective studies, the reported incidence of clinically evident thrombocytopenia after MMR vaccination ranged from 1 per 30,000 to 1 per 40,000 vaccinated children, with a temporal clustering of cases occurring 2–3 weeks after vaccination. With passive surveillance, the reported incidence ranged from 1 per 100,000 to 1 per million distributed doses. Results of one retrospective study confirmed that a causal relation exists between receipt of MMR and idiopathic thrombocytopenic purpura and indicated that the absolute risk within 6 weeks of vaccination was 1 in 22,300 doses with 2 out of 3 cases occurring in the 6-week post-vaccination period being caused by MMR. However, the incidence of thrombocytopenia reported with natural rubella or measles infection is substantially greater than that reported with vaccination, being approximately 1 per 3000 children during one measles epidemic. Evidence from case reports suggests that the risk of vaccine-induced thrombocytopenia may be increased in individuals with a history of idiopathic thrombocytopenic purpura, particularly for those who developed it with a previous dose of the vaccine (see Cautions: Precautions and Contraindications); however, results of one retrospective study indicate that children with a history of idiopathic thrombocytopenic purpura prior to the first dose of MMR are not at increased risk of vaccine-associated idiopathic thrombocytopenic purpura. In most cases, vaccine-associated thrombocytopenic purpura usually has been transient and benign, although hemorrhage occurred rarely.

Regional lymphadenopathy or leukocytosis have been reported in individuals receiving rubella virus vaccine live.

Other Adverse Systemic Effects Moderate fever (38.3–39.4°C) occurs occasionally following rubella vaccination, and higher fever occurs less frequently. Syncope, headache, dizziness, malaise, irritability, diarrhea, nausea, vomiting, sore throat, cough, and rhinitis also have been reported.

There have been isolated reports of encephalitis, polyneuritis, and polyneuropathy, including Guillain-Barré syndrome, following administration of vaccines containing rubella virus live; however, the National Academy of Sciences Institute of Medicine concluded that current evidence is insufficient to accept or reject a causal relationship. Forms of optic neuritis, including retrobulbar neuritis, papillitis, and retinitis, occur rarely following viral infections, and have been reported to occur 1–3 weeks following administration of some live virus vaccines. Nerve deafness, otitis media, and conjunctivitis have been reported.

■ **Local Effects** Burning and/or stinging of short duration may occur at the injection site because of the slightly acidic pH of rubella virus vaccine live. Induration, erythema, tenderness or pain, and wheal and flare may occur occasionally at the vaccine injection site. Such reactions usually are mild and transient.

■ **Precautions and Contraindications** MMR is contraindicated in individuals with a hypersensitivity to the vaccine or any component in the formulation, including gelatin. (See Gelatin Allergy under Cautions: Sensitivity Reactions, in Precautions and Contraindications.) In addition, MMR is contraindicated in those with a history of anaphylactic or anaphylactoid reaction to neomycin. (See Neomycin Allergy under Cautions: Sensitivity Reactions, in Precautions and Contraindications.)

MMR is contraindicated in certain other individuals, including pregnant women. (See Individuals with Altered Immunocompetence under Cautions: Precautions and Contraindications and Cautions: Pregnancy, Fertility, and Lactation.)

Sensitivity Reactions Prior to administration, the recipient and/or parent or guardian should be questioned concerning reactions to previous doses of rubella virus-containing vaccine or MMR. Individuals who have a hypersensitivity reaction to the first dose should be tested for immunity to rubella; if results indicate immunity, a second dose is not necessary. Any individual with an anaphylactic reaction to a previous dose should not receive another dose, regardless of results of serologic testing.

Although the rubella virus used in the preparation of MMR is propagated in human diploid cells, the measles and mumps virus components of MMR are propagated in chick embryo tissue culture and the usual precautions for use in individuals with allergy to egg-related antigens apply to the use of MMR. (See Allergy to Egg-related Antigens under Precautions and Contraindications: Sensitivity Reactions, in Measles Virus Vaccine Live 80:12.)

Epinephrine should be available for immediate treatment of an anaphylactic reaction if such reaction occurs.

Neomycin Allergy. Because MMR contains trace amounts of neomycin, the vaccine is contraindicated in individuals who have had an anaphylactic or anaphylactoid reaction to topically or systemically administered neomycin.

Neomycin allergy usually is characterized by a delayed-type (cell-mediated) hypersensitivity reaction, such as contact dermatitis, rather than an anaphylactic reaction. Following administration of rubella virus vaccine live to individuals who have had a delayed-type hypersensitivity reaction to neomycin, the typical adverse reaction, if any, is a contact dermatitis (e.g., characterized by an erythematous, pruritic nodule or papule) occurring within 48–96 hours.

The ACIP and the American Academy of Pediatrics (AAP) state that vaccines containing trace amounts of neomycin should *not* be used in individuals with a history of anaphylactic reaction to neomycin, but use of such vaccines may be considered in those with a history of delayed-type hypersensitivity reaction to neomycin if benefits of vaccination outweigh risks.

Gelatin Allergy. The possibility of allergic reactions to hydrolyzed gelatin, which is present in MMR as a stabilizer, should be considered since anaphylactic reactions to the vaccine have been reported rarely in individuals with anaphylactic sensitivity to gelatin. MMR should not be administered to individuals with a history of anaphylactic reactions to gelatin or gelatin-containing products. Although skin testing for gelatin sensitivity before administering the vaccine to such individuals can be considered, there are no specific protocols for this purpose. Because gelatin used in vaccines manufactured in the US usually is derived from porcine sources and food gelatin may be derived solely from bovine sources, a negative food history does not exclude the possibility of a reaction to the gelatin contained in the vaccines.

Individuals with Altered Immunocompetence MMR generally is contraindicated in individuals with primary immunodeficiencies (e.g., cellular immune deficiency, hypogammaglobulinemia, dysgammaglobulinemia) and in individuals with suppressed immune responses resulting from acquired immunodeficiency syndrome (AIDS) or other clinical manifestations of human immunodeficiency virus (HIV) infection, blood dyscrasias, leukemia, lymphomas of any type, or any other malignant neoplasms affecting the bone marrow or lymphatic systems.

Replication of rubella vaccine virus may be potentiated in individuals with primary immunodeficiencies (e.g., cellular immune deficiency, hypogammaglobulinemia, dysgammaglobulinemia) or with suppressed immune response resulting from leukemia, lymphoma, other malignancies affecting the bone marrow or lymphatic system, or blood dyscrasias. Severe immunosuppression may be caused by many disease conditions (e.g., congenital immunodeficiency, HIV infection, hematologic or generalized malignancy) and by immunosuppressive therapy. For some conditions, all infected individuals are severely immunocompromised, whereas for other conditions, the degree of immune compromise depends on the severity of the condition, which in turn depends on the disease and treatment stage. Although there is no evidence that wild rubella or rubella virus vaccine live causes serious illness in immunocompromised individuals, concern exists about the potential risk of administering any live virus vaccine to such individuals. Therefore, with the exception of individuals with HIV infection, immunocompromised individuals should not receive a rubella virus-containing vaccine, especially those who are severely immunosuppressed. Ultimately, the patient's clinician must assume responsibility for determining whether the patient is severely immunocompromised based on clinical and laboratory assessment. MMR should not be given to an individual with a family history of congenital or hereditary immunodeficiency until the immunocompetence of the individual has been documented. The greatest risk associated with administering a live rubella virus-containing vaccine in immunosuppressed patients appears to be with vaccines that also include live measles virus as a component. (See Cautions: Precautions and Contraindications in Measles Virus Vaccine Live 80:12.)

MMR generally is contraindicated in individuals receiving immunosuppressive therapy (e.g., alkylating agents, antimetabolites, corticotropin, corticosteroids [at immunosuppressive dosages], radiation therapy), although the manufacturer states that the vaccine is not contraindicated in individuals receiving corticosteroids as replacement therapy (e.g., for Addison's disease). (See Drug Interactions: Immunosuppressive Agents.)

The ACIP states that use of live virus vaccines can be considered in patients with leukemia, lymphoma, or other malignancies if the disease is in remission and chemotherapy was terminated at least 3 months prior to vaccination.

Antibody responses to MMR and efficacy may be decreased in immunocompromised individuals.

HIV-infected Individuals. The ACIP, AAP, US Centers for Disease Control and Prevention (CDC), National Institutes of Health (NIH), Infectious Diseases Society of America (IDSA), Pediatric Infectious Diseases Society, and others state that MMR should be administered to all *asymptomatic* HIV-infected individuals according to the usually recommended immunization schedules and should be considered for all symptomatic HIV-infected individuals who do *not* have evidence of severe immunosuppression and who otherwise would be eligible for such vaccination. The presence of immunocompromised or HIV-infected individuals in a household does not preclude administration of MMR to other household members.

MMR is contraindicated in HIV-infected individuals with *severe immunosuppression.* (See HIV-Infected Individuals under Uses: Primary Immunization.)

Fever Fever has been reported. Following vaccination, patients should be monitored for temperature elevations.

Risk of Transmissible Agents in Preparations Containing Albumin MMR contains *recombinant* human albumin.

Monovalent rubella virus vaccine live (no longer commercially available in the US) and the fixed-combination vaccine containing measles, mumps, rubella, and varicella antigens (MMRV; ProQuad®) contain albumin human. Since albumin human is prepared from pooled human plasma, it is a potential vehicle for transmission of human viruses, and theoretically may carry a risk of transmitting the causative agent of Creutzfeldt-Jakob disease (CJD).

For further information on precautions related to transmissible agents in plasma-derived preparations, see Risk of Transmissible Agents in Plasma-derived Preparations under Cautions: Precautions and Contraindications, in Albumin Human 16:00.

Concomitant Illness The decision whether to administer or delay administration of MMR in an individual with a current or recent acute illness depends largely on the severity of symptoms and etiology of the illness. The manufacturer states that MMR is contraindicated in patients with any febrile respiratory illness or other active febrile infections. The ACIP and AAP state that minor acute illness, such as upper respiratory infection (with or without fever) or mild diarrhea, does not preclude vaccination. However, vaccination of individuals with moderate or severe acute illness (with or without fever) generally should be deferred until they have recovered from the acute phase of the illness. This precaution avoids superimposing adverse effects of the vaccine on the underlying illness or mistakenly concluding that a manifestation of the underlying illness resulted from vaccination. However, data generally are not available on the safety and immunogenicity of measles, mumps, and rubella virus-containing vaccines in individuals with moderate or severe febrile illness.

Thrombocytopenia Individuals with thrombocytopenia may be at increased risk of developing more severe thrombocytopenia following vaccination. In addition, individuals who experienced thrombocytopenia after the first dose of monovalent rubella virus vaccine live or MMR may develop thrombocytopenia with repeat doses. Serologic evidence of immunity may be obtained in lieu of vaccination. The decision to vaccinate such individuals should depend on the benefits of immunity and the risks of recurrence or exacerbation of thrombocytopenia.

Risk of Neurodevelopmental Disorders Although it has been theorized that there is a link between the antigens contained in MMR and neurodevelopmental disorders in children (autism), evidence has been insufficient to support an association between neurodevelopmental disorders and MMR. In 2004, the Immunization Safety Review Committee of the Institute of Medicine (IOM) examined the hypothesis that MMR is causally associated with autism and concluded that the evidence favors rejection of a causal relationship between MMR and autism.

Tuberculosis Vaccination is not recommended for individuals with untreated, active tuberculosis. Vaccination in these individuals should be deferred until antituberculosis therapy has been initiated. Administration of live, attenuated vaccines is not contraindicated in individuals with a positive tuberculin skin test who do not have active tuberculosis infection. Tuberculin testing is not a prerequisite for administration of rubella virus vaccine live or MMR.

Transmission of Vaccine Virus Small amounts of the vaccine virus are excreted from the nose or throat of most susceptible individuals 7–28 days after administration of rubella virus vaccine live. While there is a theoretical possibility that the virus could be transmitted to susceptible, close, personal contacts of the vaccinated individual, there is no evidence to indicate that the vaccine virus can be transmitted to contacts and such transmission is not regarded as a significant risk. The vaccine virus can be transmitted in milk to breastfed infants. (See Lactation in Cautions: Pregnancy and Lactation.)

Limitations of Vaccine Effectiveness MMR may not protect all individuals from rubella.

Safety and efficacy of MMR have not been established for postexposure prophylaxis following exposure to rubella. (See Uses: Postexposure Vaccination.)

Improper Storage and Handling Improper storage or handling of vaccines may result in loss of vaccine potency and reduced immune response in vaccinees.

MMR that has been mishandled or has not been stored at the recommended temperature should not be administered. (See Chemistry and Stability: Stability.)

Lyophilized and reconstituted vaccine should be protected from light at all times because exposure to light may inactivate the vaccine virus.

Freezing or exposing the diluent supplied by the manufacturer to freezing temperatures should be avoided; the diluent may be refrigerated or stored at room temperature.

All vaccines should be inspected upon delivery and monitored during storage to ensure that the appropriate temperature is maintained.

■ **Pediatric Precautions** Safety and efficacy of MMR in children younger than 6 months of age have not been established, and use of the vaccine in this age group is not recommended.

■ **Geriatric Precautions** Clinical studies of MMR did not include sufficient numbers of seronegative individuals 65 years of age or older to determine whether these individuals respond differently than younger individuals. Other reported clinical experience has not identified differences in responses between geriatric and younger individuals.

■ **Mutagenicity and Carcinogenicity** The mutagenic or carcinogenic potential of MMR has not been evaluated.

■ **Pregnancy, Fertility, and Lactation** ***Pregnancy*** Although the manufacturer states that MMR should not be administered to pregnant women and that appropriate steps should be taken to prevent conception for 3 months following vaccination, the ACIP and AAP state that women vaccinated with MMR should avoid becoming pregnant for 4 weeks (i.e., 28 days) after vaccination. (See the discussion that follows for more specific details.) Natural rubella infection during pregnancy, especially during the first trimester, may cause congenital abnormalities. Although the teratogenic potential of rubella virus-containing vaccines appears to be less than that of the wild virus and normal infants have been born to women who received such vaccines during early pregnancy, rubella vaccine virus can cross the placenta and safety for the developing fetus has not been established.

When rubella virus vaccine live containing the RA 27/3 strain replaced other rubella vaccines in 1979, concern was raised that the new vaccine might have a higher affinity for fetal tissue and be associated with greater potential for teratogenic effects than previously available vaccines since the RA 27/3 rubella virus strain was derived from an aborted rubella-infected human fetus and is produced in human embryonic lung cell lines. Available data indicate that there is probably no greater risk of placental or fetal infection from RA 27/3 vaccine than from Cendehill or HPV-77 vaccines. There is *no* evidence to indicate that rubella vaccines, including the RA 27/3 vaccine, can cause defects associated with congenital rubella syndrome (CRS). Although asymptomatic glandular hypospadias has occurred in 2 infants born to rubella-susceptible women who received RA 27/3 vaccine during pregnancy and hypospadias has been noted in infants with CRS, there are *no* data to suggest that glandular hypospadias is a CRS-associated defect. Based on experience to date, the theoretical maximum risk (derived from the binomial distribution with 95% confidence limits) for serious malformations in infants born to RA 27/3 vaccinees is reported to range from 0–1.6%; however, the overall maximum risk remains far less than the 20% or greater risk of CRS associated with maternal infection with wild rubella virus during the first trimester of pregnancy.

While no cases of CRS-associated defects have been reported, rubella vaccine viruses, including the RA 27/3 strain, can cross the placenta and infect the fetus. Data collected by CDC over an 18-year period indicate that approximately 1.5% of infants born to rubella-susceptible vaccinees had serologic evidence of subclinical rubella infection, regardless of the vaccine strain administered to the mother. The CDC data also indicate that the rubella virus isolation rate from abortuses of women who received the RA 27/3 vaccine is about 3% compared with about 20% for abortuses of women who received the Cendehill or HPV-77 vaccines; this finding provides additional evidence that the RA 27/3 vaccine poses no greater risks of teratogenicity than did these latter vaccines.

The ACIP and CDC state that use of MMR is contraindicated during pregnancy because of the theoretical, albeit small, risk of CRS or other teratogenic effects in infants born to women who receive the vaccine during pregnancy. Reasonable precautions should be taken to preclude vaccination of pregnant women, including asking women if they are pregnant, excluding those who state that they are, informing the others of the theoretical risks to the fetus, and explaining the importance of not becoming pregnant for a specified period of time after vaccination. The manufacturer recommends that pregnancy be avoided for 3 months after receipt of rubella virus-containing vaccine; however while the ACIP also previously recommended that pregnancy be avoided for 3 months after receipt of rubella virus-containing vaccine or MMR, more recent data and experience prompted ACIP to shorten the length of time for this precaution. Based on data from several sources indicating that no cases of CRS have been identified among infants born to women who were inadvertently vaccinated against rubella within 3 months or early in pregnancy, the ACIP now states that pregnancy should be avoided for 28 days after receipt of MMR. The risk of CRS is considered so small as to be negligible in women who are inadvertently vaccinated during pregnancy or in women who become pregnant within 3 months after vaccination; therefore, the ACIP and CDC state that rubella vaccination in these women should not in itself necessitate interruption of pregnancy. Because birth defects, one-third of which are serious, occur in 3–5% of *all* births, confusion about the etiology of a birth defect may result when the vaccine is administered during pregnancy.

Lactation Following postpartum vaccination with rubella virus-containing vaccine, rubella vaccine virus reportedly is distributed into milk and can be transmitted to breastfed infants. At least one breastfed infant whose mother received monovalent rubella virus vaccine live exhibited mild clinical illness typical of acquired rubella; however, in other breastfed infants with serologic evidence of rubella infection, none exhibited severe disease and ACIP states that vaccine virus infections from breastfeeding remain asymptomatic. The manufacturer states that MMR should be administered with caution to nursing women. The ACIP states that breast-feeding generally is not a contraindication to administration of MMR since the vaccine appears to pose no special problems for the mother or her nursing infant.

Drug Interactions

■ **Blood Products** Blood products (e.g., whole blood, packed red blood cells, plasma) may interfere with the immune response to certain live virus vaccines, including measles, mumps, and rubella virus vaccine live (MMR; M-M-R® II); therefore, MMR should not be administered simultaneously with or for specified intervals before or after administration of blood products.

Administration of MMR should be deferred for at least 3 months following administration of red blood cells (with adenine-saline added); for at least 6 months following administration of packed red blood cells or whole blood; and for at least 7 months following administration of plasma or platelet products.

After receiving MMR, vaccinees should avoid blood products for 2 weeks; if use of a blood product is considered necessary during this period, a repeat vaccine dose should be given after the recommended interval unless serologic testing is feasible and indicates a response to the vaccine was attained.

■ **Immunosuppressive Agents** Individuals receiving immunosuppressive agents (e.g., corticotropin, corticosteroids [at immunosuppressive dosages], alkylating agents, antimetabolites, radiation therapy) may have a diminished response to rubella virus-containing vaccine, and replication of the virus may be potentiated. Vaccination with MMR should be deferred until the immunosuppressive agent is discontinued; the manufacturer states that individuals receiving corticosteroids as replacement therapy (e.g., those with Addison's disease) generally may receive the vaccine. The exact interval between discontinuance of immunosuppressive therapy and regaining the ability to respond to live virus vaccines is not known, but live viral vaccines generally should not be administered for at least 3 months after discontinuance of immunosuppressive therapy. Individuals with leukemia in remission who have not received chemotherapy for at least 3 months may receive a live virus vaccine. The precise amount and duration of systemically absorbed corticosteroid therapy needed to suppress the immune system of an otherwise healthy individual are not well defined. Although of recent theoretical concern, there is no evidence of increased severe reactions to live vaccines in individuals receiving corticosteroid aerosol therapy, and such therapy is not in itself a reason to delay vaccination. Most experts, including the US Public Health Service Advisory Committee in Immunization Practices (ACIP) and American Academy of Pediatrics (AAP), agree that short-term (less than 2 weeks), low- to moderate-dose systemic corticosteroid therapy; long-term, alternate-day, systemic corticosteroid therapy using low to moderate doses of short-acting drugs; topical corticosteroid therapy (e.g., nasal, cutaneous, ophthalmic); or aerosol corticosteroid therapy; intra-articular, bursal, or tendon injections with corticosteroids should not be immunosuppressive in usual dosages and do not necessarily contraindicate vaccination with live virus vaccines. Although the immunosuppressive effects of corticosteroid therapy vary, many clinicians consider a dose equivalent to 2 mg/kg or 20 mg total of prednisone daily for 2 weeks or longer as sufficiently immunosuppressive to raise concerns about the safety of vaccination with live virus vaccines.

■ **Immune Globulins** Antibodies contained in immune globulin preparations (e.g., immune globulin IM [IGIM], immune globulin IV [IGIV], hepatitis B immune globulin [HBIG], rabies immune globulin [RIG], tetanus immune globulin [TIG], varicella-zoster immune globulin [VZIG]) may interfere with the immune response to certain live virus vaccines, including MMR.

MMR should be deferred for at least 3 months following administration of TIG, HBIG, IGIM used for prophylaxis of tetanus, hepatitis B virus (HBV), or hepatitis A virus (HAV); for at least 4 months following administration of RIG; for at least 5 months following administration of VZIG for varicella prophylaxis or IGIM used for measles prophylaxis in immunocompetent individuals; for at least 6 months following use of cytomegalovirus immune globulin IV (CMV-IGIV) or IGIM used for measles prophylaxis in immunocompromised individuals; for at least 8 months following administration of IGIV for replacement therapy of immunodeficiencies VZIG or IGIV used for postexposure prophylaxis of severe varicella; for at least 8–10 months following administration of IGIV for the treatment of idiopathic thrombocytopenic purpura (ITP); or for at least 11 months following administration of IGIV for Kawasaki syndrome. If simultaneous administration of a vaccine containing rubella virus vaccine live and one of these immune globulin preparations or administration at less than the recommended interval is deemed necessary (e.g., because of imminent exposure to disease), the fact that vaccine-induced immunity may be compromised should be considered and, unless there is serologic evidence of an adequate antibody response to the live virus vaccine, an additional dose of vaccine should be administered at the specified interval. If administered simultaneously, the live virus vaccine and immune globulin should be administered at separate sites anatomically remote from one another. However, MMR may be given prior to discharge from the hospital to susceptible postpartum women who have received $Rh_o(D)$ immune globulin provided that serologic testing is done 8 weeks or longer after vaccination to determine if seroconversion has occurred.

The fact that revaccination may be necessary in individuals who receive an immune globulin preparation shortly after MMR should be considered. In general, vaccine virus replication and stimulation of immunity occur within 7–14 days after administration of a live virus vaccine. Therefore, if the interval between administration of measles virus vaccine live and subsequent administration of one of these preparations is less than 14 days, an additional dose of vaccine should be given after the appropriate interval previously specified, unless serologic testing indicates that an adequate antibody response to the vaccine occurred. An additional dose of vaccine generally is unnecessary if the interval between vaccination and administration of the immune globulin or blood product is longer than 2 weeks.

■ **Live Vaccines** ***Measles, Mumps, Rubella, and Varicella Vaccines*** Rubella virus vaccine live may be administered concurrently with measles virus vaccine live, mumps virus vaccine live, and varicella virus vaccine live.

Rubella virus vaccine live is commercially available in a fixed-combination vaccine containing measles virus vaccine live and mumps virus vaccine live (MMR) to facilitate concomitant administration of all 3 antigens. Administration of MMR results in immunologic responses similar to those obtained with administration of the 3 antigens at separate sites.

MMR may be administered concurrently with monovalent varicella virus vaccine live (Varivax®) at a different site using a separate syringe. Results of studies in healthy children 12–36 months of age indicate that seroconversion rates, antibody responses, and adverse effects reported with simultaneous administration of the vaccines are similar to those reported when the vaccines are administered 6 weeks apart. Because there is a theoretical concern that the immune response to one live viral vaccine may be impaired if administered within 1 month of another, if MMR and varicella virus vaccine live are not administered simultaneously then they should be administered at least 1 month apart. There is some evidence that administration of varicella virus vaccine live less than 30 days after MMR decreases the effectiveness of the varicella vaccine. Results of a retrospective cohort study that used data from the Vaccine Safety Datalink (VSD) project and included children 12 months of age or older who were vaccinated during January 1995 to December 1999 indicate that administration of varicella virus vaccine live less than 30 days after MMR results in a 2.5-fold increase in the incidence of breakthrough varicella infections. However, when the vaccines were administered concurrently, there was no increase in the risk for breakthrough infections.

Rubella virus vaccine live also is commercially available in a fixed-combination vaccine containing MMR and varicella virus vaccine live (MMRV; ProQuad®). Studies using MMRV (ProQuad®) in healthy children 1–6 years of age indicate that the antibody responses against measles, mumps, rubella, and varicella antigens following a single dose of ProQuad® are similar to those obtained after a single dose of MMR and a single dose of varicella virus vaccine live (Varivax®). However, there is some evidence that the relative risk for febrile seizures in infants may be higher with the fixed-combination vaccine MMRV than that reported when a dose of single-antigen varicella virus vaccine live (Varivax®) and a dose of MMR are given concomitantly. For information on the fixed-combination vaccine containing MMR and varicella virus vaccine live (ProQuad®; MMRV), see Varicella Virus Vaccine Live 80:12.

Influenza Vaccine Live Intranasal Because of theoretical concerns that the immune response to one live virus vaccine might be impaired if given within 30 days of another live virus vaccine, if MMR and influenza virus vaccine live intranasal are not administered on the same day, they should be administered at least 4 weeks apart.

Other Live Vaccines Some oral live vaccines (e.g., rotavirus vaccine live oral, typhoid vaccine live oral) can be administered concomitantly with or at any interval before or after MMR.

Because of theoretical concerns that the immune response to other live virus vaccines might be impaired if given within 30 days of another live virus vaccine, if MMR and yellow fever vaccine are not administered on the same day, they should be administered at least 4 weeks apart.

■ **Inactivated Vaccines and Toxoids** MMR may be administered simultaneously with (using different syringes and different injection sites) or at any interval before or after inactivated vaccines, recombinant vaccines, polysaccharide vaccines, or toxoids.

The ACIP states that MMR and *Haemophilus influenzae* type b (Hib) conjugate vaccines may be given concomitantly.

Although specific studies evaluating simultaneous administration of MMR and hepatitis B vaccine, diphtheria and tetanus toxoids and acellular pertussis vaccine adsorbed (DTaP) or tetanus toxoid and reduced diphtheria toxoid and acellular pertussis vaccine adsorbed (Tdap) are not available, the ACIP and AAP state that these vaccines may be administered concomitantly.

MMR may be given concomitantly with parenteral inactivated influenza vaccines (using different syringes and different injection sites) or at any interval before or after administration of inactivated influenza vaccines.

The ACIP and AAP state that MMR may be administered concurrently with pneumococcal vaccine, including pneumococcal conjugate vaccine (PCV) or pneumococcal 23-valent polysaccharide vaccine (PPSV23), at a different site using a separate syringe.

Laboratory Test Interferences

■ **Tuberculin** Live attenuated measles, mumps, and rubella virus vaccines have been reported to temporarily suppress tuberculin skin sensitivity; therefore, tuberculin tests (if required) should be done before, simultaneously with, or 4–6 weeks after administration of measles, mumps, and rubella virus vaccine live (MMR; M-M-R® II).

Pharmacology

Monovalent rubella virus vaccine live (no longer commercially available in the US) and the fixed-combination vaccine containing measles, mumps, and rubella antigens (measles, mumps, and rubella virus vaccine live [MMR]) stimulate immunity to rubella (German measles) by inducing production of specific antibodies, including rubella hemagglutination-inhibiting (HI) antibodies. Although vaccine-induced antibody titers generally are lower than those stimulated by natural rubella infection, vaccine-induced immunity protects against clinical illness and viremia after natural exposure. Studies using monovalent rubella virus vaccine live indicate that administration of a single dose results in serologic evidence of immunity in 95% of vaccine recipients 12 months of age or older and confers long-term, probably lifelong, protection.

■ **Rubella Virus and Infection** Rubella virus is an RNA virus classified as a Rubivirus in the Togaviridae family. Although 25–50% of rubella infections may be subclinical or asymptomatic, infection in adults and children usually is manifested as a mild, febrile, rash illness that may include lymphadenopathy, malaise, and/or conjunctivitis. Arthralgia and arthritis also can occur and has been reported in up to 70% of adolescent and adult females with the disease. Rare complications of rubella infection include thrombocytopenic purpura, encephalitis, neuritis, and orchitis. The most serious complications of rubella infection occur when women in their first trimester of pregnancy become infected with the virus.

Rubella infection during pregnancy may cause congenital rubella infection and congenital rubella syndrome (CRS). Congenital rubella infection can affect all organs in the developing fetus and result in miscarriage, abortion, stillbirth, fetal anomalies, or asymptomatic infection in the infant. Up to 85–90% of infants born to women who become infected during the first 8–11 weeks of gestation will develop a pattern of birth defects called CRS; 20–25% of infants born to women who become infected during the first 20 weeks of pregnancy develop CRS. CRS may be characterized by one or more fetal anomalies that are auditory (e.g., sensorineural deafness), ophthalmic (e.g., cataracts, microphthalmia, glaucoma, chorioretinitis), cardiac (e.g., patent ductus arteriosus, peripheral pulmonary artery stenosis, atrial or ventricular septal defects), and/or neurologic (e.g., microencephaly, meningoencephalitis, mental retardation). CRS also may result in radiolucent bone defects, hepatosplenomegaly, thrombocytopenia, and purpuric skin lesions and some infants will have both intrauterine and postnatal growth retardation. Infants infected with rubella late in gestation may not exhibit clinical manifestations of CRS; however, any infant infected with rubella in utero can shed the virus for up to 1 year or longer.

Postnatal rubella infection usually is transmitted person-to-person by direct or droplet contact from nasopharyngeal secretion. The incubation period for rubella is 12–23 days. Individuals with rubella are most infectious when rash is erupting, but virus may be shed from 7 days before until 5–7 days after rash onset.

Natural rubella infection appears to result in immunity that is long-lasting and probably life-long. However, reexposure to natural rubella occasionally results in reinfection without clinical illness or detectable viremia. The risk for CRS among infants born to women reinfected with rubella during pregnancy is minimal.

■ **Response to Rubella Virus Vaccine Live** A single subcutaneous dose of monovalent rubella virus vaccine live (no longer commercially available in the US) containing the RA 27/3 strain of live, attenuated rubella virus in susceptible individuals 12 months of age or older induces rubella HI antibodies in at least 97% of vaccinees. Protection against rubella usually is present 21–28 days after vaccination; however, a small percentage (1–5%) of vaccinees may fail to seroconvert after a single dose. Most individuals who do not respond to the first dose of rubella virus vaccine live would be expected to respond to a second dose. Seroconversion in response to rubella vaccination parallels protection from the disease.

Monovalent rubella virus vaccine live containing the RA 27/3 strain of live, attenuated rubella virus induces higher immediate post-vaccination levels of HI, complement-fixing, and neutralizing antibodies than previously available vaccines that contained other strains of rubella virus (Cendehill, HPV-77 DE-5, HPV-77 DK-12) and also induces a broader variety of antibodies, including anti-theta and anti-iota precipitating antibodies, resulting in an immunologic response that more closely resembles that induced by natural rubella infection. The increased levels and broader profile of antibodies induced appear to correlate with greater resistance to subclinical reinfection with the wild-type virus and provide greater confidence for lasting immunity.

The duration of protection from rubella infection following administration of rubella virus-containing vaccine has not been fully determined. Individuals 12 months of age or older who receive a single subcutaneous dose of rubella virus-containing vaccine can be expected to have long-term (for at least 15 years), probably life-long, protection against clinical rubella and asymptomatic viremia. Vaccine-induced rubella HI antibodies have been reported to persist at least 10 years in some individuals. Antibodies measured by neutralization assays or enzyme linked immunosorbent assays (ELISA) are still detectable in most individuals 11–13 years after vaccination. Although data from several studies indicate that levels of vaccine-induced antibodies may decline over time, data from surveillance of rubella and CRS suggest that waning immunity with increased susceptibility to rubella disease does not occur.

Chemistry and Stability

■ **Chemistry** Rubella virus vaccine live is a preparation of live, attenuated rubella virus. Monovalent rubella virus vaccine live (Meruvax® II) is no longer commercially available in the US. Rubella virus vaccine live is commercially available in the US in a fixed-combination vaccine with measles virus vaccine live and mumps virus vaccine live (MMR; M-M-R® II) and in a fixed-combination vaccine containing MMR and varicella virus vaccine live (MMRV; ProQuad®). For information on the fixed-combination vaccine containing MMR and varicella virus vaccine live, see Varicella Virus Vaccine Live 80:12.

Vaccines containing rubella virus vaccine live meet standards established by the Center for Biologics Evaluation and Research of the US Food and Drug Administration. MMR contains the Wistar Institute RA 27/3 strain of rubella virus. The virus is propagated in human diploid (WI-38) cell culture. The potency of MMR is expressed in terms of the amount of virus estimated to infect 50% of a number of standardized tissue culture preparations under specified conditions (Tissue Culture Infective Dose 50% or $TCID_{50}$). Following reconstitution with the diluent provided by the manufacturer, each 0.5-mL dose of reconstituted MMR contains not less than 1000 $TCID_{50}$ of measles virus, 12,500 $TCID_{50}$ of mumps virus, and 1000 $TCID_{50}$ of rubella virus. Each 0.5-mL dose of the MMR also contains sorbitol (14.5 mg), sodium phosphate, sucrose (1.9 mg), sodium chloride, hydrolyzed gelatin (14.5 mg), recombinant albumin human (up to 0.3 mg), fetal bovine serum (less than 1 part per million), and approximately 25 mcg of neomycin. The cells, virus pools, fetal bovine serum, and albumin human used in preparation of MMR are screened for the absence of adventitious agents; the albumin human is processed using the Cohn cold alcohol fractionation procedure.

Lyophilized MMR occurs as a light yellow compact crystalline plugs and the reconstituted vaccine occurs as a clear, yellow solutions. MMR do not contain thimerosal or any other preservative.

■ **Stability** In lyophilized form, MMR should be refrigerated at 2–8°C but may be frozen. The vials containing diluent provided by the manufacturer may be refrigerated at 2–8°C or stored at room temperature. During shipping, MMR must be stored at 10°C or less and may be packed in solid carbon dioxide (dry ice). If the vaccine is shipped with dry ice, the diluent must be shipped separately.

Following reconstitution with the diluent provided by the manufacturer, MMR should be refrigerated at 2–8°C and discarded if not used within 8 hours. Both the lyophilized and reconstituted vaccine should be protected from light, which may inactivate the virus.

Preparations

Excipients in commercially available drug preparations may have clinically important effects in some individuals; consult specific product labeling for details.

Measles, Mumps, and Rubella Virus Vaccine Live (MMR)

Parenteral

For injection, for subcutaneous use	Measles Virus Vaccine Live (More Attenuated Enders' Line) 1000 $TCID_{50}$, Mumps Virus Vaccine Live (Jeryl Lynn [B level] Strain) 12,500 $TCID_{50}$, and Rubella Virus Vaccine Live (Wistar RA 27/3 Strain) 1000 $TCID_{50}$ per 0.5 mL	**M-M-R® II,** Merck

Measles, Mumps, Rubella and Varicella Virus Vaccine Live (MMRV)

Parenteral		
For injection, for subcutaneous use	Measles Virus Vaccine Live (More Attenuated Enders' Line) ≥3 log $_{10}$ tissue culture infective dose 50% ($TCID_{50}$), Mumps Virus Vaccine Live (Jeryl Lynn [B level] Strain) ≥4.3 log $_{10}$ $TCID_{50}$, Rubella Virus Vaccine Live (Wistar RA 27/3 Strain) ≥3 log $_{10}$ $TCID_{50}$, and Varicella Virus Vaccine Live (Oka/Merck Strain) ≥3.99 log $_{10}$ plaque-forming units (PFU) per 0.5 mL	**ProQuad®**, Merck

Selected Revisions January 2010,

Varicella Virus Vaccine Live

Chickenpox Vaccine

■ Varicella virus vaccine is a live, attenuated virus vaccine that contains varicella zoster virus (VZV) of the Oka/Merck strain and is used to stimulate active immunity to varicella (chickenpox). Varicella virus vaccine is commercially available in the US as a monovalent vaccine (Varivax®) and a fixed-combination vaccine containing measles, mumps, rubella, and varicella antigens (MMRV; ProQuad®). Other varicella vaccines may be available in other countries (e.g., Oka/Biken or Oka/RIT strains) that are similar, but not identical, to the Oka/Merck strain.

Uses

Varicella virus vaccine live is used to stimulate active immunity to varicella (chickenpox). Varicella virus vaccine live is commercially available as a single-antigen vaccine (Varivax®) for use in adults, adolescents, and children 12 months of age or older and as a fixed-combination vaccine containing measles, mumps, rubella, and varicella antigens (MMRV; ProQuad®) for use in children 12 months through 12 years of age. MMRV (ProQuad®) contains the same potency of measles, mumps, and rubella antigens as commercially available measles, mumps, and rubella virus vaccine live (MMR) and contains a slightly higher potency of varicella antigen than the single-antigen varicella vaccine (Varivax®).

The US Public Health Service Advisory Committee on Immunization Practices (ACIP), the American Academy of Pediatrics (AAP), the American Academy of Family Physicians (AAFP), and the Infectious Diseases Society of America (IDSA) recommend *universal* immunization against varicella with 2 doses of a vaccine containing varicella virus vaccine live for *all* susceptible, healthy children 12 months through 12 years of age unless the vaccine is contraindicated. The ACIP, AAP, AAFP, IDSA, American College of Obstetricians and Gynecologists (ACOG), and American College of Physicians (ACP) also recommend universal immunization against varicella with 2 doses of varicella virus vaccine live for *all* adolescents and adults 13 years of age or older without evidence of immunity, unless the vaccine is contraindicated. These experts state that special consideration should be given to use of varicella virus vaccine live in susceptible adults who have close contact with individuals who are at high risk for severe varicella (e.g., health-care personnel and family contacts of immunocompromised individuals) and susceptible adults and adolescents who are at high risk for exposure or transmission of the disease (e.g., teachers of young children, child-care employees, residents and staff members of institutional settings including correctional institutions, college students, military personnel, those living in households with children, non-pregnant women of childbearing age, international travelers). Varicella virus vaccine live also has been used for postexposure vaccination† in susceptible individuals and for outbreak prevention and control in certain settings.

The ACIP states that individuals have evidence of immunity to varicella if there is written documentation of age-appropriate vaccination (one vaccine dose in preschool children 12 months of age or older or 2 doses in school-aged children, adolescents, and adults), they were born in the US before 1980 (US birth before 1980 should *not* be considered evidence of immunity for health-care providers and pregnant women), they have a history of herpes zoster based on a diagnosis by a health-care provider, or there is laboratory evidence of immunity or laboratory confirmation of varicella infection. In addition, the ACIP states that individuals with a history of *typical varicella disease* based on a diagnosis or verification of such history by any health-care provider (e.g., school or occupational clinic nurse, nurse practitioner, physician assistant, clinician) can be considered to have evidence of immunity to varicella. For those reporting a history of or presenting with *atypical and/or mild varicella*, health-care providers should seek either an epidemiologic link to a typical varicella case (e.g., case occurred in the context of an outbreak or patient had household exposure to varicella in the previous 3 weeks) or evidence of laboratory confirmation performed at the time of acute disease; when such documentation is lacking, individuals should *not* be considered as having a valid history of varicella since other diseases may mimic mild, atypical varicella.

■ **Past and Current Considerations Regarding Varicella Vaccine Recommendations** The ACIP, AAP, AAFP, and IDSA first recommended universal immunization against varicella in all healthy, susceptible children in the US in 1996; however, there has been some controversy hindering implementation of this recommendation. Results of several studies evaluating the short-term benefits and costs related to use of varicella virus vaccine live indicate that universal immunization of healthy children is cost-effective. These studies evaluated both direct medical costs related to varicella and indirect costs related to work-loss of the parents of children with varicella. However, some clinicians have expressed concerns about routine use of the vaccine in healthy children, partly because long-term efficacy and duration of protection against varicella have not been determined and because long-term epidemiologic effects of widespread use of the vaccine are unclear.

It has been suggested that universal immunization of healthy children could increase the incidence of varicella in susceptible, healthy adolescents and adults. For example, if immunity to varicella eventually wanes in immunized children who received primary immunization against varicella, there is a theoretical possibility that varicella infections will occur in these individuals later in life. Widespread (but not universal) use of varicella virus vaccine live could result in an increased incidence of varicella infections in adults who were not vaccinated as children and were not previously exposed to natural varicella infection. Such a shift in age distribution to older individuals could increase the overall morbidity associated with varicella since the disease generally is more severe in adults than in children. This concern has now been addressed with recommendations that emphasize use of varicella virus vaccine live in susceptible older children, adolescents, and adults, in addition to universal immunization of younger children. Beginning in June 2005, the ACIP expanded their varicella vaccination recommendations to promote wider use of the vaccine in adolescents and adults. Vaccination with 2 doses of varicella virus vaccine live is now recommended for adolescents and adults 13 years of age or older who do not have evidence of immunity to varicella. In addition, to prevent herpes zoster (also known as shingles or zoster) caused by reactivation of varicella zoster virus (VZV) infection, the ACIP recommends that *all* adults 60 years of age or older receive a single dose of zostervaccine live (Zostavax®), unless the vaccine is contraindicated. (See Zoster Vaccine Live 80:12.)

Another concern expressed by some clinicians is that additional long-term studies are needed to evaluate the effects of universal varicella immunization on the incidence of subsequent herpes zoster. Theoretically, individuals who receive varicella virus vaccine live and have breakthrough varicella infections caused by wild-type virus could harbor both virus types and be at risk for reactivation and herpes zoster associated with either type. (See Cautions: Latent Infections and Herpes Zoster.)

Long-term studies, including 15-year follow-up of children following administration of varicella virus vaccine live, have been initiated. The US Centers for Disease Control and Prevention (CDC) encourages all state public health agencies to continue ongoing surveillance for varicella incidence and hospitalization and death rates; investigation of all varicella-related deaths; and establishment of reporting systems for varicella cases in schools, day-care centers, health-care provider offices, and hospitals.

■ **Risks of Varicella Exposure and Infection** Varicella occurs most frequently in susceptible children, usually in those younger than 10 years of age, but has been reported with increasing frequency in susceptible adolescents and adults. Prior to licensure of varicella virus vaccine live (i.e., prior to 1995), approximately 4 million cases of varicella occurred annually in the US, with peak incidence during late winter and early spring and an average annual incidence of 15–16 cases per 1000. Age-specific incidence data for that time period indicate that more than 90% of reported cases occurred in individuals younger than 15 years of age with 33 and 44% of cases in children 1–4 and 5–9 years of age, respectively. Since 1995, when varicella virus vaccine live became commercially available, there have been substantial decreases in the incidence of varicella and varicella-associated hospitalizations in the US in all age groups, especially in children 1–9 years of age. The number of hospitalizations and deaths from varicella have decreased more than 90% in the US since 1996. Adults who immigrate to the US from tropical areas where natural exposure to the heat-labile virus is unlikely are at particular risk of infection in the US.

Varicella is highly communicable, and the secondary infection rate in healthy, susceptible individuals exposed through household contact generally is 80–90%. Although less than 5% of varicella cases in the US occur in adults older than 20 years of age, 55% of varicella-related deaths occur in this age group. Varicella is associated with severe maternal and congenital (See Cautions: Pregnancy, Fertility, and Lactation) morbidity and mortality, with approximately 10–20% of infected pregnant women developing varicella pneumonia that has a maternal mortality rate as high as 40%.

■ **Serologic Testing and Evaluation of Susceptibility** *Prevaccination* serologic testing is not required before administration of varicella virus vaccine live since the vaccine is well tolerated by immune individuals and a prior history of chickenpox is not a contraindication to the vaccine. *Prevaccination* serologic testing is not warranted in children 12 months through 12 years of age without a history of chickenpox since the majority of these children are susceptible.

Routine *postvaccination* serologic testing to confirm seroconversion following administration of varicella virus vaccine live in otherwise healthy children, adolescents, or adults is not routinely recommended because of the high rate of seroconversion in these individuals and because commercially available assays lack sensitivity to detect vaccine-induced immunity and may give false-negative results.

In health-care institutions, *prevaccination* serologic screening of personnel who have a negative or uncertain history of varicella may be cost-effective. However, the ACIP and Hospital Infection Control Practices Advisory Committee (HICPAC) state that routine *postvaccination* testing of health-care personnel probably is not recommended. (See Health-care Personnel under Uses: Primary Immunization.)

Ideally, individuals 12 months of age and older who are scheduled to undergo solid organ transplantation should be tested for serologic evidence of varicella immunity and, if susceptible, should receive varicella vaccine at least 1 month prior to the procedure.

Levels of anti-varicella zoster virus antibodies (anti-VZV) that protect against varicella infection have not been identified and seroconversion following administration of varicella virus vaccine live generally is defined as acquisition of any detectable level of anti-VZV antibodies. Although varicella is unlikely to develop in individuals who have detectable anti-VZV antibodies, breakthrough varicella infections can occur despite seroconversion and presence of such antibodies.

Many different serologic tests have been used to determine the presence or absence of anti-VZV and these tests differ in sensitivity and specificity, time required to obtain results, and availability. While fluorescent antimembrane antibody assay (FAMA), indirect fluorescent antibody (IFA), neutralization (N), and radioimmunoassay (RIA) are sensitive tests, they are time consuming and not usually appropriate for general diagnostic laboratories. The tests most widely used are latex agglutination (LA) and enzyme-linked immunosorbent assay (ELISA). The commercially available LA test uses latex particles coated with VZV glycoprotein antigens and is a sensitive and specific test requiring only 15 minutes for completion; however, the LA test is less effective for detecting antibody following vaccination than for detecting antibody response following natural varicella infection and can yield false-positive results. The commercially available ELISA test is less sensitive, but more specific, than the LA test and should be considered when screening health-care providers for varicella susceptibility.

■ **Primary Immunization** ***Children 12 Months through 12 Years of Age*** The ACIP, AAP, AAFP, IDSA, and other clinicians recommend that all healthy, susceptible children 12 months through 12 years of age without evidence of immunity receive 2 doses of a vaccine containing varicella virus vaccine live. Vaccines containing varicella virus vaccine live are not recommended in children younger than 12 months of age since safety and efficacy in this age group have not been fully evaluated. (See Cautions: Pediatric Precautions.)

The ACIP, AAP, and AAFP state that the first dose of a vaccine containing varicella virus vaccine live should be administered at 12 through 15 months of age and the second dose at 4 through 6 years of age (i.e., before the child begins kindergarten or first grade). The second dose of a vaccine containing varicella virus vaccine live may be administered prior to 4 years of age, provided at least 3 months have elapsed since the first dose was given and both doses are administered at 12 months of age or older; however, if a second dose was administered at least 28 days following the first dose, the second dose does not need to be repeated. The first dose of a vaccine containing varicella virus vaccine live ideally should be administered on or after the first birthday as soon as the child becomes eligible for vaccination.

To ensure immunization of all children, the ACIP, AAP, AAFP, and other clinicians recommend that the immunization status of children 11–12 years of age be evaluated during routine health maintenance visits and that catch-up vaccination be given to any previously unvaccinated child without a reliable history of natural varicella infection. In children younger than 13 years of age, the catch-up second dose of varicella virus vaccine live should be administered at least 3 months after the initial dose; however, if a second dose was administered at least 28 days following the first dose, the second dose does not need to be repeated. In previously unvaccinated children 13 through 18 years of age, 2 doses of single-antigen varicella virus vaccine live should be given at least 4 weeks apart.

Primary immunization against varicella can be integrated with primary immunization against measles, mumps, rubella, diphtheria, tetanus, pertussis, *Haemophilus influenzae* type b (Hib), hepatitis A, hepatitis B, human papillomavirus (HPV), influenza, pneumococcal disease, meningococcal disease, and poliomyelitis. (See Drug Interactions: Vaccines.)

Fixed-combination Vaccine Containing Varicella Vaccine and Other Antigens. When there are no contraindications to any of the individual components, the commercially available fixed-combination vaccine containing MMR and varicella virus vaccine live (MMRV; ProQuad®) can be used instead of the single-antigen varicella virus vaccine live for primary immunization in children 12 months through 12 years of age when the first dose of MMR and first dose of varicella virus vaccine live are both indicated or when a second dose of MMR and a first or second dose of varicella virus vaccine live are both indicated.

The ACIP, AAP, and AAFP state that use of a combination vaccine generally is preferred over separate injections of the equivalent component vaccines. However, although use of MMRV (ProQuad®) reduces the number of required injections when both vaccines are indicated during a single health-care visit, there is some evidence that the relative risk for febrile seizures in infants 12 through 23 months of age may be higher with the fixed-combination vaccine than that reported when a dose of single-antigen varicella virus vaccine live (Varivax®) and a dose of MMR are given concomitantly. (See Use of Fixed Combinations under Cautions: Precautions and Contraindications.)

When the first dose of MMR and first dose of varicella virus vaccine live are indicated in infants and children 12 through 47 months of age, the ACIP states that providers considering use of MMRV (ProQuad®) should advise the parent or caregiver about the benefits and risks associated with the fixed-combination vaccine compared with the individual component vaccines. Although MMRV (ProQuad®) results in 1 less injection, it is associated with a higher risk for fever and febrile seizures on days 5 through 12 after the first dose in children 12 through 23 months of age (i.e., about 1 extra febrile seizure for every 2300–2600 doses of ProQuad®). The ACIP states that if providers face any barriers to clearly communicating these benefits and risks (e.g., language barrier), then MMR and varicella virus vaccine live should be administered instead of MMRV (ProQuad®). When the first dose of MMR and first dose of varicella virus vaccine live are indicated in children 48 months of age or older and when second doses are indicated in those 15 months through 12 years of age, the ACIP states that use of MMRV (ProQuad®) generally is preferred over separate injections of the component vaccines; considerations should include provider assessment (e.g., number of injections, vaccine availability, likelihood of improved coverage, likelihood of patient return, storage and cost considerations), patient preference, and potential for adverse effects.

Safety and efficacy of MMRV (ProQuad®) have not been established in individuals with human immunodeficiency virus (HIV) infection†. Therefore, pending further accumulation of data, the fixed-combination vaccine should not be used in HIV-infected individuals. (See HIV-infected Individuals under Primary Immunization: Individuals with Altered Immunocompetence and Their Household Contacts, in Uses).

Clinical studies in healthy children 12–23 months of age indicate that those who received a single dose of MMRV (ProQuad®) developed antibody levels against measles, mumps, rubella, and varicella that were similar to levels attained in children who received a single dose of MMR and a single dose of varicella virus vaccine live concomitantly at separate sites.

Adults and Adolescents 13 Years of Age or Older The ACIP, AAP, AAFP, IDSA, ACOG, and ACP recommend that *all* healthy, susceptible adults and adolescents 13 of age or older without evidence of immunity to varicella receive primary immunization with 2 doses of varicella virus vaccine live given 4–8 weeks apart. Safety and efficacy of the fixed-combination vaccine containing MMR and varicella virus vaccine live (MMRV; ProQuad®) have *not* been established in adults and adolescents 13 years of age or older and should not be used in this age group.

Previously, it was recommended that primary immunization against varicella virus vaccine live be considered only for susceptible adults at high risk for exposure or transmission of varicella. However, beginning in June 2005, the ACIP began recommending universal immunization with varicella virus vaccine live for *all* healthy, susceptible, nonpregnant adolescents and adults 13–49 years of age unless the vaccine is contraindicated. Currently, the ACIP, AAFP, ACOG, and ACP recommend primary immunization against varicella for all adults, unless contraindicated. Primary immunization with 2 doses of varicella virus vaccine live is especially important in susceptible adults who have close contact with individuals at high risk for severe varicella (e.g., health-care personnel and family contacts of immunocompromised individuals) and those who are at high risk for exposure or transmission of varicella (e.g., teachers of young children, child-care personnel, residents and staff in institutional settings such as correctional institutions, college students, military personnel, adolescents and adults living in households with children, nonpregnant women of childbearing age, international travelers). (See Individuals with Altered Immunocompetence and their Household Contacts and see Health-Care Personnel under Uses: Primary Immunization.) To facilitate vaccination of susceptible adolescents and adults, varicella virus vaccine live should be offered during routine health-care visits.

Varicella virus vaccine live should not be used in women who are pregnant or might become pregnant within 4 weeks of receiving the vaccine. (See Cautions: Pregnancy, Fertility, and Lactation.) The ACIP, AAFP, and ACOG recommend that all pregnant women be assessed for evidence of varicella immunity and those without such evidence should receive a dose of monovalent varicella virus vaccine live administered after delivery or termination of pregnancy (before discharge) and a second dose administered 4–8 weeks after the first dose (at a postpartum or other health-care visit). The ACIP and AAP recommend the use of standing orders to ensure administration of the vaccine in health-care settings where completion or termination of pregnancy occur.

For adults 60 years of age or older, the ACIP recommends that *all* adults in this age group receive a single dose of zoster vaccine live, unless the vaccine is contraindicated. The varicella antigen contained in commercially available zoster vaccine live (Zostavax®) is the same as that contained in varicella virus vaccine live (Varivax®); however, zoster vaccine live is about 14 times more potent than varicella virus vaccine live. The dose of zoster vaccine live is used to boost active immunity to VZV in adults 60 years of age or older and prevent herpes zoster (also known as shingles or zoster) caused by reactivation of VZV infection. (See Zoster Vaccine Live 80:12.)

Internationally Adopted Children and Other Immigrants Individuals seeking an immigrant visa for permanent US residency must provide proof of age-appropriate vaccination according to the US Recommended Childhood and Adolescent Immunization Schedules or the US Recommended Adult Schedule (see Immunization Schedules, US 80:00). Although this vaccination requirement applies to all immigrant infants and children entering the US, internationally adopted children younger than 11 years of age are exempt from the overseas vaccination requirements; however, adoptive parents are required to sign a waiver indicating their intention to comply with the vaccination requirements within 30 days after the infant or child arrives in the US. The CDC states that more than 90% of newly arrived internationally adopted children need catch-up vaccinations to meet the US Recommended Immunization Schedules.

The fact that immunization schedules of other countries may differ from US schedules (e.g., different recommended vaccines, recommended ages of administration, and/or number and timing of vaccine doses) also should be considered. Vaccines administered outside the US can generally be accepted as valid if the administration schedule was similar to that recommended in the US childhood and adolescent immunization schedules. Only written vaccination records should be considered as evidence of previous vaccination since such records are more likely to accurately predict protection if the vaccines administered, intervals between doses, and child's age at the time of vaccination are similar to US recommendations; however, the extent to which an internationally adopted child's immunization record reflects their protection against disease is unclear and it is possible there may be transcription errors in such records (e.g., single-antigen vaccine may have been administered although a multiple-antigen vaccine was recorded). Although vaccines with inadequate potency have been produced in other countries, most vaccines used worldwide are immunogenic and produced with adequate quality control standards.

When the immune status of an internationally adopted child is uncertain, health-care providers can either repeat vaccinations (since this usually is safe and avoids the need to obtain and interpret serologic tests) and/or use selective serologic testing to determine the need for immunizations (helps avoid unnecessary injections). Because varicella virus vaccine live is not available in the majority of countries, especially developing countries, all internationally adopted children who lack reliable evidence of varicella immunity should be vaccinated using an age-appropriate regimen of varicella virus vaccine live according to the US recommended immunization schedule. Although serologic testing can be done to verify immunization status in children older than 12 months of age, such testing prior to vaccination is not recommended in children younger than 12 years of age coming from tropical countries, unless there is a history of the disease.

Individuals with Altered Immunocompetence and Their Household Contacts Varicella virus vaccine live, like most other live viral vaccines, generally is contraindicated in children, adolescents, and adults with altered immunocompetence, including those with primary immunodeficiencies (e.g., cellular immune deficiency, hypogammaglobulinemia, dysgammaglobulinemia), blood dyscrasias, leukemia, lymphomas of any type or any other malignant neoplasms affecting the bone marrow or lymphatic system, HIV infection, and individuals receiving immunosuppressive therapy (e.g., corticosteroids, antineoplastic agents, radiation).

Because individuals with altered immunocompetence are at high risk for serious varicella infections, vaccination of their susceptible, healthy household contacts is recommended since such a strategy provides protection for the immunocompromised individual by decreasing the likelihood that wild-type varicella virus will be introduced into the household. While vaccination of household contacts of immunocompromised individuals theoretically results in a risk of transmission of vaccine virus to the immunocompromised individual, the risk appears to be minimal and the benefits of vaccinating susceptible household contacts outweigh the potential risk for transmission of vaccine virus to immunocompromised contacts. However, if the healthy household contact develops a varicelliform rash following vaccination, they probably should avoid contact with the immunocompromised, susceptible individual. If inadvertent contact does occur, use of varicella zoster immune globulin (VZIG) for postexposure prophylaxis in the immunocompromised individual probably is unnecessary since transmission of vaccine virus is rare and disease associated with this type of transmission is expected to be mild if it occurs. However, some experts recommend that use of acyclovir should be considered in immunocompromised individuals (e.g., HIV-infected individuals) who develop skin lesions possibly related to vaccine virus after contact with a recipient of varicella virus vaccine live.

HIV-infected Individuals. Safety and efficacy of varicella virus vaccine live have not been established in children, adolescents, or adults with HIV infection†. However, because HIV-infected individuals are at increased risk for morbidity from varicella and herpes zoster, the ACIP, AAP, CDC, National Institutes of Health (NIH), HIV Medicine Association of the Infectious Diseases Society of America (IDSA), Pediatric Infectious Diseases Society, and others state that use of single-antigen varicella virus vaccine live can be considered in selected HIV-infected individuals who are asymptomatic or mildly symptomatic. These experts suggest that, after weighing risks and benefits, use of the single-antigen varicella vaccine should be considered in HIV-infected† children 1–8 years of age with age-specific $CD4^+$ T-cell percentages of at least 15% and may be considered in HIV-infected† adults, adolescents, and children older than 8 years of age with $CD4^+$ T-cell counts of 200/mm^3 or greater. Other HIV-infected children, adolescents, or adults who are more severely immunocompromised should *not* receive varicella virus vaccine live.

Routine screening for HIV prior to administration of varicella virus vaccine live is unnecessary. If varicella virus vaccine live is used in an HIV-infected individual†, the possibility that such individuals may be at increased risk for complications after vaccination with a live virus should be considered since they have impaired cellular immunity. Because individuals with impaired cellular immunity are potentially at greater risk for complications after vaccination with a live vaccine, HIV-infected children and their caregivers should be encouraged to consult their clinician if the child develops a postvaccination varicella-like rash. If an HIV-infected individual is inadvertently vaccinated and varicella develops, appropriate antiviral therapy (e.g., acyclovir) may modify the severity of the disease.

Children and Adolescents with Acute Lymphocytic Leukemia. Although monovalent varicella virus vaccine live was used in the past under an investigational protocol in certain children and adolescents with acute lymphocytic (lymphoblastic) leukemia (ALL)† in remission, this protocol has been terminated. The ACIP and AAP state that varicella virus vaccine live should *not* be used routinely in susceptible children with leukemia and use of the vaccine in leukemic children in remission who do not have evidence of immunity to varicella should only be undertaken with expert guidance and only if antiviral therapy is available in case complications occur. ACIP states that use of live virus vaccines can be considered in patients with leukemia or other malignancies if the disease is in remission and chemotherapy was terminated at least 3 months prior to vaccination.

Transplant Recipients. Information regarding use of varicella virus vaccine live in hematopoietic stem cell transplant (HSCT) or bone marrow transplant (BMT) recipients or patients who have undergone solid organ transplantation (e.g., kidney or liver transplantation) is limited.

Ideally, individuals 12 months of age or older who are scheduled to undergo solid organ transplantation should be tested for serologic evidence of immunity to varicella and, if susceptible, should receive varicella virus vaccine live at least 1 month prior to the procedure. Although some solid organ transplant recipients have received live virus vaccines (e.g., MMR, varicella virus vaccine live) after transplantation (e.g., at least 6 months after transplantation, when minimal immunosuppressive agents were being given, when there were no recent episodes of organ rejection), but data are too limited to recommend general use of the vaccines in this population. The AAP recommends that serum antibody concentrations should be measured in all solid organ transplant recipients 1 year or longer after transplantation and appropriate vaccines administered if indicated.

The AAP states that varicella virus vaccine live is contraindicated in HSCT recipients during the first 24 months after transplantation and that use of the vaccine in HSCT patients should be restricted to research protocols in which the vaccine may be considered 24 months or longer after HSCT in those presumed to be immunocompetent.

Health-care Personnel The ACIP and HICPAC state that *all* health-care personnel should ensure that they are immune to varicella and recommend that susceptible personnel receive primary immunization with 2 doses of varicella virus vaccine live as soon as possible. Immunization of susceptible personnel protects the worker following varicella exposure in the workplace and also may help reduce nosocomial transmission of VZV; this is particularly important for health-care personnel who have close contact with individuals who are at high risk for serious complications from varicella. Sources of nosocomial infections include patients, hospital staff, and visitors (e.g., children of hospital employees) who have varicella or herpes zoster; airborne transmission of the virus in hospitals has resulted in varicella infection in susceptible individuals who had no direct contact with the index case patient.

In health-care institutions, serologic screening of personnel who have a negative or uncertain history of varicella is likely to be cost-effective. However, while varicella is unlikely to develop in individuals who have detectable anti-VZV, seroconversion does not always result in full protection and varicella has occurred in health-care personnel who had previous evidence of seroconversion. The ACIP and HICPAC state that routine testing of health-care personnel for varicella immunity following administration of 2 doses of varicella virus vaccine live probably is not necessary, but that testing vaccinees for seropositivity immediately after exposure to VZV is a potentially effective strategy for identifying those who remain at risk for varicella. The ACIP states that health-care personnel who have received 2 doses of varicella virus vaccine and who are exposed to varicella should be monitored through the employee health program or by an infection control nurse daily during days 10–21 after exposure to determine clinical status (i.e., screen daily for fever, skin lesions, and systemic symptoms). The ACIP and HICPAC state that health-care workers who remain susceptible may be furloughed or, alternatively, such individuals can be monitored daily to determine clinical status and then furloughed at the onset of manifestations of varicella. Institutional guidelines are needed for the management of exposed health-care workers who have received varicella virus vaccine live but do not have detectable antibody and for health-care personnel who develop clinical varicella.

Only health-care personnel who are immune to varicella (i.e., have a positive history of varicella infection, have serologic evidence of immunity, or have received varicella virus vaccine live) should care for patients who have confirmed or suspected VZV infection. Strategies that have been used to manage clusters of VZV infection in hospitals have included isolating varicella patients and susceptible patients who have been exposed to the virus; controlling air flow; daily screening of all exposed, susceptible personnel for skin lesions, fever, and systemic symptoms; and furloughing exposed, susceptible personnel or temporarily reassigning them to locations remote from patient-care areas. However, policies of furloughing exposed, susceptible health-care personnel are disruptive (these individuals are potentially infective for 9–21 days after exposure) and costly and may be inadequate for preventing spread of the infection in the hospital setting. Although postexposure use of varicella virus vaccine live can be considered for unvaccinated health-care personnel who lack documented immunity at the time of exposure to varicella, preexposure vaccination is the preferred method for preventing varicella in health-care settings. While varicella zoster immune globulin (VZIG) can be used for postexposure prophylaxis in health-care personnel, VZIG does not necessarily prevent varicella, may prolong the incubation period by 1 week or more, and is costly. In addition, the only VZIG preparation available for use in the US (VariZIG®; Cangene) must be obtained through an investigational new drug (IND) protocol under an expanded access program. For patients who have been exposed to varicella and who are at increased risk for severe disease and complications, this VZIG preparation can be obtained by contacting FFF Enterprises (the sole authorized US distributor) at 800-843-7477 (available 24-hours daily).

Travelers The CDC and ACIP recommend primary immunization with varicella virus vaccine live in susceptible travelers. Varicella occurs throughout the world. Although vaccination against varicella is not a requirement for entry into any country (including the US), the CDC states that individuals traveling or living abroad should ensure that they are immune. Unless the vaccine is contraindicated, the CDC and ACIP recommend that susceptible adults, adolescents, and children 12 months of age or older receive primary immunization with varicella virus vaccine live prior to international travel.

■ **Postexposure Vaccination and Outbreak Control** The ACIP and AAP recommend postexposure vaccination in susceptible children, adolescents, and adults following exposure to varicella, unless contraindicated. There is some evidence that varicella virus vaccine live may be effective in preventing varicella or modifying severity of the disease if given within 3 days, and possibly up to 5 days, after exposure. In a limited study in healthy siblings of children with varicella, administration of a single dose of vaccine (approximately 4350 units of the Oka/Merck strain of live, attenuated virus) within 3 days after the onset of rash in the index case appeared to prevent infection in 90% of susceptible siblings.

If the exposure does not cause infection, postexposure vaccination should induce protection against subsequent exposure. If the exposure results in infection, no evidence indicates that administration of varicella virus vaccine live during the presymptomatic or prodromal stage of illness increases the risk for vaccine-associated adverse effects or more severe natural disease. Although postexposure use of varicella virus vaccine live can be considered for unvaccinated health-care personnel who lack documented immunity at the time of exposure to varicella, preexposure vaccination is the preferred method for preventing varicella in health-care settings. (See Health-care Personnel under Uses: Primary Immunization.)

When varicella virus vaccine live cannot be used (e.g., pregnant women, neonates, immunocompromised individuals) and postexposure prophylaxis is considered necessary, *passive* immunization with VZIG within 96 hours of exposure is recommended to prevent or reduce the severity of varicella. The only VZIG preparation available for use in the US (VariZIG®; Cangene) must be obtained through an investigational new drug (IND) protocol under an expanded access program. For patients who have been exposed to varicella and who are at increased risk for severe disease and complications (e.g., pregnant women, neonates, immunocompromised individuals), this VZIG preparation can be obtained by contacting FFF Enterprises (the sole authorized US distributor) at 800-843-7477 (available 24 hours daily). Varicella virus vaccine live should *not* be administered concomitantly with VZIG. (See Drug Interactions: Immune Globulins.) If VZIG is not available for postexposure prophylaxis, immune globulin IV (IGIV) can be used. If varicella develops despite passive immunization, therapies that reduce disease severity and complications (e.g., acyclovir) may be beneficial.

Varicella virus vaccine live can be used in the prevention and control of varicella outbreaks (e.g., in child-care facilities, schools, institutions). Varicella outbreaks can persist for up to 4–6 months. During varicella outbreaks, the ACIP and AAP recommend a second dose of varicella virus vaccine live for those who previously received only a single dose, provided the age-appropriate time interval has elapsed since the first dose (i.e., 3 months for children 12 months through 12 years of age, at least 4 weeks for adults and adolescents 13 years of age and older).

Dosage and Administration

■ **Reconstitution and Administration** Varicella virus vaccine live (Varivax®) and the fixed-combination vaccine containing measles, mumps, rubella, and varicella antigens (MMRV; ProQuad®) are administered by subcutaneous injection. These vaccines should *not* be given intravascularly.

Although some clinicians state that inadvertent IM† administration of varicella virus vaccine live does not necessitate revaccination, this route of administration is *not* recommended.

The preferred site for subcutaneous injection of Varivax® or MMRV (ProQuad®) is the outer aspect of the upper deltoid; injections also can be given into the anterolateral thigh. For children 1 year of age and older, adolescents, and adults, the upper-outer triceps area usually is preferred. To ensure appropriate delivery, subcutaneous injections should be made at a 45° angle using a 5/8-inch, 23- to 25-gauge needle. Prior to injection, care should be taken to ensure that the needle is not in a blood vessel.

When multiple vaccines are administered during a single health-care visit, each vaccine should be given with a different syringe and at different injection sites. Injection sites should be separated by at least 1 inch (if anatomically feasible) to allow appropriate attribution of any local adverse effects that may occur. If multiple vaccines must be given into a single limb, the deltoid may be used in older children and adults, but the anterolateral thigh is preferred in infants and younger children.

Since syncope may occur following vaccination, vaccinees should be observed for approximately 15 minutes after the vaccine dose is administered. If syncope occurs, the patient should be observed until symptoms resolve. Syncope after vaccination occurs most frequently in adolescents and young adults.

Varicella virus vaccine live should *not* be administered concomitantly with varicella zoster immune globulin (VZIG). (See Drug Interactions: Immune Globulins.)

Varivax® Varicella virus vaccine live (Varivax®) is reconstituted by adding 0.7 mL of the diluent provided by the manufacturer to the vial of lyophilized vaccine and gently agitating the vial. Only the diluent supplied by the manufacturer should be used to reconstitute the vaccine. Varicella virus vaccine live should be reconstituted and administered using sterile syringes and needles that are free of preservatives, antiseptics, and detergents, since these substances may inactivate live viral vaccines. The reconstituted vaccine should be inspected visually for particulate matter and discoloration whenever solution and container permit.

To minimize loss of potency and ensure an adequate immunizing dose, varicella virus vaccine live should be administered immediately following reconstitution and any reconstituted vaccine not used within 30 minutes should be discarded. (See Chemistry and Stability: Stability.)

MMRV (ProQuad®) MMRV (ProQuad®) is reconstituted by adding the entire volume of diluent provided by the manufacturer to the vial of lyophilized vaccine and gently agitating the vial. Only the diluent supplied by the manufacturer should be used to reconstitute the fixed-combination vaccine. The vaccine should be reconstituted and administered using sterile syringes and needles that are free of preservatives, antiseptics, and detergents, since these substances may inactivate live viral vaccines. The reconstituted vaccine should be inspected visually for particulate matter and discoloration whenever solution and container permit.

To minimize loss of potency and ensure an adequate immunizing dose, MMRV (ProQuad®) should be administered immediately following reconstitution and any reconstituted vaccine not used within 30 minutes should be discarded.

■ **Dosage** Single-antigen varicella virus vaccine live (Varivax®) and the fixed-combination vaccine containing measles, mumps, rubella, and varicella antigens (MMRV; ProQuad®) are administered in 0.5-mL doses.

When the single-antigen varicella vaccine (Varivax®) is administered within 30 minutes following reconstitution as specified, each 0.5-mL dose contains at least 1350 plaque-forming units (PFU) of Oka/Merck varicella virus (approximately 3.13 $\log_{10}$ PFU). (See Chemistry and Stability: Stability.)

When the fixed-combination vaccine (MMRV; ProQuad®) is reconstituted as specified, each 0.5-mL dose contains the same potency of measles, mumps, and rubella antigens as measles, mumps, and rubella virus vaccine live (MMR) and at least 3.99 $\log_{10}$ PFU of Oka/Merck varicella virus.

Children 12 Months Through 12 Years of Age **Varivax®.** For routine primary immunization in healthy children 12 months through 12 years of age, a 2-dose regimen of varicella virus vaccine live is used.

For routine childhood immunization, the US Public Health Service Advisory Committee on Immunization Practices (ACIP), American Academy of Pediatrics (AAP), and American Academy of Family Physicians (AAFP) recommend administration of the first dose at 12 through 15 months of age and the second dose at 4 through 6 years of age (i.e., before the child begins kindergarten or the first grade). The second dose may be administered prior to age 4–6 years, provided at least 3 months have elapsed since the first dose was given and both doses are administered at 12 months of age or older; however, if a second dose was administered at least 28 days following the first dose, the second dose does not need to be repeated.

Catch-up vaccination is recommended during routine preventive care visits for children without a reliable history of varicella or in those who have not previously received 2 doses of a vaccine containing varicella virus vaccine live. Children who previously received one dose should receive a second dose, preferably at least 3 months after the first dose and children who have not received any doses of the vaccine should receive 2 doses given at least 3 months apart; however, if a second dose was administered at least 28 days following the first dose, the second dose does not need to be repeated.

MMRV (ProQuad®). For routine primary immunization in healthy children 12 months through 12 years of age, MMRV (ProQuad®) is given as a 0.5-mL dose.

MMRV (ProQuad®) may be used when simultaneous administration of the first or second dose of varicella virus vaccine live and the first or second dose of measles, mumps, and rubella virus vaccine live (MMR) are both indicated in a child 12 months through 12 years of age and there are no contraindications to any of the antigens. When considering use in infants and children 12 through 47 months of age, the ACIP states that providers should advise the parent or caregiver about the benefits and risks associated with MMRV (ProQuad®) compared with the individual component vaccines. (See Fixed-combination Vaccine Containing Varicella Vaccine and Other Antigens under Primary Immunization: Children 12 Months through 12 Years of Age, in Uses.)

At least 1 month should elapse between a dose of a measles-containing vaccine (e.g., MMR) and a dose of MMRV (ProQuad®) and preferably at least 3 months should elapse between a dose of a varicella-containing vaccine (e.g., Varivax®) and a dose of MMRV (ProQuad®); however, if a second dose of a varicella-containing vaccine was administered at least 28 days following the first dose, the second dose does not need to be repeated.

Adults and Adolescents 13 Years of Age or Older Varivax®. For routine primary immunization in adults and adolescents 13 years of age or older, 2 doses of varicella virus vaccine live should be given 4–8 weeks apart. A longer interval between the first and second dose does not necessitate a third dose, but may leave the individual susceptible for the intervening months.

Catch-up vaccination is recommended during routine preventive care visits for adolescents and adults without a reliable history of varicella who have not previously received 2 doses of a vaccine containing varicella virus vaccine live. Adolescents and adults who previously received one dose should receive a second dose given at least 4 weeks after the first dose. Adolescents and adults who have not received the vaccine should receive 2 doses given 4–8 weeks apart.

HIV-infected Individuals Varivax®. When varicella virus vaccine live is used in selected children 12 months through 12 years of age who have human immunodeficiency virus (HIV) infection† and are asymptomatic or only mildly symptomatic with CD4+ T-lymphocyte percentages of at least 15%, the ACIP, AAP, Centers for Disease Control and Prevention (CDC), National Institutes of Health (NIH), HIV Medicine Association of the Infectious Diseases Society of America (IDSA), and Pediatric Infectious Diseases Society recommend that 2 doses of the vaccine be given at least 3 months apart.

If varicella virus vaccine live is used in HIV-infected adults, adolescents, and children older than 8 years of age with $CD4^+$ T-cell counts of 200/mm^3 or greater, the ACIP, AAP, NIH, CDC, and HIV Medicine Association of the IDSA recommend that 2 doses of the single-antigen vaccine be given at least 3 months apart.

Other HIV-infected children, adolescents, or adults who are more severely immunocompromised should *not* receive varicella vaccine. (See HIV-infected Individuals under Primary Immunization: Individuals with Altered Immunocompetence and Their Household Contacts, in Uses.)

MMRV (ProQuad®). Data are not available on the safety, immunogenicity, or efficacy of MMRV; ProQuad®) in HIV-infected children and the ACIP and other experts state that the fixed-combination vaccine should *not* be administered as a substitute for the component vaccines when vaccinating HIV-infected children.

Postexposure Vaccination and Outbreak Control If varicella virus vaccine live is used for postexposure prophylaxis† of varicella in susceptible children 12 months of age and older and adults, the vaccine should be given within 3–5 days after the exposure.

However, if varicella zoster immune globulin (VZIG) or immune globulin IV (IGIV) is used for postexposure prophylaxis of varicella in susceptible individuals, varicella virus vaccine live should not be administered for at least 5–8 months following the immune globulin. (See Drug Interactions: Immune Globulins.) Varicella virus vaccine live is not necessary in patients who develop varicella following exposure.

If varicella virus vaccine live is used for outbreak control during a varicella outbreak, the ACIP and AAP recommend that individuals who previously received a single dose of varicella virus vaccine live should receive a second dose of the vaccine if resources permit such a strategy and if the appropriate interval has elapsed since the first vaccine dose (i.e., at least 3 months in children 12 months through 12 years of age and at least 4 weeks in adults and adolescents 13 years of age or older).

Additional Doses or Revaccination The duration of protection following primary immunization with 2 doses of varicella virus vaccine live has not been fully established to date. Although immunity may wane as the time since primary immunization with varicella virus vaccine increases, there is some evidence from long-term efficacy studies that protection against varicella may last for at least 5–10 years after administration of a single dose of the vaccine. (See Pharmacology: Extent and Duration of Immunity.)

Cautions

Varicella virus vaccine live generally is well tolerated in healthy children, adolescents, and adults. In a placebo-controlled trial in healthy children and adolescents, pain and erythema at the injection site were the only adverse reactions that occurred more frequently in vaccine recipients than in placebo recipients. Administration of varicella virus vaccine live to individuals with serologic evidence of varicella zoster virus (VZV) antibodies (anti-VZV) elicited by previous vaccination or natural infection does not appear to be associated with a clinically important increase in the incidence of adverse effects compared with administration in susceptible individuals.

The fixed-combination vaccine containing measles, mumps, rubella, and varicella antigens (MMRV; ProQuad®) generally is well tolerated. Adverse effects reported with the fixed-combination vaccine are similar to those reported when varicella virus vaccine live and the fixed combination of measles, mumps, and rubella virus vaccine live (MMR) are administered concurrently at separate sites. In clinical studies in healthy children 12–23 months of age, fever (38.9°C or higher) and measles-like rash were the only adverse effects that occurred more frequently in those who received MMRV (ProQuad®) compared with those who received MMR and varicella virus vaccine live at separate sites. In children who received a second dose of MMRV (ProQuad®), the incidence of adverse effects reported after the second dose was similar to or lower than that reported with the first dose. (See Use of Fixed Combinations under Cautions: Precautions and Contraindications.)

■ **Local Effects** The most frequent adverse effects of varicella virus vaccine live are local reactions including pain, soreness, swelling, and erythema. Pruritus, hematoma, induration, or stiffness also has been reported. These adverse local reactions generally occur within the first 48 hours following vaccination and are more common in adolescents and adults than in children. Local effects may persist for several days following vaccination, particularly following a second dose.

In healthy children 12 months through 12 years of age who received a single dose of varicella virus vaccine live, adverse local effects (e.g., pain/soreness, swelling and/or erythema, rash, pruritus, hematoma, induration, stiffness) were reported in 2–29% of vaccinees. When a 2-dose regimen was used in children, the incidence of injection site reactions (usually erythema and swelling) observed in the first 4 days following vaccination was slightly higher after the second dose (overall incidence 25.4%) than after the first dose (overall incidence 21.7%).

In healthy adults and adolescents 13 years of age or older who received a 2-dose regimen of varicella virus vaccine live, adverse local effects occurred in 10–25% following the initial dose and in 27–47% following the second dose.

In addition to the more common local effects, a varicella-like maculopapular or papulovesicular rash composed of only a few lesions or vesicles (median: 2–5) has occurred at the injection site in 1–12% of healthy children, adolescents, or adults who received varicella virus vaccine live. The varicelliform rash at the injection site generally occurs 6–30 days after vaccination. In adults and adolescents 13 years of age or older, the varicelliform rash occurs at a peak of 6–20 days following the first dose of vaccine and 0–6 days following the second dose. While vaccine virus generally is not present in the lesions, the virus has been isolated occasionally and theoretically could be transmitted. (See Cautions: Transmission of Vaccine Virus.) A more generalized rash also can occur. (See Cautions: Systemic Effects.)

■ **Systemic Effects** ***Febrile Reactions*** In healthy children 12 months through 12 years of age who received a single dose of varicella virus vaccine live, fever (38.3°C or higher) occurred in 12–31% during the first 42 days following the dose. In a placebo-controlled study using a vaccine similar to the vaccine commercially available for use in the US, the incidence of fever was the same in children who received the vaccine and in those who received placebo. Although a causal relationship was not established, febrile seizures have occurred rarely (less than 0.1%) in children who received varicella virus vaccine live. Febrile seizures also have been reported with the fixed-combination vaccine containing measles, mumps, rubella, and varicella antigens (MMRV; ProQuad®). (See Use of Fixed Combinations under Cautions: Precautions and Contraindications.)

In healthy adults and adolescents 13 years of age or older who received a 2-dose regimen of varicella virus vaccine live, fever (37.7°C or higher) occurred during the first 42 days following vaccination in up to 10% after the first or second dose.

Rash A generalized varicella-like maculopapular or papulovesicular rash occurs in 4–10% of healthy children who receive a dose of varicella virus vaccine live at 12 months through 12 years of age; the rash generally is mild, composed of 1–30 vesicles, appears 5–41 days after administration of the vaccine, and persists for 2–8 days.

In healthy adults and adolescents 13 years of age or older, varicella-like rash occurred in 1–8% and appears within 35 days after a dose of varicella virus vaccine live. The rash generally is mild, composed of a median of 5–6 vesicles (range: 1–47 vesicles), lasts for a median of 4–8 days (range: 1–21 days), and occurs more frequently after the first dose than after the second dose. Although a generalized, typical varicelliform rash may develop, the rash also can be difficult to distinguish from other rashes and occasionally may resemble mosquito bites.

Sensitivity Reactions Adverse effects that appear to be hypersensitivity reactions to varicella virus vaccine live have been reported rarely, including anaphylaxis, rash, urticaria, hypersensitivity vasculitis, erythema multiforme, and Stevens-Johnson syndrome.

Varicella virus vaccine live contains hydrolyzed gelatin as a stabilizer, which may stimulate hypersensitivity reactions in some individuals. At least 2 healthy adults who had immediate reactions (i.e., wheezing and dyspnea with or without urticaria) within 15 minutes after receiving varicella virus vaccine live (vaccine type not identified) were found to have IgE antibodies to bovine gelatin. While IgE antibodies specific to gelatin were not found in 2 adults with nonimmediate reactions to the vaccine (i.e., erythema and swelling at the injection site), it has been suggested that these reactions may have been related to a cell-mediated immune response to gelatin since gelatin-specific T-cell responses (detected by in vitro lymphocyte proliferation assay and an assay for antigen-specific IL-2 responsiveness) have been found in individuals with nonimmediate-type reactions to live viral vaccines that contain gelatin. (See Sensitivity Reactions under Cautions: Precautions and Contraindications.)

Other Adverse Systemic Effects Other adverse systemic effects that have been reported in 1% or more of healthy children, adolescents, or adults receiving varicella virus vaccine live and may or may not be related to the vaccine include upper respiratory illness, cough, irritability/nervousness, fatigue, disturbed sleep, diarrhea, loss of appetite, nausea, vomiting, otitis, diaper rash/contact rash, headache, teething, malaise, abdominal pain, other rash, ocular complaints, chills, lymphadenopathy, myalgia, lower respiratory illness, stiff neck, heat rash/prickly heat, arthralgia, eczema/dry skin/dermatitis, cold/canker sore, constipation, and pruritus. Although a causal relationship has not been established, pneumonia, pneumonitis, encephalitis, and ataxia have been reported rarely following administration of varicella virus vaccine live. In addition, Henoch-Schönlein purpura, secondary bacterial infections of skin and soft tissue (including impetigo and cellulitis), pharyngitis, thrombocytopenia (including immune thrombocytopenic purpura), dizziness, nonfebrile seizures, aseptic meningitis, Guillain-Barré syndrome, transverse myelitis, Bell's palsy, and paresthesia have been reported during postmarketing surveillance.

■ **Breakthrough Varicella Infections** Although varicella virus vaccine live is effective in promoting immunity to varicella in most individuals, breakthrough varicella infections may occur following exposure to wild-type virus in children or adults who have seroconverted following vaccination. These infections (i.e., wild-type VZV infection occurring more than 42 days after vaccination) generally are milder than those reported in unvaccinated individuals and are associated with a low rate of fever and rapid recovery.

In studies using live, attenuated varicella vaccines containing 1000–9000 units per dose, breakthrough infections have occurred in up to 4% of healthy children or adolescents within 8 years following vaccination and in 7–9% of immunosuppressed children, including those with acute lymphoblastic leukemia (ALL). In one study in children and adolescents 12 months to 17 years of age who received varicella vaccine virus live containing 950–3265 units per dose, breakthrough infections occurred in about 19% within 10 years. Most cases of breakthrough varicella are much milder than infections reported in unvaccinated individuals. Breakthrough infections generally involve less than 100 vesicles and are associated with a low rate of fever and with rapid recovery. In one study of an outbreak of varicella at a US day-care center, the efficacy of the vaccine in preventing disease of any severity in immunized children following exposure to an index case with breakthrough varicella infection was only 44% but was 86% in preventing moderate or severe disease; the risk of breakthrough infection was greatest in children who had been vaccinated 3 or more years prior to the outbreak.

The rate of breakthrough infections in healthy adults who receive the vaccine is higher, and these infections may occur in as many as 31% of adults. Although breakthrough varicella infections in adults generally involve less than 50 vesicles, some infections may be associated with 50–300 vesicles or more.

Breakthrough infections may occur despite seroconversion and evidence of anti-VZV. However, there appears to be an inverse relationship between antibody levels and development of breakthrough varicella infections, and individuals with higher antibody levels 6 weeks after vaccination have lower rates of breakthrough disease. In children, the varicella antibody response measured by glycoprotein enzyme-linked immunosorbent assay (gpELISA) 6 weeks post-vaccination correlates with neutralizing antibody levels, VZV-specific T-cell proliferative responses, vaccine efficacy, and long-term protection against varicella after exposure to VZV. Results of some clinical trials indicate that the incidence of breakthrough infections is lower in children with postvaccination antibody titers of 5 units or greater measured by gpELISA than in children with lower postvaccination antibody titers.

The rate of disease transmission from vaccinees who develop breakthrough varicella infections appears to be low in children, but has not been studied in adults. Data from studies conducted in 1981–1989 indicate that breakthrough infections occurred in about 5% of vaccinated children 1–8 years following vaccination and resulted in secondary transmission to about 12% of their vaccinated siblings. The US Public Health Service Advisory Committee on Immunization Practices (ACIP) states that vaccinated individuals with less than 50 varicella lesions were only one third as contagious as unvaccinated individuals with varicella. However, vaccinated individuals who had more than 50 varicella lesions were as contagious as unvaccinated individuals with varicella. Vaccinated individuals with varicella tend to have milder disease, and, although they are less contagious than unvaccinated persons with varicella, they might not receive a diagnosis and be isolated; therefore, these individuals might have more opportunities to infect others in community settings and contribute to VZV transmission.

■ **Latent Infections and Herpes Zoster** Primary immunization with varicella virus vaccine live does not necessarily ensure protection against latent infection or reactivation of latent infections in those previously infected with natural wild-type VZV. Herpes zoster has been reported rarely in immunocompromised children and healthy children, adolescents, and adults who received primary immunization with varicella virus vaccine live. Herpes zoster in vaccinated individuals may be caused by vaccine virus or by wild-type virus. There is no evidence to date that latent vaccine virus infections are any more likely to reactivate than latent infections caused by wild-type virus.

Most cases of herpes zoster reported to date have occurred 3–5 years after vaccination and were mild without sequelae. The manufacturer states that 9454 healthy children 12 months to 12 years of age and 1648 adolescents and adults have received Varivax® in clinical trials and that the calculated incidence of herpes zoster has been 18.8 cases per 100,000 person years for children (8 cases during 42,556 person years) and 18.5 cases per 100,000 person years for adolescents and adults (1 case during 5410 person years). According to data from one study in children who received single-antigen varicella vaccine, the rate of herpes zoster after vaccination was 22 per 100,000 person years in those 12–24 months age, 30 per 100,000 person years in those 5–9 years of age, and 47 per 100,000 person years for those younger than 14 years of age. Cases of herpes zoster in healthy vaccine recipients have been confirmed to be caused by both vaccine virus and wild-type virus, suggesting that some herpes zoster cases in vaccinees might result from antecedent natural varicella infection that might not have been detected by the patient or from infection after vaccination.

Although further study is needed, waning cell-mediated immunity to VZV may predispose to reactivation of the virus. The long-term effect of primary immunization with varicella virus vaccine live on the incidence of subsequent herpes zoster, particularly in vaccinees exposed to natural varicella, is unknown. Although further long-term study is needed, the reported rate of herpes zoster in vaccine recipients appears to be considerably lower than that reported in population-based studies in healthy children who have had natural varicella. In children with ALL†, herpes zoster appears to occur less frequently in those who have received varicella virus vaccine live than in those who have had natural varicella infection.

■ **Transmission of Vaccine Virus** Varicella live vaccines (Varivax® and MMRV [ProQuad®]) contain live, attenuated virus. Transmission of vaccine virus may occur rarely between vaccinees and susceptible contacts. Vaccine virus has been isolated from vesicular fluid obtained from individuals who developed a varicelliform rash following primary immunization with varicella virus vaccine live, and individuals who receive the vaccine can transmit the vaccine virus to susceptible close contacts. The risk for transmission of vaccine virus to susceptible close contacts appears to be minimal following vaccination of healthy children or adults, but may be increased if the vaccine recipient develops a varicelliform rash following vaccination and/or the vaccine recipient is immunocompromised. Transmission of vaccine virus from vaccinees without a varicella-like rash has been reported, but not confirmed.

Transmission of vaccine virus to susceptible siblings following administration of the vaccine to children with leukemia in remission has been documented. Data from studies in children with leukemia who developed varicelliform rash after receiving varicella virus vaccine live indicate that the vaccine virus was transmitted to 14–17% of their healthy, susceptible siblings within 1 month. In one family, tertiary transmission to a second healthy sibling occurred, with rash developing 18 days after onset of rash in the secondary case and 33 days after onset of rash in the leukemic child; vaccine virus was isolated from all 3 siblings and the rash in the healthy siblings was mild (11 and 40 lesions).

Postmarketing surveillance suggests that transmission of vaccine virus from healthy vaccinees who develop a varicelliform rash to healthy, susceptible contacts occurs only rarely. There have been at least 5 documented cases of transmission of vaccine virus from immunocompetent vaccinated individuals to susceptible contacts; all reported cases resulted in mild disease without complications. In one documented case, vaccine virus was transmitted from a healthy child to his pregnant mother. The child received varicella virus vaccine live at 12 months of age and developed a varicelliform rash (approximately 30 lesions) 24 days later; the mother developed varicella (approximately 100 lesions) 16 days after the child's rash was evident. Results of in vitro testing confirmed that the rash in both the child and his mother was caused by vaccine virus. The mother elected to terminate the pregnancy, and fetal tissue tested by PCR was negative for varicella vaccine virus.

Vaccine-related contact infections reported to date generally have been mild or subclinical, indicating that the vaccine virus remains attenuated when transmitted. While the risk of transmission appears to be minimal when the vaccine recipient does not develop a varicelliform rash, vaccine recipients should attempt to avoid close contact with high-risk individuals (e.g., immunocompromised individuals, pregnant women without a documented history of varicella or laboratory evidence of prior infection, and neonates of such susceptible pregnant women) for up to 6 weeks following vaccination, whenever possible. If contact with high-risk individuals is unavoidable, the potential risk of transmission of vaccine virus should be weighed against the risk of acquiring and transmitting natural varicella virus.

Vaccinees who develop a rash should avoid contact with susceptible, immunocompromised individuals until the rash resolves. If contact inadvertently occurs, postexposure prophylaxis with varicella zoster immune globulin (VZIG) is unnecessary since transmission is rare and contact infections generally are mild.

■ **Precautions and Contraindications** Varicella virus vaccine live and the fixed-combination vaccine containing MMR and varicella virus vaccine live (MMRV; ProQuad®) are contraindicated in individuals who are hypersensitive to the vaccines or any component in the formulations, including gelatin. (See Sensitivity Reactions under Cautions: Precautions and Contraindications.)

The patient and/or the patient's parent or guardian should be informed of the benefits and risks of immunization with varicella virus vaccine live or MMRV (ProQuad®) and should be provided with a copy of the appropriate Vaccine Information Statement (available at the CDC website http://www.cdc.gov/vaccines/pubs/vis/default.htm). Patients and/or the patient's parent or guardian also should be instructed to report any severe or unusual adverse reactions to their health-care provider. Clinicians or individuals can report any adverse reactions that occur following vaccination to VAERS at 800-822-7967 or http://www.vaers.hhs.gov.

Sensitivity Reactions Prior to administration, the recipient and/or parent or guardian should be questioned concerning reactions to previous doses of varicella virus vaccine or similar preparations. Epinephrine should be readily available for immediate treatment of an anaphylactic reaction if such a reaction should occur.

Because varicella virus vaccine live and MMRV (ProQuad®) contain trace amounts of neomycin, the vaccines are contraindicated in individuals who have had an anaphylactic reaction to topically or systemically administered neomycin. Neomycin allergy usually is characterized by a delayed-type (cell-mediated) hypersensitivity reaction, such as contact dermatitis (e.g., characterized by an erythematous, pruritic nodule or papule) occurring within 48–96 hours. The US Public Health Service Advisory Committee on Immunization Practices (ACIP) and American Academy of Pediatrics (AAP) state that vaccines containing trace amounts of neomycin should *not* be used in individuals with a history of anaphylactic reaction to neomycin, but use of such vaccines may be considered in those with a history of a delayed-type hypersensitivity reaction to neomycin if benefits of vaccination outweigh risks.

The possibility of an allergic reaction to hydrolyzed gelatin, which is present in varicella virus vaccine live and MMRV (ProQuad®) as a stabilizer, should be considered. Although skin testing for gelatin sensitivity before administering a gelatin-containing vaccine such as varicella virus vaccine live can be considered, there are no specific protocols for this purpose. Because gelatin used in vaccines manufactured in the US usually is derived from porcine sources, and food gelatin may be derived solely from bovine sources, a negative food history does not exclude the possibility of a reaction to the gelatin contained the vaccine.

Individuals with Altered Immunocompetence Varicella virus vaccine live and MMRV (ProQuad®) generally are contraindicated in individuals with primary immunodeficiencies (e.g., cellular immune deficiency, hypogammaglobulinemia, dysgammaglobulinemia) and in individuals with suppressed immune responses resulting from acquired immunodeficiency syndrome (AIDS) or other clinical manifestations of human immunodeficiency virus (HIV) infection, blood dyscrasias, leukemia, lymphomas of any type, or any other malignant neoplasms affecting the bone marrow or lymphatic systems. (See Individuals with Altered Immunocompetence and Their Household Contacts under Uses: Primary Immunization.) The vaccines also generally are contraindicated in individuals with a family history of congenital or hereditary immunodeficiency in a first-degree relative (e.g., parents and siblings), unless the immune competence of the potential vaccine recipient has been clinically substantiated or verified by a laboratory.

Varicella virus vaccine live and MMRV (ProQuad®) are contraindicated in individuals in whom immunologic responses have been suppressed because of immunosuppressive therapy (e.g., corticosteroids, antineoplastic agents, radiation therapy). Use of the vaccine in individuals receiving corticosteroid dosages that are immunosuppressive can result in a more extensive vaccine-associated rash or disseminated disease. (See Drug Interactions: Immunosuppressive Agents.)

Contact with High-risk Individuals The fact that recipients of varicella virus vaccine live and MMRV (ProQuad®) may be capable of transmitting the vaccine viruses to close, susceptible contacts should be considered. It is recommended that vaccine recipients avoid close association with susceptible high-risk individuals for up to 6 weeks following vaccination, whenever possible. High-risk individuals include immunocompromised individuals, pregnant women without a documented history of varicella or laboratory evidence of prior infection, and neonates of such susceptible pregnant women. In circumstances when contact with high-risk individuals is unavoidable, the potential risk of transmission of vaccine virus should be weighed against the risk of acquiring and transmitting natural varicella virus. Vaccine recipients who develop a varicelliform rash should avoid contact with immunocompromised, susceptible individuals until the rash resolves. The American Academy of Pediatrics (AAP) and other clinicians state that if contact inadvertently occurs, use of varicella zoster immune globulin (VZIG) for postexposure prophylaxis is unnecessary since transmission is rare and contact infections generally are mild. However, some experts recommend that use of acyclovir be considered in immunocompromised individuals who develop skin lesions possibly related to vaccine virus after contact with a recipient of varicella virus vaccine live. The role of VZIG or acyclovir as prophylaxis for high-risk individuals exposed to vaccinated individuals with lesions will be difficult to evaluate given the rarity of transmission of vaccine virus.

Concomitant Illness The decision whether to administer or delay administration of varicella virus vaccine live or MMRV (ProQuad®) in an individual with a current or recent acute illness depends largely on the severity of symptoms and etiology of the illness. The manufacturer states that the vaccines are contraindicated in individuals with any febrile respiratory illness or other active febrile infection. ACIP and AAP state that minor acute illness, such as mild upper respiratory infection (with or without fever) or mild diarrhea, does not preclude vaccination. However, vaccination of individuals with moderate or severe acute illness (with or without fever) generally should be deferred until they have recovered from the acute phase of the illness. This precaution avoids superimposing adverse effects of the vaccine on the underlying illness or mistakenly concluding that a manifestation of the underlying illness resulted from vaccination.

Known history of varicella disease is not a contraindication to varicella vaccination.

The manufacturer states that varicella virus vaccine live and MMRV (ProQuad®) are contraindicated in individuals with active untreated tuberculosis. The ACIP states that, although no data exist regarding whether either varicella or varicella virus vaccine live exacerbates tuberculosis, vaccination is not recommended for individuals with untreated, active tuberculosis. However, tuberculin skin testing is not a prerequisite for administration of varicella virus vaccine live.

Thrombocytopenia Thrombocytopenia has been reported after administration of varicella virus vaccine live or measles, mumps, and rubella virus vaccine live (MMR); thrombocytopenia has worsened in those with preexisting thrombocytopenia and may worsen with subsequent doses.

The manufacturer of MMRV (ProQuad®) states that potential benefits and risks should be evaluated before considering use of the vaccine in patients who develop thrombocytopenia or had worsening of thrombocytopenia with a previous dose. Serologic testing for antibody to MMR should be considered to determine whether additional doses should be given.

Use of Fixed Combinations Whenever the fixed-combination vaccine containing measles, mumps, rubella, and varicella antigens (MMRV; ProQuad®) is used, the contraindications and precautions related to each antigen should be considered.

For complete information on adverse effects and precautions and contraindications related to measles, mumps, and rubella antigens (including hypersensitivity to eggs), see Cautions in the individual monographs on Measles Virus Vaccine Live, Mumps Virus Vaccine Live, and Rubella Virus Vaccine Live in 80:12.

There is some evidence that the relative risk for febrile seizures in children 12–60 months of age after a dose of MMRV (ProQuad®) is higher than that reported when a dose of monovalent varicella virus vaccine live (Varivax®) and a dose of MMR are given concomitantly. Interim results from a postmarketing observational study in children 12–60 months of age (99% were 12–23 months of age) indicate that the relative risk for febrile seizures 5–12 days after a dose of MMRV (ProQuad®) is 2.3 times higher than in historic, age- and gender-matched controls who received a dose of varicella virus vaccine live (Varivax®) and a dose of MMR concomitantly. (See Fixed-combination Vaccine Containing Varicella Vaccine and Other Antigens under Primary Immunization: Children 12 months through 12 Years of Age, in Uses.)

The manufacturer recommends that MMRV (ProQuad®) be used with caution in individuals with a history of cerebral injury, personal or family history of seizures, or any other condition in which fever-induced stress should be avoided. The ACIP states that a personal or family (i.e., sibling, parent) history of seizures is a precaution for use of MMRV (ProQuad®). Studies suggest that children with a personal or family history of febrile seizures or family history of epilepsy are at increased risk for febrile seizures compared with children who do not have such histories. ACIP states that the risks of using MMRV (ProQuad®) in children with a personal or family history of seizures generally outweigh the benefits and such children should receive a dose of MMR and a dose of varicella virus vaccine live.

Data are not available regarding safety and efficacy of MMRV (ProQuad®) in HIV-infected individuals†. The ACIP, AAP, Centers for Disease Control and Prevention (CDC), National Institutes of Health (NIH), HIV Medicine Association of the Infectious Diseases Society of America (IDSA), and the Pediatric Infectious Diseases Society state that the fixed-combination vaccine should not be used in HIV-infected individuals. When vaccination against varicella is indicated in HIV-infected individuals, monovalent varicella virus vaccine live (Varivax®) should be used. (See HIV-infected Individuals under Primary Immunization: Individuals with Altered Immunocompetence and Their Household Contacts, in Uses.)

MMRV (ProQuad®) contains albumin human. Since albumin is prepared from pooled human plasma, it is a potential vehicle for transmission of human viruses, including the causative agents of viral hepatitis and HIV infection, and theoretically may carry a risk of transmitting the causative agent of Creutzfeldt-Jakob disease (CJD) or variant CJD (vCJD).

Limitations of Vaccine Effectiveness Varicella virus vaccine live (Varivax®) and MMRV (ProQuad®) may not protect all individuals from varicella.

Safety and efficacy of varicella virus vaccine live (Varivax®) or MMRV (ProQuad®) for postexposure prophylaxis have not been established and it is not known whether administration of varicella vaccine immediately after exposure to natural varicella virus will prevent illness. However, the single-antigen varicella vaccine has been used for postexposure vaccination† in susceptible individuals and for outbreak prevention and control in certain settings. (See Uses: Postexposure Vaccination and Outbreak Control.)

Improper Storage and Handling Improper storage or handling of vaccines may result in loss of vaccine potency and reduced immune response in vaccinees.

Single-antigen varicella vaccine (Varivax®) or MMRV (ProQuad®) that has been mishandled or has not been stored at the recommended temperature should not be administered. (See Chemistry and Stability: Stability.)

The lyophilized varicella virus vaccine live should be protected from light at all times since exposure to light may inactivate the vaccine virus.

All vaccines should be inspected upon delivery and monitored during storage to ensure that the appropriate temperature is maintained. If there are concerns about mishandling, the manufacturer or state or local health departments should be contacted for guidance on whether the vaccine is usable.

Reconstituted vaccine should be discarded if not used within 30 minutes and should not be frozen. (See Chemistry and Stability: Stability.)

■ **Pediatric Precautions** Safety and efficacy of varicella virus vaccine live (Varivax®) in children younger than 12 months of age have not been established, and use of the vaccine in this age group is not recommended. Transplacental antibodies to VZV reportedly persist for no more than 6–8 months after delivery and should not interfere with the immunologic response to varicella virus vaccine live if vaccines containing the antigen are administered to children at 12 months of age or older.

A few clinicians have suggested that consideration can be given to administering Varivax® to children as young as of 6 months age† as a means of decreasing the risk of transmission of wild-type varicella infection to high-risk household members (e.g., individuals with altered immunocompetence, pregnant woman without a documented history of varicella or laboratory evidence of prior infection). However, such use is not included in current ACIP or AAP recommendations for the vaccine.

Safety and efficacy of the fixed-combination vaccine containing MMR and varicella virus vaccine live (MMRV; ProQuad®) have not been established in children younger than 12 months of age or in children or adolescents 13 years of age or older.

■ **Geriatric Precautions** Clinical studies of varicella virus vaccine live (Varivax®) did not include sufficient numbers of seronegative adults 65 years of age and older to determine whether geriatric adults respond differently than younger individuals. Other reported clinical experience has not identified differences in responses between geriatric and younger individuals.

The fixed-combination vaccine containing MMR and varicella virus vaccine live (MMRV; ProQuad®) is not indicated in adults, including geriatric adults.

■ **Mutagenicity and Carcinogenicity** The mutagenic and carcinogenic potential of varicella virus vaccine live (Varivax®) or the fixed-combination vaccine containing MMR and varicella virus vaccine live (MMRV; ProQuad®) have not been evaluated.

■ **Pregnancy, Fertility, and Lactation** ***Pregnancy*** Varicella virus vaccine live and the fixed-combination vaccine containing MMR and varicella virus vaccine live (MMRV; ProQuad®) are contraindicated in pregnant women, and pregnancy should be avoided for 1–3 months following vaccination. Natural varicella infection during pregnancy, especially during the first 2 trimesters, has been associated with congenital varicella syndrome which may result in spontaneous abortion, fetal death, or congenital abnormalities. Animal reproduction studies have not been performed to date with varicella virus vaccine live or MMRV (ProQuad®), and it is not known if the vaccines can cause fetal harm when administered to pregnant women or can affect fertility.

On theoretical grounds, live attenuated vaccines generally are avoided in pregnant women or those likely to become pregnant within 3 months of vaccination. Reasonable precautions should be taken to preclude vaccination of pregnant women, including asking postpubertal women if they are pregnant, excluding those who state that they are, informing the others of the theoretical risks to the fetus, and explaining the importance of not becoming pregnant for 1–3 months after vaccination. Although the manufacturer recommends that pregnancy be avoided for 3 months after administration of live viral vaccines, the ACIP and AAP have stated that pregnancy should be avoided for at least 1 month following administration of varicella virus vaccine live. The ACIP suggests that if a woman is pregnant when vaccinated or becomes pregnant within 1 month of vaccination, she should be counseled concerning potential effects on the fetus. Because the virulence of the attenuated varicella virus used in the vaccine is less than that of the wild-type virus, the ACIP suggests that the risk to the fetus, if any, should be lower than that following natural varicella infection and in most circumstances a decision to terminate a pregnancy should not be based on whether varicella virus vaccine live was administered during pregnancy.

The manufacturer, in collaboration with the US Centers for Disease Control and Prevention (CDC), has established a registry to monitor pregnancy outcomes in women who inadvertently receive a vaccine containing varicella virus vaccine live during pregnancy or any time during the 3 months prior to pregnancy, and clinicians and health-care providers are encouraged to register such patients at 800-986-8999.

The ACIP and AAP state that the presence of a pregnant woman in a household does not contraindicate use of varicella virus vaccine live in other household members. Vaccination of the susceptible household member will likely protect the susceptible pregnant woman from exposure to wild-type VZV. If varicella virus vaccine live is administered to a household member and the recipient develops a varicelliform rash, contact with the susceptible pregnant woman should be avoided if possible. Vaccine virus has been transmitted from a healthy 12-month-old child who developed a varicelliform rash following vaccination to his pregnant mother. (See Cautions: Transmission of Vaccine Virus.) After elective abortion, no virus was detected in the fetal tissue.

The ACIP, American Academy of Family Physicians (AAFP), and American College of Obstetricians and Gynecologists (ACOG) recommend that all pregnant women be assessed for evidence of varicella immunity and those without such evidence should receive a dose of monovalent varicella virus vaccine live administered after delivery or termination of pregnancy (before discharge) and a second dose administered 4–8 weeks after the first dose (at a postpartum or other health-care visit).

Lactation It is not known whether attenuated varicella virus contained in varicella virus vaccine live is distributed into milk following subcutaneous administration. Because some viruses are distributed into milk, the manufacturer states that the vaccine should be used with caution in nursing women. Although organisms contained in live vaccines multiply within the body and some may be distributed into milk following immunization of the mother (e.g., rubella virus vaccine live), there is no evidence that this occurs with varicella vaccine and no evidence that it would adversely affect a nursing infant. The ACIP and AAP state that use of monovalent varicella virus vaccine live in susceptible nursing women may be considered, especially if the risk for exposure to natural infection is high.

Drug Interactions

■ **Antiviral Agents** Because antiviral agents active against herpesviruses (e.g., acyclovir, famciclovir, valacyclovir) may reduce efficacy of varicella virus vaccine live, the US Public Health Service Advisory Committee on Immunization Practices (ACIP) recommends that these antiviral agents be discontinued at least 24 hours before administration of vaccines containing varicella virus vaccine live, if possible.

■ **Blood Products** Blood products (e.g., whole blood, packed red blood cells [RBCs], plasma) may interfere with the immune response to certain live virus vaccines (e.g., measles virus vaccine live); therefore, these live vaccines should not be administered simultaneously with or for specified intervals before or after administration of these preparations. Although specific studies evaluating possible interference with the immune response to varicella virus vaccine live have not been performed, use of the vaccine generally should be deferred following administration of blood products.

The ACIP recommends that administration of varicella virus vaccine live should be deferred for at least 3 months following administration of RBCs (with adenine-saline added), for at least 6 months following administration of administration of packed RBCs or whole blood, and for at least 7 months following administration of plasma or platelet products. However, because of the importance of postpartum vaccination in women without evidence of varicella immunity, vaccination of such women should not be delayed because they received a blood product. If simultaneous administration of varicella virus vaccine live and a blood product or administration at less than the recommended interval is deemed necessary, the fact that vaccine-induced immunity may be compromised should be considered and, unless there is serologic evidence of an adequate antibody response to the live virus vaccine, an additional dose of vaccine should be administered at the specified interval.

The fact that revaccination may be necessary in individuals who receive a blood product shortly after varicella virus vaccine live also should be considered. After receiving varicella virus vaccine live, vaccinees should avoid blood products for 2 weeks; if use of a blood product is considered necessary during this period, a repeat vaccine dose should be given after the recommended interval unless serologic testing is feasible and indicates a response to the vaccine was attained.

■ **Immune Globulins** Antibodies contained in immune globulin preparations (e.g., immune globulin, cytomegalovirus immune globulin, hepatitis B immune globulin, rabies immune globulin [RIG], tetanus immune globulin [TIG], varicella zoster immune globulin [VZIG]) may interfere with the immune response to certain live virus vaccines (e.g., measles virus vaccine live) and these vaccines should not be administered simultaneously with or for specified intervals before or after administration of these preparations. Although specific studies evaluating possible interference with the immune response to varicella virus vaccine live have not been performed, use of the vaccine generally should be deferred following administration of immune globulin.

The ACIP recommends that administration of varicella virus vaccine live should be deferred for at least 3 months following administration of TIG, hepatitis B immune globulin (HBIG), or IGIM used for postexposure prophylaxis of hepatitis A virus (HAV); for at least 4 months following administration of RIG; for at least 5 months following administration of IGIM used for measles prophylaxis in immunocompetent individuals; for at least 6 months following administration of cytomegalovirus immune globulin IV (CMV-IGIV), or IGIM for measles prophylaxis in immunocompromised individuals; for at least 8 months following administration of IGIV for replacement therapy of immunodeficiencies; for at least 8–10 months following administration of IGIV for the treatment of idiopathic thrombocytopenic purpura (ITP); or for at least 11 months following administration of IGIV for Kawasaki syndrome. The ACIP also recommends that administration of varicella virus vaccine live be deferred for at least 5–8 months after administration of VZIG or IGIV for postexposure prophylaxis of severe varicella. If simultaneous administration of varicella virus vaccine live and one of these immune globulin preparations or administration at less than the recommended interval is deemed necessary, the fact that vaccine-induced immunity may be compromised should be considered and, unless there is serologic evidence of an adequate antibody response to the live virus vaccine, an additional dose of vaccine should be administered at the specified interval. If administered simultaneously, the live virus vaccine and immune globulin should be administered at separate sites anatomically remote from each other.

Specific studies are not available evaluating whether passively acquired antibodies from Rho(D) immune globulin interfere with the immune response to varicella virus vaccine live. Because of the importance of postpartum varicella vaccination in women who do not have evidence of varicella immunity, vaccination of such women should not be delayed because they received Rho(D) immune globulin.

The fact that revaccination may be necessary in individuals who receive an immune globulin preparation shortly after varicella virus vaccine live also should be considered. In general, vaccine virus replication and stimulation of immunity occur within 7–14 days after administration of a live virus vaccine. Therefore, if the interval between administration of varicella virus vaccine live and subsequent administration of one of these preparations is less than 14 days, an additional dose of vaccine should be given after the appropriate interval previously specified, unless serologic testing indicates that an adequate antibody response to the vaccine occurred. An additional dose of vaccine generally is unnecessary if the interval between vaccination and administration of the immune globulin is longer than 2 weeks.

■ **Immunosuppressive Agents** Individuals receiving immunosuppressive agents (e.g., corticotropin, corticosteroid, alkylating agents, antimetabolites, radiation therapy) may have a diminished immunologic response to live vaccines such as varicella virus vaccine live, and replication of the virus may be potentiated. Administration of varicella virus vaccine live or the fixed-combination vaccine containing measles, mumps, rubella, and varicella antigens (MMRV; ProQuad®) generally should be deferred until immunosuppressive therapy is discontinued since these individuals are more susceptible to infections than healthy individuals and more extensive vaccine-associated rash or disseminated disease can occur.

While no data have been published concerning whether susceptible children who are receiving steroids by oral inhalation can be vaccinated safely, the ACIP states that the consensus of most experts based on clinical experience is that vaccination of these children is safe. Short-term (less than 2 weeks), low- to moderate-dose systemic corticosteroid therapy; long-term, alternate-day systemic corticosteroid therapy using low to moderate doses of short-acting drugs; topical corticosteroid therapy (e.g., nasal, cutaneous, ophthalmic); or intra-articular, bursal, or tendon injections with corticosteroids should *not* be immunosuppressive in usual dosages and do not necessarily contraindicate administration of live viral vaccines. However, use of live viral vaccines generally is contraindicated in patients receiving high doses of systemic corticosteroids or when systemic immunosuppression occurs with prolonged topical corticosteroid therapy. Varicella virus vaccine live, therefore, may be administered to susceptible children who are receiving topical corticosteroids or systemic corticosteroid for certain conditions (e.g., asthma, Addison's disease) and who are not otherwise immunocompromised if they are receiving such therapy in a daily dosage equivalent to less than 2 mg/kg or 20 mg of oral prednisone given for less than 2 weeks. The ACIP recommends that serologic testing be done 6 weeks following vaccination of these children, and those who have not seroconverted should be revaccinated.

The optimum interval between discontinuance of immunosuppressive therapy and subsequent administration of a live viral vaccine has not been determined. Although the ACIP recommends that live viral vaccines generally not be administered for at least 3 months after immunosuppressive therapy is discontinued in patients who received high-dose systemic corticosteroids (i.e., daily dosage equivalent to or greater than 2 mg/kg or 20 mg of oral prednisone) for 2 weeks or longer, the ACIP and American Academy of Pediatrics (AAP) suggest that delaying administration of varicella virus vaccine live for at least 1 month after high-dose immunosuppressive therapy is discontinued probably is sufficient.

Individuals with leukemia who have not received chemotherapy for at least 3 months generally can receive a live viral vaccine. However, vaccination of leukemic children who are in remission and who do not have evidence of immunity to varicella should be undertaken only with expert guidance and with the availability of antiviral therapy should complications ensue.

The manufacturer of the fixed-combination vaccine containing MMR and varicella virus vaccine live (MMRV; ProQuad®) states that the vaccine may be used in individuals receiving topical corticosteroids or low-dose corticosteroids for asthma prophylaxis or replacement therapy (e.g., for Addison's disease).

■ **Vaccines** Although specific studies may not be available evaluating concurrent administration of varicella virus vaccine live with each antigen, simultaneous administration with other age-appropriate vaccines, including live virus vaccines, toxoids, or inactivated or recombinant vaccines, during the same health-care visit is not expected to affect immunologic responses or adverse reactions to any of the preparations.

Immunization with varicella virus vaccine live can be integrated with immunization against diphtheria, tetanus, pertussis, hepatitis A, hepatitis B, human papillomavirus (HPV), influenza, poliovirus, measles, mumps, rubella, rotavirus, meningococcal disease, pneumococcal disease, and rotavirus. However, unless combination vaccines appropriate for the age and vaccination status of the recipient are used, each parenteral vaccine should be administered using a different syringe and different injection site.

Inactivated Vaccines and Toxoids **Diphtheria and Tetanus Toxoids and Pertussis Vaccines.** Varicella virus vaccine live may be administered concurrently with diphtheria and tetanus toxoids and acellular pertussis vaccines adsorbed (DTaP). Although specific studies are not available, the ACIP and AAP state that there is no reason to suspect that simultaneous administration of varicella virus vaccine live will affect the immune response to these other antigens and that, when necessary, varicella virus vaccine live may be given concurrently with or at any interval before or after these vaccines. Results of a retrospective cohort study that used data from the Vaccine Safety Datalink (VSD) project and included children 12 months of age or older who were vaccinated during January 1995 to December 1999 indicate that administration of varicella virus vaccine live less than 30 days after MMR results in a 2.5-fold increase in the incidence of breakthrough varicella infections.

The manufacturer states that data are insufficient to date to recommend concurrent administration of the fixed-combination vaccine containing measles, mumps, and rubella virus vaccine live (MMR) and varicella virus vaccine live (MMRV; ProQuad®) with DTaP.

Inactivated Vaccines. Varicella virus vaccine live may be administered concurrently with haemophilus b conjugate (Hib) vaccines or hepatitis B vaccine (recombinant). Although specific studies are not available, the ACIP and AAP state that there is no reason to suspect that simultaneous administration of varicella virus vaccine live will affect the immune response to these other vaccines and that, when necessary, varicella virus vaccine live may be given concurrently with or at any interval before or after these vaccines. The manufacturer of the fixed-combination vaccine containing MMR and varicella virus vaccine live (MMRV; ProQuad®) states that the vaccine may be administered concurrently with Hib conjugate (meningococcal protein conjugate) and hepatitis B vaccine. MMRV (ProQuad®) has been administered concomitantly with Hib vaccine and hepatitis B vaccine at separate injection sites and seroconversion rates and antibody titers for measles, mumps, rubella, varicella, anti-PRP, and hepatitis B were comparable with results obtained when the vaccines were administered 6 weeks apart.

Varicella virus vaccine live may be administered concurrently with poliovirus vaccine inactivated (IPV). The manufacturer states that data are not available to date regarding concurrent administration of the fixed-combination vaccine containing MMR and varicella virus vaccine live (MMRV; ProQuad®) with IPV.

Since parenteral influenza virus vaccines are inactivated vaccines, interactions with live vaccines such as varicella vaccine are unlikely. Parenteral influenza virus vaccine inactivated may be administered simultaneously with (using different syringes and different injection sites) or at any interval before or after varicella virus vaccine live.

Although specific studies are not available, pneumococcal vaccines are inactivated vaccines and interactions with varicella virus vaccine live are not expected. Varicella virus vaccine live may be administered concurrently with (using different syringes and different injection sites) or at any interval before or after pneumococcal vaccine. Data are not available to date regarding concurrent administration of the fixed-combination vaccine containing MMR and varicella virus vaccine live (MMRV; ProQuad®) with pneumococcal 7-valent conjugate vaccine.

Live Vaccines **Measles, Mumps, and Rubella Virus Vaccine Live.** Varicella virus vaccine live may be administered concurrently with MMR at a different site using a separate syringe. Results of studies in healthy children 12–36 months of age indicate that seroconversion rates, antibody responses, and adverse effects reported with simultaneous administration of the vaccines are similar to those reported when the vaccines are administered 6 weeks apart.

Because there is a theoretical concern that the immune response to one live viral vaccine may be impaired if administered within 1 month of another, the AAP and ACIP recommend that varicella virus vaccine live and MMR be administered at least 1 month apart if they are not administered simultaneously. There is some evidence that administration of varicella virus vaccine live less than 30 days after MMR decreases the effectiveness of the varicella vaccine. Results of a retrospective cohort study that used data from the Vaccine Safety Datalink (VSD) project and included children 12 months of age or older who were vaccinated during January 1995 to December 1999 indicate that administration of varicella virus vaccine live less than 30 days after MMR results in a 2.5-fold increase in the incidence of breakthrough varicella infections.

There is evidence that the fixed-combination vaccine containing MMR and varicella virus vaccine live (MMRV; ProQuad®) is safe and effective in healthy children 12 months through 12 years of age. Studies using MMRV (ProQuad®) in healthy children 1–6 years of age indicate that the antibody responses to measles, mumps, rubella, and varicella antigens following a single dose of the fixed-combination vaccine are similar to those obtained after a single dose of MMR and a single dose of Varivax®. However, there is some evidence that the relative risk for febrile seizures in infants may be higher with the fixed-combination vaccine than that reported when a dose of single-antigen varicella virus vaccine live (Varivax®) and a dose of MMR are given concomitantly. (See Use of Fixed Combinations under Cautions: Precautions and Contraindications.)

Intranasal Live Influenza Virus Vaccines. Studies using seasonal influenza virus vaccine live intranasal (FluMist®) indicate that simultaneous administration with varicella virus vaccine live in children 12–15 months of age did not interfere with the immune response to either vaccine and did not increase the frequency of adverse effects. If influenza virus vaccine live intranasal and varicella virus vaccine live are not given simultaneously, they should be given at least 4 weeks apart, if possible.

Other Live Vaccines. Although data are limited regarding simultaneous administration of varicella virus vaccine live and live vaccines other than MMR, the ACIP states that there is no evidence to date that parenterally administered live vaccines interfere with the immune response to other live vaccines (e.g., rotavirus vaccine live oral, typhoid vaccine live oral, yellow fever virus vaccine live) and these vaccines may be administered concurrently. The ACIP and AAP state that some live oral vaccines (e.g., rotavirus vaccine live oral, typhoid vaccine live oral, poliovirus vaccine live oral [OPV; no longer commercially available in the US]) can be administered simultaneously with or at any interval before or after live parenteral vaccines.

If varicella virus vaccine live and intranasal or other parenteral live vaccines are not administered on the same day, they should be administered at least 4 weeks (i.e., 28 days) apart to minimize the potential for interference.

■ **Salicylates** The manufacturer recommends that individuals who receive varicella virus vaccine live or the fixed-combination vaccine containing MMR and varicella virus vaccine live (MMRV; ProQuad®) avoid use of salicylates for 6 weeks following vaccination. This precaution is based on the fact that Reye's syndrome has been reported in children and adolescents who received salicylates during natural varicella infection. However, an association between Reye's syndrome, administration of varicella virus vaccine live, and use of salicylates has not been established, and the syndrome has not been reported to date in recipients of the vaccine. For children who are receiving long-term salicylate therapy, the AAP suggests that the theoretical risks associated with the vaccine be weighed against the known risks of the wild-type virus. The ACIP states that, since the risk for serious salicylate-associated complications is likely to be greater in children in whom natural varicella disease develops than in children who receive the vaccine containing attenuated virus, children who have rheumatoid arthritis or other conditions requiring therapeutic salicylate therapy probably should receive varicella virus vaccine live in conjunction with subsequent close monitoring.

Laboratory Test Interferences

■ **Tuberculin** The effect of varicella virus vaccine live, if any, on tuberculin testing has not been determined. Since measles virus vaccine live has been reported to temporarily suppress tuberculin skin sensitivity, the US Centers for Disease Control and Prevention (CDC) states that until additional information is available, tuberculin tests (if required) should be administered before, simultaneously with, or 4–6 weeks after administration of varicella virus vaccine live or the fixed-combination vaccine containing MMR and varicella virus vaccine live (MMRV; ProQuad®). The US Public Health Service Advisory Committee on Immunization Practices (ACIP) states that vaccination with varicella virus vaccine live should not be delayed based only on a theoretical concern about a possible interaction with tuberculin skin testing.

Pharmacology

Varicella virus vaccine live stimulates active immunity to varicella (chickenpox). Varicella vaccines commercially available for use in the US contains live, attenuated varicella zoster virus (VZV) of the Oka/Merck strain. This vaccine virus differs slightly from wild-type VZV circulating in the US and can be identified by distinctive DNA restrictive endonuclease cleavage patterns. Although further study is needed, it has been theorized that there may be antigenic differences between the vaccine and wild-type VZV since the immune responses elicited by varicella virus vaccine live are not identical to those elicited by the wild-type virus.

Varicella virus vaccine live can induce both humoral and cell-mediated responses in vaccinees; however, the role and relative contribution of each type of response to long-term immunity against varicella has not been fully determined. Efficacy of varicella virus vaccine live in preventing varicella infection varies depending on the age and immunocompetence of the vaccinee. In some individuals, especially healthy adults and immunocompromised children, the vaccine provides partial immunity and modification of subsequent varicella infection rather than complete protection.

■ **Varicella Zoster Virus and Infection** Varicella (chickenpox) and herpes zoster (shingles, zoster) are distinct clinical entities caused by the same virus, VZV, a member of the family Herpesviridae. Varicella is the primary infection. During varicella, the virus invades sensory neurons and becomes latent in sensory nerve ganglia, establishing a source of potential secondary infection. Herpes zoster, the secondary infection, results from reactivation of the latent virus. Natural varicella infection elicits development of specific antibodies and cell-mediated immunity and generally confers lifelong protection against subsequent varicella infection. However, in 10–20% of individuals, especially older adults and immunocompromised individuals, reactivation of the latent virus and subsequent herpes zoster (shingles) occurs, with the incidence increasing with age in adults.

In otherwise healthy children, varicella usually is an acute, self-limited disease characterized by fever, malaise, and a generalized vesicular rash consisting of 250–500 lesions. In neonates, adolescents, adults, and immunocompromised individuals, varicella may be a more serious illness associated with a greater number of lesions and an increased risk of complications (e.g., pneumonia, encephalitis, glomerulonephritis, bacterial superinfection including necrotizing fasciitis). Adults are more likely to acquire varicella pneumonia or varicella encephalitis than otherwise healthy children; pneumonia is the principal cause of death among adults with varicella.

Before licensure of varicella virus vaccine live (i.e., prior to 1995), an average of 4 million cases of varicella and 100–150 varicella-associated deaths were reported each year in the US. The rate of complications, including varicella-related death, is greatest in immunocompromised individuals and individuals who contract varicella when they are younger than 1 year of age or older than 15 years of age. Varicella-related fatality rates are reported to be 1 per 100,000 cases in children 1–14 years of age, 2.7 per 100,000 cases in adolescents and young adults 15–19 years of age, and 25.2 per 100,000 cases in adults 30–49 years of age. During the first 4 months of 1997, state health departments reported 3 varicella-related fatalities (varicella pneumonia and/or varicella encephalitis) in young adult women who were infected by exposure to unvaccinated preschool-aged children with typical cases of varicella; 2 of these women were previously in good health and contracted the disease through household exposure and the other woman had Crohn's disease. The most common complications of varicella that resulted in hospitalizations were skin and soft tissue infections (especially invasive group A streptococcal infections), pneumonia, dehydration, and encephalitis.

Varicella is highly contagious and the secondary infection rate in healthy, susceptible individuals exposed through household contact generally is 80–90%. The disease is transmitted person-to-person through airborne respiratory droplet infection or direct contact, droplet, or aerosol from vesicular fluid of skin vesicles, which contain high titers of anti-VZV. Varicella virus enters the host through the upper respiratory tract or the conjunctiva. Individuals with varicella are most contagious 1 or 2 days before the onset of rash and shortly after its onset, but continue to be contagious for 4–7 days after its onset when vesicles have dried and crusted. Following exposure to the disease or virus, the incubation period in healthy individuals averages about 14–16 days (range: 9–21 days). In immunocompromised individuals, the incubation period may be shorter and these individuals may be contagious for a longer period of time, presumably because their immune system is depressed allowing viral replication to persist. The incubation period may be prolonged (up to 28 days) in individuals who receive varicella zoster immune globulin (VZIG) of IGIV for postexposure prophylaxis. In utero infections can occur, and fetal infections occurring during the first and second trimesters may result in congenital varicella disease. Infants born to mothers with active varicella at the time of delivery may develop the disease within the first 2 weeks of life; the usual interval from onset of rash in the mother to disease onset in the neonate is 9–15 days.

■ **Response to Varicella Virus Vaccine Live** The immunologic response to varicella virus vaccine live has been evaluated using various live, attenuated vaccines containing Oka/Biken, Oka/RIT, or Oka/Merck strains in potencies ranging from 200–9000 units. The humoral and cell-mediated immune responses elicited by varicella virus vaccine live appear to be less than those elicited by natural infection with wild-type VZV. It has been suggested that potency of varicella virus vaccine live may affect both the seroconversion rate and the duration of immune response following vaccination; doses with a higher potency may induce greater immunologic responses and provide longer-lasting immunity.

Levels of specific antibodies that protect against varicella infection have not been defined and the acquisition of any detectable level of antibodies against VZV generally has been used to indicate seroconversion in individuals who receive varicella virus vaccine live. The manufacturer states that seroconversion is based on an optical density (OD) cutoff, corresponding approximately to a lower limit of 0.6 glycoprotein enzyme-linked immunosorbent assay (gpELISA) units/mL. There is some evidence that breakthrough varicella infections occur in substantially fewer children who have geometric mean antibody titers of 5 units or greater (measured by gpELISA) following receipt of varicella virus vaccine live than in those who have gpELISA titers less than 5 units.

In healthy children 12 months to 12 years of age, the seroconversion rate is 98% after a single dose of varicella vaccine and 100% after a second vaccine dose given 3 months after the first dose. In those 13 years of age and older, the seroconversion rate is 75–94% after a single dose and 99% after a second dose. Although administration of a second dose of vaccine for primary immunization in healthy adults increases the seroconversion rate, there is no evidence that the second dose affects the duration of protection against varicella. In a study that evaluated varicella virus vaccine live in healthy children 12 months to 12 years of age, a single dose (containing the Oka/Merck strain in a potency of 2900–9000 units) resulted in a seroconversion rate of 98% and geometric mean antibody titers (measured by gpELISA) of 11.4 and 19.5 at 6 weeks and 1 year, respectively, after the dose. Children who received a second dose of the vaccine 3 months after the first dose had a seroconversion rate of 100% and geometric mean antibody titers of 145.1 and 31.2 at 6 weeks and 1 year, respectively.

Varicella virus vaccine live is less immunogenic in healthy adolescents and adults than in healthy children, and there is some evidence that antibody titers induced by the vaccine are inversely related to the age of the vaccine recipient. In a study in adolescents and adults 13–49 years of age, the geometric mean titer of antibody measured by gpELISA 4 weeks after the second dose of varicella virus vaccine live was 23–30 in those 13–19 years of age, 10–18 in those 20–29 years of age, and 11–14 in those 30–49 years of age. In all age groups, antibody titers were higher in those who received the second dose 8 weeks after the initial dose than in those who received the second dose 4 weeks after the initial dose. Many healthy adults who do not seroconvert after a single dose of varicella virus vaccine live do so after a second dose.

In immunosuppressed children, including children with acute lymphocytic (lymphoblastic) leukemia (ALL) in remission, solid tumors, or renal insufficiency, the seroconversion rate following administration of a single dose of live, attenuated varicella virus vaccine containing 550–4000 units is 87–95%, and the seroconversion rate following administration of a second dose of vaccine is 95–98%.

■ **Extent and Duration of Immunity** Continued long-term studies are necessary to determine the extent and duration of protection against varicella provided by primary immunization with 1 or 2 doses of varicella virus vaccine live. Seroconversion following administration of varicella virus vaccine live does not result in complete protection in all individuals, and breakthrough varicella infections may occur in some children or adults who seroconverted following vaccination and are subsequently exposed to wild-type virus. Approximately 2–4% of healthy children, 7–9% of children with ALL, and 31% of healthy adults who initially seroconvert following primary vaccination with varicella virus vaccine live develop breakthrough varicella infections as a result of exposure to natural, wild-type virus following close contact with an individual with varicella. In one study in healthy children 12 months to 17 years of age, 19% of vaccinated children had breakthrough infections during a 10-year follow-up period and the breakthrough rate averaged 3% per year. In both healthy children and children with ALL, breakthrough varicella infections usually occur during the first 1–2 years following vaccination. These breakthrough varicella infections in vaccinated individuals generally are less severe than natural varicella infections occurring in unvaccinated, susceptible individuals. (See Cautions: Breakthrough Varicella Infections.)

In healthy children who receive the vaccine at 12 months through 12 years of age, immunity to varicella may persist at least 5–10 years. Although up to about 30% of healthy adults or children with ALL become seronegative 1 year after vaccination, it has been suggested that some of these individuals may have residual immunity (e.g., cell-mediated immunity) that is not detected with serologic tests for antibody. Further study is needed to assess the rate of protection against serious complications of varicella infection in adults (e.g., encephalitis, hepatitis, pneumonitis) or protection against congenital varicella syndrome during pregnancy.

Subsequent exposure to natural wild-type varicella infection appears to boost anti-VZV levels in vaccinated individuals, even in individuals who do not develop clinical symptoms of breakthrough infection. This boosting theoretically could contribute to long-term protection against the disease, and it is possible that varicella immunity may wane in some individuals in highly vaccinated populations because of a lack of exposure to natural varicella. The duration of protection against varicella in vaccinated individuals in the absence of such wild-type boosting is unknown.

Chemistry and Stability

■ **Chemistry** Varicella virus vaccine live is commercially available in the US as a single-antigen vaccine (Varivax®) and in a fixed-combination vaccine containing measles, mumps, rubella, and varicella antigens (MMRV; ProQuad®). When reconstituted as directed with the diluent provided by the manufacturer, Varivax® occurs as a clear, colorless to pale yellow liquid and MMRV (ProQuad®) occurs as a clear, pale yellow to light pink liquid.

Varicella virus vaccine live available for use in the US is a lyophilized preparation of live, attenuated varicella zoster virus (VZV) of the Oka/Merck strain. This vaccine is similar, but not identical, to varicella vaccines available in Japan and other countries that contain Oka/Biken or Oka/RIT strains of VZV. The vaccine commercially available for use in the US, like other live, attenuated varicella vaccines, is derived from the same strain of virus originally isolated in 1970 from a Japanese child with natural (wild-type) varicella infection. The virus was isolated in human embryonic lung cells and attenuated by serial passage in several different cell lines at different temperatures. The Oka/Merck strain contained in the US vaccine is attenuated by multiple passages through human embryonic lung cell cultures, embryonic guinea pig cell cultures, the WI-38 strain of human diploid cell cultures, and the MRC-5 strain of human diploid cell cultures (free of adventitious agents). The attenuated virus is suspended in a medium containing sucrose, phosphate, glutamate, and hydrolyzed gelatin and then lyophilized.

Vaccine containing varicella virus vaccine live commercially available for use in the US meets standards established by the Center for Biologics Evaluation and Research of the US Food and Drug Administration. Potency of the varicella component of the vaccines is expressed in terms of plaque-forming units (PFU) of OKA/Merck virus.

Following reconstitution with the diluent provided by the manufacturer and storage at room temperature (20–25°C) for 30 minutes, each 0.5-mL dose of Varivax® contains at least 1350 units of Oka/Merck varicella virus (approximately 3.13 $\log_{10}$ PFU), approximately 25 mg of sucrose, 12.5 mg of hydrolyzed gelatin, 3.2 mg of sodium chloride, 0.5 mg of monosodium glutamate, 0.45 mg of sodium phosphate dibasic, 0.08 mg of potassium phosphate monobasic, and 0.08 mg of potassium chloride and may contain residual components of MRC-5 cells (including DNA and protein) and trace quantities of sodium phosphate monobasic, edetate disodium (EDTA), neomycin, and fetal bovine serum.

Following reconstitution with the diluent provided by the manufacturer, each 0.5-mL dose of MMRV (ProQuad®) contains the same potency of measles, mumps, and rubella antigens as measles, mumps, and rubella virus vaccine live (MMR), at least 3.99 $\log_{10}$ PFU of Oka/Merck varicella virus, no more than 21 mg of sucrose, 11 mg of hydrolyzed gelatin, 2.4 mg sodium chloride, 1.8 mg sorbitol, 0.4 mg monosodium glutamate, 72 mcg of potassium phosphate monobasic, 60 mcg of potassium chloride, and 36 mcg of potassium phosphate dibasic and may contain residual components of MRC-5 cells (including DNA and protein) and less than 16 mcg of neomycin, 0.5 mcg bovine calf serum, and other buffer and media ingredients.

The vaccines do not contain thimerosal or any other preservatives.

■ **Stability** Varicella virus vaccine live is thermolabile and requires particular care to preserve its potency.

To ensure that there is no loss of potency during shipment from the manufacturer, the lyophilized single-antigen vaccine (Varivax®) and the lyophilized fixed-combination vaccine (MMRV; ProQuad®) must be maintained frozen at a temperature of −15°C or colder until delivery.

After delivery from the manufacturer, lyophilized Varivax® or lyophilized MMRV (ProQuad®) must be kept frozen at −15°C or colder and protected from light; any freezer (e.g., chest, frost-free) that reliably maintains an average temperature of −15°C or colder and has a separate sealed freezer door is acceptable. Refrigerators with ice compartments that are either not tightly enclosed or enclosed with unsealed, uninsulated doors (e.g., small, dormitory-style refrigerators) usually do not meet temperature requirements. The diluent provided by the manufacturer should be stored separately, either at room temperature (20–25°C) or in a refrigerator and should not be frozen. Varivax® retains a potency of at least 1500 units for at least 24 months when stored in a frost-free freezer with an average temperature of −15°C or colder.

Because varicella virus vaccine live is thermolabile, planning for appropriate handling and storage is necessary if varicella immunization sessions will be held at a site distant from the freezer in which vials of the vaccine are stored. The number of vials of lyophilized Varivax® vaccine required for the immunization session should be transferred in a suitable container (e.g., the original shipping container or a comparable container with a properly fitted lid) using an adequate quantity of solid carbon dioxide (dry ice) and should be delivered within 2 days.

Prior to reconstitution, Varivax® or MMRV (ProQuad®) may be stored for up to 72 continuous hours at 2–8°C. Therefore, when optimal handling conditions are not feasible (e.g., because of the location of the freezer storage area, distance to the immunization clinic site, concern for security of the room where vaccines are administered, unavailability of dry ice), potency of varicella virus vaccine live can be maintained if vials containing unreconstituted vaccine are stored for a maximum of 72 hours at a temperature of 2–8°C. However, a temperature recording device should be included in the transport container to ensure that the temperature is no warmer than 2–8°C. Any vials of lyophilized Varivax® or MMRV (ProQuad®) stored at 2–8°C should be discarded if not used within 72 hours after removal from freezer storage. For information regarding vaccine stability under conditions other than those recommended, contact the manufacturer at 800-637-2590.

Following reconstitution, potency of varicella virus vaccine live decreases rapidly at room temperature, although viral antigen content remains the same regardless of length of storage. In one stability study using a live, attenuated varicella vaccine containing the Oka/Merck strain of virus, the vaccine had an initial potency of 1770 units immediately following reconstitution; following storage at room temperature, the reconstituted vaccine had a potency of 400–500 or 80–160 units at 6 or 24 hours, respectively. To minimize loss of potency and ensure an adequate immunizing dose, reconstituted Varivax® or reconstituted MMRV (ProQuad®) should be used immediately and any unused vaccine discarded if not used within 30 minutes. Reconstituted Varivax® or MMRV (ProQuad®) should not be frozen.

Preparations

Excipients in commercially available drug preparations may have clinically important effects in some individuals; consult specific product labeling for details.

Varicella Virus Vaccine Live

Parenteral

For injection, for subcutaneous use	1350 plaque-forming units (PFU) per 0.5 mL	**Varivax®**, Merck

Measles, Mumps, Rubella and Varicella Virus Vaccine Live (MMRV)

Parenteral

For injection, for subcutaneous use	Measles Virus Vaccine Live (More Attenuated Enders' Line) ≥3 log $_{10}$ tissue culture infective dose 50% ($TCID_{50}$), Mumps Virus Vaccine Live (Jeryl Lynn [B level] Strain) ≥4.3 log $_{10}$ $TCID_{50}$, Rubella Virus Vaccine Live (Wistar RA 27/3 Strain) ≥3 log $_{10}$ $TCID_{50}$, and Varicella Virus Vaccine Live (Oka/Merck Strain) ≥3.99 log $_{10}$ plaque-forming units (PFU) per 0.5 mL	**ProQuad®**, Merck

†Use is not currently included in the labeling approved by the US Food and Drug Administration

Zoster Vaccine Live

Varicella-Zoster Virus Vaccine Live, VZV Vaccine, ZVL

■ Zoster vaccine live is a preparation of live, attenuated varicella zoster virus (VZV) of the Oka/Merck strain and is used to boost active immunity to VZV.

Uses

■ **Prevention of Herpes Zoster** Zoster vaccine live is used in immunocompetent adults 50 years of age and older to prevent herpes zoster (also known as zoster or shingles) caused by reactivation of varicella zoster virus

(VZV) infection. The vaccine also appears to reduce the frequency, severity, and/or duration of postherpetic neuralgia (PHN) in individuals who develop zoster despite vaccination.

Zoster vaccine live should *not* be used for the *treatment* of zoster or PHN. The vaccine should *not* be administered during an acute episode of zoster in an attempt to prevent development of PHN. Zoster vaccine live has no role in postexposure management of zoster.

Zoster vaccine live should *not* be used for prevention of primary varicella infection (chickenpox) or in children or adults younger than 50 years of age. Zoster vaccine live has no role in postexposure management of chickenpox.

Varicella (chickenpox) and herpes zoster (zoster, shingles) are distinct clinical entities caused by the same virus, VZV, a member of the family Herpesviridae. During primary infection, VZV causes chickenpox and the virus invades sensory neurons and becomes latent in sensory nerve ganglia, establishing a source of potential secondary infection. Natural varicella infection elicits development of specific antibodies and cell-mediated immunity and generally confers lifelong protection against subsequent varicella infection. Secondary infection results from reactivation of latent VZV and manifests as zoster. Zoster is characterized by a unilateral, painful, vesicular cutaneous eruption with a dermatomal distribution; however, the most frequently debilitating symptom is pain. Pain associated with zoster may occur during the prodrome, the acute eruptive phase, and the postherpetic phase of the infection (PHN). Serious complications, including scarring, bacterial superinfection, allodynia, cranial and motor neuron palsies, pneumonia, encephalitis, visual impairment, hearing loss, and death can occur as the result of zoster.

It is estimated that 500,000 to 1 million cases of zoster occur each year in the US; many patients develop PHN and require long-term management for refractory PHN. Over 90% of adults have been infected with VZV and are at risk of developing zoster. The risk of developing zoster increases with age and declining cell-mediated immunity to VZV. Zoster occurs principally in individuals older than 45 years of age; the lifetime risk of zoster is estimated to be at least 32%, and 50% of adults living until 85 years of age will develop zoster.

Choice of Zoster Vaccines There are 2 different types of zoster vaccine commercially available in the US for immunization against zoster in adults 50 years of age or older: zoster vaccine recombinant (RZV; Shingrix®) and zoster vaccine live (ZVL; Zostavax®).

Zoster vaccine recombinant is an inactivated (recombinant) zoster vaccine that contains recombinant VZV surface glycoprotein E (gE) antigen and an adjuvant (i.e., $AS01_B$) and is administered IM in a 2-dose series. Zoster vaccine live contains live, attenuated VZV and is administered subcutaneously as a single dose. The live, attenuated virus vaccine is contraindicated in immunocompromised adults; the US Public Health Service Advisory Committee on Immunization Practices (ACIP) states that additional data are needed regarding use of zoster vaccine recombinant in immunocompromised adults since such individuals were excluded from initial trials evaluating the safety and efficacy of the recombinant vaccine.

For prevention of zoster in immunocompetent adults 50 years of age or older, ACIP states that zoster vaccine recombinant (not zoster vaccine live) is the preferred vaccine and can be used in such individuals regardless of history of zoster or prior vaccination with varicella virus vaccine live or zoster vaccine live. ACIP states that the recombinant zoster vaccine also is preferred in adults 50 years of age or older with certain chronic medical conditions (e.g., chronic renal failure, diabetes mellitus, rheumatoid arthritis, chronic pulmonary disease). Although zoster vaccine live is labeled by FDA for use in adults 50 years of age or older, ACIP states that data to date indicate that the duration of protection is uncertain 5 years after vaccination with the live, attenuated virus vaccine and that adults who receive this vaccine at 50–59 years of age may not be protected when their risks for zoster and its complications are highest. (See Duration of Immunity under Cautions: Warnings/Precautions.)

ACIP states that either zoster vaccine recombinant or zoster vaccine live can be used for prevention of zoster in immunocompetent adults 60 years of age or older.

Clinical Experience **Adults 50–59 Years of Age.** Safety and efficacy of zoster vaccine live for prevention of zoster in adults 50–59 years of age were evaluated in a double-blind, placebo-controlled trial (Zostavax® Efficacy and Safety Trial [ZEST]) that randomized 22,439 adults in this age group to receive a single dose of zoster vaccine live or placebo. Median follow-up was 1.3 years (range 0–2 years) and cases of zoster were confirmed by polymerase chain reaction (PCR; 86%) or, in the absence of virus detection, by clinical evaluation (14%). In the intent-to-treat population, zoster vaccine live reduced the risk of developing zoster in adults 50–59 years age by 69.8% compared with placebo.

Interim analysis of data from a prospective, observational cohort study was used to estimate long-term efficacy of zoster vaccine live for prevention of zoster and PHN based on incidence rates of protocol-defined first episodes of zoster and PHN in the vaccinated and unvaccinated groups, including adjustments for calendar time, age, sex, race/ethnicity, healthcare resource utilization, comorbid conditions, and immunocompromise status. In adults who received a single dose of zoster vaccine live at 50–59 years of age, efficacy of the vaccine against zoster was 60% over the first 3 years following vaccination and 36% in the third year postvaccination. Data were insufficient at the time of the interim analysis to assess efficacy against PHN in adults who received zoster vaccine live at 50–59 years of age.

Adults 60 Years of Age or Older. Safety and efficacy of zoster vaccine live for prevention of zoster and PHN in adults 60 years of age or older have been evaluated in a randomized, placebo-controlled trial (Shingles Prevention Study [SPS]) in 38,546 adults in this age group randomized to receive a single dose of either zoster vaccine live or placebo. Study participants had a history of varicella or were US residents for at least 30 years, but had no history of zoster and had received no prior doses of a vaccine containing VZV antigen. Potency of the 12 vaccine lots of zoster vaccine live used in this trial varied and each dose contained an estimated range of 18,700–60,000 plaque-forming units (PFU) of attenuated VZV of the Oka/Merck strain. The median estimated potency at the time of vaccination was 24,600 PFU and the minimum estimated potency at the time of vaccination was 18,700 PFU; more than 90% of vaccinees received a vaccine containing 32,300 PFU or less of the Oka/Merck strain. Vaccine recipients were followed for the development of zoster for a median of 3.1 years (range: 1 day to 4.9 years). The primary end point was the burden of illness due to zoster (zoster burden-of-illness score), a severity-by-duration measure of the incidence, severity, and duration of zoster-associated pain and discomfort. A secondary endpoint was the incidence of PHN. Those who developed zoster during the study were offered antiviral treatment with famciclovir and, if indicated, adjunctive analgesic therapy (specific analgesic agents used were determined by each clinician).

Results of this placebo-controlled trial indicated that a single dose of zoster vaccine live can reduce the risk of developing zoster in adults 60 years of age or older. Efficacy of the vaccine in preventing zoster (confirmed by PCR [93%], viral culture [1%] or, in the absence of virus detection, by clinical evaluation [6%]) in vaccinees who were followed for at least 30 days postvaccination and who did not develop zoster within 30 days postvaccination (modified intent-to-treat analysis) was 51% overall. In vaccinees who developed zoster despite vaccination, pain and discomfort associated with the disease were decreased by 61%. Vaccine efficacy in preventing zoster was highest (64%) in adults 60–69 years of age and declined with increasing age; efficacy in adults 70–79 years of age or those 80 years of age or older was 41 or 18%, respectively. Study participants suspected of having zoster were monitored for the development of PHN (defined as zoster-associated pain rated by the individual as 3 or greater on a 10-point scale and occurring or persisting for at least 90 days) following the onset of localized rash. Modified intent-to-treat analysis indicated that the median duration of clinically important pain (pain score of 3 or more on a 10-point scale) among those with confirmed zoster was 20 or 22 days in those who received vaccine or placebo, respectively. The overall incidence of PHN in adults 60 years of age and older who developed zoster was 8.6% in those who received the vaccine versus 12.5% in those who received placebo. The benefits of zoster vaccine live in the prevention of PHN may be principally due to the reduced incidence of zoster.

Interim analysis of data from a prospective, observational cohort study was used to estimate long-term efficacy of zoster vaccine live for prevention of zoster and PHN based on incidence rates of protocol-defined first episodes of zoster and PHN in the vaccinated and unvaccinated groups, including adjustments for calendar time, age, sex, race/ethnicity, healthcare resource utilization, comorbid conditions, and immunocompromise status. In adults who received a single dose of zoster vaccine live at 60–69 years of age, 70–79 years of age, or 80 years of age or older, efficacy of the vaccine against zoster over the first 5 years following vaccination was 49, 46, or 44%, respectively, and efficacy in the fifth year postvaccination was 34, 29, or 36%, respectively. In addition, the average vaccine efficacy against PHN in adults who received zoster vaccine live at 60–69 years of age, 70–79 years of age, or 80 years of age or older was 72, 69, or 61%, respectively, over the first 5 years following vaccination and 61, 69, or 34%, respectively, in the fifth year postvaccination. The benefits of zoster vaccine live in the prevention of PHN can be attributed in part to the effect of the vaccine on prevention of zoster.

Dosage and Administration

■ **Reconstitution and Administration** Zoster vaccine live is administered *only* by subcutaneous injection. The vaccine should *not* be administered IM or intravascularly.

To maintain potency during shipment and storage, lyophilized zoster vaccine live should be kept frozen at −50° to −15°C and protected from light. Any freezer, including a frost-free unit, that reliably maintains an average temperature of −50° to −15°C and has a separate sealed freezer door is acceptable; use of dry ice may expose the vaccine to temperatures colder than −50°C. When optimal handling conditions are not feasible (e.g., during transportation), lyophilized zoster vaccine live may be stored for up to 72 hours at 2–8°C; however, the refrigerated vaccine should be discarded if it has not been used within 72 hours after removal from storage at −50 to −15°C. The vial containing the diluent supplied by the manufacturer should be stored separately either at room temperature (20–25°C) or in a refrigerator (2–8°C). For information regarding vaccine stability under conditions other than those recommended, the manufacturer may be contacted at 800-637-2590.

Zoster vaccine live is reconstituted immediately following removal from the freezer by adding the entire contents of the vial containing the diluent provided by the manufacturer to the vial of lyophilized vaccine. Only the diluent supplied by the manufacturer should be used to reconstitute the vaccine. To avoid excessive foaming, the diluent should be injected slowly into the vial of lyophilized vaccine and the vial gently agitated to obtain a semi-hazy to translucent off-white to pale yellow suspension.

To minimize loss of potency, zoster vaccine live should be administered immediately following reconstitution and any reconstituted vaccine not used within 30 minutes should be discarded. The reconstituted vaccine should not be frozen. Zoster vaccine live does not contain thimerosal or any other preservatives.

Zoster vaccine live should be reconstituted and administered using sterile syringes and needles that are free of preservatives, antiseptics, and detergents since these substances may inactivate live, attenuated virus vaccines.

Healthcare professionals should be aware that 2 different types of zoster vaccines are commercially available in the US (zoster vaccine live [ZVL; Zostavax®] and zoster vaccine recombinant [RZV; Shingrix®]) and these vaccines have different recommendations for dosage and administration (e.g., different routes of administration, number of required doses) and different storage requirements. FDA has received multiple reports of medication errors involving zoster vaccine (e.g., incorrect reconstitution, incorrect route of administration, incorrect interval or number of vaccine doses, inappropriate age of vaccinee, administration after incorrect storage) due to confusion about the 2 different products. *Dosage and administration recommendations for the specific zoster vaccine used must be followed.*

Subcutaneous Injection The entire contents of the single-dose vial of reconstituted zoster vaccine live should be administered subcutaneously into the deltoid region of the upper arm.

To ensure appropriate delivery of the vaccine, subcutaneous injections should be made at a 45° angle using a 5/8-inch, 23- to 25-gauge needle.

■ **Dosage** ***Adult Dosage*** **Adults 50 Years of Age or Older.** Zoster vaccine live is given as a single dose.

Adults 50 years of age or older should receive a single dose of zoster vaccine live consisting of the entire contents (0.65 mL) of a reconstituted single-dose vial of the vaccine.

The duration of protection beyond 4–5 years after vaccination with zoster vaccine live and the need for additional (booster) doses of the vaccine have not been determined. (See Duration of Immunity under Cautions: Warnings/Precautions.)

Cautions

■ **Contraindications** Zoster vaccine live is contraindicated in individuals with a history of anaphylactic/anaphylactoid reaction to gelatin, neomycin, or any other vaccine component. (See Sensitivity Reactions under Cautions: Warnings/Precautions.)

Zoster vaccine live is contraindicated in individuals who are immunodeficient or immunosuppressed due to disease or therapy. These individuals include, but are not limited to, those with primary or acquired immunodeficiency states, acquired immunodeficiency syndrome (AIDS) or other clinical manifestations of human immunodeficiency virus (HIV) infection, leukemia, lymphoma, or other malignant neoplasms affecting the bone marrow or lymphatic system (see Individuals with Altered Immunocompetence under Cautions: Warnings/Precautions) and individuals receiving immunosuppressive therapy (see Drug Interactions: Immunosuppressive Agents).

Zoster vaccine live is contraindicated in pregnant women and pregnancy should be avoided for 3 months following vaccination. (See Pregnancy under Warnings/Precautions: Specific Populations, in Cautions.)

■ **Warnings/Precautions** ***Sensitivity Reactions*** Serious adverse reactions, including anaphylaxis, have occurred following administration of zoster vaccine live.

Appropriate medical treatment (e.g., epinephrine) should be available for immediate use in case an anaphylactic/anaphylactoid reaction occurs following administration of zoster vaccine live.

Gelatin Allergy. Zoster vaccine live contains hydrolyzed porcine gelatin (15.58 mg per dose). The vaccine is contraindicated in individuals with a history of anaphylactic/anaphylactoid reactions to gelatin.

The US Public Health Service Advisory Committee on Immunization Practices (ACIP) states that individuals with a history of anaphylactic reaction to gelatin or gelatin-containing products should be evaluated by an allergist prior to receiving a gelatin-containing vaccine.

Neomycin Allergy. Zoster vaccine live contains trace amounts of neomycin. Neomycin hypersensitivity usually manifests as a delayed-type (cell-mediated) contact dermatitis.

The manufacturer states that zoster vaccine live is contraindicated in individuals with a history of anaphylactic/anaphylactoid reaction to neomycin. ACIP states that individuals with a history of anaphylactic reaction to neomycin should be evaluated by an allergist before receiving a neomycin-containing vaccine.

The manufacturer and ACIP state that a history of delayed-type allergic reaction to neomycin is not a contraindication to use of the vaccine.

Individuals with Altered Immunocompetence Because zoster vaccine live contains live, attenuated virus, it is contraindicated in individuals immunosuppressed as a result of disease (e.g., primary or acquired immunodeficiency, HIV infection, leukemia, lymphoma, other malignancies involving the bone marrow or lymphatic system) or immunosuppressive therapy.

The immune response to the vaccine and efficacy may be reduced in individuals with altered immunocompetence. In addition, use of zoster vaccine live in individuals with altered immunocompetence may result in serious or fatal disseminated varicella zoster virus (VZV) disease caused by the vaccine strain. Administration of the vaccine to an immunocompromised patient with chronic lymphocytic leukemia was associated with a fatal disseminated VZV infection complicated by meningoencephalitis.

Although HIV-infected adults, especially those with $CD4^+$ T-cell counts less than 200/mm^3, are at increased risk for zoster, zoster vaccine live is contraindicated in such individuals.

When initiation of immunosuppressive therapy is anticipated, ACIP and other experts state that administration of zoster vaccine live can be considered if the vaccine dose is administered at least 2–4 weeks prior to initiation of such therapy. (See Drug Interactions: Immunosuppressive Agents.)

ACIP and other experts state that zoster vaccine live can be administered to healthy, immunocompetent adults who reside in households with immunocompromised individuals. However, if the vaccinee develops a zoster-associated rash, they should avoid close contact with immunocompromised individuals until the lesions resolve.

Transmission of Vaccine Virus Zoster vaccine live contains live, attenuated VZV. Transmission of vaccine virus may occur between vaccinees and susceptible contacts.

Although not reported to date with zoster vaccine live, transmission of vaccine virus has occurred rarely with other vaccines containing live, attenuated VZV of the Oka/Merck strain (e.g., varicella virus vaccine live; Varivax®). In most reported cases, transmission of vaccine virus occurred between recipients of varicella virus vaccine live who developed a varicella-like rash and susceptible contacts; however, transmission of vaccine virus may also have occurred from vaccine recipients without a VZV-like rash.

The risk of possible transmission of vaccine virus to a susceptible contact (including pregnant women who have not had chickenpox) should be weighed against the risk of developing natural zoster that could be transmitted to a susceptible contact.

Concomitant Illness A decision to administer or delay vaccination in an individual with a current or recent acute illness depends on the severity of symptoms and etiology of the illness.

Zoster vaccine live should *not* be administered during an acute episode of herpes zoster (zoster, shingles); vaccination should be deferred until after the acute stage of the illness is over and symptoms have abated.

The manufacturer states that zoster vaccine live should be deferred in patients with active untreated tuberculosis.

The manufacturer suggests that zoster vaccine live be deferred in individuals with acute illness (e.g., in the presence of fever).

ACIP states that mild acute illness generally does not preclude vaccination. However, moderate or severe acute illness (with or without fever) is a precaution for vaccination and vaccine administration should be deferred until the individual has recovered from the acute phase of the illness. This precaution avoids superimposing adverse effects of the vaccine on the underlying illness or mistakenly concluding that a manifestation of the underlying illness resulted from administration of the vaccine.

Limitations of Vaccine Effectiveness Zoster vaccine live does not prevent zoster in all vaccine recipients. In vaccinated individuals who develop zoster, the duration of pain and discomfort associated with postherpetic neuralgia (PHN) may be shorter compared with that reported in those who have not been vaccinated.

Zoster vaccine live may be less effective in individuals 70 years of age or older than in those 60–69 years of age.

Duration of Immunity The duration of protection against zoster following a single dose of zoster vaccine live and the need for revaccination or additional (booster) doses are not fully determined.

Data to date indicate the duration of protection following a single dose of zoster vaccine live is at least 4–5 years, but the duration of protection beyond 5 years is uncertain. A substantial decrease in effectiveness occurs following the first year after vaccination with zoster vaccine live and there is some evidence that efficacy against zoster in vaccinees is less than 35% by 6 years postvaccination.

Although zoster vaccine live is labeled by FDA for use in adults 50 years of age or older, ACIP states that adults who receive the vaccine at 50–59 years of age may not be protected when their risk for zoster and its complications is highest.

Improper Storage and Handling Improper storage or handling of vaccines may reduce vaccine potency and can result in reduced or inadequate immune responses in vaccinees.

All vaccines should be inspected upon delivery and monitored during storage to ensure that the appropriate temperature is maintained.

Zoster vaccine live that has been mishandled or has not been stored at the recommended temperature should *not* be administered. To maintain potency, lyophilized zoster vaccine live should be stored frozen at −50 to −15°C and used within 30 minutes following reconstitution. (See Dosage and Administration: Reconstitution and Administration.)

If there are concerns about mishandling, the manufacturer or state or local immunization or health departments should be contacted for guidance on whether the vaccine is usable.

Specific Populations **Pregnancy.** Zoster vaccine live is contraindicated in pregnant women and pregnancy should be avoided for 3 months following administration of the vaccine.

Available data regarding inadvertent administration of zoster vaccine live to pregnant women are insufficient to assess vaccine-associated risks in such women.

Naturally occurring VZV infection during pregnancy can cause fetal harm (i.e., congenital varicella syndrome). Because a theoretical risk for congenital varicella syndrome cannot be ruled out, varicella zoster live should *not* be administered to pregnant women.

Vaccinees should be informed of the theoretical risk of transmitting the live, attenuated vaccine virus to varicella-susceptible individuals, including pregnant women who have not had chickenpox. (See Transmission of Vaccine Virus under Cautions: Warnings/Precautions.)

Lactation. The manufacturer states that it is not know whether live, attenuated VZV contained in zoster vaccine live is distributed into human milk.

The benefits of breast-feeding and the importance of zoster vaccine live to the woman should be considered along with the potential adverse effects on the breast-fed child from the vaccine or from the underlying maternal condition (i.e., susceptibility to reactivation of VZV infection).

ACIP states that live, attenuated virus vaccines generally do not pose any unusual risks for women who are breast-feeding or their breast-fed infants. Although live viruses in vaccines can replicate in the mother, the majority of live vaccine viruses (including varicella vaccine virus) do not appear to be distributed into milk. Therefore, ACIP states that breast-feeding is not a contraindication for zoster vaccine live.

Pediatric Use. Zoster vaccine live is *not* indicated for prevention of primary varicella infection (chickenpox) and should *not* be used in children or adolescents.

Geriatric Use. Safety and efficacy of zoster vaccine live have been established *only* in adults 50 years of age or older, including geriatric adults.

The median age of individuals enrolled in the largest clinical trial of the vaccine was 69 years (range: 59–99 years); approximately 54% of vaccine recipients were 60–69 years of age, 40% were 70–79 years of age, and 7% were 80 years of age or older.

■ **Common Adverse Effects** The most common adverse reactions to zoster vaccine live are injection site reactions (erythema, pain/tenderness, swelling, pruritus, warmth, hematoma, induration), headache, and extremity pain.

Drug Interactions

■ **Antiviral Agents** Data are not available to date regarding concurrent use of zoster vaccine live and antiviral agents active against varicella zoster virus (e.g., acyclovir, famciclovir, valacyclovir). However, the potential exists for these antiviral agents to interfere with replication of the live, attenuated varicella zoster virus (VZV) contained in zoster vaccine live and reduce efficacy of the vaccine.

The US Public Health Service Advisory Committee on Immunization Practices (ACIP) states that antiviral agents active against VZV should be discontinued at least 24 hours before administration of zoster vaccine live, if possible, and should not be administered until at least 14 days after the vaccine.

■ **Blood Products** Zoster vaccine live may be administered concurrently with or at any time before or after blood or other antibody-containing blood products (e.g., whole blood, packed red blood cells [RBCs], plasma, platelet products).

■ **Immune Globulins** Zoster vaccine live may be administered concurrently with or at any time before or after immune globulin (immune globulin IM [IGIM], immune globulin IV [IGIV], immune globulin subcutaneous) or specific hyperimmune globulin (hepatitis B immune globulin [HBIG], rabies immune globulin [RIG], tetanus immune globulin [TIG], varicella zoster immune globulin [VZIG]).

■ **Immunosuppressive Agents** Immune responses to vaccines may be reduced in individuals receiving immunosuppressive therapy. In addition, use of zoster vaccine live in individuals receiving immunosuppressive therapy may result in serious and potentially fatal disseminated VZV disease caused by the vaccine strain. Zoster vaccine live is contraindicated in individuals receiving immunosuppressive therapy. (See Individuals with Altered Immunocompetence under Cautions: Warnings/Precautions.)

Live, attenuated virus vaccines generally should be administered at least 2–4 weeks prior to initiation of immunosuppressive therapy and should not be administered during or for certain periods of time after immunosuppressive therapy is discontinued.

Live, attenuated virus vaccines generally should be administered at least 2–4 weeks prior to initiation of chemotherapy or radiation therapy or deferred until at least 3 months after such therapy is discontinued.

In solid organ transplant recipients receiving immunosuppressive anti-rejection therapies, ACIP recommends that administration of zoster vaccine live be deferred until at least 1 month following discontinuance of such therapies.

ACIP states that zoster vaccine live should be administered at least 2 week prior to treatment with anti-B-cell antibodies (e.g., rituximab) or deferred until at least 1 month after such therapy is discontinued. The optimal time to administer vaccines in patients who have received treatment with anti-B-cell antibodies is unclear. Some experts state that live, attenuated virus vaccines generally should be given at least 2–4 weeks before or deferred until at least 6 months after treatment with anti-B-cell antibodies (e.g., rituximab) has been discontinued.

ACIP states that live, attenuated virus vaccines should be administered at least 2 weeks prior to initiation of therapy with certain immunosuppressive biologic response modifiers (e.g., colony-stimulating factors, interleukins, tumor necrosis factor [TNF; TNF-α] blocking agents) or deferred until at least 3 months after such therapy is discontinued.

Because high-dose, systemic corticosteroid therapy (i.e., prednisone or equivalent in a dosage of at least 2 mg/kg daily or at least 20 mg daily given for 2 weeks or longer) is considered immunosuppressive, ACIP and other experts state that live, attenuated virus vaccines, including zoster vaccine live, should be deferred for at least 1 month after such therapy is discontinued. The vaccine does not need to be deferred in patients receiving short-term (less than 2 weeks) or low- to moderate-dose systemic corticosteroid therapy (less than 20 mg of prednisone or equivalent daily); long-term, alternate-day, systemic corticosteroid therapy using short-acting drugs; maintenance physiologic doses (replacement therapy); topical corticosteroid therapy (e.g., cutaneous, ophthalmic); or corticosteroids administered by oral inhalation or by intra-articular, bursal, or tendon injection.

■ **Vaccines** Concurrent administration of zoster vaccine live with other age-appropriate inactivated vaccines or toxoids during the same health-care visit (using separate syringes and different injection sites) generally is not expected to affect immunologic responses or adverse reactions to any of the vaccines. (See Pneumococcal Vaccine under Drug Interactions: Vaccines.)

If another parenteral live vaccine is indicated in a patient receiving zoster vaccine live, ACIP states that the vaccines should either be administered on the same day or at least 4 weeks (28 days) apart.

Influenza Vaccine Zoster vaccine live may be administered concurrently with parenteral inactivated influenza vaccine (using separate syringes and different injection sites).

Data from a double-blind, controlled study in adults 60 years of age or older indicate that concurrent administration of trivalent seasonal influenza virus vaccine inactivated and zoster vaccine live results in antibody responses that are similar to those reported when the vaccines are administered 4 weeks apart.

Data from a double-blind, controlled study in adults 50 years of age or older indicate that concurrent administration of quadrivalent seasonal influenza vaccine inactivated and zoster vaccine live results in antibody responses that are similar to those reported when the vaccines are administered 4 weeks apart.

Pneumococcal Vaccine The manufacturer of zoster vaccine live states that consideration should be given to administering zoster vaccine live and pneumococcal 23-valent vaccine (PPSV23; Pneumovax® 23) at least 4 weeks apart.

Data from a randomized, double-blind, controlled study in adults 60 years of age or older indicate that concurrent administration of zoster vaccine live and PPSV23 (Pneumovax® 23) resulted in a significantly reduced antibody response to zoster vaccine live compared with that reported when the vaccines were administered 4 weeks apart. When assessed using representative pneumococcal serotypes (3, 14, 19A, 22F), the antibody response to PPSV23 (Pneumovax® 23) following concurrent administration was similar to that reported when the vaccines were administered 4 weeks apart. Concurrent administration of zoster vaccine live and PPSV23 (Pneumovax® 23) did not result in a clinically important increase in adverse effects compared with administration during separate visits (4 weeks apart).

Description

Zoster vaccine live is a lyophilized preparation of live, attenuated varicella zoster virus (VZV) of the Oka/Merck strain and is used to boost cell-mediated immunity to VZV, thereby reducing the risk of reactivation of VZV and development of herpes zoster (also known as zoster or shingles) and complications of the disease. The varicella antigen contained in commercially available zoster vaccine live (Zostavax®) is the same as that contained in varicella virus vaccine live (Varivax®); however, zoster vaccine live is about 14 times more potent than varicella virus vaccine live.

Each dose of varicella vaccine live (Zostavax®) contains not less than 19,400 PFU of the Oka/Merck strain; each dose of varicella virus vaccine live (Varivax®) contains a minimum of 1350 PFU of the Oka/Merck strain. There is evidence that the potency of varicella antigen contained in zoster vaccine live (in contrast to that contained in varicella virus vaccine live) is required to elicit a clinically important increase in cell-mediated immunity to VZV among older adults.

Administration of a single dose of zoster vaccine live boosts VZV antibody levels 2.3-fold in adults 50–59 years of age or 1.7-fold in adults 60 years of age or older, as measured by glycoprotein enzyme-linked immunosorbent assay (gpELISA). The minimum antibody titer that correlates with protection against zoster has not been established.

Advice to Patients

Prior to administration of zoster vaccine live, provide a copy of manufacturer's patient information to the patient or patient's legal representative. Also provide a copy of the appropriate CDC Vaccine Information Statement (VIS) to the patient or patient's legal representative (VISs are available at https://www.cdc.gov/vaccines/hcp/vis/index.html).

Advise the patient of the risks and benefits of vaccination with zoster vaccine live.

Advise the patient that zoster vaccine live is used to prevent zoster (shingles) and cannot be used to treat shingles once the condition develops. Also advise the patient that the vaccine is not used to prevent primary varicella infection (chickenpox).

Advise the patient that zoster vaccine live may not provide protection against zoster (shingles) in all vaccinees.

Advise the patient that they should not receive zoster vaccine live if they have a history of anaphylactic/anaphylactoid reactions to any of its ingredients (e.g., gelatin, neomycin).

Advise the patient that they should not receive zoster vaccine live if they have a disease that weakens the immune system (e.g., human immunodeficiency virus [HIV] infection, leukemia, lymphoma) or are receiving treatment that may weaken the immune system (e.g., high-dose corticosteroids).

Advise the patient of the theoretical risk of transmitting the vaccine virus to varicella-susceptible individuals, including immunosuppressed or immunodeficient individuals or pregnant women who have not had chickenpox. Importance of patient informing clinician if they expect to be in close contact with individuals with weakened immune systems, neonates, or pregnant women who have not had chickenpox or have not been vaccinated against chickenpox.

Importance of contacting clinicians if an adverse reaction or hypersensitivity reaction (difficulty breathing or swallowing) occurs following the vaccine dose. Clinicians or individuals can report any adverse reactions that occur following vaccination to the Vaccine Adverse Event Reporting System (VAERS) at 800-822-7967 or http://www.vaers.hhs.gov/.

Importance of informing clinicians of existing or contemplated concomitant therapy, including prescription and OTC drugs, and any concomitant illnesses.

Importance of women informing clinicians if they are or plan to become pregnant or plan to breast-feed. (See Pregnancy under Warnings/Precautions: Specific Populations, in Cautions.)

Importance of informing patients of other important precautionary information. (See Cautions.)

Overview® (see Users Guide). For additional information on this drug until a more detailed monograph is developed and published, the manufacturer's labeling should be consulted. It is *essential* that the manufacturer's labeling be consulted for more detailed information on usual cautions, precautions, contraindications, potential drug interactions, laboratory test interferences, and acute toxicity.

Preparations

Excipients in commercially available drug preparations may have clinically important effects in some individuals; consult specific product labeling for details.

Zoster Vaccine Live

Parenteral

For injectable suspension, for subcutaneous use	≥19,400 plaque-forming units (PFU) of Oka/Merck strain of varicella zoster virus per 0.65 mL	**Zostavax®**, Merck

Zoster Vaccine Recombinant

RZV

■ Zoster vaccine recombinant contains recombinant varicella zoster virus (VZV) surface glycoprotein E (gE) and an adjuvant (i.e., $AS01_B$) and is used to boost active immunity to VZV.

Uses

■ Prevention of Herpes Zoster Zoster vaccine recombinant is used in adults 50 years of age and older to prevent herpes zoster (also known as zoster or shingles) caused by reactivation of varicella zoster virus (VZV) infection. The vaccine also appears to reduce the frequency and/or duration of postherpetic neuralgia (PHN) in individuals who develop zoster despite vaccination.

Zoster vaccine recombinant should *not* be used for *treatment* of zoster or PHN. The vaccine should *not* be administered during an acute episode of zoster. Zoster vaccine has no role in postexposure management of zoster.

Zoster vaccine recombinant should *not* be used for prevention of primary varicella infection (chickenpox) or in children or adults younger than 50 years of age. Zoster vaccine has no role in postexposure management of chickenpox.

Varicella (chickenpox) and herpes zoster (zoster, shingles) are distinct clinical entities caused by the same virus, VZV, a member of the family Herpesviridae. During primary infection, VZV causes chickenpox and the virus invades sensory neurons and becomes latent in sensory nerve ganglia, establishing a source of potential secondary infection. Natural varicella infection elicits development of specific antibodies and cell-mediated immunity and generally confers lifelong protection against subsequent varicella infection. Secondary infection results from reactivation of latent VZV and manifests as zoster. Zoster is characterized by a unilateral, painful, vesicular cutaneous eruption with a dermatomal distribution; however, the most frequently debilitating symptom is pain. Pain associated with zoster may occur during the prodrome, the acute eruptive phase, and the postherpetic phase of the infection (PHN). Serious complications, including scarring, bacterial superinfection, allodynia, cranial and motor neuron palsies, pneumonia, encephalitis, visual impairment, hearing loss, and death can occur as the result of zoster.

It is estimated that 500,000 to 1 million cases of zoster occur each year in the US; many patients develop PHN and require long-term management for refractory PHN. Over 90% of adults have been infected with VZV and are at risk of developing zoster. The risk of developing zoster increases with age and declining cell-mediated immunity to VZV. Zoster occurs principally in individuals older than 45 years of age; the lifetime risk of zoster is estimated to be at least 32%, and 50% of adults living until 85 years of age will develop zoster.

Choice of Zoster Vaccines There are 2 different types of zoster vaccine commercially available in the US for immunization against zoster in adults 50 years of age or older: zoster vaccine recombinant (RZV; Shingrix®) and zoster vaccine live (ZVL; Zostavax®).

Zoster vaccine recombinant is an inactivated (recombinant) zoster vaccine that contains recombinant VZV surface glycoprotein E (gE) antigen and an adjuvant (i.e., $AS01_B$) and is administered IM in a 2-dose series. Zoster vaccine live contains live, attenuated VZV and is administered subcutaneously as a single dose. The live, attenuated vaccine is contraindicated in immunocompromised adults; the US Public Health Service Advisory Committee on Immunization Practices (ACIP) states that additional data are needed regarding use of zoster vaccine recombinant in immunocompromised adults since such individuals were excluded from initial trials evaluating the safety and efficacy of the recombinant vaccine.

For prevention of zoster in immunocompetent adults 50 years of age or older, ACIP states that zoster vaccine recombinant (not zoster vaccine live) is the preferred vaccine and can be used in such individuals regardless of history of zoster or prior vaccination with varicella virus vaccine live or zoster vaccine live. ACIP states that the recombinant zoster vaccine also is preferred in adults 50 years of age or older with certain chronic medical conditions (e.g., chronic renal failure, diabetes mellitus, rheumatoid arthritis, chronic pulmonary disease). Although zoster vaccine live is labeled by FDA for use in adults 50 years of age or older, ACIP states that data to date indicate that the duration of protection is uncertain 5 years after vaccination with the live, attenuated vaccine and that adults who receive this vaccine at 50–59 years of age may not be protected when their risks for zoster and its complications are highest. (See Duration of Immunity under Cautions: Warnings/Precautions.)

ACIP states that either zoster vaccine recombinant or zoster vaccine live can be used for prevention of zoster in immunocompetent adults 60 years of age or older.

Clinical Experience **Adults 50 Years of Age or Older.** Safety and efficacy of zoster vaccine recombinant for prevention of zoster have been evaluated in 2 multicenter, randomized, double-blind, placebo-controlled, phase 3 trials (ZOE-50 [study 1] and ZOE-70 [study 2]) that included a total of 27,922 adults 50 years of age or older (modified total vaccinated cohort) from North America, Latin America, Europe, Asia, and Australia. Trial participants were randomized to receive a 2-dose series of zoster vaccine recombinant (second dose given 2 months after first dose) or placebo and stratified according to age (50–59 years of age, 60–69 years of age, 70–79 years of age, and 80 years of age or older). Individuals who had a history of zoster, history of vaccination against varicella or zoster, or were immunocompromised were excluded from ZOE-50 and ZOE-70. The primary efficacy end point in both trials was overall vaccine efficacy in reducing the risk of zoster compared with placebo. A secondary end point was the incidence of PHN. Median follow-up was 3.1 years (range: 0–3.7 years) and 3.9 years (range: 0–4.5 years) for ZOE-50 and ZOE-70, respectively. Cases of zoster were confirmed by polymerase chain reaction (PCR) or by a clinical evaluation committee.

ZOE-50 included 14,759 adults 50 years of age or older (mean age 62.3 years, 61.2% female, 72.3% white, 18.9% Asian, 1.7% black, 7% other racial/ethnic groups). Results of this placebo-controlled trial indicated that 2 doses of zoster vaccine recombinant given 2 months apart can reduce the risk of developing zoster in adults 50 years of age or older. Overall efficacy of the vaccine in preventing zoster in this age group was 97.2%. When stratified according to age, vaccine efficacy in preventing zoster was 96.6, 97.4, and 97.9% in adults 50–59 years of age, 60–69 years of age, and 70 years of age or older, respectively.

ZOE-70 included 13,163 adults 70 years of age or older (mean age 75.5 years, 54.7% female, 77.6% white, 17.1% Asian, 1% black, 4.2% other racial/ethnic groups). Results of this placebo-controlled trial indicated that 2 doses of zoster vaccine recombinant given 2 months apart can reduce the risk of developing zoster in adults 70 years of age or older. Overall efficacy of the vaccine in preventing zoster in this age group was 89.8%. When stratified according to age, vaccine efficacy in preventing zoster was 90% in adults 70–79 years of age and 89.1% in those 80 years of age or older. Among those who developed confirmed zoster, use of pain medication for zoster-associated pain was reported in 43.5% of vaccine recipients versus 71.7% of those who received placebo.

Participants in both phase 3 trials (ZOE-50 and ZOE-70) who were suspected of having zoster were monitored for the development of PHN (defined as zoster-associated pain rated by the patient as 3 or greater on a 10-point scale and occurring or persisting for at least 90 days following the onset of localized rash in those with confirmed zoster). In ZOE-50, no cases of PHN were reported in vaccine recipients 50 years of age and older versus 18 cases in those who received placebo. In ZOE-70, vaccine efficacy against PHN was 85.5%; 4 cases of PHN were reported in vaccine recipients versus 28 cases in those who received placebo. The benefits of zoster vaccine recombinant in the prevention of PHN may be principally due to the reduced incidence of zoster.

Immune response to zoster vaccine recombinant was evaluated in a random subset of patients from the phase 3 trials (ZOE-50 and ZOE-70). At baseline, more than 99% of participants in these phase 3 trials were seropositive for anti-glycoprotein E (anti-gE) antibodies and median frequencies of gE-specific CD4

T-cells expressing 2 or more activation markers ($CD4^{2+}$ T-cell frequencies) were comparable between those randomized to receive zoster vaccine recombinant or placebo. Results of the subset analysis indicated that 97.8% of vaccine recipients met the criterion for a humoral response compared with 2% of placebo recipients. A mean peak response was observed at 1 month after the second dose of zoster vaccine recombinant, and 77% of vaccine recipients remained above the humoral response threshold at 36 months; postvaccination geometric mean anti-gE antibody concentrations were 39.1- and 8.3-fold higher than baseline antibody concentrations at 1 and 36 months, respectively, after the second dose. Results of the subset analysis also indicated that the cell-mediated immune response (based on gE-specific $CD4^{2+}$ T-cell frequencies) was 93.3% at 1 month after the second dose of zoster vaccine recombinant compared with no response in placebo recipients. The minimum immune response that correlates with protection against zoster has not been established.

Immunogenicity and safety of zoster vaccine recombinant (2 doses given approximately 2 months apart) in adults 50 years of age or older with a history of zoster were evaluated in a phase 3, nonrandomized, open-label study. The mean age of the 96 study participants was 64.9 years (range: 50–89 years of age) and all were seropositive for anti-gE antibodies at baseline; 67.7% had a history of clinician-documented zoster within the past 4 years and 32.3% had a history of clinician-documented zoster more than 4 years prior to study entry. Individuals with active zoster, previous vaccination with varicella virus vaccine live or any zoster vaccine, and those with confirmed or suspected altered immunocompetence as the result of disease or immunosuppressive therapy were excluded. Results indicated that immunogenicity and safety of zoster vaccine recombinant were not adversely affected by a previous zoster episode. At 1 month after the second dose of zoster vaccine recombinant, 90.2% of vaccine recipients had a fourfold increase in anti-gE antibody concentrations compared with baseline concentrations. Postvaccination geometric mean anti-gE antibody concentrations appeared comparable across all age groups (50–59 years of age, 60–69 years of age, 70 years of age or older) and across all timeframes since the previous episode of zoster (4 years or less, 5–9 years, 10 years or more).

Dosage and Administration

■ Reconstitution and Administration Zoster vaccine recombinant is administered *only* by IM injection. The vaccine should *not* be administered subcutaneously, intradermally, or IV.

Zoster vaccine recombinant is commercially available as a kit containing single-dose vials of lyophilized varicella zoster virus (VZV) surface glycoprotein E (gE) antigen and single-dose vials of $AS01_B$ adjuvant suspension. (See Description.)

Prior to administration, a single-dose vial of lyophilized VZV gE antigen from the kit should be reconstituted by adding the entire contents of a single-dose vial of adjuvant suspension from the kit according to the manufacturer's directions. After the adjuvant suspension component is added to the VZV gE antigen component, the vaccine should be gently agitated to ensure that the powder is completely dissolved. The reconstituted vaccine should appear as an opalescent, colorless to pale brown liquid and should be discarded if it contains particulates or appears discolored. The manufacturer's labeling should be consulted for additional information regarding preparation of zoster vaccine recombinant.

Following reconstitution, zoster vaccine recombinant should be administered immediately or may be stored at 2–8°C and administered within 6 hours; any reconstituted vaccine not used within 6 hours should be discarded. Zoster vaccine recombinant does not contain any preservatives.

The kit containing the components of zoster vaccine recombinant should be stored at 2–8°C and protected from light. The kit components and the reconstituted vaccine should not be frozen and should be discarded if freezing has occurred.

Zoster vaccine recombinant may be given concurrently with other age-appropriate vaccines. When multiple vaccines are administered during a single health-care visit, each parenteral vaccine should be given using separate syringes and different injection sites. Injection sites should be separated by at least 1 inch (if anatomically feasible) to allow appropriate attribution of any local adverse effects that may occur.

Healthcare professionals should be aware that 2 different types of zoster vaccine are commercially available in the US (zoster vaccine recombinant [RZV; Shingrix®] and zoster vaccine live [ZVL; Zostavax®]) and these vaccines have different recommendations for dosage and administration (e.g., different routes of administration, different number of required doses) and different storage requirements. FDA has received multiple reports of medication errors involving zoster vaccine (e.g., incorrect reconstitution, incorrect route of administration, incorrect interval or number of vaccine doses, inappropriate age of vaccinee, administration after incorrect storage) due to confusion about the 2 different products. *Dosage and administration recommendations for the specific zoster vaccine used must be followed.*

IM Injection Reconstituted zoster vaccine recombinant should be administered IM, preferably into the deltoid region of the upper arm.

To ensure delivery of the vaccine into muscle, IM injections should be made at a 90° angle to the skin using a needle length appropriate for the individual's age and body mass, thickness of adipose tissue and muscle at the injection site, and injection technique. Anatomic variability, especially in the deltoid, should be considered and clinical judgment should be used to avoid inadvertent underpenetration or overpenetration of muscle.

■ Dosage ***Adult Dosage*** **Adults 50 Years of Age or Older.** Zoster vaccine recombinant is given in a series of 2 doses. Each dose consists of 0.5 mL of reconstituted vaccine.

Adults 50 years of age or older should receive two 0.5-mL IM doses of zoster vaccine recombinant given 2–6 months apart.

A 2-dose regimen of zoster vaccine recombinant is indicated regardless of history of herpes zoster (zoster, shingles) or prior vaccination with varicella virus vaccine live or zoster vaccine live.

The minimum interval between the 2 doses of zoster vaccine recombinant is 4 weeks. The US Public Health Service Advisory Committee on Immunization Practices (ACIP) states that the second dose should be repeated if it was inadvertently given less than 4 weeks after the first dose.

If interruptions or delays result in an interval longer than 6 months between the 2 doses of zoster vaccine recombinant, ACIP states that the vaccine series does not need to be restarted; however, efficacy of a dosing interval longer than 6 months has not been evaluated to date.

If zoster vaccine recombinant is used in adults who previously received zoster vaccine live, ACIP and other experts recommend that the recombinant vaccine should *not* be administered until at least 2 months after the live, attenuated zoster vaccine was administered.

The duration of protection against zoster following a 2-dose series of zoster vaccine recombinant has not been fully determined. (See Duration of Immunity under Cautions: Warnings/Precautions.)

Cautions

■ Contraindications Zoster vaccine recombinant is contraindicated in individuals with a history of severe allergic reaction (e.g., anaphylaxis) to any component of the vaccine or a previous dose of the vaccine. (See Sensitivity Reactions under Cautions: Warnings/Precautions.)

■ Warnings/Precautions ***Sensitivity Reactions*** Prior to administration of zoster vaccine recombinant, all known precautions should be taken to prevent adverse reactions, including a review of the patient's history with respect to possible sensitivity to the vaccine or previous vaccine-related adverse reactions.

Appropriate medical treatment should be readily available in case an anaphylactic reaction occurs following administration of zoster vaccine recombinant.

Individuals with Altered Immunocompetence Individuals with altered immunocompetence were excluded from initial clinical trials evaluating safety and efficacy of zoster vaccine recombinant.

The US Public Health Service Advisory Committee on Immunization Practices (ACIP) states that recombinant vaccines generally can be administered safely to individuals with altered immunocompetence.

Recommendations for use of recombinant vaccines in individuals with human immunodeficiency virus (HIV) infection usually are the same as those for individuals without HIV infection.

Immune responses to zoster vaccine recombinant and efficacy may be reduced in individuals receiving immunosuppressive therapy. (See Drug Interactions: Immunosuppressive Agents.)

Concomitant Illness A decision to administer or delay vaccination in an individual with a current or recent acute illness depends on the severity of symptoms and etiology of the illness.

Zoster vaccine recombinant should *not* be administered during an acute episode of herpes zoster (zoster, shingles); vaccination should be deferred until after the acute stage of the illness is over and symptoms have abated.

Zoster vaccine recombinant may be administered to age-appropriate adults with certain chronic medical conditions (e.g., chronic renal failure, diabetes mellitus, rheumatoid arthritis, chronic pulmonary disease).

ACIP states that mild acute illness generally does not preclude vaccination. However, moderate or severe acute illness (with or without fever) is a precaution for vaccination and vaccine administration should be deferred until the individual has recovered from the acute phase of the illness. This precaution avoids superimposing adverse effects of the vaccine on the underlying illness or mistakenly concluding that a manifestation of the underlying illness resulted from administration of the vaccine.

Limitations of Vaccine Effectiveness Zoster vaccine recombinant does not prevent zoster in all vaccine recipients. In vaccinated individuals who develop zoster, the duration of pain and discomfort may be reduced.

Duration of Immunity The duration of protection against zoster following a 2-dose series of zoster vaccine recombinant has not been fully determined.

Data to date indicate the duration of protection following the 2-dose series of zoster vaccine recombinant is at least 4 years. ACIP states that zoster vaccine recombinant is likely to provide substantial protection against zoster for more than 4 years.

Improper Storage and Handling Improper storage or handling of vaccines may reduce vaccine potency and can result in reduced or inadequate immune responses in vaccinees.

All vaccines should be inspected upon delivery and monitored during storage to ensure that the appropriate temperature is maintained. (See Dosage and Administration: Reconstitution and Administration.)

Vaccine that has been mishandled or has not been stored at the recommended temperature should *not* be administered.

If there are concerns about mishandling, the manufacturer or state or local immunization or health departments should be contacted for guidance on whether the vaccine is usable.

Specific Populations **Pregnancy.** Data are not available regarding use of zoster vaccine recombinant in pregnant women. In animal studies, there was no evidence that zoster vaccine recombinant or the $AS01_B$ adjuvant component of the vaccine affected fetal development or caused fetal harm.

ACIP states that consideration should be given to delaying administration of zoster vaccine recombinant in pregnant women.

Lactation. It is not known whether zoster vaccine recombinant is distributed into human milk, affects milk production, or affects the breast-fed infant. The benefits of breast-feeding and the importance of zoster vaccine recombinant to the woman should be considered along with the potential adverse effects on the breast-fed child from the vaccine or from the underlying maternal condition (i.e., susceptibility to reactivation of VZV infection).

ACIP states that administration of a recombinant vaccine to a woman who is breast-feeding generally does not pose any unusual risks for the woman or her breast-fed infant. However, these experts state that consideration should be given to deferring administration of zoster vaccine recombinant in women who are breast-feeding.

Pediatric Use. Safety and efficacy of zoster vaccine recombinant have not been established in pediatric patients and the vaccine is *not* indicated for prevention of primary varicella infection (chickenpox).

Geriatric Use. Safety and efficacy of zoster vaccine recombinant have been established *only* in adults 50 years of age or older, including geriatric adults.

In phase 3 clinical trials of zoster vaccine recombinant, 15.3% of study participants were 60–69 years of age, 46.7% were 70–79 years of age, and 13.1% were 80 years and older or older. There were no clinically meaningful differences in efficacy of the vaccine across these age groups or between adults 60 years of age and older and those 50–59 years of age; however, adverse effects were reported less frequently in vaccine recipients 70 years of age or older compared with those 50–69 years of age.

■ **Common Adverse Effects** The most common adverse reactions to zoster vaccine recombinant are injection site reactions, including pain (78%), erythema (38%), and swelling (26%), and systemic reactions, including myalgia (45%), fatigue (45%), headache (38%), shivering (27%), fever (21%), and GI symptoms (nausea, vomiting, diarrhea, and/or abdominal pain) (17%).

Drug Interactions

■ **Immunosuppressive Agents** Immune responses to zoster vaccine recombinant may be decreased in individuals receiving immunosuppressive agents.

In individuals receiving corticosteroids, the US Public Health Service Advisory Committee on Immunization Practices (ACIP) states that zoster vaccine recombinant may be used in those receiving low-dose systemic corticosteroid therapy (prednisone or equivalent in a dosage less than 20 mg daily) or inhaled or topical corticosteroid therapy. Zoster vaccine recombinant has not been evaluated to date in individuals receiving high-dose corticosteroid therapy.

■ **Vaccines** Concurrent administration of zoster vaccine recombinant with other age-appropriate vaccines or toxoids during the same health-care visit (using separate syringes and different injection sites) is not expected to affect immunologic responses or adverse reactions to any of the vaccines.

Influenza Vaccine Zoster vaccine recombinant may be administered concurrently with parenteral non-adjuvant-containing influenza virus vaccine inactivated (using separate syringes and different injection sites). Data from an open-label study in adults 50 years of age or older indicated that concomitant administration of a dose of seasonal quadrivalent influenza virus vaccine inactivated (Fluarix® Quadrivalent) and a dose of zoster vaccine recombinant does not interfere with the immune responses to either vaccine and is not associated with any safety concerns.

Safety and efficacy of concomitant or sequential administration of zoster vaccine recombinant and adjuvant-containing influenza virus vaccine inactivated (Fluad®) have not been evaluated.

Pneumococcal Vaccine Data from an open-label, randomized, controlled study in adults 50 years of age or older (mean age 63.2 years) indicate that concurrent administration of zoster vaccine recombinant (first dose of the 2-dose series) and pneumococcal 23-valent vaccine (PPSV23; Pneumovax® 23) at different sites followed by the second dose of zoster vaccine recombinant 2 months later does not interfere with the immune responses to either vaccine and does not affect the safety profile of the vaccines.

Zoster Vaccine Live Safety and immunogenicity of zoster vaccine recombinant have been evaluated in patients who previously received zoster vaccine live at least 5 years before administration of zoster vaccine recombinant; shorter intervals have not been evaluated. ACIP states that there are no data or theoretical concerns to indicate that zoster vaccine recombinant would be less effective or less safe if administered to an adult who received zoster vaccine live less than 5 years earlier.

If zoster vaccine recombinant is used in adults 50 years of age or older who previously received zoster vaccine live, ACIP and other experts recommend that the recombinant zoster vaccine should be administered at least 2 months after the live, attenuated zoster vaccine was administered.

Description

Zoster vaccine recombinant is an inactivated (recombinant) vaccine used to boost immunity to varicella zoster virus (VZV), thereby reducing the risk of reactivation of VZV and development of herpes zoster (also known as zoster or shingles) and complications of the disease. Zoster vaccine recombinant is commercially available as a kit containing single-dose vials of lyophilized VZV surface glycoprotein E (gE) antigen (sterile white powder) and single-dose vials of $AS01_B$ adjuvant suspension (opalescent, colorless to pale brown liquid). The recombinant gE antigen component is prepared using recombinant DNA technology and Chinese hamster ovary (CHO) cells in media containing amino acids (without albumin, antibiotics, or animal-derived proteins) and then purified using chromatography. The adjuvant component is a liposomal formulation of $AS01_B$ composed of 3-O-desacyl-4′-monophosphoryl lipid A (MPL) (produced from *Salmonella minnesota*) and QS-21 (a saponin purified from plant extract *Quillaja saponaria* Molina). The liposomes are composed of dioleoyl phosphatidylcholine (DOPC) and cholesterol in phosphate-buffered saline solution and water for injection. The $AS01_B$ adjuvant enhances the immune response to the recombinant VZV gE antigen.

Following reconstitution of a single-dose vial of the VZV gE antigen component with a single-dose vial of the $AS01_B$ adjuvant component, each 0.5-mL dose of zoster vaccine recombinant contains 50 mcg of recombinant gE antigen, 50 mcg of MPL, and 50 mcg of QS-21. In addition, each 0.5-mL dose of the vaccine contains 20 mg of sucrose (as stabilizer) and also contains 4.4 mg of sodium chloride, 1 mg of DOPC, 0.54 mg of potassium dihydrogen phosphate, 0.25 mg of cholesterol, 0.16 mg of sodium dihydrogen phosphate dihydrate, 0.15 mg of disodium phosphate anhydrous, 0.12 mg of dipotassium phosphate, and 0.08 mg of polysorbate 80. The vaccine may contain residual amounts of host cell proteins (3% or less) and DNA (2.1 picograms or less) from the manufacturing process.

Administration of a 2-dose vaccination series of zoster vaccine recombinant in adults 50 years of age or older boosts VZV-specific cell-mediated immune responses and VZV-specific humoral immunity resulting in a reduced risk of zoster and postherpetic neuralgia (PHN) in vaccinees. The minimum immune response that correlates with protection against zoster has not been established.

Advice to Patients

Prior to administration of zoster vaccine recombinant, provide a copy of the appropriate CDC Vaccine Information Statement (VIS) to the patient or patient's legal representative (VISs are available at https://www.cdc.gov/vaccines/hcp/vis/index.html).

Advise the patient of the risks and benefits of vaccination with zoster vaccine recombinant.

Advise the patient of the importance of receiving 2 doses of zoster vaccine recombinant given 2–6 months apart.

Advise the patient that zoster vaccine recombinant may not provide protection in all vaccinees.

Inform patients about the potential for adverse reactions temporally associated with the vaccine. Clinicians or individuals can report any adverse reactions that occur following vaccination to the Vaccine Adverse Event Reporting System (VAERS) at 800-822-7967 or http://www.vaers.hhs.gov/.

Importance of informing clinicians of existing or contemplated concomitant therapy, including prescription and OTC drugs, and any concomitant illnesses.

Importance of women informing clinicians if they are or plan to become pregnant or plan to breast-feed.

Importance of informing patients of other important precautionary information. (See Cautions.)

Overview® (see Users Guide). For additional information on this drug until a more detailed monograph is developed and published, the manufacturer's labeling should be consulted. It is *essential* that the manufacturer's labeling be consulted for more detailed information on usual cautions, precautions, contraindications, potential drug interactions, laboratory test interferences, and acute toxicity.

Preparations

Excipients in commercially available drug preparations may have clinically important effects in some individuals; consult specific product labeling for details.

Zoster Vaccine Recombinant, Adjuvanted

Parenteral

Kit, for IM use only	For injectable suspension, for IM use, 50 mcg of recombinant varicella zoster virus glycoprotein E antigen per 0.5 mL Injectable suspension, for IM use, $AS01_B$ adjuvant containing 50 mcg of 3-*O*-desacyl-4′-monophosphoryl lipid A (MPL) and 50 mcg of *Quillaja saponaria* Molina (QS21) per 0.5 mL	**Shingrix®**, GlaxoSmithKline

84:00 Skin and Mucous Membrane Agents*

84:04 Anti-infectives

84:04.04 Antibacterials

Bacitracin§
Clindamycin§
Erythromycin§
Gentamicin§
Metronidazole§
Minocycline§
Mupirocin§
Neomycin§
Ozenoxacin§
Retapamulin§
Tetracyclines§
see also:
Dapsone 84:92

84:04.06 Antivirals

Acyclovir§
Docosanol§
Penciclovir§

84:04.08 Antifungals

84:04.08.04 Allylamines

Naftifine§
Terbinafine§

84:04.08.08 Azoles

Butoconazole§
Clotrimazole§
Econazole§
Efinaconazole§
Ketoconazole§
Luliconazole§
Miconazole§
Oxiconazole§
Sertaconazole§
Sulconazole§
Terconazole§
Tioconazole§

84:04.08.12 Benzylamines

Butenafine§

84:04.08.20 Hydroxypyridones

Ciclopirox§

84:04.08.24 Oxaboroles

Tavaborole§

84:04.08.28 Polyenes

Nystatin§

84:04.08.40 Thiocarbamates

Tolnaftate§

84:04.08.92 Antifungals, Miscellaneous

Carbol-Fuchsin§
Gentian Violet§
Sodium Thiosulfate§
Undecylenic Acid§

84:04.12 Scabicides and Pediculicides

Benzyl Alcohol§
Benzyl Benzoate§
Crotamiton§
Ivermectin§
Lindane§
Malathion§
Permethrin§
Pyrethrins with Piperonyl Butoxide§
Spinosad§
see also:
Sulfur 84:28

84:04.92 Local Anti-infectives, Miscellaneous

Benzalkonium Chloride§
Boric Acid§
Chlorhexidine§
Hexachlorophene§
Iodine§
Iodoquinol§
Mafenide§
Selenium Sulfide§
Silver Sulfadiazine§

84:06 Anti-inflammatory Agents

84:06.08 Corticosteroids

Topical Corticosteroids General Statement *p. 3580*
Alclometasone§
Amcinonide§
Betamethasone§
Clobetasol§
Clocortolone§
Desonide§
Desoximetasone§
Diflorasone§
Fluocinolone§
Flurandrenolide§
Halcinonide§
Hydrocortisone§
Mometasone§
Prednicarbate§
Triamcinolone§

84:06.20 Nonsteroidal Anti-inflammatory Agents

Diclofenac§

84:06.92 Anti-inflammatory Agents, Miscellaneous

Crisaborole§

84:08 Antipruritics and Local Anesthetics

Benzocaine§
Dibucaine§
Doxepin§
Ethyl Chloride§
Phenazopyridine§
Pramoxine§
see also:
Diphenhydramine 4:04

84:12 Astringents

Aluminum Acetate§
Aluminum Chloride Hexahydrate§

84:16 Cell Stimulants and Proliferants

Becaplermin§
Palifermin§
Tretinoin§

84:20 Detergents

Green Soap§

84:24 Emollients, Demulcents, and Protectants

Vitamins A and D§

84:28 Keratolytic Agents

Salicylic Acid§
Sulfur§
Urea§

84:32 Keratoplastic Agents

Coal Tar§

84:50 Depigmenting and Pigmenting Agents

84:50.04 Depigmenting Agents

Hydroquinone§
Mequinol and Tretinoin§
Monobenzone§

84:50.06 Pigmenting Agents

Dihydroxyacetone§
Methoxsalen§

84:80 Sunscreen Agents

Sunscreens§

84:92 Skin and Mucous Membrane Agents, Miscellaneous

Acitretin§
Adapalene§
Alefacept§
Alitretinoin§
Aminolevulinic Acid§
Azelaic Acid§
Bexarotene§
Brimonidine§
Brodalumab§
Calcipotriene§
Collagenase§
Dapsone§
Dextranomer§
Doxycycline§
Dupilumab§
Eflornithine§
Fibrin Sealant§
Finasteride§
Fluorouracil§
Glycopyrronium§
Guselkumab *p. 3583*
Hydrogen Peroxide 40%§
Imiquimod§
Ingenol§
Isotretinoin§
Ixekizumab§
Mechlorethamine§
Minoxidil§
Nitroglycerin§

§ Omitted from the print version of *AHFS Drug Information*® because of space limitations. This monograph is available on the *AHFS Drug Information*® website, http://ahfsdruginformation.com. Username: ahfs2020; Password: ASHP94498.
* Please see the full *AHFS Pharmacologic-Therapeutic Classification*© on p. viii. Not all classes are used in the printed edition.

ANTI-INFLAMMATORY AGENTS 84:06
CORTICOSTEROIDS 84:06.08

Topical Corticosteroids General Statement

■ Hydrocortisone or synthetic derivatives of hydrocortisone are used topically as anti-inflammatory agents.

Uses

■ Dermatoses Topical corticosteroids are used for the symptomatic relief of inflammatory dermatoses. The cause of the dermatoses should be determined and eliminated if possible; dermatoses are controlled but not cured by these drugs. Although systemic corticosteroids are more effective in most dermatologic inflammations, topical treatment is preferred in most responsive cases because it causes fewer adverse systemic effects.

Topical corticosteroids generally are most effective in the treatment of acute or chronic dermatoses such as seborrheic or atopic dermatitis, localized neurodermatitis, anogenital pruritus, psoriasis, and the inflammatory phase of xerosis. Topical corticosteroids are effective in the late phase of allergic contact dermatitis or irritant dermatitis, but systemic corticosteroids are usually required to relieve the acute manifestations of these dermatoses.

Individual topical corticosteroid preparations vary in anti-inflammatory activity (as measured by vasoconstrictor assay) and in percutaneous penetration, but therapeutic efficacy of a particular drug can often be increased by increasing the concentration or by using occlusive dressing therapy. As with systemic use, some patients may respond better to one topical corticosteroid than to another. Topical corticosteroid preparations may be grouped according to relative anti-inflammatory activity, but *activity may vary considerably depending upon the vehicle, the site of application, disease, the individual patient, and whether or not an occlusive dressing is used.* (See Pharmacokinetics.) *Approximate* relative activity (based principally on vasoconstrictor assay and/or clinical effectiveness in psoriasis) of some topical corticosteroid preparations in decreasing order is as follows (preparations in each group are approximately equivalent):

Group I

Betamethasone dipropionate (Diprolene®) cream (optimized vehicle) or ointment (optimized vehicle) 0.05% (of betamethasone)
Betamethasone dipropionate (Diprolene® AF) cream 0.05% (of betamethasone)
Clobetasol propionate (Clobex®, Temovate®, Olux®) cream, foam, ointment, lotion, or shampoo 0.05%
Diflorasone diacetate (Psorcon®) ointment (optimized vehicle) 0.05%

Group II

Amcinonide (Cyclocort®) ointment 0.1%
Betamethasone dipropionate (Diprosone®) ointment 0.05% (of betamethasone)
Desoximetasone (Topicort®) cream or ointment 0.25%
Desoximetasone (Topicort®) gel 0.05%
Diflorasone diacetate (Florone®, Maxiflor®) ointment 0.05%
Fluocinonide (Lidex®) cream or ointment 0.05%
Fluocinonide gel 0.05%
Halcinonide (Halog®) cream 0.1%

Group III

Betamethasone benzoate gel 0.025%
Betamethasone dipropionate (Diprosone®) cream 0.05% (of betamethasone)
Betamethasone valerate (Valisone®) ointment 0.1% (of betamethasone)
Diflorasone diacetate (Florone®, Maxiflor®) cream 0.05%
Mometasone furoate (Elocon®) ointment 0.1%
Triamcinolone acetonide (Aristocort®) cream 0.5%

Group IV

Desoximetasone (Topicort® LP) cream 0.05%
Fluocinolone acetonide (Synalar-HP®) cream 0.2%
Fluocinolone acetonide (Synalar®) ointment 0.025%
Flurandrenolide (Cordran®) ointment 0.05%
Triamcinolone acetonide (Aristocort®, Kenalog®) ointment 0.1%

Group V

Betamethasone benzoate cream 0.025%
Betamethasone dipropionate (Diprosone®) lotion 0.05% (of betamethasone)
Betamethasone valerate (Valisone®) cream 0.1% (of betamethasone)
Betamethasone valerate (Valisone®) lotion 0.1% (of betamethasone)
Fluocinolone acetonide (Synalar®) cream 0.025%
Flurandrenolide (Cordran®) cream 0.05%
Hydrocortisone butyrate (Locoid®) cream 0.1%
Hydrocortisone valerate (Westcort®) cream 0.2%
Prednicarbate (Dermatop® Emollient) cream 0.1%
Triamcinolone acetonide (Kenalog®) cream 0.1%
Triamcinolone acetonide (Kenalog®) lotion 0.1%

Group VI

Alclometasone dipropionate (Aclovate®) cream or ointment 0.05%
Desonide (Tridesilon®) cream 0.05%
Fluocinolone acetonide (Synalar®) solution 0.01%

Although some dermatoses may require therapy with a relatively more active corticosteroid initially, treatment with hydrocortisone, dexamethasone (a topical preparation is no longer commercially available in the US) , methylprednisolone, or prednisolone, which are generally considered to be less active (i.e., Group VII) than preparations in groups I–VI, is often sufficient and is less likely to cause adverse reactions. Although fluorinated corticosteroids are generally more biologically active and have greater antimitotic activity than non-fluorinated drugs, fluorination is not essential for increased anti-inflammatory activity (e.g., hydrocortisone valerate has more topical anti-inflammatory activity than does betamethasone or dexamethasone). Relatively more active corticosteroids with or without occlusive dressing therapy are used for severe or resistant dermatoses such as psoriasis and chronic neurodermatitis. Dermatoses such as discoid lupus erythematosus, lichen planus, granuloma annulare, and psoriasis of palms, soles, elbows, and knees or psoriatic plaques usually require topical corticosteroids with increased anti-inflammatory activity and occlusive dressings or intralesional or sublesional corticosteroid injections. Hypertrophic lichen planus, alopecia areata, hypertrophic scars, and keloids generally require intralesional corticosteroid therapy.

■ Ulcerative Colitis and Anorectal Disorders Hydrocortisone is used as a retention enema in the adjunctive treatment of mild or moderate acute ulcerative colitis limited to the rectosigmoid or left colon and, to a lesser extent, in some patients with mild acute ulcerative colitis of the transverse or descending colon. Corticosteroid enemas are usually effective in patients with mild or moderate acute ulcerative colitis of the rectosigmoid who do not adequately respond to sulfasalazine alone or in whom sulfasalazine cannot be given; sulfasalazine is generally considered the drug of choice for maintenance therapy in mild or moderate ulcerative colitis. Systemic corticosteroids and/or corticosteroid enemas are more effective than sulfasalazine in acute attacks of ulcerative colitis but, if surgery is required, it should not be delayed in favor of corticosteroid therapy.

Hydrocortisone acetate, as rectal suppositories or a suspension (foam), may be effective in the adjunctive treatment of ulcerative colitis of the rectum. As rectal suppositories, hydrocortisone acetate is also used in the treatment of other inflammatory conditions of the anorectum (e.g., inflamed hemorrhoids, post-irradiation or factitial proctitis, cryptitis, pruritus ani).

Preparations containing a corticosteroid and local anesthetic may be useful in the symptomatic relief of anorectal disorders such as hemorrhoids, but commercially available corticosteroid combinations with antihistamines, astringents, keratolytics, and/or vasoconstrictors are of questionable efficacy.

■ **Other Uses** Topical corticosteroids are commercially available in combination with antibiotics such as neomycin and antifungals such as clioquinol (iodochlorhydroxyquin). Results of some well-controlled clinical studies using cortisol suggest that these combination preparations are more effective than either the corticosteroid or anti-infective agent alone in infected dermatoses. Combined therapy with triamcinolone and nystatin has been shown to be more effective than nystatin alone for improving the clinical severity of cutaneous candidiasis, especially during the first few days of therapy; combined therapy generally provides earlier relief of signs and symptoms of this infection than does nystatin alone. If topical corticosteroids are used in combination with topical anti-infective agents, the benefit must be weighed against the risk of contact sensitization to the anti-infective agent and suppression by the corticosteroid of manifestations of infection. (See Cautions: Precautions and Contraindications.)

For EENT uses of corticosteroids, see 52:08. For systemic and intralesional uses of corticosteroids, see 68:04.

Dosage and Administration

For dermatologic use, topical corticosteroids are available in various dosage forms including creams, dressings (tape), foams, gels, lotions, ointments, solutions, and aerosols (suspensions). The choice of a dosage form depends on the location of the lesion and the condition being treated. Lotions are probably best for the treatment of weeping eruptions, especially in areas subject to chafing such as the axilla, foot, and groin. Lotions, gels, and aerosols may be used on hairy areas, particularly the scalp. Creams are suitable for most dermatoses, but ointments, which may also provide some occlusion, are usually used for the treatment of dry, scaly lesions. Because certain areas of the body may be more susceptible to atrophic changes than others following treatment with corticosteroids, certain topical corticosteroid preparations (e.g., betamethasone dipropionate 0.05% gel; clobetasol propionate 0.05% cream, foam, gel, lotion, solution, or shampoo; hydrocortisone valerate 0.2% cream; mometasone furoate 0.1% cream, lotion, or ointment) should not be applied to the face or intertriginous areas (e.g., axilla, groin).

Because the formulation of dermatologic corticosteroid products affects percutaneous penetration and subsequent activity of the drug, extemporaneous preparation or dilution of most commercially available products with another vehicle may result in decreased effectiveness.

The area of skin to be treated may be thoroughly cleansed before topical application of corticosteroids to reduce the risk of infection. However, some clinicians believe that, unless an occlusive dressing is used, cleansing of the treated area is unnecessary and may be irritating. Topical corticosteroids are generally applied sparingly in thin films and rubbed gently into the affected area 1–4 times daily. When a favorable response is achieved, the frequency of application or concentration of the corticosteroid is reduced to the minimum necessary to maintain control and avoid relapse and, if possible, the drug should be discontinued.

For occlusive dressing therapy, the affected area is soaked or washed to remove scales and a corticosteroid cream, lotion, or ointment is applied in a thin film or is rubbed gently into the lesion and another thin film applied. After applying the corticosteroid, the affected area is covered with a thin, pliable plastic film which is sealed to adjacent normal skin with adhesive tape or held in place by a gauze or elastic bandage. If the affected area is moist, the edges of the plastic film may be incompletely sealed or the film may be punctured to allow excess moisture to escape. For added moisture in dry lesions, the corticosteroid may be covered with a dampened cloth before the plastic film is applied or the affected area may be briefly soaked in water before application of the drug and plastic film. Thin polyethylene gloves may be used on the hands and fingers, plastic garment bags may be used on the trunk or buttocks, a tight shower cap may be used for the scalp, or whole-body suits may be used instead of plastic film to provide occlusion. Flurandrenolide tape may be used alone as an occlusive dressing for small areas.

The frequency of occlusive dressing changes depends on the condition being treated; cleansing of the skin and reapplication of the corticosteroid are essential at each dressing change. The occlusive dressing is usually left in place for 12–24 hours and therapy is repeated as needed. Some manufacturers state that the occlusive dressing may be left in place for 3–4 days at a time in resistant conditions, because theoretically the longer the occlusive dressing is left in place at one time, the more rapidly the dermatoses respond to topical corticosteroid therapy. However, most clinicians recommend intermittent use of occlusive dressings for 12 hours daily to reduce the risk of adverse effects (particularly infection) and systemic absorption and for greater convenience. For example, the corticosteroid and an occlusive dressing may be used at night, and the topical corticosteroid or a bland emollient may be used without an occlusive dressing during the day. In patients with extensive lesions, sequential occlusion of only one portion of the body at a time may be preferable to whole-body occlusion.

Cautions

■ **Systemic Effects** In general, topical application of corticosteroids to the skin does not provoke clinical evidence of systemic absorption. However, adverse systemic corticosteroid effects may occur when the drugs are used on large areas of the body, for prolonged periods of time, with an occlusive dressing, and/or in infants and children or when potent agents (e.g., those in group I) are used. (See Cautions: Precautions and Contraindications.) Reversible hypothalamic-pituitary-adrenal (HPA) axis suppression, manifestations of Cushing's syndrome, hyperglycemia, and glucosuria have occurred in some patients receiving topical corticosteroids. Recovery of HPA-axis function is generally prompt and complete following discontinuance of the drug. In some patients, signs and symptoms of steroid withdrawal may occur, necessitating supplemental systemic corticosteroid therapy. Reversible HPA-axis suppression has occurred following topical dosages as low as 2 g of the 0.05% clobetasol propionate cream or ointment (1 mg of the drug) daily or 7 g of the 0.05% betamethasone dipropionate cream in an optimized vehicle (3.5 mg of betamethasone) daily or following repeated application of 14 g of the 0.05% betamethasone dipropionate ointment in an optimized vehicle (7 mg of betamethasone) daily in patients with psoriasis. Numbness of fingers has been reported in patients receiving topical clobetasol propionate preparations. In at least one patient receiving hydrocortisone buteprate cream, paresthesia has been reported.

Rectal administration or topical application of corticosteroids to the genitourinary tract for prolonged periods produces systemic effects. For cautions in the systemic use of corticosteroids, see the Corticosteroids General Statement 68:04.

■ **Local Effects** Topical corticosteroids may cause adverse dermatologic effects. Adverse dermatologic effects are most likely to occur in intertriginous and facial areas and are most severe with fluorinated corticosteroids; fluorinated derivatives should be used with caution on the face. Local adverse corticosteroid effects occur most frequently with occlusive dressings, especially with prolonged therapy, and may require discontinuing the occlusive dressing.

Topical corticosteroids may cause atrophy of the epidermis, subcutaneous tissue, and dermal collagen and drying and cracking or tightening of the skin. Epidermal thinning, telangiectasia, increased fragility of cutaneous blood vessels, purpura, and atrophic striae may also occur. Other adverse dermatologic effects of topical corticosteroids include acne, acneiform eruption, vesiculation, irritation, pruritus, hypertrichosis, rosacea-like eruptions on the face, erythema, hyperesthesia, urticaria, perioral dermatitis, burning or stinging sensation, folliculitis, hypopigmentation, and alopecia. Skin ulceration has occurred in patients with impaired circulation who were treated with topical corticosteroids. Local pain or burning and rectal bleeding have occurred rarely with rectal administration of hydrocortisone as an enema.

Adverse dermatologic effects of topical corticosteroids usually improve when the drug is discontinued but may persist for long periods; atrophic striae may be permanent. When prolonged (2 months or more) topical fluorinated corticosteroid therapy is discontinued, pustular "rebound" may occur, especially on the face, perianal region, or genitals. Although improvement usually occurs spontaneously within a few weeks, some patients may require treatment with a systemic antibiotic (e.g., tetracycline) and a topical nonfluorinated corticosteroid (e.g., hydrocortisone) and/or sulfur.

In addition to the other adverse dermatologic effects of topical corticosteroid therapy, maceration of the skin and miliaria may occur, especially when occlusive dressings are used. Stripping of the epidermis and purpura have occurred with flurandrenolide tape dressings.

Topically applied corticosteroids are generally nonsensitizing, but allergic contact dermatitis may occur rarely. Allergic contact dermatitis associated with topical corticosteroids usually is diagnosed by observing a failure to heal rather than noting a clinical exacerbation as with most topical preparations that do not contain corticosteroids; such an observation should be corroborated with appropriate diagnostic patch testing.

Dermatologic infection may occur with topical corticosteroid therapy, particularly when an occlusive dressing is used. The anti-inflammatory activity of the drugs can also mask the manifestations of infection.

■ **Precautions and Contraindications** Patients receiving large doses of a potent topical corticosteroid applied to extensive areas or under an occlusive dressing should be evaluated periodically for evidence of HPA-axis suppression by using the urinary free cortisol test, plasma cortisol test, or corticotropin (ACTH) stimulation test. If HPA-axis suppression is evident, an attempt should be made to withdraw the drug, reduce the frequency of application, or substitute a less potent topical corticosteroid.

Patients receiving topical corticosteroids should be instructed to use the preparations only as directed by the physician, only for the disorder for which it was prescribed, and for no longer than the time period prescribed. Unless occlusive dressings are part of the prescribed regimen, patients should be instructed that treated areas of skin should not be bandaged or otherwise covered or wrapped as to be occlusive. Occlusive dressings (including flurandrenolide tape) should not be used on weeping or exudative lesions, and flurandrenolide tape should not be used in intertriginous areas. Because thermal homeostasis may be impaired when occlusive dressings cover large areas, they should be removed if body temperature increases. Care should be taken to avoid the risk of suffocation with the plastic occlusive material. Some potent topical corticosteroids (e.g., betamethasone dipropionate, clobetasol propionate) should *not* be used with occlusive dressings because of the risk of adverse systemic effects. (See Dosage and Administration in the individual monographs in 84:06.08.)

Because certain areas of the body may be more susceptible to atrophic changes than others following treatment with corticosteroids, certain topical corticosteroid preparations (e.g., betamethasone dipropionate 0.05% gel; clobetasol propionate 0.05% cream, foam, gel, lotion, solution, or shampoo; hydrocortisone valerate 0.2% cream; mometasone furoate 0.1% cream, lotion, or ointment) should not be applied to the face or intertriginous areas (e.g., axilla, groin).

Patients should be carefully monitored when topical corticosteroids are used in the treatment of psoriasis, because exacerbation of the disease or development of pustular psoriasis may occur during topical corticosteroid therapy or when the drugs are withdrawn.

Some commercially available formulations of topical corticosteroids contain sulfites that may cause allergic-type reactions, including anaphylaxis and life-threatening or less severe asthmatic episodes, in certain susceptible individuals. The overall prevalence of sulfite sensitivity in the general population is unknown but probably low; such sensitivity appears to occur more frequently in asthmatic than in nonasthmatic individuals.

If skin irritation or contact dermatitis occurs during topical corticosteroid therapy, the drug should be discontinued and appropriate therapy initiated. It should be kept in mind that occlusive plastic dressings rarely may cause local or hypersensitivity reactions.

Topical corticosteroids should not be used in patients with markedly impaired circulation since skin ulceration has occurred in these patients following use of the drugs.

Topical corticosteroids should be used with caution and occlusive dressings should not be used in patients with primary skin infection. If secondary infection of the inflammatory lesion(s) develops, the occlusive dressing should be discontinued and appropriate topical anti-infective therapy initiated. If the infection does not respond promptly to such therapy, the manufacturers recommend that corticosteroid therapy be discontinued until the infection has been controlled. Some manufacturers state that topical corticosteroids are contraindicated in patients with tuberculosis of the skin, dermatologic fungal infections, and cutaneous or systemic viral infection, including vaccinia and varicella and herpes simplex of the eye or adjacent skin. However, most clinicians believe topical corticosteroids can be used with caution if the infection is treated. Corticosteroids reportedly may produce false-negative results with the nitroblue-tetrazolium test for bacterial infections.

The immunosuppressive effects of corticosteroids may be associated with impairment of the normal function of T cells and macrophages; such impairment may result in activation of latent infection or exacerbation of intercurrent infections, including those caused by *Candida*, *Mycobacterium*, *Toxoplasma*, *Strongyloides*, *Pneumocystis*, *Cryptococcus*, *Nocardia*, and ameba. Corticosteroid-containing preparations should be used with caution in patients with impaired T-cell function or in those receiving other immunosuppressive therapy.

Ocular instillation should be avoided when topical corticosteroids are applied on the eyelids or skin near the eyes because of the risk of corticosteroid-induced open-angle glaucoma.

Rectal corticosteroid therapy should be used with caution in patients with severe ulcerative disease, and only after adequate proctologic examination, because of the risk of intestinal perforation. Rectal corticosteroid therapy is contraindicated in patients with intestinal obstruction, abscess, impending perforation, peritonitis, extensive fistulas, and fresh intestinal anastomoses or sinus tracts.

Topical corticosteroid therapy is contraindicated in patients hypersensitive to any component of the preparation.

■ **Pediatric Precautions** *Pediatric patients may be more susceptible to topical corticosteroid-induced HPA-axis suppression and Cushing's syndrome than mature individuals because of a greater skin surface area-to-body weight ratio.* In open-label studies, adrenal suppression occurred in 14–17% of children 9–12 years of age, 23–32% of children 6–8 years of age, 29–38% of children 2–5 years of age, and 36–50% of infants 3 months to 1 year of age who received topical betamethasone dipropionate creams (including those formulated in an optimized [augmented] vehicle) or ointments for the treatment of atopic dermatitis. HPA-axis suppression, Cushing's syndrome, and intracranial hypertension have occurred in children receiving topical corticosteroids. Manifestations of adrenal suppression in children include retardation of linear growth, delayed weight gain, low plasma cortisol concentrations, and lack of response to corticotropin (ACTH) stimulation. Manifestations of intracranial hypertension include bulging fontanelles, headaches, and bilateral papilledema. Topical corticosteroid therapy in children should be limited to the minimum amount necessary for therapeutic efficacy; chronic topical corticosteroid therapy may interfere with growth and development. Parents should be advised not to use tight-fitting diapers or plastic pants on a child being treated in the diaper area, since such garments may constitute occlusive dressings. The manufacturer of Lotrisone® cream states that use of this preparation in the treatment of diaper dermatitis is not recommended.

■ **Pregnancy, Fertility, and Lactation** Safe use of topical corticosteroids during pregnancy has not been established. Although there are no adequate and controlled studies to date in humans, potent corticosteroids have been shown to be teratogenic in animals following topical application. Topical corticosteroids should be used during pregnancy only when the potential benefits justify the possible risks to the fetus. The drugs should not be used on extensive areas, in large amounts, or for prolonged periods in pregnant women.

It is not known whether topical corticosteroids affect fertility. However, reproduction studies in rats using subcutaneous dosages of clobetasol propionate up to 50 mcg/kg daily have revealed an increase in the incidence of fetal resorption and a decrease in the number of living fetuses at the highest dose.

It is not known whether topical corticosteroids are distributed into milk; however, systemic corticosteroids are distributed into milk. Topical corticosteroids should be used with caution in nursing women.

Pharmacology

Following topical application, corticosteroids produce anti-inflammatory, antipruritic, and vasoconstrictor actions. The activity of the drugs is thought to result at least in part from binding with a steroid receptor. Corticosteroids decrease inflammation by stabilizing leukocyte lysosomal membranes, preventing release of destructive acid hydrolases from leukocytes; inhibiting macrophage accumulation in inflamed areas; reducing leukocyte adhesion to capillary endothelium; reducing capillary wall permeability and edema formation; decreasing complement components; antagonizing histamine activity and release of kinin from substrates; reducing fibroblast proliferation, collagen deposition, and subsequent scar tissue formation; and possibly by other mechanisms as yet unknown. Corticosteroids, especially the fluorinated corticosteroids, have antimitotic activity on cutaneous fibroblasts and the epidermis.

Tachyphylaxis to the anti-inflammatory effects of the corticosteroids (as shown by vasoconstrictor assay) may occur with repeated application although the clinical importance of this effect is unknown. Following 3-times daily application to normal skin at the same site, diminished vasoconstrictor response may occur within 4–5 days. Withdrawal of the drug for 2–4 days restores response, although maximum vasoconstrictor response may be diminished; when application of the drug is reinstated, tachyphylaxis recurs.

Pharmacokinetics

Percutaneous penetration of corticosteroids varies among individual patients and can be increased by the use of occlusive dressings, by increasing the concentration of the corticosteroid, and by using different vehicles. The use of an occlusive dressing with hydrocortisone for 96 hours substantially enhances percutaneous penetration of the drug; however, such use for up to 24 hours does not appear to alter penetration of topically applied hydrocortisone. Fluorinated corticosteroids apparently do not penetrate the dermis to a greater extent than does hydrocortisone.

Following topical application of a corticosteroid to most areas of normal skin, only minimal amounts of the drug reach the dermis and subsequently the systemic circulation; however, absorption is markedly increased when the skin has lost its keratin layer and can be increased by inflammation and/or diseases of the epidermal barrier (e.g., psoriasis, eczema). The drugs are absorbed to a greater degree from the scrotum, axilla, eyelid, face, and scalp than from the forearm, knee, elbow, palm, and sole. Even after washing the area being treated, prolonged absorption of the corticosteroid occurs, possibly because the drug is retained in the stratum corneum.

Topical application of corticosteroids to the mucosa of the genitourinary or lower intestinal tract may result in substantial systemic absorption of the drugs. In healthy individuals, as much as 30–90% of rectally administered hydrocortisone as a retention enema may be absorbed. Greater amounts of hydrocortisone may be absorbed rectally if the intestinal mucosa is inflamed.

Corticosteroids vary in the extent to which they are bound to plasma proteins.

Following percutaneous penetration of a topical corticosteroid, the drug that is systemically absorbed probably follows the metabolic pathways of systemically administered corticosteroids. (See Pharmacokinetics: Elimination, in the Corticosteroids General Statement 68:04.) Corticosteroids usually are metabolized in the liver and excreted by the kidneys. Some topical corticosteroids and their metabolites are excreted in bile.

Chemistry

Hydrocortisone or synthetic derivatives of hydrocortisone are used topically as anti-inflammatory agents. These corticosteroids are 21-carbon steroids with the general structure above.

In the corticosteroids, an 11β-hydroxyl group is required for anti-inflammatory activity. Corticosteroids having a ketone group at C 11 (e.g., cortisone and prednisone) must be reduced to their corresponding 11-hydroxyl analogs (hydrocortisone and prednisolone) to be pharmacologically active. This reduction apparently does not occur quickly enough in dermal tissues for these drugs to be effective topically. Anti-inflammatory corticosteroids may have substitutions at positions 6, 9, and 16. Structural modifications of hydrocortisone affect the topical anti-inflammatory activity, and multiple modifications may produce more pronounced effects than would be predicted on the basis of individual changes. The presence of a C 1 to C 2 double bond enhances anti-inflammatory activity. Although substitution of an α-methyl group on C 6 has no consistent effect on activity, a 6α-fluoro substituent enhances anti-inflammatory activity. Substitution of a chlorine atom for the hydroxyl group at position 21 also increases anti-inflammatory activity. Substitution of a fluorine atom in the 9α-position, an acetonide group at positions 16 and 17, omission of the hydroxyl group at position 17 or 21, or esterification of the hydroxyl group at 17 or 21 profoundly increases anti-inflammatory activity. Substitution at C 16 of an α- or β-methyl group has no consistent effect on anti-inflammatory activity.

For further information on chemistry and stability, uses, and dosage and administration of topical corticosteroids, see the individual monographs in 84:06.08.

SKIN AND MUCOUS MEMBRANE AGENTS, MISCELLANEOUS 84:92

Guselkumab

■ Guselkumab, a recombinant human immunoglobulin G_1 lambda ($IgG_1\lambda$) monoclonal antibody, binds specifically to the p19 subunit of interleukin-23 (IL-23), a proinflammatory cytokine.

Uses

■ **Plaque Psoriasis** Guselkumab is used for the management of moderate to severe plaque psoriasis in patients who are candidates for systemic therapy or phototherapy. Guselkumab has been shown to reduce disease activity compared with placebo and adalimumab, as measured by the Psoriasis Area and Severity Index (PASI) and the Investigator's Global Assessment (IGA), in adults with such disease. PASI is a composite score that takes into consideration both the fraction of body surface area affected and the nature and severity of the psoriatic changes within the affected areas (i.e., induration, erythema, scaling); the IGA is a 5-point scale for rating the clinician's impression of the overall severity of psoriasis based on induration, erythema, and scaling: 0 (clear), 1 (minimal), 2 (mild disease), 3 (moderate disease), and 4 (severe disease).

Guselkumab has been evaluated in 2 multicenter, randomized, double-blind, placebo-controlled studies (VOYAGE 1 and VOYAGE 2) in 1829 adults who had moderate to severe plaque psoriasis (IGA score of at least 3) for at least 6 months with involvement of at least 10% of the body surface area, had a PASI score of at least 12, and were candidates for systemic therapy or phototherapy. Patients with guttate, erythrodermic, or pustular psoriasis were excluded from these studies. For the first phase of the studies (weeks 0–16), patients were randomized to receive guselkumab (100 mg at weeks 0 and 4 followed by 100 mg every 8 weeks), adalimumab (80 mg at week 0 followed by 40 mg once every other week beginning at week 1), or placebo. In the second (active-comparator) phase (weeks 0–48 in VOYAGE 1 and weeks 0–28 in VOYAGE 2), patients originally assigned to receive placebo crossed over to treatment with guselkumab (100 mg every 8 weeks) at week 16. FDA review of the active-comparator phase was limited to sites in the US and Canada, where patients received the US-licensed adalimumab product. The third phase of VOYAGE 2 (weeks 28–72) was a randomized withdrawal phase during which long-term responders (i.e., patients originally assigned to receive guselkumab who achieved at least 90% improvement from baseline in PASI score [PASI-90] at week 28) were rerandomized to continue receiving the drug or to receive placebo until loss of response.

In VOYAGE 1 and 2 studies, the primary outcome measures were the proportion of patients who achieved a PASI-90 response from baseline to week 16 and the proportion who achieved an IGA response of clear or minimal at week 16. In these 2 studies, a PASI-90 response at week 16 was achieved in 70–73 or 2–3% of patients who received guselkumab or placebo, respectively; an IGA response of clear or minimal at week 16 was achieved in 84–85 or 7–8% of patients who received guselkumab or placebo, respectively. FDA's review indicated that after 16 weeks, an IGA response of clear or minimal was achieved in 74–84 or 61–62% of patients who received guselkumab or adalimumab (US-licensed product), respectively; a PASI-90 response was achieved in 64–73 or 41–42% of patients who received guselkumab or adalimumab, respectively; and a PASI-75 response was achieved in 83–91 or 63–70% of patients who received guselkumab or adalimumab, respectively. Similar results were reported by study investigators for the global active-comparator evaluation. In VOYAGE 2, 89% of long-term responders who were rerandomized to guselkumab at week 28 maintained a PASI-90 response at week 48, compared with 37% of those rerandomized to receive placebo. The median time to loss of PASI-90 response among long-term responders rerandomized to receive placebo was approximately 15 weeks.

Guselkumab also was associated with improvements in region-specific (i.e., scalp, nails, hands, and feet) as well as overall measures of psoriasis severity, including improvements in symptoms (itching, pain, stinging, burning, skin tightness) and signs (skin dryness, cracking, scaling, shedding or flaking redness, bleeding) compared with placebo at week 16, as reported by patients using the Psoriasis Symptom and Signs Diary (PSSD), a daily (24-hour) recall diary that uses an 11-point scale to assess the severity of manifestations. In addition, a PPSD score of 0 (symptom free) was achieved at week 24 in 35–36 or 22–23% of patients who received guselkumab or adalimumab, respectively.

Guselkumab also has been evaluated in a multicenter, randomized, double-blind study (NAVIGATE) in adults with plaque psoriasis who had an inadequate response to treatment with ustekinumab. Patients had moderate to severe plaque psoriasis (IGA score of at least 3) for at least 6 months with involvement of at least 10% of the body surface area, had a PASI score of at least 12, and were candidates for systemic therapy or phototherapy. In the initial phase of the study, 871 patients received open-label treatment with ustekinumab (weight-based dose of 45 or 90 mg at weeks 0 and 4). Patients who did not have an adequate response (i.e., 268 patients with an IGA score of 2 or greater) at week 16 were randomized to receive guselkumab (100 mg at weeks 16 and 20, followed by 100 mg every 8 weeks) or to continue receiving ustekinumab (45 or 90 mg every 12 weeks). Among patients who did not respond to 16 weeks of ustekinumab therapy, an IGA response of clear or minimal with at least a 2-grade improvement in IGA score was achieved in 31 or 14% of patients who received guselkumab or ustekinumab, respectively, at week 28 (12 weeks after randomization).

No differences in response to guselkumab were identified in subgroups defined by age, race, gender, body weight, and prior biologic or nonbiologic systemic therapy.

Dosage and Administration

■ **Administration** Guselkumab is administered by subcutaneous injection. The manufacturer states that IV or IM use is not recommended. Guselkumab is intended for use under the guidance and supervision of a clinician; however, the drug may be *self-administered* if the clinician determines that the patient and/or their caregiver is competent to safely administer the drug after appropriate training.

Guselkumab is commercially available in single-use prefilled syringes. Guselkumab injection is a clear and colorless to slightly yellow solution that may contain small translucent particles.

Prior to administration, guselkumab solution should be inspected visually for particulate matter or discoloration; the solution should be discarded if it is cloudy or discolored or contains large particulates. Guselkumab prefilled syringes for subcutaneous administration are for single use only; unused portions of the solution should be discarded. Guselkumab prefilled syringes should be stored at 2–8°C in the original carton until administration and protected from light. The injection should not be frozen or shaken. The guselkumab prefilled syringe should be allowed to sit at room temperature inside the carton for at least 30 minutes prior to administration; guselkumab should not be warmed in any other way (e.g., microwave, hot water). The needle cap should not be removed while the prefilled syringe is warming to room temperature.

Guselkumab is administered subcutaneously into the anterior thighs (the preferred site) or lower abdomen (except for the 2-inch area around the umbilicus). Guselkumab may be administered subcutaneously into the upper arm by a caregiver or clinician. Injections should not be made into areas where the skin is tender, bruised, red, hard, thick, or scaly. Injections into psoriatic lesions also should be avoided.

■ **Dosage** For the management of moderate to severe plaque psoriasis in adults who are candidates for phototherapy or systemic therapy, the recommended dosage of guselkumab is 100 mg at weeks 0 and 4, followed by 100 mg every 8 weeks.

■ **Special Populations** Dosage adjustment of guselkumab based on body weight or age is not necessary. The manufacturer makes no specific dosage recommendations for patients with renal or hepatic impairment. (See Specific Populations under Cautions: Warnings/Precautions.)

Cautions

■ **Contraindications** The manufacturer states that there are no known contraindications to the use of guselkumab.

■ **Warnings/Precautions** ***Infectious Complications.*** Risk of infection may be increased in patients receiving guselkumab. Bacterial, fungal, and viral infections, including gastroenteritis, upper respiratory tract infections, tinea infections, and herpes simplex infections, have been observed in patients receiving guselkumab. In placebo-controlled portions of clinical studies over 16 weeks in patients with psoriasis, infections occurred in 23% of patients receiving guselkumab compared with 21% of those receiving placebo; serious infections were reported in less than 0.2% of patients receiving guselkumab or placebo.

Guselkumab should not be used in patients with any clinically important active infection and should not be administered until the infection resolves or is adequately treated. Potential risks and benefits of the drug should be considered prior to initiating therapy in patients with chronic infection or a history of recurring infections. If a serious infection develops or does not respond to standard therapy, guselkumab should be discontinued and the patient should be monitored closely until the infection resolves.

Patients should be evaluated for tuberculosis prior to initiation of guselkumab therapy. Guselkumab should not be administered to patients with active tuberculosis infection; when indicated, an appropriate antimycobacterial regimen for treatment of latent tuberculosis should be initiated prior to administration of guselkumab. Antimycobacterial therapy also should be considered prior to initiation of guselkumab in patients with a history of latent or active tuberculosis in whom an adequate course of antimycobacterial treatment for these indications cannot be confirmed. Patients receiving guselkumab should be monitored closely for signs and symptoms of active tuberculosis during and after treatment with the drug.

Immunization Administration of all age-appropriate vaccines recommended by current immunization guidelines should be considered prior to initiation of guselkumab therapy. Live vaccines should be avoided during therapy with guselkumab. Data are not available regarding response to live or inactivated vaccines.

Immunogenicity As with all therapeutic proteins, there is potential for immunogenicity in patients who receive guselkumab. In clinical studies in patients with plaque psoriasis, antibodies to guselkumab were detected in approximately 6% of patients receiving the drug for periods of up to 52 weeks. Neutralizing antibodies were detected in approximately 7% of the patients who tested positive for antibodies to the drug; lower trough concentrations of guselkumab were observed in approximately one-half of patients with antibody formation, but antibodies to the drug generally were not associated with loss of efficacy or injection site reactions.

Specific Populations **Pregnancy.** There are no adequate data regarding use of guselkumab in pregnant women. Human immunoglobulin G (IgG) is known to cross the placenta; thus, the potential exists for fetal exposure to the drug. An embryofetal development study in cynomolgus monkeys revealed no evidence of adverse developmental effects; however, when guselkumab administration was continued until parturition, an increase in neonatal deaths was observed. No guselkumab-related effects on functional or immunologic development were observed in the offspring from birth through 6 months of age.

Lactation. It is not known whether guselkumab is distributed into human milk, affects milk production, or affects the breast-fed infant. The benefits of breast-feeding and the importance of guselkumab to the woman should be considered along with potential adverse effects on the breast-fed infant from the drug or from the underlying maternal condition.

Pediatric Use. Safety and efficacy of guselkumab in pediatric patients younger than 18 years of age have not been established.

Geriatric Use. Of the 1748 patients with plaque psoriasis who received guselkumab in clinical trials, approximately 5% were 65 years of age and older, while less than 1% were 75 years of age and older. Although no overall differences in efficacy or safety between geriatric patients and younger adults were observed, the clinical trials did not include sufficient numbers of patients 65 years of age and older to determine whether geriatric patients respond differently than younger adults.

Hepatic Impairment. The pharmacokinetics of guselkumab have not been formally studied in patients with hepatic impairment.

Renal Impairment. The pharmacokinetics of guselkumab have not been formally studied in patients with renal impairment.

■ **Common Adverse Effects** Adverse effects reported in 1% or more of patients with plaque psoriasis receiving guselkumab (during the initial 16 weeks of therapy) and more frequently with the drug than with placebo include upper respiratory tract infection (e.g., nasopharyngitis, pharyngitis), headache, injection site reactions, arthralgia, elevated hepatic enzymes, diarrhea, gastroenteritis, tinea infections, and herpes simplex infections.

Drug Interactions

■ **Drugs Metabolized by Hepatic Microsomal Enzymes** Formation of cytochrome P-450 (CYP) isoenzymes can be altered by elevated levels of certain cytokines (e.g., interleukin-1 [IL-1], interleukin-6 [IL-6], interleukin-10 [IL-10], tumor necrosis factor [TNF; TNF-α], interferon) during chronic inflammation. As an antagonist of interleukin-23 (IL-23), guselkumab could normalize the formation of CYP isoenzymes. Data from an exploratory drug interaction study in a limited number of patients with moderate to severe psoriasis indicate that guselkumab is unlikely to interact with drugs metabolized by CYP isoenzymes 1A2, 2C9, 2C19, or 3A4; however, the potential for guselkumab to interact with drugs metabolized by CYP2D6 could not be excluded. Upon initiation of guselkumab in patients who are receiving CYP substrates (e.g., caffeine, midazolam, omeprazole, dextromethorphan), especially those with a narrow therapeutic index (e.g., warfarin), clinicians should consider monitoring for therapeutic effect or drug concentration and consider dosage adjustment of the CYP substrate as needed.

■ **Vaccines** Live vaccines should not be administered to patients receiving guselkumab. (See Immunization under Cautions: Warnings/Precautions.)

■ **Nonsteroidal Anti-inflammatory Agents** Concomitant use of ibuprofen or aspirin does not affect clearance of guselkumab.

■ **Acetaminophen** Concomitant use of acetaminophen does not affect clearance of guselkumab.

Description

Guselkumab is a recombinant human immunoglobulin G_1 lambda ($IgG_1\lambda$) monoclonal antibody that binds specifically to the p19 subunit of interleukin-23 (IL-23); it is produced by recombinant DNA technology in a mammalian cell line. IL-23 is a naturally occurring cytokine that is involved in normal inflammatory and immune responses. IL-23 stimulates production of proinflammatory cytokines, including interleukin-17 (IL-17) and interleukin-22 (IL-22), which contribute to chronic inflammation in individuals with psoriasis. Guselkumab binds to the p19 subunit of IL-23, disrupts IL-23-mediated signaling, and inhibits the release of proinflammatory cytokines and chemokines.

The metabolic pathway of guselkumab has not been characterized. As a human $IgG_1\lambda$ monoclonal antibody, the drug is expected to be degraded into small peptides and amino acids via catabolic pathways in the same manner as endogenous IgG. Guselkumab exhibited dose-proportional pharmacokinetics in patients with psoriasis over a subcutaneous dose range of 10–300 mg. In healthy individuals, bioavailability was approximately 49% following subcutaneous administration. In patients with psoriasis, peak serum concentrations of guselkumab were achieved by approximately 5.5 days after a single subcutaneous 100-mg dose of the drug. The mean half-life was approximately 15–18 days across all psoriasis studies. Guselkumab clearance and volume of distribution increase as body weight increases; age does not substantially alter the drug's clearance.

Advice to Patients

A copy of the manufacturer's patient information (medication guide) and instructions for use for guselkumab should be provided to all patients with each prescription of the drug. Importance of patients reading the medication guide prior to initiation of therapy and each time the prescription is refilled.

Importance of instructing patient and/or caregiver regarding proper storage, dosage, and administration of guselkumab, including the use of aseptic technique, and proper disposal of needles and syringes if it is determined that the patient and/or caregiver is competent to safely administer the drug.

Importance of informing patients that guselkumab may lower the ability of their immune system to fight infections. Importance of advising patients to promptly inform clinician if any signs or symptoms of infection (e.g., fever, sweats, or chills; muscle aches; cough, shortness of breath, or blood in the phlegm; weight loss; warm, red, or painful sores on the body; diarrhea or stomach pain; burning upon urination or increased urination) occur.

Importance of reviewing vaccination status with clinician and receiving all appropriate vaccinations prior to initiation of guselkumab.

Importance of informing clinicians of existing or contemplated concomitant therapy, including prescription and OTC drugs, as well as any concomitant illnesses (e.g., active infection) or any history of tuberculosis or other infections.

Importance of women informing clinicians if they are or plan to become pregnant or plan to breast-feed.

Importance of informing patients of other important precautionary information. (See Cautions.)

Overview® (see Users Guide). For additional information on this drug until a more detailed monograph is developed and published, the manufacturer's labeling should be consulted. It is *essential* that the manufacturer's labeling be consulted for more detailed information on usual cautions, precautions, contraindications, potential drug interactions, laboratory test interferences, and acute toxicity.

Preparations

Excipients in commercially available drug preparations may have clinically important effects in some individuals; consult specific product labeling for details.

Guselkumab

Parenteral

Injection, for subcutaneous use	100 mg/mL	**Tremfya®**, Janssen Biotech

Secukinumab

■ Secukinumab, a recombinant human immunoglobulin G_1 kappa (IgG_1 kappa) monoclonal antibody, binds specifically to and inhibits the biologic activity of interleukin-17A (IL-17A), a proinflammatory cytokine.

Uses

■ **Plaque Psoriasis** Secukinumab is used for the management of moderate to severe plaque psoriasis in patients who are candidates for phototherapy or systemic therapy. Secukinumab has been shown to reduce disease activity compared with placebo, as measured by the Psoriasis Area and Severity Index (PASI) and modified Investigator's Global Assessment (IGA), in adults with such disease. PASI is a composite score that takes into consideration both the fraction of body surface area affected and the nature and severity of the psoriatic changes within the affected areas (i.e., induration, erythema, scaling); the modified IGA is a 5-point scale for rating the clinician's impression of the overall severity of psoriasis based on induration, erythema, and scaling: 0 (clear), 1 (almost clear), 2 (mild disease), 3 (moderate disease), and 4 (severe disease).

In 4 randomized, double-blind, placebo-controlled studies (ERASURE, FIXTURE, FEATURE, and JUNCTURE), 2403 adults who had moderate to severe plaque psoriasis, involvement of at least 10% of the body surface area, and a PASI score of 12 or greater and who were candidates for phototherapy or systemic therapy were randomized to receive secukinumab 150 mg, secukinumab 300 mg, etanercept 50 mg (FIXTURE study only), or placebo. In each study, the assigned dose of secukinumab was administered subcutaneously once weekly for 5 weeks followed by once every 4 weeks. In the FIXTURE study, etanercept was administered subcutaneously at a dosage of 50 mg twice weekly for 12 weeks followed by 50 mg once weekly. In both the ERASURE and FIXTURE studies, placebo recipients who did not achieve a reduction in PASI score of at least 75% (PASI 75 response) from baseline to week 12 were rerandomized to receive either the 150- or 300-mg regimen of secukinumab beginning at week 12. Each study included a 12-week induction period followed by a 40-week maintenance period.

The pivotal studies were ERASURE and FIXTURE, with a combined enrollment of 2044 patients. FEATURE and JUNCTION were smaller studies (combined enrollment of 359 patients) that evaluated efficacy and safety of secukinumab self-administered by prefilled syringe and injection pen, respectively. Of the 2403 patients included in the 4 placebo-controlled studies, 79% had received no prior biologic therapy, and 8 or 45% had experienced treatment failure following prior biologic or nonbiologic therapy, respectively. Approximately 15–25% of patients had a history of psoriatic arthritis.

Primary end points in all 4 studies were the proportion of patients who achieved a PASI 75 response from baseline to week 12 and the proportion who achieved an IGA response of clear or almost clear at week 12.

A greater proportion of patients who received secukinumab achieved a PASI 75 response and IGA response of clear or almost clear at week 12 than did those who received placebo (all 4 studies) or etanercept (FIXTURE). Among patients receiving secukinumab 150 or 300 mg, PASI 75 response rates at week 12 were 71 or 82%, respectively, in ERASURE; 67 or 76%, respectively, in FIXTURE; 69 or 75%, respectively, in FEATURE; and 70 or 87%, respectively, in JUNCTURE. In comparison, 0–5% of patients receiving placebo in the 4 studies and 44% of patients receiving etanercept in the FIXTURE study attained a PASI 75 response at week 12. In addition, the percentages of patients receiving secukinumab 150 or 300 mg who attained an IGA response of clear or almost clear at week 12 were 51 or 65%, respectively, in ERASURE; 51 or 62%, respectively, in FIXTURE; 53 or 68%, respectively, in FEATURE; and 52 or 73%, respectively, in JUNCTURE. However, only 0–3% of patients receiving placebo in the 4 studies and 27% of patients receiving etanercept in the FIXTURE study attained an IGA response of clear or almost clear at week 12.

PASI 90 response (defined using the same criteria as PASI 75 but with a level of improvement of 90%) at week 12 was achieved in 39 or 59% of patients who received secukinumab 150 or 300 mg, respectively, compared with 1% of those who received placebo in ERASURE. In FIXTURE, 42 or 54% of patients who received secukinumab 150 or 300 mg, respectively, achieved a PASI 90 response, compared with 2 or 21% of individuals who received placebo or etanercept, respectively. Similar results were obtained in the FEATURE and JUNCTURE studies. In FEATURE, PASI 90 was achieved in 46 or 60% of patients receiving secukinumab 150 or 300 mg, respectively, compared with 0% of those receiving placebo; in JUNCTURE, PASI 90 was achieved in 40 or 55% of patients receiving secukinumab 150 or 300 mg, respectively, compared with 0% of those receiving placebo.

Clinical improvements were maintained with continued treatment over 52 weeks. In ERASURE, 72 or 81% of patients who received secukinumab 150 or 300 mg, respectively, and achieved a PASI 75 response at week 12 maintained their responses at week 52, and 59 or 74% of patients who received secukinumab 150 or 300 mg, respectively, and achieved a response of clear or almost clear on the IGA at week 12 also maintained their responses. Similarly, in FIXTURE, PASI 75 responses were maintained at week 52 in 82 or 84% of patients who received secukinumab 150 or 300 mg, respectively, and IGA responses of clear or almost clear were maintained in 68 or 80% of patients receiving these respective treatments.

Secukinumab also was associated with improvements in itching, pain, and scaling compared with placebo at week 12, as reported by patients using the Psoriasis Symptom Diary, a daily (24-hour recall) diary, to assess the severity and impact of symptoms; about 39% of patients in the ERASURE and FIXTURE studies opted to participate in these assessments.

No differences in response to secukinumab were identified in subgroups defined by age, race, and gender. Post-hoc analyses suggested that patients with lower body weight and less severe disease may achieve an acceptable response with secukinumab doses of 150 mg.

Dosage and Administration

■ **Administration** Secukinumab is administered by subcutaneous injection. The manufacturer states that IV use is not recommended. Secukinumab is intended for use under the guidance and supervision of a clinician; however, the drug may be *self-administered* if the clinician determines that the patient and/or their caregiver is competent to safely administer the drug after appropriate training.

Secukinumab is administered subcutaneously into the upper arms, thighs, or any quadrant of the abdomen; injections within 2 inches of the navel should be avoided. Injection sites should be rotated. Injections should not be made into areas where the skin is tender, bruised, erythematous, indurated, or affected by psoriasis.

Secukinumab injection is commercially available in injection pens and prefilled syringes; the drug also is commercially available as a lyophilized powder intended for institutional use only.

Cross-study comparisons suggest that trough concentrations achieved following secukinumab administration by injection pen may be 23–26% higher than those achieved following administration by prefilled syringe and 23–30% higher than those achieved following subcutaneous injection of the reconstituted powder.

Secukinumab Injection Secukinumab injection is commercially available in injection pens (Sensoready®) and prefilled syringes with a 27-gauge, ½-inch needle. Secukinumab is a clear to slightly opalescent, colorless to slightly yellow solution.

Prior to administration, secukinumab solution should be inspected visually for particulate matter or discoloration; the solution should be discarded if it is cloudy or discolored or contains particulates. Secukinumab injection pens and prefilled syringes are for single use only; the drug contains no preservatives and any unused portions of the solution should be discarded. Secukinumab injection pens and prefilled syringes should be protected from light and stored at 2–8°C in the original carton until administration; the injection should not be frozen or shaken. The injection pen or prefilled syringe should be allowed to sit at room temperature in the unopened carton for 15–30 minutes prior to subcutaneous injection. The needle cap should *not* be removed while the pen or prefilled syringe is warming to room temperature. The injection should be administered within 1 hour after the pen or prefilled syringe is removed from the refrigerator.

Secukinumab Lyophilized Powder Secukinumab also is commercially available as a lyophilized powder in single-use vials intended for institutional use only (e.g., in a hospital, clinic, or clinician's office).

Secukinumab lyophilized powder must be reconstituted prior to administration by a trained clinician using proper aseptic technique and without interruption. Preparation time from piercing the stopper until end of reconstitution averages 20 minutes and should not exceed 90 minutes. Secukinumab vials should be protected from light and stored at 2–8°C in the original carton; the drug should not be frozen or shaken. The appropriate number of vials containing secukinumab lyophilized powder should be removed from the refrigerator and allowed to sit for 15–30 minutes to reach room temperature prior to reconstitution; the sterile water for injection diluent used to reconstitute the drug also should be at room temperature.

Secukinumab lyophilized powder should be reconstituted by slowly adding 1 mL of sterile water for injection to a vial labeled as containing 150 mg of secukinumab to provide a solution containing 150 mg/mL; the stream of sterile water diluent should be directed onto the lyophilized powder. The vial should be tilted at an angle of approximately 45 degrees and gently rotated between the fingertips for approximately 1 minute and should *not* be shaken or inverted. The vial should then sit for approximately 10 minutes at room temperature to allow for dissolution; foaming of the solution may occur. The vial should again be tilted at an angle of approximately 45 degrees and gently rotated between the fingertips for approximately 1 minute and should *not* be shaken or inverted. The vial should then be allowed to sit undisturbed for approximately 5 minutes at room temperature. The reconstituted solution should be inspected visually for particulate matter and color; the solution should be free of particulate matter, clear to opalescent, and colorless to slightly yellow. The reconstituted solution should *not* be used if it has not fully dissolved, if it is discolored or cloudy, or if foreign particles are present.

Following reconstitution, the solution should be administered immediately or stored in the refrigerator at 2–8°C for up to 24 hours; the reconstituted solution should *not* be frozen. If the reconstituted solution is stored at 2–8°C, the solution should be removed from the refrigerator and allowed to sit for 15–30 minutes to reach room temperature prior to administration. The reconstituted solution should be administered within 1 hour following removal from storage at 2–8°C, as secukinumab does not contain preservatives. The vial should *not* be inverted when withdrawing the reconstituted solution for administration.

■ **Dosage** For the management of moderate to severe plaque psoriasis in adults who are candidates for phototherapy or systemic therapy, the recommended dosage of secukinumab is 300 mg at weeks 0, 1, 2, 3, and 4, followed by 300 mg every 4 weeks by subcutaneous injection. Each 300-mg dose is administered as 2 injections of 150 mg. For some patients (e.g., those with lower body weight and less severe disease), doses of 150 mg may be acceptable.

■ **Special Populations** The manufacturer makes no specific dosage recommendations for geriatric patients or for patients with renal or hepatic impairment. (See Specific Populations under Cautions: Warnings/Precautions.)

Cautions

■ **Contraindications** Secukinumab is contraindicated in patients with known hypersensitivity to the drug or any ingredient in the formulation.

■ **Warnings/Precautions** ***Sensitivity Reactions*** **Hypersensitivity Reactions.** Anaphylaxis and urticaria were reported in patients who received secukinumab in clinical studies. If an anaphylactic or other serious allergic reaction occurs, secukinumab should be discontinued immediately and appropriate supportive treatment initiated.

Latex Sensitivity. Some packaging components (i.e., removable cap) of the secukinumab injection pen and prefilled syringe contain natural latex proteins in the form of natural rubber latex and should not be handled by individuals sensitive to latex. Some individuals may be hypersensitive to natural latex proteins found in a wide range of medical devices, including such packaging components, and the level of sensitivity may vary depending on the form of natural rubber present; rarely, hypersensitivity reactions to natural latex proteins have been fatal. The manufacturer states that the safety of using secukinumab injection pens or prefilled syringes in latex-sensitive individuals has not been established.

Infectious Complications Patients receiving secukinumab may be at an increased risk of developing infections. In placebo-controlled clinical studies, higher rates of common infections (e.g., nasopharyngitis [11.4 versus 8.6%], upper respiratory tract infections [2.5 versus 0.7%], and mucocutaneous candidiasis [1.2 versus 0.3%]) were observed in patients receiving secukinumab compared with those receiving placebo. The incidence of some types of infections appeared to be dose dependent.

In the placebo-controlled phase of clinical studies (up to 12 weeks), a higher rate of infections was reported in individuals receiving secukinumab (28.7%) compared with those receiving placebo (18.9%), while serious infections were reported in 0.14 or 0.3% of those receiving secukinumab or placebo, respectively. Over the entire treatment period (up to 52 weeks for most patients), infections were reported in 47.5% of individuals receiving secukinumab (0.9 per patient-year of follow-up), and serious infections were reported in 1.2% of patients receiving the drug (0.015 per patient-year of follow-up).

Secukinumab-associated neutropenia was reported in clinical studies; however, most cases were transient and reversible, and no serious neutropenia-associated infections were reported. Clinicians should exercise caution when considering use of secukinumab in patients with a chronic infection or history of recurrent infections. If a serious infection develops, the patient should be closely monitored and secukinumab should be discontinued until the infection resolves.

Patients should be evaluated for tuberculosis prior to initiation of secukinumab therapy. Secukinumab should not be administered to patients with active tuberculosis infection; when indicated, an appropriate antimycobacterial regimen for treatment of latent tuberculosis should be initiated prior to administration of secukinumab. Antimycobacterial therapy also should be considered prior to initiation of secukinumab in patients with a history of latent or active tuberculosis in whom an adequate course of antimycobacterial treatment for these indications cannot be confirmed. Patients receiving secukinumab should be monitored closely for signs and symptoms of active tuberculosis during and after treatment with the drug.

Exacerbation of Crohn's Disease Secukinumab should be used with caution and close monitoring in patients with coexisting active Crohn's disease, as exacerbations of Crohn's disease (in some cases serious) were observed in patients receiving the drug in clinical studies. A randomized, placebo-controlled phase 2a study evaluating secukinumab in patients with active Crohn's disease was terminated early because of lack of efficacy, with the results suggesting an adverse effect on disease activity in patients with objective evidence of inflammation. Secukinumab was associated with higher rates of serious adverse effects, including drug-related worsening of Crohn's disease, and higher rates of infection compared with placebo.

Immunization Administration of all age-appropriate vaccines recommended by current immunization guidelines should be considered prior to initiation of secukinumab therapy. Live vaccines should be avoided during therapy with secukinumab. Patients receiving secukinumab may receive inactivated vaccines. (See Drug Interactions: Vaccines.)

Immunogenicity As with all therapeutic proteins, there is potential for immunogenicity in patients who receive secukinumab. In clinical studies in patients with plaque psoriasis, antibodies to secukinumab were detected in less than 1% of patients receiving the drug for periods of up to 52 weeks. Neutralizing antibodies were detected in approximately one-half of the patients who tested positive for antibodies to the drug; neutralizing antibodies were not associated with loss of efficacy.

Specific Populations **Pregnancy.** Category B. (See Users Guide.)

Lactation. It is not known whether secukinumab is distributed into human milk or if the drug is absorbed systemically after ingestion. Because many drugs are distributed into human milk, caution should be exercised when secukinumab is administered to nursing women.

Pediatric Use. Safety and efficacy of secukinumab in pediatric patients younger than 18 years of age have not been established.

Geriatric Use. Of the 3430 patients with plaque psoriasis who received secukinumab in clinical trials, 7% were 65 years of age and older, while less than 1% were 75 years of age and older. Although no overall differences in efficacy or safety between geriatric patients and younger adults were observed, the clinical trials did not include sufficient numbers of patients 65 years of age and older to determine whether geriatric patients respond differently than younger adults.

Population pharmacokinetic analysis indicated that clearance of secukinumab was not significantly influenced by age in adults with plaque psoriasis. The apparent clearance of secukinumab appears to be similar in patients 65 years of age or older and younger adults.

Hepatic Impairment. The pharmacokinetics of secukinumab have not been formally studied in patients with hepatic impairment.

Renal Impairment. The pharmacokinetics of secukinumab have not been formally studied in patients with renal impairment.

■ **Common Adverse Effects** Adverse effects reported in 1% or more of patients with plaque psoriasis receiving secukinumab (initial 12 weeks of therapy) and more frequently with the drug than with placebo include nasopharyngitis, diarrhea, upper respiratory tract infection, rhinitis, oral herpes, pharyngitis, rhinorrhea, and urticaria.

Drug Interactions

No formal drug interaction studies have been performed to date.

■ **Drugs Metabolized by Hepatic Microsomal Enzymes** The manufacturer states that the role of interleukin-17A (IL-17A) in the regulation of cytochrome P-450 (CYP) isoenzymes has not been elucidated. Formation of CYP isoenzymes can be altered by elevated levels of certain cytokines (e.g., interleukin-1 [IL-1], interleukin-6 [IL-6], interleukin-10 [IL-10], tumor necrosis factor [TNF; TNF-α], interferon) during chronic inflammation. As an antagonist of IL-17A, secukinumab could normalize the formation of CYP isoenzymes. Upon initiation or discontinuance of secukinumab in patients who are receiving concomitant CYP substrates, especially those with a narrow therapeutic index, the clinician should consider monitoring for therapeutic effect (e.g., warfarin) or drug concentration (e.g. cyclosporine) and consider dosage adjustment of the CYP substrate.

■ **Vaccines** ***Live Vaccines*** Live vaccines should *not* be administered to patients receiving secukinumab.

Inactivated Vaccines Patients receiving secukinumab may receive inactivated vaccines. Antibody responses to a meningococcal (group C) oligosaccharide diphtheria CRM_{197} conjugate vaccine (not commercially available in the US) and to an inactivated seasonal influenza virus vaccine (non-US preparation) were similar in healthy individuals who received secukinumab (single 150-mg dose) and those who received placebo 2 weeks prior to immunization. Clinical effectiveness of meningococcal and influenza vaccines in patients receiving secukinumab therapy has not been established. Inactivated vaccines received during secukinumab therapy may not elicit an immune response sufficient to prevent disease.

Description

Secukinumab is a recombinant human immunoglobulin G_1 kappa (IgG_1 kappa) monoclonal antibody that is specific for interleukin-17A (IL-17A); it is produced in a recombinant Chinese hamster ovary cell line. IL-17A is a subtype of the IL-17 family of proinflammatory cytokines secreted principally by T-helper 17 (Th17) cells. Elevated levels of IL-17A have been found in psoriatic lesions and blood of individuals with psoriasis. Secukinumab binds to IL-17A and inhibits its interaction with the IL-17 receptor, thus neutralizing the biologic activity of IL-17A and inhibiting the release of proinflammatory cytokines, chemokines, and mediators of tissue damage.

The metabolic pathway of secukinumab has not been characterized. As a human IgG_1 kappa monoclonal antibody, the drug is expected to be degraded into small peptides and amino acids via catabolic pathways in the same manner as endogenous IgG. Secukinumab exhibited dose-proportional pharmacokinetics in patients with psoriasis over a subcutaneous dose range of 25–300 mg. In healthy individuals and patients with plaque psoriasis, bioavailability ranged from 55–77% following a subcutaneous dose of 150 or 300 mg. In patients with psoriasis, peak plasma concentrations of the drug were achieved by approximately 6 days after subcutaneous administration of secukinumab 150 or 300 mg. Concentrations of the drug in interstitial fluid in lesional and nonlesional skin of patients with plaque psoriasis were 27–40% of serum concentrations at 1 and 2 weeks following a single 300-mg subcutaneous dose. The mean half-life ranged from 22–31 days in plaque psoriasis patients following IV (not recommended by manufacturer) or subcutaneous administration. Secukinumab clearance and volume of distribution increase as body weight increases.

Trough concentrations achieved following administration of the drug by injection pen may be higher than those achieved following administration by prefilled syringe or of the reconstituted powder. (See Dosage and Administration: Administration.)

Advice to Patients

A copy of the manufacturer's patient information (medication guide) for secukinumab should be provided to all patients with each prescription of the drug. Importance of advising patients about potential benefits and risks of secukinumab. Importance of patients reading the medication guide prior to initiation of therapy and each time the prescription is refilled.

Importance of instructing patient and/or caregiver regarding proper storage, dosage, and administration of secukinumab, including the use of aseptic technique, and proper disposal of needles and syringes if it is determined that the patient and/or caregiver is competent to safely administer the drug.

Importance of informing patients that secukinumab may lower the ability of their immune system to fight infections. Importance of advising patients to promptly inform clinician if any signs or symptoms of infection (e.g., fever, sweats, or chills; muscle aches; cough, shortness of breath, or blood in the phlegm; weight loss; warm, red, or painful sores on the body; diarrhea or stomach pain; burning upon urination or increased urination) occur.

Importance of advising patients with coexisting Crohn's disease to inform a clinician if they experience worsening of Crohn's disease symptoms during secukinumab therapy.

Importance of reviewing vaccination status with clinician and receiving all appropriate vaccinations prior to initiation of secukinumab.

Importance of alerting clinician if allergy to latex exists.

Importance of advising patients to seek immediate medical attention if they experience symptoms of a serious allergic reaction (e.g., feeling of faintness; swelling of eyelids, face, lips, mouth, tongue, or throat; dyspnea or throat tightness; chest tightness; rash).

Importance of informing clinicians of existing or contemplated therapy, including prescription and OTC drugs, as well as any concomitant illnesses (e.g., active infection, Crohn's disease) or any history of tuberculosis or other infections.

Importance of women informing clinicians if they are or plan to become pregnant or plan to breast-feed.

Importance of informing patients of other important precautionary information. (See Cautions.)

Overview® (see Users Guide). For additional information on this drug until a more detailed monograph is developed and published, the manufacturer's labeling should be consulted. It is *essential* that the manufacturer's labeling be consulted for more detailed information on usual cautions, precautions, contraindications, potential drug interactions, laboratory test interferences, and acute toxicity.

Preparations

Excipients in commercially available drug preparations may have clinically important effects in some individuals; consult specific product labeling for details.

Secukinumab

Parenteral		
Injection, for subcutaneous use	150 mg/mL	**Cosentyx®** (available as single-use prefilled syringes and single-use pens), Novartis
For injection, for subcutaneous use	150 mg	**Cosentyx®**, Novartis

Ustekinumab

■ Ustekinumab, a human immunoglobulin G_1 kappa (IgG_1) monoclonal antibody directed against the p40 subunit of interleukin-12 (IL-12) and interleukin-23 (IL-23), is an immunosuppressive agent.

REMS

FDA approved a REMS for ustekinumab to ensure that the benefits outweigh the risks. The REMS may apply to one or more preparations of ustekinumab and consists of the following: communication plan. See the FDA REMS page (https://www.accessdata.fda.gov/scripts/cder/rems/index.cfm).

Uses

■ **Plaque Psoriasis** Ustekinumab is used for the management of moderate to severe plaque psoriasis in adults who are candidates for systemic therapy or phototherapy.

Ustekinumab has been evaluated in 2 multicenter, randomized, double-blind, placebo-controlled studies (PHOENIX 1 and PHOENIX 2) in adults 18 years of age or older who had plaque psoriasis for at least 6 months with involvement of at least 10% of the body surface area, had a Psoriasis Area and Severity Index (PASI) score of at least 12, and were candidates for systemic therapy or phototherapy. Patients with guttate, erythrodermic, or pustular psoriasis were excluded from these studies. Both studies were conducted in 3 phases. For the first phase (weeks 0–12), patients were randomized in equal proportions, stratified by body weight, to receive ustekinumab 45 mg, ustekinumab 90 mg, or placebo. Treatment was initiated with 2 doses of the drug administered 4 weeks apart; subsequent doses were administered at 12-week intervals. In the second phase (weeks 12–40 in PHOENIX 1 and weeks 12–28 in PHOENIX 2), patients assigned to placebo crossed over to active treatment. The third phase of PHOENIX 1 (weeks 40–76) was a randomized withdrawal phase during which long-term responders (i.e., patients originally assigned to receive ustekinumab who achieved at least 75% improvement from baseline in PASI score [PASI-75] at weeks 28 and 40) were rerandomized to continue receiving the drug or to receive placebo until loss of response. In PHOENIX 2, the third phase (weeks 28–52) was a randomized dose-intensification phase during which partial responders (i.e., patients originally assigned to receive ustekinumab who achieved at least 50 but less than 75% improvement from baseline in PASI score) were rerandomized to continue receiving the drug every 12 weeks or to begin receiving the drug every 8 weeks.

In the PHOENIX 1 and 2 studies, the primary outcome measure was the proportion of patients who achieved a PASI-75 response at week 12. In these 2 studies, a PASI-75 response at 12 weeks was achieved in 67, 66–76, or 3–4% of patients who received ustekinumab 45 mg, ustekinumab 90 mg, or placebo, respectively. In addition, a status of cleared or minimal disease on the Physician's Global Assessment (PGA) scale was achieved at 12 weeks in 59–68, 61–73, or 4% of patients who received ustekinumab 45 mg, ustekinumab 90 mg, or placebo, respectively. Onset of response, as measured by PASI-75 response, was observed by 4 weeks after initiation of therapy. In patients who weighed less than 100 kg, response rates were similar for both the 45- and 90-mg doses of ustekinumab; however, in patients who weighed more than 100 kg, higher response rates were observed with 90-mg doses compared with 45-mg doses of ustekinumab. In these 2 studies, a PASI-75 response at 12 weeks was achieved in 73–74 or 65–78% of patients weighing 100 kg or less who received ustekinumab 45 or 90 mg, respectively; however, a PASI-75 response at 12 weeks was achieved in 49–54 or 68–71% of patients weighing more than 100 kg who received ustekinumab 45 or 90 mg, respectively. In PHOENIX 1, 89% of long-term responders who were rerandomized to ustekinumab at week 40 maintained a PASI-75 response at week 52, compared with 63% of those rerandomized to placebo. The median time to loss of PASI-75 response among long-term responders rerandomized to placebo was 16 weeks.

Ustekinumab also has been evaluated in a multicenter, randomized, active comparator study (ACCEPT) in adults 18 years of age or older who had plaque psoriasis for at least 6 months with involvement of at least 10% of the body surface area, had a PASI score of at least 12, had a PGA score of at least 3, and were candidates for systemic therapy or phototherapy. Patients were randomized to receive ustekinumab (45 or 90 mg at weeks 0 and 4) or etanercept (50 mg twice weekly for 12 weeks), a tumor necrosis factor (TNF; TNF-α) blocking agent. Patients in the etanercept group who did not have a response (i.e., patients who had moderate, marked, or severe psoriasis) at week 12 received 90 mg of ustekinumab at weeks 16 and 20, and patients who did not have a response to ustekinumab received one additional dose of ustekinumab at week 16. Treatment was interrupted starting at week 12 in all patients with cleared, minimal, or mild psoriasis; patients were retreated with ustekinumab if psoriasis recurred and was classified as moderate, marked, or severe. The primary outcome measure (i.e., proportion of patients who achieved a PASI-75 response at week 12) was achieved in 68 or 74% of patients who received ustekinumab 45 or 90 mg, respectively, compared with 57% of those who received etanercept. In addition, a status of cleared or minimal disease on the PGA scale at 12 weeks was achieved in 65 or 71% of patients receiving ustekinumab 45 or 90 mg, respectively, compared with 49% of those receiving etanercept. Among patients who did not respond to 12 weeks of etanercept therapy, 49% achieved a PASI-75 response and 40% had cleared or minimal disease at 12 weeks after initiating ustekinumab therapy. Retreatment of patients who experienced a recurrence of their disease after ustekinumab discontinuance resulted in responses (cleared, minimal, or mild disease) in 84% of the patients.

■ **Psoriatic Arthritis** Ustekinumab is used alone or in conjunction with methotrexate for the management of active psoriatic arthritis in adults.

Ustekinumab has been evaluated for the management of active psoriatic arthritis (5 or more swollen joints and 5 or more tender joints) in 2 randomized, double-blind, placebo-controlled studies (PSUMMIT 1 and PSUMMIT 2) in 927 adults who had an inadequate response to therapy with disease-modifying antirheumatic drugs (DMARDs) or nonsteroidal anti-inflammatory agents (NSAIAs). The studies included patients with any of the following forms of the disease: polyarticular arthritis without rheumatoid nodules, spondylitis with peripheral arthritis, asymmetric peripheral arthritis, distal interphalangeal joint arthritis, or arthritis mutilans. Patients in these studies were required to have had active psoriatic arthritis for at least 6 months. Enthesitis or dactylitis was present at baseline in more than 70 or 40%, respectively, of patients. Patients were randomized to receive ustekinumab 45 or 90 mg or placebo at weeks 0 and 4 and then every 12 weeks thereafter. At week 16, patients with less than 5% improvement from baseline in the number of both tender and swollen joints entered early escape in which their assigned treatment was adjusted in a blinded manner; among patients meeting the early escape criteria, those receiving placebo began receiving ustekinumab 45 mg, those receiving ustekinumab 45 mg began receiving ustekinumab 90 mg, and those receiving ustekinumab 90 mg continued receiving this dosage. At 24 weeks, all patients still receiving placebo began receiving ustekinumab 45 mg. Patients receiving stable dosages of methotrexate (25 mg/week or less), oral corticosteroids (equivalent to 10 mg or less of prednisone daily), or NSAIAs could continue receiving these agents during the studies. In PSUMMIT 1, 80% of patients had received prior DMARD therapy; prior treatment with tumor necrosis factor (TNF; TNF-α) blocking agents was not allowed. In PSUMMIT 2, 86% of patients had received prior treatment with DMARDs, including one or more TNF blocking agents in 58% of patients; more than 70% of these patients had discontinued treatment with TNF blocking agents because of inadequate efficacy or intolerance. About 50% of patients received stable dosages of methotrexate during the 2 studies.

The primary outcome measure was the proportion of patients achieving an American College of Rheumatology (ACR) 20 response at week 24. An ACR 20 response is achieved if the patient experiences a 20% or greater improvement in tender and swollen joint count and a 20% or greater improvement in at least 3 of the following criteria: patient pain assessment, patient global assessment, physician global assessment, patient self-assessed disability, or laboratory measures of disease activity (e.g., C-reactive protein [CRP] level). ACR 50 responses are defined using the same criteria with a level of improvement of 50%. Physical function was assessed using the disability index of the Health Assessment Questionnaire (HAQ-DI). Structural damage in the hands and feet was assessed radiographically by the change from baseline in the van der Heijde-Sharp score modified for assessment of psoriatic arthritis.

In both studies, a greater proportion of patients who received ustekinumab 45 or 90 mg achieved an ACR 20 response compared with patients who received placebo. ACR 20 responses were achieved at 24 weeks by 50 or 44% of patients receiving ustekinumab 90 mg, 42 or 44% of those receiving ustekinumab 45 mg, and 23 or 20% of those receiving placebo in PSUMMIT 1 and PSUMMIT 2, respectively. ACR 20 response was maintained through week 52. ACR 50 responses were achieved at 24 weeks by 28 or 23% of patients receiving ustekinumab 90 mg, 25 or 17% of those receiving ustekinumab 45 mg, and 9 or 7% of those receiving placebo in PSUMMIT 1 and PSUMMIT 2, respectively. In both studies, treatment with ustekinumab 45 or 90 mg was associated with greater improvement from baseline to week 24 in HAQ-DI score compared with placebo; improvements were maintained through week 52. In addition, ustekinumab was associated with greater improvement in enthesitis and dactylitis compared with placebo.

ACR responses were observed regardless of prior therapy with TNF blocking agents, although response rates tended to be lower among those who had received prior TNF blocking therapy. Among patients in PSUMMIT 2 who had received prior therapy with one or more TNF blocking agents, ACR 20 response was achieved at 24 weeks by 34, 37, or 14% of those receiving ustekinumab 90 mg, ustekinumab 45 mg, or placebo, respectively; among those who had not received prior therapy with TNF blocking agents, corresponding ACR 20 response rates were 55, 54, and 29%, respectively.

Analysis of combined radiographic data from the 2 studies indicated less progression of structural damage at 24 weeks in patients receiving ustekinumab 45 or 90 mg compared with those receiving placebo; continued inhibition of structural damage at week 52 was reported in patients receiving ustekinumab. The treatment effect observed in the combined data analysis was derived from PSUMMIT 1. Differences in treatment effect between the 2 studies may be related to the smaller size and the heterogeneity of the patient population in PSUMMIT 2 or the higher rate of missing data due to early treatment discontinuance in PSUMMIT 2, especially among placebo recipients who had received prior treatment with TNF blocking agents. Further study is needed to determine the effect of ustekinumab on progression of structural damage in patients with psoriatic arthritis who have received prior treatment with TNF blocking agents.

Dosage and Administration

■ **General** The Risk Evaluation and Mitigation Strategy (REMS) for ustekinumab includes a voluntary, disease-specific patient registry (Psoriasis Longitudinal Assessment and Registry [PSOLAR]). (See REMS.) For additional information on PSOLAR, including instructions for enrolling patients in this voluntary registry, health care providers should call 888-PSOLAR5 (888-776-5275) or access http://www.clinicaltrials.gov and search for PSOLAR.

Methotrexate, nonsteroidal anti-inflammatory agents (NSAIAs), and/or corticosteroids may be continued in patients receiving ustekinumab for the management of psoriatic arthritis.

■ **Administration** Ustekinumab is administered by subcutaneous injection. Ustekinumab is intended for use under the supervision of a clinician, but may be *self-administered* if the clinician determines that the patient and/or their caregiver is competent to prepare and safely administer the drug after appropriate training. Ustekinumab should only be administered to patients who will be closely monitored and have regular follow-up visits with a clinician.

Prior to administration, commercially available ustekinumab injection should be inspected visually for particular matter and discoloration; if either is present, the solution should be discarded. Ustekinumab vials and prefilled syringes should be stored at 2–8°C in the original carton to protect the solution from light until administration. Ustekinumab injection should not be frozen or shaken. Any unused portion remaining in the vial or syringe should be discarded since the injection for subcutaneous use contains no preservative.

The manufacturer recommends that each subcutaneous injection be administered at a different anatomic site (such as upper arms, gluteal regions, thighs, or any quadrant of the abdomen) than the previous injection, and not into areas where the skin is tender, bruised, erythematous, or indurated. The manufacturer recommends use of a 27-gauge, ½-inch needle to administer ustekinumab.

■ **Dosage** ***Plaque Psoriasis*** For the management of moderate to severe plaque psoriasis in adults, the recommended dosage of ustekinumab in patients weighing 100 kg or less is 45 mg by subcutaneous injection at 0 and 4 weeks, followed by 45 mg by subcutaneous injection every 12 weeks. The recommended dosage of ustekinumab in patients weighing more than 100 kg is 90 mg by subcutaneous injection at 0 and 4 weeks, followed by 90 mg by subcutaneous injection every 12 weeks. In patients weighing more than 100 kg, 45-mg doses were effective in clinical studies, but not as effective as 90-mg doses (see Uses: Plaque Psoriasis).

Psoriatic Arthritis For the management of active psoriatic arthritis in adults, the recommended dosage of ustekinumab is 45 mg by subcutaneous injection at 0 and 4 weeks, followed by 45 mg by subcutaneous injection every 12 weeks. The recommended dosage of ustekinumab in patients with coexisting moderate to severe plaque psoriasis who weigh more than 100 kg is 90 mg by subcutaneous injection at 0 and 4 weeks, followed by 90 mg by subcutaneous injection every 12 weeks.

■ **Special Populations** The manufacturer makes no specific dosage recommendations for geriatric patients or patients with hepatic or renal impairment.

Cautions

■ **Contraindications** Ustekinumab is contraindicated in patients with a history of clinically important hypersensitivity to the drug or any ingredient in the formulation.

■ **Warnings/Precautions** ***Infectious Complications*** Risk of infection, including reactivation of latent infections, may be increased in patients receiving ustekinumab. Serious bacterial, fungal, and viral infections have been observed in patients receiving ustekinumab. Serious infections requiring hospitalization, including cellulitis, diverticulitis, osteomyelitis, viral infections, gastroenteritis, appendicitis, cholecystitis, sepsis, pneumonia, and urinary tract infections, occurred during clinical studies in patients with psoriasis. In clinical studies in patients with psoriatic arthritis, serious infections included cholecystitis.

In placebo-controlled portions of clinical studies in patients with psoriasis (mean follow-up of approximately 13 weeks), infections and serious infections occurred in 27 and 0.3%, respectively, of patients receiving ustekinumab, compared with 24 and 0.4%, respectively, of those receiving placebo. In the controlled and uncontrolled portions of clinical studies in patients with psoriasis (median follow-up of 3.2 years), infections and serious infections were reported in 72.3 and 2.8%, respectively, of patients receiving ustekinumab.

Individuals genetically deficient in interleukin-12 (IL-12)/interleukin-23 (IL-23) are particularly vulnerable to disseminated infections caused by mycobacteria (including nontuberculous environmental mycobacteria), salmonella (including nontyphi strains), and BCG vaccine; serious, sometimes fatal, infections have been reported in such individuals. It is not known whether patients with ustekinumab-induced blockade of IL-12/IL-23 will be susceptible to these types of infections. Appropriate diagnostic testing for these infections (e.g., tissue culture, stool culture) should be considered as dictated by clinical circumstances.

Ustekinumab should not be used in patients with any clinically important active infection and should not be administered until the infection resolves or is adequately treated. If a serious infection develops, ustekinumab should be discontinued until the infection resolves. Caution is advised when considering use of ustekinumab in patients with a chronic infection or a history of recurrent infection.

Patients should be evaluated for active or latent tuberculosis prior to initiation of ustekinumab therapy. Ustekinumab should not be administered to patients with active tuberculosis. When indicated, an appropriate antimycobacterial regimen for the treatment of latent tuberculosis should be initiated prior to ustekinumab therapy. Antimycobacterial therapy also should be considered prior to initiation of ustekinumab in individuals with a history of latent or active tuberculosis in whom an adequate course of antimycobacterial treatment for these indications cannot be confirmed. Patients receiving ustekinumab should be closely monitored for signs and symptoms of active tuberculosis during and after treatment.

Malignancies Ustekinumab is an immunosuppressant and may increase the risk of malignancy. Malignancies have been reported in patients who received the drug in clinical studies. In the controlled and uncontrolled portions of clinical studies evaluating ustekinumab in patients with psoriasis (median follow-up of 3.2 years), nonmelanoma skin cancer or other malignancies were reported in 1.5 or 1.7%, respectively, of patients receiving the drug. The most frequently observed malignancies other than nonmelanoma skin cancer included prostate cancer, melanoma, colorectal cancer, and breast cancer. The incidence of malignancies other than nonmelanoma skin cancer in ustekinumab-treated patients was similar to the expected incidence in the general US population.

In animals, inhibition of the p40 subunit of IL-12/IL-23 increased the risk of malignancy. Ultraviolet (UV) radiation-induced skin cancers developed earlier and more frequently in mice genetically manipulated to be deficient in both IL-12 and IL-23 or IL-12 alone. The relevance of these experimental data to risk of malignancy in humans is unknown.

The rapid appearance of multiple cutaneous squamous cell carcinomas has been reported in ustekinumab-treated patients with preexisting risk factors for nonmelanoma skin cancer. All patients receiving ustekinumab should be monitored for the appearance of nonmelanoma skin cancer. Patients older than 60 years of age, those with a history of prolonged immunosuppressive therapy, and those with a history of psoralen and UVA radiation (PUVA) treatment should be monitored closely.

The safety of ustekinumab has not been evaluated in patients with a history of malignancy or a known malignancy.

Sensitivity Reactions **Hypersensitivity Reactions.** Hypersensitivity reactions, including anaphylaxis, angioedema, rash, and urticaria, have been reported during postmarketing experience. If an anaphylactic or other clinically important hypersensitivity reaction occurs, ustekinumab should be discontinued and appropriate therapy should be instituted.

Latex Sensitivity. The needle cover of the prefilled syringe contains dry natural rubber and should not be handled by individuals sensitive to latex.

Reversible Posterior Leukoencephalopathy Syndrome Reversible posterior leukoencephalopathy syndrome (RPLS), a neurologic syndrome characterized by reversible vasogenic subcortical edema, occurred in one patient who received 12 doses of the drug over approximately 2 years; the patient presented with headache, seizures, and confusion. No additional doses of ustekinumab were administered, and the patient fully recovered with appropriate treatment.

RPLS is associated with conditions such as preeclampsia, eclampsia, and acute hypertension and with cytotoxic or immunosuppressive therapy. The syndrome may manifest with headache, seizures, confusion, encephalopathy, blindness, and other visual and neurologic disturbances. Magnetic resonance imaging (MRI) is used to confirm the diagnosis of RPLS. RPLS is not caused by demyelination or a known infectious agent.

If RPLS is suspected, ustekinumab should be discontinued and appropriate treatment instituted.

Immunization Prior to initiation of ustekinumab therapy, patients should receive all age-appropriate vaccines as recommended by current immunization guidelines. Live vaccines should not be administered to patients receiving ustekinumab. BCG vaccine should not be administered during ustekinumab therapy or for one year before or after ustekinumab therapy. (See Drug Interactions: Vaccines.)

Immunogenicity Antibodies to ustekinumab have been detected, generally in low titers, in approximately 6% of patients with psoriasis or psoriatic arthritis receiving the drug. Neutralizing antibodies were detected in a majority of patients with psoriasis who tested positive for anti-ustekinumab antibodies. No apparent association between antibody development and injection site reactions has been observed. No serious hypersensitivity reactions to ustekinumab were observed in these studies.

Specific Populations **Pregnancy.** Category B. (See Users Guide.) Women who have been exposed to ustekinumab during pregnancy should be encouraged to enroll in a pregnancy registry for the drug by contacting 877-311-8972.

Lactation. Ustekinumab is distributed into milk in lactating monkeys. Since immunoglobulin G (IgG) is distributed into human milk, the manufacturer states that ustekinumab also is expected to distribute into human milk. It is not known whether ustekinumab is absorbed systemically following ingestion; however, published data suggest that antibodies in breast milk do not enter the neonatal and infant circulation in substantial amounts. Caution is advised if the drug is administered in nursing women. The unknown risks to the infant from GI or systemic exposure to ustekinumab should be weighed against the known benefits of breast-feeding.

Pediatric Use. Safety and efficacy of ustekinumab in pediatric patients younger than 18 years of age have not been established.

Geriatric Use. In clinical trials evaluating ustekinumab in patients with psoriasis or psoriatic arthritis, approximately 6.2% of patients receiving ustekinumab have been 65 years of age or older and about 0.7% have been 75 years of age or older. Although no differences in safety and efficacy relative to younger adults were observed, the number of patients 65 years of age or older is insufficient to determine whether they respond differently than younger adults.

About 5.5% of patients included in a population pharmacokinetic analysis of ustekinumab were 65 years of age or older; there were no apparent changes in pharmacokinetic parameters (clearance and volume of distribution) in those older than 65 years of age.

Hepatic Impairment. Pharmacokinetic data in patients with hepatic impairment are not available.

Renal Impairment. Pharmacokinetic data in patients with renal impairment are not available.

■ **Common Adverse Effects** Adverse effects reported in 1% or more of patients with psoriasis receiving ustekinumab in clinical studies and more frequently with ustekinumab than with placebo include nasopharyngitis, upper respiratory tract infection, headache, fatigue, diarrhea, back pain, dizziness, pharyngolaryngeal pain, pruritus, injection site erythema, myalgia, and depression. In clinical studies in patients with psoriatic arthritis, arthralgia, nausea, and dental infections were reported in 1% or more of patients receiving ustekinumab and more frequently with the drug than with placebo.

Drug Interactions

No formal drug interaction studies have been performed to date. Ustekinumab has been used concomitantly with methotrexate, nonsteroidal anti-inflammatory agents (NSAIAs), and/or corticosteroids in patients with psoriatic arthritis; analysis of population pharmacokinetic data indicated that concomitant use of these agents or prior use of tumor necrosis factor (TNF; TNF-α) blocking agents does not alter clearance of ustekinumab.

■ **Drugs Metabolized by Hepatic Microsomal Enzymes** Because increased levels of cytokines (e.g., interleukin-1 [IL-1], interleukin-6 [IL-6], interleukin-10 [IL-10], tumor necrosis factor [TNF; TNF-α], interferon [IFN]) during chronic inflammation may suppress the formation of cytochrome P-450 (CYP) isoenzymes, ustekinumab could normalize the formation of CYP enzymes. Although IL-12 and/or IL-23 at concentrations of 10 ng/mL did not alter the activity of CYP isoenzymes 1A2, 2B6, 2C9, 2C19, 2D6, or 3A4 in human hepatocytes in vitro, the clinical relevance of these data has not been established. Following initiation of ustekinumab therapy in patients who are receiving concomitant therapy with drugs metabolized by CYP isoenzymes (e.g., cyclosporine, warfarin), particularly those with a low therapeutic index, monitoring for therapeutic effect and/or changes in serum drug concentrations should be considered, and the dosage of the drug adjusted as needed.

■ **Allergy Immunotherapy** Ustekinumab has not been evaluated in patients who have undergone allergy immunotherapy. The drug may decrease the protective effect of allergy immunotherapy (i.e., decrease tolerance), which may increase the risk of an allergic reaction to a dose of allergen immunotherapy. Caution should be exercised in patients who are receiving or who have received allergy immunotherapy, particularly for anaphylaxis.

■ **Immunosuppressive Agents** The safety of ustekinumab in combination with other immunosuppressive agents in patients with psoriasis has not been established.

Methotrexate Concomitant use of methotrexate in patients with psoriatic arthritis does not appear to alter the safety or efficacy of ustekinumab.

■ **Phototherapy** The safety of ustekinumab in combination with phototherapy in patients with psoriasis has not been established. Ultraviolet (UV) radiation-induced skin cancers developed earlier and more frequently in mice genetically manipulated to be deficient in both IL-12 and IL-23 or IL-12 alone. (See Malignancies under Cautions: Warnings/Precautions.)

■ **Vaccines** Live vaccines should not be administered to patients receiving ustekinumab. BCG vaccine should not be administered during therapy with the drug for one year before or after ustekinumab therapy. (See Infectious Complications under Cautions: Warnings/Precautions.) Caution is advised when administering live vaccines to household contacts of patients receiving ustekinumab because of the potential risk for shedding the vaccine organism from the household contact and transmission to the patient.

Inactivated vaccines administered during a course of ustekinumab therapy may not elicit an immune response sufficient to prevent disease.

Description

Ustekinumab, a human monoclonal antibody directed against the p40 subunit of interleukin-12 (IL-12) and interleukin-23 (IL-23), is an immunosuppressive agent. Ustekinumab is produced in a recombinant cell line using recombinant DNA technology and is purified using standard bioprocessing technology.

Ustekinumab is an immunoglobulin G_1 kappa (IgG_1) monoclonal antibody that binds with high affinity and specificity to the p40 subunit of both IL-12 and IL-23. IL-12 and IL-23 are naturally occurring cytokines that are involved in inflammatory and immune responses, such as natural killer cell activation and $CD4^+$ T-cell differentiation and activation. Studies using in vitro models indicate that ustekinumab disrupts IL-12- and IL-23-mediated signaling and cytokine cascades by disrupting the interaction of these cytokines with a shared cell-surface receptor chain, IL-12 $\beta 1$.

The metabolic pathway of ustekinumab has not been characterized. As a human IgG_1 kappa monoclonal antibody, the drug is expected to be degraded into small peptides and amino acids via catabolic pathways in the same manner as endogenous IgG. The mean half-life of ustekinumab was 14.9–45.6 days across all psoriasis studies following IV and subcutaneous administration. Administration of 90-mg doses of ustekinumab in patients weighing more than 100 kg results in median trough serum concentrations of the drug that are comparable to those achieved following administration of 45-mg doses in patients weighing 100 kg or less (see Uses: Plaque Psoriasis and also see Dosage and Administration: Dosage).

Advice to Patients

Importance of patients reading the manufacturer's patient information (medication guide) prior to initiation of therapy and each time the prescription is refilled.

Importance of instructing patient and/or caregiver regarding proper dosage and administration of ustekinumab, including the use of aseptic technique, and proper disposal of needles and syringes if it is determined that the patient and/or caregiver is competent to safely administer the drug.

Importance of informing patients that ustekinumab may lower the ability of their immune system to fight infections. Importance of contacting clinicians if any signs or symptoms of infection develop.

Risk of malignancies while receiving ustekinumab.

Importance of advising patients to seek immediate medical attention if they experience any symptoms of serious allergic reactions.

Importance of alerting clinician if allergy to latex exists.

Importance of informing clinicians of existing or contemplated concomitant therapy, including prescription and OTC drugs, as well as any concomitant illnesses or any history of infection.

Importance of women informing clinicians if they are or plan to become pregnant or plan to breast-feed. Importance of encouraging women who have been exposed to ustekinumab during pregnancy to enroll in the pregnancy registry for the drug by contacting 877-311-8972.

Importance of informing patients of other important precautionary information. (See Cautions.)

Overview® (see Users Guide). For additional information on this drug until a more detailed monograph is developed and published, the manufacturer's labeling should be consulted. It is *essential* that the manufacturer's labeling be consulted for more detailed information on usual cautions, precautions, contraindications, potential drug interactions, laboratory test interferences, and acute toxicity.

Preparations

Excipients in commercially available drug preparations may have clinically important effects in some individuals; consult specific product labeling for details.

Ustekinumab

Parenteral

Injection, for subcutaneous use	45 mg/0.5 mL	**Stelara®** (available as single-use prefilled syringes and single-use vials), Janssen Biotech
	90 mg/mL	**Stelara®** (available as single-use prefilled syringes and single-use vials), Janssen Biotech

Selected Revisions December 2014, © Copyright, July 2011, American Society of Health-System Pharmacists, Inc.

86:00 Smooth Muscle Relaxants*

86:12 Genitourinary Smooth Muscle Relaxants

86:12.04 Antimuscarinics

Darifenacin§
Fesoterodine§
Flavoxate§
Oxybutynin§
Solifenacin§
Tolterodine§
Trospium§

86:12.08 β_3-Adrenergic Agonists

86:12.08.12 Selective β_3-Adrenergic Agonists

Mirabegron§

86:16 Respiratory Smooth Muscle Relaxants

Aminophylline, see Theophyllines
Diphylline, see Theophyllines
Oxtriphylline, see Theophyllines
Theophyllines§
see also:
Anticholinergic Agents 12:08
Sympathomimetic (Adrenergic) Agents 12:12
Vasodilating Agents 24:12
Vasodilating Agents 48:48

§ Omitted from the print version of *AHFS Drug Information*® because of space limitations. This monograph is available on the *AHFS Drug Information*® web site, http://www.ahfsdruginformation.com. Username: ahfs2020; Password: ASHP94498.

* Please see the full *AHFS Pharmacologic-Therapeutic Classification*© on p. viii. Not all classes are used in the printed edition.

88:00 Vitamins

88:04 Vitamin A

Beta Carotene§
Vitamin A§

88:08 Vitamin B Complex

Cyanocobalamin, see Vitamin B_{12}§
Folic Acid§
Hydroxocobalamin, see Vitamin B_{12}§
Niacin/Niacinamide§
Pantothenic Acid/Calcium Pantothenate/ Dexpanthenol§
Pyridoxine§
Riboflavin§
Thiamine§
Vitamin B_{12}§
see also:
Leucovorin 92:12

88:12 Vitamin C

Ascorbic Acid§

88:16 Vitamin D

Vitamin D Analogs General Statement§
Calcifediol§
Calcitriol§
Doxercalciferol§
Ergocalciferol§
Paricalcitol§

88:20 Vitamin E

Vitamin E§

88:24 Vitamin K Activity

Phytonadione§

88:28 Multivitamin Preparations

Multivitamins§

§ Omitted from the print version of *AHFS Drug Information*® because of space limitations. This monograph is available on the *AHFS Drug Information*® website, http://ahfsdruginformation.com. Username: ahfs2020; Password: ASHP94498.

92:00 Miscellaneous Therapeutic Agents

92:04 Alcohol Deterrents

Disulfiram§
see also:
Naltrexone 28:10

92:08 5-α-Reductase Inhibitors

Dutasteride§
Finasteride§
see also:
Finasteride 84:92

92:12 Antidotes

Acetylcysteine *p. 3592*
Fomepizole§
Glucarpidase *p. 3595*
Leucovorin *p. 3596*
Levoleucovorin *p. 3599*
Methylene Blue§
Pralidoxime *p. 3602*
Sugammadex *p. 3604*
Uridine Triacetate *p. 3607*
see also:
Amyl Nitrite 24:12.08
Antivenin (Latrodectus mactans) 80:04
Antivenin (Micrurus fulvius) 80:04
Atropine 12:08.08
Benzodiazepines General Statement 28:24.08
Botulinum Antitoxin, see Immunobiologic Agents available from the CDC 80:00
Calcium Salts 40:12
Crotalidae Polyvalent Immune Fab 80:04

92:16 Antigout Agents

92:18 Antisense Oligonucleotides

92:20 Immunomodulatory Agents

92:22 Bone Anabolic Agents

92:24 Bone Resorption Inhibitors

92:26 Carbonic Anhydrase Inhibitors

92:28 Cariostatic Agents

92:32 Complement Inhibitors

92:36 Disease-modifying Antirheumatic Drugs

92:40 Gonadotropin-releasing Hormone Antagonists

92:44 Immunosuppressive Agents

92:56 Protective Agents

92:92 Other Miscellaneous Therapeutic Agents

§ Omitted from the print version of *AHFS Drug Information*® because of space limitations. This monograph is available on the *AHFS Drug Information*® website, http://ahfsdruginformation.com. Username: ahfs2020; Password: ASHP94498.

ANTIDOTES 92:12

Acetylcysteine

N-Acetylcysteine

■ Acetylcysteine, the *N*-acetyl derivative of the naturally occurring amino acid, L-cysteine, is an antidote for acetaminophen overdosage as well as a mucolytic agent and sulfhydryl donor.

Uses

■ Antidote for Acetaminophen Overdosage Acetylcysteine is used orally or IV as an antidote for the treatment of acetaminophen overdosage. When administered within 8 hours of acetaminophen ingestion, oral or IV acetylcysteine can effectively prevent or minimize hepatotoxicity associated with acute overdosage of acetaminophen. Acetylcysteine is most effective if administered within 8 hours of ingestion; however, acetylcysteine also may be effective when given 24 hours or longer after ingestion.

The oral route was the recommended route of administration for acetylcysteine in the treatment of acetaminophen overdosage in the US before 2004, in part because an oral dosage form was the only dosage form commercially available at that time. An IV preparation became commercially available in the US in 2004; IV acetylcysteine is designated an orphan drug by the US Food and Drug Administration (FDA) for the treatment of moderate to severe acetaminophen overdosage.

Clinical studies have clearly demonstrated efficacy of orally administered acetylcysteine, and oral administration may result in higher intrahepatic concentrations of the drug than IV administration. However, oral administration often produces nausea and vomiting, and administration of antiemetic agents may be needed to complete therapy. IV administration obviates potential difficulties associated with administration of an emetic or activated charcoal and has been used in Canada and United Kingdom. IV administration achieves higher plasma concentrations compared with oral administration; it has been suggested that higher plasma concentrations may exert useful extrahepatic effects. However, anaphylactoid reactions have been reported following IV administration.

In all cases of suspected acetaminophen overdosage, a regional poison control center (800-222-1222) may be contacted immediately for assistance in diagnosis and for directions in the use of acetylcysteine as an antidote.

For further information on the manifestations and treatment of acetaminophen overdosage, see Acute Toxicity in Acetaminophen 28:08.92.

■ Prevention of Nephropathy Associated with Radiographic Contrast Media Acetylcysteine has been used to prevent radiographic contrast media-induced nephropathy†. The risk of radiographic contrast media-associated decreases in renal function appears to be increased in patients with chronic kidney disease, diabetes mellitus, older age, low hematocrit, hemodynamic instability, or conditions resulting in low effective circulating blood volume (e.g., heart failure, left ventricular systolic dysfunction). In addition, the risk of contrast media-induced decreases in renal function depends on contrast media properties (high osmolality, ionic compound, increased viscosity) and administration of a larger volume of contrast media. Various strategies have been investigated for prophylaxis of contrast media-induced nephropathy. Available evidence supports use of hydration as a prophylactic measure. Several pharmacologic agents, including acetylcysteine, have been evaluated for prophylaxis of contrast media-induced nephropathy. A review of controlled studies published in peer-reviewed journals before January 2006 identified 22 studies comparing acetylcysteine with placebo. Findings from 11 of 20 studies that reported contrast media-induced nephropathy and 13 of 20 studies that reported a change in serum creatinine concentration favored acetylcysteine prophylaxis. Most studies of acetylcysteine prophylaxis have been conducted in patients undergoing coronary angiography or percutaneous coronary interventions. Only a few studies have been conducted in patients receiving IV contrast media. Of 12 meta-analyses published as of early 2006 on the use of acetylcysteine for prevention of contrast media-induced nephropathy, 9 presented pooled risk estimates suggesting benefit; however, most of the analyses found significant unexplained heterogeneity among the studies, which limits conclusions that can be drawn. Factors that might have contributed to the observed heterogeneity included differences in contrast media used, definitions of contrast-induced nephropathy, patient selection, concomitant interventions, acetylcysteine dose and route of administration, and timing of the procedure (i.e., urgent or elective). The authors of this review of controlled studies state that available data do not support definite conclusions regarding the efficacy of acetylcysteine for the prevention of contrast media-induced nephropathy. An expert panel convened to evaluate the relevant literature and make consensus recommendations on this topic reached similar conclusions in 2005, when the panel determined that acetylcysteine has not been shown to be consistently effective in reducing the risk of contrast media-induced nephropathy. Well-designed studies with sufficient statistical power are needed to conclusively determine whether acetylcysteine prophylaxis reduces the incidence of contrast media-induced nephropathy.

■ Mucolytic Uses Acetylcysteine is used as a mucolytic agent in the adjunctive treatment of patients with abnormal, viscid, or inspissated mucous secretions in such conditions as acute and chronic bronchopulmonary disorders (e.g., pneumonia, bronchitis, emphysema, tracheobronchitis, chronic asthmatic bronchitis, tuberculosis, bronchiectasis, primary amyloidosis of the lung); atelectasis caused by mucus obstruction; pulmonary complications of cystic fibrosis; pulmonary complications of thoracic and cardiovascular surgery; and post-traumatic chest conditions. Acetylcysteine is also used during anesthesia and in the preparation of patients for bronchograms, bronchospirometry, bronchial wedge catheterization, and other diagnostic bronchial studies. The drug also is used in tracheostomy care to prevent endotracheal crusting and to reduce or eliminate the need for bronchoscopy. As with other mucolytic aerosol preparations, evaluation of the effectiveness of acetylcysteine is difficult and must be based on subjective observations. It has not been established that acetylcysteine offers any advantage over properly performed saline instillations or adequate humidification.

Dosage and Administration

■ Administration As an antidote for acetaminophen overdosage, acetylcysteine is administered orally as a 5% solution or by IV infusion. As a mucolytic agent, acetylcysteine, usually in a 10–20% solution, may be administered by nebulization, direct application, or intratracheal instillation.

Oral Administration For the treatment of acetaminophen overdosage, acetylcysteine is administered orally as a 5% solution. The commercially available 20% solution of the drug may be diluted 1:3 with a diet cola soft drink or other diet soft drink; if administered via a gastric tube or Miller-Abbott tube, water may be used as the diluent. Diluted solutions should be freshly prepared and used within 1 hour. If the patient is persistently unable to retain orally administered acetylcysteine, the drug may be administered via a duodenal tube.

IV Infusion *Acetylcysteine concentrate for injection must be diluted in 5% dextrose injection prior to infusion.* The appropriate dose of acetylcysteine should be withdrawn from the required number of vials and added to an appropriate volume of 5% dextrose injection (see table). The total volume administered should be reduced as needed for patients weighing less than 40 kg or requiring fluid restriction.

Table 1. Recommended Volumes of 5% Dextrose Injection for Dilution of IV Acetylcysteine Doses

Patient's Weight (kg)	Volume of Diluent for Indicated Dose		
	Loading Dose	First Maintenance Dose	Second Maintenance Dose
≥40	200 mL	500 mL	1 L
30	100 mL	250 mL	500 mL
25	100 mL	250 mL	500 mL
20	60 mL	140 mL	280 mL
15	45 mL	105 ml	210 mL
10	30 mL	70 ml	140 mL

When acetylcysteine is used for the treatment of acetaminophen overdosage, the manufacturer recommends that diluted solutions of the drug be infused IV as a loading dose given over 1 hour, followed by a first maintenance dose given over 4 hours, and then a second maintenance dose given over 16 hours.

Oral Inhalation and Intratracheal Instillation For oral inhalation or intratracheal instillation, the commercially available 20% solution of acetylcysteine may be used undiluted or may be diluted with 0.9% sodium chloride injection or inhalation solution or sterile water for injection or inhalation. The 10% solution of acetylcysteine may be used undiluted. Solutions of acetylcysteine do not contain a preservative and care should be taken to minimize contamination of the sterile solution.

When acetylcysteine is used as a mucolytic agent, the method of administration depends on the condition being treated. When administered by nebulization, compressed air should be used to provide pressure. Oxygen may also be used but the usual precautions in patients with severe respiratory disease and CO_2 retention should be observed. Ultrasonic nebulizers may also be used to administer acetylcysteine. Hand-bulb nebulizers are not recommended because the output is usually too small and the particle size is often too large. Acetylcysteine may be administered using conventional nebulizers made of plastic or glass; however, certain materials used in nebulization equipment react with acetylcysteine (e.g., iron, copper, rubber), and any part of the equipment that may come in contact with acetylcysteine should be made of glass, plastic, or a metal that does not react with the drug. (See Chemistry and Stability: Stability.) The nebulized solution may be breathed directly or a plastic face mask, face tent, mouthpiece, oxygen tent, or head tent may be used. Nebulizers may also be fitted to intermittent positive pressure breathing (IPPB) machines. Acetylcysteine solutions should not be placed directly into the chamber of heated (hot-pot) nebulizers. A heated nebulizer may be part of the nebulizer assembly to provide a warm saturated atmosphere if acetylcysteine is introduced by means of a separate unheated nebulizer and the usual precautions for administration of warm saturated nebulae are observed. When acetylcysteine is nebulized continuously with a dry gas, the solution may become over-concentrated and nebulization may be impaired; after three-fourths of the initial volume has been nebulized, it is advisable to dilute the remaining solution with an approximately equal volume of sterile water for injection. Nebulizing equipment should be cleaned immediately after use since residues may occlude fine orifices or corrode metal parts.

■ **Dosage** Acetylcysteine is commercially available as acetylcysteine and as the sodium salt; dosages and concentrations are expressed in terms of acetylcysteine.

Antidote for Acetaminophen Overdosage **Acute Acetaminophen Overdosage.** Because the reported or estimated amount of acetaminophen ingestion often is inaccurate and is not a reliable guide to the therapeutic management of the overdose, the preferred method to assess the risk of toxicity after acute acetaminophen ingestion usually is measurement of plasma or serum acetaminophen concentrations. Plasma or serum acetaminophen concentrations should be determined as soon as possible, but no sooner than 4 hours after ingestion (to ensure that peak concentrations have occurred). If an extended-release preparation of acetaminophen was ingested, it may be appropriate to obtain an additional sample of plasma or serum 4–6 hours after the initial sample for determination of drug concentrations. Plasma or serum acetaminophen concentrations are used in conjunction with a nomogram (see Acute Toxicity in Acetaminophen 28:08.92) to estimate the potential for hepatotoxicity and the necessity of acetylcysteine therapy. A full course of acetylcysteine therapy is indicated if initial plasma or serum acetaminophen concentrations fall on or above the dashed line on the nomogram. *If plasma or serum acetaminophen concentrations cannot be obtained, it should be assumed that the overdosage is potentially toxic, and acetylcysteine therapy should be initiated.* Acetylcysteine may be withheld until acetaminophen assay results are available provided initiation of acetylcysteine is not delayed beyond 8 hours after acetaminophen ingestion. If more than 8 hours has elapsed since acetaminophen ingestion, acetylcysteine therapy should be started immediately.

When indicated (i.e., in patients in whom the initial acetaminophen concentration is toxic on the nomogram or in those in whom a toxic dose is suspected and the time of ingestion is unknown, 8 hours have elapsed since ingestion, acetaminophen concentrations cannot be obtained, or acetaminophen concentration values will not be available within 8 hours of ingestion), acetylcysteine therapy is initiated as soon as possible with an IV or oral loading dose in adults and pediatric patients. In the event that a loading dose of acetylcysteine is administered before plasma or serum acetaminophen concentration values are available, the initial plasma or serum concentration (obtained at least 4 hours after ingestion) is used in conjunction with the nomogram to determine the necessity of completing a full course of acetylcysteine therapy. In such situations, administration of a full course of therapy is indicated if the initial plasma or serum acetaminophen concentration falls on or above the dashed line on the nomogram; acetylcysteine therapy is discontinued if the initial acetaminophen concentration falls below the dashed line on the nomogram.

Because acetylcysteine therapy may be useful even when instituted more than 24 hours after an overdose, a full course of acetylcysteine therapy is recommended for patients presenting 24 or more hours postingestion with measurable plasma or serum acetaminophen concentrations or biochemical evidence of hepatic injury.

When acetylcysteine is administered orally, a loading dose of 140 mg/kg is administered. To complete a full course of therapy, the loading dose is followed by oral maintenance doses of 70 mg/kg every 4 hours for 17 doses. If a patient receiving oral acetylcysteine vomits a loading or maintenance dose within 1 hour of administration, the dose should be repeated. If the patient is persistently unable to retain orally administered acetylcysteine, the drug may be administered via a duodenal tube. Antiemetic therapy also may be used for persistent vomiting. The usual dosage of oral acetylcysteine is appropriate in patients given activated charcoal; higher dosages are not necessary in these patients.

Alternatively, acetylcysteine can be administered by IV infusion. Acetylcysteine is administered as a loading dose of 150 mg/kg infused over 1 hour, followed by a first maintenance dose of 50 mg/kg infused over 4 hours, and then a second maintenance dose of 100 mg/kg infused over 16 hours (for a full course consisting of 300 mg/kg administered IV over 21 hours).

An IV regimen that delivers a total dose of 980 mg/kg over 48 hours† also has been used. This regimen involves IV administration of a loading dose of 140 mg/kg over 1 hour, followed by IV maintenance doses of 70 mg/kg every 4 hours for 12 additional doses. Each maintenance dose is infused over 1 hour.

The manufacturer of IV acetylcysteine states that data are not available to determine whether dosage adjustment is needed in patients with moderate or severe renal impairment. Published reports do not indicate that the dosage of acetylcysteine should be reduced in patients with hepatic impairment. Data are not available to determine whether dosage adjustment is needed in patients with hepatic cirrhosis.

In cases of acute acetaminophen ingestion, a regional poison center (800-222-1222) or an assistance line for acetaminophen overdosage (800-525-6115) can be contacted.

For further information on the manifestations and treatment of acetaminophen overdosage, including the associated nomogram relating acetaminophen concentration and hepatotoxic probability, see Acute Toxicity in Acetaminophen 28:08.92.

Multiple Supratherapeutic Acetaminophen Doses. In contrast to acute acetaminophen overdosage, guidelines for the treatment of repeated supratherapeutic acetaminophen ingestion (i.e., ingestion of multiple, higher-than-recommended doses of acetaminophen for extended periods of time) currently are not available. Some poison centers use plasma asparatate aminotransferase (AST) and/or alanine aminotransferase (ALT) concentrations and plasma or serum acetaminophen concentrations to estimate the potential for hepatotoxicity and necessity of acetylcysteine therapy. In cases of repeated supratherapeutic ingestion of acetaminophen, a regional poison center (800-222-1222) or an assistance line for acetaminophen overdosage (800-525-6115) can be contacted.

Prevention of Contrast Media-induced Nephropathy For the prevention of nephropathy associated with administration of radiographic contrast media† in adults, an oral acetylcysteine dosage of 600 mg twice daily, given the day before and on the day of the administration of contrast media, has been used, for a total of 4 doses. Other oral dosages have been investigated. IV administration of acetylcysteine also has been investigated.

Mucolytic Uses **Nebulization.** When nebulized into a face mask, mouthpiece, or tracheostomy, as in the treatment of bronchopulmonary disease or cystic fibrosis, the usual adult or pediatric dosage of acetylcysteine is 3–5 mL of the 20% solution or 6–10 mL of the 10% solution 3 or 4 times daily; however, 1–10 mL of the 20% solution or 2–20 mL of the 10% solution may be given every 2–6 hours. When a closed tent or croupette is used, maintenance of a heavy mist may require up to 300 mL of the 10 or 20% solution for a single, continuous treatment. The volume of acetylcysteine solution should be sufficient to maintain a very heavy mist in the tent or croupette for the desired period. Administration for intermittent or continuous prolonged periods, including overnight, may be desirable.

Direct Instillation. When acetylcysteine is administered by direct instillation in adults or pediatric patients, 1–2 mL of a 10–20% solution may be given as often as every hour.

Intratracheal Instillation. When acetylcysteine is administered by direct instillation in adults or pediatric patients, 1–2 mL of a 10–20% solution may be given as often as every hour.

Diagnostic Bronchial Studies. Prior to diagnostic bronchial studies in adults or pediatric patients, 2 or 3 doses of 1–2 mL of the 20% solution or 2–4 mL of the 10% solution may be administered by nebulization or intratracheal instillation.

Cautions

■ **Adverse Effects** ***Oral Administration*** Nausea, vomiting, and other GI symptoms may occur following oral administration of acetylcysteine in the treatment of acetaminophen overdosage. The drug may also aggravate vomiting associated with acetaminophen overdosage. Administration of dilute acetylcysteine solutions may minimize the tendency of the drug to aggravate vomiting.

Generalized urticaria, sometimes accompanied by mild fever, has occurred rarely following oral administration of acetylcysteine. Marked elevations in liver function test results (e.g., AST [SGOT] and ALT [SGPT]), occurred on 2 occasions following administration of high doses (total doses: 106 and 250 g over 3–4 days) of acetylcysteine rectally and via nasogastric tube in a 3-year-old boy with cystic fibrosis; these abnormalities were noted within a few days of initiation of acetylcysteine therapy and resolved gradually following discontinuance of the drug.

IV Administration Anaphylactoid reactions (i.e., acute hypersensitivity reactions such as rash, hypotension, wheezing, and/or dyspnea) have been reported in patients receiving IV acetylcysteine for the treatment of acetaminophen overdosage; in some cases, the anaphylactoid reactions were serious, including death in a patient with asthma. Rash, urticaria, and pruritus are the most frequently reported adverse reactions in patients receiving IV acetylcysteine. Acute flushing and erythema also have occurred; these reactions generally occur 30–60 minutes after initiating the infusion and resolve despite continued infusion of the drug. Reactions to acetylcysteine that involve manifestations other than flushing and erythema should be considered anaphylactoid reactions and treated as such.

No adverse effects were noted following IV infusion of acetylcysteine at a mean rate of 4.2 mg/kg per hour for 24 hours in 10 preterm infants (gestational age of 25–31 weeks and weight of 500–1380 g) or following infusion of acetylcysteine 0.1–1.3 mg/kg per hour for 6 days in 6 neonates (gestational age of 26–30 weeks and weight of 520–1335 g).

Oral Inhalation and Intratracheal Instillation Acetylcysteine appears to have a wide margin of safety. Adverse effects of acetylcysteine following oral inhalation or intratracheal instillation may include stomatitis, nausea, vomiting, drowsiness, clamminess, severe rhinorrhea, and fever. Acetylcysteine solutions have a slight, disagreeable odor which may contribute to the incidence of nausea. When a face mask is used for nebulization of acetylcysteine, there may be stickiness on the face afterwards which can be easily removed by washing with water.

Sensitization to acetylcysteine has been reported rarely, but has not been confirmed by patch testing. Sensitization to acetylcysteine and dermal eruptions have been reported in several inhalation therapists after frequent and extended exposure to the drug.

Irritation of the tracheal and bronchial tracts and hemoptysis have occurred following administration of acetylcysteine; however, such findings are not uncommon in patients with bronchopulmonary disease and a causal relationship has not been established.

Chest tightness and bronchoconstriction have been reported with acetylcysteine. Clinically overt acetylcysteine-induced bronchospasm occurs rarely and unpredictably, even in patients with asthmatic bronchitis or bronchitis complicating bronchial asthma. Occasionally, patients receiving oral inhalation of acetylcysteine develop increased airway obstruction of varying and unpredictable severity. Patients who have had such reactions to previous therapy with acetylcysteine may not react during subsequent therapy with the drug, and patients who have had inhalation treatments with acetylcysteine without incident may react to subsequent therapy.

■ **Precautions and Contraindications** ***Oral Administration*** Since oral administration of acetylcysteine may result in vomiting or aggravate vomiting associated with acetaminophen overdosage, patients at risk of gastric hemorrhage (e.g., those with esophageal varices or peptic ulcers) should be evaluated with regard to the relative risks of upper GI hemorrhage and acetaminophen-induced hepatotoxicity and treatment with acetylcysteine given accordingly. If generalized urticaria or other allergic symptoms occur during oral acetylcysteine therapy, the drug should be discontinued unless it is considered essential and the allergic symptoms can be otherwise controlled. The manufacturers state that if encephalopathy resulting from hepatic failure occurs during oral acetylcysteine therapy, the drug should be discontinued to avoid further administration of nitrogenous substances; there are no data indicating that acetylcysteine adversely affects hepatic failure, but it is a theoretical possibility.

IV Administration If an anaphylactoid reaction (rash, hypotension, wheezing, dyspnea, or any dermatologic manifestations other than flushing and erythema) occurs during IV acetylcysteine therapy, the drug should be temporarily interrupted in order to administer antihistamines and, in severe reactions, epinephrine. Once treatment of the anaphylactoid reaction has been initiated, IV acetylcysteine can be reinstituted cautiously. If the anaphylactoid reaction recurs or increases in severity, IV acetylcysteine should be discontinued and alternative management considered.

Acetylcysteine should be used with caution in patients with asthma or a history of bronchospasm.

To avoid fluid overload (which can result in hyponatremia, seizure, and death), the volume of 5% dextrose used to dilute acetylcysteine injection should be adjusted as needed. The total volume of 5% dextrose should be reduced in patients weighing less than 40 kg and those requiring fluid restriction.

IV acetylcysteine is contraindicated in patients with known hypersensitivity or previous anaphylactoid reaction to acetylcysteine or any ingredient in the formulation.

Oral Inhalation and Intratracheal Instillation Asthmatic patients receiving acetylcysteine by oral inhalation or intratracheal instillation should be observed closely during such therapy; if bronchospasm occurs, a bronchodilator should be given by nebulization. If bronchospasm progresses, acetylcysteine should be discontinued immediately.

An increased volume of liquefied bronchial secretions may develop after administration of acetylcysteine and the airway may become occluded. If cough is inadequate to maintain an open airway during acetylcysteine therapy, mechanical suction or endotracheal aspiration should be instituted.

Acetylcysteine solutions are contraindicated in patients hypersensitive to the drug.

■ **Mutagenicity and Carcinogenicity** No evidence of acetylcysteine-induced mutagenicity was seen with an in vitro microbial test system (Ames test) with or without metabolic activation.

No evidence of oncogenic activity was observed in rats given oral acetylcysteine in dosages up to 1000 mg/kg daily (5.2 times the human mucolytic dose) for 12 months. Acetylcysteine has not been evaluated in long-term carcinogenicity studies in animals.

■ **Pregnancy, Fertility, and Lactation** Reproductive studies in rabbits using oral acetylcysteine dosages of 500 mg/kg daily (2.6 times the human mucolytic dose) on days 6 through 16 of gestation revealed no teratogenicity. Studies in rabbits exposed for 30–35 minutes twice daily to a nebulized solution containing acetylcysteine and isoproterenol hydrochloride on days 16 through 18 of gestation revealed no teratogenicity. Perinatal and postnatal studies in rats exposed to a nebulized solution containing acetylcysteine and isoproterenol did not reveal harm to the fetus or newborns. Acetylcysteine has been reported to cross the placenta in humans following oral or IV administration. However, there are no adequate and controlled studies to date using acetylcysteine in pregnant women, and the drug should be used during pregnancy only when clearly needed.

Reproductive studies in rats exposed to acetylcysteine and isoproterenol and in rabbits using acetylcysteine dosages up to 2.6 times the usual human dosage have not revealed evidence of impairment of fertility. No effect on fertility was observed in male or female rats exposed to a nebulized solution containing acetylcysteine and isoproterenol hydrochloride. A slight reduction in fertility was observed in a reproductive study in rats given oral acetylcysteine dosages of 500 or 1000 mg/kg daily (2.6 or 5.2 times the human mucolytic dose, respectively).

Since it is not known if acetylcysteine is distributed into human milk, the drug should be used with caution in nursing women.

Pharmacology

The exact mechanism(s) by which acetylcysteine prevents or minimizes acetaminophen-induced hepatotoxicity has not been fully determined. In vitro and animal data indicate that small quantities of acetaminophen are metabolized by a cytochrome P-450 microsomal enzyme to a reactive intermediate metabolite (*N*)-acetyl-*p*-benzoquinoneimine, *N*-acetylimidoquinone, NAPQI), which is further metabolized via conjugation with glutathione and ultimately excreted in urine as a mercapturic acid. It has been suggested that this intermediate metabolite is responsible for acetaminophen-induced liver necrosis and that high doses of acetaminophen may deplete glutathione so that inactivation of this toxic metabolite is decreased. At high doses, the capacity of metabolic pathways for conjugation with glucuronic acid and sulfuric acid may be exceeded, resulting in increased metabolism of acetaminophen by alternate pathways. Acetylcysteine may protect the liver by maintaining or restoring glutathione levels or by acting as an alternate substrate for conjugation with (and therefore detoxification of) the toxic intermediate metabolite.

The exact mechanism(s) by which acetylcysteine might prevent radiographic contrast media-associated nephrotoxicity is unclear. It has been suggested that since radiographic contrast media-induced renal toxicity may be related to formation of reactive oxygen species or to reduced antioxidant activity, acetylcysteine, a thiol-containing antioxidant, may reduce the ability of the generated oxygen free radicals to damage cells by acting as an oxygen free-radical scavenger. In addition, the drug also may increase the biologic effects of nitric oxide by combining with the oxide to form *S*-nitrosothiol, a potent vasodilator. The interaction of acetylcysteine and nitric oxide may limit the production of the damaging peroxinitrate radical, because acetylcysteine would compete with the superoxide radical for nitric oxide. Acetylcysteine also increases the expression of nitric oxide synthase and therefore may improve blood flow.

Acetylcysteine reduces the viscosity of purulent and nonpurulent pulmonary secretions and facilitates their removal by coughing, postural drainage, or mechanical means. The mucolytic effect of the drug has been shown to depend on the free sulfhydryl group, which is thought to reduce disulfide linkages of mucoproteins through an interchange reaction, forming a mixed disulfide and a free sulfhydryl group. This action is most pronounced at pH 7–9. Acetylcysteine does not depolymerize proteins and it has no action on fibrin or on living tissue. Its activity is unaffected by DNA.

Pharmacokinetics

Following oral administration (e.g., when used as an antidote for acetaminophen overdosage), acetylcysteine is absorbed from the GI tract.

Following IV administration of acetylcysteine, mean elimination half-lives of 5.6 and 11 hours have been reported in adults and in neonates, respectively. The mean elimination half-life was increased by 80% in patients with severe liver damage (i.e., alcoholic cirrhosis [Child-Pugh score of 7–13] or primary and/or secondary biliary cirrhosis [Child-Pugh score of 5–7]).

Following oral inhalation or intratracheal instillation, most of the administered drug appears to participate in the sulfhydryl-disulfide reaction (see Pharmacology); the remainder is absorbed from the pulmonary epithelium, deacetylated by the liver to cysteine, and subsequently metabolized.

Chemistry and Stability

■ **Chemistry** Acetylcysteine is the *N*-acetyl derivative of the naturally occurring amino acid, L-cysteine. The drug occurs as a white, crystalline powder with a slight acetic odor. Acetylcysteine is freely soluble in water and in alcohol. Acetylcysteine is commercially available as aqueous solutions of the sodium salt of the drug which are colorless and have an odor and taste of hydrogen sulfide. Commercially available acetylcysteine sodium solutions are sterile; solutions are prepared from acetylcysteine with the aid of sodium hydroxide and have a pH 6–7.5.

For IV administration, acetylcysteine is commercially available as a sterile aqueous solution of acetylcysteine as a concentrate for injection; the concentrate also contains edetate disodium and sodium hydroxide and has a pH of 6–7.5.

■ **Stability** Unopened vials of acetylcysteine sodium solution should be stored at 15–30°C. Following exposure to air, oral and oral inhalation solutions should be stored at 2–8°C to retard oxidation and should be used within 96 hours.

Acetylcysteine is a reducing agent and is incompatible with oxidizing agents. Solutions of acetylcysteine become discolored and liberate hydrogen sulfide upon contact with rubber, some metals, particularly iron and copper, and/or when subjected to autoclaving. Acetylcysteine does not react with glass, plastic, aluminum, anodized aluminum, chromed metal, tantalum, sterling silver, or stainless steel. Although silver may become tarnished after exposure to acetylcysteine, this does not affect potency of the drug. The presence of a light purple color in acetylcysteine sodium oral and oral inhalation solutions does not appreciably affect potency of the drug; however, it is best to utilize equipment constructed with plastic or glass and with stainless steel or another nonreactive metal when administering acetylcysteine by nebulization. The presence of a light pink to light purple color in acetylcysteine injection does not affect the quality of the product.

The manufacturers state that solutions of acetylcysteine sodium are physically and/or chemically incompatible with solutions containing amphotericin B, tetracyclines, erythromycin lactobionate, or ampicillin sodium. When one of these anti-infectives is to be administered by aerosol inhalation, it should be nebulized separately. Acetylcysteine solutions are also physically incompatible with iodized oil, trypsin, chymotrypsin, and hydrogen peroxide.

Commercially available acetylcysteine concentrate for injection should be stored at 20–25°C. When diluted with 5% dextrose, resultant solutions are stable for 24 hours at controlled room temperature.

Preparations

Excipients in commercially available drug preparations may have clinically important effects in some individuals; consult specific product labeling for details.

Acetylcysteine Sodium

Oral Inhalation, Intratracheal Instillation, and Oral		
Solution	100 mg (of acetylcysteine) per mL (10%)*	**Acetylcysteine Sodium Solution**
		Mucomyst®, Brystol-Myers
	200 mg (of acetylcysteine) per mL (20%)*	**Acetylcysteine Sodium Solution**
		Mucomyst®, Brystol-Meyers

*available from one or more manufacturer, distributor, and/or repackager by generic (nonproprietary) name

Acetylcysteine

Parenteral		
For injection concentrate, for IV infusion	200 mg/mL	**Acetadote®**, Cumberland

†Use is not currently included in the labeling approved by the US Food and Drug Administration

Glucarpidase

■ Glucarpidase (also known as carboxypeptidase G_2 [$CPDG_2$]) is a recombinant bacterial enzyme that is used as an antidote for methotrexate toxicity.

Uses

■ **Methotrexate Toxicity** Glucarpidase is used as an adjunct to leucovorin rescue for the treatment of toxic plasma methotrexate concentrations (exceeding 0.454 mcg/mL [1 μmol/L]) in patients with delayed methotrexate clearance due to renal impairment. Glucarpidase is designated an orphan drug by the US Food and Drug Administration (FDA) for this use. Because of the potential for subtherapeutic concentrations of methotrexate, glucarpidase should *not* be used in patients who exhibit the expected clearance of methotrexate (plasma methotrexate concentrations within 2 standard deviations of the mean methotrexate excretion curve specific for the methotrexate dose administered) or in those with normal or mildly impaired renal function.

Treatment of methotrexate toxicity traditionally has included leucovorin rescue and supportive measures (IV hydration, urinary alkalinization). However, leucovorin rescue alone does not reduce systemic (i.e., extracellular) methotrexate concentrations and does not completely reverse toxicity when methotrexate concentrations are sustained above 10 μmol/L. Extracorporeal procedures (e.g., hemodialysis) have been used, although such procedures are invasive, have variable efficacy in removing systemic methotrexate, and often are associated with rebound methotrexate concentrations. Because methotrexate is excreted principally by the kidneys, high systemic concentrations of the drug (e.g., following high-dose methotrexate therapy) may cause acute renal impairment in some patients (i.e., by pH-dependent precipitation of methotrexate and its metabolites in renal tubules or by causing direct injury to the renal tubular epithelium); this causes further delay in methotrexate clearance, resulting in subsequent severe systemic toxicities (e.g., myelosuppression, mucositis, hepatotoxicity). Glucarpidase converts circulating methotrexate to inactive metabolites that are primarily eliminated hepatically, thus providing an alternative, nonrenal route for methotrexate elimination in patients with renal impairment.

The current indication for glucarpidase is based principally on data from a subset of 22 treatment-evaluable patients enrolled in a single-arm, open-label study that involved 184 patients with markedly delayed methotrexate clearance (defined as more than 2 standard deviations greater than the mean excretion curve for methotrexate) and toxic plasma methotrexate concentrations (exceeding 0.454 mcg/mL [1 μmol/L]) due to renal impairment. The primary measure of efficacy was the proportion of patients who achieved a rapid and sustained clinically important reduction (RSCIR) in plasma methotrexate concentration (defined as an attainment of plasma methotrexate concentration of 0.454 mcg/mL [1 μmol/L] or less within 15 minutes of glucarpidase administration that was sustained for up to 8 days). The median age of patients was 15.5 years (range: 5–84 years); the most common types of malignancies were osteogenic sarcoma (50%) and leukemia or lymphoma (45%). In this study, all patients received glucarpidase 50 units/kg by IV injection over 5 minutes; a second dose of glucarpidase was administered 48 hours after the initial dose in patients with pre-glucarpidase plasma methotrexate concentrations exceeding 45.4 mcg/mL (100 μmol/L). Patients continued to receive IV hydration, urinary alkalinization, and leucovorin rescue. Following administration of the first dose of glucarpidase, 10 of the 22 patients (45%) achieved RSCIR. Of the remaining 12 patients who failed to achieve RSCIR, 5 patients (23%) achieved a *transient* plasma methotrexate concentration of 0.454 mcg/mL (1 μmol/L) or less; in these 5 patients, the median increase in plasma methotrexate concentration from nadir was 0.636 mcg/mL (1.4 μmol/L). Methotrexate concentrations were reduced by at least 97% within 15 minutes in all 22 patients and were maintained at a greater than 95% reduction for up to 8 days in 20 of the 22 patients. Based on results of exploratory analyses, patients with lower pre-glucarpidase plasma methotrexate concentrations were more likely to achieve RSCIR compared with patients with higher pre-glucarpidase plasma methotrexate concentrations; RSCIR was achieved in 10 of 13 patients (77%) with pre-glucarpidase methotrexate concentrations of 22.7 mcg/mL (50 μmol/L) or less and in 0 of 9 patients (0%) with pre-glucarpidase methotrexate concentrations exceeding 22.7 mcg/mL (50 μmol/L). Despite this observation, all 9 patients with pre-glucarpidase plasma methotrexate concentrations exceeding 22.7 mcg/mL (50 μmol/L) were able to achieve a greater than 95% reduction in plasma methotrexate concentration for up to 8 days following glucarpidase administration.

There currently are no controlled trials comparing efficacy of glucarpidase plus supportive care with supportive care alone in patients with toxic plasma methotrexate concentrations due to renal impairment. Therefore, effects of glucarpidase on survival or on the risk of death associated with methotrexate toxicity have not been established. Glucarpidase did not prevent fatal methotrexate toxicity in 3% of patients receiving the drug in clinical safety studies.

Administration of a second dose of glucarpidase has *not* been shown to provide additional benefit. In the pivotal single-arm, open-label study in which patients with pre-glucarpidase methotrexate concentrations exceeding 45.4 mcg/mL (100 μmol/L) received a second dose of glucarpidase (50 units/kg administered 48 hours after the first dose), RSCIR was not achieved in any patient with pre-second-dose methotrexate concentrations exceeding 0.454 mcg/mL (1 μmol/L). In other studies, administration of a second dose of glucarpidase did not result in further reduction in plasma methotrexate concentrations. (See Methotrexate Toxicity under Dosage and Administration: Dosage.) This lack of efficacy following the second dose may be due to the presence of high concentrations of the methotrexate inactive metabolite 4-deoxy-4-amino-N^{10}-methylpteroic acid (DAMPA), which inhibits hydrolysis of methotrexate, and/or the presence of antiglucarpidase antibodies. (See Antibody Formation under Cautions: Warnings/Precautions.)

Dosage and Administration

■ **General** Glucarpidase should be used only in patients who exhibit delayed methotrexate clearance (plasma methotrexate concentrations exceeding 2 standard deviations above the mean methotrexate excretion curve specific for the methotrexate dose administered) due to renal impairment. Early recognition of delayed methotrexate clearance and renal impairment (i.e., an increase in serum creatinine concentration and/or oliguria) and urgent intervention are essential to prevent development of severe methotrexate-induced toxicities.

Glucarpidase should be used in conjunction with leucovorin rescue and supportive measures (i.e., IV hydration, urinary alkalinization with sodium bicarbonate). Because the pharmacokinetics of leucovorin and levoleucovorin are similar, the manufacturer of glucarpidase states that levoleucovorin may be substituted for leucovorin.

■ **Reconstitution and Administration** Glucarpidase is administered by direct IV injection over 5 minutes. The IV line should be flushed before and after administration of the drug.

Prior to administration, glucarpidase powder for injection should be reconstituted by adding 1 mL of sterile 0.9% sodium chloride for injection to the vial labeled as containing 1000 units of glucarpidase. The contents should be mixed by gently rolling and tilting the vial; the vial should *not* be shaken. The reconstituted solution should be inspected visually and should be discarded if the solution is not clear, colorless, and free of particulate matter. Reconstituted glucarpidase solution may be used immediately or stored at 2–8°C for up to 4 hours; unused portions of the solution should be discarded.

Unreconstituted glucarpidase powder for injection should be stored at 2–8°C and should *not* be frozen.

■ **Dosage** Dosage of glucarpidase is expressed in terms of units; a unit of glucarpidase activity is defined as the quantity of enzyme needed to catalyze the hydrolysis of 0.454 mcg/mL (1 μmol/L) of methotrexate per minute at 37°C.

Methotrexate Toxicity The recommended dosage of glucarpidase for the treatment of toxic plasma methotrexate concentrations (exceeding 0.454 mcg/mL [1 μmol/L]) in adults and pediatric patients with delayed methotrexate clearance due to renal impairment is a single IV injection of 50 units/kg.

Following administration of glucarpidase, rescue therapy with leucovorin (or levoleucovorin) should be continued. During the first 48 hours after glucarpidase administration, leucovorin (or levoleucovorin) should be administered at the same dosage administered prior to glucarpidase administration; beyond 48 hours, dosage should be based on the measured methotrexate concentration. (See Drug Interactions: Reduced Folates and also see Leucovorin Calcium 92:12.) Therapy with leucovorin (or levoleucovorin) should be continued until the methotrexate concentration has been maintained below the threshold for such treatment for at least 3 days.

Because of the lack of efficacy observed with the second dose, use of more than one dose of glucarpidase is *not* recommended. (See Uses: Methotrexate Toxicity.)

■ **Special Populations** There are no special population dosage recommendations at this time. (See Specific Populations under Cautions: Warnings/Precautions.)

Cautions

■ **Contraindications** The manufacturer states there are no known contraindications to the use of glucarpidase.

■ **Warnings/Precautions** ***Sensitivity Reactions*** Serious hypersensitivity reactions, including anaphylaxis, may occur. In clinical studies, serious hypersensitivity reactions occurred in less than 1% of patients receiving glucarpidase.

Monitoring of Methotrexate Concentrations and Assay Interference Glucarpidase converts methotrexate to 4-deoxy-4-amino-N^{10}-methylpteroic acid (DAMPA), an inactive metabolite that interferes with immunoassays and causes an overestimation of plasma methotrexate concentrations. Because of the long half-life of DAMPA (approximately 9 hours), plasma methotrexate concentrations measured by immunoassay within 48 hours following glucarpidase administration are unreliable. Therefore, the manufacturer recommends using a chromatographic method to obtain reliable measurements of plasma methotrexate concentrations within 48 hours following glucarpidase administration.

Continuation of Adjunctive Therapy Following administration of glucarpidase, rescue therapy with leucovorin (or levoleucovorin) should be continued until the methotrexate concentration has been maintained below the threshold for such treatment for at least 3 days. (See Methotrexate Toxicity under Dosage and Administration: Dosage and also see Drug Interactions: Reduced Folates.) IV hydration and urinary alkalinization should be continued as indicated.

Antibody Formation Antiglucarpidase antibodies have been detected in 16 of 96 (17%) patients receiving the drug in clinical studies. Antiglucarpidase antibodies were detected between 7 days to 7 months following exposure to glucarpidase. The incidence of antiglucarpidase antibody formation appeared to be similar in patients receiving either 1 or 2 doses of glucarpidase (12 of 78 patients [15%] or 4 of 18 patients [22%], respectively).

The development of antiglucarpidase antibodies is not expected to be clinically important considering the rapid time to maximum pharmacodynamic effect (15 minutes) and the recommended dosage regimen (i.e., single dose).

Specific Populations **Pregnancy.** Category C. (See Users Guide.)

Lactation. It is not known whether glucarpidase is distributed into human milk. Caution is advised when glucarpidase is administered in nursing women.

Pediatric Use. Efficacy of glucarpidase as adjunctive therapy for the treatment of toxic plasma methotrexate concentrations (exceeding 0.454 mcg/mL [1 μmol/L]) in pediatric patients with delayed methotrexate clearance due to renal impairment has been established in one study that included 12 patients 5–16 years of age. In this study, 3 of the 6 pediatric patients with pre-glucarpidase plasma methotrexate concentrations of 0.454–22.7 mcg/mL (1–50 μmol/L) achieved rapid and sustained clinically important reductions (RSCIR) in plasma methotrexate concentrations, while none of the remaining 6 patients with pre-glucarpidase plasma methotrexate concentrations exceeding 22.7 mcg/mL (50 μmol/L) achieved RSCIR.

In an analysis of pooled clinical safety data in 147 patients 1 month to 17 years of age, no overall difference in safety was observed between pediatric and adult patients.

Geriatric Use. In clinical studies, 15% of patients were 65 years of age or older and 4% were 75 years of age or older. No overall differences in safety or efficacy were observed between geriatric patients and younger adults.

Hepatic Impairment. Glucarpidase has not been studied in patients with hepatic impairment.

Renal Impairment. Following IV administration of glucarpidase 50 units/kg in 4 patients with severe renal impairment (creatinine clearance less than 30 mL/minute), mean pharmacokinetic parameters of glucarpidase (as assessed by enzymatic assay) were similar to those observed in healthy individuals except for a prolonged half-life (8.2 hours compared with 5.6 hours in healthy individuals).

■ **Common Adverse Effects** Adverse effects reported in 1% or more of patients receiving glucarpidase include paresthesia, flushing, nausea and/or vomiting, hypotension, and headache.

Drug Interactions

■ **Reduced Folates** Leucovorin is a substrate of glucarpidase. In patients receiving high-dose methotrexate therapy with leucovorin rescue, administration of glucarpidase 2 hours before a leucovorin dose reduced peak plasma concentrations and area under the plasma concentration-time curve (AUC) of leucovorin by 52 and 33%, respectively, and of its active metabolite (5-methyltetrahydrofolate) by 93 and 92%, respectively. Similar effects would be expected with levoleucovorin. Therefore, leucovorin or levoleucovorin should not be administered within 2 hours before or after glucarpidase administration. During the first 48 hours after glucarpidase administration, dosage adjustment of the continuing leucovorin or levoleucovorin regimen is not necessary since dosage is based on the patient's methotrexate concentration prior to glucarpidase administration. (See Methotrexate Toxicity under Dosage and Administration: Dosage.)

■ **Other Substrates of Glucarpidase** Concomitant use with other drugs that are substrates of glucarpidase (including folic acid antagonists [e.g., pyrimethamine, trimethoprim]) may result in decreased peak plasma concentrations and AUC of the glucarpidase substrate.

Description

Glucarpidase (also known as carboxypeptidase G_2 [$CPDG_2$]) is a bacterial enzyme produced by recombinant DNA technology. Glucarpidase was isolated from the *Pseudomonas* strain RS-16 and cloned, purified, and sequenced in genetically modified *Escherichia coli*. Glucarpidase rapidly hydrolyzes the carboxyl-terminal glutamate residue of folic acid, folic acid derivatives, and classic antifolates (e.g., methotrexate, leucovorin); the drug converts methotrexate to its inactive metabolites 4-deoxy-4-amino-N^{10}-methylpteroic acid (DAMPA) and glutamate, which are metabolized principally by the liver. Following administration of glucarpidase (50 units/kg) in the pivotal single-arm, open-label study, plasma methotrexate concentrations (measured by chromatographic method) were reduced by at least 97% within 15 minutes in all 22 treatment-evaluable patients and were maintained at a greater than 95% reduction for up to 8 days in 20 of the 22 patients.

Because of the large molecular size of glucarpidase, the drug is distributed primarily in the intravascular (i.e., extracellular) compartment and does not directly reduce intracellular concentrations (or interfere with intracellular antineoplastic effects) of methotrexate; therefore, rescue therapy with leucovorin must be continued following administration of glucarpidase. (See Methotrexate Toxicity under Dosage and Administration: Dosage and also see Drug Interactions: Reduced Folates.) Reductions in plasma methotrexate concentrations produced by glucarpidase are expected to cause redistribution (i.e., efflux) of intracellular methotrexate back into plasma, resulting in a rise in plasma methotrexate concentrations; as such, small rebound increases in plasma methotrexate concentrations have been observed in patients receiving glucarpidase in clinical studies.

The mean elimination half-life of glucarpidase is 5.6 hours (as assessed by enzymatic assay) or 9 hours (as assessed by enzyme-linked immunosorbent assay [ELISA]).

Advice to Patients

Risk of hypersensitivity reactions, including anaphylaxis.

Risk of infusion reactions. Importance of immediately reporting signs and symptoms of such reactions, including fever, chills, flushing, feeling hot, rash, hives, itching, throat tightness or breathing difficulty, tingling, numbness, or headache.

Importance of continued monitoring of plasma methotrexate concentrations and renal function after discharge from the hospital.

Importance of women informing clinicians if they are or plan to become pregnant or plan to breast-feed.

Importance of informing clinicians of existing or contemplated concomitant therapy, including prescription and OTC drugs, as well as any concomitant illnesses.

Importance of informing patients of other important precautionary information. (See Cautions.)

Overview® (see Users Guide). For additional information on this drug until a more detailed monograph is developed and published, the manufacturer's labeling should be consulted. It is *essential* that the manufacturer's labeling be consulted for more detailed information on usual cautions, precautions, contraindications, potential drug interactions, laboratory test interferences, and acute toxicity.

Preparations

Excipients in commercially available drug preparations may have clinically important effects in some individuals; consult specific product labeling for details.

Glucarpidase

Parenteral

For injection, for IV use only	1000 units	**Voraxaze®**, BTG

Leucovorin Calcium

Citrovorum Factor, Folinic Acid, 5-Formyl Tetrahydrofolate

■ Leucovorin calcium is the calcium salt of folinic acid, an active metabolite of folic acid.

Uses

■ **Prevention and Treatment of Toxicity Associated with Folic Acid Antagonists** Leucovorin is used as an antidote to diminish the toxicity and counteract the effect of unintentional overdosage of folic acid antagonists, such as methotrexate, trimethoprim, and pyrimethamine. Leucovorin also is used in conjunction with these folic acid antagonists for the prevention and treatment of undesired hematopoietic effects of the drugs. When used in the treatment of accidental overdosage of folic acid antagonists, leucovorin therapy should be initiated as soon as possible since the effectiveness of leucovorin in counteracting hematologic toxicity diminishes as the time period between antifolate (e.g., methotrexate) administration and leucovorin rescue increases.

Methotrexate Toxicity Leucovorin rescue has been administered in conjunction with high-dose methotrexate therapy in an effort to control the duration of exposure of sensitive cells to methotrexate. This regimen has been more effective than methotrexate alone in inducing and maintaining remissions in osteogenic sarcoma, head and neck cancer, refractory acute leukemia, and lung carcinoma; the superiority of this combination in other neoplastic diseases has not been demonstrated. Generally, leucovorin should not be administered simultaneously with systemic methotrexate because the therapeutic effect as well as the toxicity of the antimetabolite may be nullified; however, leucovorin can generally be administered 6–24 hours after methotrexate infusion. When methotrexate is administered by intra-arterial (regional perfusion) or intrathecal injection, leucovorin can be given IM, IV, or orally concomitantly to offset systemic methotrexate toxicity without abolishing the local activity of the antineoplastic drug.

Leucovorin has been used in conjunction with methotrexate in the treatment of psoriasis; however, results have been conflicting. Some investigators reported small doses of leucovorin increased the number, size, and activity of psoriasiform lesions when administered orally 24–72 hours after oral methotrexate. Other investigators have found leucovorin to decrease the adverse effects of methotrexate without decreasing the effects of the antimetabolite when leucovorin was administered IM 2 hours after IM methotrexate.

Trimetrexate Glucuronate Toxicity Leucovorin is administered concomitantly with trimetrexate glucuronate and continued for 72 hours after the last dose to prevent potentially serious or life-threatening toxicities (e.g., bone marrow suppression) associated with the drug.

Pyrimethamine Toxicity Protozoa are unable to utilize leucovorin, apparently because they require *p*-aminobenzoic acid (PABA) for biosynthesis of an active cofactor. For this reason, therapeutic doses of leucovorin have been administered at the same time as pyrimethamine to decrease the hematologic toxicity of pyrimethamine in the treatment of toxoplasmosis, *Pneumocystis carinii* pneumonia, or *Plasmodium falciparum* malaria, without nullifying the effect of pyrimethamine on the parasite.

Trimethoprim Toxicity Leucovorin has been used to antagonize the hematologic toxicity of trimethoprim without interfering with the drug's antibacterial effectiveness.

■ **Megaloblastic Anemia** Leucovorin is used in the treatment of folate deficient megaloblastic anemias of infancy, pregnancy, sprue, and nutritional deficiencies when oral folic acid therapy is not feasible. However, since the ability to convert folic acid to tetrahydrofolic acid is not impaired in these anemias, leucovorin has no advantage over folic acid injection.

In contrast to folic acid, leucovorin is also effective in the treatment of megaloblastic anemia produced by congenital dihydrofolate reductase deficiency. Leucovorin is *not* effective in and should not be used for the treatment of pernicious anemia and other megaloblastic anemias secondary to lack of vitamin B_{12}. (See Cautions: Precautions and Contraindications.)

■ **Combined Therapy with Fluorouracil for Advanced Colorectal Carcinoma** Leucovorin calcium is used to potentiate the antineoplastic activity of, and thus improve response to, fluorouracil in the palliative treatment of advanced colorectal carcinoma. Leucovorin calcium is designated an orphan drug by the US Food and Drug Administration (FDA) for such use. Such combined therapy is employed in an attempt to prolong survival relative to fluorouracil alone in patients with advanced disease. In vitro studies and clinical evidence have shown that the cytotoxicity of fluorouracil may be enhanced by leucovorin; it appears that elevated intracellular concentrations of reduced folates (e.g., leucovorin) may stabilize the covalent ternary complex formed by fluorodeoxyuridylic acid, 5,10-methylenetetrahydrofolate, and thymidylate synthase, enhancing inhibition of this enzyme and thereby increasing the efficacy of fluorouracil.

Analysis of pooled data from several randomized studies in patients with advanced colorectal carcinoma indicates that combined therapy with IV fluorouracil and IV leucovorin calcium produces higher objective response rates (i.e., tumor responses) than does IV fluorouracil alone. However, despite the superiority in objective tumor response with combined therapy, overall survival rates were not improved appreciably compared with fluorouracil alone. In this analysis, overall objective response rates were about 23% for combined fluorouracil and leucovorin therapy and 11% for fluorouracil alone, with only 3 and 2.6%, respectively, exhibiting complete responses; median durations of survival were 11.5 months for combined therapy and 11 months for fluorouracil alone. It remains unclear why the higher response rate did not result in improved survival with combination therapy. It was suggested that the low rates of response, particularly complete responses, for such advanced disease observed both in patients receiving combined therapy and in those receiving monotherapy may have been insufficient to affect overall survival. In addition, the large number of nonresponders to fluorouracil alone who subsequently received combined therapy may have obscured any potential difference in survival; however, a survival benefit also was not apparent when trials with crossovers were excluded. While it remains to be established, the possibility exists that survival differences may be more apparent with less advanced stages of disease.

Combination therapy in randomized studies in patients with advanced colorectal carcinoma consisted of regimens in which courses of IV fluorouracil and IV leucovorin calcium therapy were repeated at approximately monthly intervals and those in which courses were repeated weekly. The approximately monthly regimens included 5-day courses of fluorouracil 370 mg/m² and leucovorin calcium 200 or 500 mg/m² daily, fluorouracil 425 mg/m² and leucovorin calcium 20 mg/m² daily, or fluorouracil 400 mg/m² and leucovorin calcium 200 mg/m² daily, repeated at intervals of 4–5 weeks. Weekly dosage schedules of the combination included 600 mg/m² of fluorouracil and 25, 200, or 500 mg/m² of leucovorin administered once weekly, usually for 6 weeks. Fluorouracil alone was administered in various dosage regimens, including 5-day courses of 370, 400, or 500 mg/m² or 13.5 mg/kg daily, repeated at intervals of 4–5 weeks. Other dosage regimens of IV fluorouracil without leucovorin (i.e., fluorouracil 12 mg/kg daily for 5 days [total daily dosage did not exceed 800 mg] followed by fluorouracil 15 mg/kg once weekly, with dosage being increased by 10% weekly until dose-limiting toxicity or the desired degree of myelosuppression occurred) or 600 mg every 7 days also were used.

While analysis of almost all individual randomized studies in patients with advanced disease also failed to reveal a survival benefit, a tendency toward improved survival was observed with combined fluorouracil and leucovorin therapy in a few of these studies; however, this tendency may be lost with continued follow-up. In one study (the NCCTG/Mayo Clinic Trial) in which patients were followed for a median of 21 months (range: 14—41 months), improved survival was associated with combined regimens of fluorouracil and either high- (200 mg/m² daily for 5 days) or low- (20 mg/m² daily for 5 days) dose leucovorin; however, the survival benefit was limited to those with nonmeasurable disease. In this study, no advantage was apparent for the high-dose leucovorin regimen, but study and analysis of possible dose-response differences are continuing.

IV fluorouracil also has been used in combination with orally administered leucovorin in a limited number of patients with advanced colorectal carcinoma.

The combination of fluorouracil and leucovorin with methotrexate or cisplatin also is being studied in the treatment of advanced colorectal carcinoma. In patients with advanced colorectal carcinoma, combined therapy with fluorouracil and leucovorin was associated with higher objective response rates and longer median durations of survival than therapy with sequential methotrexate, fluorouracil, and leucovorin; objective response rates were 31–33% and median durations of survival were 402–418 days in patients receiving combined therapy with fluorouracil and leucovorin compared with objective response rates of 4% and a median duration of survival of 223 days in patients receiving sequential methotrexate, fluorouracil, and leucovorin therapy.

In addition to possible therapeutic potentiation, leucovorin may potentiate the risk of fluorouracil-induced toxicity (especially GI toxicity, including diarrhea, nausea, stomatitis, and vomiting, and, to a lesser degree, myelosuppression). A syndrome characterized by progression from mild to severe GI symptoms and rarely to potentially fatal enterocolitis has been reported in several studies of patients with advanced colorectal carcinoma receiving combined therapy with the drugs; in these studies, adverse GI effects (e.g., severe diarrhea, stomatitis) were the dose-limiting toxicity. (See Cautions: GI Effects, in Fluorouracil 10:00). Limited data suggest that once-weekly administration of fluorouracil plus leucovorin may be associated with a higher risk of developing serious adverse GI effects than 5-day regimens administered at approximately monthly intervals. Severe diarrhea appears to be the dose-limiting toxicity associated with once-weekly administration of the combination, while diarrhea and/or mucositis appear to be the dose-limiting toxicities associated with the 5-day regimens. Combined therapy with fluorouracil and leucovorin should *not* be initiated or continued in patients with symptomatic GI toxicity until such symptoms have completely resolved. Close monitoring is particularly important in patients who develop diarrhea with such combined therapy since rapid clinical deterioration and death can occur. Death secondary to severe enterocolitis, diarrhea, and dehydration has occurred in geriatric patients receiving the combination.

Dosage and Administration

■ **Reconstitution and Administration** Leucovorin calcium is administered orally or by IM or IV injection. The drug should be given parenterally rather than orally in patients with GI toxicity, nausea, or vomiting and when individual doses greater than 25 mg are to be administered. Parenteral administration generally is preferred when leucovorin is administered following chemotherapy with a folic acid antagonist and there is a possibility that the patient may vomit and not absorb oral leucovorin. Leucovorin calcium should *not* be administered intrathecally.

Leucovorin calcium powder for injection should be reconstituted by adding 5 or 10 mL of sterile water for injection or bacteriostatic water for injection containing benzyl alcohol to a vial labeled as containing 50 or 100 mg of leucovorin, respectively; the resultant solutions contain 10 mg/mL. Leucovorin calcium vials of the powder for injection labeled as containing 350 mg of leucovorin should be reconstituted by adding 17 mL of sterile water for injection or bacteriostatic water for injection containing benzyl alcohol to the vial; the resultant solution contains 20 mg/mL. When parenteral doses greater than 10 mg/m² are necessary, leucovorin calcium powder for injection reconstituted with sterile water for injection should be used; leucovorin calcium powder for injection reconstituted with bacteriostatic water containing benzyl alcohol should be used only when parenteral doses of 10 mg/m² or lower are required. Since parenteral leucovorin calcium doses exceeding 10 mg/m² are used in combination with fluorouracil for the treatment of advanced colorectal carcinoma, leucovorin calcium *powder for injection* (reconstituted with *sterile water for injection*) should be used for this indication. When leucovorin is administered by IV infusion, the infusion rate should not exceed 16 mL (160 mg of leucovorin) per minute because of the calcium concentration of the solution.

■ **Dosage** Dosage of leucovorin calcium is expressed in terms of leucovorin.

Prevention and Treatment of Hematologic Toxicity Associated with Folic Acid Antagonists As an antidote for inadvertent overdosage of folic acid antagonists, the manufacturers recommend that leucovorin be administered IM or IV in amounts equal to the weight of the antagonist given, as soon as the overdosage is detected and preferably within the first hour. When large doses or overdoses of methotrexate are given, leucovorin can be administered by IV infusion in doses up to 75 mg within 12 hours, followed by 12 mg IM every 6 hours for 4 doses. When average doses of methotrexate appear to have an adverse effect, 6–12 mg of leucovorin may be given IM every 6 hours for 4 doses. Prompt administration of leucovorin calcium is essential.

Methotrexate Toxicity. As part of a high-dose methotrexate regimen in cancer chemotherapy, leucovorin rescue therapy must begin within 24 hours of methotrexate administration. Dosage of leucovorin is approximately twice that of levoleucovorin (the active levorotatory [*l*] isomer). (See Levoleucovorin Calcium 92:12.)

The manufacturers of leucovorin calcium state that a typical leucovorin rescue dosage schedule is 10 mg/m² usually administered parenterally followed by 10 mg/m² orally (if there is adequate GI function) every 6 hours until the serum methotrexate concentration has declined to less than 10^{-8} *M*. If at 24 hours following methotrexate administration the patient's serum creatinine has increased to 50% or more above the serum creatinine prior to methotrexate or the serum methotrexate concentration is greater than 5×10^{-6} *M*, or if at 48 hours following methotrexate administration the serum methotrexate concentration is greater than 9×10^{-7} *M*, leucovorin dosage should be increased immediately to 100 mg/m² every 3 hours until the serum methotrexate concentration is less than 10^{-8} *M*. Use of high-dose methotrexate and leucovorin rescue therapy in treating certain cancers is an evolving science, and the optimum dosage and sequence of methotrexate and leucovorin calcium have not been established. Patients should not be given such therapy unless a specific formal protocol is being followed; the clinician should consult published protocols for the dosage of leucovorin calcium and the duration of methotrexate therapy before leucovorin calcium is administered.

In one study utilizing methotrexate in the treatment of psoriasis, the toxic effects of methotrexate were usually overcome by 4–8 mg of leucovorin administered IM 2 hours after IM methotrexate.

Trimetrexate Glucuronate Toxicity. The usual leucovorin dosage for the prevention of potentially serious and life-threatening toxicities in immunocompromised patients receiving trimetrexate glucuronate for the treatment of *Pneumocystis carinii* pneumonia is 20 mg/m² every 6 hours (total daily dose of 80 mg/m²). Leucovorin may be administered orally or IV (over 5–10 minutes) in these patients; if leucovorin is administered orally, the calculated dose should be rounded up to the next 25-mg increment. Leucovorin should be continued for at least 72 hours after the last trimetrexate dose. For the treatment of moderate to severe *Pneumocystis carinii* pneumonia in adults, the usual dosage of trimetrexate is 45 mg/m² given once daily. The recommended course of trimetrexate therapy is 21 days and that of leucovorin is 24 days.

Dosage of trimetrexate and leucovorin must be adjusted according to the hematologic tolerance of the patient. For patients with neutrophil counts exceeding 1000/ mm³ and platelet counts exceeding 75,000/ mm³ (grade 1 toxicity), the usual dosages of trimetrexate and leucovorin can be used. For those with neutrophil counts of 750–1000/ mm³ and platelet counts of 50,000–75,000/ mm³ (grade 2 toxicity), the usual trimetrexate dosage should be used but leucovorin dosage should be increased to 40 mg/m² every 6 hours. Trimetrexate dosage should be reduced to 22 mg/ mm² once daily and leucovorin dosage should be increased to 40 mg/m² every 6 hours for neutrophil and platelet counts of 500–749 and 25,000–49,999 per mm³ (grade 3 toxicity), respectively. When using these dosage guidelines, dosage should be modified based on the *worst* of the two blood cell counts. For patients with lower neutrophil or platelet counts (grade 4 toxicity), leucovorin dosage should be increased to 40 mg/m² every 6 hours, and trimetrexate therapy should be discontinued if such changes occur prior to day 10 of therapy, continuing the higher dosage of leucovorin for an additional 72 hours. If such low counts develop during days 10–21 of trimetrexate therapy, the drug may be withheld up to 96 hours to permit recovery of the blood count(s) to a minimum of grade 3 toxicity before reinstituting trimetrexate; dosage should be adjusted according to the grade of hematologic toxicity achieved at the time of recovery. If hematologic toxicity does not improve to a minimum of grade 3 toxicity after 96 hours, trimetrexate therapy should be discontinued; leucovorin should be continued at the higher dosage for 72 hours after the last dose of trimetrexate.

Pyrimethamine Toxicity. The dosage of leucovorin necessary to prevent hematologic toxicity associated with pyrimethamine varies depending on the dosage of the folic acid antagonist and the clinical status of the patient.

In adults or children receiving pyrimethamine in a dosage of 25–100 mg daily or 1–2 mg/kg daily for the *treatment* of toxoplasmosis, some clinicians suggest that 10–25 mg of leucovorin be administered with each dose of pyrimethamine.

When a regimen containing pyrimethamine (50 or 75 mg once weekly) and dapsone is used for the prevention of initial episodes (*primary prophylaxis*) of *P. carinii* pneumonia or *Toxoplasma gondii* infections or prevention of recurrence (*chronic maintenance therapy of secondary prophylaxis*) of *P. carinii* pneumonia in adults or adolescents with human immunodeficiency virus (HIV) infection, some clinicians recommend that oral leucovorin be administered concomitantly in a dosage of 25 mg once weekly. If adults or adolescents are receiving a regimen that contains a higher dosage of pyrimethamine (25–50 mg once daily) with clindamycin or sulfadiazine for *secondary prophylaxis* of toxoplasmosis, the dosage of leucovorin necessary to prevent hematologic toxicity may range from 10–25 mg once daily. When a regimen containing pyrimethamine 25 mg once daily and atovaquone is used for *primary* or *secondary* prophylaxis against toxoplasmosis in adults and adolescents with HIV infection, some clinicians recommend that oral leucovorin be administered concomitantly in a dosage of 10 mg daily.

In HIV-infected children receiving a regimen that contains pyrimethamine (1 mg/kg once daily) with dapsone or clindamycin for *primary or secondary prophylaxis*, respectively, of toxoplasmosis, some clinicians recommend a leucovorin dosage of 5 mg once every 3 days.

Megaloblastic Anemia In the treatment of folate deficient megaloblastic anemias, up to 1 mg of leucovorin may be given IM daily. Although doses of 10 mg daily have been recommended in the past, the manufacturers state there is no evidence that IM doses greater than 1 mg daily are more effective. The duration of leucovorin therapy for megaloblastic anemia depends on the hematologic response to the drug, as evidenced in both peripheral blood and bone marrow. In general, patient response to therapy depends on the degree and nature of the folate deficiency, but once proper corrective measures are undertaken, deficient patients will generally respond rapidly. During the first 24 hours of treatment, the patient experiences an improved sense of well-being; the bone marrow begins to become normoblastic within 48 hours. Reticulocytosis generally begins within 2–5 days after the start of therapy.

In the treatment of megaloblastic anemia resulting from a congenital deficiency of dihydrofolate reductase, 3–6 mg of leucovorin has been given IM daily.

Combined Therapy with Fluorouracil for Advanced Colorectal Carcinoma For potentiation of the antineoplastic effects of fluorouracil in the palliative treatment of advanced colorectal carcinoma, optimum dosage of leucovorin has not been clearly established. Current evidence indicates that an IV leucovorin dose of 20 mg/m² followed by an IV fluorouracil dose of 425 mg/m² can be used. Alternatively, a leucovorin dose of 200 mg/m² administered by slow IV injection (over a minimum of 3 minutes) followed by an IV fluorouracil dose of 370 mg/m² can be used, but there currently is no evidence of superiority with this leucovorin dosage. Either selected regimen is administered daily for 5 days and may be repeated at 4-week intervals for 2 additional courses; thereafter, the regimen may be repeated at intervals of 4–5 weeks provided toxicity from the previous course of combined therapy has subsided. Dosage of fluorouracil in subsequent courses of therapy should be adjusted according to patient tolerance of the prior treatment course; dosage of leucovorin in subsequent courses generally is not adjusted according to toxicity. Daily fluorouracil dosage generally is reduced by 20% in patients who experienced moderate hematologic or GI toxicity in the prior course and by 30% in those patients who experienced severe toxicity. If no toxicity occurs, fluorouracil dosage may be increased by 10%. Other combination dosage regimens also have been used. (See Uses: Combined Therapy with Fluorouracil for Advanced Colorectal Carcinoma.)

Cautions

■ **Adverse Effects** Leucovorin appears to be nontoxic in therapeutic doses, although thrombocytosis has been reported in patients receiving leucovorin during intra-arterial infusion of methotrexate. In addition, hypersensitivity reactions, including anaphylactoid reactions and urticaria, have been reported with both oral and parenteral use of leucovorin. While leucovorin can potentiate the toxic effects of fluorouracil, potentially resulting in increased severity and frequency of certain effects, the observed toxicity is that generally associated with fluorouracil. (See Uses: Combined Therapy with Fluorouracil for Advanced Colorectal Carcinoma and also see the Cautions section in the monograph on Fluorouracil 10:00.)

■ **Precautions and Contraindications** Since allergic reactions have been reported following oral and parenteral administration of folic acid, the possibility of allergic reactions to leucovorin should be considered.

There is a potential danger in administering leucovorin to patients with undiagnosed anemia, as leucovorin may obscure the diagnosis of pernicious anemia by alleviating hematologic manifestations of the disease while allowing neurologic complications to progress. This may result in severe nervous system damage before the correct diagnosis is made. Adequate doses of vitamin B_{12} may prevent, halt, or improve neurologic changes caused by pernicious anemia.

When leucovorin rescue is used in conjunction with high-dose methotrexate therapy, the drugs should be administered only by physicians experienced in cancer chemotherapy, in centers where facilities for measuring blood methotrexate concentrations are available. Leucovorin is usually effective in counteracting severe methotrexate toxicity in these regimens, but toxic reactions to methotrexate may occur despite leucovorin therapy, especially when the half-life of methotrexate is increased (e.g., renal dysfunction). Therefore, it is extremely important that leucovorin be administered until the blood concentration of methotrexate declines to nontoxic concentrations.

Since leucovorin calcium enhances the toxicity of fluorouracil, adjunctive therapy with leucovorin calcium and fluorouracil should be given only by, or under the supervision of, physicians experienced in cancer chemotherapy and in the use of antimetabolites. Hematologic indices (complete blood cell counts with differential, and quantitative platelet count) should be performed before each course of therapy with fluorouracil and leucovorin and repeated weekly during the first 2 courses of therapy and once during each subsequent course of therapy (when anticipated leukocyte nadir occurs). Determinations of serum electrolyte concentrations and liver function tests should be performed before each course of therapy for the first 3 courses of therapy and then prior to each other course of therapy. Dosage of fluorouracil should be reduced in patients who experienced moderate or severe hematologic or GI toxicity. (See Dosage and Administration: Dosage.) Therapy should be interrupted until the leukocyte count is 4000/mm^3 and the platelet count is 130,000/mm^3. If these counts do not increase to these levels within 2 weeks, therapy should be discontinued. Patients should be followed up with physical examinations before each course of therapy, and appropriate radiographic examinations should be performed as needed. Therapy should be discontinued if there is clear evidence of tumor progression.

There is some evidence to suggest that the risk of fluorouracil-induced GI toxicity may be increased in patients receiving leucovorin concomitantly with the drug. Death secondary to severe enterocolitis, diarrhea, and dehydration has occurred in geriatric patients receiving the drugs concomitantly. Concomitant granulocytopenia and fever were present in some but not all cases. (See Cautions: GI Effects, in Fluorouracil 10:00.) Combined leucovorin and fluorouracil therapy should be used with extreme caution in geriatric or debilitated patients since such patients are more likely to develop serious toxicity from fluorouracil.

■ **Pregnancy and Lactation** Animal reproduction studies have not been performed with leucovorin. It is also not known whether leucovorin can cause fetal harm when administered to pregnant women. Leucovorin should be used during pregnancy only when clearly needed.

Since it is not known if leucovorin is distributed into milk, the drug should be used with caution in nursing women.

Pharmacology

Leucovorin is a derivative of tetrahydrofolic acid, the reduced form of folic acid, which is involved as a cofactor for 1-carbon transfer reactions in the biosynthesis of purines and pyrimidines of nucleic acids. Impairment of thymidylate synthesis in patients with folic acid deficiency is thought to account for the defective DNA synthesis that leads to megaloblast formation and megaloblastic and macrocytic anemias. Because of its ready conversion to other tetrahydrofolic acid derivatives, leucovorin is a potent antidote for both the hematopoietic and reticuloendothelial toxic effects of folic acid antagonists (e.g., methotrexate, pyrimethamine, trimethoprim). It is postulated that in some cancers leucovorin enters and "rescues" normal cells from the toxic effects of folic acid antagonists, in preference to tumor cells, because of a difference in membrane transport mechanisms; this principle is the basis of high-dose methotrexate therapy with "leucovorin rescue."

Pharmacokinetics

■ **Absorption and Disribution** In vivo, leucovorin calcium is rapidly and extensively converted to other tetrahydrofolic acid derivatives including 5-methyl tetrahydrofolate, which is the major transport and storage form of folate in the body.

Normal total serum folate concentrations have been reported to range from 0.005–0.015 mcg/mL. Folate is actively concentrated in CSF, and normal CSF concentrations are reported to be about 0.016–0.021 mcg/mL. Normal erythrocyte folate concentrations range from 0.175–0.316 mcg/mL. In general, serum folate concentrations less than 0.005 mcg/mL indicate folate deficiency and concentrations less than 0.002 mcg/mL usually result in megaloblastic anemia. Following IM administration of a 15-mg (7.5 mg/m^2) dose in healthy men, mean peak serum folate concentrations of 0.241 mcg/mL occur within about 40 minutes. Following oral administration of a 15-mg (7.5 mg/m^2) dose in healthy men, mean peak serum folate concentrations of 0.268 mcg/mL occur within about 1.72 hours. Areas under the serum folate concentration-time curves (AUCs) are reported to be about 8% less following IM injection in the gluteal region than in the deltoid region and about 12% less following IM injection in the gluteal region than following IV or oral administration.

Tetrahydrofolic acid and its derivatives are distributed to all body tissues; the liver contains about one-half of total body folate stores. In a small number of patients, biliary concentration of folates was about 4.5 times the plasma folate concentration after oral administration of a 2-mg dose of leucovorin; this is believed to represent the hepatic folate pool rather than excretion of the administered dose.

■ **Elimination** Leucovorin is excreted in urine, mainly as 10-formyl tetrahydrofolate and 5,10-methenyl tetrahydrofolate. There is some evidence that 5-methyl tetrahydrofolate may be conserved by the kidneys in preference to 5-formyl tetrahydrofolate (leucovorin). Loss of folate in the urine becomes approximately logarithmic as the amount of leucovorin administered exceeds 1 mg.

Chemistry and Stability

■ **Chemistry** Leucovorin calcium is the calcium salt of folinic acid, an active metabolite of folic acid. Leucovorin consists of equal amounts of *d*- and *l*-isomers; the *l*-isomer (levoleucovorin) is the pharmacologically active isomer. (See Levoleucovorin Calcium 92:12.) Leucovorin calcium occurs as a yellowish white or yellow, odorless powder and has solubilities of more than 500 mg/mL in water and less than 1 mg/mL in alcohol. The pK_as of leucovorin are 3.1, 4.8, and 10.4.

■ **Stability** Leucovorin calcium powder for injection and tablets should be stored at 15–30°C and protected from light.

When leucovorin calcium powder for injection is reconstituted as directed, resultant solutions should be used immediately when reconstituted with sterile water for injection or within 7 days when reconstituted with bacteriostatic water for injection containing benzyl alcohol.

Leucovorin calcium solutions that have been admixed with 10% dextrose injection, 10% dextrose and 0.9% sodium chloride injection, Ringer's injection, or lactated Ringer's injection are stable for 24 hours when stored at room temperature protected from light. Although some former manufacturers of leucovorin calcium powder for injection have recommended that reconstituted solutions of the drug be protected from light, there is evidence that solutions of the drug are not adversely affected by exposure to room light. Reconstituted solutions of leucovorin calcium that have been further diluted with 50 mL of 5% dextrose injection and stored in Viaflex® or glass containers unprotected from light retain at least 90% potency for 24 hours at room temperature.

Preparations

Excipients in commercially available drug preparations may have clinically important effects in some individuals; consult specific product labeling for details.

Leucovorin Calcium

Oral		
Tablets	5 mg (of leucovorin)*	**Leucovorin Calcium Tablets** (scored)
	10 mg (of leucovorin)*	**Leucovorin Calcium Tablets** (scored)
	15 mg (of leucovorin)*	**Leucovorin Calcium Tablets** (scored)
	25 mg (of leucovorin)*	**Leucovorin Calcium Tablets** (scored)
Parenteral		
For injection	50 mg (of leucovorin)*	**Leucovorin Calcium for Injection**
	100 mg (of leucovorin)*	**Leucovorin Calcium for Injection**
	200 mg (of leucovorin)*	**Leucovorin Calcium for Injection** (preservative-free)
	350 mg (of leucovorin)*	**Leucovorin Calcium for Injection**
	500 mg (of leucovorin)*	**Leucovorin Calcium for Injection** (preservative-free)
Injection	10 mg (of leucovorin) per mL (500 mg)*	**Leucovorin Calcium Injection** (preservative-free)

*available from one or more manufacturer, distributor, and/or repackager by generic (nonproprietary) name

LEVOleucovorin Calcium

l-Leucovorin

■ Levoleucovorin calcium, the levorotatory (*l*) isomer of racemic *d,l*-leucovorin, is one of several active, chemically reduced derivatives of folic acid.

Uses

■ **Toxicity Associated with Folic Acid Antagonists** Levoleucovorin calcium rescue is used after high-dose methotrexate therapy (to control the duration of exposure of sensitive cells to methotrexate for treatment of osteosarcoma. Levoleucovorin also is used as an antidote to diminish the toxicity and counteract the effects of unintentional overdosage of methotrexate (e.g., resulting from impaired elimination) and other folic acid antagonists. Levoleucovorin is designated an orphan drug by the US Food and Drug Administration (FDA) for these uses.

Safety and efficacy of levoleucovorin rescue were evaluated in an analysis of data from 2 open-label studies and other unpublished trials in a limited number of patients (6–21 years of age) with osteogenic sarcoma. Of the 16 patients evaluated, 13 received levoleucovorin 7.5 mg every 6 hours for 60 hours or longer beginning 24 hours after completion of methotrexate (12 g/m^2 IV over 4 hours), and 3 received levoleucovorin 7.5 mg every 3 hours for 18 doses beginning 12 hours after completion of methotrexate (12.5 g/m^2 IV over 6 hours). Patients received a mean of 18.2 doses of levoleucovorin and a mean total dose of 350 mg per methotrexate course. Efficacy of levoleucovorin was determined by comparing its ability to prevent methotrexate-related toxicity with that of racemic leucovorin. In the first open-label study, 3 patients receiving a total of 22 courses of levoleucovorin following high-dose methotrexate therapy experienced fewer serious adverse events (0% of the 22 courses) compared with 6 historical control patients receiving a total of 24 courses of racemic leucovorin (10% of the 24 courses). In the second open-label study in which 15 patients received a total of 90 courses of levoleucovorin, severe adverse events were reported in 4% of the 90 courses. However, it should be noted that interpretation of these results is limited by the statistical limitations of the studies (e.g., small sample size, reliance on retrospective review of records for historical control data).

Although levoleucovorin may ameliorate the hematologic toxicity associated with high-dose methotrexate, the drug has no effect on other established toxicities of methotrexate such as the nephrotoxicity resulting from drug and/or metabolite precipitation in the kidney.

■ **Colorectal Cancer** ***Combined Therapy with Fluorouracil for Advanced-stage Colorectal Cancer*** Levoleucovorin calcium is used in combination with fluorouracil for the palliative treatment of advanced-stage colorectal cancer. Use of levoleucovorin calcium in combination with fluorouracil and other agents (i.e., irinotecan, oxaliplatin)† also has been studied for the treatment of advanced-stage colorectal cancer†; however, use of levoleucovorin in regimens containing fluorouracil and either irinotecan or oxaliplatin currently is not fully established for this indication because of inadequate data and/or experience.

Levoleucovorin and Fluorouracil. The current indication for use of levoleucovorin in combination with fluorouracil for the palliative treatment of advanced-stage colorectal cancer is based principally on the results of a phase 3, open-label, randomized study. In this study, 926 patients with advanced-stage (i.e., unresectable) colorectal cancer were randomized to receive levoleucovorin 100 mg/m² by IV injection, racemic leucovorin 125 mg/m² orally at 1-hour intervals for 4 doses, or racemic leucovorin 200 mg/m² by IV injection; fluorouracil (370 mg/m² given as an IV injection) was administered immediately following the IV dose of leucovorin or levoleucovorin or 1 hour after the fourth oral dose of leucovorin. The drugs were administered daily on days 1–5 of the treatment cycle, with dosages adjusted as needed based on toxicity and response; treatment cycles were repeated at 4 and 8 weeks and every 5 weeks thereafter until disease progression or unacceptable toxicity occurred. Overall response rates for the 3 groups did not differ significantly; 1-year survival was approximately 40% for all treatment groups. There were no substantial differences in toxicity between levoleucovorin and racemic leucovorin when used in conjunction with fluorouracil.

In a second phase 3, open-label, randomized trial in 248 patients with metastatic and/or recurrent colorectal cancer, levoleucovorin was compared with racemic leucovorin to determine if a twofold increase in leucovorin dosage (given as levoleucovorin) would result in differences in overall response rate, toxicity, and survival. Patients received either levoleucovorin (100 mg/m²) or racemic leucovorin (100 mg/m²) by IV injection, followed immediately by fluorouracil (400 mg/m² as a 2-hour IV infusion), on days 1–5 of each 4-week treatment cycle, with dosages adjusted as needed based on toxicity and response. A slight improvement in overall response rate was reported for levoleucovorin/fluorouracil compared with racemic leucovorin/fluorouracil; the overall response rate was 32% (5% complete and 27% partial responses) for patients receiving levoleucovorin/fluorouracil compared with 25% (3% complete and 21% partial responses) for those receiving racemic leucovorin/fluorouracil. Median time to progression was 8 or 6.25 months with levoleucovorin/fluorouracil or racemic leucovorin/fluorouracil treatment, respectively; overall survival (14.5 versus 15 months), 1-year survival (58.3 versus 60.6%), and estimated 2-year survival (15.3 versus 23%) for patients receiving racemic leucovorin/fluorouracil or levoleucovorin/fluorouracil, respectively, did not differ significantly. The discontinuance rates were similar (34%) for both groups. Severe adverse events were slightly more common in patients receiving racemic leucovorin/fluorouracil compared with those receiving levoleucovorin/fluorouracil (18 versus 13%). Increased incidences of granulocytopenia (all grades; 39 versus 21%), grade 3 or 4 granulocytopenia (8 versus 2%), grade 3 or 4 leukopenia (5 versus 0%), and grade 3 or 4 diarrhea (10 versus 7%) were reported with racemic leucovorin/fluorouracil compared with levoleucovorin/fluorouracil treatment; however, the investigators acknowledged that the increased incidence of granulocytopenia observed with racemic leucovorin/fluorouracil treatment may be of limited clinical importance based on a lack of complications (e.g., febrile/neutropenic events) and the low incidence of granulocytopenia overall for the study population. The incidences of grade 1 or 2 stomatitis and diarrhea were similar for both groups.

In a third study (OPTIMOX1; a study that evaluated alternative dosing sequences and regimens as a means for reducing the incidence of oxaliplatin-induced sensory neuropathy), one of the treatment regimens, the simplified de Gramont regimen, consisted of IV levoleucovorin or racemic leucovorin in combination with fluorouracil (as a continuous IV infusion). However, neither response nor toxicity results based on the leucovorin formulation used have been reported to date.

Levoleucovorin/Fluorouracil in Combination with Other Agents. Levoleucovorin has been used as a component of irinotecan/fluorouracil/levoleucovorin (FOLFIRI) or oxaliplatin/fluorouracil/levoleucovorin (FOLFOX) regimens for treatment of advanced-stage colorectal cancer; however, data are not available from randomized studies directly comparing safety and efficacy of levoleucovorin versus racemic leucovorin in such regimens. Randomized studies evaluating different schedules of various FOLFOX regimens (i.e., FOLFOX4, FOLFOX6, modified FOLFOX6, FOLFOX7), as well as the FOLFIRI regimen, have allowed use of either IV levoleucovorin or racemic leucovorin in these regimens, although the basis for selection of one leucovorin formulation over the other is unclear. Available response and toxicity data from these studies reflect the treatment schedules and sequences evaluated; analyses based on the leucovorin formulation used have not been reported.

In the FOCUS (Fluorouracil, Oxaliplatin, and CPT11[irinotecan]–Use and Sequencing) study in patients with poor-prognosis, advanced-stage colorectal cancer, levoleucovorin was used exclusively as the leucovorin component of the fluorouracil-, irinotecan-, and oxaliplatin-based regimens evaluated for first- or second-line therapy. Safety and response data have been reported from this study for the various chemotherapy sequences and combinations studied; however, the specific effects attributable to levoleucovorin have not been fully characterized.

Data are not available from randomized studies directly comparing safety and efficacy of levoleucovorin and racemic leucovorin in combination with fluorouracil and either irinotecan or oxaliplatin in patients with advanced-stage colorectal cancer. Published data describing the use of levoleucovorin as a component of combination therapy with a fluorouracil-based regimen (i.e., FOLFOX or FOLFIRI) and bevacizumab are not available; therefore, the safety of levoleucovorin in such combination regimens has not been fully established.

Dosage and Administration

■ **Reconstitution and Administration** Levoleucovorin calcium is administered by IV administration; the drug should *not* be administered intrathecally. When administered by IV injection, the injection rate should not exceed 160 mg of levoleucovorin per minute (16 mL per minute as a 10-mg/mL solution) because of the calcium concentration (4.26 mg Ca^{++} per 64 mg of levoleucovorin calcium pentahydrate) of the solution. Levoleucovorin has been administered by IV infusion in various published studies.

Levoleucovorin calcium is commercially available as a powder for injection and as an injection solution. Strict aseptic technique must be observed since the drug contains no preservative.

Levoleucovorin calcium powder for injection is reconstituted by adding 5.3 mL of 0.9% sodium chloride injection to a vial labeled as containing 50 mg of levoleucovorin to provide a solution containing 10 mg/mL. The manufacturer states that reconstitution with sodium chloride solutions containing preservatives (e.g., benzyl alcohol) has not been studied and is not recommended. Following reconstitution, levoleucovorin solution may be administered by IV injection or further diluted, immediately, in an appropriate volume of 0.9% sodium chloride injection or 5% dextrose injection to yield a concentration of 0.5–5 mg/mL. Following reconstitution or further dilution using 0.9% sodium chloride injection, levoleucovorin is stable for up to 12 hours when stored at room temperature. Following dilution in 5% dextrose injection, the drug is stable for up to 4 hours when stored at room temperature.

The commercially available levoleucovorin 10-mg/mL injection may be further diluted in an appropriate volume of 0.9% sodium chloride injection or 5% dextrose injection to yield a concentration of 0.5 mg/mL. Following dilution in 0.9% sodium chloride injection or 5% dextrose injection, the drug is stable for up to 4 hours when stored at room temperature.

Reconstituted and diluted solutions of levoleucovorin should be inspected visually for particulate matter and discoloration prior to administration whenever solution and container permit; the solutions should not be used if cloudiness or a precipitate is observed.

Because of the risk of precipitation, levoleucovorin should not be combined with other agents in the same admixture.

■ **Dosage** Levoleucovorin is commercially available as the calcium pentahydrate; dosage of the drug is expressed in terms of levoleucovorin (i.e., 64 mg of levoleucovorin calcium pentahydrate is equivalent to 50 mg of levoleucovorin).

Levoleucovorin is dosed at one-half the usual dosage of racemic leucovorin. (See Description.) The manufacturer makes no specific recommendations regarding dosage in pediatric patients; however, safety and efficacy of levoleucovorin have been evaluated in 16 patients 6–21 years of age. (See Uses: Toxicity Associated with Folic Acid Antagonists.)

Toxicity Associated with Folic Acid Antagonists **Rescue after High-dose Methotrexate Therapy.** Dosage recommendations for levoleucovorin are based on a methotrexate dosage of 12 g/m² administered by IV infusion over 4 hours; the prescribing information for methotrexate should be consulted for additional information. Dosage and duration of levoleucovorin rescue therapy should be adjusted based on the elimination pattern of methotrexate and the patient's renal function (see Table 1).

Serum creatinine and methotrexate concentrations should be monitored at least once daily. Levoleucovorin therapy should be continued, and adequate hydration and urinary alkalinization (pH of 7 or greater) maintained, until serum methotrexate concentration declines to less than 0.05 micromolar (5×10^{-8} *M*). Patients who experience delayed early methotrexate elimination are likely to develop reversible renal failure; therefore, fluid and electrolyte status also should be closely monitored in such patients until serum methotrexate concentration declines to less than 0.05 micromolar (5×10^{-8} *M*) and renal failure has resolved.

Table 1. Guidelines for Levoleucovorin Dosage Adjustment in Patients with Normal or Delayed Methotrexate Elimination

Clinical Situation	Serum Methotrexate Concentration[a]	Levoleucovorin Dosage and Monitoring
Normal methotrexate elimination[b]	Approximately 10 micromolar (10^{-5} *M*) at 24 hours, 1 micromolar (10^{-6} *M*) at 48 hours, and less than 0.2 micromolar (2 x 10^{-7} *M*) at 72 hours after methotrexate administration	7.5 mg (approximately 5 mg/m²) IV every 6 hours for 60 hours (10 doses), starting at 24 hours after initiation of methotrexate infusion[b]
Delayed late methotrexate elimination	Greater than 0.2 micromolar (2 x 10^{-7} *M*) at 72 hours and greater than 0.05 micromolar (5 x 10^{-8} *M*) at 96 hours after methotrexate administration	Continue levoleucovorin 7.5 mg IV every 6 hours until methotrexate concentration declines to less than 0.05 micromolar (5 x 10^{-8} *M*)
Delayed early methotrexate elimination and/or evidence of acute renal injury	50 micromolar (5 x 10^{-5} *M*) or greater at 24 hours or 5 micromolar (5 x 10^{-6} *M*) or greater at 48 hours after methotrexate administration, *or* a 100% or greater increase in serum creatinine concentration at 24 hours after methotrexate administration (e.g., an increase from 0.5 to 1 mg/dL or more)	75 mg IV every 3 hours until methotrexate concentration declines to less than 1 micromolar (10^{-6} *M*), then 7.5 mg IV every 3 hours until methotrexate concentration declines to less than 0.05 micromolar (5 x 10^{-8} *M*)

[a] The possibility that the patient is receiving other drugs that interact with methotrexate (e.g., by decreasing methotrexate elimination, binding to serum albumin) should always be considered when laboratory abnormalities or clinical toxicities are observed.

[b] In patients with mild abnormalities in methotrexate elimination or renal function who experience clinically important toxicity, levoleucovorin rescue should be extended for an additional 24 hours (i.e., 14 doses over 84 hours) for subsequent methotrexate courses.

Methotrexate Overdosage. Levoleucovorin rescue should begin as soon as possible following unintentional overdosage and within 24 hours of methotrexate administration if delayed elimination is detected; delayed administration of levoleucovorin may reduce its effectiveness in counteracting toxicity associated with folic acid antagonists.

The usual levoleucovorin dosage for management of methotrexate overdosage is 7.5 mg (approximately 5 mg/m²) IV every 6 hours until serum methotrexate concentration declines to less than 0.01 micromolar (10^{-8} *M*). Serum creatinine and serum methotrexate concentrations should be determined at 24-hour intervals. If the 24-hour serum creatinine concentration increases 50% over baseline, the 24-hour methotrexate concentration is greater than 5 micromolar (5 x 10^{-6} *M*), or the 48-hour methotrexate concentration is greater than 0.9 micromolar (9 x 10^{-7} *M*), levoleucovorin dosage should be increased to 50 mg/m² IV every 3 hours until serum methotrexate concentration declines to less than 0.01 micromolar (10^{-8} *M*). Hydration (3 L daily) and urinary alkalinization with sodium bicarbonate (to maintain a urinary pH of 7 or greater) should be employed concomitantly.

Colorectal Cancer **Combined Therapy with Fluorouracil for Advanced-stage Colorectal Cancer.** Regimens of levoleucovorin and fluorouracil that historically have been used for the palliative treatment of advanced-stage colorectal cancer include a levoleucovorin dose of 100 mg/m² administered by slow IV injection (over a minimum of 3 minutes) followed by an IV fluorouracil dose of 370 mg/m², or a levoleucovorin dose of 10 mg/m² administered by IV injection followed by an IV fluorouracil dose of 425 mg/m². Either regimen is administered daily for 5 days and may be repeated at 4-week intervals for 2 additional courses; thereafter, the regimen may be repeated at intervals of 4–5 weeks provided toxicity from the previous course of combined therapy has resolved completely.

Dosage of fluorouracil in subsequent courses of therapy should be adjusted according to patient tolerance of the prior treatment course; dosage of levoleucovorin in subsequent courses is not adjusted because of toxicity. Daily fluorouracil dosage generally is reduced by 20% in patients who experienced moderate hematologic or GI toxicity in the prior course and by 30% in those patients who experienced severe toxicity. If no toxicity occurs, fluorouracil dosage may be increased by 10%.

Other levoleucovorin and fluorouracil dosage regimens also have been used. (See Levoleucovorin and Fluorouracil under Colorectal Cancer: Combined Therapy with Fluorouracil for Advanced-stage Colorectal Cancer, in Uses.)

■ **Special Populations** ***Patients with Delayed Methotrexate Elimination*** Higher dosages and extended duration of levoleucovorin therapy may be required if delayed methotrexate excretion is caused by third space fluid accumulation (i.e., ascites, pleural effusion), renal impairment, or inadequate hydration.

Cautions

■ **Contraindications** Pernicious anemia or other megaloblastic anemias secondary to lack of vitamin B_{12}; such use may obscure the diagnosis of pernicious anemia by alleviating hematologic manifestations while allowing neurologic complications to progress.

Hypersensitivity to folic acid or folinic acid.

■ **Warnings/Precautions** ***Rate of Administration*** The injection rate should not exceed 160 mg of levoleucovorin per minute (16 mL per minute as a 10-mg/mL solution) because of the calcium concentration of the solution.

Toxicity Potentiation with Concomitant Therapy Levoleucovorin potentiates the toxicity of fluorouracil; therefore, fluorouracil dosage must be reduced when levoleucovorin is used concomitantly in the treatment of advanced-stage colorectal cancer. Although toxicities in patients receiving levoleucovorin in combination with fluorouracil are qualitatively similar to those in patients receiving fluorouracil alone, GI toxicities (particularly stomatitis and diarrhea) occur more frequently and may be more severe or prolonged in patients receiving combined therapy. Deaths from severe enterocolitis, diarrhea, and dehydration have been reported in geriatric patients receiving weekly racemic leucovorin concomitantly with fluorouracil. In addition, in a study evaluating higher weekly dosages of fluorouracil and racemic leucovorin, an increased risk of severe GI toxicity was observed in geriatric and/or debilitated patients.

In several clinical trials in patients with advanced-stage colorectal cancer, treatment-related toxicity occurred more frequently in patients receiving a low dose of racemic leucovorin (20 mg/m²) in combination with fluorouracil (425 mg/m²) than in patients receiving a higher dose of racemic leucovorin (200 mg/m²) in combination with fluorouracil (370 mg/m²). In one study, 20% of patients receiving fluorouracil in combination with racemic leucovorin 20 mg/m² experienced toxicity (primarily GI toxicity) requiring hospitalization, compared with 7% of those receiving fluorouracil alone or in combination with racemic leucovorin 200 mg/m². In another study, 11% of patients receiving fluorouracil in combination with racemic leucovorin 20 mg/m² required hospitalization for treatment-related toxicity, compared with 3% of those receiving fluorouracil in combination with racemic leucovorin 200 mg/m².

Combined therapy with fluorouracil and levoleucovorin should not be initiated or continued in patients with symptomatic GI toxicity until such symptoms have resolved completely. Patients who develop diarrhea should be monitored with particular care until the diarrhea has resolved, since rapid clinical deterioration and death can occur. (See Cautions: Precautions and Contraindications, in Leucovorin Calcium 92:12.)

Concomitant use of racemic leucovorin with co-trimoxazole for treatment of *Pneumocystis jiroveci* (formerly *P. carinii*) pneumonia in patients with HIV infection has been associated with increased rates of treatment failure and morbidity.

Seizures and/or syncope have occurred rarely in cancer patients receiving racemic leucovorin, usually in conjunction with fluoropyrimidine therapy; cases have occurred most commonly in patients with other predisposing factors (e.g., CNS metastasis). A causal relationship to racemic leucovorin has not been fully established.

Sensitivity Reactions Allergic reactions have been reported in patients receiving levoleucovorin.

Specific Populations **Pregnancy.** Category C. (See Users Guide.)

Lactation. It is not known whether levoleucovorin is distributed into milk; because of the potential for serious adverse reactions to levoleucovorin in nursing infants, a decision should be made whether to discontinue nursing or the drug, taking into account the importance of the drug to the woman.

Pediatric Use. Safety and efficacy of levoleucovorin have been evaluated in 16 patients 6–21 years of age. (See Uses: Toxicity Associated with Folic Acid Antagonists.) The manufacturer makes no specific recommendations regarding use in pediatric patients.

Geriatric Use. Clinical studies of levoleucovorin in the treatment of osteosarcoma did not include patients 65 years of age and older to determine whether geriatric patients respond differently than younger patients.

In a clinical trial evaluating levoleucovorin in combination with fluorouracil for the treatment of advanced-stage colorectal cancer, adverse reactions were consistent with known toxicities of fluorouracil; no overall differences in adverse effects were observed between geriatric patients (65 years of age or older) and younger adults. However, deaths from severe enterocolitis, diarrhea, and dehydration have been reported in geriatric patients receiving weekly racemic leucovorin concomitantly with fluorouracil. (See Cautions: Precautions and Contraindications, in Leucovorin Calcium 92:12.)

Renal Impairment. Renal impairment may cause delayed methotrexate elimination; higher dosages and extended duration of levoleucovorin therapy may be required in patients with renal impairment. (See Dosage and Administration: Special Populations.)

■ **Common Adverse Effects** Adverse effects reported in more than 15% of patients receiving levoleucovorin rescue following high-dose methotrexate therapy include vomiting, stomatitis, and nausea. Less frequently reported adverse effects, occurring in less than 10% of patients, include diarrhea, dyspepsia, typhlitis, dyspnea, dermatitis, confusion, neuropathy, abnormal renal function, and taste perversion.

Adverse effects reported in more than 50% of patients with advanced-stage colorectal cancer receiving levoleucovorin in combination with fluorouracil include diarrhea, nausea, and stomatitis. Other frequently reported adverse effects, occurring in 20–40% of patients, include vomiting, asthenia/fatigue/malaise, anorexia/decreased appetite, dermatitis, and alopecia. The incidence of adverse effects is similar to that reported in patients receiving an equipotent dosage of racemic leucovorin in combination with fluorouracil.

Drug Interactions

■ **Anticonvulsants** Folic acid in large amounts may counteract the anticonvulsant effect of phenobarbital, phenytoin, and primidone and increase the frequency of seizures in susceptible children. Racemic leucovorin has been shown to increase hepatic metabolism and decrease plasma concentrations of phenytoin in rats. Therefore, caution is advised when levoleucovorin is used concomitantly with anticonvulsants.

■ **Co-trimoxazole** Concomitant use of racemic leucovorin with co-trimoxazole for treatment of *Pneumocystis jiroveci* (formerly *P. carinii*) pneumonia in patients with HIV infection has been associated with increased rates of treatment failure and morbidity.

■ **Fluorouracil** Levoleucovorin potentiates the toxicity of fluorouracil. (See Toxicity Potentiation with Concomitant Therapy under Cautions: Warnings/Precautions.)

■ **Glucarpidase** In patients receiving high-dose methotrexate therapy with leucovorin rescue, administration of glucarpidase (an enzyme that converts methotrexate to inactive metabolites) 2 hours before a racemic leucovorin dose reduced systemic exposure and peak plasma concentrations of leucovorin and its active metabolite, 5-methyltetrahydrofolate. Similar effects would be expected with levoleucovorin. In addition, methotrexate concentrations measured by immunoassay within 48 hours following glucarpidase administration are unreliable. Racemic leucovorin or levoleucovorin should not be administered within 2 hours before or after glucarpidase administration. Dosage adjustment of the continuing racemic leucovorin or levoleucovorin regimen is not necessary since dosage is based on the patient's methotrexate concentration prior to glucarpidase administration. During the first 48 hours after glucarpidase administration, racemic leucovorin or levoleucovorin should be administered at the same dosage administered prior to glucarpidase administration; beyond 48 hours, dosage should be based on the measured methotrexate concentration. Therapy with racemic leucovorin or levoleucovorin should be continued until the methotrexate concentration has been maintained below the threshold for such treatment for at least 3 days.

■ **Methotrexate** High dosages of racemic leucovorin may reduce the efficacy of intrathecally administered methotrexate.

Description

Levoleucovorin is the levorotatory (*l*) isomer of racemic *d,l*-leucovorin. Levoleucovorin is the pharmacologically active isomer and constitutes approximately 50% of racemic leucovorin; therefore, the effects of levoleucovorin are observed at half the dose of racemic leucovorin. Because levoleucovorin is a reduced derivative of folic acid and does not require reduction by dihydrofolate reductase to participate in reactions utilizing folates, the drug counteracts the therapeutic and toxic effects of folic acid antagonists (e.g., methotrexate). The drug also enhances the efficacy and toxicity of fluoropyrimidines (e.g., fluorouracil) by stabilizing binding of the fluorouracil metabolite 5-fluoro-2′-deoxyuridine-5′-monophosphate (FdUMP) to thymidylate synthase (an enzyme responsible for DNA repair and replication), thus enhancing inhibition of this enzyme.

Levoleucovorin is actively and passively transported across cell membranes. In vivo, levoleucovorin is converted to 5-methyltetrahydrofolic acid (5-methyl-THF), the primary circulating form of active reduced folate. Levoleucovorin and 5-methyl-THF are polyglutamated intracellularly by the enzyme folylpolyglutamate synthetase. Folylpolyglutamates are active and participate in numerous biochemical pathways that require reduced folate.

Following IV administration of a single 15-mg dose of levoleucovorin in healthy male volunteers, peak serum concentrations of (6*S*)-5-methyl-5,6,7,8-tetrahydrofolate (the *l*-isomer of 5-methyl-THF) were reached within 0.9 hours. The mean terminal half-life of total tetrahydrofolate and (6*S*)-5-methyl-5,6,7,8-tetrahydrofolate were 5.1 and 6.8 hours, respectively. Levoleucovorin and its metabolites are excreted in urine.

Data from several crossover studies in healthy individuals and patients with colorectal cancer have shown no substantial differences in exposure to the *l*-isomer of leucovorin or to 5-methyltetrahydrofolate regardless of whether IV racemic leucovorin or an equipotent dose of IV levoleucovorin is administered.

Advice to Patients

Risk of diarrhea, vomiting, stomatitis, and nausea.

Importance of women informing clinicians immediately if they are or plan to become pregnant or plan to breast-feed.

Importance of informing clinicians of existing or contemplated concomitant therapy, including prescription and OTC drugs, as well as any concomitant illnesses (e.g., renal impairment).

Importance of informing patients of other important precautionary information. (See Cautions.)

Overview® (see Users Guide). For additional information on this drug until a more detailed monograph is developed and published, the manufacturer's labeling should be consulted. It is *essential* that the manufacturer's labeling be consulted for more detailed information on usual cautions, precautions, contraindications, potential drug interactions, laboratory test interferences, and acute toxicity.

Preparations

Excipients in commercially available drug preparations may have clinically important effects in some individuals; consult specific product labeling for details.

LEVOleucovorin Calcium

Parenteral

For injection, for IV use	50 mg (of levoleucovorin)	**Fusilev®**, Spectrum
Injection, for IV use	10 mg (of levoleucovorin) per mL (175 and 250 mg)	**Fusilev®**, Spectrum

†Use is not currently included in the labeling approved by the US Food and Drug Administration

Selected Revisions December 2012, © Copyright, January 2009, American Society of Health-System Pharmacists, Inc.

Pralidoxime Chloride

2-Pyridine Aldoxime Methochloride, 2-PAM Chloride

Uses

■ **Organophosphate Pesticide Poisoning** Pralidoxime chloride is used concomitantly with atropine and supportive measures (e.g., removal of secretions, maintenance of an adequate airway, and artificial ventilation) to reverse muscle paralysis (particularly of respiratory muscles) associated with toxic exposure to organophosphate anticholinesterase pesticides and chemicals. Pralidoxime appears to be most effective when given soon after exposure; the drug may still be effective if more than 48 hours have elapsed. Clinical cases in which atropine and pralidoxime have been used include toxic exposure to azodrin, bidrin, carbophenthion, coumaphos (Co-ral), DFP, diazinon, dichlorvos, dichlorvos with chlordane, dicrotophos, dimethoate, disulfoton, EPN, guthion, isoflurophate, Metasystox 1® and fenthion, methyl demeton, methyl parathion, mevinphos, OMPA, parathion, parathion and mevinphos, phosdrin, phosphamidon, sarin, Systox®, trithion, and TEPP. Results of animal studies indicate that pralidoxime may be an effective antidote in toxic exposure to various other organophosphates possessing anticholinesterase activity, but the drug appears to be ineffective or only marginally effective against toxic exposure to Ciodrin®, dimefox, dimethoate, methyl diazinon, methyl phencapton, mipafox, phorate, schradan, and Wepsyn®. Pralidoxime is not effective in the treatment of toxic exposure to phosphorus, inorganic phosphates, or organophosphates which do not possess anticholinesterase activity.

■ **Chemical Warfare Agent Poisoning** Pralidoxime chloride is used concomitantly with atropine for the treatment of nerve agent poisoning in the context of chemical warfare or terrorism. Pralidoxime chloride must be administered within minutes to hours following exposure to nerve agents to be effective.

The most toxic of the known chemical warfare agents are the nerve agents. Most nerve agents are liquid at room temperature (although most are volatile at ambient temperatures, the term nerve gas is a misnomer); nerve agents are readily absorbed after inhalation of aerosols (e.g., following an explosion), ingestion, or dermal contact. Nerve agents (e.g., sarin, soman, tabun, VX [methylphosphonothionic acid]) are chemically similar to the organophosphate pesticides and exert their biologic effects by inhibiting acetylcholinesterase enzymes. Nerve agents alter cholinergic synaptic transmission at neuroeffector junctions (muscarinic effects), at skeletal myoneural junctions and autonomic ganglia (nicotinic effects), and in the CNS. Manifestations of nerve agent exposure include rhinorrhea, chest tightness, pinpoint pupils, dyspnea, excessive salivation and sweating, nausea, vomiting, abdominal cramps, involuntary defecation and/or urination, muscle twitching, confusion, seizures, flaccid paralysis, coma, respiratory failure, and death. While initial effects of nerve agent exposure depend on the dose and route of exposure, signs and symptoms generally are similar regardless of the route of exposure. Manifestations may not be apparent until as long as 18 hours following dermal exposure, and CNS effects (e.g., fatigue, irritability, nervousness, memory impairment) may persist as long as 6 weeks following recovery from the acute effects of nerve agent exposure.

Initial management of nerve agent poisoning includes aggressive airway control and ventilation (administration of nebulized β-adrenergic agonist [e.g., albuterol] and antimuscarinics [e.g., ipratropium bromide] may be necessary), and administration of atropine and pralidoxime chloride. Diazepam may be needed for seizure control. Rapid decontamination using standard hazardous materials (HAZMAT) procedures is important to prevent further absorption by the victim and to prevent contamination of others (e.g., emergency personnel, health-care workers) by direct contact or off-gassing of nerve agents from contaminated clothing. Following initial therapy and decontamination, additional treatment with atropine and supportive measures in a hospital setting are likely to be necessary.

■ **Other Uses** Atropine is generally used alone in the treatment of muscarinic toxicity resulting from exposure to carbamate insecticides; pralidoxime is not generally used. Pralidoxime is contraindicated in the treatment of toxic exposure to carbaryl since it appears to increase the toxicity of carbaryl.

Pralidoxime has been used for the management of overdosage of drugs that carbamylate cholinesterase, such as ambenonium, neostigmine, and pyridostigmine, particularly in the treatment of cholinergic crisis in patients with myasthenia gravis. However, pralidoxime is reportedly less effective against these agents than against organophosphate anticholinesterases and may precipitate a myasthenic crisis in these patients. (See Cautions: Precautions and Contraindications.)

Dosage and Administration

■ **Reconstitution and Administration** Pralidoxime chloride is usually administered IV, preferably as an infusion given over 15–30 minutes. (See Cautions: Adverse Effects.) In patients with pulmonary edema or if IV infusion is not practical or a more rapid effect is desired, pralidoxime chloride solutions containing 50 mg/mL may be administered by slow IV injection over a period of at least 5 minutes. Pralidoxime chloride may also be administered by IM injection.

Pralidoxime chloride sterile powder for injection is reconstituted by adding

20 mL of sterile water for injection to the vial labeled as containing 1 g of the drug to provide a solution containing approximately 50 mg/mL. Because of the relatively large volume of diluent required, sterile water for injection containing preservatives should not be used to reconstitute pralidoxime chloride sterile powder for injection. Following reconstitution, pralidoxime chloride solutions should be used within a few hours. For IV infusion, the calculated dose of the reconstituted solution is further diluted in 100 mL with 0.9% sodium chloride injection.

To facilitate out-of-hospital IM administration in the event of pesticide or nerve agent poisoning, pralidoxime chloride injection is available as an auto-injector (pralidoxime chloride injection auto-injector). In addition, pralidoxime chloride is available in an auto-injector that also contains atropine (DuoDote® auto-injector, ATNAA auto-injector). Each prefilled DuoDote® auto-syringe and each prefilled ATNAA auto-syringe provides a single IM dose of atropine 2.1 mg and pralidoxime chloride 600 mg. When activated, the auto-injector sequentially administers atropine and pralidoxime chloride through a single needle. For *self-administration* or administration by a partner or civilian emergency responder in an out-of-hospital setting, the contents of a pralidoxime chloride auto-injector or atropine and pralidoxime chloride auto-injector (DuoDote®) should be injected IM into the anterolateral aspect of the thigh. In an out-of-hospital setting, the contents of an atropine and pralidoxime chloride auto-injector (ATNAA) should be injected IM into the anterolateral aspect of the thigh or into the buttock.

For IM administration, some authorities suggest that pralidoxime chloride sterile powder for injection be reconstituted by adding 3 mL of sterile water for injection or 0.9% sodium chloride for injection to the vial labeled as containing 1 g of the drug to provide a solution containing 300 mg/mL.

■ **Dosage** ***Organophosphate Pesticide Poisoning*** For the treatment of toxic exposure to organophosphate cholinesterase inhibitors, pralidoxime therapy should be initiated at the same time as atropine. The usual initial IV dose of pralidoxime chloride is 1–2 g given over 15 to 30 minutes for adults, or 20–40 mg/kg given over 30 minutes for children. Dosage of pralidoxime chloride should be reduced in patients with renal insufficiency. The dose of pralidoxime chloride may be repeated in about 1 hour if muscle weakness has not been relieved. Additional doses may be administered cautiously if muscle weakness continues. Alternatively, some clinicians recommend continuous IV infusion of 500 mg of the drug per hour. In severe cases, especially after ingestion of the poison, the manufacturer recommends electrocardiographic monitoring because the anticholinesterase may cause heart block. Continued absorption of the anticholinesterase from the lower bowel constitutes new exposure; in such cases, additional doses of pralidoxime may be needed every 3–8 hours. As in all cases of organophosphate poisoning, the patient should be observed closely for at least 24 hours.

To facilitate out-of-hospital administration, pralidoxime is available in a prefilled auto-injector containing atropine 2.1 mg and pralidoxime chloride 600 mg (e.g., DuoDote®); the auto-injector should be used by emergency medical service personnel. For administration in an out-of-hospital setting, the dose of pralidoxime and atropine (DuoDote®) is based on severity of symptoms. For the treatment of adults with 2 or more mild symptoms of pesticide exposure (e.g., miosis or blurred vision, tearing, runny nose, hypersalivation or drooling, wheezing, muscle fasciculations, nausea/vomiting), administer contents of one auto-injector (atropine 2.1 mg and pralidoxime chloride 600 mg) by IM injection. If the patient develops any severe symptoms (behavioral changes, severe breathing difficulty, severe respiratory secretions, severe muscle twitching, involuntary defecation or urination, seizures, unconsciousness), administer contents of two additional auto-injectors IM in rapid succession. For the treatment of adults who present with any severe symptoms, administer contents of three auto-injectors (total dose: atropine 6.3 mg and pralidoxime chloride 1800 mg) IM in rapid succession. Additional doses should not be administered unless definitive medical care is available.

Chemical Warfare Agents The dose and route of administration of pralidoxime chloride for the treatment of nerve agent (e.g., sarin, soman, tabun, VX [methylphosphonothioic acid]) poisoning in the context of chemical warfare or terrorism is based on the severity of symptoms (i.e., mild/moderate or severe), the victim's age, and the treatment setting. Mild to moderate symptoms include localized sweating, muscle fasciculations, nausea, vomiting, weakness, and/or dyspnea; severe symptoms include apnea, flaccid paralysis, seizures, and/or unconsciousness. Pralidoxime chloride must be administered within minutes to hours following exposure to nerve agents to be effective. Pralidoxime is administered concomitantly with atropine.

For the immediate treatment of nerve agent poisoning in an out-of-hospital setting, pralidoxime chloride usually is administered IM. The usual out-of-hospital IM adult dose is 600 mg for those with mild to moderate symptoms and 1800 mg for those with severe symptoms; frail geriatric adults with mild to moderate symptoms may receive 10 mg/kg and those with severe symptoms may receive 25 mg/kg. In an out-of-hospital setting, the usual IM dose of pralidoxime chloride for children 0–10 years of age and adolescents older than 10 years of age with mild to moderate symptoms is 15 mg/kg, and the usual dose for children 0–10 years of age and adolescents older than 10 years of age with severe symptoms is 25 mg/kg.

To facilitate out-of-hospital administration, pralidoxime chloride injection is available in a prefilled auto-injector; the auto-injector should be used by individuals who have received adequate training in the recognition and treatment of nerve agent poisoning. For the initial treatment of adults with symptoms of nerve agent poisoning, one 600-mg IM dose of pralidoxime chloride should be administered; pralidoxime is administered after atropine. If symptoms are still present after 15 minutes, another dose of atropine and another 600-mg dose of pralidoxime chloride should be administered. If symptoms persist after an additional 15 minutes, another dose of atropine and another 600-mg dose of pralidoxime chloride should be administered. If symptoms persist after the third doses, medical care should be sought.

Another option for out-of-hospital administration is to administer atropine and pralidoxime using a prefilled auto-injector containing atropine 2.1 mg and pralidoxime chloride 600 mg (e.g., DuoDote®, ATNAA). For the treatment of adults with 2 or more mild symptoms of nerve agent poisoning (e.g., miosis or blurred vision, tearing, runny nose, hypersalivation or drooling, wheezing, muscle fasciculations, nausea/vomiting), the contents of one auto-injector (atropine 2.1 mg and pralidoxime chloride 600 mg) should be administered by IM injection. If the patient develops any severe symptoms (behavioral changes, severe breathing difficulty, severe respiratory secretions, severe muscle twitching, involuntary defecation or urination, seizures, unconsciousness), the contents of 2 additional auto-injectors should be administered by IM injection in rapid succession. For the treatment of adults who present with any severe symptoms, the contents of 3 auto-injectors (total dose: atropine 6.3 mg and pralidoxime chloride 1800 mg) should be administered by IM injection in rapid succession. Additional doses should not be administered unless definitive medical care is available.

In an emergency department or similar setting, pralidoxime chloride generally is administered by slow IV injection. When pralidoxime chloride is administered IV in such a setting for the treatment of nerve agent poisoning, the usual adult dose is 15 mg/kg (maximum 1 g) for those with mild to moderate or severe symptoms; frail geriatric adults with mild to moderate or severe symptoms may receive 5–10 mg/kg. In an emergency department setting, the usual IV dose of pralidoxime chloride for children 0–10 years of age and adolescents older than 10 years of age with mild to moderate or severe symptoms is 15 mg/kg. Atropine is administered concomitantly with pralidoxime.

Diazepam may be administered for seizure control.

Other Uses As an antagonist to carbamate anticholinesterase agents used in the treatment of myasthenia gravis (e.g., ambenonium, neostigmine, pyridostigmine), 1–2 g of pralidoxime chloride has been given IV initially, followed by 250 mg every 5 minutes.

Cautions

■ **Adverse Effects** Although pralidoxime is generally well-tolerated, dizziness, blurred vision, diplopia and impaired accommodation, headache, drowsiness, nausea, tachycardia, hyperventilation, maculopapular rash, and muscular weakness have been reported following administration of the drug. However, it is difficult to differentiate the toxic effects produced by atropine or organophosphates from those of pralidoxime, and the condition of patients suffering from organophosphate intoxication will generally mask minor signs and symptoms reported in normal subjects who receive pralidoxime. When atropine and pralidoxime are used concomitantly, signs of atropinism may occur earlier than when atropine is used alone, especially if the total dose of atropine is large and administration of pralidoxime is delayed. Excitement, confusion, manic behavior, and muscle rigidity have been reported following recovery of consciousness, but these symptoms have also occurred in patients who were not treated with pralidoxime.

Rapid IV injection of pralidoxime has produced tachycardia, laryngospasm, muscle rigidity, and transient neuromuscular blockade; therefore, the drug should be administered slowly, preferably by IV infusion. IV administration of pralidoxime reportedly may also cause hypertension which is related to the dose and rate of infusion. Some clinicians recommend that the patient's blood pressure be monitored during pralidoxime therapy. For adults, IV administration of 5 mg of phentolamine mesylate reportedly quickly reverses pralidoxime-induced hypertension.

IM administration of pralidoxime may produce mild pain at the injection site.

■ **Precautions and Contraindications** Pralidoxime should always be used under close medical supervision.

Pralidoxime should be used with caution in patients with myasthenia gravis who are receiving anticholinesterase agents, since the drug may precipitate a myasthenic crisis.

Pralidoxime should be used with caution and in reduced dosage in patients with impaired renal function.

The use of succinylcholine, theophylline, aminophylline, reserpine, and respiratory depressants (e.g., barbiturates, morphine, phenothiazines) should be avoided in patients with toxic exposure to anticholinesterase compounds.

■ **Pregnancy** Safe use of pralidoxime during pregnancy has not been established.

Pharmacology

The principal pharmacologic effect of pralidoxime is reactivation of cholinesterase which has been recently inactivated by phosphorylation as the result of exposure to certain organophosphates. Pralidoxime removes the phosphoryl group from the active site of the inhibited enzyme by nucleophilic attack, regenerating active cholinesterase and forming an oxime complex. Pralidoxime also detoxifies certain organophosphates by direct chemical reaction and probably also reacts directly with cholinesterase to protect it from inhibition. Pralidoxime must be administered before aging of the inhibited enzyme occurs; after aging is completed, phosphorylated cholinesterase cannot be reactivated, and newly synthesized cholinesterase must replace the inhibited enzyme. Pralidoxime is not equally antagonistic to all anticholinesterases, partly because the time period required for aging of the inhibited enzyme varies and depends on the specific organophosphate bound to the cholinesterase.

Pralidoxime also reactivates cholinesterase which has been inactivated by carbamylation. However, carbamylated cholinesterase has a much faster rate of spontaneous reactivation than does phosphorylated cholinesterase.

Cholinesterase reactivation produced by pralidoxime occurs principally at the neuromuscular junction and results in reversal of anticholinesterase-induced paralysis of respiratory and other skeletal muscles. The drug also reactivates cholinesterase at autonomic effector sites and, to a lesser degree, within the CNS. Pralidoxime is effective against nicotinic manifestations of anticholinesterase poisoning (e.g., muscular twitching, fasciculation, cramps, weakness, pallor, tachycardia, elevated blood pressure). The drug does not substantially influence muscarinic effects (e.g., bronchoconstriction, dyspnea, cough, increased bronchial secretion, nausea, vomiting, abdominal cramps, diarrhea, increased sweating, salivation, lacrimation, bradycardia, fall in blood pressure, miosis, blurred vision, urinary frequency, and incontinence). Therefore, pralidoxime is used in conjunction with atropine, which ameliorates muscarinic symptoms and directly blocks the effects of accumulation of excess acetylcholine at various sites including the respiratory center.

Other reported pharmacologic effects of pralidoxime include depolarization at the neuromuscular junction, anticholinergic action, mild inhibition of cholinesterase, sympathomimetic effects, potentiation of the depressor action of acetylcholine in nonatropinized animals, and potentiation of the pressor action of acetylcholine in atropinized animals. However, the contribution of these effects to the therapeutic action of the drug has not been established.

Pharmacokinetics

■ **Absorption** Absorption of pralidoxime chloride is variable and incomplete following oral administration (oral tablets of the drug are no longer commercially available in the US). Based on results of animal studies, the minimum therapeutic plasma concentration of pralidoxime is considered to be 4 mcg/mL. Peak plasma oxime concentrations are reached 5–15 minutes after IV administration and 10–20 minutes after IM administration of pralidoxime chloride. In a study in healthy adults, IV pralidoxime chloride doses of 7.5–10 mg/kg were needed to produce plasma oxime concentrations of 4 mcg/mL or greater at 1 hour after administration; IM doses of 7.5–10 mg/kg were needed to achieve initial plasma concentrations of 4 mcg/mL or greater, and only IM doses of 10 mg/kg maintained plasma oxime concentrations at 4 mcg/mL or greater for 1 hour.

■ **Distribution** Pralidoxime is distributed throughout the extracellular water. Because of its quaternary ammonium structure, the drug is not generally believed to enter the CNS, but recent animal studies and human clinical responses observed by some investigators have raised some controversy on this point. Pralidoxime does not readily penetrate the cornea following systemic or topical administration, but therapeutic concentrations are reportedly achieved in the eye following subconjunctival injection. Pralidoxime is not appreciably bound to plasma proteins.

It is not known if pralidoxime is distributed into milk.

■ **Elimination** Although the exact metabolic fate of pralidoxime has not been completely elucidated, the drug is believed to be metabolized in the liver. The half-life of pralidoxime in patients with normal renal function varies and has been reported to range from 0.8–2.7 hours. Pralidoxime is rapidly excreted in urine as unchanged drug and as a metabolite. Approximately 80–90% of an IV or IM dose of pralidoxime chloride is excreted unchanged within 12 hours after administration. A recent study has suggested that active tubular secretion may be involved, although the specific mechanism has not been identified.

Chemistry

Pralidoxime chloride, a quaternary ammonium oxime, is a cholinesterase reactivator. The drug occurs as a white to pale yellow, crystalline powder and is freely soluble in water. Following reconstitution with sterile water for injection, pralidoxime chloride solutions containing 50 mg/mL have a pH of 3.5–4.5. The pK_a of pralidoxime is 7.8–8.

Preparations

Pralidoxime chloride injection auto-injector is supplied through the Directorate of Medical Materiel, Defense Supply Center Philadelphia or other local, state, or federal agency. ATNAA is supplied through the Directorate of Medical Material, Defense Supply Center Philadelphia. Duodote® is available for hospitals and emergency responders through Meridian Medical Technology (800-638-8093).

Excipients in commercially available drug preparations may have clinically important effects in some individuals; consult specific product labeling for details.

Pralidoxime Chloride

Parenteral		
For injection	1 g	Protopam® Chloride, Baxter
Injection	600 mg*	Pralidoxime Chloride Injection Auto-Injector

*available from one or more manufacturer, distributor, and/or repackager by generic (nonproprietary) name

Pralidoxime Chloride and Atropine

Parenteral		
Injection	600 mg/2 mL Pralidoxime Chloride and 2.1 mg/0.7 mL Atropine	ATNAA Auto-Injector (each drug is in a separate chamber), Meridian
	600 mg/2 mL Pralidoxime Chloride and 2.1 mg/0.7 mL Atropine	DuoDote® Auto-Injector (each drug is in a separate chamber), Meridian

Sugammadex Sodium

■ Sugammadex sodium, a modified γ-cyclodextrin, is a selective relaxant binding agent.

Uses

■ **Reversal of Neuromuscular Blockade** Sugammadex is used for the reversal of neuromuscular blockade induced by rocuronium bromide or vecuronium bromide in patients undergoing surgery. The drug substantially decreases the time to recovery from moderate or deep neuromuscular blockade induced by the steroidal neuromuscular blocking agents rocuronium and vecuronium. At the highest recommended dose of 16 mg/kg, sugammadex also demonstrated efficacy for rapid reversal of profound neuromuscular blockade induced by high-dose (1.2 mg/kg) rocuronium bromide when given shortly (approximately 3 minutes) after the onset of the neuromuscular block. Sugammadex is an effective reversal agent for rocuronium and vecuronium only and should *not* be used to reverse the effects of *nonsteroidal* neuromuscular blocking agents (e.g., succinylcholine, benzylisoquinolinium compounds [atracurium, mivacurium]).

Efficacy of sugammadex for reversal of *moderate* neuromuscular blockade induced by rocuronium or vecuronium was evaluated in a randomized, multicenter, active-controlled study in 189 adults (median age 50–51 years, median body weight 72–76 kg, 54% male) undergoing elective surgery under general anesthesia that required endotracheal intubation and maintenance of neuromuscular blockade. Surgical procedures were mainly endocrine, ocular, ENT (ear, nose, and throat), abdominal (gynecologic, colorectal, urologic), orthopedic, vascular, or dermatologic. Patients were first randomized to receive either rocuronium bromide (initial intubating dose of 0.6 mg/kg followed by 0.1–0.2 mg/kg as needed during surgery) or vecuronium bromide (initial intubating dose of 0.1 mg/kg followed by 0.02–0.03 mg/kg as needed during surgery) for neuromuscular blockade. The reversal agent (sugammadex 2 mg/kg or neostigmine methylsulfate 50 mcg/kg plus glycopyrrolate 10 mcg/kg) was then given at the reappearance of the second twitch (T_2) in a train-of-four (TOF) stimulation (indicating recovery to moderate neuromuscular blockade) after the last dose of rocuronium or vecuronium was administered. The primary measure of efficacy was time to recovery of the TOF twitch ratio to 0.9, which is the currently accepted standard for adequate recovery of neuromuscular function following use of neuromuscular blocking agents. Time to recovery of neuromuscular function was substantially faster following administration of sugammadex compared with neostigmine. In patients with rocuronium- or vecuronium-induced neuromuscular blockade, median time to recovery was 1.4 or 2.1 minutes, respectively, with sugammadex compared with 21.5 or 29 minutes, respectively, with neostigmine.

Efficacy of sugammadex for reversal of *deep* neuromuscular blockade induced by rocuronium or vecuronium was evaluated in a similarly designed randomized, active-controlled study in 157 adults (median age 54–56 years, median body weight 81–84 kg, 45% male) undergoing elective surgery under general anesthesia that required endotracheal intubation and maintenance of neuromuscular blockade. In this study, the surgical procedures were mainly abdominal (i.e., gynecologic, colorectal, urologic), orthopedic, reconstructive, or neurologic. Patients were randomized to receive rocuronium bromide (initial intubating dose of 0.6 mg/kg followed by 0.15 mg/kg as needed during surgery) or vecuronium bromide (initial intubating dose of 0.1 mg/kg followed by 0.015 mg/kg as needed during surgery) to maintain neuromuscular blockade. The reversal agent (sugammadex 4 mg/kg or neostigmine methylsulfate 70 mcg/kg plus glycopyrrolate 14 mcg/kg) was given at the reappearance of 1–2 posttetanic counts (indicating deep neuromuscular blockade) after the last dose of rocuronium or vecuronium was administered. The primary efficacy measure in this study also was time to recovery of the TOF twitch ratio to 0.9, although neostigmine was not expected to have an effect on recovery time since anticholinesterase agents are not effective in reversing deep neuromuscular blockade. Time to recovery of neuromuscular function was substantially faster following sugammadex administration compared with neostigmine; median time to recovery in patients receiving sugammadex was 2.7 or 3.3 minutes in the rocuronium or vecuronium groups, respectively, while time to recovery in patients receiving neostigmine was 49–50 minutes. A wider range of recovery times was observed with sugammadex in this study compared with recovery times in the study evaluating reversal from moderate neuromuscular blockade.

Efficacy of sugammadex for *rapid* reversal of rocuronium-induced neuromuscular blockade was evaluated in a randomized, active-controlled study that compared time to recovery from a profound rocuronium-induced neuromuscular block after administration of sugammadex with time to spontaneous recovery from succinylcholine. In this study, 110 patients (median age 43 years, median weight 70 kg, 42% male) undergoing elective surgery (mainly gynecologic, orthopedic, or reconstructive) that required endotracheal intubation and a short duration of neuromuscular blockade were randomized to receive high-dose rocuronium bromide (1.2 mg/kg) or succinylcholine chloride (1 mg/kg). Sugammadex was administered 3 minutes after the start of rocuronium. The primary measure of efficacy in this study was time from the start of administration of the neuromuscular blocking agent to recovery of the first twitch (T_1) in a TOF to 10% of the baseline value. Time to recovery of the TOF ratio to 0.9 was evaluated as a secondary end point. Mean time to recovery of T_1 to 10% of baseline was substantially faster with rocuronium/sugammadex than with spontaneous recovery from succinylcholine (4.4 and 7.1 minutes, respectively). In patients who received sugammadex, mean time to recovery of the TOF ratio to 0.9 was 2.2 minutes.

Sugammadex has not been studied for reversal of rocuronium- or vecuronium-induced neuromuscular blockade in the intensive care unit (ICU) setting.

Dosage and Administration

■ **General** Sugammadex should be administered only by trained clinicians experienced in the use of neuromuscular blocking agents and their reversal agents.

Patients should be monitored for adequate ventilation and maintenance of a patent airway from the time of sugammadex administration until complete recovery of neuromuscular function. (See Respiratory Function Monitoring under Cautions: Warnings/Precautions.) To ensure adequate reversal from the neuromuscular block, an objective (quantitative) method of monitoring such as peripheral nerve stimulation is recommended in conjunction with other clinical assessments (e.g., observation of skeletal muscle tone, respiratory measurements). Adequate recovery of neuromuscular function generally is defined as a train-of-four (TOF) ratio of at least 0.9 in addition to the patient's ability to maintain satisfactory ventilation and a patent airway.

If readministration of a steroidal neuromuscular blocking agent is required (e.g., for intubation) after reversal with sugammadex, a minimum wait time should be observed. (See Readministration of Neuromuscular Blocking Agents under Cautions: Warnings/Precautions.)

■ **Administration** Sugammadex is administered by direct IV ("bolus") injection over 10 seconds into an existing IV line. The manufacturer states that the drug has only been administered as a single direct IV injection in clinical trials.

Sugammadex injection should be inspected visually for particulate matter and discoloration prior to administration. The drug may be administered through an existing IV line containing the following solutions: 5% dextrose, 0.9% sodium chloride, 5% dextrose and 0.9% sodium chloride, 2.5% dextrose and 0.45% sodium chloride, Isolyte® P in 5% dextrose, Ringer's injection, or lactated Ringer's injection. The IV administration line should be adequately flushed (e.g., with 0.9% sodium chloride injection) between administration of sugammadex and other drugs. Sugammadex should not be mixed with other drugs.

Prior to use, sugammadex injection should be stored at room temperature (25°C) but may be exposed to temperatures of 15–30°C. The drug should be protected from light; if not protected from light, the vial should be used within 5 days.

■ **Dosage** Dosage of sugammadex sodium is expressed in terms of sugammadex.

The appropriate dose and timing of sugammadex should be based on twitch response monitoring and the extent of spontaneous recovery that has occurred. Recommended doses are based on actual body weight and not on the anesthetic regimen used. Use of lower than recommended doses of sugammadex may lead to an increased risk of recurrence of neuromuscular blockade and is therefore not recommended.

Routine Reversal of Rocuronium- or Vecuronium-induced Neuromuscular Blockade For reversal of rocuronium- or vecuronium-induced *moderate* neuromuscular blockade (i.e., spontaneous recovery has reached the reappearance of the second twitch [T_2] in response to TOF stimulation), the recommended adult dose of sugammadex is 2 mg/kg.

For reversal of rocuronium- or vecuronium-induced *deep* neuromuscular blockade (i.e., spontaneous recovery of the twitch response has reached 1–2 posttetanic counts and there are no twitch responses to TOF stimulation), the recommended adult dose of sugammadex is 4 mg/kg.

Immediate Reversal of Rocuronium-induced Neuromuscular Blockade If there is a clinical need for reversal of neuromuscular blockade immediately (i.e., approximately 3 minutes) following administration of a single 1.2-mg/kg dose of rocuronium bromide, the recommended adult dose of sugammadex is 16 mg/kg. Efficacy of sugammadex 16 mg/kg for immediate reversal of *vecuronium*-induced neuromuscular blockade has not been established.

■ **Special Populations** No dosage adjustment is necessary in patients with mild or moderate renal impairment. Sugammadex is not recommended in patients with severe renal impairment, including those requiring dialysis. (See Renal Impairment under Warnings/Precautions: Specific Populations, in Cautions.)

No dosage adjustment is necessary in geriatric patients with normal organ function. However, because sugammadex is substantially excreted by the kidneys and geriatric patients are more likely to have decreased renal function, the risk of adverse effects may be greater in such patients; careful dosage selection and monitoring of renal function are advised. (See Geriatric Use under Warnings/Precautions: Specific Populations, in Cautions.)

No dosage adjustment is necessary in patients with preexisting cardiac (e.g., ischemic heart disease, heart failure, arrhythmia) or pulmonary conditions.

Cautions

■ **Contraindications** Sugammadex is contraindicated in patients with known hypersensitivity to the drug or any ingredient in the formulation. (See Anaphylaxis and Hypersensitivity under Cautions: Warnings/Precautions.)

■ **Warnings/Precautions** ***Anaphylaxis and Hypersensitivity*** Serious, potentially fatal, hypersensitivity reactions (including anaphylaxis) have been reported with sugammadex in premarketing clinical trials, postmarketing reports, and the medical literature. Such reactions have occurred in patients with no prior exposure to the drug. Manifestations have ranged from isolated skin reactions (e.g., flushing, urticaria, erythematous rash) to more severe systemic reactions (e.g., anaphylaxis or anaphylactic shock with manifestations such as severe hypotension, tachycardia, swelling of the tongue or pharynx, bronchospasm, and pulmonary obstructive events). In some cases, severe hypersensitivity reactions required the use of vasopressors, prolonged hospitalization, and/or additional respiratory support (e.g., intubation, prolonged intubation, assisted ventilation). Although the risk of anaphylaxis appears to increase with higher doses, anaphylactic reactions have occurred at sugammadex doses less than 16 mg/kg in the postmarketing setting.

In a double-blind, placebo-controlled repeat-dose study evaluating hypersensitivity reactions to sugammadex, healthy individuals were randomized to receive sugammadex 4 mg/kg, sugammadex 16 mg/kg, or placebo IV with a 5-day washout period between doses. Of the 299 individuals who received sugammadex, anaphylaxis was reported in one patient (0.3%) in the 16-mg/kg group; manifestations including conjunctival edema, urticaria, erythema, swelling of the uvula, and reduction in peak expiratory flow occurred within 5 minutes after the first dose was administered. Nausea, pruritus, and urticaria were the most common non-anaphylactic hypersensitivity reactions reported in this study and appeared to be dose related; the overall incidence of hypersensitivity was 1, 7, or 9% in individuals receiving placebo, sugammadex 4 mg/kg, or sugammadex 16 mg/kg, respectively. In another study in healthy individuals, anaphylaxis occurred in 3 of 298 individuals (1%) receiving sugammadex 16 mg/kg.

Patients should be observed closely for possible hypersensitivity reactions after administration of sugammadex. Clinicians should be prepared for the possibility of such reactions and take necessary precautions.

Bradycardia Marked bradycardia, sometimes resulting in cardiac arrest, has been reported within minutes after administration of sugammadex. Patients should be closely monitored for hemodynamic changes during and after reversal of neuromuscular blockade; anticholinergic agents (e.g., atropine) should be administered if clinically important bradycardia is observed.

Respiratory Function Monitoring In clinical studies, a small number of patients experienced delayed or minimal reversal of neuromuscular blockade following sugammadex administration. Recurrence of neuromuscular blockade also is possible following extubation. Therefore, ventilatory support must be provided for all patients until adequate spontaneous respiration is restored and the ability to maintain a patent airway is assured. Ventilatory support may still be required after complete recovery of neuromuscular function because residual respiratory depression may occur due to other drugs used perioperatively or postoperatively.

If neuromuscular blockade persists after sugammadex is administered or recurs following extubation, appropriate steps should be taken to provide adequate ventilation. (See Dosage and Administration: General.)

Readministration of Neuromuscular Blocking Agents If readministration of a steroidal neuromuscular blocking agent is necessary (e.g., for intubation) after reversal with sugammadex, a minimum wait time should be observed before the neuromuscular blocking agent is administered.

Following administration of sugammadex (2 or 4 mg/kg), at least 5 minutes should elapse before administration of rocuronium bromide 1.2 mg/kg, and at least 4 hours should elapse before administration of rocuronium bromide 0.6 mg/kg or vecuronium bromide 0.1 mg/kg. If rocuronium bromide 1.2 mg/kg is administered within 30 minutes after reversal with sugammadex, the onset of neuromuscular blockade may be delayed up to approximately 4 minutes and the duration of blockade shortened by approximately 15 minutes. In patients with mild or moderate renal impairment, a minimum wait time of 24 hours is recommended between administration of sugammadex (2 or 4 mg/kg) and readministration of rocuronium bromide 0.6 mg/kg or vecuronium bromide 0.1 mg/kg; if a shorter wait time is necessary, a rocuronium bromide dose of 1.2 mg/kg should be used for a new blockade.

Following reversal of rocuronium-induced neuromuscular blockade with sugammadex 16 mg/kg, a wait time of 24 hours is recommended before readministration of rocuronium or administration of vecuronium.

If neuromuscular blockade is required before the recommended wait times have elapsed, the manufacturer states that a nonsteroidal neuromuscular blocking agent should be used. However, the onset of neuromuscular blockade may be delayed with use of a depolarizing neuromuscular blocking agent such as succinylcholine in this setting.

Recurrence of Neuromuscular Blockade The risk of recurrence of neuromuscular blockade may be increased with concurrent use of certain drugs (i.e., drugs that displace rocuronium or vecuronium from sugammadex binding sites) or use of lower than recommended doses of sugammadex. Risk also may be increased when drugs that potentiate neuromuscular blockade are used during the postoperative period; the manufacturer states that the prescribing information for rocuronium or vecuronium should be consulted for specific drugs that may potentiate neuromuscular blockade. (See Drug Interactions: Drugs that Displace Rocuronium or Vecuronium.)

Mechanical ventilation may be required if recurrence of neuromuscular blockade occurs.

Coagulopathy and Bleeding Sugammadex may alter coagulation parameters and increase the risk of bleeding. In healthy individuals, sugammadex increased activated partial thromboplastin time (aPTT), prothrombin time (PT), and the international normalized ratio (INR) by up to 25% for up to 1 hour. In vitro, sugammadex in combination with vitamin K antagonists (e.g., warfarin), unfractionated heparin, low molecular weight heparins, rivaroxaban, or dabigatran resulted in additional increases in aPTT and PT/INR of up to 25 or 50% at peak plasma concentrations of sugammadex corresponding to 4 or 16 mg/kg doses, respectively.

In a study in patients undergoing major orthopedic surgery who were receiving thromboprophylaxis with heparin or a low molecular weight heparin, increases in aPTT and PT/INR of 5.5 and 3%, respectively, were observed within 1 hour following administration of sugammadex 4 mg/kg; however, a corresponding increase in the incidence of bleeding or anemia was not observed.

The risk of bleeding has not been evaluated with sugammadex 16 mg/kg in patients receiving thromboprophylaxis drugs. Bleeding risk also has not been evaluated in patients with known coagulopathies and those receiving therapeutic anticoagulation or thromboprophylaxis with drugs other than heparin and low molecular weight heparin; coagulation parameters should be carefully monitored in such patients.

Light Anesthesia When neuromuscular blockade was reversed intentionally during anesthesia in clinical trials, signs of light anesthesia (e.g., movement, coughing, grimacing, suckling of the tracheal tube) were occasionally noted.

Specific Populations **Pregnancy.** There are no data regarding use of sugammadex in pregnant women. Animal studies revealed no evidence of teratogenicity when sugammadex was administered during the period of organogenesis in rats and rabbits at maternal exposures up to 6 and 8 times, respectively, the maximum recommended human dose. However, incomplete ossification and reduced fetal body weight were observed in rabbits at sugammadex doses 8 times the maximum recommended human dose, which corresponds to a dose level that also produced maternal toxicity.

Lactation. It is not known whether sugammadex is distributed into human milk or if the drug has any effect on milk production or the nursing infant. The drug is distributed into milk in rats. The benefits of breast-feeding and the importance of sugammadex to the woman should be considered along with the potential adverse effects on the breast-fed infant from the drug or underlying maternal condition.

Pediatric Use. The manufacturer states that safety and efficacy of sugammadex have not been established in pediatric patients; however, the drug has been used for reversal of moderate *rocuronium*-induced neuromuscular blockade in pediatric patients.

In a study evaluating sugammadex for reversal of rocuronium-induced neuromuscular blockade in pediatric and adult patients undergoing surgery, similar recovery times were observed in pediatric patients 2–17 years of age and adults. Sugammadex plasma concentrations were similar in the different age groups, and no overall difference in safety was observed.

Animal studies have demonstrated increased sugammadex bone deposition in juvenile rats compared with adult rats. Decreased bone length and tooth abnormalities (i.e., discoloration and disturbance of enamel formation) were observed in juvenile rats receiving IV sugammadex daily for 28 days at doses approximately 0.1–3 times the maximum recommended human dose; these effects were not observed with once-weekly sugammadex doses up to 1.2 times the maximum recommended human dose.

Geriatric Use. In a study evaluating use of sugammadex in geriatric patients, median time to recovery of the train-of-four (TOF) ratio to 0.9 following administration of sugammadex 2 mg/kg at the reappearance of T_2 was 2.5 and 3.6 minutes in patients 65–74 years of age and those 75 years of age or older, respectively, compared with 2.2 minutes in younger adults (18–64 years of age). Across all clinical trials, geriatric patients 65 years of age or older who received sugammadex 4 mg/kg at 1–2 posttetanic counts had a median time to recovery of 2.5 minutes compared with 2 minutes in younger adults.

Hepatic Impairment. The pharmacokinetics of sugammadex have not been studied in patients with hepatic impairment. The manufacturer states that caution should be exercised if sugammadex is used in patients with hepatic impairment accompanied by coagulopathy or severe edema.

In a small observational study in patients undergoing hepatic surgery, the mean time to recovery from rocuronium-induced neuromuscular blockade following sugammadex 2 or 4 mg/kg was not substantially different in patients with hepatic impairment compared with those with normal hepatic function.

Renal Impairment. Sugammadex is principally eliminated by renal excretion; clearance is decreased and half-life prolonged in patients with renal impairment, resulting in increased systemic exposure of the drug.

Use of sugammadex is not recommended in patients with severe renal impairment, including those requiring dialysis, because of prolonged and increased drug exposure and insufficient experience in such patients. (See Special Populations under Dosage and Administration: Dosage.)

If readministration of a neuromuscular blocking agent (e.g., for intubation) is necessary after reversal with sugammadex in patients with mild or moderate renal impairment, a minimum wait time may be necessary. (See Readministration of Neuromuscular Blocking Agents under Cautions: Warnings/Precautions.)

■ **Common Adverse Effects** Adverse effects reported in 10% or more of patients receiving sugammadex in clinical studies and with an incidence greater than that observed with placebo include vomiting, pain, nausea, hypotension, and headache.

Drug Interactions

Sugammadex is not likely to be metabolized by cytochrome P-450 (CYP) enzymes; therefore, CYP-mediated drug interactions are not expected.

Based on binding affinities between sugammadex and other drugs, pharmacokinetic-pharmacodynamic models, and data from preclinical and clinical studies, no clinically important pharmacodynamic drug interactions other than with toremifene and hormonal contraceptives are expected with sugammadex.

■ **Drugs that Displace Rocuronium or Vecuronium** Displacement of rocuronium or vecuronium from sugammadex by other drugs (e.g., toremifene) can result in recurrence of neuromuscular blockade, possibly requiring mechanical ventilation. Risk of displacement interactions is highest during the time period equivalent to 3 elimination half-lives of sugammadex. If a concomitantly administered drug causes displacement of rocuronium or vecuronium from sugammadex, administration of the concomitant drug should be stopped (in case of an infusion).

Toremifene Because toremifene has a high binding affinity for sugammadex, there is an increased likelihood that a displacement interaction may occur. In patients who have received toremifene on the same day of surgery, recovery of neuromuscular function may be delayed.

■ **Hormonal Contraceptives** Sugammadex binds to progestogen in vitro and may result in decreased exposure and reduced efficacy of hormonal contraceptives. The manufacturer states that administration of a single bolus dose of sugammadex is considered to be equivalent to missing a dose of oral contraceptive containing an estrogen or progestogen. Patients using hormonal contraceptives, including oral and non-oral forms, should use an additional, *non-hormonal* method of contraception for 7 days following sugammadex administration.

Description

Sugammadex, a modified γ-cyclodextrin, is a selective relaxant binding agent. Sugammadex reverses neuromuscular blockade by binding to and forming a complex with (i.e., encapsulating) steroidal nondepolarizing neuromuscular blocking agents (e.g., rocuronium, vecuronium), thereby reducing the amount of neuromuscular blocking agent available to bind to nicotinic cholinergic receptors in the neuromuscular junction. Sugammadex forms a complex with free rocuronium or vecuronium molecules in plasma in a 1:1 ratio; because of its cyclodextrin structure (hydrophilic molecule with a lipophilic core), the drug specifically encapsulates lipophilic (e.g., steroidal) molecules. Among the steroidal neuromuscular blocking agents, sugammadex exhibits higher binding affinity for rocuronium than vecuronium, and a much lower affinity for pancuronium. The drug does not exhibit any binding affinity for succinylcholine, mivacurium, atracurium, or cisatracurium.

Commercially available sugammadex sodium injection may contain up to 7% of the monohydroxy derivative of the drug. The binding affinity of the monohydroxy derivative for rocuronium or vecuronium is approximately half that of sugammadex; however, products with up to 7% of the monohydroxy derivative have demonstrated nearly similar efficacy in reversing rocuronium- or vecuronium-induced neuromuscular blockade.

Pharmacokinetics of sugammadex are based on the total concentration of free plus complex-bound sugammadex; the pharmacokinetic parameters of complex-bound sugammadex are assumed to be the same as those of free sugammadex. Sugammadex exhibits linear pharmacokinetics after administration of single IV doses of 1–16 mg/kg. Neither sugammadex nor the complex of sugammadex and rocuronium binds to plasma proteins or erythrocytes. Sugammadex binds to hydroxyapatite in vitro; in animal studies, the drug distributed into and was retained in sites of active mineralization with a mean half-life of 172 and 8 days in bone and teeth, respectively. Sugammadex is not metabolized. The drug is principally eliminated by the kidneys (96%), almost completely as unchanged drug; over 90% of a dose is excreted within 24 hours. Less than 0.02% of a dose is excreted in the feces or expired. The elimination half-life of sugammadex is about 2 hours in anesthetized patients with normal renal function, and 4, 6, or 19 hours in patients with mild, moderate, or severe renal impairment, respectively. Hemodialysis using a high-flux filter removes about 70% of the drug over 3–6 hours.

Pharmacokinetics of sugammadex do not appear to be affected by age, gender, or race.

Advice to Patients

Importance of informing women that sugammadex can substantially decrease the effectiveness of hormonal contraceptives, including oral and nonoral forms; women should be advised to use additional nonhormonal forms of contraception for 7 days after sugammadex administration.

Importance of women informing clinicians if they are or plan to become pregnant or plan to breast-feed.

Importance of informing patients of other important precautionary information. (See Cautions.)

Overview® (see Users Guide). For additional information on this drug until a more detailed monograph is developed and published, the manufacturer's labeling should be consulted. It is *essential* that the manufacturer's labeling be consulted for more detailed information on usual cautions, precautions, contraindications, potential drug interactions, laboratory test interferences, and acute toxicity.

Preparations

Excipients in commercially available drug preparations may have clinically important effects in some individuals; consult specific product labeling for details.

Sugammadex Sodium

Parenteral		
Injection	100 mg (of sugammadex) per mL	**Bridion®**, Merck

Uridine Triacetate

Vistonuridine

■ Uridine triacetate, an acetylated prodrug of uridine and a pyrimidine analog, is a direct biochemical antagonist of fluorouracil and a uridine replacement agent.

Uses

Uridine triacetate, formerly called vistonuridine, is commercially available in the US in 2 different oral formulations: Vistogard® granules, which are used for the treatment of fluorouracil or capecitabine overdosage or toxicity, and Xuriden® granules, which are used for the treatment of hereditary orotic aciduria.

■ **Fluorouracil or Capecitabine Overdosage or Toxicity** Uridine triacetate (Vistogard®) is used for emergency treatment of patients following fluorouracil or capecitabine overdosage regardless of the presence of symptoms. The drug also is used in patients who exhibit early onset, severe or life-threatening cardiac or CNS toxicity and/or early onset, unusually severe adverse reactions (e.g., GI toxicity, neutropenia) within 96 hours following the end of fluorouracil or capecitabine administration. Uridine triacetate is designated an orphan drug by FDA for use as an antidote in the treatment of fluorouracil or capecitabine poisoning. Uridine triacetate is *not* recommended for the nonemergency treatment of adverse reactions associated with fluorouracil or capecitabine because it may decrease the clinical efficacy of these drugs. In addition, the safety and efficacy of uridine triacetate initiated more than 96 hours following the end of fluorouracil or capecitabine administration have not been established.

Fluorouracil and capecitabine (a prodrug of fluorouracil) are antineoplastic agents that are widely used in the treatment of a variety of malignancies. Although overdosages of fluorouracil and capecitabine are quite rare, they can result in substantial morbidity and mortality. In addition, some patients, such as those with a partial or complete deficiency of the enzyme dihydropyrimidine dehydrogenase (DPYD; a rate-limiting enzyme in the catabolism of fluoropyrimidines), may have impaired elimination of these drugs and experience severe toxicity as a result. For further information concerning fluorouracil and capecitabine toxicity and overdosage, see Capecitabine 10:00 and see also Fluorouracil 10:00.

The current indication for uridine triacetate (Vistogard®) is based principally on the results of 2 single-arm, open-label studies in 135 patients (median age: 59 years [range: 1–83 years], 56% male, 72% white) with fluorouracil or capecitabine overdosage (87%) or who presented with severe or life-threatening toxicities within 96 hours following the end of fluorouracil or capecitabine administration (13%). The first study was a collection of single-patient investigational new drug applications designed to provide emergency access to uridine triacetate, and the second study was an expanded access protocol designed to provide better efficacy and safety data for the drug. Overdosage was defined as administration of fluorouracil at a dose or infusion rate greater than the intended dose or maximum tolerated dose for the patient's intended regimen; 94, 4, or 3% of such patients were overdosed by infusion rate (range: 1.3–720 times the intended infusion rate) alone, dose alone, or both dose and infusion rate, respectively. Severe or life-threatening toxicities in these patients involved the CNS (e.g., encephalopathy, acute mental status change), cardiovascular system, GI tract (e.g., mucositis), and bone marrow (e.g., neutropenia). Uridine triacetate was administered at a dosage of 10 g orally every 6 hours for 20 doses or at a body surface area-adjusted dosage of 6.2 g/m^2 per dose for 20 doses for 4 pediatric patients 1–7 years of age. The primary measure of efficacy was survival at 30 days or until the resumption of chemotherapy if prior to 30 days. Of the 135 patients treated with uridine triacetate, overall survival at 30 days was 96%, and 33% of the patients resumed chemotherapy in less than 30 days. There were 5 deaths overall; 2 of these patients were treated *after* 96 hours following the end of fluorouracil administration. In patients receiving uridine triacetate for an overdosage of fluorouracil or capecitabine in both studies, survival at 30 days was 97%. In patients receiving uridine triacetate for early-onset, severe or life-threatening toxicity, the survival at 30 days was 89%. In retrospective case reports that included 25 patients who received only supportive care following fluorouracil overdosages by infusion rate (range: 1.9–64 times the intended infusion rate), the survival rate was 16%.

■ **Hereditary Orotic Aciduria** Uridine triacetate (Xuriden®) is used for the treatment of hereditary orotic aciduria. Uridine triacetate is designated an orphan drug by the FDA for use in this condition.

Hereditary orotic aciduria (uridine monophosphate synthase deficiency) is a rare congenital autosomal recessive disorder of pyrimidine metabolism; the disorder is usually diagnosed in infants and children and has an estimated birth prevalence of less than 1:1,000,000. Hereditary orotic aciduria is caused by a defect in the uridine monophosphate synthase gene, which results in a deficiency of the bifunctional enzyme uridine 5′-monophosphate synthase. This enzyme is responsible for catalysis of the final two steps of the de novo pyrimidine biosynthetic pathway in mammalian cells and results in systemic deficiency of pyrimidine nucleotides and excretion of orotic acid in the urine. (See Description.) Clinical manifestations of hereditary orotic aciduria include hematologic abnormalities (e.g., megaloblastic anemia, decreased white blood cell and neutrophil counts), urinary tract obstruction due to formation of orotic acid crystals in the urinary tract, failure to thrive, and developmental delays.

The current indication for uridine triacetate (Xuriden®) is based principally on data from a single-arm, 6-week, open-label study with a 6-month extension phase conducted in 4 patients (age range: 3–19 years, 75% male) with hereditary orotic aciduria that demonstrated improvement or stability in hematologic parameters, urinary orotic acid and orotidine concentrations, and growth. All patients received uridine triacetate 60 mg/kg orally once daily for 6 weeks. Three of the patients had previously been treated with uridine and were switched to oral uridine triacetate at study entry. For these patients, the primary measure of efficacy was stability of the patients' prespecified hematologic parameter during the study period. For the treatment-naive (previously untreated) patient, the primary measure of efficacy was improvement of the patient's prespecified hematologic parameter during the study period. The prespecified hematologic parameters in the patients were neutrophil count and percentage of neutrophils (1 patient), white blood cell count (1 patient), and mean corpuscular volume (2 patients).

Uridine triacetate therapy resulted in stability of the hematologic parameters in all 4 patients at both the 6-week and 6-month assessments in this study; the previously untreated patient, however, did not meet the prespecified criteria for improvement of the hematologic parameter. All patients with normal urinary orotic acid and orotidine concentrations at baseline maintained such concentrations after 6 weeks of treatment with uridine triacetate. During the extension phase of the study in which patients continued to receive uridine triacetate at dosages of 60–120 mg/kg once daily, hematologic parameters and growth (as determined by height and weight percentiles for age) either improved or remained stable and urinary orotic acid and orotidine concentrations remained stable after 6 months of treatment. No adverse effects associated with uridine triacetate therapy were reported in this study.

The efficacy and safety of uridine triacetate therapy in patients with hereditary orotic aciduria are further supported by 19 case reports in the published literature. In 18 of these patients, the condition was diagnosed between the ages of 2 months and 12 years and all of these patients were treated with exogenous uridine; the remaining patient, who was diagnosed at 28 years of age, was not treated with exogenous uridine. These case reports of patients with hereditary orotic aciduria treated with exogenous sources of uridine demonstrated similar results as uridine triacetate therapy in the pivotal efficacy study.

Dosage and Administration

■ **General** Uridine triacetate is commercially available in the US as Vistogard® and Xuriden®, which have different labeled indications. (See Uses.)

Restricted Distribution Program Uridine triacetate (as Vistogard®) can only be obtained through a specialty pharmacy. For inpatient use, clinicians may contact the specialty pharmacy at 844-293-0007. For outpatient use and information on the case management program, clinicians may contact the specialty pharmacy at 844-374-0604. Ordering information also is available on the Vistogard® website (https://www.vistogard.com/Resources/How-to-Order).

Uridine triacetate (as Xuriden®) also can only be obtained through a specialty pharmacy. Clinicians may contact the manufacturer at 800-914-0071 for availability and ordering information.

■ **Administration** Uridine triacetate is administered orally as granules (e.g., Vistogard®, Xuriden®) and may be given without regard to meals (see Description).

Opened packets or mixtures of uridine triacetate with food, milk, or infant formula should not be stored. Packets of the drug are for single use only; any unused portions should be discarded. Any granules left in an open packet should not be used for subsequent dosing.

Vistogard® Granules Uridine triacetate (Vistogard®) treatment should begin as soon as possible following overdosage or early-onset toxicity of fluorouracil or capecitabine and should be given within 96 hours following the end of fluorouracil or capecitabine administration.

Pediatric doses of uridine triacetate should be weighed using a scale accurate to at least 0.1 g or measured using a graduated teaspoon accurate to one-fourth teaspoonful. For patients requiring 10-g doses of uridine triacetate, the contents of a full packet may be administered without weighing or measuring.

Each Vistogard® dose should be mixed with 3–4 ounces of soft food (e.g., applesauce, pudding, yogurt) and ingested within 30 minutes. The drug may be given without regard to meals. The granules should *not* be chewed. Patients should drink at least 120 mL (4 ounces) of water after each dose.

Nausea and vomiting may occur during Vistogard® therapy because of capecitabine or fluorouracil toxicity and, less commonly, because of the slightly bitter taste of the uridine triacetate granules. If a patient vomits within 2 hours after receiving a dose of uridine triacetate, another full dose should be administered as soon as possible after the vomiting episode. The next dose should be administered at the regularly scheduled time. Use of an antiemetic (e.g., a type 3 serotonin [5-HT_3] receptor antagonist) also may be helpful in such cases.

If a dose of uridine triacetate is missed, the missed dose should be administered as soon as possible and the next dose should be administered at the regularly scheduled time.

Nasogastric Tube or Gastrostomy Tube. Uridine triacetate (Vistogard®) may be administered via nasogastric or gastrostomy tube when necessary (e.g., severe mucositis, coma). About 100 mL (approximately 4 fluid ounces) of a food starch-based thickening product in water should be prepared and stirred briskly until the thickener has dissolved. The contents of one 10-g packet of Vistogard® granules should be crushed to a fine powder and then added to about 100 mL (4 ounces) of reconstituted food starch-based thickening product. For pediatric patients receiving doses of less than 10 g, the mixture should be prepared in a ratio not exceeding 1 g of uridine triacetate to 10 mL of reconstituted food starch-based thickening product and mixed thoroughly.

Following administration of the mixture using the nasogastric or gastrostomy tube, the tube should be flushed with water.

Xuriden® Granules Doses of uridine triacetate (Xuriden®) should be weighed using a scale accurate to at least 0.1 g or measured using a graduated teaspoon accurate to the fraction of the dose to be administered. For patients requiring doses of uridine triacetate in multiples of 2 g (i.e., three-fourths teaspoonful), the contents of the required number of 2-g packets may be administered without weighing or measuring.

Doses of uridine triacetate should be administered orally immediately after mixing with 3–4 ounces of applesauce, pudding, or yogurt. The granules should *not* be chewed. Administration of each dose should be followed with at least 120 mL (4 ounces) of water.

Xuriden® granules may be mixed with 5 mL of milk or infant formula instead of soft foods for patients receiving up to 2 g (three-fourths teaspoonful) of uridine triacetate granules. The manufacturer's instructions for preparing such doses using a medicine cup and an oral syringe in the Xuriden® prescribing information should be consulted. Doses that are mixed in milk or infant formula should be administered using an oral syringe placed between the patient's cheek and gum at the back of the mouth. A bottle of milk or infant formula may be given after administration of the drug, if desired.

■ Dosage

Dosage of uridine triacetate is expressed in terms of the salt.

Fluorouracil or Capecitabine Overdosage or Toxicity For the emergency treatment of patients following fluorouracil or capecitabine overdosage (regardless of the presence of symptoms) or patients who exhibit early onset, severe or life-threatening cardiac or CNS toxicity and/or early onset, unusually severe adverse reactions (e.g., GI toxicity, neutropenia), the recommended dosage of uridine triacetate (Vistogard®) in adults is 10 g (one packet) orally every 6 hours for a total of 20 doses for a full course of treatment.

In pediatric patients with such fluorouracil or capecitabine overdosage or toxicity, the recommended dosage of uridine triacetate is 6.2 g/m² of body surface area (not exceeding 10 g/dose) orally every 6 hours for a total of 20 doses for a full course of treatment. (See Table 1.)

Table 1. Uridine Triacetate (Vistogard®) Pediatric Dosing Based on Body Surface Area.

Body Surface Area (m²)	Vistogard® 6.2 g/m² per dose	
	Dose (g)	Dose (graduated teaspoonful)
0.34–0.44	2.1–2.7	1
0.45–0.55	2.8–3.4	1¼
0.56–0.66	3.5–4.1	1½
0.67–0.77	4.2–4.8	1¾
0.78–0.88	4.9–5.4	2
0.89–0.99	5.5–6.1	2¼
1–1.1	6.2–6.8	2½
1.11–1.21	6.9–7.5	2¾
1.22–1.32	7.6–8.1	3
1.33–1.43	8.2–8.8	3¼
1.44 or greater	10	1 full 10-g packet[a]

Note: One packet of Vistogard® granules contains 10 g of uridine triacetate. Dose by body surface area in this table was rounded to achieve the approximate dose. Each dose is administered every 6 hours for 20 doses.

[a] One entire 10-g packet may be used without weighing or measuring.

Hereditary Orotic Aciduria The recommended initial dosage of uridine triacetate (Xuriden®) for the treatment of adult and pediatric patients with hereditary orotic aciduria is 60 mg/kg orally once daily. (See Table 2.)

Table 2. *Initial* Uridine Triacetate (Xuriden®) 60 mg/kg Daily Dosage Based on Body Weight.

Patient Weight (in kg)	Xuriden® 60 mg/kg Daily Dosage	
	Dose (in grams using a scale)	Dose (in teaspoonful)
Up to 5	0.4	1/8
6–10	0.4–0.6	¼
11–15	0.7–0.9	½
16–20	1–1.2	½
21–25	1.3–1.5	½
26–30	1.6–1.8	¾[a]
31–35	1.9–2.1[a]	¾[a]
36–40	2.2–2.4	1
41–45	2.5–2.7	1
46–50	2.8–3	1
51–55	3.1–3.3	1¼
56–60	3.4–3.6	1¼
61–65	3.7–3.9[b]	1½[b]
66–70	4–4.2[b]	1½[b]
71–75	4.3–4.5	1½[b]
greater than 75	6[c]	2[c]

Note: One packet of Xuriden® granules contains 2 g (approximately three-fourths teaspoon) of uridine triacetate. Total daily dosages by weight category in this table were rounded to achieve the approximate dosage level.

[a] One entire 2-g packet may be used without weighing or measuring.

[b] Two entire 2-g packets may be used without weighing or measuring.

[c] Three entire 2-g packets may be used without weighing or measuring.

Dosage of uridine triacetate may be increased to 120 mg/kg (not to exceed 8 g) orally once daily for insufficient response. (See Table 3.) Signs of insufficient response may include urinary concentrations of orotic acid that are above normal or are increased above the usual or expected range for the patient, worsening of laboratory parameters affected by the condition (e.g., red or white blood cell indices), or worsening of other manifestations of the condition.

Table 3. *Increased* Uridine Triacetate (Xuriden®) 120 mg/kg Daily Dosage for Insufficient Response Based on Body Weight.

Patient Weight (in kg)	Xuriden® 120 mg/kg Daily Dosage	
	Dose (in grams using a scale)	Dose (in teaspoonful)
Up to 5	0.8	¼
6–10	0.8–1.2	½
11–15	1.4–1.8	¾
16–20	2–2.4	1
21–25	2.6–3	1
26–30	3.2–3.6	1¼
31–35	3.8–4.2[a]	1½[a]
36–40	4.4–4.8	1¾
41–45	5–5.4	2[b]
46–50	5.6–6	2[b]
51–55	6.2–6.6	2¼
56–60	6.8–7.2	2½
61–65	7.4–7.8	2½
66–70	8[c]	2¾[c]
71–75	8[c]	2¾[c]
greater than 75	8[c]	2¾[c]

Note: One packet of Xuriden® granules contains 2 g (approximately three-fourths teaspoon) of uridine triacetate. Total daily dosages by weight category in this table were rounded to achieve the approximate dosage level.

[a] Two entire 2-g packets may be used without weighing or measuring.

[b] Three entire 2-g packets may be used without weighing or measuring.

[c] Four entire 2-g packets may be used without weighing or measuring.

■ Special Populations

No dosage adjustment is necessary based on age, body size, race, or gender in adults.

Cautions

■ Contraindications

The manufacturer states that there are no known contraindications to the use of uridine triacetate.

■ Warnings/Precautions

Warnings and Precautions The manufacturer states that there are no warnings or precautions associated with uridine triacetate therapy.

Specific Populations **Pregnancy.** Limited case reports of uridine triacetate (Vistogard®) use during pregnancy are inadequate to inform a drug-associated risk of birth defects and miscarriage. There are no data regarding use of uridine triacetate (Xuriden®) in pregnant women to inform a drug-associated risk.

Animal studies have not revealed evidence of teratogenicity or fetal harm at uridine triacetate dosages of about one-half the maximum recommended human dosage of Vistogard® or 2.7 times the maximum recommended human dosage of Xuriden® administered to pregnant rats during the period of organogenesis.

Lactation. It is not known whether uridine triacetate is distributed into human milk; effects of the drug on breast-fed infants or milk production also are not known. The benefits of breast-feeding and the woman's clinical need for uridine triacetate should be considered along with any potential adverse effects on the breast-fed infant from the drug or from the underlying maternal condition.

Pediatric Use. Safety and efficacy of uridine triacetate (Vistogard®) for emergency treatment following fluorouracil or capecitabine overdosage or early-onset, severe or life-threatening toxicity have been established in pediatric patients. Such use is supported by an open-label study that included 6 pediatric patients 1–16 years of age. Four of these pediatric patients were 1–7 years of age and received a body surface area-adjusted dosage of the drug.

Safety and efficacy of uridine triacetate (Xuriden®) for treatment of hereditary orotic aciduria have been established in a single open-label study in 4 pediatric patients 3 years of age or older and based on case reports of 18 pediatric patients who began uridine triacetate treatment at 2 months to 12 years of age.

Clinical response and safety of uridine triacetate in adults and pediatric patients are similar; however, data are limited. (See Uses.)

Geriatric Use. In clinical studies evaluating uridine triacetate (Vistogard®) for treatment of fluorouracil or capecitabine overdosage or toxicity, 30% of patients were 65 years of age or older and 11% were 75 years of age or older. Clinical studies did not include sufficient numbers of patients 65 years of age or older to determine whether they respond differently than younger adults.

In a population pharmacokinetic analysis, patient age (range: 20–83 years) did not substantially affect uridine pharmacokinetics.

■ **Common Adverse Effects** The most common adverse effects occurring in more than 2% of patients receiving uridine triacetate (Vistogard®) for emergency treatment of fluorouracil or capecitabine overdosage or toxicity in clinical trials were vomiting, nausea, and diarrhea.

No adverse effects were reported in patients receiving uridine triacetate (Xuriden®) for the treatment of hereditary orotic aciduria in the principal efficacy study.

Drug Interactions

Clinically important drug interactions with uridine triacetate have not been identified to date.

In vitro studies indicate that uridine triacetate and uridine do not have clinically important inhibitory effects on cytochrome P-450 (CYP) isoenzymes 3A4, 1A2, 2C8, 2C9, 2C19, 2D6, or 2E1. In vitro studies also indicate that uridine triacetate and uridine do not induce CYP isoenzymes 1A2, 2B6, or 3A4.

■ **Drugs Affecting or Metabolized by Hepatic Microsomal Enzymes** Clinically important drug interactions between uridine triacetate and drugs that affect or are metabolized by CYP isoenzymes appear unlikely.

■ **Drugs Affecting or Affected by P-glycoprotein Transport System** In vitro studies indicate that uridine triacetate is a weak substrate for P-glycoprotein (P-gp). Uridine triacetate inhibited the transport of digoxin (a P-gp substrate) with an IC_{50} (concentration that inhibits activity by 50%) of 344 μM. Potential pharmacokinetic interaction of uridine triacetate with orally administered substrates of P-gp cannot be ruled out due to the potential for locally increased (gut) concentrations of uridine triacetate.

■ **Drugs Affecting GI Absorption** The manufacturer states that the expanded access protocol for uridine triacetate (Vistogard®) initially contained instructions to avoid drugs that could potentially interfere with the GI absorption of uridine triacetate (e.g., bismuth subsalicylate, cholestyramine, sucralfate). However, there currently is no evidence that these drugs can slow the absorption of uridine or uridine triacetate. In addition, formal drug interaction studies have confirmed the lack of such an interaction. Therefore, the instruction to avoid drugs that may interfere with absorption of uridine triacetate was removed from the expanded access protocol and also was not included in the Vistogard® prescribing information.

■ **Antineoplastic Agents** The effect of uridine triacetate on the antitumor activity of fluorouracil is not known. However, concomitant use of uridine triacetate potentially may result in decreased fluorouracil or capecitabine efficacy. The manufacturer states that use of uridine triacetate is *not* recommended for the *nonemergency* treatment of adverse reactions associated with fluorouracil or capecitabine.

Description

Uridine triacetate is an acetylated prodrug of uridine and a pyrimidine analog. In fluorouracil or capecitabine overdosage or toxicity, uridine triacetate is a direct biochemical antagonist of fluorouracil. Excess circulating uridine derived from uridine triacetate is converted into uridine triphosphate (UTP), which competes with 5-fluorouridine triphosphate (FUTP; a cytotoxic intermediate metabolite of fluorouracil) for incorporation into RNA, thereby inhibiting cell damage and cell death.

In hereditary orotic aciduria, uridine triacetate provides an exogenous source of uridine for replacement therapy in patients who are unable to synthesize adequate quantities of uridine. Uridine can be used for the synthesis of uridine nucleotides by essentially all cells. Restoration of intracellular uridine nucleotide concentrations to within the normal range reduces the overproduction of orotic acid by feedback inhibition, thereby also reducing the urinary excretion of orotic acid.

Following oral administration, uridine triacetate is deacetylated by nonspecific esterases present throughout the body to form uridine. Uridine triacetate has a substantially higher oral bioavailability than uridine, providing fourfold to sixfold more uridine into the systemic circulation than equimolar oral doses of uridine. Uridine triacetate crosses the intestinal mucosa much more readily than uridine, and peak plasma concentrations of uridine following single-dose oral administration of uridine triacetate are generally achieved within 2–3 hours. Administration of a slightly different formulation of uridine triacetate granules with food in healthy adults did not affect the overall rate and extent of uridine exposure compared with those observed following administration of the drug in the fasted state. Uridine crosses the blood-brain barrier. Circulating uridine is taken up by mammalian cells via specific nucleoside transporters. Uridine can be excreted by the kidneys or metabolized by normal pyrimidine catabolic pathways present in most tissues. The elimination half-life of uridine is approximately 2–2.5 hours.

Advice to Patients

Importance of providing patients or their caregivers with a copy of the manufacturer's patient information (Vistogard®) or instructions for use (Xuriden®).

For Vistogard® or Xuriden® doses less than the entire contents of a packet, importance of weighing or measuring the prescribed dose using appropriate equipment (e.g., a scale accurate to at least 0.1 g, a graduated teaspoon accurate to one-fourth teaspoonful or the fraction of the dose to be administered).

Uridine triacetate granules should *not* be chewed. Vistogard® and Xuriden® granules may be mixed with food (e.g., applesauce, pudding, yogurt). Xuriden® also may be mixed in milk or infant formula. Any unused portion of uridine triacetate granules remaining in the single-use packets after measuring out the appropriate dose should be discarded.

Importance of patients completing the full course of treatment (i.e., 20 doses) of Vistogard® even if they feel well. If a patient vomits within 2 hours after receiving a dose of Vistogard®, another full dose should be administered as a replacement as soon as possible after the vomiting episode; the next dose should be administered at the regularly scheduled time. If a dose of Vistogard® is missed, the missed dose should be administered as soon as possible and the next dose should be administered at the regularly scheduled time.

Importance of informing clinicians of existing or contemplated concomitant therapy, including prescription and OTC drugs and dietary or herbal supplements, as well as any concomitant illnesses.

Importance of advising women receiving uridine triacetate to inform clinicians if they are or plan to become pregnant or plan to breast-feed.

Importance of informing patients of other important precautionary information. (See Cautions.)

Overview® (see Users Guide). For additional information on this drug until a more detailed monograph is developed and published, the manufacturer's labeling should be consulted. It is *essential* that the manufacturer's labeling be consulted for more detailed information on usual cautions, precautions, contraindications, potential drug interactions, laboratory test interferences, and acute toxicity.

Preparations

Distribution of uridine triacetate (Vistogard® and Xuriden®) is restricted. (See Restricted Distribution Program under Dosage and Administration: General.)

Excipients in commercially available drug preparations may have clinically important effects in some individuals; consult specific product labeling for details.

Uridine Triacetate

Oral		
Granules	2 g (of uridine triacetate) per packet	**Xuriden®**, Wellstat
	10 g (of uridine triacetate) per packet	**Vistogard®**, Wellstat (marketed by BTG)

ANTIGOUT AGENTS 92:16

Allopurinol

■ Allopurinol, a structural isomer of hypoxanthine, is a xanthine oxidase inhibitor.

Uses

■ **Gout** Allopurinol is used to lower serum and urinary uric acid concentrations in the management of primary and secondary gout. The drug is indicated in patients with frequent disabling attacks of gout. Because therapy with allopurinol is not without some serious risks, the drug is *not* recommended for the management of asymptomatic hyperuricemia; however, some clinicians have suggested that therapy should be initiated when serum urate concentrations exceed 9 mg/dL (by the colorimetric method) because these concentrations are often associated with increased joint changes and renal complications. Allopurinol is used for the management of gout when uricosurics cannot be used because of adverse effects, allergy, or inadequate response; when there are visible tophi or radiographic evidence of uric acid deposits and stones; or when serum urate concentrations are greater than 8.5–9 mg/dL and a family history of tophi and low urate excretion exists. Allopurinol also is used for the management of primary or secondary gouty nephropathy with or without secondary oliguria. The goal of therapy is to lower serum urate concentration to about 6 mg/dL. Allopurinol will often promote resolution of tophi and uric acid crystals by decreasing serum urate concentrations.

Since allopurinol has no analgesic or anti-inflammatory activity, it is of no value in the treatment of acute gout attacks and will prolong and exacerbate inflammation during the acute phase. Allopurinol may increase the frequency of acute attacks during the first 6–12 months of therapy, even when normal or subnormal serum urate concentrations have been maintained. Therefore, prophylactic doses of colchicine should generally be administered concurrently during the first 3–6 months of allopurinol therapy. Acute attacks may occur in spite of such therapy, but usually become less severe and are of briefer duration after several months of allopurinol therapy. During these acute attacks, allopurinol should be continued without changing dosage and full therapeutic doses of colchicine or other anti-inflammatory agents should be administered.

In early uncomplicated gout, either allopurinol or a uricosuric agent may be used. Since uricosuric agents tend to increase urinary uric acid concentrations and the risk of stone formation, allopurinol is preferred in patients with urinary uric acid excretion of greater than 900 mg daily or with gouty nephropathy, urinary tract stones or obstruction, or azotemia. The activity of allopurinol and uricosurics is additive and, when administered concomitantly, smaller doses of each drug can be used. Combined use of the two types of drugs is especially effective in the presence of tophaceous deposits.

■ **Chemotherapy-induced Hyperuricemia** Allopurinol and allopurinol sodium are used for the management of patients with leukemia, lymphoma, and solid tumor malignancies who are undergoing chemotherapy expected to result in tumor lysis and subsequent elevations of serum and urinary uric acid concentrations. For patients unable to tolerate oral therapy, allopurinol sodium for injection may be used. Allopurinol is especially useful in preventing hyperuricemia and uric acid nephropathy resulting from tissue breakdown after cancer chemotherapy or radiation therapy. Allopurinol therapy should be discontinued when the potential for hyperuricemia is no longer present.

In one compassionate treatment program in patients undergoing chemotherapy for the management of malignancies, administration of IV allopurinol sodium was shown to reduce serum uric acid concentrations in 93% of patients with hyperuricemia (68% of whom achieved normal serum urate concentrations) and to maintain normal serum uric acid concentrations in 97% of those patients in whom the drug was initiated while having normal serum urate concentrations. However, because of study design, clinical outcome associated with IV allopurinol sodium therapy could not be assessed.

Results of a randomized, open-labeled comparative study in pediatric patients 4 months to 17 years of age with leukemia or lymphoma and a high risk for developing tumor lysis suggest that oral allopurinol may be slower and less effective in decreasing plasma uric acid concentrations than IV rasburicase. (See Uses: Chemotherapy-induced Hyperuricemia, in Rasburicase 44:00.) At the time of this study, IV allopurinol was unavailable. However, the different routes of administration for the drugs (i.e., oral versus IV) are not believed to account for the differences that were observed. Further study is needed to determine whether the more rapid control and reduction of plasma uric acid concentrations that is achieved with rasburicase therapy than is achieved with allopurinol therapy also will result in substantial decreases in metabolic complications and morbidity associated with tumor lysis syndrome, or the need for additional renal support (dialysis or hemofiltration).

■ **Recurrent Renal Calculi** Allopurinol is used in the management of recurrent calcium oxalate renal calculi in males whose urinary urate excretion exceeds 800 mg daily and in females whose urinary urate excretion exceeds 750 mg daily. Therapy with the drug has reduced the rate of calculus events (passage of a new calculus or radiographic evidence of a new or enlarged calculus) and has prolonged the time to recurrence in patients with hyperuricosuria and normocalciuria and a history of recurrent calcium oxalate renal calculi. The use of allopurinol for this disorder must be carefully evaluated initially and reevaluated periodically to determine that therapy with the drug is beneficial and outweighs the risks. Clinical experience suggests that patients with recurrent calcium oxalate renal calculi may also benefit from dietary changes such as reductions in animal protein, sodium, refined sugars, oxalate-rich foods, and excessive calcium intake, as well as increases in oral fluids and dietary fiber. Allopurinol is also used for the prevention of uric acid renal calculi in patients with a history of recurrent stone formation.

■ **Other Uses** Allopurinol has been used to reduce hyperuricemia secondary to glucose-6-phosphate dehydrogenase deficiency†, Lesch-Nyhan syndrome†, polycythemia vera†, sarcoidosis†, and secondary to the administration of thiazides† or ethambutol†.

Dosage and Administration

■ **Administration** Allopurinol is administered orally. Allopurinol also has been administered rectally†. Allopurinol sodium is administered by IV infusion. IV therapy with the drug generally is used in patients who do not tolerate oral therapy.

In all patients receiving allopurinol, fluid intake should be sufficient to yield a daily urine output of at least 2 L and maintenance of a neutral or, preferably, alkaline urine is desirable.

Pharmacogenetic Testing Because of a strong association between the presence of the variant human leukocyte antigen (HLA)-B*5801 allele and risk of developing allopurinol-induced severe hypersensitivity reactions, pharmacogenetic testing for HLA-B*5801 should be considered prior to initiation of allopurinol therapy in certain high-risk populations in which this allele is known to be highly prevalent. The American College of Rheumatology (ACR) and some clinicians state that screening for HLA-B*5801 should be considered prior to initiation of allopurinol therapy in populations in which both the HLA-B*5801 allele frequency is increased and HLA-B*5801-positive patients have a very high risk of experiencing severe hypersensitivity reactions (e.g., individuals of Korean ancestry with stage 3 or worse chronic kidney disease, individuals of Han Chinese or Thai ancestry irrespective of renal function). Genotyping results are considered positive if 1 or 2 copies of HLA-B*5801 are detected and negative if no copies of the variant allele are detected. Experts state that allopurinol therapy should be avoided in patients who have tested positive for HLA-B*5801. If use of allopurinol cannot be avoided and the benefits are considered to outweigh the risks, more intensive monitoring for manifestations of hypersensitivity reactions is required. (See Pharmacogenomics of Allopurinol-induced Serious Hypersensitivity Reactions under Cautions: Dermatologic and Sensitivity Reactions.)

Application of HLA genotyping as a screening tool has important limitations and must never substitute for appropriate clinical vigilance and patient management. Many HLA-B*5801-positive patients who are treated with allopurinol will never develop severe cutaneous reactions, and such reactions may develop in HLA-B*5801-negative patients. (See Cautions: Dermatologic and Sensitivity Reactions.) For additional information and guidance on how to interpret and apply the results of HLA-B*5801 testing, the Clinical Pharmacogenetics Implementation Consortium (CPIC) guideline for HLA genotype and allopurinol dosing should be consulted.

Oral Administration Oral allopurinol usually is administered in a single daily dose. The manufacturers recommend that oral doses greater than 300 mg be administered in divided doses. Administration of the drug after meals may minimize adverse GI effects.

IV Infusion Allopurinol sodium powder for injection is reconstituted by adding 25 mL of sterile water for injection to a vial labeled as containing allopurinol sodium equivalent to 500 mg of allopurinol to provide a solution containing 20 mg of allopurinol per mL. Reconstituted solutions should be further diluted prior to administration with 0.9% sodium chloride injection or 5% dextrose injection to a final concentration not exceeding 6 mg of allopurinol per mL Allopurinol solutions should be inspected visually for particulate matter and discoloration whenever solution and container permit. The injection should be discarded if discoloration or particulate matter is present.

Rectal Administration Extemporaneously prepared allopurinol suppositories† have been given rectally in patients unable to tolerate oral medications, particularly during cancer chemotherapy, but pharmacokinetic studies indicate that little if any of the drug is absorbed systemically following this route of administration.

■ **Dosage** Dosage of allopurinol varies with the severity of the disease and should be adjusted according to the response and tolerance of the patient. Dosage of allopurinol also may be adjusted according to results of serum uric acid concentrations, which should be maintained within the normal range.

Gout In patients with gout, allopurinol therapy should be initiated at a low dosage to reduce the possibility of early flare-up of acute gouty attacks and also because some data suggest that higher initial dosages may be associated with increased risk of severe hypersensitivity reactions. Dosage should be gradually increased to achieve target serum urate concentrations (less than 6 mg/dL), or until the maximum recommended dosage is reached.

The manufacturers recommend that patients be started on oral allopurinol dosages of 100 mg daily and that the daily dose of the drug be increased by 100 mg at weekly intervals until the serum urate concentration falls to 6 mg/dL or less, or until the maximum recommended dosage of 800 mg daily is reached. The manufacturers state that the usual dosage may range from 200–300 mg daily in adults with mild gout and from 400–600 mg daily in those with moderately severe tophaceous gout. Serum urate concentrations are often reduced more slowly with allopurinol than with uricosuric drugs and minimum concentrations may not be reached for 1–3 weeks. After serum urate concentrations are controlled, it may be possible to reduce dosage; the manufacturers state that the minimum effective dosage is 100–200 mg daily. Allopurinol therapy should be continued indefinitely; irregular dosage schedules may lead to increased serum urate concentrations.

Some experts recommend that allopurinol therapy be initiated at a dosage of 100 mg daily or less in adults with gout and that dosage be increased every 2–5 weeks in increments of 100 mg daily to achieve target serum urate concentrations or until a maximum recommended dosage of 800–900 mg daily is reached. Although a dosage of 300 mg daily is commonly used, up to one-half of patients with normal renal function will not achieve target serum urate concentrations at this dosage. In some studies utilizing dosages up to 600–800 mg daily, target serum urate concentrations were achieved in 75–80% of patients.

When allopurinol is added to a therapeutic regimen of colchicine, uricosuric agents, and/or anti-inflammatory agents, a transition period of several months may be necessary before the latter drugs can be discontinued. During this period, the drugs should be administered concomitantly, and allopurinol dosage should be adjusted until serum urate concentrations are normal and freedom from acute gouty attacks is maintained for several months. When the uricosuric agent is being withdrawn, dosage of the uricosuric agent should be gradually reduced over several weeks.

Chemotherapy-induced Hyperuricemia **Oral Dosage.** For the prevention of acute uric acid nephropathy in patients with leukemia, lymphoma, and solid tumor malignancies who are undergoing chemotherapy that is expected to result in tumor lysis and subsequent elevations of serum and urinary uric acid concentrations, adults may receive 600–800 mg of allopurinol daily for 2–3 days; most clinicians recommend that this therapy begin 1–2 days before initiating chemotherapy. When allopurinol is used with mercaptopurine or azathioprine, dosage of the latter drugs must be reduced. (See Drug Interactions: Antineoplastic Agents.) In the initial management of hyperuricemia secondary to neoplastic disease, children younger than 6 years of age may receive 150 mg of allopurinol daily and children 6–10 years of age may receive 300 mg daily. After about 48 hours of therapy, dosage should be adjusted according to the response of the patient.

IV Dosage. Dosage of allopurinol sodium is expressed in terms of allopurinol.

For patients who cannot tolerate oral allopurinol therapy, the manufacturer of allopurinol sodium for injection recommends that adults and children older than 10 years of age receive an allopurinol dosage of 200–400 mg/m² daily and children 10 years and younger receive an initial dosage of 200 mg/m² daily (both by continuous infusion or in equally divided intermittent IV infusions administered at 6-, 8-, or 12-hour intervals) beginning 24–48 hours before initiation of chemotherapy. In adults and children greater than 10 years of age daily IV allopurinol dosages should not exceed 600 mg since higher dosages do not appear to provide additional benefit.

Recurrent Calcium Oxalate Renal Calculi For the management of recurrent calcium oxalate renal calculi in patients with hyperuricosuria, the recommended initial dosage of allopurinol is 200–300 mg daily. Subsequent dosage may be increased or decreased depending on control of hyperuricosuria assessed by 24-hour urinary urate excretion determinations.

■ **Dosage in Renal Impairment** Various approaches to dosing allopurinol in patients with renal impairment have been recommended in an attempt to minimize the risk of allopurinol-induced hypersensitivity reactions. Use of a low initial dosage has been recommended to reduce the risk of such reactions; the relationship between hypersensitivity reactions and the maintenance dosage used in renal impairment is more controversial. This uncertainty is reflected in the lack of consensus on allopurinol dosage in patients with renal impairment. (See Cautions: Dermatologic and Sensitivity Reactions.)

In patients with impaired renal function, allopurinol and particularly its metabolite oxypurinol may accumulate and, thus, dosage should be reduced. Initial dosages in these patients should be lower than those used in patients with normal renal function.

The manufacturers and some experts recommend that maximum dosages of allopurinol be adjusted according to creatinine clearance. For oral dosing, the manufacturers recommend 200 mg of allopurinol daily when creatinine clearance is 10–20 mL/minute and state that dosage should not exceed 100 mg daily in patients with creatinine clearances less than 10 mL/minute. In patients with severely impaired renal function (i.e., creatinine clearance less than 3 mL/minute), the manufacturers state that use of longer dosing intervals also may be required.

Some clinicians have recommended alternative maintenance dosages of allopurinol based on the patient's creatinine clearance (see Table 1). Although such creatinine clearance-based dosing was widely adopted, this dosing strategy frequently fails to reduce serum urate concentrations to target levels, and evidence that this strategy reduces the risk of allopurinol-induced hypersensitivity reactions in patients who tolerate low initial dosages of the drug is lacking. More recent data suggest that dosage can be increased safely beyond these creatinine clearance-based maintenance dosages, with greater reduction of serum urate concentrations.

Table 1. Creatinine Clearance-based Maintenance Dosages of Allopurinol in Renal Impairment

Creatinine Clearance (mL/minute)	Maintenance Dosage
0	100 mg every 3 days
10	100 mg every 2 days
20	100 mg daily
40	150 mg daily
60	200 mg daily
80	250 mg daily

Based on data suggesting that initial dosage is a risk factor for allopurinol-induced hypersensitivity reactions, the American College of Rheumatology (ACR) and some clinicians recommend that allopurinol therapy be initiated at a reduced dosage of 50 mg daily in patients with stage 4 or worse chronic kidney disease (creatinine clearance less than 30 mL/minute). Dosage may be adjusted in increments of 50–100 mg every 2–5 weeks to achieve target serum urate concentrations. The ACR and some other clinicians state that dosage may be increased to levels exceeding 300 mg daily, even in patients with renal impairment, provided patients receive appropriate education and are monitored regularly for evidence of hypersensitivity reactions or other adverse effects.

Other experts and clinicians recommend use of even lower initial dosages (based on estimated glomerular filtration rate [eGFR]) in patients with renal impairment (see Table 2), followed by a gradual increase in dosage (e.g., in 50-mg increments at intervals of approximately every 4 weeks); although these experts state that maximum dosage in patients with renal impairment should be lower than in patients without renal impairment, target serum urate concentrations should be the same.

Table 2. GFR-based Dosages for Initiation of Allopurinol Therapy in Renal Impairment

Estimated GFR (mL/minute per 1.73 m²)	Initial Dosage
Less than 5	50 mg weekly
5–15	50 mg twice weekly
16–30	50 mg every 2 days
31–45	50 mg daily
46–60	50 and 100 mg on alternating days
61–90	100 mg daily

For IV dosing, the manufacturer states that patients with creatinine clearances of 10–20 mL/minute can receive 200 mg daily, those with creatinine clearances of 3–10 mL/minute can receive 100 mg daily, and those with creatinine clearances less than 3 mL/minute may receive 100 mg daily at extended intervals.

Cautions

Results of early clinical studies and experience suggested that some allopurinol-induced adverse effects (e.g., acute attacks of gout, rash) occurred in more than 1% of patients, but current experience suggests that adverse effects of the drug occur in less than 1% of patients. The reduced incidence in adverse effects observed with more recent experience may have resulted in part from initiating therapy with the drug more gradually and following current prescribing precautions and recommendations.

■ **Dermatologic and Local Effects** The most common adverse effect of oral allopurinol is a pruritic maculopapular rash. Dermatitides of the exfoliative, urticarial, erythematous, eczematoid, hemorrhagic, and purpuric types have also occurred. Alopecia, fever, and malaise may also occur alone or in conjunction with dermatitis. In addition, severe furunculoses of the nose, cellulitis, and ichthyosis have been reported. The incidence of rash may be increased in patients with renal insufficiency. Skin reactions may be delayed and have been reported to occur as long as 2 years after initiating allopurinol therapy. Rarely, skin rash may be followed by severe hypersensitivity reactions which may sometimes be fatal. (See Cautions: Dermatologic and Sensitivity Reactions.) Some patients who have developed severe dermatitis have also developed cataracts (including a case of toxic cataracts), but the exact relationship between allopurinol and cataracts has not been established. Pruritus, onycholysis, and lichen planus have also occurred rarely in patients receiving allopurinol. Facial edema, sweating, and skin edema have also occurred rarely, but a causal relationship to the drug has not been established.

Local injection site reactions have been reported in patients receiving allopurinol sodium IV.

■ **Dermatologic and Sensitivity Reactions** Serious and sometimes fatal hypersensitivity reactions have been reported in approximately 0.1–0.4% of patients receiving allopurinol. The reactions include a spectrum of cutaneous reactions and systemic manifestations, including toxic epidermal necrolysis (TEN), Stevens-Johnson syndrome (SJS), drug reaction with eosinophilia and systemic symptoms (DRESS), and allopurinol hypersensitivity syndrome; systemic manifestations may include fever, leukocytosis, atypical circulating lymphocytes, eosinophilia, lymphadenopathy, vasculitis, and organ system involvement such as hepatitis and acute renal failure. The reactions also have been referred to as severe cutaneous adverse reactions (SCARs). These reactions have similar clinical presentations, and some of the terms have been used interchangeably in published literature to describe the clinical syndromes. Onset typically occurs within weeks or months following initiation of allopurinol therapy, but may occur later. The mortality rate of severe allopurinol-induced hypersensitivity reactions is up to 20–30%. If such reactions occur, allopurinol should be discontinued immediately, since early diagnosis and drug discontinuance may improve prognosis.

Serious and fatal cases of hypersensitivity angiitis and allergic vasculitis involving erythematous maculopapular rash with desquamation, severe exfoliative dermatitis, vesicular bullous dermatitis, arterial nephrosclerosis, oliguria, congestive heart failure, and acute onset of permanent deafness have been reported during therapy with the drug. Allopurinol-induced hepatotoxicity may also be a hypersensitivity reaction to the drug. (See Cautions: Hepatic Effects.) A generalized hypersensitivity vasculitis has rarely led to irreversible hepatotoxicity and death.

Presence of human leukocyte antigen (HLA)-B*5801, an inherited allelic variant of the HLA-B gene, is strongly associated with severe hypersensitivity reactions to allopurinol, particularly in certain Asian populations. (See Pharmacogenomics of Allopurinol-induced Serious Hypersensitivity Reactions under Cautions: Dermatologic and Sensitivity Reactions.) However, other genetic or nongenetic factors (e.g., renal impairment, thiazide diuretic use, recent initiation of allopurinol therapy, high initial allopurinol dosage) also have been associated with an increased risk of such reactions. The magnitude of risk associated with these factors is uncertain because of the low incidence of severe allopurinol-associated hypersensitivity reactions. The frequency of allopurinol-induced hypersensitivity reactions may be increased in patients with decreased renal function who receive allopurinol and a thiazide diuretic concomitantly. (See Cautions: Precautions and Contraindications and see Drug Interactions: Diuretics.)

Some of the reported nongenetic risk factors (e.g., renal impairment, diuretic therapy, higher allopurinol dosage) are associated with increased plasma concentrations of oxypurinol, the active metabolite of allopurinol. Oxypurinol has been shown to bind to the peptide-binding groove of HLA-B*5801 and activate T cells in a dose-dependent manner, and some reports suggest that increased oxypurinol concentrations may be associated with poorer prognosis in patients who experience hypersensitivity reactions. However, evidence of a clear relationship between oxypurinol concentration and development of allopurinol-induced hypersensitivity is lacking.

There are conflicting data regarding allopurinol dosage. Some data suggest that high initial dosages are associated with increased risk of hypersensitivity reactions and that initiating allopurinol therapy at a low dosage adjusted for renal function may reduce the risk of such reactions. However, the relationship between allopurinol maintenance dosage, particularly in individuals with renal impairment, and hypersensitivity is more controversial, and this uncertainty is reflected in the lack of consensus on allopurinol dosage in renal impairment. (See Dosage and Administration: Dosage in Renal Impairment.)

Allopurinol should not be administered to patients who have previously shown hypersensitivity to it or who have had a serious reaction to the drug. (See Cautions: Precautions and Contraindications.)

Pharmacogenomics of Allopurinol-induced Serious Hypersensitivity Reactions Studies have demonstrated a strong association, particularly in certain Asian populations, between the risk of developing allopurinol-induced severe hypersensitivity reactions (SJS, TEN, DRESS, allopurinol hypersensitivity syndrome) and the presence of HLA-B*5801, an inherited allelic variant of the HLA-B gene. The HLA-B*5801 allele is found most commonly in individuals of Han Chinese, Korean, or Thai ancestry, with some estimates indicating that up to 20%, approximately 12%, or 6–15% of individuals in these respective ethnic groups may be HLA-B*5801-positive. Studies conducted in Japan and Europe suggest that 1–2% of these populations may be HLA-B*5801-positive. In the US, the allele reportedly is present in approximately 7% of individuals of Asian ancestry, 3–6% of African-Americans, and less than 2% of Caucasians and Hispanics. The strength of the association between HLA-B*5801 and hypersensitivity reactions appears to vary among ethnic groups according to the frequency of HLA-B*5801 expression. In one study in Taiwan, HLA-B*5801 was present in 100% of Han Chinese patients with allopurinol-induced hypersensitivity syndrome, SJS, or TEN, compared with 15% of allopurinol-tolerant patients and 20% of population controls. Strong associations also have been reported in Thai and Korean populations. More modest associations have been observed in Japanese and European Caucasian populations, with HLA-B*5801 present in approximately 36–56 and 55–64%, respectively, of patients with severe hypersensitivity reactions to allopurinol.

Presence of the HLA-B*5801 allele has not been found to be predictive of less severe dermatologic reactions (e.g., simple or mild rash, maculopapular eruption) associated with allopurinol.

Pharmacogenetic testing for HLA-B*5801 should be considered prior to initiation of allopurinol therapy in certain high-risk populations in which this allele is known to be highly prevalent. The American College of Rheumatology (ACR) and some clinicians state that screening for HLA-B*5801 should be considered prior to initiation of allopurinol therapy in populations in which both the HLA-B*5801 allele frequency is increased and HLA-B*5801-positive patients have a very high risk of experiencing severe hypersensitivity reactions (e.g., individuals of Korean ancestry with stage 3 or worse chronic kidney disease, individuals of Han Chinese or Thai ancestry irrespective of renal function). Experts state that allopurinol therapy should be avoided in patients who have tested positive for HLA-B*5801. If use of allopurinol cannot be avoided and the benefits of allopurinol are considered to outweigh the risks, more intensive monitoring for manifestations of hypersensitivity reactions is required.

Severe hypersensitivity reactions can occur in allopurinol-treated patients who are negative for HLA-B*5801 regardless of their ethnicity, and a substantial number of patients with the variant allele will not develop severe hypersensitivity reactions if they receive allopurinol therapy. Results of cost-effectiveness analyses conducted for some populations (mostly in Asia) suggest that screening for HLA-B*5801 prior to initiation of allopurinol therapy would be cost-effective in certain populations (e.g., Taiwanese and Thai populations, Korean patients with chronic renal insufficiency), and prospective studies evaluating HLA-B*5801 screening in Taiwanese individuals of Han Chinese ancestry and in Korean patients with chronic renal insufficiency suggest that screening these populations for HLA-B*5801 reduces the incidence of allopurinol-induced severe adverse cutaneous reactions below historically predicted rates. Additional studies are needed to assess the role of screening in other populations with lower or ill-defined frequencies of the allele. Based on estimated allele frequency and health-care costs in the US, some clinicians suggest that screening of African-Americans prior to initiation of allopurinol therapy also may be cost-effective.

Application of HLA genotyping as a screening tool has important limitations and must never substitute for appropriate clinical vigilance and patient management. Regardless of genotyping results, patients receiving allopurinol should be monitored closely.

■ **Hepatic Effects** Alterations in liver function test results, including transient elevations of serum alkaline phosphatase, urinary urobilinogen, AST, and ALT, and decreases in sulfobromophthalein excretion have occurred in some patients. Reversible hepatomegaly, hepatocellular damage (including necrosis), granulomatous changes, liver failure, hepatitis, hyperbilirubinemia, and jaundice have also occurred. The mechanism of some hepatotoxic reactions to allopurinol has been described as a hypersensitivity reaction, since fever, rash, peripheral eosinophilia, and liver biopsy findings of eosinophilia and noncaseating granulomas occurred; however, other mechanisms may also have been involved.

■ **Hematologic Effects** Leukocytosis, leukopenia, eosinophilia, thrombocytopenia, blast crisis, hemorrhage, bone marrow aplasia, neutropenia, ecchymosis, disseminated intravascular coagulation, and fatal bone marrow suppression and granulocytopenia have been reported rarely in patients receiving allopurinol. Most patients in whom bone marrow suppression was reported during allopurinol therapy were also receiving other drugs with myelosuppressive potential concomitantly. Bone marrow suppression may occur as early as 6 weeks and as late as 6 years after initiation of allopurinol. Mild reticulocytosis, lymphocytosis, agranulocytosis, pancytopenia, anemia, hemolytic anemia, aplastic anemia, decreased prothrombin levels, and eosinophilic fibrohistiocytic bone marrow lesions have also occurred rarely, but a causal relationship to allopurinol has not been established.

■ **GI Effects** Adverse GI effects of allopurinol may include nausea, vomiting, diarrhea, intermittent abdominal pain, enlarged abdomen, constipation, flatulence, intestinal obstruction, proctitis, alteration or loss of taste, gastritis, and dyspepsia. Anorexia, GI bleeding, hemorrhagic pancreatitis, stomatitis, mucositis, salivary gland swelling, and tongue edema have also occurred rarely in patients receiving allopurinol, but a causal relationship to the drug has not been established.

■ **Nervous System Effects** Peripheral neuropathy, neuritis, paresthesia, headache, generalized seizure, status epilepticus, myoclonus, hypotonia, twitching, agitation, changes in mental status, cerebral infarction, coma, dystonia, paralysis, tremor, and somnolence have occurred rarely in patients receiving allopurinol. Optic neuritis, dizziness, vertigo, depression, confusion, amnesia, insomnia, asthenia, and foot drop have also occurred rarely in patients receiving allopurinol, but a causal relationship to the drug has not been established.

■ **Other Adverse Effects** Other reported adverse effects of allopurinol include fever, diaphoresis, myopathy, arthralgias, and epistaxis. Renal failure, decreased renal function, hematuria, increased creatinine, oliguria, hyperuricemia, and urinary tract infection also have been reported. Patients receiving allopurinol also have developed lactic acidosis, metabolic acidosis, water intoxication, hyperphosphatemia, hypomagnesemia, hyponatremia, hypernatremia, hypokalemia, hyperkalemia, hypercalcemia, and other electrolyte abnormalities. Tumor lysis syndrome, sepsis, septic shock, and other infections also have been reported.

Other adverse effects reported with allopurinol include respiratory failure/insufficiency, acute respiratory distress syndrome (ARDS), increased respiratory rate, and apnea. Hypervolemia, heart failure, cardiorespiratory arrest, hypotension, hypertension, pulmonary embolism, decreased venous pressure, flushing, stroke, ECG abnormalities, ventricular fibrillation, splenomegaly, hyperglycemia, glycosuria, and uremia also have been reported. Malaise, pericarditis, peripheral vascular disease, thrombophlebitis, bradycardia, vasodilation, hypercalcemia, hyperlipidemia, gynecomastia in males, lymphadenopathy, myalgia, bronchospasm, pharyngitis, rhinitis, asthma, macular retinitis, iritis, conjunctivitis, amblyopia, tinnitus, nephritis, albuminuria, primary hematuria, and decreased libido have occurred rarely in patients receiving allopurinol, but a causal relationship to the drug has not been established.

Patients with renal disease have shown either an increase or a decrease in BUN concentrations, pyelonephritis, renal colic, bilateral ureteral obstruction, xanthine stones, and oxypurinol stones and sludge during allopurinol therapy. In cancer patients who develop hyperuricemia, changes in renal function may be associated with the underlying malignancy, rather than with administration of allopurinol. In several patients in whom renal function deteriorated during allopurinol therapy, concurrent conditions (e.g., multiple myeloma, congestive myocardial disease) were present before initiation of allopurinol therapy.

One study in rats indicated that the concentration of iron stored in the liver was increased during administration of allopurinol. This disturbance in iron storage has not been demonstrated clinically. In another study, however, a reversible rise in serum iron concentrations and decrease in total iron binding capacity occurred in patients receiving 500–600 mg of allopurinol daily; these effects reverted to normal when dosage was reduced to 300 mg daily.

■ Precautions and Contraindications Allopurinol should be discontinued at the first appearance of rash or any sign that may indicate an allergic reaction, since severe hypersensitivity reactions that may be fatal have been reported following appearance of rash. Although, in some patients with rash, allopurinol may be reinstated at a lower dosage without untoward incident, the drug should *not* be reinstituted in patients who have had a severe reaction. Patients initiating allopurinol therapy should be informed of the potential for severe hypersensitivity reactions to occur and should be advised to immediately discontinue the drug and seek medical attention at the first appearance of any signs or symptoms of hypersensitivity (e.g., rash, pruritus). Pharmacogenetic testing should be considered prior to initiation of therapy in certain high-risk patients who may have a genetic predisposition to severe allopurinol-induced hypersensitivity reactions. (See Pharmacogenetic Testing under Dosage and Administration: Administration.)

Allopurinol may increase the frequency of acute gouty attacks during the first 6–12 months of therapy; therefore, prophylactic doses of colchicine should generally be administered concurrently during the first 3–6 months of allopurinol therapy. (See Uses: Gout.)

Patients should be warned that drowsiness may occur during allopurinol therapy and may impair their ability to perform activities requiring mental alertness. Patients should also be warned to discontinue the drug and consult their physician immediately at the first sign of rash, painful urination, blood in the urine, irritation of the eyes, or swelling of the lips or mouth.

Liver function tests (particularly in patients with preexisting liver disease), renal function tests (particularly in patients with impaired renal function or concurrent illness that can affect renal function such as hypertension or diabetes mellitus), and complete blood cell counts should be performed before initiating allopurinol and periodically during therapy, especially during the first few months. If patients receiving allopurinol develop anorexia, weight loss, or pruritus, assessment of liver function should be part of the diagnostic evaluation.

Patients with impaired renal function must be carefully observed while receiving allopurinol (particularly during the early stages of therapy) and the dosage decreased or the drug discontinued if evidence of deterioration in renal function occurs and persists. Patients with impaired renal function require lower dosages of allopurinol than those with normal renal function. (See Dosage and Administration: Dosage in Renal Impairment.) The usual initial dosage of allopurinol should be reduced in patients with impaired renal function. Since concomitant therapy with allopurinol and a thiazide diuretic in patients with decreased renal function may increase the risk of allopurinol-induced hypersensitivity reactions, concomitant therapy with the drugs should be used with caution in such patients and the patients should be observed closely. (See Drug Interactions: Diuretics.)

■ Pediatric Precautions Pending further accumulation of data, the manufacturers state that allopurinol is rarely indicated in children except in those with hyperuricemia secondary to neoplastic disease, cancer chemotherapy, or genetic disorders of purine metabolism. Clinical experience in about 200 pediatric patients suggests that safety and efficacy of allopurinol sodium for injection are similar to those in adults.

■ Geriatric Precautions The manufacturer of allopurinol sodium for injection states that clinical studies of parenteral allopurinol sodium did not include a sufficient number of patients 65 years of age or older to determine whether such patients respond differently than younger individuals, but that other reported clinical experience has not identified differences in response between geriatric and younger patients. In a pharmacokinetic study, peak plasma concentrations and area under the plasma concentration-time curve (AUC) of oxypurinol (active metabolite of allopurinol) were about 50–60% higher in geriatric individuals than in younger individuals following single oral allopurinol dosing. (See Pharmacokinetics: Absorption.) Since these differences appear to be related to changes in renal function in geriatric patients, some clinicians state that adjustments in allopurinol dosage may be necessary in geriatric patients based on the degree of renal impairment. (See Dosage and Administration: Dosage in Renal Impairment.) In addition, appropriate dosage of allopurinol in geriatric patients should be selected with caution because of the greater frequency of decreased hepatic, renal, or cardiac function and of concomitant disease and drug therapy in these patients.

■ Pregnancy, Fertility, and Lactation Although there are no adequate and controlled studies to date using allopurinol in pregnant women, the drug has been shown to be teratogenic in mice using intraperitoneal allopurinol doses of 50 or 100 mg/kg (0.3 or 0.75 times the recommended human dose on a mg/m^2 basis) on gestation days 10 or 13. Allopurinol should be used during pregnancy only when clearly needed.

Reproduction studies in rats and rabbits using dosages up to 20 times the usual human dosage have not revealed evidence of impaired fertility. Infertility in human males and impotence have occurred rarely during allopurinol therapy, but a causal relationship to the drug has not been established.

Since allopurinol and oxypurinol are distributed into milk, allopurinol should be used with caution in nursing women.

Drug Interactions

The following drug interactions were observed in patients receiving oral allopurinol therapy. Although many patients received long-term oral administration of allopurinol (e.g., those with gout or renal calculi), these interactions may be relevant to allopurinol sodium for injection therapy as well.

■ Drugs that Increase Serum Urate Concentration Many drugs may increase serum urate concentrations, including most diuretics, pyrazinamide, diazoxide, alcohol, and mecamylamine. If these drugs are administered during allopurinol therapy, dosage of allopurinol may need to be increased.

■ Ampicillin and Amoxicillin An increased incidence of rash reportedly occurs in patients with hyperuricemia who are receiving allopurinol and concomitant ampicillin or amoxicillin as compared with those receiving allopurinol, ampicillin, or amoxicillin alone. Some clinicians suggest that either allopurinol or hyperuricemia may potentiate aminopenicillin allergenicity. However, other clinicians state that the rash reported in patients receiving allopurinol and aminopenicillins concomitantly is generally the delayed aminopenicillin rash that appears to be nonimmunologic. The clinical importance of this effect has not been determined; however, some clinicians suggest that concomitant use of the drugs should be avoided if possible.

■ Anticoagulants Allopurinol inhibits the hepatic microsomal drug metabolism of dicumarol. In one study, the half-life of dicumarol was increased from 51 to 152 hours when the anticoagulant was taken concurrently with allopurinol. Although the clinical importance of this effect may vary, patients taking allopurinol with dicumarol should be observed for increased anticoagulant effects and prothrombin time should be monitored periodically in these patients. Allopurinol has *not* been shown to substantially potentiate the anticoagulant effect of warfarin except in one case when warfarin, allopurinol, and indomethacin were administered concurrently.

■ Antineoplastic Agents In dosages of 300–600 mg daily, allopurinol inhibits the oxidative metabolism of azathioprine and mercaptopurine by xanthine oxidase, thus increasing the possibility of toxic effects from these drugs, particularly bone marrow depression. When allopurinol is administered concomitantly with mercaptopurine or azathioprine, the doses of the antineoplastic agents should initially be reduced to 25–33% of the usual dose and subsequent dosage adjusted according to the patient response and toxic effects. Substitution of thioguanine for mercaptopurine has also been suggested.

Concomitant administration of allopurinol with cyclophosphamide may increase the incidence of bone marrow depression as compared with cyclophosphamide alone, but the mechanism for this interaction is not known. However, results of a well-controlled study in patients with lymphoma have shown that concomitant use of allopurinol with cyclophosphamide, doxorubicin, bleomycin, procarbazine, and/or mechlorethamine did not increase the incidence of bone marrow depression in these patients.

■ Chlorpropamide Allopurinol and chlorpropamide cause adverse hepatorenal reactions. Although the combination does not enhance the occurrence of these reactions, caution is indicated if these 2 drugs are administered concomitantly. Because allopurinol or its metabolites may compete with chlorpropamide for renal tubular secretion, patients who receive these drugs concomitantly (especially those with renal insufficiency) should be observed for signs of excessive hypoglycemia.

■ Cyclosporine Increased blood concentrations of cyclosporine have been reported in patients receiving allopurinol and cyclosporine concomitantly. Therefore, blood cyclosporine concentrations should be monitored and dosage adjustments of cyclosporine should be considered when these drugs are used concomitantly.

■ Didanosine In 2 patients with renal impairment, concomitant use of allopurinol (300 mg daily) and buffered didanosine (single 200-mg dose) increased peak plasma concentrations and area under the concentration-time curve (AUC) of didanosine by 232 and 312%, respectively. In 14 healthy individuals who received allopurinol (300 mg daily) and buffered didanosine (single 400-mg dose), peak plasma concentrations and AUC of didanosine were increased by 69 and 113%, respectively. The manufacturer of didanosine states that concomitant use of allopurinol and didanosine is contraindicated since increased didanosine exposure may result in increased didanosine-associated toxicity.

■ Diuretics Diuretics such as thiazides, furosemide, and ethacrynic acid, when given with allopurinol, may increase serum oxypurinol concentrations and may thereby increase the risk of serious allopurinol toxicity, including hypersensitivity reactions (particularly in patients with decreased renal function); however, allopurinol has been used safely with thiazides to reduce hyperuricemia induced by the diuretics†. A review of reports of allopurinol toxicity in patients who were receiving concomitant therapy with allopurinol and a thiazide indicated that patients were principally receiving a thiazide for hypertension and that tests to rule out decreased renal function secondary to hypertensive nephropathy were not often performed; however, in patients in whom renal insufficiency was documented, dosage of allopurinol was not appropriately reduced. Although a causal mechanism and relationship have not been definitely established, the evidence suggests that renal function should be monitored (even in the absence of renal failure) in patients receiving allopurinol and a thiazide concomitantly and that dosage of allopurinol in such patients should be adjusted even more conservatively than usual if decreased renal function is detected. Consideration should be given to the indication for concomitant diuretic use and whether alternative agents (e.g., other antihypertensive agents) might appropriately be used. When diuretics (particularly thiazides) and allopurinol are used concomitantly, especially in patients with chronic renal impairment, more intensive monitoring for manifestations of hypersensitivity reactions is required. (See Cautions: Dermatologic and Sensitivity Reactions.)

■ Uricosuric Agents Uricosurics promote urinary excretion of oxypurinol (which also inhibits xanthine oxidase) and may thereby reduce the inhibition of xanthine oxidase produced by allopurinol therapy; however, the effects of allopurinol and a uricosuric are generally additive, and the combination is usually used to therapeutic advantage. Renal precipitation of oxypurines has not occurred to date in patients receiving allopurinol alone or in combination with a uricosuric, but the possibility should be kept in mind.

Pharmacology

Allopurinol inhibits xanthine oxidase, the enzyme that catalyzes the conversion of hypoxanthine to xanthine and of xanthine to uric acid. Oxypurinol, a metabolite of allopurinol, also inhibits xanthine oxidase. By inhibiting xanthine oxidase, allopurinol and its metabolite block conversion of the oxypurines (hypoxanthine and xanthine) to uric acid, thus decreasing serum and urine concentrations of uric acid. The drug differs, therefore, from uricosuric agents which lower serum urate concentrations by promoting urinary excretion of uric acid. Xanthine oxidase concentrations are not altered by long-term administration of the drug.

Allopurinol does not directly interfere with purine nucleotide or nucleic acid synthesis. The drug, however, indirectly increases oxypurine and allopurinol ribonucleotide concentrations and decreases phosphoribosylpyrophosphate concentrations, thus decreasing *de novo* purine biosynthesis by pseudofeedback inhibition. In addition, allopurinol increases the incorporation of hypoxanthine and xanthine into DNA and RNA, thereby further decreasing serum urate concentrations. Allopurinol may produce a deficit of total purines (uric acid and oxypurines) amounting to several hundred mg daily.

Accompanying the decrease in uric acid produced by allopurinol is an increase in serum and urine concentrations of hypoxanthine and xanthine. Plasma concentrations of these oxypurines do not, however, rise commensurately with the fall in serum urate concentrations and are often 20–30% less than would be expected in view of urate concentrations prior to allopurinol therapy. This discrepancy occurs because renal clearance of the oxypurines is at least 10 times greater than that of uric acid. In addition, normal urinary purine output is almost exclusively uric acid, but after treatment with allopurinol, it is composed of uric acid, xanthine, and hypoxanthine, each having independent solubility. Thus, the risk of crystalluria is reduced. Alkalinization of the urine increases the solubility of the purines, further minimizing the risk of crystalluria. Decreased tubular transport of uric acid also results in increased renal reabsorption of calcium and decreased calcium excretion.

Allopurinol also interferes with *de novo* pyrimidine nucleotide synthesis by inhibiting orotidine 5′-phosphate decarboxylase. Secondary orotic aciduria and orotidinuria result. Orotic acid is highly insoluble and could form a heavy sediment of urinary crystals; however, the increased excretion of orotic acid and orotidine rarely exceeds 10% of the total pyrimidines synthesized by the body. In addition, enhanced conversion of uridine to uridine 5′-monophosphate usually occurs and, therefore, this partial inhibition of pyrimidine synthesis is considered innocuous.

In rats, allopurinol reportedly increases liver storage of iron by inhibiting the ferritin-xanthine oxidase system responsible for mobilization of iron from the liver; however, this effect has not been demonstrated clinically.

Allopurinol may also inhibit hepatic microsomal enzymes. Allopurinol is not cytotoxic and has no effect on transplantable tumors. The drug has no analgesic, anti-inflammatory, or uricosuric activity.

Pharmacokinetics

■ **Absorption** Following oral administration, approximately 80–90% of a dose of allopurinol is absorbed from the GI tract. Peak plasma concentrations of allopurinol are reached 2–6 hours after a usual dose.

Following oral administration of single 100- or 300-mg dose of allopurinol in healthy adult males in one study, peak plasma allopurinol concentrations of about 0.5 or 1.4 μg/mL, respectively, occurred in about 1–2 hours, while peak oxypurinol (the active metabolite of allopurinol) concentrations of about 2.4 and 6.4 μg/mL, respectively, were reached within about 3–4 hours. In the same study, following IV infusion over 30 minutes of a single 100- or 300-mg dose of allopurinol (as allopurinol sodium), peak plasma concentrations of about 1.6 and 5.1 μg/mL, respectively, occurred in about 30 minutes, while peak oxypurinol concentrations of about 2.2 and 6.2 μg/mL, respectively, were reached within about 4 hours.

Peak plasma concentrations and the area under the plasma concentration-time curve (AUC) of oxypurinol following oral administration of allopurinol 200 mg as a single dose have been reported to be about 50–60% higher in geriatric patients (71–93 years of age) than in younger adults (24–35 years of age); these differences appear to be related to changes in renal function in geriatric patients. Some clinicians state that adjustments in allopurinol dosage may be necessary in geriatric patients based on the degree of renal impairment. (See Dosage and Administration: Dosage in Renal Impairment.)

Because allopurinol concentrations are difficult to determine and because serum concentrations may not adequately reflect the amount of drug bound to xanthine oxidase in the tissues, serum urate concentrations should be used to monitor therapy. After beginning allopurinol therapy, serum urate concentrations begin to decrease slowly within 24–48 hours and reach a nadir after 1–3 weeks of therapy. During allopurinol therapy, serum urate concentrations remain relatively constant; however, serum urate concentrations usually return to pretreatment levels within 1–2 weeks after discontinuing the drug. Because of the continued mobilization of urate deposits, substantial reduction of uric acid may be delayed 6–12 months or may not occur in some patients, particularly in those with tophaceous gout and in those who are underexcretors of uric acid.

Allopurinol is absorbed poorly following rectal administration of the drug as suppositories (in a cocoa butter or polyethylene glycol base). Plasma allopurinol or oxypurinol concentrations have been minimal or undetectable following such rectal administration.

■ **Distribution** Allopurinol is uniformly distributed in total tissue water with the exception of the brain, where concentrations of the drug are approximately 50% those of other tissues. Small amounts of oxypurinol and allopurinol crystals have been found in muscle. Allopurinol and oxypurinol are not bound to plasma proteins. Allopurinol and oxypurinol are distributed into milk.

■ **Elimination** Allopurinol and allopurinol sodium are rapidly metabolized by xanthine oxidase to oxypurinol, which is pharmacologically active. Rapid metabolism of allopurinol to oxypurinol does not seem to be affected substantially during multiple dosing. Pharmacokinetic parameters (e.g., AUC, plasma elimination half-lives) of oxypurinol appear to be similar following oral administration of allopurinol and IV administration of allopurinol sodium. The half-lives of allopurinol and oxypurinol are about 1–3 hours and 18–30 hours, respectively, in patients with normal renal function and are increased in patients with renal impairment. Patients genetically deficient in xanthine oxidase are unable to convert allopurinol to oxypurinol. Both allopurinol and oxypurinol are conjugated and form their respective ribonucleosides.

About 5–7% of an oral allopurinol dose is excreted in urine unchanged within 6 hours after ingestion and about 12% of an IV dose of the drug is excreted unchanged 5 hours after administration. After this time, the drug is excreted by the kidneys as oxypurinol and in small amounts as allopurinol and oxypurinol ribonucleosides. Unlike allopurinol, a large part of oxypurinol is reabsorbed by the renal tubules; therefore, its renal clearance is much lower than that of allopurinol. About 70% of the administered daily dose is excreted in urine as oxypurinol and an additional 20% appears in feces as unchanged drug within 48–72 hours.

Allopurinol and oxypurinol are dialyzable.

Chemistry and Stability

■ **Chemistry** Allopurinol, a structural isomer of hypoxanthine, is a xanthine oxidase inhibitor used in the treatment of gout and selected hyperuricemias. The drug occurs as a fluffy white to off-white powder having a slight odor and is very slightly soluble in water and in alcohol. The apparent pK_a of allopurinol is 9.4 and its active oxidative metabolite, oxypurinol (alloxanthine), has an apparent pK_a of 7.7.

Allopurinol sodium occurs as a white amorphous mass and has a pK_a of 9.31. Following reconstitution of the commercially available allopurinol sodium lyophilized powder with sterile water for injection to a concentration of 20 mg/mL, the solution is clear and almost colorless with no more than a slight opalescence and has a pH of 11.1–11.8.

■ **Stability** Allopurinol tablets should be stored in well-closed containers at 15–30°C. Commercially available allopurinol sodium lyophilized powder for injection should be stored at a controlled room temperature of 20–25°C. Following reconstitution of allopurinol sodium for injection with sterile water for injection, the solutions contain approximately 20 mg/mL and should be further diluted with 0.9% sodium chloride injection or 5% dextrose injection. These further diluted allopurinol sodium solutions, containing no more than 6 mg/mL, should be stored at 20–25°C and should be used within 10 hours of reconstitution. Reconstituted and/or diluted solutions should not be refrigerated.

Allopurinol sodium injection has been reported to be incompatible with various drugs (e.g., sodium bicarbonate), but the compatibility depends on several factors (e.g., concentrations of the drugs, resulting pH, temperature). Specialized references should be consulted for specific compatibility information.

An oral suspension of allopurinol containing 20 mg/mL has been prepared extemporaneously from the commercially available tablets. The tablets were crushed, mixed with a volume of suspending agent (Cologel®) equal to one-third the final volume, and then the suspension was brought to the final volume with a 2:1 mixture of simple syrup and wild cherry syrup. The resulting suspension was stable for at least 14 days when stored in an amber glass bottle at room temperature or 5°C.

Preparations

Excipients in commercially available drug preparations may have clinically important effects in some individuals; consult specific product labeling for details.

Allopurinol

Oral		
Tablets	100 mg*	**Allopurinol Tablets**
		Zyloprim® (scored), Prometheus
	300 mg*	**Allopurinol Tablets**
		Zyloprim® (scored), Prometheus

*available from one or more manufacturer, distributor, and/or repackager by generic (nonproprietary) name

Allopurinol Sodium

Parenteral		
For injection, for IV infusion only	500 mg (of allopurinol)*	**Allopurinol Sodium for Injection**
		Aloprim®, Mylan

*available from one or more manufacturer, distributor, and/or repackager by generic (nonproprietary) name

†Use is not currently included in the labeling approved by the US Food and Drug Administration

Colchicine

■ Colchicine is an antigout and antimitotic agent.

Uses

■ **Gout Flare** Colchicine is used to relieve acute gout flares (acute attacks of gouty arthritis). Nonsteroidal anti-inflammatory agents (NSAIAs) (e.g., indomethacin, ibuprofen, naproxen, sulindac, piroxicam, ketoprofen) are as effective as, and better tolerated than, usual dosages of colchicine for short-term use in relieving acute attacks of gouty arthritis. (See Indomethacin 28:08.04.24.) Corticosteroids also are used to relieve acute attacks of gouty arthritis. Colchicine is considered a second-line agent; colchicine may be used for the treatment of acute gouty arthritis in patients who have not responded to or who cannot tolerate recommended therapies (i.e., NSAIAs, corticosteroids).

Colchicine should be initiated at the first sign of an acute gout flare. When colchicine is administered orally within 12 hours of the onset of an acute gout flare, 38% of patients receiving the drug in the currently recommended dosage have a favorable response.

Colchicine also is used in the prophylactic treatment of recurrent gout flares. Colchicine has no effect on plasma concentrations or urinary excretion of uric acid; therefore, concomitant administration of allopurinol or a uricosuric agent (e.g., febuxostat, probenecid, sulfinpyrazone) is necessary to decrease serum urate concentrations. Prophylactic doses of colchicine should be administered *before* the initiation of allopurinol or uricosuric therapy because sudden changes in serum urate concentrations may precipitate acute gout attacks. After the serum urate concentration has been reduced to the desired level and acute gout attacks have not occurred for 3–6 months (some clinicians suggest 1–12 months), colchicine may be discontinued and the patient may be treated with urate-lowering agents alone. Colchicine is frequently used in combination with probenecid to facilitate prophylactic therapy in patients with chronic gouty arthritis. The usefulness of the commercially available fixed-dosage preparation is limited, however, because the colchicine present exceeds the amount required by most patients.

■ **Familial Mediterranean Fever** Colchicine is used in the management of familial Mediterranean fever. The drug has been used effectively for chronic prophylactic therapy to reduce the frequency and severity of the episodic attacks of painful serositis in patients with familial Mediterranean fever. Chronic prophylactic therapy reportedly is associated with marked amelioration of attacks (both frequency and severity) or remission in about 90% of patients with this condition, but therapy with the drug is not curative and manifestations of this condition return to pretreatment levels following discontinuance of colchicine. Chronic prophylactic therapy also appears to prevent amyloidosis, manifested by nephropathy, in patients with familial Mediterranean fever who lack evidence of amyloidosis when therapy is initiated. Colchicine appears to be effective in preventing amyloidosis regardless of whether patients continue to experience episodic attacks of serositis during chronic prophylactic therapy with the drug. Colchicine may prevent deterioration in patients in the proteinuric phase of the disease when amyloid involvement is minimal. The drug generally appears to be of limited value in altering the effects of amyloid deposits when clinical amyloidosis is evident, particularly when proteinuria has progressed to nephrosis, although a beneficial effect (e.g., restoration of serum albumin concentrations toward normal, slight improvement in renal function) may be evident in some patients.

■ **Regulatory Actions Affecting Colchicine** Colchicine injection became available in the US in the 1950s and has been used for the treatment of acute attacks of gout. Colchicine injection preparations that have been commercially available have *not* been approved by the US Food and Drug Administration (FDA). Serious adverse events, some fatal, have been reported in patients receiving colchicine injection. (See Cautions: Adverse Effects.) Because of the potentially serious health risks associated with unapproved colchicine injection, FDA announced on February 8, 2008, that it would take enforcement action (e.g., seizure, injunction, other judicial proceeding) against all firms, including compounding pharmacies, attempting to manufacture, ship, or deliver colchicine injection.

Although commercially available, single-entity, oral preparations of colchicine also lacked FDA approval, FDA did not take action against colchicine tablets in February 2008; risks associated with use of the tablets are believed to be lower than those associated with use of the injection. In July 2009, FDA approved a single-ingredient oral colchicine preparation. During the review process, FDA identified 2 safety concerns associated with use of colchicine. Reports suggested that drug interactions play an important role in the development of colchicine toxicity. There also was evidence that the dosage of colchicine previously used for treatment of acute gout flares could be reduced without reducing the drug's efficacy. The labeling now includes extensive information on drug interactions and a new (lower) dosage for acute gout flare. Colchicine in fixed combination with probenecid is approved by the FDA for the management of recurrent gouty arthritis.

Dosage and Administration

■ **Administration** Colchicine is administered orally without regard to meals. Colchicine has been administered by IV injection; however, IV preparations of colchicine have been withdrawn from the US market because of safety concerns. (See Uses: Regulatory Actions Affecting Colchicine and see Cautions.)

Patients receiving colchicine should be instructed on how to resume therapy in the event of a missed dose. Patients with gout who are receiving colchicine for treatment of an acute flare but not for prophylaxis of recurrent flares should be instructed to take the missed dose as soon as possible. Those receiving the drug to treat an acute gout flare during colchicine prophylaxis should be instructed to take the missed dose immediately and then wait 12 hours before resuming the previous dosing schedule. Patients receiving colchicine for treatment of familial Mediterranean fever or for prophylaxis of recurrent gout flares (without treatment for an acute gout flare) should be instructed to take the missed dose as soon as possible and then resume their usual dosing schedule, but not to take a double dose to make up for the missed dose.

■ **Dosage** Dosage of colchicine depends on the patient's age, renal and hepatic function, and whether the drug is administered concomitantly with or within 14 days following therapy with drugs that affect hepatic metabolism or the P-glycoprotein transport system.

Treatment of Acute Gout Flare The recommended oral dosage of colchicine for relief of an acute gout flare in patients who are *not* receiving concomitant therapy with a moderate or potent inhibitor of cytochrome P-450 (CYP) isoenzyme 3A4 or an inhibitor of the P-glycoprotein transport system, and who have not received such therapy during the prior 14 days, is 1.2 mg given at the first sign of flare followed by 0.6 mg one hour later. The maximum recommended dosage for treatment of acute gout flare is 1.8 mg administered over a one-hour period. Higher dosages of colchicine have not been shown to be more effective in relieving acute gout flares. Additional courses of colchicine therapy for treatment of an acute gout flare should not be repeated until 3 days have elapsed. Patients receiving colchicine for prevention of gout flares who are not receiving a CYP3A4 inhibitor also may receive colchicine (1.2 mg initially followed by 0.6 mg 1 hour later) to relieve an acute gout flare; following the 2-dose treatment course, 12 hours should elapse before prophylactic doses of the drug are resumed.

In patients receiving concomitant therapy with a *potent inhibitor* of CYP3A4, such as atazanavir, boceprevir, clarithromycin, darunavir with low-dose ritonavir (*ritonavir-boosted* darunavir), *ritonavir-boosted* fosamprenavir, indinavir, itraconazole, ketoconazole, nefazodone, nelfinavir, ritonavir, saquinavir, telaprevir, telithromycin, *ritonavir-boosted* tipranavir, the fixed combination of lopinavir and ritonavir (lopinavir/ritonavir), or the fixed combination of elvitegravir, cobicistat, emtricitabine, and tenofovir, and those who have received such therapy during the prior 14 days, the recommended oral dosage of colchicine for relief of an acute gout flare is 0.6 mg given at the first sign of flare followed by 0.3 mg 1 hour later. Additional courses of colchicine therapy for treatment of an acute gout flare should not be repeated until 3 days have elapsed. Use of colchicine for the treatment of acute gout flares is not recommended in individuals receiving the drug for prevention of gout flares who also are receiving therapy with a CYP3A4 inhibitor.

In patients receiving concomitant therapy with a *moderate inhibitor* of CYP3A4, such as aprepitant, diltiazem, erythromycin, fluconazole, fosamprenavir (without ritonavir), grapefruit juice, or verapamil, and those who have received such therapy during the prior 14 days, the recommended oral dosage of colchicine for relief of an acute gout flare is a single 1.2-mg dose given at the first sign of flare. Additional courses of colchicine therapy for treatment of an acute gout flare should not be repeated until 3 days have elapsed. Use of colchicine for the treatment of acute gout flare is not recommended in individuals receiving the drug for prevention of gout flares who also are receiving therapy with a CYP3A4 inhibitor.

In patients receiving concomitant therapy with a drug that inhibits the P-glycoprotein transport system, such as cyclosporine or ranolazine, and those who have received such therapy during the prior 14 days, the recommended oral dosage of colchicine for relief of an acute gout flare is a single 0.6-mg dose given at the first sign of flare. Additional courses of colchicine therapy for treatment of an acute gout flare should not be repeated until 3 days have elapsed.

The safety and efficacy of repeat courses of colchicine for treatment of acute gout flare have not been evaluated.

Prophylactic Treatment of Recurrent Gout Flare The recommended oral dosage of colchicine for prophylaxis of recurrent gout flares in adults and adolescents older than 16 years of age who are not receiving concomitant therapy with a moderate or potent inhibitor of CYP3A4 or an inhibitor of the P-glycoprotein transport system, and who have not received such therapy during the prior 14 days, is 0.6 mg once or twice daily. The maximum recommended dosage is 1.2 mg daily.

In patients receiving concomitant therapy with a *potent inhibitor* of CYP3A4, such as atazanavir, boceprevir, clarithromycin, *ritonavir-boosted* darunavir, *ritonavir-boosted* fosamprenavir, indinavir, itraconazole, ketoconazole, nefazodone, nelfinavir, ritonavir, saquinavir, telaprevir, telithromycin, *ritonavir-boosted* tipranavir, lopinavir/ritonavir, or the fixed combination of elvitegravir, cobicistat, emtricitabine, and tenofovir, and those who have received such therapy during the prior 14 days, the recommended oral dosage of colchicine for prophylaxis of recurrent gout flares is 0.3 mg daily or every other day.

In patients receiving concomitant therapy with a *moderate inhibitor* of CYP3A4, such as aprepitant, diltiazem, erythromycin, fluconazole, fosamprenavir (without ritonavir), grapefruit juice, or verapamil, and those who have received such therapy during the prior 14 days, the recommended oral dosage of colchicine for prophylaxis of recurrent gout flares is 0.3 mg twice daily, 0.6 mg once daily, or 0.3 mg once daily.

In patients receiving concomitant therapy with a drug that inhibits the P-glycoprotein transport system, such as cyclosporine or ranolazine, and those who have received such therapy during the prior 14 days, the recommended oral dosage of colchicine for prophylaxis of recurrent gout flares is 0.3 mg once daily or every other day.

Familial Mediterranean Fever For management of familial Mediterranean fever in patients who are *not* receiving concomitant therapy with a moderate or potent inhibitor of CYP3A4 or an inhibitor of the P-glycoprotein transport system, and who have not received such therapy during the prior 14 days, colchicine may be given in a dosage of 1.2–2.4 mg daily in adults and adolescents older than 12 years of age, a dosage of 0.9–1.8 mg daily in children 6–12 years of age, and a dosage of 0.3–1.8 mg daily in children 4–6 years of age. The daily dosage may be given once daily or in 2 divided doses. Dosage of the drug may be increased in increments of 0.3 mg daily to the maximum recommended dosage. Alternatively, in patients experiencing intolerable adverse effects, dosage may be decreased in increments of 0.3 mg daily.

In adults and adolescents receiving concomitant therapy with a *potent inhibitor* of CYP3A4, such as atazanavir, boceprevir, clarithromycin, *ritonavir-boosted* darunavir, *ritonavir-boosted* fosamprenavir, indinavir, itraconazole, ketoconazole, nefazodone, nelfinavir, ritonavir, saquinavir, telaprevir, telithromycin, *ritonavir-boosted* tipranavir, lopinavir/ritonavir, or the fixed combination of elvitegravir, cobicistat, emtricitabine, and tenofovir, and those who have received such therapy during the prior 14 days, the maximum recommended dosage of colchicine for the management of familial Mediterranean fever is 0.6 mg daily; the daily dosage may be given as 0.3 mg twice daily.

In adults and adolescents receiving concomitant therapy with a *moderate inhibitor* of CYP3A4, such as aprepitant, diltiazem, erythromycin, fluconazole, fosamprenavir (without ritonavir), grapefruit juice, or verapamil, and those who have received such therapy during the prior 14 days, the maximum recommended dosage of colchicine for the management of familial Mediterranean fever is 1.2 mg daily; the daily dosage may be given as 0.6 mg twice daily.

In adults and adolescents receiving concomitant therapy with a drug that inhibits the P-glycoprotein transport system, such as cyclosporine or ranolazine, and those who have received such therapy during the prior 14 days, the maximum recommended dosage of colchicine for the management of familial Mediterranean fever is 0.6 mg daily; the daily dosage may be given as 0.3 mg twice daily.

These maximum recommended dosages for patients with familial Mediterranean fever who are receiving CYP3A4 or P-glycoprotein inhibitors are intended for individuals for whom a dosage range of 1.2–2.4 mg daily would be appropriate in the absence of interacting drugs (i.e., adults and adolescents older than 12 years of age). The manufacturer currently makes no specific recommendations regarding maximum colchicine dosage in children 4–12 years of age who are receiving CYP3A4 or P-glycoprotein inhibitors.

■ Dosage in Renal and Hepatic Impairment ***Dosage in Renal Impairment*** Use of colchicine in combination with a potent CYP3A4 inhibitor, such as atazanavir, boceprevir, clarithromycin, *ritonavir-boosted* darunavir, *ritonavir-boosted* fosamprenavir, indinavir, itraconazole, ketoconazole, nefazodone, nelfinavir, ritonavir, saquinavir, telaprevir, telithromycin, *ritonavir-boosted* tipranavir, lopinavir/ritonavir, or the fixed combination of elvitegravir, cobicistat, emtricitabine, and tenofovir, or with a P-glycoprotein inhibitor, such as cyclosporine or ranolazine, in patients with renal impairment is contraindicated.

Gout Flare. Use of colchicine for the treatment of an acute gout flare is not recommended in patients with renal impairment who are receiving the drug for prevention of gout flares.

Colchicine dosage adjustment is not needed in patients with mild (creatinine clearance 50–80 mL/minute) to moderate (creatinine clearance 30–50 mL/minute) renal impairment who are receiving the drug for treatment of an acute gout flare or for prophylaxis of recurrent gout flares; however, such patients should be monitored for adverse effects.

In patients with severe renal impairment, the recommended initial dosage of colchicine for prophylaxis of recurrent gout flares is 0.3 mg daily; close monitoring is needed if the dosage is increased. When colchicine is used for the treatment of an acute gout flare in patients with severe renal impairment, dosage adjustment is not needed, but additional courses of colchicine therapy for acute gout flares should not be repeated until 2 weeks have elapsed. Alternative therapy should be considered for patients with severe renal impairment requiring repeat courses of therapy.

In patients who are undergoing dialysis, the recommended dosage of colchicine for prophylaxis of recurrent gout flares is 0.3 mg twice weekly; close monitoring is advised. When colchicine is used for the treatment of an acute gout flare in patients who are undergoing dialysis, the recommended dosage of colchicine is 0.6 mg at the first sign of flare. Additional courses of colchicine therapy for acute gout flares should not be repeated until 2 weeks have elapsed.

Familial Mediterranean Fever. Patients with mild (creatinine clearance 50–80 mL/minute) to moderate (creatinine clearance 30–50 mL/minute) renal impairment who are receiving colchicine for management of familial Mediterranean fever should be monitored for adverse effects. Dosage adjustment may be needed.

In patients with severe (creatinine clearance less than 30 mL/minute) renal impairment or undergoing dialysis, the recommended initial dosage of colchicine for management of familial Mediterranean fever is 0.3 mg daily. Dosage can be increased with careful monitoring.

Dosage in Hepatic Impairment Use of colchicine in combination with a potent CYP3A4 inhibitor, such as atazanavir, boceprevir, clarithromycin, *ritonavir-boosted* darunavir, *ritonavir-boosted* fosamprenavir, indinavir, itraconazole, ketoconazole, nefazodone, nelfinavir, ritonavir, saquinavir, telaprevir, telithromycin, *ritonavir-boosted* tipranavir, lopinavir/ritonavir, the fixed combination of elvitegravir, cobicistat, emtricitabine, and tenofovir, or with a P-glycoprotein inhibitor, such as cyclosporine or ranolazine, in patients with hepatic impairment is contraindicated.

Gout Flare. Colchicine dosage adjustment is not needed in patients with mild to moderate hepatic impairment who are receiving the drug for treatment of an acute gout flare or for prophylaxis of recurrent gout flares; however, such patients should be monitored for adverse effects.

Dosage reduction should be considered in patients with severe hepatic impairment who are receiving colchicine for prophylaxis of recurrent gout flares. When colchicine is used for the treatment of an acute gout flare in patients with severe hepatic impairment, dosage adjustment is not needed, but additional courses of colchicine therapy for acute gout flares should not be repeated until 2 weeks have elapsed. Alternative therapy should be considered for patients with severe hepatic impairment requiring repeat courses of therapy.

Familial Mediterranean Fever. Patients with mild to moderate hepatic impairment who are receiving colchicine for management of familial Mediterranean fever should be monitored for adverse effects.

Dosage adjustment should be considered for patients with severe hepatic impairment who are receiving colchicine for management of familial Mediterranean fever.

Cautions

■ Adverse Effects The most common adverse effects of oral colchicine therapy are nausea, abdominal discomfort, vomiting, and diarrhea. Pharyngolaryngeal pain has been reported.

Bladder spasm, paralytic ileus, stomatitis, hypothyroidism, nonthrombocytopenic purpura, and prostration have also been reported with colchicine therapy.

Myelosuppression, disseminated intravascular coagulation, and renal, hepatic, circulatory, and CNS cellular injury have been reported in patients receiving colchicine, generally in those receiving excessive dosages of the drug. Leukopenia, granulocytopenia, thrombocytopenia, pancytopenia, and aplastic anemia have been reported. Death has occurred in one patient with normal renal and hepatic function who developed pancytopenia and bone marrow aplasia following IV administration of 10 mg of colchicine (IV preparations are no longer commercially available in the US) over a 5-day period.

Neuromuscular toxicity and rhabdomyolysis have been reported in patients receiving long-term colchicine therapy. Patients with renal dysfunction and geriatric patients, including those with normal renal and hepatic function, are at increased risk. Concomitant therapy with an HMG-CoA reductase inhibitor (statin), fibric acid derivative, or cyclosporine also may increase the risk for development of myopathy. Following discontinuance of colchicine, symptoms generally resolve within one week to several months.

Loss of body and scalp hair, rash, vesicular dermatitis, peripheral neuritis or neuropathy, myopathy, rhabdomyolysis, anuria, renal damage, hematuria, and one case of purpura have been reported with prolonged administration of colchicine. Colchicine may also cause increased serum concentrations of alkaline phosphatase, aminotransferases (AST, ALT), and creatine kinase (CK, creatine phosphokinase, CPK). Other reported adverse effects include sensory motor neuropathy, maculopapular rash, abdominal pain or cramping, lactose intolerance, myotonia, muscle weakness or pain, azoospermia, and oligospermia.

Serious adverse events have been reported in patients receiving IV colchicine. Many of these adverse effects were the result of colchicine toxicity. As of June 2007, the US Food and Drug Administration (FDA) was aware of 50 reports of adverse effects associated with use of IV colchicine; 23 of these events were fatal. Reported adverse effects included neutropenia, acute renal failure, thrombocytopenia, congestive heart failure, and pancytopenia. Three deaths were associated with use of compounded IV colchicine. Tests of vials from the same lot used to treat these 3 patients indicated that the concentration of colchicine was 4 mg/mL; labeling on the vial indicated that the concentration of colchicine was 0.5 mg/mL. Because of the potentially serious health risks associated with colchicine injection, FDA announced on February 8, 2008, that it would take enforcement action against all firms, including compounding pharmacies, attempting to manufacture, ship, or deliver colchicine injection.

Oral preparations containing colchicine remain on the market; risks associated with use of the tablets are believed to be lower than those associated with use of the injection.

■ Precautions and Contraindications Concomitant use of colchicine with certain drugs is contraindicated or requires particular caution. (See Drug Interactions and also see Dosage and Administration: Dosage.)

Colchicine is contraindicated in patients with renal or hepatic impairment who are receiving a drug that inhibits the P-glycoprotein transport system or is a potent CYP3A4 inhibitor (see Dosage and Administration: Dosage in Renal and Hepatic Impairment); fatal or life-threatening colchicine toxicity has occurred in such patients following therapeutic doses of colchicine.

■ Pediatric Precautions Safety and efficacy of colchicine for treatment of gout in children have not been established.

Safety and efficacy of colchicine for management of familial Mediterranean fever in children have been evaluated in uncontrolled studies. Long-term use of colchicine did not appear to affect growth in children with familial Mediterranean fever.

■ **Geriatric Precautions** Clinical studies of colchicine for treatment of acute gout flares, prophylactic treatment of recurrent gout flares, or management of familial Mediterranean fever did not include sufficient numbers of patients 65 years of age and older to determine whether geriatric patients respond differently than younger patients. Drug dosage generally should be titrated carefully in geriatric patients with gout; the greater frequency of decreased renal function and of concomitant disease and drug therapy observed in geriatric patients also should be considered.

■ **Pregnancy, Fertility, and Lactation** Chromosomal aberrations have been reported in a limited number of patients receiving prolonged colchicine therapy. Colchicine crosses the placenta in humans and has been shown in animal reproduction and development studies to cause embryofetal toxicity, teratogenic effects, and altered postnatal development at exposure levels within or above the therapeutic range. Although there are no adequate and controlled studies to date in humans, results of one study suggest that patients receiving prolonged colchicine therapy may have a greater risk of producing trisomic offspring if conception occurs during therapy with the drug. Other clinicians, however, contend that this study is inconclusive and at most merely suggestive of a probable increased risk to the offspring. Data from a limited number of published studies indicate that use of colchicine for the treatment of familial Mediterranean fever in pregnant women was not associated with increased risk of miscarriage, stillbirth, or teratogenic effects. Colchicine should be used during pregnancy only if the potential benefits outweigh the risks.

The effect of colchicine on labor and delivery is not known.

Colchicine has adversely affected spermatogenesis in humans and animals. Reversible azoospermia has been reported in a 36-year-old man who received 0.6 mg of colchicine twice daily for several months.

Colchicine is distributed into milk. (See Pharmacokinetics: Distribution.) Limited information suggests that exclusively breast-fed infants receive less than 10% of the maternal weight-adjusted dose. Although the drug can affect GI cell renewal and permeability, some experts state that the actual amounts of the drug distributed into breast milk are not high enough to warrant cessation of nursing. No adverse effects have been reported to date in breast-fed infants of women receiving colchicine therapy who were observed over periods of up to 10 months. The American Academy of Pediatrics (AAP) states that the drug usually is compatible with breast-feeding. Some clinicians have suggested that exposure of the infant to the drug could be minimized by waiting 8–12 hours after a dose to breast-feed the infant. The manufacturer states that caution is advised; the infant should be observed for adverse effects.

Drug Interactions

■ **Drugs Affecting Hepatic Microsomal Enzymes** Colchicine is metabolized by cytochrome P-450 (CYP) isoenzyme 3A4. In vitro studies indicate that colchicine does not inhibit or induce CYP isoenzymes 1A2, 2A6, 2B6, 2C8, 2C9, 2C19, 2D6, 2E1, or 3A4.

Concomitant use of colchicine with potent CYP3A4 inhibitors, such as atazanavir, boceprevir, clarithromycin, *ritonavir-boosted* darunavir, *ritonavir-boosted* fosamprenavir, indinavir, itraconazole, ketoconazole, nefazodone, nelfinavir, ritonavir, saquinavir, telaprevir, telithromycin, *ritonavir-boosted* tipranavir, lopinavir/ritonavir, or the fixed combination of elvitegravir, cobicistat, emtricitabine, and tenofovir, or with moderate CYP3A4 inhibitors, such as aprepitant, diltiazem, erythromycin, fluconazole, fosamprenavir (without ritonavir), grapefruit juice, or verapamil, may result in substantially increased plasma concentrations of colchicine. If concomitant therapy is required, the dosage of colchicine must be reduced or treatment with colchicine may need to be interrupted. (See Dosage and Administration: Dosage.) Use of colchicine in combination with a potent CYP3A4 inhibitor in patients with renal or hepatic impairment is contraindicated.

Clarithromycin An increase in plasma colchicine concentrations (227% increase in peak plasma concentration, 281% increase in area under the plasma concentration-time curve [AUC]) was observed when a single 0.6-mg dose of colchicine was administered concomitantly with clarithromycin (250 mg twice daily for 7 days). Severe or fatal colchicine toxicity has been reported with concomitant clarithromycin and colchicine therapy.

Ketoconazole An increase in plasma colchicine concentrations (102% increase in peak plasma concentration, 212% increase in AUC) was observed when a single 0.6-mg dose of colchicine was administered concomitantly with ketoconazole (200 mg twice daily for 5 days).

Ritonavir An increase in plasma colchicine concentrations (184% increase in peak plasma concentration, 296% increase in AUC) was observed when a single 0.6-mg dose of colchicine was administered concomitantly with ritonavir (100 mg twice daily for 5 days).

Verapamil An increase in plasma colchicine concentrations (40% increase in peak plasma concentration, 103% increase in AUC) was observed when a single 0.6-mg dose of colchicine was administered concomitantly with verapamil (240 mg daily for 5 days). Neuromuscular toxicity has been reported with concomitant verapamil and colchicine therapy.

Diltiazem An increase in plasma colchicine concentrations (44% increase in peak plasma concentration, 93% increase in AUC) was observed when a single 0.6-mg dose of colchicine was administered concomitantly with diltiazem (240 mg daily for 7 days). Neuromuscular toxicity has been reported with concomitant diltiazem and colchicine therapy.

Grapefruit Juice No substantial change in plasma concentrations of colchicine was observed when a single 0.6-mg dose of colchicine was administered concomitantly with grapefruit juice (240 mL twice daily for 4 days). However, when colchicine was given concomitantly with other moderate CYP3A4 inhibitors (e.g., diltiazem, verapamil), substantial increases in plasma colchicine concentrations were reported. The manufacturer states that patients receiving colchicine should be advised not to consume grapefruit or grapefruit juice. If a moderate CYP3A4 inhibitor (including grapefruit juice) is given concomitantly with colchicine, the manufacturer recommends adjustment of colchicine dosage (see Dosage and Administration: Dosage).

■ **Drugs Affecting the P-glycoprotein Transport System** Concomitant use of colchicine with drugs that inhibit the P-glycoprotein transport system, such as cyclosporine or ranolazine, results in substantially increased plasma concentrations of colchicine. If use of a P-glycoprotein inhibitor is required, the dosage of colchicine must be reduced or treatment with colchicine may need to be interrupted. (See Dosage and Administration: Dosage.) Use of colchicine in combination with a P-glycoprotein inhibitor in patients with renal or hepatic impairment is contraindicated.

Cyclosporine Administration of a single 100-mg dose of cyclosporine, a P-glycoprotein inhibitor, concomitantly with a single 0.6-mg dose of colchicine resulted in increases in plasma colchicine concentrations (270% increase in peak plasma concentration, 259% increase in AUC). Fatal colchicine toxicity has been reported with concomitant cyclosporine and colchicine therapy. Concomitant use of cyclosporine and colchicine also may result in increased cyclosporine concentrations and additive nephrotoxic effects; therefore, renal function and blood concentrations of cyclosporine should be monitored and cyclosporine dosage should be adjusted accordingly if colchicine is initiated or discontinued or the colchicine dosage is altered in patients receiving cyclosporine.

■ **Antilipemic Agents** Addition of an HMG-CoA reductase inhibitor (statin) or other lipid-lowering agents (e.g., fibric acid derivatives) to long-term therapy with colchicine or addition of colchicine to long-term therapy with these antilipemic agents has resulted in myopathy and rhabdomyolysis; death has been reported. Potential benefits and risks of such concomitant therapy should be weighed. Patients should be monitored for muscle pain, tenderness, and weakness, especially during the initial phase of such concomitant therapy.

■ **Azithromycin** An increase in plasma colchicine concentrations (22% increase in peak plasma concentration, 57% increase in AUC) was observed when a single 0.6-mg dose of colchicine was administered concomitantly with azithromycin (500 mg initially, followed by 250 mg daily for 4 days).

■ **Digoxin** Digoxin is a P-glycoprotein transport system substrate. Rhabdomyolysis has been reported in an individual receiving colchicine and digoxin concomitantly. Potential benefits and risks of concomitant therapy with colchicine and digoxin should be weighed. Patients should be monitored for muscle pain, tenderness, and weakness, especially during the initial phase of such concomitant therapy.

■ **Estrogens or Progestins** Administration of an oral contraceptive (ethinyl estradiol 35 mcg with norethindrone 1 mg) concomitantly with colchicine (0.6 mg twice daily for 14 days) in healthy women did not alter the plasma concentrations of either the estrogen or the progestin.

■ **Theophylline** No change in plasma concentrations of theophylline was observed when theophylline was administered concomitantly with colchicine (0.6 mg twice daily for 14 days) in healthy individuals.

Laboratory Test Interferences

Colchicine has been reported to interfere with urinary determinations of 17-hydroxycorticosteroids using the Reddy, Jenkins, and Thorn procedure. Colchicine may cause false-positive results in urine tests for erythrocytes or hemoglobin.

Acute Toxicity

■ **Manifestations** Poisoning may occur from repeated administration of large doses or from a single toxic dose of colchicine. Death has occurred following ingestion of as little as 7 mg of colchicine, although individuals have survived larger doses. The lethal dose in humans has been estimated to be 65 mg. In individuals receiving IV colchicine, death has occurred following cumulative doses as low as 5.5 mg. The median IV lethal dose in rats is 1.7 mg/kg. There is usually a delay of a few hours between ingestion of the toxic dose of colchicine and the appearance of the first toxic symptoms, regardless of the route of administration.

The first stage of acute colchicine toxicity typically begins within 24 hours of ingestion and includes adverse GI effects resulting in fluid loss and volume depletion; peripheral leukocytosis also may occur. Life-threatening complications occur during the second stage, which occurs 24–72 hours after administration, and result from multiorgan failure.

The first symptoms of acute colchicine toxicity involve the GI tract and include nausea, anorexia, abdominal pain, vomiting, paralytic ileus, and diarrhea which may be severe and bloody due to hemorrhagic gastroenteritis. Stomatitis, arthralgia, malaise, hypocalcemia, fever, and rashes including scarlatiniform rash may also occur. Dehydration may occur resulting in oliguria. Renal damage as evidenced by hematuria and oliguria has been reported. Hepatomegaly and liver tenderness with elevated serum concentrations of AST

(SGOT) and alkaline phosphatase may occur. Extreme vascular damage may result in shock and cardiovascular collapse. Leukopenia may occur and may persist for several days followed by leukocytosis with numerous metamyelocytes and myelocytes. Other hematologic manifestations of colchicine toxicity include bone marrow depression, thrombocytopenia, granulocytopenia, immature leukocytes, pancytopenia, anemia with anisocytosis, polychromasia, and basophilic stippling. Muscular weakness is marked and an ascending paralysis of the CNS may develop, although the patient usually remains conscious. Mental confusion, delirium, and seizures may occur. There may be a loss of deep tendon and Achilles tendon reflexes, and Babinski's reflex may be elicited. Death usually occurs as a result of respiratory depression or cardiovascular collapse.

■ **Treatment** There is no specific antidote for colchicine poisoning. Gastric lavage should be performed initially and measures initiated to prevent shock. Other treatment is symptomatic and supportive. Colchicine is not removed by dialysis.

Pharmacology

■ **Gout** Colchicine possesses antigout activity. The drug also has weak anti-inflammatory activity but has no analgesic activity. The drug has no effect on urinary excretion of uric acid or on serum urate concentration, solubility, or binding to serum proteins. Although the mechanism of the antigout effect of colchicine is not completely known, the drug appears to disrupt cytoskeletal functions through inhibition of β-tubulin polymerization into microtubules, thus preventing activation, degranulation, and migration of neutrophils believed to mediate some gout symptoms.

■ **Familial Mediterranean Fever** The mechanism of colchicine's beneficial effects in familial Mediterranean fever has not been fully elucidated. Colchicine may interfere with intracellular assembly of the inflammasome complex in neutrophils and monocytes that mediates activation of interleukin-1β.

Pharmacokinetics

■ **Absorption** Following oral administration, colchicine is absorbed from the GI tract and is partially metabolized in the liver. The drug and its metabolites re-enter the intestinal tract via biliary secretions and the unchanged drug may be reabsorbed from the intestine. Following oral administration of colchicine 1.8 mg over 1 hour under fasting conditions, peak plasma concentrations of 6.2 ng/mL were reached in 1.8 hours. Following oral administration of 0.6 mg twice daily for 10 days, a mean peak plasma concentration of 3.6 ng/mL was reached at 1.3 hours after a dose. Administration of colchicine with food did not affect rate of absorption but decreased the extent of absorption by 15%. Absolute bioavailability is reported to be approximately 45%.

The presence of a secondary peak in colchicine concentrations, ranging from 39–155% of the height of the initial peak concentration, has been reported in some individuals 3–36 hours after oral administration and has been attributed to intestinal secretion and reabsorption and/or biliary circulation.

■ **Distribution** Colchicine is about 39% bound to serum proteins, mainly albumin.

Colchicine crosses the placenta. Fetal plasma concentrations of the drug are reported to be approximately 15% of the maternal concentration.

Colchicine is distributed into milk. In a limited number of nursing women receiving long-term colchicine therapy at dosages of 1–1.5 mg daily, peak concentrations of the drug in milk were similar to serum concentrations and ranged from 1.9–8.6 ng/mL. Higher concentrations of the drug in milk (31, 24–27, or 10 ng/mL at 2, 4, or 7 hours, respectively, after a dose) have been reported in the absence of concurrent serum concentration data in a nursing woman receiving colchicine 1 mg daily.

■ **Elimination** Following IV administration of a single therapeutic dose (IV preparations are no longer commercially available in the US), colchicine is rapidly removed from the plasma; plasma half-life is about 20 minutes. The drug has a half-life of about 60 hours in leukocytes.

Colchicine is demethylated in the liver by cytochrome P-450 (CYP) isoenzyme 3A4. In healthy individuals, 40–65% of an orally administered 1-mg dose of the drug is excreted unchanged in urine. Enterohepatic circulation and biliary excretion may occur. A half-life of 26.6–31.2 hours has been reported in healthy young adults receiving colchicine 0.6 mg orally twice daily. Colchicine is a substrate of the P-glycoprotein transport system. Colchicine is not removed by hemodialysis.

Clearance of colchicine is decreased in patients with renal impairment. In one study, patients with severe renal disease eliminated little or no colchicine or its metabolites in the urine, resulting in a prolonged plasma half-life. Total body clearance of colchicine was reduced by 75% in patients with end-stage renal disease requiring dialysis.

In patients with hepatic impairment, substantial interpatient variability in colchicine pharmacokinetics has been observed. In some patients with mild to moderate cirrhosis, clearance of colchicine was decreased substantially and plasma half-life was prolonged compared with healthy individuals; however, no consistent trends were observed in patients with primary biliary cirrhosis.

Chemistry and Stability

■ **Chemistry** Colchicine, a phenanthrene derivative, is an antigout drug obtained from species of *Colchicum*. Colchicine occurs as pale yellow, amorphous scales or powder and is soluble in water and freely soluble in alcohol.

■ **Stability** Colchicine darkens on exposure to light and should be stored in tight, light-resistant containers.

Preparations

Excipients in commercially available drug preparations may have clinically important effects in some individuals; consult specific product labeling for details.

Colchicine

Oral		
Tablets	0.6 mg	**Colcrys®** (scored), Takeda

Probenecid and Colchicine

Oral		
Tablets	500 mg Probenecid and Colchicine 0.5 mg*	**Probenecid and Colchicine Tablets**

*available from one or more manufacturer, distributor, and/or repackager by generic (nonproprietary) name

Febuxostat

■ Febuxostat is a xanthine oxidase inhibitor.

Uses

■ **Gout** Febuxostat is used for long-term management of hyperuricemia in patients with gout who have had an inadequate response to maximum recommended dosages of allopurinol or in whom allopurinol is not tolerated or is not recommended. Febuxostat is not recommended for the management of asymptomatic hyperuricemia. (See Cardiovascular Death under Warnings/Precautions: Warnings, in Cautions.)

The major goal in the management of hyperuricemia and gout is long-term reduction in serum urate concentrations to levels below the limit of urate solubility (about 6.8 mg/dL). Such a reduction over time will prevent or reverse the formation and deposition of urate crystals.

Efficacy of febuxostat was evaluated in 3 randomized, active-controlled studies in patients with hyperuricemia (serum urate concentrations of at least 8 mg/dL) and gout. Because initiation of therapy with urate-lowering agents is associated with an increased frequency of acute gouty attacks (gout flare), patients received concomitant therapy with naproxen or colchicine as prophylaxis against gout flares. At the final evaluation (6 months for 2 studies, 12 months for 1 study), 45%, 67–74%, or 36–42% of those receiving febuxostat 40 mg daily, febuxostat 80 mg daily, or allopurinol (300 mg daily in those with normal renal function; reduced dosage in those with renal impairment), respectively, achieved serum urate concentrations of less than 6 mg/dL.

Dosage and Administration

■ **General** Acute gout attacks (gout flare) may occur after initiation of therapy with febuxostat. Therefore, gout flare prophylaxis with a nonsteroidal anti-inflammatory agent (NSAIA) or colchicine should be considered; these agents may be started when febuxostat therapy is initiated and may be beneficial for up to 6 months. If a gout flare occurs, febuxostat may be continued, and the gout flare managed as appropriate.

Testing for target serum urate concentrations can be performed after 2 weeks of febuxostat therapy.

■ **Administration** Febuxostat is administered orally without regard to meals or antacids.

■ **Dosage** The recommended initial dosage of febuxostat for the management of hyperuricemia in patients with gout is 40 mg once daily. The dosage of febuxostat may be increased to 80 mg once daily in patients who do not achieve serum urate concentrations of less than 6 mg/dL following 2 weeks of therapy with febuxostat 40 mg once daily.

■ **Special Populations** Dosage adjustment is not needed in geriatric patients, patients with mild to moderate hepatic impairment (Child-Pugh class A or B), or those with mild to moderate renal impairment (creatinine clearance of 30–89 mL/minute). In patients with severe renal impairment (creatinine clearance of 15–29 mL/minute), the maximum recommended dosage of febuxostat is 40 mg once daily. The manufacturer makes no specific dosage recommendations for patients with severe hepatic impairment (Child-Pugh class C). (See Specific Populations under Cautions: Warnings/Precautions.)

Cautions

■ **Contraindications** Concomitant therapy with azathioprine or mercaptopurine. (See Drug Interactions: Drugs Metabolized by Xanthine Oxidase.)

■ **Warnings/Precautions** *Warnings* **Cardiovascular Death.** Results from a postmarketing randomized, double-blind, noninferiority cardiovascular outcome study (CARES) in 6190 patients with coexisting gout and cardiovascular disease indicate that cardiovascular mortality was higher in patients receiving febuxostat compared with those receiving allopurinol. All patients in this study had a history of major cardiovascular disease (e.g., myocardial infarction, unstable angina or transient ischemic attack requiring hospitalization, stroke, peripheral vascular disease, diabetes mellitus with microvascular or macrovascular disease). The cardiovascular mortality rate was 4.3% in febuxostat-treated patients versus 3.2% in patients treated with allopurinol (hazard ratio: 1.34). Sudden cardiac death was the most common cause of cardiovascular mortality in these patients. Because of the imbalance in cardiovascular mortality, overall mortality also was higher in patients receiving febuxostat compared with those receiving allopurinol (7.8 versus 6.4%, hazard ratio: 1.22). The incidence of major cardiovascular events, including nonfatal myocardial infarction, unstable angina requiring urgent coronary revascularization, and nonfatal stroke, was similar in febuxostat- and allopurinol-treated patients.

Because a higher incidence of cardiovascular mortality has been reported in patients receiving febuxostat compared with those receiving allopurinol, febuxostat should be reserved for use in patients who have had an inadequate response to maximum recommended dosages of allopurinol or in whom allopurinol is not tolerated or is not recommended; the risks and benefits of initiating or continuing febuxostat therapy should be considered.

Patients receiving febuxostat should be monitored for signs and symptoms of adverse cardiovascular events. Prophylactic low-dose aspirin therapy should be considered in patients with a history of cardiovascular disease.

Sensitivity Reactions **Dermatologic and Hypersensitivity Reactions.** Serious dermatologic reactions (including Stevens-Johnson syndrome, erythema multiforme, toxic epidermal necrolysis, and drug reaction with eosinophilia and systemic symptoms [DRESS]) and hypersensitivity reactions have been reported in patients receiving febuxostat during postmarketing experience. Many patients reporting dermatologic reactions to febuxostat also reported similar reactions to previous therapy with allopurinol. The manufacturer states that febuxostat should be used with caution in patients with history of dermatologic reactions to allopurinol.

Febuxostat therapy should be discontinued if serious dermatologic reactions (e.g., rash; red and painful skin; peeling or blistering of the skin; swelling or blistering of the lips, eyes, or mouth) are suspected.

Other Warnings and Precautions **Acute Gout.** An increased frequency of acute gout attacks (gout flare) may occur after initiation of febuxostat due to increased mobilization of urate from tissue deposits in response to reduction in serum uric acid concentrations. Gout flare prophylaxis with a nonsteroidal anti-inflammatory agent (NSAIA) or colchicine should be considered; these agents may be started when febuxostat therapy is initiated.

Hepatic Effects. Serum aminotransferase (i.e., AST, ALT) concentrations exceeding 3 times the upper limit of normal (ULN) have been reported in patients receiving febuxostat. In addition, hepatic failure, sometimes fatal, has been reported in patients receiving febuxostat during postmarketing experience; a causal relationship to the drug cannot be excluded.

Liver function tests (serum ALT, AST, alkaline phosphatase, and total bilirubin concentrations) should be performed prior to initiation of febuxostat therapy and repeated promptly in patients with manifestations suggestive of liver damage, such as fatigue, anorexia, right upper abdominal discomfort, dark-colored urine, or jaundice. If aminotransferase concentrations are elevated (ALT exceeding 3 times the ULN), febuxostat therapy should be interrupted and the cause of the abnormalities investigated. The cause should be treated, if possible, to resolution or stabilization. If an alternate etiology is not found, febuxostat therapy should not be restarted.

Patients without an alternate etiology who have serum ALT concentrations exceeding 3 times the ULN with total bilirubin concentrations exceeding 2 times the ULN are at risk for severe liver injury. Febuxostat should not be restarted in these patients. The manufacturer states that febuxostat may be used with caution in patients with lesser elevations of serum ALT or bilirubin if an alternate probable cause of the liver function test abnormalities has been determined.

Specific Populations **Pregnancy.** Data are inadequate regarding use of febuxostat in pregnant women.

Animal reproduction studies using febuxostat have not revealed evidence of fetal harm at exposures greater than those attained with the maximum recommended human dosage.

Lactation. Febuxostat is distributed into milk in rats at concentrations up to approximately 7 times plasma concentrations of the drug. It is not known whether febuxostat distributes into human milk, affects the breast-fed infant, or affects milk production.

The benefits of breast-feeding and the importance of febuxostat to the woman should be considered along with the potential adverse effects on the breast-fed child from the drug or from the underlying maternal condition.

Pediatric Use. Safety and efficacy have not been established in pediatric patients.

Geriatric Use. No substantial differences in safety and efficacy have been observed in geriatric patients relative to younger adults, but increased sensitivity of some older patients cannot be ruled out.

Pharmacokinetic values in geriatric adults were similar to those in younger adults. Dosage adjustment based on age is not needed.

Hepatic Impairment. Febuxostat has not been studied in patients with severe hepatic impairment (Child-Pugh class C); caution is advised if used in these individuals. Dosage adjustment is not needed in patients with mild to moderate hepatic impairment (Child-Pugh class A or B).

Renal Impairment. Following administration of repeated 80-mg doses of febuxostat in patients with mild or moderate renal impairment, systemic exposure to the drug was increased by 7 or 45%, respectively, compared with patients with normal renal function. Dosage adjustment is not needed in patients with mild to moderate renal impairment.

Following administration of repeated 40-mg doses of febuxostat in patients with severe renal impairment, systemic exposure to the drug was increased by 96% compared with patients with normal renal function. Dosage adjustment is recommended for patients with severe impairment. (See Dosage and Administration: Special Populations.)

Febuxostat has not been studied in individuals with end-stage renal disease who are undergoing dialysis.

Secondary Hyperuricemia. Febuxostat has not been evaluated in patients with secondary hyperuricemia. Use of febuxostat in patients whose rate of urate formation is greatly increased is not recommended.

■ **Common Adverse Effects** Adverse effects reported in 1% or more of patients receiving febuxostat include liver function abnormalities, nausea, arthralgia, and rash.

Drug Interactions

■ **Drugs Affecting Hepatic Microsomal or Other Enzymes** Febuxostat is metabolized by conjugation by uridine diphosphate-glucuronosyltransferase (UGT) enzymes, including UGT 1A1, 1A3, 1A9, and 2B7, as well as by oxidation by cytochrome P-450 (CYP) isoenzymes, including CYP 1A2, 2C8, and 2C9, and non-CYP enzymes. However, the relative contribution of each enzyme isoform to the drug's metabolism is not clear. Drug interactions generally are not expected between febuxostat and inhibitors or inducers of particular enzyme isoforms.

■ **Drugs Metabolized by Hepatic Microsomal Enzymes** Febuxostat does not inhibit CYP isoenzymes 1A2, 2C9, 2C19, or 3A4, but is a weak inhibitor of CYP2D6. Febuxostat does not induce CYP isoenzymes 1A2, 2B6, 2C9, 2C19, or 3A4. Pharmacokinetic interactions are unlikely between febuxostat and substrates of these isoenzymes.

Desipramine Effects of febuxostat on desipramine pharmacokinetics are not considered clinically important; dosage adjustment is not expected to be necessary.

■ **Drugs Metabolized by Xanthine Oxidase** Febuxostat is a xanthine oxidase inhibitor and may increase plasma concentrations of drugs metabolized by xanthine oxidase, resulting in toxicity.

Azathioprine and Mercaptopurine Increased plasma concentrations of azathioprine and mercaptopurine have been reported when these drugs were administered concomitantly with allopurinol, another xanthine oxidase inhibitor. Drug interaction studies between febuxostat and azathioprine or mercaptopurine are not available. Therefore, concomitant use of febuxostat with these drugs is contraindicated.

Theophylline Following concomitant administration of febuxostat (80 mg once daily) and theophylline in healthy individuals, peak plasma concentrations and systemic exposure to theophylline were not altered substantially, but urinary excretion of 1-methylxanthine (a major metabolite of theophylline) was increased by approximately 400-fold. The long-term safety of exposure to 1-methylxanthine is not known. If febuxostat is used concomitantly with theophylline, caution is advised. The manufacturer states that theophylline dosage adjustments are not necessary when febuxostat and theophylline are used concomitantly.

■ **Antacids** Pharmacokinetic interaction is unlikely.

■ **Antineoplastic Agents** Studies have not been conducted with antineoplastic agents; data are not available regarding safety of febuxostat in patients receiving antineoplastic agents. (See Drug Interactions: Drugs Metabolized by Xanthine Oxidase.)

■ **Colchicine** Clinically important pharmacokinetic interaction is unlikely; dosage adjustment is not needed.

■ **Hydrochlorothiazide** Clinically important pharmacokinetic interaction is unlikely; dosage adjustment is not needed.

■ **Nonsteroidal Anti-inflammatory Agents** ***Indomethacin*** Clinically important pharmacokinetic interaction is unlikely; dosage adjustment is not needed.

Naproxen Clinically important pharmacokinetic interaction is unlikely; dosage adjustment is not needed.

■ **Warfarin** Pharmacokinetic interaction is unlikely; dosage adjustment is not needed.

Description

Febuxostat inhibits xanthine oxidase, the enzyme that catalyzes the conversion of hypoxanthine to xanthine and xanthine to uric acid. By blocking uric acid production, febuxostat decreases serum concentrations of uric acid. Febuxostat has minimal effects on other enzymes involved in purine and pyrimidine synthesis and metabolism.

Febuxostat is extensively metabolized by conjugation by uridine diphosphate-glucuronosyltransferase (UGT) enzymes, including UGT 1A1, 1A3, 1A9, and 2B7, as well as by oxidation by cytochrome P-450 (CYP) isoenzymes, including CYP 1A2, 2C8, and 2C9, and non-CYP enzymes. The drug is eliminated in urine (49%) and feces (45%), principally in the form of various metabolites and their conjugates; 3 and 12% of an administered dose is recovered as unchanged drug in urine and feces, respectively.

Advice to Patients

Importance of reading the patient information (medication guide) provided by the manufacturer.

Importance of informing patients that higher cardiovascular mortality has been reported with febuxostat compared with allopurinol therapy in patients with gout and established cardiovascular disease. Instruct all patients, including those who do not have cardiovascular disease, to be alert for the development of signs and symptoms of cardiovascular events (e.g., chest pain, shortness of breath, rapid or irregular heartbeat, symptoms suggestive of stroke).

Importance of informing patients that gout flares may initially increase when starting treatment with febuxostat and that medications to help reduce flares may be taken regularly for the first few months after initiation. Advise patients that they should not discontinue febuxostat therapy if such flares occur.

Risk of adverse hepatic effects. Importance of promptly reporting any symptoms suggestive of liver injury (e.g., fatigue, anorexia, right upper abdominal discomfort, dark urine, jaundice).

Risk of severe dermatologic or hypersensitivity reactions. Importance of advising patients to notify their clinician at the earliest onset of any manifestations of severe dermatologic or hypersensitivity reactions (e.g., rash; red and painful skin; peeling or blistering of the skin; swelling or blistering of the lips, eyes, or mouth; difficulty swallowing or breathing).

Importance of informing clinicians of existing or contemplated concomitant therapy, including prescription and OTC drugs and herbal products, and any concomitant illnesses (e.g., cardiovascular or cerebrovascular disease).

Importance of women informing clinicians if they are or plan to become pregnant or plan to breast-feed.

Importance of advising patients of other important precautionary information. (See Cautions.)

Overview® (see Users Guide). For additional information on this drug until a more detailed monograph is developed and published, the manufacturer's labeling should be consulted. It is *essential* that the manufacturer's labeling be consulted for more detailed information on usual cautions, precautions, contraindications, potential drug interactions, laboratory test interferences, and acute toxicity.

Preparations

Excipients in commercially available drug preparations may have clinically important effects in some individuals; consult specific product labeling for details.

Febuxostat

Oral		
Tablets	40 mg	Uloric®, Takeda
	80 mg	Uloric®, Takeda

Pegloticase

■ Pegloticase is a pegylated biosynthetic (recombinant DNA origin) modified mammalian urate oxidase (uricase) enzyme.

REMS

FDA approved a REMS for pegloticase to ensure that the benefits outweigh the risks. The REMS may apply to one or more preparations of pegloticase and consists of the following: communication plan. See the FDA REMS page (https://www.accessdata.fda.gov/scripts/cder/rems/index.cfm).

Uses

■ **Gout** Pegloticase is used in the management of chronic gout that is refractory to conventional therapy (i.e., chronic gout in patients in whom maximum recommended dosages of xanthine oxidase inhibitors have failed to normalize serum uric acid concentrations and to adequately control clinical manifestations of the disease or in whom these drugs are contraindicated). Pegloticase is designated an orphan drug by the US Food and Drug Administration (FDA) for this use. Pegloticase is not recommended for the treatment of asymptomatic hyperuricemia.

In 2 similarly designed, multicenter, randomized, double-blind, placebo-controlled studies of 6 months' duration, efficacy of pegloticase was evaluated in a total of 212 adults with chronic gout that was refractory to conventional therapy. Patients included in these studies had a baseline serum uric acid concentration of 8 mg/dL or higher; symptomatic gout with at least 3 flares in the previous 18 months, one or more tophi, or gouty arthritis; and a contraindication to allopurinol or a history of allopurinol treatment failure (i.e., failure of a 3-month or longer course of allopurinol given at maximum recommended dosages to reduce serum uric acid concentration to less than 6 mg/dL). Patients received pegloticase 8 mg (of uricase protein) IV every 2 or 4 weeks or placebo. All patients received an oral antihistamine, IV corticosteroid, and acetaminophen prior to each infusion for prophylaxis of allergic or infusion-related reactions, as well as a regimen of nonsteroidal anti-inflammatory agents (NSAIAs) or colchicine, or both, for prophylaxis of gout flares beginning at least one week before initiation of pegloticase treatment unless contraindicated or not tolerated. The primary end point in both studies was control of plasma uric acid concentrations; the major secondary end point was resolution of tophi. Plasma uric acid concentrations were reduced to less than 6 mg/dL for at least 80% of the time during months 3 and 6 of treatment in 38–47% of patients receiving pegloticase every 2 weeks compared with none of those receiving placebo. Approximately 70% of patients had tophi at baseline; among patients with tophaceous deposits, 45% of those receiving pegloticase 8 mg (of uricase protein) every 2 weeks achieved a complete response (defined as complete resolution of at least one tophus, no new tophi, and no progression of any existing tophi) at 6 months compared with 8% of those receiving placebo. Pegloticase-treated patients who exhibited a response in uric acid concentrations were more likely than nonresponders to have a reduction in the number of tender and swollen joints and to report improved outcomes on the Health Assessment Questionnaire (HAQ) Patient Global Assessment. Preliminary data from an open-label extension of these studies in 151 patients indicated that efficacy of pegloticase therapy is maintained for periods of up to 1 year.

Pegloticase 8 mg (of uricase protein) every 4 weeks also demonstrated efficacy in controlling plasma uric acid concentrations; however, this regimen was associated with an increased frequency of anaphylaxis and infusion reactions and was less effective in reducing tophi.

Dosage and Administration

■ **General** Patients should receive an antihistamine and corticosteroid prior to each infusion of pegloticase to minimize the risk of anaphylaxis and infusion reactions. Patients should be closely monitored for such reactions for an appropriate period of time after administration of the drug. Because the risk of anaphylaxis or infusion reactions is higher in patients who have lost therapeutic response to the drug, uric acid concentration should be determined prior to each infusion of the drug. (See Sensitivity Reactions under Cautions: Warnings/Precautions.)

Because of the risk of acute gout attacks (gout flare) following initiation of pegloticase therapy, gout flare prophylaxis with a nonsteroidal anti-inflammatory agent (NSAIA) or colchicine is recommended; the prophylactic regimen should be started at least one week prior to initiation of pegloticase therapy and continued for at least 6 months unless such therapy is contraindicated or not tolerated. (See Gout Flares under Cautions: Warnings/Precautions.)

■ **Administration** Pegloticase is administered by IV infusion via gravity feed, syringe pump, or infusion pump. The drug should not be administered by rapid IV injection, such as IV push or bolus.

Dilution Commercially available pegloticase injection concentrate must be diluted prior to IV administration. Solutions for IV infusion are prepared by withdrawing 1 mL of pegloticase injection concentrate from a vial labeled as containing 8 mg/mL of uricase protein and injecting the concentrate into a 250-mL bag containing 0.45 or 0.9% sodium chloride injection. Pegloticase should not be mixed or diluted with other drugs. Any unused portion of the drug remaining in the vial should be discarded. The infusion bag containing the diluted pegloticase solution should be inverted a number of times to ensure thorough mixing; the solution should not be shaken. Pegloticase infusion solutions should be inspected visually for particulate matter and discoloration prior to administration.

Pegloticase infusion solutions should be used within 4 hours of dilution. Although the diluted drug is stable for 4 hours when stored either under refrigeration (2–8°C) or at room temperature (20–25°C), the manufacturer recommends that pegloticase infusion solutions be refrigerated and protected from light. Solutions of the drug should be allowed to reach room temperature prior to administration but should not be subjected to heating (e.g., hot water, microwave).

Rate of Administration IV infusions of pegloticase should be administered over at least 120 minutes.

If an infusion reaction occurs during administration of pegloticase, the infusion may be slowed, temporarily stopped and then restarted at a slower rate, or discontinued, depending on the severity of the reaction.

Risk Evaluation and Mitigation Strategy A Risk Evaluation and Mitigation Strategy (REMS) has been required and approved by the US Food and Drug Administration (FDA) for pegloticase. The goal of this REMS program is to inform healthcare providers and patients about the serious risks associated with pegloticase therapy, including the risks of anaphylaxis and infusion reactions and the contraindication to use of pegloticase in patients with glucose-6-phosphate dehydrogenase (G-6-PD) deficiency. (See Cautions.) The REMS program consists of a medication guide to be dispensed with every pegloticase prescription and a communication plan requiring initial and periodic communications from the manufacturer to certain targeted groups of healthcare providers.

■ **Dosage** Dosage of pegloticase is expressed in terms of the amount of uricase protein.

The recommended adult dosage of pegloticase for the management of chronic gout that is refractory to conventional therapy is 8 mg (of uricase protein) given as an IV infusion every 2 weeks. The optimum duration of therapy has not been established.

Because the risk of anaphylaxis or infusion reactions is higher in patients who have lost therapeutic response to the drug, discontinuance of therapy should be considered if uric acid concentrations rise above 6 mg/dL, particularly if 2 consecutive measurements exceed 6 mg/dL. (See Sensitivity Reactions under Cautions: Warnings/Precautions.)

■ **Special Populations** Dosage adjustment is not routinely required based on age or renal impairment.

Cautions

■ **Contraindications** Pegloticase is contraindicated in patients with glucose-6-phosphate dehydrogenase (G-6-PD) deficiency since the drug may cause hemolysis and methemoglobinemia in these individuals. Patients at higher risk for G-6-PD deficiency (e.g., patients of African or Mediterranean ancestry) should be screened for G-6-PD deficiency before initiating pegloticase therapy.

■ **Warnings/Precautions** ***Sensitivity Reactions*** **Anaphylaxis.** During clinical trials, anaphylaxis occurred despite pretreatment with an oral antihistamine, IV corticosteroid, and/or acetaminophen in 6.5% of patients receiving pegloticase 8 mg (of uricase protein) every 2 weeks, compared with none of those receiving placebo. Manifestations included wheezing, perioral or lingual edema, or hemodynamic instability, with or without rash or urticaria. Because the pretreatment regimen may have blunted symptoms or signs of anaphylaxis, the reported frequency may underestimate the drug's potential to cause such reactions.

Pegloticase should be administered in a healthcare setting by healthcare providers prepared to manage anaphylaxis. Patients should be pretreated with antihistamines and corticosteroids and should be closely monitored for an appropriate period of time after administration of pegloticase. Anaphylaxis may occur with any infusion of the drug. Although reactions generally occur within 2 hours of an infusion, delayed-type hypersensitivity reactions also have occurred. Risk of anaphylaxis is higher in patients whose uric acid concentration rises above 6 mg/dL, particularly when 2 consecutive measurements exceed 6 mg/dL. Serum uric acid concentration should be determined prior to each infusion of the drug; if concentrations rise above 6 mg/dL, discontinuance of treatment should be considered.

Infusion Reactions. During clinical trials, infusion reactions (e.g., urticaria, dyspnea, chest discomfort or pain, erythema, pruritus) occurred despite pretreatment with an oral antihistamine, IV corticosteroid, and/or acetaminophen in 26% of patients receiving pegloticase 8 mg (of uricase protein) every 2 weeks and 41% of patients receiving the drug at a dosage of 8 mg every 4 weeks, compared with 5% of patients receiving placebo. Because the pretreatment regimen may have blunted symptoms or signs of infusion reactions, the reported frequency may underestimate the drug's potential to cause such reactions.

Pegloticase should be administered in a healthcare setting by healthcare providers prepared to manage infusion reactions. Patients should be pretreated with antihistamines and corticosteroids and should be closely monitored for approximately 1 hour after pegloticase administration. Pegloticase should be infused slowly over no less than 120 minutes. In the event of an infusion reaction, the infusion should be slowed or should be stopped and then restarted at a slower rate. If a severe infusion reaction occurs, the infusion should be discontinued and appropriate treatment instituted as needed. Risk of an infusion reaction is higher in patients whose uric acid concentration rises above 6 mg/dL, particularly when 2 consecutive measurements exceed 6 mg/dL. Serum uric acid concentration should be determined prior to each infusion of the drug; if concentrations rise above 6 mg/dL, discontinuance of treatment should be considered.

Gout Flares An increase in gout flares frequently is observed upon initiation of antihyperuricemic therapy as changes in serum uric acid concentrations result in mobilization of urate from tissue deposits. During clinical trials evaluating pegloticase, 74 or 81% of patients receiving the drug at a dosage of 8 mg (of uricase protein) every 2 or 4 weeks, respectively, and 51% of those receiving placebo experienced one or more gout flares during the first 3 months of therapy despite receiving prophylaxis for such flares.

Prophylaxis with a nonsteroidal anti-inflammatory agent (NSAIA) or colchicine is recommended beginning at least one week before initiation of pegloticase therapy and continuing at least 6 months, unless contraindicated or not tolerated. Pegloticase does not need to be discontinued because of a gout flare.

Congestive Heart Failure Pegloticase has not been formally studied in patients with congestive heart failure (CHF), but exacerbation of heart failure has been reported in patients receiving the drug. Pegloticase should be used with caution and close monitoring following infusions in patients with CHF.

Retreatment with Pegloticase The safety and efficacy of resuming pegloticase therapy after treatment has been interrupted for longer than 4 weeks have not been established in controlled clinical trials. Patients reinitiating therapy with the drug after a drug-free interval may be at increased risk of anaphylaxis and infusion reactions and should be monitored closely.

Immunogenicity Antipegloticase antibodies developed in 92% of patients receiving pegloticase every 2 weeks. Antipegloticase antibodies appear to bind to the polyethylene glycol (PEG) portion of the drug, even though antibodies to PEG were detected in only 42% of patients receiving pegloticase. (See Drug Interactions.) High antipegloticase antibody titers were associated with reduced serum concentrations of the drug and failure to maintain pegloticase-induced normalization of serum uric acid. The incidence of infusion reactions was higher in patients with high antipegloticase antibody titers compared with patients who had undetectable or low antibody titers (53 versus 6% among patients receiving the drug every 2 weeks).

Specific Populations **Pregnancy.** Category C. (See Users Guide.)

Lactation. It is not known whether pegloticase is distributed into milk. Because many drugs are distributed into human milk and because of the potential for serious adverse reactions to pegloticase in nursing infants, the manufacturer recommends that the drug not be used in nursing women.

Pediatric Use. Safety and efficacy have not been established in children younger than 18 years of age.

Geriatric Use. No substantial differences in safety and efficacy relative to younger adults were observed, but increased sensitivity cannot be ruled out.

Hepatic Impairment. Pegloticase has not been studied in patients with hepatic impairment.

Renal Impairment. About 32% of patients receiving pegloticase 8 mg (of uricase protein) every 2 weeks in clinical trials had a creatinine clearance of 62.5 mL/minute or less. No substantial differences in efficacy were observed.

■ **Common Adverse Effects** Adverse effects reported in 5% or more of patients receiving pegloticase at a dosage of 8 mg (of uricase protein) every 2 weeks include gout flares, infusion reactions, nausea, contusion or ecchymosis, nasopharyngitis, constipation, chest pain, anaphylaxis, and vomiting.

Drug Interactions

No formal drug interaction studies have been conducted to date.

Because antipegloticase antibodies appear to bind to the polyethylene glycol (PEG) portion of the drug, the potential exists for the antibodies to bind with other pegylated drugs. The effect of such antibodies on the efficacy of other PEG-containing drugs is not known.

Description

Pegloticase is a biosynthetic (recombinant DNA origin) modified mammalian (porcine-like) urate oxidase (uricase, urate hydroxylase) enzyme that is covalently bound to monoethoxypolyethylene glycol (PEG). The urate oxidase protein is prepared using recombinant DNA technology and a genetically modified strain of *Escherichia coli*. Pegloticase is a uric acid-specific enzyme that catalyzes the oxidation of uric acid to allantoin, thereby lowering serum uric acid concentrations. Allantoin is an inert, water-soluble purine metabolite that is readily eliminated, mainly by renal excretion. Maintaining the serum urate concentration below the saturation point for monosodium urate (e.g., maintaining concentrations at 6 mg/dL or less) may prevent crystal formation and promote resolution of existing tophaceous crystal deposits, thus preventing long-term joint, bone, cartilage, and tissue destruction. A single dose of pegloticase rapidly suppresses plasma uric acid and generally maintains concentrations below 6 mg/dL for more than 12 days.

Advice to Patients

Pegloticase medication guide must be provided to the patient each time the drug is administered (see Risk Evaluation and Mitigation Strategy under Dosage and Administration: Administration); importance of the patient reading the medication guide before initiating therapy and before each subsequent infusion.

Importance of informing patients that anaphylaxis and infusion reactions can occur with any infusion. Importance of informing patients of the signs and symptoms of anaphylaxis (e.g., wheezing, swelling of the throat or tongue, throat tightness, hoarseness, difficulty swallowing, dizziness, fainting, fast or weak heartbeat, feelings of nervousness, rash, itching, urticaria) and infusion reactions (e.g., urticaria, erythema, difficulty breathing, flushing, chest discomfort or pain, rash). Advise patients to seek medical care immediately if they experience any symptoms of an allergic reaction during or at any time after an infusion of pegloticase. Counsel patients on the importance of adhering to therapy prescribed to prevent or lessen the severity of these reactions.

Importance of informing patients not to take pegloticase if they have glucose-6-phosphate dehydrogenase (G-6-PD) deficiency. Counsel patients that they may be tested to determine if they have G-6-PD deficiency.

Importance of informing patients that gout flares may initially increase when starting treatment with pegloticase and that medications to help reduce flares may be taken regularly for the first few months after initiation. Advise patients that they should not discontinue pegloticase therapy if such flares occur.

Importance of women informing clinicians if they are or plan to become pregnant or plan to breast-feed.

Importance of informing clinicians of existing or contemplated concomitant therapy, including prescription and OTC drugs and herbal or dietary supplements, as well as any concomitant conditions (e.g., heart failure, G-6-PD deficiency).

Importance of informing patients of other important precautionary information. (See Cautions.)

Overview® (see Users Guide). For additional information on this drug until a more detailed monograph is developed and published, the manufacturer's labeling should be consulted. It is *essential* that the manufacturer's labeling be consulted for more detailed information on usual cautions, precautions, contraindications, potential drug interactions, laboratory test interferences, and acute toxicity.

Preparations

Excipients in commercially available drug preparations may have clinically important effects in some individuals; consult specific product labeling for details.

Pegloticase

Parenteral

Injection, concentrate, for IV infusion	8 mg/mL (of uricase protein)	**Krystexxa®**, Savient

Selected Revisions December 2014, © Copyright, June 2011, American Society of Health-System Pharmacists, Inc.

IMMUNOMODULATORY AGENTS 92:20

Dimethyl Fumarate DMF

■ Dimethyl fumarate, a fumaric acid derivative, has immunomodulatory and disease-modifying activity in multiple sclerosis.

Uses

■ **Multiple Sclerosis** Dimethyl fumarate is used orally in the management of adults with relapsing forms of multiple sclerosis (MS; e.g., relapsing-remitting MS [RRMS]).

Dimethyl fumarate is one of several disease-modifying therapies used in the management of RRMS. Although not curative, these therapies have all been shown to modify several measures of disease activity, including relapse rates, new or enhancing magnetic resonance imaging (MRI) lesions, and disability progression; results of placebo-controlled studies indicate that treatment with a disease-modifying agent can reduce the frequency of MS attacks by 28–68%. The American Academy of Neurology (AAN) recommends that disease-modifying therapy be offered to patients with RRMS who have had recent relapses and/or MRI activity; these experts state that the benefits versus risks (e.g., adverse effects or burden of taking a long-term medication) of treatment in patients who have not had relapses in 2 or more years and do not have active MRI lesions are not known. Because CNS damage occurs early and continues throughout the course of MS, other clinicians recommend that disease-modifying therapy be initiated as soon as possible following diagnosis and continued indefinitely unless there is a clear lack of benefit, adverse effects are intolerable, the patient is unable to adhere to the recommended treatment regimen, or a more appropriate treatment becomes available. Clinicians should consider the adverse effects, tolerability, method of administration, safety, efficacy, and cost of the drugs in addition to patient preferences when selecting an appropriate disease-modifying therapy.

Efficacy and safety of dimethyl fumarate were principally demonstrated in 2 randomized, double-blind, placebo-controlled studies that evaluated dimethyl fumarate in adults with RRMS. Dosage of dimethyl fumarate in both studies was 120 mg given either twice or 3 times daily for the first 7 days, then 240 mg given twice or 3 times daily. Both studies included patients who had experienced at least 1 clinical relapse during the prior year or had a brain MRI scan demonstrating at least one gadolinium-enhancing lesion within 6 weeks of randomization; patients had Expanded Disability Status Scale (EDSS) scores of 0–5. Neurologic evaluations were performed at baseline, every 3 months, and at the time of suspected relapse. MRI evaluations were performed at baseline, month 6, and year 1 and 2 in a subset of patients.

The Determination of the Efficacy and Safety of Oral Fumarate in Relapsing-Remitting MS (DEFINE) trial was conducted in 1234 adults with RRMS. The median age of enrolled patients in the study was 39 years, the median time since diagnosis was 4 years, and the median EDSS score at baseline was 2. At 2 years, the proportion of patients who had an MS relapse (the primary end point) was substantially lower (relative risk reduction of 49%) in patients receiving dimethyl fumarate 240 mg twice daily than in those receiving placebo (27 and 46%, respectively). The annualized relapse rate also was substantially lower in patients receiving dimethyl fumarate 240 mg twice daily (0.17) than in those receiving placebo (0.36), representing a 53% reduction in this rate. Secondary MRI end points demonstrated substantially fewer new or enlarged T2-weighted hyperintense lesions and substantially fewer gadolinium-enhancing lesions in the dimethyl fumarate-treated patients compared with those receiving placebo; dimethyl fumarate also substantially reduced the rate of disability progression. The 240-mg 3 times daily dosage of dimethyl fumarate was found to provide no additional therapeutic benefit over the 240-mg twice daily dosage.

The Comparator and an Oral Fumarate in Relapsing-Remitting Multiple Sclerosis (CONFIRM) trial was conducted in 1417 adults with RRMS; the study included an open-label comparator arm. The primary end point in this study was the annualized relapse rate at 2 years. Patients were randomized to receive dimethyl fumarate 240 mg twice daily, dimethyl fumarate 240 mg 3 times daily, open-label glatiramer acetate 20 mg daily by subcutaneous injection, or placebo for up to 2 years. The median age of enrolled patients in the study was 37 years, the median time since diagnosis was 3 years, and the median EDSS score at baseline was 2.5. At 2 years, the annualized relapse rate was found to be substantially lower in patients receiving dimethyl fumarate 240 mg twice daily (0.22), dimethyl fumarate 240 mg 3 times daily (0.2), and glatiramer acetate (0.29) than in those receiving placebo (0.4); relative reductions were 44% with twice-daily dimethyl fumarate, 51% with thrice-daily dimethyl fumarate, and 29% with glatiramer acetate. This study was not designed to test superiority or non-inferiority of dimethyl fumarate compared with glatiramer acetate. In addition, the number of new and newly enlarging T2 hyperintense lesions and new T1 hypointense lesions was substantially lower in dimethyl fumarate- and glatiramer acetate-treated patients compared with those receiving placebo. Reductions in disability progression with twice-daily dimethyl fumarate, thrice-daily dimethyl fumarate, and glatiramer acetate relative to placebo were not found to be statistically significant in this study. In addition, the 240-mg 3 times daily dosage of dimethyl fumarate provided no additional therapeutic benefit over the 240-mg twice-daily dosage.

Subgroup analyses of both the DEFINE and CONFIRM trial data based on clinically relevant baseline patient and disease characteristics (e.g., gender, age, relapse history, McDonald criteria, treatment history, EDSS score, T2 lesion volume, gadolinium-enhancing lesions) consistently showed a treatment benefit with dimethyl fumarate across a broad range of patient subgroups.

The efficacy of dimethyl fumarate in patients with primary-progressive MS† has not been established to date.

Direct comparative studies between dimethyl fumarate and other oral drugs used in the treatment of RRMS (e.g., fingolimod, teriflunomide) have not been performed to date; however, clinical experience with these oral agents suggests that dimethyl fumarate may be more effective than teriflunomide and better tolerated than fingolimod therapy.

Dosage and Administration

■ **General** Because of the risk of lymphopenia, the manufacturer recommends obtaining a complete blood cell (CBC) count, including lymphocyte count, prior to initiation of dimethyl fumarate therapy, following 6 months of therapy, every 6–12 months thereafter, and as clinically indicated. (See Lymphopenia under Cautions: Warnings/Precautions.) Liver function tests (i.e., serum aminotransferase, alkaline phosphatase, and total bilirubin concentrations) should be performed prior to initiating dimethyl fumarate and during therapy as clinically indicated. (See Hepatic Injury under Cautions: Warnings/Precautions.)

■ **Administration** Dimethyl fumarate delayed-release capsules are administered orally twice daily with or without food. However, taking the drug with food may reduce the incidence of flushing. In addition, administration of non-enteric-coated aspirin (up to a dose of 325 mg) 30 minutes prior to dimethyl fumarate administration may reduce the incidence and severity of flushing. (See Flushing under Cautions: Warnings/Precautions and also see Drug Interactions: Aspirin.) In patients who experience troublesome adverse GI effects, taking the drug with food also may improve its tolerability.

The delayed-release capsules of dimethyl fumarate should be swallowed whole and intact, and should *not* be crushed or chewed; the contents of the capsules also should *not* be sprinkled on food.

■ **Dosage** The recommended initial dosage of dimethyl fumarate in adults with relapsing forms of multiple sclerosis (MS; e.g., relapsing-remitting MS [RRMS]) is 120 mg given twice daily (total of 240 mg daily). After 7 days, the dosage should be increased to a maintenance dosage of 240 mg given twice daily (total of 480 mg daily). The Tecfidera® 30-day Starter Pack, which contains 120-mg capsules of dimethyl fumarate for the first 7 days of therapy and 240-mg capsules of the drug for the next 23 days of therapy, is designed to be used during the first month of therapy.

A temporary reduction in the maintenance dosage of dimethyl fumarate from 240 mg twice daily to 120 mg twice daily may be considered in patients who do not tolerate the usual maintenance dosage. The recommended maintenance dosage of 240 mg twice daily should be resumed within 4 weeks. Discontinuance of the drug should be considered in patients unable to tolerate a return to the usual maintenance dosage of 240 mg given twice daily.

■ **Special Populations** Dimethyl fumarate has not been evaluated in patients with hepatic or renal impairment; however, the manufacturer states that these conditions are unlikely to affect exposure to the drug's active metabolite, monomethyl fumarate (MMF). Therefore, no dosage adjustment is necessary in such patients.

No dosage adjustment is necessary in geriatric patients. (See Geriatric Use under Warnings/Precautions: Specific Populations, in Cautions.)

Cautions

■ **Contraindications** Dimethyl fumarate is contraindicated in patients with known hypersensitivity to dimethyl fumarate or any excipients in the formulation. Hypersensitivity reactions reported in dimethyl fumarate-treated patients have included anaphylaxis and angioedema. (See Anaphylaxis and Angioedema under Cautions: Warnings/Precautions.)

■ **Warnings/Precautions** ***Anaphylaxis and Angioedema*** Dimethyl fumarate may cause anaphylaxis or angioedema after the first dose or at any time during therapy. Signs and symptoms of these hypersensitivity reactions have included difficulty breathing, urticaria, and swelling of the throat and tongue. Patients should be instructed to discontinue dimethyl fumarate and seek immediate medical care if they experience signs and symptoms of anaphylaxis or angioedema. (See Contraindications under Cautions.)

Progressive Multifocal Leukoencephalopathy Progressive multifocal leukoencephalopathy (PML), a serious opportunistic infection of the brain caused by the JC virus (JCV), has been reported in patients receiving dimethyl fumarate. PML typically occurs only in immunocompromised patients and usually leads to death or severe disability. In November 2014, the FDA alerted healthcare professionals and patients about a fatal case of PML that occurred in a patient with multiple sclerosis who had been receiving dimethyl fumarate for 4 years while enrolled in a clinical trial. The patient in the case reported by the FDA and subsequently published experienced prolonged lymphopenia (i.e., lymphocyte counts predominantly lower than 500/mm³ for 3.5 years) while receiving dimethyl fumarate; the causative role of lymphopenia in this case is unknown. (See Lymphopenia under Cautions: Warnings/Precautions.) The patient had no other known medical conditions resulting in compromised immune system function and had not previously been treated with natalizumab, which is known to be associated with PML. In addition, the patient was not concurrently receiving any immunosuppressive or immunomodulatory drugs.

PML has previously been reported in Europe in patients receiving other preparations containing dimethyl fumarate. The FDA stated that it was aware of 4 such cases at the time of approval of dimethyl fumarate in the US. Three of the cases occurred in patients with psoriasis treated with Fumaderm® (a combination preparation available in Germany that contains dimethyl fumarate and 3 different salts of its metabolite, monomethyl fumarate), and one case occurred in a patient treated with a compounded preparation that included dimethyl fumarate. The patients in 2 of these cases had previously been exposed to immunosuppressive therapy. In the other 2 cases, patients experienced prolonged lymphopenia with lymphocyte counts lower than 500/mm³. The FDA stated that the contribution of dimethyl fumarate to the development of PML in these European cases is not known. An additional case of PML that developed in a European patient receiving topical corticosteroids and a compounded psoriasis preparation containing dimethyl fumarate has since been reported; however, the patient did not develop severe lymphopenia.

Dimethyl fumarate therapy should be immediately withheld at the first sign or symptom suggestive of PML and an appropriate diagnostic evaluation should be performed. Symptoms typically associated with PML are diverse, progress over a period of days to weeks, and include progressive weakness on one side of the body or clumsiness of limbs, vision disturbance, and changes in thinking, memory, and orientation that can lead to confusion and personality changes. MRI signs of PML may be apparent before clinical manifestations develop; any suspicious findings on MRI should be followed with further investigation. Lymphocyte counts also should be monitored in patients receiving dimethyl fumarate. (See Lymphopenia under Cautions: Warnings/Precautions and also see Advice to Patients.)

For additional information on PML, see Progressive Multifocal Leukoencephalopathy under Warnings/Precautions: Warnings, in Natalizumab 92:20.

Lymphopenia Dimethyl fumarate may decrease lymphocyte counts. In placebo-controlled clinical trials, mean lymphocyte counts decreased by approximately 30% during the first year of therapy with the drug and remained stable thereafter. Mean lymphocyte counts improved 4 weeks following discontinuance of the drug, but did not return to baseline values. (See Description.)

In placebo-controlled clinical trials, 6% of dimethyl fumarate-treated patients and less than 1% of placebo recipients had lymphocyte counts lower than 500/mm³. The incidence of infections (60 and 58%) and serious infections (2 and 2%) was similar in patients receiving dimethyl fumarate and placebo, respectively. Although an increased incidence of serious infections was not observed in patients with decreased lymphocyte counts in controlled trials, one dimethyl fumarate-treated patient in an extension study developed PML in the setting of prolonged lymphopenia (i.e., lymphocyte counts predominantly lower than 500/mm³ for 3.5 years). (See Progressive Multifocal Leukoencephalopathy under Cautions: Warnings/Precautions.) In controlled and uncontrolled clinical trials, 2% of dimethyl fumarate-treated patients had lymphocyte counts lower than 500/mm³ for at least 6 months; in these patients, the majority of lymphocyte counts remained lower than 500/mm³ with continued therapy.

Dimethyl fumarate has not been studied in patients with preexisting low lymphocyte counts.

Prior to initiation of dimethyl fumarate, a complete blood cell (CBC) count, including lymphocyte count, should be obtained. A CBC should also be obtained following 6 months of dimethyl fumarate therapy, every 6–12 months thereafter, and as clinically indicated.

In patients with lymphocyte counts lower than 500/mm³ persisting for more than 6 months, interruption of dimethyl fumarate therapy should be considered. Because of the potential for a delay in lymphocyte recovery following discontinuance of dimethyl fumarate, monitoring of lymphocyte counts until lymphopenia is resolved should also be considered.

In patients with serious infections, withholding dimethyl fumarate treatment should be considered until the infection has resolved. The decision about whether or not to resume dimethyl fumarate therapy should be individualized based on clinical circumstances.

Hepatic Injury Liver function test abnormalities (e.g., elevations in serum aminotransferase concentrations to more than fivefold the upper limit of normal [ULN] and elevations in total bilirubin concentrations to more than twofold the ULN) have been reported during postmarketing experience with dimethyl fumarate. Such abnormalities occurred within a few days to several months after initiation of therapy, and resolved upon discontinuance of the drug. Although liver failure and death did not occur in any of the reported cases, marked increases in liver function tests may be indicative of serious liver injury.

Liver function tests (i.e., serum aminotransferase, alkaline phosphatase, and total bilirubin concentrations) should be performed prior to initiating dimethyl fumarate and during therapy as clinically indicated. If there is any evidence of liver injury, the drug should be discontinued. (See Advice to Patients.)

Flushing Dimethyl fumarate may cause flushing (e.g., warmth, redness, itching, and/or burning sensation). In clinical trials, 40% of patients receiving the drug experienced flushing. Symptoms generally began soon after initiating dimethyl fumarate and improved or resolved over time. In most patients, flushing was mild or moderate in severity. Discontinuance of therapy for flushing was reported in 3% of patients receiving dimethyl fumarate; less than 1% of patients had serious flushing symptoms that were not life-threatening but resulted in hospitalization.

Administration of dimethyl fumarate with food may reduce the incidence of flushing. Alternatively, administration of non-enteric-coated aspirin (up to a dose of 325 mg) 30 minutes prior to dimethyl fumarate administration may reduce the incidence and severity of flushing. (See Dosage and Administration: Administration, Drug Interactions: Aspirin, and also see Description.)

Specific Populations **Pregnancy.** There are no adequate data on the developmental risks associated with the use of dimethyl fumarate during pregnancy. Embryotoxic effects (e.g., reduced fetal body weight, delayed ossification, lethality) have been observed in animal studies.

Patients should be encouraged to enroll in the Tecfidera® pregnancy registry by calling 866-810-1462 or visiting http://www.tecfiderapregnancyregistry.com.

Lactation. It is not known whether dimethyl fumarate or its metabolites are distributed into human milk. The effects of dimethyl fumarate on the nursing infant or on milk production also are not known. The benefits of breastfeeding should be considered along with the woman's clinical need for dimethyl fumarate and any potential adverse effects on the breastfed infant from the drug or underlying maternal condition.

Pediatric Use. Safety and efficacy of dimethyl fumarate have not been established in pediatric patients younger than 18 years of age.

Geriatric Use. Clinical studies of dimethyl fumarate did not include sufficient numbers of patients 65 years of age and older to determine whether geriatric patients respond differently than younger adults. (See Dosage and Administration: Special Populations.)

Hepatic Impairment. The pharmacokinetics of dimethyl fumarate have not been studied in patients with hepatic impairment. (See Dosage and Administration: Special Populations.)

Renal Impairment. The pharmacokinetics of dimethyl fumarate have not been studied in patients with renal impairment. (See Dosage and Administration: Special Populations.)

■ **Common Adverse Effects** Adverse effects reported in 10% or more of patients with multiple sclerosis receiving dimethyl fumarate and with an incidence at least 2% greater than with placebo include flushing, abdominal pain, diarrhea, and nausea. The incidence of flushing and adverse GI effects (e.g., nausea, vomiting, diarrhea, abdominal pain, dyspepsia) generally is higher early in the course of dimethyl fumarate treatment (occurring mainly in the first month) and decreases over time with continued therapy (see Dosage and Administration: Administration).

Proteinuria, pruritus, reduced lymphocyte counts, elevations in hepatic transaminase concentrations (e.g., ALT, AST), and transient eosinophilia (during the first 2 months of therapy) also have been reported in patients receiving dimethyl fumarate.

Drug Interactions

No potential drug interactions with dimethyl fumarate or its active metabolite, monomethyl fumarate (MMF), were identified in cytochrome P-450 inhibition and induction studies, P-glycoprotein studies, or studies of protein binding.

■ **Aspirin** Non-enteric-coated aspirin 325 mg administered approximately 30 minutes prior to dimethyl fumarate over 4 days in healthy individuals did not alter the pharmacokinetic profile of dimethyl fumarate and its active metabolite, MMF, but reduced the incidence and severity of flushing. (See Dosage and Administration: Administration and also see Flushing under Cautions: Warnings/Precautions.)

■ **Glatiramer Acetate** Administration of a single IM dose of glatiramer acetate did not alter the pharmacokinetics of MMF.

■ **Interferon Beta** Administration of a single IM dose of interferon beta-1a did not alter the pharmacokinetics of MMF.

■ **Oral Contraceptives** Drug interaction studies with dimethyl fumarate and oral contraceptives have not been performed to date. However, the results of in vitro CYP induction studies suggest that clinically important pharmacokinetic interactions are unlikely with combined use.

■ **Vaccines** The effectiveness of vaccines in patients receiving dimethyl fumarate has not been evaluated to date.

Description

Dimethyl fumarate is a fumaric acid derivative; the drug is a methyl ester of fumaric acid. Dimethyl fumarate has immunomodulatory and disease-modifying activity in multiple sclerosis (MS). The exact mechanism by which dimethyl fumarate exerts therapeutic effects in MS is unknown; however, the immunomodulatory effect appears to be mediated by many cells of the immune system. Dimethyl fumarate and its active metabolite, monomethyl fumarate (MMF), have been shown to activate the nuclear factor (erythroid-derived 2)-like 2 (Nrf2) pathway in vitro and in vivo in animals and humans; the Nrf2 antioxidant response pathway is involved in the cellular response to oxidative stress. In vitro and animal studies suggest that Nrf2-dependent upregulation of antioxidant response genes by dimethyl fumarate and MMF may protect various cells and tissues, including some in the CNS, from experimental toxic oxidative stress.

Activation of the Nrf2 pathway by dimethyl fumarate and MMF also may inhibit proliferation of lymphocytes and hematopoietic stem cells. Some preliminary data indicate that subsets of peripheral blood leucocytes and lymphocytes are affected differently by dimethyl fumarate therapy; a more pronounced reduction in CD8$^+$ T-cell counts than in CD4$^+$ T-cell counts has been observed in patients receiving therapy with the drug.

In addition, MMF has been shown to be a nicotinic acid receptor agonist in vitro. Nicotinic acid and fumaric acid derivatives such as dimethyl fumarate can cause skin flushing as an adverse effect; it has been suggested that such flushing reactions may be mediated by the activation of hydroxy-carboxylic acid receptor 2 (HCA_2) and involve the formation of prostaglandins.

Following oral administration, dimethyl fumarate undergoes rapid presystemic hydrolysis by esterases and is converted to its active metabolite, MMF. Dimethyl fumarate is not quantifiable in plasma after oral administration; therefore, all pharmacokinetic analyses related to dimethyl fumarate were performed with plasma MMF concentrations. Median time to peak plasma concentrations of MMF is 2–2.5 hours. Accumulation of MMF does not occur with multiple doses of dimethyl fumarate. A high-fat, high-calorie meal did not affect the area under the concentration-time curve (AUC) of MMF, but decreased peak plasma concentrations of MMF by 40% and delayed the time to reach peak concentrations from 2 to 5.5 hours; the incidence of flushing was decreased by approximately 25% in the fed state. MMF is 27–45% protein bound; protein binding is independent of concentration. Dimethyl fumarate is extensively metabolized by esterases present in the GI tract, blood, and tissues to MMF before it reaches the systemic circulation. MMF is further metabolized by the tricarboxylic acid (TCA) cycle; the cytochrome P-450 (CYP) system is not involved in the metabolism of dimethyl fumarate. The major metabolites found in plasma include MMF, fumaric acid, citric acid, and glucose. Exhalation of carbon dioxide (CO_2) is the primary route of elimination, and accounts for approximately 60% of an orally administered dose; renal and fecal elimination are minor routes of elimination, accounting for 16 and 1% of a dose, respectively. The elimination half-life of MMF is approximately 1 hour; in the majority of individuals, no circulating MMF is present 24 hours following an oral dose of dimethyl fumarate.

Advice to Patients

Importance of reading the manufacturer's patient information prior to beginning dimethyl fumarate therapy and rereading it each time the prescription is refilled.

Risk of anaphylaxis and angioedema. Importance of advising patients to discontinue dimethyl fumarate and seek immediate medical care if they develop signs and symptoms of anaphylaxis or angioedema (e.g., difficulty breathing, urticaria, swelling of the throat and tongue).

Importance of informing patients that progressive multifocal leukoencephalopathy (PML) has occurred in a dimethyl fumarate-treated patient, and that PML is characterized by a progression of deficits and usually leads to death or severe disability over weeks to months. Importance of immediately informing clinician of any new or worsening symptoms suggestive of PML (e.g., progressive weakness on one side of the body; clumsiness of limbs; disturbance of vision; changes in thinking, memory, and orientation leading to confusion and personality changes) that have progressed over days to weeks. Importance of advising patients not to stop taking dimethyl fumarate without first consulting with their clinician.

Importance of informing patients that they will receive 2 strengths of dimethyl fumarate delayed-release capsules when starting treatment: 120-mg capsules for the 7-day initial dosage and 240-mg capsules for the maintenance dosage. Both strengths of the drug should be taken twice daily.

Importance of informing patients to swallow dimethyl fumarate delayed-release capsules whole and intact, and not to crush, chew, or sprinkle the capsule contents on food. Importance of informing patients that the capsules may be taken with or without food.

Importance of informing patients that flushing and adverse GI effects (e.g., abdominal pain, diarrhea, nausea) commonly occur during dimethyl fumarate therapy, particularly at the initiation of treatment, and that they may decrease over time. Importance of advising patients to contact their clinician if they experience persistent and/or severe flushing or GI reactions. Importance of also advising patients that taking dimethyl fumarate with food or taking non-enteric-coated aspirin prior to taking dimethyl fumarate may be helpful in such cases.

Risk of decreased lymphocyte counts. Importance of informing patients that a complete blood cell count should be obtained before starting dimethyl fumarate therapy and that complete blood counts are also recommended following 6 months of therapy, every 6–12 months thereafter, and as clinically indicated.

Risk of liver injury. Importance of advising patients to immediately report any possible manifestations, including fatigue, anorexia, right upper abdominal discomfort, dark urine, or jaundice; importance of patients receiving liver function tests prior to and during treatment as clinically indicated to monitor for such effects.

Importance of women informing their clinician if they are or plan to become pregnant or plan to breast-feed. Importance of encouraging enrollment of pregnant women in the Tecfidera® pregnancy registry at 866-810-1462 or on the website http://www.tecfiderapregnancyregistry.com.

Importance of informing clinician of existing or contemplated concomitant therapy, including prescription and OTC drugs and herbal supplements, as well as any concomitant illnesses (e.g., leukopenia, lymphopenia, infections).

Importance of informing patients of other important precautionary information. (See Cautions.)

Overview® (see Users Guide). For additional information on this drug until a more detailed monograph is developed and published, the manufacturer's labeling should be consulted. It is *essential* that the manufacturer's labeling be consulted for more detailed information on usual cautions, precautions, contraindications, potential drug interactions, laboratory test interferences, and acute toxicity.

Preparations

Excipients in commercially available drug preparations may have clinically important effects in some individuals; consult specific product labeling for details.

Dimethyl Fumarate

Oral		
Capsules, delayed-release	120 mg	**Tecfidera®**, Biogen
	240 mg	**Tecfidera®**, Biogen
Kit	7-day bottle containing 14 delayed-release capsules of dimethyl fumarate 120 mg (Tecfidera®)	**Tecfidera® 30-day Starter Pack,** Biogen
	23-day bottle containing 46 delayed-release capsules of dimethyl fumarate 240 mg (Tecfidera®)	

†Use is not currently included in the labeling approved by the US Food and Drug Administration

Fingolimod Hydrochloride

■ Fingolimod hydrochloride, a sphingosine 1-phosphate (S1P) receptor modulator, has immunomodulatory and disease-modifying activity in multiple sclerosis.

REMS

FDA approved a REMS for fingolimod to ensure that the benefits outweigh the risk. The REMS may apply to one or more preparations of fingolimod and consists of the following: communication plan. See the FDA REMS page (https://www.accessdata.fda.gov/scripts/cder/rems/index.cfm).

Uses

■ **Multiple Sclerosis** Fingolimod hydrochloride is used orally for the treatment of relapsing forms of multiple sclerosis (MS; e.g., relapsing-remitting MS [RRMS]).

Fingolimod was the first oral disease-modifying treatment for MS to become commercially available in the US and is currently one of several disease-modifying therapies that may be used in the management of patients with RRMS. Although not curative, these therapies have all been shown to modify several measures of disease activity, including relapse rates, new or enhancing magnetic resonance imaging (MRI) lesions, and disability progression; results of placebo-controlled studies indicate that treatment with a disease-modifying agent can reduce the frequency of MS attacks by 28–68%. The American Academy of Neurology (AAN) recommends that disease-modifying therapy be offered to patients with RRMS who have had recent relapses and/or MRI activity; these experts state that the benefits versus risks (e.g., adverse effects or burden of taking a long-term medication) of treatment in patients who have not had relapses in 2 or more years and do not have active MRI lesions are not known. Because CNS damage occurs early and continues throughout the course of MS, other clinicians recommend that disease-modifying therapy be initiated as soon as possible following diagnosis and continued indefinitely unless there is a clear lack of benefit, adverse effects are intolerable, the patient is unable to adhere to the recommended treatment regimen, or a more appropriate treatment becomes available. Clinicians should consider the adverse effects, tolerability, method of administration, safety, efficacy, and cost of the drugs in addition to patient preferences when selecting an appropriate disease-modifying therapy.

Efficacy of fingolimod in adults with RRMS was demonstrated in 2 clinical studies (FREEDOMS and TRANSFORMS) that evaluated daily fingolimod dosages of 0.5 mg and 1.25 mg. Both studies included patients who had experienced at least 2 clinical relapses during the previous 2 years or at least 1 clinical relapse during the prior year and had Expanded Disability Status Scale (EDSS) scores of 0–5.5. The primary efficacy endpoint for both studies was the annualized relapse rate (defined as the number of confirmed relapses per year).

The FREEDOMS trial was a randomized, double-blind, placebo-controlled study in 1272 patients with RRMS who had not received any interferon beta or glatiramer acetate for at least the previous 3 months and had not received natalizumab therapy for at least the previous 6 months. The median age of patients in this study was 37 years, median disease duration was 6.7 years, and median EDSS score at baseline was 2. Patients were randomized to receive fingolimod 0.5 or 1.25 mg once daily or placebo for up to 24 months. The annualized relapse rate was found to be substantially lower in fingolimod-treated patients than in those who received placebo. Patients receiving 0.5 mg of the drug daily had an annualized relapse rate of 0.18 compared with a relapse rate of 0.4 in placebo recipients, representing a 54% reduction in this rate. Time to onset of 3-month disability progression, which was a secondary endpoint, was also substantially delayed with fingolimod therapy compared with placebo. Secondary MRI endpoints demonstrated substantially fewer new or enlarged lesions on T2-weighted images, substantially fewer gadolinium-enhancing lesions, and substantially less brain volume loss in the fingolimod-treated patients compared with those receiving placebo. The 1.25-mg daily dosage of fingolimod provided no additional therapeutic benefit over the 0.5-mg daily dosage in this study.

The TRANSFORMS trial was a randomized, double-blind, double-dummy, active-controlled study in 1292 patients with RRMS. The median age of patients in the study was 36 years, median disease duration was approximately 6 years, and median EDSS score at baseline was 2. Patients were randomized to receive fingolimod 0.5 or 1.25 mg orally once daily or interferon beta-1a 30 mcg IM once weekly for up to 12 months. The annualized relapse rate was substantially lower in patients receiving fingolimod 0.5 mg (0.16) or fingolimod 1.25 mg (0.2) compared with those receiving interferon beta-1a (0.33). In addition, the number of new and newly enlarging T2 lesions was substantially reduced in fingolimod-treated patients compared with those receiving interferon beta-1a. No substantial differences were observed among the study groups with regard to progression of disability. The 1.25-mg daily dosage provided no additional benefit over the 0.5-mg daily dosage in this study.

Pooled results of the 2 principal efficacy studies in adults demonstrated a consistent and substantial reduction in the annualized relapse rate with fingolimod therapy compared with comparator (placebo and interferon beta-1a) in subgroups defined by gender, age, prior MS therapy, and disease activity.

Efficacy of fingolimod in pediatric patients was evaluated in a randomized, double-blind active-controlled study that compared the drug with interferon beta-1a in children 10 years of age or older with RRMS. Patients were eligible for the study if they had experienced at least 2 clinical relapses during the previous 2 years or at least 1 clinical relapse during the prior year, or had evidence of at least 1 gadolinium-enhancing lesion on MRI within 6 months prior to randomization; patients were also required to have a baseline EDSS score of 0–5.5. The annualized relapse rate (primary efficacy outcome) was substantially reduced in patients receiving fingolimod (0.122) compared with those receiving interferon beta-1a (0.675); the relative reduction was 81.9%. In addition, the number of new or newly enlarging T2 lesions and the number of gadolinium-enhancing T1 lesions were substantially reduced in fingolimod-treated patients compared with those receiving interferon beta-1a.

Fingolimod currently is not FDA-labeled for use in patients with primary-progressive MS (PPMS)† who experience steady worsening of their condition without acute attacks. In clinical trials evaluating fingolimod in patients with PPMS, the drug did not have an effect on disability progression, but substantially affected MRI measures of disease activity.

Additional studies are necessary to more clearly determine the efficacy and safety profile of fingolimod, particularly during long-term use, and the optimal role of the drug in treating MS, particularly in comparison with other disease-modifying therapies (e.g., dimethyl fumarate, glatiramer acetate, interferon beta, teriflunomide).

■ **Autoimmune Neuropathy** Fingolimod hydrochloride has been designated an orphan drug by the FDA for use in the treatment of chronic inflammatory demyelinating polyneuropathy†.

Dosage and Administration

■ **Administration** Fingolimod hydrochloride is administered orally once daily without regard to meals.

Clinical trial experience suggests that a washout period is not necessary when switching multiple sclerosis (MS) patients from interferon beta or glatiramer acetate therapy to other MS treatments, including fingolimod. However, the manufacturer and some clinicians recommend using caution when switching patients from drugs with prolonged immune effects (e.g., natalizumab, mitoxantrone, teriflunomide) to fingolimod. Some clinicians recommend that approximately 6 months elapse following discontinuance of natalizumab and initiation of fingolimod therapy. Some clinicians also recommend that 2 months elapse following discontinuance of fingolimod prior to initiation of another MS therapy, although a shorter washout period may be adequate if switching to an agent without immunosuppressant effects. (See Infectious Complications under Cautions: Warnings/Precautions and see also Immunosuppression Following Discontinuance under Cautions: Warnings/Precautions.)

First-Dose Monitoring *Initiation of fingolimod therapy results in a decrease in heart rate. After the first dose, the heart rate decrease starts within an hour and the nadir on day 1 generally occurs within about 6 hours; however, the nadir can be observed up to 24 hours after the first dose in some patients.* (See Bradyarrhythmia and Atrioventricular Block under Cautions: Warnings/Precautions.)

First-dose monitoring is recommended whenever fingolimod therapy is initiated or reinitiated (after discontinuance for more than 14 days), or when dosage is increased (in pediatric patients). The first dose of fingolimod should be administered in a setting in which resources to appropriately manage symptomatic bradycardia are available. To assess patient response to the first dose, all patients should be observed for at least 6 hours for signs and symptoms of bradycardia with hourly pulse and blood pressure measurements. An electrocardiogram (ECG) should be obtained in all patients prior to the first dose and at the end of the observation period.

Additional observation (i.e., beyond 6 hours) should be instituted until the finding has resolved in the following situations: heart rate 6 hours post-dose is less than 45 beats per minute (in adults), less than 55 beats per minute (in pediatric patients 12 years of age or older), or less than 60 beats per minute (in pediatric patients 10–11 years of age); heart rate 6 hours post-dose is at the lowest value suggesting that the maximum pharmacodynamic effect on the heart may not have occurred; or ECG 6 hours post-dose shows new-onset second-degree or higher atrioventricular (AV) block. Patients at their lowest post-dose heart rate at the end of the observation period should be monitored until their heart rate increases.

If post-dose symptomatic bradycardia occurs, appropriate management and continuous ECG monitoring should be initiated and observation continued until the symptoms have resolved. If pharmacologic intervention is required for symptomatic bradycardia, continuous overnight ECG monitoring in a medical facility should be instituted and the first-dose monitoring strategy should be repeated after the second dose of fingolimod.

Patients with some preexisting conditions (e.g., ischemic heart disease, history of myocardial infarction, congestive heart failure, history of cardiac arrest, cerebrovascular disease, uncontrolled hypertension, history of symptomatic bradycardia, history of recurrent syncope, severe untreated sleep apnea, AV block, sinoatrial heart block) may poorly tolerate fingolimod-induced bradycardia or experience serious rhythm disturbances after the first dose of the drug. Such patients should have a cardiac evaluation by an appropriately trained clinician prior to initiating fingolimod therapy; if a decision is made to initiate therapy, they should be monitored overnight with continuous ECG monitoring in a medical facility.

Because initiation of fingolimod therapy results in a decreased heart rate and may prolong the QT interval, patients with a prolonged corrected QT (QT_c) interval (i.e., exceeding 450 msec in adult and pediatric males; exceeding 470 msec in adult females; or exceeding 460 msec in pediatric females) before dosing or during the 6-hour observation period, patients at additional risk for QT prolongation (e.g., those with hypokalemia, hypomagnesemia, congenital long QT syndrome), or patients receiving concurrent therapy with QT-prolonging drugs with a known risk of torsades de pointes (e.g., citalopram, certain antipsychotic agents [e.g., chlorpromazine, haloperidol, olanzapine, pimozide, quetiapine, risperidone, thioridazine, ziprasidone], erythromycin, methadone) should be monitored overnight with continuous ECG monitoring in a medical facility.

Because of the risk of severe bradycardia or heart block, patients receiving concurrent therapy with drugs that slow heart rate or AV conduction (e.g., β-adrenergic blocking agents, digoxin, heart-rate-lowering calcium-channel blocking agents [diltiazem or verapamil]) who cannot switch to drugs that do not slow the heart rate or AV conduction should receive continuous overnight ECG monitoring after the first dose of fingolimod. (See Drug Interactions: Drugs that Slow Heart Rate or Atrioventricular Conduction.)

Reinitiation of Therapy Following Discontinuance If fingolimod therapy is discontinued for more than 14 days after the first month of treatment, the effects on heart rate and AV conduction may recur upon reintroduction of the drug; therefore, the same precautions (i.e., first-dose monitoring) as for initial dosing should apply. Within the first 2 weeks of treatment, first-dose monitoring procedures are recommended after treatment interruption of 1 day or more; during weeks 3 and 4 of treatment, first dose procedures are recommended after treatment interruption of more than 7 days. (See First-Dose Monitoring under Dosage and Administration: Administration.)

■ **Dosage** Dosage of fingolimod hydrochloride is expressed in terms of fingolimod.

The recommended dosage of fingolimod for the treatment of relapsing forms of MS (e.g., relapsing-remitting MS [RRMS]) in adults and pediatric patients 10 years of age or older weighing more than 40 kg is 0.5 mg once daily. The recommended dosage of fingolimod in pediatric patients 10 years of age or older weighing 40 kg or less is 0.25 mg once daily. Dosages higher than 0.5 mg daily are associated with a greater incidence of adverse reactions without additional benefit.

■ **Special Populations** The manufacturer states that the usual 0.5 mg once-daily dosage of fingolimod appears appropriate for adults with renal impairment; routine dosage adjustment is not necessary. (See Renal Impairment under Warnings/Precautions: Specific Populations, in Cautions.)

In patients with severe hepatic impairment, the manufacturer recommends close monitoring; however, routine dosage adjustment does not appear to be necessary. Dosage adjustment is not necessary in patients with mild or moderate hepatic impairment. (See Hepatic Impairment under Warnings/Precautions: Specific Populations, in Cautions.)

Dosage adjustment in geriatric patients does not appear to be necessary. (See Geriatric Use under Warnings/Precautions: Specific Populations, in Cautions.)

Cautions

■ **Contraindications** Fingolimod is contraindicated in patients who recently (i.e., in the past 6 months) experienced myocardial infarction, unstable angina, stroke, transient ischemic attack, decompensated heart failure requiring hospitalization, or class III or IV heart failure.

Fingolimod is contraindicated in patients with a history or presence of Mobitz type II second-degree or third-degree atrioventricular (AV) block or sick sinus syndrome unless the patient has a functioning pacemaker.

Fingolimod is contraindicated in patients with a baseline corrected QT interval (QT_c) of 500 msec or greater.

Fingolimod is contraindicated in patients concurrently receiving class Ia or class III antiarrhythmic agents. (See Drug Interactions: Drugs that Prolong the QT Interval.)

Fingolimod is contraindicated in patients with a history of hypersensitivity reaction to fingolimod or any ingredient contained in the formulation.

■ **Warnings/Precautions** ***Bradyarrhythmia and Atrioventricular Block*** Because of the risk of fingolimod-associated bradyarrhythmia and AV block, patients should be monitored during initiation of therapy. (See First-Dose Monitoring under Dosage and Administration: Administration.)

After the first dose of fingolimod, heart rate decrease starts within an hour and the maximal decline on the first day generally occurs within 6 hours; recovery (although not to baseline levels) occurs by 8–10 hours post-dose. There is a second period of heart rate decrease within 24 hours after the first dose due to physiologic diurnal variation; in some patients, the heart rate decrease during the second period is more pronounced than the decrease observed in the first 6 hours. Heart rates below 40 beats per minute in adults and below 50 beats per minute in pediatric patients were rarely observed. Patients who experience bradycardia generally are asymptomatic but some experience hypotension, dizziness, fatigue, palpitations, and chest pain, which usually resolve within the first 24 hours of therapy. Symptomatic bradycardia following the first dose was reported in 0.6% of fingolimod-treated adults in controlled studies.

Following the second dose of fingolimod, a further decrease in heart rate may occur but be of smaller magnitude than that observed after the first dose. With continued dosing, the heart rate returns to baseline within one month. Clinicians should continue to be alert to patient reports of cardiac symptoms throughout this period.

Initiation of fingolimod treatment has produced transient AV conduction delays. In controlled clinical trials in adults, first-degree AV block following the first dose was reported in 4.7% of fingolimod-treated patients and in 1.6% of patients receiving placebo. Second-degree AV block (Mobitz types I [Wenckebach] or 2:1 AV block) following the first dose was reported in 4% of fingolimod-treated patients in a study with available 24-hour Holter monitoring data. Conduction abnormalities usually are transient, asymptomatic, and resolve within the first 24 hours on treatment; however, treatment with atropine or isoproterenol is occasionally required. (See Drug Interactions.)

During postmarketing surveillance, third-degree AV block and AV block with junctional escape have been observed during the first-dose, 6-hour observation period with fingolimod. Isolated delayed-onset events, including transient asystole and unexplained death, have occurred within 24 hours of the first dose. These events were confounded by concomitant medications and/or preexisting disease, and the causal relationship to fingolimod is uncertain. Syncope also was reported after the first dose of fingolimod.

Infectious Complications Fingolimod causes a dose-dependent reduction in peripheral lymphocyte count to 20–30% of baseline values because of reversible sequestration of lymphocytes in lymphoid tissues. Fingolimod may therefore increase the risk of infections, some of which are serious, life-threatening, or fatal. (See Progressive Multifocal Leukoencephalopathy under Cautions: Warnings/Precautions.)

Before initiating fingolimod treatment, a recent complete blood count (CBC; i.e., within 6 months or after discontinuance of previous therapy) should be available. Patients with active acute or chronic infections should not begin fingolimod treatment until the infection(s) has resolved. If a patient develops a serious infection during treatment, discontinuance of fingolimod, at least temporarily, should be considered, and the benefits and risks of therapy should be reassessed prior to reinitiation of therapy. Because elimination of fingolimod after discontinuance may take up to 2 months, monitoring for infections should be continued throughout this period. (See Advice to Patients.)

In controlled studies in patients with multiple sclerosis (MS), the overall rate of infections (72%) with fingolimod was similar to placebo; however, bronchitis, herpes zoster, influenza, sinusitis, and pneumonia were more common in fingolimod-treated patients. Serious infections occurred in 2.3% of the patients receiving fingolimod compared with 1.6% of the placebo recipients.

In controlled trials, herpetic infections occurred in 9% of patients receiving fingolimod 0.5 mg daily compared with 7% of those receiving placebo. Two patients receiving fingolimod died of herpetic infections (one of disseminated primary herpes zoster and the second of herpes simplex encephalitis) during controlled studies. In both cases, the patients received a higher fingolimod dosage (1.25 mg daily) than that recommended for treatment of MS and also had received high-dose corticosteroid therapy for suspected MS relapse. Serious, life-threatening disseminated varicella zoster and herpes simplex infections, including cases of encephalitis and multiorgan failure, have occurred in patients receiving fingolimod 0.5 mg daily in the postmarketing setting; one of these events was fatal. The manufacturer states that disseminated herpetic infections should be included in the differential diagnosis of patients receiving fingolimod who present with an atypical MS relapse or multiorgan failure. Cases of Kaposi's sarcoma (a disorder associated with a particular strain of human herpes virus) have been reported during postmarketing experience with fingolimod; patients with manifestations consistent with Kaposi's sarcoma should be promptly evaluated and managed.

Cryptococcal infections, including some cases of cryptococcal meningitis and disseminated cryptococcal infections, have been reported with fingolimod during the postmarketing period. These infections generally occurred after 2 years of treatment, but can occur earlier. The manufacturer states that patients with signs and symptoms consistent with cryptococcal meningitis should undergo prompt diagnostic evaluation and treatment.

In clinical studies, fingolimod has not been administered concomitantly with antineoplastic, noncorticosteroid immunosuppressive, or immunomodulating therapies used in the treatment of MS. Concomitant use of fingolimod with any of these therapies or with corticosteroid therapy would be expected to increase the risk of immunosuppression. When switching to fingolimod from immunomodulating or immunosuppressive therapies, clinicians should consider the drugs' duration of effects and mechanism of action to avoid unintentional additive immunosuppressive effects. (See Dosage and Administration: Administration and also see Drug Interactions: Antineoplastic, Immunosuppressive, or Immunomodulating Therapies.)

Before initiating fingolimod therapy, patients without a healthcare professional-confirmed history of chickenpox or without documentation of a full course of vaccination against varicella zoster virus (VZV) should be tested for antibodies to VZV. VZV vaccination of antibody-negative patients is recommended prior to starting fingolimod therapy; initiation of treatment with the drug should then be postponed for 1 month to allow the full effect of vaccination to occur.

Progressive Multifocal Leukoencephalopathy Progressive multifocal leukoencephalopathy (PML), a serious opportunistic infection caused by the JC virus (JCV), has been reported in MS patients receiving fingolimod in the postmarketing setting. PML typically occurs in immunocompromised patients and usually leads to death or severe disability. The majority of cases have occurred in patients who received fingolimod for at least 2 years. Patients in the reported cases had no other known systemic medical conditions that would compromise immune function and had not previously received natalizumab, which is a known cause of PML; they also were not receiving concomitant therapy with any other immunosuppressive or immunomodulatory agents.

FDA previously had notified healthcare professionals and patients about a patient in Europe who developed PML while receiving fingolimod for possible MS. In that case, FDA stated that PML could not be conclusively associated with fingolimod therapy due to confounding factors (i.e., the patient had previously been treated with an immunosuppressive agent that can cause PML and also had received multiple courses of IV corticosteroids prior to and during fingolimod therapy).

Symptoms typically associated with PML are diverse, progress over a period of days to weeks, and include progressive weakness on one side of the body or clumsiness of limbs, vision disturbances, confusion, and changes in thinking, memory, orientation, or personality. At the first sign or symptom suggestive of PML, fingolimod therapy should be withheld and an appropriate diagnostic evaluation performed. MRI signs of PML may be apparent before clinical manifestations develop; any suspicious findings on MRI should be followed with further investigation.

Macular Edema Fingolimod increases the risk of macular edema. A dose-dependent increase in the risk of macular edema was observed in the clinical development program of fingolimod. In 2-year, double-blind, placebo-controlled studies in MS patients, macular edema (with or without visual symptoms) occurred in 1.5% of patients receiving fingolimod 1.25 mg daily, 0.5% of patients receiving fingolimod 0.5 mg daily, and 0.4% of those receiving placebo. Macular edema usually occurred within the first 3–4 months of therapy. These studies excluded patients with diabetes mellitus, which is a known risk factor for macular edema. Although some patients presented with blurred vision or decreased visual acuity, others were asymptomatic and diagnosed upon routine ophthalmologic examination. Macular edema generally improved or resolved with or without treatment following drug discontinuance; however, some patients had residual visual acuity loss even after resolution of the macular edema. Macular edema also has been reported in patients receiving 0.5 mg of fingolimod daily in the postmarketing setting.

An ophthalmologic examination of the fundus, including the macula, should be performed in all patients at baseline and 3–4 months after initiation of fingolimod therapy. If a patient reports visual disturbances at any time during therapy, an additional ophthalmologic examination should be performed. Continuation of fingolimod therapy in patients who develop macular edema has not been evaluated; any decision on whether to discontinue therapy should include an assessment of the potential benefits and risks for the individual patient. The risk of recurrence of macular edema after rechallenge also has not been evaluated.

Patients with a history of uveitis and patients with diabetes mellitus have an increased risk of macular edema during fingolimod therapy. The incidence of macular edema also is increased in MS patients with a history of uveitis. In the combined clinical trial experience with all dosages of fingolimod, the incidence of macular edema was approximately 20% in MS patients with a history of uveitis compared with 0.6% in those without a history of uveitis. Fingolimod has not been evaluated in MS patients with diabetes mellitus. In addition to the examination of the fundus, including the macula, prior to fingolimod treatment and 3–4 months after beginning therapy, MS patients with diabetes mellitus or a history of uveitis should have regular follow-up ophthalmologic evaluations while receiving the drug.

Posterior Reversible Encephalopathy Syndrome Rare cases of posterior reversible encephalopathy syndrome (PRES) have been reported in patients receiving fingolimod. Symptoms have included sudden onset of severe headache, altered mental status, visual disturbances, and seizure. Although the symptoms of PRES are usually reversible, they may evolve into ischemic stroke or cerebral hemorrhage. Therefore, a delay in diagnosis and treatment of PRES may lead to permanent neurologic sequelae. If PRES is suspected, fingolimod therapy should be discontinued.

Respiratory Effects Dose-dependent reductions in forced expiratory volume over 1 second (FEV_1) and diffusion lung capacity for carbon monoxide (DLCO) were observed as early as 1 month after beginning fingolimod therapy. In 2-year, placebo-controlled studies, the reduction from baseline in the percent of predicted values for FEV_1 at the time of last assessment on the drug or placebo was 2.8% for fingolimod 0.5 mg and 1% for placebo. For DLCO, the reduction from baseline in percent of predicted values at the time of last assessment was 3.3% for fingolimod 0.5 mg and 0.5% for placebo. FEV_1 changes appear to be reversible after discontinuing fingolimod; there is insufficient information to determine the reversibility of the DLCO decrease after drug discontinuance. In placebo-controlled studies in MS patients, dyspnea was reported in 9% of the fingolimod-treated patients and in 7% of those receiving placebo. Several patients discontinued fingolimod therapy because of unexplained dyspnea during the extension studies. The manufacturer states that fingolimod has not been evaluated in MS patients with compromised respiratory function.

Spirometric evaluation of respiratory function and DLCO evaluation should be performed during fingolimod therapy if clinically indicated. (See Advice to Patients.)

Liver Injury Elevations in hepatic enzyme concentrations may occur in patients receiving fingolimod. Recent (i.e., within last 6 months) transaminase and bilirubin concentrations should be available before initiation of therapy. In 2-year, placebo-controlled studies, elevations 3 times the upper limit of normal or greater in serum transaminases occurred in 14% of patients treated with fingolimod 0.5 mg daily compared with 3% of patients receiving placebo; elevations 5 times the upper limit of normal occurred in 4.5% of patients treated with fingolimod 0.5 mg daily compared with 1% of patients receiving placebo. The majority of these elevations occurred within 6–9 months. Transaminase elevations returned to normal within approximately 2 months after discontinuance of the drug. Recurrence of transaminase elevations upon rechallenge was reported in some patients.

Liver enzymes should be monitored in patients who develop symptoms suggestive of hepatic dysfunction (e.g., unexplained nausea, vomiting, abdominal pain, fatigue, anorexia, jaundice, dark urine). Fingolimod should be discontinued if clinically important liver injury is confirmed. Patients with preexisting liver disease may be at increased risk of developing elevated liver enzymes with the drug.

Fetal/Neonatal Morbidity and Mortality Results of animal studies indicate that fingolimod may cause fetal harm. Women of childbearing potential should use effective contraception during and for 2 months after discontinuance of the drug. (See Pregnancy under Warnings/Precautions: Specific Populations, in Cautions.)

Blood Pressure Effects In clinical trials, patients treated with fingolimod 0.5 mg daily had an average increase of approximately 3 mm Hg in systolic blood pressure and approximately 2 mm Hg in diastolic blood pressure. These increases were first detected approximately 2 months following treatment initiation and persisted with continued treatment. Hypertension was reported in 8% of fingolimod-treated patients (0.5 mg daily) compared with 4% of patients receiving placebo. Blood pressure should be monitored during treatment with the drug.

Cutaneous Malignancies Basal cell carcinoma was reported in 2% of adults receiving fingolimod 0.5 mg compared with 1% of those receiving placebo in clinical studies. Melanoma and Merkel cell carcinoma also have been reported during postmarketing experience with the drug.

Periodic skin examinations are recommended in all patients receiving fingolimod, particularly in those with risk factors for skin cancer. Patients should be monitored for any suspicious skin lesions, and, if observed, promptly evaluated. The usual precautions for skin cancer (e.g., limiting exposure to sunlight and UV light, using an appropriate sunscreen) should be taken. (See Advice to Patients.)

Immunosuppression Following Discontinuance Fingolimod remains in the blood and has pharmacodynamic effects, including decreased lymphocyte counts, for up to 2 months following the last dose. Because of fingolimod's continuing pharmacodynamic effects, initiating other drugs during this period warrants the same considerations needed for concomitant administration (e.g., risk of additive immunosuppressive effects). (See Drug Interactions: Antineoplastic, Immunosuppressive, or Immunomodulating Therapies.)

Sensitivity Reactions **Hypersensitivity.** Hypersensitivity reactions (e.g., rash, urticaria, angioedema) have been reported during postmarketing experience in patients receiving fingolimod. (See Cautions: Contraindications.)

Laboratory Test Interaction Because fingolimod reduces blood lymphocyte counts via redistribution into secondary lymphoid organs, peripheral blood lymphocyte counts cannot be used to evaluate the lymphocyte subset status in patients treated with the drug. A recent CBC should be available prior to initiating fingolimod therapy.

Specific Populations **Pregnancy.** There are no adequate data regarding the developmental risk associated with the use of fingolimod during pregnancy; however, teratogenic and embryolethal effects have been demonstrated in animal studies with doses similar to or less than those used clinically. Women of childbearing potential should use effective contraception during and for 2 months following fingolimod therapy. (See Advice to Patients.)

A pregnancy registry has been established to monitor the pregnancy outcomes of women exposed to fingolimod during pregnancy. Clinicians are encouraged to enroll patients in the registry by calling 877-598-7237, emailing gpr@quintiles.com, or visiting http://www.gilenyapregnancyregistry.com.

Lactation. Fingolimod is distributed into milk in rats. It is not known whether the drug is distributed into human milk. The effects of the drug on the nursing infant or on milk production also are not known. The benefits of breastfeeding should be considered along with the woman's clinical need for fingolimod and any potential adverse effects on the breastfed infant from the drug or underlying maternal condition.

Pediatric Use. Safety and efficacy of fingolimod in pediatric patients younger than 10 years of age have not been established.

In the clinical study establishing efficacy of fingolimod in pediatric patients 10 years of age or older, adverse effects were generally similar to those observed in adults, with the exception of seizures, which occurred at a higher rate (5.6%) in fingolimod-treated pediatric patients.

In juvenile animal toxicity studies, changes in bone mineral density, neurobehavioral abnormalities, delayed sexual maturation, and decreased T-cell dependent antibody response were observed when fingolimod was administered orally to young rats.

It is recommended that pediatric patients receive all age-appropriate vaccinations according to current immunization guidelines, if possible, prior to initiation of fingolimod therapy.

Geriatric Use. Experience in patients 65 years of age and over is insufficient to determine whether they respond differently than younger adults. Fingolimod should be used with caution in geriatric patients, reflecting the greater frequency of decreased hepatic and renal function and of concomitant disease and other drug therapy.

Hepatic Impairment. Exposure to fingolimod (but not to the active metabolite fingolimod-phosphate) is doubled in patients with severe hepatic impairment (Child-Pugh class C); fingolimod exposure increases to a lesser extent in patients with mild (Child-Pugh class A) or moderate (Child-Pugh class B) hepatic impairment (by 12 and 44%, respectively). The pharmacokinetics of fingolimod-phosphate in patients with mild or moderate hepatic impairment have not been evaluated. Patients with severe hepatic impairment should be closely monitored since the risk of adverse reactions is greater in such patients.

Renal Impairment. In patients with severe renal impairment, peak concentrations and AUC of fingolimod increased by 32 and 43%, respectively, and peak concentrations and AUC of fingolimod-phosphate increased by 25 and 14%, respectively, while the elimination half-life of the drug was unchanged. Systemic exposure of 2 fingolimod metabolites (M2 and M3) increased (by threefold and 13-fold, respectively) in patients with severe renal impairment; the potential toxicity of these metabolites has not been fully characterized. Pharmacokinetics of fingolimod in patients with mild or moderate renal impairment have not been evaluated.

■ **Common Adverse Effects** Adverse effects reported in 10% or more of patients receiving fingolimod (0.5 mg daily) and more frequently than with placebo include headache, elevations in serum transaminase concentrations, diarrhea, nausea, cough, influenza, sinusitis, back pain, abdominal pain, and pain in extremity.

Drug Interactions

■ **Drugs Affecting or Metabolized by Hepatic Microsomal Enzymes** Fingolimod is primarily metabolized by cytochrome P-450 (CYP) isoenzyme 4F2 and possibly other CYP4F isoenzymes; inhibitors or inducers of CYP4F2 and possibly other CYP4F isoenzymes might alter the exposure to fingolimod or fingolimod-phosphate, the active metabolite.

In vitro studies indicate that CYP3A4 may contribute to the metabolism of fingolimod in cases of potent induction of CYP3A4. Concurrent administration of potent CYP450 enzyme inducers, such as carbamazepine, phenobarbital, phenytoin, and St. John's wort (*Hypericum perforatum*), may reduce the area under the concentration-time curve (AUC) of fingolimod and fingolimod-phosphate. The clinical importance of this potential decreased exposure is unknown.

In vitro studies indicate that fingolimod has little or no inhibitory activity on CYP isoenzymes 1A2, 2A6, 2B6, 2C9, 2C19, 2D6, 2E1, 3A4/5, or 4A9/11 (fingolimod only). Similarly, fingolimod-phosphate has little or no inhibitory activity on CYP isoenzymes 1A2, 2A6, 2B6, 2C8, 2C9, 2C19, 2D6, 2E1, or 3A4. Pharmacokinetic interactions are unlikely with drugs that are mainly metabolized by these isoenzymes.

The potential of fingolimod to inhibit CYP2C8 and fingolimod-phosphate to inhibit CYP2B6 is not known.

Fingolimod does not appear to substantially induce CYP isoenzymes 1A2,

2B6, 2C8, 2C9, 2C19, 3A (including 3A4), or 4F2 or P-glycoprotein. In vitro studies with fingolimod-phosphate did not indicate induction of CYP isoenzymes 1A2, 2B6, 2C8, 2C9, 2C19, 3A, 4F2, 4F3B, or 4F12, and fingolimod-phosphate is unlikely to have clinically important induction effects on these isoenzymes at therapeutic concentrations of fingolimod.

■ **Antiarrhythmic Agents** Fingolimod is contraindicated in patients concurrently receiving class Ia (e.g., quinidine, procainamide) or class III (e.g., amiodarone, sotalol) antiarrhythmic agents.

■ **Drugs that Prolong the QT Interval** Fingolimod has not been studied in patients concurrently treated with drugs that prolong the QT interval. Because initiation of fingolimod treatment results in decreased heart rate and may prolong the QT interval, patients receiving non-antiarrhythmic drugs that prolong the QT interval with a known risk of torsades de pointes (e.g., citalopram, certain antipsychotic agents [e.g., chlorpromazine, haloperidol, olanzapine, pimozide, quetiapine, risperidone, thioridazine, ziprasidone], erythromycin, methadone) should be monitored overnight with continuous ECG monitoring in a medical facility. (See First-Dose Monitoring under Dosage and Administration: Administration and see also Drug Interactions: Antiarrhythmic Agents.)

■ **Antineoplastic, Immunosuppressive, or Immunomodulating Therapies** Antineoplastic agents, immunosuppressive agents (including corticosteroid therapy), or immunomodulating therapies are expected to increase the risk of immunosuppression in fingolimod-treated patients, and the risk of additive immune system effects must be considered if these therapies are concurrently administered with fingolimod.

The manufacturer and some clinicians recommend using caution when switching patients from drugs with prolonged immune effects, such as natalizumab, mitoxantrone, or teriflunomide, to fingolimod; the duration and mechanism of action of these drugs must be considered to avoid unintended additive immunosuppressive effects when initiating fingolimod therapy. (See Dosage and Administration: Administration, see Infectious Complications under Cautions: Warnings/Precautions, and see also Immunosuppression Following Discontinuance under Cautions: Warnings/Precautions.)

■ **Atropine** Atropine has been used to treat fingolimod-associated bradycardia in some patients. Single-dose fingolimod and fingolimod-phosphate exposure was not substantially altered during concurrent administration of atropine.

■ **Carbamazepine** Concurrent administration of carbamazepine (a potent CYP450 inducer) 600 mg twice daily at steady state and a single 2-mg dose of fingolimod decreased AUC of fingolimod and fingolimod-phosphate by approximately 40%. The manufacturer states that the clinical importance of this decrease is not known.

■ **Cyclosporine** Pharmacokinetics of single-dose fingolimod and steady-state cyclosporine were not altered during concurrent administration of the drugs.

■ **Drugs that Slow Heart Rate or Atrioventricular Conduction** Experience with fingolimod in patients concurrently receiving drugs that slow the heart rate or atrioventricular (AV) conduction (e.g., β-adrenergic blocking agents, digoxin, heart-rate-lowering calcium-channel blocking agents [e.g., diltiazem, verapamil]) is limited. Concomitant use of these drugs during fingolimod initiation may be associated with severe bradycardia or heart block. Before initiating fingolimod therapy, clinicians should consult the prescribing clinician to determine if it is possible to switch to drugs that do not slow the heart rate or AV conduction. In patients who cannot switch to another drug, extended continuous ECG monitoring, including overnight monitoring, after the first dose of fingolimod is recommended. (See First-Dose Monitoring under Dosage and Administration: Administration.)

An additional 15% reduction in heart rate has been observed upon initiation of fingolimod when given concurrently with atenolol in healthy individuals in one study; such an effect was not observed with concurrent diltiazem and fingolimod administration. The pharmacokinetics of these drugs were not substantially altered during concurrent administration and a clinically important pharmacokinetic interaction appears unlikely.

■ **Isoproterenol** Single-dose fingolimod and fingolimod-phosphate exposures were not substantially altered during concurrent administration of isoproterenol.

■ **Ketoconazole** The AUCs of fingolimod and fingolimod-phosphate increased by 70% when fingolimod was concomitantly administered with ketoconazole, a potent CYP3A4 and CYP4F inhibitor. Patients receiving fingolimod and systemic ketoconazole concomitantly should be closely monitored since the risk of adverse effects is greater; fingolimod dosage reduction should be considered if necessary.

■ **Oral Contraceptives** Fingolimod did not substantially alter the steady-state exposure of an oral contraceptive containing ethinyl estradiol and levonorgestrel in healthy women, suggesting that such oral contraceptives may provide effective contraception in women of childbearing potential who are treated with fingolimod. The manufacturer states that drug interaction studies have not been performed with oral contraceptives that contain other progestins; however, an effect of fingolimod on their exposure is considered unlikely.

■ **Selective Serotonin-reuptake Inhibitors** In a population pharmacokinetic evaluation in MS patients, fluoxetine and paroxetine, which are both potent inhibitors of CYP isoenzyme 2D6, did not substantially affect pre-dose concentrations of fingolimod and fingolimod-phosphate. (See Drug Interactions: Drugs that Prolong the QT Interval.)

■ **Other Drugs used in Multiple Sclerosis** In a population pharmacokinetic evaluation, a number of drugs that are commonly prescribed concomitantly in MS patients, including amantadine, amitriptyline, baclofen, corticosteroids, gabapentin, oxybutynin chloride, modafinil, and pregabalin, did not have a clinically important effect (i.e., less than 20% change) on fingolimod or fingolimod-phosphate pre-dose concentrations.

■ **Vaccines** Fingolimod reduces the immune response to vaccination. Vaccination may be less effective during and for up to 2 months after discontinuance of fingolimod therapy. The use of live attenuated vaccines should be avoided during and for 2 months after treatment with the drug because of the risk of infection. (See Infectious Complications under Cautions: Warnings/Precautions and see also Advice to Patients.)

Description

Fingolimod hydrochloride is derived from the fungal metabolite myriocin and is used orally as a disease-modifying treatment for multiple sclerosis (MS). The drug is metabolized by sphingosine kinase, predominantly type 2, to the active metabolite, fingolimod-phosphate. Fingolimod-phosphate is a sphingosine 1-phosphate (S1P) receptor modulator and binds with high affinity to S1P receptor subtypes 1, 3, 4, and 5. The $S1P_1$ receptor regulates lymphocyte egress from both the thymus and peripheral lymphoid organs and is essential for lymphocyte recirculation. Binding of fingolimod-phosphate to $S1P_1$ blocks the capacity of lymphocytes to egress from lymph nodes, thereby reducing the number of lymphocytes in the peripheral blood and CNS. Although the exact mechanism by which fingolimod exerts therapeutic effects in MS is unknown, it may involve reduction of lymphocyte migration into the CNS. Preclinical findings suggest that fingolimod may directly affect neuropathologic processes such as neurodegeneration, gliosis, and endogenous repair mechanisms within the CNS through modulation of S1P receptors that are expressed on neural cells.

Biotransformation of fingolimod occurs by 3 main pathways: reversible stereoselective phosphorylation to the pharmacologically active (*S*)-enantiomer of fingolimod-phosphate, oxidative biotransformation mainly via the cytochrome P-450 (CYP) 4F2 isoenzyme and possibly other CYP4F isoenzymes with subsequent fatty acid-like degradation to inactive metabolites, and formation of pharmacologically inactive nonpolar ceramide analogs of fingolimod. In vitro studies indicate that CYP3A4 also may contribute to the metabolism of fingolimod in cases of potent induction of CYP3A4. Following oral administration, approximately 81% of the dose is slowly excreted in the urine as inactive metabolites. Fingolimod and fingolimod-phosphate are not excreted intact in urine but are the principal components in feces with amounts of each representing less than 2.5% of the dose. The average elimination half-life of fingolimod is 6–9 days; fingolimod-phosphate has a similar elimination half-life.

Advice to Patients

Importance of providing a copy of the fingolimod medication guide to the patient each time the drug is dispensed; importance of patient reading the medication guide prior to initiating fingolimod therapy and each time the prescription is refilled.

Importance of advising patients that initiation of fingolimod results in a transient decrease in heart rate, particularly after the first dose, and that they will be observed in their clinician's office or other medical facility for at least 6 hours after the first dose. Advise patients that if fingolimod is discontinued for more than 14 days, heart rate effects similar to those observed on treatment initiation may be seen and observation for at least 6 hours will again be needed on treatment re-initiation; the same precautions apply if treatment is interrupted for more than 1 day within the first 2 weeks of treatment, or for more than 7 days during weeks 3 and 4 of treatment. Advise patients to immediately contact their clinician or go to the emergency room if they experience dizziness, tiredness, or a slow or irregular heartbeat during therapy.

Importance of informing patients that progressive multifocal leukoencephalopathy (PML) has occurred in fingolimod-treated patients; PML is characterized by a progression of deficits and usually leads to death or severe disability over weeks to months. Importance of informing clinician of any symptoms suggestive of PML (e.g., progressive weakness on one side of the body; clumsiness of limbs; vision disturbance; changes in thinking, memory, or orientation leading to confusion and personality changes) that have progressed over days to weeks. Importance of advising patients not to stop taking fingolimod without first consulting with their clinician.

Possible increased risk of infections. Importance of informing patients that fingolimod may lower the number of lymphocytes in their blood and that their clinician may do a blood test before initiating fingolimod therapy. Importance of advising patients to immediately contact their clinician if they develop any symptoms of infection (e.g., fever, chills, tiredness, body aches, nausea, vomiting) during and for 2 months following discontinuance of the drug. Importance of informing patients that prior or concomitant use of drugs that suppress the immune system may increase the risk of infection.

Importance of patients informing clinicians of recent vaccination (within the past 1 month) before starting fingolimod. Advise patients that some vaccines should be avoided during treatment with fingolimod and for 2 months after discontinuing the drug. Importance of advising patients to delay fingolimod therapy until after varicella zoster virus (VZV) vaccination if they have not had chickenpox or a previous VZV vaccination.

Risk of posterior reversible encephalopathy syndrome; importance of advising patients to immediately report any manifestations (e.g., sudden onset of severe headache, altered mental status, visual disturbance, or seizure) to their clinician. Any delay in treatment could lead to permanent neurologic disability.

Risk of macular edema. Importance of informing patients that macular edema can cause some of the same eye symptoms as an MS attack (optic neuritis); however, some patients may not notice any symptoms. Because macular edema usually starts in the first 3 to 4 months after beginning fingolimod therapy, importance of informing patients that their clinician should test their vision before starting fingolimod therapy and 3 to 4 months after initiating treatment as well as any time the patient notices vision changes during therapy. Advise patients to immediately contact their clinician if they experience any vision changes (e.g., blurriness or shadows in the center of vision, a blind spot in the center of vision, sensitivity to light, unusually colored or tinted vision). Inform patients that their risk of developing macular edema is higher if they have diabetes or have had uveitis.

Risk of breathing problems. Importance of advising patients to immediately contact their clinician if they experience any trouble breathing such as new onset or worsening of shortness of breath.

Risk of increased liver enzymes. Importance of advising patients to contact their clinician if they have unexplained nausea, vomiting, abdominal pain, fatigue, anorexia, jaundice, and/or dark urine.

Importance of informing patients that fingolimod may cause fetal harm. Importance of discussing this possible fetal risk with women of childbearing age whether they are pregnant, might be pregnant, or are trying to become pregnant. Advise women of childbearing age of the need for effective contraception during and for 2 months after stopping fingolimod treatment. Importance of advising patients to immediately inform their clinician if they become pregnant while taking fingolimod or within 2 months after stopping treatment. Importance of informing women who become pregnant while taking fingolimod about the existence of the pregnancy registry. (See Pregnancy under Warnings/Precautions: Specific Populations, in Cautions.)

Risk of basal cell carcinoma and melanoma; importance of advising patients that any suspicious skin lesions should be promptly evaluated. Advise patients to limit exposure to sunlight and UV light by wearing protective clothing and using a sunscreen with a high protection factor.

Risk of hypersensitivity reactions; importance of advising patients to contact their clinician if any manifestations (e.g., rash, urticaria, angioedema) occur.

Importance of women informing clinicians if they are or plan to breastfeed.

Importance of advising patients that fingolimod remains in the blood and continues to have effects, including decreased blood lymphocyte counts, for up to 2 months following the last dose.

Importance of patients informing clinicians of existing or contemplated concomitant therapy, including prescription drugs (e.g., antiarrhythmic agents, β-adrenergic blocking agents, chlorpromazine, citalopram, diltiazem, erythromycin, haloperidol, ketoconazole, methadone) and OTC drugs, vitamins, and herbal supplements, as well as any concomitant illnesses (e.g., heart disease [including cardiac arrhythmias, stroke, warning stroke, myocardial infarction, or angina], breathing problems including during sleep, liver disease, diabetes, history of uveitis).

Importance of advising patients not to discontinue fingolimod without first talking with their clinician.

Importance of informing patients of other important precautionary information. (See Cautions.)

Overview® (see Users Guide). For additional information on this drug until a more detailed monograph is developed and published, the manufacturer's labeling should be consulted. It is *essential* that the manufacturer's labeling be consulted for more detailed information on usual cautions, precautions, contraindications, potential drug interactions, laboratory test interferences, and acute toxicity.

Preparations

Excipients in commercially available drug preparations may have clinically important effects in some individuals; consult specific product labeling for details.

Fingolimod Hydrochloride

Oral

Capsules	0.25 mg (of fingolimod)	**Gilenya®**, Novartis
	0.5 mg (of fingolimod)	**Gilenya®**, Novartis

†Use is not currently included in the labeling approved by the US Food and Drug Administration

Glatiramer Acetate

■ Glatiramer acetate, a mixture of synthetic polypeptides containing 4 naturally occurring amino acids, has immunomodulatory and disease-modifying activity in multiple sclerosis.

Uses

■ **Multiple Sclerosis** Glatiramer acetate is used for the treatment of relapsing forms of multiple sclerosis (MS; relapsing-remitting MS [RRMS]); the drug has been shown to reduce the frequency of relapses in patients with RRMS and to also reduce the risk of conversion to MS in patients with an isolated clinical episode who have magnetic resonance imaging (MRI) features consistent with MS.

Glatiramer acetate is one of several disease-modifying therapies used in the management of RRMS. Although not curative, these therapies have all been shown to modify several measures of disease activity, including relapse rates, new or enhancing MRI lesions, and disability progression; results of placebo-controlled studies indicate that treatment with a disease-modifying agent can reduce the frequency of MS attacks by 28–68%. The American Academy of Neurology (AAN) recommends that disease-modifying therapy be offered to patients with RRMS who have had recent relapses and/or MRI activity; these experts state that the benefits versus risks (e.g., adverse effects or burden of taking a long-term medication) of treatment in patients who have not had relapses in 2 or more years and do not have active MRI lesions are not known. Because CNS damage occurs early and continues throughout the course of MS, other clinicians recommend that disease-modifying therapy be initiated as soon as possible following diagnosis and continued indefinitely unless there is a clear lack of benefit, adverse effects are intolerable, the patient is unable to adhere to the recommended treatment regimen, or a more appropriate treatment becomes available. Clinicians should consider the adverse effects, tolerability, method of administration, safety, efficacy, and cost of the drugs in addition to patient preferences when selecting an appropriate disease-modifying therapy.

Evidence of efficacy of glatiramer acetate in the management of RRMS is based on the results of 5 randomized, placebo-controlled studies; 4 of the studies were conducted with a dosage of 20 mg once daily and one study was conducted with a dosage of 40 mg 3 times weekly. The first 2 studies demonstrated a reduction in relapse rates with glatiramer acetate compared with placebo; patients in these studies received glatiramer acetate 20 mg or placebo once daily by subcutaneous injection, had baseline disability levels no higher than 6 (i.e., ambulatory) according to the Expanded Disability Status Scale (EDSS), and had experienced at least 2 relapses (i.e., exacerbations) of their disease during the 2 years prior to study admission. In the first study (single-center pilot study in 50 patients), relapse was defined as the rapid onset of new symptoms or worsening of existing symptoms that persisted for at least 48 hours; in the second study (multicenter study in 251 patients), relapse was defined as the appearance or reappearance of one or more neurologic abnormalities persisting for at least 48 hours and immediately preceded by at least 30 days of a relatively stable or improving neurologic state. Relapses were considered confirmed only when symptoms were accompanied by objective changes on neurologic examination consistent with a defined level of change on the EDSS.

The proportion of patients who remained relapse-free during 2 years of treatment with glatiramer acetate or placebo was 56 or 28%, respectively, in the single-center study and 34 or 27%, respectively, in the multicenter study; these differences were not statistically significant based on intent-to-treat analysis (i.e., all patients who received at least 1 dose of glatiramer acetate or placebo and who had at least 1 on-treatment assessment). However, mean relapse frequency (exacerbations per patient) was reduced with glatiramer acetate compared with placebo in both studies (based on intent-to-treat analysis), averaging 0.6 or 2.4, respectively, in the single-center study and 1.19 or 1.68, respectively, in the multicenter study.

Efficacy of glatiramer acetate in reducing relapse rates in patients with RRMS has been maintained for at least 10 years in an open-label study; data from this study suggest that early initiation of glatiramer acetate therapy reduces the risk of disease progression.

In another double-blind, placebo-controlled study, efficacy of glatiramer acetate (20 mg subcutaneously once daily) in the management of RRMS was evaluated through the use of MRI. MRI assessment detects subclinical disease activity in RRMS (number and volume of CNS lesions) more frequently than change in disability level. Inclusion criteria for this multinational study were similar to those in the multicenter clinical study but patients also had to have at least one gadolinium (Gd)-enhancing lesion on their MRI at study entry. The primary outcome measure in this study was the total number of Gd-enhancing lesions on T1-weighted images over the 9-month study period; in patients receiving glatiramer acetate, the median cumulative number of such lesions was 11 compared with 17 in patients receiving placebo. Secondary outcome measures, including number of new enhancing lesions, monthly change in volume of enhancing lesions, and change in volume and number of new lesions observed on T2-weighted images, also were improved with glatiramer acetate therapy. The observed relapse rate averaged 33% lower with glatiramer acetate than with placebo, and the total number of relapses correlated with the cumulative number of Gd-enhancing lesions in both treatment groups.

Efficacy of early glatiramer acetate therapy in delaying the onset of clinically definite MS in adult patients who have experienced a first clinical episode and have MRI features consistent with MS was evaluated in a multicenter, double-blind, placebo-controlled study (PreCISe study). In the PreCISe study, 481 patients who had recently (i.e., within 90 days) experienced an isolated demyelinating event and had 2 or more MRI brain lesions typical of MS were randomized to receive either glatiramer acetate 20 mg or placebo once daily by subcutaneous injection. The primary outcome measure was the time until the development of a second exacerbation, and secondary outcomes were brain MRI measures, including number of new T2 lesions and T2 lesion volume. Patients were followed for up to 3 years or until they developed a second clinical exacerbation. Glatiramer acetate was found to reduce the risk of developing clinically definite MS by 45% compared with placebo. The percentage of patients who experienced a relapse within 3 years in the glatiramer acetate and placebo groups was 24.7 and 42.9%, respectively. In addition, the time to development of a second exacerbation was substantially delayed with glatiramer acetate compared with placebo (722 and 336 days, respectively). The glatiramer acetate-treated patients also demonstrated fewer new T2 lesions and a lower T2 lesion volume at the last observation compared with those receiving placebo.

Efficacy of glatiramer acetate 40 mg 3 times weekly was evaluated in a double-blind, placebo-controlled study in patients who had experienced a median of 2 relapses in the 2 years prior to study entry and were not currently receiving interferon beta therapy. Patients had a median EDSS score of 2.5 at baseline. The number of confirmed relapses, the primary outcome measure, was substantially reduced (by 34%) in patients receiving glatiramer acetate compared with those receiving placebo. Glatiramer acetate therapy also substantially reduced the cumulative number of new or enlarging T2 lesions (by 35%) and the number of enhancing lesions on T1-weighted images (by 45%) at 6 and 12 months relative to placebo.

Clinical experience to date suggests that the efficacy of glatiramer acetate is generally similar to that of interferon beta in the treatment of RRMS. Efficacy of glatiramer acetate compared with other disease-modifying therapies (e.g., fingolimod, mitoxantrone, natalizumab) has not been fully evaluated to date.

Dosage and Administration

■ **General** Routine laboratory monitoring is not considered necessary in patients receiving glatiramer acetate.

■ **Administration** Glatiramer acetate is administered by subcutaneous injection only using the commercially available prefilled syringe; the drug should *not* be given IV. Subcutaneous injections of glatiramer acetate may be administered into the arm, abdomen, hip, or thigh.

To minimize the risk of localized lipoatrophy and skin necrosis, patients should be advised to follow proper injection technique and to rotate injection areas and sites with each injection. (See Lipoatrophy and Skin Necrosis under Cautions: Warnings/Precautions.) The initial self-administered dose should be administered under the supervision of a qualified clinician.

Several preparations of glatiramer acetate are commercially available (e.g., Copaxone®, Glatopa® and other generic preparations), and there are 2 commercially available dosage strengths of the drug. Glatiramer acetate 20 mg/mL is administered once daily and glatiramer acetate 40 mg/mL is administered 3 times a week; the 2 different dosage strengths are not interchangeable.

Commercially available prefilled syringes of glatiramer acetate are intended for single use only; any unused portion should be discarded. After removal from refrigerated storage, prefilled syringes should be allowed to warm to room temperature for 20 minutes before drug administration.

■ **Dosage** The recommended dosage of glatiramer acetate for the treatment of relapsing forms of multiple sclerosis (MS; e.g., relapsing-remitting MS [RRMS]) depends on the dosage strength used (20 mg/mL or 40 mg/mL); the 2 dosage strengths are not interchangeable. When using the commercially available 20-mg/mL injection, the recommended dosage is 20 mg once daily by subcutaneous injection. When using the commercially available 40-mg/mL injection, the recommended dosage is 40 mg 3 times a week by subcutaneous injection; injections should be given at least 48 hours apart.

■ **Special Populations** There are no special population dosage recommendations at this time.

Cautions

■ **Contraindications** Glatiramer acetate is contraindicated in patients with known hypersensitivity to glatiramer acetate or mannitol.

■ **Warnings/Precautions** ***Immediate Post-injection Reaction*** Immediately after subcutaneous injection of glatiramer acetate 20 mg/mL or 40 mg/mL, approximately 16 or 2%, respectively, of patients in placebo-controlled clinical trials experienced a constellation of generally transient, self-limited symptoms that did not require treatment and included at least 2 of the following symptoms: flushing, chest pain or tightness, palpitations, anxiety, dyspnea, constriction of the throat, tachycardia, and urticaria. These reactions generally occur several months after initiation of glatiramer acetate therapy (although they may occur earlier) and individual patients may experience one or several episodes of these symptoms. It is not known whether any of these symptoms actually represents a specific syndrome. During the postmarketing period, there have been reports of patients with similar symptoms who received emergency medical care. It is not currently known whether these reactions have an immunologic or nonimmunologic mechanism or whether multiple episodes in a given patient have similar mechanisms.

Injection site hypersensitivity, allergic reactions, and anaphylactic or anaphylactoid reactions have been reported during postmarketing experience with glatiramer acetate therapy, including rare cases of anaphylaxis accompanied by anti-glatiramer IgE antibodies; some of these reactions developed from one to several months or more after initiating therapy with the drug.

Chest Pain Transient chest pain occurred in approximately 13 or 2% of patients receiving glatiramer acetate 20 or 40 mg/mL, respectively, in controlled clinical studies. Some of these episodes occurred as part of immediate post-injection reactions (see Immediate Post-injection Reaction under Cautions: Warnings/Precautions), but many did not; the pathogenesis of this adverse effect is unknown. In addition, whether such episodes were temporally related to glatiramer acetate injection was not always known. Chest pain generally lasted only a few minutes, often was not associated with other symptoms, and did not appear to produce clinically important sequelae. Episodes of chest pain generally occurred at least 1 month after initiation of glatiramer acetate therapy, and some patients experienced more than one such episode.

Lipoatrophy and Skin Necrosis Localized lipoatrophy (i.e., loss of subcutaneous fat) and, rarely, skin necrosis at the subcutaneous injection site have been reported during postmarketing experience with glatiramer acetate. Lipoatrophy may occur at various times after treatment initiation, sometimes after several months, and is thought to be permanent; it has been most commonly reported on arms and thighs. There is no known treatment for lipoatrophy. Therefore, patients should be advised to follow proper injection technique and to rotate injection areas and sites daily to possibly minimize these events. Some clinicians recommend that further subcutaneous injection of glatiramer acetate be avoided in any area in which lipoatrophy is evident. (See Dosage and Administration: Administration.)

Potential Effects on Immune Response Because glatiramer acetate can modify immune response, the drug may interfere with immune functions. In theory, glatiramer acetate could interfere with the recognition of foreign antigens and undermine the body's tumor surveillance ability and defenses against infection. Although limited testing suggests no evidence of such effects, this risk has not been systematically evaluated. Therapy with glatiramer acetate is intended to minimize the autoimmune response to myelin; however, chronic administration of the drug could possibly result in untoward effects from continued alteration of cellular immunity.

Studies in animals suggest that immune complexes are deposited in the renal glomeruli. Antibodies that react to glatiramer acetate are formed in most patients receiving the drug daily at the recommended dosage; current evidence suggests that such antibodies do not neutralize the drug's therapeutic effects. These antibodies have been almost exclusively of the IgG class, predominantly the IgG-1 subclass. In a controlled study in patients with RRMS who were treated with glatiramer acetate 20 mg daily for 2 years, 80% of patients had serum IgG concentrations at least 3 times baseline values after 3 months of treatment; after 12 months of treatment, 30% of patients still had serum IgG concentrations at least 3 times baseline values and 90% of patients still had concentrations above baseline. IgE antibodies were not detected in the 94 sera studied. (See Immediate Post-injection Reaction under Cautions: Warnings/Precautions.)

Specific Populations **Pregnancy.** Category B. (See Users Guide.)

Lactation. It is not known whether glatiramer acetate is distributed into human milk. Caution should be exercised when the drug is used in nursing women.

Pediatric Use. Safety and efficacy of glatiramer acetate have not been established in pediatric patients younger than 18 years of age.

Geriatric Use. Glatiramer acetate has not been studied in geriatric patients.

Renal Impairment. The pharmacokinetics of glatiramer acetate have not been studied in patients with renal impairment.

■ **Common Adverse Effects** The most common adverse effects reported with glatiramer acetate 20 mg/mL in controlled clinical trials include injection site reactions (e.g., pain, erythema, inflammation, pruritus, mass, edema, hypersensitivity, fibrosis, atrophy or lipoatrophy, necrosis), vasodilatation, rash, dyspnea, and chest pain.

The most common adverse effect reported with glatiramer acetate 40 mg/mL in controlled clinical trials was injection site reactions.

Drug Interactions

Interactions between glatiramer acetate and other drugs have not been fully evaluated. Experience from clinical trials suggests there are no clinically important interactions between glatiramer acetate and drugs commonly used in multiple sclerosis, including concurrent corticosteroid therapy for up to 28 days. The manufacturer states that glatiramer acetate has not been formally evaluated in combination with interferon beta.

Description

Glatiramer acetate is a mixture of synthetic polypeptides containing L-glutamic acid, L-alanine, L-tyrosine, and L-lysine in a fixed molar ratio.

The mechanism of action of glatiramer acetate in multiple sclerosis currently has not been fully elucidated. However, the drug is thought to act by modifying immune processes believed to be responsible for the pathogenesis of multiple sclerosis. Such action is supported by the results of studies of the pathogenesis of experimental allergic encephalomyelitis (EAE), a condition induced in animals through immunization against CNS-derived material containing myelin. Studies in vitro and in animals suggest that glatiramer acetate therapy induces and activates drug-specific suppressor T-cells and downregulates immune response (e.g., inflammation) to myelin antigens in the periphery. The biologic activity of glatiramer acetate is determined by its ability to block the induction of EAE in mice.

Studies in animals and healthy individuals suggest that a substantial portion of a subcutaneous dose of glatiramer acetate is hydrolyzed locally to small oligopeptides and free amino acids. Some portion of the dose is presumed to enter the lymphatic circulation, including regional lymph nodes, and some may enter systemic circulation intact. The drug itself does not appear to cross the blood-brain barrier; rather, glatiramer acetate-induced T-cells that migrate into the CNS appear to be responsible for downregulation of inflammation.

Advice to Patients

Importance of reading the manufacturer's patient information prior to beginning glatiramer acetate therapy and each time the prescription is refilled.

Importance of clinicians instructing patient and/or caregivers in proper injection techniques (including use of aseptic technique) and about avoiding reuse of syringes and needles and proper disposal of such equipment.

Risk of post-injection reaction. Importance of advising patients that glatiramer acetate may cause various symptoms after injection, including flushing, chest pain, palpitations, anxiety, dyspnea, throat constriction, and urticaria. Clinicians should inform patients that these symptoms usually are transient and self-limited and do not require specific treatment. However, patients should be advised to contact their clinician immediately if any serious reactions (e.g., flushing, chest pain, tachycardia, anxiety, breathing difficulties or tightness in the throat, swelling, rash, hives, itching) occur immediately after injection. Patients also should be informed that such reactions may occur early or begin several months after initiation of treatment, and that they may experience one or several episodes of these symptoms.

Importance of advising patients that they may experience chest pain either as part of a post-injection reaction or in isolation. Patients should be informed that the pain should be transient (usually lasting only for a few minutes). Some patients may experience more than one such episode, usually beginning at least one month after beginning treatment. Importance of advising patients to seek medical attention if they experience chest pain of unusual duration or intensity.

Risk of lipoatrophy and skin necrosis at injection site. Patients should be advised to follow proper injection technique and to rotate injection areas and sites with each injection.

Importance of advising patients that the 20-mg/mL and 40-mg/mL strengths of glatiramer acetate are not interchangeable and are administered using different dosage schedules.

Importance of informing patients of the recommended storage instructions for glatiramer acetate (refrigeration at 2–8°C preferred, but may be stored for up to 1 month at room temperature [15–30°C]). Importance of advising patients not to expose the drug to higher temperatures, freezing temperatures, or to intense light.

Importance of women informing clinicians if they are or plan to become pregnant or plan to breast-feed.

Importance of patient informing clinicians of existing or contemplated concomitant therapy, including prescription and OTC drugs, as well as any concomitant illnesses.

Importance of clinicians informing patient of other important precautionary information. (See Cautions.)

Overview® (see Users Guide). For additional information on this drug until a more detailed monograph is developed and published, the manufacturer's labeling should be consulted. It is *essential* that the manufacturer's labeling be consulted for more detailed information on usual cautions, precautions, contraindications, potential drug interactions, laboratory test interferences, and acute toxicity.

Preparations

Excipients in commercially available drug preparations may have clinically important effects in some individuals; consult specific product labeling for details.

Glatiramer Acetate

Parenteral		
Injection, for subcutaneous use	20 mg/1 mL*	**Copaxone®** (available as 1-mL prefilled syringe), Teva Neuroscience
		Glatiramer Acetate Injection
		Glatopa® (available as 1-mL prefilled syringe), Sandoz
	40 mg/1 mL*	**Copaxone®** (available as 1-mL prefilled syringe), Teva Neuroscience
		Glatopa® (available as 1-mL prefilled syringe), Sandoz

*available from one or more manufacturer, distributor, and/or repackager by generic (nonproprietary) name

Interferon Beta

■ Interferon beta, a biosynthetic (recombinant DNA origin) form of endogenous human interferon beta, is a biologic response modifier that has beneficial effects in the management of multiple sclerosis. Interferon beta is available as interferon beta-1a and interferon beta-1b. Interferon beta-1a also is available covalently bound to polyethylene glycol (PEG) (i.e., peginterferon beta-1a). For information on peginterferon beta-1a, see Peginterferon Beta-1a 92:20.

Uses

■ **Multiple Sclerosis** Interferon beta (beta-1a, beta-1b) is used in the management of multiple sclerosis (MS), a chronic, immune-mediated inflammatory and degenerative disorder of the CNS that results in injury to the myelin sheaths (demyelination), the oligodendrocytes, and the axons and nerve cells themselves. Interferon beta-1a is commercially available as a once-weekly IM injection (Avonex®) or a 3-times-weekly subcutaneous injection (Rebif®). Interferon beta-1b is commercially available as a subcutaneous alternate-day injection (Betaseron®, Extavia®); the 2 currently available interferon beta-1b preparations are identical except for some packaging components (e.g., needle size). Some preparations of interferon beta have been designated orphan drugs by the US Food and Drug Administration (FDA) for the treatment of MS.

Interferon beta has been used for the management of various types of MS, including relapsing forms of MS (e.g., relapsing-remitting MS [RRMS]), secondary progressive MS†, and primary progressive MS†, and also has been used in patients with an isolated demyelinating event who are considered to be at high risk of developing clinically definite MS. Interferon beta appears to reduce the frequency of neurologic disturbances (also known as attacks or relapses) and produces a beneficial effect on several magnetic resonance imaging (MRI) measures of disease activity.

Some clinicians recommend initiating interferon beta therapy as soon as possible following onset of MS in order to maximize benefits of the drug. Immunomodulators such as interferon beta appear to be of little use once axonal degeneration has reached a critical threshold and clinical progression of the disorder is established. Although many patients subjectively report improvement in various manifestations following initiation of interferon beta therapy, the drug generally is ineffective in the treatment of some common symptoms of MS (e.g., bladder dysfunction, spasticity, fatigue), for which other pharmacologic agents (e.g., antispasmodic agents, skeletal muscle relaxants) may be indicated.

Important differences in beneficial effects (clinical, MRI measures of response) between the different types of interferon beta in the management of MS have not been reported and the existence of such differences is as yet unknown. Clinical interpretation of head-to-head comparative studies involving various interferon beta preparations is limited by methodologic problems (e.g., short duration, open-label studies, nonstandardized dosages and/or routes of administration). Some of these studies were principally designed to provide evidence to the FDA that one particular preparation of interferon beta was sufficiently different to justify overturning the Orphan Drug Act protection of another preparation.

Relapsing-Remitting Forms of Multiple Sclerosis Interferon beta (beta-1a, beta-1b) is used to reduce the frequency of clinical exacerbations and slow the accumulation of physical disability in adults with RRMS; in clinical studies, therapy with interferon beta also was shown to delay the time to conversion to clinically definite MS in patients experiencing a first clinical episode who had MRI features consistent with MS (see Patients with a First Clinical Episode under Multiple Sclerosis: Relapsing-Remitting Forms of Multiple Sclerosis, in Uses).

Approximately 85–90% of patients newly diagnosed with MS will have the relapsing-remitting form of the disorder. Such patients typically have recurrent attacks of neurologic dysfunction followed by complete or, more commonly, partial recovery. Interferon beta is one of several disease-modifying therapies used in the management of RRMS. Although not curative, these therapies have all been shown to modify several measures of disease activity, including relapse rates, new or enhancing MRI lesions, and disability progression; results of placebo-controlled studies indicate that treatment with a disease-modifying agent can reduce the frequency of MS attacks by 28–68%. The American Academy of Neurology (AAN) recommends that disease-modifying therapy be offered to patients with RRMS who have had recent relapses and/or MRI activity; these experts state that the benefits versus risks (e.g., adverse effects or burden of taking a long-term medication) of treatment in patients who have not had relapses in 2 or more years and do not have active new MRI lesions are not known. Because CNS damage occurs early and continues throughout the course of MS, other clinicians recommend that disease-modifying therapy be initiated as soon as possible following diagnosis and continued indefinitely unless there is a clear lack of benefit, adverse effects are intolerable, the patient is unable to adhere to the recommended treatment regimen, or a more appropriate treatment becomes available. Clinicians should consider the adverse effects, tolerability, method of administration, safety, efficacy, and cost of the drugs in addition to patient preferences when selecting an appropriate disease-modifying therapy.

Because permanent disability in patients with RRMS is thought to result from incomplete recovery from attacks, pivotal studies of interferon beta have focused on 2 therapeutic objectives: prevention of relapses and cumulative disability. In these studies, assessment of clinical disability principally was based on the Expanded Disability Status Scale (EDSS) and the extent of disease was based on MRI measures of disease activity (e.g., gadolinium-enhanced or T2 lesion volume). These short-term surrogate measures of underlying pathology in MS patients may not consistently predict long-term patient outcomes.

In the multicenter, placebo-controlled study that established efficacy of interferon beta-1b (Betaseron®) for the management of RRMS, ambulatory patients (EDSS score of 0–5.5) with RRMS who received high doses (0.25 mg) subcutaneously every other day for 2 years had reduced clinical relapse rates and lessened new MRI activity compared with those who received low doses (0.05 mg) subcutaneously every other day or placebo. The effect of interferon beta treatment on measures of disease severity (i.e., MRI measures of disease burden, disability progression) was less impressive. There was a robust effect of treatment on the MRI T2 disease burden, but no statistically significant effect on the measure of confirmed 1-point EDSS progression (i.e., a change of one or more EDSS point sustained on 2 consecutive assessments performed 3 months apart), which was the primary end point of the trial. Efficacy of the Extavia® preparation of interferon beta-1b in the management of RRMS is based on the efficacy study conducted with Betaseron®.

In the multicenter, placebo-controlled study that established efficacy of interferon beta-1a (Avonex®) for the management of RRMS, ambulatory patients (EDSS score up to 3.5) with RRMS who received 30 mcg IM once weekly for 2 years had decreases in confirmed 1-point EDSS progression rates, which was the primary end point of the trial, compared with those who received placebo. The clinical relapse rate and the neurologic attack rate as measured by the median number of gadolinium-enhanced lesions on MRI were reduced in patients receiving interferon beta-1a compared with those receiving placebo. The total volume of T2 disease burden seen on MRI also was reduced compared with placebo, but this difference was not statistically significant. Interferon beta-1a (Avonex®) received its orphan drug designation for the management of RRMS based on a lower incidence of an adverse local effect (i.e., skin necrosis at injection sites) compared with interferon beta-1b (Betaseron®). (See Injection Site Necrosis under Cautions: Local Effects.)

A second interferon beta-1a preparation (Rebif®) received its orphan drug designation over Avonex® for the management of RRMS based on results of a randomized, open-label, evaluator-blinded, comparative study, the Evidence for Interferon Dose Effect: European-North American Comparative Efficacy (EVIDENCE) trial. Results of this study indicated that the relative risk of experiencing a relapse at any time during the initial 24-week treatment period in patients with clinically active RRMS was approximately 32–37% lower in patients who received the higher dose (44 mcg), more frequent (3 times weekly) subcutaneous administration of Rebif® than in those who received the lower dose (30 mcg), less frequent (once weekly) IM administration of Avonex®. The number of active combined unique lesions on MRI scans (defined as active lesions on T2 or T1 post-gadolinium sequences) also was substantially reduced in patients treated with Rebif® compared with those treated with Avonex®. These results are consistent with those of the Independent Comparison of Interferon (INCOMIN) trial, in which a greater clinical benefit over a 2-year treatment period was shown in patients who received higher dose (0.25 mg subcutaneously), more frequently administered (every other day) Betaseron®, both on clinical outcomes (i.e., relapse-free status and sustained progression) and on MRI outcomes (i.e., new T2 lesions or gadolinium-enhanced lesions), compared with those who received the lower dose (30 mcg IM), less frequently administered (once weekly) Avonex®.

Although the results of these and other clinical studies suggest that there may be a dose-response curve associated with the use of high dosages and/or high frequency of interferon beta for the treatment of MS, some clinicians state that methodologic problems (e.g., short duration, open-label studies, nonstandardized dosages and/or routes of administration) in these head-to-head comparative studies limit clinical interpretation of the findings.

Patients with a First Clinical Episode. Interferon beta has been used in patients who have experienced their first clinical episode (e.g., isolated demyelinating event) and have MRI features consistent with early MS. Some clinicians recommend initiating interferon beta therapy as soon as possible following onset of MS in order to maximize benefits of such therapy. Results of several clinical studies have shown that early initiation of interferon beta therapy can substantially delay the time to a second clinical event or the development of new MRI brain lesions in patients with a first demyelinating event who are considered to be at high risk of developing MS based on MRI findings. These studies do not, however, provide evidence that the ultimate development of clinically definite MS is prevented by such treatment or that early interferon beta therapy affects long-term disability outcome in this patient population. In addition, because most clinical studies of interferon beta were conducted over a short duration (e.g., 2–3 years) using a combination of short-term clinical (e.g., EDSS disability assessments, rate of clinical attacks) and MRI measures of disease activity (e.g., T2 lesion load), it remains to be established whether interferon beta can alter the underlying disease process, including progression of the disease over the long term.

In one study in high-risk patients 18–50 years of age who had just experienced their first clinically isolated (monosymptomatic or polysymptomatic) episode of demyelinating disease (e.g., optic neuritis, spinal cord syndrome, brainstem/cerebellar syndrome) and had MRI lesions typical of MS, once-weekly IM administration of interferon beta-1a (Avonex®) 30 mcg substantially delayed the development of a second clinical exacerbation compared with placebo during a 2- to 3-year study period. All patients had received a standard corticosteroid regimen (IV followed by oral) prior to initiation of interferon beta-1a or placebo. During 3 years of follow-up, the relative risk of developing a second clinical event (exacerbation) was lower in the interferon beta-1a group than in the placebo group (35 or 50%, respectively). Compared with the placebo group, patients who received interferon beta-1a had a relative reduction in the volume of brain lesions, fewer new or enlarging lesions, and fewer gadolinium-enhanced lesions at 18 months.

In another study, patients 18–40 years of age with clinical manifestations indicating unifocal or multifocal CNS involvement who were experiencing a first neurologic episode suggesting MS (occurring within the last 3 months) and a positive MRI scan received interferon beta-1a (Rebif®) 22 mcg subcutaneously once weekly or placebo. The primary outcome measure was the conversion to clinically definite MS as defined by the occurrence of a second exacerbation (i.e., new symptom or worsening of preexisting symptoms accompanied by a corresponding new neurologic sign or focal neurologic dysfunction lasting at least 24 hours that was not associated with fever and was preceded by stability or improvement for at least 30 days). During the 2-year study, 34% of those receiving interferon beta-1a and 45% of those receiving placebo converted to clinically definite MS and there were fewer new T2 lesions in the interferon beta-1a group. However, only 16% of those receiving interferon beta-1a and 6% of those receiving placebo were free of temporal dissemination of MRI lesions in the 2 years after clinical onset of the disease.

Efficacy of interferon beta-1b (Betaseron®) in patients with a first clinical episode was evaluated in a randomized, double-blind, placebo-controlled study in 468 patients 18–45 years of age who had recently experienced an isolated demyelinating event and had at least 2 MRI brain lesions typical of MS. Patients received interferon beta-1b 0.25 mg subcutaneously every other day or placebo within 60 days of onset of the clinical event and were treated for a period of up to 2 years or until a second exacerbation occurred. The primary outcome measure was time to development of a second exacerbation with involvement of at least 2 distinct anatomical regions (i.e., conversion to clinically definite MS). Treatment with interferon beta-1b substantially delayed the time to second exacerbation compared with placebo; the relative risk of developing a second exacerbation within 2 years was substantially lower in patients receiving interferon beta-1b compared with those receiving placebo (28 versus 45%, respectively). Patients receiving interferon beta-1b also had fewer new active lesions at the end of the study compared with placebo recipients; however, the change in T2 lesion volume was not substantially different between the groups. Efficacy of the Extavia® preparation of interferon beta-1b in patients with a first clinical episode is based on the efficacy study conducted with Betaseron®.

Secondary Progressive Multiple Sclerosis Interferon beta has been used with equivocal results in the management of secondary progressive MS†. Studies generally have shown a benefit in terms of relapse rates, but not on disability progression. Secondary progressive MS generally is characterized by a decrease in the rate of neurologic attacks and steady deterioration from baseline function, unrelated to acute neurologic attacks. Approximately 80% of patients with RRMS develop secondary progressive MS over time as a natural progression of the disorder. Some experts suggest that disease-modifying therapy may be beneficial in ambulatory patients with secondary progressive MS who have relapses or active new MRI lesions, provided the benefits of such therapy outweigh the risks.

In one randomized, placebo-controlled, double-blind study evaluating interferon beta-1b 0.25 mg subcutaneously every other day for up to 3 years in patients with secondary progressive MS, there was a substantial difference in time to confirmed progression in disability (as determined by a 1-point increase on the EDSS or a 0.5-point increase if baseline EDSS was 6–6.5) in favor of interferon beta-1b. In this study, approximately 39% of patients who received interferon beta-1b had confirmed progression in disease compared with approximately 50% of those who received placebo, which represents a relative reduction of approximately 22% in the proportion of patients with sustained disease progression. In addition, clinical and MRI attack rates, and volume of white matter disease seen on MRI were all reduced in patients who received interferon beta-1b compared with those who received placebo. Interferon beta-1b therapy also reduced the likelihood of becoming wheelchair bound (i.e., a score of 7 on EDSS) during the study. Subsequent studies with interferon beta-1b in patients with secondary progressive MS also demonstrated reductions in the clinical attack rate, the MRI attack rate, and the volume of white matter disease seen on T2-weighted MRI, but reduction in the confirmed 1-point EDSS progression rate (the primary end point of the trials) was not significant.

In placebo-controlled studies evaluating interferon beta-1a preparations for the treatment of secondary progressive MS, a beneficial effect of the drug on relapse prevention was observed; however, interferon beta-1a was not more effective than placebo in delaying clinical disease progression.

The observed differences in efficacy between relapse and disability outcomes in the interferon beta studies in patients with secondary progressive MS suggest that axonal damage, which is believed to underlie progressive accumulation of disease, may result from a relatively noninflammatory process and/or may result from a time lag between inflammation and subsequent axonal destruction. The clinical course of patients with persistent disability, therefore, would not be expected to be substantially altered by currently available disease-modifying agents.

Primary Progressive Multiple Sclerosis Interferon beta has been investigated for use in the management of primary progressive MS (PPMS)†, a type of MS that affects approximately 10–15% of patients diagnosed with MS. Patients with PPMS experience a progressive, uninterrupted accumulation of neurologic deficit (without clinical attacks) from disease onset that usually results in a worse prognosis for ultimate disability compared with that of patients with RRMS. Because PPMS appears to have less of an inflammatory component than relapsing courses of MS, many clinicians believe that patients with PPMS may be less likely to respond to immunomodulators such as interferon beta. Ocrelizumab is currently the only disease-modifying therapy that has been shown to alter disease progression in patients with PPMS; studies with other disease-modifying agents generally have not demonstrated a benefit on disability progression, although some effects on MRI measures of disease activity were observed. Results of 2 randomized, double-blind, placebo-controlled studies showed no clinical benefits of interferon beta therapy in a limited number of patients with PPMS.

■ **Other Uses** Results of preliminary trials with interferon beta in the treatment of amyotrophic lateral sclerosis (ALS)†, as an adjunct to tamoxifen for the treatment of metastatic breast cancer†, or as an adjunct to radiation therapy for the treatment of patients with locally advanced, non-small cell lung cancer† have shown no clear treatment benefit with use of interferon beta. Use of interferon beta has resulted, however, in greater rates of both acute and late treatment-related toxicity in patients with locally advanced non-small cell lung cancer receiving concomitant radiation therapy.

Dosage and Administration

■ **Reconstitution and Administration** Interferon beta-1a is administered by IM injection once weekly (Avonex®) or by subcutaneous injection 3 times a week (Rebif®).

Interferon beta-1b (Betaseron®, Extavia®) is administered by subcutaneous injection every other day. The 2 commercially available beta-1b preparations (Betaseron® and Extavia®) are identical except for certain packaging components (e.g., needle size).

To prevent or reduce flu-like symptoms, patients may be premedicated with analgesic and/or antipyretic agents on treatment days. Some clinicians suggest that administering interferon beta in the evening may make some adverse effects (e.g., flu-like syndrome) more tolerable since this avoids peak serum concentrations of the drug during the day. (See Cautions: Flu-like Syndrome.)

Interferon beta is intended for use under the guidance and supervision of a clinician, but may be *self-administered* if the clinician determines that the patient and/or their caregiver is competent to prepare and safely administer the drug after appropriate training and with medical follow-up. The initial self-administered dose should be performed under the supervision of a qualified clinician. Injection technique is of particular importance when interferon beta is administered subcutaneously because of the substantial risk of developing injection site reactions (e.g., inflammation, pain, necrosis) with this route of administration. (See Cautions: Local Effects.) Patients and/or caregivers who administer interferon beta in a home setting should be trained on proper injection techniques and cautioned against reuse of syringes and needles and should be supplied with a puncture-resistant container and instructions for the proper, safe disposal of such equipment after use. Patients should be given a copy of the manufacturer's patient information (medication guide and instructions for use) for the specific preparation of interferon beta-1a (Avonex® or Rebif®) or interferon beta-1b (Betaseron® or Extavia®) used.

IM Injection **Interferon Beta-1a.** Interferon beta-1a for IM injection (Avonex®) is commercially available as a single-dose vial containing lyophilized powder, a single-use prefilled syringe, and a single-use prefilled auto-injector (i.e., Avonex Pen®). IM injections of Avonex® should be administered into the thigh or upper arm. Injections with Avonex Pen® should be made into the upper outer thigh. Injection sites should be rotated and should be free from any skin irritation, redness, bruising, infection, or scarring prior to injection. Injection sites should be inspected for any redness, swelling, or tenderness 2 hours after the drug is administered.

Avonex® lyophilized powder for IM injection is reconstituted by adding 1.1 mL of the sterile water for injection diluent supplied by the manufacturer to a vial labeled as containing 33 mcg of the drug. The diluent should be added slowly to the vial to avoid foaming. To ensure complete dissolution of the drug, the vial should be swirled gently but not shaken. The resultant solution has a concentration of 30 mcg of interferon beta-1a per mL. The manufacturer of Avonex® states that reconstituted solutions of the drug should be used as soon as possible but are stable for up to 6 hours when refrigerated at 2–8°C. Any residual solution remaining after withdrawal of a dose should be discarded since the drug contains no preservatives and is intended for single use only. Vials of Avonex® lyophilized powder are packaged with a syringe and a 23-gauge, 1¼-inch needle supplied by the manufacturer; the manufacturer states that a 25-gauge, 1-inch needle for IM injection may be substituted by the clinician if appropriate.

The prefilled syringes and auto-injectors should be removed from the refrigerator and allowed to reach room temperature (about 30 minutes) prior to administration; external heat sources (e.g., hot water) should not be used to warm the solution. Prefilled syringes are packaged with a 23-gauge, 1¼-inch needle supplied by the manufacturer; the manufacturer states that a 25-gauge, 1-inch needle for IM injection may be substituted by the clinician if appropriate. The prefilled auto-injector (Avonex Pen®) should be used only with the 25-gauge, ⅝-inch needle supplied by the manufacturer; no other needles may be substituted. Patients and/or caregivers should be advised that the needle cap of the prefilled syringe contains natural rubber latex, which may cause allergic reactions in individuals who are sensitive to latex. (See Latex Sensitivity under Cautions: Sensitivity Reactions.)

Subcutaneous Injection **Interferon Beta-1a.** Interferon beta-1a for subcutaneous injection (Rebif®) is commercially available as a prefilled syringe or auto-injector. Subcutaneous injections of Rebif® should be administered into the abdomen, thigh, upper arm, or buttocks; injections near the waistline or within 2 inches of the navel should be avoided. Injection sites should be rotated to minimize the risk of injection site reactions (e.g., infection, necrosis). Injections should *not* be made into areas where the skin is irritated, reddened, bruised, infected, or abnormal in any way. Removing the drug from the refrigerator 30 minutes prior to use may reduce the incidence of injection site pain.

Commercially available Rebif® prefilled syringes and auto-injectors contain no preservatives and are intended for single use only; any unused portions should be discarded.

Interferon Beta-1b. Interferon beta-1b for subcutaneous injection (Betaseron®, Extavia®) is commercially available as a lyophilized powder that must be reconstituted prior to use. An optional auto-injector (Betaconnect®) is available and may be obtained through the manufacturer's patient support program by calling 1-800-788-1467. The manufacturer's instructions for use should be consulted for specific information regarding use of the Betaconnect® auto-injector. Subcutaneous injections of interferon beta-1b should be administered into the abdomen, thigh, upper arm, or buttocks; injections near the waistline or navel should be avoided. Injection sites should be rotated to minimize the risk of injection site reactions (e.g., infection, necrosis). Injections should *not* be made into areas where the skin is reddened, bruised, infected, or abnormal in any way.

Interferon beta-1b lyophilized powder is reconstituted by slowly adding 1.2 mL of the 0.54% sodium chloride diluent from the prefilled diluent syringe supplied by the manufacturer to a vial labeled as containing 0.3 mg of the drug. After adding the diluent, the vial should be swirled gently but should not be shaken to avoid foaming. The resultant solution has a concentration of 0.25 mg of interferon beta-1b per mL. The reconstituted solution should be inspected visually for particulate matter and discoloration and discarded if either is present. The drug should be used immediately after reconstitution or may be refrigerated at 2–8°C for up to 3 hours. Any residual solution remaining after withdrawal of a dose should be discarded since the drug contains no preservatives and is intended for single use only. Patients and/or caregivers should be advised that the removable rubber cap of the prefilled diluent syringe supplied with Extavia® contains natural rubber latex, which may cause allergic reactions in individuals who are sensitive to latex. (See Latex Sensitivity under Cautions: Sensitivity Reactions.)

■ **Dosage** Dosage of interferon beta is expressed in terms of mg. Potency of interferon beta also has been expressed in terms of international units; each mg of interferon beta-1a is equivalent to approximately 200 million units of antiviral activity for Avonex® and 270 million units for Rebif®, and each mg of interferon beta-1b is equivalent to approximately 32 million units for Betaseron® and Extavia®. Although commercially available preparations of interferon beta-1a (Avonex®, Rebif®) generally have similar specific activities on a mcg-for-mcg basis when tested using the same assay system, dosages of these interferon beta-1a preparations and interferon beta-1b expressed in terms of units or mcg are not directly comparable. Some experts state that the conversion of interferon beta-1a doses to interferon beta-1b doses can be calculated using published data, with the result that 6 million units (30 mcg) of Avonex® is approximately equivalent to 7–9 million units (220–280 mcg) of Betaseron®. However, commercially available interferon beta preparations should not be switched in the middle of a treatment regimen, except for safety reasons, and patients should be cautioned not to change the dosage or schedule of administration of interferon beta except at the advice of their clinician.

Multiple Sclerosis **Interferon Beta-1a.** For the management of relapsing forms of multiple sclerosis (MS; e.g., relapsing-remitting MS [RRMS]), the recommended adult dosage of interferon beta-1a (Avonex®) is 30 mcg once weekly administered by IM injection. To reduce the incidence and severity of flu-like symptoms, therapy may be initiated at a dosage of 7.5 mcg once weekly, and then increased by increments of 7.5 mcg each week for the next 3 weeks to the recommended dosage of 30 mcg once weekly. If a dose is missed, the missed dose should be administered as soon as possible followed by resumption of the regular weekly schedule. The drug should *not* be administered on 2 consecutive days.

Safety and efficacy of Avonex® therapy beyond 3 years have not been established.

For the management of RRMS, the recommended adult dosage of interferon beta-1a (Rebif®) is 22 or 44 mcg 3 times weekly administered by subcutaneous injection. Injections should be administered, if possible, at the same time (preferably in the late afternoon or evening) on the same 3 days (e.g., Monday, Wednesday, and Friday) at least 48 hours apart each week. Treatment generally should be initiated at 20% of the prescribed dosage, and then gradually increased over a 4-week period to the target dosage of 22 or 44 mcg 3 times weekly using the schedule in Table 1. When titrating to the 22-mcg dose, only prefilled syringes (not auto-injectors) should be used.

Table 1. Rebif® Dosage Titration Schedule

	Percentage of Target Dose	Rebif® 22 mcg Target Dose	Rebif® 44 mcg Target Dose
Weeks 1–2	20%	4.4 mcg (use ½ of 8.8-mcg syringe)	8.8 mcg (use full 8.8-mcg syringe or auto-injector)
Weeks 3–4	50%	11 mcg (use ½ of 22-mcg syringe)	22 mcg (use full 22-mcg syringe or auto-injector)
Weeks 5+	100%	22 mcg (use full 22-mcg syringe or auto-injector)	44 mcg (use full 44-mcg syringe or auto-injector)

Safety and efficacy of Rebif® therapy beyond 2 years have not been established.

Interferon Beta-1b. For the management of RRMS, the recommended adult dosage of interferon beta-1b (e.g., Betaseron®, Extavia®) is 0.25 mg every other day administered by subcutaneous injection. The manufacturer recommends that therapy be initiated at a dosage of 0.0625 mg, and then increased gradually over a 6-week period to the recommended dosage using the schedule in Table 2.

Table 2. Betaseron® and Extavia® Dosage Titration Schedule

	Percentage of Target Dose	Betaseron® and Extavia® Dose
Weeks 1–2	25%	0.0625 mg
Weeks 3–4	50%	0.125 mg
Weeks 5–6	75%	0.1875 mg
Weeks 7+	100%	0.25 mg

If a dose of interferon beta-1b (Betaseron®, Extavia®) is missed, the missed dose should be administered as soon as possible and the next scheduled dose should be administered approximately 48 hours later. The drug should *not* be administered on 2 consecutive days.

Safety and efficacy of interferon beta-1b therapy beyond 3 years have not been established.

Cautions

Interferon beta shares some of the toxic potentials of interferon alfa, and the usual precautions of interferon therapy should be observed. (See Cautions in Interferon Alfa 8:18.20 and in 10:00.) The incidence and severity of some adverse effects reported with interferon beta therapy in patients with multiple sclerosis (MS) may be related to the dosage and duration of therapy, route of administration (subcutaneous versus IM injection), and/or performance status of the patient. Because common manifestations of MS (e.g., fatigue, malaise) often are the same as those related to the use of interferon beta, it may not always be possible to distinguish between adverse effects of the drug and the patient's underlying disorder. Some adverse nervous system effects associated with interferon beta also may result from transient pseudoexacerbations (produced either by clinical or subclinical increases in body temperature or increased spasticity) or from changes in the immune system caused by the immunomodulating effects of interferon beta. Consequently, it is not uncommon for patients to feel worse or to experience a temporary worsening of their symptoms immediately following initiation of interferon beta therapy. These effects often abate with continued therapy and should not be interpreted as an indication of treatment failure.

The most common adverse effects of interferon beta therapy are flu-like symptoms and local effects at the injection site. The incidence of injection site reactions does not appear to be related to the type of interferon beta (beta-1a, beta-1b), but is related to the route of administration; higher rates have been reported following subcutaneous administration than following IM administration of the drug.

■ **Flu-like Syndrome** Flu-like syndrome is one of the most common adverse effects associated with interferon beta therapy and has been reported in up to 59% of patients with relapsing forms of MS who received the drug in clinical studies. Symptoms reported include headache (50–70%), fatigue (33–41%), fever (20–31%), chills (19–21%), malaise (4–6%), myalgia (23–29%), rigors (6–13%), and/or arthralgia (9%). Although there is considerable interindividual variation in the development of flu-like symptoms, these symptoms occur most frequently during initiation of interferon beta therapy (e.g., within hours or days after an injection) and usually subside within a few months with continued therapy. Data from one limited study suggest that women and patients with low body weight may be at particular risk for developing flu-like symptoms.

■ **Local Effects** Following subcutaneous injection of interferon beta-1a or beta-1b, mild to moderate injection site reactions (e.g., hemorrhage, hypersensitivity, inflammation, mass, pain, edema, atrophy, redness, induration) were reported in approximately 78–92% of patients in controlled trials. Following IM injection of interferon beta-1a, mild to moderate injection site reactions (e.g., pain, inflammation) were reported in 3–8% of patients in clinical studies; ecchymosis at the injection site has been reported in 6% of patients. Injection site abscess or cellulitis, possibly requiring surgical intervention, has rarely been reported during postmarketing surveillance. These local reactions following IM or subcutaneous injection generally are more severe with more frequent and higher doses of interferon beta.

Injection Site Necrosis Necrosis, a potentially severe injection site reaction, has been reported in 1–4% of patients receiving subcutaneous injections of interferon beta-1a or beta-1b in controlled trials. Necrosis at the injection site has not been reported to date following IM injection of interferon beta-1a. Injection site necrosis usually occurs within the first 3–4 months of therapy, although there have been post-marketing surveillance reports of this adverse reaction occurring more than 2 years after initiation of therapy. Necrosis may occur at single or multiple injection sites. The necrotic lesions typically are 3 cm or less in diameter, but larger areas have been reported. While necrosis has commonly extended only to subcutaneous fat, there are reports of necrosis extending to and including fascia overlying muscle. In some lesions where biopsy results are available, vasculitis has been reported.

Factors that may be associated with the development of skin necrosis at injection sites include nonsterile injection techniques, administering cold interferon beta solutions, failure to rotate injection sites, and exposure of recent injection sites to UV light. The pathogenic mechanism of injection site necrosis is as yet unknown, but may be caused by a hypersensitivity reaction localized to the blood vessels. Antibiotic treatment and debridement and/or skin grafting have been required. In most cases, healing was associated with scarring.

■ **Nervous System Effects** Depression, suicidal ideation, and suicide attempts have been reported with increased frequency in patients receiving type I interferons (interferon alfa, interferon beta). In addition, development of new or worsening of other preexisting psychiatric disorders, including psychosis, has been reported during postmarketing surveillance. Depression, suicides, and suicide attempts have been reported during clinical studies evaluating interferon beta-1b (Betaseron®) and there have been postmarketing reports of suicide in patients receiving interferon beta-1a (Rebif®). It is not known whether these neuropsychiatric symptoms are related to the underlying neurologic basis of MS, to interferon beta therapy, or to a combination of both.

Other adverse nervous system effects that have occurred in patients receiving interferon beta in clinical studies include asthenia (24–53%), dizziness (14%), hypertonia (7–40%), incoordination (4–17%), insomnia (21%), and somnolence (4–5%). In addition, anxiety, confusion, emotional lability, convulsion, dizziness, and psychotic symptoms have been reported during postmarketing surveillance.

Seizures also have been reported in temporal association with the use of interferon beta in clinical studies and during postmarketing experience. It is not known whether these events were related to a preexisting seizure disorder, to the effects of MS, to interferon beta therapy, or to a combination of these and other potential risk factors (e.g., fever).

■ **Hematologic Effects** Decreased peripheral blood counts in all cell lines (e.g., pancytopenia, leukopenia, thrombocytopenia) have been reported in patients receiving interferon beta preparations. Leukopenia, in some cases requiring dosage reduction, was reported in 18% of patients receiving interferon beta-1b (Betaseron®) in clinical studies; lymphocyte count less than 1500/mm^3, absolute neutrophil count (ANC) less than 1500/mm^3, and white blood cell count less than 3000/mm^3 occurred in 86, 13, and 13%, respectively, of patients receiving the drug. In clinical studies of interferon beta-1a, leukopenia, thrombocytopenia, and anemia were reported in 28–36, 2–8, and 3–5%, respectively, of patients receiving Rebif®, and anemia was reported in 4% of patients receiving Avonex®. Some reported cases of thrombocytopenia involved nadirs below 10,000/mm^3, and some recurred with rechallenge.

Thrombotic microangiopathy (TMA), including sometimes fatal thrombotic thrombocytopenic purpura and hemolytic uremic syndrome, has been reported in patients receiving interferon beta therapy. The onset of TMA ranged from several weeks to years after the drug was initiated.

■ **GI Effects** Abdominal pain was reported in about 8–22% of patients receiving interferon beta in clinical studies. Nausea was reported in 23% of patients receiving IM interferon beta-1a, and dry mouth occurred in 1–5% of patients receiving subcutaneous interferon beta-1a. In addition, nausea, diarrhea, and vomiting have been reported during postmarketing experience with interferon beta-1b.

■ **Hepatic Effects** Severe hepatic injury (e.g., hepatitis, autoimmune hepatitis, liver failure sometimes requiring transplantation) has been reported rarely with interferon beta therapy. Symptoms of hepatic impairment have been reported 1–6 months following initiation of interferon beta therapy. In some cases, these events occurred in the presence of other drugs or medical conditions that have been associated with hepatic injury. Asymptomatic elevations in serum aminotransferase concentrations (particularly ALT) occur commonly with interferon beta therapy and in some cases may recur following rechallenge with the drug. Transient increases in serum AST and/or ALT concentrations have been reported in about 10–27% of patients receiving interferon beta-1a (Rebif®) in clinical studies. Increased serum ALT concentrations (greater than 5 times baseline) or increased serum AST concentrations (greater than 5 times baseline) have occurred in 12 or 4%, respectively, of patients receiving interferon beta-1b (Betaseron®) in clinical studies.

■ **Musculoskeletal Effects** Adverse musculoskeletal effects, including arthralgia, back pain, myalgia, and skeletal pain, have occurred in 9–29% of patients receiving interferon beta in clinical studies. Increased spasticity, severe enough to require use of skeletal muscle relaxants such as baclofen, also has been reported in patients receiving interferon beta, but appears to occur more frequently in patients with primary progressive MS than in those with relapsing-remitting MS.

■ **Respiratory Effects** Sinusitis and upper respiratory tract infections occurred in 14% and dyspnea and bronchitis occurred in 6–8% of patients receiving interferon beta in clinical studies. Bronchospasm also has been reported during postmarketing surveillance.

■ **Genitourinary Effects** Impotence was reported in 8% of men and metrorrhagia was reported in 9% of women receiving interferon beta in clinical studies.

Urinary tract infections, urinary urgency, urinary frequency, abnormal urine constituents, and urinary incontinence were reported in 2–17% of patients receiving interferon beta in clinical studies.

■ **Cardiovascular Effects** Peripheral edema, chest pain, vasodilation, and hypertension have occurred in 2–12% of patients receiving interferon beta in clinical studies.

Congestive heart failure, cardiomyopathy (with or without congestive heart failure), palpitations, and tachycardia have been reported with some preparations of interferon beta during postmarketing surveillance.

■ **Endocrine and Metabolic Effects** Thyroid disorder has occurred in 4–6% of patients receiving interferon beta in clinical studies, and hypothyroidism and hyperthyroidism have been reported during postmarketing surveillance.

■ **Dermatologic Effects** Skin disorders, hyperhidrosis, and alopecia have occurred in 4–10% of patients receiving interferon beta in controlled clinical trials. Other adverse dermatologic reactions that have been reported during postmarketing surveillance include pruritus, skin discoloration, and urticaria.

■ **Sensitivity Reactions** Anaphylaxis or anaphylactoid reactions have been reported rarely in patients receiving interferon beta-1a or beta-1b. Other sensitivity reactions reported in patients receiving interferon beta include dyspnea, bronchospasm, orolingual edema, mild to severe skin rash (maculopapular, erythematous, vesicular), and urticaria. Although a clear relationship to dose or duration of interferon beta therapy remains to be established, allergic reactions, some of which have been severe, have occurred after prolonged interferon beta therapy.

Latex Sensitivity Some packaging components of certain interferon beta preparations (e.g., Avonex® prefilled syringe cap, Extavia® prefilled diluent syringe cap) contain natural rubber latex. Some individuals may be hypersensitive to natural latex proteins found in a wide range of medical devices, including such packaging components, and the level of sensitivity may vary depending on the form of natural rubber present; rarely, hypersensitivity reactions to natural latex proteins have been fatal. Such packaging components should not be handled by individuals sensitive to latex. The safety of Extavia® reconstituted using the prefilled diluent syringe in latex-sensitive individuals has not been studied.

Immunogenicity As with all therapeutic proteins, there is a potential for immunogenicity with interferon beta therapy. Most patients with MS who receive long-term interferon beta therapy will develop either binding or neutralizing antibodies to the drug. Of the 2 types of antibodies, binding antibodies are the most prevalent and, in many cases, do not interfere with the receptor-mediated functions of interferon beta. It is possible, however, that these antibodies might increase the clearance of interferon beta through the reticuloendothelial system and, thereby, lower serum interferon beta concentrations. Development of binding antibodies has not been shown to be predictive of later development of neutralizing antibodies, which are capable of interfering with receptor-mediated functions and have been associated with reduced bioavailability and/or loss of biologic activity. The presence of neutralizing antibodies, particularly in persistently high titers, has been associated with reductions in radiographic and clinical efficacy of interferon beta therapy. Although patients who developed antibodies to interferon beta in some clinical studies did worse over time compared with those who did not develop these antibodies, the long-term consequences of neutralizing antibodies are as yet unknown. Neutralizing antibodies generally develop 6–24 months after initiation of therapy, after which the risk of developing such antibodies is low.

The prevalence of interferon neutralizing antibodies has not been clearly elucidated, in part because of differences in detection methods, sampling times, and differences in dosage regimens. In pivotal clinical studies in patients with MS, neutralizing antibodies were detected in 24–31% or 5% of patients receiving subcutaneous or IM interferon beta-1a, respectively, and in up to 45% of patients receiving interferon beta-1b. Because the results of antibody tests are highly dependent on the sensitivity and specificity of the assay and can be influenced by other factors, including sample handling, timing of sample collection, and the patient's concurrent drugs and comorbidities, comparison of the incidence of antibodies between different interferon beta preparations may be misleading. Type of interferon preparation, dosing frequency, total dose, and route of administration have been suggested as factors that may affect the risk of antibody development. Interferon beta-1a administered IM has been shown to be less immunogenic than subcutaneously administered interferon beta-1a or beta-1b, and some evidence also indicates that the rate of neutralizing antibody production is lower with interferon beta-1a compared with interferon beta-1b, although the persistence of these differences is difficult to determine.

Because neutralizing antibody titers fluctuate over time and may even become undetectable despite continuous treatment, the development of antibodies during interferon beta therapy should not necessarily be interpreted as indicating permanent resistance to the drug. Some clinicians recommend that patients with MS who continue to have relapses despite several months of interferon beta (beta-1a or beta-1b) be tested for neutralizing antibodies. Neutralizing antibodies to interferon beta-1a and beta-1b are cross-reactive and switching from one interferon beta preparation (beta-1a, beta-1b) to another is unlikely to benefit patients in whom antibodies already have been induced. Because the titer of serum neutralizing antibody level that is biologically important remains uncertain, the benefits of routine testing for neutralizing antibodies in patients receiving interferon beta therapy are uncertain.

■ **Ocular Effects** Abnormal vision has occurred in 7–13% of patients receiving interferon beta-1a in clinical studies. In addition, xerophthalmia and other ocular disorders have occurred in up to 4% of patients.

■ **Other Adverse Effects** Lymphadenopathy has been reported in 6–12% of patients in clinical studies of interferon beta.

Pancreatitis has been reported during postmarketing surveillance.

■ **Precautions and Contraindications** Interferon beta is contraindicated in patients with a history of hypersensitivity to natural or recombinant interferon beta or any other component of the formulations. Some interferon beta preparations (e.g., Avonex® lyophilized powder for IM injection, Betaseron®, Extavia®, Rebif®) contain albumin human and are contraindicated in patients hypersensitive to albumin.

Patients should be informed of the risk of developing depression prior to initiating interferon beta therapy and should be advised to report any symptoms of depression, suicidal ideation, and/or psychosis immediately to their clinician. Because there is a high prevalence of mood disorders in patients with MS, a history of depression is not an absolute contraindication to the use of interferon beta. However, some clinicians state that interferon beta therapy may be inappropriate in patients with a history of suicide attempts or major depressive ideation requiring psychiatric intervention or admission to a psychiatric institution. In addition, patients receiving interferon beta should be closely monitored for evidence of depression or other psychiatric symptoms; discontinuance of therapy should be considered if any such symptoms occur. Although dosage reduction or treatment cessation may lead to resolution of the depressive symptomatology, depression may persist and suicides have occurred even after withdrawing interferon beta. However, a causal relationship between these events and interferon beta has not been established. In most cases, it is difficult to separate neuropsychiatric symptoms related to interferon beta therapy to those related to the underlying neurologic basis of MS.

Because severe hepatic injury, including autoimmune hepatitis and hepatic failure requiring liver transplantation, has been reported rarely in patients receiving interferon beta (see Cautions: Hepatic Effects), the drug should be initiated with caution in patients with active liver disease, alcohol abuse, increased serum ALT concentrations (exceeding 2.5 times the upper limit of normal), or a history of clinically important liver disease. In addition, the potential risks should be considered when interferon beta is used concomitantly with other drugs associated with hepatic injury (including alcohol) or when other drugs are added to an existing interferon beta treatment regimen. Patients receiving interferon beta should be monitored for manifestations of hepatic injury. Liver function tests should be performed at regular intervals (e.g., 1, 3, and 6 months) following initiation of therapy and then periodically thereafter in the absence of clinical symptoms. Some manufacturers recommend discontinuance of therapy if substantial elevations in serum aminotransferase concentrations or clinical manifestations of liver dysfunction (e.g., jaundice) occur. The manufacturer of Rebif® recommends that dosage reduction be considered if serum ALT concentrations increase above 5 times the upper limit of normal; dosage may be gradually re-escalated when serum ALT concentrations return to normal.

Although no direct or indirect cardiotoxicity has been attributed to interferon beta therapy to date, congestive heart failure, cardiomyopathy, and cardiomyopathy with congestive heart failure have been reported during postmarketing surveillance with certain preparations of interferon beta in patients without known predisposition to these events or other known etiologies. In some cases, these events have been temporally related to the administration of the drug and have recurred upon rechallenge. Patients with preexisting congestive heart failure should be monitored for worsening of their clinical condition during initiation and continued treatment with interferon beta. Some manufacturers state that discontinuance of therapy should be considered if worsening of congestive heart failure occurs with no other etiology.

Because injection site necrosis has been reported with subcutaneous injections of interferon, patients receiving subcutaneous preparations should be periodically evaluated on their understanding and use of aseptic technique and proper procedures for self administration. Patients should be advised to promptly report any possible manifestations of injection site necrosis (e.g., any break in the skin, which may be associated with blue-black discoloration, swelling, or drainage of fluid at the injection site). Whether to discontinue therapy following a single site of necrosis depends on the extent of necrosis; if therapy is continued, the drug should not be administered into the affected area until it is fully healed. If multiple sites of necrosis occur, therapy should be discontinued until healing occurs.

To prevent or reduce flu-like symptoms, analgesic and/or antipyretic agents (e.g., nonsteroidal anti-inflammatory agents [NSAIA], acetaminophen) may be administered prophylactically on treatment days. Some experts suggest advising patients to take an NSAIA (e.g., ibuprofen) or acetaminophen 4 hours before, at the time of, and 4 hours after interferon beta injections; advising patients to administer the drug in the evenings (just prior to bedtime) may also permit patients to sleep through many of the symptoms.

Patients should be monitored for signs and symptoms of decreased blood counts. Monitoring of complete blood cell counts (CBC), including differential is recommended during treatment with interferon beta; patients with myelosuppression may require more intensive monitoring.

Cases of thrombotic microangiopathy (TMA) have been reported in patients receiving interferon beta therapy. If clinical manifestations and/or laboratory findings consistent with TMA occur, the drug should be discontinued and the patient managed as clinically indicated.

Because seizures have been reported in patients receiving interferon beta, some manufacturers recommend that the drug be used with caution in patients with preexisting seizure disorders. If patients with no seizure history develop seizures during interferon beta therapy, an etiologic basis should be established and appropriate anticonvulsant therapy instituted prior to considering resumption of therapy.

Because autoimmune disorders of multiple target organs, including idiopathic thrombocytopenia, hyperthyroidism, hypothyroidism, and autoimmune hepatitis, have been reported during postmarketing experience with interferon beta, discontinuance of the drug should be considered if a new autoimmune disorder develops. Cases of drug-induced lupus erythematosus, sometimes associated with positive autoantibody test results (i.e., antinuclear antibodies [ANA] or antibodies to double-stranded DNA [anti-dsDNA]), also have been reported in patients receiving interferon beta. Interferon beta therapy should be discontinued if patients develop any manifestations of lupus (e.g., rash, serositis, polyarthritis, nephritis, Raynaud phenomenon).

■ **Pediatric Precautions** Although the safety and efficacy of interferon beta in children younger than 18 years of age have not been established, the drug has been used with variable results for the management of childhood onset MS in children younger than 18 years of age. In one study that included a limited number of patients, treatment failure rates in children 10.5–17 years of age who received interferon beta-1a or beta-1b were higher than those reported in well-controlled studies in adults, but these results may be attributed to the selection of children with severe forms of childhood onset MS (i.e., with numerous relapses) or other unknown factors. Adverse effects reported when interferon beta was used in children younger than 18 years of age were similar to those reported in adults. Additional well-controlled studies with prolonged follow-up are needed to assess the long-term efficacy of interferon beta in pediatric patients.

■ **Geriatric Precautions** Clinical studies of interferon beta did not include sufficient numbers of patients 65 years of age and older to determine whether geriatric patients respond differently than younger patients. In general, dosage of interferon beta should be titrated carefully in geriatric patients, usually initiating therapy at the low end of the dosage range. The greater frequency of decreased hepatic, renal, and/or cardiac function and of concomitant disease and drug therapy observed in the elderly also should be considered.

■ **Mutagenicity and Carcinogenicity** Interferon beta did not exhibit mutagenic potential in in vitro chromosomal aberration studies in human lymphocytes or in microbial (Ames) test systems with or without metabolic activation. Animal studies evaluating the carcinogenic potential of interferon beta have not been performed to date.

■ **Pregnancy, Fertility, and Lactation** There are no adequate and well-controlled studies of interferon beta in pregnant women; the drug should be used during pregnancy only if the potential benefits justify the possible risks to the fetus. Interferon beta was not teratogenic in several monkey studies; it is not known if teratogenic effects would be observed in humans. Interferon beta has been shown to be associated with substantial increases in embryolethal or abortifacient effects in cynomolgus or rhesus monkeys. These effects are consistent with the abortifacient effects in monkey studies using other type 1 interferons (e.g., interferon alfa). Spontaneous abortions have been reported rarely in pregnant women who received interferon beta in clinical studies.

Studies have not been conducted to date to determine whether interferon beta affects fertility in humans. Menstrual irregularities, anovulation, and decreased serum progesterone concentrations were observed in monkeys administered interferon beta at a dosage 100 times the recommended weekly human dosage (based on body surface area), but no effects were observed at a dosage approximately 2 times the recommended weekly human dosage. These effects were reversible after discontinuance of the drug. No effects of interferon beta were observed on either the menstrual cycle or associated hormonal profiles (e.g., progesterone, estradiol) in female cynomolgus or rhesus monkeys.

Studies in male cynomolgus monkeys treated with interferon beta-1a dosages up to 9 times the recommended human dosage (based on body surface area) did not result in any demonstrable adverse effect on sperm count, motility, morphology, or reproductive function.

It is not known whether interferon beta is distributed into milk. Because of the potential for serious adverse reactions to interferon beta in nursing infants, a decision should be made whether to discontinue nursing or the drug, taking into account the importance of the drug to the woman.

Drug Interactions

Although formal drug interaction studies have not been performed to date with interferon beta, the drug has been used concomitantly with corticosteroids, corticotropin (ACTH), antidepressants, and/or oral contraceptives during placebo-controlled studies without unusual adverse effects.

The potential risks for hepatic injury should be considered when interferon beta is used in conjunction with other agents associated with hepatotoxicity (e.g., alcohol) or when another agent is added to an existing interferon beta regimen. (See Cautions: Hepatic Effects.)

Acute Toxicity

Limited information is available on the acute toxicity of interferon beta; the maximum dose of interferon beta in humans is not known.

Chronic Toxicity

There is no evidence that abuse or dependence occurs with interferon beta-therapy. However, the risk of dependence has not been systematically evaluated.

Pharmacology

Interferons are species-specific proteins, and occasionally glycoproteins, that possess complex antiviral, antineoplastic, and immunomodulating activities. Endogenous interferons (interferon alfa, interferon beta, interferon gamma) are potent cytokines produced and secreted principally by peripheral blood leukocytes, fibroblasts, and epithelial cells in response to viral infection or certain other inducers. Endogenous interferon beta is produced principally by fibroblasts (and therefore previously was referred to as fibroblast interferon) and epithelial cells in response to such inducers and, like the other interferons, is a biologic response modifier. While interferons share many actions, they can be distinguished serologically and/or by certain biologic properties; however, experimental findings may not be predictive of clinical activity. Interferon alfa and interferon beta (type I interferons) are 30–40% homologous, in terms of nucleic acid and amino acid sequences, and their genes are both encoded on the same chromosome; in addition, these interferons, unlike interferon gamma (type 2 interferon), bind to and compete for the same cell surface receptors.

Binding of interferon beta to its receptors initiates a complex cascade of intracellular events that leads to the expression of numerous interferon-induced gene products and markers, including 2', 5'-oligoadenylate synthetase (an enzyme involved in viral suppression), beta 2-microglobulin, and neopterin (a product of activated macrophages and T cells). These markers reflect a range of biologic activities of interferon beta, including effects on major histocompatibility complex (MHC) class-I gene expression, antiviral and anti-proliferative actions, and monocyte activation. In both clinical and preclinical studies, induction of biologic response markers roughly correlates with plasma activity concentrations of interferon beta. With commercially available synthetic preparations of interferon beta, the relative dose of each preparation also can be assessed from levels of antiviral protein (MxA) stimulation, in which in vitro stimulation of peripheral blood with all 3 agents resulted in a dose-dependent increase in MxA levels that was roughly equivalent for each agent on an unit-for-unit basis using the published unit values. Although results of one pharmacodynamic study suggested that IM administration of interferon beta-1a caused a substantially greater plasma area under the concentration-time curve (AUC) for interferon beta activity compared with subcutaneous administration of the drug, results of subsequent studies have failed to find differences in terms of induction of the biologic response markers between the 2 types of interferon beta or between the different routes of administration. Results of pharmacodynamic studies have shown that the production of neopterin, human Mx protein, and 2',5'-oligoadenylate synthetase were all induced in a dose-dependent manner for both interferon beta-1a and beta-1b.

■ **Effects in Multiple Sclerosis** The mechanisms of action of interferon beta in the treatment of multiple sclerosis (MS) have not been fully elucidated but may involve immunomodulating effects, including anti-inflammatory effects. It has been suggested that one mechanism may involve inhibition or suppression of the production and immunoactivating effects of interferon gamma; interferon beta inhibits the production of interferon gamma, which appears to be involved in exacerbations of MS. The mechanism of action of the drug also may involve inhibition of release of other cytokines, such as tumor necrosis factor (TNF) and lymphotoxin (which both damage oligodendrocytes); inhibition of the proliferation of T cells, which release interferon gamma and lymphotoxin; and augmentation of suppressor T-cell function, which is deficient in MS. Although the clinical importance is unclear, there is evidence that interleukin 10 (IL-10) concentrations in serum and CSF are increased in patients receiving interferon beta-1a.

There is no evidence that interferon beta acts indirectly on MS by increasing serum cortisol concentrations; dosages up to 45 million units of interferon beta every other day have been shown not to alter serum cortisol concentrations during therapy.

The contribution, if any, of the antiviral activity of interferon beta to the drug's effect in MS currently is not known. While viral infection may precipitate acute exacerbations of MS, the precise pathophysiologic role of viral infection in the disease currently is unclear.

Pharmacokinetics

The pharmacokinetics of IM interferon beta-1a (Avonex®) or subcutaneous interferon beta-1a (Rebif®) have been evaluated in healthy individuals, but not in individuals with multiple sclerosis (MS). Pharmacokinetic data in MS patients receiving usual dosages of interferon beta-1b (Betaseron®, Extavia®) are not available because serum concentrations of the drug are either low or undetectable following subcutaneous administration of 0.25 mg or less. Studies using IV interferon beta-1b (not commercially available in the US) indicate that pharmacokinetic parameters of the drug are similar in healthy individuals and individuals with diseases other than MS.

Gender-related effects on pharmacokinetic parameters have not been observed in studies using interferon beta-1a (Rebif®). Pharmacokinetics of interferon beta-1a or beta-1b in pediatric and geriatric patients or in patients with renal or hepatic insufficiency have not been established.

■ **Absorption** Systemic exposure, as determined by area under the concentration-time curve (AUC) and peak plasma concentrations, is greater following IM than subcutaneous administration of interferon beta-1a (Avonex®). Plasma concentrations of interferon beta-1a may be sustained after IM administration due to prolonged absorption from the IM site. Following a single IM dose of Avonex®, peak plasma concentrations of interferon beta-1a generally occur in 15 hours.

Following subcutaneous injection of interferon beta-1a (Rebif®) in healthy individuals, peak plasma concentrations of approximately 5 units/mL are reached 16 hours after a single dose of 60 mcg. An increase in AUC of approximately 240% was observed when doses of the drug were given subcutaneously every other day, suggesting that accumulation of interferon beta-1a occurs after repeated subcutaneous administration.

The bioavailability of interferon beta-1b (Betaseron®, Extavia®) is approximately 50%, based on a total dose of 0.5 mg of the drug given as 2 divided subcutaneous injections at different sites in healthy individuals. Following subcutaneous injection of single or multiple daily doses of 0.5 mg of interferon beta-1b to healthy individuals, plasma concentrations of the drug were generally below 100 units/mL. Mean peak plasma interferon beta-1b concentrations of 40 units/mL are reached 1–8 hours after single or multiple daily subcutaneous doses of 0.5 mg of interferon beta-1b in healthy individuals.

■ **Distribution** Information on distribution of interferon beta-1a or beta-1b is not available. It is not known whether interferon beta-1a or beta-1b cross the placenta or are distributed into milk.

■ **Elimination** Following a single IM dose of interferon beta-1a (Avonex®), serum concentrations decline at a rate consistent with an elimination half-life of 19 hours.

Studies using interferon beta-1a (Rebif®) in healthy individuals indicate that the drug has a plasma half-life of approximately 69 hours after a single subcutaneous dose. Total clearance of the drug is approximately 33–55 L/hour in these individuals.

Mean terminal elimination half-life of interferon beta-1b ranges from 8 minutes to 4.3 hours in healthy individuals.

Chemistry and Stability

■ **Chemistry** Interferon beta is a biosynthetic (recombinant DNA origin) form of naturally occurring interferon beta. There currently are 2 different types of interferon beta (recombinant) commercially available in the US, interferon beta-1a and interferon beta-1b. Commercially available interferon beta-1a preparations (Avonex®, Rebif®) are glycosylated, recombinant preparations derived from Chinese hamster ovary (CHO) cells, and have an amino acid sequence identical to that of endogenous human interferon beta. Commercially available interferon beta-1b preparations (Betaseron®, Extavia®) are nonglycosylated recombinant products derived from cultures of genetically modified *Escherichia coli.*

Potency of interferon beta (recombinant DNA origin) has been expressed in international units (IU, units) of antiviral activity using a reference standard calibrated against the standard established by the World Health Organization (WHO) for natural interferon beta.

Interferon Beta-1a Interferon beta-1a powder for IM injection (Avonex®) occurs as a sterile, white to off-white, lyophilized powder. Following reconstitution with the sterile water for injection diluent supplied by the manufacturer, each 1 mL contains 30 mcg of interferon beta-1a, 15 mg of albumin human, 5.8 mg of sodium chloride, 5.7 mg of dibasic sodium phosphate, and 1.2 mg of monobasic sodium phosphate. The reconstituted solution occurs as a clear to slightly yellow solution, has a pH of approximately 7.3, and contains no preservatives.

Each 0.5 mL of Avonex® in prefilled syringes or auto-injectors contains 30 mcg of interferon beta-1a, 0.79 mg of sodium acetate trihydrate, 0.25 mg of glacial acetic acid, 15.8 mg of arginine hydrochloride, and 0.025 mg of polysorbate 20 in water for injection. The IM injection has a pH of approximately 4.8. Using the WHO standard, Avonex® has a specific activity of approximately 200 million units of antiviral activity per mg.

Each 0.5 mL of interferon beta-1a solution for subcutaneous injection (Rebif®) in prefilled syringes or auto-injectors containing 22 or 44 mcg of interferon beta-1a contains 2 or 4 mg of albumin human, respectively, and both solutions also contain 27.3 mg of mannitol, 0.4 mg of sodium acetate, and water for injection; neither solution contains a preservative. Each 0.2 mL of Rebif® solution for subcutaneous injection in prefilled syringes or auto-injectors containing 8.8 mcg of interferon beta-1a contains 0.8 mg of albumin human, 10.9 mg of mannitol, 0.16 mg sodium acetate, and water for injection. Using the WHO standard, Rebif® has a specific activity of approximately 270 million units of antiviral activity per mg.

Interferon Beta-1b Interferon beta-1b powder for subcutaneous injection (Betaseron®, Extavia®) occurs as a white to off-white, lyophilized powder. Following reconstitution with the 0.54% sodium chloride diluent provided by the manufacturer, each 1 mL contains 0.25 mg of interferon beta-1b and also contains albumin human and mannitol as stabilizers. The reconstituted solution occurs as a clear solution, has a pH of approximately 7.4, and contains no preservatives. Using the WHO standard, Betaseron® and Extavia® have a specific activity of approximately 32 million units of antiviral activity per mg.

■ **Stability** ***Interferon Beta-1a*** Avonex® lyophilized powder for IM injection should be refrigerated at 2–8°C, but may be stored at 25°C for up to 30 days. Following reconstitution with the sterile water for injection diluent provided by the manufacturer, Avonex® solutions should be used as soon as possible, but are stable for up to 6 hours when refrigerated at 2–8°C. Lyophilized Avonex® and reconstituted solutions of the drug should be protected from light, should not be exposed to high temperatures, and should not be frozen. The prefilled syringes and auto-injectors containing Avonex® solution for IM injection should be stored at 2–8°C, but may be exposed to temperatures up to 25°C for no more than 7 days. The prefilled syringes and auto-injectors should be protected from light and should not be frozen or exposed to high temperatures; the drug should be discarded if exposed to temperatures exceeding 25°C or to conditions other than those recommended.

Rebif® solution for subcutaneous injection in prefilled syringes or auto-injectors should be stored at 2–8°C, but may be stored at temperatures up to 25°C for up to 30 days. The prefilled syringes and auto-injectors should be protected from heat and light, and should not be frozen.

Interferon Beta-1b Betaseron® and Extavia® lyophilized powder for subcutaneous injection should be stored at 20–25°C, but may be exposed to temperatures of 15–30°C for up to 3 months. Following reconstitution with the 0.54% sodium chloride diluent provided by the manufacturer, Betaseron® and Extavia® solutions should be used immediately, but may be refrigerated at 2–8°C for up to 3 hours. Both lyophilized drug and reconstituted solutions should not be frozen.

Preparations

Excipients in commercially available drug preparations may have clinically important effects in some individuals; consult specific product labeling for details.

Interferon Beta-1a

Parenteral

For injection, for IM use	30 mcg	**Avonex**® (with sterile water for injection diluent, syringe, 23-gauge needle, and vial adapter), Biogen
Injection, for IM use	30 mcg per 0.5 mL	**Avonex**® (available as prefilled syringes and prefilled auto-injectors [Avonex Pen®]), Biogen
Injection, for subcutaneous use	8.8 mcg per 0.2 mL	**Rebif**® (available as prefilled syringes and prefilled auto-injectors [Rebidose®]), EMD Serono
	22 mcg per 0.5 mL	**Rebif**® (available as prefilled syringes and prefilled auto-injectors [Rebidose®]), EMD Serono
	44 mcg per 0.5 mL	**Rebif**® (available as prefilled syringes and prefilled auto-injectors [Rebidose®]), EMD Serono

Interferon Beta-1b

Parenteral

For injection, for subcutaneous use	0.3 mg	**Betaseron**® (with prefilled syringe containing 0.54% sodium chloride diluent, 30-gauge needle, vial adapter, and alcohol swabs), Bayer
		Extavia® (with prefilled syringe containing 0.54% sodium chloride diluent, 27-gauge needle, vial adapter, and alcohol swabs), Novartis

†Use is not currently included in the labeling approved by the US Food and Drug Administration

Ocrelizumab

■ Ocrelizumab, a recombinant humanized anti-CD20 monoclonal antibody, has immunomodulatory and disease-modifying activity in multiple sclerosis (MS).

Uses

■ **Multiple Sclerosis** ***Relapsing-remitting Multiple Sclerosis*** Ocrelizumab is used in the management of relapsing forms of multiple sclerosis (MS), including clinically isolated syndrome, relapsing-remitting disease, and active secondary progressive disease.

Ocrelizumab is one of several disease-modifying therapies used in the management of relapsing forms of MS. Although not curative, these therapies have all been shown to modify several measures of disease activity, including relapse rates, new or enhancing magnetic resonance imaging (MRI) lesions, and disability progression; results of placebo-controlled studies indicate that treatment with a disease-modifying agent can reduce the frequency of MS attacks by 28–68%. The American Academy of Neurology (AAN) recommends that disease-modifying therapy be offered to patients with RRMS who have had recent relapses and/or MRI activity; these experts state that the benefits versus risks (e.g., adverse effects or burden of taking a long-term medication) of treatment in patients who have not had relapses in 2 or more years and do not have active MRI lesions are not known. Because CNS damage occurs early and continues throughout the course of MS, other clinicians recommend that disease-modifying therapy be initiated as soon as possible following diagnosis and continued indefinitely unless there is a clear lack of benefit, adverse effects are intolerable, the patient is unable to adhere to the recommended treatment regimen, or a more appropriate treatment becomes available. Clinicians should consider the adverse effects, tolerability, method of administration, safety, efficacy, and cost of the drugs in addition to patient preferences when selecting an appropriate disease-modifying therapy.

Efficacy and safety of ocrelizumab for the management of relapsing forms of MS were established in 2 identical randomized, double-blind, active-controlled studies (OPERA I and II) that compared ocrelizumab with a standard drug used in the management of MS (interferon beta-1a [Rebif®]). In these studies, ocrelizumab was more effective than interferon beta-1a in reducing relapse rates and progression of disability.

Both studies included adults with relapsing forms of MS who had experienced at least 2 clinical relapses during the previous 2 years or at least 1 clinical relapse during the prior year and had an Expanded Disability Status Scale (EDSS) score of 0–5.5 at baseline. Ocrelizumab was administered by IV infusion at a dosage of 600 mg every 24 weeks (after 2 initial doses of 300 mg were given 14 days apart) and interferon beta-1a was administered subcutaneously at a dosage of 44 mcg 3 times weekly. Neurologic examinations were performed every 12 weeks and at the time of suspected relapse, and MRI scans were performed at baseline and at weeks 24, 48, and 96. The primary efficacy end point in both studies was the annualized relapse rate at 96 weeks. Relapse was defined as new or worsening neurologic symptoms not associated with fever or infection that persisted for at least 24 hours after at least 30 days of clinical stability or improvement, and was confirmed by objective changes on neurologic examination. Secondary outcome measures included MRI findings and the proportion of patients with confirmed disability progression (defined as an increase from baseline of at least 1 EDSS point [or at least 0.5 points for patients with baseline EDSS score greater than 5.5] that was sustained for at least 12 weeks). Baseline characteristics were similar across both studies (mean age was 37 years, 66% were female, mean number of relapses in the previous year was 1.3, mean EDSS score was 2.8, and mean duration of disease was 3.8–4.1 years).

In both studies, ocrelizumab substantially reduced the annualized relapse rate and the proportion of patients with disability progression compared with interferon beta-1a therapy. The annualized relapse rate was 0.16 with ocrelizumab versus 0.29 with interferon beta-1a in both studies, corresponding to a relative risk reduction of 46–47%. The proportion of patients with confirmed disability progression based on pooled data from the 2 studies was 9.8% in the ocrelizumab group compared with 15.2% in the interferon beta-1a group (relative risk reduction of 40%). In addition to these clinical findings, ocrelizumab had a substantial effect on MRI measures of disease activity; patients who received ocrelizumab had substantially fewer T1 gadolinium-enhancing lesions (relative reduction of 94–95%) and new and/or enlarged T2-weighted hyperintense lesions (relative reduction of 77–83%) compared with those who received interferon beta-1a.

Primary Progressive Multiple Sclerosis Ocrelizumab is used in the management of primary progressive MS (PPMS). PPMS affects approximately 10–15% of patients diagnosed with MS and is characterized by progressive worsening of neurologic function from disease onset. In contrast to relapsing forms of MS, patients with PPMS generally do not experience distinct relapses or remissions, although relapses may occur. Ocrelizumab is currently the only disease-modifying therapy that has been shown to alter disease progression in patients with PPMS; other immunomodulatory agents used for the treatment of relapsing forms of MS generally have not been effective for patients with PPMS, and other drugs that have been used in PPMS (e.g., IV glucocorticoids, methotrexate, cladribine, immune globulin IV, rituximab, mitoxantrone) have only demonstrated limited efficacy in clinical studies. Because of the demonstrated benefits of ocrelizumab, experts recommend that the drug be offered to PPMS patients unless the risks outweigh the benefits.

Efficacy and safety of ocrelizumab for the management of PPMS were established in a randomized, double-blind, placebo-controlled study (ORATORIO) in 732 adults with PPMS who had a baseline EDSS score of 3–6.5 and a score of 2 or greater on the EDSS pyramidal functional scale due to lower extremity findings. Patients were randomized in a 2:1 ratio to receive ocrelizumab 600 mg (administered as two 300-mg IV infusions 14 days apart) or placebo every 24 weeks for at least 5 doses (i.e., 120 weeks) and until a prespecified number of confirmed disability progression events occurred. Neurologic examinations were performed every 12 weeks and MRI scans were performed at baseline and at weeks 24, 48, and 120. The primary efficacy end point was the time to onset of confirmed disability progression (defined as an increase from baseline of at least 1 EDSS point [or at least 0.5 points for patients with baseline EDSS score greater than 5.5] that was sustained for at least 12 weeks, or patient withdrawal from the study due to onset of disability progression). The mean age of patients in this study was 45 years, 49% were female, the mean duration of symptoms was 6.7 years, and the mean EDSS score at baseline was 4.7.

Ocrelizumab substantially delayed the time to onset of disability progression compared with placebo. At the end of the study, the proportion of patients with confirmed disability progression was 32.9% in the ocrelizumab group and 39.3% in the placebo group (relative risk reduction of 24%). Patients who received ocrelizumab also demonstrated substantial improvement in the timed 25-foot walk, a major secondary end point. In addition, a substantial reduction in T2 hyperintense lesion volume was observed with ocrelizumab compared with placebo at 120 weeks; mean T2 lesion volume decreased by 0.39 cm^3 from baseline in patients who received ocrelizumab, but increased by 0.79 cm^3 in those who received placebo. Results of an exploratory subgroup analysis suggested an apparent lack of treatment effect on the disability progression outcome in women compared with men. However, a gender imbalance was not observed with other clinical and MRI outcome measures (e.g., annualized relapse rate, T2 lesion volume, number of new or enlarging T2 lesions).

Dosage and Administration

■ General Ocrelizumab should be administered under close supervision of an experienced clinician and only in settings where appropriate medical support is available for management of serious infusion-related reactions. (See Infusion Reactions under Cautions: Warnings/Precautions.)

To reduce the incidence and/or severity of infusion-related reactions, patients should be premedicated with IV methylprednisolone 100 mg (or an equivalent corticosteroid) 30 minutes prior to each ocrelizumab infusion and an antihistamine (e.g., diphenhydramine) approximately 30–60 minutes prior to each ocrelizumab infusion. In addition, premedication with an antipyretic (e.g., acetaminophen) may be considered. Patients should be monitored for infusion-related reactions during and for at least 1 hour after each infusion.

Prior to initiating ocrelizumab therapy, all patients should be screened for hepatitis B virus (HBV) infection. (See Cautions: Contraindications and also see Infectious Complications under Cautions: Warnings/Precautions.)

Patients should complete any necessary immunizations at least 4 weeks prior to initiation of ocrelizumab for live or live attenuated vaccines, and whenever possible, at least 2 weeks prior to initiation of ocrelizumab for inactivated vaccines. (See Drug Interactions: Vaccines.)

Prior to each infusion, patients should be evaluated for active infections; ocrelizumab therapy should be delayed in patients with active infection until the infection resolves.

■ Administration Ocrelizumab is administered by IV infusion. The first 2 doses of the drug (300 mg) are administered over approximately 2.5 hours, and subsequent doses (600 mg) are administered over approximately 3.5 hours. The total duration of infusion may be increased if infusion reactions occur.

Commercially available ocrelizumab injection concentrate should be stored at 2–8°C in the original carton to protect the drug from light; the vials should not be frozen or shaken.

The injection concentrate and diluted solutions of the drug should be inspected visually for particulate matter and discoloration prior to administration. The injection concentrate should be clear or slightly opalescent, and colorless to pale brown; the drug should be discarded if visible particles or discoloration is present. Each vial is intended for single use only; any unused portions should be discarded because the drug contains no preservatives.

Dilution Prior to administration, ocrelizumab injection concentrate containing 300 mg/10 mL must be diluted in 0.9% sodium chloride injection using proper aseptic technique. No other diluents should be used.

To prepare the solution for IV infusion, the appropriate dose of ocrelizumab should be withdrawn from 1 or 2 vials of the injection concentrate and diluted in 0.9% sodium chloride injection to yield a final concentration of approximately 1.2 mg/mL. To prepare a 300-mg dose, 10 mL of ocrelizumab injection concentrate should be withdrawn and added to an infusion bag containing 250 mL of 0.9% sodium chloride injection; to prepare a 600-mg dose, 20 mL of ocrelizumab injection concentrate should be withdrawn and added to an infusion bag containing 500 mL of 0.9% sodium chloride injection.

Following dilution, ocrelizumab infusion solution should be administered immediately; if not used immediately, the solution may be stored under refrigeration (2–8°C) for up to 24 hours followed by an additional 8 hours (including infusion time) at room temperature (up to 25°C). The diluted solution should be brought to room temperature prior to the start of infusion. In the event that an infusion cannot be completed in the same day, the remaining solution should be discarded.

Ocrelizumab infusion should be administered through a separate IV line using a 0.2- or 0.22-μm inline filter. The manufacturer states that ocrelizumab solution is compatible with polyvinylchloride (PVC) and polyolefin bags and IV administration sets.

Rate of Administration The first 2 doses of ocrelizumab (300 mg) should be infused at an initial rate of 30 mL/hour; the infusion rate may be increased by 30 mL/hour every 30 minutes to a maximum rate of 180 mL/hour. Subsequent doses of ocrelizumab (600 mg) should be infused at an initial rate of 40 mL/hour; the infusion rate may be increased by 40 mL/hour every 30 minutes to a maximum rate of 200 mL/hour.

If infusion-related reactions occur, the infusion rate should be reduced or ocrelizumab therapy should be interrupted depending on the severity of the reaction. In patients experiencing a mild to moderate infusion-related reaction, the infusion rate should be reduced to half the rate at the onset of the infusion reaction, and the reduced rate should be maintained for at least 30 minutes; if this reduced rate is tolerated, the rate may be increased in the usually recommended increments and intervals. In patients experiencing a severe infusion-related reaction, the infusion should be immediately interrupted and appropriate symptomatic and supportive therapy provided; once the reaction has resolved, the infusion may be resumed at half the rate at the onset of the infusion reaction. If this reduced rate is tolerated, the rate may be increased in the usually recommended increments and intervals. If a life-threatening or disabling infusion reaction occurs, ocrelizumab therapy should be immediately and permanently discontinued and appropriate supportive treatment provided. (See Infusion Reactions under Cautions: Warnings/Precautions.)

■ **Dosage** ***Multiple Sclerosis*** For the management of relapsing or primary progressive forms of multiple sclerosis in adults, ocrelizumab therapy should be initiated with two 300-mg infusions administered 2 weeks apart. The recommended maintenance dosage of 600 mg once every 6 months should then be administered (starting 6 months after the first 300-mg dose).

If a dose is missed, the missed dose should be administered as soon as possible rather than waiting until the next scheduled dose. The schedule of administration should be adjusted to maintain the 6-month interval between maintenance doses. Doses must be separated by at least 5 months.

■ **Special Populations** The manufacturer makes no special population dosage recommendations at this time.

Dosage adjustment based on body weight is not necessary.

Cautions

■ **Contraindications** Ocrelizumab is contraindicated in patients with active hepatitis B virus (HBV) infection. Ocrelizumab also is contraindicated in patients with a history of life-threatening infusion reactions to the drug.

■ **Warnings/Precautions** ***Infusion Reactions*** Infusion-related reactions have been reported in patients receiving ocrelizumab. Such reactions can include pruritus, rash, urticaria, erythema, bronchospasm, throat irritation, oropharyngeal pain, dyspnea, pharyngeal or laryngeal edema, flushing, hypotension, pyrexia, fatigue, headache, dizziness, nausea, and tachycardia. In clinical studies of ocrelizumab for the management of multiple sclerosis (MS), infusion reactions were reported in 34–40% of patients who received the drug despite the use of premedication; serious reactions occurred in 0.3% of ocrelizumab-treated patients, in some cases requiring hospitalization. Infusion reactions occurred most commonly with the first infusion, and decreased in incidence and severity over subsequent doses.

Ocrelizumab should be administered only in settings where appropriate medical support is available for management of serious infusion-related reactions. Patients should receive appropriate premedication with a corticosteroid and an antihistamine, with or without an antipyretic. (See Dosage and Administration: General.) Patients should be monitored for infusion-related reactions during and for at least 1 hour after completion of each infusion and be advised that infusion reactions can occur up to 24 hours after the infusion. (See Advice to Patients.) Management of ocrelizumab-induced infusion reactions should be individualized based on the severity of the reaction. The drug should be immediately and permanently discontinued if a life-threatening infusion reaction occurs. For reactions of lesser severity, the infusion rate may be reduced, the infusion may be temporarily interrupted, and/or symptomatic treatment administered. (See Rate of Administration under Dosage and Administration: Administration.)

Infectious Complications Ocrelizumab may increase the risk of infection. In clinical studies, ocrelizumab increased the risk of upper and lower respiratory tract, skin, and herpes-related infections, but was not associated with an increased risk of serious infections. In active-controlled studies in patients with relapsing forms of MS, infections were reported in 58% of patients receiving ocrelizumab compared with 52% of those receiving interferon beta-1a. In the placebo-controlled study in patients with primary progressive MS (PPMS), infections were reported in 70% of patients receiving ocrelizumab compared with 68% of those receiving placebo. Infections were predominantly mild to moderate in severity. In patients with active infection, ocrelizumab therapy should be delayed until the infection resolves.

Respiratory tract infections occurred with greater frequency in ocrelizumab-treated patients than those who received interferon beta-1a or placebo and consisted mostly of mild to moderate upper respiratory infections; such infections were reported in 40 or 49% of patients with relapsing forms of MS or PPMS, respectively, who received the drug.

In clinical studies of patients with relapsing forms of MS, herpes infection was reported more frequently in patients receiving ocrelizumab than those receiving interferon beta-1a, and included oral herpes (3 versus 2.2%), herpes zoster (2.1 versus 1%), herpes simplex (0.7 versus 0.1%), and genital herpes (0.1 versus 0%). Among all herpes virus infections reported in the PPMS study, oral herpes occurred more frequently in ocrelizumab-treated patients than those who received placebo (2.7 versus 0.8%).

Although not reported in clinical studies of ocrelizumab, reactivation of HBV infection has been reported in patients receiving other anti-CD20 monoclonal antibodies and has resulted in fulminant hepatitis, hepatic failure, and death. All patients should be screened for HBV infection by testing for hepatitis B surface antigen (HBsAg) and hepatitis B core antibody (anti-HBc) before initiating treatment with ocrelizumab. Ocrelizumab is contraindicated in patients with active HBV infection confirmed by positive HBsAg and anti-HBc tests. Liver disease experts should be consulted prior to initiating and during ocrelizumab therapy in patients with any evidence of HBV infection (HBsAg-negative and anti-HBc-positive, or carriers of HBV [HBsAg-positive]).

Although not reported to date in clinical studies of ocrelizumab, progressive multifocal leukoencephalopathy (PML), an opportunistic infection of the brain caused by the JC virus, has been reported in patients receiving other anti-CD20 monoclonal antibodies and MS therapies. Patients who are immunocompromised or receiving multiple immunosuppressant therapies are at increased risk for PML. Symptoms typically associated with PML are diverse, progress over a period of days to weeks, and include progressive weakness on one side of the body or clumsiness of limbs, vision disturbances, confusion, and changes in cognition, memory, orientation, or personality. MRI signs of PML may be apparent before clinical manifestations develop. At the first sign or symptom suggestive of PML, ocrelizumab therapy should be withheld and an appropriate diagnostic evaluation performed.

Ocrelizumab may interfere with the safety and effectiveness of vaccines; patients should receive all necessary vaccinations prior to initiating the drug. (See Drug Interactions: Vaccines and also see Pregnancy under Warnings/Precautions: Specific Populations, in Cautions.)

Malignancy Ocrelizumab may increase the risk of malignancies. Malignancies, including breast cancer, were reported more frequently in patients receiving ocrelizumab (6 of 781 women) than those receiving interferon beta-1a or placebo (0 of 668 women) in controlled studies. The manufacturer recommends following standard breast cancer screening guidelines in patients receiving ocrelizumab.

Immunogenicity As with all therapeutic proteins, there is a potential for immunogenicity with ocrelizumab therapy. In controlled studies, anti-drug antibodies were detected in 12 of 1311 (approximately 1%) ocrelizumab-treated patients and neutralizing antibodies were detected in 2 of these patients. Clearance of ocrelizumab was increased and faster B-cell repletion was observed in the patients with neutralizing antibodies; however, antibody development did not appear to affect efficacy or safety of the drug.

Specific Populations **Pregnancy.** There are no adequate data regarding use of ocrelizumab in pregnant women; ocrelizumab may cause fetal harm. Increased perinatal mortality, depletion of B-cell populations, and renal, bone marrow, and testicular toxicity were observed in the offspring of monkeys administered ocrelizumab during pregnancy. Women of childbearing potential should use effective contraceptive measures during ocrelizumab therapy and for 6 months following the last dose of the drug.

Transient peripheral B-cell depletion and lymphocytopenia have been reported in infants born to women exposed to other anti-CD20 monoclonal antibodies during pregnancy. The effects of maternal exposure to ocrelizumab on infant B-cell levels are not known. However, the possibility that B-cell depletion may occur in infants born to women who received ocrelizumab during pregnancy should be considered; B-cell depletion can affect vaccine immune responses in infants. Prior to administering live or live attenuated vaccines to infants born to mothers treated with ocrelizumab during pregnancy, recovery of B-cell counts should be confirmed in these infants as measured by $CD19^+$ B cells. Inactivated vaccines may be administered as indicated to these infants prior to recovery from B-cell depletion, but consideration should be given to assessing the vaccine immune response in consultation with a qualified specialist to determine whether a protective immune response was mounted.

Lactation. It is not known whether ocrelizumab is distributed into human milk; the drug is distributed into milk in monkeys. The effects of ocrelizumab on nursing infants or on milk production are not known. The benefits of breast-feeding should be considered along with the importance of ocrelizumab to the woman and any potential adverse effects on the breast-fed infant from the drug or the underlying maternal condition.

Pediatric Use. Safety and efficacy of ocrelizumab have not been established in pediatric patients.

Geriatric Use. Clinical studies of ocrelizumab did not include sufficient numbers of patients 65 years of age or older to determine whether they respond differently than younger patients.

Hepatic Impairment. Data from clinical studies indicate that pharmacokinetics of ocrelizumab are not influenced by mild hepatic impairment.

Renal Impairment. Data from clinical studies indicate that pharmacokinetics of ocrelizumab are not influenced by mild renal impairment.

■ **Common Adverse Effects** Adverse effects reported in 5% or more of patients with relapsing forms of MS receiving ocrelizumab in clinical studies and with an incidence greater than that observed with interferon beta-1a include upper respiratory tract infection, infusion reaction, depression, lower respiratory tract infection, back pain, herpes virus infection, and pain in extremity.

Adverse effects reported in 5% or more of patients with PPMS receiving ocrelizumab in clinical studies and with an incidence greater than that observed with placebo include upper respiratory tract infection, infusion reaction, skin infection, lower respiratory tract infection, cough, diarrhea, peripheral edema, and herpes virus infection.

Drug Interactions

No formal drug interaction studies have been performed to date. Drug interactions mediated by cytochrome P-450 (CYP) enzymes, other metabolizing enzymes, or transporters are not expected.

■ **Immunosuppressive or Immunomodulatory Agents** Increased immunosuppression may occur with concomitant use of immunosuppressive or immunomodulatory agents, including immunosuppressant doses of corticosteroids. The risk of additive immune system effects must be considered if these therapies are administered concomitantly with ocrelizumab.

When switching patients from drugs with prolonged immune effects (e.g., daclizumab, fingolimod, mitoxantrone, natalizumab, teriflunomide) to ocrelizumab, the duration and mechanism of action of these drugs must be considered to avoid unintended additive immunosuppressive effects.

Ocrelizumab has not been studied in combination with other therapies for multiple sclerosis.

■ **Vaccines** Safety and effectiveness of live or live attenuated vaccines administered concomitantly with ocrelizumab have not been established; therefore, administration of these vaccines is not recommended during ocrelizumab therapy and until B-cell repletion occurs.

In a randomized open-label study, patients with relapsing forms of MS who were receiving ocrelizumab therapy at the time of vaccination with an inactivated vaccine (e.g., tetanus toxoid-containing vaccine, pneumococcal polysaccharide or conjugate vaccine, influenza virus vaccine inactivated) experienced attenuated antibody responses to the vaccine; the impact of this finding on vaccine effectiveness is not known.

Any necessary immunizations should be completed at least 4 weeks prior to initiation of ocrelizumab for live or live attenuated vaccines and, whenever possible, at least 2 weeks prior to initiation of ocrelizumab for inactivated vaccines. (See Pregnancy under Warnings/Precautions: Specific Populations, in Cautions.)

Description

Ocrelizumab, a recombinant humanized anti-CD20 monoclonal antibody, has immunomodulatory and disease-modifying activity in multiple sclerosis (MS); the drug is a glycosylated immunoglobulin G_1 (IgG_1). Although the exact mechanism of action of ocrelizumab in the management of MS has not been fully elucidated, the drug's immunomodulatory effects are thought to result from depletion of CD20-expressing B cells. There is increasing evidence suggesting that B cells play an important role in the pathogenesis of MS through various mechanisms (e.g., antigen presentation, autoantibody production, cytokine secretion). Ocrelizumab binds specifically to the large extracellular loop of CD20, a cell-surface antigen expressed on pre-B cells, mature B cells, and memory B cells; binding of ocrelizumab to CD20 triggers a host immune response consisting of antibody-dependent cell-mediated cytotoxicity (ADCC) and complement-dependent cytotoxicity (CDC), resulting in depletion of CD20-expressing B cells. Because CD20 is not expressed on lymphoid stem cells or plasma cells, B-cell reconstitution and preexisting humoral immunity are preserved.

Circulating $CD19^+$ B cells (used as a marker for B-cell counts) are depleted within 14 days of ocrelizumab infusion. In clinical studies, B-cell counts increased above baseline or the lower limit of normal (LLN) at least once between infusions of ocrelizumab in 0.3–4.1% of patients. Following completion of ocrelizumab therapy, median time to B-cell recovery to baseline or LLN was 72 weeks (range: 27–175 weeks). B-cell counts returned to baseline or LLN in 90% of patients within 2.5 years of the last infusion.

Ocrelizumab exhibits essentially linear and dose-proportional pharmacokinetics over the dosage range of 400 mg to 2 g. The metabolic pathway of ocrelizumab has not been characterized, but the drug is expected to be cleared principally by catabolism. The terminal half-life of ocrelizumab is 26 days. Pharmacokinetics of ocrelizumab are not substantially affected by gender, race, or body weight.

Advice to Patients

Importance of advising patients to read the manufacturer's patient information (medication guide).

Risk of infusion reactions; importance of informing patients that they will need to be monitored for at least 1 hour after each infusion. Patients should be advised that infusion reactions may occur up to 24 hours after each infusion and to immediately contact their clinician if they experience any manifestations of such a reaction (e.g., rash, urticaria, cough or wheezing, shortness of breath, difficulty breathing, swelling of the throat, flushing, dizziness, tachycardia).

Risk of infections; importance of advising patients to immediately contact their clinician if they develop any signs or symptoms of infection (e.g., fever, chills, cough, cold sores, shingles, genital sores) during or after ocrelizumab therapy.

Importance of informing patients that progressive multifocal leukoencephalopathy (PML) has occurred in patients treated with drugs that are similar to ocrelizumab and that the condition usually leads to death or severe disability over weeks or months. Importance of advising patients to inform their clinician if they develop any new or worsening neurologic symptoms suggestive of PML. (See Infectious Complications under Cautions: Warnings/Precautions.)

Risk of reactivation of hepatitis B virus (HBV) infection. Importance of informing patients that monitoring will be required if they are at risk.

Importance of advising patients that any necessary immunizations should be completed at least 4 weeks prior to initiation of ocrelizumab for live or live attenuated vaccines and, whenever possible, at least 2 weeks prior to initiation of ocrelizumab for inactivated vaccines. Administration of live or live attenuated vaccines is not recommended during ocrelizumab therapy and until B-cell recovery occurs.

Risk of malignancies, including breast cancer. Importance of advising patients to follow standard breast cancer screening guidelines.

Importance of women informing clinicians if they are or plan to become pregnant or plan to breast-feed. Advise women of childbearing potential of the need for effective contraception during therapy and for 6 months after the last dose of ocrelizumab.

Importance of informing clinicians of recent, existing, or contemplated concomitant therapy, including prescription and OTC drugs and dietary or herbal supplements (e.g., immunosuppressants or other treatments for multiple sclerosis), as well as any concomitant illnesses (e.g., active infections).

Importance of informing patients of other important precautionary information. (See Cautions.)

Overview® (see Users Guide). For additional information on this drug until a more detailed monograph is developed and published, the manufacturer's labeling should be consulted. It is *essential* that the manufacturer's labeling be consulted for more detailed information on usual cautions, precautions, contraindications, potential drug interactions, laboratory test interferences, and acute toxicity.

Preparations

Excipients in commercially available drug preparations may have clinically important effects in some individuals; consult specific product labeling for details.

Ocrelizumab

Parenteral

For injection concentrate, for IV Infusion	30 mg/mL (300 mg)	**Ocrevus®**, Genentech

Peginterferon Beta-1a

Pegylated interferon beta-1a
PEG-IFN beta-1a

■ Peginterferon beta-1a contains interferon beta-1a (recombinant DNA origin) covalently bound to polyethylene glycol (PEG); interferon beta-1a has immunomodulatory and disease-modifying activity in multiple sclerosis (MS).

For information on nonconjugated interferon beta, see Interferon Beta 92:20.

Uses

■ **Multiple Sclerosis** Peginterferon beta-1a is used in the management of relapsing forms of multiple sclerosis (MS; e.g., relapsing-remitting MS [RRMS]).

Peginterferon beta-1a is one of several disease-modifying therapies used in the management of RRMS. Although not curative, these therapies have all been shown to modify several measures of disease activity, including relapse rates, new or enhancing magnetic resonance imaging (MRI) lesions, and disability progression; results of placebo-controlled studies indicate that treatment with a disease-modifying agent can reduce the frequency of MS attacks by 28–68%. The American Academy of Neurology (AAN) recommends that disease-modifying therapy be offered to patients with RRMS who have had recent relapses and/or MRI activity; these experts state that the benefits versus risks (e.g., adverse effects or burden of taking a long-term medication) of treatment in patients who have not had relapses in 2 or more years and do not have active new MRI lesions are not known. Because CNS damage occurs early and continues throughout the course of MS, other clinicians recommend that disease-modifying therapy be initiated as soon as possible following diagnosis and continued indefinitely unless there is a clear lack of benefit, adverse effects are intolerable, the patient is unable to adhere to the recommended treatment regimen, or a more appropriate treatment becomes available. Clinicians should consider the adverse effects, tolerability, method of administration, safety, efficacy, and cost of the drugs in addition to patient preferences when selecting an appropriate disease-modifying therapy.

Efficacy and safety of peginterferon beta-1a have been established in a randomized, double-blind, multicenter, placebo-controlled study in approximately 1500 adults with RRMS. Results of this study demonstrated that peginterferon beta-1a was substantially more effective than placebo in reducing clinical relapse rates and also had a beneficial effect on several secondary outcome measures (i.e., disability progression, MRI findings). Patients included in this study had experienced at least 2 relapses in the previous 3 years with at least 1 relapse in the year prior to study entry; baseline characteristics were similar between the treatment groups (mean age 37 years, mean disease duration 3.6 years, mean Expanded Disability Status Scale [EDSS] score 2.46, 71% female). In the placebo-controlled portion of the study, patients received peginterferon beta-1a (125 mcg every 2 weeks or every 4 weeks) or placebo for 48 weeks; after this period, patients receiving placebo were re-randomized to one of the active peginterferon beta-1a treatment groups, and both groups continued to receive the drug for a total of 2 years. Neurologic examinations were performed at baseline, every 12 weeks, and at the time of suspected relapse, and MRI evaluations were performed at baseline and at 24 and 48 weeks. The primary efficacy end point was the annualized relapse rate over 1 year (i.e., total number of relapses divided by patient-years). Relapse was defined as new or recurrent neurologic symptoms not associated with fever or infection, not occurring within 30 days of the onset of other confirmed relapses, persisting for at least 24 hours, and accompanied by objective changes on neurologic exam.

At 48 weeks, the annualized relapse rate was substantially reduced with peginterferon beta-1a therapy compared with placebo. Although the study was not designed to compare the 2 different dosage regimens, a larger treatment effect was observed when the drug was administered every 2 weeks versus every 4 weeks. Patients who received peginterferon beta-1a 125 mcg every 2 weeks had an annualized relapse rate of 0.26 compared with a rate of 0.4 in those who received placebo (relative reduction of 36%). In addition, the proportion of patients with relapses or disability progression at 48 weeks was substantially reduced with peginterferon beta-1a compared with placebo. With regard to MRI outcomes, patients who received peginterferon beta-1a had substantially fewer new or enlarged T2-weighted hyperintense lesions and substantially fewer gadolinium-enhancing lesions than those who received placebo.

Overall results of the 2-year study demonstrated that the benefits of peginterferon beta-1a were maintained with long-term treatment. In patients who received peginterferon beta-1a 125 mcg every 2 weeks for 2 years, further reductions in the annualized relapse rate were observed in the second year of therapy.

Direct comparative studies between peginterferon beta-1a and nonconjugated interferon beta-1a or other drugs for the treatment of MS have not been performed to date; however, consistent benefits and effects generally have been observed among the various interferons used for MS.

Dosage and Administration

■ **Administration** Peginterferon beta-1a is administered by subcutaneous injection every 14 days into the abdomen, back of the upper arm, or thigh. Injection sites should be rotated to minimize the risk of injection site reactions. (See Injection Site Reactions under Cautions: Warnings/Precautions.)

Peginterferon beta-1a is commercially available as a single-dose prefilled injection pen or syringe containing 63, 94, or 125 mcg of the drug. Patients should be instructed on the proper techniques for self-administering subcutaneous injections using the prefilled injection pen or syringe. (See Advice to Patients.)

Prior to use, peginterferon beta-1a prefilled pens and syringes should be stored at 2–8°C in their original carton and protected from light; the drug should not be frozen. If refrigeration is not available, the prefilled pens and syringes may be stored at temperatures of 2–25°C for a period of up to 30 days; the drug products may be removed from and returned to refrigeration, if necessary, provided the total combined time out of refrigeration within a temperature range of 2–25°C does not exceed 30 days.

Prior to administration, peginterferon beta-1a should be allowed to reach room temperature (about 30 minutes). The prefilled pens and syringes are intended for single-use only; any unused portions should be discarded.

To prevent or reduce flu-like symptoms, analgesic and/or antipyretic agents may be administered prophylactically or concurrently with peginterferon beta-1a. (See Advice to Patients.)

■ **Dosage** Dosage of peginterferon beta-1a is expressed in terms of mcg of interferon beta-1a.

The recommended dosage of peginterferon beta-1a in adults with relapsing forms of multiple sclerosis (MS; e.g., relapsing-remitting MS [RRMS]) is 125 mcg every 14 days by subcutaneous injection. Therapy should be initiated at a low dosage and increased gradually up to this recommended maintenance dosage according to the following titration schedule: 63 mcg on the first day of therapy (day 1), 94 mcg 14 days later (day 15), and 125 mcg on day 29 and every 14 days thereafter.

The Plegridy® or Plegridy® Pen Starter Pack, which contains a 63 mcg prefilled injection pen or syringe, and a 94 mcg prefilled injection pen or syringe, is designed to be used during dosage titration.

■ **Special Populations** The manufacturer makes no specific dosage recommendations for patients with renal impairment; however, results of a pharmacokinetic study suggest that dosage adjustments are not necessary in such patients. (See Renal Impairment under Warnings/Precautions: Specific Populations, in Cautions.)

Dosage adjustments based on body weight, gender, or age are not required.

Cautions

■ **Contraindications** Peginterferon beta-1a is contraindicated in patients with known hypersensitivity to natural or recombinant interferon beta or peginterferon, or any other ingredient in the formulation.

■ **Warnings/Precautions** ***Hepatotoxicity*** Adverse hepatic effects ranging from asymptomatic, transient elevations in hepatic aminotransferases to more serious hepatic injury (e.g., hepatitis, autoimmune hepatitis, rare cases of hepatic failure) have been reported with interferon beta therapy.

Increased hepatic aminotransferase concentrations (ALT and AST) and hepatic injury were reported in patients receiving peginterferon beta-1a in controlled clinical studies. ALT elevations exceeding 5 times the upper limit of normal (ULN) occurred in 2% of patients receiving the drug (compared with 1% of placebo-treated patients), and AST elevations exceeding 5 times the ULN occurred in less than 1% of patients in both treatment groups. At least 2 patients had concurrent elevations of aminotransferase and total bilirubin concentrations, which resulted in acute liver failure in one of the cases; however, both patients recovered following discontinuance of the drug.

Patients receiving peginterferon beta-1a should be monitored for manifestations of hepatic injury.

Depression and Suicide Neuropsychiatric disorders, including depression, suicidal ideation, and suicide attempts, have been reported with increased frequency in patients receiving interferons, including interferon beta. In clinical studies of peginterferon beta-1a in patients with multiple sclerosis (MS), adverse events related to depression and suicidal ideation were reported in 8% of patients receiving the drug, but occurred with equal frequency in those receiving placebo; such events were considered serious in less than 1% of patients in both treatment groups.

Discontinuance of peginterferon beta-1a should be considered in patients who develop depression or other serious psychiatric symptoms during therapy.

Seizures Seizures have been reported in association with the use of interferon beta. In clinical studies of peginterferon beta-1a in patients with MS, seizures occurred in less than 1% of patients in both the active drug and placebo groups.

Peginterferon beta-1a should be used with caution in patients with preexisting seizure disorders.

Injection Site Reactions Injection site reactions are among the most common adverse effects associated with subcutaneous administration of interferon beta. In clinical studies, local injection site reactions (i.e., erythema, pain, pruritus, edema) occurred in 66% of patients receiving peginterferon beta-1a, and a serious injection site reaction was reported in 3% of the patients. Injection site necrosis occurred in at least one patient, but resolved with standard medical treatment.

The decision whether to discontinue therapy following a single site of necrosis should be based on the extent of necrosis. For patients who continue peginterferon beta-1a therapy after injection site necrosis has occurred, subsequent injections of the drug should not be made near the affected site until the lesion has fully healed. If multiple lesions occur, peginterferon beta-1a therapy should be discontinued until healing occurs.

Cardiovascular Effects Congestive heart failure and cardiomyopathy (with or without congestive heart failure) have occurred in patients receiving interferon beta. In clinical studies of peginterferon beta-1a in patients with MS, cardiovascular events were reported in 7% of patients in both the active drug and placebo groups. No serious cardiovascular events were reported in patients receiving peginterferon beta-1a.

Patients with substantial cardiac disease should be monitored for worsening of their condition during initiation and continued treatment with peginterferon beta-1a.

Hematologic Effects Decreased peripheral blood cell counts in all cell lines, including rare pancytopenia and thrombocytopenia, have been reported with interferon beta therapy. In clinical studies of peginterferon beta-1a, leukocyte counts less than 3000/mm^3 occurred in 7% of patients receiving the drug compared with 1% of those receiving placebo. Clinically important decreases in lymphocyte counts to below 500/mm^3, neutrophil counts to below 1000/mm^3, and platelet counts to below 100,000/mm^3 were observed in less than 1% of peginterferon beta-1a-treated patients in these studies. At least one patient had severe thrombocytopenia (platelet counts of 10,000/mm^3 or less) and one patient had severe neutropenia (neutrophil counts of 500/mm^3 or less); in both cases, the hematologic abnormality resolved after discontinuance of the drug.

Complete blood cell counts (CBC), including differential and platelets, should be monitored during peginterferon beta-1a therapy. In addition, patients receiving the drug should be monitored for infections, bleeding, and symptoms of anemia. Patients with myelosuppression may require more intensive monitoring of blood cell counts.

Thrombotic Microangiopathy Thrombotic microangiopathy (TMA), including sometimes fatal thrombotic thrombocytopenic purpura and hemolytic uremic syndrome, has been reported in patients receiving interferon beta therapy.

If clinical manifestations and/or laboratory findings consistent with TMA occur, peginterferon beta-1a should be discontinued and the patient managed as clinically indicated.

Autoimmune Diseases Autoimmune disorders of multiple target organs, including idiopathic thrombocytopenic purpura (ITP), hyperthyroidism, hypothyroidism, and autoimmune hepatitis, have been reported in patients receiving interferon beta therapy. In clinical studies of peginterferon beta-1a in patients with MS, the incidence of autoimmune disorders was less than 1% in both the active drug and placebo groups.

If a new autoimmune disorder develops in a patient receiving peginterferon beta-1a, discontinuance of the drug should be considered.

Immunogenicity As with all therapeutic proteins, there is a potential for immunogenicity with peginterferon beta-1a therapy. In the principal clinical study of peginterferon beta-1a in patients with MS, neutralizing antibodies were detected in less than 1% of patients who received the drug at the recommended dosage for 1 year. Approximately 7% of peginterferon beta-1a-treated patients developed antibodies to polyethylene glycol (PEG); however, the presence of these antibodies did not appear to affect overall exposure or pharmacodynamic response to the drug.

Sensitivity Reactions **Hypersensitivity.** Anaphylaxis and other serious allergic reactions have been reported rarely in patients receiving interferon beta, including peginterferon beta-1a. (See Cautions: Contraindications.) In clinical studies of peginterferon beta-1a, a serious allergic reaction (e.g., angioedema, urticaria) occurred in less than 1% of patients who received the drug; such reactions resolved promptly after treatment with antihistamines or corticosteroids.

Peginterferon beta-1a should be discontinued if a serious allergic reaction occurs.

Specific Populations **Pregnancy.** Category C. (See Users Guide.)

There are no adequate and well-controlled studies of peginterferon beta-1a in pregnant women; the drug should be used during pregnancy only if the potential benefits justify the possible risks to the fetus. Animal reproduction studies have not been conducted to date with peginterferon beta-1a; however, studies using nonconjugated interferon beta in pregnant monkeys demonstrated some abortifacient activity (at doses higher than recommended human doses), but no evidence of teratogenic or other adverse fetal effects.

A pregnancy registry has been established to monitor pregnancy outcomes in women exposed to peginterferon beta-1a during pregnancy. Patients should be encouraged to enroll in the registry by calling 866-810-1462 or visiting www.plegridypregnancyregistry.com.

Lactation. It is not known whether peginterferon beta-1a is distributed into human milk. Because many drugs are distributed into human milk, caution is advised when peginterferon beta-1a is used in nursing women.

Pediatric Use. Safety and efficacy of peginterferon beta-1a have not been established in pediatric patients.

Geriatric Use. Safety and efficacy of peginterferon beta-1a have not been established in geriatric patients.

Renal Impairment. Because of the possibility of increased drug exposure, patients with severe renal impairment should be monitored for adverse effects of peginterferon beta-1a. Results of a pharmacokinetic study indicated that systemic exposure to peginterferon beta-1a was increased by approximately 30, 40, or 53% in patients with mild (creatinine clearance 50–80 mL/minute), moderate (creatinine clearance 30–50 mL/minute), or severe (creatinine clearance less than 30 mL/minute) renal impairment, respectively, compared with individuals with normal renal function. However, these changes were considered to be marginal and not sufficient to warrant dosage adjustments.

In patients with end-stage renal disease undergoing hemodialysis 2 or 3 times a week, systemic exposure of peginterferon beta-1a was similar to that of individuals with normal renal function. Approximately 24% of a dose is removed during a hemodialysis session.

■ **Common Adverse Effects** Adverse effects reported in 10% or more of patients receiving peginterferon beta-1a and with an incidence at least 2% greater than placebo include injection site reactions (e.g., erythema, pain, pruritus), flu-like symptoms, pyrexia, headache, myalgia, chills, asthenia, and arthralgia.

Flu-like symptoms (reported in approximately 47% of patients) and injection site reactions (reported in approximately 66% of patients) were the most common adverse effects associated with peginterferon beta-1a.

Drug Interactions

Formal drug interaction studies have not been performed to date with peginterferon beta-1a.

Description

Peginterferon beta-1a is a biosynthetic (recombinant DNA origin) preparation of human interferon beta-1a covalently bound to polyethylene glycol (PEG). The interferon beta-1a portion of the drug is identical to that contained in commercially available interferon beta-1a (Avonex®). As a result of conjugation with PEG, clearance of the drug is reduced, systemic exposure is increased, and plasma half-life is prolonged, allowing for less frequent dosing compared with the nonconjugated interferon. According to the World Health Organization (WHO) standard, peginterferon beta-1a (Plegridy®) has a specific activity of approximately 100 million units of antiviral activity per mg of protein.

The mechanism of action of peginterferon beta-1a in the treatment of multiple sclerosis (MS) has not been fully elucidated; however, a variety of immunomodulating effects (e.g., inhibition of tumor necrosis factor or other cytokines, inhibition of T-cell proliferation, augmentation of suppressor T-cell function) have been described with interferon beta-1a.

Pharmacokinetic parameters of peginterferon beta-1a are subject to high interindividual variability. Dose-proportional increases in peak plasma concentrations and systemic exposure of the drug were observed following administration of single or multiple subcutaneous doses ranging from 63–188 mcg; accumulation of the drug did not occur after multiple-dose administration. Following subcutaneous administration of peginterferon beta-1a in patients with MS, peak plasma concentrations of the drug were achieved within 1–1.5 days. Peginterferon beta-1a is not extensively metabolized in the liver; renal excretion is the major route of elimination. The half-life of peginterferon beta-1a is approximately 78 hours in patients with MS. Body weight, gender, and age do not appear to affect pharmacokinetics of the drug.

Advice to Patients

Importance of patients reading the manufacturer's patient information (medication guide) and instructions for use before initiating treatment and each time the prescription is refilled.

Importance of taking peginterferon beta-1a exactly as prescribed. Advise patients not to change their dosage or administration schedule without consulting their clinician.

Importance of instructing patients regarding proper methods of preparation and self injection of peginterferon beta-1a, including the use of aseptic technique. Importance of providing instructions on the appropriate use, storage, and disposal of injection pens and needles.

Risk of hepatotoxicity; importance of advising patients to immediately inform their clinician if they experience any symptoms of liver injury (e.g., jaundice, nausea, loss of appetite, fatigue, unusual bleeding, confusion, somnolence, dark-colored urine, pale stools).

Risk of developing depression and suicidal ideation. Importance of patients immediately notifying their clinician if symptoms of depression or suicidal ideation occur.

Risk of seizures. Importance of patients immediately informing their clinician if a seizure occurs during therapy.

Risk of hypersensitivity reactions, including anaphylaxis. Importance of advising patients to seek immediate medical attention if any symptoms of hypersensitivity occur.

Risk of injection site reactions, including necrosis. Importance of patients immediately informing their clinician if any blue-black discoloration, swelling, or fluid drainage occurs in conjunction with skin breakage at the injection site.

Importance of informing patients that worsening of heart disease has occurred with interferon beta-1a therapy. Importance of informing patients of the symptoms of worsening heart failure and to immediately report any such symptoms to their clinician.

Importance of informing patients that flu-like symptoms (e.g., headache, muscle and joint aches, fever, chills, fatigue) are common following initiation of therapy with peginterferon beta-1a, and that concurrent administration of analgesics and/or antipyretics may minimize these symptoms.

Importance of women informing clinicians if they are or plan to become pregnant or plan to breast-feed. Encourage patients to enroll in the Plegridy® pregnancy registry if they become pregnant while taking the drug.

Importance of patients informing clinicians of existing or contemplated concomitant therapy, including prescription and OTC drugs, as well as any concomitant illnesses (e.g., liver disease, psychiatric disorders, seizures).

Importance of informing patients of other important precautionary information. (See Cautions.)

Overview® (see Users Guide). For additional information on this drug until a more detailed monograph is developed and published, the manufacturer's labeling should be consulted. It is *essential* that the manufacturer's labeling be consulted for more detailed information on usual cautions, precautions, contraindications, potential drug interactions, laboratory test interferences, and acute toxicity.

Preparations

Excipients in commercially available drug preparations may have clinically important effects in some individuals; consult specific product labeling for details.

Peginterferon Beta-1a

Parenteral

Injection, for subcutaneous use	125 mcg/0.5 mL	**Plegridy®** (available as single-dose prefilled syringe), Biogen
		Plegridy® Pen (available as single-dose prefilled pens), Biogen
Kit, injection, for subcutaneous use	1 syringe, 63 mcg/0.5 mL 1 syringe, 94 mcg/0.5 mL	**Plegridy® Starter Pack** (available as single-dose prefilled syringes), Biogen
	1 injection pen, 63 mcg/0.5 mL 1 injection pen, 94 mcg/0.5 mL	**Plegridy® Pen Starter Pack** (available as single-dose prefilled pens), Biogen

Teriflunomide

■ Teriflunomide, a pyrimidine synthesis inhibitor, has immunomodulatory and disease-modifying activity in multiple sclerosis. The drug is the active metabolite of leflunomide, an antirheumatic agent.

Uses

■ **Multiple Sclerosis** Teriflunomide is used orally to reduce the frequency of relapses in adults with relapsing forms of multiple sclerosis (MS; e.g., relapsing-remitting MS [RRMS]).

Teriflunomide is one of several disease-modifying therapies used in the management of RRMS. Although not curative, these therapies have all been shown to modify several measures of disease activity, including relapse rates, new or enhancing magnetic resonance imaging (MRI) lesions, and disability progression; results of placebo-controlled studies indicate that treatment with a disease-modifying agent can reduce the frequency of MS attacks by 28–68%. The American Academy of Neurology (AAN) recommends that disease-modifying therapy be offered to patients with RRMS who have had recent relapses and/or MRI activity; these experts state that the benefits versus risks (e.g., adverse effects or burden of taking a long-term medication) of treatment in patients who have not had relapses in 2 or more years and do not have active MRI lesions are not known. Because CNS damage occurs early and continues throughout the course of MS, other clinicians recommend that therapy be initiated as soon as possible following diagnosis and continued indefinitely unless there is a clear lack of benefit, adverse effects are intolerable, the patient is unable to adhere to the recommended treatment regimen, or a more appropriate treatment becomes available. Clinicians should consider the adverse effects, tolerability, method of administration, safety, efficacy, and cost of the drugs in addition to patient preferences when selecting an appropriate disease-modifying therapy.

Efficacy and safety of teriflunomide were demonstrated in 4 randomized, double-blind, placebo-controlled studies. The first 2 studies included patients with relapsing forms of MS who had at least 1 relapse in the previous year or at least 2 relapses in the previous 2 years. Patients were not permitted to receive interferon beta or any other MS therapy for a specified period of time prior to study entry as well as during the study. Baseline characteristics were similar in both studies; the mean age of patients was 38 years, mean disease duration was 5 years, and mean Expanded Disability Status Scale (EDSS) score at baseline was 2.7. The majority of patients had RRMS while a few patients had a progressive form of MS with relapses. Patients were randomized to receive once-daily doses of teriflunomide 7 mg, teriflunomide 14 mg, or placebo. Neurologic evaluations were performed at screening, every 12 weeks, and after suspected relapses.

In these 2 studies, teriflunomide (7 or 14 mg daily) substantially reduced the annualized relapse rate (the primary efficacy outcome) compared with placebo; relative reductions of 22–36% were observed across the studies. A consistent reduction in the annualized relapse rate also was observed in subgroups defined by gender, age group, prior MS therapy, and baseline disease activity. The risk of disability progression sustained for 12 weeks was substantially reduced in the teriflunomide 14 mg daily group compared with those receiving placebo. In one of the studies that evaluated the effect of teriflunomide on MRI measures of disease activity, both dosages were associated with substantially reduced total lesion volume and T1-weighted gadolinium-enhancing lesions compared with placebo.

In the third study, patients with a recent (within 90 days) first demyelinating event and 2 or more MRI lesions typical of MS were randomized to receive teriflunomide (7 or 14 mg daily) or placebo. The percentage of patients who remained relapse free was substantially greater in the teriflunomide-treated groups (70.5% in patients receiving the 7-mg dose and 72.2% in patients receiving the 14-mg dose) compared with those who received placebo (61.7%).

In the fourth study, the effect of teriflunomide on MRI activity was evaluated in 179 adults with relapsing MS. MRIs were performed at baseline and at 6, 12, 18, 24, 30, and 36 weeks. In this study, patients receiving teriflunomide 7 or 14 mg once daily for 36 weeks had a substantially lower mean number of unique active lesions (1.06 or 0.98, respectively) per brain MRI scan (which was the primary end point) during the 36-week treatment period compared with those receiving placebo (2.69).

Clinical experience to date suggests that teriflunomide has approximately similar efficacy and improved tolerability when compared with interferon beta in the treatment of RRMS. The efficacy of teriflunomide compared with other disease-modifying treatments for MS (e.g., dimethyl fumarate, fingolimod hydrochloride, glatiramer acetate, natalizumab) has not been fully evaluated to date.

The manufacturer states that concurrent use of teriflunomide with antineoplastic or immunosuppressive therapies (e.g., mitoxantrone, natalizumab)† used for the treatment of MS has not been evaluated to date. Safety studies in which teriflunomide was used in combination with other immunomodulating therapies (e.g., glatiramer acetate, interferon beta)† for up to one year did not reveal any specific safety concerns; however, the longer-term safety of these combinations in the treatment of MS remains to be established. (See Drug Interactions: Immunosuppressive and Immunomodulating Agents.)

Dosage and Administration

■ **Administration** Teriflunomide is administered orally once daily without regard to food.

■ **Dosage** The recommended dosage of teriflunomide in adults with relapsing forms of multiple sclerosis (MS; relapsing-remitting MS [RRMS]) is 7 or 14 mg once daily.

■ **Special Populations** The manufacturer states that no dosage adjustment is necessary for patients with mild, moderate, or severe renal impairment. Dose supplementation following hemodialysis or peritoneal dialysis also is unlikely to be necessary. (See Renal Impairment under Warnings/Precautions: Specific Populations, in Cautions.)

No dosage adjustment is necessary in patients with mild or moderate hepatic impairment. However, teriflunomide has not been studied in patients with severe hepatic impairment and use of the drug is contraindicated in such patients. (See Hepatotoxicity under Cautions: Warningsand also see Hepatic Impairment under Warnings/Precautions: Specific Populations, in Cautions.)

The manufacturer makes no specific dosage recommendations for geriatric patients. (See Geriatric Use under Warnings/Precautions: Specific Populations, in Cautions.)

■ **Accelerated Elimination Procedures** Teriflunomide is eliminated slowly from the plasma. Without an accelerated elimination procedure, it takes an average of 8 months to reach plasma concentrations less than 0.02 mcg/mL and, because of individual variations in drug clearance, it may take as long as 2 years. An accelerated elimination procedure may be used at any time following teriflunomide discontinuance. (See Accelerated Elimination Procedures under Cautions: Other Warnings and Precautions.)

The manufacturer states that elimination of teriflunomide may be accelerated by using either an oral cholestyramine or activated charcoal procedure.

Cholestyramine procedure: The manufacturer recommends that 8 g of cholestyramine be administered orally every 8 hours for 11 days. If this dosage of cholestyramine is not well tolerated, the manufacturer states that 4 g of cholestyramine may be administered orally 3 times daily instead.

Activated charcoal procedure: The manufacturer recommends that a suspension of 50 g of activated charcoal be administered orally every 12 hours for 11 days.

If either elimination procedure is poorly tolerated, the treatment days do not need to be consecutive unless teriflunomide plasma concentrations need to be reduced rapidly.

Following completion of the 11-day accelerated elimination procedures, both regimens successfully accelerated teriflunomide elimination, resulting in more than a 98% decrease in plasma concentrations of the drug.

Use of an accelerated elimination procedure may potentially result in a return of disease activity if the patient had been responding to teriflunomide therapy.

Cautions

■ **Contraindications** Teriflunomide is contraindicated in patients with severe hepatic impairment.

Teriflunomide is contraindicated in women who are pregnant and in women of childbearing potential not using reliable contraception.

Teriflunomide is contraindicated in patients with a history of hypersensitivity reaction to the drug, to leflunomide, or any ingredient in the formulations.

Because teriflunomide is the principal active metabolite of leflunomide, concurrent use of leflunomide is contraindicated in patients receiving teriflunomide therapy.

■ **Warnings/Precautions** *Warnings* **Hepatotoxicity.** Severe liver injury, including fatal liver failure and dysfunction, has been reported in some patients receiving leflunomide (an antirheumatic agent). (See Cautions: Hepatic Effects and Cautions: Precautions and Contraindications, in Leflunomide 92:36.) The manufacturer states that a similar risk is expected for teriflunomide as the recommended dosages of teriflunomide (the principal active metabolite of leflunomide) and leflunomide result in a similar range of plasma concentrations of teriflunomide. Patients with preexisting liver disease may be at increased risk of developing elevated serum transaminases when taking teriflunomide. Concomitant use of teriflunomide with potentially hepatotoxic drugs may increase the risk of severe liver injury.

In controlled clinical studies, increases in serum ALT concentrations exceeding 3 times the upper limit of normal (ULN) occurred in 5.8 and 6.2% of patients receiving teriflunomide 7 and 14 mg daily, respectively, and in 3.8% of those receiving placebo. ALT elevations usually occurred during the first year of teriflunomide therapy, and in half of the cases, returned to normal despite continued administration of the drug. In these studies, if the ALT elevation exceeded 3 times the ULN on 2 consecutive tests, teriflunomide was discontinued and patients underwent an accelerated elimination procedure. In the patients who underwent drug discontinuance and an accelerated elimination procedure, half of the cases returned to normal or near normal values within 2 months. One patient in these studies experienced ALT concentrations 32 times the ULN and jaundice for 5 months following initiation of teriflunomide 14 mg daily. The patient was hospitalized at 5 weeks and recovered following plasmapheresis and an accelerated elimination procedure with cholestyramine; teriflunomide-induced liver injury could not be ruled out.

The manufacturer states that patients with preexisting acute or chronic liver disease and those with ALT concentrations exceeding 2 times the ULN before initiating treatment should not normally be treated with teriflunomide. The drug is contraindicated in patients with severe hepatic impairment.

Transaminase and bilirubin concentrations should be obtained within 6 months prior to initiation of teriflunomide therapy. During the first 6 months of therapy, ALT concentrations should be monitored at least once monthly. Additional monitoring should be considered in patients concomitantly receiving other potentially hepatotoxic drugs. If serum transaminase concentrations exceed 3 times the ULN, discontinuance of teriflunomide should be considered. Serum transaminase and bilirubin concentrations should be monitored during teriflunomide therapy, especially in patients who develop signs or symptoms of hepatic dysfunction (e.g., unexplained nausea, vomiting, abdominal pain, fatigue, anorexia, jaundice, dark urine).

If teriflunomide-induced liver injury is suspected, the drug should be discontinued and an accelerated elimination procedure (see Dosage and Administration: Accelerated Elimination Procedures) should be initiated; liver function tests should be monitored weekly until the values return to normal. If teriflunomide is considered unlikely to have caused the ALT elevation because another probable cause of liver injury is identified, resumption of the drug may be considered.

Fetal/Neonatal Morbidity and Mortality. There are no human data regarding the developmental risks associated with use of teriflunomide during pregnancy; however, based on animal data, the drug may cause fetal harm (e.g., embryo-fetal death, skeletal variations, malformations). In animal reproductive studies, teriflunomide was shown to be teratogenic and embryolethal in multiple species when administered during pregnancy in dosages lower than those used clinically. Leflunomide (which is metabolized to teriflunomide) also has demonstrated embryolethality and teratogenic effects in animal reproduction studies. The mechanism of the drug's therapeutic effects is thought to also be involved in the mechanism of developmental toxicity. (See Description.)

Teriflunomide is contraindicated in pregnant women and women of childbearing potential who do not use effective contraception. Women of childbearing potential should use effective contraception during therapy and following discontinuance of the drug until it is verified that plasma concentrations are less than 0.02 mcg/mL. (See Pregnancy under Warnings/Precautions: Specific Populations, in Cautions.)

Teriflunomide is present in human semen; animal studies to evaluate the risk of male-mediated fetal toxicity have not been conducted to date. To minimize any possible risk, men receiving teriflunomide not wishing to father a child and their female partners should use reliable contraception. Men treated with teriflunomide who wish to father a child should discontinue the drug and either undergo an accelerated elimination procedure or wait until it is verified that plasma concentrations are less than 0.02 mcg/mL. (See Dosage and Administration: Accelerated Elimination Procedures.)

Other Warnings and Precautions **Accelerated Elimination Procedures.** Because it can take from 8 months to 2 years for plasma concentrations of teriflunomide to decrease to undetectable levels (less than 0.02 mcg/mL) following discontinuance of therapy, an accelerated elimination procedure should be used whenever faster removal of the drug is required or desirable. The manufacturer recommends use of an accelerated elimination procedure in all women of childbearing potential upon discontinuance of teriflunomide, in men who wish to father a child after discontinuance of teriflunomide, or when the drug is discontinued because of potentially serious adverse effects (e.g., suspected liver injury, serious infection, peripheral neuropathy, severe dermatologic reactions, new onset or worsening pulmonary symptoms). For more information on procedures to hasten elimination of teriflunomide following discontinuance of the drug, see Dosage and Administration: Accelerated Elimination Procedures.

If the patient responded to teriflunomide treatment, an accelerated elimination procedure may result in return of disease activity.

Hematologic Effects. A mean decrease in white blood cell count of approximately 15% (mainly neutrophils and lymphocytes) and in platelet count of approximately 10% was observed in teriflunomide-treated patients in placebo-controlled studies. In clinical studies, a neutrophil count less than 1500/mm^3 was observed in 12 and 16% of patients receiving teriflunomide 7 and 14 mg daily, respectively, compared with 7% of those receiving placebo; a lymphocyte count less than 800/mm^3 was observed in 10 and 12% of patients receiving teriflunomide 7 and 14 mg daily, respectively, compared with 6% of patients receiving placebo. Decreases in mean white blood cell count generally occurred during the first 6 weeks of therapy, and the white blood cell count remained low during treatment.

No cases of serious pancytopenia were reported in premarketing clinical trials of teriflunomide; however, rare cases of pancytopenia and agranulocytosis have been reported during postmarketing experience with leflunomide. A similar risk would be expected for teriflunomide since it is the main active metabolite of leflunomide. Thrombocytopenia (with platelet counts decreasing to less than 50,000/mm^3 in rare cases) has been reported during postmarketing experience with teriflunomide.

A complete blood cell count should be obtained within 6 months prior to initiation of treatment with teriflunomide. Further hematologic monitoring should be based on signs and symptoms suggestive of bone marrow suppression.

Risk of Infection/Tuberculosis Screening. Patients with active acute or chronic infections should not begin teriflunomide treatment until the infection is resolved. If a patient develops a serious infection during teriflunomide therapy, interruption of therapy and initiation of an accelerated elimination procedure should be considered. (See Dosage and Administration: Accelerated Elimination Procedures.) The risks and benefits of continuing teriflunomide should be reassessed prior to resumption of therapy. (See Advice to Patients.)

Teriflunomide is not recommended in patients with severe immunodeficiency, bone marrow disease, or severe, uncontrolled infections. Drugs with immunosuppressive potential, such as teriflunomide, may increase susceptibility to infections, including opportunistic infections. In clinical studies, no overall increase in the risk of serious infection was observed in patients receiving teriflunomide 7 or 14 mg daily (1.4 and 2.2%, respectively) compared with placebo (2.1%). However, one fatal case of *Klebsiella pneumoniae* sepsis occurred in a patient receiving teriflunomide 14 mg daily for 1.7 years. Reactivation of cytomegalovirus hepatitis also has been observed in clinical studies. In postmarketing experience with leflunomide, fatal infections, particularly *Pneumocystis jiroveci* (formerly *Pneumocystis carinii*) pneumonia and aspergillosis, were reported. Most of the reports were confounded by concomitant immunosuppressant therapy and/or comorbidities, in addition to rheumatoid disease, that may predispose patients to infection.

In clinical studies with teriflunomide, cases of tuberculosis were observed. Prior to initiation of teriflunomide therapy, patients should be screened for latent tuberculosis infection with a tuberculin skin test or blood test for mycobacterium tuberculosis infection. Teriflunomide has not been studied in patients with a positive tuberculosis screen and the safety of the drug in individuals with latent tuberculosis infection is unknown. Patients testing positive in tuberculosis screening should be treated with an appropriate antimycobacterial regimen prior to initiating teriflunomide therapy.

Vaccination. Limited clinical data are available regarding the efficacy and safety of vaccination in patients receiving teriflunomide. The manufacturer states that vaccination with live vaccines is not recommended in teriflunomide-treated patients. In addition, the long elimination half-life of teriflunomide should be considered when contemplating administration of a live vaccine after discontinuing the drug. (See Drug Interactions: Vaccines.)

Malignancy. The risk of malignancy, particularly lymphoproliferative disorders, is increased in patients receiving some immunosuppressant drugs. There is a potential for immunosuppression with teriflunomide. Although an increased incidence of malignancies and lymphoproliferative disorders has not been observed in patients receiving teriflunomide in clinical trials, larger and longer-term studies are needed to determine whether there is an increased risk of malignancy or lymphoproliferative disorders with the drug.

Peripheral Neuropathy. In clinical studies, peripheral neuropathy, including polyneuropathy and mononeuropathy (e.g., carpal tunnel syndrome), was reported more frequently in patients receiving teriflunomide compared with those receiving placebo; most cases were of mild or moderate severity. The incidence of peripheral neuropathy (confirmed by nerve conduction studies) was 1.4% (13 patients) in patients receiving teriflunomide 7 mg daily, 1.9% (17 patients) in patients receiving teriflunomide 14 mg daily, and 0.4% (4 patients) in those receiving placebo. Treatment was discontinued in 8 patients with peripheral neuropathy; 5 of the patients recovered following drug discontinuance. Some of the remaining cases of peripheral neuropathy did not resolve with continued teriflunomide therapy. Peripheral neuropathy also has been reported in leflunomide-treated patients.

Patients 60 years of age or older, patients receiving concomitant neurotoxic medications, and those with diabetes may have an increased risk of peripheral neuropathy. If a patient receiving teriflunomide develops symptoms consistent with peripheral neuropathy (e.g., bilateral numbness or tingling of hands or feet), discontinuance of teriflunomide and an accelerated elimination procedure should be considered. (See Dosage and Administration: Accelerated Elimination Procedures.)

Blood Pressure Increases. In placebo-controlled clinical studies, hypertension was reported in 3.1 or 4.3% of patients receiving teriflunomide 7 or 14 mg daily, respectively. Mean increases in systolic blood pressure were 2.3 and 2.7 mm Hg, and mean increases in diastolic blood pressure were 1.4 and 1.9 mm Hg in patients receiving 7 and 14 mg of the drug, respectively.

Blood pressure should be evaluated prior to initiation of teriflunomide and periodically thereafter. Elevated blood pressure should be appropriately managed during treatment with the drug.

Interstitial Lung Disease. Interstitial lung disease (including acute interstitial pneumonitis) has been reported during postmarketing experience with teriflunomide.

Interstitial lung disease and worsening of preexisting interstitial lung disease, sometimes fatal, also have been reported rarely in patients with rheumatoid arthritis receiving leflunomide. Interstitial lung disease may occur acutely at any time during therapy and has a variable clinical presentation.

In patients experiencing new or worsening pulmonary symptoms (e.g., cough, dyspnea) with or without associated fever, discontinuance of teriflunomide should be considered. If discontinuance is necessary, initiation of an accelerated elimination procedure should also be considered. (See Dosage and Administration: Accelerated Elimination Procedures.)

Sensitivity Reactions **Hypersensitivity.** Hypersensitivity reactions, including anaphylaxis and angioedema, have been reported with teriflunomide.

If any manifestations of anaphylaxis or angioedema occur during therapy, teriflunomide should be immediately discontinued and an accelerated elimination procedure performed (unless the reaction is clearly not drug related). (See Dosage and Administration: Accelerated Elimination Procedures.) Patients who experience a severe hypersensitivity reaction to teriflunomide should be not be re-exposed to the drug.

Serious Dermatologic Reactions. Serious skin reactions, including Stevens-Johnson syndrome and toxic epidermal necrolysis, have been reported in patients receiving teriflunomide; at least 1 fatality has occurred as a result.

If a serious skin reaction occurs, teriflunomide should be immediately discontinued and an accelerated elimination procedure performed (unless the reaction is clearly not drug related). (See Dosage and Administration: Accelerated Elimination Procedures.) Patients who experience a serious dermatologic reaction with teriflunomide should not be re-exposed to the drug.

Multi-organ Hypersensitivity. Multi-organ hypersensitivity (also known as drug reaction with eosinophilia and systemic symptoms [DRESS]) has been reported rarely with leflunomide (which is metabolized to teriflunomide). The clinical presentation typically includes fever associated with other organ system involvement (e.g., rash, lymphadenopathy, hepatic dysfunction, eosinophilia).

If manifestations of DRESS occur, teriflunomide should be immediately discontinued and an accelerated elimination procedure performed (unless the reaction is clearly not drug related). (See Dosage and Administration: Accelerated Elimination Procedures.) Patients who experience DRESS with teriflunomide should not be re-exposed to the drug.

Specific Populations **Pregnancy.** Because teriflunomide may cause fetal harm, the drug must not be used in pregnant women and in women of childbearing potential who are not using effective contraception. (See Cautions: Contraindications and also see Fetal/Neonatal Morbidity and Mortality under Warnings/Precautions: Warnings, in Cautions.) Pregnancy must be excluded prior to initiation of therapy in women of childbearing potential. In addition, such women should use effective contraception during and following discontinuance of therapy (until plasma concentrations of the drug are less than 0.02 mcg/mL since such concentrations are expected to have minimal embryofetal risk).

If pregnancy occurs during treatment, teriflunomide should be immediately discontinued and an accelerated elimination procedure should be performed. (See Dosage and Administration: Accelerated Elimination Procedures.) Under these conditions, the patient should be referred to an obstetrician/gynecologist, preferably with experience in reproductive toxicology, for further evaluation and counseling.

Women receiving teriflunomide who wish to become pregnant should discontinue the drug and undergo an accelerated elimination procedure; effective contraceptive methods should be used until it is verified that plasma teriflunomide concentrations are less than 0.02 mcg/mL.

A pregnancy registry has been established to monitor the pregnancy outcomes of women exposed to teriflunomide during pregnancy. Clinicians and patients are encouraged to report any such pregnancies to the registry by calling 800-745-4447, option 2.

Lactation. Teriflunomide is distributed into milk in rats. It is not known whether the drug is distributed into human milk. The benefits of breastfeeding should be considered along with the woman's clinical need for teriflunomide and any potential adverse effects on the nursing infant from the drug or underlying maternal condition.

Pediatric Use. Safety and effectiveness of teriflunomide in pediatric patients have not been established.

Geriatric Use. Clinical studies of teriflunomide did not include patients older than 65 years of age.

Hepatic Impairment. Mild and moderate hepatic impairment had no impact on the pharmacokinetics of teriflunomide. The pharmacokinetics of teriflunomide in patients with severe hepatic impairment have not been evaluated.

Because of the possible increased risk of hepatotoxicity, patients with preexisting acute or chronic liver disease or baseline serum ALT concentrations greater than 2 times the ULN before initiating therapy should not normally be treated with the drug. Teriflunomide is contraindicated in patients with severe hepatic impairment. (See Dosage and Administration: Special Populations and also see Hepatotoxicity under Warnings/Precautions: Warnings, in Cautions.)

Renal Impairment. Severe renal impairment had no clinically important effect on the pharmacokinetics of teriflunomide. In a limited number of patients receiving leflunomide, teriflunomide (leflunomide's active metabolite) was found to be only negligibly removed by peritoneal dialysis and hemodialysis. The manufacturer states that no dosage adjustment is necessary in patients with mild, moderate, or severe renal impairment.

■ **Common Adverse Effects** Adverse effects reported in 10% or more of patients receiving teriflunomide and with an incidence at least 2% greater than with placebo include increased ALT concentrations, alopecia (e.g., hair loss, hair thinning), diarrhea, influenza, nausea, and paresthesia.

If severe adverse effects (e.g., hepatotoxicity, serious skin reactions) occur, teriflunomide can be more rapidly cleared from the body by the use of an accelerated elimination procedure following discontinuance of the drug. (See Dosage and Administration: Accelerated Elimination Procedures.)

Drug Interactions

Teriflunomide is not metabolized by cytochrome P-450 (CYP) isoenzymes or flavin monoamine oxidase enzymes.

In vitro and in vivo studies suggest that teriflunomide is an inhibitor of CYP2C8 and an in vivo study suggests that the drug is a weak inducer of CYP1A2.

Teriflunomide is an inhibitor of the efflux transporter breast cancer resistant protein (BCRP), organic anion transporting polypeptide (OATP) 1B1, OATP 1B3, and organic anion transporter 3 (OAT3).

Because it can take up to 2 years for plasma concentrations of teriflunomide to decrease to undetectable concentrations following discontinuance of the drug, the possibility exists that drug interactions could occur in patients who are no longer receiving therapy with the drug. The risk of such drug interactions can be reduced by use of an accelerated elimination procedure to hasten elimination of teriflunomide after discontinuance of therapy. (See Dosage and Administration: Accelerated Elimination Procedures.)

■ **Drugs Affecting or Metabolized by Hepatic Microsomal Enzymes** Teriflunomide did not affect the pharmacokinetics of bupropion (a CYP2B6 substrate), midazolam (a CYP3A4 substrate), *S*-warfarin (a CYP2C9 substrate), omeprazole (a CYP2C19 substrate), or metoprolol (a CYP2D6 substrate).

CYP2C8 Substrates When a single dose of repaglinide (0.25 mg), a CYP2C8 substrate, was administered following repeated doses of teriflunomide, mean peak plasma concentrations and area under the plasma concentration-time curve (AUC) of repaglinide were increased 1.7- and 2.4-fold, respectively.

The manufacturer recommends that teriflunomide-treated patients receiving concomitant drugs that are metabolized by CYP2C8 (e.g., paclitaxel, pioglitazone, repaglinide, rosiglitazone) be monitored since the exposure of such drugs may be increased; dosage of the concomitant drug should be adjusted accordingly.

CYP1A2 Substrates Repeated doses of teriflunomide decreased peak concentrations and AUC of caffeine (a CYP1A2 substrate and probe) by 18 and 55%, respectively. When teriflunomide is used concomitantly with drugs metabolized by CYP1A2 (e.g., alosetron, duloxetine, theophylline, tizanidine), patients should be monitored since the exposure of such drugs may be reduced; dosage of the concomitant drug should be adjusted accordingly.

■ **Drugs Transported by Organic Anion Transporters and Organic Anion-Transporting Polypeptide** Teriflunomide can increase systemic exposure of drugs that are substrates of OAT3 (e.g., cefaclor, cimetidine, ciprofloxacin, penicillin G, ketoprofen, furosemide, methotrexate, zidovudine) or substrates of OATP (e.g., methotrexate, rifampin, atorvastatin, nateglinide, pravastatin, repaglinide, simvastatin). If used concomitantly, patients should be monitored closely for signs of increased exposure to these substrate drugs and dosage should be adjusted accordingly.

■ **Drugs Transported by Breast Cancer Resistance Protein** Teriflunomide can increase systemic exposure of drugs that are substrates of BCRP (e.g., rosuvastatin, mitoxantrone). If used concomitantly, patients should be monitored closely for signs of increased exposure to these substrate drugs and dosage should be adjusted accordingly. Dosage of rosuvastatin should not exceed 10 mg daily when used concomitantly with teriflunomide.

■ **Hepatotoxic Agents** Concomitant administration of teriflunomide with other potentially hepatotoxic drugs may increase the risk of adverse hepatic effects. The manufacturer states that additional monitoring of liver function tests should be considered when teriflunomide is administered with other potentially hepatotoxic drugs. (See Hepatotoxicity under Warnings/Precautions: Warnings, in Cautions.)

■ **Immunosuppressive and Immunomodulating Agents** The manufacturer states that concurrent use of teriflunomide with antineoplastic or immunosuppressive therapies (e.g., mitoxantrone, natalizumab) used in the treatment of multiple sclerosis (MS) has not been evaluated to date. Safety studies in which teriflunomide was used with other immunomodulating therapies (e.g., glatiramer acetate, interferon beta) for up to one year did not reveal any specific safety concerns; however, the longer-term safety of these combinations in the treatment of MS remains to be established.

In any situation in which the decision is made to switch from teriflunomide to another agent with a known potential for hematologic suppression, it would be advisable to monitor for hematologic toxicity since there will be overlapping systemic exposure to both drugs. Use of an accelerated elimination procedure may decrease this risk, but may also result in a return of disease activity if the patient was responding to teriflunomide therapy. (See Dosage and Administration: Accelerated Elimination Procedures.)

■ **Neurotoxic Agents** Concomitant administration of teriflunomide with other potentially neurotoxic drugs (e.g., bortezomib, etanercept, infliximab, ixabepilone, oxaliplatin, linezolid) may increase the risk of peripheral neuropathy. (See Peripheral Neuropathy under Cautions: Other Warnings and Precautions.)

■ **Caffeine** Repeated doses of teriflunomide decreased peak concentrations and AUC of caffeine (a CYP1A2 substrate and probe) by 18 and 55%, respectively.

■ **Cholestyramine and Activated Charcoal** Oral administration of cholestyramine or activated charcoal in teriflunomide-treated individuals reduces the plasma concentration and hastens elimination of the drug. Following completion of 11-day accelerated elimination procedures, either drug successfully accelerated teriflunomide elimination, resulting in more than a 98% decrease in plasma concentrations of teriflunomide. (See Dosage and Administration: Accelerated Elimination Procedures and also see Accelerated Elimination Procedures under Cautions: Other Warnings and Precautions.)

■ **Leflunomide** Teriflunomide is the main active metabolite of leflunomide; therefore, additive toxicity would be expected with combined use of these drugs. The manufacturer states that concurrent administration of teriflunomide and leflunomide is contraindicated.

■ **Oral Contraceptives** Repeated doses of teriflunomide increased mean peak concentrations and AUC of ethinyl estradiol by 1.58- and 1.54-fold, respectively, and levonorgestrel by 1.33- and 1.41-fold, respectively. Consideration should be given to the type or dosage of oral contraceptives used concurrently with teriflunomide. (See Pregnancy under Warnings/Precautions: Specific Populations, in Cautions.)

■ **Rifampin** Rifampin, a potent CYP and transporter inducer, does not affect the pharmacokinetics of teriflunomide.

■ **Vaccines** Limited clinical data are available on the efficacy and safety of vaccinations in patients receiving teriflunomide. The manufacturer states that vaccination with live vaccines is not recommended during teriflunomide therapy and for at least 6 months following discontinuance of the drug. The manufacturer cautions that the prolonged elimination half-life of teriflunomide should be taken into account when considering administration of a live vaccine following discontinuance of teriflunomide.

Effective influenza vaccination is important in patients with MS because influenza can cause serious complications and is associated with a higher incidence of exacerbations in such patients. In the multicenter, multinational Teriflunomide and Vaccination (TERIVA) study, 128 adults with MS receiving teriflunomide 7 mg daily, teriflunomide 14 mg daily, or a stabilized dosage of interferon beta-1 (Avonex®, Betaseron®, Genfaxone® [not commercially available in the US], or Rebif®) for more than 6 months were vaccinated with influenza virus vaccine inactivated (exact formulation was chosen based on national standards). Patients in all 3 treatment groups were generally found to mount an acceptable immune response to seasonal influenza vaccination and the vaccine was found to be well tolerated.

■ **Warfarin** Repeated dosing of teriflunomide did not affect the pharmacokinetics of *R*- and *S*-warfarin (a CYP2C9 substrate) in a study in healthy individuals. However, peak international normalized ratio (INR) was decreased by 25% during concomitant administration compared with warfarin alone. When warfarin is used concomitantly with teriflunomide, the manufacturer recommends close INR follow-up and monitoring.

Description

Teriflunomide is the principal active metabolite of leflunomide (an antirheumatic agent) and is responsible for leflunomide's pharmacologic activity in vivo. Both teriflunomide and leflunomide are pyrimidine synthesis inhibitors that act as an immunomodulatory agents with anti-inflammatory properties. Teriflunomide reversibly inhibits dihydroorotate dehydrogenase, an important mitochondrial enzyme involved in de novo pyrimidine synthesis, which results in reduced pyrimidine ribonucleotide concentrations and reduced proliferation of activated lymphocytes. Although the exact mechanism of action of teriflunomide in the management of multiple sclerosis has not been fully elucidated, it may involve, at least in part, a reduction in the number of activated lymphocytes in the CNS. For additional information on the pharmacologic effects of teriflunomide and leflunomide, see Pharmacology: Immunomodulating Effects, in Leflunomide 92:36.

At recommended dosages, teriflunomide and leflunomide produce similar plasma concentrations of teriflunomide. Following oral administration of teriflunomide, median time to achieve peak plasma concentrations of teriflunomide ranges from 1–4 hours. Steady-state concentrations of the drug are achieved in approximately 3 months. Food does not have a clinically relevant effect on teriflunomide pharmacokinetics. Teriflunomide is highly bound (greater than 99%) to plasma proteins and is mainly distributed to plasma. The primary biotransformation pathway to minor metabolites is hydrolysis; secondary pathways include oxidation, *N*-acetylation, and sulfate conjugation. The elimination half-life of teriflunomide is approximately 18 or 19 days following repeated doses of 7 or 14 mg of the drug, respectively. Because the prolonged half-life of teriflunomide is mainly due to enterohepatic recirculation, an accelerated elimination procedure may be used to shorten the effective half-life of the drug (see Dosage and Administration: Accelerated Elimination Procedures). Approximately 60% of the total administered radioactivity was recovered with 37.5% in feces (mainly as unchanged drug) and 22.6% in urine within 21 days. Following an accelerated elimination procedure with cholestyramine, an additional 23.1% of the dose was recovered (mostly in feces).

Advice to Patients

Importance of providing a copy of the teriflunomide medication guide to the patient each time the drug is dispensed; importance of patient reading the medication guide prior to initiating teriflunomide therapy and each time the prescription is refilled.

Importance of patients being counseled on and understanding the benefits and potential risks of treatment with teriflunomide. Importance of advising patients not to discontinue teriflunomide without first talking with their clinician.

Importance of informing patients of the potential for hepatotoxic effects and the need for monitoring of liver enzymes prior to initiating teriflunomide and for at least 6 months while they are receiving the drug. Importance of reporting signs or symptoms of hepatotoxicity such as unexplained nausea, vomiting, fatigue, anorexia, jaundice, and/or dark urine to their clinician.

Risk of fetal harm (based on animal studies). Importance of advising women of childbearing potential of the need for effective contraception during teriflunomide treatment and until completion of an accelerated elimination procedure. Women of childbearing potential should also be informed that an accelerated elimination procedure can be used at any time after discontinuance of teriflunomide. Women of childbearing potential should be advised to notify their clinician immediately if they experience any delay in menses or believe they may be pregnant. Importance of informing women who become pregnant while taking teriflunomide about the existence of the Aubagio® pregnancy registry. Importance of instructing men who are taking teriflunomide and wish to father a child to discontinue teriflunomide and use an accelerated elimination procedure. Importance of instructing men taking teriflunomide who do not wish to father a child that they and their female partners should use reliable contraception. (See Fetal/Neonatal Morbidity and Mortality under Warnings/Precautions: Warnings, in Cautions and see also Pregnancy under Warnings/Precautions: Specific Populations, in Cautions.)

Importance of women informing clinicians if they plan to breast-feed.

Importance of informing patients that teriflunomide may stay in the blood for up to 2 years following the last dose and that an accelerated elimination procedure may be used if needed.

Possible increased risk of infections. Importance of informing patients that teriflunomide may lower the number of leukocytes in their blood and that their clinician may check their blood counts before initiating teriflunomide therapy. Importance of advising patients to contact their clinician if they develop any symptoms of infection (e.g., fever, tiredness, body aches, chills, nausea, vomiting), particularly if they develop fever.

Advise patients that some vaccines should be avoided during treatment with teriflunomide and for at least 6 months after discontinuing the drug.

Risk of peripheral neuropathy. Patients should be advised to contact their clinician if they develop symptoms of peripheral neuropathy (e.g., numbness or tingling of the hands or feet) that are different from their multiple sclerosis symptoms.

Risk of serious allergic reactions; importance of advising patients to immediately discontinue the drug and seek medical attention if any manifestations of hypersensitivity reactions occur (e.g., dyspnea, urticaria, angioedema, skin rash).

Importance of informing patients that teriflunomide may increase blood pressure.

Risk of acute renal failure. Importance of advising patients to contact their clinician if they experience pain in their side (i.e., flank pain).

Risk of hyperkalemia. Importance of advising patients to contact their clinician if they experience persistent nausea or an increase in heart rate.

Risk of interstitial lung disease. Importance of advising patients to contact their clinician if they experience shortness of breath or coughing with or without fever.

Importance of informing clinician of existing or contemplated concomitant therapy, including prescription and OTC drugs and herbal supplements, as well as any concomitant illnesses.

Importance of informing patients of other important precautionary information. (See Cautions.)

Overview® (see Users Guide). For additional information on this drug until a more detailed monograph is developed and published, the manufacturer's labeling should be consulted. It is *essential* that the manufacturer's labeling be consulted for more detailed information on usual cautions, precautions, contraindications, potential drug interactions, laboratory test interferences, and acute toxicity.

Preparations

Excipients in commercially available drug preparations may have clinically important effects in some individuals; consult specific product labeling for details.

Teriflunomide

Oral		
Tablets, film-coated	7 mg	**Aubagio®**, Genzyme
	14 mg	**Aubagio®**, Genzyme

†Use is not currently included in the labeling approved by the US Food and Drug Administration

Thalidomide

■ Thalidomide, a synthetic glutamic acid derivative, is an immunomodulatory agent with anti-inflammatory, antiangiogenic, and sedative and hypnotic activity; the drug is also a potent teratogen.

REMS

FDA approved a REMS for thalidomide to ensure that the benefits outweigh the risks. The REMS may apply to one or more preparations of thalidomide and consists of the following: elements to assure safe use and implementation system. See the FDA REMS page (http://www.accessdata.fda.gov/scripts/cder/rems/index.cfm) or the ASHP REMS Resource Center (https://www.ashp.org/REMS).

Uses

■ **Overview** Thalidomide is labeled by the US Food and Drug Administration (FDA) for acute treatment of cutaneous manifestations of moderate to severe erythema nodosum leprosum (ENL) in leprosy patients and for maintenance therapy for prevention and suppression of cutaneous manifestations of ENL recurrence. The drug has been designated an orphan drug by FDA for the treatment of ENL and treatment and maintenance of reactional lepromatous leprosy. Thalidomide also is used for the treatment of multiple myeloma and is designated an orphan drug by FDA for use in this condition. Thalidomide also has been designated an orphan drug by FDA for treatment of wasting syndrome associated with human immunodeficiency virus (HIV) infection†; prevention and treatment of severe recurrent aphthous stomatitis in severely, terminally immunocompromised patients†; prevention and treatment of graft-versus-host disease in patients receiving bone marrow transplantation†; treatment of clinical manifestations of mycobacterial infection caused by *Mycobacterium tuberculosis* and nontuberculous mycobacteria†; treatment of Crohn's disease†; and treatment of primary brain tumors†. In addition, thalidomide has been used for the treatment of a variety of inflammatory and/or dermatologic disorders, treatment of various HIV-associated conditions, and treatment of various malignancies. Use of thalidomide may not limit disease progression and/or death.

Restricted Distribution Because thalidomide is a known human teratogen and can cause severe, life-threatening birth defects or fetal death if given during pregnancy (see Teratogenic Effects under Pregnancy, Fertility, and Lactation: Pregnancy, in Cautions), the drug was approved by the FDA for marketing in the US in 1998 only under a special restricted distribution program, the System for Thalidomide Education and Prescribing Safety (STEPS), designed to help ensure the safe and effective prescribing, dispensing, and use of commercially available thalidomide. In the US, the STEPS distribution program restricts access to commercially available thalidomide to prescribing clinicians, pharmacies, and patients who are registered in the program and mandates compliance with registration, education, and safety requirements of the program. (See Dosage and Administration: Restricted Distribution Program.) The STEPS program minimizes, but may not completely eliminate, the risk that thalidomide may inadvertently be given to a pregnant woman. Thalidomide also is available in the US for use in clinical trials under protocol conditions. *The risks versus benefits of thalidomide must be addressed each time use of the drug is being considered.*

Past and Current Therapeutic Perspective In the late 1950s, thalidomide was marketed in several other countries, including the United Kingdom and Canada, and was available over-the-counter in some countries (e.g., Germany) for use as a sedative and for the treatment of various conditions, including asthma, hypertension, migraine, and common symptoms of early pregnancy (e.g., morning sickness), often in combination with other drugs. Thalidomide was being used in clinical studies in the US, but did not receive FDA approval at that time principally because of European reports of thalidomide-associated peripheral neuropathy that may be irreversible and unanswered questions about potential adverse effects on fetuses. Because of thalidomide's prompt sedative effects, lack of hangover, and apparent safety (in regards to overdosage), the drug was considered to be a safe alternative to barbiturates, and its manufacturer at that time promoted it as a nontoxic drug with no adverse effects, and completely safe for administration to pregnant women. However, reports of serious adverse effects soon appeared and use of thalidomide was linked to an epidemic of severe and often fatal fetal and neonatal malformations (most frequently phocomelia) that affected children in 46 countries.During that time, 17 babies were born in the US with thalidomide-associated phocomelia to mothers who received the drug from overseas sources or received premarketing samples distributed by drug company representatives. In 1961, the manufacturer withdrew thalidomide from the world market.

A few years later, there were reports that leprosy patients with inflammatory lesions related to ENL reactions had experienced improvement in these lesions while receiving thalidomide as a sedative. The discovery of thalidomide's therapeutic efficacy in the treatment of ENL led to investigations that revealed the anti-inflammatory and immunomodulatory effects of the drug and prompted studies evaluating the drug in various autoimmune or inflammatory diseases and various conditions in HIV-infected patients. In addition, after in vitro and animal studies indicated that thalidomide has anti-angiogenesis activity, investigations were initiated to evaluate use of the drug for a variety of neoplastic diseases. Most information to date regarding use of thalidomide for the treatment of inflammatory or immune disorders or for the treatment of patients with HIV infection or malignancy consists of case reports or data obtained from uncontrolled studies in a limited number of patients. Well-controlled clinical studies are needed to evaluate the safety and efficacy of thalidomide for the treatment of these various indications.

■ **Erythema Nodosum Leprosum** Thalidomide is used for acute treatment of cutaneous manifestations of moderate to severe erythema nodosum leprosum (ENL) reactions (lepra type 2 reactions) in leprosy patients, and also is used for maintenance therapy for prevention and suppression of cutaneous manifestations of ENL recurrence. Thalidomide has been used in conjunction with corticosteroid therapy for the acute treatment of ENL reactions that include moderate to severe neuritis in addition to cutaneous manifestations; however, thalidomide should *not* be used alone as monotherapy for treatment of ENL reactions complicated by neuritis. In these situations, thalidomide generally is initiated in conjunction with systemic corticosteroid therapy and the corticosteroid is slowly withdrawn if neuritis resolves.

ENL is a recurrent, immunologically mediated syndrome that occurs principally in patients with multibacillary leprosy. While ENL reactions have been reported to occur in 10–50% of lepromatous leprosy patients and 25–30% of borderline lepromatous patients, these reactions are being reported less frequently in patients receiving the currently recommended multidrug antileprosy regimens that include clofazimine than in those who received dapsone monotherapy. ENL usually occurs after initiation of anti-infective therapy for leprosy (generally within the first 2 years of treatment), although occasionally it may occur spontaneously in untreated lepromatous leprosy patients or after treatment is discontinued. These reactions are considered to be a manifestation of the disease rather than an adverse reaction to antileprosy regimens. Clinical symptoms include cutaneous papules or nodules that are painful or tender, erythematous, and histologically vasculitic; the papules may pustulate and ulcerate, appear as recurrent crops, and are widely distributed, generally appearing on extensor surfaces of the extremities and on the face. Cutaneous symptoms of ENL may be accompanied by peripheral neuritis (usually of the ulnar nerve), fever, malaise, wasting, uveitis, lymphadenitis orchitis, and glomerulonephritis. Histologically, ENL is an acute vasculitis or panniculitis that is thought to be secondary to immune (i.e., antigen-antibody) complex deposition.

Depending on the severity of manifestations, ENL reactions generally are treated using analgesics, corticosteroids, and/or thalidomide; clofazimine also has anti-inflammatory effects and is beneficial in the treatment of ENL reactions. While mild ENL reactions in some patients may be adequately managed with a nonsteroidal anti-inflammatory agent (e.g., aspirin, indomethacin) and bedrest, moderate to severe ENL reactions generally are treated with corticosteroids and/or thalidomide, and hospitalization may be required. The antileprosy regimen usually is continued while the ENL reaction is treated. Corticosteroid therapy (usually prednisolone) generally is effective for the treatment of moderate and severe ENL and usually is necessary when ENL is complicated by neuritis; however, long-term therapy may be required and there is a risk that ENL patients (especially those with chronic ENL) may become steroid dependent.

In patients already receiving clofazimine as part of a multidrug antileprosy regimen, a temporary increase in clofazimine dosage may allow a reduction in corticosteroid requirements; clofazimine dosage effective for the treatment of ENL reactions is slightly higher than that usually recommended for the treatment of leprosy. However, clofazimine is not as effective or as rapidly acting as corticosteroids or thalidomide in the treatment of ENL and should not be initiated as the sole agent for the treatment of severe ENL.

Thalidomide is effective for the treatment of moderate to severe ENL reactions, and some clinicians suggest that thalidomide may be the drug of choice for the treatment of these reactions, especially severe, recurrent reactions, in part because a prompt response to thalidomide generally is obtained and because of concerns related to long-term use of corticosteroids in leprosy patients. However, the risks versus benefits of thalidomide therapy must be considered, especially in women of childbearing age. Early diagnosis and treatment of ENL is important since these reactions are associated with considerable morbidity, especially if chronic, recurrent ENL occurs. Therapy for leprosy and leprosy reactional states should be undertaken in consultation with an expert in the treatment of leprosy. In the US, the Gillis W. Long Hansen's Disease Center at 800-642-2477 should be contacted for further information on the management of leprosy reactional states.

Information regarding safety and efficacy of thalidomide for the treatment of cutaneous manifestations of moderate to severe ENL is derived from more than 30 years of experience with the drug, open-label and controlled studies and case reports involving leprosy patients from many different countries, and a retrospective study of leprosy patients treated in the US by the US Public Health Service (USPHS). There is evidence that use of thalidomide in leprosy patients with moderate to severe ENL reactions can result in prompt resolution of the signs and symptoms of ENL, and the drug has been effective in patients with severe chronic ENL refractory to corticosteroid therapy. In one controlled study in patients with ENL cutaneous lesions who received 7-day regimens of thalidomide (400 mg daily) or placebo, a response (i.e., complete remission of symptoms or advanced remission of about 50% of existing ENL skin lesions) occurred in 66 or 9% of treatment courses in patients receiving thalidomide or placebo, respectively. In a similar study, a complete response (i.e., the absence of skin lesions) occurred in 75 or 25% of treatment courses in patients receiving thalidomide or aspirin, respectively.

In a double-blind, placebo-controlled, randomized, dose-comparison study, 22 male patients with ENL received 6 capsules containing either 100 mg (group A; 12 patients) or 300 mg (group B; 10 patients) of thalidomide for 1 week. A 6-week, 4-capsules per day tapering followed in which patients in group A received a 50-mg thalidomide dosage daily in weeks 2 and 3, followed by placebo capsules in weeks 4 through 7, while patients in group B received gradual dosage decreases every 2 weeks. Comparable improvement was observed at day 7 in 12 or 7 patients in group A or B, respectively. However, slower tapering in group B was associated with less reemergence of ENL through week 7 than patients in group A. Most patients developed new lesions soon after discontinuing treatment. Some clinicians suggest that slower tapering from a higher initial thalidomide dosage may improve ENL responses, although high recurrence rates after discontinuance indicate that further studies are needed to identify better tapering regimens.

Safety and efficacy of thalidomide have been evaluated in a prospective, comparative (versus prednisolone) study in 60 patients with moderate to severe ENL. Patients were randomized to receive a thalidomide dosage of 300 mg daily for 1 week, which was gradually reduced by 50 mg every 2 weeks (30 patients), or prednisolone 40 mg daily for 2 weeks, which was subsequently tapered by 10 mg every 2 weeks (30 patients). Faster clinical response (cutaneous and systemic), fewer relapses, and longer periods of remission were observed in patients receiving thalidomide compared with those receiving prednisolone. In addition, adverse effects were more frequently observed in patients receiving prednisolone than in those receiving thalidomide.

Efficacy of thalidomide for the treatment of chronic ENL reactions has been evaluated in 2 limited crossover studies of hospitalized, corticosteroid-dependent ENL patients who were receiving dapsone and were treated with a 4- to 6-week regimen of thalidomide (300 mg daily) or placebo. In the first crossover study, the weekly corticosteroid dosage could be reduced in about 89% of patients while thalidomide was administered, but corticosteroid dosage had to be increased when placebo was administered. In the second crossover study, 100 or 12.5% of patients decreased their weekly dosage of corticosteroids while receiving a 6-week regimen of thalidomide or placebo, respectively.

Information regarding safety and efficacy of thalidomide for the prevention of ENL relapse is limited, and labeling for this use is based on data obtained from a retrospective evaluation of ENL patients treated by the USPHS. A subset of these ENL patients receiving thalidomide had repeated relapse of ENL symptoms when thalidomide was discontinued, but remission of symptoms when treatment with the drug was reinitiated.

■ **Multiple Myeloma** ***Thalidomide and Dexamethasone*** Thalidomide is used in combination with dexamethasone for the treatment of newly diagnosed multiple myeloma. The efficacy of thalidomide is based on response rates; there are no data demonstrating a clinical benefit (e.g., improvement in survival). Efficacy of thalidomide in the treatment of multiple myeloma has been studied in a randomized, multicenter, open label study in 207 newly diagnosed patients. Patients were randomized to receive thalidomide (200 mg daily; 103 patients) and dexamethasone (40 mg once daily; 104 patients) on days 1–4, 9–12, and 17–20 every 28 days) or dexamethasone alone (40 mg once daily on days 1–4, 9–12, and 17–20 every 28 days). Each study population group received four 28-day cycles. Response rates, based on serum or urine paraprotein measurements, were higher in those receiving combination therapy with thalidomide and dexamethasone compared with those receiving dexamethasone alone (51.5 vs 35.6%, respectively).

Use of thalidomide in patients with multiple myeloma is associated with increased risk of venous thromboembolic events (e.g., deep venous thrombosis, pulmonary embolus). Such risk increases substantially when thalidomide is used in combination with standard chemotherapy, including dexamethasone. (See Cautions: Thromboembolic Events.)

Thalidomide, Bortezomib, and Dexamethasone Thalidomide also has been studied in combination with bortezomib and dexamethasone† (bortezomib-thalidomide-dexamethasone) as induction therapy for newly diagnosed multiple myeloma in transplant-eligible patients in several phase 3, open-label, randomized studies. The GIMEMA and PETHEMA/GEM studies compared bortezomib-thalidomide-dexamethasone with the combination of thalidomide and dexamethasone (thalidomide-dexamethasone), whereas the IFM2013-04 study compared bortezomib-thalidomide-dexamethasone with the combination of bortezomib, cyclophosphamide, and dexamethasone (bortezomib-cyclophosphamide-dexamethasone).

In the GIMEMA study in 480 patients with previously untreated multiple myeloma, postinduction complete plus near-complete response rate was 31% in patients receiving bortezomib-thalidomide-dexamethasone compared with 11% in those receiving thalidomide-dexamethasone; improved responses also were observed with bortezomib-thalidomide-dexamethasone following first (52 versus 31%) and second (55 versus 41%) autologous stem cell transplants and subsequent consolidation therapy (62 versus 45%). The median time to best complete or near-complete response was shorter in patients receiving bortezomib-thalidomide-dexamethasone compared with those receiving thalidomide-dexamethasone (9 versus 14 months). At a median follow-up of 36 months, progression-free survival was prolonged in patients who received bortezomib-thalidomide-dexamethasone compared with those who received thalidomide-dexamethasone (hazard ratio 0.63); however, no difference in estimated 3-year overall survival (86 versus 84%, respectively) was observed between the groups. Subgroup analysis based on poor prognostic factors (i.e., older than 60 years of age, advanced disease stage, elevated serum LDH concentration, high infiltration of bone marrow plasma cells, chromosome 13q deletion [del(13q)], t(4;14) translocation with or without chromosome 17p deletion [del(17p)]) suggested that the progression-free survival benefit of bortezomib-thalidomide-dexamethasone was consistent across these subgroups; however, because the proportion of patients with the del(17p) chromosomal abnormality was substantially smaller than the proportion of patients with other high-risk cytogenetic abnormalities, the effect of bortezomib-thalidomide-dexamethasone on progression-free survival in patients with the del(17p) chromosomal abnormality was not evaluated.

In the PETHEMA/GEM study in 386 patients with newly diagnosed multiple myeloma, the complete response rate (35 versus 14%) was higher following induction therapy with bortezomib-thalidomide-dexamethasone compared with thalidomide-dexamethasone; improved complete response rates also were maintained following autologous stem cell transplantation (46 versus 24%). Among patients with high-risk cytogenetic features, complete response rate was substantially higher in patients who received bortezomib-thalidomide-dexamethasone compared with those who received thalidomide-dexamethasone (35 versus 0%); complete responses were achieved in 38 or 58% of patients receiving bortezomib-thalidomide-dexamethasone who had t(4;14) or del(17p) chromosomal abnormalities, respectively, compared with 0% of patients receiving thalidomide-dexamethasone who had either chromosomal abnormality. At a median follow-up of 35.2 months, median progression-free survival was prolonged in patients who received bortezomib-thalidomide-dexamethasone compared with those who received thalidomide-dexamethasone (56.2 versus 28.2 months); however, no difference in estimated 4-year overall survival (74 versus 65%, respectively) was observed between the treatment groups.

In the IFM2013-04 study in 340 patients with previously untreated multiple myeloma, the overall response rate (92.3 versus 83.4%) and the rate of very good partial response or better (66.3 versus 56.2%) were higher following induction therapy with bortezomib-thalidomide-dexamethasone compared with bortezomib-cyclophosphamide-dexamethasone; however, no significant difference in complete response rate was observed between the treatment groups.

Because peripheral neuropathy occurs frequently with thalidomide- and bortezomib-based induction regimens, a modified bortezomib-thalidomide-dexamethasone induction regimen using reduced dosages of thalidomide and bortezomib was compared with bortezomib-dexamethasone in another phase 3 study in 199 patients. In this study, the rate of very good partial response or better following induction therapy was higher with bortezomib-thalidomide-dexamethasone compared with bortezomib-dexamethasone (49 versus 36%); however, postinduction complete response (13 and 12%, respectively) and overall response (88 and 81%, respectively) rates were similar for both treatment groups. At a median follow-up of 32 months, median progression-free survival was similar in patients who received bortezomib-thalidomide-dexamethasone compared with those who received bortezomib-dexamethasone (26 versus 30 months, respectively).

Use of thalidomide in combination with bortezomib and dexamethasone also was investigated in an open-label, noncomparative phase 2 study in 98 patients randomized to receive bortezomib-thalidomide-dexamethasone with or without cyclophosphamide. In this study, postinduction rates of overall response and complete plus near-complete response were 100 and 51%, respectively, in patients receiving bortezomib-thalidomide-dexamethasone and 94 and 43%, respectively, in those receiving bortezomib-thalidomide-dexamethasone-cyclophosphamide. At a median follow-up of 64.8 months, median progression-free survival was 56.3 months with bortezomib-thalidomide-dexamethasone and 36.3 months with bortezomib-thalidomide-dexamethasone-cyclophosphamide; the difference was not statistically significant and was largely related to an imbalance between treatment groups in the number of patients receiving subsequent therapy for relapsed disease prior to meeting the specified criteria for disease progression.

Use of bortezomib-thalidomide-dexamethasone as induction therapy for newly diagnosed multiple myeloma in transplant-eligible patients has improved postinduction response rates and prolonged progression-free survival in several randomized controlled studies; however, the same benefits were not observed in a study evaluating a modified bortezomib-thalidomide-dexamethasone regimen (i.e., reduced thalidomide and bortezomib dosages). Therefore, the role of a modified bortezomib-thalidomide-dexamethasone regimen using reduced dosages of thalidomide and bortezomib is unclear. In addition, in the absence of studies including adequate numbers of patients with the del(17p) chromosomal abnormality, attempts to identify whether these patients might derive clinical benefit (e.g., prolonged progression-free survival) from bortezomib-thalidomide-dexamethasone induction therapy are speculative; additional studies are needed to identify subgroups of patients with high-risk cytogenetic features who might benefit from such therapy. The AHFS Oncology Expert Committee concluded that use of thalidomide in combination with bortezomib and dexamethasone as induction therapy for newly diagnosed multiple myeloma in transplant-eligible patients may be considered a reasonable choice (accepted; with possible conditions); however, use of a modified bortezomib-thalidomide-dexamethasone regimen using reduced dosages of thalidomide and bortezomib is not fully established because of unclear risk/benefit and/or inadequate experience. (See Thalidomide, Bortezomib, and Dexamethasone under Dosage: Multiple Myeloma, in Dosage and Administration.) Factors that should be considered when selecting a combination chemotherapy regimen for use as induction therapy for newly diagnosed multiple myeloma in transplant-eligible patients include performance status and preexisting conditions (e.g., peripheral neuropathy).

Use of thalidomide in patients with multiple myeloma is associated with increased risk of venous thromboembolic events (e.g., deep venous thrombosis, pulmonary embolus). Such risk increases substantially when thalidomide is used in combination with standard chemotherapy. (See Cautions: Thromboembolic Events.)

For further information on the use of combination therapy with thalidomide, bortezomib, and dexamethasone as induction therapy for newly diagnosed multiple myeloma in transplant-eligible patients, see Induction Therapy Prior to Stem Cell Transplantation in Newly Diagnosed Multiple Myeloma under Uses: Multiple Myeloma, in Bortezomib 10:00.

■ **Inflammatory and/or Dermatologic Disorders** Based on the beneficial effects of thalidomide in the treatment of inflammatory dermatoses associated with ENL, the drug has been used for the treatment of a variety of inflammatory and/or dermatologic disorders, including Behcet's syndrome†, erosive lichen planus†, erythema multiforme†, lupus erythematosus† (discoid lupus erythematosus, subacute or chronic cutaneous lupus erythematosus, cutaneous manifestations of systemic lupus erythematosus), prurigo nodularis†, actinic prurigo†, cutaneous Langerhans cell histiocytosis†, uremic pruritus†, porphyria cutanea tarda†, and pyoderma gangrenosum†. There is evidence that thalidomide can be beneficial and may result in improvements in the dermatologic and mucocutaneous manifestations of these conditions; however, there is recurrence of lesions and symptoms in many patients when the drug is discontinued and long-term maintenance therapy may be necessary. Most clinicians recommend that thalidomide be used for the treatment of inflammatory and/or dermatologic disorders only in selected patients with severe refractory disease unresponsive to other appropriate agents (e.g., corticosteroids).

Behcet's Syndrome In patients with Behcet's syndrome†, a chronic inflammatory disease of unknown etiology characterized by recurrent orogenital ulceration, skin lesions, and arthritic symptoms that may be complicated by GI, ocular, and neurologic involvement, thalidomide therapy (100–400 mg daily) has resulted in resolution of dermatologic, mucocutaneous, and arthritic manifestations of the disease. However, symptoms and/or lesions generally recur within several weeks after the drug is discontinued. In a randomized, double-blind, placebo-controlled study in adult males with Behcet's syndrome with mucocutaneous lesions (without major organ involvement), a complete response (resolution of orogenital ulcers and follicular lesions) was obtained in 6 or 16% of patients receiving thalidomide in a dosage of 100 or 300 mg daily, respectively; there were no complete responses in those receiving placebo. While there are some reports that GI, ophthalmic, and/or neurologic symptoms also may improve during thalidomide therapy, further study is needed to determine whether thalidomide has any clinically important effect on these manifestations of the disease.

In a clinical trial, thalidomide has been used in a limited number of young patients (9–34 years of age) with juvenile-onset of severe Behcet syndrome† (manifested by severe abdominal pain; intestinal ulceration, bleeding, perforation, or obstruction; recurrent stomatitis; oral aphthosis; genital ulceration; erythema nodosum in the extremities; ileocolitis; fever). All patients, but one, were receiving corticosteroids; severe steroid toxicity, osteoporosis, and/or steroid dependence was reported. The initial thalidomide dosage was 2 mg/kg daily; dosage was increased to 3 mg/kg daily or decreased to 0.5–1 mg/kg daily, according to patients' response. All patients showed improvement in clinical symptoms and all patients were able to discontinue corticosteroids. The end point of the trial was complete remission of the disease without using the drug; however, clinicians failed to withdraw thalidomide from all patients except one. Further large-scale clinical trials are needed to determine the appropriate duration of thalidomide therapy.

Other Dermatologic Disorders Thalidomide has *not* been effective when used for the treatment of toxic epidermal necrolysis†. In a limited placebo-controlled study in adults with toxic epidermal necrolysis, there was no evidence that thalidomide had any beneficial effect on necrolysis, and patients receiving thalidomide had a higher mortality rate than those receiving placebo. In another randomized placebo-controlled trial in patients with toxic epidermal necrolysis, therapy with thalidomide was not shown to be effective and was associated with substantially higher mortality than placebo. Further randomized, controlled studies are needed to understand the mechanism of toxic epidermal necrolysis and to evaluate treatments of the disease especially in patients receiving high doses of steroids and IV immunoglobulins. In addition, there have been several reported cases of patients with malignancies developing toxic epidermal necrolysis while receiving thalidomide (usually with dexamethasone.)

■ **Uses in HIV-infected Patients** Thalidomide is being investigated for a variety of uses in HIV-infected patients, including treatment of HIV-associated aphthous ulcers†, HIV-associated diarrhea†, HIV-associated wasting syndrome†, and Kaposi's sarcoma†. The drug also has been used as an adjunct to anti-infective agents in the treatment of mycobacterial infections†, including *Mycobacterium tuberculosis* and *M. avium* complex (MAC) infections, in HIV-infected patients. While evidence is accumulating that thalidomide may provide some benefits in HIV-infected patients (e.g., promote healing of aphthous ulcers, ameliorate weight loss), further study is needed to evaluate safety and efficacy of thalidomide in HIV-infected patients and to determine whether the drug may increase viral load (i.e., plasma HIV-1 RNA levels) and/or may be associated with an increased incidence of adverse effects in this patient population.

HIV-associated Aphthous Ulcers Thalidomide (100–300 mg once daily) has been effective for the treatment and prevention of oropharyngeal, esophageal, and anogenital aphthous ulcers in HIV-infected patients†. The drug has been effective for the treatment of severe recurrent aphthous stomatitis in HIV-infected patients, and also has been effective for the treatment of severe recurrent aphthous stomatitis in immunocompetent patients or patients who are immunocompromised but not HIV-infected† (see Uses: Recurrent Aphthous Stomatitis). Thalidomide is not considered a drug of first choice for the treatment of aphthous ulcers in HIV-infected patients, but may be effective in patients with recurrent ulcers refractory to other therapies (e.g., corticosteroids).

Efficacy of thalidomide for the treatment of oral and esophageal aphthous ulcers in HIV-infected patients has been evaluated in a phase II double-blind, placebo-controlled study through the National Institute of Allergy and Infectious Diseases (NIAID) AIDS Clinical Trials Group (ACTG) (study ACTG 251). HIV-infected patients with oral aphthous ulcers were randomized to receive a 4-week regimen of thalidomide (200 mg once daily) or placebo; if healing of ulcers was not complete after this regimen, an additional 4-week regimen of thalidomide was administered. At 4 weeks, a complete response was obtained in 55 or 7% of patients receiving thalidomide or placebo, respectively.

HIV-associated Wasting Syndrome Thalidomide has been used for the treatment of wasting syndrome in a limited number of HIV-infected patients† and also has been used for the treatment of cachexia in other severely immunocompromised patients† (e.g., cancer patients). There is some evidence that thalidomide therapy (50–400 mg daily) may decrease elevated TNF-α plasma concentrations and may promote weight gain in HIV-infected patients. However, thalidomide may increase plasma TNF-α concentrations in some HIV-infected patients. The precise role of TNF-α in the wasting syndrome is unclear and additional study is necessary to evaluate the safety and efficacy of thalidomide in the treatment of HIV-associated wasting syndrome.

HIV-associated Diarrhea Thalidomide has been used with some success in a limited number of patients for the treatment of HIV-associated diarrhea, including microsporidiosis†. In one group of HIV-infected patients with chronic diarrhea and weight loss caused by *Enterocytozoon bieneusi* infection that was not responsive to albendazole, use of thalidomide (100 mg daily for 4 weeks) had a beneficial effect (i.e., complete or partial clinical response including increased weight and decreased stool frequency) in 55% of patients. Although there is evidence that thalidomide may relieve some symptoms of microsporidian enteritis in some patients, results of an in vitro study indicate that the drug has no direct activity against microsporidia.

Kaposi's Sarcoma Safety and efficacy of thalidomide for the management of cutaneous Kaposi's sarcoma† have been evaluated in a phase II dose-escalating study through the National Cancer Institute (NCI). Twenty HIV-infected male patients (29–49 years of age) with biopsy-confirmed Kaposi's sarcoma (having at least 5 assessable lesions and objective evidence of tumor progression over 2 months before enrollment), received an initial thalidomide dosage of 200 mg daily; dosage was increased by 200 mg daily every 14 days up to a maximum of 1 g daily (for up to 1 year). Dosage reductions or delays in dose escalation were permitted for toxicity. To be eligible for the study, patients were required to be either on stable antiretroviral therapy for at least 4 weeks or not receiving such therapy for at least 2 weeks. Seventeen patients were assessed for response, using the NIAID ACTG criteria. Eight patients achieved partial response (defined as no progressive disease and at least a 4-week persistence of either a 50% decrease in the sum of the cross products of the lesions, a 50% reduction in the total number of lesions, or flattening of 50% or more of the nodular lesions) for an overall major response rate of 47%. When all 20 patients were assessed on an intent-to-treat basis, the response rate (partial and complete [defined as the absence of any evident disease for 4 weeks] responses) was 40%. Seven of the 20 patients achieved the maximum thalidomide dosage of 1 g daily used for a median of 19.9 weeks. Overall, the results suggest that thalidomide has activity against Kaposi's sarcoma at dosages that can be tolerated for 6 months or more. The severity of adverse effects was graded according to toxicity criteria established by the NCI. The principal toxicity that limited dose escalation was drowsiness.

Preliminary results from a case report and 2 small trials have suggested that Kaposi's sarcoma may respond to thalidomide dosages as low as 100 mg daily. Further studies are needed to assess the dose-response relationship of thalidomide for this condition.

■ **Neoplastic Diseases** Because there is evidence that thalidomide is an inhibitor of angiogenesis, the drug is being evaluated for the treatment of a variety of malignancies, including advanced or metastatic breast cancer†, Kaposi's sarcoma† (see Kaposi's Sarcoma under Uses: Use in HIV-infected Patients), melanoma†, ovarian cancer†, myelodysplastic syndrome (MDS)†, advanced pancreatic cancer†, primary brain tumors† (recurrent high-grade astrocytomas and mixed gliomas), androgen-independent prostate cancer†, and renal carcinoma†. There is some evidence that thalidomide may have antitumor activity; however, further study is needed to establish safety and efficacy of the drug in the treatment of various malignancies and identify optimal dosages of the drug in patients with cancer.

Cachexia Thalidomide also has been used for the treatment of cachexia† in patients with advanced cancer, and there is some evidence that the drug may provide benefits in these patients in terms of improvement in symptoms of insomnia, nausea, appetite, and feelings of well-being. (See Uses in HIV-infected Patients: HIV-associated Wasting Syndrome, in Uses.)

■ **Graft-versus-host Disease** Thalidomide has been used with some success for the *treatment* of graft-versus-host disease† (GVHD) in adult and pediatric bone marrow transplant recipients, but has been associated with increased morbidity and mortality when used for *prophylaxis* of chronic GVHD in adult bone marrow transplant recipients.

Thalidomide generally has been used in allogeneic bone marrow transplant recipients for the *treatment* of chronic or refractory GVHD unresponsive to other therapies (e.g., corticosteroids, azathioprine, tacrolimus, cyclosporine, antithymocyte globulin); only limited information is available regarding use of the drug for the treatment of acute GVHD. In a study in adult and pediatric patients with chronic or refractory GVHD who received thalidomide therapy (800–1600 mg daily for a median duration of 240 days), a complete response was obtained in 32% and a partial response was obtained in 27%; the overall survival rate was 64%. Thalidomide has been effective when used for the treatment of chronic or corticosteroid-dependent GVHD in pediatric patients 0.5–17 years of age†.

When thalidomide was used for *prophylaxis* of chronic GVHD in a controlled study of adult allogeneic bone marrow transplant patients who had no evidence of active acute GVHD at study entry, those receiving thalidomide (200 mg twice daily beginning 80 days after transplant) experienced a higher incidence of chronic GVHD and had a substantially higher mortality rate compared with those receiving placebo. Chronic GVHD occurred in 64 or 38% of patients receiving thalidomide or placebo, respectively; overall mortality was about 39 or 8%, and mortality from GVHD was about 21 or 4% in those receiving thalidomide or placebo, respectively.

Thalidomide also has been used with some success in the *treatment* of GVHD† in adult peripheral blood stem cell transplant recipients.

■ **Recurrent Aphthous Stomatitis** Thalidomide has been effective when used for the treatment of severe aphthous oral ulcers in patients with recurrent aphthous stomatitis† (RAS). The drug has been used effectively for the treatment of RAS in immunocompetent adults and pediatric patients and also has been effective when used in immunocompromised patients, including cancer patients and HIV-infected patients (see Uses in HIV-infected Patients: HIV-associated Aphthous Ulcers, in Uses).In a placebo-controlled cross-over study in patients with severe RAS, a complete clinical remission was obtained in 48 or 9% of patients receiving thalidomide or placebo, respectively. Oral ulcers generally heal within 1–6 weeks after initiation of thalidomide therapy (100–300 mg daily), but higher dosage may be needed in some patients (400–600 mg daily) and ulcers may relapse when the drug is discontinued. In some patients, relapse may be prevented or treated using thalidomide maintenance therapy (50–100 mg daily).

■ **GI Disorders** ***Crohn's Disease*** Thalidomide has been used with some success in a limited number of patients for the treatment of refractory Crohn's disease† (e.g., in those with moderately to severely, chronically active or fistulizing disease). In patients who did not respond to or were intolerant of usually recommended therapies (e.g., corticosteroids, sulfasalazine, azathioprine, mercaptopurine, methotrexate), thalidomide therapy (50–300 mg daily) resulted in resolution of small bowel ulceration, bleeding, or pain and improvement related to quality of life or symptoms associated with fistulas. In at least one patient with Crohn's disease, thalidomide therapy also resulted in resolution of severe, recurrent oral aphthous ulcers. Thalidomide has been used in a limited number patients with Crohn's disease (i.e., active fistulous disease, luminal disease) who developed infliximab-induced delayed hypersensitivity reactions. Complete closure was observed in 2 patients, one with a single perirectal fistula, the other with 5 perianal fistulae at 4 or 12 weeks of thalidomide therapy, respectively. Two patients who continued thalidomide for more than 3 months remained in remission at 5 and 7 months.

Limited data indicate that thalidomide (100 mg daily) may be effective in maintaining response in patients with chronically active and fistulizing refractory Crohn's disease whose disease has responded to infliximab (dosage of 5 mg/kg administered as one or more infusions in patients with chronically active disease and 3 or more infusions in those with fistulizing disease). The median follow-up was 238 days from initiation of thalidomide therapy and 265 days after the last infusion of infliximab. Remission rates (full improvement) with thalidomide were 92, 83, or 83% at 3, 6, or 12 months, respectively, after the last dose of infliximab.

Results of a 12-week, open-label study in a limited number of patients (20–77 years of age) with chronic inflammatory bowel disease† (IBD; 5 with Crohn's disease, 2 with ulcerative colitis, and 1 with indeterminate colitis) indicate that use of thalidomide can result in clinical response in patients with chronically active Crohn's disease who have not responded to prior therapy (e.g., 5-amino-salicylic acid preparations, prednisone, azathioprine). Initially, patients were receiving 100 mg of thalidomide daily after which the daily dosage was increased to a maximum of 400 mg according to patients' response or adverse effect profile. Patients continued to receive other drugs for IBD during the duration of the trial. The Crohn's Disease Activity Index (CDAI) decreased from 117 to 48; improvement included decreased stool frequency, erythrocyte sedimentation rate (ESR), and inflammation and histological grades. Two months after the trial, stool frequency returned to pretreatment levels indicating that the effect of thalidomide is of short duration. Long term studies are needed; minimizing the dosage over an extended period may be a potential solution.

(For further information on the management of Crohn's disease, see Uses: Crohn's Disease, in Mesalamine 56:36).

Other GI Disorder Thalidomide also has been used with some success in a limited number of patients for the treatment of ulcerative colitis†, but additional study is needed.

■ **Other Uses** Thalidomide has been used in a limited number of patients for the treatment of refractory ankylosing spondylitis†, refractory rheumatoid arthritis†, or sarcoidosis†, but additional study and experience are needed.

Because thalidomide is an inhibitor of angiogenesis and there is some evidence that loss of vision in the severe, wet form of macular degeneration may be related to angiogenesis in the blood vessels behind the macula, the drug is being investigated for the treatment of macular degeneration†.

Dosage and Administration

■ **Administration** Thalidomide is administered orally. Because administration with a high-fat meal substantially delays the time to peak plasma concentrations of thalidomide, the drug should be administered with water at least 1 hour after a meal.

When thalidomide is given as a single daily dose, the manufacturer recommends that the dose preferably be given at bedtime (to minimize the sedative effects of the drug) with water and at least 1 hour after the evening meal. When high daily dosage of thalidomide is necessary (e.g., 400 mg daily), the daily dose may be given as a single dose at bedtime or, alternatively, in divided doses given with water at least 1 hour after meals.

■ **Dosage** ***Erythema Nodosum Leprosum*** For acute treatment of cutaneous manifestations of moderate to severe erythema nodosum leprosum (ENL) in adults and children 12 years of age or older, thalidomide should be initiated at a dosage of 100–300 mg daily. Patients weighing less than 50 kg should receive a low initial dosage of thalidomide (e.g., 100 mg daily). For the treatment of severe cutaneous ENL reactions or in patients who previously required high thalidomide dosages to control an ENL reaction, the drug may be initiated at a dosage up to 400 mg daily.

Thalidomide generally should be continued until signs and symptoms of active ENL reaction have subsided (usually at least 2 weeks), and dosage should then be gradually reduced. The manufacturer recommends that daily dosage of thalidomide be reduced in 50-mg increments every 2–4 weeks until the drug is discontinued or recurrence of ENL occurs. Patients who have recurrence of ENL while thalidomide dosage is being reduced and those who have a documented history indicating that prolonged maintenance treatment is necessary to prevent recurrence of cutaneous ENL should be maintained on the minimum dosage of the drug required to control the reaction. Thereafter, gradual decrease and discontinuance of maintenance dosage should be attempted every 3–6 months.

Patients with moderate to severe neuritis associated with severe ENL reactions may receive corticosteroid therapy concomitantly with thalidomide; corticosteroid dosage may be tapered and the corticosteroid discontinued when neuritis has ameliorated.

Multiple Myeloma **Thalidomide and Dexamethasone.** Thalidomide in combination with dexamethasone (in 28-day treatment cycles) is used for the treatment of newly diagnosed multiple myeloma in adults. The usual dosage of thalidomide is 200 mg given once daily. (See Dosage and Administration: Administration.) Dexamethasone is administered orally as 40-mg doses on days 1–4, 9–12, and 17–20 every 28 days.

The manufacturer states that thalidomide may be discontinued temporarily or dosage decreased in patients who develop adverse effects (e.g., constipation, oversedation, peripheral neuropathy). Once such effects have subsided, thalidomide may be reinitiated at a lower or previously used dosage based on clinical judgment.

Thalidomide, Bortezomib, and Dexamethasone. Thalidomide has been used in several regimens in combination with bortezomib and dexamethasone† as induction therapy for newly diagnosed multiple myeloma in transplant-eligible patients.

When thalidomide has been used in combination with bortezomib and dexamethasone as induction therapy for newly diagnosed multiple myeloma in transplant-eligible patients, thalidomide 200 mg was administered orally daily (after initial dosage escalation during cycle 1 with 100 mg orally on days 1–14 followed by 200 mg orally daily thereafter) along with bortezomib 1.3 mg/m^2 by IV injection twice weekly for 2 weeks (days 1, 4, 8, and 11) and dexamethasone 40 mg orally on days 1, 2, 4, 5, 8, 9, 11, and 12. Treatment cycles were repeated every 21 days for 3 cycles.

Thalidomide 200 mg also has been administered orally daily (after initial dosage escalation during cycle 1 with 50 mg orally on days 1–14 followed by 100 mg orally on days 15–28) along with bortezomib 1.3 mg/m^2 by IV injection twice weekly for 2 weeks (days 1, 4, 8, and 11) and dexamethasone 40 mg orally on days 1–4 and 9–12. Treatment cycles were repeated every 4 weeks for 6 cycles.

Thalidomide 100 mg has been administered orally daily along with bortezomib 1.3 mg/m^2 by subcutaneous or IV injection twice weekly for 2 weeks (days 1, 4, 8, and 11) and dexamethasone 40 mg orally on days 1–4 and 9–12. Treatment cycles were repeated every 3 weeks for 4 cycles.

A modified regimen using reduced dosages of thalidomide and bortezomib is not fully established.

Recurrent Aphthous Stomatitis For the treatment of recurrent aphthous stomatitis† in adults, including those who are HIV-infected, thalidomide dosages of 100–300 mg daily have been used. However, higher dosages (e.g., 400–600 mg daily) may be necessary in some patients. The optimum duration of thalidomide therapy has not been elucidated, but ulcers may relapse following discontinuance of the drug.

Crohn's Disease For the management of refractory Crohn's disease† in adults, thalidomide dosages of 50–300 mg daily have been used. Thalidomide dosages of 100 mg daily have been used in maintenance therapy of chronically active or fistulizing refractory Crohn's disease† in patients whose disease has responded to infliximab.

Graft-versus-host Disease For the *treatment* of graft-versus-host disease† (GVHD), thalidomide dosages of 800–1600 mg daily have been used. The drug should *not* be used for prophylaxis of chronic GVHD. (See Uses: Graft-versus-host Disease.)

■ **Restricted Distribution Program** *Because thalidomide is a known human teratogen and can cause severe, life-threatening birth defects if administered during pregnancy, commercially available thalidomide must be obtained through a restricted distribution program, the System for Thalidomide Education and Prescribing Safety (STEPS), designed to help ensure that fetal exposure to the drug does not occur.* Clinicians, pharmacies, and patients must be registered in the STEPS program before they can prescribe, dispense, and receive thalidomide, and compliance with all terms outlined in the program is mandatory. The STEPS program controls access to thalidomide; educates STEPS participants (clinicians, pharmacists, patients) about the risks associated with thalidomide and the procedural requirements for safe use of the drug; and monitors compliance with the registration, education, and safety requirements of the program.

The STEPS program was created by Celgene in collaboration with the US Food and Drug Administration (FDA), the Birth Defects Branch of the US Centers for Disease Control and Prevention (CDC), and patient advocacy groups (e.g., the Thalidomide Victims Association of Canada). While the program was based on safety models currently in use for isotretinoin and clozapine, it incorporates additional controls and compliance monitoring not included in prior drug distribution programs. For information regarding the STEPS program, Celgene's customer service department should be contacted at 888-423-5436.

Prescribing Clinicians Before prescribing thalidomide, clinicians must be registered in the STEPS Prescriber Registry and must agree to prescribe the drug in accordance with the STEPS patient eligibility criteria and monitoring procedures. Clinicians can be registered by returning a completed, signed registration card to Celgene. Clinicians must agree to provide comprehensive patient counseling on the benefits and risks of thalidomide as outlined in the STEPS informed consent document; provide appropriate contraception counseling and pregnancy testing or refer the patient to a qualified obstetrics-gynecology specialist for such counseling; complete the prescriber portion of the patient monitoring survey; and submit a copy of the completed informed consent document (signed by the patient and prescriber) and a copy of the patient monitoring survey.

Clinicians must agree to write each prescription for no more than a 28-day supply of thalidomide at a time (with no refills), inform the patient that each prescription must be filled within 7 days of being written, and encourage the patient to return all unused thalidomide to the dispensing pharmacy. The STEPS program does not allow automatic prescription refills, and the clinician must ensure that patients return for monthly office visits to obtain subsequent prescriptions for thalidomide. At each monthly visit and before a new prescription for the drug is issued, the clinician must provide the patient with additional counseling about adverse effects of thalidomide and the use of appropriate contraceptive measures; ensure that a serum pregnancy test is performed in any female patient of childbearing potential; ask the patient to complete a patient survey form about their compliance with contraceptive measures, pregnancy testing, and drug therapy; and submit the completed patient survey form as directed by the STEPS program.

Dispensing Pharmacies To receive thalidomide from the manufacturer for dispensing, pharmacies must be registered in the STEPS Pharmacy Dispensing Registry and agree to comply with all requirements of the program. The director of pharmacy or head pharmacist registers the pharmacy by returning a completed, signed pharmacy registration card to Celgene. After the manufacturer enters all of the information provided by the pharmacist into the dispensing database, the pharmacy will be eligible to dispense thalidomide, and the manufacturer will provide a continuing education monograph to the pharmacy. The registering pharmacist must agree to inform all staff pharmacists of the dispensing procedures for thalidomide.

When a new patient presents an initial prescription for thalidomide to the pharmacy, the pharmacist must collect from the patient a copy of the STEPS informed consent document (signed by the patient and a registered prescriber) and a copy of the completed patient monitoring survey. The pharmacist will then register the patient into the STEPS distribution database using a patient registration form provided by the manufacturer. Subsequent to successful patient registration, the manufacturer will ship the drug to the registered pharmacy for arrival within 2 days.

All prescriptions for thalidomide must be presented to the pharmacist in person, and may not be communicated to the pharmacist over the phone. Before dispensing thalidomide, the pharmacist must activate the authorization number on every prescription by calling the Celgene® Customer Care Center at 1-888-423-5436 and obtaining a confirmation number; this number must be written on the thalidomide prescription.

The pharmacist may not fill a single thalidomide prescription for more than a 28-day supply of the drug; automatic refills are not allowed. The pharmacist must verify that each prescription was written within the preceding 7 days, and must *not* dispense the drug if the prescription was written more than 7 days previously, or if there is (or should be) more than a 7-day supply of the drug remaining from the preceding prescription. Blister packs containing the drug must be dispensed intact (i.e., the drug may *not*be repackaged). Pharmacists must encourage all patients to return all unused drug to the dispensing pharmacy, where it will be accepted and destroyed or returned to the manufacturer.

Patients To receive commercially available thalidomide, a patient must be registered in the STEPS program and agree to comply with all requirements of the program, including mandatory contraceptive measures, and participation in a telephone survey and patient registry while taking thalidomide. Patients can receive a prescription for thalidomide from the prescribing clinician only after the patient has received comprehensive counseling on the benefits and risks of thalidomide as outlined in the STEPS informed consent document, has demonstrated to the clinician that they are capable of understanding the risks associated with thalidomide and instructions on use of the drug, has received appropriate contraception counseling and pregnancy testing either from the prescribing clinician or a qualified obstetrics-gynecology specialist, has had any questions answered by the clinician, and has signed the informed consent document and completed the patient monitoring survey. As part of the educational requirements of the program, the patient must view the patient-oriented video titled *Important Information for Men and Women Taking Thalomid® (thalidomide)* and/or read the patient brochure provided by the manufacturer and must understand their contents, including other possible health problems resulting from thalidomide adverse effects. The patient also must understand that thalidomide must be kept out of the reach of children, and must *never* be given to women who are able to have children. The patient must have been warned by the clinician that an unborn baby will almost certainly have serious birth defects and even die if a woman becomes pregnant or is pregnant while taking thalidomide. For minors 18 years of age or younger, a parent or legal guardian must be educated concerning the hazards of thalidomide and agree to ensure that the minor complies with all requirements of the STEPS program.

Female patients in the STEPS program who are of childbearing potential (i.e., adolescents and women who are sexually mature, have had menses at some time in the 24 consecutive months preceding initiation of thalidomide, have not undergone a hysterectomy) must agree to use effective contraceptive measures (which may include abstinence) for at least 4 weeks prior to, throughout, and for at least 4 weeks after completion of thalidomide therapy. These women must have a confirmed negative pregnancy test result prior to initiation of thalidomide therapy and also must agree to have regular, repeat pregnancy tests throughout therapy (i.e., once weekly during the first month and monthly or every 2 weeks in women with regular or irregular menstrual cycles, respectively). (See Pregnancy under Cautions: Pregnancy, Fertility, and Lactation.) Male patients in the STEPS program must agree to use a latex condom every time they have sexual contact with a woman of childbearing potential. All patients must agree to *not* share their thalidomide with anyone else (even if the other individual has similar symptoms); to keep the drug out of the reach of children; and to not donate blood or semen while receiving thalidomide.

The patient must present a copy of the completed informed consent document (signed by the patient and registered prescriber) and patient monitoring survey to the dispensing pharmacist who then registers the patient with Celgene. Once a patient is registered in the STEPS distribution database and has received their first 28-day supply of thalidomide, they must return to the prescribing clinician at monthly intervals to receive subsequent prescriptions for thalidomide; the program does not allow automatic refills. At each monthly visit to the prescribing clinician and before a new prescription for the drug is issued, the patient must receive additional counseling about adverse effects of thalidomide and the use of appropriate contraception, receive a serum pregnancy test (if female and of childbearing potential), and complete a patient monitoring survey.

Monitoring and Compliance Compliance with the educational, informed consent, and pregnancy-testing components of the STEPS program is monitored through the patient surveys that must be completed by prescribing clinicians and patients when each initial and subsequent prescription of thalidomide is written. The surveys are designed to monitor compliance with, and implementation and execution of STEPS safety procedures, and to analyze outcomes.

The STEPS program also is monitored by a quality assurance committee composed of Celgene employees, agents, and consultants. In addition, all aspects of the STEPS program are subject to FDA audits. Although the FDA is not directly responsible for the operation of the STEPS program registry, the FDA can verify that the STEPS program is operating appropriately by conducting periodic inspections of pharmacies, and by reviewing data from and procedures of the clinicians and patient registry. State boards of pharmacy have no regulatory oversight of the registry process.

The STEPS program is *not* designed to restrict prescribing and dispensing of commercially available thalidomide to only the FDA-labeled use of the drug. The registration system will collect information regarding any disease for which the drug is being used, regardless of FDA-approved labeling; therefore, clinicians registered in the STEPS program are not restricted from prescribing the drug for unlabeled (off-label) uses.

Although the STEPS program is highly restrictive and minimizes the risk that thalidomide may inadvertently be given to a pregnant woman, the risk of such exposure may not be completely eliminated. The FDA states that if there is even *one* fetal exposure to thalidomide, the entire distribution system will be reevaluated, and steps will be taken to ensure that all deficiencies are corrected.

Cautions

Thalidomide is a known human teratogen and has caused severe, life-threatening birth defects or fetal death when used during pregnancy. (See Precautions and Contraindications: Teratogenicity Precautions and Contraindications, in Cautions.) Another potentially serious adverse effect reported with thalidomide is peripheral neuropathy that may be irreversible. Other adverse effects reported with thalidomide generally are mild to moderate in severity, and usually do not require discontinuance of the drug. The most common adverse effects of thalidomide are CNS effects (e.g., drowsiness, somnolence, dizziness) and dermatologic effects (e.g., rash).

Information on adverse effects of thalidomide reported by the manufacturer was obtained principally from controlled clinical studies in leprosy patients who received thalidomide in a dosage of 50–300 mg daily for the treatment of erythema nodosum leprosum (ENL) and controlled clinical studies in patients with human immunodeficiency virus (HIV) infection who received thalidomide in a dosage of 100–200 mg daily. Additional information on adverse effects of thalidomide reported by the manufacturer was obtained from uncontrolled clinical studies in ENL patients, uncontrolled studies or case reports involving patients who received thalidomide for a wide variety of investigational uses, and spontaneous reports from other sources. The manufacturer states that the incidence of adverse effects reported in these uncontrolled studies and other sources is unknown, and a causal relationship between some of these effects and thalidomide has not been established. Although thalidomide received approval by the US Food and Drug Administration (FDA) in 1998 for use in the treatment of ENL in leprosy patients, data regarding the safety and efficacy of the drug have been accumulating since the drug first became available for use in Europe in the late 1950s.

■ **Thromboembolic Events** Use of thalidomide in patients with multiple myeloma is associated with increased risk of venous thromboembolic events (e.g., deep venous thrombosis, pulmonary embolus). Such risk increases substantially when thalidomide is used in combination with standard chemotherapy, including dexamethasone. In a controlled clinical trial, an increased incidence of venous thromboembolic events was observed in patients receiving thalidomide in combination with dexamethasone compared with those receiving dexamethasone alone (22.5 versus 4.9%). Patients and clinicians are advised to watch for signs and symptoms of thromboembolism. Patients should be instructed to notify a clinician if they develop shortness of breath, chest pain, and/or arm or leg swelling.

The manufacturer and some experts state that decisions regarding use of thromboprophylaxis and selection of an appropriate thromboprophylaxis regimen (e.g., aspirin, anticoagulant) should be based on careful assessment of the patient's risk factors for thromboembolism. The International Myeloma Working Group (IMWG) currently recommends thromboprophylaxis with aspirin for multiple myeloma patients receiving thalidomide who have one or no underlying individual and/or myeloma-related risk factors for venous thromboembolism and thromboprophylaxis with a low molecular weight heparin for those with 2 or more individual and/or myeloma-related risk factors. The IMWG also recommends that thromboprophylaxis with a low molecular weight heparin be considered in thalidomide-treated patients receiving high-dose dexamethasone, doxorubicin, or multiple antineoplastic agents, independent of additional risk factors. The IMWG states that although full-dose warfarin (international normalized ratio [INR] 2–3) is an alternative to low molecular weight heparins, there is limited clinical experience with this approach. The American Society of Clinical Oncology (ASCO) currently recommends pharmacologic thromboprophylaxis for multiple myeloma patients receiving thalidomide in conjunction with dexamethasone or antineoplastic agents, and states that those at lower risk for thromboembolism may receive either aspirin or a low molecular weight heparin, while those at higher risk should receive a low molecular weight heparin.

Deep venous thrombosis and pulmonary embolism also have been reported in patients with ENL.

■ **Nervous System Effects** ***Peripheral Neuropathy*** Thalidomide may cause potentially severe nerve damage (i.e., polyneuritis or peripheral neuropathy) that may be irreversible. The incidence of peripheral neuropathy in patients receiving thalidomide has been reported to range from less than 1% to more than 70%. Incidence data regarding this adverse effect has been difficult to obtain, in part because the drug often is used in patients with diseases that may be associated with neuropathy (e.g., leprosy patients with ENL, patients with HIV infection) and it may be difficult to differentiate the neuropathologic symptoms and changes caused by the underlying disease from those caused by the drug.

Despite long-term experience with use of thalidomide in leprosy patients with ENL, there have been few reports of thalidomide-associated peripheral neuropathy in these patients; in some studies, less than 1% of patients receiving the drug for treatment of ENL experienced peripheral neuropathy. It has been suggested that this may not be an accurate reflection of the incidence of this adverse effect in these patients since peripheral neuritis was not recognized as a potential adverse effect of thalidomide in early studies of the drug, in part because ENL patients frequently have neuropathy in association with their disease and may not have reported such effects while receiving the drug. Therefore, preexisting neuropathy in ENL patients may complicate recognition of thalidomide-associated peripheral neuropathy. In addition, such symptoms may be difficult to monitor since ENL neuritis may improve during thalidomide therapy, but relapse after therapy with the drug is discontinued.

In controlled studies in HIV-infected patients, neuropathy occurred in 7–8% of those receiving thalidomide. In one limited study in HIV-infected patients receiving thalidomide 400 mg daily for 3 months, 7% of patients experienced neuropathy symptoms requiring discontinuance of the drug. In other limited studies, 4% of HIV infected patients receiving 200–300 mg of thalidomide for 14–21 days experienced severe symptoms of neuropathy. It has been suggested that HIV-infected patients may be particularly susceptible to the development of thalidomide-associated polyneuritis. However, since axonal degeneration with clinical and electrophysiologic symptoms resembling those of thalidomide-associated polyneuropathies may occur in HIV-infected patients and other forms of polyneuropathy (including demyelinating and polyradiculopathy) also are reported in such patients, it may be difficult to differentiate neuropathologic changes caused by the underlying disease from those caused by thalidomide.

In a retrospective study of patients receiving thalidomide for a variety of dermatologic conditions, thalidomide-associated peripheral neuropathy occurred in 21–50% of patients and was most frequent in women and geriatric patients. Limited data indicate that peripheral neuropathy occurs in up to 75% of patients receiving thalidomide for the treatment of prurigo nodularis†.

Thalidomide-associated peripheral neuropathy generally has been reported with chronic use of the drug over a period of months, but also has been reported with relatively short-term use of the drug. The correlation between peripheral neuropathy and the cumulative thalidomide dose is unclear; symptoms have been reported to begin after a cumulative dose of 40–50 g in some patients, but also have occurred with no apparent relationship to cumulative dose. There have been some cases when symptoms of thalidomide-associated peripheral neuropathy were not apparent until after the drug was discontinued.

Polyneuropathic symptoms may improve in some patients when thalidomide is discontinued, but symptoms may resolve slowly or not at all after discontinuance of the drug. In a study of patients with thalidomide-induced peripheral neuropathy who were followed for 4–6 years after discontinuing the drug, 25% experienced full recovery, 25% had some improvement of symptoms, and 50% had no improvement in signs and symptoms of neuropathy.

Clinical symptoms of thalidomide-induced neuropathy include predominantly symmetric painful paresthesia of the hands and feet, often accompanied by sensory loss in lower limbs. Muscle weakness and cramps, signs of pyramidal tract involvement, and carpal tunnel syndrome have been reported often. An unpleasant pedal symptom, described as "tightness around the feet," was reported in 8–47% of patients in some studies. In early reports, thalidomide-associated peripheral neuropathies were characterized mostly by sensory symptoms, including hypoesthesia and hyperesthesia, hyperalgesia, impaired temperature sensitivity, and impaired vegetative (i.e., autonomic) nervous functions. These symptoms occasionally were accompanied by mild proximal muscle weakness, or evidence of pyramidal tract damage, but motor disturbances appeared to occur rarely. Muscle weakness rapidly improved after discontinuance of the drug, but sensory deficits were slow to improve, and occasionally worsened even while the patient was not receiving thalidomide. Because there was no substantial correlation between the severity of the condition and the total dose of the drug, and because discontinuance of thalidomide did not result in improvement in many cases, initially it could not be established that such neurologic disturbances were actually caused by thalidomide. Subsequently, the association between thalidomide and peripheral neuropathies was established in clinical studies of patients with discoid lupus erythematosus, prurigo nodularis, and aphthous stomatitis; in these studies, the neurologic status of patients was assessed before and after initiation of thalidomide therapy.

Physiologically, thalidomide polyneuropathy is characterized by axonal degeneration without demyelinization (i.e., a "dying back process"). Electrophysiologic alteration principally is characterized by a decreased sensory action potential amplitude on medial nerves of the arm, and peroneal and sural (medial cutaneous) nerves of the leg, with relative conservation of conduction velocities; however, decreased sensory and motor conduction velocities have been observed. Also, increased somatosensory latency of activation after sural nerve stimulation may occur in the absence of clinical abnormalities in patients receiving thalidomide. Because electrophysiologic alterations may occur before the onset of subjective symptoms, the reported incidence of neuropathy in thalidomide studies is higher if neurophysiologic tests, rather than clinical symptoms, are used for diagnosis.

Other Nervous System Effects Thalidomide exhibits sedative and hypnotic effects, and drowsiness and somnolence are common during therapy with the drug. In controlled clinical studies, adverse nervous system effects (other than peripheral neuritis) occurred in 54% of ENL patients receiving thalidomide, and 34–56 or 34% of HIV-infected patients receiving thalidomide or placebo, respectively. Drowsiness occurred in 38% and malaise occurred in 8% of ENL patients receiving thalidomide, and drowsiness occurred in 36–38 or 11% of HIV-infected patients receiving thalidomide or placebo, respectively. Headache occurred in about 12% of leprosy ENL patients receiving thalidomide, and 17–19 or 11% of HIV-infected patients receiving thalidomide or placebo, respectively. Vertigo occurred in 8% and dizziness occurred in 4–25% of ENL patients receiving thalidomide; dizziness occurred in 19% of HIV-infected patients receiving the drug. Paresthesia occurred in 6–16 or 11% of HIV-infected patients receiving thalidomide or placebo, respectively, and also has been reported when the drug was used in ENL patients. Tremor occurred in 4% of leprosy patients with ENL receiving thalidomide, and agitation or nervousness occurred in 3–9% of HIV-infected patients receiving the drug. Insomnia occurred in 9 or 6% of HIV-infected patients receiving thalidomide or placebo, respectively.

Adverse nervous system effects reported in patients with ENL or HIV infection receiving thalidomide in uncontrolled studies include abnormal gait, abnormal thinking, amnesia, anxiety, ataxia, causalgia, circumoral paresthesia, confusion, decreased libido, decreased reflexes, dementia, dysesthesia, depression, emotional lability, euphoria,hypalgesia, hyperesthesia, hostility, hyperkinesia, incoordination, meningitis, neuralgia, neuritis, neurologic disorder, neuropathy, peripheral neuritis, and psychosis. Carpal tunnel disorder, foot drop, hangover effect, migraine, or suicide attempt was reported in at least one patient receiving thalidomide. Disturbance of consciousness (e.g., lethargy, syncope, loss of consciousness, stupor) have been reported.

Seizures, including tonic-clonic (grand mal) seizures, have been reported during postmarketing experience with thalidomide. Because the reports of seizures in patients receiving thalidomide were submitted voluntarily from a population of unknown size, their frequency cannot be estimated. Most of the patients in whom seizures were reported had disorders that may have predisposed them to seizure activity, and it currently is not known whether thalidomide has any epileptogenic activity.

■ **Dermatologic and Sensitivity Reactions** Adverse dermatologic effects occur commonly in patients receiving thalidomide. In controlled clinical studies, adverse dermatologic effects occurred in 42% of ENL patients receiving thalidomide, and 47–56 or 54% of HIV-infected patients receiving thalidomide or placebo, respectively. Rash occurred in 21% of ENL patients receiving thalidomide, and 25 or 31% of HIV-infected patients receiving thalidomide or placebo, respectively. Maculopapular rash occurred in 4% of ENL patients receiving thalidomide, and 17–19 or 6% of HIV-infected patients receiving thalidomide or placebo, respectively. Pruritus occurred in 3–8% of ENL patients receiving thalidomide, and 3–6 or 6% of HIV-infected patients receiving thalidomide or placebo, respectively. Fungal dermatitis or nail disorder occurred in 4% of ENL patients receiving thalidomide, and 3–9% of HIV-infected patients receiving thalidomide. Peripheral edema occurred in 4–8% of ENL patients and 3–8% of HIV-infected patients receiving thalidomide. Facial edema occurred in 4% and urticaria occurred in 1–2% of ENL patients receiving thalidomide. Sweating occurred in 12 or 11% of HIV-infected patients receiving thalidomide or placebo, respectively. Acne occurred in 3–11% of HIV-infected patients receiving thalidomide.

Severe, potentially fatal skin reactions including Stevens-Johnson syndrome and toxic epidermal necrolysis, which may be fatal, have been reported. In one limited study in HIV-infected patients, 14% of those receiving thalidomide (400 mg daily for 3 months) experienced severe skin reactions; these reactions resulted in discontinuance of drug in 7%. In another limited study in HIV-infected patients (with or without tuberculosis) who received thalidomide (300 mg daily for 3 weeks), 30% experienced severe rash that was associated with low CD4$^+$ T-cell counts. The mean CD4$^+$ T-cell count was 17 or 216 cells/mm^3 in those with or without rash, respectively. Thalidomide was discontinued and rash resolved in 25% of patients. However, one patient with rash continued to receive thalidomide because of a missed appointment and subsequently developed Stevens-Johnson syndrome with desquamation that resolved after discontinuance of the drug.

Hypersensitivity reactions characterized by cutaneous and/or febrile symptoms have been reported in HIV-infected patients receiving thalidomide. In some of these HIV-infected patients, rechallenge with thalidomide resulted in accelerated hypersensitivity, including hypotension. Therefore, some clinicians state that if thalidomide rechallenge in an HIV-infected patient is unavoidable (e.g., to elucidate a drug reaction in a patient receiving a complex drug regimen), the patient should be hospitalized when the drug is administered and for at least 24 hours following the rechallenge.

Adverse dermatologic and hypersensitivity reactions reported in patients with ENL or HIV infection receiving thalidomide in uncontrolled studies include allergic reaction, alopecia, angioedema, benign skin neoplasm, dry skin, eczema, exfoliative dermatitis, herpes simplex, ichthyosis, incomplete Stevens-Johnson syndrome, perifollicular thickening, photosensitivity, psoriasis, seborrhea, skin discoloration, skin disorder, skin necrosis, urticaria, and vesiculobullous rash. Erythema nodosum, myxedema, petechiae, or purpura was reported in at least one patient receiving thalidomide.

■ **GI Effects** In controlled clinical studies, adverse GI effects occurred in 21% of ENL patients receiving thalidomide, and 44–50 or 43% of HIV-infected patients receiving thalidomide or placebo, respectively. Diarrhea occurred in 4% and nausea occurred in 4–6% of ENL patients receiving thalidomide; diarrhea and nausea occurred in 17 and 12% of HIV-infected patients, respectively, receiving the drug. Vomiting has been reported in 1–2% of ENL patients receiving the drug. Abdominal pain and constipation occurred in 4–11% of ENL patients and 3–19% of HIV-infected patients receiving thalidomide. Oral candidiasis occurred in 4% of ENL patients and 6–11% of HIV-infected patients receiving thalidomide. Tooth pain occurred in 4% of ENL patients receiving thalidomide. Dry mouth occurred in 8–9 or 6–72% of HIV-infected patients receiving thalidomide or placebo, respectively. Anorexia occurred in 3–9 or 6% of HIV-infected patients receiving thalidomide or placebo, respectively. Flatulence occurred in 8 or 6% of HIV-infected patients receiving thalidomide or placebo, respectively.

Adverse GI effects reported in patients with ENL or HIV infection receiving thalidomide in uncontrolled studies include enlarged abdomen, increased appetite and weight gain, colitis, dry mouth, dyspepsia, dysphagia, eructation, esophagitis, flatulence, gastroenteritis, GI disorder, GI hemorrhage, gum disorder, intestinal obstruction, intestinal perforation, parotid gland enlargement, periodontitis, stomatitis, taste perversion, tongue discoloration, tooth disorder, and vomiting. Aphthous stomatitis or stomach ulcer has been reported in at least one patient receiving thalidomide.

■ **Respiratory Effects** In controlled clinical studies, adverse respiratory effects occurred in 12% of ENL patients receiving thalidomide, and 19–25 or 26% of HIV-infected patients receiving thalidomide or placebo, respectively. Pharyngitis occurred in 4% of ENL patients, and 6–8 or 6% of HIV-infected patients receiving thalidomide or placebo, respectively. Sinusitis or rhinitis occurred in 4% of ENL patients, and sinusitis occurred in 3–8 or 6% of HIV-infected patients receiving thalidomide or placebo, respectively.

Adverse respiratory effects reported in patients with ENL or HIV infection receiving thalidomide in uncontrolled studies include apnea, bronchitis, cough, emphysema, epistaxis, lung disorder, lung edema, pneumonia (including that caused by *Pneumocystis carinii*), pulmonary embolus, rales, upper respiratory infection, pleural effusion, and voice alteration. Also, dyspnea has been reported in at least one patient receiving thalidomide.

■ **Genitourinary Effects** In controlled clinical studies, adverse genitourinary effects occurred in 8% of ENL patients receiving thalidomide, and 6–17 or 11% of HIV-infected patients receiving thalidomide or placebo, respectively. Impotence occurred in 8% of ENL patients and 3–12% of HIV-infected patients receiving thalidomide. Albuminuria occurred in 3–8 or 6% of HIV-infected patients receiving thalidomide or placebo, respectively. Hematuria occurred in 11 or 3% of HIV-infected patients receiving thalidomide or placebo, respectively.

Adverse genitourinary effects reported in patients with ENL or HIV infection receiving thalidomide in uncontrolled studies include hematuria, orchitis, proteinuria, pyuria, and urinary frequency. Acute renal failure, amenorrhea, enuresis, metrorrhagia, or oliguria has been reported in at least one patient receiving thalidomide.

■ **Hematologic Effects** In controlled clinical studies, adverse hematologic effects occurred in 22–41 or 29% of HIV-infected patients receiving thalidomide or placebo, respectively. Leukopenia occurred in 17–25 or 9% of HIV-infected patients receiving thalidomide or placebo, respectively; in one study, leukopenia occurred in 14% of ENL patients receiving the drug. Lymphadenopathy occurred in 6–12 or 9% of HIV-infected patients receiving thalidomide or placebo, respectively. Anemia occurred in 6–12 or 9% of HIV-infected patients receiving thalidomide or placebo, respectively.

Adverse hematologic effects reported in patients with ENL or HIV infection receiving thalidomide in uncontrolled studies include aplastic anemia, cyanosis, decreased CD4$^+$ T-cell count, erythrocyte sedimentation rate increase, eosinophilia, granulocytopenia, hypochromic anemia, leukemia, leukocytosis, leukopenia, neutropenia, macrocytic anemia, megaloblastic anemia, microcytic anemia, elevated mean corpuscular volume, abnormal erythrocyte count, thrombocytopenia, and changes in prothrombin time. Chronic myelogenous leukemia, erythroleukemia, nodular sclerosing Hodgkin's disease, lymphopenia, or pancytopenia has been reported in at least one patient receiving thalidomide.

■ **Musculoskeletal Effects** In controlled clinical studies, asthenia occurred in 8% of ENL patients receiving thalidomide, and 6–22 or 3% of HIV-infected patients receiving or placebo, respectively. Back pain occurred in 4% of ENL patients and 6% of HIV-infected patients receiving thalidomide. Neck pain and neck rigidity each occurred in 4% of patients with ENL receiving thalidomide.

Adverse musculoskeletal effects reported in patients with ENL or HIV infection receiving thalidomide in uncontrolled studies include arthritis, bone tenderness, hypertonia, joint disorder, leg cramps, myalgia, myasthenia, periosteal disorder, and upper extremity pain.

■ **Cardiovascular Effects** Adverse cardiovascular effects reported in patients with ENL or HIV infection receiving thalidomide in uncontrolled studies include angina pectoris, arrhythmia, atrial fibrillation, bradycardia, cerebral ischemia, cerebrovascular accident, chest pain, congestive heart failure, deep thrombophlebitis, heart arrest, heart failure, hypertension, hypotension, murmur, myocardial infarction,palpitation, pericarditis, peripheral vascular disorder, postural (orthostatic) hypotension, syncope, tachycardia, thrombophlebitis, thrombosis, and vasodilation. Raynaud's syndrome has been reported in at least one patient receiving thalidomide. Sick sinus syndrome and ECG abnormalities also have been reported.

The manufacturer states that some patients who developed bradycardia required medical intervention; the clinical importance and underlying etiology of bradycardia in these patients are unknown.

■ **Hepatic Effects** In controlled clinical studies, increased serum AST (SGOT) concentrations occurred in 3–12 or 6% of HIV-infected patients receiving thalidomide or placebo, respectively; multiple abnormalities in liver function test results occurred in 9% of HIV-infected patients receiving thalidomide.

Adverse hepatic effects reported in patients with ENL or HIV infection receiving thalidomide in uncontrolled studies include increased liver function test results, increased serum ALT (SGPT) concentrations, bilirubinemia, cholangitis, cholestatic jaundice, enlarged liver, and hepatitis. Bile duct obstruction has occurred in at least one patient receiving thalidomide.

■ **Ocular and Otic Effects** Adverse ocular and otic effects reported in patients with ENL or HIV infection receiving thalidomide in uncontrolled studies include amblyopia, conjunctivitis, dry eye, ocular disorder, ocular pain, lacrimation disorder, retinitis, deafness, and tinnitus. Diplopia or nystagmus has occurred in at least one patient receiving thalidomide.

■ **Effects on HIV Viral Load and Tumor Necrosis Factor** Increased HIV viral load (i.e., increased plasma HIV-1 RNA levels) and increased levels of plasma tumor necrosis factor alpha (TNF-α) and soluble TNF-α receptor type II have been reported in some HIV-infected patients receiving thalidomide. In one controlled study in HIV-infected patients, median plasma HIV-1 RNA levels increased by 0.42 $\log_{10}$ copies/mL in patients receiving thalidomide compared with a 0.05 $\log_{10}$-copies/mL increase in those receiving placebo. A similar trend of increased HIV load was reported in another study in HIV-infected patients. However, the clinical importance of these effects is unknown since the patients involved were not receiving the potent antiretroviral agent combination regimens currently recommended for HIV-infected patients. (See Pharmacology: Immunomodulatory Effects.)

■ **Other Adverse Effects** In controlled clinical studies, accidental injury occurred in 4% of ENL patients, and 6 or 3% of HIV-infected patients receiving thalidomide or placebo, respectively. Chills occurred in 4% of ENL patients, and 9 or 11% of HIV-infected patients receiving thalidomide or placebo, respectively. Pain occurred in 8% of ENL patients, and 3 or 6% of HIV-infected patients receiving thalidomide or placebo, respectively. Fever occurred in 19–22 or 17% of HIV-infected patients receiving thalidomide or placebo, respectively. Infection occurred in 6–8 or 3% of HIV-infected patients receiving thalidomide or placebo, respectively. Hyperlipidemia occurred in 6–9 or 3% of HIV-infected patients receiving thalidomide or placebo, respectively.

Other adverse effects reported in patients with ENL or HIV infection receiving thalidomide in uncontrolled studies include avitaminosis, altered hormone concentrations, altered alkaline phosphatase concentrations, dehydration, increased BUN, decreased creatinine clearance, inappropriate antidiuretic hormone concentrations, increased serum creatinine, electrolyte abnormalities, tumor lysis syndrome, hypocalcemia, hypercalcemia, hypercholesterolemia, hyperglycemia, hypokalemia, hyperkalemia, hyponatremia, hyperlipidemia, hypoproteinemia, hyperuricemia, increased lactic dehydrogenase, increased lipase, decreased phosphorus, amyloidosis, ascites, chills and fever, cellulitis, cyst, diabetes, fever, flu-like syndrome, hernia, moniliasis, palpable spleen, pancreatitis, sarcoma, sepsis, and viral infection. Galactorrhea, gynecomastia, hypomagnesemia, hypothyroidism, and lymphedema have occurred in at least one patient receiving thalidomide.

■ Precautions and Contraindications

Teratogenicity Precautions and Contraindications Because thalidomide is a known human teratogen (see Teratogenic Effects under Pregnancy, Fertility, and Lactation: Pregnancy), the drug is commercially available in the US only through a restricted distribution program, the System for Thalidomide Education and Prescribing Safety (STEPS) designed to minimize the chance of fetal exposure and help ensure the safe and effective prescribing, dispensing, and use of thalidomide. Thalidomide may be prescribed only by licensed physicians who are registered in the STEPS program and understand the risk of teratogenicity if thalidomide is used during pregnancy. For information on the distribution program, see Dosage and Administration: Restricted Distribution Program.

Thalidomide is contraindicated in pregnant women and should be used in females of childbearing potential only when alternative therapies are considered inappropriate and the patient is capable of understanding and complying with the patient registration, education, and safety requirements of the STEPS program, including mandatory contraceptive measures and pregnancy testing. Female patients should be advised to immediately discontinue taking thalidomide and inform their clinician if they become pregnant (or for any reason they think they might be pregnant), miss a menstrual period, experience unusual menstrual bleeding, or stop using contraceptive measures. (See Pregnancy, Fertility, and Lactation: Pregnancy, in Cautions.)

Thalidomide should be used in sexually mature males only when the patient is capable of understanding and complying with the patient registration, education, and safety requirements of the STEPS program, including mandatory contraceptive measures for men. Male patients receiving thalidomide should be instructed to inform their clinician if they have unprotected heterosexual sexual contact while receiving thalidomide or during the first 4 weeks after discontinuing the drug or if they think that their sexual partner may be pregnant.

Patients should be advised to take thalidomide only as prescribed, and in compliance with the requirements of the STEPS program. Patients should be warned not to share thalidomide with anyone else and to keep the drug out of the reach of children. In addition, patients should be instructed not to donate blood and male patients should be warned not to donate semen while taking thalidomide.

Contraceptive Measures. All women and adolescent females of childbearing potential and all sexually mature males receiving thalidomide must use effective contraceptive measures (which may include abstinence) to help ensure that fetal exposure to thalidomide does not occur. Contraceptive measures are indicated even in females with a history of infertility. The only females who do not need to observe mandatory contraceptive measures are those who have undergone hysterectomy or who are postmenopausal and have had no menses for at least 24 consecutive months.

All women and adolescent females of childbearing potential *must* use 2 reliable forms of contraception simultaneously (unless the patient chooses to remain continuously abstinent from engaging in heterosexual sexual contact) beginning 4 weeks prior to initiating thalidomide therapy and continuing until 4 weeks after thalidomide therapy is discontinued. The patient must use at least 2 birth control methods; preferably one should be a highly effective birth control method (intrauterine device [IUD]; oral, injectable, or implanted hormonal contraceptives; tubal ligation; vasectomized partner) *and* one should be an effective barrier method (latex condom, diaphragm, cervical cap). However, if either IUD or hormonal contraceptive use is contraindicated in the female, 2 other effective methods may be used. Females of childbearing potential receiving thalidomide concomitantly with any other drug that can reduce efficacy of oral contraceptives must use 2 *other* effective methods of contraception or abstain from heterosexual sexual contact. Drugs that may interfere with the effectiveness of oral contraceptives include protease inhibitors (e.g., amprenavir, indinavir, nelfinavir, ritonavir, saquinavir), griseofulvin, rifampin, rifabutin, phenytoin, or carbamazepine. (See Drug Interactions: Hormonal Contraceptives and Drugs that Interfere with Hormonal Contraceptives.)

Sexually mature males (including those who have successfully undergone vasectomy) receiving thalidomide must completely avoid unprotected sexual contact with women of childbearing potential because thalidomide is present in semen. While receiving thalidomide and for at least 4 weeks after discontinuing the drug, sexually mature males must use a latex condom each time they have sexual contact with a woman of childbearing potential. The risk to the fetus from the semen of male patients receiving thalidomide is not known.

All females of childbearing potential must be tested for pregnancy within the 24 hours immediately prior to the first dose of thalidomide using a reliable serum pregnancy test with the sensitivity to detect human serum chorionic gonadotropin (HCG) concentrations of 50 mIU/mL. The prescribing clinician should not provide the woman with a prescription for thalidomide until a written report of the pregnancy test is available indicating that results are negative. Serum pregnancy tests must then be repeated at regular intervals during thalidomide therapy (i.e., weekly during the first month, then every 2 or 4 weeks in women with irregular or regular menstrual cycles, respectively). Pregnancy tests also should be performed if a patient misses her period or if there is any abnormality in menstrual bleeding. If pregnancy occurs during thalidomide therapy, the drug should be discontinued immediately. (See Pregnancy under Cautions: Pregnancy, Fertility, and Lactation.)

Thromboembolic Events Since use of thalidomide in patients with multiple myeloma is associated with increased risk of venous thromboembolic events (e.g., deep venous thrombosis, pulmonary embolism) in patients receiving thalidomide in combination with dexamethasone therapy compared with those receiving dexamethasone alone, the manufacturer recommends that patients and clinicians observe for signs and symptoms of thromboembolism and patients notify a clinician if they develop shortness of breath, chest pain, and/or arm or leg swelling. Decisions regarding use of thromboprophylaxis should be based on careful assessment of the patient's risk factors for thromboembolism. (See Cautions: Thromboembolic Events.)

Peripheral Neuropathy Precautions and Contraindications Because thalidomide may cause peripheral neuropathy that can be irreversible, patients should be instructed to immediately report initial symptoms (e.g., numbness, tingling, pain or a burning sensation in the hands and feet) of peripheral neuropathy to their prescribing clinician. To ensure that early signs of neuropathy are detected, patients should be examined, counseled, and questioned regularly during thalidomide therapy (i.e., monthly for the first 3 months of thalidomide treatment, and periodically thereafter).

Early detection and differential diagnosis of thalidomide-induced neuritis may be difficult in leprosy patients with ENL and in HIV-infected patients because neuritis associated with these diseases may be similar to that caused by thalidomide.

To assist in detection of asymptomatic neuropathy, the manufacturer states that consideration should be given to using electrophysiologic testing, consisting of sensory nerve action potential (SNAP) amplitude measurement at baseline and every 6 months thereafter. If manifestations of peripheral neuropathy develop, thalidomide should be discontinued immediately (if clinically appropriate) to minimize further damage. Usually, treatment with thalidomide should be resumed only if manifestations of neuropathy return to baseline.

Drugs known to be associated with peripheral neuropathy should be used with caution in patients receiving thalidomide. (See Drug Interactions: Drugs Associated with Peripheral Neuropathy.)

CNS Precautions and Contraindications Patients should be warned that thalidomide frequently causes drowsiness and somnolence, and may impair their ability to perform hazardous activities requiring mental alertness or physical coordination (e.g., operating machinery, driving a motor vehicle). Patients also should be warned not to take any other drugs that may cause drowsiness without consulting their clinician. Patients should be advised that thalidomide may potentiate the drowsiness caused by alcohol. (See Drug Interactions: CNS Agents.)

Because seizures, including tonic-clonic (grand mal) seizures, have been reported during postmarketing experience with thalidomide, the manufacturer states that patients with a history of seizures or other risk factors for the development of seizures should be monitored closely for clinical changes that could precipitate acute seizure activity.

Other Precautions and Contraindications Because thalidomide may cause dizziness and orthostatic hypotension, patients receiving the drug should be instructed to sit upright for a few minutes before standing up from a reclining position.

Because decreased leukocyte counts, including neutropenia, have been reported in patients receiving thalidomide, the drug should not be initiated in patients with absolute neutrophil counts (ANC) less than 750/mm^3. Leukocyte counts and differentials should be routinely monitored, especially in patients who are prone to neutropenia (e.g., HIV-infected patients). If the ANC decreases to less than 750/mm^3 while the patient is receiving thalidomide, the patient's drug regimen should be reevaluated and consideration given to withholding thalidomide if clinically appropriate.

Because increases in viral load (i.e., increased plasma HIV-1 RNA levels) have been reported when thalidomide was used in some HIV-infected patients, the manufacturer states that plasma HIV-1 RNA levels should be measured after the first and third months of thalidomide treatment and every 3 months thereafter.

Since thalidomide has been shown to be present in the serum and semen of patients receiving thalidomide, healthcare providers or other care givers who have been exposed to body fluids from patients receiving thalidomide should take appropriate precautions (e.g., wearing gloves to prevent potential cutaneous exposure to thalidomide, washing the exposed area with soap and water). (See Teratogenic Effects under Pregnancy, Fertility, and Lactation: Pregnancy, in Cautions.)

Thalidomide is contraindicated in patients who are hypersensitive to the drug or any ingredient in the formulation. The drug should be discontinued if signs and symptoms of hypersensitivity (e.g., erythematous macular rash associated with fever, tachycardia, hypotension) occur and are severe; if thalidomide therapy is resumed and the reaction recurs, thalidomide should be permanently discontinued. Because hypersensitivity reactions characterized by cutaneous and/or febrile manifestations have been reported in HIV-infected patients receiving thalidomide and because rechallenge with the drug resulted in accelerated hypersensitivity (including hypotension) in some of these patients, some clinicians recommend that if thalidomide rechallenge is unavoidable in an HIV-infected patient (e.g., to elucidate a drug reaction in a patient receiving a complex drug regimen), the patient should be hospitalized when the drug is administered and for at least 24 hours following the rechallenge.

Because severe, potentially fatal skin reactions, including Stevens-Johnson syndrome and toxic epidermal necrolysis, have been reported with thalidomide therapy, the drug should be discontinued if a rash occurs and should be resumed only after appropriate clinical evaluation. If the rash is exfoliative, purpuric, or bullous or if Stevens-Johnson syndrome or toxic epidermal necrolysis is suspected, use of thalidomide should *not* be resumed. Some clinicians state that thalidomide should not be used to treat toxic epidermal necrolysis.

■ **Pediatric Precautions** Although safety and efficacy of thalidomide in pediatric patients younger than 12 years of age have not been established, the drug has been used in a limited number of children 6 months to 12 years of age†. The manufacturer states that when thalidomide was used in a limited number of patients 11–17 years of age (usually in a dosage of 100 mg daily), response rates and safety profile were similar to those observed in adults. When thalidomide was used for the treatment of graft-versus-host disease in a limited number of bone marrow transplant recipients 1.5–17 years of age†, adverse effects of the drug included somnolence (which required discontinuance of the drug in at least one child), constipation, and a syndrome of rash, eosinophilia, and pancreatitis (which resolved after the drug was discontinued).

Thalidomide is contraindicated in adolescent females of childbearing potential (i.e., those who are sexually mature, have had menses at some time during the 24 consecutive months preceding initiation of treatment with thalidomide, have not undergone a hysterectomy) unless alternative therapies are considered inappropriate and the patient is capable of complying with the contraceptive measures (which may include abstinence) designed to help ensure that fetal exposure to thalidomide does not occur. (See Teratogenic Precautions and Contraindications: Contraceptive Measures, in Cautions.)

For males and females 18 years of age and younger, a parent or legal guardian must be educated concerning the hazards of thalidomide and agree to ensure that the minor complies with all requirements of the STEPS program.

■ **Geriatric Precautions** No overall differences in efficacy or safety were observed between geriatric and younger patients. Other clinical experience has not revealed age-related differences in response; however, the possibility of greater sensitivity of some older patients cannot be ruled out.

■ **Mutagenicity and Carcinogenicity** There was no evidence of mutagenic effects when thalidomide was evaluated in vitro using bacterial test systems (Ames test using *Salmonella typhimurium* and *Escherichia coli*), in vitro using mammalian test systems (Chinese hamster ovary cells, AS52/XPRT mammalian cell forward gene mutation assay), in vitro using human lymphocytes (chromosome aberration assay, micronucleus assay), or in vivo using mammalian test systems (CD-1 mice, micronucleus test). While there have been a few unsubstantiated reports that positive results were obtained when thalidomide was tested for mutagenicity in *Salmonella* and mouse bone marrow cells, these results have not been confirmed.

Although thalidomide is teratogenic, the drug is *not* considered to be mutagenic in humans. A report that 2 men with birth defects attributed to thalidomide exposure each fathered a child with birth defects resulted in speculation that thalidomide may be mutagenic in addition to teratogenic and capable of causing second generation birth defects. However, there is no evidence to support such a hypothesis and experts state that the birth defects in both these children were *not* the result of parental thalidomide exposure but probably occurred because of genetic abnormalities related to spontaneous mutations that occurred in the parents. The fathers of both children may have had malformations caused in part by thalidomide exposure, but the father of one child had anomalies that were quite atypical from those associated with thalidomide exposure. While only limited information is available about one of the children, both appeared to have limb formation abnormalities similar to those of their respective fathers. Since mutagens attack genes at random, if thalidomide did have a mutagenic effect distinct from its teratogenic effect, it is unlikely that the mutations would result specifically in limb malformations. There is no evidence that the incidence of birth defects in children born to parents with birth defects related to thalidomide exposure is any higher than that reported in the general population and no evidence that thalidomide-associated birth defects are inheritable.

Long-term studies to evaluate the carcinogenic potential of thalidomide have not been performed to date.

■ **Pregnancy, Fertility, and Lactation** ***Pregnancy*** Thalidomide is a known human teratogen, and can cause severe, life-threatening birth defects or fetal death if taken during pregnancy. The drug can cause teratogenic effects even if only a single dose of the drug (e.g., 50–100 mg; regardless of strength) is taken during pregnancy. Since the risks clearly outweigh any possible benefits in women who are or may become pregnant, thalidomide is contraindicated in such women. If the drug is inadvertently administered during pregnancy or if a patient becomes pregnant while receiving the drug, the drug should be discontinued immediately and the patient referred to an obstetrician-gynecologist experienced in reproductive toxicity for further evaluation and counseling. The patient should be informed that if their clinician is not available, information about emergency contraception (including information regarding clinicians who provide emergency contraceptive services) can be obtained by calling 888-668-2528 or by using other sources (e.g., http://www.opr.princeton.edu/ec). For information about postcoital contraception, see Estrogen-Progestin Combinations and Progestins in Contraceptives 68:12.Any suspected exposure of a fetus to thalidomide should be reported to the FDA MedWatch Program (800-FDA-1088) and also to the manufacturer, Celgene Corporation (1-888-423-5436).

To minimize the chance of fetal exposure and help ensure the safe and effective use of thalidomide in the US, patients must be registered in the STEPS program before they can receive commercially available drug. (See Dosage and Administration: Restricted Distribution Program.) The STEPS program includes mandatory contraceptive measures for both men and women, as well as mandatory pregnancy testing to confirm that a woman is not pregnant before thalidomide therapy is initiated and did not become pregnant during or immediately after therapy with the drug. (See Contraceptive Measures under Precautions and Contraindications: Teratogenicity Precautions and Contraindications, in Cautions.)

Thalidomide is contraindicated in women of childbearing potential unless alternative therapies are considered to be inappropriate and the patient is capable of understanding and following the conditions of the STEPS program, including mandatory contraceptive measures designed to ensure that the woman is essentially unable to become pregnant while receiving thalidomide. Women of childbearing potential are considered to be women and adolescent females who are sexually mature, have had menses at some time in the 24 consecutive months preceding initiation of treatment with thalidomide (i.e., are not postmenopausal), and have not undergone a hysterectomy. It is mandatory that such women (even if they are infertile) agree *not* to try to become pregnant for at least 4 weeks after discontinuing thalidomide treatment, and comply with effective contraceptive measures (which may include abstinence) for at least 4 weeks prior to, throughout, and for at least 4 weeks after completion of thalidomide therapy. In addition, a reliable serum pregnancy test with the sensitivity to detect human serum chorionic gonadotropin (HCG) concentrations of 50 mIU/mL must be performed within 24 hours prior to beginning thalidomide therapy, and results must be negative. Serum pregnancy tests must then be repeated at regular intervals during thalidomide therapy (i.e., weekly during the first month, then every 2 or 4 weeks in women with irregular or regular menstrual cycles, respectively). Pregnancy testing and counseling should be performed if a patient misses her period or if there is any abnormality in menstrual bleeding during thalidomide therapy.

Thalidomide is contraindicated in sexually mature males unless the patient is capable of understanding and following the conditions of the STEPS program, including mandatory contraceptive measures. Because thalidomide is present in semen, sexually mature males (including those who have successfully undergone vasectomy) receiving thalidomide must not have unprotected sexual contact with women of childbearing potential. These males must use a latex condom each time sexual contact with a woman occurs during and for at least 4 weeks after discontinuing the drug. The risk to the fetus from the semen of male patients receiving thalidomide is not known.

Teratogenic Effects. It has been estimated that there were more than 10,000 reported cases of infants born with birth defects related to use of thalidomide in pregnant women in other countries between 1957 (when thalidomide was first introduced in the world market) and 1963 (several years after the drug was removed from the world market). Although thalidomide was not commercially available in the US at that time, there were at least 17 reports of infants with thalidomide-associated birth defects being born to women in the US during those years; these women had received the drug from overseas sources or received premarketing samples distributed by drug company representatives.

A variety of human fetal abnormalities related to thalidomide administration during pregnancy have been documented. The most common birth defects reported following fetal exposure to thalidomide are musculoskeletal fetal abnormalities involving the loss of all or part of one or more bones; however, fetal deformities may occur in almost any organ of the body and defects of internal organs have been reported with some skeletal deformities. The mortality rate at or shortly after birth in infants born with thalidomide-induced abnormalities has been reported to be about 40%; most fatalities are related to serious malformations of internal organs.

Skeletal deformities caused by thalidomide include amelia (absence of legs and/or arms) and absence of bones; phocomelia (short legs and/or arms) and bone hypoplasia; hand deformities (e.g., radial club hand); thumb aplasia, hypoplasia, triphalangia, and nonopposability; finger aplasia, hypoplasia, fixed flexion, and syndactyly; and hip dysplasia and dislocation. Skeletal deformities appear to follow the craniocaudal progression of fetal morphogenesis. Most individuals with thalidomide defects of the upper limbs have normal lower limbs, some have defects of all limbs, but those with normal upper limbs and deformed lower limbs are rare. When substantial parts of bones are missing, the muscles normally attached to them are hypoplastic, but the degree of muscle hypoplasia does not always correspond to the level of bone loss (e.g., marked hypoplasia of shoulder and upper arm muscles may occur in a patient with a humerus of normal length). In general, more pronounced shortness of stature than that associated only with short leg bones occurs, resulting from poor growth, spinal osteochondritis, and progressive kyphosis. Thalidomide-induced skeletal deformities usually are bilaterally symmetric, similar to malformations reported with other teratogenic drugs. However, the extent of symmetry varies with the nature of the defect, both in the number of appreciably asymmetric deformities and in the closeness of the match between left and right.

The next most common group of abnormalities reported following fetal exposure to thalidomide are craniofacial and orofacial fetal abnormalities involving the ear, eye, and nerve supplies to the face, external ocular muscles, and lacrimal glands; these deformities tend to occur in a variety of combinations and permutations. External ear deformities tend to be bilateral and symmetric, and include anotia, microtia or micropinna, and small or absent auditory canals. Individuals with anotia and a blind or absent external auditory canal (meatus) are profoundly deaf in the affected ear. Facial palsy may occur (usually unilaterally rather than bilaterally) and almost always is associated with anotia or microtia on the same side. Abnormalities of ocular structures occur frequently, including anophthalmos, microphthalmos coloboma of the iris and retina, and conjunctival dermoid cyst. Microphthalmos and coloboma often occur together, and are predominantly bilateral. Restricted ocular movements may occur; ocular movement defects are nearly always associated with otic defects, often associated with facial weakness, and tend to be bilateral. Tear-saliva syndrome (crocodile tears) has been reported, in which tears are secreted in association with eating (rather than saliva) but may not be secreted in association with crying. This syndrome results from incorrect neural connections (probably in the brain stem), is bilateral or unilateral, and usually is associated with otic abnormalities and ocular movement defects. Less common orofacial defects that have reported include cleft palate, high arched palate, bifid uvula, palatal palsy, cleft lip,choanal atresia, and mandibular and dental abnormalities.

Other fetal deformities that have been associated with thalidomide exposure during pregnancy include congenital heart defects and other cardiovascular malformations (e.g., patent ductus arteriosus, ventricular and/or atrial septal defects, pulmonary stenosis); renal and urinary tract malformations (e.g., defects of the kidney, ureter, and bladder); genital malformations (e.g., hypospadias, vaginal atresia, fallopian tube interruption, bicornate uterus, hypoplasia of the scrotum or labia, and undescended, small, or absent testis); GI tract malformations (e.g., duodenal atresia, duodenal stenosis, pyloric stenosis, anorectal stenosis, imperforate anus with fistula, anteriorly placed anus); gallbladder aplasia; and respiratory tract malformations.

Most teratogenic effects appear to have occurred as the result of exposure to thalidomide early in pregnancy, and there is some evidence that a distinct window of embryonic sensitivity to thalidomide's teratogenic effects exists (i.e., from about 34–50 days after the beginning of the last menstrual period). Some malformations appear to be associated with particular periods of embryonic exposure, including aplasia of the ear or stenosis of the rectum which appear to be associated with exposure to thalidomide at 34–38 or 49–50 days, respectively, after the beginning of the last menstrual period. However, incorrect reporting of the dates of last menstrual periods and/or thalidomide administration dates as well as atypical menstrual cycle duration may have resulted in considerable inaccuracy in these data. It has been suggested that limb defects may be secondary to an inhibition of blood vessel growth in the developing fetal limb bud, and studies of thalidomide's effects in fetal animal tissues have suggested that neural as well as limb development effects occur. The risk of potentially severe birth defects occurring following fetal thalidomide exposure later in pregnancy is unknown, but may be substantial. Animal studies to characterize the effects of thalidomide on late stage pregnancy have not been conducted. While numerous mechanisms for thalidomide-induced fetal abnormality and mortality have been proposed, some have been refuted and others have not been adequately studied; additional study is required to elucidate how thalidomide causes teratogenic effects in fetuses.

The only type of thalidomide exposure known to have resulted in drug-associated birth defects was related to oral administration of the drug. Currently no specific data are available regarding cutaneous absorption or inhalation of thalidomide in women of childbearing potential and whether such exposures may result in any birth defect. Patients should be instructed *not* to handle extensively or open thalidomide capsules and to maintain capsules stored in blister packs until ingestion. If there has been contact with a non-intact thalidomide capsule or the powder contents, the exposed area should be washed with soap and water. Thalidomide has been shown to be present in the serum and semen of patients receiving thalidomide. If healthcare providers or other care givers are exposed to body fluids from patients receiving thalidomide, appropriate precautions should be taken (e.g., wearing gloves to prevent the potential cutaneous exposure to thalidomide, washing the exposed area with soap and water).

Fertility In fertility studies in male and female rabbits receiving daily thalidomide dosages of 500 or 100 mg/kg, respectively, no impaired mating performance or fertility was observed. However, slight testicular pathological and histopathological effects were observed in male rabbits receiving daily dosages of the drug of 30 mg/kg or more.

The effect of thalidomide on fertility in humans has not been determined. Thalidomide is present in semen. The risk to the fetus from the semen of male patients receiving thalidomide is not known.

Lactation It is not known whether thalidomide is distributed into human milk. Because many drugs are distributed into milk, and because of the potential for serious thalidomide-related adverse effects in nursing infants, a decision should be made whether to discontinue nursing or the drug, taking into account the importance of the drug to the mother.

Drug Interactions

■ Hormonal Contraceptives and Drugs that Interfere with Hormonal Contraceptives Concomitant administration of thalidomide and oral contraceptives containing ethinyl estradiol and norethindrone does not appear to affect the pharmacokinetics of the hormones. In 2 studies in healthy women 21–45 years of age who received a 3-week regimen of thalidomide (200 mg of thalidomide daily) followed by a single oral dose of an estrogen-progestin combination oral contraceptive (70 mcg of ethinyl estradiol and 2 mg of norethindrone), the pharmacokinetics of both ethinyl estradiol and norethindrone were the same as those obtained in these women when the contraceptive was administered without thalidomide.

While it is unlikely that thalidomide would affect efficacy of oral contraceptives since the drug does not appear to affect the pharmacokinetics of the hormones, other drugs that the patient may be receiving, including HIV protease inhibitors (e.g., amprenavir, indinavir, nelfinavir, ritonavir, saquinavir), griseofulvin, rifampin, rifabutin, phenytoin, carbamazepine, or herbal supplements such as St. John's wort, may reduce efficacy of oral contraceptives up to 1 month after discontinuance of these agents. Because it is mandatory that women of childbearing potential receiving thalidomide use *effective* contraceptive measures for at least 4 weeks prior to, throughout, and for at least 4 weeks after completion of thalidomide therapy, women of childbearing potential receiving thalidomide concomitantly with any other drug that can reduce efficacy of oral contraceptives must use 2 *other* effective methods of contraception or abstain from heterosexual sexual contact. (See: Contraceptive Measures under Precautions and Contraindications: Teratogenicity Precautions and Contraindications, in Cautions.)

■ CNS Agents Thalidomide has been reported to enhance the sedative effects of some drugs, including barbiturates, chlorpromazine, and reserpine, and may potentiate the somnolence caused by alcohol.

■ Drugs Associated with Peripheral Neuropathy Because of the potential for additive effects, drugs known to be associated with peripheral neuropathy (e.g., certain antiretroviral agents [e.g., didanosine], certain antineoplastic agents [e.g., paclitaxel; platinum-containing drugs such as cisplatin; vinca alkaloids such as vincristine]) should be used with caution in patients receiving thalidomide.

Acute Toxicity

■ Pathogenesis Limited information is available on the acute toxicity of thalidomide in humans. The commercially available racemic mixture of thalidomide appears to have a low potential for acute toxicity, principally because racemic thalidomide has poor aqueous solubility and limited absorption as the result of interaction (i.e., hydrogen bonding) between carboxyl groups of the racemates. In addition, the drug is rapidly and spontaneously hydrolyzed in vivo to numerous metabolites and accumulation of the drug does not occur, even in patients with severe renal impairment. Although the LD_{50} of either the levorotatory or dextrorotatory enantiomers of thalidomide is about 0.5 g/kg in rodents, animal studies indicate that racemic thalidomide is not fatal when given in doses of 10 g/kg.

■ Manifestations Overdosage of thalidomide may cause prolonged sleep as a result of the drug's sedative and hypnotic effects, but fatalities are unlikely since the drug does not cause respiratory depression. In 3 reported suicide attempts involving deliberate ingestion of up to 14.4 g of thalidomide, all 3 individuals recovered without reported sequelae.

Chronic Toxicity

Physical and/or psychologic dependence have not been reported in individuals receiving thalidomide. However, the manufacturer states that, like other anxiolytic, sedative, and hypnotic drugs, it is possible that habituation to the sedative and hypnotic effects of thalidomide could occur.

Chronic use of thalidomide may result in potentially severe peripheral neuropathy, which can be irreversible. (See Nervous System Effects: Peripheral Neuropathy, in Cautions.) To ensure early detection of thalidomide-induced neuropathy, patients should be examined regularly (i.e., monthly for the first 3 months of thalidomide therapy, and periodically thereafter). Consideration should be given to using electrophysiologic testing, consisting of sensory nerve action potential (SNAP) amplitude measurement at baseline and every 6 months thereafter.

Pharmacology

■ Mechanism of Action Thalidomide has immunomodulatory, anti-inflammatory, and antiangiogenic activities. The drug also has sedative and hypnotic effects.

The mechanism(s) of action of the immunomodulatory and anti-inflammatory effects of thalidomide are complex and have not been fully determined; these effects appear to result in part from modulation of tumor necrosis factor alpha (TNF-α) levels, costimulatory or adjuvant effect on T-cells resulting in increased T-cell proliferation and increased production of interleukin-2 and interferon-γ, and/or modulation of leukocyte migration and chemotaxis. Other anti-inflammatory and immunomodulatory effects of the drug may include suppression of macrophage involvement of prostaglandin synthesis and modulation of interleukin-10 and interleukin-12 production by peripheral blood mononuclear cells.

The immunomodulatory and anti-inflammatory effects of thalidomide differ from those of other immunosuppressive agents, including corticosteroids, cyclosporin (e.g., cyclosporine) or macrolide (e.g., tacrolimus) immunosuppressants, pentoxifylline, immunosuppressive purine analogs (e.g. azathioprine) and purine metabolism inhibitors (e.g., mycophenolic acid), and also differ from those of nonsteroidal anti-inflammatory agents. Thalidomide does not appear to interfere with important host antimicrobial mechanisms; the drug has no substantial inhibitory effect on lymphocyte proliferation, does not impair delayed-type hypersensitivity reactions, and does not impair granuloma formation.

Thalidomide has no direct antibacterial activity against *Mycobacterium leprae*. In addition, results of an in vitro study using *Enterocytozoon bieneusi*, *Encephalitozoon intestinalis*, and *E. cuniculi* indicate that thalidomide has no direct activity against microsporidia.

■ **Immunomodulatory Effects** Use of thalidomide in the management of multiple myeloma, erythema nodosum leprosum (ENL], and various inflammatory and/or dermatologic disorders is based on the drug's immunomodulatory effects. Thalidomide's immunomodulatory effects may result from modulation of TNF-α levels, costimulatory or adjuvant effect on T-cells resulting in increased T-cell proliferation and increased production of interleukin-2 and interferon-γ, and/or modulation of leukocyte extravascular migration mechanisms. However, in vitro studies and preliminary clinical studies indicate that the immunomodulatory effects of thalidomide vary considerably under different conditions, and some evidence indicates that effects of the drug may be species specific.

Treatment of thalidomide in patients with multiple myeloma is accompanied by an increase in the number of circulating natural killer cells, and an increase in plasma levels of interleukin-2 and interferon-gamma (T cell derived cytokines associated with cytotoxic activity). In patients with multiple myeloma, thalidomide inhibits TNF-α expression by bone marrow stromal cells, resulting in inhibition of growth of multiple myeloma cells. Thalidomide enhances T cell activation, releasing cytokines IL-2 and interferon-γ. These cytokines activate natural killer cells causing lysis of multiple myeloma cells.

The difficulty in characterizing thalidomide's mechanism of action has been attributed in part to numerous in vivo metabolites that result from the combination of optical enantiomerism, hydrolysis, and hydroxylation of the drug. In studies of enantiomerically stable thalidomide analogs (with an α-methyl group attached to the chiral carbon), levorotatory analogs demonstrated more immunomodulatory, sedative, and teratogenic activity, and more inhibition of TNF-α release, than dextrorotatory analogs. Although apparent enantiomer-specific effects of thalidomide have been reported from in vitro and in vivo studies, data from such studies are limited by rapid racemization and the pharmacokinetics of the drug in the system being studied, and should be interpreted with caution. Spontaneous hydrolysis of thalidomide yields products that do not appear to have immunomodulatory activity; the extent of hepatic metabolism of the drug appears to be limited, and some experts state that insufficient evidence exists to support speculation that formation of active metabolites is required for thalidomide's effects.

The immunomodulatory effects of thalidomide may be related to suppression of excessive TNF-α production; however, there also is some evidence that thalidomide is capable of enhancing TNF-α synthesis. The drug selectively inhibits the production of TNF-α by cultured human monocytes (possibly by inhibiting production and/or enhancing the degradation of TNF-α messenger RNA) without influencing either general protein synthesis or the expression of other monocyte-derived cytokines (e.g., IL-1, IL-6, GM-CSF). Administration of thalidomide has been reported to decrease circulating TNF-α levels in patients with erythema nodosum leprosum (ENL).

Wasting syndrome and the associated systemic symptoms (e.g., anorexia, fever) also may be mediated by excessive TNF-α production, and there is limited evidence that thalidomide may reduce plasma TNF-α concentrations and ameliorate wasting in patients with HIV infection and/or tuberculosis. However, the role of TNF-α in HIV infection is unclear because evidence of TNF-α production in patients with HIV infection is inconsistent and includes reports of undetected, increased, or unchanged production of the cytokine. Also, serum and plasma TNF-α levels fluctuate because of the cytokine's short half-life, and may not accurately reflect the actual extent of TNF-α production and/or the degree of TNF-α-related toxicities. Such discrepancies in apparent TNF-α levels may result from the different assays used, or from defects in the methods used to determine in vitro and in vivo cytokine production. In addition, cytokines may be produced and act locally in tissue, and it is possible that circulating levels of TNF-α do not reflect tissue activity.

The effect of thalidomide on TNF-α levels, HIV replication, and HIV disease manifestations such as wasting is unclear. In one limited controlled study of patients with wasting syndrome associated with HIV-1 infection (with or without tuberculosis), those receiving thalidomide experienced a substantially greater weight gain than those receiving placebo; however, only the patients with HIV and tuberculosis experienced decreased plasma TNF-α and decreased plasma HIV-1 RNA levels while receiving thalidomide, and these patients experienced a higher mean weight gain than those with HIV infection alone. Data from some studies in patients with HIV infection indicate that thalidomide inhibited TNF-α activation of latent HIV-1 in monocytes and reduced replication of the virus; however, some evidence indicates that thalidomide *increases* plasma TNF-α and soluble TNF-α type II receptor levels in patients with HIV infection, and may increase HIV replication. In a placebo-controlled study in HIV-infected patients, thalidomide therapy (200 mg daily for 4 weeks) apparently had no inhibitory effect on HIV replication and no effect on plasma TNF-α levels, but did increase plasma levels of soluble IL-2 receptor, soluble CD8 antigen, and IL-12. In addition, in vitro studies using purified T-cells from these patients indicated that exposure to thalidomide resulted in a costimulatory effect resulting in increased production of IL-2 and interferon-γ.

There is evidence that thalidomide induces down-modulation of selected cell surface adhesion molecules involved in leukocyte migration, and the drug's immunomodulatory mechanism of action may result in part from modulation of cellular interactions involving direct physical contact (i.e., adhesion and detachment) of leukocytes with endothelial cells. Limited data indicate that thalidomide may modulate TNF-α induction of endothelial cell adhesion molecules; this effect may interfere with leukocyte adhesion to endothelium, and prevent the initiation of leukocytic extravasation into inflammatory foci. Also, once adhesion of leukocytes to vascular endothelium occurs, thalidomide may interfere with their detachment, and impede transmigration of leukocytes into extravascular tissue. Although thalidomide may up- or down-modulate different adhesion receptors, and its effects on various types of leukocytes is variable, treatment with thalidomide induces a prompt reduction in the number of neutrophils and CD4$^+$ T-cells in the lesions of patients with ENL. Leukocyte infiltration and cytokine (especially TNF-α) responses are present in focal inflammatory lesions characterized by post-capillary vasculitis (e.g., ENL lesions and mucocutaneous aphthae), and these immunopathologic conditions are those most clearly responsive to thalidomide. Such antivasculitic effects also may be enhanced by thalidomide's modulation of TNF-α synthesis or release. However, the exact mechanism of action for the drug's clinical immunomodulatory activity is unclear, and further study is required to elucidate the drug's mechanism of action.

■ **Effects on Angiogenesis** Thalidomide inhibits angiogenesis, and it has been suggested that the teratogenic effects of thalidomide on fetal limbs may be related to inhibition of blood vessel growth in the developing fetal limb bud. Thalidomide's anti-angiogenic effects have been demonstrated in several animal angiogenesis models; however, there is evidence that the drug's anti-angiogenic effects may be species specific and possibly may be related to a species-specific metabolite and/or metabolic activation. Thalidomide reduced the area of vascularization in a rabbit corneal model of induced neovascularization. The drug also inhibited angiogenesis in a rat aorta model and in human aortic endothelial cells when human or rabbit microsomes were present, but not when rat microsomes were present.

The mechanism of thalidomide's anti-angiogenic effects is unknown. It has been suggested that inhibition of cytokine synthesis (especially that of TNF-α) may contribute to thalidomide's anti-angiogenic effect; however, there is some evidence from animal models that thalidomide's effect on angiogenesis is independent of the drug's effect on TNF-α and possibly may result from a direct inhibitory effect on some component of angiogenesis.

■ **Sedative and Hypnotic Effects** Thalidomide has CNS depressant effects and causes sedation. The drug has a prompt sedative effect, and does not cause a hangover. The glutarimide ring contained in thalidomide appears to be responsible for the sedative and hypnotic effects of the drug; the ring is structurally similar to ring moieties contained in some other sedative and hypnotic drugs (e.g., glutethimide). Thalidomide may activate a sleep center in the forebrain, a mechanism of action unlike that of barbiturates. Thalidomide has little acute CNS toxicity, and does not cause incoordination or respiratory depression even at large doses. (See Acute Toxicity.) While thalidomide initially was investigated for use as a sedative and hypnotic in the late 1950s, the drug is no longer promoted for use as a sedative and hypnotic because of its teratogenic risk. (See Uses: Overview.)

Pharmacokinetics

The pharmacokinetics of thalidomide have been studied in healthy adults, adults with leprosy, adults with human immunodeficiency virus (HIV) infection, and geriatric men with prostate cancer. While there is some evidence that bioavailability of oral thalidomide (i.e., peak plasma concentrations, area under the plasma concentration-time curve [AUC]) may be greater in leprosy patients than in healthy individuals, results of a single-dose study indicate that the pharmacokinetics of thalidomide in HIV-infected individuals are similar to those in healthy individuals. Age-related changes in the pharmacokinetics of thalidomide have not been observed in healthy individuals, leprosy patients 20–69 years of age, or prostate cancer patients 55–80 years of age. The pharmacokinetics of thalidomide have not been studied to date in individuals younger than 18 years of age. While limited data indicate that the pharmacokinetics of thalidomide are similar in males and females, specific comparative studies have not been performed to determine whether there are any gender- or race-related differences in the pharmacokinetics of the drug. The pharmacokinetics of thalidomide in patients with renal (except those with end-stage renal disease) or hepatic impairment have not been determined.

Based on studies in healthy adults and HIV-infected patients, the pharmacokinetics of thalidomide can best be described by a single-compartment model with first-order absorption and elimination. Results of studies in healthy adults indicate that accumulation of thalidomide does not occur, and pharmacokinetic parameters are similar following single or multiple doses of the drug.

■ **Absorption** The absolute bioavailability of thalidomide administered as the commercially available racemic mixture of the drug has not been determined to date, in part because racemic thalidomide has poor aqueous solubility.

The limited aqueous solubility of racemic thalidomide does not appear to be due to a lipophilic structure, since the drug has a relative distribution between lipid and aqueous phases of about 2:1. However, the 4 carboxyl groups of the racemic form of the drug appear to interact through hydrogen bonding to result in relative aqueous insolubility. In contrast, the pure levorotatory or dextrorotatory enantiomers of thalidomide are 3–5 times more soluble than the racemic drug and are more readily absorbed.

Following oral administration of racemic thalidomide, the drug is slowly absorbed from the GI tract, and some interindividual variation in absorption has been reported. The relative bioavailability of thalidomide capsules compared with an oral polyethylene glycol (PEG) solution of the drug is 90%. When thalidomide is administered in increasing doses in healthy individuals, the extent of absorption (as measured by the AUC) increases proportionally with increasing dose; however, peak plasma concentrations of the drug increase in a less than proportional manner and the time to peak plasma concentrations is delayed, indicating that thalidomide's poor aqueous solubility affects the rate of oral absorption.

Mean peak plasma concentrations of thalidomide generally are attained 2.5–6 hours after an oral dose. In a study in healthy men 21–43 years of age who received a single 200-mg dose of thalidomide given as tablets (not commercially available in the US), mean peak plasma concentrations of 1.15 mcg/mL were attained at a mean of 4.4 hours. In healthy women 21–45 years of age who received a single 200-mg dose of thalidomide given as 50- or 100-mg capsules (100-mg capsules not commercially available in the US), mean peak plasma concentrations of 2.3–3.2 mcg/mL were attained within about 6 hours. In healthy adults who received a single 50-, 200-, or 400-mg oral dose of thalidomide as 50-mg capsules, mean peak plasma concentrations of 0.62, 1.76, or 2.82 mcg/mL, respectively, were attained at 2.9, 3.5, or 4.3 hours, respectively, after the dose.

In adults with leprosy who received a single 400-mg oral dose of thalidomide as 50-mg capsules, peak plasma concentrations of 3.44 mcg/mL were attained 5.7 hours after the dose.

In adults with HIV infection (without active opportunistic infections or concomitant disease that potentially could alter drug absorption) who received a single 100- or 300-mg dose of thalidomide as capsules, mean peak plasma concentrations of the drug were 1.2 or 3.5 mcg/mL, respectively, and were attained at a mean of 3.4 hours after either dose. In another study in asymptomatic HIV-infected adults who received single 100- or 200-mg doses of the drug, peak plasma concentrations averaged 1.2 or 1.9 mcg/mL, respectively, and were attained at 2.5 or 3.3 hours, respectively.

In men 55–80 years of age with prostate cancer who received a single 200- or 800-mg oral dose of thalidomide as 50-mg capsules, median peak plasma concentrations were 1.97 or 4.42 mcg/mL, respectively, and were attained at a median of 3.32 or 4.42 hours, respectively, after the dose. When these patients received multiple doses of thalidomide, mean peak plasma concentrations at steady state were 1.8 mcg/mL in those receiving 200 mg once daily and 7.57 mcg/mL in those receiving 800 mg daily.

Food may delay but does not appear to substantially affect the extent of absorption of thalidomide. Administration of thalidomide with a high-fat meal increased the time to peak plasma concentration to approximately 6 hours, but resulted in less than a 10% change in either the AUC or peak plasma concentration of the drug.

■ Distribution Information on distribution of thalidomide in humans is not available. Although pharmacologic and adverse effects of thalidomide appear to be organ specific, such effects do not correspond well with pharmacokinetic distribution data obtained in animals. While results of some animal studies indicate that high concentrations of thalidomide are found in the GI tract, liver, and kidneys, and lower concentrations are found in muscle, brain, and adipose tissue, other distribution studies in animals have failed to detect substantial accumulation of the drug in any particular organ. When radiolabeled thalidomide was administered to animals in one study, there was an even distribution of radioactivity, except for slight enhancement of radioactivity in kidneys, liver, biliary tissue, white (but not grey) matter of the CNS, and peripheral nerve trunks. In rabbits, thalidomide concentrations in CSF are about 50% of concurrent plasma concentrations of the drug. Thalidomide is present in semen; in at least one study, the drug was detectable in the semen of HIV-infected men receiving thalidomide 100 mg daily.

Thalidomide crosses the placenta in humans and in animals. Malformations of human fetuses exposed to thalidomide during the first trimester of pregnancy exhibit striking organ specificity. Fetal skeletal deformities involving the loss of part or all of one or more bones are most common, but fetal deformities may occur in almost any organ of the body and defects of internal organs accompany some skeletal deformities (e.g., amelia, phocomelia). Seemingly isolated neurodevelopmental regions (e.g., the eyes, ears, and possibly some brain stem neurons innervating facial muscles) are affected in cases of thalidomide embryopathy, but other neurodevelopmental defects rarely occur, and the skin and the lymphatic organs are notably not affected by fetal exposure to thalidomide. (See Teratogenic Effects under Pregnancy, Fertility, and Lactation: Pregnancy, in Cautions.)

The apparent volume of distribution of thalidomide has been reported to be 69.9–82.7 L in HIV-infected adults.

Results of an in vitro study indicate that the dextrorotatory and levorotatory enantiomers of thalidomide are 55 and 66%, respectively, bound to plasma proteins.

■ Elimination The mean elimination half-life of thalidomide following a single 200-mg oral dose ranges from 3–6.7 hours, and the elimination half-life appears to be similar following multiple doses of the drug. In a study in healthy adults who received a single 50-, 200-, or 400-mg oral dose of the drug, the mean elimination half-life of thalidomide was 5.5, 5.5, or 7.3 hours, respectively. The mean elimination half-life of thalidomide was 6.9 hours in adults with leprosy who received a single 400-mg oral dose and 4.6–6.5 hours in HIV-infected adults who received a single 100- to 300-mg dose.

While the exact metabolic fate of thalidomide in humans is not known, numerous metabolites may be formed as a result of optical enantiomerism and hydrolysis and hydroxylation of the drug. Commercially available thalidomide is a 1:1 racemic mixture of the dextrorotatory and levorotatory enantiomers of the drug, and chiral inversion and spontaneous hydrolysis of the enantiomers occurs in vivo or in vitro. The half-life for racemization of an enantiomer in whole blood is about 2.25 hours. In vivo, chiral inversion appears to occur principally in the circulation and in albumin-rich extravascular sites. Chiral inversion and hydrolysis of thalidomide apparently occur by several different mechanisms.

Thalidomide does not induce or inhibit its own metabolism; when the drug was administered to healthy women at a dosage of 200 mg once daily for 18 days, similar pharmacokinetics were observed on the first and last day of dosage. Hepatic metabolism of thalidomide is limited, and only the parent compound appears to be metabolized by cytochrome P-450 (CYP) isoenzymes.

The principal metabolic pathway of thalidomide appears to be nonenzymatic spontaneous hydrolysis. All 4 amide bonds in thalidomide are susceptible to hydrolytic cleavage and, under physiologic conditions, ring opening occurs first in the phthalimide moiety. Spontaneous hydrolysis to form more than 10 metabolites occurs rapidly in vitro, with a mean half-life (dependent on incubation temperature and pH) of 2–5 hours for both optical isomers. There is evidence that thalidomide metabolites formed by spontaneous hydrolysis in vitro have no immunomodulatory activity; however, further study is required to characterize the pharmacologic activity, if any, of metabolites formed in vivo.

Hydroxylation can occur at 4 sites in thalidomide (i.e., 2 sites in each of the phthalimide and glutarimide moieties). Metabolism and some pharmacologic effects of thalidomide may be species specific. Hydroxylated metabolites have been identified in species sensitive to the teratogenic effects of thalidomide (e.g., rabbit), and there is evidence that rat (a species *not* sensitive to teratogenic effects of the drug) microsomes are not able to produce a metabolite that is toxic to lymphocytes in other species. Intermediary forms (i.e., arene oxides or epoxides) proposed to be responsible for the teratogenic effects of the drug have not been demonstrated, hydroxylated metabolites resulting from epoxide activation have not been confirmed in human samples, and in vitro human microsomal preparations do not appear to catalyze the formation of hydroxylated metabolites.

The exact route of elimination of thalidomide in humans is unknown. Thalidomide is not appreciably excreted via the kidneys (less than 1%) in humans; some of the drug may be eliminated in the bile. Although total body clearance of the drug is about 170–207 mL/minute, unmetabolized thalidomide has a renal clearance of 1.15–1.38 mL/minute and less than 0.7% of the drug is excreted in urine as unchanged drug. Thalidomide is thought to be hydrolyzed to numerous metabolites; however, in individuals who received a single oral dose of the drug, only 0.02% of the dose was eliminated in urine as 4-hydroxy thalidomide 12–24 hours after administration. At 48 hours after a single oral dose, thalidomide is not detectable in urine.

In a study of 6 patients with end-stage renal disease, thalidomide (200 mg) was administered on a nondialysis and a dialysis day. Comparison of concentration-time profiles on a non dialysis and a dialysis day showed that the mean total clearance increased by a factor of 2.5 during hemodialysis; blood samples were collected at least 10 hours following administration of the drug. Since dialysis was performed 10 hours after the thalidomide dose was given, there were no statistically significant differences in the AUC of patients receiving the drug on a non dialysis or dialysis day. Therefore, no dosage adjustment was necessary in patients with end-stage renal disease undergoing dialysis.

Chemistry and Stability

■ Chemistry Thalidomide, a synthetic glutamic acid derivative, is an immunomodulatory agent. The drug is structurally similar to, but pharmacologically different from, glutethimide. Thalidomide contains a phthalimide ring and a glutarimide ring; the glutarimide ring is similar to that contained in glutethimide and may be responsible for the sedative and hypnotic effects of thalidomide. Because the glutarimide ring has a single asymmetric carbon (chiral center), thalidomide may exist as either an optically active levorotatory or dextrorotatory enantiomer. The enantiomers rapidly interconvert in vivo and in vitro; it is unknown whether the enantiomers have distinct pharmacologic properties. Thalidomide is commercially available as a 1:1 racemic mixture of the 2 enantiomers with a net optical rotation of zero.

Thalidomide occurs as a white to off-white, nearly odorless, crystalline powder. The drug has a solubility of 45–60 mcg/mL in water at 25°C. Thalidomide enantiomers are 3–5 times more soluble than the racemic drug. While the aqueous solubility of racemic thalidomide has been reported to be 50 mcg/mL, the aqueous solubility of the separate enantiomers has been reported to be 250 mcg/mL.

■ Stability Commercially available thalidomide capsules should be stored at 15–30°C and protected from light.

Since currently there are no specific data regarding cutaneous absorption or inhalation of thalidomide in women of childbearing potential and whether such exposures may result in any birth defect, patients should be instructed *not* to handle extensively or open thalidomide capsules and to maintain capsules stored in blister packs until ingestion. (See Teratogenic Effects under Pregnancy, Fertility, and Lactation: Pregnancy, in Cautions.)

In vitro in whole blood, serum, or plasma, thalidomide undergoes chiral inversion and spontaneous hydrolysis. All 4 amide bonds of the drug are susceptible to hydrolytic cleavage at pH exceeding 6. Inversion of the enantiomers occurs at a greater rate in vitro in blood at 37°C than in vivo. The rate of inversion and hydrolysis of thalidomide is pH dependent and increases with pH over the range of 7–7.5.

Preparations

Because thalidomide is a known human teratogen and can cause severe, life-threatening birth defects if administered during pregnancy, commercially available thalidomide must be obtained through a restricted distribution program, the System for Thalidomide Education and Prescribing Safety (STEPS), designed to help ensure that fetal exposure to the drug does not occur. See Restricted Distribution Program under Dosage and Administration.

Excipients in commercially available drug preparations may have clinically important effects in some individuals; consult specific product labeling for details.

Thalidomide

Oral		
Capsules	50 mg	Thalomid®, Celgene
	100 mg	Thalomid®, Celgene
	150 mg	Thalomid®, Celgene
	200 mg	Thalomid®, Celgene

†Use is not currently included in the labeling approved by the US Food and Drug Administration

Selected Revisions August 2018,

BONE RESORPTION INHIBITORS 92:24

Alendronate Sodium

■ Alendronate sodium, a synthetic bisphosphonate analog of pyrophosphate, is a bone resorption inhibitor.

Uses

■ **Osteoporosis** Alendronate is used in the treatment and prevention of osteoporosis in postmenopausal women; the drug also is used to increase bone mass in men with osteoporosis.

Osteoporosis, a systemic skeletal disease characterized by low bone mass and microarchitectural deterioration of bone tissue with consequent increased bone fragility and susceptibility to fracture (usually of the spine, hip, and wrist), is observed in a large proportion of postmenopausal women. Adult women have less bone mass than men at all ages, and decreased production of estrogen at menopause is associated with accelerated bone loss, particularly from the lumbar spine, for about 5 years, during which time skeletal mass loss averages 3% per year. Osteoporosis from age-related bone loss can also develop in men. While the risk of osteoporosis and resulting fractures cannot be quantified by a single clinical finding or test result, many risk factors have been identified, with the probability of developing osteoporosis increasing with multiple risk factors. Risk factors include early menopause, advanced age, low bone mineral density (BMD), low body mass index (BMI), previous fracture or family history of fracture/osteoporosis, excessive alcohol intake, smoking, inadequate physical activity, low calcium and vitamin D intake, certain drugs (e.g., glucocorticoids), and medical conditions or diseases (e.g., rheumatoid arthritis, diabetes mellitus, Cushing syndrome, hyperparathyroidism).

In addition to lifestyle modifications (e.g., regular weight-bearing exercise, avoidance of excessive alcohol and tobacco use), adequate intake of calcium (1–1.2 g daily) and vitamin D (800–1000 units daily) is essential in the prevention and treatment of osteoporosis and is recommended for all postmenopausal women and men 50 years of age or older. Additional pharmacologic therapy should be considered in such patients with high risk of fractures (generally those who have experienced a previous hip or vertebral fracture or who have low BMD). Pharmacologic therapy also may be considered in postmenopausal women and in men 50 years of age or older who have low bone mass, although there is less evidence supporting overall fracture risk reduction in such patients. When selecting an appropriate pharmacologic agent, experts recommend use of a drug with proven antifracture efficacy; available options include bisphosphonates (e.g., alendronate, risedronate, zoledronic acid, ibandronate), denosumab, raloxifene, calcitonin, or teriparatide with varying levels of recommendation given in expert guidelines based on the evidence supporting fracture risk reduction for each drug. While estrogen/hormone therapy was commonly used in the past for the treatment of osteoporosis in postmenopausal women, there is some evidence indicating that such therapy is associated with an increased risk of breast cancer, cardiovascular, cerebrovascular, and thromboembolic events. Choice of osteoporosis therapy should be individualized based on the potential benefits and adverse effects of therapy as well as patient preferences, comorbidities, and risk factors.

Prevention in Postmenopausal Women Alendronate is used for the prevention of osteoporosis in postmenopausal women. The drug is used adjunctively with other measures (e.g., diet, calcium, vitamin D, weight-bearing exercise, physical therapy, avoidance of excessive cigarette smoking and/or alcohol consumption) to retard further bone loss and the progression of osteoporosis in postmenopausal women. The goal of preventive therapy is preservation of bone mass and a resultant decrease in fracture risk.

Alendronate has been evaluated for the prevention of osteoporosis in postmenopausal women in 2 double-blind, placebo-controlled studies of 2 or 3 years' duration that included 2056 women (40–60 years of age). In these studies, therapy with alendronate 5 mg daily increased BMD, as determined by dual-energy radiographic absorption (DXA) measurements, in the lumbar spine, femoral neck, trochanter bone, and total body. While women receiving placebo lost approximately 1% of BMD per year, substantial increases in BMD were observed in women receiving alendronate. In one of the studies that included postmenopausal women who had experienced menopause 6–36 months before initiation of the study, administration of alendronate (5 or 10 mg daily given for 3 years or, alternatively, 20 mg daily given for 2 years, followed by administration of placebo daily for 1 year) at 3 years was associated with a 1–4% increase in lumbar spine, femoral neck, and trochanter BMD and 0.3–1% increase in total body BMD compared with baseline, while placebo recipients lost about 2–4% BMD in these sites; a lower dosage (1 mg daily) of alendronate for 3 years attenuated but did not fully prevent losses in BMD relative to those in women receiving placebo. Limited data indicate that alendronate (5 mg daily) reduced the rate of bone loss on forearm by about half relative to placebo. In a 1-year controlled study in postmenopausal women with osteoporosis, alendronate 70 mg once weekly produced increases in BMD similar to those observed with a dosage of 10 mg daily.

In osteoporosis prevention studies that evaluated alendronate therapy (Early Postmenopausal Intervention Cohort Study) for 24 months, raloxifene (European trial), or various estrogen/progestin combinations for hormone replacement therapy (HRT), alendronate (5 mg daily) therapy was associated with 1.3–1.9% increases in hip BMD compared with baseline, raloxifene hydrochloride therapy (60 mg daily) was associated with 1.6% increases, and HRT was associated with 1.8–3.2% increases. In these studies, alendronate, raloxifene, or HRT was associated with increases in BMD of lumbar spine of 2.9–3.5%, 1.6%, or 4–5.1%, respectively, compared with baseline.

Treatment in Postmenopausal Women Alendronate is used alone or in fixed combination with cholecalciferol (vitamin D_3) for the treatment of osteoporosis in postmenopausal women.

In several double-blind, placebo-controlled trials in postmenopausal women with osteoporosis (defined as lumbar spine BMD values at least 2 standard deviations below premenopausal mean values), therapy with alendronate 10 mg daily for 2–3 years substantially increased BMD in the lumbar spine, femoral neck, and trochanter; total body BMD also increased, suggesting that BMD increases in the spine and hip did not occur at the expense of other skeletal sites. In long-term trials (e.g., 3 years with several extensions up to 10 years), increases in BMD were apparent as early as 3 months after initiation of alendronate therapy and continued throughout therapy. Results of some studies indicate that some therapeutic effects on bone mass are maintained for up to 5 years following withdrawal of alendronate therapy (following 5 years of treatment) at the lumbar spine, trochanter, and total body; after discontinuance of therapy, BMD decreased appreciably at the femoral neck and forearm over the next 5 years of follow-up. Bone histology studies in postmenopausal women with osteoporosis treated with alendronate 1–20 mg daily for 1, 2, or 3 years indicate that bone formed during treatment with the drug is of normal quality. Among women who had sustained a vertebral fracture, alendronate therapy reduced the risk of new vertebral fractures, including women at high risk for further vertebral fractures (e.g., those with severe osteoporosis, those 75 years or older).

Analysis of pooled data from several US and multinational placebo-controlled trials in postmenopausal women indicates that alendronate therapy (5 or 10 mg daily for 3 years, or 20 mg daily for 2 years followed by 5 mg daily for 1 year) was associated with a reduced incidence of vertebral fractures (a 48% relative risk reduction) and, because of a reduction in the frequency and severity of fractures, less height loss than that occurring with placebo, even among patients who sustained a vertebral fracture. Several large, placebo-controlled clinical trials have noted a reduced incidence of vertebral and other types of fractures (e.g., hip, wrist) in postmenopausal women, most of whom had osteoporosis. In a large, placebo-controlled clinical trial in women with osteoporosis who had an existing vertebral fracture, alendronate therapy (5 or 10 mg once daily given concomitantly with calcium and vitamin D supplementation) reduced the incidence of hip fracture by 51% and wrist fracture by 48% at 3 years; the proportion of patients requiring hospitalization also was reduced (31 or 25% with placebo or alendronate, respectively). The frequency of adverse effects, including GI disorders, also was similar between alendronate or placebo. In another large, long-term (4-year), placebo-controlled trial in women with low BMD but without vertebral fractures, alendronate (5 mg daily for 2 years, then 10 mg daily thereafter) reduced the risk of clinical fractures in women with osteoporosis (baseline femoral neck BMD exceeding 2.5 standard deviations below the normal adult mean) but not in those with higher

BMDs. The incidence of atrial fibrillation in these 2 placebo-controlled trials was numerically higher in the alendronate-treated groups compared with that observed in the placebo-treated groups. (See Atrial Fibrillation under Warnings/Precautions: General Precautions, in Cautions in Zoledronic Acid 92:24.)

Combination Therapy Alendronate has been used concomitantly with various estrogen or estrogen/progestin combinations and calcium to increase bone mass in postmenopausal women with osteoporosis. In several clinical trials in postmenopausal women with osteoporosis, the combination of estrogen-containing hormone replacement therapy (HRT) and alendronate resulted in a greater degree of suppression of bone turnover than either therapy given alone. In a long-term, placebo-controlled trial comparing therapy with alendronate (10 mg once daily), conjugated estrogens (0.625 mg daily), or the combination of these drugs in postmenopausal women with osteoporosis who had undergone hysterectomy and were not currently receiving antiresorptive therapy, combination therapy increased lumbar spine and femoral neck BMD to a greater degree than either agent alone or placebo at 2 years. All women received supplementation with calcium 500 mg daily. Bone histology studies in these patients indicated that the bone formed during therapy was of normal quality. Compared with placebo, bone turnover after 18 months was suppressed by 98% with combined alendronate and HRT, 94% with alendronate therapy alone, and 78% with HRT alone. In another comparative study in postmenopausal women who had osteoporosis despite receiving estrogen or estrogen plus progestin (medroxyprogesterone) HRT for at least 1 year (mean duration almost 10 years), the addition of alendronate (10 mg once daily) to supplementation with daily vitamin D and calcium (if baseline calcium intake was less than 1000 mg daily) increased BMD in the lumbar spine and hip trochanter compared with HRT alone. In either trial, the incidence of new fractures was similar across treatment groups. However, the size and duration of these studies may have been inadequate to detect differences in fracture incidence for combination therapy compared with alendronate or placebo, and further studies are needed. The safety of combination therapy reportedly was consistent with that of each antiresorptive agent alone. However, some clinicians state that concomitant hormone replacement therapy currently is not recommended in patients receiving alendronate because of lack of clinical experience with such use.

Treatment in Men Alendronate also is used alone or in fixed combination with cholecalciferol (vitamin D_3) for the treatment of osteoporosis in men. In a double-blind, placebo-controlled trial in men 31–87 years of age (mean age: 63) with hypogonadal or idiopathic osteoporosis, therapy with alendronate (10 mg daily) substantially increased BMD in the lumbar spine, hip, femoral neck, and trochanter; total body BMD also increased, suggesting that BMD increases in the spine and hip did not occur at the expense of other skeletal sites. Osteoporosis in these men was defined as a femoral neck BMD value at least 2 standard deviations below the mean in healthy young men and a lumbar spine BMD value at least 1 standard deviation below the mean in healthy young men, or a femoral neck BMD of at least 1 standard deviation below the mean value in healthy young men and at least one sustained fracture. All patients in the study received supplemental calcium (500 mg daily as calcium carbonate) and vitamin D (400–450 units daily). Increases in BMD were apparent as early as 6 months after initiation of alendronate therapy and continued throughout therapy. Alendronate therapy was associated with a reduced incidence of new vertebral fractures and, because of a reduction in the frequency of fractures, less height loss than that occurring with calcium and vitamin D supplementation only.

In another double-blind, placebo-controlled trial in men 38–91 years of age (mean age: 66 years) with hypogonadal or idiopathic osteoporosis, therapy with alendronate (70 mg once weekly for 1 year) substantially increased BMD in the lumbar spine, femoral neck, trochanter, and total body. Osteoporosis in these men was defined as a femoral neck BMD value at least 2 standard deviations below the mean for healthy young men and a lumbar spine BMD value at least 1 standard deviation below the mean for healthy young men; a lumbar spine BMD of at least 2 standard deviations below the mean value for healthy young men and a femoral neck BMD value at least 1 standard deviation below the mean for healthy young men; or at least one sustained fracture and a femoral neck BMD value at least 1 standard deviation below the mean for healthy young men. The increases in BMD with weekly therapy were similar to those seen at 1 year in patients receiving 10 mg of alendronate daily. Among men receiving alendronate in both studies (daily or weekly therapy), response to therapy was similar regardless of age (65 years of age or older, younger than 65 years of age), gonadal function (baseline testosterone concentrations of at least 9 ng/dL, less than 9 ng/dL), or baseline BMD (femoral neck and lumbar spine BMD at least 2.5 standard deviations from the mean for young men, less than 2.5 standard deviations from the mean).

■ **Glucocorticoid-induced Osteoporosis** Alendronate is used in the treatment of glucocorticoid-induced osteoporosis. The manufacturer recommends use of alendronate in men and women receiving a daily dosage equivalent to at least 7.5 mg of prednisone who have low BMD; risks versus benefits of alendronate therapy in patients receiving a lower dosage of glucocorticoids have not been established. Alendronate also has been used in the prevention of glucocorticoid-induced osteoporosis†.

Osteoporosis and related fractures are some of the most serious complications of long-term glucocorticoid therapy. More than 10% of patients are diagnosed with a fracture and 30–40% have radiographic evidence of vertebral fractures during long-term glucocorticoid use. The risk of fracture is both dose and duration dependent, with higher daily or cumulative doses of glucocorticoids and longer durations of use associated with greater risk. A high glucocorticoid dosage generally is considered a daily dosage equivalent to more than 7.5 mg of prednisone. However, some studies have reported an increased risk of fracture with daily dosages as low as 2.5–7.5 mg of prednisolone or equivalent, while others have found no appreciable decline in bone density with prednisone dosages averaging 8 mg daily or dosages of less than 5 mg daily. Because glucocorticoid-induced osteoporosis can be effectively prevented, the American College of Rheumatology (ACR) recommends that appropriate preventive therapy be considered for patients in whom the benefits of such therapy outweigh the potential harms. ACR recommendations are based on a risk-stratification approach in which an individual's risk level for developing a fracture (low, moderate, or high) is determined based on predisposing factors including the individual's preexisting or anticipated glucocorticoid dosage. An initial clinical fracture risk assessment is recommended within 6 months of initiating long-term glucocorticoid therapy with reassessments recommended every 12 months during continued treatment. Lifestyle modifications (e.g., diet, smoking cessation, weight-bearing or resistance-training exercise) and calcium/vitamin D intake should be optimized in all patients receiving long-term (at least 3 months) glucocorticoid therapy at a daily dosage equivalent to at least 2.5 mg of prednisone. The need for additional pharmacologic therapy should be determined based on the patient's risk for fractures. ACR recommends an oral bisphosphonate in adults receiving long-term glucocorticoid therapy who are considered to be at moderate-to-high risk of fracture. Oral bisphosphonates generally are preferred because of their demonstrated benefits in reducing fracture risk as well as their safety and low cost; other options include IV bisphosphonates, teriparatide, denosumab, and raloxifene (for postmenopausal women if no other therapy is appropriate). ACR states that the available data on fracture risk and risk reduction are more limited in children and adults younger than 40 years of age; however, treatment with oral bisphosphonates and calcium/vitamin D is recommended because the possible benefits appear to outweigh the risks. For additional information on the prevention and treatment of glucocorticoid-induced osteoporosis, see Osteoporosis under Cautions: Musculoskeletal Effects, in the Corticosteroids General Statement 68:04

Alendronate has been evaluated for the treatment of glucocorticoid-induced osteoporosis in men and women with a variety of underlying diseases (e.g., rheumatoid arthritis, systemic lupus erythematosus, polymyalgia rheumatica, inflammatory myopathy, inflammatory bowel disease, asthma) and usually with low bone mineral density (e.g., 1–2 standard deviations below the mean for healthy young adults in more than 70% of those studied) who were receiving glucocorticoid therapy (e.g., a daily dosage of at least 7.5 mg of prednisone or equivalent) in 2 placebo-controlled, double-blind, randomized studies of 1 year's duration and an extension of one of these studies for a total duration of 2 years. In these studies, therapy with alendronate 5 or 10 mg daily (given concomitantly with calcium and vitamin D supplementation) increased BMD, as determined by DXA measurements in the lumbar spine, femoral neck, trochanter bone, and total body; 2 years after initiating alendronate therapy, lumbar BMD was increased by 2.8–3.9 and trochanter BMD also was increased and femoral neck BMD maintained relative to baseline values. While patients receiving placebo lost approximately 0.4, 0.7, or 1.2% of BMD within about 1 year at the lumbar spine, trochanter bone, or femoral neck, respectively, and 0.8% with 2 years at the lumbar spine; BMD either increased or was maintained in these sites in patients receiving alendronate for such periods of time. Administration of alendronate 5 mg daily was associated with a 2.1, 1.1, or 1.2% increase in lumbar spine, trochanter bone, or femoral neck, respectively, and administration of alendronate 10 mg daily was associated with a 2.9, 2.7, or 1% increase in lumbar spine, trochanter bone, and femoral neck, respectively, after 1 year. Total body BMD was maintained with 5 mg of alendronate daily after 1 year but was increased with 5 or 10 mg of the drug daily after 2 years.

The increases in BMD in patients receiving 10 mg of alendronate daily were similar to those receiving alendronate 5 mg except in postmenopausal women not receiving estrogen replacement therapy. In these women, BMD increases (relative to placebo) at the lumbar spine were 4.1 or 1.6% in patients receiving 10 or 5 mg of alendronate daily, respectively, while at the trochanter bone, BMD increases were 2.8 or 1.7% in patients receiving 10 or 5 mg of alendronate daily, respectively; at other sites, increases in BMD were similar when using the different dosages of alendronate. In these studies, greatest increase in BMD occurred in the first year of therapy and only maintenance or smaller increases in BMD were reported in the second year of therapy with alendronate. In addition, the efficacy of alendronate reportedly was not affected by age, gender, race, underlying disease, previous duration or current dosage of corticosteroid therapy, baseline BMD, baseline bone turnover or concomitant administration of other drugs. Bone histology was normal in several patients (receiving alendronate 10 mg daily for 1 year) who underwent bone biopsy. In these studies after 1 year of therapy, patients receiving alendronate (5 or 10 mg daily), had fewer new vertebral fractures than those receiving placebo (2.3 versus 3.7%, respectively), but the difference was not significant. Analysis of pooled data indicates that after 2 years of therapy, the incidence of a new vertebral fracture was 0.7 or 6.8% in patients receiving alendronate (5 or 10 mg daily for 2 years, or 2.5 mg for 1 year followed by 10 mg for the second year) or placebo, respectively. However, these findings were based on very few fractures occurring mainly in postmenopausal women.

■ **Paget Disease of Bone** Alendronate also is used orally in the treatment of moderate to severe Paget disease of bone (osteitis deformans). In most patients with Paget disease, only small areas of bone are involved and patients are usually asymptomatic; mild symptoms in these patients usually can be controlled with analgesics. Treatment with alendronate should be considered in patients with serum alkaline phosphatase concentrations at least twice the upper limit of normal, those who are symptomatic, or those at risk for future complications from their disease.

In clinical trials in males and females with moderate to severe Paget disease of bone (serum alkaline phosphatase concentrations at least twice the upper limit of normal), suppression of alkaline phosphatase (i.e., either normalization of serum concentrations or a decrease of at least 60% compared with baseline concentrations) after 6 months of therapy occurred in a substantially greater percentage of patients receiving alendronate (40 mg daily) than in those receiving etidronate disodium (400 mg daily) or placebo. Bone histology studies in patients with Paget disease of bone treated with alendronate 40 mg daily for 6 months indicate that bone formed during treatment with the drug is of normal quality. In placebo-controlled trials, the decreased bone turnover associated with bisphosphonate therapy has resulted in pain relief.

Retreatment with alendronate may be considered, following a 6-month posttreatment evaluation period, in patients with Paget disease of bone who have relapsed (as determined by an increase in serum alkaline phosphatase concentration). The manufacturer states that while clinical data on retreatment with alendronate currently are lacking, responses to initial therapy with the drug in patients who had or had not received prior bisphosphonate therapy have been similar.

Dosage and Administration

■ **General** Hypocalcemia and other disturbances of bone and mineral metabolism must be corrected before alendronate therapy is initiated. Patients should receive supplemental calcium and vitamin D if their dietary intake is inadequate. Supplemental vitamin D is recommended in patients at increased risk for vitamin D insufficiency (e.g., those older than 70 years of age; those who are nursing home bound or chronically ill; patients with GI malabsorption syndrome). The recommended intake of vitamin D is 400–800 units daily; a once-weekly dose of alendronate/cholecalciferol fixed-combination preparation containing cholecalciferol 2800 or 5600 units provides the equivalent of 400 or 800 units, respectively, of vitamin D daily.

■ **Administration** Alendronate sodium is administered orally as tablets or oral solution. The drug should be taken only upon rising for the day. Alendronate tablets and oral solution have equivalent bioavailability.

The fixed combination of alendronate sodium and cholecalciferol is administered orally as tablets.

To facilitate absorption of alendronate (alone or in fixed combination with cholecalciferol), the drug should be taken with a full glass (180–240 mL) of plain water at least 30 minutes before the first food, beverage, or other orally administered drug of the day; waiting longer than 30 minutes before eating, drinking, or ingesting another drug will improve absorption of alendronate. To facilitate gastric emptying when alendronate oral solution is given, the patient should drink at least 60 mL (2 ounces, ¼ cup) of water following administration of the drug. Because of the potential for oropharyngeal irritation or ulceration, patients should be instructed not to suck or chew alendronate tablets. Alendronate (alone or in combination with cholecalciferol) should be administered in an upright position (sitting or standing). Patients should be instructed to avoid lying down for at least 30 minutes following administration and until after the first food of the day to facilitate delivery of the drug to the stomach and minimize potential esophageal irritation. (See Upper GI Effects under Cautions: Warning/Precautions.) In addition, patients should be instructed not to take alendronate (alone or in fixed combination with cholecalciferol) at bedtime or before arising for the day.

If a patient misses a weekly dose of alendronate or alendronate/cholecalciferol, the missed dose should be taken the morning after it is remembered, followed by resumption of the regular weekly schedule. Patients should not take 2 tablets on the same day.

■ **Dosage** Dosage of alendronate sodium, which is present as the monosodium trihydrate, is expressed in terms of alendronate.

Osteoporosis The safety and efficacy of alendronate for the treatment of osteoporosis are based on clinical data supporting fracture reduction over 4 years of treatment. The optimal duration of bisphosphonate treatment for osteoporosis has not been established. Some evidence suggests that increased durations of bisphosphonate use may be associated with a higher risk of some adverse effects (e.g., jaw osteonecrosis). All patients receiving bisphosphonates should have periodic evaluations to determine the need for continued therapy. Discontinuance of bisphosphonate therapy may be considered after 3–5 years of use for patients who are assessed to be at low risk of fracture. Risk of fracture should be evaluated periodically in patients who discontinue therapy.

Prevention in Women. For the prevention of osteoporosis, the usual dosage of alendronate in postmenopausal women who are at risk for developing osteoporosis is 5 mg once *daily* as a tablet. Alternatively, these women may receive 35 mg once *weekly* as a tablet.

Treatment in Women and Men. For the treatment of osteoporosis in postmenopausal women, the usual dosage of alendronate is 10 mg once *daily* as a tablet or 70 mg once *weekly* as a tablet or the oral solution. If the fixed combination of alendronate and cholecalciferol is used in postmenopausal women, the usual dosage is alendronate 70 mg and cholecalciferol 5600 units once *weekly*; alternatively, a dosage of alendronate 70 mg and cholecalciferol 2800 units once *weekly* may be given.

For increasing bone mass in men with osteoporosis, the usual dosage of alendronate is 10 mg once *daily* as a tablet. Alternatively, a dosage of 70 mg once *weekly* as a tablet or the oral solution may be considered for men. If the fixed combination of alendronate and cholecalciferol is used in men with osteoporosis, the usual dosage is alendronate 70 mg and cholecalciferol 5600 units once *weekly*; alternatively, a dosage of alendronate 70 mg and cholecalciferol 2800 units once *weekly* may be given.

Glucocorticoid-induced Osteoporosis. For the treatment of glucocorticoid-induced osteoporosis, the usual dosage of alendronate in postmenopausal women receiving hormone replacement therapy (HRT), premenopausal women, and men is 5 mg once daily. In postmenopausal women who are not receiving HRT, the recommended dosage of alendronate is 10 mg once daily. Dosage recommendations for the prevention of glucocorticoid-induced osteoporosis† generally are the same as those for treatment of this condition.

The manufacturer states that bone mineral density (BMD) should be measured prior to initiation of alendronate therapy and repeated after 6–12 months in patients receiving the drug for glucocorticoid-induced osteoporosis. Before initiating alendronate therapy in patients receiving long-term glucocorticoid therapy, the manufacturer recommends that gonadal hormone status be evaluated and replacement therapy given, if appropriate.

Paget Disease For the treatment of Paget disease of bone, the usual dosage of alendronate in adults is 40 mg once daily for 6 months. Retreatment with alendronate may be considered after a 6-month posttreatment evaluation period if relapse occurs (i.e., based on increased serum alkaline phosphatase concentrations) or if initial treatment failed to normalize serum alkaline phosphatase concentrations.

■ **Special Populations** No dosage adjustments are necessary for patients with mild to moderate renal insufficiency (creatinine clearance of 35–60 mL/minute). Safety and efficacy of alendronate and the fixed combination of alendronate and cholecalciferol have not been established in patients with severe renal insufficiency (creatinine clearance less than 35 mL/minute); use is not recommended in such patients.

Dosage modifications of alendronate based solely on age are not necessary in geriatric patients.

Cautions

■ **Contraindications** Esophageal abnormalities that delay esophageal emptying (e.g., stricture, achalasia).

Use of alendronate oral solution is contraindicated in patients at increased risk of aspiration.

Inability to stand or sit upright for at least 30 minutes.

Hypocalcemia.

Known hypersensitivity to alendronate or any ingredient in the formulation.

■ **Warnings/Precautions** ***Upper GI Effects*** Because severe adverse esophageal effects including esophagitis, esophageal ulcers, perforations, and/or erosions (occasionally with bleeding and rarely followed by esophageal stricture or perforation) have been reported in patients receiving oral bisphosphonates, clinicians should be alert to any sign or symptom associated with such adverse effects. (See Cautions: Contraindications.) Patients should be instructed to discontinue alendronate and contact a clinician if dysphagia, odynophagia, new or worsening heartburn, or retrosternal pain occurs. It appears that gastric antisecretory agents (e.g., omeprazole), while beneficial in the management of esophagitis, show no benefit for treatment of alendronate-induced esophagitis. The incidence of these esophageal effects is greater in patients who do not drink a full (180–240 mL) glass of water when taking oral bisphosphonates and in those who do not avoid lying down for at least 30 minutes following administration or who continue to take the drugs after experiencing symptoms suggestive of esophageal irritation; therefore, patients should be instructed carefully about proper administration of alendronate. Alendronate should be used with caution in patients with active upper GI disease (e.g., Barrett's esophagus, dysphagia, other esophageal diseases, gastritis, duodenitis, ulcers).

Gastric or duodenal ulcers, including some that were severe and with complications, have been reported in patients receiving oral bisphosphonates during postmarketing experience, although no increased risk was observed in controlled clinical trials.

Although data are conflicting, there is some evidence suggesting a possible association between use of oral bisphosphonates and an increased risk of esophageal cancer. During the period of postmarketing surveillance from October 1995 (initial marketing of alendronate) through mid-May 2008, FDA received reports of esophageal cancer in 23 patients in the US receiving alendronate (as the suspect drug in 21 cases and the concomitant drug in 2 cases); 8 deaths were reported. The histologic diagnosis was adenocarcinoma in 7 patients and squamous-cell carcinoma in 1 patient. At least 1 patient received alendronate despite having a diagnosis of Barrett's esophagus, a precursor of esophageal carcinoma. The median time from initiation of alendronate to diagnosis of esophageal cancer was 2.1 years (range 5–10 years, based on 16 patients). The most common site of cancer was the distal esophagus, with gastric involvement in some patients. Reports of esophageal cancer in the US in patients receiving other oral bisphosphonates were not found in the FDA's adverse-event reporting database at the time of analysis. However, esophageal cancer was reported in 31 patients in Europe and Japan receiving bisphosphonates, including alendronate, risedronate, ibandronate, and etidronate. Alendronate was the suspect drug in 21 of these cases, with risedronate, ibandronate, and/or etidronate identified as suspect drugs in 6 cases; a bisphosphonate was the concomitant drug in 4 cases. Six patients were reported to have adenocarcinoma, while 5 patients had squamous-cell carcinoma; 6 deaths were reported. Barrett's esophagus was reported in 3 patients and appeared to have been diagnosed near the time of diagnosis of esophageal cancer and after alendronate use. The median time from drug exposure to diagnosis of esophageal cancer was 1.3 years (range 0.3–8 years, based on 21 patients). In a large case-control study in a cohort of patients from the UK General Practice Research Database, risk of esophageal cancer was increased by 30% in patients who had at least one prescription issued for an oral bisphosphonate (alendronate, etidronate, or risedronate) compared with those not receiving such prescriptions; the risk was approximately doubled among patients who had 10 or more prescriptions issued for an oral bisphosphonate or who had an estimated duration of bisphosphonate use (calculated as the time between the first and last prescription issued during the observation period) of more than 3 years. However, another retrospective cohort study using the same database found no evidence of an increased risk of esophageal cancer in patients receiving oral bisphosphonates. Other observational studies, including a study in patients receiving long-term alendronate therapy and a cohort study of Danish patients with fractures, have shown either no risk or a reduced risk of esophageal cancer following use of oral bisphosphonates. Because of conflicting findings and limitations of currently available data, additional study is needed to determine the association, if any, between oral bisphosphonate use and esophageal cancer. FDA states that benefits of oral bisphosphonates in reducing the risk of serious fractures continue to outweigh their potential risks in patients with osteoporosis and that it is important to consider that esophageal cancer is rare, especially in women. FDA also states that there is insufficient information at this time to recommend routine endoscopic screening in asymptomatic patients receiving oral bisphosphonates. Avoidance of oral bisphosphonates in patients with Barrett's esophagus, a known precursor to esophageal adenocarcinoma, has been recommended.

Metabolic Effects Hypocalcemia and other disturbances of bone and mineral metabolism must be corrected before alendronate therapy is initiated. Supplemental calcium and vitamin D should be administered if dietary intake is inadequate. Serum calcium and symptoms of hypocalcemia should be monitored during therapy.

Possible asymptomatic decreases in serum calcium and phosphate concentrations may occur, particularly in patients with Paget disease and in those receiving glucocorticoids; ensure adequate calcium and vitamin D intake in such patients.

The fixed combination of alendronate and cholecalciferol (vitamin D_3) is not recommended for the treatment of vitamin D deficiency (i.e., 25-hydroxyvitamin D concentration below 9 ng/mL). Patients at risk for vitamin D insufficiency (e.g., GI malabsorption syndromes) may require higher doses of vitamin D supplementation; measurement of 25-hydroxyvitamin D should be considered in such patients.

Vitamin D_3 supplementation may increase the risk of hypercalcemia and/or hypercalciuria in patients with diseases associated with unregulated overproduction of 1,25-dihydroxyvitamin D (e.g., leukemia, lymphoma, sarcoidosis). Urine and serum calcium should be monitored in these patients.

Osteonecrosis of the Jaw Osteonecrosis and osteomyelitis of the jaw have been reported in patients receiving bisphosphonates. Most instances have occurred in association with tooth extraction and/or local infection with delayed wound healing. (See Osteonecrosis of the Jaw under Cautions: Warnings/Precautions, in Zoledronic Acid 92:24.)

While the mechanism by which these adverse effects occur has not been elucidated, it has been suggested that suppression of bone turnover and remodeling by bisphosphonates impairs the ability to repair microfractures in the maxilla and mandible that occur with daily mastication. Known risk factors for osteonecrosis of the jaw include invasive dental procedures (e.g., tooth extraction, dental implants, boney surgery), cancer, concomitant therapies (e.g., chemotherapy, glucocorticoids, angiogenesis inhibitors), poor oral hygiene, and comorbid disorders (e.g., periodontal and/or other preexisting dental disease, anemia, coagulopathy, infection, ill-fitting dentures). Risk also may be increased with increased duration of bisphosphonate use. Discontinuance of bisphosphonate treatment may reduce the risk for osteonecrosis of the jaw in patients requiring invasive dental procedures. Clinical judgment of the treating clinician and/or oral surgeon should guide the management of each patient based on individual benefit/risk assessment. Patients who develop osteonecrosis of the jaw while receiving bisphosphonate therapy should receive care by an oral surgeon. In these patients, extensive dental surgery to treat osteonecrosis of the jaw may exacerbate the condition. Discontinuance of bisphosphonate therapy should be considered based on assessment of benefits and risks in individual patients.

Atypical Fracture of the Femur Atypical, low-energy, or low-trauma femoral fractures have been reported in bisphosphonate-treated patients. These fractures can occur anywhere in the femoral shaft from the subtrochanteric region of the hip (i.e., below the lesser trochanter) to above the supracondylar flare and are transverse or short oblique in orientation without evidence of comminution. Such fractures generally have occurred with use of bisphosphonate therapy for more than 3 years (median 7 years in one analysis of available data). The magnitude of this risk is unclear, although such fractures appear to be rare; in addition, causality has not been established since atypical fractures also have occurred in patients not receiving bisphosphonates. Most cases of atypical femoral fractures with bisphosphonate therapy have been reported in individuals receiving treatment for osteoporosis. Such fractures most commonly occur in individuals with minimal or no trauma. Most individuals have reported prodromal symptoms presenting as dull, aching thigh pain for weeks to months prior to the occurrence of an atypical fracture. Bilateral involvement (i.e., a fracture in the contralateral limb) and evidence of delayed healing of the fracture also may be present. Concomitant use of glucocorticoid, estrogen, and proton-pump inhibitor therapy may increase the risk of an atypical fracture.

Individuals with a history of bisphosphonate exposure presenting with new thigh or groin pain should be evaluated for possible atypical femoral fracture; an assessment of the contralateral limb also should be performed to rule out possible bilateral involvement (i.e., presence of radiographic change or fracture). Interruption of bisphosphonate therapy should be considered in individuals presenting with symptoms suggestive of a possible femoral fracture following completion of a comprehensive risk-benefit assessment performed on an individualized basis. Bisphosphonate therapy should be *discontinued* if a femoral shaft fracture is confirmed. (See Atypical Fracture of the Femur under Cautions: Warnings/Precautions, in Zoledronic Acid 92:24.)

Musculoskeletal Pain Severe, occasionally incapacitating bone, joint, and/or muscle pain has been reported infrequently during postmarketing experience in patients receiving bisphosphonates, including alendronate. The time to onset of symptoms varied from 1 day to years (mean onset about 3 months) after treatment initiation. Such pain has improved following discontinuance of the drug in most patients; however, other patients have reported slow or incomplete resolution of severe musculoskeletal pain. In some patients, symptoms recurred upon subsequent rechallenge with the same drug or another bisphosphonate. The manufacturer states that alendronate should be discontinued if severe symptoms develop.

Atrial Fibrillation While data are conflicting, a possible increased risk of atrial fibrillation has been identified with use of bisphosphonates. (See Atrial Fibrillation under Cautions: Warnings/Precautions, in Zoledronic Acid 92:24.)

Use of Fixed Combinations When alendronate is used in fixed combination with cholecalciferol, the cautions, precautions, and contraindications associated with cholecalciferol should be considered.

Specific Populations **Pregnancy.** There are no studies of alendronate in pregnant women; the drug should be used during pregnancy only if the potential benefits justify the potential risks to the mother and fetus.

Lactation. It is not known whether alendronate is distributed into human milk. Because many drugs are distributed into human milk, caution is advised when alendronate is used in nursing women.

Pediatric Use. The manufacturer states that safety and efficacy of alendronate have not been established in children. In a randomized trial in pediatric patients (4–18 years of age) with osteogenesis imperfecta, treatment with alendronate did not reduce the risk of fracture or bone pain; there was an increased incidence of vomiting in children receiving alendronate compared with placebo.

Geriatric Use. No substantial differences in safety and efficacy have been observed in geriatric patients relative to younger adults. However, the possibility that some older patients may exhibit increased sensitivity to the drug cannot be ruled out.

Hepatic Impairment. Alendronate has not been evaluated in patients with hepatic impairment.

Renal Impairment. Alendronate should not be used in patients with severe renal impairment (creatinine clearance less than 35 mL/minute).

■ **Common Adverse Effects** The most common adverse effects reported in 3% or more of patients receiving alendronate in clinical studies include abdominal pain, acid regurgitation, constipation, diarrhea, dyspepsia, musculoskeletal pain, and nausea.

Drug Interactions

■ **Antacids or Mineral Supplements Containing Divalent Cations** Pharmacokinetic interaction (decreased alendronate absorption) is possible when alendronate is used concomitantly with antacids, mineral supplements, or oral drugs containing multivalent cations (e.g., calcium). Patients should wait at least 30 minutes after alendronate is administered to take any other oral medications.

■ **Nonsteroidal Anti-inflammatory Agents** Concomitant use of aspirin and alendronate (at dosages greater than 10 mg daily) was associated with increased GI toxicity in clinical studies. Although adverse GI effects did not appear to be increased with concomitant use of nonsteroidal anti-inflammatory agents (NSAIAs) and lower dosages of alendronate (5 or 10 mg daily) in one study, caution is advised during such concomitant therapy.

■ **Prednisone** No change in alendronate bioavailability was observed with concomitant use of prednisone.

■ **Ranitidine** IV ranitidine has been shown to double alendronate bioavailability; however, the clinical importance of this interaction and whether the same effects will occur in patients receiving oral histamine H_2-receptor antagonists are not known.

Description

Alendronate sodium, a synthetic bisphosphonate (also referred to as diphosphonate) analog of pyrophosphate, is an inhibitor of osteoclast-mediated bone resorption. Alendronate is structurally and pharmacologically related to etidronate and pamidronate. Unlike pyrophosphate but like etidronate and pamidronate, alendronate is resistant to enzymatic hydrolysis by phosphatases.

Alendronate appears to inhibit bone resorption in a dose-dependent manner and is 100–1000 times more potent than etidronate in this effect. In addition, alendronate is a highly selective inhibitor of bone resorption; data from animals indicate that the dose of alendronate that inhibits bone mineralization is up to 6000 times greater than the dose that inhibits resorption. Alendronate is incorporated into bone and has an estimated terminal elimination half-life of at least 10 years in humans; however, while incorporated into bone matrix, the drug is not pharmacologically active.

Advice to Patients

Importance of providing a copy of the manufacturer's patient information.

Importance of correct administration (e.g., avoiding foods and beverages other than plain water, not lying down for at least 30 minutes following administration, avoiding administering at bedtime or before arising for the day).

Importance of swallowing tablets whole, without chewing or sucking.

Importance of discontinuing and informing clinician if symptoms of esophageal disease (e.g., difficulty or pain on swallowing; retrosternal, abdominal or esophageal pain; new or worsening heartburn) develop.

Importance of adhering to recommended lifestyle modifications (e.g., weight-bearing exercise, calcium and vitamin D consumption, avoidance of excessive cigarette smoking and/or alcohol consumption).

Importance of women informing clinicians if they are or plan to become pregnant or plan to breast-feed.

Importance of informing clinicians of existing or contemplated concomitant therapy, including prescription and OTC drugs, as well as any concomitant illnesses.

Importance of advising patients of other important precautionary information. (See Cautions.)

Overview® (see Users Guide). For additional information on this drug until a more detailed monograph is developed and published, the manufacturer's labeling should be consulted. It is *essential* that the manufacturer's labeling be consulted for more detailed information on usual cautions, precautions, contraindications, potential drug interactions, laboratory test interferences, and acute toxicity.

Preparations

Excipients in commercially available drug preparations may have clinically important effects in some individuals; consult specific product labeling for details.

Alendronate Sodium

Oral		
Solution	70 mg (of alendronate)/75 mL*	Alendronate Sodium Oral Solution
Tablets	5 mg (of alendronate)*	Alendronate Sodium Tablets
	10 mg (of alendronate)*	Alendronate Sodium Tablets
	35 mg (of alendronate)*	Alendronate Sodium Tablets
	40 mg (of alendronate)*	Alendronate Sodium Tablets
	70 mg (of alendronate)*	Alendronate Sodium Tablets Fosamax®, Merck
Tablets, for solution	70 mg (of alendronate)	Binosto®, Mission

*available from one or more manufacturer, distributor, and/or repackager by generic (nonproprietary) name

Alendronate Sodium and Cholecalciferol

Oral		
Tablets	70 mg (of alendronate) and Cholecalciferol 2800 units	Fosamax Plus D®, Merck
	70 mg (of alendronate) and Cholecalciferol 5600 units	Fosamax Plus D®, Merck

†Use is not currently included in the labeling approved by the US Food and Drug Administration

Denosumab

■ Denosumab, a fully human monoclonal antibody that is specific for the receptor activator of nuclear factor kappa-B ligand (RANKL) and acts as a RANKL inhibitor, is a bone resorption inhibitor.

REMS

FDA approved a REMS for denosumab to ensure that the benefits outweigh the risk. The REMS may apply to one or more preparations of denosumab and consists of the following: medication guide and communication plan. See the FDA REMS page (https://www.accessdata.fda.gov/scripts/cder/rems/index.cfm).

Uses

Denosumab (Prolia®) is used in the treatment of osteoporosis in postmenopausal women and men at high risk for fracture, in the treatment of glucocorticoid-induced osteoporosis in patients at high risk for fracture, and to increase bone mass in patients at high risk for fracture who are receiving androgen deprivation or aromatase inhibitor therapy.

Denosumab (Xgeva®) is used to prevent skeletal-related events (SREs) in patients with multiple myeloma or with bone metastases from solid tumors. Denosumab (Xgeva®) also is used for the treatment of giant cell tumor of bone and for the treatment of bisphosphonate-refractory hypercalcemia associated with malignant neoplasms; denosumab has been designated an orphan drug by FDA for these uses.

■ **Osteoporosis** Denosumab is used for the treatment of osteoporosis in postmenopausal women and men who are at high risk of fractures. In addition to adequate intake of calcium/vitamin D and other lifestyle modifications (e.g., exercise, avoidance of excessive alcohol and tobacco use), experts recommend that pharmacologic therapy for osteoporosis be considered in postmenopausal women and in men 50 years of age or older who are at high risk of fractures (generally those who have experienced a previous hip or vertebral fracture or who have low bone mineral density [BMD]); pharmacologic therapy also may be considered in postmenopausal women and in men 50 years of age or older who have low bone mass, although there is less evidence supporting overall fracture risk reduction in such patients. When selecting an appropriate pharmacologic agent, use of a drug with proven antifracture efficacy is recommended. Experts recommend denosumab as one of several first-line drugs that may be used. Choice of therapy should be individualized based on the potential benefits (with respect to fracture risk reduction) and adverse effects of therapy as well as patient preferences, comorbidities, and risk factors. For additional information on the treatment of osteoporosis, see Uses: Osteoporosis, in Alendronate 92:24.

Treatment in Postmenopausal Women at High Risk for Fracture Denosumab is used in the treatment of osteoporosis in postmenopausal women at high risk for fracture, defined as a history of osteoporotic fracture or multiple risk factors for fracture. Denosumab also is used in the treatment of osteoporosis in postmenopausal women following failure of or intolerance to other osteoporosis therapies. For information on osteoporosis, including information on risk factors, see Uses: Osteoporosis, in Alendronate 92:24.

Clinical Experience. Efficacy of denosumab in preventing fractures in postmenopausal women with osteoporosis was established in the Fracture Reduction Evaluation of Denosumab in Osteoporosis Every 6 Months (FREEDOM) study. In this double-blind, multinational study, 7808 postmenopausal women 60–91 years of age with baseline BMD T-scores between −2.5 and −4 (measured at the lumbar spine or total hip) were randomized to receive either 60 mg of denosumab or placebo subcutaneously once every 6 months for 3 years. Women were excluded from the study if they had diseases that influence bone metabolism (e.g., rheumatoid arthritis, osteogenesis imperfecta, Paget disease) or were receiving other drugs that affect bone metabolism. Women with a history of more than 3 years of oral bisphosphonate therapy or any history of IV bisphosphonate therapy were excluded from the study; those who had received oral bisphosphonates for less than 3 years and had not received such therapy for at least 12 months could be included. All patients were instructed to take at least 1 g of calcium and at least 400 international units (IU, units) of vitamin D daily (at least 400 units daily in those with baseline 25-hydroxyvitamin D concentrations exceeding 20 ng/mL; at least 800 units daily in those with baseline concentrations of 12–20 ng/mL).

Denosumab was more effective than placebo in reducing the rate of new morphometric vertebral fractures at 1, 2, and 3 years. Treatment with denosumab was associated with a 68% relative risk reduction in new vertebral fractures diagnosed using semiquantitative radiographic assessments. At 3 years, 2.3% of women receiving denosumab had experienced a new vertebral fracture compared with 7.2% of women receiving placebo. In addition, at 3 years, treatment with denosumab was associated with a 20% relative risk reduction in new nonvertebral fractures and a 40% relative risk reduction in new hip fractures.

At 3 years, patients receiving denosumab had substantial increases in BMD at all anatomic sites measured. The mean percent change from baseline BMD was determined in denosumab- and placebo-treated patients, and the mean difference in BMD in those receiving denosumab compared with those receiving placebo (treatment difference) was 8.8% at the lumbar spine, 6.4% at total hip, and 5.2% at the femoral neck. Qualitative histology assessments of bone biopsy specimens obtained from a subset of the women who received denosumab showed normal bone architecture with no evidence of mineralization defects, woven bone, or marrow fibrosis. Histomorphometry assessments revealed markedly reduced bone formation rates. (See Suppression of Bone Turnover under Cautions: Warnings/Precautions.)

Treatment in Men at High Risk for Fracture Denosumab is used in the treatment of osteoporosis in men at high risk for fracture, defined as a history of osteoporotic fracture or multiple risk factors for fracture. Denosumab also is used in the treatment of osteoporosis in men following failure of or intolerance to other osteoporosis therapies. For information on osteoporosis, including information on risk factors, see Uses: Osteoporosis, in Alendronate 92:24.

Clinical Experience. In a 1-year, randomized, double-blind, placebo-controlled study in men with osteoporosis, those receiving denosumab had greater increases in BMD than those receiving placebo. A total of 242 men 31–84 years of age (mean age 65 years) with baseline BMD T-scores between −2 and −3.5 (lumbar spine or femoral neck) or baseline lumbar spine BMD T-scores between −1 and −3.5 and a history of major osteoporotic fracture were randomized to receive either denosumab (60 mg) or placebo subcutaneously every 6 months. Men were excluded from the study if they had diseases that affect bone (e.g., rheumatoid arthritis, osteogenesis imperfecta, Paget disease) or were receiving other drugs that affect bone. All patients were instructed to take at least 1 g of calcium and 800 units of vitamin D daily. The treatment difference in mean lumbar spine BMD from baseline to 1 year was 4.8% (5.7% increase in those receiving denosumab versus 0.9% increase in those receiving placebo). The treatment difference in mean BMD at the total hip or femoral neck from baseline to 1 year in those receiving denosumab versus placebo was 2 or 2.2%, respectively. Consistent effects on BMD at the lumbar spine were reported regardless of age, race, baseline BMD, testosterone concentrations, and level of bone turnover.

■ **Glucocorticoid-induced Osteoporosis** Denosumab is used in the treatment of glucocorticoid-induced osteoporosis in men and women at high risk for fracture, defined as a history of osteoporotic fracture or multiple risk factors for fracture. Denosumab also is used in the treatment of glucocorticoid-induced osteoporosis following failure of or intolerance to other osteoporosis therapies. The manufacturer recommends use of denosumab in patients who are either initiating or continuing long-term (at least 6 months) systemic glucocorticoid therapy in a dosage equivalent to at least 7.5 mg daily of prednisone.

The American College of Rheumatology (ACR) recommends optimizing calcium and vitamin D intake and lifestyle modifications (e.g., diet, smoking cessation, weight-bearing or resistance-training exercise) in all patients receiving long-term glucocorticoid therapy; in addition, pharmacologic therapy with an oral bisphosphonate is recommended in patients who are considered to be at moderate-to-high risk of fracture. Oral bisphosphonates generally are preferred because of their demonstrated antifracture benefits, safety, and cost; denosumab is suggested as an alternative. For additional information on the management of glucocorticoid-induced osteoporosis, see Cautions: Musculoskeletal Effects in the Corticosteroids General Statement 68:04.

Clinical Experience In a randomized, double-blind, active-controlled study in 795 adults receiving glucocorticoid therapy (dosage of at least 7.5 mg daily of prednisone or equivalent) for a planned duration of at least 6 months, patients receiving denosumab had greater increases in lumbar spine BMD from baseline to one year compared with those receiving risedronate. Patient enrollment was stratified by duration of glucocorticoid use at study entry: less than 3 months (glucocorticoid-initiating group) or 3 months or longer (glucocorticoid-continuing group). Patients younger than 50 years of age were required to have a history of osteoporotic fracture, while those 50 years of age or older who were continuing glucocorticoid therapy were required to have a baseline BMD T-score of −2 or less at the lumbar spine, total hip, or femoral neck (or a history of osteoporotic fracture and a BMD T-score of −1 or less). Patients were randomized (stratified by gender) to receive denosumab (60 mg by subcutaneous injection every 6 months) or risedronate (5 mg orally daily) for 24 months. All patients were instructed to take at least 1 g of calcium and 800 units of vitamin D daily. The mean age of patients in the study was 63 years (range: 20–94 years); 70% of patients were women, and approximately 77% of patients were receiving glucocorticoid therapy for a rheumatologic disorder. At study entry, approximately 63% of patients had received glucocorticoid therapy for at least 3 months.

At 12 months, denosumab increased lumbar spine BMD to a greater extent than risedronate; lumbar spine BMD was increased by an average of 3.8 or 0.8% with denosumab or risedronate treatment, respectively, in the group initiating glucocorticoid therapy and by an average of 4.4 or 2.3% with these respective treatments in the group continuing glucocorticoid therapy. Within both of these subgroups, effects on lumbar spine BMD were consistent regardless of gender; race; menopausal status; baseline age, lumbar spine BMD T-score, or glucocorticoid dosage; or geographic region.

Qualitative histology assessments in a limited number of patients revealed normal architecture with no evidence of mineralization defects or bone marrow abnormality. However, suppression of bone remodeling was observed in 2 of 3 biopsy specimens obtained from denosumab-treated patients, whereas active bone remodeling was evident in all specimens obtained from risedronate-treated patients. (See Suppression of Bone Turnover under Cautions: Warnings/Precautions.)

■ **Bone Loss Associated with Androgen Deprivation Therapy**

Treatment in Men with Nonmetastatic Prostate Cancer at High Risk for Fracture Denosumab is used to increase bone mass in men at high risk for fracture receiving androgen deprivation therapy for nonmetastatic prostate cancer. Denosumab also has reduced the incidence of vertebral fractures in these patients.

Clinical Experience. In a 3-year, randomized, double-blind, placebo-controlled, phase 3 study in men receiving androgen deprivation therapy for nonmetastatic prostate cancer, those receiving denosumab had greater increases in lumbar spine BMD from baseline to 2 years than those receiving placebo. A total of 1468 men who were either 70 years of age or older or younger than 70 years of age with baseline BMD T-scores below −1 or history of prior osteoporotic fracture (mean age 75 years, mean baseline lumbar spine BMD T-score −0.4) were randomized to receive subcutaneous denosumab (60 mg) or placebo once every 6 months for a total of 6 doses. All patients were instructed to take at least 1 g of calcium and 400 units of vitamin D daily. The treatment difference in mean lumbar spine BMD from baseline to 2 years was 6.7% (5.6% increase in those receiving denosumab versus 1% decrease in those receiving placebo). At 3 years, the treatment difference in BMD from baseline in those receiving denosumab versus placebo was 7.9, 5.7, and 4.9% at the lumbar spine, total hip, and femoral neck, respectively. In addition, at 3 years, the cumulative incidence of new vertebral fractures was lower in men receiving denosumab (1.5%) than in those receiving placebo (3.9%).

■ **Bone Loss Associated with Aromatase Inhibitor Therapy**

Treatment in Women with Breast Cancer at High Risk for Fracture Denosumab is used to increase bone mass in women at high risk for fracture receiving adjuvant aromatase inhibitor therapy for breast cancer.

Clinical Experience. In a 2-year, randomized, double-blind, placebo-controlled, phase 3 study in women receiving adjuvant aromatase inhibitor therapy for breast cancer who had low bone mass (BMD T-score −2.5 to −1), those receiving denosumab had greater increases in lumbar spine BMD from baseline to 1 year than those receiving placebo. A total of 252 women (median age 59 years, mean baseline lumbar spine BMD T-score −1.1) were randomized to receive subcutaneous denosumab (60 mg) or placebo once every 6 months for a total of 4 doses. All patients were instructed to take at least 1 g of calcium and 400 units of vitamin D daily. The treatment difference in BMD at the lumbar spine from baseline to 1 year was 5.5% (4.8% increase in those receiving denosumab versus 0.7% decrease in those receiving placebo). At 2 years, the treatment difference in BMD from baseline in those receiving denosumab versus placebo was 7.6, 4.7, and 3.6% at the lumbar spine, total hip, and femoral neck, respectively. A subsequent analysis revealed that the beneficial effects of denosumab were consistent across key clinical subgroups (i.e., duration of aromatase inhibitor therapy, type of aromatase inhibitor, prior tamoxifen use, age, time since menopause, baseline body mass index, baseline T-scores).

■ **Multiple Myeloma and Bone Metastases of Solid Tumors**

Prevention of Skeletal-related Events Denosumab is used to prevent skeletal-related events (SREs; pathologic fracture, radiation therapy to bone, surgery to bone, spinal cord compression) in patients with bone metastases from solid tumors and in patients with multiple myeloma.

Clinical Experience. In 3 similarly designed randomized, double-blind, active-controlled, phase 3 studies (trials 1, 2, and 3) in adults with bone metastases from solid tumors, denosumab was noninferior to zoledronic acid in delaying time to first SRE. Denosumab also was noninferior to zoledronic acid in delaying time to first SRE in a subsequent randomized, double-blind, active-controlled, phase 3 study in adults with newly diagnosed multiple myeloma and at least one osteolytic lesion. These studies randomized patients to receive subcutaneous denosumab (120 mg once every 4 weeks) or IV zoledronic acid (4 mg once every 4 weeks; dosage adjusted based on renal function); all patients were instructed to take at least 500 mg of calcium and 400 units of vitamin D daily.

Trial 1 included 2046 adults (80% white, 99% female, median age 57 years) with advanced breast cancer and at least one bone metastasis. Results indicated that treatment with denosumab was superior to zoledronic acid in delaying time to first on-study SRE in these patients. Patients receiving zoledronic acid (median of 17 doses) experienced a first on-study SRE at a median of 26.4 months; this primary end point had not yet been reached in patients receiving denosumab (median of 18 doses). Denosumab also reduced the risk of developing multiple SREs (secondary end point of time to first and subsequent on-study SREs) by 23% compared with zoledronic acid. Although overall survival or disease progression was similar in both treatment groups, patients receiving denosumab had a lower mean skeletal morbidity rate (i.e., the ratio of the number of SREs per patient divided by the patient's time at risk) and greater suppression of bone turnover markers (urine N-telopeptide, adjusted for urine creatinine levels [uNTx/Cr] and bone-specific alkaline phosphatase [BSAP]) from baseline to 13 weeks.

Trial 2 included 1776 adults (87% white, median age 60 years) with solid tumors other than breast or castration-resistant prostate cancer (40% non-small cell lung cancer, 9% renal cell carcinoma, 6% small cell lung cancer) or multiple myeloma (10%) and with at least one bone metastasis or osteolytic lesion. Results indicated that denosumab was noninferior to zoledronic acid in delaying time to first SRE. Patients received a median of 7 doses of study drug and the median time to first on-study SRE in patients receiving denosumab was 20.5 months versus 16.3 months in those receiving zoledronic acid. Time to first and subsequent SREs (risk of developing multiple SREs) was similar with both drugs. Although there were no differences in overall survival or disease progression between the 2 treatment groups, patients receiving denosumab had greater suppression of bone turnover markers (uNTx/Cr and BSAP) from baseline to 13 weeks. When results were stratified by tumor type (non-small cell lung cancer, multiple myeloma, or other solid tumor), denosumab was superior to zoledronic acid in delaying time to first on-study SRE only among patients with other solid tumors. Subgroup analysis also revealed that there was an increased risk of mortality in patients with multiple myeloma receiving denosumab compared with those receiving zoledronic acid. However, potential confounding factors included imbalances in baseline prognostic factors, myeloma treatments, and early study withdrawals between denosumab- and zoledronic acid-treated patients with multiple myeloma, which tended to favor zoledronic acid.

Trial 3 included 1901 men (86% white, median age 71 years) with castration-resistant prostate cancer and at least one bone metastasis. Results indicated that denosumab was superior to zoledronic acid in delaying time to first on-study SRE in these patients. The median time to first on-study SRE was 20.7 months in those receiving denosumab (median 13 doses) versus 17.1 months in those receiving zoledronic acid (median 11 doses). Time to first and subsequent on-study SREs also was substantially delayed in men receiving denosumab compared with those receiving zoledronic acid. Overall survival, disease progression, and prostate-specific antigen levels were similar between the 2 treatment groups. Those receiving denosumab had greater suppression of bone turnover markers (uNTx/Cr and BSAP) from baseline to 13 weeks than those receiving zoledronic acid.

The fourth study included 1718 adults (82% white, 46% female, median age 63 years) with newly diagnosed multiple myeloma with at least one osteolytic lesion. Because of zoledronic acid dosage restrictions, the study excluded patients with severe renal impairment (creatinine clearance less than 30 mL/minute). Randomization was stratified by the therapy selected for first-line treatment of myeloma, intent to undergo autologous peripheral blood stem cell (PBSC) transplantation, prior occurrence of an SRE, International Staging System (ISS) stage at diagnosis, and geographic region. At study entry, 96% of patients were receiving or planned to receive novel therapy as first-line treatment for myeloma; 55% intended to undergo autologous PBSC transplantation; 61% previously had experienced an SRE; and 32, 38, or 29% had ISS stage I, II, or III disease, respectively, at diagnosis. The median baseline creatinine clearance was 77 mL/minute; 27% of patients had a baseline creatinine clearance of 60 mL/minute or less. Results indicated that denosumab was noninferior to zoledronic acid in delaying the time to first on-study SRE. The median time to first on-study SRE was 22.8 months in those receiving denosumab (median 16 doses) versus 24 months in those receiving zoledronic acid (median 15 doses); 60% of all first on-study SREs occurred within the first 3 months of the study, and 81% occurred within the first 6 months. Overall survival was similar between the 2 treatment groups. Adverse renal effects occurred more frequently in patients receiving zoledronic acid, whereas hypocalcemia was more frequent in those receiving denosumab.

■ **Giant Cell Tumor of Bone** Denosumab is used for the treatment of giant cell tumor of bone in adults and skeletally mature adolescents when the disease is unresectable or surgical resection is likely to result in severe morbidity.

Clinical Experience Objective response to denosumab was observed in 2 open-label trials in adults or skeletally mature adolescents with histologically confirmed measurable giant cell tumor of bone that was recurrent, unresectable, or likely to result in severe morbidity if surgically resected (trials 4 and 5). Patients received denosumab in a dosage of 120 mg subcutaneously once every 4 weeks with an additional dose on days 8 and 15 of the first month of treatment. Trial 4 was a single arm trial in 37 adults and trial 5 was a parallel cohort trial in 282 adults or skeletally mature adolescents (10 patients were 13–17 years of age). Patients in trial 5 were enrolled in 3 cohorts: those with surgically unsalvageable disease (e.g., sacral or spinal disease sites or pulmonary metastases), those with surgically salvageable disease for which surgical intervention was likely to result in severe morbidity (e.g., joint resection, limb amputation, hemipelvectomy), or patients who previously participated in trial 4.

Objective response was evaluated by an independent review committee using modified Response Evaluation Criteria in Solid Tumors (RECIST 1.1). The overall objective response rate was 25% for evaluable patients in trials 4 and 5. All responses were partial responses, and the estimated median time to response was 3 months. In 47 patients with an objective response, the median duration of follow-up was 20 months (range 2–44 months) and 51% had a duration of response lasting at least 8 months.

■ **Hypercalcemia Associated with Malignancy** Denosumab is used for the treatment of bisphosphonate-refractory hypercalcemia of malignancy.

Use of denosumab in the treatment of hypercalcemia of malignancy is supported by results of an open-label, noncomparative, phase 2 study in 33 patients with bisphosphonate-refractory hypercalcemia of malignancy (with or without bone metastasis). The study included patients with an albumin-corrected serum calcium concentration exceeding 12.5 mg/dL despite IV bisphosphonate therapy within 7–30 days prior to initiation of denosumab (120 mg subcutaneously once every 4 weeks with an additional dose on day 8 and day 15 of the first month of treatment). In this study, 64 or 70% of patients achieved a response (albumin-corrected serum calcium concentration of 11.5 mg/dL or less) by day 10 or day 57, respectively, and 36 or 64% of patients achieved a complete response (albumin-corrected serum calcium concentration of 10.8 mg/dL or less) by day 10 or day 57, respectively. The median time to response or complete response was 9 or 23 days, respectively, and the median duration of response or complete response was 104 or 34 days, respectively. Concurrent cancer chemotherapy did not appear to affect response.

Dosage and Administration

■ **Administration** Denosumab is administered by subcutaneous injection.

Subcutaneous injections of denosumab should be made into the upper arm, upper thigh, or abdomen. The drug should not be administered IV or by IM or intradermal injection.

For treatment of osteoporosis or treatment of bone loss associated with androgen deprivation or aromatase inhibitor therapy, denosumab is available as a preservative-free 60-mg/mL solution (Prolia®) in single-use prefilled syringes for administration by a health-care provider.

For prevention of skeletal-related events (SREs) in patients with multiple myeloma or bone metastases from solid tumors, for treatment of bisphosphonate-refractory hypercalcemia of malignancy, or for treatment of giant cell tumor of bone, denosumab is available as a preservative-free 120-mg/1.7-mL solution (Xgeva®) in single-use vials.

Denosumab should be stored at 2–8°C and must be used within 14 days after removal from refrigeration. The drug should not be exposed to temperatures exceeding 25°C or to direct light or heat. Denosumab should not be shaken vigorously.

Prior to administration, denosumab may be warmed to room temperature by allowing the drug to stand in the original container at room temperature (up to 25°C) for approximately 15–30 minutes; other methods should not be used to warm the drug.

Denosumab should appear clear, colorless to pale yellow and may contain trace amounts of translucent to white proteinaceous particles; the solution should not be used if it is discolored, cloudy, or contains many particles or foreign matter.

When denosumab is administered using the prefilled syringe, the gray needle cap should be removed and all of the solution should be administered by subcutaneous injection. After the injection is complete, the needle guard should be activated to prevent accidental needle sticks. The clear plastic finger grip should be held with one hand, with the needle pointed away from the body; the green safety guard should be grasped at its base with the other hand and gently slid toward the needle until the safety guard has locked securely in place. The needle guard will render the unit useless if activated prior to administering the injection. The needle cap of the prefilled syringe contains dry natural rubber (latex) and should not be handled by individuals sensitive to latex. (See Latex Sensitivity under Warnings/Precautions: Sensitivity Reactions, in Cautions.)

When denosumab is administered using the single-use vial, a 27-gauge needle should be used to withdraw and inject the entire contents of the vial subcutaneously. The vial should not be re-entered, and any remaining solution should be discarded along with the vial.

■ **Dosage** Preexisting hypocalcemia must be corrected prior to initiation of denosumab treatment. Supplementation with calcium and vitamin D may be required during denosumab treatment. (See Hypocalcemia and Mineral Metabolism under Cautions: Warnings/Precautions.)

Osteoporosis **Treatment in Postmenopausal Women at High Risk for Fracture.** The usual dosage of denosumab in postmenopausal women with osteoporosis at high risk for fracture is 60 mg as a single subcutaneous injection once every 6 months.

If a dose is missed, it should be administered as soon as it is convenient for the patient. Thereafter, denosumab doses should be given every 6 months from the date of the last dose.

Treatment in Men at High Risk for Fracture. The usual dosage of denosumab in men with osteoporosis at high risk for fracture is 60 mg as a single subcutaneous injection once every 6 months.

If a dose is missed, it should be administered as soon as it is convenient for the patient. Thereafter, denosumab doses should be given every 6 months from the date of the last dose.

Glucocorticoid-induced Osteoporosis The usual dosage of denosumab for the treatment of glucocorticoid-induced osteoporosis in adults at high risk for fracture is 60 mg as a single subcutaneous injection once every 6 months.

If a dose is missed, it should be administered as soon as it is convenient for the patient. Thereafter, denosumab doses should be given every 6 months from the date of the last dose.

Bone Loss Associated with Androgen Deprivation Therapy **Treatment in Men with Nonmetastatic Prostate Cancer at High Risk for Fracture.** The usual dosage of denosumab to increase bone mass in men with nonmetastatic prostate cancer receiving androgen deprivation therapy and at high risk for fracture is 60 mg as a single subcutaneous injection once every 6 months.

If a dose is missed, it should be administered as soon as it is convenient for the patient. Thereafter, denosumab doses should be given every 6 months from the date of the last dose.

Bone Loss Associated with Aromatase Inhibitor Therapy **Treatment in Women with Breast Cancer at High Risk for Fracture.** The usual dosage of denosumab to increase bone mass in women with breast cancer receiving adjuvant aromatase inhibitor therapy and at high risk for fracture is 60 mg as a single subcutaneous injection once every 6 months.

If a dose is missed, it should be administered as soon as it is convenient for the patient. Thereafter, denosumab doses should be given every 6 months from the date of the last dose.

Multiple Myeloma and Bone Metastases of Solid Tumors **Prevention of Skeletal-related Events.** The usual dosage of denosumab for prevention of SREs in adults with multiple myeloma or with bone metastases from solid tumors is 120 mg as a single subcutaneous injection once every 4 weeks.

Giant Cell Tumor of Bone The usual dosage of denosumab for treatment of giant cell tumor of bone in adults and skeletally mature adolescents is 120 mg as a single subcutaneous injection once every 4 weeks. In addition, a

120-mg dose should be given on day 8 and day 15 during the first month of treatment.

Hypercalcemia Associated with Malignancy The usual dosage of denosumab for treatment of bisphosphonate-refractory hypercalcemia of malignancy in adults is 120 mg as a single subcutaneous injection once every 4 weeks. In addition, a 120-mg dose should be given on day 8 and day 15 during the first month of treatment.

■ **Special Populations** No dosage adjustment is necessary when denosumab is used in patients with renal impairment. However, clinical trial data indicate that patients with severe renal impairment (creatinine clearance less than 30 mL/minute) or receiving dialysis are at greater risk of developing hypocalcemia. (See Renal Impairment under Warnings/Precautions: Specific Populations, in Cautions and also see Hypocalcemia and Mineral Metabolism under Cautions: Warnings/Precautions.)

Cautions

■ **Contraindications** Denosumab is contraindicated in patients with hypocalcemia (preexisting hypocalcemia must be corrected prior to initiating denosumab) or a history of clinically important hypersensitivity (e.g., systemic hypersensitivity) to denosumab or any component in the formulation. The manufacturer states that denosumab (Prolia®) is contraindicated in pregnant women. (See Fetal/Neonatal Morbidity and Mortality under Cautions: Warnings/Precautions.)

■ **Warnings/Precautions** ***Choice of Denosumab Products*** Denosumab is commercially available as Prolia® and Xgeva®; these products are labeled by FDA for different indications. (See Uses.) Prolia® and Xgeva® should *not* be used concomitantly.

Fetal/Neonatal Morbidity and Mortality Adequate data are not available regarding denosumab use in pregnant women; however, based on findings of animal studies and its mechanism of action, denosumab may cause fetal harm if administered during pregnancy. Fetal loss, stillbirths, postnatal mortality, and evidence of absent lymph nodes, abnormal bone growth, reduced bone strength, reduced hematopoiesis, dental dysplasia, tooth malalignment, and decreased neonatal growth have been reported in reproduction studies in monkeys; some of the observed bone abnormalities have recovered once drug exposure ceased following birth.

Pregnancy testing should be performed prior to initiation of denosumab therapy in women with reproductive potential. (See Cautions: Contraindications.) Women with reproductive potential should be advised to use effective methods of contraception during denosumab therapy and for at least 5 months after the last dose of the drug. Patients should be apprised of the potential hazard to the fetus if denosumab is used during pregnancy.

The manufacturer states that use of a condom during sexual encounters is not necessary by men receiving denosumab (Prolia®). Although denosumab is present in low concentrations (maximum concentration of approximately 2% of serum concentrations) in seminal fluid in men receiving a single 60-mg dose of the drug, the manufacturer states that it is unlikely that a female partner of the patient or a partner's fetus would be exposed to pharmacologically relevant concentrations of the drug. The maximum amount of denosumab (administered as a 60-mg dose) delivered to a female partner during vaginal intercourse would result in exposure levels approximately 11,000 times lower than those in a patient receiving a 60-mg dose of the drug and at least 38 times lower than the no observed effect level in monkeys.

Sensitivity Reactions **Hypersensitivity.** Systemic hypersensitivity reactions (e.g., anaphylaxis, hypotension, dyspnea, throat tightness, facial and upper airway edema, lip swelling, rash, pruritus, urticaria) have been reported in patients receiving denosumab.

If anaphylaxis or other clinically important hypersensitivity reaction occurs, denosumab should be discontinued and appropriate therapy initiated. The drug should not be reinitiated in such patients.

Latex Sensitivity. Some packaging components (i.e., needle cap) of denosumab (Prolia®) prefilled syringes contain natural latex proteins in the form of dry natural rubber (latex), and should not be handled by individuals sensitive to latex. Some individuals may be hypersensitive to natural latex proteins found in a wide range of medical devices, including such packaging components, and the level of sensitivity may vary depending on the form of natural rubber present; rarely, hypersensitivity reactions to natural latex proteins have been fatal.

Hypocalcemia and Mineral Metabolism Decreased serum calcium concentrations can occur during denosumab therapy, and preexisting hypocalcemia may be exacerbated by the drug. Severe, symptomatic hypocalcemia (including some fatalities) has been reported.

In postmenopausal women receiving denosumab for treatment of osteoporosis, hypocalcemia (serum calcium less than 8.5 mg/dL) was reported in 1.7% of patients, and the nadir in serum calcium was observed approximately 10 days after a dose in those with normal renal function. In patients receiving denosumab for treatment of bone loss associated with androgen deprivation or aromatase inhibitor therapy, hypocalcemia (serum calcium less than 8.4 mg/dL) was reported in 2.4% of patients at 1 month.

Severe hypocalcemia (corrected serum calcium less than 7 mg/dL) occurred in 3.1% of patients with bone metastases receiving denosumab for prevention of SREs versus 1.3% of patients receiving zoledronic acid; 33% of those who developed severe hypocalcemia while receiving denosumab had 2 or more episodes of severe hypocalcemia. Severe hypophosphatemia (serum phosphorous less than 2 mg/dL) occurred in 15.4% of patients receiving denosumab for prevention of SREs compared with 7.4% of patients receiving zoledronic acid. Severe hypocalcemia or hypophosphatemia occurred in 2 or 21%, respectively, of patients with multiple myeloma receiving denosumab, while moderate hypocalcemia (corrected serum calcium of 7 to less than 8 mg/dL) or severe hypophosphatemia occurred in 2.6 or 9.5%, respectively, of those with giant cell tumor of bone receiving the drug.

Preexisting hypocalcemia must be corrected prior to initiating denosumab therapy. In addition, patients receiving denosumab should be monitored for hypocalcemia and receive calcium, vitamin D, and magnesium supplementation as clinically indicated.

The manufacturer states that *all* patients receiving denosumab for treatment of osteoporosis or treatment of bone loss associated with androgen deprivation or aromatase inhibitor therapy should receive 1 g of calcium and at least 400 units of vitamin D daily during denosumab therapy. In addition, clinical monitoring of calcium, phosphorus, and magnesium is highly recommended within 14 days of denosumab administration in those predisposed to hypocalcemia and disturbances of mineral metabolism (e.g., history of hypoparathyroidism, thyroid surgery, parathyroid surgery, malabsorption syndromes, excision of small intestine, severe renal impairment, receiving dialysis). In some patients, hypocalcemia has persisted for weeks or months and has required frequent monitoring and IV and/or oral calcium replacement therapy, with or without vitamin D supplementation.

The manufacturer states that serum calcium concentrations should be monitored throughout denosumab therapy, but particularly during the first weeks following initiation of therapy, in patients receiving the drug for prevention of SREs or treatment of giant cell tumor of bone; monitoring should be more frequent in those receiving concomitant therapy with other drugs that may reduce serum calcium concentrations. Patients should receive calcium, vitamin D, and magnesium supplementation as necessary.

The risk of hypocalcemia is greater in patients receiving inadequate or no calcium supplementation and in those with increasing renal impairment, particularly those with severe renal impairment (creatinine clearance less than 30 mL/minute) or receiving dialysis. (See Renal Impairment under Warnings/Precautions: Specific Populations, in Cautions.)

Osteonecrosis of the Jaw Osteonecrosis of the jaw (ONJ) has been reported in patients receiving denosumab. ONJ may occur spontaneously, but is generally associated with tooth extraction and/or local infection with delayed healing. The condition may manifest as jaw pain, osteomyelitis, osteitis, bone erosion, tooth or periodontal infection, toothache, gingival ulceration, or gingival erosion.

Risk factors for ONJ include invasive dental procedures (e.g., tooth extraction, dental implants, oral surgery), diagnosis of cancer, concomitant therapies (e.g., chemotherapy, immunosuppressive therapy, angiogenesis inhibitors, corticosteroids), poor oral hygiene, and comorbidities (e.g., preexisting dental disease, anemia, coagulopathy, diabetes mellitus, infection, ill-fitting dentures). In clinical trials in patients with cancer, longer durations of denosumab use were associated with a higher incidence of ONJ. The risk of ONJ also may be increased in patients receiving concomitant therapy with other drugs known to cause ONJ.

Prior to initiating denosumab, a routine oral examination and appropriate preventative dentistry should be performed, especially in patients with risk factors for ONJ. All patients should maintain good oral hygiene and receive appropriate preventive dentistry during denosumab therapy.

Invasive dental procedures should be avoided during denosumab treatment. For patients requiring invasive dental procedures, the prescriber and/or oral surgeon should use clinical judgment and an assessment of the risks and benefits to guide the management plan. Temporary discontinuance of denosumab therapy should be considered; however, the optimal duration of treatment interruption is unknown.

Patients who develop or are suspected of having ONJ while receiving denosumab should be referred to a dentist or oral surgeon. Extensive dental surgery to treat ONJ may exacerbate the condition. Discontinuance of denosumab should be considered in such patients based on patient-specific risk-benefit assessment.

Atypical Subtrochanteric and Diaphyseal Femoral Fracture Atypical low energy or low trauma fractures of the femur have been reported in patients receiving denosumab. Such fractures can occur anywhere along the femoral shaft from just below the lesser trochanter to above the supracondylar flare and have a transverse or short oblique orientation without evidence of comminution. They may be bilateral and often occur with minimal or no trauma to the affected area. Many patients report prodromal pain in the affected area (usually dull or aching thigh pain) that presents weeks to months before a complete fracture occurs. In some cases, patients had been receiving concomitant glucocorticoid (prednisone) treatment at the time of fracture.

Patients receiving denosumab should be advised to report new or unusual pain in the thigh, hip, or groin. Patients reporting such symptoms should be suspected of having an atypical fracture and should be evaluated to rule out an incomplete femur fracture. Because atypical fractures may occur bilaterally, the contralateral limb also should be evaluated for fracture.

Interruption of denosumab treatment should be considered pending an assessment of the risks and benefits of the drug for the individual patient.

Hypercalcemia Following Discontinuance of Therapy Severe, symptomatic hypercalcemia requiring hospitalization and complicated by acute renal injury has been reported following discontinuance of denosumab therapy in patients with giant cell tumor of bone and in pediatric patients with growing skeletons. (See Pediatric Use under Warnings/Precautions: Specific Populations, in Cautions.) Hypercalcemia has been reported within the first year following treatment discontinuance. Following discontinuance of denosumab therapy, patients should be monitored for manifestations of hypercalcemia, serum calcium concentrations should be monitored periodically, requirements for calcium and vitamin D supplementation should be reevaluated, and patients should be managed as clinically appropriate.

Multiple Vertebral Fractures Following Discontinuance of Therapy Cases of multiple vertebral fractures have been reported following discontinuance of denosumab therapy. Patients at increased risk for multiple vertebral fractures include those with risk factors for or a history of osteoporosis and those with prior vertebral fractures. When denosumab therapy is discontinued, the risk of fractures, including multiple vertebral fractures, increases. Following discontinuance of therapy, markers of bone resorption initially increase above pretreatment values and then return to pretreatment values 24 months after the last dose of the drug; bone mineral density (BMD) returns to pretreatment values within 18 months after the last dose. In a phase 3 clinical study evaluating denosumab in postmenopausal women with osteoporosis (Fracture Reduction Evaluation of Denosumab in Osteoporosis Every 6 Months [FREEDOM] study), 6% of women who discontinued denosumab therapy and remained in the study experienced new vertebral fractures and 3% experienced multiple new vertebral fractures. New vertebral fractures have occurred as early as 7 months (mean: 19 months) after the last dose of the drug.

Prior to initiation of denosumab therapy in patients with osteoporosis or bone loss associated with androgen deprivation or aromatase inhibitor therapy, benefits and risks of the drug for the individual patient should be assessed; if denosumab therapy is discontinued, initiation of an alternative bone resorption inhibitor should be considered. When denosumab therapy is discontinued in patients with bone metastases from solid tumors, multiple myeloma, giant cell tumor of bone, or hypercalcemia of malignancy, the patient's risk for vertebral fractures should be evaluated.

Serious Infections Denosumab may increase the risk of infection.

In the FREEDOM study evaluating efficacy and safety of denosumab in postmenopausal women with osteoporosis, serious infections leading to hospitalization were reported more frequently in patients receiving denosumab than placebo. Serious skin infections (e.g., cellulitis, erysipelas), endocarditis, and infections of the abdomen, urinary tract, and ear were reported. The overall incidence of infections and the incidence of opportunistic infections reported in denosumab-treated patients were similar to rates reported in placebo-treated patients.

Patients receiving concomitant therapy with immunosuppressive agents or those with impaired immune systems may be at greater risk of serious infections during denosumab therapy. The need for continued denosumab therapy should be assessed in patients who develop serious infections while receiving the drug.

Dermatologic Reactions In the FREEDOM study evaluating denosumab in postmenopausal women with osteoporosis, adverse epidermal and dermal events were reported more frequently in denosumab-treated patients than in placebo-treated patients. Dermatologic reactions included dermatitis, eczema, and rash; most of these reactions were not specific to the injection site.

Discontinuance of denosumab therapy should be considered if severe dermatologic symptoms develop.

Musculoskeletal Pain Severe and occasionally incapacitating bone, joint, and/or muscle pain has been reported during postmarketing experience in patients receiving denosumab. Symptoms reportedly have recurred in some patients following rechallenge with the drug. The time to onset of symptoms has ranged from one day to several months after initiation of therapy. Discontinuance of the drug should be considered if severe musculoskeletal pain develops.

Suppression of Bone Turnover Significant suppression of bone remodeling, as evidenced by biochemical markers of bone turnover and bone histomorphometry, was reported in clinical trials of denosumab in patients with osteoporosis.

When biochemical markers of bone turnover (i.e., serum C-telopeptide of type I collagen [CTX] and serum procollagen type I N-terminal propeptide [PINP]) were measured in a subset of patients in the FREEDOM study (postmenopausal women with osteoporosis), suppression was evident shortly after denosumab was initiated and continued for the duration of the 3-year study. The CTX was 86, 72, and 72% lower and the PINP was 18, 50, and 76% lower at 1 month, 6 months (immediately prior to a dose), and 3 years, respectively, in those who received denosumab compared with those who received placebo.

In addition, tetracycline labeling studies have shown substantial decreases in bone formation rates in denosumab-treated patients compared with placebo-treated patients. In a study where bone biopsies were obtained at 3 years in postmenopausal women with osteoporosis, 100% of patients receiving placebo had double tetracycline labeling, indicating active bone remodeling; however, 38% of patients receiving denosumab had no tetracycline labeling, suggesting that bone formation was suppressed in these patients. In a study where bone biopsies were obtained at 1 year in men with osteoporosis, 100% of those receiving placebo had double tetracycline labeling, while 6% of those receiving denosumab had no tetracycline labeling. In a study where bone biopsies were obtained at 1 year from a limited number of patients with glucocorticoid-induced osteoporosis, all patients receiving risedronate had tetracycline labeling, whereas 2 of 3 denosumab-treated patients had no tetracycline labeling.

The long-term effects of the degree of bone remodeling suppression seen with denosumab are unknown. Because these effects may contribute to adverse outcomes, such as ONJ, atypical fractures, and delayed fracture healing, patients receiving denosumab should be monitored for such events.

Immunogenicity and Antibody Formation Denosumab-binding antibodies have been reported in less than 1% of patients who received denosumab therapy for periods of up to 5 years. Denosumab-neutralizing antibodies have not been reported to date, and antibody formation does not appear to affect denosumab pharmacokinetics, toxicity, or efficacy.

Specific Populations **Pregnancy.** Based on animal findings and its mechanism of action, denosumab may cause fetal harm if administered to pregnant women. (See Fetal/Neonatal Morbidity and Mortality under Cautions: Warnings/Precautions, in Cautions.) Pregnancy status should be confirmed prior to initiation of denosumab therapy in women with reproductive potential.

Lactation. It is not known whether denosumab is distributed into human milk, affects breast-fed infants, or affects milk production. Denosumab is distributed into milk in monkeys in concentrations of up to 0.5% of those attained in serum at up to one month after the last dose. Studies in pregnant mice indicate that denosumab exposure during pregnancy may impair maternal mammary gland development and lactation; however, no impairment of maternal mammary gland development or lactation was observed in monkeys. The manufacturer states that the developmental and health benefits of breast-feeding should be considered along with the mother's clinical need for denosumab (Xgeva®) and any potential adverse effects on the breast-fed infant from the drug or from the underlying maternal condition.

Pediatric Use. Safety and efficacy of denosumab have been established for treatment of giant cell tumor of bone in skeletally mature adolescents. Safety and efficacy of denosumab have not been established for any other indication in pediatric patients. Clinically important hypercalcemia has been reported following discontinuance of denosumab therapy in pediatric patients with growing skeletons who received the drug for treatment of giant cell tumor of bone or for other unlabeled (off-label) uses. Denosumab potentially may impair bone growth in children with open growth plates and may inhibit eruption of dentition. The manufacturer states that denosumab (Prolia®) is not recommended in pediatric patients younger than 4 years of age because of the high rates of skeletal growth in this age group and the potential for the drug to adversely affect long-bone growth and dentition.

Geriatric Use. When the total number of patients studied in clinical trials of denosumab (Prolia®) is considered, 76% were 65 years of age or older, while 27% were 75 years of age or older; in clinical trials in men with osteoporosis or in patients with glucocorticoid-induced osteoporosis, 55 or 47%, respectively, of patients were 65 years of age or older, while 16 or 17%, respectively, were 75 years of age or older. Of the total number of patients studied in clinical trials of denosumab (Xgeva®) for prevention of skeletal-related events in patients with multiple myeloma or with bone metastases from solid tumors, 44–45% were 65 years of age or older, while 16–17% were 75 years of age or older. Although no overall differences in efficacy or safety were observed between geriatric and younger patients and other clinical experience has revealed no evidence of age-related differences, the possibility that some older patients may exhibit increased sensitivity to the drug cannot be ruled out.

Hepatic Impairment. Clinical studies have not been conducted to evaluate the effect of hepatic impairment on the pharmacokinetics of denosumab.

Renal Impairment. Pharmacokinetics of denosumab are not affected by renal impairment, and dosage adjustment is not necessary in patients with renal impairment. However, in one study in patients with various degrees of renal function who received a single 60-mg dose of denosumab and in a second study in patients with severe renal impairment (creatinine clearance less than 30 mL/minute) or requiring dialysis who received two 120-mg doses of the drug, the risk of hypocalcemia increased with increasing renal impairment (occurring most commonly in those with severe renal impairment or receiving dialysis) and with inadequate or no calcium supplementation. Hypocalcemia was mild to moderate in severity in 96% of patients in these studies. Patients with severe renal impairment or receiving dialysis may exhibit marked elevations in serum parathyroid hormone (PTH) concentrations.

The manufacturer states that the benefits and risks should be considered when using denosumab in patients with severe renal impairment or patients receiving dialysis. Clinical monitoring of calcium, phosphorus, and magnesium is highly recommended, and adequate calcium and vitamin D supplementation is important. (See Hypocalcemia and Mineral Metabolism under Cautions: Warnings/Precautions.)

■ **Common Adverse Effects** Adverse effects reported in clinical trials in more than 5% of patients receiving denosumab for the treatment of osteoporosis and reported more frequently with the drug than with placebo include back pain, extremity pain, musculoskeletal pain, hypercholesterolemia, and cystitis (in postmenopausal women) or back pain, arthralgia, and nasopharyngitis (in men).

Adverse effects reported in clinical trials in more than 3% of patients receiving denosumab for the treatment of glucocorticoid-induced osteoporosis and reported more frequently with denosumab than with risedronate include back pain, hypertension, bronchitis, and headache.

In clinical trials in patients receiving androgen deprivation or aromatase inhibitor therapy, adverse effects reported in 10% or more of patients receiving denosumab for treatment of bone loss and reported more frequently with the drug than with placebo include arthralgia and back pain.

Adverse effects reported in clinical trials in 25% or more of patients with bone metastases receiving denosumab for prevention of SREs include fatigue/asthenia, hypophosphatemia, and nausea. Adverse events reported in these clinical trials in 10% or more of patients receiving denosumab and more frequently with denosumab than with zoledronic acid include dyspnea, diarrhea, hypocalcemia, and hypophosphatemia.

Adverse effects reported in clinical trials in 10% or more of patients with multiple myeloma receiving denosumab for prevention of SREs include diarrhea, nausea, anemia, back pain, thrombocytopenia, peripheral edema, hypocalcemia, upper respiratory infection, rash, and headache. Severe hypophosphatemia occurred in 21% of patients.

Adverse effects reported in clinical trials in 10% or more of patients receiving denosumab for treatment of giant cell tumor of bone include arthralgia, headache, nausea, back pain, fatigue, and extremity pain. Severe hypophosphatemia occurred in approximately 10% of patients.

Adverse effects reported in clinical trials in more than 20% of patients receiving denosumab for bisphosphonate-refractory hypercalcemia of malignancy include nausea, dyspnea, decreased appetite, headache, peripheral edema, vomiting, anemia, constipation, and diarrhea. Grade 3 hypophosphatemia occurred in 76% of patients.

Drug Interactions

■ **Drugs Metabolized by Hepatic Microsomal Enzymes** Clinically important drug interactions are not expected when denosumab is used concomitantly with drugs metabolized by cytochrome P-450 isoenzyme 3A4 (CYP3A4) in postmenopausal women with osteoporosis. (See Drug Interactions: Midazolam.)

■ **Drugs Affecting Serum Calcium Concentrations** Because hypocalcemia has been reported in patients receiving denosumab, serum calcium concentrations should be monitored more frequently than usual in patients receiving concomitant therapy with other drugs that may also decrease calcium concentrations. (See Hypocalcemia and Mineral Metabolism under Cautions: Warnings/Precautions.)

■ **Antineoplastic Agents** In clinical trials evaluating denosumab for prevention of skeletal-related events (SREs) in patients with bone metastases, there was no evidence that antineoplastic treatment (chemotherapy and/or hormone therapy) affected systemic exposure or pharmacodynamic effects of denosumab. Serum denosumab concentrations at 1 and 3 months and the median reduction in urine N-terminal telopeptide corrected for urine creatinine (uNTx/Cr) from baseline to 3 months were similar in patients receiving concomitant chemotherapy and/or hormone therapy.

■ **Etanercept** In postmenopausal women with rheumatoid arthritis and low bone mineral density (BMD), the pharmacokinetics of etanercept (50 mg once weekly by subcutaneous injection) were not altered by denosumab (single 60-mg dose administered by subcutaneous injection 7 days after an etanercept dose).

■ **Immunosuppressive Agents** Concomitant use with immunosuppressive agents may increase the risk of serious infections. Risks and benefits should be assessed to guide use of denosumab in patients receiving immunosuppressive agents. (See Serious Infections under Cautions: Warnings/Precautions.)

■ **Midazolam** Administration of oral midazolam (single 2-mg dose) 2 weeks after a 60-mg subcutaneous dose of denosumab in postmenopausal women with osteoporosis did not affect the pharmacokinetics of midazolam, a drug that is metabolized by CYP3A4.

Description

Denosumab, a fully human monoclonal immunoglobulin G_2 (IgG_2) antibody, is a bone resorption inhibitor. The drug has affinity and specificity for human receptor activator of nuclear factor kappa-B (RANK) ligand (RANKL) and acts as a RANKL inhibitor. A member of the tumor necrosis factor (TNF) superfamily, membrane-bound RANKL is expressed by osteoblasts. Its receptor (RANK) is expressed on the cell surfaces of osteoclasts and osteoclast precursors. The interaction between RANK and RANKL is integral to the normal bone resorption process as it promotes osteoclast differentiation and activation and inhibits osteoclast apoptosis. The actions of denosumab are similar to those of osteoprotegerin, a decoy receptor for RANKL that is principally secreted by osteoblasts and bone marrow stromal cells. Denosumab (like osteoprotegerin) binds RANKL, preventing interaction with RANK. This inhibits osteoclast formation, function, and survival and, ultimately, bone resorption. In contrast to osteoprotegerin, however, denosumab is specific for RANKL and does not appear to bind to other members of the TNF superfamily.

Denosumab therapy results in reduced bone resorption markers and increased cortical and trabecular bone mass and strength. Reductions in bone formation markers are also seen, presumably due to the natural coupling of bone formation and resorption processes. The effects of denosumab are considered reversible since bone turnover markers and bone mineral density (BMD) return to baseline within 12 months after the drug is discontinued. When rechallenged with denosumab, patients exhibit reproducible suppression of bone remodeling and increases in BMD.

In giant cell tumors of bone, stromal cells express RANKL and osteoclast-like giant cells express RANK receptor; signaling through the RANK receptor contributes to osteolysis and tumor growth. Denosumab prevents RANKL from activating the receptor on the surfaces of osteoclast, their precursors, and osteoclast-like giant cells.

Following subcutaneous administration, bioavailability of denosumab is 61–62%. The drug exhibits a prolonged absorption phase; the median time to peak serum concentrations after a single 60-mg subcutaneous dose is 10 days (range 3–21 days). Denosumab also exhibits a prolonged β-phase and a more rapid terminal elimination phase, resulting in a mean half-life of approximately 25–28 days.

Studies in postmenopausal women with osteoporosis indicate that biochemical bone turnover markers are suppressed within days after a 60-mg dose of denosumab and maximal reductions generally occur by 1 month; toward the end of the recommended 6-month dosing interval in such women, serum concentrations of denosumab decrease with subsequent increases in bone turnover markers.

In patients with bone metastases receiving subcutaneous denosumab in a dosage of 120 mg once every 4 weeks, serum denosumab concentrations accumulated up to 2.8-fold and steady state was achieved by 6 months. In patients with breast cancer and bone metastases, the median reduction in urine N-telopeptide adjusted for urine creatinine (uNTx/Cr) was 82% within 1 week following the initial 120-mg dose; in several trials in patients with bone metastases from solid tumors, the median reduction in uNTx/Cr from baseline to 3 months was approximately 80%. In patients with newly diagnosed multiple myeloma receiving subcutaneous denosumab in a dosage of 120 mg once every 4 weeks, steady-state concentrations of the drug appeared to be achieved by 6 months; the median reduction in uNTx/Cr was approximately 75% by week 5 and 74–79% during weeks 9–49 of therapy.

When administered at the recommended dosage in patients with giant cell tumor of bone (120 mg once every 4 weeks, with an additional 120-mg dose given on day 8 and day 15 during the first month), steady state was achieved in 3 months.

The pharmacokinetics of denosumab are not affected by age, race, or gender. Studies using denosumab in a dosage of 60 mg once every 6 months indicate that pharmacokinetics are not affected by body weight. Studies using denosumab in a dosage of 120 mg once every 4 weeks indicate that steady-state exposure is lower in 120-kg patients compared with 66-kg patients. Characterization of other monoclonal antibodies indicates that absorption is probably mediated by the lymphatic system. Denosumab clearance is thought to occur via the reticuloendothelial system and renal excretion is not expected.

Advice to Patients

Denosumab (Prolia®) medication guide must be provided to the patient each time the drug is administered; importance of reading the medication guide prior to initiating therapy and prior to each subsequent dose. (See REMS.)

Importance of receiving adequate calcium and vitamin D supplementation during denosumab therapy, and importance of seeking medical attention if signs or symptoms of hypocalcemia develop (e.g., spasms, twitches, muscle cramps, numbness or tingling in fingers, toes, or near mouth).

Advise patients to seek prompt medical attention if they develop symptoms of hypersensitivity (e.g., rash, urticaria, pruritus, lip swelling, shortness of breath, hypotension, respiratory tract edema). Advise such patients they should not receive further doses of denosumab.

Advise patients to seek prompt medical attention if they develop signs or symptoms of infection, including cellulitis (e.g., fever, chills, severe abdominal pain, frequent or urgent need to urinate or burning feeling when urinating, skin that is red, swollen, hot, or tender to touch).

Advise patients to seek prompt medical attention if they develop signs or symptoms of dermatologic reactions (e.g., redness, itching, rash, dry skin, blisters that ooze or crust, peeling skin).

Importance of maintaining good oral hygiene during denosumab treatment; importance of informing dentist about denosumab treatment prior to dental procedures. Advise patients to inform clinician or dentist if persistent pain and/or slow healing of mouth or jaw occurs after dental surgery, or if symptoms of osteonecrosis of the jaw (pain, numbness, swelling of or drainage from the jaw, mouth, or teeth) occur at any time.

Advise patients to report new or unusual thigh, hip, or groin pain since these may be symptoms of atypical femoral fracture.

Advise patients that the risk for multiple vertebral fractures may be increased after denosumab therapy is discontinued, particularly in those with a history of osteoporosis or vertebral fractures. Advise patients not to interrupt denosumab therapy without consulting their clinician.

Advise patients of the potential for hypercalcemia following discontinuance of denosumab therapy in patients with giant cell tumor of bone and in pediatric patients with growing skeletons. Advise patients to report symptoms of hypercalcemia (e.g., nausea, vomiting, headache, decreased alertness) following denosumab discontinuance.

Advise patients to inform their clinician if severe bone, joint, and/or muscle pain occurs.

Advise patients that denosumab is commercially available as Prolia® and Xgeva®; patients should not receive concomitant treatment with both drugs.

Importance of informing clinicians about latex allergy. (See Latex Sensitivity under Warnings/Precautions: Sensitivity Reactions, in Cautions.)

Inform patients receiving denosumab for treatment of osteoporosis or treatment of bone loss associated with androgen deprivation or aromatase inhibitor therapy that if a dose is missed, the dose should be given as soon as convenient and subsequent dose should be scheduled for 6 months from date of last dose.

Importance of informing clinicians of existing or contemplated concomitant therapy, including prescription and OTC drugs, as well as any concomitant illnesses.

Importance of women informing clinicians if they are or plan to become pregnant or plan to breast-feed. Advise female patients with reproductive potential that a pregnancy test is recommended prior to initiation of denosumab therapy and that they should use effective methods of contraception during therapy and for at least 5 months after the last dose of the drug. (See Fetal/Neonatal Morbidity and Mortality under Cautions: Warnings/Precautions and also see Lactation under Warnings/Precautions: Specific Populations, in Cautions.)

Importance of informing patients of other important precautionary information. (See Cautions.)

Overview® (see Users Guide). For additional information on this drug until a more detailed monograph is developed and published, the manufacturer's labeling should be consulted. It is *essential* that the manufacturer's labeling be consulted for more detailed information on usual cautions, precautions, contraindications, potential drug interactions, laboratory test interferences, and acute toxicity.

Preparations

Excipients in commercially available drug preparations may have clinically important effects in some individuals; consult specific product labeling for details.

Denosumab

Parenteral		
Injection, for subcutaneous use	60 mg/mL	**Prolia®**, Amgen
	120 mg/1.7 mL	**Xgeva®**, Amgen

Selected Revisions August 2019,

Ibandronate Sodium

■ Ibandronate sodium, a synthetic bisphosphonate analog of pyrophosphate, is a bone resorption inhibitor.

Uses

■ **Osteoporosis** Ibandronate sodium is used for the prevention and treatment of postmenopausal osteoporosis. In addition to adequate intake of calcium/vitamin D and other lifestyle modifications (e.g., exercise, avoidance of excessive alcohol and tobacco use), experts recommend that pharmacologic therapy for osteoporosis be considered in postmenopausal women who are at high risk of fractures (generally those who have experienced a previous hip or vertebral fracture or who have low bone mineral density [BMD]); pharmacologic therapy also may be considered in postmenopausal women who have low bone mass, although there is less evidence supporting overall fracture risk reduction in such patients. When selecting an appropriate pharmacologic agent, use of a drug with proven antifracture efficacy is recommended. Available options include bisphosphonates (e.g., alendronate, risedronate, zoledronic acid, ibandronate), denosumab, raloxifene, calcitonin, or teriparatide with varying levels of recommendation given in expert guidelines based on the available evidence supporting fracture risk reduction for each drug. Choice of therapy should be individualized based on the potential benefits and adverse effects of therapy as well as patient preferences, comorbidities, and risk factors. For additional information on the prevention and treatment of osteoporosis, see Uses: Osteoporosis, in Alendronate 92:24.

Prevention in Postmenopausal Women Ibandronate is used for the prevention of osteoporosis in postmenopausal women. Risk factors for postmenopausal osteoporosis and related fractures include early menopause, decreased BMD, low body mass index (BMI), previous fracture or family history of fracture/osteoporosis, excessive alcohol intake, smoking, inadequate physical activity, low calcium and vitamin D intake, certain drugs (e.g., glucocorticoids), and medical conditions or diseases (e.g., rheumatoid arthritis, diabetes mellitus, Cushing syndrome, hyperparathyroidism).

Efficacy of oral ibandronate in the prevention of osteoporosis was established in a 2-year, randomized, double-blind, placebo-controlled, dose-ranging study in 653 postmenopausal women (41–82 years of age) who were in menopause for 8.5 years on average. All patients were receiving supplementation with 500 mg of calcium daily. In this study, ibandronate given at a dosage of 2.5 mg daily was more effective than placebo in increasing BMD of the lumbar spine and total hip.

Efficacy of oral ibandronate given once monthly for the prevention of osteoporosis has been demonstrated in a 1-year, randomized, double-blind, placebo-controlled study in 160 postmenopausal women (46–60 years of age) with low baseline bone mass. Women in the study were 5.4 years postmenopause on average, and all women received supplementation with 400 units of vitamin D and 500 mg of calcium daily. Therapy with ibandronate 150 mg once monthly was associated with a mean increase in lumbar spine BMD of 4.12% from baseline relative to placebo; BMD at other skeletal sites also increased relative to baseline values.

Treatment in Postmenopausal Women Ibandronate is used in the treatment of osteoporosis in postmenopausal women.

Efficacy of ibandronate given as a daily or once-monthly oral regimen has been established in several randomized, double-blind, multinational, dose-comparison studies in postmenopausal women with osteoporosis.

In a placebo-controlled study in postmenopausal women with osteoporosis, the rate of new vertebral fractures after 3 years of treatment (the primary end point) was substantially reduced in women receiving oral ibandronate daily (2.5 mg once daily) or intermittently (20 mg every other day for 12 doses every 3 months) compared with that in patients receiving placebo. The diagnosis of a vertebral fracture was based on qualitative diagnosis by a radiologist and on quantitative morphometric criteria (an absolute decrease in height of at least 4 mm and a relative height ratio or relative height reduction in a vertebral body of at least 20%). Over the course of the 3-year study, new vertebral fractures were found in 4.7, 4.9, or 9.6% of women receiving ibandronate 2.5 mg daily, 20 mg every other day, or placebo, respectively (relative risk reduction of 52% with daily or 50% with intermittent ibandronate, respectively, compared with placebo). The incidence of nonvertebral fractures at 3 years (a secondary end point) was similar with the active treatments; 9.1 or 8.9% with daily or intermittent ibandronate, respectively, compared with 8.2% with placebo. BMD at 3 years relative to baseline BMD (a secondary end point) increased appreciably at the lumbar spine, total hip, femoral neck, and trochanter with either daily or intermittent ibandronate therapy compared with placebo.

In a 2-year noninferiority trial comparing oral ibandronate administered monthly (100 or 150 mg once monthly) or daily (2.5 mg once daily), an ibandronate dosage of 150 mg once monthly was at least as effective as 2.5 mg once daily in increasing BMD of the lumbar spine (primary end point at 1 year) in postmenopausal women with osteoporosis. Analysis of other skeletal sites (secondary end points) indicated consistently higher BMDs of the total hip, femoral neck, and trochanter with a dosage of 150 mg once monthly compared with 2.5 mg once daily.

In a trial comparing IV ibandronate administered quarterly (3 mg once every 3 months) or bimonthly (2 mg every 2 months) with daily oral ibandronate (2.5 mg once daily), both IV regimens were more effective than the daily oral regimen in increasing BMD of the lumbar spine at 1 year compared with baseline (the primary end point) in postmenopausal women with osteoporosis.

Bone histology studies in a limited number of postmenopausal women with osteoporosis treated with oral ibandronate (2.5 mg daily for 34 months), quarterly IV ibandronate (3 mg every 3 months for 22 months), or bimonthly IV ibandronate (2 mg every 2 months for 23 months) indicated bone formation of normal quality without evidence of mineralization defects or osteomalacia during treatment with the drug. (See Musculoskeletal Pain under Cautions: Warnings/Precautions, in Cautions.)

■ **Glucocorticoid-induced Osteoporosis** Ibandronate also has been used in the management of glucocorticoid-induced osteoporosis†.

The American College of Rheumatology (ACR) recommends optimizing calcium and vitamin D intake and lifestyle modifications (e.g., diet, smoking cessation, weight-bearing or resistance-training exercise) in all patients receiving long-term glucocorticoid therapy; in addition, pharmacologic therapy with an oral bisphosphonate is recommended in patients who are considered to be at moderate-to-high risk of fracture. Oral bisphosphonates generally are preferred because of their demonstrated antifracture benefits as well as their safety and low cost; other options include IV bisphosphonates, teriparatide, denosumab, and raloxifene (for postmenopausal women if no other therapy is appropriate). For additional information on the use of bisphosphonates for prevention and treatment of glucocorticoid-induced osteoporosis, see Uses: Glucocorticoid-induced Osteoporosis, in Alendronate 92:24.

Dosage and Administration

■ **General** Hypocalcemia and other disturbances of bone and mineral metabolism must be corrected before ibandronate sodium therapy is initiated; patients should receive supplemental calcium and vitamin D if their dietary intake is inadequate.

■ **Administration** Ibandronate sodium is administered orally or by IV injection.

Oral Administration To facilitate oral absorption and reduce the potential for esophageal irritation, ibandronate should be taken with a full glass (180–240 mL) of plain water at least 60 minutes prior to the first food, beverage (other than plain water), or other orally administered drug or supplement (including vitamins, antacids, and calcium) of the day. Such supplements should be taken at a different time of the day than when ibandronate is taken. Because of the potential for oropharyngeal ulceration, patients should be instructed not to suck or chew ibandronate tablets; the tablets should be swallowed whole. Patients should be instructed to avoid lying down for at least 60 minutes following oral administration of ibandronate.

If a daily oral dose is not taken in the morning, the dose should not be taken later that same day; the next dose should be taken the next day at the regularly scheduled time.

When administered monthly, patients should take the oral dose in the morning on the same day each month. If a monthly dose is missed and the next scheduled dose is more than 7 days away, patients should take the missed dose the next morning after it is remembered and resume the regular schedule. If the next scheduled dose is 1–7 days away, patients should wait until the next regularly scheduled time to take the next dose (i.e., maintain the regular schedule); more than one 150-mg tablet should not be taken within the same week.

IV Administration IV ibandronate must be administered by a health-care professional. Ibandronate injection should be administered IV over a period of 15–30 seconds once every 3 months. If a dose is missed, the dose should be rescheduled and administered as soon as possible. Subsequent injections should be scheduled at 3-month intervals; the drug should not be administered more often than once every 3 months.

Ibandronate injection must only be administered IV. The safety and efficacy of ibandronate injection administered by routes other than IV injection have not been established. Care should be taken not to administer ibandronate injection intra-arterially or paravenously as such administration could result in tissue damage. Because of the risk of anaphylaxis or other severe hypersensitivity reactions, appropriate medical support should be readily available during IV administration of the drug. (See Hypersensitivity under Warnings/Precautions: Sensitivity Reactions, in Cautions.)

Ibandronate injection must not be mixed with calcium-containing solutions or other IV drugs.

Ibandronate injection should be inspected visually for particulate matter and discoloration before administration. Prefilled syringes of the drug should be discarded if the solution is discolored or contains a precipitate.

■ **Dosage** Dosage of ibandronate sodium, which is commercially available as the monosodium monohydrate, is expressed in terms of ibandronate.

The optimal duration of bisphosphonate therapy for osteoporosis has not been established. Safety and efficacy of ibandronate for the management of osteoporosis are based on clinical data over 3 years (for the oral formulation) or 1 year (for the IV formulation). Some evidence suggests that increased durations of bisphosphonate use may be associated with a higher risk of some adverse effects (e.g., jaw osteonecrosis, atypical fractures). (See Cautions.) All patients receiving a bisphosphonate should have periodic evaluations to determine the need for continued therapy with the drug. Discontinuance of bisphosphonate therapy may be considered after 3–5 years of use for patients who are assessed to be at low risk of fracture. Risk of fracture should be evaluated periodically in patients who discontinue therapy.

Osteoporosis **Prevention in Postmenopausal Women.** The recommended oral dosage of ibandronate for prevention of osteoporosis is 150 mg once monthly.

Treatment in Postmenopausal Women. The recommended oral dosage of ibandronate for treatment of osteoporosis is 150 mg once monthly.

The recommended IV dosage of ibandronate for treatment of osteoporosis is 3 mg once every 3 months. The dose should be injected IV over a period of 15–30 seconds.

Special Populations **Renal Impairment.** Dosage adjustments are not necessary in patients with mild to moderate renal impairment; use of ibandronate is not recommended in patients with severe renal impairment (creatinine clearance less than 30 mL/minute).

Cautions

■ **Contraindications** Hypocalcemia or known hypersensitivity to ibandronate or any ingredient in the formulation.

With oral ibandronate, abnormalities of the esophagus that delay esophageal emptying, such as stricture or achalasia.

With oral ibandronate, inability to stand or sit upright for at least 60 minutes.

■ **Warnings/Precautions** ***GI Effects*** Since severe adverse esophageal effects including esophagitis, esophageal ulcers, and/or erosions (occasionally with bleeding and rarely followed by esophageal stricture or perforation) have been reported in patients receiving oral bisphosphonates, clinicians should be alert to any sign or symptom associated with such adverse effects. Patients should be instructed to discontinue ibandronate and contact a clinician if dysphagia, odynophagia, retrosternal pain, or new or worsening heartburn occurs. Since the incidence of severe adverse esophageal effects is greater in patients who do not drink a full (180–240 mL) glass of water when taking oral bisphosphonates and in those who lie down following administration of the drugs or who continue to take the drugs after experiencing symptoms suggestive of esophageal irritation, patients should be instructed carefully about proper administration of ibandronate. Ibandronate should be used with caution in patients with active upper GI disease (e.g., Barrett's esophagus, dysphagia, other esophageal diseases, gastritis, duodenitis, ulcers).

Gastric or duodenal ulcers also have been reported in patients receiving oral bisphosphonates during postmarketing experience, although no increased risk was observed in controlled clinical trials.

Although data are conflicting, there is some evidence suggesting a possible association between use of oral bisphosphonates and an increased risk of esophageal cancer. During the period of postmarketing surveillance from October 1995 (initial marketing of alendronate) through mid-May 2008, FDA received reports of esophageal cancer in 23 patients in the US receiving alendronate (as the suspect drug in 21 cases and the concomitant drug in 2 cases); 8 deaths were reported. An additional 31 cases of esophageal cancer were reported at the time in patients in Europe and Japan who had received an oral bisphosphonate, including alendronate, risedronate, ibandronate, and etidronate. (See Upper GI Effects under Cautions: Warnings/Precautions, in Alendronate 92:24.) In a large case-control study in a cohort of patients from the UK General Practice Research Database, risk of esophageal cancer was increased by 30% in patients who had at least one prescription issued for an oral bisphosphonate (alendronate, etidronate, or risedronate) compared with those not receiving such prescriptions; the risk was approximately doubled among patients who had 10 or more prescriptions issued for an oral bisphosphonate or who had an estimated duration of bisphosphonate use (calculated as the time between the first and last prescription issued during the observation period) of more than 3 years. However, another retrospective cohort study that used the same database found no evidence of an increased risk of esophageal cancer in patients receiving oral bisphosphonates. Other observational studies, including a study in patients receiving long-term alendronate therapy and a cohort study of Danish patients with fractures, have shown either no risk or a reduced risk of esophageal cancer following use of oral bisphosphonates. Because of conflicting findings and limitations of currently available data, additional study is needed to determine the association, if any, between oral bisphosphonate use and esophageal cancer. FDA states that the benefits of oral bisphosphonates in reducing the risk of serious fractures continue to outweigh their potential risks in patients with osteoporosis and that it is important to consider that esophageal cancer is rare, especially in women. FDA also states that there is insufficient information at this time to recommend routine endoscopic screening in asymptomatic patients receiving oral bisphosphonates. Avoidance of oral bisphosphonates in patients with Barrett's esophagus, a known precursor to esophageal adenocarcinoma, has been recommended.

Route of Administration Ibandronate injection must be administered IV by a health-care professional; the drug should not be administered by non-IV (e.g., intra-arterial) routes of administration. (See IV Administration under Dosage and Administration: Administration.)

Renal Effects Use of ibandronate is not recommended in patients with severe renal impairment (creatinine clearance less than 30 mL/minute).

Bisphosphonates have been associated with renal toxicity, manifested as deterioration of renal function and rarely, acute renal failure. The risk of adverse renal effects during parenteral therapy with bisphosphonates depends on coexisting conditions associated with renal impairment, concomitant therapy with other nephrotoxic drugs, preexisting renal disease, dehydration, dosage, infusion volume and rate, and multiple cycles of treatment. Acute renal failure has not been observed with IV ibandronate in controlled clinical trials following administration of recommended doses administered over 15–30 seconds.

Renal function should be assessed in patients with concomitant diseases or receiving drugs with nephrotoxic effects. Serum creatinine concentrations should be measured prior to administration of each dose of ibandronate injection. Treatment should be withheld in patients with deterioration of renal function.

Osteonecrosis of the Jaw Osteonecrosis and osteomyelitis of the jaw have been reported in patients, principally in those with cancer, who have received IV bisphosphonates. Most instances have been observed in cancer patients receiving IV bisphosphonate therapy, but some patients have experienced this adverse effect during oral bisphosphonate therapy. While the mechanism by which these adverse effects occur has not been elucidated, it has been suggested that suppression of bone turnover and remodeling by bisphosphonates impairs the ability to repair microfractures in the maxilla and mandible that occur with daily mastication. Most cases of osteonecrosis with bisphosphonate therapy have been associated with tooth extraction and/or local infection with delayed healing. (See Osteonecrosis of the Jaw under Cautions: Warnings/Precautions, in Zoledronic Acid 92:24.) Known risk factors for osteonecrosis of the jaw include invasive dental procedures (e.g., tooth extraction, dental implants, boney surgery), cancer, concomitant therapies (e.g., chemotherapy, corticosteroids, angiogenesis inhibitors), poor oral hygiene, and comorbid disorders (e.g., periodontal and/or other preexisting dental disease, anemia, coagulopathy, infection, ill-fitting dentures). Risk also may be increased with increased duration of bisphosphonate use. Discontinuance of bisphosphonate treatment may reduce the risk for osteonecrosis of the jaw in patients requiring invasive dental procedures. Clinical judgment of the treating clinician and/or oral surgeon should guide the management of each patient based on individual benefit/risk assessment. Patients who develop osteonecrosis of the jaw while receiving bisphosphonate therapy should receive care by an oral surgeon. In these patients, extensive dental surgery to treat osteonecrosis of the jaw may exacerbate the condition. Discontinuance of bisphosphonate therapy should be considered based on assessment of benefits and risks in individual patients.

Atypical Fracture of the Femur Atypical, low-energy, or low-trauma femoral fractures have been reported in bisphosphonate-treated patients. These fractures can occur anywhere in the femoral shaft from the subtrochanteric region of the hip (i.e., below the lesser trochanter) to above the supracondylar flare and are transverse or short oblique in orientation without evidence of comminution. Such fractures generally have occurred with use of bisphosphonate therapy for more than 3 years (median 7 years in one analysis of available data). The magnitude of this risk is unclear, although such fractures appear to be rare; in addition, causality has not been established since atypical fractures also have occurred in patients not receiving bisphosphonates. Most cases of atypical femoral fractures with bisphosphonate therapy have been reported in individuals receiving treatment for osteoporosis. Such fractures most commonly occur in individuals with minimal or no trauma. Many individuals have reported prodromal symptoms presenting as dull, aching thigh pain for weeks to months prior to the occurrence of an atypical fracture. Bilateral involvement (i.e., a fracture in the contralateral limb) and evidence of delayed healing of the fracture also may be present. Concomitant use of glucocorticoid, estrogen, and proton-pump inhibitor therapy may increase the risk of an atypical fracture.

Individuals with a history of bisphosphonate exposure presenting with new thigh or groin pain should be evaluated for possible atypical femoral fracture; an assessment of the contralateral limb also should be performed to rule out possible bilateral involvement (i.e., presence of radiographic change or fracture). Interruption of bisphosphonate therapy should be considered in individuals presenting with symptoms suggestive of a possible femoral fracture following completion of a comprehensive risk-benefit assessment performed on an individualized basis. Bisphosphonate therapy should be *discontinued* if a femoral shaft fracture is confirmed. (See Atypical Fracture of the Femur under Cautions: Warnings/Precautions, in Zoledronic Acid 92:24.)

Musculoskeletal Pain Severe, occasionally incapacitating bone, joint, and/or muscle pain has been reported infrequently during postmarketing experience in patients receiving bisphosphonates. The time to onset of symptoms varied from 1 day to years (mean onset about 3 months) after treatment initiation. Musculoskeletal pain has improved following discontinuance of the drug in most patients; however, some patients have reported slow or incomplete resolution of such pain. In some patients, musculoskeletal pain recurred upon subsequent rechallenge with the same drug or another bisphosphonate. Discontinuance of ibandronate should be considered if severe symptoms develop.

Metabolic Effects Hypocalcemia, hypovitaminosis D, and other disturbances of bone and mineral metabolism should be corrected before ibandronate therapy is initiated, and patients with osteoporosis receiving oral ibandronate should receive supplemental calcium and vitamin D if their daily dietary intake is inadequate.

Atrial Fibrillation While data are conflicting, a possible increased risk of atrial fibrillation has been identified with use of bisphosphonates. (See Atrial Fibrillation under Cautions: Warnings/Precautions, in Zoledronic Acid 92:24.)

Sensitivity Reactions **Hypersensitivity.** Hypersensitivity reactions, including fatal anaphylaxis following ibandronate injection, have been reported. (See Cautions: Contraindications and see IV Administration under Dosage and Administration: Administration.)

Specific Populations **Pregnancy.** There are no data in pregnant women to inform any drug-associated risks with ibandronate. The drug is not indicated for use in women of childbearing potential. In reproductive animal studies, maternal and fetal toxicity (including postimplantation loss, developmental anomalies, and deaths) have been observed.

Lactation. Ibandronate is distributed into milk in rats at concentrations averaging 1.5 times that in plasma; it is not known whether the drug is distributed into milk in humans. It is not known whether ibandronate has any effects on the nursing infant or on milk production.

Pediatric Use. Safety and efficacy have not been established in children. Ibandronate is not indicated for use in children.

Geriatric Use. No overall differences in safety and efficacy relative to younger adults have been observed. However, the possibility that some older patients may exhibit increased sensitivity to the drug cannot be ruled out. The greater frequency of decreased renal function observed in the elderly also should be considered.

Renal Impairment. Ibandronate should not be used in patients with severe renal impairment (creatinine clearance less than 30 mL/minute).

■ **Common Adverse Effects** Adverse effects occurring in at least 2% of patients receiving *daily* oral ibandronate therapy in osteoporosis treatment or prevention studies and in more patients than with placebo include upper respiratory tract infection, back pain, dyspepsia, bronchitis, pain in the extremities, diarrhea, headache, pneumonia, myalgia, urinary tract infection, hypercholesterolemia, infection (unspecified), dizziness, joint disorder, asthenia, tooth disorder, arthritis, vertigo, vomiting, allergic reaction, pharyngitis, gastritis, and nerve root lesion.

Adverse effects occurring in at least 2% of patients receiving *once-monthly* oral ibandronate include upper abdominal or abdominal pain, hypertension, dyspepsia, arthralgia, nausea, diarrhea, back pain, constipation, influenza, pain in the extremities, nasopharyngitis, headache, influenza-like illness and acute phase inflammatory reaction, localized osteoarthritis, bronchitis, urinary tract infection, dizziness, rash (including pruritic, macular, papular, erythematous, or generalized rash; dermatitis or allergic dermatitis; exanthem; erythema; and dermatitis medicamentosa), myalgia, upper respiratory tract infection, and insomnia.

Adverse effects occurring in at least 2% of patients receiving *quarterly* IV ibandronate therapy for the treatment of osteoporosis include arthralgia, back pain, cystitis, gastroenteritis, upper abdominal or abdominal pain, influenza-like illness and acute phase inflammatory reaction, headache, dyspepsia, nasopharyngitis, constipation, fatigue, diarrhea, pain in the extremities, myalgia, urinary tract infection, osteoarthritis, rash (including pruritic, macular, papular, erythematous, or generalized rash, dermatitis or allergic dermatitis, exanthem, erythema, and dermatitis medicamentosa), bronchitis, and nausea.

Drug Interactions

■ **Antacids or Mineral Supplements Containing Divalent Cations** Pharmacokinetic interaction (decreased absorption of ibandronate) when oral ibandronate is used concomitantly with antacids or vitamin or mineral supplements containing multivalent cations (e.g., aluminum, calcium, magnesium, iron). Oral ibandronate should be administered at least 60 minutes prior to taking any other oral drugs.

■ **Drugs Affecting Hepatic Microsomal Enzymes** Ibandronate does not induce or inhibit cytochrome P-450 (CYP) isoenzymes and is not metabolized. Pharmacokinetic interactions unlikely.

■ **Drugs Excreted through Renal Tubular Transport** Based on limited data in animals, ibandronate is not excreted through renal tubular transport. Pharmacokinetic interaction is unlikely.

■ **Nonsteroidal Anti-inflammatory Agents** Because aspirin, nonsteroidal anti-inflammatory agents (NSAIAs), and bisphosphonates are all associated with GI irritation, caution should be exercised in the concomitant use of NSAIAs and oral ibandronate.

■ **Histamine H_2-Receptor Antagonists, Proton Pump Inhibitors** Pharmacokinetic interaction (increased oral bioavailability of ibandronate) has been observed when IV ranitidine is administered before (15 or 90 minutes) and after (30 minutes) oral ibandronate; however, the interaction is not considered to be clinically important.

Among patients receiving histamine H_2-receptor antagonists or proton pump inhibitors in clinical trials of ibandronate, no evidence of increased adverse upper GI effects was observed with ibandronate compared with placebo.

■ **Melphalan** Pharmacokinetic interaction unlikely with concomitant IV melphalan and IV ibandronate.

■ **Prednisolone** Pharmacokinetic interaction unlikely with concomitant oral prednisolone and IV ibandronate.

■ **Tamoxifen** Pharmacokinetic interaction unlikely with concomitant oral tamoxifen and IV ibandronate.

Description

Ibandronate sodium, a synthetic bisphosphonate analog of pyrophosphate, is an inhibitor of osteoclast-mediated bone resorption. Ibandronate decreases bone resorption and turnover in a dose-dependent manner, resulting in maintenance of or increases in bone mineral density (BMD) and a net increase in bone mass compared with placebo in postmenopausal women. Ibandronate is structurally and pharmacologically related to other bisphosphonates (e.g., alendronate, etidronate, pamidronate, risedronate, zoledronic acid).

About 50–60% of an absorbed oral or IV dose of ibandronate sodium is eliminated in urine as unchanged drug. Nonrenal clearance is believed to result from uptake of the drug by bone. Unabsorbed drug is excreted unchanged in feces. Ibandronate is not metabolized and does not inhibit cytochrome P-450 (CYP) enzymes 1A2, 2A6, 2C9, 2C19, 2D6, 2E1, or 3A4 in vitro.

Advice to Patients

A copy of the manufacturer's patient information (i.e., medication guide) should be provided with each dispensed prescription and/or prior to each injection.

Importance of adhering to recommended lifestyle modifications (e.g., exercise, calcium and vitamin D supplementation).

Importance of correct oral administration (e.g., avoiding foods and beverages other than plain water [including mineral water] prior to administration, not lying down for at least 60 minutes following administration) in order to minimize the risk of upper GI effects. Importance of *not* taking vitamins, calcium, or antacids within 60 minutes of taking oral ibandronate. Necessity of swallowing tablets whole, without chewing or sucking, to avoid possibility of oropharyngeal ulceration. Importance of reviewing how to resume therapy in the event of a missed dose. Importance of discontinuing oral ibandronate and informing clinician if symptoms of esophageal disease (e.g., new or worsening dysphagia, difficulty or pain on swallowing, retrosternal pain, heartburn) develop.

Importance of informing a clinician if severe bone pain, joint pain, muscular pain, or jaw disease develops.

Importance of informing a clinician if new thigh or groin pain develops.

Importance of women informing clinicians if they are or plan to become pregnant or plan to breast-feed.

Importance of informing clinicians of existing or contemplated concomitant therapy, including prescription and OTC drugs (vitamins, supplements, antacids), as well as any concomitant illnesses (e.g., preexisting dysphagia, esophageal disorders, renal impairment). Importance of advising patients of other important precautionary information. (See Cautions.)

Overview® (see Users Guide). For additional information until a more detailed monograph is developed and published, the manufacturer's labeling should be consulted. It is *essential* that the manufacturer's labeling be consulted for more detailed information on usual uses, cautions, pre-

cautions, contraindications, potential drug interactions, laboratory test interferences, and acute toxicity.

Preparations

Excipients in commercially available drug preparations may have clinically important effects in some individuals; consult specific product labeling for details.

Ibandronate Sodium

Oral		
Tablets, film-coated	150 mg (of ibandronate)*	**Boniva**®, Genentech **Ibandronate Sodium Tablets**
Parenteral		
Injection, for IV use only	1 mg (of ibandronate) per mL*	**Boniva**® (available in prefilled syringe with needle and swabs), Genentech **Ibandronate Sodium Injection**

*available from one or more manufacturer, distributor, and/or repackager by generic (nonproprietary) name

†Use is not currently included in the labeling approved by the US Food and Drug Administration

Selected Revisions March 2018,

Risedronate Sodium

■ Risedronate sodium, a synthetic pyridinyl bisphosphonate analog, is a bone resorption inhibitor.

Uses

■ **Osteoporosis** Risedronate sodium is used for the prevention and treatment of postmenopausal osteoporosis; the drug also is used in men with osteoporosis to increase bone mass.

In addition to adequate intake of calcium/vitamin D and other lifestyle modifications (e.g., exercise, avoidance of excessive alcohol and tobacco use), experts recommend that pharmacologic therapy for osteoporosis be considered in postmenopausal women and in men 50 years of age or older who are at high risk of fractures (generally those who have experienced a previous hip or vertebral fracture or who have low bone mineral density [BMD]); pharmacologic therapy also may be considered in postmenopausal women and in men 50 years of age or older who have low bone mass, although there is less evidence supporting overall fracture risk reduction in such patients. When selecting an appropriate pharmacologic agent, use of a drug with proven antifracture efficacy is recommended. Available options include bisphosphonates (e.g., alendronate, risedronate, zoledronic acid, ibandronate), denosumab, raloxifene, calcitonin, or teriparatide with varying levels of recommendation given in expert guidelines based on the available evidence supporting fracture risk reduction for each drug. Choice of therapy should be individualized based on the potential benefits and adverse effects of therapy as well as patient preferences, comorbidities, and risk factors. For additional information on the prevention and treatment of osteoporosis, see Uses: Osteoporosis, in Alendronate 92:24.

Prevention in Postmenopausal Women Risedronate is used for the prevention of osteoporosis in postmenopausal women. Risk factors for postmenopausal osteoporosis and related fractures include early menopause, advanced age, low BMD, low body mass index (BMI), previous fracture or family history of fracture/osteoporosis, excessive alcohol intake, smoking, inadequate physical activity, low calcium and vitamin D intake, certain drugs (e.g., glucocorticoids), and medical conditions or diseases (e.g., rheumatoid arthritis, diabetes mellitus, Cushing syndrome, hyperparathyroidism).

In a double-blind, placebo-controlled study in early postmenopausal women (42–63 years of age), risedronate sodium administration (5 mg daily for 2 years) was associated with an increase in BMD in the lumbar spine, femoral neck, and trochanter bone compared with placebo. In another study, increases in BMD in the femoral neck and midshaft radius were observed in postmenopausal women (37–82 years of age) with osteopenia who received risedronate sodium (5 mg daily for 1 year) and conjugated estrogens (0.625 mg daily) compared with those who received conjugated estrogens without risedronate. Bone histology studies in postmenopausal women treated with risedronate sodium 5 mg daily plus estrogen indicate that the bone formed had normal lamellar structure and mineralization.

Efficacy of risedronate 35 mg once weekly for the prevention of osteoporosis was evaluated in a randomized, double-blind, placebo-controlled study in 278 postmenopausal women. All women received daily supplementation with vitamin D (400 units) and calcium (1 g). After 1 year of treatment, risedronate substantially increased BMD at the lumbar spine, total proximal femur, femoral neck, and trochanter compared with placebo (least-square mean increase in BMD of 2.9, 1.5, 1.2, and 1.8%, respectively).

Treatment in Postmenopausal Women Risedronate is used in the treatment of osteoporosis in postmenopausal women.

In placebo-controlled studies in postmenopausal women with osteoporosis, therapy with risedronate sodium 5 mg daily for 2–3 years substantially increased BMD in the lumbar spine, femoral neck, and femoral trochanter and maintained BMD at the midshaft radius while patients treated with placebo lost BMD at all sites. Bone histology studies in postmenopausal women with osteoporosis treated with risedronate sodium 5 mg daily indicate that bone formed during treatment with the drug is of normal quality. Risedronate therapy reduced the incidence of vertebral and nonvertebral (e.g., wrist, humerus, hip, pelvis, leg) fractures among postmenopausal women with osteoporosis who had previously sustained vertebral fractures.

In a 1-year controlled study in postmenopausal women with osteoporosis, risedronate sodium 35 or 50 mg once weekly (as immediate-release tablets) produced increases in lumbar spine and hip BMD similar to those observed with a dosage of 5 mg daily.

In a 1-year double-blind, active-controlled study, risedronate sodium 35 mg once weekly (as delayed-release tablets) was found to be noninferior to a dosage of 5 mg daily (as immediate-release tablets) with respect to mean change in BMD from baseline.

In 2 double-blind trials, risedronate sodium in a monthly dosage of 150 mg was found to be noninferior to a regimen of 5 mg daily in increasing BMD. Risedronate was administered as a single 150-mg tablet once a month in one of the studies and as a 75-mg tablet on 2 consecutive days each month in the other study. In both studies, the mean change in BMD for the lumbar spine and other skeletal sites was similar between the monthly and daily dosing regimens.

Treatment in Men Risedronate is used for the treatment of osteoporosis in men to increase bone mass.

Efficacy and safety of the drug for this use is based principally on results of a double-blind, placebo-controlled study in men 36–84 years of age (mean age: 60.6 years) with osteoporosis (defined as a femoral neck BMD of at least 2 standard deviations below the normal adult mean and a lumbar spine BMD of at least 1 standard deviation below the normal adult mean, or a femoral neck BMD of at least 1 standard deviation below the normal adult mean and a lumbar spine BMD of at least 2.5 standard deviations below the normal adult mean). All patients received supplemental calcium (1 g daily) and vitamin D (400–500 units daily). Treatment with risedronate sodium 35 mg once weekly substantially increased BMD in the lumbar spine, femoral neck, trochanter, and total hip compared with placebo (mean treatment differences of 4.5, 1.1, 2.2, and 1.5%, respectively). Increases in BMD were apparent as early as 6 months (the earliest time point tested) after initiation of risedronate therapy. Few vertebral and nonvertebral fractures were reported in this study, and no difference in fracture rates was observed between the treatment groups.

■ **Glucocorticoid-induced Osteoporosis** Risedronate is used for the prevention and treatment of glucocorticoid-induced osteoporosis. The manufacturer recommends use of risedronate in men and women who are either initiating or continuing systemic glucocorticoid therapy for chronic disease in a daily dosage equivalent to at least 7.5 mg of prednisone.

The American College of Rheumatology (ACR) recommends optimizing calcium and vitamin D intake and lifestyle modifications (e.g., diet, smoking cessation, weight-bearing or resistance-training exercise) in all patients receiving long-term glucocorticoid therapy; in addition, pharmacologic therapy with an oral bisphosphonate is recommended in patients who are considered to be at moderate-to-high risk of fracture. Oral bisphosphonates generally are preferred because of their demonstrated antifracture benefits as well as their safety and low cost; other options include IV bisphosphonates, teriparatide, denosumab, and raloxifene (for postmenopausal women if no other therapy is appropriate). For additional information on the use of bisphosphonates for prevention and treatment of glucocorticoid-induced osteoporosis, see Uses: Glucocorticoid-induced Osteoporosis, in Alendronate 92:24.

Prevention In a placebo-controlled, double-blind, randomized study, risedronate sodium 5 mg daily for 1 year prevented bone loss in men and women with a variety of underlying diseases (e.g., rheumatoid arthritis, temporal arteritis, polymyalgia rheumatica, systemic lupus erythematosus, asthma) who had initiated glucocorticoid therapy within 3 months of study entry and had normal mean lumbar spine BMD. BMD was maintained or increased in patients receiving risedronate while patients receiving placebo experienced decreases in BMD at the lumbar spine, femoral neck, and trochanter. In patients who underwent bone biopsies at the end of the study, bone histology was normal in patients receiving risedronate and corticosteroids.

Treatment In patients with glucocorticoid-induced osteopenia or osteoporosis who had been receiving glucocorticoids for at least 6 months before study entry, therapy with risedronate sodium (5 mg daily for 1 year) was associated with a 2.7 or 1.9% increase in BMD at the lumbar spine or femoral neck, respectively, compared with placebo. A dosage of 2.5 daily of risedronate sodium was not substantially more effective than placebo in this study. When both risedronate dosage groups were combined, risedronate therapy also was associated with a decreased incidence of vertebral fractures relative to placebo.

■ **Paget Disease of Bone** Risedronate is used in the treatment of Paget disease of bone (osteitis deformans).

Six months after initiation of therapy in a clinical study in men and women with moderate to severe Paget disease of bone (serum alkaline phosphatase concentrations at least twice the upper limit of normal), normalization of serum alkaline phosphatase concentrations occurred in 77% of patients receiving risedronate sodium (30 mg daily for 2 months) and in 11% of those receiving etidronate disodium (400 mg daily for 6 months). At month 18 (16 and 12 months after discontinuance of risedronate and etidronate, respectively), 53%

of those who had received risedronate remained in biochemical remission, compared with 14% of those treated with etidronate. Risedronate has been effective in a limited number of patients with refractory Paget disease who had not responded to prior therapy with etidronate or calcitonin. Bone biopsies of non-Pagetic bone in patients with Paget disease of bone treated with risedronate did not reveal evidence of osteomalacia, impairment of bone remodeling, or an appreciable decline in bone turnover.

Dosage and Administration

■ **General** Hypocalcemia and other disturbances of bone and mineral metabolism must be corrected before risedronate therapy is initiated. Patients should receive supplemental calcium and vitamin D if their dietary intake is inadequate, particularly in patients with Paget disease of bone.

■ **Administration** Risedronate sodium is administered orally.

Immediate-release Tablets To facilitate absorption, risedronate immediate-release tablets should be taken with a full glass (180–240 mL) of plain water at least 30 minutes before the first food, beverage, or other orally administered drug or supplement (including calcium, antacids, or vitamins) of the day. Because of the potential for oropharyngeal irritation, patients should be instructed not to suck or chew the tablets. Patients should be instructed to avoid lying down for at least 30 minutes following administration of risedronate to facilitate delivery of the drug to the stomach and minimize potential esophageal irritation.

Delayed-release Tablets Risedronate 35 mg delayed-release tablets should be taken in the morning immediately following breakfast; delayed-release tablets should not be administered under fasting conditions to minimize the risk of abdominal pain when using this formulation. The tablets should be swallowed whole with at least 120 mL of plain water (and not chewed, cut, or crushed). Patients should be instructed to avoid lying down for at least 30 minutes following administration of risedronate to facilitate delivery of the drug to the stomach and minimize potential esophageal irritation.

■ **Dosage** ***Osteoporosis*** For *treatment* of osteoporosis in postmenopausal women, the usual dosage of risedronate sodium is 5 mg once *daily*, 35 mg (given as immediate-release or delayed-release tablets) once *weekly*, or 150 mg *monthly* (given as a 150-mg tablet once monthly or a 75-mg tablet on 2 consecutive days per month).

For the *prevention* of osteoporosis in postmenopausal women, the usual dosage of risedronate sodium is 5 mg once *daily* or 35 mg once *weekly* as immediate release tablets. Alternatively, a dosage of 150 mg once *monthly* (given as a 150-mg tablet or as a 75-mg tablet on 2 consecutive days) may be considered.

For the *treatment* of osteoporosis in men, the recommended dosage of risedronate sodium is 35 mg once weekly.

If a weekly 35-mg dose of risedronate sodium is missed, the missed dose should be taken the next morning after the day it is remembered, followed by resumption of the regular weekly schedule on the originally chosen day. Patients should *not* take 2 risedronate sodium 35-mg tablets on the same day.

If a monthly 150-mg dose of risedronate sodium is missed and the next scheduled dose is more than 7 days away, patients should take the missed dose the next morning after it is remembered and resume the regular schedule. If the next scheduled dose is within 7 days, patients should wait until the next month's scheduled dose and resume their regular dosing schedule at that time; more than one 150-mg tablet should not be taken within the same week.

If one or both doses are missed in patients receiving the consecutive-day dosing schedule (i.e., risedronate sodium 75 mg on 2 consecutive days per month) and the next month's scheduled dose is more than 7 days away, patients should be instructed as follows: if both 75-mg doses are missed, one dose should be taken the next morning after it is remembered followed by the second dose the next consecutive morning; if only one 75-mg dose is missed, the missed dose should be taken the next morning after it is remembered. The regular dosing schedule should then be resumed; more than two 75-mg tablets should not be taken within the same week. If one or both doses are missed in patients receiving the consecutive-day dosing schedule and the next month's scheduled doses are within 7 days, patients should wait until the time of the next month's scheduled dose and resume their regular dosing schedule at that time.

The optimal duration of bisphosphonate treatment for osteoporosis has not been established. Safety and efficacy of risedronate for the treatment of osteoporosis are based on clinical data over 3 years (for the immediate-release tablets) or 1 year (for the 35-mg delayed-release tablets). Some evidence suggests that increased durations of bisphosphonate use may be associated with an increased risk of some adverse effects (e.g., atypical fractures, jaw osteonecrosis). All patients receiving a bisphosphonate should have periodic evaluations to determine the need for continued therapy. Discontinuance of bisphosphonate therapy may be considered after 3–5 years of use for patients who are assessed to be at low risk of fracture. Risk of fracture should be evaluated periodically in patients who discontinue therapy.

Glucocorticoid-induced Osteoporosis For the prevention or treatment of glucocorticoid-induced osteoporosis, the usual adult dosage of risedronate sodium is 5 mg once daily. The manufacturer states that safety and efficacy of risedronate when given for periods exceeding 1 year in the prevention or treatment of glucocorticoid-induced osteoporosis have not been established.

Paget Disease For the treatment of Paget disease of bone, the usual dosage of risedronate sodium in adults is 30 mg administered once daily for 2 months. After a post-treatment observation period of at least 2 months, a second course of risedronate sodium at the same dosage should be considered if there is evidence of recurrence of the disease process or if the initial treatment fails to normalize serum alkaline phosphatase concentrations. No data are available on the safety and efficacy of more than one course of retreatment with risedronate sodium for Paget disease.

■ **Special Populations** Risedronate should not be used in patients with severe renal impairment (creatinine clearance less than 30 mL/minute). Adjustments in risedronate sodium dosage are not necessary in patients with mild-to-moderate renal impairment (creatinine clearance 30 mL/minute or greater), geriatric patients, or in patients with hepatic impairment.

Cautions

■ **Contraindications** Hypocalcemia, known hypersensitivity to risedronate or any ingredient in the formulation, inability to stand or sit upright for at least 30 minutes, or abnormalities of the esophagus that delay esophageal emptying (e.g., stricture, achalasia).

■ **Warnings/Precautions** ***Formulation Considerations*** Risedronate immediate-release tablets (e.g., Actonel®) and risedronate delayed-release tablets (Atelvia®) contain the same active ingredient; patients should not receive both formulations concomitantly.

Upper GI Effects Because severe adverse esophageal effects including esophagitis, esophageal ulcers, and/or erosions (occasionally with bleeding and rarely followed by esophageal stricture or perforation) have been reported in patients receiving oral bisphosphonates, clinicians should be alert to any sign or symptom associated with such adverse effects. Patients should be instructed to discontinue risedronate and contact a clinician if dysphagia, odynophagia, retrosternal pain, or new or worsening heartburn occurs. The incidence of severe adverse esophageal effects is greater in patients who do not drink the recommended amount of water when taking oral bisphosphonates and in those who do not avoid lying down for at least 30 minutes following administration or who continue to take the drugs after experiencing symptoms suggestive of esophageal irritation; therefore, patients should be instructed carefully about proper administration of risedronate. (See Dosage and Administration: Administration.) Risedronate should be used with caution in patients with active upper GI disease (e.g., Barrett's esophagus, dysphagia, other esophageal diseases, gastritis, duodenitis, ulcers).

Gastric or duodenal ulcers, including some that were severe and with complications, have been reported in patients receiving oral bisphosphonates during postmarketing experience, although no increased risk was observed in controlled clinical trials.

Although data are conflicting, there is some evidence suggesting a possible association between use of oral bisphosphonates and an increased risk of esophageal cancer. During the period of postmarketing surveillance from October 1995 (initial marketing of alendronate) through mid-May 2008, FDA received reports of esophageal cancer in 23 patients in the US receiving alendronate (as the suspect drug in 21 cases and the concomitant drug in 2 cases); 8 deaths were reported. An additional 31 cases of esophageal cancer were reported at the time in patients in Europe and Japan who had received an oral bisphosphonate, including alendronate, risedronate, ibandronate, and etidronate. (See Upper GI Effects under Cautions: Warnings/Precautions, in Alendronate Sodium 92:24.) In a large case-control study in a cohort of patients from the UK General Practice Research Database, risk of esophageal cancer was increased by 30% in patients who had at least one prescription issued for an oral bisphosphonate (alendronate, etidronate, or risedronate) compared with those not receiving such prescriptions; the risk was approximately doubled among patients who had 10 or more prescriptions issued for an oral bisphosphonate or who had an estimated duration of bisphosphonate use (calculated as the time between the first and last prescription issued during the observation period) of more than 3 years. However, another retrospective cohort study that used the same database found no evidence of an increased risk of esophageal cancer in patients receiving oral bisphosphonates. Other observational studies, including a study in patients receiving long-term alendronate therapy and a cohort study of Danish patients with fractures, have shown either no risk or a reduced risk of esophageal cancer following use of oral bisphosphonates. Because of conflicting findings and limitations of currently available data, additional study is needed to determine the association, if any, between oral bisphosphonate use and esophageal cancer. FDA states that benefits of oral bisphosphonates in reducing the risk of serious fractures continue to outweigh their potential risks in patients with osteoporosis and that it is important to consider that esophageal cancer is rare, especially in women. FDA also states that there is insufficient information at this time to recommend routine endoscopic screening in asymptomatic patients receiving oral bisphosphonates. Avoidance of oral bisphosphonates in patients with Barrett's esophagus, a known precursor to esophageal adenocarcinoma, has been recommended.

Osteonecrosis of the Jaw Osteonecrosis and osteomyelitis of the jaw have been reported in patients, principally in those with cancer, who have received bisphosphonates. Most instances of jaw osteonecrosis have occurred in association with tooth extraction and/or local infection with delayed healing. (See Osteonecrosis of the Jaw under Cautions: Warnings/Precautions, in Zoledronic Acid 92:24.) Known risk factors for osteonecrosis of the jaw include invasive dental procedures (e.g., tooth extraction, dental implants, boney surgery), cancer, concomitant therapies (e.g., chemotherapy, corticosteroids, angiogenesis inhibitors), poor oral hygiene, and comorbid disorders (e.g., periodontal and/or other preexisting dental disease, anemia, coagulopathy, infection, ill-fitting dentures). Risk also may be increased with increased duration of bisphosphonate use. Discontinuance of bisphosphonate treatment may reduce the risk for osteonecrosis of the jaw in patients requiring invasive dental procedures. Clinical judgment of the treating clinician and/or oral surgeon should guide the management of each patient based on individual benefit/risk assessment. Patients who develop osteonecrosis of the jaw while receiving bisphosphonate therapy should receive care by an oral surgeon. In these patients, extensive dental surgery to treat osteonecrosis of the jaw may exacerbate the condition. Discontinuance of bisphosphonate therapy should be considered based on assessment of benefits and risks in individual patients.

Atypical Fracture of the Femur Atypical, low-energy, or low-trauma femoral fractures have been reported in bisphosphonate-treated patients. These fractures can occur anywhere in the femoral shaft from the subtrochanteric region of the hip (i.e., below the lesser trochanter) to above the supracondylar flare and are transverse or short oblique in orientation without evidence of comminution. Such fractures generally have occurred with use of bisphosphonate therapy for more than 3 years (median 7 years in one analysis of available data). The magnitude of this risk is unclear, although such fractures appear to be rare; in addition, causality has not been established since atypical fractures also have occurred in patients not receiving bisphosphonates. Most cases of atypical femoral fractures with bisphosphonate therapy have been reported in individuals receiving treatment for osteoporosis. Such fractures most commonly occur in individuals with minimal or no trauma. Most individuals have reported prodromal symptoms presenting as dull, aching thigh pain for weeks to months prior to the occurrence of an atypical fracture. Bilateral involvement (i.e., a fracture in the contralateral limb) and evidence of delayed healing of the fracture also may be present. Concomitant use of glucocorticoid, estrogen, and proton-pump inhibitor therapy may increase the risk of an atypical fracture.

Individuals with a history of bisphosphonate exposure presenting with new thigh or groin pain should be evaluated for possible atypical femoral fracture; an assessment of the contralateral limb also should be performed to rule out possible bilateral involvement (i.e., presence of radiographic change or fracture). Interruption of bisphosphonate therapy should be considered in individuals presenting with symptoms suggestive of a possible femoral fracture following completion of a comprehensive risk-benefit assessment performed on an individualized basis. Bisphosphonate therapy should be *discontinued* if a femoral shaft fracture is confirmed. (See Atypical Fracture of the Femur under Cautions: Warnings/Precautions, in Zoledronic Acid 92:24.)

Musculoskeletal Pain Severe, occasionally incapacitating bone, joint, and/or muscle pain have been reported infrequently during postmarketing experience in patients receiving bisphosphonates, including risedronate. The time to onset of symptoms varied from 1 day to years (mean onset about 3 months) after treatment initiation. Musculoskeletal pain has improved following discontinuance of the drug in most patients; however, some patients have reported slow or incomplete resolution of severe musculoskeletal pain. In some patients, musculoskeletal pain recurred upon subsequent rechallenge with the same drug or another bisphosphonate. The risk factors for and incidence of severe musculoskeletal pain associated with bisphosphonates are unknown. The association between bisphosphonates and severe musculoskeletal pain may be overlooked by clinicians, which may delay diagnosis, prolong pain and/or impairment, and necessitate the use of analgesics. Clinicians should evaluate whether bisphosphonate use might be responsible for severe musculoskeletal pain in patients who present with these symptoms; temporary or permanent discontinuance of therapy should be considered in such cases.

Metabolic Effects Hypocalcemia and other disturbances of bone and mineral metabolism must be corrected before risedronate therapy is initiated, and patients with osteoporosis or Paget disease of bone should receive supplemental calcium and vitamin D if their daily dietary intake is inadequate.

Endocrine Effects Before initiating risedronate therapy in patients receiving long-term glucocorticoid therapy, sex hormones should be measured and replacement therapy considered, if appropriate.

Atrial Fibrillation While data are conflicting, a possible increased risk of atrial fibrillation has been identified with use of bisphosphonates. (See Atrial Fibrillation under Cautions: Warnings/Precautions, in Zoledronic Acid 92:24.)

Specific Populations **Pregnancy.** Category C. (See Users Guide.)

Lactation. Risedronate is distributed into milk in rats; it is not known whether the drug is distributed into human milk. Because of the potential for serious adverse effects from risedronate in nursing infants, a decision should be made whether to discontinue nursing or the drug.

Pediatric Use. Risedronate is not indicated for use in pediatric patients. Efficacy and safety of the drug in pediatric patients were evaluated in a 1-year, randomized, double-blind, placebo-controlled study in 143 pediatric patients 4 to less than 16 years of age with osteogenesis imperfecta. Although risedronate was effective in increasing lumbar spine bone mineral density (BMD) compared with placebo, therapy with the drug was not associated with a reduction in fracture risk. Adverse effects reported in the pediatric patients evaluated in this study generally were similar to those reported in adults with osteoporosis; however, an increased risk of vomiting relative to placebo was observed with risedronate.

Geriatric Use. No substantial differences in safety and efficacy have been observed in geriatric patients relative to younger adults.

Hepatic Impairment. Efficacy and safety of risedronate have not been evaluated in patients with hepatic impairment. Because the drug is not metabolized in the liver, the manufacturer states that dosage adjustments are not likely to be necessary in patients with hepatic impairment.

Renal Impairment. Risedronate is not recommended in patients with severe renal impairment (creatinine clearance less than 30 mL/minute). No dosage adjustments are necessary in patients with mild to moderate renal impairment (creatinine clearance of at least 30 mL/minute).

■ **Common Adverse Effects** Adverse effects occurring in more than 5% of patients receiving *daily* risedronate therapy include back, chest or abdominal pain, pain (unspecified), hypertension, flu-like syndrome, peripheral edema, nausea, diarrhea, constipation, arthralgia, joint disorder,depression, headache, dizziness, myalgia, rash, cataract, pharyngitis, rhinitis, urinary tract infection, and infection (unspecified). Adverse effects occurring in more than 5% of patients receiving *once-weekly* risedronate include back or abdominal pain, pain (unspecified), hypertension, flu syndrome, infection (unspecified), accidental injury, overdose, nausea, constipation, dyspepsia, arthralgia, traumatic bone fracture, myalgia, headache, asthenia, and urinary tract infection.

Drug Interactions

■ **Antacids or Mineral Supplements Containing Divalent Cations** Pharmacokinetic interaction (decreased risedronate absorption) is possible when risedronate is used concomitantly with antacids or mineral supplements containing divalent cations (e.g., calcium, magnesium, iron). Patients should not administer these supplements and antacids at the same time as risedronate.

■ **Drugs Affecting Hepatic Microsomal Enzymes** Risedronate does not induce or inhibit cytochrome P-450 (CYP) isoenzymes and is not metabolized. Pharmacokinetic interaction unlikely.

■ **Nonsteroidal Anti-inflammatory Agents** There is no evidence of increased adverse upper GI effects when risedronate is administered concomitantly with nonsteroidal anti-inflammatory agents (NSAIAs).

■ **Histamine H_2-receptor Antagonists, Proton Pump Inhibitors** There is no evidence of increased adverse upper GI effects when risedronate is administered concomitantly with histamine H_2-receptor antagonists or proton pump inhibitors.

Description

Risedronate sodium, a synthetic pyridinyl bisphosphonate analog of pyrophosphate, is an inhibitor of osteoclast-mediated bone resorption.

Advice to Patients

A copy of the manufacturer's patient information (i.e., medication guide) should be provided with each dispensed prescription if risedronate is used for osteoporosis.

Importance of reviewing manufacturer's instructions for correct administration of risedronate, including importance of avoiding foods and beverages other than plain water or lying down for 30 minutes following administration of risedronate and of how to resume therapy in the event of a missed dose. Necessity of swallowing tablets whole, without crushing, chewing, or sucking.

Importance of discontinuing risedronate and contacting a clinician if symptoms of severe esophageal adverse effects (e.g., difficulty or pain with swallowing, retrosternal, abdominal or esophageal pain, severe or persistent heartburn) develop.

Importance of adherence to any recommended lifestyle modifications (e.g., weight-bearing exercise, calcium and vitamin D supplementation, avoidance of excessive cigarette smoking and/or alcohol consumption).

Importance of informing a clinician if severe bone pain, joint pain, muscular pain, or jaw disease develops.

Importance of informing a clinician if new thigh or groin pain develops.

Importance of women informing clinicians if they are or plan to become pregnant or plan to breast-feed.

Importance of informing clinicians of existing or contemplated concomitant therapy, including prescription and OTC drugs, as well as any concomitant illnesses (e.g., kidney disease).

Overview® (see Users Guide.). For additional information on this drug until a more detailed monograph is developed and published, the manufacturer's labeling should be consulted. It is *essential* that the manufacturer's labeling be consulted for more detailed information on usual cautions, precautions, contraindications, potential drug interactions, laboratory test interferences, and acute toxicity.

Preparations

Excipients in commercially available drug preparations may have clinically important effects in some individuals; consult specific product labeling for details.

Risedronate Sodium

Oral

Tablets, film-coated	5 mg*	**Actonel®**, Warner Chilcott
		Risedronate Sodium Tablets

	30 mg*	**Actonel®**, Warner Chilcott **Risedronate Sodium Tablets**
	35 mg*	**Actonel®**, Warner Chilcott **Risedronate Sodium Tablets**
	75 mg*	**Actonel®**, Warner Chilcott **Risedronate Sodium Tablets**
	150 mg*	**Actonel®**, Warner Chilcott **Risedronate Sodium Tablets**
Tablets, delayed-release	35 mg*	**Atelvia®**, Warner Chilcott **Risedronate Sodium Delayed-release Tablets**

*available from one or more manufacturer, distributor, and/or repackager by generic (nonproprietary) name

Zoledronic Acid

■ Zoledronic acid, a synthetic imidazole bisphosphonate analog of pyrophosphate, is a bone resorption inhibitor.

Uses

■ **Hypercalcemia Associated with Malignancy** Zoledronic acid is used in conjunction with achievement and maintenance of adequate hydration for the treatment of hypercalcemia (albumin-corrected serum calcium concentration of 12 mg/dL or greater) associated with malignant neoplasms. For the treatment of mild or asymptomatic hypercalcemia, measures more conservative (e.g., hydration alone or combined with loop diuretics) than therapy with agents such as zoledronic acid generally are used.

Controlled clinical studies have shown that single-dose IV zoledronic acid (4 mg infused over 5 minutes) is more effective in the treatment of moderate to severe malignancy-associated hypercalcemia (albumin-corrected serum calcium concentration of 12 mg/dL or greater) than single-dose IV pamidronate disodium (90 mg infused over 2 hours). In these studies, patients received zoledronic acid or pamidronate disodium in conjunction with IV hydration (750 mL of fluid, of which 250 mL was administered prior to study drug administration). Normocalcemia (corrected serum calcium concentrations not exceeding 10.8 mg/dL) was attained more quickly and maintained for a longer period of time in patients receiving zoledronic acid than in those receiving pamidronate. Analysis of pooled data from these studies indicates that 70 or 88% of patients receiving pamidronate disodium or zoledronic acid, respectively, achieved a normal serum calcium concentration within 10 days of treatment. For responders, the median duration of complete response (defined as the time from onset of normocalcemia until the last corrected serum calcium concentration of 10.8 mg/dL or less) following a single dose was approximately 32 or 18 days for zoledronic acid or pamidronate, respectively. The median time to recurrence (defined as the time from drug administration until the last corrected serum calcium concentration of less than 11.6 mg/dL) was longer with zoledronic acid (30 days) than with pamidronate (17 days). Subgroup analysis indicates that complete response rates were not affected by cancer type, the presence or absence of bone metastases, baseline blood parathyroid hormone-related protein concentrations, baseline BUN-to-creatinine ratio, age, sex, or race.

Retreatment with zoledronic acid may be considered in patients with recurrent or refractory hypercalcemia of malignancy. Data from a limited number of patients indicate that a second course of IV zoledronic acid therapy can normalize serum calcium concentrations when malignancy-associated hypercalcemia is refractory to or recurs following an adequate response to an initial course of therapy. A second course of therapy with zoledronic acid at a higher than recommended dose (8 mg) returned corrected serum calcium concentrations to normal within 10 days after retreatment in 52% of patients whose hypercalcemia was refractory to or recurred following an adequate response to an initial dose of zoledronic acid 4 mg. For responders, the median duration of complete response following retreatment was 11 days. The median time to recurrence following retreatment was 8 days.

■ **Bone Metastases of Solid Tumors and Osteolytic Lesions of Multiple Myeloma** Zoledronic acid is used as an adjunct to antineoplastic therapy for the treatment of bone metastases of solid tumors and osteolytic lesions of multiple myeloma. In patients with bone metastases associated with prostate cancer, zoledronic acid should be used as second-line therapy and is reserved for those with disease progression following one or more hormonal therapies.

The efficacy of zoledronic acid in combination with antineoplastic therapy (e.g., chemotherapy or hormonal therapy) for the treatment of bone metastases in patients with advanced solid tumors or osteolytic bone lesions associated with multiple myeloma has been demonstrated in several large clinical trials. In a long-term (12 months' duration) comparative study in patients with breast cancer and bone metastases or with stage III multiple myeloma and at least one osteolytic bone lesion, combined zoledronic acid (4 mg, administered as a 5- or 15-minute IV infusion once every 3–4 weeks) and antineoplastic therapy (chemotherapy or hormonal therapy) was as effective as combined pamidronate disodium (90 mg, administered as a 2-hour IV infusion once every 3–4 weeks) and antineoplastic therapy in reducing the incidence of bone-related complications (e.g., fractures or spinal cord compression, bone deterioration requiring radiotherapy or orthopedic surgery) and in delaying the development of such complications. The median time to the first bone-related complication was 373 days in patients receiving zoledronic acid and 363 days in patients receiving pamidronate. Patients with pain experienced a decrease in pain during adjunctive zoledronic acid or pamidronate therapy, while the need for supplemental analgesic therapy decreased or remained relatively unchanged. Secondary end points such as change in performance status or median time to overall disease progression or death did not differ between the treatment groups.

In a long-term (10.5 months' duration) placebo-controlled trial, patients with hormone-refractory prostate cancer and bone metastases who were receiving combined zoledronic acid (4 mg, administered as a 5- or 15-minute IV infusion once every 3 weeks) and hormonal therapy showed a decrease in the incidence and a delay in the development of bone-related complications (e.g., fractures or spinal cord compression, bone deterioration requiring radiotherapy or orthopedic surgery, bone pain necessitating a change in hormonal therapy) compared with those receiving hormonal therapy alone. The incidence of bone-related complications was lower in patients receiving adjunctive zoledronic acid (33%) than in those receiving hormonal therapy alone (44%). The first bone-related complication was observed at 321 days in those receiving hormonal therapy alone and such complications were not observed at that time in those receiving adjunctive zoledronic acid.

Data from a long-term placebo-controlled trial in patients with bone metastases and solid tumors other than breast or prostate cancer showed no appreciable difference in the incidence of bone-related complications (e.g., fractures or spinal cord compression, bone deterioration requiring radiotherapy or orthopedic surgery, bone pain necessitating a change in antineoplastic therapy) in patients receiving combined zoledronic acid (4 mg, administered as a 15-minute IV infusion once every 3 weeks) and antineoplastic therapy compared with those receiving antineoplastic therapy alone; however, there was a median delay of 67 days in the development of such complications in the group receiving zoledronic acid. Bone-related complications were observed in 38% of patients receiving adjunctive zoledronic acid compared with 44% of those receiving antineoplastic therapy alone. The median time to the first bone-related complication was 230 or 163 days, respectively, in patients receiving adjunctive zoledronic acid or antineoplastic therapy alone. More than two-thirds of the patients had preexisting bone-related complications; the median survival of patients enrolled in the trial (6 months) was less than the planned trial duration (9 months).

■ **Osteoporosis** Zoledronic acid is used for the prevention and treatment of postmenopausal osteoporosis; the drug also is used to increase bone mass in men with osteoporosis.

In addition to adequate intake of calcium/vitamin D and other lifestyle modifications (e.g., exercise, avoidance of excessive alcohol and tobacco use), experts recommend that pharmacologic therapy for osteoporosis be considered in postmenopausal women and in men 50 years of age or older who are at high risk of fractures (generally those who have experienced a previous hip or vertebral fracture or who have low bone mineral density [BMD]); pharmacologic therapy also may be considered in postmenopausal women and in men 50 years of age or older who have low bone mass, although there is less evidence supporting overall fracture risk reduction in such patients. When selecting an appropriate pharmacologic agent, use of a drug with proven antifracture efficacy is recommended. Available options include bisphosphonates (e.g., alendronate, risedronate, zoledronic acid, ibandronate), denosumab, raloxifene, calcitonin, or teriparatide with varying levels of recommendation given in expert guidelines based on the available evidence supporting fracture risk reduction for each drug. Choice of therapy should be individualized based on the potential benefits and adverse effects of therapy as well as patient preferences, comorbidities, and risk factors. For additional information on the prevention and treatment of osteoporosis, see Uses: Osteoporosis, in Alendronate 92:24.

Prevention in Postmenopausal Women Zoledronic acid is used for the prevention of osteoporosis in postmenopausal women. Risk factors for postmenopausal osteoporosis and related fractures include early menopause, decreased BMD, low body mass index (BMI), previous fracture or family history of fracture/osteoporosis, excessive alcohol intake, smoking, inadequate physical activity, low calcium and vitamin D intake, certain drugs (e.g., glucocorticoids), and medical conditions or diseases (e.g., rheumatoid arthritis, diabetes mellitus, Cushing syndrome, hyperparathyroidism).

In a 2-year, double-blind, placebo-controlled study in postmenopausal women 45 years of age or older with osteopenia, treatment with zoledronic acid resulted in a substantial increase in total hip and lumbar spine BMD compared with placebo at 2 years. In this study, zoledronic acid 5 mg was administered as a once-yearly IV infusion (total of 2 doses) or as a single IV infusion at study randomization (total of 1 dose); both dosage regimens were effective in preventing bone loss over the 2-year study period. Levels of bone turnover markers were reduced at all time points in both zoledronic acid treatment groups, but the effect was more sustained with the once-yearly regimen.

Treatment in Postmenopausal Women Zoledronic acid is used for the treatment of osteoporosis in postmenopausal women. Efficacy of zoledronic acid given as a once-yearly IV infusion has been established in 2 long-term (3 years' duration) randomized, double-blind, placebo-controlled, multinational studies in postmenopausal women with osteoporosis (diagnosed by BMD with or without vertebral fracture[s]). In each study, zoledronic acid was given as a single 5-mg dose by IV infusion over at least 15 minutes. In these studies, the incidence of new fractures (hip, vertebral, non-vertebral fractures) was reduced among patients receiving zoledronic acid compared with that observed with placebo with or without background therapies for osteoporosis (excluding bisphosphonates). Bone histology studies of patients from one of the studies indicated that the bone formed during therapy with zoledronic acid had normal architecture and mineralization. In patients at high risk of fractures (defined as those with a history of a recent, low-trauma hip fracture), zoledronic acid reduced the incidence of subsequent fractures.

Treatment in Men Zoledronic acid is used to increase bone mass in men with osteoporosis. Efficacy of zoledronic acid given as a once-yearly IV infusion was established in a long-term (2 years' duration) randomized, double-blind, active-controlled, multicenter study in men with osteoporosis or osteoporosis secondary to hypogonadism. Zoledronic acid was given as a single 5-mg dose by IV infusion over at least 15 minutes; this dose could be repeated once. The active control was an oral bisphosphonate administered once weekly for up to 2 years. All patients received elemental calcium 1 g and vitamin D 800–1000 international units (IU, units) daily. In this study, once-yearly zoledronic acid by IV infusion was noninferior to the once-weekly oral bisphosphonate based on the percent change in lumbar spine BMD at month 24 compared with baseline (6.1 versus 6.2% increase in BMD with zoledronic acid versus oral bisphosphonate, respectively).

■ **Glucocorticoid-induced Osteoporosis** Zoledronic acid is used in the treatment and prevention of glucocorticoid-induced osteoporosis. The manufacturer recommends use of zoledronic acid in men and women who are either initiating or receiving long-term (at least 12 months) systemic glucocorticoid therapy in a daily dosage equivalent to at least 7.5 mg of prednisone.

The American College of Rheumatology (ACR) recommends optimizing calcium and vitamin D intake and lifestyle modifications (e.g., diet, smoking cessation, weight-bearing or resistance-training exercise) in all patients receiving long-term glucocorticoid therapy; in addition, pharmacologic therapy with an oral bisphosphonate is recommended in patients who are considered to be at moderate-to-high risk of fracture. Oral bisphosphonates generally are preferred because of their antifracture benefits as well as their safety and low cost; other options include IV bisphosphonates, teriparatide, denosumab, and raloxifene (for postmenopausal women if no other therapy is appropriate). For additional information on the use of bisphosphonates for prevention and treatment of glucocorticoid-induced osteoporosis, see Uses: Glucocorticoid-induced Osteoporosis, in Alendronate 92:24.

Safety and efficacy of zoledronic acid for the treatment and prevention of glucocorticoid-induced osteoporosis were evaluated in a randomized, double-blind, active-controlled study in men and women receiving glucocorticoid therapy (daily dosage of at least 7.5 mg of prednisone or equivalent). Patients were stratified according to their duration of glucocorticoid use: up to 3 months (prevention group) or more than 3 months (treatment group). In this study, zoledronic acid was administered in a single 5-mg dose by IV infusion over 15–20 minutes, and the active control (risedronate) was administered orally in a dosage of 5 mg once daily. At 12 months, zoledronic acid increased lumbar spine BMD to a greater extent than risedronate; lumbar BMD increased by an average of 4.1 versus 2.7%, respectively, in the treatment group and by an average of 2.6 versus 0.6%, respectively, in the prevention group. Qualitative histology assessments in a subset of patients who received zoledronic acid revealed normal architecture with no evidence of mineralization defects. However, there was an apparent reduction in activation frequency and bone remodeling rates when compared with histomorphometry results seen with zoledronic acid in the postmenopausal osteoporosis population; the long-term consequences of such effects are unknown.

■ **Paget Disease of Bone** Zoledronic acid is used for the management of moderate-to-severe Paget disease of bone (osteitis deformans). Efficacy of the drug in the treatment of Paget disease of bone has been established in 2 randomized, double-blind studies of 6 months' duration, in which zoledronic acid 5 mg as a single dose by IV infusion produced a more rapid and effective therapeutic response (as defined by either normalization of serum alkaline phosphatase concentrations or a reduction of at least 75% from baseline in total serum alkaline phosphatase excess [i.e., "excess" being defined as the difference between the measured concentration and the midpoint of the normal range] at the end of 6 months) than risedronate 30 mg orally once daily for 2 months. Most patients achieved a response to zoledronic acid by day 63 of the study.

Treatment with zoledronic acid should be considered in patients with serum alkaline phosphatase concentrations of at least twice the age-specific upper limit of normal, in those who are symptomatic, or in those at risk for future complications from their disease. After a single treatment of zoledronic acid in patients with Paget disease of bone, an extended remission period is observed. Specific data on retreatment of the disease are not available. However, retreatment may be considered in patients who have relapsed based on increases in serum alkaline phosphatase concentrations, in those who failed to achieve normalization of serum alkaline phosphatase concentrations, or in patients who are symptomatic, according to current standards of medical care.

■ **Prevention of Aromatase Inhibitor-associated Bone Loss** Zoledronic acid has been studied for the prevention of aromatase inhibitor-associated bone loss in women receiving adjuvant hormonal therapy for early-stage breast cancer†.

Prevention in Postmenopausal Women Efficacy and safety of zoledronic acid for the prevention of aromatase inhibitor-associated bone loss in women receiving adjuvant hormonal therapy for early-stage breast cancer† have been studied in several phase 3, open-label, randomized studies (Zometa-Femara Adjuvant Synergy Trial [Z-FAST], ZO-FAST, E-ZO-FAST, and North Central Cancer Treatment Group [NCCTG]-N03CC study). The Z-FAST, ZO-FAST, and E-ZO-FAST studies included postmenopausal women with stage I–IIIa estrogen receptor-positive and/or progesterone receptor-positive breast cancer; patients had a baseline T-score of −2 standard deviations (SD) from normal or better and did not have a history of a low-intensity fracture or evidence of an existing fracture. Patients enrolled in these studies were randomized to receive upfront or delayed zoledronic acid. Women in the upfront group received zoledronic acid following randomization; women in the delayed group did not begin treatment with zoledronic acid until their T-score declined to less than −2 standard deviations or after occurrence of a nontraumatic fracture or evidence of an asymptomatic fracture. Patients received zoledronic acid 4 mg by IV infusion over 15 minutes every 6 months for 5 years in addition to oral calcium and vitamin D. All patients received letrozole 2.5 mg orally daily for 5 years. Patients enrolled in these studies were not permitted to receive other drugs known to affect the skeleton (e.g., IV bisphosphonates, chronic corticosteroids) during the study or for a specified period of time prior to study entry.

In the Z-FAST study, BMD in both the lumbar spine and total hip sites was improved at 61 months for the upfront group but declined in the delayed group in women still remaining in the study at that time (approximately 60% of those initially enrolled), regardless of baseline T-score, clinically important risk factors, or chemotherapy status. A decline in BMD of at least 8% in the lumbar spine in women with a normal BMD at baseline (defined as T-score better than −1 SD from normal) occurred more frequently in those receiving delayed treatment than in those receiving upfront treatment (20 versus 1.7%, respectively, based on intent-to-treat analysis). In women with preexisting mild to moderate osteopenia (i.e., a decline to a T-score between −1 and −2 SD), a BMD decrease of at least 8% in the lumbar spine occurred in 5.7 and 0.3% of patients in the delayed and upfront treatment groups, respectively, based on intent-to-treat analysis. At 61 months, upfront administration of zoledronic acid reduced progression to mild to moderate osteopenia in women with a normal BMD at baseline compared with delayed administration of the drug (2 versus 11%, respectively), and reduced progression to severe osteopenia (i.e., a decline to a T-score below −2 SD) in women with preexisting mild to moderate osteopenia (0 versus 4.9%, respectively). The 2-year fracture rate was similar (4.3 and 4%) for both treatment groups, with an increase at 5 years to 9.3 and 11% in the upfront and delayed groups, respectively. The mean difference in percentage change from baseline BMD for the lumbar spine and total hip sites at 61 months was 8.9 and 6.7%, respectively, between the upfront treatment and delayed treatment groups. At the time of the final analysis at a follow-up of 61 months, 24.6% of the women in the delayed group had begun treatment with zoledronic acid; 66.2% of these women had met protocol-defined criteria to receive zoledronic acid. Bone turnover marker analysis at 61 months revealed lower serum N-telopeptide (NTx) and bone-specific alkaline phosphatase (BSAP) concentrations in the upfront group than those in the delayed group. Renal impairment occurred at a similar rate in both treatment groups; however, potential osteonecrosis of the jaw occurred more frequently in women receiving upfront therapy than in those receiving delayed therapy (2 versus 0 cases).

Data from the ZO-FAST study also demonstrated improvement of BMD in both the lumbar spine and total hip sites at 60 months for the upfront group but BMD declined in the delayed group. Upfront administration of zoledronic acid increased BMD in the lumbar spine by 3.9% in women with a normal BMD at baseline, but a 7.1% decrease occurred in those receiving delayed administration of the drug. Upfront zoledronic acid substantially improved BMD in the lumbar spine by 5.3% compared with delayed administration, which resulted in a 4.2% decrease in women with established (natural) postmenopausal status. In women who were newly (induced) postmenopausal, a decrease of 0.3 or 9.3% in BMD in the lumbar spine was reported in the upfront or delayed treatment groups, respectively. At the time of the final analysis, the mean difference in percentage change from baseline BMD in the lumbar spine and total hip sites was 9.7 and 5.8%, respectively, between the upfront treatment and delayed treatment groups. At the time of the final analysis at a follow-up of 60 months, 27% of the women in the delayed group had met criteria to receive zoledronic acid. Renal impairment occurred at a similar rate in both treatment groups, and 9 potential osteonecrosis of the jaw events were reported in the overall study population.

Data from the E-ZO-FAST study were consistent with the Z-FAST and ZO-FAST studies. Improvement of BMD at both the lumbar spine and total hip sites was observed at 12 months for the upfront group, but BMD declined in the delayed group regardless of baseline T-score, postmenopausal status, or chemotherapy status. At 12 months, 13% of the women in the delayed group had met criteria to receive zoledronic acid. In this study, upfront administration of zoledronic acid reduced progression to osteopenia in women with a normal BMD at baseline compared with delayed administration of the drug (2.1 versus 12.5%, respectively). In women with preexisting osteopenia, improvement to a normal BMD occurred more frequently in women receiving upfront administration of zoledronic acid compared with those receiving delayed administration of the drug (18.3 versus 8%, respectively), and maintenance of a normal BMD in women with a normal BMD at baseline occurred more frequently in those receiving upfront therapy than in those receiving delayed therapy (71.1 versus 57.2%, respectively). The 1-year fracture rate was 0.8 and 1.9% in the upfront and delayed groups, respectively. At 12 months, the mean difference in percentage change from baseline BMD in the lumbar spine and total hip sites was 5.4 and 3.3%, respectively, between the upfront and delayed treatment groups. Among women with established postmenopausal status and those who were recently (induced) menopausal, the percentage change from baseline BMD between the upfront and delayed treatment groups was 5.2 and 6.8%, respectively. Adverse effects generally were similar in both treatment groups, although bone pain (8.3 versus 4.1%), pyrexia (6.7 versus 0%), and influenza-like illness (6 versus 1.1%) occurred more frequently in women in the upfront group compared with those in the delayed group. Osteonecrosis of the jaw occurred in 0.4% of women receiving upfront therapy compared with none of those receiving delayed therapy.

Data from a similarly designed study (NCCTG-N03CC) also demonstrated an improvement in lumbar spine BMD in postmenopausal women treated with letrozole who had received prior tamoxifen therapy and were randomized to receive upfront zoledronic acid therapy. At the time of the final analysis at a follow-up of 60 months, 42% of women initially enrolled in the study were evaluable for the primary BMD end point and 14.7% of women in the delayed group crossed over to receive zoledronic acid. Clinically important lumbar spine bone loss (i.e., BMD decrease of 5% or greater from baseline) occurred more frequently in women receiving delayed therapy compared with those receiving upfront therapy (41.2 versus 10.2%), and clinically important total hip and femoral neck bone loss was reported in 45.8 or 7.6% of those receiving delayed or upfront therapy, respectively; a BMD decrease of 10% from baseline in the lumbar spine occurred in 16.8 and 5.1% of women in the delayed and upfront treatment groups, respectively. The mean difference in BMD for the lumbar spine was 9.4% between the upfront treatment and delayed treatment groups. However, there was no difference between the groups in the 5-year fracture rate. Adverse effects generally were similar between both treatment groups, although pyrexia (9 versus 3%) and elevated serum creatinine concentrations (9 versus 5%) occurred more frequently in women receiving upfront therapy compared with those receiving delayed therapy. Osteonecrosis of the jaw occurred in 2 or 1% of women receiving upfront or delayed therapy, respectively.

Although longer-term follow-up of the 3 companion Zometa-Femara Adjuvant Synergy Trials (Z-FAST, ZO-FAST, E-ZO-FAST) and NCCTG-N03CC study is needed to further clarify between-treatment differences in fracture incidence, upfront administration of zoledronic acid in postmenopausal women receiving aromatase inhibitor therapy significantly prevented lumbar spine and total hip BMD losses compared with those whose therapy was delayed until a decline in T-score to less than −2 SD, nontraumatic fracture, or evidence of an asymptomatic fracture occurred. Based on current evidence, use of zoledronic acid in postmenopausal women receiving aromatase inhibitor therapy may be considered a reasonable choice (accepted, with possible conditions); factors that should be considered when determining the optimal time to initiate therapy are baseline BMD and history of prior fractures.

Prevention in Premenopausal Women Efficacy and safety of zoledronic acid for the prevention of aromatase inhibitor-associated bone loss in premenopausal women receiving adjuvant hormonal therapy plus a gonadotropin-releasing hormone (GnRH, luteinizing hormone-releasing hormone) agonist (e.g., goserelin) for stage I or II estrogen receptor-positive or progesterone receptor-positive breast cancer† were studied in a BMD substudy of a phase 3, open-label, randomized study (Austrian Breast and Colorectal Cancer Study Group-12 [ABCSG-12]). The ABCSG-12 study included premenopausal women with early-stage estrogen receptor-positive and/or progesterone receptor-positive breast cancer. In this substudy, 401 patients were randomized in a 1:1:1:1 ratio to receive hormonal therapy with tamoxifen (20 mg orally daily) or anastrozole (1 mg orally daily) plus a GnRH agonist (goserelin acetate 3.6 mg by subcutaneous injection every 28 days) to induce ovarian suppression with or without zoledronic acid. An initial zoledronic acid dosage of 8 mg IV every 6 months was used; the protocol was subsequently amended to reduce the dosage to 4 mg by IV infusion over 15 minutes every 6 months following reports of increased toxicity (e.g., nephrotoxicity) with the higher dose. Therapy was continued for a duration of 3 years in all treatment groups.

A lower rate of decline in bone loss after 3 years of treatment was reported in those premenopausal women still remaining in the study at that time (about one-third of those initially enrolled) who were receiving zoledronic acid with anastrozole-goserelin or tamoxifen-goserelin compared with those receiving anastrozole-goserelin or tamoxifen-goserelin alone. The incidence of osteopenia at 3 years in the lumbar spine was 44 or 54% in patients receiving zoledronic acid-anastrozole-goserelin or anastrozole-goserelin alone, respectively. Osteoporosis was not reported in patients receiving zoledronic acid-anastrozole-goserelin, but 25% of women receiving anastrozole-goserelin alone became osteoporotic. Two years after the completion of the study treatment, partial improvement in BMD at both the lumbar spine and trochanter sites was observed in those receiving anastrozole-goserelin or tamoxifen-goserelin alone, although BMD had not fully recovered to the baseline measurement; in contrast, an improvement in BMD was reported in those receiving zoledronic acid with anastrozole-goserelin or tamoxifen-goserelin. Although not specific for the anastrozole-goserelin regimen, no fractures were reported in patients receiving zoledronic acid at 5 years; 2 fractures occurred in women receiving anastrozole-goserelin or tamoxifen-goserelin alone.

Improvements in BMD were observed in premenopausal women with early-stage breast cancer when zoledronic acid was administered concurrently with an aromatase inhibitor and GnRH agonist. However, longer-term follow-up of this study is needed, especially as these women enter menopause, to further clarify lasting clinical efficacy (i.e., clinically important fracture reduction) and late adverse effects of zoledronic acid therapy. Based on current evidence, use of zoledronic acid for the prevention of aromatase inhibitor-associated bone loss in premenopausal women is not fully established because of unclear risk/benefit.

■ **Breast Cancer** Efficacy and safety of zoledronic acid in combination with adjuvant systemic therapy in postmenopausal women with early or locally advanced breast cancer† have been studied in 2 open-label, randomized phase 3 studies (Austrian Breast and Colorectal Cancer Study Group-12 [ABCSG-12] and Adjuvant Zoledronic Acid to Reduce Recurrence [AZURE]-BIG 01/04 study), with supportive data from a meta-analysis and 3 open-label, randomized phase 3 studies evaluating the use of zoledronic acid for the prevention of aromatase inhibitor-associated bone loss†.

In the ABCSG-12 study, 1803 premenopausal women with estrogen receptor-positive and/or progesterone receptor-positive stage I or II breast cancer were randomized in a 1:1:1:1 ratio to receive hormonal therapy with tamoxifen (20 mg orally daily) or anastrozole (1 mg orally daily) plus a GnRH agonist (goserelin acetate 3.6 mg by subcutaneous injection every 28 days) to induce ovarian suppression with or without zoledronic acid. An initial zoledronic acid dosage of 8 mg IV every 6 months was used; the protocol was subsequently amended to reduce the dosage to 4 mg by IV infusion over 15 minutes every 6 months following reports of increased toxicity (e.g., nephrotoxicity) with the higher dose. Therapy was continued for a duration of 3 years in all treatment groups. In this study, the primary measure of efficacy was disease-free survival. The median age of patients enrolled in the study was 45 years (range: 25–58); 31% had positive lymph node involvement and 85% did not receive neoadjuvant chemotherapy. All patients enrolled in the study had hormone receptor-positive tumors. At a median follow-up of 62 months, addition of zoledronic acid to hormonal therapy improved the rate of disease-free survival compared with hormonal therapy alone (92 versus 88%; hazard ratio of 0.68). Similar results were observed but predefined statistical significance was not achieved at a median follow-up of 94.4 months. Zoledronic acid administered concurrently with hormonal therapy was associated with numerically, but not significantly, improved overall survival compared with hormonal therapy alone (96.7 versus 94.5%). A subset analysis of disease-free survival and overall survival based on clinically relevant baseline patient and disease characteristics demonstrated consistent treatment benefit with zoledronic acid regardless of lymph node status and disease stage (T1 or T2/3), but no difference in disease-free survival or overall survival was apparent in patients 40 years of age or younger receiving zoledronic acid compared with those receiving hormonal therapy alone. Adverse effects generally were consistent with known safety profiles of each agent, although arthralgia (24 versus 18%), bone pain (35 versus 25%), nausea/vomiting (8.6 versus 6.1%), pyrexia (8.9 versus 2.2%), dermatologic effects (6.5 versus 4.3%), peripheral nerve disease (5.7 versus 3.4%), tachycardia (2.1 versus 0.8%), cognitive disorder (1.4 versus 0.3%), and hypocalcemia (0.4 versus 0%) occurred more frequently in women receiving zoledronic acid concurrently with hormonal therapy compared with those receiving hormonal therapy alone. No confirmed cases of osteonecrosis of the jaw were reported.

In the AZURE-BIG 01/04 study, 3360 patients with stage II or III invasive breast cancer were randomized to receive zoledronic acid in addition to adjuvant antineoplastic therapy (i.e., hormonal therapy, chemotherapy, or both) or adjuvant antineoplastic therapy alone. Patients randomized to receive zoledronic acid received 4 mg by IV infusion every 3–4 weeks for 6 doses, then every 3 months for 8 doses, followed by every 6 months for 5 doses (for a total duration of 5 years). The majority of patients had positive lymph node involvement (98%), 78% had estrogen receptor-positive tumors, 45% were premenopausal, 31% had been postmenopausal for greater than 5 years, and 15% had been postmenopausal for 5 years or less. Most patients (74%) enrolled in the study planned to receive hormonal therapy in combination with chemotherapy. The majority of patients enrolled in the study planned to receive an anthracycline-containing regimen (93%) and 23% planned to receive a taxane-containing regimen. In this study, the primary measure of efficacy was disease-free survival. At median follow-up times of 59 and 84 months, no significant difference in disease-free survival (hazard ratios of 0.98 and 0.94, respectively) or overall survival (hazard ratios of 0.85 and 0.93, respectively) was observed between patients receiving zoledronic acid and antineoplastic therapy and those receiving antineoplastic therapy alone; however, zoledronic acid substantially reduced the incidence of bone fractures and bone metastasis by 31 and 19–22%, respectively, compared with antineoplastic therapy alone. A preplanned subset analysis of invasive disease-free survival based on menopausal status suggested a treatment benefit, primarily a reduction in extraskeletal invasive disease-free events, with the addition of zoledronic acid to antineoplastic therapy in women who had experienced menopause at least 5 years before study entry (hazard ratio of 0.77), but not in women in other menopausal groups (e.g., premenopausal, perimenopausal, unknown menopausal status) (hazard ratio of 1.03). Adverse effects were similar between both treatment groups, although 33 cases (confirmed in 26 cases) of potential osteonecrosis of the jaw occurred in women receiving zoledronic acid plus antineoplastic therapy compared with no cases in those receiving antineoplastic therapy alone.

Use of zoledronic acid in combination with adjuvant endocrine therapy in postmenopausal women also has been evaluated in several phase 3, open-label, randomized bone mineral density (BMD) studies (Z-FAST, ZO-FAST, and E-ZO-FAST). (See Prevention in Postmenopausal Women under Uses: Prevention of Aromatase Inhibitor-associated Bone Loss.) Women enrolled in these studies were postmenopausal with stage I to IIIa estrogen receptor-positive and/or progesterone receptor-positive breast cancer. Patients enrolled in these studies were randomized to receive zoledronic acid as either upfront therapy or delayed therapy (based on decline in BMD). Patients received zoledronic acid 4 mg by IV infusion over 15 minutes every 6 months for 5 years. All patients received letrozole 2.5 mg orally daily for 5 years. In the E-ZO-FAST study at a median follow-up of 12 months, no difference in disease-free survival rate was observed between women receiving upfront or delayed zoledronic acid (97.2 versus 98.1%, respectively). Although no difference in disease-free survival was observed between the 2 treatment groups in the Z-FAST study at a median follow-up of 61 months (absolute difference of 0.7%), upfront administration of zoledronic acid therapy prolonged disease-free survival compared with delayed administration of the drug (hazard ratio of 0.66) in the ZO-FAST study. In the ZO-FAST study, breast cancer-related events in patients receiving upfront administration versus delayed administration of zoledronic acid included locoregional recurrence (0.9 versus 2.3%), distant recurrence (5.5 versus 7.7%), and bone metastases (2.6 versus 4.5%). No difference in overall survival was observed between the 2 treatment groups in the Z-FAST and ZO-FAST studies. At the time of analysis in the Z-FAST, ZO-FAST, and E-ZO-FAST studies, 25, 27, and 13%, respectively, of women in the delayed treatment group had begun treatment with zoledronic acid.

The Early Breast Cancer Trialists' Collaborative Group (EBCTCG) conducted a meta-analysis of individual patient data from 26 randomized clinical trials evaluating addition of bisphosphonate (any drug, dose, and schedule) therapy to standard adjuvant systemic therapy in women with early-stage breast cancer. This meta-analysis indicated that addition of bisphosphonate therapy to standard systemic therapy (median duration of therapy of 3.4 years) modestly reduced the risk of bone recurrence (rate ratio of 0.83) and bone fractures (rate ratio of 0.85) at 10 years compared with standard systemic therapy alone. Addition of bisphosphonate therapy to adjuvant systemic therapy also resulted in small reductions in the risk of recurrence (rate ratio of 0.94, which corresponded to an absolute difference in recurrence rate of 1.1% at 10 years), distant recurrence (rate ratio of 0.92, which corresponded to an absolute difference in rate of distance recurrence of 1.4% at 10 years), and breast cancer mortality (rate ratio 0.91, which corresponded to an absolute difference in breast cancer mortality rate of 1.7% at 10 years). However, consistent with data from the ABCSG-12 and AZURE-BIG 01/04 studies, subset analysis based on menopausal status suggested clinical benefit with adjuvant bisphosphonate therapy in postmenopausal women but not in premenopausal women. In postmenopausal women, the addition of bisphosphonate therapy to adjuvant systemic therapy reduced the risk of bone recurrence (rate ratio of 0.72, which corresponded to an absolute difference in bone recurrence rate of 2.2% at 10 years) and breast cancer mortality (rate ratio of 0.82, which corresponded to an absolute difference in breast cancer mortality rate of 3.3% at 10 years).

Based on current evidence, use of zoledronic acid in combination with adjuvant systemic therapy may be considered a reasonable choice (accepted) in postmenopausal women with early or locally advanced breast cancer. The American Society of Clinical Oncology (ASCO) and Cancer Care Ontario (CCO) state that postmenopausal women who are candidates for adjuvant systemic therapy for the treatment of breast cancer should consider receiving a bisphosphonate (i.e., zoledronic acid) during the course of adjuvant therapy for up to 5 years. Although some clinicians state that any bone-modifying agent that has demonstrated a reduction in the risk of fragility fractures in at-risk populations (e.g., postmenopausal women, drug-induced osteoporosis) may be effective as adjuvant therapy for breast cancer, sufficient data are only available from clinical trials evaluating zoledronic acid or clodronate (not commercially available in the US); additional data are needed to further elucidate clinical benefit of other bone-modifying agents. The optimal time for initiating bisphosphonates is not known; however, bisphosphonate therapy was generally initiated soon after surgery or chemotherapy in most clinical trials. The optimal duration of adjuvant bisphosphonate therapy is not known; however, the duration should not exceed 5 years since toxicity of long-term (e.g., beyond 5 years) use of bisphosphonates, including zoledronic acid, has not been determined. ASCO states that clinicians should consider patient and disease characteristics (e.g., risk of recurrence) and adverse effects when deciding whether bisphosphonate therapy should be added to adjuvant systemic therapy.

Dosage and Administration

■ **General** Hypocalcemia and other disturbances of bone and mineral metabolism must be corrected before zoledronic acid therapy is initiated for the management of osteoporosis or Paget disease.

Renal function should be evaluated (with creatinine clearance or serum creatinine concentrations) prior to each dose of zoledronic acid; more frequent monitoring is recommended in patients at high risk of acute renal failure (e.g., geriatric patients, those receiving diuretic therapy). (See Renal Effects under Cautions: Warnings/Precautions.) Zoledronic acid should not be administered for prevention or treatment of osteoporosis or for treatment of Paget disease of bone in patients who have severe renal impairment (creatinine clearance less than 35 mL/minute) or evidence of acute renal impairment.

■ **Administration** Zoledronic acid is administered by IV infusion over *no less than* 15 minutes. (See Renal Effects under Cautions: Warnings/Precautions.)

Zoledronic acid is commercially available as a *solution concentrate* containing 4 mg of the drug per 5 mL (Zometa® concentrate or generic equivalents) and as a *ready-to-use injection* containing 4 mg of the drug per 100 mL (Zometa® ready-to-use or generic equivalents) for use in patients with cancer-related indications. Zoledronic acid also is available as a *ready-to-use injection* containing 5 mg of the drug per 100 mL (Reclast® or generic equivalents) for use in the prevention or treatment of osteoporosis or for treatment of Paget disease of bone.

Zoledronic acid should be administered through separate vented infusion lines apart from other drugs and should not be allowed to come in contact with any solutions containing calcium or other divalent cations.

Zoledronic Acid for Cancer-related Indications *The concentrated zoledronic acid solution (Zometa® concentrate or generic equivalents) must be diluted in 100 mL of 0.9% sodium chloride or 5% dextrose injection prior to IV administration.* The commercially available 5-mL vial of injection concentrate is formulated to provide the full labeled dose of zoledronic acid (4 mg) when diluted as directed for patients with normal renal function (baseline creatinine clearance exceeding 60 mL/minute). For preparation of reduced doses in patients with mild to moderate renal impairment (baseline creatinine clearance of 30–60 mL/minute), the appropriate volume of drug concentrate should be withdrawn from the vial and *further diluted* as directed. For patients with a baseline creatinine clearance of 50–60 mL/minute, 4.4 mL of the concentrated drug solution should be withdrawn from the 5-mL vial to obtain a dose of 3.5 mg (for subsequent dilution). For patients with a baseline creatinine clearance of 40–49 mL/minute, 4.1 mL of the concentrated drug solution should be withdrawn to obtain a dose of 3.3 mg (for subsequent dilution). For patients with a baseline creatinine clearance of 30–39 mL/minute, 3.8 mL of the concentrated drug solution should be withdrawn to obtain a dose of 3 mg (for subsequent dilution). The withdrawn amount of drug concentrate should then be diluted in 100 mL of 0.9% sodium chloride or 5% dextrose injection. (See Bone Metastases of Solid Tumors and Osteolytic Lesions of Multiple Myeloma under Dosage and Administration: Dosage.) *To avoid inadvertent injection of the concentrated solution, the undiluted drug concentrate should not be stored in a syringe.*

The ready-to-use 4-mg/100-mL formulation of zoledronic acid (Zometa® ready-to-use or generic equivalents) may be administered directly without further dilution in patients with normal renal function (baseline creatinine clearance greater than 60 mL/minute). For preparation of reduced doses of the drug for patients with mild to moderate renal impairment (baseline creatinine clearance of 30–60 mL/minute), the appropriate volume of the drug solution should be withdrawn from the 100-mL bottle and replaced with an equal volume of 0.9% sodium chloride or 5% dextrose injection. For patients with a baseline creatinine clearance of 50–60 mL/minute, 12 mL of the drug solution should be withdrawn from the 100-mL bottle (and replaced with 12 mL of 0.9% sodium chloride or 5% dextrose injection) to obtain the recommended dose of 3.5 mg. For patients with a baseline creatinine clearance of 40–49 mL/minute, 18 mL of the drug solution should be withdrawn (and replaced with 18 mL of 0.9% sodium chloride or 5% dextrose injection) to obtain the recommended dose of 3.3 mg. For patients with a baseline creatinine clearance of 30–39 mL/minute, 25 mL of the drug solution should be withdrawn (and replaced with 25 mL of 0.9% sodium chloride or 5% dextrose injection) to obtain the recommended dose of 3 mg.

Zoledronic acid should *not* be mixed or diluted with calcium-containing solutions (e.g., lactated Ringer's solution).

Strict adherence to administration recommendations for diluted zoledronic acid concentrate (Zometa® concentrate or generic equivalents) is important, since smaller infusion volumes (e.g., 50 mL) and rapid (over 5 minutes) IV infusion rates have been associated with an increased risk of renal impairment, which may progress to renal failure.

Prior to initiating zoledronic acid therapy in the treatment of malignancy-associated hypercalcemia, it is important to establish adequate hydration and urinary output in order to increase renal excretion of calcium; adequate hydration should be maintained throughout therapy with the drug. Overhydration should be avoided, especially in those with heart failure. An attempt should be made to achieve and maintain a urinary output of 2 L per day throughout therapy with zoledronic acid.

Zoledronic Acid for Osteoporosis and Paget Disease of Bone To minimize risk of renal toxicity, patients receiving zoledronic acid for prevention or treatment of osteoporosis or for treatment of Paget disease of bone must be appropriately hydrated prior to administration of the drug. Zoledronic acid therapy should be withheld in such patients with evidence of dehydration and may be resumed once normovolemic status has been achieved. Each dose of zoledronic acid should be followed by a flush with 10 mL of 0.9% sodium chloride.

Administration of acetaminophen following zoledronic acid administration may reduce the incidence of acute-phase inflammatory reactions (e.g., fever, myalgia, flu-like symptoms, headache, arthralgia).

■ **Dosage** Dosage of zoledronic acid, which is commercially available for parenteral use as the monohydrate, is calculated on the anhydrous basis.

Hypercalcemia Associated with Malignancy For the treatment of hypercalcemia (albumin-corrected serum calcium concentration of at least 12 mg/dL) associated with malignancy in adults, the manufacturer recommends that zoledronic acid (Zometa®) be infused IV as a single dose of 4 mg over no less than 15 minutes.

Single doses of the drug should not exceed 4 mg since renal impairment, which may progress to renal failure has occurred following administration of zoledronic acid in recommended or higher than recommended dosages.

After a post-treatment observation period of at least 7 days, a second course of zoledronic acid *at the same dosage* may be considered if there is evidence of recurrence of the disease process or if the initial treatment fails to normalize serum calcium concentrations. If patients with hypercalcemia of malignancy experience a deterioration of renal function during therapy with zoledronic acid, the possible risk of renal failure with subsequent doses of the drug must be carefully weighed against the potential benefits of treatment. No data are available to date on the safety and efficacy of more than one course of retreatment with zoledronic acid or of the recommended retreatment dosage of 4 mg of zoledronic acid in patients with hypercalcemia of malignancy.

Bone Metastases of Solid Tumors and Osteolytic Lesions of Multiple Myeloma For the treatment of bone metastases associated with solid tumors or the treatment of osteolytic lesions associated with multiple myeloma in adults, the manufacturer-recommended dosage of zoledronic acid is 4 mg given IV over no less than 15 minutes once every 3–4 weeks. Single doses of the drug should not exceed 4 mg since renal impairment, which may progress to renal failure has occurred following administration of zoledronic acid in recommended or higher than recommended dosages. The optimum duration of such therapy is not known.

In patients with bone metastases of solid tumors and osteolytic lesions of multiple myeloma and mild to moderate renal impairment (baseline creatinine clearance of 30–60 mL/minute), lower initial dosages of zoledronic acid are recommended. The following dosages are recommended:

Table 1. Initial Dosage of Zoledronic Acid in Adults with Bone Metastases of Solid Tumors and Osteolytic Lesions of Multiple Myeloma Based on Renal Function

Calculated Creatinine Clearance (mL/minute)	IV Dosage (Infused over no less than 15 minutes)
>60	4 mg every 3–4 weeks
50–60	3.5 mg every 3–4 weeks
40–49	3.3 mg every 3–4 weeks
30–39	3 mg every 3–4 weeks

If patients with bone metastases associated with solid tumors or with osteolytic lesions associated with multiple myeloma experience a deterioration of renal function during therapy with zoledronic acid (defined as an increase in serum creatinine concentration of at least 0.5 or 1 mg/dL, respectively, in patients with normal [less than 1.4 mg/dL] or elevated [1.4 mg/dL or greater] baseline serum creatinine concentrations), the drug should be withheld until serum creatinine concentrations return to within 10% of baseline concentrations. Zoledronic acid should be reinitiated at the same dosage that was used prior to the treatment interruption. Studies in this patient population included individuals with serum creatinine concentrations up to 3 mg/dL.

Patients with multiple myeloma or bone metastases associated with solid tumors who are receiving zoledronic acid therapy should receive supplemental therapy with oral calcium (500 mg of elemental calcium daily) and a multivitamin containing vitamin D (400 international units [IU, units] daily).

Osteoporosis in Postmenopausal Women For *prevention* of osteoporosis in postmenopausal women, the recommended dosage of zoledronic acid is 5 mg by IV infusion over no less than 15 minutes every 2 years in patients with a creatinine clearance of at least 35 mL/minute. (See Renal Impairment under Warnings/Precautions: Specific Populations, in Cautions.) Patients must receive supplemental calcium and vitamin D if dietary intake is inadequate; postmenopausal women generally require at least 800–1000 units of vitamin D and 1.2 g of calcium daily.

For *treatment* of osteoporosis in postmenopausal women, the manufacturer recommends that zoledronic acid be infused IV as a single 5-mg dose over no less than 15 minutes once yearly in patients with a creatinine clearance of at least 35 mL/minute. (See Renal Impairment under Warnings/Precautions: Specific Populations, in Cautions.) For treatment of osteoporosis and to reduce the risk of hypocalcemia, patients must receive supplemental calcium and vitamin D if dietary intake is inadequate; generally, women older than 50 years of age require 800–1000 units of vitamin D daily and at least 1.2 g of elemental calcium daily.

The optimal duration of bisphosphonate treatment for osteoporosis has not been established. Safety and efficacy of zoledronic acid for the treatment of osteoporosis is based on clinical data supporting fracture reduction over 3 years of treatment. Some evidence suggests that increased durations of bisphosphonate use may be associated with an increased risk of some adverse effects (e.g., atypical fractures, jaw osteonecrosis). All patients receiving a bisphosphonate should have periodic evaluations to determine the need for continued therapy with the drug. Discontinuance of bisphosphonate therapy may be considered after 3–5 years of use for patients who are assessed to be at low risk of fracture. Patients who discontinue therapy should have their risk for fracture evaluated periodically.

Osteoporosis in Men For the treatment of osteoporosis or osteoporosis secondary to hypogonadism in men, the manufacturer recommends that zoledronic acid be infused IV as a single 5-mg dose over no less than 15 minutes once yearly in patients with a creatinine clearance of at least 35 mL/minute. (See Renal Impairment under Warnings/Precautions: Specific Populations, in Cautions.) For treatment of osteoporosis and to reduce the risk of hypocalcemia, patients must receive supplemental calcium and vitamin D if dietary intake is inadequate; generally, 800–1000 units of vitamin D daily and at least 1.2 g of elemental calcium daily is recommended.

The optimal duration of bisphosphonate treatment for osteoporosis has not been established. Some evidence suggests that bisphosphonate therapy for more than 3 years (median 7 years in one analysis of available data) in patients with osteoporosis may be associated with an increased risk of atypical fracture of the femur. (See Atypical Fracture of the Femur under Cautions: Warnings/Precautions.) All patients receiving a bisphosphonate should have periodic evaluations to determine the need for continued therapy with the drug.

Glucocorticoid-induced Osteoporosis For the treatment or prevention of glucocorticoid-induced osteoporosis, the manufacturer recommends that zoledronic acid be infused IV as a single 5-mg dose over no less than 15 minutes once yearly in patients with a creatinine clearance of at least 35 mL/minute. (See Renal Impairment under Warnings/Precautions: Specific Populations, in Cautions.) Patients must receive supplemental calcium and vitamin D if dietary intake is inadequate; an average of at least 800–1000 units of vitamin D and 1.2 g of calcium daily is recommended.

Paget Disease of Bone For the treatment of Paget disease of bone, the initial adult dosage of zoledronic acid is 5 mg, infused IV over at least 15 minutes, in patients with a creatinine clearance of at least 35 mL/minute. (See Renal Impairment under Warnings/Precautions: Specific Populations, in Cautions.) Retreatment with zoledronic acid may be considered if relapse occurs based on increases in serum alkaline phosphatase, if initial treatment failed to normalize serum alkaline phosphatase concentrations, or if the patient is symptomatic, according to current standards of medical care. However, no data are available to date on the safety and efficacy of more than one course of treatment with zoledronic acid in patients with Paget disease of bone. To reduce the risk for hypocalcemia, all patients with Paget disease of bone should receive 1.5 g of elemental calcium daily in divided doses (750 mg twice daily or 500 mg 3 times daily) and 800 units of vitamin D daily, particularly in the first 2 weeks following zoledronic acid administration.

Prevention of Aromatase Inhibitor-associated Bone Loss in Postmenopausal Women When zoledronic acid has been used for prevention of bone loss associated with use of aromatase inhibitor therapy in postmenopausal women†, zoledronic acid 4 mg has been administered by IV infusion over 15 minutes every 6 months for 5 years. In clinical trials, patients were encouraged to take supplemental oral calcium (500 mg to 1.2 g daily) and vitamin D (400–800 units daily). (See Prevention in Postmenopausal Women under Uses: Prevention of Aromatase Inhibitor-associated Bone Loss.)

Adjuvant Therapy for Early or Locally Advanced Breast Cancer When zoledronic acid has been used in combination with adjuvant systemic therapy in postmenopausal women with early or locally advanced breast cancer†, zoledronic acid 4 mg has been administered by IV infusion over 15 minutes every 6 months for 3–5 years. In clinical trials, patients were encouraged to take supplemental oral calcium (400 mg to 1.2 g daily) and vitamin D (200–800 units daily). (See Uses: Breast Cancer.)

■ **Special Populations** The manufacturer states that dosage adjustments of zoledronic acid are not necessary in patients with hypercalcemia of malignancy who have mild to moderate renal impairment (serum creatinine concentrations less than 4.5 mg/dL) prior to initiation of therapy.

In patients with bone metastases of solid tumors and osteolytic lesions of multiple myeloma and mild to moderate renal impairment (baseline creatinine clearance of 30–60 mL/minute), lower initial dosages of zoledronic acid are recommended. (See Bone Metastases of Solid Tumors and Osteolytic Lesions of Multiple Myeloma under Dosage and Administration: Dosage.)

The manufacturer states that dosage adjustments of zoledronic acid are not necessary in patients receiving the drug for prevention or treatment of osteoporosis or for treatment of Paget's disease of bone who have a creatinine clearance of 35 mL/minute or greater.

Cautions

■ **Contraindications** Known hypersensitivity to zoledronic acid, other bisphosphonates, or any ingredient in the formulations.

Hypocalcemia.

Use of zoledronic acid for prevention or treatment of osteoporosis or for treatment of Paget disease of bone is contraindicated in patients with creatinine clearance of less than 35 mL/minute or those with evidence of acute renal impairment.

■ **Warnings/Precautions** ***Osteonecrosis of the Jaw*** Osteonecrosis and osteomyelitis of the jaw have been reported in patients receiving bisphosphonates. Most of these patients had neoplasms and were receiving IV bisphosphonates and concurrent chemotherapy, head and neck radiation therapy, or corticosteroids, and most cases have been associated with dental procedures such as tooth extraction. Some cases also have occurred in patients with postmenopausal osteoporosis treated with oral or IV bisphosphonate therapy. Other risk factors for the development of osteonecrosis of the jaw may include coexisting infection(s), anemia, coagulation disorders, preexisting oral disease, and/or trauma. Risk also may be increased with increased duration of bisphosphonate use.

A dental examination (panoramic jaw radiograph) to detect dental and periodontal infections with appropriate preventive dentistry (e.g., removal of abscessed and nonrestorable teeth and involved periodontal tissues, rehabilitation of salvageable dentition, dental prophylaxis, caries control, restorative dental care) should be considered prior to treatment with bisphosphonates in patients with risk factors (e.g. cancer; concomitant chemotherapy, corticosteroids, angiogenesis inhibitors, or radiation therapy; poor oral hygiene). Follow-up hard and soft tissue oral assessment should be performed every 3–4 months, depending on risk, and oncologists should briefly inspect the oral cavity of prospective candidates for bisphosphonate therapy at baseline and at every follow-up visit. If bisphosphonate therapy can be briefly delayed without risk of a skeletal-related complication, teeth with a poor prognosis should be extracted and other dental surgeries should be completed prior to initiation of bisphosphonate therapy. The benefit or risk of withholding bisphosphonate therapy in cancer patients requiring dental surgery has not been evaluated to date. The decision to withhold bisphosphonate therapy in such patients must be made by an oncologist in consultation with an oral maxillofacial surgeon or another dental specialist. During treatment with bisphosphonates in cancer patients with risk factors for osteonecrosis, dentists should check and adjust removable dentures for potential soft-tissue injury, especially tissue overlying bone. Such patients should avoid invasive dental procedures if possible during treatment with bisphosphonates, as dental surgery may exacerbate the condition. In patients requiring dental procedures during bisphosphonate treatment or patients with established osteonecrosis, no data are available to suggest whether discontinuance of therapy reduces the risk of osteonecrosis of the jaw or disease progression, respectively. Management of patients requiring dental treatment should be based on an individual assessment of risks and benefits. Dental infections should be managed aggressively nonsurgically with root canal treatment if possible or with minimal surgical intervention.

In patients with established osteonecrosis requiring dental surgery, cessation or interruption of therapy may be considered taking into account the potential risk of further osteonecrosis versus the risk of skeletal complication or hypercalcemia of malignancy. The decision to withdraw bisphosphonate therapy may be coordinated between the oncologist and an oral surgeon.

Atypical Fracture of the Femur Findings from several case reports and case series suggest that therapy with bisphosphonates, particularly when used for more than 3 years (median 7 years in this analysis), may be associated with an increased risk of atypical fractures of the femur. The magnitude of this risk with bisphosphonate therapy is unclear, although such fractures appear to be rare; in addition, causality has not been established since atypical fractures also have occurred in patients not receiving bisphosphonates. Most cases of atypical femoral fractures with bisphosphonate therapy have been reported in individuals receiving treatment for osteoporosis.

Atypical femoral fractures represent a subset of femoral fractures occurring in the subtrochanteric region (i.e. below the lesser trochanter) or femoral diaphysis (or shaft) of the femur, which are *not* common sites associated with osteoporosis-related hip fractures. Such fractures often occur with minimal or no trauma, are referred to as low-energy or low-trauma fractures (i.e., equivalent to a fall from a standing height or less), and may be associated with activities of normal daily living. Radiographically, these fractures have unique characteristics described as a transverse or short oblique configuration and often lack evidence of comminution; both complete (extension through both cortices) and incomplete (involving only the lateral cortex) fractures have been reported with bisphosphonate therapy.

The pathophysiology of bisphosphonate-associated atypical femoral fractures is not fully known; however, severely suppressive (or oversuppressive) effects on both bone turnover and bone remodeling, leading to accumulation of localized microdamage and a subsequent impairment in bone repair have been proposed as possible mechanisms. Reports of atypical fractures in the general population and in individuals receiving bisphosphonate therapy are rare, accounting for less than 1% of all reported hip and femur fractures.

In a report published by the Task Force of the American Society for Bone and Mineral Research (ASBMR), 310 cases of bisphosphonate-associated atypical femoral fractures were identified through case reports/series; the majority (286 of 310) of reported cases involved the use of bisphosphonate therapy for an osteoporosis-related condition. The age range of individuals was 36–92 years; the median duration of bisphosphonate therapy at the time of fracture was 7 years (range: 1.3–17 years). Most individuals, including 70% of cases reported in the ASBMR analysis, reported prodromal symptoms presenting as a dull, aching thigh pain, weeks to months prior to occurrence of an atypical fracture. Bilateral involvement, either as a confirmed fracture (i.e., a simultaneous or sequential fracture) or the presence of a radiographic change in the contralateral limb, also may be present at the time of diagnosis of an atypical femoral fracture and was reported in 28% (60 of 215) of cases in the ASBMR analysis. Delayed healing of the fracture site, possibly related to suppressive effects on bone turnover associated with bisphosphonate therapy, has been described with atypical femoral fractures and was reported in 26% (29 of 112) of cases in the ASBMR analysis. Concomitant use of glucocorticoid, estrogen, and proton-pump inhibitor therapy may increase the risk of an atypical fracture. In the ASBMR analysis, 34% of cases occurred in individuals receiving concomitant glucocorticoids (i.e., prednisone) at the time of fracture; in one series, the risk of subtrochanteric fracture was increased in individuals receiving concomitant bisphosphonate and glucocorticoid therapy. Use of concomitant proton-pump inhibitor therapy was reported in 39% of evaluable cases. Vitamin D deficiency, defined as a serum 25-hydroxyvitamin D (25-OHD) concentration of 20 ng/mL or less, also has been identified as a risk factor in some patients experiencing a bisphosphonate-related fracture.

The safety and efficacy of zoledronic acid for the treatment of osteoporosis are based on clinical data supporting fracture reduction over 3 years of treatment. The optimal duration of bisphosphonate treatment for osteoporosis has not been established. The US Food and Drug Administration (FDA) is continuing to collect data on the safety and efficacy of long-term bisphosphonate use (i.e., greater than 3 to 5 years) when used for the prevention and treatment of osteoporosis. FDA and some experts recommend reevaluation of the need for continued bisphosphonate therapy in individuals receiving treatment for 5 years or longer, taking into consideration bone mineral density (particularly in the hip region), fracture history, and possible risk factors (i.e., a co-morbid condition and/or use of concomitant drugs known to adversely affect bone integrity); some experts recommend an annual evaluation in such patients. Because atypical fractures also have been reported in some individuals receiving bisphosphonate therapy in combination with other drugs known to affect bone integrity and/or bone remodeling (i.e., glucocorticoids, proton pump inhibitors, estrogen, tamoxifen), some experts recommend performing a risk-benefit assessment in individuals determined to have a low or slightly elevated fracture risk, to determine the need for continued bisphosphonate therapy in light of the potential increased risk associated with the use of required concomitant therapy.

Individuals with a history of bisphosphonate exposure presenting with new thigh or groin pain should be evaluated for possible atypical femur fracture; an assessment of the contralateral limb also should be performed to rule out possible bilateral involvement (i.e., presence of a radiographic change or fracture). Interruption of bisphosphonate therapy should be considered in individuals presenting with symptoms suggestive of a possible femoral fracture following completion of a comprehensive risk-benefit assessment performed on an individualized basis. Bisphosphonate therapy should be *discontinued* if a femoral shaft fracture is confirmed.

Musculoskeletal Pain Severe, occasionally incapacitating bone, joint, and/or muscle pain have been reported infrequently through postmarketing experience in patients receiving bisphosphonates, including zoledronic acid. The time to the onset of symptoms varied from 1 day to years after treatment initiation. Musculoskeletal pain has improved following discontinuance of the drug in some patients, whereas other patients have reported slow or incomplete resolution of such pain. In some patients, musculoskeletal pain recurred upon subsequent rechallenge with the same drug or another bisphosphonate. The risk factors for and incidence of severe musculoskeletal pain associated with bisphosphonates are unknown. The association between bisphosphonates and severe musculoskeletal pain may be overlooked by clinicians, which may delay diagnosis, prolong pain and/or impairment, and necessitate the use of analgesics. Clinicians should evaluate whether bisphosphonate use might be responsible for severe musculoskeletal pain in patients who present with these symptoms; temporary or permanent discontinuance of therapy should be considered in such cases.

Fetal/Neonatal Morbidity and Mortality Although no data are available on the fetal risk of bisphosphonates in humans, these drugs do cause fetal harm in animals. Data from animals suggest that uptake of bisphosphonates into fetal bone is greater than that into maternal bone. A theoretical risk to the fetus (e.g., skeletal and other abnormalities) exists if a woman becomes pregnant after completing a course of bisphosphonate therapy. The impact of variables such as time between cessation of bisphosphonate therapy to conception, the particular bisphosphonate used, and the route of administration (IV versus oral) on this risk has not been established.

Renal Effects Bisphosphonates, including zoledronic acid, have been associated with renal toxicity, manifested as deterioration of renal function and potential renal failure. Acute renal failure requiring dialysis and sometimes resulting in hospitalization and/or death, has occurred rarely in patients receiving zoledronic acid (Reclast®), mostly for osteoporosis indications. At least 24 cases of renal impairment and acute renal failure were identified in an FDA postmarketing safety review of Reclast® in 2009; 7 deaths were reported. Since the initial safety review, additional reports of renal toxicity associated with the use of Reclast® have been received by the FDA. The time to onset of renal toxicity was approximately 11 days following infusion of the drug. More than half of the patients in these reports also experienced a transient increase in serum creatinine concentrations following infusion of zoledronic acid; the median increase in serum creatinine concentration was 4 mg/dL. Many of the patients had underlying renal disease or other risk factors (e.g., dehydration, advanced age, concomitant use of nephrotoxic agents) that may have contributed to their risk of renal impairment. Renal function deterioration progressing to renal failure and dialysis also has been observed in clinical trials and during postmarketing experience in patients receiving Zometa®. Such renal function deterioration has occurred following administration of higher than recommended doses, but also after administration of the usual dose of 4 mg infused over the recommended infusion period (15 minutes). In some cases, renal impairment occurred after administration of the initial zoledronic acid dose.

Renal function should be evaluated (with creatinine clearance or serum creatinine concentrations) prior to administering each dose of zoledronic acid and more frequently in patients at high risk of acute renal failure, including geriatric patients and those receiving diuretic therapy. Interim monitoring of renal function also should be considered in patients receiving concomitant drugs (e.g., digoxin) that are primarily eliminated by the kidneys. (See Drug Interactions: Drugs Eliminated by Renal Excretion.) Use of zoledronic acid for prevention or treatment of osteoporosis or for treatment of Paget disease of bone is contraindicated in patients with creatinine clearance less than 35 mL/minute and in those with evidence of acute renal impairment; the drug should be used with caution in patients with chronic renal impairment. Risk factors predisposing patients to renal deterioration, such as dehydration (e.g., secondary to fever, sepsis, GI loss, or diuretic therapy) or use of other nephrotoxic agents, should be identified and managed. To help prevent renal impairment, patients should be appropriately hydrated prior to administration of zoledronic acid, especially geriatric patients and those receiving concomitant diuretic therapy. Transient increases in serum creatinine concentrations during therapy may be corrected with administration of IV fluids.

Administration of zoledronic acid 4 mg by IV infusion over a period of 5 minutes has been shown to increase the risk of renal toxicity (i.e., increases in serum creatinine), which can progress to renal failure. The incidence of renal toxicity and renal failure is reduced when the same dose is administered IV over a period of 15 minutes. *Zoledronic acid should be administered by IV infusion over no less than 15 minutes.* (See Dosage and Administration: Administration.)

Metabolic Effects Hypocalcemia and other factors affecting bone and mineral metabolism (e.g., hypoparathyroidism, thyroid surgery, parathyroid surgery, malabsorption syndromes, excision of small intestine) must be corrected before zoledronic acid therapy is initiated in patients with Paget's disease of bone or postmenopausal osteoporosis. Serum calcium, phosphorus, and magnesium concentrations should be monitored in such patients. Standard hypercalcemia-related metabolic parameters, including serum concentrations of calcium, phosphate, magnesium, potassium, and other electrolytes, should be monitored carefully following initiation of zoledronic acid therapy in patients with hypercalcemia of malignancy. If hypocalcemia, hypophosphatemia, or hypomagnesemia occurs, short-term supplemental therapy may be necessary.

Respiratory Effects Bisphosphonates have been associated with bronchoconstriction in aspirin-sensitive asthmatic patients. Zoledronic acid should be used with caution in such patients.

Atrial Fibrillation While data are conflicting, a possible increased risk of atrial fibrillation has been identified with use of bisphosphonates. In 1 of the 2 pivotal preapproval studies in women with postmenopausal osteoporosis, an increased incidence of serious (i.e., events resulting in hospitalization or disability or considered life-threatening) atrial fibrillation was observed in patients receiving zoledronic acid compared with that in placebo recipients. Most of these cases occurred more than 1 month after infusion of zoledronic acid. However, an increased incidence of serious atrial fibrillation with zoledronic acid was not confirmed in a second preapproval study in women with osteoporosis or in a study in men with osteoporosis. Among patients with postmenopausal osteoporosis with or without vertebral fractures who received alendronate, another bisphosphonate drug, in 2 randomized, placebo-controlled trials, the incidence of atrial fibrillation was numerically higher in the alendronate-treated groups compared with that observed in the placebo-treated groups.

To further evaluate the potential for increased risk of atrial fibrillation with certain bisphosphonates, the FDA reviewed data from long-term (6 months' to 3 years' duration) placebo-controlled clinical trials from the sponsors of alendronate, ibandronate, risedronate, and zoledronic acid. Analysis of data from approximately 19,700 patients receiving bisphosphonates and approximately 18,300 patients receiving placebo indicated a difference in event rates of 0–3 events per 1000 patients between bisphosphonates and placebo. The occurrence of atrial fibrillation was rare in each study; 2 or fewer instances of atrial fibrillation occurred in most studies. Across all studies reviewed, no clear association was observed between overall bisphosphonate exposure, dosage, or duration of bisphosphonate therapy and the rate of atrial fibrillation. FDA is continuing to monitor postmarketing adverse event reports of atrial fibrillation and is exploring the feasibility of conducting additional epidemiologic studies to examine the incidence and clinical course of atrial fibrillation in patients exposed to bisphosphonates.

Formulation Considerations Patients receiving Zometa® should not receive Reclast® or other bisphosphonates, nor should patients receiving Reclast® be treated concomitantly with Zometa® or other bisphosphonates.

Specific Populations **Pregnancy.** Category D. (See Users Guide and see Fetal/Neonatal Morbidity and Mortality under Cautions: Warnings/Precautions.)

Lactation. It is not known whether zoledronic acid is distributed into milk; because of the potential for serious adverse effects in nursing infants from zoledronic acid, a decision should be made whether to discontinue nursing or the drug, taking into account the importance of the drug to the woman. It is also important to consider that zoledronic acid is retained by bone for prolonged periods and may be released over weeks to years, possibly affecting nursing infants.

Pediatric Use. Zoledronic acid is not indicated for use in children.

Geriatric Use. No overall differences in safety and efficacy of zoledronic acid relative to younger adults; however, the incidence of acute-phase inflammatory reactions was less in geriatric patients with osteoporosis or Paget disease of bone than in younger adults. Because of the greater frequency of impaired renal function in geriatric patients, the manufacturer states that renal function should be monitored with particular care in this age group.

Renal Impairment. In clinical studies of zoledronic acid in patients with multiple myeloma or bone metastases associated with solid tumors or in those with hypercalcemia associated with malignancy, individuals with severe renal impairment (serum creatinine concentrations exceeding 3 or 4.5 mg/dL, respectively) were excluded. Limited data are available in patients with a baseline serum creatinine concentration exceeding 2 mg/dL or with a creatinine clearance of less than 30 mL/minute. The drug should be used in patients with hypercalcemia of malignancy and severe renal impairment only after consideration of other treatment options and only when the potential benefit from the drug outweighs the possible risk of worsening renal function. Zoledronic acid is not recommended in patients with bone metastases associated with solid tumors or multiple myeloma and severe renal impairment. Use of zoledronic acid for prevention or treatment of osteoporosis or for treatment of Paget disease of bone is contraindicated in patients who have severe renal impairment (creatinine clearance of less than 35 mL/minute); the drug should be used with caution in such patients with chronic renal impairment.

■ Common Adverse Effects

Hypercalcemia of Malignancy Fever, nausea, constipation, anemia, dyspnea, diarrhea, progression of cancer, abdominal pain, insomnia, vomiting, urinary tract infection, anxiety, hypophosphatemia, confusion, agitation, moniliasis, hypokalemia, skeletal pain, cough, hypotension, hypomagnesemia.

Bone Metastases of Solid Tumors and Osteolytic Lesions of Multiple Myeloma Nausea, fatigue, anemia, vomiting, fever, constipation, dyspnea, diarrhea, myalgia, cough, edema of the lower extremities, arthralgia, headache, dizziness, weight loss, paresthesia, back pain, depression, abdominal pain, dehydration, limb pain, decreased appetite, neutropenia, urinary tract infection, hypoesthesia, anxiety, alopecia, dermatitis, rigors, thrombocytopenia, dyspepsia, upper respiratory tract infection.

Osteoporosis Treatment in Postmenopausal Women Arthralgia, fever, headache, hypertension, myalgia, extremity pain, flu-like illness, dizziness, shoulder pain, diarrhea, bone pain, fatigue, chills, asthenia.

Osteoporosis Prevention in Postmenopausal Women Headache, dizziness, hypoesthesia, hypertension, nausea, diarrhea, vomiting, dyspepsia, abdominal pain, constipation, arthralgia, myalgia, back pain, extremity pain, muscle spasms, musculoskeletal pain, bone pain, neck pain, generalized pain, pyrexia, chills fatigue, asthenia, peripheral edema, non-cardiac chest pain.

Osteoporosis Treatment in Men Myalgia, fatigue, headache, musculoskeletal pain, pain (unspecified), chills, flu-like illness, abdominal pain, malaise, dyspnea.

Glucocorticoid-induced Osteoporosis Adverse effects are generally similar to those reported in the postmenopausal osteoporosis population. Common adverse effects that were either not observed in the postmenopausal osteoporosis treatment trial or reported more frequently in the corticosteroid-induced osteoporosis trial included abdominal pain, musculoskeletal pain, back pain, bone pain, extremity pain, nausea, and dyspepsia.

Paget Disease of Bone Headache, nausea, dizziness, arthralgia, bone pain, influenza/flu-like illness, fever, fatigue, rigors, myalgia, diarrhea, constipation, lethargy, dypsnea, dyspepsia, pain.

Drug Interactions

■ Drugs Eliminated by Renal Excretion

When zoledronic acid is used concomitantly with drugs eliminated renally (e.g., digoxin), increased exposure of the concomitantly administered drug is possible.

■ Loop Diuretics

Pharmacologic interaction (increased risk of hypocalcemia) is possible when zoledronic acid is used with loop diuretics. Caution is advised.

■ Aminoglycosides

Pharmacologic interaction (additive effect in lowering serum calcium concentrations for prolonged periods) is possible when zoledronic acid is used with aminoglycosides. Caution is advised.

■ Nephrotoxic Agents

Pharmacologic interaction (increased risk of renal dysfunction) is possible when zoledronic acid is used with nephrotoxic agents. The drugs should be used concomitantly with caution.

■ Thalidomide

No substantial changes in pharmacokinetics of zoledronic acid or in creatinine clearance were observed with concomitant administration of thalidomide. Dosage adjustments are not necessary.

Description

Zoledronic acid, a synthetic imidazole bisphosphonate analog of pyrophosphate, is an inhibitor of osteoclast-mediated bone resorption. Zoledronic acid is structurally and pharmacologically related to alendronate, risedronate, and pamidronate.

Zoledronic acid inhibits increased osteoclastic activity and skeletal calcium release induced by tumors. In patients with hypercalcemia of malignancy, zoledronic acid decreases serum calcium and phosphorus and increases urinary calcium and phosphorus excretion.

Zoledronic acid is eliminated in urine as unchanged drug. In patients with cancer and bone metastases, an average of 39% of an IV dose of zoledronic acid was excreted in urine within 24 hours. Nonrenal clearance is believed to result from uptake of the drug by bone; subsequently, the drug is released systemically via bone turnover. Results of in vitro studies indicate that zoledronic acid does not inhibit the cytochrome P-450 (CYP) enzyme system.

Advice to Patients

Importance of calcium and vitamin D supplementation for maintenance of serum calcium concentrations in patients with Paget's disease of bone, multiple myeloma and bone metastasis of solid tumors, or osteoporosis. Importance of contacting a clinician promptly if symptoms of hypocalcemia (e.g., numbness or tingling feeling [especially in or around the mouth], muscle spasms) occur.

Importance of informing a clinician if severe bone pain, joint pain, muscular pain, or jaw disease develops.

Importance of informing a clinician if new thigh or groin pain develops.

Importance of informing patients that zoledronic acid should not be used for prevention or treatment of osteoporosis or for treatment of Paget's disease of bone in patients with severe renal impairment. Patients should be advised of the importance of monitoring kidney function during therapy.

Importance of informing clinicians of existing or contemplated concomitant therapy, including prescription and OTC drugs (e.g., diuretics, nonsteroidal anti-inflammatory agents, antibiotics), as well as any concomitant conditions (e.g., kidney disease, aspirin sensitivity). Importance of women informing clinicians if they are or plan to become pregnant or plan to breast-feed. Advise women of childbearing potential to avoid pregnancy. Apprise pregnant patients of potential fetal hazard. Importance of advising patients of other important precautionary information. (See Cautions.)

Overview® (see Users Guide.). For additional information on this drug until a more detailed monograph is developed and published, the manufacturer's labeling should be consulted. It is *essential* that the manufacturer's labeling be consulted for more detailed information on usual cautions, precautions, contraindications, potential drug interactions, laboratory test interferences, and acute toxicity.

Preparations

Excipients in commercially available drug preparations may have clinically important effects in some individuals; consult specific product labeling for details.

Zoledronic Acid

Parenteral

For injection, concentrate, for IV infusion	0.8 mg (of anhydrous zoledronic acid) per mL*	**Zoledronic Acid Injection** **Zometa®**, Novartis
For injection, for IV infusion	0.05 mg (of anhydrous zoledronic acid) per mL*	**Zoledronic Acid Injection** **Reclast®**, Novartis
	0.04 mg (of anhydrous zoledronic acid) per mL*	**Zoledronic Acid Injection** **Zometa®**, Novartis

*available from one or more manufacturer, distributor, and/or repackager by generic (nonproprietary) name

†Use is not currently included in the labeling approved by the US Food and Drug Administration

DISEASE-MODIFYING ANTIRHEUMATIC DRUGS 92:36

Adalimumab

■ Adalimumab, a recombinant DNA-derived human immunoglobulin G_1 (IgG_1) monoclonal antibody specific for human tumor necrosis factor (TNF; TNF-α), is a biologic response modifier and is a disease-modifying antirheumatic drug (DMARD).

Uses

■ **Rheumatoid Arthritis in Adults** Adalimumab is used for the management of the signs and symptoms of rheumatoid arthritis, to induce a major clinical response, to improve physical function, and to inhibit progression of structural damage associated with the disease in adults with moderate to severe active rheumatoid arthritis. Adalimumab can be used alone or in combination with methotrexate or other nonbiologic disease-modifying antirheumatic drugs (DMARDs).

Adalimumab has been evaluated for the management of rheumatoid arthritis in 5 randomized, double-blind clinical trials in adults with active disease as defined by the American College of Rheumatology (ACR). Adults included in these trials had 6 or more swollen joints and 9 or more tender joints. Adalimumab was administered in combination with methotrexate, in combination with a DMARD and/or other antirheumatic agents, or as monotherapy in these trials.

The ACR criteria for improvement (ACR response) in measures of disease activity was used as the principal measure of clinical response in trials evaluating the efficacy of adalimumab. An ACR 20 response is achieved if the patient experiences a 20% improvement in tender and swollen joint count and a 20% or greater improvement in at least 3 of the following criteria: patient pain assessment, patient global assessment, physician global assessment, patient self-assessed disability, or laboratory measures of disease activity (i.e., erythrocyte sedimentation rate [ESR] or C-reactive protein [CRP] level). ACR 50 and ACR 70 responses are defined using the same criteria with a level of improvement of 50 and 70%, respectively. Major clinical response is defined as achieving an ACR 70 response for a continuous 6-month period. The Sharp score, a composite score of erosions and joint space narrowing in hands, wrists, and forefeet, was used as the principal measure of structural damage.

Results of clinical studies indicate that usual dosages of adalimumab are more effective than placebo in the treatment of rheumatoid arthritis. Clinical evaluations of adalimumab suggest that therapy with adalimumab in conjunction with methotrexate is more effective than therapy with either agent alone. Therapy with adalimumab reduces the number of swollen and tender joints, reduces pain, improves the quality of life, and reduces disease activity as assessed by laboratory measures (i.e., CRP, ESR). Response to adalimumab can occur within 1 week following initiation of therapy. Durable responses have been maintained for up to 4 years in adults receiving adalimumab.

Results of 2 randomized, placebo-controlled trials in adults with active rheumatoid arthritis despite methotrexate therapy indicate that addition of adalimumab to the methotrexate regimen was associated with greater clinical benefit than use of methotrexate alone. In patients receiving adalimumab 40 mg once every other week in combination with their usual dosage of methotrexate, an ACR 20 was achieved 63–65 or 59% of patients at 24 or 52 weeks, respectively; an ACR 50 was achieved in 39–52 or 42% of patients at 24 or 52 weeks, respectively; and an ACR 70 was achieved in 21–24 or 23% of patients at 24 or 52 weeks, respectively. In patients receiving placebo in combination with their usual methotrexate regimen, an ACR 20 was achieved in 13–30 or 24% of patients at 24 or 52 weeks, respectively; an ACR 50 was achieved in 7–10 or 10% of patients at 24 or 52 weeks, respectively; and an ACR 70 was achieved in 3 or 5% of patients at 24 or 52 weeks, respectively. One trial included radiographic assessment of structural joint damage at baseline and 12 months. In this trial, there was more progression of joint damage from baseline in the group of patients who received placebo with methotrexate compared with those who received adalimumab with methotrexate.

In a randomized, placebo-controlled trial in adults with active rheumatoid arthritis receiving antirheumatic therapy (e.g., a DMARD, nonsteroidal anti-inflammatory agents [NSAIAs], corticosteroid) at study entry and during the study, adalimumab given at a dosage of 40 mg once every other week for 24 weeks was associated with an ACR 20 in 53% of patients; an ACR 20 was reported in 35% of placebo-treated patients.

In another randomized, placebo-controlled trial in adults with active rheumatoid arthritis who had not responded adequately to one or more DMARDs, therapy with adalimumab 40 mg once every other week (as monotherapy) for 26 weeks was associated with an ACR 20, 50, or 70 in 46, 22, or 12% of patients, respectively, and therapy with adalimumab 40 mg every week for 26 weeks was associated with an ACR 20, 50, or 70 in 53, 35, or 18% of patients, respectively. In this trial, an ACR 20, 50, or 70 was reported in 19, 8, or 2% of patients receiving placebo, respectively.

Adalimumab also has been evaluated in adults with early active rheumatoid arthritis (i.e., duration less than 3 years) who had never received therapy with methotrexate. Patients were randomized to receive adalimumab (40 mg every other week), methotrexate (20 mg once weekly by week 8) , or adalimumab in conjunction with methotrexate. Evaluation at 52 weeks indicated that treatment with adalimumab in conjunction with methotrexate was associated with a greater percentage of patients achieving an ACR response than treatment with adalimumab or methotrexate alone. In patients receiving adalimumab alone, an ACR 20 was achieved in 54 or 49% of patients at 52 or 104 weeks, respectively; an ACR 50 was achieved in 41 or 37% of patients at 52 or 104 weeks, respectively; and an ACR 70 was achieved in 26 or 28% of patients at 52 or 104 weeks, respectively. In patients receiving methotrexate alone, an ACR 20 was achieved in 63 or 56% of patients at 52 or 104 weeks, respectively; an ACR 50 was achieved in 46 or 43% of patients at 52 or 104 weeks, respectively; and an ACR 70 was achieved in 27 or 28% of patients at 52 or 104 weeks, respectively. In patients receiving adalimumab in conjunction with methotrexate, an ACR 20 was achieved in 73 or 69% of patients at 52 or 104 weeks, respectively; an ACR 50 was achieved in 62 or 59% of patients at 52 or 104 weeks, respectively; and an ACR 70 was achieved in 46 or 47% of patients at 52 or 104 weeks, respectively. A major clinical response was achieved in 25, 28, or 49% of those receiving adalimumab, methotrexate, or adalimumab in conjunction with methotrexate, respectively. There was more progression of joint damage from baseline in the group of patients who received adalimumab or methotrexate alone compared with those who received adalimumab in conjunction with methotrexate.

For further information on the treatment of rheumatoid arthritis, including the role of tissue necrosis factor (TNF) blocking agents, see Uses: Rheumatoid Arthritis, in Methotrexate 10:00.

■ **Juvenile Arthritis** Adalimumab is used for the management of the signs and symptoms of moderately to severely active polyarticular juvenile idiopathic arthritis (formerly known as juvenile rheumatoid arthritis) in pediatric patients 4 years of age or older. Adalimumab can be used with or without methotrexate.

Adalimumab has been evaluated in a randomized, double-blind, multicenter study in 171 pediatric patients (4–17 years of age) with polyarticular juvenile idiopathic arthritis. Patients had signs of moderately to severely active disease that did not respond adequately to treatment with nonsteroidal anti-inflammatory agents (NSAIAs), analgesics, corticosteroids, or DMARDs. Patients were stratified to 2 groups, those receiving methotrexate (at a dosage of at least 10 mg/m^2 weekly) and those not receiving methotrexate; patients also continued to receive stable dosages of NSAIAs and/or prednisone (up to 0.2 mg/kg daily; maximum dosage of 10 mg daily). In the initial phase of the study, patients received open-label treatment with adalimumab at a dosage of 24 mg/m^2 (up to a maximum of 40 mg) by subcutaneous injection once every other week for 16 weeks. At the end of the 16-week initial open-label phase, an ACR Pediatric 30% (ACR Pedi 30) response (defined as an improvement of 30% or more in at least 3 of the 6 core criteria for juvenile rheumatoid arthritis and a worsening of 30% or more in no more than 1) was observed in 94% of patients receiving adalimumab in combination with methotrexate and in 74% of patients receiving adalimumab without methotrexate. Patients who achieved an ACR Pedi 30 response were randomized to receive double-blinded treatment with adalimumab 24 mg/m^2 (up to a maximum of 40 mg) by subcutaneous injection or placebo once every other week for 32 weeks or until disease flare (primary outcome; defined as a worsening of at least 30% from baseline in at least 3 of 6 ACR Pedi 30 core criteria, at least 2 active joints, and improvement of at least 30% in no more than 1 of the 6 core criteria). During the double-blind phase, fewer patients receiving adalimumab experienced disease flare than those receiving placebo. Among patients not receiving methotrexate, disease flares occurred in 43% of those receiving adalimumab and in 71% of those receiving placebo, while in those receiving methotrexate, disease flares occurred in 37% of those receiving adalimumab and in 65% of those receiving placebo. Rates of ACR Pedi 30, 50, or 70 responses (ACR Pedi 50 and 70 responses are defined using the same criteria as Pedi 30 with a level of improvement of 50 and 70%, respectively) at week 48 were higher in patients receiving adalimumab and methotrexate than in those receiving placebo and methotrexate; in the subset of patients not receiving concomitant methotrexate therapy, significant differences in ACR response rates between patients who received adalimumab and those who received placebo were not observed. After the 32-week double-blind phase or at the time of disease flare (during double-blind phase), patients were eligible to receive open-label treatment with adalimumab at a dosage of 24 mg/m^2 (up to a maximum of 40 mg) by subcutaneous injection once every other week for up to 136 weeks. Afterward, patients were converted to a fixed-dose adalimumab regimen based on body weight (20 mg by subcutaneous injection once every other week in patients weighing less than 30 kg and 40 mg of adalimumab by subcutaneous injection once every other week in patients weighing 30 kg or more) for 16 weeks. ACR Pedi responses were maintained for up to 2 years in the open-label extension phase in patients who received adalimumab throughout the study.

■ Psoriatic Arthritis Adalimumab is used for the management of signs and symptoms of psoriatic arthritis, to improve physical function, and to inhibit the progression of structural damage associated with the disease in adults with active psoriatic arthritis. Adalimumab can be used alone or in combination with nonbiologic DMARDs. Clinical evaluations of adalimumab have shown that the drug is more effective than placebo in the management of psoriatic arthritis.

Adalimumab has been evaluated for the management of psoriatic arthritis in a randomized, double-blind, placebo-controlled study in adults with active psoriatic arthritis (3 or more swollen joints and 3 or more tender joints) who had an inadequate response to therapy with a NSAIA. The study included patients with any of the following forms of the disease: distal interphalangeal involvement, polyarticular arthritis, arthritis mutilans, asymmetric psoriatic arthritis, or ankylosing spondylitis-like. Patients receiving stable dosages of methotrexate at study enrollment could continue methotrexate during the study. The ACR criteria for improvement in measures of disease activity were used to measure clinical response and the Psoriasis Area and Severity Index (PASI) was used to evaluate skin lesions. Physical function and disability were assessed using the Health Assessment Questionnaire Disability Index (HAQ-DI) and the general health-related quality of life questionnaire SF-36. A modified total Sharp score that included distal interphalangeal joints was used to measure structural damage. At week 12, an ACR 20, 50, or 70 was achieved in 58, 36, or 20%, respectively, of patients who received adalimumab compared with 14, 4, or 1%, respectively, of patients receiving placebo. At week 24, an ACR 20, 50, or 70 was achieved in 57, 39, or 23%, respectively, of patients who received adalimumab compared with 15, 6, or 1%, respectively, of patients receiving placebo. At week 24, 59 or 42% of adalimumab-treated patients achieved a 75 or 90% improvement in PASI, respectively, compared with 1 or 0% of placebo-treated patients, respectively.

Response to adalimumab can occur within 2 weeks following initiation of therapy. ACR and PASI responses in patients not receiving methotrexate were similar to the responses in those receiving methotrexate; clinical response in patients with each of the subtypes of psoriatic arthritis (only a few patients had the arthritis mutilans or ankylosing spondylitis-like subtypes) appeared to be similar. Adalimumab therapy was associated with greater improvement from baseline in the HAQ-DI and the SF-36 physical component summary score at 12 and 24 weeks compared with placebo. Adalimumab therapy was not associated with deterioration in the SF-36 mental component summary score. Improvement in physical function based on the HAQ-DI was maintained for up to 84 weeks. At week 24, adalimumab therapy was more effective than placebo in retarding radiographic progression. Inhibition of progression was maintained through week 48 in adalimumab-treated patients. ACR and PASI responses reported in a smaller 12-week study in adults with active psoriatic arthritis who had not responded adequately to DMARD therapy were similar to those reported in the study in patients with an inadequate response to NSAIAs.

■ Ankylosing Spondylitis Adalimumab is used for the management of the signs and symptoms of ankylosing spondylitis in adults with active disease. In one study in patients with active ankylosing spondylitis, 20, 50, or 70% improvement in the Assessment in Ankylosing Spondylitis (ASAS) response criteria was achieved at 12 weeks in 58, 38, or 23%, respectively, of those receiving adalimumab compared with 21, 10, or 5%, respectively, of those receiving placebo. Response to adalimumab was observed at week 2; responses have been maintained for up to 1 year. A greater proportion of patients receiving adalimumab (22%) achieved a low level of disease activity (assessed using each of the 4 ASAS response parameters) compared with those receiving placebo (6%). At week 24, adalimumab therapy was associated with greater improvement from baseline in the Ankylosing Spondylitis Quality of Life Questionnaire score and SF-36 physical component summary score compared with treatment with placebo. Results reported from a smaller study in patients with ankylosing spondylitis were similar to the ASAS responses observed in this controlled study.

■ Crohn's Disease Adalimumab is used to reduce the signs and symptoms of Crohn's disease and to induce and maintain clinical remission in adults with moderately to severely active disease who have had an inadequate response to conventional therapy. Adalimumab also is used to reduce the signs and symptoms of Crohn's disease and to induce clinical remission in adults with moderately to severely active Crohn's disease who have lost response to or are intolerant to infliximab.

Safety and efficacy of adalimumab in the management of Crohn's disease were evaluated in randomized, double-blind, placebo-controlled studies in adults with moderately to severely active Crohn's disease (Crohn's disease activity index [CDAI] 220–450). The CDAI score is based on the daily number of liquid or very soft stools, severity of abdominal pain or cramping, general well-being, presence or absence of extraintestinal manifestations, presence or absence of an abdominal mass, use or nonuse of antidiarrheal drugs, the hematocrit, and body weight; scores below 150 indicate clinical remission and scores above 450 indicate severe illness. Patients who were receiving fixed dosages of aminosalicylates, corticosteroids, and/or immunomodulatory agents were permitted to continue receiving these drugs during the studies (79% of patients continued to receive one or more of these drugs). Two studies evaluated the use of adalimumab for induction of remission; one study evaluated patients who had not previously received an agent that blocks tumor necrosis factor (TNF) while a second study evaluated patients who had lost response to or were intolerant to infliximab therapy. In both studies, clinical remission by week 4 was reported in more patients receiving adalimumab than in those receiving placebo. A clinical response (defined as a reduction from baseline CDAI score of at least 70 points) at 4 weeks was observed in 58 or 34% of TNF blocking agent-naive patients receiving subcutaneous adalimumab (160 mg once at week 0 and 80 mg once at week 2) or placebo (once at week 0 and once at week 2), respectively, and in 52 or 34%, respectively, of infliximab resistant or intolerant patients receiving adalimumab (160 mg once at week 0 and 80 mg once at week 2) or placebo (once at week 0 and once at week 2), respectively. Clinical remission (defined as CDAI score less than 150) was observed in 36 or 12%, respectively, of TNF blocking agent-naive patients receiving adalimumab or placebo, and in 21 or 7%, respectively, of infliximab resistant or intolerant patients receiving adalimumab or placebo.

Safety and efficacy of adalimumab for maintenance of remission in patients with moderately to severely active Crohn's disease were evaluated in a randomized, double-blind, placebo-controlled study that included 854 adults. Initially, patients received open-label treatment with subcutaneous adalimumab (80 mg once at week 0 and 40 mg once at week 2). After 4 weeks, clinical response (defined as a reduction from baseline CDAI score of at least 70 points) occurred in 58% (499 out of 854) of patients; these patients were assessed in the primary analysis of maintenance of clinical response or remission. Patients were then randomized to receive subcutaneous adalimumab (40 mg once every other week), adalimumab (40 mg once every week), or placebo. Patients who were receiving fixed dosages of aminosalicylates, corticosteroids, and/or immunomodulatory agents were permitted to continue receiving these drugs during the study (79% of patients continued to receive one or more of these drugs). Among adults who achieved clinical response at week 4, a greater proportion of patients receiving adalimumab achieved clinical remission at weeks 26 and 56 compared with those receiving placebo. At week 26, the clinical response was maintained in 54 or 28% of patients receiving adalimumab (40 mg once every other week) or placebo, respectively, while clinical remission (defined as CDAI score less than 150) was maintained in 40 or 17% of patients receiving adalimumab (40 mg once every other week) or placebo, respectively. At week 56, the clinical response was maintained in 43 or 18% of patients receiving adalimumab (40 mg once every other week) or placebo, while clinical remission was maintained in 36 or 12% of patients receiving adalimumab (40 mg once every other week) or placebo, respectively. Treatment with adalimumab 40 mg once every week was not associated with higher remission rates than adalimumab 40 mg once every other week. Among patients who achieved clinical response at week 4, a longer time in remission was reported in patients receiving adalimumab (40 mg once every other week) compared with those receiving placebo. Among patients who were not in response by week 12, continued treatment beyond 12 weeks did not result in more responses.

■ **Ulcerative Colitis** Adalimumab is used to induce and sustain clinical remission in adults with moderately to severely active ulcerative colitis who have had an inadequate response to immunosuppressive agents such as corticosteroids, azathioprine, or mercaptopurine. Efficacy of adalimumab in patients with ulcerative colitis who have lost response to or were intolerant to TNF blocking agents has not been established.

Efficacy and safety of adalimumab in the management of ulcerative colitis were evaluated in 2 randomized, double-blind, placebo-controlled studies (ULTRA 1 and ULTRA 2) in adults with moderately to severely active ulcerative colitis despite current or prior therapy with immunosuppressive agents such as corticosteroids, azathioprine, or mercaptopurine. Patients who had received prior therapy with TNF blocking agents were excluded from ULTRA 1; however, patients who had lost response to or were intolerant to TNF blocking agents could be enrolled in ULTRA 2. Among patients enrolled in ULTRA 2, 40% had received prior treatment with another TNF blocking agent.

In ULTRA 1, a total of 390 patients were randomized to receive one of 2 adalimumab regimens (adalimumab 160 mg at week 0, 80 mg at week 2, then 40 mg at weeks 4 and 6 [160 mg/80 mg]; adalimumab 80 mg at week 0, 40 mg at week 2, then 40 mg at weeks 4 and 6 [80 mg/40 mg]) or placebo for the primary analysis. In ULTRA 2, a total of 518 patients were randomized to receive either adalimumab (160 mg at week 0, 80 mg at week 2, then 40 mg every 2 weeks from weeks 4–50) or placebo. In both studies, patients receiving stable dosages of aminosalicylates and immunosuppressive agents could continue receiving these agents; tapering of corticosteroid dosage was permitted after week 8. In the 2 study populations combined, 69% of patients received aminosalicylates, 59% received corticosteroids, and 37% received azathioprine or mercaptopurine concomitantly with their assigned treatment; 92% of patients received at least one of these agents.

Efficacy of adalimumab for induction of clinical remission (defined as Mayo score of 2 or less with no individual subscore exceeding 1) was evaluated at week 8 in both studies. Clinical remission at week 52 and sustained clinical remission (defined as clinical remission at both weeks 8 and 52) also were evaluated in ULTRA 2. In both studies, a greater proportion of patients receiving adalimumab 160 mg/80 mg achieved clinical remission at week 8 compared with patients receiving placebo (16.5–18.5 versus 9.2–9.3%). In ULTRA 1, clinical remission rates were similar in patients receiving adalimumab 80 mg/40 mg and those receiving placebo (10 and 9.2%, respectively). In ULTRA 2, clinical remission rates at week 52 (17.3 versus 8.5%) and sustained remission rates (8.5 versus 4.1%) also were higher in patients receiving adalimumab 160 mg/80 mg compared with those receiving placebo.

The treatment effect at week 8 appeared to be smaller among patients who had received prior treatment with other TNF blocking agents than for the overall ULTRA 2 study population. In the subgroup of patients who had received prior treatment with TNF blocking agents, clinical remission was achieved at week 8 by similar proportions of patients receiving adalimumab and those receiving placebo (9 and 7%, respectively); however, in this subgroup of patients, clinical remission was achieved at week 52 by 10% of those receiving adalimumab compared with 3% of those receiving placebo, and sustained clinical remission rates were 5 and 1%, respectively. Additional studies are needed to more fully evaluate the effects of adalimumab in patients with ulcerative colitis who lost response to or did not tolerate prior treatment with TNF blocking agents.

An open-label follow-up study was conducted upon completion of ULTRA 1. At week 8 (the end of the blinded study), adalimumab therapy (40 mg every 2 weeks) was initiated in placebo recipients and continued in both groups of patients currently receiving the drug; beginning at week 12, patients with an inadequate response could begin receiving weekly 40-mg doses of the drug. At week 52, the clinical remission rate was 25.6% with every-2-week dosing and 29.5% with either weekly or every-2-week dosing.

■ **Plaque Psoriasis** Adalimumab is used for the treatment of moderate to severe chronic plaque psoriasis in adults who are candidates for systemic therapy or phototherapy and in whom other systemic therapies are medically less appropriate. Adalimumab should be used only in patients who will be closely monitored and who will have regular follow-up visits with a clinician.

Safety and efficacy of adalimumab were assessed in several randomized, double-blind, placebo-controlled studies in 1696 adults with moderate to severe chronic plaque psoriasis who were candidates for systemic therapy or phototherapy. In one study, 1212 patients with chronic plaque psoriasis involving at least 10% of body surface area (BSA) who had a baseline Physician's Global Assessment (PGA) of at least moderate disease severity and Psoriasis Area and Severity Index (PASI) score of at least 12 within 3 treatment periods were randomized to receive subcutaneous adalimumab (80 mg once at week 0 followed by 40 mg once every other week beginning at week 1) or placebo for 16 weeks. After 16 weeks, a PASI 75 (defined as a PASI score improvement of at least 75% compared with baseline) response was reported in 71 or 7% of patients receiving adalimumab or placebo, respectively. A status of clear or minimal disease on the PGA scale after 16 weeks of treatment was achieved in 62 or 4% of patients receiving adalimumab or placebo, respectively. Patients with a PASI 75 response then received open-label treatment with adalimumab 40 mg once every other week for 17 weeks. After 17 weeks of open-label adalimumab therapy, patients who maintained a PASI 75 response at week 33 and originally were randomized to active treatment were re-randomized to receive adalimumab 40 mg once every other week or placebo for an additional 19 weeks. Continued efficacy of adalimumab after 52 weeks of treatment was observed: PASI 75 response was reported in 79 or 43% of patients receiving adalimumab or placebo, respectively, while "clear" or "minimal" disease was reported in 68 or 28% of patients receiving the drug or placebo, respectively.

In another study, 147 patients with chronic plaque psoriasis involving at least 10% of BSA who had a PASI score of at least 12 were randomized to receive subcutaneous adalimumab (80 mg once at week 0 followed by 40 mg once every other week beginning at week 1) or placebo for 16 weeks. After 16 weeks, a PASI 75 response was reported in 78 or 19% of patients receiving adalimumab or placebo, respectively. "Clear" or "minimal" disease after 16 weeks of treatment was observed in 71 or 10% of patients receiving adalimumab or placebo, respectively.

During an open-label extension of phase 2 and 3 studies, 1468 adults with moderate to severe chronic plaque psoriasis received adalimumab for periods of about 2–5 years; those with a stable response ("clear" or "minimal" disease) at the end of the open-label treatment period discontinued adalimumab and were monitored for relapse ("moderate" or worse disease), at which time adalimumab therapy was reinitiated. Of the initial group of 1468 patients, 347 patients had a stable response to adalimumab and discontinued therapy; 178 of those patients subsequently relapsed (median time of relapse: approximately 5 months after drug discontinuance) and reinitiated therapy with the drug. Of the patients who relapsed and reinitiated adalimumab therapy (80 mg once at week 0 followed by 40 mg once every other week beginning at week 1), 69% had "clear" or "minimal" disease after 16 weeks of retreatment. No patients experienced transformation of their condition to pustular or erythrodermic psoriasis during the drug withdrawal period.

Dosage and Administration

■ **Administration** Adalimumab is administered by subcutaneous injection. Adalimumab is intended for use under the guidance and supervision of a clinician; however, the drug may be *self-administered* if the clinician determines that the patient and/or their caregiver is competent to safely administer the drug after appropriate training and with medical follow-up as necessary.

Adalimumab is commercially available in single-use prefilled syringes equipped with a 27-gauge, ½-inch needle and in single-use prefilled injection pens. Adalimumab also is commercially available in single-use vials intended for institutional use only (e.g., in a hospital, clinic, or clinician's office). Prior to administration, adalimumab solutions should be inspected visually for particulate matter or discoloration; if either is present, the solution should be discarded. Adalimumab injection contains no preservative, and any unused portions of solution should be discarded. Once adalimumab solution has been withdrawn from the vial into a syringe for administration, it should be used promptly. Adalimumab injection should be stored at 2–8°C and protected from light; the prefilled syringes should be stored in the original carton until administration. The injection should not be frozen; solutions that have been frozen should not be used. During travel, adalimumab should be stored in a cool carrier with an ice pack.

Subcutaneous injections of adalimumab should be made into the thighs or abdomen; however, abdominal injections should not be made within 5.18 cm (2 inches) of the umbilicus. Injection sites should be rotated. New injections should be given at least 2.54 cm (1 inch) from an old site, and injections should not be made into areas where the skin is tender, bruised, red, or hard, or into scars or stretch marks. Injections into psoriatic lesions also should be avoided.

Methotrexate, other nonbiologic disease-modifying antirheumatic drugs (DMARDs), corticosteroids, nonsteroidal anti-inflammatory agents (NSAIAs), and/or analgesics may be continued in adults receiving adalimumab for the management of rheumatoid arthritis, psoriatic arthritis, or ankylosing spondylitis.

Methotrexate, corticosteroids, NSAIAs, and/or analgesics may be continued in pediatric patients receiving adalimumab for the management of juvenile idiopathic arthritis.

Aminosalicylates and/or corticosteroids may be continued in adults receiving adalimumab for the treatment of Crohn's disease or ulcerative colitis. Azathioprine, mercaptopurine, or methotrexate may be continued, if necessary, in adults receiving adalimumab for the treatment of Crohn's disease. Azathioprine and mercaptopurine may be continued, if necessary, in adults receiving adalimumab for the treatment of ulcerative colitis. (See Malignancies and Lymphoproliferative Disorders under Warnings/Precautions: Warnings, in Cautions.)

■ **Dosage** ***Rheumatoid Arthritis in Adults*** For the management of rheumatoid arthritis in adults, the usual dosage of adalimumab is 40 mg once every other week by subcutaneous injection. Patients *not* receiving methotrexate may obtain additional benefit if the interval between adalimumab doses is shortened and adalimumab 40 mg is administered once weekly.

Juvenile Arthritis For the management of juvenile idiopathic arthritis in pediatric patients 4–17 years of age, the recommended dosage of adalimumab is 20 mg once every other week by subcutaneous injection in patients weighing 15 kg to less than 30 kg and 40 mg once every other week by subcutaneous injection in patients weighing 30 kg or more.

Psoriatic Arthritis For the management of psoriatic arthritis in adults, the usual dosage of adalimumab is 40 mg once every other week by subcutaneous injection.

Ankylosing Spondylitis For the management of ankylosing spondylitis in adults, the usual dosage of adalimumab is 40 mg once every other week by subcutaneous injection.

Crohn's Disease For the treatment of Crohn's disease in adults, the recommended initial dosage of adalimumab is 160 mg by subcutaneous injection once on day 1 (given as four 40-mg injections in one day or as two 40-mg injections per day for 2 consecutive days), followed by 80 mg once 2 weeks later (on day 15). A maintenance dosage of 40 mg once every other week should be started on day 29 (2 weeks after the 80-mg dose). The use of adalimumab therapy beyond 1 year has not been evaluated in controlled clinical studies in patients with Crohn's disease.

Ulcerative Colitis For the treatment of ulcerative colitis in adults, the recommended initial dosage of adalimumab is 160 mg by subcutaneous injection on day 1 (given as four 40-mg injections in one day or as two 40-mg injections per day for 2 consecutive days), followed by 80 mg once 2 weeks later (on day 15). A maintenance dosage of 40 mg once every other week should be started on day 29 (2 weeks after the 80-mg dose). If clinical remission is not achieved by 8 weeks (day 57), adalimumab should be discontinued.

Plaque Psoriasis For the management of plaque psoriasis in adults, the recommended initial dosage of adalimumab is 80 mg by subcutaneous injection, followed by 40 mg once every other week starting 1 week after the initial dose. The use of adalimumab therapy beyond 1 year has not been evaluated in controlled clinical studies in patients with plaque psoriasis.

■ **Special Populations** No special population dosage recommendations at this time.

Cautions

■ **Contraindications** Known hypersensitivity to adalimumab or any ingredient in the formulation.

■ **Warnings/Precautions** ***Warnings*** **Infectious Complications.** Patients receiving tumor necrosis factor (TNF) blocking agents, including adalimumab, are at increased risk of developing serious infections involving various organ systems and sites that may require hospitalization or result in death. Opportunistic infections caused by bacterial, mycobacterial, invasive fungal, viral, parasitic, or other opportunistic pathogens—including aspergillosis, blastomycosis, candidiasis, coccidioidomycosis, histoplasmosis, legionellosis, listeriosis, pneumocystosis, and tuberculosis—have been reported in patients receiving TNF blocking agents. Infections frequently have been disseminated rather than localized. Patients should be closely monitored during and after treatment with TNF blocking agents for the development of signs or symptoms of infection (e.g., fever, malaise, weight loss, sweats, cough, dyspnea, pulmonary infiltrates, serious systemic illness including shock). Most patients who developed serious infections were receiving concomitant therapy with immunosuppressive agents such as methotrexate or corticosteroids.

In controlled trials in adults with rheumatoid arthritis, psoriatic arthritis, ankylosing spondylitis, Crohn's disease, ulcerative colitis, or plaque psoriasis, the rate of serious infection was 4.6 per 100 patient-years in adalimumab-treated patients and 3.1 per 100 patient-years in control patients. Serious infections included pneumonia, septic arthritis, prosthetic infection, postsurgical infection, erysipelas, cellulitis, diverticulitis, and pyelonephritis. Tuberculosis (frequently disseminated or extrapulmonary at clinical presentation), invasive fungal infections, and other opportunistic infections also have occurred in patients receiving adalimumab or other TNF blocking agents. Most of the cases of tuberculosis occurred within the first 8 months following initiation of adalimumab therapy; these cases may reflect recrudescence of latent tuberculosis infection. As of September 2011, the US Food and Drug Administration (FDA) had identified 103 reports of *Legionella* pneumonia associated with TNF blocking agents, including adalimumab. The 103 cases of *Legionella* pneumonia occurred in patients 25–85 years of age, many of whom received concomitant therapy with immunosuppressive agents (e.g., corticosteroids and/or methotrexate); 17 deaths were reported. In 78% of the cases of *Legionella* pneumonia, the median duration of TNF blocker therapy prior to the onset of *Legionella* pneumonia was 10.4 months (range: less than 1 month to 73 months). As of September 2011, FDA also had identified 26 published reports of *Listeria* infections, including meningitis, bacteremia, endophthalmitis, and sepsis, in patients who received TNF blocking agents; 7 deaths were reported. Many of the *Listeria* infections occurred in patients who had received concomitant therapy with immunosuppressive agents. In addition, FDA identified fatal *Listeria* infections during a review of data regarding laboratory-confirmed infections that occurred in premarketing clinical studies and during postmarketing surveillance.

An increased incidence of serious infections also was observed in clinical studies in patients with rheumatoid arthritis when a TNF blocking agent was used concomitantly with anakinra (a human interleukin-1 receptor antagonist) or abatacept (a selective costimulation modulator). (See Drug Interactions: Biologic Antirheumatic Agents.)

Adalimumab therapy should not be initiated in patients with active infections, including localized infections. Patients older than 65 years of age, patients with comorbid conditions, and/or patients receiving concomitant therapy with immunosuppressive agents such as corticosteroids or methotrexate may be at increased risk of infection. Clinicians should consider potential risks and benefits of the drug prior to initiating therapy in patients with a history of chronic, recurring, or opportunistic infections; patients with underlying conditions that may predispose them to infections; and patients who have been exposed to tuberculosis or who have resided or traveled in regions where tuberculosis or mycoses such as histoplasmosis, coccidioidomycosis, and blastomycosis are endemic. Any patient who develops a new infection while receiving adalimumab should undergo a thorough diagnostic evaluation (appropriate for an immunocompromised patient); appropriate anti-infective therapy should be initiated, and the patient should be closely monitored. The drug should be discontinued in patients who develop serious infection or sepsis.

Because tuberculosis has been reported in patients receiving adalimumab, all patients should be evaluated for active or latent tuberculosis and for the presence of risk factors for tuberculosis prior to and periodically during therapy with the drug. When indicated, an appropriate antimycobacterial regimen for the treatment of latent tuberculosis infection should be initiated prior to adalimumab therapy. Antimycobacterial treatment lowers the risk of latent tuberculosis infection progressing to active disease (i.e., reactivation) in patients receiving adalimumab. Antimycobacterial therapy also should be considered prior to initiation of adalimumab in individuals with a history of latent or active tuberculosis in whom an adequate course of antimycobacterial treatment cannot be confirmed and in individuals with a negative tuberculin skin test who have risk factors for tuberculosis. Consultation with a tuberculosis specialist is recommended when deciding whether antimycobacterial therapy should be initiated. Active tuberculosis has developed in adalimumab-treated patients who previously received antimycobacterial therapy for latent or active tuberculosis. Patients receiving adalimumab, including individuals with a negative tuberculin skin test, should be monitored for signs and symptoms of active tuberculosis. A diagnosis of tuberculosis should be strongly considered in patients who develop new infections while receiving adalimumab, especially in those who previously have traveled to countries where tuberculosis is highly prevalent or who have been in close contact with an individual with active tuberculosis.

Invasive fungal infections often are not recognized in patients receiving TNF blocking agents; this has led to delays in appropriate treatment. Clinicians should ascertain if patients receiving TNF blocking agents who present with signs and symptoms suggestive of systemic fungal infection reside or have traveled in regions where mycoses are endemic. Empiric antifungal therapy should be considered in patients at risk of histoplasmosis or other invasive fungal infections who develop severe systemic illness. Following resolution of an invasive fungal infection, the decision regarding whether to reinitiate TNF blocking agent therapy should involve reevaluation of the risks and benefits of such therapy, particularly in patients who reside in regions where mycoses are endemic. Whenever feasible, decisions regarding initiation and duration of antifungal therapy and reinitiation of TNF blocking agent therapy should be made in consultation with a specialist in the diagnosis and management of fungal infections.

Malignancies and Lymphoproliferative Disorders. Malignancies, some fatal, have been reported in children, adolescents, and young adults who received treatment with TNF blocking agents beginning when they were 18 years of age or younger. In August 2009, FDA reported the results of an analysis of reports of lymphoma and other malignancies in children and adolescents who had received TNF blocking agents. These cases were reported postmarketing and were derived from various sources, including registries and spontaneous postmarketing reports. FDA identified 48 cases of malignancies in children and adolescents in the analysis.

Of the 48 cases reviewed by FDA, approximately 50% were lymphomas, including Hodgkin's disease and non-Hodgkin's lymphoma. The other cases represented a variety of malignancies, including rare malignancies that are usually associated with immunosuppression and malignancies that are not usually observed in children and adolescents. Other malignancies reported included leukemia, melanoma, and solid organ cancers; malignancies such as leiomyosarcoma, hepatic malignancies, and renal cell carcinoma, which rarely occur in children, also were reported. The malignancies occurred after a median of 30 months (range: 1–84 months) following the first dose of therapy with TNF blocking agents. Of the 48 cases of malignancies, 11 deaths were reported; causes of death included hepatosplenic T-cell lymphoma (9 cases), T-cell lymphoma (1 case), and sepsis following remission of lymphoma (1 case). The reporting rates for cases of malignancy with adalimumab were not calculated during the analysis because of minimal use in pediatric patients. Most of the 48 patients (88%) also were receiving other immunosuppressive drugs such as azathioprine and methotrexate; these agents also are associated with an increased risk of lymphoma. Although there were other contributory factors, the role of TNF blocking agents in the development of malignancies in children and adolescents could not be excluded. Therefore, FDA has concluded that there is an increased risk of malignancy with TNF blocking agents. However, due to the relatively rare occurrence of these cancers, the limited number of pediatric patients who received TNF blocking agents, and the possible role of other immunosuppressive drugs used concomitantly with TNF blocking agents, FDA was unable to fully characterize the strength of the association between use of TNF blocking agents and the development of a malignancy. Additional data are expected from ongoing, long-term, observational, postmarketing studies and registries that are being created by the manufacturers of TNF blocking agents.

Hepatosplenic T-cell lymphoma, a rare, aggressive, usually fatal type of T-cell lymphoma, has been reported during postmarketing experience mainly in adolescents and young adults with Crohn's disease or ulcerative colitis who received treatment with TNF blocking agents and/or thiopurine analogs (mercaptopurine or azathioprine). Most of the reported cases of hepatosplenic T-cell lymphoma occurred in patients who had received a combination of immunosuppressive agents, including TNF blocking agents and thiopurine analogs (azathioprine or mercaptopurine). It is not clear whether the occurrence of hepatosplenic T-cell lymphoma was related to use of a TNF blocking agent or use of a TNF blocking agent in conjunction with other immunosuppressive agents. In some cases, potential confounding factors could not be excluded because complete medical histories were not available. As of December 31, 2010, FDA had identified 7 cases of hepatosplenic T-cell lymphoma in patients with Crohn's disease, ulcerative colitis, or rheumatoid arthritis who had received adalimumab (2 cases) or both adalimumab and infliximab (5 cases); in 4 of these cases, a thiopurine analog (mercaptopurine or azathioprine) was used concomitantly. These 7 cases of hepatosplenic T-cell lymphoma occurred in patients 21–70 years of age following adalimumab therapy for periods ranging from 3 doses up to 1 year of therapy; most of the patients were men, and 5 of the 7 cases were fatal. Since patients with certain conditions (e.g., rheumatoid arthritis, Crohn's disease, ankylosing spondylitis, psoriatic arthritis, plaque psoriasis) may be at increased risk for lymphoma, it may be difficult to measure the added risk of treatment with TNF blocking agents, azathioprine, and/or mercaptopurine.

In clinical studies, lymphoma has been observed more frequently in patients receiving agents that block TNF than in control patients. In controlled and uncontrolled studies evaluating adalimumab in adults with rheumatoid arthritis, psoriatic arthritis, ankylosing spondylitis, Crohn's disease, ulcerative colitis, or plaque psoriasis, the rate of lymphoma in adalimumab-treated patients was approximately 0.11 per 100 patient-years. This rate is approximately threefold higher than the rate expected in the general US population. Patients with rheumatoid arthritis or other chronic inflammatory diseases, especially those with highly active disease and/or chronic exposure to immunosuppressive therapies, may be at increased risk of lymphoma, even in the absence of TNF blocking agent therapy.

In addition to lymphoma, various other malignancies including breast cancer, colorectal cancer, lung cancer, melanoma, nonmelanoma skin cancer, and prostate cancer have been reported in patients receiving adalimumab in clinical trials. In controlled studies evaluating adalimumab in adults with rheumatoid arthritis, psoriatic arthritis, ankylosing spondylitis, Crohn's disease, ulcerative colitis, or plaque psoriasis, the rate of malignancies other than nonmelanoma skin cancer was 0.6 per 100 patient-years in adalimumab-treated patients and 0.6 per 100 patient-years in control patients; the rate of nonmelanoma skin cancer was 0.7 per 100 patient-years in adalimumab-treated patients and 0.2 per 100 patient-years in control patients. Some immune related diseases, such as Crohn's disease, have been shown to increase the risk of cancer independent of treatment with TNF blocking agents, while for others, such as juvenile idiopathic arthritis, it is unknown whether there is an increased risk of cancer.

In controlled studies of other TNF blocking agents in adults at increased risk of malignancies (e.g., patients with chronic obstructive pulmonary disease [COPD] who have a substantial history of smoking, patients with Wegener's granulomatosis receiving concomitant cyclophosphamide), a greater proportion of malignancies occurred in patients receiving the TNF blocking agent compared with control patients.

Cases of acute and chronic leukemia have been reported during postmarketing surveillance of TNF blocking agents used in the management of rheumatoid arthritis and other conditions. In August 2009, FDA reported the results of a review of 147 cases of leukemia in adults and pediatric patients who received TNF blocking agents; these cases had been identified during postmarketing surveillance. Of the 147 cases, acute myeloid leukemia (44 cases), chronic lymphocytic leukemia (31 cases), and chronic myeloid leukemia (23 cases) were the most frequent types of leukemia reported. Four cases of leukemia were reported in children. Most patients (61%) also were receiving other immunosuppressive drugs. There were a total of 30 deaths reported; leukemia was reported as the cause of 26 of the 30 deaths, and the event was associated with the use of TNF blocking agents. Leukemia generally occurred during the first 2 years of therapy. The interpretation of these findings was complicated by the fact that published epidemiologic studies suggest that patients with rheumatoid arthritis may be at increased risk of leukemia, independent of any treatment with TNF blocking agents. However, based on the available data, FDA has concluded that there is a possible association between treatment with TNF blocking agents and the development of leukemia in patients receiving these drugs.

Clinicians should consider the possibility of and monitor for the occurrence of malignancies during and following treatment with TNF blocking agents. The risks and benefits of TNF blocking agents, including adalimumab, should be considered prior to initiating therapy in patients with a known malignancy (other than a successfully treated nonmelanoma skin cancer) or when considering whether to continue TNF blocking agent therapy in patients who develop a malignancy. Because therapy with TNF blocking agents and/or thiopurine analogs (azathioprine or mercaptopurine) may increase the risk of malignancies, including hepatosplenic T-cell lymphoma, the risks and benefits of these agents should be carefully considered, especially in adolescents and young adults and especially in the treatment of Crohn's disease or ulcerative colitis. All patients, but particularly those with a history of prior prolonged immunosuppressive therapy or a history of psoralen and UVA light (PUVA) therapy, should be examined for the presence of nonmelanoma skin cancer prior to and during therapy with adalimumab.

Other Warnings/Precautions

Sensitivity Reactions. Anaphylaxis, angioedema, and other allergic reactions (e.g., allergic rash, anaphylactoid reactions, fixed drug eruption, nonspecified drug reaction, urticaria) have occurred in patients receiving adalimumab. If a serious allergic reaction or anaphylaxis occurs, adalimumab should be discontinued immediately and appropriate therapy initiated.

The needle cover of prefilled syringes of adalimumab contains dry natural rubber (latex) and should not be handled by individuals sensitive to latex.

Patients Infected with Hepatitis B Virus. Use of TNF blocking agents, including adalimumab, may increase the risk of reactivation of hepatitis B virus (HBV) infection in patients who are chronic carriers of this virus (i.e., hepatitis B surface antigen-positive [HBsAg-positive]). HBV reactivation has resulted in death in a few individuals receiving TNF blocking agent therapy. Most patients experiencing HBV reactivation were receiving concomitant therapy with other immunosuppressive agents; use of multiple immunosuppressive agents may have contributed to HBV reactivation.

Patients at risk for HBV infection should be screened before initiation of adalimumab therapy. Chronic carriers of HBV should be appropriately evaluated and monitored prior to the initiation of therapy, during treatment, and for up to several months following therapy with adalimumab. Safety and efficacy of antiviral therapy for prevention of viral reactivation in HBV carriers receiving a TNF blocking agent have not been established. Adalimumab should be discontinued if HBV reactivation occurs, and appropriate treatment, including antiviral therapy, should be initiated. It has not been established whether adalimumab can be safely readministered once control of the reactivated HBV infection has been achieved; caution is advised if adalimumab therapy is resumed in such a situation.

Nervous System Effects. New onset or exacerbation of clinical manifestations and/or radiographic evidence of central or peripheral nervous system demyelinating disorders (e.g., multiple sclerosis, optic neuritis, Guillain-Barré syndrome) has been reported rarely in patients receiving adalimumab or other TNF blocking agents. Clinicians should exercise caution when considering adalimumab therapy in patients with preexisting or recent-onset central or peripheral nervous system demyelinating disorders.

Hematologic Effects. Pancytopenia including aplastic anemia has been reported rarely in patients receiving agents that block TNF. Adverse hematologic effects, including leukopenia and thrombocytopenia, have occurred rarely in adalimumab-treated patients. Whether these hematologic abnormalities are directly attributable to adalimumab remains to be determined. If substantial hematologic abnormalities occur, discontinuance of adalimumab should be considered.

Cardiovascular Effects. There have been reports of worsening heart failure and new-onset heart failure in patients receiving agents that block TNF, including adalimumab. While adalimumab has not been formally studied in patients with heart failure, other agents that block TNF (i.e., etanercept, infliximab) have been associated with adverse cardiovascular effects in patients with heart failure. If adalimumab is used in patients with heart failure, caution and careful monitoring are recommended.

Immunologic Reactions and Antibody Formation. Adalimumab therapy may result in the formation of autoimmune antibodies. In controlled clinical trials in patients with rheumatoid arthritis, 12% of those receiving adalimumab developed new positive antinuclear antibodies (ANA) compared with 7% of those receiving placebo. A lupus-like syndrome has occurred in at least 2 patients receiving adalimumab; symptoms resolved following discontinuance of the drug. If a patient develops manifestations suggestive of a lupus-like syndrome, adalimumab should be discontinued.

Patients receiving adalimumab may develop antibodies to the drug. In clinical studies that evaluated adalimumab in patients with rheumatoid arthritis, approximately 5% of adalimumab-treated patients who were tested for the presence of antibodies at multiple time points over 6–12 months developed low-titer neutralizing antibodies to the drug at least once during therapy. The incidence of antibody formation was lower in patients receiving adalimumab in conjunction with methotrexate than in patients receiving adalimumab monotherapy (1 versus 12%). The incidence of antibody formation may be lower in patients receiving adalimumab (as monotherapy) every week compared with patients receiving the drug every other week. In addition, clinical response (ACR 20) in patients receiving adalimumab (as monotherapy) every other week was achieved in fewer antibody-positive patients than antibody-negative patients. A relationship between the development of antibodies to adalimumab and the incidence of adverse effects has not been observed. The long-term immunogenicity of adalimumab remains to be determined.

In a clinical study in pediatric patients receiving adalimumab for the treatment of juvenile idiopathic arthritis, approximately 16% of adalimumab-treated children developed neutralizing antibodies to the drug at least once during therapy. The incidence of antibody formation was lower in patients receiving adalimumab in conjunction with methotrexate than in patients receiving adalimumab monotherapy (6 versus 26%).

The incidence of antibody formation to adalimumab in patients receiving the drug for the treatment of ankylosing spondylitis was similar to the incidence reported in patients receiving the drug for rheumatoid arthritis. The incidence of antibody formation in patients receiving adalimumab monotherapy for the treatment of psoriatic arthritis was similar to the incidence reported in adalimumab-treated patients with rheumatoid arthritis; however, the incidence of antibody formation in patients with psoriatic arthritis receiving adalimumab in conjunction with methotrexate was higher than the incidence reported in patients with rheumatoid arthritis receiving adalimumab in conjunction with methotrexate (7 versus 1%). The incidence of antibody formation in patients receiving the drug for Crohn's disease or ulcerative colitis was 3 or 5%, respectively. In patients receiving adalimumab monotherapy for the treatment of plaque psoriasis, the incidence of antibody formation was 8%. However, because of assay limitations, antibodies to adalimumab could be detected only when serum adalimumab concentrations were less than 2 mcg/mL; the incidence of antibody formation in patients with serum adalimumab concentrations of less than 2 mcg/mL (approximately 40% of patients with psoriasis and 25% of patients with ulcerative colitis who were studied) was 20.7%. When adalimumab monotherapy for plaque psoriasis was withdrawn and subsequently reinitiated, the incidence of antibody formation following retreatment was similar to that observed prior to drug withdrawal.

Immunization. Live vaccines should be avoided during therapy with adalimumab. Patients receiving adalimumab may receive inactivated vaccines. (See Drug Interactions: Vaccines.)

Psoriasis. Cases of new-onset psoriasis, including pustular and palmoplantar psoriasis, have been reported with the use of TNF blocking agents, including adalimumab. In August 2009, FDA reported the results of a review of 69 cases of new-onset psoriasis, including pustular (17 cases) and palmoplantar (15 cases) psoriasis, in patients receiving TNF blocking agents for the management of autoimmune and rheumatic conditions other than psoriasis and psoriatic arthritis. None of the patients reported having psoriasis prior to initiation of the TNF blocking agent. However, exacerbation of preexisting psoriasis has been reported with the use of TNF blocking agents. Two of the 69 cases of new-onset psoriasis included in FDA's review occurred in pediatric patients. The development of psoriasis during treatment with TNF blocking agents occurred from weeks to years following initiation of the drug. Twelve of the psoriasis cases resulted in hospitalization, which was the most severe outcome reported. Most patients experienced improvement of their psoriasis following discontinuance of the TNF blocking agent. Due to the number of reported cases and the temporal relationship between the initiation of TNF blocking agents and the development of psoriasis, FDA has concluded that there is a possible association between the development of psoriasis and use of TNF blocking agents. Clinicians should consider the possibility of and monitor for manifestations (e.g., new rash) of new or worsening psoriasis, particularly pustular and palmoplantar psoriasis, during treatment with TNF blocking agents.

Hepatic Effects. Severe hepatic reactions, including acute liver failure, have been reported in patients receiving TNF blocking agents. In phase 3 clinical studies evaluating adalimumab in patients with rheumatoid arthritis, psoriatic arthritis, or ankylosing spondylitis, increased serum ALT concentrations of 3 or more times the upper limit of normal occurred in 3.5% of adalimumab-treated patients compared with 1.5% of control patients. Because many of the patients in these studies received concomitant therapy with drugs known to increase liver enzyme concentrations (e.g., methotrexate, nonsteroidal anti-inflammatory agents [NSAIAs]), the relationship between adalimumab and increased liver enzyme concentrations is not clear. In phase 3 studies in patients with Crohn's disease or plaque psoriasis, serum ALT elevations of 3 or more times the upper limit of normal were observed in equal proportions of adalimumab-treated patients and control patients with Crohn's disease (0.9%) or plaque psoriasis (1.8%). In phase 3 studies in patients with ulcerative colitis, serum ALT elevations of 3 or more times the upper limit of normal were observed in 1.5% of patients receiving adalimumab at the recommended dosage and 1% of patients receiving placebo.

Specific Populations **Pregnancy.** Category B. (See Users Guide and see Pediatric Use under Warnings/Precautions: Specific Populations, in Cautions.)

Lactation. Limited data indicate that small amounts of adalimumab distribute into human milk and suggest that the drug is not likely to be absorbed by breast-fed infants. Although adalimumab was used in 2 nursing women without apparent adverse effects on their breast-fed infants, systemic bioavailability of the drug from milk has not been determined and any effect of this exposure on nursing infants is unknown. (See Pediatric Use under Warnings/Precautions: Specific Populations, in Cautions.) In addition, the potential for neonates and preterm infants to absorb the drug from breast milk is unknown. The drug should be used with caution in nursing women.

Pediatric Use. Safety and efficacy of adalimumab for uses other than juvenile idiopathic arthritis have not been established in pediatric patients.

Safety and efficacy of adalimumab for the management of juvenile idiopathic arthritis have been evaluated in pediatric patients 4–17 years of age. Adalimumab has not been studied in patients younger than 4 years of age, and data in patients weighing less than 15 kg are limited.

When use of adalimumab is being considered for pediatric patients, the vaccination status of the child should be reviewed and all age-appropriate vaccines included in the current Recommended Childhood Immunization Schedule (see Immunization Schedules, US 80:00) should be administered.

Malignancies, some fatal, have been reported in children and adolescents who received treatment with TNF blocking agents, including adalimumab. (See Malignancies and Lymphoproliferative Disorders under Warnings/Precautions: Warnings, in Cautions.)

Neonates and infants who were exposed to adalimumab in utero may have impaired immune responses. Data from 8 infants exposed to adalimumab in utero suggest that the drug crosses the placenta; the clinical importance of elevated adalimumab concentrations in infants is unknown. The risks and benefits of administering live vaccines to infants who were exposed to adalimumab in utero should be considered, since the safety of live vaccines in these infants is unknown.

Geriatric Use. No substantial differences in efficacy have been observed in geriatric patients relative to younger adults. The incidence of serious infection and malignancy in adalimumab-treated patients older than 65 years of age is higher than the incidence in younger adults receiving the drug. Because the overall incidence of infection and malignancy is higher in the geriatric population in general than in younger adults, adalimumab should be used with caution in geriatric patients.

■ **Common Adverse Effects** Adverse effects reported in 5% or more of patients receiving adalimumab for the management of rheumatoid arthritis include upper respiratory tract infection, headache, rash, sinusitis, accidental injury, nausea, injection site reaction, urinary tract infection, flu syndrome, abdominal pain, hyperlipidemia, hypercholesterolemia, back pain, hematuria, increase in alkaline phosphatase, and hypertension. Adverse effects reported in patients with psoriatic arthritis, Crohn's disease, ulcerative colitis, or ankylosing spondylitis are similar to those in patients with rheumatoid arthritis. In clinical studies in patients with plaque psoriasis, arthralgia was observed in a greater proportion of patients receiving adalimumab than in patients receiving placebo.

Adverse effects reported in patients with juvenile idiopathic arthritis receiving adalimumab generally are similar in frequency and type to those in adults. Severe adverse reactions reported in pediatric patients include neutropenia, streptococcal pharyngitis, increased serum concentrations of aminotransferases, herpes zoster, myositis, metrorrhagia, appendicitis, and infection. Adverse reactions reported in 5% or more of patients receiving adalimumab for the management of juvenile idiopathic arthritis include infection, injection site pain, injection site reaction, hypersensitivity reaction (e.g., localized allergic sensitivity reaction, rash), and mild to moderate increases in creatine kinase (CK, creatine phosphokinase, CPK) concentration.

Drug Interactions

■ **Drugs Metabolized by Hepatic Microsomal Enzymes** Because increased levels of cytokines (e.g., tumor necrosis factor [TNF; TNF-α]) during chronic inflammation may suppress the formation of cytochrome P-450 (CYP) isoenzymes, it is possible that a drug that antagonizes cytokine activity, such as adalimumab, could normalize the formation of CYP enzymes. Following initiation or discontinuance of adalimumab therapy, patients receiving certain drugs metabolized by CYP isoenzymes (i.e., those with a low therapeutic index [e.g., cyclosporine, theophylline, warfarin]) should be monitored for therapeutic effect and/or changes in serum concentrations, and dosages of these drugs may be adjusted as needed.

■ **Biologic Antirheumatic Agents** Concomitant use of adalimumab and other biologic disease-modifying antirheumatic drugs (DMARDs) is not recommended.

Caution should be exercised when switching from one biologic DMARD to another, since overlapping biologic activity may further increase the risk of infection.

Abatacept When abatacept (a selective costimulation modulator) and a TNF blocking agent were used concomitantly in patients with rheumatoid arthritis, an increased incidence of infection and serious infection was observed, with no substantial improvement in efficacy over that observed with a TNF blocking agent alone. Concomitant use of adalimumab and abatacept is not recommended.

Anakinra When anakinra (a human interleukin-1 receptor antagonist) and etanercept (another TNF blocking agent) were used concomitantly in patients with rheumatoid arthritis, an increased incidence of serious infection and neutropenia was observed, with no substantial improvement in efficacy over that observed with etanercept alone. Concomitant use of adalimumab and anakinra is not recommended.

Rituximab An increased risk of serious infection has been observed in patients with rheumatoid arthritis who received rituximab (an anti-CD20 monoclonal antibody) and subsequently received therapy with a TNF blocking agent.

Tocilizumab Concomitant use of tocilizumab (an anti-interleukin-6-receptor monoclonal antibody) and biologic DMARDs such as TNF blocking agents has not been studied and should be avoided because of the possibility of increased immunosuppression and increased risk of infection.

Other TNF Blocking Agents Concomitant use of adalimumab and other TNF blocking agents is not recommended.

Other Biologic Antirheumatic Agents The manufacturer states that insufficient data are available regarding the concomitant use of adalimumab and other biologic agents used in the management of rheumatoid arthritis, psoriatic arthritis, ankylosing spondylitis, Crohn's disease, ulcerative colitis, or plaque psoriasis.

■ **Methotrexate** Methotrexate decreased clearance of adalimumab after single or multiple doses by 29 or 44%, respectively, in patients with rheumatoid arthritis; dosage adjustment is not necessary.

■ **Natalizumab** Concomitant use of natalizumab (an anti-α4-integrin monoclonal antibody) and TNF blocking agents in the management of Crohn's disease should be avoided since such use may result in increased risk of progressive multifocal leukoencephalopathy (PML) or other serious infections.

■ **Vaccines** Live vaccines should not be administered to patients receiving adalimumab. Information is not available regarding whether adalimumab would affect the rate of secondary transmission of infection following administration of a live vaccine.

Patients receiving adalimumab may receive inactivated vaccines. Antibody response to inactivated vaccines (i.e., pneumococcal polysaccharide vaccine, influenza virus vaccine inactivated) has been investigated in patients receiving adalimumab. In patients with rheumatoid arthritis, no difference in antibody response to pneumococcal polysaccharide vaccine was detected between patients receiving adalimumab and patients receiving placebo. Adalimumab-treated rheumatoid arthritis patients receiving influenza virus vaccine inactivated have developed protective antibody titers; however, titers to influenza antigens were lower in patients receiving adalimumab than in placebo-treated patients.

Description

Adalimumab, a human monoclonal antibody specific for human tumor necrosis factor (TNF; TNF-α), is a biologic response modifier. Adalimumab is an immunoglobulin G_1 (IgG_1) made by phage display technology with amino acid sequences from the human germline; adalimumab does not contain nonhuman components or artificially fused human peptide sequences. Adalimumab is indistinguishable in structure and function from naturally occurring human IgG_1 and has a terminal half-life comparable to that of human IgG_1 (about 2 weeks). Adalimumab is produced by recombinant DNA technology in a mammalian cell expression system and is purified by a process that includes specific viral inactivation and removal steps.

Adalimumab has high specificity and affinity for TNF (TNF-α); adalimumab does not bind to or inactivate lymphotoxin α (TNF-β). Adalimumab binds to TNF before TNF can interact with the p55 and p75 cell surface tumor necrosis factor receptors (TNFRs). By preventing the binding of TNF to cell surface TNFRs, adalimumab blocks the biologic activity of TNF. In vitro, adalimumab lyses surface TNF-expressing cells in the presence of complement.

TNF, a naturally occurring cytokine, has a broad spectrum of biologic activities; TNF is involved in normal inflammatory and immune responses and also plays a role in a number of autoimmune and inflammatory diseases, including rheumatoid arthritis, juvenile idiopathic arthritis, psoriatic arthritis, and ankylosing spondylitis. While the causes of rheumatoid arthritis have not been fully elucidated, increased concentrations of TNF in the synovial fluid of rheumatoid arthritis patients play a critical role in the progression of inflammatory synovitis and articular matrix degradation in these patients. TNF promotes the synthesis of other proinflammatory cytokines, stimulates endothelial cells to express adhesion molecules that attract leukocytes into affected joints, accelerates the production of metalloproteinases, and inhibits the synthesis of cartilage proteoglycans. Increased concentrations of TNF also are found in psoriatic plaques. Adalimumab treatment may reduce epidermal thickness and infiltration of inflammatory cells in plaque psoriasis. Adalimumab modulates responses that are induced or regulated by TNF, including expression of adhesion molecules, serum concentrations of matrix metalloproteinase, and serum concentrations of cytokines.

Advice to Patients

Importance of advising patients about potential benefits and risks of adalimumab. Importance of patients reading the manufacturer's patient information (medication guide) prior to initiation of therapy and each time the prescription is refilled.

Importance of instructing patient and/or caregiver regarding proper dosage and administration of adalimumab, including the use of aseptic technique, and proper disposal of needles and syringes if it is determined that the patient and/or caregiver is competent to safely administer the drug.

Increased susceptibility to infection. Importance of seeking immediate medical attention if signs and symptoms suggestive of infection (e.g., fever; fatigue; cough; warm, red, or painful skin; sores on the body; muscle aches; diarrhea; stomach pain; shortness of breath; weight loss; burning on urination; urinary frequency) develop.

Risk of lymphoma, including hepatosplenic T-cell lymphoma, leukemia, or other malignancies with use of tumor necrosis factor (TNF) blocking agents. Importance of informing patients and caregivers about the increased risk of cancer development in children, adolescents, and young adults, taking into account the clinical utility of TNF blocking agents, the relative risks and benefits of these and other immunosuppressive drugs, and the risks associated with untreated disease. Importance of promptly informing clinicians if signs and symptoms of malignancies (e.g., unexplained weight loss; fatigue; abdominal pain; persistent fever; night sweats; easy bruising or bleeding; swollen lymph nodes in the neck, underarm, or groin; hepatomegaly or splenomegaly) occur.

Importance of informing clinician of any new or worsening medical conditions (e.g., neurologic conditions [e.g., demyelinating disorders], heart failure, autoimmune disorders [e.g., lupus-like syndrome], psoriasis, cytopenias).

Importance of alerting clinician if allergy to latex exists.

Importance of promptly contacting a clinician if manifestations of an allergic reaction (e.g., urticaria, facial swelling, difficulty breathing) occur.

Importance of taking the drug as prescribed and of not altering or discontinuing therapy without first consulting with a clinician.

Importance of informing clinicians of existing or contemplated concomitant therapy, including prescription and OTC drugs, as well as any concomitant illnesses or any history of cancer, tuberculosis, hepatitis B virus infection, or other chronic or recurring infections.

Importance of women informing clinicians if they are or plan to become pregnant or plan to breast-feed.

Importance of informing patients of other important precautionary information. (See Cautions.)

Preparations

Excipients in commercially available drug preparations may have clinically important effects in some individuals; consult specific product labeling for details.

Adalimumab

Parenteral

Injection, for subcutaneous use	20 mg/0.4 mL	**Humira®** (available as disposable prefilled syringes with alcohol swabs), Abbott
	40 mg/0.8 mL	**Humira®** (available as disposable prefilled syringes and prefilled injection pens with alcohol swabs, and as single-use vials), Abbott

Selected Revisions May 2018, © Copyright, September 2003, American Society of Health-System Pharmacists, Inc.

Apremilast

■ Apremilast, a selective phosphodiesterase type 4 (PDE4) inhibitor, is a disease-modifying antirheumatic drug (DMARD).

Uses

■ **Psoriatic Arthritis** Apremilast is used for the management of active psoriatic arthritis in adults. The drug has been shown to reduce the signs and symptoms of active arthritis and to improve physical function in patients with the disease.

Safety and efficacy of apremilast for the management of active psoriatic arthritis were evaluated in 3 randomized, double-blind, placebo-controlled studies (PALACE-1, PALACE-2, and PALACE-3) in 1493 adults with active psoriatic arthritis (as defined by the Classification Criteria for Psoriatic Arthritis [CASPAR], with 3 or more swollen joints and 3 or more tender joints) who had an inadequate response to therapy with biologic and/or nonbiologic disease-modifying antirheumatic drugs (DMARDs). Patients also were required to have had a diagnosis of psoriatic arthritis for at least 6 months and, in PALACE-3, to have plaque psoriasis with a qualifying skin lesion (diameter of 2 cm or greater). Patients were randomized to receive apremilast 20 or 30 mg twice daily (initiated at 10 mg daily and titrated in increments of 10 mg each day to the assigned dosage) or placebo and were stratified by baseline DMARD treatment. Patients receiving stable dosages of methotrexate (25 mg/week or less), leflunomide (20 mg/day or less), sulfasalazine (2 g/day or less), low-dose oral corticosteroids (equivalent to 10 mg of prednisone daily or less), and/or nonsteroidal anti-inflammatory agents (NSAIAs) could continue such agents during the studies. Prior DMARD therapy included only nonbiologic agents in 76% of patients; 22% of patients had received prior therapy with biologic DMARDs. Patients who had experienced treatment failure following use of more than 3 biologic or nonbiologic DMARDs or more than 1 tumor necrosis factor (TNF; TNF-α) blocking agent were excluded, and no more than 10% of patients enrolled in the studies were allowed to have a history of TNF blocker failure. During the studies, 65% of patients received concomitant therapy with at least one DMARD, with 55, 7, or 9% of patients receiving stable dosages of methotrexate, leflunomide, or sulfasalazine, respectively; in addition, 14 or 71% of patients received stable dosages of low-dose oral corticosteroids or NSAIAs, respectively. The median duration of psoriatic arthritis was 5 years; most patients had either the symmetric polyarthritis (62%) or asymmetric oligoarthritis (27%) form of the disease.

The primary outcome measure in all 3 studies was the proportion of patients achieving an American College of Rheumatology (ACR) 20 response (modified for psoriatic arthritis) at week 16. An ACR 20 response was achieved if the patient experienced a 20% improvement in tender and swollen joint count and a 20% or greater improvement in at least 3 of the following criteria: patient pain assessment, patient global assessment, physician global assessment, patient self-assessed disability, or laboratory measures of disease activity (i.e., C-reactive protein [CRP] level). ACR 50 and 70 responses are defined using the same criteria with a level of improvement of 50 or 70%, respectively. Physical function was assessed using the Health Assessment Questionnaire Disability Index (HAQ-DI).

In all 3 studies, a greater proportion of patients who received apremilast achieved an ACR 20 response at week 16 than did those who received placebo. Among patients receiving apremilast 20 or 30 mg twice daily, ACR 20 response rates at week 16 were 30 or 38%, respectively, in PALACE-1; 37 or 32%, respectively, in PALACE-2; and 28 or 41%, respectively, in PALACE-3; in comparison, 18–19% of patients receiving placebo in the 3 studies attained ACR 20 responses at week 16. The response data indicated a small numerical advantage for the 30-mg dosage over the 20-mg dosage, but results of the 3 studies did not show a clear, consistent statistical or clinical advantage for the higher dosage.

ACR 50 and 70 responses at week 16 generally supported the primary efficacy results. ACR 50 response rates at week 16 for patients receiving apremilast 20 or 30 mg twice daily were 16 or 16%, respectively, in PALACE-1; 15 or 11%, respectively, in PALACE-2; and 12 or 15%, respectively, in PALACE-3; 5–8% of patients receiving placebo in the 3 studies attained ACR 50 responses at week 16. ACR 70 response rates at week 16 for patients receiving apremilast 20 or 30 mg twice daily were 6 or 4%, respectively, in PALACE-1; 4 or 1%, respectively, in PALACE-2; and 5 or 4%, respectively, in PALACE-3; 1–2% of patients receiving placebo in the 3 studies attained ACR 70 responses at week 16. Apremilast also improved dactylitis and enthesitis in patients with these manifestations of the disease.

Improvements in physical function (as measured by change in HAQ-DI score) from baseline to week 16 were greater in all 3 studies for patients receiving apremilast 30 mg twice daily compared with those receiving placebo and also were greater in 2 of the 3 studies (PALACE-1 and PALACE-2) for patients receiving apremilast 20 mg twice daily compared with those receiving placebo.

■ **Plaque Psoriasis** Apremilast is used for the management of moderate to severe plaque psoriasis in adults who are candidates for phototherapy or systemic therapy. Apremilast has been shown to reduce disease activity, as measured by the Psoriasis Area and Severity Index (PASI) and the static Physician Global Assessment (sPGA) score, in such patients. PASI is a composite score that takes into consideration both the fraction of body surface area affected and the nature and severity of the psoriatic changes within the affected areas (i.e., induration, erythema, scaling); the sPGA measures the clinician's impression of disease severity at a single time point.

In 2 randomized, double-blind, placebo-controlled studies (ESTEEM 1 and ESTEEM 2), 1257 adults who had moderate to severe plaque psoriasis, with involvement of at least 10% of the body surface area, an sPGA score of 3 or greater, and a PASI score of 12 or greater, and who were candidates for phototherapy or systemic therapy were randomized to receive apremilast 30 mg twice daily or placebo. Patients could receive concurrent therapy with certain topical treatments (i.e., low-potency topical corticosteroids on the face, axilla, and groin; coal tar shampoo and/or salicylic acid preparations for psoriatic scalp lesions). Approximately 30% of patients enrolled in the study had received prior phototherapy and 54% had received prior conventional systemic and/or biologic therapy for psoriasis; approximately one-third of the patients had received no prior phototherapy or systemic or biologic therapy. The mean baseline PASI score was 19.07, and approximately 70 or 30% of patients had baseline sPGA scores of 3 (indicating moderate disease) or 4 (indicating severe disease), respectively. At week 16, 28.8–33.1% of patients receiving apremilast achieved a reduction in PASI score of at least 75% from baseline (PASI 75 response), compared with 5.3–5.8% of those receiving placebo. In addition, 20.4–21.7% of patients receiving apremilast achieved a status of clear (0) or almost clear (1) on the sPGA scale at week 16, compared with 3.9–4.4% of those receiving placebo. Among patients who responded to apremilast and were rerandomized at week 32 to receive placebo, the median time to loss of PASI 75 response following treatment withdrawal was 5.1 weeks.

Dosage and Administration

■ **Administration** Apremilast is administered orally without regard to meals. Apremilast tablets should *not*be crushed, split, or chewed.

■ **Dosage** ***Psoriatic Arthritis*** For the management of active psoriatic arthritis in adults, the recommended maintenance dosage of apremilast is 30 mg twice daily. Therapy should be initiated at a low dosage and increased gradually (over 5 days in increments of 10 mg daily) to reduce the risk of GI symptoms. The recommended titration schedule is as follows: 10 mg in the morning on day 1, 10 mg in the morning and 10 mg in the evening on day 2, 10 mg in the morning and 20 mg in the evening on day 3, 20 mg in the morning and 20 mg in the evening on day 4, 20 mg in the morning and 30 mg in the evening on day 5, and 30 mg twice daily thereafter.

Plaque Psoriasis For the management of moderate to severe plaque psoriasis in adults, the recommended maintenance dosage of apremilast is 30 mg twice daily. Therapy should be initiated at a low dosage and increased gradually (over 5 days in increments of 10 mg daily) to reduce the risk of GI symptoms. The recommended titration schedule is as follows: 10 mg in the morning on day 1, 10 mg in the morning and 10 mg in the evening on day 2, 10 mg in the morning and 20 mg in the evening on day 3, 20 mg in the morning and 20 mg in the evening on day 4, 20 mg in the morning and 30 mg in the evening on day 5, and 30 mg twice daily thereafter.

■ **Special Populations** In adults with severe renal impairment (creatinine clearance less than 30 mL/minute), a reduced maintenance apremilast dosage of 30 mg once daily is recommended for the management of active psoriatic arthritis or moderate to severe plaque psoriasis; the recommended dosage titration schedule for initiation of therapy in adults with severe renal impairment is as follows: 10 mg in the morning for 3 days (days 1, 2, and 3), followed by 20 mg in the morning for 2 days (days 4 and 5), and then 30 mg once daily thereafter. Dosage adjustments are not necessary in patients with hepatic impairment. The manufacturer makes no specific dosage recommendations for geriatric patients. (See Specific Populations under Cautions: Warnings/Precautions.)

Cautions

■ **Contraindications** Apremilast is contraindicated in patients with known hypersensitivity to the drug or any ingredient in the formulation.

■ **Warnings/Precautions** ***Depression and Suicidality*** Apremilast therapy is associated with an increase in depression. In clinical trials in patients with psoriatic arthritis, depression or depressed mood was reported in 1% of patients receiving apremilast compared with 0.8% of those receiving placebo and resulted in discontinuance of the assigned treatment in 0.3% of those receiving the drug compared with none of those receiving placebo; depression was considered serious in 0.2% of apremilast-treated patients and no placebo recipients. In clinical trials in patients with psoriasis, depression was reported in 1.3% of patients receiving apremilast compared with 0.4% of those receiving placebo and resulted in discontinuance of the assigned treatment in 0.1% of patients receiving the drug and none of those receiving placebo; depression was considered serious in 0.1% of apremilast-treated patients and no placebo recipients.

Suicidal ideation and behavior, including completed suicide, also have been observed in clinical trials. In clinical trials in patients with psoriatic arthritis, suicidal ideation and behavior were observed in 3 patients (0.2%) receiving apremilast and in no patients receiving placebo; completed suicide was reported in no patients receiving apremilast but in 2 patients receiving placebo. In clinical trials in patients with psoriasis, suicidal behavior was observed in 1 patient (0.1%) receiving apremilast and in 1 patient (0.2%) receiving placebo; 1 patient receiving apremilast attempted suicide and 1 patient receiving placebo completed suicide.

Clinicians should carefully weigh the risks and benefits of apremilast therapy prior to using the drug in patients with a history of depression and/or suicidal thoughts or behavior. In addition, clinicians should carefully evaluate the risks and benefits of continuing therapy with apremilast if such effects occur. (See Advice to Patients.)

Weight Loss Weight loss has been reported in patients receiving recommended dosages of apremilast. In clinical trials in patients with psoriatic arthritis, weight loss of 5–10% of body weight was reported in 10% of patients receiving apremilast (30 mg twice daily) compared with 3.3% of those receiving placebo. In clinical trials in patients with psoriasis, weight loss of 5–10% of body weight was reported in 12% of patients receiving apremilast (30 mg twice daily) compared with 5% of those receiving placebo, while loss of 10% or more of body weight was reported in 2% of patients receiving apremilast (30 mg twice daily) and 1% of those receiving placebo.

Weight should be monitored regularly in patients receiving apremilast. If unexplained or clinically important weight loss occurs, weight loss should be evaluated and discontinuance of apremilast should be considered.

Interactions Concomitant use of cytochrome P-450 (CYP) enzyme inducers (e.g., carbamazepine, phenobarbital, phenytoin, rifampin) with apremilast is not recommended because loss of apremilast efficacy may occur. (See Drug Interactions: Drugs Affecting Hepatic Microsomal Enzymes.)

Specific Populations **Pregnancy.** Category C. (See Users Guide.)

Reproduction studies in cynomolgus monkeys receiving apremilast during organogenesis resulted in dose-related increases in spontaneous abortion and embryofetal death at doses equivalent to 2.1 times the maximum recommended human dose. To monitor pregnancy outcomes in women who have been exposed to apremilast, a pregnancy registry has been established. Information about the registry can be obtained by calling 877-311-8972.

Lactation. Apremilast is distributed into milk in mice; it is not known whether the drug is distributed into human milk. Apremilast should be used with caution in nursing women.

Pediatric Use. Safety and efficacy of apremilast have not been established in pediatric patients younger than 18 years of age.

Geriatric Use. In controlled clinical trials evaluating apremilast for the management of psoriatic arthritis, about 10% of patients were 65 years of age and older, while about 1% were 75 years of age and older. No overall differences in safety were observed between geriatric and younger adults.

In controlled clinical trials evaluating apremilast for the management of psoriasis, about 9% of patients were 65 years of age and older, while less than 1% were 75 years of age and older. No overall differences in efficacy and safety were observed between geriatric and younger adults.

Following oral administration of a single 30-mg dose of apremilast, area under the concentration-time curve (AUC) and peak plasma concentrations of the drug were approximately 13 and 6% higher, respectively, in patients 65–85 years of age compared with those 18–55 years of age.

Hepatic Impairment. Moderate or severe hepatic impairment (Child-Pugh class B or C) does not alter the pharmacokinetics of apremilast. No dosage adjustment is necessary in these patients.

Renal Impairment. Following administration of a single 30-mg dose of apremilast in patients with severe renal impairment (creatinine clearance less than 30 mL/minute), AUC and peak plasma concentrations of the drug were increased by approximately 88 and 42%, respectively. Dosage adjustment is recommended in patients with severe renal impairment. (See Dosage and Administration: Special Populations.) The effects of mild or moderate renal impairment on the pharmacokinetics of the drug have not been determined to date.

■ **Common Adverse Effects** Adverse effects reported in 2% or more of patients receiving apremilast 30 mg twice daily for active psoriatic arthritis (and at a frequency that was at least 1% higher than that reported for placebo) include diarrhea, nausea, headache, upper respiratory tract infection, vomiting, nasopharyngitis, and upper abdominal pain.

Adverse effects reported in 2% or more of patients receiving apremilast for psoriasis (and with greater frequency than in patients receiving placebo) include diarrhea, nausea, upper respiratory tract infection, tension headache, headache, abdominal pain, vomiting, fatigue, dyspepsia, decreased appetite, insomnia, back pain, migraine, and frequent bowel movements.

Drug Interactions

Apremilast undergoes cytochrome P-450 (CYP)-mediated oxidative metabolism, with subsequent glucuronidation, and non-CYP-mediated hydrolysis. In vitro, oxidative metabolism is mediated principally by CYP3A4, with minor contributions from CYP1A2 and CYP2A6.

In vitro, apremilast does not inhibit CYP isoenzyme 1A2, 2A6, 2B6, 2C8, 2C9, 2C19, 2D6, 2E1, or 3A4, nor does apremilast induce CYP isoenzyme 1A2, 2B6, 2C9, 2C19, or 3A4.

In vitro data indicate that apremilast is a substrate but not an inhibitor of P-glycoprotein (P-gp) and that the drug is neither a substrate nor an inhibitor of organic anion transporters (OAT) 1 and 3, organic anion transporting polypeptides (OATP) 1B1 and 1B3, organic cation transporter (OCT) 2, or breast cancer resistance protein (BCRP).

■ **Drugs Affecting Hepatic Microsomal Enzymes** Systemic exposure of apremilast is reduced when the drug is used concomitantly with potent CYP inducers (see Drug Interactions: Rifampin). Concomitant use of apremilast with potent CYP inducers (e.g., carbamazepine, phenobarbital, phenytoin, rifampin) may result in loss of apremilast efficacy and is not recommended.

■ **Estrogens/Progestins** In healthy women, concomitant administration of apremilast (30 mg twice daily) with an oral contraceptive containing the CYP3A4 substrates ethinyl estradiol and norgestimate did not substantially affect the pharmacokinetics of the oral contraceptive components; pharmacokinetics of apremilast also were unchanged.

■ **Ketoconazole** In healthy individuals, concomitant administration of ketoconazole (400 mg daily for 7 days) (an inhibitor of both CYP3A and P-gp) with apremilast (single 20-mg dose) appeared to have some effects on apremilast disposition, but overall did not result in clinically important effects on exposure to the drug.

■ **Methotrexate** In patients receiving stable weekly methotrexate therapy, concomitant use of apremilast (30 mg twice daily) with methotrexate (15 or 20 mg once weekly) did not substantially affect the pharmacokinetics of either drug.

■ **Rifampin** When the potent CYP inducer rifampin (600 mg once daily for 15 days) was administered concomitantly with apremilast (single 30-mg dose) in healthy individuals, area under the concentration-time curve (AUC) and peak plasma concentration of apremilast were reduced by 72 and 43%, respectively. Concomitant use may result in loss of apremilast efficacy and is not recommended.

Description

Apremilast, a selective inhibitor of phosphodiesterase type 4 (PDE4), is a disease-modifying antirheumatic drug (DMARD). PDE4 is the dominant phosphodiesterase expressed in immune cells and a major enzyme involved in metabolism of cyclic adenosine-3',5'-monophosphate (cAMP). Thus, selective inhibition of PDE4 results in accumulation of intracellular cAMP, a modulator of inflammatory responses, which can down-regulate inflammatory responses by increasing expression of anti-inflammatory mediators and partially inhibiting expression of inflammatory cytokines that are thought to play a role in the pathogenesis of psoriasis and active psoriatic arthritis. The exact mechanism(s) of action of apremilast in the management of these conditions has not been fully elucidated.

Following oral administration, apremilast has an absolute bioavailability of approximately 73%. Administration with food does not alter the extent of absorption. Apremilast is extensively metabolized; up to 23 metabolites have been identified in plasma, urine, and feces. The major circulating forms of the drug are apremilast (45%) and the inactive glucuronide conjugate M12 (39%). Apremilast undergoes cytochrome P-450 (CYP)-mediated oxidative metabolism, with subsequent glucuronidation, and non-CYP-mediated hydrolysis; in vitro, oxidative metabolism is mediated principally by CYP3A4, with minor contributions from CYP1A2 and CYP2A6. The terminal elimination half-life of apremilast is approximately 6–9 hours. Following oral administration of radiolabeled apremilast, approximately 58% of radioactivity was recovered in urine and 39% was recovered in feces; unchanged drug in urine and feces accounted for only 3 and 7%, respectively, of the radiolabeled dose.

Advice to Patients

Importance of instructing patients that apremilast should be taken only as prescribed. Importance of advising patients that apremilast tablets should *not* be crushed, split, or chewed. Importance of informing patients that apremilast may be taken without regard to meals.

Risk of emergence or worsening of depression. Importance of instructing patients and their caregivers or families to be alert for the emergence or worsening of depression, suicidal thoughts, or other mood changes and to contact a clinician if such changes occur.

Risk of weight loss. Importance of regular monitoring for weight loss and of informing a clinician if substantial or unexplained weight loss occurs.

Risk of interactions with drugs that are potent inducers of cytochrome P-450 (CYP) enzymes (e.g., carbamazepine, phenobarbital, phenytoin, rifampin). Importance of informing clinician of existing or contemplated concomitant therapy, including prescription and OTC drugs and dietary or herbal supplements, as well as any concomitant illnesses.

Importance of women informing their clinician if they are or plan to become pregnant or plan to breast-feed.

Importance of informing patients of other precautionary information. (See Cautions.)

Overview® (see Users Guide). For additional information on this drug until a more detailed monograph is developed and published, the manufacturer's labeling should be consulted. It is *essential* that the manufacturer's labeling be consulted for more detailed information on usual cautions, precautions, contraindications, potential drug interactions, laboratory test interferences, and acute toxicity.

Preparations

Excipients in commercially available drug preparations may have clinically important effects in some individuals; consult specific product labeling for details.

Apremilast

Oral		
Kit	4 Tablets, film-coated, Apremilast 10 mg (Otezla®) 4 Tablets, film-coated, Apremilast 20 mg (Otezla®) 19 Tablets, film-coated, Apremilast 30 mg (Otezla®)	**Otezla® Starter Pack** (available as blister pack containing tablets for first 2 weeks of therapy), Celgene
Tablets, film-coated	30 mg	**Otezla®**, Celgene

Selected Revisions May 2018, © Copyright, March 2015, American Society of Health-System Pharmacists, Inc.

Baricitinib

■ Baricitinib, a Janus kinase (JAK) inhibitor, is an immunomodulating agent and a disease-modifying antirheumatic drug (DMARD).

Uses

■ **Rheumatoid Arthritis in Adults** Baricitinib is used for the management of moderately to severely active rheumatoid arthritis in adults who have had an inadequate response to one or more tumor necrosis factor (TNF; TNF-α) blocking agents. Baricitinib has been shown to induce clinical responses and improve physical function in patients with rheumatoid arthritis when administered at the recommended dosage.

Baricitinib can be used alone or in combination with methotrexate or other nonbiologic disease-modifying antirheumatic drugs (DMARDs; examples include hydroxychloroquine, leflunomide, and sulfasalazine). Concomitant use of baricitinib with other Janus kinase (JAK) inhibitors (e.g., tofacitinib) or biologic DMARDs, such as TNF blocking agents (e.g., adalimumab, certolizumab pegol, etanercept, golimumab, infliximab), interleukin-1 (IL-1) receptor antagonists (e.g., anakinra), anti-CD20 monoclonal antibodies (e.g., rituximab), selective costimulation modulators (e.g., abatacept), and anti-interleukin-6-receptor monoclonal antibodies (e.g., sarilumab, tocilizumab), is not recommended. Concomitant use of baricitinib with potent immunosuppressive agents (e.g., azathioprine, cyclosporine) also is not recommended.

Efficacy and safety of baricitinib at a dosage of 2 mg daily have been evaluated in 2 randomized, double-blind, controlled studies (RA-BUILD and RA-BEACON) in adults with active rheumatoid arthritis, as defined by the American College of Rheumatology (ACR)/European League Against Rheumatism (EULAR) 2010 rheumatoid arthritis classification criteria. Patients had moderately to severely active disease with 6 or more tender joints, 6 or more swollen joints, and elevated C-reactive protein (CRP) concentrations at baseline. In RA-BUILD, patients who had an inadequate response or intolerance to at least one conventional nonbiologic DMARD were randomized to receive baricitinib 2 mg daily, baricitinib 4 mg daily, or placebo for 24 weeks either alone or in addition to a stable background regimen of up to 2 nonbiologic DMARDs; most patients were receiving methotrexate with or without another nonbiologic DMARD (23 or 49%, respectively) and only 7% were not receiving any other DMARDs concomitantly with baricitinib. Patients who had received prior biologic DMARD therapy were excluded from RA-BUILD. In RA-BEACON, patients who had an inadequate response or intolerance to at least one TNF blocking agent and were receiving a stable dosage of one or more nonbiologic DMARDs at study entry were randomized to receive baricitinib 2 mg daily, baricitinib 4 mg daily, or placebo for 24 weeks in addition to their existing nonbiologic DMARD therapy; approximately 38% of patients in RA-BEACON also had received prior therapy with at least one biologic DMARD that was not a TNF blocking agent. Patients in RA-BEACON were required to have discontinued biologic DMARDs at least 4 weeks before randomization (or at least 6 months for rituximab). In both studies, those receiving low stable dosages of corticosteroids (equivalent to 10 mg or less of prednisone daily) and/or stable dosages of nonsteroidal anti-inflammatory agents (NSAIAs) or analgesics could continue such agents. Patients who failed to achieve at least 20% reduction in tender and swollen joint counts by week 16 were switched from their assigned treatment to baricitinib 4 mg daily.

The ACR criteria for improvement (ACR response) in measures of disease activity were used as the principal measure of clinical response; an ACR 20 response is achieved if the patient experiences a 20% or greater improvement in tender and swollen joint count and a 20% or greater improvement in at least 3 of the following criteria: patient pain assessment, patient global assessment, physician global assessment, patient self-assessed disability, or laboratory measures of disease activity (i.e., erythrocyte sedimentation rate [ESR] or CRP level). An ACR 50 or ACR 70 response is defined using the same criteria but with a level of improvement of 50 or 70%, respectively. The primary end point in RA-BUILD and RA-BEACON was the proportion of patients who achieved an ACR 20 response at week 12.

In both studies, a substantially greater proportion of patients treated with baricitinib 2 or 4 mg daily achieved an ACR 20 response at weeks 12 and 24 compared with those receiving placebo. ACR 20 response was achieved at 12 weeks by 66, 62, or 39% of patients receiving baricitinib 2 mg daily, baricitinib 4 mg daily, or placebo, respectively, in RA-BUILD and by 49, 55, or 27% of patients receiving these respective treatments in RA-BEACON. ACR 50 and ACR 70 responses also were achieved in a greater proportion of baricitinib-treated patients compared with placebo recipients. In addition, a greater proportion of patients receiving baricitinib 2 or 4 mg daily in both studies achieved a low level of disease activity at week 12, as measured by a 28-joint Disease Activity Score using CRP (DAS 28 [CRP]) of less than 2.6, compared with those receiving placebo. Patients receiving baricitinib also demonstrated greater improvements in physical function as measured by the Health Assessment Questionnaire-Disability Index (HAQ-DI) at week 24.

Because a clear relationship between dosage and ACR response has not been established and because the risk of serious adverse events appears to be dose related, only the 2-mg daily dosage of baricitinib currently is recommended for management of rheumatoid arthritis in FDA-approved labeling. In addition, because of uncertain risk-benefit assessment, baricitinib currently is FDA-labeled only for patients who have had an inadequate response to one or more TNF blocking agents.

Dosage and Administration

■ **General** Baricitinib therapy should not be initiated in patients with an absolute lymphocyte count of less than 500/mm^3, an absolute neutrophil count (ANC) of less than 1000/mm^3, or hemoglobin concentration of less than 8 g/dL.

Baricitinib should not be used concomitantly with other Janus kinase (JAK) inhibitors, biologic disease-modifying antirheumatic drugs (DMARDs), or potent immunosuppressive agents. (See Uses: Rheumatoid Arthritis in Adults.)

Prior to initiation of baricitinib therapy, patients should be evaluated for latent tuberculosis infection; appropriate antimycobacterial treatment should be initiated if indicated. Baricitinib should not be used in patients with active tuberculosis or other serious active infection. (See Infectious Complications under Warnings/Precautions: Warnings, in Cautions.)

Restricted Distribution Baricitinib can only be obtained through specialty pharmacies. Clinicians may consult the Olumiant® website (https://www.olumiant.com) for specific information regarding distribution of the drug.

■ **Administration** Baricitinib is administered orally without regard to food.

■ **Dosage** ***Rheumatoid Arthritis in Adults*** For the management of rheumatoid arthritis in adults who have had an inadequate response or intolerance to one or more tumor necrosis factor (TNF; TNF-α) blocking agents, the recommended dosage of baricitinib is 2 mg once daily.

Treatment Interruption for Toxicity. If a serious infection develops, baricitinib therapy should be interrupted until the infection has been controlled.

Baricitinib therapy also should be interrupted in patients with lymphopenia, neutropenia, or anemia. (See Hematologic Effects under Warnings/Precautions: Other Warnings and Precautions, in Cautions.) If absolute lymphocyte count decreases to less than 500/mm^3, baricitinib therapy should be interrupted until lymphocyte count recovers to at least 500/mm^3. If ANC decreases to less than 1000/mm^3, baricitinib therapy should be interrupted until ANC recovers to at least 1000/mm^3. If hemoglobin concentration decreases to less than 8 g/dL, baricitinib therapy should be interrupted until hemoglobin concentration recovers to at least 8 g/dL. Following treatment interruption for lymphopenia, neutropenia, or anemia, baricitinib may be resumed at the recommended dosage of 2 mg daily.

■ **Special Populations** Dosage adjustment is not necessary in patients with mild renal impairment; however, baricitinib should not be used in patients with moderate to severe renal impairment (estimated glomerular filtration rate [eGFR] less than 60 mL/minute per 1.73 m^2). (See Renal Impairment under Warnings/Precautions: Specific Populations, in Cautions.)

Dosage adjustment is not necessary in patients with mild or moderate hepatic impairment. Use of the drug in patients with severe hepatic impairment has not been evaluated and is not recommended. (See Hepatic Impairment under Warnings/Precautions: Specific Populations, in Cautions.)

Dosage adjustments based on body weight, ethnicity, gender, or age are not required. (See Geriatric Use under Warnings/Precautions: Specific Populations, in Cautions.)

Cautions

■ **Contraindications** The manufacturer states that there are no known contraindications to the use of baricitinib.

■ **Warnings/Precautions** ***Warnings*** **Infectious Complications.** Serious and sometimes fatal infections, including bacterial, mycobacterial, invasive fungal, viral, or other opportunistic infections, have been reported in patients with rheumatoid arthritis receiving baricitinib. The most common serious infections reported in patients receiving baricitinib have included pneumonia, herpes zoster, and urinary tract infection. Tuberculosis may present with pulmonary or extrapulmonary disease. Opportunistic infections (e.g., multidermatomal herpes zoster, esophageal candidiasis, pneumocystosis, histoplasmosis, cryptococcosis, cytomegalovirus [CMV] infection, BK virus infection) have been reported in patients receiving baricitinib. Some patients have presented with disseminated rather than local disease. Most patients who experienced serious infections were receiving concomitant therapy with immunosuppressive agents such as methotrexate or corticosteroids.

In controlled clinical trials in patients with rheumatoid arthritis, the rate of infections during the first 16 weeks of treatment was approximately 99, 100, or 82 events per 100 patient-years in patients receiving baricitinib 2 mg daily, baricitinib 4 mg daily, or placebo, respectively. Serious infections during the first 16 weeks were reported at a rate of 3.6, 3.7, or 4.2 events per 100 patient-years in patients receiving baricitinib 2 mg daily, baricitinib 4 mg daily, or placebo, respectively.

Patients should be closely monitored during and after treatment with baricitinib for the development of signs or symptoms of infection.

Baricitinib therapy should not be initiated in patients with serious active infections, including localized infections. Clinicians should consider potential risks and benefits of the drug prior to initiating therapy in patients with a history of chronic, recurring, serious, or opportunistic infections; patients with underlying conditions that may predispose them to infections; and patients who have been exposed to tuberculosis or who reside or have traveled in regions where tuberculosis or mycoses are endemic. Any patient who develops a new infection while receiving baricitinib should undergo a thorough diagnostic evaluation (appropriate for an immunocompromised patient), appropriate anti-infective therapy should be initiated, and the patient should be closely monitored. Baricitinib therapy should be interrupted in patients who develop an infection that fails to respond to anti-infective therapy, a serious infection, an opportunistic infection, or sepsis and should not be resumed until the infection is controlled.

Because tuberculosis has been reported in patients receiving baricitinib, all patients should be evaluated for active or latent tuberculosis prior to and periodically during therapy with the drug. Patients with active tuberculosis should not receive baricitinib. When indicated, an appropriate antimycobacterial regimen for the treatment of latent tuberculosis infection should be initiated prior to baricitinib therapy. Antimycobacterial therapy also should be considered prior to initiation of baricitinib in individuals with a history of latent or active tuberculosis in whom an adequate course of antimycobacterial therapy cannot be confirmed and in individuals with a negative test for latent tuberculosis who have risk factors for tuberculosis. Consultation with a tuberculosis specialist is recommended when deciding whether antimycobacterial therapy should be initiated. Patients receiving baricitinib, including individuals with a negative test for latent tuberculosis, should be monitored for signs and symptoms of active tuberculosis.

Viral reactivation can occur in patients receiving baricitinib. Herpes zoster reactivation has been reported in patients receiving the drug. If herpes zoster reactivation occurs, baricitinib therapy should be interrupted until the episode has resolved.

The risk of reactivation of chronic viral hepatitis in patients receiving baricitinib is not known. Patients with evidence of active hepatitis B virus (HBV) or hepatitis C virus (HCV) infection were excluded from clinical trials of baricitinib. All patients should be screened for viral hepatitis in accordance with current standards of care before initiation of baricitinib therapy. Patients testing positive for hepatitis C antibody but negative for HCV RNA may receive baricitinib. Patients testing positive for hepatitis B surface antibody (anti-HBs) and hepatitis B core antibody (anti-HBc) but negative for hepatitis B surface antigen (HBsAg) also may receive baricitinib but should be monitored for expression of HBV DNA; consultation with liver disease experts is recommended if HBV DNA is detected.

Malignancies and Lymphoproliferative Disorders. Lymphoma and other malignancies have been observed in patients receiving baricitinib.

In controlled clinical trials in patients with moderately to severely active rheumatoid arthritis, malignancies (excluding nonmelanoma skin cancer) were reported during the first 16 weeks of treatment at a rate of 0.7 or 0.3 events per 100 patient-years in patients receiving baricitinib 2 or 4 mg daily, respectively, and at a rate of 0 events per 100 patient-years in placebo recipients. In a long-term extension study, malignancies (excluding nonmelanoma skin cancer) were reported at a rate of 0.6 or 0.7 events per 100 patient-years in patients receiving baricitinib 2 or 4 mg daily, respectively, for periods of up to 52 weeks.

The risks and benefits of baricitinib should be considered prior to initiating therapy in patients with a known malignancy (other than successfully treated nonmelanoma skin cancer) or when considering whether to continue baricitinib in patients who develop a malignancy.

Because nonmelanoma skin cancers have been reported in patients receiving baricitinib, periodic dermatologic examinations are recommended for patients receiving the drug who are at increased risk for skin cancer.

Thromboembolic Events. Serious and sometimes fatal thromboembolic events, including deep-vein thrombosis, pulmonary embolism, and arterial thrombosis in the extremities, have been reported in patients receiving baricitinib in controlled clinical trials. A relationship between platelet count elevation and thromboembolic events has not been established. (See Hematologic Effects under Warnings/Precautions: Other Warnings and Precautions, in Cautions.)

In controlled clinical trials in patients with moderately to severely active rheumatoid arthritis, venous thromboembolic events (i.e., deep-vein thrombosis or pulmonary embolism) were reported during the first 16 weeks of treatment at a rate of 1.7 events per 100 patient-years in patients receiving baricitinib 4 mg daily and in none of the patients receiving baricitinib 2 mg daily or placebo. In a long-term extension study, venous thromboembolic events were reported at a rate of 0.6 or 0.8 events per 100 patient-years in patients receiving baricitinib 2 or 4 mg daily, respectively, for periods of up to 52 weeks. Arterial thromboembolic events were reported during the first 16 weeks of treatment at a rate of 1.4 or 0.7 events per 100 patient-years in patients receiving baricitinib 2 or 4 mg daily, respectively, and at a rate of 0.3 events per 100 patient-years in placebo recipients; following treatment for periods of up to 52 weeks, the rate of arterial thromboembolic events was 0.9 or 0.3 events per 100 patient-years in patients receiving baricitinib 2 or 4 mg daily, respectively.

Baricitinib should be used with caution in patients who are at increased risk of thrombosis. Patients with signs or symptoms suggestive of deep-vein thrombosis, pulmonary embolism, or arterial thrombosis should be evaluated promptly and treated appropriately.

Other Warnings and Precautions **GI Perforation.** Cases of GI perforation have been reported in patients receiving baricitinib in controlled clinical trials. The role of Janus kinase (JAK) inhibition by baricitinib in these cases is not known. Baricitinib should be used with caution in patients who may be at increased risk for GI perforation (e.g., patients with a history of diverticulitis). Patients with new onset of abdominal symptoms should be evaluated promptly for early identification of GI perforation.

Hematologic Effects. Lymphopenia with absolute lymphocyte count less than 500/mm^3 has been reported in patients receiving baricitinib. Lymphocyte counts below the lower limit of normal were associated with infection in patients receiving baricitinib in controlled clinical trials. Lymphocyte counts should be monitored at baseline and periodically during treatment. Baricitinib therapy should not be initiated in patients with lymphocyte counts less than 500/mm^3, and treatment should be interrupted if lymphocyte count decreases to less than 500/mm^3.

Neutropenia with absolute neutrophil count (ANC) less than 1000/mm^3 has been reported in patients receiving baricitinib. Neutrophil counts should be monitored at baseline and periodically during treatment. Baricitinib therapy should not be initiated in patients with ANC less than 1000/mm^3, and treatment should be interrupted if ANC decreases to less than 1000/mm^3.

Anemia with hemoglobin concentration less than 8 g/dL has been reported in patients receiving baricitinib. Hemoglobin concentrations should be monitored at baseline and periodically during treatment. Baricitinib therapy should not be initiated in patients with hemoglobin concentrations less than 8 g/dL, and treatment should be interrupted if hemoglobin concentration decreases to less than 8 g/dL.

Dose-related increases in platelet count have been reported in patients receiving baricitinib. In controlled clinical trials in patients with rheumatoid arthritis, mean platelet counts at 16 weeks were increased by 15,000 or 23,000/mm^3 in patients receiving baricitinib 2 or 4 mg daily, respectively, compared with a mean increase of 3000/mm^3 in those who received placebo. A relationship between platelet count elevation and thromboembolic events has not been established. (See Thromboembolic Events under Warnings/Precautions: Warnings, in Cautions.)

Hepatic Effects. Baricitinib has been associated with elevated hepatic enzyme concentrations. AST and ALT elevations of at least 5 or at least 10 times the upper limit of normal (ULN) have been observed in controlled clinical trials.

Liver function tests should be monitored at baseline and periodically during treatment. In case of elevated hepatic enzyme concentrations, patients should be evaluated promptly for drug-induced hepatotoxicity. If drug-induced hepatic injury is suspected, baricitinib therapy should be interrupted until such diagnosis has been excluded.

Metabolic Effects. Dose-related increases in total cholesterol, low-density lipoprotein (LDL)-cholesterol, high-density lipoprotein (HDL)-cholesterol, and triglyceride concentrations have been observed in patients receiving baricitinib. Increases in these parameters were observed at 12 weeks of baricitinib therapy and concentrations remained stable thereafter. In controlled clinical trials, mean concentrations of LDL-cholesterol and HDL-cholesterol increased by 8 and 7 mg/dL, respectively, in patients receiving baricitinib 2 mg daily and by 14 and 9 mg/dL, respectively, in patients receiving baricitinib 4 mg daily. Mean ratios of LDL-cholesterol to HDL-cholesterol were essentially unchanged. Mean triglyceride concentrations increased by 7 or 15 mg/dL in patients receiving baricitinib 2 or 4 mg daily, respectively.

Lipid concentrations should be monitored approximately 12 weeks after initiation of baricitinib therapy. Dyslipidemia should be managed according to current standards of care.

Immunization. Administration of live vaccines should be avoided during therapy with baricitinib. Immunizations should be updated according to current administration guidelines prior to initiation of baricitinib therapy.

Specific Populations **Pregnancy.** Adequate data are not available regarding use of baricitinib in pregnant women.

Reduced fetal body weight, dose-related increases in skeletal malformations, and embryolethality (in rabbits only) have been observed in rats and rabbits given baricitinib at dosages producing exposures of 20 and 84 times, respectively, the exposure at the maximum recommended human dosage. However, there was no evidence of developmental toxicity in rats and rabbits at exposure levels approximately 5 and 13 times, respectively, the exposure at the maximum recommended human dosage.

Lactation. It is not known whether baricitinib is distributed into human milk; the drug is distributed into milk in rats. The effects of baricitinib on nursing infants or on milk production are not known. Because of the potential for serious adverse reactions to baricitinib in nursing infants, women should be advised not to breast-feed while receiving the drug.

Pediatric Use. Safety and efficacy of baricitinib have not been established in pediatric patients.

Geriatric Use. In controlled clinical trials of baricitinib in patients with rheumatoid arthritis, 17% of patients were 65 years of age or older, while 2% were 75 years of age and older. No overall differences in safety or efficacy relative to younger adults were observed, but increased sensitivity in some older individuals cannot be ruled out.

Dosage in geriatric patients should be selected with caution because of possible age-related decreases in renal function. Monitoring of renal function may be useful in such patients.

Hepatic Impairment. Systemic exposure to baricitinib is not substantially increased in individuals with moderate hepatic impairment. Therefore, no dosage adjustment is recommended in patients with mild or moderate hepatic impairment. Use of baricitinib has not been studied and is not recommended in patients with severe hepatic impairment.

Renal Impairment. Systemic exposure to baricitinib is increased by 1.41-, 2.22-, or 4.05-fold in individuals with mild, moderate, or severe renal impairment, respectively, and by 2.41-fold in individuals with end-stage renal disease receiving hemodialysis. Dosage adjustment is not necessary in patients with mild renal impairment; however, use of baricitinib is not recommended in patients with moderate to severe renal impairment (estimated glomerular filtration rate [eGFR] less than 60 mL/minute per 1.73 m^2).

■ **Common Adverse Effects** Adverse effects occurring in 1% or more of patients with rheumatoid arthritis receiving baricitinib (at a dosage of 2 or 4 mg daily) in clinical trials and more commonly with the drug than with placebo include upper respiratory tract infection, nausea, herpes simplex, and herpes zoster.

Drug Interactions

In vitro studies suggest that baricitinib is a substrate for organic anion transporter (OAT) 3, P-glycoprotein (P-gp), breast cancer resistance protein (BCRP), and multidrug and toxin extrusion transporter (MATE) 2K.

In vitro studies also suggest that baricitinib is a substrate for cytochrome P-450 (CYP) isoenzyme 3A4; however, concomitant administration of a CYP3A inducer (i.e., rifampin) or CYP3A inhibitors (i.e., fluconazole, ketoconazole) did not result in clinically important changes in the pharmacokinetics of baricitinib.

Baricitinib neither inhibits nor induces CYP isoenzymes 1A2, 2B6, 2C8, 2C9, 2C19, 2D6, or 3A in vitro. Baricitinib also does not inhibit P-gp or organic anion transporting polypeptide (OATP) 1B1 in vitro.

In vitro, baricitinib inhibits OAT1, OAT2, OAT3, organic cation transporter (OCT) 1, OCT2, OATP1B3, BCRP, MATE1, and MATE2K; however clinically important changes in the pharmacokinetics of drugs that are substrates of these transporters is unlikely.

■ **Drugs Affecting Organic Anion Transport** Concomitant use of baricitinib with potent inhibitors of OAT3 (e.g., probenecid) may result in substantially increased exposure to baricitinib. However, pharmacokinetic simulations using less-potent OAT3 inhibitors (e.g., diclofenac, ibuprofen) predicted minimal effect on the pharmacokinetics of baricitinib. Concomitant use of baricitinib and potent OAT3 inhibitors is not recommended. Dosage adjustment is not necessary with concomitant use of baricitinib and OAT3 inhibitors that are less potent than probenecid.

■ **Biologic Antirheumatic Agents** Baricitinib should not be used concomitantly with biologic disease-modifying antirheumatic drugs (DMARDs). (See Uses: Rheumatoid Arthritis in Adults.)

■ **Immunosuppressive Agents** Concomitant use of baricitinib with other immunosuppressive agents may increase the risk of serious infection. Concomitant use with potent immunosuppressive agents (e.g., azathioprine, cyclosporine) is not recommended.

Concomitant administration of baricitinib and cyclosporine (an inhibitor of P-gp and BCRP) had no clinically important effect on the pharmacokinetics of baricitinib.

■ **Antifungal Agents** Concomitant administration of baricitinib and ketoconazole (a CYP3A inhibitor) or fluconazole (an inhibitor of CYP3A, 2C9, and 2C19) had no clinically important effects on the pharmacokinetics of baricitinib. Dosage adjustment of baricitinib is not necessary if used concomitantly with ketoconazole or fluconazole.

■ **Digoxin** Concomitant administration of baricitinib and digoxin (a P-gp substrate) had no clinically important effect on the pharmacokinetics of digoxin. Dosage adjustment of digoxin is not necessary with concomitant use.

■ **Methotrexate** Concomitant administration of baricitinib and methotrexate did not have clinically important effects on the pharmacokinetics of either drug. Dosage adjustments are not necessary if baricitinib is used concomitantly with methotrexate.

■ **Omeprazole** Concomitant administration of baricitinib and omeprazole had no clinically important effects on the pharmacokinetics of baricitinib. Dosage adjustment of baricitinib is not necessary if used concomitantly with omeprazole.

■ **Oral Contraceptives** Concomitant administration of baricitinib and an oral contraceptive containing ethinyl estradiol and levonorgestrel (CYP3A substrates) had no clinically important effects on the pharmacokinetics of the oral contraceptive components.

■ **Probenecid** Concomitant administration of baricitinib and probenecid (a potent OAT3 inhibitor) resulted in an approximately twofold increase in the area under the concentration-time curve (AUC) of baricitinib; peak plasma concentration of baricitinib was not affected. Concomitant use of baricitinib and probenecid is not recommended.

■ **Rifampin** Concomitant administration of baricitinib and rifampin (a CYP inducer) had no clinically important effect on the pharmacokinetics of baricitinib. Dosage adjustment of baricitinib is not necessary if used concomitantly with rifampin.

■ **Simvastatin** Concomitant administration of baricitinib and simvastatin (a CYP3A substrate) had no clinically important effect on the pharmacokinetics of simvastatin. Dosage adjustment of simvastatin is not necessary with concomitant use.

■ **Vaccines** Live vaccines should not be administered to patients receiving baricitinib.

Description

Baricitinib, a Janus kinase (JAK) inhibitor, is an immunomodulating agent and a disease-modifying antirheumatic drug (DMARD). JAKs are a family of intracellular tyrosine kinases consisting of JAK1, JAK2, JAK3, and tyrosine kinase (TYK) 2 that mediate the signaling of cytokines and growth factors that are important for hematopoiesis and immune function. Binding of cytokines to receptors on the cell surface activates pairing of JAKs (e.g., JAK1/JAK2, JAK1/JAK3, JAK1/TYK2, JAK2/JAK2, JAK2/TYK2), which leads to phosphorylation and subsequent localization of signal transducer and activator of transcription (STAT) proteins to the nucleus and modulation of gene expression. Baricitinib modulates the cytokine signaling pathway at the point of JAKs, preventing the phosphorylation and activation of STATs. In vitro, baricitinib has greater inhibitory potency at JAK1 and JAK2 and, to a lesser extent, TYK2 relative to JAK3, and the drug inhibits cytokine-induced STAT phosphorylation mediated by JAK1/JAK2, JAK1/JAK3, JAK1/TYK2, or JAK2/TYK2 combinations with comparable potencies. The relevance of inhibition of specific JAKs to the therapeutic efficacy of baricitinib is not known.

Baricitinib has been shown to cause dose-dependent inhibition of interleukin-6 (IL-6)-induced STAT3 phosphorylation in whole blood of healthy individuals, with maximal inhibition observed approximately 1 hour after dosing and a return to near baseline activity by 24 hours.

In clinical trials, mean serum concentrations of IgG, IgM, and IgA decreased within 12 weeks of initiation of baricitinib and then remained stable through 52 weeks of therapy; changes in concentrations of these immunoglobulins generally occurred within normal reference ranges. Decreases in serum C-reactive protein (CRP) concentrations were observed as early as 1 week in patients with rheumatoid arthritis receiving baricitinib; these decreases were maintained throughout treatment.

Following oral administration, peak plasma concentrations of baricitinib are achieved in approximately 1 hour. Following repeated once-daily dosing, steady-state concentrations of the drug are attained in 2–3 days with minimal accumulation. Administration with a high-fat meal delays time to peak plasma concentration by 0.5 hours and reduces the area under the concentration-time curve (AUC) and peak plasma concentrations of the drug by 11 and 18%, respectively; these effects on drug exposure are not considered clinically important. The absolute oral bioavailability of baricitinib is approximately 80%. Baricitinib is approximately 50% bound to plasma proteins and 45% bound to serum proteins. Baricitinib is eliminated principally by renal filtration and active secretion. Approximately 69% of an orally administered dose is eliminated in urine as unchanged drug, 15% is eliminated in feces as unchanged drug, and 6% is eliminated as metabolites. Metabolism of the drug is mediated mainly by cytochrome P-450 (CYP) isoenzyme 3A4. The elimination half-life of baricitinib is approximately 12 hours in patients with rheumatoid arthritis. The pharmacokinetics of baricitinib are not affected by age, gender, body weight, or race.

Advice to Patients

Importance of advising patients about potential benefits and risks of baricitinib. Importance of patients reading the medication guide prior to initiation of therapy and each time the prescription is refilled.

Increased susceptibility to infection. Risk of herpes zoster, which may be serious. Importance of promptly informing clinicians if any signs or symptoms of infection (e.g., fever, sweating, chills, myalgia, cough, dyspnea, fatigue, diarrhea, dysuria, erythema) develop.

Risk of lymphoma and other malignancies.

Risk of thromboembolic events. Importance of contacting clinicians if symptoms of thromboembolism (e.g., shortness of breath; chest pain; swelling, pain, or tenderness in the leg) develop.

Risk of GI perforation. Importance of promptly notifying clinicians of persistent fever and abdominal pain or changes in bowel function.

Importance of informing clinicians of existing or contemplated concomitant therapy, including prescription and OTC drugs, as well as any concomitant illnesses or any history of cancer, thromboembolism, diverticulitis, gastric or intestinal ulcers, tuberculosis, hepatitis B virus or hepatitis C virus infection, or other chronic or recurring infections.

Importance of periodic laboratory monitoring.

Importance of women informing clinicians if they are or plan to become pregnant or plan to breast-feed.

Importance of informing patients of other important precautionary information. (See Cautions.)

Overview® (see Users Guide). For additional information on this drug until a more detailed monograph is developed and published, the manufacturer's labeling should be consulted. It is *essential* that the manufacturer's labeling be consulted for more detailed information on usual cautions, precautions, contraindications, potential drug interactions, laboratory test interferences, and acute toxicity.

Preparations

Distribution of baricitinib is restricted. (See Restricted Distribution under Dosage and Administration: General.)

Excipients in commercially available drug preparations may have clinically important effects in some individuals; consult specific product labeling for details.

Baricitinib

Oral

Tablets, film-coated	2 mg	**Olumiant®**, Lilly

Certolizumab Pegol

■ Certolizumab pegol, a pegylated recombinant humanized Fab′ fragment of a monoclonal antibody that is specific for tumor necrosis factor (TNF; TNF-α), is a biologic response modifier and a disease-modifying antirheumatic drug (DMARD).

Uses

■ **Crohn's Disease** Certolizumab pegol is used to reduce the signs and symptoms of Crohn's disease and to maintain clinical response in adults with moderately to severely active Crohn's disease who have had an inadequate response to conventional therapies.

Efficacy of certolizumab pegol has been evaluated in several double-blind, placebo-controlled, randomized studies in patients with moderately to severely active Crohn's disease. In these studies, the Crohn's Disease Activity Index (CDAI) was used for clinical assessment. The CDAI score is based on observations by the patient (e.g., the daily number of liquid or very soft stools, severity of abdominal pain, general well-being) and objective evidence (e.g., number of extraintestinal manifestations, presence of an abdominal mass, use or nonuse of antidiarrheal drugs, hematocrit, body weight).

Safety and efficacy of certolizumab pegol was evaluated in a 26-week multicenter, randomized, double-blind, placebo-controlled study in 662 adults with moderately to severely active Crohn's disease. To be included in the study, patients had to have had Crohn's disease for a minimum of 3 months and have a CDAI score of 220–450. Patients receiving stable dosages of 5-aminosalicylates, corticosteroids, azathioprine, 6-mercaptopurine, methotrexate, or anti-infective agents could continue such agents. Patients were randomized at week 0 to receive certolizumab pegol (400 mg given subcutaneously) or placebo at weeks 0, 2, 4, and then every 4 weeks. Primary end points were response at week 6 and response at both weeks 6 and 26. Clinical response (defined as a reduction from baseline CDAI of at least 100 points) was observed in 35 or 27% of those receiving certolizumab pegol or placebo, respectively, at week 6. At both weeks 6 and 26, clinical response was observed in 23 or 16% of patients receiving certolizumab pegol or placebo, respectively. At week 6 and both weeks 6 and 26, rates of remission (defined as an absolute CDAI score of 150 points or less) did not differ between those receiving certolizumab pegol and those receiving placebo. Remission was observed in 22 or 17% of those receiving certolizumab pegol or placebo, respectively, at week 6 and in 14 or 10% of patients, respectively, at both weeks 6 and 26.

Safety and efficacy of certolizumab pegol for maintenance therapy was evaluated in a 26-week multicenter, randomized, double-blind, placebo-controlled study in 668 adults with moderately to severely active Crohn's disease. To be included in the study, patients had to have had Crohn's disease for a minimum of 3 months and have a CDAI score of 220–450. Patients receiving stable dosages of 5-aminosalicylates, corticosteroids, azathioprine, 6-mercaptopurine, methotrexate, or anti-infective agents could continue such agents. Patients received induction therapy (i.e., certolizumab pegol 400 mg given subcutaneously at weeks 0, 2, and 4); patients who responded (defined as a reduction from baseline CDAI of at least 100 points) at week 6 were randomized to receive certolizumab pegol (400 mg given subcutaneously) or placebo at weeks 8, 12, 16, 20, and 24. The primary end point was response at week 26. At week 26, response was observed in 63 or 36% of patients receiving certolizumab pegol or placebo, respectively. Remission (defined as an absolute CDAI score of 150 points or less) was observed in 48 or 29% of patients receiving certolizumab pegol or placebo, respectively, at week 26.

For information on Crohn's disease and its treatment, see Mesalamine 56:36.

■ Rheumatoid Arthritis in Adults Certolizumab pegol is used for the management of moderately to severely active rheumatoid arthritis in adults. Certolizumab can be used alone or in combination with methotrexate or other nonbiologic disease-modifying antirheumatic drugs (DMARDs).

Safety and efficacy of certolizumab pegol were evaluated in 4 randomized, double-blind, placebo-controlled studies in 2068 adults with moderately to severely active rheumatoid arthritis (as defined by the American College of Rheumatology [ACR]) for at least 6 months prior to the start of the study. To be included in these studies, patients were required to have at least 9 swollen and 9 tender joints. Certolizumab pegol was administered in combination with methotrexate (stable dosage of at least 10 mg weekly) in 3 of these studies (studies RA-1, RA-2, and RA-3) and was administered as monotherapy in one study (RA-4). Efficacy data were collected and analyzed through week 24 (studies RA-2, RA-3, and RA-4) or week 52 (study RA-1). Patients receiving stable dosages of low-dose corticosteroids (equivalent to 10 mg of prednisone daily or less), nonsteroidal anti-inflammatory agents (NSAIAs), and/or other analgesics could continue these agents.

In studies RA-1 and RA-2, 1601 patients (982 patients in study RA-1 and 619 patients in study RA-2) who had active rheumatoid arthritis despite receiving methotrexate therapy were randomized to receive one of 2 regimens of certolizumab pegol (400 mg at 0, 2, and 4 weeks, followed by either 200 or 400 mg every 2 weeks thereafter) or placebo, each given in conjunction with a stable methotrexate regimen. Exclusion criteria included, but were not limited to, use of etanercept or anakinra within the previous 3 months or use of another biologic DMARD within the previous 6 months and failure to respond to prior therapy with a TNF blocking agent. Other DMARDs (excluding methotrexate) were discontinued prior to the study. The mean number of prior DMARDs (excluding methotrexate) was 1.2–1.4. In study RA-2, 1.3% of patients had received prior TNF blocking agent therapy.

In study RA-3, 247 patients who had active rheumatoid arthritis despite receiving methotrexate therapy were randomized to receive certolizumab pegol (400 mg every 4 weeks) or placebo, each given in conjunction with a stable methotrexate regimen.

In study RA-4, 220 patients who had not achieved an adequate response to or had not tolerated prior DMARD therapy were randomized to receive certolizumab pegol (400 mg every 4 weeks) or placebo. Exclusion criteria included, but were not limited to, use of a biologic DMARD within the previous 6 months or prior therapy with a TNF blocking agent. Other DMARDs were discontinued prior to the study. Patients had received an average of 2 prior DMARDs; approximately 82% of patients in the study had received prior methotrexate therapy.

The primary outcome measure in studies RA-2, RA-3, and RA-4 was ACR 20 response at 24 weeks; in study RA-1, the primary outcome measures were ACR 20 response at 24 weeks and change from baseline in the modified total Sharp score at 52 weeks. An ACR 20 response is achieved if the patient experiences a 20% improvement in tender and swollen joint count and a 20% or greater improvement in at least 3 of the following criteria: patient pain assessment, patient global assessment, physician global assessment, patient self-assessed disability, or laboratory measures of disease activity (e.g., C-reactive protein [CRP] level). The modified total Sharp score is a composite measure of radiographically assessed structural damage (i.e., joint erosion and joint space narrowing).

In studies RA-1 and RA-2, a greater proportion of patients who received certolizumab pegol in conjunction with methotrexate achieved an ACR 20 response at 24 weeks than did patients who received methotrexate alone. In these 2 studies, an ACR 20 response at 24 weeks was reported in 57–59% of patients who received combined therapy with certolizumab pegol 200 mg every 2 weeks and methotrexate, 58–61% of those who received combined therapy with certolizumab pegol 400 mg every 2 weeks and methotrexate, and 9–14% of those who received methotrexate and placebo. Results of study RA-1 also indicated that certolizumab pegol and methotrexate inhibited progression of structural damage, as measured by the modified total Sharp score, to a greater extent than did methotrexate alone. In this study, 69 or 72% of patients receiving combined therapy with certolizumab pegol 200 or 400 mg, respectively, and methotrexate, compared with 52% of those receiving methotrexate and placebo, experienced no radiographic progression at 52 weeks. The mean change in modified total Sharp score from baseline to week 52 was smaller in patients receiving certolizumab pegol 200 or 400 mg (0.4 or 0.2 Sharp units, respectively) in conjunction with methotrexate compared with patients receiving methotrexate and placebo (2.8 Sharp units).

In study RA-4, 46% of patients receiving certolizumab pegol (400 mg every 4 weeks) as monotherapy achieved an ACR 20 response at 24 weeks compared with 9% of patients receiving placebo.

The manufacturer states that responses in study RA-3 were similar to those observed in study RA-4.

In these 4 studies, patients receiving certolizumab pegol, either alone or in conjunction with methotrexate, had greater improvements in physical function, as assessed using the disability index of the Health Assessment Questionnaire (HAQ-DI), from baseline to week 24 (studies RA-2, RA-3, and RA-4) or week 52 (study RA-1) than did control patients receiving placebo or methotrexate.

■ Ankylosing Spondylitis Certolizumab pegol is used for the management of active ankylosing spondylitis in adults.

Safety and efficacy of certolizumab pegol were evaluated in a randomized, double-blind, placebo-controlled study (RAPID-axSpA) in 325 patients with adult-onset active axial spondyloarthritis (including 178 patients with ankylosing spondylitis) who had not achieved an adequate response to or had not tolerated prior NSAIA therapy. Patients were excluded if they had received prior treatment with certolizumab pegol or more than 2 other biologic agents (including more than one TNF blocking agent) or had not responded to prior TNF blocking agent therapy. The subset of patients with ankylosing spondylitis met modified New York criteria for ankylosing spondylitis in addition to Assessment of SpondyloArthritis International Society (ASAS) criteria for axial spondyloarthritis. Patients were randomized to receive one of 2 regimens of certolizumab pegol (400 mg at 0, 2, and 4 weeks, followed by either 200 mg every 2 weeks or 400 mg every 4 weeks) or placebo. Placebo recipients who did not achieve an ASAS 20 response at weeks 14 and 16 were rerandomized at week 16 to receive one of the 2 certolizumab pegol regimens. The median duration of symptoms in patients with ankylosing spondylitis was 9.1 years; 91% of patients with ankylosing spondylitis received concomitant therapy with NSAIAs, 35% received concomitant DMARD (sulfasalazine or methotrexate) therapy, and 20% had received prior therapy with a TNF blocking agent.

The primary outcome measure was the proportion of patients achieving an ASAS 20 response at week 12. An ASAS 20 response is achieved if the patient experiences at least a 20% improvement and an absolute improvement of at least 1 unit (on a scale of 0–10) in at least 3 of the following criteria without worsening by at least 20% or 1 unit in the fourth criterion: patient global assessment, pain, function, or inflammation. ASAS 40 response is defined as at least a 40% improvement and an absolute improvement of at least 2 units in at least 3 of these criteria without any worsening in the fourth criterion.

A greater proportion of patients who received certolizumab pegol achieved an ASAS 20 response compared with patients who received placebo; response rates for the 2 certolizumab pegol regimens were similar. ASAS 20 responses were achieved at 12 or 24 weeks by 57 or 68%, respectively, of patients receiving certolizumab pegol 200 mg every 2 weeks; 64 or 70%, respectively, of those receiving certolizumab pegol 400 mg every 4 weeks; and 37 or 33%, respectively, of those receiving placebo. ASAS 40 responses were achieved at 12 or 24 weeks by 40 or 48%, respectively, of patients receiving certolizumab pegol 200 mg every 2 weeks; 50 or 59%, respectively, of those receiving certolizumab pegol 400 mg every 4 weeks; and 19 or 16%, respectively, of those receiving placebo.

■ Psoriatic Arthritis Certolizumab pegol is used for the management of active psoriatic arthritis in adults.

Safety and efficacy of certolizumab pegol were evaluated in a randomized, double-blind, placebo-controlled study (RAPID-PsA) in 409 patients with adult-onset active psoriatic arthritis (as defined by Classification Criteria for Psoriatic Arthritis [CASPAR] criteria, with 3 or more swollen joints and 3 or more tender joints) of at least 6 months' duration who had an inadequate response to treatment with one or more DMARDs. Up to 40% of patients enrolled in the study were allowed to have received prior therapy with a TNF blocking agent. Individuals who had received more than 2 biologic DMARDs or more than one TNF blocking agent for treatment of psoriasis or psoriatic arthritis and those who had not responded to prior therapy with a TNF blocking agent were excluded. Enthesitis or dactylitis was present at baseline in approximately 64 or 26%, respectively, of patients. Patients were randomized to receive one of 2 regimens of certolizumab pegol (400 mg at 0, 2, and 4 weeks, followed by either 200 mg every 2 weeks or 400 mg every 4 weeks) or placebo. Placebo recipients who did not achieve at least 10% improvement from baseline in the number of both tender and swollen joints at weeks 14 and 16 were rerandomized at week 16 to receive one of the 2 certolizumab pegol regimens. Patients receiving stable dosages of a nonbiologic DMARD (methotrexate [25 mg/week or less], sulfasalazine, or leflunomide) and/or oral corticosteroid (equivalent to 10 mg of prednisone daily or less) could continue these agents. Approximately 70% of patients received concomitant DMARD therapy (generally methotrexate), 73% received concomitant NSAIA therapy, and 20% had received prior therapy with a TNF blocking agent.

The primary clinical outcome measure was the proportion of patients achieving an ACR 20 response (See Uses: Rheumatoid Arthritis in Adults) at week 12. Physical function was assessed using the HAQ-DI. Structural damage in the hands and feet was assessed radiographically by the change from baseline in the van der Heijde-modified total Sharp score, adapted for assessment of psoriatic arthritis.

A greater proportion of patients who received certolizumab pegol (200 mg every 2 weeks or 400 mg every 4 weeks) achieved an ACR 20 response compared with patients who received placebo. ACR 20 responses were achieved at 12 or 24 weeks by 58 or 64%, respectively, of patients receiving certolizumab pegol 200 mg every 2 weeks; 52 or 56%, respectively, of patients receiving certolizumab pegol 400 mg every 4 weeks; and 24 or 24% of patients receiving placebo. Improved ACR 20 response rates were observed in patients receiving certolizumab pegol compared with those receiving placebo irrespective of concurrent DMARD or prior TNF blocking agent use. ACR 50 responses (defined using the same criteria with a level of improvement of 50%) were achieved at 12 or 24 weeks by 36 or 44%, respectively, of patients receiving certolizumab pegol 200 mg every 2 weeks; 33 or 40%, respectively, of patients receiving certolizumab pegol 400 mg every 4 weeks; and 11 or 13%, respectively, of patients receiving placebo. Both certolizumab pegol dosage regimens were associated with greater improvement from baseline to week 24 in HAQ-DI score compared with placebo. In addition, certolizumab pegol was associated with greater improvement in enthesitis and dactylitis compared with placebo. Certolizumab pegol 200 mg every 2 weeks was more effective than placebo in inhibiting radiographic progression at 24 weeks; however, certolizumab pegol 400 mg every 4 weeks did not demonstrate greater inhibition of radiographic progression compared with placebo at 24 weeks.

Although treatment with certolizumab pegol resulted in improvements in skin manifestations in patients with psoriatic arthritis, the manufacturer states that safety and efficacy of the drug in the management of plaque psoriasis have not been established.

Dosage and Administration

■ **General** Certolizumab pegol may be used alone or in combination with methotrexate or other nonbiologic disease-modifying antirheumatic drugs (DMARDs). Concomitant use with biologic DMARDs, including other tumor necrosis factor (TNF; TNF-α) blocking agents, is not recommended. Corticosteroids, nonsteroidal anti-inflammatory agents (NSAIAs), and/or other analgesics may be continued in adults receiving certolizumab pegol for the management of rheumatoid arthritis, ankylosing spondylitis, or psoriatic arthritis. In clinical studies in patients with Crohn's disease, certolizumab pegol could be used concomitantly with aminosalicylates, corticosteroids, azathioprine, mercaptopurine, methotrexate, or anti-infective agents. (See Malignancies and Lymphoproliferative Disorders under Warnings/Precautions: Warnings, in Cautions.)

■ **Reconstitution and Administration** Certolizumab pegol is administered by subcutaneous injection. Commercially available certolizumab pegol lyophilized powder should be reconstituted and administered by a healthcare professional. Certolizumab pegol solution supplied in prefilled syringes may be *self-administered* if the clinician determines that the patient and/or their caregiver is competent to safely administer the drug after appropriate training.

Certolizumab pegol lyophilized powder is supplied in a kit containing components (e.g., diluent, syringes, needles) for reconstitution and administration. The kit should be brought to room temperature prior to reconstitution. The commercially available certolizumab pegol lyophilized powder should be reconstituted by adding 1 mL of sterile water for injection (provided by the manufacturer) to the vial labeled as containing 200 mg of the drug to produce a solution containing approximately 200 mg/mL. Each vial should be gently swirled to ensure that all of the lyophilized powder comes into contact with the diluent; the vial should not be shaken. The vial should then be left undisturbed to fully reconstitute; this may take up to 30 minutes. The reconstituted solution may be stored at room temperature for up to 2 hours or refrigerated at 2–8°C for up to 24 hours; the reconstituted solution should be protected from freezing. The reconstituted solution should be at room temperature prior to administration.

Certolizumab pegol solution in prefilled syringes should be allowed to reach room temperature prior to administration; this may take about 30 minutes.

Solutions of the drug should be a clear to opalescent, colorless to pale yellow liquid and essentially free of particulate matter. Solutions of the drug should be inspected visually for particulate matter and discoloration prior to administration; if either is present, the solution should be discarded. Because the drug contains no preservative, the vials and prefilled syringes are for single use only.

Certolizumab pegol is administered subcutaneously into the thighs or abdomen. Injection sites should be rotated. Injections should not be made into areas where the skin is tender, bruised, red, or hard. When a dose of 400 mg is to be administered, the dose should be given as 2 separate injections of 200 mg each at separate sites.

The intact kit containing certolizumab pegol lyophilized powder or certolizumab pegol solution in prefilled syringes should be stored at 2–8°C and protected from freezing. Certolizumab pegol solution should be protected from light.

■ **Dosage** ***Crohn's Disease*** For the treatment of moderately to severely active Crohn's disease in adults, the usual dosage is 400 mg of certolizumab pegol (given as 2 divided subcutaneous injections at different sites). The manufacturer recommends that adults receive the initial 3 doses of certolizumab pegol at 0, 2, and 4 weeks (induction regimen); patients who respond may receive additional doses every 4 weeks (maintenance regimen).

Rheumatoid Arthritis in Adults For the management of moderately to severely active rheumatoid arthritis in adults, the usual dosage of certolizumab pegol is 400 mg (given as 2 divided subcutaneous injections at separate sites) at 0, 2, and 4 weeks, followed by 200 mg every 2 weeks. For maintenance therapy, a dosage of 400 mg every 4 weeks may be considered.

Ankylosing Spondylitis For the management of ankylosing spondylitis in adults, the usual dosage of certolizumab pegol is 400 mg (given as 2 divided subcutaneous injections at separate sites) at 0, 2, and 4 weeks, followed by 200 mg every 2 weeks or 400 mg every 4 weeks.

Psoriatic Arthritis For the management of psoriatic arthritis in adults, the usual dosage of certolizumab pegol is 400 mg (given as 2 divided subcutaneous injections at separate sites) at 0, 2, and 4 weeks, followed by 200 mg every 2 weeks. For maintenance therapy, a dosage of 400 mg every 4 weeks may be considered.

■ **Special Populations** The manufacturer makes no special population dosage recommendations at this time. The manufacturer states that there are insufficient data to provide dosage recommendations for patients with moderate or severe renal impairment. (See Renal Impairment and also Geriatric Use under Warnings/Precautions: Specific Populations, in Cautions.)

Cautions

■ **Contraindications** The manufacturer states that there are no known contraindications to the use of certolizumab pegol.

■ **Warnings/Precautions** ***Warnings*** **Infectious Complications.** Patients receiving tumor necrosis factor (TNF; TNF-α) blocking agents, including certolizumab pegol, are at increased risk of developing serious infections involving various organ systems and sites that may require hospitalization or result in death. Opportunistic infections caused by bacterial, mycobacterial, invasive fungal, viral, parasitic, or other opportunistic pathogens—including aspergillosis, blastomycosis, candidiasis, coccidioidomycosis, histoplasmosis, legionellosis, listeriosis, pneumocystosis, and tuberculosis—have been reported in patients receiving TNF blocking agents. Infections frequently have been disseminated rather than localized. Patients should be closely monitored during and after treatment with TNF blocking agents for the development of signs or symptoms of infection (e.g., fever, malaise, weight loss, sweats, cough, dyspnea, pulmonary infiltrates, serious systemic illness including shock). Most patients who developed serious infections were receiving concomitant therapy with immunosuppressive agents such as methotrexate or corticosteroids.

In placebo-controlled trials in adults with moderately to severely active Crohn's disease, the rate of infection was 38 or 30% in patients receiving certolizumab pegol or placebo, respectively; the rate of serious infection was 3 or 1%, respectively. In controlled clinical trials in adults with rheumatoid arthritis, the rate of infection was 0.91 or 0.72 per patient-year in patients receiving certolizumab pegol or placebo, respectively. The rate of serious infection was increased in certolizumab pegol-treated patients compared with placebo-treated patients, with serious infection occurring at a rate of 0.06, 0.04, or 0.02 per patient-year in patients receiving certolizumab pegol 200 mg every 2 weeks, certolizumab pegol 400 mg every 4 weeks, or placebo, respectively. Serious infections in patients with Crohn's disease or rheumatoid arthritis have included bacterial and viral infections, pneumonia, pyelonephritis, cellulitis, and tuberculosis. As of September 2011, the US Food and Drug Administration (FDA) had identified 103 reports of *Legionella* pneumonia associated with TNF blocking agents. The 103 cases of *Legionella* pneumonia occurred in patients 25–85 years of age, many of whom received concomitant therapy with immunosuppressive agents (e.g., corticosteroids and/or methotrexate); 17 deaths were reported. In 78% of the cases of *Legionella* pneumonia, the median duration of TNF blocker therapy prior to the onset of *Legionella* pneumonia was 10.4 months (range: less than 1 month to 73 months). As of September 2011, FDA also had identified 26 published reports of *Listeria* infections, including meningitis, bacteremia, endophthalmitis, and sepsis, in patients who received TNF blocking agents; 7 deaths were reported. Many of the *Listeria* infections occurred in patients who had received concomitant therapy with immunosuppressive agents. In addition, FDA identified fatal *Listeria* infections during a review of data regarding laboratory-confirmed infections that occurred in premarketing clinical studies and during postmarketing surveillance.

An increased incidence of serious infections also was observed in clinical studies in patients with rheumatoid arthritis when a TNF blocking agent was used concomitantly with anakinra (a human interleukin-1 receptor antagonist) or abatacept (a selective costimulation modulator). (See Drug Interactions: Biologic Antirheumatic Agents.)

Certolizumab pegol therapy should not be initiated in patients with active infections, including clinically important localized infections. Patients older than 65 years of age, patients with comorbid conditions, and/or patients receiving concomitant therapy with immunosuppressive agents such as corticosteroids or methotrexate may be at increased risk of infection. Clinicians should consider potential risks and benefits of the drug prior to initiating therapy in patients with a history of chronic, recurring, or opportunistic infections; patients with underlying conditions that may predispose them to infections; and patients who have been exposed to tuberculosis or who have resided or traveled in regions where tuberculosis or mycoses such as histoplasmosis, coccidioidomycosis, and blastomycosis are endemic. Any patient who develops a new infection while receiving certolizumab pegol should undergo a thorough diagnostic evaluation (appropriate for an immunocompromised patient), appropriate anti-infective therapy should be initiated, and the patient should be closely monitored. The drug should be discontinued in patients who develop serious infection or sepsis.

Because tuberculosis has been reported in patients receiving certolizumab pegol, all patients should be evaluated for active or latent tuberculosis and for the presence of risk factors for tuberculosis prior to and periodically during therapy with the drug. When indicated, an appropriate antimycobacterial regimen for the treatment of latent tuberculosis infection should be initiated prior to certolizumab pegol therapy. Antimycobacterial treatment lowers the risk of latent tuberculosis infection progressing to active disease (i.e., reactivation) in patients receiving certolizumab pegol. Antimycobacterial therapy also should be considered prior to initiation of certolizumab pegol in individuals with a history of latent or active tuberculosis in whom an adequate course of antimycobacterial treatment cannot be confirmed and in individuals with a negative tuberculin skin test who have risk factors for tuberculosis. Consultation with a tuberculosis specialist is recommended when deciding whether antimycobacterial therapy should be initiated. Patients receiving certolizumab pegol, including individuals with a negative tuberculin skin test, should be monitored for signs and symptoms of active tuberculosis. A diagnosis of tuberculosis should be strongly considered in patients who develop new infections while receiving certolizumab pegol, especially in those who previously have traveled to countries where tuberculosis is highly prevalent or who have been in close contact with an individual with active tuberculosis.

Invasive fungal infections often are not recognized in patients receiving TNF blocking agents; this has led to delays in appropriate treatment. Clinicians should ascertain whether patients receiving TNF blocking agents who present with signs and symptoms suggestive of systemic fungal infection reside or have traveled in regions where mycoses are endemic. Empiric antifungal therapy should be considered in patients at risk of histoplasmosis or other invasive fungal infections who develop severe systemic illness. Following resolution of an invasive fungal infection, the decision regarding whether to reinitiate TNF blocking agent therapy should involve reevaluation of the risks and benefits of such therapy, particularly in patients who reside in regions where mycoses are endemic. Whenever feasible, decisions regarding initiation and duration of antifungal therapy and reinitiation of TNF blocking agent therapy should be made in consultation with a specialist in the diagnosis and management of fungal infections.

Malignancies and Lymphoproliferative Disorders. The possibility exists for agents that block TNF, including certolizumab pegol, to affect host defenses against malignancies since TNF mediates inflammation and modulates cellular immune responses.

Malignancies, some fatal, have been reported in children, adolescents, and young adults who received treatment with TNF blocking agents beginning when they were 18 years of age or younger. In August 2009, FDA reported the results of an analysis of reports of lymphoma and other malignancies in children and adolescents who had received TNF blocking agents. These cases were reported postmarketing and were derived from various sources, including registries and spontaneous postmarketing reports. FDA identified 48 cases of malignancies in children and adolescents in the analysis.

Of the 48 cases reviewed by FDA, approximately 50% were lymphomas, including Hodgkin's disease and non-Hodgkin's lymphoma. The other cases represented a variety of malignancies, including rare malignancies that are usually associated with immunosuppression and malignancies that are not usually observed in children and adolescents. Other malignancies reported included leukemia, melanoma, and solid organ cancers; malignancies such as leiomyosarcoma, hepatic malignancies, and renal cell carcinoma, which rarely occur in children, also were reported. The malignancies occurred after a median of 30 months (range: 1–84 months) following the first dose of therapy with TNF blocking agents. Of the 48 cases of malignancies, 11 deaths were reported; causes of death included hepatosplenic T-cell lymphoma (9 cases), T-cell lymphoma (1 case), and sepsis following remission of lymphoma (1 case). The reporting rates for cases of malignancy with certolizumab pegol were not calculated during the analysis because of minimal use in pediatric patients. Most of the 48 patients (88%) also were receiving other immunosuppressive drugs such as azathioprine and methotrexate; these agents also are associated with an increased risk of lymphoma. Although there were other contributory factors, the role of TNF blocking agents in the development of malignancies in children and adolescents could not be excluded. Therefore, FDA has concluded that there is an increased risk of malignancy with TNF blocking agents. However, due to the relatively rare occurrence of these cancers, the limited number of pediatric patients who received TNF blocking agents, and the possible role of other immunosuppressive drugs used concomitantly with TNF blocking agents, FDA was unable to fully characterize the strength of the association between use of TNF blocking agents and the development of a malignancy. Additional data are expected from ongoing, long-term, observational, postmarketing studies and registries that are being created by the manufacturers of TNF blocking agents.

Hepatosplenic T-cell lymphoma, a rare, aggressive, usually fatal type of T-cell lymphoma, has been reported during postmarketing experience mainly in adolescents and young adults with Crohn's disease or ulcerative colitis who received treatment with TNF blocking agents and/or thiopurine analogs (mercaptopurine or azathioprine). Most of the reported cases of hepatosplenic T-cell lymphoma occurred in patients who had received a combination of immunosuppressive agents, including TNF blocking agents and thiopurine analogs (azathioprine or mercaptopurine). In some cases, potential confounding factors could not be excluded because complete medical histories were not available. As of December 31, 2010, FDA had not identified any cases of hepatosplenic T-cell lymphoma in patients who had received certolizumab pegol. Since patients with certain conditions (e.g., rheumatoid arthritis, Crohn's disease) may be at increased risk for lymphoma, it may be difficult to measure the added risk of treatment with TNF blocking agents, azathioprine, and/or mercaptopurine.

In clinical studies, lymphoma has been observed more frequently in patients receiving TNF blocking agents than in control patients. Several cases of lymphoma have been reported during clinical studies in patients receiving certolizumab pegol. Patients with Crohn's disease or other diseases requiring long-term treatment with immunosuppressive agents may be at increased risk of lymphoma compared with the general population. Patients with rheumatoid arthritis, especially those with highly active disease, also may be at increased risk of lymphoma.

During controlled and uncontrolled phases of studies evaluating certolizumab pegol in patients with Crohn's disease and other diseases, the rate of malignancies other than nonmelanoma skin cancer was 0.5 or 0.6 per 100 patient-years in patients receiving certolizumab pegol or placebo, respectively. The size of the control group and the duration of the controlled phases of these studies were insufficient to permit definitive conclusions regarding an association between certolizumab pegol use and development of malignancies.

In controlled studies of other TNF blocking agents in adults at increased risk of malignancies (e.g., patients with chronic obstructive pulmonary disease [COPD] who have a substantial history of smoking, patients with Wegener's granulomatosis receiving concomitant cyclophosphamide), a greater proportion of malignancies occurred in patients receiving the TNF blocking agent compared with control patients.

Cases of acute and chronic leukemia have been reported during postmarketing surveillance of TNF blocking agents used in the management of rheumatoid arthritis and other conditions. In August 2009, FDA reported the results of a review of 147 cases of leukemia in adults and pediatric patients who received TNF blocking agents; these cases had been identified during postmarketing surveillance. Of the 147 cases, acute myeloid leukemia (44 cases), chronic lymphocytic leukemia (31 cases), and chronic myeloid leukemia (23 cases) were the most frequent types of leukemia reported. Four cases of leukemia were reported in children. Most patients (61%) also were receiving other immunosuppressive drugs. There were a total of 30 deaths reported; leukemia was reported as the cause of 26 of the 30 deaths, and the event was associated with the use of TNF blocking agents. Leukemia generally occurred during the first 2 years of therapy. The interpretation of these findings was complicated by the fact that published epidemiologic studies suggest that patients with rheumatoid arthritis may be at increased risk of leukemia, independent of any treatment with TNF blocking agents. However, based on the available data, FDA has concluded that there is a possible association between treatment with TNF blocking agents and the development of leukemia in patients receiving these drugs.

The role of TNF blocking agents in the development of malignancies has not been fully determined. Clinicians should consider the possibility of and monitor for the occurrence of malignancies during and following treatment with TNF blocking agents. Periodic dermatologic evaluations are recommended for all patients, but particularly for those with risk factors for skin cancer. Because therapy with TNF blocking agents and/or thiopurine analogs (azathioprine or mercaptopurine) may increase the risk of malignancies, including hepatosplenic T-cell lymphoma, the risks and benefits of these agents should be carefully considered, especially in adolescents and young adults and especially in the treatment of Crohn's disease or ulcerative colitis.

Other Warnings/Precautions

Cardiovascular Effects. There have been reports of worsening heart failure and new-onset heart failure in patients receiving TNF blocking agents, including certolizumab pegol. While certolizumab pegol has not been formally studied in patients with heart failure, other TNF blocking agents have been associated with worsening heart failure and increased mortality due to heart failure. If certolizumab pegol is used in patients with heart failure, caution and careful monitoring are recommended.

Sensitivity Reactions. Allergic reactions (e.g., angioedema, dyspnea, hypotension, rash, serum sickness, urticaria) have been reported rarely in patients receiving certolizumab pegol, sometimes after the first dose of the drug. If an allergic reaction occurs, certolizumab pegol should be discontinued immediately and appropriate therapy initiated.

Patients Infected with Hepatitis B Virus. Use of TNF blocking agents may increase the risk of reactivation of hepatitis B virus (HBV) infection in patients who are chronic carriers of this virus (i.e., hepatitis B surface antigen-positive [HBsAg-positive]). HBV reactivation has resulted in death in a few individuals receiving TNF blocking agent therapy. Most patients experiencing HBV reactivation were receiving concomitant therapy with other immunosuppressive agents; use of multiple immunosuppressive agents may have contributed to HBV reactivation.

All patients should be screened for HBV infection before initiation of certolizumab pegol therapy. In patients who test positive for HBV infection, consultation with an HBV infection specialist is recommended before initiation of TNF blocking agent therapy. Chronic carriers of HBV should be appropriately evaluated and monitored prior to the initiation of therapy, during treatment, and for up to several months following therapy with certolizumab pegol. Safety and efficacy of antiviral therapy for prevention of viral reactivation in HBV carriers receiving a TNF blocking agent have not been established. Certolizumab pegol should be discontinued if HBV reactivation occurs, and appropriate treatment, including antiviral therapy, should be initiated. It has not been established whether certolizumab pegol can be safely readministered once control of the reactivated HBV infection has been achieved; caution is advised if certolizumab pegol therapy is resumed in such a situation.

Nervous System Effects. New onset or exacerbation of clinical manifestations and/or radiographic evidence of central or peripheral nervous system demyelinating disorders (e.g., multiple sclerosis, Guillain-Barré syndrome) has been reported rarely in patients receiving TNF blocking agents, including certolizumab pegol. Clinicians should exercise caution when considering certolizumab pegol therapy in patients with preexisting or recent-onset central or peripheral nervous system demyelinating disorders.

Seizure disorder, optic neuritis, and peripheral neuropathy also have been reported rarely.

Hematologic Effects. Pancytopenia, including aplastic anemia, has been reported rarely in patients receiving TNF blocking agents. Adverse hematologic effects, including leukopenia, pancytopenia, and thrombocytopenia, have occurred rarely in certolizumab pegol-treated patients. Whether these hematologic abnormalities are directly attributable to certolizumab pegol remains to be determined. If substantial hematologic abnormalities occur, discontinuance of certolizumab pegol should be considered.

Immunologic Reactions and Antibody Formation. Certolizumab pegol therapy may result in the formation of autoimmune antibodies. In clinical trials in patients with Crohn's disease, 4% of those receiving certolizumab pegol developed new positive antinuclear antibodies (ANA) compared with 2% of those receiving placebo; development of ANA also has been reported in patients with rheumatoid arthritis receiving the drug. A lupus-like syndrome has occurred rarely in patients receiving certolizumab pegol. If a patient develops manifestations suggestive of a lupus-like syndrome, certolizumab pegol should be discontinued. The effect of long-term certolizumab pegol treatment on the development of autoimmune diseases remains to be determined.

Antibodies to certolizumab pegol were detected during clinical studies in about 8% of patients with Crohn's disease and 7% of patients with rheumatoid arthritis who received the drug. Antibodies with neutralizing activity to certolizumab pegol were detected in about 6% of patients with Crohn's disease and 3% of those with rheumatoid arthritis who received the drug. The incidence of antibody formation was lower in patients receiving concomitant therapy with other immunosuppressive agents (e.g., methotrexate) than in those not receiving immunosuppressive agents at baseline (see Drug Interactions: Methotrexate). In patients with rheumatoid arthritis, antibody formation was associated with lower plasma concentrations of certolizumab pegol and reduced efficacy (i.e., American College of Rheumatology [ACR] 20 response). In patients with Crohn's disease, there was no apparent association between antibody development and efficacy or adverse events. In patients with rheumatoid arthritis, use of a loading dose of certolizumab pegol (400 mg administered every 2 weeks for 3 doses) and concomitant use of methotrexate were associated with reduced immunogenicity.

Immunization. Live vaccines should be avoided during therapy with certolizumab pegol. (See Drug Interactions: Vaccines.)

Immunosuppression. Safety and efficacy of certolizumab pegol in patients with immunosuppression have not been evaluated.

Psoriasis. Cases of new-onset psoriasis, including pustular and palmoplantar psoriasis, have been reported with the use of TNF blocking agents. In August 2009, FDA reported the results of a review of 69 cases of new-onset psoriasis, including pustular (17 cases) and palmoplantar (15 cases) psoriasis, in patients receiving TNF blocking agents for the management of autoimmune and rheumatic conditions other than psoriasis and psoriatic arthritis. None of the patients reported having psoriasis prior to initiation of the TNF blocking agent. However, exacerbation of preexisting psoriasis has been reported with the use of TNF blocking agents. Two of the 69 cases of new-onset psoriasis included in FDA's review occurred in pediatric patients. The development of psoriasis during treatment with TNF blocking agents occurred at intervals ranging from weeks to years following initiation of the drug. Twelve of the psoriasis cases resulted in hospitalization, which was the most severe outcome reported. Most patients experienced improvement of their psoriasis following discontinuance of the TNF blocking agent. Due to the number of reported cases and the temporal relationship between the initiation of TNF blocking agents and the development of psoriasis, FDA has concluded that there is a possible association between the development of psoriasis and use of TNF blocking agents. Clinicians should consider the possibility of and monitor for manifestations (e.g., new rash) of new or worsening psoriasis, particularly pustular and palmoplantar psoriasis, during treatment with TNF blocking agents.

Specific Populations **Pregnancy.** Category B. (See Users Guide.) A pregnancy registry has been established to monitor fetal outcomes of pregnant women exposed to certolizumab pegol; patients or clinicians may contact the registry at 877-311-8972 to report any exposures to the drug that occur during pregnancy.

Lactation. It is not known whether certolizumab pegol is distributed into human milk. A decision should be made whether to discontinue nursing or the drug, taking into account the importance of the drug to the woman.

Pediatric Use. Safety and efficacy of certolizumab pegol have not been established in pediatric patients.

Malignancies, some fatal, have been reported in children and adolescents who received treatment with TNF blocking agents. (See Malignancies and Lymphoproliferative Disorders under Warnings/Precautions: Warnings, in Cautions.)

Neonates and infants who were exposed to certolizumab pegol in utero may have impaired immune responses. Although certolizumab pegol concentrations in 12 infants exposed to the drug in utero were low, the clinical importance of these low concentrations is unknown. Data from one exposed infant suggested that the drug may be eliminated more slowly in infants than in adults. The risks and benefits of administering live vaccines to infants who were exposed to certolizumab pegol in utero should be considered, since the safety of live vaccines in these infants is unknown.

Geriatric Use. The manufacturer states that clinical studies of certolizumab pegol did not include a sufficient number of patients 65 years of age or older to determine whether such patients respond differently than younger individuals, but that other reported clinical experience has not identified differences in response between geriatric and younger patients. The pharmacokinetic profile in geriatric adults does not appear to differ from that in younger adults. Because the overall incidence of infection is higher in the geriatric population than in younger adults, certolizumab pegol should be used with caution in geriatric patients.

Renal Impairment. The effect of renal impairment on the pharmacokinetics of certolizumab pegol has not been specifically studied to date; however, the pharmacokinetics of the polyethylene glycol fraction of the drug are expected to be dependent on renal function. The manufacturer states that data are insufficient to provide dosage recommendations for patients with moderate to severe renal impairment.

■ **Common Adverse Effects** Adverse effects reported in 5% or more of patients receiving certolizumab pegol for the management of Crohn's disease and at an incidence higher than that reported with placebo included upper respiratory infection, urinary tract infection, and arthralgia.

Adverse effects reported in 5% or more of patients receiving certolizumab pegol for the management of rheumatoid arthritis include upper respiratory infection, headache, hypertension, and nasopharyngitis.

Adverse effects in patients with ankylosing spondylitis or psoriatic arthritis are similar to those reported in patients with rheumatoid arthritis.

Drug Interactions

Certolizumab pegol has been used concomitantly with corticosteroids, nonsteroidal anti-inflammatory agents (NSAIAs), and/or other analgesics in clinical studies; however, formal drug interaction studies with these agents have not been performed to date. Certolizumab pegol also has been used concomitantly with aminosalicylates, azathioprine, mercaptopurine, methotrexate or other nonbiologic disease-modifying antirheumatic drugs (DMARDs), and/or anti-infective agents. (See Dosage and Administration: General.)

■ **Biologic Antirheumatic Agents** Concomitant use of certolizumab pegol and other biologic disease-modifying antirheumatic drugs (DMARDs) is not recommended.

Caution should be exercised when switching from one biologic DMARD to another, since overlapping biologic activity may further increase the risk of infection.

Abatacept When abatacept (a selective costimulation modulator) and a tumor necrosis factor (TNF; TNF-α) blocking agent were used concomitantly in patients with rheumatoid arthritis, an increased incidence of infection and serious infection was observed, with no substantial improvement in efficacy over that observed with a TNF blocking agent alone. Concomitant use of certolizumab pegol and abatacept is not recommended.

Anakinra When anakinra (a human interleukin-1 receptor antagonist) and etanercept (another TNF blocking agent) were used concomitantly in patients with active rheumatoid arthritis, an increased incidence of serious infection and increased risk of neutropenia were observed, with no substantial improvement in efficacy over that observed with etanercept alone. Similar toxicities would be expected with concomitant use of anakinra and other TNF blocking agents, including certolizumab pegol. Concomitant use of certolizumab pegol and anakinra is not recommended.

Rituximab Formal drug interaction studies between rituximab (an anti-CD20 monoclonal antibody) and certolizumab pegol have not been performed; however, concomitant use of these drugs is not recommended since such use may result in increased risk of serious infection. An increased risk of serious infection has been observed in patients with rheumatoid arthritis who received rituximab and subsequently received therapy with a TNF blocking agent.

Tocilizumab Concomitant use of tocilizumab (an anti-interleukin-6-receptor monoclonal antibody) and biologic DMARDs such as TNF blocking agents has not been studied and should be avoided because of the possibility of increased immunosuppression and increased risk of infection.

■ **Methotrexate** Methotrexate has been used concomitantly with certolizumab pegol in clinical studies. Methotrexate pharmacokinetics were not altered by certolizumab pegol administration in patients with rheumatoid arthritis; the effect of methotrexate on certolizumab pharmacokinetics was not determined.

In placebo-controlled studies in patients with rheumatoid arthritis, use of methotrexate concomitantly with certolizumab pegol was associated with reduced immunogenicity. The incidence of formation of antibodies to certolizumab pegol was lower in those receiving the drug in conjunction with methotrexate than in those not receiving immunosuppressive agents at baseline. The rate of neutralizing antibody formation also was lower in those receiving certolizumab pegol and methotrexate than in those receiving certolizumab pegol alone. In patients with rheumatoid arthritis, antibody formation was associated with lower plasma concentrations and reduced efficacy of certolizumab. (See Immunologic Reactions and Antibody Formation under Warnings/Precautions: Other Warnings/Precautions, in Cautions.)

■ **Natalizumab** Formal drug interaction studies between natalizumab (an anti-α4-integrin monoclonal antibody) and certolizumab pegol have not been performed; however, concomitant use of natalizumab and TNF blocking agents, including certolizumab pegol, should be avoided since such use may result in increased risk of progressive multifocal leukoencephalopathy (PML) or other serious infections.

■ **Vaccines** Live vaccines should not be administered to patients receiving certolizumab pegol. Information is not available regarding whether certolizumab pegol would affect the rate of secondary transmission of infection following administration of a live vaccine or regarding the effects of vaccination with live vaccine in patients receiving the drug. (See also Pediatric Use under Warnings/Precautions: Specific Populations, in Cautions.)

In patients with rheumatoid arthritis, no difference in immune response to pneumococcal polysaccharide vaccine or influenza virus vaccine was detected between patients receiving the vaccines concurrently with certolizumab pegol and those receiving the vaccines with placebo; similar proportions of placebo- and certolizumab pegol-treated patients developed protective antibody titers. However, patients receiving methotrexate concomitantly with certolizumab pegol had a lower immune response to the vaccines than did those receiving certolizumab pegol alone; the clinical importance of this finding is not known.

■ **Laboratory Test Interferences** Erroneously elevated activated partial thromboplastin time (aPTT) assay results may be reported in certolizumab pegol-treated patients who do not have coagulation abnormalities; use of certolizumab does not appear to affect thrombin time (TT) or prothrombin time (PT). There is no evidence that certolizumab pegol has any effect on blood coagulation in vivo.

Description

Certolizumab pegol is a recombinant humanized Fab′ fragment of an anti-tumor necrosis factor (TNF; TNF-α) monoclonal antibody conjugated to an approximately 40-kilodalton polyethylene glycol (PEG2MAL40K). Therapeutic use of Fabs have been limited by their short half-lives; attachment of a polyethylene glycol moiety to the Fab′ fragment increases the half-life of certolizumab to a value similar to that of a whole antibody product.

Certolizumab pegol binds with high affinity to TNF-α, a cytokine involved in the regulation of immune response. The drug does not contain a fragment crystallizable (Fc) region; certolizumab pegol does not induce complement activation, antibody-dependent cellular cytotoxicity, apoptosis, or neutrophil degranulation in vitro.

Advice to Patients

Importance of advising patients about potential benefits and risks of certolizumab pegol. Importance of patients reading the manufacturer's patient information (medication guide) prior to initiation of therapy and before each injection of the drug.

Importance of instructing patient and/or caregiver regarding proper dosage and administration of certolizumab pegol, including the use of aseptic technique, and proper disposal of needles and syringes if it is determined that the patient and/or caregiver is competent to safely administer the drug.

Increased susceptibility to infection. Importance of informing clinicians promptly if any signs or symptoms suggestive of infection (e.g., persistent fever, sweating, cough, dyspnea, fatigue) occur.

Risk of lymphoma, including hepatosplenic T-cell lymphoma, leukemia, and other malignancies with use of tumor necrosis factor (TNF; TNF-α) blocking agents. Importance of informing patients and caregivers about the increased risk of cancer development in children, adolescents, and young adults, taking into account the clinical utility of TNF blocking agents, the relative risks and benefits of these and other immunosuppressive drugs, and the risks associated with untreated disease. Importance of promptly informing clinicians if signs and symptoms of malignancies (e.g., unexplained weight loss; fatigue; abdominal pain; persistent fever; night sweats; easy bruising or bleeding; swollen lymph nodes in the neck, underarm, or groin; hepatomegaly or splenomegaly) occur.

Importance of informing clinician of any new or worsening medical conditions (e.g., heart failure, neurologic disease [e.g., demyelinating disorders], autoimmune disorders [e.g., lupus-like syndrome], cytopenias, psoriasis).

Importance of promptly contacting a clinician if manifestations of an allergic reaction (e.g., urticaria, facial swelling, difficulty breathing) occur.

Importance of taking the drug as prescribed and of not altering or discontinuing therapy without first consulting with a clinician.

Importance of informing clinicians of existing or contemplated concomitant therapy, including prescription and OTC drugs, as well as any concomitant illnesses or any history of cancer, tuberculosis, hepatitis B virus infection, or other chronic or recurrent infections.

Importance of women informing clinicians if they are or plan to become pregnant or plan to breast-feed.

Importance of informing patients of other important precautionary information. (See Cautions.)

Overview® (see Users Guide). For additional information on this drug until a more detailed monograph is developed and published, the manufacturer's labeling should be consulted. It is *essential* that the manufacturer's labeling be consulted for more detailed information on usual cautions, precautions, contraindications, potential drug interactions, laboratory test interferences, and acute toxicity.

Preparations

Excipients in commercially available drug preparations may have clinically important effects in some individuals; consult specific product labeling for details.

Certolizumab Pegol

Parenteral

For injection, for subcutaneous use	2 vials (200 mg each)	**Cimzia®** (available as kit with sterile water for injection diluent, needles, syringes, and alcohol swabs), UCB
Injection, for subcutaneous use	2 syringes (200 mg/1 mL each)	**Cimzia®** (available as disposable prefilled syringes), UCB

Etanercept

Recombinant Human TNF Receptor (p75) Fc Fusion Protein, TNFR:Fc, TNR 001

■ Etanercept is a biologic response modifier that blocks the biologic activity of tumor necrosis factor (TNF) and is a disease-modifying antirheumatic drug.

Uses

Etanercept is used for the management of the signs and symptoms of rheumatoid arthritis, to induce a major clinical response, to improve physical function, and to inhibit progression of structural damage associated with the disease in adults with moderate to severe active rheumatoid arthritis. Etanercept therapy can be initiated in combination with methotrexate or alone. Etanercept also is used for the management of the signs and symptoms of moderate to severe active polyarticular course juvenile idiopathic arthritis in children 2 years of age or older.

Etanercept is used for the management of the signs and symptoms of active arthritis, to improve physical function, and to inhibit progression of structural damage in adults with psoriatic arthritis. Etanercept can be used with or without methotrexate.

Etanercept is used for the management of the signs and symptoms of ankylosing spondylitis in adults.

Etanercept is used for the management of moderate to severe chronic plaque psoriasis in adults 18 years of age or older who are candidates for systemic therapy or phototherapy.

■ **Rheumatoid Arthritis in Adults** Etanercept is used for the management of the signs and symptoms of rheumatoid arthritis, to induce a major clinical response, to improve physical function, and to inhibit progression of structural damage associated with the disease in adults with moderate to severe active rheumatoid arthritis. Etanercept therapy can be initiated in combination with methotrexate or alone. Results of several clinical trials indicate that use of a tumor necrosis factor (TNF) blocking agent (e.g., adalimumab, etanercept, infliximab) in combination with methotrexate is more effective that therapy with either drug alone, particularly with respect to clinical responses and radiographic outcome. Additional study is needed regarding several issues related to use of TNF blocking agents in the management of rheumatoid arthritis, including evaluation of potential long-term consequences of TNF blockade.

Rheumatoid arthritis, an autoimmune disorder, produces a complicated lesion in the synovium characterized by inflammation, proliferation, and destruction of cartilage and bone. Therapy for rheumatoid arthritis includes agents that block inflammation, retard synovial proliferation, and prevent joint erosion and usually consists of combinations of nonsteroidal anti-inflammatory agents (NSAIAs), DMARDs, and/or corticosteroids. The ultimate goal in managing rheumatoid arthritis is to prevent or control joint damage, prevent loss of function, and decrease pain. Although NSAIAs may be useful for initial symptomatic treatment of rheumatoid arthritis, these drugs do not alter the course of the disease or prevent joint destruction. DMARDs have the potential to reduce or prevent joint damage, preserve joint integrity and function, and reduce total health-care costs, and all patients with rheumatoid arthritis are candidates for DMARD therapy. DMARDs should be initiated early in the disease course and should not be delayed beyond 3 months in patients with active disease (i.e., ongoing joint pain, substantial morning stiffness, fatigue, active synovitis, persistent elevation of erythrocyte sedimentation rate [ESR] or C-reactive protein [CRP], radiographic evidence of joint damage) despite an adequate regimen of NSAIAs. DMARDs commonly used in the treatment of rheumatoid arthritis include etanercept, hydroxychloroquine, infliximab, leflunomide, methotrexate, and sulfasalazine. Less frequently used DMARDs include azathioprine, cyclosporine, minocycline, penicillamine, and/or oral or injectable gold compounds.

While many factors influence the choice of a DMARD, methotrexate has substantially greater long-term efficacy than other DMARDs and is used as the initial or anchor DMARD in many patients with rheumatoid arthritis. Because residual inflammation generally persists in patients receiving maximum dosages of a single DMARD, many rheumatoid arthritis patients are candidates for combination therapy to achieve optimum control. Although the most effective combination regimen of DMARDs has not been determined, regimens that have been found efficacious in clinical studies include combinations of methotrexate and cyclosporine, etanercept, adalimumab, hydroxychloroquine, infliximab, or sulfasalazine.

Low-dose oral corticosteroids and local injection of corticosteroids are effective in relieving symptoms in patients with active rheumatoid arthritis. In addition, limited evidence indicates that low-dose corticosteroids slow the rate of joint damage.

Several international groups of rheumatologists have issued consensus reports that address the role of TNF blocking agents (e.g., adalimumab, etanercept, infliximab) in the management of rheumatoid arthritis. These groups state that use of TNF blocking agents is most appropriate in patients with active disease (5 swollen joints and elevated acute-phase response [ESR of 28 mm/hour or greater, or CRP level of 2 mg/dL or greater]) despite adequate exposure to methotrexate or other effective DMARD. A course of methotrexate in a dosage of at least 20 mg weekly (or lower dosage if toxicity develops) for 3 months is considered an adequate course of DMARD therapy, and failure with such a course should prompt consideration of modification of the therapeutic regimen (e.g., initiation of an TNF blocking agent). TNF blocking agents can be added to preexisting therapy or replace existing DMARDs. While TNF blocking agents are effective in patients with rheumatoid arthritis who have never received methotrexate, use of a TNF blocking agent as the first DMARD should be limited because long-term safety and efficacy of these agents have not been established and because of cost considerations. Other factors to consider when deciding whether to use a TNF blocking agent in the treatment of rheumatoid arthritis are differences in the aggressiveness of the disease, extent of structural damage, effects of the disease on quality of life, and toxicity of previously used DMARDs. Once therapy with a TNF blocking agent has been started, patients should be assessed for therapeutic response (e.g., a 20% reduction in swollen joint count with a 20% reduction in acute-phase response). While therapy should be continued indefinitely in those who have responded to therapy and are not experiencing substantial adverse effects, therapy with the TNF blocking agent should be discontinued in patients who have not responded after 12 weeks.

Clinical Experience Clinical evaluations of etanercept have shown that usual dosages of the drug (50 mg once weekly or 25 mg twice weekly) are more effective than placebo in the treatment of rheumatoid arthritis. In addition, current data suggest that etanercept is at least as effective as methotrexate for the management of rheumatoid arthritis in adults. Clinical evaluations of etanercept indicate that therapy with etanercept in conjunction with methotrexate is more effective than therapy with either agent alone. Response to etanercept can occur within 1–2 weeks following initiation of therapy and maximum improvement usually is achieved within 3 months in adults. Durable responses have been maintained for up to 60 months in adults receiving etanercept. Some adults receiving etanercept in conjunction with methotrexate or corticosteroids have maintained clinical response following dosage reduction or discontinuance of concomitant corticosteroid and/or methotrexate therapy. Symptoms of arthritis generally return within 1 month following discontinuance of etanercept; however, in patients who have discontinued etanercept therapy for up to 18 months, reintroduction of the drug has been associated with the same magnitude of symptomatic response as that observed in patients who received continuous therapy. Therapy with etanercept reduces the number of swollen and tender joints, pain, and duration of morning stiffness, improves the quality of life, and reduces disease activity as assessed by laboratory measures (i.e., ESR, CRP).

Therapy with a Single Disease-modifying Antirheumatic Drug. Etanercept has been evaluated for the management of rheumatoid arthritis in several double-blind, placebo-controlled studies in adults with active disease (American Rheumatism Association criteria for rheumatoid arthritis with American College of Rheumatology [ACR] functional class I, II, or III) who had not responded adequately to one or more DMARDs (i.e. hydroxychloroquine, oral or injectable gold, methotrexate, azathioprine, penicillamine, sulfasalazine). Etanercept also has been evaluated in an active-controlled phase III study in adults with early active rheumatoid arthritis (i.e., duration 3 years or less) who had never received therapy with methotrexate. Adults included in these studies had 12 or more tender joints, 10 or more swollen joints, and either an ESR of 28 mm/hour or greater, a CRP of 2 mg/dL or greater, or morning stiffness for 45 minutes or longer. Patients receiving stable dosages of NSAIAs and/or prednisone (10 mg daily or less) at study enrollment could continue such agents during these studies.

The ACR criteria for improvement (ACR response) in measures of disease activity was used as the principal measure of clinical response in studies evaluating the efficacy of etanercept. An ACR 20 response is achieved if the patient experiences a 20% improvement in tender and swollen joint count and a 20% or greater improvement in at least 3 of the following criteria: patient pain assessment, patient global assessment, physician global assessment, patient self-assessed disability, or laboratory measures of disease activity (i.e., ESR or CRP level). ACR 50 and ACR 70 responses are defined using the same criteria with a level of improvement of 50 and 70%, respectively. Major clinical response is defined as achieving an ACR 70 response for a continuous 6-month period. Physical function and disability were assessed using the Health Assessment Questionnaire (HAQ). The Sharp score, a composite score of erosions and joint space narrowing in hands, wrists, and forefeet, was used as the principal measure of structural damage.

In a randomized, placebo-controlled phase III study in 234 adults with active rheumatoid arthritis who had not responded adequately to one or more (up to 4) DMARDs, an ACR 20, 50, or 70 was achieved in 62, 41, or 15% of patients, respectively, who received etanercept (25 mg subcutaneously twice weekly) for 3 months, compared with 23, 8, or 4%, respectively, of placebo-treated patients. At 6 months, an ACR 20, 50, or 70 was achieved in 59, 40, or 15%, respectively, of patients who received etanercept compared with 11, 5, or 1%, respectively, of patients receiving placebo. Evaluation at 3 months indicated that etanercept therapy was associated with greater decreases in the number of tender joints (from 31.2 at baseline to 10), number of swollen joints (from 23.5 at baseline to 12.6), pain (from 6.9 at baseline to 2.4), HAQ disability index (from 1.6 at baseline to 1), ESR (from 28 mm/hour at baseline to 15.5 mm/hour), and CRP (from 3.5 mg/dL at baseline to 0.9 mg/dL) and in greater improvement in physician and patient assessments (from 7 at baseline to 3; sliding scale from 10 [worst] to 0 [best]) than placebo; results at 6 months were essentially the same as those at 3 months. When patients in this study were stratified according to age, results indicated that etanercept is as effective in geriatric patients 65 years of age or older as in younger adults.

In another randomized, placebo-controlled study in 180 adults with active rheumatoid arthritis who had not responded adequately to one or more DMARDs, therapy with etanercept (16 mg/m^2 subcutaneously twice weekly) for 3 months was associated with an ACR 20 or 50 in 75 or 57% of patients, respectively; an ACR 20 or 50 was reported in 14 or 7%, respectively, of placebo-treated patients.

Efficacy of etanercept compared with methotrexate has been evaluated in a study that included 632 adults with early active rheumatoid arthritis (i.e., duration 3 years or less) who had not previously received methotrexate; patients in this study were randomized to receive etanercept or methotrexate for 12 months. In those receiving etanercept (25 mg subcutaneously twice weekly), an ACR 20, 50, or 70 was achieved in 65, 40, or 21% of patients, respectively, at 6 months and in 72, 49, or 25% of patients, respectively, at 12 months. In patients receiving methotrexate (7.5 mg once weekly initially increased over the first 8 weeks of the study to a maximum of 20 mg once weekly), an ACR 20, 50, or 70 was achieved in 58, 32, or 14% of patients, respectively, at 6 months and in 65, 43, or 22% of patients, respectively, at 12 months. ACR response rates were maintained through 24 months of therapy with etanercept. A major clinical response was achieved in 23% of patients receiving etanercept over the 24-month study period. Etanercept therapy was associated with reductions in the HAQ disability index (from 1.5 at baseline to 0.7 at 6 months). Radiographic analysis at months 6, 12, and 24 indicates that etanercept is at least as effective as methotrexate in delaying joint damage. Inhibition of progression of structural damage has been maintained through month 60 in some etanercept-treated patients.

Combination Therapy with Methotrexate. Etanercept can be used in combination with methotrexate for the management of rheumatoid arthritis in adults who have not responded adequately to methotrexate therapy.Current data indicate that etanercept may be particularly useful in combination with methotrexate in patients who have a suboptimal response to methotrexate; however, additional study is needed to clarify the role of etanercept used in combination with methotrexate versus other possible strategies in these patients (e.g., changing to a different DMARD, adding another DMARD).

Results of a randomized, controlled study in adults who had persistently active rheumatoid arthritis despite methotrexate therapy indicate that addition of etanercept to the regimen was associated with greater clinical benefit than use of methotrexate alone. Patients included in the study had received methotrexate for at least 6 months (stable dosage of 15–25 mg weekly for the preceding 4 weeks) and had 6 or more tender or painful joints. Patients receiving stable dosages of NSAIAs and/or prednisone (10 mg daily or less) at study enrollment could continue such agents during the study. In patients receiving etanercept (25 mg subcutaneously twice weekly) in combination with their usual methotrexate dosage, an ACR 20 was achieved in 66 or 71% of patients at 3 or 6 months, respectively; an ACR 50 was achieved in 42 or 39% at 3 or 6 months, respectively; and an ACR 70 was achieved in 15% of patients at 3 and 6 months. In patients who continued their usual methotrexate dosage, an ACR 20 was achieved in 33 or 27% of patients at 3 or 6 months, respectively, and an ACR 50 was attained in 0 or 3% at 3 or 6 months, respectively. At 6 months, the HAQ disability index had decreased from 1.5 at baseline to 0.9 in patients receiving etanercept in combination with methotrexate.

Etanercept also has been evaluated in adults with active rheumatoid arthritis (mean duration: 7 years) who had not responded adequately to at least one DMARD other than methotrexate. Patients were randomized to receive etanercept (25 mg subcutaneously twice weekly), methotrexate (7.5 mg once weekly, increased up to 20 mg once weekly), or etanercept in conjunction with methotrexate. Patients who previously received methotrexate were included in the study provided they had not received the drug within 6 months of study enrollment and had not experienced clinically important toxic effects or lack of response to the drug. In this study, treatment with etanercept in conjunction with methotrexate was more effective in reducing disease activity, improving physical function, and retarding radiographic progression than treatment with etanercept or methotrexate alone. At 52 weeks, an ACR 20, 50, or 70 was achieved in 66, 43, or 22%, respectively, of patients receiving etanercept; in

59, 36, or 17%, respectively, of those receiving methotrexate; and in 75, 63, or 40%, respectively, of those receiving etanercept in conjunction with methotrexate. A major clinical response was achieved in 10, 6, or 24% of those receiving etanercept, methotrexate, or etanercept in conjunction with methotrexate, respectively. All regimens were associated with improvement from baseline in HAQ score. Improvement in HAQ score of at least 1 unit was achieved in 40, 29, or 51% of patients receiving etanercept, methotrexate, or etanercept in conjunction with methotrexate, respectively.There was more progression of joint damage from baseline in the group of patients who received etanercept or methotrexate alone compared with those who received etanercept in conjunction with methotrexate.

■ **Juvenile Arthritis** Etanercept is used for the management of the signs and symptoms of moderate to severe active polyarticular course juvenile idiopathic arthritis (formerly known as juvenile rheumatoid arthritis) in children 2 years of age or older. Although clinical studies indicate that therapy with etanercept is associated with substantial symptomatic improvement in children and adolescents with polyarticular course juvenile idiopathic arthritis, the role of etanercept in the management of this disease relative to other available agents remains to be determined. Whether etanercept arrests or reverses the underlying disease process in pediatric patients remains to be determined; etanercept delays joint damage in adults. Etanercept has been used in conjunction with methotrexate in a limited number of children and adolescents with polyarticular course juvenile idiopathic arthritis.

Etanercept has been evaluated for the management of polyarticular course rheumatoid arthritis in children 4–17 years of age with juvenile idiopathic arthritis in a 2-part study. Children enrolled in this study included those with moderate to severe active polyarticular course juvenile idiopathic arthritis who had not responded adequately to or were intolerant of methotrexate. Methotrexate was discontinued, but those receiving stable dosages of NSAIAs and/or prednisone (0.2 mg or less/kg daily; maximum 10 mg daily) at study enrollment could continue these drugs during the study. In part 1 (open-label study), patients (median age: 11 years, range: 4–17 years, mean disease duration: 5.9 years, 62% female, 75% white) with juvenile idiopathic arthritis received etanercept 0.4 mg/kg (up to 25 mg per dose) subcutaneously twice weekly for 90 days. In part 2 (placebo-controlled study), patients with a clinical response at day 90 were randomized to continue etanercept or receive placebo for 4 months.

The principal measure of clinical response in part 1 of this study was the juvenile idiopathic arthritis definition of improvement (i.e., 30% or greater improvement in at least 3 of 6 and 30% or greater deterioration in no more than 1 of 6 core set criteria that include physician and patient/parent global assessments, active joint count, limitation of motion, functional assessment, and ESR). In part 2, disease activity was assessed by disease flare (defined as a 30% or greater deterioration in 3 of 6 and a 30% or greater improvement in no more than 1 of 6 core set criteria and a minimum of 2 active joints).

Evaluation at month 3 (i.e., completion of part 1) indicated that positive clinical response as measured by the juvenile idiopathic arthritis definition of improvement was achieved in 74% of children receiving etanercept. Response to etanercept was observed within 2 weeks following initiation of therapy. Of those children who responded (i.e., study part 2), 24% of children remaining on etanercept experienced disease flare compared with 77% of children switched to placebo. The median time to disease flare after initiation of part 2 of the study was 116 days or longer in children receiving etanercept or 28 days in placebo-treated children. Some data suggest that the incidence of flare may be higher in patients with a higher baseline ESR. Each component of the juvenile idiopathic arthritis core set deteriorated in children receiving placebo and remained stable or improved in children receiving etanercept. In children with a clinical response at month 3, continued etanercept therapy was associated with further improvement from month 3 to 7 in some children while children receiving placebo did not improve. Durable responses have been maintained for up to 48 months in children receiving etanercept. In children who experienced disease flare while receiving placebo in part 2, reintroduction of etanercept within 4 months was associated with positive clinical response in most children. The effect of continued etanercept therapy in children with polyarticular course juvenile idiopathic arthritis who did not respond within 3 months of initiating such therapy has not been precisely determined.

■ **Psoriatic Arthritis** Etanercept is used for the management of the signs and symptoms of active arthritis, to improve physical function, and to inhibit structural damage associated with the disease in adults with psoriatic arthritis. Etanercept can be used with or without methotrexate. Etanercept has been evaluated for the management of psoriatic arthritis in a randomized, double-blind, placebo-controlled study in adults with active psoriatic arthritis (3 or more swollen joints and 3 or more tender joints) in one of the following forms: distal interphalangeal involvement; polyarticular arthritis; arthritis mutilans; asymmetric psoriatic arthritis; or ankylosing spondylitis-like. Patients also had plaque psoriasis with a qualifying target lesion (diameter of 2 cm or greater). Patients receiving stable dosages of methotrexate (25 mg/week or less) at study enrollment could continue methotrexate during the study. The ACR criteria for improvement in measures of disease activity was used to measure clinical response and the Psoriasis Area and Severity Index (PASI) was used to evaluate skin lesions. Physical function and disability were assessed using the Health Assessment Questionnaire (HAQ) and the general health-related quality of life questionnaire SF-36. A modified total Sharp score which included distal interphalangeal joints was used as the principal measure of structural damage. At 6 months, an ACR 20, 50, or 70 was achieved in 50, 37, or 9%, respectively, of patients who received etanercept (25 mg subcutaneously twice weekly) compared with 13, 4, or 1%, respectively, of patients receiving placebo. At 6 months, 47 or 23% of etanercept-treated patients achieved a 50 or 75% improvement in PASI, respectively, compared with 18 or 3% of placebo-treated patients, respectively. ACR and PASI responses in patients not receiving methotrexate were similar to the responses in those receiving methotrexate; ACR responses in patients with each of the subtypes of psoriatic arthritis (only a few patients had the arthritis mutilans or ankylosing spondylitis-like subtypes) were similar. Etanercept therapy was associated with greater improvement from baseline in the HAQ disability index and the SF-36 physical component summary score at 3 and 6 months compared with placebo. Most patients in this study had little or no change in the modified total Sharp score during the 24-month study. At 12 months, more placebo-treated patients (12%) had increases of 3 or more points in the total Sharp score than etanercept-treated patients (0%). Inhibition of progression of structural damage was maintained during the second year in etanercept-treated patients.

In another double-blind, placebo-controlled study in adults with active psoriatic arthritis, 87% of patients who received etanercept (25 mg subcutaneously twice weekly for 12 weeks) met the Psoriatic Arthritis Response Criteria (a composite measure of patient and clinician global assessments and tender and swollen joint scores) compared with 23% of those who received placebo. An ACR 20 was achieved in 73% of patients who received etanercept for 12 weeks compared with 13% of placebo-treated patients. In addition, etanercept improved psoriasis skin lesions in many patients.

■ **Ankylosing Spondylitis** Etanercept is used for the management of the signs and symptoms of ankylosing spondylitis in adults with active disease. In one study in patients with active ankylosing spondylitis, evaluation at 12 weeks indicated that improvement as assessed by a 20% improvement in the Assessment in Ankylosing Spondylitis (ASAS) response criteria was achieved in 60% of those receiving etanercept compared with 27% of those receiving placebo. Patients receiving stable dosages of hydroxychloroquine, sulfasalazine, methotrexate, or prednisone (10 mg daily or less) at study entry could continue such agents during the study.

■ **Psoriasis** Etanercept is used for the management of moderate to severe chronic plaque psoriasis in adults 18 years of age or older who are candidates for systemic therapy or phototherapy. Etanercept has been evaluated for the management of chronic plaque psoriasis in several randomized, placebo-controlled, double-blind studies in adults with chronic stable plaque psoriasis. Patients enrolled in these studies were candidates for or had previously received systemic therapy or phototherapy, previously received systemic therapy or phototherapy, had involvement of at least 10% of body surface area, and had a score of 10 or greater (indicating moderate or severe disease) on the Psoriasis Area and Severity Index (PASI; a composite score that takes into consideration both the fraction of body surface area affected and the nature and severity of the psoriatic changes within the affected areas [e.g., induration, erythema, scaling]). Patients were randomized to receive low-dose etanercept (25 mg subcutaneously once weekly), medium-dose etanercept (25 mg subcutaneously twice weekly), high-dose etanercept (50 mg subcutaneously twice weekly), or placebo for 3 months; patients could continue therapy with the same or a different regimen during an open-label phase for an additional 3–9 months. The median baseline PASI score was 15–17; many patients (44–75%) had previously received systemic therapy or phototherapy. Although the concomitant use of low- or moderate-potency topical corticosteroids was permitted, use of other therapies for psoriasis was not allowed during the study.

The primary measure of efficacy in these studies was the proportion of patients achieving a reduction in PASI score of at least 75% (PASI-75) from baseline. At 3 months, a PASI-75 was achieved in 14, 32, and 46–47% of those receiving low-, medium-, and high-dose etanercept, respectively, and in 3–4% of placebo-treated patients. In addition, 21, 32–37, and 47–54% of those receiving low-, medium-, and high-dose etanercept, respectively, and 3–5% of those receiving placebo achieved a status of minimal or clear on the static Physician Global Assessment (sPGA) scale. Onset of response (reduction in PASI score of at least 75% compared with baseline) was observed 2 months after initiation of medium- or high-dose etanercept therapy. The median duration of PASI-75 response following a 6-month course of etanercept therapy was 1–2 months. In one study, retreatment (with the same dosage used in the initial randomized period) of patients who achieved a PASI-75 response during the initial 3-month treatment phase and then discontinued therapy for up to 5 months resulted in a similar proportion of responders as observed during the initial phase of the study. In the other study, most patients (77%) who achieved a PASI-75 response after 3 months of treatment with high-dose etanercept and then received 3 months of medium-dose etanercept maintained their PASI-75 response during therapy with the medium-dose regimen.

■ **Wegener's Granulomatosis** Etanercept has been investigated for the management of Wegener's granulomatosis†, and has been designated as an orphan drug by the US Food and Drug Administration (FDA) for this use. In an open-label study in a limited number of patients with Wegener's granulomatosis who had not responded adequately to standard therapy (i.e., prednisone, cyclophosphamide, methotrexate, azathioprine, cyclosporine), addition of etanercept (25 mg subcutaneously twice weekly) for a mean of 21 weeks resulted in a positive clinical response in most patients, although limited flares and persistent minor features of active disease occurred frequently. In a randomized, placebo-controlled study in patients with Wegener's granulomatosis, the rates of sustained remission, sustained periods of low-level disease activity, and time needed to achieve these measures in patients receiving etanercept in combination with standard therapy (corticosteroids plus cyclophosphamide or methotrexate) were similar to those in patients who received standard therapy alone (placebo-treated patients). In addition, the relative risk of disease flares did not differ significantly between the etanercept and placebo groups. Solid malignant tumors developed in 6 of 89 etanercept-treated patients and in none of those who received placebo (92 enrolled). Based on results of this study and the increased incidence of malignancy associated with etanercept, some clinicians state that use of the drug in regimens to induce or maintain remissions in patients with Wegener's granulomatosis is not justified. The manufacturer of etanercept states that use of etanercept is not recommended in patients with Wegener's granulomatosis who are receiving immunosuppressive therapy. (See Cautions: Malignancies and Lymphoproliferative Disorders and see Drug Interactions: Cyclophosphamide.)

■ **Crohn's Disease** Although certain tumor necrosis factor (TNF) blocking agents (e.g., adalimumab, certolizumab pegol, infliximab) have been found effective in the management of Crohn's disease, etanercept (25 mg subcutaneously twice weekly) was not effective in reducing the signs and symptoms of Crohn's disease† in a randomized, double-blind, placebo-controlled study in adults with moderate to severe disease. Whether higher doses or more frequent dosing of etanercept would be effective in the management of Crohn's disease has not been established, although some evidence from an in vitro study indicates that the effects of infliximab on lesional T cells from patients with Crohn's disease differ from the effects of etanercept. The manufacturer states that etanercept is not effective in the treatment of inflammatory bowel disease†.

■ **Other Uses** Etanercept has been investigated in the treatment of septic shock†; however, at single IV infusion doses of 0.15–1.5 mg/kg, treatment with the drug did *not* reduce mortality and the higher doses (0.45 and 1.5 mg/kg) appeared to be associated with increased mortality.

Etanercept has been investigated for the treatment of heart failure† in 2 clinical studies; these studies were terminated early because of a lack of efficacy of the drug. Results of one of the studies suggested that the mortality rate was higher in etanercept-treated patients compared with placebo recipients.

Dosage and Administration

■ **Reconstitution and Administration** Etanercept is administered by subcutaneous injection. Etanercept is commercially available as a single-use prefilled syringe, a single-use prefilled auto-injector, and a multidose vial containing lyophilized powder. Etanercept is intended for use under the guidance and supervision of a clinician, but may be *self-administered* if the clinician determines that the patient and/or their caregiver is competent to prepare and safely administer the drug after appropriate training and with medical follow-up as necessary.

For greater patient comfort, the etanercept single-use prefilled syringe or the dose tray containing etanercept lyophilized powder and diluent may be allowed to reach room temperature (about 15–30 minutes) prior to administration. The manufacturer states that the prefilled auto-injector should be left at room temperature for at least 30 minutes prior to administration. The needle cover should not be removed from the prefilled syringe or auto-injector until immediately prior to administration.

Commercially available etanercept lyophilized powder should be reconstituted by adding 1 mL of bacteriostatic water for injection (containing 0.9% benzyl alcohol) provided by the manufacturer to a vial labeled as containing 25 mg of the drug to provide a solution containing 25 mg/mL. During reconstitution, the diluent should be very slowly added to the vial and the contents gently swirled to minimize foaming during dissolution; some foaming will occur. To avoid excessive foaming, the vial should not be shaken and excessive or vigorous agitation should be avoided. The final volume in the vial will be about 1 mL. Dissolution usually takes less than 10 minutes.

Solutions of etanercept prepared with bacteriostatic water for injection supplied by the manufacturer may be stored in the original vial at 2–8°C for up to 14 days; solutions of etanercept not used within 14 days of reconstitution should be discarded. Only the volume of solution corresponding to the correct dose should be removed from the vial into a syringe; some foam or bubbles may remain in the vial. Contents of one vial of etanercept solution should not be mixed with or transferred into the contents of another vial of etanercept solution.

If only one dose will be withdrawn from the 25-mg vial, the vial adapter supplied by the manufacturer may be used to facilitate reconstitution of the drug and withdrawal of the dose from the vial. If multiple doses will be withdrawn from the vial, the manufacturer states that a syringe with a 25-gauge needle should be used to reconstitute the lyophilized powder and withdraw the dose from the vial. A 27-gauge needle should be used to administer the dose.

Etanercept solutions should not be filtered during preparation or administration. Prior to administration, solutions of etanercept should be inspected visually for particulate matter or discoloration. The solution may contain small, white, proteinaceous particles. The solution should be discarded if discolored or cloudy, or if foreign particulate matter is present.

Subcutaneous injections of etanercept should be made into the thighs, abdomen, or upper arm. Injection sites should be rotated. Injections should not be made into areas where skin is tender, bruised, red, or hard or into scars, stretch marks, or psoriatic lesions. The development of local reactions at the injection site does not preclude continued therapy with etanercept. (See Cautions: Local Reactions.)

A 50-mg dose of etanercept may be administered as a single subcutaneous injection; the recommended preparations for this dosage schedule are the 50-mg prefilled syringe and the prefilled auto-injector. Alternatively, a 50-mg dose may be administered as 2 subcutaneous injections on the same day or 3–4 days apart in adults and children; the recommended preparations for this dosage schedule are the multidose vial and the 25-mg prefilled syringe.

If it is determined that the patient and/or their caregiver is competent to safely prepare and administer etanercept, they should be given a copy of the patient information provided by the manufacturer and should receive careful instructions on the proper methods to prepare and administer the drug, including aseptic techniques. The initial self-administered dose should be made under the supervision of an appropriately qualified health-care professional. Patients and/or their caregivers should be cautioned against reuse of syringes and needles, carefully instructed on the proper, safe disposal of needles, syringes, and unused drug, and supplied with a puncture-resistant container for the proper, safe disposal of such equipment after use.

Methotrexate, glucocorticoids, salicylates, nonsteroidal anti-inflammatory agents (NSAIAs), and analgesics may be continued in adults receiving etanercept for the management of rheumatoid arthritis, ankylosing spondylitis, or psoriatic arthritis; glucocorticoids, NSAIAs, and analgesics may be continued in pediatric patients with juvenile idiopathic arthritis who are receiving etanercept.

■ **Dosage** ***Rheumatoid Arthritis in Adults*** For the management of rheumatoid arthritis in adults, the usual dosage of etanercept is 50 mg per week. Etanercept dosages exceeding 50 mg weekly are not recommended since dosages of 50 mg twice weekly have been associated with a higher incidence of adverse effects than recommended dosages (50 mg weekly). In addition, the American College of Rheumatology (ACR) response in rheumatoid arthritis patients receiving dosages of 50 mg twice weekly were similar to ACR response in patients receiving the recommended dosage.

If etanercept is used in combination with methotrexate for the treatment of rheumatoid arthritis in adults, the usual dosage of etanercept is used.

Juvenile Arthritis For the management of juvenile idiopathic arthritis in children 2–17 years of age, the usual dosage of etanercept is 0.8 mg/kg per week (maximum dosage: 50 mg per week). The 50-mg prefilled syringe or prefilled auto-injector can be used for pediatric patients weighing 63 kg or more. The manufacturer states that the 25-mg prefilled syringe should not be used for pediatric patients weighing less than 31 kg.

Psoriatic Arthritis For the management of psoriatic arthritis in adults, the usual dosage of etanercept is 50 mg per week. Etanercept dosages exceeding 50 mg weekly are not recommended. In patients with rheumatoid arthritis, dosages of 50 mg twice weekly have been associated with a higher incidence of adverse effects and similar ACR response rates compared with dosages of 50 mg once weekly.

If etanercept is used in combination with methotrexate for the treatment of psoriatic arthritis in adults, the usual dosage of etanercept is used.

Ankylosing Spondylitis For the management of ankylosing spondylitis in adults, the usual dosage of etanercept is 50 mg per week. Etanercept dosages exceeding 50 mg weekly are not recommended. In patients with rheumatoid arthritis, dosages of 50 mg twice weekly have been associated with a higher incidence of adverse effects and similar ACR response rates compared with dosages of 50 mg once weekly.

Psoriasis For the management of plaque psoriasis in adults, the usual recommended initial dosage of etanercept is 50 mg twice weekly for 3 months. Then, the etanercept dosage is reduced to 50 mg once weekly. Initial etanercept dosages of 25 mg once or twice weekly also have been effective; the proportion of responders in clinical studies was related to etanercept dosage.

■ **Dosage in Renal and Hepatic Impairment** Pharmacokinetic studies of etanercept have not been conducted in patients with hepatic failure. The manufacturer makes no specific recommendation for dosage adjustment in patients with renal and/or hepatic impairment.Limited data indicate that adjustment of the dosage of etanercept is not necessary in patients with renal failure.

Cautions

Information on the safety of etanercept has been obtained principally from clinical studies in adults with rheumatoid arthritis who received the drug for up to 80 months. Information on the safety of the drug also has been obtained from a study in 69 children 4–17 years of age with juvenile idiopathic arthritis who received the drug for up to 12 months, from a study in adults with psoriatic arthritis who received the drug for up to 2 years, from a study in adults with ankylosing spondylosis who received the drug for up to 6 months, and from studies in adults with plaque psoriasis who received the drug for up to 18 months. Adverse effects reported in clinical studies in patients with rheumatoid arthritis generally are similar to those reported in clinical studies in patients with psoriatic arthritis or ankylosing spondylitis. Etanercept generally is well tolerated; the most common adverse effects of etanercept are infection and injection site reactions. The most serious adverse effects associated with the drug are infection, neurologic events, congestive heart failure, and hematologic events. About 4% of adults receiving etanercept in clinical studies discontinued therapy because of adverse effects.

In a randomized controlled study in patients with rheumatoid arthritis, therapy with etanercept dosages of 50 mg twice weekly was associated with several serious adverse events including GI bleeding, normal pressure hydrocephalus, seizures, and stroke. In this study, serious adverse events were not observed in individuals receiving etanercept 25 mg twice weekly. In placebo-controlled trials in patients with plaque psoriasis, the proportion of patients reporting adverse effects was similar among those receiving an etanercept dosage of 50 mg twice weekly and those receiving etanercept 25 mg twice weekly or placebo.

■ Infectious Complications Patients receiving tumor necrosis factor (TNF) blocking agents, including etanercept, are at increased risk of developing serious infections involving various organ systems and sites that may require hospitalization or result in death. Opportunistic infections caused by bacterial, mycobacterial, invasive fungal, viral, parasitic, or other opportunistic pathogens—including aspergillosis, blastomycosis, candidiasis, coccidioidomycosis, histoplasmosis, legionellosis, listeriosis, pneumocystosis, and tuberculosis—have been reported in patients receiving TNF blocking agents. (See Precautions and Contraindications Related to Infectious Complications under Cautions: Precautions and Contraindications.) Infections frequently have been disseminated rather than localized. Most patients who developed serious infections were receiving concomitant therapy with immunosuppressive agents such as methotrexate or corticosteroids.

Reported incidences of serious infection in controlled trials evaluating etanercept in patients with rheumatoid arthritis, psoriatic arthritis, ankylosing spondylitis, or plaque psoriasis were similar; in these trials, serious infection occurred in 1.4% of patients receiving etanercept alone or in conjunction with methotrexate, 3.6% of those receiving methotrexate, and 0.8% of those receiving placebo. Serious infections have included pyelonephritis, bronchitis, septic arthritis, abscess, cellulitis, osteomyelitis, pneumonia, sepsis, and gastroenteritis. Invasive fungal infections have occurred in patients receiving TNF blocking agents. Fungal infections often are not recognized in these patients; this has led to delays in appropriate treatment.

Infectious complications are the most frequent adverse systemic effects reported in patients receiving etanercept. In placebo-controlled studies in adults with rheumatoid arthritis, upper respiratory tract infection (e.g., cough, rhinitis, sinusitis, influenza, pharyngitis) occurred in 38% of those receiving etanercept and 30% of those receiving placebo; infection not involving the upper respiratory tract occurred in 21% of those receiving the drug and 15% of those receiving placebo. In a comparative study in adults with rheumatoid arthritis, upper respiratory tract infection was reported in 65 or 70% of patients receiving etanercept or methotrexate, respectively, and infection not involving the upper respiratory tract was reported in 54 or 59%, respectively. In placebo-controlled trials in adults with plaque psoriasis, upper respiratory tract infection (e.g., nasopharyngitis, sinusitis) occurred in 17% of patients receiving either etanercept or placebo and infection not involving the upper respiratory tract occurred in 12 or 14% of patients receiving etanercept or placebo, respectively. In controlled studies in adults with rheumatoid arthritis, psoriatic arthritis, ankylosing spondylitis, or plaque psoriasis, the types and severity of infection were similar between etanercept-treated patients and placebo- or methotrexate-treated patients.

Various infections (viral, bacterial, fungal [histoplasmosis]) have been observed in adults and pediatric patients receiving etanercept alone or in conjunction with immunosuppressive agents; infections have been noted in all organ systems. Opportunistic infections, including atypical mycobacterial infection, herpes zoster, aspergillosis, *Pneumocystis jiroveci* (formerly *Pneumocystis carinii*) pneumonia, and other protozoal infections, have been reported during postmarketing surveillance in patients receiving etanercept. Reactivation of latent tuberculosis and new tuberculosis infections have been reported in patients receiving TNF blocking agents, including etanercept. Although data from clinical and preclinical studies suggest that the risk of reactivation of latent tuberculosis is lower in patients receiving etanercept than in those receiving TNF-blocking monoclonal antibodies, reactivation of latent tuberculosis has been reported. Tuberculosis has developed in patients who tested negative for latent tuberculosis prior to initiation of therapy. As of September 2011, the US Food and Drug Administration (FDA) had identified 103 reports of *Legionella* pneumonia associated with TNF blocking agents, including etanercept. The 103 cases of *Legionella* pneumonia occurred in patients 25–85 years of age, many of whom received concomitant therapy with immunosuppressive agents (e.g., corticosteroids and/or methotrexate); 17 deaths were reported. In 78% of the cases of *Legionella* pneumonia, the median duration of TNF blocker therapy prior to the onset of *Legionella* pneumonia was 10.4 months (range: less than 1 month to 73 months). As of September 2011, FDA also had identified 26 published reports of *Listeria* infections, including meningitis, bacteremia, endophthalmitis, and sepsis, in patients who received TNF blocking agents; 7 deaths were reported. Many of the *Listeria* infections occurred in patients who had received concomitant therapy with immunosuppressive agents. In addition, FDA identified fatal *Listeria* infections during a review of data regarding laboratory-confirmed infections that occurred in premarketing clinical studies and during postmarketing surveillance.

An increased incidence of serious infections was observed when etanercept and anakinra (a human interleukin-1 receptor antagonist) were used concurrently in patients with active rheumatoid arthritis; the incidence of serious infections was 7% among those receiving etanercept and anakinra compared with 0% among those receiving etanercept. The most common infections were bacterial pneumonia and cellulitis; one patient with pulmonary fibrosis and pneumonia died of respiratory failure. In addition, an increased incidence of serious infection was observed when a TNF blocking agent, including etanercept, was used concomitantly with abatacept (a selective costimulation modulator) in patients with rheumatoid arthritis. (See Drug Interactions: Biologic Antirheumatic Agents.)

In an open-label clinical study evaluating safety and efficacy of etanercept in pediatric patients with juvenile idiopathic arthritis, upper respiratory tract infection or GI infection was reported in 35 or 12%, respectively, of children receiving the drug. Infections reported in pediatric patients generally have been mild and similar to those commonly observed in the general pediatric population. However, serious infections (including septic shock caused by group A *β*-hemolytic streptococci, soft tissue and postoperative wound infection) have been reported in children receiving etanercept. Varicella infection associated with aseptic meningitis also has been reported in at least 2 children receiving etanercept; the infections resolved without sequelae. The manufacturer recommends that etanercept be discontinued temporarily and use of varicella-zoster immune globulin (VZIG) considered in children receiving etanercept who are susceptible to varicella and have a significant exposure to varicella virus. (See Cautions: Pediatric Precautions.)

■ Immunologic Reactions and Antibody Formation Patients receiving etanercept may develop nonneutralizing antibodies to the drug; however, a relationship between development of such antibodies and clinical response or adverse effects (e.g., injection site reactions) has not been observed. In clinical studies evaluating etanercept, patients were tested for the presence of nonneutralizing antibodies at multiple time points and such antibodies were detected at least once in the sera of 6% of etanercept-treated adults with rheumatoid arthritis, psoriatic arthritis, ankylosing spondylitis, or plaque psoriasis; similar results have been obtained in studies in children with juvenile idiopathic arthritis. In patients with plaque psoriasis, nonneutralizing antibodies to the drug were detected at week 24, 48, 72, or 96 of therapy in 3.6–8.7% of patients; the proportion of patients testing positive for antibodies to the drug increased as the duration of therapy increased. The clinical importance of these findings remains to be determined. The possibility that antibodies formed in patients receiving etanercept may interfere with assays employing murine monoclonal antibodies should be considered. (See Laboratory Test Interferences.)

Etanercept therapy may result in the formation of autoimmune antibodies. Patients receiving etanercept were tested for the presence of autoantibodies at multiple time points. While the incidence of new antibody formation in placebo-controlled studies was higher in patients receiving etanercept than in those receiving placebo, results of a study comparing etanercept and methotrexate did not reveal a pattern of increased autoantibody development in those receiving etanercept compared with those receiving methotrexate.

In adults evaluated for antinuclear antibodies (ANA) in placebo-controlled studies, 11% of those receiving etanercept developed new positive ANA (greater than or equal to 1:40) compared with 5% of those receiving placebo. New positive anti-double stranded DNA antibodies were detected in 15% (radioimmunoassay) or 3% (Crithidia lucilae assay) of those receiving etanercept compared with 4% (radioimmunoassay) or none (Crithidia lucilae assay) of placebo-treated patients. Anticardiolipin antibodies also have been detected in more etanercept-treated than placebo-treated patients.

During postmarketing surveillance, autoimmune hepatitis, cutaneous lupus, or a systemic lupus erythematosus-like syndrome has been reported rarely in patients receiving etanercept; symptoms may resolve following discontinuance of the drug. (See Precautions Related to Immunologic or Hypersensitivity Reactions under Cautions: Precautions and Contraindications.) Macrophage activation syndrome, systemic vasculitis, and sarcoidosis also have been reported during postmarketing surveillance in patients receiving etanercept.

No evidence of diminished delayed hypersensitivity, decrease in immunoglobulin concentrations, or change in the enumeration of effector cell populations was observed in a limited number of etanercept-treated rheumatoid arthritis patients.

■ Malignancies and Lymphoproliferative Disorders The possibility exists for agents that block TNF, including etanercept, to affect host defenses against malignancies since TNF mediates inflammation and modulates cellular immune responses.

Malignancies, some fatal, have been reported in children, adolescents, and young adults who received treatment with TNF blocking agents beginning when they were 18 years of age or younger. In August 2009, the US Food and Drug Administration (FDA) reported the results of an analysis of reports of lymphoma and other malignancies in children and adolescents who had received TNF blocking agents. These cases were reported postmarketing and were derived from various sources, including registries and spontaneous postmarketing reports. FDA identified 48 cases of malignancies in children and adolescents in the analysis.

Of the 48 cases reviewed by FDA, approximately 50% were lymphomas, including Hodgkin's disease and non-Hodgkin's lymphoma. The other cases represented a variety of malignancies, including rare malignancies that are usually associated with immunosuppression and malignancies that are not usually observed in children and adolescents. Other malignancies reported included leukemia, melanoma, and solid organ tumors; malignancies such as leiomyosarcoma, hepatic malignancies, and renal cell carcinoma, which rarely occur in children, also were reported. The malignancies occurred after a median of 30 months (range: 1–84 months) following the first dose of therapy with TNF blocking agents. Of the 48 cases of malignancies, 11 deaths were reported; causes of death included hepatosplenic T-cell lymphoma (9 cases), T-cell lymphoma (1 case), and sepsis following remission of lymphoma (1 case). The observed US reporting rates for cases of malignancy with etanercept in the analysis were higher compared with background rates for lymphomas, but were similar to background rates for all malignancies. The observed reporting rates offer limited inference into the potential differences in risk of malignancy among TNF blocking agents because of uncertainties about actual patient exposure to treatment and the possibility of underreporting of cases of malignancy. Most of the 48 patients (88%) also were receiving other immunosuppressive drugs such as azathioprine and methotrexate; these agents also are associated with an increased risk of lymphoma. Although there were other contributory factors, the role of TNF blocking agents in the development of malignancies in children and adolescents could not be excluded. Therefore, FDA has concluded that there is an increased risk of malignancy with TNF blocking agents. However, due to the relatively rare occurrence of these cancers, the limited number of pediatric patients who received TNF blocking agents, and the possible role of other immunosuppressive drugs used concomitantly with TNF blocking agents, FDA was unable to fully characterize the strength of the association between use of TNF blocking agents and the development of a malignancy. Additional data are expected from ongoing, long-term, observational, postmarketing studies and registries that are being created by the manufacturers of TNF blocking agents. (See Malignancy-related Precautions under Cautions: Precautions and Contraindications.)

Hepatosplenic T-cell lymphoma, a rare, aggressive, usually fatal type of T-cell lymphoma, has been reported during postmarketing experience mainly in adolescents and young adults with Crohn's disease or ulcerative colitis who received treatment with TNF blocking agents and/or thiopurine analogs (mercaptopurine or azathioprine). Although certain TNF blocking agents (e.g., adalimumab, certolizumab pegol, infliximab) are effective in the management of Crohn's disease and/or ulcerative colitis, etanercept is not effective in the management of inflammatory bowel disease. Most of the reported cases of hepatosplenic T-cell lymphoma occurred in patients who had received a combination of immunosuppressive agents, including TNF blocking agents and thiopurine analogs (azathioprine or mercaptopurine). In some cases, potential confounding factors could not be excluded because complete medical histories were not available. As of December 31, 2010, FDA had identified 1 case of hepatosplenic T-cell lymphoma in a patient with psoriasis who had received etanercept; cyclosporine and methotrexate were used concomitantly. Since patients with certain conditions (e.g., rheumatoid arthritis, Crohn's disease, ankylosing spondylitis, psoriatic arthritis, plaque psoriasis) may be at increased risk for lymphoma, it may be difficult to measure the added risk of treatment with TNF blocking agents, azathioprine, and/or mercaptopurine. (See Malignancy-related Precautions under Cautions: Precautions and Contraindications.)

In clinical studies, lymphoma has been observed more frequently in patients receiving agents that block TNF than in control patients. In clinical studies evaluating etanercept in adults with rheumatoid arthritis, psoriatic arthritis, or ankylosing spondylitis, the rate of lymphoma in etanercept-treated patients was 0.1 per 100 patient-years. This rate is approximately threefold higher than the rate expected for the general population. Patients with rheumatoid arthritis, especially those with highly active disease, may be at increased risk of lymphoma. In clinical studies evaluating etanercept in adults with plaque psoriasis, the rate of lymphoma in etanercept-treated patients was 0.05 per 100 patient-years, which was similar to the rate expected for the general population.

Cases of acute and chronic leukemia have been reported during postmarketing surveillance of TNF blocking agents used in the management of rheumatoid arthritis and other conditions. In August 2009, FDA reported the results of a review of 147 cases of leukemia in adults and pediatric patients who received TNF blocking agents; these cases had been identified during postmarketing surveillance. Of the 147 cases, acute myeloid leukemia (44 cases), chronic lymphocytic leukemia (31 cases), and chronic myeloid leukemia (23 cases) were the most frequent types of leukemia reported. Four cases of leukemia were reported in children. Most patients (61%) also were receiving other immunosuppressive drugs. There were a total of 30 deaths reported; leukemia was reported as the cause of 26 of the 30 deaths, and the event was associated with the use of TNF blocking agents. Leukemia generally occurred during the first 2 years of therapy. The interpretation of these findings was complicated by the fact that published epidemiologic studies suggest that patients with rheumatoid arthritis may be at increased risk of leukemia, independent of any treatment with TNF blocking agents. However, based on the available data, FDA has concluded that there is a possible association between treatment with TNF blocking agents and the development of leukemia in patients receiving these drugs. (See Malignancy-related Precautions under Cautions: Precautions and Contraindications.) In clinical studies evaluating etanercept, the observed rate of leukemia was 0.03 per 100 patient-years.

Melanoma and nonmelanoma skin cancer have been reported in patients receiving TNF blocking agents, including etanercept. In controlled and open-label phases of clinical studies evaluating etanercept, the rate of melanoma was 0.043 per 100 patient-years. In clinical studies evaluating etanercept in adults with rheumatoid arthritis, psoriatic arthritis, or ankylosing spondylitis, the rate of nonmelanoma skin cancer was 0.41 per 100 patient-years in etanercept-treated patients and 0.37 per 100 patient-years in control patients. In clinical studies evaluating etanercept in adults with psoriasis, the rate of nonmelanoma skin cancer was 3.54 per 100 patient-years in etanercept-treated patients and 1.28 per 100 patient-years in control patients. Merkel cell carcinoma has been reported very infrequently during postmarketing surveillance in patients who received etanercept.

In controlled clinical trials evaluating etanercept, there were no differences in exposure-adjusted occurrence rates of malignancies other than lymphoma and nonmelanoma skin cancer between etanercept-treated patients and control patients. Analysis of data from both controlled and uncontrolled phases of clinical studies of etanercept indicate that the types and rates of malignancies are similar to what would be expected in the general population, and the rates do not appear to increase over time. It has not been established whether etanercept influences the development and course of malignancies in adults.

Some immune-related diseases, such as Crohn's disease, have been shown to increase the risk of cancer independent of treatment with TNF blocking agents, while for others, such as juvenile idiopathic arthritis, it is unknown whether there is an increased risk of cancer. The role of TNF blocking agents in the development of malignancies has not been fully determined.

In a randomized, placebo-controlled study in patients with Wegener's granulomatosis†, solid malignant tumors developed in 6 of 89 patients (adenocarcinoma of the colon occurring in 2 patients and metastatic cholangiocarcinoma, renal cell carcinoma, breast cancer, and recurrent liposarcoma each occurring in one patient) receiving etanercept in conjunction with standard therapy (corticosteroids plus cyclophosphamide or methotrexate) and in none of those who received standard therapy alone. In this study, all of the etanercept-treated patients who developed a solid tumor were receiving cyclophosphamide. Because of the increased incidence of malignancies associated with etanercept and data indicating that use of etanercept in conjunction with standard therapy is not associated with improved clinical benefit for this indication compared with standard therapy alone, some clinicians state that use of the drug in regimens to induce or maintain remissions in patients with Wegener's granulomatosis is not justified. The manufacturer of etanercept states that use of etanercept is not recommended in patients with Wegener's granulomatosis who are receiving immunosuppressive therapy. (See Drug Interactions: Cyclophosphamide.)

In controlled studies of other TNF blocking agents in adults at increased risk of malignancies (e.g., patients with chronic obstructive pulmonary disease [COPD] who have a substantial history of smoking), a greater proportion of malignancies occurred in patients receiving the TNF blocking agent compared with control patients.

■ **Hepatic Effects** Use of TNF blocking agents, including etanercept, has been associated with reactivation of hepatitis B virus (HBV) infection in patients who were previously infected with this virus. HBV reactivation has resulted in death in a few individuals receiving a TNF blocking agent. Most patients experiencing HBV reactivation were receiving concomitant therapy with other immunosuppressive agents; use of multiple immunosuppressive agents may have contributed to HBV reactivation. (See Precautions Related to Hepatitis B Virus Reactivation under Cautions: Precautions and Contraindications.)

Serum transaminase elevations and autoimmune hepatitis have been reported during postmarketing surveillance in patients receiving etanercept. (See Precautions Related to Immunologic or Hypersensitivity Reactions and see Other Precautions under Cautions: Precautions and Contraindications.)

■ **Local Reactions** Subcutaneous injection of etanercept has been associated with mild to moderate reactions at the site of administration (e.g., erythema, pruritus, pain, bleeding, bruising, or swelling; annular, indurated, erythematous reaction with a raised border) in about 37% of patients with rheumatoid arthritis, psoriatic arthritis, or ankylosing spondylitis and 15% of patients with plaque psoriasis, although such reactions have been reported more frequently in some studies.

Injection site reactions generally occur in the first month of therapy and the frequency of such reactions decreases after the first month. If adverse local effects occur, they generally are evident within 1–2 days of the injection, persist for 3–5 days, and generally do not require discontinuance of therapy. Skin biopsy in one patient revealed presence of superficial, perivascular infiltrate with lymphocytes and eosinophils; direct immunofluorescence showed weak staining of IgM and C3 at the dermoepidermal junction. Although most reactions resolve without treatment, topical corticosteroids, topical antihistamines, and/or oral antihistamines have been used for the management of injection site reaction in some patients. In clinical trials, such reactions did not result in skin ulceration, require plastic surgery, or require discontinuance of etanercept. The pattern of these reactions does *not* appear to be consistent with sensitization, but rather simply may be a mild transient inflammatory reaction. About 7% of patients experienced redness at a previous injection site when subsequent injections were given.

■ **Dermatologic and Sensitivity Reactions** Allergic reactions have been reported in less than 2% of patients. Rashes occurred in 3–14% of etanercept-treated adults with rheumatoid arthritis, 1% of adults with plaque psoriasis, and 10% of etanercept-treated children. Pruritus or urticaria has been reported in 2–5 or up to 2%, respectively, of adults with rheumatoid arthritis receiving etanercept, and each of these effects has been reported in 1% of adults with plaque psoriasis receiving the drug. Cutaneous vasculitis (including leukocytoclastic vasculitis), subcutaneous nodules, angioedema, cutaneous lupus erythematosus, erythema multiforme, Stevens-Johnson syndrome, and toxic epidermal necrolysis have been reported during postmarketing surveillance in patients receiving etanercept. In one patient who experienced leukocytoclastic vasculitis, pain and swelling developed on the thigh at the etanercept injection site and then progressed to tender erythema with a purpuric, nonpalpable rash and purpuric lesions on other areas of the trunk and extremities.

New onset or worsening of psoriasis has been reported in patients receiving etanercept. In August 2009, FDA reported the results of a review of 69 cases of new-onset psoriasis, including pustular (17 cases) and palmoplantar (15 cases) psoriasis, in patients receiving TNF blocking agents for the management of autoimmune and rheumatic conditions other than psoriasis and psoriatic arthritis. None of the patients reported having psoriasis prior to initiation of the TNF blocking agent. Two of the 69 cases of new-onset psoriasis occurred in pediatric patients. The development of psoriasis during treatment with TNF blocking agents occurred from weeks to years following initiation of the drug. Twelve of the psoriasis cases resulted in hospitalization, which was the most severe outcome reported. Most patients experienced improvement of their psoriasis following discontinuance of the TNF blocking agent. Due to the number of reported cases and the temporal relationship between the initiation of TNF blocking agents and the development of psoriasis, FDA has concluded that there is a possible association between the development of psoriasis and use of TNF blocking agents. (See Other Precautions under Cautions: Precautions and Contraindications.)

■ **Nervous System Effects** Headache, dizziness, and asthenia have been reported in adults receiving etanercept for the management of rheumatoid arthritis. Headache also has occurred in children receiving etanercept in clinical studies. Paresthesia and seizures (including new onset or exacerbation of seizure disorders) have been reported during postmarketing surveillance. Depression or personality disorder has been reported in at least one child receiving the drug.

New onset or exacerbation of CNS demyelinating disorders (some presenting with mental status changes and some associated with permanent disability) and peripheral nervous system demyelinating disorders have been reported rarely with etanercept or other TNF blocking agents. Use of TNF blocking agents in patients with multiple sclerosis has been associated with increases in disease activity. During postmarketing surveillance, multiple sclerosis, transverse myelitis, optic neuritis, Guillain-Barré syndrome, demyelination, and peripheral demyelinating neuropathies have been reported in patients receiving etanercept. (See Neurologic Precautions under Cautions: Precautions and Contraindications.)

■ **Hematologic Effects** Pancytopenia including aplastic anemia, sometimes with a fatal outcome, has been reported rarely in adults or pediatric patients receiving etanercept. Whether this hematologic abnormality is directly attributable to etanercept remains to be determined. (See Other Precautions under Cautions: Precautions and Contraindications.) Anemia, leukopenia, lymphadenopathy, thrombocytopenia, and neutropenia have occurred in patients receiving etanercept.

■ **GI Effects** Diarrhea was reported in 8–16% of adults with rheumatoid arthritis and 3% of adults with plaque psoriasis receiving etanercept during clinical trials. Adverse GI effects including abdominal pain, dyspepsia, nausea, vomiting, and mouth ulcer also have been reported in patients receiving etanercept for the management of rheumatoid arthritis. Abdominal pain, vomiting, nausea, and gastroenteritis or esophagitis/gastritis have been reported in etanercept-treated children. Inflammatory bowel disease has been reported rarely during postmarketing surveillance in patients with juvenile idiopathic arthritis receiving etanercept (see Uses: Crohn's Disease).

■ **Cardiovascular Effects** Chest pain, congestive heart failure, and hypertension, have been reported in patients receiving etanercept. (See Cardiac Precautions under Cautions: Precautions and Contraindications.)

■ **Respiratory Effects** There are rare reports of pulmonary disease developing in patients receiving etanercept. Interstitial lung disease has been reported during postmarketing surveillance.

■ **Other Adverse Effects** Pyrexia has been reported in 2–3% of patients with rheumatoid arthritis receiving etanercept in controlled clinical trials. Pancreatitis, uveitis (including recurrent uveitis), and scleritis also have occurred in patients receiving etanercept.

■ **Precautions and Contraindications** A copy of the medication guide for etanercept should be provided to all patients with each prescription of the drug. Patients should review the etanercept medication guide prior to initiating therapy with the drug and each time the prescription is refilled. Patients should be advised about potential benefits and risks of etanercept therapy and instructed on the importance of taking the drug as prescribed and of not altering or discontinuing therapy without first consulting with a clinician.

Precautions and Contraindications Related to Infectious Complications Agents that block TNF, including etanercept, affect host defenses against infections since TNF mediates inflammation and modulates cellular immune responses. Patients receiving TNF blocking agents, including etanercept, are at increased risk of developing serious infections involving various organ systems and sites that may require hospitalization or result in death. Etanercept is contraindicated in patients with sepsis, and the drug should be discontinued in patients who develop a serious infection or sepsis. Patients should be closely monitored during and after treatment with TNF blocking agents for the development of signs or symptoms of infection (e.g., fever, malaise, weight loss, sweats, cough, dyspnea, pulmonary infiltrates, serious systemic illness including shock). Any patient who develops a new infection while receiving etanercept should undergo a thorough diagnostic evaluation (appropriate for an immunocompromised patient), appropriate anti-infective therapy should be initiated, and the patient should be closely monitored. Patients should be instructed to inform their clinician immediately if they experience symptoms of infection, are receiving treatment for an infection, or have recurring infections.

Etanercept therapy should not be initiated in patients with active infections, including clinically important localized infections. Patients older than 65 years of age, patients with comorbid conditions, and/or patients receiving concomitant therapy with immunosuppressive agents such as corticosteroids or methotrexate may be at increased risk of infection. Clinicians should consider the potential risks and benefits of the drug prior to initiating therapy in patients with a history of chronic, recurring, or opportunistic infections; patients with underlying conditions that may predispose them to infections; and patients who have been exposed to tuberculosis or who reside or have traveled in regions where tuberculosis or mycoses such as histoplasmosis, coccidioidomycosis, and blastomycosis are endemic. The fact that many patients who receive etanercept also are receiving concomitant therapy with immunosuppressive agents that, in addition to their underlying condition, could increase susceptibility to infection should be considered.

Because tuberculosis has been reported in patients receiving etanercept, all patients should be evaluated for active or latent tuberculosis and for risk factors for tuberculosis prior to and periodically during etanercept therapy. When indicated, an appropriate antimycobacterial regimen for the treatment of latent tuberculosis infection should be initiated prior to etanercept therapy. Antimycobacterial treatment lowers the risk of latent tuberculosis infection progressing to active disease (i.e., reactivation) in patients receiving TNF blocking agents. Antimycobacterial therapy also should be considered prior to initiation of etanercept therapy in individuals with a history of latent or active tuberculosis in whom an adequate course of antimycobacterial treatment cannot be confirmed and in individuals with a negative tuberculin skin test who have risk factors for tuberculosis. Consultation with a tuberculosis specialist is recommended when deciding whether to initiate antimycobacterial therapy. Active tuberculosis has developed in etanercept-treated patients whose latent tuberculosis screening results were negative. Patients receiving etanercept, including individuals with a negative tuberculin skin test, should be monitored for signs and symptoms of active tuberculosis. The possibility of tuberculosis should be strongly considered in patients who develop new infections while receiving etanercept, especially if they previously have traveled to countries where tuberculosis is highly prevalent or have been in close contact with an individual with active tuberculosis.

Because fungal infections have occurred in patients receiving TNF blocking agents, clinicians should ascertain if patients receiving such therapy who present with signs and symptoms suggestive of systemic fungal infection reside or have traveled in regions where mycoses are endemic. Empiric antifungal therapy should be considered in patients at risk of histoplasmosis or other invasive fungal infections who develop severe systemic illness. Whenever feasible, a specialist in fungal infections should be consulted when making decisions regarding initiation and duration of antifungal therapy. When deciding whether TNF blocking agent therapy should be reinitiated following resolution of an invasive fungal infection, the risks and benefits of such therapy should be reevaluated, particularly in patients who reside in regions where mycoses are endemic. Whenever feasible, a specialist in fungal infections should be consulted.

Malignancy-related Precautions The effect of TNF inhibition on the development and course of malignancies has not been fully elucidated. Caution is advised if etanercept is used in patients with lymphoma or lymphoproliferative disease, and possibly in those with other malignancies since the effect of blocking TNF in these individuals is unknown. Clinicians should consider the possibility of and monitor for the occurrence of malignancies during and following treatment with TNF blocking agents. Because therapy with TNF blocking agents and/or thiopurine analogs (azathioprine or mercaptopurine) may increase the risk of malignancies, including hepatosplenic T-cell lymphoma, the risks and benefits of these agents should be carefully considered, especially in adolescents and young adults and especially in the treatment of Crohn's disease or ulcerative colitis. Although certain TNF blocking agents (e.g., adalimumab, certolizumab pegol, infliximab) are effective in the management of Crohn's disease and/or ulcerative colitis, etanercept is not effective in the management of inflammatory bowel disease.

Patients and their caregivers should be informed of the increased risk of lymphoma, including hepatosplenic T-cell lymphoma, leukemia, and other malignancies associated with TNF blocking agents, as well as the increased risk of cancer development in children, adolescents, and young adults, taking into account the clinical utility of TNF blocking agents, the relative risks and benefits of these and other immunosuppressive drugs, and the risks associated with untreated disease. Patients and their caregivers should be informed of signs and symptoms of malignancies (e.g., unexplained weight loss; fatigue; abdominal pain; persistent fever; night sweats; easy bruising or bleeding; swollen lymph nodes in the neck, underarm, or groin; easy bruising or bleeding; hepatomegaly or splenomegaly) and advised to promptly inform a clinician if such signs or symptoms occur. Patients should be advised not to discontinue therapy without consulting a clinician. (See Cautions: Malignancies and Lymphoproliferative Disorders.)

Because skin cancer has been reported in patients receiving TNF blocking agents, including etanercept, periodic dermatologic examinations should be considered in all patients at increased risk.

Neurologic Precautions Because peripheral nervous system demyelinating disorders and new onset or exacerbation of CNS demyelinating disorders have been reported in patients receiving etanercept or other TNF blocking agents, clinicians should exercise caution when considering etanercept therapy in patients with preexisting or recent-onset central or peripheral nervous system demyelinating disorders. Patients should be advised to inform a clinician if signs or symptoms of new or worsening neurologic conditions (e.g., numbness, tingling, changes in vision, weakness in arms and legs) occur.

Precautions Related to Hepatitis B Virus Reactivation Hepatitis B virus (HBV) reactivation has been reported in patients receiving TNF blocking agents, including etanercept. Patients at risk for HBV infection should be screened before initiation of etanercept therapy. Patients who were previously infected with HBV should be appropriately evaluated and monitored prior to the initiation of therapy, during treatment, and for up to several months following therapy with etanercept. Safety and efficacy of antiviral therapy for prevention of viral reactivation in HBV carriers receiving a TNF blocking agent have not been established. Etanercept should be discontinued if HBV reactivation occurs, and appropriate treatment, including antiviral therapy, should be initiated.

It has not been established whether etanercept can be safely readministered once control of the reactivated HBV infection has been achieved; caution is advised if etanercept therapy is resumed in such a situation.

Precautions Related to Immunologic or Hypersensitivity Reactions During postmarketing surveillance, autoimmune hepatitis, cutaneous lupus, or a systemic lupus erythematosus-like syndrome has been reported rarely in patients receiving etanercept. If a patient develops symptoms and findings suggestive of autoimmune hepatitis or a lupus-like syndrome, etanercept should be discontinued and the patient carefully evaluated. Presence of a positive ANA or positive anticardiolipin test result without clinical symptoms suggestive of lupus-like disease does not preclude therapy with an agent that blocks TNF since presence of these antibodies does not appear to predispose patients to lupus-like syndromes. Patients should be advised to inform a clinician if signs or symptoms of an autoimmune disorder such as autoimmune hepatitis (e.g., fatigue, jaundice, poor appetite, vomiting, right-sided abdominal pain) or a lupus-like syndrome (e.g., rash on face and arms) occur.

Some packaging components (e.g., needle covers of the prefilled single-use syringe and prefilled auto-injector) of etanercept contain natural latex proteins in the form of dry natural rubber (latex). Some individuals may be hypersensitive to natural latex proteins found in a wide range of medical devices, including such packaging components, and the level of sensitivity may vary depending on the form of natural rubber present; rarely, hypersensitivity reactions to natural latex proteins have been fatal. The needle cover of the prefilled single-use syringe and the prefilled auto-injector of etanercept should not be handled by individuals sensitive to latex.

If serious allergic reaction or anaphylaxis occurs, etanercept should be discontinued immediately and appropriate therapy initiated.

Cardiac Precautions During postmarketing surveillance, there have been reports describing worsening congestive heart failure (with and without identifiable precipitating factors) and rare reports of new-onset congestive heart failure (including some reports in patients without known cardiovascular disease) in patients receiving etanercept; some of these patients have been younger than 50 years of age. In addition, in one study investigating use of the drug for the treatment of heart failure, there was a suggestion of higher mortality rates in patients receiving etanercept. Etanercept should be used with caution and careful monitoring in patients with heart failure. Patients should be advised to inform a clinician if signs or symptoms of new or worsening heart failure (e.g., shortness of breath, swelling of the feet or lower legs) occur.

Other Precautions Pancytopenia including aplastic anemia has occurred in patients receiving etanercept. Although a high risk group for this adverse effect has not been identified, caution is advised if etanercept is used in patients with a history of substantial hematologic abnormalities. Patients receiving etanercept should be advised that if they develop signs and symptoms suggestive of blood dyscrasias (e.g., persistent fever, bruising, bleeding, pallor), they should seek immediate medical attention. If substantial hematologic abnormalities are confirmed, discontinuance of etanercept should be considered.

New-onset psoriasis has been reported in patients receiving TNF blocking agents for the management of autoimmune and rheumatic conditions other than psoriasis and psoriatic arthritis. Clinicians should consider the possibility of and monitor for manifestations (e.g., new rash) of new or worsening psoriasis, particularly pustular and palmoplantar psoriasis, during treatment with TNF blocking agents. Patients should be informed of the increased risk of psoriasis or worsening of existing psoriasis with TNF blocking agents. Patients should be advised to inform a clinician if signs and symptoms of new or worsening psoriasis occur. (See Cautions: Dermatologic and Sensitivity Reactions.)

Because use of etanercept in patients with moderate to severe alcoholic hepatitis has been associated with increased mortality following 6 months of use, etanercept should be used with caution in such patients.

Hypoglycemia has been reported following initiation of etanercept therapy in patients with diabetes mellitus who were receiving antidiabetic agents. Some patients have required a reduction in dosage of the antidiabetic agent.

■ **Pediatric Precautions** Etanercept is indicated for the management of the signs and symptoms of moderate to severe active polyarticular course juvenile idiopathic arthritis in children 2 years of age or older. Etanercept has not been studied in children younger than 2 years of age with juvenile idiopathic arthritis.

Malignancies, some fatal, have been reported in children and adolescents who received treatment with TNF blocking agents. (See Cautions: Malignancies and Lymphoproliferative Disorders.)

The adverse effect profile of etanercept in pediatric patients appears to be similar to that in adults. In open-label clinical trials in children with juvenile idiopathic arthritis, adverse effects reported in children 2–4 years of age were similar to those reported in older children.

When use of etanercept is being considered for pediatric patients, the vaccination status of the child should be reviewed and all age-appropriate vaccines included in the current Recommended Childhood Immunization Schedule (see Immunization Schedules, US 80:00) should be administered, if possible, prior to initiation of etanercept therapy. (See Drug Interactions: Vaccines.) The risks and benefits of administering live vaccines to infants who were exposed to etanercept in utero should be considered prior to immunization, since the safety of live vaccines in these infants is unknown. (See Pregnancy under Cautions: Pregnancy, Fertility, and Lactation.)

Varicella infection associated with septic meningitis has been reported in 2 children receiving etanercept; the infection resolved without sequelae. If a varicella-susceptible child has a significant exposure to varicella while receiving etanercept, the manufacturer recommends that the drug be discontinued temporarily and use of varicella-zoster immune globulin (VZIG) considered.

Inflammatory bowel disease has been reported rarely during postmarketing surveillance in patients with juvenile idiopathic arthritis receiving etanercept; the drug is not effective in the management of inflammatory bowel disease. (See Uses: Crohn's Disease.)

Safety and efficacy of etanercept has not been established in pediatric patients with plaque psoriasis.

■ **Geriatric Precautions** While safety and efficacy of etanercept in geriatric patients have not been studied specifically to date, some patients with rheumatoid arthritis or plaque psoriasis who received the drug in clinical studies have been 65 years of age or older. Etanercept appears to be well tolerated in geriatric patients, and age-related differences in safety or efficacy of the drug have not been observed in clinical studies. However, the manufacturer cautions that clinical studies of the drug in patients with psoriasis did not include sufficient numbers of geriatric patients to determine whether they respond differently than younger adults. Because the geriatric population in general may have a higher incidence of infections than younger adults, etanercept should be used with caution in this age group.

■ **Mutagenicity and Carcinogenicity** The effect of etanercept on the development and course of malignancies has not been fully evaluated. Lymphoproliferative disorders and new malignancies (see Cautions: Malignancies and Lymphoproliferative Disorders) have been observed in patients receiving etanercept.

No evidence of mutagenicity was observed in in vitro or in vivo studies evaluating etanercept. Long-term animal studies have not been conducted to evaluate the carcinogenic potential of etanercept.

■ **Pregnancy, Fertility, and Lactation** Reproduction studies in rats and rabbits using etanercept doses 60–100 times higher than the usual human dose have not revealed evidence of harm to the fetus. There are no adequate and well-controlled studies to date using etanercept in pregnant women, and the drug should be used during pregnancy only when clearly needed. Limited data suggest that etanercept crosses the placenta in small amounts; in 3 neonates whose mothers received etanercept during pregnancy, concentrations of the drug in cord blood at the time of delivery were 3–32% of maternal serum concentrations. The clinical implications of in utero exposure to etanercept are unknown. (See Cautions: Pediatric Precautions.)

To monitor maternal-fetal outcomes of pregnant women exposed to etanercept, a pregnancy registry has been established. Women who become pregnant during etanercept therapy are encouraged to enroll. Patients or clinicians may contact the registry at 800-772-6436.

Studies have not been conducted to date to determine whether etanercept affects fertility in males or females.

Limited data indicate that etanercept is distributed into human milk in low concentrations and is minimally absorbed by breast-fed infants. Caution should be exercised when etanercept is used in nursing women. The manufacturer states that the benefits of breast-feeding and the importance of etanercept to the woman should be considered along with the potential adverse effects on the breast-fed child from the drug or from the underlying maternal condition. Women who choose to continue etanercept therapy while nursing are encouraged to enroll in the manufacturer's lactation surveillance program. Patients or clinicians may contact the surveillance program at 800-772-6436.

Drug Interactions

While specific drug interaction studies evaluating concomitant use of etanercept and other drugs have not been conducted to date, etanercept has been used concomitantly with methotrexate, glucocorticoids, salicylates, nonsteroidal anti-inflammatory agents (NSAIAs), and/or analgesics in clinical studies and the manufacturer of etanercept states that these drugs may be continued in patients receiving etanercept.

■ **Biologic Antirheumatic Agents** Caution should be exercised when switching from one biologic disease-modifying antirheumatic drug (DMARD) to another, since overlapping biologic activity may further increase the risk of infection.

Abatacept When abatacept (a selective costimulation modulator) and a tumor necrosis factor (TNF) blocking agent were used concomitantly in patients with rheumatoid arthritis, an increased incidence of infection and serious infection was observed, with no substantial improvement in efficacy over that observed with a TNF blocking agent alone. Concomitant use of etanercept and abatacept is not recommended.

Anakinra When etanercept and anakinra (a human interleukin-1 receptor antagonist) were used concomitantly in patients with active rheumatoid arthritis, an increased incidence of serious infections was observed, with no substantial improvement in efficacy over that observed with etanercept alone. Neutropenia was observed in 2% of patients receiving etanercept concomitantly with anakinra. Concomitant use of etanercept with anakinra is not recommended.

Rituximab An increased risk of serious infection has been observed in patients with rheumatoid arthritis who received rituximab (an anti-CD20 monoclonal antibody) and subsequently received therapy with a TNF blocking agent.

Tocilizumab Concomitant use of tocilizumab (an anti-interleukin-6-receptor monoclonal antibody) and biologic DMARDs such as TNF blocking agents has not been studied and should be avoided because of the possibility of increased immunosuppression and increased risk of infection.

■ **Cyclophosphamide** In a study in patients with Wegener's granulomatosis, addition of etanercept to standard therapy that included cyclophosphamide was associated with a higher incidence of solid malignant tumors compared with standard therapy alone. Concomitant use of etanercept and cyclophosphamide is not recommended.

■ **Methotrexate** Concomitant use of etanercept and methotrexate in patients with rheumatoid arthritis does not appear to alter the pharmacokinetics of etanercept, result in additive toxicity, or affect the pattern, frequency, or severity of the established toxicities associated with either drug.

■ **Sulfasalazine** Addition of etanercept to established therapy that included sulfasalazine has resulted in decreases in mean neutrophil counts. The clinical importance of this finding is unknown.

■ **Vaccines** Only limited data are available regarding administration of inactivated vaccines in adults receiving etanercept; data are not available to date regarding administration of vaccines in pediatric patients receiving etanercept. Although etanercept is a biologic response modifier, it is unclear whether the drug would affect the immune response to vaccines or the incidence and severity of adverse effects reported with vaccines.

A limited number of adults with rheumatoid arthritis have received inactivated vaccines (e.g., influenza virus vaccine, polyvalent pneumococcal vaccine) while receiving etanercept without evidence of unusual adverse effects. In addition, an appropriate antibody response to at least one of the antigens tested was documented in 17/17 adults with rheumatoid arthritis who received polyvalent pneumococcal vaccine and influenza virus vaccine while receiving etanercept. An effective B-cell immune response to pneumococcal 23-valent polysaccharide vaccine has been reported in etanercept-treated psoriatic arthritis patients; however, antibody titers in aggregate were moderately lower in these adults compared with adults not receiving the drug, and fewer etanercept-treated adults had twofold increases in antibodies compared with adults not receiving the drug.

Information is not available regarding whether etanercept would affect the rate of secondary transmission of infection following administration of a live vaccine. The manufacturer of etanercept states that live vaccines (e.g., measles virus vaccine live, mumps virus vaccine live, rubella virus vaccine live, poliovirus vaccine live oral, typhoid vaccine live oral, varicella virus vaccine live, yellow fever vaccine) should not be administered to patients receiving the drug.

When use of etanercept is being considered for pediatric patients with juvenile idiopathic arthritis, the vaccination status of the child should be reviewed and all age-appropriate vaccines included in the current Recommended Childhood Immunization Schedule (see Recommended Childhood Immunization Schedule at the beginning of section 80:00) should be administered, if possible, prior to initiation of etanercept therapy. (See Cautions: Pediatric Precautions.) The risks and benefits of administering live vaccines to infants who were exposed to etanercept in utero should be considered prior to immunization, since the safety of live vaccines in these infants is unknown. (See Pregnancy under Cautions: Pregnancy, Fertility, and Lactation.)

Laboratory Test Interferences

■ **Troponin** Etanercept may interfere with troponin determinations, potentially complicating interpretation of findings for myocardial disease. False-positive troponin determinations using a murine monoclonal antibody based assay (i.e., AxSym® Troponin, Abbott) have been reported in 2 patients receiving etanercept. While the mechanism responsible for these false-positive determinations has not been established, it has been suggested that this may result from cross-reactivity of antibodies formed in response to etanercept administration and the murine anti-human troponin used in the assay. Use of the currently available reformulated AxSym® Troponin I assay that contains goat protein may eliminate this interference.

■ **Other Assays Using Murine Monoclonal Antibodies** Based on reported interference with troponin determinations (see Laboratory Test Interferences: Troponin), it has been postulated that etanercept may interfere with other assays that employ murine monoclonal antibodies, including those for creatine kinase-MB fraction, folate, β-human chorionic gonadotropin, thyrotropin, thyroxine, and vancomycin.

Acute Toxicity

Limited data are available on the acute toxicity of etanercept. Toxicology studies in monkeys using etanercept doses 30 times the usual human dose have not revealed evidence of dose-limiting toxicity, and dose-limiting toxicities have not been observed in clinical studies in humans. Etanercept 60 mg/m^2 (approximately twice the recommended dose) has been administered as a single IV dose in healthy individuals without evidence of dose-limiting toxicity.

Pharmacology

■ **Immunomodulating and Anti-inflammatory Effects** Etanercept, a biosynthetic tumor necrosis factor receptor fusion protein, is a biologic response modifier. Etanercept binds to tumor necrosis factor (TNF) before TNF can interact with cell surface tumor necrosis factor receptors (TNFRs). By preventing the binding of TNF to cell surface TNFRs, etanercept blocks the biologic activity of TNF.

TNF, a naturally occurring cytokine, has a broad spectrum of biologic activity. TNF is involved in the normal inflammatory and immune responses, and also plays a role in the systemic toxicity associated with sepsis and in a number of autoimmune and inflammatory diseases, including rheumatoid arthritis. The biologic activity of TNF is mediated by specific TNF transmembrane receptors. Two TNFRs have been identified: the 75-kilodalton or p75 receptor and the 55-kilodalton or p55 receptor (formerly referred to as p80 and p60, respectively). Both TNFRs are present as soluble forms and on cell surfaces of almost all types of cells including neutrophils, vascular endothelial cells, and fibroblasts; soluble TNFRs have been detected in synovial tissue and in the cartilage-pannus junction. To initiate biologic activity, soluble TNF must bind to 2 or 3 cell surface TNFRs to initiate intracellular signal transmission.

While the causes of rheumatoid diseases or psoriasis have not been fully elucidated, proinflammatory cytokines, particularly TNF (TNF-α), have an important role in the pathogenesis of rheumatoid arthritis, polyarticular course juvenile idiopathic arthritis, ankylosing spondylitis, psoriatic arthritis, and plaque psoriasis. Cytokines such as TNF are mediators involved in the inflammatory, adhesive, angiogenic, and bone-resorbing mechanisms associated with rheumatoid arthritis. TNF induces the release of metalloproteinases (i.e., metalloproteinase-3 [stromelysin-1]) from neutrophils, fibroblasts, and chrondrocytes; induces the expression of endothelial adhesion molecules (intracellular adhesion molecule [ICAM-1], E-selectin) involved in the migration of leukocytes to extravascular sites of inflammation; and stimulates release of other proinflammatory cytokines (i.e., interleukin-1 [IL-1], IL-6). Additional evidence supporting the role of TNF in the pathogenesis of rheumatoid arthritis includes the presence of TNF at the cartilage-pannus junction and increased TNF concentrations in the synovial fluid of patients with active rheumatoid arthritis. In addition, TNF and lymphotoxin-α (TNF-β) are expressed in the synovial fluid of individuals with juvenile idiopathic arthritis or juvenile spondylarthropathy. Increased TNF concentrations have been found in the synovium and psoriatic plaques in patients with psoriatic arthritis. While other proinflammatory cytokines (i.e., IL-1) contribute to the pathogenesis of rheumatoid arthritis, TNF plays a central role because of its prominent role in the cytokine cascade.

Because of the central role of TNF in the inflammatory cascade in the rheumatoid joint, a variety of approaches have been investigated to reduce the functional level of TNF in the rheumatoid joint. The identification of soluble TNFRs present in a number of body compartments (including serum and synovial fluid) that retain TNF binding capacity has led to the development of drugs based on soluble TNFRs. Soluble TNFRs serve as physiologic regulators of the inflammatory response by inhibiting TNF activity. Levels of soluble TNFR are increased in the sera and synovial fluid of patients with rheumatoid arthritis; however, endogenous soluble TNFRs cannot adequately regulate the high levels of bioactive TNF in patients with rheumatoid arthritis.

Etanercept, a recombinant form of the p75 TNFR fused to the Fc fragment of human immunoglobulin G_1 (IgG_1), is a potent antagonist of TNF biologic activity. Etanercept has high binding affinity for TNF and lymphotoxin-α (TNF-β); each molecule of etanercept can bind to 2 TNF molecules. The binding affinity of etanercept for TNF is $10^{-10}M$. Results of in vitro studies and animal models of inflammation (e.g., murine collagen-induced arthritis) indicate that etanercept inhibits TNF activity. Following IV administration of a single dose of etanercept 5 mg/m^2 or higher in healthy adults, serum at 1.5 hours (diluted 1:6) inhibited the cytotoxic effects of rTNF (1 ng/mL) by 90–95%. In addition, etanercept can modulate biologic responses that are induced or regulated by TNF, including expression of adhesion molecules, serum concentrations of matrix metalloproteinase-3, and serum concentrations of cytokines.

While the precise mechanism of action of etanercept in the management of rheumatoid arthritis remains to be determined, the drug inhibits TNF binding to cell surface TNFR, rendering TNF biologically inactive. While etanercept prolonged the half-life of TNF in animal and human studies, the TNF was not biologically active. Therefore, etanercept is a cytokine "carrier" and a TNF antagonist. Etanercept neutralizes circulating TNF, a mechanism of action that differs from that of a receptor antagonist (receptor antagonists block activity by interacting with the receptor but leave the ligand in circulation).

Whether etanercept can exert activity through binding to Fc receptors is unknown. In vitro, cells expressing transmembrane TNF that bind etanercept are not lysed in the presence or absence of complement.

Because TNF mediates inflammation and modulates cellular immune responses, the possibility exists that TNF blocking agents, including etanercept, could affect host defenses against infections and malignancies. (See Cautions:

Infectious Complications and Cautions: Malignancies and Lymphoproliferative Disorders.)

Pharmacokinetics

The pharmacokinetics of etanercept have been studied in healthy adults and adults with rheumatoid arthritis who received single doses of the drug, adults with rheumatoid arthritis who received the drug for up to 6 months, and children 4–17 years of age with juvenile idiopathic arthritis who received the drug for up to 18 weeks. Studies in adults have not revealed differences in the pharmacokinetics of etanercept based on gender or age. The manufacturer states that the pharmacokinetics of etanercept have not been systematically evaluated in patients with hepatic impairment. Limited data in patients with chronic renal failure undergoing hemodialysis indicate that pharmacokinetic values in patients with chronic renal failure are similar to those in patients with normal renal function.

■ **Absorption** Because of its protein nature, etanercept is destroyed in the GI tract and must be administered parenterally. Bioavailability following a single subcutaneous dose of etanercept is approximately 60%. Following subcutaneous injection of a single 25-mg dose of etanercept in a limited number of healthy adults or adults with rheumatoid arthritis, peak serum etanercept concentrations of 1.46 mcg/mL (range: 0.37–3.47 mcg/mL) or 1.1 mcg/mL were achieved within 51 hours (range: 25–78 hours) or 69 hours, respectively. Following long-term administration (i.e., 6 months) of etanercept 25 mg subcutaneously twice weekly in adults with rheumatoid arthritis, peak serum concentrations were 2.4 mcg/mL. In another study in patients with rheumatoid arthritis, serum concentrations of etanercept at steady state in patients receiving etanercept 50 mg subcutaneously once weekly were essentially the same as values in patients receiving etanercept 25 mg subcutaneously twice weekly. Based on available data, peak serum concentration of etanercept following repeated dosing is about 2–7 times higher than that achieved with a single dose of the drug and $AUC_{0-72\text{ hours}}$ about 4 times higher. In most adults with rheumatoid arthritis receiving etanercept 25 mg subcutaneously twice weekly, steady-state concentrations are expected to be achieved approximately 3 weeks after initiation of therapy.

Following IV infusion† over 30 minutes of a single dose of etanercept of 5, 10, 15, or 30 mg/m² in a limited number of healthy adults, peak serum concentrations of etanercept averaged 2.1, 3.8, 8.8, or 14.3 mcg/mL, respectively. Following IV infusion over 30 minutes of a single dose of etanercept of 4, 8, 16, or 32 mg/m² in a limited number of adults with rheumatoid arthritis, serum concentrations averaged 1.54, 1.99, 4.78, or 12.9 mcg/mL, respectively, 1 hour post dose, and 0.597, 0.934, 1.64, or 3.61 mcg/mL 72 hours post dose.

In children 4–17 years of age with juvenile idiopathic arthritis who received etanercept 0.4 mg/kg subcutaneously twice weekly (up to a maximum dosage of 50 mg per week), serum concentrations after repeated dosing averaged 2.1 mcg/mL (range: 0.7–4.3 mcg/mL). Population pharmacokinetic data suggest that the pharmacokinetic differences between regimens of 0.4 mg/kg twice weekly and 0.8 mg/kg once weekly in pediatric patients with juvenile idiopathic arthritis are of the same magnitude as differences between twice-weekly and once-weekly regimens in adults with rheumatoid arthritis.

■ **Distribution** Distribution of etanercept into body tissues and fluids, including partition of the drug into synovial fluid, has not been well characterized. Nuclear imaging in one patient with active Crohn's disease indicates that etanercept is distributed into bone, liver, lung, spleen, and kidneys. An apparent volume of distribution of 12 L (range: 5–25 L) has been reported following subcutaneous injection of a single 25-mg dose of etanercept in healthy adults.

It is not known if etanercept crosses the placenta or is distributed into milk.

■ **Elimination** The metabolic fate of etanercept remains to be determined. Because etanercept is a large molecule, the drug may be eliminated by the reticuloendothelial system. Following subcutaneous administration of a single 25-mg dose of etanercept in a limited number of healthy adults or adults with rheumatoid arthritis, half-life of the drug averaged 68 hours (range: 28–100 hours) or 102 hours, respectively. An apparent clearance of 132 mL/hour was reported in healthy adults; a clearance of 160 mL/hour was reported in patients with rheumatoid arthritis. There was considerable interindividual variation in clearance in healthy individuals.

Preliminary data indicate that clearance of etanercept is reduced to a small extent in children 4–8 years of age compared with adults.

Chemistry and Stability

■ **Chemistry** Etanercept, a biologic response modifier, is a recombinant form of the human 75 kilodalton (p75) tumor necrosis factor receptor (TNFR) fused to the Fc fragment of human immunoglobulin G_1 (IgG_1). The TNFR component of etanercept contains the soluble extracellular ligand-binding domain of human TNFR p75; the Fc component contains the C_H2 domain, the C_H3 domain, and the hinge region, but not the C_H1 domain of IgG_1. Etanercept is a dimer consisting of 2 copies of the TNFR component linked by the Fc portion. The drug is composed exclusively of human amino acid sequences, contains 934 amino acids, and has an apparent molecular weight of about 150 kilodaltons.

Etanercept is prepared from mammalian cells using DNA recombinant technology. DNA encoding the soluble portion of human TNFR p75 is linked to DNA encoding the Fc portion of human IgG_1, and the combined DNA is expressed using Chinese hamster ovary (CHO) cells.

Etanercept is commercially available in a single-use prefilled syringe containing 25 or 50 mg of etanercept and a single-use prefilled auto-injector containing 50 mg of etanercept. The preservative-free etanercept solution also contains sucrose, sodium chloride, L-arginine, and phosphate buffers. The solution is clear and colorless and has a pH of about 6.3.

Etanercept also is commercially available as a sterile, white, lyophilized powder for injection. Vials labeled as containing 25 mg of etanercept also contain 40 mg of mannitol, 10 mg of sucrose, and 1.2 mg of tromethamine. Following reconstitution with 1 mL of bacteriostatic water for injection (containing 0.9% benzyl alcohol), etanercept solutions are clear and colorless and have a pH of about 7.4. Etanercept has a solubility in water exceeding 50 mg/mL at 25°C.

■ **Stability** Commercially available etanercept prefilled syringes and prefilled auto-injectors should be refrigerated at 2–8°C and stored in the original carton for protection from light and physical damage. Storage under conditions of extreme heat or cold should be avoided. Prefilled syringes and auto-injectors should not be frozen or shaken. The manufacturer states that individual prefilled syringes or auto-injectors may be stored at room temperature (20–25°C) for a maximum single period of 14 days, with protection from light and heat. Once a prefilled syringe or auto-injector has been stored at room temperature, it should not be placed back in a refrigerator. If not used within 14 days when stored at room temperature, the prefilled syringe or auto-injector should be discarded.

Commercially available lyophilized etanercept powder for injection should be refrigerated at 2–8°C and stored in the original carton for protection from light and physical damage. Storage under conditions of extreme heat or cold should be avoided. The drug should not be frozen or shaken. Etanercept powder for injection is shipped from the manufacturer on ice packs. When stored at 2–8°C, the lyophilized powder is stable for 24 months following the date of manufacture. The manufacturer states that individual dose trays containing etanercept powder for injection and diluent may be stored at room temperature (20–25°C) for a maximum single period of 14 days, with protection from light, heat, and humidity. Once a dose tray has been stored at room temperature, it should not be placed back in a refrigerator. If not used within 14 days when stored at room temperature, the dose tray should be discarded.

Following reconstitution with bacteriostatic water for injection (containing 0.9% benzyl alcohol), etanercept solutions may be stored in the vial at 2–8°C for up to 14 days; solutions of etanercept not used within 14 days of reconstitution should be discarded. Reconstituted solutions of etanercept should not be frozen or stored at room temperature. Studies conducted by the manufacturer indicate that etanercept reconstituted with bacteriostatic water for injection (containing 0.9% benzyl alcohol) is stable for 21 days at 2–8°C in the original vial; for 24 or 12 hours at 2–8 or 25°C, respectively, in glass syringes (Becton-Dickinson Hypak®); or for 12 hours at 2–8 or 25°C in plastic syringes (Becton-Dickinson).

Etanercept should not be filtered during preparation or administration and should not be admixed with other drugs.

Preparations

Excipients in commercially available drug preparations may have clinically important effects in some individuals; consult specific product labeling for details.

Etanercept

Parenteral		
For injection, for subcutaneous use	25 mg	**Enbrel®** (with prefilled syringe containing 1 mL bacteriostatic water for injection [with benzyl alcohol 0.9%] diluent, plunger, and vial adapter), Amgen
Injection, for subcutaneous use	25 mg/0.5 mL	**Enbrel®** (available as disposable prefilled syringes), Amgen
	50 mg/mL	**Enbrel®** (available as disposable prefilled syringes and prefilled auto-injectors [SureClick®]), Amgen

†Use is not currently included in the labeling approved by the US Food and Drug Administration

Golimumab

■ Golimumab, a human immunoglobulin G_1 kappa (IgG_1) monoclonal antibody specific for human tumor necrosis factor (TNF; TNF-α), is a biologic response modifier and a disease-modifying antirheumatic drug (DMARD).

Uses

■ **Rheumatoid Arthritis in Adults** Golimumab is used in conjunction with methotrexate for the management of moderately to severely active rheumatoid arthritis in adults. Golimumab has been shown to induce a major clinical response, improve physical function, and inhibit progression of structural damage in adults with rheumatoid arthritis.

Clinical Experience with Subcutaneous Golimumab Safety and efficacy of subcutaneous golimumab were evaluated in 3 multicenter, randomized, double-blind studies (RA-1 [GO-AFTER], RA-2 [GO-FORWARD], and RA-3 [GO-BEFORE]) in 1542 adults with moderately to severely active rheumatoid arthritis (as defined by the American College of Rheumatology [ACR]) for at least 3 months prior to administration of the study drug. To be included in these studies, patients were required to have at least 4 swollen and 4 tender joints. Golimumab was administered subcutaneously at dosages of 50 or 100 mg once every 4 weeks. Patients receiving stable dosages of low-dose corticosteroids (equivalent to 10 mg of prednisone daily or less) and/or nonsteroidal anti-inflammatory agents (NSAIAs) could continue such agents, and some patients received oral methotrexate during these studies. Approximately 77 and 57% of patients received concomitant NSAIAs and low-dose corticosteroids, respectively, in the 3 studies.

In study RA-1, 461 patients who previously received one or more doses of a tumor necrosis factor (TNF) blocking agent (i.e., adalimumab or etanercept discontinued at least 8 weeks or infliximab discontinued at least 12 weeks prior to administration of the study drug) were randomized to receive golimumab (50 or 100 mg once every 4 weeks) or placebo. Patients receiving stable dosages of methotrexate, sulfasalazine, and/or hydroxychloroquine could continue such agents or discontinue the agents prior to study start; the use of other disease-modifying antirheumatic drugs (DMARDs), including cytotoxic agents or other biologic agents, was prohibited. At week 16, patients in certain treatment groups with less than 20% improvement from baseline in the number of both tender and swollen joints entered early escape in which their study drug was adjusted in a double-blind manner (i.e., those meeting the early escape criteria who were receiving golimumab 50 mg had their golimumab dosage increased to 100 mg and those who were receiving placebo began receiving golimumab 50 mg every 4 weeks). At week 24, all remaining patients who had been receiving placebo initiated golimumab 50 mg every 4 weeks. During the unblinded long-term extension period (beginning at week 24 of the 5-year study), golimumab dosage could be adjusted (increased to 100 mg or, after week 160, decreased to 50 mg) at the clinician's discretion. The median duration of rheumatoid arthritis disease prior to study enrollment was 9.4 years, and 99% of patients previously received at least one DMARD.

In study RA-2, 444 patients who had active rheumatoid arthritis despite receiving a stable dosage of methotrexate (15–25 mg/week) and who had not previously been treated with a TNF blocking agent were randomized to receive one of 4 regimens: golimumab 100 mg every 4 weeks and placebo, golimumab 50 mg every 4 weeks and methotrexate, golimumab 100 mg every 4 weeks and methotrexate, or methotrexate and placebo. The use of other DMARDs, including sulfasalazine, hydroxychloroquine, cytotoxic agents, or other biologic agents, was prohibited. At week 16, patients in certain treatment groups with less than 20% improvement from baseline in the number of both tender and swollen joints entered early escape in which their study drug was adjusted in a double-blind manner (i.e., those meeting the early escape criteria who were receiving golimumab 100 mg and placebo began receiving methotrexate at the same stable dosage at study screening instead of placebo and continued to receive golimumab 100 mg; those meeting the early escape criteria who were receiving golimumab 50 mg and methotrexate had their golimumab dosage increased to 100 mg and continued to receive methotrexate at the same stable dosage; those meeting the early escape criteria who were receiving methotrexate and placebo began receiving golimumab 50 mg every 4 weeks instead of placebo and continued to receive methotrexate at the same stable dosage). At week 24, all remaining patients who had been receiving methotrexate and placebo discontinued placebo, initiated golimumab 50 mg every 4 weeks, and continued to receive methotrexate; patients receiving golimumab 100 mg and placebo, golimumab 50 mg and methotrexate, or golimumab 100 mg and methotrexate continued to receive their originally assigned treatment unless they entered early escape, in which case they continued to receive their modified dosage. Golimumab continued to be administered in a blinded manner every 4 weeks through week 48. During the unblinded long-term extension period (beginning at week 52 of the 5-year study), certain adjustments of golimumab dosage (increase to 100 mg or decrease to 50 mg) and concomitant therapies could be made at the clinician's discretion. The median duration of rheumatoid arthritis disease prior to study enrollment was 5.7 years, and 75% of patients previously received at least one DMARD.

In study RA-3, 637 patients with active rheumatoid arthritis who were methotrexate-naive and had not previously been treated with a TNF blocking agent were randomized to receive one of 4 regimens: golimumab 100 mg every 4 weeks and placebo, golimumab 50 mg every 4 weeks and methotrexate, golimumab 100 mg every 4 weeks and methotrexate, or methotrexate and placebo. In this study, methotrexate was administered at a dosage of 10 mg weekly beginning at week 0 and increased to 20 mg weekly by week 8. The use of other DMARDs, including sulfasalazine, hydroxychloroquine, cytotoxic agents, or other biologic agents, was prohibited. After week 24, patients in certain treatment groups with less than 20% improvement from baseline in the number of both tender and swollen joints entered early escape in which their study drug was adjusted in a blinded manner (i.e., those meeting the early escape criteria who were receiving either golimumab 50 mg and methotrexate or golimumab 100 mg and placebo switched to golimumab 100 mg every 4 weeks and methotrexate, while those receiving placebo and methotrexate switched to golimumab 50 mg every 4 weeks and methotrexate). At week 52, all remaining patients who had been receiving placebo and methotrexate and had at least one tender or swollen joint switched to therapy with golimumab 50 mg every 4 weeks and methotrexate. During the unblinded long-term extension period (beginning at week 52 of the 5-year study), certain adjustments of golimumab dosage (increase from 50 mg to 100 mg) and concomitant therapies could be made at the clinician's discretion. The median duration of rheumatoid arthritis disease prior to study enrollment was 1.2 years, and 54% of patients previously received at least one DMARD.

The primary outcome measures in these 3 studies were the proportion of patients achieving an ACR 20 response at week 14 (studies RA-1 and RA-2) or an ACR 50 response at week 24 (study RA-3) and the change from baseline to week 52 in the van der Heijde-modified Sharp score (study RA-3). An ACR 20 response is achieved if the patient experiences a 20% improvement in tender and swollen joint count and a 20% or greater improvement in at least 3 of the following criteria: patient pain assessment, patient global assessment, physician global assessment, patient self-assessed disability, or laboratory measures of disease activity (e.g., C-reactive protein [CRP] level). ACR 50 responses are defined using the same criteria with a level of improvement of 50%. The van der Heijde-modified Sharp score is a composite measure of radiographically assessed structural damage (i.e., joint erosion and joint space narrowing) in the hands and feet. Physical function was assessed using the disability index of the Health Assessment Questionnaire [HAQ-DI].

In these 3 studies, a greater proportion of patients who received golimumab in conjunction with methotrexate achieved an ACR 20 response at week 14 (studies RA-1 and RA-2) and an ACR 50 response at week 24 (studies RA-2 and RA-3) than patients who received methotrexate alone. The proportion of patients who achieved ACR responses was similar for the golimumab 50- and 100-mg dosage groups. In study RA-1, the difference between the proportion of patients who achieved an ACR 20 response with golimumab as compared with placebo was greater for patients who received concomitant DMARDs than for patients who did not receive concomitant DMARDs. In study RA-1, 40% of patients who received golimumab 50 mg every 4 weeks in conjunction with methotrexate achieved an ACR 20 response at week 14 compared with 17% of patients who received methotrexate and placebo. In study RA-2, 55% of patients who received golimumab 50 mg every 4 weeks in conjunction with methotrexate achieved an ACR 20 response at week 14 compared with 33% of patients who received methotrexate and placebo; the ACR 20 response rates for these 2 groups of patients were 60 and 28%, respectively, at week 24 and 64 and 44%, respectively, at week 52. In study RA-3, 40% of patients who received golimumab 50 mg every 4 weeks in conjunction with methotrexate achieved an ACR 50 response at week 24 compared with 29% of patients who received methotrexate and placebo. In studies RA-2 and RA-3, ACR responses were similar for both the golimumab and methotrexate monotherapy groups. Although a control group was lacking during the extended-treatment periods of these 3 studies, long-term (2–5 years) follow-up data indicated that ACR responses to golimumab were maintained during continued treatment.

In studies RA-1 and RA-2, patients receiving golimumab 50 mg every 4 weeks had greater improvements in physical function, as assessed using the HAQ-DI, from baseline to week 24 compared with those receiving placebo; a greater proportion of patients receiving golimumab 50 mg every 4 weeks in studies RA-1 (43 versus 27%) and RA-2 (65 versus 35%) also achieved a HAQ-DI response (defined as a change from baseline exceeding 0.22) at week 24.

In study RA-3, progression of structural damage, as measured by change from baseline to week 52 in the total van der Heijde-modified Sharp score, was inhibited in patients who received golimumab in combination with methotrexate but not in those who received golimumab as monotherapy, as compared with those who received methotrexate monotherapy; 71% of patients receiving golimumab 50 mg every 4 weeks and methotrexate had no progression of structural damage as assessed by total van der Heijde-modified Sharp score at week 52, compared with 54% of those receiving methotrexate monotherapy. The 100-mg dosage did not provide benefits over the 50-mg dosage for inhibiting progression of structural damage.

Clinical Experience with IV Golimumab Safety and efficacy of IV golimumab were evaluated in a randomized, double-blind, controlled study (GO-FURTHER) in 592 adults with moderately to severely active rheumatoid arthritis (as defined by the ACR) despite methotrexate therapy for at least 3 months prior to the study; patients had not received prior therapy with TNF blocking agents. To be included in the study, patients were required to have at least 6 swollen and 6 tender joints. Patients were randomized in a 2:1 ratio to receive either golimumab (2 mg/kg by IV infusion over 30 minutes at weeks 0 and 4 and every 8 weeks thereafter) or placebo, each given in conjunction with a stable methotrexate regimen (15–25 mg weekly). Patients assigned to receive placebo in conjunction with methotrexate were switched to combination therapy with golimumab and methotrexate at week 24 (or at week 16 in those with less than 10% improvement from baseline in the number of tender and swollen joints); however, the study remained blinded until completion of therapy. The final infusion was administered at week 100 and patients were followed for an additional 12 weeks. The median duration of rheumatoid arthritis disease prior to study enrollment was 4.7 years, and 50% of patients had previously received at least one DMARD other than methotrexate. Patients receiving stable dosages of low-dose corticosteroids (equivalent to 10 mg of prednisone daily or less) and/or NSAIAs could continue such agents; after week 52, another DMARD (e.g., sulfasalazine) could be substituted for methotrexate if required for patient tolerance, but use of cytotoxic agents and other biologic agents was prohibited throughout the study. NSAIAs and low-dose corticosteroids were each used in 81% of patients at baseline.

The primary outcome measure was the proportion of patients attaining an

ACR 20 response at week 14. Additional measures of clinical response and disease activity included ACR 50 and ACR 70 responses and 28-joint Disease Activity Score using C-reactive protein (DAS 28 [CRP]). A greater proportion of patients receiving golimumab and methotrexate attained an ACR 20 response at weeks 14 and 24 (59 and 63%, respectively, versus 25 and 32%, respectively), an ACR 50 response at weeks 14 and 24 (30 and 35%, respectively, versus 9 and 13%, respectively), and an ACR 70 response at weeks 14 and 24 (12 and 18%, respectively, versus 3 and 4%, respectively) compared with those receiving placebo and methotrexate. Improvements in all components of the ACR response criteria from baseline to week 14 were greater in patients receiving golimumab and methotrexate compared with those receiving placebo and methotrexate. In addition, a greater proportion of patients receiving golimumab and methotrexate attained a low level of disease activity as measured by DAS 28 (CRP) (i.e., score of less than 2.6) at week 14 compared with those receiving placebo and methotrexate (15 versus 5%). Clinical response to combined therapy with golimumab and methotrexate was maintained during 100 weeks of treatment. At week 100, ACR 20, ACR 50, and ACR 70 response rates for patients receiving combined therapy with golimumab and methotrexate throughout the study were 69, 45, and 23%, respectively; 29% of these patients had a low level of disease activity as measured by DAS 28 (CRP).

Structural joint damage was assessed radiographically as the change from baseline in the total van der Heijde-modified Sharp score and its component scores (i.e., joint erosion and joint space narrowing). At week 24, progression of structural damage was inhibited in patients who received golimumab and methotrexate compared with those who received placebo and methotrexate; 71% of patients receiving golimumab and methotrexate had no progression of structural damage as assessed by total van der Heijde-modified Sharp score at week 24, compared with 57% of those receiving placebo and methotrexate. Patients who received placebo and methotrexate before crossing over to combined therapy with golimumab and methotrexate at week 16 or 24 exhibited more progression, as measured by change from baseline in total van der Heijde-modified Sharp score, at weeks 52 and 100 than did those who received golimumab and methotrexate throughout the study; however, between weeks 24 and 100, progression was limited in both groups of patients.

Patients receiving golimumab in conjunction with methotrexate also had greater improvements in physical function (as assessed using the HAQ-DI) from baseline to week 14 and in quality-of-life measures (physical component summary score, mental component summary score, and all 8 domains of the Short Form-36 Health Survey [SF-36]) compared with patients receiving placebo in conjunction with methotrexate. Among patients receiving combined therapy with golimumab and methotrexate throughout the study, improvements in physical function and quality of life generally were maintained at weeks 100 and 112, respectively.

■ Psoriatic Arthritis Golimumab is used alone or in conjunction with methotrexate for the management of active psoriatic arthritis in adults.

Safety and efficacy of subcutaneous golimumab were evaluated in a multicenter, randomized, double-blind, placebo-controlled study (GO-REVEAL) in 405 adults with moderately to severely active psoriatic arthritis (3 or more swollen joints and 3 or more tender joints) who were receiving an NSAIA and/or DMARDs. In addition, patients were required to have a diagnosis of psoriatic arthritis for at least 6 months and plaque psoriasis with a qualifying target lesion (diameter of 2 cm or greater). Patients were randomized to receive golimumab (50 or 100 mg subcutaneously once every 4 weeks) or placebo. The study included patients with any of the following forms of the disease: polyarticular arthritis without rheumatoid nodules, asymmetric peripheral arthritis, distal interphalangeal joint arthritis, spondylitis with peripheral arthritis, or arthritis mutilans. Patients receiving stable dosages of methotrexate (25 mg/week or less), low-dose oral corticosteroids (equivalent to 10 mg of prednisone daily or less), and/or NSAIAs could continue such agents. Previous treatment with a TNF blocking agent was not allowed; the use of other DMARDs, including sulfasalazine, hydroxychloroquine, cytotoxic agents, or other biologic agents, was prohibited. At week 16, patients with less than 10% improvement from baseline in both swollen and tender joint counts entered early escape in which their study drug was adjusted in a double-blind manner (i.e., those meeting the early escape criteria who were receiving golimumab 50 mg had their golimumab dosage increased to 100 mg and those who were receiving placebo began receiving golimumab 50 mg every 4 weeks). At week 24, all remaining patients who had been receiving placebo initiated golimumab 50 mg every 4 weeks. Golimumab continued to be administered in a blinded manner every 4 weeks to week 52. During the unblinded long-term extension period (weeks 52–256), certain adjustments of golimumab dosage (increase to 100 mg or decrease to 50 mg) and concomitant therapies could be made at the clinician's discretion. The median duration of psoriatic arthritis disease prior to study enrollment was 5.1 years, and 78% of patients previously received at least one DMARD; 48, 16, or 72% of patients received stable dosages of methotrexate, low-dose oral corticosteroids, or NSAIAs, respectively, during the blinded study period.

The primary outcome measures were the proportion of patients achieving an ACR 20 response at week 14 and the change from baseline to week 24 in the van der Heijde-Sharp score modified for assessment of psoriatic arthritis. Physical function and health-related quality of life were assessed using the HAQ-DI and SF-36. A greater proportion of patients who received golimumab 50 mg every 4 weeks, with or without methotrexate, achieved an ACR 20 response at week 14 than did patients who received placebo, with or without methotrexate (51 versus 9%, respectively). The proportion of patients who achieved ACR responses was similar for the golimumab 50- and 100-mg dosage groups, as well as for patients who received golimumab with and without methotrexate. At week 24, progression of structural damage, as assessed by the modified van der Heijde-Sharp score, was inhibited in patients who received golimumab 50 mg every 4 weeks compared with those who received placebo. Golimumab therapy also was associated with greater improvements from baseline in the HAQ-DI at week 24 and in the SF-36 physical component summary at week 14 compared with placebo. Although a control group was lacking after week 24, follow-up at 5 years indicated that 63–70% of patients across all randomized groups had ACR 20 responses and the mean change from baseline in the modified van der Heijde-Sharp score was minimal. Concomitant use of golimumab with methotrexate appeared to reduce progression of structural damage compared with use of golimumab without methotrexate.

The safety and efficacy of golimumab in the management of plaque psoriasis have not been established.

■ Ankylosing Spondylitis Golimumab is used for the management of ankylosing spondylitis in adults with active disease.

Safety and efficacy of subcutaneous golimumab were evaluated in a multicenter, randomized, double-blind, placebo-controlled study (GO-RAISE) in 356 adults with active ankylosing spondylitis (as defined by the modified New York criteria) for at least 3 months prior to administration of the study drug. To be included in these studies, patients were required to have symptoms of active disease (defined as a Bath Ankylosing Spondylitis Disease Activity Index [BASDAI] score of 4 or more and a visual analog scale [VAS] score for total back pain of 4 or more, on scales of 0–10) and an inadequate response to current or previous NSAIA or DMARD therapy. Patients ineligible for participation in the study included, but were not limited to, patients with complete ankylosis of the spine and patients who had previously received treatment with a TNF blocking agent. Patients were randomized to receive golimumab (50 or 100 mg subcutaneously once every 4 weeks) or placebo. Patients receiving stable dosages of methotrexate (25 mg/week or less), sulfasalazine, hydroxychloroquine, low-dose corticosteroids (equivalent to 10 mg of prednisone daily or less), and/or NSAIAs could continue such agents; the use of other DMARDs, including cytotoxic agents or other biologic agents, was prohibited. At week 16, patients with less than 20% improvement from baseline in total back pain and morning stiffness entered early escape in which their study drug was adjusted in a double-blind manner (i.e., those meeting the early escape criteria who were receiving golimumab 50 mg had their golimumab dosage increased to 100 mg and those who were receiving placebo began receiving golimumab 50 mg every 4 weeks). At week 24, all remaining patients who had been receiving placebo initiated golimumab 50 mg every 4 weeks. Golimumab continued to be administered in a blinded manner every 4 weeks through week 100. During the unblinded long-term extension period (weeks 104–252), certain adjustments of golimumab dosage (increase to 100 mg or decrease to 50 mg) and concomitant therapies could be made at the clinician's discretion. The median duration of ankylosing spondylitis disease prior to study enrollment was 5.6 years, and 55% of patients previously received at least one DMARD; 20, 26, 1, 16, or 90% of patients received stable dosages of methotrexate, sulfasalazine, hydroxychloroquine, low-dose oral corticosteroids, or NSAIAs, respectively, during the blinded study period.

The primary outcome measure was the proportion of patients achieving an Assessment in Ankylosing Spondylitis (ASAS) 20 response at week 14. An ASAS 20 response is achieved if the patient experiences at least a 20% improvement and an absolute improvement of at least 10 units (on a scale of 0–100) in at least 3 of the following criteria without worsening in the fourth criterion: patient global assessment, pain, function, or inflammation. A greater proportion of patients who received golimumab 50 mg every 4 weeks, with or without DMARDs, achieved an ASAS 20 response at week 14 than did patients who received placebo, with or without DMARDs (59 versus 22%, respectively). At week 24, 56% of those receiving golimumab 50 mg every 4 weeks, with or without DMARDs, achieved an ASAS 20 response; 23% of those receiving placebo, with or without DMARDs, achieved an ASAS 20 response. The proportion of patients who achieved ASAS responses was similar for the golimumab 50- and 100-mg dosage groups. Clinical improvements observed in patients receiving golimumab at week 24 were maintained through up to 5 years of treatment.

■ Ulcerative Colitis Golimumab is used in patients with moderately to severely active ulcerative colitis who require continuous corticosteroid therapy or who have had an inadequate response to or were intolerant to conventional therapies (oral aminosalicylates, oral corticosteroids, azathioprine, or mercaptopurine) to induce and maintain clinical response, to improve endoscopic appearance of the mucosa during induction therapy, to induce clinical remission, and to achieve and sustain clinical remission in those who have responded to induction therapy.

Safety and efficacy of subcutaneous golimumab were established in 2 randomized, double-blind, placebo-controlled studies (PURSUIT-SC and PURSUIT-M) in adults with ulcerative colitis. PURSUIT-SC evaluated golimumab induction therapy and included a dose-finding phase 2 study followed by a dose-confirming phase 3 study. PURSUIT-M evaluated golimumab maintenance therapy in patients who had responded to induction therapy with the drug. Induction therapy with IV† golimumab (single 1-, 2-, or 4-mg/kg induction dose) also has been evaluated (PURSUIT-IV); however, the study failed to establish efficacy of these induction regimens.

Patients enrolled in PURSUIT-SC had moderately to severely active ulcerative colitis (as defined by a Mayo score of 6–12 with an endoscopy subscore of 2 or 3) and were corticosteroid dependent or had an inadequate response or intolerance to one or more conventional therapies (i.e., oral aminosalicylates, oral corticosteroids, azathioprine, mercaptopurine). Those who had received prior therapy with TNF blocking agents were excluded from the study. The Mayo score ranges from 0–12 and includes 4 subscales (i.e., stool frequency, rectal bleeding, findings on endoscopy, and physician global assessment), each scored from 0–3 (normal to most severe, respectively). An endoscopy subscore of 2 is defined by marked erythema, lack of vascular pattern, friability, and erosions, whereas an endoscopy subscore of 3 is defined by spontaneous bleeding and ulceration.

Two of the induction regimens evaluated in the dose-finding phase 2 study (golimumab 400 mg at week 0 and 200 mg at week 2 [400 mg/200 mg], golimumab 200 mg at week 0 and 100 mg at week 2 [200 mg/100 mg]) were selected for further evaluation in the phase 3 study. The phase 3 evaluation included data for 761 patients. Patients receiving stable dosages of oral aminosalicylates, oral corticosteroids (equivalent to 40 mg of prednisone daily or less), azathioprine, mercaptopurine, and/or methotrexate were permitted to continue receiving these drugs throughout the study. The median baseline Mayo score for the phase 2 and 3 studies combined was 8. The primary outcome measure in the phase 3 study was the proportion of patients in clinical response at week 6; clinical response was defined as a decrease in Mayo score of at least 3 points and at least 30% from baseline score, with a reduction in rectal bleeding subscore of at least 1 point or an absolute rectal bleeding subscore of 0 (no blood seen) or 1 (streaks of blood with stool less than half the time). Other outcome measures included clinical remission and improved mucosal appearance. Clinical remission was defined as a Mayo score of 0–2 with no individual subscore exceeding 1. Improved mucosal appearance was defined as a Mayo endoscopy subscore of 0 (normal mucosa or inactive disease) or 1 (erythema, decreased vascular pattern, mild friability). At week 6, clinical response rates (51 versus 30%), clinical remission rates (18 versus 6%), and rates of improved mucosal appearance (42 versus 29%) were higher in patients receiving induction therapy with golimumab 200 mg/100 mg compared with those receiving placebo. Induction therapy with golimumab 400 mg/200 mg provided no additional benefit beyond that provided by a dosage of 200 mg/100 mg.

PURSUIT-M was a randomized-withdrawal study that evaluated 456 patients who had attained clinical response with golimumab induction therapy and had tolerated the drug during either the PURSUIT-SC or PURSUIT-IV study. Approximately 35% of these patients were in clinical remission at the start of the PURSUIT-M maintenance study. Patients who had responded to golimumab induction therapy were randomized to receive maintenance therapy with subcutaneous golimumab (50 or 100 mg every 4 weeks) or placebo. Those receiving stable dosages of oral aminosalicylates, azathioprine, mercaptopurine, and/or methotrexate could continue such agents. At the start of the maintenance study, approximately 52% of patients who had responded to golimumab induction therapy were receiving corticosteroids, 31% were receiving azathioprine or mercaptopurine, less than 1% were receiving methotrexate, and 80% were receiving aminosalicylates. In patients receiving corticosteroids, a corticosteroid-tapering regimen was initiated at the start of the maintenance trial. The primary outcome measure was the proportion of patients maintaining clinical response through week 54. In PURSUIT-M, clinical response was maintained through week 54 in 50, 47, or 31% of those receiving golimumab 100 mg every 4 weeks, golimumab 50 mg every 4 weeks, or placebo, respectively. A greater proportion of patients receiving golimumab 100 mg every 4 weeks, compared with those receiving placebo (28 versus 16%), achieved clinical remission at both weeks 30 and 54 without demonstrating a loss of response at any time point through week 54; although golimumab 50 mg every 4 weeks showed a numerical advantage over placebo for this outcome measure (23% of patients in clinical remission), the difference was not statistically significant.

Dosage and Administration

■ General Golimumab is used in conjunction with methotrexate for the management of moderately to severely active rheumatoid arthritis in adults; the drug may be used with or without methotrexate in adults with psoriatic arthritis or ankylosing spondylitis. Corticosteroids, other nonbiologic disease-modifying antirheumatic drugs (DMARDs), and nonsteroidal anti-inflammatory agents (NSAIAs) or analgesics may be continued in adults receiving golimumab for the management of rheumatoid arthritis, psoriatic arthritis, or ankylosing spondylitis.

Aminosalicylates, corticosteroids, azathioprine, mercaptopurine, and/or methotrexate could be continued during pivotal trials of golimumab in patients with ulcerative colitis. However, the possibility of an increased risk of hepatosplenic T-cell lymphoma with combination immunosuppressive therapy in such patients should be considered carefully. (See Malignancies and Lymphoproliferative Disorders under Warnings/Precautions: Warnings, in Cautions.)

■ Administration Golimumab is administered by subcutaneous injection; the drug also may be administered by IV infusion in adults with rheumatoid arthritis. Golimumab is intended for use under the guidance and supervision of a clinician; however, subcutaneous golimumab may be *self-administered* if the clinician determines that the patient and/or their caregiver is competent to safely administer the drug after appropriate training. Efficacy and safety of switching between IV and subcutaneous golimumab formulations and routes of administration have not been established.

Subcutaneous Administration For subcutaneous administration, golimumab is commercially available in prefilled syringes and in prefilled auto-injectors (SmartJect®) equipped with a 27-gauge, ½-inch needle. Prior to subcutaneous administration, golimumab solutions should be inspected visually for particulate matter or discoloration; if either is present, the solution should be discarded. Golimumab prefilled syringes and auto-injectors for subcutaneous administration are for single use only; unused portions of the solution should be discarded. Golimumab injection should be stored at 2–8°C in the original carton until administration and protected from light. The injection should not be frozen or shaken. The golimumab prefilled syringe or auto-injector should be allowed to sit at room temperature outside of the carton for 30 minutes prior to subcutaneous injection; golimumab should *not* be warmed in any other way (e.g., microwave, hot water). The syringe needle cover or auto-injector cap should *not* be removed while the prefilled syringe or auto-injector is warming to room temperature.

Golimumab is administered subcutaneously into the thighs. Golimumab also may be administered subcutaneously into the lower abdomen below the umbilicus; however, abdominal injections should not be made within 5.08 cm (2 inches) of the umbilicus. Golimumab may be administered subcutaneously into the upper arm by a caregiver. If multiple injections are required to administer a single dose, separate injection sites should be used. Injection sites should be rotated. Injections should not be made into areas where the skin is tender, bruised, red, or hard or into scars or stretch marks.

IV Administration For IV infusion, golimumab is commercially available as an injection concentrate containing 12.5 mg/mL. IV golimumab should be stored at 2–8°C in the original carton until administration and protected from light. The vials should not be frozen or shaken.

Prior to IV administration, golimumab injection concentrate must be diluted in 0.45 or 0.9% sodium chloride injection to provide a total volume of 100 mL (i.e., if a 100-mL bottle or bag of 0.45 or 0.9% sodium chloride injection is used, a volume of diluent equal to the total required volume of golimumab injection concentrate should be removed from the infusion container prior to addition of the golimumab injection concentrate). The total required volume of golimumab injection concentrate should be added slowly to the infusion container, and the diluted solution gently mixed. Any unused portion of drug should be discarded since the injection concentrate contains no preservative. Golimumab solutions should be inspected visually for particulate matter and discoloration prior to dilution and administration. The injection concentrate should appear colorless to light yellow and should not be used if discoloration or particulates other than a few fine translucent particles are present. The diluted solution may be stored for 4 hours at room temperature. Diluted golimumab solutions should be infused IV over 30 minutes using an inline nonpyrogenic, low-protein-binding filter with a pore size not exceeding 0.22 μm. Golimumab should not be infused simultaneously through the same IV line with any other drug. The diluted solution should not be used if discoloration or particulate matter is present.

■ Dosage ***Rheumatoid Arthritis in Adults*** For the management of moderately to severely active rheumatoid arthritis in adults, the usual dosage of golimumab is 50 mg once monthly by subcutaneous injection or 2 mg/kg given by IV infusion over 30 minutes at weeks 0 and 4 and then every 8 weeks thereafter; golimumab should be used in conjunction with methotrexate for the management of rheumatoid arthritis.

Psoriatic Arthritis For the management of active psoriatic arthritis in adults, the usual dosage of golimumab is 50 mg once monthly by subcutaneous injection.

Ankylosing Spondylitis For the management of active ankylosing spondylitis in adults, the usual dosage of golimumab is 50 mg once monthly by subcutaneous injection.

Ulcerative Colitis For the management of moderately to severely active ulcerative colitis in adults, the recommended dosage of golimumab is 200 mg at week 0 followed by 100 mg at week 2 (induction therapy) and then 100 mg every 4 weeks thereafter (maintenance therapy), with all doses given by subcutaneous injection.

■ Special Populations Dosage adjustment of subcutaneous golimumab based on weight or gender is not necessary. The manufacturer makes no specific dosage recommendations for geriatric patients or patients with hepatic or renal impairment.

Cautions

■ Contraindications The manufacturer states that there are no known contraindications to the use of golimumab.

■ Warnings/Precautions ***Warnings*** **Infectious Complications.** Patients receiving tumor necrosis factor (TNF) blocking agents, including golimumab, are at increased risk of developing serious infections involving various organ systems and sites that may require hospitalization or result in death. Opportunistic infections caused by bacterial, mycobacterial, invasive fungal, viral, or parasitic organisms—including aspergillosis, blastomycosis, candidiasis, coccidioidomycosis, histoplasmosis, legionellosis, listeriosis, pneumocystosis, and tuberculosis—have been reported in patients receiving TNF blocking agents. Infections frequently have been disseminated rather than localized. Patients should be closely monitored during and after treatment with TNF blocking agents for the development of signs or symptoms of infection (e.g., fever, malaise, weight loss, sweats, cough, dyspnea, pulmonary infiltrates, serious systemic illness including shock). Most patients who developed serious infections were receiving concomitant therapy with immunosuppressive agents such as methotrexate or corticosteroids.

In controlled trials evaluating subcutaneous golimumab in adults with rheumatoid arthritis, psoriatic arthritis, or ankylosing spondylitis, infection was reported in 28 or 25% of golimumab-treated or control patients, respectively, following 16 weeks of treatment; the rate of serious infection was 1.4 or 1.3%, respectively. In a controlled trial evaluating IV golimumab in adults with rheumatoid arthritis, infection was reported following 24 weeks of treatment in 27% of patients receiving golimumab and methotrexate compared with 24% of those receiving placebo and methotrexate; the rate of serious infection was 0.9 or 0%, respectively. In controlled trials in patients with ulcerative colitis, rates of infection and serious infection during the induction period (through week 6) were similar in patients receiving subcutaneous golimumab (200 mg at week 0 and 100 mg at week 2) and those receiving placebo; infection was reported in approximately 12% of patients. Among patients who received golimumab induction therapy, rates of infection and serious infection through 60 weeks of treatment were similar in those who received a maintenance regimen of golimumab 100 mg every 4 weeks and those who received placebo.

Serious infections reported in patients receiving golimumab have included sepsis, pneumonia, cellulitis, opportunistic infections, abscess, tuberculosis, invasive fungal infections, and hepatitis B virus (HBV) infection. As of September 2011, FDA had identified 103 reports of *Legionella* pneumonia associated with TNF blocking agents, including golimumab. The 103 cases of *Legionella* pneumonia occurred in patients 25–85 years of age, many of whom received concomitant therapy with immunosuppressive agents (e.g., corticosteroids and/or methotrexate); 17 deaths were reported. In 78% of the cases of *Legionella* pneumonia, the median duration of TNF blocker therapy prior to the onset of *Legionella* pneumonia was 10.4 months (range: less than 1 month to 73 months). As of September 2011, FDA also had identified 26 published reports of *Listeria* infections, including meningitis, bacteremia, endophthalmitis, and sepsis, in patients who received TNF blocking agents; 7 deaths were reported. Many of the *Listeria* infections occurred in patients who had received concomitant therapy with immunosuppressive agents. In addition, FDA identified fatal *Listeria* infections during a review of data regarding laboratory-confirmed infections that occurred in premarketing clinical studies and during postmarketing surveillance.

An increased incidence of serious infections also was observed in clinical studies in patients with rheumatoid arthritis when a TNF blocking agent was used concomitantly with anakinra (a human interleukin-1 receptor antagonist) or abatacept (a selective costimulation modulator). (See Drug Interactions: Biologic Antirheumatic Agents.)

Golimumab therapy should not be initiated in patients with active infections, including clinically important localized infections. Patients older than 65 years of age, patients with comorbid conditions, and/or patients receiving concomitant therapy with immunosuppressive agents such as corticosteroids or methotrexate may be at increased risk of infection. Clinicians should consider potential risks and benefits of the drug prior to initiating therapy in patients with a history of chronic, recurring, or opportunistic infections; patients with underlying conditions that may predispose them to infections; and patients who have been exposed to tuberculosis or who reside or have traveled in regions where tuberculosis or mycoses such as histoplasmosis, coccidioidomycosis, and blastomycosis are endemic. Any patient who develops a new infection while receiving golimumab should undergo a thorough diagnostic evaluation (appropriate for an immunocompromised patient), appropriate anti-infective therapy should be initiated, and the patient should be closely monitored. The drug should be discontinued in patients who develop a serious infection, an opportunistic infection, or sepsis.

Because tuberculosis has been reported in patients receiving golimumab, including in patients who received golimumab during and following treatment for latent tuberculosis, all patients should be evaluated for active or latent tuberculosis and for the presence of risk factors for tuberculosis prior to and periodically during therapy with the drug. When indicated, an appropriate antimycobacterial regimen for the treatment of latent tuberculosis infection should be initiated prior to golimumab therapy. Antimycobacterial treatment lowers the risk of latent tuberculosis infection progressing to active disease (i.e., reactivation) in patients receiving golimumab. Antimycobacterial therapy also should be considered prior to initiation of golimumab in individuals with a history of latent or active tuberculosis in whom an adequate course of antimycobacterial treatment cannot be confirmed and in individuals with a negative tuberculin skin test who have risk factors for tuberculosis. Consultation with a tuberculosis specialist is recommended when deciding whether antimycobacterial therapy should be initiated. Patients receiving golimumab, including individuals with a negative tuberculin skin test, patients who are receiving treatment for latent tuberculosis, and patients who previously were treated for tuberculosis infection, should be monitored for signs and symptoms of active tuberculosis. A diagnosis of tuberculosis should be considered in patients who develop new infections while receiving golimumab, especially in those who previously have traveled to countries where tuberculosis is highly prevalent or who have been in close contact with an individual with active tuberculosis.

Failure to recognize invasive fungal infections in patients receiving TNF blocking agents has led to delays in appropriate treatment. Clinicians should ascertain whether patients receiving TNF blocking agents who present with signs and symptoms suggestive of systemic fungal infection reside or have traveled in regions where mycoses are endemic. Empiric antifungal therapy should be considered in patients at risk of histoplasmosis or other invasive fungal infections who develop severe systemic illness, taking into account both the risk for severe fungal infection and the risks associated with antifungal therapy. Serologic tests for histoplasmosis may be negative in some patients with active infection. Following resolution of an invasive fungal infection, the decision regarding whether to reinitiate TNF blocking agent therapy should involve reevaluation of the risks and benefits of such therapy, particularly in patients who reside in regions where mycoses are endemic. Whenever feasible, decisions regarding initiation and duration of antifungal therapy and reinitiation of TNF blocking agent therapy should be made in consultation with a specialist in the diagnosis and management of fungal infections.

Malignancies and Lymphoproliferative Disorders. Malignancies, some fatal, have been reported in children, adolescents, and young adults who received treatment with TNF blocking agents beginning when they were 18 years of age or younger. In August 2009, FDA reported the results of an analysis of reports of lymphoma and other malignancies in children and adolescents who had received TNF blocking agents. These cases were reported postmarketing and were derived from various sources, including registries and spontaneous postmarketing reports. Golimumab was not FDA-approved at the time of the analysis and, therefore, was not included in the analysis. The FDA identified 48 cases of malignancies in children and adolescents in the analysis.

Of the 48 cases reviewed by FDA, approximately 50% were lymphomas, including Hodgkin's disease and non-Hodgkin's lymphoma. The other cases represented a variety of malignancies, including rare malignancies that are usually associated with immunosuppression and malignancies that are not usually observed in children and adolescents. Other malignancies reported included leukemia, melanoma, and solid organ cancers; malignancies such as leiomyosarcoma, hepatic malignancies, and renal cell carcinoma, which rarely occur in children, also were reported. The malignancies occurred after a median of 30 months (range: 1–84 months) following the first dose of therapy with TNF blocking agents. Of the 48 cases of malignancies, 11 deaths were reported; causes of death included hepatosplenic T-cell lymphoma (9 cases), T-cell lymphoma (1 case), and sepsis following remission of lymphoma (1 case). Most of the 48 patients (88%) also were receiving other immunosuppressive drugs such as azathioprine and methotrexate; these agents also are associated with an increased risk of lymphoma. Although there were other contributory factors, the role of TNF blocking agents in the development of malignancies in children and adolescents could not be excluded. Therefore, FDA concluded that there is an increased risk of malignancy with TNF blocking agents. However, due to the relatively rare occurrence of these cancers, the limited number of pediatric patients who received TNF blocking agents, and the possible role of other immunosuppressive drugs used concomitantly with TNF blocking agents, FDA was unable to fully characterize the strength of the association between use of TNF blocking agents and the development of a malignancy.

Hepatosplenic T-cell lymphoma, a rare, aggressive, usually fatal type of T-cell lymphoma, has been reported during postmarketing experience mainly in adolescent and young adult males with Crohn's disease or ulcerative colitis who received treatment with TNF blocking agents and/or thiopurine analogs (mercaptopurine or azathioprine). Most of the reported cases of hepatosplenic T-cell lymphoma occurred in patients who had received a combination of immunosuppressive agents, including TNF blocking agents and thiopurine analogs (azathioprine or mercaptopurine), at or prior to diagnosis. In some cases, potential confounding factors could not be excluded because complete medical histories were not available. Since patients with certain conditions (e.g., rheumatoid arthritis, Crohn's disease, ankylosing spondylitis, psoriatic arthritis) may be at increased risk for lymphoma, it may be difficult to measure the added risk of treatment with TNF blocking agents, azathioprine, and/or mercaptopurine.

In clinical studies, lymphoma has been observed more frequently in patients receiving TNF blocking agents than in control patients. In controlled studies evaluating golimumab in patients with rheumatoid arthritis, psoriatic arthritis, or ankylosing spondylitis, the incidence of lymphoma was 0.21 per 100 patient-years in golimumab-treated patients and 0 per 100 patient-years in placebo-treated patients. In these studies (including during uncontrolled phases of the studies), the incidence of lymphoma in golimumab-treated patients was approximately 3.8-fold higher than the expected incidence in the general US population. Through week 60 of controlled studies evaluating golimumab in patients with ulcerative colitis, no cases of lymphoma were reported in patients receiving the drug. Patients with rheumatoid arthritis and other chronic inflammatory diseases, especially those with highly active disease and/or long-term exposure to immunosuppressive therapies, may be at increased risk of lymphoma, even in the absence of TNF blocking agent therapy.

Cases of acute and chronic leukemia have been reported in patients receiving TNF blocking agents, including golimumab, for the management of rheumatoid arthritis and other conditions. In August 2009, FDA reported the results of a review of 147 cases of leukemia in adults and pediatric patients who received TNF blocking agents. Of the 147 cases, acute myeloid leukemia (44 cases), chronic lymphocytic leukemia (31 cases), and chronic myeloid leukemia (23 cases) were the most frequent types of leukemia reported. Four cases of leukemia were reported in children. Most patients (61%) also were receiving other immunosuppressive drugs. There were a total of 30 deaths reported; leukemia was reported as the cause of 26 of the 30 deaths, and the event was associated with the use of TNF blocking agents. Leukemia generally occurred during the first 2 years of therapy. The interpretation of these findings was complicated by the fact that published epidemiologic studies suggest that patients with rheumatoid arthritis may be at increased risk of leukemia, independent of any treatment with TNF blocking agents. However, based on the available data, FDA concluded that there is a possible association between treatment with TNF blocking agents and the development of leukemia in patients receiving these drugs.

In a controlled study evaluating IV golimumab in patients with rheumatoid arthritis, one case of malignancy other than lymphoma and nonmelanoma skin cancer was reported in a patient receiving the drug during the 24-week controlled phase of the study; over approximately 92 weeks of treatment (including both controlled and uncontrolled periods of study), the incidence of such malignancies per 100 patient-years of IV golimumab use was 0.31, and the incidence of nonmelanoma skin cancer was 0.1 per 100 patient-years of exposure. In controlled studies evaluating subcutaneous golimumab in patients with rheumatoid arthritis, psoriatic arthritis, or ankylosing spondylitis, the incidence of malignancies other than lymphoma was not increased in golimumab-treated patients compared with placebo-treated patients. In these studies (including during uncontrolled phases of the studies), the incidence of malignancies other than lymphoma in golimumab-treated patients was similar to the expected incidence in the general US population. Through week 60 of controlled studies evaluating golimumab in patients with ulcerative colitis, the incidence of malignancies other than lymphoma and nonmelanoma skin cancer was similar to the expected incidence in the general US population. Short follow-up periods (e.g., 1 year or less) may not accurately reflect the true incidence of malignancies.

Melanoma and Merkel cell carcinoma have been reported in patients receiving TNF blocking agents, including cases of melanoma in golimumab-treated patients.

In controlled studies of other TNF blocking agents in patients at increased risk of malignancies (e.g., patients with chronic obstructive pulmonary disease [COPD], patients with Wegener's granulomatosis receiving concomitant cyclophosphamide), a greater proportion of malignancies occurred in patients receiving the TNF blocking agent compared with control patients. In a phase 2, dose-ranging, randomized, placebo-controlled study evaluating the safety and efficacy of golimumab (50, 100, or 200 mg once every 4 weeks) in 309 patients with uncontrolled, severe persistent asthma†, malignancies developed in 8 golimumab-treated patients and in none of the control patients; 6 of the 8 golimumab-treated patients developed malignancies other than nonmelanoma skin cancer, and 5 of the 8 golimumab-treated patients received 200-mg doses of the drug. The malignancies in golimumab-treated patients were diagnosed between days 76–448 of the study. Study drug administration was discontinued early as a result of the unfavorable risk-to-benefit profile observed in patients who received golimumab.

Clinicians should consider the possibility of and monitor for the occurrence of malignancies during and following treatment with TNF blocking agents. Periodic dermatologic evaluations are recommended for all patients receiving TNF blocking agents, but particularly for those with risk factors for skin cancer. The risks and benefits of TNF blocking agents, including golimumab, should be considered prior to initiating therapy in patients with a known malignancy (other than a successfully treated nonmelanoma skin cancer) or when considering whether to continue TNF blocking agent therapy in patients who develop a malignancy. Because therapy with TNF blocking agents and/or thiopurine analogs (azathioprine or mercaptopurine) may increase the risk of malignancies, including hepatosplenic T-cell lymphoma, the risks and benefits of these agents should be carefully considered, especially in adolescents and young adults and especially in the treatment of Crohn's disease or ulcerative colitis.

Because it remains to be established whether golimumab affects the risk for development of dysplasia or colon cancer, all patients with ulcerative colitis who have a history of dysplasia or colon carcinoma, or are at increased risk for these conditions (e.g., those with long-standing ulcerative colitis or primary sclerosing cholangitis), should be screened for dysplasia at regular intervals, both before therapy and throughout their disease, in accordance with current standards of care. In patients with newly diagnosed dysplasia, the risks and benefits of continued golimumab therapy must be carefully considered.

Other Warnings/Precautions **Patients Infected with Hepatitis B Virus.** Use of TNF blocking agents, including golimumab, may increase the risk of reactivation of hepatitis B virus (HBV) infection in patients who are chronic carriers of this virus (i.e., hepatitis B surface antigen-positive [HBsAg-positive]). HBV reactivation has resulted in death in a few individuals receiving TNF blocking agent therapy. Most patients experiencing HBV reactivation were receiving concomitant therapy with other immunosuppressive agents.

The manufacturer states that all patients should be screened for HBV infection before initiation of golimumab therapy. In patients who test positive for HBsAg, consultation with an HBV infection specialist is recommended before initiation of TNF blocking agent therapy. Chronic carriers of HBV should be appropriately evaluated and monitored prior to the initiation of therapy, during treatment, and for up to several months following therapy with golimumab. Safety and efficacy of antiviral therapy for prevention of viral reactivation in HBV carriers receiving a TNF blocking agent have not been established. Golimumab should be discontinued if HBV reactivation occurs, and appropriate treatment, including antiviral therapy, should be initiated. It has not been established whether golimumab can be safely readministered once control of the reactivated HBV infection has been achieved; caution is advised if golimumab therapy is resumed in such a situation.

Cardiovascular Effects. New-onset or worsening heart failure, sometimes fatal, has been reported in patients receiving TNF blocking agents, including golimumab. While golimumab has not been studied in patients with a history of heart failure, other TNF blocking agents have been associated with increased morbidity (exacerbations requiring hospitalization) or mortality in patients with heart failure. If golimumab is used in patients with heart failure, caution and careful monitoring are recommended. Golimumab should be discontinued if new or worsening symptoms of heart failure occur.

Nervous System Effects. New onset or exacerbation of central or peripheral nervous system demyelinating disorders (e.g., multiple sclerosis, Guillain-Barré syndrome) has been reported rarely in patients receiving golimumab or other TNF blocking agents. Central demyelination, multiple sclerosis, optic neuritis, and peripheral demyelinating polyneuropathy have been reported rarely in patients receiving golimumab. Clinicians should exercise caution when considering therapy with TNF blocking agents, including golimumab, in patients with central or peripheral nervous system demyelinating disorders. Discontinuance of golimumab should be considered if these disorders develop.

Hematologic Effects. Pancytopenia, leukopenia, neutropenia, aplastic anemia, and thrombocytopenia have been reported in patients receiving golimumab or other TNF blocking agents. TNF blocking agents, including golimumab, should be used with caution in patients who have or have had substantial cytopenias.

Immunization and Use of Therapeutic Infectious Agents. Live vaccines and therapeutic infectious agents should be avoided during therapy with golimumab. Administration of live vaccines to infants who were exposed to golimumab in utero is not recommended for 6 months following the last golimumab dose given to the infant's mother during pregnancy. (See Pregnancy under Warnings/Precautions: Specific Populations, in Cautions.) Patients receiving golimumab may receive inactivated vaccines. (See Drug Interactions: Vaccines and Therapeutic Infectious Agents.)

Immunologic Reactions and Antibody Formation. The use of TNF blocking agents, including golimumab, has been associated with the formation of antinuclear antibodies (ANA) and, rarely, with the development of a lupus-like syndrome. Golimumab should be discontinued in patients who develop symptoms suggestive of a lupus-like syndrome. Development of antibodies to double-stranded DNA (anti-dsDNA) also has been reported in patients receiving golimumab.

In phase 3 clinical studies evaluating subcutaneous golimumab in patients with rheumatoid arthritis, psoriatic arthritis, or ankylosing spondylitis, antibodies to the drug were detected in about 4% of golimumab-treated patients across all studies; the incidence of antibody formation was similar for each of the 3 indications for treatment. The incidence of antibody formation was lower in patients receiving golimumab concomitantly with methotrexate than in patients receiving golimumab without methotrexate (2 versus 7%). Antibodies to golimumab were detected in approximately 3% of patients receiving the drug in ulcerative colitis studies. The incidence of antibody formation was lower in patients receiving golimumab concomitantly with other immunosuppressive agents (i.e., azathioprine, mercaptopurine, methotrexate) than in patients who received golimumab without such concomitant therapy (2 versus 4%). Antibodies to golimumab also were detected in 3% of patients who received golimumab in combination with methotrexate through week 24 in a clinical study evaluating IV golimumab in patients with rheumatoid arthritis. Patients who developed antibodies to golimumab generally had lower steady-state trough serum concentrations of the drug. Most patients with an antibody response to golimumab in phase 2 and 3 studies had neutralizing antibodies to golimumab, as measured by cell-based functional assay. However, the small number of patients who formed antibodies to golimumab limits the ability to draw definitive conclusions regarding the relationship between the presence of antibodies to the drug and efficacy or safety of the drug.

Psoriasis. Cases of new-onset psoriasis, including pustular and palmoplantar psoriasis, have been reported with the use of TNF blocking agents, including golimumab. In August 2009, FDA reported the results of a review of 69 cases of new-onset psoriasis, including pustular (17 cases) and palmoplantar (15 cases) psoriasis, in patients receiving TNF blocking agents for the management of autoimmune and rheumatic conditions other than psoriasis and psoriatic arthritis. None of the patients reported having psoriasis prior to initiation of the TNF blocking agent. However, exacerbation of preexisting psoriasis has been reported with the use of TNF blocking agents, including golimumab. Two of the 69 cases of new-onset psoriasis occurred in pediatric patients. The development of psoriasis during treatment with TNF blocking agents occurred at intervals ranging from weeks to years following initiation of the drug. Twelve of the psoriasis cases resulted in hospitalization, which was the most severe outcome reported. Most patients experienced improvement of their psoriasis following discontinuance of the TNF blocking agent. Due to the number of reported cases and the temporal relationship between the initiation of TNF blocking agents and the development of psoriasis, FDA concluded that there is a possible association between the development of psoriasis and use of TNF blocking agents. Clinicians should consider the possibility of and monitor for manifestations (e.g., new rash) of new or worsening psoriasis, particularly pustular and palmoplantar psoriasis, during treatment with TNF blocking agents. Discontinuance of golimumab therapy may be considered if new-onset or worsening psoriasis occurs.

Hepatic Effects. Severe hepatic reactions, including acute liver failure, have been reported in patients receiving TNF blocking agents.

In phase 3 clinical studies evaluating subcutaneous golimumab in patients with rheumatoid arthritis, psoriatic arthritis, or ankylosing spondylitis, increased serum ALT and AST concentrations have been reported in 4 and 3%, respectively, of golimumab-treated patients, compared with 3 and 2%, respectively, of placebo-treated patients; increases in serum ALT concentrations of 3 or more times the upper limit of normal (ULN) or 5 or more times the ULN occurred in 2 or 0.7%, respectively, of golimumab-treated patients, compared with 2 or 0.2%, respectively, of control patients. In a clinical trial evaluating IV golimumab in patients with rheumatoid arthritis, increases in serum ALT concentrations of 3 or more times the ULN or 5 or more times the ULN occurred during 24 weeks of treatment in 2.3 or 0.8%, respectively, of golimumab-treated patients and in 2.5 or 0%, respectively, of control patients. In clinical studies evaluating golimumab in patients with ulcerative colitis, increases in serum ALT concentrations of 3 or more times the ULN or 5 or more times the ULN were reported in 2 or 1%, respectively, of golimumab-treated patients during 46 weeks of follow-up, compared with 1.5 or 1%, respectively, of placebo-treated patients during 18 weeks of follow-up. Because many of the patients in these studies received concomitant therapy with drugs known to increase liver enzyme concentrations (e.g., methotrexate, nonsteroidal anti-inflammatory agents [NSAIAs]), the relationship between golimumab and increased liver enzyme concentrations is not clear.

Sensitivity Reactions. Serious systemic hypersensitivity reactions (e.g., anaphylactic reactions) have been reported during postmarketing surveillance in patients receiving golimumab, sometimes after the first dose of the drug. In patients receiving IV golimumab, hypersensitivity reactions including urticaria, pruritus, dyspnea, and nausea have been reported during and generally within one hour following IV infusion of the drug. If an anaphylactic or other serious allergic reaction occurs, golimumab should be discontinued immediately and appropriate therapy initiated.

The needle cover of the prefilled syringe and the syringe in the auto-injector contain dry natural rubber; these items should not be handled by individuals sensitive to latex.

Specific Populations **Pregnancy.** Category B. (See Users Guide.)

Immunoglobulin G (IgG) antibodies are known to cross the placenta during pregnancy and have been detected in the serum of infants born to women who received IgG antibodies. Since golimumab is an IgG antibody, infants born to women who received golimumab during their pregnancy may be at increased risk of infection for up to 6 months. Administration of live vaccines to infants who were exposed to golimumab in utero is not recommended for 6 months following the last golimumab dose given to the infant's mother during pregnancy. (See Drug Interactions: Vaccines and Therapeutic Infectious Agents.)

Lactation. Golimumab is distributed into milk in lactating cynomolgus monkeys. It is not known whether golimumab is distributed into human milk or absorbed systemically following ingestion. A decision should be made whether to discontinue nursing or the drug, taking into account the importance of the drug to the woman.

Pediatric Use. Safety and efficacy of golimumab have not been established in children younger than 18 years of age.

Malignancies, some fatal, have been reported in children and adolescents who received treatment with TNF blocking agents. (See Malignancies and Lymphoproliferative Disorders under Warnings/Precautions: Warnings, in Cautions.)

Geriatric Use. In phase 3 clinical studies evaluating subcutaneous golimumab in patients with rheumatoid arthritis, psoriatic arthritis, or ankylosing spondylitis, there were no overall differences in serious adverse events, serious infections, and adverse events in those 65 years of age or older compared with younger adults. Clinical studies evaluating subcutaneous golimumab in patients with ulcerative colitis or evaluating IV golimumab in patients with rheumatoid arthritis did not include sufficient numbers of patients 65 years of age or older to determine whether geriatric patients respond differently than younger adults. Because the overall incidence of infection is higher in the geriatric population than in younger adults, golimumab should be used with caution in geriatric patients.

The pharmacokinetics of subcutaneous golimumab do not appear to be influenced by age in adults. The apparent clearance of subcutaneous golimumab in patients 65 years of age or older appears to be similar to that in younger adults.

Hepatic Impairment. The pharmacokinetics of golimumab have not been formally studied in patients with hepatic impairment.

Renal Impairment. The pharmacokinetics of golimumab have not been formally studied in patients with renal impairment.

■ **Common Adverse Effects** Adverse effects reported in 3% or more of patients receiving subcutaneous golimumab for the management of rheumatoid arthritis, psoriatic arthritis, or ankylosing spondylitis and occurring at an incidence that is at least 1% higher than that reported with placebo include upper respiratory infection (nasopharyngitis, pharyngitis, laryngitis, rhinitis), injection site reactions (injection site erythema, urticaria, induration, pain, bruising, pruritus, irritation, paresthesia), viral infections (e.g., herpes, influenza), increased aminotransferase (ALT, AST) concentrations, and hypertension. The adverse effect profile in patients with ulcerative colitis is similar to that observed in patients with rheumatologic conditions.

Adverse effects reported in 3% or more of patients receiving IV golimumab for the management of rheumatoid arthritis and occurring at an incidence that is at least 1% higher than that reported with placebo include upper respiratory infection (e.g., nasopharyngitis, pharyngitis, laryngitis, rhinitis), viral infection (e.g., influenza, herpes), bronchitis, hypertension, and rash.

Drug Interactions

■ **Drugs Metabolized by Hepatic Microsomal Enzymes** Because increased levels of cytokines (e.g., tumor necrosis factor [TNF]-α) during chronic inflammation may suppress the formation of cytochrome P-450 (CYP) isoenzymes, it is expected that a drug that antagonizes cytokine activity, such as golimumab, could normalize the formation of CYP enzymes. Following initiation or discontinuance of golimumab therapy, patients receiving certain drugs metabolized by CYP isoenzymes (i.e., those with a low therapeutic index [e.g., cyclosporine, theophylline, warfarin]) should be monitored for therapeutic effect and/or changes in serum concentrations, and dosages of these drugs may be adjusted as needed.

■ **Biologic Antirheumatic Agents** Caution should be exercised when switching from one biologic disease-modifying antirheumatic drug (DMARD) to another, since overlapping biologic activity may further increase the risk of infection. Concomitant use of golimumab and other biologic agents used in the management of rheumatoid arthritis, psoriatic arthritis, or ankylosing spondylitis is not recommended because of the possibility of an increased risk of infection.

Abatacept When abatacept (a selective costimulation modulator) and a TNF blocking agent were used concomitantly in patients with rheumatoid arthritis, an increased incidence of infection and serious infection was observed, with no substantial improvement in efficacy over that observed with a TNF blocking agent alone. Concomitant use of golimumab and abatacept is not recommended.

Anakinra When anakinra (a human interleukin-1 receptor antagonist) and etanercept (another TNF blocking agent) were used concomitantly in patients with active rheumatoid arthritis, an increased incidence of serious infection and neutropenia was observed, with no substantial improvement in efficacy over that observed with etanercept alone. Concomitant use of golimumab and anakinra is not recommended.

Rituximab An increased risk of serious infection has been observed in patients with rheumatoid arthritis who received rituximab (an anti-CD20 monoclonal antibody) and subsequently received therapy with a TNF blocking agent. Concomitant use of golimumab and rituximab is not recommended.

■ **Corticosteroids** Concomitant use of golimumab and oral corticosteroids does not appear to influence the apparent clearance of golimumab.

■ **Methotrexate** For the management of rheumatoid arthritis, golimumab should be used in conjunction with methotrexate. (See Uses: Rheumatoid Arthritis in Adults and also see Dosage and Administration: General.)

Since concomitant use or nonuse of methotrexate does not appear to influence the efficacy or safety of golimumab for the management of psoriatic arthritis or ankylosing spondylitis, golimumab may be used with or without methotrexate for the management of psoriatic arthritis or ankylosing spondylitis. (See Psoriatic Arthritis and also see Ankylosing Spondylitis under Uses and also see Dosage and Administration: General.)

Patients with rheumatoid arthritis, psoriatic arthritis, or ankylosing spondylitis receiving subcutaneous golimumab concomitantly with methotrexate had approximately 52, 36, or 21% higher mean steady-state trough concentrations of golimumab, respectively, than those receiving subcutaneous golimumab without methotrexate. A population pharmacokinetic analysis indicated that concomitant use of methotrexate with IV golimumab in patients with rheumatoid arthritis decreased the clearance of golimumab by about 9%. In addition, methotrexate may decrease clearance of golimumab by reducing the development of antigolimumab antibodies. (See Immunologic Reactions and Antibody Formation under Warnings/Precautions: Other Warnings/Precautions, in Cautions.)

■ **Nonsteroidal Anti-inflammatory Agents** Concomitant use of golimumab and nonsteroidal anti-inflammatory agents (NSAIAs) does not appear to influence the apparent clearance of golimumab.

■ **Sulfasalazine** Concomitant use of golimumab and sulfasalazine does not appear to influence the apparent clearance of golimumab.

■ **Vaccines and Therapeutic Infectious Agents** Live vaccines and therapeutic infectious agents (e.g., BCG for intravesical instillation) should not be administered to patients receiving golimumab since such concomitant use could result in infections, including disseminated infections. Limited data are available regarding whether TNF blocking agents would affect the rate of secondary transmission of infection following administration of a live vaccine or regarding the response to live vaccines in patients receiving the drug. Administration of live vaccines to infants who were exposed to golimumab in utero is not recommended for 6 months following the last golimumab dose given to the infant's mother during pregnancy. (See Pregnancy under Warnings/Precautions: Specific Populations, in Cautions.)

Patients receiving golimumab may receive inactivated vaccines. In a clinical study in patients with psoriatic arthritis, the proportion of patients who had an adequate immune response (at least a twofold increase in antibody titers) to pneumococcal polysaccharide vaccine was similar in golimumab-treated and placebo-treated patients; however, the proportion of patients exhibiting a response to pneumococcal vaccine was lower among patients receiving methotrexate compared with patients not receiving methotrexate in both golimumab-treated and placebo-treated patients. These data suggest that golimumab does not suppress the humoral immune response to pneumococcal polysaccharide vaccine.

Description

Golimumab, a human monoclonal antibody specific for human tumor necrosis factor (TNF; TNF-α), is a biologic response modifier and a disease-modifying antirheumatic drug (DMARD). Golimumab is an immunoglobulin G_1 kappa (IgG_1) that was created using genetically engineered mice immunized with human TNF, resulting in an antibody with human-derived antibody variable and constant regions. Golimumab is produced by a recombinant cell line cultured by continuous perfusion and is purified by a process that includes specific viral inactivation and removal steps.

Golimumab binds to both soluble and transmembrane bioactive forms of human TNF-α, which prevents the binding of TNF-α to its receptors. By preventing the binding of TNF-α to its receptors, golimumab inhibits the biologic activity of TNF-α. Golimumab does not appear to bind to other TNF superfamily ligands; golimumab does not bind to or neutralize human lymphotoxin. Golimumab does not lyse human monocytes expressing transmembrane TNF in the presence of complement or effector cells.

Increased concentrations of TNF-α, a cytokine protein, in the blood, synovium, and joints have been implicated in the pathophysiology of several chronic inflammatory diseases such as rheumatoid arthritis, psoriatic arthritis, and ankylosing spondylitis. TNF-α is an important mediator of the articular inflammation that is characteristic of these diseases. In vitro, golimumab modulated the biologic effects mediated by TNF in several bioassays, including the expression of adhesion proteins responsible for leukocyte infiltration and secretion of proinflammatory cytokines. The exact mechanism of action of golimumab in the treatment of ulcerative colitis is unknown.

Golimumab exhibits dose-proportional pharmacokinetics when given IV or subcutaneously within the clinical dosage range. The absolute bioavailability of golimumab following subcutaneous injection is approximately 53%; peak serum concentrations of the drug are attained in approximately 2–6 days in healthy individuals and in patients with active rheumatoid arthritis. Steady-state concentrations of the drug are attained by week 12 in patients with rheumatoid arthritis, psoriatic arthritis, or ankylosing spondylitis receiving the recommended subcutaneous dosage (50 mg every 4 weeks); by week 8 after the first maintenance dose in patients with ulcerative colitis receiving the recommended subcutaneous dosage (induction dosage of 200 mg at week 0 and 100 mg at week 2 and maintenance dosage of 100 mg every 4 weeks thereafter); and by week 12 in patients with rheumatoid arthritis receiving the recommended IV dosage (2 mg/kg at weeks 0 and 4 and every 8 weeks thereafter). Data directly comparing a 2-mg/kg IV dose with a 50-mg subcutaneous dose are not available to date. Patients who developed antigolimumab antibodies generally had lower steady-state serum trough concentrations of the drug. Elimination pathways for golimumab have not been characterized. The terminal half-life of the drug is estimated to be approximately 2 weeks.

Advice to Patients

A copy of the manufacturer's patient information (medication guide) for golimumab should be provided to all patients with each prescription of the drug. Importance of advising patients about potential benefits and risks of golimumab. Importance of patients reading the medication guide prior to initiation of therapy and each time the prescription is refilled.

Importance of instructing patient and/or caregiver regarding proper dosage and administration of subcutaneous golimumab, including the use of aseptic technique, and proper disposal of needles and syringes if it is determined that the patient and/or caregiver is competent to safely administer the drug.

Increased susceptibility to infection. Importance of promptly informing clinicians if any signs or symptoms of infection (e.g., persistent fever, sweating, cough, dyspnea, fatigue, diarrhea, burning upon urination, warm, red or painful skin) develop.

Risk of lymphoma, including hepatosplenic T-cell lymphoma, leukemia, and other malignancies with use of tumor necrosis factor (TNF) blocking agents. Importance of informing patients and caregivers about the increased risk of cancer development in children, adolescents, and young adults, taking into account the clinical utility of TNF blocking agents, the relative risks and benefits of these and other immunosuppressive drugs, and the risks associated with untreated disease. Importance of promptly informing clinicians if signs and symptoms of malignancies (e.g., unexplained weight loss; fatigue; abdominal pain; persistent fever; night sweats; swollen lymph nodes in the neck, underarm, or groin; easy bruising or bleeding; hepatomegaly or splenomegaly; changes in appearance of skin or growths on skin) occur.

Importance of alerting clinician if allergy to latex exists.

Importance of informing clinician of any new or worsening medical conditions (e.g., heart failure, neurologic disease [e.g., demyelinating disorders], autoimmune disorders [e.g., lupus-like syndrome], liver disease, cytopenias, psoriasis).

Importance of taking the drug as prescribed and of not altering or discontinuing therapy without first consulting with a clinician.

Importance of informing clinicians of existing or contemplated concomitant therapy, including prescription and OTC drugs, as well as any concomitant illnesses or any history of cancer, tuberculosis, hepatitis B virus infection, or other chronic or recurring infections.

Importance of women informing clinicians if they are or plan to become pregnant or plan to breast-feed.

Importance of informing patients of other important precautionary information. (See Cautions.)

Overview® (see Users Guide). For additional information on this drug until a more detailed monograph is developed and published, the manufacturer's labeling should be consulted. It is *essential* that the manufacturer's labeling be consulted for more detailed information on usual cautions, precautions, contraindications, potential drug interactions, laboratory test interferences, and acute toxicity.

Preparations

Excipients in commercially available drug preparations may have clinically important effects in some individuals; consult specific product labeling for details.

Golimumab

Parenteral		
Injection, for subcutaneous use	50 mg/0.5 mL	**Simponi®** (available as disposable prefilled syringes and prefilled auto-injectors [SmartJect®]), Janssen Biotech
	100 mg/mL	**Simponi®** (available as disposable prefilled syringes and prefilled auto-injectors [SmartJect®]), Janssen Biotech
Concentrate, for Injection, for IV use	12.5 mg/mL (50 mg)	**Simponi Aria®**, Janssen Biotech

†Use is not currently included in the labeling approved by the US Food and Drug Administration

inFLIXimab, inFLIXimab-dyyb

Anti-tumor Necrosis Factor-alpha, Anti-TNF-α, cA2, Infliximab-dyyb, CT-P13

■ Infliximab and infliximab-dyyb, chimeric human-murine immunoglobulin G_1 kappa (IgG_1 kappa) monoclonal antibodies that have a high affinity for human tumor necrosis factor (TNF; TNF-α), are biologic response modifiers.

Infliximab-dyyb is biosimilar to infliximab (Remicade®). FDA defines a biosimilar as a biological that is highly similar to an FDA-licensed reference biological with the exception of minor differences in clinically inactive components and for which there are no clinically meaningful differences in safety, purity, or potency. The claim of biosimilarity is based on a totality-of-evidence approach, which includes consideration of data from analytical, animal, and clinical studies. Therefore, biosimilarity of 2 drugs may be established even when there are formulation or minor structural differences or minor differences in rates of adverse effects between the drugs as long as these differences are not clinically meaningful. Clinical studies for demonstration of biosimilarity include assessment of immunogenicity and pharmacokinetics/pharmacodynamics and address at least one indication licensed for the reference biological. Biosimilars are approved through an abbreviated licensure pathway that establishes biosimilarity between the proposed biological and the reference biological but does not independently establish safety and effectiveness of the proposed biological.

While infliximab-dyyb is biosimilar to the reference biological (Remicade®), these drugs are *not* interchangeable; instead, they are considered therapeutic alternatives. Biosimilarity of infliximab-dyyb and infliximab (Remicade®) was established through advanced analytical studies evaluating structural and functional similarity, pharmacokinetic studies, clinical efficacy and safety studies in patients with rheumatoid arthritis and in those with ankylosing spondylitis, and long-term extensions of these clinical studies evaluating the safety of switching from infliximab to infliximab-dyyb.

In this monograph, unless otherwise stated, the term "infliximab products" refers to infliximab (the reference drug), infliximab-dyyb (the biosimilar), or both drugs.

Uses

Infliximab or infliximab-dyyb is used to reduce the signs and symptoms of Crohn's disease and to induce and maintain clinical remission in adults and pediatric patients with moderately to severely active disease who have had an inadequate response to conventional therapies. Infliximab or infliximab-dyyb also is used to reduce the number of draining enterocutaneous and rectovaginal fistulas and maintain fistula closure in adults with fistulizing Crohn's disease.

In adults with moderately to severely active ulcerative colitis who have had an inadequate response to conventional therapies, infliximab or infliximab-dyyb is used to reduce the signs and symptoms of the disease, to induce and maintain clinical remission and mucosal healing, and to eliminate use of corticosteroids. In pediatric patients with moderately to severely active ulcerative colitis who have had an inadequate response to conventional therapies, infliximab is used to reduce the signs and symptoms of the disease and to induce and maintain clinical remission. Although safety and efficacy of infliximab-dyyb also have been established in pediatric patients with ulcerative colitis, the labeled indication for infliximab in these patients was still protected by the exclusivity provisions of orphan drug designation when FDA approved the infliximab-dyyb biosimilar.

Infliximab or infliximab-dyyb is used in combination with methotrexate for the management of the signs and symptoms of rheumatoid arthritis, to improve physical function, and to inhibit progression of structural damage associated with the disease in patients with moderately to severely active rheumatoid arthritis.

Infliximab or infliximab-dyyb is used to reduce the signs and symptoms of ankylosing spondylitis in patients with active disease.

Infliximab or infliximab-dyyb is used to reduce the signs and symptoms of active arthritis, inhibit the progression of structural damage, and improve physical function in patients with psoriatic arthritis.

Infliximab or infliximab-dyyb is used for the treatment of chronic, severe (i.e., extensive and/or disabling) plaque psoriasis in adults who are candidates for systemic therapy and when other systemic therapies are medically less appropriate.

Infliximab is being investigated for the treatment of juvenile arthritis† and Behcet's syndrome†.

■ **Crohn's Disease** Infliximab or infliximab-dyyb is used to reduce the signs and symptoms of Crohn's disease and to induce and maintain clinical remission in adults and pediatric patients with moderately to severely active disease who have had an inadequate response to conventional therapies (e.g., corticosteroids, mesalamine or sulfasalazine, azathioprine or mercaptopurine). Infliximab or infliximab-dyyb also is used to reduce the number of draining enterocutaneous and rectovaginal fistulas and to maintain fistula closure in adults with fistulizing Crohn's disease. Infliximab has been designated as an orphan drug by FDA for these uses.

Active Crohn's Disease Results of several open-label and at least one double-blind, placebo-controlled study in adults indicate that a single dose of infliximab can result in a clinical response (including clinical remission) in patients with moderately to severely active Crohn's disease who have not responded to prior therapies. In addition, there is evidence that the drug can result in improvements in systemic measures of inflammation (e.g., C-reactive protein [CRP], erythrocyte sedimentation rate [ESR]) and can result in a reduction in the severity of intestinal mucosal ulceration and inflammation as demonstrated by endoscopy and biopsy. In patients who respond to infliximab, the reduction in signs and symptoms of Crohn's disease may allow dosage reduction or withdrawal of oral corticosteroid therapy in steroid-dependent patients.

Safety and efficacy of infliximab in the management of active Crohn's disease were evaluated in a double-blind, placebo-controlled, dose-ranging study that included 108 adults with moderately to severely active Crohn's disease who had an inadequate response to conventional therapies (e.g., corticosteroids, mesalamine, azathioprine or mercaptopurine). To be included in the study, patients had to have had Crohn's disease for a minimum of 6 months and have a Crohn's Disease Activity Index (CDAI) of 220–400 at the time of study entry. The CDAI score is based on the daily number of liquid or very soft stools, severity of abdominal pain or cramping, general well-being, presence or absence of extraintestinal manifestations, presence or absence of an abdominal mass, use or nonuse of antidiarrheal drugs, the hematocrit, and body weight; scores below 150 indicate clinical remission and scores above 450 indicate severe illness. Patients were randomized to receive placebo or a single dose of 5, 10, or 20 mg/kg of infliximab given by IV infusion over 2 hours. Those who were receiving fixed dosages of oral corticosteroids, oral mesalamine, and/or azathioprine or mercaptopurine continued to receive these drugs during the study (92% continued to receive one or more of these drugs). A clinical response (defined as a reduction from baseline CDAI of 70 points or more at 4 weeks after the dose without an increased need for other Crohn's drugs or surgical intervention) was observed in 81, 50, or 64% of patients receiving 5, 10, or 20 mg/kg of infliximab, respectively, compared with 16% of patients receiving placebo. At 4 weeks after the dose, 33% of those who received infliximab and 4% of those who received placebo were in clinical remission based on the CDAI. There was no evidence of a dose-response relationship (doses exceeding 5 mg/kg did not result in a greater response rate) and, at all 3 infliximab dosages, the maximum response was observed within 2–4 weeks after the IV infusion. At 12 weeks after the dose, the overall rate of clinical response or clinical remission based on the CDAI was 41 or 24%, respectively, in those who received infliximab compared with 12 or 8%, respectively, in those who received placebo.

To determine whether patients with moderately or severely active Crohn's disease who do not respond to a single dose of infliximab would respond to an additional dose of the drug, the subset of patients in the above study who did not have a clinical response 4 weeks after the initial infliximab or placebo dose were enrolled in an open-label follow-up study and given a single 10-mg/kg dose of infliximab. In those who had received placebo in the original study, the rate of clinical response or remission was 58 or 47%, respectively, 4 weeks following this 10-mg/kg infliximab dose. However, in those who had already received a dose of infliximab in the first phase of the study, the rate of clinical response or remission was only 34 or 17%, respectively, 4 weeks following the second dose of the drug. These results indicate that patients who do not respond to an initial infliximab dose may be less likely to respond to a second dose of the drug.

Maintenance of Remission of Crohn's Disease. Safety and efficacy of infliximab for maintenance therapy in patients with moderately or severely active Crohn's disease were evaluated in a preliminary study and in a double-blind, multidose, multicenter study (ACCENT I) that included more than 500 adults. The duration of response to infliximab usually ranges from 4–12 weeks in patients who experience a clinical benefit after a single dose of the drug. In one preliminary study, a subset of 73 adults from a double-blind, placebo-controlled study who had maintained a clinical response 8 weeks after an initial placebo or infliximab dose were re-randomized at week 12 to receive 4 doses of placebo or infliximab (10 mg/kg) given by IV infusion at 8-week intervals (i.e., weeks 12, 20, 28, 36). Those who were receiving fixed dosages of oral corticosteroids, oral mesalamine or sulfasalazine, and/or azathioprine or mercaptopurine continued to receive these drugs during the study; patients receiving oral corticosteroids where allowed to taper dosage if they responded to treatment. Patients were assessed every 4 weeks through week 48. The clinical response was maintained through week 44 (8 weeks after the fourth infusion) in 62 or 37% of patients receiving infliximab or placebo, respectively. In those randomized to receive infliximab for maintenance therapy, 37.8% were in clinical remission at week 12 and 52.9% were in clinical remission at week 44. In contrast, 44.4% of those randomized to receive placebo for maintenance therapy were in clinical remission at week 12 and only 20% were in clinical remission at week 44. Although further study is needed to determine the relative benefits of concomitant use of infliximab and azathioprine or mercaptopurine for maintenance of remission, 75% of patients receiving one of these drugs concomitantly with infliximab had a clinical response at 44 weeks compared with 50% of those not receiving one of these drugs concomitantly.

In a double-blind study of 573 adults with moderately to severely active Crohn's disease that was designed to compare the safety and efficacy of a maintenance regimen of infliximab to a single dose of the drug (ACCENT I), all patients received an initial 5-mg/kg dose of infliximab; following assessment of clinical response at week 2 (defined as a CDAI decrease of at least 70 points and at least a 25% decrease from baseline CDAI), patients were randomized to receive placebo or an infliximab induction regimen (5-mg/kg doses given at weeks 2 and 6 followed by either 5- or 10-mg/kg maintenance doses given once every 8 weeks) for up to 1 year. Those who were receiving fixed dosages of oral corticosteroids (prednisone 40 mg or less daily or equivalent), oral mesalamine, sulfasalazine, anti-infective agents, azathioprine, mercaptopurine, or methotrexate continued to receive these drugs during the study; patients receiving oral corticosteroids were allowed to taper the dosage after week 6 if they responded to treatment. Among adults who responded to the initial dose of infliximab, 39 or 46% of those receiving 5- or 10-mg maintenance doses of infliximab, respectively, were in clinical remission at week 30 compared with 25% of those receiving maintenance doses of placebo. In addition, among patients receiving corticosteroids at baseline, 25 or 34% of those receiving 5- or 10-mg maintenance doses of infliximab, respectively, were in clinical remission and were able to discontinue corticosteroid use at week 54 compared with 11% of those receiving maintenance doses of placebo. The median time to loss of response in those receiving maintenance doses of infliximab or placebo was 46 or 19 weeks, respectively.

Although the relative benefits of concomitant use of infliximab and an immunosuppressant agent (e.g., methotrexate, azathioprine) for maintenance therapy remain to be determined, 50% of those receiving immunosuppressive therapy at baseline maintained clinical response at week 54 compared with 41% of those not receiving such therapy.

Patients in this study who responded initially but subsequently lost response were eligible to receive infliximab at a higher dose than the dose they had been receiving; these patients were eligible to receive infliximab on an episodic basis at a dose 5 mg/kg higher than the dose they had been receiving in the study. Most patients responded to the higher dose.

Among adults who did not respond to the initial dose of infliximab, 59% of those receiving maintenance doses of infliximab responded by week 14 compared with 51% of those receiving maintenance doses of placebo. In patients who did not respond to infliximab by week 14, additional doses of infliximab did not result in clinically important response.

In a subset of patients with mucosal ulceration at baseline who participated in an endoscopic study, 13 of 43 patients receiving maintenance doses of infliximab had endoscopic evidence of mucosal healing at week 10 compared with 1 of 28 patients receiving placebo for maintenance therapy. Nine of 12 patients receiving maintenance doses of infliximab with mucosal healing at week 10 also had mucosal healing at week 54.

Fistulizing Crohn's Disease Infliximab or infliximab-dyyb is used to reduce the number of draining enterocutaneous and rectovaginal fistulas and to maintain fistula closure in patients with fistulizing Crohn's disease. Further study is needed to determine the relative safety and efficacy of infliximab and other therapies used for the management of fistulizing Crohn's disease (e.g., ciprofloxacin and/or metronidazole; azathioprine or mercaptopurine; surgical intervention). Some clinicians suggest that, although data are not available to date to support use of infliximab as first-line therapy for fistulizing Crohn's disease, use of the drug should be considered when fistulas have not responded to appropriate anti-infective regimens (e.g., ciprofloxacin and/or metronidazole) and/or immunosuppressive therapy (e.g., azathioprine or mercaptopurine). In addition, because therapy with infliximab can result in complete closure of all fistula tracks in many patients with complex fistulas, most clinicians now suggest use of infliximab as first-line therapy in these patients. Whether infliximab or surgery (placing noncutting setons) is the initial treatment of choice for patients with complex perianal fistulas who do not have active rectal disease is unknown.

Safety and efficacy of infliximab in the management of fistulizing Crohn's disease have been evaluated in a double-blind, placebo-controlled study involving 94 adults with one or more cutaneously draining fistulas of at least 3 months' duration (90% had perianal fistulas, 10% had abdominal fistulas, 55%

had multiple cutaneously draining fistulas). Patients were randomized to receive placebo or infliximab (5 or 10 mg/kg) given by IV infusion over 2 hours at weeks 0, 2, and 6 and were followed for up to 26 weeks. Those who were receiving fixed dosages of oral corticosteroids, oral mesalamine or sulfasalazine, anti-infectives, and/or methotrexate, azathioprine, or mercaptopurine continued to receive these drugs during the study (83% continued to receive one or more of these drugs). A clinical response (defined as a 50% or greater reduction from baseline in the number of fistulas draining after gentle compression during at least 2 consecutive visits without an increased need for other drugs used for the treatment of Crohn's disease or surgical intervention) occurred in 68 or 56% of patients receiving infliximab in a dosage of 5 or 10 mg/kg, respectively, versus 26% of those receiving placebo. Closure of all fistulas was attained in 52% of patients receiving infliximab versus 13% of those receiving placebo. In patients receiving infliximab, the median time to onset of response was 2 weeks and the median duration of response was 12 weeks; there was no evidence of a dose-response relationship. New fistula(s) occurred in approximately 15% of patients receiving infliximab or placebo.

Long-term safety and efficacy of infliximab in the management of fistulizing Crohn's disease have been evaluated in a multicenter, double-blind, randomized, placebo-controlled trial (A Crohn's Disease Clinical Trial Evaluating Infliximab in a New Long-Term Treatment Regimen in Patients with Fistulizing Crohn's Disease; [ACCENT II]) in adults with at least one draining fistula (e.g., perianal, enterocutaneous, or rectovaginal fistulas) for at least 3 months. In the initial phase of this study, all 282 patients received infliximab (5 mg/kg) at weeks 0, 2, and 6; those with a clinical response (defined as a 50% or greater reduction from baseline in the number of fistulas draining after gentle compression during at least 2 consecutive visits without an increased need for other drugs used for the treatment of Crohn's disease or surgical intervention) at both week 10 and 14 were randomized (195 patients) to receive placebo (99 patients) or infliximab (96 patients; 5 mg/kg) at week 14 and then every 8 weeks through week 46 (maintenance treatment). Those who were receiving stable dosages of 5-aminosalicylates, oral corticosteroids, methotrexate, azathioprine, mercaptopurine, mycophenolate mofetil, or anti-infective agents continued to receive these drugs during the study. At week 14, 65% of patients had a clinical response to the initial 3 doses of infliximab; in the group of responders, 87% had perianal fistulas, 14% had abdominal fistulas, 8% had rectovaginal fistulas. During the maintenance treatment phase of the study, time to loss of clinical response was longer in patients who received infliximab every 8 weeks than in those receiving placebo (14 weeks for placebo versus 40 weeks for infliximab). At week 54, 46 or 23% of patients receiving infliximab or placebo, respectively, had a response, while 36 or 19% of patients receiving infliximab or placebo, respectively, had complete response (defined as absence of draining fistulas). There was a trend toward fewer hospitalizations in those receiving infliximab maintenance compared with those receiving placebo. Patients who initially had a clinical response but lost response (defined as recrudescence of draining fistulas, need for a change in a drug used for the disease, need for additional therapy for persistent or worsening luminal disease activity, need for surgery, or discontinuance of infliximab because of perceived lack of efficacy) were eligible to receive infliximab maintenance treatment using a dosage 5 mg/kg higher than the dosage they originally received; 66% of patients originally randomized to placebo responded to infliximab 5 mg/kg and 57% of patients originally randomized to infliximab 5 mg/kg responded to infliximab 10 mg/kg. Although 87 patients who did not have an initial response to infliximab at both weeks 10 and 14 were also randomized to receive placebo (44 patients) or infliximab (43 patients) at week 14 and then every 8 weeks through week 46, patients who did not respond by week 14 were unlikely to respond to additional doses of infliximab. In patients who did not have an initial response to infliximab, 16 (7 out of 44 patients) or 21% (9 out of 43 patients) of those receiving placebo or infliximab, respectively, had response. At week 22, patients who were receiving placebo for maintenance and who had a loss of response were eligible to cross over to maintenance therapy with infliximab (5 mg/kg) while those who were receiving maintenance therapy with infliximab (5 mg/kg) could cross over to receive infliximab (10 mg/kg). In patients who crossed over from placebo to maintenance therapy with infliximab, response was reestablished in 61% (25 out of 41 patients) of individuals. Overall, a similar number of patients in the infliximab or placebo groups developed new fistulas (17%) and new abscesses (15%).

Crohn's Disease in Pediatric Patients Infliximab or infliximab-dyyb is used to reduce the signs and symptoms of Crohn's disease and to induce and maintain clinical remission in pediatric patients with moderately to severely active disease who have had an inadequate response to conventional therapy. The current indication for use in children with Crohn's disease is based principally on the results of a randomized, open-label study (Study Peds Crohn's) of infliximab in 112 pediatric patients 6–17 years of age (median age, 13 years) with moderately to severely active disease having a median Pediatric Crohn's Disease Activity Index (PCDAI) of 40 (on a scale of 0–100) and an inadequate response to conventional therapy. Prior to enrollment in the study, patients were required to be on a stable dosage of mercaptopurine, azathioprine, or methotrexate; 35% of the patients also were receiving corticosteroids at baseline. All patients received infliximab induction therapy with 5 mg/kg administered at weeks 0, 2, and 6. At week 10, 103 patients were randomized to receive maintenance therapy of 5 mg/kg of infliximab every 8 or 12 weeks. At week 10, 88% of patients had clinical response (defined as a decrease in PCDAI score of 15 or more points from baseline and a total PCDAI score of 30 points or less), and 59% of patients were in clinical remission (defined as a PCDAI score of 10 points or less). The proportion of pediatric patients achieving a clinical response at week 10 compared favorably with the rate of clinical response reported in adults with active Crohn's disease who received infliximab in a clinical trial. The clinical response rate both at week 30 (73 versus 47%) and week 54 (64 versus 33%) was higher in pediatric patients receiving infliximab every 8 weeks than in those receiving the drug every 12 weeks. In addition, the clinical remission rate both at week 30 (60 versus 35%) and week 54 (56 versus 24%) was higher in patients receiving infliximab every 8 weeks than in those receiving the drug every 12 weeks. Among patients receiving corticosteroids at baseline, 46 or 33% of those receiving maintenance doses of infliximab every 8 or 12 weeks, respectively, were in clinical remission and were able to discontinue corticosteroid use at week 30, while at week 54, 46 or 17% of those receiving maintenance doses of infliximab every 8 or 12 weeks, respectively, were in clinical remission and were able to discontinue corticosteroid use.

In another open-label study in 15 pediatric patients 6–18 years of age with medically refractory Crohn's disease (unable to tolerate corticosteroid taper; PCDAI score of 30 or greater; no improvement despite use of mercaptopurine, methotrexate, and/or cyclosporine for 4 months or longer), a single 5-mg/kg dose of infliximab was administered by IV infusion. At 4 weeks after the dose, 14/15 (94%) had responded to infliximab with a decrease in the PCDAI score of 25 points or greater; at 10 weeks, 10/15 (67%) were in clinical remission (PCDAI score of 15 or less). All patients continued mercaptopurine or methotrexate therapy during and after the infliximab infusion, but oral corticosteroid dosage was tapered in most patients. During the 52-week follow-up of the 14 responders, 11 (78%) had clinical relapse that required additional drug therapy or surgical intervention. When these children were subdivided based on disease duration, the relapse rate was 50% in those who had been diagnosed with Crohn's disease less than 2 years previously; however, the relapse rate was 100% in those who had been diagnosed more than 2 years previously.

In an open-label study in 19 pediatric patients 9–19 years of age with moderately or severely active Crohn's disease, 1–3 doses of infliximab (5 mg/kg) were given by IV infusion usually at 4-week intervals. At 4 weeks after the initial dose, all 19 pediatric patients had a clinical response documented by physician global assessment and PCDAI score; at 12 weeks after the initial dose, only 4 patients maintained a clinical response to the drug.

(For further information on the management of Crohn's disease, see Uses; Crohn's Disease, in Mesalamine 56:36).

■ **Ulcerative Colitis** In adults with moderately to severely active ulcerative colitis who have had an inadequate response to conventional therapies, infliximab or infliximab-dyyb is used to reduce the signs and symptoms of the disease, to induce and maintain clinical remission and mucosal healing, and to eliminate use of corticosteroids. In pediatric patients with moderately to severely active ulcerative colitis who have had an inadequate response to conventional therapies, infliximab is used to reduce the signs and symptoms of the disease and to induce and maintain clinical remission. Although safety and efficacy of infliximab-dyyb also have been established in pediatric patients with ulcerative colitis, the labeled indication for infliximab in these patients was still protected by the exclusivity provisions of orphan drug designation when FDA approved the infliximab-dyyb biosimilar.

Safety and efficacy of infliximab in the management of ulcerative colitis in adults were evaluated in 2 randomized, double-blind, placebo-controlled studies (the Active Ulcerative Colitis Trials 1 and 2; ACT 1 and ACT 2, respectively) in 728 patients with moderately to severely active ulcerative colitis who had an inadequate response to conventional therapies. In the ACT 1 study, patients had an inadequate response to or were intolerant of corticosteroids alone or in combination with azathioprine or mercaptopurine, while in the ACT 2 study, patients had an inadequate response to or were intolerant of corticosteroids alone or in combination with azathioprine or mercaptopurine and/or to preparations containing 5-aminosalicylates. Patients were randomized to receive placebo or a 5- or 10-mg/kg dose of infliximab at weeks 0, 2, and 6 and then every 8 weeks through week 22 in the ACT 2 study or week 46 in the ACT 1 study. Patients in the ACT 2 study were allowed to continue blinded therapy to week 46 at the investigator's discretion. Those who were receiving fixed dosages of azathioprine or mercaptopurine, and/or 5-aminosalicylates, continued to receive these drugs during the study. Corticosteroids were tapered gradually until discontinuance. In both studies, the proportions of patients who had a clinical response or remission at weeks 8 and 30, and at week 54 in the ACT 1 study, were higher by a factor of 1.7 to more than 2 in patients receiving infliximab than in those receiving placebo. Clinical response (defined as a reduction from baseline Mayo score of at least 3 points and at least 30%, with an accompanying decrease in the subscore for rectal bleeding of at least 1 point or an absolute rectal-bleeding subscore of 0 or 1) at week 30 in the ACT 1 study was reported in 52 or 51% of patients receiving 5 or 10 mg of infliximab, respectively, compared with 30% patients receiving placebo, while in the ACT 2 study such response was observed in 47 or 60% of patients receiving 5 or 10 mg of infliximab, respectively, compared with 26% of patients receiving placebo. At week 54 in the ACT 1 study, clinical response was reported in 46 or 44% of patients receiving 5 or 10 mg of infliximab, respectively, compared with 20% of patients receiving placebo. The rates of clinical response were similar between the subpopulations of patients who were refractory to corticosteroids and those who were not refractory to corticosteroids. In the ACT 1 study, in patients refractory to corticosteroids, clinical response at week 8 was reported in 77 or 68% of those receiving 5 or 10 mg of infliximab, respectively, and in 35% of those receiving placebo, while in patients not refractory to corticosteroids, such response was reported in 67 or 59% of those receiving 5 or 10 mg of infliximab, respectively, and in 38% of those receiving placebo. In the ACT 2 study, in patients refractory to corticosteroids, clinical response at week 8 was reported in 63 or 66% of those receiving 5 or 10 mg of infliximab, respectively, and in 38% of those receiving placebo, while in patients not refractory to corticosteroids, such response was reported in 65 or 70% of those receiving 5 or 10 mg of infliximab, respectively, and in 26% of those receiving placebo. At week 30, clinical remission was reported in 34 and 37% of patients receiving 5 or 10 mg of infliximab, respectively, compared with 16% of those receiving placebo in the ACT 1 study, while such remission was observed in 26 or 36% of patients receiving 5 or 10 mg of infliximab, respectively, compared with 11% of patients receiving placebo. At week 54 in the ACT 1 study, clinical remission was reported in 35 or 34% of patients receiving 5 or 10 mg of infliximab, respectively, compared with 17% of patients receiving placebo. The proportions of patients with a sustained clinical response or sustained remission were significantly higher in patients receiving infliximab than in those receiving placebo. In addition, mucosal healing at weeks 8 and 30 in both studies (ACT 1 and ACT 2) and at week 54 in ACT 1 occurred in significantly more patients receiving infliximab than in those receiving placebo. At baseline, 61 and 51% of patients were receiving corticosteroids in the ACT 1 and ACT 2 studies, respectively. The proportions of patients who were in clinical remission and had discontinued corticosteroids at week 30 in both studies and at week 54 in the ACT 1 study, were higher in those receiving infliximab that in those receiving placebo.

Ulcerative Colitis in Pediatric Patients Infliximab is used to reduce the signs and symptoms of ulcerative colitis and to induce and maintain clinical remission in pediatric patients with moderately to severely active ulcerative colitis who have had an inadequate response to conventional therapy. Infliximab has been designated as an orphan drug by FDA for the treatment of ulcerative colitis in pediatric patients. Although safety and efficacy of infliximab-dyyb for such use also have been established, the labeled indication for infliximab in pediatric patients with ulcerative colitis was still protected by the exclusivity provisions of orphan drug designation when FDA approved the infliximab-dyyb biosimilar.

Efficacy and safety of infliximab for this indication are supported by evidence from controlled clinical studies in adults and by an uncontrolled study in 60 pediatric patients 6–17 years of age with moderately to severely active ulcerative colitis (Mayo score of 6–12, endoscopic subscore of 2 or greater) and an inadequate response to conventional therapies. At the start of the study in pediatric patients, 53% of patients were receiving immunosuppressive therapy with mercaptopurine, azathioprine, or methotrexate, and 62% were receiving corticosteroids; discontinuance of immunosuppressive agents and tapering of corticosteroid dosage was permitted after week 0. All patients received induction therapy with infliximab (5 mg/kg at weeks 0, 2, and 6); those who exhibited a response at week 8 were randomized to receive a maintenance regimen of 5 mg/kg every 8 weeks through week 46 or 5 mg/kg every 12 weeks through week 42. Patients who experienced loss of response during maintenance therapy were allowed to receive higher and/or more frequent doses of the drug.

At week 8 of the pediatric study, approximately 73% of patients exhibited a clinical response (defined as a reduction from baseline Mayo score of at least 3 points and at least 30%, with an accompanying decrease in the subscore for rectal bleeding of at least 1 point or achievement of an absolute rectal-bleeding subscore of 0 or 1); 40% of patients were in clinical remission as defined by Mayo score (2 points or less, with no individual subscore exceeding 1), and approximately 33% of patients were in clinical remission as measured by the Pediatric Ulcerative Colitis Activity Index (PUCAI) (score less than 10 points). Clinical response at 8 weeks was observed in 23 of 32 patients (72%) receiving concomitant immunosuppressive therapy at baseline and in 21 of 28 patients (75%) not receiving such therapy at baseline.

At week 54 of the pediatric study, clinical remission (as measured by PUCAI score) was observed in 8 of 21 patients receiving infliximab every 8 weeks and 4 of 22 patients receiving the drug every 12 weeks. Of the 45 patients randomized to receive maintenance therapy, 23 patients (including 9 patients receiving infliximab every 8 weeks and 14 patients receiving the drug every 12 weeks) required higher and/or more frequent doses of the drug because of loss of response, and 9 of those patients (including 7 patients who received the drug every 8 weeks) achieved remission at week 54. Efficacy of infliximab in inducing and maintaining mucosal healing could not be established because the study was uncontrolled and few patients underwent endoscopy at week 54.

■ **Rheumatoid Arthritis in Adults** Infliximab or infliximab-dyyb is used in conjunction with methotrexate for the management of the signs and symptoms of rheumatoid arthritis, to improve physical function, and to inhibit progression of structural damage associated with the disease in adults with moderately to severely active rheumatoid arthritis. Results of several clinical trials indicate that use of a tumor necrosis factor (TNF) blocking agent (e.g., adalimumab, etanercept, infliximab) in combination with methotrexate is more effective that therapy with either drug alone, particularly with respect to clinical responses and radiographic outcome. Additional study is needed regarding several issues related to use of TNF blocking agents in the management of rheumatoid arthritis, including evaluation of potential adverse consequences of long-term TNF blockade. Only limited data are available to date regarding the efficacy of infliximab used without concomitant methotrexate in adults with rheumatoid arthritis, and the manufacturers state that infliximab or infliximab-dyyb should be used in conjunction with methotrexate for the management of this disease.

Rheumatoid arthritis, an autoimmune disorder, produces a complicated lesion in the synovium characterized by inflammation, proliferation, and destruction of cartilage and bone. Therapy for rheumatoid arthritis includes agents that block inflammation, retard synovial proliferation, and prevent joint erosion and usually consists of combinations of nonsteroidal anti-inflammatory agents (NSAIAs), DMARDs, and/or corticosteroids. The ultimate goal in managing rheumatoid arthritis is to prevent or control joint damage, prevent loss of function, and decrease pain. Although NSAIAs may be useful for initial symptomatic treatment of rheumatoid arthritis, these drugs do not alter the course of the disease or prevent joint destruction. DMARDs have the potential to reduce or prevent joint damage, preserve joint integrity and function, and reduce total health-care costs, and all patients with rheumatoid arthritis are candidates for DMARD therapy. DMARDs should be initiated early in the disease course.

While many factors influence the choice of a DMARD, methotrexate is used as the initial or anchor DMARD in many patients with rheumatoid arthritis. Because residual inflammation generally persists in patients receiving maximum dosages of a single DMARD, many rheumatoid arthritis patients are candidates for combination therapy to achieve optimum control.

Low-dose oral corticosteroids and local injection of corticosteroids are effective in relieving symptoms in patients with active rheumatoid arthritis.

Use of TNF blocking agents is most appropriate in patients with active disease despite adequate exposure to methotrexate or other effective conventional DMARD. A course of methotrexate in a dosage of at least 20 mg weekly (or lower dosage if toxicity develops) for 3 months is considered an adequate course of DMARD therapy, and failure with such a course should prompt consideration of the therapeutic regimen (e.g., initiation of a TNF blocking agent). TNF blocking agents can be added to preexisting therapy or replace existing DMARDs. Once therapy with a TNF blocking agent has been started, patients should be assessed for therapeutic response. Therapy with the TNF blocking agent should be discontinued in patients who have not responded after 12 weeks.

Combination Therapy with Methotrexate Safety and efficacy of infliximab used in conjunction with methotrexate for the management of rheumatoid arthritis in adults have been evaluated in several open-label and double-blind, placebo-controlled studies in adults with active disease as defined by the American College of Rheumatology (ACR) who had not responded adequately to methotrexate. Infliximab in conjunction with methotrexate also has been evaluated in a controlled study in adults with early active rheumatoid arthritis (i.e., duration of 3 years or less) who had not previously received therapy with methotrexate. Results indicate that addition of infliximab to a methotrexate regimen can result in decreases in the signs and symptoms of rheumatoid arthritis. For patients with early active rheumatoid arthritis, concomitant use of infliximab and methotrexate is more effective than methotrexate (as the sole DMARD) for the management of rheumatoid arthritis in adults. In addition, infliximab used concomitantly with methotrexate can improve physical function and inhibit the progression of structural damage in patients with rheumatoid arthritis.

Concomitant use of infliximab and methotrexate for the management of rheumatoid arthritis was evaluated in a large double-blind, placebo-controlled, phase III, international study that involved 428 patients (Anti-TNF Trial in Rheumatoid Arthritis with Concomitant Therapy [ATTRACT]). At study entry, patients had active rheumatoid arthritis (defined as 6 or more swollen or tender joints and at least 2 additional manifestations, including morning stiffness for 45 minutes or longer, ESR of 28 mm/hour or greater, or CRP level of 2 mg/dL or greater) despite having received methotrexate (oral or parenteral) and folic acid consistently for at least 3 months. Study patients were a median age of 51 years old, had a median disease duration of 11 years, and previously received treatment with 2.5–2.8 DMARDs other than methotrexate. These patients had median swollen and tender joint counts of 21 and 31, respectively; 77% were rheumatoid factor positive; 37% had undergone a joint surgery; 25% had joint replacement surgery; and approximately 40% were classified as ACR functional class III.

Patients were randomized to receive placebo or 3 or 10 mg/kg of infliximab by IV infusion at weeks 0, 2 and 6, followed by additional doses given once every 4 or 8 weeks. Patients continued to receive stable weekly dosages of methotrexate (median dosage 16 mg once weekly) beginning 4 weeks before and throughout the study. Those who were receiving stable dosages of NSAIAs and/or oral corticosteroids (oral prednisone 10 mg or less daily or equivalent) for at least 4 weeks prior to study entry were permitted to continue these drugs; patients who had not received such therapy were not permitted to initiate these drugs after entering the study. Patient evaluations were performed every 4 weeks and assessed according to ACR criteria for improvement (ACR response); the primary end point was the proportion of patients at week 30 who experienced a 20% improvement in rheumatoid disease activity (ACR 20 response). The ACR 20 response is achieved if the patient experiences a 20% or greater improvement in both tender and swollen joint counts and a 20% or greater improvement in at least 3 of the following criteria: patient pain assessment, patient global assessment, physician global assessment, patient self-assessed disability, or laboratory indicators of disease activity (i.e., ESR or CRP level). Patients also were evaluated for ACR 50 and 70 responses (these are defined using the same criteria as ACR 20 with a level of improvement of 50 or 70%, respectively); reductions in individual measures of disease activity; and a general health assessment.

At 30 weeks, an ACR 20 response was attained in 50% of patients who received 3 mg/kg of infliximab every 8 weeks concomitantly with weekly methotrexate compared with 20% of patients who received placebo and weekly methotrexate. Similar response rates were observed in patients receiving the higher infliximab dosage (10 mg/kg) and/or more frequent doses (every 4 weeks). At 30 weeks, an ACR 50 response was attained in 26–31% and an ACR 70 response was attained in 8–18% of patients who received infliximab in a dosage of 3 or 10 mg/kg every 4 or 8 weeks concomitantly with once weekly methotrexate; an ACR 50 or 70 response was attained at week 30 in only 5 or 0%, respectively, of patients who received placebo with once weekly methotrexate.

At 54 weeks, 42–59% of those who received 3 or 10 mg/kg of infliximab once every 4 or 8 weeks concomitantly with once weekly methotrexate maintained an ACR 20 response compared with 17% of patients who received placebo concomitantly with once weekly methotrexate. At 54 weeks, an ACR 50 or 70 response was maintained in 21–40% or 11–26%, respectively, of those receiving infliximab concomitantly with once weekly methotrexate compared with only 9 or 2%, respectively, of patients receiving placebo concomitantly with once weekly methotrexate.

Physical function and disability were assessed using the Health Assessment Questionnaire (HAQ) and the general health-related quality-of-life questionnaire SF-36. All 4 dosage regimens of infliximab and weekly methotrexate were associated with greater improvement from baseline in the HAQ and SF-36 physical component summary score averaged over time through week 54 compared with the placebo plus methotrexate regimen; in addition, the infliximab regimens were not associated with deterioration in the SF-36 mental component summary score. Improvements in HAQ and SF-36 were maintained through week 102.

Structural damage in the hands and feet of patients in this study was assessed radiographically at baseline and at weeks 54 and 102 using the van der Heijde-modified Sharp score (a composite score of structural damage that measures the number and size of joint erosions and the degree of joint space narrowing in hands/wrists and feet). At 54 weeks, there was more progression of joint damage from baseline in the group of patients who received placebo with once weekly methotrexate compared with those who received infliximab with once weekly methotrexate. The inhibition of progression of structural damage reported in patients receiving infliximab at week 54 was maintained through week 102. There also was evidence that infliximab had a benefit on both erosions and joint-space narrowing when these scores were examined independently and when the hands and feet were examined separately.

Efficacy of infliximab in conjunction with methotrexate has been evaluated in a study that included 1004 adults with early active rheumatoid arthritis (i.e., duration of 3 years or less) who had not previously received methotrexate. The median age of study patients was 51 years, and the median disease duration was 0.6 years. These patients had median swollen and tender joint counts of 19 and 31, respectively; greater than 80% of these individuals had joint damage at baseline. Patients were randomized to receive placebo or 3 or 6 mg/kg of infliximab by IV infusion at weeks 0, 2, and 6, followed by additional doses given once every 8 weeks. All patients received methotrexate (optimized to a dosage of 20 mg each week by week 8 of the study); patients receiving stable dosages of NSAIAs and/or oral corticosteroids (oral prednisone 10 mg or less daily or equivalent) at study entry were permitted to continue these drugs. Reduction in the signs and symptoms of rheumatoid arthritis were evaluated using ACR criteria, physical function and disability was assessed using HAQ scores, and joint damage was assessed using the van der Heijde-modified Sharp score. At 54 weeks, 62–66% of patients receiving 3 or 6 mg/kg of infliximab with once-weekly methotrexate attained an ACR 20 response compared with 54% of those who received placebo concomitantly with once weekly methotrexate. At 54 weeks, an ACR 50 or 70 response was attained by 46–50 or 33–37%, respectively, of patients receiving infliximab concomitantly with weekly methotrexate compared with 32 or 21%, respectively, of those receiving placebo with once-weekly methotrexate. Both dosage regimens of infliximab and weekly methotrexate were associated with greater improvement from baseline in the HAQ averaged over time through week 54 compared with the placebo plus methotrexate regimen. Radiographic analysis at week 54 indicates that infliximab in conjunction with methotrexate is more effective than methotrexate alone in delaying joint damage.

Therapy with a Single Disease-modifying Antirheumatic Drug There are limited data available regarding efficacy of infliximab without concurrent methotrexate for the management of rheumatoid arthritis in adults†. Although infliximab was used without concomitant methotrexate in several early studies evaluating the safety and efficacy of the drug for the management of rheumatoid arthritis, long-term experience with other DMARDs indicates that combination therapy with 2 DMARDs often is necessary to achieve optimum control in patients with moderately to severely active disease. Therefore, subsequent studies evaluated the safety and efficacy of infliximab used concomitantly with methotrexate. (See Combination Therapy with Methotrexate under Uses: Rheumatoid Arthritis in Adults.) The manufacturers state that infliximab or infliximab-dyyb should be used in combination with methotrexate for the management of rheumatoid arthritis.

Results of early open-label and placebo-controlled studies using infliximab as the only DMARD in adults with rheumatoid arthritis indicated that the drug could result in clinical improvement in patients who had not responded adequately to other DMARDs. In one multicenter, placebo-controlled, double-blind study, 73 adults with rheumatoid arthritis were randomized to receive a single dose of placebo or 1 or 10 mg/kg of infliximab given by IV infusion. Patients were not allowed to receive any other DMARDs beginning 4 weeks before the study; however, those receiving stable dosages of oral corticosteroids or NSAIAs were allowed to continue these drugs. At 4 weeks after the dose, a clinical response (defined as a Paulus 20% response) was reported in 44 or 79% of patients who received a 1- or 10-mg/kg infliximab dose, respectively, compared with 8% of those who received placebo. A Paulus 50% response was reported at 4 weeks in 28 or 58% of patients who received 1 or 10 mg/kg of the drug, respectively, compared with 8% of those who received placebo. Although there was no evidence of a dose-response relationship based on results at 2 weeks, the higher dose (10 mg/kg) was associated with significantly higher response rates and greater responses (e.g., improvements in pain score, grip strength, CRP, ESR) than the lower dose (1 mg/kg) at week 4. There also was some evidence that the higher dose resulted in a more prolonged response than the lower dose.

■ **Ankylosing Spondylitis** Infliximab or infliximab-dyyb is used to reduce the signs and symptoms of ankylosing spondylitis in patients with active disease. In one placebo-controlled study in adults with ankylosing spondylitis, 53% of those receiving infliximab (5-mg/kg doses given at 0, 2, and 6 weeks) experienced at least a 50% reduction in disease activity (assessed using the Bath Ankylosing Spondylitis Disease Activity Index [BASDAI]) compared with 9% of those receiving placebo. In addition, infliximab therapy was associated with improvements in physical function and quality of life.

■ **Psoriatic Arthritis** Infliximab or infliximab-dyyb is used to reduce the signs and symptoms of active arthritis, inhibit the progression of structural damage, and improve physical function in patients with psoriatic arthritis.

Safety and efficacy of infliximab in the management of active psoriatic arthritis (i.e., at least 5 swollen joints and at least 5 tender joints, with one or more of the following subtypes: arthritis involving DIP joints, arthritis mutilans, asymmetric peripheral arthritis, polyarticular arthritis, spondylitis with peripheral arthritis) were evaluated in a multicenter, double-blind, placebo-controlled study in 200 adult patients who had an inadequate response to therapy with DMARDs or NSAIAs. Patients also had plaque psoriasis with qualifying target lesion of at least 2 cm in diameter. During the 24-week double-blind phase, patients were randomized to receive infliximab 5 mg/kg by IV infusion (100 patients) or placebo (100 patients) at weeks 0, 2, 6, 14, and 22. Forty-six percent of patients continued to receive stable doses of methotrexate (up to 25 mg weekly). Patient evaluations were assessed according to ACR criteria for improvement (ACR response). Patients receiving placebo, who achieved less than 10% improvement from baseline at week 16, were switched to induction therapy with infliximab (early escape). At week 24, all patients receiving placebo were switched to induction therapy with infliximab. Infliximab therapy was continued through week 46 for all patients. At 14 weeks, an ACR 20 response was attained in 58% of patients who received infliximab compared with 11% of patients who received placebo. (For definition of ACR responses, see Combination Therapy with Methotrexate under Uses: Rheumatoid Arthritis in Adults.) The response was similar regardless of concomitant use with methotrexate. Improvement has been observed in some patients as early as week 2. At 6 months, ACR 20, 50, or 70 response was attained in 54, 41, or 27% of patients, respectively, who received infliximab, compared with 16, 4, or 2% of patients receiving placebo. Similar responses were seen in patients with each of the subtypes of psoriatic arthritis, although few patients were enrolled with arthritis mutilans and spondylitis with peripheral arthritis subtypes. Infliximab therapy resulted in improvements in the components of the ACR response criteria and in dactylitis and enthesopathy compared with placebo. The clinical response was maintained through week 54.

Among the 170 patients who had baseline affected body surface area (BSA) of 3% or more, improvement in the Psoriasis Area and Severity Index (PASI) of at least 75% (PASI 75) from baseline was achieved at week 14 (regardless of concomitant methotrexate use) in 64% of patients receiving infliximab and in 2% of patients receiving placebo. Improvement was observed in some patients as early as week 2. At 6 months, PASI 75 and PASI 90 responses were achieved in 60 and 39%, respectively, of patients receiving infliximab and in 1 and 0%, respectively, of patients receiving placebo. The PASI response generally was maintained through week 54.

Structural damage in the hands and feet was assessed radiographically by the change from baseline in the van der Heijde-Sharp (vdH-S) score, modified by the addition of hand distal interphalangeal (DIP) joints. The total modified vdH-S score was a composite score of structural damage measuring the number and size of joint erosions and the degree of joint space narrowing (JSN) in the hands and feet. At week 24, less radiographic progression (mean change of −0.7 versus 0.82), less progression in erosion scores (−0.56 versus 0.51), and less progression in JSN scores (−0.14 versus 0.31) were observed in patients receiving infliximab compared with those receiving placebo. Continued inhibition of structural damage at week 54 was reported in patients receiving infliximab. A median change of 0 in the vdH-S score was reported during the 12-month study in patients initially randomized to either infliximab or placebo. Readily apparent radiographic progression was observed in a higher percentage of patients receiving placebo than in those receiving infliximab (12 versus 3%).

Patients receiving infliximab experienced substantial improvement in physical function as assessed by the HAQ Disability Index (HAQ-DI), with median improvement of 43% from baseline to week 14 and week 24 in patients receiving infliximab compared with 0% in those receiving placebo. During the 24-week placebo-controlled portion of the trial, a clinically meaningful improvement in HAQ-DI (decrease of at least 0.3 units) was reported in 54% of patients receiving infliximab and in 22% of those receiving placebo. Patients receiving infliximab also achieved a greater improvement in the physical and mental component summary scores of the SF-36 Health Survey compared with patients receiving placebo. These responses were maintained for up to 2 years in an open-label extension study.

■ **Plaque Psoriasis** Infliximab or infliximab-dyyb is used for the treatment of chronic, severe (i.e., extensive and/or disabling) plaque psoriasis in adults who are candidates for systemic therapy when other systemic therapies are medically less appropriate. Infliximab products should only be used in patients who will be closely monitored and will have regular follow-up visits with a clinician.

Safety and efficacy of infliximab were assessed in 3 randomized, double-blind, placebo-controlled studies (EXPRESS, EXPRESS II, SPIRIT) in adults (18 years of age or older) with chronic, stable plaque psoriasis involving at least 10% of body surface area (BSA), who had a Psoriasis Area and Severity Index (PASI) score of at least 12, and who were candidates for systemic therapy or phototherapy. Patients with guttate, pustular, or erythrodermic psoriasis were excluded from the studies. With the exception of low-dependency topical corticosteroids on the face and groin after week 10, no concomitant psoriasis treatments were allowed during the studies. The primary end point in all 3 studies was the proportion of patients who achieved a reduction in PASI score of at least 75% from baseline to week 10 (PASI 75). Efficacy and safety of infliximab treatment beyond 50 weeks have not been evaluated in patients with plaque psoriasis.

In the EXPRESS study, 378 patients were randomized to receive placebo or a 5-mg/kg dose of infliximab by IV infusion at weeks 0, 2, and 6 (induction therapy) and then every 8 weeks through week 46 (maintenance therapy). At week 24, patients who were randomized to receive placebo were crossed over to receive 5 mg/kg dose of infliximab (induction therapy) by IV infusion and then maintenance therapy (every 8 weeks). Patients had a median baseline PASI score of 21 and a baseline static Physician Global Assessment (sPGA) score ranging from moderate (52% of patients) to marked (36%) to severe (2%). Chronic, stable plaque psoriasis involving at least 20% of BSA was present in 75% of patients. 71 or 82% of patients had received prior systemic therapy or phototherapy, respectively. PASI 75 was achieved in 80 or 3% of patients receiving infliximab or placebo, respectively. Patients also were evaluated by the sPGA score (a 6-category scale ranging from "5=severe" to "0=cleared") according to the physician's overall assessment of the psoriasis severity focusing on induration, erythema, and scaling. "Cleared" or "minimal" score (consisting of none or minimal elevation in plaque, up to faint red coloration in erythema, and none or minimal fine scale over less than 5% of the plaque) was achieved in 80 or 4% of patients receiving the drug or placebo, respectively. In the subgroup of patients with more extensive psoriasis who previously had received phototherapy, PASI 75 was achieved at week 10 in 85% of patients receiving infliximab compared with 4% of those receiving placebo.

In the EXPRESS II study, 835 patients (having a median baseline PASI score of 18, 63% having psoriasis involving at least 20% of BSA, and 55 or 64% having received prior systemic or phototherapy, respectively) were randomized to receive placebo or a 3- or 5-mg/kg dose of infliximab at weeks 0, 2, or 6 (induction therapy). At week 14, patients randomized to receive a 3- or 5-mg/kg dose of infliximab were randomized to receive either scheduled (every 8 weeks) or "as needed" maintenance treatment through week 46. At week 16, patients who were randomized to receive placebo were crossed over to receive a 5-mg/kg dose of infliximab induction therapy followed by maintenance therapy every 8 weeks. PASI 75 was achieved in 2, 70, or 75%, respectively, of patients receiving placebo or a dose of 3 or 5 mg/kg of infliximab. Patients also were evaluated by the rPGA score (a 6-category scale ranging from "6=severe" to "1=clear") assessed relative to baseline in which overall lesions were graded with consideration to the percent of body involvement as well as overall induration, scaling, and erythema. "Clear" or "excellent" score (consisting of some residual pinkness or pigmentation to marked improvement [nearly normal skin texture; some erythema may have been present]) was achieved in 1, 69, or 75% of patients receiving placebo or a dose of 3 or 5 mg/kg of infliximab, respectively. In the subgroup of patients with more extensive psoriasis who previously had received phototherapy, PASI 75 was achieved at week 10 in 1, 72, or 77% of patients receiving placebo or a dose of 3 or 5 mg/kg of infliximab, respectively. In the subgroup of patients with more extensive psoriasis who had failed or were intolerant to phototherapy, PASI 75 was achieved at week 10 in 2, 70, or 78% of patients receiving placebo or a dose of 3 or 5 mg/kg of infliximab, respectively. Maintenance of response was studied in 292 (out of 313) patients randomized to receive infliximab 3 mg/kg and in 297 (out of the 314) patients randomized to receive infliximab 5 mg/kg. At week 14, patients were stratified by PASI response at week 10 and by investigational site and were then randomized to receive either scheduled or as needed maintenance therapy. A higher percentage of patients receiving scheduled maintenance therapy (every 8 weeks) appeared to maintain a PASI 75 through week 50 compared with patients receiving as needed maintenance therapy, with the best response maintained with a dosage of 5 mg/kg every 8 weeks. In a subset of patients who had achieved a response at week 10, maintenance of response appeared to be greater in patients receiving infliximab 5 mg/kg every 8 weeks. A decline in response in a subpopulation of patients in each group over time was observed in patients receiving either as needed or scheduled maintenance therapy.

In the SPIRIT study, 249 patients who previously had received either psoralen plus ultraviolet A treatment (PUVA) or other systemic psoriasis therapy were randomized to receive placebo or a 3- or 5-mg/kg dose of infliximab at weeks 0, 2, and 6 (induction therapy). At week 26, patients with an sPGA score of "moderate" or "worse" (a score of at least 3 on a scale of 0–5) received an additional dose of the randomized treatment. Patients had a median baseline PASI score of 19 and a baseline sPGA score of moderate (62% of patients), marked (22%), or severe (3%); BSA of at least 20% was present in 75% of patients. At week 26, 46% of enrolled patients received an additional infliximab dose. PASI 75 was achieved in 6, 72, or 88% of patients receiving placebo or a dose of 3 or 5 mg/kg of infliximab, respectively. In addition, a score of "cleared" or "minimal" by the sPGA score was achieved in 10, 72, or 90% of patients receiving placebo or a dose of 3 or 5 mg/kg of infliximab, respectively.

■ **Juvenile Arthritis** Infliximab has been used in a limited number of pediatric patients with juvenile rheumatoid arthritis† (also known as juvenile idiopathic arthritis); however, further study is needed to evaluate the safety and efficacy of the drug for juvenile rheumatoid arthritis.

Safety and efficacy of infliximab for the management of juvenile rheumatoid arthritis† have been evaluated in children 4–17 years of age with juvenile arthritis who had not responded adequately to methotrexate. Pediatric patients were randomized to receive placebo or 3 mg/kg of infliximab by IV infusion at weeks 0, 2, 6, and 14. Patients continued to receive oral or parenteral methotrexate (10–15 mg/m² per week); study participants also could receive folic acid prophylaxis (required for methotrexate), oral corticosteroids, NSAIAs, and/or other analgesics. At week 14, those who received placebo crossed over to all active treatment; these individuals received 6 mg/kg of infliximab by IV infusion at weeks 14, 16, and 20, followed by additional doses given once every 8 weeks concomitantly with weekly methotrexate through week 44 . Children who received infliximab during the initial 14 weeks of the study continued to receive 3 mg/kg of infliximab once every 8 weeks concomitantly with weekly methotrexate through week 44.

The primary end point of this study was the American College of Rheumatology (ACR) Pediatric 30 (Pedi 30) criteria for improvement (i.e., 30% or greater improvement in at least 3 of 6 and 30% or greater deterioration in no more than 1 of 6 core set criteria that include physician and patient/parent global assessments, active joint count, limitation of motion, functional assessment, and ESR) at week 14. An ACR Pedi 30 was achieved by 63.8% of patients who received infliximab concomitantly with methotrexate compared with 49.2% of patients who received placebo and methotrexate at week 14. Achievement of the primary end point did not differ significantly between infliximab-treated children and placebo-treated children. At week 16 when all study participants were receiving infliximab, an ACR Pedi 30 was achieved by 73.2% of patients. At week 52, an ACR Pedi 50 or 70 (defined using the same criteria as Pedi 30 with a level of improvement of 50 or 70%, respectively) was achieved by 69.6 or 51.8%, respectively, of study participants. Other observations from this study include a higher rate of immunogenic reactions in study participants than has been observed in infliximab-treated adults. (See Cautions: Pediatric Precautions.)

■ **Behcet's Syndrome** Infliximab has been used in a limited number of patients with Behcet's syndrome†; however, further study is needed to evaluate safety and efficacy of the drug in this disease. Behcet's syndrome is a chronic inflammatory disorder of unknown etiology characterized by recurrent orogenital ulceration, skin lesions, and arthritic symptoms that may be complicated by GI, ocular, and neurologic involvement. Proinflammatory cytokines, including TNF, are produced by monocytes as part of the inflammatory cascade in Behcet's disease. Use of infliximab in an adult with Behcet's disease who was receiving maintenance therapy with oral prednisone resulted in improvement in GI symptoms and discontinuance of the corticosteroid. In addition, use of infliximab (5-mg/kg doses given at 0, 2, and 6 weeks) resulted in improvements in both oral and genital lesions in an adult with Behçet's disease who had recalcitrant orogenital ulceration and a single 5-mg/kg dose of infliximab decreased acute ocular inflammation and improved visual acuity in several adults with panuveitis associated with Behçet's disease.

■ **Other Uses** Because of evidence that TNF may play a role in progression of heart failure, infliximab has been investigated for the management of congestive heart failure† in patients with moderate to severe (New York Heart Association [NYHA] class III or IV) congestive heart failure. In a phase II, double-blind, placebo-controlled study, patients with stable NYHA class III or IV congestive heart failure (left ventricular ejection fraction 35% or less) were randomized to receive placebo, infliximab 5 mg/kg, or infliximab 10 mg/kg at 0, 2, and 6 weeks. However, there was no evidence that infliximab improved clinical status of these patients and those receiving infliximab (especially those receiving 10 mg/kg) had a higher incidence of mortality and hospitalization for worsening heart failure compared with those receiving placebo. (See Cardiac Precautions and Contraindications under Cautions: Precautions and Contraindications.)

Dosage and Administration

■ **Reconstitution and Administration** Infliximab or infliximab-dyyb is administered by IV infusion.

Commercially available infliximab or infliximab-dyyb lyophilized powder must be reconstituted and diluted prior to administration using proper aseptic technique.

Infliximab or infliximab-dyyb lyophilized powder should be reconstituted by adding 10 mL of sterile water for injection to a vial labeled as containing 100 mg of infliximab or infliximab-dyyb, respectively, to provide a solution containing 10 mg/mL. Based on the indicated dosage of infliximab or infliximab-dyyb, the appropriate number of vials of the drug should be reconstituted. During reconstitution, the sterile water diluent should be directed toward the side of the vial using a sterile syringe with a 21-gauge or smaller needle and the contents gently swirled to minimize foaming during dissolution; some foaming will occur. To avoid excessive foaming, the vial should not be shaken and excessive or vigorous agitation should be avoided. The reconstituted solution should be inspected visually for particulate matter. The reconstituted solution should be colorless to light yellow and opalescent and should not be used if discolored or opaque or if foreign particles other than a few translucent proteinaceous particles are present. The reconstituted solution should be allowed to stand for 5 minutes before being diluted for administration. Reconstituted infliximab or infliximab-dyyb should then be diluted in 0.9% sodium chloride injection to provide a total volume of 250 mL (i.e., if a 250-mL bottle or bag of 0.9% sodium chloride injection is used, a volume of the diluent equal to the total required volume of reconstituted infliximab or infliximab-dyyb solution should be removed from the bag or bottle prior to addition of the infliximab or infliximab-dyyb solution). The total required volume of reconstituted infliximab or infliximab-dyyb solution should be added slowly to the diluent and the diluted solution should be gently mixed.

The final concentration of the reconstituted and diluted infliximab or infliximab-dyyb solution should be 0.4–4 mg/mL. Infliximab or infliximab-dyyb infusion should begin within 3 hours of reconstitution and dilution of the drug. This solution should be infused IV over a period of at least 2 hours.

An in-line, sterile, nonpyrogenic, low-protein-binding filter with a pore diameter of 1.2 μm or less should be used for administration. As with all parenteral products, diluted solutions of infliximab or infliximab-dyyb should be inspected visually for particulate matter and discoloration prior to administration whenever solution and container permit. Any unused portions should be discarded since the lyophilized drug does not contain any preservatives or bacteriostatic agents. The manufacturers recommend that infliximab products not be admixed with other drugs or infused in the same IV line with other drugs.

Pretreatment Regimen, Rate Titration Schedule, and Patient Monitoring To prevent or ameliorate acute infusion reactions to infliximab products, the manufacturers and some clinicians suggest that use of a pretreatment regimen be considered prior to each dose of the drug. For patients who are receiving an initial infliximab dose and patients without a history of acute infusion reactions with prior doses of the drug, the manufacturer of infliximab suggests that clinicians consider using a regimen of oral diphenhydramine (25–50 mg) and/or oral acetaminophen (650 mg); for those with a history of acute infusion reactions with prior doses of infliximab, clinicians can consider a regimen of oral or IV diphenhydramine (25–50 mg), oral acetaminophen (650 mg), and oral or, alternatively, IV prednisone (40 mg) or hydrocortisone (100 mg).

Infliximab or infliximab-dyyb infusions should be administered IV over at least 2 hours. The manufacturer of infliximab states that IV infusions can be given at a rate of 2 mL/minute or, alternatively, a rate titration schedule may be used in an attempt to prevent or ameliorate acute infusion reactions. If a rate titration schedule is used in patients who are receiving an initial infliximab dose, those without a history of acute infusion reactions to prior doses of the drug, or those with a history of such reactions, the manufacturer of infliximab recommends that the IV infusion be initiated at a rate of 10 mL/hour for the first 15 minutes followed by 20 mL/hour for 15 minutes, 40 mL/hour for 15 minutes, 80 mL/hour for 15 minutes, 150 mL/hour for 30 minutes, and then 250 mL/hour for 30 minutes.

The manufacturers state that, in general, the risks and benefits of readministration of infliximab or infliximab-dyyb after a period without treatment (especially readministration as a reinduction regimen at 0, 2, and 6 weeks) should be carefully considered. If maintenance therapy with infliximab products for the management of psoriasis is interrupted, infliximab or infliximab-dyyb therapy should be reinitiated as a single dose followed by maintenance therapy. (See Cautions: Sensitivity Reactions and Antibody Formation.)

Patients should be monitored closely (including measurement of vital signs) during and for at least 30 minutes after each IV infusion of the drug. Trained personnel and appropriate drugs should be available to treat anaphylaxis if it occurs. The manufacturer of infliximab recommends that vital signs (pulse, blood pressure) be measured immediately prior to initiating an IV infusion of the drug, frequently during the infusion (every 30 minutes in those without a history of acute infusion reactions with prior doses of the drug and every 15 minutes in those with a history of such reactions), and 30 minutes after completion of the infusion. If a patient experiences a clinically important change in vital signs (e.g., diastolic blood pressure drops 15–20 mm Hg) or any symptoms of hypersensitivity (e.g., urticaria, shortness of breath) while receiving an IV infusion of an infliximab product, the infusion should be stopped immediately, manifestations evaluated, and appropriate therapy initiated. If the reaction is not severe and can be controlled with a regimen of oral diphenhydramine (25–50 mg), oral acetaminophen (650 mg), and oral or IV prednisone (40 mg), then the infusion may be resumed with caution using a rate titration procedure starting at 10 mL/hour. However, the infliximab product infusion should be discontinued and not completed if the reaction does not resolve with this regimen or is more severe and requires treatment with epinephrine.

■ **Dosage** ***Crohn's Disease*** Nonbiologic agents used for the management of Crohn's disease (e.g., corticosteroids, mesalamine, sulfasalazine, azathioprine, mercaptopurine, methotrexate, anti-infective agents) may be continued in patients receiving infliximab products. However, when deciding whether infliximab products should be used alone or in combination with other immunosuppressive agents such as azathioprine or mercaptopurine, clinicians should consider both the possibility of an increased risk of hepatosplenic T-cell lymphoma with combination therapy and the observed (in infliximab studies) increase in immunogenicity and hypersensitivity reactions associated with infliximab products given as monotherapy. (See Cautions: Sensitivity Reactions and Antibody Formation and also Cautions: Malignancies and Lymphoproliferative Disorders.)

Adult Dosage. The usual adult dosage of infliximab or infliximab-dyyb for the management of moderately or severely active Crohn's disease or fistulizing Crohn's disease is 5 mg/kg given by IV infusion over a period of at least 2 hours.

The manufacturers recommend that adults with moderately to severely active Crohn's disease or with fistulizing Crohn's disease receive the initial 3 doses of infliximab or infliximab-dyyb at 0, 2, and 6 weeks (induction regimen) and that additional doses be given once every 8 weeks thereafter (maintenance regimen). An increase in infliximab or infliximab-dyyb dose to 10 mg/kg may be considered in patients who respond initially but subsequently lose response. Patients who do not respond to infliximab or infliximab-dyyb by week 14 are unlikely to respond with continued administration; discontinuance of the drug should be considered in these patients.

Pediatric Dosage. The recommended dosage of infliximab or infliximab-dyyb in pediatric patients 6 years of age or older with moderately to severely active Crohn's disease is 5 mg/kg given by IV infusion over a period of at least 2 hours at 0, 2, and 6 weeks (induction therapy) followed by a maintenance regimen of 5 mg/kg every 8 weeks.

Ulcerative Colitis Nonbiologic agents used for the management of ulcerative colitis (e.g., corticosteroids, azathioprine, mercaptopurine, 5-aminosalicylates) may be continued in patients receiving infliximab products. However, when deciding whether infliximab products should be used alone or in combination with other immunosuppressive agents such as azathioprine or mercaptopurine, clinicians should consider both the possibility of an increased risk of hepatosplenic T-cell lymphoma with combination therapy and the observed (in infliximab studies) increase in immunogenicity and hypersensitivity reactions associated with infliximab products given as monotherapy. (See Cautions: Sensitivity Reactions and Antibody Formation and also Cautions: Malignancies and Lymphoproliferative Disorders.)

Adult Dosage. The usual adult dosage of infliximab or infliximab-dyyb for the management of moderately or severely active ulcerative colitis is 5 mg/kg given by IV infusion over a period of at least 2 hours.

The manufacturers recommend that adults with moderately to severely active ulcerative colitis receive the initial 3 doses of infliximab or infliximab-dyyb at 0, 2, and 6 weeks (induction regimen) and that additional doses be given once every 8 weeks thereafter (maintenance regimen).

Pediatric Dosage. The recommended dosage of infliximab in pediatric patients 6 years of age or older with moderately to severely active ulcerative colitis is 5 mg/kg given by IV infusion over a period of at least 2 hours at 0, 2, and 6 weeks (induction regimen) followed by a maintenance regimen of 5 mg/kg every 8 weeks.

Rheumatoid Arthritis in Adults Infliximab or infliximab-dyyb is used in conjunction with methotrexate for the management of rheumatoid arthritis; only limited data are available to date regarding safety and efficacy of infliximab products used without concomitant methotrexate in the management of this disease. Other nonbiologic agents used for the management of rheumatoid arthritis (e.g., corticosteroids, nonsteroidal anti-inflammatory agents [NSAIAs]) may be continued in patients receiving infliximab products.

For the management of moderately to severely active rheumatoid arthritis in adults, the usual dosage of infliximab or infliximab-dyyb is 3 mg/kg given by IV infusion over a period of at least 2 hours. The manufacturers recommend that adults with rheumatoid arthritis receive the initial 3 doses of infliximab or infliximab-dyyb at 0, 2, and 6 weeks (induction regimen) and that additional doses be given once every 8 weeks thereafter (maintenance regimen). For patients who have an incomplete response to this 3-mg/kg regimen, consideration can be given to increasing the infliximab or infliximab-dyyb dosage up to 10 mg/kg and/or administering infliximab or infliximab-dyyb doses as often as once every 4 weeks.

Ankylosing Spondylitis For the management of ankylosing spondylitis in adults, the usual dosage of infliximab or infliximab-dyyb is 5 mg/kg given by IV infusion over a period of at least 2 hours. The manufacturers recommend that adults with ankylosing spondylitis receive the initial 3 doses of infliximab or infliximab-dyyb at 0, 2, and 6 weeks (induction regimen) and that additional doses be given once every 6 weeks thereafter (maintenance regimen).

Psoriatic Arthritis For the management of psoriatic arthritis in adults, the usual dosage of infliximab or infliximab-dyyb is 5 mg/kg given by IV infusion over a period of at least 2 hours. The manufacturers recommend that adults with psoriatic arthritis receive the initial 3 doses of infliximab or infliximab-dyyb at 0, 2, and 6 weeks (induction regimen) and that additional doses be given once every 8 weeks thereafter (maintenance regimen).

Plaque Psoriasis For the management of chronic severe plaque psoriasis in adults, the usual dosage of infliximab or infliximab-dyyb is 5 mg/kg given by IV infusion over a period of at least 2 hours. The manufacturers recommend that adults with plaque psoriasis receive the initial 3 doses of infliximab or infliximab-dyyb at 0, 2, and 6 weeks (induction regimen) and that additional doses be given once every 8 weeks thereafter (maintenance regimen). If maintenance therapy with infliximab or infliximab-dyyb for the management of psoriasis is interrupted, infliximab or infliximab-dyyb therapy should be reinitiated as a single dose followed by maintenance therapy. (See Cautions: Sensitivity Reactions and Antibody Formation.)

■ **Dosage in Renal and Hepatic Impairment** Pharmacokinetic studies of infliximab or infliximab-dyyb have not been conducted in patients with renal and/or hepatic impairment, and the manufacturers do not make specific recommendations for dosage adjustment in such patients.

Cautions

Information on the safety of infliximab has been obtained principally from clinical studies in adults with Crohn's disease, rheumatoid arthritis, ankylosing spondylitis, psoriatic arthritis, ulcerative colitis, and plaque psoriasis; information has been obtained from 2625 patients who received infliximab for at least 30 weeks and from 374 of these patients who received the drug for at least 1 year. Infliximab generally is well tolerated; however, serious infectious complications, including some fatalities, have been reported in some patients receiving the drug. In addition, some patients receiving infliximab have experienced acute or delayed infusion reactions that may require discontinuance of the drug. The most common adverse effects resulting in discontinuance were infusion-related reactions, dyspnea, rash, flushing, and headache. In clinical studies in patients with psoriasis, serious adverse reactions were reported during up to 16 weeks of treatment in 0.5 or 1.6% of patients receiving 3- or 5-mg/kg doses of infliximab, respectively, compared with 1.9% of those receiving placebo.

Based on demonstration of biosimilarity, FDA considers that no clinically meaningful differences in safety exist between infliximab and infliximab-dyyb. No substantial differences in the frequencies of adverse effects have been observed between infliximab and infliximab-dyyb. In addition, no substantial changes in antidrug antibody responses have been observed in patients following a single switch from infliximab to infliximab-dyyb, and no new safety concerns have been identified in these patients compared with those receiving continuous infliximab-dyyb therapy.

■ **Infectious Complications** Patients receiving tumor necrosis factor (TNF) blocking agents, including infliximab products, are at increased risk of developing serious infections involving various organ systems and sites that may require hospitalization or result in death. Opportunistic infections caused by bacterial, mycobacterial, invasive fungal, viral, or parasitic organisms—including aspergillosis, blastomycosis, candidiasis, coccidioidomycosis, histoplasmosis, legionellosis, listeriosis, pneumocystosis, and tuberculosis—have been reported in patients receiving TNF blocking agents. (See Precautions and Contraindications Related to Infectious Complications, under Cautions: Precautions and Contraindications.) Infections frequently have been disseminated rather than localized. Most patients who developed serious infections were receiving concomitant therapy with immunosuppressive agents such as corticosteroids or methotrexate.

In clinical studies evaluating infliximab in patients with rheumatoid arthritis, serious infection was reported in 5.3% of patients who received infliximab in conjunction with methotrexate and in 3.4% of those who received methotrexate and placebo (follow-up: 52 weeks for both groups). Serious infections reported in patients receiving infliximab have included pneumonia, cellulitis, abscess, skin ulceration, sepsis, and bacterial infection. Extrapulmonary and disseminated tuberculosis, including fatal miliary tuberculosis, have been reported in patients receiving infliximab products. During clinical trials, tuberculosis was reported in 14 patients receiving infliximab, and there were 4 fatalities related to miliary tuberculosis. During postmarketing surveillance, other cases of tuberculosis have been reported. Reactivation of latent tuberculosis and new tuberculosis infections have been reported in patients receiving infliximab products, including in patients who previously received antimycobacterial therapy for latent or active tuberculosis. Cases of active tuberculosis also have been reported in patients receiving infliximab products while they were receiving antimycobacterial therapy for latent tuberculosis. As of September 2002, FDA had received 335 reports of infliximab-associated tuberculosis. Most of the cases of tuberculosis occurred within the first 2 months following initiation of infliximab therapy; these cases may reflect recrudescence of latent tuberculosis infection. As of September 2011, FDA had identified 103 reports of *Legionella* pneumonia associated with TNF blocking agents, including infliximab. The 103 cases of *Legionella* pneumonia occurred in patients 25–85 years of age, many of whom received concomitant therapy with immunosuppressive agents (e.g., corticosteroids and/or methotrexate); 17 deaths were reported. In 78% of the cases of *Legionella* pneumonia, the median duration of TNF blocker therapy prior to the onset of *Legionella* pneumonia was 10.4 months (range: less than 1 month to 73 months). As of September 2011, FDA also had identified 26 published reports of *Listeria* infections, including meningitis, bacteremia, endophthalmitis, and sepsis, in patients who received TNF blocking agents; 7 deaths were reported. Many of the *Listeria* infections occurred in patients who had received concomitant therapy with immunosuppressive agents. In addition, FDA identified fatal *Listeria* infections during a review of data regarding laboratory-confirmed infections that occurred in premarketing clinical studies and during postmarketing surveillance. Invasive fungal infections have occurred in patients receiving TNF blocking agents. Failure to recognize fungal infections has led to delays in appropriate treatment.

An increased incidence of serious infections also was observed in clinical studies in patients with rheumatoid arthritis when a TNF blocking agent was used concomitantly with anakinra (a human interleukin-1 receptor antagonist) or abatacept (a selective costimulation modulator). (See Drug Interactions: Biologic Agents.)

In clinical studies in adults with Crohn's disease or rheumatoid arthritis, infections requiring treatment were reported in 36% of those receiving infliximab (average follow-up: 53 weeks) and 28% of those receiving placebo (average follow-up: 47 weeks). The most frequently reported infections involved the upper respiratory tract (e.g., sinusitis, pharyngitis, bronchitis) or urinary tract. In clinical studies in adults with rheumatoid arthritis, upper respiratory tract infections occurred in 32% of patients receiving infliximab compared with 25% of those receiving placebo.

In a study in adults with fistulizing Crohn's disease (ACCENT II), 15% of patients developed a new fistula-related abscess.

In clinical studies in patients with ulcerative colitis, infections requiring antimicrobial therapy were reported in 27% of those receiving infliximab (average follow-up: 41 weeks) and 18% of those receiving placebo (average follow-up: 32 weeks).

In pediatric patients receiving infliximab for the treatment of Crohn's disease, infections were reported more frequently in patients receiving the drug every 8 weeks than in those receiving the drug every 12 weeks (74 versus 38%). The most commonly reported infections were upper respiratory tract infection and pharyngitis, and the most commonly reported serious infection was abscess. Pneumonia and herpes zoster also have been reported in pediatric patients receiving infliximab for the treatment of Crohn's disease.

In pediatric patients receiving infliximab for the treatment of ulcerative colitis, infection, infection requiring antimicrobial therapy, and serious infection were reported in 52, 37, and 12%, respectively, of patients. Infection occurred in 59% of pediatric patients receiving the recommended maintenance regimen of 5 mg/kg every 8 weeks. The most commonly reported infections were upper respiratory tract infection and pharyngitis.

Fatal disseminated BCG infection has been reported during postmarketing experience in an infant who received BCG vaccine after having been exposed to infliximab in utero.

■ **Sensitivity Reactions and Antibody Formation** Hypersensitivity reactions have been reported in patients receiving infliximab products; these reactions vary in their time to onset and have required hospitalization in some patients. Erythema multiforme, Stevens-Johnson syndrome, and toxic epidermal necrolysis have been reported during postmarketing experience in patients receiving infliximab products.

Acute Infusion Reactions Acute infusion reactions that appear to be hypersensitivity reactions to the drug have been reported during or within 1–2 hours after an IV infusion of infliximab products. In phase 3 clinical studies, infusion reactions were reported in 18% of patients receiving infliximab compared with 5% of patients receiving placebo. In these studies, 27% of patients who experienced an infusion reaction during infliximab induction therapy also experienced an infusion reaction during maintenance therapy with the drug, whereas 9% of patients who had no infusion reactions during infliximab induction therapy experienced an infusion reaction during maintenance therapy. Infusion reaction rates remained stable through 1 year in patients receiving infliximab in the psoriasis EXPRESS study. Infusion reaction rates in the psoriasis EXPRESS II study were variable over time and were somewhat higher following the final infusion than after the initial infusion. In the 3 psoriasis studies, acute infusion reactions were reported in 7, 4, or 1%, respectively, of patients receiving a 3- or 5-mg/kg dose of infliximab or placebo.

Acute infusion reactions to infliximab products usually consist of urticaria, dyspnea, and/or hypotension; however, fever, chills, headache, pruritus, chest pain, and/or hypertension also have been reported. Most acute infusion reactions have been mild and transient, and symptoms have been controlled by slowing the infusion rate, discontinuing the infusion, or treatment (e.g., with antihistamines). Serious infusion reactions, including anaphylaxis, seizures, erythematous rash, and/or hypotension have been reported in less than 1% of patients receiving infliximab. Anaphylactic reactions, including laryngeal/pharyngeal edema and severe bronchospasm, and seizure have occurred during postmarketing experience in patients receiving infliximab products. Myocardial ischemia/infarction and transient vision loss have been reported rarely in patients receiving infliximab products, either during or within 2 hours of infusion.

Infusion reactions that were not serious (including nonserious anaphylactoid reactions) were reported in 18% of pediatric patients receiving infliximab for the treatment of Crohn's disease. About 13% of pediatric patients receiving infliximab for the treatment of ulcerative colitis experienced one or more nonserious infusion reactions, including 18% of pediatric patients receiving the recommended maintenance regimen of 5 mg/kg every 8 weeks.

Infusion reactions were reported in 35 or 18%, respectively, of children receiving 3- or 6-mg/kg doses of infliximab for the treatment of juvenile rheumatoid arthritis. The most frequently reported infusion-related events were vomiting, fever, headache, and hypotension. Serious infusion reactions occurred in a few patients.

Patients who develop antibodies to infliximab appear to be 2–3 times more likely to have an infusion reaction than patients who do not develop antibodies to the drug. There is some evidence from studies of infliximab that the incidence of acute infusion reactions to infliximab products is lower in patients who are receiving concomitant therapy with immunosuppressive agents (e.g., azathioprine, mercaptopurine, methotrexate) than in those not receiving such therapy.

The manufacturers and some clinicians suggest that use of a pretreatment regimen (e.g., acetaminophen, antihistamines, prednisone) be considered prior to each infusion of the drug to prevent or ameliorate these acute infusion reactions. In addition, use of a rate titration schedule to administer IV infusions of infliximab can be considered. (See Pretreatment Regimen, Rate Titration Schedule, and Patient Monitoring, under Dosage and Administration: Reconstitution and Administration.)

Although safety and efficacy of the procedure have not been established, at least 2 Crohn's disease patients with a history of anaphylactic/anaphylactoid reactions to infliximab have received a subsequent dose of the drug using a desensitization procedure that involved dose escalation in an intensive care setting.

In clinical studies in patients with rheumatoid arthritis, Crohn's disease, or psoriasis, readministration of infliximab after a period without treatment resulted in a higher incidence of infusion reactions as compared to regular maintenance treatment. In a clinical trial evaluating 2 long-term treatment strategies (i.e., long-term maintenance therapy with infliximab versus retreatment with an induction regimen of infliximab following disease flare) in patients with moderate to severe psoriasis, serious infusion reactions were reported in 4% of patients receiving retreatment following disease flare compared with less than 1% of those receiving long-term maintenance therapy. Patients in this study did not receive other immunosuppressive agents concomitantly with infliximab. Most of the serious infusion reactions occurred during the second infusion at week 2 and manifestations included, but were not limited to, dyspnea, urticaria, facial edema, and hypotension. In all cases, infliximab therapy was discontinued and/or other treatment was instituted with complete resolution of signs and symptoms.

Delayed Infusion Reactions Infusion reactions that appear to be delayed hypersensitivity or serum sickness-like reactions have occurred after initial therapy with infliximab products (i.e., as early as after the second dose) and when therapy with infliximab products was reinstituted following an extended period without such treatment. Delayed infusion reactions to infliximab were first reported in a study in adults with moderately to severely active Crohn's disease or fistulizing Crohn's disease who were receiving retreatment with infliximab after an interval of 2–4 years. Delayed hypersensitivity reactions (generally reported as serum sickness or a combination of arthralgia and/or myalgia with fever and/or rash) have been reported in about 1% of patients with plaque psoriasis receiving infliximab in clinical studies; these reactions generally occurred within 2 weeks after repeat infusion of the drug.

There is some evidence that patients who have received at least 3 months of therapy with an immunosuppressive agent (e.g., azathioprine, mercaptopurine, methotrexate) prior to administration of infliximab have a lower rate of development of human antichimeric antibodies (HACA) and a lower rate of infusion reactions than patients not receiving such therapy.

Human Antichimeric Antibodies Infliximab and infliximab-dyyb are chimeric human-murine monoclonal antibodies, and patients receiving these products may develop infliximab-specific antibodies (HACA). The clinical importance of the development of antibodies to infliximab relative to the safety and efficacy of the drug have not been fully determined to date. There is some evidence from clinical studies that the presence of such antibodies may be associated with an increase in the incidence of infusion reactions, a decrease in infliximab half-life, and a decrease in clinical efficacy.

Data are limited regarding the overall incidence of infliximab antibodies in patients receiving the drug. The presence of infliximab in the serum sample may interfere with enzyme immunoassay (EIA) methods used to measure antibodies to infliximab and result in underestimation of the prevalence of antibody development to the drug. EIA methods were used to assess antibody development in the following studies; however, in pediatric patients with ulcerative colitis, a second assay method, an electrochemiluminescence immunoassay (ECLIA) method (which is 60-fold more sensitive than the original EIA method and permits classification of patient samples as either positive or negative for antibodies to the drug without the need for an inconclusive category) also was used. In patients receiving a 3-dose infliximab induction regimen followed by maintenance therapy who were evaluated over 1–2 years of treatment, 10% of patients were antibody-positive by EIA; most patients had low antibody titers. Patients with Crohn's disease who had a drug-free interval longer than 16 weeks were more likely to be antibody-positive than patients who received the usually recommended maintenance regimen of infliximab (i.e., doses every 8 weeks). EIA antibody test results were inconclusive (because infliximab was present in the serum sample) in approximately 77% of pediatric patients receiving infliximab in conjunction with stable dosages of mercaptopurine, azathioprine, or methotrexate for the treatment of Crohn's disease; following exclusion of these inconclusive samples, 3 of 24 patients (12.5%) had antibodies to infliximab. Antibodies to infliximab were detected by EIA in 38 or 12%, respectively, of children receiving 3- or 6-mg/kg doses of infliximab for the treatment of juvenile rheumatoid arthritis. In pediatric patients with ulcerative colitis, antibodies to the drug were detected by EIA or ECLIA in 7 or 52%, respectively, of patients.

Patients with Crohn's disease or rheumatoid arthritis receiving concomitant immunosuppressive therapy (e.g., methotrexate, azathioprine, mercaptopurine) were less likely to be antibody-positive. In patients who received infliximab in a dosage of 1, 3, or 10 mg/kg without concomitant methotrexate, infliximab antibodies were detected by EIA in 53, 21, or 7%, respectively; in those who received the same dosages of infliximab with concomitant methotrexate therapy (7.5 mg once weekly), infliximab antibodies were present in 15, 7, or 0%, respectively. Although further study is needed, it has been suggested that these data indicate that higher infliximab dosages and concomitant methotrexate therapy may induce a degree of immunologic tolerance to infliximab. (See Drug Interactions: Methotrexate.)

In one study, development of antibodies to infliximab was detected by EIA in 15% of 191 patients with psoriatic arthritis receiving infliximab 5 mg/kg with or without methotrexate. In the psoriasis EXPRESS II study in patients who received infliximab for 1 year at a dosage of 5 or 3 mg/kg, antibodies to infliximab were detected by EIA in 36 or 51% of patients, respectively, while in the psoriasis SPIRIT study in patients who received infliximab induction therapy at a dosage of 5 or 3 mg/kg, antibodies to infliximab were detected by EIA in 20 or 27%, respectively. Despite the increase in antibody formation, serious infusion reaction rates in patients receiving infliximab induction therapy at a dosage of 5 mg/kg followed by maintenance therapy every 8 weeks in the psoriasis EXPRESS and EXPRESS II studies and in patients receiving induction therapy at a dosage of 5 mg/kg in the psoriasis SPIRIT study were similar to those observed in other study populations (less than 1%). The effects of the apparent increased immunogenicity in patients with psoriasis on efficacy and infusion reaction rates with chronic infliximab therapy compared with patients with other disease states receiving infliximab products are not known.

No clinically meaningful differences have been found between infliximab-dyyb and infliximab with respect to antidrug antibody response resulting from administration of these drugs.

Autoantibodies and Lupus-like Syndrome Therapy with infliximab products may induce formation of autoantibodies and rarely may result in development of a lupus-like syndrome.

Adults with moderately to severely active Crohn's disease receiving infliximab have been tested for the presence of autoantibodies at baseline and at multiple time points during follow-up in clinical studies. When patients receiving infliximab in clinical studies were evaluated for the presence of antinuclear antibodies (ANA) and antibodies to double stranded DNA (anti-dsDNA), about 50 or 17 % had developed ANA or anti-dsDNA antibodies, respectively, between study entry and final evaluation. In these studies, about 20 or 0% of patients receiving placebo developed ANA or anti-dsDNA antibodies, respectively. When data from several studies in adults with rheumatoid arthritis were combined, approximately 30% of the study population had ANA at the time of study entry and 0% had anti-dsDNA. After infliximab treatment, 53% had ANA and 14% had anti-dsDNA. The mean time to detection of anti-dsDNA following initiation of infliximab therapy was 6.3 weeks (range: 4–10 weeks); in most patients, anti-dsDNA antibodies resolved within 4–6 weeks after induction. With the exception of one patient who had immunoglobulin G (IgG), IgA, and IgM class anti-dsDNA antibodies and who had clinical manifestations suggestive of a drug-induced lupus syndrome, anti-dsDNA antibodies in all other patients were of the IgM class only.

Children receiving infliximab for the treatment of juvenile arthritis have been tested for the presence of ANA and anti-dsDNA antibodies. The 3-mg/kg dose of infliximab was associated with a substantially higher risk of ANAs and anti-dsDNA antibodies than the 6-mg/kg dose. Approximately 14.8 or 13% of children receiving the 3-mg/kg dose of infliximab developed ANA or anti-dsDNA antibodies, respectively, between study entry and final evaluation. Only 2.2% of children receiving the 6-mg/kg dose of infliximab developed ANA antibodies during the study; 0% of children receiving this dose developed anti-dsDNA antibodies.

Clinical symptoms consistent with a lupus-like syndrome (e.g., rash on face, hands, or forearms, exacerbation of joint pains, fever, dyspnea, pleuropericarditis) have occurred rarely in patients receiving infliximab products; these manifestations improved or resolved following discontinuance of the drug and appropriate medical therapy. One rheumatoid arthritis patient receiving infliximab in a clinical study developed a vasculitic rash and became positive for anti-dsDNA antibodies after the second infliximab dose; however, the rash and antibodies resolved spontaneously 11 weeks later. Current data are insufficient to determine whether induction of anti-dsDNA antibodies is associated with an increased risk of developing a lupus-like syndrome if infliximab therapy is continued for prolonged periods. The manufacturers recommend that infliximab products be discontinued in patients who develop a lupus-like syndrome. (See Precautions and Contraindications Related to Sensitivity Reactions and Antibody Formation, under Cautions: Precautions and Contraindications.)

Development of anticardiolipin antibodies has been reported rarely in patients with rheumatoid arthritis receiving infliximab.

■ **Malignancies and Lymphoproliferative Disorders** Malignancies, some fatal, have been reported in children, adolescents, and young adults who received treatment with TNF blocking agents beginning when they were 18 years of age or younger. In August 2009, FDA reported the results of an analysis of reports of lymphoma and other malignancies in children and adolescents who had received TNF blocking agents. These cases were reported postmarketing and were derived from various sources, including registries and spontaneous postmarketing reports. FDA identified 48 cases of malignancies in children and adolescents in the analysis.

Of the 48 cases reviewed by FDA, approximately 50% were lymphomas, including Hodgkin's disease and non-Hodgkin's lymphoma. The other cases represented a variety of malignancies, including rare malignancies that are usually associated with immunosuppression and malignancies that are not usually observed in children and adolescents. Other malignancies reported included leukemia, melanoma, and solid organ tumors; malignancies such as leiomyosarcoma, hepatic malignancies, and renal cell carcinoma, which rarely occur in children, also were reported. The malignancies occurred after a median of 30 months (range: 1–84 months) following the first dose of therapy with TNF blocking agents. Of the 48 cases of malignancies, 11 deaths were reported; causes of death included hepatosplenic T-cell lymphoma (9 cases), T-cell lymphoma (1 case), and sepsis following remission of lymphoma (1 case). The observed US reporting rates for cases of malignancy with infliximab were consistently higher compared with expected background rates for lymphomas and all malignancies. The observed reporting rates offer limited inference into the potential differences in risk of malignancy among TNF blocking agents because of uncertainties about actual patient exposure to treatment and the possibility of underreporting of cases of malignancy. Most of the 48 patients (88%) also were receiving other immunosuppressive drugs such as azathioprine and methotrexate, which also are associated with an increased risk of lymphoma. Although there were other contributory factors, the role of TNF blocking agents in the development of malignancies in children and adolescents could not be excluded. Therefore, FDA has concluded that there is an increased risk of malignancy with TNF blocking agents. However, due to the relatively rare occurrence of these cancers, the limited number of pediatric patients who received TNF blocking agents, and the possible role of other immunosuppressive drugs used concomitantly with TNF blocking agents, FDA was unable to fully characterize the strength of the association between use of TNF blocking agents and the development of a malignancy. (See Malignancy-related Precautions under Cautions: Precautions and Contraindications.)

Hepatosplenic T-cell lymphoma, a rare, aggressive, usually fatal type of T-cell lymphoma, has been reported during postmarketing experience mainly in adolescent and young adult males with Crohn's disease or ulcerative colitis who received treatment with TNF blocking agents and/or thiopurine analogs (mercaptopurine or azathioprine). Most of the reported cases of hepatosplenic T-cell lymphoma occurred in patients who had received a combination of immunosuppressive agents, including TNF blocking agents and thiopurine analogs (azathioprine or mercaptopurine). In some cases, potential confounding factors could not be excluded because complete medical histories were not available. As of December 31, 2010, FDA had identified 25 cases of hepatosplenic T-cell lymphoma in patients with Crohn's disease or ulcerative colitis who had received infliximab (20 cases) or both infliximab and adalimumab (5 cases); in 22 of these cases, a thiopurine analog (mercaptopurine or azathioprine) was used concomitantly. These 25 cases of hepatosplenic T-cell lymphoma occurred in patients 12–74 years of age (median age: 29–30 years) following infliximab therapy for periods ranging from 1 dose to 8 years of intermittent therapy; 22 of the patients were males and 21 of the cases were fatal. It is not clear whether the occurrence of hepatosplenic T-cell lymphoma is related to use of TNF blocking agents or use of TNF blocking agents in conjunction with other immunosuppressive agents. Since patients with certain conditions (e.g., rheumatoid arthritis, Crohn's disease, ankylosing spondylitis, psoriatic arthritis, plaque psoriasis) may be at increased risk for lymphoma, it may be difficult to measure the added risk of treatment with TNF blocking agents, azathioprine, and/or mercaptopurine. (See Malignancy-related Precautions under Cautions: Precautions and Contraindications.)

In clinical studies, lymphoma occurred more frequently in patients receiving TNF blocking agents than in controls. Lymphoproliferative disorders, including lymphoma (e.g., non-Hodgkin's lymphoma, Hodgkin's disease) and myeloma, have been reported in patients receiving infliximab. In the controlled and open-label portions of infliximab clinical trials, 5 out of 5707 patients receiving infliximab (median duration of follow-up: 1 year) developed lymphomas compared with no cases of lymphoma in 1600 control patients (median duration of follow-up: 0.4 years). In rheumatoid arthritis patients, 2 lymphomas were observed for a rate of 0.08 cases per 100 patient-years of follow-up, which is approximately threefold higher than expected in the general population. In the combined clinical trial population for rheumatoid arthritis, Crohn's disease, psoriatic arthritis, ankylosing spondylitis, ulcerative colitis, and plaque psoriasis, 5 lymphomas were observed for a rate of 0.1 cases per 100 patient-years of follow-up, which is approximately fourfold higher than expected in the general population. Patients with rheumatoid arthritis, Crohn's disease, or plaque psoriasis (especially those with highly active disease and/or chronic exposure to immunosuppressive therapies) may be at increased risk of lymphoma (even in the absence of TNF blocking agent therapy); the role of TNF blocking agents in the development of lymphoma or other malignancies has not been fully determined. Lymphadenopathy has been reported in patients receiving infliximab in clinical studies.

In addition to lymphoma, various other malignancies, including basal cell carcinoma, breast cancer, melanoma, Merkel cell carcinoma, rectal adenocarcinoma, and squamous cell carcinoma, have been reported in patients receiving infliximab products.

In the controlled portions of clinical trials of some TNF blocking agents, including infliximab products, more malignancies (excluding lymphoma and nonmelanoma skin cancer [NMSC]) have been observed in patients receiving TNF blocking agents compared with control patients. During the controlled portions of infliximab trials in patients with moderately to severely active rheumatoid arthritis, Crohn's disease, psoriatic arthritis, ankylosing spondylitis, ulcerative colitis, and plaque psoriasis receiving infliximab, 14 of 4019 patients were diagnosed with malignancies (excluding lymphoma and NMSC) compared with 1 patient among 1597 control patients (a rate of 0.52/100 patient-years among patients receiving infliximab compared with a rate of 0.11/100 patient-years among control patients), with a median duration of follow-up of 0.5 years for patients receiving the drug and 0.4 years for control patients. The most common malignancies reported were breast and colorectal cancer and melanoma. The rate of malignancies in patients receiving infliximab was similar to that expected in the general population, while the rate in the control patients was lower than expected in the general population. The role of TNF blocking agents in the development of malignancies has not been fully determined. Rates of malignancy in clinical trials for infliximab cannot be compared with rates in clinical trials of other TNF blocking agents and such rates may not predict rates in a broader population of patients receiving the drug. (See Cautions: Mutagenicity and Carcinogenicity.)

Cases of acute and chronic leukemia have been reported during postmarketing surveillance of TNF blocking agents used in the management of rheumatoid arthritis and other conditions. In August 2009, FDA reported the results of a review of 147 cases of leukemia in adults and pediatric patients who received TNF blocking agents; these cases had been identified during postmarketing surveillance. Of the 147 cases, acute myeloid leukemia (44 cases), chronic lymphocytic leukemia (31 cases), and chronic myeloid leukemia (23 cases) were the most frequent types of leukemia reported. Four cases of leukemia were reported in children. Most patients (61%) also were receiving other immunosuppressive drugs. There were a total of 30 deaths reported; leukemia was reported as the cause of 26 of the 30 deaths, and the event was associated with the use of TNF blocking agents. Leukemia generally occurred during the first 2 years of therapy. The interpretation of these findings was complicated by the fact that published epidemiologic studies suggest that patients with rheumatoid arthritis may be at increased risk of leukemia, independent of any treatment with TNF blocking agents. However, based on the available data, FDA has concluded that there is a possible association between treatment with TNF blocking agents and the development of leukemia in patients receiving these drugs. (See Malignancy-related Precautions under Cautions: Precautions and Contraindications.)

In the maintenance portion of clinical trials evaluating infliximab for treatment of psoriasis, NMSC was more common in patients who had received prior phototherapy.

In a randomized, controlled clinical trial investigating the use of infliximab in patients with moderate to severe chronic obstructive pulmonary disease† (COPD) who were or had been heavy smokers, patients received infliximab at dosages similar to those used in rheumatoid arthritis and Crohn's disease. Nine (out of 157) patients receiving the drug developed a malignancy, including 1 case of lymphoma, for a rate of 7.67 cases per 100 patient-years of follow-up (median duration of follow-up 0.8 years). One malignancy was reported in 77 control patients, for a rate of 1.63 cases per 100 patient-years of follow-up (median duration of follow-up 0.8 years). The most frequent malignancies were lung or head and neck cancer.

In controlled studies of other TNF blocking agents in adults at increased risk of malignancies (e.g., patients with Wegener's granulomatosis receiving concomitant cyclophosphamide), a greater proportion of malignancies occurred in patients receiving the TNF blocking agent compared with control patients.

■ **Respiratory Effects** Upper respiratory infection occurred in 32% of adults with rheumatoid arthritis receiving infliximab in clinical studies compared with 25% of patients receiving placebo. Cough, sinusitis, pharyngitis, and bronchitis have been reported in 8–14% of patients receiving infliximab; these adverse effects were reported in 5–9% of patients receiving placebo.

Other adverse respiratory effects reported in patients receiving infliximab include pleurisy, lower respiratory tract infection, dyspnea, and pulmonary edema. Interstitial pulmonary disease, including pneumonitis/fibrosis and, very rarely, rapidly progressive disease, has occurred during postmarketing experience in patients receiving infliximab products.

■ **GI Effects** The incidence of most adverse GI effects (except abdominal pain) in infliximab-treated patients with rheumatoid arthritis is similar to the incidence in those with Crohn's disease. Nausea, diarrhea, abdominal pain, or dyspepsia has been reported in 21, 12, 12, or 10% of patients receiving infliximab (at least 4 doses) for the treatment of rheumatoid arthritis; the incidence of these adverse GI effects in rheumatoid arthritis patients receiving placebo was similar to the incidence in those receiving infliximab. Abdominal pain occurred in 26% of patients receiving infliximab for the treatment of Crohn's disease.

Other adverse GI effects occurring in patients receiving infliximab include constipation, hematochezia, intestinal obstruction, and peptic ulcer.

Although a causal relationship has not been established, there have been rare reports of the development or further narrowing of intestinal strictures and/or intestinal obstruction in patients with Crohn's disease who received infliximab. Infliximab has been used in some patients with ulcerated or nonulcerated stenosis in the ileum or transverse or sigmoid colon without stricture-related adverse effects; however, a new rectal stricture requiring multiple endoscopic dilatations has been reported in at least one patient who received infliximab and there has been at least one report of an ulcerated stenosis in the sigmoid area that became a nonulcerated stricture after therapy with the drug. There have been several reports of patients becoming obstructed at sites of previously documented intestinal strictures after infliximab therapy; obstructions in these patients occurred 1–12 weeks after an initial dose or 0.5–8 weeks after the last dose of infliximab. (See GI Precautions and Contraindications, under Cautions: Precautions and Contraindications.)

■ **Hepatic Effects** Severe hepatic reactions (e.g., acute liver failure, jaundice, hepatitis, cholestasis, autoimmune hepatitis) have been reported rarely during postmarketing surveillance in patients receiving infliximab products. These reactions occurred between 2 weeks to longer than 1 year after initiation of therapy with the drug; hepatic aminotransferase elevations were not observed prior to discovery of the liver injury in many of these cases. Some of these cases were fatal or needed liver transplantation.

In clinical trials in patients with rheumatoid arthritis, Crohn's disease, ulcerative colitis, ankylosing spondylitis, plaque psoriasis, and psoriatic arthritis, increases in serum AST (SGOT) and/or ALT (SGPT) concentrations were observed in a greater proportion of patients receiving infliximab than in controls, both when infliximab was given as monotherapy and when it was used in combination with other immunosuppressive agents. In these patient populations, increases in serum ALT concentrations of 5 or more times the upper limit of normal (ULN) were observed in less than 1 to 4% of patients receiving infliximab. In general, patients who developed hepatic aminotransferase elevations were asymptomatic, and such increases either decreased or resolved with either continuation or discontinuance of infliximab or modification of concomitant drug therapy.

In clinical trials in adults with rheumatoid arthritis, mild (less than 2 times the ULN) or moderate (2–3 times the ULN) transient increases in serum ALT concentrations have occurred in 34% of patients receiving infliximab in conjunction with methotrexate and in 24% of patients receiving placebo in conjunction with methotrexate. Increases in serum ALT concentrations of 3 or more times the ULN were observed in 3.9 or 3.2% of patients receiving infliximab in conjunction with methotrexate or methotrexate without infliximab, respectively (median follow-up about 1 year).

In clinical trials in patients with Crohn's disease (median follow-up 54 weeks), mild to moderate increases in serum ALT concentrations have been observed in 39 or 34% of patients receiving maintenance therapy with infliximab or placebo, respectively. In addition, increases in serum ALT concentrations of 3 or more times the ULN were observed in 5 or 4% of patients receiving maintenance therapy with infliximab or placebo, respectively.

In a clinical trial in pediatric patients with Crohn's disease (median follow-up 53 weeks), mild to moderate increases in serum ALT concentrations have been observed in 18% of patients receiving infliximab. In addition, increases in serum ALT concentrations of 3 or more and 5 or more times the ULN were observed in 4 and 1% of patients receiving infliximab, respectively.

In a clinical trial in patients with ankylosing spondylitis (who were not receiving methotrexate), mild to moderate increases in ALT concentrations occurred in 40 or 13% of patients receiving infliximab or placebo, respectively. In addition, increases in serum ALT concentrations of 3 or more times the ULN were observed in 6 or 0% of patients receiving infliximab or placebo, respectively.

In a clinical trial in patients with ulcerative colitis, mild to moderate increases in ALT concentrations have occurred in 17 or 12% of patients receiving infliximab or placebo, respectively. In addition, increases in serum ALT concentrations of 3 or more times the ULN were observed in 2 or 1% of patients receiving infliximab or placebo, respectively.

In a clinical trial in pediatric patients with ulcerative colitis (median follow-up of 49 weeks), increases in serum ALT concentrations of up to 3 times the ULN occurred in 17% of patients receiving infliximab, while increases of 3 or more times the ULN or 5 or more times the ULN occurred in 7 or 2%, respectively, of patients receiving the drug.

In a clinical trial in patients with psoriatic arthritis, mild to moderate increases in ALT concentrations occurred in 42 or 16% of patients receiving infliximab or placebo, respectively. In addition, increases in serum ALT concentrations of 3 or more times the ULN were observed in 5 or 0% of patients receiving infliximab or placebo, respectively.

In clinical trials in patients with plaque psoriasis, mild to moderate increases in ALT concentrations have occurred in 49 or 24% of patients receiving infliximab or placebo, respectively. In addition, increases in serum ALT concentrations of 3 or more times the ULN were observed in 8 or less than 1% of patients receiving infliximab or placebo, respectively.

■ **Patients Infected with Hepatitis B Virus** Use of TNF blocking agents, including infliximab products, has been associated with reactivation of hepatitis B virus (HBV) infection in patients who are chronic carriers of this virus (i.e., hepatitis B surface antigen-positive [HBsAg-positive]). HBV reactivation has resulted in death in a few individuals receiving a TNF blocking agent. Most patients experiencing HBV reactivation were receiving concomitant therapy with other immunosuppressive agents; use of multiple immunosuppressive agents may have contributed to HBV reactivation.

■ **Nervous System Effects** Headache was reported in approximately 18% of patients receiving infliximab in clinical studies for the treatment of rheumatoid arthritis compared with 14% of those receiving placebo. Dizziness, vertigo, and seizure have been reported in infliximab-treated patients. Transient vision loss has been reported rarely in patients receiving infliximab products, either during or within 2 hours of infusion.

CNS manifestations of systemic vasculitis and new onset or exacerbation of clinical manifestations and/or radiographic evidence of central or peripheral nervous system demyelinating disorders (e.g., multiple sclerosis, optic neuritis, Guillain-Barré syndrome) have been reported rarely in patients receiving infliximab products or other TNF blocking agents. Transverse myelitis, chronic inflammatory demyelinating polyneuropathy, and multifocal motor neuropathy have been reported during postmarketing surveillance in patients receiving infliximab products. Aseptic meningitis has occurred in one patient receiving infliximab.

■ **Dermatologic and Local Effects** Rash or pruritus has been reported in 10 or 7%, respectively, of patients receiving infliximab for the treatment of rheumatoid arthritis. Increased sweating has been reported in patients receiving infliximab. Cutaneous vasculitis has been reported during postmarketing experience in patients receiving infliximab products.

New onset or worsening of psoriasis has been reported in patients receiving infliximab products. In August 2009, FDA reported the results of a review of 69 cases of new-onset psoriasis, including pustular (17 cases) and palmoplantar (15 cases) psoriasis, in patients receiving TNF blocking agents for the management of autoimmune and rheumatic conditions other than psoriasis and psoriatic arthritis. None of the patients reported having psoriasis prior to initiation of the TNF blocking agent. Two of the 69 cases of new-onset psoriasis occurred in pediatric patients. The development of psoriasis during treatment with TNF blocking agents occurred at varying intervals, ranging from weeks to years following initiation of the drug. Twelve of the psoriasis cases resulted in hospitalization, which was the most severe outcome reported. Most patients experienced improvement of their psoriasis following discontinuance of the TNF blocking agent. Due to the number of reported cases and the temporal relationship between the initiation of TNF blocking agents and the development of psoriasis, FDA has concluded that there is a possible association between the development of psoriasis and use of TNF blocking agents. (See Other Precautions and Contraindications under Cautions: Precautions and Contraindications.)

■ **Musculoskeletal Effects** Arthralgia has been reported in 8% of patients receiving infliximab for the treatment of rheumatoid arthritis in clinical studies.

■ **Cardiovascular Effects** Hypertension has occurred in 7% of patients receiving infliximab in clinical studies for the treatment of rheumatoid arthritis. Hypotension and bradycardia also have occurred in infliximab-treated patients. Pericardial effusion has been reported during postmarketing experience in patients receiving infliximab products; myocardial ischemia/infarction also has been reported rarely in patients receiving infliximab products, either during or within 2 hours of infusion.

Use of infliximab in patients with moderate to severe (New York Heart Association [NYHA] class III or IV) congestive heart failure† was associated with higher incidences of mortality and hospitalization for worsening heart failure compared with similar patients receiving placebo. In a phase II study involving use of infliximab (5 or 10 mg/kg given at 0, 2, and 6 weeks) in patients with NYHA class III or IV congestive heart failure, at week 28, 4 of 101 patients receiving infliximab had died versus 0 of 49 patients receiving placebo. At week 28, 14 of 101 patients receiving infliximab had been hospitalized for worsening congestive heart failure versus 5 of 49 patients receiving placebo. Results of this study suggest that infliximab dosages of 10 mg/kg are associated with higher rates of mortality and dosages of 5 and 10 mg/kg are associated with higher rates of adverse cardiovascular effects. There have been postmarketing reports of worsening heart failure, with or without identifiable precipitating factors, in patients receiving infliximab. New-onset heart failure, including heart failure in patients without known cardiovascular disease, has been reported rarely in infliximab-treated patients. (See Cardiac Precautions and Contraindications, under Cautions: Precautions and Contraindications.)

■ **Hematologic Effects** Cases of leukopenia, neutropenia, thrombocytopenia, and pancytopenia, some with fatal outcome, and idiopathic or thrombotic thrombocytopenic purpura have been reported in patients receiving infliximab products. Anemia or hemolytic anemia has occurred in patients receiving infliximab.

■ **Other Adverse Effects** Fatigue or fever has been reported in 7–9% of patients receiving infliximab in clinical studies. Other adverse effects reported in infliximab-treated patients include allergic reaction, edema, dehydration, thrombophlebitis, sarcoidosis, and sudden death. Systemic vasculitis has been reported during postmarketing experience in patients receiving infliximab products.

■ **Precautions and Contraindications** A copy of the medication guide for infliximab or infliximab-dyyb should be provided to all patients prior to each infusion of the drug. Patients should be instructed to read the medication guide prior to initiation of therapy and each time they receive an infusion of the drug. Patients should be advised about potential benefits and risks of infliximab or infliximab-dyyb therapy and should be instructed on the importance of taking the drug as prescribed and of not altering or discontinuing therapy without first consulting with a clinician.

Precautions and Contraindications Related to Infectious Complications Patients receiving TNF blocking agents, including infliximab products, are at increased risk of developing serious infections that may require hospitalization or result in death. Therapy with infliximab products should be discontinued in patients who develop a serious infection or sepsis. Patients should be closely monitored during and after treatment with TNF blocking agents for the development of signs or symptoms of infection (e.g., fever, malaise, weight loss, sweats, cough, dyspnea, pulmonary infiltrates, serious systemic illness including shock). Any patient who develops a new infection while receiving an infliximab product should undergo a thorough diagnostic evaluation (appropriate for an immunocompromised patient), appropriate anti-infective therapy should be initiated, and the patient should be closely monitored. Patients should be instructed to inform their clinician immediately if they experience symptoms of infection, are receiving treatment for an infection, or have recurring infections.

Therapy with infliximab products should not be initiated in patients with active infections, including clinically important localized infections. Patients older than 65 years of age, patients with comorbid conditions, and/or patients receiving concomitant therapy with immunosuppressive agents such as corticosteroids or methotrexate may be at increased risk of infection. Clinicians should consider the potential risks and benefits of the drug prior to initiating therapy in patients with a history of chronic, recurring, or opportunistic infections; patients with underlying conditions that may predispose them to infections; and patients who have been exposed to tuberculosis or who reside or have traveled in regions where tuberculosis or mycoses such as histoplasmosis, coccidioidomycosis, and blastomycosis are endemic. The fact that many patients who receive infliximab products also are receiving concomitant therapy with immunosuppressive agents that, in addition to their underlying condition (e.g., Crohn's disease, rheumatoid arthritis), could increase susceptibility to infection should be considered.

Because tuberculosis has been reported in patients receiving infliximab products, including in patients who received infliximab products during treatment for latent tuberculosis or following treatment for active or latent tuberculosis, all patients should be evaluated for active or latent tuberculosis and for risk factors for tuberculosis prior to and periodically during therapy with the drug. When indicated, an appropriate antimycobacterial regimen for the treatment of latent tuberculosis should be initiated prior to therapy with infliximab products. Antimycobacterial treatment lowers the risk of latent tuberculosis infection progressing to active disease (i.e., reactivation) in patients receiving TNF blocking agents. Antimycobacterial therapy also should be considered prior to initiation of infliximab product therapy in individuals with a history of latent or active tuberculosis in whom an adequate course of antimycobacterial treatment cannot be confirmed and in individuals with a negative tuberculin skin test who have risk factors for tuberculosis. Consultation with a tuberculosis specialist is recommended when deciding whether to initiate antimycobacterial therapy. Patients receiving infliximab products, including individuals with a negative tuberculin skin test, should be monitored for signs and symptoms of active tuberculosis. If active tuberculosis is diagnosed during therapy with infliximab products, the drug should be discontinued and an appropriate antimycobacterial regimen initiated. The possibility of tuberculosis should be strongly considered in patients who develop new infections while receiving infliximab products, especially if they previously have traveled to countries where tuberculosis is highly prevalent or have been in close contact with an individual with active tuberculosis. (See the Antituberculosis Agents General Statement 8:16.04.)

Infection with *Histoplasma capsulatum*, *Coccidioides immitis*, *Legionella*, *Listeria*, *Pneumocystis jiroveci* (formerly *Pneumocystis carinii*) and other bacterial, mycobacterial, or fungal infections have been reported in patients receiving infliximab products. The potential risks and benefits of therapy with infliximab products should be carefully evaluated before the drug is initiated in individuals who reside or have traveled in areas where mycoses are endemic. Clinicians should ascertain if patients receiving TNF blocking agents who present with signs and symptoms suggestive of systemic fungal infection reside or have traveled in regions where mycoses are endemic. Empiric antifungal therapy should be considered in patients at risk of histoplasmosis or other invasive fungal infections who develop severe systemic illness, taking into account both the risk for severe fungal infection and the risks associated with antifungal therapy. Serologic tests for histoplasmosis may be negative in some patients with active infection. When deciding whether TNF blocking agent therapy should be reinitiated following resolution of an invasive fungal infection, the risks and benefits of such therapy should be reevaluated, particularly in patients who reside in regions where mycoses are endemic. Whenever feasible, decisions regarding initiation and duration of antifungal therapy and reinitiation of TNF blocking agent therapy should be made in consultation with a specialist in fungal infections.

Precautions Related to Hepatotoxicity Since severe hepatic reactions (e.g., acute liver failure, jaundice, hepatitis, cholestasis, autoimmune hepatitis) have been reported rarely in patients receiving infliximab products, patients with signs or symptoms of hepatic dysfunction should be evaluated for evidence of liver injury. Patients should be instructed to inform a clinician if they develop symptoms of possible hepatotoxicity (e.g., jaundice, dark brown-colored urine, right-sided abdominal pain, fever, severe fatigue). If jaundice and/or marked hepatic aminotransferase elevations (5 or more times the ULN) develop, the infliximab product should be discontinued and the hepatic abnormality investigated.

Hepatitis B virus (HBV) reactivation has been reported in patients receiving TNF blocking agents. All patients should be screened before initiation of therapy with infliximab products. Consultation with an expert in the treatment of hepatitis B is recommended for patients who test positive for hepatitis B surface antigen. Chronic carriers of HBV should be appropriately evaluated and monitored prior to the initiation of therapy, during treatment, and for up to several months following therapy with infliximab products. Safety and efficacy of antiviral therapy for prevention of viral reactivation in HBV carriers receiving a TNF blocking agent have not been established. Therapy with the infliximab product should be discontinued if HBV reactivation occurs, and appropriate treatment, including antiviral therapy, should be initiated. It has not been established whether an infliximab product can be safely readministered once control of the reactivated HBV infection has been achieved; caution is advised if infliximab products are resumed in such a situation.

Precautions and Contraindications Related to Sensitivity Reactions and Antibody Formation Infliximab products are contraindicated in patients with known hypersensitivity to murine proteins or any ingredient in the formulation. In addition, infliximab products should not be readministered to patients who have experienced a severe hypersensitivity reaction to these products.

If a severe hypersensitivity reaction occurs during therapy with infliximab or infliximab-dyyb, the drug should be discontinued immediately and appropriate therapy initiated. Drugs for the treatment of hypersensitivity reactions (e.g., acetaminophen, antihistamines, corticosteroids, and/or epinephrine) should be immediately available. The fact that both acute infusion reactions (occurring during or within 1–2 hours after IV infusion) and delayed infusion reactions (occurring 3–12 days after IV infusion) have been reported in patients receiving infliximab products should be considered. (See Acute Infusion Reactions and see Delayed Infusion Reactions, under Cautions: Sensitivity Reactions and Antibody Formation.)

Because acute infusion reactions have been reported with infliximab products, patients should be monitored closely (including measurement of vital signs) during and for at least 30 minutes after each IV infusion of the drug. In addition, to prevent or ameliorate acute infusion reactions, use of a pretreatment regimen (e.g., acetaminophen, antihistamines, prednisone) prior to each infliximab product dose and use of a rate titration schedule to administer IV infusions of the drug can be considered. (See Pretreatment Regimen, Rate Titration Schedule, and Patient Monitoring, under Dosage: Reconstitution and Administration.) If a patient experiences a clinically important change in vital signs (e.g., diastolic blood pressure drops 15–20 mm Hg) or any symptoms of hypersensitivity (e.g., urticaria, shortness of breath) while receiving an IV infusion of an infliximab product, the infusion should be stopped immediately, manifestations evaluated, and appropriate therapy initiated. The manufacturer of infliximab states that if the infusion is stopped because of an acute infusion reaction but the reaction is not severe and can be controlled with the use of drugs other than epinephrine (e.g., diphenhydramine, acetaminophen, prednisone), then the infusion may be restarted with caution using a rate titration schedule. If the infusion can be completed in these patients, then they may receive additional indicated doses of the infliximab product with caution and in the presence of appropriately trained medical personnel. However, if the acute infusion reaction is more serious and requires treatment with epinephrine or if symptoms increase in severity, then the infusion of the infliximab product should be discontinued.

Because delayed infusion reactions have occurred 3–12 days after an infliximab dose in patients who received retreatment with the drug after a period of 2–4 years, caution should be exercised when retreating patients with infliximab products following an extended period of time (e.g., after 1 year or longer). The manufacturers state that, in general, the risks and benefits of readministration of infliximab or infliximab-dyyb after a period without treatment (especially readministration as a reinduction regimen at 0, 2 and 6 weeks) should be carefully considered, since such retreatment regimens have resulted in a higher incidence of infusion reactions as compared to regular maintenance treatment. If maintenance therapy with infliximab or infliximab-dyyb for the management of psoriasis is interrupted, the drug should be reinitiated as a single dose followed by maintenance therapy. Patients should be advised to seek medical advice and treatment in the event they develop manifestations suggestive of a delayed infusion reaction after receiving an infliximab product.

Therapy with infliximab products may result in the development of human antichimeric antibodies [HACA], and there is some evidence that patients who develop these antibodies have a higher rate of infusion reactions than other patients.

Therapy with infliximab products may result in formation of autoantibodies and, rarely, a lupus-like syndrome. The drug should be discontinued in any patient who develops manifestations consistent with systemic lupus erythematosus (SLE) or a lupus-like syndrome. However, use of infliximab products is not necessarily contraindicated in patients who develop ANA or anticardiolipin antibodies without lupus-like manifestations since these autoantibodies do not appear to indicate that these patients are at increased risk of developing lupus-like syndromes.

GI Precautions and Contraindications Information on the safety and efficacy of infliximab in Crohn's disease patients who have intestinal strictures is limited to date since patients with symptomatic stenosis or ileal strictures were excluded from most clinical studies of the drug. Intestinal strictures develop as a complication of Crohn's disease in some patients as the result of chronic inflammation and/or mucosal healing and fibrous tissue deposition. The development or further narrowing of intestinal strictures and/or intestinal obstruction have been reported rarely in Crohn's disease patients who received infliximab, and it has been suggested that the rapid healing in response to infliximab may possibly have contributed to luminal stenosis and/or obstruction in these patients. The manufacturer of infliximab and some clinicians suggest that the drug be used with caution in Crohn's disease patients who have a history of intestinal strictures.

Cardiac Precautions and Contraindications Infliximab or infliximab-dyyb doses exceeding 5 mg/kg are contraindicated in patients with moderate to severe (NYHA class III or IV) heart failure. Infliximab has been associated with adverse outcomes in patients with heart failure; treatment options other than infliximab products should be considered in these patients. If infliximab products are used in patients with heart failure, caution and careful monitoring are recommended. Patients with heart failure should be instructed to inform a clinician in case of new or worsening heart failure symptoms (e.g., shortness of breath, swelling of ankles or feet, sudden weight gain). The drug should be discontinued in any patient who develops new or worsening symptoms of heart failure.

Malignancy-related Precautions Clinicians should consider the possibility of and monitor for the occurrence of malignancies during and following treatment with TNF blocking agents. Clinicians should exercise caution when considering therapy with infliximab products in patients with a history of malignancy or when deciding whether to continue therapy in patients who develop a malignancy while receiving an infliximab product. Because therapy with TNF blocking agents and/or thiopurine analogs (azathioprine or mercaptopurine) may increase the risk of malignancies, including hepatosplenic T-cell lymphoma, the risks and benefits of these agents should be carefully considered, especially in adolescent and young adult males and in the treatment of Crohn's disease or ulcerative colitis. When deciding whether infliximab products should be used alone or in combination with other immunosuppressive agents, clinicians should consider both the possibility of an increased risk of hepatosplenic T-cell lymphoma with combination therapy and the observed (in infliximab studies) increase in immunogenicity and hypersensitivity reactions associated with infliximab products given as monotherapy.

Patients and their caregivers should be informed of the increased risk of lymphoma, including hepatosplenic T-cell lymphoma, leukemia, and other malignancies associated with TNF blocking agents, as well as the increased risk of cancer development in children, adolescents, and young adults, taking into account the clinical utility of TNF blocking agents, the relative risks and benefits of these and other immunosuppressive agents, and the risks associated with untreated disease. Patients and their caregivers should be informed of the signs and symptoms of malignancies (e.g., unexplained weight loss; fatigue; abdominal pain; persistent fever; night sweats; easy bruising or bleeding; swollen lymph nodes in the neck, underarm, or groin; easy bruising or bleeding; hepatomegaly or splenomegaly) and advised to promptly inform a clinician if such signs or symptoms occur. Patients should be advised not to discontinue therapy without consulting a clinician. (See Cautions: Malignancies and Lymphoproliferative Disorders.)

Because melanoma and Merkel cell carcinoma have been reported in patients receiving infliximab products, periodic skin examination is recommended for all patients, particularly those with risk factors for skin cancer.

Because nonmelanoma skin cancer has been reported in patients with psoriasis receiving infliximab, patients with psoriasis who are receiving infliximab products, particularly those who received prior prolonged phototherapy for their disease, should be monitored for nonmelanoma skin cancer.

Because malignancies (mainly lung cancer or head and neck malignancies) were reported more frequently in infliximab-treated than placebo-treated patients with moderate to severe COPD, clinicians should exercise caution when considering therapy with infliximab products in such patients.

Other Precautions and Contraindications New-onset psoriasis has been reported in patients receiving TNF blocking agents for the management of autoimmune and rheumatic conditions other than psoriasis and psoriatic arthritis. Clinicians should consider the possibility of and monitor for manifestations (e.g., new rash) of new or worsening psoriasis, particularly pustular and palmoplantar psoriasis, during treatment with TNF blocking agents. Patients should be informed of the increased risk of psoriasis or worsening of existing psoriasis with TNF blocking agents. Patients should be advised to inform a clinician if signs and symptoms of new or worsening psoriasis occur. (See Cautions: Dermatologic and Local Effects.)

Because CNS manifestations of systemic vasculitis, seizures, and new onset or exacerbation of demyelinating disorders have been reported rarely in patients receiving infliximab products or other TNF blocking agents, clinicians should exercise caution when considering use of infliximab products in patients with these neurologic disorders and should consider discontinuance of the infliximab product if these disorders develop. Patients receiving infliximab products should be advised to inform a clinician if they develop signs and symptoms suggestive of nervous system disorders (e.g., vision changes, weakness in arms and/or legs, numbness or tingling, seizures).

Leukopenia, neutropenia, thrombocytopenia, and pancytopenia have occurred in patients receiving infliximab products. Although a high-risk group for these adverse effects has not been identified, caution is advised if infliximab products are used in patients with a history of substantial hematologic abnormalities. Patients receiving infliximab products should be advised to seek immediate medical attention if they develop signs and symptoms suggestive of blood dyscrasias or infection (e.g., persistent fever, bruising, bleeding, pallor). If substantial hematologic abnormalities are confirmed, discontinuance of the infliximab product should be considered.

■ **Pediatric Precautions** Safety and efficacy of infliximab products in pediatric patients with plaque psoriasis have not been established.

Safety and efficacy of infliximab or infliximab-dyyb have been established in pediatric patients 6 years of age and older with Crohn's disease. The manufacturer states that infliximab has been studied in this population only in conjunction with conventional immunosuppressive therapy. Safety and efficacy of long-term therapy (exceeding 1 year) with infliximab products in pediatric patients with Crohn's disease have not been established. Adverse effects reported more frequently in pediatric patients with Crohn's disease than in adults with Crohn's disease receiving infliximab include anemia, leukopenia, flushing, viral infection, neutropenia, bone fracture, infection, bacterial infection, and respiratory tract allergy. The most common serious adverse effects reported during postmarketing use of infliximab products for the treatment of Crohn's disease in pediatric patients include infections (some fatal), including opportunistic infections and tuberculosis, infusion reactions, and hypersensitivity reactions. Other serious adverse effects reported during postmarketing use of infliximab products for the treatment of Crohn's disease in pediatric patients include malignancies (including hepatosplenic T-cell lymphomas), transient hepatic enzyme abnormalities, lupus-like syndromes, and the development of autoantibodies. Acute infusion reactions consisting of dyspnea with or without diffuse erythema and facial swelling have been reported in at least 3 pediatric patients who received infliximab. In one 10-year-old child with Crohn's disease who received a second dose of infliximab 3 weeks after the initial dose, a reaction consisting of chest tightness, cough, shortness of breath, and a sense of impending doom associated with tachycardia, systolic blood pressure drop of 30 mm Hg and pulse oximetry decreasing to 85% occurred 10 minutes after initiation of the infusion.

Safety and efficacy of infliximab in pediatric patients 6 years of age and older with ulcerative colitis are supported by clinical studies in adults and additional safety and pharmacokinetic data from an uncontrolled study in pediatric patients 6–17 years of age (see Ulcerative Colitis in Pediatric Patients, under Uses: Ulcerative Colitis). Safety and efficacy of long-term infliximab therapy (exceeding 1 year) in pediatric patients with ulcerative colitis have not been established. Adverse effects reported in the uncontrolled study evaluating infliximab in pediatric patients with ulcerative colitis generally were similar to those reported in adults with ulcerative colitis and most commonly included upper respiratory tract infection, pharyngitis, abdominal pain, fever, and headache. The proportion of patients with infections was similar to that reported for pediatric patients with Crohn's disease but greater than that reported for adults with ulcerative colitis. Limited data suggested that the overall rate of adverse effects, including infusion reactions, in children 6–11 years of age was similar to that in adolescents 12–17 years of age; however, greater proportions of children 6–11 years of age experienced serious adverse effects or discontinued therapy because of adverse effects. The proportion of patients with infections was higher in the younger age group, but similar proportions of patients in both age groups had serious infections.

Although safety and efficacy of infliximab-dyyb for use in pediatric patients with ulcerative colitis also have been established, the labeled indication for infliximab in pediatric patients with ulcerative colitis was still protected by the exclusivity provisions of orphan drug designation when FDA approved the infliximab-dyyb biosimilar.

Malignancies, some fatal, have been reported in children and adolescents who received treatment with TNF blocking agents. (See Cautions: Malignancies and Lymphoproliferative Disorders.)

The manufacturer states that infliximab has been studied in pediatric patients with Crohn's disease only in conjunction with conventional immunosuppressive therapy. In the study evaluating infliximab in pediatric patients with ulcerative colitis, approximately half of the patients were receiving concomitant therapy with immunosuppressive agents (azathioprine, mercaptopurine, or methotrexate) at the start of the study. Use of infliximab products in the absence of other immunosuppressive agents may increase the likelihood of infliximab-specific antibody formation and increase the risk of hypersensitivity reactions. (See Cautions: Sensitivity Reactions and Antibody Formation.) It is unclear whether reported cases of hepatosplenic T-cell lymphoma in patients receiving infliximab products have been related to use of the TNF blocking agent or use of the TNF blocking agent in conjunction with other immunosuppressive agents. (See Cautions: Malignancies and Lymphoproliferative Disorders.) Therefore, risks and benefits should be carefully assessed when deciding whether to use infliximab products alone or in combination with other immunosuppressive agents.

Pharmacokinetic values for infliximab in pediatric patients 6–17 years of age with Crohn's disease or ulcerative colitis are similar to values in adults with these diseases.

Safety and efficacy of infliximab for the management of juvenile rheumatoid arthritis† have been evaluated in children 4–17 years of age with juvenile arthritis who had not responded adequately to methotrexate. While infliximab in combination with methotrexate produced important and durable clinical effects in children, the primary efficacy end point (i.e., the American College of Rheumatology [ACR] Pediatric 30 [Pedi 30] criteria for improvement) measured at week 14 did not differ between infliximab-treated children and placebo recipients. A 3-mg/kg dose of infliximab was associated with a higher risk of serious adverse events, infusion reactions, and development of antibodies to infliximab, antinuclear antibodies (ANAs), and antibodies to double stranded DNA (anti-ds DNA) compared with a 6-mg/kg dose. Further study is needed to evaluate the safety and efficacy of the drug for juvenile rheumatoid arthritis.

All pediatric patients should be brought up to date with all vaccinations prior to initiation of therapy with infliximab products.

Infliximab has been detected for up to 6 months in the serum of infants whose mothers received infliximab products during pregnancy. Infants who were exposed to infliximab products in utero may be at increased risk of infection. Fatal disseminated BCG infection has been reported in an infant who received BCG vaccine after having been exposed to infliximab in utero. Infants exposed to infliximab products in utero should not receive live vaccines for at least 6 months following birth. Women who received infliximab or infliximab-dyyb during pregnancy should be advised to inform their infant's clinician of this use since alteration of the infant's vaccination schedule may be indicated.

■ **Geriatric Precautions** Clinical studies evaluating infliximab for the management of Crohn's disease, ulcerative colitis, ankylosing spondylitis, and psoriatic arthritis have included an insufficient number of patients 65 years of age and older to make a valid comparison of the drug's safety and efficacy in geriatric patients compared with younger adults. In clinical studies in adults with rheumatoid arthritis or plaque psoriasis, there were no overall differences in the safety and efficacy of infliximab in those 65 years of age or older compared with younger adults; however, the incidence of serious adverse effects was higher in infliximab-treated and control patients 65 years of age or older compared with younger adults. Because serious infectious complications have been reported in some patients receiving infliximab products (see Cautions: Infectious Complications) and because the overall incidence of infection is higher in geriatric adults than in younger individuals, the manufacturers state that infliximab products should be used with caution in geriatric patients.

■ **Mutagenicity and Carcinogenicity** The effect of infliximab products on the development and course of malignancies has not been fully evaluated. Lymphoproliferative disorders and new malignancies, including hepatosplenic T-cell lymphoma (see Cautions: Malignancies and Lymphoproliferative Disorders and see Cautions: Pediatric Precautions), have been observed in patients receiving infliximab products. Patients with Crohn's disease, rheumatoid arthritis, or plaque psoriasis, particularly patients with highly active disease and/or chronic exposure to immunosuppressive therapies, appear more prone to develop lymphomas (even in the absence of TNF blocking agent therapy); while for patients with other immune-related diseases, such as juvenile idiopathic arthritis, it is unknown whether there is an increased risk of cancer.

Infliximab did not have clastogenic or mutagenic effects in the in vivo mouse micronucleus test or the Ames assay (*Salmonella-Escherichia coli*), respectively, and did not induce chromosomal aberrations in a human lymphocyte assay. No evidence of tumorigenicity was observed in mice given CV1q (an analogous antibody that inhibits the function of murine TNF-α) 10 or 40 mg/kg (2 or 8 times, respectively, the human dose of 5 mg/kg for Crohn's disease) weekly for 6 months. The relevance of these findings to clinical use of infliximab products is unknown.

■ **Pregnancy, Fertility, and Lactation** There are no adequate and controlled studies to date using infliximab or infliximab-dyyb in pregnant women, and the drugs should be used during pregnancy only when clearly needed. Infliximab products cross the placenta and infliximab has been detected for up to 6 months in the serum of infants whose mothers received infliximab products during pregnancy (see Cautions: Pediatric Precautions). Some clinicians suggest that pregnancy be ruled out (i.e., negative pregnancy test) before initiating therapy with TNF inhibitors in women of childbearing potential and that these women use an effective contraceptive while receiving these drugs. Reproduction studies using infliximab products in animals have not been conducted since the drug only binds TNF from humans and other primates and does not cross-react with TNF from other species. In a developmental toxicity study conducted in mice using a murine anti-TNF antibody that selectively inhibits murine TNF, no evidence of maternal toxicity, embryotoxicity, or teratogenicity was observed. In pharmacodynamic animal models using an analogous anti-TNF antibody, doses of 10–15 mg/kg produced maximal pharmacologic effectiveness; in animal reproduction studies, doses up to 40 mg/kg produced no adverse effects.

The effect of infliximab products on human fertility or reproductive capacity is not known. In a fertility and reproduction study in mice using a murine anti-TNF antibody that selectively inhibits murine TNF, no impairment of fertility was observed.

It is not known whether infliximab products are distributed into milk or absorbed systemically following ingestion. Because many drugs and immunoglobulins are distributed into milk, and because of the potential for adverse reactions to infliximab products in nursing infants, women should not breast-feed while taking infliximab or infliximab-dyyb. A decision should be made whether to discontinue nursing or the drug, taking into account the importance of the drug to the woman.

Drug Interactions

Although specific drug interaction studies evaluating concomitant use of infliximab or infliximab-dyyb and other drugs have not been conducted to date, most patients in clinical studies evaluating infliximab received one or more concomitant drugs. Patients with Crohn's disease usually received infliximab concomitantly with corticosteroids, mesalamine or sulfasalazine, azathioprine or mercaptopurine, and/or anti-infective agents; patients with rheumatoid arthritis usually received infliximab concomitantly with methotrexate and may also have received corticosteroids, nonsteroidal anti-inflammatory agents (NSAIAs), folic acid, or narcotics.

In patients with Crohn's disease, serum concentrations of infliximab do not appear to be affected by baseline use of corticosteroids, mesalamine or sulfasalazine, or anti-infectives (ciprofloxacin, metronidazole). There is some evidence from studies of infliximab that the incidence of some adverse immunologic reactions to infliximab products (e.g., infusion reactions, formation of antibodies to infliximab) is lower in patients receiving infliximab products concomitantly with immunosuppressive agents (e.g., corticosteroids, azathioprine, mercaptopurine, methotrexate) compared with those receiving infliximab products without such agents. (See Cautions: Sensitivity Reactions and Antibody Formation.) There is some evidence that concomitant use of methotrexate may affect the pharmacokinetics of infliximab. (See Drug Interactions: Methotrexate.)

When deciding whether infliximab products should be used alone or in combination with other immunosuppressive agents, clinicians should consider both the possibility of an increased risk of hepatosplenic T-cell lymphoma with combination therapy and the observed (in infliximab studies) increase in immunogenicity and hypersensitivity reactions associated with infliximab products given as monotherapy. (See Cautions: Sensitivity Reactions and Antibody Formation and also Cautions: Malignancies and Lymphoproliferative Disorders.)

■ **Drugs Metabolized by Hepatic Microsomal Enzymes** Because increased levels of cytokines (e.g., tumor necrosis factor [TNF]-α, interferon, interleukin-1, interleukin-6, interleukin-10) during chronic inflammation may suppress the formation of cytochrome P-450 (CYP) isoenzymes, it is expected that a drug that antagonizes cytokine activity, such as an infliximab product, could normalize the formation of CYP enzymes. Following initiation or discontinuance of therapy with infliximab products, patients receiving certain drugs metabolized by CYP isoenzymes (i.e., those with a low therapeutic index [e.g., cyclosporine, theophylline, warfarin]) should be monitored for therapeutic effect and/or changes in serum concentrations, and dosages of these drugs may be adjusted as needed.

■ **Biologic Agents** Caution should be exercised when switching from one biologic disease-modifying antirheumatic drug (DMARD) to another, since overlapping biologic activity may further increase the risk of infection.

Insufficient data are available regarding concomitant use of infliximab products with other biologic agents used to treat the same conditions. Concomitant use of infliximab products with these agents is not recommended because of an increased risk of infection.

Abatacept When abatacept (a selective costimulation modulator) and a TNF blocking agent were used concomitantly in patients with rheumatoid arthritis, an increased incidence of infection and serious infection was observed, with no substantial improvement in efficacy over that observed with a TNF blocking agent alone. Similar toxicities would be expected with concomitant use of abatacept and infliximab products. Concomitant use of infliximab products and abatacept is not recommended.

Anakinra When anakinra (a human interleukin-1 receptor antagonist) and etanercept (another agent that blocks TNF) were used concomitantly in patients with rheumatoid arthritis, an increased incidence of serious infection and neutropenia was observed, with no substantial improvement in efficacy over that observed with etanercept alone. Similar toxicities would be expected with concomitant use of anakinra and other agents that block TNF, including infliximab products. Concomitant use of infliximab products and anakinra is not recommended.

Natalizumab Concomitant use of natalizumab (an anti-α4-integrin monoclonal antibody) and TNF blocking agents in the management of Crohn's disease should be avoided since such use may result in increased risk of progressive multifocal leukoencephalopathy (PML) or other serious infections.

Rituximab An increased risk of serious infection has been observed in patients with rheumatoid arthritis who received rituximab (an anti-CD20 monoclonal antibody) and subsequently received therapy with a TNF blocking agent.

Tocilizumab Concomitant use of tocilizumab (an anti-interleukin-6-receptor monoclonal antibody) and biologic DMARDs such as TNF blocking agents, including infliximab products, has not been studied and should be avoided because of the possibility of increased immunosuppression and increased risk of infection.

■ **Methotrexate** Although specific pharmacokinetic interaction studies have not been performed, data from one double-blind, placebo-controlled study in adults with rheumatoid arthritis suggest that concomitant use of methotrexate may affect the pharmacokinetics of infliximab. In this study, patients who received infliximab in a dosage of 1 mg/kg (given by IV infusion over 2 hours at weeks 0, 2, 6, 10, and 14) concomitantly with oral placebo (once weekly) had mean serum infliximab concentrations that decreased to 0.1 mcg/mL (the limits of detection) by the fourth week after the second infusion and by the second week after each subsequent infusion; however, patients who received the same dosage of infliximab concomitantly with oral methotrexate (7.5 mg once weekly) had mean serum infliximab concentrations that were maintained at approximately 2–20 mcg/mL during each interval. Although patients receiving infliximab in a dosage of 3 or 10 mg/kg had serum infliximab concentrations that were similar regardless of whether they were receiving the drug alone or in conjunction with methotrexate (7.5 mg once weekly), serum infliximab concentrations after the final infusion were consistently higher and decreased at a slower rate in those receiving methotrexate than in those receiving placebo.

The mechanisms and clinical importance of this possible pharmacokinetic interaction have not been determined. There is some evidence that development of antibodies to infliximab occurs less frequently in patients receiving infliximab in conjunction with methotrexate than in those receiving infliximab alone.

(See Cautions: Sensitivity Reactions and Antibody Formation.) It has been suggested that methotrexate, by decreasing the immunogenic potential of infliximab, may result in a slower rate of clearance of infliximab.

■ **Vaccines and Therapeutic Infectious Agents** The interval between vaccination and initiation of therapy with infliximab products should be in accordance with current vaccination guidelines.

Live vaccines (e.g., measles virus vaccine live, mumps virus vaccine live, rubella virus vaccine live, poliovirus vaccine live oral [OPV; no longer commercially available in the US], rotavirus vaccine live oral, typhoid vaccine live oral, varicella virus vaccine live, yellow fever vaccine) and other live therapeutic infectious agents (e.g., BCG for intravesical instillation) should not be administered to patients receiving infliximab products. Use of live vaccines or live therapeutic infectious agents could result in infections, including disseminated infections. Limited data are available regarding whether infliximab products would affect the rate of secondary transmission of infection following administration of a live vaccine or regarding the response to live vaccines in patients receiving the drug. Fatal disseminated BCG infection has been reported in an infant who received BCG vaccine after having been exposed to infliximab in utero. Infants exposed to infliximab products in utero should not receive live vaccines for at least 6 months following birth. (See Cautions: Pediatric Precautions.)

Acute Toxicity

There are limited data available on the acute toxicity of infliximab; the maximum tolerated dose of the drug in humans has not been established. No direct toxic effect was observed in patients who received single infliximab doses of 20 mg/kg (approximately 2–7 times the usual dose). If overdosage of infliximab or infliximab-dyyb occurs, the patient should be monitored for adverse effects and appropriate symptomatic treatment should be initiated.

Pharmacology

■ **Immunomodulating and Anti-inflammatory Effects** Infliximab and infliximab-dyyb, chimeric human-murine anti-human tumor necrosis factor (TNF; TNF-α) monoclonal antibodies, are biologic response modifiers. Infliximab products have a high affinity for and bind specifically to soluble and transmembrane forms of TNF thereby inhibiting binding of TNF to cell surface tumor necrosis factor receptors (TNFRs). The association constant (K_a) of infliximab for TNF is $10^{10}M^{-1}$. By binding to TNF, infliximab and infliximab-dyyb neutralize the cytokine. Although the exact mechanism(s) of the anti-inflammatory effects of infliximab products in the management of Crohn's disease or rheumatoid arthritis remains to be more fully determined, binding and neutralization of TNF appears to be the principal mechanism. There also is some evidence that infliximab may inhibit expression of TNF by binding soluble TNF attached to TNF receptors present on activated macrophages and T cells. The prolonged (6–12 weeks) anti-inflammatory effect of infliximab appears attributable to decreased leukocyte trafficking and IgG-mediated neutralization and initiation of the apoptotic lysis of activated macrophages and T cells.

While infliximab products specifically bind to and neutralize TNF, etanercept (a biosynthetic tumor necrosis factor receptor fusion protein) neutralizes both TNF and lymphotoxin α (TNF-β), a related cytokine that utilizes the same receptors as TNF. The clinical importance of the specificity of infliximab products compared with that of etanercept is unknown. Although both TNF inhibitors appear to provide similar clinical benefits in patients with rheumatoid arthritis, the safety and efficacy of the drugs have not been directly compared in clinical studies.

The TNF precursor, a 26 kilodalton (kDa) transmembrane protein, is expressed in many cell-types throughout the human body; however, macrophages, monocytes, and T cells appear to be the principal sites of production of TNF and other proinflammatory cytokines, chemokines, proteases, oxygen radicals, and nitric oxide. The active form of TNF is a 17 kDa soluble protein fragment formed when the TNF converting enzyme (TACE) cleaves a 26 kDa precursor molecule. After separating from the cell membrane, these soluble TNF molecules aggregate into trimolecular complexes (51 kD homotrimers) that subsequently bind 2 receptors (type I or p55 [also called p60] and type II or p75 [also called p80]) that are expressed on many cell types, including fibroblasts, leukocytes, and endothelial cells. TACE also cleaves the extracellular domain of its complementary ligand of TNF, forming soluble TNF receptors (sTNFRs). These circulating sTNFRs are then free to bind the trimolecular TNF complexes, rendering them biologically inactive; thus, the sTNFRs function as natural inhibitors of TNF-mediated inflammation.

While it is clear that chronic inflammatory processes are not due solely to overexpression of TNF, the regulatory cytokine plays a critical role in the control of the production of other cytokines involved in the pathogenesis of inflammation of Crohn's disease and rheumatoid arthritis. A variety of physiologic and pathologic functions have been ascribed to TNF-TNF receptor interactions and the effects of TNF include induction of proinflammatory cytokines such as interleukin 1(IL-1), IL-6 and IL-8, enhancement of leukocyte migration by increasing endothelial layer permeability and expression of adhesion molecules by endothelial cells and leukocytes, activation of neutrophil and eosinophil functional activity, induction of acute phase proteins (C-reactive protein, serum amyloid A [SAA] haptoglobin, fibrinogen) and tissue degrading enzymes produced by synoviocytes and/or chondrocytes. TNF blocks the action of lipoprotein lipase, causing severe cachexia in experimental models of chronic infection. In addition, TNF induces programmed cell death (apoptosis), stimulates the release matrix metalloproteinases from fibroblasts, chondrocytes, and neutrophils, and up-regulates the expression of endothelial adhesion molecules, leading to the migration of leukocytes into extravascular tissues. TNF also mediates pain, fever, shock, and anemia.

The complex interactions of paracrine or autocrine pathways mediated by networks of pro- and anti-inflammatory cytokines are implicated in many chronic inflammatory disorders and TNF plays a prominent role in the pathogenesis of Crohn's disease, rheumatoid arthritis, multiple sclerosis, systemic vasculitis, allograft rejection, and graft-versus-host disease. Mucosal biopsies from patients with Crohn's disease demonstrate increased TNF concentrations and intestinal mononuclear cell infiltrates in the lamina propria. Increased concentrations of TNF have been measured in fecal samples from Crohn's disease patients and in the joints of patients with rheumatoid arthritis and levels correlated with disease manifestations in these patients. Increased concentrations of TNF also have been reported in involved tissues and fluids of patients with ulcerative colitis, ankylosing spondylitis, psoriatic arthritis, and plaque psoriasis.

The ability of infliximab and infliximab-dyyb to inhibit the functional activity of TNF has been demonstrated in a variety of in vitro bioassays utilizing human fibroblasts, endothelial and epithelial cells, neutrophils, and B and T cells. The relationship of these biological response markers to the mechanism(s) of infliximab products' clinical effects is not known. In addition, cell lysis by complement or effector cells has been observed in vitro in cells that express transmembrane TNF and are bound by infliximab. In vivo studies have shown that anti-TNF antibodies reduce GI manifestations in a nonhuman primate model of colitis (cotton-top tamarin) and reduce synovitis and joint erosions in a murine model of collagen-induced arthritis.

In patients with Crohn's disease, infliximab products have been shown to reduce inflammatory cell migration, reduce TNF production in areas of intestinal inflammation, and reduce the proportion of lamina propria mononuclear cells able to express TNF and interferon.

In patients with rheumatoid arthritis, infliximab products reduce infiltration of inflammatory cells into inflamed areas of the joint and downregulate expression of molecules that mediate cellular adhesion (E-selectin, intercellular adhesion molecule-1 [ICAM-1], vascular cell adhesion molecule-1 [VCAM-1]), chemoattraction (IL-8 and monocyte chemotactic protein [MCP-1]), and tissue degradation (MMP 1 and 3). Infliximab also has been shown to inhibit pannus neoangiogenesis and proliferation through down-regulation of vascular endothelial growth factor (VEGF). Results of studies in transgenic mice that develop polyarthritis as the result of constitutive expression of TNF indicate that infliximab products can prevent such disease in these mice and, if administered after disease onset, allow eroded joints to heal. There is evidence that infliximab can prevent or inhibit progression of structural damage in patients with rheumatoid arthritis.

In patients with Crohn's disease or rheumatoid arthritis, therapy with infliximab products may result in decreases in proinflammatory cytokines (IL-1, IL-6) and decreases in systemic measures of inflammation, including C-reactive protein (CRP) levels and erythrocyte sedimentation rate (ESR). Peripheral blood lymphocytes from patients treated with infliximab products exhibit a normal proliferative response to in vitro mitogenic stimulation and lymphocyte counts are not decreased in patients who receive the drugs.

In patients with psoriatic arthritis, therapy with infliximab products results in a reduction in the number of T-cells and blood vessels in the synovium and psoriatic skin lesions and a reduction of macrophages in the synovium. In patients with plaque psoriasis, therapy with infliximab products may reduce the epidermal thickness and infiltration of inflammatory cells.

Pharmacokinetics

The pharmacokinetics of infliximab have been studied in adults with rheumatoid arthritis and adults with Crohn's disease. These studies have not revealed differences in the pharmacokinetics of the drug based on age or weight. The effects of gender or hepatic and/or renal impairment on the pharmacokinetics of infliximab have not been systematically evaluated.

In studies evaluating the pharmacokinetics of infliximab, most patients received the drug concomitantly with stable dosages of one or more other drugs used in the treatment of Crohn's disease (e.g., corticosteroids, mesalamine or sulfasalazine, azathioprine or mercaptopurine) or rheumatoid arthritis (e.g., corticosteroids, methotrexate, nonsteroidal anti-inflammatory agents [NSAIAs]).

Pharmacokinetic similarity between infliximab and infliximab-dyyb has been demonstrated, and FDA considers that the pharmacokinetic data provide support for a totality-of-evidence determination of biosimilarity between the 2 drugs.

■ **Absorption** Data from adults who received single IV infusions of 1–20 mg/kg of infliximab indicate a predictable and linear relationship between the dose administered and the maximum serum concentration and area under the serum concentration-time curve (AUC). In one study in adults with rheumatoid arthritis who received single 5-, 10-, or 20-mg/kg doses of infliximab given by IV infusion over 2 hours, peak serum concentrations 1–4 hours after the start of the infusion averaged 192.1, 426.7, or 907.4 mcg/mL, respectively; serum concentrations of the drug then decreased exponentially from day 3 through week 12 and were still detectable in most patients at week 10.

Systemic accumulation of infliximab does not appear to occur in adults receiving multiple doses of the drug given by IV infusion once every 4 or 8 weeks following an initial 3-dose induction regimen (doses at 0, 2, and 6 weeks).

In adults 20–65 years of age with moderately to severely active Crohn's disease who received a series of 4 doses of infliximab (10 mg/kg given once every 8 weeks), median serum infliximab concentrations 8 weeks after each dose were 7.9–10 mcg/mL; serum concentrations were still detectable 12 weeks after the final dose (median concentration: 2.2 mcg/mL).

In a phase 3 study in adults 19–80 years of age with active rheumatoid arthritis (the Anti-TNF Trial in Rheumatoid Arthritis with Concomitant Therapy [ATTRACT]), infliximab doses of 3 or 10 mg/kg were given by IV infusion over 2 hours at weeks 0, 2, and 6, followed by additional doses given once every 4 or 8 weeks. All patients included in the study were receiving stable dosages of methotrexate (at least 12.5 mg of oral or parenteral methotrexate once weekly) and folic acid that were continued during infliximab therapy; in addition, some also were receiving stable dosages of NSAIAs and/or oral corticosteroids (oral prednisone 10 mg or less daily or equivalent). Prior to the scheduled infliximab dose at 30 weeks, mean serum infliximab concentrations in those receiving a dosage of 3 mg/kg once every 4 or 8 weeks were 9.7 or 1.5 mcg/mL, respectively, and mean serum concentrations in those receiving 10 mg/kg once every 4 or 8 weeks were 35.8 or 8.9 mcg/mL, respectively.

Following administration of infliximab 5 mg/kg, peak and trough concentrations of the drug in pediatric patients 6–17 years of age with Crohn's disease or ulcerative colitis were similar to those in adults with these diseases.

Steady-state AUCs in children with juvenile arthritis who weighed 35 kg or less given 6 mg/kg of infliximab were similar to those reported in adults given infliximab 3 mg/kg. In addition, steady-state AUCs in children who weighed more than 35 kg given 3 mg/kg of infliximab were similar to those reported in adults given infliximab 3 mg/kg.

■ **Distribution** Distribution of infliximab into body tissues and fluids, including joints, has not been characterized. The volume of distribution of infliximab at steady state is independent of dose, indicating that the drug is distributed principally within the vascular compartment. In one study in adults with rheumatoid arthritis, the apparent volume of distribution of infliximab at steady state was 3.1–4.3 L.

Infliximab products cross the placenta. It is not known if infliximab products are distributed into milk.

■ **Elimination** The terminal elimination half-life of infliximab in adults with Crohn's disease, rheumatoid arthritis, or plaque psoriasis has been reported to be about 8–12 days. The terminal elimination half-life in pediatric patients 6–17 years of age with Crohn's disease or ulcerative colitis was similar to that reported in adults with these diseases.

The metabolic fate of infliximab has not been determined to date, but the drug may be eliminated by the reticuloendothelial system. Infliximab is not metabolized by hepatic cytochrome P-450 (CYP) enzymes.

Following IV infusion of infliximab doses of 5–20 mg/kg in adults with rheumatoid arthritis, the apparent clearance of the drug is 11–11.4 mL/hour. While differences in clearance of infliximab have not been observed in patient subgroups defined by age, weight, or gender, clearance of infliximab is increased in patients who have developed antibodies to the drug. Whether renal or hepatic impairment affects infliximab clearance has not been determined.

Chemistry and Stability

■ **Chemistry** Infliximab and infliximab-dyyb, biologic response modifiers, are chimeric human-murine immunoglobulin G_1 kappa (IgG_1 kappa) monoclonal antibodies that have a high affinity for human tumor necrosis factor (TNF; TNF-α). Infliximab and infliximab-dyyb consist of the constant region of human IgG_1 kappa coupled to the variable region of a high-affinity neutralizing murine anti-human TNF antibody. Because of the presence of human constant region sequences, the chimeric antibody is less immunogenic, has a longer half-life, and is more potent in binding and neutralizing human TNF compared with the murine antibody. The molecular weight of infliximab or infliximab-dyyb is approximately 149,100.

Infliximab is produced by continuous fermentation of a mouse myeloma cell line that has been transfected with cloned DNA coding for the chimeric antibody. The drug is purified from the culture supernatant using column chromatography and undergoes measures to inactivate and remove viruses.

Infliximab and infliximab-dyyb are commercially available as sterile, white, lyophilized powders for IV infusion. Vials labeled as containing 100 mg of infliximab or infliximab-dyyb also contain 500 mg of sucrose, 0.5 mg of polysorbate (Tween®) 80, 2.2 mg of monobasic sodium phosphate, and 6.1 mg of dibasic sodium phosphate. Following reconstitution with 10 mL of sterile water for injection, infliximab or infliximab-dyyb solutions are colorless to light yellow and opalescent; the solutions may contain a few translucent particles since the drug is a protein. Reconstituted solutions of infliximab or infliximab-dyyb have a pH of approximately 7.2.

■ **Stability** Commercially available infliximab or infliximab-dyyb lyophilized powder should be stored at 2–8°C. Unopened vials of infliximab may be stored at temperatures up to 30°C for a single period of up to 6 months; following removal from refrigerated storage, the drug cannot be returned to refrigerated storage. Since the lyophilized drugs do not contain a preservative, the manufacturers recommend that IV infusions of infliximab or infliximab-dyyb be initiated within 3 hours of preparation; any unused portions should be discarded.

Preparations

Excipients in commercially available drug preparations may have clinically important effects in some individuals; consult specific product labeling for details.

inFLIXimab

Parenteral

For injection, for IV infusion	100 mg	**Remicade®**, Janssen

inFLIXimab-dyyb

Parenteral

For injection, for IV infusion	100 mg	**Inflectra®**, Pfizer

†Use is not currently included in the labeling approved by the US Food and Drug Administration

Sarilumab

■ Sarilumab, a recombinant human immunoglobulin G_1 (IgG_1) kappa monoclonal antibody specific for interleukin-6 (IL-6) receptor, is a biologic response modifier and a disease-modifying antirheumatic drug (DMARD).

Uses

■ **Rheumatoid Arthritis in Adults** Sarilumab is used for the management of moderately to severely active rheumatoid arthritis in adults who have had an inadequate response or intolerance to one or more disease-modifying antirheumatic drugs (DMARDs). Sarilumab may be used alone or in combination with methotrexate or other nonbiologic DMARDs (examples include hydroxychloroquine, leflunomide, and sulfasalazine). Concomitant use of sarilumab with other biologic DMARDs, such as tumor necrosis factor (TNF; TNF-α) blocking agents (e.g., adalimumab, certolizumab pegol, etanercept, golimumab, infliximab), interleukin-1 (IL-1) receptor antagonists (e.g., anakinra), anti-CD20 monoclonal antibodies (e.g., rituximab), and selective costimulation modulators (e.g., abatacept), should be avoided. Concomitant use of these biologic agents with sarilumab has not been studied, and there is a possibility of increased immunosuppression and increased risk of infection with concomitant use. Sarilumab has been shown to induce clinical responses, improve physical function, and inhibit progression of structural damage in adults with rheumatoid arthritis.

Safety and efficacy of sarilumab have been evaluated in 2 randomized, double-blind, placebo-controlled, multicenter studies in adults (18 years of age or older) with moderately to severely active rheumatoid arthritis (as defined by the American College of Rheumatology [ACR]). In these studies, sarilumab was administered in combination with methotrexate in patients with an inadequate response to this drug (MOBILITY study) or in combination with methotrexate and/or other nonbiologic DMARDs (hydroxychloroquine, leflunomide, and/or sulfasalazine) in patients who had an inadequate response to, or had not tolerated, one or more TNF blocking agents (TARGET study). Patients included in these studies had 8 or more tender joints and 6 or more swollen joints. Those receiving low stable dosages of corticosteroids (equivalent to 10 mg or less of prednisone daily) could continue such therapy. Sarilumab was administered subcutaneously at a dosage of 150 or 200 mg once every 2 weeks.

The ACR criteria for improvement (ACR response) in measures of disease activity were used as the principal measure of clinical response in studies evaluating the efficacy of sarilumab. An ACR 20 response is achieved if the patient experiences a 20% or greater improvement in tender and swollen joint count and a 20% or greater improvement in at least 3 of the following criteria: patient pain assessment, patient global assessment, physician global assessment, patient self-assessed disability, or laboratory measures of disease activity (i.e., erythrocyte sedimentation rate [ESR] or C-reactive protein [CRP] level). An ACR 70 response is defined using the same criteria but with a level of improvement of 70%. The proportion of patients who achieved an ACR 20 response at week 24 was the primary end point in the studies of sarilumab. In addition, the total van der Heijde-modified Sharp score (a composite score of erosions and joint space narrowing in hands and feet) was used as the principal measure of joint damage and the Health Assessment Questionnaire Disability Index (HAQ-DI) was used to assess physical function and disability.

In the MOBILITY study, 1197 patients who had active rheumatoid arthritis for at least 3 months despite receiving a stable dosage of methotrexate (10–25 mg/week) were randomized to receive one of 3 regimens: sarilumab 150 mg every 2 weeks, sarilumab 200 mg every 2 weeks, or placebo, each given in combination with methotrexate for 52 weeks. At week 16, patients previously randomized to receive sarilumab 150 mg every 2 weeks or placebo who achieved less than 20% improvement from baseline in the number of tender or swollen joints were permitted to cross over to open-label therapy with sarilumab 200 mg every 2 weeks. Approximately 20% of patients in the study had previously received a biologic DMARD; patients with a history of nonresponse to prior biologic DMARD therapy were excluded from the study.

In the MOBILITY study, ACR 20 responses were achieved at 24 weeks in 58, 66.4, or 33.4% of patients receiving sarilumab 150 mg and methotrexate, sarilumab 200 mg and methotrexate, or placebo and methotrexate, respectively, while ACR 70 responses were achieved at 24 weeks in 19.8, 24.8, or 7.3% of patients receiving these respective treatment regimens. ACR responses observed at 24 weeks were maintained through 1 year. At 1 year, 12.8, 14.8, or 3% of patients receiving sarilumab 150 mg and methotrexate, sarilumab 200 mg and methotrexate, or placebo and methotrexate, respectively, had achieved major clinical responses (defined as ACR 70 responses for a continuous 24-week period). At 24 weeks, a greater proportion of patients receiving sarilumab 150 or 200 mg and methotrexate (27.8 or 34.1%, respectively) had a low level of disease activity, as defined by a 28-joint Disease Activity Score using CRP (DAS 28 [CRP]) of less than 2.6, compared with patients who received placebo and methotrexate (10.1%). However, this criterion does not preclude residual disease activity, and 33.1, 37.8, or 20% of patients in these respective treatment groups who achieved a DAS 28 (CRP) of less than 2.6 still had 3 or more active joints. Findings at 1 year indicated that treatment with sarilumab 150 or 200 mg and methotrexate inhibited progression of structural damage compared with placebo and methotrexate. At 1 year, 47.8 or 55.6% of patients receiving sarilumab 150 or 200 mg and methotrexate, respectively, exhibited no radiographic progression, as determined by change in the total van der Heijde-modified Sharp score, compared with 38.7% of patients receiving placebo and methotrexate. Patients receiving sarilumab 150 or 200 mg and methotrexate also experienced greater improvements in physical function and disability, as assessed using HAQ-DI scores, at 16 weeks compared with those who received placebo and methotrexate.

In the TARGET study, 546 patients who had active rheumatoid arthritis for at least 6 months and who had an inadequate response to, or had not tolerated, one or more TNF blocking agents were randomized to receive one of 3 regimens: sarilumab 150 mg every 2 weeks, sarilumab 200 mg every 2 weeks, or placebo, each given in combination with methotrexate and/or other nonbiologic DMARDs for 24 weeks. At week 12, patients with less than 20% improvement from baseline in the number of both tender or swollen joints were permitted to cross over to open-label therapy with sarilumab 200 mg every 2 weeks. ACR 20 responses were achieved at 24 weeks in 55.8, 60.9, or 33.7% of patients receiving sarilumab 150 mg and nonbiologic DMARDs, sarilumab 200 mg and nonbiologic DMARDs, or placebo and nonbiologic DMARDs, respectively, while ACR 70 responses were achieved at 24 weeks in 19.9, 16.3, or 7.2% of patients receiving these respective treatment regimens. At 24 weeks, a greater proportion of patients receiving sarilumab 150 or 200 mg (24.9 or 28.8%, respectively) had a low level of disease activity, as defined by a DAS 28 (CRP) of less than 2.6, compared with patients who received placebo (7.2%). Patients receiving sarilumab 150 or 200 mg and nonbiologic DMARDs also experienced greater improvements in physical function and disability, as assessed using HAQ-DI scores, at 12 weeks compared with those who received placebo and nonbiologic DMARDs.

For further information on the treatment of rheumatoid arthritis, see Uses: Rheumatoid Arthritis, in Methotrexate 10:00.

Dosage and Administration

■ **General** Therapy with sarilumab should not be initiated in patients with an absolute neutrophil count (ANC) of less than 2000 cells/mm³, platelet count of less than 150,000 cells/mm³, or ALT or AST concentration exceeding 1.5 times the upper limit of normal (ULN). (See Hematologic Effects and also Hepatic Effects under Warnings/Precautions: Other Warnings and Precautions, in Cautions.)

Methotrexate, other nonbiologic disease-modifying antirheumatic drugs (DMARDs), and corticosteroids may be continued in adults receiving sarilumab for the management of rheumatoid arthritis. Sarilumab should not be used concomitantly with other biologic DMARDs, such as tumor necrosis factor (TNF; TNF-α) blocking agents, interleukin-1 (IL-1) receptor antagonists, anti-CD20 monoclonal antibodies, and selective costimulation modulators. (See Uses: Rheumatoid Arthritis in Adults.)

Prior to initiation of sarilumab therapy, patients should be evaluated for tuberculosis infection and antimycobacterial therapy should be initiated if indicated. (See Infectious Complications under Warnings/Precautions: Warnings, in Cautions.)

■ **Administration** Sarilumab is administered by subcutaneous injection only. Sarilumab is intended for use under the guidance and supervision of a clinician; however, the drug may be *self-administered* if the clinician determines that the patient and/or their caregiver is competent to safely administer the drug after appropriate training.

Sarilumab is commercially available in single-use prefilled syringes. Each syringe delivers 150 or 200 mg of sarilumab in 1.14 mL. The entire contents of the prefilled syringe should be administered as a single dose.

Sarilumab injection is a clear and colorless to pale yellow solution. Prior to administration, sarilumab solution should be inspected visually for particulate matter or discoloration; if the syringe appears to be damaged or the solution contains particulates or is cloudy or discolored, the solution should be discarded. Sarilumab prefilled syringes should be stored at 2–8°C in the original carton until administration and protected from light. The injection should not be frozen or shaken. If refrigeration is not available, the prefilled syringes may be stored at room temperatures up to 25°C in the original carton for a period of up to 14 days. At least 30 minutes prior to administration, the prefilled syringe should be removed from the refrigerator and allowed to reach room temperature; the syringe should not be warmed in any other way (e.g., microwave, hot water).

Sarilumab is administered subcutaneously into the anterior thigh or abdomen (except for the 2-inch area around the umbilicus). Sarilumab may be administered subcutaneously into the upper arm by a caregiver or clinician. Injection sites should be rotated. Injections should not be made into areas where the skin is tender, bruised, or damaged or into scars.

■ **Dosage** ***Rheumatoid Arthritis in Adults*** For the management of moderately to severely active rheumatoid arthritis in adults who have had an inadequate response or intolerance to one or more DMARDs, the recommended dosage of sarilumab is 200 mg by subcutaneous injection once every 2 weeks.

Dosage Modification or Discontinuance for Toxicity If a serious infection or an opportunistic infection develops, sarilumab should be interrupted until the infection is controlled.

If certain dose-related laboratory changes (i.e., neutropenia, thrombocytopenia, elevated liver enzyme concentrations) occur, reduction in sarilumab dosage to 150 mg every 2 weeks or temporary interruption or discontinuance of sarilumab therapy is recommended (see tables).

Table 1. Recommended Dosage Adjustment Based on Absolute Neutrophil Count (ANC) in Adults with Rheumatoid Arthritis.

ANC (cells/mm³)	Recommendation
>1000	Maintain current dosage
500–1000	Interrupt sarilumab therapy until ANC is >1000; resume sarilumab at 150 mg every 2 weeks and increase to 200 mg every 2 weeks as clinically indicated
<500	Discontinue sarilumab

Table 2. Recommended Dosage Adjustment Based on Platelet Count in Adults with Rheumatoid Arthritis.

Platelet Count (cells/mm³)	Recommendation
50,0000–100,000	Interrupt sarilumab therapy until platelet count is >100,000; resume sarilumab at 150 mg every 2 weeks and increase to 200 mg every 2 weeks as clinically indicated
<50,000	Repeat platelet count; discontinue sarilumab if results are confirmed

Table 3. Recommended Dosage Adjustment Based on Changes in Liver Enzyme Laboratory Value in Adults with Rheumatoid Arthritis.

ALT Value	Recommendation
>1 to 3 times ULN	Modify dosage of concomitant DMARDs if appropriate
>3 to 5 times ULN	Interrupt sarilumab therapy until ALT values are <3 times ULN; resume sarilumab at 150 mg every 2 weeks and increase to 200 mg every 2 weeks as clinically indicated
>5 times ULN	Discontinue sarilumab

■ **Special Populations** Dosage adjustment is not necessary in patients with mild or moderate renal impairment; use of sarilumab in patients with severe renal impairment has not been evaluated. Use of the drug in patients with hepatic impairment is not recommended. (See Hepatic Impairment under Warnings/Precautions: Specific Populations, in Cautions.) The manufacturer makes no specific dosage recommendations for geriatric patients.

Cautions

■ **Contraindications** Sarilumab is contraindicated in patients with known hypersensitivity to the drug or any ingredient in the formulation.

■ **Warnings/Precautions** ***Warnings*** **Infectious Complications.** Serious and sometimes fatal infections, including bacterial, mycobacterial, invasive fungal, viral, or other opportunistic infections, have been reported in patients with rheumatoid arthritis receiving immunosuppressive agents including sarilumab. The most common serious infections reported in patients with rheumatoid arthritis receiving sarilumab have included pneumonia and cellulitis. Opportunistic infections (e.g., tuberculosis, candidiasis, pneumocystosis) also have been reported in patients receiving sarilumab. Other serious infections (e.g., aspergillosis, cryptococcal infection, histoplasmosis) may occur. Patients have presented with disseminated rather than local disease; patients often were receiving concomitant therapy with immunosuppressive agents (e.g., methotrexate, corticosteroids) that, in addition to their underlying condition, could have predisposed them to infections.

Patients should be closely monitored during treatment with sarilumab for the development of signs or symptoms of infection.

Sarilumab therapy should not be initiated in patients with active infections, including localized infections. Clinicians should consider potential risks and benefits of the drug prior to initiating therapy in patients with a history of chronic, recurring, serious, or opportunistic infections; patients with underlying conditions that may predispose them to infections; and patients who have been exposed to tuberculosis or who reside or have traveled in regions where tuberculosis or mycoses are endemic. Any patient who develops a new infection while receiving sarilumab should undergo a thorough diagnostic evaluation (appropriate for an immunocompromised patient), appropriate anti-infective therapy should be initiated, and the patient should be closely monitored. If a serious infection or an opportunistic infection develops, sarilumab should be interrupted until the infection is controlled.

All patients should be evaluated for latent tuberculosis and for the presence of risk factors for tuberculosis prior to and periodically during therapy with sarilumab. When indicated, an appropriate antimycobacterial regimen for the treatment of latent tuberculosis infection should be initiated prior to sarilumab therapy. Antimycobacterial therapy should be considered prior to initiation of sarilumab in individuals with a history of latent or active tuberculosis in whom an adequate course of antimycobacterial treatment cannot be confirmed and in individuals with a negative test for latent tuberculosis who have risk factors for tuberculosis. Consultation with a tuberculosis specialist is recommended when deciding whether antimycobacterial therapy should be initiated. Patients receiving sarilumab, including individuals with a negative test for latent tuberculosis, should be monitored for signs and symptoms of active tuberculosis.

Viral reactivation can occur in patients receiving immunosuppressive therapies. Herpes zoster exacerbation has been reported in patients receiving sarilumab. The risk of reactivation of hepatitis B virus (HBV) infection in patients receiving sarilumab is not known.

Sensitivity Reactions **Hypersensitivity Reactions.** Hypersensitivity reactions (e.g., injection site rash or erythema, rash, pruritus, urticaria) have been reported in patients receiving sarilumab. During clinical trials of sarilumab, hypersensitivity reactions requiring treatment discontinuance have been reported.

Patients receiving sarilumab should be advised to seek medical attention if they experience symptoms of a hypersensitivity reaction (see Advice to Patients). If a hypersensitivity reaction occurs, administration of the drug should be stopped immediately. Sarilumab is contraindicated in patients with known hypersensitivity to the drug.

Other Warnings and Precautions **Hematologic Effects.** Neutropenia and thrombocytopenia have been reported during clinical trials in patients receiving sarilumab, but decreases in neutrophil counts were not associated with infection, including serious infection, and decreases in platelet counts were not associated with bleeding.

Neutrophil and platelet counts should be evaluated prior to initiation of sarilumab therapy, 4–8 weeks after initiation of therapy, and every 3 months thereafter. In patients with neutropenia or thrombocytopenia, dosage adjustment, treatment interruption, or discontinuance of the drug may be necessary. Neutrophil counts should be evaluated at the end of the 2-week dosing interval because the neutrophil nadir generally occurs 3–4 days following sarilumab administration and the neutrophil count then recovers toward baseline. (See Dosage and Administration: General and also see Dosage Modification or Discontinuance for Toxicity under Dosage and Administration: Dosage.)

Hepatic Effects. Sarilumab has been associated with elevated aminotransferase concentrations. In clinical trials, these changes were reversible following reduction of the sarilumab dosage or interruption of sarilumab therapy and were not associated with clinical evidence of hepatic injury. The incidence and magnitude of aminotransferase elevations were increased when sarilumab was used in conjunction with a hepatotoxic drug (e.g., methotrexate).

Serum ALT and AST concentrations should be evaluated prior to initiation of sarilumab therapy, 4–8 weeks after initiation of therapy, and every 3 months thereafter. Other liver function tests (e.g., bilirubin) should be monitored when clinically indicated. In patients with elevated aminotransferase concentrations, dosage adjustment, treatment interruption, or discontinuance of sarilumab or concomitantly administered disease-modifying antirheumatic drugs (DMARDs) may be necessary. (See Dosage and Administration: General and also see Dosage Modification or Discontinuance for Toxicity under Dosage and Administration: Dosage.)

Effects on Serum Lipids. Increased serum concentrations of total cholesterol, triglycerides, low-density lipoprotein (LDL)-cholesterol, and/or high-density lipoprotein (HDL)-cholesterol have been reported in patients receiving sarilumab.

Lipoprotein concentrations should be monitored 4–8 weeks after initiation of sarilumab therapy and approximately every 6 months thereafter. Lipid disorders should be managed as clinically appropriate.

GI Perforation. GI perforation has been reported in patients receiving sarilumab, usually as a complication of diverticulitis. Most patients who experienced GI perforation were receiving concomitant therapy with nonsteroidal anti-inflammatory agents (NSAIAs) or corticosteroids. The relative contribution of these agents versus sarilumab to the occurrence of GI perforation remains to be determined.

Patients who experience new-onset abdominal symptoms should be promptly evaluated.

Malignancies. Immunosuppressive therapy may increase the risk of malignancies. Whether treatment with sarilumab affects development of malignancies remains to be determined. Malignancies were reported in clinical trials of the drug.

Immunization. Live vaccines should be avoided during therapy with sarilumab. (See Drug Interactions: Vaccines.)

Immunogenicity. As with all therapeutic proteins, there is potential for immunogenicity in patients who receive sarilumab. In clinical studies in patients with rheumatoid arthritis, antibodies to sarilumab were detected in approximately 4, 6, or 2% of patients receiving sarilumab 200 mg every 2 weeks, 150 mg every 2 weeks, or placebo, respectively, in combination with a DMARD. Neutralizing antibodies were detected in 1 or approximately 2% of patients receiving the drug at these respective dosages in combination with a DMARD. Antibodies to sarilumab were detected in approximately 9% of patients receiving sarilumab alone; neutralizing antibodies developed in about 7% of such patients. Population pharmacokinetic analysis suggested that clearance of sarilumab was increased in patients with neutralizing antibodies. However, no relationship between antibody development and adverse effects or loss of clinical response was observed.

Specific Populations **Pregnancy.** There are no adequate data regarding use of sarilumab in pregnant women. As pregnancy progresses, monoclonal antibodies are increasingly transported across the placenta, with the largest amount transferred during the third trimester. However, there was no evidence of embryotoxicity or fetal malformations in cynomolgus monkeys following administration of sarilumab during organogenesis at dosages producing exposures up to 84 times the exposure at the maximum recommended human dosage. Because interleukin-6 (IL-6) is increased in cervical and myometrial tissues during parturition, sarilumab may delay parturition by interfering with cervical ripening and myometrial contractions. Sarilumab should be used during pregnancy only when the potential benefits to the woman justify the potential risk to the fetus.

Infants exposed to sarilumab in utero may have impaired immune responses. The risks and benefits of administering live vaccines to such infants should be considered. (See Drug Interactions: Vaccines.)

A pregnancy registry has been established to monitor fetal outcomes of pregnant women exposed to sarilumab; patients or clinicians may contact the registry at 877-311-8972 to report any exposures to the drug that occur during pregnancy.

Lactation. It is not known whether sarilumab is distributed into milk or is absorbed from the GI tract in breast-fed infants. Because immunoglobulin G (IgG) is distributed into human milk, it is possible that sarilumab is distributed into milk. Potential effects of the drug on milk production or on breast-fed infants are unknown. The benefits of breast-feeding and the importance of sarilumab to the woman should be considered along with potential adverse effects on the breast-fed infant from the drug or from the underlying maternal condition.

Pediatric Use. Safety and efficacy of sarilumab in pediatric patients younger than 18 years of age have not been established.

Neonates and infants who were exposed to sarilumab in utero may have impaired immune responses; the risks and benefits of administering live vaccines to such infants should be considered.

Geriatric Use. Of the total number of patients with rheumatoid arthritis studied in clinical trials of sarilumab, 15% were 65 years of age or older while 1.6% were 75 years of age or older. Although no overall differences in safety and efficacy were observed between geriatric and younger patients, serious infections occurred more frequently in those 65 years of age or older. Because the geriatric population in general may have a higher incidence of infections than younger adults, sarilumab should be used with caution in this age group.

Hepatic Impairment. Safety and efficacy of sarilumab have not been established in patients with hepatic impairment, including those with serologic evidence of hepatitis B virus (HBV) or hepatitis C virus (HCV) infection. Use of the drug in patients with active hepatic disease or hepatic impairment is not recommended. (See Hepatic Effects under Warnings/Precautions: Other Warnings and Precautions, in Cautions.)

Renal Impairment. The effect of renal impairment on the pharmacokinetics of sarilumab has not been specifically studied to date. Although population pharmacokinetic data suggest an increase in exposure to sarilumab in patients with mild to moderate renal impairment (creatinine clearance of 30 to less than 90 mL/minute), sarilumab is not expected to undergo substantial renal elimination and dosage adjustment is not necessary. Sarilumab has not been evaluated in patients with severe renal impairment.

■ **Common Adverse Effects** Adverse effects reported in 3% or more of patients receiving sarilumab include neutropenia, increased ALT concentrations, injection site reactions (e.g., erythema, pruritus), upper respiratory tract infection, and urinary tract infection.

Drug Interactions

■ **Drugs Metabolized by Hepatic Microsomal Enzymes** Because increased levels of cytokines including interleukin-6 (IL-6) in inflammatory conditions such as rheumatoid arthritis may suppress the formation of cytochrome P-450 (CYP) enzymes, inhibition of IL-6 activity by sarilumab may restore CYP enzyme activity to higher levels. Effects of sarilumab on CYP enzyme activity may persist for several weeks after the drug is discontinued. Following initiation or discontinuance of sarilumab therapy, patients receiving certain drugs metabolized by CYP isoenzymes (i.e., those with a low therapeutic index that require individualized dosing [e.g., theophylline, warfarin]) should be monitored for therapeutic effect and/or changes in serum concentrations, and dosages of these drugs should be adjusted as needed. Caution also is advised when sarilumab is used concomitantly with CYP3A4 substrates (e.g., oral contraceptives, atorvastatin, lovastatin) for which a reduction in efficacy would be undesirable.

Simvastatin Subcutaneous administration of a single 200-mg dose of sarilumab one week prior to oral administration of a single 40-mg dose of simvastatin (a substrate of CYP3A4 and organic anion transport protein [OATP] 1B1) in patients with rheumatoid arthritis reduced systemic exposures to simvastatin and simvastatin acid by 45 and 36%, respectively, compared with administration of simvastatin alone.

■ **Antirheumatic Drugs** Concomitant use of methotrexate does not appear to affect clearance of sarilumab. Sarilumab has not been studied in conjunction with biologic disease-modifying antirheumatic drugs (DMARDs), including tumor necrosis factor (TNF; TNF-α) blocking agents, or with Janus kinase (JAK) inhibitors (e.g., tofacitinib). Concomitant use of sarilumab with biologic DMARDs should be avoided. (See Uses: Rheumatoid Arthritis in Adults.)

■ **Vaccines** Safety of live vaccines in patients receiving sarilumab has not been established and there is a possibility of increased risk of infection with concomitant use. Live vaccines should be avoided during therapy with sarilumab. The interval between administration of live vaccines and initiation of sarilumab therapy should be in accordance with current vaccination guidelines regarding immunosuppressive agents. Information is not available regarding secondary transmission of infection from individuals receiving live vaccines to patients receiving sarilumab. (See also Pediatric Use under Warnings/Precautions: Specific Populations, in Cautions.)

Description

Sarilumab, a recombinant human monoclonal antibody specific for interleukin-6 (IL-6) receptor, is a biologic response modifier and a disease-modifying antirheumatic drug (DMARD). Sarilumab is an IgG_1 kappa immunoglobulin that binds specifically to both soluble and membrane-bound IL-6 receptors and inhibits IL-6-mediated signaling through these receptors, thereby resulting in a reduction in inflammatory mediator production.

IL-6, a pleiotropic proinflammatory cytokine, is produced by various cell types, including T cells, B lymphocytes, monocytes, fibroblasts, synoviocytes, and endothelial cells, and has a broad spectrum of biologic activities. IL-6 is involved in T-cell activation, induction of immunoglobulin secretion, initiation of hepatic acute phase protein synthesis, stimulation of hematopoietic precursor cell proliferation and differentiation, and induction of osteoclast differentiation and activation. While the causes of rheumatoid arthritis have not been fully elucidated, proinflammatory cytokines, including IL-6, appear to play critical roles in the disease process. IL-6 is overexpressed in synovial tissue in patients with rheumatoid arthritis and is thought to contribute to synovial proliferation and joint destruction in patients with the disease. Elevated levels of IL-6 in serum and synovial fluid have been shown to correlate with clinical and laboratory measures of disease activity in patients with rheumatoid arthritis.

The absolute bioavailability of sarilumab following subcutaneous injection is approximately 80%. Following repeated subcutaneous administration of sarilumab 150 or 200 mg every 2 weeks, peak serum concentrations of the drug are attained in approximately 2–4 days and steady-state concentrations of the drug are attained within 14–16 weeks; systemic accumulation of the drug is twofold to threefold. With an increase in dosage from 150 mg every 2 weeks to 200 mg every 2 weeks, steady-state concentrations of the drug increase by approximately twofold. Although systemic exposure to sarilumab tends to decrease as body weight increases, differences in exposure based on body weight are not associated with clinically important effects on efficacy or safety of the drug in patients with rheumatoid arthritis. The metabolic pathway of sarilumab has not been characterized; as with other therapeutic proteins, the drug is expected to be catabolized into peptides and amino acids in the same manner as endogenous IgG. Sarilumab exhibits concentration-dependent clearance. At low sarilumab concentrations, target-mediated nonlinear clearance plays a major role in determining total drug clearance; at higher concentrations, the nonlinear pathway is saturated and clearance is determined mainly by linear clearance. The apparent steady-state half-life of sarilumab in adults with rheumatoid arthritis is up to 8 or up to 10 days following subcutaneous administration of sarilumab 150 or 200 mg, respectively, every 2 weeks. Patients who developed antisarilumab antibodies generally had increased apparent clearance of the drug. The pharmacokinetics of sarilumab are not affected by age, gender, or race.

Advice to Patients

A copy of the manufacturer's patient information (medication guide and instructions for use) for sarilumab should be provided to all patients. Importance of patients and/or caregivers reading the patient information prior to initiation of therapy and each time the prescription is refilled.

Importance of instructing patient regarding proper dosage and administration of sarilumab, including the use of aseptic technique, and proper disposal of the prefilled syringes if it is determined that the patient is competent to safely administer the drug.

Risk of increased susceptibility to infection. Importance of informing clinicians immediately if any signs or symptoms suggestive of infection (e.g., fever, sweating, or chills; cough, dyspnea, or blood in the phlegm; diarrhea; weight loss; burning upon urination or increased frequency of urination; warm, red, or painful skin) develop.

Risk of GI perforation, usually as a complication of diverticulitis and more commonly in those receiving concomitant therapy with nonsteroidal anti-inflammatory agents (NSAIAs) or corticosteroids. Importance of informing clinician immediately if severe, persistent abdominal pain occurs.

Risk of hypersensitivity reactions. Importance of contacting a clinician prior to administering the next dose if manifestations of an allergic reaction (e.g., urticaria, rash, flushing) occur; importance of seeking immediate medical attention if manifestations of a serious allergic reaction (e.g., difficulty breathing, chest pain, feelings of faintness or dizziness, abdominal pain or vomiting, swelling of the lips, tongue, or face) occur.

Importance of patients informing clinicians that they are receiving sarilumab therapy before scheduling any surgery or medical procedures.

Importance of informing clinicians of existing or contemplated concomitant therapy, including prescription (e.g., biologic antirheumatic drugs, immunizations) and OTC drugs and dietary or herbal supplements, as well as any concomitant illnesses (e.g., active infection, liver disease, diverticulitis, stomach ulcers) or any history of tuberculosis or other chronic or recurring infections.

Importance of periodic laboratory monitoring.

Importance of women informing clinicians if they are or plan to become pregnant or plan to breast-feed. Importance of clinicians informing women about the existence of and encouraging enrollment in the pregnancy registry for sarilumab.

Importance of informing patients of other important precautionary information. (See Cautions.)

Overview® (see Users Guide). For additional information on this drug until a more detailed monograph is developed and published, the manufacturer's labeling should be consulted. It is *essential* that the manufacturer's labeling be consulted for more detailed information on usual cautions, precautions, contraindications, potential drug interactions, laboratory test interferences, and acute toxicity.

Preparations

Excipients in commercially available drug preparations may have clinically important effects in some individuals; consult specific product labeling for details.

Sarilumab

Parenteral		
Injection, for subcutaneous use	150 mg/1.14 mL	**Kevzara®** (available as single-use prefilled syringes), Sanofi-Aventis and Regeneron
	200 mg/1.14 mL	**Kevzara®** (available as single-use prefilled syringes), Sanofi-Aventis and Regeneron

Selected Revisions July 2018, © Copyright, June 2017, American Society of Health-System Pharmacists, Inc.

Tocilizumab

■ Tocilizumab, a recombinant humanized immunoglobulin G_1 (IgG_1) monoclonal antibody specific for interleukin-6 (IL-6) receptor, is a biologic response modifier and a disease-modifying antirheumatic drug (DMARD).

Uses

Tocilizumab is used alone or in combination with methotrexate or other nonbiologic disease-modifying antirheumatic drugs (DMARDs) for the management of moderately to severely active rheumatoid arthritis in adults who have had an inadequate response to one or more DMARDs. Tocilizumab also is used alone or in combination with methotrexate for the management of active systemic or polyarticular juvenile idiopathic arthritis (JIA).

■ **Rheumatoid Arthritis in Adults** Tocilizumab is used for the management of moderately to severely active rheumatoid arthritis in adults who have had an inadequate response to one or more DMARDs. Tocilizumab can be used alone or in combination with methotrexate or other nonbiologic DMARDs (examples include hydroxychloroquine, leflunomide, minocycline, and sulfasalazine). Concomitant use of tocilizumab with other biologic DMARDs, such as tumor necrosis factor (TNF; TNF-α) blocking agents (e.g., adalimumab, certolizumab pegol, etanercept, golimumab, infliximab), interleukin-1 (IL-1) receptor antagonists (e.g., anakinra), anti-CD20 monoclonal antibodies (e.g., rituximab), and selective costimulation modulators (e.g., abatacept), should be avoided. Concomitant use of these biologic agents with tocilizumab has not been studied, and there is a possibility of increased immunosuppression and increased risk of infection with concomitant use. Tocilizumab has been shown to induce clinical responses, improve physical function, and inhibit progression of structural damage in adults with rheumatoid arthritis.

Clinical Experience with IV Tocilizumab Safety and efficacy of IV tocilizumab have been evaluated in 5 randomized, double-blind studies in adults (18 years of age or older) with moderate to severe active rheumatoid arthritis. In these studies, tocilizumab was administered as monotherapy, in combination with methotrexate or other nonbiologic DMARDs in patients with an inadequate response to these drugs, or in combination with methotrexate in patients with an inadequate response to TNF blocking agents. Patients included in these studies had 8 or more tender joints and 6 or more swollen joints. Those receiving low stable dosages of corticosteroids (equivalent to 10 mg or less of prednisone daily) and/or stable dosages of nonsteroidal anti-inflammatory agents (NSAIAs) could continue such agents. Tocilizumab was administered IV at a dosage of 4 or 8 mg/kg once every 4 weeks.

The American College of Rheumatology (ACR) criteria for improvement (ACR response) in measures of disease activity were used as the principal measure of clinical response in studies evaluating the efficacy of tocilizumab. An ACR 20 response is achieved if the patient experiences a 20% improvement in tender and swollen joint count and a 20% or greater improvement in at least 3 of the following criteria: patient pain assessment, patient global assessment, physician global assessment, patient self-assessed disability, or laboratory measures of disease activity (i.e., erythrocyte sedimentation rate [ESR] or C-reactive protein [CRP] level). An ACR 70 response is defined using the same criteria but with a level of improvement of 70%. The proportion of patients who achieved an ACR 20 response at week 24 was the primary end point in the studies of tocilizumab. In one longer-term study, the total Sharp-Genant score (a composite score of erosions and joint space narrowing in hands, wrists, and forefeet) was used as the principal measure of joint damage, and the Health Assessment Questionnaire Disability Index (HAQ-DI) was used to assess physical function and disability.

Clinical evaluations of tocilizumab indicate that, in adults with active rheumatoid arthritis despite therapy with methotrexate or other nonbiologic DMARD(s), the addition of tocilizumab to the DMARD regimen is associated with greater efficacy than use of the nonbiologic DMARD(s) alone. In addition, therapy with tocilizumab in conjunction with methotrexate has been more effective than methotrexate alone in patients with an inadequate response to prior therapy with TNF blocking agents. In patients with an inadequate response to prior therapy with nonbiologic DMARDs or TNF blocking agents, response rates were higher in those receiving tocilizumab 8 mg/kg IV every 4 weeks compared with those receiving 4 mg/kg IV every 4 weeks. When tocilizumab was compared with methotrexate as monotherapy in patients with active rheumatoid arthritis, tocilizumab was more effective than methotrexate. Response to tocilizumab can occur 2–4 weeks following initiation of therapy in some patients.

In the study evaluating efficacy of tocilizumab as monotherapy (AMBITION), patients were randomized to receive either tocilizumab (8 mg/kg IV every 4 weeks) or methotrexate (7.5 mg weekly, increased up to 20 mg weekly). Patients were excluded if they had received methotrexate in the past 6 months, had previously discontinued methotrexate because of lack of response or clinically important toxicity, or had previously discontinued therapy with a TNF blocking agent because of inadequate response. About two-thirds of the patients in the study had never received methotrexate therapy. An ACR 20 response was achieved in 70% of patients receiving tocilizumab and 53% of those receiving methotrexate for 24 weeks.

In 2 studies (OPTION and LITHE), therapy with tocilizumab given in combination with methotrexate was evaluated in patients who had not responded adequately to methotrexate; patients in these studies were randomized to receive tocilizumab 4 mg/kg IV every 4 weeks, tocilizumab 8 mg/kg IV every 4 weeks, or placebo, each given in conjunction with a stable dosage of methotrexate (10–25 mg weekly). Patients who had been treated unsuccessfully with a TNF blocking agent were excluded from these studies. In one study (OPTION), ACR 20 responses were achieved at 24 weeks in 59, 48, or 27% of those receiving tocilizumab 8 mg/kg and methotrexate, tocilizumab 4 mg/kg and methotrexate, or placebo and methotrexate, respectively. The other study (LITHE) was longer term (2 years with an optional 3-year extension phase) and was designed to assess changes in signs and symptoms of rheumatoid arthritis at 24 weeks, with subsequent assessments of joint damage and physical functioning at 1 and 2 years of treatment. Following 1 year of treatment with the randomly assigned regimen, patients received open-label treatment with tocilizumab 8 mg/kg for an additional year or had the option to continue their double-blind treatment if improvement in swollen and tender joint count was maintained above 70%. Planned interim analyses indicated that ACR 20 responses were achieved at 24 weeks in 56, 51, or 27% and at 1 year in 56, 47, or 25% of those receiving tocilizumab 8 mg/kg and methotrexate, tocilizumab 4 mg/kg and methotrexate, or placebo and methotrexate, respectively. At 1 year, 7, 4, or 1% of patients receiving tocilizumab 8 mg/kg and methotrexate, tocilizumab 4 mg/kg and methotrexate, or placebo and methotrexate, respectively, had achieved major clinical responses (defined as ACR 70 responses for a continuous 24-week period). Findings at 1 year also indicated that treatment with tocilizumab 4 or 8 mg/kg and methotrexate inhibited progression of structural damage compared with placebo and methotrexate. At 1 year, 78 or 83% of patients receiving tocilizumab 4 or 8 mg/kg and methotrexate, respectively, exhibited no radiographic progression, as determined by change in total Sharp-Genant score, compared with 66% of patients receiving placebo and methotrexate. Patients receiving tocilizumab 4 or 8 mg/kg and methotrexate also experienced greater improvements in physical function and disability, as assessed using HAQ-DI scores, at 1 year compared with those who received placebo and methotrexate. By the end of the 2-year study, most patients in the placebo and methotrexate group had crossed over to tocilizumab and methotrexate treatment.

In one study (TOWARD) in patients who had not responded adequately to treatment with one or more nonbiologic DMARDs, tocilizumab (8 mg/kg IV weekly) or placebo was added to the stable background DMARD regimen. For 76% of patients in the study, the background regimen contained one DMARD, most commonly methotrexate (mean dosage of 15 mg weekly). Patients who had been treated unsuccessfully with a TNF blocking agent or had previously received any cell-depleting therapy were excluded. At 24 weeks, an ACR 20 response was achieved in 61 or 24% of those receiving tocilizumab or placebo, respectively, in conjunction with the nonbiologic DMARD(s).

Tocilizumab, given in combination with methotrexate, also was evaluated in one study (RADIATE) in patients with rheumatoid arthritis who had not responded adequately to, or who had not tolerated, one or more TNF blocking agents. Patients in this study were randomized to receive tocilizumab 4 mg/kg IV every 4 weeks, tocilizumab 8 mg/kg IV every 4 weeks, or placebo, each given in combination with methotrexate 10–25 mg weekly; tocilizumab was initiated following discontinuance of any other DMARDs and stabilization of the methotrexate dosage. At 24 weeks, an ACR 20 response was achieved in 50, 30, or 10% of those receiving tocilizumab 8 mg/kg and methotrexate, tocilizumab 4 mg/kg and methotrexate, or placebo and methotrexate, respectively.

Analysis of long-term data from the 5 studies showed that improvements from baseline in clinical measures of efficacy generally were sustained through at least 4.2 years of tocilizumab therapy.

Clinical Experience with Subcutaneous Tocilizumab Efficacy and safety of subcutaneous tocilizumab have been evaluated in 2 double-blind, controlled studies in adults with moderate to severe active rheumatoid arthritis. One study was a noninferiority study that compared tocilizumab 162 mg subcutaneously every week with tocilizumab 8 mg/kg IV every 4 weeks. The other study was a placebo-controlled superiority study evaluating tocilizumab 162 mg subcutaneously every other week. In these studies, the effects of subcutaneously administered tocilizumab on clinical response and progression of joint damage were consistent with the effects observed in studies evaluating IV administration of the drug.

In the active-control study (SUMMACTA), 1262 patients with moderate to severe active rheumatoid arthritis were randomized in a 1:1 ratio to receive subcutaneous tocilizumab (162 mg every week) or IV tocilizumab (8 mg/kg every 4 weeks) for 24 weeks in conjunction with a stable dosage of one or more nonbiologic DMARDs. To be included in the study, patients were required to have at least 4 tender and 4 swollen joints and to have had an inadequate response to at least one DMARD. Patients receiving stable dosages of NSAIAs and/or low stable dosages of corticosteroids (equivalent to 10 mg or less of prednisone daily) could continue such agents. Approximately 21% of patients included in the study had experienced an inadequate response to prior TNF-blocking agent therapy. ACR 20 response at 24 weeks (the primary measure of efficacy) was observed in 69 or 73% of patients receiving subcutaneous or IV tocilizumab, respectively, establishing noninferiority of the subcutaneous regimen. ACR 50 and ACR 70 responses were observed in 47 and 24%, respectively, of those receiving subcutaneous tocilizumab and 49 and 28%, respectively, of those receiving IV tocilizumab. At 24 weeks, similar proportions of patients receiving subcutaneous or IV tocilizumab (38 or 37%, respectively) had a low level of disease activity, as defined by a Disease Activity Score in 28 joints (DAS 28) of less than 2.6. The mean decrease in HAQ-DI score from baseline to week 24 was 0.6 in both treatment groups, and similar proportions of patients receiving subcutaneous or IV tocilizumab (65 or 67%, respectively) achieved clinically important improvement in HAQ-DI score (change from baseline of at least 0.3 units).

Following the 24-week double-blind period in the SUMMACTA study, patients who had received subcutaneous tocilizumab were randomized in an 11:1 ratio to receive subcutaneous or IV tocilizumab, while those who had received IV tocilizumab were randomized in a 2:1 ratio to receive IV or subcutaneous tocilizumab in a 72-week open-label extension of the study. The proportions of patients who achieved ACR responses, DAS 28 score indicating a low level of disease activity, and clinically important improvement in HAQ-DI score were maintained through week 72 (97 weeks of tocilizumab treatment) and were similar across treatment groups.

In the placebo-controlled study (BREVACTA), 656 patients with moderate to severe active rheumatoid arthritis were randomized in a 2:1 ratio to receive subcutaneous tocilizumab (162 mg every other week) or placebo for 24 weeks in conjunction with a stable dosage of one or more nonbiologic DMARDs. To be included in the study, patients were required to have at least 8 tender and 6 swollen joints and to have had an inadequate response to at least one DMARD. Patients receiving stable dosages of NSAIAs and/or low stable dosages of corticosteroids (equivalent to 10 mg or less of prednisone daily) could continue such agents. Approximately 21% of patients included in the study had experienced an inadequate response to prior TNF-blocking agent therapy. ACR 20 response at 24 weeks (the primary measure of efficacy) was observed in 61% of patients receiving tocilizumab compared with 32% of those receiving placebo. In addition, ACR 50 and ACR 70 responses were observed at 24 weeks in 40 and 20%, respectively, of tocilizumab-treated patients compared with 12 and 5%, respectively, of placebo recipients. At 24 weeks, 32 or 4% of patients receiving tocilizumab or placebo, respectively, had a low level of disease activity, as defined by a DAS 28 score of less than 2.6. Less progression of joint damage, as assessed radiographically by the change in van der Heijde-modified Sharp score (a composite score of structural damage that measures joint erosions and joint space narrowing in the hands, wrists, and feet), was observed in patients receiving tocilizumab compared with those receiving placebo. The mean decrease in HAQ-DI score from baseline to week 24 was 0.4 or 0.3, and the proportion of patients who achieved clinically important improvement in HAQ-DI score (change from baseline of at least 0.3 units) was 58 or 47% for patients receiving tocilizumab or placebo, respectively.

In the SUMMACTA study, the proportion of patients achieving responses (ACR responses and DAS 28 scores indicating low disease activity) to either IV tocilizumab (8 mg/kg every 4 weeks) or subcutaneous tocilizumab (162 mg every week) generally were similar regardless of body weight, but tended to be lower and more variable in the small subset of patients weighing 100 kg or more. However, in the BREVACTA study, patients weighing 100 kg or more had poorer ACR responses to subcutaneous tocilizumab (162 mg every *other* week) than did patients in 2 lower-weight categories.

For further information on the treatment of rheumatoid arthritis, see Uses: Rheumatoid Arthritis, in Methotrexate 10:00.

■ **Juvenile Idiopathic Arthritis** Tocilizumab is used for the management of active systemic or polyarticular juvenile idiopathic arthritis (JIA). Tocilizumab can be used alone or in combination with methotrexate. Concomitant use of tocilizumab with other biologic DMARDs should be avoided. Such concomitant use has not been studied, and there is a possibility of increased immunosuppression and increased risk of infection with concomitant use.

Polyarticular Juvenile Idiopathic Arthritis Tocilizumab is used for the management of active polyarticular JIA. Tocilizumab can be used alone or in combination with methotrexate. Tocilizumab has been shown to produce clinical improvement in patients 2–17 years of age with active polyarticular JIA.

Tocilizumab has been evaluated in a randomized, double-blind treatment-withdrawal study (CHERISH) in patients 2–17 years of age with active polyarticular JIA who had not responded adequately to or had not tolerated treatment with methotrexate. Patients included in this study had at least 6 months of active disease, with at least 5 joints with active arthritis (swollen or limitation of movement with pain and/or tenderness) and limitation of motion in at least 3 of the active joints. Disease subtypes included rheumatoid factor-positive or -negative polyarticular JIA and extended oligoarticular JIA. Patients receiving low stable dosages of corticosteroids (equivalent to 0.2 mg/kg or less [maximum of 10 mg] of prednisone daily) and/or a stable dosage of NSAIAs or methotrexate (10–20 mg/m^2 per week) could continue such therapy; however, concomitant use of other nonbiologic or biologic DMARDs was not permitted. Approximately 32% of patients had received prior biologic DMARD therapy.

During a 16-week lead-in period, all 188 patients enrolled in the study received IV tocilizumab; those weighing 30 kg or more received a dosage of 8 mg/kg every 4 weeks, while those weighing less than 30 kg were randomized to receive a dosage of either 8 or 10 mg/kg every 4 weeks. At week 16, all patients with JIA-ACR 30 response were randomly assigned in a 1:1 ratio (stratified by concomitant methotrexate and corticosteroid use) to continue receiving tocilizumab at the previously assigned dosage or to receive placebo for 24 weeks. JIA-ACR responses are defined as the percentage improvement (e.g., 30, 50, 70, or 90%) in 3 of any 6 core outcome variables compared with baseline, with worsening in no more than 1 of the remaining variables by 30% or more. Core outcome variables consist of physician global assessment, parent or patient global assessment, number of joints with active arthritis, number of joints with limitation of movement, erythrocyte sedimentation rate (ESR), and physical function (as assessed using the disability index of the Childhood Health Assessment Questionnaire [CHAQ-DI]).

At the end of the lead-in period, 91% of patients receiving tocilizumab in combination with methotrexate and 83% of those receiving tocilizumab monotherapy (a total of 163 patients) achieved a JIA-ACR 30 response and entered the treatment-withdrawal period; JIA-ACR 50 and JIA-ACR 70 responses were observed at the end of the lead-in period in 84 and 64%, respectively, of patients receiving tocilizumab in combination with methotrexate and 80 and 55%, respectively, of those receiving tocilizumab monotherapy. Response rates for children weighing less than 30 kg and receiving the 8-mg/kg dose were numerically lower than those for the other 2 treatment groups.

During the treatment-withdrawal period, a greater proportion of patients receiving placebo (48%) compared with those receiving tocilizumab (26%) experienced a JIA-ACR 30 flare (the primary measure of efficacy). JIA-ACR 30 flare was defined as 3 or more of the 6 core outcome variables worsening by at least 30% with no more than 1 of the remaining variables improving by more than 30% relative to the start of the treatment-withdrawal period. At the end of the treatment-withdrawal evaluation period, JIA-ACR 30, 50, and 70 responses were observed in a greater proportion of patients receiving tocilizumab compared with those receiving placebo.

Follow-up of patients in a subsequent open-label extension period is ongoing.

Systemic Juvenile Idiopathic Arthritis Tocilizumab is used for the management of active systemic JIA. Tocilizumab can be used alone or in combination with methotrexate. Tocilizumab has been shown to produce clinical improvement and to improve physical function in patients 2–17 years of age with active systemic JIA.

Tocilizumab has been evaluated in a 12-week randomized, double-blind, placebo-controlled study in 112 patients 2–17 years of age with active systemic JIA that had not responded adequately to treatment with NSAIAs and corticosteroids. Patients included in this study had at least 6 months of active disease, with either 5 or more active joints or 2 or more active joints and fever. Patients were randomized in a 2:1 ratio to receive tocilizumab (administered IV every 2 weeks at a weight-adjusted dosage [8 mg/kg in those weighing 30 kg or more, 12 mg/kg in those weighing less than 30 kg]) or placebo and were stratified according to body weight, disease duration, corticosteroid dosage, and methotrexate use. Those receiving stables dosages of NSAIAs, corticosteroids (equivalent to 0.5 mg/kg or less [maximum of 30 mg] of prednisone daily), and methotrexate (20 mg/m^2 or less per week) could continue such therapy; however, concomitant use of other nonbiologic or biologic DMARDs was not permitted. Approximately 82% of patients had received prior biologic DMARD therapy. Tapering of the corticosteroid dosage was permitted beginning at week 6 in patients who achieved a JIA-ACR 70 response. At week 12, the combined primary end point of JIA-ACR 30 response and absence of fever was observed in 85% of patients receiving tocilizumab compared with 24% of those receiving placebo. JIA-ACR 30, 50, and 70 responses were observed at week 12 in 91, 85, and 71%, respectively, of patients receiving tocilizumab, compared with 24, 11, and 8%, respectively, of those receiving placebo. Tocilizumab therapy also was associated with improvement in systemic manifestations (fever and rash). A greater proportion of patients receiving tocilizumab reduced their corticosteroid dosage by at least 20% without experiencing a subsequent occurrence of systemic symptoms or JIA-ACR 30 flare, compared with placebo recipients (24 versus 3%). In addition, a greater proportion of patients receiving tocilizumab had clinically important improvements in physical function, as assessed using the CHAQ-DI, from baseline to week 12, compared with those receiving placebo (77 versus 19%).

A total of 110 patients subsequently were entered into a long-term, single-group, open-label extension study. At 44 weeks of follow-up, responses to tocilizumab therapy (absence of fever, JIA-ACR response rates, systemic symptoms) were similar to those observed in the 12-week randomized study. By week 44, 43% of patients had discontinued oral corticosteroid therapy; about 50% of these patients had discontinued corticosteroid use for 18 weeks or longer. At 52 weeks of follow-up, 80% of patients had JIA-ACR 70 response and no fever, 59% had JIA-ACR 90 response and no fever, 48% had no joints with active arthritis, and 52% had discontinued oral corticosteroid therapy; the proportion of patients with moderate or severe functional impairment was 38%, compared with 82% at study baseline.

Dosage and Administration

■ **General** Therapy with tocilizumab should not initiated in patients with an absolute neutrophil count (ANC) of less than 2000/mm^3, platelet count of less than 100,000/mm^3, or ALT or AST concentration exceeding 1.5 times the upper limit of normal (ULN).

Methotrexate, other nonbiologic disease-modifying antirheumatic drugs (DMARDs), nonsteroidal anti-inflammatory agents (NSAIAs), and corticosteroids may be continued in adults receiving tocilizumab for the management of rheumatoid arthritis. Methotrexate, NSAIAs, and corticosteroids may be continued in patients with juvenile idiopathic arthritis (JIA). Tocilizumab should not be used concomitantly with other biologic DMARDs, such as tumor necrosis factor (TNF; TNF-α) blocking agents, interleukin-1 (IL-1) receptor antagonists, anti-CD20 monoclonal antibodies, and selective costimulation modulators. (See Uses.)

■ **Administration** Tocilizumab is administered by IV infusion over 60 minutes; the drug should not be administered by rapid IV injection (e.g., IV push or bolus). The drug also may be administered by subcutaneous injection in the management of rheumatoid arthritis in adults. Tocilizumab currently is not FDA-labeled for subcutaneous use in the management of polyarticular or systemic JIA.

IV Administration Tocilizumab injection concentrate (containing 20 mg/mL) must be diluted prior to IV administration. The appropriate dose of the injection concentrate should be diluted in 0.9% sodium chloride injection to provide a final volume of 50 mL for administration in patients with polyarticular or systemic JIA who weigh less than 30 kg and to a final volume of 100 mL for administration in adults with rheumatoid arthritis or patients with polyarticular or systemic JIA who weigh 30 kg or more. A volume of diluent equal to the total required volume of tocilizumab injection concentrate should be removed from the bag or bottle of 0.9% sodium chloride injection prior to the addition of tocilizumab injection concentrate. The total required volume of tocilizumab injection concentrate (0.2, 0.4, 0.5, or 0.6 mL/kg for a dose of 4, 8, 10, or 12 mg/kg, respectively) should be added slowly to the diluent, and the bag or bottle should be inverted gently to mix the solution. The manufacturer states that tocilizumab infusion solutions are compatible with polypropylene, polyethylene, and polyvinyl chloride infusion bags and polypropylene, polyethylene, and glass infusion bottles. Prior to administration, tocilizumab infusion solutions should be inspected visually for particulate matter and discoloration; if either is present, the solution should be discarded. Tocilizumab infusion solutions may be stored at 2–8°C or room temperature for up to 24 hours and should be protected from light. Any unused portion remaining in the vial should be discarded since the injection concentrate contains no preservative.

Tocilizumab infusion solutions should be allowed to reach room temperature prior to administration. Tocilizumab should not be infused simultaneously through the same IV line with other drugs.

Subcutaneous Administration Tocilizumab is administered by subcutaneous injection. Tocilizumab is intended for use under the guidance and supervision of a clinician; however, the drug may be *self-administered* if the clinician determines that the patient and/or their caregiver is competent to safely administer the drug after appropriate training.

Tocilizumab for subcutaneous use is commercially available in prefilled single-use syringes equipped with a needle safety device. Each syringe delivers 162 mg of tocilizumab in 0.9 mL. The entire contents of the prefilled syringe should be administered as a single dose. Prior to administration, tocilizumab solutions should be inspected visually for particulate matter or discoloration; if the syringe appears to be damaged or the solution contains particulates or is cloudy or discolored, the solution should be discarded. Tocilizumab injection for subcutaneous use should be protected from light and stored at 2–8°C in the original carton until administration. The injection should not be frozen and the prefilled syringes should be kept dry. The syringe should be allowed to sit at room temperature outside of the carton for 30 minutes prior to subcutaneous injection; tocilizumab should not be warmed in any other way (e.g., microwave, hot water). The commercially available subcutaneous injection should not be used for IV administration.

Tocilizumab is administered subcutaneously into the anterior thigh or abdomen (except for the 2-inch area around the umbilicus). Tocilizumab may be administered subcutaneously into the upper arm by a caregiver. Injection sites should be rotated. Injections should not be made into areas where the skin is tender, bruised, red, hard, or nonintact or into scars or moles.

■ **Dosage** ***Rheumatoid Arthritis in Adults*** For the management of rheumatoid arthritis in adults who have had an inadequate response to one or more DMARDs, the recommended initial dosage of tocilizumab is 4 mg/kg IV once every 4 weeks; the dosage can be increased to 8 mg/kg IV once every 4 weeks based on clinical response. Doses exceeding 800 mg are not recommended (see Description).

Alternatively, adults with rheumatoid arthritis who weigh less than 100 kg may receive tocilizumab 162 mg subcutaneously every other week; the dosage can be increased to 162 mg every week based on clinical response. Patients who weigh 100 kg or more may receive tocilizumab 162 mg subcutaneously every week. (See Description and also see Clinical Experience with Subcutaneous Tocilizumab under Uses: Rheumatoid Arthritis in Adults.)

When switching from IV to subcutaneous administration, the first subcutaneous dose may be administered in place of the next scheduled IV dose.

Dosage Modification or Discontinuance for Toxicity. If a serious infection, an opportunistic infection, or sepsis develops, tocilizumab should be discontinued until the infection is controlled.

If certain dose-related laboratory changes (i.e., elevated liver enzyme concentrations, neutropenia, thrombocytopenia) occur in patients with rheumatoid arthritis receiving tocilizumab 8 mg/kg IV every 4 weeks, reduction in tocilizumab dosage to 4 mg/kg IV every 4 weeks or temporary interruption or discontinuance of tocilizumab therapy is recommended (see tables). If such dose-related laboratory changes occur in patients with rheumatoid arthritis receiving subcutaneous tocilizumab, reduction in the frequency of tocilizumab administration from weekly to every other week or temporary interruption or discontinuance of therapy is recommended (see tables).

Table 1. Recommended Dosage Adjustment Based on Changes in Liver Enzyme Laboratory Value in Adults with Rheumatoid Arthritis

ALT or AST Value	Recommendation
>1 to 3 times ULN	Modify dosage of concomitant DMARDs if appropriate For persistent increases within this range: IV: Reduce tocilizumab dosage to 4 mg/kg every 4 weeks or interrupt tocilizumab therapy until ALT/AST values have returned to normal Subcutaneous: Reduce frequency of tocilizumab administration to every other week or interrupt tocilizumab therapy until ALT/AST values have returned to normal; resume tocilizumab with administration every other week and then increase frequency to every week as clinically indicated
>3 to 5 times ULN (confirmed by repeat testing)	Interrupt tocilizumab therapy until ALT/AST values are <3 times ULN and follow recommendations for ALT/AST values of >1 to 3 times ULN For persistent increases of >3 times ULN, discontinue tocilizumab
>5 times ULN	Discontinue tocilizumab

Table 2. Recommended Dosage Adjustment Based on Absolute Neutrophil Count (ANC) in Adults with Rheumatoid Arthritis

ANC (cells/mm³)	Recommendation
>1000	Maintain current dosage
500–1000	Interrupt tocilizumab therapy When ANC is >1000/mm³: IV: Resume tocilizumab at 4 mg/kg every 4 weeks and increase to 8 mg/kg every 4 weeks as clinically indicated Subcutaneous: Resume tocilizumab with administration every other week and then increase frequency to every week as clinically indicated
<500	Discontinue tocilizumab

Table 3. Recommended Dosage Adjustment Based on Platelet Count in Adults with Rheumatoid Arthritis

Platelet Count (cells/mm³)	Recommendation
50,0000–100,000	Interrupt tocilizumab therapy When platelet count is >100,000/mm³: IV: Resume tocilizumab at 4 mg/kg every 4 weeks and increase to 8 mg/kg every 4 weeks as clinically indicated Subcutaneous: Resume tocilizumab with administration every other week and then increase frequency to every week as clinically indicated
<50,000	Discontinue tocilizumab

Juvenile Idiopathic Arthritis Tocilizumab is administered in a weight-adjusted dosage once every 4 weeks in patients with polyarticular JIA and once every 2 weeks in those with systemic JIA. For the management of polyarticular JIA in patients 2 years of age or older, the recommended dosage of tocilizumab is 10 mg/kg IV once every 4 weeks in those weighing less than 30 kg and 8 mg/kg IV once every 4 weeks in those weighing 30 kg or more. For the management of systemic JIA in patients 2 years of age or older, the recommended dosage of tocilizumab is 12 mg/kg IV once every 2 weeks in those weighing less than 30 kg and 8 mg/kg IV once every 2 weeks in those weighing 30 kg or more. Because the patient's weight may fluctuate, dosage should not be adjusted based solely on the patient's weight as measured at a single visit. If certain dose-related laboratory changes (i.e., elevated liver enzyme concentrations, neutropenia, thrombocytopenia) occur, interruption of therapy may be required.

Treatment Interruptions or Discontinuance for Toxicity. If a serious infection, an opportunistic infection, or sepsis develops, tocilizumab should be discontinued until the infection is controlled.

Tocilizumab dosage reductions have not been evaluated in patients with polyarticular or systemic JIA. However, interruption of tocilizumab therapy is recommended for certain dose-related laboratory changes (i.e., elevated liver enzyme concentrations, neutropenia, thrombocytopenia) at values similar to those considered in adults with rheumatoid arthritis (see tables). If clinically appropriate, dosage reduction or discontinuance of concomitant therapy with methotrexate and/or other agents should be considered and tocilizumab withheld pending clinical evaluation. The decision to discontinue tocilizumab therapy because of a laboratory abnormality should be individualized.

■ **Special Populations** Dosage adjustment is not necessary in patients with mild renal impairment; use of tocilizumab in patients with moderate or severe renal impairment has not been evaluated. Use of the drug in patients with hepatic impairment is not recommended. (See Hepatic Impairment under Warnings/Precautions: Specific Populations, in Cautions.) The manufacturer makes no specific dosage recommendations for geriatric patients.

Cautions

■ **Contraindications** Tocilizumab is contraindicated in patients with known hypersensitivity to the drug. (See Sensitivity Reactions under Warnings/Precautions: Other Warnings and Precautions, in Cautions.)

■ **Warnings/Precautions** ***Warnings*** **Infectious Complications.** Serious and sometimes fatal infections, including bacterial, mycobacterial, invasive fungal, viral, protozoal, or other opportunistic infections, have been reported in patients with rheumatoid arthritis receiving immunosuppressive agents including tocilizumab. Serious infections reported in patients with rheumatoid arthritis receiving tocilizumab have included pneumonia, urinary tract infection, cellulitis, herpes zoster, gastroenteritis, diverticulitis, sepsis, and septic (bacterial) arthritis. Opportunistic infections (e.g., tuberculosis, cryptococcal infection, aspergillosis, candidiasis, pneumocystosis) also have been reported in patients receiving tocilizumab. Other serious infections may occur. Patients have presented with disseminated rather than local disease; patients often were receiving concomitant therapy with immunosuppressive agents (e.g., methotrexate, corticosteroids) that, in addition to their underlying condition, could have predisposed them to infections.

Serious infections, including pneumonia, bronchitis, otitis media, upper respiratory tract infection, gastroenteritis, cellulitis, varicella, and herpes zoster, also have been reported in patients with polyarticular or systemic juvenile idiopathic arthritis (JIA) receiving tocilizumab.

Patients should be closely monitored during and after treatment with tocilizumab for the development of signs or symptoms of infection.

Tocilizumab therapy should not be initiated in patients with active infections, including localized infections. Clinicians should consider potential risks and benefits of the drug prior to initiating therapy in patients with a history of chronic, recurring, serious, or opportunistic infections; patients with underlying conditions that may predispose them to infections; and patients who have been exposed to tuberculosis or who reside or have traveled in regions where tuberculosis or mycoses are endemic. Any patient who develops a new infection while receiving tocilizumab should undergo a thorough diagnostic evaluation (appropriate for an immunocompromised patient), appropriate anti-infective therapy should be initiated, and the patient should be closely monitored. If a serious infection, an opportunistic infection, or sepsis develops, tocilizumab should be discontinued until the infection is controlled.

All patients should be evaluated for latent tuberculosis and for the presence of risk factors for tuberculosis prior to and periodically during therapy with tocilizumab. When indicated, an appropriate antimycobacterial regimen for the treatment of latent tuberculosis infection should be initiated prior to tocilizumab therapy. Antimycobacterial therapy should be considered prior to initiation of tocilizumab in individuals with a history of latent or active tuberculosis in whom an adequate course of antimycobacterial treatment cannot be confirmed and in individuals with a negative test for latent tuberculosis who have risk factors for tuberculosis. Consultation with a tuberculosis specialist is recommended when deciding whether antimicrobial therapy should be initiated. Patients receiving tocilizumab, including individuals with a negative test for latent tuberculosis, should be monitored for signs and symptoms of active tuberculosis.

Viral reactivation can occur in patients receiving immunosuppressive therapies. Herpes zoster exacerbation has been reported in patients receiving tocilizumab.

Other Warnings and Precautions **GI Perforation.** GI perforation has been reported in patients receiving tocilizumab, usually as a complication of diverticulitis in patients with rheumatoid arthritis. Most patients who experienced GI perforation were receiving concomitant therapy with nonsteroidal anti-inflammatory agents (NSAIAs), corticosteroids, or methotrexate. The relative contribution of these agents versus IV tocilizumab to the occurrence of GI perforation remains to be determined.

Caution is advised if tocilizumab is used in patients at risk for GI perforation. Patients who experience new-onset abdominal symptoms should be promptly evaluated for GI perforation.

Hematologic Effects. Reduction in neutrophil count to less than 1000/mm^3 has been reported during clinical trials in patients receiving tocilizumab. Decreases in neutrophil counts to below 1000/mm^3 did not appear to be associated with serious infection.

Reductions in platelet counts also have been reported in patients receiving tocilizumab. In clinical trials of the drug, decreases in platelet counts were not associated with severe bleeding.

Neutrophil and platelet counts should be monitored 4–8 weeks after initiation of tocilizumab therapy and every 3 months thereafter in adults with rheumatoid arthritis, at the time of the second tocilizumab infusion and every 4–8 weeks thereafter in patients with polyarticular JIA, and at the time of the second infusion and every 2–4 weeks thereafter in patients with systemic JIA. In patients with neutropenia or thrombocytopenia, dosage adjustment, treatment interruption, or discontinuance of the drug may be necessary. (See Dosage and Administration: Dosage.)

Hepatic Effects. Tocilizumab has been associated with elevated aminotransferase concentrations. In clinical trials, these changes were reversible following reduction of the tocilizumab or concomitant DMARD dosage or interruption of tocilizumab therapy and were not associated with clinical evidence of hepatic injury. The incidence and magnitude of aminotransferase elevations were increased when tocilizumab was used in conjunction with a hepatotoxic drug (e.g., methotrexate). In one patient, aminotransferase values were normal during tocilizumab therapy but increased substantially when methotrexate was added to the regimen. Aminotransferase values returned to normal once therapy with both drugs was discontinued.

Serum ALT and AST concentrations should be monitored 4–8 weeks after initiation of tocilizumab therapy and every 3 months thereafter in adults with rheumatoid arthritis, at the time of the second tocilizumab infusion and every 4–8 weeks thereafter in patients with polyarticular JIA, and at the time of the second infusion and every 2–4 weeks thereafter in patients with systemic JIA. Other liver function tests should be monitored when clinically indicated. In patients with elevated aminotransferase concentrations, dosage adjustment, treatment interruption, or discontinuance of tocilizumab or concomitantly administered DMARDs may be necessary. (See Dosage and Administration: Dosage.)

Effects on Serum Lipids. Increased serum concentrations of total cholesterol, triglycerides, low-density lipoprotein (LDL)-cholesterol, and/or high-density lipoprotein (HDL)-cholesterol have been reported in patients receiving tocilizumab.

In adults with rheumatoid arthritis or patients with polyarticular or systemic JIA, lipoprotein concentrations should be monitored 4–8 weeks after initiation of tocilizumab therapy and approximately every 24 weeks thereafter. Lipid disorders should be managed as clinically appropriate.

Malignancies. Immunosuppressive therapy may increase the risk of malignancies. Whether treatment with tocilizumab affects development of malignancies remains to be determined. Malignancies were reported in clinical trials of the drug.

Sensitivity Reactions. Hypersensitivity reactions, including anaphylaxis, have been reported in patients receiving tocilizumab; fatal anaphylactic reactions have occurred in those receiving IV infusions of the drug. During clinical trials of tocilizumab, hypersensitivity reactions requiring treatment discontinuance (e.g., anaphylaxis, generalized erythema, rash, urticaria) have been reported in various patient populations and with either IV or subcutaneous therapy. During postmarketing experience, hypersensitivity reactions, including anaphylaxis and death, have occurred in patients receiving various IV dosages, either with or without concomitant antirheumatic therapy, including in patients who received premedication. Hypersensitivity reactions, including anaphylaxis, have occurred both with and without prior hypersensitivity reactions and as early as the first IV infusion of the drug.

Appropriate agents and equipment should be available for immediate use in case a serious hypersensitivity reaction occurs during IV infusion of the drug. Patients receiving subcutaneous therapy with tocilizumab should be advised to seek medical attention if they experience symptoms of a hypersensitivity reaction (see Advice to Patients). If a hypersensitivity reaction occurs, administration of the drug should be stopped immediately and the drug should be permanently discontinued. Tocilizumab is contraindicated in patients with known hypersensitivity to the drug.

Nervous System Effects. The effect of tocilizumab on demyelinating disorders remains to be determined. Multiple sclerosis and chronic inflammatory demyelinating polyneuropathy have been reported rarely in patients with rheumatoid arthritis receiving tocilizumab in clinical trials. Patients receiving tocilizumab should be monitored for signs and symptoms suggestive of a demyelinating disorder. Clinicians should exercise caution when considering tocilizumab therapy in patients with preexisting or recent-onset demyelinating disorders.

Immunization. Live vaccines should be avoided in patients receiving tocilizumab. Vaccinations should be brought up to date prior to initiation of the drug. (See Drug Interactions: Vaccines.)

Immunogenicity. In clinical trials evaluating IV tocilizumab in patients with rheumatoid arthritis, antibodies to the drug were detected in about 2% of tocilizumab-treated patients; about 11% of these patients experienced hypersensitivity reactions resulting in drug discontinuance. Neutralizing antibodies developed in about 1% of such patients receiving the drug IV. In clinical trials evaluating subcutaneous tocilizumab in patients with rheumatoid arthritis, antibodies to the drug were detected in 0.9% of patients receiving the subcutaneous formulation; neutralizing antibodies developed in about 0.8% of patients receiving this formulation of the drug. No relationship between antibody development and adverse effects or loss of clinical response was observed, and detection rates were similar with IV or subcutaneous therapy. In clinical trials evaluating IV tocilizumab in patients with JIA, antibodies to the drug were detected in 3 patients and were associated with angioedema and urticaria in 1 patient.

Specific Populations **Pregnancy.** Category C. (See Users Guide.) Pregnancy registry at 877-311-8972.

Lactation. It is not known whether tocilizumab is distributed into milk or absorbed from the GI tract in breast-fed infants. Because immunoglobulin G (IgG) is distributed into human milk, it is possible that tocilizumab is distributed into milk. A decision should be made whether to discontinue nursing or the drug, taking into account the importance of the drug to the woman.

Pediatric Use. Safety and efficacy of IV tocilizumab for the management of active polyarticular or systemic JIA have been established in pediatric patients 2 years of age and older. Safety and efficacy of the drug in children younger than 2 years of age or for the management of conditions other that polyarticular or systemic JIA in children have not been established. Safety and efficacy of subcutaneous administration of the drug also have not been established in pediatric patients. In patients with polyarticular or systemic JIA, the pattern of adverse effects, including liver enzyme elevations, neutropenia, thrombocytopenia, and lipid abnormalities, is similar to that observed in adults with rheumatoid arthritis. In studies of a murine analog of tocilizumab in juvenile mice, no evidence of toxicity, including no impairment of skeletal growth, immune function, and sexual maturation, was observed.

Geriatric Use. Approximately 16% of patients with rheumatoid arthritis who received IV tocilizumab in clinical trials have been 65 years of age or older and about 2% have been 75 years of age or older. Approximately 28% of patients with rheumatoid arthritis who received subcutaneous tocilizumab in clinical trials have been 65 years of age or older and about 4% have been 75 years of age or older. Serious infection occurred with greater frequency in those 65 years of age or older relative to younger adults. Because the geriatric population in general may have a higher incidence of infections than younger adults, tocilizumab should be used with caution in this age group.

Hepatic Impairment. Safety and efficacy of tocilizumab have not been established in patients with hepatic impairment, including those with serologic evidence of hepatitis B virus (HBV) or hepatitis C virus (HCV) infection. Use of the drug in patients with active hepatic disease or hepatic impairment is not recommended.

Renal Impairment. Tocilizumab has not been evaluated in patients with moderate to severe renal impairment. Mild renal impairment (creatinine clearance less than 80 mL/minute but not less than 50 mL/minute) does not appear to alter the pharmacokinetics of the drug.

■ **Common Adverse Effects** Adverse effects reported in 5% or more of patients receiving tocilizumab include upper respiratory tract infection, nasopharyngitis, headache, hypertension, increased ALT concentrations, and reactions at the subcutaneous injection site (e.g., erythema, pruritus, pain, hematoma). The adverse effect profiles of IV and subcutaneous tocilizumab are similar except for a higher frequency of injection site reactions with subcutaneous administration.

Drug Interactions

■ **Drugs Metabolized by Hepatic Microsomal Enzymes** Possible increased metabolism of drugs that are metabolized by cytochrome P-450 (CYP) isoenzymes. Because cytokines such as interleukin-6 (IL-6) may down-regulate CYP enzymes, inhibition of IL-6 by tocilizumab in patients with rheumatoid arthritis may restore CYP enzyme activity to higher levels. In vitro studies indicate that tocilizumab may alter expression of CYP isoenzymes including 1A2, 2B6, 2C9, 2C19, 2D6, and 3A4; effects of the drug on CYP2C8 or transporters (e.g., P-glycoprotein) have not been elucidated. Effects of tocilizumab on CYP enzyme activity may persist for several weeks after the drug is discontinued.

Following initiation or discontinuance of tocilizumab therapy, patients receiving certain drugs metabolized by CYP isoenzymes (i.e., those with a low therapeutic index that require individualized dosing [e.g., cyclosporine, theophylline, warfarin]) should be monitored for therapeutic effect and/or changes in serum concentrations, and dosages of these drugs should be adjusted as needed. Caution also is advised when tocilizumab is used concomitantly with CYP3A4 substrates (e.g., oral contraceptives, atorvastatin, lovastatin) for which a reduction in efficacy would be undesirable.

Dextromethorphan Pharmacokinetic interaction (possible decreased exposure to dextromethorphan and/or dextrorphan). In patients with rheumatoid arthritis who are not receiving tocilizumab, administration of dextromethorphan

30 mg results in systemic exposure to dextromethorphan (a substrate of CYP2D6 and CYP3A4) that is similar to that observed in healthy individuals; however, exposure to the dextrorphan metabolite (a substrate of CYP3A4) is substantially reduced in rheumatoid arthritis patients. One week following IV administration of a single 8-mg/kg dose of tocilizumab, exposures to dextromethorphan and dextrorphan were decreased by 5 and 29%, respectively.

Omeprazole Pharmacokinetic interaction (possible decreased exposure to omeprazole following initiation of tocilizumab therapy). In patients with rheumatoid arthritis who are not receiving tocilizumab, administration of omeprazole 10 mg results in systemic exposure to omeprazole (a substrate of CYP2C19 and CYP3A4) that is approximately twofold higher than values observed in healthy individuals. In patients with rheumatoid arthritis who received 10 mg of omeprazole before and one week after IV administration of an 8-mg/kg dose of tocilizumab, systemic exposure to omeprazole (as measured by area under the plasma concentration-time curve [AUC]) decreased by 12% in poor and intermediate metabolizers of the drug and by 28% in extensive metabolizers; AUC values for omeprazole observed following the tocilizumab dose were slightly higher than values observed after omeprazole administration in healthy individuals.

Simvastatin Pharmacokinetic interaction (possible decreased exposure to simvastatin and simvastatin acid following initiation of tocilizumab therapy). In patients with rheumatoid arthritis who are not receiving tocilizumab, administration of simvastatin 40 mg results in systemic exposures to simvastatin (a substrate of CYP3A4 and organic anion transporter [OATP] 1B1) and its metabolite, simvastatin acid, that are approximately fourfold to tenfold higher and twofold higher, respectively, than values observed in healthy individuals. One week after rheumatoid arthritis patients received a single 10-mg/kg IV dose of tocilizumab, systemic exposures to simvastatin and simvastatin acid decreased by 57 and 39%, respectively, and values in the tocilizumab-treated patients were similar to or slightly higher than values observed after simvastatin administration in healthy individuals. Following discontinuance of tocilizumab in rheumatoid arthritis patients, systemic exposure to simvastatin and simvastatin acid increased. When selecting simvastatin dosages for patients with rheumatoid arthritis, clinicians should consider the potential for altered systemic exposure to the drug following initiation or discontinuance of tocilizumab therapy.

■ **Antirheumatic Drugs** Concomitant use of methotrexate, corticosteroids, and/or nonsteroidal anti-inflammatory agents (NSAIAs) does not appear to affect clearance of tocilizumab. Concomitant use of methotrexate (10–25 mg once weekly) and tocilizumab (single 10-mg/kg IV dose) did not affect exposure to methotrexate.

Tocilizumab has not been studied in conjunction with biologic disease-modifying antirheumatic drugs (DMARDs), including tumor necrosis factor (TNF; TNF-α) blocking agents. Concomitant use of tocilizumab with biologic DMARDs should be avoided. (See Uses.)

■ **Vaccines** Live vaccines should not be administered to patients receiving tocilizumab. Because inhibition of interleukin-6 (IL-6) may interfere with the normal immune response to new antigens, all patients (but particularly those with polyarticular or systemic juvenile idiopathic arthritis [JIA]) should receive all appropriate vaccines recommended by current immunization guidelines prior to initiation of tocilizumab therapy. The interval between administration of live vaccines and initiation of tocilizumab therapy should be in accordance with current vaccination guidelines regarding immunosuppressive agents. Information is not available regarding immune response to vaccines in patients receiving tocilizumab, nor is information available regarding secondary transmission of infection from individuals receiving live vaccines to patients receiving tocilizumab.

Description

Tocilizumab, a recombinant humanized monoclonal antibody specific for interleukin-6 (IL-6) receptor, is a biologic response modifier and a disease-modifying antirheumatic drug (DMARD). Tocilizumab is an IgG_1 kappa immunoglobulin that binds specifically to both soluble and membrane-bound IL-6 receptors and inhibits IL-6-mediated signaling through these receptors, thereby resulting in a reduction in inflammatory mediator production.

IL-6, a pleiotropic proinflammatory cytokine, is produced by various cell types, including T-cells, B-lymphocytes, monocytes, fibroblasts, synoviocytes, and endothelial cells, and has a broad spectrum of biologic activities. IL-6 is involved in T-cell activation, induction of immunoglobulin secretion, initiation of hepatic acute phase protein synthesis, stimulation of hematopoietic precursor cell proliferation and differentiation, and induction of osteoclast differentiation and activation. While the causes of rheumatoid arthritis have not been fully elucidated, proinflammatory cytokines, including IL-6, appear to play critical roles in the disease process. IL-6 is overexpressed in synovial tissue in patients with rheumatoid arthritis and is thought to contribute to synovial proliferation and joint destruction in patients with the disease. Elevated levels of IL-6 in serum and synovial fluid have been shown to correlate with clinical and laboratory measures of disease activity in patients with rheumatoid arthritis. IL-6 also is elevated in serum and synovial fluid in patients with polyarticular or systemic juvenile idiopathic arthritis (JIA), and the elevated levels of IL-6 have been correlated with disease activity.

Tocilizumab exhibits concentration-dependent clearance. At low tocilizumab concentrations, concentration-dependent nonlinear clearance plays a major role in determining total drug clearance; at higher concentrations, the nonlinear pathway is saturated and clearance is determined mainly by linear clearance. Linear clearance increases as body size increases; thus, following administration of a weight-based IV dose of 8 mg/kg in adults with rheumatoid arthritis, systemic drug exposure is substantially greater in individuals weighing more than 100 kg than in those weighing less than 60 kg (see Dosage and Administration: Dosage). At a fixed subcutaneous dosage, tocilizumab exposure is inversely related to body weight. The apparent steady-state half-life of tocilizumab in adults with rheumatoid arthritis is up to 11 or up to 13 days following IV administration of tocilizumab 4 or 8 mg/kg, respectively, every 4 weeks and up to 13 or up to 5 days after subcutaneous administration of tocilizumab 162 mg every week or every other week, respectively. The reported half-life in pediatric patients with polyarticular or systemic juvenile idiopathic arthritis (JIA) is up to 16 or up to 23 days, respectively.

Advice to Patients

A copy of the manufacturer's patient information (medication guide) for tocilizumab must be provided to all patients and/or caregivers prior to each infusion of the drug. Importance of advising patients and/or caregivers about potential benefits and risks of tocilizumab. Importance of patients and/or caregivers reading the medication guide prior to initiation of therapy and each time the drug is infused or the prescription is refilled.

Importance of instructing patient and/or caregiver regarding proper dosage and administration of tocilizumab, including the use of aseptic technique, and proper disposal of needles and syringes if it is determined that the patient and/or caregiver is competent to safely administer the drug.

Importance of consulting clinician if the subcutaneous injection does not deliver the full dose.

Risk of hypersensitivity reactions. Importance of contacting a clinician prior to administering the next dose if manifestations of an allergic reaction (e.g., urticaria, rash, flushing) occur; importance of seeking immediate medical attention if manifestations of a serious allergic reaction (e.g., difficulty breathing, chest pain, feelings of faintness or dizziness, abdominal pain or vomiting, swelling of the lips, tongue, or face) occur.

Risk of increased susceptibility to infection. Importance of informing clinicians immediately if any signs or symptoms suggestive of infection (e.g., fever; sweating; cough; dyspnea; diarrhea; burning or pain upon urination; warm, red, or painful skin) develop.

Risk of GI perforation. Importance of informing clinician immediately if severe, persistent abdominal pain occurs.

Importance of informing clinicians of existing or contemplated concomitant therapy, including prescription (e.g., biologic antirheumatic drugs, immunizations) and OTC drugs, as well as any concomitant illnesses or any history of tuberculosis or other chronic or recurring infections.

Importance of periodic laboratory monitoring.

Importance of women informing clinicians if they are or plan to become pregnant or plan to breast-feed.

Importance of informing patients of other important precautionary information. (See Cautions.)

Overview® (see Users Guide). For additional information on this drug until a more detailed monograph is developed and published, the manufacturer's labeling should be consulted. It is *essential* that the manufacturer's labeling be consulted for more detailed information on usual cautions, precautions, contraindications, potential drug interactions, laboratory test interferences, and acute toxicity.

Preparations

Excipients in commercially available drug preparations may have clinically important effects in some individuals; consult specific product labeling for details.

Tocilizumab (recombinant)

Parenteral

Injection, for subcutaneous use	162 mg/0.9 mL	**Actemra®** (available as single-use prefilled syringe), Genentech
Injection concentrate, for IV infusion	20 mg/mL	**Actemra®**, Genentech

Tofacitinib Citrate

Tasocitinib

■ Tofacitinib citrate, a Janus kinase (JAK) inhibitor, is an immunomodulating agent and a disease-modifying antirheumatic drug (DMARD).

Uses

■ **Rheumatoid Arthritis in Adults** Tofacitinib citrate (as conventional or extended-release tablets) is used for the management of moderately to severely active rheumatoid arthritis in adults who have had an inadequate response or intolerance to methotrexate. Tofacitinib has been shown to induce clinical responses, improve physical function, and inhibit progression of structural damage in patients with rheumatoid arthritis.

Tofacitinib can be used alone or in combination with methotrexate or other nonbiologic disease-modifying antirheumatic drugs (DMARDs; examples include hydroxychloroquine, leflunomide, minocycline, and sulfasalazine). Concomitant use of tofacitinib with biologic DMARDs, such as tumor necrosis factor (TNF) blocking agents (e.g., adalimumab, certolizumab pegol, etanercept, golimumab, infliximab), interleukin-1 (IL-1) receptor antagonists (e.g., anakinra), anti-CD20 monoclonal antibodies (e.g., rituximab), selective costimulation modulators (e.g., abatacept), and anti-interleukin-6-receptor monoclonal antibodies (e.g., sarilumab, tocilizumab), is not recommended. Concomitant use of tofacitinib with potent immunosuppressive agents (e.g., azathioprine, cyclosporine) also is not recommended.

Safety and efficacy of tofacitinib have been evaluated in 5 randomized, double-blind, controlled studies of 6–24 months' duration in adults (18 years of age or older) with moderate to severe active rheumatoid arthritis. In these studies, tofacitinib was administered as monotherapy in patients with an inadequate response to at least one biologic or nonbiologic DMARD, in combination with methotrexate in patients with an inadequate response to methotrexate or at least one TNF blocking agent, or in combination with nonbiologic DMARD(s) in patients with an inadequate response to at least one biologic or nonbiologic DMARD. Patients in these studies generally had 6 or more tender joints and 6 or more swollen joints. Those receiving low stable dosages of corticosteroids (equivalent to 10 mg or less of prednisone daily) and/or stable dosages of nonsteroidal anti-inflammatory agents (NSAIAs) generally could continue such agents. In some studies, patients also were allowed to continue stable dosages of antimalarial agents. Tofacitinib was administered orally at a dosage of 5 or 10 mg twice daily. In all 5 studies, patients randomized to receive placebo were subsequently advanced in a blinded manner to a second predetermined treatment of tofacitinib 5 or 10 mg twice daily. Advancement to tofacitinib therapy occurred at 3 months in clinical studies of 6 months' duration. In studies of at least 12 months' duration, treatment was advanced at 3 months in placebo recipients who were nonresponders and at 6 months in all other placebo recipients.

The principal measures of clinical response in studies evaluating the efficacy of tofacitinib were the American College of Rheumatology criteria for improvement (ACR response) in measures of disease activity, changes in the Health Assessment Questionnaire–Disability Index (HAQ-DI, a measure of physical function and disability), and achievement of a Disease Activity Score (DAS28 [ESR]) of less than 2.6 (i.e., DAS-defined remission) at 3 or 6 months. DAS28 (ESR) is a composite index of 4 weighted variables: swollen and tender counts for 28 joints, patient global assessment, and erythrocyte sedimentation rate (ESR). An ACR 20 response is achieved if the patient experiences a 20% or greater improvement in tender and swollen joint count and a 20% or greater improvement in at least 3 of the following criteria: patient pain assessment, patient global assessment, physician global assessment, patient self-assessed disability, or laboratory measures of disease activity (i.e., ESR or C-reactive protein [CRP] level). An ACR 50 or ACR 70 response is defined using the same criteria but with a level of improvement of 50 or 70%, respectively. Structural damage, as measured by changes in the total modified Sharp/van der Heijde score, a composite measure of radiographically assessed structural damage (i.e., joint erosion and joint space narrowing), also was assessed in the 2-year study.

Clinical evaluations of tofacitinib indicate that, in adults with active rheumatoid arthritis despite therapy with methotrexate or other DMARD(s), administration of tofacitinib (alone or in combination with methotrexate or other nonbiologic DMARDs) at a dosage of 5 or 10 mg twice daily results in higher ACR 20, ACR 50, and ACR 70 response rates at 3 and 6 months compared with placebo. In clinical trials, higher ACR 20 response rates compared with placebo were observed within 2 weeks. In clinical trials with a duration of at least 12 months, ACR response rates and HAQ-DI results were consistent at 6 and 12 months in patients receiving tofacitinib. Across the 5 clinical trials, improvements in HAQ-DI scores for tofacitinib versus placebo were similar.

In a 6-month study evaluating tofacitinib as monotherapy, 610 patients who had an inadequate response to prior DMARD therapy (biologic or nonbiologic) received tofacitinib 5 mg twice daily, tofacitinib 10 mg twice daily, or placebo. An ACR 20 response at 3 months was achieved in 59, 65, or 26% of patients receiving tofacitinib 5 mg twice daily, tofacitinib 10 mg twice daily, or placebo, respectively. The ACR 20 response rate following 6 months of therapy with tofacitinib 5 or 10 mg twice daily was 69 or 70%, respectively. Patients receiving tofacitinib experienced greater improvements in physical functioning (as measured by change in HAQ-DI score) from baseline to 3 months, but were not substantially more likely to achieve DAS-defined remission at 3 months, compared with patients receiving placebo.

In a 12-month clinical study evaluating concomitant therapy with tofacitinib and methotrexate, 717 patients with an inadequate response to prior methotrexate therapy were randomized to receive tofacitinib 5 or 10 mg twice daily, adalimumab 40 mg subcutaneously every other week, or placebo, each given in conjunction with a stable dosage of methotrexate. Patients receiving tofacitinib 5 or 10 mg twice daily demonstrated greater improvement from baseline in physical functioning at 3 months compared with patients receiving placebo. The mean difference from placebo in HAQ-DI improvement from baseline was −0.22 or −0.32 in patients receiving tofacitinib 5 or 10 mg twice daily, respectively. At 6 months, an ACR 20 response was achieved in 52, 53, 47, or 28% and DAS-defined remission was achieved in 6, 13, 7, or 1% of patients assigned to receive tofacitinib 5 mg twice daily, tofacitinib 10 mg twice daily, adalimumab, or placebo, respectively; in these analyses, in order to account for patients who switched from placebo to tofacitinib at 3 months, patients who did not respond by 3 months were considered nonresponders even if they responded after 3 months.

In a 24-month clinical study evaluating concomitant therapy with tofacitinib and methotrexate, 797 patients with an inadequate response to prior methotrexate therapy were randomized to receive tofacitinib 5 or 10 mg twice daily or placebo, each given in conjunction with a stable dosage of methotrexate. Patients receiving tofacitinib 10 mg twice daily, but not those receiving tofacitinib 5 mg twice daily, demonstrated greater improvement from baseline in HAQ-DI scores at 3 months compared with patients receiving placebo. An ACR 20 response at 3 months was achieved in 55, 67, or 27% of patients receiving tofacitinib 5 mg twice daily, tofacitinib 10 mg twice daily, or placebo, respectively; at 6 months, ACR 20 response rates were 50, 62, and 25%, respectively. DAS-defined remission at 6 months was reported in 6, 13, or 1% of patients assigned to receive tofacitinib 5 mg twice daily, tofacitinib 10 mg twice daily, or placebo, respectively. In these analyses, patients who did not achieve a response by month 3 were considered nonresponders even if they achieved a response after month 3. At 6 months, tofacitinib 10 mg twice daily inhibited progression of structural damage, as measured by mean change in the total modified Sharp/van der Heijde score, compared with placebo; the difference between tofacitinib 5 mg twice daily and placebo did not reach statistical significance. At 6 months, 84 or 79% of patients receiving tofacitinib 5 or 10 mg twice daily, respectively, had no progression of structural damage compared with 74% of those receiving placebo. Although radiographic findings from this study suggested that tofacitinib slows progression of joint damage, interpretation of the results is complicated because the proportion of study patients with radiographic progression of structural damage during this time period was small, approximately one-half of placebo recipients were considered nonresponders at 3 months and were advanced to a tofacitinib regimen, and missing data created problems with analysis.

Another 6-month clinical study evaluated concomitant therapy with tofacitinib and methotrexate in 399 patients with an inadequate response to prior therapy with at least one TNF blocking agent; patients were randomized to receive tofacitinib 5 or 10 mg twice daily or placebo, each given in conjunction with a stable dosage of methotrexate. An ACR 20 response at 3 months was achieved in 41, 48, or 24% of patients receiving tofacitinib 5 mg twice daily, tofacitinib 10 mg twice daily, or placebo, respectively. The ACR 20 response rate following 6 months of therapy with tofacitinib 5 or 10 mg twice daily was 51 or 54%, respectively. Patients receiving tofacitinib experienced greater improvements in physical functioning (as measured by change in HAQ-DI score) from baseline to 3 months and were substantially more likely to achieve DAS-defined remission at 3 months compared with patients receiving placebo. DAS-defined remission was reported at 3 months in 7, 9, or 2% of patients receiving tofacitinib 5 mg twice daily, tofacitinib 10 mg twice daily, or placebo, respectively. The DAS-defined remission rate following 6 months of therapy with tofacitinib 5 or 10 mg twice daily was 8 or 15%, respectively.

In a 12-month study in 792 patients with an inadequate response to at least one biologic or nonbiologic DMARD, tofacitinib 5 or 10 mg twice daily or placebo was added to a stable dosage of a nonbiologic DMARD (excluding potent immunosuppressive agents such as azathioprine or cyclosporine). ACR responses and improvements in physical functioning generally were similar to those observed in other clinical studies evaluating tofacitinib for management of rheumatoid arthritis.

A sixth clinical study, which was conducted in 952 adults with moderately to severely active rheumatoid arthritis who had never received methotrexate therapy, provided additional evidence that tofacitinib inhibits progression of joint damage. In this 2-year study, patients were randomized to receive tofacitinib 5 or 10 mg twice daily or methotrexate (initiated at a dosage of 10 mg weekly and increased to 20 mg weekly, if tolerated, by week 8). At 6 and 12 months, tofacitinib 5 or 10 mg twice daily inhibited progression of structural damage, as measured by the mean change from baseline in the total modified Sharp/van der Heijde score, compared with methotrexate. At 6 months, 73 or 77% of patients receiving tofacitinib 5 or 10 mg twice daily, respectively, had no progression of structural damage compared with 55% of patients receiving methotrexate.

Although other dosages of tofacitinib have been studied, the recommended dosage of tofacitinib for the management of rheumatoid arthritis in adults is 5 mg twice daily. A dosage of 10 mg twice daily is *not* recommended for the management of rheumatoid arthritis. (See Warnings under Cautions: Warnings/Precautions.)

For further information on the treatment of rheumatoid arthritis, see Uses: Rheumatoid Arthritis, in Methotrexate 10:00.

■ **Psoriatic Arthritis** Tofacitinib citrate (as conventional or extended-release tablets) is used for the management of active psoriatic arthritis in adults who have had an inadequate response or intolerance to methotrexate or other DMARDs. Tofacitinib has been shown to induce clinical responses and improve physical functioning in patients with psoriatic arthritis. Concomitant use of tofacitinib with biologic DMARDs (see Uses: Rheumatoid Arthritis in Adults) or with potent immunosuppressive agents (e.g., azathioprine, cyclosporine) is not recommended.

Efficacy and safety of tofacitinib for the management of psoriatic arthritis in adults have been established in 2 randomized, double-blind studies. OPAL Broaden was a 12-month active-and placebo-controlled study in 422 patients who had not responded adequately to at least one nonbiologic DMARD and had not received prior therapy with a TNF blocking agent. OPAL Beyond was a 6-month placebo-controlled study in 394 patients with a history of inadequate response or intolerance to at least one TNF blocking agent. Patients in both studies had active psoriatic arthritis (with at least 3 tender/painful joints and at least 3 swollen joints) and active plaque psoriasis. In OPAL Broaden, patients were randomized in a 2:2:2:1:1 ratio to receive tofacitinib 5 mg twice daily, tofacitinib 10 mg twice daily, adalimumab 40 mg every 2 weeks, placebo for 3 months followed by tofacitinib 5 mg twice daily, or placebo for 3 months followed by tofacitinib 10 mg twice daily. In OPAL Beyond, patients were randomized in 2:2:1:1 ratio to receive tofacitinib 5 mg twice daily, tofacitinib 10 mg twice daily, placebo for 3 months followed by tofacitinib 5 mg twice daily, or placebo for 3 months followed by tofacitinib 10 mg twice daily. Patients in both studies received concomitant therapy with a stable dosage of a single conventional nonbiologic DMARD, most commonly methotrexate, throughout the study. The primary measures of efficacy were the proportion of patients achieving an ACR 20 response at 3 months and the change from baseline in HAQ-DI score at 3 months; ACR 50 and ACR 70 responses also were assessed. OPAL Broaden was not designed to evaluate noninferiority or superiority of tofacitinib compared with adalimumab.

Patients enrolled in the 2 studies had various manifestations of psoriatic arthritis: involvement of more than 5 joints (90%), distal interphalangeal joint involvement (61%), involvement of fewer than 5 joints or asymmetric involvement (21%), spondylitis (19%), and arthritis mutilans (8%). Enthesitis or dactylitis was present in 80 or 53% of patients, respectively. The mean duration of the disease prior to enrollment in OPAL Broaden or OPAL Beyond was 6 or 9.4 years, respectively. In OPAL Beyond, 66, 19, or 15% of patients had experienced treatment failure following use of 1, 2, or at least 3 TNF blocking agents, respectively.

A greater proportion of patients receiving tofacitinib (5 or 10 mg twice daily) compared with those receiving placebo achieved ACR 20, ACR 50, and ACR 70 responses at 3 months in OPAL Broaden and ACR 20 and ACR 50 responses in OPAL Beyond. In these 2 studies, ACR 20, ACR 50, and ACR 70 responses were achieved at 3 months in 50, 28–30, and 17%, respectively, of patients receiving tofacitinib 5 mg twice daily; 47–61, 28–40, and 14%, respectively, of patients receiving tofacitinib 10 mg twice daily; 52, 33, and 19%, respectively, of those receiving adalimumab 40 mg every 2 weeks (in OPAL Broaden); and 24–33, 10–15, and 5–10%, respectively, of those receiving placebo. Improvement in ACR 20 response was observed within 2 weeks following initiation of tofacitinib therapy. ACR responses were maintained through the end of the studies (6 or 12 months), but could not be compared with placebo because of the advancement from placebo to tofacitinib at 3 months. Improvements in dactylitis and enthesitis also were observed in tofacitinib-treated patients.

Improvements in physical function, as measured by change in HAQ-DI score from baseline to 3 months, were greater in both studies for patients receiving tofacitinib 5 or 10 mg twice daily compared with those receiving placebo. In the 2 studies, 50–53 of patients receiving tofacitinib 5 mg twice daily and 41–55% of those receiving tofacitinib 10 mg twice daily achieved a HAQ-DI response (defined as improvement from baseline to 3 months of 0.35 or greater) compared with 28–31% of those receiving placebo.

Although radiographic evaluations were performed at baseline and 12 months in OPAL Broaden, all placebo recipients were advanced to tofacitinib therapy at 3 months and mean change in total modified Sharp/van der Heijde score from baseline to 12 months was minimal in all treatment groups in this study. Comparisons between the tofacitinib groups and the placebo or adalimumab groups were insufficient to establish an effect of tofacitinib on progression of structural damage in patients with psoriatic arthritis.

Although other dosages of tofacitinib have been studied, the recommended dosage of tofacitinib for the management of psoriatic arthritis in adults is 5 mg twice daily. A dosage of 10 mg twice daily is *not* recommended for the management of psoriatic arthritis. (See Warnings under Cautions: Warnings/Precautions.)

■ **Ulcerative Colitis** Tofacitinib citrate (as conventional tablets) is used for the management of moderately to severely active ulcerative colitis in adults who have had an inadequate response to or have not tolerated therapy with TNF blocking agents. Tofacitinib has been shown to induce clinical remission, improve endoscopic appearance of the mucosa, and produce sustained corticosteroid-free remission during maintenance therapy in patients with ulcerative colitis. Concomitant use of tofacitinib with biologic therapies for ulcerative colitis or with potent immunosuppressive agents (e.g., azathioprine, cyclosporine) is not recommended.

Efficacy and safety of tofacitinib for the management of ulcerative colitis in adults have been established in 3 randomized, double-blind, placebo-controlled studies, including 2 identically designed studies (OCTAVE Induction studies 1 and 2) evaluating tofacitinib as induction therapy in a total of 1139 patients and one study (OCTAVE Sustain) evaluating tofacitinib as maintenance therapy in 593 patients who achieved a clinical response upon completion of an OCTAVE Induction study.

Patients enrolled in the induction studies had moderately to severely active ulcerative colitis (as defined by a Mayo score of 6–12 with an endoscopy subscore of at least 2 and rectal bleeding subscore of at least 1) and had a history of inadequate response or intolerance (i.e., treatment failure) to at least 1 of the following drugs: oral or IV corticosteroids, azathioprine, mercaptopurine, or a TNF blocking agent. The Mayo score ranges from 0–12 and includes 4 subscales (i.e., stool frequency, rectal bleeding, findings on endoscopy, and physician global assessment), each scored from 0–3 (normal to most severe, respectively). An endoscopy subscore of 2 is defined by marked erythema, lack of vascular pattern, friability, and erosions, whereas an endoscopy subscore of 3 is defined by spontaneous bleeding and ulceration. The median baseline Mayo score for the induction studies was 9. Patients were randomized in a 4:1 ratio to receive tofacitinib (10 mg twice daily) or placebo for 8 weeks. Stable dosages of oral aminosalicylates and corticosteroids (up to 25 mg daily of prednisone or equivalent) were permitted during the induction studies, but concomitant therapy with immunosuppressive agents (oral immunomodulators or biologic therapies) was not allowed. In the 2 induction studies combined, 52, 73, or 72% of patients had a history of treatment failure with TNF blocking agents, corticosteroids, or immunosuppressive agents, respectively. During the induction studies, 47% of patients received concomitant therapy with oral corticosteroids and 71% received aminosalicylates.

In the induction studies, the primary measure of efficacy was the proportion of patients achieving clinical remission at 8 weeks; other outcome measures included clinical response and improved or normalized mucosal appearance at 8 weeks. Clinical remission was defined as a Mayo score of 0–2 with no individual subscore exceeding 1 and a rectal bleeding subscore of 0. Clinical response was defined as a decrease in Mayo score of at least 3 points and at least 30% from baseline score, with a reduction in rectal bleeding subscore of at least 1 point or an absolute rectal bleeding subscore of 0 (no blood seen) or 1 (streaks of blood with stool less than half the time). Improved mucosal appearance was defined as a Mayo endoscopy subscore of 0 (normal mucosa or inactive disease) or 1 (erythema, decreased vascular pattern), and normalized mucosal appearance was defined as a Mayo endoscopy subscore of 0.

In both induction studies, clinical remission rates and rates of improved mucosal appearance were higher in patients receiving tofacitinib compared with those receiving placebo. Clinical remission was achieved in 17–18 or 4–8% of patients receiving tofacitinib or placebo, respectively, and improved mucosal appearance was observed in 28–31 or 12–16% of those receiving tofacitinib or placebo, respectively. In addition, clinical response was achieved in 55–60 or 29–33% of patients receiving tofacitinib or placebo, respectively, and mucosal appearance was normalized in 7% of patients receiving tofacitinib and 2% of those receiving placebo in both studies. Decreases in subscores for rectal bleeding and stool frequency were observed as early as 2 weeks in patients receiving tofacitinib.

In OCTAVE Sustain, patients who achieved a clinical response at 8 weeks in OCTAVE Induction study 1 or 2 were re-randomized in a 1:1:1 ratio to receive tofacitinib (5 or 10 mg twice daily) or placebo for 52 weeks. Approximately 30% of patients were in clinical remission at the start of the maintenance study; 49% were receiving oral corticosteroids; and 45, 75, or 70% had a history of treatment failure with TNF blocking agents, corticosteroids, or immunosuppressive agents, respectively. In patients receiving corticosteroids, a corticosteroid-tapering regimen was initiated at the start of the maintenance trial. As in the induction studies, concomitant therapy with oral aminosalicylates was permitted, but concomitant therapy with immunosuppressive agents (oral immunomodulators or biologic therapies) was not allowed. The primary measure of efficacy was the proportion of patients in clinical remission at 52 weeks. Other outcome measures included improved or normalized mucosal appearance at 52 weeks, maintenance of clinical response (i.e., clinical response at both baseline and 52 weeks), maintenance of clinical remission (i.e., clinical remission at both baseline and 52 weeks), and sustained corticosteroid-free remission (i.e., corticosteroid-free remission at baseline, 24 weeks, and 52 weeks).

In the maintenance study, both dosages of tofacitinib were more effective than placebo for achieving remission at 52 weeks, improved mucosal appearance at 52 weeks, and sustained corticosteroid-free remission. Clinical remission was achieved at 52 weeks in 34 or 41% of patients receiving tofacitinib 5 or 10 mg twice daily, respectively, compared with 11% of those receiving placebo. Improved mucosal appearance was observed at 52 weeks in 37 or 46% of patients receiving tofacitinib 5 or 10 mg twice daily, respectively, compared with 13% of those receiving placebo. Sustained corticosteroid-free remission was achieved in 35 or 47% of patients receiving tofacitinib 5 or 10 mg twice daily, respectively, compared with 5% of those receiving placebo. In addition, maintenance of clinical remission or clinical response was observed in 46 or 52%, respectively, of patients receiving tofacitinib 5 mg twice daily; 56 or 62%, respectively, of those receiving tofacitinib 10 mg twice daily, and 10 or 20%, respectively, of those receiving placebo. Mucosal appearance was normalized at 52 weeks in 15, 17, or 4% of patients receiving these respective treatments.

Exploratory subgroup analysis demonstrated treatment effects regardless of prior failure of TNF blocking agent therapy, but suggested that response and remission rates tended to be higher in patients without a history of failed therapy with TNF blocking agents.

Data are available from an open-label extension study for a subset of 291 patients who did not achieve a clinical response upon completion of an OCTAVE Induction study but continued to receive tofacitinib at a dosage of 10 mg twice daily; after a total of 16 weeks of tofacitinib therapy, 149 of these patients (51%) achieved a clinical response and 25 patients (8.6%) achieved clinical remission. Data available at 52 weeks (for 144 of these patients) indicated that 65 patients were in clinical remission following 52 weeks of treatment with tofacitinib 10 mg twice daily.

Dosage and Administration

■ **General** Tofacitinib therapy should not be initiated in patients with a lymphocyte count of less than 500/mm³, an absolute neutrophil count (ANC) of less than 1000/mm³, or a hemoglobin concentration of less than 9 g/dL.

Tofacitinib should not be used concomitantly with biologic disease-modifying antirheumatic drugs (DMARDs) or potent immunosuppressive agents. (See Uses: Rheumatoid Arthritis in Adults.)

Concomitant use of tofacitinib with potent inducers of cytochrome P-450 (CYP) isoenzyme 3A4 (e.g., rifampin) may result in loss of or reduced clinical response to tofacitinib.

■ **Administration** Tofacitinib citrate conventional or extended-release tablets are administered orally without regard to meals. The extended-release tablets should be swallowed intact and should not be crushed, split, or chewed.

■ **Dosage** Dosage of tofacitinib citrate is expressed in terms of tofacitinib.

Dosage recommendations specific to the condition being treated should be followed. (See Warnings under Cautions: Warnings/Precautions.)

Rheumatoid Arthritis or Psoriatic Arthritis in Adults For the management of rheumatoid arthritis in adults who have had an inadequate response or intolerance to methotrexate or for the management of psoriatic arthritis in adults who have had an inadequate response or intolerance to methotrexate or other DMARDs, the recommended dosage of tofacitinib is 5 mg twice daily (as conventional tablets) or 11 mg once daily (as extended-release tablets). Patients receiving tofacitinib 5 mg twice daily (as conventional tablets) may be switched to tofacitinib 11 mg once daily (as extended-release tablets) the day following the last dose of the conventional tablets. A dosage of 10 mg twice daily (as conventional tablets) is *not* recommended for the management of rheumatoid arthritis or psoriatic arthritis. (See Warnings under Cautions: Warnings/Precautions.)

In patients receiving concomitant therapy with potent inhibitors of CYP3A4 (e.g., ketoconazole) and in patients receiving concomitant therapy with one or more drugs that result in both moderate inhibition of CYP3A4 and potent inhibition of CYP2C19 (e.g., fluconazole), dosage of tofacitinib should be reduced to 5 mg once daily (as conventional tablets).

Dosage Modifications for Toxicity. If a serious infection develops, tofacitinib therapy should be interrupted until the infection has been controlled.

Tofacitinib therapy also should be interrupted or discontinued in patients with lymphopenia, neutropenia, or anemia. (See Hematologic Effects under Warnings/Precautions: Other Warnings/Precautions, in Cautions.)

In patients who develop a lymphocyte count of less than 500/mm³ (confirmed by repeat testing), tofacitinib should be discontinued.

In patients with a persistent decrease in ANC to 500–1000/mm³, tofacitinib therapy should be interrupted until the ANC exceeds 1000/mm³; tofacitinib therapy then may be resumed at the usual dosage of 5 mg twice daily (as conventional tablets) or 11 mg once daily (as extended-release tablets). Tofacitinib therapy should be discontinued in patients with an ANC of less than 500/mm³.

In patients with a decrease in hemoglobin concentration of more than 2 g/dL or with a hemoglobin concentration of less than 8 g/dL, tofacitinib therapy should be interrupted until the hemoglobin concentration has normalized.

Ulcerative Colitis For the management of ulcerative colitis in adults who have had an inadequate response or intolerance to tumor necrosis factor (TNF) blocking agents, the recommended dosage of tofacitinib (as conventional tablets) for induction therapy is 10 mg twice daily for 8 weeks; patients should then be evaluated and, depending on therapeutic response, may begin maintenance therapy with the drug. If necessary, the induction dosage of 10 mg twice daily may be administered for a maximum of 16 weeks. If adequate therapeutic benefit is not achieved after 16 weeks of treatment with tofacitinib 10 mg twice daily, this dosage should be discontinued.

The recommended adult maintenance dosage is 5 mg twice daily. Use of 10 mg twice daily beyond the induction period should be reserved for patients with loss of response and should be limited to the shortest duration needed, with careful consideration of potential benefits and risks for the individual patient. (See Warnings under Cautions: Warnings/Precautions.) The lowest effective dosage that maintains response should be used.

In patients receiving concomitant therapy with potent inhibitors of CYP3A4 (e.g., ketoconazole) and in patients receiving concomitant therapy with one or more drugs that result in both moderate inhibition of CYP3A4 and potent inhibition of CYP2C19 (e.g., fluconazole), dosage of tofacitinib should be reduced from 10 mg twice daily to 5 mg twice daily or from 5 mg twice daily to 5 mg once daily.

Dosage Modifications for Toxicity. If a serious infection develops, tofacitinib therapy should be interrupted until the infection has been controlled.

Tofacitinib therapy also should be interrupted or discontinued in patients with lymphopenia, neutropenia, or anemia. (See Hematologic Effects under Warnings/Precautions: Other Warnings/Precautions, in Cautions.)

In patients who develop a lymphocyte count of less than 500/mm³ (confirmed by repeat testing), tofacitinib should be discontinued.

In patients with a persistent decrease in ANC to 500–1000/mm³ on a dosage of 10 mg twice daily, dosage of the drug should be reduced to 5 mg twice daily; when the ANC exceeds 1000/mm³, dosage may be returned to 10 mg twice daily based on clinical response. In patients with a persistent decrease in ANC to 500–1000/mm³ on a dosage of 5 mg twice daily, tofacitinib therapy should be interrupted until the ANC exceeds 1000/mm³; tofacitinib therapy then may be resumed at a dosage of 5 mg twice daily. Tofacitinib therapy should be discontinued in patients with an ANC of less than 500/mm³.

In patients with a decrease in hemoglobin concentration of more than 2 g/dL or with a hemoglobin concentration of less than 8 g/dL, tofacitinib therapy should be interrupted until the hemoglobin concentration has normalized.

■ **Special Populations** Tofacitinib should not be used in patients with severe hepatic impairment. For the management of rheumatoid arthritis or psoriatic arthritis in patients with moderate or severe renal impairment (including those receiving hemodialysis) and in patients with moderate hepatic impairment, dosage of tofacitinib should be reduced to 5 mg once daily (as conventional tablets); those receiving tofacitinib extended-release tablets should be switched to therapy with the conventional tablets at a dosage of 5 mg once daily. For the management of ulcerative colitis in patients with moderate or severe renal impairment (including those receiving hemodialysis) and in patients with moderate hepatic impairment, dosage of tofacitinib (as conventional tablets) should be reduced from 10 mg twice daily to 5 mg twice daily or from 5 mg twice daily to 5 mg once daily. In patients with renal impairment receiving hemodialysis, the dose should be administered after the dialysis session on dialysis days; if a dose is taken before the dialysis procedure, administration of a supplemental dose following dialysis is not necessary. Dosage adjustment is not necessary in patients with mild renal or hepatic impairment. In addition, dosage adjustments based on body weight, ethnicity, gender, or age are not required.

Cautions

■ **Contraindications** The manufacturer states that there are no known contraindications to the use of tofacitinib.

■ **Warnings/Precautions** ***Warnings*** **Infectious Complications.** Patients receiving tofacitinib are at increased risk of developing serious infections that may require hospitalization or result in death. Serious and sometimes fatal infections caused by bacterial, mycobacterial, invasive fungal, viral, or other opportunistic organisms—including cryptococcosis, pneumocystosis, histoplasmosis, tuberculosis and other mycobacterial infections, esophageal candidiasis, multidermatomal herpes zoster, cytomegalovirus infection, listeriosis, and BK virus infection—have been reported in patients receiving tofacitinib. The most common serious infections reported in patients receiving tofacitinib included pneumonia, cellulitis, herpes zoster, urinary tract infection, diverticulitis, and appendicitis. Other serious infections (e.g., coccidioidomycosis) also may occur. Patients may present with disseminated rather than localized disease. Most patients who developed serious infections were receiving concomitant therapy with immunosuppressive agents such as methotrexate or corticosteroids.

In controlled clinical trials in patients with rheumatoid arthritis, the overall frequency of infections during the first 3 months of treatment was 20, 22, or 18% in patients receiving tofacitinib 5 mg twice daily, tofacitinib 10 mg twice daily, or placebo, respectively. Serious infections were reported at a rate of 1.7 events per 100 patient-years in tofacitinib-treated patients and 0.5 events per 100 patient-years in placebo-treated patients during the first 3 months of therapy. The rate of serious infections during the first 12 months of tofacitinib therapy was 2.7 events per 100 patient-years.

In patients with ulcerative colitis, the risk of serious infections and herpes zoster (including meningoencephalitis and ophthalmologic and disseminated cutaneous infections) was dose dependent, occurring more frequently in patients receiving tofacitinib 10 mg twice daily compared with those receiving tofacitinib 5 mg twice daily.

The risk of infection may be higher with increasing degrees of lymphopenia. (See Hematologic Effects under Warnings/Precautions: Other Warnings/Precautions, in Cautions.) Lymphocyte counts should be considered when assessing an individual patient's risk of infection.

Because of the higher incidence of infections generally observed in patients with diabetes mellitus, tofacitinib should be used with caution in diabetic patients. In addition, because patients with a history of chronic lung disease and those who develop interstitial lung disease may be more susceptible to infections, caution is advised in these patients.

Patients should be closely monitored during and after treatment with tofacitinib for the development of signs or symptoms of infection (e.g., fever, malaise, weight loss, sweats, cough, dyspnea, pulmonary infiltrates, serious systemic illness including shock).

Tofacitinib therapy should not be initiated in patients with serious active infections, including localized infections. Tofacitinib should be discontinued in patients who develop a serious infection, opportunistic infection, or sepsis and should not be resumed until the infection is controlled. Clinicians should consider potential risks and benefits of tofacitinib prior to initiating therapy in patients with a history of chronic, recurring, serious, or opportunistic infections; patients with underlying conditions that may predispose them to infections; and patients who have been exposed to tuberculosis or who reside or have traveled in regions where tuberculosis or mycoses are endemic. Any patient who develops a new infection while receiving tofacitinib should undergo a thorough diagnostic evaluation (appropriate for an immunocompromised patient), appropriate anti-infective therapy should be initiated, and the patient should be closely monitored.

Because tuberculosis has been reported in patients receiving tofacitinib, all patients should be evaluated for active or latent tuberculosis and for the presence of risk factors for tuberculosis prior to and periodically during therapy with the drug. When indicated, an appropriate antimycobacterial regimen for the treatment of latent tuberculosis infection should be initiated prior to tofacitinib therapy. Antimycobacterial therapy also should be considered prior to initiation of tofacitinib in individuals with a history of latent or active tuberculosis in whom an adequate course of antimycobacterial therapy cannot be confirmed and in individuals with a negative test for latent tuberculosis who have risk factors for tuberculosis. Consultation with a tuberculosis specialist is recommended when deciding whether antimycobacterial therapy should be initiated. Patients receiving tofacitinib, including individuals with a negative test for latent tuberculosis, should be monitored for signs and symptoms of active tuberculosis, which may present with pulmonary or extrapulmonary disease.

Viral reactivation can occur in patients receiving tofacitinib. Herpes zoster reactivation has been reported in patients receiving the drug. The risk of herpes zoster is increased in patients receiving tofacitinib and appears to be increased in patients treated in Japan or Korea.

Reactivation of hepatitis B virus (HBV) infection also has been reported during postmarketing experience. The effect of tofacitinib on the risk of reactivation of chronic viral hepatitis is not known; patients with serologic evidence of HBV or hepatitis C virus (HCV) infection were excluded from clinical trials of the drug. All patients should be screened for viral hepatitis in accordance with clinical guidelines before initiation of tofacitinib therapy.

Mortality. In an ongoing postmarketing study evaluating safety of tofacitinib in patients with rheumatoid arthritis, interim analysis revealed a higher overall mortality rate, including sudden cardiovascular death, in patients receiving tofacitinib 10 mg twice daily compared with those receiving either tofacitinib 5 mg twice daily or a tumor necrosis factor (TNF) blocking agent, each given in combination with methotrexate. Because the study was designed to assess cardiovascular risks as well as risks of cancer and opportunistic infections, enrolled patients were 50 years of age or older and had at least one cardiovascular risk factor. Interim analysis revealed 45 deaths during 3884 patient-years of follow-up in patients receiving tofacitinib 10 mg twice daily compared with 25 deaths during 3982 patient-years of follow-up in those receiving TNF blocking agents. FDA will reassess this safety concern when final study results are available. (See Thromboembolic Complications under Warnings/Precautions: Warnings, in Cautions.)

The 10-mg twice-daily dosage of tofacitinib is FDA-labeled only for the management of ulcerative colitis for use as induction therapy and in limited situations during maintenance therapy. (See Ulcerative Colitis under Dosage and Administration: Dosage.) Tofacitinib at a dosage of 10 mg twice daily (as conventional tablets) or 22 mg once daily (as extended-release tablets) is *not* recommended for the management of rheumatoid arthritis or psoriatic arthritis. In patients with ulcerative colitis, tofacitinib should be used at the lowest effective dosage and for the shortest duration needed to achieve and maintain therapeutic response.

Malignancies and Lymphoproliferative Disorders. Lymphoma and other malignancies (e.g., lung cancer, breast cancer, melanoma, prostate cancer, pancreatic cancer) have been observed in patients receiving tofacitinib. In addition, an increased incidence of Epstein Barr virus (EBV)-associated posttransplant lymphoproliferative disorder has been observed in renal allograft recipients receiving tofacitinib concomitantly with immunosuppressive agents.

Among 3328 patients with rheumatoid arthritis receiving tofacitinib with or without other disease-modifying antirheumatic drugs (DMARDs) in clinical trials, 11 solid tumors and one lymphoma were diagnosed during the first 12 months of treatment compared with no cases of solid tumors or lymphoma in 809 patients receiving placebo with or without other DMARDs. Lymphomas and solid tumors also have been observed in long-term extension studies in patients with rheumatoid arthritis receiving tofacitinib.

In controlled clinical trials in patients with rheumatoid arthritis, malignancies (excluding nonmelanoma skin cancer) were reported at a rate of 0.3 events per 100 patient-years in tofacitinib-treated patients and 0 events per 100 patient-years in placebo-treated patients during the first 3 months of treatment. The rate of malignancies (excluding nonmelanoma skin cancer) during the first 12 months of treatment in patients receiving tofacitinib in clinical trials was 0.6 events per 100 patient-years in patients receiving 10 mg twice daily and 0.4 events per 100 patient-years in patients receiving 5 mg twice daily. The most common malignancies reported, including those reported during long-term extension studies, were lung and breast cancer, followed by gastric, colorectal, renal cell, and prostate cancer, lymphoma, and malignant melanoma.

Studies of longer duration are needed to evaluate the risk of malignancy associated with tofacitinib; however, current data suggest that the incidence rates for all malignancies in patients receiving tofacitinib for the treatment of rheumatoid arthritis are consistent with published estimates in patients with rheumatoid arthritis receiving biologic or nonbiologic DMARDs.

In controlled clinical trials in patients with psoriatic arthritis, 3 malignancies (excluding nonmelanoma skin cancer) were diagnosed in 474 patients receiving tofacitinib with nonbiologic DMARDs for 6–12 months compared with no malignancies in 236 patients receiving placebo with nonbiologic DMARDs for 3 months and no malignancies in 106 patients receiving adalimumab with nonbiologic DMARDs for 12 months. Malignancies also have been observed in a long-term extension study in patients with psoriatic arthritis receiving tofacitinib.

In controlled clinical trials in 1220 patients with ulcerative colitis (including both 8-week induction and 52-week maintenance trials), no cases of solid tumors or lymphoma were diagnosed in tofacitinib-treated patients. In a long-term extension study, malignancies (including solid tumors and lymphoma) were observed more frequently in patients receiving a tofacitinib dosage of 10 mg twice daily. The occurrence of nonmelanoma skin cancer in tofacitinib-treated patients with ulcerative colitis was dose dependent; a tofacitinib dosage of 10 mg twice daily was associated with increased risk.

EBV-associated posttransplant lymphoproliferative disorder was observed in 5 of 218 patients (2.3%) receiving tofacitinib compared with 0 of 111 patients receiving cyclosporine in dose-ranging trials in de novo renal transplant recipients; all patients had received induction therapy with basiliximab, high-dose corticosteroids, and mycophenolate.

The risks and benefits of tofacitinib should be considered prior to initiating therapy in patients with a known malignancy (other than successfully treated nonmelanoma skin cancer) or when considering whether to continue tofacitinib in patients who develop a malignancy.

Because nonmelanoma skin cancers have been reported in patients receiving tofacitinib, periodic dermatologic examinations are recommended for patients receiving the drug who are at increased risk for skin cancer.

Thromboembolic Complications. In an ongoing postmarketing study evaluating safety of tofacitinib in patients with rheumatoid arthritis, interim analysis revealed higher incidences of thromboembolic events, including pulmonary embolism, deep-vein thrombosis, and arterial thrombosis, in patients receiving tofacitinib 10 mg twice daily compared with those receiving either tofacitinib 5 mg twice daily or a TNF blocking agent, each given in combination with methotrexate. Many of these events were serious and some were fatal. (See Mortality under Warnings/Precautions: Warnings, in Cautions.) Because the study was designed to assess cardiovascular risks as well as risks of cancer and opportunistic infections, enrolled patients were 50 years of age or older and had at least one cardiovascular risk factor. Interim analysis revealed 19 cases of pulmonary embolism during 3884 patient-years of follow-up in patients receiving tofacitinib 10 mg twice daily compared with 3 cases during 3982 patient-years of follow-up in those receiving TNF blocking agents. Based on these interim findings, patients enrolled in the safety study who were receiving tofacitinib 10 mg twice daily for the management of rheumatoid arthritis were switched to the labeled dosage of 5 mg twice daily. FDA will reassess these safety concerns when final study results are available.

In a long-term extension study in patients with ulcerative colitis, 4 cases of pulmonary embolism were reported in patients receiving tofacitinib 10 mg twice daily, including one death in a patient with advanced cancer.

The 10-mg twice-daily dosage of tofacitinib is FDA-labeled only for the management of ulcerative colitis for use as induction therapy and in limited situations during maintenance therapy. (See Ulcerative Colitis under Dosage and Administration: Dosage.) Tofacitinib at a dosage of 10 mg twice daily (as conventional tablets) or 22 mg once daily (as extended-release tablets) is *not* recommended for the management of rheumatoid arthritis or psoriatic arthritis. In patients with ulcerative colitis, tofacitinib should be used at the lowest effective dosage and for the shortest duration needed to achieve and maintain therapeutic response.

Patients receiving tofacitinib should be advised to seek immediate medical attention if symptoms of thrombosis occur. (See Advice to Patients.) The drug should be discontinued in patients experiencing such symptoms, and the patient should be evaluated promptly. Use of tofacitinib should be avoided in patients who may be at increased risk of thrombosis.

Sensitivity Reactions Serious hypersensitivity reactions, including angioedema and urticaria, have been reported in patients receiving tofacitinib. If a serious hypersensitivity reaction occurs, tofacitinib should be discontinued promptly while the potential cause is investigated.

Other Warnings/Precautions **GI Perforation.** Cases of GI perforation have been reported in patients receiving tofacitinib in clinical trials. In clinical trials in patients with rheumatoid arthritis, many of the patients were receiving concomitant therapy with nonsteroidal anti-inflammatory agents (NSAIAs). In clinical trials in patients with ulcerative colitis, GI perforation appeared to occur at similar frequencies in patients receiving tofacitinib and those receiving placebo; many of the patients with ulcerative colitis were receiving concomitant corticosteroid therapy. The role of Janus kinase (JAK) inhibition by tofacitinib in these cases is not known.

Tofacitinib should be used with caution in patients who may be at increased risk for GI perforation (e.g., patients with a history of diverticulitis or receiving NSAIAs). Patients with new onset of abdominal symptoms should be evaluated promptly for early identification of GI perforation.

Hematologic Effects. Initial lymphocytosis (e.g., at one month following initiation of treatment) followed by gradual development of lymphopenia, with a decrease from baseline lymphocyte count of about 10% at 12 months, has been observed in patients receiving tofacitinib. Confirmed lymphocyte counts below 500/mm^3 were associated with an increased incidence of treated and serious infections. Initiation of tofacitinib therapy should be avoided in patients with lymphocyte counts of less than 500/mm^3. Lymphocyte counts should be monitored at baseline and every 3 months during treatment. Tofacitinib therapy should be interrupted or discontinued based on lymphocyte counts (see Dosage and Administration: Dosage).

Treatment with tofacitinib is associated with an increased incidence of neutropenia (neutrophil count less than 2000/mm^3) compared with placebo. A clear relationship between neutropenia and the occurrence of serious infection has not been demonstrated. Initiation of tofacitinib therapy should be avoided in patients with an ANC of less than 1000/mm^3. Neutrophil counts should be monitored at baseline, at 4–8 weeks after initiation of therapy, and every 3 months thereafter. Tofacitinib therapy should be interrupted or discontinued based on ANC measurements (see Dosage and Administration: Dosage).

Anemia has been reported in patients receiving tofacitinib. Initiation of tofacitinib therapy should be avoided in patients with hemoglobin concentrations of less than 9 g/dL. Hemoglobin concentrations should be monitored at baseline, at 4–8 weeks after initiation of therapy, and every 3 months thereafter. Tofacitinib therapy should be interrupted or discontinued based on hemoglobin concentration (see Dosage and Administration: Dosage).

Hepatic Effects. Tofacitinib has been associated with an increased incidence of elevated hepatic aminotransferase concentrations compared with placebo. These increases, which included elevations exceeding 3 times the upper limit of normal (ULN), were observed predominately in patients who were receiving concomitant therapy with other DMARDs, primarily methotrexate. Hepatic enzyme elevations were reversible upon modification of the treatment regimen (e.g., dosage reduction of concomitant DMARD or tofacitinib; interruption of tofacitinib therapy). Drug-induced hepatic injury was reported in one patient who received tofacitinib 10 mg twice daily for approximately 2.5 months. The patient developed symptomatic elevations of AST and ALT to greater than 3 times the ULN and elevation of bilirubin concentration to greater than 2 times the ULN; hospitalization and liver biopsy were required.

Hepatic aminotransferase concentrations should be routinely monitored in patients receiving tofacitinib. In case of elevations, patients should be evaluated promptly for drug-induced hepatotoxicity. If drug-induced hepatic injury is suspected, tofacitinib therapy should be interrupted until such diagnosis has been excluded.

Metabolic Effects. Dose-related increases in concentrations of total cholesterol, low-density lipoprotein (LDL)-cholesterol, high-density lipoprotein (HDL)-cholesterol, and triglycerides have been observed in patients receiving tofacitinib. Increases in these parameters were observed following one month of tofacitinib therapy and remained stable thereafter, with maximum increases generally occurring within the first 6 weeks of therapy. The effect of these increases on cardiovascular morbidity and mortality has not been determined.

In controlled clinical trials, mean concentrations of LDL-cholesterol and HDL-cholesterol increased during the first 3 months of therapy by 15 and 10%, respectively, in patients receiving tofacitinib 5 mg twice daily and by 19 and 12%, respectively, in patients receiving tofacitinib 10 mg twice daily. Mean ratios of LDL-cholesterol to HDL-cholesterol were essentially unchanged. In a controlled clinical trial, elevated concentrations of LDL-cholesterol and apolipoprotein B decreased to pretreatment levels in response to treatment with a hydroxymethylglutaryl-CoA (HMG-CoA) reductase inhibitor (statin).

Lipid concentrations should be measured approximately 4–8 weeks after initiation of tofacitinib therapy. Hyperlipidemia should be managed according to current standards of care.

Immunizations. Administration of live vaccines should be avoided during therapy with tofacitinib. (See Drug Interactions: Vaccines.) Immunizations should be updated according to current administration guidelines prior to initiation of tofacitinib therapy.

GI Obstruction. Because symptoms of GI obstruction have been reported rarely following administration of nondeformable extended-release drug formulations in patients with known GI strictures, tofacitinib extended-release tablets should be used with caution in patients with preexisting, severe, pathologic or iatrogenic narrowing of the GI tract.

Effects on Fertility. Findings of animal studies suggest that tofacitinib may reduce fertility in females; it is not known whether this effect is reversible.

Specific Populations **Pregnancy.** Adequate data are not available regarding use of tofacitinib in pregnant women. Fetocidal and teratogenic effects have been observed in rats and rabbits. In addition, reductions in live litter size, postnatal survival, and pup body weights have been observed in rats. Because the applicability of these findings to women receiving recommended dosages of tofacitinib is uncertain, pregnancy planning and prevention should be considered in females with reproductive potential.

Data suggest that increased disease activity in women with rheumatoid arthritis or ulcerative colitis is associated with an increased risk of adverse pregnancy outcomes (e.g., preterm delivery, low birthweight, small for gestational age at birth).

A pregnancy registry has been established to monitor fetal outcomes of pregnant women exposed to tofacitinib; patients or clinicians may contact the registry at 877-311-8972 to report any exposures to the drug that occur during pregnancy.

Lactation. Tofacitinib is distributed into milk in rats; it is not known whether the drug is distributed into human milk, affects milk production, or affects nursing infants. Because of the serious adverse effects (e.g., serious infections) observed in tofacitinib-treated adults, breast-feeding is not recommended during tofacitinib therapy and for at least 18 hours after the last dose of the drug administered as conventional tablets or 36 hours after the last dose administered as extended-release tablets.

Pediatric Use. Safety and efficacy have not been established in children.

Geriatric Use. In controlled trials of tofacitinib in patients with rheumatoid arthritis, 15% of patients were 65 years of age or older, while 2% were 75 years of age and older. In these studies, a higher incidence of serious infections was reported in patients 65 years of age or older compared with younger patients. Clinical studies of tofacitinib in patients with ulcerative colitis did not include sufficient numbers of patients 65 years of age or older to determine whether geriatric patients respond differently than younger adults. Tofacitinib should be used with caution in geriatric patients, taking into consideration the higher incidence of infections generally observed in geriatric patients. Age does not substantially alter pharmacokinetics of the drug.

Hepatic Impairment. Use of tofacitinib is not recommended in patients with severe hepatic impairment. Dosage adjustment is recommended in patients with moderate hepatic impairment since increased drug exposure may increase the risk of adverse effects; patients receiving tofacitinib extended-release tablets who develop moderate hepatic impairment should switch to therapy with a reduced dosage of the conventional tablets (see Dosage and Administration: Special Populations). Systemic exposure to tofacitinib is increased by 3 or 65% in patients with mild or moderate hepatic impairment, respectively.

Safety and efficacy of tofacitinib have not been evaluated in patients with serologic evidence of HBV or HCV infection.

Renal Impairment. Systemic exposure to tofacitinib is increased by 41, 71, or 156% in patients with mild, moderate, or severe renal impairment, respectively. In patients with end-stage renal disease receiving hemodialysis, systemic exposure to tofacitinib is increased by approximately 40%. Dosage adjustment is recommended in patients with moderate to severe renal impairment, including those receiving hemodialysis; patients receiving tofacitinib extended-release tablets who develop moderate or severe renal impairment should switch to therapy with a reduced dosage of the conventional tablets (see Dosage and Administration: Special Populations).

■ **Common Adverse Effects** Adverse effects occurring in 2% or more of patients with rheumatoid arthritis receiving tofacitinib 5 or 10 mg twice daily and more commonly than in patients receiving placebo include diarrhea, nasopharyngitis, upper respiratory tract infection, headache, and hypertension. Adverse effects in patients with psoriatic arthritis are similar to those observed in patients with rheumatoid arthritis.

Adverse effects occurring in 5% or more of patients with ulcerative colitis receiving tofacitinib for either induction therapy (10 mg twice daily) or maintenance therapy (5 or 10 mg twice daily) and more commonly than in patients receiving placebo include nasopharyngitis, elevated cholesterol concentrations, headache, upper respiratory tract infection, increased blood creatine kinase (CK, creatine phosphokinase, CPK) concentrations, rash, diarrhea, and herpes zoster.

Drug Interactions

■ **Drugs Affecting Hepatic Microsomal Enzymes** Metabolism of tofacitinib is mediated primarily by cytochrome P-450 (CYP) isoenzyme 3A4, with a minor contribution from CYP2C19. Concomitant administration of tofacitinib with a potent inhibitor of CYP3A4 (e.g., ketoconazole) or with one or more drugs that result in both moderate inhibition of CYP3A4 and potent inhibition of CYP2C19 (e.g., fluconazole) results in increased tofacitinib exposure. (See Drug Interactions: Antifungal Agents.) Reduction of tofacitinib dosage is recommended when such drugs are used concomitantly; tofacitinib dosage in patients with rheumatoid arthritis or psoriatic arthritis should be reduced to 5 mg once daily (as conventional tablets), while tofacitinib dosage (as conventional tablets) in patients with ulcerative colitis should be reduced from 10 mg twice daily to 5 mg twice daily or from 5 mg twice daily to 5 mg once daily. Patients with rheumatoid arthritis or psoriatic arthritis receiving therapy with tofacitinib extended-release tablets should be switched to therapy with the conventional tablets at a dosage of 5 mg once daily. Concomitant administration of drugs that inhibit only CYP2C19 is unlikely to substantially alter the pharmacokinetics of tofacitinib.

Concomitant administration of potent inducers of CYP3A4 (e.g., rifampin) results in decreased tofacitinib exposure and may result in decreased efficacy or loss of efficacy of tofacitinib. (See Drug Interactions: Rifampin.)

■ **Drugs Metabolized by Hepatic Microsomal Enzymes** Tofacitinib does not substantially inhibit or induce the activity of CYP isoenzymes 1A2, 2B6, 2C8, 2C9, 2C19, 2D6, or 3A4 in vitro at clinically relevant concentrations. In addition, tofacitinib does not appear to normalize CYP enzyme activity over time in patients with rheumatoid arthritis. Therefore, tofacitinib is not expected to alter metabolism of CYP substrates.

■ **Drugs Metabolized by Uridine Diphosphate-glucuronosyltransferase** In vitro studies indicate that tofacitinib does not substantially inhibit the activity of uridine diphosphate-glucuronosyltransferase (UGT) isoenzymes 1A1, 1A4, 1A6, 1A9, or 2B7.

■ **Drugs Affecting or Affected by Transport Systems** Pharmacokinetic interactions are unlikely with drugs that inhibit the P-glycoprotein transport system.

In vitro studies indicate that tofacitinib is unlikely to inhibit transporter proteins such as P-glycoprotein or organic anion or cation transport proteins at clinically relevant concentrations.

■ **Antifungal Agents** In healthy individuals, the potent CYP3A4 inhibitor ketoconazole (400 mg orally once daily for 3 days) increased peak plasma concentrations and area under the concentration-time curve (AUC) of tofacitinib (single oral dose of 10 mg) by 16 and 103%, respectively. Oral administration of fluconazole (a moderate CYP3A4 and potent CYP2C19 inhibitor) under steady-state conditions (400-mg loading dose followed by 200 mg once daily) increased peak plasma concentrations and AUC of tofacitinib (single oral dose of 30 mg) by 27 and 78%, respectively. Reduction of tofacitinib dosage is recommended when ketoconazole or fluconazole is used concomitantly. In patients with rheumatoid arthritis or psoriatic arthritis, tofacitinib dosage should be reduced to 5 mg once daily (as conventional tablets), while tofacitinib dosage (as conventional tablets) in patients with ulcerative colitis should be reduced from 10 mg twice daily to 5 mg twice daily or from 5 mg twice daily to 5 mg once daily. Patients with rheumatoid arthritis or psoriatic arthritis receiving therapy with tofacitinib extended-release tablets should be switched to therapy with the conventional tablets at a dosage of 5 mg once daily.

■ **Biologic Antirheumatic Agents** Tofacitinib should not be used concomitantly with biologic disease-modifying antirheumatic drugs (DMARDS). (See Uses: Rheumatoid Arthritis in Adults.) Concomitant use of tofacitinib with such drugs in patients with rheumatoid arthritis, psoriatic arthritis, or ulcerative colitis has not been studied to date.

■ **Immunosuppressive Agents** Concomitant use of tofacitinib with potent immunosuppressive agents (e.g., azathioprine, cyclosporine, tacrolimus) increases the risk of immunosuppression and is not recommended. Concomitant use of tofacitinib with such agents in patients with rheumatoid arthritis, psoriatic arthritis, or ulcerative colitis has not been studied to date.

In healthy individuals, cyclosporine (200 mg orally every 12 hours for 5 days) decreased the clearance of tofacitinib (single oral dose of 10 mg), resulting in a 73% increase in the AUC of tofacitinib, accompanied by a 17% decrease in peak plasma tofacitinib concentrations.

In healthy individuals, tacrolimus (5 mg orally every 12 hours for 7 days) slightly decreased the clearance of tofacitinib (single oral dose of 10 mg), resulting in a 21% increase in the AUC of tofacitinib, accompanied by a 9% decrease in peak plasma tofacitinib concentrations.

■ **Metformin** Metformin (a substrate of organic cation transporter [OCT] and multidrug and toxin extrusion transporter [MATE] proteins) does not substantially alter peak plasma concentrations or AUC of tofacitinib. No dosage adjustment is required when the drugs are used concomitantly.

■ **Methotrexate** Tofacitinib pharmacokinetics were not substantially altered by methotrexate administration in patients with rheumatoid arthritis; tofacitinib decreased peak plasma concentrations and AUC of methotrexate by 13 and 10%, respectively. Dosage adjustments are not necessary when tofacitinib is used concomitantly with methotrexate.

■ **Midazolam** In healthy individuals, tofacitinib (30 mg orally twice daily for 6 days) did not substantially alter peak plasma concentrations or AUC of the CYP3A substrate midazolam (single oral dose of 2 mg). No dosage adjustment is required when the drugs are used concomitantly.

■ **Oral Contraceptives** In healthy women, tofacitinib (30 mg orally twice daily for 9 days) did not substantially alter exposure to a single dose of an oral contraceptive containing ethinyl estradiol 30 mcg and levonorgestrel 0.15 mg. Tofacitinib increased AUCs of ethinyl estradiol and levonorgestrel by 7 and 1%, respectively; decreased peak plasma concentrations of ethinyl estradiol by 10%; and increased peak plasma concentrations of levonorgestrel by 12%. No dosage adjustment is required.

■ **Rifampin** In healthy individuals, the CYP3A inducer rifampin (600 mg orally once daily for 7 days) decreased peak plasma concentrations and AUC of tofacitinib (single oral dose of 30 mg) by 74 and 84%, respectively. Concomitant use of rifampin may decrease efficacy of tofacitinib.

■ **Vaccines** Live vaccines should not be administered to patients receiving tofacitinib. The interval between administration of live vaccines and initiation of tofacitinib therapy should be in accordance with current vaccination guidelines for patients receiving immunosuppressive agents.

Dissemination of the vaccine virus strain from zoster vaccine live (a vaccine containing live, attenuated varicella zoster virus) in a patient initiating tofacitinib therapy has been reported. Dissemination of the vaccine strain occurred 16 days after vaccine administration and 2 days after initiation of tofacitinib therapy (5 mg twice daily). The patient had no history of varicella infection and no anti-varicella antibodies at baseline. Tofacitinib was discontinued and the patient recovered following standard antiviral therapy.

Description

Tofacitinib citrate, a Janus kinase (JAK) inhibitor, is an immunomodulating agent and a disease-modifying antirheumatic drug (DMARD). JAKs are a family of intracellular tyrosine kinases consisting of JAK1, JAK2, JAK3, and tyrosine kinase (TYK) 2 that mediate the signaling of cytokines and growth factors that are important for hematopoiesis and immune function. Binding of cytokines to receptors on the cell surface activates pairing of JAKs (e.g., JAK1/JAK2, JAK1/JAK3, JAK1/TYK2, JAK2/JAK2, JAK2/TYK2), which leads to phosphorylation and subsequent localization of signal transducer and activator of transcription (STAT) proteins to the nucleus and modulation of gene expression. Tofacitinib modulates the signaling pathway at the point of JAKs, preventing the phosphorylation and activation of STATs. Tofacitinib inhibits JAK1 and JAK3 and, to a lesser extent, JAK2. In vitro, tofacitinib inhibited the activity of JAK1/JAK2, JAK1/JAK3, and JAK2/JAK2 combinations with IC_{50} (concentration that inhibits activity by 50%) values of 406, 56, and 1377 nM, respectively. The relevance of inhibition of specific JAK combinations to the therapeutic efficacy of tofacitinib is not known.

Treatment with tofacitinib has been shown to cause dose-dependent decreases in circulating CD16/56$^+$ natural killer cells, with estimated maximum reductions occurring after approximately 8–10 weeks of therapy; these decreases resolved approximately 2–6 weeks following discontinuance of tofacitinib. Dose-dependent increases in B-cell counts also have been observed with tofacitinib therapy; however, changes in circulating T-lymphocyte counts and T-lymphocyte subsets (CD3$^+$, CD4$^+$, and CD8$^+$) were small and inconsistent. The clinical importance of these changes in cell counts is unknown.

After 6 months of treatment, total serum concentrations of IgG, IgM, and IgA were lower in patients with rheumatoid arthritis receiving tofacitinib compared with patients receiving placebo; however, the changes in these concentrations were small and were not dose dependent.

Rapid decreases in serum C-reactive protein (CRP) concentrations have been observed in patients with rheumatoid arthritis receiving tofacitinib; these decreases were maintained throughout dosing. Changes in CRP concentrations are not reversed fully within 2 weeks following discontinuance of tofacitinib, indicating a longer duration of pharmacodynamic activity compared with the pharmacokinetic half-life of the drug.

Similar changes in T-cell and B-cell counts and CRP concentrations have been observed in patients with active psoriatic arthritis although reversibility was not assessed.

The absolute bioavailability of tofacitinib following oral administration as conventional tablets is approximately 74%. Peak plasma concentrations of the drug are achieved within 0.5–1 or 4 hours following oral administration as conventional or extended-release tablets, respectively. Peak concentrations and area under the serum concentration-time curve (AUC) are equivalent following oral administration of tofacitinib 5 mg twice daily as conventional tablets or 11 mg once daily as extended-release tablets. Administration of tofacitinib conventional tablets with a high-fat meal reduces peak plasma concentrations of the drug by 32% but does not substantially alter the AUC. Administration of tofacitinib extended-release tablets with a high-fat meal increases peak plasma concentrations of the drug by 27% and delays the time to peak plasma concentrations by approximately 1 hour, but does not alter AUC. The elimination half-life of tofacitinib is approximately 3 or 6 hours following oral administration as conventional or extended-release tablets, respectively. Tofacitinib is eliminated mainly by hepatic metabolism (70%) and, to a lesser extent, by renal excretion as unchanged drug (30%). Metabolism of the drug is mediated mainly by cytochrome P-450 (CYP) isoenzyme 3A4, with a minor contribution by CYP2C19.

Advice to Patients

Importance of discussing potential risks and benefits of therapy with the patient; importance of the patient reading the medication guide prior to initiation of therapy and each time the prescription is refilled.

Importance of storing tofacitinib conventional or extended-release tablets in the original container.

Increased susceptibility to infection. Risk of herpes zoster, which may be serious. Importance of not initiating tofacitinib therapy if active infection is present. Importance of promptly informing clinicians if any signs or symptoms of infection (e.g., persistent fever, sweating, chills, myalgia, cough, dyspnea, fatigue, diarrhea, dysuria, erythema) develop.

Risk of lymphoma and other malignancies. Risk of lymphoproliferative disorder in patients receiving tofacitinib in combination with drugs for prevention of renal allograft rejection.

Importance of discontinuing tofacitinib therapy and seeking immediate medical attention if signs or symptoms suggestive of thrombosis (e.g., sudden shortness of breath; chest pain exacerbated by breathing; leg pain or tenderness; redness, swelling, or discoloration of a leg or arm) occur.

Importance of discontinuing tofacitinib therapy and promptly notifying clinician if manifestations of a hypersensitivity reaction (e.g., swelling of the lips, tongue, or throat; urticaria) occur.

Risk of GI perforation. Importance of promptly notifying clinicians of persistent fever and abdominal pain or changes in bowel function.

Importance of informing clinicians of existing or contemplated concomitant therapy, including prescription and OTC drugs, as well as any concomitant illnesses or any history of cancer, tuberculosis, hepatitis B virus or hepatitis C virus infection, other chronic or recurring infections, or thrombotic or cardiac disease.

Importance of periodic laboratory monitoring.

Importance of women informing clinicians if they are or plan to become pregnant or plan to breast-feed. Women with reproductive potential should be advised of the potential risk to the fetus, and those who become pregnant while receiving tofacitinib should be advised that a pregnancy registry is available. Women should be advised to avoid breast-feeding during tofacitinib therapy and for at least 18 hours after the last dose is given as conventional tablets or 36 hours after the last dose is given as extended-release tablets.

Potential for tofacitinib to impair fertility in females. It is not known whether this effect is reversible.

Potential for the inert shell of the extended-release tablets to be eliminated in the stool or via colostomy after the drug has been absorbed.

Importance of informing patients of other important precautionary information. (See Cautions.)

Overview® (see Users Guide). For additional information on this drug until a more detailed monograph is developed and published, the manufacturer's labeling should be consulted. It is *essential* that the manufacturer's labeling be consulted for more detailed information on usual cau-

tions, precautions, contraindications, potential drug interactions, laboratory test interferences, and acute toxicity.

Preparations

Excipients in commercially available drug preparations may have clinically important effects in some individuals; consult specific product labeling for details.

Tofacitinib Citrate

Oral		
Tablets, extended-release, film-coated	11 mg (of tofacitinib)	**Xeljanz® XR**, Pfizer
Tablets, film-coated	5 mg (of tofacitinib)	**Xeljanz®**, Pfizer
	10 mg (of tofacitinib)	**Xeljanz®**, Pfizer

IMMUNOSUPPRESSIVE AGENTS 92:44

azaTHIOprine
azaTHIOprine Sodium

■ Azathioprine, a chemical analog of the physiologic purines adenine, guanine, and hypoxanthine, is a purine antagonist antimetabolite and an immunosuppressive agent.

Uses

■ **Renal Allotransplantation** Azathioprine is used as an adjunct for prevention of the rejection of kidney allografts. The drug is usually used in conjunction with other immunosuppressive therapy including local radiation therapy, corticosteroids, and other cytotoxic agents.

The maximum effectiveness of azathioprine occurs when the drug is administered during the induction period of the antibody response, starting either at the time of antigenic stimulation or within 2 days following. Under certain conditions of pretreatment with mercaptopurine, followed by an interval of at least 5 days before administration of the antigen and no subsequent treatment, a paradoxical enhancement of antibody formation has been observed. The effects of azathioprine and its active metabolite, mercaptopurine, may not be observed until several days after initiation of therapy and may persist for several days after clearance of the compounds is completed.

■ **Rheumatoid Arthritis** Azathioprine is used for the management of the signs and symptoms of rheumatoid arthritis in adults. Azathioprine is one of several disease modifying antirheumatic drugs (DMARDs) that can be used when DMARD therapy is appropriate. (For further information on the treatment of rheumatoid arthritis, see Uses: Rheumatoid Arthritis, in Methotrexate 10:00.) Nonsteroidal anti-inflammatory agents (NSAIAs), including aspirin, and/or corticosteroids may be continued when treatment with azathioprine is initiated. The manufacturers state that combined use of azathioprine and other DMARDS has not been studied and is not recommended.

■ **Crohn's Disease** Azathioprine has been used in the management of moderately to severely or chronically active Crohn's disease†, and to maintain clinical remission in corticosteroid-dependent patients, and to provide benefit in patients with fistulizing Crohn's disease†.

Azathioprine (e.g., 2–3 mg/kg daily) has been used in conjunction with corticosteroids to induce remission in patients with mildly to severely active refractory Crohn's disease; however, onset of action of azathioprine is slow and several months usually are required to achieve clinical response. Therefore, the role, if any, of azathioprine in the management of acute disease activity is uncertain. Azathioprine is used in patients with chronically active corticosteroid-dependent Crohn's disease. Results of several placebo-controlled trials indicate that azathioprine may be effective in maintaining remission in patients with corticosteroid-induced clinical remissions and in allowing reduction of oral corticosteroid therapy in corticosteroid-dependent patients. In several studies, frequency of relapse associated with azathioprine has been substantially lower than that associated with placebo. Results of long-term follow-up studies indicate that treatment with azathioprine may be effective for up to 4 years. Limited data indicate that relapse rates after 4 years of immunosuppressive therapy may be similar whether therapy has been maintained or discontinued; however, further larger studies are needed to confirm such data.

Azathioprine also has been found effective in the management of fistulizing Crohn's disease. Current clinical practice concerning use of azathioprine is based on a point analysis of 5 controlled trials in which fistula closure was considered a secondary end point and on several uncontrolled case studies. Data from these studies indicate that long-term (several years) therapy with azathioprine may be effective in the management of fistulizing Crohn's disease. However, because there currently are no controlled studies employing fistula closure as a primary end point, additional study is needed to more clearly establish efficacy.

Azathioprine (1.5–2 mg/kg daily) has been used effectively in pediatric patients with refractory or corticosteroid-dependent Crohn's disease†. In these patients, therapy with azathioprine may result in improvement of disease symptoms and reduction of corticosteroid dosage, and frequency of hospitalization.

Risks and benefits of azathioprine therapy should be carefully considered in patients with inflammatory bowel disease†, especially in adolescents and young adults with the disease. Cases of hepatosplenic T-cell lymphoma have been reported in patients receiving azathioprine for the management of inflammatory bowel disease. (See Cautions: Malignancies and Lymphoproliferative Disorders.)

(For more information on the management of Crohn's disease, see Uses: Crohn's Disease, in Mesalamine 56:36).

Dosage and Administration

■ **Reconstitution and Administration** Azathioprine is usually administered orally. Following renal transplantation, azathioprine may initially be given IV to patients unable to tolerate oral medication. Oral therapy should replace parenteral therapy as soon as possible.

Since azathioprine is an antimetabolite, the manufacturer states that consideration should be given to handling and disposal according to guidelines issued for hazardous drugs (see the ASHP Guidelines on Handling Hazardous Drugs at http://www.ahfsdruginformation.com), although there is no general agreement that all of the procedures recommended in such guidelines are necessary or appropriate.

Azathioprine sodium powder for injection is reconstituted by adding 10 mL of sterile water for injection to a vial labeled as containing 100 mg of the drug. The resultant solution contains 10 mg/mL, and may be given by direct IV injection or further diluted in 0.9% sodium chloride or 5% dextrose injection for IV infusion. IV infusions of the drug are usually administered over 30–60 minutes; however, infusions have been given over periods ranging from 5 minutes to 8 hours.

Reconstituted solutions of azathioprine should be inspected visually prior to administration, whenever solution and container permit.

■ **Dosage** Dosage of azathioprine must be carefully adjusted and individualized according to the patient's response and tolerance. Dosage may need to be reduced in patients with impaired renal function. (See Cautions: Precautions and Contraindications.) Dosage of azathioprine sodium is expressed in terms of azathioprine. Azathioprine may be given as a single daily dose or in divided doses.

The manufacturers and some clinicians recommend that thiopurine methyl transferase (TPMT) phenotype or genotype be determined prior to initiation of azathioprine therapy, since risk of hematologic toxicity may be increased in patients with intermediate, low, or absent activity of the enzyme and decreased dosage or alternative therapy should be considered in these individuals. (See Pharmacokinetics: Elimination and see Cautions: Precautions and Contraindications.)

Renal Allotransplantation The usual oral dosage of azathioprine in adults undergoing renal transplantation is 3–5 mg/kg daily beginning on the day of (and in some cases 1–3 days before) transplantation. Following transplantation, the drug may be given IV in the same dosage until the patient can tolerate oral therapy (usually 1–4 days). Dosage reduction to maintenance levels of 1–3 mg/kg daily is usually possible. When severe hematologic or other toxicity occurs, discontinuance of azathioprine therapy may be required even if rejection of the allograft may be a consequence of drug withdrawal.

Rheumatoid Arthritis For the treatment of severe, active rheumatoid arthritis, the usual initial oral adult dosage of azathioprine is 1 mg/kg (approximately 50–100 mg) daily. If the initial response is unsatisfactory and no serious adverse effects occur after 6–8 weeks of therapy, daily dosage may be increased by 0.5 mg/kg; daily dosage may then be increased as necessary at 4-week intervals by 0.5 mg/kg up to a maximum of 2.5 mg/kg. A therapeutic response usually occurs after 6–8 weeks of therapy; an adequate trial should be a minimum of 12 weeks. Patients who do not respond after 12 weeks can be considered unresponsive to the drug. Therapy may be continued in patients who respond, but patients must be closely monitored and gradual dosage reduction to the lowest possible effective level should be attempted. Daily maintenance dosage may be reduced to the lowest possible effective level in increments of 0.5 mg/kg (or approximately 25 mg) every 4 weeks, while keeping other therapy constant. The optimum duration of maintenance therapy has not been determined. Azathioprine may be administered in a single or twice-daily doses.

Crohn's Disease For the management of Crohn's disease†, adults have received an oral azathioprine dosage of 2–4 mg/kg daily, while pediatric patients have received 1.5–2 mg/kg daily.

Cautions

■ **Malignancies and Lymphoproliferative Disorders** Chronic immunosuppression with azathioprine increases the risk of malignancy. Patients receiving immunosuppressive drugs, including azathioprine, are at increased risk of developing lymphoma and other malignancies, particularly of the skin. Malignancies, including posttransplant lymphoma and hepatosplenic T-cell lymphoma in patients with inflammatory bowel disease, have been reported. (See Cautions: Precautions and Contraindications.)

Renal transplant recipients have an increased risk of developing malignancy (e.g., skin cancer, reticulum cell sarcoma, lymphomas). The risk of posttransplant lymphomas may be increased in patients who receive aggressive treatment with immunosuppressive drugs, including azathioprine. Therefore, therapy with immunosuppressive drugs should be maintained at the lowest effective dosage.

The incidence of lymphoproliferative disease in patients with rheumatoid arthritis appears to be substantially higher than that in the general population. The precise risk of malignancy associated with azathioprine is unknown; however, evidence suggests that the risk may be elevated in patients with rheumatoid arthritis, although to a lesser extent than in renal transplant patients. Limited data are available on the incidence and risk of malignancy in patients with rheumatoid arthritis receiving azathioprine. In one study, the incidence of lymphoproliferative disease in patients with rheumatoid arthritis receiving higher-than-recommended doses of azathioprine was 1.8 cases per 1000 patient-years of follow-up compared with 0.8 cases per 1000 patient-years of follow-up in those not receiving the drug. However, the proportion of risk attributable to the azathioprine dosage or to other therapies (e.g., alkylating agents) in these patients has not been determined. Acute myelogenous leukemia and solid tumors have been reported in patients with rheumatoid arthritis who received the drug. Patients with rheumatoid arthritis who have previously been treated with alkylating agents (e.g., cyclophosphamide, chlorambucil, melphalan) may have a prohibitive risk of malignancy if treated with azathioprine.

Hepatosplenic T-cell lymphoma, a rare, aggressive, usually fatal type of T-cell lymphoma, has been reported during postmarketing experience mainly in adolescent and young adult males with Crohn's disease or ulcerative colitis who received treatment with thiopurine analogs (azathioprine or mercaptopurine) and/or tumor necrosis factor (TNF) blocking agents. Although most of the reported cases occurred in patients who had received a combination of immunosuppressive agents, including TNF blocking agents and thiopurine analogs (azathioprine or mercaptopurine), cases have been reported in patients receiving azathioprine or mercaptopurine alone. As of December 31, 2010, the US Food and Drug Administration (FDA) had identified 12 cases of hepatosplenic T-cell lymphoma in patients with Crohn's disease or ulcerative colitis who had received azathioprine without concomitant or sequential immunosuppressive therapy. These 12 cases of hepatosplenic T-cell lymphoma occurred mostly in patients 15–45 years of age (median age: 21 years) following 4–17 years of azathioprine therapy; most of the patients were males, and 10 of the 12 cases were fatal. In addition, FDA identified 25 cases of hepatosplenic T-cell lymphoma in patients with Crohn's disease or ulcerative colitis who had received a TNF blocking agent (infliximab or both infliximab and adalimumab); in 22 of these cases, a thiopurine analog (azathioprine or mercaptopurine) was used concomitantly. In some cases, potential confounding factors could not be excluded because complete medical histories were not available. Since patients with certain conditions (e.g., Crohn's disease, rheumatoid arthritis) may be at increased risk for lymphoma, it may be difficult to measure the added risk of treatment with TNF blocking agents, azathioprine, and/or mercaptopurine. (See Cautions: Precautions and Contraindications.)

■ **Hematologic Effects** The principal toxic effect of azathioprine is bone marrow depression manifested by leukopenia, anemias including macrocytic anemia, pancytopenia, and thrombocytopenia, which may result in prolongation of clotting time and eventual hemorrhage. Hematologic effects are dose related and may be more severe in renal transplant patients whose allograft is undergoing rejection. Delayed hematologic suppression may occur. Hematologic status must be carefully monitored. (See Cautions: Precautions and Contraindications.)

When receiving usual dosages of azathioprine, patients with intermediate levels of thiopurine methyl transferase (TPMT) activity (about 10–11% of the population) may be at increased risk of developing myelotoxicity, while those with low or absent levels of the enzyme (0.3% of the population) are at increased risk of life-threatening myelotoxicity. Reduced dosage is recommended in patients with intermediate TPMT activity, while alternative therapy may be considered in those with low or absent levels of TPMT.

■ **GI Effects** Nausea, vomiting, anorexia, and diarrhea may occur in patients receiving large doses of azathioprine. Adverse GI effects may be minimized by giving the drug in divided doses and/or after meals. Vomiting with abdominal pain may occur rarely with a hypersensitivity pancreatitis.

A GI hypersensitivity reaction characterized by severe nausea and vomiting has been reported. This reaction also may be accompanied by diarrhea, rash, fever, malaise, myalgias, elevations in liver enzymes, and, occasionally, hypotension. Symptoms of GI toxicity most often develop within the first several weeks of azathioprine therapy and are reversible upon discontinuance of the drug. The reaction can occur within several hours after rechallange with a single dose of the drug.

Other adverse GI effects include ulceration of the mucous membranes of the mouth, esophagitis with possible ulceration, and steatorrhea.

■ **Hepatic Effects** Hepatotoxicity manifested by increased serum alkaline phosphatase, bilirubin, and/or aminotransferase concentrations may occur in patients receiving azathioprine, principally in allograft recipients. Azathioprine-induced hepatotoxicity following transplantation occurs most frequently within 6 months of transplantation and is generally reversible following discontinuance of the drug. Rare, but life-threatening hepatic veno-occlusive disease has occurred during chronic azathioprine therapy in several renal allograft recipients and in a patient with panuveitis; serious complications, including progressive portal hypertension, progressive liver failure requiring a portacaval shunt, progressive chronic liver failure with portal hypertension and esophageal varices, and/or rapid deterioration resulting in death, occurred in most of these patients. Veno-occlusive disease was associated with cytomegalovirus infection in some of these patients and with use of azathioprine but not with dosage of the drug, type or duration of renal allograft, or type of underlying renal disease. Reports to date suggest that the onset of hepatic veno-occlusive disease generally occurs after 1–2 years of therapy and that the disease occurs principally in males. The clinical syndrome is usually manifested initially by jaundice, often followed by the development of ascites and other signs of portal hypertension. Serum alkaline phosphatase and bilirubin concentrations are usually elevated. Prognosis is poor. Because hepatic veno-occlusive disease may result in rapid clinical deterioration, prompt diagnosis and therapeutic intervention are necessary. Many clinicians suggest that liver biopsy to diagnose veno-occlusive disease should be performed in renal allograft recipients receiving azathioprine at the first sign of mild hepatic dysfunction. If veno-occlusive disease is evident, azathioprine therapy should be promptly and permanently discontinued; alternative immunosuppressive therapy should be considered and, if liver failure is progressive, anticoagulation, a portacaval shunt, or hepatic allotransplantation should be considered.

Hepatotoxicity occurs in less than 1% of patients with rheumatoid arthritis who receive azathioprine.

■ **Other Adverse Effects** Azathioprine may also cause rash, infection, drug fever, serum sickness, alopecia, arthralgia, retinopathy, Raynaud's disease, reversible interstitial pneumonitis, and pulmonary edema. Some of these adverse effects can occur as manifestations of rare hypersensitivity reactions. Azathioprine-induced hypersensitivity reactions are often characterized by a combination of symptoms, including fever, rigors, musculoskeletal symptoms (arthralgias, myalgias), and/or cutaneous effects (generalized erythematous or maculopapular rash with nonspecific inflammatory changes demonstrated on biopsy); pulmonary manifestations (e.g., cough and/or dyspnea) and hypotension (which may be severe and, in the presence of fever, mimic septic shock) may also occur. Sweet's syndrome (acute febrile neutrophilic dermatosis) also has been reported.

■ **Precautions and Contraindications** Azathioprine is a toxic drug and must be used only under close medical supervision. Clinicians using azathioprine should be thoroughly familiar with the risks for development of malignancy, the mutagenic potential of the drug in female and male patients, and the possible hematologic toxicities associated with the immunosuppressant. Other immunosuppressive therapy given concomitantly with azathioprine therapy may increase the toxic potential of the drug.

Patients who have received azathioprine therapy should be monitored for the occurrence of malignancies since these patients are at increased risk for developing lymphoma and other malignancies, particularly of the skin. Because therapy with thiopurine analogs (azathioprine or mercaptopurine) and/or TNF blocking agents may increase the risk of malignancies, including hepatosplenic T-cell lymphoma, the risks and benefits of these agents should be carefully considered, especially in adolescents and young adults with Crohn's disease or ulcerative colitis. Patients and caregivers should be informed of the increased risk of malignancy associated with azathioprine, including the potential increased risk of hepatosplenic T-cell lymphoma, especially in adolescents and young adults with inflammatory bowel disease who receive treatment with thiopurine analogs (azathioprine or mercaptopurine) and/or TNF blocking agents, and should be advised of the relative risks and benefits of these and other immunosuppressive agents. Patients and caregivers should be informed of the signs and symptoms of malignancies such as hepatosplenic T-cell lymphoma (e.g., splenomegaly, hepatomegaly, abdominal pain, persistent fever, night sweats, weight loss) and advised to contact a clinician if such signs or symptoms occur. Patients should be advised not to discontinue therapy without consulting a clinician. Because therapy with azathioprine increases the risk for skin cancer, patients receiving the drug should be advised to limit exposure to sunlight and UV light by wearing protective clothing and using a sunscreen with a high protection factor. (See Cautions: Malignancies and Lymphoproliferative Disorders.)

Because patients with intermediate levels of thiopurine methyl transferase (TPMT; an enzyme involved in the methylation of 6-mercaptopurine, a metabolite of azathioprine) may be at increased risk of developing hematologic toxicity and those with low or absent levels of the enzyme are at increased risk of life-threatening hematologic toxicity, the manufacturers and some clinicians recommend that TPMT phenotype or genotype be determined prior to initiation of azathioprine therapy. (See Pharmacokinetics: Elimination.) TPMT testing should be considered in patients with abnormal complete blood cell count (CBC) results that persist despite dosage reduction of azathioprine.

Hematologic status must be carefully monitored in patients receiving azathioprine. When azathioprine therapy is initiated, patients should be informed of the need for periodic blood counts while receiving the drug and encouraged to report any unusual bleeding or bruising to their clinician. Complete blood counts, including platelet counts, should be monitored weekly during the first month of therapy, twice monthly for the second and third months of therapy, and monthly thereafter (or more frequently if dosage alterations or other therapy changes are necessary). Since the drug effect may continue for several days after the last dose of azathioprine, to avoid irreversible depression of the bone marrow, dosage of azathioprine should be reduced or therapy interrupted from the first sign of abnormal depression of the bone marrow until the count stabilizes. Since azathioprine-induced leukopenia does not correlate with therapeutic effect, dosage of the drug should not be increased intentionally to decrease the leukocyte count.

Hepatic function must be carefully monitored in patients receiving azathioprine. Serum alkaline phosphatase, bilirubin, and aminotransferase concentrations should be determined periodically for early detection of possible hepatotoxicity. Consideration should be given to discontinuing the drug if jaundice occurs. If hepatic veno-occlusive disease is clinically suspected, azathioprine therapy should be promptly and permanently discontinued; appropriate diagnostic and therapeutic measures should be initiated. (See Cautions: Hepatic Effects.) In patients with preexisting liver dysfunction, azathioprine should be administered with caution.

Despite the use of immunosuppressive therapy, the successful outcome of renal transplantation is largely dependent on careful donor selection. Although acute rejection of kidney transplants may be prevented or treated by the use of immunosuppressive therapy, signs of chronic rejection of the organ may occur; these changes may not be apparent until several months or years after transplantation.

Infection, which may be fatal, is a common hazard during therapy with immunosuppressive agents. Fungal, protozoal, viral, and uncommon bacterial infections may occur. Patients receiving azathioprine should be advised of the danger of infection during therapy with the drug and encouraged to report signs and symptoms of infection to their clinician. When infection occurs, dosage of azathioprine and/or other drugs used to prevent rejection should be reduced, and appropriate therapy for the infection instituted.

Patients receiving azathioprine, particularly those with impaired renal function or those receiving allopurinol concomitantly, should be given careful dosage instructions. (See Drug Interactions: Allopurinol.) Only small initial doses of azathioprine should be administered to patients with renal impairment, since the drug and its metabolites may be excreted more slowly in these patients and result in a greater cumulative effect. Because cadaveric kidneys often develop tubular necrosis and delayed onset of adequate function, clearance of azathioprine and mercaptopurine may be impaired; dosage should be appropriately reduced in these patients.

Persistent negative nitrogen balance and/or muscle wasting have been reported in some patients receiving prolonged therapy with azathioprine and corticosteroids; dosage should be reduced if this occurs.

Azathioprine is contraindicated in patients who are hypersensitive to the drug. If severe, continuous rejection occurs, it is probably preferable to allow the allograft to be rejected than to increase the dosage of azathioprine to very toxic levels.

■ **Pediatric Precautions** Safety and efficacy of azathioprine have not been established in pediatric patients.

Cases of hepatosplenic T-cell lymphoma have been reported in adolescents receiving azathioprine for the management of inflammatory bowel disease. (See Cautions: Malignancies and Lymphoproliferative Disorders.)

■ **Mutagenicity and Carcinogenicity** Chronic immunosuppression with azathioprine increases the risk of malignancy in humans; malignancies, including posttransplant lymphoma and hepatosplenic T-cell lymphoma in patients with inflammatory bowel disease, have been reported. (See Cautions: Malignancies and Lymphoproliferative Disorders.)

Azathioprine is mutagenic in humans. Chromosomal abnormalities have been documented in humans receiving azathioprine, but the abnormalities were reversed following discontinuance of the drug.

■ **Pregnancy, Fertility, and Lactation** Azathioprine is teratogenic in rabbits and mice when given in dosages equivalent to the human dosage (5 mg/kg daily). Abnormalities included skeletal malformations and visceral anomalies.

Azathioprine can cause fetal harm when administered to a pregnant woman. Limited immunologic and other abnormalities have occurred in some infants born to renal transplant recipients who received azathioprine. Lymphopenia, decreased IgG and IgM concentrations, cytomegalovirus infection, and a decreased thymic shadow were observed in one infant whose mother had received 150 mg of azathioprine and 30 mg of prednisone daily throughout pregnancy; most of these findings had apparently normalized by 10 weeks of age. Pancytopenia and severe immunodeficiency were reported in a premature infant whose mother received 125 mg of azathioprine and 12.5 mg of prednisone throughout pregnancy. Preaxial polydactyly was observed in one infant whose mother received 200 mg of azathioprine daily and 20 mg of prednisone every other day during pregnancy, while a large myelomeningocele in the upper lumbar region and bilateral lower limb deformities were reported in another infant whose father was receiving long-term azathioprine therapy. Azathioprine should not be used during pregnancy unless the potential benefits outweigh the possible risks; whenever possible, use of the drug during pregnancy should be avoided. If azathioprine is used during pregnancy or if the patient becomes pregnant while taking the drug, the patient should be informed about the potential hazard to the fetus. Women of childbearing potential should be advised to avoid becoming pregnant. The manufacturer states that azathioprine should not be used for the treatment of rheumatoid arthritis in pregnant women. Some clinicians state that, because of the potential for carcinogenesis and unknown long-term effects on fetal immunosuppression, use of azathioprine in pregnancy should be limited to women with severe or life-threatening rheumatoid arthritis. If azathioprine is administered during pregnancy, serious neonatal leukopenia and thrombocytopenia may be prevented by reducing the azathioprine dosage at 32 weeks' gestation; close prenatal monitoring for growth and long-term follow-up of offspring are essential.

Azathioprine has been reported to cause temporary depression in spermatogenesis and reduction in sperm viability and sperm count in mice at doses 10 times the usual human dose; a reduced percentage of fertile matings occurred when animals received 5 mg/kg.

Azathioprine or its metabolites are distributed into milk. Because of the potential for tumorigenicity associated with the drug, a decision should be made whether to discontinue nursing or the drug taking into account the importance of the drug to the woman.

Drug Interactions

■ **Allopurinol** Allopurinol inhibits one of the metabolic pathways of azathioprine (i.e., the oxidative metabolism of mercaptopurine by xanthine oxidase), thus increasing the possibility of toxic effects of azathioprine, particularly bone marrow depression. When azathioprine and allopurinol are administered concomitantly, dosage of azathioprine should be reduced to 25–33% of the usual dosage, and subsequent dosage adjusted according to the patient response and toxic effects.

■ **Angiotensin-converting Enzyme Inhibitors** Anemia and severe leukopenia may occur when angiotensin-converting enzyme (ACE) inhibitors are administered concomitantly with azathioprine.

■ **Aminosalicylates** In vitro, aminosalicylates (mesalamine, olsalazine, sulfasalazine) have been shown to inhibit the enzyme thiopurine methyl transferase (TPMT), an enzyme involved in the methylation of 6-mercaptopurine (a metabolite of azathioprine). Caution should be used during concomitant administration of azathioprine with aminosalicylates.

■ **Drugs affecting Myelopoiesis** Concomitant use of drugs affecting myelopoiesis (e.g., co-trimoxazole) with azathioprine may result in severe leukopenia, especially in patients who have undergone renal transplantation.

■ **Ribavirin** Use of ribavirin for the treatment of hepatitis C virus (HCV) infection in patients receiving azathioprine has been reported to result in severe pancytopenia and may increase the risk of azathioprine-related myelotoxicity. Ribavirin inhibits inosine monophosphate dehydrogenase, an enzyme required for one of the metabolic pathways of azathioprine; this leads to accumulation of an azathioprine metabolite, 6-methylthiopurine ribonucleoside-5′-phosphate (6-methylthioinosine monophosphate), that is associated with myelotoxicity (e.g., neutropenia, thrombocytopenia, anemia). Patients receiving azathioprine concomitantly with ribavirin should have complete blood counts, including platelet counts, monitored weekly for the first month of therapy, twice monthly for the second and third months of therapy, and monthly thereafter (or more frequently if dosage or other therapy changes are necessary).

■ **Warfarin** Azathioprine may inhibit the anticoagulant effect of warfarin.

Pharmacology

Azathioprine mainly exhibits immunosuppressive activity. The exact mechanism of immunosuppressive activity of the drug has not been determined. The action of azathioprine probably depends on several factors. Azathioprine, which is an antagonist to purine metabolism, may inhibit RNA and DNA synthesis. The drug may also be incorporated into nucleic acids resulting in chromosome breaks, malfunctioning of the nucleic acids, or synthesis of fraudulent proteins. The drug may also inhibit coenzyme formation and functioning, thereby interfering with cellular metabolism. Mitosis may also be inhibited by the drug.

In patients who undergo renal transplantation, azathioprine suppresses hypersensitivities of the cell-mediated type and causes variable alterations in antibody production. Suppression of T-cell effects depends on the temporal relationship to antigenic stimulus and engraftment; azathioprine has little effect on established transplant rejections or secondary responses. In animal models of autoimmune disease, the drug suppresses disease manifestations and underlying pathology.

Pharmacokinetics

■ **Absorption** Azathioprine is readily absorbed from the GI tract. Following oral administration of usual doses of azathioprine, blood concentrations of the drug are usually less than 1 mcg/mL; however, because purine antagonists rapidly enter into anabolic and catabolic pathways of purines, blood measurements actually represent several compounds and the importance of blood concentrations is questionable.

■ **Distribution** Distribution of azathioprine has not been fully characterized, but the drug is rapidly cleared from blood. Both mercaptopurine and azathioprine are approximately 30% bound to serum proteins, but both appear to be dialyzable. Azathioprine and its metabolites have been shown to cross the placenta.

■ **Elimination** Azathioprine is metabolized in vivo to 6-mercaptopurine, apparently by sulfhydryl compounds such as glutathione. The metabolites of azathioprine are excreted by the kidneys; only small amounts of azathioprine and mercaptopurine are excreted intact. 6-Mercaptopurine is metabolized by 2 major competing metabolic pathways in erythrocytes and liver or, alternatively, 6-mercaptopurine is incorporated as cytotoxic 6-thioguanine nucleotides into

DNA. The proportion of metabolites varies among individuals. 6-Mercaptopurine is oxidized to 6-thiouric acid by the enzyme xanthine oxidase. In addition, the sulfhydryl group of 6-mercaptopurine undergoes methylation, catalyzed by thiopurine methyl transferase (TPMT) to form the inactive metabolite methyl-6-mercaptopurine. The degree of activity of TPMT is under genetic control and is subject to individual variation. The most common nonfunctional alleles associated with reduced TPMT activity are TPMT*2, TPMT*3A, and TPMT*3C. Approximately 10% of Caucasians and African Americans inherit 1 nonfunctional allele (heterozygous) and have intermediate TPMT activity while about 0.3% of such populations inherit 2 nonfunctional alleles (homozygous) and have low or absent TPMT activity. Nonfunctional alleles are less common in the Asian population. There is an inverse relationship between TPMT activity and 6-thioguanine nucleotide concentrations in erythrocytes and, possibly, other hematopoietic tissues, because these cells have negligible amounts of xanthine oxidase (the enzyme involved in the other [oxidative] metabolism of 6-mercaptopurine), leaving TPMT methylation as the only inactivation pathway in these cells. Patients who have low TPMT activity have increased concentrations of the immunosuppressive 6-thioguanine nucleotides in erythrocytes and, therefore, they may develop myelotoxicity. (See Cautions: Hematologic Effects and see Cautions: Precautions and Contraindications.) The fate of the nitromethylimidazole portion of azathioprine has not been completely elucidated. Small amounts of azathioprine are also split to give 1-methyl-4-nitro-5-thioimidazole. azathioprine is only partially dialyzable.

Chemistry and Stability

■ **Chemistry** Azathioprine is a chemical analog of the physiologic purines—adenine, guanine, and hypoxanthine. Azathioprine, like mercaptopurine and thioguanine, is a purine antagonist antimetabolite. The drug is used mainly for its immunosuppressive activity. Azathioprine occurs as a pale yellow, odorless powder and is insoluble in water and very slightly soluble in alcohol. Azathioprine sodium powder for injection is a sterile, bright yellow, amorphous mass or cake prepared by lyophilization of an aqueous solution of azathioprine and sodium hydroxide. Some manufacturers may add hydrochloric acid to the commercially available azathioprine sodium powder for injection to adjust the pH. Following reconstitution of azathioprine sodium powder for injection with sterile water for injection to a concentration of 10 mg/mL, the solution has a pH of approximately 9.6.

■ **Stability** Azathioprine tablets should be protected from light and stored in well-closed containers, usually at 15–25°C; one manufacturer states that the tablets should be stored at a controlled room temperature between 20–25°C. Azathioprine sodium powder for injection should be protected from light and stored at 15–25°C in the carton until time of use.

Azathioprine is stable in solution at neutral or acid pH but is hydrolyzed to mercaptopurine at alkaline pH. Hydrolysis to mercaptopurine also occurs in the presence of sulfhydryl compounds such as cysteine, glutathione, or hydrogen sulfide. Following reconstitution of azathioprine sodium powder for injection with sterile water for injection to a concentration of 10 mg/mL, the solution is reportedly stable for approximately 2 weeks at room temperature; however, the reconstituted solution contains no preservatives, and it is recommended that the solution be used within 24 hours after reconstitution.

An oral suspension of azathioprine containing 50 mg/mL has been prepared extemporaneously from the commercially available tablets. The tablets were crushed, mixed with a volume of suspending agent (Cologel®) equal to one-third the final volume, and then the suspension was brought to the final volume with a 2:1 mixture of simple syrup and wild cherry syrup. The resulting suspension was stable for at least 56 or 84 days when stored in an amber glass bottle at room temperature or 5°C, respectively.

Preparations

Excipients in commercially available drug preparations may have clinically important effects in some individuals; consult specific product labeling for details.

azaTHIOprine

Oral		
Tablets	50 mg*	**azaTHIOprine Tablets** (scored)
		Imuran® (scored), Prometheus
	75 mg	**Azasan®** (scored), Salix
	100 mg	**Azasan®** (scored), Salix

*available from one or more manufacturer, distributor, and/or repackager by generic (nonproprietary) name

azaTHIOprine Sodium

Parenteral		
For injection, for IV use	100 mg (of azathioprine)*	**azaTHIOprine Sodium for Injection**

*available from one or more manufacturer, distributor, and/or repackager by generic (nonproprietary) name

†Use is not currently included in the labeling approved by the US Food and Drug Administration

Basiliximab

■ Basiliximab, a recombinant DNA-derived chimeric (human-murine) monoclonal antibody, is an immunosuppressive agent.

Uses

■ **Renal Allotransplantation** Basiliximab is used for the prevention of rejection of renal allografts. The manufacturer recommends that basiliximab be used in conjunction with cyclosporine and corticosteroids.

Efficacy and safety of basiliximab in adults have been evaluated in 4 randomized, double-blind, placebo-controlled studies in patients undergoing cadaveric or living-donor renal transplantation. In these studies, the basiliximab regimen consisted of two 20-mg IV doses, a dosage chosen to provide saturation of IL-2Rα for 30–45 days. The first dose of basiliximab was given within 2 hours prior to transplantation (day 0) and the second dose on day 4 following transplantation.

In 2 of the clinical trials in adults (18–75 years of age) who underwent a first renal transplantation and who had at least one HLA mismatch, the incidences of an episode of acute rejection, death, or graft loss during the first 6 months after renal transplantation (the primary end point) were reduced in patients receiving basiliximab by IV infusion in conjunction with a standard immunosuppressive regimen of oral cyclosporine (modified) (Neoral®) and corticosteroids (e.g., methylprednisolone, prednisolone); the primary end point occurred in 38–42% of patients receiving basiliximab compared with 55–57% of patients receiving placebo. Basiliximab therapy also was associated with a lower incidence of biopsy-confirmed renal allograft rejection at both 6 and 12 months posttransplantation (a secondary end point) in both studies; however, there were no differences at 12 months in the rate of delayed graft function, patient survival, or graft survival between basiliximab- and placebo-treated patients in either study.

In the 2 other clinicial trials in adults (18–70 years of age) who underwent a first or second renal transplantation from a cadaveric or living donor (not necessarily related to the patient), basiliximab was administered by IV injection in conjunction with a standard triple-drug (triple) immunosuppressive regimen consisting of cyclosporine (modified), corticosteroids, and either azathioprine or mycophenolate mofetil. In the study in which patients received basiliximab and the azathioprine-containing triple immunosuppressive regimen, the incidence of a first episode of acute rejection (the primary end point) at 6 months was reduced with basiliximab compared with placebo; the primary end point occurred in 21 or 35% of patients receiving basiliximab or placebo, respectively.

Efficacy of basiliximab in preventing acute rejection has not been demonstrated in recipients of a second renal allograft or other solid organ transplants (e.g., liver transplantation).

Dosage and Administration

■ **Reconstitution and Administration** Basiliximab is administered only by direct IV injection (IV "bolus") or IV infusion via a central or peripheral line. Patients receiving basiliximab by IV bolus injection may experience nausea, vomiting, and local reactions, including pain. When given by IV infusion, the diluted drug should be infused over 20–30 minutes.

Basiliximab is reconstituted using aseptic technique by adding 5 mL of sterile water for injection to a vial labeled as containing 20 mg of the drug. The vial should be shaken gently to dissolve the contents into a clear to opalescent, colorless solution that is isotonic. This solution may either be administered by IV injection or diluted to a volume of 50 mL with 0.9% sodium chloride or 5% dextrose injection to produce the admixture for IV infusion. To avoid foaming, the diluted IV solution should be mixed by gently inverting the bag; the admixture should *not* be shaken.

Because commercially available basiliximab does not contain antimicrobial preservatives or bacteriostatic agents, IV solutions of the drug should be prepared with care to assure sterility. The manufacturer recommends that the reconstituted solution of basiliximab be used immediately following preparation, although this solution may be stored at 2–8°C for up to 24 hours or at room temperature (15–30°C for up to 4 hours. The reconstituted solution should be discarded if not used within 24 hours. Reconstituted and diluted IV solutions of basiliximab should be inspected visually for particulate matter and discoloration prior to administration whenever solution and container permit; such solutions should not be used if color or particulate matter is present.

Incompatibility was not observed between basiliximab and polyvinyl chloride bags or infusion sets. No data are available regarding the compatibility of basiliximab with other IV drugs. Basiliximab should not be admixed with other drugs nor should other drugs be infused simultaneously through the same IV line.

■ **General Dosage** The manufacturer recommends that basiliximab be given in conjunction with cyclosporine and corticosteroid therapy. Basiliximab should be administered only when it has been determined that the patient will receive the graft and concomitant immunosuppressive therapy. If complications (e.g., severe hypersensitivity reactions to basiliximab, graft loss) occur after the initial dose of basiliximab, the second dose should be withheld.

For prevention of renal allograft rejection in adults, the recommended regimen of basiliximab consists of 2 doses of 20 mg each, with the first dose given within 2 hours prior to transplantation and the second dose given 4 days after transplantation.

■ **Special Populations** For prevention of renal allograft rejection in pediatric patients (1–16 years of age) who weigh less than 35 kg, the recommended regimen of basiliximab consists of 2 doses of 10 mg each; pediatric patients who weigh 35 kg or more should receive the usual adult regimen. The first dose should be given within 2 hours prior to transplantation and the second dose 4 days after transplantation.

Cautions

■ **Contraindications** Known hypersensitivity to basiliximab or any ingredient in the formulation.

■ **Warnings/Precautions** ***Warnings*** **Basiliximab should be used only by clinicians experienced in immunosuppressive therapy and the management of organ transplant patients. The clinician responsible for the administration of basiliximab should have complete information necessary for follow-up of the patient. Management of patients receiving basiliximab should be performed in facilities equipped with adequate laboratory and supportive medical equipment and staffed with adequate medical personnel.**

Clinicians should inform patients about the potential benefits of basiliximab and attendant risks of immunosuppressive therapy. The risk of lymphoproliferative disorders or opportunistic infections is increased in patients receiving immunosuppressive therapy and patients should be monitored accordingly, although neither complication occurred more often in patients treated with basiliximab than with placebo.

Sensitivity Reactions Anaphylaxis and other severe, acute (onset within 24 hours) hypersensitivity reactions have been observed upon initial exposure to basiliximab and/or upon subsequent exposure after several months. Drugs to treat severe hypersensitivity reactions, including anaphylaxis, should be immediately available during basiliximab therapy. Severe, acute hypersensitivity reactions to basiliximab may include hypotension, tachycardia, cardiac failure, dyspnea, wheezing, bronchospasm, pulmonary edema, respiratory failure, urticaria, rash, pruritus, and/or sneezing. Patients who have a severe hypersensitivity reaction to basiliximab should not receive the drug again. Patients who have previously received basiliximab should be given a subsequent course of therapy with the drug only with extreme caution. The potential risks of such subsequent administration of basiliximab, specifically those that involve immunosuppression, are not known.

General Precautions **Immune Response.** It is not known whether therapy with basiliximab has a long-term effect on the ability of the immune system to respond to antigens first encountered during immunosuppression induced by the drug.

Immunogenicity. An anti-idiotype antibody response without deleterious clinical effect was detected in 4 of 339 renal-transplant patients who had been treated with basiliximab. None of these patients showed evidence of faster clearance of basiliximab or a shorter duration of IL-2Rα saturation with the drug in the presence of anti-idiotype antibody. In a US clinical trial in patients who had undergone renal transplantation and were receiving basiliximab, human anti-murine antibody was detected in 2 of 138 patients not exposed to muromonab-CD3 and in 4 of 34 patients who subsequently received muromonab-CD3. Clinical data on the use of muromonab-CD3 in patients treated previously with basiliximab suggest that subsequent use of muromonab-CD3 or other murine anti-lymphocytic antibody preparations is not precluded.

These data are based on the percentage of patients with tests considered positive for basiliximab antibodies detected with ELISA; these results are highly dependent on the sensitivity and specificity of the ELISA assay. Other factors that may influence the observed incidence of positive assay results for an antibody include the manner in which samples are handled, concomitant therapy with other drugs, and underlying disease. Therefore, comparing the incidence of antibodies to basiliximab versus that with other drugs may be misleading.

Specific Populations **Pregnancy.** Category B. (See Users Guide.) Women of childbearing potential should use effective contraception before, during, and for 4 months following basiliximab therapy.

Lactation. Not known whether basiliximab is distributed in milk; discontinue nursing or the drug because of potential for serious adverse effects in infants.

Pediatric Use. Limited data are available concerning use of basiliximab in pediatric patients. In a study evaluating the safety and pharmacokinetics of basiliximab, a limited number of patients 1–16 years of age received the drug by direct IV injection (IV bolus) in addition to therapy with standard immunosuppressive agents, including cyclosporine (modified), corticosteroids, azathioprine, and mycophenolate mofetil. Acute rejection at 6 months occurred at a rate comparable to the incidence in adults in studies of basiliximab administered in conjunction with a triple immunosuppressive regimen. The most frequent adverse effects in these pediatric patients were hypertension, hypertrichosis, and rhinitis (49% each), urinary tract infections (46%), and fever (39%). The overall profile of adverse effects with basiliximab in these patients was consistent with general clinical experience in pediatric renal transplant patients and with controlled studies of the drug in adult renal transplant recipients.

It is not known whether the immune response to vaccines, infection, and other antigens is impaired during therapy with basiliximab or whether the immune response will remain impaired following therapy with basiliximab.

Geriatric Use. Available limited data in patients 65 years of age or older suggest that the adverse effect profile for basiliximab in geriatric patients is similar to that in younger adults and that adjustment of dosage based solely on age is not required. Use immunosuppressive drugs with caution in geriatric patients.

■ **Common Adverse Effects** GI effects were reported most frequently (69% with basiliximab and 67% with placebo) and included constipation, nausea, diarrhea, abdominal pain, vomiting, and dyspepsia. Other adverse effects occurring in at least 10% of patients receiving basiliximab were hyperkalemia, hypokalemia, hyperglycemia, hyperuricemia, hypophosphatemia, hypercholesterolemia, headache, tremor, urinary tract infection, pain, peripheral edema, fever, viral infection, hypertension, dyspnea, upper respiratory tract infection, surgical wound complications, acne, insomnia, and anemia. Adverse effects in clinical trials with basiliximab or placebo were similar in incidence and type.

The overall incidence of cytomegalovirus infection in patients receiving dual or triple immunosuppressive regimens was similar with basiliximab (15%) or placebo (17%). However, in patients treated with a triple immunosuppressive regimen, serious cytomegalovirus infections occurred at a higher incidence with basiliximab (11%) than with placebo (5%).

Drug Interactions

Adjustment of the dosage of basiliximab is not necessary when administered in conjunction with a triple immunosuppressive regimen of cyclosporine, corticosteroids, and either azathioprine or mycophenolate mofetil. Although total body clearance of basiliximab was reduced by 22 or 51% in patients receiving either azathioprine or mycophenolate mofetil, respectively, with cyclosporine (modified) and corticosteroids in clinical trials, the variation in clearance of basiliximab among individual patients appeared to be consistent with observations in individuals receiving the drug in dual immunosuppressive regimens. An increase in adverse effects was not observed in clinical studies of basiliximab in patients who received concomitant therapy with antithymocyte globulin or antilymphocyte globulin, azathioprine, corticosteroids, cyclosporine, mycophenolate mofetil, or muromonab-CD3.

Description

Basiliximab, a recombinant DNA-derived chimeric (human-murine) monoclonal antibody, is an immunosuppressive agent. This glycoprotein is obtained through fermentation of an established mouse myeloma cell line genetically engineered to express plasmids containing the human heavy- and light-chain constant region genes and murine heavy- and light-chain variable region genes encoding the RFT5 antibody that binds selectively to IL-2Rα (i.e., CD25 antigen), the α-chain of the interleukin-2 (IL-2) receptor. IL-2Rα is selectively expressed on the surface of antigenically stimulated (activated) T-lymphocytes.

Acute rejection epidoses occur in 30–50% of patients who have undergone renal transplantation and result in a substantial reduction in long-term (5 years or more) graft survival. By binding with high affinity ($K_a = 1 \times 10^{10}$ *M*) to IL-2Rα and inhibiting binding of IL-2 to antigenically stimulated T lymphocytes, basiliximab competitively inhibits IL-2-mediated lymphocyte activation, which is integral to the cell-mediated immune response involved in allograft rejection. At recommended dosages, basiliximab serum concentrations are sufficient for saturation of IL-2Rα for an average of 36 days.

Advice to Patients

Importance of understanding potential benefits of basiliximab and risks of immunosuppressive therapy. Importance of women informing clinicians if they are or plan to become pregnant or to breast-feed.

Overview® (see Users Guide). For additional information on this drug until a more detailed monograph is developed and published, the manufacturer's labeling should be consulted. Is is *essential* that the manufacturer's labeling be consulted for more detailed information on usual cautions, precautions, contraindications, potential drug interactions, laboratory test interferences, and acute toxicity.

Preparations

Excipients in commercially available drug preparations may have clinically important effects in some individuals; consult specific product labeling for details.

Basiliximab

Parenteral

Injection	20 mg	**Simulect®**, Novartis

Belatacept

■ Belatacept, a recombinant fusion protein and selective T-cell costimulation blocker, is an immunosuppressive agent.

REMS

FDA approved a REMS for belatacept to ensure that the benefits outweigh the risks. The REMS may apply to one or more preparations of belatacept and consists of the following: medication guide and communication plan. See the FDA REMS page (https://www.accessdata.fda.gov/scripts/cder/rems/index.cfm).

Uses

■ **Renal Allotransplantation** Belatacept is used for the prevention of rejection of renal allografts in adults receiving renal transplants. The drug has been designated as an orphan drug by the US Food and Drug Administration (FDA) for this use. The manufacturer recommends that belatacept be used in conjunction with basiliximab induction, mycophenolate mofetil, and corticosteroids. In addition, the manufacturer states that belatacept should be used only in patients who are Epstein-Barr virus (EBV)-seropositive. (See Cautions: Contraindications and see also Posttransplant Lymphoproliferative Disorder under Warnings/Precautions: Warnings, in Cautions.)

The efficacy and safety of belatacept in adults undergoing de novo renal transplantation were evaluated in 2 randomized, open-label, multicenter, active-controlled (cyclosporine), 3-year studies. In both of these studies, belatacept was given in 2 different dosage regimens: the currently recommended dosage regimen (less intensive regimen) and a regimen with higher cumulative doses and more frequent dosing than the recommended dosage regimen (more intensive regimen). All patients also received an immunosuppressive regimen consisting of basiliximab induction, mycophenolate mofetil, and corticosteroids.

Study 1 (the BENEFIT trial) was conducted in 666 adults receiving a kidney transplant from living or standard-criteria deceased donors. Efficacy outcomes at 12 months included composite patient and graft survival, composite renal impairment end point, and incidence of acute rejection. The efficacy failure rates (defined as the occurrence of biopsy-proven acute rejection, graft loss, death, or lost to follow-up) at 1 year for the recommended belatacept regimen and cyclosporine were approximately 22 and 17%, respectively, and at 3 years were approximately 26% in both groups. The incidence of biopsy-proven acute rejection was higher in patients treated with the recommended belatacept regimen than in those treated with the cyclosporine, regimen (20 and 10% in patients receiving the recommended belatacept regimen and the cyclosporine regimen respectively, at 1 year; 22 and 14% in patients receiving the recommended belatacept regimen and the cyclosporine regimen, respectively, at 3 years). At 1 year, both belatacept regimens had similar patient and graft survival (97% for the recommended regimen and 95% for the more intensive regimen) compared with the cyclosporine regimen (93%). At 3 years, patient and graft survival was 91% with the recommended belatacept regimen and 87% with the cyclosporine regimen. Approximately 87% of the patients in the BENEFIT trial were EBV seropositive prior to transplantation, and the efficacy results in EBV-seropositive patients were consistent with those in the total study population. Tolerability was generally similar between the belatacept- and the cyclosporine-based regimens. However, belatacept was associated with better renal function; measured and calculated glomerular filtration rates (GFR) were both higher in patients treated with the recommended belatacept regimen compared with those treated with the cyclosporine regimen.

Study 2 (the BENEFIT-EXT trial) was conducted in 543 adults receiving extended-criteria donor organs (i.e., donors 60 years of age and older or donors 50 years of age and older with at least 2 other risk factors [cerebrovascular accident, hypertension, or serum creatinine greater than 1.5 mg/dL] or an anticipated cold ischemia time of 24 hours or more or donation after cardiac death). Primary outcomes at 12 months were composite patient and graft survival and composite renal impairment. The incidence of biopsy-proven acute rejection at 1 year and 3 years was found to be similar in patients treated with belatacept and cyclosporine in this study. At 1 year, patient and graft survival also was similar in the 3 treatment groups (89% with the recommended belatacept regimen, 86% with the more intensive belatacept regimen, and 85% with the cyclosporine regimen). At 3 years, patient and graft survival was 82% for the recommended belatacept regimen and 78% for the cyclosporine regimen. The efficacy failure rates (defined as the occurrence of biopsy-proven acute rejection, graft loss, death, or lost to follow-up) at 1 year for the recommended belatacept regimen and the cyclosporine regimen were 29 and 28%, respectively, and at 3 years were 36 and 37%, respectively. Approximately 91% of the patients in the BENEFIT-EXT trial were EBV seropositive prior to transplantation, and the efficacy failure rates in EBV-seropositive patients were similar to those in the total study population. Renal function was better in the belatacept-treated patients; measured and calculated GFR were both higher in patients treated with the recommended belatacept regimen compared with those treated with cyclosporine.

In an open-label extension analysis of a phase 2 clinical trial comparing belatacept- and cyclosporine-based regimens in renal transplantation, renal function remained stable in the belatacept-treated patients over the 5-year study period.

The manufacturer warns that use of belatacept for the prevention of organ rejection in transplanted organs other than the kidney (e.g., liver transplants) has not been established. (See Uses: Hepatic Allotransplantation and see also Use in Liver Transplantation under Warnings/Precautions: Warnings, in Cautions.)

■ **Hepatic Allotransplantation** Although belatacept has been used for the prevention of rejection of liver allografts†, the manufacturer states that use of the drug in liver transplant recipients is *not* recommended. In a clinical trial involving liver transplant patients, use of belatacept regimens with more frequent administration than any of those studied in kidney transplantation in conjunction with mycophenolate mofetil and corticosteroids was associated with a higher incidence of graft loss and death compared with the tacrolimus control regimens. (See Use in Liver Transplantation under Warnings/Precautions: Warnings, under Cautions.)

Dosage and Administration

■ **Administration** Belatacept is administered only by IV infusion. Premedication is not required prior to administration of the drug.

Commercially available belatacept lyophilized powder for injection must be reconstituted and diluted prior to administration using proper aseptic technique. IV infusion of the drug must be completed within 24 hours of reconstitution of the belatacept lyophilized powder.

The belatacept infusion must be administered with an infusion set and a sterile, nonpyrogenic, low-protein-binding filter (with a pore diameter of 0.2–1.2 μm). Diluted solutions of the drug should be inspected visually for particulate matter and discoloration prior to administration.

Information on physical and/or chemical compatibility of belatacept with other drugs is not available; the manufacturer recommends that belatacept not be infused through the same IV line as other drugs.

Reconstitution Belatacept must be reconstituted/prepared using only the *silicone-free disposable syringe* provided with each vial. If belatacept powder is accidentally reconstituted using a different syringe, translucent particles may develop in the solution; any solutions prepared using siliconized syringes should be discarded.

Belatacept lyophilized powder should be reconstituted by adding 10.5 mL of a suitable diluent (sterile water for injection, 0.9% sodium chloride injection, or 5% dextrose injection) to a vial labeled as containing 250 mg of the drug to produce a solution containing 25 mg/mL. Based on the total infusion dose of belatacept, the appropriate number of vials of the drug should be reconstituted. During reconstitution, the diluent should be directed toward the side of the vial using the *silicone-free disposable syringe* provided by the manufacturer and an 18- to 21-gauge needle, and the vial rotated and inverted with gentle swirling to minimize foaming during dissolution. Prolonged and vigorous agitation of the vial should be avoided, and the vial also should not be shaken. The reconstituted solution should be clear to slightly opalescent and colorless to pale yellow and should not be used if opaque particles, discoloration, or other foreign particles are present.

Dilution Reconstituted belatacept solution must be diluted with a suitable infusion fluid (0.9% sodium chloride injection or 5% dextrose injection) prior to IV infusion. Belatacept reconstituted with either sterile water for injection or 0.9% sodium chloride injection should be further diluted with 0.9% sodium chloride injection. Belatacept reconstituted with either sterile water for injection or 5% dextrose injection should be further diluted with 5% dextrose injection. From the appropriate size infusion container, a volume of infusion fluid that is equal to the volume of the reconstituted belatacept solution required to provide the prescribed dose should be withdrawn. The required volume of reconstituted solution should then be injected into the infusion container using the same *silicone-free disposable syringe* used for reconstitution, and the infusion container gently rotated to ensure mixing. The final belatacept concentration in the infusion container should range from 2–10 mg/mL. An infusion volume of 100 mL is appropriate for most patients and doses, but total infusion volumes ranging from 50–250 mL may be used.

Rate of Administration IV infusions of belatacept solution should be given over 30 minutes.

■ **Dosage** Because of an increased risk of posttransplant lymphoproliferative disorder (PTLD) predominantly involving the CNS, progressive multifocal leukoencephalopathy (PML), and serious CNS infections, administration of higher than recommended dosages or more frequent administration of belatacept is not recommended. (See Cautions.)

The total infusion dose of belatacept should be based on the actual body weight of the patient at the time of transplantation, and should not be modified during the course of therapy unless body weight changes by more than 10%.

The actual prescribed dose of belatacept must be evenly divisible by 12.5 mg to be prepared accurately using the reconstituted solution and the silicone-free disposable syringe. For example, if a patient weighs 64 kg and the dosage is 10 mg/kg, then the calculated dose is 640 mg. The closest doses that are evenly divisible by 12.5 below and above 640 mg are 637.5 mg and 650 mg; the nearest dose to 640 mg is 637.5 mg. Therefore, the actual prescribed dose for the patient should be 637.5 mg.

For the prevention of renal allograft rejection in adults undergoing renal transplantation, the recommended initial dose of belatacept is 10 mg/kg administered by IV infusion over 30 minutes on the day of transplantation (prior to implantation, day 1), day 5 (approximately 96 hours after day 1 dose), and at the end of weeks 2, 4, 8, and 12 after transplantation.

During the maintenance phase of treatment, 5 mg/kg of belatacept should be administered by IV infusion over 30 minutes at the end of week 16 after transplantation and then every 4 weeks (plus or minus 3 days) thereafter.

■ Special Populations The manufacturer currently makes no special population dosage recommendations. However, pharmacokinetic studies in kidney transplant recipients indicate that age, gender, race, renal function, hemodialysis, and hepatic function do not affect clearance of belatacept.

Cautions

■ Contraindications Belatacept is contraindicated in transplant recipients who are Epstein-Barr virus (EBV) seronegative or with unknown EBV serostatus because of the risk of posttransplant lymphoproliferative disorder (PTLD), which predominantly involves the CNS. (See Posttransplant Lymphoproliferative Disorder under Warnings/Precautions: Warnings, under Cautions.)

■ Warnings/Precautions ***Warnings*** **Posttransplant Lymphoproliferative Disorder.** Patients receiving belatacept are at increased risk of developing posttransplant lymphoproliferative disorder (PTLD), predominantly involving the CNS, compared with patients receiving a cyclosporine-based regimen. In a pooled analysis of 3 clinical studies involving 472 patients treated with the recommended dosage regimen of belatacept or a very similar regimen, there were 5 cases of PTLD (including 2 cases with CNS involvement) reported up to 3 years following transplantation. In 477 patients treated with a belatacept regimen with a higher cumulative dose and more frequent administration, there were 8 reported cases of PTLD (including 6 cases with CNS involvement). The rate of PTLD in 949 patients treated with any of the belatacept regimens in this analysis was ninefold higher in those who were Epstein-Barr virus (EBV) seronegative or serostatus unknown compared with those who were EBV seropositive. All cases of PTLD in this analysis occurred within the first 18 months of belatacept therapy, although a case of PTLD has been reported in a patient who was treated with the drug for over 4 years. Clinicians should consider the possibility of PTLD in belatacept-treated patients who are experiencing new or worsening neurologic, cognitive, or behavioral signs and symptoms (see Advice to Patients).

Because the total burden of immunosuppression is a risk factor for PTLD, higher than recommended doses or more frequent administration of belatacept and higher than recommended doses of concomitant immunosuppressive agents are not recommended. In addition, the risk of PTLD is higher in EBV-seronegative patients; therefore, patients who are EBV-seronegative or with unknown EBV serostatus should *not* receive belatacept. EBV serology should be determined before initiating treatment with belatacept, and only patients who are EBV seropositive should receive the drug.

Other known risk factors for PTLD include cytomegalovirus (CMV) infection and concurrent T-cell-depleting therapy. Therefore, T-cell-depleting therapies (e.g., antithymocyte globulin) used to treat acute rejection should be used cautiously in patients receiving belatacept. CMV prophylaxis is recommended for at least 3 months after transplantation in patients receiving the drug. Patients who are EBV seropositive and CMV seronegative also may be at increased risk for PTLD compared with patients who are EBV seropositive and CMV seropositive. CMV-seronegative patients are at increased risk for CMV disease (a known risk factor for PTLD); the clinical importance of CMV serology for PTLD remains to be determined. Clinicians should consider these findings when prescribing belatacept.

Management of Immunosuppression. Belatacept should be used only by clinicians experienced in immunosuppressive therapy and the management of kidney transplant patients. Patients receiving the drug should be managed in facilities equipped and staffed with adequate laboratory and supportive medical resources, and the clinician responsible for maintenance therapy should have complete information requisite for follow-up of the patient.

Other Malignancies. Patients receiving immunosuppressants, including belatacept, are at an increased risk of developing malignancies, in addition to PTLD, including those affecting the skin. (See Posttransplant Lymphoproliferative Disorder under Warnings/Precautions: Warnings, in Cautions.) In the BENEFIT and BENEFIT-EXT trials, malignancies (excluding non-melanoma skin cancer and PTLD) were reported in 3.5 and 3.7% of patients receiving the recommended belatacept regimen and the cyclosporine control regimen, respectively. Exposure to sunlight and UV light should be limited during belatacept therapy by wearing protective clothing and using a sunscreen with a high protection factor. (See Advice to Patients.)

Progressive Multifocal Leukoencephalopathy. Cases of progressive multifocal leukoencephalopathy (PML; an opportunistic viral infection of the brain), sometimes fatal, have been reported in patients treated with immunosuppressive agents, including belatacept. PML is caused by the polyomavirus JC (also called the JC virus) and risk factors include high levels of overall immunosuppression and impairment of immune function. In clinical trials with belatacept, 2 cases of PML were reported in patients receiving belatacept at higher cumulative doses and more frequently than recommended, mycophenolate mofetil, and corticosteroids; one case occurred in a kidney transplant recipient and the other case occurred in a liver transplant recipient. Because PML has been associated with high levels of overall immunosuppression, recommended doses and frequency of administration of belatacept and concomitant immunosuppressives, including mycophenolate mofetil, should not be exceeded.

PML should be considered in the differential diagnosis of patients with new or worsening neurologic, cognitive, or behavioral signs or symptoms. PML is usually diagnosed by brain imaging, CSF testing for JC viral DNA by polymerase chain reaction, and/or brain biopsy. Consultation with a specialist (e.g., neurologist and/or infectious disease specialist) should be considered in any suspected or confirmed case of PML. If PML is diagnosed, clinicians should consider reduction or withdrawal of immunosuppression taking into account that this may also increase the risk of graft rejection in transplant recipients. Although the optimal pharmacologic treatment of PML remains to be established, antiviral agents (e.g., cidofovir) have reportedly been successfully used in the treatment of PML in several transplant recipients to date. Early diagnosis and rapid initiation of treatment appear to be essential for patient recovery from this progressive viral disease.

Other Serious Infections. Patients receiving immunosuppressants, including belatacept, are at an increased risk of developing bacterial, viral (e.g., CMV, herpes), fungal, and protozoal infections, including opportunistic infections. These infections may lead to serious, including fatal, outcomes. Prophylaxis for CMV is recommended for at least 3 months after transplantation in belatacept-treated patients. Prophylaxis for *Pneumocystis jiroveci* also is recommended after transplantation in patients receiving the drug.

Tuberculosis was observed more frequently in patients receiving belatacept than in those receiving cyclosporine in clinical trials. Patients should be evaluated for tuberculosis and tested for latent infection prior to initiating belatacept. Latent tuberculosis infection treatment, if necessary, should be initiated prior to belatacept administration.

Cases of polyoma virus-associated nephropathy (PVAN), mainly due to BK virus infection, have been reported. PVAN is associated with serious outcomes, including deteriorating renal function and kidney graft loss. Patient monitoring may help detect patients at risk for PVAN. Decreasing total immunosuppression should be considered for patients who develop evidence of PVAN, but the risk that reduced immunosuppression represents to the functioning allograft should also be considered.

Use in Liver Transplantation. Use of belatacept in liver transplant patients is *not* recommended. In a clinical study in liver transplant patients, use of belatacept with more frequent administration than studied in renal transplantation in combination with mycophenolate mofetil and corticosteroids was associated with a higher rate of mortality and graft loss compared with the tacrolimus control regimens. In addition, 2 cases (one fatal) of PTLD involving the liver allograft and one fatal case of PML were reported in the 147 patients randomized to belatacept. The 2 cases of PTLD were reported among the 140 EBV-seropositive patients (1.4%). (See Posttransplant Lymphoproliferative Disorder under Warnings/Precautions: Warnings, under Cautions.) The fatal case of PML was reported in a patient receiving higher than recommended doses of belatacept and mycophenolate mofetil. (See Progressive Multifocal Leukoencephalopathy under Warnings/Precautions: Warnings, under Cautions.)

Other Warnings and Precautions **Immunization.** Use of live vaccines should be avoided during belatacept therapy. (See Drug Interactions: Vaccines and see also Advice to Patients.)

Specific Populations **Pregnancy.** Category C. (See Users Guide.)

Autoimmunity has been observed in animal offspring exposed to abatacept (a drug closely related to belatacept) in utero; the clinical relevance of this finding to patients or a fetus exposed in utero to belatacept is unknown.

To monitor maternal-fetal outcomes of pregnant women exposed to belatacept or whose partners have received the drug, clinicians are encouraged to enroll pregnant women in the National Transplantation Pregnancy Registry (NTPR) by telephone at 877-955-6877 or via their website at http://www.tju.edu/ntpr/index.cfm. Women also may enroll themselves in the registry.

Lactation. It is not known whether belatacept is distributed into human milk or absorbed systemically after ingestion by a nursing infant. However, the drug is distributed into milk in rats. Because many drugs are distributed into human milk and because of the potential for serious adverse reactions from belatacept in nursing infants, a decision should be made whether to discontinue nursing or the drug, taking into account the importance of the drug to the woman.

Pediatric Use. Safety and efficacy of belatacept have not been established in pediatric patients younger than 18 years of age.

Because T-cell development continues into the teenage years, the manufacturer states that the potential concern for autoimmunity in neonates also applies to pediatric use of belatacept.

Geriatric Use. Approximately 15% of renal transplant recipients who received belatacept in clinical trials were 65 years of age or older and about 3% were 75 years of age or older. No overall differences in safety or efficacy relative to younger adults were observed, but increased sensitivity or reduced efficacy in older individuals cannot be ruled out.

In population pharmacokinetic analyses in kidney transplant recipients, patient age did not affect the clearance of belatacept. (See Dosage and Administration: Special Populations.)

Hepatic Impairment. In population pharmacokinetic analyses in kidney transplant recipients, hepatic function (measured by albumin concentrations) did not affect the clearance of belatacept. (See Dosage and Administration: Special Populations.)

Renal Impairment. In population pharmacokinetic analyses in kidney transplant recipients, renal function (measured by calculated glomerular filtration rate) and concurrent hemodialysis did not affect the clearance of belatacept. (See Dosage and Administration: Special Populations.)

■ **Common Adverse Effects** Adverse effects reported in 20% or more of patients treated with the recommended dosage and frequency of belatacept in clinical trials include anemia, diarrhea, urinary tract infection, peripheral edema, constipation, hypertension, pyrexia, graft dysfunction, cough, nausea, vomiting, headache, hypokalemia, hyperkalemia, and leukopenia.

Drug Interactions

No formal drug interaction studies have been conducted with belatacept to date.

■ **Drugs Affecting or Metabolized by Hepatic Microsomal Enzymes** In vitro studies have shown that belatacept inhibits production of certain cytokines during an autoimmune response. Other biologic therapies that are cytokines or cytokine modulators have been shown to affect the expression and/or functional activities of cytochrome P-450 (CYP) enzymes in vitro and/or in vivo. If patients receiving belatacept exhibit signs and symptoms of altered efficacy or adverse events associated with concurrently administered drugs that are metabolized by CYP, clinicians should be aware of the potentially altered CYP-mediated metabolism of these drugs.

■ **Immunosuppressive Agents** Concurrent administration of other immunosuppressive agents during belatacept therapy is associated with an increased susceptibility to infection, an increased risk of malignancies, and some other adverse effects (including posttransplant lymphoproliferative disorder [PTLD] and progressive multifocal leukoencephalopathy [PML]). (See Cautions.)

Because concurrent use of T-cell-depleting therapy increases the risk of PTLD, T-cell-depleting agents used in the treatment of acute rejection (e.g., antithymocyte globulin) should be used cautiously in patients receiving belatacept.

■ **Mycophenolate Mofetil** In a pharmacokinetic substudy of the BENEFIT and BENEFIT-EXT trials (see Uses: Renal Allotransplantation), patients received mycophenolate mofetil (500–1500 mg twice daily) concurrently with either belatacept (5 mg/kg) or cyclosporine. Mean, dose-normalized peak plasma concentrations and area under the concentration-time curve (AUC) of mycophenolic acid (MPA) were approximately 20 and 40% higher, respectively, with concurrent use of belatacept compared with concurrent cyclosporine. Clinicians should be aware that exposure to mycophenolic acid also may be altered after switching from cyclosporine to belatacept and vice versa in patients concomitantly receiving mycophenolate mofetil.

■ **Vaccines** The possibility that immune response to vaccination may be diminished in patients receiving belatacept should be considered.

The manufacturer states that live vaccines (including influenza virus vaccine live intranasal, measles virus vaccine live, mumps virus vaccine live, rubella virus vaccine live, poliovirus vaccine live oral [OPV; no longer commercially available in the US], BCG vaccine, yellow fever vaccine, varicella virus vaccine live, typhoid vaccine live oral) should be avoided in patients receiving belatacept therapy.

Description

Belatacept, a recombinant fusion protein and selective T-cell costimulation blocker, is an immunosuppressive agent. The drug consists of the modified extracellular domain of cytotoxic T-lymphocyte-associated antigen (CTLA)-4 fused to a portion of the Fc domain of human immunoglobulin G_1 (IgG_1). Belatacept is structurally and pharmacologically related to abatacept, but binds CD80 and CD86 more avidly than abatacept. Belatacept binds to CD80 and CD86 on antigen-presenting cells thereby blocking CD28-mediated costimulation of T lymphocytes. In vitro, the drug inhibits T lymphocyte proliferation and the production of the cytokines interleukin-2, interferon gamma, interleukin-4, and tumor necrosis factor-α (TNF-α). Activated T lymphocytes are the principal mediators of immunologic rejection. In nonhuman primate models of renal transplantation, belatacept monotherapy prolonged graft survival and decreased the production of anti-donor antibodies.

The pharmacokinetics of belatacept were found to be linear in healthy individuals, with exposure increasing proportionally after a single IV infusion dose ranging from 1–20 mg/kg. When the recommended dosage regimen of belatacept is administered, mean serum concentrations of the drug reach steady state by week 8 in the initial phase following transplantation and by month 6 during the maintenance phase. Population pharmacokinetic analyses in kidney transplant recipients revealed a trend toward higher clearance of belatacept with increasing body weight. However, patient age, gender, race, renal function, hepatic function, diabetes, and concurrent hemodialysis did not affect clearance of the drug. The terminal elimination half-life of belatacept averages 9.8 days following single-dose administration in healthy individuals. Following multiple-dose administration of 5 and 10 mg/kg of the drug in renal transplant recipients, the terminal half-life averages 8.2 and 9.8 days, respectively.

Advice to Patients

Importance of providing copy of manufacturer's written patient information (medication guide) each time belatacept is dispensed, and importance of reading this information before beginning therapy with the drug and before each treatment. (See REMS.)

Importance of informing patients of the increased risk of posttransplant lymphoproliferative disorder (PTLD), especially CNS PTLD, with belatacept therapy and the risk of progressive multifocal leukoencephalopathy (PML). Patients should be instructed to immediately report any of the following neurologic, cognitive, or behavioral signs and symptoms: changes in mood or usual behavior; confusion, problems thinking, or loss of memory; changes in walking or talking; decreased strength or weakness on one side of the body; and changes in vision during or after belatacept therapy.

Patients receiving belatacept should be informed about the increased risk of malignancies, in addition to PTLD, in patients receiving immunosuppressive therapy, especially skin cancer. Importance of limiting exposure to sunlight and other UV light by wearing protective clothing and using sunscreens with a high protection factor. Patients should also be instructed to watch for any signs or symptoms of skin cancer, such as suspicious moles or lesions.

Importance of informing patients of the increased risk of infection while receiving immunosuppressive therapy and the importance of taking antimicrobial prophylaxis regimens as prescribed. Instruct patients to immediately report any signs and symptoms of infection during belatacept therapy.

Importance of informing patients that vaccinations may be less effective while receiving belatacept. Patients should be instructed to avoid receiving live vaccines during belatacept therapy.

Importance of informing patients that belatacept has not been studied in pregnant or nursing women, and that the effects of the drug on pregnant women or nursing infants are not known. Importance of women informing their clinician if they are or plan to become pregnant or plan to breast-feed. Importance of encouraging enrollment of pregnant women in the National Transplantation Pregnancy Registry (see Pregnancy under Warnings/Precautions: Specific Populations, under Cautions).

Importance of informing clinicians of existing or contemplated concomitant therapy, including prescription (e.g., immunizations) and OTC drugs and dietary or herbal supplements, as well as any concomitant illnesses.

Importance of advising patients of other important precautionary information. (See Cautions.)

Overview® (see Users Guide). For additional information on this drug until a more detailed monograph is developed and published, the manufacturer's labeling should be consulted. It is *essential* that the manufacturer's labeling be consulted for more detailed information on usual cautions, precautions, contraindications, potential drug interactions, laboratory test interferences, and acute toxicity.

Preparations

Excipients in commercially available drug preparations may have clinically important effects in some individuals; consult specific product labeling for details.

Belatacept

Parenteral		
For injection, for IV infusion only	250 mg	Nulojix® (available in single-use vials with a silicone-free disposable syringe), Bristol-Myers Squibb

†Use is not currently included in the labeling approved by the US Food and Drug Administration

Belimumab

■ Belimumab, a recombinant fully human immunoglobulin G_1 lambda (IgG_1 lambda) monoclonal antibody, inhibits soluble human B-lymphocyte stimulator (BLyS) and is an immunosuppressive agent.

Uses

■ **Systemic Lupus Erythematosus** Belimumab is used in conjunction with other standard therapies in the management of active, autoantibody-positive systemic lupus erythematosus (SLE). Efficacy of belimumab has not been established in patients with severe active lupus nephritis or severe active CNS lupus, and belimumab has not been studied in combination with other biologic agents or IV cyclophosphamide. Therefore, use of belimumab is not recommended in these situations. In addition, efficacy of the drug in black patients with SLE remains to be definitively established.

In 3 randomized, double-blind, placebo-controlled studies, efficacy and safety of belimumab were evaluated in a total of 2133 adults with SLE. Patients with severe active lupus nephritis or severe active CNS lupus were excluded from the studies. Patients enrolled in these studies were receiving stable, standard regimens of corticosteroids, antimalarials, nonsteroidal anti-inflammatory agents (NSAIAs), and/or immunosuppressive agents (e.g., azathioprine, methotrexate, mycophenolate) upon study entry. Use of other biologic agents and IV cyclophosphamide was not permitted.

The first study (a phase 2 study) evaluated belimumab (1, 4, or 10 mg/kg IV on days 0, 14, and 28 and then every 28 days) plus standard care compared with placebo plus standard care over 52 weeks in 449 patients with active SLE and a history of measurable autoantibodies (28% of the patients were autoantibody negative at baseline). The primary end points were percent change in Safety of Estrogens in Lupus Erythematosus National Assessment-Systemic Lupus Erythematosus Disease Activity Index (SELENA-SLEDAI) score from baseline to week 24 and time to first disease flare over 52 weeks. The SELENA-SLEDAI score reflects disease activity based on the presence or absence of 24 manifestations of SLE; scoring is weighted by the organ system involved. Response, as assessed by these end points, did not differ significantly between belimumab (any dosage) and placebo. However, exploratory analysis suggested that autoantibody-positive SLE patients responded better to belimumab plus standard care than to standard care alone. In an open-label extension of this study, treatment with belimumab for periods of up to 4 years resulted in sustained improvement in disease activity and reductions in disease flares in patients with serologically active disease.

As a result of these phase 2 findings, enrollment in 2 subsequent phase 3 studies (BLISS-76 and BLISS-52) was limited to patients with autoantibody-positive SLE. BLISS-76 and BLISS-52 were randomized, double-blind, placebo-controlled studies with similar designs except for study duration (76 and 52 weeks, respectively). Patients included in these studies had active SLE (SELENA-SLEDAI score of 6 or more) and positive autoantibody test results (i.e., antinuclear antibodies [ANA] or antibodies to double-stranded DNA [anti-dsDNA]) at screening. Treatment consisted of belimumab (1 or 10 mg/kg IV on days 0, 14, and 28 and then every 28 days up to 48 weeks in BLISS-52 and 72 weeks in BLISS-76) plus standard care or placebo plus standard care. The primary measure of efficacy was a composite end point (SLE Responder Index [SRI]) that defined response as meeting each of the following criteria at week 52: a reduction of 4 or more points from baseline in the SELENA-SLEDAI score; no new "A" rating (reflecting very active disease) and no more than 1 new "B" rating (reflecting moderately active disease) on assessments of the 8 organ systems included in the British Isles Lupus Assessment Group (BILAG) disease activity index; and no worsening (i.e., no increase of 0.3 or more points from baseline) on the 4-point Physician's Global Assessment (PGA) visual analog scale. In this composite end point, the SELENA-SLEDAI score measured global improvement, while the other measures were intended to ensure that improvement in disease activity was not offset by worsening of the patient's overall condition (PGA) or by worsening in previously unaffected organ systems (BILAG).

Results of BLISS-76 and BLISS-52 suggest that belimumab can modestly reduce disease activity in patients with severe autoantibody-positive SLE. In both studies, the proportion of patients achieving an SRI response at week 52 was significantly higher in the belimumab 10-mg/kg group (43–58%) than in the placebo group (34–44%). Only one of the 2 studies demonstrated a significant difference in SRI response rate between belimumab 1 mg/kg and placebo; therefore, use of the 1-mg/kg dose is not recommended. Reductions in disease activity were related mainly to improvements in the most commonly involved organ systems, namely, the mucocutaneous, musculoskeletal, and immunologic systems. Analyses of the drug's corticosteroid-sparing effects and its efficacy in preventing severe disease flares failed to show consistent, statistically significant effects across both studies. During weeks 40–52 of treatment, 19–21% of patients receiving belimumab 1 mg/kg, 17–19% of those receiving belimumab 10 mg/kg, and 12–13% of those receiving placebo were able to reduce their average prednisone dosage by at least 25% to 7.5 mg or less daily. At least one severe disease flare occurred over 52 weeks of treatment in 16–18% of patients receiving belimumab 1 mg/kg, 14–18% of those receiving belimumab 10 mg/kg, and 23–24% of those receiving placebo.

A limited number of black patients with SLE were enrolled in these 2 phase 3 studies. Exploratory analysis of combined data from the 2 studies indicated that SRI response rates were lower for black patients receiving belimumab 1 or 10 mg/kg (31 or 36%, respectively) than for black patients receiving placebo (44%). However, in the phase 2 study, black patients and patients of other racial groups did not appear to respond differently to belimumab. No definitive conclusions can be drawn from these subgroup analyses; caution should be used when considering belimumab for treatment of SLE in black patients.

Dosage and Administration

■ **General** Premedication (e.g., an antihistamine) should be considered before each infusion of the drug to minimize the risk of infusion and hypersensitivity reactions. (See Infusion Reactions and also see Sensitivity Reactions under Cautions: Warnings/Precautions.)

■ **Administration** Belimumab is administered by IV infusion only. The drug should not be administered by rapid IV injection, such as IV push or bolus. Belimumab should not be infused simultaneously through the same IV line with other agents. Administration of the drug should be completed within 8 hours of reconstitution.

Reconstitution Commercially available belimumab lyophilized powder must be reconstituted and diluted prior to IV administration. Belimumab should be removed from the refrigerator and allowed to stand at room temperature for 10–15 minutes prior to reconstitution. Vials labeled as containing 120 or 400 mg of belimumab should be reconstituted by adding 1.5 or 4.8 mL, respectively, of sterile water for injection, to provide a solution containing 80 mg/mL. During reconstitution, the sterile water diluent should be directed toward the side of the vial to minimize foaming. The vial should be gently swirled for 60 seconds every 5 minutes until the powder is dissolved. The vial should not be shaken. Dissolution usually occurs within 10–15 minutes but may require up to 30 minutes. The reconstituted solution should be protected from direct sunlight. If the reconstituted solution is not used immediately, the manufacturer recommends that it be stored under refrigeration (2–8°C).

Dilution Reconstituted belimumab solutions should be further diluted with 0.9% sodium chloride injection to a final volume of 250 mL prior to administration. Belimumab is incompatible with dextrose-containing solutions and should not be diluted with these solutions. The manufacturer states that only 0.9% sodium chloride injection should be used for dilution. Prior to addition of belimumab to the infusion bag or bottle, a volume of 0.9% sodium chloride injection equal to the volume of belimumab to be added should be removed and discarded. The appropriate volume of reconstituted belimumab should then be added to the diluent, and the infusion bag or bottle should be gently inverted to ensure thorough mixing. Commercially available belimumab for injection contains no preservatives and is intended for single use; any unused solution in the vial must be discarded. Belimumab infusion solutions may be stored at 2–8°C or room temperature. Belimumab infusion solutions should be inspected visually for particulate matter and discoloration prior to administration.

Rate of Administration IV infusions of belimumab should be administered over 1 hour. If an infusion reaction occurs during administration, the infusion may be slowed or interrupted. If a serious hypersensitivity reaction occurs, the infusion should be discontinued immediately.

■ **Dosage** The recommended adult dosage of belimumab for the management of systemic lupus erythematosus (SLE) is 10 mg/kg at 2-week intervals for the first 3 doses and at 4-week intervals thereafter. Belimumab should be used in conjunction with other standard therapies for SLE (see Uses: Systemic Lupus Erythematosus).

■ **Special Populations** Dosage adjustment is not required in patients with renal impairment. The manufacturer makes no specific dosage recommendations for geriatric patients or patients with hepatic impairment. (See Specific Populations under Cautions: Warnings/Precautions.)

Cautions

■ **Contraindications** History of anaphylactic reaction to belimumab.

■ **Warnings/Precautions** ***Mortality*** More deaths were reported with belimumab than with placebo during clinical trials in patients with systemic lupus erythematosus (SLE). A total of 14 deaths occurred during the placebo-controlled, double-blind periods of these trials, including 3 deaths (0.4%) among placebo recipients, 5 deaths (0.7%) among patients receiving belimumab 1 mg/kg, no deaths among patients receiving belimumab 4 mg/kg, and 6 deaths (0.9%) among patients receiving belimumab 10 mg/kg. Etiologies included infection, cardiovascular disease, and suicide; however, no single cause of death predominated.

Infectious Complications Serious and sometimes fatal infections have been reported in patients receiving immunosuppressive agents, including belimumab. Clinicians should exercise caution when considering the use of belimumab in patients with chronic infections. Patients receiving any therapy for chronic infection should not begin therapy with belimumab. If a patient develops a new infection during treatment, interruption of belimumab therapy should be considered and the patient should be monitored closely.

Infections, including upper respiratory tract infection, urinary tract infection, nasopharyngitis, sinusitis, bronchitis, and influenza, occurred in 71% of patients receiving belimumab compared with 67% of those receiving placebo in controlled clinical studies. Serious infections, including pneumonia, urinary tract infection, cellulitis, and bronchitis, occurred in 6% of patients receiving belimumab and 5.2% of those receiving placebo. Fatal infections occurred in 0.3% of patients receiving belimumab and 0.1% of those receiving placebo.

Malignancy Immunosuppressive therapy may increase the risk of malignancies. Whether treatment with belimumab affects development of malignancies remains to be determined. Malignancies were reported in clinical trials of the drug.

Sensitivity Reactions Hypersensitivity reactions, including anaphylaxis, hypotension, angioedema, urticaria or other rash, pruritus, and dyspnea, were reported on the day of an infusion in 13% of patients receiving belimumab and 11% of those receiving placebo. Anaphylaxis was observed in 0.6% of patients receiving belimumab and 0.4% of those receiving placebo. Because of overlapping clinical manifestations, it was not possible to distinguish between hypersensitivity reactions and infusion reactions in all cases. Although some patients (13%) received premedication regimens, there was insufficient experience to establish whether premedication reduced the frequency or severity of hypersensitivity reactions.

Belimumab should be administered by healthcare providers prepared to manage anaphylaxis. If a serious hypersensitivity reaction occurs, the infusion should be discontinued immediately and appropriate supportive care should be provided. Patients should be monitored during and for an appropriate period of time after administration of belimumab.

Infusion Reactions Infusion-related reactions, most commonly including headache, nausea, and skin reactions, were reported in 17% of patients receiving belimumab and 15% of those receiving placebo. Serious infusion reactions (excluding hypersensitivity reactions) were reported in 0.5% of patients receiving belimumab and 0.4% of those receiving placebo and included bradycardia, myalgia, headache, rash, urticaria, and hypotension. Although some patients (13%) received premedication regimens, there was insufficient experience to establish whether premedication reduced the frequency or severity of infusion reactions.

Belimumab should be administered by healthcare providers prepared to manage infusion reactions. In the event of an infusion reaction, the infusion should be slowed or interrupted.

Psychiatric Effects Psychiatric events, including depression, insomnia, and anxiety, were reported more frequently in patients receiving belimumab than in those receiving placebo (16 versus 12%). Serious psychiatric events or serious depression was reported in 0.8 or 0.4%, respectively, of patients receiving belimumab and in 0.4 or 0.1%, respectively, of patients receiving placebo; suicide has been reported. Most patients who reported serious depression or suicidal behavior had a history of depression or other serious psychiatric disorders, and most were receiving psychoactive drugs. It is unknown if belimumab increases the risk for these events.

Immunization Live vaccines should be avoided during and for 30 days prior to initiation of belimumab therapy. (See Drug Interactions: Vaccines.)

Concomitant Therapy Belimumab has not been studied in combination with other biologic therapies, including B-cell-targeted therapies, or IV cyclophosphamide. The manufacturer states that use of belimumab in combination with biologic therapies or IV cyclophosphamide is not recommended.

Immunogenicity In 2 clinical trials, antibodies to belimumab were detected in 4.8% of patients receiving belimumab doses of 1 mg/kg. Antibodies to the drug also were detected in 0.7% of those receiving belimumab doses of 10 mg/kg; however, because of the potential for high drug concentrations to reduce assay sensitivity, the actual frequency of antibody positivity in patients receiving doses of 10 mg/kg may exceed 0.7%. Neutralizing antibodies have been detected in several patients receiving the drug. Mild infusion-related reactions have been reported in several patients with antibody formation; however, the clinical importance of antibelimumab antibodies is not known.

Specific Populations **Pregnancy.** Category C. (See Users Guide.) Women of childbearing potential should use effective contraceptive methods during belimumab therapy and for at least 4 months after discontinuance of the drug.

To monitor maternal-fetal outcomes of pregnant women exposed to belimumab, a pregnancy registry has been established. Clinicians are encouraged to enroll pregnant women receiving belimumab in the registry; women also may enroll themselves in the registry by calling 877-681-6296.

Lactation. Belimumab is distributed into milk in cynomolgus monkeys. It is not known whether the drug is distributed into human milk or is absorbed systemically following ingestion. Because maternal antibodies are distributed into human milk, a decision should be made whether to discontinue nursing or the drug, taking into account the importance of breast-feeding to the infant and the importance of the drug to the woman.

Pediatric Use. Safety and efficacy have not been established in children.

Geriatric Use. Experience in patients 65 years of age and older is insufficient to determine whether they respond differently than younger adults; belimumab should be used with caution in geriatric patients.

Hepatic Impairment. The effect of hepatic impairment on the pharmacokinetics of belimumab has not been formally studied. However, in population pharmacokinetic analyses, interindividual variability in belimumab clearance was not explained by baseline transaminase (AST, ALT) or bilirubin concentration. Belimumab has not been studied in patients with severe hepatic impairment.

Renal Impairment. The effect of renal impairment on the pharmacokinetics of belimumab has not been formally studied. However, clinical studies of the drug in patients with SLE included a limited number of patients with moderate to severe renal impairment (creatinine clearance of 15–59 mL/minute). Although population pharmacokinetic analyses showed that belimumab clearance was increased at higher creatinine clearances and in the presence of proteinuria in excess of 2 g daily, belimumab clearance in patients with renal impairment was within the expected range of values and effects are unlikely to be clinically important.

Blacks. Exploratory analyses of data from two phase 3 studies of belimumab in patients with SLE indicated that response rates were lower for black patients receiving belimumab than for black patients receiving placebo. (See Uses: Systemic Lupus Erythematosus.) Belimumab should be used with caution in black patients.

■ **Common Adverse Effects** Adverse effects reported in 5% or more of patients receiving belimumab include nausea, diarrhea, pyrexia, nasopharyngitis, bronchitis, insomnia, pain in extremity, depression, migraine, and pharyngitis.

Drug Interactions

No formal drug interaction studies have been performed with belimumab to date.

■ **Angiotensin-converting Enzyme (ACE) Inhibitors** Concomitant use of belimumab and ACE inhibitors resulted in increased systemic clearance of belimumab; however, the effect was not considered clinically important.

■ **Antimalarials** Concomitant use of antimalarial agents (e.g., chloroquine, hydroxychloroquine) and belimumab did not substantially alter the pharmacokinetics of belimumab.

■ **Corticosteroids** Concomitant use of belimumab and corticosteroids resulted in increased systemic clearance of belimumab; however, the effect was not considered clinically important.

■ **HMG-CoA Reductase Inhibitors** Concomitant use of hydroxymethylglutaryl-coenzyme A (HMG-CoA) reductase inhibitors (statins) and belimumab did not substantially alter the pharmacokinetics of belimumab.

■ **Immunomodulatory or Immunosuppressive Agents** Concomitant use of belimumab with other immunosuppressive agents may increase the risk of infection. The manufacturer states that use of belimumab in conjunction with IV cyclophosphamide or other biologic agents, including B-cell-targeted therapies, is not recommended.

Concomitant use of azathioprine, methotrexate, or mycophenolate with belimumab did not substantially alter the pharmacokinetics of belimumab.

■ **Nonsteroidal Anti-inflammatory Agents** Concomitant use of aspirin or other nonsteroidal anti-inflammatory agents (NSAIAs) with belimumab did not substantially alter the pharmacokinetics of belimumab.

■ **Vaccines** Live vaccines should not be administered during or within 30 days prior to initiation of belimumab therapy since safety has not been established. No data are available on secondary transmission of infection from persons receiving live vaccines to patients receiving belimumab or on the effects of immunization in patients receiving belimumab. Belimumab may interfere with the immune response to vaccines.

Description

Belimumab is a recombinant fully human immunoglobulin G_1 lambda (IgG_1 lambda) monoclonal antibody that specifically binds to and inhibits the biologic effects of soluble human B-lymphocyte stimulator (BLyS). BLyS is a cytokine in the tumor necrosis factor (TNF) ligand family that contributes to B-lymphocyte differentiation and survival. BLyS binds to 3 receptors on B lymphocytes: transmembrane activator and calcium modulator and cyclophilin ligand interactor (TACI), B-cell maturation antigen (BCMA), and B-cell-activating factor receptor/BLyS receptor 3 (BAFF-R/BR3). BLyS inhibits B-cell apoptosis and stimulates differentiation of B cells into immunoglobulin-producing plasma cells. Selective inhibition of BLyS reduces the number of B cells, with preferential reduction of naive and transitional B cells. BLyS is overexpressed in patients with systemic lupus erythematosus (SLE) and other autoimmune diseases. Belimumab inhibits the binding of soluble BLyS to its receptors on B cells, thereby inhibiting the survival of B cells, including autoreactive B cells, and reducing the differentiation of B cells into immunoglobulin-producing plasma cells.

In clinical trials in patients with SLE, treatment with belimumab significantly reduced circulating $CD19^+$, $CD20^+$, naive, and activated B cells, plasmacytoid cells, and the SLE B-cell subset at week 52. Memory cells increased initially and slowly declined toward baseline levels by week 52. Treatment also led to reductions in IgG and antibodies to double-stranded DNA (anti-dsDNA) and to increases in complement (C3 and C4). Clinical relevance of these effects has not been definitively established.

Advice to Patients

Importance of reading the manufacturer's patient information (medication guide) before initiating therapy and before each subsequent infusion.

Importance of informing patients that there were more deaths among belimumab-treated patients than among placebo recipients during clinical trials in patients with systemic lupus erythematosus.

Risk of increased susceptibility to infection. Importance of promptly informing clinicians if any signs or symptoms suggestive of infection (e.g., fever, chills, pain or burning upon urination, frequent urination, bloody diarrhea, cough) develop.

Risk of hypersensitivity reactions, including anaphylaxis. Importance of seeking immediate medical care if signs or symptoms of hypersensitivity reactions (e.g., wheezing, difficulty breathing, perioral or lingual edema, rash) occur.

Importance of promptly reporting new or worsening depression, suicidal thoughts, or other mood changes.

Importance of not receiving live vaccines during belimumab therapy.

Importance of promptly reporting any symptoms suggestive of cardiac disease (e.g., chest discomfort or pain, shortness of breath, cold sweats, nausea, dizziness).

Importance of women informing clinicians if they are or plan to become pregnant or plan to breast-feed. Advise women of childbearing potential to use an effective contraceptive method during belimumab therapy and for at least 4 months following discontinuance of the drug. (See Pregnancy under Warnings/Precautions: Specific Populations, in Cautions).

Importance of informing clinicians of existing or contemplated concomitant therapy, including prescription and OTC drugs and herbal or dietary supplements, as well as any concomitant illnesses or any history of chronic infections.

Importance of informing patients of other important precautionary information. (See Cautions.)

Overview® (see Users Guide). For additional information on this drug until a more detailed monograph is developed and published, the manufacturer's labeling should be consulted. It is *essential* that the manufacturer's labeling be consulted for more detailed information on usual cau-

tions, precautions, contraindications, potential drug interactions, laboratory test interferences, and acute toxicity.**

Preparations

Excipients in commercially available drug preparations may have clinically important effects in some individuals; consult specific product labeling for details.

Belimumab

Parenteral

For injection, for IV infusion	120 mg	**Benlysta®**, Human Genome Sciences (also promoted by GlaxoSmithKline)
	400 mg	**Benlysta®**, Human Genome Sciences (also promoted by GlaxoSmithKline)

cycloSPORINE

Cyclosporin A

■ Cyclosporine is a cyclosporin immunosuppressive agent and disease-modifying antirheumatic drug.

Uses

Cyclosporine is used for the prevention of rejection of kidney, liver, or heart allografts. The manufacturers and some clinicians recommend that cyclosporine be used in conjunction with corticosteroid therapy, at least initially. Cyclosporine is also used for the treatment of chronic allograft rejection in patients previously treated with other immunosuppressive agents (e.g., azathioprine).

■ **Renal Allotransplantation** Cyclosporine is used to prolong graft survival of allogeneic renal transplants. Therapy with cyclosporine alone has achieved graft survival rates ranging from 71–91% 1 year after renal transplantation. In a retrospective study, patient and graft survival rates were 86 and 70%, respectively, 4 years after transplantation in cyclosporine-treated patients.

Concomitant administration of cyclosporine and corticosteroids in some studies has resulted in reduction of cyclosporine dosage and decreased frequency of cyclosporine's nephrotoxic effects while continuing to optimally prolong graft survival; however, some clinicians suggest that concomitant administration of cyclosporine and corticosteroids does not increase effectiveness and may increase the frequency of adverse systemic effects (e.g., lymphoma). In a study in renal allograft recipients receiving cyclosporine alone or in combination with corticosteroids, graft survival rates after 1 year were 88 vs 84%, respectively; infectious complications and hypertension occurred more frequently in patients receiving combined therapy with cyclosporine and a corticosteroid than in those receiving cyclosporine alone. Concomitant administration of cyclosporine and corticosteroids did not improve renal function and was associated with increased frequency of lymphoma, probably resulting from excessive immunosuppression. Although the manufacturers recommend that cyclosporine be used in conjunction with corticosteroid therapy, at least initially, further study is needed to determine the role of concomitant therapy in renal allograft recipients.

When immunosuppressive therapy with cyclosporine alone or combined with corticosteroids has been compared with combined azathioprine and corticosteroid therapy, graft survival rates generally were equivalent or higher in patients receiving cyclosporine with or without corticosteroids. In patients with renal allografts, the 1-year actuarial graft survival rates for cyclosporine vs combined azathioprine and corticosteroid therapy have been reported to be 72–77 vs 52–62%, respectively; the 1-year patient survival rates for cyclosporine vs combined azathioprine and corticosteroid therapy were 88–94 vs 76–92%, respectively. Some cyclosporine-treated patients also received periodic corticosteroid therapy for acute rejection episodes. The 4-year actuarial graft survival rates for these therapies have been reported to be 76 vs 62%, respectively, and the 4-year actuarial patient survival rates were 86 vs 70%, respectively. In one study, graft survival rate in cyclosporine-treated patients was higher in patients receiving first renal allografts than in those receiving second ones and in patients receiving HLA-A and/or B mismatched allografts than in those receiving allografts matched at HLA-A and B loci; there was no correlation in graft survival with warm or cold ischemia or with anti-HLA antibodies. Cyclosporine-treated patients generally have had higher serum creatinine concentrations than those receiving combined azathioprine and corticosteroid therapy. The relative effects of prophylactic immunosuppressive regimens containing cyclosporine and/or equine antithymocyte globulin (ATG) on graft survival rates remain to be determined. Results of several comparative studies indicate that the effects on graft survival rates of prophylactic immunosuppressive regimens containing cyclosporine or equine antilymphocyte globulin (ALG) are similar.

Although cyclosporine prolongs graft survival, the drug may not prevent acute episodes of renal allograft rejection. The number of patients experiencing acute episodes of renal allograft rejection and the median time to onset of these episodes (about 1 week) have been reported to be similar for cyclosporine- or combined azathioprine/corticosteroid-treated patients. However, in one study, first acute episodes of rejection were substantially less severe in patients receiving cyclosporine than in those receiving combined azathioprine and corticosteroid therapy. In some cyclosporine-treated patients, renal graft losses resulting from irreversible acute graft rejection may be associated with persistently low trough serum concentrations of the drug; however, optimum therapeutic trough concentrations have not been determined. The occurrence of graft rejection is difficult to differentiate from cyclosporine-induced nephrotoxicity. (See Cautions: Renal Effects.) Rapid increases in serum creatinine concentration that occur simultaneously with low blood or plasma cyclosporine concentrations may indicate graft rejection.

Some clinicians recommend that cyclosporine generally be discontinued and combined therapy with azathioprine and corticosteroids be initiated in patients who do not tolerate cyclosporine (e.g., nephrotoxicity) or in whom intractable rejection occurs. In one study, the 1-year actuarial graft survival rate in patients switched from cyclosporine to combined azathioprine and corticosteroid therapy was 60%. Conversion to immunosuppressive therapy with azathioprine and corticosteroids usually results in decreased serum creatinine concentrations; however, complications, including acute rejection episodes, serious infections, or azathioprine-induced leukopenia, may occur. In one study, the need to switch from cyclosporine to combined azathioprine and corticosteroid therapy because of cyclosporine-induced nephrotoxicity or intractable rejection was eliminated when routine (3 times weekly) monitoring of trough serum cyclosporine concentrations was initiated; however, optimum trough concentrations have not been determined.

■ **Hepatic Allotransplantation** Cyclosporine is used to prolong graft and patient survival in hepatic allograft recipients. Administration of cyclosporine and low-dose prednisone has resulted in 1-year actuarial patient survival rates of 60–80% in a limited number of hepatic allograft recipients. However, response rates may be variable and may depend on the underlying condition of the patient or the immunosuppressive regimen used. Cyclosporine's effectiveness in hepatic allotransplantation has been shown in children and adults. Decreased frequency of postoperative infectious complications may be observed in hepatic allograft recipients who have received cyclosporine compared with those treated with other immunosuppressive therapy.

■ **Cardiac Allotransplantation** Cyclosporine is used to prolong graft and patient survival in cardiac allograft recipients. The drug has been used concomitantly with low-dose corticosteroid therapy to decrease the frequency and clinical severity of rejection episodes, reduce infectious complications compared with other immunosuppressive agents, and facilitate early patient rehabilitation following cardiac transplantation. Two-year actuarial patient survival rates for cardiac allograft recipients receiving cyclosporine vs combined azathioprine and corticosteroid therapy have been reported to be 77 vs 58%, respectively, in a limited number of patients.

Cyclosporine has also been used in a limited number of patients with combined heart-lung transplantation†.

■ **Bone Marrow Allotransplantation** The value of cyclosporine in the prevention of acute graft-vs-host disease following bone marrow transplantation† remains to be clearly established. Results of studies to date suggest that prophylaxis with cyclosporine is comparable to, but not more effective than, prophylaxis with methotrexate for the prevention or amelioration of acute graft-vs-host disease or improving survival in patients undergoing bone marrow transplantation for leukemias. Limited data suggest that prophylactic combination therapy with cyclosporine and methotrexate is more effective for the prevention or amelioration of acute graft-vs-host disease and possibly improves survival compared with cyclosporine alone. Cyclosporine has also been used with some success for the treatment of moderate to severe, acute graft-vs-host disease following bone marrow transplantation. Limited data suggest that cyclosporine may be as effective as corticosteroid therapy. Corticosteroids are generally considered the initial therapy of choice for the treatment of acute graft-vs-host disease.

■ **Rheumatoid Arthritis** Oral cyclosporine is used in the management of the active stage of severe rheumatoid arthritis in selected adults who have an inadequate therapeutic response to methotrexate; the drug may be used in combination with methotrexate in those who do not respond adequately to methotrexate monotherapy. Oral cyclosporine also has been useful in the treatment of rheumatoid arthritis in adults who had an insufficient therapeutic response to, or who did not tolerate nonsteroidal anti-inflammatory agents† (NSAIAs) and other† disease-modifying antirheumatic drugs (DMARDs) (e.g., gold compounds, penicillamine). Cyclosporine is one of several DMARDs that can be used when DMARD therapy is appropriate. (For further information on the treatment of rheumatoid arthritis, see Uses: Rheumatoid Arthritis, in Methotrexate 10:00.)

In a placebo-controlled study, cyclosporine administered for 6 months was more effective than placebo in decreasing the number of painful and tender or swollen joints. Results of an uncontrolled clinical study of patients treated with cyclosporine for a median of 29 months showed in comparison to baseline articular index that at 18 months pain (as rated on a visual analog scale) and the duration of morning stiffness were decreased, while functional capacity (as rated on a visual analog scale) was improved. After 24 months of therapy, articular index, pain, and duration of morning stiffness remained decreased. Although few comparative studies with other DMARDs have been published, cyclosporine appears to be as effective as azathioprine, chloroquine, or methotrexate in the management of rheumatoid arthritis. Cyclosporine, azathioprine, and methotrexate did not differ in global assessment of efficacy based on the number of clinical and laboratory variables that improved after 1 year of therapy. The decrease in the number of swollen joints did not differ between cyclosporine and chloroquine after 24 weeks of therapy with either drug as the initial DMARD. The difference between groups in radiologic evidence of progression of disease, as indicated by the increase in the number of target joints with juxtaarticular erosions at 12 months compared with baseline, favored patients who were receiving cyclosporine over the controls who were receiving another DMARD (e.g., chloroquine, hydroxychloroquine, sulfasalazine, auranofin, parenteral gold compounds, penicillamine).

Combined use of cyclosporine and methotrexate appears to improve therapeutic response in patients with rheumatoid arthritis that had improved partially with methotrexate alone. After 6 months of therapy, improvement in the tender-joint count was greater with combined cyclosporine (mean dosage: 3 mg/kg daily) and methotrexate than with methotrexate alone. In addition, more patients treated with cyclosporine and methotrexate had improvement in rheumatoid arthritis, based on criteria of the American College of Rheumatology (i.e., improvement by at least 20% in the number of tender joints, number of swollen joints, and in 3 of 5 other clinical measures including pain, physician's global assessment, patient's global assessment, degree of disability, erythrocyte sedimentation rate). Complete blood cell count and liver function should be monitored at least monthly in patients receiving cyclosporine and methotrexate therapy concomitantly.

■ **Psoriasis** Oral cyclosporine is used in immunocompetent adults with severe (i.e., extensive and/or disabling), recalcitrant plaque psoriasis that is not adequately responsive to at least one systemic therapy (e.g., retinoids, methotrexate, psoralen and UVA light [PUVA therapy]) or in patients for whom other systemic therapy is contraindicated or cannot be tolerated. Discontinuance of therapy with cyclosporine, as with other therapies, will result in relapse of psoriasis in most patients, while rebound occurs rarely.

■ **Crohn's Disease** Cyclosporine has been used in the management of refractory inflammatory, fistulizing, and chronically active Crohn's disease.†

Efficacy of cyclosporine has been evaluated in several uncontrolled studies in patients with refractory (e.g., to corticosteroids, anti-infective agents, mercaptopurine, azathioprine, surgery) inflammatory or fistulizing Crohn's disease†. In these studies, a limited number of patients with inflammatory or fistulizing disease (who continued to receive anti-infective agents, corticosteroids, azathioprine, mercaptopurine, and/or mesalamine) initially received a continuous IV infusion of cyclosporine over 24 hours (4 mg/kg daily for about 2–10 days) until clinical response (complete response in inflammatory disease usually was defined as resolution of diarrhea and abdominal pain, while partial response was defined as a decrease in stool frequency and/or abdominal pain; complete response in fistulizing disease was defined as closure of the fistulas and cessation of drainage, while partial response was defined as reduction in the size, drainage, and discomfort associated with fistulas) was achieved. About 78–88% of patients responded while receiving IV cyclosporine and most of those who responded were switched to oral cyclosporine (5–8 mg/kg daily) for a mean duration of about 2.5–12.2 (range: 0.5–37 months) months. However, only about 29–71% of the patients who responded to IV cyclosporine, continued to respond while receiving oral cyclosporine and in 1 study (patients receiving oral cyclosporine for a median of 10.5 weeks), 71% of patients who responded to IV cyclosporine, relapsed after discontinuance of cyclosporine therapy. Some clinicians suggest, however, that a short course (about 4–6 months) of therapy with cyclosporine (administered as an IV infusion initially and followed by an oral course of the drug) given concomitantly with mercaptopurine or azathioprine (drugs associated with long-term improvement in fistulizing Crohn's disease) may be effective in some patients with refractory inflammatory or fistulizing Crohn's disease. Because both mercaptopurine and azathioprine have a slow onset of action (17 weeks or more) and cyclosporine has a faster onset, such an overlap of therapies (for about 4 months) may be beneficial in the fistulizing disease; however, additional well-controlled studies are needed to evaluate the clinical efficacy of these combinations. It also should be considered, that IV administration of cyclosporine may be associated with severe adverse effects and many clinicians state that the drug should be reserved for the management of severe refractory disease.

Results of several uncontrolled and some placebo-controlled trials indicate that oral cyclosporine (5–15 mg/kg daily) has not been consistently effective for inducing or maintaining remission in refractory chronically active Crohn's disease†. In a placebo-controlled, double-blind, randomized trial in patients with refractory, chronically active Crohn's disease, clinical improvement has been reported in more patients receiving oral cyclosporine (5–7.5 mg/kg daily) than in those receiving placebo (59% for cyclosporine versus 32% for placebo) at the end of a 3-month treatment period. However, during a subsequent 3-month tapering period, 36 or 55% of patients receiving cyclosporine or placebo, respectively, whose disease improved during the initial 3-month therapy, have relapsed; no substantial difference in disease improvement between cyclosporine therapy and placebo has been observed during the 6-month follow-up period.

For further information about the management of Crohn's disease, see Uses: Crohn's Disease, in Mesalamine 56:36.

■ **Ophthalmic Uses** For ophthalmic uses of cyclosporine, see 52:08.92.

■ **Other Uses** Cyclosporine potentially may be useful for the treatment of various other conditions that have an immunologic basis†.

Cyclosporine also has been used to decrease the frequency of pancreatic† or corneal allograft rejection†.

Dosage and Administration

■ **Administration** Cyclosporine is administered orally as conventional (nonmodified) or modified formulations; the drug also is administered by IV infusion.

Oral Administration Cyclosporine may be administered orally as the conventional liquid-filled capsules or the conventional oral solution. Alternatively, the drug may be administered orally as modified, liquid formulations (Gengraf®, Neoral®) that form emulsions in aqueous fluids; the modified formulations are available as oral solutions for emulsion and as oral liquid-filled capsules. When exposed to an aqueous environment, Neoral® oral solution forms a homogenous transparent emulsion with a droplet size smaller than 100 nm in diameter, which has been referred to as a microemulsion. Gengraf® also is described as forming a microemulsion when exposed to an aqueous environment. The 2 commercially available modified oral formulations of cyclosporine, Neoral® and Gengraf®, have been demonstrated to be bioequivalent to each other.

Modified formulations of cyclosporine (Gengraf®, Neoral®), both as the solution and in the liquid-filled capsules, have increased oral bioavailability compared with the conventional oral solution and liquid-filled capsules of the drug, and therefore the conventional (nonmodified) and modified formulations are *not* bioequivalent and cannot be used interchangeably without appropriate medical supervision. (See Pharmacokinetics: Absorption.) Patients should be informed that any change in the formulation of cyclosporine that they are receiving should be performed under the supervision of a clinician since adjustment of the dosage may be necessary and caution should be observed during such a transition.

Patients should be advised that oral formulations of cyclosporine should be administered on a consistent schedule with regard to time of day and in relation to meals. When an oral solution formulation is used, doses of cyclosporine should be measured carefully. A graduated oral syringe is provided for proper measurement of a dose of cyclosporine oral solution formulations. When measuring a dose of an oral solution formulation, the protective cover of the oral syringe should be removed, if present, and the prescribed dose of the drug withdrawn from the bottle of oral solution and transferred to a glass (not plastic) container of suitable beverage to enhance palatability. To increase the palatability of the conventional (nonmodified) oral solution, the measured dose of cyclosporine may be mixed with milk, chocolate milk, or orange juice, preferably at room temperature but not hot. To increase palatability of the modified oral solution of Gengraf® or Neoral®, the measured dose of the oral cyclosporine solution preferably should be mixed with orange or apple juice at room temperature; milk should *not* be used for dilution of the solution since the resultant mixture can be unpalatable. The manufacturers recommend that frequent changing of the diluting beverage be avoided. The diluted solution or emulsion containing cyclosporine should be stirred well and administered immediately, not allowing the mixture to stand before administration. Use of a glass container may minimize adherence of the drug to the walls of the container; styrofoam containers should *not* be used because they are porous and may absorb the drug. After the initial diluted solution or emulsion has been administered, the container should be rinsed with additional diluent (e.g., juice) and the remaining mixture administered to ensure that the entire dose of the drug has been given. After use of Neoral® oral solution, the manufacturer states that the outside of the dosing syringe should be dried with a clean, dry towel and the syringe replaced in its protective cover. After use of Gengraf® oral solution, the manufacturer states that the outside of the dosing syringe should be dried with a clean, dry towel and the syringe stored in a clean, dry place. To avoid turbidity, the dosing syringes for Gengraf® and Neoral® oral solution should not be rinsed with water, alcohol, or other cleaning agents. If the syringes require cleaning, they must be completely dry before reuse. Introduction of water into the product by any means will cause variation in dose.

Concomitant oral administration of cyclosporine conventional (nonmodified) or modified capsules or solutions with grapefruit juice should be avoided since unpredictable but potentially clinically important increases in oral bioavailability of the drug can result. Although some evidence suggested that patients who wished to continue consumption of grapefruit juice during cyclosporine therapy could do so if at least 90 minutes elapsed between administration of the drug and such consumption, other evidence indicates that such separation in timing may not be adequate, and additional study is needed. (See Drugs and Foods Affecting Hepatic Microsomal Enzymes: Grapefruit Juice, in Drug Interactions.)

IV Infusion Because of the risk of anaphylaxis, IV administration of cyclosporine should be reserved for patients in whom oral administration of the drug is not tolerated or is contraindicated. (See Cautions: Precautions and Contraindications.) *Cyclosporine concentrate for injection must be diluted prior to IV infusion.* For IV infusion, each mL of the concentrate should be diluted in 20–100 mL of 0.9% sodium chloride or 5% dextrose injection immediately before administration. Diluted solutions that have not been administered within 24 hours should be discarded. The required dose of diluted solution is infused over 2–6 hours.

Cyclosporine concentrate for injection and the diluted solution for infusion should be inspected visually for particulate matter and discoloration prior to administration whenever solution and container permit.

■ **Dosage** ***Transplant Recipients*** Dosage of cyclosporine should be individualized. Monitoring blood or plasma, but preferably whole blood, concentrations of cyclosporine has an essential role in individualizing dosage and managing transplant recipients during therapy with the drug. However, optimum concentrations have not been precisely defined, and suggested ranges vary depending on the assay method and body fluid employed as well as the patient population treated and therapeutic regimen used. Therefore, the type of assay used (See Pharmacokinetics), organ transplanted, time since transplantation, other immunosuppressive agents administered concurrently, and other factors are important considerations in the assessment of cyclosporine blood concentrations. The clinical evaluation of rejection and toxicity, adjustment of dosage, and assessment of compliance may be assisted by monitoring blood concentrations of cyclosporine; however, recommended ranges of cyclosporine concentrations that are consistent with optimum efficacy for *all* patients currently cannot be defined. Therefore, it is preferable that patients be managed using a center experienced in the use and interpretation of cyclosporine concentrations and their application to dosage adjustment.

Laboratory Monitoring. Most clinicians currently base monitoring on trough (predose) concentrations of the drug. It is important that the sampling time for a given patient be standardized and that consideration be given to the effect of once- versus twice-daily dosing of cyclosporine. While most recent experience has been with assays that are specific for unchanged cyclosporine (See Pharmacokinetics), data are accumulating on the use of total drug (both cyclosporine and metabolites) concentrations, and some centers may have switched to such monitoring methods. The frequency of monitoring depends in part on the time that has elapsed since transplantation, intercurrent illness, and concomitant drugs. While there are no hard and fast rules, and monitoring should be performed whenever clinical manifestations suggest that dosage adjustment might be necessary, some clinicians generally monitor frequently (e.g., 3 or 4 times weekly to daily) during the early posttransplantation period, reducing monitoring to once monthly by 6 months to 1 year after transplantation. Timing of determinations also should take into account the time to pharmacokinetic reequilibration following recent dosage changes; in general, determinations made within 3 days of a dosage change (2 days for children) will not reflect steady state. If management with a center experienced in therapeutic drug monitoring of cyclosporine is not possible, specialized references can be consulted for general monitoring and dosing guidelines. Results obtained with various methods are not interchangeable, and specialized references and/or the assay manufacturer's labeling should be consulted for interpretative guidelines.

If plasma assay methods are used, the possibility that concentrations may vary with temperature at the time of plasma separation from whole blood and that cyclosporine plasma concentrations may be about 20–50% of cyclosporine blood concentrations should be considered. In addition, monitoring of blood or plasma cyclosporine concentrations does not obviate monitoring of renal function (e.g., serum creatinine and creatinine clearance determination) or tissue biopsies in patients receiving the drug. Periodic determination of blood or plasma cyclosporine concentrations and adjustment in dosage, when necessary, are especially important in patients, particularly hepatic allograft recipients, receiving long-term oral therapy since absorption of the drug may be erratic.

In one suggested regimen employing a highly specific assay (high-pressure liquid chromatography [HPLC]), dosage of cyclosporine in renal allograft recipients was adjusted to achieve trough blood concentrations determined just prior to the next dose (24 hours after the previous dose) of 100–200 ng/mL. Blood concentrations determined by HPLC are unchanged cyclosporine alone, and they have been shown to correlate directly to those determined by monoclonal specific radioimmunoassays (m-RIA-sp). Nonspecific assay methods that detect both unchanged drug and its metabolites also are available, and such assay methods generally were employed in older studies; blood cyclosporine concentrations determined by these methods were about twice those reported with specific assay methods. Therefore, comparing concentrations reported in the published literature with those for a given patient using current assays must employ a detailed knowledge of the assay method used. Although several assays and assay matrices are available, the current consensus is that assays specific for unchanged cyclosporine correlate best with clinical events. Such assays include HPLC, monoclonal antibody RIAs, monoclonal antibody FPIA, and EMIT, which have sensitivity and are reproducible and convenient.

Usual Dosage. For prevention of allograft rejection in adults and children, the usual initial oral dose of conventional (nonmodified) formulations of cyclosporine is 15 mg/kg administered as a single dose 4–12 hours before transplantation. Although this initial dose varied from 14–18 mg/kg in most clinical studies, the highest dose continues to be used in only a few transplant centers, while doses at the lower end of the range have been favored. Administration of even lower initial dosages (e.g., 10–14 mg/kg daily) is the trend for renal allotransplantation. Postoperatively, the usual dosage of 15 mg/kg (range: 14–18 mg/kg) daily, administered as a single daily dose, is continued for 1–2 weeks and then tapered by 5% per week (over about 6–8 weeks) to a maintenance dosage of 5–10 mg/kg daily. In several studies, pediatric patients have required and tolerated higher dosages. Some clinicians have successfully tapered maintenance dosage to as low as 3 mg/kg daily in selected renal allograft recipients without an apparent increase in graft rejection rate.

Therapy with modified oral cyclosporine formulations (Gengraf®, Neoral®) can be started with an initial dose given 4–12 hours before transplantation or postoperatively. The initial dosage of the modified formulations varies depending on the organ transplanted and the other immunosuppressive agents included in the immunosuppressive protocol. Newly transplanted patients may receive a modified oral formulation at the same initial dose as for the conventional (nonmodified) oral formulation. A survey conducted in 1994 on the use of the conventional oral formulation in American transplant centers provides additional information on suggested initial dosages. Renal allograft recipients received an average initial dosage of 9 mg/kg in 2 equally divided doses daily at 75 centers. Hepatic allograft recipients received an average initial dosage of 8 mg/kg in 2 equally divided doses daily at 30 centers, and cardiac allograft recipients received an average initial dosage of 7 mg/kg in 2 equally divided doses daily at 24 centers. The dosage of the modified oral formulation subsequently is adjusted to attain a predefined blood cyclosporine concentration. The therapeutic range of *trough* blood concentrations of cyclosporine is the same for both the modified oral formulations and the conventional oral formulations. However, attainment of therapeutic trough blood concentrations of cyclosporine with the modified oral formulations will result in greater exposure (AUC) to the drug than would occur with conventional oral formulations. Titration of dosage should be based on clinical evaluation of rejection and patient tolerability. Lower maintenance dosages may be possible with the modified oral formulations.

If consideration is given to conversion of an allograft recipient from a conventional oral formulation of cyclosporine to a modified oral one, therapy with the modified oral formulation should be initiated at the same dosage that the patient is receiving of the conventional oral formulation (1:1 conversion). After conversion to the modified oral formulation, the increase in trough blood concentrations may be more pronounced and clinically important in some patients. The initial dosage subsequently should be adjusted to attain trough blood concentrations that are similar to those achieved with the conventional oral formulation. However, attainment of therapeutic trough blood concentrations will result in greater exposure (AUC) to cyclosporine than would occur with the conventional oral formulation. Monitoring of trough blood cyclosporine concentrations every 4–7 days after conversion to the modified oral formulation is recommended strongly until this measure is the same as it was with the conventional oral formulation. Safety of the patient also should be monitored with evaluation of such measures as the serum creatinine concentration and blood pressure every 2 weeks for the first 2 months after conversion to the modified oral formulation. The dosage must be adjusted appropriately if trough blood concentrations are outside of the range desired and/or if the measures of safety worsen.

Different strategies in dosage with the modified oral formulations are required for patients suspected of having poor absorption of cyclosporine from the conventional oral formulation. When trough blood concentrations are lower than expected relative to the dosage of the conventional oral formulation, the patient may have poor or inconsistent absorption of cyclosporine from this formulation. Patients tend to have higher blood cyclosporine concentrations after conversion to the modified oral formulations. The higher bioavailability of cyclosporine from the modified oral formulations may result in excessive trough blood concentrations after conversion to these formulations. Clinicians should be particularly cautious with conversional dosages exceeding 10 mg/kg daily. Individual titration of the dosage should be guided by trough blood concentrations, tolerability, and clinical response. After conversion to the modified oral formulation in patients who may have poor absorption of cyclosporine from the conventional oral formulation, trough blood concentrations should be measured more frequently, at least twice weekly, while such monitoring should be done daily in patients receiving more than 10 mg/kg daily, until the trough blood cyclosporine concentration is maintained in the desired range.

In patients unable to take the drug orally, cyclosporine may be administered by IV infusion at about one-third the recommended oral dosage. The usual initial IV dose of cyclosporine for adults and children is 5–6 mg/kg administered as a single dose 4–12 hours before transplantation. Postoperatively, the usual IV dosage of 5–6 mg/kg once daily is continued until the patient is able to tolerate oral administration of the drug. Pediatric patients may require higher dosages. Patients should be switched to an oral formulation of cyclosporine as soon as possible after surgery.

Concomitant Corticosteroid Therapy. For the prevention of allograft rejection, the manufacturer states that corticosteroid therapy should always be used concomitantly with IV cyclosporine. For the prevention of allograft rejection, the manufacturers recommend that corticosteroid therapy be administered concomitantly with conventional (nonmodified) oral formulations and be administered concomitantly, at least initially, with the modified oral formulations. Dosage of corticosteroids should be adjusted individually according to the clinical situation. Various schedules to taper corticosteroid dosage appear to yield similar results. Prednisone may be administered orally at an initial dosage of 2 mg/kg daily for 4 days and then tapered to 1 mg/kg daily by day 7, to 0.6 mg/kg daily by day 14, to 0.3 mg/kg daily by the end of the first month, and to a maintenance dosage of 0.15 mg/kg daily by the end of the second month. Corticosteroid dosage may be tapered further based on individual consideration of patient status and allograft function. Alternatively, an initial oral prednisone dose of 200 mg may be given and then tapered by 40 mg daily until a maintenance dosage of 20 mg daily is achieved; this maintenance dosage is then continued for 60 days and tapered to 10 mg daily during subsequent months.

Some clinicians believe that routine concomitant use of corticosteroids during cyclosporine therapy is not necessary and that their use should be reserved for acute periods of allograft rejection. Some clinicians suggest that if an acute rejection episode occurs in renal allograft recipients, 1 g of methylprednisolone be administered IV daily for 3 days; this dosage may be continued for an additional 3 days if rejection does not resolve following the initial course. If rejection continues after two 3-day courses of therapy, switching the patient to therapy with azathioprine and corticosteroids should be considered. Alternatively, some clinicians suggest that methylprednisolone be administered IV in a dosage of 0.5 or 1 g daily for 3 days for the management of an acute rejection reaction in renal allograft recipients. If necessary, courses of methylprednisolone therapy may be repeated until a total dosage of 6 g has been administered. If rejection continues, cyclosporine should be discontinued and switching the patient to therapy with azathioprine and corticosteroids should be considered.

Rheumatoid Arthritis For the management of rheumatoid arthritis in adults and children 18 years of age and older, the usual initial dosage of a modified oral cyclosporine formulation (e.g., Gengraf®, Neoral®) is 2.5 mg/kg daily given in 2 divided doses. Therapeutic response in patients with rheumatoid arthritis generally is apparent after 4–8 weeks of therapy. In patients with insufficient therapeutic response who have good tolerance to the drug (including serum creatinine concentration less than 30% above baseline), the dosage may be increased by 0.5–0.75 mg/kg daily after 8 weeks and, again, after 12 weeks to a maximum of 4 mg/kg daily. Lack of benefit by the 16th week of therapy should be considered a therapeutic failure and cyclosporine should be discontinued. Therapy with salicylates, other nonsteroidal anti-inflammatory agents (NSAIAs), or oral corticosteroids may be continued during cyclosporine therapy. To control adverse effects (e.g., hypertension, elevations in serum creatinine concentration to 30% above baseline, clinically important laboratory test abnormalities) that occur at any time during cyclosporine therapy, the cyclosporine dosage should be decreased by 25–50%. Cyclosporine should be discontinued if adverse effects are severe or do not respond to reduction of dosage.

When cyclosporine is used concomitantly with methotrexate for the management of rheumatoid arthritis, cyclosporine should be administered at the same initial dosage and range of adjustment as when administered alone. Administration of a modified oral cyclosporine formulation at 3 mg/kg daily or less generally is applicable in patients also receiving methotrexate at up to 15 mg weekly. There currently is only limited experience with long-term treatment of rheumatoid arthritis with the modified oral cyclosporine formulations. Following discontinuance of the drug, control of rheumatoid arthritis usually wanes within 4 weeks.

Use of cyclosporine for rheumatoid arthritis should be preceded by careful physical examination of the patient, including measurement of blood pressure on at least 2 occasions and determination of serum creatinine concentration twice for a baseline. During the first 3 months of therapy with cyclosporine, blood pressure and serum creatinine concentration should be evaluated every 2 weeks; thereafter, patients should be evaluated monthly if they are stable. Hypertension that develops during therapy with cyclosporine should elicit reduction of the dosage by 25–50%. Persistent hypertension should be managed by further reduction of the dosage of cyclosporine or use of antihypertensive agents. Withdrawal of cyclosporine generally results in return of blood pressure to baseline. Serum creatinine concentration and blood pressure should always be monitored after concomitant NSAIA therapy is modified by an increase in dosage and after initiation of new NSAIA therapy during cyclosporine therapy. Monthly evaluation with complete blood cell count and liver function tests is recommended in patients who also are receiving methotrexate concomitantly with cyclosporine.

Psoriasis For the management of psoriasis in adults and children 18 years of age and older, the usual initial dosage of a modified oral cyclosporine formulation (e.g., Gengraf®, Neoral®) is 1.25 mg/kg twice daily. This dosage should be continued for at least 4 weeks unless prohibited by adverse effects. Some improvement in clinical manifestations of psoriasis generally is observed after 2 weeks of therapy. If the initial cyclosporine dosage does not produce substantial clinical improvement within 4 weeks, dosage should be increased by approximately 0.5 mg/kg daily once every 2 weeks. Dosage may be increased in these increments to a maximum of 4 mg/kg daily based on the patient's tolerance and response.

Cyclosporine may not produce satisfactory control and stabilization of psoriasis until after 12–16 weeks of therapy. In a clinical study that evaluated titration of the dosage of cyclosporine, improvement of psoriasis by at least 75%, as indicated by scores on the Psoriasis Area and Severity Index, was observed in 51 or 79% of patients after 8 or 16 weeks of therapy, respectively. Lack of satisfactory response after patients receive 6 weeks of cyclosporine at the maximum dosage tolerated, up to 4 mg/kg daily, should lead to discontinuance of therapy.

In patients whose disease is controlled adequately and who appear stable, the regimen of cyclosporine should be adjusted so that the patient receives the lowest dosage that maintains an adequate response, which would not necessarily be total clearance of psoriasis. A satisfactory response was maintained in 60% of patients in clinical studies with dosages at the lower end of the recommended range. Dosages less than 2.5 mg/kg daily also may be equally effective.

To control adverse effects (e.g., hypertension, elevations in serum creatinine concentration to 25% or more above baseline, clinically important laboratory test abnormalities) that occur at any time during cyclosporine therapy, the dosage should be decreased by 25–50%. Cyclosporine should be discontinued if adverse effects are severe or do not respond to reduction of the dosage.

Discontinuance of cyclosporine therapy will result in relapse after several weeks, with approximately 50 or 75% of patients experiencing relapse within 6 or 16 weeks of discontinuance, respectively. Rebound does not occur in most patients after withdrawal of cyclosporine. Transformation of chronic plaque psoriasis to more severe forms of psoriasis that included pustular and erythrodermic psoriasis reportedly has occurred in some patients. There currently is only limited experience with the long-term treatment of psoriasis with modified oral cyclosporine formulations, and the manufacturers do not recommend continuous therapy with the drug for extended periods exceeding 1 year. Strategies in the long-term management of psoriasis should include consideration of alternation of cyclosporine with other therapies.

Use of cyclosporine for psoriasis should be preceded by careful dermatologic and physical examination of the patient, including measurement of blood pressure on at least 2 occasions. Physical examination should include evaluation for the presence of occult infection because cyclosporine is an immunosuppressive agent. The patient also should be evaluated for the presence of tumors at this initial examination and throughout therapy with cyclosporine. A biopsy should be obtained from dermatologic lesions that do not typify psoriasis before therapy with cyclosporine commences. Cyclosporine should be administered only after malignant or premalignant dermatologic lesions have been treated appropriately and only if other therapies for psoriasis are not an option.

During the first 3 months of therapy with cyclosporine in the management of psoriasis, blood pressure should be evaluated every 2 weeks; thereafter, patients should be evaluated monthly if they are stable or more frequently if their dosage is adjusted. Hypertension may occur at recommended dosages, with risk increased as the dosage and duration of therapy with the drug increases. If hypertension develops during therapy with cyclosporine, dosage should be reduced by 25–50% in patients without a history of hypertension prior to receiving the drug. Cyclosporine should be withdrawn if hypertension fails to respond to multiple reductions in dosage. Antihypertensive therapy of patients being managed for hypertension prior to initiation of cyclosporine therapy should be adjusted for effectiveness during cyclosporine therapy. When adequate adjustment of antihypertensive therapy is not possible or is not tolerated, cyclosporine should be withdrawn.

Measurements that should be obtained for baseline include serum creatinine concentration determined on 2 occasions, BUN, complete blood cell count, and serum concentrations of magnesium, potassium, uric acid, and lipoproteins. Serum creatinine must be monitored frequently. During the first 3 months of therapy with cyclosporine in the management of psoriasis, serum creatinine concentration and BUN should be evaluated every 2 weeks; thereafter, stable patients should be evaluated monthly. When the serum creatinine concentration exceeds baseline by 25% or more, repeated measurement should be obtained within 2 weeks. The dosage of cyclosporine should be reduced by 25–50% if the serum creatinine concentration on repeated measurement continues to exceed baseline by 25% or more. Such reduction of the dosage also is necessary if serum creatinine concentration exceeds baseline by 50% or more at *any time*. If the serum creatinine concentration does not decrease to within 25% of baseline after the dosage was modified twice, the drug should be withdrawn. Serum creatinine concentration also should be monitored after concomitant therapy with a NSAIA is modified by an increase in dosage and after initiation of new NSAIA therapy.

Complete blood cell count and serum concentrations of magnesium, potassium, uric acid, and lipids should be monitored every 2 weeks during the first 3 months of therapy with cyclosporine in the management of psoriasis; thereafter, these values should be monitored monthly in stable patients or more frequently when the dosage is adjusted. Mild hypomagnesemia and hyperkalemia that are asymptomatic and increases in the serum concentration of uric acid may occur with cyclosporine. Serum concentrations of triglycerides or cholesterol may be increased modestly during therapy with cyclosporine. The dosage of cyclosporine should be reduced by 25–50% in response to any abnormality of clinical concern.

Patients receiving cyclosporine to treat psoriasis should be warned about appropriate protection from the sun and avoidance of excessive solar exposure.

Crohn's Disease. For the management of refractory, inflammatory or fistulizing Crohn's disease†, cyclosporine has been administered initially in a dosage of 4 mg/kg daily for about 2–10 days, as a continuous IV infusion over 24 hours. Most of those who responded were switched to oral cyclosporine (5–8 mg/kg daily) for a mean duration of about 2.5–12.2 (range: 0.5–37 months) months.

Cautions

Patients who experienced adverse effects during treatment with cyclosporine for rheumatoid arthritis were affected principally by renal dysfunction, hypertension, headache, hirsutism/hypertrichosis, and GI disturbances. Therapy with cyclosporine was discontinued in clinical studies because of elevated serum creatinine concentration or hypertension in about 7 or 5% of patients, respectively, treated with the drug for rheumatoid arthritis at dosages within the recommended range. Reversibility of these changes generally occurred with timely reduction of the dosage or withdrawal of cyclosporine. Elevation of serum creatinine concentration increases in frequency and severity as the dosage of cyclosporine and its duration of administration increase. Maintenance of the regimen is likely to result in more pronounced increases in serum creatinine concentration.

Patients who experienced adverse effects during treatment with cyclosporine for psoriasis were affected principally by renal dysfunction, hypertension, headache, paresthesia or hyperesthesia, hirsutism/hypertrichosis, abdominal discomfort, diarrhea, nausea/vomiting, influenza-like symptoms, hypertriglyceridemia, lethargy, and musculoskeletal or joint pain. Therapy with cyclosporine was discontinued in clinical studies because of elevated serum creatinine concentration or hypertension in about 5 or 1% of patients, respectively, treated with the drug for psoriasis at dosages within the range recommended. Elevation of blood pressure or serum creatinine concentration in patients receiving cyclosporine for the management of psoriasis generally was reversible after dosage reduction or withdrawal of the drug. Elevation of serum creatinine concentration increases in frequency and severity as the dosage of cyclosporine and its duration of therapy increase. Maintenance of the regimen is likely to result in more pronounced increases in serum creatinine concentration that may lead to irreversible renal damage. Progressive renal failure led to the death of a patient who developed renal deterioration while receiving cyclosporine for the treatment of psoriasis and continued to receive the drug.

■ **Renal Effects** The most frequent and clinically important adverse effect of cyclosporine is nephrotoxicity. Nephrotoxic effects (usually manifested as increased BUN and serum creatinine concentrations) of cyclosporine have been observed in 25–32, 38, or 37% of patients receiving the drug for kidney, heart, or liver allografts, respectively. Elevations of BUN and serum creatinine concentrations resulting from cyclosporine therapy appear to be dose related, may be associated with high trough concentrations of the drug, and are usually reversible upon discontinuance of the drug. Clinical manifestations of cyclosporine-induced nephrotoxicity may include fluid retention, dependent edema, and, in some cases, a hyperchloremic, hyperkalemic metabolic acidosis. The risk of cyclosporine-induced nephrotoxicity may be increased in patients receiving other potentially nephrotoxic agents. (See Drug Interactions: Nephrotoxic Drugs.) Mild cyclosporine-induced nephrotoxicity generally occurs within 2–3 months after transplantation. Although some decline from preoperative levels generally occurs in patients with mild nephrotoxicity, the BUN and serum creatinine concentrations reportedly become stabilized in the range of 35–45 mg/dL and 2–2.5 mg/dL, respectively, in these patients; however, these elevations often respond to dosage reduction. In some patients, more severe nephrotoxic effects have been observed early after transplantation and have been characterized by rapid increases in BUN and serum creatinine concentrations; these elevations usually respond to dosage reduction.

Differentiation of Nephrotoxicity and Allograft Rejection In patients with renal allografts, acute episodes of allograft rejection must be differentiated from nephrotoxic effects of cyclosporine. When increased serum creatinine concentrations occur without the usual symptoms of renal allograft rejection (e.g., fever, graft tenderness or enlargement), cyclosporine-induced nephrotoxicity is likely. Although reliable and sensitive differentiation of cyclosporine-induced nephrotoxicity from renal allograft rejection through specific diagnostic criteria currently is not possible, and nephrotoxicity and rejection may coexist in up to 20% of patients, either adversity has been associated with various parameters (e.g., history, clinical, laboratory, biopsy, aspiration cytology, urine cytology, manometry, ultrasonography, magnetic resonance imagery, radionuclide scan, and response to therapy) that can be used in an attempt to differentiate between the two. For example, nephrotoxicity from cyclosporine has been associated with a history of having undergone a transplant involving prolonged kidney preservation time or prolonged anastomosis time, having received concomitant therapy with nephrotoxic drugs (e.g., an aminoglycoside, a nonsteroidal anti-inflammatory agent), or having received an organ from a donor who was older than 50 years of age or who was hypotensive, whereas renal allograft rejection has been associated with a history of antidonor immune response or previous renal allotransplantation. Nephrotoxicity often becomes apparent clinically more than 6 weeks postoperatively in patients whose allograft functioned initially or as prolonged initial nonfunction of the allograft that resembles acute tubular necrosis, whereas renal allograft rejection often becomes apparent clinically less than 4 weeks postoperatively and manifests with signs such as fever exceeding 37.5°C, swelling and tenderness of the graft, weight gain exceeding 0.5 kg, and a decrease in daily urine volume by more than 500 mL or 50%.

In some studies, patients with nephrotoxicity had high trough concentrations of cyclosporine in biologic fluid, as measured with a nonspecific (e.g., polyclonal radioimmunoassay [RIA] now obsolete) or a specific (e.g., high-performance liquid chromatography [HPLC]) assay for cyclosporine. The manufacturers state that a trough serum concentration of cyclosporine, as measured by polyclonal RIA, exceeding 200 ng/mL has been associated with the occurrence of nephrotoxicity. However, the relationship between nephrotoxicity and trough or other concentrations of cyclosporine in biologic fluid (e.g., whole blood) measured with specific monoclonal RIA or HPLC has not been fully established. (See Pharmacokinetics.) By comparison, allograft rejection has been associated with low trough concentrations of cyclosporine in biologic fluid, as measured with a nonspecific (e.g., polyclonal RIA) or a specific (e.g., monoclonal RIA, HPLC) assay for cyclosporine. The manufacturers state that a trough serum concentration of cyclosporine, as measured by polyclonal RIA, of less than 150 ng/mL has been associated with the occurrence of rejection. Other concentrations of the drug in biologic fluid (e.g., whole blood) at which rejection occurred have been reported with the use of specific assays for cyclosporine.

Common laboratory findings associated with cyclosporine-induced nephrotoxicity include a gradual increase in serum creatinine concentration (e.g., less than 0.15 mg/dL daily) that reaches a plateau of less than 25% above baseline, and a ratio of blood urea nitrogen (BUN) to serum creatinine of at least 20. By comparison, laboratory findings associated with allograft rejection include a rapid increase in serum creatinine concentration (e.g., exceeding 0.3 mg/dL daily) that reaches a plateau exceeding 25% above baseline, or a BUN to creatinine ratio of less than 20.

The histologic features of allograft biopsies in patients with cyclosporine-induced nephrotoxicity include effects on the arterioles, tubules, and interstitium. Such findings include arteriolopathy manifested as medial hypertrophy and hyalinosis, nodular deposits, intimal thickening, endothelial vacuolization, and progressive scarring. Renal tubular effects of nephrotoxicity include atrophy, isometric vacuolization, and isolated calcifications. Interstitial effects of nephrotoxicity include minimal edema, mild focal infiltrates of mononuclear cells, and diffuse interstitial fibrosis that often is the striped form. The histologic features of allograft biopsies in patients with rejection include effects on the arterioles and arteries, tubules, interstitium, and glomeruli. Such findings include endovasculitis manifested as arteriolar and arterial endothelial cell proliferation, intimal arteritis, fibrinoid necrosis, and sclerosis. Renal tubular effects of rejection include tubulitis with erythrocyte and leukocyte casts and some irregular vacuolization. Interstitial effects of rejection include a diffuse moderate to severe infiltrate of mononuclear cells, edema, and hemorrhage. Glomerulitis, manifested as infiltration of glomerular capillaries by mononuclear cells, is associated with rejection. Histologic changes, including thromboses of arteriolar and glomerular capillaries and mesangial sclerosis, also have occurred in cyclosporine-treated patients with renal dysfunction following bone marrow transplantation.

With cyclosporine-induced nephrotoxicity, renal allograft evaluation with aspiration cytology reveals deposits of the drug in tubular and endothelial cells and fine isometric vacuolization of tubular cells; urine cytology reveals tubular cells with vacuolization of cytoplasm and granularization. Manometry shows an intracapsular pressure of less than 40 mm Hg, and ultrasonography shows the renal cross-sectional area to be unchanged. With rejection, aspiration cytology shows that the graft generally is affected by an inflammatory infiltrate of mononuclear cells that includes phagocytes, macrophages, lymphoblastoid cells, and activated T-cells; HLA-DR antigens are expressed strongly by these mononuclear cells. Urine cytology in rejection may show degenerative renal tubular cells, plasma cells, and lymphocyturia exceeding 20% of the urinary sediment. Intrarenal manometry shows an intracapsular pressure exceeding 40 mm Hg in many patients with rejection, and ultrasonography shows an increase in graft cross-sectional area; the anteroposterior diameter is equal to or greater than the transverse diameter.

In most patients with nephrotoxicity, magnetic resonance imagery shows normal renal appearance, and radionuclide scans performed with technetium Tc 99m pentetate (DTPA) and iodohippurate sodium I 131 to evaluate renal perfusion and tubular function, respectively, show renal perfusion to be normal (although a generally decreased perfusion is observed occasionally) and tubular function to be decreased. While the decrease in tubular function is a deteriorative effect, renal perfusion is not decreased to a deleterious extent. With rejection, findings of magnetic resonance imagery include loss of distinct corticomedullary junction, swelling of the allograft, image intensity of parenchyma that approaches the image intensity of psoas, and loss of hilar fat; radionuclide scans may show patchy arterial flow. Evaluation of renal perfusion and tubular function with technetium Tc 99m pentetate or iodohippurate sodium I 131, respectively, shows that renal perfusion is decreased to a greater extent than is tubular function in patients with rejection; uptake of indium In 111-labeled platelets or technetium Tc 99m in colloid is increased.

Limited data suggest that some of the variables associated with nephrotoxicity actually may be risk factors for the development of nephrotoxicity from cyclosporine. The number of episodes of acute deterioration of renal function induced by cyclosporine (e.g., increase in serum creatinine concentration corrected by a decrease in the dose of cyclosporine), trough concentrations of cyclosporine during the second and third months after transplantation, the number of episodes of unexplained acute deterioration of renal function (e.g., increase in serum creatinine concentration unresponsive to a decrease in the dose of cyclosporine), and the number of treatments for rejection (e.g., corticosteroids) were correlated with chronic nephrotoxicity (e.g., arteriolopathy, striped form of interstitial fibrosis, tubular atrophy). The variables that were discriminative of nephrotoxicity included the number of episodes of acute deterioration of renal function induced by cyclosporine, the number of episodes of unexplained acute deterioration of renal function, the number of episodes of rejection, and the number of treatments for rejection, with patients with nephrotoxicity having experienced more episodes of acute deterioration of renal function, whether induced by the drug or unexplained, than patients with rejection, and those with rejection exhibiting a stronger history of multiple episodes of rejection and being treated for such more often. Some patients with chronic nephrotoxicity did not exhibit acute cyclosporine-induced deterioration of renal function. Poor primary function of the allograft occurred more often in these patients than in patients who had both acute deterioration of renal function induced by cyclosporine and chronic nephrotoxicity.

Response to a reduction in cyclosporine dosage generally can distinguish nephrotoxicity from rejection since the renal function of patients with nephrotoxicity usually recovers with such dosage modification. By comparison, response (e.g., in renal function) to an increase in dosage of concomitant corticosteroids or to antithymocyte globulin generally indicates the presence of rejection rather than nephrotoxicity.

A form of cyclosporine-associated nephropathy that is characterized by serial deterioration in renal function and changes in renal morphology also has been described. In this nephropathy, the rise in serum creatinine concentration does not diminish in response to a decrease in the dosage of, or discontinuance of therapy with, cyclosporine in 5–15% of allograft recipients. Renal biopsy in such patients will show one or more morphologic changes, none of which is entirely specific to structural nephrotoxicity associated with cyclosporine, although diagnosis of such nephropathy requires evidence of these changes. The morphologic changes include renal tubular vacuolization, tubular microcalcifications, peritubular capillary congestion, arteriolopathy, and a striped form of interstitial fibrosis with tubular atrophy. Of interest in the consideration of the development of cyclosporine-associated nephropathy is that the appearance of interstitial fibrosis reportedly is associated with higher cumulative doses of cyclosporine or persistently high circulating trough concentrations of the drug, particularly during the first 6 months after transplantation when dosages tend to be highest. Furthermore, renal allografts appear to be most vulnerable to the toxic effects of cyclosporine during this time. Other factors that contribute to the development of interstitial fibrosis include prolonged perfusion time, warm ischemia time, and episodes of acute toxicity and acute or chronic rejection. Whether interstitial fibrosis is reversible and its correlation to renal function are not known. Arteriolopathy reportedly was reversible when the dosage of cyclosporine was decreased or therapy with the drug was discontinued.

Management of Nephrotoxicity Gradual reduction of cyclosporine dosage is recommended for the management of nephrotoxicity, with careful patient assessment for several days to weeks. When patients are unresponsive to reduction of cyclosporine dosage and the possibility of allograft rejection has been excluded, switching from cyclosporine to therapy with alternative immunosuppressants (e.g., azathioprine and prednisone) should be considered. Concomitant use of corticosteroids with cyclosporine does not appear to improve renal function.

Other Renal Effects Hyperkalemia (that may be associated with hyperchloremic metabolic acidosis), hypomagnesemia, and decreased serum bicarbonate concentration have been reported frequently in patients receiving cyclosporine; these effects may result from nephrotoxic effects of the drug. Hyperuricemia also occurs commonly in cyclosporine-treated patients, particularly in those receiving diuretics concurrently, and may result in gout in some patients. Although not clearly established, hyperuricemia appears to result at least in part from decreased renal clearance of uric acid. Hematuria has occurred rarely in patients receiving cyclosporine.

Impairment of renal function (e.g., increased BUN and serum creatinine concentrations, decreased glomerular filtration rate (GFR) and effective renal plasma flow) and morphologic evidence of renal injury (e.g., renal tubular atrophy, interstitial fibrosis, arteriolar hyalinosis) have been observed in some patients who received short- or long-term treatment with cyclosporine for psoriasis. Elevated serum creatinine concentrations occurred in about 20% of patients. Elevations of BUN and serum creatinine concentrations resulting from cyclosporine at dosages used for psoriasis may be associated with relatively high trough concentrations of the drug but usually are reversible after discontinuance of the drug. Although limited data suggested the reversibility of decreases in GFR and effective renal plasma flow resulting from cyclosporine therapy for psoriasis, these manifestations of renal impairment may persist despite discontinuance of the drug. In patients who developed nephrotoxicity, as indicated by a decrease of more than 20% in GFR or a decrease of more than 25% in total renal blood flow, after 3 months of treatment with cyclosporine, evaluation at 3 months subsequent to discontinuance of the drug showed recovery of GFR but not of renal blood flow. GFR and effective renal plasma flow continued to be decreased below baseline 4 months after discontinuance of cyclosporine in patients who received the drug for a median of 12 months at a dosage of 5 mg/kg daily for 3 months that was then reduced by 0.35 mg/kg daily every month until the minimum effective dose was achieved. In some patients who received cyclosporine for an average of 30 months at a dosage of up to 5 mg/kg daily, GFR and renal plasma flow rate were below the lower 2.5 percentile of normal compared with the renal function of healthy individuals matched for age and gender 1 month after discontinuance of the drug. Biopsies occasionally showed kidneys with structural damage manifested as renal tubular atrophy, interstitial fibrosis, and hyaline arteriolopathy that were graded as moderate. Mild tubulointerstitial scarring and glomerulosclerosis were observed in the other patients but a relationship to cyclosporine was not certain. A correlation between severity of renal injury and severity of recurrent acute nephrotoxicity was found, which suggests recurrent severe acute nephrotoxicity (i.e., serum creatinine increased by more than 90% above baseline) to be a risk factor for chronic nephrotoxicity from cyclosporine. Histologic evidence of renal tubular atrophy, arteriolar hyalinosis, and increases above normal in interstitium and obsolescent glomeruli have been observed in patients who received cyclosporine at a mean dosage of 3 mg/kg daily for an average of 5 years.

Cyclosporine administered to treat rheumatoid arthritis resulted in serum creatinine concentrations increasing by at least 30 or 50% in up to 43–48 or 18–24% of patients, respectively. Maintenance of the regimen is likely to result in more pronounced increases in serum creatinine concentration that may lead to irreversible renal damage. The maximal increase in serum creatinine concentration may be a predictor of nephropathy from cyclosporine. Features suggesting nephropathy were observed in the renal biopsies of some patients with rheumatoid arthritis treated with cyclosporine for an average of 19 months. The dosage was 4 mg/kg daily or less in one of the patients. Dosage reduction or withdrawal of cyclosporine resulted in improvement in serum creatinine concentrations in most of these patients. Morphologic features that are identified with nephropathy induced by cyclosporine generally were not observed in renal biopsies from patients who had mostly completed 6 months of therapy with the drug and who did not appear to have renal dysfunction. Renal biopsies obtained by the 20th month of therapy with cyclosporine for rheumatoid arthritis and after 30–46 months of treatment showed morphologic changes compared with baseline that were not considered to be specific to nephropathy induced by the drug. In a limited study, differences in renal biopsies were not observed between patients with rheumatoid arthritis treated with cyclosporine at dosages less than 5 mg/kg daily for an average of 26 months and controls derived from autopsies of patients with rheumatoid arthritis. In the patients treated with cyclosporine, creatinine clearance that was measured or calculated was decreased from baseline by 26 or 24%, respectively, after 24 months of therapy. Cyclosporine administered to treat rheumatoid arthritis resulted in elevated BUN in 1% to less than 3% of patients.

Renal tubular atrophy and interstitial fibrosis was observed in 21% of patients with psoriasis who received cyclosporine dosages of 1.2–7.6 mg/kg daily for an average of 23 months. Such structural damage to the kidney was shown on repeated biopsy in some of the patients who were maintained on various dosages of cyclosporine for an additional period averaging 2 years, so that 30% of patients were affected overall. Most of these patients were receiving at least 5 mg/kg daily of cyclosporine, which exceeds the highest dosage recommended, had been taking the drug for more than 15 months, and/or had a clinically important increase in serum creatinine concentration for more than 1 month. Discontinuance of therapy with cyclosporine resulted in normalization of serum creatinine concentration in most patients. Quantitative digital morphometric analysis showed an increase in the percentage of fibrotic area in the tubular interstitium after 3.5 years of therapy with 3–6 mg/kg daily of cyclosporine compared with evaluation 1 year earlier. After 2 years of receiving cyclosporine generally at a dosage of 2.5–6 mg/kg daily, all patients had abnormal renal morphology, although the renal biopsy was normal at baseline in many of the patients. Evaluation of biopsies for focal interstitial fibrosis and arteriolar hyaline wall thickening showed increases compared with baseline. The percentage of sclerotic glomeruli was increased compared with baseline after 4 years of therapy with cyclosporine.

■ **Cardiovascular Effects** The manufacturers state that mild to moderate hypertension occurs in about 50% of renal transplant recipients who receive cyclosporine and in most cardiac transplant patients receiving the drug. In one study in renal allograft recipients, hypertension occurred in about 40% of cyclosporine-treated patients; 2 of these patients developed malignant hypertension with associated seizures. In some patients with cardiac allografts who developed hypertension while receiving cyclosporine, therapy with hypotensive agents has been required.

Hypertension generally develops within a few weeks after beginning cyclosporine therapy and affects both the systolic and diastolic blood pressure. Although the mechanism has not been clearly established, there is some evidence that hypertension may result from the renal vasoconstrictive effects of the drug. The manufacturers state that hypertension associated with cyclosporine therapy may respond to dosage reduction and/or antihypertensive therapy. However, some evidence from clinical studies suggests that response to antihypertensive therapy may be variable and that elevations in diastolic blood pressure may be more resistant to treatment than elevations in systolic pressure.

Myocardial infarction has occurred rarely in patients receiving the drug.

Cyclosporine administered to treat rheumatoid arthritis resulted in hypertension in up to about 26% of patients. Systolic hypertension (i.e., measurement of systolic blood pressure that twice exceeded 140 mm Hg) and diastolic hypertension (i.e., measurement of diastolic blood pressure that twice exceeded 90 mm Hg) developed in 33 and 19% of patients, respectively. Arrhythmia occurred in up to about 5% of patients. Abnormal heart sounds, cardiac failure, myocardial infarction, and peripheral ischemia each occurred in 1% to less then 3% of patients.

Cyclosporine administered to treat psoriasis resulted in the development of hypertension (i.e., systolic blood pressure of 160 mm Hg or greater and/or diastolic blood pressure of 90 mm Hg or greater) in about 28% of patients.

■ **Nervous System Effects** Adverse nervous system effects occur frequently in patients receiving cyclosporine. Tremor reportedly occurs in 12–21, 31, or 55% of patients with kidney, heart, or liver allografts, respectively, who receive cyclosporine. In one study in renal allograft recipients, however, tremor occurred in about 40% of cyclosporine-treated patients. Cyclosporine-induced tremor may be manifested as a fine hand tremor, usually is mild in severity, may improve despite continued therapy, and/or may be alleviated by a decrease in dosage of the drug.

Seizures (particularly when cyclosporine was used in combination with high-dose corticosteroids), headache, paresthesia, hyperesthesia, flushing, and confusion have been reported occasionally in patients receiving cyclosporine. There is some evidence that cyclosporine-induced seizures and other neurotoxicity may be associated with high blood or plasma concentrations of the drug, concurrent high-dose corticosteroid therapy, hypertension, and/or hypomagnesemia. Encephalopathy, manifested by impaired consciousness, seizures, visual changes (e.g., blindness), loss of motor function, movement disorders, and psychiatric disturbances, has been described in patients receiving cyclosporine; in many cases, such manifestations were accompanied by white-matter changes (documented by imaging procedures and pathologic findings). Adverse neurologic effects in most cases are reversible upon discontinuance of the drug or in some patients following dosage reduction.

Optic disc edema with possible visual impairment secondary to benign intracranial hypertension has been reported rarely in patients receiving cyclosporine; this complication occurred more frequently in transplant recipients than in patients receiving the drug for other indications.

Psychiatric disorders including anxiety, flat affect, and depression have occurred rarely in patients receiving the drug.

Cyclosporine administered to treat rheumatoid arthritis resulted in headache in up to about 25% of patients. Tremor or paresthesia occurred in up to about 13 or 11% of patients, respectively. Dizziness, depression, flushing, insomnia, or migraine occurred in up to about 8, 6, 5, 4, or 3% of patients, respectively. Hypoesthesia, neuropathy, and vertigo each occurred in 1% to less than 3% of patients. Psychiatric disorders that occurred in 1% to less than 3% of patients include anxiety, impaired concentration, confusion, emotional lability, decreased libido, increased libido, nervousness, paroniria, and somnolence.

Cyclosporine administered to treat psoriasis resulted in adverse effects of the central and peripheral nervous system in about 26% of patients. Headache occurred in about 16% of patients. Paresthesia occurred in about 7% of patients. Dizziness, flushes, insomnia, nervousness, and vertigo each occurred in 1% to less than 3% of patients. Adverse psychiatric effects occurred in about 5% of patients.

■ **Dermatologic Effects** Adverse dermatologic effects including hirsutism and gingival hyperplasia have occurred frequently during cyclosporine therapy. The manufacturers state that hirsutism occurs in 21, 28, or 45% of patients with kidney, heart, or liver allografts, respectively, who received cyclosporine; however, hirsutism reportedly has been observed in 30–45% of renal allograft recipients in some studies. Hirsutism usually develops within 2–4 weeks after transplantation, is mild, and involves the face, arms, eyebrows, and back. Although most patients can tolerate cyclosporine-induced hirsutism, occasionally it can be severe and some patients may prefer cosmetic alleviation of the excess hair (e.g., by shaving or use of depilatories). In addition, although development of hirsutism does not appear to be dose related, improvement may occur following a decrease in dosage of the drug.

Gingival hyperplasia reportedly occurs in 4–9, 5, or 16% of cyclosporine-treated patients with kidney, heart, or liver allografts, respectively, although in one study, gingival hyperplasia occurred in 30% of cyclosporine-treated patients. Cyclosporine-induced gingival hyperplasia is clinically similar to that observed with phenytoin therapy and appears to occur more frequently in pediatric patients. To reduce the risk of developing cyclosporine-induced gingival hyperplasia, careful oral hygiene should be maintained before and following transplantation. Gingival hyperplasia generally resolves 1–2 months following discontinuance of the drug; gingivectomy has been required rarely in patients with severe hyperplasia.

Acne and brittle and abnormal fingernails occur occasionally in patients receiving cyclosporine.

Cyclosporine administered to treat rheumatoid arthritis resulted in hypertrichosis or rash in up to about 19 or 12% of patients. Alopecia, gingival hyperplasia, or gingivitis each occurred in up to about 4% of patients. Bullous eruption or skin ulceration each occurred in up to about 1% of patients. Angioedema, dermatitis, dry skin, eczema, folliculitis, gingival bleeding, nail disorder, abnormal pigmentation, pruritus, skin disorder, and urticaria each occurred in 1% to less than 3% of patients.

Cyclosporine administered to treat psoriasis resulted in adverse effects of the skin and appendages in about 18% of patients. Hypertrichosis occurred in about 7% of patients. Gingival hyperplasia occurred in about 4% of patients. Acne, dry skin, folliculitis, gingival bleeding, keratosis, pruritus, and rash each occurred in 1% to less than 3% of patients.

■ **Hepatic Effects** Hepatotoxicity has reportedly occurred in 4 or less, 7, or 4% of patients with kidney, heart, or liver allografts, respectively, usually during the first month of therapy with cyclosporine when higher dosages of the drug are used. Abnormalities of liver function test results (e.g., increased serum aminotransferase [transaminase] and gamma-glutamyl transferase concentrations) and increased serum bilirubin concentration are signs of cyclosporine hepatotoxicity. Reduction of cyclosporine dosage usually reverses the hepatotoxic effects of the drug; in one study, hepatotoxicity was associated with trough serum concentrations (determined by RIA) greater than 1000 ng/mL. Although increased serum alkaline phosphatase concentration has also been reported, it appears to be from bone rather than liver origin.

Hyperbilirubinemia occurred in 1% to less than 3% of patients with psoriasis receiving cyclosporine. Hyperbilirubinemia that was minor and related to dosage has been observed without evidence of hepatocellular damage.

■ **GI Effects** Adverse GI effects, including diarrhea, nausea and vomiting, anorexia, and abdominal discomfort have occurred frequently during cyclosporine therapy. Gastritis, hiccups, and peptic ulcer have occurred less frequently. Constipation, difficulty in swallowing, and upper GI bleeding have been reported rarely in patients receiving the drug.

Cyclosporine administered to treat rheumatoid arthritis resulted in nausea, abdominal pain, diarrhea, or dyspepsia in up to about 23, 15, 13, or 12% of patients, respectively. Vomiting, flatulence, or GI disorder that was not otherwise specified occurred in up to about 9, 5, or 4% of patients, respectively. Anorexia or rectal hemorrhage each occurred in up to about 3% of patients. Stomatitis occurred in up to about 7% of patients. Constipation, dysphagia, eructation, esophagitis, gastritis, gastroenteritis, glossitis, salivary gland enlargement, tongue disorder, tooth disorder, gastric ulcer, and peptic ulcer each occurred in 1% to less than 3% of patients.

Cyclosporine administered to treat psoriasis resulted in adverse GI effects in about 20% of patients. Nausea, diarrhea, abdominal pain, or dyspepsia occurred in about 6, 5, 3, or 2% of patients. Abdominal distention, increased appetite, and constipation each occurred in 1% to less than 3% of patients.

■ **Infectious Complications** Infectious complications, including pneumonia, septicemia, abscesses, and urinary tract, viral, local and systemic fungal, and skin and wound infections, have occurred frequently during cyclosporine therapy. When infectious complications occurring during cyclosporine therapy were compared with those occurring during combined azathioprine and corticosteroid therapy in one study, the frequency of bacterial, viral, and fungal infections was similar in both groups. However, in another study, septicemia, abscesses, and cytomegalovirus infections occurred less frequently in patients receiving cyclosporine than in those receiving azathioprine and corticosteroids; the frequency of other viral infections, local fungal infections, urinary tract infections, pneumonia, and wound and skin infections was similar in both groups.

Cyclosporine administered to treat rheumatoid arthritis resulted in respiratory infection that was not otherwise specified, influenza-like symptoms, urinary tract infection, or pneumonia in up to about 9, 6, 3 or 1% of patients, respectively. Abscess, bacterial infection, cellulitis, fungal infection, herpes simplex, herpes zoster, moniliasis, renal abscess, and viral infection each occurred in 1% to less than 3% of patients.

Cyclosporine administered to treat psoriasis resulted in infection or potential infection in about 25% of patients. Influenza-like symptoms or upper respiratory tract infections occurred in about 10 or 8% of patients, respectively. In addition, respiratory infection or viral and other infections of the respiratory system occurred in 1% to less than 3% of patients.

■ **Hematologic Effects** Adverse hematologic effects of cyclosporine reportedly occurring occasionally include leukopenia, anemia, and thrombocytopenia. Renal and other (e.g., bone marrow) allograft recipients who received cyclosporine as well as some patients who received the drug for other conditions (e.g., uveitis) have developed a syndrome of thrombocytopenia and microangiopathic hemolytic anemia. This vasculopathy is pathologically similar to the hemolytic uremic syndrome, with manifestations that include thrombosis of the renal microvasculature with platelet-fibrin thrombi occluding glomerular capillaries and afferent arterioles, microangiopathic hemolytic anemia, thrombocytopenia and decreased renal function, and such findings are generalizable to other immunosuppressive agents used after transplantation. Although graft failure can result from this syndrome, rejection is not conditional to such vasculopathy, which occurs with avid platelet consumption within the allograft, as shown by indium-111 labeled platelet studies. Neither the pathogenesis nor optimal management of the syndrome are clear. Although resolution has occurred after reduction of the dosage or discontinuance of cyclosporine, and therapy with streptokinase and heparin or with plasmapheresis, the efficacy of such interventions appears to depend on early detection with indium-111 labeled platelet scans. Lymphoma has also occurred occasionally. (See Cautions: Mutagenicity and Carcinogenicity.) Evidence from animal studies and clinical studies in humans indicates that cyclosporine does not appear to depress bone marrow function. In one study, bone marrow depression occurred in 12% of patients receiving azathioprine and corticosteroids but did not occur in cyclosporine-treated patients. In another study, leukopenia (leukocyte count less than 2000/mm^3) occurred in only one cyclosporine-treated patient while it occurred in about 10% of patients receiving azathioprine and corticosteroids.

Cyclosporine administered to treat rheumatoid arthritis resulted in anemia, leukopenia, or lymphadenopathy in 1% to less than 3% of patients.

Cyclosporine administered to treat psoriasis resulted in adverse effects related to leukocytes and the reticuloendothelial system in about 4% of patients. Platelet, bleeding, and clotting disorders or red blood cell disorder occurred in 1% to less than 3% of patients.

■ **Sensitivity Reactions** Sensitivity reactions (including anaphylaxis) have reportedly occurred in 2% or less of patients receiving cyclosporine. Anaphylaxis has been reported in 0.1% of patients receiving the drug IV. There have been no reports to date of anaphylaxis following administration of cyclosporine as conventional (nonmodified) liquid-filled capsules or oral solution (which do *not* contain polyoxyl 35 castor oil); in addition, some patients who developed anaphylaxis while receiving the drug IV subsequently received the conventional oral solution without unusual adverse effect. Anaphylactic reactions to IV cyclosporine include flushing of the face and upper thorax, acute respiratory distress with dyspnea and wheezing, hypotension, tachycardia, and, rarely, death. Although the exact mechanism of these reactions is not known, an association with polyoxyl 35 castor oil in the vehicle of the commercially available concentrate for injection has been suggested. Polyoxyl 35 castor oil has been shown to cause anaphylactoid reactions in animals, including stimulation of histamine release and a hypotensive effect; death has occurred in some animals. An immunologic mechanism (e.g., antibody production, complement activation) has been suggested in some studies and case reports; it has also been suggested that polyoxyl 35 castor oil may enhance the immunogenicity of other agents such as drugs. Anaphylactic reactions have been associated with administration of other drugs in a polyoxyl 35 castor oil-containing vehicle; other reactions (e.g., severe edema, abnormal liver function test results, hyperlipidemia, decreased plasma viscosity) have also been associated with IV use of polyoxyl 35 castor oil-containing preparations. Although IV cyclosporine-induced anaphylactic reactions may subside in some patients when IV infusion of the drug is stopped, death resulting from respiratory arrest and aspiration pneumonia has occurred in at least one patient.

Allergic reactions occurred in 1% to less than 3% of patients who received cyclosporine to treat rheumatoid arthritis.

■ **Other Adverse Effects** Hyperlipidemia and abnormalities in electrophoresis may occur in patients receiving IV cyclosporine, since the vehicle in the commercially available cyclosporine concentrate for injection (polyoxyl 35 castor oil) has been associated with the development of these effects. Although hyperlipidemia and lipoprotein abnormalities are reversible following discontinuance of the drug, their occurrence during cyclosporine therapy usually does not require discontinuance of the drug.

Benign fibroadenoma of the breast has been reported in a few renal allograft recipients receiving cyclosporine alone. Although a definite causal relationship to the drug has not been established, fibroadenoma resolved in one patient following dosage reduction of cyclosporine.

Other adverse effects reportedly occurring in at least 3% of patients receiving cyclosporine include sinusitis and gynecomastia. Conjunctivitis, edema, fever, hearing loss, hyperglycemia (possibly induced by concomitant corticosteroid therapy), muscle pain, and tinnitus have occurred in 2% or less of patients receiving the drug. Chest pain, hair breaking, joint pain, aseptic necrosis, lethargy, mouth sores, night sweats, pancreatitis, visual disturbances, weakness, musculoskeletal abnormalities, and weight loss have been reported rarely in patients receiving cyclosporine.

Cyclosporine administered to treat rheumatoid arthritis resulted in increases in nonprotein nitrogen (NPN) in up to about 19% of patients. Edema that was not otherwise specified, pain, or leg cramps/involuntary muscle contractions occurred in up to about 14, 13, or 12% of patients, respectively. Upper respiratory tract disorders occurred in up to 14% of patients, respectively. Fatigue, chest pain, or hypomagnesemia each occurred in up to about 6% of patients. Arthropathy, coughing, dyspnea, ear disorder that was not otherwise specified, or pharyngitis each occurred in up to about 5% of patients. Micturition frequency, purpura, sinusitis, or accidental trauma each occurred in up to 4% of patients. Bronchitis, fever, rhinitis, or rigors each occurred in up to about 3% of patients. Menstrual disorder or leukorrhea occurred in up to about 3 or 1% of female patients; breast fibroadenosis, breast pain, and uterine hemorrhage each occurred in 1% to less than 3% of patients. Dysuria occurred in up to about 1% of patients. Other adverse effects that occurred in 1% to less than 3% of patients include arthralgia, asthenia, bilirubinemia, bone fracture, bronchospasm, bursitis, cataract, abnormal chest sounds, conjunctivitis, deafness, diabetes mellitus, dry mouth, enanthema, epistaxis, ocular pain, goiter, hematuria, hot flushes, hyperkalemia, hyperuricemia, hypoglycemia, joint dislocation, malaise, micturition urgency, myalgia, nocturia, overdose, polyuria, procedure not otherwise specified, pyelonephritis, stiffness, increased sweating, synovial cyst, taste perversion, tendon disorder, tinnitus, tonsillitis, urinary incontinence, abnormal urine, vestibular disorder, abnormal vision, weight decrease, and weight increase.

Cyclosporine administered to treat psoriasis resulted in adverse effects in the body as a whole in about 29% of patients. Pain occurred in about 4% of patients. Chest pain, fever, and hot flushes each occurred in 1% to less than 3% of patients. Adverse effects of the urinary system occurred in about 24% of patients. Micturition frequency occurred in 1 to less than 3% of patients. Adverse effects related to resistance mechanism occurred in about 19% of patients. Serum concentrations of triglycerides increased to more than 750 mg/dL in about 15% of patients and serum concentrations of cholesterol increased to more than 300 mg/dL in less than 3% of patients. Elevated serum concentrations of triglycerides or cholesterol generally are reversible after dosage reduction or discontinuance of cyclosporine. Adverse effects of the musculoskeletal system occurred in about 13% of patients. Arthralgia occurred in about 6% of patients. Adverse metabolic and nutritional effects occurred in about 9% of patients. Adverse reproductive effects occurred in about 9% of female patients. Adverse effects of the respiratory system (e.g., bronchospasm, coughing, dyspnea, rhinitis) occurred in about 5% of patients. Abnormal vision occurred in 1% to less than 3% of patients. Uric acid may increase in concentration and attacks of gout occurred rarely with cyclosporine.

■ **Precautions and Contraindications** Cyclosporine should be used for therapeutic applications other than transplantation only by clinicians experienced in such use of immunosuppressive therapy. The risks and benefits of cyclosporine in the management of psoriasis should be weighed carefully since the drug is a potent immunosuppressive agent with a number of potentially serious adverse effects. At dosages used in organ transplant recipients, cyclosporine should be used only under the supervision of a clinician experienced in immunosuppressive therapy and the management of organ transplant patients. Management of patients during initiation of, or any major change in, cyclosporine therapy should be performed in facilities equipped with adequate laboratory and supportive medical equipment and staffed with adequate medical personnel. Although patients who are stabilized on cyclosporine may receive the drug as outpatients, periodic laboratory monitoring is required. The clinician responsible for cyclosporine maintenance therapy should have complete information necessary for appropriate follow-up of the patient.

Immunosuppression with cyclosporine may result in increased susceptibility to infection, including serious infections with fatal outcomes, and the possible development of lymphoma. (See Cautions: Mutagenicity and Carcinogenicity.) The increased risk of developing lymphomas and other malignancies, especially of the skin, associated with cyclosporine or other immunosuppressive therapy appears to be related to the degree and duration of immunosuppression irrespective of the specific drugs. Because of the increased risk for skin cancer, patients should be advised to limit ultraviolet light exposure. The manufacturer cautions that, although cyclosporine should be administered with corticosteroids, conventional (nonmodified) oral formulations of the drug and the concentrate for injection should not be administered concomitantly with other immunosuppressive agents since increased susceptibility to infection and risk of lymphoma may result. However, the manufacturers of the modified oral formulations (Gengraf®, Neoral®) state that these modified formulations may be administered with other immunosuppressives, although the degree of immunosuppression produced may result in an increased risk of lymphoma and other neoplasms and in susceptibility to infection. In addition, such potential danger for oversuppression of the immune system requires that the benefits versus risks of therapeutic regimens containing multiple immunosuppressive agents be weighed carefully.

Comparative risk remains to be elucidated as to whether the risk of developing lymphomas is greater, in general, in patients with rheumatoid arthritis receiving cyclosporine than in rheumatoid arthritis patients who are untreated or being treated with cytotoxic agents. Before therapy with cyclosporine for rheumatoid arthritis is initiated, as well as during its course, patients should be evaluated thoroughly for the presence of malignancies. The risk for malignancies may be increased with concurrent use of cyclosporine and other immunosuppressive agents through induction of excessive immunosuppression.

The risk of developing malignancies of the skin and lymphoproliferative disorders is increased in patients receiving cyclosporine to treat psoriasis, although the relative risk of such occurrence with cyclosporine or other immunosuppressive agents is comparable. In addition, previous therapy with PUVA and, to a lesser extent, with methotrexate or other immunosuppressive agents, coal tar, UVB light, or other radiation increases the risk of developing malignancies of the skin. Before therapy with cyclosporine is initiated, as well as during its course, patients should be evaluated thoroughly for the presence of malignancies with consideration that psoriatic plaques may obscure malignant lesions. A biopsy should be obtained from dermatologic lesions that do not typify psoriasis, before therapy with cyclosporine commences. Cyclosporine should be administered only after suspicious lesions resolve completely and only if other therapies are not an option. Because excessive immunosuppression is possible that would place the patient at risk for malignancies to develop, therapy with methotrexate or other immunosuppressive agents, PUVA, UVB, or other radiation should *not* be administered concurrently with cyclosporine in the management of psoriasis. In addition, therapy with coal tar should not be administered concurrently with cyclosporine.

Immunosuppressed patients are at an increased risk for opportunistic infections, including reactivation of latent viral infections. These include BK virus-associated nephropathy (BKVN), which has been reported in patients receiving immunosuppressants, including cyclosporine, mycophenolate, sirolimus, and tacrolimus. Primary infection with polyoma BK virus typically occurs in childhood; following initial infection, the virus remains latent, but reactivation may occur in immunocompromised patients. BKVN has principally been observed in renal transplant patients (usually within the first year post-transplantation) and may result in serious outcomes, including deterioration of kidney function and renal allograft loss. Risk of BK virus reactivation appears to be related to the degree of overall immunosuppression rather than use of any specific immunosuppressive agent; patients receiving a maintenance immunosuppressive regimen of at least 3 drugs appear to be at highest risk. Patients should be monitored for possible signs of BKVN, including deterioration in renal function, during therapy with cyclosporine; screening assays for polyomavirus replication also have been recommended by some clinicians. Early intervention in patients who develop BKVN is critical; a reduction in immunosuppressive therapy should initially be considered in such patients. Although a variety of other treatment approaches have been used anecdotally in patients with BKVN, including antiviral therapy (e.g., cidofovir), leflunomide, IV immunoglobulins, and fluoroquinolone antibiotics, additional experience and well-controlled studies are necessary to more clearly establish the optimal treatment of such patients.

Cyclosporine should not be administered as therapy for psoriasis in patients with abnormal renal function, hypertension that is uncontrolled, or malignancies because such conditions may increase the risk for nephrotoxicity and hypertension. The presence of these conditions also contraindicates therapy with cyclosporine to manage rheumatoid arthritis.

Because of the risk of anaphylaxis (see Cautions: Sensitivity Reactions), IV cyclosporine should be reserved for patients unable to tolerate oral formulations of the drug. Patients receiving IV cyclosporine should be under continuous observation for at least the first 30 minutes following initiation of the IV infusion and should be closely monitored at frequent intervals thereafter for possible allergic manifestations. Appropriate equipment for maintenance of an adequate airway and other supportive measures and agents for the treatment of anaphylactic reactions (e.g., epinephrine, oxygen) should be readily available whenever cyclosporine is administered IV. If anaphylaxis occurs, IV infusion of cyclosporine should be discontinued immediately and the patient given appropriate therapy (e.g., epinephrine, oxygen) as indicated.

Any cyclosporine preparation is contraindicated in patients with known hypersensitivity to the drug, and the concentrate for injection or modified oral formulations also are contraindicated in those with known hypersensitivity to any ingredient in the formulation (e.g., polyoxyl 35 castor oil [Cremophor® EL] or polyoxyl 40 hydrogenated castor oil [Cremophor® RH40]).

Blood or plasma concentrations of the drug should be monitored periodically in patients receiving conventional (nonmodified) oral formulations of cyclosporine (liquid-filled capsules or oral solution), since absorption of orally administered cyclosporine is reportedly erratic during long-term therapy. Because of the highly variable GI absorption of cyclosporine and the accumulation of data relating trough concentrations with efficacy, predose (trough) concentrations should be monitored. However, monitoring of blood or plasma concentrations of cyclosporine is not a substitute for renal function monitoring or tissue biopsies. When necessary (e.g., because of changes in oral absorption of the drug), dosage adjustment should be made to avoid toxicity resulting from high blood or plasma concentrations of the drug or to prevent possible organ rejection resulting from low concentrations. Monitoring of blood or plasma cyclosporine concentrations may be especially important in hepatic allograft recipients, since absorption of the drug in these patients may be erratic, especially during the first few weeks of the posttransplantation period because of surgical techniques (e.g., bile duct management) or surgically induced liver dysfunction. In addition, patients with GI malabsorption syndromes may have difficulty in achieving therapeutic blood or plasma concentrations when the drug is administered orally. Blood or plasma concentrations of cyclosporine also should be monitored routinely in allograft recipients receiving modified oral formulations and periodically in patients with rheumatoid arthritis being treated with these preparations of cyclosporine so that toxicity secondary to high concentrations of the drug is avoided.

Patients receiving cyclosporine should be informed of the necessity of routine laboratory testing (e.g., BUN and serum creatinine, bilirubin, and liver enzyme concentrations) for the assessment of renal and hepatic function. Patients should also be given careful dosage instructions, advised of the potential risks during pregnancy, and informed of the increased risk of neoplasia during cyclosporine therapy. In addition, they should be advised that oral formulations of cyclosporine should be administered on a consistent schedule with regard to time of day and in relation to meals, and that any change in oral formulation of the drug requires the supervision of a clinician and should be done cautiously.

At high dosages, cyclosporine may cause nephrotoxicity and/or hepatotoxicity. Renal allograft recipients who develop increased BUN and serum creatinine concentrations should be carefully evaluated before adjustment of cyclosporine dosage is initiated, since these increases do not necessarily indicate that organ rejection has occurred. The development of renal dysfunction at any time during the course of cyclosporine therapy requires close monitoring of the patient and frequent dosage adjustment may be required. In patients with persistently high elevations of BUN and serum creatinine concentrations who are unresponsive to adjustment of cyclosporine dosage, switching to other immunosuppressive therapy should be considered. (See Cautions: Renal Effects.) If severe, intractable renal allograft rejection occurs and does not respond to rescue therapy with corticosteroids and monoclonal antibodies, it may be preferable to switch to alternative immunosuppressive therapy or to allow the kidney to be rejected and removed rather than to increase cyclosporine dosage to an excessive level in an attempt to reverse the rejection episode.

During therapy with cyclosporine in the management of psoriasis, renal function must be monitored since renal dysfunction and structural damage to the kidney are potential adverse effects. Nephrotoxicity may occur at recommended dosages, with increasing risk as the dosage and duration of therapy with the drug increases. The serum creatinine concentration and BUN may increase in patients receiving cyclosporine, reflecting a decrease in the glomerular filtration rate. The maximal increase in serum creatinine concentration may be a predictive factor for cyclosporine-induced nephropathy. Structural damage to the kidney and persistent renal dysfunction may result from cyclosporine when patients are monitored inadequately and adjustment of the dosage is improper. Geriatric patients should be monitored with particular care because renal function also decreases with age. Monitoring the serum creatinine concentration regularly and reducing the dosage when values exceed baseline by 25% or more help to lower the risk of nephropathy from cyclosporine. Elevated serum creatinine concentrations generally reverse upon timely cyclosporine dosage reduction or disontinuance. The risk of nephropathy from cyclosporine in patients with psoriasis also is decreased by initiating therapy with the drug at 2.5 mg/kg daily and not exceeding a maximum dosage of 4 mg/kg daily.

■ Pediatric Precautions Although there are no adequate and controlled studies to date in children, cyclosporine has been used in children as young as 6 months of age without unusual adverse effects; the modified oral formulations have been used in children as young as 1 year of age. Cyclosporine has been used in hepatic and renal allograft recipients 7.5 months to 18 years of age. Children receiving cyclosporine and low-dose corticosteroid therapy have shown increased patient and graft survival rates and fewer adverse systemic effects on growth and development than those receiving therapy with other immunosuppressive agents; however, some clinicians have reported an increased frequency of seizures, possibly related to concomitant hypertension or high-dose corticosteroid therapy, in children receiving cyclosporine. The possibility that serious nephrotoxicity, hypertension, and/or seizures may occur in children receiving the drug should be considered.

The safety and efficacy of cyclosporine for the management of juvenile rheumatoid arthritis or psoriasis in children younger than 18 years of age have not been established.

■ Geriatric Precautions Although safety and efficacy of cyclosporine have not been specifically studied in geriatric patients, 17.5% of patients treated with the drug for rheumatoid arthritis in clinical studies were 65 years of age and older. Patients 65 years of age or older were more likely to develop systolic hypertension while receiving cyclosporine to treat rheumatoid arthritis in clinical studies. This age group also was more likely to have elevated serum creatinine concentrations that were 50% or more above baseline after 3–4 months of receiving cyclosporine.

■ Mutagenicity and Carcinogenicity Various tests have not shown cyclosporine to be mutagenic. No evidence of cyclosporine-induced mutagenesis or genotoxicity was observed with the Ames microbial mutagen test, the V-79-HGPRT test, the micronucleus assay in mice and Chinese hamsters, chromosome-aberration tests in Chinese hamster bone marrow, the mouse dominant lethal assay, or the DNA-repair test in sperm from mice treated with the drug. However, in an in vitro study that used human lymphocytes, high concentrations of cyclosporine appeared to induce sister chromatid exchange.

In a long-term study, the frequency of lymphocytic lymphomas was increased in female mice and that of hepatocellular adenomas was increased in male mice receiving 4 mg/kg daily. Following long-term administration in rats, the frequency of pancreatic islet cell adenomas was higher than the control rate in rats receiving 0.5 mg/kg of cyclosporine daily. In these studies, cyclosporine was administered in doses 0.01–0.16 times the maintenance dose for humans. The development of hepatocellular carcinomas and pancreatic islet cell adenomas in mice and rats did not appear to be dose related.

An increase in the incidence of malignancy is a recognized complication of immunosuppression in allograft recipients and patients with psoriasis or rheumatoid arthritis. Skin cancers and non-Hodgkin's lymphoma develop most commonly. Lesions may regress after reduction or discontinuance of immunosuppression. Patients treated with cyclosporine are at greater risk for the development of malignancies than is the normal, healthy population, although such risk is similar to patients treated with other immunosuppressive therapies.

Lymphomas have developed in patients receiving cyclosporine alone or in combination with other immunosuppressive agents, and some patients have developed a lymphoproliferative disorder that resolved following discontinuance of the drug. The lymphomas and lymphoproliferative disorders appear to be associated with Epstein-Barr virus (EBV) infections. It has been suggested that cyclosporine may cause alteration of the antibody for EBV or may inhibit the cell-mediated response to EBV, resulting in the development of lymphoma. With the exception of corticosteroids, the manufacturer states that conventional (nonmodified) oral formulations of cyclosporine or the concentrate for injection should not be used concomitantly with other immunosuppressive agents, since the risk of lymphoma may be increased. However, the manufacturers of the modified oral formulations (Gengraf®, Neoral®) state that these modified formulations may be administered with other immunosuppressives, although the degree of immunosuppression produced may result in an increased risk of lymphoma and other neoplasms and in susceptibility to infection. In addition, such potential danger for oversuppression of the immune system requires that the benefits versus risks of therapeutic regimens containing multiple immunosuppressive agents be weighed carefully.

Although the risk of lymphoma appears to be greatest when there is substantial immunosuppression (i.e., concomitant use of multiple immunosuppressive agents), all immunosuppressed patients should be considered at risk for developing lymphoma. The nature and optimum management of posttransplant lymphomas and lymphoproliferative disorders in allograft recipients remain to be clearly established, and clinicians should consult specialized references for current methods of evaluation and management. Some clinicians suggest that immunosuppressive therapy with cyclosporine and corticosteroids should be reduced or discontinued in patients who develop posttransplant lymphomas or lymphoproliferative disorders. In one study, reduction of cyclosporine and/or prednisone dosage resulted in resolution of lymphomas but was not associated with allograft rejection. Squamous cell carcinoma occurred in one patient receiving cyclosporine following renal transplantation but has not been directly attributed to the drug.

Lymphoma developed in several patients who received cyclosporine to treat rheumatoid arthritis. Epidemiologic analyses indicated a relationship between cyclosporine and lymphoma, but no relationship to other malignancies that have been reported, including skin cancers, diverse types of solid tumors, and multiple myeloma. Carcinoma or tumor not otherwise specified each occurred in 1% to less than 3% of patients who received cyclosporine.

Patients receiving cyclosporine to treat psoriasis have developed malignancies, especially of the skin. Squamous cell carcinoma or basal cell carcinoma occurred in 0.9 or 0.4% of patients, respectively, who received the drug. In another aggregate of clinical studies, tumors were reported in about 2% of patients who received the drug. Malignancies of the skin that included squamous cell and basal cell carcinomas were reported in about 1% of patients who received cyclosporine. Most of these patients had been treated previously with PUVA and some had received prior therapy with methotrexate, coal tar, or UVB. A history of previous cancer of the skin or a lesion that was a potential predisposition to such cancer was present in some of the patients before therapy with cyclosporine began. The lymphoproliferative disorders that developed in patients receiving cyclosporine for psoriasis included in one patient each non-Hodgkin's lymphoma that required chemotherapy and mycosis fungoides that regressed spontaneously after withdrawal of cyclosporine. Benign lymphocytic infiltration occurred in some patients with spontaneous regression occurring after withdrawal of cyclosporine or, in one patient, while administration of the drug continued. Malignancies that involved various organs accounted for the rest of the patients affected to yield an incidence of about 1%. During post-marketing surveillance, several more patients were reported to have developed tumors while receiving cyclosporine for psoriasis. Cervical intraepithelial neoplasia developed in a patient with chronic plaque psoriasis treated for over 3 years with 3 mg/kg daily of cyclosporine.

■ **Pregnancy, Fertility, and Lactation** Although there are no adequate and well-controlled studies using cyclosporine in pregnant women, the drug has been shown to be embryotoxic and fetotoxic in rats and rabbits when administered orally at maternally toxic doses. Fetal toxicity was observed in these animals at doses 0.8–5.4 times (corrected for body surface area) the human maintenance dose of 6 mg/kg. Cyclosporine caused increased prenatal and postnatal mortality and reduced fetal weight with related skeletal retardation in these rats and rabbits. In women who received cyclosporine therapy throughout pregnancy, premature birth (gestational age of 28–36 weeks) and reduced neonatal weight occurred consistently. Most of the pregnancies also were complicated by growth retardation (which may be severe), fetal loss, preeclampsia, eclampsia, premature labor, abruptio placentae, oligohydramnios, Rh incompatibility, and fetoplacental dysfunction. Premature birth was the most frequent complication, while being small for gestational age and neonatal complications were less common. Malformations occurred in some neonates and in a few cases of fetal loss. A full-term neonate was born to a woman who underwent a renal transplant prior to conception and received 450 mg of cyclosporine alone daily throughout pregnancy, and other successful pregnancies have been reported in allograft recipients who received the drug daily during pregnancy. Abnormalities in renal function or blood pressure were not observed in a limited number of children 7 years of age or younger exposed to cyclosporine in utero.

Cyclosporine should be used during pregnancy only when the potential benefits justify the possible risks to the fetus. In patients with psoriasis, the risks and benefits of therapy with cyclosporine during pregnancy should be evaluated carefully, with discontinuance of therapy considered seriously because of possible disruption of the interaction between the mother and fetus.

Reproduction studies in rats receiving cyclosporine have not revealed evidence of impaired fertility.

Since cyclosporine is distributed into milk, nursing should be avoided in women receiving the drug.

Drug Interactions

■ **Nephrotoxic Drugs** Interactions that may potentiate renal dysfunction are well substantiated between cyclosporine and various drugs, including aminoglycosides, vancomycin, co-trimoxazole, ciprofloxacin, melphalan, amphotericin B, ketoconazole, certain nonsteroidal anti-inflammatory agents (NSAIAs) (e.g., azapropazon [not commercially available in the US], diclofenac, naproxen, sulindac), cimetidine, ranitidine, fibric acid derivatives (e.g., fenofibrate, bezafibrate), methotrexate, colchicine, and tacrolimus; in some cases, the resultant potentiation of renal dysfunction resulted from the nephrotoxic potential of the interacting drug while in others it resulted from accumulation of cyclosporine induced by the interacting drug. If concomitant use of cyclosporine with such drugs is unavoidable, renal function should be monitored carefully.

Since nephrotoxic effects may be additive, concomitant use of cyclosporine with potentially nephrotoxic drugs (e.g., acyclovir, aminoglycoside antibiotics, amphotericin B) should be avoided.

Concomitant administration of cyclosporine and amphotericin B has produced additive nephrotoxicity. In bone marrow allograft recipients receiving cyclosporine alone, cyclosporine and amphotericin B, or amphotericin B and methotrexate, increases in serum creatinine concentration were substantially greater in patients receiving cyclosporine and amphotericin B compared with those receiving cyclosporine alone or amphotericin B and methotrexate. Since it may be dangerous (i.e., risk of allograft rejection) to completely discontinue cyclosporine therapy when serum creatinine increases in allograft recipients, it has been suggested that if concomitant amphotericin B therapy is necessary in these patients, cyclosporine be temporarily withheld until the trough serum cyclosporine concentration (determined by RIA) is less than 150 ng/mL and that subsequent dosage be adjusted accordingly; this reduction in cyclosporine dosage may decrease the risk of nephrotoxicity while maintaining adequate immunosuppression.

Concomitant administration of cyclosporine and gentamicin has resulted in an increased risk of acute tubular necrosis in renal allograft recipients when compared with concomitant administration of ampicillin and cyclosporine or gentamicin alone. Therefore, administration of aminoglycosides should be avoided in renal allograft recipients who are receiving cyclosporine.

Concomitant administration of cyclosporine and co-trimoxazole has resulted in increases in serum creatinine concentrations. Concomitant administration of cyclosporine and melphalan has resulted in renal failure, and plasma creatinine concentrations and BUN were within normal limits or did not deteriorate in patients treated with melphalan without subsequent administration of cyclosporine.

In patients with rheumatoid arthritis, the combination of cyclosporine and naproxen or sulindac resulted in additive decreases in renal function, as determined with technetium Tc 99m pentatate (DTPA) and iodohippurate sodium I 131 or *p*-aminohippuric acid (PAH) clearances. However, calculated creatinine clearance did not distinguish NSAIAs from acetaminophen in patients receiving cyclosporine in a dosage stabilized to treat rheumatoid arthritis and 4 weeks of concomitant therapy with 200 mg daily of indomethacin, 200 mg daily of ketoprofen, 400 mg daily of sulindac, or 4 g daily of acetaminophen. Creatinine clearance differed between indomethacin and acetaminophen but the increase of 6% observed with acetaminophen compared with indomethacin was not considered clinical in magnitude.

Concomitant administration of cyclosporine and diclofenac may increase the nephrotoxic potential of cyclosporine. In addition to increases in serum creatinine concentration, increased serum potassium concentrations and/or blood pressure have occurred in some patients receiving the drugs concomitantly. In patients with rheumatoid arthritis, concomitant administration of cyclosporine and diclofenac resulted in elevation of the AUC of diclofenac but did not affect blood concentrations of cyclosporine. Because blood concentrations of diclofenac have been observed to increase by approximately double with concomitant administration of cyclosporine and diclofenac, a lower dosage in the therapeutic range of diclofenac should be used in patients receiving this combination. Pharmacokinetic interactions of clinical importance have not been observed between cyclosporine and aspirin, indomethacin, ketoprofen, or piroxicam. However, because of the risk of additive decreases in renal function, patients with rheumatoid arthritis who are receiving concurrent therapy with cyclosporine and any NSAIA should be monitored with close attention to clinical status and serum creatinine concentration.

Concomitant administration of cyclosporine and colchicine may increase concentrations of cyclosporine, resulting in additive nephrotoxic effects. Cyclosporine also may reduce clearance of colchicine increasing the potential for enhanced colchicine toxicity (myopathy, neuropathy), particularly in patients with renal impairment. Patients should be monitored closely for colchicine toxicity during concurrent administration with cyclosporine; colchicine should be discontinued or dosage of the drug reduced if toxicity occurs.

■ **Immunosuppressive and Antineoplastic Agents** With the exception of corticosteroids, the manufacturer states that conventional (nonmodified) oral formulations of cyclosporine or the concentrate for injection should not be used concomitantly with other immunosuppressive agents since the risk of lymphoma (see Cautions: Mutagenicity and Carcinogenicity) and susceptibility to infection may be increased. However, the manufacturers of the modified oral formulations (Gengraf®, Neoral®) state that these modified formulations may be administered with other immunosuppressives, although the degree of immunosuppression produced may result in an increased risk of lymphoma and other neoplasms and in susceptibility to infection. In addition, such potential danger for oversuppression of the immune system requires that the benefits versus risks of therapeutic regimens containing multiple immunosuppressive agents be weighed carefully. The manufacturers state that patients with psoriasis should not receive cyclosporine concomitantly with other immunosuppressive agents since excessive immunosuppression may result.

Concomitant administration of cyclosporine and sirolimus substantially increases blood sirolimus concentrations. Sirolimus should be given 4 hours following cyclosporine administration to minimize the effect on sirolimus concentrations. Elevated serum creatinine concentrations also have been reported in patients receiving sirolimus and full dosages of cyclosporine concurrently; such increases generally are reversible following cyclosporine dosage reduction.

Concomitant administration of cyclosporine and methotrexate resulted in elevation of the AUC of methotrexate in patients with rheumatoid arthritis. In a limited study, the AUC of methotrexate increased by approximately 30% and the AUC of the metabolite, 7-hydroxymethotrexate, decreased by approximately 80% during coadministration of cyclosporine and methotrexate to patients with rheumatoid arthritis. However, the clinical importance of these observations is not known. Blood concentrations of cyclosporine did not appear to be affected by coadministration of cyclosporine and methotrexate.

■ **Potassium-sparing Drugs** Because cyclosporine may cause hyperkalemia, the manufacturers state that the drug should not be used concomitantly with potassium-sparing diuretics. Caution is advised and control of potassium concentrations recommended when cyclosporine is administered concomitantly with potassium-sparing drugs (e.g., angiotensin-converting enzyme [ACE] inhibitors, angiotensin II receptor antagonists) or potassium-containing drugs or in patients receiving a potassium-rich diet.

■ **Drugs and Foods Affecting Hepatic Microsomal Enzymes** Because cyclosporine is extensively metabolized, the concentration of drug in biologic fluid (e.g., plasma, blood) may be altered by drugs or foods (e.g., grapefruit juice) that affect hepatic microsomal enzymes, especially cytochrome P-450 isoenzyme subfamily CYP3A. Drugs and foods that inhibit hepatic microsomal enzymes could decrease the metabolism of cyclosporine and increase its concentration in biologic fluid. This potential interaction has been well substantiated to occur between cyclosporine and diltiazem, nicardipine, verapamil, mibefradil, fluconazole, itraconazole, ketoconazole, voriconazole, clarithromycin, erythromycin, quinupristin/dalfopristin, methylprednisolone, allopurinol, amiodarone, bromocriptine, colchicine, imatinib, danazol, oral contraceptives, or metoclopramide. Drugs that induce cytochrome P-450 activity could increase the metabolism of cyclosporine and decrease its concentration in biologic fluid. This potential interaction has been well substantiated to occur between cyclosporine and nafcillin, rifampin, carbamazepine, oxcarbazepine, phenobarbital, phenytoin, octreotide, sulfinpyrazone, terbinafine, or ticlopidine. In addition, clinicians should be cautious about concurrent administration of cyclosporine with rifabutin. Although the effect of rifabutin on the metabolism of cyclosporine has not been studied, the metabolism of other drugs by the cytochrome P-450 system has increased with rifabutin. Concomitant administration of cyclosporine with drugs that affect its metabolism requires monitoring of the concentration of cyclosporine in biologic fluid with appropriate adjustment of cyclosporine dosage.

Azole-derivative Antifungal Agents Concomitant administration of cyclosporine and ketoconazole has been reported to increase plasma concentrations of cyclosporine and serum creatinine concentrations. It has been suggested that ketoconazole may interfere with the metabolism of cyclosporine via hepatic microsomal enzyme inhibition, although other mechanisms may also be involved. When ketoconazole therapy is initiated in patients receiving cyclosporine, renal function and blood or plasma cyclosporine concentrations should be monitored; some clinicians also recommend that reduction in cyclosporine dosage or replacement of cyclosporine with another immunosuppressive agent be considered. Patients stabilized on both drugs may require an increase in cyclosporine dosage when ketoconazole is discontinued.

Concomitant administration of cyclosporine and fluconazole has been reported to increase whole blood concentrations of cyclosporine, and such increase may be associated with nephrotoxic effects. Serum creatinine concentration increased in at least one patient receiving cyclosporine following initiation of fluconazole therapy at a dosage of 200 mg every other day. However, such changes were not observed in several other patients receiving fluconazole 100 or 200 mg daily. Increases in trough cyclosporine concentrations and serum creatinine concentration also occurred when fluconazole dosage was increased from 100 to 300 mg daily. Evidence suggests that fluconazole interferes with the metabolism of cyclosporine via hepatic microsomal enzyme inhibition.

Concomitant administration of cyclosporine and itraconazole has been reported to increase whole blood or serum concentrations of cyclosporine and serum creatinine concentrations. Evidence indicates that itraconazole competitively inhibits the hydroxylation of cyclosporine via hepatic microsomal enzyme inhibition.

Concomitant administration of cyclosporine and voriconazole also may increase blood or plasma cyclosporine concentrations.

Macrolides Concomitant use of cyclosporine and erythromycin may result in substantial increases in blood or plasma concentrations of cyclosporine and subsequent signs of cyclosporine toxicity (e.g., nephrotoxicity). Studies in healthy adults indicate that erythromycin can substantially decrease plasma clearance of cyclosporine, presumably by inhibiting hepatic metabolism of the drug, although the exact mechanism remains to be clearly determined. Cyclosporine and erythromycin should be used concomitantly with caution, and patients should be monitored for evidence of cyclosporine toxicity. Renal function and blood or plasma concentrations of cyclosporine should be monitored when erythromycin therapy is administered or discontinued in patients receiving cyclosporine or vice versa, and cyclosporine dosage adjusted appropriately as necessary.

Concomitant use of cyclosporine and clarithromycin has resulted in increases in the whole blood concentration of cyclosporine. Elevation in serum creatinine concentration was uncommon.

Corticosteroids Concomitant administration of prednisolone with cyclosporine may result in decreased plasma clearance of prednisolone, and plasma concentrations of cyclosporine may be increased during concomitant therapy with cyclosporine and methylprednisolone. In addition, seizures have reportedly occurred in adult and pediatric patients receiving cyclosporine and high-dose corticosteroid therapy concurrently with cyclosporine. The mechanism for this interaction may involve competitive inhibition of hepatic microsomal enzymes. The potential drug interaction between cyclosporine and prednisolone or methylprednisolone and the possibility of exacerbated toxicity, as well as the need for appropriate dosage adjustment, should be considered when these drugs are administered concomitantly.

Calcium-Channel Blocking Agents Mibefradil (no longer commercially available in the US) inhibits the metabolism of cyclosporine, with resultant increased blood concentrations of the immunosuppressive agent; the possible need for cyclosporine dosage adjustment should be considered during concomitant mibefradil therapy. In addition, when cyclosporine is used in combination with mibefradil and an HMG-CoA reductase inhibitor (e.g., lovastatin, simvastatin), increased blood concentrations of cyclosporine and the HMG-CoA reductase inhibitor also may occur which potentially could lead to HMG-CoA reductase inhibitor-induced rhabdomyolysis; therefore, concomitant use of the drugs should be avoided.

Concomitant administration of cyclosporine and verapamil has resulted in increased whole blood concentrations of cyclosporine. It has been suggested that verapamil may interfere with metabolism of cyclosporine via hepatic microsomal enzyme inhibition. However, evaluation of the effect of verapamil on the pharmacokinetics of the major metabolites of cyclosporine indicated that the interaction between cyclosporine and verapamil was not secondary to interference with *N*-demethylation.

Concomitant administration of cyclosporine and nicardipine has resulted in increased whole blood or plasma cyclosporine concentrations. Concomitant administration of cyclosporine and nifedipine resulted in more frequent occurrence of gingival hyperplasia compared with cyclosporine alone.

Concomitant administration of cyclosporine and diltiazem has resulted in increased blood cyclosporine concentrations and consequent cyclosporine-induced nephrotoxicity. Although further study is needed, it has been suggested that diltiazem may interfere with metabolism of cyclosporine via hepatic microsomal enzyme inhibition.

Other Drugs Affecting Hepatic Microsomal Enzymes Concomitant administration of cyclosporine and rifampin, phenytoin, phenobarbital, or a combination of IV sulfamethazine and trimethoprim (co-trimoxazole) reportedly has resulted in decreased cyclosporine concentrations, probably by increasing hepatic metabolism of the drug. Monitoring of plasma or blood cyclosporine concentrations and appropriate dosage adjustment are necessary when any of these drugs is used concomitantly with cyclosporine.

Concomitant administration of cyclosporine and cimetidine has resulted in increased serum creatinine concentrations, although some evidence suggests that renal function may not be adversely affected despite a decrease in creatinine clearance. An increase in whole blood concentrations of cyclosporine occurred with concomitant administration of cyclosporine, cimetidine, and metronidazole. Concomitant administration of cyclosporine and ranitidine also has resulted in an increase in serum creatinine concentrations. However, some evidence indicates that serum creatinine concentration, creatinine clearance, and inulin clearance are affected minimally by the combination of cyclosporine and ranitidine.

Clearance of lovastatin reportedly was reduced with concomitant administration of cyclosporine, and such alterations could result in toxic effects of the antilipemic agent. Adverse effects observed during concomitant cyclosporine and lovastatin therapy have included myositis, myolysis, or rhabdomyolysis. Manifestations of such myopathy included myalgia and/or muscle weakness and increases in serum creatine kinase concentration. Acute renal failure has occurred concurrently with myopathy.

Combined use of mibefradil (no longer commercially available in the US), cyclosporine, and an HMG-CoA reductase inhibitor (e.g., lovastatin, simvastatin) can result in a potentially serious interaction and therefore should be avoided. (See Drugs and Foods Affecting Hepatic Microsomal Enzymes: Calcium-Channel Blocking Agents, in Drug Interactions.)

Concomitant use of cyclosporine and allopurinol has resulted in increases in the whole blood concentration of cyclosporine. Serum creatinine concentration may also be elevated. Concomitant administration of cyclosporine and danazol also has resulted in increased blood cyclosporine concentrations and serum creatinine concentrations.

Concomitant administration of cyclosporine and carbamazepine has resulted in decreased concentrations of cyclosporine in biologic fluid (e.g., whole blood) that were subtherapeutic in adults. In children whose dosage of cyclosporine was stabilized, trough concentrations of cyclosporine in whole blood were lower compared with control in patients treated concurrently with carbamazepine.

Grapefruit Juice Concomitant oral administration of grapefruit juice with cyclosporine has been reported to increase bioavailability of the drug. The interaction does *not* appear to occur with sweet ("common") orange juice, but some evidence indicates that it is likely with sour (Seville) orange juice.

In several studies in healthy adults or renal transplant recipients receiving cyclosporine as conventional (nonmodified) oral capsules with 175–250 mL of oral grapefruit juice, oral bioavailability of the drug increased by about 20–200%. Although it has been suggested that separating oral administration of cyclosporine and the juice by at least 90 minutes may minimize the effect on bioavailability, peak serum cyclosporine concentrations still may be increased, and other evidence suggests that the effect of grapefruit juice on drug bioavailability may persist much longer (e.g., for at least 10 hours), possibly secondary to a prolonged effect of the interacting constituent(s) on enzymes in the gut wall. Therefore, additional study is needed to determine whether separation of cyclosporine and grapefruit juice administration during the day can adequately minimize the potential interaction.

The interaction between grapefruit juice and cyclosporine bioavailability appears to result from inhibition, probably prehepatic, of the cytochrome P-450 enzyme system by some constituent(s) in the juice; grapefruit juice does not interfere appreciably with metabolism following IV drug administration. Both fresh and frozen grapefruit juice have been shown to inhibit first-pass metabolism of drugs metabolized by various cytochrome P-450 isoenzymes, including CYP1A2, CYP2A6, and the CYP3A subfamily (e.g., CYP3A4); these enzymes are present in the liver and/or extrahepatic tissues such as intestinal mucosa. Following oral administration of cyclosporine, certain benzodiazepines (e.g., midazolam, triazolam), and certain calcium-channel blocking agents (e.g., 1,4-dihydropyridine derivatives), such prehepatic inhibition of drug metabolism by grapefruit juice appears mainly to involve the CYP3A4 isoenzyme, principally within the small intestinal wall (e.g., in the jejunum), thus increasing systemic availability of these drugs. The magnitude of this interaction may be particularly notable for drugs such as cyclosporine that exhibit poor oral bioavailability when administered alone and in individuals in whom oral bioavailability is already relatively low.

The constituent(s) of grapefruit juice principally responsible for this interaction has not been elucidated fully. In addition, the composition of grapefruit juice is variable depending on natural and commercial factors. Such factors influencing individual concentrations of various grapefruit constituents include fruit variety, environmental conditions (e.g., temperature, humidity, location), fruit maturity, and juicing procedures (e.g., extraction pressure, method and extent of debittering, final adjustments of the juice product such as addition of essential oils and pulp). Grapefruit juice contains high concentrations of bioflavonoids, which have been shown to inhibit cytochrome P-450 microsomal enzymes. Although naringin, a bioflavonoid that gives grapefruit its characteristic bitter taste, has been a principal suspect because of the relatively high concentrations present in the fruit, in vitro and in vivo evidence indicates that this bioflavonoid probably has little or no effect on the inhibition of cytochrome P-450 enzymes. Naringenin, the aglycone metabolite of naringin, is a more potent inhibitor of cytochrome enzymes, but recent evidence suggests that this constituent may only contribute to, not be principally responsible for, grapefruit juice-induced drug interactions. Complicating interpretation of these data, however, are methodologic limitations of human studies that currently cannot elucidate the extent to which these or other flavonoids may contribute to the metabolic interactions. Further complicating interpretation are potential problems with extrapolating results obtained with hepatic microsomes to extrahepatic cytochromes since the interaction probably is prehepatic (i.e., involving the small intestine). In addition, the effects of flavonoids on metabolic reactions can be complex and, in some cases, the same flavonoid or possibly a metabolite can inhibit one reaction and stimulate another or even the same reaction in a concentration-dependent manner. Alternatively, some evidence indicates that 6′,7′-dihydroxybergamottin, a furanocoumarin (psoralen) compound present in grapefruit juice but not in sweet orange juice, may be the main constituent responsible for such drug interactions involving cytochrome P-450 enzymes.

Cyclosporine concentrations ideally are maintained in a relatively narrow range to prevent transplant rejection and minimize toxicity. Because concomitant oral administration of cyclosporine and grapefruit juice can result in clinically important increases in systemic concentrations of the drug, such administration should be avoided. Although some clinicians have suggested that grapefruit juice may provide a nontoxic and inexpensive alternative to drugs that have been used to improve oral bioavailability of cyclosporine and thus reduce the required dose of this expensive drug, others have cautioned that the resultant effects would be unpredictable since the composition of this juice is not standardized. The effect of grapefruit juice on oral bioavailability of the drug from the more bioavailable modified oral formulations (i.e., Gengraf®, Neoral®) remains to be established, but the manufacturers recommend that concomitant use of these formulations and the juice also be avoided.

■ St. John's Wort (Hypericum perforatum) Concomitant use of cyclosporine and St. John's wort (*Hypericum perforatum*) has resulted in marked reduction in the blood concentrations of cyclosporine, leading to subtherapeutic levels, rejection of transplanted organs, and graft loss.

■ Vaccines The possibility that the immune response to vaccination may be diminished in patients receiving cyclosporine should be considered. In addition, because of the immunosuppressive effects of cyclosporine, the manufacturers recommend that live vaccines be avoided during therapy with the drug.

■ Other Drugs Concomitant administration of cyclosporine and metoclopramide has resulted in increased area under the blood concentration-time curve of cyclosporine. It has been suggested that absorption of cyclosporine increased through acceleration of gastric emptying of the drug stimulated by metoclopramide. Concomitant use of cyclosporine and orlistat should be avoided because of the potential for decreased cyclosporine absorption.

Concomitant use of bosentan and cyclosporine has resulted in decreased plasma cyclosporine concentrations by approximately 50% and increased steady-state plasma bosentan concentrations by about 3- to 4-fold. The manufacturer of bosentan states that concomitant use of bosentan and cyclosporine is contraindicated.

Concomitant administration of cyclosporine and digoxin has resulted in decreases in apparent volume of distribution and serum clearance of digoxin. Cardiac glycoside toxicity (e.g., bidirectional ventricular tachycardia, anorexia, nausea, vomiting, diarrhea) occurred and serum digoxin concentrations were increased within a few days after patients already receiving digoxin began receiving cyclosporine. The mechanism of this interaction may involve the decrease in glomerular filtration rate induced by cyclosporine, since in dogs concomitant administration of cyclosporine and digoxin resulted in acute decreases in the renal clearance of the glycoside, glomerular filtration, and renal perfusion.

For information on potential interactions between cyclosporine and NSAIAs, see Drug Interactions: Nephrotoxic Drugs.

Acute Toxicity

■ Pathogenesis Limited information is available on the acute toxicity of cyclosporine. The oral LD_{50} of cyclosporine is about 2.3, 1.5, or greater than 1 g/kg in mice, rats, and rabbits, respectively. The IV LD_{50} is 148, 104, or 46 mg/kg in mice, rats, and rabbits, respectively.

■ Manifestations Overdosage of cyclosporine is likely to produce symptoms that are mainly extensions of common adverse reactions. Transient hepatotoxicity and nephrotoxicity may occur but should resolve following elimination or discontinuance of the drug.

■ Treatment In acute oral cyclosporine overdose, the stomach should be emptied by inducing emesis. Induction of emesis is probably useful up to 2 hours after ingestion. If the patient is comatose, having seizures, or lacks the gag reflex, gastric lavage may be performed if an endotracheal tube with cuff inflated is in place to prevent aspiration of gastric contents. Supportive and symptomatic treatment should be initiated. Hemodialysis and charcoal hemoperfusion reportedly are not useful for enhancing the elimination of cyclosporine following overdosage. When overdosage occurs in patients prescribed cyclosporine therapy, the drug may be withheld for a few days or alternate-day therapy may be initiated until the patient is stabilized.

Pharmacology

■ Immunosuppressive Effects Cyclosporine mainly exhibits immunosuppressive activity. In vivo studies in animals have shown that cyclosporine inhibits cell-mediated immune responses such as allograft rejection, delayed hypersensitivity (e.g., tuberculin-induced), experimental allergic encephalomyelitis, Freund's adjuvant-induced arthritis, and graft-vs-host disease. Cyclosporine has also been shown to inhibit primary and secondary responses to T cell-dependent antigens (e.g., xenogeneic [heterologous]erythrocytes) in animals. The drug may also inhibit humoral immune responses to some extent. Increased survival of allogeneic (homologous) transplants involving skin, heart, kidney, liver, pancreas, bone marrow, small intestine, and lung has been shown in animals receiving the drug.

The exact mechanism(s) of immunosuppressive action of cyclosporine has not been fully elucidated but appears to mainly involve inhibition of lymphocytic proliferation and function. It has been suggested that the immunosuppressive action of cyclosporine results from specific and reversible inhibition of immunocompetent T cells (T-lymphocytes) in the G_0 (resting) or G_1 (first "gap," postmitotic, or presynthetic) phase of the cell cycle. Cyclosporine mainly inhibits T-helper (inducer) cells; some inhibition of T-suppressor cells may also be involved. The drug also inhibits T-cytotoxic cells and interleukin-2-producing T cells. Cyclosporine inhibits production and/or release of lymphokines including interleukin-2 (T-cell growth factor) and interleukin-1 (lymphocyte-activating factor). Cyclosporine inhibits the release of interleukin-2 from activated T cells and also inhibits interleukin-2-induced activation of resting T cells; the drug does not appear to inhibit activation of resting T cells that is induced by exogenous interleukin-2.

There is conflicting evidence to date whether cyclosporine affects B cells (B-lymphocytes). In some studies, cyclosporine inhibited B-cell responses to macrophage-processed antigens and directly suppressed B cells in the blastogenic phase. In other studies, cyclosporine did not inhibit B-cell antibody production. In animals, cyclosporine does *not* affect the function of phagocytic cells (enzyme secretion, chemotactic migration of granulocytes, macrophage migration, in vivo carbon clearance) or that of tumor cells (growth rate, metastasis).

Unlike other currently available immunosuppressive agents (e.g., azathioprine), cyclosporine lacks clinically important myelosuppressive activity. In one study following administration of high dosages of cyclosporine, bone marrow cell counts (i.e., granulocytes, monocytes, stem cells) showed only slight reductions in cell numbers; proliferation of bone marrow stem cells was normal or enhanced.

■ Renal Effects Cyclosporine produces nephrotoxic effects which generally appear to be dose dependent and reversible. (See Cautions: Renal Effects.) Increased BUN and/or serum creatinine concentrations have been observed during therapy with the drug. In some patients following bone marrow or renal transplantation, histologic evidence of nephrotoxicity has been observed including arteriolar and glomerular thrombi, marked tubular injury, and interstitial fibrosis. Ischemically injured kidneys may be particularly sensitive to the nephrotoxic effects of the drug. Hypertension, hyperkalemia, and hyperuricemia frequently result from therapy with cyclosporine and may be caused directly by the drug's nephrotoxic effects. Increased plasma renin activity has been reported in animals receiving cyclosporine and may contribute to the development of hypertension.

■ Other Effects There is some evidence that cyclosporine may have antimalarial, antineoplastic, and antischistosomal activity; however, the clinical importance of these findings has not been determined.

Pharmacokinetics

Cyclosporine as unchanged drug is chiefly responsible for immunosuppressive activity, although certain metabolites (e.g., AM1, AM9, AM4N) appear to contribute, at least in part, to this activity. Determination of the pharmacokinetics of cyclosporine appears to be biologic fluid dependent (blood vs plasma or serum) and assay-method dependent (radioimmunoassay vs high-pressure liquid chromatography). Because of these apparent differences, interpretation of pharmacokinetic data and determination of a relationship between biologic fluid concentrations and therapeutic and/or toxic effects of the drug are difficult. Although the most appropriate biologic fluid and assay method for determining cyclosporine concentrations have not been fully established, most experts currently recommend that whole blood preferably be used since the higher cyclosporine concentrations present in this fluid (relative to plasma or serum) can be measured more precisely and accurately than with these other fluids. In addition, there is some evidence from renal allograft recipients that whole blood rather than plasma determinations may be a more useful guide to efficacy and/or toxicity of cyclosporine, although precise relationships remain to be established. In addition, these experts currently recommend that an assay method with high specificity for unchanged cyclosporine preferably be used. Some laboratories may continue to report, and clinicians to use, cyclosporine concentrations determined in plasma or serum, and, while the benefits remain unclear,some centers advocate the use of both nonspecific and specific assays in order to gain insight into the proportion of immunoreactivity resulting from metabolites of the drug. In addition, interpretation of results can be difficult, in part because of the complex pharmacokinetics of the drug, variety of assay methods used, and the broad range of acceptable values, depending on the clinical indication for cyclosporine use and time since transplantation. Therefore, all values for cyclosporine concentration must be qualified by the biologic fluid and assay method used, and any guidance regarding possible dosage adjustment should include information on appropriate reference ranges and be tailored to the patient population being treated and any associated treatment protocols.

Distribution of cyclosporine into erythrocytes is temperature and concentration dependent; therefore, reported plasma concentrations are affected by temperature during the separation of plasma and may also be affected by concentration of the drug. Variability of plasma cyclosporine concentrations may be minimized by allowing the sample to equilibrate at room temperature for at least 1 hour prior to centrifugation. Determinations of drug concentration using anticoagulated, hemolyzed whole blood may avoid the problem of temperature-dependent redistribution of the drug between plasma and erythrocytes. Plasma concentrations of the drug may also be affected by the patient's lipoprotein concentration and hematocrit. Following administration of the same dose, blood concentrations of cyclosporine are higher than plasma concentrations since the drug is distributed into erythrocytes. Plasma and serum cyclosporine concentrations are comparable.

Although both RIA and HPLC have been used to determine biologic fluid cyclosporine concentrations, RIA has been used most extensively since HPLC determination of cyclosporine concentrations is technically difficult and variable; the 2 assays do not yield comparable results. Both specific (for unchanged drug) and nonspecific RIA methods are available. When RIA methods that employ nonspecific monoclonal or polyclonal antibodies are used for monitoring cyclosporine concentrations, cross-reactivity of the antisera with circulating metabolites of cyclosporine has resulted in higher cyclosporine concentrations than when HPLC is used. The ratio of specific (either RIA or HPLC) to nonspecific assays of blood cyclosporine concentrations has varied from 1:1 to 1:8; however, for nonspecific immunoassays, the ratio usually is 1:2 to 1:3 for stable renal allograft patients several months after surgery but is 1:3 to 1:4 for cardiac or hepatic allograft recipients, and may be as great as 1:19 in hepatic allograft recipients with severe cholestasis. The ratio may remain constant for fixed points of comparison during the dosing interval. Additional study is needed to determine whether a similar constancy for these fixed-point ratios exists in patients with impaired hepatic function, especially during the early posttransplantation period in hepatic allograft recipients, since cyclosporine is metabolized principally in the liver and undergoes substantial biliary elimination. In addition to RIA, immunoassay methods currently employed include a nonspecific or specific fluorescence polarization immunoassay (FPIA) and a specific enzyme multiplied immunoassay technique (EMIT). Even with specific immunoassays, some cross-reactivity with cyclosporine metabolites may exist, resulting in slightly different reference ranges for cyclosporine concentrations. Therefore, it is important that consistent laboratories and methods be used and that the reference ranges for each group of organ transplant recipients and method of assay be known; in addition, any attempt at comparing these ranges with other institutions generally should be limited to circumstances in which the same assay method and therapeutic regimens are employed.

At present, use of any of the currently available specific immunoassays (RIA, FPIA, FPIA) is acceptable for routine monitoring of whole blood trough cyclosporine concentrations. Although use of HPLC also may be appropriate for determining trough cyclosporine concentrations, differences in the results obtained with this assay method relative to immunoassays should be considered when monitoring cyclosporine therapy.

■ **Absorption** Following oral administration, cyclosporine is variably and incompletely absorbed. The extent of absorption depends on the individual patient, patient population (e.g., transplant type), posttransplantation time (e.g., increasing during the early posttransplantation period in renal transplant recipients), bile flow (micellar absorption of the drug involving bile), GI state (e.g., decreased with diarrhea), and the formulation administered. Absorption of orally administered cyclosporine from conventional (nonmodified) oral formulations reportedly is erratic during long-term therapy. In hepatic allograft recipients, GI absorption of cyclosporine also may be erratic, especially during the first few weeks of the posttransplantation period because of surgical techniques (e.g., bile duct management with resultant reductions in bile flow) or surgically induced liver dysfunction.

Peak blood and plasma cyclosporine concentrations occur at about 3.5 hours following oral administration of conventional (nonmodified) formulations of the drug. Following oral administration, cyclosporine is metabolized on first pass through the liver. (See Pharmacokinetics: Elimination.) Although oral bioavailability of cyclosporine administered as conventional oral formulations averages 30% across various allograft recipients, it exhibits considerable interindividual variation, ranging from 2–89%, depending on numerous variables including organ transplant type; in hepatic or renal allograft recipients, estimates range from less than 10% to as high as 89%, respectively. Following oral administration of a single 600-mg dose of cyclosporine as a conventional solution in one study, the mean absolute bioavailability was about 30% (range: 10–60%) and a mean peak plasma concentration of about 540 ng/mL (range: 240–1250 ng/mL) was reached at about 3–4 hours. Limited data indicate that the bioavailability of the conventional liquid-filled capsules of cyclosporine is equivalent to that of the conventional oral solution. In a small number of renal transplant patients who received a mean daily cyclosporine dosage of 3.9 mg/kg (range: 2.2–6.6 mg/kg), given as the conventional oral solution for 1 week followed by the same dosage as the capsules for 1 week, the relative bioavailability of the conventional liquid-filled capsules was 111% (based on the area under the blood concentration-time curve from 0–12 hours) of the oral solution. The manufacturer states that peak plasma or blood concentrations of cyclosporine (as determined by HPLC) are approximately 1 or 1.4–2.7 ng/mL per mg of an orally administered dose from a conventional formulation, respectively, in healthy adults.

Although the absolute oral bioavailability of cyclosporine administered as the modified oral formulations (Gengraf®, Neoral®) has not been determined in adults, these formulations have greater bioavailability than the conventional (nonmodified) oral formulations of cyclosporine. In addition, while the peak blood or plasma concentration and area under the concentration-time curve (AUC) of cyclosporine increase with the dose administered, with a curvilinear (parabolic) relationship observed at doses between 0–1.4 g of conventional (nonmodified) oral formulations when the biologic fluid used is blood, the AUC of cyclosporine is linearly related to usual doses of the drug administered as the modified oral formulations; a linear relationship also has been described for conventional oral formulations when plasma and HPLC were used. Despite the increased AUC and peak blood concentrations of cyclosporine associated with the modified oral formulations, dose-normalized trough concentrations of the drug are similar for both the conventional and modified formulations. The AUC of cyclosporine differed between individuals by a percent coefficient of variation of approximately 20–50% in renal transplant patients administered cyclosporine as the conventional (nonmodified) oral formulation or a modified oral formulation. Such a factor makes individualization of dosage necessary for optimal therapy. Intraindividual variability in the AUC of cyclosporine and time to peak blood concentration of the drug is reduced with the modified oral formulations compared with the conventional oral formulation. Some evidence indicates that intraindividual variability in peak and trough blood concentrations of cyclosporine also is less with the modified oral formulations. In renal allograft recipients, the percent coefficients of variation within individuals in the AUC of cyclosporine for modified and conventional (nonmodified) oral formulations were 9–21 and 19–26%, respectively. Intraindividual variabilities in the trough concentration of cyclosporine from modified and conventional oral formulations were 17–30 and 16–38%, respectively, in these patients. Limited data in children also show that the bioavailability of cyclosporine is higher with the modified oral formulations. The modified oral capsules of Neoral® are bioequivalent with Neoral® oral solution. The modified oral capsules of Gengraf® also are bioequivalent with the modified oral solution of Gengraf®. In addition, the 2 commercially available modified oral formulations of cyclosporine, Neoral® and Gengraf®, have been demonstrated to be bioequivalent to each other.

The higher bioavailability of the modified oral formulations relative to the conventional (nonmodified) oral formulation varies across patient populations. The mean relative AUC of cyclosporine for a modified oral formulation (Neoral®) compared with the conventional oral formulation ranged from 1.2–1.5 in crossover studies of stable renal transplant patients. In de novo renal transplant patients administered either formulation of cyclosporine, the dose-normalized AUC was 23% greater with the modified oral formulation. In de novo hepatic allograft recipients administered either formulation of cyclosporine 28 days after transplantation, the dose-normalized AUC was 50% greater with the modified oral formulation. The absolute oral bioavailability of cyclosporine was 43% (range: 30–68%) from the modified oral formulation compared with 28% (range: 17–42%) from the conventional oral formulation in de novo hepatic transplant patients aged 1.4–10 years old. In a limited number of hepatic allograft recipients with external biliary diversion, the oral bioavailability of cyclosporine was 6.5 times greater with the modified oral formulation (Neoral®) administered during the first month after transplantation than with the conventional oral formulation. In a limited number of cardiac allograft recipients, the AUC of cyclosporine was greater with the modified oral formulation (Neoral®) relative to the conventional oral formulation. In a limited number of patients with rheumatoid arthritis, the AUC of cyclosporine was about 20% greater with the modified oral formulation (Neoral®) compared with the conventional oral formulation. Peak blood concentrations are increased by 40–106% in renal transplant patients and by approximately 90% in hepatic transplant patients. Peak blood concentrations of cyclosporine occur from 1.5–2 hours following oral administration of the modified formulations to renal transplant patients.

Food decreases the AUC and peak blood concentration of cyclosporine attained with the modified oral formulations. In healthy individuals, the AUC and peak blood concentration of cyclosporine were decreased by 15 and 26%, respectively, when the oral formulation of Neoral® was administered 30 minutes after the start of consumption of a high-fat meal (e.g., 960 calories, 54.4 g of fat). In another study, the AUC and peak blood concentration of cyclosporine decreased by 13 and 33%, respectively, when a high-fat meal (e.g., 669 calories, 45 g of fat) was eaten within 30 minutes before administration of this modified oral formulation. Similar effects occurred with a low-fat meal (e.g., 667 calories, 15 g of fat). However, other data have not shown the AUC of cyclosporine from the modified oral formulation of Neoral® to be affected by a high-fat meal (45 g) or a low-fat meal (15 g). Similar discordance of data on the effect of food on cyclosporine absorption with conventional formulations has been described, although high-fat meals and meals given early postoperatively appear most likely to enhance absorption.

External biliary diversion in de novo hepatic transplant patients had very little effect on the absorption of cyclosporine from the oral formulation of Neoral®. The change from the trough to the maximal blood concentration of cyclosporine when the T-tube was closed differed by 6.9% from when it was open. In adult de novo renal transplant patients being treated with this modified oral formulation at a dosage of 597 mg (7.95 mg/kg) daily, the AUC over one dosing interval of cyclosporine was 8772 ng •h/mL at 4 weeks. The peak and trough (obtained prior to the morning dose, approximately 12 hours after last dose) blood concentrations of cyclosporine were 1802 and 361 ng/mL, respectively, as determined by specific monoclonal fluorescence polarization immunoassay. In stable adult renal transplant patients being treated with this modified oral formulation at a dosage of 344 mg (4.1 mg/kg) daily, the AUC over one dosing interval was 6035 ng•h/mL. The peak and trough blood concentrations of cyclosporine in these patients were 1333 and 251 ng/mL, respectively, as determined by specific monoclonal fluorescence polarization immunoassay. In adult de novo hepatic transplant patients being treated with this formulation at a dosage of 458 mg (6.9 mg/kg) daily, the AUC over one dosing interval was 7187 ng•h/mL at 4 weeks. The peak and trough blood concentrations of the drug in these patients were 1555 and 268 ng/mL, respectively, as determined by specific monoclonal RIA.

In stable hepatic transplant patients 2–8 years of age being treated with the oral formulation of Neoral® at a dosage of 101 mg (5.95 mg/kg) in 3 divided doses daily, the peak blood concentration of cyclosporine was 629 ng/mL, as determined by specific monoclonal RIA, and the AUC over one dosing interval was 2163 ng•h/mL. In stable hepatic transplant patients 8–15 years of age being treated with this modified formulation at a dosage of 188 mg (4.96 mg/kg) in 2 divided doses daily, the peak blood concentration of the drug was 975 ng/mL, as determined by specific monoclonal RIA, and the AUC over one dosing interval was 4272 ng•h/mL. In a stable hepatic transplant patient 3 years of age being treated with this modified oral formulation at a dosage of 120 mg (8.3 mg/kg) in 2 divided doses daily, the peak blood concentration was 1050 ng/mL, as determined by specific monoclonal fluorescence polarization immunoassay, and the AUC over one dosing interval was 5832 ng•h/mL. In stable hepatic transplant patients 8–15 years of age being treated with this modified formulation at a dosage of 158 mg (5.5 mg/kg) in 2 divided doses daily, the peak blood cyclosporine concentration was 1013 ng/mL, as determined by specific monoclonal fluorescence polarization immunoassay, and the AUC over one dosing interval was 4452 ng•h/mL. In stable renal transplant patients 7–15 years of age being treated with the modified oral formulation at a dosage of 328 mg (7.4 mg/kg) in 2 divided doses daily, the peak blood concentration was 1827 ng/mL, as determined by specific monoclonal fluorescence polarization immunoassay, and the AUC over one dosing interval was 6922 ng•h/mL.

Blood or plasma concentrations of cyclosporine required for therapeutic effect or associated with toxicity have not been established precisely. (See introductory paragraphs in Pharmacokinetics.) Organ rejection has reportedly occurred less frequently when trough blood concentrations of the drug (determined by HPLC) were greater than 100 ng/mL. Although optimum trough cyclosporine concentrations have not been determined, trough blood or plasma concentrations (i.e., at 24 hours) of 250–800 or 50–300 ng/mL, respectively, as determined by RIA, appear to minimize the frequency of graft rejection and cyclosporine-induced adverse effects. An association between trough serum concentrations (determined by RIA) greater than 500 ng/mL and cyclosporine-induced nephrotoxicity has been reported.

■ **Distribution** Cyclosporine is widely distributed into body fluids and tissues, with most of the drug being distributed outside the blood volume. Following oral administration of a single 600-mg dose as a conventional formulation in adults with normal renal and hepatic function, the apparent volume of distribution (V_d) of cyclosporine has been reported to be 13 L/kg. The drug has a volume of distribution at steady-state (V_{ss}) of 3–5 L/kg following IV administration in solid organ allograft recipients. In one study following IV administration of cyclosporine in patients with severely impaired renal function (i.e., creatinine clearance less than 5 mL/minute), V_{ss} ranged from 1.45–7.26 L/kg.

Approximately 90–98% of cyclosporine in plasma is protein bound, mainly to lipoproteins (85–90% of total protein binding). Of lipoprotein binding, 43–57% is to high-density lipoproteins (HDLs), 25% to low-density lipoproteins (LDLs), and 2% to very-low-density lipoproteins (VLDLs). Distribution of the drug in blood is dose dependent; in vitro in blood, 33–47% of the drug is distributed into plasma, 4–9% into lymphocytes, 4–12% into granulocytes, and 41–58% into erythrocytes. At high concentrations, distribution of cyclosporine into leukocytes and erythrocytes becomes saturated. Concentrations of the drug achieved in mononuclear cells have been reported to be 1000 times greater than those achieved in erythrocytes.

Cyclosporine crosses the placenta in animals and humans. In a renal allograft recipient who received 450 mg of cyclosporine daily throughout pregnancy, the drug was not present in amniotic fluid at 36 weeks or at amniotomy, but maternal and cord blood concentrations at delivery were 86 and 54 mcg/L, respectively.

Cyclosporine is distributed into milk. Cyclosporine concentrations in milk reportedly were 101, 109, and 263 mcg/L on the second, third, and fourth days of the postpartum period, respectively, in a patient who received 450 mg of the drug daily throughout pregnancy and the postpartum period. Studies in animals have shown that cyclosporine is distributed into milk at a maximum concentration of 2% of the maternal dose.

■ **Elimination** Blood concentrations of cyclosporine generally appear to decline in a biphasic manner, although a triphasic disposition also has been described. In adults with normal renal and hepatic function, the half-life in the initial phase ($t_{1/2\alpha}$) has been reported to average 1.2 hours and the half-life in the terminal elimination phase ($t_{1/2\beta}$) has averaged 8.4–27 hours (range: 4–50 hours). In one study following IV administration of cyclosporine in patients with severely impaired renal function (i.e., creatinine clearance less than 5 mL/minute), $t_{1/2\beta}$ averaged 15.8 or 16.5 hours based on blood cyclosporine concentrations determined by HPLC or RIA, respectively.

Clearance of cyclosporine from blood following IV administration is approximately 5–7 mL/minute per kg as determined with data (using HPLC) from adult renal or hepatic transplant patients. Clearance of the drug in infants may be up to severalfold higher and in older children twice as high as that in adults. Cardiac transplant patients appear to have slightly slower blood cyclosporine clearance.

The apparent clearance of cyclosporine administered as a modified oral formulation was 593 mL/minute (7.8 mL/minute per kg) after 4 weeks of therapy and 492 mL/minute (5.9 mL/minute per kg) as determined with data (using monoclonal fluorescence polarization immunoassay) from adult de novo renal transplant patients who received a dosage of 597 mg (7.95 mg/kg) daily and from stable adult renal transplant patients who received a dosage of 344 mg (4.1 mg/kg) daily, respectively; after 4 weeks of therapy clearance was 577 mL/minute (8.6 mL/minute per kg) as determined with data (using monoclonal RIA) from de novo hepatic transplant patients who received a dosage of 458 mg (6.89 mg/kg) daily. Limited data are available for pediatric patients. Clearance of cyclosporine from blood averaged 10.6 mL/minute per kg in a study (using specific monoclonal RIA) of renal transplant patients 3–16 years of age administered the drug IV. The range in cyclosporine clearance was 9.8–15.5 mL/minute per kg in a study of renal transplant patients 2–16 years old. Data (using HPLC) from hepatic transplant patients 0.6–5.6 years of age revealed an average clearance of 9.3 mL/minute per kg. The clearance of cyclosporine administered as a modified oral formulation was 285 mL/minute (16.6 mL/minute per kg) or 378 mL/minute (10.2 mL/minute per kg) as determined with data (specific monoclonal RIA used) from stable hepatic transplant patients 2–8 or 8–15 years of age, respectively, who received a dosage of 101 mg (5.95 mg/kg) or 188 mg (4.96 mg/kg) daily, respectively; clearance was 171 mL/minute (11.9 mL/minute per kg) and 328 mL/min (11 mL/minute per kg) as determined with data (using specific monoclonal fluorescence polarization immunoassay) from stable hepatic transplant patients 3 years of age or 8–15 years old, respectively, who received a dosage of 120 mg (8.3 mg/kg) or 158 mg (5.5 mg/kg) daily, respectively. In stable renal transplant patients 7–15 years of age who received cyclosporine as a modified oral formulation at a dosage of 328 mg (7.4 mg/kg) daily, clearance of the drug was 418 mL/minute (8.7 mL/minute per kg) as determined with specific monoclonal fluorescence polarization immunoassay. The clearance of cyclosporine reportedly is not changed substantially by renal failure or dialysis.

Cyclosporine is extensively metabolized in the liver via the cytochrome P-450 enzyme system, principally by the CYP3A isoenzyme, and less extensively in the GI tract and the kidney to at least 30 metabolites found in bile, feces, blood, and urine. The pharmacologic and toxicologic activities of cyclosporine's metabolites are considerably less than those of the parent drug. The drug undergoes extensive first-pass metabolism following oral administration. Several major metabolic pathways, including hydroxylation of the C_γ-carbon of 2 leucine residues, C_λ-carbon hydroxylation and cyclic ether formation (with oxidation of the double bond) in the side chain of the amino acid 3-hydroxyl-*N*,4-dimethyl-l-2-amino-6-octenoic acid, and *N*-demethylation of *N*-methyl leucine residues, are involved. Conjugation of these metabolites or hydrolysis of the cyclic peptide chain does not appear to be an important pathway for cyclosporine metabolism. Oxidation of cyclosporine at its 1-λ, 4-*N*-desmethylated, and 9-γ positions yields the major metabolites known as AM1 (M17), AM4N (M21), and AM9 (M1), respectively. The AUCs at steady state of AM1, AM4N, and AM9 were approximately 70, 7.5, and 21%, respectively, of the blood AUC for cyclosporine in renal transplant patients treated with a conventional oral formulation of the drug. The manufacturers state that the percentages of a dose present as AM1, AM4N, and AM9 are similar after administration of the conventional (nonmodified) oral formulation or the modified oral formulations, as indicated by blood or biliary concentrations in stable renal or de novo hepatic transplant patients, respectively. In stable renal transplant patients, the ratio of AUC at steady state for AM1 and AM9 to that for cyclosporine did not differ between the conventional oral formulation and the modified oral formulation.

Cyclosporine is principally excreted via bile, almost entirely as metabolites. Only about 6% of a dose of the drug is excreted in urine, with 0.1% of a dose being excreted unchanged. However, urinary excretion of unchanged drug may be increased in certain patient populations (e.g., early posttransplant period in bone marrow allograft recipients) and in younger patients.

Chemistry and Stability

■ **Chemistry** Cyclosporine (cyclosporin A) is a cyclosporin immunosuppressive agent produced as a metabolite of the fungus species *Aphanocladium album* or *Beauveria nivea*. The drug is a nonpolar, cyclic polypeptide antibiotic consisting of 11 amino acids. Cyclosporine is one of several biologically active antibiotics (cyclosporins) produced by these fungi; cyclosporin A and C are the major metabolites.

Cyclosporine occurs as a white or essentially white, finely crystalline powder. The drug is relatively insoluble in water, having an aqueous solubility of 0.04 mg/mL at 25°C, and is generally soluble in lipids and organic solvents, having a solubility of more than 80 mg/mL in alcohol at 25°C. The potency of cyclosporine is determined on the anhydrous basis; each mcg of cyclosporine is defined as the activity (potency) contained in 1.0173 mcg of the FDA's cyclosporine master standard.

Commercially available cyclosporine conventional (nonmodified) oral solution has a clear, yellow, oily appearance. Cyclosporine conventional oral solution contains the drug in an olive oil and peglicol 5 oleate (Labrafil® M 1944CS) vehicle with 12.5% (v/v) alcohol. Commercially available cyclosporine concentrate for injection occurs as a clear, faintly brownish-yellow solution. Cyclosporine concentrate for injection is a sterile solution of the drug in polyoxyl 35 castor oil (Cremophor® EL, polyethoxylated castor oil) with 32.9% (v/v) alcohol. At the time of manufacture, the air in the ampuls of cyclosporine concentrate for injection is replaced with nitrogen. The concentrate for injection contains no more than 42 USP endotoxin units per mL. Cyclosporine also is commercially available as 25-, 50-, and 100-mg conventional (nonmodified) liquid-filled, soft gelatin capsules.

Cyclosporine also is commercially available as a modified, nonaqueous liquid formulation (Neoral®) of the drug that immediately forms an emulsion in aqueous fluids; the formulation is available as an oral solution for emulsion and as oral 25- and 100-mg liquid-filled soft gelatin capsules containing the oral solution for emulsion. When exposed to an aqueous environment, the oral solution for emulsion forms a homogenous transparent emulsion with a droplet size smaller than 100 nm in diameter; as a result, the formulation has been referred to as an oral solution for microemulsion. In this formulation, the molecular structure of cyclosporine is unaltered, and aqueous dilution results in formation of an emulsion without reprecipitation of the drug. Cyclosporine is dispersed in a mixture of propylene glycol (hydrophilic solvent) and corn oil monoglycerides, diglycerides, and triglycerides (lipophilic solvent); when dispersed, polyoxyl 40 hydrogenated castor oil serves as a surfactant, and d,l-α-tocopherol is present as an antioxidant. Neoral® oral solution and liquid-filled capsules also contains dehydrated alcohol in a maximum concentration of 11.9% (v/v).

In addition, cyclosporine is commercially available as a modified liquid formulation (Gengraf®) of the drug that forms an aqueous dispersion (also referred to as a microemulsion) of the drug in an aqueous environment; this formulation is available as both an oral solution and as oral 25- and 100-mg liquid-filled capsules. Cyclosporine is dispersed in a mixture of propylene glycol, sorbitan monooleate, and either polyoxyl 40 hydrogenated castor oil (in the oral solution) or polyoxyl 35 castor oil and polyethylene glycol (in the capsules). Gengraf® liquid-filled capsules also contain alcohol 12.8% (v/v).

The modified oral formulations of cyclosporine (Neoral® and Gengraf®), both as the oral solution and the oral capsules, have increased oral bioavailability compared with the conventional (nonmodified) oral solution and liquid-filled capsules of the drug (i.e., Sandimmune®). Therefore, the conventional (nonmodified) and modified formulations are *not* bioequivalent and cannot be used interchangeably without appropriate medical supervision. (See Pharmacokinetics: Absorption.)

■ **Stability** Cyclosporine conventional (nonmodified) oral solution should be stored in the original container at temperature less than 30°C and protected from freezing; refrigeration should be avoided since coalescence and separation of the oral solution could occur. Opened containers of cyclosporine conventional oral solution must be used within 2 months. Cyclosporine concentrate for injection should be stored at a temperature less than 30°C and protected from freezing and light. Cyclosporine conventional liquid-filled capsules should be stored in their original unit-dose container at a controlled room temperature of 25°C but may be exposed to temperatures ranging from 15–30°C. When stored as directed, the capsules have an expiration date of 3 years from the date of manufacture. An odor may be detected when the unit-dose container is opened, which will dissipate shortly thereafter, but this odor does not affect the quality of the preparation.

Cyclosporine (modified) liquid-filled, soft gelatin capsules (commercially available as Neoral®) should be stored in their original unit-dose packaging at 20–25°C, and Neoral® oral solution also should be stored in the original container at 20–25°C. At temperatures less than 20°C, Neoral® oral solution may gel, and light flocculation and/or the formation of a light sediment also may occur; however, such changes do not affect dosing with the syringe provided or efficacy and can be reversed by allowing the solution to warm to a room temperature of 25°C. Neoral® oral solution should not be refrigerated, and once opened, containers of the oral solution must be used within 2 months.

Cyclosporine (modified) liquid-filled capsules commercially available as Gengraf® should be stored in their original unit-dose packaging at 15–30°C, and Gengraf® oral solution also should be stored in the original container at 15–30°C. At temperatures less than 20°C, Gengraf® oral solution may gel, and light flocculation and/or the formation of a light sediment also may occur; however, such changes do not affect dosing with the syringe provided or efficacy and can be reversed by allowing the solution to warm to a room temperature of 15–30°C. Gengraf® oral solution should not be refrigerated, and once opened, containers of the oral solution must be used within 2 months.

Cyclosporine concentrate for injection that has been diluted to a final concentration of approximately 2 mg/mL is stable for 24 hours in 5% dextrose or 0.9% sodium chloride injection in glass or PVC containers. Diluted solutions of the drug in 5% dextrose or 0.9% sodium chloride injection do not require protection from light. There is some evidence that substantial amounts of cyclosporine may be lost during infusion through plastic tubing in IV administration sets. Because of combined loss during storage and administration via plastic IV tubing, it has been suggested that dilutions in 0.9% sodium chloride injection be considered stable for no longer than 6 or 12 hours in PVC or glass containers, respectively. Polyoxyl 35 castor oil can cause leaching of bis(2-ethylhexyl) phthalate (BEHP, DEHP) from PVC containers and, following dilution of cyclosporine concentrate for injection in PVC containers, substantial leaching of DEHP occurs in a time-dependent manner. The manufacturer makes no specific recommendations regarding the compatibility of the concentrate for injection with plastic containers; however, to minimize exposure of the patient to leached DEHP, some clinicians recommend that diluted solutions of the drug in PVC containers be administered immediately after preparation.

Preparations

Excipients in commercially available drug preparations may have clinically important effects in some individuals; consult specific product labeling for details.

cycloSPORINE

Oral		
Capsules, liquid-filled (nonmodified)	25 mg	**SandIMMUNE®**, Novartis
	50 mg	**SandIMMUNE®**, Novartis
	100 mg	**SandIMMUNE®**, Novartis
Capsules, liquid-filled, for emulsion (modified)	25 mg	**Gengraf®**, Abbott **Neoral®**, Novartis
	100 mg	**Gengraf®**, Abbott **Neoral®**, Novartis
For emulsion, solution (modified)	100 mg/mL	**Gengraf®**, Abbott **Neoral®**, Novartis
For solution, concentrate (nonmodified)	100 mg/mL	**SandIMMUNE®**, Novartis
Parenteral		
For injection, concentrate for IV infusion only	50 mg/mL	**SandIMMUNE® I.V.**, Novartis

†Use is not currently included in the labeling approved by the US Food and Drug Administration

Mycophenolate Mofetil Mycophenolate Sodium

■ Mycophenolate mofetil and mycophenolate sodium are used as immunosuppressive agents. Mycophenolate mofetil is a prodrug that has little pharmacologic activity until hydrolyzed in vivo to mycophenolic acid, the pharmacologically active metabolite. Mycophenolate sodium delayed-release tablets release the active moiety, mycophenolic acid, in the small intestine.

Uses

Mycophenolate mofetil (CellCept®) is used for the prevention of rejection of kidney, heart, or liver allografts. The manufacturer recommends that mycophenolate mofetil be used in conjunction with cyclosporine and corticosteroid therapy. Mycophenolate mofetil also has been used in the management of Crohn's disease†.

Mycophenolate sodium (Myfortic®) is used in conjunction with cyclosporine and corticosteroid therapy for the prevention of rejection of kidney allografts.

Mycophenolate mofetil and mycophenolate sodium have been used in the management of systemic sclerosis (often called scleroderma)†.

■ **Renal Allotransplantation** ***Adult Patients*** Mycophenolate mofetil is used for the prevention of rejection of renal allografts in adults and pediatric patients 3 months to 18 years of age. In clinical trials in renal transplant patients, a regimen consisting of mycophenolate mofetil, cyclosporine, and corticosteroids was more effective than regimens consisting of either azathioprine or placebo in combination with cyclosporine and corticosteroids in preventing acute rejection, graft loss, or death at 6 months following transplantation.

Efficacy and safety of mycophenolate mofetil has been evaluated in 3 randomized, double-blind, multicenter trials in adults undergoing cadaveric renal transplantation. In each trial, mycophenolate mofetil was given in 2 different dosages (1 or 1.5 g twice daily) in immunosuppressive regimens that included cyclosporine, corticosteroids, and (in one study) antithymocyte globulin. Mycophenolate mofetil was compared with azathioprine (1–2 mg/kg daily or 100–150 mg daily) in 2 studies and with placebo in a third study; patients receiving azathioprine or placebo in these studies also received cyclosporine and corticosteroids. In these trials, the primary efficacy end point was the rate of treatment failure, defined as the first occurrence of an acute episode of biopsy-proven acute rejection, death, graft loss, or early termination of the study for any reason without a prior biopsy-proven acute rejection episode, in the first 6 months after transplantation. Results of these studies indicate that mycophenolate mofetil was more effective than azathioprine or placebo in reducing the incidence of treatment failure at 6 months following transplantation. When mycophenolate mofetil was compared with azathioprine, the treatment failure rates at 6 months for mycophenolate mofetil 2 g, mycophenolate mofetil 3 g, azathioprine (1–2 mg/kg daily), and azathioprine (100–150 mg daily) were 31.1–38.2, 31.3–34.8, 47.6, and 50%, respectively.When mycophenolate mofetil was compared with placebo, treatment failure rates at 6 months for mycophenolate mofetil 2 g, mycophenolate mofetil 3 g, and placebo were 30.3, 38.8, and 56%, respectively. The cumulative incidence of combined 1-year graft loss or patient death for mycophenolate mofetil 2 g, mycophenolate mofetil 3 g, and control (placebo or azathioprine), were 8.5–11.7%, 10–11.5, and 11.5–13.6%, respectively.

Mycophenolate sodium is used for the prevention of rejection of renal allographs in adults and pediatric patients 5–16 years of age. In clinical trials in *de novo* or stable renal transplant patients, a regimen consisting of mycophenolate sodium, cyclosporine, and/or corticosteroids was as effective as a regimen consisting of mycophenolate mofetil, cyclosporine, and corticosteroids in preventing acute rejection, graft loss, or death.

Mycophenolate mofetil therapy has been associated with a high incidence of adverse GI effects and a high proportion of patients receiving the drug required dosage reductions, interruptions in therapy, or discontinuance of the immunosuppressant due to adverse effects. Such changes in drug therapy have a negative impact on transplant outcomes (higher incidence of acute rejection, decreased graft survival). Mycophenolate sodium delayed-release tablets were designed to improve GI tolerance by delaying release of mycophenolic acid until the drug reaches the small intestine. However, results of comparative clinical studies have shown that incidence of adverse GI effects reported in patients receiving mycophenolate sodium have been similar to those in patients receiving mycophenolate mofetil.

Safety and efficacy of mycophenolate sodium delayed-release tablets have been evaluated in 2 multicenter, randomized, double-blind, comparative trials. In one 12-month study, 423 *de novo* renal transplant patients (18–75 years of age) who were receiving their first cadaveric (84%), living- unrelated, or human leukocyte antigen (HLA)-mismatched living-related donor kidney transplant, were randomized to receive (within 24–48 hours of transplantation) mycophenolate sodium (mycophenolic acid 720 mg twice daily) or mycophenolate mofetil (1 g twice daily) in conjunction with cyclosporine and corticosteroids. Patients undergoing transplantation at centers that routinely used induction therapy with antithymocyte or antilymphocyte antibody preparations (about 41%) were allowed to receive such therapy. The primary efficacy end point was the rate of treatment failure, defined as the first occurrence of acute rejection episode (biopsy-proven), graft loss, death, or loss to follow-up, in the first 6 months after transplantation. Mycophenolate sodium was as effective as mycophenolate mofetil in reducing the incidence of treatment failure rates at 6 and 12 months following transplantation. The treatment failure rates at 6 months for mycophenolate sodium and mycophenolate mofetil in this study were 25.8 and 26.2%, respectively, while at 12 months, treatment failure rates were 28.6 and 28.1%, respectively.

In the other 12-month study, maintenance therapy with mycophenolate sodium delayed-release tablets has been evaluated in 322 renal transplant patients (18–75 years of age) who had undergone primary or secondary cadaveric or living donor kidney transplantation, were at least 6 months posttransplant, and were receiving immunosuppressive regimens that included mycophenolate mofetil and cyclosporine, with or without corticosteroids, for at least 2 weeks before study entry. Patients were randomized to continue mycophenolate mofetil (1 g twice daily) or to switch to mycophenolate sodium (mycophenolic acid 720 mg twice daily). The incidence of treatment failure (defined as the first occurrence of acute rejection episode [biopsy-proven], graft loss, death, or loss to follow-up) at 6 and 12 months in patients receiving mycophenolate sodium was similar to that in patients receiving mycophenolate mofetil. The treatment failure rates at 6 months for mycophenolate sodium and mycophenolate mofetil in this study were 4.4 and 6.7%, respectively, while at 12 months, treatment failure rates were 7.5 and 12.3%, respectively. Results of this and other studies indicate that mycophenolate sodium can be substituted for mycophenolate mofetil without loss of efficacy.

Pediatric Patients In an open-label multicenter study in pediatric patients 3 months to 18 years of age who underwent cadaveric renal transplantation, mycophenolate mofetil was administered by oral suspension in a dosage of 600 mg/m^2 twice daily (maximum daily dosage 1 g twice daily) in conjunction with cyclosporine and corticosteroids. In this study, the overall biopsy-proven rejection rate at 6 months was comparable to that reported in adults. In addition, the rate of biopsy-proven rejection was similar across the various age groups (i.e., 3 months to younger than 6 years of age, 6 years to younger than 12 years of age; 12–18 years of age). At 12 months, the combined incidence of graft loss (5%) and patient death (2%) in children was similar to that observed in adults.

Safety and efficacy of mycophenolate sodium have been established in stable renal transplant pediatric patients 5–16 years of age. Use of mycophenolate sodium in this age group is supported by evidence from adequate and well controlled studies in stable adult renal transplant patients (who received mycophenolate sodium therapy) and limited pharmacokinetic data in stable renal transplant pediatric patients 5–16 years of age. Safety and efficacy of mycophenolate sodium in pediatric *de novo* renal transplant patients have not been established .

■ **Cardiac Allotransplantation** Mycophenolate mofetil is used in adults for the prevention of rejection of cardiac allografts. This indication for mycophenolate mofetil is based on the results of one double-blind, randomized, multicenter active-controlled trial that enrolled 650 adults (578 of whom received at least one dose of either study drug) undergoing their first cardiac transplantation. Patients were randomized to receive oral mycophenolate mofetil (1.5 g twice daily) or oral azathioprine (1.5–3 mg/kg daily) in immunosuppressive regimens that included cyclosporine and corticosteroids. In this study, there were 2 primary efficacy end points; the first one was defined as the proportion of patients who had at least one endomyocardial biopsy-proven rejection with hemodynamic compromise after transplantation, underwent retransplantation, or died within the first 6 months, while the second primary efficacy end point was defined as the proportion of patients who died or underwent retransplantation during the first 12 months after the original transplantation. At 6 months, the incidence of biopsy-proven rejection accompanied by hemodynamic compromise in patients receiving mycophenolate mofetil (35%) was similar to that seen in patients receiving azathioprine (32%). At 12 months, mycophenolate mofetil was at least as effective as azathioprine in preventing death or retransplantation (6.2 vs 11.4%, respectively).

Use of an immunosuppressive regimen consisting of mycophenolate mofetil in conjunction with sirolimus and a corticosteroid following 12 weeks of therapy with a regimen consisting of mycophenolate mofetil, cyclosporine or tacrolimus, and a corticosteroid was investigated in the Heart Spare the Nephron (HSN) clinical trial in patients undergoing cardiac transplantation. The trial was designed to investigate whether switching from cyclosporine or tacrolimus to sirolimus at 12 weeks after transplantation would be associated with beneficial effects on renal function. The study was terminated early due to a higher than expected incidence of acute rejection in patients switched to sirolimus.

■ **Hepatic Allotransplantation** Mycophenolate mofetil is used in adults for the prevention of rejection of liver allografts. This indication for mycophenolate mofetil is based on the results of one double-blind, randomized, active-controlled, multicenter trial that enrolled 565 adults undergoing primary hepatic allotransplantation. Patients were randomized to receive mycophenolate mofetil (1 g IV twice daily for up to 14 days, followed by 1.5 g given orally twice daily) or azathioprine (1–2 mg/kg IV daily followed by the same dosage orally) in immunosuppressive regimens that included cyclosporine and corticosteroids. In this study, there were 2 primary efficacy end points; the first was defined as the proportion of patients who had one or more biopsy-proven and treated rejection, who underwent retransplantation, or who died, while the second primary efficacy point was defined as the proportion of patients who experienced graft loss (by death or undergoing retransplantation) during the first 12 months after the primary transplantation. At 6 months, the incidence of one or more episodes of biopsy-proven and treated rejection, retransplantation, or death was 38.5 or 47.7% in those receiving mycophenolate mofetil or azathioprine, respectively. At 12 months, mycophenolate mofetil and azathioprine were similarly effective in preventing retransplantation or death.

■ **Crohn's Disease** Mycophenolate mofetil has been used in the management of Crohn's disease†. The comparative efficacy of mycophenolate mofetil versus azathioprine has been investigated in several studies. In a randomized, comparative, prospective trial that included 70 patients with moderately to severely active Crohn's disease, efficacy of mycophenolate mofetil was evaluated in the management of corticosteroid-dependent chronically active Crohn's disease. In this study, the Crohn's Disease Activity Index (CDAI) was used for clinical assessment. The CDAI score is based on subjective observations by the patient (e.g., the daily number of liquid or very soft stools, severity of abdominal pain, general well-being) and objective evidence (e.g., number of extraintestinal manifestations, presence of an abdominal mass, use or nonuse of antidiarrheal drugs, the hematocrit, body weight). Patients with a CDAI score of 150 to greater than 300 were randomized to receive prednisolone (50 mg daily initially and tapered to a maintenance dosage of 5 mg daily) concomitantly with mycophenolate mofetil (15 mg/kg daily; approximately 1.5 g daily) or azathioprine (2.5 mg/kg daily). One month after randomization, efficacy of mycophenolate mofetil was similar to that of azathioprine (median reduction of 120 points for mycophenolate mofetil versus 97 points for azathioprine) in patients with moderately active disease (CDAI of 150–300), while in patients with severely active disease (CDAI exceeding 300), use of mycophenolate mofetil was associated with substantially greater reduction in CDAI scores than azathioprine (median reduction of 265 points for mycophenolate mofetil versus 117 points for azathioprine). During 2–6 months of therapy, CDAI scores remained stable and at comparable levels in mycophenolate-treated patients with moderately and severely active disease. However, after 6 months of therapy, there was a clear trend for a continuous decrease in CDAI scores in patients with severely active disease who were receiving azathioprine.

Efficacy of mycophenolate mofetil also has been evaluated in several small uncontrolled trials in patients with refractory Crohn's disease. While results of some clinical studies have indicated that mycophenolate mofetil may be beneficial in some patients with chronically active disease (including those with fistulizing disease) who did not respond or were intolerant of other immunosuppressants, results of other clinical trials in patients with chronically active disease refractory to corticosteroids, mercaptopurine, or azathioprine have not demonstrated such benefit. Although mycophenolate has been well tolerated in many of these studies, it should be considered that the drug has been associated rarely with an increased incidence of adverse GI effects (e.g., ulceration, hemorrhage, perforation) and mycophenolate should be used with caution in patients with active serious GI disease. In general, mycophenolate mofetil should be reserved for patients with Crohn's disease who are refractory to or intolerant of azathioprine, mercaptopurine, methotrexate, or infliximab. Additional well-controlled studies are needed to define the role, if any, of mycophenolate mofetil in the management of refractory Crohn's disease.

For further information on the management of Crohn's disease, see Uses: Crohn's Disease, in Mesalamine 56:36.

■ **Systemic Sclerosis** Mycophenolate mofetil and mycophenolate sodium have been used in the management of systemic sclerosis (often called scleroderma)†. Systemic sclerosis is a rare and heterogeneous autoimmune connective tissue disease and fibrosing disorder; the disease most commonly affects women and often develops during middle age. Systemic sclerosis is characterized by immune dysregulation, microvascular disease, and excess collagen deposition. The disease can impair organ function, reduce physical function, decrease quality of life, and result in premature mortality. Although sclerosis of the skin (i.e., fibrosis and thickening) is a hallmark of the diffuse cutaneous form of the disease and skin involvement is usually extensive, progressive, and debilitating, cardiopulmonary involvement, particularly interstitial lung disease (ILD) and pulmonary arterial hypertension (PAH), accounts for most of the increased mortality in patients with this condition. The etiology of systemic sclerosis is not fully understood at this time.

Treatment of systemic sclerosis should be individualized and usually is based on the disease comorbidities (i.e., clinical manifestations, organ involvement). Prevention of progression of the disease is an important goal of treatment, and early diagnosis and intervention appear to be essential in achieving this goal. Because of the clinical complexity in diagnosing and treating systemic sclerosis, some experts state that referral to a specialized treatment center with expertise in treating systemic sclerosis should be strongly considered. A variety of immunosuppressants have been used in the clinical management of skin and lung involvement associated with systemic sclerosis to date, including azathioprine, cyclophosphamide, methotrexate, mycophenolate mofetil or mycophenolate sodium, rituximab, and corticosteroids. However, because of the heterogeneity and variable course of this rare disease, it is difficult to fully assess the relative clinical efficacy of various therapeutic interventions, including immunosuppressant therapy.

Based on encouraging results in a number of uncontrolled clinical studies and case series as well as a randomized, controlled clinical trial, which are summarized below, many experts currently recommend mycophenolate (i.e., mycophenolate mofetil and mycophenolate sodium) as one of several immunosuppressants that can be used as first-line therapy in the initial management (i.e., induction therapy) of patients with systemic sclerosis, particularly for those with early and active systemic sclerosis and with active skin involvement or ILD. Longer-term mycophenolate therapy also is used and recommended by some experts to maintain improvement and prevent progression of skin involvement and/or ILD in patients with systemic sclerosis. Although mycophenolate mofetil and mycophenolate sodium are considered therapeutically equivalent, some clinicians consider mycophenolate sodium to be better tolerated than mycophenolate mofetil, particularly in terms of adverse GI effects. Some clinicians feel more comfortable and have greater experience prescribing mycophenolate mofetil in patients with systemic sclerosis but would consider switching to mycophenolate sodium in patients who are unable to tolerate mycophenolate mofetil at the recommended target dosage while other clinicians prefer to initiate and maintain therapy with mycophenolate sodium because of its potential for improved tolerability.

In a randomized, double-blind, multicenter clinical trial (the Scleroderma Lung Study II [SLS-II]), efficacy and tolerability of oral cyclophosphamide and mycophenolate mofetil therapy were compared in 126 adults with scleroderma-associated ILD. Mycophenolate mofetil therapy was initiated at a dosage of 500 mg given twice daily and the dosage was increased over time up to a maximum target dosage of 1.5 g twice daily; therapy was continued for 2 years. In the other treatment arm, cyclophosphamide therapy was initiated at a dosage of 50–150 mg once daily (based on weight) and was titrated up to a target dosage of 2 mg/kg (range: 1.8–2.3 mg/kg) once daily for 12 months followed by matching placebo for the next 12 months. The principal study end point was the change in forced vital capacity (FVC) from baseline as a percentage of the predicted normal value (FVC %) over the 24-month course of the study. Although no significant difference was noted between the treatment groups for the primary end point in post-hoc analyses, both 24-month mycophenolate mofetil treatment and 12-month cyclophosphamide treatment produced substantial improvement in lung function (as assessed by the adjusted FVC %) over 24 months. Both mycophenolate and cyclophosphamide therapy also resulted in significant improvements in skin scores and dyspnea over the 2-year course of the study. Responses to therapy occurred mainly between 9 and 24 months, suggesting slow onset of the potential disease-modifying effects of these drugs in patients with scleroderma-associated lung disease. Overall, mycophenolate mofetil therapy appeared to be better tolerated and resulted in fewer withdrawals from therapy than oral cyclophosphamide.

Mycophenolate therapy (given as either mycophenolate mofetil or mycophenolate sodium) also has been evaluated in the treatment of systemic sclerosis in a number of prospective and retrospective observational studies and case series to date. The results from these studies suggest that mycophenolate therapy may help improve skin involvement and stabilize or improve pulmonary function and fibrosis in patients with the disease. Mycophenolate therapy generally has been well tolerated in these clinical studies and case series and appears to be better tolerated than some other immunosuppressants that have been used to treat systemic sclerosis (e.g., cyclophosphamide, azathioprine).

In an observational study evaluating the long-term efficacy and tolerability of mycophenolate mofetil in the management of skin disease in a cohort of 42 adults with diffuse scleroderma from the Australian Scleroderma Cohort Study, mycophenolate therapy (mean dosage of 1.9 g daily) for a minimum of 12 months was associated with modest improvements in modified Rodnan skin score (mRSS). After 1 year of therapy, 43% of the patients demonstrated clinically important improvement (defined as a reduction in mRSS of 5 or more from baseline); 92% of the patients demonstrated such improvement after 4 years of mycophenolate therapy. In a retrospective study, data from 12 patients with scleroderma-associated ILD who did not adequately respond to IV cyclophosphamide and who were treated with mycophenolate mofetil therapy for 2 years were reviewed. Overall, pulmonary function tests improved in approximately 42% of these patients following mycophenolate mofetil therapy; 25% of the patients demonstrated improved FVC values and about 17% of the patients demonstrated improved diffusing capacity of the lung for carbon monoxide (DLCO) values.

In a retrospective study in 98 patients with diffuse cutaneous systemic sclerosis who received long-term mycophenolate mofetil therapy (i.e., 12 months), improvement in skin disease (as assessed by the mRSS) was observed as early as 3 months after initiating therapy and continued throughout the 12-month follow-up period. Improved general and muscle severity scores as well as improved subjective quality-of-life measures and stable pulmonary disease were also observed in the mycophenolate-treated patients. In a prospective, open-label study in 15 adults with early diffuse systemic sclerosis who received mycophenolate mofetil therapy (500 mg twice daily for week 1, then 1 g twice daily for week 2, and, if tolerated, 1.5 g twice daily by week 4 and thereafter) for over 12 months, significantly improved mRSS and Medsger severity scores in the general, peripheral vascular, and skin organ system categories were reported. In addition, pulmonary function did not worsen in the mycophenolate-treated patients and showed a trend toward improvement.

In a retrospective study, 109 patients with systemic sclerosis who were treated with mycophenolate mofetil therapy for 5 years were compared to a cohort of 63 patients receiving other immunosuppressants. A substantially lower frequency of clinically important pulmonary fibrosis and substantially higher 5-year survival from disease onset and from initiation of therapy were observed in the mycophenolate-treated cohort compared with the cohort receiving other immunosuppressants. There was no significant difference in the change in mRSS or FVC between the 2 treatment cohorts. In another retrospective study in 13 patients with recent-onset scleroderma-associated ILD who had received mycophenolate mofetil in dosages higher than 1 g daily for at least 6 months, a small but statistically significant improvement in vital capacity (VC) was observed (a mean increase of 4% of the predicted normal value after 12 months of treatment). These patients had demonstrated a substantial decline in VC (mean decrease of 5% of the predicted normal value) in the 12 months prior to initiation of mycophenolate mofetil therapy. DLCO did not change significantly during mycophenolate therapy (mean increase of 1% of the predicted normal value after 12 months of treatment) but had decreased significantly in the 12 months prior to mycophenolate treatment (a mean decrease of 5% of the predicted normal value).

In a prospective, observational study of mycophenolate mofetil in 25 previously untreated patients with diffuse progressive cutaneous systemic sclerosis of recent onset (i.e., within 24 months), patients treated with a median mycophenolate mofetil dosage of 2 g daily for an average of about 8 months demonstrated substantial improvement in skin involvement (as measured by the mRSS and affected body surface area) and stabilization of pulmonary function. In addition, skin biopsies from 3 of the patients revealed histopathological improvement and decreased expression of fibrosis-related genes.

Further controlled clinical studies are needed to more clearly determine the optimal role of mycophenolate therapy and other immunosuppressants in the clinical management of patients with systemic sclerosis-associated skin and lung disease.

Dosage and Administration

■ **Reconstitution and Administration** Mycophenolate mofetil and mycophenolate sodium are administered orally; mycophenolate mofetil hydrochloride is administered by IV infusion. When mycophenolate is used for the prevention of rejection of organ allographs, the drug is used concomitantly with an immunosuppressive regimen that includes cyclosporine and corticosteroids; other immunosuppressive agents, including antithymocyte globulin, antilymphocyte globulin, muromonab-CD3, basiliximab, or daclizumab (no longer commercially available in the US), also have been used.

The US Food and Drug Administration (FDA) currently requires that the manufacturer's patient information (medication guide) for mycophenolate mofetil or mycophenolate sodium be distributed to every patient each time the drug is dispensed. Because of the teratogenic potential of the drug, mycophenolate oral and parenteral preparations should be handled and prepared with care. Mycophenolate mofetil tablets should not be crushed and capsules should not be opened or crushed. Mycophenolate sodium delayed-release tablets should not be crushed, chewed, or cut. Inhalation of mycophenolate mofetil powder contained in the oral capsules or in the oral suspension (before and after reconstitution) and contact with the skin or mucous membranes should be avoided. In addition, contact with mycophenolate mofetil hydrochloride IV solution should be avoided. In case of accidental skin or mucous membrane contact, the affected area should be washed thoroughly with soap and water. If contact with the eyes occurs, they should be washed with water. The manufacturer recommends wiping up any spilled drug with a wet paper towel.

IV mycophenolate mofetil hydrochloride, which should be initiated within 24 hours following transplantation, generally is reserved for patients who cannot tolerate or are unable to take an oral dosage form. The drug can be administered IV for up to 14 days. Oral therapy should replace parenteral therapy as soon as possible.

Mycophenolate mofetil hydrochloride powder for injection is reconstituted by adding 14 mL of 5% dextrose injection to a vial labeled as containing 500 mg of mycophenolate mofetil; the vial should be gently shaken. The reconstituted solution is slightly yellow. For a 1-g infusion dose, the contents of 2 such reconstituted vials are added to 140 mL of 5% dextrose injection while for a 1.5-g infusion dose, the contents of 3 such reconstituted vials are added to 210 mL of 5% dextrose injection; the concentration of mycophenolate mofetil in the resulting solutions is 6 mg/mL. IV administration of mycophenolate mofetil hydrochloride should be started within 4 hours of reconstitution and dilution of the drug; solutions should be stored at 25°C with excursions of 15–30°C permitted. Strict aseptic technique must be observed since the drug contains no preservative. Mycophenolate mofetil hydrochloride should not be admixed with other drugs nor should other drugs be infused simultaneously through the same IV line. Prior to administration, reconstituted and diluted solutions of mycophenolate mofetil hydrochloride should be inspected visually for particulate matter and discoloration; if particulate matter or discoloration is evident, the solution should be discarded.

Mycophenolate mofetil hydrochloride should be infused IV over at least 2 hours by either a peripheral or central vein; the drug should *not* be administered by rapid IV ("bolus") injection or rapid IV infusion.

Oral mycophenolate mofetil should be administered as soon as possible following renal, cardiac, or hepatic transplantation.

Administration of mycophenolate mofetil with food does not affect the area under the plasma concentration-time curve (AUC) of mycophenolic acid; however, decreases (by about 40%) of peak plasma concentrations of mycophenolic acid have been observed. Therefore, the manufacturer recommends that mycophenolate mofetil tablets, capsules, and oral suspension be administered on an empty stomach (e.g., 1 hour before or 2 hours after a meal); however, in stable renal transplant recipients, the drug may be given with food, if necessary. If a dose is missed, the dose should be taken as soon as it is remembered unless it is time for the next dose; a double dose should not be taken to make up for a missed dose.

Mycophenolate sodium may be administered as soon as possible following renal transplantation in adults.

Mycophenolate sodium delayed-release tablets are administered on an empty stomach, 1 hour before or 2 hours after food. If a dose is missed, the dose should be taken as soon as it is remembered unless it is time for the next dose; a double dose should not be taken to make up for a missed dose. Administration of mycophenolate sodium with food does not affect the AUC of mycophenolic acid; however, decreases in peak plasma concentration (by about 33%) and delay in time to peak plasma concentrations (from 1.5–2.75 hours to 5 hours) have been observed. To reduce variability in mycophenolic acid absorption between doses, mycophenolate sodium should be taken on an empty stomach.

It is recommended that mycophenolate mofetil powder for oral suspension be reconstituted at the time of dispensing by adding 94 mL of water (about 47 mL initially followed by another 47 mL after vigorous shaking for 1 minute) to provide a suspension containing 200 mg/mL. The bottle should be shaken well again for 1 minute to suspend the powder. Mycophenolate mofetil oral suspension also can be administered by a nasogastric tube (minimum 1.7 mm in interior diameter; minimum French size number 8).

■ General Dosage

Dosage of mycophenolate mofetil and mycophenolate mofetil hydrochloride are both expressed in terms of mycophenolate mofetil. Dosage of mycophenolate sodium is expressed in terms of mycophenolic acid.

Commercially available mycophenolate mofetil tablets, capsules, and oral suspension reportedly are bioequivalent. Mycophenolate sodium delayed-release tablets should not be used interchangeably with mycophenolate mofetil tablets, capsules, or oral suspension without supervision of a clinician, because absorption of the drug from these preparations is not equivalent. In a study in stable renal transplant recipients, administration of single oral doses of mycophenolate sodium delayed-release tablets (mycophenolic acid 720 mg) or mycophenolate mofetil 1-g oral preparations resulted in bioequivalent mycophenolic acid exposure.

Adults

Renal Allotransplantation. For the prevention of renal allograft rejection in adults, the usual dosage of mycophenolate mofetil is 1 g administered IV or orally twice daily. Although 2- and 3-g daily dosages of mycophenolate mofetil have been used in clinical trials, no efficacy advantage could be shown for the higher dosage in the overall renal transplant patient population. In addition, 2-g daily dosages of mycophenolate mofetil were associated with a superior safety profile when compared with the 3-g daily dosage.

When mycophenolate sodium delayed-release tablets are used for the prevention of renal allograft rejection in adults, the usual dosage is 720 mg of mycophenolic acid twice daily.

Cardiac Allotransplantation. For the prevention of cardiac allograft rejection in adults, the usual dosage of mycophenolate mofetil is 1.5 g administered IV or orally twice daily (3 g total daily dosage).

Hepatic Allotransplantation. For the prevention of hepatic allograft rejection in adults, the usual dosage of mycophenolate mofetil hydrochloride is 1 g administered IV twice daily or 1.5 g administered orally twice daily.

Crohn's Disease. For the management of Crohn's disease† in adults who do not respond to or were intolerant of other immunosuppressants (e.g., azathioprine, mercaptopurine), mycophenolate mofetil dosages of 1–2 g daily have been used.

Systemic Sclerosis. For the treatment of systemic sclerosis† in adults, an initial mycophenolate mofetil dosage of 500 mg given orally twice daily (1 g total daily dosage) for the first 1–4 weeks has been used. The dosage has then been gradually increased up to a target maintenance dosage of 1–1.5 g given orally twice daily (total daily dosage of 2–3 g) based on clinical response and tolerability. Although many patients can tolerate a total daily dosage of 3 g, some patients may require somewhat lower maintenance dosages because of adverse effects, particularly adverse GI effects (see Cautions).

When mycophenolate sodium delayed-release tablets have been used for the treatment of systemic sclerosis† in adults, initial dosages of 360 mg of mycophenolic acid once or twice daily have been used. The dosage has then been increased to 720 or 1080 mg of mycophenolic acid twice daily if tolerated.

Although the optimal duration of mycophenolate therapy in the treatment of systemic sclerosis is not fully known, the drug has been used for up to 5 years in some patients with the disease. Some clinical experience to date suggests that long-term immunosuppressant therapy may be necessary to stabilize and prevent progression of the disease.

Pediatric Patients

Renal Allotransplantation. For the prevention of renal allograft rejection in pediatric patients 3 months to 18 years of age, the usual dosage of mycophenolate mofetil (as the oral suspension) is 600 mg/m^2 administered orally twice daily, up to a maximum dosage of 1 g twice daily. Children with a body surface area of 1.25–1.5 m^2 can receive 750 mg (as capsules) twice daily for a total daily mycophenolate mofetil dosage of 1.5 g, while children with a body surface area greater than 1.5 m^2 can receive a dosage of 1 g (as capsules or tablets) twice daily for a total daily mycophenolate mofetil dosage of 2 g.

Mycophenolate sodium should be administered as maintenance therapy *only* in stable pediatric renal transplant recipients; safety and efficacy of the drug in *de novo* pediatric renal transplant recipients have not been established.

For the prevention of renal allograft rejection in pediatric patients 5–16 years of age, the usual dosage of mycophenolic acid (administered as mycophenolate sodium delayed-release tablets) is 400 mg/m^2 twice daily (up to a maximum of 720 mg twice daily). Pediatric patients with a body surface area of 1.19–1.58m^2 may receive a daily dosage of 1080 mg (administered as three 180-mg tablets or one 180-mg tablet and one 360-mg tablet twice daily). Pediatric patients with a body surface area greater than 1.58m^2 may receive a daily dosage of 1440 mg (administered as four 180-mg tablets or two 360-mg tablets twice daily). A mycophenolate sodium dosage form suitable for providing an appropriate dosage for pediatric patients with a body surface area less than 1.19 m^2 is not commercially available in the US.

■ Special Populations

Dosage adjustment of mycophenolate mofetil preparations or mycophenolic acid (administered as mycophenolate sodium delayed-release tablets) is not necessary in renal transplant recipients experiencing postoperative delayed graft function. No dosage adjustment is necessary in renal transplant recipients with severe hepatic parenchymal disease; however, it is not known whether dosage adjustment is needed in hepatic impairment of other etiologies.

Mycophenolate mofetil dosages exceeding 1 g twice daily should be avoided in renal transplant recipients with severe chronic renal impairment (GFR less than 25 mL/minute per 1.73 m^2) beyond the immediate posttransplant period.

If neutropenia (absolute neutrophil count [ANC] of less than 1300/mm^3) develops, mycophenolate therapy should be temporarily discontinued or the dosage reduced, suitable diagnostic tests be performed, and appropriate patient management be instituted.

Mycophenolate mofetil dosage adjustment based solely on age is not necessary in geriatric patients 65 years of age or older.

When mycophenolate sodium is used in geriatric adults, the maximum recommended dosage is mycophenolic acid 720 mg twice daily.

Cautions

■ Contraindications

Known hypersensitivity to mycophenolate mofetil, mycophenolate sodium, mycophenolic acid, or any ingredient in the formulation. Mycophenolate mofetil hydrochloride for IV injection contains polysorbate (Tween®) 80 and should not be used in patients with known severe hypersensitivity to the surfactant.

■ Warnings/Precautions

Warnings

Mycophenolate shares the toxic potentials of currently available immunosuppressive agents. Immunosuppression with the drug may result in increased susceptibility to infection (e.g., infectious complications) and the possible development of lymphoma. Such risk appears to be related to the intensity and duration of immunosuppression rather than to the use of any specific immunosuppressive agent. Mycophenolate mofetil and mycophenolate sodium should be used by clinicians experienced in immunosuppressive therapy and the management of patients receiving these drugs. Patients receiving the drug should be managed in facilities equipped with adequate laboratory and supportive medical resources, and the clinician responsible for maintenance therapy should have complete information requisite for follow-up of the patients. Patients should be advised to read the medication guide for mycophenolate mofetil or mycophenolate sodium that is provided each time the drug is dispensed.

Carcinogenicity. Potential for the development of lymphoma and other malignancies, particularly of the skin, which may result from immunosuppression. Because of the increased risk for skin cancer, patients should be advised to limit their exposure to sunlight or other UV light by wearing protective clothing and using sunscreen with a high protection factor.

Lymphoproliferative disease or lymphoma occurred in 0.4–1.3% of allograft recipients receiving mycophenolate in conjunction with other immunosuppressive agents in clinical studies. Non-melanoma skin carcinoma was reported in 0.9–4.2% of patients while other types of malignancy were reported in 0.5–2.1% of patients.

Fetal/Neonatal Morbidity and Mortality. Mycophenolate may cause fetal toxicity when administered to pregnant women. Use of mycophenolate mofetil has been associated with increased risk of first-trimester pregnancy loss and serious congenital malformations. Information on pregnancy outcome in transplant recipients has been compiled by the National Transplantation Pregnancy Registry (NTPR). Information on 33 pregnancies in transplant recipients who received mycophenolate mofetil during pregnancy has been reported to the registry; there were 15 spontaneous abortions (45%) and 18 live-born infants; 4 of these infants had structural abnormalities (22%). NTPR data indicate that congenital abnormalities have occurred in 4–5% of neonates born to transplant recipients receiving other immunosuppressive agents. Postmarketing data are available on 77 women exposed to mycophenolate mofetil during pregnancy; 25 had a spontaneous abortion and 14 had a malformed infant or fetus. Fetal anomalies reported include ear abnormalities (43%, from postmarketing data), other orofacial deformities (e.g., cleft lip, cleft palate), and malformations of the limbs, heart, esophagus, and kidneys.

Teratogenic and embryocidal effects have been observed in animals receiving mycophenolate at doses 0.02–0.9 times the recommended human dose. Fetal anomalies have included anophthalmia, agnathia, and hydrocephaly in rats, and ectopia cordis, ectopic kidneys, diaphragmatic hernia, and umbilical hernia in rabbits.

Mycophenolate should be used during pregnancy only when the potential benefits justify the possible risks to the fetus. Women of childbearing potential should be informed of the potential risks of fetal toxicity prior to the initiation of therapy. A reliable blood or urine pregnancy test (i.e., having a sensitivity of at least 25 mIU/mL for human chorionic gonadotropin [HCG]) should be performed within 1 week prior to beginning mycophenolate therapy, and therapy with the drug should not be initiated until a report of the pregnancy test is available indicating that results are negative. Women of childbearing potential should use 2 reliable forms of contraception for at least 4 weeks prior to, throughout, and for at least 6 weeks after discontinuance of mycophenolate, unless the patient commits to continuous abstinence from heterosexual contact. Concomitant use of mycophenolate and certain oral hormonal contraceptives may result in decreased concentrations of the oral hormonal contraceptive. (See Drug Interactions: Oral Contraceptives.)

If mycophenolate is administered during pregnancy or if a patient becomes pregnant while receiving the drug, the patient should be informed of the potential hazard to the fetus. In certain situations, maternal benefits may outweigh the risks to the fetus. Women exposed to mycophenolate during pregnancy should be encouraged to enroll in the NTPR.

Infectious Complications. Use of immunosuppressive agents, including mycophenolate, may result in increased susceptibility to infection (i.e., opportunistic infections, sepsis, life-threatening/fatal infections). In clinical studies, serious infections (e.g., sepsis, fatal infections) occurred in 2% of renal and cardiac allograft recipients and in 5% of hepatic allograft recipients receiving mycophenolate mofetil. In one clinical study, the overall incidence of opportunistic infections in cardiac allograft recipients receiving mycophenolate mofetil was about 10% higher than in those receiving azathioprine; however, such difference was not associated with excess mortality associated with the infection or sepsis in patients receiving mycophenolate mofetil. Viral infections (e.g., cytomegalovirus [CMV] infections, herpes simplex, herpes zoster) have been reported more frequently in cardiac transplant recipients receiving mycophenolate mofetil than in those receiving azathioprine. Meningitis, infectious endocarditis, tuberculosis, and atypical mycobacterial infections have been reported during postmarketing surveillance of the drug.

Latent Viral Infections. Immunosuppressed patients are at an increased risk for opportunistic infections, including reactivation of latent viral infections. These include BK virus-associated nephropathy (BKVN), which has been reported in patients receiving immunosuppressants, including mycophenolate mofetil, cyclosporine, sirolimus, and tacrolimus. Primary infection with polyoma BK virus typically occurs in childhood; following initial infection, the virus remains latent, but reactivation may occur in immunocompromised patients. BKVN has principally been observed in renal transplant patients (usually within the first year posttransplantation), and may result in serious outcomes, including deterioration of kidney function and renal allograft loss. Risk of BK virus reactivation appears to be related to the degree of overall immunosuppression rather than use of any specific immunosuppressive agent; patients receiving a maintenance immunosuppressive regimen of at least 3 drugs appear to be at highest risk. Patients should be monitored for possible signs of BKVN, including deterioration in renal function, during therapy with mycophenolate mofetil or mycophenolate sodium; screening assays for polyomavirus replication also have been recommended by some clinicians. Early intervention in patients who develop BKVN is critical; a reduction in immunosuppressive therapy should initially be considered in such patients. Although a variety of other treatment approaches have been used anecdotally in patients with BKVN, including antiviral therapy (e.g., cidofovir), leflunomide, IV immunoglobulins, and fluoroquinolone antibiotics, additional experience and well-controlled studies are necessary to more clearly establish the optimal treatment of such patients.

Progressive multifocal leukoencephalopathy (PML), an opportunistic viral infection of the brain, has been reported during postmarketing experience with mycophenolate mofetil (CellCept®). PML is caused by the JC virus and typically occurs in immunocompromised patients. At least 17 cases (10 confirmed, 7 possible) of PML have been reported in patients receiving mycophenolate mofetil; death occurred in at least 7 patients. Most reported cases of PML have occurred in patients who were receiving mycophenolate mofetil for the prevention of rejection of a solid organ transplant or for the management of systemic lupus erythematosus (SLE)†. These patients also were receiving other immunosuppressants (i.e., corticosteroids, cyclosporine, tacrolimus, and azathioprine in transplant recipients; corticosteroids, cyclophosphamide, and cyclosporine in SLE patients) or had compromised immune function. Hemiparesis, apathy, confusion, cognitive impairment, and ataxia were the most common manifestations of PML observed in these patients.

To date, no cases of PML have been reported in patients receiving mycophenolate sodium (Myfortic®). Because mycophenolate sodium is converted to the same active metabolite (mycophenolic acid) as mycophenolate mofetil, use of mycophenolate sodium is expected to be associated with the same risk of PML as use of mycophenolate mofetil.

The possible diagnosis of PML should be considered in immunocompromised patients receiving mycophenolate who experience neurologic manifestations. Consultation with a neurologist is advised as clinically indicated. Decreasing total immunosuppression may improve the outcome of PML, but also may increase the risk of graft rejection in transplant recipients. Clinicians should consider the potential risks versus benefits of reduced immunosuppression.

Hematologic Effects. Severe neutropenia (i.e., absolute neutrophil counts [ANC] of less than 500/mm^3) has been reported in up to 2, 2.8, or 3.6% of renal, cardiac, or hepatic allograft recipients, respectively, receiving 3-g daily dosages of mycophenolate mofetil.

Neutropenia has been observed most frequently between 31–180 days posttransplant in patients receiving immunosuppressive therapy for the prevention of rejection of kidney, heart, or liver allograft. Neutropenia may be related to mycophenolate, concomitant therapies, viral infection, or a combination of these causes.

Complete blood cell counts (CBCs) should be performed weekly during the first month of therapy, twice monthly during the second and third month, and then monthly thereafter, during the first year. If neutropenia (ANC of less than 1300/mm^3) develops, mycophenolate therapy be temporarily discontinued or the dosage reduced, suitable diagnostic tests be performed, and appropriate patient management be instituted.

Pure red cell aplasia (PRCA), a condition in which red blood cell precursors in the bone marrow are absent or nearly absent, has been reported in patients receiving immunosuppressive regimens containing mycophenolate mofetil. At least 41 cases of PRCA have been reported in patients receiving mycophenolate mofetil. Some of these patients also were receiving other immunosuppressants, including alemtuzumab, azathioprine, and tacrolimus. Because these patients were receiving multiple immunosuppressive agents, the relative contribution of mycophenolate mofetil and other immunosuppressants to the development of PRCA is not known. Risk of PRCA also should be considered in patients receiving mycophenolate sodium, because this drug is converted to the same active metabolite (mycophenolic acid) as mycophenolate mofetil. PRCA can produce varying degrees of anemia from subclinical to severe; manifestations may include fatigue, lethargy, pallor, weakness, tachycardia, and/or dyspnea. Although the mechanism for mycophenolate-induced PRCA has not been determined, immunosuppression may play a role. In some cases, PRCA was found to be reversible with dosage reduction or discontinuance of mycophenolate mofetil. However, clinicians should consider the possibility of graft rejection if immunosuppression is reduced in transplant patients; any changes in immunosuppressive therapy should be implemented under appropriate medical supervision.

Major Toxicities **GI Effects.** Severe GI bleeding (requiring hospitalization) has occurred in 3, 1.7, or 5.4% of renal, cardiac, or hepatic transplant recipients, respectively, receiving 3-g daily dosages of mycophenolate mofetil in clinical studies. In studies evaluating safety of mycophenolate sodium, severe GI bleeding was reported in 1% of *de novo* renal transplant patients and 1.3% of those receiving maintenance therapy. Mycophenolate mofetil therapy is associated with a high incidence of adverse GI effects; mycophenolate sodium delayed-release tablets were developed to improve GI tolerance. However, adverse GI effects in patients receiving mycophenolate sodium in comparative clinical studies have been similar to those in patients receiving mycophenolate mofetil. Because mycophenolate mofetil and mycophenolate sodium have been associated with adverse GI effects and rarely with serious GI effects (ulceration, hemorrhage, or perforation), the drugs should be administered with caution in patients with active serious GI disease.

General Precautions **Hypoxanthine Phosphoribosyltransferase Deficiency.** Because mycophenolic acid inhibits inosine monophosphate dehydrogenase, mycophenolate mofetil and mycophenolate sodium should be avoided, on theoretical grounds, in patients with rare hereditary deficiency of hypoxanthine-guanine phosphoribosyltransferase (HGPRT), including Kelley-Seegmiller or Lesch-Nyhan syndrome.

Phenylketonuria. Individuals with phenylketonuria and those who must restrict their intake of phenylalanine should be warned that mycophenolate mofetil oral suspension contains aspartame (NutraSweet®), which is metabolized in the GI tract to provide about 0.56 mg of phenylalanine per 5 mL of the suspension.

Specific Populations **Pregnancy.** Category D. See Users Guide, and see Fetal/Neonatal Morbidity and Mortality under Warnings/Precautions: Warnings, in Cautions.

Lactation. Mycophenolic acid is distributed into milk in rats; not known whether this drug is distributed into milk in humans. Discontinue nursing or the drug, taking into account the importance of the drug to the woman. Women should not breast-feed for at least 6 weeks after discontinuance of mycophenolate sodium therapy.

Pediatric Use. Safety of mycophenolate mofetil for the prevention of rejection of renal allografts in children 3 months to 18 years of age is based on data from a pediatric pharmacokinetic and safety study. The manufacturer states that safety and efficacy of mycophenolate mofetil in pediatric patients younger than 3 months of age receiving renal allografts have not been established. In addition, safety and efficacy have not been established in pediatric patients younger than 18 years of age receiving allogenic cardiac or hepatic transplants.

Limited data are available concerning use of mycophenolate mofetil in pediatric patients. In one study in children 1–18 years of age receiving mycophenolate mofetil 600 mg/m^2 (oral suspension) twice daily following renal transplantation, pharmacokinetic parameters, including the area under the plasma concentration-time curve (AUC), were similar to those reported in adult renal transplant recipients receiving mycophenolate mofetil 1 g twice daily. Results of several pediatric studies and analysis of an open-label study in children 3 months to 18 years of age undergoing renal transplantation suggest that the safety profile in children generally is similar to that in adults, although a difference in the incidence of certain adverse effects (e.g. abdominal pain, fever, infection, pain, sepsis, diarrhea, vomiting, pharyngitis, respiratory tract infection, hypertension, and anemia) has been higher in pediatric patients than in adults. In clinical studies in pediatric patients, lymphoproliferative malignancies have been reported rarely (about 1.4%), while other types of malignancies were not observed in children in these studies. Severe GI bleeding (requiring hospitalization) has been reported in 3.4% of pediatric patients undergoing renal transplantation.

Safety and efficacy of mycophenolate sodium in stable renal transplant pediatric patients 5–16 years of age is based on evidence from adequate and well controlled studies in stable adult renal transplant patients receiving mycophenolate sodium and limited pharmacokinetic data in stable renal transplant pediatric patients 5–16 years of age. Safety and efficacy of mycophenolate sodium have not been established in pediatric *de novo* renal transplant patients.

Limited data are available concerning use of mycophenolate sodium in pediatric patients. Following administration of a single dose of mycophenolate sodium (mycophenolic acid 450 mg/m^2) in stable pediatric renal transplant patients 5–16 years of age, peak plasma concentrations and AUC of mycophenolic acid were 33 and 18% higher, respectively, than those reported in adults receiving the same dose based on body surface area (720 mg). The clinical importance of these findings remains to be determined. Pharmacokinetic data are not available in pediatric patients younger than 5 years of age.

Geriatric Use. Clinical studies of mycophenolate did not include sufficient numbers of patients 65 years of age or older to determine whether they respond differently than younger adults. While other clinical experience has not revealed differences in response, drug dosages should be selected cautiously in geriatric patients. The greater frequency of decreased hepatic, renal, and/or cardiac function and of concomitant diseases and drug therapy observed in the elderly also should be considered. Geriatric patients may be at increased risk of developing GI hemorrhage, pulmonary edema, or certain infections (e.g., invasive CMV infection) than younger patients.

Hepatic Impairment. No dosage adjustment for mycophenolate preparations is necessary for renal transplant recipients with severe hepatic parenchymal disease; not known whether dosage adjustment is needed for other hepatic diseases. No data are available for cardiac transplant recipients with severe hepatic parenchymal disease.

Renal Impairment. Administration of a single dose of mycophenolate mofetil in individuals with severe long-term renal impairment (glomerular filtration rate less than 25 mL/minute per 1.73 m^2) has resulted in higher AUC values for mycophenolic acid and the phenolic glucuronide of mycophenolic acid than values in individuals with less severe impairment or no impairment.

Patients receiving mycophenolate mofetil who experience posttransplant delay in graft function generally have AUC values for mycophenolic acid that are similar to those not experiencing graft function delay; however, the AUC for the phenolic glucuronide of mycophenolic acid is increased twofold to threefold in patients experiencing delayed graft function compared with those not experiencing delayed function. Dosage adjustment does not appear to be necessary in these patients; however, patients should be carefully observed.

No data are available on the use of mycophenolate mofetil in cardiac or hepatic transplant recipients with severe chronic renal impairment; mycophenolate mofetil may be used in these patients if the potential benefits outweigh the potential risks.

Studies evaluating the pharmacokinetics of mycophenolate sodium have not been conducted in patients with renal impairment. AUC values for mycophenolic acid in patients with renal impairment receiving mycophenolate sodium are not expected to increase appreciably relative to values in patients with normal renal function; however, AUC values for the phenolic glucuronide metabolite of mycophenolic acid are expected to increase substantially with decreased renal function. Plasma concentrations of mycophenolic acid and the phenolic glucuronide of mycophenolic acid may be increased in patients with severe renal impairment (glomerular filtration rate less than 25 mL/minute per 1.73 m^2) compared with plasma concentrations of healthy individuals and those with mild to moderate renal impairment. Patients with severe renal impairment should be carefully observed for possible adverse effects associated with increased plasma concentrations of free (unbound) mycophenolic acid and the phenolic glucuronide of mycophenolic acid. Safety of long-term exposure to increased concentrations of the phenolic glucuronide of mycophenolic acid remains to be determined.

■ **Common Adverse Effects** The most frequently reported adverse effects associated with mycophenolate mofetil therapy are diarrhea, leukopenia, sepsis, vomiting, higher frequency of infections, including opportunistic infections (e.g., CMV infections, herpes zoster, herpes simplex, candidal infections, aspergillosis, and *Pneumocystis carinii* pneumonia). Adverse reactions occurring in 20% or more of patients receiving mycophenolate mofetil include pain (e.g., abdominal, chest, back), fever, headache, anemia (e.g., hypochromic), thrombocytopenia, leukocytosis, urinary tract infection, abnormal renal function, hypertension, hypotension, cardiovascular disorder, tachycardia, edema (e.g., peripheral) hypercholesterolemia, hypokalemia, hyperkalemia, hyperglycemia, increases in blood urea nitrogen (BUN) and serum creatinine concentration, increased lactic dehydrogenase, hypomagnesemia, hypocalcemia, constipation, dyspepsia, nausea, vomiting, anorexia, abnormal liver function test results, cough, dyspnea, lung disorder, sinusitis, pleural effusion, rash, tremor, insomnia, dizziness, anxiety, and paresthesia.

The adverse effect profile in patients receiving IV mycophenolate mofetil hydrochloride is similar to that in patients receiving oral mycophenolate mofetil; phlebitis and thrombosis have been reported in 4% of patients receiving IV infusion of the drug.

In controlled studies in patients undergoing renal transplantation, the overall safety profile in those receiving mycophenolate mofetil 2 g daily was better than in those receiving 3 g daily. The types of adverse effects reported in renal, cardiac, or hepatic transplant studies generally are similar (except for those unique to the specific organ involved).

The most frequent adverse effects reported in patients receiving mycophenolate sodium include constipation, nausea, diarrhea, urinary tract infection, and nasopharyngitis. Adverse reactions occurring in 20% or more of patients receiving mycophenolate sodium include leukopenia, vomiting, dyspepsia, CMV infections, insomnia, and postoperative pain. In controlled studies in patients undergoing renal transplantation, the incidence of adverse effects reported in patients receiving mycophenolate sodium was similar to that reported in patients receiving mycophenolate mofetil.

Drug Interactions

■ **Immunosuppressants** In clinical trials in patients undergoing transplant procedures, mycophenolate mofetil has been administered concurrently with cyclosporine, antithymocyte globulin (equine), muromonab-CD3, and/or corticosteroids; the manufacturer states that safety and efficacy of mycophenolate mofetil in combination with immunosuppressive agents other than these agents have not been determined.

In clinical trials in patients undergoing renal transplantation, mycophenolate sodium has been administered concurrently with cyclosporine, antithymocyte globulin, antilymphocyte globulin, muromonab-CD3, basiliximab, daclizumab (no longer commercially available in the US), and/or corticosteroids; the manufacturer states that safety and efficacy of mycophenolate sodium in combination with immunosuppressive agents other than these agents have not been determined.

Potential pharmacodynamic interaction (bone marrow suppression) with azathioprine. Concomitant use not recommended.

Concomitant use of mycophenolate mofetil with mycophenolate sodium is not recommended. Potential pharmacodynamic interaction (bone marrow suppression).

Concomitant use of mycophenolate mofetil without cyclosporine results in increased systemic exposure to mycophenolic acid compared with use of mycophenolate mofetil with cyclosporine. The lower systemic exposure to mycophenolic acid when mycophenolate mofetil is used with cyclosporine has been attributed to cyclosporine-induced inhibition of multidrug-resistance-associated protein 2 transporter in the biliary tract; inhibition of this transporter prevents excretion of the phenolic glucuronide of mycophenolic acid into bile (the phenolic glucuronide of mycophenolic acid is converted to mycophenolic acid via enterohepatic recirculation). Use of mycophenolate mofetil or mycophenolate sodium with or without cyclosporine does not affect plasma cyclosporine concentrations.

■ **Anti-infective Agents** Pharmacokinetic interaction with co-trimoxazole unlikely.

Potential pharmacokinetic interaction with concomitant use of rifampin with mycophenolate mofetil (decreased systemic exposure to mycophenolic acid). Concomitant use of mycophenolate mofetil and rifampin not recommended unless benefit outweighs risk.

Concomitant use of mycophenolate mofetil and the anti-infective combination of norfloxacin and metronidazole not recommended due to potential pharmacokinetic interaction (decreased systemic exposure to mycophenolic acid); however, no substantial effect on systemic exposure to mycophenolic acid was observed when mycophenolate mofetil was administered with norfloxacin or metronidazole.

Concomitant administration of mycophenolate mofetil and oral ciprofloxacin or amoxicillin plus clavulanic acid decreased median trough concentrations of mycophenolic acid (active metabolite of mycophenolate mofetil) by approximately 50% in 3 days following initiation of antibiotic therapy in one study in renal transplant recipients. The potential mechanism for this drug interaction may be an antibiotic-induced reduction in glucuronidase-possessing enteric bacteria resulting in decreased enterohepatic recirculation of mycophenolic acid. Because changes in mycophenolic acid concentrations did not necessarily correlate with overall drug exposure, the clinical importance of these findings is not clear.

■ **Antiviral Agents** Potential pharmacokinetic interaction with concomitant use of acyclovir with mycophenolate mofetil (increased plasma concentrations of acyclovir and the phenolic glucuronide of mycophenolic acid). Potential pharmacokinetic interaction with ganciclovir and valganciclovir in patients with renal impairment (increased plasma concentrations of the metabolites of the drugs). If acyclovir or ganciclovir is used in patients receiving mycophenolate sodium, blood cell counts should be monitored during treatment with the antiviral agent.

■ **Antacids** Potential pharmacokinetic interaction (decreased plasma concentrations of mycophenolic acid) with antacids containing aluminum and magnesium hydroxides. Mycophenolate mofetil or mycophenolate sodium may be used in patients receiving these antacids; however, the immunosuppressant should not be administered simultaneously with the antacids.

■ **Salicylates** Potential pharmacokinetic interaction based on in vitro data (increased free fraction of mycophenolic acid).

■ **Cholestyramine** Potential pharmacokinetic interaction (decreased plasma concentrations of mycophenolic acid). Administration of mycophenolate mofetil or mycophenolate sodium with cholestyramine or other agents that interfere with enterohepatic recirculation of the drug is not recommended.

■ **Oral Contraceptives** Potential pharmacokinetic interaction with concomitant use of levonorgestrel with mycophenolate mofetil (decreased plasma concentrations of levonorgestrel). Pharmacokinetic interaction unlikely with concomitant use of mycophenolate mofetil with ethinyl estradiol, desogestrel, or gestodene. Pharmacokinetic interaction unlikely with mycophenolate sodium. Oral contraceptives should be administered with caution in patients receiving mycophenolate and additional methods of birth control methods should be used.

■ **Phosphate Binders** Potential pharmacokinetic interaction with concomitant administration of sevelamer and mycophenolate mofetil (decreased plasma concentrations of mycophenolic acid). The manufacturer recommends that sevelamer or other non-calcium-containing phosphate binders be given 2 hours after the administration of mycophenolate mofetil.

■ **Probenecid and other Inhibitors of Tubular Secretion** Potential pharmacokinetic interaction based on animal data (increased plasma concentrations of mycophenolic acid and the phenolic glucuronide of mycophenolic acid).

■ **Drugs that Alter Intestinal Flora** Drugs that alter intestinal flora may interfere with mycophenolate mofetil or mycophenolate sodium by disrupting enterohepatic recirculation; interference with the hydrolysis of the phenolic glucuronide metabolite of mycophenolic acid to mycophenolic acid may decrease the amount of mycophenolic acid available for absorption.

■ **Vaccines** Potential interaction with live virus vaccine (decreased response to vaccination). Avoid use of live virus vaccine in patients receiving mycophenolate mofetil or mycophenolate sodium. Vaccination with influenza virus vaccine inactivated may be of value.

Pharmacokinetics

■ **Absorption** Mycophenolate mofetil is rapidly absorbed following oral administration; bioavailability is 94%. Following oral and IV administration, mycophenolate mofetil undergoes rapid and complete metabolism to mycophenolic acid, the active metabolite. Mycophenolate mofetil tablets, capsules, and oral suspension are bioequivalent.

Following oral administration of the delayed-release tablets (mycophenolate sodium), mycophenolic acid is released in the small intestine; bioavailability is 72%.

Mycophenolate sodium delayed-release tablets cannot be used interchangeably with mycophenolate mofetil tablets, capsules, or oral suspension without clinician supervision. Single oral doses of mycophenolate sodium delayed-release tablets (mycophenolic acid 720 mg) and mycophenolate mofetil 1 g result in bioequivalent mycophenolic acid exposure.

Food decreases peak plasma concentrations of mycophenolic acid (by 33–40%); no effect on the mycophenolic acid AUC.

Plasma concentrations of free (unbound) mycophenolic acid and total mycophenolic acid glucuronide have increased in nontransplant individuals with severe chronic renal impairment (GFR <25 mL/minute per 1.73 m^2). Plasma mycophenolic acid concentrations in patients with delayed graft function similar to values in patients not experiencing delayed graft function.

Pharmacokinetic parameters, including AUC, in children 1–18 years of age receiving mycophenolate mofetil 600 mg/m^2 (oral suspension) twice daily following renal transplantation, are similar to values in adult renal transplant recipients receiving 1 g twice daily. Peak plasma concentrations and AUC of mycophenolic acid in stable pediatric renal transplant patients 5–16 years of age receiving a single dose of mycophenolate sodium (mycophenolic acid 450 mg/m^2) increased (33 and 18%, respectively) relative to adults receiving the same dose based on body surface area. Clinical importance not determined.

■ **Distribution** Mycophenolic acid is ≥97–98% bound to plasma protein (mainly albumin).

■ **Elimination** Mycophenolate mofetil undergoes complete metabolism to mycophenolic acid; metabolism occurs presystemically following oral administration. Mycophenolic acid is metabolized by glucuronyl transferase to the phenolic glucuronide of mycophenolic acid. The phenolic glucuronide is converted to mycophenolic acid via enterohepatic recirculation.

Mycophenolate mofetil is excreted in urine (93%) as the phenolic glucuronide of mycophenolic acid (87%) and in feces (6%). Mycophenolate sodium is excreted principally in urine as phenolic glucuronide of mycophenolic acid (>60%) and as unchanged mycophenolic acid (3%).

The half-life of mycophenolic acid is 8–17.9 hours.

Plasma concentrations of mycophenolic acid glucuronide are higher in nontransplant subjects with severe renal impairment than in those with mild impairment or normal renal function. Plasma concentrations of mycophenolic acid glucuronide are higher in transplant patients with delayed renal graft function than in patients not experiencing delayed graft function. Dialysis does not remove mycophenolic acid. Pharmacokinetic studies in patients with alcoholic cirrhosis indicate that hepatic mycophenolic acid glucuronidation is not affected by hepatic parenchymal disease; hepatic disease with other etiologies (e.g., biliary cirrhosis) may show a different effect.

Description

Mycophenolate mofetil, the 2-morpholinoethyl ester of mycophenolic acid, is an immunosuppressive agent. Mycophenolate mofetil is a prodrug that has little pharmacologic activity until it is rapidly and completely hydrolyzed in vivo to the pharmacologically active metabolite, mycophenolic acid. Mycophenolate mofetil differs structurally and pharmacologically from other immunosuppressive agents.

Mycophenolate sodium also is an immunosuppressive agent. Following oral administration of mycophenolate sodium delayed-release tablets, mycophenolic acid (the active moiety) is released in the small intestine.

Acute rejection episodes occur in up to 60% or more of patients who have undergone renal transplantation and result in a substantial reduction in long-term (5 years or longer) graft survival. Although the exact mechanism of the immunosuppressive effect of action of mycophenolic acid has not been fully elucidated, it appears to be related to inhibition of lymphocyte production. Mycophenolic acid is a potent, selective, noncompetitive, reversible inhibitor of inosine monophosphate dehydrogenase (IMPDH), an essential enzyme in *de novo* guanosine synthesis. Because T- and B-cells are dependent on *de novo* synthesis of purines (e.g., guanosine), mycophenolic acid selectively inhibits proliferation of T- and B-cells. The drug inhibits proliferative responses of T- and B-cells to both mitogenic and allospecific stimulation. Mycophenolic acid suppresses antibody formation by B-cells. By preventing glycosylation of lymphocyte and monocyte glycoproteins involved in intercellular adhesion to endothelial cells, mycophenolic acid may inhibit recruitment of leukocytes to sites of inflammation and graft rejection.

Mycophenolate mofetil is well absorbed following oral administration, having an absolute bioavailability of approximately 94% (based on mycophenolic acid). The absolute bioavailability of mycophenolic acid following oral administration of mycophenolate sodium delayed-release tablets in stable renal transplant patients has been reported to be approximately 72%, Following oral administration of mycophenolate sodium delayed-release (enteric-coated) tablets, the median time to peak plasma concentrations of the drug is 1.5–2.75 hours compared with 0.5–1 hour reported with conventional preparations of mycophenolate mofetil. Administration of mycophenolate sodium (as delayed-release tablets) or mycophenolate mofetil with food does not affect the AUC of mycophenolic acid; however, decreases by about 33 or 40% of the peak plasma concentrations of mycophenolic acid have been observed, respectively.

The pharmacologically active metabolite, mycophenolic acid, is metabolized principally by glucuronyl transferase to form the phenolic glucuronide metabolite of mycophenolic acid, which is not pharmacologically active. In vivo, the phenolic glucuronide metabolite is converted back to mycophenolic acid via enterohepatic recirculation; concurrent administration of drugs that interfere with such recirculation may decrease plasma concentrations of mycophenolic acid. (See Drug Interactions: Cholestyramine.) Ninety-three percent of an orally administered dose of mycophenolate mofetil is excreted in urine (mainly [about 87%] as the phenolic glucuronide of mycophenolic acid) and 6% is excreted in feces. Following administration of mycophenolate sodium, most of the dose (greater than 60%) of mycophenolic acid is excreted in urine as the phenolic glucuronide of mycophenolic acid and 3% is excreted in urine as mycophenolic acid. Mycophenolic acid and the phenolic glucuronide of mycophenolic acid usually are not removed by dialysis.

Advice to Patients

Importance of taking mycophenolate as directed. Importance of reading manufacturer's patient information (medication guide) before initiating therapy and each time drug is refilled. Importance in following patient instructions for administration, handling, and storage of mycophenolate mofetil oral suspension.

Patients should be informed about the risk of lymphoproliferative disease and other malignancies (particularly skin cancer). Importance of informing clinician of any unexplained fever, prolonged tiredness, weight loss, swelling of lymph nodes, or unusual skin changes (e.g., new lesions or bumps, discoloration, brown or black lesions with uneven borders). Importance of limiting sunlight or other UV light exposure by wearing protective clothing and using sunscreens with a high protection factor; importance of avoiding tanning beds or sunlamps.

Patients receiving mycophenolate should be informed of the necessity of routine laboratory testing (e.g., complete blood cell count).

Importance of informing a clinician immediately of any evidence of infection (e.g., temperature elevations of 100.5°F or greater, cold or flu symptoms, earache, headache, pain on urination, white patches in the mouth or throat), unexpected bruising, bleeding, or other manifestations of bone marrow depression. Importance of also informing a clinician of any unusual tiredness, lack of energy, dizziness, or fainting.

Inform women of childbearing potential of possible risk to fetus prior to initiating therapy. Importance of women informing clinicians if they are or plan to become pregnant or plan to breast-feed. Advise women of childbearing potential to avoid pregnancy and to use 2 methods of effective contraception for at least 4 weeks before, during, and for at least 6 weeks after discontinuance of the drug. Advise such women that mycophenolate may decrease effectiveness of certain oral contraceptives. When the drug is administered during pregnancy, or if the patient becomes pregnant while receiving the drug, the patient should be informed of the potential hazard to the fetus and the potential risk for loss of the pregnancy, especially in the first trimester.

Women receiving mycophenolate sodium should avoid breast-feeding for at least 6 weeks after discontinuance of the drug.

Importance of patients informing a clinician if they plan on receiving any vaccines while taking mycophenolate; patients should be instructed to avoid live virus vaccines.

Importance of informing clinicians of concomitant conditions (e.g., ulcers, Lesch-Nyhan or Kelley-Seegmiller syndrome, phenylketonuria) and existing or contemplated concomitant therapy, including prescription and OTC drugs.

Importance of informing patients of other important precautionary information. (See Cautions.)

Overview® (see Users Guide). For additional information on this drug until a more detailed monograph is developed and published, the manufacturer's labeling should be consulted. It is *essential* that the manufacturer's labeling be consulted for more detailed information on usual cautions, precautions, contraindications, potential drug interactions, laboratory test interferences, and acute toxicity.

Preparations

Excipients in commercially available drug preparations may have clinically important effects in some individuals; consult specific product labeling for details.

Mycophenolate Mofetil

Oral		
Capsules	250 mg	**CellCept®**, Roche
For oral suspension	200 mg/mL	**CellCept®**, Roche
Tablets	500 mg	**CellCept®**, Roche

Mycophenolate Mofetil Hydrochloride

Parenteral		
For injection, for IV infusion only	500 mg (of mycophenolate mofetil)	**CellCept® Intravenous**, Roche

Mycophenolate Sodium

Oral		
Tablets, delayed-release, (enteric-coated) film-coated	180 mg (of mycophenolic acid)	**Myfortic®**, Novartis
	360 mg (of mycophenolic acid)	**Myfortic®**, Novartis

†Use is not currently included in the labeling approved by the US Food and Drug Administration

Sirolimus

Rapamycin

■ Sirolimus, a macrolide antibiotic, is a potent immunosuppressive agent.

Uses

■ **Renal Allotransplantation** Sirolimus is used for the prevention of rejection of renal allografts in patients 13 years of age or older receiving renal transplants. The manufacturer recommends therapeutic drug monitoring in all patients receiving the drug.

Sirolimus is used initially in conjunction with both cyclosporine and corticosteroid therapy. The manufacturer cautions that safety and efficacy of de novo use of sirolimus without cyclosporine have not been established in renal transplant patients. (See De Novo Use Without Cyclosporine under Warnings/Precautions: Other Warnings and Precautions, in Cautions.)

In clinical trials in renal transplant patients, a regimen consisting of sirolimus, cyclosporine, and corticosteroids was more effective than regimens consisting of either azathioprine or placebo in combination with cyclosporine and corticosteroids in preventing acute rejection, graft loss, or death at 6 months following transplantation. Concomitant therapy with sirolimus and cyclosporine appears to provide additive immunosuppressive effects while allowing reduced dosages of cyclosporine and/or a reduction in dosage or discontinuance of corticosteroids. However, long-term combined use of sirolimus and cyclosporine has been associated with deterioration of renal allograft function. Therefore, in patients with low to moderate immunologic risk, the manufacturer recommends that, at 2–4 months posttransplantation, cyclosporine be gradually withdrawn over a 4- to 8-week period and that the sirolimus dosage be adjusted to achieve recommended blood concentrations of the drug. In patients with high immunologic risk (e.g., black recipients, repeat renal transplant patients who lost a previous allograft for immunologic reason, and/or patients with a high level of panel-reactive antibodies [PRA; peak PRA level of more than 80%]), the manufacturer recommends that sirolimus be used in combination with cyclosporine and corticosteroids for the first year following transplantation. However, safety and efficacy of sirolimus in combination with cyclosporine and corticosteroids have not been studied beyond one year in high immunologic risk patients; therefore, any adjustments to the immunosuppressive regimen in these patients should be considered based on the clinical status of the patient.

The current indication for sirolimus in the prevention of organ rejection is based on the results of several randomized, double-blind, multicenter controlled studies involving renal allograft recipients. In 2 studies, sirolimus was given in 2 different dosages (2 and 5 mg once daily) as the oral solution in immunosuppressive regimens that included both cyclosporine and corticosteroids (e.g., prednisone). Sirolimus was compared with azathioprine (2–3 mg/kg daily) in one study (study 1) and with placebo in the other (study 2). In both studies, the primary efficacy end point was the rate of treatment failure, defined as the first occurrence of an acute rejection episode (biopsy confirmed), graft loss, or death, in the first 6 months after transplantation. Sirolimus was more effective than azathioprine or placebo in reducing the incidence of treatment failure at 6 months following transplantation. In addition, antibody therapy (i.e., with muromonab-CD3 or antithymocyte globulin) for treatment of acute rejection was required less frequently in patients receiving sirolimus than in azathioprine or placebo recipients. The treatment failure rates at 6 months for sirolimus 2 mg, sirolimus 5 mg, and azathioprine 2–3 mg/kg daily in study 1 were 18.7, 16.8, and 32.3%, respectively; failure rates at 6 months for sirolimus 2 mg, sirolimus 5 mg, and placebo in study 2 were 30, 25.6, and 47.7%, respectively. Following 24 months of therapy, treatment failure rates for sirolimus 2 mg, sirolimus 5 mg, and azathioprine 2–3 mg/kg in study 1 were 32.8, 25.9, and 36%, respectively; failure rates at 36 months for sirolimus 2 mg, sirolimus 5 mg, and placebo in study 2 were 44.1, 41.6, and 54.6%, respectively. In both studies, long-term (24 or 36 months) follow-up indicated that graft survival rates were similar in patients receiving sirolimus and those receiving azathioprine or placebo, but renal function declined at a greater rate and glomerular filtration rates were lower in patients receiving sirolimus and cyclosporine than in those receiving azathioprine or placebo and cyclosporine. In study 1, which was prospectively stratified by race within treatment centers, treatment failure in black patients was lower with the 5-mg daily dosage of sirolimus compared with azathioprine but similar to azathioprine in those receiving sirolimus 2 mg daily. In study 2, which was not prospectively stratified by race, treatment failure was similar for both sirolimus dosages compared with placebo in black patients. (See Dosage and Administration: Special Populations.)

In another multicenter clinical study (study 3), safety and efficacy of maintenance therapy with sirolimus following discontinuation of cyclosporine at 3–4 months following renal transplantation were evaluated in patients with low to moderate immunologic risk (i.e., patients without Banff grade III acute rejection or vascular rejection episodes in the 4-week period before randomization, patients with serum creatinine concentrations of 4.5 mg/dL or less, and patients with adequate renal function to support cyclosporine withdrawal [based on clinician judgment]). All patients received standard sirolimus therapy (sirolimus given as tablets, cyclosporine, and corticosteroids) for the first 3 months following transplantation and then were randomized to continue standard therapy or to receive sirolimus in dosages adjusted based on target sirolimus trough concentrations following gradual withdrawal of cyclosporine. Allograft survival rates at 12, 24, and 36 months following transplantation were similar in both treatment groups. Although the incidence of biopsy-proven acute rejection from randomization through 12 months was 4.2% in the group receiving standard therapy compared with 9.8% in the group receiving sirolimus following cyclosporine withdrawal, patients receiving sirolimus following cyclosporine withdrawal had higher mean glomerular filtration rates at 12, 24, and 36 months than did those who continued to receive standard therapy. In the subset of patients receiving renal allografts with 4 or more HLA mismatches, patients who received sirolimus following cyclosporine withdrawal had higher rates of acute rejection (15.3%) than did patients who continued to receive standard therapy (3%); however, among those receiving renal allografts with 3 or fewer HLA mismatches, rates of acute rejection were similar in both treatment groups. In a subsequent extension of this cyclosporine withdrawal study, the results for the cyclosporine withdrawal group at 48 and 60 months following transplantation were consistent with those observed at month 36; 52% of the patients in the sirolimus with cyclosporine withdrawal group remained on therapy through month 60 and demonstrated sustained glomerular filtration rates. The manufacturer states that cyclosporine withdrawal has not been studied in patients with Banff grade III acute rejection or vascular rejection prior to cyclosporine withdrawal, those who are dialysis dependent, those with serum creatinine concentrations greater than 4.5 mg/dL, black patients, multiorgan transplant recipients, secondary transplant recipients, or patients with a high level of panel-reactive antibodies.

Use of sirolimus in high immunologic risk renal transplant patients was studied in a multicenter clinical trial (study 4) of one year's duration in high risk patients (defined as black ethnicity, repeat transplant following loss of a previous allograft for immunologic reasons, and/or recipients with a high level of panel-reactive antibodies [PRA; peak PRA level over 80%]). Patients in the sirolimus plus cyclosporine arm of this study received an immunosuppressive regimen consisting of concentration-controlled sirolimus, concentration-controlled cyclosporine, and corticosteroids; antibody induction therapy was used in 88.4% of the patients. The sirolimus and cyclosporine immunosuppressive regimen was found to be effective in these high risk patients in the first year following renal transplantation, with an efficacy failure rate of 23.2%, a biopsy-proven acute rejection rate of 17.4%, and a graft survival rate of 90.2%.

Conversion from calcineurin inhibitors (e.g., cyclosporine, tacrolimus) to sirolimus has been evaluated in maintenance renal transplant recipients 6 months to 10 years following renal transplantation in a randomized, multicenter, and controlled study (study 5). The Sirolimus Renal Conversion Trial (CONVERT) was designed to determine whether renal function improved following conversion from a calcineurin inhibitor-based to a sirolimus-based immunosuppressive regimen. In this study, 830 patients 13 years of age or older who had been receiving maintenance therapy with either cyclosporine or tacrolimus along with corticosteroids and azathioprine or mycophenolate mofetil for at least 12 weeks were randomly assigned to continue the calcineurin inhibitor or to convert from the calcineurin inhibitor to sirolimus. The patients were stratified into 2 subsets according to their baseline glomerular filtration rate (GFR): 20–40 mL/minute or more than 40 mL/minute. In this trial, there was no benefit associated with conversion to sirolimus with regard to improvement in renal function, and a higher incidence of proteinuria was observed in the sirolimus conversion arm. In addition, enrollment of patients with a baseline GFR of 40 mL/minute or less was discontinued because of a higher incidence of serious adverse effects (including pneumonia, acute rejection, graft loss, and death). In the remaining group of patients with a baseline GFR greater than 40 mL/minute, sirolimus conversion at 2 years was associated with excellent patient and graft survival, no difference in acute rejection rate, increased urinary protein excretion, and a lower incidence of malignancy compared with calcineurin inhibitor continuation. (See Proteinuria under Warnings/Precautions: Other Warnings and Precautions, in Cautions.)

The manufacturer states that safety and efficacy of conversion from calcineurin inhibitors (e.g., cyclosporine, tacrolimus) to sirolimus in maintenance renal transplant patients have not been established. In addition, the manufacturer recommends that the clinical results of the CONVERT trial be taken into account when considering a conversion from calcineurin inhibitors to sirolimus in stable renal transplant recipients because of the lack of evidence showing improved renal function following conversion and the increased urinary protein excretion and increased incidence of treatment-emergent nephrotic-range proteinuria following conversion, particularly in patients with preexisting abnormal urinary protein excretion prior to conversion.

■ **Hepatic Allotransplantation** Although sirolimus has been used for the prevention of rejection of liver allografts†, the manufacturer states that safety and efficacy of the drug as immunosuppressive therapy have not been established in liver transplant patients and that such use is therefore *not* recommended. Sirolimus has been associated with adverse outcomes in patients following liver transplantation, including excess mortality, graft loss, and hepatic artery thrombosis when used in combination with other immunosuppressants (e.g., cyclosporine, tacrolimus). (See Excess Mortality, Graft Loss, and Hepatic Artery Thrombosis in Liver Transplant Patients under Warnings/Precautions: Warnings, in Cautions.)

■ **Lung Allotransplantation** Although sirolimus has been used for the prevention of rejection of lung allografts†, the manufacturer states that safety and efficacy of the drug as immunosuppressive therapy have not been established in lung transplant patients and that such use is therefore *not* recommended. Cases of bronchial anastomotic dehiscence, most of which were fatal, have been reported in de novo lung transplant patients who received sirolimus in combination with other immunosuppressants. (See Bronchial Anastomotic Dehiscence in Lung Transplant Patients under Warnings/Precautions: Warnings, in Cautions.)

Dosage and Administration

■ **Administration** Sirolimus is administered orally as tablets or oral solution. To minimize variability in systemic exposure to sirolimus, the drug should be given once daily, consistently with or without food. Grapefruit juice reduces cytochrome P-450 (CYP) 3A4 (CYP3A4)-mediated metabolism of sirolimus and should not be administered with or used for dilution of the drug. (See Drug Interactions: Grapefruit Juice.)

Sirolimus tablets should not be crushed, chewed, or split; the oral solution should be used in patients who are unable to take the tablets.

For dilution and administration of sirolimus oral solution, the prescribed amount of oral solution should be withdrawn from the bottle using the amber oral dose syringe supplied by the manufacturer and then the correct amount of the drug emptied into a glass or plastic container that holds at least 2 ounces (1/4 cup or 60 mL) of water or orange juice. Other liquids, including grapefruit juice, should *not* be used for dilution. The diluted oral solution should be stirred vigorously and drunk at once. The container should be refilled with an additional volume (minimum of 4 ounces [½ cup or 120 mL]) of water or orange juice, stirred vigorously, and then drunk at once.

Sirolimus therapy should be initiated as soon as possible following renal transplantation as part of an initial immunosuppressive regimen that includes both cyclosporine and corticosteroids. At 2–4 months following transplantation, gradual discontinuance of cyclosporine and adjustment of the sirolimus dosage to achieve recommended blood concentrations of the drug are recommended in patients at low to moderate immunologic risk. In patients at high immunologic risk (defined as black ethnicity, repeat transplant following loss of a previous allograft for immunologic reasons, and/or recipients with a high level of panel-reactive antibodies [PRA; peak PRA level over 80%]), the manufacturer recommends that sirolimus be used in combination with cyclosporine and corticosteroids for the first 12 months following renal transplantation.

■ **Dosage** Commercially available sirolimus tablets and oral solution are not bioequivalent. However, the manufacturer states that because 2-mg doses of sirolimus given as conventional tablets and as the oral solution have been shown to be therapeutically equivalent, such formulations may be interchangeable on a mg-per-mg basis at doses that do not exceed 2 mg. It is not known whether the commercially available sirolimus tablets and the oral solution are therapeutically equivalent at doses exceeding 2 mg.

Renal Allotransplantation When sirolimus is used for the prevention of renal allograft rejection in patients who have undergone renal transplantation, the manufacturer cautions that frequent sirolimus dosage adjustments based on non-steady-state sirolimus concentrations can lead to overdosing or underdosing since sirolimus has a long half-life. Once the maintenance dosage is adjusted, the renal transplant recipient should be maintained on the new sirolimus dosage for at least 7–14 days before subsequent dosage adjustment is made based on drug concentrations. If subsequent dosage adjustment is required, the manufacturer states that the new dosage can be estimated in most patients based on the following equation:

$$\text{new sirolimus dosage} = \text{current sirolimus dosage} \times \frac{\text{target concentration}}{\text{current concentration}}$$

A loading dose may be necessary in addition to a new maintenance dosage if an increase in trough sirolimus concentrations is required and can be estimated based on the following equation:

$$\text{sirolimus loading dose} = 3 \times (\text{new maintenance dosage} - \text{current maintenance dosage})$$

The manufacturer states that no more than 40 mg of sirolimus should be given within any one-day period. If an estimated daily dose exceeds 40 mg because of the addition of a loading dose, the loading dose should be given in divided doses over a 2-day period. The manufacturer recommends that trough whole blood concentrations of sirolimus be monitored for at least 3–4 days after a loading dose is administered.

Therapeutic Drug Monitoring. Monitoring of trough whole blood sirolimus concentrations is recommended in *all* renal transplant patients receiving sirolimus for the prevention of renal allograft rejection, particularly in those patients likely to have altered drug metabolism, patients 13 years of age or older who weigh less than 40 kg, patients with hepatic impairment, when a change in sirolimus dosage form has been made, and during concurrent therapy with potent inhibitors or inducers of CYP3A4 (see Drug Interactions). However, therapeutic drug monitoring should not be the sole basis for adjusting sirolimus therapy; careful attention to clinical signs and symptoms, tissue biopsy findings, and laboratory results is also necessary during therapy.

The recommended 24-hour trough concentration ranges for sirolimus are based on chromatographic methods. In clinical practice, sirolimus whole blood concentrations currently are being measured by both chromatographic and immunoassay methodologies. However, the measured concentrations of sirolimus in whole blood depend on the type of assay used, and the concentrations obtained by these different methodologies are not interchangeable. Since results are assay and laboratory dependent and the results may change over time, any adjustments to the targeted therapeutic range must therefore be made with a detailed knowledge of the site-specific assay used to determine sirolimus trough concentrations. The manufacturer recommends that clinicians involved in the management of patients receiving sirolimus therapy determine the following: which assay is being used in their laboratories; whether there is any change to the assay used; and whether there is a change to the laboratory's reference range and/or a subsequent change to the institution's or referring center's recommended therapeutic range for sirolimus. With this information, target sirolimus levels can be appropriately adjusted to achieve optimal clinical results. It is essential that communication be maintained with the laboratory performing the sirolimus assays. Specialized references should be consulted for additional information on sirolimus therapeutic drug monitoring.

Patients at Low to Moderate Immunologic Risk. For the prevention of renal allograft rejection in renal transplant patients at low to moderate immunologic risk, sirolimus is administered orally once daily, with the initial dose administered as soon as possible after transplantation. The initial immunosuppressive regimen should include both cyclosporine and corticosteroids. De novo renal transplant recipients at low to moderate immunologic risk should receive a sirolimus loading dose equivalent to 3 times the maintenance dosage; for example, a 6-mg loading dose of sirolimus should be followed by a maintenance dosage of 2 mg daily. Although a regimen consisting of higher loading and maintenance doses (loading dose of 15 mg followed by a maintenance dosage of 5 mg daily) was used in clinical trials and found to be safe and effective, no efficacy advantage could be shown for the higher dosage in the overall patient population. (See Dosage and Administration: Special Populations.) In addition, sirolimus 2 mg daily demonstrated a superior safety profile compared with the 5-mg daily dosage. Therapeutic drug monitoring of sirolimus blood concentrations is recommended in all renal transplant patients to maintain drug concentrations within the recommended range. (See Therapeutic Drug Monitoring under Dosage: Renal Allotransplantation, in Dosage and Administration.)

Since concomitant administration of oral cyclosporine (modified) (e.g., Neoral®) increases the rate and extent of sirolimus absorption (i.e., increased peak blood concentrations and AUC, respectively), the manufacturer recommends that sirolimus be taken 4 hours after administration of cyclosporine (modified) oral solution (e.g., Neoral® oral solution, SangCya® [no longer commercially available in the US] oral solution) or liquid-filled capsules (modified) (e.g., Neoral® soft gelatin capsules).

In patients at low to moderate immunologic risk who have received concomitant sirolimus and cyclosporine therapy for 2–4 months following renal transplantation, gradual discontinuance of cyclosporine over a 4- to 8-week period is recommended by the manufacturer. Sirolimus dosage should be adjusted to maintain trough whole blood concentrations of the drug in the range of 16–24 ng/mL (based on chromatographic assay method) for the first year following transplantation; thereafter, trough concentrations of 12–20 ng/mL are recommended. (See Therapeutic Drug Monitoring under Dosage: Renal Allotransplantation, in Dosage and Administration.)

Patients at High Immunologic Risk. For the prevention of renal allograft rejection in renal transplant patients at high immunologic risk (defined as black ethnicity, repeat transplant following loss of a previous allograft for immunologic reasons, and/or recipient with a high level of panel-reactive antibodies [PRA; peak PRA level over 80%]), sirolimus is administered orally once daily, with the initial dose administered as soon as possible after transplantation. The initial immunosuppressive regimen should include both cyclosporine and corticosteroids. The manufacturer recommends that sirolimus be used in combination with cyclosporine and corticosteroids for the first 12 months following renal transplantation; however, safety and efficacy of this combined regimen have not been studied beyond 12 months following transplantation. Therefore, the manufacturer states that any adjustments to the immunosuppressive regimen after the first 12 months following transplantation should be considered based on the clinical status of the patient. Therapeutic drug monitoring of sirolimus blood concentrations is recommended in all renal transplant patients to maintain drug concentrations within the recommended range. (See Therapeutic Drug Monitoring under Dosage: Renal Allotransplantation, in Dosage and Administration.)

Since concomitant administration of oral cyclosporine (modified) (e.g., Neoral®) increases the rate and extent of sirolimus absorption (i.e., increased peak blood concentrations and AUC, respectively), the manufacturer recommends that sirolimus be taken 4 hours after administration of cyclosporine (modified) oral solution (e.g., Neoral® oral solution, SangCya® [no longer commercially available in the US] oral solution) or liquid-filled capsules (modified) (e.g., Neoral® soft gelatin capsules).

For renal transplant patients at high immunologic risk receiving combined sirolimus and cyclosporine therapy, the manufacturer states that sirolimus should be initiated with a loading dose of up to 15 mg on day 1 posttransplantation. Beginning on day 2, an initial maintenance dosage of 5 mg daily should be given. A trough level should be obtained between days 5 and 7, and the daily dosage of sirolimus should thereafter be adjusted. The initial dosage of cyclosporine should be up to 7 mg/kg daily given in divided doses and the dosage should subsequently be adjusted to achieve target whole blood trough concentrations. Prednisone should be administered at a dosage of at least 5 mg daily. Antibody induction therapy may be used.

■ **Special Populations** The initial dosage of sirolimus for the prevention of renal allograft rejection in patients 13 years of age or older who weigh less than 40 kg should be 1 mg/m² daily based on body surface area, with a loading dose of 3 mg/m².

Sirolimus is not extensively eliminated by the kidneys, and the manufacturer states that adjustment of sirolimus dosage is not necessary in renal transplant patients with impaired renal function receiving the drug.

Sirolimus is extensively metabolized by the liver, and the manufacturer recommends a reduction of approximately one-third in the maintenance dosage of sirolimus in renal transplant patients with mild or moderate hepatic impairment and a reduction of approximately one-half in renal transplant patients with severe hepatic impairment; the loading dose in these patients does not require modification.

The manufacturer states that routine dosage adjustment in geriatric patients receiving sirolimus for the prevention of renal allograft rejection is not necessary; however, dosage selection in geriatric patients should be cautious, usually starting at the lower end of the dosage range, reflecting the greater frequency of decreased hepatic or cardiac function and of concomitant diseases or other drug therapy in this population.

Cautions

■ **Contraindications** Known hypersensitivity to sirolimus or its derivatives or any ingredient in the sirolimus formulation.

■ **Warnings/Precautions** ***Warnings*** *Sirolimus should be used only by clinicians experienced in immunosuppressive therapy and the management of renal transplant patients. Patients receiving the drug should be managed in facilities equipped and staffed with adequate laboratory and supportive medical resources, and the clinician responsible for maintenance therapy should have complete information requisite for follow-up of the patient.*

Increased Susceptibility to Infection and Possible Development of Lymphoma. Immunosuppression may result in increased susceptibility to infection (including opportunistic infections [e.g., tuberculosis], fatal infections, and sepsis) and possible development of lymphoma and other malignancies, particularly of the skin. Lymphoma/lymphoproliferative disease was reported in 0.7–3.2% of sirolimus-treated patients and 0.6–0.8% of patients receiving azathioprine and placebo in studies 1 and 2. (See Uses: Renal Allotransplantation.)

Excess Mortality, Graft Loss, and Hepatic Artery Thrombosis in Liver Transplant Patients. Use of sirolimus in combination with tacrolimus has been associated with excess mortality and graft loss in a study in de novo liver transplant patients (22% in combination compared with 9% on tacrolimus alone). Many of these patients had evidence of infection at or near the time of death. In this and another study in de novo liver transplant recipients, concurrent use of sirolimus with cyclosporine or tacrolimus was associated with an increased risk of hepatic artery thrombosis (HAT; 7% in combination compared with 2% in the control arm). Most cases of HAT occurred within 30 days posttransplantation and most resulted in graft loss or death. In a clinical study in stable liver transplant patients 6–144 months after transplantation and receiving a calcineurin inhibitor-based regimen, an increased number of deaths was observed in the group converted to a sirolimus-based regimen compared with those continued on a calcineurin-based regimen (3.8 and 1.4%, respectively; difference not statistically significant). (See Uses: Hepatic Allotransplantation and also see Drug Interactions: Cyclosporine and Other Immunosuppressants.) Because safety and efficacy of sirolimus as immunosuppressive therapy in liver transplant patients have not been established, such use is *not* recommended by the manufacturer.

Bronchial Anastomotic Dehiscence in Lung Transplant Patients. Cases of bronchial anastomotic dehiscence, most of which were fatal, have been reported in de novo lung transplant patients who received sirolimus in combination with other immunosuppressants. Because safety and efficacy of sirolimus as immunosuppressive therapy in lung transplant patients have not been established, such use is *not* recommended by the manufacturer.

Sensitivity Reactions Hypersensitivity reactions, including anaphylactic or anaphylactoid reactions, angioedema, exfoliative dermatitis, and hypersensitivity vasculitis, have been associated with sirolimus administration.

Sirolimus has been associated with angioedema. Concurrent use of other drugs known to cause angioedema (e.g., angiotensin-converting enzyme [ACE] inhibitors, angiotensin II receptor antagonists, nonsteroidal anti-inflammatory agents) may increase the risk of developing angioedema.

Other Warnings and Precautions **Fluid Accumulation and Abnormal Wound Healing.** Impaired or delayed wound healing, including lymphocele and wound dehiscence, has been reported in sirolimus-treated patients. Lymphocele, a known surgical complication of renal transplantation, occurred more often in sirolimus-treated patients and appeared to be dose-related. In addition, abnormal wound healing following transplant surgery, including fascial dehiscence, incisional hernia, and anastomotic disruption (e.g., wound, vascular, airway, ureteral, biliary), has been reported in patients receiving the drug. Clinicians should consider appropriate measures to minimize such complications (i.e., patient selection based on body mass index [BMI], reduced sirolimus dosage, use of closed suction drains, modifications of surgical technique). Patients with a BMI greater than 30 kg/m² may be at increased risk of abnormal wound healing.

Fluid accumulation, including peripheral edema, lymphedema, pleural effusion, ascites, and pericardial effusions (including hemodynamically important effusions and tamponade requiring intervention [e.g., pericardial drainage] in children and adults), also has been reported in patients receiving sirolimus.

Hyperlipidemia. Increased serum cholesterol and triglycerides requiring treatment occurred more frequently in sirolimus-treated patients compared with those receiving azathioprine or placebo in studies 1 and 2. (See Uses: Renal Allotransplantation.) Increased incidences of hypercholesterolemia (43–46%) and/or hypertriglyceridemia (45–57%) were reported in patients receiving sirolimus compared with those receiving placebo (each 23%). Immunosuppressed renal transplant patients have a higher prevalence of clinically important hyperlipidemia than the general population, and the manufacturer states that the risks and benefits of sirolimus therapy in patients with preexisting hyperlipidemia should be carefully considered before initiating an immunosuppressive regimen containing sirolimus.

Patients receiving sirolimus should be monitored for hyperlipidemia. If hyperlipidemia is detected, interventions such as diet, exercise, and use of antilipemic agents should be initiated based on current clinical guidelines.

In clinical trials, concomitant use of sirolimus and HMG-CoA reductase inhibitors and/or fibric acid derivatives has generally been well tolerated. However, the manufacturer recommends that patients receiving sirolimus and cyclosporine therapy who are concurrently receiving an HMG-CoA reductase inhibitor and/or fibric acid derivative should be monitored for the possible development of rhabdomyolysis and other adverse effects (e.g., hepatic toxicity), which are described in the prescribing information for these antilipemic agents. (See Drug Interactions: Antilipemic Agents.)

Renal Function. Mean serum creatinine concentrations were increased and mean glomerular filtration rate (GFR) was decreased in patients receiving cyclosporine and sirolimus compared with those receiving cyclosporine with placebo or azathioprine. In addition, the rate of decline in renal function in these studies was greater in patients receiving sirolimus and cyclosporine compared with those receiving control therapies. Renal function should be closely monitored in patients receiving maintenance immunosuppression with regimens that include sirolimus and cyclosporine, since long-term combined use of these drugs has been associated with deterioration of renal function.

Appropriate adjustment of the immunosuppressive regimen, including discontinuance of sirolimus and/or cyclosporine, should be considered in patients with elevated or increasing serum creatinine concentrations. In patients at low to moderate immunologic risk, continuation of combination therapy with cyclosporine for longer than 4 months posttransplantation should be considered only in patients in whom the potential benefits outweigh the possible risks. Caution should be exercised when using other drugs (e.g., aminoglycosides, amphotericin B) that are known to have a deleterious effect on renal function in patients receiving sirolimus.

In patients with delayed graft function, sirolimus may delay recovery of renal function.

Proteinuria. The manufacturer recommends periodic quantitative monitoring of urinary protein excretion in patients receiving sirolimus. In a study evaluating conversion from calcineurin inhibitors to sirolimus for maintenance immunosuppression 6–120 months following renal transplantation, increased urinary protein excretion was commonly observed from 6 through 24 months after conversion to sirolimus compared with continuation of calcineurin inhibitors. Protein excretion increased the most following conversion in patients with the greatest amount of urinary protein excretion prior to sirolimus conversion. New-onset nephrosis (nephrotic syndrome) was reported in 2.2% of patients in the sirolimus conversion group compared with 0.4% of patients in the calcineurin inhibitor continuation group. Nephrotic-range proteinuria (defined as urinary protein to creatinine ratio higher than 3.5) was reported in 9.2% of patients in the sirolimus conversion group compared with 3.7% of patients in the calcineurin inhibitor continuation group. In some patients, reduction in the degree of urinary protein excretion was observed following sirolimus discontinuance. Early treatment of proteinuria may help prevent long-term adverse effects on graft survival.

The manufacturer states that safety and efficacy of conversion from calcineurin inhibitors to sirolimus in maintenance renal transplant patients have not been established. (See Uses: Renal Allotransplantation.)

Latent Viral Infections. Immunosuppressed patients are at an increased risk for opportunistic infections, including reactivation of latent viral infections. These include BK virus-associated nephropathy (BKVN), which has been reported in patients receiving immunosuppressants, including sirolimus, cyclosporine, mycophenolate mofetil, and tacrolimus. Primary infection with polyoma BK virus typically occurs in childhood; following initial infection, the virus remains latent but reactivation may occur in immunocompromised patients. BKVN has principally been observed in renal transplant patients (usually within the first year posttransplantation) and may result in serious outcomes, including deterioration of kidney function and renal allograft loss. Risk of BK virus reactivation appears to be related to the degree of overall immunosuppression rather than use of any specific immunosuppressive agent; patients receiving a maintenance immunosuppressive regimen of 4 or more drugs appear to be at highest risk.

Patients should be monitored for possible signs of BKVN, including deterioration in renal function, during sirolimus therapy; screening assays for polyomavirus replication also have been recommended by some clinicians. Early intervention in patients who develop BKVN is critical; a reduction in immunosuppressive therapy should initially be considered in such patients. Although a variety of other treatment approaches have been used anecdotally in patients with BKVN, including antiviral therapy (e.g., cidofovir), leflunomide, IV immunoglobulins, and fluoroquinolone antibiotics, additional experience and well-controlled studies are necessary to more clearly establish the optimal treatment of such patients.

Cases of progressive multifocal leukoencephalopathy (PML; an opportunistic viral infection of the brain), sometimes fatal, have been reported in patients treated with immunosuppressive agents, including sirolimus. PML is caused by the polyomavirus JC (also called the JC virus) and risk factors include treatment with immunosuppressive therapies and impairment of immune function. PML commonly presents with hemiparesis, apathy, confusion, cognitive impairment, and ataxia, and the possible diagnosis of PML should be considered in immunocompromised patients receiving sirolimus who experience neurologic manifestations. Consultation with a neurologist is advised as clinically indicated. Decreasing total immunosuppression may improve the outcome of PML, but also may increase the risk of graft rejection in transplant recipients. Clinicians should consider the potential risks versus benefits of reduced immunosuppression in such cases. Although the optimal pharmacologic treatment of PML remains to be established, antiviral agents (e.g., cidofovir) have reportedly been successfully used in the treatment of PML in several transplant recipients to date. Early diagnosis of PML and rapid initiation of treatment appear to be essential for patient recovery from this progressive viral disease.

Interstitial Lung Disease. Cases of interstitial lung disease (including pneumonitis, bronchiolitis obliterans organizing pneumonia, and pulmonary fibrosis), some fatal, with no identified infectious etiology have occurred in patients receiving immunosuppressive regimens including sirolimus. Symptoms associated with interstitial pneumonitis have included dry cough, exertional dyspnea, and fatigue. The risk for such adverse effects may be increased with increased trough blood concentrations of sirolimus. In some cases, interstitial lung disease has resolved upon discontinuance or dosage reduction of sirolimus.

De Novo Use Without Cyclosporine. Safety and efficacy of de novo use of sirolimus without cyclosporine are not established in renal transplant patients. In a multicenter clinical study, de novo renal transplant patients treated with sirolimus, mycophenolate mofetil, corticosteroids, and an interleukin-2 (IL-2) receptor antagonist had substantially higher acute rejection rates and numerically higher death rates compared with those treated with cyclosporine, mycophenolate mofetil, corticosteroids, and an IL-2 receptor antagonist. A benefit in terms of better renal function was not apparent in the treatment arm with de novo use of sirolimus without cyclosporine. These findings were also noted in a similar treatment group of another clinical trial.

Increased Risk of Calcineurin Inhibitor-induced Hemolytic Uremic Syndrome/Thrombotic Thrombocytopenic Purpura/Thrombotic Microangiopathy. Concurrent use of sirolimus and a calcineurin inhibitor (e.g., cyclosporine, tacrolimus) may increase the risk of calcineurin inhibitor-induced hemolytic uremic syndrome (HUS)/thrombotic thrombocytopenic purpura (TTP)/thrombotic microangiopathy (TMA).

Antimicrobial Prophylaxis. Cases of *Pneumocystis jiroveci* (formerly *Pneumocystis carinii*) pneumonia have been reported in sirolimus-treated patients not receiving antimicrobial prophylaxis. Therefore, the manufacturer states that antimicrobial prophylaxis for *P. jiroveci* pneumonia should be administered for 1 year following transplantation.

Cytomegalovirus (CMV) prophylaxis is recommended for 3 months following transplantation, particularly in patients at increased risk for CMV disease.

Assays for Sirolimus Therapeutic Drug Monitoring. The manufacturer states that the 24-hour trough concentration ranges for sirolimus recommended in the prescribing information for Rapamune® are based on chromatographic methods. In current clinical practice, however, whole blood concentrations of sirolimus are being measured by both chromatographic and immunoassay methodologies. Because measured whole blood concentrations depend on the type of assay used, concentrations obtained by these different methodologies are not interchangeable. (See Therapeutic Drug Monitoring under Dosage: Renal Allotransplantation, in Dosage and Administration.)

Skin Cancer. Patients receiving immunosuppressive therapy are at increased risk for skin cancer. Patients should be advised to limit exposure to sunlight and ultraviolet (UV) light by wearing protective clothing and using a sunscreen with a high protection factor. (See Advice to Patients.)

Interaction with Potent Inhibitors and Inducers of Cytochrome P-450 Isoenzyme 3A4 and/or P-glycoprotein. Concurrent administration of sirolimus with potent inhibitors of cytochrome P-450 (CYP) isoenzyme 3A4 (CYP3A4) and/or P-glycoprotein (including ketoconazole, voriconazole, itraconazole, erythromycin, telithromycin, and clarithromycin) or potent inducers of CYP3A4 and/or P-glycoprotein (including rifampin and rifabutin) is not recommended. (See Drug Interactions: Inhibitors or Inducers of Cytochrome P-450 Isoenzyme 3A4 and P-glycoprotein.)

Specific Populations **Pregnancy.** Category C. (See Users Guide.) Women of childbearing potential should use effective contraception before, during, and for 12 weeks after discontinuance of sirolimus therapy.

The National Transplantation Pregnancy Registry (NTPR) is a pregnancy registry for pregnant women receiving immunosuppressants following any solid organ transplantation; the NTPR encourages reporting of all immunosuppressant exposures during pregnancy in transplant patients by telephone at 877-955-6877 or via their website: https://www.transplantpregnancyregistry.org/.

Lactation. Sirolimus is distributed into milk in trace amounts in rats; not known whether the drug is distributed into milk in humans. Discontinue nursing or the drug because of potential for serious adverse effects in infants.

Pediatric Use. Safety and efficacy of sirolimus have not been established in pediatric patients younger than 13 years of age.

Safety and efficacy of sirolimus have been established in pediatric and adolescent renal transplant patients 13 years of age and older judged to be at low to moderate immunologic risk. Use of sirolimus in this subpopulation of pediatric patients is supported by evidence from adequate and well-controlled trials of sirolimus in adults with additional pharmacokinetic data in pediatric renal transplant patients. (See Uses: Renal Allotransplantation and also see Dosage and Administration: Special Populations.)

Safety and efficacy data from a controlled, multicenter clinical trial of 36 months' duration in pediatric and adolescent renal transplant patients younger than 18 years of age judged to be at high immunologic risk (i.e., history of one or more acute rejection episodes and/or presence of chronic allograft nephropathy) did not support the chronic use of sirolimus in combination with calcineurin inhibitors and corticosteroids because of the higher incidence of lipid abnormalities and deterioration of renal function and the lack of a demonstrated therapeutic benefit compared with a calcineurin inhibitor-based regimen.

Geriatric Use. Clinical studies of sirolimus did not include a sufficient number of patients 65 years of age or older to determine whether they respond differently than younger patients. Differences in responses between geriatric patients and younger patients have not been identified. Following administration of sirolimus oral solution or tablets, sirolimus trough concentrations in renal transplant patients over 65 years of age were similar to those observed in adults 18–65 years of age. These data suggest that dosage adjustments based solely on age are not necessary in geriatric renal transplant patients. The manufacturer states that dosage selection in geriatric patients should generally be cautious, usually starting at the low end of the dosage range, reflecting the greater frequency of decreased hepatic or cardiac function and of concomitant disease or other drug therapy.

Hepatic Impairment. In pharmacokinetic studies, patients with hepatic impairment had higher mean sirolimus area under the plasma concentration-time curve (AUC) values compared with individuals with normal hepatic function; as severity of hepatic impairment increased, steady increases in mean sirolimus elimination half-lives and decreases in mean sirolimus clearance normalized for body weight were observed. Therefore, maintenance dosage adjustment of sirolimus and therapeutic drug monitoring are recommended in all patients with hepatic impairment. (See Dosage and Administration: Special Populations.)

The safety and efficacy of sirolimus as immunosuppressive therapy in liver transplant patients have not been established, and therefore such use is not recommended. (See Dosage and Administration: Special Populations and also see Excess Mortality, Graft Loss, and Hepatic Artery Thrombosis in Liver Transplant Patients under Warnings/Precautions: Warnings, in Cautions.)

■ **Common Adverse Effects** Adverse reactions occurring in 20% or more of patients receiving sirolimus in clinical trials include peripheral edema, hypercholesterolemia, hypertriglyceridemia, hypertension, increased serum creatinine concentrations, constipation, abdominal pain, diarrhea, headache, fever, urinary tract infection, anemia, nausea, arthralgia, pain, acne or acne-like eruption, rash, and thrombocytopenia. Adverse reactions that resulted in sirolimus discontinuance in more than 5% of patients in clinical trials were increased serum creatinine concentrations, hypertriglyceridemia, and thrombotic thrombocytopenic purpura (TTP).

Drug Interactions

■ **Inhibitors or Inducers of Cytochrome P-450 Isoenzyme 3A4 and P-glycoprotein** Sirolimus is a known substrate for both cytochrome P-450 (CYP) isoenzyme 3A4 (CYP3A4) and P-glycoprotein. Inducers of CYP3A4 and P-glycoprotein may decrease sirolimus blood concentrations while inhibitors of CYP3A4 and P-glycoprotein may increase sirolimus concentrations.

The manufacturer states that concomitant use of sirolimus with potent inducers (e.g., rifampin, rifabutin) and potent inhibitors (e.g., itraconazole, ketoconazole, voriconazole, clarithromycin, erythromycin, telithromycin) of CYP3A4 and P-glycoprotein should be avoided. Alternative agents with lesser drug interaction potential should be considered.

Caution is advised when sirolimus is used with other drugs or other agents that are modulators of CYP3A4 and P-glycoprotein. The dosage of sirolimus and/or the concurrently administered drug(s) may require adjustment. The following drugs potentially may increase sirolimus blood concentrations: bromocriptine, cimetidine, cisapride, clotrimazole, danazol, diltiazem, dronedarone, fluconazole, HIV protease inhibitors (e.g., indinavir, ritonavir), metoclopramide, nicardipine, troleandomycin, and verapamil. The following drugs and other agents potentially may decrease sirolimus concentrations: carbamazepine, phenobarbital, phenytoin, rifapentine, and St. John's wort (*Hypericum perforatum*). When given concurrently with sirolimus, verapamil concentrations also may increase. (See Drug Interactions: Verapamil.)

■ **Cyclosporine and Other Immunosuppressants** Cyclosporine, a substrate and inhibitor of CYP3A4 and P-glycoprotein, has been shown to increase sirolimus concentrations during concurrent administration. To minimize such potential increases, sirolimus should be taken 4 hours after administration of oral cyclosporine. If cyclosporine is withdrawn from combination therapy with sirolimus, a higher sirolimus dosage is necessary to maintain the recommended sirolimus trough concentration ranges.

Potential pharmacologic interaction when sirolimus is given with other immunosuppressants (increased risk of infectious complications and malignancies), particularly with more potent immunosuppressive regimens (see Cautions).

Potential pharmacologic interaction with cyclosporine or tacrolimus (increased risk of hepatic artery thrombosis) in de novo liver transplant recipients. Most cases of hepatic artery thrombosis occurred within 30 days posttransplantation and led to graft loss or death. In one study reporting excess mortality and graft loss in association with combined use of sirolimus and tacrolimus in de novo liver transplant recipients, many of the patients had evidence of infection at or near the time of death.

Possible decreased exposure to tacrolimus during concurrent administration of sirolimus. Potential pharmacologic interaction with concurrent sirolimus and tacrolimus administration (increased risk of wound healing complications, impaired renal function, and insulin-dependent posttransplant diabetes mellitus in heart transplant† recipients). The manufacturer of tacrolimus recommends avoiding concomitant use of sirolimus and tacrolimus.

Concomitant use of sirolimus and a calcineurin inhibitor (e.g., cyclosporine, tacrolimus) may increase the risk of calcineurin inhibitor-induced hemolytic uremic syndrome/thrombotic thrombocytopenic purpura/thrombotic microangiopathy.

■ **Diltiazem** Pharmacokinetic interaction (increased bioavailability of sirolimus). Sirolimus concentration monitoring is recommended, with adjustment of sirolimus dosage if needed.

■ **Dronedarone** Concomitant use of sirolimus and dronedarone potentially may increase plasma concentrations of sirolimus. In one case report, a more than threefold increase in trough sirolimus concentration compared with baseline was reported 3 days following initiation of dronedarone therapy in a renal transplant recipient. The manufacturer of dronedarone currently recommends monitoring plasma concentrations of sirolimus, with adjustment of sirolimus dosage, if needed, during concurrent administration. Some clinicians have suggested that combined dronedarone and sirolimus therapy be avoided, if possible. If concurrent use cannot be avoided, they recommend reducing the sirolimus dosage by 50–75% prior to initiating dronedarone therapy and close monitoring of sirolimus trough levels, particularly during the titration phase.

■ **Ketoconazole** Pharmacokinetic interaction (increased bioavailability of sirolimus). Concomitant use should be avoided; alternative anti-infective therapy with less potential for enzyme induction should be considered.

■ **Rifampin** Pharmacokinetic interaction (enzyme induction and decreased bioavailability of sirolimus). Concomitant use should be avoided; alternative anti-infective therapy with less potential for enzyme induction should be considered.

■ **Verapamil** Pharmacokinetic interaction (increased bioavailability of sirolimus and verapamil). Caution is advised during concurrent administration; sirolimus concentration monitoring is recommended with adjustment of sirolimus dosage if needed. Adjustment of verapamil dosage is also recommended if needed.

■ **Antilipemic Agents** Antilipemic agents are often used to treat hyperlipidemia in renal transplant recipients. In clinical trials, concurrent administration of sirolimus and antilipemic agents (i.e., HMG-CoA reductase inhibitors and/or fibric acid derivatives) appeared to be well tolerated. The manufacturer recommends monitoring for possible development of rhabdomyolysis and other adverse effects (e.g., hepatic toxicity) associated with HMG-CoA reductase inhibitors and/or fibric acid derivatives in patients receiving such concomitant therapy. (See Hyperlipidemia under Warnings/Precautions: Other Warnings and Precautions, in Cautions.)

A clinically important pharmacokinetic interaction between sirolimus and atorvastatin appears unlikely.

■ **Nephrotoxic Drugs** The manufacturer recommends exercising caution when using drugs that may adversely affect renal function in patients receiving sirolimus (e.g., aminoglycosides, amphotericin B). (See Renal Function under Warnings/Precautions: Other Warnings and Precautions, in Cautions.)

■ **Vaccines** The possibility that immune response to vaccination may be diminished in patients receiving sirolimus should be considered. The manufacturer recommends that live vaccines (e.g., measles, mumps, rubella, oral polio, BCG, yellow fever, varicella, typhoid vaccine live oral [containing the Ty21a strain of *Salmonella typhi*]) be avoided during therapy with the drug.

■ **Grapefruit Juice** Grapefruit juice reduces CYP3A4-mediated metabolism of sirolimus and should not be administered with or used for dilution of the drug.

Description

Sirolimus, a macrolide antibiotic produced by *Streptomyces hygroscopicus* and structurally similar to tacrolimus, is a potent immunosuppressive agent. Sirolimus has been estimated to be about 27 times as potent as tacrolimus in animal models of heart, kidney, and small bowel transplantation.

While the precise mechanism of action of sirolimus is uncertain, the drug appears to have immunosuppressive actions distinct from those of other immunosuppressants such as cyclosporine and tacrolimus. Cyclosporine and tacrolimus bind to cytosolic receptors known as immunophilins (i.e., cyclophilin and FK binding protein-12 [FKBP-12], respectively), forming complexes that inhibit the production of cytokines (e.g., interleukin-2 , interleukin-4) via the calcineurin pathway. Inhibition of calcineurin activity by these drugs inhibits early activation of T-cells by these cytokines and ultimately blocks cell-cycle progression in the G_0 and G_1 phases. While sirolimus binds to the same immunophilin (FKBP-12) as tacrolimus to generate an immunosuppressive complex, the sirolimus/FKBP-12 complex has no effect on the calcineurin pathway. The sirolimus/FKBP-12 complex binds to and inhibits the activation of the mammalian target of rapamycin (mTOR), a key regulatory kinase. This inhibition results in suppression of cytokine-driven T-cell proliferation. Sirolimus appears to inhibit cell-cycle progression at a later stage (mid-to-late G_1 phase) than tacrolimus. Sirolimus also inhibits interleukin-2-dependent and independent proliferation of B-lymphocytes and the production of antibodies (e.g., immunoglobulins A, M, and G).

In animals, sirolimus reverses acute rejection of heart and kidney allografts and suppresses immune-mediated events associated with systemic lupus erythematosus, collagen-induced arthritis, autoimmune type 1 diabetes mellitus, autoimmune myocarditis, experimental allergic encephalomyelitis, graft-versus-host disease, and autoimmune uveoretinitis. Increased survival of transplanted kidney, heart, skin, islet, small bowel, pancreaticoduodenal, and bone marrow allografts has been shown in animals receiving the drug.

Sirolimus is rapidly but poorly absorbed from the GI tract, with an apparent systemic bioavailability of about 15% following oral administration as a solution. The mean bioavailability of sirolimus tablets is about 27% greater than that of sirolimus oral solution. The manufacturer states that tablets and solutions of sirolimus are not bioequivalent; however, therapeutic equivalence has been demonstrated at the 2-mg dose level. Administration of the drug with a high-fat breakfast results in a reduction in peak blood concentration and an increase in time to peak concentration and total systemic exposure (area under the blood concentration-time curve [AUC]). (See Dosage and Administration: Administration.)

Sirolimus is a substrate for cytochrome P-450 (CYP) isoenzyme 3A4 and P-glycoprotein and is extensively metabolized in the liver by *O*-methylation and/or hydroxylation. While 7 major metabolites of sirolimus have been identified, sirolimus is the principal species in whole blood and is responsible for greater than 90% of immunosuppressive activity. The drug has an elimination half-life of 57–63 hours in kidney transplant recipients.

Advice to Patients

Importance of providing copy of manufacturer's written patient information (medication guide) each time sirolimus is dispensed, and importance of reading this information prior to taking the drug.

Sirolimus may increase risk of skin cancer. Importance of avoiding sunlight or other UV light by wearing protective clothing and sunglasses and using sunscreens with a high protection factor.

Importance of following manufacturer's instructions for dilution and administration of sirolimus oral solution.

Importance of informing women of childbearing age of potential risks and that they should use effective contraception prior to initiation of sirolimus therapy, during therapy, and for 12 weeks after discontinuance of therapy. Importance of women informing their clinician if they are breast-feeding or plan to breast-feed.

Importance of informing clinicians of existing or contemplated concomitant therapy, including prescription and OTC drugs and dietary or herbal supplements.

Importance of avoiding ingestion of grapefruit juice during sirolimus therapy unless otherwise instructed.

Importance of advising patients of other important precautionary information. (See Cautions.)

Overview® (see Users Guide). For additional information until a more detailed monograph is developed and published, the manufacturer's labeling should be consulted. It is *essential* that the manufacturer's labeling be consulted for more detailed information on usual cautions, precautions, contraindications, potential drug interactions, laboratory test interferences, and acute toxicity.

Preparations

Excipients in commercially available drug preparations may have clinically important effects in some individuals; consult specific product labeling for details.

Sirolimus

Oral		
Solution	1 mg/mL	**Rapamune®**, Wyeth
Tablets	0.5 mg	**Rapamune®**, Wyeth
	1 mg	**Rapamune®**, Wyeth
	2 mg	**Rapamune®**, Wyeth

†Use is not currently included in the labeling approved by the US Food and Drug Administration

Tacrolimus

■ Tacrolimus, a macrolide antibiotic, is a potent immunosuppressive agent.

Uses

Tacrolimus is used for the prevention of rejection of liver, kidney, or heart allografts. Tacrolimus also has been used in the management of Crohn's disease†.

■ Hepatic Allotransplantation Tacrolimus is used for the prevention of rejection of liver allografts. The manufacturer recommends that tacrolimus be used in conjunction with corticosteroid therapy.

The indication for tacrolimus in hepatic allograft transplantation is based on data from 2 prospective, randomized, non-blinded multicenter studies involving hepatic allograft recipients. Patients received an immunosuppressive regimen that included corticosteroids and either tacrolimus or cyclosporine. Tacrolimus and cyclosporine were comparably effective in these patients in terms of survival of patients and of grafts 1 year after transplantation. In the study that excluded patients with renal dysfunction, fulminant hepatic failure with stage IV encephalopathy, and cancers but that included patients 12 years old and younger, patient and graft survival rates 1 year after transplantation for both groups combined were 88 and 81%, respectively. In the study that included patients with renal dysfunction, fulminant hepatic failure in stage IV encephalopathy, and cancers other than primary hepatic with metastases but that excluded pediatric patients, patient and graft survival rates 1 year after transplantation for both groups combined were 78 and 73%, respectively.

■ Renal Allotransplantation Tacrolimus is used for the prevention of rejection of renal allografts. The manufacturer recommends that tacrolimus be used in conjunction with corticosteroid therapy.

The indication for tacrolimus in renal allograft transplantation is based on data from a randomized, multicenter, non-blinded, prospective study of tacrolimus-based immunosuppression compared with a cyclosporine-based regimen. Patients younger than 6 years of age were excluded. Study therapy was initiated when posttransplant renal function was stable (i.e., serum creatinine of 4 mg/dL or less), which was a median of 4 days after transplant (range: 1–14 days). All patients received prophylactic induction therapy consisting of antilymphocyte antibody therapy, corticosteroids, and azathioprine. Overall 1-year patient and graft survival were 96.1 and 89.6%, respectively, and were equivalent in the 2 treatment arms. Although data on secondary outcomes (e.g., incidence of acute rejection, use of muromonab-CD3 [OKT3] for corticosteroid-resistant rejection, incidence of refractory rejection) were collected, the manufacturer states that because of the nature of the study design, differences in secondary outcomes could not be assessed reliably.

Other studies also have demonstrated the safety and efficacy of tacrolimus as primary therapy in prolonging survival of renal allografts; tacrolimus therapy has been administered in combination with corticosteroids and/or azathioprine in several studies. One-year graft and patient survival rates of 82–99% and 93–100%, respectively, have been reported; tacrolimus and cyclosporine appear to be comparably effective as therapy for this indication.

Tacrolimus also has been used in the secondary prevention of renal allograft transplant rejection† (i.e., "rescue" therapy) in case of acute or chronic allograft rejection or cyclosporine toxicity. Overall graft survival following such therapy has been reported to range from 59–86%.

■ Cardiac Allotransplantation Tacrolimus is used for the prevention of rejection of cardiac allografts. The manufacturer recommends that tacrolimus be used in conjunction with corticosteroid therapy and either azathioprine or mycophenolate mofetil.

The indication for tacrolimus in cardiac allograft transplantation is based on data from 2 open-label, randomized, multicenter studies comparing the safety and efficacy of tacrolimus-based immunosuppression and cyclosporine-based immunosuppression in primary orthotopic heart transplantation. In the first study, which was conducted in Europe, 314 adults received a regimen of antibody induction therapy, corticosteroids, and azathioprine in combination with either tacrolimus or modified cyclosporine for 18 months. The incidence of biopsy-proven acute rejection at 6 months was substantially lower in the tacrolimus-based group of patients than in those receiving the cyclosporine-based regimen (ISHLT grade 1B acute rejection or greater: 54 versus 66%, respectively; grade 3A or greater: 28 versus 42%, respectively). Tacrolimus and cyclosporine were comparably effective in these 2 groups in terms of survival of patients and of grafts 18 months after transplantation (92 and 89%, respectively).

In the second study, which was conducted in the US and consisted of 3 treatment arms, 331 adults undergoing de novo cardiac transplantation received an immunosuppressive regimen containing corticosteroids and either tacrolimus with sirolimus, tacrolimus with mycophenolate mofetil, or modified cyclosporine with mycophenolate mofetil for 1 year; antibody induction therapy also was allowed. The incidence of biopsy-proven acute rejection (ISHLT grade 3A or greater) or hemodynamic compromise requiring treatment was lower in the tacrolimus-treated patients at 6 months (22–24 versus 32%, respectively) and was significantly lower at 1 year in patients treated with tacrolimus and mycophenolate mofetil compared with patients treated with cyclosporine and mycophenolate mofetil (23 versus 37%, respectively). Similar patient and graft survival rates 1 year after transplantation were evident in the 2 mycophenolate mofetil-treated groups with approximately 94% survival reported in the tacrolimus plus mycophenolate mofetil group and 86% survival in the modified cyclosporine plus mycophenolate mofetil group. However, patients in the tacrolimus and sirolimus group exhibited an increased risk of wound healing complications, renal impairment, and insulin-dependent posttransplant diabetes mellitus; the manufacturer states that this combination is therefore not recommended.

■ Crohn's Disease Tacrolimus has been used in the management of fistulizing Crohn's disease†. Administration of oral tacrolimus has been effective for fistula improvement, but not for fistula remission in patients with perianal Crohn's disease. Efficacy of tacrolimus in the management of fistulizing Crohn's disease has been evaluated in a randomized, double-blind, placebo-controlled study involving 48 patients (12 years of age and older) with one or more open draining enterocutaneous fistulas that had not closed with administration of at least one anti-infective agent. Patients were randomized to receive placebo (26 patients) or oral tacrolimus (22 patients) 200 mcg/kg daily for 10 weeks. Those who were receiving stable dosages of corticosteroids, oral or rectal 5-aminosalicylic acid derivatives, oral anti-infective agents, azathioprine, mercaptopurine, methotrexate, or mycophenolate mofetil continued to receive these drugs during the study. The primary outcome was fistula improvement (defined as closure of 50% or more of particular fistulas that were open and draining at baseline and maintenance of such closures for at least 4 weeks), while secondary outcome was fistula remission (defined as closure of all fistulas and maintenance of such closures for at least 4 weeks). Fistula improvement was attained in 43% of patients receiving tacrolimus versus 8% of those receiving placebo, while fistula remission was attained in 10 or 8% of patients receiving tacrolimus or placebo, respectively; the difference in fistula remission was not considered statistically significant. Some clinicians state that because of the potential for tacrolimus-associated nephrotoxicity (especially at high doses) and because complete fistula remission has not been achieved with the drug, tacrolimus should be reserved for patients who do not respond to or are intolerant of all other therapies used for the management of fistulizing Crohn's disease (e.g., ciprofloxacin and/or metronidazole, azathioprine or mercaptopurine, infliximab).

Although there are no controlled or dose-response studies, limited data indicate that patients with severe fulminant Crohn's disease† who do not respond to parenteral corticosteroids may respond to IV tacrolimus.

For more information on the management of Crohn's disease, see Uses: Crohn's Disease, in Mesalamine 56:36.

For topical uses of tacrolimus, see 84:92.

Dosage and Administration

■ **Administration** Tacrolimus is administered orally or by IV infusion. However, because of the risk of anaphylaxis, IV administration of the drug should be reserved for patients who cannot accommodate oral administration. Although food can reduce both the rate and extent of GI absorption of tacrolimus, the manufacturer makes no specific recommendations regarding administration of the drug with meals. Because grapefruit juice affects CYP3A-mediated metabolism and has been reported to increase blood trough concentrations of tacrolimus in hepatic transplant patients when co-administered with the drug, the manufacturer recommends that such co-administration be avoided.

Tacrolimus therapy generally should be initiated no earlier than 6 hours after liver or heart transplantation and within 24 hours of kidney transplantation. Initiation of tacrolimus therapy, however, should be delayed in renal transplant patients until renal function has been recovered (e.g., as indicated by a serum creatinine concentration of 4 mg/dL or less). It is recommended that patients initiate tacrolimus therapy with the oral capsules, if possible. In patients receiving cyclosporine, initiation of tacrolimus therapy should be delayed at least 24 hours after discontinuance of cyclosporine to minimize the risk of excess nephrotoxicity; the manufacturer recommends that these drugs *not* be used concomitantly. Similarly, patients receiving tacrolimus should not be transferred to cyclosporine until at least 24 hours after discontinuance of tacrolimus. Such substitution should be delayed further if blood concentrations of cyclosporine or tacrolimus are elevated.

Tacrolimus for injection concentrate must be diluted prior to IV infusion. For IV infusion, the concentrate is diluted with 0.9% sodium chloride or 5% dextrose injection to a concentration of 4–20 mcg (0.004–0.02 mg) per mL. Preparation of the solution in polyethylene or glass containers allows storage for 24 hours beyond which unused solution should be discarded. A plasticized polyvinyl chloride (PVC) container should *not* be used because stability of the solution is decreased and polyoxyl 60 hydrogenated castor oil contained in the formulation may leach phthalates (e.g., bis(2-ethylhexyl)phthalate [BEHP, DEHP]) from PVC containers. Because of the chemical instability of tacrolimus in alkaline media, the injection should not be mixed or co-infused with solutions of pH 9 or greater (e.g., ganciclovir or acyclovir).

Each required daily dose of diluted tacrolimus injection is infused IV continuously over 24 hours.

Tacrolimus for injection concentrate and diluted solutions of the drug should be inspected visually for particulate matter and discoloration prior to administration whenever solution and container permit.

■ **Dosage** Dosage of tacrolimus is expressed in terms of anhydrous drug. Dosage titration, including that during maintenance, should be individualized and guided by clinical assessments of organ rejection and patient tolerability. Patients should be given complete dosing instructions. The manufacturer recommends concomitant corticosteroid therapy during the early posttransplantation period.

Therapeutic Drug Monitoring Monitoring blood tacrolimus concentrations may be useful in assessing organ rejection and toxicity, adjusting dosage, and determining compliance. Factors influencing frequency of monitoring include, but are not limited to, hepatic or renal dysfunction, the addition or discontinuance of potentially interacting drugs, and the time since transplant. The manufacturer states that therapeutic blood monitoring is not a replacement for renal and hepatic function monitoring and tissue biopsies. Although there is a lack of direct correlation between blood tacrolimus concentrations and efficacy, the relative risk of drug toxicity (e.g., nephrotoxicity, posttransplant diabetes mellitus) appears to be increased with higher trough concentrations. Therefore, the monitoring of trough whole blood concentrations is recommended to assist in the clinical evaluation of toxicity.

Most hepatic transplant patients appear to be most stable when trough whole blood tacrolimus concentrations are maintained between 5–20 ng/mL; long-term, posttransplant patients are maintained at the lower end of this range. Children generally appear to require higher tacrolimus dosages than adults on a weight basis to achieve comparable blood concentrations. In renal transplant patients, data from the US trial indicate that trough whole blood concentrations of tacrolimus (as measured by IMx®) are most variable during the first week of dosing. During the first 3 months, 80% of the patients maintained trough concentrations between 7–20 ng/mL and between 5–15 ng/mL through 1 year. In cardiac transplant patients, data from the European trial indicate that trough whole blood concentrations of tacrolimus (as measured by IMx®) are most variable during the first week of dosing. During the first 3 months, approximately 80% of the patients maintained trough concentrations between 8–20 ng/mL and between 6–18 ng/mL through 18 months.

Two methods have been used for the assay of tacrolimus: a microparticle enzyme immunoassay (MEIA) and an enzyme-linked immunosorbent assay (ELISA). Both methods use the same monoclonal antibody for tacrolimus. Comparison of the concentrations reported in the published literature using the current assays must be made with detailed knowledge of the assay methods and biologic matrices employed. Whole blood is the matrix of choice and specimens should be collected into tubes containing ethylene diamine tetraacetic acid (EDTA) anticoagulant. Heparin anticoagulant is not recommended because of the tendency of the sample to form clots on storage. Samples which are not analyzed immediately should be stored at room temperature or in a refrigerator and assayed within 7 days; if samples are to be kept longer, they should be frozen at −20°C for up to 12 months.

Specialized sources regarding the therapeutic monitoring of tacrolimus should be consulted for further discussion of the clinical utility of tacrolimus monitoring.

Other Considerations Because of the risk of potentially life-threatening hypersensitivity reactions (e.g., anaphylaxis) associated with the parenteral formulation, tacrolimus therapy should be initiated orally whenever possible. However, during the initial posttransplantation period, it often is not possible to administer the drug orally. Therefore, a period of parenteral therapy with the drug often cannot be avoided. If tacrolimus therapy is initiated IV, oral therapy with the drug should be substituted as soon as tolerated.

Patients receiving tacrolimus IV should be under continuous observation for at least the first 30 minutes following initiation of the IV infusion and should be monitored closely at frequent intervals for possible allergic manifestations. In addition, appropriate equipment and agents for the management of anaphylactic reactions (e.g., epinephrine, oxygen) should be readily available. If anaphylaxis occurs, IV infusion of the drug should be discontinued and appropriate therapy instituted. The oral formulation of tacrolimus does not contain polyoxyl 60 hydrogenated castor oil, and therefore a history of anaphylaxis with the parenteral formulation does not necessarily preclude oral therapy with the drug.

In patients unable to take the drug orally, the usual initial IV dosage of tacrolimus is 10 mcg/kg (0.01 mg/kg) daily for cardiac transplantation and 30–50 mcg/kg (0.03–0.05 mg/kg) daily for hepatic and renal transplantation commencing no earlier than 6 hours after transplantation. Adults should receive a dosage at the lower end of the dosage range. Concomitant corticosteroid therapy is recommended early posttransplantation. IV infusion of tacrolimus should continue only until the patient can tolerate oral therapy. In most cases, therapy with the drug can be switched to the oral route within 2–4 days. Oral tacrolimus should start 8–12 hours after IV infusion is discontinued. While higher IV doses administered in divided 2- to 4-hour infusions have been employed, such dosages no longer are recommended because of the increased risk of adverse effects associated with high plasma concentrations of the drug.

Oral Dosage Dosage requirements generally decline with continued therapy, and long-term administration is necessary to prevent rejection. In general, children require and tolerate higher tacrolimus maintenance dosages than adults.

Hepatic Allograft Transplantation. The usual initial oral tacrolimus dosage in adult hepatic transplant patients is 100–150 mcg/kg (0.1–0.15 mg/kg) daily, administered in 2 divided daily doses every 12 hours. The usual initial oral tacrolimus dose in pediatric hepatic transplant patients is 150–200 mcg/kg (0.15–0.2 mg/kg) daily, administered in 2 divided daily doses every 12 hours. In both adult and pediatric hepatic transplant patients, the typical trough whole blood tacrolimus concentrations should be 5–20 ng/mL when measured at months 1–12 posttransplant.

Renal Allograft Transplantation. The usual initial oral tacrolimus dosage in renal transplant patients is 200 mcg/kg (0.2 mg/kg) daily, administered in 2 divided daily doses every 12 hours. Patients receiving this tacrolimus dosage should have typical whole blood tacrolimus concentrations of 7–20 ng/mL and 5–15 ng/mL when measured at months 1–3 or 4–12 months posttransplant, respectively. Black renal transplant patients may require higher tacrolimus doses to maintain comparable whole blood trough drug concentrations.

Cardiac Allograft Transplantation. The usual initial oral tacrolimus dosage in cardiac transplant patients is 75 mcg/kg (0.075 mg/kg) daily, administered in 2 divided daily doses every 12 hours. Patients receiving this tacrolimus dosage should have typical trough whole blood tacrolimus concentrations of 10–20 ng/mL and 5–15 ng/mL when measured at months 1–3 or on or after 4 months posttransplant, respectively.

Crohn's Disease. If tacrolimus is used for the management of fistulizing Crohn's disease†, an oral dosage of 200 mcg/kg daily administered in 2 divided daily doses for 10 weeks was used in one study in patients 12 years of age and older.

■ **Dosage in Renal and Hepatic Impairment** Because of reduced clearance and prolonged half-life of tacrolimus in patients with severe hepatic impairment (Child-Pugh score of 10 or higher), lower dosages of tacrolimus and close monitoring of blood concentrations may be required in these patients. The drug's nephrotoxic potential also necessitates administering the lowest dosage in the respective ranges of dosages recommended for oral and IV administration in patients with renal or hepatic impairment. This dosage may need to be further decreased. Initiation of tacrolimus therapy generally should be delayed for up to 48 hours or longer in patients who develop postoperative oliguria.

Cautions

Tacrolimus shares the toxic potentials of currently available immunosuppressive agents. Because most transplant patients receiving tacrolimus have had multiple baseline symptomatology and clinical abnormalities and were receiving multiple drugs, some reported effects may not be directly attributable to tacrolimus and it is difficult to determine whether a causal relationship exists for some reported adverse effects. In addition, a variety of dosage regimens has been used in clinical trials to determine the therapeutic dosage, making interpretation of adverse effects difficult. More than one adverse effect was reported in virtually all (99.8%) patients receiving tacrolimus in clinical trials. The most common adverse effects of the drug include renal dysfunction, those involving the nervous system (e.g., tremor, headache) and GI tract (e.g., diarrhea, nausea), hypertension, alterations in glucose metabolism, hyperkalemia, and infectious complications. These effects may occur following oral or IV administration of tacrolimus and, with the exception of altered glucose metabolism, may be dose related and respond to reduction in dosage. The tolerability profile of tacrolimus appears to be similar in adults and children.

■ **Renal Effects** Nephrotoxicity is among the most common adverse effects of tacrolimus, especially at high doses. Nephrotoxicity occurred in approximately 36–40%, 52%, and 59% of patients receiving the drug following hepatic, renal, and cardiac transplantation, respectively, in clinical trials. Increased serum creatinine concentration occurred in 24–45% and increased BUN in 12–30% of patients receiving tacrolimus in clinical trials. Nephrotoxicity may be dose related and may respond to dosage reduction. Urinary tract infection occurred in 16–34% and oliguria in 18–19% of patients receiving the drug in clinical trials. Hematuria, renal failure, albuminuria, cystitis, dysuria, hydronephrosis, renal tubular necrosis, nocturia, pyuria, toxic nephropathy, urinary frequency, and urinary incontinence each were reported in more than 3% of patients receiving tacrolimus in clinical trials. In addition, acute renal failure, hemorrhagic cystitis, hemolytic-uremic syndrome, micturition disorder, bladder spasm, urge incontinence, urinary retention, and glycosuria also have been reported.

■ **Nervous System Effects** Neurotoxicity may occur in patients receiving tacrolimus, especially at high doses. Headache and tremor are the most frequent adverse nervous system effects and among the most common adverse effects of tacrolimus. Headache occurred in 37–64% and tremor in 15–56% of patients receiving the drug in clinical trials. Tremor occurred more frequently in tacrolimus-treated renal transplant and cardiac transplant patients than in cyclosporine-treated patients in clinical trials; the incidence of other neurologic events was otherwise similar in the 2 treatment groups. In some patients, tremor may be accentuated with voluntary movement and interfere with performance of motor skills. Headache and tremor have been associated with elevated whole blood tacrolimus concentrations and may respond to dosage reduction.

Insomnia occurred in 32–64%, paresthesia in 17–40%, dizziness in up to 19%, and asthenia in 11–52% of patients receiving tacrolimus in clinical trials. In addition, abnormal dreams, agitation, amnesia, anxiety, confusion, seizures (which may be focal or tonic-clonic), mental depression, expressive dysphasia, emotional lability, encephalopathy, hallucinations, hypertonia, incoordination, myoclonic reactions, nervousness, neuropathy, psychosis, somnolence, and abnormal thinking each were reported in more than 3% of patients receiving tacrolimus in clinical trials. Coma, delirium, aphasia, hyperesthesia, focal weakness, fatigue, malaise, impairment of psychomotor function, vertigo, akinetic mutism (speech apraxia), impaired writing, sleep disturbances, elevated mood, numbness, hemiplegia, monoparesis, peripheral neurotoxicity (including fluctuating flaccid quadriparesis, symmetrical facial weakness, neuralgia, nerve compression, bilateral ptosis, and lethargy), hemorrhagic stroke, leukoencephalopathy, and meningitis also have been reported. Coma and delirium have been associated with elevated plasma concentrations of tacrolimus.

■ **GI Effects** Diarrhea is among the most common adverse effects of tacrolimus, occurring in 37–72% of patients receiving the drug in clinical trials. Other common adverse GI effects include nausea, which occurred in 32–46% of patients, constipation, which occurred in 23–35% of patients, anorexia, which occurred in up to 34% of patients, vomiting, which occurred in 14–29% of patients, dyspepsia, which occurred in up to 28% of patients, and abdominal pain, which occurred in 29–59% of patients receiving the drug in clinical trials. Diarrhea may be dose related and is sometimes associated with other adverse GI effects such as nausea and vomiting. Diarrhea may respond to dosage reduction. Occasionally, GI toxicity may be severe and require discontinuance of tacrolimus. Dysphagia, esophagitis, flatulence, gastritis, GI hemorrhage, GI perforation, ileus, increased appetite, enlarged abdomen, peritonitis, oral candidiasis, rectal disorder, and stomatitis each were reported in more than 3% of patients receiving tacrolimus in clinical trials. Colitis, enterocolitis, intra-abdominal abscess, acute pancreatitis with hyperamylasemia, stomach ulcer, GI disorder, gastroenteritis, duodenitis, ulcerative esophagitis, and cytomegalovirus (CMV) enteritis also have been reported.

■ **Cardiovascular Effects** Hypertension is among the most common adverse effects of tacrolimus, occurring in 38–89% of patients receiving the drug in clinical trials. Hypertension usually is mild to moderate in severity and can be controlled by concomitant administration of antihypertensive agents. (See Cautions: Precautions and Contraindications.) Chest pain has been reported in up to 19% of patients receiving the drug in clinical trials.

Myocardial hypertrophy has been reported in association with the administration of tacrolimus and generally is manifested by echocardiographically demonstrated increases in left ventricular posterior wall and interventricular septum thickness. In addition, myocardial hypertrophy associated with clinically manifested ventricular dysfunction has been reported rarely in patients receiving the drug. Hypertrophy has been observed in infants, children, and adults receiving the drug. This condition appears to be reversible in most cases following dose reduction or discontinuance of therapy. In a group of 20 patients with pretreatment and posttreatment echocardiograms showing evidence of myocardial hypertrophy, mean tacrolimus whole blood concentrations during the period prior to diagnosis of hypertrophy ranged from 11–53 ng/mL in infants (age 0.4–2 years), 4–46 ng/mL in children (age 2–15 years), and 11–24 ng/mL in adults (age 37–53 years).

Adverse cardiovascular effects of tacrolimus that occurred in more than 3% of patients receiving the drug in clinical trials include abnormal ECG, angina pectoris, hypotension, postural hypotension, vasodilatation, and tachycardia. Palpitations, prolongation of the QT interval and cardiac arrhythmias (including atrial flutter, atrial fibrillation, and torsades de pointes), bradycardia or decreased heart rate, pericardial effusion or fluid collection, congestive heart failure, cardiopulmonary failure, syncope, flushing, and hypertrophic obstructive cardiomyopathy also have been reported.

■ **Metabolic and Electrolyte Effects** Hyperglycemia is the most common adverse metabolic effect of tacrolimus, occurring in 22–70% of patients receiving the drug in clinical trials; this effect may develop more commonly in adults than in children. Hyperglycemia may require insulin therapy and may be associated with new-onset insulin-dependent diabetes mellitus, which was reported in up to 24% of patients receiving the drug in clinical trials. Insulin dependence was reversible in 15 and 50% of renal transplant patients at 1 and 2 years posttransplant, respectively, and in 31–45% and 17–30% of liver and heart transplant patients, respectively, at 1 year posttransplant. In some cases, peripheral insulin resistance may occur. As has been observed in association with the administration of other immunosuppressant drugs, black and Hispanic renal transplant patients were at an increased risk of development of posttransplant diabetes mellitus. The risk of development of posttransplant diabetes mellitus increased with increasing whole blood trough concentrations of tacrolimus and with increasing steroid doses. A change in pancreatic sensitivity to hyperglycemia and in peripheral sensitivity to insulin also appears to be involved in the diabetogenic effect of tacrolimus. In animals, the drug causes substantial hyperglycemia, with selective depletion in insulin-producing pancreatic β-cells and decreased glucose-induced insulin release.

Another common adverse metabolic effect of tacrolimus is hyperkalemia, which occurred in 8–45% of patients receiving the drug in clinical trials. Hyperkalemia may result from a relative hyporenin-aldosterone status induced by the drug, and is not always associated with nephrotoxicity. Hyperkalemia generally responds to dosage reduction or treatment with sodium polystyrene sulfonate or fludrocortisone. Hypokalemia also occurred in 13–29%, hypophosphatemia in up to 49%, and hypomagnesemia in 16–48% of patients receiving tacrolimus in clinical trials. Edema has been reported in 18% and hyperlipemia has been reported in up to 34% of patients receiving tacrolimus in clinical trials. Other adverse metabolic and electrolyte effects that occurred in more than 3% of patients receiving tacrolimus in clinical trials include acidosis, alkalosis, hyperphosphatemia, hyperuricemia, hypocalcemia, hyponatremia, decreased bicarbonate, dehydration, hypervolemia, hypercholesterolemia, hypoglycemia, hypoproteinemia, and Cushing's syndrome.

■ **Infectious Complications** Infectious complications, including pneumonia, sepsis, meningitis, and urinary tract, intra-abdominal, viral (e.g., cytomegalovirus), local and systemic fungal, upper respiratory tract, and skin and wound infections, have occurred frequently (e.g., in up to 45% of patients in clinical trials) during tacrolimus therapy. When infectious complications occurring during tacrolimus therapy are compared with those occurring during cyclosporine therapy, the frequency of bacterial, viral, and fungal infections with tacrolimus is similar to or less than that with cyclosporine. Patients with recurrent hepatitis C appear to have a higher risk of major infections with tacrolimus therapy.

■ **Hepatic Effects** Abnormal liver function test results, including increased serum AST (SGOT), ALT (SGPT), and LDH concentrations, occurred in up to 36% of patients receiving tacrolimus in clinical trials. Ascites occurred in up to 27% of patients receiving the drug in clinical trials. Cholangitis, jaundice (including cholestatic jaundice), increased serum γ-glutamyltransferase (γ-glutamyltranspeptidase, GT, GGTP) concentration, hepatitis or granulomatous hepatitis (which may be secondary to CMV infection), increased serum alkaline phosphatase concentration, liver damage, and bilirubinemia each were reported in more than 3% of patients receiving tacrolimus in clinical trials. Hypoalbuminemia also has been reported.

■ **Hematologic Effects** Anemia (which may result from acute hemolysis) is the most common adverse hematologic effect of tacrolimus, occurring in 5–65% of patients receiving the drug in clinical trials. Leukocytosis and thrombocytopenia occurred in up to 32 and up to 24%, respectively, of patients receiving tacrolimus in clinical trials; leukopenia was reported in up to 48% of patients receiving the drug in clinical trials. Hemorrhage, coagulation disorders, ecchymosis, hypochromic anemia, deep thrombophlebitis, thrombosis, polycythemia, decreased serum iron, and decreased prothrombin each were reported in more than 3% of patients receiving tacrolimus in clinical trials. Purpura, thrombocytopenic purpura, thrombotic thrombocytopenic purpura, peripheral vascular disorder, and phlebitis also have been reported.

■ **Respiratory Effects** Pleural effusion occurred in 30–36% of patients receiving tacrolimus in clinical trials. Atelectasis and dyspnea occurred in 5–28% and 5–29%, respectively, of patients receiving the drug in clinical trials; increased cough was reported in up to 18% of patients receiving the drug in clinical trials. Asthma, bronchitis, pneumothorax, lung disorders, pulmonary edema, pharyngitis, pneumonia, respiratory disorder, rhinitis, sinusitis, and voice alteration each were reported in more than 3% of patients receiving tacrolimus in clinical trials. Pulmonary fungal infections (including aspergillosis and cryptococcosis) also have been reported.

■ **Dermatologic Effects** Pruritus occurred in 15–36% and rash in 10–24% of patients receiving tacrolimus in clinical trials. Other adverse dermatologic effects of tacrolimus that occurred in more than 3% of patients receiving the drug in clinical trials include acne, alopecia, exfoliative dermatitis, fungal dermatitis, mucocutaneous herpes simplex infections, hirsutism, skin discoloration, skin ulcer, skin disorder, sweating, and photosensitivity reaction. Fungal cellulitis, cutaneous cryptococcus infection, herpes zoster infections, toxic epidermal necrolysis, and Stevens-Johnson syndrome also have been reported.

■ **Musculoskeletal Effects** Back pain is a common adverse musculoskeletal effect of tacrolimus, occurring in 17–30% of patients receiving the drug in clinical trials. Arthralgia has been reported in up to 25% of patients receiving tacrolimus therapy. Cramps, generalized spasm, leg cramps, myalgia, myasthenia, joint disorder, and osteoporosis each were reported in more than 3% of patients receiving tacrolimus in clinical trials. Septic fungal arthritis also has been reported.

■ **Ocular and Otic Effects** Abnormal vision, amblyopia, ear pain, otitis media, and tinnitus each were reported in more than 3% of patients receiving tacrolimus in clinical trials. Photophobia, cytomegalovirus (CMV) retinitis, blurred vision, and hearing loss including deafness also have been reported.

■ **Sensitivity Reactions** Anaphylactic reactions have occurred in some patients receiving IV tacrolimus. The exact cause of these reactions is not known, but tacrolimus for injection concentrate contains polyoxyl 60 hydrogenated castor oil (HCO-60), which may in part be responsible for hypersensitivity reactions (e.g., anaphylaxis) reported with use of the injection. Drugs with other castor oil derivatives (e.g., polyoxyl 35 castor oil [Cremophor® EL, polyethoxylated castor oil]) in their formulation also have been associated with anaphylaxis in a small proportion of treated patients. (For information on hypersensitivity reactions associated with castor oil-derivative vehicles, see Cautions: Sensitivity Reactions in Cyclosporine 92:44.)

■ **Other Adverse Effects** Pain occurred in 24–63%, fever in 19–48%, and peripheral edema in 12–36% of patients receiving tacrolimus in clinical trials. Abnormal healing, abscess, chills, hernia, vaginitis, weight gain, enlarged abdomen, accidental injury, allergic reaction, cellulitis, flu-like syndrome, generalized edema, peritonitis, and photosensitivity reaction each were reported in more than 3% of patients receiving the drug in clinical trials. Night sweats, weight loss, acute pancreatitis with hyperamylasemia, pancreatic pseudocyst, and abnormal menstruation also have been reported.

■ **Precautions and Contraindications** Tacrolimus should be used only under the supervision of a clinician experienced in immunosuppressive therapy and the management of organ transplant patients. Management of patients during initiation of, or any major change in, tacrolimus therapy should be performed in facilities equipped with adequate laboratory and supportive medical equipment and staffed with adequate medical personnel. Although patients who are stabilized on tacrolimus may receive the drug as outpatients, periodic laboratory monitoring is required. The clinician responsible for tacrolimus maintenance therapy should have complete information necessary for appropriate follow-up of the patient. Patients receiving tacrolimus should be informed of the necessity of routine laboratory testing (e.g., BUN, serum creatinine, bilirubin, and liver enzyme concentrations) for the assessment of renal and hepatic function. Patients should be informed that tacrolimus can cause diabetes mellitus and should be advised to see their clinician if they develop frequent urination or increased thirst or hunger. Patients also should be given careful dosage instructions, advised not to change the drug dosage without first consulting their clinician, advised of the potential risks during pregnancy, and informed of the increased risk of neoplasia during tacrolimus therapy.

Immunosuppression with tacrolimus may result in increased susceptibility to infection and the possible development of lymphoma or other neoplasms. (See Cautions: Mutagenicity and Carcinogenicity.) Because of the risk of oversuppression of the immune system and associated susceptibility to infection and risk of lymphoma, the manufacturer recommends that combination immunosuppressant therapy be used with caution. (See Drug Interactions: Immunosuppressants.)

Immunosuppressed patients are at an increased risk for opportunistic infections, including reactivation of latent viral infections. These include BK virus-associated nephropathy (BKVN), which has been reported in patients receiving immunosuppressants, including tacrolimus, cyclosporine, mycophenolate, and sirolimus. Primary infection with polyoma BK virus typically occurs in childhood; following initial infection, the virus remains latent, but reactivation may occur in immunocompromised patients. BKVN has principally been observed in renal transplant patients (usually within the first year posttransplantation) and may result in serious outcomes, including deterioration of kidney function and renal allograft loss. Risk of BK virus reactivation appears to be related to the degree of overall immunosuppression rather than use of any specific immunosuppressive agent; patients receiving a maintenance immunosuppressive regimen of at least 3 drugs appear to be at highest risk. Patients should be monitored for possible signs of BKVN, including deterioration in renal function, during therapy with tacrolimus; screening assays for polyomavirus replication also have been recommended by some clinicians. Early intervention in patients who develop BKVN is critical; a reduction in immunosuppressive therapy should initially be considered in such patients. Although a variety of other treatment approaches have been used anecdotally in patients with BKVN, including antiviral therapy (e.g., cidofovir), leflunomide, IV immunoglobulins, and fluoroquinolone antibiotics, additional experience and well-controlled studies are necessary to more clearly establish the optimal treatment of such patients.

Progressive multifocal leukoencephalopathy (PML), an opportunistic viral infection of the brain, also has been reported during postmarketing experience with tacrolimus. PML is caused by the JC virus and typically occurs in immunocompromised patients. In many cases, patients were receiving multiple immunosuppressive agents that may have contributed to the risk of PML. The possible diagnosis of PML should be considered in any immunocompromised patient who develops progressive neurologic deficits.

Tacrolimus may cause nephrotoxicity, especially at high doses, and serum creatinine concentration should be monitored regularly in patients receiving the drug. (See Cautions: Renal Effects.) More overt nephrotoxicity, characterized by increased serum creatinine concentration and decreased urinary output, is observed during the period immediately following hepatic transplantation. The development of renal dysfunction at any time during the course of tacrolimus therapy requires close monitoring of the patient, and frequent dosage adjustment may be required. In patients with persistently high elevations of BUN and serum creatinine concentrations who are unresponsive to adjustment of tacrolimus dosage, switching to other immunosuppressive therapy (e.g., cyclosporine and corticosteroids) should be considered. Tacrolimus should be used with caution when administered concomitantly with other nephrotoxic agents (e.g., aminoglycosides, amphotericin B, cisplatin). To avoid excessive nephrotoxicity, tacrolimus should not be used concomitantly with cyclosporine. In patients receiving cyclosporine, tacrolimus therapy should not be initiated for at least 24 hours after discontinuance of cyclosporine to minimize the risk of excess nephrotoxicity. Similarly, patients receiving tacrolimus should not be transferred to cyclosporine until at least 24 hours after discontinuance of tacrolimus. Transfers to the alternative agent should be delayed further if blood concentrations of cyclosporine or tacrolimus are elevated. Because an increased risk of renal impairment was associated with the combined use of tacrolimus and sirolimus in cardiac allograft recipients, tacrolimus should not be used concomitantly with sirolimus.

Because of the risk of myocardial hypertrophy in patients receiving tacrolimus, echocardiographic evaluation should be considered in patients who develop renal failure or clinical manifestations of ventricular dysfunction while receiving the drug. If myocardial hypertrophy is diagnosed, dosage reduction or discontinuance of tacrolimus therapy should be considered.

Neurotoxicity, including tremor, headache, seizures, changes in motor function, altered mental status, and altered sensory function may occur in patients receiving tacrolimus, especially at high doses. (See Cautions: Nervous System Effects.) Neurologic function and status should be monitored closely in patients receiving the drug.

Because hypertension is a common adverse effect of tacrolimus, patients may require antihypertensive therapy while receiving the drug. Because of the risk of hyperkalemia, concomitant use of potassium-sparing diuretics should be avoided. Calcium-channel blocking agents should be used with caution in the management of tacrolimus-induced hypertension since these agents may interfere with tacrolimus metabolism. Patients receiving tacrolimus and a calcium-channel blocking agent concomitantly should be monitored closely for increased blood tacrolimus concentrations and may require dosage reduction of tacrolimus during concomitant therapy.

Because tacrolimus may interfere with glucose metabolism and cause hyperglycemia (see Cautions: Metabolic Effects), fasting blood glucose concentrations should be determined regularly and monitoring of metabolic function should be performed as clinically warranted in patients receiving the drug; insulin therapy may be necessary in some patients receiving tacrolimus. Because tacrolimus also may cause anemia or other adverse hematologic effects, hematologic function should be monitored as clinically warranted.

Because tacrolimus may result in hyperkalemia (sometimes severe), serum potassium concentrations should be monitored regularly during therapy with the drug and concomitant use of potassium-sparing diuretics or potassium supplements should be avoided. If hyperkalemia occurs during tacrolimus therapy, appropriate management should be instituted (e.g., restriction of potassium intake, administration of a potassium-binding resin or a mineralocorticoid).

Liver transplant patients receiving tacrolimus who develop posttransplant hepatic impairment may be at increased risk of developing renal insufficiency associated with high whole blood concentrations of the drug. These patients should be monitored closely, and dosage adjustments should be considered. Some evidence suggests that lower dosages of tacrolimus should be used in these patients. (See Dosage and Administration: Dosage in Renal and Hepatic Impairment.)

Because of the risk of anaphylaxis, IV tacrolimus should be reserved for patients who cannot accommodate oral administration. Patients receiving IV tacrolimus should be under continuous observation for at least the first 30 minutes following initiation of the IV infusion and should be monitored closely at frequent intervals thereafter for possible allergic manifestations. Appropriate equipment for maintenance of an adequate airway and other supportive measures and agents for the treatment of anaphylactic reactions (e.g., epinephrine, oxygen) should be readily available whenever tacrolimus is administered IV. If anaphylaxis occurs, IV infusion of tacrolimus should be discontinued immediately and the patient given appropriate therapy (e.g., epinephrine, oxygen) as indicated. Tacrolimus is contraindicated in patients with hypersensitivity to the drug, and tacrolimus for injection concentrate is contraindicated in patients with hypersensitivity to polyoxyl 60 hydrogenated castor oil (HCO-60).

■ **Pediatric Precautions** The manufacturer states that successful hepatic transplants have been performed in pediatric patients (up to 16 years of age) receiving tacrolimus.Two randomized, active-controlled studies of tacrolimus in primary liver transplantation included 56 pediatric patients; 31 of these patients were randomized to tacrolimus-based therapy and 25 to cyclosporine-based therapy. In addition, at least 122 pediatric patients received tacrolimus in an uncontrolled trial in living related-donor liver transplantation. Published reports also indicate that hepatic allografts and living related-donor hepatic transplants have been performed successfully in pediatric patients younger than 12 years of age receiving tacrolimus. Clinical experience in children suggests that safety and efficacy of tacrolimus are similar to those in adults. In general, children without preexisting renal or hepatic impairment require and tolerate higher tacrolimus dosages after hepatic transplantation than adults, but pediatric transplant patients may be more susceptible to lymphoproliferative disorders associated with tacrolimus use. (See Cautions: Mutagenicity and Carcinogenicity.)

The manufacturer states that experience with tacrolimus therapy in pediatric renal and cardiac allografts is limited. Several clinical trials and case reports of tacrolimus in pediatric renal allograft patients have described similar safety and efficacy as that reported in adult patients. Several clinical trials and case report series also have demonstrated efficacy and safety of tacrolimus for the prevention of rejection of cardiac allografts in pediatric patients. In addition, some pediatric patients receiving other immunosuppressants (e.g., cyclosporine) have been successfully converted to tacrolimus therapy because of refractory rejection or because they could not tolerate the initial immunosuppressant. The manufacturer states that some of the earlier cardiac transplantation pediatric studies may have employed higher dosages and target trough concentrations of tacrolimus and other immunosuppressive agents whereas some of the more recent studies employ the use of induction agents and/or mycophenolate mofetil, which may allow for reduced tacrolimus dosages and target trough concentrations at the lower end of the commonly used ranges.

■ **Geriatric Precautions** Safety and efficacy of tacrolimus in geriatric patients have not been studied specifically to date. Because geriatric patients frequently have decreased renal function (e.g., glomerular filtration), particular attention should be paid to evaluating renal function prior to initiation of tacrolimus and subsequently thereafter in this age group. If evidence of renal impairment exists or develops, appropriate adjustments in dosage should be made. (See Dosage and Administration: Dosage in Renal and Hepatic Impairment.)

■ **Mutagenicity and Carcinogenicity** Tacrolimus did not exhibit genotoxic activity in vitro in bacterial (*Salmonella* and *E. coli*) or mammalian (Chinese hamster lung-derived cells) assays. No evidence of mutagenicity was observed in vitro in the CHO/HGPRT assay or in vivo in clastogenicity assays performed in mice. Tacrolimus also did not cause unscheduled DNA synthesis in rodent hepatocytes.

Carcinogenicity studies of tacrolimus have been carried out in male and female rats and mice. In both the mouse and rat studies (duration: 80 and 104 weeks, respectively), tacrolimus doses (corrected for body surface area) of 0.8–2.5 times (mice) and 3.5–7.1 times (rats) the recommended human clinical dosage range of 0.1–0.2 mg/kg per day were not associated with a relationship to tumor incidence.

An increased incidence of malignancy is recognized to occur with immunosuppression in transplant recipients. Patients receiving immunosuppressive agents, including tacrolimus, are at increased risk of developing lymphomas and other malignancies, particularly of the skin. The risk appears to be related to the intensity and duration of immunosuppression rather than to the use of any specific immunosuppressive agent. In addition, some organ transplant patients receiving immunosuppressive agents have developed a lymphoproliferative disorder that appears to be associated with Epstein-Barr virus (EBV) infections. The risk of lymphoproliferative disorder appears greatest in young children who are at risk for primary EBV infections while immunosuppressed or whose immunosuppressive regimen is changed to tacrolimus following long-term immunosuppressive therapy. With the exception of corticosteroids, tacrolimus should not be used concomitantly with other immunosuppressive agents, since the risk of lymphoma may be increased. Although the risk of lymphoma appears to be greatest when there is substantial immunosuppression (i.e., concomitant use of multiple immunosuppressive agents), all immunosuppressed patients should be considered at risk for developing lymphoma. The nature and optimum management of posttransplant lymphomas and lymphoproliferative disorders in allograft recipients remain to be clearly established, and clinicians should consult specialized references for current methods of evaluation and management.

■ **Pregnancy, Fertility, and Lactation** Reproduction studies using tacrolimus in rats and rabbits have demonstrated maternal and fetal toxic effects. Tacrolimus, at oral doses of 0.32 and 1 mg/kg (0.5–1 and 1.6–3.3 times the recommended human clinical dose of 0.1–0.2 mg/kg based on body surface area corrections, respectively) during organogenesis in rabbits, was associated with maternal toxicity and an increased incidence of abortions. The higher dose also was associated with an increased incidence of fetal malformations and developmental variations. Tacrolimus, at oral doses of 3.2 mg/kg during organogenesis in rats, was associated with maternal toxicity, increased number of late resorptions, decreased number of live births, and decreased pup weight and viability.

Tacrolimus was associated with reduced pup weights when administered orally to pregnant rats following organogenesis and during lactation at doses of 1 and 3.2 mg/kg (0.7–1.4 and 2.3–4.6 times the recommended human clinical dose based on body surface area corrections, respectively). Tacrolimus crosses the placenta in humans. There have been reports of successful pregnancies in women receiving liver transplants whose immunosuppressive therapy was tacrolimus, with and without corticosteroids. Of ten pregnancies described, 9 healthy full-term infants were delivered; one infant conceived within 1 month of maternal liver transplantation was born at 22 weeks and died within 2 hours following delivery. There are no adequate and controlled studies to date using tacrolimus in pregnant women, and the drug should be used during pregnancy only when the potential benefits justify the possible risks to the fetus.

In reproduction studies in animals, tacrolimus did not impair male or female fertility.

Tacrolimus is distributed into milk. Because of the potential for serious adverse reactions to tacrolimus in nursing infants, nursing should be avoided in women receiving the drug.

Drug Interactions

■ **Drugs Affecting Hepatic Microsomal Enzymes** Because tacrolimus is metabolized principally by the cytochrome P-450 (CYP) 3A4 isoenzyme, blood concentrations of the drug or its active metabolites are likely to be altered by potent inhibitors or inducers of this enzyme in patients who were previously stabilized on tacrolimus therapy. Concomitant use of tacrolimus with such agents requires monitoring of the concentration of tacrolimus in whole blood with appropriate adjustment of tacrolimus dosage. Therefore, whole blood or plasma concentrations of tacrolimus should be monitored with appropriate adjustment of tacrolimus dosages when such drugs are used concomitantly. The following drugs or herbal preparations reportedly may *increase* or *decrease* blood tacrolimus concentrations:

Table 1. Drugs That May Increase Blood Tacrolimus Concentrations[a]

aluminum hydroxide-magnesium hydroxide	itraconazole
bromocriptine	ketoconazole[b]
chloramphenicol	lansoprazole[c]
cimetidine	methylprednisolone
cisapride	metoclopramide
clarithromycin	nefazodone
clotrimazole	nicardipine
cyclosporine	nifedipine
danazol	omeprazole
erythromycin	troleandomycin
ethinyl estradiol	verapamil
fluconazole	voriconazole
HIV protease inhibitors	

[a] This table is not all inclusive.

[b] Concomitant oral use substantially decreases apparent clearance of oral tacrolimus; clearance of IV tacrolimus is not substantially altered.

[c] Concomitant administration may inhibit tacrolimus metabolism and substantially increase whole blood concentrations of the drug, particularly in poor CYP2C19 metabolizers.

Table 2. Drugs That May Decrease Blood Tacrolimus Concentrations[a]

carbamazepine	rifabutin
caspofungin	rifampin
phenobarbital	sirolimus[b]
phenytoin	St. John's wort

[a] This table is not all inclusive.

[b] Because of an increased risk of hepatic artery thrombosis, graft loss, and death, concomitant use of tacrolimus and sirolimus is not recommended in de novo liver transplant recipients. Because of an increased risk of impaired renal function, concomitant use of tacrolimus and sirolimus also is not recommended in heart transplant recipients.

Antiretroviral Agents Although formal drug interaction studies of tacrolimus and antiretroviral agents have not been conducted, the manufacturer states that tacrolimus should be used with caution in patients receiving antiretroviral agents that are metabolized by CYP3A (e.g., nelfinavir, ritonavir). In a clinical study of 5 liver transplant recipients, concomitant administration of tacrolimus and nelfinavir resulted in substantial increases in blood tacrolimus concentrations that necessitated on average a 16-fold reduction in the tacrolimus dose in order to maintain mean trough tacrolimus blood concentrations of 9.7 ng/mL. Therefore, frequent monitoring of blood tacrolimus concentrations and appropriate dosage adjustment are essential when tacrolimus and nelfinavir are used concomitantly.

■ **Drugs Metabolized by Hepatic Microsomal Enzymes** Concomitant use of tacrolimus and phenytoin may result in increased plasma concentrations of phenytoin.

■ **Immunosuppressants** Because of the risk of oversuppression of the immune system and associated susceptibility to infection and risk of lymphoma, the manufacturer recommends that combination immunosuppressant therapy be used with caution.

Concomitant use of tacrolimus and sirolimus in de novo liver transplant recipients has been associated with an increased risk of hepatic artery thrombosis, graft loss, and death. Most cases of hepatic artery thrombosis occurred within 30 days posttransplantation and led to graft loss or death. In one study reporting excess mortality and graft loss in association with combined use of sirolimus and tacrolimus in de novo liver transplant recipients, many of the patients had evidence of infection at or near the time of death. In addition, concomitant use of tacrolimus and sirolimus in cardiac transplant recipients in one arm of the US clinical trial was associated with an increased risk of wound healing complications, renal function impairment, and insulin-dependent posttransplant diabetes mellitus. Therefore, the manufacturer states that concurrent administration of tacrolimus and sirolimus is not recommended.

■ **Nephrotoxic Drugs** Because of the potential for additive or synergistic impairment of renal function, tacrolimus should be used with caution in patients receiving other nephrotoxic drugs (e.g., aminoglycoside antibiotics, amphotericin B, cisplatin, ganciclovir).

Cyclosporine Concomitant administration of tacrolimus and cyclosporine has resulted in additive/synergistic nephrotoxicity. To avoid excessive nephrotoxicity, tacrolimus should not be used concomitantly with cyclosporine. The manufacturer recommends delaying initiation of tacrolimus therapy for at least 24 hours after discontinuance of cyclosporine therapy. Initiation of tacrolimus therapy may be further delayed in the presence of elevated cyclosporine levels.

■ **Grapefruit Juice** Because grapefruit juice affects CYP3A-mediated metabolism of tacrolimus, patients should be instructed to avoid grapefruit-containing foods and beverages.

■ **Potassium-sparing Diuretics** Concomitant use of tacrolimus and potassium-sparing diuretics or potassium supplements may result in potentially severe hyperkalemia and should be avoided.

■ **Vaccines** The possibility that the immune response to vaccination may be diminished in patients receiving tacrolimus should be considered. In addition, the manufacturer recommends that live vaccines (e.g., measles, mumps, rubella, oral polio, BCG, yellow fever, TY 21a typhoid) be avoided during therapy with the drug.

Description

Tacrolimus is a macrolide antibiotic produced by *Streptomyces tsukubaensis*. The drug is a potent immunosuppressive agent that is pharmacologically but *not* structurally related to cyclosporine and that exhibits only limited antimicrobial activity. Tacrolimus is approximately 10- to 200-fold more potent than cyclosporine on a weight basis in various in vitro T-cell test systems of immune function.

In animals, tacrolimus inhibits cell-mediated immune responses such as allograft rejection, delayed hypersensitivity, collagen-induced arthritis, experimental allergic encephalomyelitis, and graft-vs-host disease while humoral immunity is inhibited to a lesser extent. Increased survival of the host and of the transplanted graft of liver, kidney, heart, bone marrow, small bowel, pancreas, lung, trachea, skin, cornea, and limb has been shown in animals receiving the drug.

The exact mechanism(s) of immunosuppressive action of tacrolimus has not been elucidated but appears to involve inhibition of the activation of T cells. Studies suggest that tacrolimus binds to an intracellular protein, FKBP-12. Binding of the complex of tacrolimus and FKBP-12 with calcium, calmodulin, and calcineurin inhibits the phosphatase activity of calcineurin, which may prevent the dephosphorylation and translocation of nuclear factor of activated T cells (NF-AT). NF-AT putatively initiates gene transcription for the formation of lymphokines (e.g., interleukin-2, gamma interferon) involved in the activation of T cells.

SumMon® (see Users Guide). For additional information on this drug until a more detailed monograph is developed and published, the manufacturer's labeling should be consulted. It is *essential* that the labeling be consulted for detailed information on the usual cautions, precautions, and contraindications concerning potential drug interactions and/or laboratory test interferences and for information on acute toxicity.

Preparations

Excipients in commercially available drug preparations may have clinically important effects in some individuals; consult specific product labeling for details.

Tacrolimus

Oral		
Capsules	0.5 mg (of anhydrous tacrolimus)	**Prograf®**, Astellas
	1 mg (of anhydrous tacrolimus)	**Prograf®**, Astellas
	5 mg (of anhydrous tacrolimus)	**Prograf®**, Astellas
Parenteral		
For injection, concentrate, for IV infusion only	5 mg (of anhydrous tacrolimus) per mL	**Prograf®**, Astellas

†Use is not currently included in the labeling approved by the US Food and Drug Administration

INDEX

Synonyms, pharmacy equivalent names (PENs) (e.g., co-careldopa), and acronyms (e.g., AZT) for drugs usually appear in regular type and are cross-referenced ("*see*") to the appropriate monograph title. **Boldface** type is used for the title of the monograph, the proprietary (trade, brand) names, and *AHFS*® Pharmacologic-Therapeutic classes. In some index entries, "tall man" (mixed case) lettering is used for drug names or synonyms (e.g., diazePAM) when recommended by FDA or the Institute for Safe Medication Practices (ISMP).

The monograph title listed in boldface type following "*see*" usually is the corresponding nonproprietary (generic) name for the index entry (e.g., **Abelcet**®, see **Amphotericin B**); however, the monograph title may indicate that information about a drug can be found in a monograph about a group of drugs (e.g., **Colace**®, see **Stool Softeners** [Colace® is a proprietary name for docusate sodium, which is described in the monograph titled Stool Softeners]).

Some monographs have been omitted from the print edition of *AHFS Drug Information*® because of space limitations. Copies of these monographs are available on the "For Subscribers" page of the *AHFS Drug Information*® website, www.ahfsdruginformation.com, in the "Electronic Only Monographs" section. **(Username: ahfs2020; Password: ASHP94498)** Associated index entries for these monographs are followed by a symbol ("§") rather than by a page number. This symbol refers the user to a footnote that also provides the above username and password for the 2020 edition.

A

§ Electronic-only monographs at ahfsdruginformation.com. Username: ahfs2020; Password: ASHP94498

§ Electronic-only monographs at ahfsdruginformation.com. Username: ahfs2020; Password: ASHP94498

§ Electronic-only monographs at ahfsdruginformation.com. Username: ahfs2020; Password: ASHP94498

§ Electronic-only monographs at ahfsdruginformation.com. Username: ahfs2020; Password: ASHP94498

B

§ Electronic-only monographs at ahfsdruginformation.com. Username: ahfs2020; Password: ASHP94498

§ Electronic-only monographs at ahfsdruginformation.com. Username: ahfs2020; Password: ASHP94498

C

§ Electronic-only monographs at ahfsdruginformation.com. Username: ahfs2020; Password: ASHP94498

§ Electronic-only monographs at ahfsdruginformation.com. Username: ahfs2020; Password: ASHP94498

§ Electronic-only monographs at ahfsdruginformation.com. Username: ahfs2020; Password: ASHP94498

D

§ Electronic-only monographs at ahfsdruginformation.com. Username: ahfs2020; Password: ASHP94498

§ Electronic-only monographs at ahfsdruginformation.com. Username: ahfs2020; Password: ASHP94498

§ Electronic-only monographs at ahfsdruginformation.com. Username: ahfs2020; Password: ASHP94498

§ Electronic-only monographs at ahfsdruginformation.com. Username: ahfs2020; Password: ASHP94498

§ Electronic-only monographs at ahfsdruginformation.com. Username: ahfs2020; Password: ASHP94498

§ Electronic-only monographs at ahfsdruginformation.com. Username: ahfs2020; Password: ASHP94498

G

§ Electronic-only monographs at ahfsdruginformation.com. Username: ahfs2020; Password: ASHP94498

H

§ Electronic-only monographs at ahfsdruginformation.com. Username: ahfs2020; Password: ASHP94498

I

§ Electronic-only monographs at ahfsdruginformation.com. Username: ahfs2020; Password: ASHP94498

J

K

§ Electronic-only monographs at ahfsdruginformation.com. Username: ahfs2020; Password: ASHP94498

L

§ Electronic-only monographs at ahfsdruginformation.com. Username: ahfs2020; Password: ASHP94498

M

§ Electronic-only monographs at ahfsdruginformation.com. Username: ahfs2020; Password: ASHP94498

§ Electronic-only monographs at ahfsdruginformation.com. Username: ahfs2020; Password: ASHP94498

§ Electronic-only monographs at ahfsdruginformation.com. Username: ahfs2020; Password: ASHP94498

O

§ Electronic-only monographs at ahfsdruginformation.com. Username: ahfs2020; Password: ASHP94498

P

§ Electronic-only monographs at ahfsdruginformation.com. Username: ahfs2020; Password: ASHP94498

§ Electronic-only monographs at ahfsdruginformation.com. Username: ahfs2020; Password

§ Electronic-only monographs at ahfsdruginformation.com. Username: ahfs2020; Password: ASHP94498

Q

§ Electronic-only monographs at ahfsdruginformation.com. Username: ahfs2020; Password: ASHP94498

R

§ Electronic-only monographs at ahfsdruginformation.com. Username: ahfs2020; Password: ASHP94498

§ Electronic-only monographs at ahfsdruginformation.com. Username: ahfs2020; Password: ASHP94498

§ Electronic-only monographs at ahfsdruginformation.com. Username: ahfs2020; Password: ASHP94498

§ Electronic-only monographs at ahfsdruginformation.com. Username: ahfs2020; Password: ASHP94498

T

§ Electronic-only monographs at ahfsdruginformation.com. Username: ahfs2020; Password: ASHP94498

§ Electronic-only monographs at ahfsdruginformation.com. Username: ahfs2020; Password: ASHP94498

U

V

§ Electronic-only monographs at ahfsdruginformation.com. Username: ahfs2020; Password: ASHP94498

W

X

Y

§ Electronic-only monographs at ahfsdruginformation.com. Username: ahfs2020; Password: ASHP94498

Z

§ Electronic-only monographs at ahfsdruginformation.com. Username: ahfs2020; Password: ASHP94498